MEDICAL ECONOMICS

W9-ARP-107

Today's top source of definitve medical information

Medical Economics has long been the most respected, most trusted publisher of essential medical information in the country. Thousands of professionals regularly rely on these vital publications in their day-to-day work.

For over 50 years, PHYSICIANS' DESK REFERENCE® has been universally recognized as the "last word" on prescription medicines and their effects. Medical Economics has proudly continued this tradition of providing resources for the entire healthcare industry in all its publications.

Every edition is guaranteed to be:

COMPREHENSIVE—Complete coverage of all the essential details assures you of getting all the facts.

AUTHORITATIVE—FDA-approved information gives you the confidence of always getting the official data you need.

UP-TO-DATE–We pride ourselves on our widespread network which allows us to constantly gather, organize and publish critical medical information in easy-to-use formats. Our full-time staff verifies all data before it is published.

EASY-TO-USE—Organized and indexed for quick, easy access, all publications are ready for fast reference.

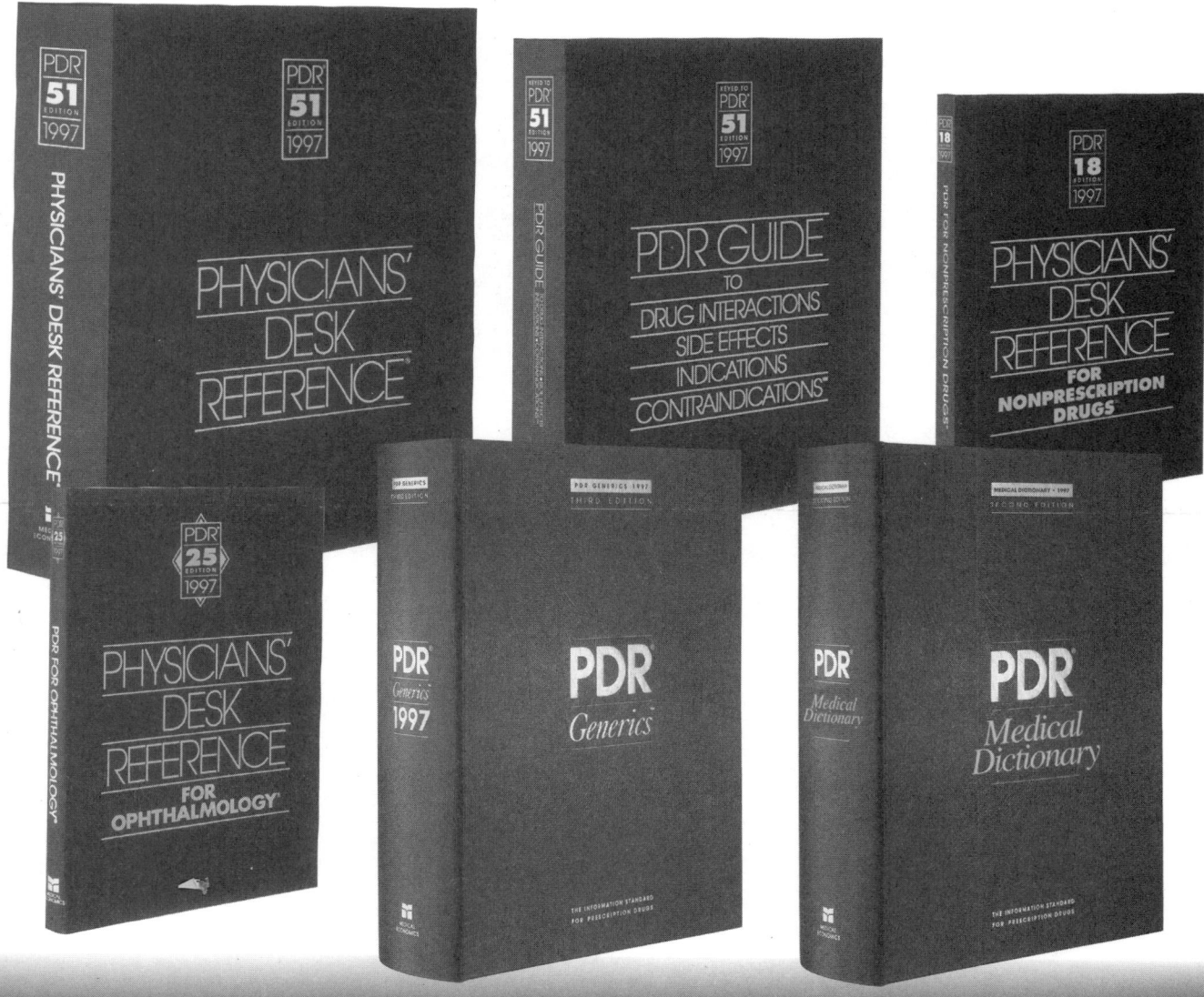

KEEP YOUR ENTIRE DRUG REFERENCE LIBRARY COMPLETELY UP-TO-DATE WITH THESE KEY VOLUMES!

1997 PHYSICIANS' DESK REFERENCE®

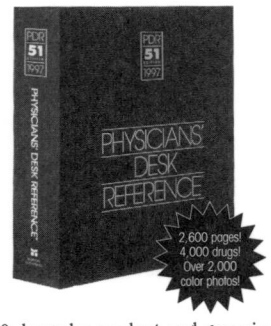

Physicians have turned to PDR® for the latest word on prescription drugs for over 50 years! Today, PDR is still considered the standard prescription drug reference and can be found in virtually every physician's office, hospital, and pharmacy in the United States. In fact, nine out of ten doctors consider PDR their most important reference source. Now the 51st Edition will soon be available and your old edition will be obsolete.

You'll find the most complete data on over 4,000 drugs by product and generic name (both in the same convenient index), manufacturer, and category. PDR provides complete medical information, usage and warnings, and product overviews that summarize listings, plus more than 2,000 full-size, full-color photos cross-referenced to the drug. $71.95

1997 PDR GUIDE TO DRUG INTERACTIONS, SIDE EFFECTS, INDICATIONS, CONTRAINDICATIONS™

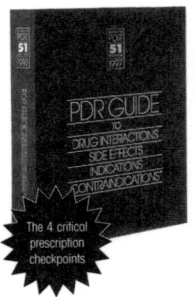

The most up-to-date listings in four vital areas: **Interactions:** identify potential problems with drug combinations by brand and generic name. **Side Effects:** look up specific sign, symptom, or abnormality to see if any drugs the patient is taking might be the problem. **Indications:** a complete list of all drugs indicated—all cross-referenced to your 1997 PDR! The new *Contraindications Index* lists all drugs that must not be prescribed in the presence of a given medical condition. $49.95

PDR® MEDICAL DICTIONARY

More than 100,000 entries! 1,900+ pages include a complete Medical Etymology section to help the reader understand medical/scientific word formation. Includes a comprehensive cross-reference table of generic and brand-name pharmaceuticals and manufacturers, plus a 31-page appendix containing useful charts on scales, temperatures, temperature equivalents, metric and SI units, weights and measures, laboratory and reference values, blood groups and much more. $44.95

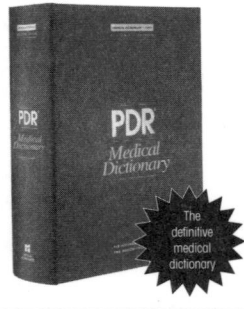

PDR® GENERICS™

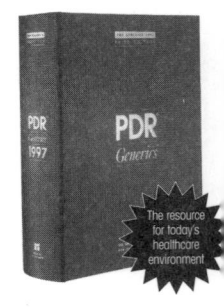

Here is the most comprehensive reference of its kind, providing complete prescribing and pricing information on nearly 40,000 medications, both brand and generic.

Compiled, edited, and reviewed by a team of 400 pharmacists and physicians, it includes complete pricing data–including average package prices—the average unit cost of each dosage form and strength, each alternative's therapeutic equivalency, and identification of companies approved to manufacture the drug. $79.95

1997 PDR FOR NONPRESCRIPTION DRUGS®

The acknowledged authority offers full FDA-approved descriptions of the most commonly used OTC medicines, four separate indices and in-depth data on ingredients, indications, and drug interactions. Includes a valuable new *Companion Drug Index* that lists common diseases and frequently encountered side effects, along with the prescription drugs associated with them, plus OTC products recommended for symptomatic relief. $44.95

1997 PDR FOR OPHTHALMOLOGY®

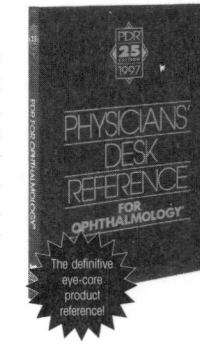

The definitive reference filled with accurate, up-to-date information specifically for the eye-care professional. It provides detailed reference data on drugs and equipment used in the fields of ophthalmology and optometry. Its comprehensive coverage includes lens types and their uses... specialized instrumentation... color product photographs... a detailed encyclopedia of pharmaceuticals in ophthalmology... five full indices... an extensive bibliography... and much more. $46.95

Complete your 1997 PDR® Library NOW! Enclose payment and save shipping costs.

(P7) _____ copies 1997 Physicians' Desk Reference
$71.95 ea. ....$_____

(T7) _____ copies 1997 PDR Supplements A&B
(payment must be enclosed) $21.95 set ....$_____

(N7) _____ copies 1997 PDR for Nonprescription Drugs
$44.95 ea. ....$_____

(G7) _____ copies 1997 PDR Guide to Drug Interactions,
Side Effects, Indications, Contraindications
$49.95 ea. ....$_____

(O7) _____ copies 1997 PDR for Ophthalmology
$46.95 ea. ....$_____

(J7) _____ copies PDR Medical Dictionary
$44.95 ea. ....$_____

(X7) _____ copies 1997 PDR Generics
$79.95 ea. ....$_____

Shipping & handling ....$_____

Sales Tax (FL, GA, IA, & NJ)..........................$_____

TOTAL AMOUNT OF ORDER........................$_____

Prices slightly higher outside U.S. and all customs, duty and other taxes are the customer's responsibility.
We cannot ship to P.O. box numbers.

PLEASE INDICATE METHOD OF PAYMENT:

☐ **PAYMENT ENCLOSED** (shipping & handling FREE)

☐ Check payable to PDR   ☐ VISA   ☐ MasterCard   ☐ Discover   ☐ American Expr

Account No. _____   Exp. Date _____

Telephone No. _____   Signature _____

☐ **BILL ME LATER** (Add $6.25 per book for shipping and handling)

☐ **SAVE TIME AND MONEY EVERY YEAR AS A SUBSCRIBER.** Check here to enter a standing order for editions of publications ordered. They will be shipped to you automatically, after advance notice, a you are guaranteed earliest delivery and free shipping and handling.

Name _____

Address _____

City/State/Zip _____

Mail this order form to: Physicians' Desk Reference, P.O. Box 10689, Des Moines, IA 50336

PDR® Electronic Library™ on CD-ROM

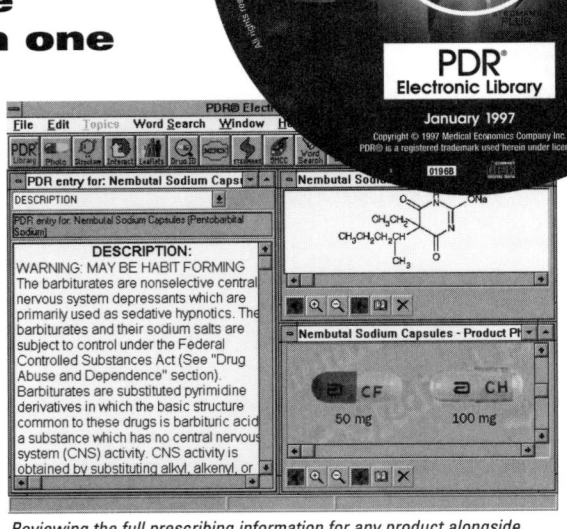

Speed diagnosis and prescribing with fast, flexible access to the medical references you need in one fully integrated system.

PDR Electronic Library on CD-ROM is a Windows-based system that instantly gives you all the information you need from the most current editions of Physician's Desk Reference®, PDR® Supplements, PDR for Nonprescription Drugs®, PDR for Ophthalmology®, and PDR Guide to Drug Interactions, Side Effects, Indications, Contraindications™. The system also includes a powerful multi-drug interaction screening module.

Choose from the large and growing selection of optional modules available on the PDR Electronic Library CD-ROM:

 The Merck Manual. The most widely-used medical text in the world integrated with PDR and Stedman's Medical Dictionary.

 Stedman's Medical Dictionary. The most comprehensive medical dictionary available fully integrated with PDR and the Merck Manual.

 PDR® Family Guide to Prescription Drugs Patient Leaflets. Print easy-to-follow patient handouts, including photos, for nearly 1,000 products.

 PDR® Drug ID. Fast and accurate identification of virtually any tablet or capsule.

 Griffith's 5-Minute Clinical Consult. Provides quick access to diagnoses and treatments for over 1,000 medical problems.

Reviewing the full prescribing information for any product alongside available product images and chemical structures is a snap with PDR Electronic Library on CD-ROM.

 Stedman's PLUS Spell Checker. 300,000+ medical and pharmaceutical terms added to your word processor's spell checker. (Not available for free trial.)

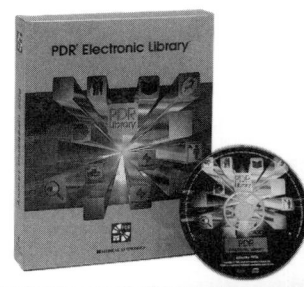

Equipment Required:
IBM PC compatible computer, MS windows 3.1 or higher, 8MB RAM, 10MB available on hard drive, VGA color monitor, Double-speed CD-ROM drive.

Provided under terms of one-year single-user license agreement.

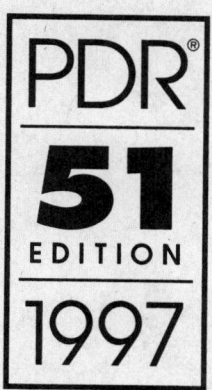

PDR 51 EDITION 1997

PHYSICIANS' DESK REFERENCE®

Medical Consultant
Ronald Arky, MD, Charles S. Davidson Professor of Medicine and Master, Francis Weld Peabody Society, Harvard Medical School

Executive Vice President, Directory Services: Paul A. Konowitch

Vice President of Product Management: Stephen B. Greenberg
Product Managers: Cy S. Caine, Mark A. Friedman
National Sales Manager: Dikran N. Barsamian
Senior Account Manager: Anthony Sorce
Account Managers
Donald V. Bruccoleri
Lawrence C. Keary
Jeffrey M. Keller
Jeffrey F. Pfohl
P. Anthony Pinsonault
Trade Sales Manager: Robin B. Bartlett
Trade Sales Account Executive: Bill Gaffney
Direct Marketing Manager: Robert W. Chapman
Marketing Communications Manager: Maryann Malorgio
Director, Professional Support Services: Mukesh Mehta, RPh
Drug Information Specialists: Thomas Fleming, RPh, Marion Gray, RPh
Editor, Special Projects: David W. Sifton

Vice President of Production: David A. Pitler
Vice President, Contract Services/Fulfillment: Steven R. Andreazza
Contracts and Support Services Director: Marjorie A. Duffy
Manager, Database Administration: Lynne Handler
Director of Production, Annuals: Carrie Williams
Manager of Production, Annuals: Kimberly Hiller-Vivas
Senior Production Coordinators: Amy B. Brooks, Dawn B. McCall
Production Coordinator: Mary Ellen R. Breun
Index/Format Manager: Jeffrey D. Schaefer
Senior Format Editor: Gregory J. Westley
Assistant Index Editor: Eileen C. Idzik
Art Associate: Joan K. Akerlind
Electronic Publishing Coordinator: Joanne M. Pearson
Senior Digital Imaging Coordinator: Shawn W. Cahill
Digital Imaging Coordinator: Frank J. McElroy, III

ISBN: 1-56363-201-2

MEDICAL ECONOMICS

The leader in healthcare information products and services

FOREWORD TO THE FIFTY-FIRST EDITION

Providing healthcare professionals with easy access to the latest, most authoritative drug information possible: That's PDR's fundamental mission. Over the years, we've refined, enhanced, and expanded PDR's many products and services to better meet this goal; and this year we're once again pleased to introduce several significant additions in the constellation of reference works that have come to constitute the PDR database.

For starters, you'll see an important expansion of the popular *PDR Guide*. In the 1997 edition, this invaluable companion to PHYSICIANS' DESK REFERENCE will include an index of every contraindication cited in PDR, providing you with a handy list of drugs to avoid in any given situation. With this addition, the guide now becomes the *PDR Guide to Drug Interactions, Side Effects, Indications, Contraindications*—a truly unique database of the major prescribing considerations that are among every physician's greatest concerns.

You can also look forward to an important new feature in the 1997 edition of *PDR For Nonprescription Drugs*: A convenient Companion Drug Index that lists over-the-counter products used in conjunction with prescription drug therapy, either to reverse drug-induced side effects or to relieve symptoms of the illness itself. For each problem, this new index will list the categories of prescription drugs that may be implicated, as well as the over-the-counter preparations that can provide relief.

Starting in 1997, you also might want to consider a visit to PDRNET.COM on the World Wide Web. This exciting new on-line service will offer registered users full MEDLINE service, as well as instant access to PDR prescribing information.

The new PDRNET.COM service is the latest member of the growing PDR family of medical references available in both traditional and electronic form. The list of printed references from PDR now includes:

- *Physicians' Desk Reference®*
- *PDR Guide to Drug Interactions, Side Effects, Indications, Contraindications™*
- *PDR For Nonprescription Drugs®*
- *PDR For Ophthalmology®*
- *PDR® Generics™*
- *PDR® Medical Dictionary™*
- *PDR® Nurse's Handbook™*
- *PDR® Nurse's Dictionary™*
- *PDR Supplements*

PDR and its major companion volumes are also found in the *PDR® Electronic Library™* on CD-ROM, now used in over 30,000 practices. This Windows-compatible disc provides users with a complete database of PDR prescribing information, electronically searchable for instant retrieval. A standard subscription includes PDR's sophisticated prescription-screening program and an exhaustive file of chemical structures, illustrations, and full-color product photographs. Optional enhancements include the complete contents of *The Merck Manual* and *Stedman's Medical Dictionary*, as well as a handy file of patient handouts drawn from PDR's consumer handbook, *The PDR® Family Guide to Prescription Drugs®*. The disc is available for use on individual PCs and PC networks.

For personal use—on rounds or on the go—there's also *Pocket PDR®*, a unique handheld electronic database of prescribing information that literally fits in your pocket. And for facilities with large, mainframe-based information systems, PDR information is also available as a preformatted text file on magnetic tape. For more information on these or any other members of the growing family of PDR products, please call, toll-free, 1-800-232-7379 or fax 201-573-4956.

PHYSICIANS' DESK REFERENCE is published by Medical Economics Company in cooperation with participating manufacturers. The 1997 edition provides the latest available information on more than 3,500 specific pharmaceutical products, including over 300 completely new listings. Each full-length entry provides you with an exact copy of the product's FDA-approved labeling.

Under the federal Food, Drug and Cosmetics (FD&C) Act, a drug approved for marketing may be labeled, promoted, and advertised by the manufacturer for only those uses for which the drug's safety and effective-

ness have been established. The Code of Federal Regulations 201.100(d)(1) pertaining to labeling for prescription products requires that for PDR content "indications, effects, dosages, routes, methods, and frequency and duration of administration and any relevant warnings, hazards, contraindications, side effects, and precautions" must be "*same in language and emphasis*" as the approved labeling for the products. The Food and Drug Administration (FDA) regards the words *same in language and emphasis* as requiring VERBATIM use of the approved labeling providing such information. Furthermore, information that is emphasized in the approved labeling by the use of type set in a box, or in capitals, boldface, or italics, must be given the same emphasis in PDR.

The FDA has also recognized that the FD&C Act does not, however, limit the manner in which a physician may use an approved drug. Once a product has been approved for marketing, a physician may choose to prescribe it for uses or in treatment regimens or patient populations that are not included in approved labeling. The FDA also observes that accepted medical practice includes drug use that is not reflected in approved drug labeling. For products that do not have official package circulars, the publisher has emphasized the necessity of describing such products comprehensively, so that physicians can have access to all information essential for intelligent and informed decision-making.

The function of the publisher is the compilation, organization, and distribution of this information. Each product description has been prepared by the manufacturer, and edited and approved by the manufacturer's medical department, medical director, and/or medical consultant. In organizing and presenting the material in PHYSICIANS' DESK REFERENCE, the publisher does not warrant or guarantee any of the products described, or perform any independent analysis in connection with any of the product information contained herein. PHYSICIANS' DESK REFERENCE does not assume, and expressly disclaims, any obligation to obtain and include any information other than that provided to it by the manufacturer. It should be understood that by making this material available the publisher is not advocating the use of any product described herein, nor is the publisher responsible for misuse of a product due to typographical error. Additional information on any product may be obtained from the manufacturer.

CONTENTS

SECTION 1

MANUFACTURERS' INDEX

Listed in this index are all manufacturers participating in PHYSICIANS' DESK REFERENCE. It is through their courtesy that PDR is brought to the medical profession.

Each company's entry includes the address, phone, and fax number of its headquarters and regional offices, as well as contacts for inquiries, orders, and medical emergency information. Products with entries in the Product Information or Diagnostic Product Information sections are listed with their page numbers. Other products available from the manufacturer are listed following the described products.

If an entry in the index lists multiple page numbers, the first ones shown refer to photographs of the product, the last one to its prescribing information.

■ **Bold page numbers** indicate full prescribing information.
■ *Italic page numbers* signify partial information.
■ The ◆ symbol marks drugs shown in the Product Identification Guide.
■ The ◉◻ symbol means product information is located in *PDR For Nonprescription Drugs*.
■ The © symbol means product information is located in PDR For Ophthalmology.

**ABANA PHARMACEUTICALS,   303, 402
INC.**
1 Chase Corporate Drive, Suite 260
Birmingham, AL 35244

Direct Inquiries to:
Customer Service
(205) 988-4588
FAX: (205) 988-3294

For Medical Information Contact:
In Emergencies:
(205) 988-4588
FAX: (205) 988-3294

Products Described:
◆Nasabid SR Caplets   303,   *402*
◆Obenix Capsules   303,   *402*
◆Otocain Drops   303,   *402*
◆Vanex Forte Caplets   303,   *402*
◆Vanex Grape Liquid   303,   *402*
◆Vanex-HD Liquid   303,   *402*

Other Products Available:
Endagen-HD Liquid
Nasatuss Liquid

ABBOTT LABORATORIES   303, 402
100 Abbott Park Rd.
Abbott Park, IL 60064

Pharmaceutical Products Division—
Direct Inquiries to:
Customer Service
(800) 255-5162
Technical Services:
(800) 441-4987
Physician Services:
(800) 222-6885
For Medical Information Contact:
Generally:
(800) 633-9110
Adverse Drug Experiences:
(800) 633-9110
Sales and Ordering:
(800) 255-5162

Hospital Products Division—
Direct Inquiries to:
Customer Service
(800) 222-6883
For Medical Information Contact:
(708) 937-3806
Sales and Ordering:
(800) 222-6883

Products Described:
Abbo-Code Index *402*
◆Abbokinase   303,   **403**
◆Abbokinase Open-Cath   303,   **405**
Abbo-Pac *402*
◆Biaxin Filmtab   303,   **406**
◆Biaxin Granules   303,   **406**
Calcijex Injection   412
Cartrol Tablets   413
Cefol Filmtab   415
◆Cylert Chewable Tablets   303,   415
◆Cylert Tablets   303,   415
◆Depakene Capsules   303,   416
Depakene Syrup   416
◆Depakote Sprinkle Capsules . .   303
◆Depakote Tablets   303,   418
◆Desoxyn Gradumet Tablets .   303,   422
Dical-D Tablets & Wafers   424
E.E.S. 200 Liquid   427
◆E.E.S. 400 Filmtab   303,   427
E.E.S. 400 Liquid   427

E.E.S. Granules **427**
Enduron Tablets **424**
◆EryPed Drops and Chewable
   Tablets   303,   **425**
◆EryPed 200 & EryPed 400
   Granules   303,   **425**
◆Ery-Tab Tablets   303,   **426**
◆Erythrocin Stearate Filmtab .   303,   **429**
◆Erythromycin Base Filmtab .   303,   **430**
◆Erythromycin Delayed-Release
   Capsules, USP   303,   **431**
Fero-Folic-500 Filmtab **433**
Fero-Grad-500 Filmtab **434**
Fero-Gradumet Filmtab **434**
◆Hytrin Capsules   303,   **434**
Iberet Filmtab **437**
Iberet-500 Filmtab **437**
Iberet-500 Liquid **438**
Iberet-Folic-500 Filmtab **433**
Iberet-Liquid **438**
◆K-Lor Powder Packets   303,   **438**
◆K-Tab Filmtab   303,   **439**
◆Nembutal Sodium Capsules .   303,   **440**
Nembutal Sodium Solution **442**
Nembutal Sodium
   Suppositories **444**
Norisodrine with Calcium
   Iodide Syrup **446**
◆Norvir Capsules   303,   **447**
◆Norvir Oral Solution   303,   **447**
Oretic Tablets **450**
◆PCE Dispertab Tablets   303,   **453**
Panhematin **452**
Peganone Tablets **455**
Phenurone Tablets **455**
◆Placidyl Capsules   303,   **456**
◆ProSom Tablets   303,   **457**
◆Tranxene T-TAB Tablets . . .   304,   **459**
◆Tranxene-SD Half Strength
   Tablets   304,   **459**
◆Tranxene-SD Tablets   304,   **459**

Other Products Available:
0.25% Acetic Acid Irrigation, USP
   (Aqualite)
Sterile A-hydroCort
5% Alcohol & 5% Dextrose Injection
Sterile A-methaPred
Amidate (Etomidate Injection) Ampul,
   Abboject
Aminophylline 250 mg, 10 mL, Ampul &
   Vial
Aminophylline 500 mg, 20 mL, Ampul &
   Vial
Aminosyn 3.5% M
Aminosyn 5%
Aminosyn 7%
Aminosyn II 7%
Aminosyn 7% TPN Kit
Aminosyn 7% with Electrolytes
Aminosyn 7% with Electrolytes TPN Kit
Aminosyn 8.5%
Aminosyn II 8.5%
Aminosyn 8.5% TPN Kit
Aminosyn 8.5% with Electrolytes
Aminosyn 10%
Aminosyn II 10%
Aminosyn 10% TPN Kit
Aminosyn with Dextrose, Nutrimix Dual
   Chamber
Aminosyn II in Dextrose, Nutrimix
   Dual Chamber
Aminosyn-HBC 7%
Aminosyn-PF 7% and 10%
Ammonium Chloride
Anticoagulant Citrate Phosphate
   Dextrose Solution, USP
Atropine 0.1 mg/mL, 5 mL, Abboject
   Syringe

Atropine 0.1 mg/mL, 10 mL, Abboject
   Syringe
Balanced Salt Solution
Bretylium Tosylate in 5% Dextrose
   Injection (2 mg/mL and 4 mg/mL)
Bupivacaine Hydrochloride Injection,
   USP, 0.25%, 0.5%, 0.75%, Ampul,
   Abboject Syringe
Butensin Picrate Ointment
Calcidrine Syrup
Calcium Acetate 0.5 mEq/mL Injection
Calcium Chloride 10%, Abboject
Calcium Gluceptate Injection Ampul &
   Abboject
Cecon Solution
Cenolate Ampules
Chromium 10 mL (4 mg/mL)
Colchicine Tablets
Copper 10 mL (4 mg/mL)
Cysteine Hydrochloride Injection
Dayalets Filmtab
Dayalets Plus Iron Filmtab
Dehydrated Alcohol Injection, USP
Desoxyn Tablets
6% Dextran 75 w/v & 5% Dextrose
   Injection
6% Dextran 75 w/v & 0.9% Sodium
   Chloride Injection
2.5% Dextrose & ½ Str Lactated
   Ringer's Injection
5% Dextrose & Lactated Ringer's
   Injection
5% Dextrose & Ringer's Injection
2.5% Dextrose & 0.45% Sodium
   Chloride Injection, USP
5% Dextrose & 0.225% Sodium
   Chloride Injection, USP
5% Dextrose & 0.3% Sodium Chloride
   Injection, USP
5% Dextrose & 0.45% Sodium Chloride
   Injection, USP
5% Dextrose & 0.9% Sodium Chloride
   Injection, USP
10% Dextrose & 0.9% Sodium Chloride
   Injection, USP
2.5% Dextrose Injection, USP
5% Dextrose Injection, USP
5% Dextrose Injection, USP
   (ADD-Vantage)
5% Dextrose Injection, USP (Partial fill)
5% Dextrose & 0.15% Pot Chl Injection
   (20 mEq)
5% Dextrose & 0.224% Pot Chl
   Injection (30 mEq)
5% Dextrose & 0.3% Pot Chl Injection
   (40 mEq)
5% Dextrose & 0.225% Sodium
   Chloride with 0.075% Potassium
   Chloride Injection (10 mEq)
5% Dextrose & 0.225% Sodium
   Chloride with 0.15% Potassium
   Chloride Injection (20 mEq)
5% Dextrose & 0.225% Sodium
   Chloride with 0.224% Potassium
   Chloride Injection (30 mEq)
5% Dextrose & 0.225% Sodium
   Chloride with 0.3% Potassium
   Chloride Injection (40 mEq)
5% Dextrose & 0.3% Sodium Chloride
   with 0.075% Potassium Chloride
   Injection (10 mEq)
5% Dextrose & 0.3% Sodium Chloride
   with 0.15% Potassium Chloride
   Injection (20 mEq)
5% Dextrose & 0.3% Sodium Chloride
   with 0.224% Potassium Chloride
   Injection (30 mEq)

5% Dextrose & 0.45% Sodium Chloride
   with 0.075% Potassium Chloride
   Injection (10 mEq)
5% Dextrose & 0.45% Sodium Chloride
   with 0.15% Potassium Chloride
   Injection (20 mEq)
5% Dextrose & 0.45% Sodium Chloride
   with 0.224% Potassium Chloride
   Injection (30 mEq)
5% Dextrose & 0.45% Sodium Chloride
   with 0.3% Potassium Chloride
   Injection (40 mEq)
10% Dextrose Injection, USP
20% Dextrose Injection, USP
30% Dextrose Injection, USP
40% Dextrose Injection, USP
50% Dextrose Injection, USP
60% Dextrose Injection, USP
70% Dextrose Injection, USP
Dicumarol Tablets
Dopamine Hydrochloride in 5% Dextrose
   Injection (800, 1600, 3200 mcg/mL)
Empty Evacuated Container
Endrate Solution, Ampoules
Enduronyl Tablets
Enduronyl Forte Tablets
Ephedrine Sulfate, Injection
Epinephrine 1:10,000, 10 mL., Abboject
Ery Derm Topical Solution
Erythrocin ADD-Vantage Kits
Erythrocin-I.V.
Erythrocin Lactobionate-I.V.
Erythrocin Piggyback
Fentanyl Injection, Ampul, Vial
Gentamicin Premix ADD-Vantage
   Products
Gentamicin Sulfate in 0.9% Sodium
   Chloride Injection (0.8, 0.9, 1.0, 1.2,
   1.4 mg/mL)
1.5% Glycine Irrigation/Aqualite
1.5% Glycine Irrigation, USP
   (Flex & Aqualite)
Glycopyrrolate Injection
Heparin Sodium in 5% Dextrose
   Injection (50 & 100 Units/mL)
Heparin Sodium in 0.45% Sodium
   Chloride Injection (50 & 100
   Units/mL)
Hydroxyzine HCl Injection, Abbojects,
   Ampuls, Vials, Syringes
Inpersol & 1.5% Dextrose
Inpersol & 2.5% Dextrose
Inpersol & 4.25% Dextrose
Inpersol-LM with 1.5% Dextrose
Inpersol-LM with 2.5% Dextrose
Inpersol-LM with 4.25% Dextrose
Isoproterenol HCl 1:5,000 5 mL,
   Universal Add Syringe
Isoproterenol HCl 1:5,000 10 mL,
   Universal Add Syringe
Isoproterenol HCl 1:50,000, 10 mL,
   Abboject
10% LMD w/v and 5% Dextrose
   Injection
10% LMD w/v and 0.9% Sodium
   Chloride Injection
LTA Kit, Preattached
LTA II Kit
LTA Pediatric Kit
Lactated Ringers for Irrigation (Flex)
Lactated Ringer's Injection, USP
Lidocaine HCl Injection, 0.2% in 5%
   Dextrose
Lidocaine HCl Injection, 0.4% in 5%
   Dextrose
Lidocaine HCl Injection, 0.8% in 5%
   Dextrose
Lidocaine HCl Injection, USP, 1%, 5 mL,
   Abboject

◆ **Shown in Product Identification Section**   *Italic Page Number* **Indicates Brief Listing**   **Described in PDR For Nonprescription Drugs** ◉◻

Lidocaine HCl Injection, USP, 1%, 5 mL,
Sterile Pack Abboject
Lidocaine HCl Injection, USP, 2%, 5 mL,
Abboject
Lidocaine HCl Injection, USP, 2%, 5 mL,
Sterile Pack Abboject
Lidocaine HCl Injection, USP, 20%, 5
mL, 1 gram-Pintop, U.A.S.
Lidocaine HCl Injection, USP, 20%, 10
mL, 2 gram-Pintop, U.A.S.
Lidocaine HCl Injection, USP, 5% with
7.5% Dextrose
Liposyn II 10% and 20%
Magnesium Sulfate 12.5%, 8 mL, Pintop
Magnesium Sulfate 50% w/v Ampoules,
Vials & Abboject
Mammol Ointment
Manganese 10 mL (1 mg/mL)
5% Mannitol Injection, USP
10% Mannitol Injection, USP
15% Mannitol Injection, USP
20% Mannitol Injection, USP
25% Mannitol Injection, USP
Meperidine HCl Injection (10 mg/mL,
PCA Vials)
Metronidazole Injection, USP (5 mg/mL)
Morphine Sulfate Injection, USP
(1 & 5 mg/mL, PCA Vials)
Nalbuphine Hydrochloride Injection, USP
Nembutal Elixir
Neut Abbo-Vial & Pintop
Nitropress
Normosol-M 900 CAL
Normosol-M & 5% Dextrose Injection
Normosol-R
Normosol-R pH 7.4
Normosol-R & 5% Dextrose Injection
Optilets-500 Filmtab
Optilets-M-500 Filmtab
Penthrane
Pentothal (Sterile Powder)
Pentothal (Thiopental Sodium for
Injection)
Pentothal Kit
Pentothal RTM Syringe
Pentothal Rectal Suspension in Syringe
Phenobarbital Sodium Ampoules
Physiosol Irrigation (Aqualite)
Plegisol
Potassium Acetate 40 mEq Vial, Pintop
& Fliptop
Potassium Chloride Injection Ampoules
& Vials, Pintop & Universal Additive
Syringe
Potassium Chloride 20 mEq. in D-5 W in
Abbo-Vac
Potassium Phosphate 15 mM Vial,
Pintop & Fliptop
Potassium Phosphate 45 mM Vial
Procainamide Hydrochloride Injection,
USP
Procaine Hydrochloride Injection 1% &
2% Vial
Quelicin (Succinylcholine Chloride
Injection) Ampul & Vial, Pintop
Ringer's Injection, USP
Ringer's Irrigation, USP (Aqualite)
Sodium Acetate 40 mEq, 100 mEq and
200 mEq Vials
5% Sodium Bicarbonate Injection, USP
4.2% Sodium Bicarbonate Injection, 10
mEq in 10 mL Abboject (Neonatal)
7.5% Sodium Bicarbonate Injection,
44.6 mEq in 50 mL ampul or
Abboject
8.4% Sodium Bicarbonate Injection, 50
mEq in 50 mL Abboject or Fliptop Vial
8.4% Sodium Bicarbonate Injection,
10 mEq in 10 mL Abboject (Pediatric)
0.45% Sodium Chloride Injection, USP
5% Sodium Chloride
0.9% Sodium Chloride Injection
0.9% Sodium Chloride Injection, USP
(ADD-Vantage)
0.9% Sodium Chloride Injection,
USP (Partial Fill)
0.9% Sodium Chloride Irrigation, USP
(Flex and Aqualite)
0.45% Sodium Chloride Irrigation, USP
(Aqualite)
Sodium Lactate Injection, USP, 1/6
Molar
Sodium Phosphate 45 mg/15 mL
Sorbitol-Mannitol Irrigation (Flex &
Aqualite)
Sterile Urea
Surbex-T Filmtab
Surbex with C Filmtab
Surbex 750 with Iron Filmtab
Surbex 750 with Zinc Filmtab
TPN Electrolytes
Tham-E
Tham Solution
Theophylline in 5% Dextrose Injection
(0.4, 0.8, 1.6, 2, 4 mg/mL)
Tubocurarine Chloride Injection, USP
Ureaphil
Urologic G Irrigation (Aqualite)
Water for Injection, Ampoules, Vial
Water for Injection Bacteriostatic 30 mL
Fliptop
Water for Injection, Sterile, USP
Water, for Irrigation, Sterile, USP (Flex
and Aqualite)
Water for Respiratory Therapy, Sterile
(Flex)
Zinc 10 mL (1 mg/1 mL)

AC LABORATORY   461
750 Stimson Ave.
City of Industry, CA 91745

Direct Inquiries to:
Yung Feng Hung
(818) 336-8889
FAX: (818) 336-1299

ADAMS LABORATORIES, INC.
(See MEDEVA PHARMACEUTICALS,
INC.)

ADVANCED NUTRITIONAL   461
TECHNOLOGY, INC.
6988 Sierra Ct.
Dublin, CA 94568

Direct Inquiries to:
(800) 624-6543
(510) 828-2128
FAX: (510) 828-6848

AKORN, INC.   462
100 Akorn Drive
Abita Springs, LA 70420

Direct Inquiries to:
Customer Service
(800) 535-7155
(504) 893-9300

(For information on Akorn ophthalmic
pharmaceutical products, please
consult PDR FOR
OPHTHALMOLOGY)

ALCON LABORATORIES, INC.   465
Alcon Laboratories, Inc.
And its affiliates Inc.
Corporate Headquarters
P.O. Box 6600
6201 South Freeway
Fort Worth, TX 76134

Direct Inquiries to:
Sales Services
(817) 293-0450

Other Products Available:
A.C.S. Closure System Needles and
Sutures
A-OK Ophthalmic Knives
Alcon Surgical System
(Irrigation/Aspiration Kits;
Phacoemulsification Kits)
Bion Tears
BSS Irrigation Solution (15mL, 30mL,
250mL, 500mL)
BSS Plus Irrigation Solution (30mL,
500mL)
BSS and BSS Plus Irrigation Solution
Administration Set
Cetamide Ointment
Cetapred Ointment
Cryophake Sterile, Disposable
Cryoextractor
Cyclogyl Ophthalmic Solution
Cyclomydril Ophthalmic Solution
Cystitomes & Cannulas
DUOVISC Viscoelastic System
Duratears Naturale Lubricant Eye
Ointment
Enuclene Ophthalmic Solution
Epinal Ophthalmic Solution
Eye Pak Surgical Drape
Fluorescite Injection
Gonioscopic Prism Solution
I-Knife Ophthalmic Knife
Intraocular Lenses
Iopidine Ophthalmic Solution
Ismotic Solution
I-SPEAR Miniature Surgical Sponge
Maxidex Ophthalmic Solution
Maxitrol Ointment
Microphake Sterile Disposable
Cryoextractor
Microsponge Miniature Surgical Sponge
Miostat Intraocular Solution
Natacyn Ophthalmic Suspension
Optemp Sterile Disposable Cautery
Osmoglyn Oral Osmotic Agent
Pilopine HS Gel
Post-Operative Kits
Procedure Packs
PROFENAL Ophthalmic Solution
PROVISC Viscoelastic Material
PTG, Alcon Applanation
Pneumatonograph
Steri-Units Sterile Ophthalmic Units for
Single Use Only
Vexol
VISCOAT Viscoelastic Solution
Zolyse Ophthalmic Solution

ALCON (PUERTO RICO) INC.
P.O. Box 3000
Humacao, Puerto Rico 00661

For Medical Information Contact:
Medical Department
P.O. Box 6380
Fort Worth, TX 76115
(817) 293-0450

Products Available:
Adsorbocarpine
Adsorbonac
Adsorbotear
Alcaine
Econopred
Econopred Plus
Glaucon
Isopto Atropine
Isopto Carbachol
Isopto Carpine
Isopto Cetamide
Isopto Cetapred
Isopto Homatropine
Isopto Hyoscine
Maxidex Suspension
Maxitrol Suspension
Mydfrin 2.5%
Mydrapred
Mydriacyl
Naphcon
Naphcon Forte
Zincfrin

ALLERGAN, INC.   304, 470
2525 Dupont Drive
P.O. Box 19534
Irvine, CA 92623-9534

Direct Inquiries to:
(714) 752-4500

Other Products Available:
Albalon Solution with Liquifilm
Betagan Liquifilm Sterile Ophthalmic
Solution with C Cap Compliance Cap
Q.D. and B.I.D.
Chloroptic S.O.P. Sterile Ophthalmic
Ointment
Chloroptic Sterile Ophthalmic Solution
Epifrin Sterile Ophthalmic Solution
FML Forte Liquifilm Sterile Ophthalmic
Suspension
FML Liquifilm Sterile Ophthalmic
Suspension
FML S.O.P. Sterile Ophthalmic Ointment
FML-S Sterile Ophthalmic Suspension
Genoptic Liquifilm Sterile Ophthalmic
Solution
Genoptic S.O.P. Sterile Ophthalmic
Ointment
HMS Liquifilm Sterile Ophthalmic
Suspension
Ophthetic Sterile Ophthalmic Solution
Paremyd Sterile Ophthalmic Solution
Pilagan Liquifilm Sterile Ophthalmic
Solution with C Cap Compliance Cap
Q.I.D.
Poly-Pred Liquifilm Sterile Ophthalmic
Suspension
Pred Forte Sterile Ophthalmic
Suspension
Pred-G Liquifilm Sterile Ophthalmic
Suspension
Pred-G S.O.P. Sterile Ophthalmic
Ointment
Pred Mild Sterile Ophthalmic Suspension
Propine Ophthalmic Solution, USP, 0.1%
Sterile with C Cap Compliance Cap
B.I.D.

ALLERGAN HERBERT
(See ALLERGAN, INC.)

ALPHA THERAPEUTIC   480
CORPORATION
5555 Valley Boulevard
Los Angeles, CA 90032

Direct Inquiries to:
(213) 225-2221
(800) 421-0008
FAX: (213) 227-7027

For Medical Information Contact:
In Emergencies:
Jonathan Goldsmith, M.D., Medical
Director
(213) 227-7210
After Hours Emergency Orders:
(800) 421-0008

ALPHARMA   481
U.S. Pharmaceuticals Division
7205 Windsor Blvd.
Baltimore, MD 21244

Direct Inquiries to:
Customer Service
(800) 638-9096

ALRA LABORATORIES, INC.   484

3850 Clearview Court
Gurnee, IL 60031

Direct Inquiries to:
Professional Services
(847) 244-9440
(800) 248-ALRA
FAX: (847) 244-9464

Products Described:

Other Products Available:
AZM-TAB, Acetazolamide Tablets
Chlordiazepoxide Capsules
Ferrous Sulfate Drops
Hydrochlorothiazide Tablets
IMP-TAB, Imipramine Tablets
Methalgen Cream
Multi Vitamin Drops
Multi Vitamin Drops With Fluoride
Multi Vitamin Drops With Iron
SS-TAB, Sulfisoxazole Tablets
TOL-TAB, Tolbutamide Tablets
Vitamin Drops With Fluoride

ALZA PHARMACEUTICALS   304, 485

A Division of Alza Corporation
950 Page Mill Road
P.O. Box 10950
Palo Alto, California 94303-0802

Direct Inquiries to:
Customer Service
(800) 227-9953
FAX: (415) 962-4212

**For Medical Information or
Emergencies Contact:**
**For Testoderm, Progestasert,
Ocusert:**
Medical Communications
(800) 634-8977
FAX: (415) 962-2488
For Ethyol:
Medical Communications
(800) 506-4959
FAX: (415) 962-2488

Products Described:

Other Products Available:
Progestasert Intrauterine Progesterone
Contraceptive System

AMERICAN LECITHIN COMPANY   488

115 Hurley Rd.
Unit 2 B
Oxford, CT 06478

Direct Inquiries to:
Randall E. Zigmont
(203) 262-7100
FAX: (203) 262-7101

For Medical Information Contact:
Randall E. Zigmont
(203) 262-7100
FAX: (203) 262-7101

Products Described:

Other Products Available:
PhosChol Gold

AMERICAN RED CROSS   488

National Headquarters
Biomedical Services
431 18th St. NW
Washington, DC 20006-5306

Direct Inquiries to:
Professional Services Department:
(703) 312-8737
FAX: (703) 312-8742
Customer Service Department:
(800) 446-8883
FAX: (703) 312-8746

Products Described:

AMGEN INC.   304, 489

1840 Dehavilland Drive
Thousand Oaks, CA 91230-1789

Direct Inquiries to:
Customer Services Department
(800) 282-6436
FAX: (800) 292-6436

For Medical Information Contact:
Generally:
Professional Services Department
(800) 772-6436
FAX: (818) 865-3707

In Emergencies:
(800) 772-6436
After Hours and Weekends:
(800) 772-6436

Sales and Ordering:
Customer Services Department
(800) 282-6436
FAX: (800) 292-6436

Products Described:

ANAQUEST INC.*
(See OHMEDA PHARMACEUTICAL
PRODUCTS DIVISION INC.)

APOTHECON
(See BRISTOL-MYERS SQUIBB
COMPANY)

ARCO PHARMACEUTICALS, INC.   513

105 Orville Drive
Bohemia, NY 11716

Direct Inquiries to:
Professional Service Department
(516) 567-9500

Products Described:

Other Products Available:
Arco-Cee Tablets
Arcoret Tablets
Arcoret w/Iron Tablets
Arcotinic Liquid
Arcotinic Tablets
C-B Time Capsules
C-B Time Liquid
C-B Time 500 Tablets
Co-Gel Tablets
Mega-B with C
Spantuss Liquid
Spantuss Tablets

ARMOUR PHARMACEUTICAL COMPANY
(See CENTEON)

B. F. ASCHER & COMPANY, INC.   514

15501 W 109th St.
Lenexa, KS 66219-1308

Direct Inquiries to:
Product Information Department
(913) 888-1880

Products Described:

Other Products Available:
Ayr Saline Nasal Drops
Ayr Saline Nasal Gel
Ayr Saline Nasal Mist
Cough-X Lozenges
Hy-Phen Tablets
Itch-X Gel
Itch-X Spray
Mobidin Tablets
Mobigesic Pain Reliever - Fever Reducer
Tablets
Mobisyl Pain Relieving Creme
Pen•Kera Creme
Pretty Feet & Hands Rough Skin
Remover
Tolfrinic Tablets

ASTRA MERCK INC.   304, 514

725 Chesterbrook Boulevard
Wayne, PA 19087-5677

For Medical Information Contact:
Generally:
(800) 236-9933
Adverse Drug Experiences:
(800) 236-9933

Products Described:

**Products listed are
manufactured by Merck &
Co. Inc., West Point, PA
19486.**

ASTRA USA, INC.   304, 522

50 Otis Street
Westborough, MA 01581-4500

Direct Inquiries to:
(508) 366-1100

Kenalog-10 and Kenalog-40 Suspension
Metoprolol Tartrate Tablets
Mucomyst and Mucomyst-10
Mycolog-II Cream and Ointment
Mycostatin Oral Suspension
Mycostatin Oral Tablets
Nadolol Tablets
Nafcillin Sodium for Injection USP and in ADD-Vantage Vials
Naldecon Syrup, Tablets, Pediatric Drops and Pediatric Syrup
Naturetin-5 Tablets and Naturetin-10 Tablets
Neostigmine Methylsulfate Injection USP
Niacin Tablets USP
Nitrazine Paper
Ophthaine Solution
Oxacillin Capsules USP and for Oral Solution
Oxacillin for Injection USP and in ADD-Vantage Vials
Penicillin G Potassium for Injection USP
Penicillin G Sodium for Injection USP
Polycillin Capsules and Oral Suspension (see Principen)
Potassium Cl Extended Release Tablets
Principen Capsules, for Oral Suspension, and Pediatric Drops
Prolixin Tablets
Pronestyl Capsules, Tablets and Injection
Pronestyl-SR Tablets
Rauzide Tablets
SMZ-TMP Oral Solution and Tablets
Spec-T Sore Throat Anesthetic Lozenges
Spec-T Sore Throat/Cough Suppressant Lozenges
Spec-T Sore Throat/Decongestant Lozenges
Sumycin Tablets, Capsules and Syrup
Theragran Hematinic
Tobramycin Sulfate Injection USP
Trimox Capsules and for Oral Suspension
Tubocurarine Chloride Injection USP
Vasodilan
Veetids Tablets and for Oral Suspension
Velosef Capsules and for Oral Suspension
Vesprin Injection

APOTHECON/INVAMED

Products Not Described:
Amantadine Hydrochloride Capsules, USP
Atenolol Tablets
Benztropine Mesylate Tablets, USP
Cimetidine Tablets, USP
Cyclobenzaprine Hydrochloride Tablets, USP
Gemfibrozil Tablets, USP
Glipizide Tablets, USP
Hydroxychloroquine Sulfate Tablets, USP
Indapamide Tablets, USP
Metoclopramide Tablets, USP
Naproxen Sodium Tablets, USP
Orphenadrine Citrate/Aspirin/Caffeine
Prochlorperazine Maleate Tablets, USP

BRISTOL-MYERS SQUIBB ONCOLOGY/IMMUNOLOGY DIVISION **307, 696**
A Bristol-Myers Squibb Company
P.O. Box 4500
Princeton, NJ 08543-4500
(609) 897-2000

For Medical Information Contact:
Generally:
Bristol-Myers Squibb Drug Information Department
P.O. Box 4500
Princeton, NJ 08543-4500
(800) 426-7644
Adverse Drug Experiences
and Product Defects Reporting call during business hours only:
(609) 252-3737

Sales and Ordering:
Orders may be placed by:

1. Calling the following toll-free number between 8:30 AM-6:00 PM EST:
Continental U.S.: (800) 631-5244
Alaska-Hawaii: (800) 631-5244

2. Mail orders and all inquiries should be sent to:
Bristol-Myers Squibb Oncology Division
Attn: Customer Service
P.O. Box 5250
Princeton, NJ 08543-5250

3. Faxing your purchase orders to:
(800) 523-2965

4. Transmitting computer-to-computer on the NWDA and UCS formats through Ordernet Services use: DEA # PE0048579

Products Described:
BiCNU . . . 696
◆Blenoxane . . . 307, 697
CeeNU Capsules . . . 699
◆Cytoxan for Injection . . . 307, 700
◆Cytoxan Tablets . . . 307, 700
◆Etopophos for Injection . . . 307, 701
◆Fungizone Oral Suspension . . . 307, 704
Hydrea Capsules . . . 705
◆IFEX . . . 307, 706
Lysodren Tablets . . . 707
◆Megace Oral Suspension . . . 307, 708
◆Megace Tablets . . . 307, 710
◆Mesnex Injection . . . 307, 711
◆Mutamycin for Injection . . . 307, 712
Mycostatin Pastilles . . . 713
◆Paraplatin for Injection . . . 307, 713
Platinol for Injection . . . 717
◆Platinol-AQ Injection . . . 307, 719
Rubex for Injection . . . 721
◆Taxol Injection . . . 307, 723
Teslac Tablets . . . 727
◆VePesid Capsules and Injection . . . 307,308, 727
◆Videx Tablets, Powder for Oral Solution, & Pediatric Powder for Oral Solution . . . 308, 2980
Vumon for Injection . . . 729
◆Zerit Capsules . . . 308, 731

BRISTOL-MYERS PRODUCTS **306, 734**
A Bristol-Myers Squibb Company
345 Park Avenue
New York, NY 10154

Direct Inquiries to:
Products Division
Consumer Affairs Department
1350 Liberty Avenue
Hillside, NJ 07207
(800) 468-7746

Products Described:
Alpha Keri Moisture Rich Body Oil . . . ◙
Backache Caplets . . . ◙
Arthritis Strength Bufferin Analgesic Caplets . . . ◙
Extra Strength Bufferin Analgesic Tablets . . . ◙
Bufferin Analgesic Tablets and Caplets . . . ◙
Allergy-Sinus Comtrex Multi-Symptom Allergy Sinus Formula Tablets and Day-Night Tablet/Caplet . . . ◙
Comtrex Maximum Strength Multi-Symptom Cold Reliever Tablets/Caplets/Liqui-Gels/Liquid . . . ◙
Non-Drowsy Comtrex Maximum Strength Caplets . . . ◙
◆Aspirin Free Excedrin Analgesic Caplets and Geltabs . . . 306, 734
◆Excedrin Extra-Strength Analgesic Tablets, Caplets, and Geltabs . . . 306, 734
Excedrin P.M. Analgesic/Sleeping Aid Tablets, Caplets, Liquigels . . . 735
4-Way Fast Acting Nasal Spray - Original Formula (regular & mentholated) & Metered Spray Pump (regular) . . . ◙
4-Way Long Lasting Nasal Spray . . . ◙
Keri Lotion - Original Formula . . . ◙
Keri Lotion - Silky Smooth Formula . . . ◙
Keri Lotion - Sensitive Skin, Fragrance-Free Formula . . . ◙
Therapeutic Mineral Ice, Pain Relieving Gel . . . ◙

Other Products Available:
Alpha Keri Moisture Rich Cleansing Bar
Ammens Medicated Powder
B.Q. Cold Tablets
Ban Antiperspirant Cream Deodorant
Ban Basic Non-aerosol Antiperspirant Spray
Ban Clear Antiperspirant
Ban Clear Roll-On
Ban For Men Clear Antiperspirant
Ban For Men Deodorant
Ban Fresh & Dry Roll-On Antiperspirant Deodorant
Ban Roll-on Antiperspirant Deodorant
Ban Sensitive Touch Roll-On Antiperspirant Deodorant
Ban Sensitive Touch Solid Antiperspirant Deodorant
Ban Solid Antiperspirant Deodorant
Day/Night Comtrex
Sinus Excedrin Caplets and Liquigels
Fisherman's Friend Lozenges Extra Strong and Original
Fisherman's Friend Lozenges, Sugar Free Extra Strong and Refreshing Mint
Fostex 10% Benzoyl Peroxide Bar
Fostex 10% Benzoyl Peroxide (Vanish) Gel
Fostex 10% Benzoyl Peroxide Wash
Fostex Medicated Cleansing Bar
Fostex Medicated Cleansing Cream
4 Way Cold Tablets
Keri Cort-10 Cream
Keri Cream
Minit-Rub Analgesic Ointment
Mum Antiperspirant Cream Deodorant
No Doz Chewable Tablets
No Doz Maximum Strength Caplets
Nuprin Tablets and Caplets
Pazo Hemorrhoid Ointment and Suppositories
Therapeutic Mineral Ice Exercise Formula

WESTWOOD-SQUIBB PHARMACEUTICALS INC. **2791**
A Bristol-Myers Squibb Company
100 Forest Avenue
Buffalo, NY 14213
(716) 887-3400

For Medical Information Contact:
Generally:
Consumer Affairs Department:
(716) 887-7667
Adverse Drug Experiences
and Product Defects Reporting call during business hours only:
(716) 887-7667

Products Described:
Capitrol Shampoo . . . 2791
Desquam-E 2.5 Emollient Gel . . . 2792
Desquam-E 5 Emollient Gel . . . 2792
Desquam-E 10 Emollient Gel . . . 2792
Desquam-X 5 Gel . . . 2792
Desquam-X 10 Gel . . . 2792
Desquam-X 10 Bar . . . 2792
Desquam-X 5 Wash . . . 2792
Desquam-X 10 Wash . . . 2792
Dovonex Cream 0.005% . . . 2792
Dovonex Ointment 0.005% . . . 2793
Eurax Cream & Lotion . . . 2794
Exelderm Cream 1.0% . . . 2794
Exelderm Solution 1.0% . . . 2795
Halog Cream, Ointment & Solution 0.1% . . . 2795
Halog-E Cream 0.1% . . . 2795
Lac-Hydrin 12% Lotion . . . 2796
Moisturel Cream . . . 2796
Moisturel Lotion . . . 2797
Mycostatin Cream & Topical Powder . . . 2797
T-Stat 2.0% Topical Solution and Pads . . . 2797
Ultravate Cream 0.05% . . . 2797
Ultravate Ointment 0.05% . . . 2798
Westcort Cream 0.2% . . . 2799
Westcort Ointment 0.2% . . . 2800

Other Products Available:
Balnetar
Estar Gel
Fostril
Lac-Hydrin Five Lotion
Lowila Cake
Maxivate Cream, Lotion & Ointment 0.05%
Moisturel Sensitive Skin Cleanser
Pernox Scrub Cleanser
PreSun Active 15 and 30 Clear Gel Sunscreens
PreSun 15 and 29 Sensitive Skin Sunscreens
PreSun 21 Block
PreSun 23 and For Kids Spray Mist Sunscreens
PreSun 29 For Kids Lotion Sunscreen
PreSun 46 Moisturizing Sunscreen
Sebulex Dandruff Shampoo
Sebulex Dandruff Shampoo with Conditioners
Sebulon Shampoo
Sebutone and Sebutone Cream Antiseborrheic Tar Shampoos

BIO-TECHNOLOGY GENERAL CORP. **783**
BTG PHARMACEUTICALS
70 Wood Avenue South
Iselin, NJ 08830

Direct Inquiries to:
(908) 632-8800

For Medical Information or Emergencies Contact:
(800) 741-2698

For Customer Service and Ordering:
(800) 741-2698
FAX: (800) 741-2696

Products Described:
Delatestryl Injection . . . *783*
Oxandrin . . . 783

J. R. CARLSON LABORATORIES, INC. **784**
15 College Drive
Arlington Heights, IL 60004-1985

Direct Inquiries to:
Customer Service
(847) 255-1600
FAX: (847) 255-1605

For Medical Information Contact:
In Emergencies:
Customer Service
(847) 255-1600
FAX: (847) 255-1605

Products Described:
ACES Antioxidant Soft Gels . . . *784*
Co-Q10 . . . *785*
E-Gems Soft Gels . . . *785*

CARNRICK LABORATORIES, INC. **308, 785**
65 Horse Hill Road
Cedar Knolls, NJ 07927

Direct Inquiries to:
(201) 267-2670
FAX: (201) 267-2728

For Medical Information Contact:
Medical Director
(201) 267-2670
FAX: (201) 267-2728

Products Described:
◆Amen Tablets . . . 308, 785
◆Bontril PDM Tablets . . . 308, *786*
◆Bontril Slow-Release Capsules 308, 786
◆Capital And Codeine Suspension . . . 308, *787*
◆Exgest LA Tablets . . . 308, 787
◆Hydrocet Capsules . . . 308, 787
◆Midrin Capsules . . . 308, 788
◆Motofen Tablets . . . 308, 789
◆Nolahist Tablets . . . 308, 790
◆Nolamine Timed-Release Tablets . . . 308, 790
◆Phrenilin Forte Capsules . . . 308, 790
◆Phrenilin Tablets . . . 308, 790
◆Propagest Tablets . . . 308, 791
◆Salflex Tablets . . . 308, 791
◆Sinulin Tablets . . . 308, 792
◆Skelaxin Tablets . . . 308, 793
◆Theo-X Extended-Release Tablets . . . 308, 793

CENTEON **795**
1020 First Avenue
King of Prussia, PA 19406-1310

Direct Inquiries to:
(610) 878-4000

For Medical Information Contact:
(800) 504-5434

Sales and Ordering:
Customer Support Center
(800) 683-1288
FAX: (610) 878-4888

Products Described:
Albuminar-5, Albumin (Human) U.S.P. 5% . . . 795
Albuminar-25, Albumin (Human) U.S.P. 25% . . . 796
Bioclate, Antihemophilic Factor (Recombinant) . . . 797
Gammar-P I.V., Immune Globulin Intravenous (Human) . . . 798
Helixate, Antihemophilic Factor (Recombinant) . . . 799
Humate-P, Antihemophilic Factor (Human), Dried Pasteurized . . . 801
Monoclate-P, Factor VIII:C Pasteurized, Monoclonal Antibody Purified Antihemophilic Factor (Human) . . . 802
Mononine, Coagulation Factor IX (Human), Monoclonal Antibody Purified . . . 804
Plasma-Plex, Plasma Protein Fraction (Human) U.S.P. 5% Solution Heat-Treated . . . 806
Stimate, (desmopressin acetate) Nasal Spray, 1.5 mg/mL . . . 806

CENTER LABORATORIES **808**
Division of EM Industries, Inc.
35 Channel Drive
Port Washington, NY 11050

Direct Inquiries to:
Customer Services
(800) 223-6837
FAX: (516) 767-4229

For Medical Information Contact:
In Emergencies:
Technical Services
(516) 767-1800

Products Described:
EpiPen - Epinephrine Auto-Injector . . . 808
EpiPen Jr.- Epinephrine Auto-Injector . . . 808

Other Products Available:
Ace Spacer (Holding Chamber)
Astech Peak Flow Meter
Center-Al - Allergenic Extracts Alum-Precipitated
Epi EZ Pen-Epinephrine Auto-Injector
Epi EZ Pen, Jr.-Epinephrine Auto-Injector

CENTOCOR B.V.
Einsteinweg 101
233 CB Leiden, The Netherlands
Subsidiary of Centocor Inc.

Products Described:
◆ ReoPro Vials 322, 1526

CENTRAL   308, 808
PHARMACEUTICALS, INC.
120 East Third St.
Seymour, IN 47274

Direct Inquiries to:
Schwarz Pharma Drug Safety and
Information
P.O. Box 2038
Milwaukee, WI 53201
(800) 558-5114

Products Described:
◆ Azdone Tablets 308, 808
Codiclear DH Syrup 808
Codimal DH Syrup 809
Codimal DM Syrup 809
◆ Codimal-L.A. Capsules . . . 308, 809
◆ Codimal-L.A. HALF Capsules . 308, 809
Codimal PH Syrup 809
◆ Co-Gesic Tablets 308, 809
◆ Guaimax-D Tablets 308, 809
◆ Mono-Gesic Tablets 308, 810
◆ Niferex-150 Capsules 308, 811
◆ Niferex-150 Forte Capsules . 308, 811
Niferex Elixir 811
Niferex Tablets 811
Niferex w/Vitamin C Tablets 811
◆ Niferex-PN Forte Tablets . . 308, 811
◆ Niferex-PN Tablets 308, 811
PEDIAPAP Oral Solution 811
Prednicen-M 21-Pak 811
Theoclear-80 Syrup 811

Other Products Available:
Codimal Tablets & Capsules
GG-Cen Capsules

CETUS ONCOLOGY CORPORATION
(See CHIRON THERAPEUTICS)

CETYLITE INDUSTRIES, INC.   812
9051 River Road
Pennsauken, NJ 08110-3293
Mailing address:
P.O. Box 90006
Pennsauken, NJ 08110-0700

Direct Inquiries to:
Mr. Stanley L. Wachman, President
(609) 665-6111
(800) 257-7740
FAX: (609) 665-5408

Products Described:
Cetacaine Topical Anesthetic 812

Other Products Available:
Cetylite Skin Screen Protective Skin
Lotion
Protexin Oral Breath Spray
Protexin Oral Rinse Concentrate

CHATTEM, INC.   812
1715 West 38th Street
Chattanooga, TN 37409

Direct Inquiries to:
Gary Galante
(423) 821-4571, Ext. 336

Products Described:
Herpecin-L Cold Sore Lip
Balm Stick 812

CHIRON THERAPEUTICS   812
4560 Horton Street
Emeryville, CA 94608-2997

For Medical Information Contact:
Generally:
Professional Services (6:00 AM to
5:00 PM PST):
(800) CHIRON-8
(800) 244-7668
FAX: (510) 601-3435
In Emergencies:
(6:00 AM to 5:00 PM PST):
(800) CHIRON-8
(800) 244-7668
**After Hours and Weekend
Emergencies:**
(415) 885-8777

Sales and Ordering:
(800) CHIRON-8
(800) 244-7668
FAX: (510) 601-3434

Products Described:
Proleukin for Injection 812

CIBAGENEVA   308, 816
PHARMACEUTICALS

Ciba-Geigy Corporation
556 Morris Avenue
Summit, NJ 07901
(for branded products)

For Information Contact:
Consumer Affairs Department:
(800) 742-2422
Medical Services Department:
556 Morris Avenue
Summit, NJ 07901

Geneva Pharmaceuticals, Inc.
2655 West Midway Boulevard
P.O. Box 446
Broomfield, CO 80038-0446
(for branded generic products)

For Information Contact:
Customer Support Department:
(800) 525-8747
(303) 466-2400
FAX: (303) 469-6467

Products Described:
◆ Actigall Capsules 308, 818
◆ Anafranil Capsules 308, 819
◆ Anturane Capsules 309, 823
◆ Anturane Tablets 309, 823
◆ Apresazide Capsules 309, 824
◆ Apresoline Hydrochloride
Tablets 309, 826
Aredia for Injection 827
◆ Brethaire Inhaler 309, 830
◆ Brethine Ampuls 309, 832
◆ Brethine Tablets 309, 831
◆ Cataflam Tablets 309, 833
◆ Cytadren Tablets 309, 837
Desferal Vials 838
◆ Esidrix Tablets 309, 839
◆ Esimil Tablets 309, 840
◆ Estraderm Transdermal
System 309, 842
◆ Ismelin Tablets 309, 845
◆ Lamprene Capsules 309, 846
◆ Lioresal Tablets 309, 847
Lopressor Injection 848
◆ Lopressor Tablets 309, 848
◆ Lopressor HCT Tablets 309, 850
◆ Lotensin Tablets 309, 852
◆ Lotensin HCT Tablets 309, 855
◆ Lotrel Capsules 309, 858
◆ Ludiomil Tablets 309, 861
◆ PBZ Tablets 309, 863
◆ PBZ-SR Tablets 309, 862
Priscoline Hydrochloride
Ampuls 864
Regitine Vials 864
◆ Rimactane Capsules 309, 865
◆ Ritalin Hydrochloride Tablets . 309, 866
◆ Ritalin-SR Tablets 309, 866
◆ Ser-Ap-Es Tablets 309, 867
◆ Slow-K Extended-Release
Tablets 309, 869
◆ Tegretol Chewable Tablets . . 309, 870
Tegretol Suspension 870
◆ Tegretol Tablets 309, 870
◆ Tegretol-XR Tablets 309, 870
Tofranil Ampuls 873
◆ Tofranil Tablets 309, 875
◆ Tofranil-PM Capsules 309, 876
◆ Transderm-Nitro Transdermal
Therapeutic System 309, 878
◆ Vivelle Transdermal System . . 310, 880
◆ Voltaren Tablets 310, 833
◆ Voltaren-XR Tablets 310, 833

Other Products Available:
Albuterol Sulfate Tablets
Allopurinol Tablets
Alprazolam Tablets
Amiloride/HCTZ Tablets
Amitriptyline Tablets
Amoxapine Tablets
APAP/Codeine Tablets
Atenolol Tablets
Captopril Tablets
Carbidopa/Levodopa Tablets
Carisoprodol Tablets
Chlorpromazine HCl Tablets
Chlorzoxazone Tablets
Cimetidine Tablets
Clemastine Tablets
Clindamycin Phosphate Topical Solution
Clonidine Tablets
Cyclobenzaprine HCl Tablets
Decongestant Sr Tablets
Desipramine HCl Tablets
Diazepam Tablets
Diclofenac Sodium Tablets
Diphenhydramine HCl Capsules
Disobrom Tablets
Disopyramide Phosphate Capsules
Doxepin HCl Capsules
Ercaf Tablets
Fenoprofen Calcium Capsules
Fenoprofen Calcium Tablets
Fluphenazine HCl Tablets
Flurbiprofen Tablets
Furosemide Tablets
Glipizide Tablets
Glyburide Tablets
Haloperidol Tablets
Hydroxychloroquine Tablets
Imipramine HCl Tablets
Indomethacin Capsules
Isosorbide Dinitrate Tablets
Isoxsuprine Tablets
Ketoprofen Capsules
Lonox Tablets
Loperamide Capsules
Lorazepam Tablets
Meclizine HCl Tablets
Meclofenamate Sodium Capsules
Meprobamate Tablets
Methazolamide Tablets
Methocarbamol Tablets
Methyclothiazide Tablets
Methyldopa Tablets
Methyldopa/HCTZ Tablets
Metoclopramide Tablets
Metoprolol Tartrate Tablets
Metronidazole Tablets
Naproxen Sodium Tablets
Naproxen Tablets
Nitrofurantoin Macrocrystals Capsules
Nortriptyline Capsules
Oxazepam Capsules
Perphenazine Tablets
Perphenazine/Amitriptyline HCl Tablets
Pindolol Tablets
Prednisone Tablets
Promethazine Tablets
Propoxyphene/APAP Tablets
Propoxyphene/NAP/APAP Tablets
Propoxyphene HCl Capsules
Propanolol/HCTZ Tablets
Pseudoephedrine Tablets
Quinidine Gluconate Tablets
Quinidine Sulfate Tablets
Resaid S.R. Capsules
Spironolactone Tablets
Sulindac Tablets
Temazepam Capsules
Thioridazine Tablets
Thiothixene Capsules
Timolol Maleate Tablets
Trazodone HCl Tablets
Triam/HCTZ Capsules
Triam/HCTZ (Dyazide) Capsules
Triam/HCTZ (Maxzide) Tablets
Triam/HCTZ (mini-Maxzide) Tablets
Triazolam Tablets
Trifluoperazine HCl Tablets
Verapamil Tablets

CIBA PHARMACEUTICAL COMPANY
(See CIBAGENEVA PHARMACEUTICALS)

CIBA SELF-MEDICATION, INC.   308, 883
581 Main Street
Woodbridge, NJ 07095

Direct Inquiries to:
Consumer Affairs
(800) 452-0051

After Hours and Weekend Emergencies:
(908) 277-5000

Products Described:
Dulcolax Suppositories 883
◆ Dulcolax Tablets 308, 883
◆ Habitrol Nicotine Transdermal
System 308, 884
Maalox Antacid/Anti-Gas
Tablets 889
Maalox Antacid Liquid 888
Extra Strength Maalox
Antacid/Anti-Gas Liquid
and Tablets 888
Perdiem 889
Perdiem Fiber 889
◆ Slow Fe Tablets 308, 889
◆ Slow Fe with Folic Acid 308, 890
◆ Transderm Scop Transdermal
Therapeutic System 308, 890

Other Products Available:
Acutrim 16 Hour Steady Control
Appetite Suppressant
Acutrim Late Day Strength Appetite
Suppressant
Acutrim Maximum Strength Appetite
Suppressant
Allerest Eye Drops
Allerest No Drowsiness Tablets
Allerest Tablets Maximum Strength
Americaine Aerosol and First Aid
Ointment
Americaine Hemorrhoidal Ointment
Arthritis Pain Ascriptin
Maximum Strength Ascriptin
Regular Strength Ascriptin
Bacid Capsules
Caldecort 1% Hydrocortisone Cream
Caldesene Ointment
Caldesene Powder
Prescription Strength Cruex Cream
Prescription Strength Cruex Spray
Powder
Cruex Spray Powder
Cruex Squeeze Powder
Prescription Strength Desenex Cream
Prescription Strength Desenex Spray
Powder
Prescription Strength Desenex Spray
Liquid
Desenex Ointment
Desenex Spray Powder
Desenex Shake Powder
Desenex Foot and Sneaker Spray Powder
Desenex Foot and Sneaker Shake Powder
Doan's Extra Strength Analgesic
Extra Strength Doan's P.M.
Doan's Regular Strength Analgesic
Efidac 24 Chlorpheniramine Tablets
Efidac 24 Pseudoephedrine Tablets
Eucalyptamint 100% All Natural
Ointment
Eucalyptamint Muscle Pain Alpine Breeze
Eucalyptamint Muscle Pain Powder Fresh
Fiberall Fiber Wafers - Fruit & Nut
Fiberall Fiber Wafers - Oatmeal Raisin
Fiberall Powder, Natural Flavor
Fiberall Powder, Orange Flavor
Kondremul Plain
Maalox Anti-Gas Tablets, Regular
Strength and Extra Strength
Maalox Heartburn Relief Suspension
Myoflex Analgesic Cream
Nostrilla 12 Hour
Nupercainal HC 1%
Nupercainal Hemorrhoidal and
Anesthetic Ointment
Nupercainal Pain Relief Cream
Nupercainal Suppositories
Otrivin Nasal Drops
Otrivin Pediatric Nasal Drops
Otrivin Nasal Spray
Privine Nasal Drops
Privine Nasal Spray
Sinarest Extra Strength Tablets
Sinarest No Drowsiness Tablets
Sinarest Tablets
Sunkist Children's Chewable
Multivitamins - Complete
Sunkist Children's Chewable
Multivitamins - Plus Extra C
Sunkist Children's Chewable
Multivitamins - Plus Iron
Sunkist Children's Chewable
Multivitamins - Regular
Sunkist Vitamin C - Chewable
Sunkist Vitamin C - Easy to Swallow
Ting Cream
Ting Spray Powder
Ting Spray Liquid
Vitron-C Tablets

COLGATE ORAL   891
PHARMACEUTICALS, INC.
a subsidiary of Colgate-Palmolive
Company
One Colgate Way
Canton, MA 02021 USA

Direct Inquiries to:
Professional Services Department
(800) 226-5428

For Medical Information Contact:
In Emergencies:
Pittsburgh Poison Control
(412) 692-5596

Products Described:
Luride Drops 50 ml 891
Luride Lozi-Tabs Tablets 892
Periogard Oral Rinse 892
PreviDent 5000 Plus Cream 893

CONNAUGHT   893, 2988
LABORATORIES, INC.
A Pasteur Merieux Company
Swiftwater, PA 18370

For Medical Information Contact:
Generally:
Medical Affairs
(800) VACCINE
(800) 822-2463
Adverse Drug Experiences:
Medical Director
(717) 839-7187
(800) 835-3592

Sales and Ordering:
Connaught Laboratories, Inc.
Customer Service
(800) VACCINE
(800) 822-2463
(717) 839-7187

Products Described:
ActHIB 893
Diphtheria and Tetanus
Toxoids and Pertussis
Vaccine Adsorbed USP (For
Pediatric Use) 897
Fluzone 897
Imogam Rabies Immune
Globulin (Human) 897
Imovax Rabies I.D. Rabies
Vaccine (See Rabies
Vaccine, Imovax Rabies I.D.)
Imovax Rabies Vaccine 899
IPOL Poliovirus Vaccine
Inactivated 903
JE-VAX 904
Menomune-A/C/Y/W-135 906
Mono-Vacc Test (O.T.) 2988
MSTA Mumps Skin Test
Antigen 2988
ProHIBiT Haemophilus b
Conjugate Vaccine
(Diphtheria Toxoid
Conjugate) 911
Rabies Immune Globulin
(Human), Imogam Rabies
Vaccine (See Imogam
Rabies Immune Globulin
(Human))

CPH INTERNATIONAL 916
P.O. Box 11439
Oakland, CA 94611

For Medical Information Contact:
FAX: (510) 352-6009

CURATEK PHARMACEUTICALS 917
1965 Pratt Boulevard
Elk Grove Village, IL 60007

Direct Inquiries to:
Professional Services Department
(800) 332-7680

For Medical Information Contact:
In Emergencies:
Robert J. Borgman, Ph.D.
(847) 806-7680

DANIELS PHARMACEUTICALS, 310, 918
INC.
2517 25th Avenue North
St. Petersburg, FL 33713-3918

Direct Inquiries to:
(800) 237-7427

DERMIK LABORATORIES, INC. 919
500 Arcola Road, P.O. Box 1200
Collegeville, PA 19426-0107

Direct Inquiries to:
P.O. Box 1200
Collegeville, PA 19426-0107

Manufacturing and Distribution:
Tinley Park, IL 60477
18504 N. Creek Drive West
Sparks, NV 89431
655 Spice Islands Drive, Suite 101
(702) 353-4100
Decatur, GA 30034
3310 Colonial Parkway

DEY LABORATORIES 310, 926
2751 Napa Valley Corporate Drive
Napa, CA 94558
(800) 869-9005

Direct Inquiries to:
Russ Johnston
(800) 755-5560
FAX: (707) 224-8918

For Medical Information Contact:
In Emergencies:
Allan Kaplan
(707) 224-3200
FAX: (707) 224-3235

DISTA PRODUCTS AND ELI 310, 926
LILLY AND COMPANY

For Medical Information Contact:
Lilly Research Laboratories
Lilly Corporate Center
Indianapolis, IN 46285
(800) 545-5979

Direct Inquiries to:
Lilly Corporate Center
Indianapolis, IN 46285
(317) 276-2000

AREA SALES OFFICES:
Atlanta, GA 30328
North Park Town Center
Building 500, Suite 710
1100 Abernathy Road, NE
(770) 551-5360
Bala Cynwyd, PA 19004
401 City Avenue
Suite 400
(610) 617-1150
Birmingham, AL 35243
3800 Colonade Parkway
Suite 250
(205) 967-0103
Brea, CA 92621
Three Pointe Drive
Suite 300
(714) 257-2200
Chicago, IL 60631
Suite 810, O'Hare Plaza
8725 West Higgins Road
(312) 693-8740
Dallas, TX 75248
15301 Dallas Parkway
Suite 960, Box 66
(214) 960-6737
Indianapolis, IN 46268
Suite 203, 10 Fortune Park
3905 Vincennes Road
(317) 276-5770
Stamford, CT 06902
300 First Stamford Place
(203) 357-1422

DORSEY LABORATORIES
(See SANDOZ
PHARMACEUTICALS/CONSUMER
DIVISION)

DORSEY PHARMACEUTICALS
(See SANDOZ PHARMACEUTICALS
CORPORATION, DORSEY DIVISION)

DOW HICKAM PHARMACEUTICALS 940
INC.
P.O. Box 2006
Sugar Land, TX 77487-2006

Direct Inquiries to:
Professional Service Department
(713) 240-1000

DUPONT PHARMA 310, 941
DuPont Merck Plaza
Hickory Run
P.O. Box 80723
Wilmington, DE 19880-0723
(302) 992-5000

Direct All Product-Related Inquiries to:
Medical Affairs Department

**For Product Information/Adverse Drug
Experience Reporting Contact:**
Product Information
(302) 992-4240

DURA PHARMACEUTICALS, INC 968
5880 Pacific Center Blvd.
San Diego, CA 92121-4204

Direct Inquiries to:
Ginny Halvorsen, Marketing Services
Coordinator
(619) 457-2553 ext. 172
FAX: (619) 457-2299

For Medical Information Contact:
Medical Affairs Department
(619) 457-2553
FAX: 619-457-2555

DURAMED PHARMACEUTICALS, 979
INC.
5040 Duramed Drive
Cincinnati, OH 45213

Direct Inquiries to:
Philip J. Rose R.Ph.
V.P. Marketing and Managed Care
(513) 731-9900
(800) 543-3763

For Medical Information Contact:
In Emergencies:
Bill Stoltman
(800) 543-8338

ECR PHARMACEUTICALS 979
Distributor of ECR Pharmaceuticals &
Wm. P. Poythress Products
3981 Deep Rock Road, P.O. Box 71600
Richmond, VA 23255

Direct Inquiries to:
Professional Services Department
(804) 527-1950
FAX: (804) 527-1959

For Medical Information Contact:
In Emergencies:
Professional Services Department
(804) 527-1950
FAX: (804) 527-1959

ELKINS-SINN, INC. 980
2 Esterbrook Lane
Cherry Hill, NJ 08003-4099

Direct General Inquiries to:
(610) 688-4400

**For Emergency Medical Information
Contact:**
Day: (800) 934-5556 (8:30 AM to
4:30 PM, Eastern Standard Time,
Weekdays only)
Night: (610) 688-4400 (Emergencies
only; non-emergencies should wait
until the next day)

**For Medical/Pharmacy Inquiries on
Marketed Products Contact:**
(800) 934-5556 (8:30 AM to 4:30 PM,
Eastern Standard Time, Weekdays
only)

Other Products Available:
Almora Tablets
Ambenyl Cough Syrup
Andro L.A. "200" Injectable
Anergan "50" Injectable
Banalg Hospital Strength Arthritic Pain Reliever
Banalg Liniment
Banflex Injectable
Brompheniramine Maleate Injection
Cebocap Capsules
Conex with Codeine Liquid
Cyomin Injectable
Dalalone Injectable
Dalalone L.A. Injectable
depAndrogyn Injectable
depGynogen Injectable
depMedalone "40" Injectable
depMedalone "80" Injectable
Disotate Injectable
Endal Expectorant
Endal-HD Plus
Lidocaine 1% & 2% Injectable
Pedameth Capsules
Pedameth Liquid
Predalone "50" Injectable
Solu-Eze Solvent
Triamcinolone Diacetate Injectable
Triamonide "40" Injectable
Verazinc Capsules

FUJISAWA USA, INC. 311, 1021
Parkway North Center
3 Parkway North
Deerfield, IL 60015-2548

For Medical Information Contact:
Generally:
Medical and Scientific Information
(800) 727-7003
In Emergencies:
Medical and Scientific Information
(800) 727-7003

Products Described:
Adenocard Injection ... **1021**
Adenoscan ... **1022**
Aristocort Suspension (Forte Parenteral) ... *1024*
Aristocort Suspension (Intralesional) ... *1023*
Aristocort A 0.025% Cream ... *1023*
Aristocort A 0.5% Cream ... *1024*
Aristocort A 0.1% Cream ... *1024*
Aristocort A 0.1% Ointment ... *1024*
Aristospan Suspension (Intra-articular) ... *1025*
Aristospan Suspension (Intralesional) ... *1024*
Cefizox for Intramuscular or Intravenous Use ... **1025**
Cefizox for Intramuscular or Intravenous Use Pharmacy Bulk Package ... *1027*
Cefizox for Intravenous Infusion ... *1027*
Cefizox for Intravenous Use in Galaxy Plastic Container ... *1027*
Cyclocort Topical Cream 0.1% ... **1028**
Cyclocort Topical Lotion 0.1% ... *1028*
Cyclocort Topical Ointment 0.1% ... *1028*
Elase Ointment ... *1028*
Elase-Chloromycetin Ointment ... *1028*
◆Prograf ... **311, 1028**

GALDERMA LABORATORIES, INC. 1031
P.O. Box 331329
Fort Worth, TX 76163

Direct Inquiries to:
(817) 263-2600

Products Described:
Benzac 5 & 10 Gel ... **1031**
Benzac AC 2½%, 5%, and 10% Water-Base Gel ... **1031**
Benzac AC Wash 2½%, 5%, 10% Water-Base Cleanser ... **1031**
Benzac W Wash 5 & 10 Water-Base Cleanser ... **1031**
Benzac W 2½, 5 & 10 Water-Base Gel ... **1031**
Cetaphil Gentle Cleansing Bar ... **1032**
Cetaphil Moisturizing Cream ... **1032**
Cetaphil Moisturizing Lotion ... **1032**
Cetaphil Skin Cleanser ... **1032**
DesOwen Cream, Ointment and Lotion ... **1032**
Differin Gel ... **1033**
MetroCream ... **1034**
MetroGel ... **1034**

GATE PHARMACEUTICALS 311, 1035
650 Cathill Road
Sellersville, PA 18960
(See also TEVA PHARMACEUTICALS USA)

Direct Inquiries to:
(800) 292-4283

Products Described:
◆Adipex-P Tablets and Capsules ... **311, 1035**
◆Moban Tablets and Concentrate ... **311, 1036**
◆Orap Tablets ... **311, 1037**

GEBAUER COMPANY 1040
9410 St. Catherine Avenue
Cleveland, OH 44104

Direct Inquiries to:
(800) 321-9348
(216) 271-5252

For Medical Information Contact:
In Emergencies:
(800) 321-9348
(216) 271-5252
After Hours and Weekend Emergencies:
Chemtrec:
(800) 424-9300

Products Described:
Ethyl Chloride, U.S.P. ... **1040**
Fluori-Methane ... **1040**

Other Products Available:
Salivart

GEIGY PHARMACEUTICALS
(See CIBAGENEVA PHARMACEUTICALS)

GENDERM CORPORATION 1041
600 Knightsbridge Parkway
Lincolnshire, IL 60069

Direct Inquiries to:
Medical Information Department
(847) 634-7373

Products Described:
Dolorac Cream ... **1041**
Novacet Lotion ... **1041**
Occlusal-HP ... **1041**
Pentrax Shampoo ... **1042**
PrameGel ... **1042**
SalAc ... **1042**
Zonalon Cream ... **1042**
Zostrix Cream ... **1043**
Zostrix-HP Cream ... **1043**

Other Products Available:
A-Fil
Meted Shampoo
Pentrax Gold
Texacort Topical Solution 1%
Texacort Topical Solution 2.5%

GENENTECH, INC. 311, 1043
460 Point San Bruno Blvd.
South San Francisco, CA 94080-4990
(415) 225-1000

For Medical Information Contact:
Medical Information or Drug Experience Departments (24 hours):
(800) 821-8590
(415) 225-1000
Or write:
Medical Information or Drug Experience Departments
Genetech, Inc.
460 Point San Bruno Blvd.
South San Francisco, CA 94080-4990

Products Described:
◆Actimmune ... **311, 1043**
◆Activase ... **311, 1045**
◆Nutropin ... **311, 1049**
◆Nutropin AQ Injection ... **311, 1051**
◆Protropin ... **311, 1053**
◆Pulmozyme Inhalation ... **311, 1054**

GENEVA PHARMACEUTICALS, INC.
(See CIBAGENEVA PHARMACEUTICALS)

GENZYME CORPORATION 1055
One Kendall Square
Cambridge, MA 02139

Direct Inquiries to:
Clinical Services
(800) 745-4447
FAX: (617) 252-7700

For Medical Information Contact:
In Emergencies:
(800) 745-4447

Products Described:
Ceredase ... **1055**
Cerezyme ... **1056**

GILEAD SCIENCES 1057
333 Lakeside Drive
Foster City, CA 94404

Direct Inquiries to:
Customer Service
(800) GILEAD5

For Medical Information Contact:
Director, Medical Information
(800) GILEAD5
FAX: (800) 693-9009

Products Described:
Vistide Injection ... **1057**

GLAXO WELLCOME INC. 312, 1061
Five Moore Drive
Research Triangle Park
North Carolina 27709
(919) 483-2100

Direct Inquiries to:
Medical Services Department
(919) 483-2100

For Medical or Drug Information (Healthcare Professionals) Contact:
Medical Services Department
(800) 334-0089
In Emergencies:
(800) 334-0089

For Consumer Inquiries Contact:
(800) 722-9292

Products Described:
◆Aclovate Cream ... **312, 1061**
◆Aclovate Ointment ... **312, 1061**
◆Anectine Injection ... **312, 1062**
◆Anectine Sterile Powder Flo-Pack ... **312, 1062**
◆Beclovent Inhalation Aerosol and Refill ... **312, 1063**
◆Beconase AQ Nasal Spray ... **312, 1065**
◆Beconase Inhalation Aerosol ... **312, 1065**
◆Ceftin for Oral Suspension ... **312, 1067**
◆Ceftin Tablets ... **312, 1067**
◆Ceptaz ... **312, 1070**
◆Cortisporin Cream ... **312, 1073**
◆Cortisporin Ointment ... **312, 1074**
◆Cortisporin Ophthalmic Ointment Sterile ... **312, 1074**
◆Cortisporin Ophthalmic Suspension Sterile ... **312, 1075**
◆Cortisporin Otic Solution Sterile ... **312, 1076**
◆Cortisporin Otic Suspension Sterile ... **312, 1077**
◆Cutivate Cream ... **312, 1078**
◆Cutivate Ointment ... **312, 1078**
◆Digibind ... **312, 1079**
◆Emgel 2% Topical Gel ... **312, 1081**
◆Exosurf Neonatal for Intratracheal Suspension ... **312, 1081**
◆Flolan for Injection ... **313, 1085**
◆Flonase Nasal Spray ... **313, 1088**
◆Flovent 44 mcg Inhalation Aerosol ... **313, 1089**
◆Flovent 110 mcg Inhalation Aerosol ... **313, 1089**
◆Flovent 220 mcg Inhalation Aerosol ... **313, 1089**
◆Fortaz ... **313, 1092**
◆Imitrex Injection ... **313, 1095**
◆Imitrex Tablets ... **313, 1099**
◆Imuran Injection ... **313, 1103**
◆Imuran Tablets ... **313, 1103**
◆Kemadrin Tablets ... **313, 1105**
◆Lamictal Tablets ... **313, 1105**
◆Lanoxicaps ... **313, 1110**
◆Lanoxin Elixir Pediatric ... **313, 1113**
◆Lanoxin Injection ... **313, 1116**
◆Lanoxin Injection Pediatric ... **313, 1119**
◆Lanoxin Tablets ... **313, 1121**
◆Mantadil Cream ... **313, 1124**
◆Mivacron Injection ... **313, 1125**
◆Mivacron Premixed Infusion ... **313, 1125**
◆Neosporin G.U. Irrigant Sterile ... **313, 1130**
◆Neosporin Ophthalmic Ointment Sterile ... **314, 1130**
◆Neosporin Ophthalmic Solution Sterile ... **314, 1131**
◆Nimbex Injection ... **314, 1131**
◆Nuromax Injection ... **314, 1136**
◆Oxistat Cream ... **314, 1139**
◆Oxistat Lotion ... **314, 1139**
◆Pediotic Suspension Sterile ... **314, 1140**
◆Polysporin Ophthalmic Ointment Sterile ... **314, 1140**
◆Proloprim Tablets ... **314, 1141**
◆Septra DS Tablets ... **314, 1146**
◆Septra Grape Suspension ... **314, 1146**
◆Septra I.V. Infusion ... **314, 1142**
◆Septra I.V. Infusion ADD-Vantage Vials ... **314, 1144**
◆Septra Suspension ... **314, 1146**
◆Septra Tablets ... **314, 1146**
◆Serevent Inhalation Aerosol ... **314, 1149**
◆Temovate Cream ... **314, 1152**
◆Temovate E Emollient ... **314, 1154**
◆Temovate Gel ... **314, 1153**
◆Temovate Ointment ... **314, 1152**
◆Temovate Scalp Application ... **314, 1153**
◆Tracrium Injection ... **314, 1155**
◆Trandate Injection ... **314, 1158**
◆Trandate Tablets ... **314, 1158**
◆T.R.U.E. Test ... **314, 1162**
◆Valtrex Caplets ... **314, 1167**
◆Vasoxyl Injection ... **315, 1169**
◆Ventolin Inhalation Aerosol and Refill ... **315, 1170**
◆Ventolin Inhalation Solution ... **315, 1171**
◆Ventolin Nebules Inhalation Solution ... **315, 1172**
◆Ventolin Rotacaps for Inhalation ... **315, 1173**
◆Ventolin Syrup ... **315, 1175**
◆Ventolin Tablets ... **315, 1176**
◆Viroptic Ophthalmic Solution, 1% Sterile ... **315, 1177**
◆Wellbutrin Tablets ... **315, 1177**
◆Zantac 150 EFFERdose Granules ... **315, 1182**
◆Zantac 150 EFFERdose Tablets ... **315, 1182**
◆Zantac 150 GELdose Capsules ... **315, 1182**
◆Zantac 300 GELdose Capsules ... **315, 1182**
◆Zantac 150 Tablets ... **315, 1182**
◆Zantac 300 Tablets ... **315, 1182**
◆Zantac Injection ... **315, 1180**
◆Zantac Injection Premixed ... **315, 1180**
◆Zantac Syrup ... **315, 1182**
◆Zinacef ... **315, 1184**
◆Zovirax Capsules ... **315, 1187**
◆Zovirax Ointment 5% ... **315, 1190**
◆Zovirax Sterile Powder ... **316, 1191**
◆Zovirax Suspension ... **315, 1187**
◆Zovirax Tablets ... **315, 1187**
◆Zyloprim Tablets ... **316, 1194**

GLAXO WELLCOME ONCOLOGY/HIV 316, 1196
A Division of Glaxo Wellcome Inc.
Five Moore Drive
Research Triangle Park, NC 27709

For Medical Information Contact:
Generally:
Medical Services Department
(800) 334-0089
In Emergencies:
Medical Services Department
(800) 334-0089

For Consumer Inquiries Contact:
(800) 722-9292

Products Described:
◆Alkeran for Injection ... **316, 1196**
◆Alkeran Tablets ... **316, 1198**
◆Daraprim Tablets ... **316, 1199**
◆Epivir Oral Solution ... **316, 1200**
◆Epivir Tablets ... **316, 1200**
◆Leucovorin Calcium for Injection, Wellcovorin Brand ... **316, 1203**
◆Leucovorin Calcium Tablets, Wellcovorin Brand ... **316, 1204**
◆Leukeran Tablets ... **316, 1205**
◆Mepron Suspension ... **316, 1206**
◆Myleran Tablets ... **316, 1209**
◆Navelbine Injection ... **316, 1212**
◆Purinethol Tablets ... **316, 1214**
◆Retrovir Capsules ... **316, 1216**
◆Retrovir I.V. Infusion ... **316, 1221**
◆Retrovir Syrup ... **316, 1216**
◆Thioguanine Tablets, Tabloid Brand ... **316, 1225**
◆Zofran Injection ... **316, 1227**
◆Zofran Injection Premixed ... **316, 1227**
◆Zofran Tablets ... **316, 1231**

GLENWOOD, INC.
(See GLENWOOD-PALISADES)

GLENWOOD-PALISADES 316, 1233
82 North Summit Street
Tenafly, NJ 07670

Direct Inquiries to:
Professional Services Department
(800) 237-9083
(201) 569-0050
FAX: (201) 567-4443

For Medical Emergencies Contact:
Professional Services Department
(800) 237-9083
(201) 569-0050
FAX: (201) 567-4443

Products Described:
Bichloracetic Acid Kahlenberg ... **1233**
Calphosan Injection ... **1234**
PALS Internal Deodorant ... *1234*
◆Potaba Capsules, Envules, Powder, and Tablets ... **316, 1234**
◆Scleromate Injection ... **316, 1234**
◆Yocon Tablets ... **316, 1235**
Yodoxin Tablets ... **1235**

Other Products Available:
Bar-Test
Boropak
Carbiset
Carbiset-TR
Isocom
Klerist-D
Myotonachol
Renoquid
X-Wax
ZBT Baby Powder

A.C. GRACE CO. 1236
1100 Quitman Road
P.O. Box 570
Big Sandy, TX 75755

Direct Inquiries to:
Roy Erickson
(903) 636-4368
FAX: (903) 636-4051

For Medical Emergencies Contact:
Roy Erickson
(903) 636-4368
FAX: (903) 636-4051

Products Described:
Unique E Vitamin E Capsules 1236

GRAY PHARMACEUTICAL CO. 1236
Affiliate, The Purdue Frederick Company
100 Connecticut Avenue
Norwalk, CT 06850-3590

For Medical Information Contact:
Medical Department
(203) 853-0123

Products Described:
Senna X-Prep Bowel Evacuant
Liquid 1236

Other Products Available:
X-Prep Kit 1
X-Prep Kit 2

GUARDIAN LABORATORIES 1236
A Division of United-Guardian, Inc.
230 Marcus Boulevard
Hauppauge, NY 11788
P.O. Box 18050
Hauppauge, NY 11788
(516) 273-0900
(800) 645-5566

For Medical Information Contact:
Director of Medical Research
(516) 273-0900
(800) 645-5566

Products Described:
Clorpactin WCS-90 1236
Renacidin Irrigation 1236
Renacidin Powder 1236

HAUCK PHARMACEUTICALS
(See ROBERTS PHARMACEUTICAL
CORPORATION)

HEALTHPOINT MEDICAL 316, 1236
2400 Handley-Ederville Road
Fort Worth, TX 76118

Direct Inquiries to:
(800) 441-8227

Products Described:
◆ Accuzyme Ointment 316, 1236

HEEL/BHI, INC. 1237
11600 Cochiti SE
Albuquerque, NM 87123

Direct Inquiries to:
Medical Department
(800) 621-7644
(505) 293-3843
FAX: (505) 275-1672

Products Described:
Traumeel Injection Solution 1237
Traumeel Ointment 1237
Traumeel Oral Drops 1237
Traumeel Oral Liquid in Vials 1237
Traumeel Tablets 1237

Other Products Available:
Engystol Tablets
Euphorbium Nasal Spray
Galium-Heel Liquid
Gripp-Heel Tablets
Lymphomyosot Liquid
Lymphomyosot Tablets
Vertigoheel Liquid
Vertigoheel Tablets
Zeel Ointment
Zeel Tablets

HIGH CHEMICAL CO. 1237
3901-A Nebraska Street
Levittown, PA 19056

Direct Inquiries to:
Nalin Parikh
(800) 447-8792
FAX: (215) 788-3148

Products Described:
Sarapin 1237

HILL DERMACEUTICALS, INC. 1238
505 West Robinson Street
Orlando, Florida 32801

Direct Inquiries to:
Rosario G. Ramirez
(407) 896-8280
FAX: (407) 246-1520

Products Described:
Derma-Smoothe/FS Topical
Oil 1238
FS Shampoo 1238

HOECHST MARION ROUSSEL 316, 1238
10236 Marion Park Drive
Mail: P.O. Box 9627
Kansas City, MO 64134-0627

Direct Inquiries to:
Customer Information Center,
K1-MO928
P.O. Box 9627
Kansas City, MO 64134-0627
(800) 552-3656

For Medical Information Contact:
Generally:
Medical Informatics
P.O. Box 9627
Kansas City, MO 64134-0627
(800) 633-1610
After Hours and Weekend
Emergencies:
(816) 966-5000

Products Described:
◆ Altace Capsules 316, 1238
◆ Amaryl Tablets 316, 1241
◆ A/T/S 2% Acne Topical Gel 316, 1244
◆ A/T/S 2% Acne Topical
Solution 316, 1244
AVC Cream 1245
AVC Suppositories 1245
◆ Bentyl 10 mg Capsules . . . 316, 1246
Bentyl Injection 1246
Bentyl Syrup 1246
◆ Bentyl 20 mg Tablets 316, 1246
◆ Bricanyl Subcutaneous
Injection 317, 1247
◆ Bricanyl Tablets 317, 1248
◆ Cantil Tablets 317
Carafate Suspension 1250
◆ Carafate Tablets 317, 1249
◆ Cardizem CD Capsules . . . 317, 1251
◆ Cardizem SR Capsules . . . 317, 1255
◆ Cardizem Injectable 1253
Cardizem Lyo-Ject Syringe 1253
◆ Cardizem Tablets 317, 1257
◆ Cephulac Solution 317
◆ Chronulac Solution 317
◆ Claforan Sterile and Injection 317, 1259
◆ Clomid 317, 1262
◆ Dermatop Emollient Cream
0.1% 317, 1264
◆ DiaBeta Tablets 317, 1265
Ditropan Syrup 1267
◆ Ditropan Tablets 317, 1267
◆ Hiprex 317
◆ Lasix Injection, Oral Solution
and Tablets 317, 1267
◆ Loprox 1% Cream and Lotion 317, 1269
Nitro-Bid IV 1270
Nitro-Bid Ointment 1272
◆ Norpramin Tablets 317, 1273
◆ Pavabid Plateau Caps 317
◆ Pentasa 317, 1275
◆ Rifadin Capsules 317, 1276
Rifadin I.V. 1276
◆ Rifamate Capsules 317, 1278
◆ Rifater 317, 1280
◆ Seldane Tablets 318, 1284
◆ Seldane-D Extended-Release
Tablets 318, 1286
◆ Silvadene Cream 1% 318, 1288
◆ Tace 318
◆ Tenuate and Tenuate Dospan
Tablets 318
◆ Topicort Emollient Cream
0.25% 318, 1289
◆ Topicort Gel 0.05% 318, 1290
◆ Topicort LP Emollient Cream
0.05% 318, 1289
◆ Topicort Ointment 0.25% . . 318, 1291
◆ Trental Tablets 318, 1291

Other Products Available:
Metatensin Tablets
Metahydrin Tablets
Novafed A Capsules

**HOECHST-ROUSSEL PHARMACEUTICALS
INC.**
(See HOECHST MARION ROUSSEL)

HORUS THERAPEUTICS, INC. 1293
2320 Brighton-Henrietta Town Line
Road
Rochester, NY 14623

Direct Inquiries to:
Bernard Ouellette
(716) 292-4820
FAX: (716) 292-4836

Products Described:
Thalitone 1293

HYLAND DIVISION
(See BAXTER HEALTHCARE
CORPORATION)

ICN PHARMACEUTICALS, 318, 1294
INC.
ICN Plaza
3300 Hyland Avenue
Costa Mesa, CA 92626

Direct Inquiries to:
Customer Service Department
(800) 556-1937
(714) 545-0100
FAX: (714) 641-7289

Products Described:
Android Capsules, 10 mg 1297
Benoquin Cream 20% 1298
◆ 8-MOP Capsules 318, 1294
Eldopaque 4% Cream 1299
Eldoquin Forte 4% Cream 1299
Fototar Cream 1300
Mestinon Injectable 1300
Mestinon Syrup 1300
◆ Mestinon Tablets 318, 1300
◆ Mestinon Timespan Tablets 318, 1300
Oxsoralen Lotion 1% 1301
◆ Oxsoralen-Ultra Capsules . 318, 1302
Prostigmin Injectable 1305
◆ Prostigmin Tablets 318, 1306
Solaquin Forte 4% Cream 1299
Solaquin Forte 4% Gel 1299
Tensilon Injectable 1307
◆ Testred Capsules, 10 mg . . 318, 1308
◆ Trisoralen Tablets 318, 1309
Viquin Forte 4% Cream 1299
Virazole 1310

Other Products Available:
Eldopaque 2% Cream
Eldoquin 2% Cream
GlyDerm AHA's
Insta-Glucose
RVPaque Cream
Solaquin 2% Cream
Vitadye Lotion

IMMUNEX CORPORATION 1312
51 University Street
Seattle, WA 98101

Direct Inquiries to:
Customer Service
(800) 466-8639
FAX: (800) 441-6303

For Medical Information Contact:
Generally:
Professional Services
(800) 466-8639
FAX: (800) 221-6820
FAX: (206) 223-5525
In Emergencies:
Professional Services
(800) 466-8639
FAX: (800) 221-6820
FAX: (206) 223-5525

Products Described:
Amicar Syrup, Tablets, and
Injection 1312
Leucovorin Calcium for
Injection 1313
Leucovorin Calcium Tablets . . . 1315
Leukine 1317
Levoprome 1321
Methotrexate Sodium Tablets,
Injection, for Injection and
LPF Injection 1322
Novantrone for Injection 1327
Thioplex (Thiotepa For
Injection) 1329

IMMUNO-U.S., INC. 1330
1200 Parkdale Road
Rochester, MI 48307-1744

Direct Inquiries to:
(810) 652-7872
FAX: (810) 652-6810

Products Described:
Albumin (Human) 5% 1330
Albumin (Human) 25% 1330
Bebulin VH Immuno 1330
Feiba VH Immuno 1330
Iveegam 1331

INTERFERON SCIENCES, INC.
783 Jersey Avenue
New Brunswick, NJ 08901-3660

Alferon N Injection (See Purdue
Frederick Company)

INTERNATIONAL ETHICAL LABS. 1331
1021 Avenue Americo Miranda
Reparto Metropolitano
San Juan, PR 00921

Direct Inquiries to:
Mr. Sammy Diaz, President
(787) 765-3510
(787) 763-8414
FAX: (787) 767-1110

Products Described:
Aflaxen Tablets 1331
Biocef Capsules and Oral
Suspension 1331
Bio-Tab Tablets 1331
Despec SR Caplets 1331
Despec Liquid 1331
Despec SF 1331
Mio-Rel Injectable 1331
Neuroforte-R Vial 1331

Neuroforte-Six Monovial 1331
Redutemp 500 mg O/S 1331
Relagesic 1331
Remular-S 1331
Tencon Capsules 1331
Tuss-DA RX 1331

ION LABORATORIES, INC. 1331
7431 Pebble Drive
Fort Worth, TX 76118

Direct Inquiries to:
David E. Brown or Judy Martin
(817) 589-7257
FAX: (817) 590-0973

For Medical Information Contact:
In Emergencies:
David E. Brown
(817) 589-7257
FAX: (817) 590-0973

Products Described:
E.N.T. Tablets 1331
E.N.T. Plus Treatment
Package 1331
Erex Tablets 1331
Liquibid Tablets 1331
Liquibid-D Tablets 1331
Rescon Capsules 1331
Rescon Liquid 1331
Rescon-DM Liquid 1331
Rescon-ED Capsules 1331
Rescon-GG Liquid 1331
Rescon JR Capsules 1331
Sinupan Capsules 1331
Zantryl Capsules 1331

JACOBUS PHARMACEUTICAL CO., 1331
INC.
37 Cleveland Lane
P.O. Box 5290
Princeton, NJ 08540

Direct Inquiries to:
Professional Services
(609) 921-7447
FAX: (609) 799-1176

For Medical Information Contact:
In Emergencies:
Medical Department
(609) 921-7447
FAX: (609) 799-1176

Products Described:
Dapsone Tablets USP 1331
PASER Granules 1333

JANSSEN PHARMACEUTICA 318, 1334
INC.
1125 Trenton-Harbourton Road
P.O. Box 200
Titusville, NJ 08560-0200

For Medical Information Contact:
Generally:
Professional Services
(800) JANSSEN
(609) 730-2000
FAX: (609) 730-3044
After Hours and Weekends:
(800) JANSSEN
Holidays:
Routine: (800) 253-3682
Emergencies: (908) 524-0400

Products Described:
◆ Alfenta Injection 318, 1334
◆ Duragesic Transdermal
System 318, 1336
◆ Ergamisol Tablets 318, 1340
◆ Hismanal Tablets 318, 1341
◆ Imodium Capsules 318, 1343
◆ Nizoral 2% Cream 318, 1344
◆ Nizoral 2% Shampoo 318, 1344
◆ Nizoral Tablets 318, 1345
◆ Propulsid Tablets 318, 1346
◆ Propulsid Suspension . . . 318, 1346
◆ Risperdal Tablets 318, 1348
◆ Sporanox Capsules 318, 1352
◆ Sufenta Injection 318, 1355
◆ Vermox Chewable Tablets . 318, 1357

JOHNSON & JOHNSON • 318, 1358
**MERCK CONSUMER
PHARMACEUTICALS CO.**
Camp Hill Road
Ft. Washington, PA 19034

Direct Inquiries to:
Consumer Affairs Department
Fort Washington, PA 19034
(215) 233-7000

For Medical Information Contact:
In Emergencies:
(215) 233-7000

Products Described:
◆ ALternaGEL Liquid 318, 1358
◆ Dialose Tablets 318, 1358
◆ Dialose Plus Tablets 318, 1358

MEAD JOHNSON PHARMACEUTICALS
(See BRISTOL-MYERS SQUIBB COMPANY)

MEDEVA PHARMACEUTICALS, INC.   **1602**
14801 Sovereign Road
Fort Worth, TX 76155-2645

Direct Inquiries to:
Customer Service Department
P.O. Box 1766
Rochester, NY 14603
(716) 274-5300
(888) 9-MEDEVA

For Emergency Medical Information Contact:
(800) 932-1950 (24 hours)
(888) 9-MEDEVA (24 hours)

For Educational Information Contact:
Medeva Pharmaceuticals, Inc.
P.O. Box 1766
Rochester, NY 14603

Products Described:

MEDICIS DERMATOLOGICS, INC.   **1627**
4343 East Camelback Road
Phoenix, AZ 85018

For Medical Information Contact:
  Generally:
  Medical Affairs Department
  (602) 808-8800
  FAX: (602) 808-0822
  In Emergencies:
  (602) 808-8800

Products Described:

MEDIMMUNE, INC.   **1630**
35 West Watkins Mill Road
Gaithersburg, MD 20878

Direct Inquiries to:
Professional Services:
(800) 949-3789
Customer Services:
(301) 527-4300

For Medical Information Contact:
  In Emergencies:
  (301) 527-4300

Products Described:

MEDISAN PHARMACEUTICALS INC.   **1633**
400 Lanidex Plaza
Parsippany, NJ 07054

Direct Inquiries to:
Jane Flynn
(800) 763-3472
FAX: (201) 515-9799

Products Described:

MEDTRONIC, INC.   **1634**
NEUROLOGICAL DIVISION
800 53rd Avenue, NE
Minneapolis, MN 55421

Direct Inquiries to:
(800) 328-0810
(612) 572-5000

Products Described:

MERCK & CO., INC.   **324, 1638**
P.O. Box 4
West Point, PA 19486-0004

For Medical Information Contact:
  Generally:
  Product and service information:
  Call the Merck National Service
  Center, 8:00 AM to 7:00 PM (ET),
  Monday through Friday:
    (800) NSC-MERCK
    (800) 672-6372
    FAX: (800) MERCK-68
    FAX: (800) 637-2568
  Adverse Drug Experiences:
  Call the Merck National Service
  Center, 8:00 AM to 7:00 PM (ET),
  Monday through Friday:
    (800) NSC-MERCK
    (800) 672-6372
  In Emergencies:
  24-hour emergency information for
  healthcare professionals:
    (800) NSC-MERCK
    (800) 672-6372

Sales and Ordering:
For product orders and direct account
inquiries only, call the Order
Management Center, 8:00 AM to 7:00
PM (ET), Monday through Friday:
  (800) MERCK RX
  (800) 637-2579

Products Described:

MERICON INDUSTRIES, INC.   **1825**
8819 N. Pioneer Road
Peoria, IL 61615

Direct Inquiries to:
William R. Connelly
(309) 693-2150
FAX: (309) 693-2158

Products Described:

MERIEUX INSTITUTE, INC.
(See CONNAUGHT LABORATORIES, INC.)

MERZ PHARMACEUTICALS   **1825**
(Formerly Mayrand Pharmaceuticals)
Division of Merz, Inc.
4215 Tudor Lane
Greensboro, NC 27410

Direct Inquiries to:
Dr. Robert P. Halliday
(910) 856-2003
FAX: (910) 856-0107

For Medical Information Contact:
  In Emergencies:
  Dr. Robert P. Halliday
  (910) 856-2003
  FAX: (910) 856-0107

BRANCH OFFICE:
4 Dundas Circle
Greensboro, NC 27407
(910) 292-5347
FAX: (910) 855-8011

Products Described:

Other Products Available:
Anamine Syrup
Anamine T. D. Capsules
Anatuss Syrup
Anatuss Tablets
Becomject-100
Cyanoject-10
Cyanoject-30
Decaject-5
Decaject-10
Decaject-L.A.
Depoject-40
Depoject-80
Flexoject
Glytuss Tabs
Kenaject-40
Lidoject-1
Lidoject-2
Phenoject-50
Predaject-50
Tristoject
Vistaject-50

MILEX PRODUCTS, INC.   **1827**
5915 Northwest Highway
Chicago, IL 60631

Direct Inquiries to:
(312) 631-6484
FAX: (312) 631-8156

Manufacturing and Distribution:
SHIPPING OFFICES:
Milex Carolinas
  Post Office Box 23060
  Charlotte, NC 28212
  (704) 545-4567
Milex Puerto Rico
  GPO Box 554
  San Juan, PR 00936
  (809) 764-8602
Milex Southern
  Post Office Drawer "M"
  Weathersford, TX 76086
  (817) 599-7604
Milex Western
  Post Office Box 46305
  Los Angeles, CA 90046
  (213) 651-4301
Milex Hawaii
  Box 6337
  Honolulu, HI 96818
  (808) 422-9581

Products Described:

MISSION PHARMACAL COMPANY   **1828**
10999 IH 10 West, Suite 1000
San Antonio, TX 78230-1355

Direct Inquiries to:
P.O. Box 786099
San Antonio, TX 78278-6099
(210) 696-8400
FAX: (210) 696-6010

For Medical Information Contact:
  In Emergencies:
  George Alexandrides
  (210) 533-7118
  FAX: (210) 533-4487

Products Described:

Other Products Available:
Compete
Supac

MONARCH PHARMACEUTICALS   **325, 1830**
355 Beecham Street
Bristol, TN 37620

Direct Inquiries to:
(800) 776-3637
FAX: (423) 989-6279

For Medical Emergencies Contact:
Dr. Henry Richards, M.D.
(800) 546-4906
FAX: (423) 989-6137

Products Described:

ODYSSEY NUTRICEUTICAL SCIENCES 1860
60 Hamilton Street
Cambridge, MA 02139

Direct Inquiries to:
(617) 497-5100
(800) 790-8378
FAX: (617) 497-6990

Products Described:
Healthy Heart 1860

OHMEDA PHARMACEUTICAL PRODUCTS DIVISION INC. 1860
110 Allen Road
Box 804
Liberty Corner, NJ 07938-0804

BRANCH OFFICES:
Western Region:
1848 Norwood Plaza, Suite 109
Hurst, TX 76054
(817) 282-1767

Eastern Region:
1375 Plainfield Avenue
Watchung, NJ 07060
(908) 322-8272

Direct Inquiries to:
Professional Services Department
(800) ANA-DRUG
(800) 262-3784

For Medical Information Contact:
In Emergencies:
Lawrence McKay, M.D.
Vice President, Clinical Development
(800) ANA-DRUG
(800) 262-3784

Sales and Ordering:
To place an order between 8:00 AM and 4:00 PM:
(800) 345-2700

Products Described:
Brevibloc (esmolol HCl) Injection 1860
Dizac (diazepam injectable emulsion) CIV 1862
Enlon (edrophonium chloride injection, USP) *1863*
Enlon-Plus (edrophonium chloride, USP and atropine sulfate, USP) Injection *1863*
Ethrane (enflurane, USP) *1863*
Forane (isoflurane, USP) *1863*
Revex (nalmefene hydrochloride injection) 1863
Suprane (desflurane, USP) 1865
Dizac is a trademark of Pharmacia AB Sweden
Revex is a registered trademark of Baker Norton Pharmaceuticals, Inc.

ORGANON INC. 325, 1866
375 Mt. Pleasant Ave.
West Orange, NJ 07052

Direct Inquiries to:
(201) 325-4500

For Medical Inquiries Contact:
(800) 631-1253
FAX: (201) 325-4699

Products Described:
Arduan for Injection *1866*
◆BCG VACCINE, USP (TICE) . . 326, *1866*
◆Calderol Capsules 325, *1866*
Cortrosyn for Injection *1866*
◆Cotazym Capsules 325, 1866
◆Cotazym-S Capsules 325, *1867*
Deca-Durabolin Injection *1867*
◆Desogen Tablets 325, 1867
Durabolin Injection *1873*
◆Humegon for Injection 325, 1873
◆Jenest-28 326
Norcuron for Injection 1875
Pavulon Injection *1878*
Pregnyl for Injection 1878
Regonol Injection *1878*
◆Remeron Tablets 326, 1878
Reversol Injection *1881*
Succinylcholine Chloride Injection *1881*
◆TICE BCG, USP 326, 1881
◆Wigraine Tablets 326, 1884
◆Zemuron Injection 326, 1885
◆Zymase Capsules 326, 1889

ORTHO BIOTECH INC. 326, 1889
P.O. Box 300
Raritan, NJ 08869-0602

Direct Inquiries to:
Customer Services
(800) 325-7504
FAX: (908) 526-6457

Products Described:
Leustatin 1889
Orthoclone OKT3 Sterile Solution 1892
◆Procrit for Injection 326, 1896

ORTHO DIAGNOSTIC SYSTEMS INC. 1902
A Johnson & Johnson Company
1001 US Hwy 202
Raritan, NJ 08869-0606

Direct Inquiries to:
Customer Service
(800) 322-6374 (ODSI)

Products Described:
MICRhoGAM Rh_o(D) Immune Globulin (Human) 1902
RhoGAM Rh_o(D) Immune Globulin (Human) 1902

ORTHO PHARMACEUTICAL CORPORATION 326, 1903
Route 202, P. O. Box 300
Raritan, NJ 08869-0602

For Medical Information Contact:
Generally:
(800) 682-6532
In Emergencies:
(908) 218-7325

Products Described:
Aci-Jel Therapeutic Vaginal Jelly 1903
◆All-Flex Arcing Spring Diaphragm (See also Ortho Diaphragm Kits) 326, 1921
◆Micronor Tablets 326, 1903
◆Modicon 21 Tablets 326, 1928
Modicon 28 Tablets 1928
◆Monistat Dual-Pak 326, 1906
◆Monistat 3 Vaginal Suppositories 326, 1905
◆Ortho-Cept 21 Tablets 326, 1907
Ortho-Cept 28 Tablets 1907
◆Ortho-Cyclen 21 Tablets . . . 326, 1914
Ortho-Cyclen 28 Tablets 1914
Ortho Diaphragm Kits—All-Flex Arcing Spring; Ortho Coil Spring; Ortho-White Flat Spring 1921
Ortho Diaphragm Kit-Coil Spring 1921
Ortho Dienestrol Cream 1922
◆Ortho-Est .625 Tablets 326, 1925
◆Ortho-Est 1.25 Tablets 326, 1925
◆Ortho-Novum 1/35□21 Tablets 326, 1928
Ortho-Novum 1/35□28 Tablets 1928
◆Ortho-Novum 1/50□21 Tablets 326, 1928
Ortho-Novum 1/50□28 Tablets 1928
◆Ortho-Novum 7/7/7 □21 Tablets 327, 1928
Ortho-Novum 7/7/7 □28 Tablets 1928
◆Ortho-Novum 10/11□21 Tablets 327, 1928
Ortho-Novum 10/11□28 Tablets 1928
◆Ortho Tri-Cyclen 21 Tablets . 326, 1914
Ortho Tri-Cyclen 28 Tablets . . . 1914
Ortho-White Diaphragm Kit-Flat Spring (See also Ortho Diaphragm Kits) 1921
◆ParaGard T 380A Intrauterine Copper Contraceptive 327, 1936
◆Protostat Tablets 327, 1939
Sultrin Triple Sulfa Cream 1941
Sultrin Triple Sulfa Vaginal Tablets 1941
◆Terazol 3 Vaginal Cream . . . 327, 1941
◆Terazol 3 Vaginal Suppositories 327, 1942
◆Terazol 7 Vaginal Cream . . . 327, 1943

ORTHO PHARMACEUTICAL CORPORATION DERMATOLOGICAL DIVISION 326, 1943
1000 U.S Hwy. Route 202
P.O. Box 300
Raritan, NJ 08869-0602

For Medical Information Contact:
Dermatological Medical Information
(800) 426-7762

Products Described:
◆Erycette (erythromycin 2%) Topical Solution 326, 1943
◆Grifulvin V (griseofulvin tablets) Microsize (griseofulvin oral suspension) Microsize . . . 326, 1944
◆Monistat-Derm (miconazole nitrate 2%) Cream 326, 1944
◆Renova (tretinoin emollient cream) 0.05% 326, 1945
◆Retin-A (tretinoin) Cream/Gel/Liquid 326, 1947
◆Spectazole (econazole nitrate 1%) Cream 326, 1947

PADDOCK LABORATORIES, INC. 1948
3940 Quebec Avenue North
Minneapolis, MN 55427

Direct Inquiries to:
Martin A. Erickson, III, R.Ph.
(612) 546-4676
FAX: (612) 548-4842

For Medical Information Contact:
In Emergencies:
Carol Anding, Regulatory Affairs
(800) 328-5113
FAX: (612) 546-4842

Products Described:
Actidose with Sorbitol *1948*
Actidose-Aqua *1948*
Clinda-Derm *1948*
Diabe-Tuss DM Syrup 1948
Erythra-Derm *1948*
Glutose 15, Glutose 45 (Oral Glucose Gel) *1948*
Glutose Tablets *1948*
Nystatin Paddock, USP for Extemporaneous Preparation of Oral Suspension *1948*
Nystop (Nystatin Topical Powder, USP) 1948
Podocon-25 1949

Other Products Available:
Acetaminophen Tablets 325 mg
Albuterol Sulfate, USP
Aluminum Paste
5-Aminosalicylic Acid Powder
Aquabase
Ascorbic Acid Tablets 500 mg
Aspirin Suppositories 125 mg, 300 mg, 600 mg
Aspirin Tablets 325 mg
Aspirin Tablets, Enteric-Coated 325 mg, 650 mg
Bacitracin Powder, USP
Belladonna and Opium Suppositories CII
Benzoin Compound Tincture, USP
Betamethasone Valerate Powder, USP
Bisacodyl Suppositories 10 mg
Bisacodyl Tablets 5 mg
Castor Oil, USP
Clindamycin Phosphate Powder, USP
Colistin Sulfate Powder, USP
Dermabase
Dexamethasone Acetate Powder USP
Dexamethasone Sodium Phosphate Powder, USP, Micronized
Docusate Calcium Capsules 240 mg
Docusate Sodium Capsules 100 mg, 250 mg
Docusate Sodium Capsules w/Casanthranol Capsules 100 mg/30 mg
Emulsoil (Self-Emulsifying Castor Oil)
Erythromycin Powder, USP
Fattibase
Ferrous Gluconate Tablets
Ferrous Sulfate Tablets
Folic Acid Tablets
Gentamicin Sulfate Powder, USP
Glutol
Green Soap Tincture, USP
Hydrocortisone Acetate Powder, USP
Hydrocortisone Acetate Suppositories 25 mg
Hydrocortisone Powder, USP
Hydrocream Base
Hydromorphone HCl Suppositories CII
Hydromorphone HCl Powder USP CII
Ipecac Syrup, USP
Isoniazid Tablets USP 300 mg
Liqua-Gel
Liquaderm-A
Milk of Magnesia, USP
Morphine Sulfate Powder USP CII
Morphine Sulfate Suppositories 5 mg, 10 mg, 20 mg, 30 mg CII
Neomycin Sulfate Powder, USP
Ora-Plus
Ora-Sweet
Ora-Sweet SF
Podophyllum Resin, USP
Polybase
Polymyxin B Sulfate Powder, USP
Progesterone Injectable, USP
Progesterone Powder, USP, Micronized
Progesterone Powder, USP, Wettable, Microcrystalline
Retinoic Acid, USP
Schamberg Lotion
Sorbitol Solution, 70%
Suspendol-S
Testosterone Powder, USP CIII
Testosterone Propionate Powder, USP CIII
Triamcinolone Acetonide Powder, USP
Trimethobenzamide Suppositories 100 mg, 200 mg
Zincate Capsules 220 mg

PALISADES PHARMACEUTICALS, INC.
(See GLENWOOD-PALISADES)

PAR PHARMACEUTICAL, INC. 1949
One Ram Ridge Road
Spring Valley, NY 10977

Direct Inquiries to:
Customer Service
(800) 828-9393
(914) 425-7100

Products Described:
Albuterol Sulfate Syrup 2mg/5mL *1949*
Allopurinol Tablets *1949*
Alprazolam Tablets *1949*
Amiloride HCl Tablets *1949*
Atenolol Tablets *1949*
Benztropine Mesylate Tablets . . . *1949*
Captopril Tablets *1949*
Carisoprodol and Aspirin Tablets *1949*
Chlorzoxazone Tablets *1949*
Cimetidine Tablets *1949*
Clonidine HCl and Chlorthalidone Tablets *1949*
Cyproheptadine HCl Tablets *1949*
Dexamethasone Tablets *1949*
Doxepin HCl Capsules *1949*
Fluphenazine HCl Tablets *1949*
Flurazepam HCl Capsules *1949*
Glipizide Tablets *1949*
Haloperidol Tablets *1949*
Hydralazine HCl Tablets *1949*
Hydra-Zide (Hydralazine HCl and Hydrochlorothiazide) Capsules *1949*
Ibuprofen Tablets *1949*
Imipramine HCl Tablets *1949*
Isosorbide Dinitrate Oral Tablets *1949*
Meclizine HCl Tablets *1949*
Megestrol Acetate Tablets *1949*
Melatonin *1949*
Melatonin SR *1949*
Metaproterenol Sulfate Tablets *1949*
Methocarbamol and Aspirin Tablets *1949*
Methyldopa and Hydrochlorothiazide Tablets . . . *1949*
Metoprolol Tartrate Tablets *1949*
Metronidazole Tablets *1949*
Minoxidil Tablets *1949*
Nystatin Oral Tablets *1949*
Pindolol Tablets *1949*
Piroxicam Capsules *1949*
Temazepam Capsules *1949*
Thermazene Cream 1% (Silver Sulfadiazine Cream, 1%) *1949*
Triamterene and Hydrochlorothiazide Tablets . . . *1949*
Triazolam Tablets *1949*

PARKE-DAVIS 327, 1950
Division of Warner-Lambert Company
201 Tabor Rd
Morris Plains, NJ 07950

For Medical Information Contact:
Generally:
During working hours:
Customer Service
Product/Medical Information
(800) 223-0432
FAX: (201) 540-2248
After Hours and Weekend Emergencies:
(201) 540-6089

Products Described:
◆Accupril Tablets 327, 1950
◆Anusol-HC Cream 2.5% 327, 1953
◆Anusol-HC Suppositories . . . 327, 1954
Benadryl Parenteral 1955
Benadryl Steri-Vials, Ampoules, and Steri-Dose Syringe 1955
◆Celontin Kapseals 327, 1955
Cerebyx Injection 1956
Chloromycetin Sodium Succinate 1960
◆Cognex Capsules 327, 1961
Coly-Mycin M Parenteral
Coly-Mycin S Otic w/Neomycin & Hydrocortisone 1965
◆Dilantin Infatabs 327, 1967
◆Dilantin Kapseals 327, 1965
Dilantin-125 Suspension 1969
◆Doryx Capsules 327, 1970
◆Easprin 327, 1971
◆ERYC 327, 1972
◆Lopid Tablets 327, 1974
◆Nardil 327, 1977
◆Neurontin Capsules 327, 1978
◆Nitrostat Tablets 327, 1981
◆Ponstel 327, 1982
◆Procanbid Extended-Release Tablets 327, 1983
◆Pyridium 327, 1985
◆Zarontin Capsules 327, 1986
Zarontin Syrup 1986

Other Products Available:
ACTH Steri-Vial
Adrenalin Chloride Solution 1:100 & 1:1,000
Antibiotics
Chloromycetin Products
Coly-Mycin Products
Humatin
Aplisol (tuberculin PPD, diluted)

PRINCETON PHARMACEUTICAL PRODUCTS
(See BRISTOL-MYERS SQUIBB COMPANY)

PROCTER & GAMBLE   2124
(For Rx products, also see Procter & Gamble Pharmaceuticals)
P.O. Box 5516
Cincinnati, OH 45201

Direct Inquiries to:
Charles E. Lambert
(800) 358-8707

For Medical Information Contact:
In Emergencies, call collect:
(513) 558-4422

Products Described:
Aleve 2124
Children's Vicks Chloraseptic
  Sore Throat Lozenges . . . . . . ◧
Children's Vicks Chloraseptic
  Sore Throat Spray . . . . ◧
Children's Vicks DayQuil
  Allergy Relief . . . . ◧
Children's Vicks NyQuil
  Cold/Cough Relief . . . . ◧
Femstat 3 2124
Head & Shoulders Dandruff
  Shampoo . . . . ◧
Head & Shoulders Dandruff
  Shampoo Dry Scalp . . . . ◧
Head & Shoulders Intensive
  Treatment Dandruff and
  Seborrheic Dermatitis
  Shampoo . . . . ◧
Metamucil Powder, Orange
  Flavor 2125
Metamucil Original Texture
  Powder, Regular Flavor 2125
Metamucil Smooth Texture
  Powder, Orange Flavor 2125
Metamucil Smooth Texture
  Powder, Sugar-Free, Orange
  Flavor 2125
Metamucil Smooth Texture
  Sugar-Free, Regular Flavor . . .2125
Metamucil Wafers, Apple
  Crisp and Cinnamon Spice
  Flavors 2125
Oil of Olay Daily UV
  Protectant SPF 15 Beauty
  Fluid-Regular and Fragrance
  Free (Olay Co. Inc.) . . . . . . ◧
Oil of Olay Daily UV
  Protectant SPF 15 Moisture
  Replenishing Cream . . . . . . ◧
Pediatric Vicks 44d Cough &
  Head Congestion RELIEF . . . . . ◧
Pediatric Vicks 44e Chest
  Cough & Chest Congestion
  RELIEF . . . . ◧
Pediatric Vicks 44m Cough &
  Cold RELIEF . . . . ◧
Pepto-Bismol Original Liquid,
  Original and Cherry Tablets
  and Easy-To-Swallow
  Caplets 2126
Pepto-Bismol Maximum
  Strength Liquid 2126
Pepto Diarrhea Control 2127
Percogesic Analgesic Tablets . ◧
Peridex 2127
Vicks Chloraseptic Cough and
  Throat Drops: Cherry,
  Menthol & Honey Lemon
  Flavors . . . . ◧
Vicks Chloraseptic Gargle &
  Mouth Rinse . . . . ◧
Vicks Chloraseptic Sore
  Throat Spray: Cherry and
  Menthol Flavors . . . . ◧
Vicks Chloraseptic Sore
  Throat Lozenges: Cherry
  and Menthol Flavors . . . . . . ◧
Original Vicks Cough Drops:
  Cherry and Menthol Flavors . . . ◧
Vicks Cough Drops: Cherry
  and Menthol Flavors . . . . . . ◧
Vicks DayQuil Allergy Relief 4
  Hour . . . . ◧
Vicks DayQuil Allergy Relief
  12-Hour Extended Release . . . ◧
Vicks DayQuil Liquid &
  LiquiCaps Multi-Symptom
  Cold/Flu Relief . . . . ◧
Vicks DayQuil SINUS Pressure
  & CONGESTION Relief . . . . . . ◧
Vicks Dayquil SINUS Pressure
  & PAIN Relief with
  IBUPROFEN . . . . ◧
Vicks 44 LiquiCaps Cough,
  Cold & Flu Relief . . . . ◧
Vicks 44 LiquiCaps
  Non-Drowsy Cough and
  Cold Relief . . . . ◧
Vicks 44 Cough RELIEF . . . . . ◧
Vicks 44D Cough & Head
  Congestion RELIEF . . . . ◧
Vicks 44E Chest Cough &
  Chest Congestion RELIEF . . . . ◧
Vicks 44M Cough, Cold & Flu
  RELIEF . . . . ◧
Vicks Nyquil Hot Therapy . . . ◧
Vicks NyQuil Multi-Symptom
  Cold/Flu Relief (Liquid) . . . . ◧

Vicks NyQuil LiquiCaps
  Multi-Symptom Cold/Flu
  Relief . . . . ◧
Vicks Sinex Nasal Spray and
  Ultra Fine Mist for Sinus
  Relief . . . . ◧
Vicks Sinex 12 Hour Nasal
  Spray and Ultra Fine Mist
  for Sinus Relief . . . . ◧
Vicks Vapor Inhaler . . . . . . ◧
Vicks VapoRub (cream) . . . . . ◧
Vicks VapoRub (ointment) . . . ◧
Vicks VapoSteam . . . . ◧

PROCTER & GAMBLE   329, 2128
PHARMACEUTICALS, INC.
Sharon Woods Technical Center
11450 Grooms Road
Cincinnati, OH 45242-1434

Direct Inquiries to:
Customer Service
(800) 448-4878

For Medical Information Contact:
Generally:
Medical Communications
(800) 836-0658
FAX: (800) 438-0138
Or Write:
Procter & Gamble Pharmaceuticals
Medical Communications Department
11450 Grooms Road
Cincinnati, OH 45242-1434
In Emergencies:
Medical Communications
(800) 836-0658

Products Described:
◆Asacol Delayed-Release
  Tablets 329, 2129
Brontex Liquid 2130
◆Brontex Tablets 329, 2130
Dantrium Capsules 2131
Dantrium Intravenous 2132
◆Didronel Tablets 329, 2133
Helidac Therapy 2135
◆Macrobid Capsules 329, 2138
◆Macrodantin Capsules . . . 329, 2140

Other Products Available:
Furadantin Oral Suspension

THE PURDUE FREDERICK   329, 2142
COMPANY
100 Connecticut Avenue
Norwalk, CT 06850-3590

For Medical Information Contact:
Medical Department
(203) 853-0123

Products Described:
Alferon N Injection 2142
Betadine Brand First Aid
  Antibiotics & Moisturizer
  Ointment 2144
Betadine Disposable
  Medicated Douche 2144
Betadine First Aid Cream 2144
Betadine Medicated Douche . . . 2144
Betadine Medicated Gel 2144
Betadine Medicated Vaginal
  Suppositories 2145
Betadine Ointment 2145
Betadine Pre-Mixed Medicated
  Disposable Douche 2144
Betadine Skin Cleanser 2145
Betadine Solution 2145
Betadine Surgical Scrub 2145
Betasept Surgical Scrub 2145
Cardioquin Tablets 2146
Cerumenex Drops 2148
◆DHCplus Capsules 329, 2148
◆MS Contin Tablets 329, 2149
◆MSIR Oral Capsules 329, 2152
◆MSIR Oral Solution 329, 2152
◆MSIR Oral Solution
  Concentrate 329, 2152
◆MSIR Tablets 330, 2152
Senokot Children's Syrup 2154
Senokot Granules 2154
Senokot Syrup 2154
Senokot Tablets 2154
SenokotXTRA Tablets 2154
Senokot-S Tablets 2154
◆Trilisate Liquid 330, 2155
◆Trilisate Tablets 330, 2155
◆Uniphyl 400 mg and 600 mg
  Tablets 330, 2157

Other Products Available:
Arthropan Liquid
Betadine Aerosol Spray
Betadine Antiseptic Gauze Pad
Betadine Antiseptic Lubricating Gel
Betadine Medicated Douche Kit
Betadine Mouthwash/Gargle
Betadine Perineal Wash Concentrate Kit
Betadine Shampoo
Betadine Skin Cleanser Foam
Betadine Solution Swab Aid
Betadine Solution Swabsticks
Betadine Surgi-Prep Sponge-Brush
Betadine Viscous Formula Antiseptic
  Gauze Pad
Senokot Suppositories

Senokot Tablets Unit Strip Pack
T-Phyl Tablets

PURDUE PHARMA L.P.   330, 2163
100 Connecticut Avenue
Norwalk, CT 06850-3590

For Medical Information Contact:
Medical Department
(203) 853-0123

Products Described:
◆OxyContin Tablets 330, 2163
◆OxyIR Capsules 330, 2167

R&D LABORATORIES, INC.   2168
4640 Admiralty Way, Suite 710
Marina del Rey, CA 90292

Direct Inquiries to:
Rhoda Makoff, PhD
(310) 305-8053
(800) 338-9066
FAX: (310) 305-8103

For Medical Information Contact:
In Emergencies:
Dwight Makoff, M.D.
(310) 652-9162

Products Described:
Amin-Aid Instant Drink 2168
d-Biotin Capsules 2168
Calci-Chew Tablets 2168
Calci-Mix Capsules 2168
L-Carnitine Capsules 2168
DiabeVite Tablets 2168
Mag-Carb Capsules 2168
NephrAmine Injection 2169
Nephro-Calci Tablets 2168
Nephro-Derm Cream 2168
Nephro-Fer Tablets 2168
Nephro-Fer Rx Tablets 2168
Nephro-Vite Tablets 2170
Nephro-Vite + Fe Tablets 2170
Nephro-Vite Rx Tablets 2170
Regain Medical Nutrition Bar . .2170

RECKITT & COLMAN   330, 2170
PHARMACEUTICALS, INC.
1909 Huguenot Road
Richmond, VA 23235

Direct Inquiries to:
Professional Services
(804) 379-1090
FAX: (804) 379-1215

For Medical Information Contact:
In Emergencies:
Medical Department
(804) 379-1090
FAX: (804) 379-1215

Manufacturing and Distribution:
Distribution Center
3 Boulden Circle
New Castle, DE 19720
(302) 328-4578
FAX: (302) 323-3222

Products Described:
◆Buprenex Injectable 330, 2170

REED & CARNRICK
(See REEDCO, INC.)

REEDCO, INC.   2172
Road #3, KM 76.9
HCO4 Box 4013
Humacao, Puerto Rico 00791-9502

Direct Inquiries to:
Block Drug Company, Inc.
Consumer Affairs
(201) 434-3000, Ext. 1308
FAX: (201) 434-5739

For Medical Information Contact:
In Emergencies:
Block Drug Company, Inc.
Consumer Affairs
(800) 365-6500, Ext. 1308
FAX: (201) 434-5739

Products Described:
Kwell Cream & Lotion 2172
Kwell Shampoo 2173
Phazyme . . . . ◧

Other Products Available:
Proxigel

REID-ROWELL
(See SOLVAY PHARMACEUTICALS,
INC.)

RESPA PHARMACEUTICALS, INC.   2174
P.O. Box 88222
Carol Stream, IL 60188

Direct Inquiries to:
(630) 462-9986
FAX: (630) 462-9934

Products Described:
Respa-1st Tablets 2174
Respa-A.R.M. Tablets 2174
Respa-DM Tablets 2174
Respa-GF Tablets 2174
Respahist Capsules 2174

REXAR PHARMACAL
(See RICHWOOD PHARMACEUTICAL
CO.)

RHÔNE-POULENC RORER   330, 2174
PHARMACEUTICALS INC.
500 Arcola Road
Collegeville, PA 19426-0107
(610) 454-8000

Direct Inquiries to:
QUALITY ASSURANCE QUESTIONS:
John Chiles, Manager, Quality Control
(610) 454-3130
REGULATORY AFFAIRS QUESTIONS:
Ron Panner, Director, Regulatory Affairs
(610) 454-3026

For Medical Information Contact:
PRODUCT INFORMATION/ADVERSE
DRUG EXPERIENCES/EMERGENCIES
Medical Information and Education
(800) 340-7502
(610) 454-8110

Products Described:
◆Azmacort Oral Inhaler 330, 2175
Barotrast 2174
Calcimar Injection, Synthetic . . . 2176
Calel-D Tablets 2174
◆DDAVP Injection 330, 2178
◆DDAVP Injection 15 mcg/mL . 330, 2179
◆DDAVP Nasal Spray 330, 2180
◆DDAVP Rhinal Tube 330, 2180
◆DDAVP Tablets 330, 2182
Dialume Capsules 2174
◆Dilacor XR Extended-release
  Capsules 330, 2183
Esophotrast Cream 2174
HP Acthar Gel 2174
Hygroton Tablets 2174
◆Intal Inhaler 330, 2185
◆Intal Nebulizer Solution . . . 330, 2186
◆Lovenox Injection 330, 2187
Lozol Tablets 2174
◆Nasacort AQ Nasal Spray . . 330, 2191
◆Nasacort Nasal Inhaler . . . 330, 2189
Nasalcrom Nasal Solution 2192
Nicobid Tempules 2174
Nicolar Tablets 2174
◆Nitrolingual Spray 330, 2193
◆Oncaspar 330, 2194
Oratrast 2174
Parepectolin Suspension 2174
◆Penetrex Tablets 330, 2196
Regroton Tablets 2174
Demi-Regroton Tablets 2174
◆Rilutek Tablets 330, 2198
◆Slo-bid Gyrocaps 330, 2201
Slo-Phyllin GG Capsules 2174
Slo-Phyllin GG Syrup 2174
Slo-Phyllin 80 Syrup 2174
Slo-Phyllin Tablets 2174
◆Taxotere for Injection
  Concentrate 331, 2204
◆Tilade Inhaler 330, 2207
Tussar-2 Syrup 2174
Tussar DM Syrup 2174
Tussar SF Syrup 2174

RICHARDSON-VICKS INC
(See PROCTER & GAMBLE)

RICHWOOD   331, 2209
PHARMACEUTICAL
COMPANY, INC.
7900 Tanners Gate Drive, Suite 200
Florence, KY 41042

Direct Inquiries to:
(606) 282-2100
FAX: (606) 282-2103

Products Described:
Acuprin 81-Adult Low Dose
  Aspirin 2209
◆Adderall Tablets 331, 2209
Bellatal-Belladonna with
  Phenobarbital Alkaloids
  Tablets 2211
◆DextroStat-Dextroamphetamine-
  Sulfate Tablets 331, 2211
Dosaflex-Liquid Laxative 2212
MS/L-Morphine Sulfate Liquid . . 2212
MS/L Concentrate-Morphine
  Sulfate Liquid Concentrate . . . 2212
MS/S-Morphine Sulfate
  Suppositories 2212
Oby-Cap-Phentermine HCl
  Capsules 2212

Other Products Available:
Bismuth Subgallate-Colostomy or
  Ileostomy Deodorant

Isoxsuprine HCl-Peripheral Vasodilators
X-TROZINE L.A.-Phendimetrazine Tartrate Extended Release Capsules

RIKER LABORATORIES, INC.
(See 3M PHARMACEUTICALS)

ROBERTS PHARMACEUTICAL CORPORATION 331, 2212
4 Industrial Way West
Eatontown, NJ 07724 U.S.A.

Direct Inquiries to:
Customer Service
(908) 389-1182
(800) 828-2088
FAX: (908) 389-1014

For Medical Information Contact:
(800) 992-9306

Products Described:
Cheracol *2212*
Cheracol-D Cough Formula . . . . ◘
Cheracol Nasal Spray Pump . . . . ◘
Cheracol Plus Cough/Cold . . . . ◘
Cheracol Sore Throat Spray . . . . ◘
Citrocarbonate Antacid . . . . ◘
Clocream Skin Cream . . . . ◘
Colace Capsules, Syrup, Liquid 2212
Colace Microenema 2213
Colace-T 50 mg Tablets 2213
Colace-T 100 mg Tablets 2213
Comhist LA Capsules *2213*
Comhist Tablets *2213*
Dopar Capsules *2214*
Eltroxin Tablets 2214
◆Eminase 331, 2215
Entuss Liquid *2217*
Entuss Tablets *2217*
Entuss-D Liquid *2217*
Entuss-D Jr. Liquid *2217*
Entuss-D Tablets *2217*
◆Ethmozine Tablets 331, 2217
Furacin Soluble Dressing 2220
Furacin Topical Cream 2220
Furoxone Liquid 2221
Furoxone Tablets 2221
Haltran Tablets . . . . ◘
Kasof Capsules . . . . ◘
Norethin 1/35E *2222*
Norethin 1/50M *2222*
◆Noroxin Tablets 331, 2222
Nucofed Expectorant 2225
Nucofed Pediatric Expectorant 2225
Nucofed Syrup and Capsules 2225
Orthoxicol Cough Syrup . . . . ◘
P-A-C (Revised Formula) Analgesic Tablets . . . . ◘
Peri-Colace Capsules and Syrup 2226
Pro-Banthine Tablets 2226
Pyrroxate Capsules . . . . ◘
Quibron Capsules 2227
Quibron-300 Capsules 2227
Quibron-T Tablets 2227
Quibron-T/SR Tablets 2227
Saluron Tablets *2229*
Salutensin Tablets *2230*
Salutensin-Demi Tablets *2230*
Sigtab Tablets . . . . ◘
◆Supprelin Injection 331, 2230
◆Tigan Capsules 331, 2231
Tigan Injectable 2231
Tigan Suppositories 2231
◆Topicycline for Topical Solution 331, *2232*
Zymacap Capsules . . . . ◘

Other Products Available:
Alkets Tablets
Calcium Lactate Tablets, USP
Cevi-Fer Capsules (sustained release)
Cheracol Cough Syrup
Cheracol Sinus 12-hour Tablets
Cheracol Sore Throat Discs
Chlorafed H.S. Timecelles
Chlorafed Liquid
Chlorafed Timecelles
Clomycin Antibiotic Ointment
D-Vert Capsules
Diostate D Tablets
Dolacet Capsules
Duvoid
Duvoid Tablets
Entuss Expectorant
Entuss Tablets
Entuss-D Jr. Liquid
Entuss-D Liquid
Entuss-D Tablets
Gastrosed Drops
Gastrosed Tablets
Histor-D Timecelles
Lipomul Oral Liquid
Niacels Capsules
Nitrodisc
Orexin Tablets
Probec-T Tablets
Procort Cream
Romycin Topical Solution
Sinufed Timecelles
Sinumist-SR Caplets
Super D Perles
Tencet Capsules

A. H. ROBINS COMPANY, INC. 331, 2232
1407 Cummings Drive
Richmond, VA 23220

Direct General Inquiries to:
(610) 688-4400

For Emergency Medical Information Contact:
Medical Affairs
Day: (800) 934-5556 (8:30 AM to 4:30 PM, Eastern Standard Time, Weekdays only)
Night: (610) 688-4400 (Emergencies only; non-emergencies should wait until the next day)

For Medical/Pharmacy Inquiries on Marketed Products Contact:
(800) 934-5556 (8:30 AM to 4:30 PM, Eastern Standard Time, Weekdays only)

Products Described:
Dimetane-DC Cough Syrup 2232
Dimetane-DX Cough Syrup 2233
◆Donnatal Capsules 331, 2234
Donnatal Elixir 2234
◆Donnatal Extentabs 331, 2234
◆Donnatal Tablets 331, 2234
◆Donnazyme Tablets 331, 2235
Dopram Injectable 2235
◆Micro-K Extencaps 331, 2237
◆Micro-K 10 Extencaps 331, 2237
Micro-K LS Packets 2238
Phenaphen with Codeine Capsules *2239*
◆Pondimin Tablets 331, 2239
◆Quinidex Extentabs 331, 2240
◆Reglan Injectable 331, 2243
Reglan Syrup 2243
◆Reglan Tablets 331, 2243
◆Robaxin Injectable 331, 2245
◆Robaxin Tablets 331, 2246
◆Robaxin-750 Tablets 331, 2246
◆Robaxisal Tablets 331, 2246
◆Robinul Forte Tablets 331, 2247
◆Robinul Injectable 331, 2247
◆Robinul Tablets 331, 2247
Robitussin A-C Syrup 2248
Robitussin-DAC Syrup 2249
◆Tenex Tablets 331, 2249
Viokase Powder 2251
◆Viokase Tablets 331, 2251

Other Products Available:
Mitrolan Tablets

ROCHE PHARMACEUTICALS 331, 2252
Roche Laboratories Inc.
340 Kingsland Street
Nutley, New Jersey 07110-1199

For Medical Information Contact:
Generally:
Write: Professional Product Information Department
Call: (800) 526-6367
In Emergencies:
(800) 526-6367
(24-hour service)
Adverse Drug Experiences:
(800) 526-6367

Customer Service (Distribution):
(800) 526-0625

Products Described:
◆Accutane Capsules 331, 2252
◆Anaprox Tablets 331, 2277
◆Anaprox DS Tablets 331, 2277
◆Ancobon Capsules 331, 2254
◆Bactrim DS Tablets 331, 2257
Bactrim I.V. Infusion 2255
Bactrim Pediatric Suspension 2257
◆Bactrim Tablets 331, 2257
◆Berocca Plus Tablets 331, 2259
◆Berocca Tablets 331, 2259
Bumex Injection 2260
◆Bumex Tablets 331, 2260
◆Cardene Capsules 331, 2261
◆Cardene SR Capsules 332, 2264
◆CellCept Capsules 331, 2265
◆Cytovene Capsules 332, 2270
Cytovene-IV 2270
◆EC-Naprosyn Delayed-Release Tablets 332, 2277
Efudex Cream 2280
Efudex Topical Solutions 2280
◆Fansidar Tablets 332, 2281
Fluorouracil Injection 2282
Sterile FUDR 2284
◆Gantanol Tablets 332, 2285
Gantrisin Pediatric Suspension 2286
Gantrisin Syrup 2286
Gantrisin Tablets 2286
◆Hivid Tablets 332, 2287
◆Invirase Capsules 332, 2291
◆Klonopin Tablets 332, 2294
◆Lariam Tablets 332, 2295
◆Larodopa Tablets 332, 2296
Levo-Dromoran Injectable 2297
◆Levo-Dromoran Tablets 332, 2297
Lidex Cream 0.05% 2299
Lidex Gel 0.05% 2299
Lidex Ointment 0.05% 2299
Lidex Topical Solution 0.05% 2299
Lidex-E Cream 0.05% 2299
◆Matulane Capsules 332, 2300
Naprosyn Suspension 2277
◆Naprosyn Tablets 332, 2277
Nasalide Nasal Solution 0.025% 2301
Nasarel Nasal Solution 2302
◆Rocaltrol Capsules 332, 2303
Rocephin Injectable Vials, ADD-Vantage, Galaxy Container 2305
Roferon-A Injection 2308
Romazicon 2311
Synalar Cream 0.025% 2299
Synalar Topical Solution 0.01% 2299
◆Tegison Capsules 332, 2314
◆Tel-E-Ject Product: Versed Injection 332, *2317*
◆Ticlid Tablets 332, 2317
Toradol IM Injection, IV Injection 2319
◆Toradol Tablets 332, 2319
◆Trimpex Tablets 332, 2323
Versed Injection 2324
◆Vesanoid Capsules 332, 2327

ROCHE PRODUCTS INC. 332, 2329
Manati, Puerto Rico

For Medical Information Contact:
Roche Laboratories
(800) 526-6367

Customer Service (Distribution):
Roche Laboratories
(800) 526-0625

Products Described:
◆Dalmane Capsules 332, 2329
◆Librax Capsules 332, 2330
◆Librium Capsules 332, 2331
Librium Injectable 2332
◆Limbitrol DS Tablets 332, 2333
◆Limbitrol Tablets 332, 2333
◆Tel-E-Ject Product: Valium Injectable 332, *2334*
Valium Injectable 2336
◆Valium Tablets 332, 2335

ROERIG DIVISION
(See PFIZER INC)

RORER CONSUMER PHARMACEUTICALS
(See RHÔNE-POULENC RORER PHARMACEUTICALS INC., CONSUMER PHARMACEUTICAL PRODUCTS)

RORER PHARMACEUTICALS
(See RHÔNE-POULENC RORER PHARMACEUTICALS INC.)

ROSS PRODUCTS DIVISION 2337
Abbott Laboratories
Columbus, OH 43215-1724

Direct Inquiries to:
(800) 227-5767

Products Described:
Advera Specialized Complete Nutrition 2337
Alimentum Protein Hydrolysate Formula With Iron *2337*
AlitraQ Specialized Elemental Nutrition With Glutamine 2337
Clear Eyes ACR Astringent/Lubricant Eye Redness Reliever Drops . . . . ◘
Clear Eyes CLR Soothing Drops . . . . ◘
Clear Eyes Lubricant Eye Redness Reliever Drops . . . . ◘
Ear Drops by Murine—(See Murine Ear Wax Removal System/Murine Ear Drops) . . . . ◘
Ensure Complete Balanced Nutrition 2338
Ensure High Protein Complete Balanced Nutrition 2337
Ensure Light Complete, Balanced Nutrition 2338
Ensure Plus High Calorie Complete Nutrition 2338
Ensure With Fiber Complete, Balanced Nutrition 2338
Glucerna Specialized Nutrition with Fiber for Patients with Abnormal Glucose Tolerance 2338
Isomil DF Soy Formula For Diarrhea *2339*
Isomil SF Sucrose-Free Soy Formula with Iron *2339*
Isomil Soy Formula with Iron *2339*
Jevity Isotonic Liquid Nutrition with Fiber 2339
Jevity Plus 1.2 Cal/mL, High-Nitrogen Liquid Nutrition With Patented Fiber Blend 2339
Murine Ear Wax Removal System/Murine Ear Drops . . . . ◘
Murine Tears Lubricant Eye Drops . . . . ◘
Murine Tears Plus Lubricant Redness Reliever Eye Drops . . . . ◘
Nepro Specialized Liquid Nutrition 2339
Osmolite Isotonic Liquid Nutrition 2339
Osmolite HN High Nitrogen Isotonic Liquid Nutrition 2339
Osmolite HN Plus 1.2 Cal/mL, High-Nitrogen Liquid Nutrition 2340
Pediaflor Drops *2348*
Pedialyte Oral Electrolyte Maintenance Solution 2340
PediaSure Complete Liquid Nutrition 2342
PediaSure With Fiber Complete Liquid Nutrition 2343
Pediazole Suspension 2340
Perative Specialized Liquid Nutrition 2343
Polycose Glucose Polymers 2343
Pramilet FA *2348*
Promote High Protein Liquid Nutrition 2343
Promote With Fiber, High-Protein Liquid Nutrition 2343
Pulmocare Specialized Nutrition for Pulmonary Patients 2344
Rehydralyte Oral Electrolyte Rehydration Solution 2344
Ross Hospital Formula System *2344*
- Alimentum Protein Hydrolysate Formula With Iron *2344*
- Isomil 20 Soy Formula With Iron *2344*
- Pedialyte Oral Electrolyte Maintenance Solution *2344*
- Similac 20 Low-Iron Infant Formula *2344*
- Similac With Iron 20 Infant Formula *2344*
- Similac 24 Low-Iron Infant Formula *2344*
- Similac With Iron 24 Infant Formula *2344*
- Similac 27 Low-Iron Infant Formula *2344*
- Similac Natural Care Low-Iron Human Milk Fortifier *2344*
- Similac NeoCare Infant Formula With Iron *2344*
- Similac PM 60/40 Low-Iron Infant Formula *2344*
- Similac Special Care 20 Low-Iron Premature Infant Formula *2344*
- Similac Special Care With Iron 20 Premature Infant Formula *2344*
- Similac Special Care 24 Low-Iron Premature Infant Formula *2344*
- Similac Special Care With Iron 24 Premature Infant Formula *2344*
- Similac 5% Glucose Water *2344*
- Similac 10% Glucose Water *2344*
- Sterilized Water *2344*

Ross Metabolic Formula System *2344*
- Calcilo XD Low-Calcium/Vitamin D-Free Infant Formula With Iron *2344*
- Cyclinex-1 Amino Acid-Modified Medical Food With Iron *2344*
- Cyclinex-2 Amino Acid-Modified Medical Food *2344*
- Flavonex Flavored Energy Supplement *2344*
- Glutarex-1 Amino Acid-Modified Medical Food With Iron *2344*
- Glutarex-2 Amino Acid-Modified Medical Food *2344*
- Hominex-1 Amino Acid-Modified Medical Food With Iron *2344*
- Hominex-2 Amino Acid-Modified Medical Food *2344*
- I-Valex-1 Amino Acid-Modified Medical Food With Iron *2344*
- I-Valex-2 Amino Acid-Modified Medical Food *2344*
- Ketonex-1 Amino Acid-Modified Food With Iron *2344*
- Ketonex-2 Amino Acid-Modified Food *2344*
- Phenex-1 Amino Acid-Modified Medical Food With Iron *2344*
- Phenex-2 Amino Acid-Modified Medical Food *2344*
- Pro-Phree Protein-Free Energy Module With Iron/Vitamins/Minerals *2344*
- Propimex-1 Amino Acid-Modified Medical Food With Iron *2344*

◆ **Shown in Product Identification Section** *Italic Page Number* **Indicates Brief Listing** **Described in PDR For Nonprescription Drugs** ◘

◆ **Shown in Product Identification Section**   *Italic Page Number* **Indicates Brief Listing**   **Described in PDR For Nonprescription Drugs**

Sales and Ordering:
(800) 323-1603

Products Described:
◆Aldactazide Tablets 335, 2556
◆Aldactone Tablets 335, 2558
◆Ambien Tablets 335, 2559
◆Brevicon 21-Day Tablets . . . 335, 2563
◆Brevicon 28-Day Tablets . . . 335, 2563
◆Calan SR Caplets 335, 2571
◆Calan Tablets 335, 2568
◆Covera-HS Tablets 335, 2573
◆Cytotec 335, 2576
◆Daypro Caplets 335, 2578
◆Demulen 1/35-21 . . . . 335, 2580
◆Demulen 1/35-28 . . . . 335, 2580
◆Demulen 1/50-21 . . . . 335, 2580
◆Demulen 1/50-28 . . . . 335, 2580
◆Flagyl 375 Capsules 335, 2587
◆Kerlone Tablets 335, 2588
Lomotil Liquid 2591
◆Lomotil Tablets 335, 2591
◆Maxaquin Tablets 335, 2593
◆Norinyl 1+35 21-Day Tablets 335, 2563
◆Norinyl 1+35 28-Day Tablets 335, 2563
◆Norinyl 1+50 21-Day Tablets 335, 2563
◆Norinyl 1+50 28-Day Tablets 335, 2563
◆Norpace Capsules 335, 2596
◆Norpace CR Capsules 335, 2596
◆Nor-Q D Tablets 335, 2598
Synarel Nasal Solution for Central Precocious Puberty . . . 2603
Synarel Nasal Solution for Endometriosis 2605
◆Tri-Norinyl 21-Day Tablets . . . 335, 2607
◆Tri-Norinyl 28-Day Tablets . . . 335, 2607

Other Products Available:
Flagyl Tablets

SEATRACE PHARMACEUTICALS, INC. 2612
P.O. Box 363
Gadsden, AL 35902

Direct Inquiries to:
Hugh Campbell, C.E.O.
(205) 442-5023
FAX: (205) 442-5075

For Medical Emergencies Contact:
Hugh Campbell, C.E.O.
(205) 442-5023
FAX: (205) 442-5075

Products Described:
Banobese Tablets *2612*
Ceta Plus Capsules *2612*
Dyline GG Liquid *2612*
Dyline GG Tablets *2612*
G-Tuss Liquid *2612*
Gua-SR Tablets *2612*
Lobac Capsules *2612*
Lobac Tablets *2612*
Meni-D Capsules *2612*
ND Clear Capsules *2613*
Tenake Capsules *2613*
Tuss-DM Liquid *2613*
Tuss-DS Liquid *2613*
Tuss-HC Liquid *2613*
Tuss-PD Liquid *2613*
V-Dec-M Tablets *2613*
Versacaps Capsules *2613*

SEQUUS PHARMACEUTICALS, INC. 335, 2613
960 Hamilton Court
Menlo Park, CA 94025

Direct Inquiries to:
Department of Professional Services
(800) 323-9049

For Medical Emergencies Contact:
Ed Schnipper, M.D., or
Ron Lewis, M.D.
(800) 323-9051

Products Described:
◆Doxil 335, 2613

SERONO LABORATORIES, INC. 2616, 2995
100 Longwater Circle
Norwell, MA 02061

Direct Inquiries to:
Customer Service, Sales and Ordering
(800) 283-8088 x5141
(617) 982-9000 x5141

For Medical Information or to Report Adverse Drug Experiences Contact:
Drug Information and Surveillance Group
(800) 283-8088 x5562
(617) 982-9000 x5562

Products Described:
Geref (sermorelin acetate for injection) 2995
Metrodin (urofollitropin for injection) 2616
Pergonal (menotropins for injection, USP) 2618
Profasi (chorionic gonadotropin for injection, USP) 2620
Serophene (clomiphene citrate tablets, USP) 2621

SIGMA-TAU PHARMACEUTICALS, INC. 2623
800 South Frederick Avenue
Gaithersburg, MD 20877

Direct Inquiries to:
(301) 948-1041

Products Described:
Carnitor Injection 2623
Carnitor Tablets and Solution 2624

SMITHKLINE BEECHAM CONSUMER HEALTHCARE, L.P. 2625
Unit of SmithKline Beecham Inc.
P.O. Box 1467
Pittsburgh, PA 15230

Direct Inquiries to:
Professional Services Department
(800) BEECHAM
PA Residents: (800) 242-1718

Products Described:
Cepastat Lozenges
Contac Continuous Action Decongestant/Antihistamine-Capsules
Contac Maximum Strength Continuous Action Decongestant/Antihistamine-Caplets
Contac Severe Cold and Flu Formula Caplets
Contac Severe Cold & Flu Nighttime
Debrox Drops
Ecotrin Enteric Coated Aspirin Low Strength Tablets 2625
Ecotrin Enteric Coated Aspirin Maximum Strength Tablets and Caplets 2625
Ecotrin Enteric Coated Aspirin Regular Strength Tablets 2625
Feosol Caplets 2626
Feosol Elixir 2627
Feosol Tablets 2627
Gaviscon Regular Strength Antacid Tablets
Gaviscon Extra Strength Antacid Tablets
Gaviscon Extra Strength Liquid Antacid
Gaviscon Regular Strength Liquid Antacid
Gly-Oxide Liquid
Massengill Disposable Douche . . . 2627
Massengill Feminine Cleansing Wash 2628
Massengill Fragrance-Free Soft Cloth Towelette & Baby Powder Scent 2628
Massengill Liquid Concentrate . . . 2627
Massengill Medicated Disposable Douche 2628
Massengill Medicated Soft Cloth Towelettes 2628
Massengill Powder 2627
Nicorette 2 mg
Nicorette 4 mg
Os-Cal 250+D Tablets
Os-Cal 500 Chewable Tablets
Os-Cal 500 Tablets
Os-Cal 500+D Tablets
Os-Cal Fortified Tablets
Oxy Medicated Cleanser
Oxy Medicated Pads - Regular, Sensitive Skin and Maximum Strength
Oxy Medicated Soap
Oxy Night Watch Nighttime Acne Medication - Maximum Strength and Sensitive Skin Formulas
Oxy 10 Benzoyl Peroxide Wash
Oxy-5 and Oxy-10 Tinted and Vanishing
Sine-Off Maximum Strength Allergy/Sinus Formula Caplets
Sine-Off Maximum Strength No Drowsiness Formula Caplets
Sine-Off Sinus Medicine Tablets-Aspirin Formula
Singlet Tablets
Tagamet HB Acid Reducer
Tums, Tums EX, Tums ULTRA Antacid/Calcium Supplement Tablets
Tums Anti-gas/Antiacid

SMITHKLINE BEECHAM PHARMACEUTICALS 335, 2629
One Franklin Plaza
P.O. Box 7929
Philadelphia, PA 19101

For Medical Information Contact:
Medical Department
(800) 366-8900, Ext. 5231

Products Described:
Albenza Tablets 2629
◆Amoxil Capsules and Chewable Tablets 335, 2631
Amoxil Pediatric Drops, Powder for Oral Suspension . . . 2631
◆Ancef Injection 336, 2632
◆Androderm Testosterone Transdermal System 336, 2634
◆Augmentin Chewable Tablets . 336, 2637
◆Augmentin Powder for Oral Suspension 336, 2637
◆Augmentin Tablets 336, 2640
Bactroban Nasal 2643
Bactroban Ointment 2642
◆Compazine Injection 336, 2644
◆Compazine Multi-dose Vials . . . 336, 2644
◆Compazine Spansule Capsules . 336, 2644
◆Compazine Suppositories . . . 336, 2644
◆Compazine Syrup 336, 2644
◆Compazine Tablets 336, 2644
◆Cytomel Tablets 336, 2647
◆Dexedrine Spansule Capsules . 336, 2648
◆Dexedrine Tablets 336, 2648
◆Dibenzyline Capsules 336, 2650
◆Diphtheria and Tetanus Toxoids and Pertussis Vaccine Adsorbed 336, 2650
◆Dyazide Capsules 336, 2653
◆Dycill Capsules 336
◆Dyrenium Capsules 336, 2655
◆Engerix-B Unit-Dose Vials . . . 336, 2656
◆Eskalith Capsules 336, 2658
◆Eskalith CR Controlled Release Tablets 336, 2658
◆Famvir Tablets 336, 2660
◆Fastin Capsules 336, 2662
◆Havrix 336, 2663
◆Hycamtin for Injection 336, 2665
◆Kytril Injection 337, 2667
◆Kytril Tablets 337, 2669
◆Menest Tablets 337, 2671
◆Monocid Injection 337, 2674
◆OmniHIB 337, 2676
◆Ornade Spansule Capsules . . . 337, 2678
◆Parnate Tablets 337, 2679
◆Paxil Tablets 337, 2681
◆Rabies Vaccine Adsorbed . . . 337, 2686
◆Relafen Tablets 337, 2688
◆Ridaura Capsules 337, 2691
◆Stelazine Concentrate 337, 2692
◆Stelazine Multi-dose Vials . . . 337, 2692
◆Stelazine Tablets 337, 2692
◆Tagamet Injection 337, 2694
◆Tagamet Liquid 337, 2694
◆Tagamet Tablets 337, 2694
Tazicef for Injection 2697
◆Thorazine Ampuls 337, 2701
◆Thorazine Concentrate 337, 2701
◆Thorazine Multi-dose Vials . . . 337, 2701
◆Thorazine Spansule Capsules . 337, 2701
◆Thorazine Suppositories 337, 2701
◆Thorazine Syrup 337, 2701
◆Thorazine Tablets 337, 2701
Ticar for Injection 2704
◆Timentin for Injection 338, 2706
◆Triostat Injection 338, 2708
◆Urispas Tablets 338, 2710

Other Products Available:
Beepen-VK Powder for Oral Solution and Tablets
Nallpen for Injection
Totacillin Capsules
Totacillin Powder for Oral Suspension
Totacillin-N Injectable

SMITHKLINE CONSUMER PRODUCTS
(See SMITHKLINE BEECHAM CONSUMER HEALTHCARE, L.P.)

SOLOPAK PHARMACEUTICAL INC. 338, 2711
6001 Broken Sound Parkway
Boca Raton, FL 33487

Direct Inquiries to:
(800) 276-5672
FAX: (561) 998-3059

Products Described:
◆Ganite 338, 2711
◆Hydralazine Hydrochloride Injection USP 338, 2712

Other Products Available:
Amikacin Sulfate Injection USP
Cefazolin Sodium Injection USP
Clindamycin Phosphate Injection USP
Dextrose Injection USP
Dopamine Hydrochloride Injection USP
Droperidol Injection USP
Fluorouracil Injection USP
Gentamycin Sulfate Injection USP
Haloperidol Injection USP
Heparin Lock Flush Solution USP
Heparin Sodium Injection USP
Hydroxyzine Hydrochloride Injectionn USP
Kanamycin Sulfate Injection USP
Magnesium Sulfate Injectionn USP
Metoclopramide Injection USP
Morphine Sulfate Injection USP CII
Naloxone Hydrochloride Injection USP
Nitroglycerin Injection USP
Phenytoin Sodium Injection USP
Prochlorperazine Edisylate Injection USP
Propanolol Hydrochloride Injection USP
Sodium Chloride Injection USP
Tobramycin Sulfate Injection USP
Trimethobenzamide Hydrochloride Injection USP
Verapamil Hydrochloride Injection USP

SOLVAY PHARMACEUTICALS, INC. 338, 2713
901 Sawyer Road
Marietta, GA 30062
(770) 578-9000

For Medical Information Contact:
Generally:
Medical Services Department
(770) 578-9000
FAX: (770) 578-5586
In Emergencies:
(800) 241-1643

Sales and Ordering:
Orders may be placed by calling this toll free number:
(800) 241-1643
FAX: (770) 578-5901
Ordernet access is available.
Mail orders should be sent to:
Solvay Pharmaceuticals
Order Entry Department
901 Sawyer Road
Marietta, GA 30062

Products Described:
CORTENEMA 2713
◆CREON 5 Capsules 338, 2714
◆CREON 10 Capsules 338, 2714
◆CREON 20 Capsules 338, 2714
DUPHALAC Solution 2714
◆ESTRATAB Tablets (0.3, 0.625, 1.25, 2.5 mg) 338, 2715
◆ESTRATEST Tablets 338, 2718
◆ESTRATEST H.S. Tablets 338, 2718
◆LITHOBID Slow-Release Tablets 338, 2721
◆LITHONATE Capsules 338, 2721
◆LITHOTABS Tablets 338, 2721
◆LUVOX Tablets 338, 2723
◆ROWASA Rectal Suppositories, 500 mg 338, 2727
◆ROWASA Rectal Suspension Enema 4.0 grams/unit (60 mL) 338, 2727
◆Advanced Formula ZENATE Tablets 338, 2728

Other Products Available:
Curretab Tablets
Dermacort Cream
Dermacort Lotion 1%
Dexone (0.5, 0.75, 1.5, 4mg)
Orasone 1, 5, 10, 20, 50

SOMERSET PHARMACEUTICALS, INC. 338, 2729
5215 West Laurel Street
Tampa, FL 33607

For Medical Information Contact:
Generally:
Professional Services Department
(813) 288-0040
FAX: (813) 288-0085
In Emergencies:
Cheryl D. Blume, Ph.D.
(800) 892-8889
FAX: (813) 288-0085

Products Described:
◆Eldepryl Capsules 338, 2729

SPEYWOOD PHARMACEUTICALS, INC. 2731
27 Maple Street
Milford, MA 01757-3650

Direct Inquiries to:
Customer Service:
(508) 478-8900
Educational Information:
(508) 478-8900

For Medical Information Contact:
In Emergencies:
(800) 456-7322

Sales and Ordering:
(800) 456-7322
Reimbursement Services:
(800) 334-1142

Products Described:
HYATE:C Antihemophilic Factor (Porcine) *2731*

E. R. SQUIBB & SONS, INC.
(See BRISTOL-MYERS SQUIBB COMPANY)

STAR PHARMACEUTICALS, INC. 2731
1990 N.W. 44th Street
Pompano Beach, FL 33064-8712

Direct Inquiries to:
Scott L. Davidson, President
(954) 971-9704

Sales and Ordering:
(800) 845-7827
FAX: (954) 971-7718

Products Described:
Aphrodyne 2731
Prosed/DS 2731
Uro-KP-Neutral 2731
Urolene Blue 2731
Virilon 2731
Virilon IM 2732

STIEFEL LABORATORIES, INC. 2732
255 Alhambra Circle
Coral Gables, FL 33134

BRANCH OFFICES:
Georgia
500 Satellite Blvd.
Suwanee, GA 30174
(770) 945-0101
Nevada
P.O. Box 2387
Sparks, NV 89432
New York
Route 145
Oak Hill, NY 12460
(518) 239-6901

Direct Inquiries to:
Professional Services Department
(305) 443-3800

Products Described:
Brevoxyl-4 Gel 2732
Brevoxyl-8 Gel 2732
Brevoxyl Cleansing Lotion . . . 2732
LactiCare-HC Lotion, 1% . . . 2732
LactiCare-HC Lotion, 2 ½% . . 2732
PanOxyl 5 Acne Gel 2732
PanOxyl 10 Acne Gel 2732
PanOxyl AQ 2 ½ Acne Gel . . 2732
PanOxyl AQ 5 Acne Gel 2732
PanOxyl AQ 10 Acne Gel . . . 2732
Sulfoxyl Lotion Regular 2733
Sulfoxyl Lotion Strong 2733

Other Products Available:
Acne-Aid Cleansing Bar
Benoxyl-5 Lotion
Benoxyl-10 Lotion
Brasivol Base
Brasivol Fine
Brasivol Medium
Brasivol Rough
Epilyt Lotion
LactiCare Lotion
Oilatum Soap (Scented)
Oilatum Soap (Unscented)
PanOxyl Bar 5
PanOxyl Bar 10
Polytar Shampoo
Polytar Soap
SFC Lotion
Salicylic Acid Cleansing Bar
Salicylic Acid & Sulfur Soap
Sarna Lotion
SAStid Soap
Sulfur Soap
ZNP Bar
Zeasorb Powder
Zeasorb-AF Powder

STUART PHARMACEUTICALS
(See ZENECA PHARMACEUTICALS)

SUMMIT PHARMACEUTICALS
(See CIBAGENEVA PHARMACEUTICALS)

SUPERGEN, INC. 2733
6540 Hollis Street
Emeryville, CA 94608

Direct Inquiries to:
Customer Service
(800) 905-5474
FAX: (800) 903-5474

For Medical Information Contact:
Generally:
Professional Services Department
(888) 43-SUPER
(888) 437-8737
FAX: (510) 655-1098
In Emergencies:
(415) 749-7897

Sales and Ordering:
Customer Service
(800) 905-5474
FAX: (800) 903-5474

Products Described:
Etoposide Injection 2733
Leucovorin Calcium Tablets 2733
Megestrol Acetate Tablets,
USP 2733
Methotrexate Tablets, USP 2733
Nipent for Injection 2733

SYNTEX (F.P.) INC. 2736
Humacao, Puerto Rico 00791

SYNTEX LABORATORIES, INC. 2736
3401 Hillview Ave.
P.O. Box 10850
Palo Alto, CA 94303

SYNTEX PUERTO RICO, INC. 2736
Humacao, Puerto Rico 00791

**For Medical Information Contact Roche
Laboratories:**
Generally:
Write: Professional Product
Information Department
340 Kingsland Street
Nutley, NJ 07110-1199
Call: (800) 526-6367
In Emergencies:
(800) 526-6367
(24-hour service)
Adverse Drug Experiences:
(800) 526-6367

Customer Service (Distribution):
(800) 526-0625

(For Products Described, see ROCHE
LABORATORIES)

TAP PHARMACEUTICALS 338, 2736
INC.
2355 Waukegan Road
Deerfield, IL 60015

Direct Inquiries to:
Customer Service
(800) 621-1020

For Medical Information Contact:
Generally:
Medical Department
(800) 622-2011 (LUPRON)
(800) 478-9526 (PREVACID)
In Emergencies:
Medical Department
(800) 622-2011 (LUPRON)
(800) 478-9526 (PREVACID)

Products Described:
◆ Lupron Depot 3.75 mg . . 338, 2739
◆ Lupron Depot 7.5 mg . . . 338, 2741
◆ Lupron Depot - 3 Month 22.5
mg 338, 2743
Lupron Depot-PED 7.5 mg,
11.25 mg and 15 mg 2744
Lupron Injection 2736
Lupron Injection Pediatric . . . 2737
◆ Prevacid Delayed-Release
Capsules 338, 2746

TEVA PHARMACEUTICALS USA 2748
650 Cathill Road
Sellersville, PA 18960
(See also GATE PHARMACEUTICALS)

Direct Inquiries to:
(888) TEVA-USA

Products Described:
Acetaminophen and Codeine
Phosphate Tablets (CIII) 2748
Albuterol Tablets 2748
Albuterol Sulfate Syrup 2748
Amitriptyline HCl Tablets 2748
Amoxicillin Capsules,
Chewable Tablets, and Oral
Suspension 2748
Ampicillin Capsules 2748
Atenolol Tablets 2748
Baclofen Tablets 2748
Benzonatate Capsules 2748
Betamethasone Dipropionate
Lotion 2748
Beta-Val (betamethasone
valerate) Cream, Lotion 2748
Butalbital, Acetaminophen and
Caffeine Tablets 2748
Captopril Tablets 2748
Carbamazepine Tablets and
Chewable Tablets 2748
Carbidopa and Levodopa
Tablets 2748
Cephalexin Capsules, Tablets,
and Oral Suspension 2748
Cephradine Capsules and Oral
Suspension 2748
Chlorhexidine Gluconate Oral
Rinse 2748
Chlorzoxazone Tablets 2748
Cimetidine Tablets 2748
Cinoxacin Capsules 2748
Clemastine Fumarate Tablets
and Syrup 2748
Clomiphene Citrate Tablets . . . 2748
Clotrimazole Topical Solution . . 2748
Cloxacillin Sodium Capsules
and Oral Solution 2748
Cotrim (sulfamethoxazole and
trimethoprim) Tablets, D.S.
Tablets and Pediatric
Suspension 2748

Dicloxacillin Sodium Capsules . . 2748
Diflunisal Tablets 2748
Diltiazem HCl Tablets and
Extended-Release Capsules . . . 2748
Disopyramide Phosphate
Capsules 2748
Doxycycline Hyclate Capsules
and Tablets 2748
Epitol Tablets 2748
Fluocinonide Cream, Gel,
Ointment, Topical Solution
and Emulsified-Base Cream . . . 2748
Flurbiprofen Tablets 2748
Gemfibrozil Tablets 2748
Haloperidol Oral Solution 2748
Hydrocodone Bitartrate and
Acetaminophen Tablets
(CIII) 2748
Imipramine HCl Tablets 2748
Indomethacin
Extended-Release Capsules . . . 2748
Ketoprofen Capsules 2748
Loperamide HCl Capsules 2748
Megestrol Acetate Tablets 2748
Metaproterenol Sulfate
Tablets and Syrup 2748
Metoclopramide Tablets and
Oral Solution 2748
Metoprolol Tartrate Tablets . . . 2748
Metronidazole Tablets 2748
Minocycline HCl Capsules 2748
Minoxidil Topical Solution 2748
Myco-Triacet II (nystatin and
triamcinolone acetonide)
Cream and Ointment 2748
Naproxen Tablets 2748
Naproxen Sodium Tablets 2748
Neomycin Sulfate Tablets 2748
Nortriptyline HCl Capsules . . . 2748
Nystatin Oral Tablets and Oral
Suspension 2748
Otocort (neomycin and
polymyxin B sulfates and
hydrocortisone) Sterile
Solution and Suspension . . . 2748
Oxacillin Sodium Capsules
and Oral Solution 2748
Penicillin V Potassium Tablets
and Oral Solution 2748
Piroxicam Capsules 2748
Propacet 100 (propoxyphene
napsylate and
acetaminophen) Tablets
(CIV) 2748
Propoxyphene Compound 65
Capsules (CIV) 2748
Propoxyphene HCl Capsules
(CIV) 2748
Propoxyphene Napsylate and
Acetaminophen Tablets
(CIV) 2748
Propranolol HCl
Extended-Release Capsules . . . 2748
Sucralfate Tablets 2748
Sulfamethoxazole and
Trimethoprim Tablets and
Oral Suspension 2748
Sulfanilamide Vaginal Cream . . . 2748
Theochron (theophylline
anhydrous) Extended
Release Tablets 2748
Theophylline
Extended-Release Capsules . . . 2748
Trazodone HCl Tablets 2748
Triacet (triamcinolone
acetonide) Cream 2748
Trimethoprim Tablets 2748

TYSON AND ASSOCIATES, INC. 2749
12832 Chadron Avenue
Hawthorne, CA 90250

Direct Inquiries to:
Customer Service Department
(310) 675-1080
(800) 318-9766

Products Described:
Aminomine Capsules 2749
Aminoplex Capsules 2749
Aminostasis Capsules 2749
Aminotate Capsules 2749
Aminovirox Capsules 2749
Aminoxin Enteric Tablets
(Coenzymatic B$_6$) 2749
Arginine HCl Capsules 2749
ATP (Enteric Adenosine
Triphosphate) 2749
L-Carnitine Capsules 2749
Catemine Enteric Tablets
(Tyrosine) 2750
Co-Q-10 Capsules 2749
Endorphenyl Capsules
(D-Phenylalanine) 2749
MVM Capsules (Multivitamin
Mineral) 2749
Nutrox Capsules (Anti-Oxidant
Formula) 2749
Ribo-2 Enteric Tablets
(Riboflavin 5' Phosphate) . . . 2749
Thiamilate Enteric Tablets
(Thiamine Pyrophosphate) . . . 2749
Threostat Capsules
(Threonine) 2749

Other Products Available:
Alpha-Ketoglutaric Acid

Amino-CR
Amino-Min-D
Amino-Opti-C
Camsin
Gaba
Glutathione Reduced
Iso-B
L-Arginine HCl
L-Citrulline
L-Cyseine HCl
L-Glutamine
L-Ornithine
L-Taurine
Lysinyl
Maxovite
Melatonin
Metozan
Proline
Rxosine
Sof-Gel EFA
Stasis Canister
Theradophilus
Ultracholine
Zinc Picolinate

UAD LABORATORIES
(See FOREST PHARMACEUTICALS, INC.)

UCB PHARMA, INC. 338, 2750
1950 Lake Park Drive
Smyrna (Atlanta), GA 30080

Direct Inquiries to:
(800) 477-7877

For Medical Information Contact:
Suzan E. Leake
Manager, Medical Affairs
(770) 437-5558
In Emergencies:
Medical Affairs
(800) 477-7877

Products Described:
◆ Duratuss Tablets 338, 2750
◆ Duratuss HD Elixir 338, 2750
Fe-50 Caplets 2751
◆ Lortab ASA Tablets 338, 2753
◆ Lortab 2.5/500 Tablets . . 338, 2751
◆ Lortab 5/500 Tablets . . . 338, 2751
◆ Lortab 7.5/500 Tablets . . 338, 2751
◆ Lortab 10/500 Tablets . . 338, 2751
◆ Lortab Elixir 338, 2751
Precare Prenatal
Multi-Vitamin/Mineral 2753
◆ Theo-24 Extended Release
Capsules 338, 2753
◆ Trinsicon Capsules 338, 2759
◆ Vicon Forte Capsules . . . 338, 2760

Other Products Available:
Corticaine Cream
Theo-Bid Duracap Capsules
Vicon Plus Capsules
Vicon-C Capsules
Vi-Zac Capsules

U.S. BIOSCIENCE, INC. 338, 2760
One Tower Bridge
100 Front Street
West Conshohocken, PA 19428

Direct Inquiries to:
U.S. Bioscience
(610) 832-0570

**For Medical Information or
Emergencies Contact:**
(800) 872-4672

Products Described:
◆ Hexalen Capsules 338, 2760
◆ Neutrexin for Injection 339, 2761

U. S. ETHICALS INC.
(See RHÔNE-POULENC RORER
PHARMACEUTICALS INC.)

U.S. PHARMACEUTICAL 2764
CORPORATION
2401C Mellon Court
Decatur, GA 30035
(800) 330-3040
FAX: (404) 987-4860

MAILING ADDRESS:
2401C Mellon Court
Decatur, GA 30035

Direct Inquiries to:
Raymond F. Meyer, R.Ph.,
Marketing Director
(800) 330-3040

Products Described:
Hemocyte Plus Tabules 2764
Hemocyte Tablets 2764
Hemocyte-C Tablets 2764
Hemocyte-F Elixir 2764
Hemocyte-F Tablets 2764
Magsal Tablets 2765
Medigesic Capsules 2765

UNIVAX BIOLOGICALS, INC.
(See NABI)

THE UPJOHN COMPANY
(See PHARMACIA & UPJOHN COMPANY)

UPSHER-SMITH   **339, 2765**
LABORATORIES, INC.
14905 23rd Avenue North
Minneapolis, MN 55447

For Medical Information Contact:
Write: Professional Services Department
or call: (800) 654-2299
(during business hours-8:00 am to 5:00
pm CST)

Products Described:

Other Products Available:
Bisacodyl Tablets
Bisacodyl Uniserts Suppositories
Feratab Tablets
Ferrous Gluconate Tablets
Hemorrhoidal-HC Uniserts Suppositories
  (Hemril-HC)
Hexavitamin Tablets
Sorbitol Solution
Stress-600 Tablets
Stress-600 with Zinc Tablets
Therapeutic B Complex with Vitamin C
  Capsules
Therapeutic Multivitamin Tablets
Therapeutic Multivitamin with Minerals
  Tablets
Zinc Sulfate Capsules

VITALINE CORPORATION   **2767**
385 Williamson Way
Ashland, OR 97520

Direct Inquiries to:
Jed D. Meese, Technical Director
(541) 482-9231
FAX: (541) 482-9112

Products Described:

Other Products Available:
Alka-Aid (antacid)
Antioxidant Formula
B Complex "50"
B Complex "100"
Betazyme (Betaine HCl)
Biotin-Forte 3 mg
Biotin-Forte 5 mg
Boron
Bromelain 500 mg
Cal-Carb Forte
Calcium Citrate
Cal-Mag Aspartate
C Ascorbate Plus
Catalytic Formula (proteolytic enzymes)
Chromium IMG GTF
Chromium Picolinate 200 mcg
CNS Formula
CV CoFactors
Digestive Enzymes
Enviro Stress
E-Pherol (d-alpha tocopherol)
Folic Acid/B12 Powder
Free Form Amino Acid Complex
Garlic Forte
Herbal Antioxidant with Pycnogenol
Iron Plus
K Mag Aspartate (potassium &
  magnesium)
L-Glutamine & Choline
L-Glutamine Powder
L-Lysine
Manganese
Marine Lipid Concentrate
Maximum Formula
  (multivitamin-multimineral)
Multimineral Plus Advanced Formula
Ox-Absorb
Pancreatin 4X
Pancreatin 8X
Pancrezyme 4X (vegetarian pancreatin)
Pantothenic Acid
Polysaccharide Iron Complex 150 mg
Pros-Forte

Proteolytic Formula (proteolytic
  enzymes)
Renal Vitamin Formula
Renal Vitamin Formula with Zinc
Renal Vitamins plus Iron
Selenium 200 mcg
S.O.D. (SUPEROXIDE DISMUTASE)
Thymus 200
Total Formula
  (multivitamin-multimineral)
Vita-Calcium
Vita-Mag
Vitamin A
Vitamin B-12 2500 mcg Sublingual
  Tablets
Vitamin B6 Controlled Time Release
Vitamin C Controlled Time Release
Vitamin C Powder
Vitamine C with Citrus Bioflavonoids
Vitamin D3 400 I.U.
Vitamin E 400 I.U. Oil Capsules
Zinc 220 (50 mg elemental zinc)

WAKEFIELD PHARMACEUTICALS,   **2768**
INC.
1050 Cambridge Square, Suite C
Alpharetta, GA 30201

Direct Inquiries to:
(707) 664-1661
FAX: (707) 664-1126

Products Described:

WALLACE LABORATORIES   **339, 2768**
P.O. Box 1001
Cranbury, NJ 08512

For Medical Information Contact:
Generally:
Professional Services
(609) 655-6000
**After Hours and Weekend
  Emergencies:**
(609) 655-6474

Sales and Ordering:
Wallace Laboratories
Div. of Carter-Wallace, Inc.
P.O. Box 1001
Cranbury, NJ 08512

Products Described:

Other Products Available:
Barbidonna Tablets
Barbidonna No. 2 Tablets
Butibel Elixir & Tablets
Lufyllin-EPG Elixir & Tablets
Micrainin Tablets
Vascor Tablets (See McNeil
  Pharmaceutical)

WARNER CHILCOTT INC.   **2787**
182 Tabor Road
Morris Plains, NJ 07950
(800) 521-8813

Direct Inquiries to:
(800) 521-8813

**For Product/Medical Information
Contact:**
(800) 521-8813
FAX: (201) 540-7181

**After Hours and Weekend Medical
  Emergencies:**
(303) 739-1110

Products Described:

WARNER WELLCOME   **2788**
201 Tabor Road
Morris Plains, NJ 07950

**Direct Inquiries and For Medical
  Information Contact:**
Consumer Affairs
1-(800) 524-2624
1-(800) 223-0182

Products Described:

WATSON LABORATORIES, INC.   **2790**
311 Bonnie Circle
Corona, CA 91720

Direct Inquiries to:
Customer Service Department
(800) 272-5525
FAX: (909) 270-1096

For Medical Information Contact:
In Emergencies:
(800) 272-5525
FAX: (909) 270-1096

Products Described:

WE PHARMACEUTICALS, INC. **2791**
P.O. Box 1142
Ramona, CA 92065

Direct Inquiries to:
(619) 788-9155

For Medical Emergencies Contact:
(619) 788-9155

Products Described:

WESTWOOD-SQUIBB PHARMACEUTICALS INC.
(See BRISTOL-MYERS SQUIBB COMPANY)

WHARTON LABORATORIES INC.
(See RHÔNE-POULENC RORER PHARMACEUTICALS INC.)

WHITBY PHARMACEUTICALS, INC.
(See UCB PHARMA, INC.)

WILLEN DRUG COMPANY
(See BAKER NORTON PHARMACEUTICALS, INC.)

WINTHROP PHARMACEUTICALS
90 Park Avenue
New York, NY 10016
(212) 907-2000

(See SANOFI WINTHROP PHARMACEUTICALS)

WYETH-AYERST **339, 2801, 2996**
LABORATORIES
Division of American Home Products
Corporation
P.O. Box 8299
Philadelphia, PA 19101

Direct General Inquiries to:
(610) 688-4400

For Medical Information Contact:
Medical Affairs
Day: (800) 934-5556 (8:30 AM to
4:30 PM, Eastern Standard Time,
Weekdays only)

In Emergencies:
Day: (800) 934-5556 (8:30 AM to
4:30 PM, Eastern Standard Time,
Weekdays only)
Night: (610) 688-4400 (Emergencies
only; non-emergencies should wait
until the next day)

Manufacturing and Distribution:
(Do not use freight addresses for mailing
of orders.)

Atlanta, GA--
P.O. Box 1773
Paoli, PA 19301-1773
(800) 666-7248
Freight address:
1000 Union Court
Kennesaw, GA 30144
Mail DEA order forms to:
P.O. Box 4365
Atlanta, GA 30302

Boston, MA--
P.O. Box 1773
Paoli, PA 19301-1773
(800) 666-7248
Freight address:
7 Connector Road
Andover, MA 01810
Mail DEA order forms to:
P.O. Box 9776
Andover, MA 01810-0976

Chicago, IL--
P.O. Box 1773
Paoli, PA 19301-1773
(800) 666-7248
Freight address:
745 N. Gary Avenue
Carol Stream, IL 60188
Mail DEA order forms to:
745 N. Gary Avenue
Carol Stream, IL 60188

Dallas, TX--
P.O. Box 1773
Paoli, PA 19301-1773
(800) 666-7248
Freight address:
11240 Petal Street
Dallas, TX 75238
Mail DEA order forms to:
P.O. Box 650231
Dallas, TX 75265-0231

Hawaii--
P.O. Box 1773
Paoli, PA 19301-1773
(800) 666-7248
Mail DEA order forms to:
96-1185 Waihona St., Unit C1
Pearl City, HI 96782

Kansas City, MO--
P.O. Box 1773
Paoli, PA 19301-1773
(800) 666-7248
Freight address:
1340 Taney Street
N. Kansas City, MO 64116
Mail DEA order forms to:
P.O. Box 7588
N. Kansas City, MO 64116-0288

Los Angeles, CA--
P.O. Box 1773
Paoli, PA 19301-1773
(800) 666-7248
Freight address:
6530 Altura Blvd.
Buena Park, CA 90620
Mail DEA order forms to:
P.O. Box 5000
Buena Park, CA 90622-5000

Philadelphia, PA--
P.O. Box 1773
Paoli, PA 19301-1773
(800) 666-7248
Freight address:
31 Morehall Road
Frazer, PA 19355
Mail DEA order forms to:
P.O. Box 61
Paoli, PA 19301

San Juan, Puerto Rico--
GPO Box 362917
San Juan, PR 00936
(800) 462-4748
Freight address:
Wyeth-Ayerst Laboratories P.R. Inc.
Amelia Distribution Center
Street D
Lots 32 & 35
Guaynabo, Puerto Rico 00657
Mail DEA order forms to:
GPO Box 362917
San Juan, PR 00936

Seattle, WA--
P.O. Box 1773
Paoli, PA 19301-1773
(800) 666-7248
Freight address:
19255 80th Ave. So.
Kent, WA 98032
Mail DEA order form to:
P.O. Box 5690
Kent, WA 98064-5609

Products Described:

Other Products Available:
Benzathine Penicillin G (see Bicillin)
Codeine Phosphate Injection
Cyclospasmol Capsules
Dicloxacillin Sodium Monohydrate (see
Pathocil)
Digoxin Injection
Dimenhydrinate Injection
Diphenhydramine HCl Injection
Diphtheria & Tetanus Toxoids Adsorbed,
Pediatric
Epinephrine Injection (1:1000)
Heparin Flush Kits
Heparin Flush 2 mL Kits
Hydromorphone HCl Injection
Mepergan Fortis Capsules
Meperidine HCl Injection
Meperidine HCl Injection, Redipak
Morphine Sulfate Injection
Naloxone HCl Injection
Opium & Belladonna Rectal
Suppositories
Pentobarbital Sodium Injection
Phenobarbital Sodium Injection
Prochlorperazine Edisylate Injection
Redipak Unit Dose Medications
Redipak Unit Dose Medications (Strip
Pack and/or Individually Wrapped)
Products:
Ativan Tablets, 2 mg
Effexor Tablets, 25 mg
Effexor Tablets, 37.5 mg
Effexor Tablets, 50 mg
Effexor Tablets, 75 mg
Effexor Tablets, 100 mg
Isordil Sublingual Tablets,
2.5 mg
Isordil Sublingual Tablets, 5
mg
Isordil 5 Titradose Tablets,
5 mg
Isordil 10 Titradose
Tablets, 10 mg
Isordil 20 Titradose
Tablets, 20 mg
Isordil 30 Titradose
Tablets, 30 mg
Isordil 40 Titradose
Tablets, 40 mg
Lodine Tablets, 200 mg
Lodine Tablets, 400 mg
Meperidine HCl Tablets
Mysoline Tablets, 250 mg
Orudis Capsules, 75 mg
Oruvail Capsules, 100 mg
Oruvail Capsules, 150 mg
Oruvail Capsules, 200 mg
Pen•Vee K Tablets, 250 mg
Pen•Vee K Tablets, 500
mg
Phenergan Tablets, 25 mg
Sectral Capsules, 200 mg
Serax Capsules, 10 mg
Serax Capsules, 15 mg
Serax Capsules, 30 mg
Redipak (Respiratory Therapy Unit)
Products:
Sodium Chloride 0.9%
Saline Solution (see Sodium Chloride
Injection)
Secobarbital Sodium Injection
Sodium Chloride Injection, Bacteriostatic
Sodium Chloride Solution, 0.9%
Sonacide
Sparine Injection
Sparine Tablets
Testuria
Thiamine Hydrochloride Injection
Vitamin B_{12} Injection
Wyamine Sulfate Injection
Wydase, Stabilized Solution

ZENECA PHARMACEUTICALS 341, 2932
A Business Unit of Zeneca Inc.
Wilmington, DE 19850-5437 USA
General Number: (302) 886-3000

For Medical Information Contact:
Generally:
(302) 886-8000
**After Hours and Weekend
Emergencies:**
(302) 886-3000
Adverse Drug Experiences:
(302) 886-8100

Sales and Ordering:
(800) 842-9920

Products Described:
◆Arimidex Tablets 341, 2932
◆Casodex Tablets 341, 2934
◆Cefotan for Injection 341, 2936
◆Cefotan Injection 341, 2936
◆Diprivan Injectable Emulsion . 341, 2939
  Elavil Injection 2945
◆Elavil Tablets 341, 2945
◆Hibiclens Antimicrobial Skin
  Cleanser 342, 2947

◆Hibiclens Sponge/Brush with
  Nail Cleaner 341
◆Hibistat Germicidal Hand
  Rinse 342, 2948
◆Hibistat Towelette 342, 2948
  Kadian Capsules 2948
  Merrem I.V. 2952
◆Nolvadex Tablets 342, 2957
◆Sorbitrate Chewable Tablets . 342, 2959
◆Sorbitrate Oral Tablets 342, 2959
◆Sorbitrate Sublingual Tablets . 342, 2959
◆Sular Tablets 342, 2961
◆Tenoretic Tablets 342, 2963

◆Tenormin Tablets and I.V.
  Injection 342, 2965
◆Zestoretic Tablets 342, 2968
◆Zestril Tablets 342, 2972
◆Zoladex 342, 2976
  Zoladex 3-month 2978

Other Products Available:
Metastron
  (see under Medi-Physics, Inc.,
  Amersham Healthcare)

HOW TO USE THE BRAND AND GENERIC NAME INDEX

This index lists every product alphabetically by both brand and generic name. Generic names are underlined; brand names are not.

Under each generic name, you will find a list of the brands that contain it. This enables you to find a particular product by either of its names. For example, "Ativan Injection" is listed once alphabetically and again under its generic name, lorazepam.

Each time a brand name appears, it is followed by the manufacturer's name and the page to consult for further information. Under a generic heading, all fully described brands are listed first, followed by those with only partial information. In each case, the brands are listed alphabetically.

Brand name ——————————— **ATIVAN INJECTION**
(Wyeth-Ayerst).............................**2805**
◆ **ATIVAN TABLETS**
(Wyeth-Ayerst)......................**339, 2807**
ATIVAN IN TUBEX
(Wyeth-Ayerst)..............................*2926*
ATNATIV, ANTITHROMBIN III (HUMAN) HEAT TREATED (Baxter Healthcare)...........*577*

Generic name ——————————— **LORAZEPAM**   Manufacturer
Ativan Injection
(Wyeth-Ayerst)......................**2805**
Ativan Tablets (Wyeth-Ayerst) .**339, 2807**
Ativan in Tubex
(Wyeth-Ayerst) .... *2926* —— Italic page number Indicates partial prescribing information
Brands of lorazepam
Lorazepam Tablets (Mylan) *1836*
Lorazepam Tablets (Warner Chilcott)................................... *2787*
Lorazepam Tablets USP (Watson) *2790*
Indicates photo in Product Identification Guide
◆ **LORCET 10/650 TABLETS**
(Forest).............................. **311, 1016** —— Bold page number Indicates complete prescribing information
◆ **LORCET PLUS TABLETS**
(Forest) *311, 1016*

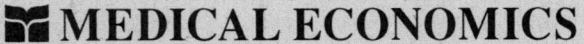

MEDICAL ECONOMICS
The leader in healthcare information products and services

SECTION 2

BRAND AND GENERIC NAME INDEX

This index includes all entries in the Product Information and Diagnostic Product Information sections. Products are listed alphabetically by both brand and generic name.

- An <u>underline</u> denotes a generic name.
- **Bold page numbers** indicate full prescribing information.
- *Italic page numbers* signify partial information.
- The ◆ symbol marks drugs shown in the Product Identification Guide.

- The ▣ symbol means product information is located in *PDR For Nonprescription Drugs*.
- The ☉ symbol means product information is located in *PDR For Ophthalmology*.

If an entry in the index lists multiple page numbers, the first ones shown refer to photographs of the product, the last one to its prescribing information. For more on this index, see "How to Use the Brand and Generic Name Index" on the preceding page.

A

ABBO-CODE INDEX (Abbott) *402*
◆**ABBOKINASE** (Abbott) **303, 403**
◆**ABBOKINASE OPEN-CATH**
(Abbott) **303, 405**
ABBO-PAC (Abbott) *402*

<u>ABCIXIMAB</u>
ReoPro Vials (Lilly) **322, 1526**

◆**ABELCET INJECTION**
(Liposome) **322, 1540**
AC SLIM CAP (AC Laboratory) . . . *461*

<u>ACARBOSE</u>
Precose (Bayer
Pharmaceutical) **305, 604**

◆**ACCUPRIL TABLETS**
(Parke-Davis) **327, 1950**

◆**ACCUTANE CAPSULES**
(Roche Pharmaceuticals) **331, 2252**

◆**ACCUZYME OINTMENT**
(Healthpoint) **316, 1236**
**ACEBUTOLOL
HYDROCHLORIDE
CAPSULES** (Mylan) *1836*

<u>ACEBUTOLOL HYDROCHLORIDE</u>
Sectral Capsules
(Wyeth-Ayerst) **341, 2914**
Acebutolol Hydrochloride
Capsules (Mylan) *1836*
Acebutolol Hydrochloride
Capsules (Watson) *2790*

◆**ACEL-IMUNE DIPHTHERIA
AND TETANUS TOXOIDS
AND ACELLULAR
PERTUSSIS VACCINE
ADSORBED** (Lederle) **320, 1415**

**ACES ANTIOXIDANT SOFT
GELS** (Carlson) *784*

<u>ACETAMINOPHEN</u>
Axocet Capsules (Savage) . . **333, 2469**
Children's TYLENOL
acetaminophen Chewable
Tablets, Elixir, Suspension
Liquid, and Suspension
Drops (McNeil Consumer) . **322, 1559**
Children's TYLENOL Cold
Multi-Symptom Chewable
Tablets and Liquid (McNeil
Consumer) **322, 1559**
Children's TYLENOL Flu
Suspension Liquid (McNeil
Consumer) **323, 1560**
DHCplus Capsules (Purdue
Frederick) **329, 2148**
Darvocet-N 50 Tablets (Lilly) . . . *1473*
Darvocet-N 100 Tablets
(Lilly) **322, 1473**
Esgic-plus Capsules (Forest) . **311, 1012**
Esgic-plus Tablets (Forest) . . **311, 1012**

**Aspirin Free Excedrin
Analgesic Caplets and
Geltabs** (Bristol-Myers
Products) **306, 734**
**Excedrin Extra-Strength
Analgesic Tablets,
Caplets, and Geltabs**
(Bristol-Myers Products) . . . **306, 734**
**Excedrin P.M.
Analgesic/Sleeping Aid
Tablets, Caplets, Liquigels**
(Bristol-Myers Products) **735**
Fioricet Tablets (Sandoz
Pharmaceuticals) **332, 2386**
**Fioricet with Codeine
Capsules** (Sandoz
Pharmaceuticals) **333, 2387**
**Hycomine Compound
Tablets** (DuPont) **948**
Hydrocet Capsules (Carnrick) . **308, 787**
**Infants' TYLENOL
acetaminophen
Suspension Drops** (McNeil
Consumer) **322, 1559**
**Infants' TYLENOL Cold
Decongestant &
Fever-Reducer Drops**
(McNeil Consumer) **322, 1561**
**Junior Strength TYLENOL
acetaminophen Coated
Caplets and Chewable
Tablets** (McNeil Consumer) . **323, 1562**
Lorcet 10/650 Tablets
(Forest) **311, 1016**
Lortab 2.5/500 Tablets
(UCB) **338, 2751**
Lortab 5/500 Tablets (UCB) . **338, 2751**
Lortab 7.5/500 Tablets
(UCB) **338, 2751**
Lortab 10/500 Tablets
(UCB) **338, 2751**
Lortab Elixir (UCB) **338, 2751**
Lurline PMS Tablets
(Fielding) *1000*
Midrin Capsules (Carnrick) . . **308, 788**
Percocet Tablets (DuPont) . . . **310, 955**
Phrenilin Forte Capsules
(Carnrick) **308, 790**
Phrenilin Tablets (Carnrick) . . **308, 790**
**Sedapap Tablets 50
mg/650 mg** (Merz) *1826*
**Sine-Aid Maximum Strength
Sinus Headache Gelcaps,
Caplets and Tablets**
(McNeil Consumer) **323, 1570**
Sinulin Tablets (Carnrick) . . . **308, 792**
Talacen Caplets (Sanofi
Winthrop) **333, 2464**
**TYLENOL acetaminophen
Extended Relief Caplets**
(McNeil Consumer) **322, 1570**
**TYLENOL acetaminophen,
Extra Strength Adult
Liquid Pain Reliever**
(McNeil Consumer) *1570*
**TYLENOL acetaminophen,
Extra Strength Gelcaps,
Geltabs, Caplets, Tablets**
(McNeil Consumer) **322, 1570**

**TYLENOL acetaminophen,
Regular Strength Caplets
and Tablets** (McNeil
Consumer) **322, 1570**
**TYLENOL Allergy Sinus,
Maximum Strength
Caplets and Gelcaps**
(McNeil Consumer) **323, 1571**
**TYLENOL Allergy Sinus
NightTime, Maximum
Strength Caplets** (McNeil
Consumer) **323, 1571**
**TYLENOL Cold Medication,
Multi-Symptom Formula
Tablets and Caplets**
(McNeil Consumer) **323, 1572**
**TYLENOL Cold Medication,
Multi-Symptom Hot Liquid
Packets** (McNeil Consumer) . **323, 1572**
**TYLENOL Cold Medication,
No Drowsiness Formula
Caplets and Gelcaps**
(McNeil Consumer) **323, 1572**
**TYLENOL Cold Severe
Congestion Caplets**
(McNeil Consumer) **323, 1573**
**TYLENOL Cough
Medication, Multi
Symptom** (McNeil
Consumer) **323, 1574**
**TYLENOL Cough
Medication with
Decongestant, Multi
Symptom** (McNeil
Consumer) **323, 1574**
**TYLENOL Flu No
Drowsiness Formula,
Maximum Strength
Gelcaps** (McNeil Consumer) . **323, 1575**
**TYLENOL Flu NightTime,
Maximum Strength
Gelcaps** (McNeil Consumer) . **323, 1575**
**TYLENOL Flu NightTime,
Maximum Strength Hot
Medication Packets**
(McNeil Consumer) **323, 1575**
**TYLENOL PM Pain
Reliever/Sleep Aid, Extra
Strength Gelcaps,
Caplets, Geltabs** (McNeil
Consumer) **323, 1576**
**TYLENOL Severe Allergy
Medication Caplets**
(McNeil Consumer) **323, 1571**
**TYLENOL Sinus, Maximum
Strength Geltabs,
Gelcaps, Caplets and
Tablets** (McNeil Consumer) . **323, 1576**
Tylenol with Codeine Elixir
(McNeil Pharmaceutical) . . . **324, 1592**
**Tylenol with Codeine
Phosphate Tablets** (McNeil
Pharmaceutical) **324, 1592**
Tylox Capsules (McNeil
Pharmaceutical) **324, 1593**
**Unisom With Pain
Relief-Nighttime Sleep Aid
and Pain Reliever** (Pfizer
Consumer) *1991*

Vicodin Tablets (Knoll
Laboratories) **320, 1404**
Vicodin ES Tablets (Knoll
Laboratories) **320, 1405**
Vicodin HP Tablets (Knoll
Laboratories) **320, 1403**
Wygesic Tablets
(Wyeth-Ayerst) **341, 2930**
Zydone Capsules (DuPont) *967*
Acetaminophen Elixir
(Pharmaceutical Associates) . . . *2056*
Acetaminophen and
Codeine Phosphate Oral
Soln. USP (Alpharma) *481*
Acetaminophen and
Codeine Phosphate Oral
Solution USP
(Pharmaceutical Associates) . . . *2055*
Acetaminophen and
Codeine Phosphate
Tablets (Duramed) *979*
Acetaminophen and
Codeine Phosphate
Tablets (Roxane) *2348*
Acetaminophen and
Codeine Phosphate
Tablets (CIII) (Teva) *2748*
Acetaminophen Elixir,
Tablets (Roxane) *2348*
Actifed Cold & Sinus
Tablets and Caplets
(Warner Wellcome) *2788*
Actifed Sinus
Daytime/Nighttime
Caplets and Tablets
(Warner Wellcome) *2788*
Anolor 300 (Blansett) *666*
APAP Drops (Alpharma) *481*
APAP Elixir-Cherry or Grape
(Alpharma) *481*
Benadryl Allergy/Cold
Tablets (Warner Wellcome) . . . *2788*
Benadryl Allergy/Sinus
Headache Caplets (Warner
Wellcome) *2788*
Bupap Tablets (ECR) *979*
Butalbital, Acetaminophen
and Caffeine Tablets
(Teva) *2748*
Butalbital, Acetaminophen
and Caffeine Tablets,
USP (Warner Chilcott) *2787*
Capital And Codeine
Suspension (Carnrick) **308, 787**
Ceta Plus Capsules
(Seatrace) *2612*
Co-Gesic Tablets (Central) . . . **308, 809**
Duradrin Capsules (Duramed) . . . *979*
Endocet Tablets USP CII
(Oxycodone HCl 5mg,
Acetaminophen 325mg)
(Endo) *988*
Esgic Capsules (Forest) **311, 1012**
Esgic Tablets (Forest) *1012*
Gelpirin Tablets (Alra) *484*
Hydrocodone Bitartrate and
Acetaminophen Tablets,
USP (Warner Chilcott) *2787*
Hydrocodone Bitartrate and
Acetaminophen Tablets
(CIII) (Teva) *2748*

BREVIBLOC (ESMOLOL HCL) INJECTION (Ohmeda) 1860
◆ BREVICON 21-DAY TABLETS (Searle) 335, 2563
◆ BREVICON 28-DAY TABLETS (Searle) 335, 2563
BREVITAL SODIUM FOR INJECTION, USP (Jones Medical Industries) 1361
BREVOXYL-4 GEL (Stiefel) . . . 2732
BREVOXYL-8 GEL (Stiefel) . . . 2732
BREVOXYL CLEANSING LOTION (Stiefel) 2732
BREXIN L.A. CAPSULES (Savage) 2470
◆ BRICANYL SUBCUTANEOUS INJECTION (Hoechst Marion Roussel) 317, 1247
◆ BRICANYL TABLETS (Hoechst Marion Roussel) 317, 1248
BROMANATE DC COUGH SYRUP (Alpharma) 481
BROMANATE DM (Alpharma) 481
BROMANATE ELIXIR (Alpharma) 481
BROMANYL COUGH SYRUP (Alpharma) 481
BROMFED CAPSULES (EXTENDED-RELEASE) (Muro) 1832
BROMFED SYRUP (Muro) 80
BROMFED TABLETS (Muro) . . . 1832
BROMFED-DM COUGH SYRUP (Muro) 1832
BROMFED-PD CAPSULES (EXTENDED-RELEASE) (Muro) 1832
BROMOCRIPTINE MESYLATE
Parlodel Capsules (Sandoz Pharmaceuticals) 333, 2411
Parlodel SnapTabs (Sandoz Pharmaceuticals) 333, 2411
Bromocriptine Mesylate Tablets and Capsules (Athena) 571
BROMPHENIRAMINE MALEATE
Bromfed Capsules (Extended-Release) (Muro) . . . 1832
Bromfed Tablets (Muro) 1832
Bromfed-DM Cough Syrup (Muro) 1832
Bromfed-PD Capsules (Extended-Release) (Muro) . . . 1832
Dimetane-DC Cough Syrup (Robins) 2232
Dimetane-DX Cough Syrup (Robins) 2233
Rondec Chewable Tablets (Dura) 974
Dallergy-JR Capsules (Laser) . . . 1414
E.N.T. Tablets (Ion) 1331
E.N.T. Plus Treatment Package (Ion) 1331
Lodrane LD Capsules (ECR) . . . 979
Lodrane Liquid (ECR) 979
Poly-Histine CS (Bock) 671
Poly-Histine DM Syrup (Bock) 672
Respahist Capsules (Respa) . . . 2174
ULTRABROM Capsules (WE) 2791
ULTRABROM PD Capsules (WE) 2791
BRONCHOLATE SYRUP (Bock) 666
BRONDELATE ELIXIR (Alpharma) 481
BRONKOMETER AEROSOL (Sanofi Winthrop) 2432
BRONKOSOL SOLUTION (Sanofi Winthrop) 2432
BRONTEX LIQUID (Procter & Gamble Pharmaceuticals) 2130
◆ BRONTEX TABLETS (Procter & Gamble Pharmaceuticals) . . 329, 2130
BUDESONIDE
Rhinocort Nasal Inhaler (Astra) 304, 552
ARTHRITIS STRENGTH BUFFERIN ANALGESIC CAPLETS (Bristol-Myers Products) 80

EXTRA STRENGTH BUFFERIN ANALGESIC TABLETS (Bristol-Myers Products) 80
BUFFERIN ANALGESIC TABLETS AND CAPLETS (Bristol-Myers Products) 80
BUMETANIDE
Bumex Injection (Roche Pharmaceuticals) 2260
Bumex Tablets (Roche Pharmaceuticals) 331, 2260
Bumetanide Tablets (Mylan) . . . 1836
BUMEX INJECTION (Roche Pharmaceuticals) 2260
◆ BUMEX TABLETS (Roche Pharmaceuticals) 331, 2260
BUMINATE 5%, ALBUMIN (HUMAN), USP, 5% SOLUTION (Baxter Healthcare) . .577
BUMINATE 25%, ALBUMIN (HUMAN), USP, 25% SOLUTION (Baxter Healthcare) . .577
BUPAP TABLETS (ECR) 979
BUPIVACAINE HYDROCHLORIDE
Marcaine with Epinephrine (Sanofi Winthrop) 2446
Marcaine Injection (Sanofi Winthrop) 2446
Marcaine Spinal (Sanofi Winthrop) 2449
Sensorcaine with Epinephrine Injection (Astra) 304, 554
Sensorcaine Injection (Astra) . 304, 554
Sensorcaine-MPF with Epinephrine Injection (Astra) 554
Sensorcaine-MPF Injection (Astra) 554
Sensorcaine-MPF Spinal (Astra) 557
◆ BUPRENEX INJECTABLE (Reckitt & Colman) 330, 2170
BUPRENORPHINE HYDROCHLORIDE
Buprenex Injectable (Reckitt & Colman) 330, 2170
BUPROPION HYDROCHLORIDE
Wellbutrin Tablets (Glaxo Wellcome) 315, 1177
BUROW'S SOLUTION
Pedi-Boro Soak Paks (Pedinol) 1988
◆ BUSPAR TABLETS (Bristol-Myers Squibb) 306, 738
BUSPIRONE HYDROCHLORIDE
BuSpar Tablets (Bristol-Myers Squibb) 306, 738
BUSULFAN
Myleran Tablets (Glaxo Wellcome Oncology/HIV) 316, 1209
BUTABARBITAL SODIUM
Butisol Sodium Elixir & Tablets (Wallace) 2768
Butabarbital Sodium Elixir USP 30 mg/5 mL (Alpharma) 481
BUTALBITAL
Axocet Capsules (Savage) . . 333, 2469
Esgic-plus Capsules (Forest) .311, 1012
Esgic-plus Tablets (Forest) . 311, 1012
Fioricet Tablets (Sandoz Pharmaceuticals) 332, 2386
Fioricet with Codeine Capsules (Sandoz Pharmaceuticals) 333, 2387
Fiorinal Capsules (Sandoz Pharmaceuticals) 333, 2388
Fiorinal with Codeine Capsules (Sandoz Pharmaceuticals) 333, 2390
Fiorinal Tablets (Sandoz Pharmaceuticals) 333, 2388
Phrenilin Forte Capsules (Carnrick) 308, 790
Phrenilin Tablets (Carnrick) . . 308, 790
Sedapap Tablets 50 mg/650 mg (Merz) 1826
Anolor 300 (Blansett) 666
Bupap Tablets (ECR) 979
Butalbital, Acetaminophen and Caffeine Tablets (Teva) 2748

Butalbital, Acetaminophen and Caffeine Tablets, USP (Warner Chilcott) 2787
Butalbital, Aspirin, Caffeine, and Codeine Phosphate Capsules, USP (Watson) 2790
Butalbital, Aspirin, Caffeine and Codeine Phosphate Capsules, USP (Warner Chilcott) 2787
Esgic Capsules (Forest) . . . 311, 1012
Esgic Tablets (Forest) 1012
Medigesic Capsules (U.S. Pharmaceutical) 2765
Pacaps Capsules (Lunsco) 1544
Repan-CF Tablets (Everett) . . . 992
Tenake Capsules (Seatrace) . . . 2613
Tencon Capsules (International Ethical) 1331
BUTISOL SODIUM ELIXIR & TABLETS (Wallace) 2768
BUTOCONAZOLE NITRATE
Femstat 3 (Procter & Gamble) . . . 2124
BUTORPHANOL TARTRATE
Stadol Injectable (Bristol-Myers Squibb) 779
Stadol NS Nasal Spray (Bristol-Myers Squibb) . . . 307, 779
Stadol Injection (Apothecon) . . . 513
BUTYL AMINOBENZOATE
Cetacaine Topical Anesthetic (Cetylite) 812

C

CAFERGOT SUPPOSITORIES (Sandoz Pharmaceuticals) 2376
CAFERGOT TABLETS (Sandoz Pharmaceuticals) 2376
CAFFEINE
Cafergot Suppositories (Sandoz Pharmaceuticals) 2376
Cafergot Tablets (Sandoz Pharmaceuticals) 2376
Darvon Compound-65 (Lilly) 1475
DHCplus Capsules (Purdue Frederick) 329, 2148
Esgic-plus Capsules (Forest) .311, 1012
Esgic-plus Tablets (Forest) . 311, 1012
Aspirin Free Excedrin Analgesic Caplets and Geltabs (Bristol-Myers Products) 306, 734
Excedrin Extra-Strength Analgesic Tablets, Caplets, and Geltabs (Bristol-Myers Products) 306, 734
Fioricet Tablets (Sandoz Pharmaceuticals) 332, 2386
Fioricet with Codeine Capsules (Sandoz Pharmaceuticals) 333, 2387
Fiorinal Capsules (Sandoz Pharmaceuticals) 333, 2388
Fiorinal with Codeine Capsules (Sandoz Pharmaceuticals) 333, 2390
Fiorinal Tablets (Sandoz Pharmaceuticals) 333, 2388
Norgesic Forte Tablets (3M Pharmaceuticals) 322, 1554
Norgesic Tablets (3M Pharmaceuticals) 322, 1554
Wigraine Tablets (Organon) . 326, 1884
Anolor 300 (Blansett) 666
Butalbital, Acetaminophen and Caffeine Tablets (Teva) 2748
Butalbital, Acetaminophen and Caffeine Tablets, USP (Warner Chilcott) 2787
Butalbital, Aspirin, Caffeine, and Codeine Phosphate Capsules, USP (Watson) 2790
Butalbital, Aspirin, Caffeine and Codeine Phosphate Capsules, USP (Warner Chilcott) 2787
Esgic Capsules (Forest) . . . 311, 1012
Esgic Tablets (Forest) 1012
Gelpirin Tablets (Alra) 484
Medigesic Capsules (U.S. Pharmaceutical) 2765
Pacaps Capsules (Lunsco) 1544
Propoxyphene Compound 65 Capsules (CIV) (Teva) . . . 2748
Synalgos-DC Capsules (Wyeth-Ayerst) 2919
Tenake Capsules (Seatrace) . . . 2613

CALADRYL CLEAR LOTION (Warner Wellcome) 2789
CALADRYL CREAM FOR KIDS (Warner Wellcome) 2789
CALADRYL LOTION (Warner Wellcome) 2789
CALAMINE
Caladryl Cream For Kids (Warner Wellcome) 2789
Caladryl Lotion (Warner Wellcome) 2789
◆ CALAN SR CAPLETS (Searle) 335, 2571
◆ CALAN TABLETS (Searle) . . . 335, 2568
CALCET TABLETS (Mission) 1828
CALCET PLUS TABLETS (Mission) 1828
CALCIBIND ORAL POWDER (Mission) 1829
CALCI-CHEW TABLETS (R&D) 2168
CALCIFEDIOL
Calderol Capsules (Organon) .325, 1866
CALCIFEROL DROPS (Schwarz) 2540
CALCIFEROL IN OIL INJECTION (Schwarz) 2540
CALCIFEROL TABLETS (Schwarz) 2540
CALCIJEX INJECTION (Abbott) 412
CALCIMAR INJECTION, SYNTHETIC (Rhone-Poulenc Rorer Pharmaceuticals) 2176
CALCI-MIX CAPSULES (R&D) 2168
CALCIPOTRIENE
Dovonex Cream 0.005% (Westwood-Squibb) 2792
Dovonex Ointment 0.005% (Westwood-Squibb) 2793
CALCITONIN-SALMON
Calcimar Injection, Synthetic (Rhone-Poulenc Rorer Pharmaceuticals) 2176
Miacalcin Injection (Sandoz Pharmaceuticals) 2402
Miacalcin Nasal Spray (Sandoz Pharmaceuticals) . . . 333, 2403
Calcitonin-Salmon Injection, Synthetic (Astra) 528
CALCITRIOL
Calcijex Injection (Abbott) 412
Rocaltrol Capsules (Roche Pharmaceuticals) 332, 2303
CALCIUM
Calcet Tablets (Mission) 1828
Fosfree Tablets (Mission) 1828
Mucos (CPH International) 916
CALCIUM ACETATE
PhosLo Tablets (Braintree) . . . 306, 695
CALCIUM CARBONATE
Calci-Chew Tablets (R&D) 2168
Calci-Mix Capsules (R&D) 2168
Cotazym Capsules (Organon) 325, 1866
Florical Capsules and Tablets (Mericon Industries) . . . 1825
Gerimed Tablets (Fielding) 1000
Materna Tablets (Lederle) . . .320, 1427
Monocal Tablets (Mericon Industries) 1825
Fast-Acting Mylanta Antacid Tablets (J&J•Merck Consumer) 1359
Maximum Strength Fast-Acting Mylanta Antacid Tablets (J&J•Merck Consumer) . . . 1359
Mylanta Soothing Lozenges (J&J•Merck Consumer) . . . 319, 1360
Nephro-Calci Tablets (R&D) . . . 2168
Calcet Plus Tablets (Mission) . . . 1828
Calcium Carbonate Tablets & Oral Suspension (Roxane) 2348
Calel-D Tablets (Rhone-Poulenc Rorer Pharmaceuticals) 2174
CALCIUM CHLORIDE
Calcium Chloride 10% Injection, USP (Astra) 528

◆**GLUCOTROL XL EXTENDED RELEASE TABLETS** (Pfizer Inc) **328, 2012**

L-GLUTAMINE

AlitraQ Specialized Elemental Nutrition With Glutamine (Ross) **2337**

GLUTOSE 15, GLUTOSE 45 (ORAL GLUCOSE GEL) (Paddock) *1948*

GLUTOSE TABLETS (Paddock) . . . *1948*

GLYBURIDE

DiaBeta Tablets (Hoechst Marion Roussel) **317, 1265**
Glynase PresTab Tablets (Pharmacia & Upjohn) **2091**
Micronase Tablets (Pharmacia & Upjohn) **2099**
Glyburide Tablets USP, 1.25 mg, 2.5 mg + 5 mg (Novopharm USA) *1852*

GLYCERIN

Auralgan Otic Solution (Wyeth-Ayerst) **2810**
DML Facial Moisturizer with Sunscreen (Persön & Covey) **1989**
Fleet Babylax (Fleet) **1000**
Fleet Glycerin Laxative Rectal Applicators (Fleet) **1000**
Fleet Pain Relief Pads (Fleet) **1001**
Tucks Clear Gel (Warner Wellcome) *2790*

GLYCERYL GUAIACOLATE (see under GUAIFENESIN)

GLYCERYL TRINITRATE (see under NITROGLYCERIN)

GLYCOPYRROLATE

Robinul Forte Tablets (Robins) **331, 2247**
Robinul Injectable (Robins) . **331, 2247**
Robinul Tablets (Robins) . . . **331, 2247**

GLYNASE PRESTAB TABLETS (Pharmacia & Upjohn) . . . **2091**

GLY-OXIDE LIQUID (SmithKline Beecham) . . . . ⊙

G-MYTICIN CREME 0.1% (Pedinol) *1988*

GOLD SODIUM THIOMALATE

Myochrysine Injection (Merck & Co., Inc.) **1754**

◆**GOLYTELY** (Braintree) **306, 694**

GONADORELIN ACETATE

Lutrepulse for Injection (Ferring) **998**

GONADORELIN HYDROCHLORIDE

Factrel (Wyeth-Ayerst) **2996**

GOSERELIN ACETATE

Zoladex (Zeneca) **342, 2976**
Zoladex 3-month (Zeneca) **2978**

GRAMICIDIN

Neosporin Ophthalmic Solution Sterile (Glaxo Wellcome) **314, 1131**

GRANISETRON HYDROCHLORIDE

Kytril Injection (SmithKline Beecham Pharmaceuticals) . . **337, 2667**
Kytril Tablets (SmithKline Beecham Pharmaceuticals) . . **337, 2669**

GRANULEX (Dow Hickam) **940**

◆**GRIFULVIN V TABLETS/SUSPENSION** (Ortho Dermatological) **326, 1944**

◆**GRISACTIN CAPSULES** (Wyeth-Ayerst) *339, 2830*

◆**GRISACTIN TABLETS** (Wyeth-Ayerst) *339, 2830*

◆**GRISACTIN ULTRA TABLETS** (ESI Lederle) *310, 992*

GRISEOFULVIN

Fulvicin P/G Tablets (Schering) **334, 2499**
Fulvicin P/G 165 & 330 Tablets (Schering) **334, 2500**
Grifulvin V Tablets/Suspension (Ortho Dermatological) **326, 1944**
Gris-PEG Tablets, 125 mg & 250 mg (Allergan) **476**
Grisactin Capsules (Wyeth-Ayerst) *339, 2830*
Grisactin Tablets (Wyeth-Ayerst) *339, 2830*
Grisactin Ultra Tablets (ESI Lederle) *310, 992*

GRIS-PEG TABLETS, 125 MG & 250 MG (Allergan) **476**

G-TUSS LIQUID (Seatrace) *2612*

GUAIFED CAPSULES (EXTENDED-RELEASE) (Muro) **1833**

GUAIFED-PD CAPSULES (EXTENDED-RELEASE) (Muro) **1833**

GUAIFED SYRUP (Muro) . . . . ⊙

GUAIFENESIN

Brontex Liquid (Procter & Gamble Pharmaceuticals) **2130**
Brontex Tablets (Procter & Gamble Pharmaceuticals) . . . **329, 2130**
Codiclear DH Syrup (Central) **808**
Congess Jr. T.D. Capsules (Fleming) **1003**
Congess Sr. T.D. Capsules (Fleming) **1003**
Deconsal II Tablets (Medeva) . . . **1605**
Dilaudid Cough Syrup (Knoll Laboratories) **1383**
Duratuss Tablets (UCB) **338, 2750**
Duratuss HD Elixir (UCB) **338, 2750**
Dura-Vent Tablets (Dura) **971**
Entex LA Tablets (Dura) **972**
Entex PSE Tablets (Dura) **973**
Exgest LA Tablets (Carnrick) . . **308, 787**
Guaifed Capsules (Extended-Release) (Muro) . . . **1833**
Guaifed-PD Capsules (Extended-Release) (Muro) . . . **1833**
Guaimax-D Tablets (Central) . **308, 809**
Humibid DM Tablets (Medeva) **1612**
Humibid L.A. Tablets (Medeva) **1612**
Humibid Pediatric Capsules (Medeva) **1612**
Hycotuss Expectorant Syrup (DuPont) **950**
Lufyllin-GG Elixir & Tablets (Wallace) **2779**
Nucofed Expectorant (Roberts) **2225**
Nucofed Pediatric Expectorant (Roberts) **2225**
Organidin NR Tablets and Liquid (Wallace) **339, 2781**
Quibron Capsules (Roberts) **2227**
Quibron-300 Capsules (Roberts) **2227**
Robitussin A-C Syrup (Robins) **2248**
Robitussin-DAC Syrup (Robins) **2249**
Safe Tussin 30 Liquid (Kramer) **1413**
Syn-Rx Tablets (Medeva) **1622**
Syn-Rx DM Tablets (Medeva) . . . **1623**
Tussend Expectorant (Monarch) **325, 1831**
Tussi-Organidin DM NR Liquid and DM-S NR Liquid (Wallace) **339, 2786**
TYLENOL Cold Severe Congestion Caplets (McNeil Consumer) **323, 1573**
Vicodin Tuss Expectorant (Knoll Laboratories) **320, 1406**
Anatuss DM Syrup (Merz) *1825*
Anatuss DM Tablets (Merz) *1825*
Anatuss LA Tablets (Merz) *1825*
Benylin Expectorant (Warner Wellcome) *2788*
Benylin Multi-Symptom (Warner Wellcome) *2788*
Broncholate Syrup (Bock) *666*
Cheracol (Roberts) *2212*
D-FEDA II Tablets (WE) *2791*
Despec SR Caplets (International Ethical) *1331*
Despec Liquid (International Ethical) *1331*
Despec SF (International Ethical) *1331*
Dilor-G Tablets & Liquid (Savage) *2472*
Donatussin DC Syrup (Laser) *1414*
Donatussin Drops (Laser) *1414*
Donatussin Syrup (Laser) *1414*
Dura-Gest Capsules (Dura) *970*
Duratex Capsules (Duramed) *979*
Dyline GG Liquid (Seatrace) *2612*
Dyline GG Tablets (Seatrace) . . . *2612*
Elixophyllin-GG Oral Solution (Forest) *1011*
Entex Capsules (Dura) *972*
Entex Liquid (Dura) *972*
E.N.T. Plus Treatment Package (Ion) *1331*
Entuss Tablets (Roberts) *2217*
Entuss-D Jr. Liquid (Roberts) *2217*
Entuss-D Tablets (Roberts) *2217*
Fenesin Tablets (Dura) *974*
Fenesin DM Tablets (Dura) *974*
G-Tuss Liquid (Seatrace) *2612*
Guaifenesin Syrup (Roxane) *2348*
Guaifenesin Syrup USP (Pharmaceutical Associates) *2056*
Guaifenesin Syrup with Codeine (Pharmaceutical Associates) *2056*
Guaifenesin Syrup with Dextromethorphan (Pharmaceutical Associates) *2056*
Guaifenesin Tablets (Duramed) *979*
Guai-Vent/PSE Tablets (Dura) *974*
Gua-SR Tablets (Seatrace) *2612*
Guiatuss (Alpharma) *481*
Guiatuss AC Syrup (Alpharma) *481*
Guiatuss CF (Alpharma) *481*
Guiatuss DAC (Alpharma) *481*
Guiatuss DM (Alpharma) *481*
Guiatuss PE (Alpharma) *481*
HUMAvent L.A. Tablets (WE) *2791*
Kwelcof Liquid (Ascher) *514*
Liquibid Tablets (Ion) *1331*
Liquibid-D Tablets (Ion) *1331*
Muco-Fen DM (Wakefield) *2768*
Muco-Fen-LA Tablets (Wakefield) *2768*
Mudrane GG Tablets (ECR) *979*
Nalex Capsules (Blansett) *666*
Nalex JR Capsules (Blansett) *666*
Nasabid SR Caplets (Abana) . *303, 402*
Nasatab LA Tablets (ECR) *979*
Norel (U.S. Pharmaceutical) *2765*
Phenylpropanolamine HCl and Guaifenesin Long Acting Tablets (Duramed) *979*
Pneumomist Tablets (ECR) *979*
Pneumotussin HC Cough Syrup (ECR) *979*
Profen-LA Tablets (Wakefield) *2768*
Profen II Tablets (Wakefield) *2768*
Pseudoephedrine HCl and Guaifenesin Extended Release Tablets (Duramed) *979*
Rescon-GG Liquid (Ion) *1331*
Respa-1st Tablets (Respa) *2174*
Respa-DM Tablets (Respa) *2174*
Respa-GF Tablets (Respa) *2174*
Respaire-SR Capsules 60, 120 (Laser) *1414*
Sinupan Capsules (Ion) *1331*
Sinutab Non Drying Liquid Caps (Warner Wellcome) *2789*
SINUVENT Tablets (WE) *2791*
Slo-Phyllin GG Capsules (Rhone-Poulenc Rorer Pharmaceuticals) *2174*
Slo-Phyllin GG Syrup (Rhone-Poulenc Rorer Pharmaceuticals) *2174*
Sudafed Cold & Cough Liquid Caps (Warner Wellcome) *2789*
Sudafed Non-Drying Sinus Liquid Caps (Warner Wellcome) *2789*
Children's Sudafed Cold & Cough (Warner Wellcome) *2790*
Theolate Liquid (Alpharma) *481*
Triaminic Expectorant DH (Sandoz Consumer) *2375*
Tussafed-HC (Everett) *993*
Tussar-2 Syrup (Rhone-Poulenc Rorer Pharmaceuticals) *2174*
Tussar SF Syrup (Rhone-Poulenc Rorer Pharmaceuticals) *2174*
V-Dec-M Tablets (Seatrace) *2613*
Versacaps Capsules (Seatrace) *2613*
Zephrex Tablets (Bock) *306, 672*
Zephrex LA Tablets (Bock) . . *306, 672*

◆**GUAIMAX-D TABLETS** (Central) **308, 809**

GUAI-VENT/PSE TABLETS (Dura) *974*

GUANABENZ ACETATE

Guanabenz Acetate Tablets (Warner Chilcott) *2787*
Guanabenz Acetate Tablets, USP (Watson) *2790*
Wytensin Tablets (Wyeth-Ayerst) *2932*

GUANADREL SULFATE

Hylorel Tablets (Medeva) **1613**

GUANETHIDINE MONOSULFATE

Esimil Tablets (CibaGeneva) . . **309, 840**
Ismelin Tablets (CibaGeneva) . **309, 845**

GUANFACINE HYDROCHLORIDE

Tenex Tablets (Robins) **331, 2249**
Guanfacine Hydrochloride Tablets (Watson) *2790*
Guanfacine Hydrochloride Tablets (Warner Chilcott) *2787*

GUA-SR TABLETS (Seatrace) *2612*

GUIATUSS (Alpharma) *481*

GUIATUSS AC SYRUP (Alpharma) *481*

GUIATUSS CF (Alpharma) *481*

GUIATUSS DAC (Alpharma) *481*

GUIATUSS DM (Alpharma) *481*

GUIATUSS PE (Alpharma) *481*

H

H-BIG (NABI) *1839*

HP ACTHAR GEL (Rhone-Poulenc Rorer Pharmaceuticals) *2174*

◆**HABITROL NICOTINE TRANSDERMAL SYSTEM** (Ciba Self-Medication) **308, 884**

HAEMOPHILUS B CONJUGATE VACCINE

ActHIB (Connaught) **893**
HibTITER (Lederle) **320, 1423**
OmniHIB (SmithKline Beecham Pharmaceuticals) **337, 2676**
PedvaxHIB (Merck & Co., Inc.) **1761**
ProHIBiT Haemophilus b Conjugate Vaccine (Diphtheria Toxoid Conjugate) (Connaught) *911*

HALCINONIDE

Halog Cream, Ointment & Solution 0.1% (Westwood-Squibb) **2795**
Halog-E Cream 0.1% (Westwood-Squibb) **2795**

◆**HALCION TABLETS** (Pharmacia & Upjohn) **329, 2093**

◆**HALDOL DECANOATE 50 (50 MG/ML) INJECTION** (McNeil Pharmaceutical) **323, 1587**

◆**HALDOL DECANOATE 100 (100 MG/ML) INJECTION** (McNeil Pharmaceutical) **323, 1587**

◆**HALDOL INJECTION, TABLETS AND CONCENTRATE** (McNeil Pharmaceutical) **323, 1585**

HALFPRIN TABLETS (Kramer) **1413**

HALOBETASOL PROPIONATE

Ultravate Cream 0.05% (Westwood-Squibb) **2797**
Ultravate Ointment 0.05% (Westwood-Squibb) **2798**

HALOG CREAM, OINTMENT & SOLUTION 0.1% (Westwood-Squibb) **2795**

HALOG-E CREAM 0.1% (Westwood-Squibb) **2795**

HALOPERIDOL

Haldol Injection, Tablets and Concentrate (McNeil Pharmaceutical) **323, 1585**
Haloperidol Oral Solution USP (Pharmaceutical Associates) *2056*
Haloperidol Oral Solution (Teva) *2748*
Haloperidol Oral Soln. USP 2 mg/mL (Alpharma) *481*
Haloperidol Tablets (Mylan) *1836*

MECHLORETHAMINE HYDROCHLORIDE
Mustargen (Merck & Co., Inc.) 1752

MECLIZINE HYDROCHLORIDE
Antivert, Antivert/25 Tablets, & Antivert/50 Tablets (Pfizer Inc) 327, 1992
Bonine Tablets (Pfizer Consumer) 1990
Meclizine HCl Tablets (Par) . . . 1949
Meni-D Capsules (Seatrace) 2612

MECLOFENAMATE SODIUM
Meclofenamate Sodium Capsules (Mylan) 1836

MEDICATED BLUE SHAMPOO (Alpharma) 481

MEDIGESIC CAPSULES (U.S. Pharmaceutical) 2765

MEDIHALER-ISO AEROSOL (3M Pharmaceuticals) 1553

MEDIPLEX (U.S. Pharmaceutical) 2765

MEDROXYPROGESTERONE ACETATE
Amen Tablets (Carnrick) . . . 308, 785
Cycrin Tablets (ESI Lederle) . 310, 991
Depo-Provera Contraceptive Injection (Pharmacia & Upjohn) . . 329, 2079
Depo-Provera (Pharmacia & Upjohn) 2083
Premphase (Wyeth-Ayerst) . . 341, 2900
Prempro (Wyeth-Ayerst) . . . 341, 2905
Provera Tablets (Pharmacia & Upjohn) 329, 2110
Medroxyprogesterone Tablets (Warner Chilcott) 2787

MEFENAMIC ACID
Ponstel (Parke-Davis) 327, 1982

MEFLOQUINE HYDROCHLORIDE
Lariam Tablets (Roche Pharmaceuticals) 332, 2295

MEFOXIN (Merck & Co., Inc.) 1734

MEFOXIN PREMIXED INTRAVENOUS SOLUTION (Merck & Co., Inc.) 1737

MEGA-B (Arco) 513

◆ MEGACE ORAL SUSPENSION (Bristol-Myers Squibb Oncology/Immunology) . . . 307, 708

◆ MEGACE TABLETS (Bristol-Myers Squibb Oncology/Immunology) 307, 710

MEGADOSE (Arco) 513

MEGESTROL ACETATE
Megace Oral Suspension (Bristol-Myers Squibb Oncology/Immunology) 307, 708
Megace Tablets (Bristol-Myers Squibb Oncology/Immunology) 307, 710
Megestrol Acetate Tablets (Teva) 2748
Megestrol Acetate Tablets (Par) 1949
Megestrol Acetate Tablets, USP (SuperGen) 2733
Megestrol Acetate Tablets, USP (Warner Chilcott) 2787

◆ MELANEX TOPICAL SOLUTION (Neutrogena) 325, 1842

MELATONIN
Melatonin Tablets (AC Laboratory) 461
Melatonin (Par) 1949
Melatonin Spray (AC Laboratory) 461
Melatonin SR (Par) 1949
Vitatonin (CPH International) 916

MELLARIL CONCENTRATE (Sandoz Pharmaceuticals) 2398

◆ MELLARIL TABLETS (Sandoz Pharmaceuticals) 333, 2398

MELLARIL-S SUSPENSION (Sandoz Pharmaceuticals) 2398

MELPHALAN
Alkeran Tablets (Glaxo Wellcome Oncology/HIV) . . . 316, 1198

MELPHALAN HYDROCHLORIDE
Alkeran for Injection (Glaxo Wellcome Oncology/HIV) . . . 316, 1196

◆ MENEST TABLETS (SmithKline Beecham Pharmaceuticals) 337, 2671

MENI-D CAPSULES (Seatrace) 2612

MENINGOCOCCAL POLYSACCHARIDE VACCINE
Menomune-A/C/Y/W-135 (Connaught) 906

MENOMUNE-A/C/Y/W-135 (Connaught) 906

MENOTROPINS
Humegon for Injection (Organon) 325, 1873
Pergonal (menotropins for injection, USP) (Serono) 2618

MENTHOL
PrameGel (GenDerm) 1042
Thera-Gesic (Mission) 1830
Cool Mint Listerine (Warner Wellcome) 2789
FreshBurst Listerine (Warner Wellcome) 2789
Listerine Antiseptic (Warner Wellcome) 2789
Nephro-Derm Cream (R&D) 2168
Panalgesic Gold Cream (ECR) 979
Panalgesic Gold Liniment (ECR) 979

MEPERGAN INJECTION (Wyeth-Ayerst) 2859

MEPERGAN IN TUBEX (Wyeth-Ayerst) 2926

MEPERIDINE HYDROCHLORIDE
Demerol Carpuject (Sanofi Winthrop) 2438
Demerol Injection (Sanofi Winthrop) 2438
Demerol Syrup (Sanofi Winthrop) 2438
Demerol Tablets (Sanofi Winthrop) 333, 2438
Demerol Uni-Amp (Sanofi Winthrop) 2438
Mepergan Injection (Wyeth-Ayerst) 2859
Mepergan in Tubex (Wyeth-Ayerst) 2926
Meperidine Hydrochloride Injection (Astra) 547
Meperidine Hydrochloride Injection (Elkins-Sinn) 980
Meperidine Hydrochloride in Tubex (Wyeth-Ayerst) 2926

MEPHENYTOIN
Mesantoin Tablets (Sandoz Pharmaceuticals) 2400

MEPHOBARBITAL
Mebaral Tablets (Sanofi Winthrop) 2452

◆ MEPHYTON TABLETS (Merck & Co., Inc.) 324, 1739

MEPIVACAINE HYDROCHLORIDE
Carbocaine Injection (Sanofi Winthrop) 2432
Polocaine Injection, USP (Astra) 552
Polocaine-MPF Injection, USP (Astra) 552

MEPROBAMATE
Miltown Tablets (Wallace) 2780
PMB 200 and PMB 400 (Wyeth-Ayerst) 340, 2890
Equagesic Tablets (Wyeth-Ayerst) 2829
Equanil Tablets (Wyeth-Ayerst) 2829

◆ MEPRON SUSPENSION (Glaxo Wellcome Oncology/HIV) . . 316, 1206

MERCAPTOPURINE
Purinethol Tablets (Glaxo Wellcome Oncology/HIV) . . . 316, 1214

MEROPENEM
Merrem I.V. (Zeneca) 2952

MERREM I.V. (Zeneca) 2952

MERUVAX II (Merck & Co., Inc.) . . 1740

MESALAMINE
Asacol Delayed-Release Tablets (Procter & Gamble Pharmaceuticals) 329, 2129
Pentasa (Hoechst Marion Roussel) 317, 1275

ROWASA Rectal Suppositories, 500 mg (Solvay) 338, 2727
ROWASA Rectal Suspension Enema 4.0 grams/unit (60 mL) (Solvay) 338, 2727

MESANTOIN TABLETS (Sandoz Pharmaceuticals) 2400

MESNA
Mesnex Injection (Bristol-Myers Squibb Oncology/Immunology) 307, 711

◆ MESNEX INJECTION (Bristol-Myers Squibb Oncology/Immunology) 307, 711

MESORIDAZINE BESYLATE
Serentil Ampuls (Boehringer Ingelheim) 689
Serentil Concentrate (Boehringer Ingelheim) 689
Serentil Tablets (Boehringer Ingelheim) 306, 689

MESTINON INJECTABLE (ICN) 1300

MESTINON SYRUP (ICN) 1300

◆ MESTINON TABLETS (ICN) . . 318, 1300

◆ MESTINON TIMESPAN TABLETS (ICN) 318, 1300

MESTRANOL
Norinyl 1+50 21-Day Tablets (Searle) 335, 2563
Norinyl 1+50 28-Day Tablets (Searle) 335, 2563
Ortho-Novum 1/50□21 Tablets (Ortho Pharmaceutical) 326, 1928
Ortho-Novum 1/50□28 Tablets (Ortho Pharmaceutical) 1928
Nelova (Warner Chilcott) 2787
Norethin 1/50M (Roberts) 2222
Norethindrone and Mestranol Tablets, USP (NECON) (Watson) 2791

METAMUCIL POWDER, ORANGE FLAVOR (Procter & Gamble) 2125

METAMUCIL ORIGINAL TEXTURE POWDER, REGULAR FLAVOR (Procter & Gamble) 2125

METAMUCIL SMOOTH TEXTURE POWDER, ORANGE FLAVOR (Procter & Gamble) 2125

METAMUCIL SMOOTH TEXTURE POWDER, SUGAR-FREE, ORANGE FLAVOR (Procter & Gamble) . . . 2125

METAMUCIL SMOOTH TEXTURE, SUGAR-FREE, REGULAR FLAVOR (Procter & Gamble) 2125

METAMUCIL WAFERS, APPLE CRISP AND CINNAMON SPICE FLAVORS (Procter & Gamble) . . 2125

METAPROTERENOL SULFATE
Alupent Inhalation Aerosol (Boehringer Ingelheim) . . 306, 672
Alupent Inhalation Solution (Boehringer Ingelheim) . . 306, 672
Alupent Syrup (Boehringer Ingelheim) 672
Alupent Tablets (Boehringer Ingelheim) 672
Metaproterenol Sulfate Inhalation Solution, USP, Arm-a-Med (Astra) 547
Metaproterenol Sulfate Inhalation Solution, USP (Dey) 310, 926
Metaproterenol Sulfate Inhalation Soln. USP 0.4% (Alpharma) 481
Metaproterenol Sulfate Inhalation Soln. USP 0.6% (Alpharma) 481
Metaproterenol Sulfate Tablets (Par) 1949
Metaproterenol Sulfate Tablets and Syrup (Teva) 2748

METARAMINOL BITARTRATE
Aramine Injection (Merck & Co., Inc.) 1649

METAXALONE
Skelaxin Tablets (Carnrick) . . . 308, 793

METFORMIN HYDROCHLORIDE
Glucophage Tablets (Bristol-Myers Squibb) 307, 754

METHADONE HYDROCHLORIDE
Methadone Hydrochloride Oral Concentrate (Roxane) . . 2356
Methadone Hydrochloride Oral Solution & Tablets (Roxane) 2357
Dolophine Hydrochloride Tablets and Injection (Roxane) 2352
Methadone Hydrochloride Diskets (Dispersible Tablets) (Roxane) 2355

METHAMPHETAMINE HYDROCHLORIDE
Desoxyn Gradumet Tablets (Abbott) 303, 422

METHAZOLAMIDE
Methazolamide Tablets (Lederle Standard) 1467

METHENAMINE
Urised Tablets (PolyMedica) . . . 2123
Prosed/DS (Star) 2731
Uro-Phosphate Tablets (ECR) 979

METHENAMINE HIPPURATE
Urex Tablets (3M Pharmaceuticals) 1557

METHENAMINE MANDELATE
Uroqid-Acid No. 2 Tablets (Beach) 305, 633
Methenamine Mandelate Oral Susp. USP 500 mg/5 mL (Alpharma) 481

METHERGINE INJECTION (Sandoz Pharmaceuticals) 2401

METHERGINE TABLETS (Sandoz Pharmaceuticals) 2401

METHIMAZOLE
Tapazole Tablets (Jones Medical Industries) 1361

METHIONINE
Amino-Cerv (Milex) 1827

METHOCARBAMOL
Robaxin Injectable (Robins) . 331, 2245
Robaxin Tablets (Robins) . . . 331, 2246
Robaxin-750 Tablets (Robins) 331, 2246
Robaxisal Tablets (Robins) . . 331, 2246
Methocarbamol Tablets (Lederle Standard) 1467
Methocarbamol and Aspirin Tablets (Par) 1949

METHOHEXITAL SODIUM
Brevital Sodium for Injection, USP (Jones Medical Industries) 1361

METHOCARBAMOL AND ASPIRIN TABLETS (Par) 1949

METHOTREXATE SODIUM
Methotrexate Sodium Tablets, Injection, for Injection and LPF Injection (Immunex) 1322
Methotrexate Tablets (Mylan) 1836
Methotrexate Tablets (Roxane) 2348
Methotrexate Tablets, USP (SuperGen) 2733
Rheumatrex Methotrexate Dose Pack (Lederle) 321, 1443

METHOTRIMEPRAZINE
Levoprome (Immunex) 1321

METHOXAMINE HYDROCHLORIDE
Vasoxyl Injection (Glaxo Wellcome) 315, 1169

METHOXSALEN
8-MOP Capsules (ICN) 318, 1294
Oxsoralen Lotion 1% (ICN) . . . 1301
Oxsoralen-Ultra Capsules (ICN) 318, 1302

METHSCOPOLAMINE NITRATE
D.A. II Tablets (Dura) 972
D.A. Chewable Tablets (Dura) 970
Dura-Vent/DA Tablets (Dura) 972

Extendryl Chewable Tablets
(Fleming) 1003
Extendryl Sr. & Jr. T.D.
Capsules (Fleming) 1003
Extendryl Syrup (Fleming) 1003
AH-CHEW Chewable
Tablets (WE) 2791
Dallergy Caplets, Syrup,
Tablets (Laser) 1414
OMNIHIST L.A. Tablets
(WE) 2791

METHSUXIMIDE

Celontin Kapseals
(Parke-Davis) 327, 1955

METHYCLOTHIAZIDE

Enduron Tablets (Abbott) 424
Aquatensen Tablets
(Wallace) 2768
Diutensen-R Tablets
(Wallace) 2773
Methyclothiazide Tablets
(Mylan) 1836

METHYL SALICYLATE

Thera-Gesic (Mission) 1830
Cool Mint Listerine (Warner
Wellcome) 2789
FreshBurst Listerine (Warner
Wellcome) 2789
Listerine Antiseptic (Warner
Wellcome) 2789
Panalgesic Gold Cream
(ECR) 979
Panalgesic Gold Liniment
(ECR) 979

METHYLDOPA

Aldoclor Tablets (Merck &
Co., Inc.) 324, 1638
Aldomet Oral Suspension
(Merck & Co., Inc.) 1640
Aldomet Tablets (Merck &
Co., Inc.) 324, 1640
Aldoril Tablets (Merck & Co.,
Inc.) 324, 1644
Methyldopa &
Hydrochlorothiazide
Tablets (Lederle Standard) 1467
Methyldopa and
Hydrochlorothiazide
Tablets (Par) 1949
Methyldopa Tablets (Lederle
Standard) 1467
Methyldopa Tablets (Mylan) 1836
Methyldopa Tablets, USP
125mg, 250mg, 500mg
(Endo) 988
Methyldopa Tablets USP,
250 mg, 500 mg
(Novopharm USA) 1852
Methyldopa and
Hydrochlorothiazide
Tablets (Mylan) 1836
Methyldopa/HCTZ Tablets,
USP 250/15mg,
250/25mg (Endo) 988

**METHYLDOPATE
HYDROCHLORIDE**

Aldomet Ester HCl Injection
(Merck & Co., Inc.) 1642

METHYLENE BLUE

Urised Tablets (PolyMedica) 2123
Prosed/DS (Star) 2731
Urolene Blue (Star) 2731

METHYLERGONOVINE MALEATE

Methergine Injection (Sandoz
Pharmaceuticals) 2401
Methergine Tablets (Sandoz
Pharmaceuticals) 2401

**METHYLPHENIDATE
HYDROCHLORIDE**

Ritalin Hydrochloride
Tablets (CibaGeneva) 309, 866
Ritalin-SR Tablets
(CibaGeneva) 309, 866
Methylphenidate Tablets, 5
mg, 10 mg, 20 mg, 20 mg
ER (Novopharm USA) 1852

METHYLPREDNISOLONE

Methylprednisolone Tablets
(Duramed) 979

METHYLTESTOSTERONE

Android Capsules, 10 mg
(ICN) 1297
ESTRATEST Tablets
(Solvay) 338, 2718
ESTRATEST H.S. Tablets
(Solvay) 338, 2718
Testred Capsules, 10 mg
(ICN) 318, 1308
Virilon (Star) 2731

METHYSERGIDE MALEATE

Sansert Tablets (Sandoz
Pharmaceuticals) 2424

METOCLOPRAMIDE

Metoclopramide Oral
Solution (Roxane) 2348
Metoclopramide Oral Soln.
USP 5 mg/5 mL (Alpharma) 481
Metoclopramide Tablets
(Duramed) 979
Metoclopramide Tablets
(Lederle Standard) 1467
Metoclopramide Tablets
and Oral Solution (Teva) 2748

**METOCLOPRAMIDE
HYDROCHLORIDE**

Reglan Injectable (Robins) . . 331, 2243
Reglan Syrup (Robins) 2243
Reglan Tablets (Robins) . . . 331, 2243
Metoclopramide Oral
Solution USP
(Pharmaceutical Associates) 2056
Metoclopramide
Hydrochloride Tablets
(Watson) 2790

METOCURINE IODIDE

Metubine Iodide (Dista) 932

METOLAZONE

Mykrox Tablets (Medeva) 1617
Zaroxolyn Tablets (Medeva) 1625

METOPROLOL SUCCINATE

Toprol-XL Tablets (Astra) . . .304, 560

METOPROLOL TARTRATE

Lopressor Injection
(CibaGeneva) 848
Lopressor Tablets
(CibaGeneva) 309, 848
Lopressor HCT Tablets
(CibaGeneva) 309, 850
Metoprolol Tartrate Tablets
(Mylan) 1836
Metoprolol Tartrate Tablets
(Par) 1949
Metoprolol Tartrate Tablets
(Teva) 2748
Metoprolol Tartrate Tablets,
USP (Watson) 2790
Metoprolol Tartrate Tablets,
50 mg, 100 mg (Novopharm
USA) 1852

METROCREAM (Galderma) 1034

**METRODIN
(UROFOLLITROPIN FOR
INJECTION)** (Serono) 2616

METROGEL (Galderma) 1034

METROGEL-VAGINAL
(Curatek) 917

METRONIDAZOLE

Flagyl 375 Capsules (Searle) .335, 2587
Flagyl I.V. RTU (SCS) 2373
Helidac Therapy (Procter &
Gamble Pharmaceuticals) 2135
MetroCream (Galderma) 1034
MetroGel (Galderma) 1034
MetroGel-Vaginal (Curatek) 917
Protostat Tablets (Ortho
Pharmaceutical) 327, 1939
Metronidazole Redi-Infusion
(Preservative-Free)
(Elkins-Sinn) 980
Metronidazole Tablets (Par) 1949
Metronidazole Tablets
(Teva) 2748

**METRONIDAZOLE
HYDROCHLORIDE**

Flagyl I.V. (SCS) 2373

METUBINE IODIDE (Dista) 932

METYROSINE

Demser Capsules (Merck &
Co., Inc.) 324, 1690

◆ **MEVACOR TABLETS** (Merck
& Co., Inc.) 324, 1742

MEXILETINE HYDROCHLORIDE

Mexitil Capsules (Boehringer
Ingelheim) 306, 684
Mexiletine Capsules, 150
mg, 200 mg, 250 mg
(Novopharm USA) 1852
Mexiletine Hydrochloride
Capsules (Roxane) 2348

◆ **MEXITIL CAPSULES**
(Boehringer Ingelheim) 306, 684

MEZLIN (Bayer Pharmaceutical) 594

**MEZLIN PHARMACY BULK
PACKAGE** (Bayer
Pharmaceutical) 597

MEZLOCILLIN SODIUM

Mezlin (Bayer Pharmaceutical) 594
Mezlin Pharmacy Bulk
Package (Bayer
Pharmaceutical) 597

MIACALCIN INJECTION
(Sandoz Pharmaceuticals) 2402

◆ **MIACALCIN NASAL SPRAY**
(Sandoz Pharmaceuticals) . . . 333, 2403

MICONAZOLE NITRATE

Monistat Dual-Pak (Ortho
Pharmaceutical) 326, 1906
Monistat 3 Vaginal
Suppositories (Ortho
Pharmaceutical) 326, 1905
Monistat-Derm (miconazole
nitrate 2%) Cream (Ortho
Dermatological) 326, 1944
Miconazole Nitrate Cream
2% (Alpharma) 481
Miconazole Nitrate Vaginal
Cream 2% (Alpharma) 481
Miconazole Nitrate 100mg
Vaginal Suppositories
(Alpharma) 481
Miconazole Nitrate 200 mg
Vaginal Suppositories
(Alpharma) 481

MICRHOGAM (Ortho Diagnostic) . . . 1902

◆ **MICRO-K EXTENCAPS**
(Robins) 331, 2237

◆ **MICRO-K 10 EXTENCAPS**
(Robins) 331, 2237

MICRO-K LS PACKETS
(Robins) 2238

MICRONASE TABLETS
(Pharmacia & Upjohn) 2099

◆ **MICRONOR TABLETS** (Ortho
Pharmaceutical) 326, 1903

◆ **MIDAMOR TABLETS** (Merck
& Co., Inc.) 325, 1746

MIDAZOLAM HYDROCHLORIDE

Versed Injection (Roche
Pharmaceuticals) 2324

MICANOL CREAM (Bioglan
Pharma) 665

◆ **MIDRIN CAPSULES** (Carnrick) . 308, 788

**MILITARY DEPOT
PHARMACEUTICAL
PRODUCTS** (3M
Pharmaceuticals) 1547

**MILK OF MAGNESIA
(see under MAGNESIUM
HYDROXIDE)**

MILK OF MAGNESIA USP
(Pharmaceutical Associates) 2056

**MILK OF MAGNESIA
CONCENTRATE**
(Pharmaceutical Associates) 2056

**MILK OF MAGNESIA,
MILK OF
MAGNESIA-CONCENTRATED**
(Roxane) 2348

**MILK OF MAGNESIA
CASCARA SUSPENSION**
(Pharmaceutical Associates) 2056

**MILK OF MAGNESIA
CASCARA CONCENTRATE
SUSPENSION** (Pharmaceutical
Associates) 2056

**MILK OF
MAGNESIA-CASCARA
SUSPENSION
CONCENTRATED** (Roxane) 2348

**MILK OF
MAGNESIA-MINERAL OIL
EMULSION & EMULSION
(FLAVORED)** (Roxane) 2348

MILRINONE LACTATE

Primacor Injection (Sanofi
Winthrop) 2461

MILTOWN TABLETS
(Wallace) 2780

MINERAL OIL

Aquaphor Healing Ointment
(Beiersdorf) 636
Aquaphor Healing
Ointment, Original
Formula (Beiersdorf) 636
Eucerin Original
Moisturizing Creme
(Unscented) (Beiersdorf) 636
Eucerin Original
Moisturizing Lotion
(Beiersdorf) 636
Eucerin Plus Dry Skin Care
Moisturizing Lotion
(Beiersdorf) 636
Eucerin Plus Moisturizing
Creme (Beiersdorf) 636
Fleet Mineral Oil Enema
(Fleet) 1001
Anusol Hemorrhoidal
Ointment (Warner
Wellcome) 2788
Milk of Magnesia-Mineral
Oil Emulsion & Emulsion
(Flavored) (Roxane) 2348
Mineral Oil USP
(Pharmaceutical Associates) 2056
Mineral Oil and Mineral Oil,
Topical Light (Roxane) 2348

MINERAL WAX

Aquaphor Healing
Ointment, Original
Formula (Beiersdorf) 636

◆ **MINIPRESS CAPSULES**
(Pfizer Inc) 328, 2015

**MINITRAN TRANSDERMAL
DELIVERY SYSTEM** (3M
Pharmaceuticals) 1553

◆ **MINIZIDE CAPSULES** (Pfizer
Inc) 328, 2016

◆ **MINOCIN INTRAVENOUS**
(Lederle) 320, 1428

◆ **MINOCIN ORAL
SUSPENSION** (Lederle) 320, 1431

◆ **MINOCIN PELLET-FILLED
CAPSULES** (Lederle) 320, 1429

MINOCYCLINE HYDROCHLORIDE

DYNACIN Capsules
(Medicis) 1627
Minocin Intravenous
(Lederle) 320, 1428
Minocin Oral Suspension
(Lederle) 320, 1431
Minocin Pellet-Filled
Capsules (Lederle) 320, 1429
Minocycline HCl Capsules
(Warner Chilcott) 2787
Minocycline HCl Capsules
(Teva) 2748

MINOXIDIL

Minoxidil Tablets (Par) 1949
Minoxidil Topical Solution
2% (Alpharma) 481
Minoxidil Topical Solution
(Teva) 2748

◆ **MINTEZOL CHEWABLE
TABLETS** (Merck & Co., Inc.) . . 324, 1747

MINTEZOL SUSPENSION
(Merck & Co., Inc.) 1747

MIO-REL INJECTABLE
(International Ethical) 1331

MIRTAZAPINE

Remeron Tablets (Organon) . 326, 1878

MISOPROSTOL

Cytotec (Searle) 335, 2576

**MISSION PRENATAL
TABLETS** (Mission) 1828

**MISSION PRENATAL F.A.
TABLETS** (Mission) 1828

**MISSION PRENATAL H.P.
TABLETS** (Mission) 1828

**MISSION PRENATAL RX
TABLETS** (Mission) 1828

MITHRACIN (Bayer
Pharmaceutical) 599

PRODUCT CATEGORY INDEX

For 1997, PDR is pleased to introduce a substantially improved version of the Product Category Index. Designed for speedier, easier use, the revised index features a streamlined system of headings based on the latest medical terminology.

The index cross-references each brand by prescribing category. As always, it covers all fully described products in both the Product Information and Diagnostic Product Information sections.

If an entry in the index lists multiple page numbers, the first ones shown refer to photographs of the product, the last one to its prescribing information. The Quick-Reference Guide below will introduce you to the new system of headings and subheadings.

PRODUCT CATEGORY QUICK-REFERENCE GUIDE

A

ACROMEGALY AGENTS
ALCOHOL ABUSE PREPARATIONS
  ALCOHOL DEPENDENCE
  ALCOHOL WITHDRAWAL
ALZHEIMER'S DISEASE MANAGEMENT
AMYOTROPHIC LATERAL SCLEROSIS THERAPEUTIC AGENTS
ANALGESICS
  ACETAMINOPHEN & COMBINATIONS
  CENTRALLY ACTING ANALGESICS
  MISCELLANEOUS ANALGESICS
  NARCOTICS
    NARCOTIC AGONIST-ANTAGONIST COMBINATIONS
    NARCOTICS & COMBINATIONS
  NON-NARCOTIC & ANXIOLYTIC COMBINATIONS
  NONSTEROIDAL ANTI-INFLAMMATORY AGENTS (NSAIDS)
  SALICYLATES
    ASPIRIN & COMBINATIONS
    OTHER SALICYLATES & COMBINATIONS
ANESTHETICS
  GENERAL ANESTHETICS
  LOCAL ANESTHETICS
ANTICONVULSANTS
  BARBITURATES
  BENZODIAZEPINES
  DICARBAMATES
  GABA ANALOGUES
  HYDANTOINS
  MISCELLANEOUS ANTICONVULSANTS
  PHENYLTRIAZINES
  SUCCINIMIDES
ANTIDIABETIC AGENTS
  BIGUANIDES
  GLUCOSIDASE INHIBITORS
  INSULINS
    INTERMEDIATE ACTING INSULINS
    LONG ACTING INSULINS
    RAPID ACTING INSULINS
  SULFONYLUREAS
ANTIDOTES
  ANTICHOLINERGIC ANTAGONISTS
  ANTICHOLINESTERASE ANTAGONISTS
  BENZODIAZEPINE ANTAGONISTS
  CHELATING AGENTS
    COPPER
    IRON
    LEAD
  DIGOXIN ANTAGONISTS
  FOLIC ACID ANTAGONISTS
  HEPARIN ANTAGONISTS
  NARCOTIC ANTAGONISTS
  NONDEPOLARIZING MUSCLE RELAXANT ANTAGONISTS
ANTIFIBROSIS THERAPY, SYSTEMIC
ANTIHISTAMINES & COMBINATIONS
ANTI-INFECTIVE AGENTS, SYSTEMIC
  AIDS ADJUNCT THERAPY
  AIDS CHEMOTHERAPEUTIC AGENTS
    NON-NUCLEOSIDE REVERSE TRANSCRIPTASE INHIBITORS
    NUCLEOSIDE REVERSE TRANSCRIPTASE INHIBITORS
    PROTEASE INHIBITORS
  AMEBICIDES
  ANTHELMINTICS
  ANTIBIOTICS
    AMINOGLYCOSIDES
    B-LACTAM ANTIBIOTICS, MISCELLANEOUS
    CEPHALOSPORINS
    MACROLIDES & COMBINATIONS
    MISCELLANEOUS ANTIBIOTICS
    PENICILLINS
    TETRACYCLINES

  ANTIFUNGALS
  ANTIMALARIAL AGENTS
  ANTITUBERCULOSIS AGENTS
  ANTIVIRALS
  LEPROSTATICS
  MISCELLANEOUS ANTI-INFECTIVES
  QUINOLONES
  SULFONAMIDES & COMBINATIONS
  URINARY ANTI-INFECTIVES & COMBINATIONS
ANTINEOPLASTICS
  ADJUNCT THERAPY
  ALKYLATING AGENTS
    MISCELLANEOUS ALKYLATING AGENTS
    NITROGEN MUSTARDS
    NITROSOUREAS
  ANTIBIOTICS
  ANTIMETABOLITES
  HORMONES
    ANDROGENS
    ANTIANDROGENS
    ANTIESTROGENS
    ESTROGEN & NITROGEN MUSTARD COMBINATIONS
    ESTROGENS
    GONADOTROPIN RELEASING HORMONE (GnRH) ANALOGUES
    PROGESTINS
  IMMUNOMODULATORS
  MISCELLANEOUS ANTINEOPLASTICS
ANTIPARKINSONIAN AGENTS
ANTIRHEUMATIC AGENTS
  GOLD COMPOUNDS
  MISCELLANEOUS ANTIRHEUMATIC AGENTS
APPETITE SUPPRESSANTS

B

BIOLOGICAL RESPONSE MODIFIERS
  ALPHA₁-PROTEINASE INHIBITOR
  ANTITOXINS & ANTIVENINS
  IMMUNE SERUMS
  MISCELLANEOUS BIOLOGICALS
  SKIN TEST ANTIGENS
  TOXOIDS
  VACCINES
BLOOD MODIFIERS
  ANTICOAGULANTS
  ANTIPLATELET AGENTS
  COLONY STIMULATING FACTORS
    GRANULOCYTE (G-CSF)
    GRANULOCYTE MACROPHAGE (GM-CSF)
  HEMATINICS
    CYANOCOBALAMIN (VITAMIN B_{12}) & COMBINATIONS
    ERYTHROPOIETIN
    FOLIC ACID DERIVATIVES & COMBINATIONS
    IRON & COMBINATIONS
    LIVER & COMBINATIONS
  HEMORRHEOLOGIC AGENTS
  HEMOSTATICS
    SYSTEMIC HEMOSTATICS
  HEPARIN ANTAGONISTS
  LEUKAPHERESIS ADJUNCT
  PLASMA EXTENDERS & EXPANDERS
  PLASMA FRACTIONS, HUMAN
    ALBUMIN
    ANTIHEMOPHILIC FACTOR
    ANTITHROMBIN III
    FACTOR IX COMPLEX
    PLASMA PROTEIN FRACTION
  THROMBOLYTIC AGENTS
  VITAMIN K

C

CARDIOPROTECTIVE AGENTS
  ADRENERGIC BLOCKERS, PERIPHERAL & COMBINATIONS
  ADRENERGIC STIMULANTS, CENTRAL & COMBINATIONS

  ALPHA/BETA ADRENERGIC BLOCKERS
  ANGIOTENSIN II RECEPTOR ANTAGONISTS
  ANGIOTENSIN II RECEPTOR ANTAGONISTS WITH DIURETICS
  ANGIOTENSIN-CONVERTING ENZYME (ACE) INHIBITORS
  ANGIOTENSIN CONVERTING ENZYME (ACE) INHIBITORS WITH CALCIUM CHANNEL BLOCKERS
  ANGIOTENSIN CONVERTING ENZYME (ACE) INHIBITORS WITH DIURETICS
  ANTIARRHYTHMICS
    GROUP I
    GROUP II
    GROUP III
    GROUP IV
    MISCELLANEOUS ANTIARRHYTHMICS
  ANTILIPEMIC AGENTS
    BILE ACID SEQUESTRANTS
    FIBRIC ACID DERIVATIVES
    HMG-CoA REDUCTASE INHIBITORS
  BETA ADRENERGIC BLOCKING AGENTS
  BETA ADRENERGIC BLOCKING AGENTS WITH DIURETICS
  CALCIUM CHANNEL BLOCKERS
  DIURETICS
    CARBONIC ANHYDRASE INHIBITORS
    COMBINATION DIURETICS
    LOOP DIURETICS
    POTASSIUM-SPARING DIURETICS
    THIAZIDES & RELATED DIURETICS
  HYPERTENSIVE EMERGENCY AGENTS
  INOTROPIC AGENTS
  MISCELLANEOUS CARDIOVASCULAR AGENTS
  RAUWOLFIA DERIVATIVES & COMBINATIONS
  VASODILATORS
    CORONARY VASODILATORS
    PERIPHERAL VASODILATORS & COMBINATIONS
  VASOPRESSORS
CENTRAL NERVOUS SYSTEM STIMULANTS
  AMPHETAMINES
  MISCELLANEOUS CENTRAL NERVOUS SYSTEM STIMULANTS
CEREBRAL METABOLIC ENHANCERS
CHOLINESTERASE INHIBITORS
CONTRACEPTIVES
  DEVICES
  IMPLANTS
  INJECTABLE CONTRACEPTIVES
  ORAL CONTRACEPTIVES
CYSTIC FIBROSIS MANAGEMENT

D

DEODORANTS
  INTERNAL DEODORANTS
DIAGNOSTICS
  ADRENOCORTICAL FUNCTION
  ALLERGY, SKIN TESTS
  CUSHING'S SYNDROME
  GASTRIC ACID TEST
  GONADOTROPIC FUNCTION TEST
  HYPOTHALAMIC DYSFUNCTION TEST
  HYSTEROSALPINGOGRAPHY
  HYSTEROSCOPIC FLUID
  LYMPHOGRAPHY
  MYOCARDIAL PERFUSION SCINTIGRAPHY ADJUNCT
  PANCREATIC FUNCTION TEST
  PHEOCHROMOCYTOMA TEST
  RENAL FUNCTION TEST
  THYROID FUNCTION TEST
    THYROTROPIN
  TUBERCULIN TEST
    TUBERCULIN, OLD
    TUBERCULIN, P.P.D.
  ZOLLINGER-ELLISON SYNDROME
DOPAMINE RECEPTOR AGONISTS

E

EMERGENCY KITS
ENDOMETRIOSIS MANAGEMENT
ENZYMES
ERECTILE DYSFUNCTION THERAPY

F

FERTILITY AGENTS

G

GALACTORRHEA INHIBITORS
GASTROINTESTINAL AGENTS
  ANTACID & ANTIFLATULENT COMBINATIONS
  ANTACIDS
    ALUMINUM ANTACIDS & COMBINATIONS
    CALCIUM ANTACIDS & COMBINATIONS
    COMBINATION ANTACIDS
    MAGNESIUM ANTACIDS & COMBINATIONS
  ANTIDIARRHEALS
  ANTIEMETICS
  ANTIFLATULENTS
  ANTI-INFLAMMATORY AGENTS
  ANTISPASMODICS & ANTICHOLINERGICS
  BOWEL EVACUANTS
  CYTOPROTECTIVE AGENTS
  DIGESTIVE ENZYMES
  DUODENAL ULCER ADHERENT COMPLEX
  GALLSTONE DISSOLUTION AGENTS
  GASTROINTESTINAL STIMULANTS
  HISTAMINE H_2 RECEPTOR ANTAGONISTS
  LAXATIVES
    BULK-PRODUCING LAXATIVES
    EMOLLIENT LAXATIVES
    ENEMAS
    FECAL SOFTENERS & COMBINATIONS
    HYPEROSMOLAR AGENTS
    LAXATIVE COMBINATIONS
    MISCELLANEOUS LAXATIVES
    SALINE LAXATIVES
    STIMULANT LAXATIVES & COMBINATIONS
  MISCELLANEOUS GASTROINTESTINAL AGENTS
  PROSTAGLANDINS
  PROTON PUMP INHIBITORS
GAUCHER'S DISEASE MANAGEMENT
GOUT PREPARATIONS
  MISCELLANEOUS GOUT PREPARATIONS
  NONSTEROIDAL ANTI-INFLAMMATORY AGENTS (NSAIDS)
  URICOSURIC AGENTS & COMBINATIONS

H

HOMEOPATHIC PREPARATIONS
HORMONES
  ADRENAL CORTICAL STEROID INHIBITORS
  ANABOLIC STEROIDS
  ANDROGEN & ESTROGEN COMBINATIONS
  ANDROGENS
  BIPHOSPHONATES
  CALCITONIN
  ESTROGENS & COMBINATIONS
  GLUCOCORTICOIDS
  GLUCOSE ELEVATING AGENTS
  GONADOTROPIN INHIBITORS
  GONADOTROPIN RELEASING HORMONES (GnRH)
    GONADOTROPIN RELEASING HORMONE (GnRH) ANALOGUES
    MISCELLANEOUS GONADOTROPIN RELEASING HORMONES (GnRH)
  GONADOTROPINS
    CHORIONIC GONADOTROPIN
    MENOTROPINS
    UROFOLLITROPIN
  GROWTH HORMONE
  MINERALOCORTICOIDS
  MISCELLANEOUS HORMONES

PROGESTIN & ESTROGEN COMBINATIONS
PROGESTINS & COMBINATIONS
SOMATOSTATIN ANALOGUES
THYROID PREPARATIONS
    ANTITHYROID AGENTS
IODINE PRODUCTS
SYNTHETIC T3
SYNTHETIC T4
VASOPRESSIN & DERIVATIVES

HYPERCALCEMIA MANAGEMENT

HYPOCALCEMIA MANAGEMENT

I

IMMUNODILATORS

IMMUNOSUPPRESSIVES

M

MAST CELL STABILIZERS

MIGRAINE PREPARATIONS
BETA ADRENERGIC BLOCKING AGENTS
ERGOT DERIVATIVES & COMBINATIONS
ISOMETHEPTENE & COMBINATIONS
MISCELLANEOUS MIGRAINE PREPARATIONS
SEROTONIN (5-HT) RECEPTOR AGONISTS

MOTION SICKNESS PRODUCTS

MULTIPLE SCLEROSIS MANAGEMENT

MUSCLE RELAXANTS
NEUROMUSCULAR BLOCKING AGENTS
SKELETAL MUSCLE RELAXANTS & COMBINATIONS
SMOOTH MUSCLE RELAXANTS

N

NARCOTIC DETOXIFICATION

NASAL PREPARATIONS
ANALGESICS
ANTIBIOTICS & COMBINATIONS
ANTICHOLINERGICS
ANTI-INFLAMMATORY AGENTS
    MISCELLANEOUS ANTI-INFLAMMATORY AGENTS
    STEROIDAL ANTI-INFLAMMATORY AGENTS
HORMONES
SMOKING CESSATION AIDS

NUCLEOSIDE ANALOGUES

NUTRITIONALS
AMINO ACIDS & COMBINATIONS
MINERALS & ELECTROLYTES
    CALCIUM & COMBINATIONS
    FLUORIDE & COMBINATIONS
    MAGNESIUM & COMBINATIONS
    ORAL ELECTROLYTE MIXTURES
    PHOSPHOROUS & COMBINATIONS
    POTASSIUM & COMBINATIONS
    SYSTEMIC ALKALINIZERS
MISCELLANEOUS NUTRITIONAL SUPPLEMENTS
NUTRITIONAL THERAPY, ENTERAL
    CARBOHYDRATES
    COMPLETE THERAPEUTIC
    FIBER SUPPLEMENTS
    HIGH CALORIE
    HIGH FAT
    HIGH NITROGEN
    LACTOSE FREE
    LOW NITROGEN

LOW PROTEIN
LOW RESIDUE
MEDIUM CHAIN TRIGLYCERIDES
METABOLIC DYSFUNCTION
VITAMINS & COMBINATIONS
    GERIATRIC FORMULATIONS
    MISCELLANEOUS VITAMIN PREPARATIONS
    MULTIVITAMINS & COMBINATIONS
    MULTIVITAMINS WITH MINERALS
    PEDIATRIC FORMULATIONS WITH FLUORIDE
    PRENATAL FORMULATIONS
    RENAL FORMULATIONS
    THERAPEUTIC FORMULATIONS
    VITAMIN A & COMBINATIONS
    B VITAMINS & COMBINATIONS
    VITAMIN D ANALOGUES & COMBINATIONS
    VITAMIN E & COMBINATIONS

O

OPHTHALMIC PREPARATIONS
ACETYLCHOLINE BLOCKING AGENTS
ANTIHISTAMINES & COMBINATIONS
ANTI-INFECTIVES
    ANTIBIOTICS & COMBINATIONS
    ANTIVIRALS
    QUINOLONES
    SULFONAMIDES & COMBINATIONS
ANTI-INFLAMMATORY AGENTS
    MISCELLANEOUS ANTI-INFLAMMATORY AGENTS
    NON-STEROIDAL ANTI-INFLAMMATORY AGENTS
        (NSAIDS)
    STEROIDAL ANTI-INFLAMMATORY AGENTS &
        COMBINATIONS
ARTIFICIAL TEARS/LUBRICANTS & COMBINATIONS
BETA ADRENERGIC BLOCKING AGENTS
CARBONIC ANHYDRASE INHIBITORS
IRRIGATING SOLUTIONS
MIOTICS
    CHOLINESTERASE INHIBITORS
MYDRIATICS & CYCLOPLEGICS
SYMPATHOMIMETICS & COMBINATIONS

OSTEOPOROSIS PREPARATIONS

OTIC PREPARATIONS
ANALGESICS & ANESTHETICS
ANTIBIOTIC & STEROID COMBINATIONS
CERUMENOLYTICS
MISCELLANEOUS OTIC PREPARATIONS
STEROIDS & COMBINATIONS

OXYTOCICS
ERGOT DERIVATIVES
OXYTOCIN

P

PARASYMPATHOLYTICS

PARASYMPATHOMIMETICS

PATENT DUCTUS ARTERIOSUS AGENTS

PHOSPHATE BINDERS

PORPHYRIA AGENTS

PROSTAGLANDINS

PSYCHOTHERAPEUTIC AGENTS
ANTIANXIETY AGENTS
    BENZODIAZEPINES & COMBINATIONS
    MISCELLANEOUS ANTIANXIETY AGENTS
ANTIDEPRESSANTS
    MISCELLANEOUS ANTIDEPRESSANTS

MONOAMINE OXIDASE INHIBITORS (MAOI)
SELECTIVE SEROTONIN REUPTAKE INHIBITORS
    (SSRI)
TETRACYCLIC ANTIDEPRESSANTS
TRICYCLIC ANTIDEPRESSANTS & COMBINATIONS
ANTIMANIC AGENTS
ANTIPANIC AGENTS
ANTIPSYCHOTIC AGENTS
    MISCELLANEOUS ANTIPSYCHOTIC AGENTS
    PHENOTHIAZINES
OBSESSIVE-COMPULSIVE DISORDER MANAGEMENT
    SELECTIVE SEROTONIN REUPTAKE INHIBITORS
        (SSRI)
    TRICYCLIC ANTIDEPRESSANTS

R

RADIOPAQUE AGENTS

RESINS, ION EXCHANGE

RESPIRATORY DRUGS
ANTI-INFLAMMATORY AGENTS
    MISCELLANEOUS ANTI-INFLAMMATORY AGENTS
    STEROIDAL ANTI-INFLAMMATORY AGENTS
ANTITUSSIVES
    NARCOTIC ANTITUSSIVES & COMBINATIONS
    NON-NARCOTIC ANTITUSSIVES & COMBINATIONS
BRONCHODILATORS
    ANTICHOLINERGICS
    SYMPATHOMIMETICS & COMBINATIONS
    XANTHINE DERIVATIVES & COMBINATIONS
DECONGESTANTS & COMBINATIONS
DECONGESTANTS, EXPECTORANTS & COMBINATIONS
ENZYMES
EXPECTORANTS & COMBINATIONS
LUNG SURFACTANTS
MISCELLANEOUS COLD & COUGH PRODUCTS WITH
    ANALGESICS
MISCELLANEOUS RESPIRATORY DRUGS
RESPIRATORY STIMULANTS

S

SALT SUBSTITUTES

SCLEROSING AGENTS

SEDATIVES & HYPNOTICS
BARBITURATES
BENZODIAZEPINES
MISCELLANEOUS SEDATIVES & HYPNOTICS

SKIN & MUCOUS MEMBRANE AGENTS
ACNE PREPARATIONS
ALLERGANS FOR EPICUTANEOUS TESTING
ANALGESICS & COMBINATIONS
ANESTHETICS & COMBINATIONS
ANORECTAL PREPARATIONS
ANTIHISTAMINES & COMBINATIONS
ANTI-INFECTIVES
    ANTIBIOTICS & COMBINATIONS
    ANTIFUNGALS & COMBINATIONS
    ANTIVIRALS
    MISCELLANEOUS ANTI-INFECTIVES &
        COMBINATIONS
    SCABICIDES & PEDICULICIDES
ANTINEOPLASTICS
ANTIPERSPIRANTS
ANTIPRURITICS
ANTIPSORIATIC AGENTS
ANTISEBORRHEIC AGENTS

BURN PREPARATIONS
CAUTERIZING AGENTS
CLEANSING AGENTS
DEODORANTS
DEPIGMENTING AGENTS
DIAPER RASH PRODUCTS
EMOLLIENTS & MOISTURIZERS
ENZYMES & COMBINATIONS
KERATOLYTICS
MISCELLANEOUS SKIN & MUCOUS MEMBRANE
    AGENTS
MOUTH & THROAT PRODUCTS
    ANTIFUNGALS
    COLD SORE PREPARATIONS
    DENTAL PREPARATIONS
    LIP BALMS
    MISCELLANEOUS MOUTH & THROAT PRODUCTS
    SALIVA STIMULANTS
PHOTOSENSITIZERS
POISON IVY, OAK OR SUMAC PRODUCTS
SHAMPOOS
SHAVE CREAMS
SKIN PROTECTANTS
STEROIDS & COMBINATIONS
SUNBURN PREPARATIONS
SUNSCREENS
TAR-CONTAINING PREPARATIONS
WART PREPARATIONS
WET DRESSINGS
WOUND CARE PRODUCTS

SMOKING CESSATION AIDS

SYMPATHOLYTICS

T

TOURETTE'S SYNDROME AGENTS

TREMOR PREPARATIONS

U

URINARY TRACT AGENTS
ACIDIFIERS
ALKALINIZERS
ANALGESICS & COMBINATIONS
ANTISPASMODICS
BENIGN PROSTATIC HYPERPLASIA (BPH) THERAPY
CALCIUM OXALATE STONE PREVENTION
CYTOPROTECTIVE AGENTS
ENURESIS MANAGEMENT
MISCELLANEOUS URINARY TRACT AGENTS

UTERINE RELAXANTS

V

VAGINAL PREPARATIONS
ANTI-INFECTIVES
    ANTIFUNGALS & COMBINATIONS
    MISCELLANEOUS ANTI-INFECTIVES &
        COMBINATIONS
CLEANSERS AND DOUCHES
ESTROGENS
MISCELLANEOUS VAGINAL PREPARATIONS
PROSTAGLANDINS

VASODILATORS
CEREBRAL VASODILATORS

VERTIGO AGENTS

PRODUCT CATEGORY INDEX

DRUG INFORMATION CENTERS

ALABAMA

BIRMINGHAM
Drug Information Service
University of Alabama Hospital
619 S. 19th Street
1720 Jefferson Tower
Birmingham, AL 35233
Mon.-Fri. 8 AM-5 PM
Tel: 205-934-2162
Fax: 205-934-3501

Global Drug Information Center
Samford University
McWhorter School of Pharmacy
800 Lakeshore Drive
Birmingham, AL 35229-7027
Mon.-Fri. 8 AM-5 PM
Tel: 205-870-2891
Fax: 205-414-4012

HUNTSVILLE
Huntsville Hospital Drug
Information Center
101 Sivley Road
Huntsville, AL 35801
Mon.-Fri. 8 AM-5 PM
Tel: 205-517-8288
Fax: 205-517-6558

ARIZONA

TUCSON
Arizona Poison and Drug
Information Center
Arizona Health Sciences Center
University Medical Center
1501 N. Campbell Ave.
Rm 1156
Tucson, AZ 85724
7 days/week, 24 hours
Tel: 520-626-6016
    800-362-0101 (AZ)
Fax: 520-626-2720

ARKANSAS

LITTLE ROCK
Arkansas Poison and Drug
Information Center
College of Pharmacy-UAMS
4301 W. Markham Street
Little Rock, AR 72205
7 days/week, 24 hours
Tel: 800-376-4766 (AR)
Fax: 501-686-7357

CALIFORNIA

LOS ANGELES
Los Angeles Regional Drug and
Poison Information Center
LAC & USC Medical Center
1200 N. State Street
Room 1107 A & B
Los Angeles, CA 90033
7 days/week, 24 hours
Tel: 213-226-2622
    800-777-6476 (CA)
Fax: 213-226-4194
Poison Control Hotline:
    213-222-3212

SAN DIEGO
Drug Information
Analysis Service
Veterans Administration
Medical Center
3350 La Jolla Village Drive
San Diego, CA 92161
Mon-Fri. 8 AM-4:30 PM
Tel: 619-552-8585
Fax: 619-552-7582

Drug Information Center
U.S. Naval Hospital
34800 Bob Wilson Drive
San Diego, CA 92134-5000
Mon.-Fri. 8 AM-4 PM
Tel: 619-532-8414

Drug Information Service
University of California
San Diego Medical Center
200 West Arbor Drive
San Diego, CA 92103-8925
Mon.-Fri. 9 AM-5 PM
Tel: 900-288-8273
Fax: 619-692-1867

STANFORD
Drug Information Center
Stanford University Hospital
Dept. of Pharmacy H0301
300 Pasteur Drive
Stanford, CA 94305
Mon.-Fri. 9 AM-5 PM
Tel: 415-723-6422
Fax: 415-725-5028

COLORADO

DENVER
Rocky Mountain Drug
Consultation Center
8802 E. 9th Avenue
Denver, CO 80220
Mon.-Fri. 8 AM-4:30 PM
Tel: 303-893-3784
    900-370-3784
    (Outside Denver
    County, $1.99
    per minute)

Drug Information Center
University of Colorado Health
Science Center
4200 E. 9th Avenue, Box C239
Denver, CO 80262
Mon.-Fri. 8:30 AM-4:30 PM
Tel: 303-270-8489
Fax: 303-270-3353

CONNECTICUT

FARMINGTON
Drug Information Service
University of Connecticut
Health Center
263 Farmington Ave.
Farmington, CT 06030
Mon.-Fri. 8 AM-4:30 PM
Tel: 203-679-3783

HARTFORD
Drug Information Center
Hartford Hospital
P.O. Box 5037
80 Seymour Street
Hartford, CT 06102
Mon-Fri. 8:30 AM-5 PM
Tel: 860-545-2221
    860-545-2961
    (main pharmacy)
    after hours
Fax: 860-545-2415

NEW HAVEN
Drug Information Center
Yale-New Haven Hospital
20 York Street
New Haven, CT 06504
Mon.-Fri. 8:15 AM-4:45 PM
Tel: 203-785-2248
Fax: 203-737-4229

DISTRICT OF COLUMBIA

Drug Information Center
Washington Hospital Center
110 Irving St., NW
Washington, DC 20010
Mon.- Fri. 7:30 AM-4 PM
Tel: 202-877-6646
Fax: 202-877-8925

Drug Information Service
Howard University Hospital
2041 Georgia Ave. NW
Washington, DC 20060
Mon.-Fri. 9 AM-5 PM
Tel: 202-865-1325
Fax: 202-745-3731

FLORIDA

GAINESVILLE
Drug Information &
Pharmacy Resource Center
Shands Hospital at
University of Florida
P.O. Box 100316
Gainesville, FL 32610-0316
Mon.-Fri. 9 AM- 5 PM
Tel: 352-395-0408
(for healthcare professionals only)
Fax: 352-338-9860

JACKSONVILLE
Drug Information Service
University Medical Center
655 W. 8th Street
Jacksonville, FL 32209
Mon.-Fri. 8 AM-5 PM
Tel: 904-549-4095
Fax: 904-549-4272

MIAMI
Drug Information Center (119)
Miami VA Medical Center
1201 NW 16th Street
Miami, FL 33125
Mon-Fri. 7:30 AM-4:30 PM
Tel: 305-324-3237
Fax: 305-324-3394

NORTH MIAMI BEACH
Drug Information Service
NOVA Southeastern University
College of Pharmacy
1750 NE 167th Street
N. Miami Beach, FL 33162
Mon.-Fri. 9 AM-5 PM
Tel: 305-948-8255

GEORGIA

ATLANTA
Emory University Hospital
Dept. of Pharmaceutical Services
1364 Clifton Rd. NE
Atlanta, GA 30322
Mon.-Fri. 8:30 AM-5 PM
Tel: 404-712-4640
Fax: 404-712-7577

Drug Information Service
Northside Hospital
1000 Johnson Ferry Road
Atlanta, GA 30342
Mon.-Fri. 9 AM-4 PM
Tel: 404-851-8676
Fax: 404-851-8682

Drug Information Center
Grady Memorial Hospital and Mercer University
80 Butler St., SE
P.O. Box 26041
Atlanta, GA 30335-3801
Mon.-Fri. 8 AM-4 PM
Tel: 404-616-7725
Fax: 404-616-7727

AUGUSTA
Drug Information Center
University of Georgia
Medical College of GA
Room BIW201
1120 15th Street
Augusta, GA 30912-5600
Mon.-Fri. 8:30 AM-5 PM
Tel: 706-721-2887
Fax: 706-721-3827

IDAHO

POCATELLO
Idaho Drug Information Service
Box 8092
Pocatello, ID 83209
Mon.-Fri. 8 AM-5 PM
Tel: 208-236-4689
Fax: 208-236-4687

ILLINOIS

BLOOMINGTON
Drug Information Center
BroMenn Life Care Center
807 N. Main Street
Bloomington, IL 61701
7 days/week, 24 hours
Tel: 309-829-0755
Fax: 309-829-0760

CHICAGO
Drug Information Center
Northwestern Memorial Hospital
250 E. Superior Street
Wesley 153
Chicago, IL 60611
Tel: 312-908-7573
Fax: 312-908-7956

Saint Joseph Hospital
2900 N. Lake Shore Drive
Chicago, IL 60657
Tel: 312-665-3140
Fax: 312-665-3462

Drug Information Services
University of Chicago
5841 S. Maryland Ave.
MC 0010
Chicago, IL 60637
Mon.-Fri. 8 AM-5 PM
Tel: 312-702-1388
Fax: 312-702-6631

Drug Information Center
University of Illinois at Chicago
Room C300, MC 883
1740 W. Taylor St.
Chicago, IL 60612
Mon.-Fri. 8 AM-4 PM
Tel: 312-996-0209
Fax: 312-413-4146

HARVEY
Drug Information Center
Ingalls Memorial Hospital
1 Ingalls Drive
Harvey, IL 60426
Mon.-Fri. 8 AM-4:30 PM
Tel: 708-333-2300
Fax: 708-210-3108

HINES
Drug Information Service
Hines Veterans Administration Hospital
Inpatient Pharmacy (119B)
Hines, IL 60141
Mon.-Fri. 8 AM-4:30 PM
Tel: 708-343-7200

PARK RIDGE
Drug Information Center
Lutheran General Hospital
1775 Dempster St.
Park Ridge, IL 60068
Mon-Fri. 7:30 AM-4 PM
Tel: 847-696-8128

INDIANA

INDIANAPOLIS
Drug Information Center
St. Vincent Hospital
and Health Services
2001 W. 86th St.
P.O. Box 40970
Indianapolis, IN 46260
Mon-Fri. 8 AM-4 PM
Tel: 317-338-3200
Fax: 317-338-6547

Indiana University Medical Center/Pharmacy
Dept. UH1410
550 N. University Blvd.
Indianapolis, IN 46202
Mon.-Fri. 8 AM-4:30 PM
Tel: 317-274-3581
Fax: 317-274-2327

IOWA

DES MOINES
Regional Drug Information Center
Mercy Hospital Medical Center
400 University Ave.
Des Moines, IA 50314
Mon.-Fri. 8 AM-4:30 PM
Tel: 515-247-3286
(answered 7 days/week, 24 hours)
Fax: 515-247-3966

Mid-Iowa Poison and Drug Information Center
Iowa Methodist Medical Center
1200 Pleasant St.
Des Moines, IA 50309
7 days/week, 24 hours
Tel: 515-241-6254
     800-362-2327 (IA)
Fax: 515-241-5085

IOWA CITY
Drug Information Center
University of Iowa Hospitals and Clinics
200 Hawkins Dr.
Iowa City, IA 52242
Mon.-Fri. 8 AM-5 PM
Tel: 319-356-2600
Fax: 319-356-4545

KANSAS

KANSAS CITY
Drug Information Center
University of Kansas
Medical Center
3901 Rainbow Blvd.
Kansas City, KS 66160
Mon.-Fri. 8 AM-5 PM
Tel: 913-588-2328
Fax: 913-588-2350

KENTUCKY

LEXINGTON
Drug Information Center
Chandler Medical Center,
College of Pharmacy,
University of Kentucky
800 Rose St., C-117
Lexington, KY 40536-0084
Mon.-Fri. 8 AM-5 PM
Tel: 606-323-5320
Fax: 606-323-2049

LOUISIANA

MONROE
Drug Information Center
St. Francis Medical Center
309 Jackson St.
Monroe, LA 71201
Tel: 318-327-4250
Fax: 318-327-4125

NEW ORLEANS
Xavier University Drug Information Center
Tulane University Hospital and Clinic
Box HC12
1415 Tulane Ave.
New Orleans, LA 70112
Mon.- Fri. 9 AM-5 PM
Tel: 504-588-5670
Fax: 504-588-5862

MARYLAND

ANDREWS AFB
Drug Information Services
89th Med Gp/SGSAP
1050 W. Perimeter Rd.
Suite B1-39
Andrews AFB, MD 20331
Mon.-Fri. 7:30 AM-6 PM
Tel: 301-981-4209
Fax: 301-981-4544

ANNAPOLIS
Drug Information Services
The Anne Arundel Medical Center
Franklin & Cathedral Streets
Annapolis, MD 21401
7 days/week, 24 hours
Tel: 410-267-1130
     410-267-1000
Fax: 410-267-1628

BALTIMORE
Drug Information Services
Franklin Square Hospital Center
9000 Franklin Square Dr.
Baltimore, MD 21237
7 days/week, 24 hours
Tel: 410-682-7744
Fax: 410-682-8181

Drug Information Service
John Hopkins Medical Center
600 N. Wolfe St., Halsted 503
Baltimore, MD 21287-6180
Mon.-Fri. 8:30 AM-5 PM
Tel: 410-955-6348
Fax: 410-955-8283

Drug Information Center
University of Maryland
at Baltimore
School of Pharmacy
506 W. Fayette, 3rd Floor
Baltimore, MD 21201
Mon.-Fri. 8:30 AM-5 PM
Tel: 410-706-7568
Fax: 410-706-0897

BETHESDA
Drug Information Center
Pharmacy Dept.
Warren G. Magnuson Clinic Ctr.
National Institutes of Health
9000 Rockville Pike
Bldg 10, Room IN-257
Bethesda, MD 20892-1196
Mon.-Fri. 8:30 AM-5 PM
Tel: 301-496-2407
Fax: 301-496-0210

EASTON
Drug Information Center
Memorial Hospital
219 S. Washington St.
Easton, MD 21601
7 days/week, 7 AM - Midnight
Tel: 410-822-1000
Fax: 410-820-9489

MASSACHUSETTS
BOSTON
Drug Information Services
Brigham and Women's Hospital
75 Frances St.
Boston, MA 02115
Mon.-Fri. 7 AM-3:30 PM
Tel: 617-732-7166
Fax: 617-732-7497

Drug Information Service
New England Medical
Center Pharmacy
750 Washington St., Box 420
Boston, MA 02111
Mon.-Fri. 8 AM-4:30 PM
Tel: 617-636-8985
Fax: 617-636-5638

WORCESTER
Drug Information Center
U.M.M.C. Hospital
55 Lake Ave. North
Worcester, MA 01655
Mon.-Fri. 8:30 AM-5 PM
Tel: 508-856-3456
      508-856-2775
Fax: 508-856-1850

MICHIGAN
ANN ARBOR
Drug Information Service
University of Michigan
Medical Center
1500 East Medical Center Dr.
UHB2 D301 Box 0008
Ann Arbor, MI 48109
Mon.-Fri. 8 AM-5 PM
Tel: 313-936-8200
      313-936-8251
      313-936-7027
      (after hours)
Fax: 313-923-7027

DETROIT
Drug Information Services
Harper Hospital
3990 John R. St.
Detroit, MI 48201
Mon.-Fri. 8 AM-5 PM
Tel: 313-745-2006
      313-745-8216
      (after hours)
Fax: 313-745-1795

LANSING
Drug Information Center
Sparrow Hospital
1215 E. Michigan Ave.
Lansing, MI 48912
Mon.-Fri. 8 AM-4:30 PM
Tel: 517-483-2444
Fax: 517-483-2088

PONTIAC
Drug Information Center
St. Joseph Mercy Hospital
900 Woodward
Pontiac, MI 48341
Mon.-Fri. 8 AM-4:30 PM
Tel: 810-858-3055
Fax: 810-858-3010

ROYAL OAK
Drug Information Services
William Beaumont Hospital
3601 West 13 Mile Road
Royal Oak, MI 48073-6769
Mon.-Fri. 8 AM-4:30 PM
Tel: 810-551-4077
Fax: 810-551-4046

SOUTHFIELD
Drug Information Service
Providence Hospital
16001 West 9 Mile Rd.
P.O. Box 2043
Southfield, MI 48075
Mon.-Fri. 8 AM-4 PM
Tel: 810-424-3125
Fax: 810-424-5364

MINNESOTA
ROCHESTER
Drug Information Service
Mayo Clinic
1216 2nd St., SW
Rochester, MN 55902
Mon.-Fri. 8 AM-5 PM
Tel: 507-255-5062
      507-255-5732
      (after hours)
Fax: 507-255-7556

MISSISSIPPI
JACKSON
Drug Information Center
University of Mississippi
Medical Center
2500 N. State St.
Jackson, MS 39216
Mon.-Fri. 8 AM-5 PM
Tel: 601-984-2060
      (on call 24 hours)
Fax: 601-984-2063

MISSOURI
SPRINGFIELD
Drug Information & Clinical
Research Services
1235 E. Cherokee
Springfield, MO 65804
Mon.-Fri. 7:30 AM-4:30 PM
Tel: 417-885-3488
Fax: 417-888-7788

ST. JOSEPH
Drug Information Service
Heartland Hospital West
801 Faraon St.
St. Joseph, MO 64501
Mon.-Sat. 8 AM-8 PM
Tel: 816-271-7582
Fax: 816-271-7590

NEBRASKA
OMAHA
Drug Information Service
School of Pharmacy
Creighton University
2500 California Plaza
Omaha, NE 68178
Mon.-Fri. 8:30 AM-4:30 PM
Tel: 402-280-5101
Fax: 402-280-5149

Drug Information and
Education Services
University of Nebraska
Medical Center
600 S. 42nd Street
Omaha, NE 68178
Mon.-Fri. 8 AM-4:30 PM
Fax: 402-559-4907

NEW MEXICO
ALBUQUERQUE
New Mexico Poison & Drug
Information Center
University of New Mexico
Albuquerque, NM 87131
7 days/week, 24 hours
Tel: 505-843-2551
      800-432-6866 (NM)
Fax: 505-277-5892

NEW YORK
BRONX
Drug Information Center
Jacobi Medical Center
Dept. of Pharmacy
Room BN32
Pelham Pkwy South
and Eastchester Rd.
Bronx, NY 10461
Mon.-Fri. 9 AM-5 PM
Tel: 718-918-4556
Fax: 718-918-7848

BROOKLYN
International Drug
Information Center
Long Island University
Arnold & Marie Schwartz
College of Pharmacy
1 University Plaza
Brooklyn, NY 11201
Mon.-Fri. 9 AM-5 PM
Tel: 718-488-1064
Fax: 718-780-4056

COOPERSTOWN
Drug Information Center
The Mary Imogene Bassett
Hospital
1 Atwell Rd.
Cooperstown, NY 13326
Mon.-Fri 8:30 AM-5 PM
Tel: 607-547-3686
Fax: 607-547-3629

NEW HYDE PARK
Drug Information Center
St. John's University at Long
Island Jewish Medical Center
270-05 76th Ave
New Hyde Park, NY 11042
Mon.-Fri. 9 AM-3 PM
Tel: 718-470-DRUG
Fax: 718-470-1742

NEW YORK CITY
Drug Information Center
Memorial Sloan-Kettering
Cancer Center
1275 York Ave.
New York, NY 10021
Mon.-Fri. 9 AM-5 PM
Tel: 212-639-7552
Fax: 212-639-2171

Drug Information Center
Mount Sinai Medical Center
1 Gustave Levy Place
New York, NY 10029
Mon.-Fri. 9 AM-5 PM
Tel: 212-241-6619
Fax: 212-348-7927

Drug Information Center
Bellevue Hospital Center
462 1st Ave.
New York, NY 10016
Mon.-Fri. 9 AM-5 PM
Tel: 212-562-6504
Fax: 212-562-6503

Drug Information Service
The New York Hospital
525 E. 68th St.
New York, NY 10021
Mon.-Fri. 9 AM-5 PM
Tel: 212-746-0741
Fax: 212-746-8506

ROCHESTER
Drug Information Service
Dept. of Pharmacy
University of Rochester
601 Elmwood Ave.
Rochester, NY 14642
Mon.-Fri. 8 AM-5 PM
Tel: 716-275-3718
      716-275-2681
      (after hours)
Fax: 716-473-9842

STONY BROOK
Suffolk Drug Information Center
University Hospital
S.U.N.Y. - Stony Brook
Room 3-559, Z7310
Stony Brook, NY 11794
Mon.-Fri. 8 AM-4:30 PM
Tel: 516-444-2672
      516-444-2680
      (after hours)
Fax: 516-444-7935

NORTH CAROLINA

BUIES CREEK
Drug Information Center
School of Pharmacy Campbell
University
P.O. Box 1090
Buies Creek, NC 27506
Mon.-Fri. 8:30 AM - 4:30 PM
Tel: 910-893-1200
    800-327-5467 (NC)
Fax: 910-893-1476

CHAPEL HILL
Drug Information Center
University of North Carolina
Hospitals
101 Manning Drive
Chapel Hill, NC 27514
Mon.-Fri. 8 AM-5 PM
Tel: 919-966-2373
Fax: 919-966-1791

GREENSBORO
Triad Poison Center
Moses H. Cone Memorial
Hospital
1200 N. Elm St.
Greensboro, NC 27401
7 days/week, 24 hours
Tel: 910-574-8105
Fax: 910-574-7910

GREENVILLE
Eastern Carolina Drug
Information Center
Pitt County Memorial Hospital
Dept. of Pharmacy Service
2100 Stantonsburg Rd.
Greenville, NC 27835
Mon.-Fri. 8 AM- 5 PM
Tel: 919-816-4257
Fax: 919-816-7425

WINSTON-SALEM
Drug Information Service Center
NC Baptist Hospital
Bowman-Gray Medical Center
Medical Center Blvd.
Winston-Salem, NC 27157
Mon.-Fri 8 AM-5 PM
Tel: 910-716-2037
Fax: 910-716-2186

OHIO

ADA
Drug Information Center
Raabe College of Pharmacy
Ohio Northern University
Ada, OH 45810
Mon.-Fri. 9 AM - 5 PM
Tel: 419-772-2307
Fax: 419-772-2289

CLEVELAND
Drug Information Center
Cleveland Clinic Foundation
9500 Euclid Avenue
Cleveland, OH 44195
Mon.-Fri. 8 AM - 4:30 PM
Tel: 216-444-6456
Fax: 216-445-6221

COLUMBUS
Central Ohio Poison Center
700 Children's Drive
Columbus, OH 43205
Tel: 513-222-2227
    800-682-7625 (OH)
Fax: 614-221-2672

Drug Information Center
Ohio State University Hospital
Dept. of Pharmacy
Doan Hall 368
410 W. 10th Avenue
Columbus, OH 43210-1228
Mon.-Fri. 8 AM - 4 PM
Tel: 614-293-8679
Fax: 614-293-3264

Drug Information Center
Riverside Methodist Hospital
3535 Olantangy River Road
Columbus, OH 43214
Tel: 614-566-5425
Fax: 614-566-5447

TOLEDO
Drug Information Center The
Toledo Hospital
2142 N. Cove Blvd.
Toledo, OH 43606
Mon.-Fri. 8 AM-4:30 PM
Tel: 419-471-2171
    419-471-5637
    (after hours)
Fax: 419-479-6926

OKLAHOMA

OKLAHOMA CITY
Drug Information Center
Baptist Medical Center
3300 Northwest Expressway
Oklahoma City, OK 73112
Mon.-Fri. 8 AM-4:30 PM
Tel: 405-949-3660
Fax: 405-945-5858

Drug Information Center
Presbyterian Hospital
700 NE 13th St.
Oklahoma City, OK 73104
Mon.-Fri. 7 AM-3:30 PM
Tel: 405-271-6226
Fax: 405-271-6281

Drug Information Service
University of Oklahoma
Health Sciences Center
Room LIB-380A
1000 S. L. Young Blvd.
Oklahoma City, OK 73117
Mon.-Fri. 8 AM-5 PM

TULSA
Drug Information Service
St. Francis Hospital
6161 S. Yale Ave.
Tulsa, OK 74136
Mon.-Fri. 9 AM-5:30 PM
Tel: 918-494-6339
Fax: 918-494-1893

PENNSYLVANIA

ERIE
Pharmacy and Drug
Information Services
Hamot Medical Center
201 State St.
Erie, PA 16550
7 days/week, 24 hours
Tel: 814-877-6022
Fax: 814-877-6108

PHILADELPHIA
Drug Information Center
Temple University Hospital
Dept. of Pharmacy
Broad and Ontario St.
Philadelphia, PA 19140
Mon.-Fri. 8 AM-4:30 PM
Tel: 215-707-4644
Fax: 215-707-3463

Drug Information Center
Thomas Jefferson University
Hospital
111 S. 11th and Walnut St.
Philadelphia, PA 19107
Mon.-Fri. 8 AM-5 PM
Tel: 215-955-8877

PITTSBURGH
The Center for Drug Information
The Mercy Hospital
of Pittsburgh
1400 Locust St.
Pittsburgh, PA 15219-5166
Mon.-Fri. 8 AM-4:30 PM
Tel: 412-232-7903
    412-232-7907
Fax: 412-232-8422

Drug Information and
Pharmacoepidemiology Center
University of Pittsburgh
Medical Center
137 Victoria Hall
Pittsburgh, PA 15261
Mon-Fri. 8 AM-6 PM
Tel: 412-624-3784
Fax: 412-624-6350

UPLAND
Drug Information Center
Crozer-Chester Medical Center
1 Medical Center Blvd.
Upland, PA 19013
Mon.-Fri. 8 AM-4:30 PM
Tel: 610-447-2851
    610-447-2862
    (after hours)
Fax: 215-447-2820

WILLIAMSPORT
Drug Information Center
Susquehanna Health System
Rural Avenue Campus
Williamsport, PA 17701
Mon.-Fri. 8 AM-4 PM
Tel: 717-321-3289
Fax: 717-321-3230

PUERTO RICO

SAN JUAN
Centro Information
Medicamentos
Escuela de Farmacia RCM
P.O. Box 365067
San Juan, PR 00936-5067
Mon.-Fri. 8 AM-4:30 PM
Tel: 787-763-0196
Fax: 787-763-0196

RHODE ISLAND

PROVIDENCE
Drug Information Service
Dept. of Pharmacy Rhode
Island Hospital
593 Eddy Street
Providence, RI 02903
7 days/week, 24 hours
Tel: 401-444-5547
Fax: 401-444-8062

Drug Information Service
University of Rhode Island
Roger Williams Medical Center
825 Chalkstone Ave.
Providence, RI 02908
Mon.-Fri. 8 AM-4 PM
Tel: 401-456-2260
Fax: 401-456-2377

SOUTH CAROLINA

CHARLESTON
Drug Information Service
Medical University of
South Carolina
171 Ashley Ave.
Room 515-SFX
Charleston, SC 29425-0810
Mon.-Fri. 8 AM-5:30 PM
Tel: 803-792-3896
    800-922-5250
Fax: 803-792-5532

SPARTANBURG
Drug Information Center
Spartanburg Regional
Medical Center
101 E. Wood St.
Spartanburg, SC 29303
Mon.-Fri. 8 AM-5 PM
Tel: 864-560-6910
Fax: 864-560-6017

SOUTH DAKOTA

BROOKINGS
South Dakota Drug
Information Center
300 22nd Ave.
Brookings, SD 57006
7 days/week, 8 AM-4:30 PM
Tel: 800-456-1004 (SD)

SIOUX FALLS
Drug Information Center
McKennan Hospital
800 E. 21st St.
Sioux Falls, SD 57117-5045
7 days/week, 24 hours
Tel: 605-336-3894
    800-952-0123 (SD)
    800-843-0505
    (MN, IA, NE)
Fax: 605-322-8378

TENNESSEE
KNOXVILLE
Drug Information Center
University of Tennessee
Medical Center
1924 Alcoa Highway
Knoxville, TN 37920-6999
Mon.-Fri. 8 AM-4:30 PM
Tel: 423-544-9125

MEMPHIS
South East Regional Drug
Information Center
VA Medical Center
1030 Jefferson Ave
Memphis, TN 38104
Mon.-Fri. 7:30 AM-4 PM
Tel: 901-523-8990

Drug Information Center
University of Tennessee
847 Monroe Avenue
Suite 238, Memphis, TN 38163
Mon.-Fri. 8:30 AM - 4:30 PM
Tel: 901-448-5555
Fax: 901-448-5419

TEXAS
GALVESTON
Drug Information Center
University of Texas
Medical Branch
301 University Blvd. - G01
Galveston, TX 77555-0701
Mon.-Fri. 8 AM-5 PM
Tel: 409-772-2734
Fax: 409-747-9919

HOUSTON
Drug Information Center
Ben Taub General Hospital
Texas Southern
University/HCHD
1504 Taub Loop
Houston, TX 77030
Mon.-Fri. 8 AM-5 PM
Tel: 713-793-2920
Fax: 713-793-2937

Drug Information Center
Methodist Hospital
6565 Fannin (DB1-09)
Houston, TX 77030
Mon.-Fri. 8 AM-5 PM
Tel: 713-790-4190
Fax: 713-793-1224

LACKLAND A.F.B.
Drug Information Center
Dept. of Pharmacy Wilford Hall
Medical Center
2200 Berquist Dr., Suite 1
Lackland A.F.B., TX 78236
Mon.-Fri. 7:30 AM-5 PM
Tel: 210-670-6291
    210-670-5408

LUBBOCK
Methodist Hospital
Drug Information and
Consultation Service
3615 19th St.
Lubbock, TX 79410
Mon.-Fri. 8 AM-5 PM
Tel: 806-793-4012
    (Attn: Pharmacy)
Fax: 806-784-5323

TEMPLE
Drug Information Center
Scott and White Memorial
Hospital
2401 S. 31st St.
Temple, TX 76508
Mon.-Fri. 8 AM-6 PM
Tel: 817-724-4636
Fax: 817-724-1731

UTAH
SALT LAKE CITY
Drug Information Center
Dept. of Pharmacy Services,
Room A-050
University of Utah Hospital
50 N. Medical Dr.
Salt Lake City, UT 84132
Mon.-Fri. 8:30 AM-4:30 PM
Tel: 801-581-2073
Fax: 801-585-6688

VIRGINIA
RICHMOND
Drug Information Center
St. Mary's Hospital
5801 Bremo Rd.
Richmond, VA 23226
7 days/week, 24 hours
Tel: 804-281-8058
Fax: 804-281-4411

WEST VIRGINIA
MORGANTOWN
West Virginia Drug
Information Center
WV University-Robert C. Byrd
Health Sciences Center
1124 HSN, P.O. Box 9520
Morgantown, WV 26506
Tel: 304-293-6640
    800-352-2501 (WV)
Fax: 304-293-5483

WISCONSIN
MADISON
University of Wisconsin
Hospital & Clinics
600 Highland Ave.
Madison, WI 53792
Voice mail/24 hrs a day,
responses in 3 days
Tel: 608-262-1315
Fax: 608-263-9424

WYOMING
LARAMIE
Drug Information Center
University of Wyoming
P.O. Box 3375
Laramie, WY 82071
Mon.-Fri. 8 AM-5 PM
Tel: 307-766-2953
Fax: 307-766-6128

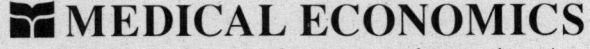

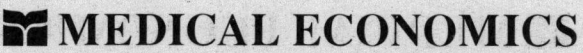

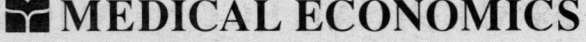

PRODUCT IDENTIFICATION GUIDE

To aid in quick identification, this section provides full-color, actual-size photographs of tablets and capsules. A variety of other dosage forms and packages are shown at less than actual size. In all, the guide contains more than 2,300 photos.

Products in this section are arranged alphabetically by manufacturer. In some instances, not all dosage forms and sizes are pictured. If others are available, a † symbol precedes the product's name. Letters or numbers representing the manufacturer's identification code are followed by an asterisk.

For more information on any of the products in this section, please turn to the Product Information Section, or check directly with the manufacturer. The page number of each product's text entry appears with its photographs.

While every effort has been made to guarantee faithful reproduction of the photos in this section, changes in size, color, and design are always a possibility. Be sure to confirm a product's identity with the manufacturer or your pharmacist.

INDEX BY MANUFACTURER

This section is made possible through the courtesy of the manufacturers whose products appear on the following pages.

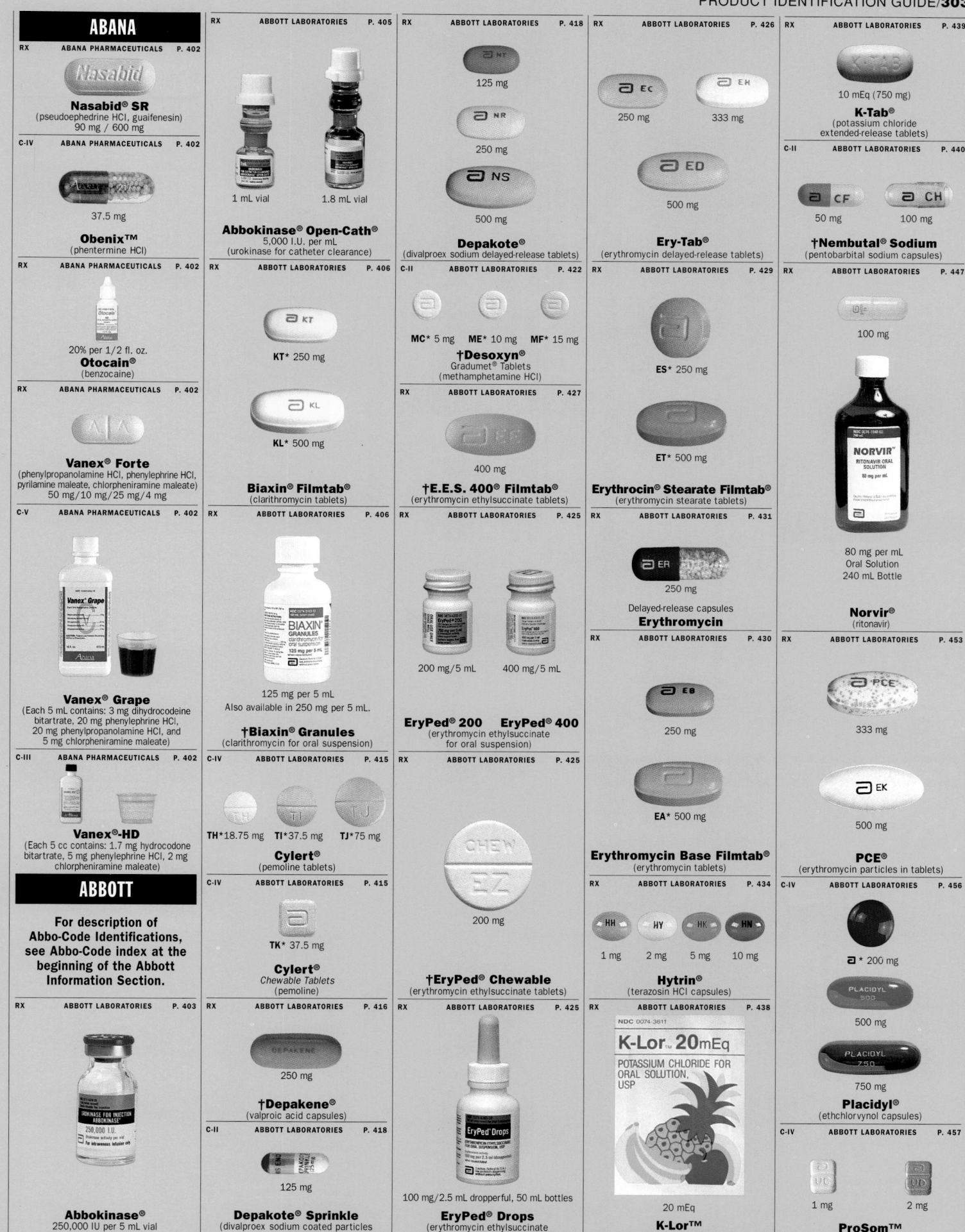

ABANA

RX   ABANA PHARMACEUTICALS   P. 402

Nasabid® SR
(pseudoephedrine HCl, guaifenesin)
90 mg / 600 mg

C-IV   ABANA PHARMACEUTICALS   P. 402

37.5 mg
Obenix™
(phentermine HCl)

RX   ABANA PHARMACEUTICALS   P. 402

20% per 1/2 fl. oz.
Otocain®
(benzocaine)

RX   ABANA PHARMACEUTICALS   P. 402

Vanex® Forte
(phenylpropanolamine HCl, phenylephrine HCl,
pyrilamine maleate, chlorpheniramine maleate)
50 mg/10 mg/25 mg/4 mg

C-V   ABANA PHARMACEUTICALS   P. 402

Vanex® Grape
(Each 5 mL contains: 3 mg dihydrocodeine
bitartrate, 20 mg phenylephrine HCl,
20 mg phenylpropanolamine HCl, and
5 mg chlorpheniramine maleate)

C-III   ABANA PHARMACEUTICALS   P. 402

Vanex®-HD
(Each 5 cc contains: 1.7 mg hydrocodone
bitartrate, 5 mg phenylephrine HCl, 2 mg
chlorpheniramine maleate)

ABBOTT

**For description of
Abbo-Code Identifications,
see Abbo-Code index at the
beginning of the Abbott
Information Section.**

RX   ABBOTT LABORATORIES   P. 403

Abbokinase®
250,000 IU per 5 mL vial
(urokinase for injection)

RX   ABBOTT LABORATORIES   P. 405

1 mL vial   1.8 mL vial

Abbokinase® Open-Cath®
5,000 I.U. per mL
(urokinase for catheter clearance)

RX   ABBOTT LABORATORIES   P. 406

KT* 250 mg

KL* 500 mg

Biaxin® Filmtab®
(clarithromycin tablets)

RX   ABBOTT LABORATORIES   P. 406

BIAXIN GRANULES
125 mg per 5 mL
Also available in 250 mg per 5 mL.

†Biaxin® Granules
(clarithromycin for oral suspension)

C-IV   ABBOTT LABORATORIES   P. 415

TH*18.75 mg   **TI***37.5 mg   **TJ***75 mg

Cylert®
(pemoline tablets)

C-IV   ABBOTT LABORATORIES   P. 415

TK* 37.5 mg

Cylert®
Chewable Tablets
(pemoline)

RX   ABBOTT LABORATORIES   P. 416

250 mg
†Depakene®
(valproic acid capsules)

C-II   ABBOTT LABORATORIES   P. 418

125 mg

Depakote® Sprinkle
(divalproex sodium coated particles
in capsules)

RX   ABBOTT LABORATORIES   P. 418

125 mg

250 mg

500 mg

Depakote®
(divalproex sodium delayed-release tablets)

C-II   ABBOTT LABORATORIES   P. 422

MC* 5 mg   **ME*** 10 mg   **MF*** 15 mg

†Desoxyn®
Gradumet® Tablets
(methamphetamine HCl)

RX   ABBOTT LABORATORIES   P. 427

400 mg
†E.E.S. 400® Filmtab®
(erythromycin ethylsuccinate tablets)

RX   ABBOTT LABORATORIES   P. 425

200 mg/5 mL   400 mg/5 mL

EryPed® 200   EryPed® 400
(erythromycin ethylsuccinate
for oral suspension)

RX   ABBOTT LABORATORIES   P. 425

CHEW EZ

200 mg

†EryPed® Chewable
(erythromycin ethylsuccinate tablets)

RX   ABBOTT LABORATORIES   P. 425

EryPed® Drops

100 mg/2.5 mL dropperful, 50 mL bottles
EryPed® Drops
(erythromycin ethylsuccinate
for oral suspension)

RX   ABBOTT LABORATORIES   P. 426

250 mg   333 mg

500 mg

Ery-Tab®
(erythromycin delayed-release tablets)

RX   ABBOTT LABORATORIES   P. 429

ES* 250 mg

ET* 500 mg

Erythrocin® Stearate Filmtab®
(erythromycin stearate tablets)

RX   ABBOTT LABORATORIES   P. 431

250 mg
Delayed-release capsules
Erythromycin

RX   ABBOTT LABORATORIES   P. 430

250 mg

EA* 500 mg

Erythromycin Base Filmtab®
(erythromycin tablets)

RX   ABBOTT LABORATORIES   P. 434

HH 1 mg   **HY** 2 mg   **HK** 5 mg   **HN** 10 mg

Hytrin®
(terazosin HCl capsules)

RX   ABBOTT LABORATORIES   P. 438

K-Lor™ 20 mEq
NDC 0074-3611
POTASSIUM CHLORIDE FOR
ORAL SOLUTION, USP

20 mEq
K-Lor™
(potassium chloride for oral solution)

RX   ABBOTT LABORATORIES   P. 439

10 mEq (750 mg)
K-Tab®
(potassium chloride
extended-release tablets)

C-II   ABBOTT LABORATORIES   P. 440

CF 50 mg   **CH** 100 mg

†Nembutal® Sodium
(pentobarbital sodium capsules)

RX   ABBOTT LABORATORIES   P. 447

100 mg

NORVIR RITONAVIR ORAL SOLUTION
80 mg per mL
Oral Solution
240 mL Bottle

Norvir®
(ritonavir)

RX   ABBOTT LABORATORIES   P. 453

PCE 333 mg

EK 500 mg

PCE®
(erythromycin particles in tablets)

C-IV   ABBOTT LABORATORIES   P. 456

* 200 mg

PLACIDYL 500
500 mg

PLACIDYL 750
750 mg

Placidyl®
(ethchlorvynol capsules)

C-IV   ABBOTT LABORATORIES   P. 457

UC 1 mg   **UD** 2 mg

ProSom™
(estazolam tablets)

---

*Abbott Abbo-Code identification letters. Filmtab® – Film sealed tablets, Abbott. **Grooved tablets.

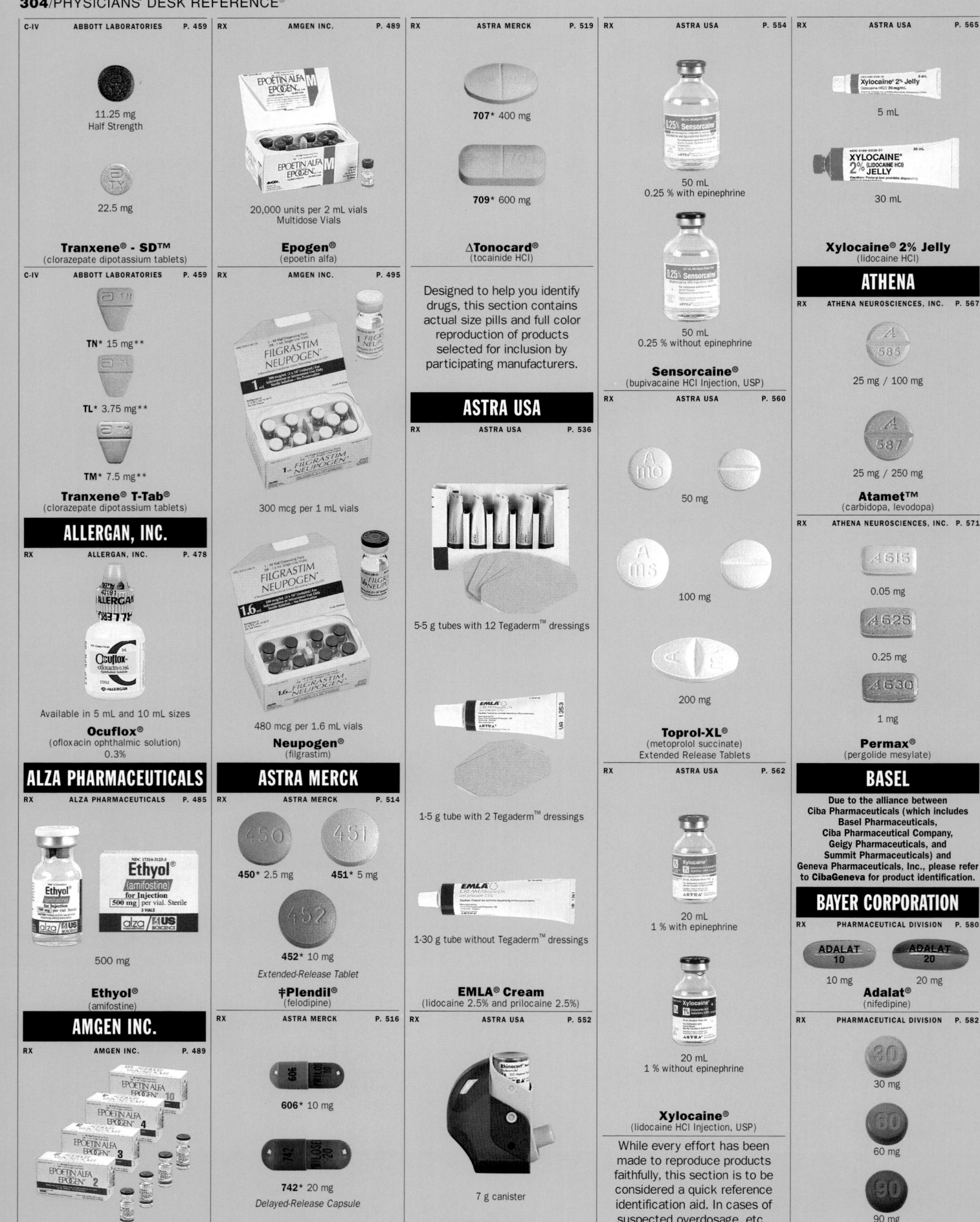

| C-IV | ABBOTT LABORATORIES | P. 459 |

11.25 mg
Half Strength

22.5 mg

Tranxene® - SD™
(clorazepate dipotassium tablets)

| C-IV | ABBOTT LABORATORIES | P. 459 |

TN* 15 mg**

TL* 3.75 mg**

TM* 7.5 mg**

Tranxene® T-Tab®
(clorazepate dipotassium tablets)

ALLERGAN, INC.

| RX | ALLERGAN, INC. | P. 478 |

Available in 5 mL and 10 mL sizes

Ocuflox®
(ofloxacin ophthalmic solution)
0.3%

ALZA PHARMACEUTICALS

| RX | ALZA PHARMACEUTICALS | P. 485 |

500 mg

Ethyol®
(amifostine)

AMGEN INC.

| RX | AMGEN INC. | P. 489 |

Epogen®
(epoetin alfa)

| RX | AMGEN INC. | P. 489 |

20,000 units per 2 mL vials
Multidose Vials

Epogen®
(epoetin alfa)

| RX | AMGEN INC. | P. 495 |

300 mcg per 1 mL vials

480 mcg per 1.6 mL vials

Neupogen®
(filgrastim)

ASTRA MERCK

| RX | ASTRA MERCK | P. 514 |

450* 2.5 mg   451* 5 mg

452* 10 mg
Extended-Release Tablet

‡Plendil®
(felodipine)

| RX | ASTRA MERCK | P. 516 |

606* 10 mg

742* 20 mg
Delayed-Release Capsule

‡Prilosec®
(omeprazole)

| RX | ASTRA MERCK | P. 519 |

707* 400 mg

709* 600 mg

ΔTonocard®
(tocainide HCl)

Designed to help you identify drugs, this section contains actual size pills and full color reproduction of products selected for inclusion by participating manufacturers.

ASTRA USA

| RX | ASTRA USA | P. 536 |

5-5 g tubes with 12 Tegaderm™ dressings

1-5 g tube with 2 Tegaderm™ dressings

1-30 g tube without Tegaderm™ dressings

EMLA® Cream
(lidocaine 2.5% and prilocaine 2.5%)

| RX | ASTRA USA | P. 552 |

7 g canister

**Rhinocort®
Nasal Inhaler**
(budesonide)

| RX | ASTRA USA | P. 554 |

50 mL
0.25 % with epinephrine

50 mL
0.25 % without epinephrine

Sensorcaine®
(bupivacaine HCl Injection, USP)

| RX | ASTRA USA | P. 560 |

50 mg

100 mg

200 mg

Toprol-XL®
(metoprolol succinate)
Extended Release Tablets

| RX | ASTRA USA | P. 562 |

20 mL
1 % with epinephrine

20 mL
1 % without epinephrine

Xylocaine®
(lidocaine HCl Injection, USP)

While every effort has been made to reproduce products faithfully, this section is to be considered a quick reference identification aid. In cases of suspected overdosage, etc., chemical analysis of the product should be done.

| RX | ASTRA USA | P. 565 |

5 mL

30 mL

Xylocaine® 2% Jelly
(lidocaine HCl)

ATHENA

| RX | ATHENA NEUROSCIENCES, INC. | P. 567 |

25 mg / 100 mg

25 mg / 250 mg

Atamet™
(carbidopa, levodopa)

| RX | ATHENA NEUROSCIENCES, INC. | P. 571 |

0.05 mg

0.25 mg

1 mg

Permax®
(pergolide mesylate)

BASEL

Due to the alliance between Ciba Pharmaceuticals (which includes Basel Pharmaceuticals, Ciba Pharmaceutical Company, Geigy Pharmaceuticals, and Summit Pharmaceuticals) and Geneva Pharmaceuticals, Inc., please refer to CibaGeneva for product identification.

BAYER CORPORATION

| RX | PHARMACEUTICAL DIVISION | P. 580 |

10 mg   20 mg

Adalat®
(nifedipine)

| RX | PHARMACEUTICAL DIVISION | P. 582 |

30 mg

60 mg

90 mg

Adalat® CC
(nifedipine)

*Abbott Abbo-Code identification letters.   Filmtab® - Film sealed tablets, Abbott.   **Grooved tablet.   ‡Registered trademark of Astra AB and ΔRegistered trademark of Astra Pharmaceutical Products, Inc.

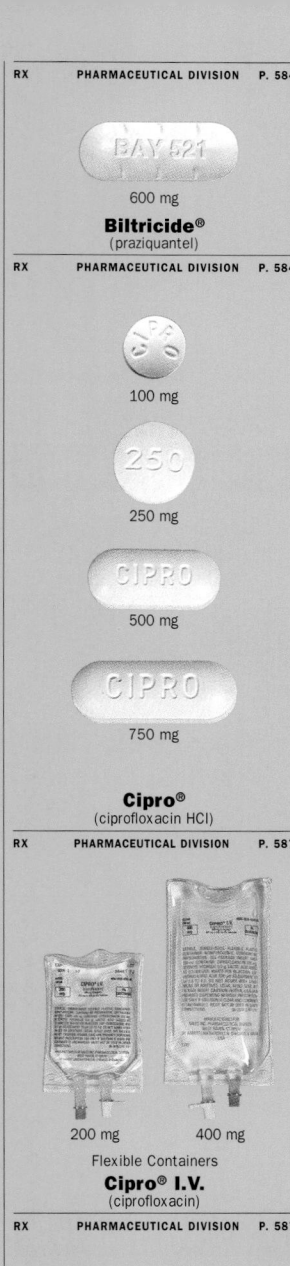

RX · PHARMACEUTICAL DIVISION · P. 584

600 mg
Biltricide®
(praziquantel)

RX · PHARMACEUTICAL DIVISION · P. 584

100 mg

250 mg

500 mg

750 mg

Cipro®
(ciprofloxacin HCl)

RX · PHARMACEUTICAL DIVISION · P. 587

200 mg   400 mg
Flexible Containers
Cipro® I.V.
(ciprofloxacin)

RX · PHARMACEUTICAL DIVISION · P. 587

20 mL   40 mL

Cipro® I.V.
(ciprofloxacin)

RX · PHARMACEUTICAL DIVISION · P. 590

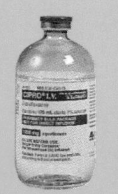

1200 mg
Pharmacy Bulk Package

Cipro® I.V.
(ciprofloxacin)

RX · PHARMACEUTICAL DIVISION · P. 601

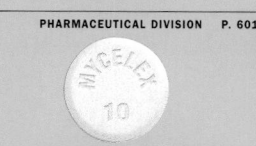

10 mg
Mycelex® Troche
(clotrimazole)

RX · PHARMACEUTICAL DIVISION · P. 602

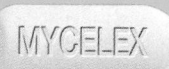

500 mg Vaginal Tablet
Mycelex®-G
(clotrimazole)

RX · PHARMACEUTICAL DIVISION · P. 603

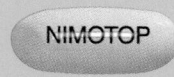

30 mg
Nimotop® Capsules
(nimodipine)

RX · PHARMACEUTICAL DIVISION · P. 604

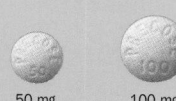

50 mg   100 mg

Precose®
(acarbose)

BAYER CORPORATION

RX · PHARMACEUTICAL DIVISION · P. 611
ALLERGY PRODUCTS

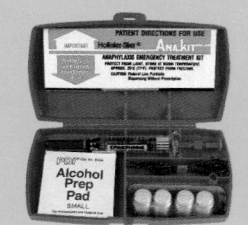

Anakit®

BAYER CORPORATION

RX · PHARMACEUTICAL DIVISION, · P. 612
BIOLOGICAL PRODUCTS

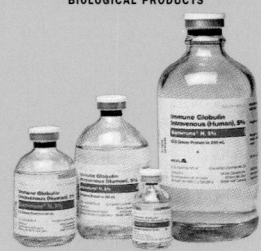

Gamimune® N, 5%
Immune Globulin Intravenous
(Human), 5%

RX · PHARMACEUTICAL DIVISION, · P. 615
BIOLOGICAL PRODUCTS

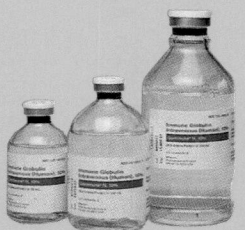

Gamimune® N, 10%
Immune Globulin Intravenous
(Human), 10%

BEACH

RX · BEACH PHARMACEUTICALS · P. 633

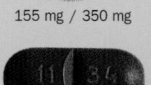

155 mg / 350 mg

305 mg / 700 mg
K-Phos® M.F.   K-Phos® No. 2**
(potassium acid phosphate,
sodium acid phosphate)

OTC · BEACH PHARMACEUTICALS · P. 632

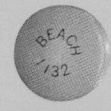

Beelith
(magnesium oxide, vitamin B6)
600 mg / 25 mg

RX · BEACH PHARMACEUTICALS · P. 633

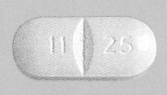

K-Phos® Neutral**
(phosphorus, sodium, potassium)
250 mg / 298 mg / 45 mg

RX · BEACH PHARMACEUTICALS · P. 633

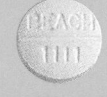

500 mg
K-Phos® Original
(potassium acid phosphate)

RX · BEACH PHARMACEUTICALS · P. 633

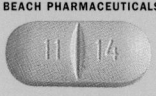

500 mg / 500 mg
Uroqid®-Acid No. 2**
(methenamine mandelate,
sodium acid phosphate)

Designed to help you identify
drugs, this section contains
actual size pills and full color
reproduction of products
selected for inclusion by
participating manufacturers.

BERLEX

RX · BERLEX LABORATORIES · P. 637

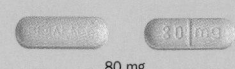

80 mg

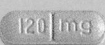

120 mg

160 mg

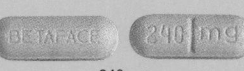

240 mg
Betapace®
(sotalol HCl)

RX · BERLEX LABORATORIES · P. 653

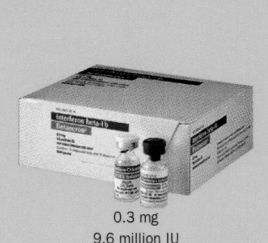

0.3 mg
9.6 million IU
Betaseron®
(Interferon beta-1b)

RX · BERLEX LABORATORIES · P. 640

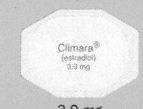

3.9 mg
(0.05 mg/day)

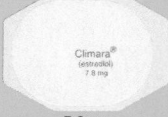

7.8 mg
(0.1 mg/day)
Climara®
(estradiol transdermal system)

RX · BERLEX LABORATORIES · P. 658

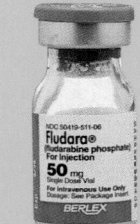

50 mg
Single dose vial
Fludara®
(fludarabine phosphate for injection)

RX · BERLEX LABORATORIES · P. 646

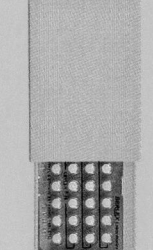

**Levlen® 28 Tablets
28-Day Regimen**
(Each light-orange tablet contains 0.15
mg levonorgestrel and 0.03 mg ethinyl
estradiol. Each pink tablet is inert.)
Also available in 21-day regimen.

Because tablets and capsules
are shown in this section,
do not infer that these are
the only dosage forms
available. Where a product
name is preceded by the
symbol †, refer to the description in the Product Information
(White Section) for other forms.

RX · BERLEX LABORATORIES · P. 646

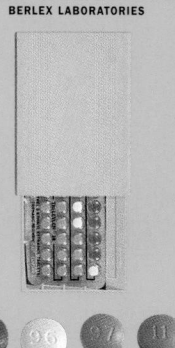

**Tri-Levlen® 28 Tablets
28-Day Regimen**
(Each brown tablet contains 0.050 mg
levonorgestrel and 0.030 mg ethinyl
estradiol. Each white tablet contains
0.075 mg levonorgestrel and 0.040 mg
ethinyl estradiol. Each light-yellow tablet
contains 0.125 mg levonorgestrel and
0.030 mg ethinyl estradiol.
Each light-green tablet is inert.)
Also available in 21-day regimen.

RX · BERLEX LABORATORIES · P. 644

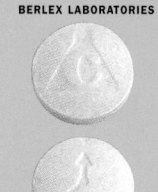

324 mg
Quinaglute Dura-Tabs®
(quinidine gluconate)
Sustained-release tablets
*The tablet designs are trademarks
of Berlex Laboratories*

BERNA

RX · BERNA PRODUCTS, CORP. · P. 660

Vivotif Berna™ Vaccine
(Typhoid Vaccine Live Oral,
Attenuated Ty 21a)

BIOGEN, INC

RX · BIOGEN, INC · P. 662

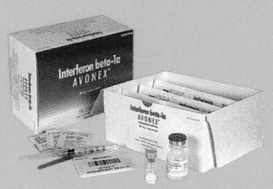

30 mcg
A four-week supply contains four Adminis-
tration Dose Packs with contents as shown.
Avonex™
(Interferon beta-1a)

BOCK PHARMACAL

RX · BOCK PHARMACAL · P. 666

100 mg
Chemet®
(succimer)

RX · BOCK PHARMACAL · P. 668

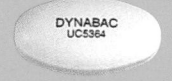

250 mg
Dynabac®
(dirithromycin)

**The name BEACH appears on the reverse side of these tablets.

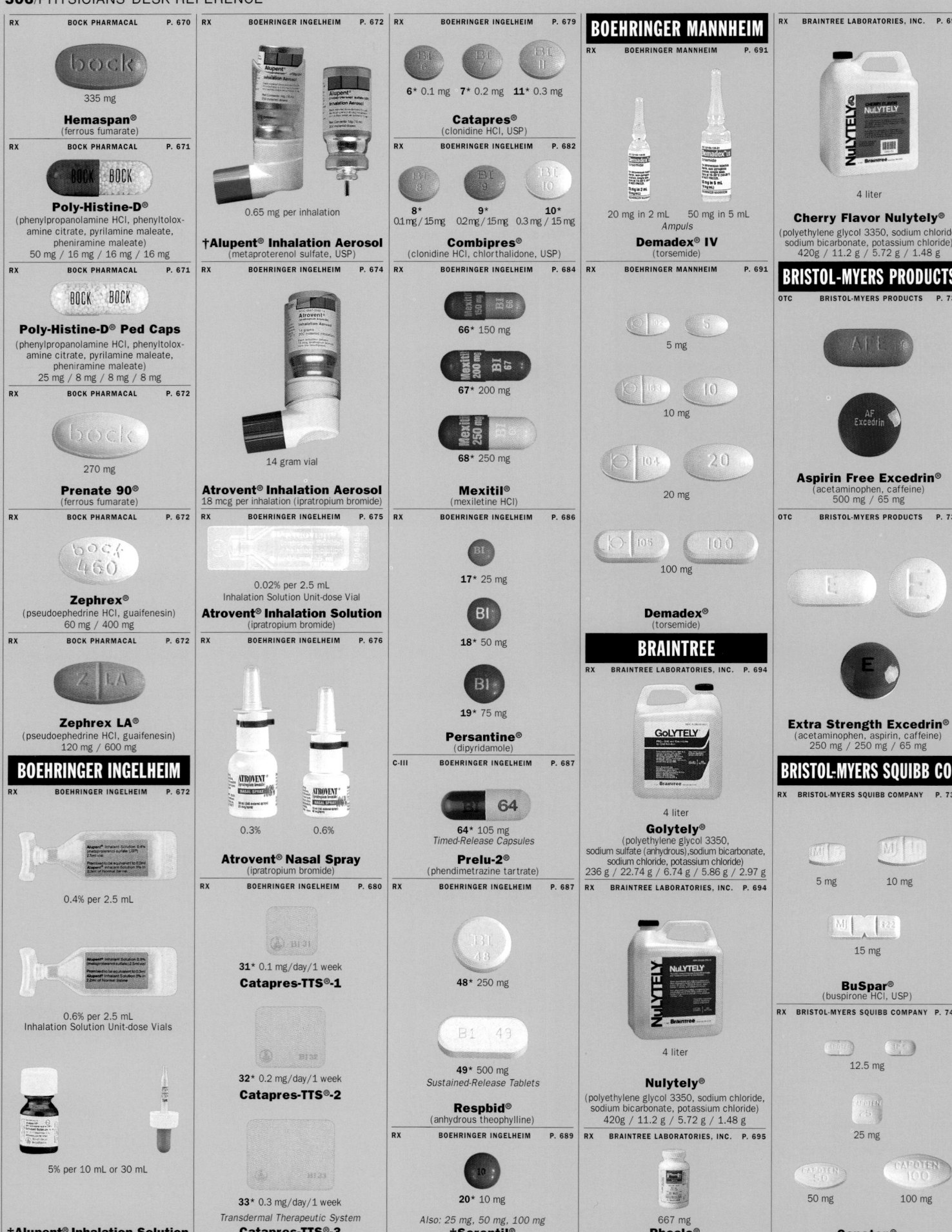

RX   BOCK PHARMACAL   P. 670

335 mg

Hemaspan®
(ferrous fumarate)

RX   BOCK PHARMACAL   P. 671

Poly-Histine-D®
(phenylpropanolamine HCl, phenyltoloxamine citrate, pyrilamine maleate,
pheniramine maleate)
50 mg / 16 mg / 16 mg / 16 mg

RX   BOCK PHARMACAL   P. 671

Poly-Histine-D® Ped Caps
(phenylpropanolamine HCl, phenyltoloxamine citrate, pyrilamine maleate,
pheniramine maleate)
25 mg / 8 mg / 8 mg / 8 mg

RX   BOCK PHARMACAL   P. 672

270 mg

Prenate 90®
(ferrous fumarate)

RX   BOCK PHARMACAL   P. 672

Zephrex®
(pseudoephedrine HCl, guaifenesin)
60 mg / 400 mg

RX   BOCK PHARMACAL   P. 672

Zephrex LA®
(pseudoephedrine HCl, guaifenesin)
120 mg / 600 mg

BOEHRINGER INGELHEIM

RX   BOEHRINGER INGELHEIM   P. 672

0.4% per 2.5 mL

0.6% per 2.5 mL
Inhalation Solution Unit-dose Vials

5% per 10 mL or 30 mL

†Alupent® Inhalation Solution
(metaproterenol sulfate, USP)

RX   BOEHRINGER INGELHEIM   P. 672

0.65 mg per inhalation

†Alupent® Inhalation Aerosol
(metaproterenol sulfate, USP)

RX   BOEHRINGER INGELHEIM   P. 674

14 gram vial

Atrovent® Inhalation Aerosol
18 mcg per inhalation (ipratropium bromide)

RX   BOEHRINGER INGELHEIM   P. 675

0.02% per 2.5 mL
Inhalation Solution Unit-dose Vial

Atrovent® Inhalation Solution
(ipratropium bromide)

RX   BOEHRINGER INGELHEIM   P. 676

0.3%   0.6%

Atrovent® Nasal Spray
(ipratropium bromide)

RX   BOEHRINGER INGELHEIM   P. 680

31* 0.1 mg/day/1 week
Catapres-TTS®-1

32* 0.2 mg/day/1 week
Catapres-TTS®-2

33* 0.3 mg/day/1 week
Transdermal Therapeutic System
Catapres-TTS®-3
(clonidine)

RX   BOEHRINGER INGELHEIM   P. 679

6* 0.1 mg   **7*** 0.2 mg   **11*** 0.3 mg

Catapres®
(clonidine HCl, USP)

RX   BOEHRINGER INGELHEIM   P. 682

8*
0.1mg/15mg

9*
0.2mg/15mg

10*
0.3 mg / 15 mg

Combipres®
(clonidine HCl, chlorthalidone, USP)

RX   BOEHRINGER INGELHEIM   P. 684

66* 150 mg

67* 200 mg

68* 250 mg

Mexitil®
(mexiletine HCl)

RX   BOEHRINGER INGELHEIM   P. 686

17* 25 mg

18* 50 mg

19* 75 mg

Persantine®
(dipyridamole)

C-III   BOEHRINGER INGELHEIM   P. 687

64* 105 mg
Timed-Release Capsules
Prelu-2®
(phendimetrazine tartrate)

RX   BOEHRINGER INGELHEIM   P. 687

48* 250 mg

49* 500 mg
Sustained-Release Tablets
Respbid®
(anhydrous theophylline)

RX   BOEHRINGER INGELHEIM   P. 689

20* 10 mg

Also: 25 mg, 50 mg, 100 mg
†Serentil®
(mesoridazine) besylate USP

BOEHRINGER MANNHEIM

RX   BOEHRINGER MANNHEIM   P. 691

20 mg in 2 mL   50 mg in 5 mL
Ampuls

Demadex® IV
(torsemide)

RX   BOEHRINGER MANNHEIM   P. 691

5 mg

10 mg

20 mg

100 mg

Demadex®
(torsemide)

BRAINTREE

RX   BRAINTREE LABORATORIES, INC.   P. 694

4 liter

Golytely®
(polyethylene glycol 3350,
sodium sulfate (anhydrous),sodium bicarbonate,
sodium chloride, potassium chloride)
236 g / 22.74 g / 6.74 g / 5.86 g / 2.97 g

RX   BRAINTREE LABORATORIES, INC.   P. 694

4 liter

Nulytely®
(polyethylene glycol 3350, sodium chloride,
sodium bicarbonate, potassium chloride)
420g / 11.2 g / 5.72 g / 1.48 g

RX   BRAINTREE LABORATORIES, INC.   P. 695

667 mg

Phoslo®
(calcium acetate tablets)

RX   BRAINTREE LABORATORIES, INC.   P. 694

4 liter

Cherry Flavor Nulytely®
(polyethylene glycol 3350, sodium chloride,
sodium bicarbonate, potassium chloride)
420g / 11.2 / 5.72 / 1.48 g

BRISTOL-MYERS PRODUCTS

OTC   BRISTOL-MYERS PRODUCTS   P. 734

Aspirin Free Excedrin®
(acetaminophen, caffeine)
500 mg / 65 mg

OTC   BRISTOL-MYERS PRODUCTS   P. 734

Extra Strength Excedrin®
(acetaminophen, aspirin, caffeine)
250 mg / 250 mg / 65 mg

BRISTOL-MYERS SQUIBB CO.

RX   BRISTOL-MYERS SQUIBB COMPANY   P. 738

5 mg   10 mg

15 mg

BuSpar®
(buspirone HCl, USP)

RX   BRISTOL-MYERS SQUIBB COMPANY   P. 740

12.5 mg

25 mg

50 mg   100 mg

Capoten®
(captopril)

RX BRISTOL-MYERS SQUIBB COMPANY P. 744

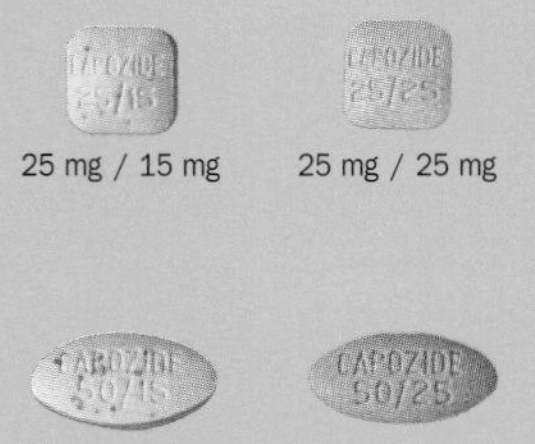

25 mg / 15 mg 25 mg / 25 mg

50 mg / 15 mg 50 mg / 25 mg

Capozide®
(captopril-hydrochlorothiazide)

RX BRISTOL-MYERS SQUIBB COMPANY P. 747

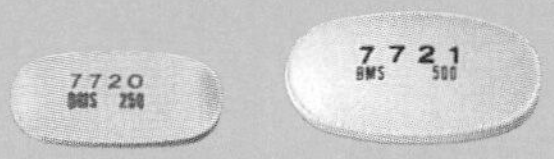

250 mg 500 mg

Cefzil®
(cefprozil)

RX BRISTOL-MYERS SQUIBB COMPANY P. 750

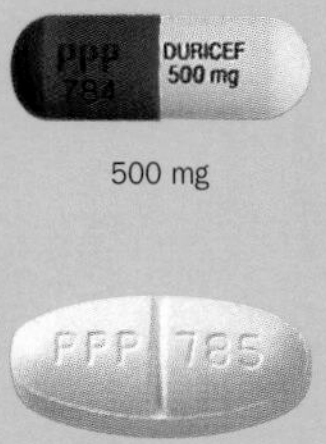

ppp 784 DURICEF 500 mg

500 mg

PPP 785

1 g

Duricef®
(cefadroxil monohydrate, USP)

RX BRISTOL-MYERS SQUIBB COMPANY P. 751

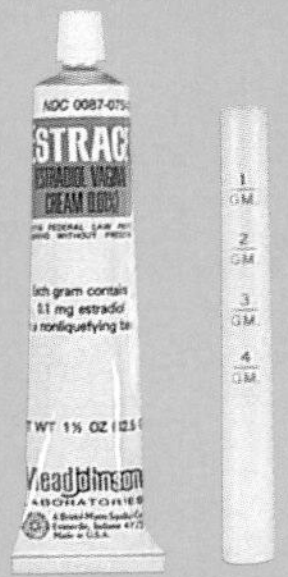

1 1/2 oz tube

Estrace® Vaginal Cream
(estradiol vaginal cream USP, 0.01%)

RX BRISTOL-MYERS SQUIBB COMPANY P. 751

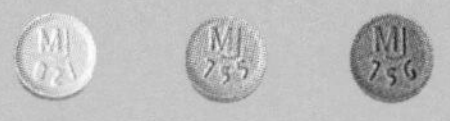

0.5 mg 1 mg 2 mg

Estrace®
(estradiol tablets, USP)

RX BRISTOL-MYERS SQUIBB COMPANY P. 754

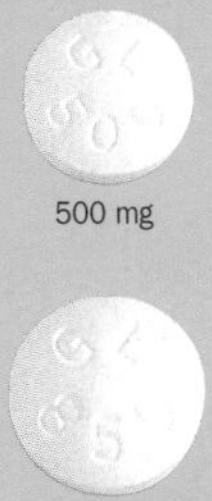

500 mg

850 mg

Glucophage®
(metformin HCl)

RX BRISTOL-MYERS SQUIBB COMPANY P. 758

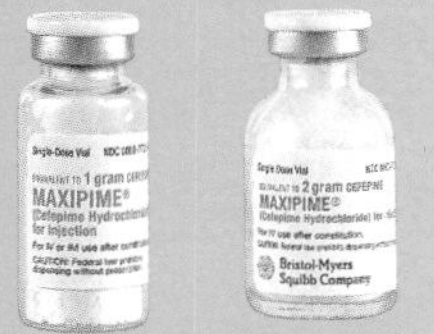

1 g 2 g

Refer to the product information section
for size and delivery systems available.

Maxipime®
(cefepime HCl for injection)

RX BRISTOL-MYERS SQUIBB COMPANY P. 762

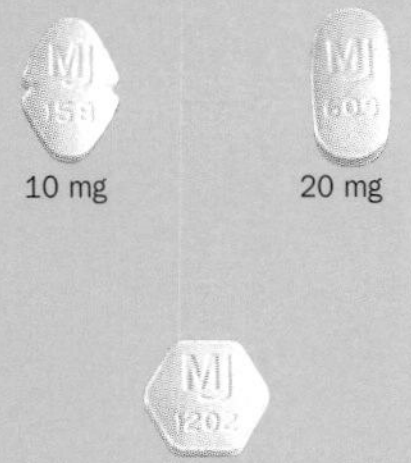

10 mg 20 mg

40 mg

Monopril®
(fosinopril sodium)

RX BRISTOL-MYERS SQUIBB COMPANY P. 765

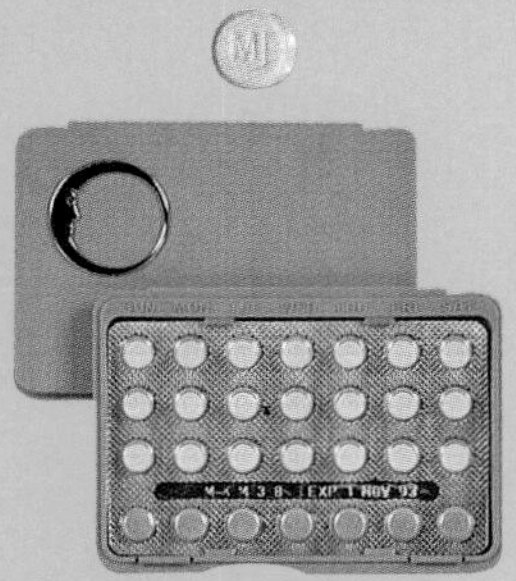

Ovcon® 35
(norethindrone and ethinyl estradiol, USP)

RX BRISTOL-MYERS SQUIBB COMPANY P. 765

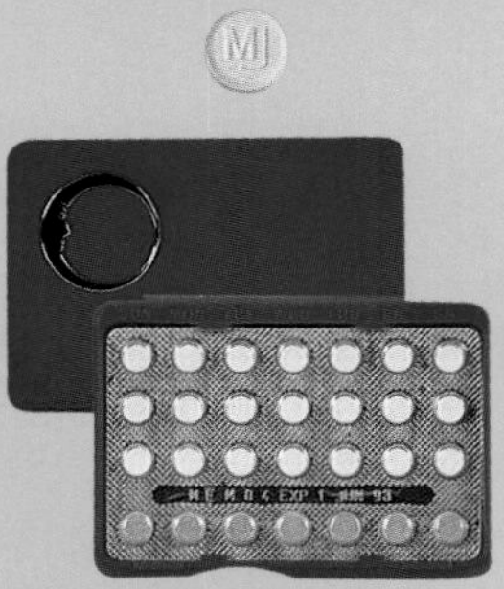

Ovcon® 50
(norethindrone and ethinyl estradiol, USP)

RX BRISTOL-MYERS SQUIBB COMPANY P. 770

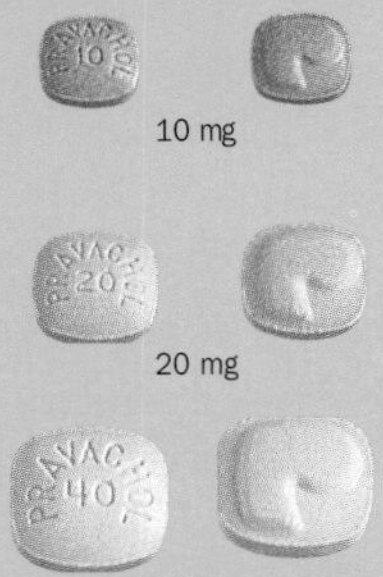

10 mg

20 mg

40 mg

Pravachol®
(pravastatin sodium)

RX BRISTOL-MYERS SQUIBB COMPANY P. 774

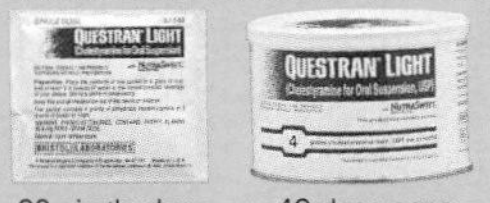

60 single dose 42 dose cans
5-gram packets 210 grams

Questran® Light
(cholestyramine for oral suspension, USP)

RX BRISTOL-MYERS SQUIBB COMPANY P. 774

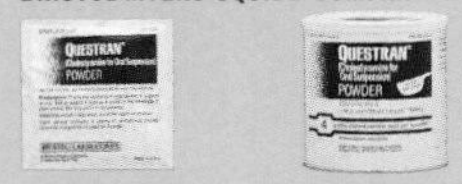

60 single dose 42 dose cans
9-gram packets 378 grams

Questran® Powder
(cholestyramine for oral suspension, USP)

RX BRISTOL-MYERS SQUIBB COMPANY P. 776

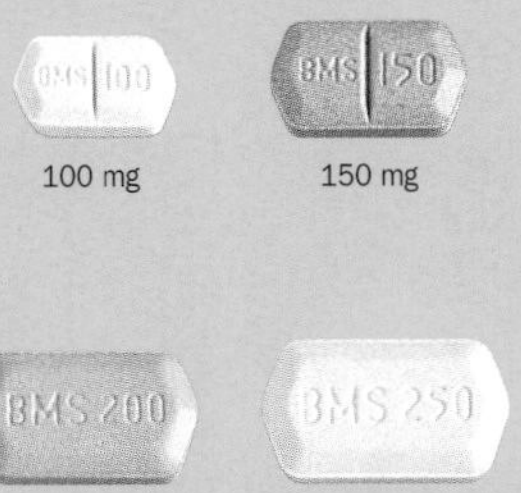

100 mg 150 mg

200 mg 250 mg

Serzone®
(nefazodone HCl tablets)

RX BRISTOL-MYERS SQUIBB COMPANY P. 779

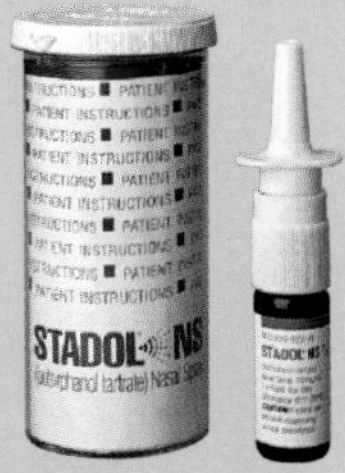

10 mg per mL

Stadol NS®
(butorphanol tartrate)

Because tablets and capsules
are shown in this section,
do not infer that these are
the only dosage forms
available. Where a product
name is preceded by the
symbol †, refer to the description in the Product Information
(White Section) for other forms.

BRISTOL-MYERS SQUIBB ONC.

RX BRISTOL-MYERS SQUIBB ONCOLOGY P. 697

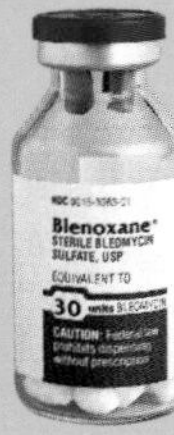

30 units per vial
Also available in 15 units per vial.

Blenoxane®
(sterile bleomycin sulfate, USP)

RX BRISTOL-MYERS SQUIBB ONCOLOGY P. 700

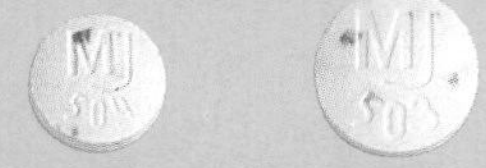

25 mg 50 mg

Cytoxan®
(cyclophosphamide tablets, USP)

RX BRISTOL-MYERS SQUIBB ONCOLOGY P. 700

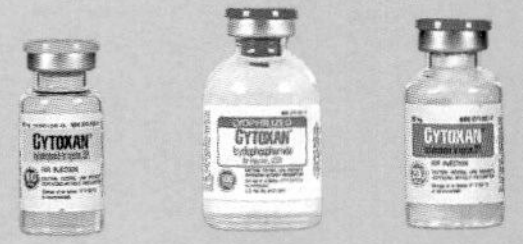

100 mg 500 mg 200 mg

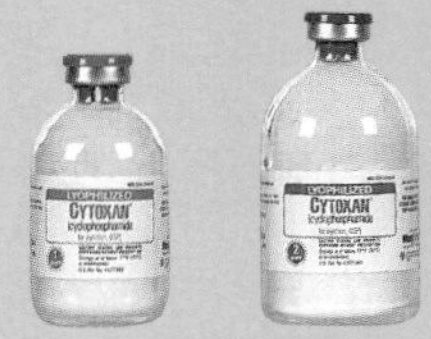

1 g 2 g

For injection

Lyophilized Cytoxan®
(cyclophosphamide for injection, USP)

RX BRISTOL-MYERS SQUIBB ONCOLOGY P. 701

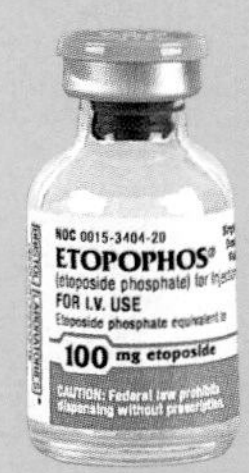

100 mg
Single-dose vial

Etopophos®
(etoposide phosphate for injection)

RX BRISTOL-MYERS SQUIBB ONCOLOGY P. 704

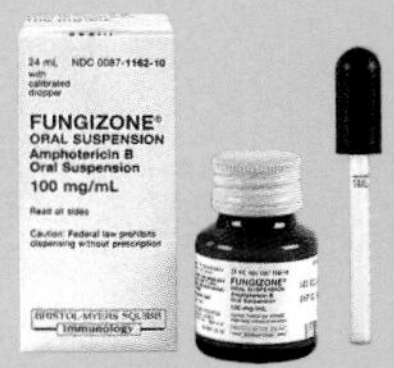

24 mL

100 mg per mL

Fungizone® Oral Suspension
(amphotericin B oral suspension)

RX BRISTOL-MYERS SQUIBB ONCOLOGY P. 706

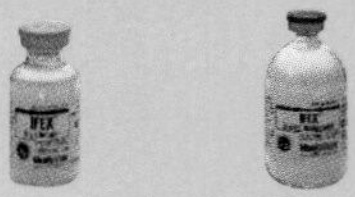

1 g 3 g

Ifex®
(sterile ifosfamide)

RX BRISTOL-MYERS SQUIBB ONCOLOGY P. 708

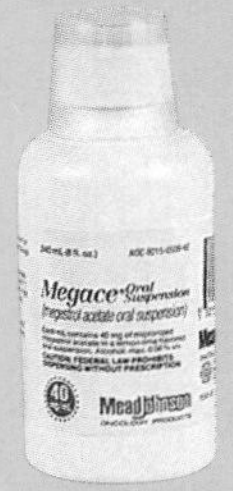

40 mg/mL

Megace® Oral Suspension
(megestrol acetate)

RX BRISTOL-MYERS SQUIBB ONCOLOGY P. 710

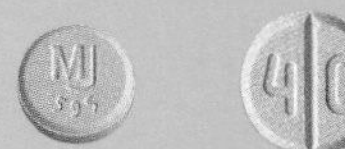

20 mg 40 mg

Megace®
(megestrol acetate tablets, USP)

RX BRISTOL-MYERS SQUIBB ONCOLOGY P. 711

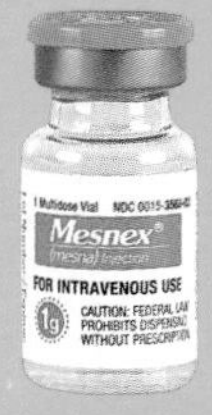

1-gm multi-dose vial

Mesnex®
(mesna injection)

RX BRISTOL-MYERS SQUIBB ONCOLOGY P. 712

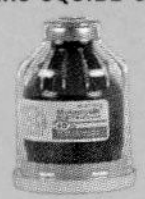

40 mg
Also available in 5 mg and 20 mg

Mutamycin®
(mitomycin for injection, USP)

RX BRISTOL-MYERS SQUIBB ONCOLOGY P. 713

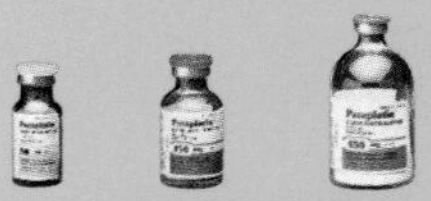

50 mg 150 mg 450 mg

Paraplatin®
(carboplatin for injection)

RX BRISTOL-MYERS SQUIBB ONCOLOGY P. 719

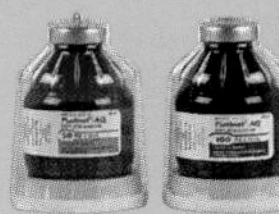

50 mg/100 mg

Platinol®-AQ
(cisplatin injection)

RX BRISTOL-MYERS SQUIBB ONCOLOGY P. 723

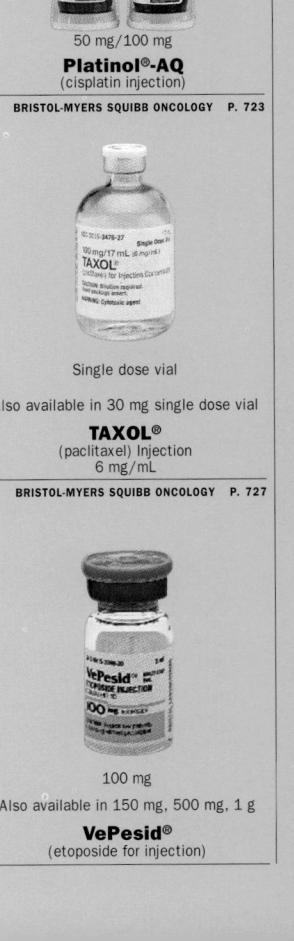

Single dose vial

Also available in 30 mg single dose vial

TAXOL®
(paclitaxel) Injection
6 mg/mL

RX BRISTOL-MYERS SQUIBB ONCOLOGY P. 727

100 mg
Also available in 150 mg, 500 mg, 1 g

VePesid®
(etoposide for injection)

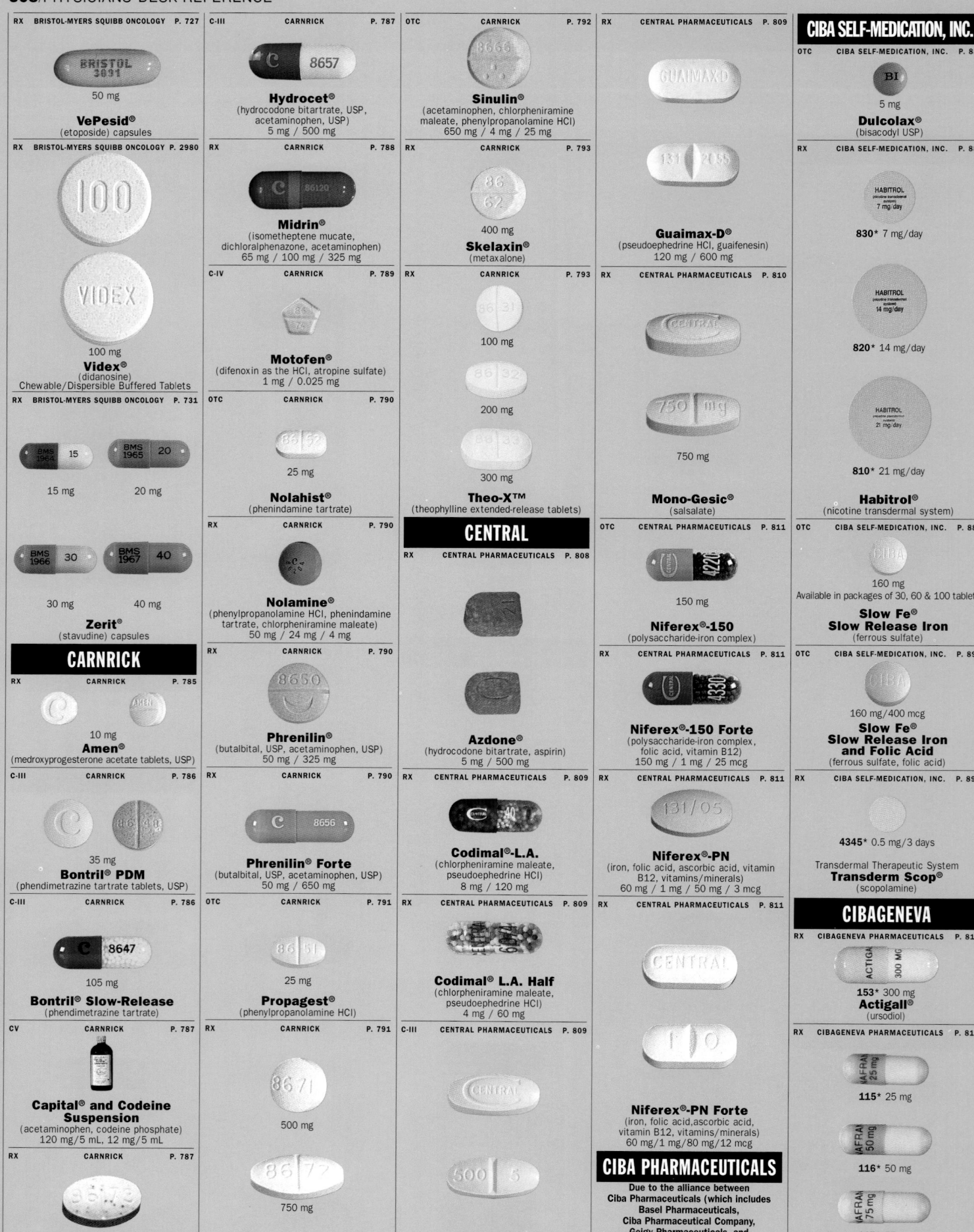

RX   BRISTOL-MYERS SQUIBB ONCOLOGY   P. 727

50 mg

VePesid®
(etoposide) capsules

RX   BRISTOL-MYERS SQUIBB ONCOLOGY   P. 2980

100 mg

Videx®
(didanosine)
Chewable/Dispersible Buffered Tablets

RX   BRISTOL-MYERS SQUIBB ONCOLOGY   P. 731

15 mg   20 mg

30 mg   40 mg

Zerit®
(stavudine) capsules

CARNRICK

RX   CARNRICK   P. 785

10 mg
Amen®
(medroxyprogesterone acetate tablets, USP)

C-III   CARNRICK   P. 786

35 mg
Bontril® PDM
(phendimetrazine tartrate tablets, USP)

C-III   CARNRICK   P. 786

105 mg
Bontril® Slow-Release
(phendimetrazine tartrate)

CV   CARNRICK   P. 787

**Capital® and Codeine
Suspension**
(acetaminophen, codeine phosphate)
120 mg/5 mL, 12 mg/5 mL

RX   CARNRICK   P. 787

Exgest® LA
(phenylpropanolamine HCl, guaifenesin)
75 mg / 400 mg

C-III   CARNRICK   P. 787

8657
Hydrocet®
(hydrocodone bitartrate, USP,
acetaminophen, USP)
5 mg / 500 mg

RX   CARNRICK   P. 788

86120
Midrin®
(isometheptene mucate,
dichloralphenazone, acetaminophen)
65 mg / 100 mg / 325 mg

C-IV   CARNRICK   P. 789

Motofen®
(difenoxin as the HCl, atropine sulfate)
1 mg / 0.025 mg

OTC   CARNRICK   P. 790

25 mg
Nolahist®
(phenindamine tartrate)

RX   CARNRICK   P. 790

Nolamine®
(phenylpropanolamine HCl, phenindamine
tartrate, chlorpheniramine maleate)
50 mg / 24 mg / 4 mg

RX   CARNRICK   P. 790

8650
Phrenilin®
(butalbital, USP, acetaminophen, USP)
50 mg / 325 mg

RX   CARNRICK   P. 790

8656
Phrenilin® Forte
(butalbital, USP, acetaminophen, USP)
50 mg / 650 mg

OTC   CARNRICK   P. 791

25 mg
Propagest®
(phenylpropanolamine HCl)

RX   CARNRICK   P. 791

500 mg

750 mg
Salflex®
(salsalate tablets, USP)

OTC   CARNRICK   P. 792

8666
Sinulin®
(acetaminophen, chlorpheniramine
maleate, phenylpropanolamine HCl)
650 mg / 4 mg / 25 mg

RX   CARNRICK   P. 793

86
62
400 mg
Skelaxin®
(metaxalone)

RX   CARNRICK   P. 793

86 31
100 mg

86 32
200 mg

86 33
300 mg
Theo-X™
(theophylline extended-release tablets)

CENTRAL

RX   CENTRAL PHARMACEUTICALS   P. 808

Azdone®
(hydrocodone bitartrate, aspirin)
5 mg / 500 mg

RX   CENTRAL PHARMACEUTICALS   P. 809

Codimal®-L.A.
(chlorpheniramine maleate,
pseudoephedrine HCl)
8 mg / 120 mg

RX   CENTRAL PHARMACEUTICALS   P. 809

Codimal® L.A. Half
(chlorpheniramine maleate,
pseudoephedrine HCl)
4 mg / 60 mg

C-III   CENTRAL PHARMACEUTICALS   P. 809

500 5
Co-Gesic®
(hydrocodone bitartrate, acetaminophen)
5 mg / 500 mg

RX   CENTRAL PHARMACEUTICALS   P. 809

131 265
Guaimax-D®
(pseudoephedrine HCl, guaifenesin)
120 mg / 600 mg

RX   CENTRAL PHARMACEUTICALS   P. 810

750 mg
Mono-Gesic®
(salsalate)

OTC   CENTRAL PHARMACEUTICALS   P. 811

150 mg
Niferex®-150
(polysaccharide-iron complex)

RX   CENTRAL PHARMACEUTICALS   P. 811

4330
Niferex®-150 Forte
(polysaccharide-iron complex,
folic acid, vitamin B12)
150 mg / 1 mg / 25 mcg

RX   CENTRAL PHARMACEUTICALS   P. 811

131/05
Niferex®-PN
(iron, folic acid, ascorbic acid, vitamin
B12, vitamins/minerals)
60 mg / 1 mg / 50 mg / 3 mcg

RX   CENTRAL PHARMACEUTICALS   P. 811

Niferex®-PN Forte
(iron, folic acid, ascorbic acid,
vitamin B12, vitamins/minerals)
60 mg/1 mg/80 mg/12 mcg

CIBA PHARMACEUTICALS

Due to the alliance between
Ciba Pharmaceuticals (which includes
Basel Pharmaceuticals,
Ciba Pharmaceutical Company,
Geigy Pharmaceuticals, and
Summit Pharmaceuticals) and
Geneva Pharmaceuticals, Inc., please refer
to CibaGeneva for product identification.

CIBA SELF-MEDICATION, INC.

OTC   CIBA SELF-MEDICATION, INC.   P. 883

BI
5 mg
Dulcolax®
(bisacodyl USP)

RX   CIBA SELF-MEDICATION, INC.   P. 884

HABITROL
7 mg/day
830* 7 mg/day

HABITROL
14 mg/day
820* 14 mg/day

HABITROL
21 mg/day
810* 21 mg/day

Habitrol®
(nicotine transdermal system)

OTC   CIBA SELF-MEDICATION, INC.   P. 889

160 mg
Available in packages of 30, 60 & 100 tablets
**Slow Fe®
Slow Release Iron**
(ferrous sulfate)

OTC   CIBA SELF-MEDICATION, INC.   P. 890

160 mg/400 mcg
**Slow Fe®
Slow Release Iron
and Folic Acid**
(ferrous sulfate, folic acid)

RX   CIBA SELF-MEDICATION, INC.   P. 890

4345* 0.5 mg/3 days
Transdermal Therapeutic System
Transderm Scop®
(scopolamine)

CIBAGENEVA

RX   CIBAGENEVA PHARMACEUTICALS   P. 818

ACTIGALL 300 MG
153* 300 mg
Actigall®
(ursodiol)

RX   CIBAGENEVA PHARMACEUTICALS   P. 819

ANAFRANIL 25 mg
115* 25 mg

ANAFRANIL 50 mg
116* 50 mg

ANAFRANIL 75 mg
117* 75 mg
Anafranil®
(clomipramine hydrochloride)

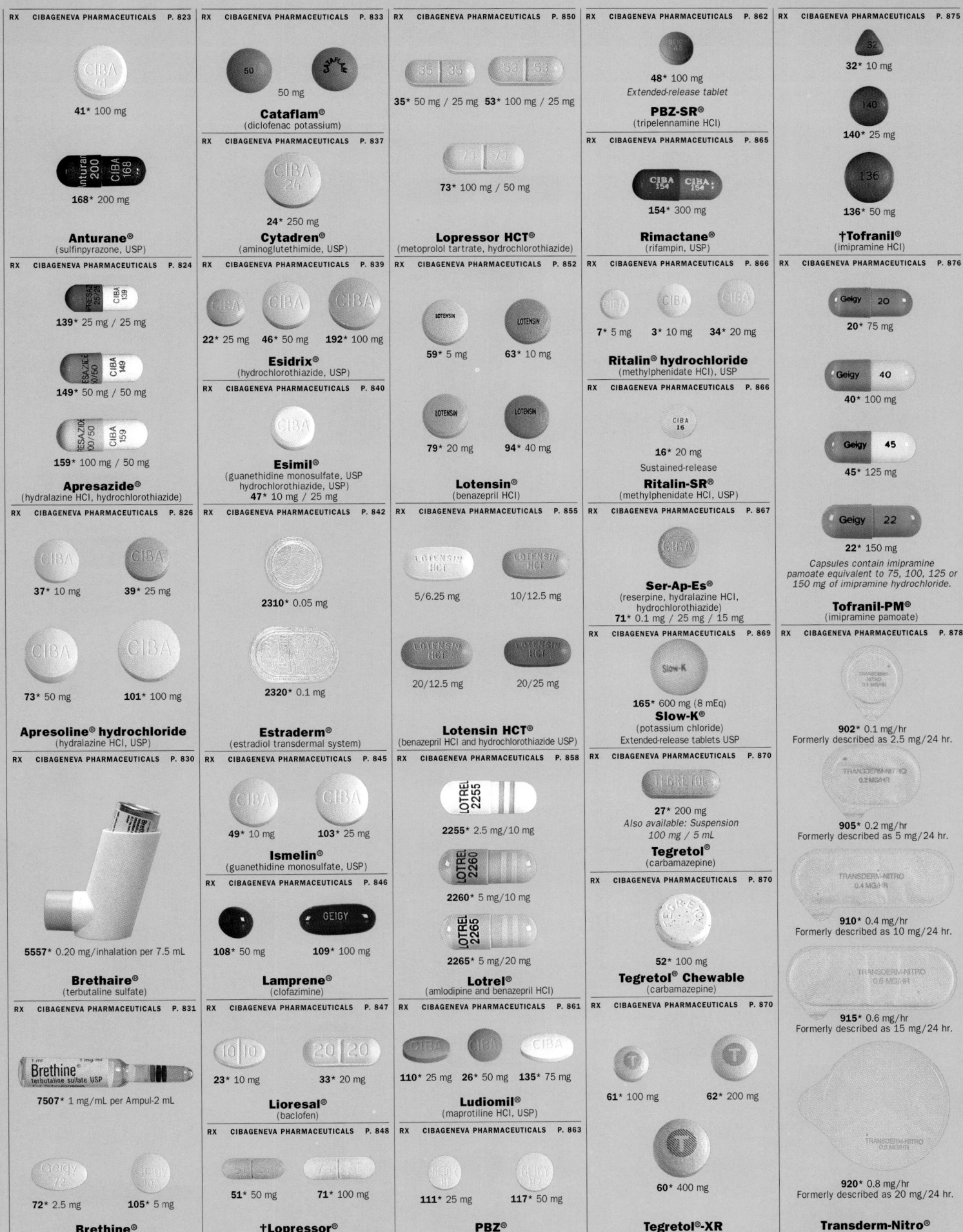

RX CIBAGENEVA PHARMACEUTICALS P. 823

41* 100 mg

168* 200 mg

Anturane®
(sulfinpyrazone, USP)

RX CIBAGENEVA PHARMACEUTICALS P. 824

139* 25 mg / 25 mg

149* 50 mg / 50 mg

159* 100 mg / 50 mg

Apresazide®
(hydralazine HCl, hydrochlorothiazide)

RX CIBAGENEVA PHARMACEUTICALS P. 826

37* 10 mg   **39*** 25 mg

73* 50 mg   **101*** 100 mg

Apresoline® hydrochloride
(hydralazine HCl, USP)

RX CIBAGENEVA PHARMACEUTICALS P. 830

5557* 0.20 mg/inhalation per 7.5 mL

Brethaire®
(terbutaline sulfate)

RX CIBAGENEVA PHARMACEUTICALS P. 831

7507* 1 mg/mL per Ampul-2 mL

Brethine®
(terbutaline sulfate)

72* 2.5 mg   **105*** 5 mg

Brethine®
(terbutaline sulfate)

RX CIBAGENEVA PHARMACEUTICALS P. 833

50 mg

Cataflam®
(diclofenac potassium)

RX CIBAGENEVA PHARMACEUTICALS P. 837

24* 250 mg

Cytadren®
(aminoglutethimide, USP)

RX CIBAGENEVA PHARMACEUTICALS P. 839

22* 25 mg   **46*** 50 mg   **192*** 100 mg

Esidrix®
(hydrochlorothiazide, USP)

RX CIBAGENEVA PHARMACEUTICALS P. 840

Esimil®
(guanethidine monosulfate, USP
hydrochlorothiazide, USP)
47* 10 mg / 25 mg

RX CIBAGENEVA PHARMACEUTICALS P. 842

2310* 0.05 mg

2320* 0.1 mg

Estraderm®
(estradiol transdermal system)

RX CIBAGENEVA PHARMACEUTICALS P. 845

49* 10 mg   **103*** 25 mg

Ismelin®
(guanethidine monosulfate, USP)

RX CIBAGENEVA PHARMACEUTICALS P. 846

108* 50 mg   **109*** 100 mg

Lamprene®
(clofazimine)

RX CIBAGENEVA PHARMACEUTICALS P. 847

23* 10 mg   **33*** 20 mg

Lioresal®
(baclofen)

RX CIBAGENEVA PHARMACEUTICALS P. 848

51* 50 mg   **71*** 100 mg

†Lopressor®
(metoprolol tartrate)

RX CIBAGENEVA PHARMACEUTICALS P. 850

35* 50 mg / 25 mg   **53*** 100 mg / 25 mg

73* 100 mg / 50 mg

Lopressor HCT®
(metoprolol tartrate, hydrochlorothiazide)

RX CIBAGENEVA PHARMACEUTICALS P. 852

59* 5 mg   **63*** 10 mg

79* 20 mg   **94*** 40 mg

Lotensin®
(benazepril HCl)

RX CIBAGENEVA PHARMACEUTICALS P. 855

5/6.25 mg   10/12.5 mg

20/12.5 mg   20/25 mg

Lotensin HCT®
(benazepril HCl and hydrochlorothiazide USP)

RX CIBAGENEVA PHARMACEUTICALS P. 858

2255* 2.5 mg/10 mg

2260* 5 mg/10 mg

2265* 5 mg/20 mg

Lotrel®
(amlodipine and benazepril HCl)

RX CIBAGENEVA PHARMACEUTICALS P. 861

110* 25 mg   **26*** 50 mg   **135*** 75 mg

Ludiomil®
(maprotiline HCl, USP)

RX CIBAGENEVA PHARMACEUTICALS P. 863

111* 25 mg   **117*** 50 mg

PBZ®
(tripelennamine HCl)

RX CIBAGENEVA PHARMACEUTICALS P. 862

48* 100 mg
Extended-release tablet
PBZ-SR®
(tripelennamine HCl)

RX CIBAGENEVA PHARMACEUTICALS P. 865

154* 300 mg

Rimactane®
(rifampin, USP)

RX CIBAGENEVA PHARMACEUTICALS P. 866

7* 5 mg   **3*** 10 mg   **34*** 20 mg

Ritalin® hydrochloride
(methylphenidate HCl), USP

RX CIBAGENEVA PHARMACEUTICALS P. 866

16* 20 mg
Sustained-release
Ritalin-SR®
(methylphenidate HCl, USP)

RX CIBAGENEVA PHARMACEUTICALS P. 867

Ser-Ap-Es®
(reserpine, hydralazine HCl,
hydrochlorothiazide)
71* 0.1 mg / 25 mg / 15 mg

RX CIBAGENEVA PHARMACEUTICALS P. 869

165* 600 mg (8 mEq)
Slow-K®
(potassium chloride)
Extended-release tablets USP

RX CIBAGENEVA PHARMACEUTICALS P. 870

27* 200 mg
*Also available: Suspension
100 mg / 5 mL*
Tegretol®
(carbamazepine)

RX CIBAGENEVA PHARMACEUTICALS P. 870

52* 100 mg
Tegretol® Chewable
(carbamazepine)

RX CIBAGENEVA PHARMACEUTICALS P. 870

61* 100 mg   **62*** 200 mg

60* 400 mg

Tegretol®-XR
(carbamazepine extended-release tablets)

RX CIBAGENEVA PHARMACEUTICALS P. 875

32* 10 mg

140* 25 mg

136* 50 mg

†Tofranil®
(imipramine HCl)

RX CIBAGENEVA PHARMACEUTICALS P. 876

20* 75 mg

40* 100 mg

45* 125 mg

22* 150 mg

*Capsules contain imipramine
pamoate equivalent to 75, 100, 125 or
150 mg of imipramine hydrochloride.*

Tofranil-PM®
(imipramine pamoate)

RX CIBAGENEVA PHARMACEUTICALS P. 878

902* 0.1 mg/hr
Formerly described as 2.5 mg/24 hr.

905* 0.2 mg/hr
Formerly described as 5 mg/24 hr.

910* 0.4 mg/hr
Formerly described as 10 mg/24 hr.

915* 0.6 mg/hr
Formerly described as 15 mg/24 hr.

920* 0.8 mg/hr
Formerly described as 20 mg/24 hr.

Transderm-Nitro®
(nitroglycerin)

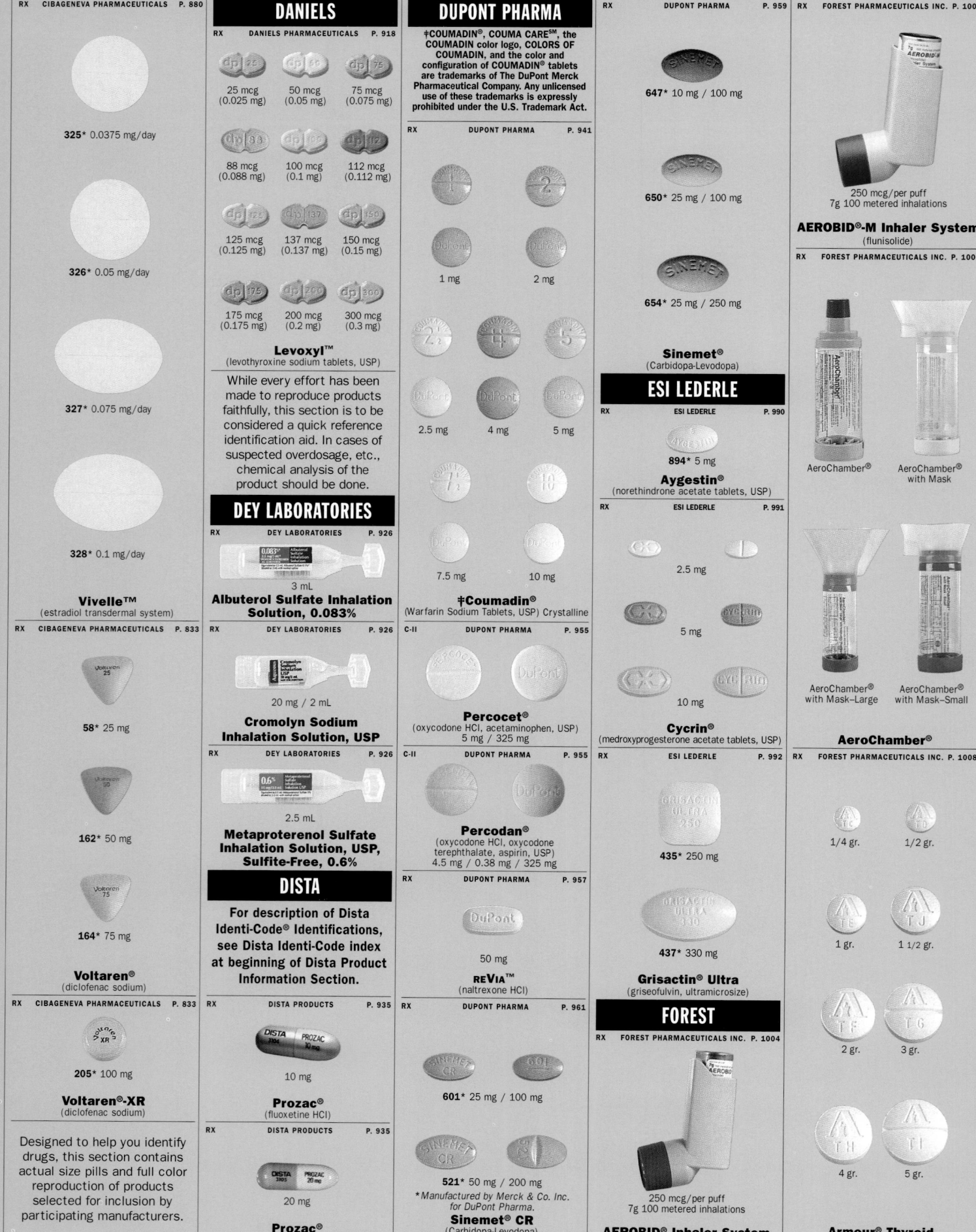

RX CIBAGENEVA PHARMACEUTICALS P. 880

325* 0.0375 mg/day

326* 0.05 mg/day

327* 0.075 mg/day

328* 0.1 mg/day

Vivelle™
(estradiol transdermal system)

RX CIBAGENEVA PHARMACEUTICALS P. 833

58* 25 mg

162* 50 mg

164* 75 mg

Voltaren®
(diclofenac sodium)

RX CIBAGENEVA PHARMACEUTICALS P. 833

205* 100 mg

Voltaren®-XR
(diclofenac sodium)

Designed to help you identify drugs, this section contains actual size pills and full color reproduction of products selected for inclusion by participating manufacturers.

DANIELS

RX DANIELS PHARMACEUTICALS P. 918

25 mcg (0.025 mg) | 50 mcg (0.05 mg) | 75 mcg (0.075 mg)

88 mcg (0.088 mg) | 100 mcg (0.1 mg) | 112 mcg (0.112 mg)

125 mcg (0.125 mg) | 137 mcg (0.137 mg) | 150 mcg (0.15 mg)

175 mcg (0.175 mg) | 200 mcg (0.2 mg) | 300 mcg (0.3 mg)

Levoxyl™
(levothyroxine sodium tablets, USP)

While every effort has been made to reproduce products faithfully, this section is to be considered a quick reference identification aid. In cases of suspected overdosage, etc., chemical analysis of the product should be done.

DEY LABORATORIES

RX DEY LABORATORIES P. 926

3 mL

Albuterol Sulfate Inhalation Solution, 0.083%

RX DEY LABORATORIES P. 926

20 mg / 2 mL

Cromolyn Sodium Inhalation Solution, USP

RX DEY LABORATORIES P. 926

2.5 mL

Metaproterenol Sulfate Inhalation Solution, USP, Sulfite-Free, 0.6%

DISTA

For description of Dista Identi-Code® Identifications, see Dista Identi-Code index at beginning of Dista Product Information Section.

RX DISTA PRODUCTS P. 935

10 mg

Prozac®
(fluoxetine HCl)

RX DISTA PRODUCTS P. 935

20 mg

Prozac®
(fluoxetine HCl)

DUPONT PHARMA

‡COUMADIN®, COUMA CARE℠, the COUMADIN color logo, COLORS OF COUMADIN, and the color and configuration of COUMADIN® tablets are trademarks of The DuPont Merck Pharmaceutical Company. Any unlicensed use of these trademarks is expressly prohibited under the U.S. Trademark Act.

RX DUPONT PHARMA P. 941

1 mg | 2 mg

2.5 mg | 4 mg | 5 mg

7.5 mg | 10 mg

‡Coumadin®
(Warfarin Sodium Tablets, USP) Crystalline

C-II DUPONT PHARMA P. 955

Percocet®
(oxycodone HCl, acetaminophen, USP)
5 mg / 325 mg

C-II DUPONT PHARMA P. 955

Percodan®
(oxycodone HCl, oxycodone terephthalate, aspirin, USP)
4.5 mg / 0.38 mg / 325 mg

RX DUPONT PHARMA P. 957

50 mg

reVia™
(naltrexone HCl)

RX DUPONT PHARMA P. 961

601* 25 mg / 100 mg

521* 50 mg / 200 mg

*Manufactured by Merck & Co. Inc. for DuPont Pharma.

Sinemet® CR
(Carbidopa-Levodopa)
Sustained-Release

RX DUPONT PHARMA P. 959

647* 10 mg / 100 mg

650* 25 mg / 100 mg

654* 25 mg / 250 mg

Sinemet®
(Carbidopa-Levodopa)

ESI LEDERLE

RX ESI LEDERLE P. 990

894* 5 mg

Aygestin®
(norethindrone acetate tablets, USP)

RX ESI LEDERLE P. 991

2.5 mg

5 mg

10 mg

Cycrin®
(medroxyprogesterone acetate tablets, USP)

RX ESI LEDERLE P. 992

435* 250 mg

437* 330 mg

Grisactin® Ultra
(griseofulvin, ultramicrosize)

FOREST

RX FOREST PHARMACEUTICALS INC. P. 1004

250 mcg/per puff
7g 100 metered inhalations

AEROBID® Inhaler System
(flunisolide)

RX FOREST PHARMACEUTICALS INC. P. 1004

250 mcg/per puff
7g 100 metered inhalations

AEROBID®-M Inhaler System
(flunisolide)

RX FOREST PHARMACEUTICALS INC. P. 1006

AeroChamber® | AeroChamber® with Mask

AeroChamber® with Mask–Large | AeroChamber® with Mask–Small

AeroChamber®

RX FOREST PHARMACEUTICALS INC. P. 1008

1/4 gr. | 1/2 gr.

1 gr. | 1 1/2 gr.

2 gr. | 3 gr.

4 gr. | 5 gr.

Armour® Thyroid
(thyroid USP)

FOREST PHARMACEUTICALS INC. P. 1008

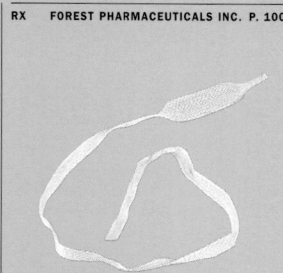

Cervidil™ Vaginal Insert
(dinoprostone 10 mg)

RX FOREST PHARMACEUTICALS INC. P. 1012

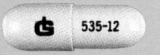
535-12

Esgic®
(butalbital*, acetaminophen,
caffeine USP)
50 mg / 325 mg / 40 mg
*[Warning: May be habit forming]

RX FOREST PHARMACEUTICALS INC. P. 1012

Esgic*plus*™
(butalbital*, acetaminophen,
caffeine USP)
50 mg / 500 mg / 40 mg
*[Warning: May be habit forming]

RX FOREST PHARMACEUTICALS INC. P. 1012

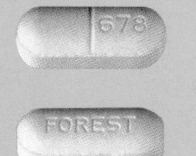
678

FOREST

Esgic*plus*™
(butalbital*, acetaminophen,
caffeine USP)
50 mg / 500 mg / 40 mg
*[Warning: May be habit forming]

RX FOREST PHARMACEUTICALS INC. P. 1013

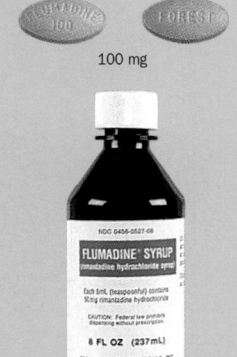
100 mg

237 mL
50 mg/5 mL

Flumadine®
(rimantadine HCl)

Because tablets and capsules
are shown in this section,
do not infer that these are
the only dosage forms
available. Where a product
name is preceded by the
symbol †, refer to the description in the Product Information
(White Section) for other forms.

FOREST PHARMACEUTICALS INC. P. 1015

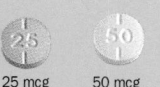
25 mcg   50 mcg   75 mcg

88 mcg   100 mcg   112 mcg

125 mcg   137 mcg   150 mcg

175 mcg   200 mcg   300 mcg

Levothroid®
(levothyroxine sodium)

C-III FOREST PHARMACEUTICALS INC. P. 1016

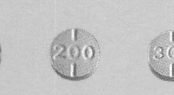
UAD

6350

Lorcet® 10/650
(hydrocodone* bitartrate,
acetaminophen USP)
10 mg/650 mg *[Warning: May be habit forming]

RX FOREST PHARMACEUTICALS INC. P. 1016

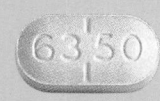
U   U

Lorcet® Plus
(hydrocodone* bitartrate,
acetaminophen USP)
7.5 mg/650 mg *[Warning: May be habit forming]

RX FOREST PHARMACEUTICALS INC. P. 1019

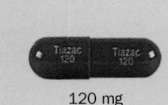
Tiazac 120   Tiazac 120
120 mg

Tiazac 180   Tiazac 180
180 mg

Tiazac 240   Tiazac 240
240 mg

Tiazac 300   Tiazac 300
300 mg

Tiazac 360   Tiazac 360
360 mg

Tiazac™
(diltiazem HCl)
Extended-Release Capsules

FOREST PHARMACEUTICALS INC. P. 1018

100 mg

Tessalon®
(benzonatate USP)

RX FOREST PHARMACEUTICALS INC. P. 1019

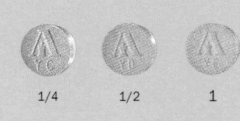
1/4   1/2   1

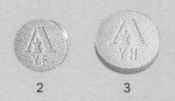
2   3

Thyrolar®
(liotrix)

FUJISAWA USA, INC.

RX FUJISAWA USA, INC. P. 1028

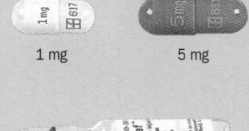
1 mg   5 mg

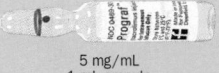
5 mg/mL
1 mL ampule

Prograf®
(tacrolimus)

GATE PHARMACEUTICALS

C-IV GATE PHARMACEUTICALS P. 1035

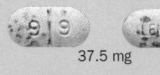
37.5 mg

†Adipex-P®
(phentermine HCl)

RX GATE PHARMACEUTICALS P. 1036

5 mg   10 mg   25 mg

50 mg   100 mg

Moban®
(molindone HCl)

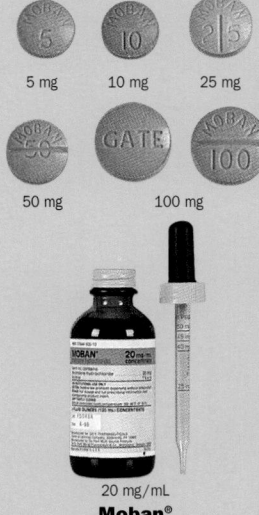
20 mg/mL

RX GATE PHARMACEUTICALS P. 1037

2 mg

Orap®
(pimozide)

GEIGY

Due to the alliance between
Ciba Pharmaceuticals (which includes
Basel Pharmaceuticals,
Ciba Pharmaceutical Company,
Geigy Pharmaceuticals, and
Summit Pharmaceuticals) and
Geneva Pharmaceuticals, Inc., please refer
to CibaGeneva for product identification.

GENENTECH, INC.

RX GENENTECH, INC. P. 1043

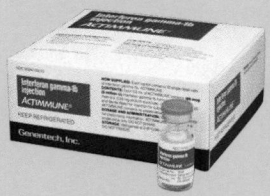
100 mcg (0.5 mL)
Each carton contains 12 single-dose vials

Actimmune®
(Interferon gamma-1b)

RX GENENTECH, INC. P. 1045

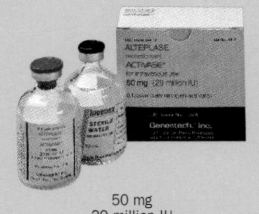
50 mg
29 million IU
Packaged with diluent

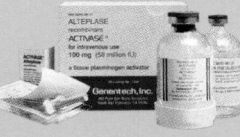
100 mg
58 million IU
Packaged with diluent and double-sided
sterile, siliconized transfer device

Activase®
(Alteplase, recombinant)

RX GENENTECH, INC. P. 1049

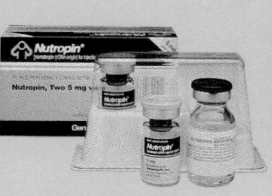
5 mg
approx. 15 IU
Packaged with 10 mL multi-dose vial of
bacteriostatic water
(benzyl alcohol preserved)

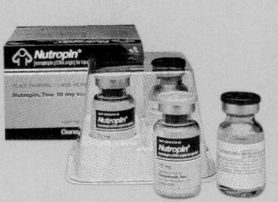
10 mg
approx. 30 IU
Packaged with 10 mL multi-dose vial of
bacteriostatic water
(benzyl alcohol preserved)

Nutropin®
(somatropin [rDNA origin] for injection)

GENENTECH, INC. P. 1051

Nutropin AQ

10 mg (5mg/mL)
approx. 30 IU
Each carton contains six (2 mL) vials

Nutropin AQ™
(somatropin [rDNA origin] injection)

RX GENENTECH, INC. P. 1053

Protropin

5 mg
approx. 15 IU
Packaged with 10 mL multi-dose vial of
bacteriostatic water
(benzyl alcohol preserved)

Protropin

10 mg
approx. 30 IU
Packaged with 10 mL multi-dose vial of
bacteriostatic water
(benzyl alcohol preserved)

Protropin®
(somatrem for injection)

RX GENENTECH, INC. P. 1054

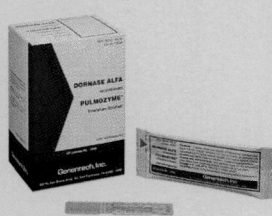
2.5 mL
(1.0 mg/mL dornase alfa)
Each carton contains 14 single-use
ampules

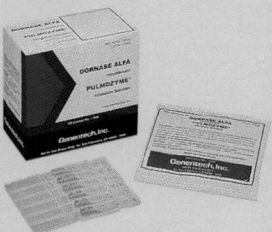
2.5 mL
(1.0 mg/mL dornase alfa)
Each carton contains 30 single-use
ampules

Pulmozyme®
(dornase alfa) recombinant,
Inhalation Solution

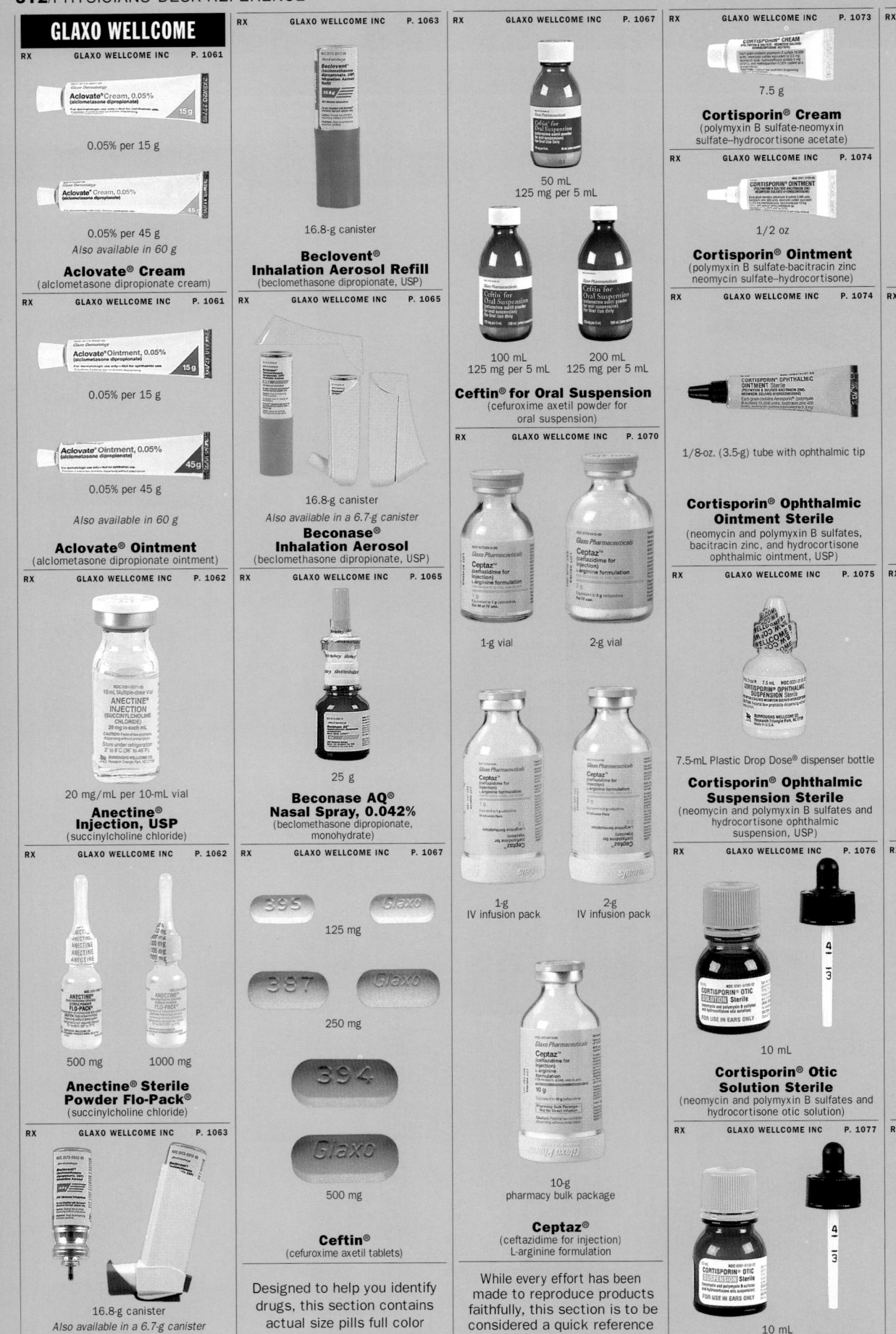

GLAXO WELLCOME

RX   GLAXO WELLCOME INC   P. 1061

0.05% per 15 g

0.05% per 45 g
Also available in 60 g

Aclovate® Cream
(alclometasone dipropionate cream)

RX   GLAXO WELLCOME INC   P. 1061

0.05% per 15 g

0.05% per 45 g

Also available in 60 g

Aclovate® Ointment
(alclometasone dipropionate ointment)

RX   GLAXO WELLCOME INC   P. 1062

20 mg/mL per 10-mL vial

**Anectine®
Injection, USP**
(succinylcholine chloride)

RX   GLAXO WELLCOME INC   P. 1062

500 mg   1000 mg

**Anectine® Sterile
Powder Flo-Pack®**
(succinylcholine chloride)

RX   GLAXO WELLCOME INC   P. 1063

16.8-g canister
*Also available in a 6.7-g canister
The appearance of this inhaler is a
trademark of Glaxo Wellcome.*

**Beclovent®
Inhalation Aerosol**
(beclomethasone dipropionate, USP)

RX   GLAXO WELLCOME INC   P. 1063

16.8-g canister

**Beclovent®
Inhalation Aerosol Refill**
(beclomethasone dipropionate, USP)

RX   GLAXO WELLCOME INC   P. 1065

16.8-g canister
Also available in a 6.7-g canister

**Beconase®
Inhalation Aerosol**
(beclomethasone dipropionate, USP)

RX   GLAXO WELLCOME INC   P. 1065

25 g

**Beconase AQ®
Nasal Spray, 0.042%**
(beclomethasone dipropionate,
monohydrate)

RX   GLAXO WELLCOME INC   P. 1067

395   Glaxo
125 mg

387   Glaxo
250 mg

394

Glaxo
500 mg

Ceftin®
(cefuroxime axetil tablets)

Designed to help you identify
drugs, this section contains
actual size pills full color
reproduction of products
selected for inclusion by
participating manufacturers.

RX   GLAXO WELLCOME INC   P. 1067

50 mL
125 mg per 5 mL

100 mL   200 mL
125 mg per 5 mL   125 mg per 5 mL

Ceftin® for Oral Suspension
(cefuroxime axetil powder for
oral suspension)

RX   GLAXO WELLCOME INC   P. 1070

1-g vial   2-g vial

1-g   2-g
IV infusion pack   IV infusion pack

10-g
pharmacy bulk package

Ceptaz™
(ceftazidime for injection)
L-arginine formulation

While every effort has been
made to reproduce products
faithfully, this section is to be
considered a quick reference
identification aid. In cases of
suspected overdosage, etc.,
chemical analysis of the
product should be done.

RX   GLAXO WELLCOME INC   P. 1073

7.5 g

Cortisporin® Cream
(polymyxin B sulfate-neomyxin
sulfate–hydrocortisone acetate)

RX   GLAXO WELLCOME INC   P. 1074

1/2 oz

Cortisporin® Ointment
(polymyxin B sulfate-bacitracin zinc
neomyxin sulfate–hydrocortisone)

RX   GLAXO WELLCOME INC   P. 1074

1/8-oz. (3.5-g) tube with ophthalmic tip

**Cortisporin® Ophthalmic
Ointment Sterile**
(neomycin and polymyxin B sulfates,
bacitracin zinc, and hydrocortisone
ophthalmic ointment, USP)

RX   GLAXO WELLCOME INC   P. 1075

7.5-mL Plastic Drop Dose® dispenser bottle

**Cortisporin® Ophthalmic
Suspension Sterile**
(neomycin and polymyxin B sulfates and
hydrocortisone ophthalmic
suspension, USP)

RX   GLAXO WELLCOME INC   P. 1076

10 mL

**Cortisporin® Otic
Solution Sterile**
(neomycin and polymyxin B sulfates and
hydrocortisone otic solution)

RX   GLAXO WELLCOME INC   P. 1077

10 mL

**Cortisporin® Otic
Suspension Sterile**
(neomycin and polymyxin B sulfates and
hydrocortisone otic suspension)

RX   GLAXO WELLCOME INC   P. 1078

0.05% per 15 g

0.05% per 60 g
Also available in 30 g

Cutivate® Cream
(fluticasone propionate cream)

RX   GLAXO WELLCOME INC   P. 1078

0.005% per 15 g

0.005% per 60 g
Also available in 30 g

Cutivate® Ointment
(fluticasone propionate ointment)

RX   GLAXO WELLCOME INC   P. 1079

**Digibind® Digoxin
Immune Fab**
(Ovine)

RX   GLAXO WELLCOME INC   P. 1081

2% per 27 g
Also available in 50 g

Emgel® 2% Topical Gel
(erythromycin)

RX   GLAXO WELLCOME INC   P. 1081

10 mL

**Exosurf Neonatal® For
Intratracheal Suspension**
(colfosceril palmitate, cetyl alcohol,
tyloxapol)

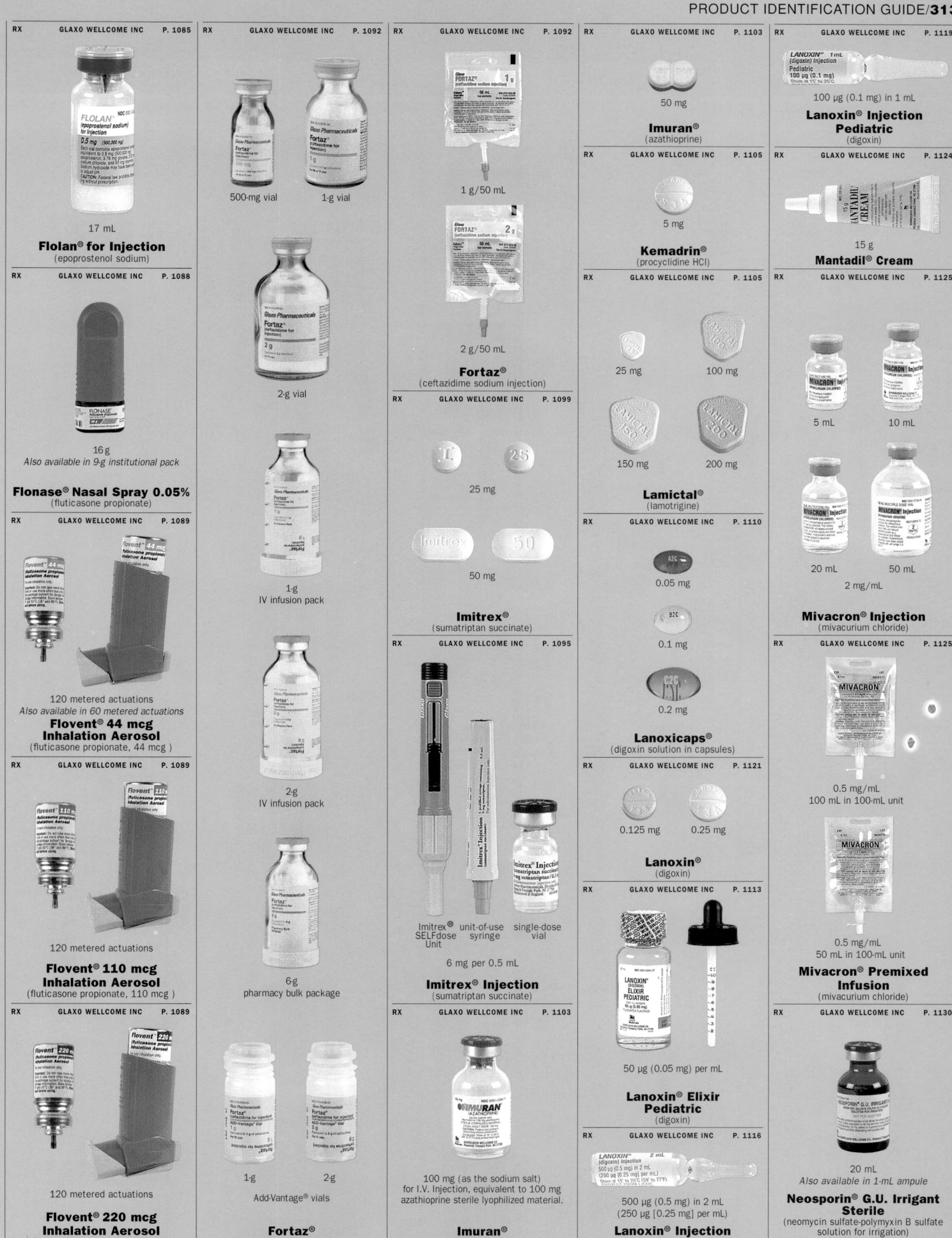

RX GLAXO WELLCOME INC P. 1085

17 mL

Flolan® for Injection
(epoprostenol sodium)

RX GLAXO WELLCOME INC P. 1088

16 g
Also available in 9-g institutional pack

Flonase® Nasal Spray 0.05%
(fluticasone propionate)

RX GLAXO WELLCOME INC P. 1089

120 metered actuations
Also available in 60 metered actuations

**Flovent® 44 mcg
Inhalation Aerosol**
(fluticasone propionate, 44 mcg)

RX GLAXO WELLCOME INC P. 1089

120 metered actuations

**Flovent® 110 mcg
Inhalation Aerosol**
(fluticasone propionate, 110 mcg)

RX GLAXO WELLCOME INC P. 1089

120 metered actuations

**Flovent® 220 mcg
Inhalation Aerosol**
(fluticasone propionate, 220 mcg)

RX GLAXO WELLCOME INC P. 1092

500-mg vial   1-g vial

2-g vial

1-g
IV infusion pack

2-g
IV infusion pack

6-g
pharmacy bulk package

Fortaz®
(ceftazidime for injection)

1-g   2-g
Add-Vantage® vials

Fortaz®
(ceftazidime for injection)

RX GLAXO WELLCOME INC P. 1092

1 g/50 mL

2 g/50 mL

Fortaz®
(ceftazidime sodium injection)

RX GLAXO WELLCOME INC P. 1099

25 mg

50 mg

Imitrex®
(sumatriptan succinate)

RX GLAXO WELLCOME INC P. 1095

Imitrex®   unit-of-use   single-dose
SELFdose   syringe   vial
Unit

6 mg per 0.5 mL

Imitrex® Injection
(sumatriptan succinate)

RX GLAXO WELLCOME INC P. 1103

100 mg (as the sodium salt)
for I.V. Injection, equivalent to 100 mg
azathioprine sterile lyophilized material.

Imuran®
(azathioprine)

RX GLAXO WELLCOME INC P. 1103

50 mg

Imuran®
(azathioprine)

RX GLAXO WELLCOME INC P. 1105

5 mg

Kemadrin®
(procyclidine HCl)

RX GLAXO WELLCOME INC P. 1105

25 mg   100 mg

150 mg   200 mg

Lamictal®
(lamotrigine)

RX GLAXO WELLCOME INC P. 1110

0.05 mg

0.1 mg

0.2 mg

Lanoxicaps®
(digoxin solution in capsules)

RX GLAXO WELLCOME INC P. 1121

0.125 mg   0.25 mg

Lanoxin®
(digoxin)

RX GLAXO WELLCOME INC P. 1113

50 µg (0.05 mg) per mL

**Lanoxin® Elixir
Pediatric**
(digoxin)

RX GLAXO WELLCOME INC P. 1116

500 µg (0.5 mg) in 2 mL
(250 µg [0.25 mg] per mL)

Lanoxin® Injection
(digoxin)

RX GLAXO WELLCOME INC P. 1119

100 µg (0.1 mg) in 1 mL

**Lanoxin® Injection
Pediatric**
(digoxin)

RX GLAXO WELLCOME INC P. 1124

15 g

Mantadil® Cream

RX GLAXO WELLCOME INC P. 1125

5 mL   10 mL

20 mL   50 mL

2 mg/mL

Mivacron® Injection
(mivacurium chloride)

RX GLAXO WELLCOME INC P. 1125

0.5 mg/mL
100 mL in 100-mL unit

0.5 mg/mL
50 mL in 100-mL unit

**Mivacron® Premixed
Infusion**
(mivacurium chloride)

RX GLAXO WELLCOME INC P. 1130

20 mL
Also available in 1-mL ampule

**Neosporin® G.U. Irrigant
Sterile**
(neomycin sulfate-polymyxin B sulfate
solution for irrigation)
NOT FOR INJECTION

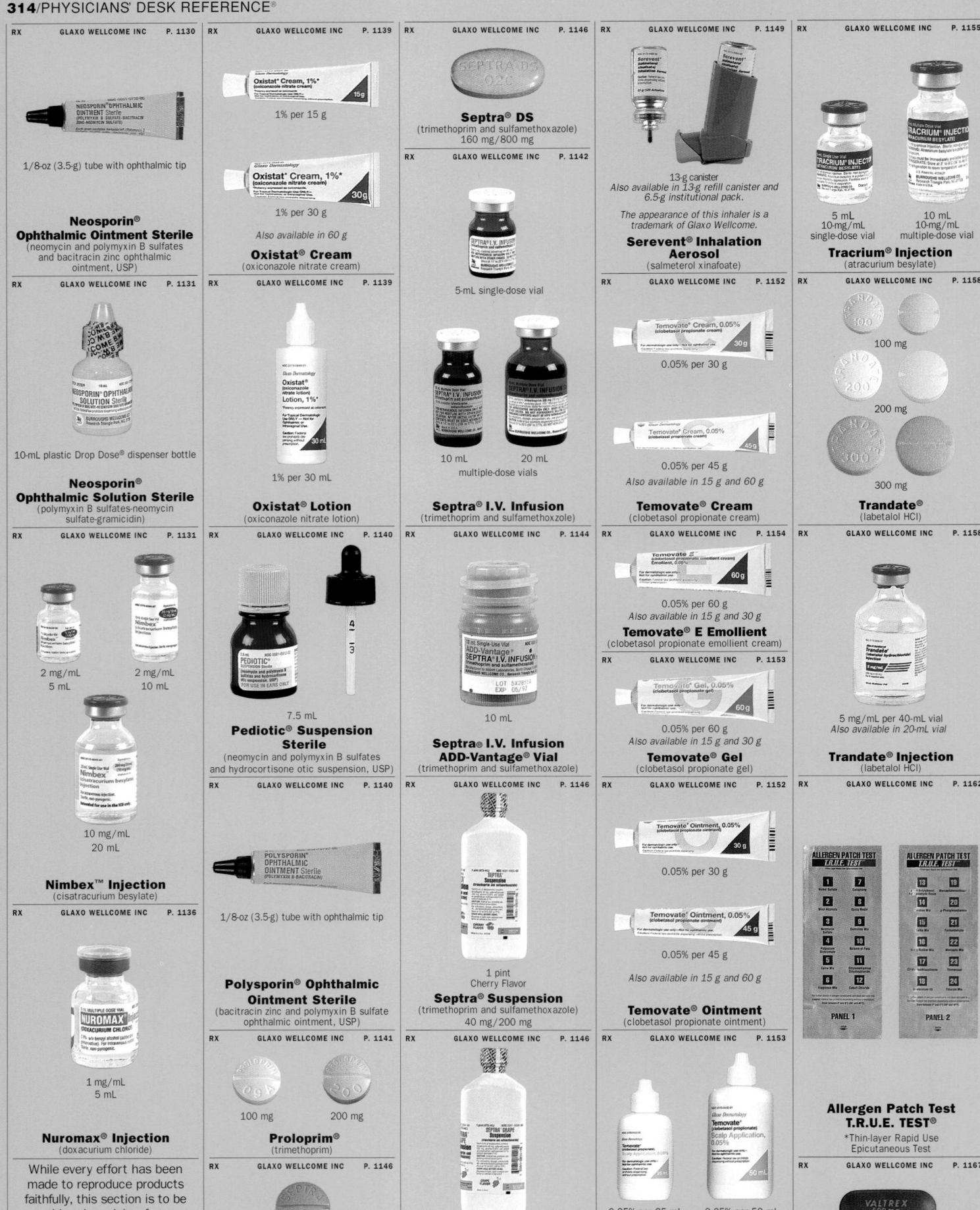

RX   GLAXO WELLCOME INC   P. 1130

1/8-oz (3.5-g) tube with ophthalmic tip

Neosporin®
Ophthalmic Ointment Sterile
(neomycin and polymyxin B sulfates
and bacitracin zinc ophthalmic
ointment, USP)

RX   GLAXO WELLCOME INC   P. 1131

10-mL plastic Drop Dose® dispenser bottle

Neosporin®
Ophthalmic Solution Sterile
(polymyxin B sulfates-neomycin
sulfate-gramicidin)

RX   GLAXO WELLCOME INC   P. 1131

2 mg/mL   2 mg/mL
5 mL   10 mL

10 mg/mL
20 mL

Nimbex™ Injection
(cisatracurium besylate)

RX   GLAXO WELLCOME INC   P. 1136

1 mg/mL
5 mL

Nuromax® Injection
(doxacurium chloride)

While every effort has been
made to reproduce products
faithfully, this section is to be
considered a quick reference
identification aid. In cases of
suspected overdosage, etc.,
chemical analysis of the
product should be done.

RX   GLAXO WELLCOME INC   P. 1139

Oxistat® Cream, 1%*
(oxiconazole nitrate cream)
1% per 15 g

Oxistat® Cream, 1%*
(oxiconazole nitrate cream)
1% per 30 g

Also available in 60 g

Oxistat® Cream
(oxiconazole nitrate cream)

RX   GLAXO WELLCOME INC   P. 1139

Oxistat®
(oxiconazole
nitrate lotion)
Lotion, 1%*
1% per 30 mL

Oxistat® Lotion
(oxiconazole nitrate lotion)

RX   GLAXO WELLCOME INC   P. 1140

7.5 mL
Pediotic® Suspension
Sterile
(neomycin and polymyxin B sulfates
and hydrocortisone otic suspension, USP)

RX   GLAXO WELLCOME INC   P. 1140

POLYSPORIN®
OPHTHALMIC
OINTMENT Sterile
(POLYMYXIN B-BACITRACIN)

1/8-oz (3.5-g) tube with ophthalmic tip

Polysporin® Ophthalmic
Ointment Sterile
(bacitracin zinc and polymyxin B sulfate
ophthalmic ointment, USP)

RX   GLAXO WELLCOME INC   P. 1141

100 mg   200 mg

Proloprim®
(trimethoprim)

RX   GLAXO WELLCOME INC   P. 1146

Septra®
(trimethoprim and sulfamethoxazole)
80 mg/400 mg

RX   GLAXO WELLCOME INC   P. 1146

Septra® DS
(trimethoprim and sulfamethoxazole)
160 mg/800 mg

RX   GLAXO WELLCOME INC   P. 1142

5-mL single-dose vial

Septra® I.V. Infusion
(trimethoprim and sulfamethoxzole)

RX   GLAXO WELLCOME INC   P. 1144

10 mL   20 mL
multiple-dose vials

Septra® I.V. Infusion
(trimethoprim and sulfamethoxzole)

RX   GLAXO WELLCOME INC   P. 1144

10 mL
Septra® I.V. Infusion
ADD-Vantage® Vial
(trimethoprim and sulfamethoxazole)

RX   GLAXO WELLCOME INC   P. 1146

1 pint
Cherry Flavor
Septra® Suspension
(trimethoprim and sulfamethoxazole)
40 mg/200 mg

RX   GLAXO WELLCOME INC   P. 1146

1 pint
Grape Flavor
Septra® Grape Suspension
(trimethoprim and sulfamethoxazole)
40 mg/ 200 mg

RX   GLAXO WELLCOME INC   P. 1149

13-g canister
*Also available in 13-g refill canister and
6.5-g institutional pack.*

*The appearance of this inhaler is a
trademark of Glaxo Wellcome.*

Serevent® Inhalation
Aerosol
(salmeterol xinafoate)

RX   GLAXO WELLCOME INC   P. 1152

Temovate® Cream, 0.05%
(clobetasol propionate cream)
0.05% per 30 g

Temovate® Cream, 0.05%
(clobetasol propionate cream)
0.05% per 45 g

Also available in 15 and 60 g

Temovate® Cream
(clobetasol propionate cream)

RX   GLAXO WELLCOME INC   P. 1154

Temovate E®
clobetasol propionate emollient cream
Emollient, 0.05%
0.05% per 60 g
Also available in 15 g and 30 g

Temovate® E Emollient
(clobetasol propionate emollient cream)

RX   GLAXO WELLCOME INC   P. 1153

Temovate® Gel, 0.05%
(clobetasol propionate gel)
0.05% per 60 g
Also available in 15 g and 30 g

Temovate® Gel
(clobetasol propionate gel)

RX   GLAXO WELLCOME INC   P. 1152

Temovate® Ointment, 0.05%
(clobetasol propionate ointment)
0.05% per 30 g

Temovate® Ointment, 0.05%
(clobetasol propionate ointment)
0.05% per 45 g

Also available in 15 and 60 g

Temovate® Ointment
(clobetasol propionate ointment)

RX   GLAXO WELLCOME INC   P. 1153

Temovate®
(clobetasol propionate)
Scalp Application,
0.05%

0.05% per 25 mL   0.05% per 50 mL

Temovate®
Scalp Application
(clobetasol propionate scalp application)

RX   GLAXO WELLCOME INC   P. 1155

5 mL   10 mL
10-mg/mL   10-mg/mL
single-dose vial   multiple-dose vial

Tracrium® Injection
(atracurium besylate)

RX   GLAXO WELLCOME INC   P. 1158

100 mg

200 mg

300 mg

Trandate®
(labetalol HCl)

RX   GLAXO WELLCOME INC   P. 1158

5 mg/mL per 40-mL vial
Also available in 20-mL vial

Trandate® Injection
(labetalol HCl)

RX   GLAXO WELLCOME INC   P. 1162

PANEL 1   PANEL 2

Allergen Patch Test
T.R.U.E. TEST®
*Thin-layer Rapid Use
Epicutaneous Test*

RX   GLAXO WELLCOME INC   P. 1167

VALTREX 500 mg

500 mg

Valtrex®
(valacyclovir HCl)

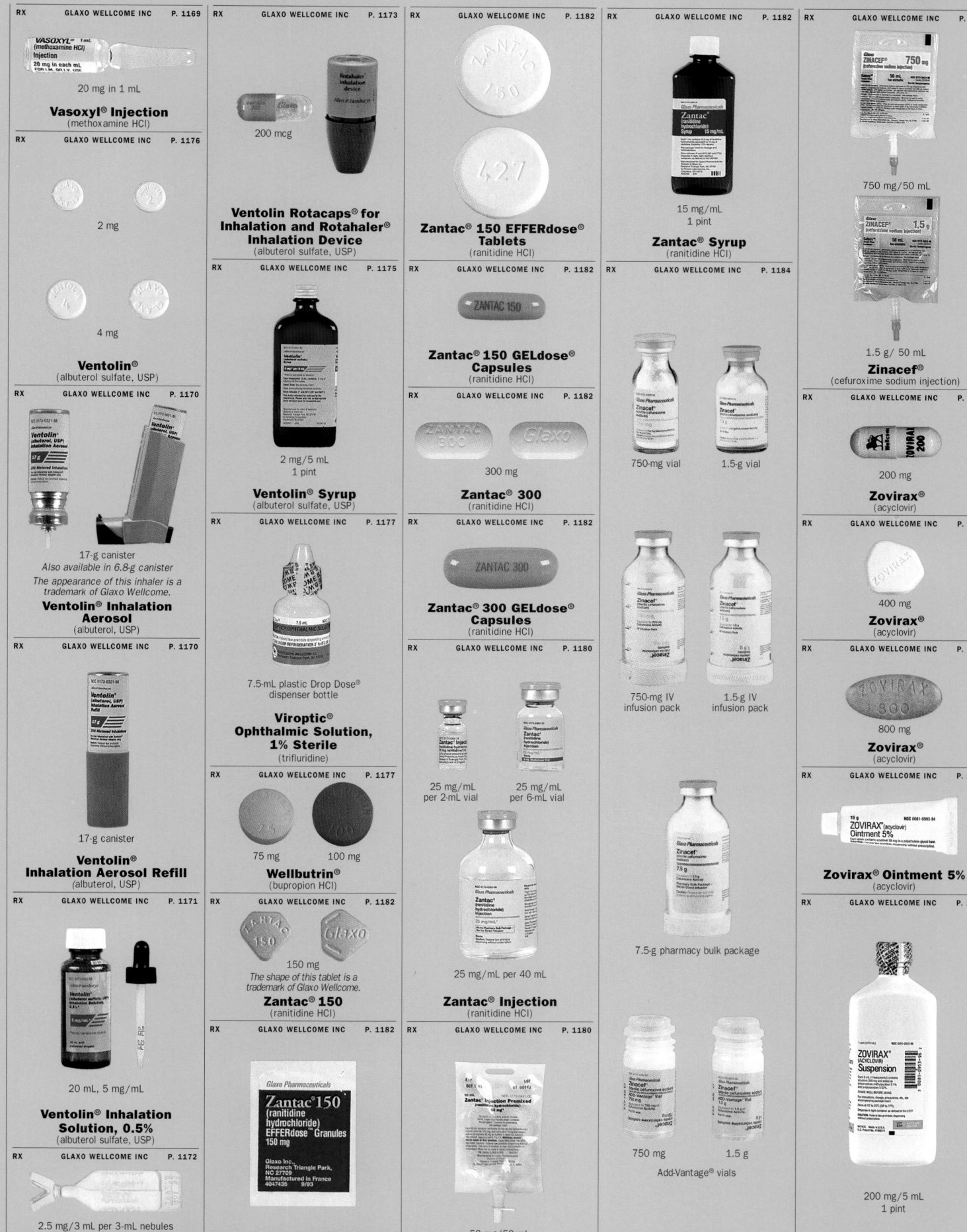

RX — GLAXO WELLCOME INC — P. 1169

20 mg in 1 mL

Vasoxyl® Injection
(methoxamine HCl)

RX — GLAXO WELLCOME INC — P. 1176

2 mg

4 mg

Ventolin®
(albuterol sulfate, USP)

RX — GLAXO WELLCOME INC — P. 1170

17-g canister
Also available in 6.8-g canister
The appearance of this inhaler is a trademark of Glaxo Wellcome.

Ventolin® Inhalation Aerosol
(albuterol, USP)

RX — GLAXO WELLCOME INC — P. 1170

17-g canister

Ventolin® Inhalation Aerosol Refill
(albuterol, USP)

RX — GLAXO WELLCOME INC — P. 1171

20 mL, 5 mg/mL

Ventolin® Inhalation Solution, 0.5%
(albuterol sulfate, USP)

RX — GLAXO WELLCOME INC — P. 1172

2.5 mg/3 mL per 3-mL nebules

Ventolin Nebules® Inhalation Solution, 0.083%
(albuterol sulfate, USP)

RX — GLAXO WELLCOME INC — P. 1173

200 mcg

Ventolin Rotacaps® for Inhalation and Rotahaler® Inhalation Device
(albuterol sulfate, USP)

RX — GLAXO WELLCOME INC — P. 1175

2 mg/5 mL
1 pint

Ventolin® Syrup
(albuterol sulfate, USP)

RX — GLAXO WELLCOME INC — P. 1177

7.5-mL plastic Drop Dose® dispenser bottle

Viroptic® Ophthalmic Solution, 1% Sterile
(trifluridine)

RX — GLAXO WELLCOME INC — P. 1177

75 mg

100 mg

Wellbutrin®
(bupropion HCl)

RX — GLAXO WELLCOME INC — P. 1182

150 mg
The shape of this tablet is a trademark of Glaxo Wellcome.

Zantac® 150
(ranitidine HCl)

RX — GLAXO WELLCOME INC — P. 1182

Glaxo Pharmaceuticals
Zantac®150
(ranitidine hydrochloride)
EFFERdose® Granules
150 mg
Glaxo Inc.,
Research Triangle Park,
NC 27709
Manufactured in France
4047435   9/93

Zantac® 150 EFFERdose® Granules
(ranitidine HCl)

RX — GLAXO WELLCOME INC — P. 1182

Zantac® 150 EFFERdose® Tablets
(ranitidine HCl)

RX — GLAXO WELLCOME INC — P. 1182

Zantac® 150 GELdose® Capsules
(ranitidine HCl)

RX — GLAXO WELLCOME INC — P. 1182

300 mg

Zantac® 300
(ranitidine HCl)

RX — GLAXO WELLCOME INC — P. 1182

Zantac® 300 GELdose® Capsules
(ranitidine HCl)

RX — GLAXO WELLCOME INC — P. 1180

25 mg/mL
per 2-mL vial

25 mg/mL
per 6-mL vial

25 mg/mL per 40 mL

Zantac® Injection
(ranitidine HCl)

RX — GLAXO WELLCOME INC — P. 1180

50 mg/50 mL

Zantac® Injection Premixed
(ranitidine HCl)

RX — GLAXO WELLCOME INC — P. 1182

15 mg/mL
1 pint

Zantac® Syrup
(ranitidine HCl)

RX — GLAXO WELLCOME INC — P. 1184

750-mg vial

1.5-g vial

RX — GLAXO WELLCOME INC — P. 1184

750-mg IV
infusion pack

1.5-g IV
infusion pack

7.5-g pharmacy bulk package

750 mg

1.5 g

Add-Vantage® vials

Zinacef®
(sterile cefuroxime sodium)

RX — GLAXO WELLCOME INC — P. 1184

750 mg/50 mL

1.5 g/ 50 mL

Zinacef®
(cefuroxime sodium injection)

RX — GLAXO WELLCOME INC — P. 1187

200 mg

Zovirax®
(acyclovir)

RX — GLAXO WELLCOME INC — P. 1187

400 mg

Zovirax®
(acyclovir)

RX — GLAXO WELLCOME INC — P. 1187

800 mg

Zovirax®
(acyclovir)

RX — GLAXO WELLCOME INC — P. 1190

Zovirax® Ointment 5%
(acyclovir)

RX — GLAXO WELLCOME INC — P. 1187

200 mg/5 mL
1 pint

Zovirax® Suspension
(acyclovir)

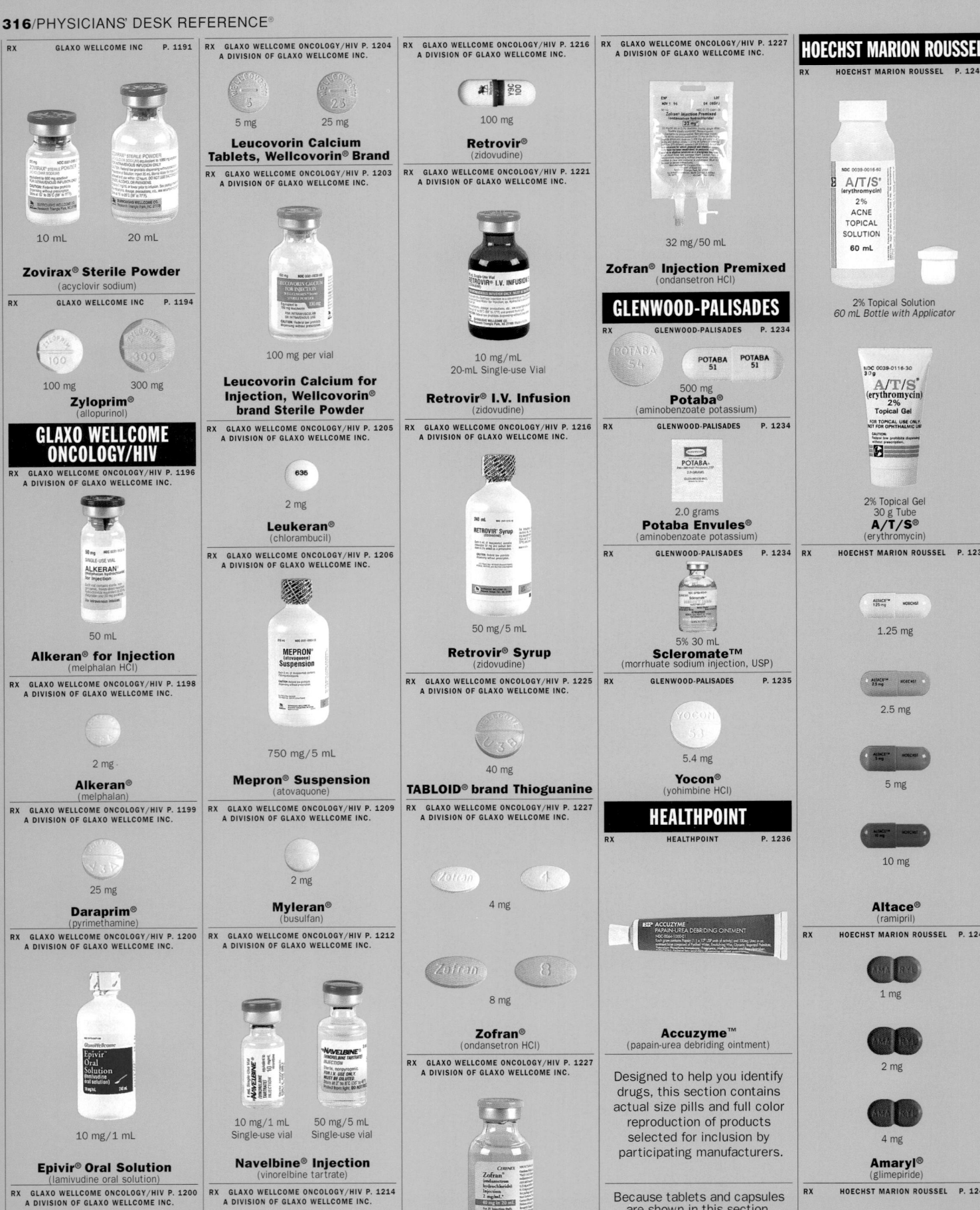

RX   GLAXO WELLCOME INC   P. 1191

10 mL   20 mL

Zovirax® Sterile Powder
(acyclovir sodium)

RX   GLAXO WELLCOME INC   P. 1194

100 mg   300 mg

Zyloprim®
(allopurinol)

GLAXO WELLCOME ONCOLOGY/HIV

RX   GLAXO WELLCOME ONCOLOGY/HIV P. 1196
A DIVISION OF GLAXO WELLCOME INC.

50 mL

Alkeran® for Injection
(melphalan HCl)

RX   GLAXO WELLCOME ONCOLOGY/HIV P. 1198
A DIVISION OF GLAXO WELLCOME INC.

2 mg

Alkeran®
(melphalan)

RX   GLAXO WELLCOME ONCOLOGY/HIV P. 1199
A DIVISION OF GLAXO WELLCOME INC.

25 mg

Daraprim®
(pyrimethamine)

RX   GLAXO WELLCOME ONCOLOGY/HIV P. 1200
A DIVISION OF GLAXO WELLCOME INC.

10 mg/1 mL

Epivir® Oral Solution
(lamivudine oral solution)

RX   GLAXO WELLCOME ONCOLOGY/HIV P. 1200
A DIVISION OF GLAXO WELLCOME INC.

150 mg

Epivir®
(lamivudine tablets)

RX   GLAXO WELLCOME ONCOLOGY/HIV P. 1204
A DIVISION OF GLAXO WELLCOME INC.

5 mg   25 mg

**Leucovorin Calcium
Tablets, Wellcovorin® Brand**

RX   GLAXO WELLCOME ONCOLOGY/HIV P. 1203
A DIVISION OF GLAXO WELLCOME INC.

100 mg per vial

**Leucovorin Calcium for
Injection, Wellcovorin®
brand Sterile Powder**

RX   GLAXO WELLCOME ONCOLOGY/HIV P. 1205
A DIVISION OF GLAXO WELLCOME INC.

635

2 mg

Leukeran®
(chlorambucil)

RX   GLAXO WELLCOME ONCOLOGY/HIV P. 1206
A DIVISION OF GLAXO WELLCOME INC.

750 mg/5 mL

Mepron® Suspension
(atovaquone)

RX   GLAXO WELLCOME ONCOLOGY/HIV P. 1209
A DIVISION OF GLAXO WELLCOME INC.

2 mg

Myleran®
(busulfan)

RX   GLAXO WELLCOME ONCOLOGY/HIV P. 1212
A DIVISION OF GLAXO WELLCOME INC.

10 mg/1 mL   50 mg/5 mL
Single-use vial   Single-use vial

Navelbine® Injection
(vinorelbine tartrate)

RX   GLAXO WELLCOME ONCOLOGY/HIV P. 1214
A DIVISION OF GLAXO WELLCOME INC.

50 mg

Purinethol®
(mercaptopurine)

RX   GLAXO WELLCOME ONCOLOGY/HIV P. 1216
A DIVISION OF GLAXO WELLCOME INC.

100 mg

Retrovir®
(zidovudine)

RX   GLAXO WELLCOME ONCOLOGY/HIV P. 1221
A DIVISION OF GLAXO WELLCOME INC.

10 mg/mL
20-mL Single-use Vial

Retrovir® I.V. Infusion
(zidovudine)

RX   GLAXO WELLCOME ONCOLOGY/HIV P. 1216
A DIVISION OF GLAXO WELLCOME INC.

50 mg/5 mL

Retrovir® Syrup
(zidovudine)

RX   GLAXO WELLCOME ONCOLOGY/HIV P. 1227
A DIVISION OF GLAXO WELLCOME INC.

40 mg

TABLOID® brand Thioguanine

RX   GLAXO WELLCOME ONCOLOGY/HIV P. 1227
A DIVISION OF GLAXO WELLCOME INC.

4 mg

8 mg

Zofran®
(ondansetron HCl)

RX   GLAXO WELLCOME ONCOLOGY/HIV P. 1227
A DIVISION OF GLAXO WELLCOME INC.

2 mg/mL per 20-mL vial
Also available in 2-mL vial

Zofran® Injection
(ondansetron HCl)

RX   GLAXO WELLCOME ONCOLOGY/HIV P. 1227
A DIVISION OF GLAXO WELLCOME INC.

32 mg/50 mL

Zofran® Injection Premixed
(ondansetron HCl)

GLENWOOD-PALISADES

RX   GLENWOOD-PALISADES   P. 1234

500 mg

Potaba®
(aminobenzoate potassium)

RX   GLENWOOD-PALISADES   P. 1234

2.0 grams

Potaba Envules®
(aminobenzoate potassium)

RX   GLENWOOD-PALISADES   P. 1234

5% 30 mL

Scleromate™
(morrhuate sodium injection, USP)

RX   GLENWOOD-PALISADES   P. 1235

5.4 mg

Yocon®
(yohimbine HCl)

HEALTHPOINT

RX   HEALTHPOINT   P. 1236

Accuzyme™
(papain-urea debriding ointment)

Designed to help you identify
drugs, this section contains
actual size pills and full color
reproduction of products
selected for inclusion by
participating manufacturers.

Because tablets and capsules
are shown in this section,
do not infer that these are
the only dosage forms
available. Where a product
name is preceded by the
symbol †, refer to the description in the Product Information
(White Section) for other forms.

HOECHST MARION ROUSSEL

RX   HOECHST MARION ROUSSEL   P. 1244

60 mL

2% Topical Solution
60 mL Bottle with Applicator

2% Topical Gel
30 g Tube
A/T/S®
(erythromycin)

RX   HOECHST MARION ROUSSEL   P. 1238

1.25 mg

2.5 mg

5 mg

10 mg

Altace®
(ramipril)

RX   HOECHST MARION ROUSSEL   P. 1241

1 mg

2 mg

4 mg

Amaryl®
(glimepiride)

RX   HOECHST MARION ROUSSEL   P. 1246

10 mg   20 mg

Bentyl®
(dicyclomine HCl USP)

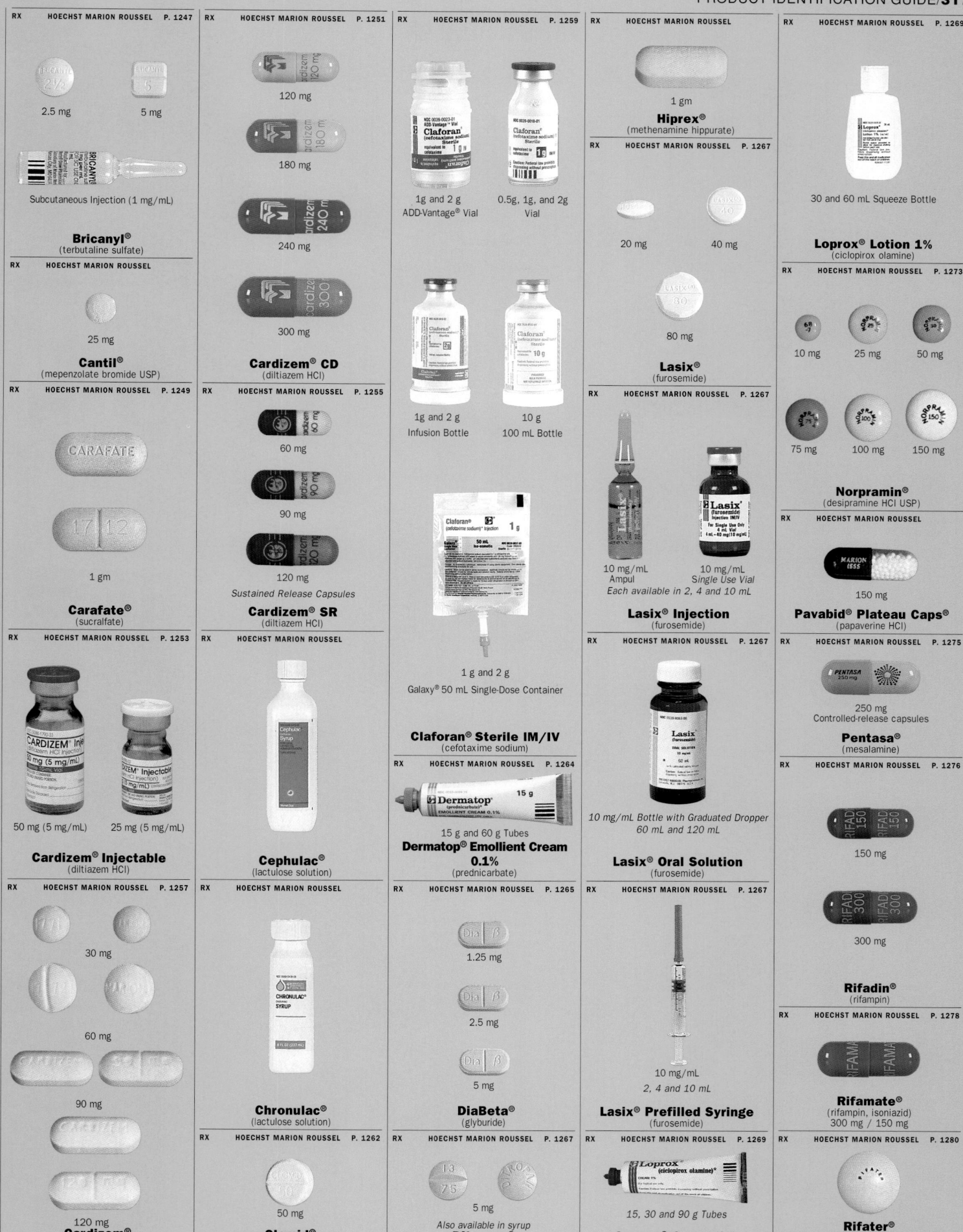

RX   HOECHST MARION ROUSSEL   P. 1247

2.5 mg   5 mg

Subcutaneous Injection (1 mg/mL)

Bricanyl®
(terbutaline sulfate)

RX   HOECHST MARION ROUSSEL

25 mg

Cantil®
(mepenzolate bromide USP)

RX   HOECHST MARION ROUSSEL   P. 1249

CARAFATE

17 12

1 gm

Carafate®
(sucralfate)

RX   HOECHST MARION ROUSSEL   P. 1253

50 mg (5 mg/mL)   25 mg (5 mg/mL)

Cardizem® Injectable
(diltiazem HCl)

RX   HOECHST MARION ROUSSEL   P. 1257

30 mg

60 mg

90 mg

120 mg

Cardizem®
(diltiazem HCl)

RX   HOECHST MARION ROUSSEL   P. 1251

120 mg

180 mg

240 mg

300 mg

Cardizem® CD
(diltiazem HCl)

RX   HOECHST MARION ROUSSEL   P. 1255

60 mg

90 mg

120 mg

Sustained Release Capsules

Cardizem® SR
(diltiazem HCl)

RX   HOECHST MARION ROUSSEL

CHRONULAC®
SYRUP

Chronulac®
(lactulose solution)

RX   HOECHST MARION ROUSSEL   P. 1262

50 mg

Clomid®
(clomiphene citrate USP)

RX   HOECHST MARION ROUSSEL   P. 1259

Claforan®
(cefotaxime sodium)
Sterile

1g and 2 g
ADD-Vantage® Vial

Claforan®
(cefotaxime sodium)
Sterile

0.5g, 1g, and 2g
Vial

Claforan
Sterile

1g and 2 g
Infusion Bottle

Claforan®
(cefotaxime sodium)
Sterile
10 g

10 g
100 mL Bottle

Claforan®
(cefotaxime sodium)¹ Injection
1 g

1 g and 2 g
Galaxy® 50 mL Single-Dose Container

Claforan® Sterile IM/IV
(cefotaxime sodium)

RX   HOECHST MARION ROUSSEL   P. 1264

Dermatop®
(prednicarbate)
EMOLLIENT CREAM 0.1%   15 g

15 g and 60 g Tubes

Dermatop® Emollient Cream 0.1%
(prednicarbate)

RX   HOECHST MARION ROUSSEL   P. 1265

Dia | β
1.25 mg

Dia | β
2.5 mg

Dia | β
5 mg

DiaBeta®
(glyburide)

RX   HOECHST MARION ROUSSEL   P. 1267

5 mg
Also available in syrup

Ditropan®
(oxybutynin chloride)

RX   HOECHST MARION ROUSSEL

1 gm

Hiprex®
(methenamine hippurate)

RX   HOECHST MARION ROUSSEL   P. 1267

20 mg   40 mg

80 mg

Lasix®
(furosemide)

RX   HOECHST MARION ROUSSEL   P. 1267

Lasix®

Lasix®
(furosemide)
Injection IM/IV

10 mg/mL
Ampul

10 mg/mL
Single Use Vial
Each available in 2, 4 and 10 mL

Lasix® Injection
(furosemide)

RX   HOECHST MARION ROUSSEL   P. 1267

Lasix®
(furosemide)
ORAL SOLUTION
10 mg/mL

10 mg/mL Bottle with Graduated Dropper
60 mL and 120 mL

Lasix® Oral Solution
(furosemide)

RX   HOECHST MARION ROUSSEL   P. 1267

10 mg/mL
2, 4 and 10 mL

Lasix® Prefilled Syringe
(furosemide)

RX   HOECHST MARION ROUSSEL   P. 1269

Loprox®
(ciclopirox olamine)

15, 30 and 90 g Tubes

Loprox® Cream 1%
(ciclopirox olamine)

RX   HOECHST MARION ROUSSEL   P. 1269

30 and 60 mL Squeeze Bottle

Loprox® Lotion 1%
(ciclopirox olamine)

RX   HOECHST MARION ROUSSEL   P. 1273

10 mg   25 mg   50 mg

75 mg   100 mg   150 mg

Norpramin®
(desipramine HCl USP)

RX   HOECHST MARION ROUSSEL

MARION 1555

150 mg

Pavabid® Plateau Caps®
(papaverine HCl)

RX   HOECHST MARION ROUSSEL   P. 1275

PENTASA 250 mg

250 mg
Controlled-release capsules

Pentasa®
(mesalamine)

RX   HOECHST MARION ROUSSEL   P. 1276

RIFAD 150

150 mg

RIFAD 300

300 mg

Rifadin®
(rifampin)

RX   HOECHST MARION ROUSSEL   P. 1278

RIFAMA

Rifamate®
(rifampin, isoniazid)
300 mg / 150 mg

RX   HOECHST MARION ROUSSEL   P. 1280

RIFATE

Rifater®
(rifampin, isoniazid, pyrazinamide)
120 mg / 50 mg / 300 mg

RX   HOECHST MARION ROUSSEL   P. 1253

Cephulac
Syrup

Cephulac®
(lactulose solution)

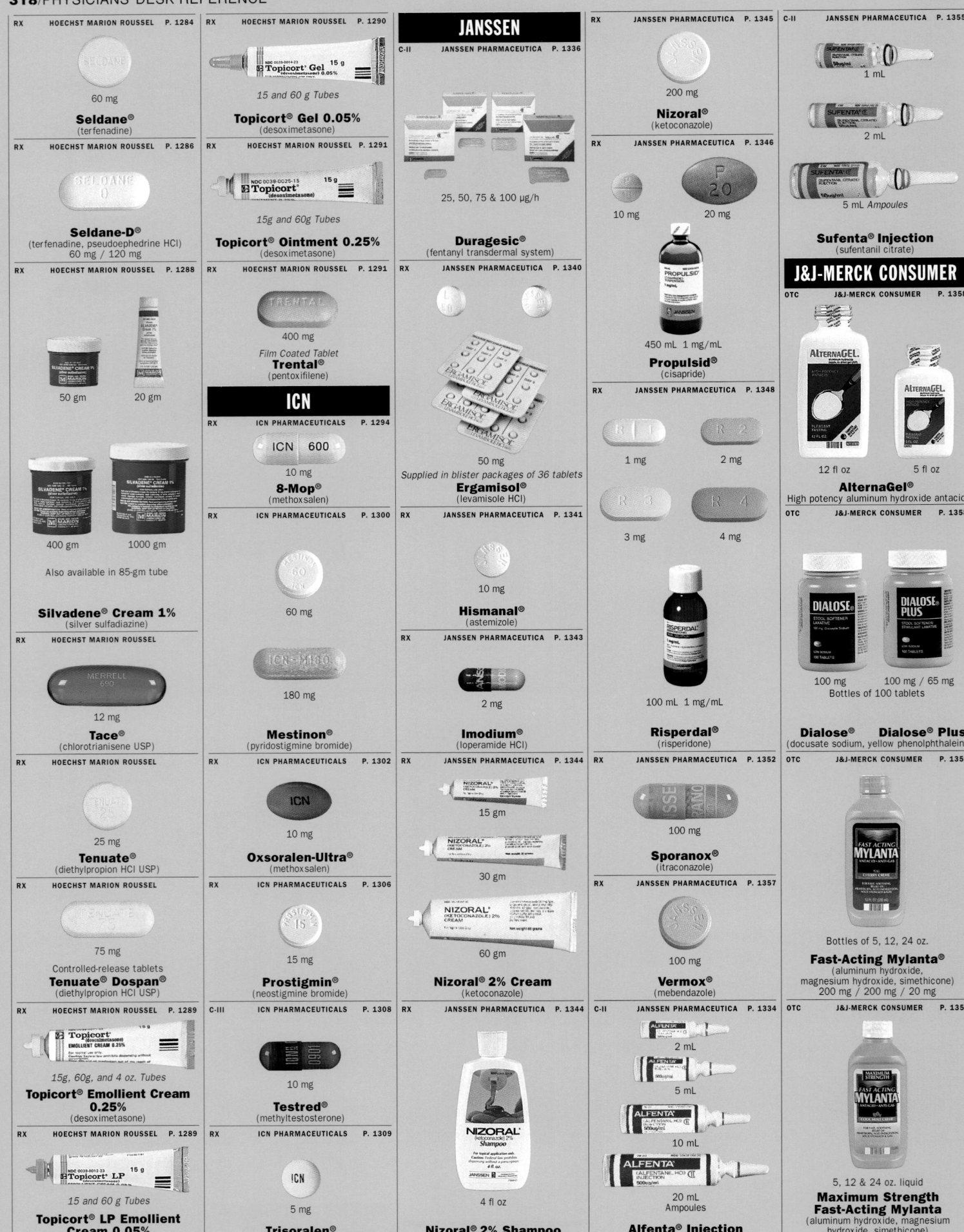

RX HOECHST MARION ROUSSEL P. 1284

60 mg

Seldane®
(terfenadine)

RX HOECHST MARION ROUSSEL P. 1286

Seldane-D®
(terfenadine, pseudoephedrine HCl)
60 mg / 120 mg

RX HOECHST MARION ROUSSEL P. 1288

50 gm   20 gm

400 gm   1000 gm

Also available in 85-gm tube

Silvadene® Cream 1%
(silver sulfadiazine)

RX HOECHST MARION ROUSSEL

12 mg

Tace®
(chlorotrianisene USP)

RX HOECHST MARION ROUSSEL

25 mg

Tenuate®
(diethylpropion HCl USP)

RX HOECHST MARION ROUSSEL

75 mg

Controlled-release tablets
Tenuate® Dospan®
(diethylpropion HCl USP)

RX HOECHST MARION ROUSSEL P. 1289

15g, 60g, and 4 oz. Tubes
**Topicort® Emollient Cream
0.25%**
(desoximetasone)

RX HOECHST MARION ROUSSEL P. 1289

15 and 60 g Tubes
**Topicort® LP Emollient
Cream 0.05%**
(desoximetasone)

RX HOECHST MARION ROUSSEL P. 1290

15 and 60 g Tubes
Topicort® Gel 0.05%
(desoximetasone)

RX HOECHST MARION ROUSSEL P. 1291

15g and 60g Tubes
Topicort® Ointment 0.25%
(desoximetasone)

RX HOECHST MARION ROUSSEL P. 1291

400 mg
Film Coated Tablet
Trental®
(pentoxifilene)

ICN

RX ICN PHARMACEUTICALS P. 1294

ICN 600
10 mg
8-Mop®
(methoxsalen)

RX ICN PHARMACEUTICALS P. 1300

60 mg

180 mg
Mestinon®
(pyridostigmine bromide)

RX ICN PHARMACEUTICALS P. 1302

10 mg
Oxsoralen-Ultra®
(methoxsalen)

RX ICN PHARMACEUTICALS P. 1306

15 mg
Prostigmin®
(neostigmine bromide)

C-III ICN PHARMACEUTICALS P. 1308

10 mg
Testred®
(methyltestosterone)

RX ICN PHARMACEUTICALS P. 1309

5 mg
Trisoralen®
(trioxsalen)

JANSSEN

C-II JANSSEN PHARMACEUTICA P. 1336

25, 50, 75 & 100 µg/h
Duragesic®
(fentanyl transdermal system)

RX JANSSEN PHARMACEUTICA P. 1340

50 mg
Supplied in blister packages of 36 tablets
Ergamisol®
(levamisole HCl)

RX JANSSEN PHARMACEUTICA P. 1341

10 mg
Hismanal®
(astemizole)

RX JANSSEN PHARMACEUTICA P. 1343

2 mg
Imodium®
(loperamide HCl)

RX JANSSEN PHARMACEUTICA P. 1344

15 gm

30 gm

60 gm
Nizoral® 2% Cream
(ketoconazole)

RX JANSSEN PHARMACEUTICA P. 1344

4 fl oz
Nizoral® 2% Shampoo
(ketoconazole)

RX JANSSEN PHARMACEUTICA P. 1345

200 mg
Nizoral®
(ketoconazole)

RX JANSSEN PHARMACEUTICA P. 1346

10 mg   20 mg
P 20

450 mL 1 mg/mL
Propulsid®
(cisapride)

RX JANSSEN PHARMACEUTICA P. 1348

R 1   R 2
1 mg   2 mg

R 3   R 4
3 mg   4 mg

100 mL 1 mg/mL
Risperdal®
(risperidone)

RX JANSSEN PHARMACEUTICA P. 1352

100 mg
Sporanox®
(itraconazole)

RX JANSSEN PHARMACEUTICA P. 1357

100 mg
Vermox®
(mebendazole)

C-II JANSSEN PHARMACEUTICA P. 1334

2 mL

5 mL

10 mL

20 mL
Ampoules
Alfenta® Injection
(alfentanil HCl)

C-II JANSSEN PHARMACEUTICA P. 1355

1 mL

2 mL

5 mL Ampoules
Sufenta® Injection
(sufentanil citrate)

J&J-MERCK CONSUMER

OTC J&J-MERCK CONSUMER P. 1358

12 fl oz   5 fl oz
AlternaGel®
High potency aluminum hydroxide antacid

OTC J&J-MERCK CONSUMER P. 1358

100 mg   100 mg / 65 mg
Bottles of 100 tablets
Dialose®   Dialose® Plus
(docusate sodium, yellow phenolphthalein)

OTC J&J-MERCK CONSUMER P. 1359

Bottles of 5, 12, 24 oz.
Fast-Acting Mylanta®
(aluminum hydroxide,
magnesium hydroxide, simethicone)
200 mg / 200 mg / 20 mg

OTC J&J-MERCK CONSUMER P. 1359

5, 12 & 24 oz. liquid
**Maximum Strength
Fast-Acting Mylanta**
(aluminum hydroxide, magnesium
hydroxide, simethicone)
400 mg / 400 mg / 40 mg

OTC   J&J-MERCK CONSUMER   P. 1360

80 mg
12 & 30 tablet convenience packs,
bottles of 60 and 100

Mylanta® Gas
(simethicone)

OTC   J&J-MERCK CONSUMER   P. 1360

125 mg
12 & 24 tablet convenience packs

**Maximum Strength
Mylanta® Gas**
(simethicone)

OTC   J&J-MERCK CONSUMER   P. 1360

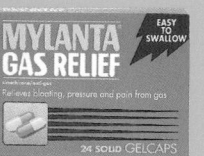

Boxes of 24 and 60 gelcaps

**Mylanta® Gas Relief
Gelcaps**
(simethicone, 62.5 mg)

OTC   J&J-MERCK CONSUMER

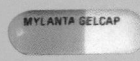

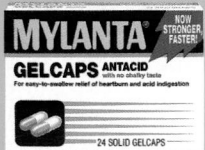

Available in 6's, 12's, 50's and 80's

Mylanta® Gelcaps Antacid
(calcium carbonate, magnesium carbonate)
311 mg / 232 mg

OTC   J&J-MERCK CONSUMER   P. 1360

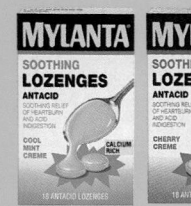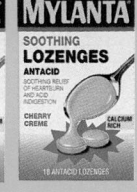

Available in boxes of 18 Lozenges
and bottles of 50

Mylanta® Soothing Lozenges
(calcium carbonate, 600 mg)

OTC   J&J-MERCK CONSUMER

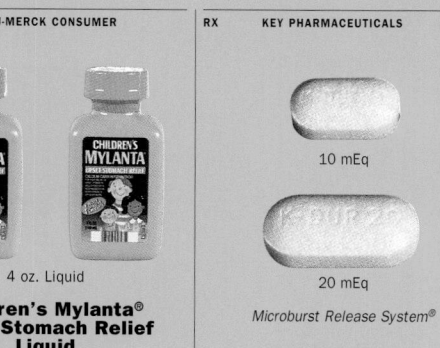

4 oz. Liquid

**Children's Mylanta®
Upset Stomach Relief
Liquid**
(calcium carbonate)
400 mg / 5 mL

OTC   J&J-MERCK CONSUMER

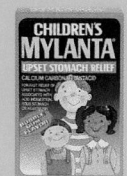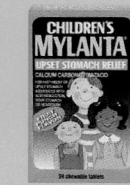

Boxes of 24 tablets.

**Children's Mylanta®
Upset Stomach Relief
Tablets**
(calcium carbonate, 400 mg)

OTC   J&J-MERCK CONSUMER   P. 1358

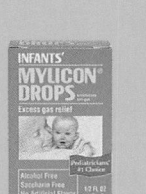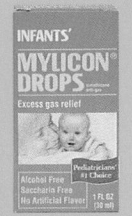

Available in 0.5 oz and 1.0 oz bottles

Infants Mylicon® Drops
(simethicone)

OTC   J&J-MERCK CONSUMER   P. 1360

**Pepcid
AC® Acid
Controller.**

Available in 6's, 12's, 50's and 80's

Pepcid AC®
(famotidine)

KEY

RX   KEY PHARMACEUTICALS   P. 1362

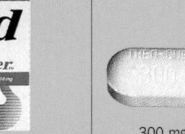
30 mg

60 mg

120 mg

Imdur™
(isosorbide mononitrate)

RX   KEY PHARMACEUTICALS   P. 1364

10 mEq

20 mEq

Microburst Release System®

K-Dur®
(potassium chloride USP)

RX   KEY PHARMACEUTICALS   P. 1365

0.1 mg/hr   0.2 mg/hr

0.3 mg/hr   0.4 mg/hr

0.6 mg/hr

Transdermal Infusion System

Nitro Dur®
(nitroglycerin)

RX   KEY PHARMACEUTICALS   P. 1367

100 mg   200 mg

300 mg   450 mg

Extended release tablets

Theo-Dur®
(theophylline anhydrous)

RX   KEY PHARMACEUTICALS   P. 1373

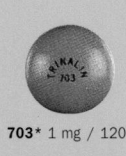

703* 1 mg / 120 mg

*Long acting
antihistamine/decongestant*

Trinalin® Repetabs®
(azatadine maleate USP,
pseudoephedrine sulfate USP)

KEY PHARMACEUTICALS   P. 1374

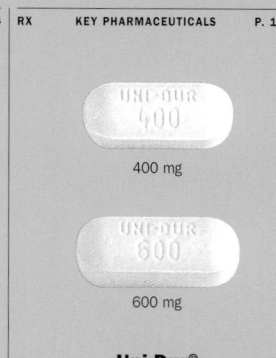
400 mg

600 mg

Uni-Dur®
(theophylline)

KNOLL LABORATORIES

C-II   KNOLL LABORATORIES   P. 1380

2 mg

†Akineton®
(biperiden HCl)

C-II   KNOLL LABORATORIES   P. 1382

2 mg   4 mg   8 mg

†Dilaudid®
(hydromorphone HCl)

C-II   KNOLL LABORATORIES   P. 1384

10 mg/mL

Dilaudid-HP®
(hydromorphone HCl)

C-II   KNOLL LABORATORIES   P. 1384

50 mg/5 mL

Dilaudid-HP®
(hydromorphone HCl)

C-II   KNOLL LABORATORIES   P. 1384

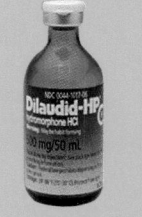
500 mg/50 mL

Dilaudid-HP®
(hydromorphone HCl)

RX   KNOLL LABORATORIES   P. 1384

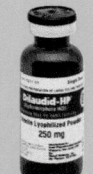
250 mg
Sterile Lyophilized Powder

Dilaudid-HP®
(hydromorphone HCl)

RX   KNOLL LABORATORIES   P. 1388

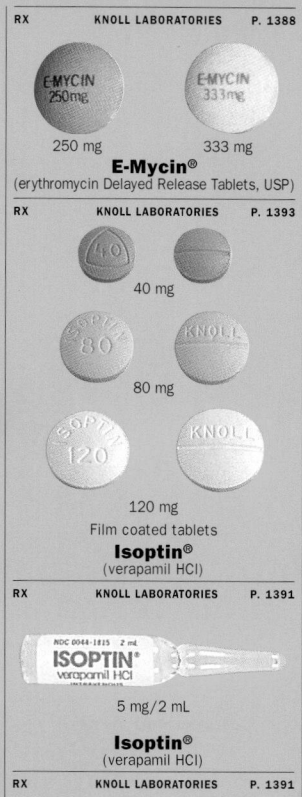
250 mg   333 mg

E-Mycin®
(erythromycin Delayed Release Tablets, USP)

RX   KNOLL LABORATORIES   P. 1393

40 mg

80 mg

120 mg

Film coated tablets

Isoptin®
(verapamil HCl)

RX   KNOLL LABORATORIES   P. 1391

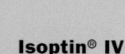
5 mg/2 mL

Isoptin®
(verapamil HCl)

RX   KNOLL LABORATORIES   P. 1391

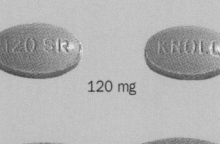
5 mg/2 mL
Single dose vial

Isoptin® IV
(verapamil HCl)

RX   KNOLL LABORATORIES   P. 1395

120 mg

180 mg

240 mg

Film-coated tablets sustained
release oral tablets

Isoptin® SR
(verapamil HCl)

RX   KNOLL LABORATORIES   P. 1398

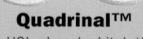

Quadrinal™
(ephedrine HCl, phenobarbital, theophylline
calcium salicylate, potassium iodide)
24 mg/24 mg/130 mg/320 mg

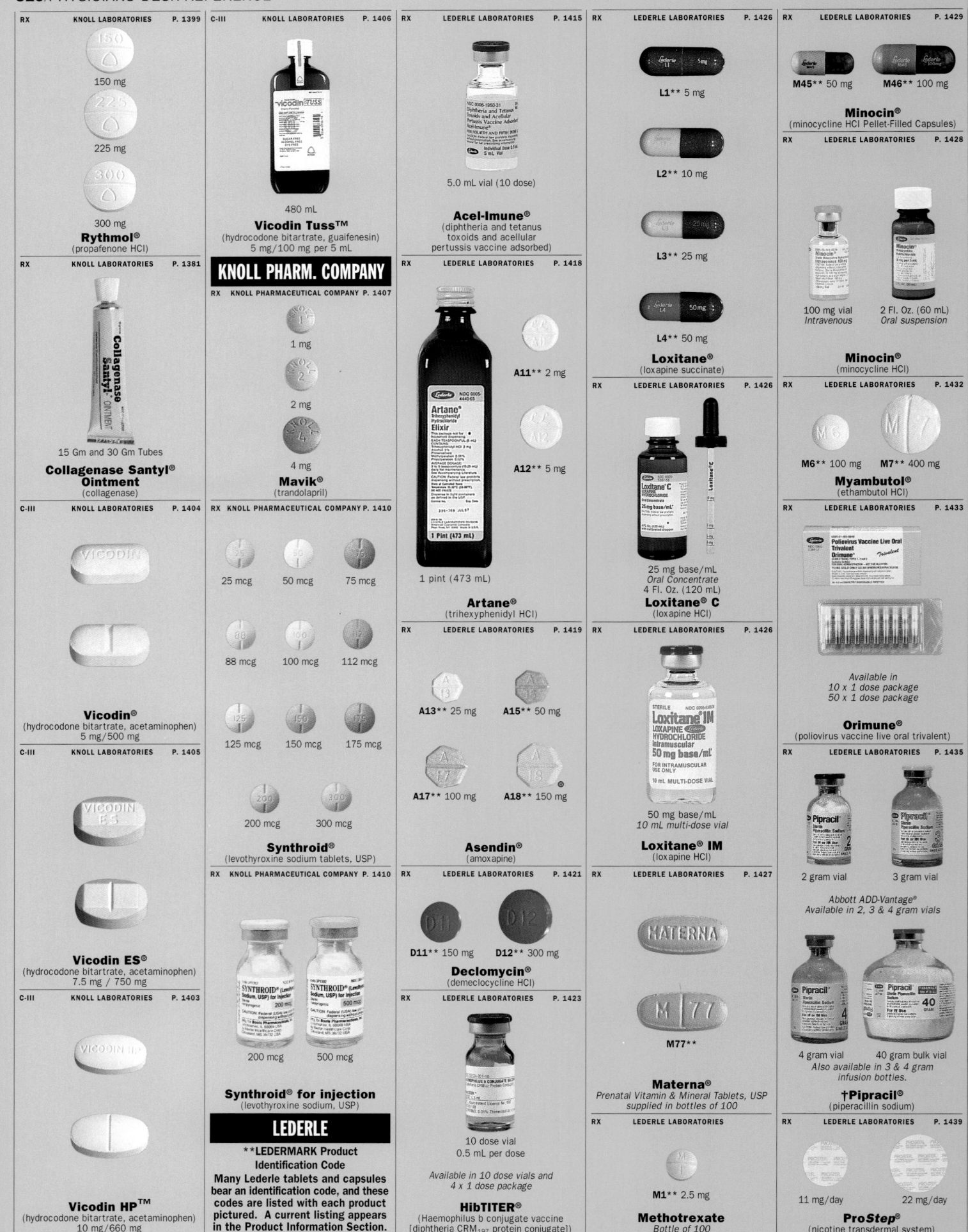

RX KNOLL LABORATORIES P. 1399

150 mg

225 mg

300 mg

Rythmol®
(propafenone HCl)

RX KNOLL LABORATORIES P. 1381

15 Gm and 30 Gm Tubes

**Collagenase Santyl®
Ointment**
(collagenase)

C-III KNOLL LABORATORIES P. 1404

VICODIN

Vicodin®
(hydrocodone bitartrate, acetaminophen)
5 mg/500 mg

C-III KNOLL LABORATORIES P. 1405

VICODIN ES

Vicodin ES®
(hydrocodone bitartrate, acetaminophen)
7.5 mg / 750 mg

C-III KNOLL LABORATORIES P. 1403

VICODIN HP

Vicodin HP™
(hydrocodone bitartrate, acetaminophen)
10 mg/660 mg

C-III KNOLL LABORATORIES P. 1406

480 mL

Vicodin Tuss™
(hydrocodone bitartrate, guaifenesin)
5 mg/100 mg per 5 mL

KNOLL PHARM. COMPANY

RX KNOLL PHARMACEUTICAL COMPANY P. 1407

1 mg

2 mg

4 mg

Mavik®
(trandolapril)

RX KNOLL PHARMACEUTICAL COMPANY P. 1410

25 mcg   50 mcg   75 mcg

88 mcg   100 mcg   112 mcg

125 mcg   150 mcg   175 mcg

200 mcg   300 mcg

Synthroid®
(levothyroxine sodium tablets, USP)

RX KNOLL PHARMACEUTICAL COMPANY P. 1410

200 mcg   500 mcg

Synthroid® for injection
(levothyroxine sodium, USP)

LEDERLE

RX LEDERLE LABORATORIES P. 1415

5.0 mL vial (10 dose)

Acel-Imune®
(diphtheria and tetanus
toxoids and acellular
pertussis vaccine adsorbed)

RX LEDERLE LABORATORIES P. 1418

A11** 2 mg

A12** 5 mg

Artane®
(trihexyphenidyl HCl)

RX LEDERLE LABORATORIES P. 1419

A13** 25 mg   **A15**** 50 mg

A17** 100 mg   **A18**** 150 mg ®

Asendin®
(amoxapine)

RX LEDERLE LABORATORIES P. 1421

D11** 150 mg   **D12**** 300 mg

Declomycin®
(demeclocycline HCl)

RX LEDERLE LABORATORIES P. 1423

10 dose vial
0.5 mL per dose

*Available in 10 dose vials and
4 x 1 dose package*

HibTITER®
(Haemophilus b conjugate vaccine
[diphtheria CRM$_{197}$ protein conjugate])

RX LEDERLE LABORATORIES P. 1426

L1** 5 mg

L2** 10 mg

L3** 25 mg

L4** 50 mg

Loxitane®
(loxapine succinate)

RX LEDERLE LABORATORIES P. 1426

25 mg base/mL
Oral Concentrate
4 Fl. Oz. (120 mL)

Loxitane® C
(loxapine HCl)

RX LEDERLE LABORATORIES P. 1426

50 mg base/mL
10 mL multi-dose vial

Loxitane® IM
(loxapine HCl)

RX LEDERLE LABORATORIES P. 1427

MATERNA

M|77

M77**

Materna®
*Prenatal Vitamin & Mineral Tablets, USP
supplied in bottles of 100*

RX LEDERLE LABORATORIES

M1** 2.5 mg

Methotrexate
Bottle of 100

RX LEDERLE LABORATORIES P. 1429

M45** 50 mg   **M46**** 100 mg

Minocin®
(minocycline HCl Pellet-Filled Capsules)

RX LEDERLE LABORATORIES P. 1428

100 mg vial
Intravenous

2 Fl. Oz. (60 mL)
Oral suspension

Minocin®
(minocycline HCl)

RX LEDERLE LABORATORIES P. 1432

M6** 100 mg   **M7**** 400 mg

Myambutol®
(ethambutol HCl)

RX LEDERLE LABORATORIES P. 1433

*Available in
10 x 1 dose package
50 x 1 dose package*

Orimune®
(poliovirus vaccine live oral trivalent)

RX LEDERLE LABORATORIES P. 1435

2 gram vial   3 gram vial

*Abbott ADD-Vantage®
Available in 2, 3 & 4 gram vials*

4 gram vial   40 gram bulk vial
*Also available in 3 & 4 gram
infusion bottles.*

†Pipracil®
(piperacillin sodium)

RX LEDERLE LABORATORIES P. 1439

11 mg/day   22 mg/day

ProStep®
(nicotine transdermal system)

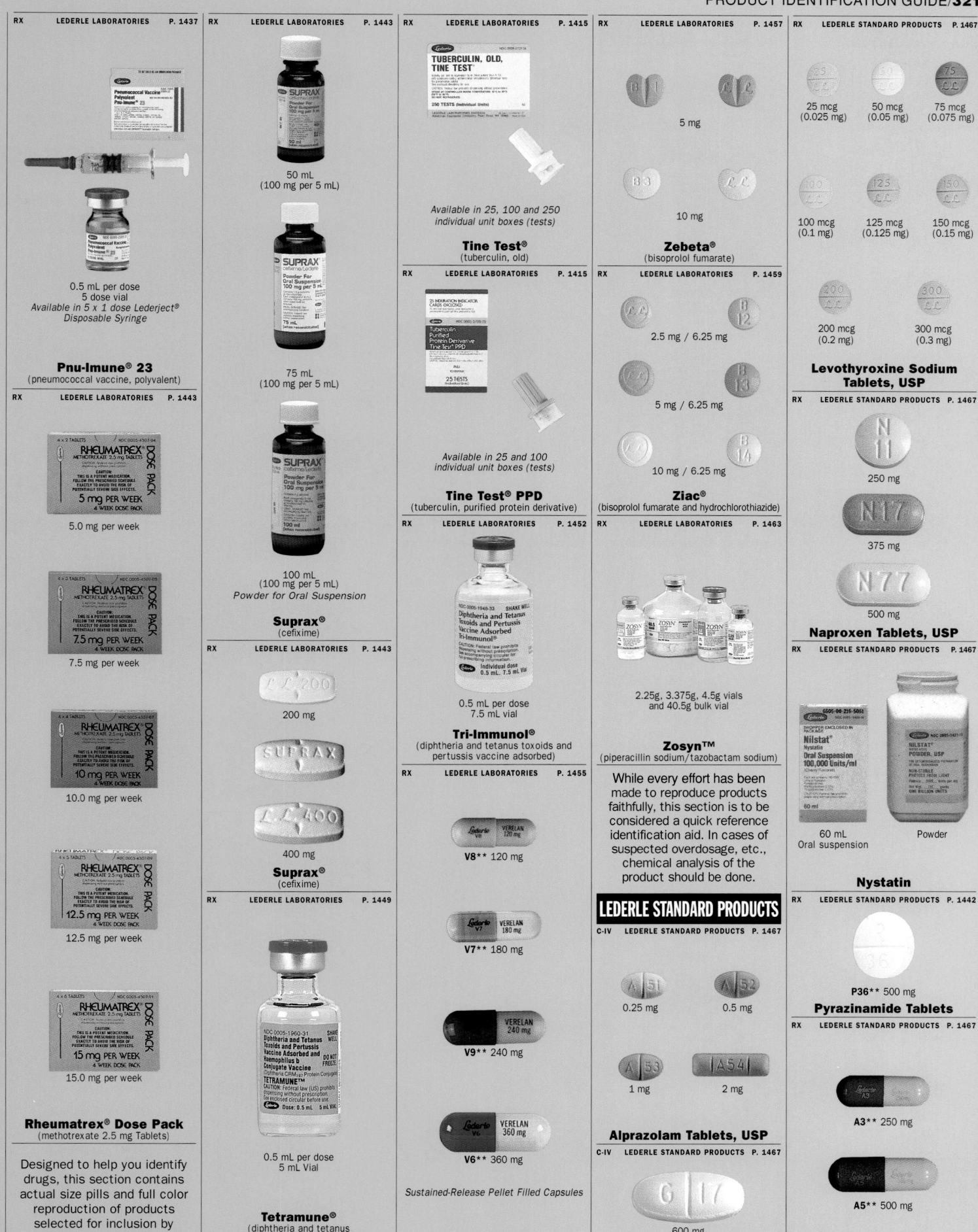

RX LEDERLE LABORATORIES P. 1437

0.5 mL per dose
5 dose vial
*Available in 5 x 1 dose Lederject®
Disposable Syringe*

Pnu-Imune® 23
(pneumococcal vaccine, polyvalent)

RX LEDERLE LABORATORIES P. 1443

5 mg PER WEEK
4 WEEK DOSE PACK
5.0 mg per week

7.5 mg PER WEEK
4 WEEK DOSE PACK
7.5 mg per week

10 mg PER WEEK
4 WEEK DOSE PACK
10.0 mg per week

12.5 mg PER WEEK
4 WEEK DOSE PACK
12.5 mg per week

15 mg PER WEEK
4 WEEK DOSE PACK
15.0 mg per week

Rheumatrex® Dose Pack
(methotrexate 2.5 mg Tablets)

Designed to help you identify drugs, this section contains actual size pills and full color reproduction of products selected for inclusion by participating manufacturers.

RX LEDERLE LABORATORIES P. 1443

50 mL
(100 mg per 5 mL)

75 mL
(100 mg per 5 mL)

100 mL
(100 mg per 5 mL)
Powder for Oral Suspension

Suprax®
(cefixime)

RX LEDERLE LABORATORIES P. 1443

200 mg

400 mg

Suprax®
(cefixime)

RX LEDERLE LABORATORIES P. 1449

0.5 mL per dose
5 mL Vial

Tetramune®
(diphtheria and tetanus toxoids and pertussis vaccine adsorbed and Haemophilus b conjugate vaccine [diphtheria CRM$_{197}$ protein conjugate])

RX LEDERLE LABORATORIES P. 1415

TUBERCULIN, OLD, TINE TEST®

250 TESTS (Individual Units)

Available in 25, 100 and 250 individual unit boxes (tests)

Tine Test®
(tuberculin, old)

RX LEDERLE LABORATORIES P. 1415

Available in 25 and 100 individual unit boxes (tests)

Tine Test® PPD
(tuberculin, purified protein derivative)

RX LEDERLE LABORATORIES P. 1452

0.5 mL per dose
7.5 mL vial

Tri-Immunol®
(diphtheria and tetanus toxoids and pertussis vaccine adsorbed)

RX LEDERLE LABORATORIES P. 1455

V8** 120 mg

V7** 180 mg

V9** 240 mg

V6** 360 mg

Sustained-Release Pellet Filled Capsules

Verelan®
(verapamil HCl)

RX LEDERLE LABORATORIES P. 1457

5 mg

10 mg

Zebeta®
(bisoprolol fumarate)

RX LEDERLE LABORATORIES P. 1459

2.5 mg / 6.25 mg

5 mg / 6.25 mg

10 mg / 6.25 mg

Ziac®
(bisoprolol fumarate and hydrochlorothiazide)

RX LEDERLE LABORATORIES P. 1463

2.25g, 3.375g, 4.5g vials and 40.5g bulk vial

Zosyn™
(piperacillin sodium/tazobactam sodium)

While every effort has been made to reproduce products faithfully, this section is to be considered a quick reference identification aid. In cases of suspected overdosage, etc., chemical analysis of the product should be done.

LEDERLE STANDARD PRODUCTS

C-IV LEDERLE STANDARD PRODUCTS P. 1467

0.25 mg

0.5 mg

1 mg

2 mg

Alprazolam Tablets, USP

C-IV LEDERLE STANDARD PRODUCTS P. 1467

600 mg

Gemfibrozil Tablets, USP

RX LEDERLE STANDARD PRODUCTS P. 1467

25 mcg
(0.025 mg)

50 mcg
(0.05 mg)

75 mcg
(0.075 mg)

100 mcg
(0.1 mg)

125 mcg
(0.125 mg)

150 mcg
(0.15 mg)

200 mcg
(0.2 mg)

300 mcg
(0.3 mg)

Levothyroxine Sodium Tablets, USP

RX LEDERLE STANDARD PRODUCTS P. 1467

250 mg

375 mg

500 mg

Naproxen Tablets, USP

RX LEDERLE STANDARD PRODUCTS P. 1467

60 mL
Oral suspension

Powder

Nystatin

RX LEDERLE STANDARD PRODUCTS P. 1442

P36** 500 mg

Pyrazinamide Tablets

RX LEDERLE STANDARD PRODUCTS P. 1467

A3** 250 mg

A5** 500 mg

†Tetracycline HCl Capsules

**LEDERMARK Product Identification Code / ®: Unique tablet shapes are trademarks of American Cyanamid Company.

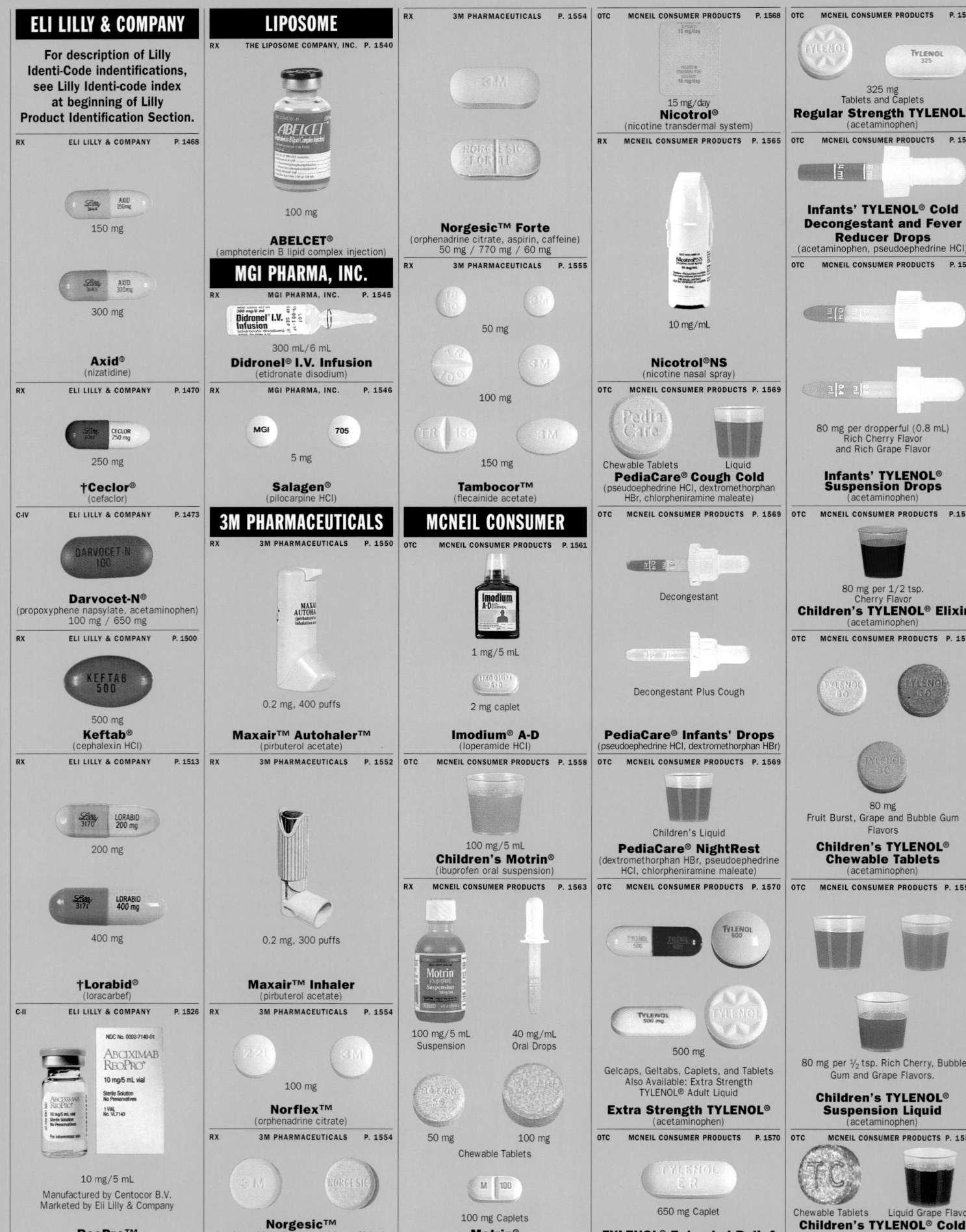

ELI LILLY & COMPANY

For description of Lilly
Identi-Code indentifications,
see Lilly Identi-code index
at beginning of Lilly
Product Identification Section.

RX   ELI LILLY & COMPANY   P. 1468

150 mg

300 mg

Axid®
(nizatidine)

RX   ELI LILLY & COMPANY   P. 1470

250 mg

†Ceclor®
(cefaclor)

C-IV   ELI LILLY & COMPANY   P. 1473

Darvocet-N®
(propoxyphene napsylate, acetaminophen)
100 mg / 650 mg

RX   ELI LILLY & COMPANY   P. 1500

500 mg

Keftab®
(cephalexin HCl)

RX   ELI LILLY & COMPANY   P. 1513

200 mg

400 mg

†Lorabid®
(loracarbef)

C-II   ELI LILLY & COMPANY   P. 1526

10 mg/5 mL
Manufactured by Centocor B.V.
Marketed by Eli Lilly & Company

ReoPro™
(abciximab)

LIPOSOME

RX   THE LIPOSOME COMPANY, INC.   P. 1540

100 mg

ABELCET®
(amphotericin B lipid complex injection)

MGI PHARMA, INC.

RX   MGI PHARMA, INC.   P. 1545

300 mL/6 mL
Didronel® I.V. Infusion
(etidronate disodium)

RX   MGI PHARMA, INC.   P. 1546

5 mg

Salagen®
(pilocarpine HCl)

3M PHARMACEUTICALS

RX   3M PHARMACEUTICALS   P. 1550

0.2 mg, 400 puffs

Maxair™ Autohaler™
(pirbuterol acetate)

RX   3M PHARMACEUTICALS   P. 1552

0.2 mg, 300 puffs

Maxair™ Inhaler
(pirbuterol acetate)

RX   3M PHARMACEUTICALS   P. 1554

100 mg

Norflex™
(orphenadrine citrate)

RX   3M PHARMACEUTICALS   P. 1554

Norgesic™
(orphenadrine citrate, aspirin, caffeine)
25 mg / 385 mg / 30 mg

RX   3M PHARMACEUTICALS   P. 1554

Norgesic™ Forte
(orphenadrine citrate, aspirin, caffeine)
50 mg / 770 mg / 60 mg

RX   3M PHARMACEUTICALS   P. 1555

50 mg

100 mg

150 mg

Tambocor™
(flecainide acetate)

MCNEIL CONSUMER

OTC   MCNEIL CONSUMER PRODUCTS   P. 1561

1 mg/5 mL

2 mg caplet

Imodium® A-D
(loperamide HCl)

OTC   MCNEIL CONSUMER PRODUCTS   P. 1558

100 mg/5 mL

Children's Motrin®
(ibuprofen oral suspension)

RX   MCNEIL CONSUMER PRODUCTS   P. 1563

100 mg/5 mL
Suspension

40 mg/mL
Oral Drops

50 mg   100 mg
Chewable Tablets

100 mg Caplets

Motrin®
(ibuprofen)

OTC   MCNEIL CONSUMER PRODUCTS   P. 1568

15 mg/day
Nicotrol®
(nicotine transdermal system)

RX   MCNEIL CONSUMER PRODUCTS   P. 1565

10 mg/mL

Nicotrol®NS
(nicotine nasal spray)

OTC   MCNEIL CONSUMER PRODUCTS   P. 1569

Chewable Tablets   Liquid

PediaCare® Cough Cold
(pseudoephedrine HCl, dextromethorphan
HBr, chlorpheniramine maleate)

OTC   MCNEIL CONSUMER PRODUCTS   P. 1569

Decongestant

Decongestant Plus Cough

PediaCare® Infants' Drops
(pseudoephedrine HCl, dextromethorphan HBr)

OTC   MCNEIL CONSUMER PRODUCTS   P. 1569

Children's Liquid

PediaCare® NightRest
(dextromethorphan HBr, pseudoephedrine
HCl, chlorpheniramine maleate)

OTC   MCNEIL CONSUMER PRODUCTS   P. 1570

500 mg
Gelcaps, Geltabs, Caplets, and Tablets
Also Available: Extra Strength
TYLENOL® Adult Liquid

Extra Strength TYLENOL®
(acetaminophen)

OTC   MCNEIL CONSUMER PRODUCTS   P. 1570

650 mg Caplet

TYLENOL® Extended Relief
(acetaminophen extended release)

OTC   MCNEIL CONSUMER PRODUCTS   P. 1570

325 mg
Tablets and Caplets
Regular Strength TYLENOL®
(acetaminophen)

OTC   MCNEIL CONSUMER PRODUCTS   P. 1561

**Infants' TYLENOL® Cold
Decongestant and Fever
Reducer Drops**
(acetaminophen, pseudoephedrine HCl)

OTC   MCNEIL CONSUMER PRODUCTS   P. 1559

80 mg per dropperful (0.8 mL)
Rich Cherry Flavor
and Rich Grape Flavor

**Infants' TYLENOL®
Suspension Drops**
(acetaminophen)

OTC   MCNEIL CONSUMER PRODUCTS   P.1559

80 mg per 1/2 tsp.
Cherry Flavor
Children's TYLENOL® Elixir
(acetaminophen)

OTC   MCNEIL CONSUMER PRODUCTS   P. 1559

80 mg
Fruit Burst, Grape and Bubble Gum
Flavors
**Children's TYLENOL®
Chewable Tablets**
(acetaminophen)

OTC   MCNEIL CONSUMER PRODUCTS   P. 1559

80 mg per ½ tsp. Rich Cherry, Bubble
Gum and Grape Flavors.
**Children's TYLENOL®
Suspension Liquid**
(acetaminophen)

OTC   MCNEIL CONSUMER PRODUCTS   P. 1559

Chewable Tablets   Liquid Grape Flavor
Children's TYLENOL® Cold
(acetaminophen, chlorpheniramine
maleate, pseudoephedrine HCl)

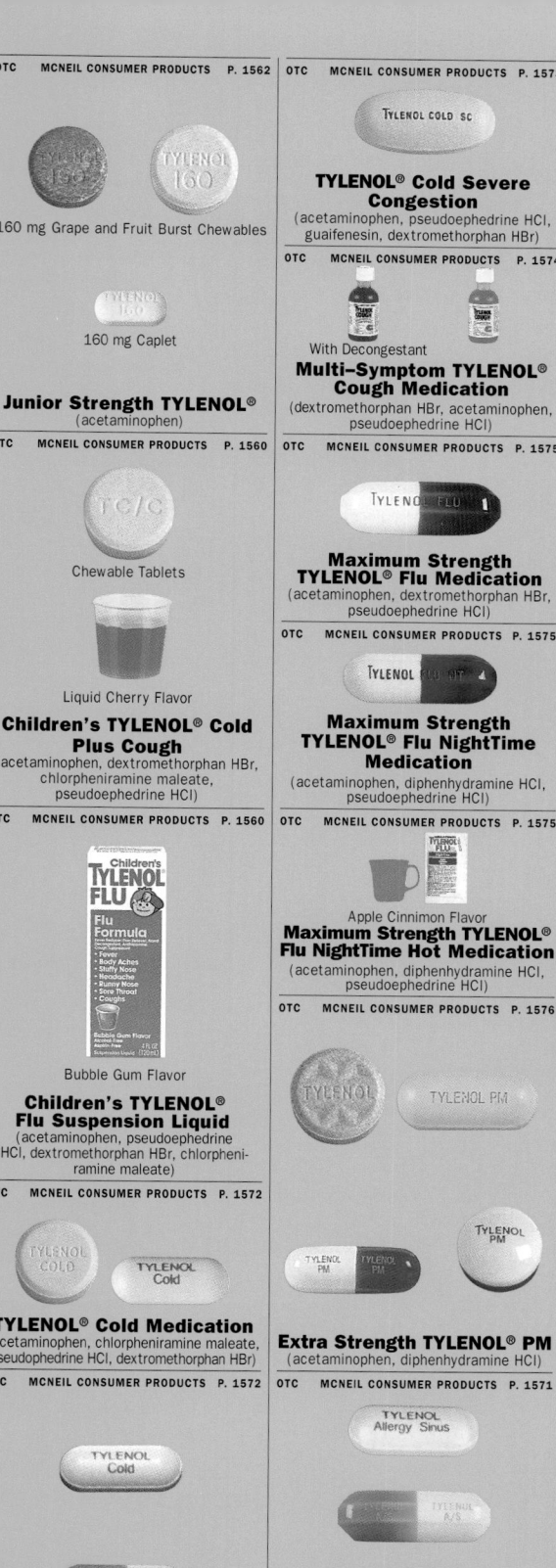

OTC   MCNEIL CONSUMER PRODUCTS   P. 1562

160 mg Grape and Fruit Burst Chewables

160 mg Caplet

Junior Strength TYLENOL®
(acetaminophen)

OTC   MCNEIL CONSUMER PRODUCTS   P. 1560

Chewable Tablets

Liquid Cherry Flavor

Children's TYLENOL® Cold Plus Cough
(acetaminophen, dextromethorphan HBr, chlorpheniramine maleate, pseudoephedrine HCl)

OTC   MCNEIL CONSUMER PRODUCTS   P. 1560

Bubble Gum Flavor

Children's TYLENOL® Flu Suspension Liquid
(acetaminophen, pseudoephedrine HCl, dextromethorphan HBr, chlorpheniramine maleate)

OTC   MCNEIL CONSUMER PRODUCTS   P. 1572

TYLENOL® Cold Medication
(acetaminophen, chlorpheniramine maleate, pseudophedrine HCl, dextromethorphan HBr)

OTC   MCNEIL CONSUMER PRODUCTS   P. 1572

TYLENOL® Cold Medication No Drowsiness Formula
(acetaminophen, pseudophedrine HCl, dextromethorphan HBr)

OTC   MCNEIL CONSUMER PRODUCTS   P. 1572

Honey Lemon Flavor
TYLENOL® Cold Hot Medication
(acetaminophen, chlorpheniramine maleate, pseudoephedrine HCl, dextromethorphan HBr)

OTC   MCNEIL CONSUMER PRODUCTS   P. 1573

TYLENOL® Cold Severe Congestion
(acetaminophen, pseudoephedrine HCl, guaifenesin, dextromethorphan HBr)

OTC   MCNEIL CONSUMER PRODUCTS   P. 1574

With Decongestant
Multi–Symptom TYLENOL® Cough Medication
(dextromethorphan HBr, acetaminophen, pseudoephedrine HCl)

OTC   MCNEIL CONSUMER PRODUCTS   P. 1575

Maximum Strength TYLENOL® Flu Medication
(acetaminophen, dextromethorphan HBr, pseudoephedrine HCl)

OTC   MCNEIL CONSUMER PRODUCTS   P. 1575

Maximum Strength TYLENOL® Flu NightTime Medication
(acetaminophen, diphenhydramine HCl, pseudoephedrine HCl)

OTC   MCNEIL CONSUMER PRODUCTS   P. 1575

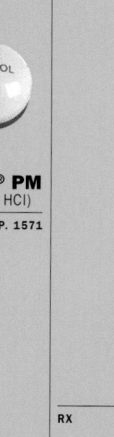

Apple Cinnimon Flavor
Maximum Strength TYLENOL® Flu NightTime Hot Medication
(acetaminophen, diphenhydramine HCl, pseudoephedrine HCl)

OTC   MCNEIL CONSUMER PRODUCTS   P. 1576

Extra Strength TYLENOL® PM
(acetaminophen, diphenhydramine HCl)

OTC   MCNEIL CONSUMER PRODUCTS   P. 1571

TYLENOL® Allergy Sinus

Maximum Strength TYLENOL® Allergy Sinus
(acetaminophen, chlorpheniramine maleate, pseudoephedrine HCl)

OTC   MCNEIL CONSUMER PRODUCTS   P. 1571

TYLENOL A/S Night Time

Maximum Strength TYLENOL® Allergy Sinus NightTime
(acetaminophen, diphenhydramine HCl, pseudoephedrine HCl)

OTC   MCNEIL CONSUMER PRODUCTS   P. 1571

TYLENOL® Severe Allergy
(acetaminophen, diphenhydramine HCl)

OTC   MCNEIL CONSUMER PRODUCTS   P. 1576

TYLENOL SINUS

Maximum Strength TYLENOL® Sinus
(acetaminophen, pseudoephedrine HCl)

OTC   MCNEIL CONSUMER PRODUCTS   P. 1570

Maximum Strength Sine-Aid®
(acetaminophen, pseudoephedrine HCl)

MCNEIL PHARMACEUTICAL

RX   MCNEIL PHARMACEUTICAL   P. 1577

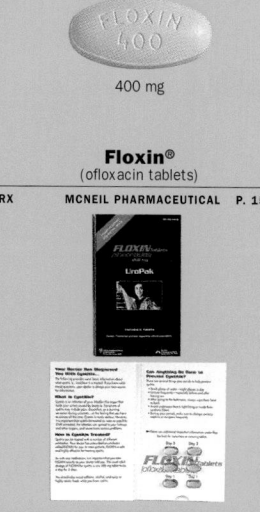

200 mg

300 mg

400 mg

Floxin®
(ofloxacin tablets)

RX   MCNEIL PHARMACEUTICAL   P. 1577

FLOXIN UroPak

6 tablets 200 mg each
Floxin® UroPak
(ofloxacin tablets)

RX   MCNEIL PHARMACEUTICAL   P. 1580

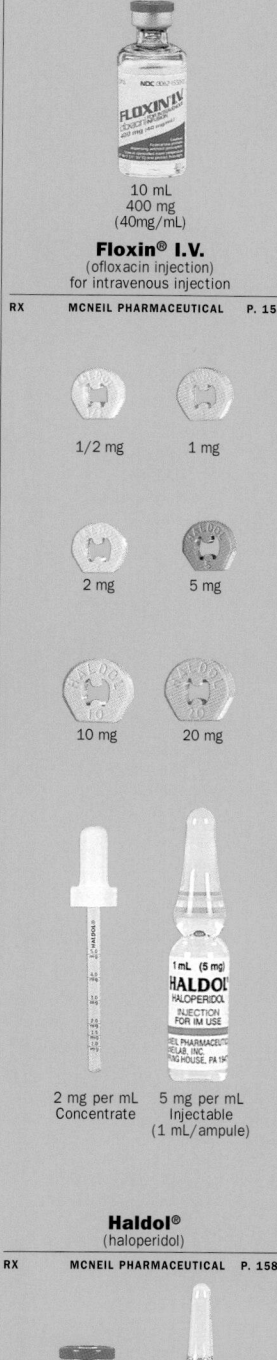

50 mL
200 mg
(4mg/mL)

100 mL
400 mg
(4mg/mL)

10 mL
400 mg
(40mg/mL)

Floxin® I.V.
(ofloxacin injection)
for intravenous injection

RX   MCNEIL PHARMACEUTICAL   P. 1585

1/2 mg   1 mg

2 mg   5 mg

10 mg   20 mg

Haldol®
(haloperidol)

RX   MCNEIL PHARMACEUTICAL   P. 1587

2 mg per mL
Concentrate

5 mg per mL
Injectable
(1 mL/ampule)

RX   MCNEIL PHARMACEUTICAL   P. 1587

50 mg/mL*
5 mL Vial

50 mg/mL*
1 mL Ampule

*as 70.05 mg per mL haloperidol decanoate

Haldol® Decanoate 50
(haloperidol decanoate)

RX   MCNEIL PHARMACEUTICAL   P. 1587

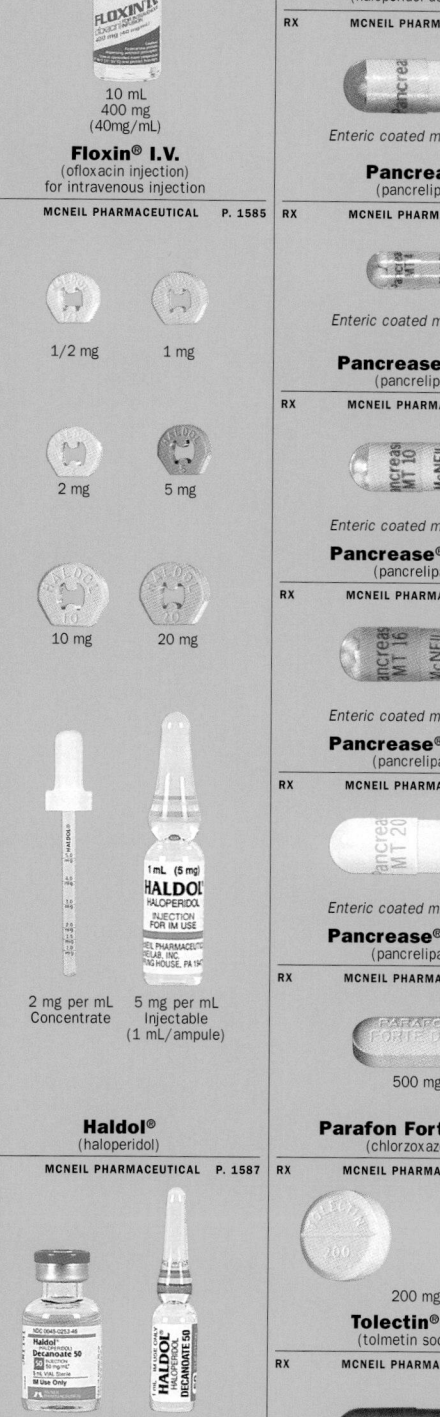

100 mg/mL*
5 mL Vial

100 mg/mL*
1 mL Ampule

*as 141.04 mg per mL
haloperidol decanoate

Haldol® Decanoate 100
(haloperidol decanoate)

RX   MCNEIL PHARMACEUTICAL   P. 1589

Enteric coated microspheres

Pancrease®
(pancrelipase)

RX   MCNEIL PHARMACEUTICAL   P. 1589

Enteric coated microtablets

Pancrease® MT 4
(pancrelipase)

RX   MCNEIL PHARMACEUTICAL   P. 1589

Enteric coated microtablets

Pancrease® MT 10
(pancrelipase)

RX   MCNEIL PHARMACEUTICAL   P. 1589

Enteric coated microtablets

Pancrease® MT 16
(pancrelipase)

RX   MCNEIL PHARMACEUTICAL   P. 1589

Enteric coated microtablets

Pancrease® MT 20
(pancrelipase)

RX   MCNEIL PHARMACEUTICAL   P. 1590

500 mg

Parafon Forte® DSC
(chlorzoxazone)

RX   MCNEIL PHARMACEUTICAL   P. 1591

200 mg

Tolectin® 200
(tolmetin sodium)

RX   MCNEIL PHARMACEUTICAL   P. 1591

400 mg

Tolectin® 400
(tolmetin sodium)

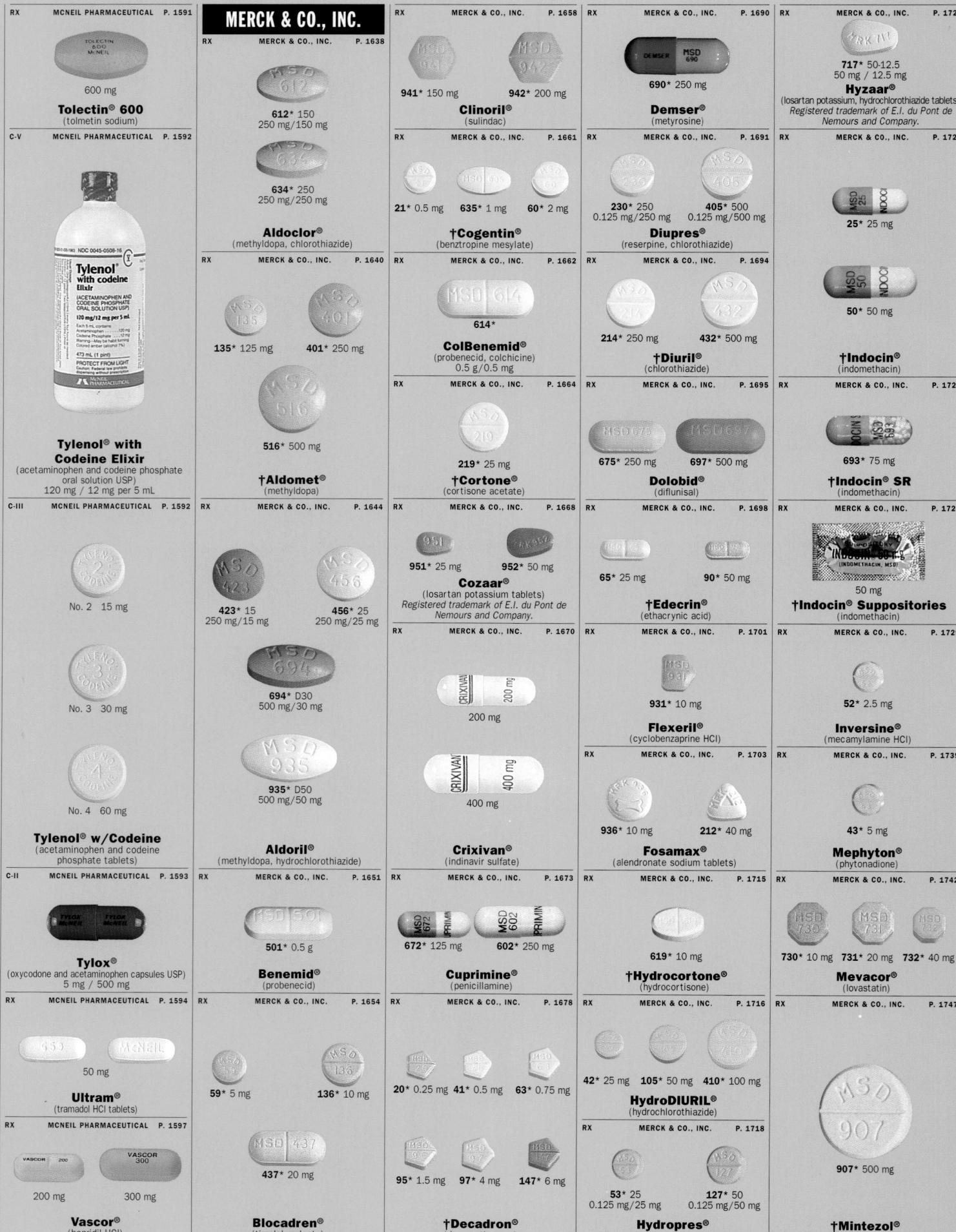

RX | MCNEIL PHARMACEUTICAL | P. 1591

600 mg
Tolectin® 600
(tolmetin sodium)

C-V | MCNEIL PHARMACEUTICAL | P. 1592

Tylenol® with Codeine Elixir
(acetaminophen and codeine phosphate oral solution USP)
120 mg / 12 mg per 5 mL

C-III | MCNEIL PHARMACEUTICAL | P. 1592

No. 2   15 mg
No. 3   30 mg
No. 4   60 mg
Tylenol® w/Codeine
(acetaminophen and codeine phosphate tablets)

C-II | MCNEIL PHARMACEUTICAL | P. 1593

Tylox®
(oxycodone and acetaminophen capsules USP)
5 mg / 500 mg

RX | MCNEIL PHARMACEUTICAL | P. 1594

50 mg
Ultram®
(tramadol HCl tablets)

RX | MCNEIL PHARMACEUTICAL | P. 1597

200 mg   300 mg
Vascor®
(bepridil HCl)

MERCK & CO., INC.

RX | MERCK & CO., INC. | P. 1638

612* 150
250 mg/150 mg

634* 250
250 mg/250 mg
Aldoclor®
(methyldopa, chlorothiazide)

RX | MERCK & CO., INC. | P. 1640

135* 125 mg   **401*** 250 mg

516* 500 mg
†Aldomet®
(methyldopa)

RX | MERCK & CO., INC. | P. 1644

423* 15
250 mg/15 mg

456* 25
250 mg/25 mg

694* D30
500 mg/30 mg

935* D50
500 mg/50 mg
Aldoril®
(methyldopa, hydrochlorothiazide)

RX | MERCK & CO., INC. | P. 1651

501* 0.5 g
Benemid®
(probenecid)

RX | MERCK & CO., INC. | P. 1654

59* 5 mg   **136*** 10 mg

437* 20 mg
Blocadren®
(timolol maleate)

RX | MERCK & CO., INC. | P. 1658

941* 150 mg   **942*** 200 mg
Clinoril®
(sulindac)

RX | MERCK & CO., INC. | P. 1661

21* 0.5 mg **635*** 1 mg **60*** 2 mg
†Cogentin®
(benztropine mesylate)

RX | MERCK & CO., INC. | P. 1662

614*
ColBenemid®
(probenecid, colchicine)
0.5 g/0.5 mg

RX | MERCK & CO., INC. | P. 1664

219* 25 mg
†Cortone®
(cortisone acetate)

RX | MERCK & CO., INC. | P. 1668

951* 25 mg   **952*** 50 mg
Cozaar®
(losartan potassium tablets)
Registered trademark of E.I. du Pont de Nemours and Company.

RX | MERCK & CO., INC. | P. 1670

200 mg

400 mg
Crixivan®
(indinavir sulfate)

RX | MERCK & CO., INC. | P. 1673

672* 125 mg   **602*** 250 mg
Cuprimine®
(penicillamine)

RX | MERCK & CO., INC. | P. 1678

20* 0.25 mg **41*** 0.5 mg **63*** 0.75 mg

95* 1.5 mg   **97*** 4 mg   **147*** 6 mg
†Decadron®
(dexamethasone)

RX | MERCK & CO., INC. | P. 1690

690* 250 mg
Demser®
(metyrosine)

RX | MERCK & CO., INC. | P. 1691

230* 250
0.125 mg/250 mg

405* 500
0.125 mg/500 mg
Diupres®
(reserpine, chlorothiazide)

RX | MERCK & CO., INC. | P. 1694

214* 250 mg   **432*** 500 mg
†Diuril®
(chlorothiazide)

RX | MERCK & CO., INC. | P. 1695

675* 250 mg   **697*** 500 mg
Dolobid®
(diflunisal)

RX | MERCK & CO., INC. | P. 1698

65* 25 mg   **90*** 50 mg
†Edecrin®
(ethacrynic acid)

RX | MERCK & CO., INC. | P. 1701

931* 10 mg
Flexeril®
(cyclobenzaprine HCl)

RX | MERCK & CO., INC. | P. 1703

936* 10 mg   **212*** 40 mg
Fosamax®
(alendronate sodium tablets)

RX | MERCK & CO., INC. | P. 1715

619* 10 mg
†Hydrocortone®
(hydrocortisone)

RX | MERCK & CO., INC. | P. 1716

42* 25 mg   **105*** 50 mg   **410*** 100 mg
HydroDIURIL®
(hydrochlorothiazide)

RX | MERCK & CO., INC. | P. 1718

53* 25
0.125 mg/25 mg

127* 50
0.125 mg/50 mg
Hydropres®
(reserpine, hydrochlorothiazide)

RX | MERCK & CO., INC. | P. 1720

717* 50-12.5
50 mg / 12.5 mg
Hyzaar®
(losartan potassium, hydrochlorothiazide tablets)
Registered trademark of E.I. du Pont de Nemours and Company.

RX | MERCK & CO., INC. | P. 1723

25* 25 mg

50* 50 mg
†Indocin®
(indomethacin)

RX | MERCK & CO., INC. | P. 1723

693* 75 mg
†Indocin® SR
(indomethacin)

RX | MERCK & CO., INC. | P. 1723

50 mg
†Indocin® Suppositories
(indomethacin)

RX | MERCK & CO., INC. | P. 1729

52* 2.5 mg
Inversine®
(mecamylamine HCl)

RX | MERCK & CO., INC. | P. 1739

43* 5 mg
Mephyton®
(phytonadione)

RX | MERCK & CO., INC. | P. 1742

730* 10 mg   **731*** 20 mg   **732*** 40 mg
Mevacor®
(lovastatin)

RX | MERCK & CO., INC. | P. 1747

907* 500 mg
†Mintezol®
(thiabendazole)

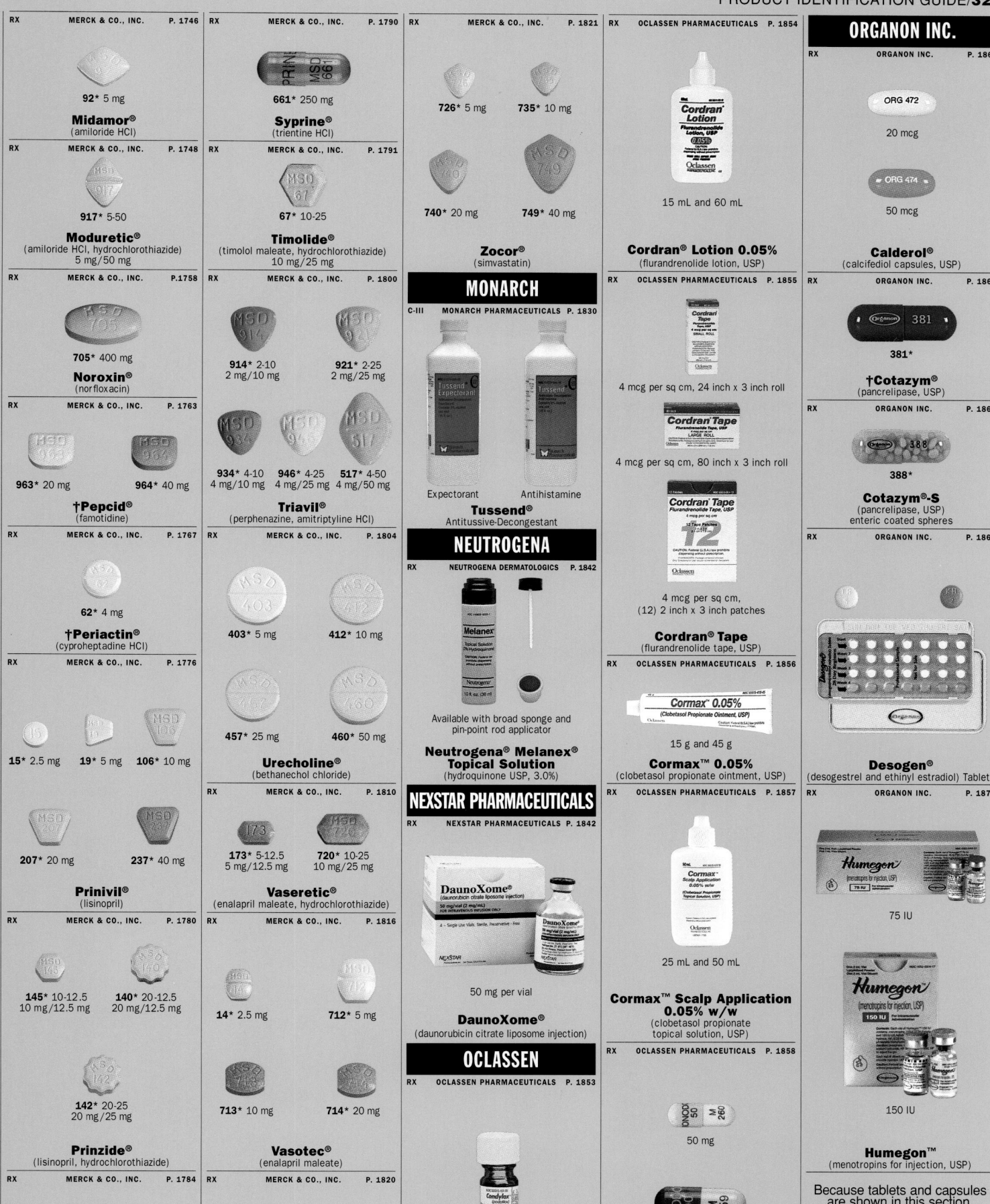

RX MERCK & CO., INC. P. 1746

92* 5 mg

Midamor®
(amiloride HCl)

RX MERCK & CO., INC. P. 1748

917* 5-50

Moduretic®
(amiloride HCl, hydrochlorothiazide)
5 mg/50 mg

RX MERCK & CO., INC. P.1758

705* 400 mg

Noroxin®
(norfloxacin)

RX MERCK & CO., INC. P. 1763

963* 20 mg   **964*** 40 mg

†Pepcid®
(famotidine)

RX MERCK & CO., INC. P. 1767

62* 4 mg

†Periactin®
(cyproheptadine HCl)

RX MERCK & CO., INC. P. 1776

15* 2.5 mg   **19*** 5 mg   **106*** 10 mg

207* 20 mg   **237*** 40 mg

Prinivil®
(lisinopril)

RX MERCK & CO., INC. P. 1780

145* 10-12.5   **140*** 20-12.5
10 mg/12.5 mg   20 mg/12.5 mg

142* 20-25
20 mg/25 mg

Prinzide®
(lisinopril, hydrochlorothiazide)

RX MERCK & CO., INC. P. 1784

72* 5 mg

Proscar®
(finasteride)

RX MERCK & CO., INC. P. 1790

661* 250 mg

Syprine®
(trientine HCl)

RX MERCK & CO., INC. P. 1791

67* 10-25

Timolide®
(timolol maleate, hydrochlorothiazide)
10 mg/25 mg

RX MERCK & CO., INC. P. 1800

914* 2-10   **921*** 2-25
2 mg/10 mg   2 mg/25 mg

934* 4-10   **946*** 4-25   **517*** 4-50
4 mg/10 mg   4 mg/25 mg   4 mg/50 mg

Triavil®
(perphenazine, amitriptyline HCl)

RX MERCK & CO., INC. P. 1804

403* 5 mg   **412*** 10 mg

457* 25 mg   **460*** 50 mg

Urecholine®
(bethanechol chloride)

RX MERCK & CO., INC. P. 1810

173* 5-12.5   **720*** 10-25
5 mg/12.5 mg   10 mg/25 mg

Vaseretic®
(enalapril maleate, hydrochlorothiazide)

RX MERCK & CO., INC. P. 1816

14* 2.5 mg   **712*** 5 mg

713* 10 mg   **714*** 20 mg

Vasotec®
(enalapril maleate)

RX MERCK & CO., INC. P. 1820

26* 5 mg   **47*** 10 mg

Vivactil®
(protriptyline HCl)

RX MERCK & CO., INC. P. 1821

726* 5 mg   **735*** 10 mg

740* 20 mg   **749*** 40 mg

Zocor®
(simvastatin)

MONARCH

C-III MONARCH PHARMACEUTICALS P. 1830

Expectorant   Antihistamine

Tussend®
Antitussive-Decongestant

NEUTROGENA

RX NEUTROGENA DERMATOLOGICS P. 1842

Available with broad sponge and
pin-point rod applicator

**Neutrogena® Melanex®
Topical Solution**
(hydroquinone USP, 3.0%)

NEXSTAR PHARMACEUTICALS

RX NEXSTAR PHARMACEUTICALS P. 1842

50 mg per vial

DaunoXome®
(daunorubicin citrate liposome injection)

OCLASSEN

RX OCLASSEN PHARMACEUTICALS P. 1853

3.5 mL

**Condylox® Topical
Solution 0.5%**
(podofilox)

RX OCLASSEN PHARMACEUTICALS P. 1854

15 mL and 60 mL

Cordran® Lotion 0.05%
(flurandrenolide lotion, USP)

RX OCLASSEN PHARMACEUTICALS P. 1855

4 mcg per sq cm, 24 inch x 3 inch roll

4 mcg per sq cm, 80 inch x 3 inch roll

4 mcg per sq cm,
(12) 2 inch x 3 inch patches

Cordran® Tape
(flurandrenolide tape, USP)

RX OCLASSEN PHARMACEUTICALS P. 1856

15 g and 45 g

Cormax™ 0.05%
(clobetasol propionate ointment, USP)

RX OCLASSEN PHARMACEUTICALS P. 1857

25 mL and 50 mL

**Cormax™ Scalp Application
0.05% w/w**
(clobetasol propionate
topical solution, USP)

RX OCLASSEN PHARMACEUTICALS P. 1858

50 mg

100 mg

Monodox®
(doxycycline monohydrate)

ORGANON INC.

RX ORGANON INC. P. 1866

ORG 472
20 mcg

ORG 474
50 mcg

Calderol®
(calcifediol capsules, USP)

RX ORGANON INC. P. 1866

381*

†Cotazym®
(pancrelipase, USP)

RX ORGANON INC. P. 1867

388*

Cotazym®-S
(pancrelipase, USP)
enteric coated spheres

RX ORGANON INC. P. 1867

Desogen®
(desogestrel and ethinyl estradiol) Tablets

RX ORGANON INC. P. 1873

75 IU

150 IU

Humegon™
(menotropins for injection, USP)

Because tablets and capsules
are shown in this section,
do not infer that these are
the only dosage forms
available. Where a product
name is preceded by the
symbol †, refer to the description in the Product Information
(White Section) for other forms.

RX ORGANON INC.

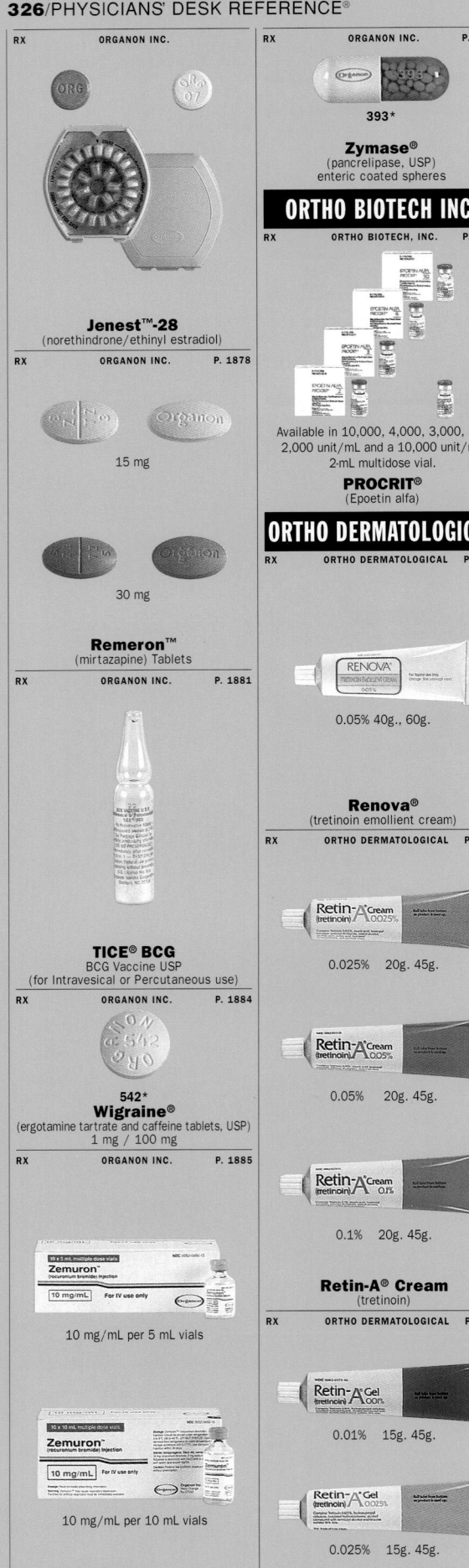

Jenest™-28
(norethindrone/ethinyl estradiol)

RX ORGANON INC. P. 1878

15 mg

30 mg

Remeron™
(mirtazapine) Tablets

RX ORGANON INC. P. 1881

TICE® BCG
BCG Vaccine USP
(for Intravesical or Percutaneous use)

RX ORGANON INC. P. 1884

542*
Wigraine®
(ergotamine tartrate and caffeine tablets, USP)
1 mg / 100 mg

RX ORGANON INC. P. 1885

10 mg/mL per 5 mL vials

10 mg/mL per 10 mL vials

Zemuron™
(rocuronium bromide)
Injection

RX ORGANON INC. P. 1889

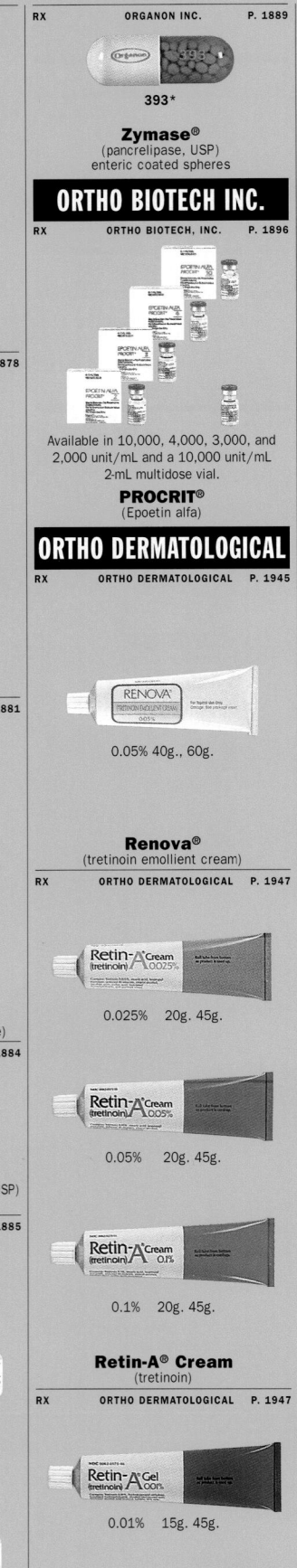

393*

Zymase®
(pancrelipase, USP)
enteric coated spheres

ORTHO BIOTECH INC.

RX ORTHO BIOTECH, INC. P. 1896

Available in 10,000, 4,000, 3,000, and
2,000 unit/mL and a 10,000 unit/mL
2-mL multidose vial.

PROCRIT®
(Epoetin alfa)

ORTHO DERMATOLOGICAL

RX ORTHO DERMATOLOGICAL P. 1945

0.05% 40g., 60g.

Renova®
(tretinoin emollient cream)

RX ORTHO DERMATOLOGICAL P. 1947

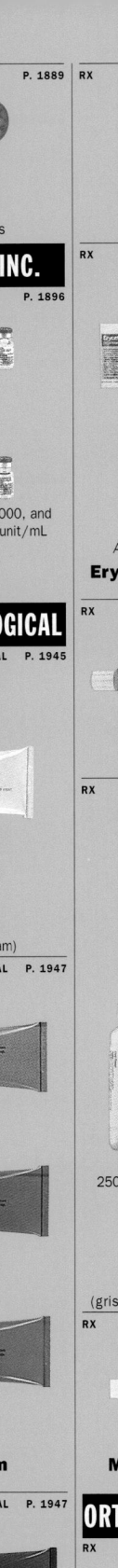

0.025% 20g. 45g.

0.05% 20g. 45g.

0.1% 20g. 45g.

Retin-A® Cream
(tretinoin)

RX ORTHO DERMATOLOGICAL P. 1947

0.01% 15g. 45g.

0.025% 15g. 45g.

Retin-A® Gel
(tretinoin)

RX ÓRTHO DERMATOLOGICAL P. 1947

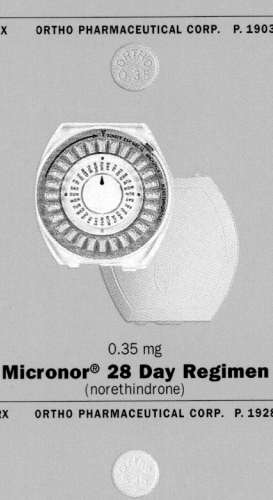

0.05% 28 mL

Retin-A® Liquid
(tretinoin)

RX ORTHO DERMATOLOGICAL P. 1943

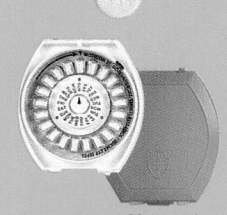

Available in 60-pledgets per box

Erycette® Topical Solution
(erythromycin 2%)

RX ORTHO DERMATOLOGICAL P. 1945

Cream 1% 15g. 30g. 85g.

Spectazole®
(econazole nitrate)

RX ORTHO DERMATOLOGICAL P. 1944

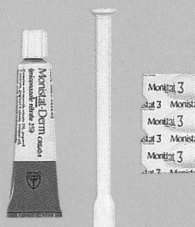

Grifulvin V®
(griseofulvin tablets) microsize
(griseofulvin oral suspension) microsize

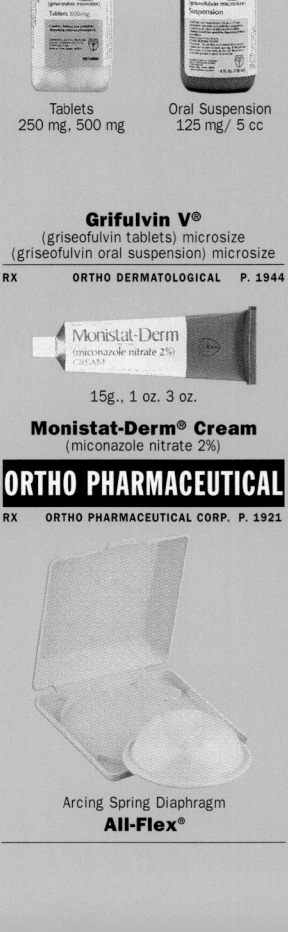

Tablets
250 mg, 500 mg

Oral Suspension
125 mg/ 5 cc

RX ORTHO DERMATOLOGICAL P. 1944

15g., 1 oz. 3 oz.

Monistat-Derm® Cream
(miconazole nitrate 2%)

ORTHO PHARMACEUTICAL

RX ORTHO PHARMACEUTICAL CORP. P. 1921

Arcing Spring Diaphragm
All-Flex®

RX ORTHO PHARMACEUTICAL CORP. P. 1903

0.35 mg
Micronor® 28 Day Regimen
(norethindrone)

RX ORTHO PHARMACEUTICAL CORP. P. 1928

Also available in 28-day regimen
containing 7 inert green tablets

Modicon® 21 Day Regimen
(norethindrone, ethinyl estradiol)

RX ORTHO PHARMACEUTICAL CORP. P. 1905

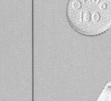

200 mg Vaginal Suppositories

Monistat® 3
(miconazole nitrate)

RX ORTHO PHARMACEUTICAL CORP. P. 1906

Monistat® Dual-Pak®
(miconazole nitrate)

RX ORTHO PHARMACEUTICAL CORP. P. 1914

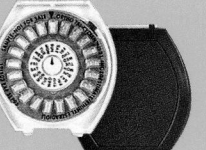

Each white tablet contains 0.180 mg
of norgestimate and 0.035 mg of
ethinyl estradiol. Each light blue tablet
contains 0.215 mg of norgestimate and
0.035 mg of ethinyl estradiol. Each blue
tablet contains 0.250 mg of norgestimate
and 0.035 mg of ethinyl estradiol.

Also available in 28 day regimen

Ortho Tri-Cyclen® 21 Day Regimen
(norgestimate, ethinyl estradiol)

RX ORTHO PHARMACEUTICAL CORP. P. 1925

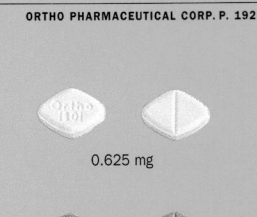

0.625 mg

1.25 mg

Ortho-EST® .625 and 1.25
(estropipate)

RX ORTHO PHARMACEUTICAL CORP. P. 1928

Also available in 28 Day Regimen

Ortho-Cept® 21 Day Regimen
(desogestrel, ethinyl estradiol)

RX ORTHO PHARMACEUTICAL CORP. P. 1914

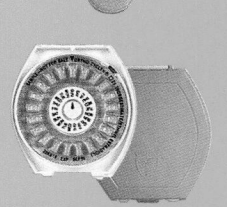

Also available in 28-day regimen

Ortho-Cyclen® 21 Day Regimen
(norgestimate, ethinyl estradiol)

RX ORTHO PHARMACEUTICAL CORP. P. 1928

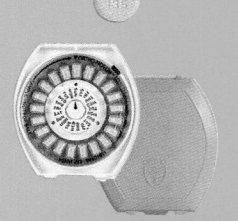

Also available in 28-Day Regimen
containing 7 inert green tablets

Ortho-Novum® 1/35 21 Day Regimen
(norethindrone, ethinyl estradiol)

RX ORTHO PHARMACEUTICAL CORP. P. 1928

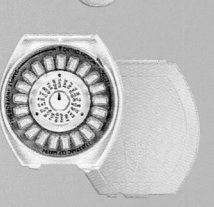

Also available in 28-day regimen
containing 7 inert green tablets

Ortho-Novum® 1/50 21 Day Regimen
(norethindrone, mestranol)

Column 1 — ORTHO PHARMACEUTICAL CORP.

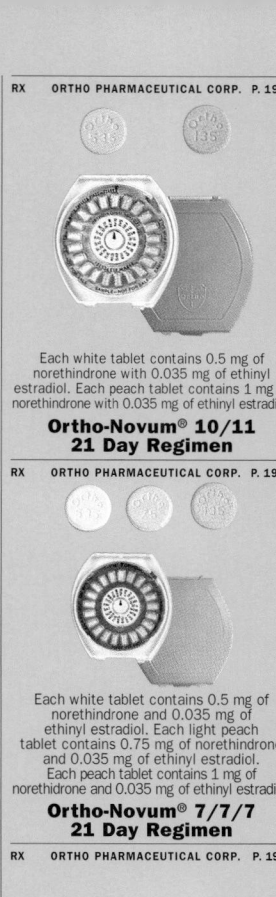

RX   ORTHO PHARMACEUTICAL CORP. P. 1928

Each white tablet contains 0.5 mg of norethindrone with 0.035 mg of ethinyl estradiol. Each peach tablet contains 1 mg of norethindrone with 0.035 mg of ethinyl estradiol.

Ortho-Novum® 10/11
21 Day Regimen

RX   ORTHO PHARMACEUTICAL CORP. P. 1928

Each white tablet contains 0.5 mg of norethindrone and 0.035 mg of ethinyl estradiol. Each light peach tablet contains 0.75 mg of norethindrone and 0.035 mg of ethinyl estradiol. Each peach tablet contains 1 mg of norethindrone and 0.035 mg of ethinyl estradiol.

Ortho-Novum® 7/7/7
21 Day Regimen

RX   ORTHO PHARMACEUTICAL CORP. P. 1936

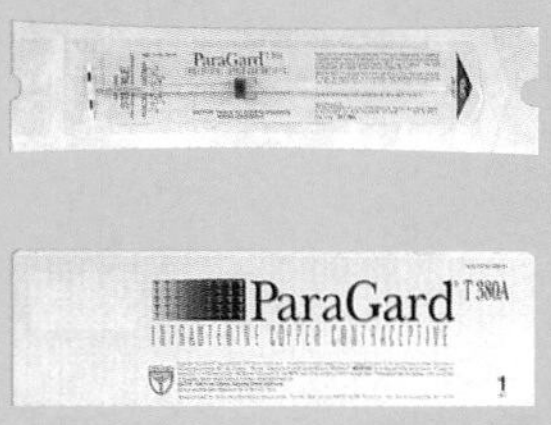

Intrauterine Copper Contraceptive

ParaGard® T 380A

RX   ORTHO PHARMACEUTICAL CORP. P. 1939

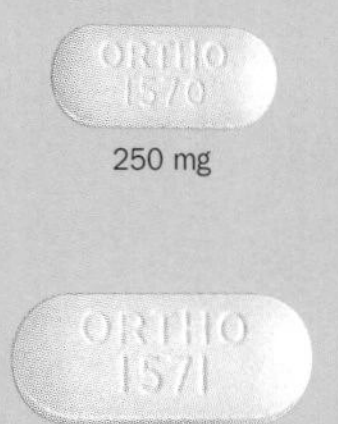

250 mg

500 mg

Protostat®
(metronidazole)

RX   ORTHO PHARMACEUTICAL CORP. P. 1941

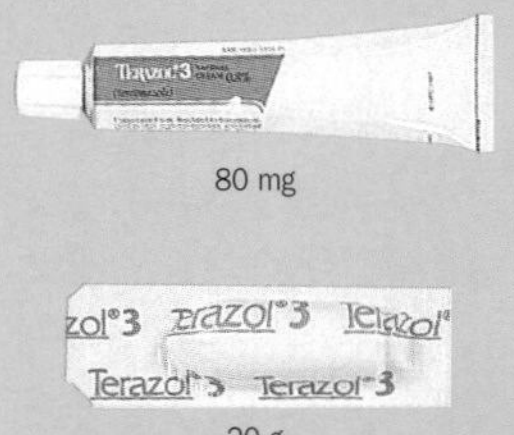

80 mg

20 g

Terazol® 3
(terconazole)

Column 2 — PARKE-DAVIS

RX   ORTHO PHARMACEUTICAL CORP. P. 1943

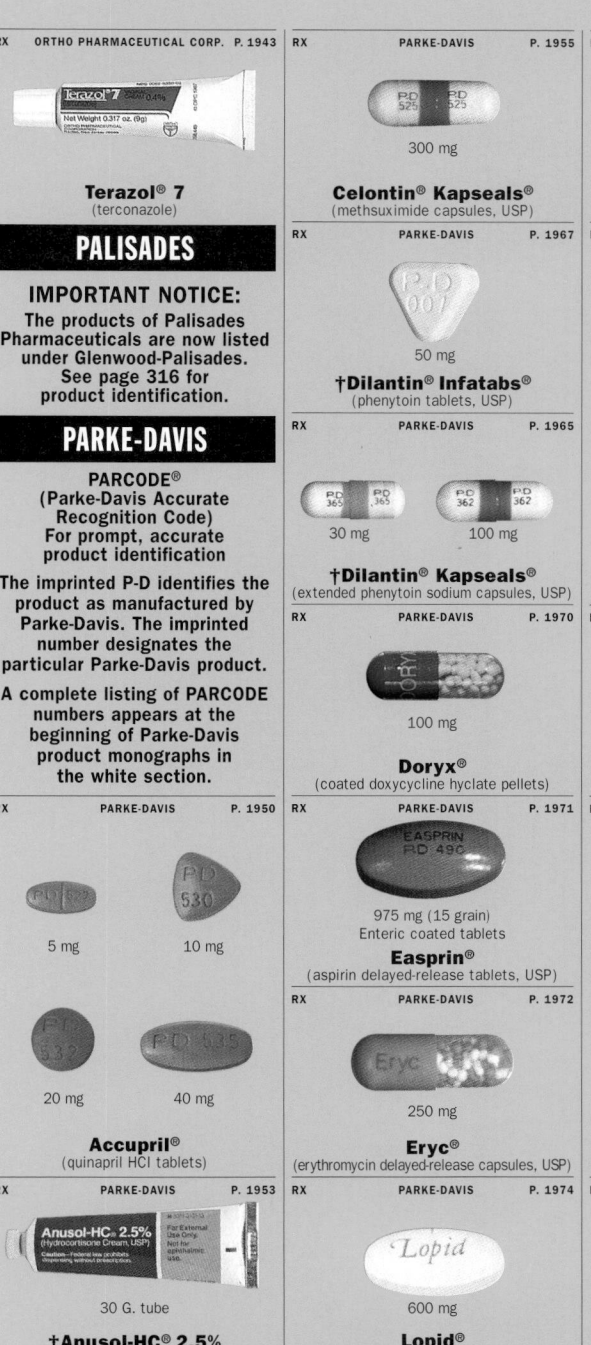

Net Weight 0.317 oz. (9g)

Terazol® 7
(terconazole)

PALISADES

IMPORTANT NOTICE:
The products of Palisades Pharmaceuticals are now listed under Glenwood-Palisades. See page 316 for product identification.

PARKE-DAVIS

PARCODE®
(Parke-Davis Accurate Recognition Code) For prompt, accurate product identification

The imprinted P-D identifies the product as manufactured by Parke-Davis. The imprinted number designates the particular Parke-Davis product.

A complete listing of PARCODE numbers appears at the beginning of Parke-Davis product monographs in the white section.

RX   PARKE-DAVIS P. 1950

5 mg   10 mg

20 mg   40 mg

Accupril®
(quinapril HCl tablets)

RX   PARKE-DAVIS P. 1953

Anusol-HC® 2.5% (Hydrocortisone Cream, USP)

30 G. tube

†Anusol-HC® 2.5%
(hydrocortisone cream, USP)

RX   PARKE-DAVIS P. 1954

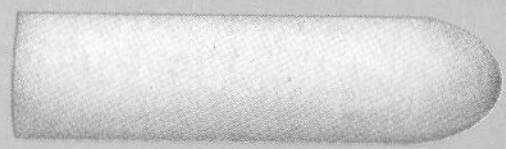

†Anusol-HC® Suppositories w/Hydrocortisone

RX   PARKE-DAVIS P. 1961

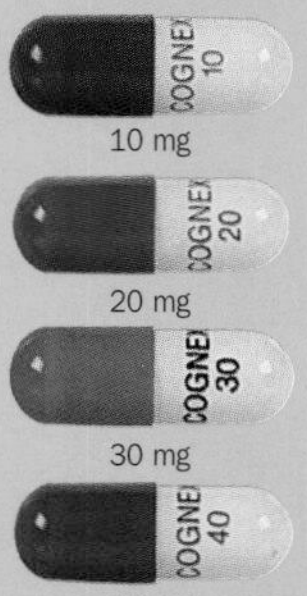

10 mg

20 mg

30 mg

40 mg

Cognex®
(tacrine HCl)

Column 3 — PARKE-DAVIS

RX   PARKE-DAVIS P. 1955

300 mg

Celontin® Kapseals®
(methsuximide capsules, USP)

RX   PARKE-DAVIS P. 1967

50 mg

†Dilantin® Infatabs®
(phenytoin tablets, USP)

RX   PARKE-DAVIS P. 1965

30 mg   100 mg

†Dilantin® Kapseals®
(extended phenytoin sodium capsules, USP)

RX   PARKE-DAVIS P. 1970

100 mg

Doryx®
(coated doxycycline hyclate pellets)

RX   PARKE-DAVIS P. 1971

975 mg (15 grain)
Enteric coated tablets

Easprin®
(aspirin delayed-release tablets, USP)

RX   PARKE-DAVIS P. 1972

250 mg

Eryc®
(erythromycin delayed-release capsules, USP)

RX   PARKE-DAVIS P. 1974

600 mg

Lopid®
(gemfibrozil tablets)

RX   PARKE-DAVIS P. 1981

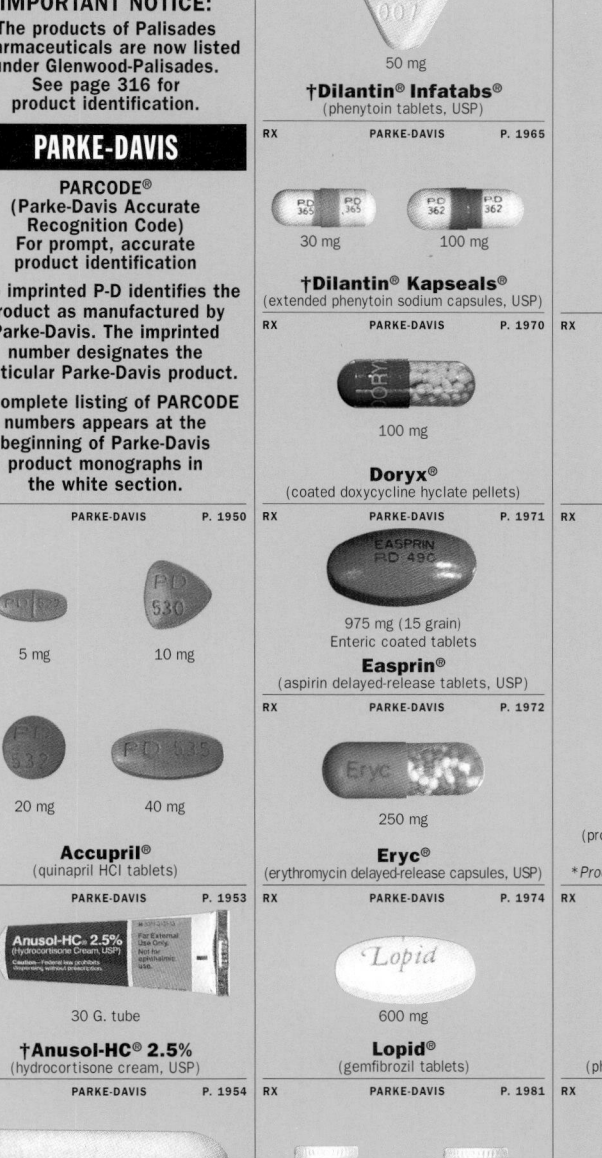

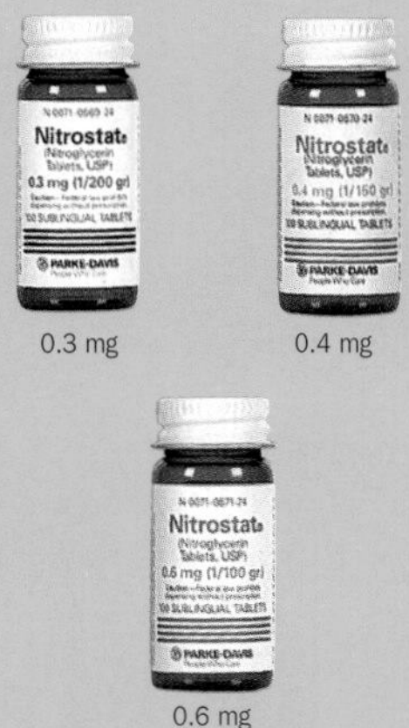

0.3 mg   0.4 mg

0.6 mg
Sublingual tablets

Nitrostat®
(nitroglycerin tablets, USP)

Column 4 — PARKE-DAVIS

RX   PARKE-DAVIS P. 1977

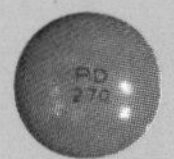

15 mg

Nardil®
(phenelzine sulfate tablets, USP)

RX   PARKE-DAVIS P. 1978

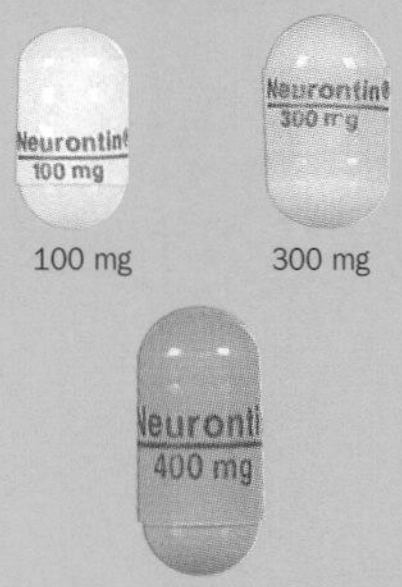

Neurontin® 100 mg   Neurontin® 300 mg

100 mg   300 mg

Neurontin® 400 mg

400 mg

Neurontin®
(gabapentin)

RX   PARKE-DAVIS P. 1982

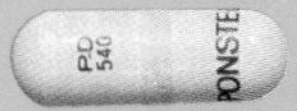

250 mg

Ponstel® Kapseals®
(mefenamic acid)

RX   PARKE-DAVIS P. 1983

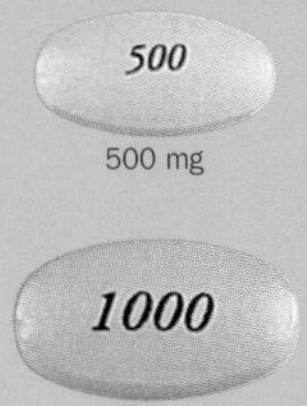

500

500 mg

1000

1000 mg

Procanbid™
(procainamide HCl extended-release tablets*)

*Procanbid™ is not USP for dissolution

RX   PARKE-DAVIS P. 1985

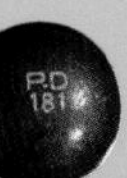

200 mg

Pyridium®
(phenazopyridine HCl tablets, USP)

RX   PARKE-DAVIS P. 1986

250 mg

†Zarontin®
(ethosuximide, USP)
Capsules

PFIZER INC

RX   ROERIG DIVISION P. 1992

210* 12.5 mg

Antivert®
(meclizine HCl)

RX   ROERIG DIVISION P. 1992

211* 25 mg

Antivert®/25
(meclizine HCl)

Column 5 — ROERIG DIVISION / PFIZER LABS

RX   ROERIG DIVISION P. 1992

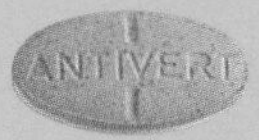

214* 50 mg

Antivert®/50
(meclizine HCl)

RX   ROERIG DIVISION P. 1992

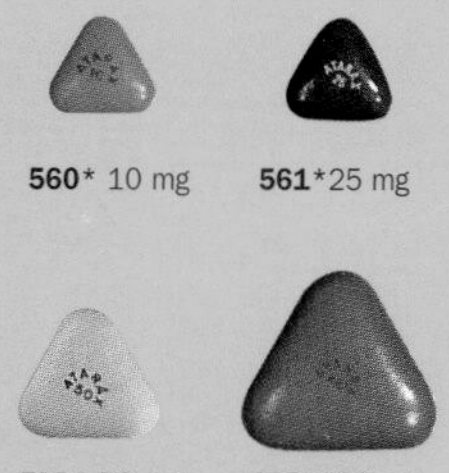

560* 10 mg   561* 25 mg

562* 50 mg   563* 100 mg

†Atarax®
(hydroxyzine HCl)

RX   ROERIG DIVISION P. 1993

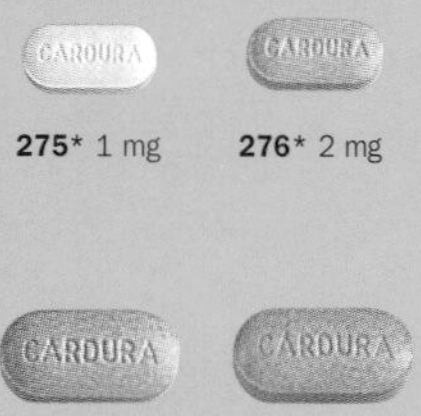

275* 1 mg   276* 2 mg

277* 4 mg   278* 8 mg

Cardura®
(doxazosin mesylate)

RX   PFIZER LABS P. 2002

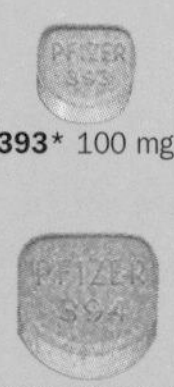

393* 100 mg

394* 250 mg
Scored tablets

Diabinese®
(chlorpropamide)

RX   ROERIG DIVISION P. 2003

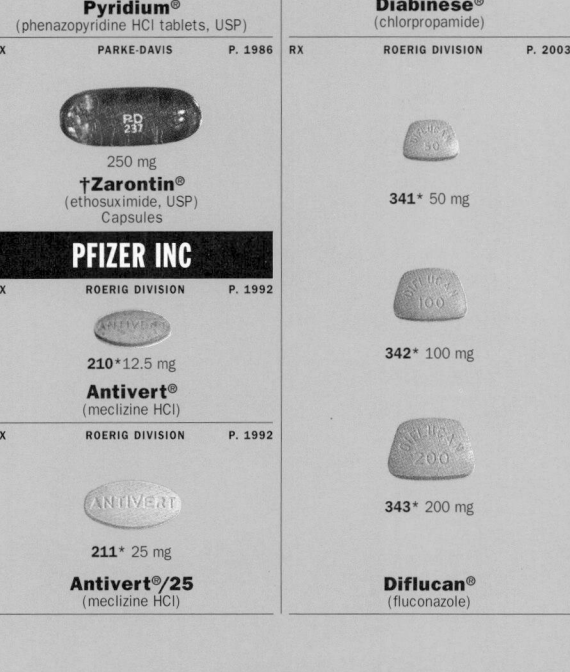

341* 50 mg

342* 100 mg

343* 200 mg

Diflucan®
(fluconazole)

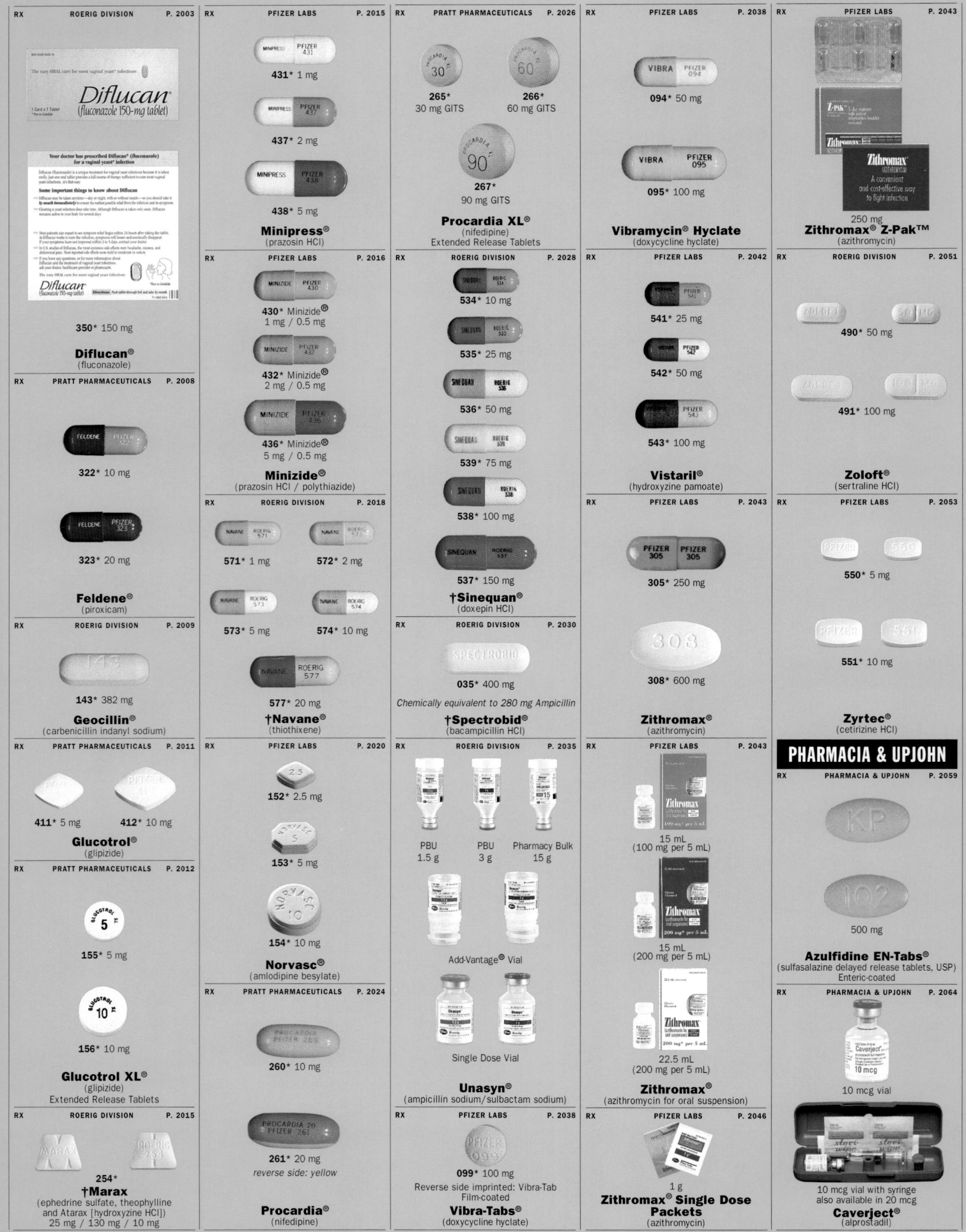

RX ROERIG DIVISION P. 2003

350* 150 mg
Diflucan®
(fluconazole)

RX PRATT PHARMACEUTICALS P. 2008

322* 10 mg

323* 20 mg
Feldene®
(piroxicam)

RX ROERIG DIVISION P. 2009

143* 382 mg
Geocillin®
(carbenicillin indanyl sodium)

RX PRATT PHARMACEUTICALS P. 2011

411* 5 mg   **412*** 10 mg
Glucotrol®
(glipizide)

RX PRATT PHARMACEUTICALS P. 2012

155* 5 mg

156* 10 mg
Glucotrol XL®
(glipizide)
Extended Release Tablets

RX ROERIG DIVISION P. 2015

254*
†Marax
(ephedrine sulfate, theophylline
and Atarax [hydroxyzine HCl])
25 mg / 130 mg / 10 mg

RX PFIZER LABS P. 2015

431* 1 mg

437* 2 mg

438* 5 mg
Minipress®
(prazosin HCl)

RX PFIZER LABS P. 2016

430* Minizide®
1 mg / 0.5 mg

432* Minizide®
2 mg / 0.5 mg

436* Minizide®
5 mg / 0.5 mg
Minizide®
(prazosin HCl / polythiazide)

RX ROERIG DIVISION P. 2018

571* 1 mg   **572*** 2 mg

573* 5 mg   **574*** 10 mg

577* 20 mg
†Navane®
(thiothixene)

RX PFIZER LABS P. 2020

152* 2.5 mg

153* 5 mg

154* 10 mg
Norvasc®
(amlodipine besylate)

RX PRATT PHARMACEUTICALS P. 2024

260* 10 mg

261* 20 mg
reverse side: yellow
Procardia®
(nifedipine)

RX PRATT PHARMACEUTICALS P. 2026

265*   **266***
30 mg GITS   60 mg GITS

267*
90 mg GITS
Procardia XL®
(nifedipine)
Extended Release Tablets

RX ROERIG DIVISION P. 2028

534* 10 mg

535* 25 mg

536* 50 mg

539* 75 mg

538* 100 mg

537* 150 mg
†Sinequan®
(doxepin HCl)

RX ROERIG DIVISION P. 2030

035* 400 mg
Chemically equivalent to 280 mg Ampicillin
†Spectrobid®
(bacampicillin HCl)

RX ROERIG DIVISION P. 2035

PBU   PBU   Pharmacy Bulk
1.5 g   3 g   15 g

Add-Vantage® Vial

Single Dose Vial
Unasyn®
(ampicillin sodium/sulbactam sodium)

RX PFIZER LABS P. 2038

099* 100 mg
Reverse side imprinted: Vibra-Tab
Film-coated
Vibra-Tabs®
(doxycycline hyclate)

RX PFIZER LABS P. 2038

094* 50 mg

095* 100 mg
Vibramycin® Hyclate
(doxycycline hyclate)

RX PFIZER LABS P. 2042

541* 25 mg

542* 50 mg

543* 100 mg
Vistaril®
(hydroxyzine pamoate)

RX PFIZER LABS P. 2043

305* 250 mg

308* 600 mg
Zithromax®
(azithromycin)

RX PFIZER LABS P. 2043

15 mL
(100 mg per 5 mL)

15 mL
(200 mg per 5 mL)

22.5 mL
(200 mg per 5 mL)
Zithromax®
(azithromycin for oral suspension)

RX PFIZER LABS P. 2046

1 g
**Zithromax® Single Dose
Packets**
(azithromycin)

RX PFIZER LABS P. 2043

250 mg
Zithromax® Z-Pak™
(azithromycin)

RX ROERIG DIVISION P. 2051

490* 50 mg

491* 100 mg
Zoloft®
(sertraline HCl)

RX PFIZER LABS P. 2053

550* 5 mg

551* 10 mg
Zyrtec®
(cetirizine HCl)

PHARMACIA & UPJOHN

RX PHARMACIA & UPJOHN P. 2059

500 mg
Azulfidine EN-Tabs®
(sulfasalazine delayed release tablets, USP)
Enteric-coated

RX PHARMACIA & UPJOHN P. 2064

10 mcg vial

10 mcg vial with syringe
also available in 20 mcg
Caverject®
(alprostadil)

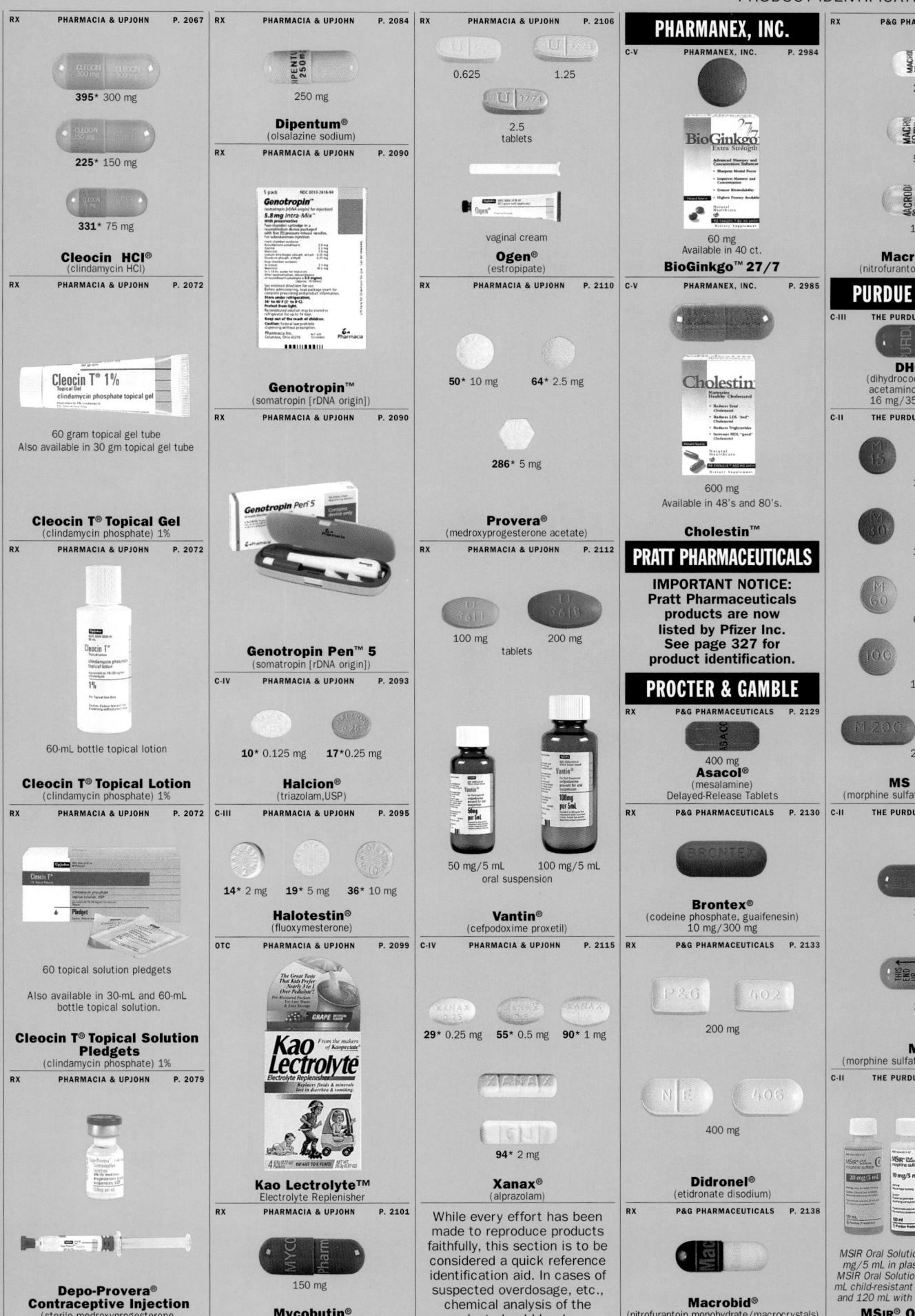

395* 300 mg

225* 150 mg

331* 75 mg

Cleocin HCl®
(clindamycin HCl)

60 gram topical gel tube
Also available in 30 gm topical gel tube

Cleocin T® Topical Gel
(clindamycin phosphate) 1%

60-mL bottle topical lotion

Cleocin T® Topical Lotion
(clindamycin phosphate) 1%

60 topical solution pledgets

Also available in 30-mL and 60-mL
bottle topical solution.

**Cleocin T® Topical Solution
Pledgets**
(clindamycin phosphate) 1%

**Depo-Provera®
Contraceptive Injection**
(sterile medroxyprogesterone
acetate suspension)

250 mg

Dipentum®
(olsalazine sodium)

Genotropin™
(somatropin [rDNA origin])

Genotropin Pen™ 5
(somatropin [rDNA origin])

10* 0.125 mg   **17***0.25 mg

Halcion®
(triazolam, USP)

14* 2 mg   **19*** 5 mg   **36*** 10 mg

Halotestin®
(fluoxymesterone)

**Kao
Lectrolyte™**
Electrolyte Replenisher

150 mg

Mycobutin®
(rifabutin capsules, USP)

0.625   1.25

2.5
tablets

vaginal cream

Ogen®
(estropipate)

50* 10 mg   **64*** 2.5 mg

286* 5 mg

Provera®
(medroxyprogesterone acetate)

100 mg   200 mg
tablets

50 mg/5 mL   100 mg/5 mL
oral suspension

Vantin®
(cefpodoxime proxetil)

29* 0.25 mg   **55*** 0.5 mg   **90*** 1 mg

94* 2 mg

Xanax®
(alprazolam)

While every effort has been
made to reproduce products
faithfully, this section is to be
considered a quick reference
identification aid. In cases of
suspected overdosage, etc.,
chemical analysis of the
product should be done.

PHARMANEX, INC.

60 mg
Available in 40 ct.

BioGinkgo™ 27/7

600 mg
Available in 48's and 80's.

Cholestin™

PRATT PHARMACEUTICALS

**IMPORTANT NOTICE:
Pratt Pharmaceuticals
products are now
listed by Pfizer Inc.
See page 327 for
product identification.**

PROCTER & GAMBLE

400 mg

Asacol®
(mesalamine)
Delayed-Release Tablets

Brontex®
(codeine phosphate, guaifenesin)
10 mg/300 mg

200 mg

400 mg

Didronel®
(etidronate disodium)

Macrobid®
(nitrofurantoin monohydrate/macrocrystals)
75 mg/25 mg

25 mg

50 mg

100 mg

Macrodantin®
(nitrofurantoin macrocrystals)

PURDUE FREDERICK

DHCplus®
(dihydrocodeine bitartrate,
acetaminophen, caffeine)
16 mg/356.4 mg/30 mg

15 mg

30 mg

60 mg

100 mg

200 mg

MS Contin®
(morphine sulfate controlled-release)

15 mg

30 mg

MSIR®
(morphine sulfate) immediate-release

*MSIR Oral Solution 10 mg/5 mL and 20
mg/5 mL in plastic bottles of 120 mL.
MSIR Oral Solution Concentrate 20 mg/1
mL child-resistant plastic bottles of 30 mL
and 120 mL with child-resistant droppers*

MSIR® Oral Solution
(morphine sulfate) immediate-release

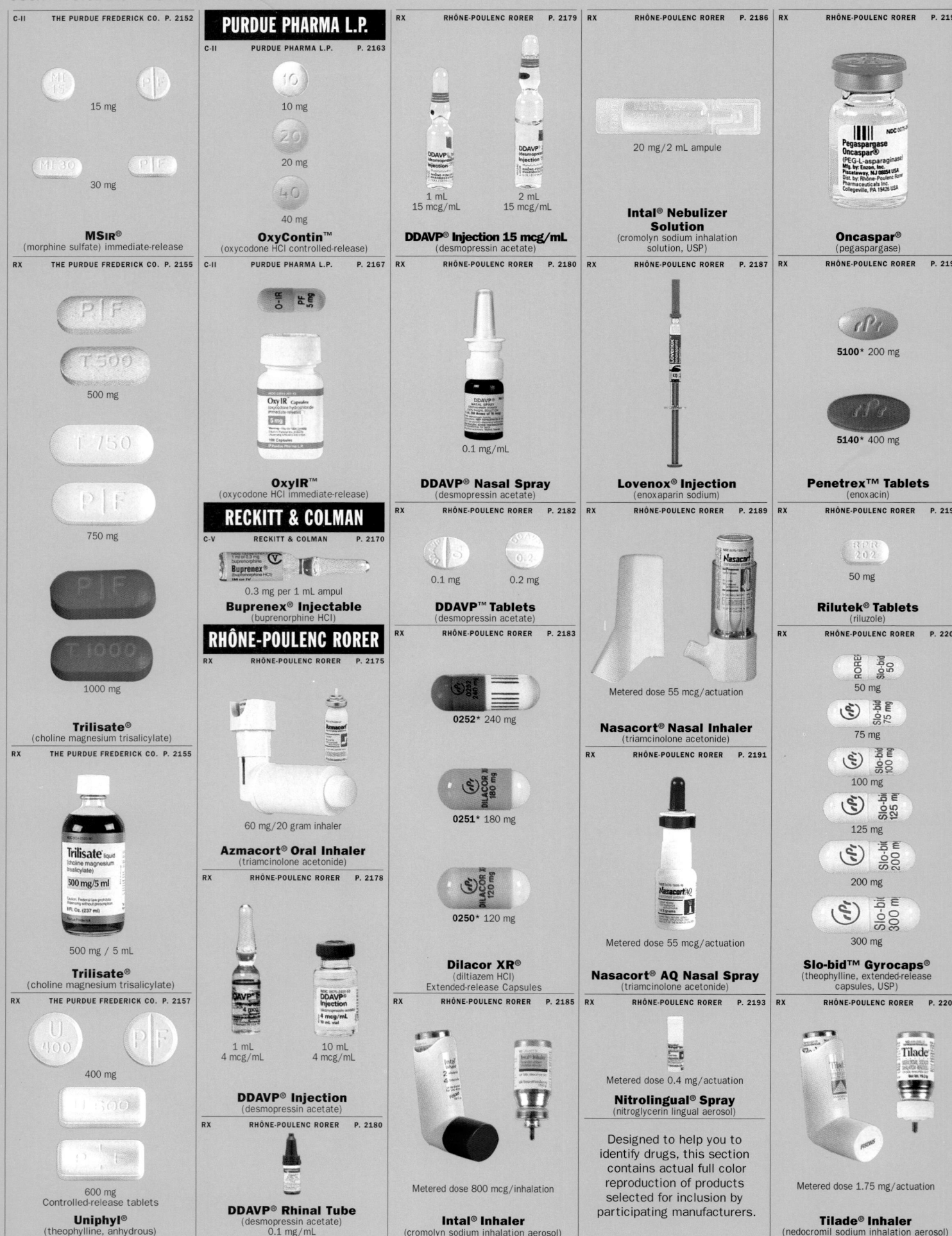

C-II   THE PURDUE FREDERICK CO. P. 2152

15 mg

30 mg

MSIR®
(morphine sulfate) immediate-release

RX   THE PURDUE FREDERICK CO. P. 2155

500 mg

750 mg

1000 mg

Trilisate®
(choline magnesium trisalicylate)

RX   THE PURDUE FREDERICK CO. P. 2155

Trilisate® liquid
(choline magnesium trisalicylate)
500 mg/5 ml

500 mg / 5 mL

Trilisate®
(choline magnesium trisalicylate)

RX   THE PURDUE FREDERICK CO. P. 2157

400 mg

600 mg
Controlled-release tablets

Uniphyl®
(theophylline, anhydrous)

PURDUE PHARMA L.P.

C-II   PURDUE PHARMA L.P. P. 2163

10 mg

20 mg

40 mg

OxyContin™
(oxycodone HCl controlled-release)

C-II   PURDUE PHARMA L.P. P. 2167

O-IR   PF
5 mg

OxyIR Capsules
5 mg

OxyIR™
(oxycodone HCl immediate-release)

RECKITT & COLMAN

C-V   RECKITT & COLMAN P. 2170

Buprenex®
(buprenorphine HCl)
0.3 mg per 1 mL ampul

Buprenex® Injectable
(buprenorphine HCl)

RHÔNE-POULENC RORER

RX   RHÔNE-POULENC RORER P. 2175

Azmacort

60 mg/20 gram inhaler

Azmacort® Oral Inhaler
(triamcinolone acetonide)

RX   RHÔNE-POULENC RORER P. 2178

1 mL
4 mcg/mL

10 mL
4 mcg/mL

DDAVP® Injection
(desmopressin acetate)

RX   RHÔNE-POULENC RORER P. 2180

0.1 mg/mL

DDAVP® Rhinal Tube
(desmopressin acetate)
0.1 mg/mL

RX   RHÔNE-POULENC RORER P. 2179

1 mL
15 mcg/mL

2 mL
15 mcg/mL

DDAVP® Injection 15 mcg/mL
(desmopressin acetate)

RX   RHÔNE-POULENC RORER P. 2180

DDAVP® Nasal Spray
(desmopressin acetate)

RX   RHÔNE-POULENC RORER P. 2182

0.1 mg   0.2 mg

DDAVP™ Tablets
(desmopressin acetate)

RX   RHÔNE-POULENC RORER P. 2183

0252* 240 mg

0251* 180 mg

0250* 120 mg

Dilacor XR®
(diltiazem HCl)
Extended-release Capsules

RX   RHÔNE-POULENC RORER P. 2185

Metered dose 800 mcg/inhalation

Intal® Inhaler
(cromolyn sodium inhalation aerosol)

RX   RHÔNE-POULENC RORER P. 2186

20 mg/2 mL ampule

**Intal® Nebulizer
Solution**
(cromolyn sodium inhalation
solution, USP)

RX   RHÔNE-POULENC RORER P. 2187

Lovenox® Injection
(enoxaparin sodium)

RX   RHÔNE-POULENC RORER P. 2189

Metered dose 55 mcg/actuation

Nasacort® Nasal Inhaler
(triamcinolone acetonide)

RX   RHÔNE-POULENC RORER P. 2191

Nasacort AQ

Metered dose 55 mcg/actuation

Nasacort® AQ Nasal Spray
(triamcinolone acetonide)

RX   RHÔNE-POULENC RORER P. 2193

Metered dose 0.4 mg/actuation

Nitrolingual® Spray
(nitroglycerin lingual aerosol)

Designed to help you to
identify drugs, this section
contains actual full color
reproduction of products
selected for inclusion by
participating manufacturers.

RX   RHÔNE-POULENC RORER P. 2194

Pegaspargase
Oncaspar®
(PEG-L-asparaginase)
Mfg. by: Enzon, Inc.
Piscataway, NJ 08854 USA
Dist. by: Rhône-Poulenc Rorer
Pharmaceuticals Inc.
Collegeville, PA 19426 USA

Oncaspar®
(pegaspargase)

RX   RHÔNE-POULENC RORER P. 2196

5100* 200 mg

5140* 400 mg

Penetrex™ Tablets
(enoxacin)

RX   RHÔNE-POULENC RORER P. 2198

RPR
202

50 mg

Rilutek® Tablets
(riluzole)

RX   RHÔNE-POULENC RORER P. 2201

50 mg

75 mg

100 mg

125 mg

200 mg

300 mg

Slo-bid™ Gyrocaps®
(theophylline, extended-release
capsules, USP)

RX   RHÔNE-POULENC RORER P. 2207

Tilade

Metered dose 1.75 mg/actuation

Tilade® Inhaler
(nedocromil sodium inhalation aerosol)

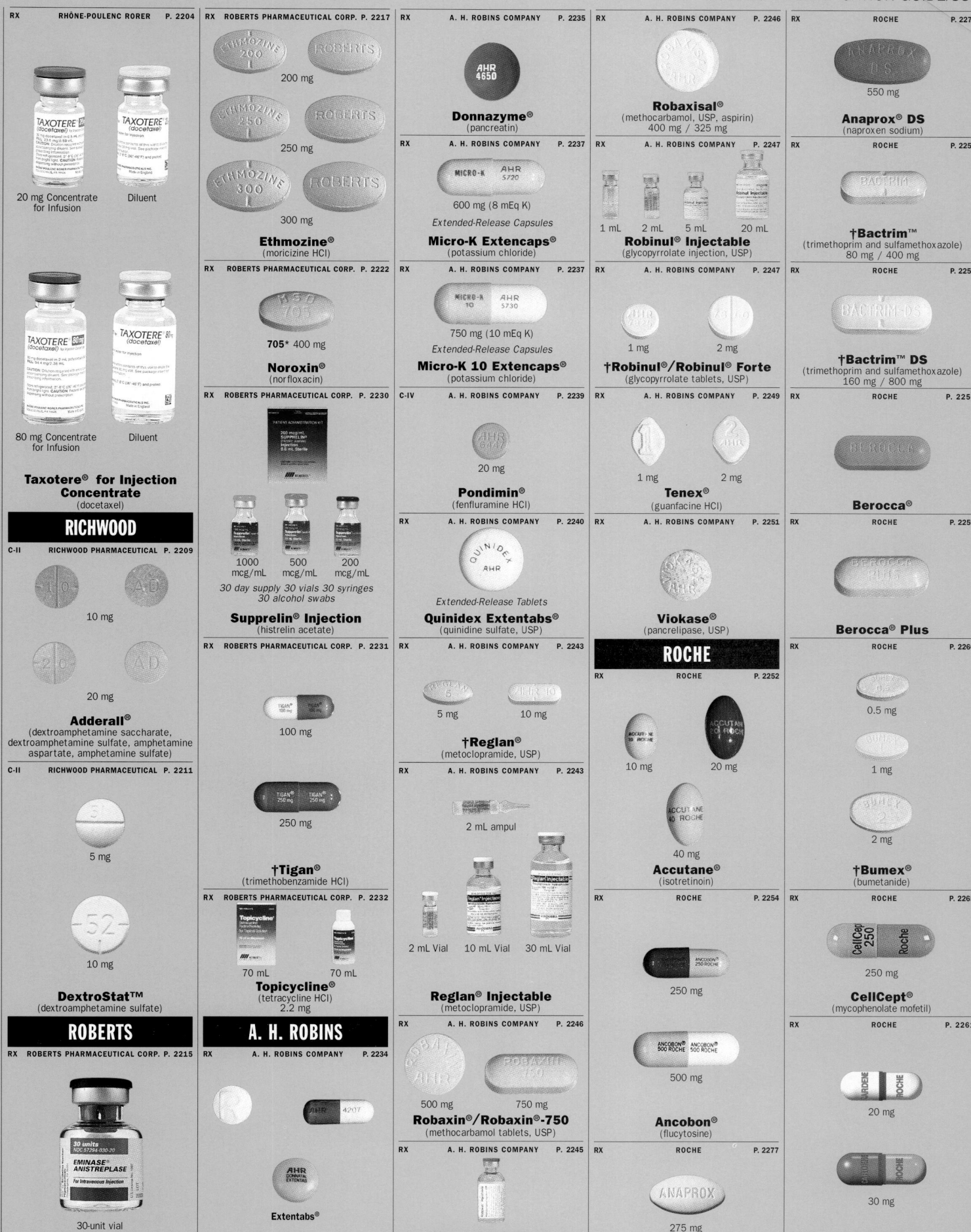

RX   RHÔNE-POULENC RORER   P. 2204

20 mg Concentrate for Infusion   Diluent

80 mg Concentrate for Infusion   Diluent

Taxotere® for Injection Concentrate
(docetaxel)

RICHWOOD

C-II   RICHWOOD PHARMACEUTICAL   P. 2209

10 mg

20 mg

Adderall®
(dextroamphetamine saccharate, dextroamphetamine sulfate, amphetamine aspartate, amphetamine sulfate)

C-II   RICHWOOD PHARMACEUTICAL   P. 2211

5 mg

10 mg

DextroStat™
(dextroamphetamine sulfate)

ROBERTS

RX   ROBERTS PHARMACEUTICAL CORP.   P. 2215

30-unit vial

Eminase®
(anistreplase)

RX   ROBERTS PHARMACEUTICAL CORP.   P. 2217

200 mg

250 mg

300 mg

Ethmozine®
(moricizine HCl)

RX   ROBERTS PHARMACEUTICAL CORP.   P. 2222

705* 400 mg

Noroxin®
(norfloxacin)

RX   ROBERTS PHARMACEUTICAL CORP.   P. 2230

1000 mcg/mL   500 mcg/mL   200 mcg/mL

30 day supply 30 vials 30 syringes
30 alcohol swabs

Supprelin® Injection
(histrelin acetate)

RX   ROBERTS PHARMACEUTICAL CORP.   P. 2231

100 mg

250 mg

†Tigan®
(trimethobenzamide HCl)

RX   ROBERTS PHARMACEUTICAL CORP.   P. 2232

70 mL   70 mL

Topicycline®
(tetracycline HCl)
2.2 mg

A. H. ROBINS

RX   A. H. ROBINS COMPANY   P. 2234

Extentabs®

†Donnatal®

RX   A. H. ROBINS COMPANY   P. 2235

AHR 4650

Donnazyme®
(pancreatin)

RX   A. H. ROBINS COMPANY   P. 2237

MICRO-K AHR 5720

600 mg (8 mEq K)
Extended-Release Capsules

Micro-K Extencaps®
(potassium chloride)

RX   A. H. ROBINS COMPANY   P. 2237

MICRO-K 10 AHR 5730

750 mg (10 mEq K)
Extended-Release Capsules

Micro-K 10 Extencaps®
(potassium chloride)

C-IV   A. H. ROBINS COMPANY   P. 2239

20 mg

Pondimin®
(fenfluramine HCl)

RX   A. H. ROBINS COMPANY   P. 2240

Extended-Release Tablets

Quinidex Extentabs®
(quinidine sulfate, USP)

RX   A. H. ROBINS COMPANY   P. 2243

5 mg   10 mg

†Reglan®
(metoclopramide, USP)

RX   A. H. ROBINS COMPANY   P. 2243

2 mL ampul

2 mL Vial   10 mL Vial   30 mL Vial

Reglan® Injectable
(metoclopramide, USP)

RX   A. H. ROBINS COMPANY   P. 2246

500 mg   750 mg

Robaxin®/Robaxin®-750
(methocarbamol tablets, USP)

RX   A. H. ROBINS COMPANY   P. 2245

Robaxin® Injectable
(methocarbamol injection, USP)
100 mg/mL

RX   A. H. ROBINS COMPANY   P. 2246

Robaxisal®
(methocarbamol, USP, aspirin)
400 mg / 325 mg

RX   A. H. ROBINS COMPANY   P. 2247

1 mL   2 mL   5 mL   20 mL

Robinul® Injectable
(glycopyrrolate injection, USP)

RX   A. H. ROBINS COMPANY   P. 2247

1 mg   2 mg

†Robinul®/Robinul® Forte
(glycopyrrolate tablets, USP)

RX   A. H. ROBINS COMPANY   P. 2249

1 mg   2 mg

Tenex®
(guanfacine HCl)

RX   A. H. ROBINS COMPANY   P. 2251

Viokase®
(pancrelipase, USP)

ROCHE

RX   ROCHE   P. 2252

10 mg   20 mg

40 mg

Accutane®
(isotretinoin)

RX   ROCHE   P. 2254

250 mg

500 mg

Ancobon®
(flucytosine)

RX   ROCHE   P. 2277

275 mg

Anaprox®
(naproxen sodium)

RX   ROCHE   P. 2277

550 mg

Anaprox® DS
(naproxen sodium)

RX   ROCHE   P. 2257

†Bactrim™
(trimethoprim and sulfamethoxazole)
80 mg / 400 mg

RX   ROCHE   P. 2257

†Bactrim™ DS
(trimethoprim and sulfamethoxazole)
160 mg / 800 mg

RX   ROCHE   P. 2259

Berocca®

RX   ROCHE   P. 2259

Berocca® Plus

RX   ROCHE   P. 2260

0.5 mg

1 mg

2 mg

†Bumex®
(bumetanide)

RX   ROCHE   P. 2265

250 mg

CellCept®
(mycophenolate mofetil)

RX   ROCHE   P. 2261

20 mg

30 mg

Cardene®
(nicardipine HCl)

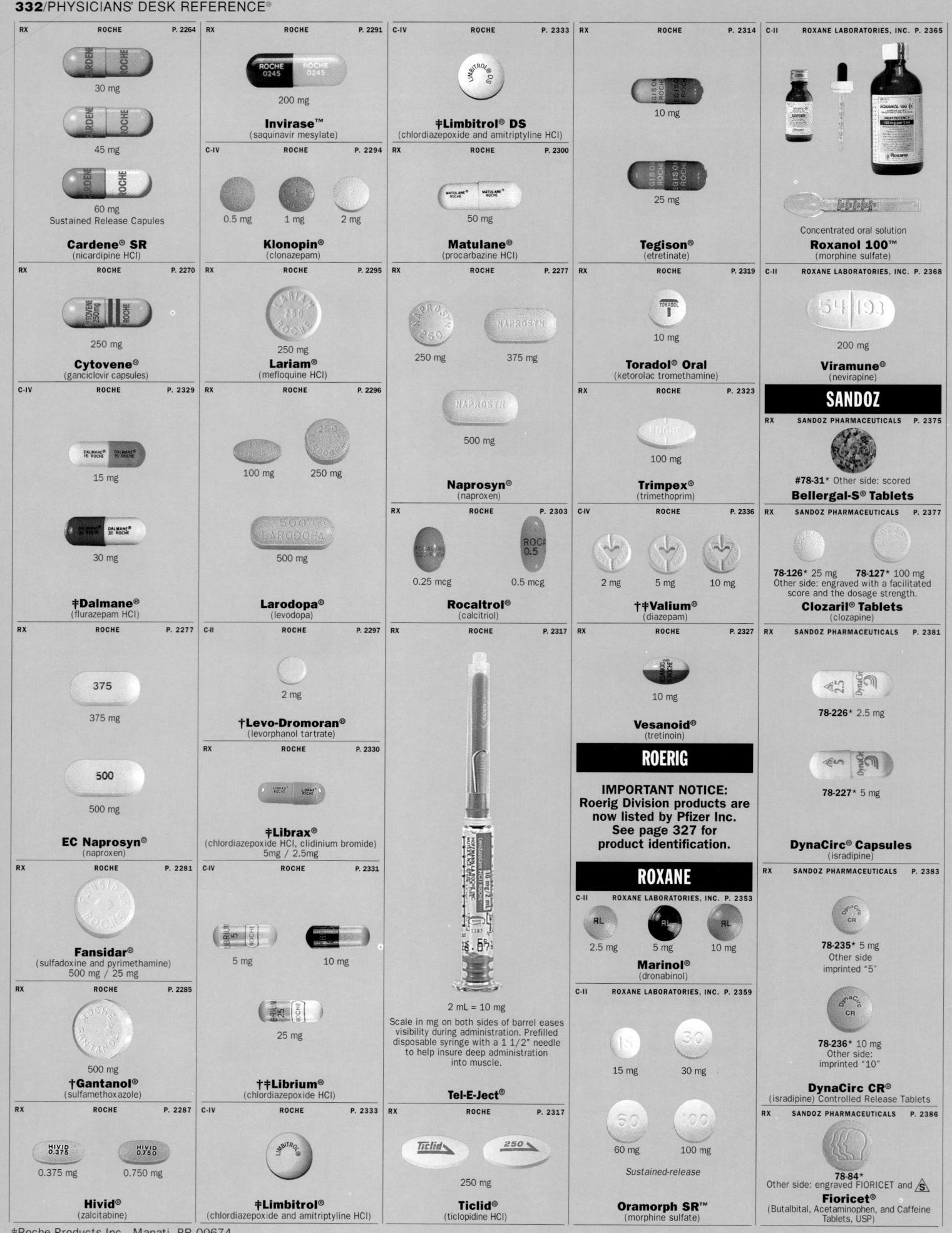

RX · ROCHE · P. 2264

30 mg

45 mg

60 mg
Sustained Release Capsules

Cardene® SR
(nicardipine HCl)

RX · ROCHE · P. 2270

250 mg

Cytovene®
(ganciclovir capsules)

C-IV · ROCHE · P. 2329

15 mg

30 mg

‡Dalmane®
(flurazepam HCl)

RX · ROCHE · P. 2277

375
375 mg

500
500 mg

EC Naprosyn®
(naproxen)

RX · ROCHE · P. 2281

Fansidar®
(sulfadoxine and pyrimethamine)
500 mg / 25 mg

RX · ROCHE · P. 2285

500 mg

†Gantanol®
(sulfamethoxazole)

RX · ROCHE · P. 2287

0.375 mg   0.750 mg

Hivid®
(zalcitabine)

C-IV · ROCHE · P. 2291

200 mg

Invirase™
(saquinavir mesylate)

C-IV · ROCHE · P. 2294

0.5 mg   1 mg   2 mg

Klonopin®
(clonazepam)

RX · ROCHE · P. 2295

250 mg

Lariam®
(mefloquine HCl)

RX · ROCHE · P. 2296

100 mg   250 mg

500 mg

Larodopa®
(levodopa)

C-II · ROCHE · P. 2297

2 mg

†Levo-Dromoran®
(levorphanol tartrate)

RX · ROCHE · P. 2330

‡Librax®
(chlordiazepoxide HCl, clidinium bromide)
5mg / 2.5mg

C-IV · ROCHE · P. 2331

5 mg   10 mg

25 mg

†‡Librium®
(chlordiazepoxide HCl)

C-IV · ROCHE · P. 2333

‡Limbitrol®
(chlordiazepoxide and amitriptyline HCl)

C-IV · ROCHE · P. 2333

‡Limbitrol® DS
(chlordiazepoxide and amitriptyline HCl)

RX · ROCHE · P. 2300

50 mg

Matulane®
(procarbazine HCl)

RX · ROCHE · P. 2277

250 mg   375 mg

500 mg

Naprosyn®
(naproxen)

RX · ROCHE · P. 2303

0.25 mcg   0.5 mcg

Rocaltrol®
(calcitriol)

RX · ROCHE · P. 2317

2 mL = 10 mg
Scale in mg on both sides of barrel eases
visibility during administration. Prefilled
disposable syringe with a 1 1/2" needle
to help insure deep administration
into muscle.

Tel-E-Ject®

RX · P. 2317

250 mg

Ticlid®
(ticlopidine HCl)

RX · ROCHE · P. 2314

10 mg

25 mg

Tegison®
(etretinate)

RX · ROCHE · P. 2319

10 mg

Toradol® Oral
(ketorolac tromethamine)

RX · ROCHE · P. 2323

100 mg

Trimpex®
(trimethoprim)

C-IV · ROCHE · P. 2336

2 mg   5 mg   10 mg

†‡Valium®
(diazepam)

RX · ROCHE · P. 2327

10 mg

Vesanoid®
(tretinoin)

ROERIG

IMPORTANT NOTICE:
Roerig Division products are
now listed by Pfizer Inc.
See page 327 for
product identification.

ROXANE

C-II · ROXANE LABORATORIES, INC. P. 2353

RL
2.5 mg   RL
5 mg   RL
10 mg

Marinol®
(dronabinol)

C-II · ROXANE LABORATORIES, INC. P. 2359

15 mg   30 mg

60 mg   100 mg

Sustained-release

Oramorph SR™
(morphine sulfate)

C-II · ROXANE LABORATORIES, INC. P. 2365

Concentrated oral solution
Roxanol 100™
(morphine sulfate)

C-II · ROXANE LABORATORIES, INC. P. 2368

54 193
200 mg

Viramune®
(nevirapine)

SANDOZ

RX · SANDOZ PHARMACEUTICALS · P. 2375

#78-31* Other side: scored
Bellergal-S® Tablets

RX · SANDOZ PHARMACEUTICALS · P. 2377

78-126* 25 mg   78-127* 100 mg
Other side: engraved with a facilitated
score and the dosage strength.
Clozaril® Tablets
(clozapine)

RX · SANDOZ PHARMACEUTICALS · P. 2381

78-226* 2.5 mg

78-227* 5 mg

DynaCirc® Capsules
(isradipine)

RX · SANDOZ PHARMACEUTICALS · P. 2383

78-235* 5 mg
Other side
imprinted "5"

78-236* 10 mg
Other side:
imprinted "10"

DynaCirc CR®
(isradipine) Controlled Release Tablets

RX · SANDOZ PHARMACEUTICALS · P. 2386

78-84*
Other side: engraved FIORICET and /S\
Fioricet®
(Butalbital, Acetaminophen, and Caffeine
Tablets, USP)

C-III   SANDOZ PHARMACEUTICALS P. 2387

78-243*

Fioricet® with Codeine Capsules
(butalbital, acetaminophen, caffeine, and codeine phosphate)

C-III   SANDOZ PHARMACEUTICALS P. 2388

78-103*

78-104*
Other side: tablets engraved SANDOZ

Fiorinal®
(butalbital, aspirin, caffeine) Capsules, USP
(butalbital, aspirin, caffeine) Tablets, USP

C-III   SANDOZ PHARMACEUTICALS P. 2390

78-107*

Fiorinal® with Codeine Capsules, USP
(butalbital, aspirin, caffeine, and codeine phosphate)

RX   SANDOZ PHARMACEUTICALS P. 2392

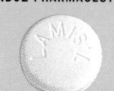

78-70* 1 mg
Other side: engraved Ⓢ

Hydergine®
(ergoloid mesylates) Tablets, USP (ORAL)

RX   SANDOZ PHARMACEUTICALS P. 2392

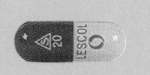

78-101* 1 mg
Other side: branded Ⓢ

Hydergine® LC
(ergoloid mesylates, USP) liquid capsules

RX   SANDOZ PHARMACEUTICALS P. 2394

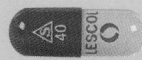

78-179* 250 mg
Other side: imprinted "250".

†Lamisil®
(terbinafine HCl tablets) Tablets

RX   SANDOZ PHARMACEUTICALS P. 2395

78-176* 20 mg

78-234* 40 mg

Lescol®
(fluvastatin sodium) Capsules

Because tablets and capsules are shown in this section, do not infer that these are the only dosage forms available. Where a product name is preceded by the symbol †, refer to the description in the Product Information (White Section) for other forms.

RX   SANDOZ PHARMACEUTICALS P. 2398

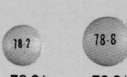

78-2* 10 mg   **78-8*** 15 mg   **78-3*** 25 mg
scored

78-4* 50 mg   **78-5*** 100 mg

78-6* 150 mg

78-7* 200 mg
Other side: imprinted Ⓢ

†Mellaril®
(thioridazine HCl) Tablets, USP

RX   SANDOZ PHARMACEUTICALS P. 2403

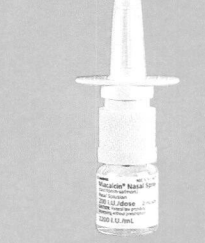

78-149*
2200 I.U./ML

Miacalcin® Nasal Spray
(calcitonin-salmon)
Nasal Solution

RX   SANDOZ PHARMACEUTICALS P. 2405

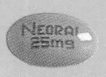

78-246* 25 mg

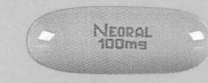

78-248* 100 mg

Neoral® Soft Gelatin Capsules
(cyclosporine capsules for microemulsion)

RX   SANDOZ PHARMACEUTICALS P. 2405

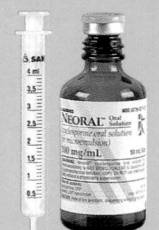

78-274* 100 mg/mL

Neoral® Oral Solution
(cyclosporine oral solution for microemulsion)

RX   SANDOZ PHARMACEUTICALS P. 2411

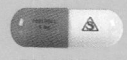

78-102* 5 mg

Parlodel® Capsules
(bromocriptine mesylate) Capsules, USP

RX   SANDOZ PHARMACEUTICALS P. 2411

78-17* 2 1/2 mg
Other side: scored

Parlodel® SnapTabs®
(bromocriptine mesylate) Tablets, USP

RX   SANDOZ PHARMACEUTICALS P. 2409

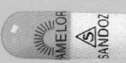

78-86* 10 mg
Other side: printed 10 mg

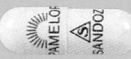

78-87* 25 mg
Other side: printed 25 mg

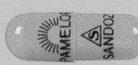

78-78* 50 mg
Other side: printed 50 mg

78-79* 75 mg
Other side: printed 75 mg

†Pamelor®
(nortriptyline HCl) Capsules, USP

C-IV   SANDOZ PHARMACEUTICALS P. 2413

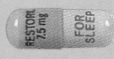

78-140* 7.5 mg

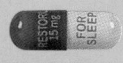

78-98* 15 mg

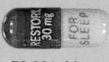

78-99* 30 mg

Restoril®
(temazepam) Capsules, USP

RX   SANDOZ PHARMACEUTICALS P. 2416

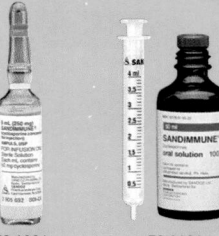

78-109*
I.V. 5 mL (250 mg)

78-110*
Oral Solution & Pipette
50 mL 100 mg/mL

Sandimmune®
(cyclosporine)

RX   SANDOZ PHARMACEUTICALS P. 2416

78-240* 25 mg

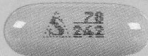

78-242* 50 mg

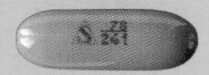

78-241* 100 mg

Sandimmune®
Soft Gelatin Capsules
(cyclosporine capsules, USP)

RX   SANDOZ PHARMACEUTICALS P. 2427

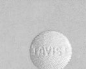

78-72* 2.68 mg
Other side: engraved 78/72

Tavist®
(clemastine fumarate tablets, USP, 2.68 mg)

RX   SANDOZ PHARMACEUTICALS P. 2428

78-111* 5 mg   **78-73*** 10 mg
Other side: embossed with "V"

Visken®
(pindolol) Tablets, USP

SANOFI WINTHROP

RX   SANOFI WINTHROP PHARMACEUTICALS P. 2437

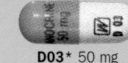

D03* 50 mg

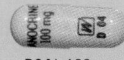

D04* 100 mg

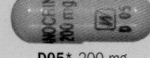

D05* 200 mg

Danocrine®
(danazol capsules, USP)

RX   SANOFI WINTHROP PHARMACEUTICALS P. 2431

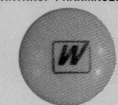

A77* 500 mg

†Aralen® Phosphate
(chloroquine phosphate tablets, USP)

C-II   SANOFI WINTHROP PHARMACEUTICALS P. 2438

D35*50 mg   **D37***100 mg
Scored tablet

†Demerol®
(meperidine HCl, USP)

RX   SANOFI WINTHROP PHARMACEUTICALS P. 2453

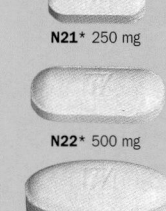

N21* 250 mg

N22* 500 mg

N23* 1 gram
Scored tablets

†NegGram®
(nalidixic acid, USP)

RX   SANOFI WINTHROP PHARMACEUTICALS P. 2459

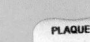

P62* 200 mg

Plaquenil® Sulfate
(hydroxychloroquine sulfate tablets, USP)

C-IV   SANOFI WINTHROP PHARMACEUTICALS

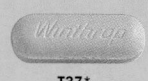

T37*
Scored tablet

Talacen®
(pentazocine HCl, USP, equivalent to 25 mg base and acetaminophen, USP, 650 mg)

C-IV   SANOFI WINTHROP PHARMACEUTICALS P. 2467

T51*
Scored tablet

†Talwin® Nx
(pentazocine HCl, USP, equivalent to 50 mg base and naloxone HCl, USP, equivalent to 0.5 mg base)

C-III   SANOFI WINTHROP PHARMACEUTICALS P. 2468

W53* 2 mg
Scored tablet

Winstrol®
(stanozolol tablets, USP)

SAVAGE LABORATORIES

RX   SAVAGE LABORATORIES P. 2469

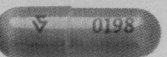

Axocet®
(butalbital, acetaminophen)
50 mg/650 mg

RX   SAVAGE LABORATORIES P. 2470

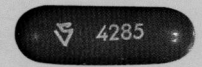

Liquid Iron Supplement in Soft Gelatin Capsule

Chromagen®
(ferrous fumarate, USP, 200 mg)

RX   SAVAGE LABORATORIES P. 2471

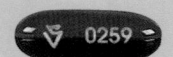

Liquid Iron Supplement in Soft Gelatin Capsule

Chromagen® FA
(ferrous fumarate, USP, folic acid, USP)
200 mg/1 mg

RX   SAVAGE LABORATORIES P. 2471

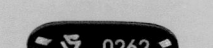

Liquid Iron Supplement in Soft Gelatin Capsule

Chromagen® Forte
(ferrous fumarate, USP, 460 mg)

RX   SAVAGE LABORATORIES P. 2475

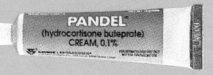

Pandel®
(hydrocortisone buteprate)
Cream 0.1%

RX   SAVAGE LABORATORIES P. 2476

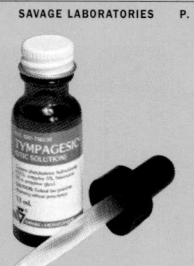

Tympagesic® Otic Solution
(phenylephrine HCl, USP, antipyrine, USP, benzocaine, USP)
0.25% / 5% / 5%

SCANDIPHARM

RX   SCANDIPHARM INC. P. 2476

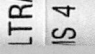

Enteric Coated Microspheres

ULTRASE®
(pancrelipase)

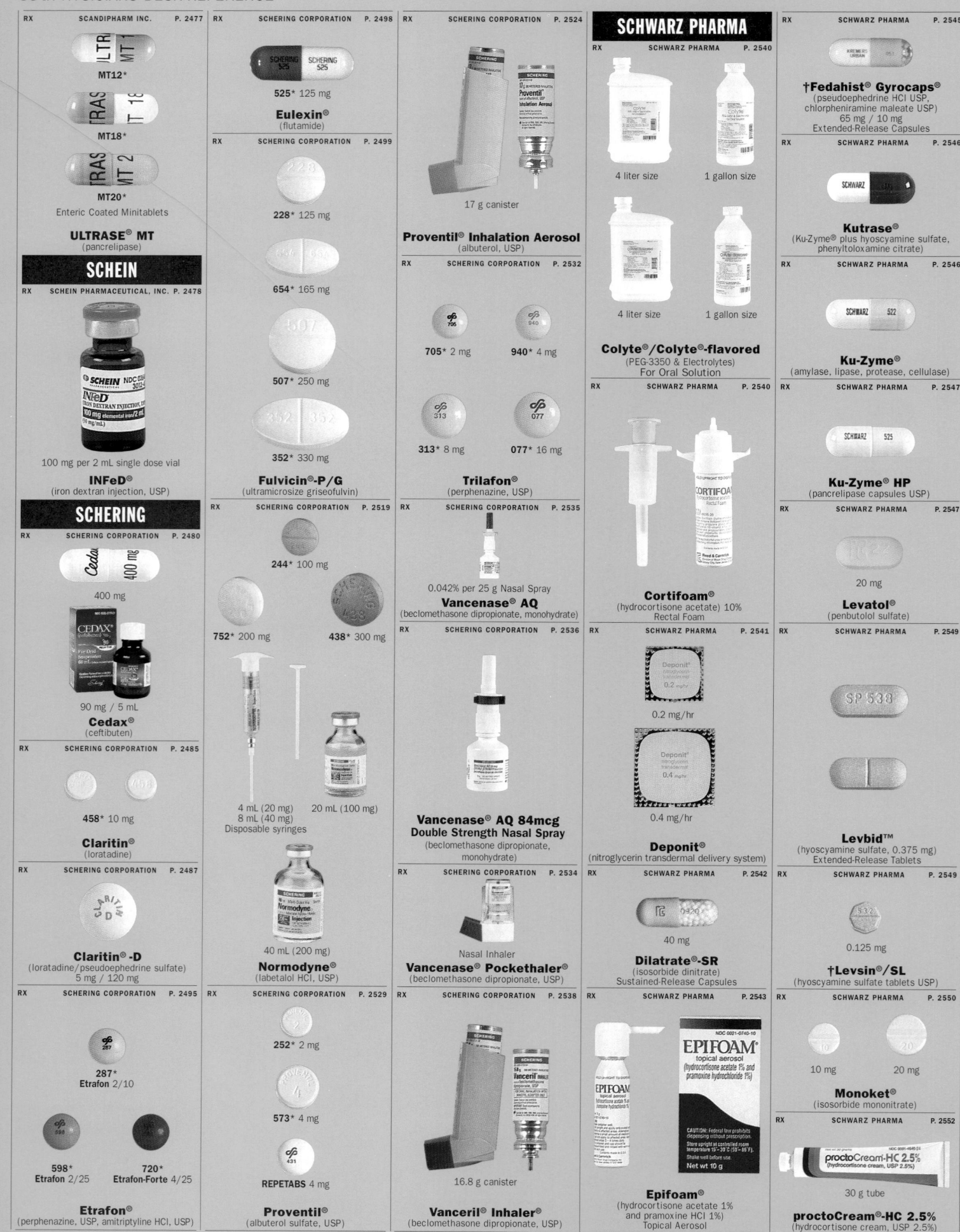

RX   SCANDIPHARM INC.   P. 2477

MT12*

MT18*

MT20*

Enteric Coated Minitablets

ULTRASE® MT
(pancrelipase)

SCHEIN

RX   SCHEIN PHARMACEUTICAL, INC. P. 2478

100 mg per 2 mL single dose vial

INFeD®
(iron dextran injection, USP)

SCHERING

RX   SCHERING CORPORATION   P. 2480

400 mg

90 mg / 5 mL

Cedax®
(ceftibuten)

RX   SCHERING CORPORATION   P. 2485

458* 10 mg

Claritin®
(loratadine)

RX   SCHERING CORPORATION   P. 2487

Claritin®-D
(loratadine/pseudoephedrine sulfate)
5 mg / 120 mg

RX   SCHERING CORPORATION   P. 2495

287*
Etrafon 2/10

598*
Etrafon 2/25

720*
Etrafon-Forte 4/25

Etrafon®
(perphenazine, USP, amitriptyline HCl, USP)

RX   SCHERING CORPORATION   P. 2498

525* 125 mg

Eulexin®
(flutamide)

RX   SCHERING CORPORATION   P. 2499

228* 125 mg

654* 165 mg

507* 250 mg

352* 330 mg

Fulvicin®-P/G
(ultramicrosize griseofulvin)

RX   SCHERING CORPORATION   P. 2519

244* 100 mg

752* 200 mg

438* 300 mg

4 mL (20 mg)
8 mL (40 mg)
Disposable syringes

20 mL (100 mg)

40 mL (200 mg)

Normodyne®
(labetalol HCl, USP)

RX   SCHERING CORPORATION   P. 2529

252* 2 mg

573* 4 mg

REPETABS 4 mg

Proventil®
(albuterol sulfate, USP)

RX   SCHERING CORPORATION   P. 2524

17 g canister

Proventil® Inhalation Aerosol
(albuterol, USP)

RX   SCHERING CORPORATION   P. 2532

705* 2 mg

940* 4 mg

313* 8 mg

077* 16 mg

Trilafon®
(perphenazine, USP)

RX   SCHERING CORPORATION   P. 2535

0.042% per 25 g Nasal Spray

Vancenase® AQ
(beclomethasone dipropionate, monohydrate)

RX   SCHERING CORPORATION   P. 2536

Vancenase® AQ 84mcg
Double Strength Nasal Spray
(beclomethasone dipropionate,
monohydrate)

RX   SCHERING CORPORATION   P. 2534

Nasal Inhaler

Vancenase® Pockethaler®
(beclomethasone dipropionate, USP)

RX   SCHERING CORPORATION   P. 2538

16.8 g canister

Vanceril® Inhaler®
(beclomethasone dipropionate, USP)

SCHWARZ PHARMA

RX   SCHWARZ PHARMA   P. 2540

4 liter size

1 gallon size

4 liter size

1 gallon size

Colyte®/Colyte®-flavored
(PEG-3350 & Electrolytes)
For Oral Solution

RX   SCHWARZ PHARMA   P. 2540

Cortifoam®
(hydrocortisone acetate) 10%
Rectal Foam

RX   SCHWARZ PHARMA   P. 2541

0.2 mg/hr

0.4 mg/hr

Deponit®
(nitroglycerin transdermal delivery system)

RX   SCHWARZ PHARMA   P. 2542

40 mg

Dilatrate®-SR
(isosorbide dinitrate)
Sustained-Release Capsules

RX   SCHWARZ PHARMA   P. 2543

EPIFOAM®
topical aerosol
(hydrocortisone acetate 1% and
pramoxine hydrochloride 1%)
Net wt 10 g

Epifoam®
(hydrocortisone acetate 1%
and pramoxine HCl 1%)
Topical Aerosol

RX   SCHWARZ PHARMA   P. 2545

†Fedahist® Gyrocaps®
(pseudoephedrine HCl USP,
chlorpheniramine maleate USP)
65 mg / 10 mg
Extended-Release Capsules

RX   SCHWARZ PHARMA   P. 2546

Kutrase®
(Ku-Zyme® plus hyoscyamine sulfate,
phenyltoloxamine citrate)

RX   SCHWARZ PHARMA   P. 2546

Ku-Zyme®
(amylase, lipase, protease, cellulase)

RX   SCHWARZ PHARMA   P. 2547

Ku-Zyme® HP
(pancrelipase capsules USP)

RX   SCHWARZ PHARMA   P. 2547

20 mg

Levatol®
(penbutolol sulfate)

RX   SCHWARZ PHARMA   P. 2549

SP 538

Levbid™
(hyoscyamine sulfate, 0.375 mg)
Extended-Release Tablets

RX   SCHWARZ PHARMA   P. 2549

0.125 mg

†Levsin®/SL
(hyoscyamine sulfate tablets USP)

RX   SCHWARZ PHARMA   P. 2550

10 mg

20 mg

Monoket®
(isosorbide mononitrate)

RX   SCHWARZ PHARMA   P. 2552

proctoCream®-HC 2.5%
(hydrocortisone cream, USP 2.5%)
30 g tube

proctoCream®-HC 2.5%
(hydrocortisone cream, USP 2.5%)

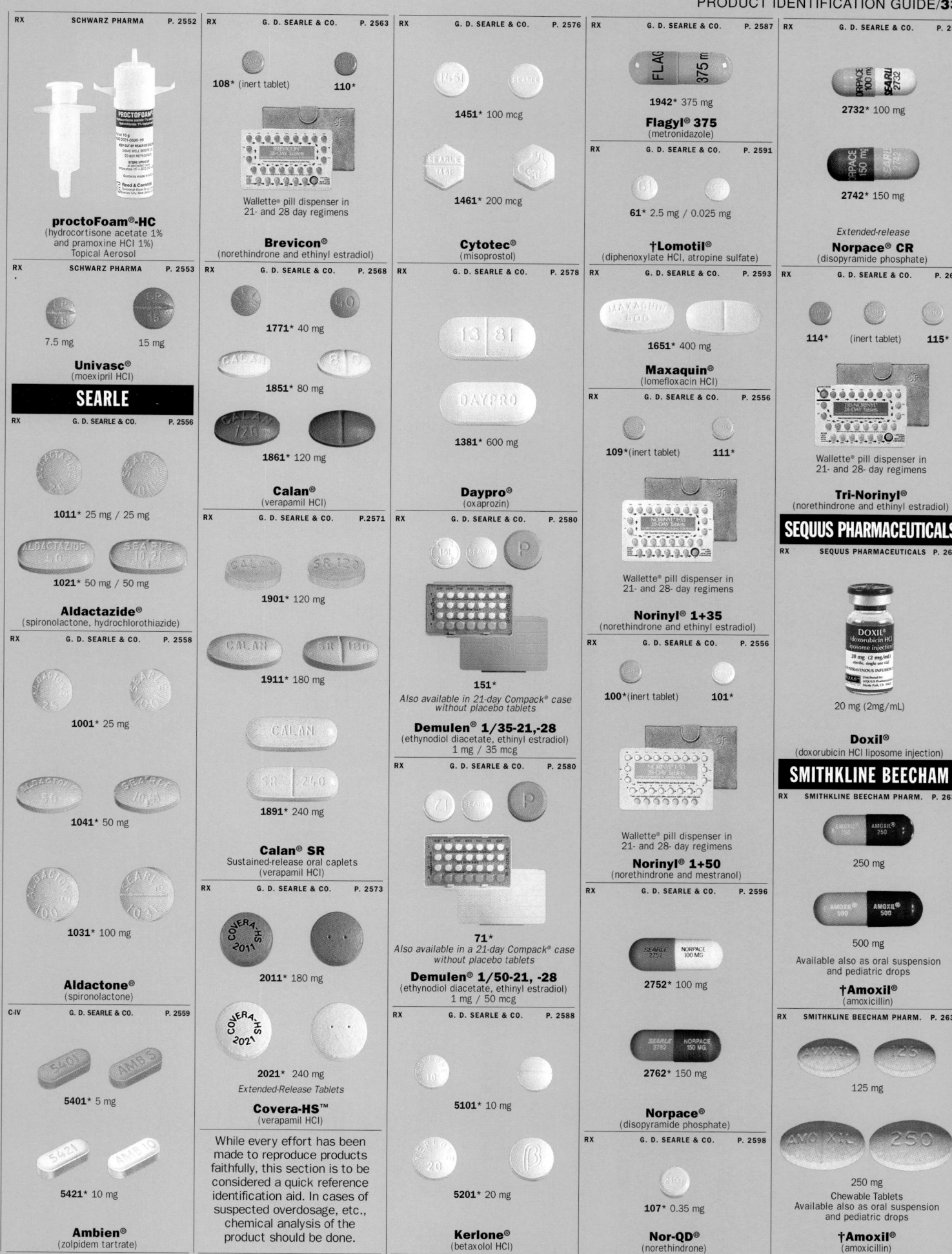

RX   SCHWARZ PHARMA   P. 2552

proctoFoam®-HC
(hydrocortisone acetate 1%
and pramoxine HCl 1%)
Topical Aerosol

RX   SCHWARZ PHARMA   P. 2553

7.5 mg   15 mg

Univasc®
(moexipril HCl)

SEARLE

RX   G. D. SEARLE & CO.   P. 2556

1011* 25 mg / 25 mg

1021* 50 mg / 50 mg

Aldactazide®
(spironolactone, hydrochlorothiazide)

RX   G. D. SEARLE & CO.   P. 2558

1001* 25 mg

1041* 50 mg

1031* 100 mg

Aldactone®
(spironolactone)

C-IV   G. D. SEARLE & CO.   P. 2559

5401* 5 mg

5421* 10 mg

Ambien®
(zolpidem tartrate)

RX   G. D. SEARLE & CO.   P. 2563

108* (inert tablet)   110*

Wallette® pill dispenser in
21- and 28 day regimens

Brevicon®
(norethindrone and ethinyl estradiol)

RX   G. D. SEARLE & CO.   P. 2568

1771* 40 mg

1851* 80 mg

1861* 120 mg

Calan®
(verapamil HCl)

RX   G. D. SEARLE & CO.   P.2571

1901* 120 mg

1911* 180 mg

1891* 240 mg

Calan® SR
Sustained-release oral caplets
(verapamil HCl)

RX   G. D. SEARLE & CO.   P. 2573

2011* 180 mg

2021* 240 mg
Extended-Release Tablets

Covera-HS™
(verapamil HCl)

While every effort has been
made to reproduce products
faithfully, this section is to be
considered a quick reference
identification aid. In cases of
suspected overdosage, etc.,
chemical analysis of the
product should be done.

RX   G. D. SEARLE & CO.   P. 2576

1451* 100 mcg

1461* 200 mcg

Cytotec®
(misoprostol)

RX   G. D. SEARLE & CO.   P. 2578

13 81

DAYPRO

1381* 600 mg

Daypro®
(oxaprozin)

RX   G. D. SEARLE & CO.   P. 2580

151*
*Also available in 21-day Compack® case
without placebo tablets*

Demulen® 1/35-21,-28
(ethynodiol diacetate, ethinyl estradiol)
1 mg / 35 mcg

RX   G. D. SEARLE & CO.   P. 2580

71*
*Also available in a 21-day Compack® case
without placebo tablets*

Demulen® 1/50-21, -28
(ethynodiol diacetate, ethinyl estradiol)
1 mg / 50 mcg

RX   G. D. SEARLE & CO.   P. 2588

5101* 10 mg

5201* 20 mg

Kerlone®
(betaxolol HCl)

RX   G. D. SEARLE & CO.   P. 2587

FLAG   375 m

1942* 375 mg

Flagyl® 375
(metronidazole)

RX   G. D. SEARLE & CO.   P. 2591

61* 2.5 mg / 0.025 mg

†Lomotil®
(diphenoxylate HCl, atropine sulfate)

RX   G. D. SEARLE & CO.   P. 2593

1651* 400 mg

Maxaquin®
(lomefloxacin HCl)

RX   G. D. SEARLE & CO.   P. 2556

109*(inert tablet)   111*

Wallette® pill dispenser in
21- and 28- day regimens

Norinyl® 1+35
(norethindrone and ethinyl estradiol)

RX   G. D. SEARLE & CO.   P. 2556

100*(inert tablet)   101*

Wallette® pill dispenser in
21- and 28- day regimens

Norinyl® 1+50
(norethindrone and mestranol)

RX   G. D. SEARLE & CO.   P. 2596

2752* 100 mg

2762* 150 mg

Norpace®
(disopyramide phosphate)

RX   G. D. SEARLE & CO.   P. 2598

107* 0.35 mg

Nor-QD®
(norethindrone)

RX   G. D. SEARLE & CO.   P. 2596

2732* 100 mg

2742* 150 mg

Extended-release
Norpace® CR
(disopyramide phosphate)

RX   G. D. SEARLE & CO.   P. 2607

114*   (inert tablet)   115*

Wallette® pill dispenser in
21- and 28- day regimens

Tri-Norinyl®
(norethindrone and ethinyl estradiol)

SEQUUS PHARMACEUTICALS

RX   SEQUUS PHARMACEUTICALS   P. 2613

DOXIL
doxorubicin HCl
liposome injection

20 mg (2mg/mL)

Doxil®
(doxorubicin HCl liposome injection)

SMITHKLINE BEECHAM

RX   SMITHKLINE BEECHAM PHARM.   P. 2631

250 mg

500 mg

Available also as oral suspension
and pediatric drops

†Amoxil®
(amoxicillin)

RX   SMITHKLINE BEECHAM PHARM.   P. 2631

125 mg

250 mg
Chewable Tablets
Available also as oral suspension
and pediatric drops

†Amoxil®
(amoxicillin)

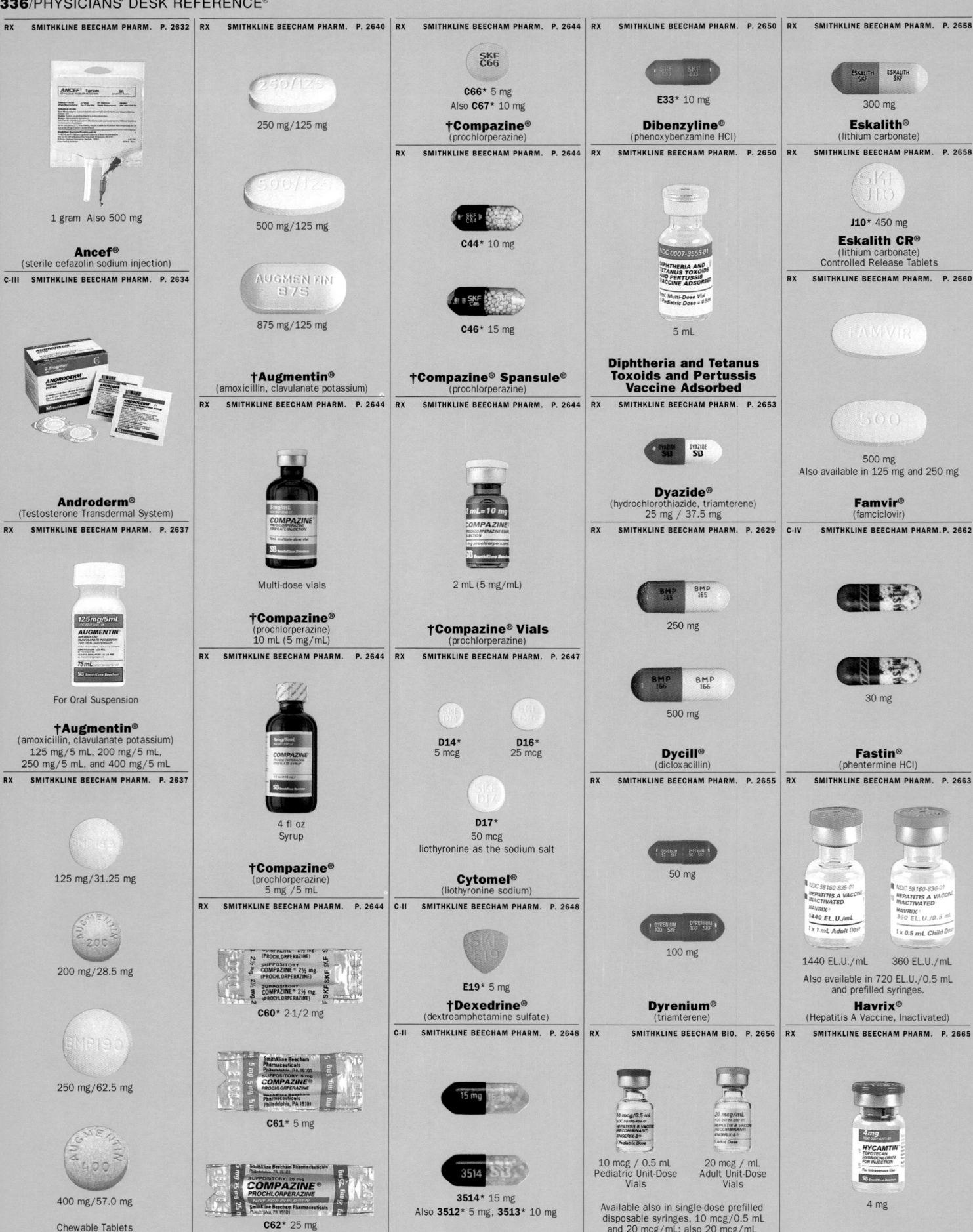

RX   SMITHKLINE BEECHAM PHARM.   P. 2632

1 gram Also 500 mg

Ancef®
(sterile cefazolin sodium injection)

C-III   SMITHKLINE BEECHAM PHARM.   P. 2634

Androderm®
(Testosterone Transdermal System)

RX   SMITHKLINE BEECHAM PHARM.   P. 2637

125mg/5mL

For Oral Suspension

†Augmentin®
(amoxicillin, clavulanate potassium)
125 mg/5 mL, 200 mg/5 mL,
250 mg/5 mL, and 400 mg/5 mL

RX   SMITHKLINE BEECHAM PHARM.   P. 2637

125 mg/31.25 mg

200 mg/28.5 mg

250 mg/62.5 mg

400 mg/57.0 mg

Chewable Tablets

†Augmentin®
(amoxicillin, clavulanate potassium)

RX   SMITHKLINE BEECHAM PHARM.   P. 2640

250 mg/125 mg

500 mg/125 mg

AUGMENTIN 875

875 mg/125 mg

†Augmentin®
(amoxicillin, clavulanate potassium)

RX   SMITHKLINE BEECHAM PHARM.   P. 2644

Multi-dose vials

†Compazine®
(prochlorperazine)
10 mL (5 mg/mL)

RX   SMITHKLINE BEECHAM PHARM.   P. 2644

4 fl oz
Syrup

†Compazine®
(prochlorperazine)
5 mg /5 mL

RX   SMITHKLINE BEECHAM PHARM.   P. 2644

C60* 2-1/2 mg

C61* 5 mg

C62* 25 mg
Suppositories

†Compazine®
(prochlorperazine)

RX   SMITHKLINE BEECHAM PHARM.   P. 2644

C66* 5 mg
Also **C67*** 10 mg

†Compazine®
(prochlorperazine)

RX   SMITHKLINE BEECHAM PHARM.   P. 2644

C44* 10 mg

C46* 15 mg

†Compazine® Spansule®
(prochlorperazine)

RX   SMITHKLINE BEECHAM PHARM.   P. 2644

2 mL (5 mg/mL)

†Compazine® Vials
(prochlorperazine)

RX   SMITHKLINE BEECHAM PHARM.   P. 2647

D14* 5 mcg   **D16*** 25 mcg

D17* 50 mcg
liothyronine as the sodium salt

Cytomel®
(liothyronine sodium)

C-II   SMITHKLINE BEECHAM PHARM.   P. 2648

E19* 5 mg

†Dexedrine®
(dextroamphetamine sulfate)

C-II   SMITHKLINE BEECHAM PHARM.   P. 2648

15 mg

3514* 15 mg
Also **3512*** 5 mg, **3513*** 10 mg

†Dexedrine® Spansule®
(dextroamphetamine sulfate)

RX   SMITHKLINE BEECHAM PHARM.   P. 2650

E33* 10 mg

Dibenzyline®
(phenoxybenzamine HCl)

RX   SMITHKLINE BEECHAM PHARM.   P. 2650

5 mL

**Diphtheria and Tetanus
Toxoids and Pertussis
Vaccine Adsorbed**

RX   SMITHKLINE BEECHAM PHARM.   P. 2653

Dyazide®
(hydrochlorothiazide, triamterene)
25 mg / 37.5 mg

RX   SMITHKLINE BEECHAM PHARM.   P. 2629

250 mg

500 mg

Dycill®
(dicloxacillin)

RX   SMITHKLINE BEECHAM PHARM.   P. 2655

50 mg

100 mg

Dyrenium®
(triamterene)

RX   SMITHKLINE BEECHAM BIO.   P. 2656

10 mcg / 0.5 mL
Pediatric Unit-Dose
Vials

20 mcg / mL
Adult Unit-Dose
Vials

Available also in single-dose prefilled
disposable syringes, 10 mcg/0.5 mL
and 20 mcg/mL; also 20 mcg/mL
in 10 mL multi-dose vials.

Engerix-B®
(Hepatitis B Vaccine [Recombinant])

RX   SMITHKLINE BEECHAM PHARM.   P. 2658

300 mg

Eskalith®
(lithium carbonate)

RX   SMITHKLINE BEECHAM PHARM.   P. 2658

J10* 450 mg

Eskalith CR®
(lithium carbonate)
Controlled Release Tablets

RX   SMITHKLINE BEECHAM PHARM.   P. 2660

500 mg

Also available in 125 mg and 250 mg

Famvir®
(famciclovir)

C-IV   SMITHKLINE BEECHAM PHARM.   P. 2662

30 mg

Fastin®
(phentermine HCl)

RX   SMITHKLINE BEECHAM PHARM.   P. 2663

1440 EL.U./mL   360 EL.U./mL

Also available in 720 EL.U./0.5 mL
and prefilled syringes.

Havrix®
(Hepatitis A Vaccine, Inactivated)

RX   SMITHKLINE BEECHAM PHARM.   P. 2665

4 mg

Hycamtin™
(topotecan HCl)

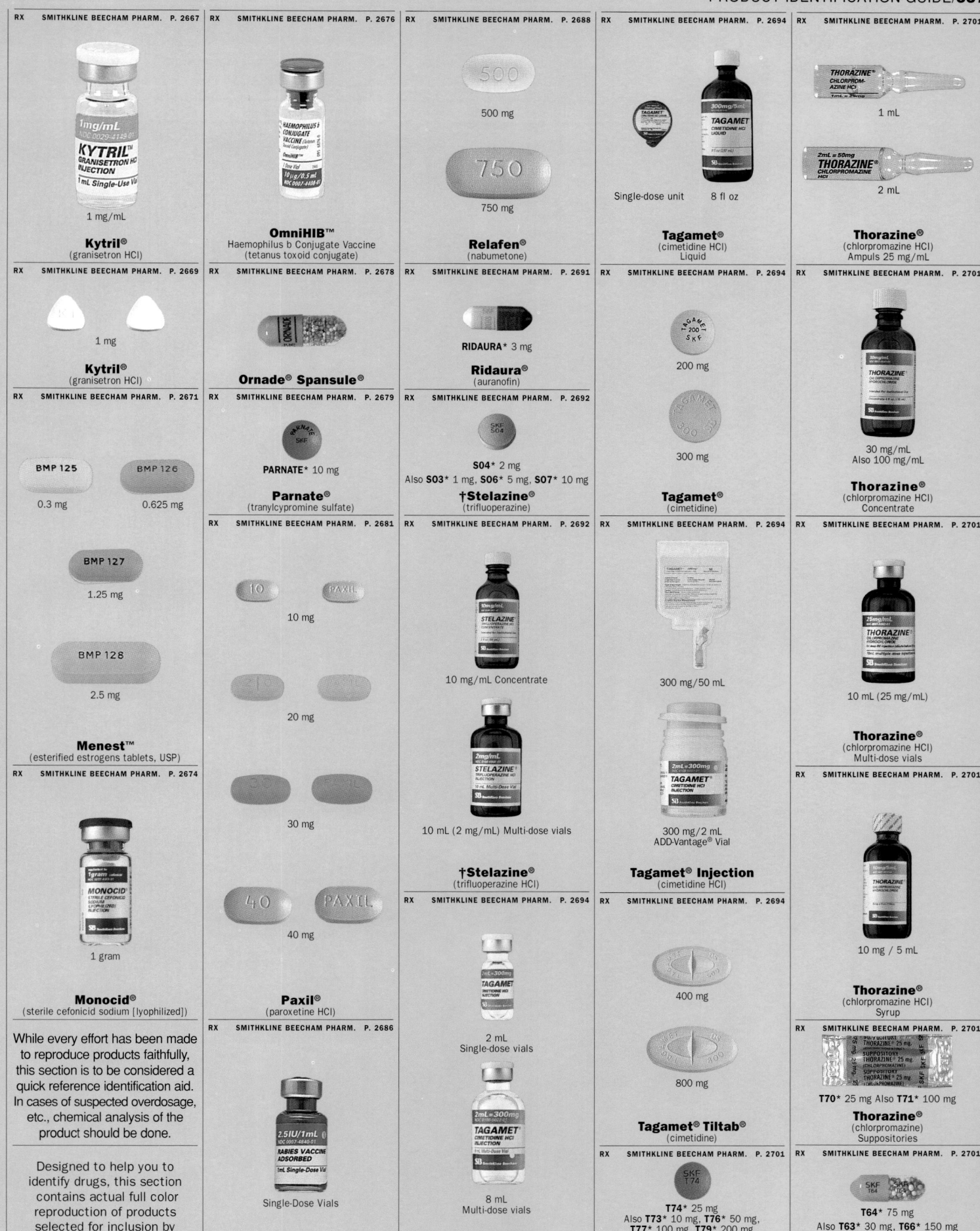

RX   SMITHKLINE BEECHAM PHARM.   P. 2667

1mg/mL
NDC 0029-4149-01
KYTRIL™
GRANISETRON HCl
INJECTION
1 mL Single-Use Vial

1 mg/mL

Kytril®
(granisetron HCl)

RX   SMITHKLINE BEECHAM PHARM.   P. 2669

1 mg

Kytril®
(granisetron HCl)

RX   SMITHKLINE BEECHAM PHARM.   P. 2671

BMP 125   BMP 126

0.3 mg   0.625 mg

BMP 127

1.25 mg

BMP 128

2.5 mg

Menest™
(esterified estrogens tablets, USP)

RX   SMITHKLINE BEECHAM PHARM.   P. 2674

1gram
MONOCID®
STERILE CEFONICID
SODIUM
[LYOPHILIZED]
INJECTION

1 gram

Monocid®
(sterile cefonicid sodium [lyophilized])

While every effort has been made
to reproduce products faithfully,
this section is to be considered a
quick reference identification aid.
In cases of suspected overdosage,
etc., chemical analysis of the
product should be done.

Designed to help you to
identify drugs, this section
contains actual full color
reproduction of products
selected for inclusion by
participating manufacturers.

RX   SMITHKLINE BEECHAM PHARM.   P. 2676

HAEMOPHILUS b
CONJUGATE
VACCINE (tetanus
Toxoid Conjugate)
OmniHIB™
10 µg/0.5 mL
1 Dose Vial
NDC 0007-4408-01

OmniHIB™
Haemophilus b Conjugate Vaccine
(tetanus toxoid conjugate)

RX   SMITHKLINE BEECHAM PHARM.   P. 2678

ORNADE

Ornade® Spansule®

RX   SMITHKLINE BEECHAM PHARM.   P. 2679

PARNATE
SKF

PARNATE* 10 mg

Parnate®
(tranylcypromine sulfate)

RX   SMITHKLINE BEECHAM PHARM.   P. 2681

10   PAXIL

10 mg

20 mg

30 mg

40   PAXIL

40 mg

Paxil®
(paroxetine HCl)

RX   SMITHKLINE BEECHAM PHARM.   P. 2686

2.5IU/1mL
NDC 0007-4840-01
**RABIES VACCINE
ADSORBED**
1mL Single-Dose Vials

Single-Dose Vials

Rabies Vaccine Adsorbed

RX   SMITHKLINE BEECHAM PHARM.   P. 2688

500

500 mg

750

750 mg

Relafen®
(nabumetone)

RX   SMITHKLINE BEECHAM PHARM.   P. 2691

RIDAURA* 3 mg

Ridaura®
(auranofin)

RX   SMITHKLINE BEECHAM PHARM.   P. 2692

SKF
S04

S04* 2 mg
Also **S03*** 1 mg, **S06*** 5 mg, **S07*** 10 mg

†Stelazine®
(trifluoperazine)

RX   SMITHKLINE BEECHAM PHARM.   P. 2692

10mg/mL
STELAZINE
TRIFLUOPERAZINE HCl
CONCENTRATE

10 mg/mL Concentrate

2mg/mL
NDC 0007-4907-01
STELAZINE
TRIFLUOPERAZINE HCl
INJECTION
10 mL Multi-Dose Vial

10 mL (2 mg/mL) Multi-dose vials

†Stelazine®
(trifluoperazine HCl)

RX   SMITHKLINE BEECHAM PHARM.   P. 2694

TAGAMET
CIMETIDINE HCl
INJECTION

2 mL
Single-dose vials

2mL=300mg
NDC 0007-0000-00
TAGAMET®
CIMETIDINE HCl
INJECTION
8mL Multi-Dose Vial

8 mL
Multi-dose vials

Tagamet® Injection
(cimetidine HCl)
300 mg/2 mL

RX   SMITHKLINE BEECHAM PHARM.   P. 2694

TAGAMET
ONE DOSE SKF

300mg/5mL
TAGAMET
CIMETIDINE HCl
LIQUID
8 fl oz (237 mL)

Single-dose unit   8 fl oz

Tagamet®
(cimetidine HCl)
Liquid

RX   SMITHKLINE BEECHAM PHARM.   P. 2694

TAGAMET
200
SKF

200 mg

TAGAMET
300 SKF

300 mg

Tagamet®
(cimetidine)

RX   SMITHKLINE BEECHAM PHARM.   P. 2694

TAGAMET

300 mg/50 mL

2mL=300mg
TAGAMET®
CIMETIDINE HCl
INJECTION

300 mg/2 mL
ADD-Vantage® Vial

Tagamet® Injection
(cimetidine HCl)

RX   SMITHKLINE BEECHAM PHARM.   P. 2694

400 mg

800 mg

Tagamet® Tiltab®
(cimetidine)

RX   SMITHKLINE BEECHAM PHARM.   P. 2701

THORAZINE®
CHLORPROM-
AZINE HCl
1mL = 25mg

1 mL

2mL = 50mg
THORAZINE®
CHLORPROMAZINE
HCl

2 mL

Thorazine®
(chlorpromazine HCl)
Ampuls 25 mg/mL

RX   SMITHKLINE BEECHAM PHARM.   P. 2701

30mg/mL
THORAZINE®
CHLORPROMAZINE
HYDROCHLORIDE ORAL
Intended For Institutional Use
SmithKline Beecham

30 mg/mL
Also 100 mg/mL

Thorazine®
(chlorpromazine HCl)
Concentrate

RX   SMITHKLINE BEECHAM PHARM.   P. 2701

25mg/mL
THORAZINE®
CHLORPROMAZINE
HYDROCHLORIDE ORAL
10mL multiple dose injection

10 mL (25 mg/mL)

Thorazine®
(chlorpromazine HCl)
Multi-dose vials

RX   SMITHKLINE BEECHAM PHARM.   P. 2701

THORAZINE®
CHLORPROMAZINE
HYDROCHLORIDE

10 mg / 5 mL

Thorazine®
(chlorpromazine HCl)
Syrup

RX   SMITHKLINE BEECHAM PHARM.   P. 2701

THORAZINE® 25 mg
SUPPOSITORY
THORAZINE® 25 mg
(CHLORPROMAZINE)
SUPPOSITORY
THORAZINE® 25 mg
(CHLORPROMAZINE)

T70* 25 mg Also **T71*** 100 mg

Thorazine®
(chlorpromazine)
Suppositories

RX   SMITHKLINE BEECHAM PHARM.   P. 2701

SKF
T74

T74* 25 mg
Also **T73*** 10 mg, **T76*** 50 mg,
T77* 100 mg, **T79*** 200 mg

Thorazine®
(chlorpromazine HCl)
Tablets

RX   SMITHKLINE BEECHAM PHARM.   P. 2701

SKF
T64

T64* 75 mg
Also **T63*** 30 mg, **T66*** 150 mg

Thorazine® Spansule®
(chlorpromazine HCl)

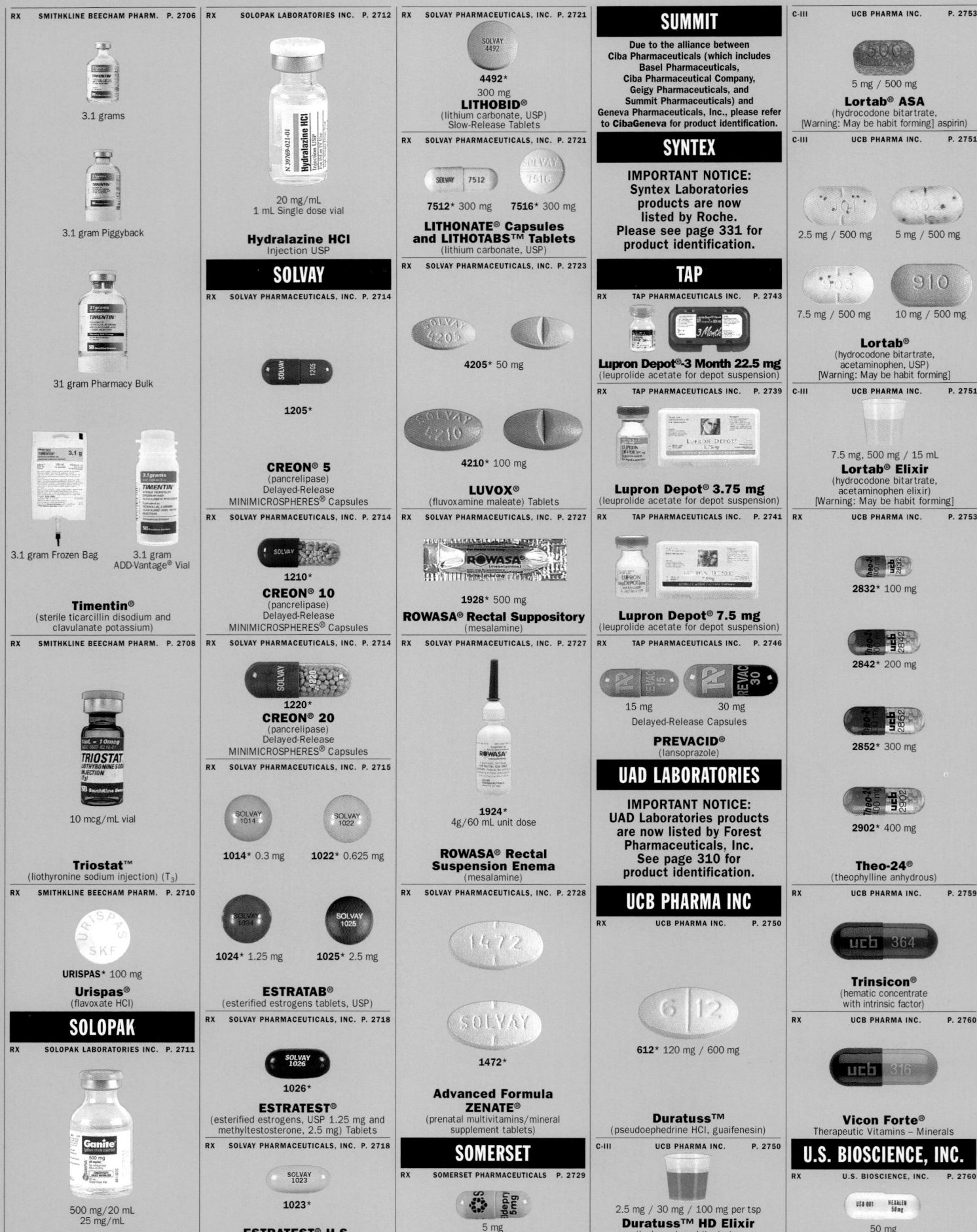

RX   SMITHKLINE BEECHAM PHARM.   P. 2706

3.1 grams

3.1 gram Piggyback

31 gram Pharmacy Bulk

3.1 gram Frozen Bag   3.1 gram
                         ADD-Vantage® Vial

Timentin®
(sterile ticarcillin disodium and
clavulanate potassium)

RX   SMITHKLINE BEECHAM PHARM.   P. 2708

10 mcg/mL vial

Triostat™
(liothyronine sodium injection) (T₃)

RX   SMITHKLINE BEECHAM PHARM.   P. 2710

URISPAS* 100 mg

Urispas®
(flavoxate HCl)

SOLOPAK

RX   SOLOPAK LABORATORIES INC.   P. 2711

500 mg/20 mL
25 mg/mL

Ganite®
(gallium nitrate injection)

RX   SOLOPAK LABORATORIES INC.   P. 2712

20 mg/mL
1 mL Single dose vial

Hydralazine HCl
Injection USP

SOLVAY

RX   SOLVAY PHARMACEUTICALS, INC.   P. 2714

1205*

CREON® 5
(pancrelipase)
Delayed-Release
MINIMICROSPHERES® Capsules

RX   SOLVAY PHARMACEUTICALS, INC.   P. 2714

1210*

CREON® 10
(pancrelipase)
Delayed-Release
MINIMICROSPHERES® Capsules

RX   SOLVAY PHARMACEUTICALS, INC.   P. 2714

1220*

CREON® 20
(pancrelipase)
Delayed-Release
MINIMICROSPHERES® Capsules

RX   SOLVAY PHARMACEUTICALS, INC.   P. 2715

1014* 0.3 mg   1022* 0.625 mg

1024* 1.25 mg   1025* 2.5 mg

ESTRATAB®
(esterified estrogens tablets, USP)

RX   SOLVAY PHARMACEUTICALS, INC.   P. 2718

1026*

ESTRATEST®
(esterified estrogens, USP 1.25 mg and
methyltestosterone, 2.5 mg) Tablets

RX   SOLVAY PHARMACEUTICALS, INC.   P. 2718

1023*

ESTRATEST® H.S.
(esterified estrogens, USP 0.625 mg and
methyltestosterone, 1.25 mg) Tablets

4492*
300 mg
LITHOBID®
(lithium carbonate, USP)
Slow-Release Tablets

RX   SOLVAY PHARMACEUTICALS, INC.   P. 2721

7512* 300 mg   7516* 300 mg

**LITHONATE® Capsules
and LITHOTABS™ Tablets**
(lithium carbonate, USP)

RX   SOLVAY PHARMACEUTICALS, INC.   P. 2723

4205* 50 mg

4210* 100 mg

LUVOX®
(fluvoxamine maleate) Tablets

RX   SOLVAY PHARMACEUTICALS, INC.   P. 2727

1928* 500 mg

ROWASA® Rectal Suppository
(mesalamine)

RX   SOLVAY PHARMACEUTICALS, INC.   P. 2727

1924*
4g/60 mL unit dose

**ROWASA® Rectal
Suspension Enema**
(mesalamine)

RX   SOLVAY PHARMACEUTICALS, INC.   P. 2728

1472*

**Advanced Formula
ZENATE®**
(prenatal multivitamins/mineral
supplement tablets)

SOMERSET

RX   SOMERSET PHARMACEUTICALS   P. 2729

5 mg

ELDEPRYL®
(selegiline HCl)

SUMMIT

Due to the alliance between
Ciba Pharmaceuticals (which includes
Basel Pharmaceuticals,
Ciba Pharmaceutical Company,
Geigy Pharmaceuticals, and
Summit Pharmaceuticals) and
Geneva Pharmaceuticals, Inc., please refer
to CibaGeneva for product identification.

SYNTEX

IMPORTANT NOTICE:
Syntex Laboratories
products are now
listed by Roche.
Please see page 331 for
product identification.

TAP

RX   TAP PHARMACEUTICALS INC.   P. 2743

Lupron Depot®-3 Month 22.5 mg
(leuprolide acetate for depot suspension)

RX   TAP PHARMACEUTICALS INC.   P. 2739

Lupron Depot® 3.75 mg
(leuprolide acetate for depot suspension)

RX   TAP PHARMACEUTICALS INC.   P. 2741

Lupron Depot® 7.5 mg
(leuprolide acetate for depot suspension)

RX   TAP PHARMACEUTICALS INC.   P. 2746

15 mg   30 mg
Delayed-Release Capsules

PREVACID®
(lansoprazole)

UAD LABORATORIES

IMPORTANT NOTICE:
UAD Laboratories products
are now listed by Forest
Pharmaceuticals, Inc.
See page 310 for
product identification.

UCB PHARMA INC

RX   UCB PHARMA INC.   P. 2750

612* 120 mg / 600 mg

Duratuss™
(pseudoephedrine HCl, guaifenesin)

C-III   UCB PHARMA INC.   P. 2750

2.5 mg / 30 mg / 100 mg per tsp
Duratuss™ HD Elixir
(hydrocodone bitartrate,
[Warning: May be habit forming]
pseudoephedrine HCl, guaifenesin)

C-III   UCB PHARMA INC.   P. 2753

5 mg / 500 mg
Lortab® ASA
(hydrocodone bitartrate,
[Warning: May be habit forming] aspirin)

C-III   UCB PHARMA INC.   P. 2751

2.5 mg / 500 mg   5 mg / 500 mg

7.5 mg / 500 mg   10 mg / 500 mg

Lortab®
(hydrocodone bitartrate,
acetaminophen, USP)
[Warning: May be habit forming]

C-III   UCB PHARMA INC.   P. 2751

7.5 mg, 500 mg / 15 mL
Lortab® Elixir
(hydrocodone bitartrate,
acetaminophen elixir)
[Warning: May be habit forming]

RX   UCB PHARMA INC.   P. 2753

2832* 100 mg

2842* 200 mg

2852* 300 mg

2902* 400 mg

Theo-24®
(theophylline anhydrous)

RX   UCB PHARMA INC.   P. 2759

Trinsicon®
(hematic concentrate
with intrinsic factor)

RX   UCB PHARMA INC.   P. 2760

Vicon Forte®
Therapeutic Vitamins – Minerals

U.S. BIOSCIENCE, INC.

RX   U.S. BIOSCIENCE, INC.   P. 2760

50 mg

Hexalen®
(altretamine)

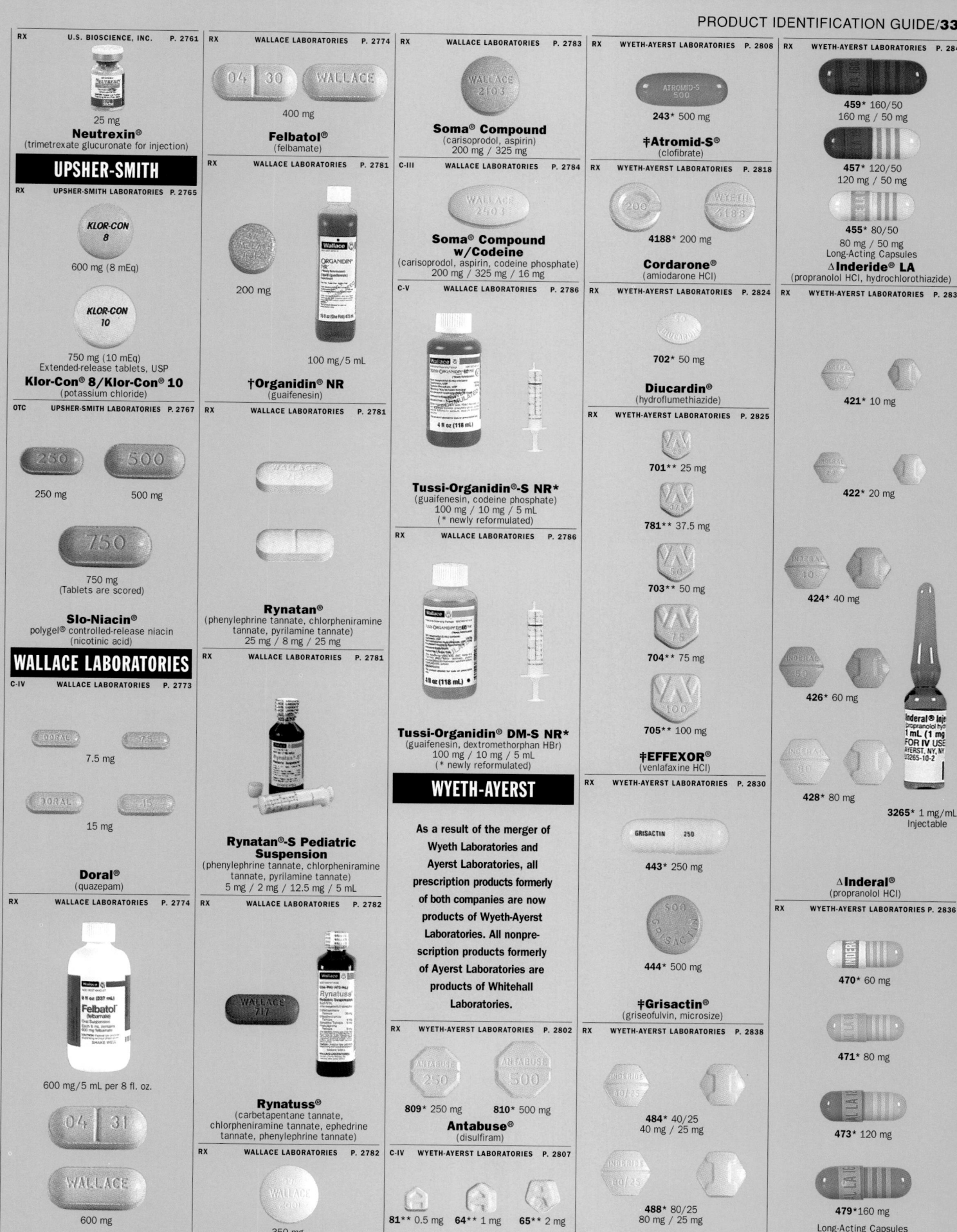

RX   U.S. BIOSCIENCE, INC.   P. 2761

25 mg
Neutrexin®
(trimetrexate glucuronate for injection)

UPSHER-SMITH

RX   UPSHER-SMITH LABORATORIES   P. 2765

KLOR-CON 8
600 mg (8 mEq)

KLOR-CON 10
750 mg (10 mEq)
Extended-release tablets, USP
Klor-Con® 8/Klor-Con® 10
(potassium chloride)

OTC   UPSHER-SMITH LABORATORIES   P. 2767

250 mg   500 mg

750 mg
(Tablets are scored)
Slo-Niacin®
polygel® controlled-release niacin
(nicotinic acid)

WALLACE LABORATORIES

C-IV   WALLACE LABORATORIES   P. 2773

DORAL 7.5 mg

DORAL 15 mg

Doral®
(quazepam)

RX   WALLACE LABORATORIES   P. 2774

04 31

WALLACE
600 mg

Felbatol®
(felbamate)

RX   WALLACE LABORATORIES   P. 2774

04 30   WALLACE
400 mg
Felbatol®
(felbamate)

RX   WALLACE LABORATORIES   P. 2781

200 mg

Wallace ORGANIDIN NR
100 mg/5 mL
†Organidin® NR
(guaifenesin)

RX   WALLACE LABORATORIES   P. 2781

WALLACE

Rynatan®
(phenylephrine tannate, chlorpheniramine
tannate, pyrilamine tannate)
25 mg / 8 mg / 25 mg

RX   WALLACE LABORATORIES   P. 2781

**Rynatan®-S Pediatric
Suspension**
(phenylephrine tannate, chlorpheniramine
tannate, pyrilamine tannate)
5 mg / 2 mg / 12.5 mg / 5 mL

RX   WALLACE LABORATORIES   P. 2782

WALLACE 717

Rynatuss®
(carbetapentane tannate,
chlorpheniramine tannate, ephedrine
tannate, phenylephrine tannate)

RX   WALLACE LABORATORIES   P. 2782

WALLACE 350 mg

Soma®
(carisoprodol)

RX   WALLACE LABORATORIES   P. 2783

WALLACE 2103

Soma® Compound
(carisoprodol, aspirin)
200 mg / 325 mg

C-III   WALLACE LABORATORIES   P. 2784

WALLACE 2403

**Soma® Compound
w/Codeine**
(carisoprodol, aspirin, codeine phosphate)
200 mg / 325 mg / 16 mg

C-V   WALLACE LABORATORIES   P. 2786

4 fl oz (118 mL)
Tussi-Organidin®-S NR*
(guaifenesin, codeine phosphate)
100 mg / 10 mg / 5 mL
(* newly reformulated)

RX   WALLACE LABORATORIES   P. 2786

4 fl oz (118 mL)
Tussi-Organidin® DM-S NR*
(guaifenesin, dextromethorphan HBr)
100 mg / 10 mg / 5 mL
(* newly reformulated)

WYETH-AYERST

As a result of the merger of
Wyeth Laboratories and
Ayerst Laboratories, all
prescription products formerly
of both companies are now
products of Wyeth-Ayerst
Laboratories. All nonpre-
scription products formerly
of Ayerst Laboratories are
products of Whitehall
Laboratories.

RX   WYETH-AYERST LABORATORIES   P. 2802

ANTABUSE 250
809* 250 mg

ANTABUSE 500
810* 500 mg
Antabuse®
(disulfiram)

C-IV   WYETH-AYERST LABORATORIES   P. 2807

81** 0.5 mg   **64**** 1 mg   **65**** 2 mg
ΔAtivan®
(lorazepam)

RX   WYETH-AYERST LABORATORIES   P. 2808

ATROMID-S 500
243* 500 mg
‡Atromid-S®
(clofibrate)

RX   WYETH-AYERST LABORATORIES   P. 2818

200   WYETH 4188
4188* 200 mg
Cordarone®
(amiodarone HCl)

RX   WYETH-AYERST LABORATORIES   P. 2824

702* 50 mg
Diucardin®
(hydroflumethiazide)

RX   WYETH-AYERST LABORATORIES   P. 2825

701** 25 mg

781** 37.5 mg

703** 50 mg

704** 75 mg

705** 100 mg
‡EFFEXOR®
(venlafaxine HCl)

RX   WYETH-AYERST LABORATORIES   P. 2830

GRISACTIN 250
443* 250 mg

500 GRISACTIN
444* 500 mg
‡Grisactin®
(griseofulvin, microsize)

RX   WYETH-AYERST LABORATORIES   P. 2838

INDERIDE 40/25
484* 40/25
40 mg / 25 mg

INDERIDE 80/25
488* 80/25
80 mg / 25 mg
ΔInderide®
(propranolol HCl, hydrochlorothiazide)

RX   WYETH-AYERST LABORATORIES   P. 2840

459* 160/50
160 mg / 50 mg

457* 120/50
120 mg / 50 mg

455* 80/50
80 mg / 50 mg
Long-Acting Capsules
ΔInderide® LA
(propranolol HCl, hydrochlorothiazide)

RX   WYETH-AYERST LABORATORIES   P. 2834

421* 10 mg

422* 20 mg

424* 40 mg

426* 60 mg

428* 80 mg

Inderal® Inj
propranolol hyd
1 mL (1 mg
FOR IV USE
AYERST, NY, NY
03265-10-2
3265* 1 mg/mL
Injectable

ΔInderal®
(propranolol HCl)

RX   WYETH-AYERST LABORATORIES   P. 2836

INDERAL
470* 60 mg

471* 80 mg

WALLA
473* 120 mg

WALLA
479* 160 mg
Long-Acting Capsules
ΔInderal® LA
(propranolol HCl)

---

† The appearance of these tablets and capsules is a trademark of Wyeth-Ayerst Laboratories.   Δ The appearance of these tablets and capsules is a registered trademark of Wyeth-Ayerst Laboratories.
**Product identification number on reverse side.

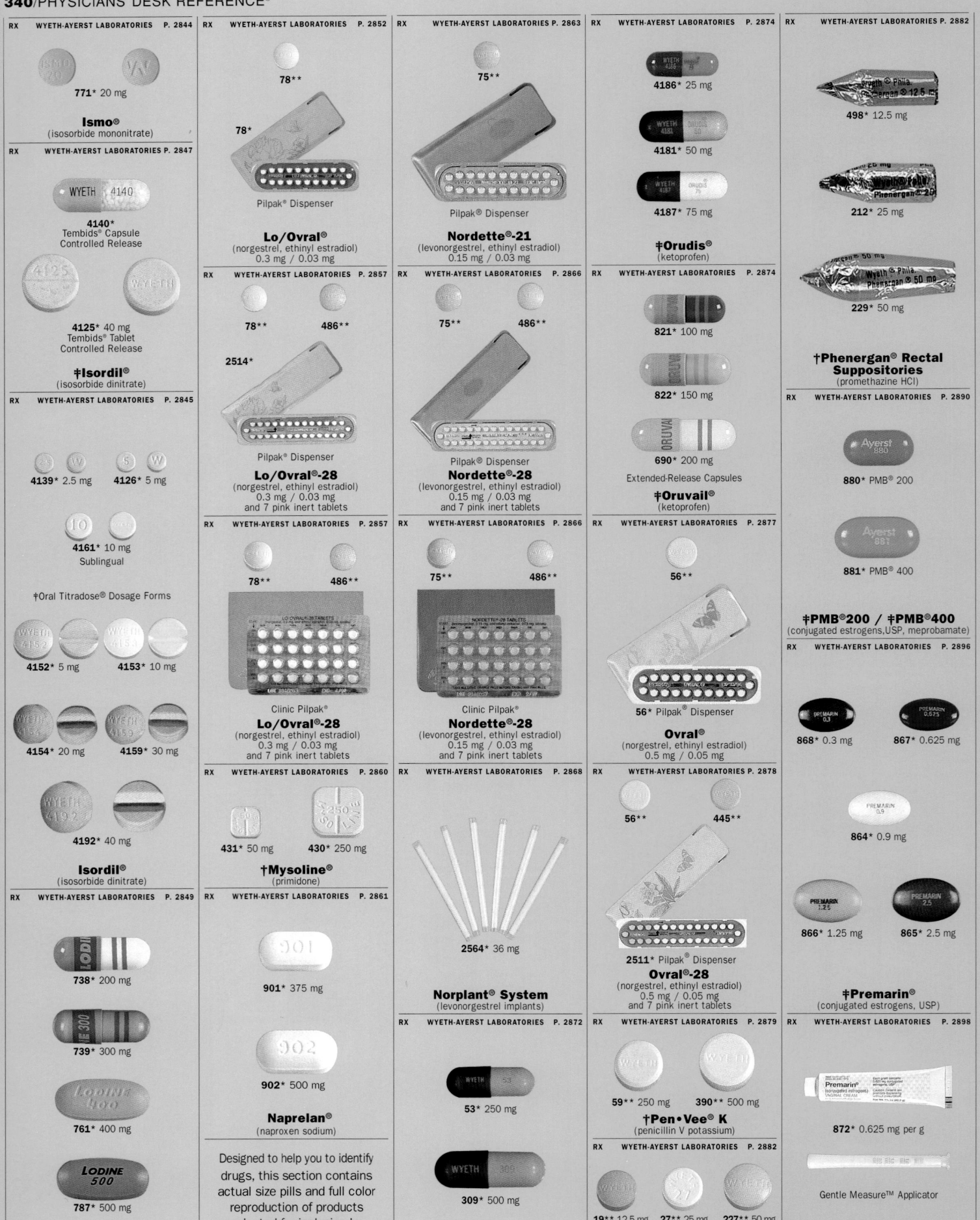

| RX | WYETH-AYERST LABORATORIES | P. 2844 |

771* 20 mg

Ismo®
(isosorbide mononitrate)

RX WYETH-AYERST LABORATORIES P. 2847

4140*
Tembids® Capsule
Controlled Release

4125* 40 mg
Tembids® Tablet
Controlled Release

‡Isordil®
(isosorbide dinitrate)

RX WYETH-AYERST LABORATORIES P. 2845

4139* 2.5 mg **4126*** 5 mg

4161* 10 mg
Sublingual

†Oral Titradose® Dosage Forms

4152* 5 mg **4153*** 10 mg

4154* 20 mg **4159*** 30 mg

4192* 40 mg

Isordil®
(isosorbide dinitrate)

RX WYETH-AYERST LABORATORIES P. 2849

738* 200 mg

739* 300 mg

761* 400 mg

787* 500 mg

‡Lodine®
(etodolac)

RX WYETH-AYERST LABORATORIES P. 2852

78**

78*

Pilpak® Dispenser

Lo/Ovral®
(norgestrel, ethinyl estradiol)
0.3 mg / 0.03 mg

RX WYETH-AYERST LABORATORIES P. 2857

78** **486****

2514*

Pilpak® Dispenser
Lo/Ovral®-28
(norgestrel, ethinyl estradiol)
0.3 mg / 0.03 mg
and 7 pink inert tablets

RX WYETH-AYERST LABORATORIES P. 2857

78** **486****

Clinic Pilpak®
Lo/Ovral®-28
(norgestrel, ethinyl estradiol)
0.3 mg / 0.03 mg
and 7 pink inert tablets

RX WYETH-AYERST LABORATORIES P. 2860

431* 50 mg **430*** 250 mg

†Mysoline®
(primidone)

RX WYETH-AYERST LABORATORIES P. 2861

901* 375 mg

902* 500 mg

Naprelan®
(naproxen sodium)

Designed to help you to identify
drugs, this section contains
actual size pills and full color
reproduction of products
selected for inclusion by
participating manufacturers.

RX WYETH-AYERST LABORATORIES P. 2863

75**

Pilpak® Dispenser

Nordette®-21
(levonorgestrel, ethinyl estradiol)
0.15 mg / 0.03 mg

RX WYETH-AYERST LABORATORIES P. 2866

75** **486****

Pilpak® Dispenser
Nordette®-28
(levonorgestrel, ethinyl estradiol)
0.15 mg / 0.03 mg
and 7 pink inert tablets

RX WYETH-AYERST LABORATORIES P. 2866

75** **486****

Clinic Pilpak®
Nordette®-28
(levonorgestrel, ethinyl estradiol)
0.15 mg / 0.03 mg
and 7 pink inert tablets

RX WYETH-AYERST LABORATORIES P. 2868

2564* 36 mg

Norplant® System
(levonorgestrel implants)

RX WYETH-AYERST LABORATORIES P. 2872

53* 250 mg

309* 500 mg

‡†Omnipen®
(ampicillin)

RX WYETH-AYERST LABORATORIES P. 2874

4186* 25 mg

4181* 50 mg

4187* 75 mg

‡Orudis®
(ketoprofen)

RX WYETH-AYERST LABORATORIES P. 2874

821* 100 mg

822* 150 mg

690* 200 mg

Extended-Release Capsules
‡Oruvail®
(ketoprofen)

RX WYETH-AYERST LABORATORIES P. 2877

56**

56* Pilpak® Dispenser

Ovral®
(norgestrel, ethinyl estradiol)
0.5 mg / 0.05 mg

RX WYETH-AYERST LABORATORIES P. 2878

56** **445****

2511* Pilpak® Dispenser
Ovral®-28
(norgestrel, ethinyl estradiol)
0.5 mg / 0.05 mg
and 7 pink inert tablets

RX WYETH-AYERST LABORATORIES P. 2879

59** 250 mg **390**** 500 mg

†Pen•Vee® K
(penicillin V potassium)

RX WYETH-AYERST LABORATORIES P. 2882

19** 12.5 mg **27**** 25 mg **227**** 50 mg

†Phenergan®
(promethazine HCl)

RX WYETH-AYERST LABORATORIES P. 2882

498* 12.5 mg

212* 25 mg

229* 50 mg

**†Phenergan® Rectal
Suppositories**
(promethazine HCl)

RX WYETH-AYERST LABORATORIES P. 2890

880* PMB® 200

881* PMB® 400

‡PMB®200 / ‡PMB®400
(conjugated estrogens,USP, meprobamate)

RX WYETH-AYERST LABORATORIES P. 2896

868* 0.3 mg **867*** 0.625 mg

864* 0.9 mg

866* 1.25 mg **865*** 2.5 mg

‡Premarin®
(conjugated estrogens, USP)

RX WYETH-AYERST LABORATORIES P. 2898

872* 0.625 mg per g

Gentle Measure™ Applicator

Premarin® Vaginal Cream
(conjugated estrogens)
Net Wt. 1 1/2 oz. (42.5 g)

† The appearance of these tablets and capsules is a trademark of Wyeth-Ayerst Laboratories.   ∆ The appearance of these tablets and capsules is a registered trademark of Wyeth-Ayerst Laboratories.
***Product identification number on reverse side

RX WYETH-AYERST LABORATORIES P. 2900

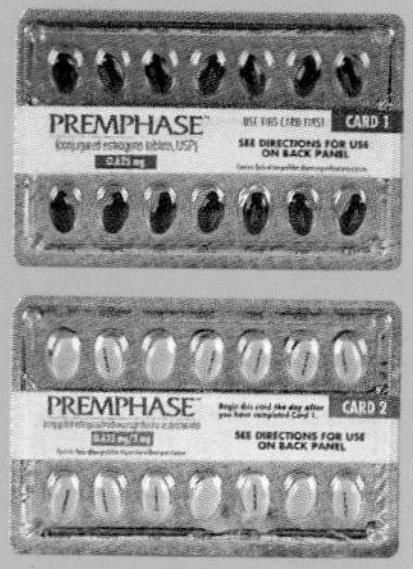

Premphase®
(conjugated estrogens tablets/
medroxyprogesterone acetate tablets, USP)
0.625 mg / 5.0 mg

RX WYETH-AYERST LABORATORIES P. 2905

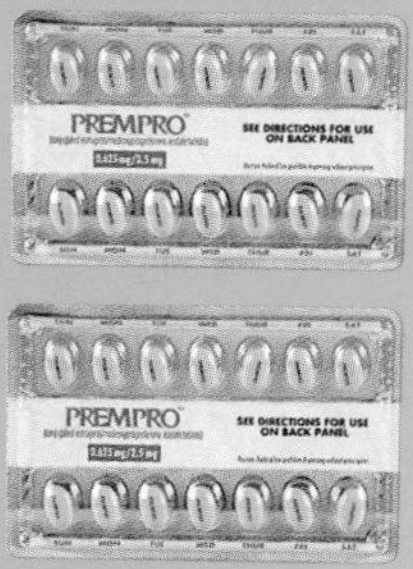

Prempro™
(conjugated estrogens tablets/
medroxyprogesterone acetate tablets, USP)
0.625 mg / 2.5 mg

RX WYETH-AYERST LABORATORIES P. 2911

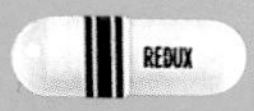

904* 15 mg

Redux™
(dexfenfluramine)

RX WYETH-AYERST LABORATORIES P. 2914

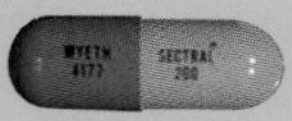

4177* 200 mg

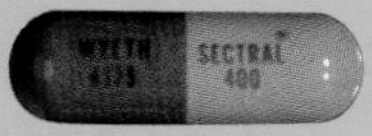

4179* 400 mg

‡†Sectral®
(acebutolol HCl)

RX WYETH-AYERST LABORATORIES

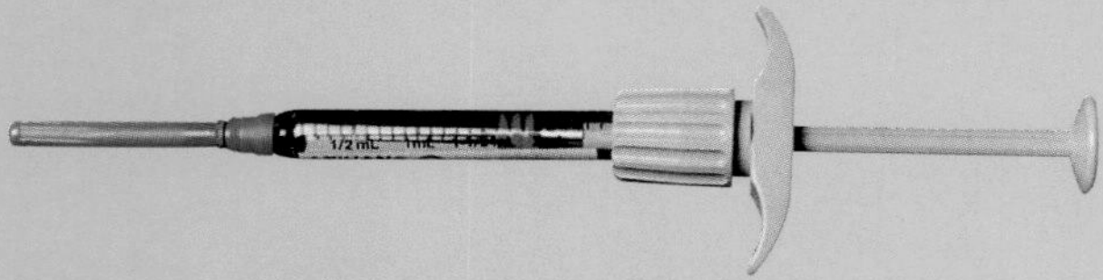

Tubex® Injector and Sterile Cartridge–Needle Unit
with hard cannula cover ready for injection.

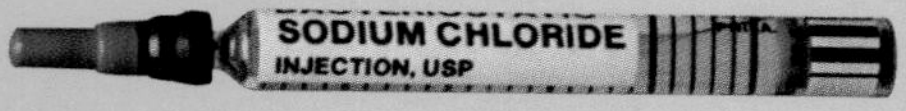

SODIUM CHLORIDE
INJECTION, USP

Tubex® Blunt Pointe™ Sterile Cartridge–Needle Unit
for use in selected "needle–less" IV port systems*

(*Consult product prescribing information for compatibility
information in the Product Information section of this PDR.)

Tubex® Closed Injection System

Examples of Tubex® Sterile Cartridge–Needle Units, Tubex® Blunt Pointe™ Sterile Cartridge–Unit, and Tubex® Injector,
components of the Tubex Closed Injection System, the most comprehensive line of small–volume unit–dose prefilled
syringe injectibles. For complete list of products available, consult Tubex listing in the Product Information Section.

C-IV WYETH-AYERST LABORATORIES P. 2916

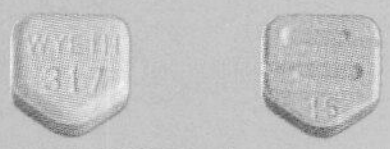

317* 15 mg

‡†Serax®
(oxazepam)

C-IV WYETH-AYERST LABORATORIES P. 2916

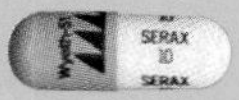

51* 10 mg

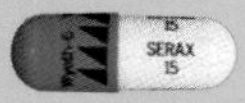

6* 15 mg

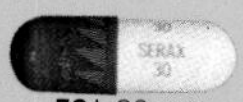

52* 30 mg

‡†Serax®
(oxazepam)

RX WYETH-AYERST LABORATORIES P. 2917

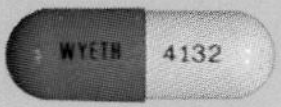

4132* 25 mg

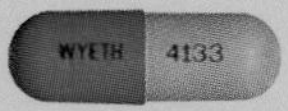

4133* 50 mg

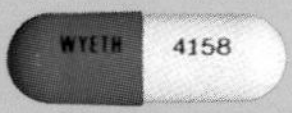

4158* 100 mg

‡Surmontil®
(trimipramine maleate)

RX WYETH-AYERST LABORATORIES P. 2932

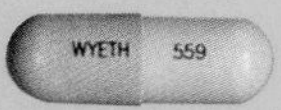

559* 250 mg

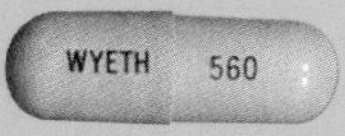

560* 500 mg

†Wymox®
(amoxicillin)

P. 2926

C-IV WYETH-AYERST LABORATORIES P. 2930

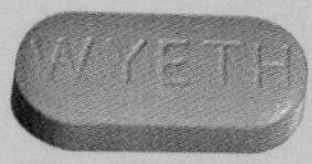

WYETH

85*
Wygesic®
(propoxyphene HCl, USP, acetaminophen, USP)
65 mg /650 mg

RX WYETH-AYERST LABORATORIES P. 2919

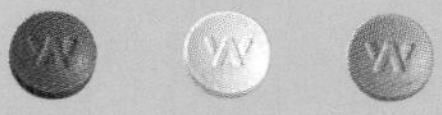

641* ** **642*** ** **643*** **

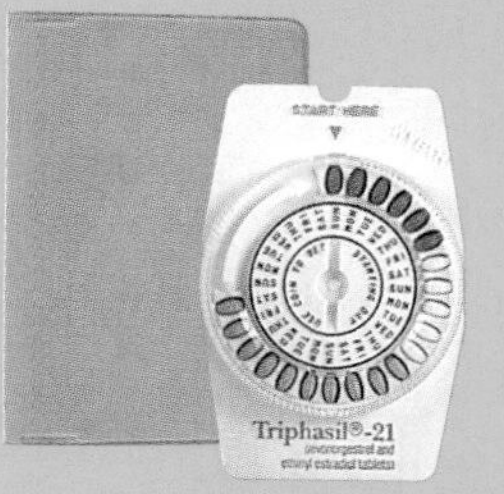

2535*

Triphasil®-21
(21 tablets containing the following:
6 brown tablets - 0.050 mg levonorgestrel
+ 0.030 mg ethinyl estradiol; 5 white
tablets - 0.075 mg levonorgestrel + 0.040 mg
ethinyl estradiol; 10 light-yellow tablets -
0.125 mg levonorgestrel + 0.030 mg
ethinyl estradiol)

RX WYETH-AYERST LABORATORIES P. 2924

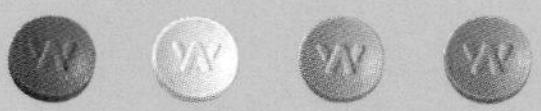

641* ** **642*** ** **643*** ** **650*** **

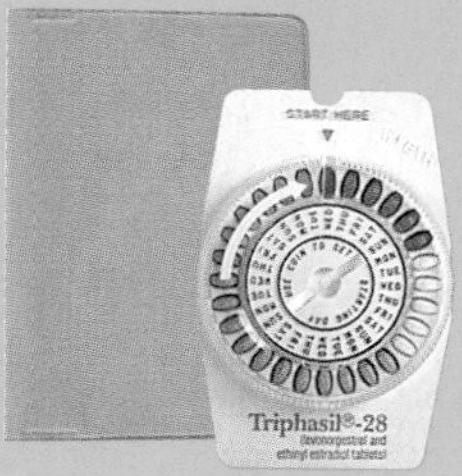

2536*

Triphasil®-28
(28 tablets containing the following: 6 brown tablets - 0.050 mg levonorgestrel
+ 0.030 mg ethinyl estradiol; 5 white
tablets - 0.075 mg levonorgestrel + 0.040 mg
ethinyl estradiol; 10 light-yellow tablets -
0.125 mg levonorgestrel + 0.030 mg
ethinyl estradiol; 7 light-green inert tablets)

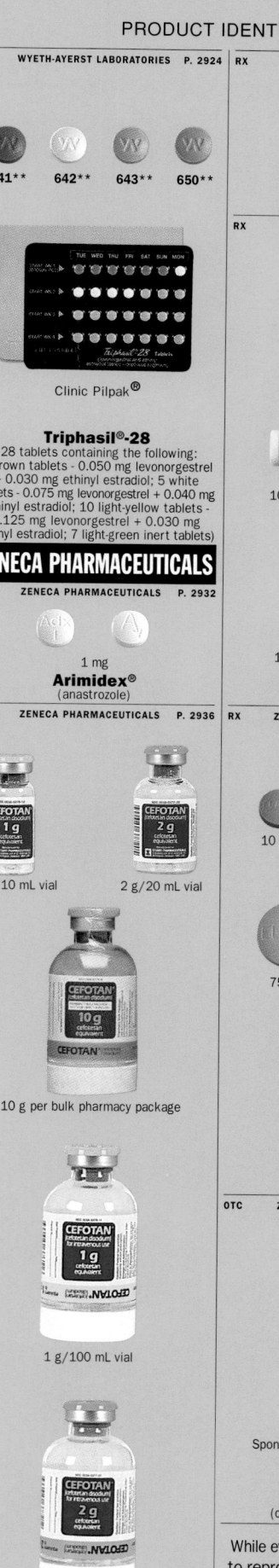

RX WYETH-AYERST LABORATORIES P. 2924

641* ** **642*** ** **643*** ** **650*** **

Clinic Pilpak®

Triphasil®-28
(28 tablets containing the following:
6 brown tablets - 0.050 mg levonorgestrel
+ 0.030 mg ethinyl estradiol; 5 white
tablets - 0.075 mg levonorgestrel + 0.040 mg
ethinyl estradiol; 10 light-yellow tablets -
0.125 mg levonorgestrel + 0.030 mg
ethinyl estradiol; 7 light-green inert tablets)

ZENECA PHARMACEUTICALS

RX ZENECA PHARMACEUTICALS P. 2932

1 mg

Arimidex®
(anastrozole)

RX ZENECA PHARMACEUTICALS P. 2936

1 g/10 mL vial   2 g/20 mL vial

CEFOTAN 10 g
10 g per bulk pharmacy package

1 g/100 mL vial

2 g/100 mL vial

Cefotan® IM/IV
(sterile cefotetan disodium)

RX ZENECA PHARMACEUTICALS P. 2934

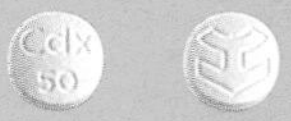

50 mg

Casodex®
(bicalutamide)

RX ZENECA PHARMACEUTICALS P. 2939

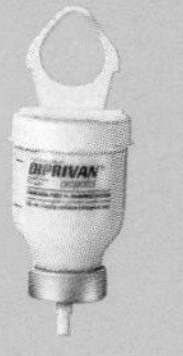

10 mg/mL per 50 mL vial

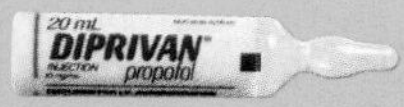

10 mg/mL per 20 mL ampules

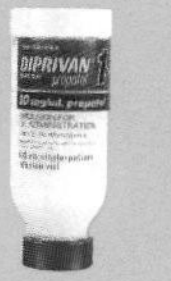

10 mg/mL per 100 mL vial

Diprivan®
(propofol)

RX ZENECA PHARMACEUTICALS P. 2945

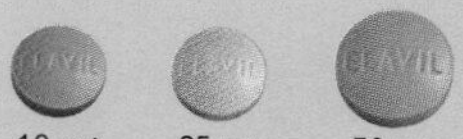

10 mg   25 mg   50 mg

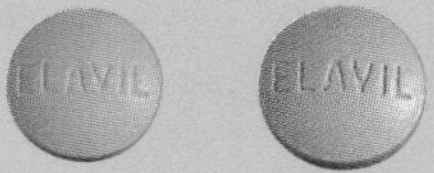

75 mg   100 mg

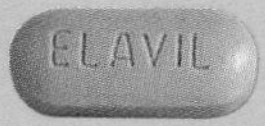

ELAVIL
150 mg

Elavil®
(amitriptyline HCl)

OTC ZENECA PHARMACEUTICALS P. 2947

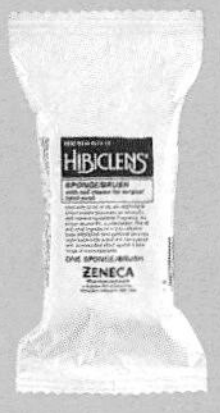

22 mL
Sponge/Brush with nail cleaner

Hibiclens®
(chlorhexidine gluconate)

While every effort has been made
to reproduce products faithfully,
this section is to be considered a
quick reference identification aid.
In cases of suspected overdosage,
etc., chemical analysis of the
product should be done.

---

† The appearance of these tablets and capsules is a trademark of Wyeth-Ayerst Laboratories   Δ The appearance of these tablets and capsules is a registered trademark of Wyeth-Ayerst Laboratories.
**Product identification number on reverse side

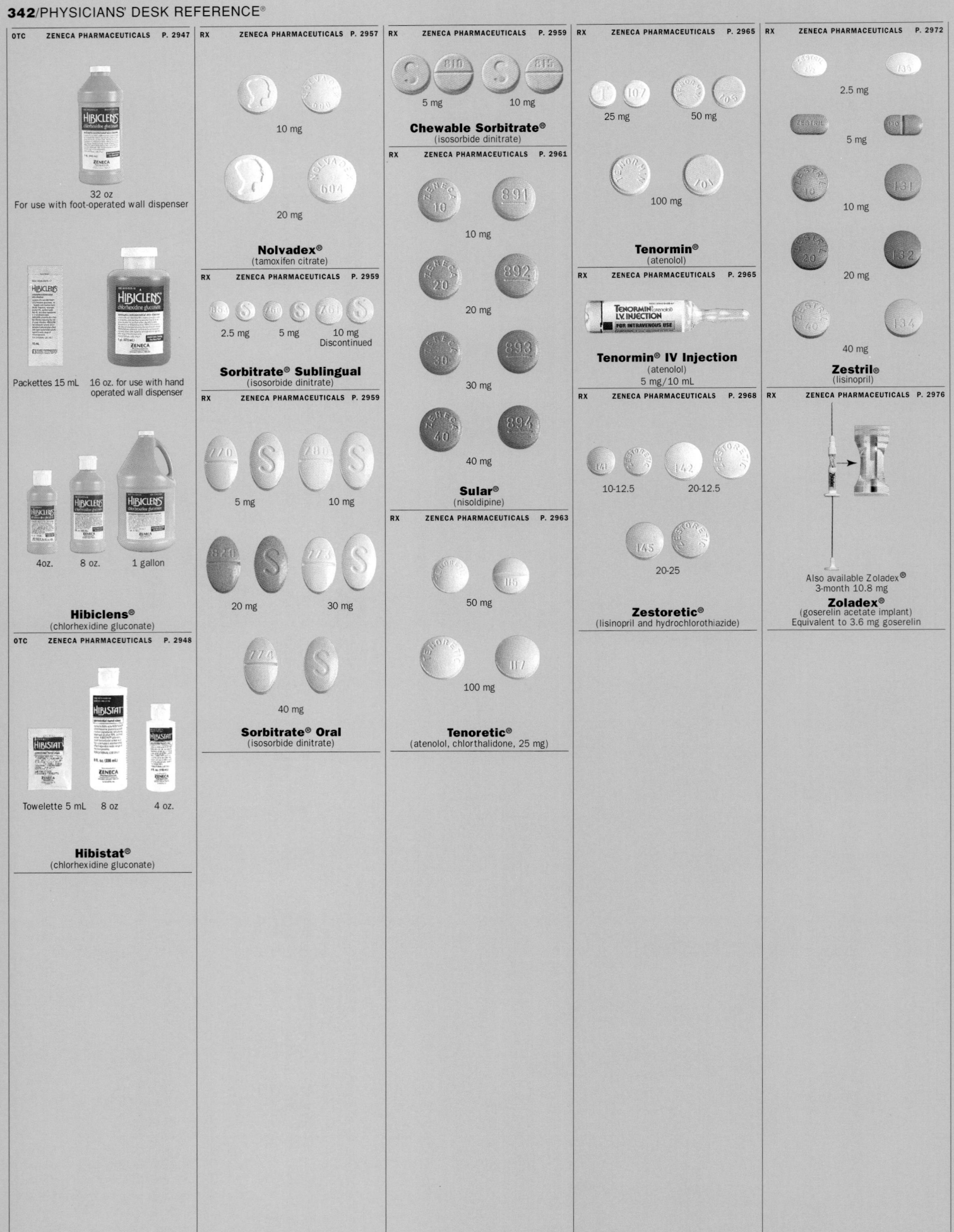

OTC   ZENECA PHARMACEUTICALS   P. 2947

32 oz
For use with foot-operated wall dispenser

Packettes 15 mL   16 oz. for use with hand operated wall dispenser

4 oz.   8 oz.   1 gallon

Hibiclens®
(chlorhexidine gluconate)

OTC   ZENECA PHARMACEUTICALS   P. 2948

Towelette 5 mL   8 oz   4 oz.

Hibistat®
(chlorhexidine gluconate)

RX   ZENECA PHARMACEUTICALS   P. 2957

10 mg

20 mg

Nolvadex®
(tamoxifen citrate)

RX   ZENECA PHARMACEUTICALS   P. 2959

2.5 mg   5 mg   10 mg
Discontinued

Sorbitrate® Sublingual
(isosorbide dinitrate)

RX   ZENECA PHARMACEUTICALS   P. 2959

5 mg   10 mg

20 mg   30 mg

40 mg

Sorbitrate® Oral
(isosorbide dinitrate)

RX   ZENECA PHARMACEUTICALS   P. 2959

5 mg   10 mg

Chewable Sorbitrate®
(isosorbide dinitrate)

RX   ZENECA PHARMACEUTICALS   P. 2961

10 mg

20 mg

30 mg

40 mg

Sular®
(nisoldipine)

RX   ZENECA PHARMACEUTICALS   P. 2963

50 mg

100 mg

Tenoretic®
(atenolol, chlorthalidone, 25 mg)

RX   ZENECA PHARMACEUTICALS   P. 2965

25 mg   50 mg

100 mg

Tenormin®
(atenolol)

RX   ZENECA PHARMACEUTICALS   P. 2965

Tenormin® IV Injection
(atenolol)
5 mg/10 mL

RX   ZENECA PHARMACEUTICALS   P. 2968

10-12.5   20-12.5

20-25

Zestoretic®
(lisinopril and hydrochlorothiazide)

RX   ZENECA PHARMACEUTICALS   P. 2972

2.5 mg

5 mg

10 mg

20 mg

40 mg

Zestril®
(lisinopril)

RX   ZENECA PHARMACEUTICALS   P. 2976

Also available Zoladex®
3-month 10.8 mg

Zoladex®
(goserelin acetate implant)
Equivalent to 3.6 mg goserelin

SECTION 5

PRODUCT INFORMATION

This section is made possible through the courtesy of the manufacturers whose products appear on the following pages. The information concerning each product has been prepared, edited, and approved by the medical department, medical director, and/or medical counsel of each manufacturer.

When a product appearing in PHYSICIANS' DESK REFERENCE® has an official package circular, its description must be in full compliance with Food & Drug Administration regulations pertaining to labeling for prescription drugs. These regulations require that in PDR® "indications, effects, dosages, routes, methods, and frequency and duration of administration, and any relevant warnings, hazards, contraindications, side effects, and precautions" must be "same in language and emphasis" as the approved labeling for the product. The FDA regards the words "same in language and emphasis" as requiring VERBATIM use of the approved labeling providing such information. Furthermore, information in the approved labeling that is emphasized by the use of type set in a box or in capitals, boldface, or italics must be given the same emphasis in PDR.

For products that do not have official package circulars, the publisher has emphasized the necessity of describing such products comprehensively, so that physicians have access to all information essential for intelligent and informed decision making.

The product descriptions in PHYSICIANS' DESK REFERENCE include all information made available to PDR by the manufacturer. The publisher does not warrant or guarantee any product, and does not perform any independent analysis of the information provided. Inclusion of a product in PDR does not represent an endorsement, and the publisher does not necessarily advocate the use of any product listed.

This edition of PHYSICIANS' DESK REFERENCE contains the latest information available when the book went to press. As new drugs are released, and new research data and clinical findings become available throughout the year, the information in the PDR database is revised accordingly. These revisions are published twice annually in the PDR Supplements. To be certain that you have the most current data, always consult the supplements before prescribing or administering any product described in the following pages.

Abana Pharmaceuticals, Inc.
1 CHASE CORPORATE DRIVE SUITE 260
BIRMINGHAM, AL 35244

Direct Inquiries to:
Customer Service
(205) 988-4588
FAX: (205) 998-3294

For Medical Information Contact:
In Emergencies:
(205) 988-4588
FAX: (205) 998-3294

NASABID® SR   ℞
Pseudoephedrine HCl,
guaifenesin 90 mg/600 mg
No generic

NDC # 12463-0600–01
Shown in Product Identification Guide, page 303

OBENIX™ Capsules   ℅
[ŏ-bē-nĭks]
Phentermine Hydrochloride USP, 37.5 mg

DESCRIPTION
Each green and clear capsule is imprinted in white with the name "ABANA" and the number "217" and contains:
Phentermine HCl 37.5mg

HOW SUPPLIED
Bottles of 100's (NDC 12463-0217-01).
Shown in Product Identification Guide, page 303

OTOCAIN™ Drops   ℞
[ŏ'tĭ-kān]
Benzocaine, 20%
Topical Anesthetic Ear Drops

DESCRIPTION
OTOCAIN™, a clear topical anesthetic liquid contains:
Benzocaine, 20% (weight/volume)

HOW SUPPLIED
Bottles of ½ fluid ounce dropper-top bottles
(NDC 12463-0218-05).
Shown in Product Identification Guide, page 303

VANEX® FORTE   ℞
[văn-ĕks' for'tā]
Antihistamine Decongestant
Long-Acting Caplet

DESCRIPTION
Each pink scored caplet is imprinted with an "A" and contains:
Phenylpropanolamine HCl .... 50 mg
Phenylephrine HCl .... 10 mg
Pyrilamine Maleate .... 25 mg
Chlorpheniramine Maleate .... 4 mg

HOW SUPPLIED
Bottles of 100's (NDC 12463-0125-01).
Shown in Product Identification Guide, page 303

VANEX® Grape Liquid   ℅
[văn-ĕks']

Each 5 mL (teaspoon) contains:
Dihydrocodeine Bitartrate 3 mg
Phenylephrine HCl 20 mg
Phenylpropanolamine HCl 20 mg
Chlorpheniramine Maleate 5 mg
Shown in Product Identification Guide, page 303

VANEX®–HD   ℅
[văn-ĕks']
Hydrocodone Bitartrate, Phenylephrine Hydrochloride, and Chlorpheniramine Maleate

DESCRIPTION
Each fluid ounce (30ml) contains:

Hydrocodone Bitartrate* .... 10 mg
*WARNING: May be habit forming
Phenylephrine HCl .... 30 mg
Chlorpheniramine Maleate .... 12 mg

HOW SUPPLIED
Bottles of one pint (473ml). (NDC 12463-0300-16).
Shown in Product Identification Guide, page 303

Abbott Laboratories
Pharmaceutical Products Division
NORTH CHICAGO, IL 60064, U.S.A.

Pharmaceutical Products Division—
Direct Inquiries to:
Customer Service:
(800) 255-5162
Technical Services:
(800) 441-4987
Physician Services:
(800) 222-6885
For Medical Information Contact:
Generally:
(800) 633-9110
Adverse Drug Experiences:
(800) 633-9110
Sales and Ordering:
(800) 255-5162

Hospital Products Division—
Direct Inquiries to:
Customer Service
(800) 222-6883
For Medical Information Contact:
(708) 937-3806
Sales and Ordering:
(800) 222-6883

ABBO–CODE™ INDEX

The Abbo-Code identification system provides positive identification of a drug and dosage strength. The following Abbott products are imprinted or debossed with an Abbo-Code designation:

PRODUCT	ABBO-CODE
Biaxin® Filmtab® Tablets (clarithromycin tablets)	
250 mg	KT
500 mg	KL
Cartrol® (carteolol hydrochloride) Filmtab® Tablets	
2.5 mg	IA
5 mg	IC
Cefol® Filmtab® Tablets B-complex vitamins with folic acid, vitamin E, and vitamin C	NJ
Colchicine Tablets, USP	
0.6 mg	AF
Cylert® Tablets ℅ (pemoline)	
18.75 mg	TH
37.5 mg	TI
75 mg	TJ
37.5 mg Chewable	TK
Depakene® Capsules (valproic acid capsules, USP)	
250 mg	DEPAKENE
Depakote® Sprinkle Capsules (divalproex sodium coated particles in capsules)	
125 mg	DEPAKOTE SPRINKLE
Depakote® Tablets (divalproex sodium delayed-release tablets)	
125 mg	NT
250 mg	NR
500 mg	NS
Desoxyn® Tablets ℅ (methamphetamine hydrochloride)	
5 mg Tablet	TE
5 mg Gradumet®	MC
10 mg Gradumet	ME
15 mg Gradumet	MF
Dicumarol Tablets	
25 mg	AN
E.E.S. 400® Filmtab® Tablets (erythromycin ethylsuccinate tablets, USP)	
400 mg erythromycin activity	EE
EryPed® Chewable Tablets (erythromycin ethylsuccinate tablets, USP)	
200 mg erythromycin activity	EZ
Enduron® Tablets (methyclothiazide tablets, USP)	
2.5 mg	ENDURON
5 mg	ENDURON

PRODUCT	ABBO-CODE
Enduronyl® Tablets 5 mg methyclothiazide and 0.25 mg deserpidine	LS
Enduronyl® Forte Tablets 5 mg methyclothiazide and 0.5 mg deserpidine	LT
Ery-Tab® Enteric-Coated Tablets (erythromycin delayed-release tablets, USP)	
250 mg	EC
333 mg	EH
500 mg	ED
Erythrocin® Stearate Filmtab® Tablets (erythromycin stearate tablets, USP)	
250 mg erythromycin activity	ES
500 mg erythromycin activity	ET
Erythromycin Base Filmtab® Tablets (erythromycin tablets, USP)	
250 mg	EB
500 mg	EA
Erythromycin Delayed-release Capsules, USP	
250 mg	ER
Fero-Folic-500® Filmtab® Tablets controlled-release iron, folic acid, and vitamin C	AJ
Hytrin® Capsules (terazosin hydrochloride capsules)	
1 mg	HH
2 mg	HY
5 mg	HK
10 mg	HN
Iberet-Folic-500® Filmtab® Tablets controlled-release iron, B-complex vitamins with folic acid, and vitamin C	AK
K · Tab® Filmtab® Tablets (potassium chloride extended-release tablets, USP)	
10 mEq (750 mg)	K-TAB
Nembutal® Sodium Capsules ℅ (pentobarbital sodium capsules, USP)	
50 mg	CF
100 mg	CH
Norvir™ Capsules (ritonavir capsules)	
100 mg	PI
Oretic® Tablets (hydrochlorothiazide tablets, USP)	
25 mg	ORETIC
50 mg	ORETIC
PCE® Dispertab® Tablets (erythromycin particles in tablets)	
333 mg	PCE
500 mg	EK
Peganone® Tablets (ethotoin tablets, USP)	
250 mg	AD
500 mg	AE
Phenurone® Tablets (phenacemide tablets, USP)	
500 mg	II
Placidyl® Capsules ℅ (ethchlorvynol capsules, USP)	
200 mg	
500 mg	PLACIDYL 500
750 mg	PLACIDYL 750
ProSom™ Tablets ℅ (estazolam tablets)	
1 mg	UC
2 mg	UD
Tranxene® T-Tab® Tablets ℅ (clorazepate dipotassium)	
3.75 mg Tablet	TL
7.5 mg Tablet	TM
15 mg Tablet	TN
Tranxene-SD™ ℅ Single Dose Tablets (clorazepate dipotassium)	
11.25 mg Half Strength	TX
22.5 mg	TY

ABBO-PAC®
Unit Dose Packages

The Abbo-Pac unit dose system from Abbott Laboratories offers a wide range of products.
Each individual dose is clearly identified by generic name, Abbott trademark name, strength, product list number, expiration date and lot number. Abbo-Pac unit dose containers are designed to accommodate virtually all hospital pharmacy storage racks and to provide maximum accessibility and ease of handling.

The following is a list of products which are now available:

PRODUCT	DOSAGE STRENGTH
Biaxin® Filmtab® Tablets (clarithromycin tablets)	250 mg
Biaxin Filmtab Tablets	500 mg
Depakote® Sprinkle Capsules (divalproex sodium coated particles in capsules)	125 mg
Depakote® Tablets (divalproex sodium delayed-release tablets)	125 mg
Depakote Tablets	250 mg
Depakote Tablets	500 mg
Enduron® Tablets (methyclothiazide tablets, USP)	5 mg
Enduronyl® Tablets (methyclothiazide 5 mg and deserpidine 0.25 mg)	
E.E.S. 400® Filmtab® Tablets (erythromycin ethylsuccinate tablets, USP)	400 mg
EryPed® Chewable Tablets (erythromycin ethylsuccinate tablets, USP)	200 mg
EryPed® 200 Granules (erythromycin ethylsuccinate for oral suspension, USP)	200 mg/5 mL
EryPed® 400 Granules (erythromycin ethylsuccinate for oral suspension, USP)	400 mg/5 mL
Ery-Tab® Enteric-Coated Tablets (erythromycin delayed-release tablets, USP)	250 mg
Ery-Tab Tablets	333 mg
Ery-Tab Tablets	500 mg
Erythrocin® Stearate Filmtab (erythromycin stearate tablets, USP)	250 mg
Erythromycin Base Filmtab® (erythromycin tablets, USP)	250 mg
Fero-Grad-500® Filmtab® Tablets Controlled-Release Iron plus Vitamin C	
Hytrin® Capsules (terazosin hydrochloride capsules)	1 mg
Hytrin Capsules	2 mg
Hytrin Capsules	5 mg
Hytrin Capsules	10 mg
Iberet®-500 Filmtab® Tablets Controlled-Release Iron plus B-Complex and Vitamin C	
K-Lor™ 20 mEq (potassium chloride for oral solution, USP)	20 mEq Potassium 20 mEq Chloride/Packet
K-Tab® Filmtab® Tablets (potassium chloride extended-release tablets, USP)	10 mEq (750 mg)
Nembutal® Sodium Capsules Ⓒ II (pentobarbital sodium capsules, USP)	100 mg
Oretic® Tablets (hydrochlorothiazide tablets, USP)	25 mg
Oretic® Tablets	50 mg
Placidyl® Capsules Ⓒ IV (ethchlorvynol capsules, USP)	500 mg
ProSom™ Tablets Ⓒ IV (estazolam tablets)	1 mg
ProSom™ Tablets Ⓒ IV	2 mg
Surbex-T® Filmtab® Tablets High-Potency B-Complex with Vitamin C	
Tranxene® T-Tab® Tablets Ⓒ IV (clorazepate dipotassium)	3.75 mg
Tranxene® T-Tab® Tablets Ⓒ IV	7.5 mg
Tranxene® T-Tab® Tablets Ⓒ IV	15 mg

ABBOKINASE® UROKINASE FOR INJECTION ℞

ABBOKINASE (urokinase for injection) should be used in hospitals where the recommended diagnostic and monitoring techniques are available. Thrombolytic therapy should be considered in all situations where the benefits to be achieved outweigh the risk of potentially serious hemorrhage. When internal bleeding does occur, it may be more difficult to manage than that which occurs with conventional anticoagulant therapy.

Urokinase treatment should be instituted as soon as possible after onset of pulmonary embolism, preferably no later than seven days after onset. Any delay in instituting lytic therapy to evaluate the effect of heparin decreases the potential for optimal efficacy.[1]

When urokinase is used for treatment of coronary artery thrombosis associated with evolving transmural myocardial infarction, therapy should be instituted within six hours of symptom onset.

DESCRIPTION

Urokinase is an enzyme (protein) produced by the kidney, and found in the urine. There are two forms of urokinase differing in molecular weight but having similar clinical effects. ABBOKINASE (urokinase for injection) is a thrombolytic agent obtained from human kidney cells by tissue culture techniques and is primarily the low molecular weight form. It is supplied as a sterile lyophilized white powder containing mannitol (25 mg/vial), Albumin (Human) (250 mg/vial), and sodium chloride (50 mg/vial).

Thin translucent filaments may occasionally occur in reconstituted ABBOKINASE vials, but do not indicate any decrease in potency of this product. No clinical problems have been associated with these filaments. See "Dosage and Administration" section.

Following reconstitution with 5 mL of Sterile Water for Injection, USP, it is a clear, slightly straw-colored solution; each mL contains 50,000 IU of urokinase activity, 0.5% mannitol, 5% Albumin (Human), and 1% sodium chloride. The pH is adjusted with sodium hydroxide and/or hydrochloric acid prior to lyophilization.

ABBOKINASE is for intravenous and intracoronary infusion only.

CLINICAL PHARMACOLOGY

Urokinase acts on the endogenous fibrinolytic system. It converts plasminogen to the enzyme plasmin. Plasmin degrades fibrin clots as well as fibrinogen and other plasma proteins.

Intravenous infusion of urokinase in doses recommended for lysis of pulmonary embolism is followed by increased fibrinolytic activity. This effect disappears within a few hours after discontinuation, but a decrease in plasma levels of fibrinogen and plasminogen and an increase in the amount of circulating fibrin (ogen) degradation products may persist for 12–24 hours.[2,3] There is a lack of correlation between embolus resolution and changes in coagulation and fibrinolytic assay results.

Information is incomplete about the pharmacokinetic properties in man. Urokinase administered by intravenous infusion is cleared rapidly by the liver. The serum half-life in man is 20 minutes or less. Patients with impaired liver function (e.g., cirrhosis) would be expected to show a prolongation in half-life. Small fractions of an administered dose are excreted in bile and urine.

INDICATIONS AND USAGE

Pulmonary Embolism

ABBOKINASE (urokinase for injection) is indicated in adults:

- For the lysis of acute massive pulmonary emboli, defined as obstruction of blood flow to a lobe or multiple segments.
- For the lysis of pulmonary emboli accompanied by unstable hemodynamics, i.e., failure to maintain blood pressure without supportive measures.

The diagnosis should be confirmed by objective means, such as pulmonary angiography via an upper extremity vein, or non-invasive procedures such as lung scanning.

Angiographic and hemodynamic measurements demonstrate a more rapid improvement with lytic therapy than with heparin therapy.[4-8]

Coronary Artery Thrombosis

ABBOKINASE has been reported to lyse acute thrombi obstructing coronary arteries, associated with evolving transmural myocardial infarction.[9] The majority of patients who received ABBOKINASE by intracoronary infusion within six hours following onset of symptoms showed recanalization of the involved vessel.

IT HAS NOT BEEN ESTABLISHED THAT INTRACORONARY ADMINISTRATION OF ABBOKINASE DURING EVOLVING TRANSMURAL MYOCARDIAL INFARCTION RESULTS IN SALVAGE OF MYOCARDIAL TISSUE, NOR THAT IT REDUCES MORTALITY. THE PATIENTS WHO MIGHT BENEFIT FROM THIS THERAPY CANNOT BE DEFINED.

I.V. Catheter Clearance

ABBOKINASE is indicated for the restoration of patency to intravenous catheters, including central venous catheters, obstructed by clotted blood or fibrin[10,11] (See separate section at end of insert concerning I.V. catheter clearance for information regarding warnings, precautions, adverse reactions, and dosage and administration.)

CONTRAINDICATIONS

Because thrombolytic therapy increases the risk of bleeding, urokinase is contraindicated in the following situations: (See WARNINGS.)

- Active internal bleeding
- History of cerebrovascular accident
- Recent (within two months) intracranial or intraspinal surgery
- Recent trauma including cardiopulmonary resuscitation
- Intracranial neoplasm, arteriovenous malformation, or aneurysm
- Known bleeding diathesis
- Severe uncontrolled arterial hypertension

WARNINGS

Bleeding

The aim of urokinase is the production of sufficient amounts of plasmin for lysis of intravascular deposits of fibrin; however, fibrin deposits which provide hemostasis, for example, at sites of needle puncture, will also lyse, and bleeding from such sites may occur.

Intramuscular injections and nonessential handling of the patient must be avoided during treatment with urokinase. Venipunctures should be performed carefully and as infrequently as possible.

Should an arterial puncture be necessary (except for intracoronary administration), upper extremity vessels are preferable. Pressure should be applied for at least 30 minutes, a pressure dressing applied, and the puncture site checked frequently for evidence of bleeding.

In the following conditions, the risks of therapy may be increased and should be weighed against the anticipated benefits:

- Recent (within 10 days) major surgery, obstetrical delivery, organ biopsy, previous puncture of non-compressible vessels
- Recent (within 10 days) serious gastrointestinal bleeding
- High likelihood of a left heart thrombus, e.g., mitral stenosis with atrial fibrillation
- Subacute bacterial endocarditis
- Hemostatic defects including those secondary to severe hepatic or renal disease
- Pregnancy
- Cerebrovascular disease
- Diabetic hemorrhagic retinopathy
- Any other condition in which bleeding might constitute a significant hazard or be particularly difficult to manage because of its location

Should serious spontaneous bleeding (not controllable by local pressure) occur, the infusion of urokinase should be terminated immediately, and treatment instituted as described under ADVERSE REACTIONS.

Use of Anticoagulants

Concurrent use of anticoagulants with intravenous administration of ABBOKINASE is not recommended. However, concurrent use of heparin may be required during intracoronary administration of ABBOKINASE. A clinical study[9] with concurrent use of heparin and ABBOKINASE during intracoronary administration has demonstrated no tendency toward increased bleeding that would not be attributable to the procedure or ABBOKINASE alone. Nevertheless, careful monitoring for excessive bleeding is advised.

Arrhythmias

Rapid lysis of coronary thrombi has been reported occasionally to cause atrial or ventricular dysrhythmias as a result of reperfusion requiring immediate treatment. Careful monitoring for arrhythmias should be maintained during and immediately following intracoronary administration of ABBOKINASE.

PRECAUTIONS

Laboratory Tests

Before commencing thrombolytic therapy, obtain a hematocrit, platelet count, and a thrombin time (TT), activated partial thromboplastin time (APTT), or prothrombin time (PT). If heparin has been given, it should be discontinued unless it is to be used in conjunction with ABBOKINASE for intracoronary administration. TT or APTT should be less than twice the normal control value before thrombolytic therapy is started.

During the infusion, coagulation tests and/or measures of fibrinolytic activity may be performed if desired. Results do not, however, reliably predict either efficacy or a risk of bleeding. The clinical response should be observed frequently, and vital signs, i.e., pulse, temperature, respiratory rate and blood pressure, should be checked at least every four hours. The blood pressure should not be taken in the lower extremities to avoid dislodgment of possible deep vein thrombi.

Following the intravenous infusion, *before (re)instituting heparin*, the TT or APTT should be less than twice the upper limits of normal. Following intracoronary infusion of ABBOKINASE, blood coagulation parameters should be determined and heparin therapy continued as appropriate.

Drug Interactions

The interaction of urokinase with other drugs has not been studied. Drugs that alter platelet function should not be used. Common examples are: aspirin, indomethacin and phenylbutazone.

Although a bolus dose of heparin is recommended prior to intracoronary use of urokinase, oral anticoagulants or heparin should not be given concurrently with large doses of urokinase such as those used for pulmonary embolism. Concomitant use of intravenous urokinase and oral anticoagulants or heparin may increase the risk of hemorrhage. (See "WARNINGS" section.)

Carcinogenicity

Adequate data are not available on the long-term potential for carcinogenicity in animals or humans.

Pregnancy

Pregnancy category B. Reproduction studies have been performed in mice and rats at doses up to 1,000 times the human dose and have revealed no evidence of impaired fertility or

Continued on next page

Abbott Laboratories—Cont.

harm to the fetus due to urokinase. There are, however, no adequate and well-controlled studies in pregnant women. Because animal reproduction studies are not always predictive of human response, this drug should be used during pregnancy only if clearly needed.

Nursing Mothers
It is not known whether this drug is excreted in human milk. Because many drugs are excreted in human milk, caution should be exercised when urokinase is administered to a nursing woman.

Pediatric Use
Safety and effectiveness in children have not been established.

ADVERSE REACTIONS

The following adverse reactions have been associated with intravenous therapy but may also occur with intracoronary artery infusion.

Bleeding
The type of bleeding associated with thrombolytic therapy can be placed into two broad categories:

—Superficial or surface bleeding, observed mainly at invaded or disturbed sites (e.g., venous cutdowns, arterial punctures, sites of recent surgical intervention, etc.).

—Internal bleeding, involving, e.g., the gastrointestinal tract, genitourinary tract, vagina, or intramuscular, retroperitoneal, or intracranial sites.

Several fatalities due to intracranial or retroperitoneal hemorrhage have occurred during thrombolytic therapy.

Should serious bleeding occur, urokinase infusion should be discontinued and, if necessary, blood loss and reversal of the bleeding tendency can be effectively managed with whole blood (fresh blood preferable), packed red blood cells and cryoprecipitate or fresh frozen plasma. Dextran should not be used. Although the use of aminocaproic acid (ACA, AMICAR®) in humans as an antidote for urokinase has not been documented, it may be considered in an emergency situation.

Allergic Reactions
In vitro tests with urokinase, as well as intradermal tests in humans, gave no evidence of induced antibody formation. Relatively mild allergic type reactions, e.g., bronchospasm and skin rash, have been reported. When such reactions occur, they usually respond to conventional therapy. In addition, rare cases of anaphylaxis have been reported.

Miscellaneous
Fever and chills, including shaking chills (rigors), nausea and/or vomiting, transient hypotension or hypertension, dyspnea, tachycardia, cyanosis, back pain, hypoxemia, and acidosis have been reported together and separately. Rare cases of myocardial infarction have also been reported. A cause and effect relationship has not been established. Aspirin is not recommended for treatment of fever.

DOSAGE AND ADMINISTRATION
ABBOKINASE IS INTENDED FOR INTRAVENOUS AND INTRACORONARY INFUSION ONLY.

A. Pulmonary Embolism:
Preparation
Reconstitute ABBOKINASE (urokinase for injection) by aseptically adding 5 mL of Sterile Water for Injection, USP, to the vial. (It is important that ABBOKINASE be reconstituted *only* with Sterile Water for Injection, USP, *without* preservatives. Bacteriostatic Water for Injection should *not* be used.) Each vial should be visually inspected for discoloration (slightly straw-colored solution) and for the presence of particulate material. Highly colored solutions should not be used. Because ABBOKINASE contains no preservatives, it should not be reconstituted until immediately before using. Any unused portion of the reconstituted material should be discarded.

To minimize formation of filaments, avoid shaking the vial during reconstitution. Roll and tilt the vial to enhance reconstitution. The solution may be terminally filtered, e.g., through a 0.45 micron or smaller cellulose membrane filter. No other medication should be added to this solution.

Reconstituted ABBOKINASE is diluted with 0.9% Sodium Chloride Injection, USP or 5% Dextrose Injection, USP, prior to intravenous infusion. (See Table I, **Dose Preparation-Pulmonary Embolism.**)

Administration
Administer ABBOKINASE (urokinase for injection) by means of a constant infusion pump that is capable of delivering a total volume of 195 mL. The following table may be used as an aid in the preparation of ABBOKINASE (urokinase for injection) for administration.

[See table I below.]

A priming dose of 2,000 IU/lb (4,400 IU/kg) of ABBOKINASE is given as the ABBOKINASE-0.9% Sodium Chloride Injection or 5% Dextrose Injection admixture at a rate of 90 mL/hour over a period of 10 minutes. This is followed by a continuous infusion of 2,000 IU/lb/hr (4,400 IU/kg/hr) of ABBOKINASE at a rate of 15 mL/hour for 12 hours. Since some ABBOKINASE admixture will remain in the tubing at the end of an infusion pump delivery cycle, the following flush procedure should be performed to insure that the total dose of ABBOKINASE is administered. A solution of 0.9% Sodium Chloride Injection or 5% Dextrose Injection approximately equal in amount to the volume of the tubing in the infusion set should be administered via the pump to flush the ABBOKINASE admixture from the entire length of the infusion set. The pump should be set to administer the flush solution at the continuous infusion rate of 15 mL/hour.

Anticoagulation After Terminating Urokinase Treatment
At the end of urokinase therapy, treatment with heparin by continuous intravenous infusion is recommended to prevent recurrent thrombosis. Heparin treatment, without a loading dose, should not begin until the thrombin time has decreased to *less than twice* the normal control value (approximately 3 to 4 hours after completion of the infusion). See manufacturer's prescribing information for proper use of heparin. This should then be followed by oral anticoagulants in the conventional manner.

B. Lysis of Coronary Artery Thrombi:[9]
Preparation
Reconstitute three (3) 250,000 IU vials of ABBOKINASE by aseptically adding 5 mL of Sterile Water for Injection, USP,

to each vial. (It is important that ABBOKINASE be reconstituted *only* with Sterile Water for Injection, USP, *without* preservatives. Bacteriostatic Water for Injection should *not* be used.) Each vial should be visually inspected for discoloration (slightly straw-colored solution) and for the presence of particulate material. Highly colored solutions should not be used. Because ABBOKINASE contains no preservatives, it should not be reconstituted until immediately before using. Any unused portion of the reconstituted material should be discarded.

To minimize formation of filaments, avoid shaking the vial during reconstitution. Roll and tilt the vial to enhance reconstitution. The solution may be terminally filtered, e.g., through a 0.45 micron or smaller cellulose membrane filter. Add the contents of the three (3) reconstituted ABBOKINASE vials to 500 mL of 5% Dextrose Injection, USP. The resulting solution admixture will have a concentration of approximately 1500 IU per mL. No other medication should be added to the solution.

The admixture should be administered immediately as described under Administration. Any solution remaining after administration should be discarded.

NOTE: Adsorption of drug from dilute protein solutions to various materials has been reported in the literature. Therefore, the directions for Preparation and Administration must be followed to assure that significant drug loss does not occur.

Administration
Prior to the infusion of ABBOKINASE, a bolus dose of heparin ranging from 2500 to 10,000 units should be administered intravenously. Prior heparin administration should be considered when calculating the heparin dose for this procedure. Following the bolus dose of heparin, the prepared ABBOKINASE solution should be infused into the occluded artery at a rate of 4 mL per minute (6000 IU per minute) for periods up to 2 hours. In a clinical study, the average total dose of ABBOKINASE utilized for lysis of coronary artery thrombi was 500,000 IU.[9]

To determine response to ABBOKINASE therapy, periodic angiography during the infusion is recommended. It is suggested that the angiography be repeated at approximately 15 minute intervals. ABBOKINASE therapy should be continued until the artery is maximally opened, usually 15 to 30 minutes after the initial opening. Following the infusion, coagulation parameters should be determined. It is advisable to continue heparin therapy after the artery is opened by ABBOKINASE.

When ABBOKINASE was administered selectively into thrombosed coronary arteries via coronary catheter within 6 hours following onset of symptoms of acute transmural myocardial infarction, 60% of the occlusions were opened.[9]

I.V. CATHETER CLEARANCE
Warnings
Excessive pressure should be avoided when ABBOKINASE is injected into the catheter. Such force could cause rupture of the catheter or expulsion of the clot into the circulation.

Precautions
Catheters may be occluded by substances other than blood products, such as drug precipitate. ABBOKINASE is not effective in such a case, and there is the possibility that the precipitate may be forced into the vascular system.

Adverse Reactions
Although there have been no adverse reactions reported as a result of using ABBOKINASE for the removal of clot obstruction from I.V. catheters, the possibility of reactions should nevertheless be considered.

Dosage and Administration
Preparation: Reconstitute ABBOKINASE (urokinase for injection) by aseptically adding 5 mL of Sterile Water for Injection, USP, to the vial. (It is important that ABBOKINASE be reconstituted *only* with Sterile Water for Injection, USP, *without* preservatives. Bacteriostatic Water for Injection should *not* be used.) Add 1 mL of the reconstituted drug to 9 mL Sterile Water for Injection, USP, to make a final dilution equivalent to 5,000 IU/mL. One mL of this preparation is to be utilized for each catheter clearing procedure. BECAUSE ABBOKINASE CONTAINS NO PRESERVATIVES, IT SHOULD NOT BE RECONSTITUTED UNTIL IMMEDIATELY BEFORE USING.

Administration: NOTE: When the following procedure is used to clear a central venous catheter, the patient should be instructed to exhale and hold his breath any time the catheter is not connected to I.V. tubing or a syringe. This is to prevent air from entering the open catheter.

Aseptically disconnect the I.V. tubing connection at the catheter hub and attach a 10 mL syringe. Determine occlusion of the catheter by *gently* attempting to aspirate blood from the catheter with the 10 mL syringe. If aspiration is not possible, remove the 10 mL syringe and attach a 1 mL tuberculin syringe filled with prepared ABBOKINASE to the catheter. Slowly and gently inject an amount of ABBOKINASE equal to the volume of the catheter. Aseptically remove the tuberculin syringe and connect a 5 mL syringe to the catheter. Wait at least 5 minutes before attempting to aspirate the drug and residual clot with the 5 mL syringe. Repeat aspiration attempts every 5 minutes. If the catheter is not open

TABLE I
Dose Preparation–Pulmonary Embolism

Weight (pounds)	Total Dose* Urokinase (IU)	Number Vials ABBOKINASE (urokinase for injection)	Volume of ABBOKINASE After Reconstitution (mL)**	+	Volume of Diluent (mL)	=	Final Volume (mL)
81–90	2,250,000	9	45		150		195
91–100	2,500,000	10	50		145		195
101–110	2,750,000	11	55		140		195
111–120	3,000,000	12	60		135		195
121–130	3,250,000	13	65		130		195
131–140	3,500,000	14	70		125		195
141–150	3,750,000	15	75		120		195
151–160	4,000,000	16	80		115		195
161–170	4,250,000	17	85		110		195
171–180	4,500,000	18	90		105		195
181–190	4,750,000	19	95		100		195
191–200	5,000,000	20	100		95		195
201–210	5,250,000	21	105		90		195
211–220	5,500,000	22	110		85		195
221–230	5,750,000	23	115		80		195
231–240	6,000,000	24	120		75		195
241–250	6,250,000	25	125		70		195

	Priming Dose	Dose for 12-Hour Period
Infusion Rate:	15 mL/10 min***	15 mL/hr for 12 hrs

*Priming dose + dose administered during 12-hour period.
**After addition of 5 mL of Sterile Water for Injection, USP, per vial. (See Preparation.)
***Pump rate = 90 mL/hr

within 30 minutes, the catheter may be capped allowing ABBOKINASE to remain in the catheter for 30 to 60 minutes before again attempting to aspirate. A second injection of ABBOKINASE may be necessary in resistant cases. When patency is restored, aspirate 4 to 5 mL of blood to assure removal of all drug and clot residual. Remove the blood-filled syringe and replace it with a 10 mL syringe filled with 0.9% Sodium Chloride Injection, USP. The catheter should then be gently irrigated with this solution to assure patency of the catheter. After the catheter has been irrigated, remove the 10 mL syringe and aseptically reconnect sterile I.V. tubing to the catheter hub.

HOW SUPPLIED
ABBOKINASE (urokinase for injection) is supplied as a sterile lyophilized preparation (**NDC** 0074-6109-05). Each vial contains 250,000 IU urokinase activity, 25 mg mannitol, 250 mg Albumin (Human), and 50 mg sodium chloride. Store ABBOKINASE powder at 2° to 8°C.

REFERENCES
1. Sherry S, et al. Thrombolytic therapy in thrombosis: A National Institutes of Health consensus development conference. *Ann Intern Med.* 1980;93:141–144.
2. Bang NU. Physiology and biochemistry of fibrinolysis. In: Bang NU, Beller FK, Deutsch E, Mammen EF, eds. *Thrombosis and Bleeding Disorders.* New York, NY: Academic Press; 1971:292–327.
3. McNicol GP. The fibrinolytic enzyme system. *Postgrad Med J.* August 1973;49 (suppl 5):10–12.
4. Sasahara AA, Hyers TM, Cole CM, et al. The urokinase pulmonary embolism trial. *Circulation.* 1973;47 (suppl 2):1–108.
5. Urokinase pulmonary embolism trial study group: Urokinase-streptokinase embolism trial. *JAMA.* 1974;229:1606–1613.
6. Sasahara AA, Bell WR, Simon TL, et al. The Phase II urokinase-streptokinase pulmonary embolism trial, *Thrombos Diathes Haemorrh* (Stuttg). 1975;33:464–476.
7. Bell WR. Thrombolytic therapy: A comparison between urokinase and streptokinase, *Sem Thromb Hemost.* 1975;2:1–13.
8. Fratantoni JC, Ness P, Simon TL. Thrombolytic therapy: Current status. *N Eng J Med.* 1975;293:1073–1078.
9. Tennant SN, Campbell WB, et al. Intracoronary thrombolysis in acute myocardial infarction: Comparison of the efficacy of urokinase to streptokinase. *Circulation.* 1984;69:756–760.
10. Lawson M, et al. The use of urokinase to restore the patency of occluded central venous catheters. *Am J Intravenous Therapy and Clinical Nutrition.* 1982;9:29–32.
11. Glynn MFX, et al. Therapy for thrombotic occlusion of long-term intravenous alimentation catheters. *Journal of Parenteral and Enteral Nutrition.* 1980;4:387–390.

Revised Aug., 1994
Ref. 06-9129-R11-Rev. August, 1994
Abbott Laboratories
North Chicago, IL 60064, U.S.A.   601-49R-5837A
Shown in Product Identification Guide, page 303

ABBOKINASE® OPEN-CATH®   ℞
(Urokinase for Catheter Clearance)

DESCRIPTION
Urokinase is an enzyme (protein) produced by the kidney, and found in the urine. There are two forms of urokinase differing in molecular weight but having similar clinical effects. Urokinase is a thrombolytic agent obtained from human kidney cells by tissue culture techniques and is primarily the low molecular weight form. It is supplied as a sterile lyophilized white powder. Following reconstitution ABBOKINASE OPEN-CATH solution is clear and essentially colorless.
Each mL of reconstituted ABBOKINASE OPEN-CATH solution contains 5000 IU of urokinase activity, 5 mg gelatin, 15 mg mannitol, 1.7 mg sodium chloride and 4.6 mg monobasic sodium phosphate anhydrous. The pH is adjusted with sodium hydroxide and/or hydrochloric acid prior to lyophilization.

CLINICAL PHARMACOLOGY
Urokinase acts on the endogenous fibrinolytic system. It converts plasminogen to the enzyme plasmin. Plasmin degrades fibrin clots as well as fibrinogen and other plasma proteins.
When used as directed for I.V. catheter clearance, only small amounts of urokinase may reach the circulation; therefore, therapeutic serum levels are not expected to be achieved. Nevertheless, one should be aware of the clinical pharmacology of urokinase.
Intravenous infusion of urokinase in doses recommended for lysis of pulmonary embolism is followed by increased fibrinolytic activity. This effect disappears within a few hours after discontinuation, but a decrease in plasma levels of fibrinogen and plasminogen and an increase in the amount of circulating fibrin (ogen) degradation products may persist for 12–24 hours.[1,2] There is a lack of correlation between embolus resolution and changes in coagulation and fibrinolytic assay results.
Information is incomplete about the pharmacokinetic properties in man. Urokinase administered by intravenous infusion is cleared rapidly by the liver. The serum half-life in man is 20 minutes or less. Patients with impaired liver function (e.g., cirrhosis) would be expected to show a prolongation in half-life. Small fractions of an administered dose are excreted in bile and urine.

INDICATIONS AND USAGE
ABBOKINASE OPEN-CATH (urokinase for catheter clearance) is indicated for the restoration of patency to intravenous catheters, including central venous catheters, obstructed by clotted blood or fibrin.[3,4,5]

CONTRAINDICATIONS
Because thrombolytic therapy increases the risk of bleeding, urokinase is contraindicated in the following situations:
—Active internal bleeding
—History of cerebrovascular accident
—Recent (within two months) intracranial or intraspinal surgery
—Recent trauma including cardiopulmonary resuscitation
—Intracranial neoplasm, arteriovenous malformation, or aneurysm
—Known bleeding diathesis
—Severe uncontrolled arterial hypertension
There have been no reports, however, which would suggest a contraindication for the use of urokinase for I.V. catheter clearance.

WARNINGS
Excessive pressure should be avoided when ABBOKINASE solution is injected into the catheter. Such force could cause rupture of the catheter or expulsion of the clot into the circulation. During attempts to determine catheter occlusion, vigorous suction should not be applied due to possible damage to the vascular wall or collapse of soft-wall catheters. Catheters may be occluded by substances other than fibrin clots such as drug precipitates. ABBOKINASE solution is not effective in such cases and there is the possibility that the substances may be forced into the vascular system.

PRECAUTIONS
Carcinogenicity
Adequate data is not available on the long-term potential for carcinogenicity in animals or humans.
Pregnancy
Pregnancy Category B. Reproduction studies have been performed in mice and rats at doses up to 1,000 times the human therapeutic dose and have revealed no evidence of impaired fertility or harm to the fetus due to urokinase. There are, however, no adequate and well-controlled studies in pregnant women. Because animal reproduction studies are not always predictive of human response, this drug should be used during pregnancy only if clearly needed.
Nursing Mothers
It is not known whether this drug is excreted in human milk. Because many drugs are excreted in human milk, caution should be exercised when urokinase is administered to a nursing woman.
Pediatric Use
Safety and effectiveness in children have not been established.

ADVERSE REACTIONS
The following reactions have been associated with ABBOKINASE (urokinase for injection) in doses recommended for lysis of pulmonary embolism.
Bleeding
The type of bleeding associated with thrombolytic therapy can be placed into two broad categories:
—Superficial or surface bleeding, observed mainly at invaded or disturbed sites (e.g., venous cutdowns, arterial punctures, sites of recent surgical intervention, etc.).
—Internal bleeding, involving, e.g., the gastrointestinal tract, genitourinary tract, vagina, or intramuscular, retroperitoneal, or intracranial sites.
Several fatalities due to intracranial or retroperitoneal hemorrhage have occurred during thrombolytic therapy.
Should serious bleeding occur, urokinase infusion should be discontinued and, if necessary, blood loss and reversal of the bleeding tendency can be effectively managed with whole blood (fresh blood preferable), packed red blood cells and cryoprecipitate or plasma. Dextran and hetastarch should not be used. Although the use of aminocaproic acid (ACA, AMICAR®) in humans as an antidote for urokinase has not been documented, it may be considered in an emergency situation.
Allergic Reactions
In vitro tests with urokinase, as well as intradermal tests in humans, gave no evidence of induced antibody formation. Relatively mild allergic type reactions, e.g., bronchospasm and skin rash, have been reported. When such reactions occur, they usually respond to conventional therapy. In addition, rare cases of anaphylaxis have been reported.
Miscellaneous
Fever and chills, including shaking chills (rigors), nausea and/or vomiting, transient hypotension or hypertension, dyspnea, tachycardia, cyanosis, back pain, hypoxemia, and acidosis have been reported together and separately. Rare cases of myocardial infarction have also been reported. A cause and effect relationship has not been established. Aspirin is not recommended for treatment of fever.

DOSAGE AND ADMINISTRATION
BECAUSE ABBOKINASE OPEN-CATH POWDER CONTAINS NO PRESERVATIVE, RECONSTITUTED SOLUTION SHOULD BE USED IMMEDIATELY AFTER RECONSTITUTION. DISCARD ANY UNUSED PORTION.
Preparation of Solution:
Univial:
1. Remove protective cap. Turn plunger-stopper a quarter turn and press to force diluent into lower chamber.
2. Roll and tilt to effect solution. Use only a clear, essentially colorless solution.
3. Sterilize top of stopper with a suitable germicide.
4. Insert needle through the center of stopper until tip is barely visible. Withdraw dose.
It is recommended that vigorous shaking be avoided during reconstitution; roll and tilt to enhance reconstitution.
Parenteral drug products should be inspected visually for particulate matter and discoloration prior to administration, whenever solution and container permit.
Administration:
When the following procedure is used to clear a central venous catheter, the patient should be instructed to exhale and hold his breath any time the catheter is not connected to I.V. tubing or a syringe. This is to prevent air from entering the open catheter.
Aseptically disconnect the I.V. tubing connection at the catheter hub and attach an empty 10 mL syringe. Determine occlusion of the catheter by *gently* attempting to aspirate blood from the catheter with the 10 mL syringe. If aspiration is not possible, remove the 10 mL syringe and attach a syringe filled with an amount of prepared ABBOKINASE OPEN-CATH solution equal to the internal volume of the catheter. Slowly and gently inject the ABBOKINASE solution into the catheter. Aseptically remove the syringe and connect a 5 mL syringe to the catheter. Wait at least 5 minutes before attempting to aspirate the drug and residual clot with the empty syringe. Repeat aspiration attempts every 5 minutes. If the catheter is not open within 30 minutes, the catheter may be capped allowing ABBOKINASE solution to remain in the catheter for an additional 30 to 60 minutes before again attempting to aspirate. A second injection of ABBOKINASE (urokinase for catheter clearance) may be necessary in resistant cases.
When patency is restored, aspirate 4 to 5 mL of blood to assure removal of all drug and residual clot. Remove the blood-filled syringe and replace it with a 10 mL syringe filled with 0.9% Sodium Chloride Injection, USP. The catheter should then be gently irrigated with this solution to assure patency of the catheter. After the catheter has been irrigated, remove the 10 mL syringe and aseptically reconnect sterile I.V. tubing to the catheter hub.

HOW SUPPLIED
ABBOKINASE OPEN-CATH (urokinase for catheter clearance) is supplied as a sterile lyophilized preparation in single dose Univial® packages of 1 mL (**NDC** 0074-6111-01) and 1.8 mL (**NDC** 0074-6145-02). Store powder below 77°F (25°C). Avoid freezing.

REFERENCES
1. Bang NU. Physiology and biochemistry of fibrinolysis. In: Bang NU, Beller FK, Deutsch E, Mammen EF, eds. *Thrombosis and Bleeding Disorders.* New York, NY: Academic Press; 1971: 292-327.
2. McNicol GP. The fibrinolytic enzyme system. *Postgrad Med J.* August 1973; 49 (suppl 5):10-12.
3. Hurtubise MR, Bottino JC, Lawson M, et al. Restoring patency of occluded central venous catheters. *Arch Surg.* 1980; 115:212-213.
4. Glynn MFX, et al. Therapy for thrombotic occlusion of long-term intravenous alimentation catheters. *Journal of Parenteral and Enteral Nutrition.* 1980; 4:387-390.
5. Lawson M, Bottino JC, Hurtubise MR, et al. The use of urokinase to restore the patency of occluded central venous catheters. *Am J IV Ther and Clin Nutr.* 1982; 9:29-30,32.

Revised: Aug., 1994
Univial-Sterile two-compartment vial, Abbott.
Ref. 06-9128-R8-Rev. August, 1994
Abbott Laboratories
North Chicago, IL 60064   509-081-5164 **MASTER**
Shown in Product Identification Guide, page 303

Continued on next page

Abbott Laboratories—Cont.

BIAXIN® Filmtab® ℞
(clarithromycin tablets)

BIAXIN® Granules ℞
(clarithromycin for oral suspension)

DESCRIPTION

Clarithromycin is a semi-synthetic macrolide antibiotic. Chemically, it is 6-*O*-methylerythromycin. The molecular formula is $C_{38}H_{69}NO_{13}$, and the molecular weight is 747.96. The structural formula is:

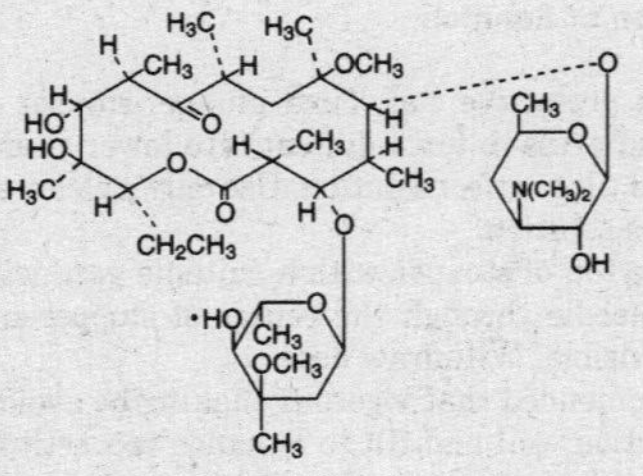

Clarithromycin is a white to off-white crystalline powder. It is soluble in acetone, slightly soluble in methanol, ethanol, and acetonitrile, and practically insoluble in water.
BIAXIN is available as tablets and granules for oral suspension.
Each yellow oval film-coated BIAXIN tablet contains 250 mg or 500 mg of clarithromycin and the following inactive ingredients: cellulosic polymers, croscarmellose sodium, D&C Yellow No. 10, FD&C Blue No. 1, magnesium stearate, povidone, propylene glycol, silicon dioxide, sorbic acid, sorbitan monooleate, stearic acid, talc, titanium dioxide, and vanillin. The 250-mg tablet also contains pregelatinized starch.
After constitution, each 5 mL of BIAXIN suspension contains 125 mg or 250 mg of clarithromycin. Each bottle of BIAXIN granules contains 1250 mg (50 mL size), 2500 mg (50 and 100 mL sizes) or 5000 mg (100 mL size) of clarithromycin and the following inactive ingredients: carbomer, caster oil, citric acid, hydroxypropyl methylcellulose phthalate, maltodextrin, potassium sorbate, povidone, silicon dioxide, sucrose, xanthan gum, titanium dioxide and fruit punch flavor.

CLINICAL PHARMACOLOGY

Pharmacokinetics:
Clarithromycin is rapidly absorbed from the gastrointestinal tract after oral administration. The absolute bioavailability of 250-mg clarithromycin tablets was approximately 50%. Food slightly delays both the onset of clarithromycin absorption and the formation of the antimicrobially active metabolite, 14-OH clarithromycin, but does not affect the extent of bioavailability. Therefore, BIAXIN tablets may be given without regard to food.
In fasting healthy human subjects, peak serum concentrations were attained within 2 hours after oral dosing. Steady-state peak serum clarithromycin concentrations were attained in 2 to 3 days and were approximately 1 μg/mL with a 250-mg dose administered every 12 hours, 2 to 3 μg/mL with a 500-mg dose administered every 12 hours, and 3 to 4 μg/mL with a 500-mg dose administered every 8 hours. The elimination half-life of clarithromycin was about 3 to 4 hours with 250 mg administered every 12 hours but increased to 5 to 7 hours with 500 mg administered every 8 to 12 hours. The nonlinearity of clarithromycin pharmacokinetics is slight at the recommended doses of 250 mg and 500 mg administered every 8 to 12 hours. With a 250 mg every 12 hours dosing, the principal metabolite, 14-OH clarithromycin, attains a peak steady-state concentration of about 0.6 μg/mL and has an elimination half-life of 5 to 6 hours. With a 500 mg every 8 to 12 hours dosing, the peak steady-state concentration of 14-OH clarithromycin is slightly higher (up to 1 μg/mL), and its elimination half-life is about 7 to 9 hours. With any of these dosing regimens, the steady-state concentration of this metabolite is generally attained within 2 to 3 days.
After a 250-mg tablet every 12 hours, approximately 20% of the dose is excreted in the urine as clarithromycin, while after a 500-mg tablet every 12 hours, the urinary excretion of clarithromycin is somewhat greater, approximately 30%. In comparison, after an oral dose of 250-mg (125 mg/5 mL) suspension every 12 hours, approximately 40% is excreted in urine as clarithromycin. The renal clearance of clarithromycin is, however, relatively independent of the dose size and approximates the normal glomerular filtration rate. The major metabolite found in urine is 14-OH clarithromycin, which accounts for an additional 10% to 15% of the dose with either a 250-mg or a 500-mg tablet administered every 12 hours.
Steady-state concentrations of clarithromycin and 14-OH clarithromycin observed following administration of 500-mg doses of clarithromycin every 12 hours to adult patients with HIV infection were similar to those observed in healthy volunteers. In adult HIV-infected patients taking 500- or 1000-mg doses of clarithromycin every 12 hours, steady-state clarithromycin C_{max} values ranged from 2-4 μg/mL and 5–10 μg/mL, respectively.
The steady-state concentrations of clarithromycin in subjects with impaired hepatic function did not differ from those in normal subjects; however, the 14-OH clarithromycin concentrations were lower in the hepatically impaired subjects. The decreased formation of 14-OH clarithromycin was at least partially offset by an increase in renal clearance of clarithromycin in the subjects with impaired hepatic function when compared to healthy subjects.
The pharmacokinetics of clarithromycin was also altered in subjects with impaired renal function. (See **PRECAUTIONS** and **DOSAGE AND ADMINISTRATION.**)
Clarithromycin and the 14-OH clarithromycin metabolite distribute readily into body tissues and fluids. There are no data available on cerebrospinal fluid penetration. Because of high intracellular concentrations, tissue concentrations are higher than serum concentrations. Examples of tissue and serum concentrations are presented below.

CONCENTRATION
(after 250 mg q 12 h)

Tissue Type	Tissue (μg/g)	Serum (μg/mL)
Tonsil	1.6	0.8
Lung	8.8	1.7

When 250-mg doses of clarithromycin as BIAXIN suspension were administered to fasting healthy adult subjects, peak plasma concentrations were attained around 3 hours after dosing. Steady-state peak plasma concentrations were attained in 2 to 3 days and were approximately 2 μg/mL for clarithromycin and 0.7 μg/mL for 14-OH clarithromycin when 250-mg doses of the clarithromycin suspension were administered every 12 hours. Elimination half-life of clarithromycin (3 to 4 hours) and that of 14-OH clarithromycin (5 to 7 hours) were similar to those observed at steady state following administration of equivalent doses of BIAXIN tablets.
For adult patients, the bioavailability of 10 mL of the 125-mg/5 mL suspension or 10 mL of the 250-mg/5 mL suspension is similar to a 250-mg or 500-mg tablet, respectively.
In children requiring antibiotic therapy, administration of 7.5 mg/kg q 12 h doses of clarithromycin as the suspension generally resulted in steady-state peak plasma concentrations of 3 to 7 μg/mL for clarithromycin and 1 to 2 μg/mL for 14-OH clarithromycin.
In HIV-infected children taking 15 mg/kg every 12 hours, steady-state clarithromycin peak concentrations generally ranged from 6-15 μg/mL.
Clarithromycin penetrates into the middle ear fluid of children with secretory otitis media.

CONCENTRATION
(after 7.5 mg/kg q 12 h for 5 doses)

Analyte	Middle Ear Fluid (μg/mL)	Serum (μg/mL)
Clarithromycin	2.5	1.7
14-OH Clarithromycin	1.3	0.8

In adults given 250 mg clarithromycin as suspension (n = 22), food appeared to decrease mean peak plasma clarithromycin concentrations from 1.2 (± 0.4) μg/mL to 1.0 (± 0.4) μg/mL and the extent of absorption from 7.2 (± 2.5) hr·μg/mL to 6.5 (± 3.7) hr·μg/mL.

Clarithromycin Tissue Concentrations 2 hours after Dose (μg/mL)/(μg/g)

Treatment	N	antrum	fundus	N	mucus
Clarithromycin	5	10.48 ± 2.01	20.81 ± 7.64	4	4.15 ± 7.74
Clarithromycin + Omeprazole	5	19.96 ± 4.71	24.25 ± 6.37	4	39.29 ± 32.79

When children (n = 10) were administered a single oral dose of 7.5 mg/kg suspension, food increased mean peak plasma clarithromycin concentration from 3.6 (± 1.5) μg/mL to 4.6 (± 2.8) μg/mL and the extent of absorption from 10.0 (± 5.5) hr·μg/mL to 14.2 (± 9.4) hr·μg/mL.
Clarithromycin 500 mg every 8 hours was given in combination with omeprazole 40 mg daily to healthy adult males. The plasma levels of clarithromycin and 14-hydroxy-clarithromycin were increased by the concomitant administration of omeprazole. For clarithromycin, the mean C_{max} was 10% greater, the mean C_{min} was 27% greater, and the mean AUC_{0-8} was 15% greater when clarithromycin was administered with omeprazole than when clarithromycin was administered alone. Similar results were seen for 14-hydroxy-clarithromycin, the mean C_{max} was 45% greater, the mean C_{min} was 57% greater, and the mean AUC_{0-8} was 45% greater. Clarithromycin concentrations in the gastric tissue and mucus were also increased by concomitant administration of omeprazole.
[See table on bottom of page.]
For Information on omeprazole, refer to the CLINICAL PHARMACOLOGY section of the PRILOSEC package insert.

Microbiology:
Clarithromycin exerts its antibacterial action by binding to the 50S ribosomal subunit of susceptible microorganisms resulting in inhibition of protein synthesis.
Clarithromycin is active *in vitro* against a variety of aerobic and anaerobic gram-positive and gram-negative microorganisms as well as most *Mycobacterium avium* complex (MAC) microorganisms.
Additionally, the 14-OH clarithromycin metabolite also has clinically significant antimicrobial activity. The 14-OH clarithromycin is twice as active against *Haemophilus influenzae* microorganisms as the parent compound. However, for *Mycobacterium avium* complex (MAC) isolates the 14-OH metabolite is 4 to 7 times less active than clarithromycin. The clinical significance of this activity against *Mycobacterium avium* complex is unknown.
Clarithromycin has been shown to be active against most strains of the following microorganisms both *in vitro* and in clinical infections as described in the **INDICATIONS AND USAGE** section:

Aerobic Gram-positive microorganisms
Staphylococcus aureus
Streptococcus pneumoniae
Streptococcus pyogenes
Aerobic Gram-negative microorganisms
Haemophilus influenzae
Moraxella catarrhalis
Other microorganisms
Mycoplasma pneumoniae
Mycobacteria
Mycobacterium avium complex (MAC) consisting of:
Mycobacterium avium
Mycobacterium intracellulare

Beta-lactamase production should have no effect on clarithromycin activity.
NOTE: Most strains of methicillin-resistant and oxacillin-resistant staphylococci are resistant to clarithromycin.
Clarithromycin has been shown to be active against most strains of *Helicobacter pylori in vitro* and in clinical infections when combined with omeprazole as described in the **INDICATIONS AND USAGE** section.

Helicobacter
Helicobacter pylori
Some *Helicobacter pylori* isolates obtained from patients treated with clarithromycin plus omeprazole demonstrated an increase in clarithromycin MIC's over time, indicating decreasing susceptibility and increasing resistance. In the two U.S. clarithromycin plus omeprazole clinical trials, 104 patients had *H. pylori* isolated and clarithromycin MIC's determined pre-treatment. Of these, 4 patients had resistant strains, 2 patients had strains with intermediate susceptibility, and 98 patients had susceptible strains. Of the patients with susceptible *H. pylori* pre-treatment, 72 patients were eradicated of the *H. pylori* and 26 patients had *H. pylori* present post-treatment. Isolates from 25 of these 26 patients became resistant to clarithromycin. The six patients with resistant or intermediate *H. pylori* strains pre-treatment had resistant strains isolated post-treatment.
The following *in vitro* data are available, **but their clinical significance is unknown.** Clarithromycin exhibits *in vitro* activity against most strains of the following microorganisms; however, the safety and effectiveness of clarithromycin in treating clinical infections due to these microorganisms have not been established in adequate and well-controlled clinical trials.

Aerobic Gram-positive microorganisms
Listeria monocytogenes
Streptococcus agalactiae
Streptococci (Groups C, F, G)
Viridans group streptococci
Aerobic Gram-negative microorganisms
Bordetella pertussis
Campylobacter jejuni

Legionella pneumophila
Neisseria gonorrhoeae
Pasteurella multocida
Other microorganisms
Chlamydia trachomatis
Anaerobic Gram-positive microorganisms
Clostridium perfringens
Peptococcus niger
Propionibacterium acnes
Anaerobic Gram-negative microorganisms
Prevotella melaninogenica (formerly *Bacteriodes melaninogenicus*)

Susceptibility Testing Excluding Mycobacteria and Helicobacter:

Dilution Techniques:

Quantitative methods are used to determine antimicrobial minimum inhibitory concentrations (MIC's). These MIC's provide estimates of the susceptibility of bacteria to antimicrobial compounds. The MIC's should be determined using a standardized procedure. Standardized procedures are based on a dilution method[1] (broth or agar) or equivalent with standardized inoculum concentrations and standardized concentrations of clarithromycin powder. The MIC values should be interpreted according to the following criteria:

MIC (μg/mL)	Interpretation
≤2.0	Susceptible (S)
4.0	Intermediate (I)
≥8.0	Resistant (R)

A report of "Susceptible" indicates that the pathogen is likely to be inhibited if the antimicrobial compound in the blood reaches the concentrations usually achievable.

A report of "Intermediate" indicates that the result should be considered equivocal, and, if the microorganism is not fully susceptible to alternative, clinically feasible drugs, the test should be repeated. This category implies possible clinical applicability in body sites where the drug is physiologically concentrated or in situations where high dosage of drug can be used. This category also provides a buffer zone which prevents small uncontrolled technical factors from causing major discrepancies in interpretation.

A report of "Resistant" indicates that the pathogen is not likely to be inhibited if the antimicrobial compound in the blood reaches the concentrations usually achievable; other therapy should be selected.

Standardized susceptibility test procedures require the use of laboratory control microorganisms to control the technical aspects of the laboratory procedures. Standard clarithromycin powder should provide the following MIC values:

Microorganism	MIC (μg/mL)
S. aureus ATCC 29213	0.12–0.5

Diffusion Techniques:

Quantitative methods that require measurement of zone diameters also provide reproducible estimates of the susceptibility of bacteria to antimicrobial compounds. One such standardized procedure[2] requires the use of standardized inoculum concentrations. This procedure uses paper disks impregnated with 15-μg clarithromycin to test the susceptibility of microorganisms to clarithromycin.

Reports from the laboratory providing results of the standard single-disk susceptibility test with a 15-μg clarithromycin disk should be interpreted according to the following criteria:

Zone Diameter (mm)	Interpretation
≥18	Susceptible (S)
14–17	Intermediate (I)
≤13	Resistant (R)

Interpretation should be as stated above for results using dilution techniques. Interpretation involves correlation of the diameter obtained in the disk test with the MIC for clarithromycin. However, standardized diffusion methods for routine *in vitro* susceptibility testing, using the 15-μg clarithromycin disk, do not measure the additive antimicrobial activity of the 14-OH metabolite and, thus, may underestimate the drug's potential activity against *Haemophilus influenzae*. *Haemophilus influenzae* isolates falling into the "Intermediate" category often respond to treatment.

As with standardized dilution techniques, diffusion methods require the use of laboratory control microorganisms that are used to control the technical aspects of the laboratory procedures. For the diffusion technique, the 15-μg clarithromycin disk should provide the following zone diameters in this laboratory test quality control strain:

Microorganism	Zone diameter (mm)
S. aureus ATCC 25923	26–32

***In vitro* Activity of Clarithromycin against Mycobacteria:**

Clarithromycin has demonstrated *in vitro* activity against *Mycobacterium avium* complex (MAC) microorganisms isolated from both AIDS and non-AIDS patients. While gene probe techniques may be used to distinguish *M. avium* species from *M. intracellulare*, many studies only reported results on *M. avium* complex (MAC) isolates.

Various *in vitro* methodologies employing broth or solid media at different pH's, with and without oleic acid-albumin-dextrose-catalase (OADC), have been used to determine clarithromycin MIC values for mycobacterial species. In general, MIC values decrease more than 16-fold as the pH of Middlebrook 7H12 broth media increases from 5.0 to 7.4. At pH 7.4, MIC values determined with Mueller-Hinton agar were 4- to 8-fold higher than those observed with Middlebrook 7H12 media. Utilization of oleic acid-albumin-dextrose-catalase (OADC) in these assays has been shown to further alter MIC values.

Clarithromycin activity against 80 MAC isolates from AIDS patients and 211 MAC isolates from non-AIDS patients was evaluated using a microdilution method with Middlebrook 7H9 broth. Results showed an MIC value of ≤4.0 μg/mL in 81% and 89% of the AIDS and non-AIDS MAC isolates, respectively. Twelve percent of the non-AIDS isolates had an MIC value ≤ 0.5 μg/mL. Clarithromycin was also shown to be active against phagocytized *M. avium* complex (MAC) in mouse and human macrophage cell cultures as well as in the beige mouse infection model.

Clarithromycin activity was evaluated against *Mycobacterium tuberculosis* microorganisms. In one study utilizing the agar dilution method with Middlebrook 7H10 media, 3 of 30 clinical isolates had an MIC of 2.5 μg/mL. Clarithromycin inhibited all isolates at >10.0 μg/mL.

Susceptibility Testing for *Mycobacterium avium* Complex (MAC):

The disk diffusion and dilution techniques for susceptibility testing against gram-positive and gram-negative bacteria should not be used for determining clarithromycin MIC values against mycobacteria. *In vitro* susceptibility testing methods and diagnostic products currently available for determining minimum inhibitory concentration (MIC) values against *Mycobacterium avium* complex (MAC) organisms have not been standardized or validated. Clarithromycin MIC values will vary depending on the susceptibility testing method employed, composition and pH of the media, and the utilization of nutritional supplements. Breakpoints to determine whether clinical isolates of *M. avium* or *M. intracellulare* are susceptible or resistant to clarithromycin have not been established.

***In vitro* Activity of Clarithromycin against *Helicobacter pylori*:**

Clarithromycin has demonstrated *in vitro* activity against *Helicobacter pylori* isolated from patients with duodenal ulcers. *In vitro* susceptibility testing methods (broth microdilution, agar dilution, E-test, and disk diffusion) and diagnostic products currently available for determining minimum inhibitory concentrations (MIC's) and zone sizes have not been standardized, validated, or approved for testing *H. pylori*. The clarithromycin MIC values and zone sizes will vary depending on the susceptibility testing methodology employed, media, growth additives, pH, inoculum concentration tested, growth phase, incubation atmosphere, and time.

Susceptibility Test for *Helicobacter pylori*:

In vitro susceptibility testing methods and diagnostic products currently available for determining minimum inhibitory concentrations (MIC's) and zone sizes have not been standardized, validated, or approved for testing *H. pylori* microorganisms. MIC values for *H. pylori* isolates collected during the two U.S. clinical trials evaluating clarithromycin plus omeprazole, were determined by broth microdilution MIC methodology[3]. Results obtained during the clarithromycin plus omeprazole clinical trials fell into a distinct bimodal distribution of susceptible and resistant clarithromycin MIC's.

If the broth microdilution MIC methodology published in Hachem, et. al.[3] is used and the following tentative breakpoints are employed, there should be reasonable correlation between MIC results and clinical and microbiological outcomes for patients treated with clarithromycin plus omeprazole.

MIC (μg/mL)	Interpretation
≤0.06	Susceptible (S)
0.12–2.0	Intermediate (I)
≥4	Resistant (R)

These breakpoints should not be used to interpret results obtained using alternative methods.

INDICATIONS AND USAGE

BIAXIN Filmtab tablets and BIAXIN Granules for oral suspension are indicated for the treatment of mild to moderate infections caused by susceptible strains of the designated microorganisms in the conditions listed below:

Adults:

Pharyngitis/Tonsillitis due to *Streptococcus pyogenes* (The usual drug of choice in the treatment and prevention of streptococcal infections and the prophylaxis of rheumatic fever is penicillin administered by either the intramuscular or the oral route. Clarithromycin is generally effective in the eradication of *S. pyogenes* from the nasopharynx; however, data establishing the efficacy of clarithromycin in the subsequent prevention of rheumatic fever are not available at present.)

Acute maxillary sinusitis due to *Haemophilus influenzae, Moraxella catarrhalis,* or *Streptococcus pneumoniae*

Acute bacterial exacerbation of chronic bronchitis due to *Haemophilus influenzae, Moraxella catarrhalis,* or *Streptococcus pneumoniae*

Pneumonia due to *Mycoplasma pneumoniae,* or *Streptococcus pneumoniae*

Uncomplicated skin and skin structure infections due to *Staphylococcus aureus,* or *Streptococcus pyogenes* (Abscesses usually require surgical drainage.)

Disseminated mycobacterial infections due to *Mycobacterium avium,* or *Mycobacterium intracellulare*

BIAXIN (clarithromycin) Filmtab tablets in combination with PRILOSEC (omeprazole) capsules is indicated for the treatment of patients with an active duodenal ulcer associated with *H. pylori* infection. The eradication of *H. pylori* has been demonstrated to reduce the risk of duodenal ulcer recurrence.

In patients who fail therapy, susceptibility testing should be done if possible. If resistance is demonstrated, alternative therapy is recommended. (For information on development of resistance see **Microbiology** section.)

Children:

Pharyngitis/Tonsillitis due to *Streptococcus pyogenes*

Acute maxillary sinusitis due to *Haemophilus influenzae, Moraxella catarrhalis,* or *Streptococcus pneumoniae*

Acute otitis media due to *Haemophilus influenzae, Moraxella catarrhalis,* or *Streptococcus pneumoniae*

NOTE: For information on otitis media, see **CLINICAL STUDIES: Otitis Media.**

Uncomplicated skin and skin structure infections due to *Staphylococcus aureus,* or *Streptococcus pyogenes* (Abscesses usually require surgical drainage.)

Disseminated mycobacterial infections due to *Mycobacterium avium,* or *Mycobacterium intracellulare*

Prophylaxis:

BIAXIN Filmtab tablets and BIAXIN Granules for oral suspension are indicated for the prevention of disseminated *Mycobacterium avium* complex (MAC) disease in patients with advanced HIV infection.

CONTRAINDICATIONS

Clarithromycin is contraindicated in patients with a known hypersensitivity to clarithromycin, erythromycin, or any of the macrolide antibiotics.

Clarithromycin is contraindicated in patients receiving terfenadine therapy who have preexisting cardiac abnormalities (arrhythmia, bradycardia, QT interval prolongation, ischemic heart disease, congestive heart failure, etc.) or electrolyte disturbances. (See **PRECAUTIONS**-*Drug Interactions.*)

For information on omeprazole, refer to the CONTRAINDICATIONS section of the PRILOSEC package insert.

WARNINGS

CLARITHROMYCIN SHOULD NOT BE USED IN PREGNANT WOMEN EXCEPT IN CLINICAL CIRCUMSTANCES WHERE NO ALTERNATIVE THERAPY IS APPROPRIATE. IF PREGNANCY OCCURS WHILE TAKING THIS DRUG, THE PATIENT SHOULD BE APPRISED OF THE POTENTIAL HAZARD TO THE FETUS. CLARITHROMYCIN HAS DEMONSTRATED ADVERSE EFFECTS OF PREGNANCY OUTCOME AND/OR EMBRYO-FETAL DEVELOPMENT IN MONKEYS, RATS, MICE, AND RABBITS AT DOSES THAT PRODUCED PLASMA LEVELS 2 TO 17 TIMES THE SERUM LEVELS ACHIEVED IN HUMANS TREATED AT THE MAXIMUM RECOMMENDED HUMAN DOSES (See. PRECAUTIONS—*Pregnancy.*)

Pseudomembranous colitis has been reported with nearly all antibacterial agents, including clarithromycin, and may range in severity from mild to life threatening. Therefore, it is important to consider this diagnosis in patients who present with diarrhea subsequent to the administration of antibacterial agents.

Treatment with antibacterial agents alters the normal flora of the colon and may permit overgrowth of clostridia. Studies indicate that a toxin produced by *Clostridium difficile* is a primary cause of "antibiotic-associated colitis".

After the diagnosis of pseudomembranous colitis has been established, therapeutic measures should be initiated. Mild cases of pseudomembranous colitis usually respond to discontinuation of the drug alone. In moderate to severe cases, consideration should be given to management with fluids and electrolytes, protein supplementation, and treatment

Continued on next page

Abbott Laboratories—Cont.

with an antibacterial drug clinically effective against *Clostridium difficile* colitis.

For information on omeprazole, refer to the WARNINGS section of the PRILOSEC package insert.

PRECAUTIONS

General: Clarithromycin is principally excreted via the liver and kidney. Clarithromycin may be administered without dosage adjustment to patients with hepatic impairment and normal renal function. However, in the presence of severe renal impairment with or without coexisting hepatic impairment, decreased dosage or prolonged dosing intervals may be appropriate.

For information on omeprazole, refer to the PRECAUTIONS section of the PRILOSEC package insert.

Information to Patients: BIAXIN tablets and oral suspension can be taken with or without food and can be taken with milk. Do NOT refrigerate the suspension.

Drug Interactions: Clarithromycin use in patients who are receiving theophylline may be associated with an increase of serum theophylline concentrations. Monitoring of serum theophylline concentrations should be considered for patients receiving high doses of theophylline or with baseline concentrations in the upper therapeutic range. In two studies in which theophylline was administered with clarithromycin (a theophylline sustained-release formulation was dosed at either 6.5 mg/kg or 12 mg/kg together with 250 or 500 mg q12h clarithromycin), the steady-state levels of C_{max}, C_{min}, and the area under the serum concentration time curve (AUC) of theophylline increased about 20%.

Concomitant administration of single doses of clarithromycin and carbamazepine has been shown to result in increased plasma concentrations of carbamazepine. Blood level monitoring of carbamazepine may be considered.

When clarithromycin and terfenadine were coadministered, plasma concentrations of the active acid metabolite of terfenadine were threefold higher, on average, than the values observed when terfenadine was administered alone. The pharmacokinetics of clarithromycin and the 14-hydroxy-clarithromycin were not significantly affected by co-administered of terfenadine once clarithromycin reached steady-state conditions. The increase in the QT interval seen in association with the elevated terfenadine acid metabolite level is unlikely to be of clinical significance in healthy individuals. Clarithromycin should not be given to patients receiving terfenadine therapy who have preexisting cardiac abnormalities (arrhythmia, bradycardia, QT interval prolongation, ischemic heart disease, congestive heart failure, etc.) or electrolyte disturbances. (See **CONTRAINDICATIONS**.)

Clarithromycin 500 mg every 8 hours was given in combination with omeprazole 40 mg daily to healthy adult subjects. The steady-state plasma concentrations of omeprazole were increased (C_{max}, AUC_{0-24}, and $T_{1/2}$ increases of 30%, 89%, and 34%, respectively), by the concomitant administration of clarithromycin. The mean 24-hour gastric pH value was 5.2 when omeprazole was administered alone and 5.7 when co-administered with clarithromycin.

Simultaneous oral administration of BIAXIN tablets and zidovudine to HIV-infected adult patients resulted in decreased steady-state zidovudine concentrations. When 500 mg of clarithromycin were administered twice daily, steady-state zidovudine AUC was reduced by a mean of 12% (n=4). Individual values ranged from a decrease of 34% to an increase of 14%. Based on limited data in 24 patients, when BIAXIN tablets were administered two to four hours prior to oral zidovudine, the steady-state zidovudine C_{max} was increased by approximately 2-fold, whereas the AUC was unaffected.

Simultaneous administration of BIAXIN tablets and didanosine to 12 HIV-infected adult patients resulted in no statistically significant change in didanosine pharmacokinetics.

Concomitant administration of fluconazole 200 mg daily and clarithromycin 500 mg twice daily to 21 healthy volunteers led to increases in the mean steady-state clarithromycin C_{min} and AUC of 33% and 18%, respectively. Steady-state concentrations of 14-OH clarithromycin were not significantly affected by concomitant administration of fluconazole.

Spontaneous reports in the post-marketing period suggest that concomitant administration of clarithromycin and oral anticoagulants may potentiate the effects of the oral anticoagulants. Prothrombin times should be carefully monitored while patients are receiving clarithromycin and oral anticoagulants simultaneously.

Elevated digoxin serum concentrations in patients receiving clarithromycin and digoxin concomitantly have also been reported in post-marketing surveillance. Some patients have shown clinical signs consistent with digoxin toxicity, including arrhythmias. Serum digoxin levels should be carefully monitored while patients are receiving digoxin and clarithromycin simultaneously.

The following drug interactions, other than increased serum concentrations of carbamazepine and active acid metabolite of terfenadine, have not been reported in clinical trials with clarithromycin; however, they have been observed with erythromycin products and/or with clarithromycin in post-marketing experience.

Concurrent use of erythromycin or clarithromycin and ergotamine or dihydroergotamine has been associated in some patients with acute ergot toxicity characterized by severe peripheral vasospasm and dysesthesia.

Erythromycin has been reported to decrease the clearance of triazolam and, thus, may increase the pharmacologic effect of triazolam. There have been post-marketing reports of drug interactions and CNS effects (e.g., somnolence and confusion) with the concomitant use of clarithromycin and triazolam.

The use of erythromycin and clarithromycin in patients concurrently taking drugs metabolized by the cytochrome P450 system may be associated with elevations in serum levels of these other drugs. There have been reports of interactions of erythromycin and/or clarithromycin with carbamazepine, cyclosporine, hexobarbital, phenytoin, alfentanil, disopyramide, lovastatin, bromocriptine, valproate, terfenadine, cisapride, pimozide, and astemizole. Serum concentrations of drugs metabolized by the cytochrome P450 system should be monitored closely in patients concurrently receiving these drugs.

Carcinogenesis, Mutagenesis, Impairment of Fertility:
The following *in vitro* mutagenicity tests have been conducted with clarithromycin:

Salmonella/Mammalian Microsomes Test
Bacterial Induced Mutation Frequency Test
In Vitro Chromosome Aberration Test
Rat Hepatocyte DNA Synthesis Assay
Mouse Lymphoma Assay
Mouse Dominant Lethal Study
Mouse Micronucleus Test

All tests had negative results except the *In Vitro* Chromosome Aberration Test which was weakly positive in one test and negative in another.

In addition, a Bacterial Reverse-Mutation Test (Ames Test) has been performed on clarithromycin metabolites with negative results.

Fertility and reproduction studies have shown that daily doses of up to 160 mg/kg/day (1.3 times the recommended maximum human dose based on mg/m²) to male and female rats caused no adverse effects on the estrous cycle, fertility, parturition, or number and viability of offspring. Plasma levels in rats after 150 mg/kg/day were 2 times the human serum levels.

In the 150 mg/kg/day monkey studies, plasma levels were 3 times the human serum levels. When given orally at 150 mg/kg/day (2.4 times the recommended maximum human dose based on mg/m²), clarithromycin was shown to produce embryonic loss in monkeys. This effect has been attributed to marked maternal toxicity of the drug at this high dose.

In rabbits, *in utero* fetal loss occurred at an intravenous dose of 33 mg/m², which is 17 times less than the maximum proposed human oral daily dose of 618 mg/m².

Long-term studies in animals have not been performed to evaluate the carcinogenic potential of clarithromycin.

Pregnancy: Teratogenic Effects. Pregnancy Category C.
Four teratogenicity studies in rats (three with oral doses and one with intravenous doses up to 160 mg/kg/day administered during the period of major organogenesis) and two in rabbits at oral doses up to 125 mg/kg/day (approximately 2 times the recommended maximum human dose based on mg/m²) or intravenous doses of 30 mg/kg/day administered during gestation days 6 to 18 failed to demonstrate any teratogenicity from clarithromycin. Two additional oral studies in a different rat strain at similar doses and similar conditions demonstrated a low incidence of cardiovascular anomalies at doses of 150 mg/kg/day administered during gestation days 6 to 15. Plasma levels after 150 mg/kg/day were 2 times the human serum levels. Four studies in mice revealed a variable incidence of cleft palate following oral doses of 1000 mg/kg/day (2 and 4 times the recommended maximum human dose based on mg/m², respectively) during gestation days 6 to 15. Cleft palate was also seen at 500 mg/kg/day. The 1000 mg/kg/day exposure resulted in plasma levels 17 times the human serum levels. In monkeys, an oral dose of 70 mg/kg/day (an approximate equidose of the recommended maximum human dose based on mg/m²) produced fetal growth retardation at plasma levels that were 2 times the human serum levels.

There are no adequate and well-controlled studies in pregnant women. Clarithromycin should be used during pregnancy only if the potential benefit justifies the potential risk to the fetus. (See **WARNINGS**.)

Nursing Mothers: It is not known whether clarithromycin is excreted in human milk. Because many drugs are excreted in human milk, caution should be exercised when clarithromycin is administered to a nursing woman. It is known that clarithromycin is excreted in the milk of lactating animals and that other drugs of this class are excreted in human milk. Preweaned rats, exposed indirectly via consumption of milk from dams treated with 150 mg/kg/day for 3 weeks, were not adversely affected, despite data indicating higher drug levels in milk than in plasma.

Pediatric Use: Safety and effectiveness of clarithromycin in children under 6 months of age have not been established. The safety of clarithromycin has not been studied in MAC patients under the age of 20 months. Neonatal and juvenile animals tolerated clarithromycin in a manner similar to adult animals. Young animals were slightly more intolerant to acute overdosage and to subtle reductions in erythrocytes, platelets and leukocytes but were less sensitive to toxicity in the liver, kidney, thymus, and genitalia.

Geriatric Use: In a steady-state study in which healthy elderly subjects (age 65 to 81 years old) were given 500 mg every 12 hours, the maximum serum concentrations and area under the curves of clarithromycin and 14-OH clarithromycin were increased compared to those achieved in healthy young adults. These changes in pharmacokinetics parallel known age-related decreases in renal function. In clinical trials, elderly patients did not have an increased incidence of adverse events when compared to younger patients. Dosage adjustment should be considered in elderly patients with severe renal impairment.

ADVERSE REACTIONS

The majority of side effects observed in clinical trials were of a mild and transient nature. Fewer than 3% of adult patients without mycobacterial infections and fewer than 2% of pediatric patients without mycobacterial infections discontinued therapy because of drug-related side effects.

The most frequently reported events in adults were diarrhea (3%), nausea (3%), abnormal taste (3%), dyspepsia (2%), abdominal pain/discomfort (2%), and headache (2%). In pediatric patients, the most frequently reported events were diarrhea (6%), vomiting (6%), abdominal pain (3%), rash (3%), and headache (2%). Most of these events were described as mild or moderate in severity. Of the reported adverse events, only 1% was described as severe.

In pneumonia studies conducted in adults comparing clarithromycin to erythromycin base or erythromycin stearate, there were fewer adverse events involving the digestive system in clarithromycin-treated patients compared to erythromycin-treated patients (13% vs 32%; p < 0.01). Twenty percent of erythromycin-treated patients discontinued therapy due to adverse events compared to 4% of clarithromycin-treated patients.

In two U.S. studies of acute otitis media comparing clarithromycin to amoxicillin/potassium clavulanate in pediatric patients, there were fewer adverse events involving the digestive system in clarithromycin-treated patients compared to amoxicillin/potassium clavulanate-treated patients (21% vs. 40%, p < 0.001). One-third as many clarithromycin-treated patients reported diarrhea as did amoxicillin/potassium clavulanate-treated patients.

Post-Marketing Experience:
Allergic reactions ranging from urticaria and mild skin eruptions to rare cases of anaphylaxis and Stevens-Johnson syndrome have occurred. Other spontaneously reported adverse events include glossitis, stomatitis, oral moniliasis, vomiting and dizziness. There have been isolated reports of hearing loss, which is usually reversible, occurring chiefly in elderly women. Reports of alterations of the sense of smell, usually in conjunction with taste perversion have also been reported.

Transient CNS events including behavioral changes, confusional states, depersonalization, disorientation, hallucinations, insomnia, nightmares, tinnitus, and vertigo have been reported during post-marketing surveillance. Events usually resolve quickly with discontinuation of the drug.

Hepatic dysfunction, including increased liver enzymes, and hepatocellular and/or cholestatic hepatitis, with or without jaundice, has been infrequently reported with clarithromycin. This hepatic dysfunction may be severe and is usually reversible. In very rare instances, hepatic failure with fatal outcome has been reported and generally has been associated with serious underlying diseases and/or concomitant medications.

Rarely, erythromycin and clarithromycin have been associated with ventricular arrhythmias, including ventricular tachycardia and torsades de pointes, in individuals with prolonged QT_c intervals.

Changes in Laboratory Values: Changes in laboratory values with possible clinical significance were as follows:
Hepatic—elevated SGPT (ALT) <1%; SGOT (AST) <1%; GGT <1%; alkaline phosphatase <1%; LDH <1%; total bilirubin <1%
Hematologic—decreased WBC <1%; elevated prothrombin time 1%
Renal—elevated BUN 4%; elevated serum creatinine <1%
GGT, alkaline phosphatase, and prothrombin time data are from adult studies only.

DOSAGE AND ADMINISTRATION

BIAXIN® Filmtab® (clarithromycin tablets) and BIAXIN® Granules (clarithromycin for oral suspension) may be given with or without food.
[See table at top right of next page.]

Active Duodenal Ulcer Associated with
***H. pylori* Infection**
(28 day therapy)

Days 1–14	Days 15–28
Clarithromycin 500 mg tablet t.i.d. plus	
Omeprazole 2 × 20 mg capsules q AM	Omeprazole 20 mg capsule q AM

For information on omeprazole, refer to the DOSAGE AND ADMINISTRATION section of the PRILOSEC package insert.

Children - The usual recommended daily dosage is 15 mg/kg/day divided q12h for 10 days.

[See table on bottom of page.]

Clarithromycin may be administered without dosage adjustment in the presence of hepatic impairment if there is normal renal function. However, in the presence of severe renal impairment ($CR_{CL} < 30$ mL/min), with or without coexisting hepatic impairment, the dose should be halved or the dosing interval doubled.

Mycobacterial infections:

Prophylaxis: The recommended dose of BIAXIN for the prevention of disseminated *Mycobacterium avium* disease is 500 mg b.i.d. In children, the recommended dose is 7.5 mg/kg b.i.d. up to 500 mg b.i.d. No studies of clarithromycin for MAC prophylaxis have been performed in pediatric populations and the doses recommended for prophylaxis are derived from MAC treatment studies in children. Dosing recommendations for children are in the table above.

Treatment: Clarithromycin is recommended as the primary agent for the treatment of disseminated infection due to *Mycobacterium avium* complex. Clarithromycin should be used in combination with other antimycobacterial drugs that have shown *in vitro* activity against MAC, including ethambutol, clofazimine, and rifampin. Although no controlled clinical trial information is available for combination therapy with clarithromycin, the U.S. Public Health Service Task Force has provided recommendations for the treatment of MAC.[4] The recommended dose for mycobacterial infections in adults is 500 mg b.i.d. In children, the recommended dose is 7.5 mg/kg b.i.d. up to 500 mg b.i.d. Dosing recommendations for children are in the table above.

Clarithromycin therapy should continue for life if clinical and mycobacterial improvements are observed.

Constituting Instructions

The table below indicates the volume of water to be added when constituting:

Total volume after constitution	Clarithromycin concentration after constitution	Amount of water to be added*
50 mL	125 mg/5 mL	27 mL
100 mL	125 mg/5 mL	55 mL
50 mL	250 mg/5 mL	27 mL
100 mL	250 mg/5 mL	55 mL

* see instructions below.

Add half the volume of water to the bottle and shake vigorously. Add the remainder of water to the bottle and shake. Shake well before each use. Oversize bottle provides shake space. Keep tightly closed.

Do not refrigerate. After mixing, store at 15° to 30°C (59° to 86°F) and use within 14 days.

HOW SUPPLIED

BIAXIN® Filmtab® (clarithromycin tablets) are supplied as yellow oval film-coated tablets imprinted (on one side) in blue with the Abbott logo and a two-letter Abbo-Code designation, KT for the 250 mg tablet and KL for the 500 mg tablet, in the following packaging sizes:

250 mg tablets:
Bottles of 60 (**NDC** 0074-3368-60) and ABBO-PAC unit dose strip packages of 100 (**NDC** 0074-3368-11).

500 mg tablets:
Bottles of 60 (**NDC** 0074-2586-60) and ABBO-PAC unit dose strip packages of 100 (**NDC** 0074-2586-11).

BIAXIN® Granules (clarithromycin for oral suspension) is supplied in the following strengths and sizes:
[See table at bottom of next page.]

Store tablets and granules for oral suspension at controlled room temperature 15° to 30°C (59° to 86°F) in a well-closed container. Protect from light. Do not refrigerate BIAXIN suspension.

CLINICAL STUDIES

Mycobacterial Infections
Prophylaxis:
A randomized, double-blind study (561) compared clarithromycin 500 mg b.i.d. to placebo in patients with CDC-defined AIDS and CD_4 counts < 100 cells/μL. This study accrued

---

ADULT DOSAGE GUIDELINES

Infection	Dosage (q 12 h)	Normal Duration (days)
Pharyngitis/Tonsillitis	250 mg	10
Acute maxillary sinusitis	500 mg	14
Acute exacerbation of chronic bronchitis due to:		
S. pneumoniae	250 mg	7–14
M. catarrhalis	250 mg	7–14
H. influenzae	500 mg	7–14
Pneumonia due to:		
S. pneumoniae	250 mg	7–14
M. pneumoniae	250 mg	7–14
Uncomplicated skin and skin structure	250 mg	7–14

682 patients from November 1992 to January 1994, with a median CD_4 cell count at study entry of 30 cells/μL. Median duration of clarithromycin was 10.6 months vs. 8.2 months for placebo. More patients in the placebo arm than the clarithromycin arm discontinued prematurely from the study (75.6% and 67.4%, respectively). However, if premature discontinuations due to MAC or death are excluded, approximately equal percentages of patients on each arm (54.8% on clarithromycin and 52.5% on placebo) discontinued study drug early for other reasons. The study was designed to evaluate the following endpoints:

1. MAC bacteremia, defined as at least one positive culture for *M. avium* complex bacteria from blood or another normally sterile site.
2. Survival.
3. Clinically significant disseminated MAC disease, defined as MAC bacteremia accompanied by signs or symptoms of serious MAC infection, including fever, night sweats, weight loss, anemia, or elevations in liver function tests.

MAC bacteremia:

In patients randomized to clarithromycin, the risk of MAC bacteremia was reduced by 69% compared to placebo. The difference between groups was statistically significant (p < 0.001). On an intent-to-treat basis, the one-year cumulative incidence of MAC bacteremia was 5.0% for patients randomized to clarithromycin and 19.4% for patients randomized to placebo. While only 19 of the 341 patients randomized to clarithromycin developed MAC, 11 of these cases were resistant to clarithromycin. The patients with resistant MAC bacteremia had a median baseline CD_4 count of 10 cells/mm³ (range 2 –25 cells/mm³). Information regarding the clinical course and response to treatment of the patients with resistant MAC bacteremia is limited. The 8 patients who received clarithromycin and developed susceptible MAC bacteremia had a median baseline CD_4 count of 25 cells/mm³ (range 10 - 80 cells/mm³). Comparatively, 53 of the 341 placebo patients developed MAC; none of these isolates were resistant to clarithromycin. The median baseline CD_4 count was 15 cells/mm³ (range 2–130 cells/mm³) for placebo patients that developed MAC.

Survival:

A statistically significant survival benefit was observed.

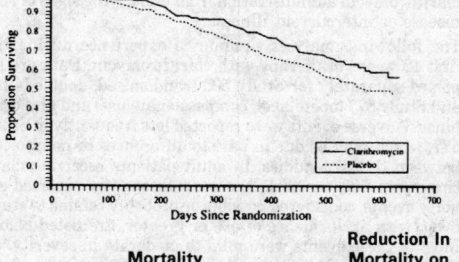

Survival
All Randomized Patients

	Mortality		Reduction In Mortality on Clarithromycin
	Placebo	Clarithromycin	
6 month	9.4%	6.5%	31%
12 month	29.7%	20.5%	31%
18 month	46.4%	37.5%	20%

Since the analysis at 18 months includes patients no longer receiving prophylaxis the survival benefit of clarithromycin may be underestimated.

Clinically significant disseminated MAC disease:

In association with the decreased incidence of bacteremia, patients in the group randomized to clarithromycin showed reductions in the signs and symptoms of disseminated MAC disease, including fever, night sweats, weight loss, and anemia.

Safety:

In AIDS patients treated with clarithromycin over long periods of time for prophylaxis against *M. avium*, it was often difficult to distinguish adverse events possibly associated with clarithromycin administration from underlying HIV disease or intercurrent illness. Median duration of treatment was 10.6 months for the clarithromycin group and 8.2 months for the placebo group.

Treatment-related* Adverse Event Incidence Rates (%) in Immunocompromised Adult Patients Receiving Prophylaxis Against *M. avium* Complex

Body System‡ Adverse Event	Clarithromycin (n = 339) %	Placebo (n = 339) %
Body as a Whole		
Abdominal pain	5.0%	3.5%
Headache	2.7%	0.9%
Digestive		
Diarrhea	7.7%	4.1%
Dyspepsia	3.8%	2.7%
Flatulence	2.4%	0.9%
Nausea	11.2%	7.1%
Vomiting	5.9%	3.2%
Skin & Appendages		
Rash	3.2%	3.5%
Special Senses		
Taste Perversion	8.0%	0.3%

* Includes those events possibly or probably related to study drug and excludes concurrent conditions.
‡ ≥ 2% Adverse Event Incidence Rates for either treatment group.

Among these events, taste perversion was the only event that had significantly higher incidence in the clarithromycin-treated group compared to the placebo-treated group. Discontinuation due to adverse events was required in 18% of patients receiving clarithromycin compared to 17% of patients receiving placebo in this trial. Primary reasons for discontinuation in clarithromycin-treated patients include headache, nausea, vomiting, depression and taste perversion.

Changes in Laboratory Values of Potential Clinical Importance:

In immunocompromised patients receiving prophylaxis against *M. avium*, evaluations of laboratory values were made by analyzing those values outside the seriously abnormal value (i.e., the extreme high or low limit) for the specified test.

PEDIATRIC DOSAGE GUIDELINES

Based on Body Weight

Dosing Calculated on 7.5 mg/kg q12h

Weight Kg	lbs	Dose (q12h)	125 mg/ 5 mL	250 mg/ 5 mL
9	20	62.5 mg	2.5 mL q12h	1.25 mL q12h
17	37	125 mg	5 mL q12h	2.5 mL q12h
25	55	187.5 mg	7.5 mL q12h	3.75 mL q12h
33	73	250 mg	10 mL q12h	5 mL q12h

Continued on next page

Abbott Laboratories—Cont.

Percentage of Patients[(a)] Exceeding Extreme Laboratory Value in Patients Receiving Prophylaxis Against *M. avium* Complex

		Clarithromycin 500 mg b.i.d.		Placebo	
Hemoglobin	<8 g/dL	4/118	3%	5/103	5%
Platelet Count	$<50 \times 10^9$/L	11/249	4%	12/250	5%
WBC Count	$<1 \times 10^9$/L	2/103	4%	0/95	0%
SGOT	>5 x ULN[b]	7/196	4%	5/208	2%
SGPT	>5 x ULN[b]	6/217	3%	4/232	2%
Alk. Phos.	>5 x ULN[b]	5/220	2%	5/218	2%

(a) Includes only patients with baseline values within the normal range or borderline high (hematology variables) and within the normal range or borderline low (chemistry variables).
(b) ULN=Upper Limit of Normal

Treatment:
Three randomized studies (500, 577, and 521) compared different dosages of clarithromycin in patients with CDC-defined AIDS and CD_4 counts <100 cells/μL. These studies accrued patients from May 1991 to March 1992. Study 500 was randomized, double-blind; Study 577 was open-label compassionate use. Both studies used 500 and 1000 mg b.i.d. doses; Study 500 also had a 2000 mg b.i.d. group. Study 521 was a pediatric study at 3.75, 7.5, and 15 mg/kg b.i.d. Study 500 enrolled 154 adult patients, Study 577 enrolled 469 adult patients, and Study 521 enrolled 25 patients between the ages of 1-20. The majority of patients had CD_4 cell counts <50/μL at study entry. The studies were designed to evaluate the following end points:

1. Change in MAC bacteremia or blood cultures negative for *M. avium*.
2. Change in clinical signs and symptoms of MAC infection including one or more of the following: fever, night sweats, weight loss, diarrhea, splenomegaly, and hepatomegaly.

The results for the 500 study are described below. The 577 study results were similar to the results of the 500 study. Results with the 7.5 mg/kg b.i.d. dose in the pediatric study were comparable to those for the 500 mg b.i.d. regimen in the adult studies.

MAC bacteremia:
Decreases in MAC bacteremia or negative blood cultures were seen in the majority of patients in all dose groups. Mean reductions in colony forming units (CFU) are shown below. Included in the table are results from a separate study with a four drug regimen[5] (ciprofloxacin, ethambutol, rifampicin, and clofazimine). Since patient populations and study procedures may vary between these two studies, comparisons between the clarithromycin results and the combination therapy results should be interpreted cautiously.

Mean Reductions in Log CFU from Baseline (After 4 Weeks of Therapy)

500 mg b.i.d (N=35)	1000 mg b.i.d. (N=32)	2000 mg b.i.d. (N=26)	Four Drug Regimen (N=24)
1.5	2.3	2.3	1.4

Although the 1000 mg and 2000 mg b.i.d. doses showed significantly better control of bacteremia during the first four weeks of therapy, no significant differences were seen beyond that point. The percent of patients whose blood was sterilized as shown by one or more negative cultures at any time during acute therapy was 61% (30/49) for the 500 mg b.i.d. group and 59% (29/49) and 52% (25/48) for the 1000 and 2000 mg b.i.d. groups, respectively. The percent of patients who had 2 or more negative cultures during acute therapy that were sustained through study Day 84 was 25% (12/49) in both the 500 and 1000 mg b.i.d. groups and 8% (4/48) for the 2000 mg b.i.d. group. By Day 84, 23% (11/49), 37% (18/49), and 56% (27/48) of patients had died or discontinued from the study, and 14% (7/49), 12% (6/49), and 13% (6/48) of patients had relapsed in the 500, 1000, and 2000 mg b.i.d. dose groups, respectively. All of the isolates had an MIC < 8 μg/mL at pre-treatment. Relapse was almost always accompanied by an increase in MIC. The median time to first negative culture was 54, 41, and 29 days for the 500, 1000, and 2000 mg b.i.d. groups, respectively. The time to first decrease of at least 1 log in CFU count was significantly shorter with the 1000 and 2000 mg b.i.d. doses (median equal to 16 and 15 days, respectively) in comparison to the 500 mg b.i.d. group (median equal to 29 days). The median time to first positive culture or study discontinuation following the first negative culture was 43, 59 and 43 days for the 500, 1000, and 2000 mg b.i.d. groups, respectively.

Clinically significant disseminated MAC Disease:
Among patients experiencing night sweats prior to therapy, 84% showed resolution or improvement at some point during the 12 weeks of clarithromycin at 500-2000 mg b.i.d. doses. Similarly, 77% of patients reported resolution or improvement in fevers at some point. Response rates for clinical signs of MAC are given below:

Resolution of Fever			Resolution of Night Sweats		
b.i.d. dose (mg)	% ever afebrile	% afebrile ≥6 weeks	b.i.d. dose (mg)	% ever resolving	% resolving ≥6 weeks
500	67%	23%	500	85%	42%
1000	67%	12%	1000	70%	33%
2000	62%	22%	2000	72%	36%

Weight Gain >3%			Hemoglobin Increase >1 gm		
b.i.d. dose (mg)	% ever gaining	% gaining ≥6 weeks	b.i.d. dose (mg)	% ever increasing	% increasing ≥6 weeks
500	33%	14%	500	58%	26%
1000	26%	17%	1000	37%	6%
2000	26%	12%	2000	62%	18%

The median duration of response, defined as improvement or resolution of clinical signs and symptoms, was 2-6 weeks. Since the study was not designed to determine the benefit of monotherapy beyond 12 weeks, the duration of response may be underestimated for the 25-33% of patients who continued to show clinical response after 12 weeks.

Survival:
Median survival time from study entry (Study 500) was 249 days at the 500 mg b.i.d. dose compared to 215 days with the 1000 mg b.i.d. dose. However, during the first 12 weeks of therapy, there were 2 deaths in 53 patients in the 500 mg b.i.d. group versus 13 deaths in 51 patients in the 1000 mg b.i.d. group. The reason for this apparent mortality difference is not known. Survival in the two groups was similar beyond 12 weeks. The median survival times for these dosages were similar to recent historical controls with MAC when treated with combination therapies.[5]
Median survival time from study entry in Study 577 was 199 days for the 500 mg b.i.d. dose and 179 days for the 1000 mg b.i.d. dose. During the first four weeks of therapy, while patients were maintained on their originally assigned dose, there were 11 deaths in 255 patients taking 500 mg b.i.d. and 18 deaths in 214 patients taking 1000 mg b.i.d.

Safety:
The adverse event profiles showed that both the 500 and 1000 mg b.i.d. doses were well tolerated. The 2000 mg b.i.d. dose was poorly tolerated and resulted in a higher proportion of premature discontinuations.

In AIDS patients and other immunocompromised patients treated with the higher doses of clarithromycin over long periods of time for mycobacterial infections, it was often difficult to distinguish adverse events possibly associated with clarithromycin administration from underlying signs of HIV disease or intercurrent illness.

The following analyses summarize experience during the first 12 weeks of therapy with clarithromycin. Data are reported separately for Study 500 (randomized, double-blind) and Study 577 (open-label, compassionate use) and also combined. Adverse events were reported less frequently in Study 577, which may be due in part to differences in monitoring between the two studies. In adult patients receiving clarithromycin 500 mg b.i.d., the most frequently reported adverse events, considered possibly or probably related to study drug, with an incidence of 5% or greater, are listed below. Most of these events were mild to moderate in severity, although 5% (Study 500: 8%; Study 577: 4%) of patients receiving 500 mg b.i.d. and 5% (Study 500: 4%; Study 577: 6%) of patients receiving 1000 mg b.i.d. reported severe adverse events. Excluding those patients who discontinued therapy or died due to complications of their underlying non-mycobacterial disease, approximately 8% (Study 500: 15%; Study 577: 7%) of the patients who received 500 mg b.i.d. and 12% (Study 500: 14%; Study 577: 12%) of the patients who received 1000 mg b.i.d. discontinued therapy due to drug-related events during the first 12 weeks of therapy. Overall, the 500 and 1000 mg b.i.d. doses had similar adverse event profiles.

Treatment-related* Adverse Event Incidence Rates (%) in Immunocompromised Adult Patients During the First 12 Weeks of Therapy with 500 mg b.i.d. Clarithromycin Dose

Adverse Event	Study 500 (n=53)	Study 577 (n=255)	Combined (n=308)
Abdominal Pain	7.5	2.4	3.2
Diarrhea	9.4	1.6	2.9
Flatulence	7.5	0.0	1.3
Headache	7.5	0.4	1.6
Nausea	28.3	9.0	12.3
Rash	9.4	2.0	3.2
Taste Perversion	18.9	0.4	3.6
Vomiting	24.5	3.9	7.5

*Includes those events possibly or probably related to study drug and excludes concurrent conditions.

A limited number of pediatric AIDS patients have been treated with clarithromycin suspension for mycobacterial infections. The most frequently reported adverse events, excluding those due to the patient's concurrent condition, were consistent with those observed in adult patients.

Changes in Laboratory Values:
In immunocompromised patients treated with clarithromycin for mycobacterial infections, evaluations of laboratory values were made by analyzing those values outside the seriously abnormal level (i.e., the extreme high or low limit) for the specified test.

Percentage of Patients[(a)] Exceeding Extreme Laboratory Value Limits During First 12 Weeks of Treatment 500 mg b.i.d. Dose[(b)]

		Study 500	Study 577	Combined
BUN	>50 mg/dL	0%	<1%	<1%
Platelet Count	$<50 \times 10^9$/L	0%	<1%	<1%
SGOT	>5 × ULN[c]	0%	3%	2%
SGPT	>5 × ULN[c]	0%	2%	1%
WBC	$<1 \times 10^9$/L	0%	1%	1%

(a) Includes only patients with baseline values within the normal range or borderline high (hematology variables) and within the normal range or borderline low (chemistry variables)
(b) Includes all values within first 12 weeks for patients who start on 500 mg b.i.d.
(c) ULN=Upper Limit of Normal

Otitis Media
In a controlled clinical study of acute otitis media performed in the United States, where significant rates of beta-lactamase producing organisms were found, clarithromycin was compared to an oral cephalosporin. In this study, very strict evaluability criteria were used to determine clinical response. For the 223 patients who were evaluated for clinical efficacy, the clinical success rate (i.e., cure plus improvement) at the post-therapy visit was 88% for clarithromycin and 91% for the cephalosporin.
In a smaller number of patients, microbiologic determinations were made at the pre-treatment visit. The following presumptive bacterial eradication/clinical cure outcomes (i.e., clinical success) were obtained:

U.S. Acute Otitis Media Study Clarithromycin vs. Oral Cephalosporin EFFICACY RESULTS

PATHOGEN	OUTCOME
S. pneumoniae	clarithromycin success rate, 13/15 (87%), control 4/5
*H. influenzae**	clarithromycin success rate, 10/14 (71%), control 3/4
M. catarrhalis	clarithromycin success rate, 4/5, control 1/1
S. pyogenes	clarithromycin success rate, 3/3, control 0/1
Overall	clarithromycin success rate, 30/37 (81%), control 8/11 (73%)

*None of the *H. influenzae* isolated pre-treatment was resistant to clarithromycin; 6% were resistant to the control agent.

Total volume after constitution	Clarithromycin concentration after constitution	Clarithromycin contents per bottle	NDC
50 mL	125 mg/5 mL	1250 mg	0074-3163-50
100 mL	125 mg/5 mL	2500 mg	0074-3163-13
50 mL	250 mg/5 mL	2500 mg	0074-3188-50
100 mL	250 mg/5 mL	5000 mg	0074-3188-13

Safety:
The incidence of adverse events in all patients treated, primarily diarrhea and vomiting, did not differ clinically or statistically for the two agents.

In two other controlled clinical trials of acute otitis media performed in the United States, where significant rates of beta-lactamase producing organisms were found, clarithromycin was compared to an oral antimicrobial agent that contained a specific beta-lactamase inhibitor. In these studies, very strict evaluability criteria were used to determine the clinical responses. In the 233 patients who were evaluated for clinical efficacy, the combined clinical success rate (i.e., cure and improvement) at the post-therapy visit was 91% for both clarithromycin and the control.

For the patients who had microbiologic determinations at the pre-treatment visit, the following presumptive bacterial eradication/clinical cure outcomes (i.e., clinical success) were obtained:

Two U.S. Acute Otitis Media Studies Clarithromycin vs. Antimicrobial/Beta-lactamase Inhibitor EFFICACY RESULTS

PATHOGEN	OUTCOME
S. pneumoniae	clarithromycin success rate, 43/51 (84%), control 55/56 (98%)
*H. influenzae**	clarithromycin success rate, 36/45 (80%), control 31/33 (94%)
M. catarrhalis	clarithromycin success rate, 9/10 (90%), control 6/6
S. pyogenes	clarithromycin success rate, 3/3, control 5/5
Overall	clarithromycin success rate, 91/109 (83%), control 97/100 (97%)

*Of the *H. influenzae* isolated pre-treatment, 3% were resistant to clarithromycin and 10% were resistant to the control agent.

Safety:
The incidence of adverse events in all patients treated, primarily diarrhea (15% vs. 38%) and diaper rash (3% vs. 11%) in young children, was clinically and statistically lower in the clarithromycin arm versus the control arm.

Duodenal Ulcer Associated with *H. pylori* Infection
Four randomized, double-blind, multi-center studies (067, 100, 812b, and 058) evaluated clarithromycin 500 mg t.i.d. plus omeprazole 40 mg q.d. for 14 days, followed by omeprazole 20 mg q.d. (067, 100, and 058) or by omeprazole 40 mg q.d. (812b) for an additional 14 days in patients with active duodenal ulcer associated with *H. pylori*. Studies 067 and 100 were conducted in the U.S. and Canada and enrolled 242 and 256 patients, respectively. *H. pylori* infection and duodenal ulcer were confirmed in 219 patients in Study 067 and 228 patients in Study 100. These studies compared the combination regimen to omeprazole and clarithromycin monotherapies. Studies 812b and 058 were conducted in Europe and enrolled 154 and 215 patients, respectively. *H. pylori* infection and duodenal ulcer were confirmed in 148 patients in Study 812b and 208 patients in Study 058. These studies compared the combination regimen to omeprazole monotherapy. The results for the efficacy analyses for these studies are described below.

Duodenal Ulcer Healing:
The combination of clarithromycin and omeprazole was as effective as omeprazole alone for healing duodenal ulcer.
[See table below.]

End-of-Treatment Ulcer Healing Rates

Study	Clarithromycin + Omeprazole	Omeprazole	Clarithromycin
U.S. Studies			
Study 100	94% (58/62)†	88% (60/68)	71% (49/69)
Study 067	88% (56/64)†	85% (55/65)	64% (44/69)
Non-U.S. Studies			
Study 058	99% (84/85)	95% (82/86)	N/A
Study 812b[1]	100% (64/64)	99% (71/72)	N/A

† p < 0.05 for clarithromycin + omeprazole versus clarithromycin monotherapy.
[1] In Study 812b patients received omeprazole 40 mg daily for days 15 to 28.

H. pylori Eradication Rates (Per-Protocol Analysis)

Study	Clarithromycin + Omeprazole	Omeprazole	Clarithromycin
U.S. Studies			
Study 100			
4–6 Weeks	64% (39/61)†‡	0% (0/59)	39% (17/44)
3 Months	70% (37/53)†‡	0% (0/42)	40% (16/40)
Study 067			
4–6 Weeks	74% (39/53)†‡	0% (0/54)	31% (13/42)
3 Months	75% (33/44)†‡	3% (1/37)	33% (11/33)
Non-U.S. Studies			
Study 058			
4–6 Weeks	74% (64/86)‡	1% (1/90)	N/A
Study 812b			
4–6 Weeks	83% (50/60)‡	1% (1/74)	N/A

† Statistically significantly higher than clarithromycin monotherapy (p < 0.05).
‡ Statistically significantly higher than omeprazole monotherapy (p < 0.05).

Eradication of H. pylori Associated with Duodenal Ulcer:
The combination of clarithromycin and omeprazole was effective in eradicating *H. pylori*.
[See table above.]

H. pylori eradication was defined as no positive test (culture or histology) at 4 weeks following the end of treatment, and two negative tests were required to be considered eradicated. In the per-protocol analysis, the following patients were excluded: dropouts, patients with major protocol violations, patients with missing *H. pylori* tests post-treatment, and patients that were not assessed for *H. pylori* eradication at 4 weeks after the end of treatment because they were found to have an unhealed ulcer at the end of treatment.
Ulcer recurrence at 6-months following the end of treatment was assessed for patients in whom ulcers were healed post-treatment.

Ulcer Recurrence at 6 months by H. pylori Status at 4–6 Weeks

	H. pylori Negative	H. pylori Positive
U.S. Studies		
Study 100		
Clarithromycin + Omeprazole	6% (2/34)	56% (9/16)
Omeprazole	— (0/0)	71% (35/49)
Clarithromycin	12% (2/17)	32% (7/22)
Study 067		
Clarithromycin + Omeprazole	38% (11/29)	50% (6/12)
Omeprazole	— (0/0)	67% (31/46)
Clarithromycin	18% (2/11)	52% (14/27)
Non-U.S. Studies		
Study 058		
Clarithromycin + Omeprazole	6% (3/53)	24% (4/17)
Omeprazole	0% (0/3)	55% (39/71)
Study 812b*		
Clarithromycin + Omeprazone	5% (2/42)	0% (0/7)
Omeprazole	0% (0/1)	54% (32/59)
* 12-month recurrence rates:		
Clarithromycin + Omeprazole	3% (1/40)	0% (0/6)
Omeprazole	0% (0/1)	67% (29/43)

Thus, in patients with duodenal ulcer associated with *H. pylori* infection, eradication of *H. pylori* reduced ulcer recurrence.

Safety:
The adverse event profiles for the four studies showed that the combination of clarithromycin 500 mg t.i.d. and omeprazole 40 mg q.d. for 14 days, followed by omeprazole 20 mg q.d. (067, 100, and 058) or 40 mg q.d. (812b) for an additional 14 days was well tolerated. Of the 346 patients who received the combination, 12 (3.5%) patients discontinued study drug due to adverse events.

Adverse Events with an Incidence of 3% or Greater

Adverse Events	Clarithromycin + Omeprazole (N=346) % of Patients	Omeprazole (N=355) % of Patients	Clarithromycin (N=166) % of Patients*
Taste Perversion	15%	1%	16%
Nausea	5%	1%	3%
Headache	5%	6%	9%
Diarrhea	4%	3%	7%
Vomiting	4%	<1%	1%
Abdominal Pain	3%	2%	1%
Infection	3%	4%	2%

*Studies 067 and 100, only

Most of these events were mild to moderate in severity.
Changes in Laboratory Values:
Changes in laboratory values with possible clinical significance in patients taking clarithromycin and omeprazole were as follows:
Hepatic - elevated direct bilirubin <1%; GGT <1%; SGOT (AST) <1%; SGPT (ALT) <1%.
Renal - elevated serum creatinine <1%.
For information on omeprazole, refer to the ADVERSE REACTIONS section of the PRILOSEC package insert.

ANIMAL PHARMACOLOGY AND TOXICOLOGY

Clarithromycin is rapidly and well-absorbed with dose-linear kinetics, low protein binding, and a high volume of distribution. Plasma half-life ranged from 1–6 hours and was species dependent. High tissue concentrations were achieved, but negligible accumulation was observed. Fecal clearance predominated. Hepatotoxicity occurred in all species tested (i.e., in rats and monkeys at doses 2 times greater than and in dogs at doses comparable to the maximum human daily dose, based on mg/m²). Renal tubular degeneration (calculated on a mg/m² basis) occurred in rats at doses 2 times, in monkeys at doses 8 times, and in dogs at doses 12 times greater than the maximum human daily dose. Testicular atrophy (on a mg/m² basis) occurred in rats at doses 7 times, in dogs at doses 3 times, and in monkeys at doses 8 times greater than the maximum human daily dose. Corneal opacity (on a mg/m² basis) occurred in dogs at doses 12 times and in monkeys at doses 8 times greater than the maximum human daily dose. Lymphoid depletion (on a mg/m² basis) occurred in dogs at doses 3 times greater than and in monkeys at doses 2 times greater than the maximum human daily dose. These adverse events were absent during clinical trials.

REFERENCES
1. National Committee for Clinical Laboratory Standards, Methods for Dilution Antimicrobial Susceptibility Tests for Bacteria that Grow Aerobically—Third Edition. Approved

Continued on next page

Abbott Laboratories—Cont.

Standard NCCLS Document M7-A3, Vol. 13, No. 25, NCCLS, Villanova, PA, December, 1993.
2. National Committee for Clinical Laboratory Standards, Performance Standards for Antimicrobial Disk Susceptibility Tests—Fifth Edition. Approved Standard NCCLS Document M2-A5, Vol. 13, No. 24, NCCLS, Villanova, PA, December, 1993.
3. Hachem, C. Y., J. E. Clarridge, R. Reddy, R. Flamm, D. G. Evans, S. K. Tanaka, and D. Y. Graham. Antimicrobial susceptibility testing of *Helicobacter pylori*: comparison of E-test, broth microdilution, and disk diffusion for ampicillin, clarithromycin, and metronidazole. *Diagnost. Microbiol. Infect. Dis.* 1996; 24:37-41.
4. Public Health Service Task Force on Prophylaxis and Therapy for Disseminated *Mycobacterium avium* complex. Recommendations on Prophylaxis and Therapy for *Mycobacterium avium* Complex Disease in Patients Infected With The Human Immunodeficiency Virus. *NEJM.* 1993;329:898-904.
5. Kemper CA, et al. Treatment of *Mycobacterium avium* Complex Bacteremia in AIDS with a Four-Drug Oral Regimen. *Ann Intern Med.* 1992;116:466-472.
Filmtab—Film-sealed tablets, Abbott
Ref. 03-4659-R9-Rev. April, 1996
Abbott Laboratories
North Chicago, IL 60064
Shown in Product Identification Guide, page 303

CALCIJEX® ℞
CALCITRIOL INJECTION
1 mcg and 2 mcg/mL

DESCRIPTION
Calcijex® (calcitriol injection) is synthetically manufactured calcitriol and is available as a sterile, isotonic, clear, aqueous solution for intravenous injection. Calcijex is available in 1 mL ampuls. Each 1 mL contains calcitriol, 1 or 2 mcg; Polysorbate 20, 4 mg; sodium chloride 1.5 mg; sodium ascorbate 10 mg added; dibasic sodium phosphate, anhydrous 7.6 mg; monobasic sodium phosphate, monohydrate 1.8 mg; edetate disodium, dihydrate 1.1 mg added. pH 7.2 (6.5 to 8.0).
Calcitriol is a colorless, crystalline compound which occurs naturally in humans. It is soluble in organic solvents but relatively insoluble in water. Calcitriol is chemically designated (5Z,7E)-9, 10-secocholesta-5,7,10(19)-triene-1α,3β,25-triol and has the following structural formula:

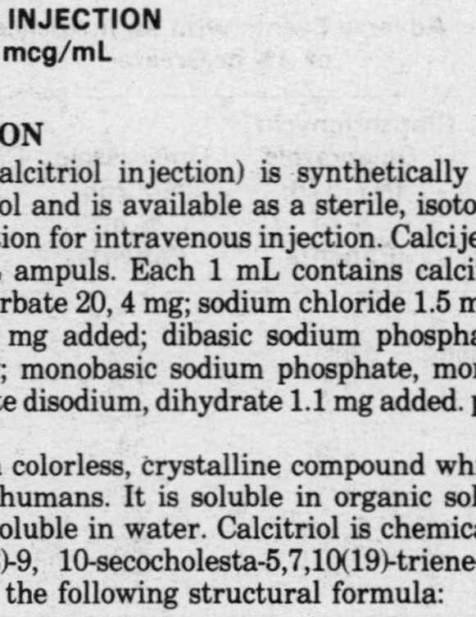

Molecular Formula: $C_{27}H_{44}O_3$
The other names frequently used for calcitriol are 1α, 25-dihydroxycholecalciferol, 1α,25-dihydroxyvitamin D_3, 1,25-DHCC, 1,25$(OH)_2D_3$ and 1,25-diOHC.

CLINICAL PHARMACOLOGY
Calcitriol is the active form of vitamin D_3 (cholecalciferol). The natural or endogenous supply of vitamin D in man mainly depends on ultraviolet light for conversion of 7-dehydrocholesterol to vitamin D_3 in the skin. Vitamin D_3 must be metabolically activated in the liver and the kidney before it is fully active on its target tissues. The initial transformation is catalyzed by a vitamin D_3-25-hydroxylase enzyme present in the liver, and the product of this reaction is 25-$(OH)D_3$ (calcifediol). The latter undergoes hydroxylation in the mitochondria of kidney tissue, and this reaction is activated by the renal 25-hydroxyvitamin D_3-1-α-hydroxylase to produce 1,25-$(OH)_2D_3$ (calcitriol), the active form of vitamin D_3.
The known sites of action of calcitriol are intestine, bone, kidney and parathyroid gland. Calcitriol is the most active known form of vitamin D_3 in stimulating intestinal calcium transport. In acutely uremic rats, calcitriol has been shown to stimulate intestinal calcium absorption. In bone, calcitriol, in conjunction with parathyroid hormone, stimulates resorption of calcium; and in the kidney, calcitriol increases the tubular reabsorption of calcium. In-vitro and in-vivo studies have shown that calcitriol directly suppresses secretion and synthesis of PTH. A vitamin D-resistant state may exist in uremic patients because of the failure of the kidney to adequately convert precursors to the active compound, calcitriol.
Calcitriol when administered by bolus injection is rapidly available in the blood stream. Vitamin D metabolites are known to be transported in blood, bound to specific plasma proteins. The pharmacologic activity of an administered dose of calcitriol is about 3 to 5 days. Two metabolic pathways for calcitriol have been identified, conversion to 1,24,25-$(OH)_3D_3$ and to calcitroic acid.

INDICATIONS AND USAGE
Calcijex® (calcitriol injection) is indicated in the management of hypocalcemia in patients undergoing chronic renal dialysis. It has been shown to significantly reduce elevated parathyroid hormone levels. Reduction of PTH has been shown to result in an improvement in renal osteodystrophy.

CONTRAINDICATIONS
Calcijex® (calcitriol injection) should not be given to patients with hypercalcemia or evidence of vitamin D toxicity.

WARNINGS
Since calcitriol is the most potent metabolite of vitamin D available, vitamin D and its derivatives should be withheld during treatment.
A non-aluminum phosphate-binding compound should be used to control serum phosphorus levels in patients undergoing dialysis.
Overdosage of any form of vitamin D is dangerous (see also OVERDOSAGE). Progressive hypercalcemia due to overdosage of vitamin D and its metabolites may be so severe as to require emergency attention. Chronic hypercalcemia can lead to generalized vascular calcification, nephrocalcinosis and other soft-tissue calcification. The serum calcium times phosphate (Ca × P) product should not be allowed to exceed 70. Radiographic evaluation of suspect anatomical regions may be useful in the early detection of this condition.

PRECAUTIONS
1. **General**
Excessive dosage of Calcijex® (calcitriol injection) induces hypercalcemia and in some instances hypercalciuria; therefore, early in treatment during dosage adjustment, serum calcium and phosphorus should be determined at least twice weekly. Should hypercalcemia develop, the drug should be discontinued immediately.
Calcijex should be given cautiously to patients on digitalis, because hypercalcemia in such patients may precipitate cardiac arrhythmias.
2. **Information for the Patient**
The patient and his or her parents should be informed about adherence to instructions about diet and calcium supplementation and avoidance of the use of unapproved nonprescription drugs, including magnesium-containing antacids. Patients should also be carefully informed about the symptoms of hypercalcemia (see ADVERSE REACTIONS).
3. **Essential Laboratory Tests**
Serum calcium, phosphorus, magnesium and alkaline phosphatase and 24-hour urinary calcium and phosphorus should be determined periodically. During the initial phase of the medication, serum calcium and phosphorus should be determined more frequently (twice weekly).
4. **Drug Interactions**
Magnesium-containing antacid and Calcijex should not be used concomitantly, because such use may lead to the development of hypermagnesemia.
5. **Carcinogenesis, Mutagenesis, Impairment of Fertility**
Long-term studies in animals have not been performed to evaluate the carcinogenic potential of Calcijex (calcitriol injection). There was no evidence of mutagenicity as studied by the Ames Method. No significant effects of calcitriol on fertility were reported using oral Calcitriol.
6. **Use in Pregnancy:** *Pregnancy Category C:*
Calcitriol given orally has been reported to be teratogenic in rabbits when given in doses 4 and 15 times the dose recommended for human use.
All 15 fetuses in 3 litters at these doses showed external and skeletal abnormalities. However, none of the other 23 litters (156 fetuses) showed significant abnormalities compared with controls.
Teratology studies in rats showed no evidence of teratogenic potential. There are no adequate and well-controlled studies in pregnant women. Calcijex should be used during pregnancy only if the potential benefit justifies the potential risk to the fetus.
7. **Nursing Mothers**
It is not known whether this drug is excreted in human milk. Because many drugs are excreted in human milk and because of the potential for serious adverse reactions in nursing infants from calcitriol, a decision should be made whether to discontinue nursing or to discontinue the drug, taking into account the importance of the drug to the mother.
8. **Pediatric Use**
Safety and efficacy of Calcijex in pediatric patients have not been established.

ADVERSE REACTIONS
Adverse effects of Calcijex® (calcitriol injection) are, in general, similar to those encountered with excessive vitamin D intake. The early and late signs and symptoms of vitamin D intoxication associated with hypercalcemia include:
1. **Early**
Weakness, headache, somnolence, nausea, vomiting, dry mouth, constipation, muscle pain, bone pain and metallic taste.
2. **Late**
Polyuria, polydipsia, anorexia, weight loss, nocturia, conjunctivitis (calcific), pancreatitis, photophobia, rhinorrhea, pruritus, hyperthermia, decreased libido, elevated BUN, albuminuria, hypercholesterolemia, elevated SGOT and SGPT, ectopic calcification, hypertension, cardiac arrhythmias and, rarely, overt psychosis.

Occasional mild pain on injection has been observed.

OVERDOSAGE
Administration of Calcijex® (calcitriol injection) to patients in excess of their requirements can cause hypercalcemia, hypercalciuria and hyperphosphatemia. High intake of calcium and phosphate concomitant with Calcijex may lead to similar abnormalities.
1. **Treatment of Hypercalcemia and Overdosage in Patients on Hemodialysis**
General treatment of hypercalcemia (greater than 1 mg/dl above the upper limit of normal range) consists of immediate discontinuation of Calcijex therapy, institution of a low calcium diet and withdrawal of calcium supplements. Serum calcium levels should be determined daily until normocalcemia ensues. Hypercalcemia usually resolves in two to seven days. When serum calcium levels have returned to within normal limits, Calcijex therapy may be reinstituted at a dose 0.5 mcg less than prior therapy. Serum calcium levels should be obtained at least twice weekly after all dosage changes.
Persistent or markedly elevated serum calcium levels may be corrected by dialysis against a calcium-free dialysate.
2. **Treatment of Accidental Overdosage of Calcitriol Injection**
The treatment of acute accidental overdosage of Calcijex should consist of general supportive measures. Serial serum electrolyte determinations (especially calcium), rate of urinary calcium excretion and assessment of electrocardiographic abnormalities due to hypercalcemia should be obtained. Such monitoring is critical in patients receiving digitalis. Discontinuation of supplemental calcium and low calcium diet are also indicated in accidental overdosage. Due to the relatively short duration of the pharmacological action of calcitriol, further measures are probably unnecessary. Should, however, persistent and markedly elevated serum calcium levels occur, there are a variety of therapeutic alternatives which may be considered, depending on the patients' underlying condition. These include the use of drugs such as phosphates and corticosteroids as well as measures to induce an appropriate forced diuresis. The use of peritoneal dialysis against a calcium-free dialysate has also been reported.

DOSAGE AND ADMINISTRATION
The optimal dose of Calcijex® (calcitriol injection) must be carefully determined for each patient.
The effectiveness of Calcijex therapy is predicated on the assumption that each patient is receiving an adequate and appropriate daily intake of calcium. The RDA for calcium in adults is 800 mg. To ensure that each patient receives an adequate daily intake of calcium, the physician should either prescribe a calcium supplement or instruct the patient in proper dietary measures.
The recommended initial dose of Calcijex is 0.5 mcg (0.01 mcg/kg) administered three times weekly, approximately every other day. Calcijex can be administered as a bolus dose intravenously through the catheter at the end of hemodialysis. If a satisfactory response in the biochemical parameters and clinical manifestations of the disease state is not observed, the dose may be increased by 0.25 to 0.50 mcg at two to four week intervals. During this titration period, serum calcium and phosphorus levels should be obtained at least twice weekly, and if hypercalcemia is noted, the drug should be immediately discontinued until normocalcemia ensues. Most patients undergoing hemodialysis respond to doses between 0.5 and 3.0 mcg (0.01 to 0.05 mcg/kg) three times per week.
Parenteral drug products should be inspected visually for particulate matter and discoloration prior to administration, whenever solution and container permit.
Discard unused portion.

HOW SUPPLIED
Calcijex® (calcitriol injection) is supplied in 1 mL ampuls containing 1 mcg (List No. 1200) and 2 mcg (List No. 1210).
Protect from light.
Store at controlled room temperature 15° to 30°C (59° to 86°F).
Caution: Federal (USA) law prohibits dispensing without prescription.

ABBOTT LABORATORIES, NORTH CHICAGO, IL 60064, USA

CARTROL® ℞
[*kär 'trōl*]
(Carteolol Hydrochloride)
Filmtab® Tablets

DESCRIPTION

CARTROL (carteolol hydrochloride) is a synthetic, nonselective, beta-adrenergic receptor blocking agent with intrinsic sympathomimetic activity. It is chemically described as 5-[3-[(1,1-dimethylethyl)amino]-2-hydroxypropoxy]-3,4-dihydro-2(1H)-quinolinone monohydrochloride. The structural formula is:

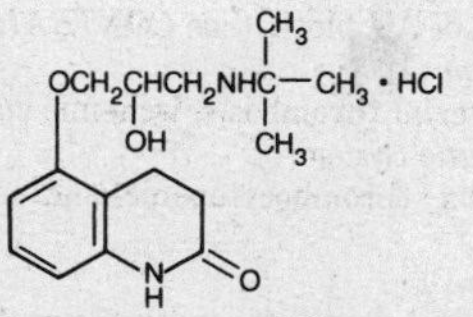

Carteolol hydrochloride is a stable, white crystalline powder which is soluble in water and slightly soluble in ethanol. The molecular weight is 328.84 and $C_{16}H_{24}N_2O_3 \cdot HCl$ is the empirical formula.
CARTROL (carteolol hydrochloride) is available as tablets containing either 2.5 mg or 5 mg of carteolol hydrochloride for oral administration.

INACTIVE INGREDIENTS

2.5 mg Tablet: Cellulosic polymers, corn starch, iron oxide, lactose, magnesium stearate, microcrystalline cellulose, polyethylene glycol, propylene glycol, and titanium dioxide.
5 mg Tablet: Cellulosic polymers, corn starch, lactose, magnesium stearate, microcrystalline cellulose, polyethylene glycol, propylene glycol, and titanium dioxide.

CLINICAL PHARMACOLOGY

CARTROL (carteolol hydrochloride) is a long-acting, nonselective, beta-adrenergic receptor blocking agent with intrinsic sympathomimetic activity (ISA) and without significant membrane stabilizing (local anesthetic) activity.
Pharmacodynamics:
Carteolol specifically competes with beta-adrenergic receptor agonists for both $beta_1$-receptors located principally in cardiac muscle and $beta_2$-receptors located in the bronchial and vascular musculature, blocking the chronotropic, inotropic, and vasodilator responses to beta-adrenergic stimulation proportionately. Because of its partial agonist activity, however, carteolol does not reduce resting beta-agonist activity as much as beta-adrenergic blockers lacking this activity. Thus, in clinical trials in man, the decreases in resting pulse rate produced by carteolol (2–5 beats per minute in various studies) were less than those produced by beta-blockers (nadolol and propranolol) without ISA (10–12 beats per minute). There are also equivocal effects on renin secretion, in contrast to beta-blockers without ISA, which inhibit renin secretion.
In controlled clinical trials carteolol, at doses up to 20 mg as monotherapy or in combination with thiazide type diuretics, produced significantly greater reductions in blood pressure than did placebo, with the full effect seen between two and four weeks. The observed differences from placebo ranged from 3.1 to 6.7 mmHg for supine diastolic blood pressure. The antihypertensive effects of carteolol are smaller in black populations but do not seem to be affected by age or sex.
Doses of carteolol greater than 10 mg once a day did not produce greater reductions in blood pressure. In fact, doses of 20 mg and above appeared to produce blood pressure reductions less than those produced by 10 mg and below. When carteolol was compared to nadolol and propranolol, although the differences were not statistically significant in relatively small studies, carteolol at doses up to 20 mg produced supine diastolic blood pressure changes consistently 2 mmHg less than that produced by either nadolol or propranolol.
Although the mechanism of the antihypertensive effect of beta-adrenergic blocking agents has not been established, multiple factors are thought to contribute to the lowering of blood pressure, including diminished response to sympathetic nerve outflow from vasomotor centers in the brain, diminished release of renin from the kidneys, and decreased cardiac output. Carteolol does not have a consistent effect on renin and other agents with ISA have been shown to have less effect than other beta-blockers on resting cardiac output (although they cause the usual decrease in exercise cardiac output so that the difference is of uncertain clinical importance), so that the mechanism of its action is particularly uncertain.
Beta-blockade interferes with endogenous adrenergic bronchodilator activity and diminishes the response to exogenous bronchodilators. This is especially important in patients subject to bronchospasm.
Single intravenous doses of carteolol (0.5 mg, 1 mg, 2.5 mg and 5 mg) produced statistically, but not clinically, significant increases from baseline in AV node conduction time and RR and PR intervals.
CARTROL (carteolol hydrochloride) induced no significant alteration in total serum cholesterol and triglycerides.
Following discontinuation of carteolol treatment in man, pharmacologic activity (evaluated by blockade of the tachycardia induced by isoproterenol or postural changes) is present for 2 to 21 days (median 14 days) after the last dose of carteolol. Following administration of recommended doses of CARTROL (carteolol hydrochloride), both beta-blocking and antihypertensive effects persist for at least 24 hours.
Pharmacokinetics and Metabolism:
Following oral administration in man, peak plasma concentrations of carteolol usually occur within one to three hours. Carteolol is well absorbed when administered orally as CARTROL (carteolol hydrochloride) tablets. The presence of food in the gastrointestinal tract somewhat slows the rate of absorption, but the extent of absorption is not appreciably affected. Compared to intravenous administration, the absolute bioavailability of carteolol from CARTROL (carteolol hydrochloride) tablets is approximately 85%.
The plasma half-life of carteolol averages approximately six hours. Steady-state serum levels are achieved within one to two days after initiating therapeutic doses of carteolol in persons with normal renal function. Since approximately 50 to 70% of a carteolol dose is eliminated unchanged by the kidneys, the half-life is increased in patients with impaired renal function. Significant reductions in the rate of carteolol elimination (and prolongations of the half-life) occur in patients as creatinine clearance decreases. Therefore, a reduction in maintenance dose and/or prolongation in dosing interval is appropriate (see DOSAGE and ADMINISTRATION).
Carteolol is 23–30% bound to plasma proteins in humans. The major metabolites of carteolol are 8-hydroxycarteolol and the glucuronic acid conjugates of both carteolol and 8-hydroxycarteolol. In man, 8-hydroxycarteolol is an active metabolite with a half-life of approximately 8 to 12 hours and represents approximately 5% of the administered dose excreted in the urine.

INDICATIONS AND USAGE

CARTROL (carteolol hydrochloride) is indicated in the management of hypertension. It may be used alone or in combination with other antihypertensive agents, especially thiazide diuretics. Preliminary data indicate that carteolol does not have a favorable effect on arrhythmias.

CONTRAINDICATIONS

CARTROL (carteolol hydrochloride) is contraindicated in patients with: 1) bronchial asthma, 2) severe bradycardia, 3) greater than first degree heart block, 4) cardiogenic shock, and 5) clinically evident congestive heart failure (see WARNINGS).

WARNINGS

Congestive Heart Failure:
Sympathetic stimulation may be a vital component supporting circulatory function in patients with congestive heart failure, and impairing that support by beta-blockade may precipitate more severe decompensation. Although CARTROL (carteolol hydrochloride) should be avoided in clinically evident congestive heart failure, it can be used with caution, if necessary, in patients with a history of failure who are well-compensated and are receiving digitalis and diuretics. Beta-adrenergic blocking agents do not abolish the inotropic action of digitalis on heart muscle.
IN PATIENTS WITHOUT A HISTORY OF CONGESTIVE HEART FAILURE, the use of beta-blockers can, in some instances, lead to congestive heart failure. Therefore, at the first sign or symptom of cardiac decompensation, discontinuation of beta-blocker therapy should be considered. The patient should be closely observed and treatment should include a diuretic and/or digitalization as necessary.
Exacerbation of Angina Pectoris Upon Withdrawal:
In patients with angina pectoris, exacerbation of angina and, in some cases, myocardial infarction have been reported following abrupt discontinuation of therapy with some beta-blockers. Therefore such patients should be cautioned against interruption of therapy without a physician's advice. The long persistence of beta-adrenergic blockade following abrupt discontinuation of CARTROL (carteolol hydrochloride), however, might be expected to minimize the possibility of this complication. When discontinuation of CARTROL (carteolol hydrochloride) is planned, dosage should be tapered gradually, as it is with other beta-blockers. If exacerbation of angina occurs when CARTROL (carteolol hydrochloride) therapy is interrupted, it is advisable to reinstitute CARTROL (carteolol hydrochloride) or other beta-blocker therapy, at least temporarily, and to take other measures appropriate for the management of unstable angina pectoris.
PATIENTS WITHOUT CLINICALLY RECOGNIZED ANGINA PECTORIS should be carefully monitored after withdrawal of CARTROL (carteolol hydrochloride) therapy, since coronary artery disease may be unrecognized.
Nonallergic Bronchospasm (e.g., chronic bronchitis, emphysema):
Patients with bronchospastic disease generally should not receive beta-blocker therapy and carteolol is contraindicated in patients with bronchial asthma. If use of CARTROL (carteolol hydrochloride) is essential, it should be administered with caution since it may block bronchodilation produced by endogenous catecholamine stimulation of $beta_2$-receptors or diminish response to therapy with a beta-receptor agonist.
Major Surgery:
The necessity, or desirability, of withdrawal of beta-blocking therapy prior to major surgery is controversial. Because beta-blockade impairs the ability of the heart to respond to reflex stimuli and may increase risks of general anesthesia and surgical procedures resulting in protracted hypotension or low cardiac output, and difficulty in restarting or maintaining a heartbeat, it has been suggested that beta-blocker therapy should be withdrawn several days prior to surgery. It is also recognized, however, that increased sensitivity to catecholamines of patients recently withdrawn from beta-blocker therapy could increase certain risks. Given the persistence of the beta-blocking activity of CARTROL (carteolol hydrochloride), effective withdrawal would take several weeks and would ordinarily be impractical. When beta-blocker therapy is not discontinued, anesthetic agents that depress the myocardium should be avoided. In one study using intravenous carteolol during surgery, recovery from anesthesia was somewhat delayed in three patients who received carteolol near the end of anesthesia, and respiratory arrest occurred in one of these patients immediately following administration of intravenous carteolol.
In the event that CARTROL (carteolol hydrochloride) treatment is not discontinued before surgery, the anesthesiologist should be informed that the patient is receiving CARTROL (carteolol hydrochloride). The effects on the heart of beta-adrenergic blocking agents, such as CARTROL (carteolol hydrochloride), may be reversed by cautious administration of isoproterenol or dobutamine.
Diabetes Mellitus and Hypoglycemia:
Beta-adrenergic blockade may prevent the appearance of premonitory signs and symptoms (e.g., tachycardia and blood pressure changes) of acute hypoglycemia, and it inhibits glycogenolysis, a normal compensatory mechanism for hypoglycemia. This is especially important for patients with labile diabetes mellitus. Beta-blockade also reduces the release of insulin in response to hyperglycemia; therefore, it may be necessary to adjust the dose of antidiabetic agents used to treat hyperglycemia.
Thyrotoxicosis:
Beta-adrenergic blockade may mask certain clinical signs of hyperthyroidism such as tachycardia. Patients suspected of having thyrotoxicosis should be managed carefully to avoid abrupt withdrawal of beta-adrenergic blockade which might precipitate a thyroid storm.

PRECAUTIONS

General:
Impaired Renal Function:
CARTROL (carteolol hydrochloride) should be used with caution in patients with impaired renal function. Patients with impaired renal function clear carteolol at a reduced rate, and dosage should be reduced accordingly (see Dosage and Administration).
Beta-adrenoreceptor blockade can cause reduction in intraocular pressure. Therefore, CARTROL (carteolol hydrochloride) may interfere with glaucoma testing. Withdrawal may lead to a return of increased intraocular pressure.
Information for Patients:
Patients, especially those with evidence of coronary artery insufficiency, should be warned against interruption or discontinuation of CARTROL (carteolol hydrochloride) therapy without the physician's advice. Although cardiac failure rarely occurs in properly selected patients, patients being treated with beta-adrenergic blocking agents should be advised to consult the physician at the first sign or symptom of impending failure (i.e., fatigue with exertion, difficulty breathing, cough or unusually fast heartbeat).
Drug Interactions:
Catecholamine-depleting drugs (e.g., reserpine) may have an additive effect when given with beta-blocking agents. Therefore, patients treated with CARTROL (carteolol hydrochloride) plus a catecholamine-depleting agent must be observed carefully for evidence of hypotension and/or excessive bradycardia, which may produce syncope or postural hypotension.
Risk of Anaphylactic Reaction: While taking beta-blockers, patients with a history of severe anaphylactic reaction to a variety of allergens may be more reactive to repeated challenge, either accidental, diagnostic, or therapeutic. Such patients may be unresponsive to the usual doses of epinephrine used to treat allergic reaction.

Continued on next page

Abbott Laboratories—Cont.

Concurrent administration of *general anesthetics* and beta-blocking agents may result in exaggeration of the hypotension induced by general anesthetics (see WARNINGS, Major Surgery).
Blunting of the antihypertensive effect of beta-adrenoreceptor blocking agents by *non-steroidal anti-inflammatory drugs* has been reported. When using these agents concomitantly, patients should be observed carefully to confirm that the desired therapeutic effect has been obtained.
Literature reports suggest that *oral calcium antagonists* may be used in combination with beta-adrenergic blocking agents when heart function is normal, but should be avoided in patients with impaired cardiac function. Hypotension, AV conduction disturbances, and left ventricular failure have been reported in some patients receiving beta-adrenergic blocking agents when an oral calcium antagonist was added to the treatment regimen. Hypotension was more likely to occur if the calcium antagonist were a dihydropyridine derivative, e.g., nifedipine, while left ventricular failure and AV conduction disturbances were more likely to occur with either verapamil or diltiazem.
Intravenous calcium antagonists should be used with caution in patients receiving beta-adrenergic blocking agents. The concomitant use of beta-adrenergic blocking agents with digitalis and either diltiazem or verapamil may have additive effects in prolonging AV conduction time.
Concomitant use of oral antidiabetic agents or *insulin* with beta-blocking agents may be associated with hypoglycemia or possibly hyperglycemia. Dosage of the antidiabetic agent should be adjusted accordingly (see WARNINGS, Diabetes Mellitus and Hypoglycemia).

Carcinogenesis, Mutagenesis, Impairment of Fertility:
CARTROL (carteolol hydrochloride) did not produce carcinogenic effects at doses 280 times the maximum recommended human dose (10 mg/70 kg/day) in two-year oral rat and mouse studies.
Tests of mutagenicity, including the Ames Test, recombinant (rec)-assay, *in vivo* cytogenetics and dominant lethal assay demonstrated no evidence for mutagenic potential.
Fertility of male and female rats and male and female mice was unaffected by administration of CARTROL (carteolol hydrochloride) at dosages up to 150 mg/kg/day. This dosage is approximately 1052 times the maximum recommended human dose.

Pregnancy:
Teratogenic Effects: Pregnancy Category C. CARTROL (carteolol hydrochloride) increased resorptions and decreased fetal weights in rabbits and rats at maternally toxic doses approximately 1052 and 5264 times the maximum recommended human dose (10 mg/70 kg/day), respectively. A dose-related increase in wavy ribs was noted in the developing rat fetus when pregnant females received daily doses of approximately 212 times the maximum recommended human dose. No such effects were noted in pregnant mice subjected to up to 1052 times the maximum recommended human dose. There are no adequate and well-controlled studies in pregnant women. CARTROL (carteolol hydrochloride) should be used during pregnancy only if the potential benefit justifies the potential risk to the fetus.

Nursing Mothers:
Studies have not been conducted in lactating humans and, therefore, it is not known whether carteolol is excreted in human milk. Studies in lactating rats indicate that CARTROL (carteolol hydrochloride) is excreted in milk. Because many drugs are excreted in human milk, caution should be exercised when CARTROL (carteolol hydrochloride) is administered to a nursing woman.

Pediatric Use:
Safety and effectiveness in children have not been established.

ADVERSE REACTIONS

The prevalence of adverse reactions has been ascertained from clinical studies conducted primarily in the United States. All adverse experiences (events) reported during these studies were recorded as adverse reactions. The prevalence rates presented below are based on combined data from nineteen placebo-controlled studies of patients with hypertension, angina or dysrhythmias, using once-daily carteolol at doses up to 60 mg. Table 1 summarizes those adverse experiences reported for patients in these studies where the prevalence in the carteolol group is 1% or greater and exceeds the prevalence in the placebo group. Asthenia and muscle cramps were the only symptoms that were significantly more common in patients receiving carteolol than in patients receiving placebo. Patients in clinical trials were carefully selected to exclude those, such as patients with asthma or known bronchospasm, or congestive heart failure, who would be at high risk of experiencing beta-adrenergic blocker adverse effect (See WARNINGS and CONTRAINDICATIONS):

TABLE 1
Adverse Reactions During
Placebo-Controlled Studies

	Placebo (n=448) %	Carteolol (n=761) %
Body as a Whole		
†Asthenia	4.0	7.1*
Abdominal Pain	0.4	1.3
Back Pain	1.6	2.1
Chest Pain	1.8	2.2
Digestive System		
Diarrhea	2.0	2.1
Nausea	1.8	2.1
Metabolic/Nutritional Disorders		
Abnormal Lab Test	1.1	1.2
Peripheral Edema	1.1	1.7
Musculoskeletal System		
Arthralgia	1.1	1.2
Muscle Cramps	0.2	2.6*
Lower Extremity Pain	0.2	1.2
Nervous System		
Insomnia	0.7	1.7
Paresthesia	1.1	2.0
Respiratory System		
Nasal Congestion	0.9	1.1
Pharyngitis	0.9	1.1
Skin and Appendages		
Rash	1.1	1.3

† Includes weakness, tiredness, lassitude and fatigue.
* Statistically significant at p=0.05 level.

The adverse experiences were usually mild or moderate in intensity and transient, but sometimes were serious enough to interrupt treatment. The adverse reactions that were most bothersome, as judged by their being reported as reasons for discontinuation of therapy by at least 0.4% of the carteolol group are shown in Table 2.

TABLE 2
Discontinuations During
Placebo-Controlled Studies

	Placebo (n=448) %	Carteolol (n=761) %
Body as a Whole		
Asthenia	0.2	0.5
Headache	0.7	0.7
Chest Pain	0.2	0.4
Skin and Appendages		
Rash	0.0	0.4
Sweating	0.2	0.4
Digestive System		
Nausea	0.0	0.4
Overall Adverse Reactions	4.2	3.3

Additional adverse reactions have been reported, but these are, in general, not distinguishable from symptoms that might have occurred in the absence of exposure to carteolol. The following additional adverse reactions were reported by at least 1% of 1568 patients who received carteolol in controlled or open, short- or long-term clinical studies, or represent less common, but potentially important, reactions reported in clinical studies or marketing experience (these rarer reactions are shown in italics): *Body as a Whole:* fever, infection, injury, malaise, pain, neck pain, shoulder pain; *Cardiovascular System:* angina pectoris, arrhythmia, *heart failure,* palpitations, *second degree heart block,* vasodilation; *Digestive System: acute hepatitis with jaundice,* constipation, dyspepsia, flatulence, gastrointestinal disorder; *Metabolic/Nutritional Disorder:* gout; *Musculoskeletal System:* pain in extremity, joint disorder, arthritis; *Nervous System: abnormal dreams,* anxiety, depression, dizziness, nervousness, somnolence; *Respiratory System:* bronchitis, *bronchospasm,* cold symptoms, cough, dyspnea, flu symptoms, lung disorder, rhinitis, sinusitis, *wheezing; Skin and Appendages:* sweating; *Special Senses:* blurred vision, conjunctivitis, eye disorder, tinnitus; *Urogenital:* impotence, urinary frequency, urinary tract infection.
In studies of patients with hypertension or angina pectoris where carteolol and positive reference beta-adrenergic blocking agents [nadolol (n=82) and propranolol (n=50)] have been compared, the differences in prevalence rates between the carteolol group and the reference agent group were statistically significant (p≤0.05) for the adverse reactions listed in Table 3. [See top of next column.]

TABLE 3
Adverse Reactions During
Positive-Controlled Studies

	Reference Agents (n=132) %	Carteolol (n=135) %
Body as a Whole		
Chest Pain	5.3	0.7
Cardiovascular System		
Bradycardia	4.5	0.0
Digestive System		
Diarrhea	11.4	4.4
Nervous System		
Somnolence	0.8	7.4
Skin and Appendages		
Sweating	5.3	0.7

POTENTIAL ADVERSE REACTIONS

In addition, other adverse reactions not listed above have been reported with other beta-adrenergic blocking agents and should be considered potential adverse reactions of CARTROL (carteolol hydrochloride).
Body as a Whole:
Fever combined with aching and sore throat.
Cardiovascular System:
Intensification of AV block. (See *CONTRAINDICATIONS*).
Digestive System:
Mesenteric arterial thrombosis, ischemic colitis.
Hemic/Lymphatic System:
Agranurocytosis, thrombocytopenic and nonthrombocytopenic purpura.
Nervous System:
Reversible mental depression progressing to catatonia; an acute reversible syndrome characterized by disorientation to time and place, short-term memory loss, emotional lability, slightly clouded sensorium, and decreased performance on neuropsychometric testing.
Respiratory System: Laryngospasm, respiratory distress.
Skin and Appendages: Erythematous rash, reversible alopecia.
Urogenital System: Peyronie's disease.
The oculomucocutaneous syndrome associated with the beta-adrenergic blocking agent practolol has not been reported with carteolol.

OVERDOSAGE

No specific information on emergency treatment of overdosage in humans is available. The most common effects expected with overdosage of a beta-adrenergic blocking agent are bradycardia, bronchospasm, congestive heart failure and hypotension.
In case of overdosage, treatment with CARTROL (carteolol hydrochloride) should be discontinued and gastric lavage considered. The patient should be closely observed and vital signs carefully monitored. The prolonged effects of carteolol must be considered when determining the duration of corrective therapy. On the basis of the pharmacologic profile, the following additional measures should be considered as appropriate.
Symptomatic Bradycardia:
Administer atropine. If there is no response to vagal blockade, administer isoproterenol cautiously.
Bronchospasm:
Administer a $beta_2$-stimulating agent such as isoproterenol and/or a theophylline derivative.
Congestive Heart Failure:
Administer diuretics and digitalis glycosides as necessary.
Hypotension:
Administer vasopressors such as intravenous dopamine, epinephrine or norepinephrine bitartrate.

DOSAGE AND ADMINISTRATION

Dosage must be individualized. The initial dose of CARTROL (carteolol hydrochloride) is 2.5 mg given as a single daily oral dose either alone or added to diuretic therapy. If an adequate response is not achieved, the dose can be gradually increased to 5 mg and 10 mg as single daily doses. Increasing the dose above 10 mg per day is unlikely to produce further substantial benefits and, in fact, may decrease the response. The usual maintenance dose of carteolol is 2.5 or 5 mg once daily.
Dosage Adjustment in Renal Impairment:
Carteolol is excreted principally by the kidneys. When administering CARTROL (carteolol hydrochloride) to patients with renal impairment, the dosage regimen should be adjusted individually by the physician. Guidelines for dose interval adjustment are shown below:

Creatinine Clearance (mL/min)	Dosage Interval (hours)
>60	24
20–60	48
<20	72

HOW SUPPLIED

CARTROL (carteolol hydrochloride) is supplied as:
2.5 mg gray tablets:
Bottles of 100 ....(**NDC** 0074-1664-13).
5 mg white tablets:
Bottles of 100 ....(**NDC** 0074-1665-13).
Recommended storage: Store under controlled room temperature, 59°–86°F (15°–30°C).
Ref. 01-2531-R3

CEFOL® Filmtab® Tablets ℞
[*c′full*]
(B-Complex, Folic Acid, Vitamin E with 750 mg Vitamin C)

DESCRIPTION

Each oral tablet provides:

Ascorbic Acid (C) (as sodium ascorbate)	750 mg
Niacinamide	100 mg
Calcium Pantothenate	20 mg
Thiamine Mononitrate (B_1)	15 mg
Riboflavin (B_2)	10 mg
Pyridoxine Hydrochloride (B_6)	5 mg
Folic Acid	500 mcg
Cyanocobalamin (B_{12})	6 mcg
Vitamin E (as dl-alpha tocopheryl acetate)	30 IU

Inactive Ingredients: Cellulosic polymers, colloidal silicon dioxide, corn starch, D&C Yellow No. 10, FD&C Blue No. 1, magnesium stearate, microcrystalline cellulose, polyethylene glycol, povidone, titanium dioxide, and vanillin.

CLINICAL PHARMACOLOGY

The vitamin components of Cefol are absorbed by the active transport process. All but Vitamin E are rapidly eliminated and not stored in the body. Vitamin E is stored in body tissues.

INDICATIONS AND USAGE

Indicated in non-pregnant* adults for treatment of Vitamin C deficiency states with associated deficient intake or increased need for Vitamin B-Complex, Folic Acid, and Vitamin E.

*Pregnancy may require greater Folic Acid intake.

CONTRAINDICATIONS

Rare hypersensitivity to Folic Acid.

WARNINGS

Folic Acid alone is improper treatment of pernicious anemia and other megaloblastic anemias where Vitamin B_{12} is deficient.

PRECAUTIONS

Folic Acid above 0.1 mg daily may obscure pernicious anemia (hematologic remission may occur while neurological manifestations remain progressive).

ADVERSE REACTIONS

Allergic sensitization has been reported following oral and parenteral administration of Folic Acid.

DOSAGE

Usual adult dose is one tablet daily.

HOW SUPPLIED

Green tablets in bottles of 100.
Filmtab—Film-sealed tablets, Abbott.
Store below 77°F (25°C).
Ref. 03-2062-3/R24

CYLERT® Ⓒ IV ℞
[*cī′ lert*]
(PEMOLINE)

DESCRIPTION

CYLERT (pemoline) is a central nervous system stimulant. Pemoline is structurally dissimilar to the amphetamines and methylphenidate.

It is an oxazolidine compound and is chemically identified as 2-amino-5-phenyl-2-oxazolin-4-one. Pemoline has the following structural formula:

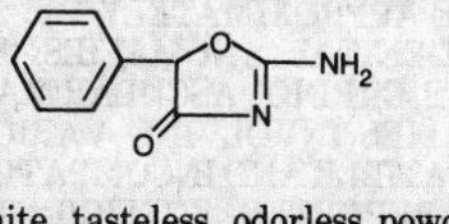

Pemoline is a white, tasteless, odorless powder, relatively insoluble (less than 1 mg/mL) in water, chloroform, ether, acetone, and benzene; its solubility in 95% ethyl alcohol is 2.2 mg/mL.

CYLERT (pemoline) is supplied as tablets containing 18.75 mg, 37.5 mg or 75 mg of pemoline for oral administration. CYLERT is also available as chewable tablets containing 37.5 mg of pemoline.

Inactive Ingredients

18.75 mg tablet: corn starch, gelatin, lactose, magnesium hydroxide, polyethylene glycol and talc.

37.5 mg tablet: corn starch, FD&C Yellow No. 6, gelatin, lactose, magnesium hydroxide, polyethylene glycol and talc.

37.5 mg chewable tablet: corn starch, FD&C Yellow No. 6, magnesium hydroxide, magnesium stearate, mannitol, polyethylene glycol, povidone, talc and artificial flavor.

75 mg tablet: corn starch, gelatin, iron oxide, lactose, magnesium hydroxide, polyethylene glycol and talc.

CLINICAL PHARMACOLOGY

CYLERT (pemoline) has a pharmacological activity similar to that of other known central nervous system stimulants; however, it has minimal sympathomimetic effects. Although studies indicate that pemoline may act in animals through dopaminergic mechanisms, the exact mechanism and site of action of the drug in man is not known.

There is neither specific evidence which clearly establishes the mechanism whereby CYLERT produces its mental and behavioral effects in children, nor conclusive evidence regarding how these effects relate to the condition of the central nervous system.

Pemoline is rapidly absorbed from the gastrointestinal tract. Approximately 50% is bound to plasma proteins. The serum half-life of pemoline is approximately 12 hours. Peak serum levels of the drug occur within 2 to 4 hours after ingestion of a single dose. Multiple dose studies in adults at several dose levels indicate that steady state is reached in approximately 2 to 3 days. In animals given radiolabeled pemoline, the drug was widely and uniformly distributed throughout the tissues, including the brain.

Pemoline is metabolized by the liver. Metabolites of pemoline include pemoline conjugate, pemoline dione, mandelic acid, and unidentified polar compounds. CYLERT is excreted primarily by the kidneys with approximately 50% excreted unchanged and only minor fractions present as metabolites.

CYLERT (pemoline) has a gradual onset of action. Using the recommended schedule of dosage titration, significant clinical benefit may not be evident until the third or fourth week of drug administration.

INDICATIONS AND USAGE

CYLERT (pemoline) is indicated in Attention Deficit Disorder (ADD) with hyperactivity as an integral part of a total treatment program which typically includes other remedial measures (psychological, educational, social) for a stabilizing effect in children with a behavioral syndrome characterized by the following group of developmentally inappropriate symptoms: moderate to severe distractibility, short attention span, hyperactivity, emotional lability, and impulsivity. The diagnosis of this syndrome should not be made with finality when these symptoms are only of comparatively recent origin. Nonlocalizing (soft) neurological signs, learning disability, and abnormal EEG may or may not be present, and a diagnosis of central nervous system dysfunction may or may not be warranted.

CONTRAINDICATIONS

CYLERT (pemoline) is contraindicated in patients with known hypersensitivity or idiosyncrasy to the drug. CYLERT should not be administered to patients with impaired hepatic function (see **ADVERSE REACTIONS**).

WARNINGS

Decrements in the predicted growth (i.e., weight gain and/or height) rate have been reported with the long-term use of stimulants in children. Therefore, patients requiring long-term therapy should be carefully monitored.

PRECAUTIONS

General:
Clinical experience suggests that in psychotic children, administration of CYLERT may exacerbate symptoms of behavior disturbance and thought disorder.

CYLERT should be administered with caution to patients with significantly impaired renal function.

Laboratory Tests:
Liver function tests should be performed prior to and periodically during therapy with CYLERT. The drug should be discontinued if abnormalities are revealed and confirmed by follow-up tests. (See **ADVERSE REACTIONS** regarding reports of abnormal liver function tests, hepatitis and jaundice.)

Drug Interactions:
The interaction of CYLERT (pemoline) with other drugs has not been studied in humans. Patients who are receiving CYLERT concurrently with other drugs, especially drugs with CNS activity, should be monitored carefully.

Decreased seizure threshold has been reported in patients receiving CYLERT concomitantly with *antiepileptic medications.*

Carcinogenesis:
Long-term studies have been conducted in rats with doses as high as 150 mg/kg/day for eighteen months. There was no significant difference in the incidence of any neoplasm between treated and control animals.

Mutagenesis:
Data are not available concerning long-term effects on mutagenicity in animals or humans.

Impairment of Fertility:
The results of studies in which rats were given 18.75 and 37.5 mg/kg/day indicated that pemoline did not affect fertility in males or females at those doses.

Pregnancy:
Teratogenic effects: Pregnancy Category B. Reproduction studies have been performed in rats and rabbits at doses of 18.75 and 37.5 mg/kg/day and have revealed no evidence of impaired fertility or harm to the fetus. There are, however, no adequate and well-controlled studies in pregnant women. Because animal reproduction studies are not always predictive of human response, this drug should be used during pregnancy only if clearly needed.

Nonteratogenic effects:
Studies in rats have shown an increased incidence of stillbirths and cannibalization when pemoline was administered at a dose of 37.5 mg/kg/day. Postnatal survival of offspring was reduced at doses of 18.75 and 37.5 mg/kg/day.

Nursing Mothers:
It is not known whether this drug is excreted in human milk. Because many drugs are excreted in human milk, caution should be exercised when CYLERT is administered to a nursing woman.

Pediatric Use:
Safety and effectiveness in children below the age of 6 years have not been established.

Long-term effects of CYLERT in children have not been established (see **WARNINGS**).

CNS stimulants, including pemoline, have been reported to precipitate motor and phonic tics and Tourette's syndrome. Therefore, clinical evaluation for tics and Tourette's syndrome in children and their families should precede use of stimulant medications.

Drug treatment is not indicated in all cases of ADD with hyperactivity and should be considered only in light of complete history and evaluation of the child. The decision to prescribe CYLERT (pemoline) should depend on the physician's assessment of the chronicity and severity of the child's symptoms and their appropriateness for his/her age. Prescription should not depend solely on the presence of one or more of the behavioral characteristics.

ADVERSE REACTIONS

The following are adverse reactions in decreasing order of severity within each category associated with CYLERT:

Hepatic: There have been reports of hepatic dysfunction including elevated liver enzymes, hepatitis and jaundice in patients taking CYLERT. The occurrence of elevated liver enzymes is not rare and these reactions appear to be reversible upon drug discontinuance. Most patients with elevated liver enzymes were asymptomatic. Although no causal relationship has been established, there have been rare reports of hepatic-related fatalities involving patients taking CYLERT.

Hematopoietic: There have been isolated reports of aplastic anemia.

Central Nervous System: The following CNS effects have been reported with the use of CYLERT: convulsive seizures; literature reports indicate that CYLERT may precipitate attacks of Gilles de la Tourette syndrome; hallucinations; dyskinetic movements of the tongue, lips, face and extremities; abnormal oculomotor function including nystagmus and oculogyric crisis; mild depression; dizziness; increased irritability; headache; and drowsiness.

Insomnia is the most frequently reported side effect of CYLERT; it usually occurs early in therapy prior to an optimum therapeutic response. In the majority of cases it is transient in nature or responds to a reduction in dosage.

Gastrointestinal: Anorexia and weight loss may occur during the first weeks of therapy. In the majority of cases it is transient in nature; weight gain usually resumes within three to six months.

Nausea and stomach ache have also been reported.

Genitourinary: A case of elevated acid phosphatase in association with prostatic enlargement has been reported in a 63 year old male who was treated with CYLERT for sleepiness. The acid phosphatase normalized with discontinuation of CYLERT and was again elevated with rechallenge.

Miscellaneous: Suppression of growth has been reported with the long-term use of stimulants in children. (See **WARNINGS.**) Skin rash has been reported with CYLERT.

Mild adverse reactions appearing early during the course of treatment with CYLERT often remit with continuing therapy. If adverse reactions are of a significant or protracted nature, dosage should be reduced or the drug discontinued.

DRUG ABUSE AND DEPENDENCE

Controlled Substance: CYLERT is subject to control under DEA schedule IV.

Abuse: CYLERT failed to demonstrate a potential for self-administration in primates. However, the pharmacologic similarity of pemoline to other psychostimulants with known dependence liability suggests that psychological and/or physical dependence might also occur with CYLERT. There have been isolated reports of transient psychotic symptoms occurring in adults following the long-term misuse of excessive oral doses of pemoline. CYLERT should be given with caution to emotionally unstable patients who may increase the dosage on their own initiative.

OVERDOSAGE

Signs and symptoms of acute overdosage, resulting principally from overstimulation of the central nervous system

Continued on next page

Abbott Laboratories—Cont.

and from excessive sympathomimetic effects, may include the following: vomiting, agitation, tremors, hyperreflexia, muscle twitching, convulsions (may be followed by coma), euphoria, confusion, hallucinations, delirium, sweating, flushing, headache, hyperpyrexia, tachycardia, hypertension and mydriasis. Consult with a Certified Poison Control Center regarding treatment for up to date guidance and advice. Treatment consists of appropriate supportive measures. The patient must be protected against self-injury and against external stimuli that would aggravate overstimulation already present. Gastric contents may be evacuated by gastric lavage. Other measures to detoxify the gut include administration of activated charcoal and a cathartic. Chlorpromazine has been reported in the literature to be useful in decreasing CNS stimulation and sympathomimetic effects. Efficacy of peritoneal dialysis or extracorporeal hemodialysis for CYLERT overdosage has not been established.

DOSAGE AND ADMINISTRATION

CYLERT (pemoline) is administered as a single oral dose each morning. The recommended starting dose is 37.5 mg/day. This daily dose should be gradually increased by 18.75 mg at one week intervals until the desired clinical response is obtained. The effective daily dose for most patients will range from 56.25 to 75 mg. The maximum recommended daily dose of pemoline is 112.5 mg.

Clinical improvement with CYLERT is gradual. Using the recommended schedule of dosage titration, significant benefit may not be evident until the third or fourth week of drug administration.

Where possible, drug administration should be interrupted occasionally to determine if there is a recurrence of behavioral symptoms sufficient to require continued therapy.

HOW SUPPLIED

CYLERT (pemoline) is supplied as monogrammed, grooved tablets in three dosage strengths:
18.75 mg tablets (white) in bottles of 100
(**NDC** 0074-6025-13);
37.5 mg tablets (orange-colored) in bottles of 100
(**NDC** 0074-6057-13);
75 mg tablets (tan-colored) in bottles of 100
(**NDC** 0074-6073-13).
CYLERT (pemoline) Chewable is supplied as 37.5 mg monogrammed, grooved tablets (orange-colored) in bottles of 100 (**NDC** 0074-6088-13).
Recommended Storage: Store below 86°F (30°C).
Ref. 03-4633-R17-Rev. December, 1995
Abbott Laboratories
North Chicago, IL 60064, U.S.A.

Shown in Product Identification Guide, page 303

DEPAKENE® Capsules and Syrup ℞
[*dep 'a-kāne*]
(Valproic Acid)

> **WARNING:**
> HEPATIC FAILURE RESULTING IN FATALITIES HAS OCCURRED IN PATIENTS RECEIVING VALPROIC ACID. EXPERIENCE HAS INDICATED THAT CHILDREN UNDER THE AGE OF TWO YEARS ARE AT A CONSIDERABLY INCREASED RISK OF DEVELOPING FATAL HEPATOTOXICITY. ESPECIALLY THOSE ON MULTIPLE ANTICONVULSANTS, THOSE WITH CONGENITAL METABOLIC DISORDERS, THOSE WITH SEVERE SEIZURE DISORDERS ACCOMPANIED BY MENTAL RETARDATION, AND THOSE WITH ORGANIC BRAIN DISEASE. WHEN DEPAKENE PRODUCTS ARE USED IN THIS PATIENT GROUP, IT SHOULD BE USED WITH EXTREME CAUTION AND AS A SOLE AGENT. THE BENEFITS OF SEIZURE CONTROL SHOULD BE WEIGHED AGAINST THE RISKS. ABOVE THIS AGE GROUP, EXPERIENCE HAS INDICATED THAT THE INCIDENCE OF FATAL HEPATOTOXICITY DECREASES CONSIDERABLY IN PROGRESSIVELY OLDER PATIENT GROUPS.
> THESE INCIDENTS USUALLY HAVE OCCURRED DURING THE FIRST SIX MONTHS OF TREATMENT. SERIOUS OR FATAL HEPATOTOXICITY MAY BE PRECEDED BY NON-SPECIFIC SYMPTOMS SUCH AS LOSS OF SEIZURE CONTROL, MALAISE, WEAKNESS, LETHARGY, FACIAL EDEMA, ANOREXIA, AND VOMITING. PATIENTS SHOULD BE MONITORED CLOSELY FOR APPEARANCE OF THESE SYMPTOMS. LIVER FUNCTION TESTS SHOULD BE PERFORMED PRIOR TO THERAPY AND AT FREQUENT INTERVALS THEREAFTER, ESPECIALLY DURING THE FIRST SIX MONTHS.

DESCRIPTION

DEPAKENE (valproic acid) is a carboxylic acid designated as 2-propylpentanoic acid. It is also known as dipropylacetic acid. Valproic acid has the following structure:

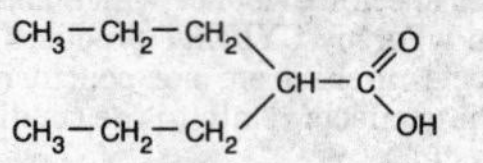

CH3—CH2—CH2
CH—C
O
CH3—CH2—CH2
OH

Valproic acid (pKa 4.8) has a molecular weight of 144 and occurs as a colorless liquid with a characteristic odor. It is slightly soluble in water (1.3 mg/mL) and very soluble in organic solvents.

DEPAKENE capsules and syrup are antiepileptics for oral administration. Each soft elastic capsule contains 250 mg valproic acid. The syrup contains the equivalent of 250 mg valproic acid per 5 mL as the sodium salt.

Inactive Ingredients

250 mg capsules: corn oil, FD&C Yellow No. 6, gelatin, glycerin, iron oxide, methylparaben, propylparaben, and titanium dioxide.

Syrup: FD&C Red No. 40, glycerin, methylparaben, propylparaben, sorbitol, sucrose, water, and natural and artificial flavors.

CLINICAL PHARMACOLOGY

Valproic acid is an antiepileptic agent which dissociates to the valproate ion in the gastrointestinal tract. The mechanism by which valproate exerts its antiepileptic effects has not been established. It has been suggested that its activity is related to increased brain levels of gamma-aminobutyric acid (GABA).

Valproic acid is rapidly absorbed after oral administration. Peak plasma concentrations of valproate ion are observed 1 to 4 hours after a single oral dose of valproic acid. A slight delay in absorption occurs when the drug is administered with meals, but this does not affect the total absorption.

Accordingly, administration of oral valproate products with food and substitution among the various DEPAKENE (valproic acid) and DEPAKOTE® (divalproex sodium) products should be without consequence. Nonetheless, any changes in dosage administration, or the addition or discontinuance of concomitant drugs should ordinarily be accompanied by close monitoring of clinical status and valproate plasma concentrations.

The plasma half-life of valproate is typically in the range of 6 to 16 hours. Half-lives in the lower part of the range are usually found in patients taking other antiepileptic drugs capable of enzyme induction.

Valproate is primarily metabolized in the liver. The major metabolic routes are glucuronidation, mitochrondrial beta oxidation, and microsomol oxidation. The major metabolites formed are the glucuronide conjugate, 2-propyl-3-keto-pentanoic acid, and 2-propyl-hydroxypentanoic acids. Other unsaturated metabolites have been reported. The major route of elimination of these metabolites is in the urine.

Patients on monotherapy will generally have longer half-lives and higher concentrations of valproate at a given dosage than patients receiving polytherapy. This is primarily due to enzyme induction caused by other antiepileptics, which results in enhanced clearance of valproate by glucuronidation and microsomal oxidation. Because of these changes in valproate clearance, monitoring of antiepileptic concentrations should be intensified whenever concomitant antiepileptics are introduced or withdrawn.

The therapeutic range is commonly considered to be 50 to 100 μg/mL of total valproate, although some patients may be controlled with lower or higher plasma concentrations.[4]

Valproate is highly bound (90%) to plasma proteins in the therapeutic range; however, protein binding is concentration-dependent and decreases at high valproate concentrations. The binding is variable among patients and may be affected by fatty acids or by highly bound drugs such as salicylate. Some clinicians favor monitoring free valproate concentrations, which may more accurately reflect CNS penetration of valproate. As yet, a consensus on the therapeutic range of free concentrations has not been established; however, monitoring total and free valproate may be informative when there are changes in clinical status, concomitant medication, or valproate dosage.

INDICATIONS AND USAGE

DEPAKENE (valproic acid) is indicated for use as sole and adjunctive therapy in the treatment of simple and complex absence seizures, and adjunctively in patients with multiple seizure types which include absence seizures.

Simple absence is defined as very brief clouding of the sensorium or loss of consciousness accompanied by certain generalized epileptic discharges without other detectable clinical signs. Complex absence is the term used when other signs are also present.

SEE WARNINGS FOR STATEMENT REGARDING FATAL HEPATIC DYSFUNCTION.

CONTRAINDICATIONS

VALPROIC ACID SHOULD NOT BE ADMINISTERED TO PATIENTS WITH HEPATIC DISEASE OR SIGNIFICANT DYSFUNCTION.

Valproic acid is contraindicated in patients with known hypersensitivity to the drug.

WARNINGS

Hepatic failure resulting in fatalities has occurred in patients receiving valproic acid. These incidents usually have occurred during the first six months of treatment. Serious or fatal hepatotoxicity may be preceded by nonspecific symptoms such as loss of seizure control, malaise, weakness, lethargy, facial edema, anorexia, and vomiting. Patients should be monitored closely for appearance of these symptoms. Liver function tests should be performed prior to therapy and at frequent intervals thereafter, especially during the first six months. However, physicians should not rely totally on serum biochemistry since these tests may not be abnormal in all instances, but should also consider the results of careful interim medical history and physical examination. Caution should be observed when administering DEPAKENE (valproic acid) to patients with a prior history of hepatic disease. Patients on multiple anticonvulsants, children, those with congenital metabolic disorders, those with severe seizure disorders accompanied by mental retardation, and those with organic brain disease may be at particular risk. Experience has indicated that children under the age of two years are at considerably increased risk of developing fatal hepatotoxicity, especially those with the aforementioned conditions. When DEPAKENE products are used in this patient group, it should be used with extreme caution and as a sole agent. The benefits of seizure control should be weighed against the risks. Above this age group, experience has indicated that the incidence of fatal hepatotoxicity decreases considerably in progressively older patient groups.

The drug should be discontinued immediately in the presence of significant hepatic dysfunction, suspected or apparent. In some cases, hepatic dysfunction has progressed in spite of discontinuation of drug.

The frequency of adverse effects (particularly elevated liver enzymes) may be dose-related. The benefit of improved seizure control which may accompany the higher doses should be weighed against the possibility of a greater incidence of adverse effects.

Usage in Pregnancy: ACCORDING TO PUBLISHED AND UNPUBLISHED REPORTS, VALPROIC ACID MAY PRODUCE TERATOGENIC EFFECTS IN THE OFFSPRING OF HUMAN FEMALES RECEIVING THE DRUG DURING PREGNANCY.

THERE ARE MULTIPLE REPORTS IN THE CLINICAL LITERATURE WHICH INDICATE THAT THE USE OF ANTIEPILEPTIC DRUGS DURING PREGNANCY RESULTS IN AN INCREASED INCIDENCE OF BIRTH DEFECTS IN THE OFFSPRING. ALTHOUGH DATA ARE MORE EXTENSIVE WITH RESPECT TO TRIMETHADIONE, PARAMETHADIONE, PHENYTOIN, AND PHENOBARBITAL, REPORTS INDICATE A POSSIBLE SIMILAR ASSOCIATION WITH THE USE OF OTHER ANTIEPILEPTIC DRUGS. THEREFORE, ANTIEPILEPTIC DRUGS SHOULD BE ADMINISTERED TO WOMEN OF CHILDBEARING POTENTIAL ONLY IF THEY ARE CLEARLY SHOWN TO BE ESSENTIAL IN THE MANAGEMENT OF THEIR SEIZURES.

THE INCIDENCE OF NEURAL TUBE DEFECTS IN THE FETUS MAY BE INCREASED IN MOTHERS RECEIVING VALPROATE DURING THE FIRST TRIMESTER OF PREGNANCY. THE CENTERS FOR DISEASE CONTROL (CDC) HAS ESTIMATED THE RISK OF VALPROIC ACID EXPOSED WOMEN HAVING CHILDREN WITH SPINA BIFIDA TO BE APPROXIMATELY 1 to 2%.[1]

OTHER CONGENITAL ANOMALIES (EG, CRANIOFACIAL DEFECTS, CARDIOVASCULAR MALFORMATIONS AND ANOMALIES INVOLVING VARIOUS BODY SYSTEMS), COMPATIBLE AND INCOMPATIBLE WITH LIFE, HAVE BEEN REPORTED. SUFFICIENT DATA TO DETERMINE THE INCIDENCE OF THESE CONGENITAL ANOMALIES IS NOT AVAILABLE.

THE HIGHER INCIDENCE OF CONGENITAL ANOMALIES IN ANTIEPILEPTIC DRUG-TREATED WOMEN WITH SEIZURE DISORDERS CANNOT BE REGARDED AS A CAUSE AND EFFECT RELATIONSHIP. THERE ARE INTRINISIC METHODOLOGIC PROBLEMS IN OBTAINING ADEQUATE DATA ON DRUG TERATOGENICITY IN HUMANS; GENETIC FACTORS OR THE EPILEPTIC CONDITION ITSELF, MAY BE MORE IMPORTANT THAN DRUG THERAPY IN CONTRIBUTING TO CONGENITAL ANOMALIES.

PATIENTS TAKING VALPROATE MAY DEVELOP CLOTTING ABNORMALITIES. A PATIENT WHO HAD LOW FIBROGEN WHEN TAKING MULTIPLE ANTICONVULSANTS INCLUDING VALPROATE GAVE BIRTH TO AN INFANT WITH AFIBRINOGENEMIA WHO SUBSE-

QUENTLY DIED OF HEMORRHAGE. IF VALPROATE IS USED IN PREGNANCY, THE CLOTTING PARAMETERS SHOULD BE MONITORED CAREFULLY.

HEPATIC FAILURE, RESULTING IN THE DEATH OF A NEWBORN AND OF AN INFANT, HAVE BEEN REPORTED FOLLOWING THE USE OF VALPROATE DURING PREGNANCY.

ANIMAL STUDIES ALSO HAVE DEMONSTRATED VALPROATE INDUCED TERATOGENICITY. Studies in rats and human females demonstrated placental transfer of the drug. Doses greater than 65 mg/kg/day given to pregnant rats and mice produced skeletal abnormalities in the offspring, primarily involving ribs and vertebrae; doses greater than 150 mg/kg/day given to pregnant rabbits produced fetal resorptions and (primarily) soft-tissue abnormalities in the offspring. In rats a dose-related delay in the onset of parturition was noted. Postnatal growth and survival of the progeny were adversely affected, particularly when drug administration spanned the entire gestation and early lactation period.

Antiepileptic drugs should not be discontinued in patients in whom the drug is administered to prevent major seizures because of the strong possibility of precipitating status epilepticus with attendant hypoxia and threat to life. In individual cases where the severity and frequency of the seizure disorder are such that the removal of medication does not pose a serious threat to the patient, discontinuation of the drug may be considered prior to and during pregnancy, although it cannot be said with any confidence that even minor seizures do not pose some hazard to the developing embryo or fetus.

The prescribing physician will wish to weigh these considerations in treating or counseling epileptic women of childbearing potential.

Tests to detect neural tube and other defects using current accepted procedures should be considered a part of routine prenatal care in childbearing women receiving valproate.

PRECAUTIONS

Hepatic Dysfunction: See BOXED WARNING, CONTRAINDICATIONS, AND WARNINGS.

General: Because of reports of thrombocytopenia, inhibition of the secondary phase of platelet aggregation, and abnormal coagulation parameters (eg, low fibrinogen), platelet counts and coagulation tests are recommended before initiating therapy and at periodic intervals. It is recommended that patients receiving DEPAKENE (valproic acid) be monitored for platelet count and coagulation parameters prior to planned surgery. Evidence of hemorrhage, bruising, or a disorder of hemostasis/coagulation is an indication for reduction of the dosage or withdrawal of therapy.

Hyperammonemia with or without lethargy or coma has been reported and may be present in the absence of abnormal liver function tests. Asymptomatic elevations of ammonia are more common and when present require more frequent monitoring. If clinically significant symptoms occur, DEPAKENE therapy should be modified or discontinued.

Since valproate may interact with concurrently administered antiepileptic drugs, periodic plasma concentration determinations of concomitant antiepileptic drugs are recommended during the early course of therapy (see PRECAUTIONS—*Drug Interactions*).

Valproate is partially eliminated in the urine as a keto-metabolite which may lead to a false interpretation of the urine ketone test.

There have been reports of altered thyroid function tests associated with valproate. The clinical significance of these is unknown.

Information for Patients: Since DEPAKENE products may produce CNS depression, especially when combined with another CNS depressant (eg, alcohol), patients should be advised not to engage in hazardous activities, such as driving an automobile or operating dangerous machinery, until it is known that they do not become drowsy from the drug.

Drug Interactions: Valproate may potentiate the action of CNS depressants (ie, alcohol, benzodiazepines, etc).

The concomitant administration of valproate with drugs that exhibit extensive protein binding (eg, aspirin, carbamazepine, dicumarol, and phenytoin) may result in alteration of serum drug concentrations.

There is evidence that valproate can cause an increase in serum phenobarbital concentrations by impairment of nonrenal clearance. This phenomenon can result in severe CNS depression. The combination of valproate and phenobarbital has also been reported to produce CNS depression without significant elevations of barbiturate or valproate serum concentrations. All patients receiving concomitant barbiturate therapy should be closely monitored for neurological toxicity. Serum barbiturate concentrations should be obtained, if possible, and the barbiturate dosage decreased, if appropriate.

Primidone is metabolized into a barbiturate and, therefore, may also be involved in a similar or identical interaction.

There have been reports of breakthrough seizures occurring with the combination of valproate and phenytoin. Most reports have noted a decrease in total plasma phenytoin concentration. However, increases in total phenytoin serum concentration have been reported. An initial fall with subsequent increase in total phenytoin concentrations has also been reported. In addition, a decrease in total serum phenytoin with an increase in the free vs. protein bound phenytoin concentrations has been reported. The dosage of phenytoin should be adjusted as required by the clinical situation.

The concomitant use of valproic acid and clonazepam may induce absence status in patients with a history of absence type seizures.

There is inconclusive evidence regarding the effects of valproate on serum ethosuximide concentrations. Patients receiving valproate and ethosuximide, especially along with other anticonvulsants, should be monitored for alterations in serum concentrations of both drugs.

Caution is recommended when valproate is used with drugs affecting coagulation (eg, aspirin, warfarin). See ADVERSE REACTIONS.

Evidence suggests that there is an association between the use of certain antiepileptics and failure of oral contraceptives. One explanation for this interaction is that enzyme-inducing antiepileptics effectively lower plasma concentrations of the relevant steroid hormones, resulting in unimpaired ovulation. However, other mechanisms, not related to enzyme induction may contribute to the failure of oral contraceptives. While valproate is not a significant enzyme inducer, and, therefore, would not be expected to decrease concentrations of steroid hormones, clinical data about the interaction of valproate with oral contraceptives is minimal.[2]

Carcinogenesis: Valproic acid was administered to Sprague Dawley rats and ICR (HA/ICR) mice at doses of 0, 80 and 170 mg/kg/day for two years. A variety of neoplasms were observed in both species. The chief findings were a statistically significant increase in the incidence of subcutaneous fibrosarcomas in high dose male rats receiving valproic acid and a statistically significant dose-related trend for benign pulmonary adenomas in male mice receiving valproic acid. The significance of these findings for man is unknown.

Mutagenesis: Studies of valproate have been performed using bacterial and mammalian systems. These studies have provided no evidence of a mutagenic potential for valproate.

Fertility: Chronic toxicity studies in juvenile and adult rats and dogs demonstrated reduced spermatogenesis and testicular atrophy at doses greater than 200 mg/kg/day in rats and greater than 90 mg/kg/day in dogs. Segment I fertility studies in rats have shown doses up to 350 mg/kg/day for 60 days to have no effect on fertility. THE EFFECT OF VALPROATE ON TESTICULAR DEVELOPMENT AND ON SPERM PRODUCTION AND FERTILITY IN HUMANS IS UNKNOWN.

Pregnancy: Pregnancy Category D: See WARNINGS.

Nursing Mothers: Valproate is excreted in breast milk. Concentrations in breast milk have been reported to be 1 to 10% of serum concentrations. It is not known what effect this would have on a nursing infant. Caution should be exercised when valproic acid is administered to a nursing woman.

ADVERSE REACTIONS

Since DEPAKENE (valproic acid) has usually been used with other antiepileptic drugs, it is not possible, in most cases, to determine whether the following adverse reactions can be ascribed to valproic acid alone, or the combination of drugs.

Gastrointestinal: The most commonly reported side effects at the initiation of therapy are nausea, vomiting, and indigestion. These effects are usually transient and rarely require discontinuation of therapy. Diarrhea, abdominal cramps, and constipation have been reported. Both anorexia with some weight loss and increased appetite with weight gain have also been reported. Some patients experiencing gastrointestinal side effects may benefit by converting therapy from DEPAKENE (valproic acid) to Depakote® (divalproex sodium).[3]

CNS Effects: Sedative effects have occurred in patients receiving valproate alone but occur most often in patients receiving combination therapy. Sedation usually abates upon reduction of other antiepileptic medication. Tremor (may be dose-related), hallucinations, ataxia, headache, nystagmus, diplopia, asterixis, "spots before eyes", dysarthria, dizziness, and incoordination. Rare cases of coma have been noted in patients receiving valproic acid alone or in conjunction with phenobarbital. In rare instances encephalopathy with fever has developed shortly after the introduction of valproate monotherapy without evidence of hepatic dysfunction or inappropriate plasma levels; all patients recovered after the drug was withdrawn.

Dermatologic: Transient hair loss, skin rash, photosensitivity, generalized pruritus, erythema multiforme, and Stevens-Johnson syndrome. A case of fatal epidermal necrolysis has been reported in a 6 month old infant taking valproate and several other concomitant medications.

Psychiatric: Emotional upset, depression, psychosis, aggression, hyperactivity and behavioral deterioration.

Musculoskeletal: Weakness.

Hematologic: Thrombocytopenia and inhibition of the secondary phase of platelet aggregation may be reflected in altered bleeding time, petechiae, bruising, hematoma formation and frank hemorrhage (see PRECAUTIONS—*General and Drug Interactions*). Relative lymphocytosis, macrocytosis, hypofibrinogenemia, leukopenia, eosinophilia, anemia including macrocytic with or without folate deficiency, bone marrow suppression, and acute intermittent porphyria.

Hepatic: Minor elevations of transaminases (eg, SGOT and SGPT) and LDH are frequent and appear to be dose-related. Occasionally, laboratory test results include increases in serum bilirubin and abnormal changes in other liver function tests. These results may reflect potentially serious hepatotoxicity. (See WARNINGS).

Endocrine: Irregular menses, secondary amenorrhea, breast enlargement, galactorrhea, and parotid gland swelling. Abnormal thyroid function tests (see PRECAUTIONS).

Pancreatic: Acute pancreatitis, including fatalities.

Metabolic: Hyperammonemia (see PRECAUTIONS), hyponatremia, and inappropriate ADH secretion.

There have been rare reports of Fanconi's Syndrome occurring chiefly in children.

Decreased carnitine concentrations have been reported although the clinical relevance is undetermined.

Hyperglycinemia has occurred and was associated with a fatal outcome in a patient with preexistent nonketotic hyperglycinemia.

Genitourinary: Enuresis.

Special Senses: Hearing loss, either reversible or irreversible, has been reported; however, a cause and effect relationship has not been established.

Other: Edema of the extremities, lupus erythematosus, and fever.

OVERDOSAGE

Overdosage with valproate may result in somnolence, heart block, and deep coma. Fatalities have been reported.

Since valproic acid is absorbed very rapidly, the benefit of gastric lavage or emesis will vary with the time since ingestion. General supportive measures should be applied with particular attention to the maintenance of adequate urinary output.

Naloxone has been reported to reverse the CNS depressant effects of valproate overdosage. Because naloxone could theoretically also reverse the antiepileptic effects of valproate, it should be used with caution.

DOSAGE AND ADMINISTRATION

DEPAKENE (valproic acid) is administered orally. The recommended initial dose is 15 mg/kg/day, increasing at one week intervals by 5 to 10 mg/kg/day, until seizures are controlled or side effects preclude further increases. The maximum recommended dosage is 60 mg/kg/day. If the total daily dose exceeds 250 mg, it should be given in a divided regimen.

The following table is a guide for the initial daily dose of DEPAKENE (valproic acid) (15 mg/kg/day):
[See table above.]

Weight (kg)	Weight (lb)	Total Daily Dose (mg)	Number of Capsules or Teaspoonfuls of Syrup: Dose 1	Dose 2	Dose 3
10—24.9	22— 54.9	250	0	0	1
25—39.9	55— 87.9	500	1	0	1
40—59.9	88— 131.9	750	1	1	1
60—74.9	132— 164.9	1,000	1	1	2
75—89.9	165— 197.9	1,250	2	1	2

The frequency of adverse effects (particularly elevated liver enzymes) may be dose-related. The benefit of improved seizure control with higher doses should be weighed against the possibility of a greater incidence of adverse reactions.

A good correlation has not been established between daily dose, serum concentration and therapeutic effect. However, therapeutic valproate serum concentrations for most patients will range from 50 to 100 μg/mL. Some patients may be controlled with lower or higher serum concentrations (see CLINICAL PHARMACOLOGY).

As the DEPAKENE dosage is titrated upward, blood concentrations of phenobarbital and/or phenytoin may be affected. (See PRECAUTIONS).

Patients who experience G.I. irritation may benefit from administration of the drug with food or by slowly building up the dose from an initial low level.

Continued on next page

Abbott Laboratories—Cont.

THE CAPSULES SHOULD BE SWALLOWED WITHOUT CHEWING TO AVOID LOCAL IRRITATION OF THE MOUTH AND THROAT.

HOW SUPPLIED

DEPAKENE (valproic acid) is available as orange-colored soft gelatin capsules of 250 mg valproic acid bearing the trademark DEPAKENE for product identification, in bottles of 100 capsules (**NDC** 0074-5681-13), and as a red syrup containing the equivalent of 250 mg valproic acid per 5 mL as the sodium salt in bottles of 16 ounces (**NDC** 0074-5682-16). Store capsules at 59–77°F (15–25°C). Store syrup below 86°F (30°C).

REFERENCES

1. Centers for Disease Control, valproate: a new cause of birth defects—report from Italy and follow-up from France, *Morbidity and Mortality Weekly Report.* 1983;32(33):438–439.
2. Mattson, RH, et al. Use of oral contraceptives by women with epilepsy. *JAMA.* 1986;256(2):238–240.
3. Wilder, BJ, et al. Gastrointestinal tolerance of divalproex sodium. *Neurology.* 1983;33:808–811.
4. Hurst DL. Expanded therapeutic range of valproate. *Pediatr Neurol.* 1987;3:342–344.

Caution—Federal (USA) Law prohibits dispensing without prescription.

Ref. 03-4581-R24

Shown in Product Identification Guide, page 303

DEPAKOTE® Tablets ℞
DIVALPROEX SODIUM
DELAYED-RELEASE TABLETS

BOX WARNING:

HEPATIC FAILURE RESULTING IN FATALITIES HAS OCCURRED IN PATIENTS RECEIVING VALPROIC ACID AND ITS DERIVATIVES. EXPERIENCE HAS INDICATED THAT CHILDREN UNDER THE AGE OF TWO YEARS ARE AT A CONSIDERABLY INCREASED RISK OF DEVELOPING FATAL HEPATOTOXICITY, ESPECIALLY THOSE ON MULTIPLE ANTICONVULSANTS, THOSE WITH CONGENITAL METABOLIC DISORDERS, THOSE WITH SEVERE SEIZURE DISORDERS ACCOMPANIED BY MENTAL RETARDATION, AND THOSE WITH ORGANIC BRAIN DISEASE. WHEN DEPAKOTE IS USED IN THIS PATIENT GROUP, IT SHOULD BE USED WITH EXTREME CAUTION AND AS A SOLE AGENT. THE BENEFITS OF THERAPY SHOULD BE WEIGHED AGAINST THE RISKS. ABOVE THIS AGE GROUP, EXPERIENCE IN EPILEPSY HAS INDICATED THAT THE INCIDENCE OF FATAL HEPATOTOXICITY DECREASES CONSIDERABLY IN PROGRESSIVELY OLDER PATIENT GROUPS.

THESE INCIDENTS USUALLY HAVE OCCURRED DURING THE FIRST SIX MONTHS OF TREATMENT. SERIOUS OR FATAL HEPATOTOXICITY MAY BE PRECEDED BY NON-SPECIFIC SYMPTOMS SUCH AS MALAISE, WEAKNESS, LETHARGY, FACIAL EDEMA, ANOREXIA, AND VOMITING. IN PATIENTS WITH EPILEPSY, A LOSS OF SEIZURE CONTROL MAY ALSO OCCUR. PATIENTS SHOULD BE MONITORED CLOSELY FOR APPEARANCE OF THESE SYMPTOMS. LIVER FUNCTION TESTS SHOULD BE PERFORMED PRIOR TO THERAPY AND AT FREQUENT INTERVALS THEREAFTER, ESPECIALLY DURING THE FIRST SIX MONTHS.

TERATOGENICITY:

VALPROATE CAN PRODUCE TERATOGENIC EFFECTS SUCH AS NEURAL TUBE DEFECTS (E.G., SPINA BIFIDA), ACCORDINGLY, THE USE OF DEPAKOTE TABLETS IN WOMEN OF CHILDBEARING POTENTIAL REQUIRES THAT THE BENEFITS OF ITS USE BE WEIGHED AGAINST THE RISK OF INJURY TO THE FETUS. THIS IS ESPECIALLY IMPORTANT WHEN THE TREATMENT OF A SPONTANEOUSLY REVERSIBLE CONDITION NOT ORDINARILY ASSOCIATED WITH PERMANENT INJURY OR RISK OF DEATH (E.G., MIGRAINE) IS CONTEMPLATED. SEE WARNINGS, INFORMATION FOR PATIENTS.

AN INFORMATION SHEET DESCRIBING THE TERATOGENIC POTENTIAL OF VALPROATE IS AVAILABLE FOR PATIENTS.

DESCRIPTION

Divalproex sodium is a stable co-ordination compound comprised of sodium valproate and valproic acid in a 1:1 molar relationship and formed during the partial neutralization of valproic acid with 0.5 equivalent of sodium hydroxide. Chemically it is designated as sodium hydrogen bis(2-propylpentanoate). Divalproex sodium has the following structure:

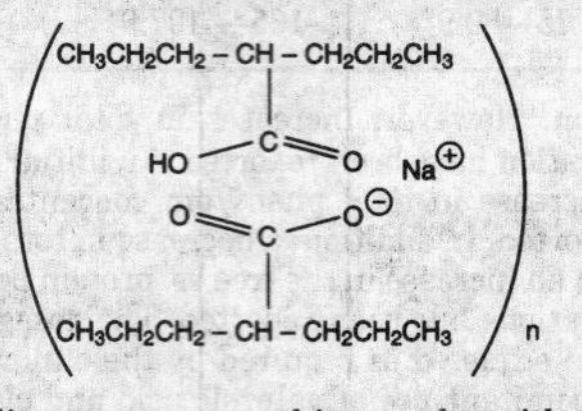

Divalproex sodium occurs as a white powder with a characteristic odor.

DEPAKOTE tablets are for oral administration. DEPAKOTE tablets are supplied in three dosage strengths containing divalproex sodium equivalent to 125 mg, 250 mg, or 500 mg of valproic acid.

Inactive Ingredients

DEPAKOTE tablets: cellulosic polymers, diacetylated monoglycerides, povidone, pregelatinized starch (contains corn starch), silica gel, talc, titanium dioxide, and vanillin.

In addition, individual tablets contain:
125 mg tablets: FD&C Blue No. 1 and FD&C Red No. 40.
250 mg tablets: FD&C Yellow No. 6 and iron oxide.
500 mg tablets: D&C Red No. 30, FD&C Blue No. 2, and iron oxide.

CLINICAL PHARMACOLOGY

Pharmacodynamics

Divalproex sodium dissociates to the valproate ion in the gastrointestinal tract. The mechanisms by which valproate exerts its therapeutic effects have not been established. It has been suggested that its activity in epilepsy is related to increased brain concentrations of gamma-aminobutyric acid (GABA).

Pharmacokinetics

Absorption/Bioavailability

Equivalent oral doses of DEPAKOTE (divalproex sodium) products and DEPAKENE (valproic acid) capsules deliver equivalent quantities of valproate ion systemically. Although the rate of valproate ion absorption may vary with the formulation administered (liquid, solid, or sprinkle), conditions of use (e.g., fasting or postprandial) and the method of administration (e.g., whether the contents of the capsule are sprinkled on food or the capsule is taken intact), these differences should be of minor clinical importance under the steady state conditions achieved in chronic use in the treatment of epilepsy.

However, it is possible that differences among the various valproate products in T_{max} and C_{max} could be important upon initiation of treatment. For example, in single dose studies, the effect of feeding had a greater influence on the rate of absorption of the tablet (increase in T_{max} from 4 to 8 hours) than on the absorption of the sprinkle capsules (increase in T_{max} from 3.3 to 4.8 hours).

While the absorption rate from the G.I. tract and fluctuation in valproate plasma concentrations vary with dosing regimen and formulation, the efficacy of valproate as an anticonvulsant in chronic use is unlikely to be affected. Experience employing dosing regimens from once-a-day to four-times-a-day, as well as studies in primate epilepsy models involving constant rate infusion, indicate that total daily systemic bioavailability (extent of absorption) is the primary determinant of seizure control and that differences in the ratios of plasma peak to trough concentrations between valproate formulations are inconsequential from a practical clinical standpoint. Whether or not rate of absorption influences the efficacy of valproate as an antimanic or antimigraine agent is unknown.

Co-administration of oral valproate products with food and substitution among the various DEPAKOTE and DEPAKENE formulations should cause no clinical problems in the management of patients with epilepsy (see **DOSAGE AND ADMINISTRATION**). Nonetheless, any changes in dosage administration, or the addition or discontinuance of concomitant drugs should ordinarily be accompanied by close monitoring of clinical status and valproate plasma concentrations.

Distribution

Protein Binding:

The plasma protein binding of valproate is concentration dependent and the free fraction increases from approximately 10% at 40 μg/mL to 18.5% at 130 μg/mL. Protein binding of valproate is reduced in the elderly, in patients with chronic hepatic diseases, in patients with renal impairment, and in the presence of other drugs (e.g., aspirin). Conversely, valproate may displace certain protein-bound drugs (e.g., phenytoin, carbamazepine, warfarin, and tolbutamide). (See **PRECAUTIONS, Drug Interactions** for more detailed information on the pharmacokinetic interactions of valproate with other drugs.)

CNS Distribution:

Valproate concentrations in cerebrospinal fluid (CSF) approximate unbound concentrations in plasma (about 10% of total concentration).

Metabolism

Valproate is metabolized almost entirely by the liver. In adult patients on monotherapy, 30-50% of an administered dose appears in urine as a glucuronide conjugate. Mitochondrial β-oxidation is the other major metabolic pathway, typically accounting for over 40% of the dose. Usually, less than 15-20% of the dose is eliminated by other oxidative mechanisms. Less than 3% of an administered dose is excreted unchanged in urine.

The relationship between dose and total valproate concentration is nonlinear; concentration does not increase proportionally with the dose, but rather, increases to a lesser extent due to saturable plasma protein binding. The kinetics of unbound drug are linear.

Elimination

Mean plasma clearance and volume of distribution for total valproate are 0.56 L/hr/1.73 m^2 and 11 L/1.73 m^2, respectively. Mean plasma clearance and volume of distribution for free valproate are 4.6 L/hr/1.73 m^2 and 92 L/1.73 m^2. Mean terminal half-life for valproate monotherapy ranged from 9 to 16 hours following oral dosing regimens of 250 to 1000 mg.

The estimates cited apply primarily to patients who are not taking drugs that affect hepatic metabolizing enzyme systems. For example, patients taking enzyme-inducing antiepileptic drugs (carbamazepine, phenytoin, and phenobarbital) will clear valproate more rapidly. Because of these changes in valproate clearance, monitoring of antiepileptic concentrations should be intensified whenever concomitant antiepileptics are introduced or withdrawn.

Special Populations

Effect of Age:

Neonates - Children within the first two months of life have a markedly decreased ability to eliminate valproate compared to older children and adults. This is a result of reduced clearance (perhaps due to delay in development of glucuronosyl transferase and other enzyme systems involved in valproate elimination) as well as increased volume of distribution (in part due to decreased plasma protein binding). For example, in one study, the half-life in children under 10 days ranged from 10 to 67 hours compared to a range of 7 to 13 hours in children greater than 2 months.

Children - Pediatric patients (i.e., between 3 months and 10 years) have 50% higher clearances expressed on weight (i.e., mL/min/kg) than do adults. Over the age of 10 years, children have pharmacokinetic parameters that approximate those of adults.

Elderly - The capacity of elderly patients (age range: 68 to 89 years) to eliminate valproate has been shown to be reduced compared to younger adults (age range: 22 to 26). Intrinsic clearance is reduced by 39%; the free fraction is increased by 44%. Accordingly, the initial dosage should be reduced in the elderly. (See **DOSAGE AND ADMINISTRATION**).

Effect of Gender:

There are no differences in the body surface area adjusted unbound clearance between males and females (4.8±0.17 and 4.7±0.07 L/hr per 1.73 m^2, respectively).

Effect of Race:

The effects of race on the kinetics of valproate have not been studied.

Effect of Disease:

Liver Disease - (See **BOXED WARNING, CONTRAINDICATIONS**, and **WARNINGS**). Liver disease impairs the capacity to eliminate valproate. In one study, the clearance of free valproate was decreased by 50% in 7 patients with cirrhosis and by 16% in 4 patients with acute hepatitis, compared with 6 healthy subjects. In that study, the half-life of valproate was increased from 12 to 18 hours. Liver disease is also associated with decreased albumin concentrations and larger unbound fractions (2 to 2.6 fold increase) of valproate. Accordingly, monitoring of total concentrations may be misleading since free concentrations may be substantially elevated in patients with hepatic disease whereas total concentrations may appear to be normal.

Renal Disease - A slight reduction (27%) in the unbound clearance of valproate has been reported in patients with renal failure (creatinine clearance < 10 mL/minute); however, hemodialysis typically reduces valproate concentrations by about 20%. Therefore, no dosage adjustment appears to be necessary in patients with renal failure. Protein binding in these patients is substantially reduced; thus, monitoring total concentrations may be misleading.

Plasma Levels and Clinical Effect

The relationship between plasma concentration and clinical response is not well documented. One contributing factor is the nonlinear, concentration dependent protein binding of valproate which affects the clearance of the drug. Thus, monitoring of total serum valproate cannot provide a reliable index of the bioactive valproate species.

For example, because the plasma protein binding of valproate is concentration dependent, the free fraction increases

from approximately 10% at 40 μg/mL to 18.5% at 130 μg/mL. Higher than expected free fractions occur in the elderly, in hyperlipidemic patients, and in patients with hepatic and renal diseases.

Epilepsy:

The therapeutic range in epilepsy is commonly considered to be 50 to 100 μg/mL of total valproate, although some patients may be controlled with lower or higher plasma concentrations.

Mania:

In placebo-controlled clinical trials of acute mania, patients were dosed to clinical response with trough plasma concentrations between 50 and 125 μg/mL (See **DOSAGE AND ADMINISTRATION**).

Clinical Trials

Mania

The effectiveness of DEPAKOTE for the treatment of acute mania was demonstrated in two 3-week, placebo controlled, parallel group studies.

(1) Study 1: The first study enrolled adult patients who met DSM-III-R criteria for Bipolar Disorder and who were hospitalized for acute mania. In addition, they had a history of failing to respond to or not tolerating previous lithium carbonate treatment. DEPAKOTE was initiated at a dose of 250 mg tid and adjusted to achieve serum valproate concentrations in a range of 50-100 μg/mL by day 7. Mean DEPAKOTE doses for completers in this study were 1118, 1525, and 2402 mg/day at days 7, 14, and 21, respectively. Patients were assessed on the Young Mania Rating Scale (YMRS; score ranges from 0-60), an augmented Brief Psychiatric Rating Scale (BPRS-A), and the Global Assessment Scale (GAS). Baseline scores and change from baseline in the week 3 endpoint (last-observation-carry-forward) analysis were as follows:

Study 1
YMRS Total Score

Group	Baseline[1]	BL to Wk 3[2]	Difference[3]
Placebo	28.8	+0.2	
DEPAKOTE	28.5	−9.5	9.7

BPRS-A Total Score

Group	Baseline[1]	BL to Wk 3[2]	Difference[3]
Placebo	76.2	+1.8	
DEPAKOTE	76.4	−17.0	18.8

GAS Score

Group	Baseline[1]	BL to Wk 3[2]	Difference[3]
Placebo	31.8	0.0	
DEPAKOTE	30.3	+18.1	18.1

[1] Mean score at baseline
[2] Change from baseline to week 3 (LOCF)
[3] Difference in change from baseline to week 3 endpoint (LOCF) between DEPAKOTE and placebo

DEPAKOTE was statistically significantly superior to placebo on all three measures of outcome.

(2) Study 2: The second study enrolled adult patients who met Research Diagnostic Criteria for manic disorder and who were hospitalized for acute mania. DEPAKOTE was initiated at a dose of 250 mg tid and adjusted within a dose range of 750-2500 mg/day to achieve serum valproate concentrations in a range of 40-150 μg/mL. Mean DEPAKOTE doses for completers in this study were 1116, 1683, and 2006 mg/day at days 7, 14, and 21, respectively. Study 2 also included a lithium group for which lithium doses for completers were 1312, 1869, and 1984 mg/day at days 7, 14, and 21, respectively. Patients were assessed on the Manic Rating Scale (MRS; score ranges from 11-63), and the primary outcome measures were the total MRS score, and scores for two subscales of the MRS, i.e., the Manic Syndrome Scale (MSS) and the Behavior and Ideation Scale (BIS). Baseline scores and change from baseline in the week 3 endpoint (last-observation-carry-forward) analysis were as follows:

Study 2
MRS Total Score

Group	Baseline[1]	BL to Day 21[2]	Difference[3]
Placebo	38.9	−4.4	
Lithium	37.9	−10.5	6.1
DEPAKOTE	38.1	−9.5	5.1

MSS Total Score

Group	Baseline[1]	BL to Day 21[2]	Difference[3]
Placebo	18.9	−2.5	
Lithium	18.5	−6.2	3.7
DEPAKOTE	18.9	−6.0	3.5

BIS Total Score

Group	Baseline[1]	BL to Day 21[2]	Difference[3]
Placebo	16.4	−1.4	
Lithium	16.0	−3.8	2.4
DEPAKOTE	15.7	−3.2	1.8

[1] Mean score at baseline
[2] Change from baseline to day 21 (LOCF)
[3] Difference in change from baseline to day 21 endpoint (LOCF) between DEPAKOTE and placebo and lithium and placebo

DEPAKOTE was statistically significantly superior to placebo on all three measures of outcome. An exploratory analysis for age and gender effects on outcome did not suggest any differential responsiveness on the basis of age or gender.

A comparison of the percentage of patients showing ≥ 30% reduction in the symptom score from baseline in each treatment group, separated by study, is shown in Figure 1.

Figure 1
Percentage of Patients Achieving ≥ 30% Reduction in Symptom Score From Baseline

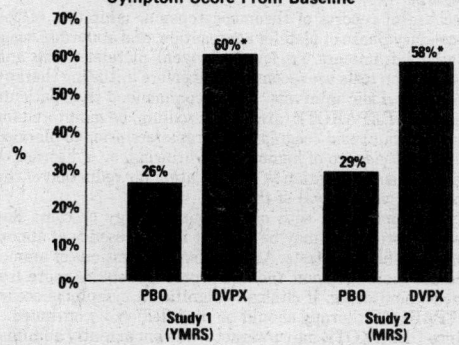

* $p < 0.05$
PBO = placebo, DVPX = DEPAKOTE

Migraine

The results of two multicenter, randomized, double-blind, placebo-controlled clinical trials established the effectiveness of DEPAKOTE in the prophylactic treatment of migraine headache.

Both studies employed essentially identical designs and recruited patients with a history of migraine with or without aura (of at least 6 months in duration) who were experiencing at least 2 migraine headaches a month during the 3 months prior to enrollment. Patients with cluster headaches were excluded. Women of childbearing potential were excluded entirely from one study, but were permitted in the other if they were deemed to be practicing an effective method of contraception.

In each study following a 4-week single-blind placebo baseline period, patients were randomized, under double blind conditions, to DEPAKOTE or placebo for a 12-week treatment phase, comprised of a 4-week dose titration period followed by an 8-week maintenance period. Treatment outcome was assessed on the basis of 4-week migraine headache rates during the treatment phase.

In the first study, a total of 107 patients (24 M, 83 F), ranging in age from 26 to 73 were randomized 2:1, DEPAKOTE to placebo. Ninety patients completed the 8-week maintenance period. Drug dose titration, using 250 mg tablets, was individualized at the investigator's discretion. Adjustments were guided by actual/sham trough total serum valproate levels in order to maintain the study blind. In patients on DEPAKOTE doses ranged from 500 to 2500 mg a day. Doses over 500 mg were given in three divided doses (TID). The mean dose during the treatment phase was 1087 mg/day resulting in a mean trough total valproate level of 72.5 μg/mL, with a range of 31 to 133 mg/mL.

The mean 4-week migraine headache rate during the treatment phase was 5.7 in the placebo group compared to 3.5 in the DEPAKOTE group (see Figure 2). These rates were significantly different.

In the second study, a total of 176 patients (19 males and 157 females), ranging in age from 17 to 76 years, were randomized equally to one of three DEPAKOTE dose groups (500, 1000, or 1500 mg/day) or placebo. The treatments were given in two divided doses (BID). One hundred thirty-seven patients completed the 8-week maintenance period. Efficacy was to be determined by a comparison of the 4-week migraine headache rate in the combined 1000/1500 mg/day group and placebo group.

The initial dose was 250 mg daily. The regimen was advanced by 250 mg every 4 days (8 days for 500 mg/day group), until the randomized dose was achieved. The mean trough total valproate levels during the treatment phase were 39.6, 62.5, and 72.5 μg/mL in the DEPAKOTE 500, 1000, and 1500 mg/day groups, respectively.

The mean 4-week migraine headache rates during the treatment phase, adjusted for differences in baseline rates, were

4.5 in the placebo group, compared to 3.3, 3.0, and 3.3 in the DEPAKOTE 500, 1000, and 1500 mg/day groups, respectively, based on intent-to-treat results (see Figure 2). Migraine headache rates in the combined DEPAKOTE 1000/1500 mg group were significantly lower than in the placebo group.

Figure 2
Mean 4-week Migraine Rates

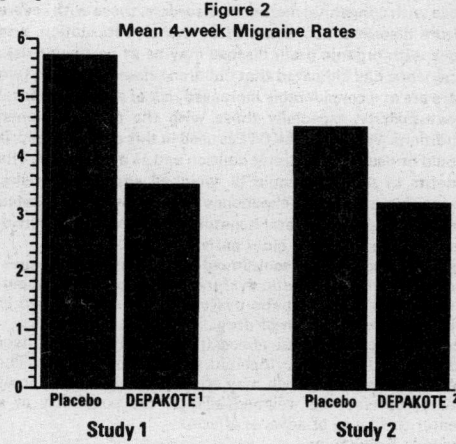

[1] Mean dose of DEPAKOTE was 1087 mg/day.
[2] Dose of DEPAKOTE was 500 or 1000 mg/day.

INDICATIONS AND USAGE

Mania

DEPAKOTE (divalproex sodium) is indicated for the treatment of the manic episodes associated with bipolar disorder. A manic episode is a distinct period of abnormally and persistently elevated, expansive, or irritable mood. Typical symptoms of mania include pressure of speech, motor hyperactivity, reduced need for sleep, flight of ideas, grandiosity, poor judgement, aggressiveness, and possible hostility.

The efficacy of DEPAKOTE was established in 3-week trials with patients meeting DSM-III-R criteria for bipolar disorder who were hospitalized for acute mania (See **Clinical Trials** under **CLINICAL PHARMACOLOGY**).

The safety and effectiveness of DEPAKOTE for long-term use in mania, i.e., more than 3 weeks, has not been systematically evaluated in controlled clinical trials. Therefore, physicians who elect to use DEPAKOTE for extended periods should continually reevaluate the long-term usefulness of the drug for the individual patient.

Epilepsy

DEPAKOTE (divalproex sodium) is indicated for use as sole and adjunctive therapy in the treatment of simple and complex absence seizures, and adjunctively in patients with multiple seizure types that include absence seizures.

Simple absence is defined as very brief clouding of the sensorium or loss of consciousness accompanied by certain generalized epileptic discharges without other detectable clinical signs. Complex absence is the term used when other signs are also present.

Migraine

DEPAKOTE is indicated for prophylaxis of migraine headaches. There is no evidence that DEPAKOTE is useful in the acute treatment of migraine headaches. Because valproic acid may be a hazard to the fetus, DEPAKOTE should be considered for women of childbearing potential only after this risk has been thoroughly discussed with the patient and weighed against the potential benefits of treatment (see **WARNINGS - Usage In Pregnancy**, **PRECAUTIONS - Information for Patients**).

SEE WARNINGS FOR STATEMENT REGARDING FATAL HEPATIC DYSFUNCTION.

CONTRAINDICATIONS

DIVALPROEX SODIUM SHOULD NOT BE ADMINISTERED TO PATIENTS WITH HEPATIC DISEASE OR SIGNIFICANT HEPATIC DYSFUNCTION.

Divalproex sodium is contraindicated in patients with known hypersensitivity to the drug.

WARNINGS

Hepatic failure resulting in fatalities has occurred in patients receiving valproic acid. These incidents usually have occurred during the first six months of treatment. Serious or fatal hepatotoxicity may be preceded by non-specific symptoms such as malaise, weakness, lethargy, facial edema, anorexia, and vomiting. In patients with epilepsy, a loss of seizure control may also occur. Patients should be monitored closely for appearance of these symptoms. Liver function tests should be performed prior to therapy and at frequent intervals thereafter, especially during the first six months. However, physicians should not totally on serum biochemistry since these tests may not be abnormal in all instances, but should also consider the results of careful interim medical history and physical examination.

Continued on next page

Abbott Laboratories—Cont.

Caution should be observed when administering DEPAKOTE products to patients with a prior history of hepatic disease. Patients on multiple anticonvulsants, children, those with congenital metabolic disorders, those with severe seizure disorders accompanied by mental retardation, and those with organic brain disease may be at particular risk. Experience has indicated that children under the age of two years are at a considerably increased risk of developing fatal hepatotoxicity, especially those with the aforementioned conditions. When DEPAKOTE is used in this patient group, it should be used with extreme caution and as a sole agent. The benefits of therapy should be weighed against the risks. Above this age group, experience in epilepsy has indicated that the incidence of fatal hepatotoxicity decreases considerably in progressively older patient groups.

The drug should be discontinued immediately in the presence of significant hepatic dysfunction, suspected or apparent. In some cases, hepatic dysfunction has progressed in spite of discontinuation of drug.

The frequency of adverse effects (particularly elevated liver enzymes and thrombocytopenia) may be dose-related. The therapeutic benefit which may accompany the higher doses should therefore be weighed against the possibility of a greater incidence of adverse effects.

Usage In Pregnancy

ACCORDING TO PUBLISHED AND UNPUBLISHED REPORTS, VALPROIC ACID MAY PRODUCE TERATOGENIC EFFECTS IN THE OFFSPRING OF HUMAN FEMALES RECEIVING THE DRUG DURING PREGNANCY.

THERE ARE MULTIPLE REPORTS IN THE CLINICAL LITERATURE WHICH INDICATE THAT THE USE OF ANTIEPILEPTIC DRUGS DURING PREGNANCY RESULTS IN AN INCREASED INCIDENCE OF BIRTH DEFECTS IN THE OFFSPRING. ALTHOUGH DATA ARE MORE EXTENSIVE WITH RESPECT TO TRIMETHADIONE, PARAMETHADIONE, PHENYTOIN, AND PHENOBARBITAL, REPORTS INDICATE A POSSIBLE SIMILAR ASSOCIATION WITH THE USE OF OTHER ANTIEPILEPTIC DRUGS.

THE INCIDENCE OF NEURAL TUBE DEFECTS IN THE FETUS MAY BE INCREASED IN MOTHERS RECEIVING VALPROATE DURING THE FIRST TRIMESTER OF PREGNANCY. THE CENTERS FOR DISEASE CONTROL (CDC) HAS ESTIMATED THE RISK OF VALPROIC ACID EXPOSED WOMEN HAVING CHILDREN WITH SPINA BIFIDA TO BE APPROXIMATELY 1 TO 2%.[1]

OTHER CONGENITAL ANOMALIES (EG, CRANIOFACIAL DEFECTS, CARDIOVASCULAR MALFORMATIONS AND ANOMALIES INVOLVING VARIOUS BODY SYSTEMS), COMPATIBLE AND INCOMPATIBLE WITH LIFE, HAVE BEEN REPORTED. SUFFICIENT DATA TO DETERMINE THE INCIDENCE OF THESE CONGENITAL ANOMALIES IS NOT AVAILABLE.

THE HIGHER INCIDENCE OF CONGENITAL ANOMALIES IN ANTIEPILEPTIC DRUG-TREATED WOMEN WITH SEIZURE DISORDERS CANNOT BE REGARDED AS A CAUSE AND EFFECT RELATIONSHIP. THERE ARE INTRINSIC METHODOLOGIC PROBLEMS IN OBTAINING ADEQUATE DATA ON DRUG TERATOGENICITY IN HUMANS; GENETIC FACTORS OR THE EPILEPTIC CONDITION ITSELF, MAY BE MORE IMPORTANT THAN DRUG THERAPY IN CONTRIBUTING TO CONGENITAL ANOMALIES.

PATIENTS TAKING VALPROATE MAY DEVELOP CLOTTING ABNORMALITIES. A PATIENT WHO HAD LOW FIBRINOGEN WHEN TAKING MULTIPLE ANTICONVULSANTS INCLUDING VALPROATE GAVE BIRTH TO AN INFANT WITH AFIBRINOGENEMIA WHO SUBSEQUENTLY DIED OF HEMORRHAGE. IF VALPROATE IS USED IN PREGNANCY, THE CLOTTING PARAMETERS SHOULD BE MONITORED CAREFULLY.

HEPATIC FAILURE, RESULTING IN THE DEATH OF A NEWBORN AND OF AN INFANT, HAVE BEEN REPORTED FOLLOWING THE USE OF VALPROATE DURING PREGNANCY.

ANIMAL STUDIES ALSO HAVE DEMONSTRATED VALPROATE INDUCED TERATOGENICITY. Studies in rats and human females demonstrated placental transfer of the drug. Doses greater than 65 mg/kg/day given to pregnant rats and mice produced skeletal abnormalities in the offspring, primarily involving ribs and vertebrae; doses greater than 150 mg/kg/day given to pregnant rabbits produced fetal resorptions and (primarily) soft-tissue abnormalities in the offspring. In rats a dose-related delay in the onset of parturition was noted. Postnatal growth and survival of the progeny were adversely affected, particularly when drug administration spanned the entire gestation and early lactation period.

The prescribing physician will wish to weigh the benefits of therapy against the risks in treating or counseling women of childbearing potential. If this drug is used during pregnancy, or if the patient becomes pregnant while taking this drug, the patient should be apprised of the potential hazard to the fetus.

Antiepileptic drugs should not be discontinued abruptly in patients in whom the drug is administered to prevent major seizures because of the strong possibility of precipitating status epilepticus with attendant hypoxia and threat to life. In individual cases where the severity and frequency of the seizure disorder are such that the removal of medication does not pose a serious threat to the patient, discontinuation of the drug may be considered prior to and during pregnancy, although it cannot be said with any confidence that even minor seizures do not pose some hazard to the developing embryo or fetus.

Tests to detect neural tube and other defects using current accepted procedures should be considered a part of routine prenatal care in childbearing women receiving valproate.

PRECAUTIONS

Hepatic Dysfunction

See **BOXED WARNING, CONTRAINDICATIONS** and **WARNINGS**.

General

Because of reports of thrombocytopenia, inhibition of the secondary phase of platelet aggregation, and abnormal coagulation parameters, (eg, low fibrinogen), platelet counts and coagulation tests are recommended before initiating therapy and at periodic intervals. It is recommended that patients receiving DEPAKOTE (divalproex sodium) be monitored for platelet count and coagulation parameters prior to planned surgery. Evidence of hemorrhage, bruising, or a disorder of hemostasis/coagulation is an indication for reduction of the dosage or withdrawal of therapy.

Hyperammonemia with or without lethargy or coma has been reported and may be present in the absence of abnormal liver function tests. Asymptomatic elevations of ammonia are more common and when present require more frequent monitoring. If clinically significant symptoms occur, DEPAKOTE therapy should be modified or discontinued.

Since DEPAKOTE may interact with concurrently administered drugs which are capable of enzyme induction, periodic plasma concentration determinations of valproate and concomitant drugs are recommended during the early course of therapy. (See **PRECAUTIONS-Drug Interactions**.)

Valproate is partially eliminated in the urine as a keto-metabolite which may lead to a false interpretation of the urine ketone test.

There have been reports of altered thyroid function tests associated with valproate. The clinical significance of these is unknown.

Suicidal ideation may be a manifestation of certain psychiatric disorders, and may persist until significant remission of symptoms occurs. Close supervision of high risk patients should accompany initial drug therapy.

Information for Patients

Since DEPAKOTE products may produce CNS depression, especially when combined with another CNS depressant (eg, alcohol), patients should be advised not to engage in hazardous activities, such as driving an automobile or operating dangerous machinery, until it is known that they do not become drowsy from the drug.

Migraine Patients: Since DEPAKOTE has been associated with certain types of birth defects, female patients of childbearing age considering the use of DEPAKOTE for the prevention of migraine should be advised to read the **Patient Information Leaflet**, which appears as the last section of the labeling.

Drug Interactions

Effects of Co-Administered Drugs on Valproate Clearance

Drugs that affect the level of expression of hepatic enzymes, particularly those that elevate levels of glucuronosyl transferases, may increase the clearance of valproate. For example, phenytoin, carbamazepine, and phenobarbital (or primidone) can double the clearance of valproate. Thus, patients on monotherapy will generally have longer half-lives and higher concentrations than patients receiving polytherapy with antiepilepsy drugs.

In contrast, drugs that are inhibitors of cytochrome P450 isozymes, e.g., antidepressants, may be expected to have little effect on valproate clearance because cytochrome P450 microsomal mediated oxidation is a relatively minor secondary metabolic pathway compared to glucuronidation and beta-oxidation.

Because of these changes in valproate clearance, monitoring of valproate and concomitant drug concentrations should be increased whenever enzyme inducing drugs are introduced or withdrawn.

The following list provides information about the potential for an influence of several commonly prescribed medications on valproate pharmacokinetics. The list is not exhaustive nor could it be, since new interactions are continuously being reported.

Drugs for which a potentially important interaction has been observed:

Aspirin - A study involving the co-administration of aspirin at antipyretic doses (11 to 16 mg/kg) with valproate to pediatric patients (n=6) revealed a decrease in protein binding and an inhibition of metabolism of valproate. Valproate free fraction was increased 4-fold in the presence of aspirin compared to valproate alone. The β-oxidation pathway consisting of 2-E-valproic acid, 3-OH-valproic acid, and 3-keto valproic acid was decreased from 25% of total metabolites excreted on valproate alone to 8.3% in the presence of aspirin. Caution should be observed if valproate and aspirin are to be co-administered.

Felbamate - A study involving the co-administration of 1200 mg/day of felbamate with valproate to patients with epilepsy (n=10) revealed an increase in mean valproate peak concentration by 35% (from 86 to 115 μg/mL) compared to valproate alone. Increasing the felbamate dose to 2400 mg/day increased the mean valproate peak concentration to 133 μg/mL (another 16% increase). A decrease in valproate dosage may be necessary when felbamate therapy is initiated.

Rifampin - A study involving the administration of a single dose of valproate (7 mg/kg) 36 hours after 5 nights of daily dosing with rifampin (600 mg) revealed a 40% increase in the oral clearance of valproate. Valproate dosage adjustment may be necessary when it is co-administered with rifampin.

Drugs for which either no interaction or a likely clinically unimportant interaction has been observed:

Antacids - A study involving the co-administration of valproate 500 mg with commonly administered antacids (Maalox, Trisogel, and Titralac - 160 mEq doses) did not reveal any effect on the extent of absorption of valproate.

Chlorpromazine - A study involving the administration of 100 to 300 mg/day of chlorpromazine to schizophrenic patients already receiving valproate (200 mg BID) revealed a 15% increase in trough plasma levels of valproate.

Haloperidol - A study involving the administration of 6 to 10 mg/day of haloperidol to schizophrenic patients already receiving valproate (200 mg BID) revealed no significant changes in valproate trough plasma levels.

Cimetidine and Ranitidine - Cimetidine and ranitidine do not affect the clearance of valproate.

Effects of Valproate on Other Drugs

Valproate has been found to be a weak inhibitor of some P450 isozymes, epoxide hydrase, and glucuronyl transferases.

The following list provides information about the potential for an influence of valproate co-administration on the pharmacokinetics or pharmacodynamics of several commonly prescribed medications. The list is not exhaustive, since new interactions are continuously being reported.

Drugs for which a potentially important valproate interaction has been observed:

Carbamazepine/carbamazepine-10,11-Epoxide - Serum levels of carbamazepine (CBZ) decreased 17% while that of carbamazepine-10,11-epoxide (CBZ-E) increased by 45% upon co-administration of valproate and CBZ to epileptic patients.

Clonazepam - The concomitant use of valproic acid and clonazepam may induce absence status in patients with a history of absence type seizures.

Diazepam - Valproate displaces diazepam from its plasma albumin binding sites and inhibits its metabolism. Co-administration of valproate (1500 mg daily) increased the free fraction of diazepam (10 mg) by 90% in healthy volunteers (n=6). Plasma clearance and volume of distribution for free diazepam were reduced by 25% and 20%, respectively, in the presence of valproate. The elimination half-life of diazepam remained unchanged upon addition of valproate.

Ethosuximide - Valproate inhibits the metabolism of ethosuximide. Administration of a single ethosuximide dose of 500 mg with valproate (800 to 1600 mg/day) to healthy volunteers (n=6) was accompanied by a 25% increase in elimination half-life of ethosuximide and a 15% decrease in its total clearance as compared to ethosuximide alone. Patients receiving valproate and ethosuximide, especially along with other anticonvulsants, should be monitored for alterations in serum concentrations of both drugs.

Lamotrigine - In a steady-state study involving 10 healthy volunteers, the elimination half-life of lamotrigine increased from 26 to 70 hours with valproate co-administration (a 165% increase). The dose of lamotrigine should be reduced when co-administered with valproate.

Phenobarbital - Valproate was found to inhibit the metabolism of phenobarbital. Co-administration of valproate (250 mg BID for 14 days) with phenobarbital to normal subjects (n=6) resulted in a 50% increase in half-life and a 30% decrease in plasma clearance of phenobarbital (60 mg single-dose). The fraction of phenobarbital dose excreted unchanged increased by 50% in presence of valproate.

There is evidence for severe CNS depression, with or without significant elevations of barbiturate or valproate serum concentrations. All patients receiving concomitant barbiturate therapy should be closely monitored for neurological toxicity. Serum barbiturate concentrations should be obtained, if possible, and the barbiturate dosage decreased, if appropriate.

Primidone, which is metabolized to a barbiturate, may be involved in a similar interaction with valproate.

Phenytoin - Valproate displaces phenytoin from its plasma albumin binding sites and inhibits its hepatic metabolism. Co-administration of valproate (400 mg TID) with phenytoin (250 mg) in normal volunteers (n=7) was associated with a 60% increase in the free fraction of phenytoin. Total plasma clearance and apparent volume of distribution of phenytoin increased 30% in the presence of valproate. Both the clearance and apparent volume of distribution of free phenytoin were reduced by 25%.

In patients with epilepsy, there have been reports of breakthrough seizures occurring with the combination of valproate and phenytoin. The dosage of phenytoin should be adjusted as required by the clinical situation.

Tolbutamide - From in vitro experiments, the unbound fraction of tolbutamide was increased from 20% to 50% when added to plasma samples taken from patients treated with valproate. The clinical relevance of this displacement is unknown.

Warfarin - In an in vitro study, valproate increased the unbound fraction of warfarin by up to 32.6%. The therapeutic relevance of this is unknown; however, coagulation tests should be monitored if DEPAKOTE therapy is instituted in patients taking anticoagulants.

Zidovudine - In six patients who were seropositive for HIV, the clearance of zidovudine (100 mg q8h) was decreased by 38% after administration of valproate (250 or 500 mg q8h); the half-life of zidovudine was unaffected.

Drugs for which either no interaction or a likely clinically unimportant interaction has been observed:

Acetaminophen - Valproate had no effect on any of the pharmacokinetic parameters of acetaminophen when it was concurrently administered to three epileptic patients.

Amitriptyline/Nortriptyline - Administration of a single oral 50 mg dose of amitriptyline to 15 normal volunteers (10 males and 5 females) who received valproate (500 mg BID) resulted in a 21% decrease in plasma clearance of amitriptyline and a 34% decrease in the net clearance of nortriptyline.

Clozapine - In psychotic patients (n=11), no interaction was observed when valproate was co-administered with clozapine.

Lithium - Co-administration of valproate (500 mg BID) and lithium carbonate (300 mg TID) to normal male volunteers (n=16) had no effect on the steady-state kinetics of lithium.

Lorazepam - Concomitant administration of valproate (500 mg BID) and lorazepam (1 mg BID) in normal male volunteers (n=9) was accompanied by a 17% decrease in the plasma clearance of lorazepam.

Oral Contraceptive Steroids - Administration of a single-dose of ethinyloestradiol (50 μg)/levonorgestrel (250 μg) to 6 women on valproate (200 mg BID) therapy for 2 months did not reveal any pharmacokinetic interaction.

Carcinogenesis
Valproic acid was administered to Sprague Dawly rats and ICR (HA/ICR) mice at doses of 0, 80, and 170 mg/kg/day for two years. A variety of neoplasms were observed in both species. The chief findings were a statistically significant increase in the incidence of subcutaneous fibrosarcomas in high dose male rats receiving valproic acid and a statistically significant dose-related trend for benign pulmonary adenomas in male mice receiving valproic acid. The significance of these findings for humans is unknown.

Mutagenesis
Studies on valproate have been performed using bacterial and mammalian systems. These studies have provided no evidence of a mutagenic potential for valproate.

Fertility
Chronic toxicity studies in juvenile and adult rats and dogs demonstrated reduced spermatogenesis and testicular atrophy at doses greater than 200 mg/kg/day in rats and greater than 90 mg/kg/day in dogs. Segment I fertility studies in rats have shown doses up to 350 mg/kg/day for 60 days to have no effect on fertility. THE EFFECT OF VALPROATE ON TESTICULAR DEVELOPMENT AND ON SPERM PRODUCTION AND FERTILITY IN HUMANS IS UNKNOWN.

Pregnancy
Pregnancy Category D: See **WARNINGS.**

Nursing Mothers
Valproate is excreted in breast milk. Concentrations in breast milk have been reported to be 1-10% of serum concentrations. It is not known what effect this would have on a nursing infant. Caution should be exercised when divalproex sodium is administered to a nursing woman.

Pediatric
Experience has indicated that children under the age of two years are at a considerably increased risk of developing fatal hepatotoxicity, especially those with the aforementioned conditions (see **BOXED WARNING**). When DEPAKOTE is used in this patient group, it should be used with extreme caution and as a sole agent. The benefits of therapy should be weighed against the risks. Above the age of 2 years, experience in epilepsy has indicated that the incidence of fatal hepatotoxicity decreases considerably in progressively older patient groups.

Younger children, especially those receiving enzyme-inducing drugs, will require larger maintenance doses to attain targeted total and unbound valproic acid concentrations. The variability in free fraction limits the clinical usefulness of monitoring total serum valproic acid concentrations. Interpretation of valproic acid concentrations in children should include consideration of factors that affect hepatic metabolism and protein binding.

The safety and effectiveness of DEPAKOTE for the treatment of acute mania has not been studied in individuals below the age of 18 years.

The safety and effectiveness of DEPAKOTE for the prophylaxis of migraines has not been studied in individuals below the age of 16 years.

Geriatric
No patients above the age of 65 years were enrolled in double-blind prospective clinical trials of mania associated with bipolar illness. In a case review study of 583 patients, 72 patients (12%) were greater than 65 years of age. A higher percentage of patients above 65 years of age reported accidental injury, infection, pain, somnolence, and tremor. Discontinuation of valproate was occasionally associated with the latter two events. It is not clear whether these events indicate additional risk or whether they result from preexisting medical illness and concomitant medication use among these patients.

There is insufficient information available to discern the safety and effectiveness of DEPAKOTE for the prophylaxis of migraines in patients over 65.

ADVERSE REACTIONS

Mania
The incidence of treatment-emergent events has been ascertained based on combined data from two placebo-controlled clinical trials of DEPAKOTE in the treatment of manic episodes associated with bipolar disorder. The adverse events were usually mild or moderate in intensity, but sometimes were serious enough to interrupt treatment. In clinical trials, the rates of premature termination due to intolerance were not statistically different between placebo, DEPAKOTE, and lithium carbonate. A total of 4%, 8% and 11% of patients discontinued therapy due to intolerance in the placebo, DEPAKOTE, and lithium carbonate groups, respectively.

Table 1 summarizes those adverse events reported for patients in these trials where the incidence rate in the DEPAKOTE-treated group was greater than 5% and greater than the placebo incidence, or where the incidence in the DEPAKOTE-treated group was statistically significantly greater than the placebo group. Vomiting was the only event that was reported by significantly (p ≤ 0.05) more patients receiving DEPAKOTE compared to placebo.

Table 1
Adverse Events Reported by > 5% of DEPAKOTE-Treated Patients During Placebo-Controlled Trials of Acute Mania[1]

Adverse Event	DEPAKOTE (n =89)	Placebo (n =97)
Nausea	22%	15%
Somnolence	19%	12%
Dizziness	12%	4%
Vomiting	12%	3%
Accidental injury	11%	5%
Asthenia	10%	7%
Abdominal pain	9%	8%
Dyspepsia	9%	8%
Rash	6%	3%

[1] The following adverse events occurred at an equal or greater incidence for placebo than for DEPAKOTE: back pain, headache, pain (unspecified), constipation, diarrhea, tremor, and pharyngitis.

The following additional adverse events were reported by greater than 1% but not more than 5% of the 89 divalproex sodium-treated patients in controlled clinical trials:
Body as a Whole: Chest pain, chills, chills and fever, cyst, fever, infection, neck pain, neck rigidity.
Cardiovascular System: Hypertension, hypotension, palpitations, postural hypotension, tachycardia, vascular anomaly, vasodilation.
Digestive System: Anorexia, fecal incontinence, flatulence, gastroenteritis, glossitis, periodontal abscess.
Hemic and Lymphatic System: Ecchymosis.
Metabolic and Nutritional Disorders: Edema, peripheral edema.
Musculoskeletal System : Arthralgia, arthrosis, leg cramps, twitching.
Nervous System: Abnormal dreams, abnormal gait, agitation, ataxia, catatonic reaction, confusion, depression, diplopia, dysarthria, hallucinations, hypertonia, hypokinesia, insomnia, paresthesia, reflexes increased, tardive dyskinesia, thinking abnormalities, vertigo.

Respiratory System: Dyspnea, rhinitis.
Skin and Appendages: Alopecia, discoid lupus erythematosis, dry skin, furunculosis, maculopapular rash, seborrhea.
Special Senses: Abnormal vision, amblyopia, conjunctivitis, deafness, dry eyes, ear disorder, ear pain, eye pain, tinnitus.
Urogenital System: Dysmenorrhea, dysuria, urinary incontinence.

Migraine
Based on two placebo-controlled clinical trials and their long term extension, DEPAKOTE was generally well tolerated with most adverse events rated as mild to moderate in severity. Of the 202 patients exposed to DEPAKOTE in the placebo-controlled trials, 17% discontinued for intolerance. This is compared to a rate of 5% for the 81 placebo patients. Including the long term extension study, the adverse events reported as the primary reason for discontinuation by ≥ 1% of 248 DEPAKOTE-treated patients were alopecia (6%), nausea and/or vomiting (5%), weight gain (2%), tremor (2%), somnolence (1%), elevated SGOT and/or SGPT (1%), and depression (1%).

Table 2 includes those adverse events reported for patients in the placebo-controlled trials where the incidence rate in the DEPAKOTE-treated group was greater than 5% and was greater than that for placebo patients.

This is table for DEPAKOTE

Table 2
Adverse Events Reported by > 5% of DEPAKOTE-treated Patients During Migraine Placebo-Controlled Trials with a Greater Incidence Than Patients Taking Placebo[1]

Body System Event	Depakote (N=202)	Placebo (N=81)
Gastrointestinal System		
Nausea	31%	10%
Dyspepsia	13%	9%
Diarrhea	12%	7%
Vomiting	11%	1%
Abdominal pain	9%	4%
Increased appetite	6%	4%
Nervous System		
Asthenia	20%	9%
Somnolence	17%	5%
Dizziness	12%	6%
Tremor	9%	0%
Other		
Weight gain	8%	2%
Back pain	8%	6%
Alopecia	7%	1%

[1] The following adverse events occurred in at least 5% of DEPAKOTE-treated patients and at an equal or greater incidence for placebo than for DEPAKOTE: pain (unspecified), infection, flu syndrome, and pharyngitis.

The following additional adverse events were reported by greater than 1% but not more than 5% of the 202 divalproex sodium-treated patients in the controlled clinical trials:
Body as a Whole: Accidental injury, allergic reaction, chest pain, chills, face edema, fever, malaise, and neck pain.
Cardiovascular System: Vasodilatation.
Digestive System: Anorexia, constipation, dry mouth, flatulence, gastrointestinal disorder (unspecified), and stomatitis.
Hemic and Lymphatic System: Ecchymosis.
Metabolic and Nutritional Disorders: Peripheral edema, SGOT increase, and SGPT increase.
Musculoskeletal System: Leg cramps and myalgia.
Nervous System: Abnormal dreams, amnesia, confusion, depression, emotional lability, insomnia, nervousness, paresthesia, speech disorder, thinking abnormalities, and vertigo.
Respiratory System: Cough increased, dyspnea, rhinitis, and sinusitis.
Skin and Appendages: Pruritus and rash.
Special Senses: Conjunctivitis, ear disorder, taste perversion, and tinnitus.
Urogenital System: Cystitis, metrorrhagia, and vaginal hemorrhage.

Other Patient Populations
Adverse events that have been reported with valproate from epilepsy trials, spontaneous reports, and other sources are listed below by body system.
Since divalproex sodium has usually been used with antiepilepsy drugs, in the treatment of epilepsy, it is not possible, in most cases, to determine whether the following adverse reactions can be ascribed to divalproex sodium alone, or the combination of drugs.

Gastrointestinal: The most commonly reported side effects at the initiation of therapy are nausea, vomiting, and indigestion. These effects are usually transient and rarely require discontinuation of therapy. Diarrhea, abdominal cramps, and constipation have been reported. Both anorexia with some weight loss and increased appetite with weight gain have also been reported. The administration of delayed-

Continued on next page

Abbott Laboratories—Cont.

release divalproex sodium may result in reduction of gastrointestinal side effects in some patients.[2]
CNS Effects: Sedative effects have occurred in patients receiving valproate alone but occur most often in patients receiving combination therapy. Sedation usually abates upon reduction of other antiepileptic medication. Tremor (may be dose-related), hallucinations, ataxia, headache, nystagmus, diplopia, asterixis, "spots before eyes", dysarthria, dizziness and incoordination. Rare cases of coma have occurred in patients receiving valproate alone or in conjunction with phenobarbital. In rare instances encephalopathy with fever has developed shortly after the introduction of valproate monotherapy without evidence of hepatic dysfunction or inappropriate plasma levels; all patients recovered after the drug was withdrawn.
Dermatologic: Transient hair loss, skin rash, photosensitivity, generalized pruritus, erythema multiforme, and Stevens-Johnson syndrome. A case of fatal epidermal necrolysis has been reported in a 6 month old infant taking valproate and several other concomitant medications.
Psychiatric: Emotional upset, depression, psychosis, aggression, hyperactivity, and behavioral deterioration.
Musculoskeletal: Weakness.
Hematologic: Thrombocytopenia and inhibition of the secondary phase of platelet aggregation may be reflected in altered bleeding time, petechiae, bruising, hematoma formation, and frank hemorrhage (see **PRECAUTIONS - General and Drug Interactions**). Relative lymphocytosis, macrocytosis, hypofibrinogenemia, leukopenia, eosinophilia, anemia including macrocytic with or without folate deficiency, bone marrow suppression, and acute intermittent porphyria.
Hepatic: Minor elevations of transaminases (eg, SGOT and SGPT) and LDH are frequent and appear to be dose-related. Occasionally, laboratory test results include increases in serum bilirubin and abnormal changes in other liver function tests. These results may reflect potentially serious hepatotoxicity (see **WARNINGS**).
Endocrine: Irregular menses, secondary amenorrhea, breast enlargement, galactorrhea, and parotid gland swelling. Abnormal thyroid function tests (see **PRECAUTIONS**).
Pancreatic: Acute pancreatitis including fatalities.
Metabolic: Hyperammonemia (see **PRECAUTIONS**), hyponatremia, and inappropriate ADH secretion.
There have been rare reports of Fanconi's syndrome occurring chiefly in children.
Decreased carnitine concentrations have been reported although the clinical relevance is undetermined.
Hyperglycinemia has occurred and was associated with a fatal outcome in a patient with preexistent nonketotic hyperglycinemia.
Genitourinary: Enuresis.
Special Senses: Hearing loss, either reversible or irreversible, has been reported; however, a cause and effect relationship has not been established.
Other: Edema of the extremities, lupus erythematosus, and fever.

OVERDOSAGE

Overdosage with valproate may result in somnolence, heart block, and deep coma. Fatalities have been reported; however patients have recovered from valproate levels as high as 2120 μg/mL.
In overdose situations, the fraction of drug not bound to protein is high and hemodialysis or tandem hemodialysis plus hemoperfusion may result in significant removal of drug. The benefit of gastric lavage or emesis will vary with the time since ingestion. General supportive measures should be applied with particular attention to the maintenance of adequate urinary output.
Naloxone has been reported to reverse the CNS depressant effects of valproate overdosage. Because naloxone could theoretically also reverse the antiepileptic effects of valproate, it should be use with caution in patients with epilepsy.

DOSAGE AND ADMINISTRATION

Mania
DEPAKOTE tablets are administered orally. The recommended initial dose is 750 mg daily in divided doses. The dose should be increased as rapidly as possible to achieve the lowest therapeutic dose which produces the desired clinical effect or the desired range of plasma concentrations. In placebo-controlled clinical trials of acute mania, patients were dosed to a clinical response with a trough plasma concentration between 50 and 125 μg/mL. Maximum concentrations were generally achieved within 14 days. The maximum recommended dosage is 60 mg/kg/day.
There is no body of evidence available from controlled trials to guide a clinician in the longer term management of a patient who improves during DEPAKOTE treatment of an acute manic episode. While it is generally agreed that pharmacological treatment beyond an acute response in mania is desirable, both for maintenance of the initial response and for prevention of new manic episodes, there are no systematically obtained data to support the benefits of DEPAKOTE in such longer-term treatment. Although there are no efficacy data that specifically address longer-term antimanic treatment with DEPAKOTE, the safety of DEPAKOTE in long-term use is supported by data from record reviews involving approximately 360 patients treated with DEPAKOTE for greater than 3 months.

Epilepsy
DEPAKOTE tablets are administered orally. The recommended initial dose is 15 mg/kg/day, increasing at one week intervals by 5 to 10 mg/kg/day until seizures are controlled or side effects preclude further increases. The maximum recommended dosage is 60 mg/kg/day. If the total daily dose exceeds 250 mg, it should be given in a divided regimen.
A good correlation has not been established between daily dose, serum concentration, and therapeutic effect. However, therapeutic valproate serum concentrations for most patients with epilepsy will range from 50 to 100 μg/mL. Some patients may be controlled with lower or higher serum concentrations (see **CLINICAL PHARMACOLOGY**).
As the DEPAKOTE dosage is titrated upward, blood concentrations of phenobarbital and/or phenytoin may be affected (see **PRECAUTIONS**).
Antiepilepsy drugs should not be abruptly discontinued in patients in whom the drug is administered to prevent major seizures because of the strong possibility of precipitating status epilepticus with attendant hypoxia and threat to life.
In epileptic patients previously receiving DEPAKENE (valproic acid) therapy, DEPAKOTE tablets should be initiated at the same daily dose and dosing schedule. After the patient is stabilized on DEPAKOTE tablets, a dosing schedule of two or three times a day may be elected in selected patients.[3]

Migraine
DEPAKOTE tablets are administered orally. The recommended starting dose is 250 mg twice daily. Some patients may benefit from doses up to 1000 mg/day. In the clinical trials, there was no evidence that higher doses led to greater efficacy.

General Dosing Advice
Dosing in Elderly Patients - Due to a decrease in unbound clearance of valproate, the starting dose should be reduced; the ultimate therapeutic dose should be achieved on the basis of clinical response.
Dose-Related Adverse Events - The frequency of adverse effects (particularly elevated liver enzymes and thrombocytopenia) may be dose-related. The benefit of improved therapeutic effect with higher doses should be weighed against the possibility of a greater incidence of adverse reactions.
G.I. Irritation - Patients who experience G.I. irritation may benefit from administration of the drug with food or by slowly building up the dose from an initial low level.

HOW SUPPLIED

DEPAKOTE tablets (divalproex sodium delayed-release tablets) are supplied as:

125 mg salmon pink-colored tablets:
Bottles of 100 .... (**NDC** 0074-6212-13)
Abbo-Pac® unit dose packages of 100.......... (**NDC** 0074-6212-11).

250 mg peach-colored tablets:
Bottles of 100 .... (**NDC** 0074-6214-13)
Bottles of 500 .... (**NDC** 0074-6214-53)
Abbo-Pac® unit dose packages of 100 .... (**NDC** 0074-6214-11)

500 mg lavender-colored tablets:
Bottles of 100 .... (**NDC** 0074-6215-13)
Bottles of 500 .... (**NDC** 0074-6215-53)
Abbo-Pac® unit dose packages of 100 .... (**NDC** 0074-6215-11).

Recommended storage: Store tablets below 86°F (30°C).

REFERENCES

1. Centers for Disease Control, Valproate: a new cause of birth defects—report from Italy and follow-up from France. *Morbidity and Mortality Weekly Report.* 1983; 32(33): 438-439.
2. Wilder, BJ, et al. Gastrointestinal tolerance of divalproex sodium. *Neurology.* 1983; 33: 808-811.
3. Wilder, BJ, et al. Twice-daily dosing of valproate with divalproex. *Clin Pharmacol Ther.* 1983; 34(4): 501-504.

Caution—Federal (U.S.A.) Law prohibits dispensing without prescription.

Patient Information Leaflet
Important Information for Women Who Could Become Pregnant
About the Use of Depakote® (divalproex sodium) Tablets for Migraine

Please read this leaflet carefully before you take Depakote® (divalproex sodium) tablets. This leaflet provides a summary of important information about taking Depakote for migraine to women who could become pregnant. Depakote is also prescribed for uses other than those discussed in this leaflet. If you have any questions or concerns, or want more information about Depakote, contact your doctor or pharmacist.

Information For Women Who Could Become Pregnant
Depakote is used to prevent or reduce the number of migraines you experience. Depakote can be obtained only by prescription from your doctor. The decision to use Depakote for the prevention of migraine is one that you and your doctor should make together, taking into account your individual needs and medical condition.
Before using Depakote, women who can become pregnant should consider the fact that **Depakote has been associated with birth defects, in particular, with spina bifida and other defects related to failure of the spinal canal to close normally. Although the incidence is unknown in migraine patients treated with Depakote, approximately 1 to 2% of children born to women with epilepsy taking Depakote in the first 12 weeks of pregnancy had these defects (based on data from the Centers for Disease Control, a U.S. agency based in Atlanta). The incidence in the general population is 0.1 to 0.2%.**

Information For Women Who Are Planning to Get Pregnant
- Women taking Depakote for the prevention of migraine who are planning to get pregnant should discuss with their doctor temporarily stopping Depakote, before and during their pregnancy.

Information For Women Who Become Pregnant While Taking Depakote
- If you become pregnant while taking Depakote for the prevention of migraine, you should contact your doctor immediately.

Other Important Information About Depakote Tablets
- Depakote tablets should be taken exactly as it is prescribed by your doctor to get the most benefits from Depakote and reduce the risk of side effects.
- If you have taken more than the prescribed dose of Depakote, contact your hospital emergency room or local poison center immediately.
- This medication was prescribed for your particular condition. Do not use it for another condition or give the drug to others.

Facts About Birth Defects
It is important to know that birth defects may occur even in children of individuals not taking any medications or without any additional risk factors.

Facts About Migraine
About 23 million Americans suffer from migraine headaches. About 75% of migraine sufferers are women. A migraine is described as a throbbing headache that gets worse with activity. Migraine may also include nausea and/or vomiting as well as sensitivity to light and sound. Migraine usually happens about once a month, but some people may have them as often as once or twice a week. Often, the symptoms from a migraine can cause people to miss work or school. If you have frequent migraines, or if acute treatment is not working for you, your doctor may prescribe a preventative therapy. Preventative (prophylactic) treatment is used to prevent attacks and reduce the frequency and severity of headache events.
This summary provides important information about the use of Depakote for migraine to women who could become pregnant. If you would like more information about the other potential risks and benefits of Depakote, ask your doctor or pharmacist to let you read the professional labeling and then discuss it with them. If you have any questions or concerns about taking Depakote, you should discuss them with your doctor.

Revised: March, 1996
Ref. 03-4663-R2
Abbott Laboratories
North Chicago, IL 60064, U.S.A.

Shown in Product Identification Guide, page 303

DESOXYN® C-II ℞
(methamphetamine hydrochloride)
Gradumet® Tablets

METHAMPHETAMINE HAS A HIGH POTENTIAL FOR ABUSE. IT SHOULD THUS BE TRIED ONLY IN WEIGHT REDUCTION PROGRAMS FOR PATIENTS IN WHOM ALTERNATIVE THERAPY HAS BEEN INEFFECTIVE. ADMINISTRATION OF METHAMPHETAMINE FOR PROLONGED PERIODS OF TIME IN OBESITY MAY LEAD TO DRUG DEPENDENCE AND MUST BE AVOIDED. PARTICULAR ATTENTION SHOULD BE PAID TO THE POSSIBILITY OF SUBJECTS OBTAINING METHAMPHETAMINE FOR NON-THERAPEUTIC USE OR DISTRIBUTION TO OTHERS, AND THE DRUG SHOULD BE PRESCRIBED OR DISPENSED SPARINGLY.

DESCRIPTION

Methamphetamine hydrochloride, chemically known as (S)-N, α-dimethylbenzeneethanamine hydrochloride, is a member of the amphetamine group of sympathomimetic amines. It has the following structural formula:

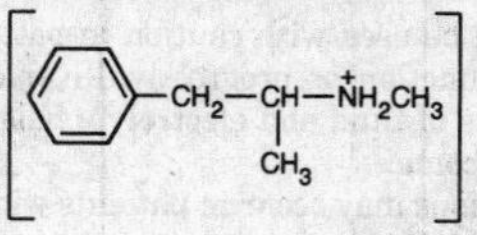

$$\left[C_6H_5 - CH_2 - CH - \overset{+}{N}H_2CH_3 \right] Cl^- \\ \qquad\qquad\quad CH_3$$

DESOXYN GraduMet sustained-release tablets are available containing 5 mg, 10 mg or 15 mg of methamphetamine hydrochloride for oral administration. The GraduMet is an inert, porous, plastic matrix, which is impregnated with methamphetamine hydrochloride. The drug is leached slowly from the GraduMet as it passes through the gastrointestinal tract. The expended matrix is not absorbed and is excreted in the stool.

Inactive Ingredients: 5 mg GraduMet tablet: magnesium stearate, methyl acrylate-methyl methacrylate copolymer, povidone and talc.

10 mg GraduMet tablet: FD&C Yellow No. 6 (sunset yellow), magnesium stearate, methyl acrylate-methyl methacrylate copolymer, povidone and talc.

15 mg GraduMet tablet: FD&C Yellow No. 5 (tartrazine), magnesium stearate, methyl acrylate-methyl methacrylate copolymer, povidone and talc.

CLINICAL PHARMACOLOGY

Methamphetamine is a sympathomimetic amine with CNS stimulant activity. Peripheral actions include elevation of systolic and diastolic blood pressures and weak bronchodilator and respiratory stimulant action. Drugs of this class used in obesity are commonly known as "anorectics" or "anorexigenics." It has not been established, however, that the action of such drugs in treating obesity is primarily one of appetite suppression. Other central nervous system actions, or metabolic effects, may be involved, for example.

Adult obese subjects instructed in dietary management and treated with "anorectic" drugs, lose more weight on the average than those treated with placebo and diet, as determined in relatively short-term clinical trials.

The magnitude of increased weight loss of drug-treated patients over placebo-treated patients is only a fraction of a pound a week. The rate of weight loss is greatest in the first weeks of therapy for both drug and placebo subjects and tends to decrease in succeeding weeks. The origins of the increased weight loss due to the various possible drug effects are not established. The amount of weight loss associated with the use of an "anorectic" drug varies from trial to trial, and the increased weight loss appears to be related in part to variables other than the drug prescribed, such as the physician-investigator, the population treated, and the diet prescribed. Studies do not permit conclusions as to the relative importance of the drug and non-drug factors on weight loss.

The natural history of obesity is measured in years, whereas the studies cited are restricted to a few weeks duration; thus, the total impact of drug-induced weight loss over that of diet alone must be considered clinically limited.

The mechanism of action involved in producing the beneficial behavioral changes seen in hyperkinetic children receiving methamphetamine is unknown.

In humans, methamphetamine is rapidly absorbed from the gastrointestinal tract. The primary site of metabolism is in the liver by aromatic hydroxylation, N-dealkylation and deamination. At least seven metabolites have been identified in the urine. The biological half-life has been reported in the range of 4 to 5 hours. Excretion occurs primarily in the urine and is dependent on urine pH. Alkaline urine will significantly increase the drug half-life. Approximately 62% of an oral dose is eliminated in the urine within the first 24 hours with about one-third as intact drug and the remainder as metabolites.

INDICATIONS AND USAGE

Attention Deficit Disorder with Hyperactivity—DESOXYN GraduMet tablets are indicated as an integral part of a total treatment program which typically includes other remedial measures (psychological, educational, social) for a stabilizing effect in children over 6 years of age with a behavioral syndrome characterized by the following group of developmentally inappropriate symptoms: moderate to severe distractibility, short attention span, hyperactivity, emotional lability, and impulsivity. The diagnosis of this syndrome should not be made with finality when these symptoms are only of comparatively recent origin. Nonlocalizing (soft) neurological signs, learning disability, and abnormal EEG may or may not be present, and a diagnosis of central nervous system dysfunction may or may not be warranted.

Exogenous Obesity—as a short-term (i.e., a few weeks) adjunct in a regimen of weight reduction based on caloric restriction, for patients in whom obesity is refractory to alternative therapy, e.g., repeated diets, group programs, and other drugs. The limited usefulness of DESOXYN GraduMet

tablets (see **CLINICAL PHARMACOLOGY**) should be weighed against possible risks inherent in use of the drug, such as those described below.

CONTRAINDICATIONS

DESOXYN GraduMet tablets are contraindicated during or within 14 days following the administration of monoamine oxidase inhibitors; hypertensive crises may result. It is also contraindicated in patients with glaucoma, advanced arteriosclerosis, symptomatic cardiovascular disease, moderate to severe hypertension, hyperthyroidism or known hypersensitivity or idiosyncrasy to sympathomimetic amines. Methamphetamine should not be given to patients who are in an agitated state or who have a history of drug abuse.

WARNINGS

Tolerance to the anorectic effect usually develops within a few weeks. When this occurs, the recommended dose should not be exceeded in an attempt to increase the effect; rather, the drug should be discontinued (see **DRUG ABUSE AND DEPENDENCE**).

Decrements in the predicted growth (i.e., weight gain and/or height) rate have been reported with the long-term use of stimulants in children. Therefore, patients requiring long-term therapy should be carefully monitored.

Usage in Nursing Mothers: Amphetamines are excreted in human milk. Mothers taking amphetamines should be advised to refrain from nursing.

PRECAUTIONS

General: DESOXYN (methamphetamine hydrochloride) GraduMet tablets should be used with caution in patients with even mild hypertension.

Methamphetamine should not be used to combat fatigue or to replace rest in normal persons.

Prescribing and dispensing of methamphetamine should be limited to the smallest amount that is feasible at one time in order to minimize the possibility of overdosage.

The 15 mg dosage strength of DESOXYN GraduMet tablets contains FD&C Yellow No. 5 (tartrazine) which may cause allergic-type reactions (including bronchial asthma) in certain susceptible individuals. Although the overall incidence of FD&C Yellow No. 5 (tartrazine) sensitivity in the general population is low, it is frequently seen in patients who also have aspirin hypersensitivity.

Information for Patients: The patient should be informed that methamphetamine may impair the ability to engage in potentially hazardous activities, such as, operating machinery or driving a motor vehicle.

The patient should be cautioned not to increase dosage, except on advice of the physician.

Drug Interactions: Insulin requirements in diabetes mellitus may be altered in association with the use of methamphetamine and concomitant dietary regimen.

Methamphetamine may decrease the hypotensive effect of *guanethidine.*

DESOXYN should not be used concurrently with *monoamine oxidase inhibitors* (see **CONTRAINDICATIONS**).

Concurrent administration of *tricyclic antidepressants* and indirect-acting sympathomimetic amines such as amphetamines, should be closely supervised and dosage carefully adjusted.

Phenothiazines are reported in the literature to antagonize the CNS stimulant action of the amphetamines.

Drug/Laboratory Test Interactions: Literature reports suggest that amphetamines may be associated with significant elevation of plasma corticosteroids. This should be considered if determination of plasma corticosteroid levels is desired in a person receiving amphetamines.

Carcinogensis, Mutagenesis, Impairment of Fertility: Data are not available on long-term potential for carcinogenicity, mutagenicity, or impairment of fertility.

Pregnancy: Teratogenic effects: Pregnancy Category C. Methamphetamine has been shown to have teratogenic and embryocidal effects in mammals given high multiples of the human dose. There are no adequate and well-controlled studies in pregnant women. DESOXYN GraduMet tablets should not be used during pregnancy unless the potential benefit justifies the potential risk to the fetus.

Nonteratogenic effects: Infants born to mothers dependent on amphetamines have an increased risk of premature delivery and low birth weight. Also, these infants may experience symptoms of withdrawal as demonstrated by dysphoria, including agitation and significant lassitude.

Nursing Mothers: See **WARNINGS.**

Pediatric Use: Safety and effectiveness for use as an anorectic agent in children below the age of 12 years have not been established.

Long-term effects of methamphetamine in children have not been established (see **WARNINGS**).

Drug treatment is not indicated in all cases of the behavioral syndrome characterized by moderate to severe distractibility, short attention span, hyperactivity, emotional lability and impulsivity. It should be considered only in light of the complete history and evaluation of the child. The decision to prescribe DESOXYN GraduMet tablets should depend on the physician's assessment of the chronicity and severity of the

child's symptoms and their appropriateness for his/her age. Prescription should not depend solely on the presence of one or more of the behavioral characteristics.

When these symptoms are associated with acute stress reactions, treatment with DESOXYN GraduMet tablets is usually not indicated.

Clinical experience suggests that in psychotic children, administration of DESOXYN GraduMet tablets may exacerbate symptoms of behavior disturbance and thought disorder.

Amphetamines have been reported to exacerbate motor and phonic tics and Tourette's syndrome. Therefore, clinical evaluation for tics and Tourette's syndrome in children and their families should precede use of stimulant medications.

ADVERSE REACTIONS

The following are adverse reactions in decreasing order of severity within each category that have been reported:

Cardiovascular: Elevation of blood pressure, tachycardia and palpitation.

Central Nervous System: Psychotic episodes have been rarely reported at recommended doses. Dizziness, dysphoria, overstimulation, euphoria, insomnia, tremor, restlessness and headache. Exacerbation of motor and phonic tics and Tourette's syndrome.

Gastrointestinal: Diarrhea, constipation, dryness of mouth, unpleasant taste and other gastrointestinal disturbances.

Hypersensitivity: Urticaria.

Endocrine: Impotence and changes in libido.

Miscellaneous: Suppression of growth has been reported with the long-term use of stimulants in children (see **WARNINGS**).

DRUG ABUSE AND DEPENDENCE

Controlled Substance: DESOXYN GraduMet tablets are subject to control under DEA schedule II.

Abuse: Methamphetamine has been extensively abused. Tolerance, extreme psychological dependence, and severe social disability have occurred. There are reports of patients who have increased the dosage to many times that recommended. Abrupt cessation following prolonged high dosage administration results in extreme fatigue and mental depression; changes are also noted on the sleep EEG. Manifestations of chronic intoxication with methamphetamine include severe dermatoses, marked insomnia, irritability, hyperactivity, and personality changes. The most severe manifestation of chronic intoxication is psychosis often clinically indistinguishable from schizophrenia.

OVERDOSAGE

Manifestations of acute overdosage with methamphetamine include restlessness, tremor, hyperreflexia, rapid respiration, confusion, assaultiveness, hallucinations, panic states, hyperpyrexia, and rhabdomyolysis. Fatigue and depression usually follow the central stimulation. Cardiovascular effects include arrhythmias, hypertension or hypotension, and circulatory collapse. Gastrointestinal symptoms include nausea, vomiting, diarrhea, and abdominal cramps. Fatal poisoning usually terminates in convulsions and coma.

Consult with a Certified Poison Control Center regarding treatment for up to date guidance and advice.

Management of acute methamphetamine intoxication is largely symptomatic and includes gastric evacuation, administration of activated charcoal, and sedation. Experience with hemodialysis or peritoneal dialysis is inadequate to permit recommendations in this regard.

Acidification of urine increases methamphetamine excretion, but is believed to increase risk of acute renal failure if myoglobinuria is present. Intravenous phentolamine (Regitine®) has been suggested for possible acute, severe hypertension, if this complicates methamphetamine overdosage. Usually a gradual drop in blood pressure will result when sufficient sedation has been achieved. Chlorpromazine has been reported to be useful in decreasing CNS stimulation and sympathomimetic effects.

Since the GraduMet tablet releases methamphetamine gradually, therapy should be directed at reversing the effects of the ingested drug and at supporting the patient until symptoms subside. Saline cathartics are useful for hastening the evacuation of the tablets that have not already released medication.

DOSAGE AND ADMINISTRATION

DESOXYN GraduMet tablets are given orally.

Methamphetamine should be administered at the lowest effective dosage, and dosage should be individually adjusted. Late evening medication should be avoided because of the resulting insomnia.

Attention Deficit Disorder with Hyperactivity:

For treatment of children 6 years or older with a behavioral syndrome characterized by moderate to severe distractibility, short attention span, hyperactivity, emotional lability and impulsivity: an initial dose of 5 mg DESOXYN once or twice a day is recommended. Daily dosage may be raised in increments of 5 mg at weekly intervals until optimum clinical response is achieved. The usual effective dose is 20 to 25 mg

Continued on next page

Abbott Laboratories—Cont.

daily. The total daily dose may be given once daily using the Gradumet tablet. The Gradumet form should not be utilized for initiation of dosage nor until the titrated daily dosage is equal to or greater than the dosage provided in a Gradumet tablet.
Where possible, drug administration should be interrupted occasionally to determine if there is a recurrence of behavioral symptoms sufficient to require continued therapy.
For obesity: one Gradumet tablet, 10 or 15 mg, once a day in the morning. Treatment should not exceed a few weeks in duration. Methamphetamine is not recommended for use as an anorectic agent in children under 12 years of age.

HOW SUPPLIED

DESOXYN (methamphetamine hydrochloride) Gradumet tablets are supplied as follows:
5 mg, white, in bottles of 100 (**NDC** 0074-6941-04); 10 mg, orange, in bottles of 100 (**NDC** 0074-6948-08); and 15 mg, yellow, in bottles of 100 (**NDC** 0074-6959-07).
® GRADUMET—Long-release dose form, Abbott.
Recommended Storage: Store below 86°F (30°C).
Ref. 03-4654-R3

Shown in Product Identification Guide, page 303

DICAL-D® TABLETS—WAFERS — OTC

[dī 'cal-d]
(Dibasic Calcium Phosphate with Vitamin D)

DESCRIPTION

Tablets
Daily dosage (three tablets) provides:

Vitamin D	399 IU (10 mcg)	99% USRDA*
Calcium	0.35 g	35% USRDA*
Phosphorus	0.27 g	27% USRDA*

Each tablet contains:
Dibasic Calcium Phosphate, hydrous (as anhydrous form) .... 500 mg
Cholecalciferol .... (133 IU) .... 3.33 mcg
Microcrystalline cellulose, sodium starch glycolate, corn starch, hydrogenated vegetable oil wax, magnesium stearate and talc added.
Calcium to phosphorus ratio 1.3 to 1.

Wafers
Daily dosage (two wafers) provides:

Vitamin D	400 IU (10 mcg)	100% USRDA*
Calcium	.464 g	46% USRDA*
Phosphorus	.36 g	36% USRDA*

Calcium to phosphorous ratio 1.29 to 1.
Each wafer contains:
Cholecalciferol .... 5 mcg (200 IU)
Dibasic Calcium Phosphate, hydrous .... 1 g
Added dextrose, sucrose, talc, stearic acid, mineral oil, salt, and natural and artificial flavorings.

*% U.S. Recommended Daily Allowance for adults and children 4 or more years of age.

INDICATIONS

Wafers:
For those individuals who must restrict their intake of dairy products.
Tablets:
For individuals with deficient intake of dairy products.

DOSAGE AND ADMINISTRATION

Usual dose for adults and children 4 years and older:
Tablets—1 tablet 3 times daily with meals, or as directed by the physician or dentist.
Wafers—Chew 1 wafer twice daily with meals, or as directed by the physician or dentist.

HOW SUPPLIED

Dical-D Tablets in bottles of 100 (**NDC** 0074-3741-13) and 500 (**NDC** 0074-3741-53).
Dical-D Wafers in boxes of 51 (**NDC** 0074-3589-01).
Recommended storage: Store in tight container below 77°F (25°C).
Ref. 03-1924-2/R4, 03-2009-2/R3 and 09-6484-5/R10

ENDURON® — ℞

[en 'de-ron]
(methyclothiazide tablets, USP)

DESCRIPTION

Methyclothiazide is a member of the benzothiadiazine (thiazide) class of drugs. It is an analogue of hydrochlorothiazide and occurs as a white to practically white crystalline powder which is basically odorless. Methyclothiazide is very slightly soluble in water and chloroform, and slightly soluble in alcohol. Chemically, methyclothiazide is represented as 6-chloro-3-(chloromethyl)-3,4-dihydro-2-methyl-2H-1,2,4-benzothiadiazine-7-sulfonamide 1,1-dioxide. The structural formula is:

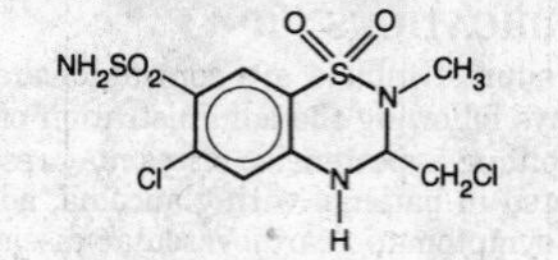

Clinically, ENDURON (methyclothiazide) is an oral diuretic-antihypertensive agent. ENDURON tablets are available in two dosage strengths containing 2.5 mg and 5 mg of methyclothiazide.

Inactive Ingredients
2.5 mg tablets: corn starch, FD&C Yellow No. 6, lactose, magnesium stearate and talc.
5 mg tablets: corn starch, D&C Red No. 36, lactose, magnesium stearate and talc.

CLINICAL PHARMACOLOGY

The diuretic and saluretic effects of methyclothiazide result from a drug-induced inhibition of the renal tubular reabsorption of electrolytes. The excretion of sodium and chloride is greatly enhanced. Potassium excretion is also enhanced to a variable degree, as it is with the other thiazides. Although urinary excretion of bicarbonate is increased slightly, there is usually no significant change in urinary pH. Methyclothiazide has a per mg natriuretic activity approximately 100 times that of the prototype thiazide, chlorothiazide. At maximal therapeutic dosages, all thiazides are approximately equal in their diuretic/natriuretic effects.
There is significant natriuresis and diuresis within two hours after administration of a single dose of methyclothiazide. These effects reach a peak in about six hours and persist for 24 hours following oral administration of a single dose.
Like other benzothiadiazines, methyclothiazide also has antihypertensive properties, and may be used for this purpose either alone or to enhance the antihypertensive action of other drugs. The mechanism by which the benzothiadiazines, including methyclothiazide, produce a reduction of elevated blood pressure is not known. However, sodium depletion appears to be involved.
Methyclothiazide is rapidly absorbed and slowly eliminated by the kidneys as intact drug but primarily as an inactive metabolite. Additional information on the pharmacokinetics is not known at this time.

INDICATIONS AND USAGE

ENDURON (methyclothiazide) is indicated in the management of hypertension either as the sole therapeutic agent or to enhance the effect of other antihypertensive drugs in the more severe forms of hypertension.
ENDURON tablets are indicated as adjunctive therapy in edema associated with congestive heart failure, hepatic cirrhosis, and corticosteroid and estrogen therapy.
ENDURON tablets have also been found useful in edema due to various forms of renal dysfunction such as the nephrotic syndrome, acute glomerulonephritis, and chronic renal failure.
Usage in Pregnancy: The routine use of diuretics in an otherwise healthy pregnant woman is inappropriate and exposes mother and fetus to unnecessary hazard. Diuretics do not prevent development of toxemia of pregnancy, and there is no satisfactory evidence that they are useful in the treatment of developed toxemia.
Edema during pregnancy may arise from pathological causes or from the physiological and mechanical consequences of pregnancy. Thiazides are indicated in pregnancy when edema is due to pathological causes, just as they are in the absence of pregnancy (see PRECAUTIONS—Pregnancy). Dependent edema in pregnancy, resulting from restriction of venous return by the expanded uterus, is properly treated through elevation of the lower extremities and use of support hose; use of diuretics to lower intravascular volume in this case is illogical and unnecessary. There is hypervolemia during normal pregnancy that is harmful to neither the fetus nor the mother (in the absence of cardiovascular disease), but that is associated with edema, including generalized edema, in the majority of pregnant women. If this edema produces discomfort, increased recumbency will often provide relief. In rare instances, this edema may cause extreme discomfort that is not relieved by rest. In these cases, a short course of diuretics may provide relief and may be appropriate.

CONTRAINDICATIONS

Methyclothiazide is contraindicated in patients with anuria and in patients with a history of hypersensitivity to this compound or other sulfonamide-derived drugs.

WARNINGS

Methyclothiazide shares with other thiazides the propensity to deplete potassium reserves to an unpredictable degree.
There have been isolated reports that certain nonedematous individuals developed severe fluid and electrolyte derangements after only brief exposure to normal doses of thiazide and non-thiazide diuretics.
Thiazides should be used with caution in patients with renal disease or significant impairment of renal function, since azotemia may be precipitated and cumulative drug effects may occur.
Thiazides should be used with caution in patients with impaired hepatic function or progressive liver disease, since minor alterations of fluid and electrolyte balance may precipitate hepatic coma.
Sensitivity reactions may occur in patients with a history of allergy or bronchial asthma.
The possibility of exacerbation or activation of systemic lupus erythematosus has been reported.
Hyperuricemia may occur or frank gout may be precipitated in certain patients receiving thiazide therapy.

PRECAUTIONS

Laboratory Tests: Initial and periodic determinations of serum electrolytes should be performed at appropriate intervals for the purpose of detecting possible electrolyte imbalances such as hyponatremia, hypochloremic alkalosis, and hypokalemia. Serum and urine electrolyte determinations are particularly important when a patient is vomiting excessively or receiving parenteral fluids.
General: All patients should be observed for clinical signs of electrolyte imbalances such as dryness of mouth, thirst, weakness, lethargy, drowsiness, restlessness, muscle pains or cramps, muscular fatigue, hypotension, oliguria, tachycardia, and gastrointestinal disturbances such as nausea and vomiting.
Hypokalemia may develop, especially with brisk diuresis, when severe cirrhosis is present, during concomitant use of corticosteroids or ACTH, or after prolonged therapy.
Interference with adequate oral electrolyte intake will also contribute to hypokalemia. Hypokalemia may be avoided or treated by use of potassium supplements or foods with a high potassium content.
Any chloride deficit is generally mild and usually does not require specific treatment except under extraordinary circumstances (as in liver disease or renal disease). Dilutional hyponatremia may occur in edematous patients in hot weather; appropriate therapy is water restriction rather than administration of salt, except in rare instances when the hyponatremia is life threatening. In actual salt depletion, appropriate replacement is the therapy of choice.
Latent diabetes mellitus may become manifest during thiazide administration.
The antihypertensive effects of the drug may be enhanced in the postsympathectomy patient.
If progressive renal impairment becomes evident as indicated by a rising nonprotein nitrogen or blood urea nitrogen, a careful reappraisal of therapy is necessary with consideration given to withholding or discontinuing diuretic therapy.
Thiazides may decrease urinary calcium excretion. Thiazides may cause intermittent and slight elevation of serum calcium in the absence of known disorders of calcium metabolism. Marked hypercalcemia may be evidence of hidden hyperparathyroidism. Thiazides should be discontinued before carrying out tests for parathyroid function.
Thiazides may cause increased concentrations of total serum cholesterol, total triglycerides, and low-density lipoproteins in some patients. Use thiazides with caution in patients with moderate or high cholesterol concentrations and in patients with elevated triglyceride levels.
Information for Patients: Patients should inform their doctor if they have: 1) had an allergic reaction to methyclothiazide or other diuretics 2) asthma 3) kidney disease 4) liver disease 5) gout 6) systemic lupus erythematosus, or 7) been taking other drugs such as cortisone, digitalis, lithium carbonate, or drugs for diabetes.
The physician should inform patients of possible side effects and caution the patient to report any of the following symptoms of electrolyte imbalance; dryness of mouth, thirst, weakness, tiredness, drowsiness, restlessness, muscle pains or cramps, nausea, vomiting or increased heart rate.
The physician should advise the patient to take this medication every day as directed. Physicians should also caution patients that drinking alcohol can increase the chance of dizziness.
Drug Interactions: Hypokalemia can sensitize or exaggerate the response of the heart to the toxic effects of *digitalis* (e.g., increased ventricular irritability).
Hypokalemia may develop during concomitant use of *steroids* or *ACTH.*
Insulin requirements in diabetic patients may be increased, decreased, or unchanged.
Thiazides may decrease arterial responsiveness to *norepinephrine.* This diminution is not sufficient to preclude effectiveness of the pressor agent for therapeutic use.
Thiazide drugs may increase the responsiveness to *tubocurarine.*
Lithium renal clearance is reduced by thiazides, increasing the risk of lithium toxicity.

Thiazides may add to or potentiate the action of *other antihypertensive drugs.* Potentiation occurs with ganglionic or peripheral adrenergic blocking drugs.

Drug/Laboratory Test Interactions: Thiazides may decrease serum PBI levels without signs of thyroid disturbance.

Thiazides should be discontinued before carrying out tests for parathyroid function.

Carcinogenesis, Mutagenesis, Impairment of Fertility: No data are available concerning the potential for carcinogenicity or mutagenicity in animals or humans. Methyclothiazide did not impair fertility in rats receiving up to 4 mg/kg/day (at least 20 times the maximum recommended human dose of 10 mg, assuming patient weight equal to or greater than 50 kg).

Pregnancy—Teratogenic Effects: Pregnancy Category B. Reproduction studies performed in rats and rabbits at doses up to 4 mg/kg/day have revealed no evidence of harm to the fetus due to methyclothiazide. There are, however, no adequate and well-controlled studies in pregnant women. Because animal reproduction studies are not always predictive of human response, this drug should be used during pregnancy only if clearly needed.

Nonteratogenic Effects: Thiazides cross the placental barrier and appear in cord blood. The use of thiazides in pregnant women requires that the anticipated benefit be weighed against possible hazards to the fetus. These hazards include fetal or neonatal jaundice, thrombocytopenia and possible other adverse reactions that have occurred in the adult.

Nursing Mothers: Thiazides are excreted in breast milk. Because of the potential for serious adverse reactions in nursing infants, a decision should be made whether to discontinue nursing or to discontinue the drug taking into account the importance of the drug to the mother.

Pediatric Use: Safety and effectiveness in children have not been established.

ADVERSE REACTIONS

Adverse reactions are usually reversible upon reduction of dosage or discontinuation of ENDURON tablets. Whenever adverse reactions are moderate or severe, it may be necessary to discontinue the drug.

The following adverse reactions have been observed, but there has not been enough systematic collection of data to support an estimate of their frequency. Consequently the reactions are categorized by organ system and are listed in decreasing order of severity and not frequency.

Body as a Whole: Headache, cramping, weakness.

Cardiovascular System: Orthostatic hypotension (may be potentiated by alcohol, barbiturates, or narcotics).

Digestive System: Pancreatitis, jaundice (intrahepatic cholestatic), sialadenitis, vomiting, diarrhea, nausea, gastric irritation, constipation, anorexia.

Hemic and Lymphatic System: Aplastic anemia, hemolytic anemia, agranulocytosis, leukopenia, thrombocytopenia.

Hypersensitivity Reactions: Anaphylactic reactions, necrotizing angiitis (vasculitis, cutaneous vasculitis), Stevens-Johnson syndrome, respiratory distress including pneumonitis and pulmonary edema, fever, purpura, urticaria, rash, photosensitivity.

Metabolic and Nutritional Disorders: Hyperglycemia, hyperuricemia, electrolyte imbalance (see PRECAUTIONS section), hypercalcemia.

Nervous System: Vertigo, dizziness, paresthesias, muscle spasm, restlessness.

Special Senses: Transient blurred vision, xanthopsia.

Urogenital System: Glycosuria.

OVERDOSAGE

Symptoms of overdosage include electrolyte imbalance and signs of potassium deficiency such as confusion, dizziness, muscular weakness, and gastrointestinal disturbances. General supportive measures including replacement of fluids and electrolytes may be indicated in treatment of overdosage.

DOSAGE AND ADMINISTRATION

ENDURON (methyclothiazide) is administered orally. Therapy should be individualized according to patient response. This therapy should be titrated to gain maximal therapeutic response as well as the minimal dose possible to maintain that therapeutic response.

For edematous conditions: The usual adult dose ranges from 2.5 to 10 mg once daily. Maximum effective single dose is 10 mg; larger single doses do not accomplish greater diuresis, and are not recommended.

For the treatment of hypertension: The usual adult dose ranges from 2.5 to 5 mg once daily.

If control of blood pressure is not satisfactory after 8 to 12 weeks of therapy with 5 mg once daily, another antihypertensive drug should be added. Increasing the dosage of methyclothiazide will usually not result in further lowering of blood pressure.

Methyclothiazide may be either employed alone for mild to moderate hypertension or concurrently with other antihypertensive drugs in the management of more severe forms of hypertension. Combined therapy may provide adequate control of hypertension with lower dosage of the component drugs and fewer or less severe side effects. An enhanced response frequently follows its concurrent administration with Harmonyl® (deserpidine) so that dosage of both drugs may be reduced.

When other antihypertensive agents are to be added to the regimen, this should be accomplished gradually. Ganglionic blocking agents should be given at only half the usual dose since their effect is potentiated by pretreatment with ENDURON tablets.

HOW SUPPLIED

ENDURON (methyclothiazide tablets, USP) is provided in two dosage sizes as monogrammed, grooved, square-shaped tablets:

2.5 mg, orange-colored:
- bottles of 100 (**NDC** 0074-6827-01),
- bottles of 1000 (**NDC** 0074-6827-02).

5 mg, salmon-colored:
- bottles of 100 (**NDC** 0074-6812-01),
- bottles of 1000 (**NDC** 0074-6812-02),
- bottles of 5000 (**NDC** 0074-6812-03),
- Abbo-Pac® unit dose packages of 100 (**NDC** 0074-6812-10).

Dispense in a USP tight container.
Recommended storage: Store below 86°F (30°C).
Ref. 03-4404-R9

ERY-PED® ℞
[erē ′ped]
(erythromycin ethylsuccinate, USP)

DESCRIPTION

Erythromycin is produced by a strain of *Streptomyces erythraeus* and belongs to the macrolide group of antibiotics. It is basic and readily forms salts with acids. The base, the stearate salt, and the esters are poorly soluble in water. Erythromycin ethylsuccinate is an ester of erythromycin suitable for oral administration.

EryPed 200 and EryPed Drops (erythromycin ethylsuccinate for oral suspension) when reconstituted with water, forms a suspension containing erythromycin ethylsuccinate equivalent to 200 mg erythromycin per 5 mL (teaspoonful) or 100 mg per 2.5 mL (dropperful) with an appealing fruit flavor. EryPed 400 when reconstituted with water, forms a suspension containing erythromycin ethylsuccinate equivalent to 400 mg of erythromycin per 5 mL (teaspoonful) with an appealing banana flavor. After mixing, EryPed must be stored below 77°F (25°C) and used within 35 days; refrigeration is not required.

Fruit-flavored EryPed Chewable tablets are easily ingested and are particularly acceptable for the administration of antibiotic medication to young children who are unable to swallow regular tablets or in whom persuasion of a pleasant taste insures cooperation. Each chewable tablet contains the equivalent of 200 mg of erythromycin activity and is scored for division into half-dose (100 mg) portions.

These products are intended primarily for pediatric use but can also be used in adults.

Inactive Ingredients: EryPed 200, EryPed 400 and EryPed Drops: Caramel, polysorbate, sodium citrate, sucrose, xanthan gum and artificial flavors.

EryPed Chewable Tablets: Citric acid, confectioner's sugar (contains corn starch), magnesium aluminum silicate, magnesium stearate, sodium carboxymethylcellulose, sodium citrate and artificial flavor.

ACTIONS

Microbiology

Biochemical tests demonstrate that erythromycin inhibits protein synthesis of the pathogen without directly affecting nucleic acid synthesis. Antagonism has been demonstrated between clindamycin and erythromycin.

NOTE: Many strains of *Hemophilus influenzae* are resistant to erythromycin alone, but are susceptible to erythromycin and sulfonamides together. Staphylococci resistant to erythromycin may emerge during a course of erythromycin therapy. Culture and susceptibility testing should be performed.

Disc Susceptibility Tests: Quantitative methods that require measurement of zone diameters give the most precise estimates of antibiotic susceptibility. One recommended procedure (21 CFR section 460.1) uses erythromycin class discs for testing susceptibility; interpretations correlate zone diameters of this disc test with MIC values for erythromycin. With this procedure, a report from the laboratory of "susceptible" indicates that the infecting organism is likely to respond to therapy. A report of "resistant" indicates that the infective organism is not likely to respond to therapy. A report of "intermediate susceptibility" suggests that the organism would be susceptible if higher doses were used.

Clinical Pharmacology

Erythromycin binds to the 50 S ribosomal subunits of susceptible bacteria and suppresses protein synthesis.

Orally administered erythromycin ethylsuccinate suspension is readily and reliably absorbed under both fasting and nonfasting conditions.

Erythromycin diffuses readily into most body fluids. Only low concentrations are normally achieved in the spinal fluid, but passage of the drug across the blood-brain barrier increases in meningitis. In the presence of normal hepatic function, erythromycin is concentrated in the liver and excreted in the bile; the effect of hepatic dysfunction on excretion of erythromycin by the liver into the bile is not known. Less than 5 percent of the orally administered dose of erythromycin is excreted in active form in the urine.

Erythromycin crosses the placental barrier and is excreted in breast milk.

INDICATIONS

Streptococcus pyogenes (Group A beta-hemolytic streptococcus): Upper and lower respiratory tract, skin, and soft tissue infections of mild to moderate severity.

Injectable benzathine penicillin G is considered by the American Heart Association to be the drug of choice in the treatment and prevention of streptococcal pharyngitis and in long-term prophylaxis of rheumatic fever.

When oral medication is preferred for treatment of the above conditions, penicillin G, V, or erythromycin are alternate drugs of choice.

When oral medication is given, the importance of strict adherence by the patient to the prescribed dosage regimen must be stressed. A therapeutic dose should be administered for at least 10 days.

Alpha-hemolytic streptococci (viridans group): Although no controlled clinical efficacy trials have been conducted, oral erythromycin has been suggested by the American Heart Association and American Dental Association for use in a regimen for prophylaxis against bacterial endocarditis in patients hypersensitive to penicillin who have congenital heart disease, or rheumatic or other acquired valvular heart disease when they undergo dental procedures and surgical procedures of the upper respiratory tract.[1] Erythromycin is not suitable prior to genitourinary or gastrointestinal tract surgery. NOTE: When selecting antibiotics for the prevention of bacterial endocarditis the physician or dentist should read the full joint statement of the American Heart Association and the American Dental Association.[1]

Staphylococcus aureus: Acute infections of skin and soft tissue of mild to moderate severity. Resistant organisms may emerge during treatment.

Streptococcus pneumoniae (Diplococcus pneumoniae): Upper respiratory tract infections (e.g., otitis media, pharyngitis) and lower respiratory tract infections (e.g., pneumonia) of mild to moderate degree.

Mycoplasma pneumoniae (Eaton agent, PPLO): For respiratory infections due to this organism.

Hemophilus influenzae: For upper respiratory tract infections of mild to moderate severity when used concomitantly with adequate doses of sulfonamides. (See sulfonamide labeling for appropriate prescribing information). The concomitant use of the sulfonamides is necessary since not all strains of *Hemophilus influenzae* are susceptible to erythromycin at the concentrations of the antibiotic achieved with usual therapeutic doses.

Chlamydia trachomatis: For the treatment of urethritis in adult males due to *Chlamydia trachomatis.*

Ureaplasma urealyticum: For the treatment of urethritis in adult males due to *Ureaplasma urealyticum.*

Treponema pallidum: Erythromycin is an alternate choice of treatment for primary syphilis in patients allergic to the penicillins. In treatment of primary syphilis, spinal fluid examinations should be done before treatment and as part of follow-up after therapy.

Corynebacterium diphtheriae: As an adjunct to antitoxin, to prevent establishment of carriers, and to eradicate the organism in carriers.

Corynebacterium minutissimum: For the treatment of erythrasma.

Entamoeba histolytica: In the treatment of intestinal amebiasis only. Extraenteric amebiasis requires treatment with other agents.

Listeria monocytogenes: Infections due to this organism.

Bordetella pertussis: Erythromycin is effective in eliminating the organism from the nasopharynx of infected individuals, rendering them non-infectious. Some clinical studies suggest that erythromycin may be helpful in the prophylaxis of pertussis in exposed susceptible individuals.

Legionnaires' Disease: Although no controlled clinical efficacy studies have been conducted, *in vitro* and limited preliminary clinical data suggest that erythromycin may be effective in treating Legionnaires' Disease.

CONTRAINDICATIONS

Erythromycin is contraindicated in patients with known hypersensitivity to this antibiotic.

Continued on next page

Abbott Laboratories—Cont.

WARNINGS
There have been reports of hepatic dysfunction with or without jaundice, occurring in patients receiving oral erythromycin products.

PRECAUTIONS
General: Erythromycin is principally excreted by the liver. Caution should be exercised when erythromycin is administered to patients with impaired hepatic function. (See "Clinical Pharmacology" and "Warnings" sections).

Prolonged or repeated use of erythromycin may result in an overgrowth of nonsusceptible bacteria or fungi. If superinfection occurs, erythromycin should be discontinued and appropriate therapy instituted.

When indicated, incision and drainage or other surgical procedures should be performed in conjunction with antibiotic therapy.

Laboratory Tests: Erythromycin interferes with the fluorometric determination of urinary catecholamines.

Drug Interactions: Erythromycin use in patients who are receiving high doses of theophylline may be associated with an increase in serum theophylline levels and potential theophylline toxicity. In case of theophylline toxicity and/or elevated serum theophylline levels, the dose of theophylline should be reduced while the patient is receiving concomitant erythromycin therapy.

Concomitant administration of erythromycin and digoxin has been reported to result in elevated digoxin serum levels.

There have been reports of increased anticoagulant effects when erythromycin and oral anticoagulants were used concomitantly.

Concurrent use of erythromycin and ergotamine or dihydroergotamine has been associated in some patients with acute ergot toxicity characterized by severe peripheral vasospasm and dysesthesia.

Erythromycin has been reported to decrease the clearance of triazolam and thus may increase the pharmacologic effect of triazolam.

The use of erythromycin in patients concurrently taking drugs metabolized by the cytochrome P450 system may be associated with elevations in serum erythromycin with carbamazepine, cyclosporine, hexobarbital and phenytoin. Serum concentrations of drugs metabolized by the cytochrome P450 system should be monitored closely in patients concurrently receiving erythromycin.

Troleandomycin significantly alters the metabolism of terfenadine when taken concomitantly; therefore, observe caution when erythromycin and terfenadine are used concurrently.

Patients receiving concomitant lovastatin and erythromycin should be carefully monitored; cases of rhabdomyolysis have been reported in seriously ill patients.

Carcinogenesis, Mutagenesis, Impairment of Fertility: Long-term (2-year) oral studies conducted in rats with erythromycin base did not provide evidence of tumorigenicity. Mutagenicity studies have not been conducted. There was no apparent effect on male or female fertility in rats fed erythromycin (base) at levels up to 0.25 percent of diet.

Pregnancy: Pregnancy Category B: There is no evidence of teratogenicity or any other adverse effect on reproduction in female rats fed erythromycin base (up to 0.25 percent of diet) prior to and during mating, during gestation, and through weaning of two successive litters. There are, however, no adequate and well-controlled studies in pregnant women. Because animal reproduction studies are not always predictive of human response, this drug should be used during pregnancy only if clearly needed. Erythromycin has been reported to cross the placental barrier in humans, but fetal plasma levels are generally low.

Labor and Delivery: The effect of erythromycin on labor and delivery is unknown.

Nursing Mothers: Erythromycin is excreted in breast milk, therefore, caution should be exercised when erythromycin is administered to a nursing woman.

Pediatric Use: See "Indications and Usage" and "Dosage and Administration" sections.

ADVERSE REACTIONS
The most frequent side effects of oral erythromycin preparations are gastrointestinal and are dose-related. They include nausea, vomiting, abdominal pain, diarrhea and anorexia. Symptoms of hepatic dysfunction and/or abnormal liver function test results may occur (see "Warnings" section).

Pseudo-membranous colitis has been rarely reported in association with erythromycin therapy.

There have been isolated reports of transient central nervous system side effects including confusion, hallucinations, seizures, and vertigo; however, a cause and effect relationship has not been established.

Occasional case reports of cardiac arrhythmias such as ventricular tachycardia have been documented in patients receiving erythromycin therapy. There have been isolated reports of other cardiovascular symptoms such as chest pain, dizziness, and palpitations; however, a cause and effect relationship has not been established.

Allergic reactions ranging from urticaria and mild skin eruptions to anaphylaxis have occurred.

There have been isolated reports of reversible hearing loss occurring chiefly in patients with renal insufficiency and in patients receiving high doses of erythromycin.

OVERDOSAGE
In case of overdosage, erythromycin should be discontinued. Overdosage should be handled with the prompt elimination of unabsorbed drug and all other appropriate measures.

Erythromycin is not removed by peritoneal dialysis or hemodialysis.

DOSAGE AND ADMINISTRATION
EryPed (erythromycin ethylsuccinate) oral suspensions and chewable tablets may be administered without regard to meals.

Children: Age, weight, and severity of the infection are important factors in determining the proper dosage. In mild to moderate infections, the usual dosage of erythromycin ethylsuccinate for children is 30 to 50 mg/kg/day in equally divided doses every 6 hours. For more severe infections this dosage may be doubled. If twice-a-day dosage is desired, one-half of the total daily dose may be given every 12 hours. Doses may also be given three times daily by administering one-third of the total daily dose every 8 hours.

The following dosage schedule is suggested for mild to moderate infections:

Body Weight	Total Daily Dose
Under 10 lbs	30-50 mg/kg/day 15-25 mg/lb/day
10 to 15 lbs	200 mg
16 to 25 lbs	400 mg
26 to 50 lbs	800 mg
51 to 100 lbs	1200 mg
over 100 lbs	1600 mg

Adults: 400 mg erythromycin ethylsuccinate every 6 hours is the usual dose. Dosage may be increased up to 4 g per day according to the severity of the infection. If twice-a-day dosage is desired, one-half of the total daily dose may be given every 12 hours. Doses may also be given three times daily by administering one-third of the total daily dose every 8 hours.

For adult dosage calculation, use a ratio of 400 mg of erythromycin activity as the ethylsuccinate to 250 mg of erythromycin activity as the stearate, base or estolate.

In the treatment of streptococcal infections, a therapeutic dosage of erythromycin ethylsuccinate should be administered for at least 10 days. In continuous prophylaxis against recurrences of streptococcal infections in persons with a history of rheumatic heart disease, the usual dosage is 400 mg twice a day.

For prophylaxis against bacterial endocarditis[1] in patients with congenital heart disease, or rheumatic or other acquired valvular heart disease when undergoing dental procedures or surgical procedures of the upper respiratory tract, give 1.6 g (20 mg/kg for children) orally 1 1/2 to 2 hours before the procedure, and then, 800 mg (10 mg/kg for children) orally every 6 hours for 8 doses.

For treatment of urethritis due to *C. trachomatis* or *U. urealyticum:* 800 mg three times a day for 7 days.

For treatment of primary syphilis: Adults: 48 to 64 g given in divided doses over a period of 10 to 15 days.

For intestinal amebiasis: Adults: 400 mg four times daily for 10 to 14 days. Children: 30 to 50 mg/kg/day in divided doses for 10 to 14 days.

For use in pertussis: Although optimal dosage and duration have not been established, doses of erythromycin utilized in reported clinical studies were 40 to 50 mg/kg/day, given in divided doses for 5 to 14 days.

For treatment of Legionnaires' Disease: Although optimal doses have not been established, doses utilized in reported clinical data were 1.6 to 4 g daily in divided doses.

HOW SUPPLIED
EryPed 200 (erythromycin ethylsuccinate for oral suspension, USP) is supplied in bottles of 100 mL (**NDC** 0074-6302-13), 200 mL (**NDC** 0074-6302-53), and 5 mL unit dose in ABBO-PAC® packages (**NDC** 0074-6302-05). Each 5 mL (teaspoonful) of reconstituted suspension contains activity equivalent to 200 mg erythromycin.

EryPed 400 (erythromycin ethylsuccinate for oral suspension, USP) is supplied in bottles of 60 mL (**NDC** 0074-6305-60), 100 mL (**NDC** 0074-6305-13), 200 mL (**NDC** 0074-6305-53), and 5 mL unit dose in ABBO-PAC packages (**NDC** 0074-6305-05). Each 5 mL (teaspoonful) of reconstituted suspension contains activity equivalent to 400 mg erythromycin.

EryPed Drops (erythromycin ethylsuccinate for oral suspension) is supplied in 50 mL bottles (**NDC** 0074-6303-50). Each 2.5 mL dropperful (1/2 teaspoonful) of reconstituted suspension contains activity equivalent to 100 mg of erythromycin.

Recommended Storage: Before mixing, store EryPed granules below 86°F (30°C).

After reconstitution, EryPed must be stored below 77°F (25°C) and used within 35 days; refrigeration not required.

EryPed Chewable (erythromycin ethylsuccinate tablets, USP) are fruit-flavored wafers containing activity equivalent to 200 mg of erythromycin and are available in packages of 40 (**NDC** 0074-6314-40). Each wafer is individually sealed in a blister package.

Recommended Storage: Store EryPed Chewable below 86°F (30°C).

Reference

1. American Heart Association. 1977. Prevention of bacterial endocarditis. Circulation 56:139A-143A.

Ref. 03-2119-R7

Shown in Product Identification Guide, page 303

ERY-TAB® ℞
[*ērē'tab*]
(erythromycin delayed-release tablets, USP)
Enteric-Coated

DESCRIPTION
Erythromycin is produced by a strain of *Streptomyces erythraeus* and belongs to the macrolide group of antibiotics. It is basic and readily forms salts with acids. The base is white to off-white crystals or powder slightly soluble in water, soluble in alcohol, in chloroform, and in ether. ERY-TAB (erythromycin delayed-release tablets) is specially enteric-coated to protect the contents from the inactivating effects of gastric acidity and to permit efficient absorption of the antibiotic in the small intestine.

ERY-TAB is available in three dosage strengths, each tablet containing either 250 mg, 333 mg, or 500 mg of erythromycin as the free base.

Inactive Ingredients: 250 mg tablet: cellulosic polymers, corn starch, diacetylated monoglycerides, D&C red No. 30, iron oxide, magnesium hydroxide, magnesium stearate, sodium starch glycolate, titanium dioxide and vanillin.

333 mg tablet: cellulosic polymers, diacetylated monoglycerides, FD&C blue No. 1, magnesium stearate, microcrystalline cellulose, povidone, sodium citrate, soybean derivatives, talc, titanium dioxide and vanillin.

500 mg tablet: cellulosic polymers, diacetylated monoglycerides, FD&C red No. 40, iron oxide, magnesium stearate, microcrystalline cellulose, povidone, sodium citrate, soybean derivatives, talc, titanium dioxide and vanillin.

ACTIONS
The mode of action of erythromycin is inhibition of protein synthesis without affecting nucleic acid synthesis. Resistance to erythromycin of some strains of *Hemophilus influenzae* and staphylococci has been demonstrated. Culture and susceptibility testing should be done. If the Kirby-Bauer method of disc susceptibility is used, a 15 mcg erythromycin disc should give a zone diameter of at least 18 mm when tested against an erythromycin susceptible organism.

Bioavailability data are available from Abbott Laboratories, Dept. 355.

ERY-TAB is well absorbed and may be given without regard to meals.

After absorption, erythromycin diffuses readily into most body fluids. In the absence of meningeal inflammation, low concentrations are normally achieved in the spinal fluid but passage of the drug across the blood-brain barrier increases in meningitis. In the presence of normal hepatic function, erythromycin is concentrated in the liver and excreted in the bile; the effect of hepatic dysfunction on excretion of erythromycin by the liver into the bile is not known. After oral administration, less than 5 percent of the activity of the administered dose can be recovered in the urine.

Erythromycin crosses the placental barrier but fetal plasma levels are low.

INDICATIONS
Streptococcus pyogenes (Group A beta hemolytic streptococcus): For upper and lower respiratory tract, skin, and soft tissue infections of mild to moderate severity.

Injectable benzathine penicillin G is considered by the American Heart Association to be the drug of choice in the treatment and prevention of streptococcal pharyngitis and in long-term prophylaxis of rheumatic fever.

When oral medication is preferred for treatment of the above conditions, penicillin G, V, or erythromycin are alternate drugs of choice.

When oral medication is given, the importance of strict adherence by the patient to the prescribed dosage regimen must be stressed. A therapeutic dose should be administered for at least 10 days.

Alpha-hemolytic streptococci (viridans group): Although no controlled clinical efficacy trials have been conducted, oral erythromycin has been suggested by the American Heart

Association and American Dental Association for use in a regimen for prophylaxis against bacterial endocarditis in patients hypersensitive to penicillin who have congenital heart disease, or rheumatic or other acquired valvular heart disease when they undergo dental procedures and surgical procedures of the upper respiratory tract.[1] Erythromycin is not suitable prior to genitourinary or gastrointestinal tract surgery. NOTE: When selecting antibiotics for the prevention of bacterial endocarditis the physician or dentist should read the full joint statement of the American Heart Association and the American Dental Association.[1]

Staphylococcus aureus: For acute infections of skin and soft tissue of mild to moderate severity. Resistant organisms may emerge during treatment.

Streptococcus pneumoniae (Diplococcus pneumoniae): For upper respiratory tract infections (e.g., otitis media, pharyngitis) and lower respiratory tract infection (e.g., pneumonia) of mild to moderate degree.

Mycoplasma pneumoniae (Eaton agent, PPLO): For respiratory infections due to this organism.

Hemophilus influenzae: For upper respiratory tract infections of mild to moderate severity when used concomitantly with adequate doses of sulfonamides. Not all strains of this organism are susceptible at the erythromycin concentrations ordinarily achieved (see appropriate sulfonamide labeling for prescribing information).

Chlamydia trachomatis: Erythromycin is indicated for treatment of the following infections caused by *Chlamydia trachomatis:* conjunctivitis of the newborn, pneumonia of infancy and urogenital infections during pregnancy. When tetracyclines are contraindicated or not tolerated, erythromycin is indicated for the treatment of uncomplicated urethral, endocervical, or rectal infections in adults due to *Chlamydia trachomatis.*[2]

Treponema pallidum: Erythromycin is an alternate choice of treatment for primary syphilis in patients allergic to the penicillins. In treatment of primary syphilis, spinal fluid examinations should be done before treatment and as part of follow-up after therapy.

Corynebacterium diphtheriae and C. minutissimum: As an adjunct to antitoxin, to prevent establishment of carriers, and to eradicate the organism in carriers.
In the treatment of erythrasma.

Entamoeba histolytica: In the treatment of intestinal amebiasis only. Extra-enteric amebiasis requires treatment with other agents.

Listeria monocytogenes: Infections due to this organism.

Neisseria gonorrhoeae: Erythrocin® Lactobionate-I.V. (erythromycin lactobionate for injection, USP) in conjunction with erythromycin base orally, as an alternative drug in treatment of acute pelvic inflammatory disease caused by *N. gonorrhoeae* in female patients with a history of sensitivity to penicillin. Before treatment of gonorrhea, patients who are suspected of also having syphilis should have a microscopic examination for *T. pallidum* (by immunofluorescence or darkfield) before receiving erythromycin, and monthly serologic tests for a minimum of 4 months.

Bordetella pertussis: Erythromycin is effective in eliminating the organism from the nasopharynx of infected individuals, rendering them non-infectious. Some clinical studies suggest that erythromycin may be helpful in the prophylaxis of pertussis in exposed susceptible individuals.

Legionnaires' Disease: Although no controlled clinical efficacy studies have been conducted, *in vitro* and limited preliminary clinical data suggest that erythromycin can be effective in treating Legionnaires' Disease.

CONTRAINDICATIONS

Erythromycin is contraindicated in patients with known hypersensitivity to this antibiotic.

WARNINGS

There have been reports of hepatic dysfunction with or without jaundice, occurring in patients receiving oral erythromycin products.

PRECAUTIONS

General: Erythromycin is principally excreted by the liver. Caution should be exercised when erythromycin is administered to patients with impaired hepatic function. (See "Clinical Pharmacology" and "Warnings" sections).

Prolonged or repeated use of erythromycin may result in an overgrowth of nonsusceptible bacteria or fungi. If superinfection occurs, erythromycin should be discontinued and appropriate therapy instituted.

When indicated, incision and drainage or other surgical procedures should be performed in conjunction with antibiotic therapy.

Laboratory Tests: Erythromycin interferes with the fluorometric determination of urinary catecholamines.

Drug Interactions: Erythromycin use in patients who are receiving high doses of theophylline may be associated with an increase in serum theophylline levels and potential theophylline toxicity. In case of theophylline toxicity and/or elevated serum theophylline levels, the dose of theophylline should be reduced while the patient is receiving concomitant erythromycin therapy.

Concomitant administration of erythromycin and digoxin has been reported to result in elevated digoxin serum levels. There have been reports of increased anticoagulant effects when erythromycin and oral anticoagulants were used concomitantly.

Concurrent use of erythromycin and ergotamine or dihydroergotamine has been associated in some patients with acute ergot toxicity characterized by severe peripheral vasospasm and dysesthesia.

Erythromycin has been reported to decrease the clearance of triazolam and thus may increase the pharmacologic effect of triazolam.

The use of erythromycin in patients concurrently taking drugs metabolized by the cytochrome P450 system may be associated with elevations in serum erythromycin with carbamazepine, cyclosporine, hexobarbital and phenytoin. Serum concentrations of drugs metabolized by the cytochrome P450 system should be monitored closely in patients concurrently receiving erythromycin.

Troleandomycin significantly alters the metabolism of terfenadine when taken concomitantly; therefore, observe caution when erythromycin and terfenadine are used concurrently.

Patients receiving concomitant lovastatin and erythromycin should be carefully monitored; cases of rhabdomyolysis have been reported in seriously ill patients.

Carcinogenesis, Mutagenesis, Impairment of Fertility: Long-term (2-year) oral studies conducted in rats with erythromycin base did not provide evidence of tumorigenicity. Mutagenicity studies have not been conducted. There was no apparent effect on male or female fertility in rats fed erythromycin (base) at levels up to 0.25 percent of diet.

Pregnancy: Pregnancy Category B: There is no evidence of teratogenicity or any other adverse effect on reproduction in female rats fed erythromycin base (up to 0.25 percent of diet) prior to and during mating, during gestation, and through weaning of two successive litters. There are, however, no adequate and well-controlled studies in pregnant women. Because animal reproduction studies are not always predictive of human response, this drug should be used during pregnancy only if clearly needed. Erythromycin has been reported to cross the placental barrier in humans, but fetal plasma levels are generally low.

Labor and Delivery: The effect of erythromycin on labor and delivery is unknown.

Nursing Mothers: Erythromycin is excreted in breast milk, therefore, caution should be exercised when erythromycin is administered to a nursing woman.

Pediatric Use: See "Indications and Usage" and "Dosage and Administration" sections.

ADVERSE REACTIONS

The most frequent side effects of oral erythromycin preparations are gastrointestinal and are dose-related. They include nausea, vomiting, abdominal pain, diarrhea and anorexia. Symptoms of hepatic dysfunction and/or abnormal liver function test results may occur (see "Warnings" section). Pseudomembranous colitis has been rarely reported in association with erythromycin therapy.

There have been isolated reports of transient central nervous system side effects including confusion, hallucinations, seizures, and vertigo; however, a cause and effect relationship has not been established.

Occasional case reports of cardiac arrhythmias such as ventricular tachycardia have been documented in patients receiving erythromycin therapy. There have been isolated reports of other cardiovascular symptoms such as chest pain, dizziness, and palpitations; however, a cause and effect relationship has not been established.

Allergic reactions ranging from urticaria and mild skin eruptions to anaphylaxis have occurred.

There have been isolated reports of reversible hearing loss occurring chiefly in patients with renal insufficiency and in patients receiving high doses of erythromycin.

OVERDOSAGE

In case of overdosage, erythromycin should be discontinued. Overdosage should be handled with the prompt elimination of unabsorbed drug and all other appropriate measures. Erythromycin is not removed by peritoneal dialysis or hemodialysis.

DOSAGE AND ADMINISTRATION

ERY-TAB (erythromycin delayed-release tablets) is well absorbed and may be given without regard to meals.

Adults: The usual dose is 250 mg four times daily in equally spaced doses. The 333 mg tablet is recommended if dosage is desired every 8 hours. If twice-a-day dosage is desired, the recommended dose is 500 mg every 12 hours.

Dosage may be increased up to 4 or more grams per day according to the severity of the infection. Twice-a-day dosing is not recommended when doses larger than 1 gram daily are administered.

Children: Age, weight, and severity of the infection are important factors in determining the proper dosage. 30 to 50 mg/kg/day, in divided doses, is the usual dose. For more severe infections, this dose may be doubled.

In the treatment of streptococcal infections, a therapeutic dosage of erythromycin should be administered for at least 10 days. In continuous prophylaxis of streptococcal infections in persons with a history of rheumatic heart disease, the dose is 250 mg twice a day.

For prophylaxis against bacterial endocarditis[1] in patients with congenital heart disease, or rheumatic or other acquired valvular heart disease when undergoing dental procedures or surgical procedures of the upper respiratory tract, give 1 g (20 mg/kg for children) orally $1^{1}/_{2}$ to 2 hours before the procedure, and then, 500 mg (10 mg/kg in children) orally every 6 hours for 8 doses.

For conjunctivitis of the newborn caused by *Chlamydia trachomatis:* Oral erythromycin suspension 50 mg/kg/day in 4 divided doses for at least 2 weeks.[2]

For pneumonia of infancy caused by *Chlamydia trachomatis:* Although the optimal duration of therapy has not been established, the recommended therapy is oral erythromycin suspension 50 mg/kg/day in 4 divided doses for at least 3 weeks.[2]

For urogenital infections during pregnancy due to *Chlamydia trachomatis:* Although the optimal dose and duration of therapy have not been established, the suggested treatment is erythromycin 500 mg, by mouth, 4 times a day for at least 7 days. For women who cannot tolerate this regimen, a decreased dose of 250 mg, by mouth, 4 times a day should be used for at least 14 days.[2]

For adults with uncomplicated urethral, endocervical, or rectal infections caused by *Chlamydia trachomatis* in whom tetracyclines are contraindicated or not tolerated: 500 mg, by mouth, 4 times a day for at least 7 days.[2]

For treatment of primary syphilis: 30 to 40 grams given in divided doses over a period of 10 to 15 days.

For treatment of acute pelvic inflammatory disease caused by *N. gonorrhoeae:* After initial treatment with Erythrocin® Lactobionate-I.V. (erythromycin lactobionate for injection, USP) 500 mg every 6 hours for 3 days, the oral dosage recommendation is 250 mg every 6 hours for 7 days.

For dysenteric amebiasis: 250 mg four times daily for 10 to 14 days, for adults; 30 to 50 mg/kg/day in divided doses for 10 to 14 days, for children.

For use in pertussis: Although optimal dosage and duration have not been established, doses of erythromycin utilized in reported clinical studies were 40 to 50 mg/kg/day, given in divided doses for 5 to 14 days.

For treatment of Legionnaires' Disease: Although optimal doses have not been established, doses utilized in reported clinical data were 1 to 4 grams erythromycin base daily in divided doses.

HOW SUPPLIED

ERY-TAB (erythromycin delayed-release tablets, USP), 250 mg, is supplied as pink tablets in bottles of 100 (**NDC** 0074-6304-13), bottles of 500 (**NDC** 0074-6304-53), and Abbo-Pac® unit dose packages of 100 (**NDC** 0074-6304-11).

ERY-TAB, 333 mg, is supplied as white tablets in bottles of 100 (**NDC** 0074-6320-13), bottles of 500 (**NDC** 0074-6320-53), and Abbo-Pac® unit dose packages of 100 (**NDC** 0074-6320-11).

ERY-TAB, 500 mg, is supplied as pink tablets in bottles of 100 (**NDC** 0074-6321-13) and Abbo-Pac® unit dose packages of 100 (**NDC** 0074-6321-11).

Recommended Storage: Store below 86°F (30°C).

REFERENCES

1. American Heart Association, 1977. Prevention of bacterial endocarditis, Circulation 56: 139A-143A.
2. CDC Sexually Transmitted Diseases Treatment Guidelines 1982.

333 mg and 500 mg tablets—U.S. Pat. No. 4,340,582.
Ref. 01-2526-R6
Shown in Product Identification Guide, page 303

E.E.S.® ℞
[ē-ē-s]
(erythromycin ethylsuccinate)

DESCRIPTION

Erythromycin is produced by a strain of *Streptomyces erythraeus* and belongs to the macrolide group of antibiotics. It is basic and readily forms salts with acids. The base, the stearate salt, and the esters are poorly soluble in water. Erythromycin ethylsuccinate is an ester of erythromycin suitable for oral administration.

Erythromycin ethylsuccinate is known chemically as erythromycin 2'-(ethylsuccinate). The molecular formula is $C_{43}H_{75}NO_{16}$ and the molecular weight is 862.06. The structural formula is:
[See chemical structure at top of next column.]

Continued on next page

Abbott Laboratories—Cont.

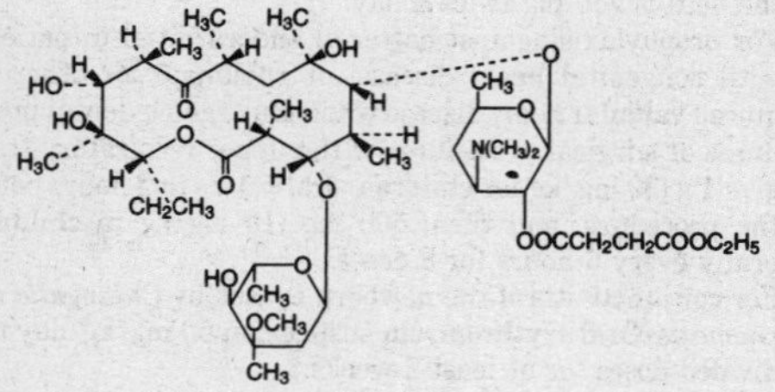

The granules are intended for reconstitution with water. When reconstituted, they are palatable cherry-flavored suspensions.

The pleasant tasting, fruit-flavored liquids are supplied ready for oral administration.

Granules and ready-made suspensions are intended primarily for pediatric use but can also be used in adults.

E.E.S. 400® Filmtab® Tablets: Each tablet contains erythromycin ethylsuccinate equivalent to 400 mg of erythromycin.

The Filmtab® tablets are intended primarily for adults or older children.

Inactive Ingredients: E.E.S. 200 Liquid: FD&C Red No. 40, methylparaben, polysorbate 60, propylparaben, sodium citrate, sucrose, water, xanthan gum and natural and artificial flavors.

E.E.S. 400 Liquid: D&C Yellow No. 10, FD&C Yellow No. 6, methylparaben, polysorbate 60, propylparaben, sodium citrate, sucrose, water, xanthan gum and natural and artificial flavors.

E.E.S. Granules: Citric acid, FD&C Red No. 3, magnesium aluminum silicate, sodium carboxymethylcellulose, sodium citrate, sucrose and artificial flavor.

E.E.S. 400 Filmtab Tablets: Cellulosic polymers, confectioner's sugar (contains corn starch), corn starch, D&C Red No. 30, D&C Yellow No. 10, FD&C Red No. 40, magnesium stearate, polacrilin potassium, polyethylene glycol, propylene glycol, sodium citrate, sorbic acid, and titanium dioxide.

ACTIONS

Microbiology: Biochemical tests demonstrate that erythromycin inhibits protein synthesis of the pathogen without directly affecting nucleic acid synthesis. Antagonism has been demonstrated between clindamycin and erythromycin.

NOTE: Many strains of *Hemophilus influenzae* are resistant to erythromycin alone, but are susceptible to erythromycin and sulfonamides together. Staphylococci resistant to erythromycin may emerge during a course of erythromycin therapy. Culture and susceptibility testing should be performed.

Disc Susceptibility Tests: Quantitative methods that require measurement of zone diameters give the most precise estimates of antibiotic susceptibility. One recommended procedure (21 CFR section 460.1) uses erythromycin class discs for testing susceptibility; interpretations correlate zone diameters of this disc test with MIC values for erythromycin. With this procedure, a report from the laboratory of "susceptible" indicates that the infecting organism is likely to respond to therapy. A report of "resistant" indicates that the infective organism is not likely to respond to therapy. A report of "intermediate susceptibility" suggests that the organism would be susceptible if higher doses were used.

Clinical Pharmacology: Erythromycin binds to the 50 S ribosomal subunits of susceptible bacteria and suppresses protein synthesis.

Orally administered erythromycin ethylsuccinate suspensions and Filmtab tablets are readily and reliably absorbed. Comparable serum levels of erythromycin are achieved in the fasting and nonfasting states.

Erythromycin diffuses readily into most body fluids. Only low concentrations are normally achieved in the spinal fluid, but passage of the drug across the blood-brain barrier increases in meningitis. In the presence of normal hepatic function, erythromycin is concentrated in the liver and excreted in the bile; the effect of hepatic dysfunction on excretion of erythromycin by the liver into the bile is not known. Less than 5 percent of the orally administered dose of erythromycin is excreted in active form in the urine.

Erythromycin crosses the placental barrier and is excreted in breast milk.

INDICATIONS

Streptococcus pyogenes (Group A beta-hemolytic streptococcus): Upper and lower respiratory tract, skin, and soft tissue infections of mild to moderate severity.

Injectable benzathine penicillin G is considered by the American Heart Association to be the drug of choice in the treatment and prevention of streptococcal pharyngitis and in long-term prophylaxis of rheumatic fever.

When oral medication is preferred for treatment of the above conditions, penicillin G, V, or erythromycin are alternate drugs of choice.

When oral medication is given, the importance of strict adherence by the patient to the prescribed dosage regimen must be stressed. A therapeutic dose should be administered for at least 10 days.

Alpha-hemolytic streptococci (viridans group): Although no controlled clinical efficacy trials have been conducted, oral erythromycin has been suggested by the American Heart Association and American Dental Association for use in a regimen for prophylaxis against bacterial endocarditis in patients hypersensitive to penicillin who have congenital heart disease, or rheumatic or other acquired valvular heart disease when they undergo dental procedures and surgical procedures of the upper respiratory tract.[1] Erythromycin is not suitable prior to genitourinary or gastrointestinal tract surgery. NOTE: When selecting antibiotics for the prevention of bacterial endocarditis the physician or dentist should read the full joint statement of the American Heart Association and the American Dental Association.[1]

Staphylococcus aureus: Acute infections of skin and soft tissue of mild to moderate severity. Resistant organisms may emerge during treatment.

Streptococcus pneumoniae (Diplococcus pneumoniae): Upper respiratory tract infections (e.g., otitis media, pharyngitis) and lower respiratory tract infections (e.g., pneumonia) of mild to moderate degree.

Mycoplasma pneumoniae (Eaton agent, PPLO): For respiratory infections due to this organism.

Hemophilus influenzae: For upper respiratory tract infections of mild to moderate severity when used concomitantly with adequate doses of sulfonamides. (See sulfonamide labeling for appropriate prescribing information). The concomitant use of the sulfonamides is necessary since not all strains of *Hemophilus influenzae* are susceptible to erythromycin at the concentrations of the antibiotic achieved with usual therapeutic doses.

Chlamydia trachomatis: For the treatment of urethritis in adult males due to *Chlamydia trachomatis.*

Ureaplasma urealyticum: For the treatment of urethritis in adult males due to *Ureaplasma urealyticum.*

Treponema pallidum: Erythromycin is an alternate choice of treatment for primary syphilis in patients allergic to the penicillins. In treatment of primary syphilis, spinal fluid examinations should be done before treatment and as part of follow-up after therapy.

Corynebacterium diphtheriae: As an adjunct to antitoxin, to prevent establishment of carriers, and to eradicate the organism in carriers.

Corynebacterium minutissimum: For the treatment of erythrasma.

Entamoeba histolytica: In the treatment of intestinal amebiasis only. Extraenteric amebiasis requires treatment with other agents.

Listeria monocytogenes: Infections due to this organism.

Bordetella pertussis: Erythromycin is effective in eliminating the organism from the nasopharynx of infected individuals, rendering them non-infectious. Some clinical studies suggest that erythromycin may be helpful in the prophylaxis of pertussis in exposed susceptible individuals.

Legionnaires' Disease: Although no controlled clinical efficacy studies have been conducted, *in vitro* and limited preliminary clinical data suggest that erythromycin may be effective in treating Legionnaires' Disease.

CONTRAINDICATIONS

Erythromycin is contraindicated in patients with known hypersensitivity to this antibiotic.

WARNINGS

There have been reports of hepatic dysfunction with or without jaundice, occurring in patients receiving oral erythromycin products.

PRECAUTIONS

General: Erythromycin is principally excreted by the liver. Caution should be exercised when erythromycin is administered to patients with impaired hepatic function. (See "Clinical Pharmacology" and "Warnings" sections).

Prolonged or repeated use of erythromycin may result in an overgrowth of nonsusceptible bacteria or fungi. If superinfection occurs, erythromycin should be discontinued and appropriate therapy instituted.

When indicated, incision and drainage or other surgical procedures should be performed in conjunction with antibiotic therapy.

Laboratory Tests: Erythromycin interferes with the fluorometric determination of urinary catecholamines.

Drug Interactions: Erythromycin use in patients who are receiving high doses of theophylline may be associated with an increase in serum theophylline levels and potential theophylline toxicity. In case of theophylline toxicity and/or elevated serum theophylline levels, the dose of theophylline should be reduced while the patient is receiving concomitant erythromycin therapy.

Concomitant administration of erythromycin and digoxin has been reported to result in elevated digoxin serum levels.

There have been reports of increased anticoagulant effects when erythromycin and oral anticoagulants were used concomitantly.

Concurrent use of erythromycin and ergotamine or dihydroergotamine has been associated in some patients with acute ergot toxicity characterized by severe peripheral vasospasm and dysesthesia.

Erythromycin has been reported to decrease the clearance of triazolam and thus may increase the pharmacologic effect of triazolam.

The use of erythromycin in patients concurrently taking drugs metabolized by the cytochrome P450 system may be associated with elevations in serum erythromycin with carbamazepine, cyclosporine, hexobarbital and phenytoin. Serum concentrations of drugs metabolized by the cytochrome P450 system should be monitored closely in patients concurrently receiving erythromycin.

Troleandomycin significantly alters the metabolism of terfenadine when taken concomitantly; therefore, observe caution when erythromycin and terfenadine are used concurrently.

Patients receiving concomitant lovastatin and erythromycin should be carefully monitored; cases of rhabdomyolysis have been reported in seriously ill patients.

Carcinogenesis, Mutagenesis, Impairment of Fertility: Long-term (2-year) oral studies conducted in rats with erythromycin base did not provide evidence of tumorigenicity. Mutagenicity studies have not been conducted. There was no apparent effect on male or female fertility in rats fed erythromycin (base) at levels up to 0.25 percent of diet.

Pregnancy: Pregnancy Category B: There is no evidence of teratogenicity or any other adverse effect on reproduction in female rats fed erythromycin base (up to 0.25 percent of diet) prior to and during mating, during gestation, and through weaning of two successive litters. There are, however, no adequate and well-controlled studies in pregnant women. Because animal reproduction studies are not always predictive of human response, this drug should be used during pregnancy only if clearly needed. Erythromycin has been reported to cross the placental barrier in humans, but fetal plasma levels are generally low.

Labor and Delivery: The effect of erythromycin on labor and delivery is unknown.

Nursing Mothers: Erythromycin is excreted in breast milk, therefore, caution should be exercised when erythromycin is administered to a nursing woman.

Pediatric Use: See "Indications and Usage" and "Dosage and Administration" sections.

ADVERSE REACTIONS

The most frequent side effects of oral erythromycin preparations are gastrointestinal and are dose-related. They include nausea, vomiting, abdominal pain, diarrhea and anorexia. Symptoms of hepatic dysfunction and/or abnormal liver function test results may occur (see "Warnings" section). Pseudomembranous colitis has been rarely reported in association with erythromycin therapy.

There have been isolated reports of transient central nervous system side effects including confusion, hallucinations, seizures, and vertigo; however, a cause and effect relationship has not been established.

Occasional case reports of cardiac arrhythmias such as ventricular tachycardia have been documented in patients receiving erythromycin therapy. There have been isolated reports of other cardiovascular symptoms such as chest pain, dizziness, and palpitations; however, a cause and effect relationship has not been established.

Allergic reactions ranging from urticaria and mild skin eruptions to anaphylaxis have occurred.

There have been isolated reports of reversible hearing loss occurring chiefly in patients with renal insufficiency and in patients receiving high doses of erythromycin.

OVERDOSAGE

In case of overdosage, erythromycin should be discontinued. Overdosage should be handled with the prompt elimination of unabsorbed drug and all other appropriate measures.

Erythromycin is not removed by peritoneal dialysis or hemodialysis.

DOSAGE AND ADMINISTRATION

Erythromycin ethylsuccinate suspensions and Filmtab tablets may be administered without regard to meals.

Children: Age, weight, and severity of the infection are important factors in determining the proper dosage. In mild to moderate infections the usual dosage of erythromycin ethylsuccinate for children is 30 to 50 mg/kg/day in equally divided doses every 6 hours. For more severe infections this dosage may be doubled. If twice-a-day dosage is desired, one-half of the total daily dose may be given every 12 hours. Doses may also be given three times daily by administering one-third of the total daily dose every 8 hours.

The following dosage schedule is suggested for mild to moderate infections:

Body Weight	Total Daily Dose
Under 10 lbs	30–50 mg/kg/day 15–25 mg/lb/day
10 to 15 lbs	200 mg
16 to 25 lbs	400 mg
26 to 50 lbs	800 mg
51 to 100 lbs	1200 mg
over 100 lbs	1600 mg

Adults: 400 mg erythromycin ethylsuccinate every 6 hours is the usual dose. Dosage may be increased up to 4 g per day according to the severity of the infection. If twice-a-day dosage is desired, one-half of the total daily dose may be given every 12 hours. Doses may also be given three times daily by administering one-third of the total daily dose every 8 hours. For adult dosage calculation, use a ratio of 400 mg of erythromycin activity as the ethylsuccinate to 250 mg of erythromycin activity as the stearate, base or estolate.

In the treatment of streptococcal infections, a therapeutic dosage of erythromycin ethylsuccinate should be administered for at least 10 days. In continuous prophylaxis against recurrences of streptococcal infections in persons with a history of rheumatic heart disease, the usual dosage is 400 mg twice a day.

For prophylaxis against bacterial endocarditis[1] in patients with congenital heart disease, or rheumatic or other acquired valvular heart disease when undergoing dental procedures or surgical procedures of the upper respiratory tract, give 1.6 g (20 mg/kg for children) orally $1^1/_2$ to 2 hours before the procedure, and then, 800 mg (10 mg/kg for children) orally every 6 hours for 8 doses.

For treatment of urethritis due to *C. trachomatis* or *U. urealyticum:* 800 mg three times a day for 7 days.

For treatment of primary syphilis: Adults: 48 to 64 g given in divided doses over a period of 10 to 15 days.

For intestinal amebiasis: Adults: 400 mg four times daily for 10 to 14 days. Children: 30 to 50 mg/kg/day in divided doses for 10 to 14 days.

For use in pertussis: Although optimal dosage and duration have not been established, doses of erythromycin utilized in reported clinical studies were 40 to 50 mg/kg/day, given in divided doses for 5 to 14 days.

For treatment of Legionnaires' Disease: Although optimal doses have not been established, doses utilized in reported clinical data were those recommended above (1.6 to 4 g daily in divided doses).

HOW SUPPLIED

E.E.S. 200 Liquid (erythromycin ethylsuccinate oral suspension, USP) is supplied in 1 pint bottles (**NDC** 0074-6306-16) and in packages of six 100-mL bottles (**NDC** 0074-6306-13). Each 5-mL teaspoonful of fruit-flavored suspension contains activity equivalent to 200 mg of erythromycin.

E.E.S. 400® Liquid (erythromycin ethylsuccinate oral suspension, USP) is supplied in 1 pint bottles (**NDC** 0074-6373-16) and in packages of six 100-mL bottles (**NDC** 0074-6373-13). Each 5-mL teaspoonful of orange, fruit-flavored suspension contains activity equivalent to 400 mg of erythromycin. Both liquid products require refrigeration to preserve taste until dispensed. Refrigeration by patient is not required if used within 14 days.

E.E.S. Granules (erythromycin ethylsuccinate for oral suspension, USP) is supplied in 100-mL (**NDC** 0074-6369-02) and 200-mL (**NDC** 0074-6369-10) size bottles. Each 5-mL teaspoonful of reconstituted cherry-flavored suspension contains activity equivalent to 200 mg of erythromycin.

E.E.S. 400 Filmtab tablets (erythromycin ethylsuccinate tablets, USP) 400 mg, are supplied as pink tablets imprinted with the Abbott Logo, ⊐ , and two letter Abbo-Code designation, EE, in bottles of 100 (**NDC** 0074-5729-13), 500 (**NDC** 0074-5729-53) and 1000 (**NDC** 0074-5729-19) and in Abbo-Pac unit dose strip packages of 100 (**NDC** 0074-5729-11).

Recommended Storage: Store tablets and granules (prior to mixing) below 86°F (30°C) .

REFERENCE

1. American Heart Association. 1977. Prevention of bacterial endocarditis. Circulation 56: 139A-143A.

Filmtab—Film-sealed tablets, Abbott.
Ref. 03-4580-R18
Shown in Product Identification Guide, page 303

ERYTHROCIN® STEARATE   ℞
[e-ry'thrō-sin]
(erythromycin stearate tablets, USP)
Filmtab® Tablets

DESCRIPTION

Erythromycin is produced by a strain of *Streptomyces erythraeus* and belongs to the macrolide group of antibiotics. It is basic and readily forms salts with acids. The base, the stearate salt, and the esters are poorly soluble in water, and are suitable for oral administration.

Erythrocin Stearate Filmtab tablets (erythromycin stearate tablets, USP) contain the stearate salt of the antibiotic in a unique film coating.

Inactive Ingredients: 250 mg tablet: Cellulosic polymers, corn starch, D&C Red No. 7, polacrilin potassium, polyethylene glycol, povidone, propylene glycol, sodium carboxymethylcellulose, sodium citrate, sorbic acid, sorbitan monooleate and titanium dioxide.

500 mg tablet: Cellulosic polymers, corn starch, FD&C Red No. 3, magnesium hydroxide, polacrilin potassium, povidone, propylene glycol, sorbitan monooleate, titanium dioxide and vanillin.

ACTIONS

Microbiology

Biochemical tests demonstrate that erythromycin inhibits protein synthesis of the pathogen without directly affecting nucleic acid synthesis. Antagonism has been demonstrated between clindamycin and erythromycin.

NOTE: Many strains of *Hemophilus influenzae* are resistant to erythromycin alone, but are susceptible to erythromycin and sulfonamides together. Staphylococci resistant to erythromycin may emerge during a course of erythromycin therapy. Culture and susceptibility testing should be performed.

Disc Susceptibility Tests:

Quantitative methods that require measurement of zone diameters give the most precise estimates of antibiotic susceptibility. One recommended procedure (21 CFR section 460.1) uses erythromycin class discs for testing susceptibility; interpretations correlate zone diameters of this disc test with MIC values for erythromycin. With this procedure, a report from the laboratory of "susceptible" indicates that the infecting organism is likely to respond to therapy. A report of "resistant" indicates that the infective organism is not likely to respond to therapy. A report of "intermediate susceptibility" suggests that the organism would be susceptible if higher doses were used.

Clinical Pharmacology

Erythromycin binds to the 50 S ribosomal subunits of susceptible bacteria and suppresses protein synthesis.

Orally administered Erythrocin Stearate tablets are readily and reliably absorbed. Optimal serum levels of erythromycin are reached when the drug is taken in the fasting state or immediately before meals.

Erythromycin diffuses readily into most body fluids. Only low concentrations are normally achieved in the spinal fluid, but passage of the drug across the blood-brain barrier increases in meningitis. In the presence of normal hepatic function, erythromycin is concentrated in the liver and excreted in the bile; the effect of hepatic dysfunction on excretion of erythromycin by the liver into the bile is not known. Less than 5 percent of the orally administered dose of erythromycin is excreted in active form in the urine.

Erythromycin crosses the placental barrier and is excreted in breast milk.

INDICATIONS

Streptococcus pyogenes (Group A betahemolytic streptococcus): Upper and lower respiratory tract, skin, and soft tissue infections of mild to moderate severity.

Injectable benzathine penicillin G is considered by the American Heart Association to be the drug of choice in the treatment and prevention of streptococcal pharyngitis and in long-term prophylaxis of rheumatic fever.

When oral medication is preferred for treatment of the above conditions, penicillin G, V, or erythromycin are alternate drugs of choice.

When oral medication is given, the importance of strict adherence by the patient to the prescribed dosage regimen must be stressed. A therapeutic dose should be administered for at least 10 days.

Alpha-hemolytic streptococci (viridans group):

Although no controlled clinical efficacy trials have been conducted, oral erythromycin has been suggested by the American Heart Association and American Dental Association for use in a regimen for prophylaxis against bacterial endocarditis in patients hypersensitive to penicillin who have congenital heart disease, or rheumatic or other acquired valvular heart disease when they undergo dental procedures and surgical procedures of the upper respiratory tract.[1] Erythromycin is not suitable prior to genitourinary or gastrointestinal tract surgery. NOTE: When selecting antibiotics for the prevention of bacterial endocarditis the physician or dentist should read the full joint statement of the American Heart Association and the American Dental Association.[1]

Staphylococcus aureus: Acute infections of skin and soft tissue of mild to moderate severity. Resistant organisms may emerge during treatment.

Streptococcus pneumoniae (Diplococcus pneumoniae): Upper respiratory tract infections (e.g., otitis media, pharyngitis) and lower respiratory tract infections (e.g., pneumonia) of mild to moderate degree.

Mycoplasma pneumoniae (Eaton agent, PPLO): For respiratory infections due to this organism.

Hemophilus influenzae: For upper respiratory tract infections of mild to moderate severity when used concomitantly with adequate doses of sulfonamides. (See sulfonamide labeling for appropriate prescribing information). The concomitant use of the sulfonamides is necessary since not all strains of *Hemophilus influenzae* are susceptible to erythromycin at the concentrations of the antibiotic achieved with usual therapeutic doses.

Chlamydia trachomatis: Erythromycin is indicated for treatment of the following infections caused by *Chlamydia trachomatis:* conjunctivitis of the newborn, pneumonia of infancy and urogenital infections during pregnancy. When tetracyclines are contraindicated or not tolerated, erythromycin is indicated for the treatment of uncomplicated urethral, endocervical, or rectal infections in adults due to *Chlamydia trachomatis.*[2]

Treponema pallidum: Erythromycin is an alternate choice of treatment for primary syphilis in patients allergic to the penicillins. In treatment of primary syphilis, spinal fluid examinations should be done before treatment and as part of follow-up after therapy.

Corynebacterium diphtheriae: As an adjunct to antitoxin, to prevent establishment of carriers, and to eradicate the organism in carriers.

Corynebacterium minutissimum: For the treatment of erythrasma.

Entamoeba histolytica: In the treatment of intestinal amebiasis only. Extra-enteric amebiasis requires treatment with other agents.

Listeria monocytogenes: Infections due to this organism.

Neisseria gonorrhoeae: Erythrocin Lactobionate-I.V. (erythromycin lactobionate for injection) in conjunction with erythromycin stearate orally, as an alternative drug in treatment of acute pelvic inflammatory disease caused by *N. gonorrhoeae* in female patients with a history of sensitivity to penicillin. Before treatment of gonorrhea, patients who are suspected of also having syphilis should have a microscopic examination for *T. pallidum* (by immunofluorescence or darkfield) before receiving erythromycin, and monthly serologic tests for a minimum of 4 months.

Bordetella pertussis: Erythromycin is effective in eliminating the organism from the nasopharynx of infected individuals, rendering them non-infectious. Some clinical studies suggest that erythromycin may be helpful in the prophylaxis of pertussis in exposed susceptible individuals.

Legionnaires' Disease: Although no controlled clinical efficacy studies have been conducted, *in vitro* and limited preliminary clinical data suggest that erythromycin may be effective in treating Legionnaires' Disease.

CONTRAINDICATIONS

Erythromycin is contraindicated in patients with known hypersensitivity to this antibiotic.

WARNINGS

There have been reports of hepatic dysfunction with or without jaundice, occurring in patients receiving oral erythromycin products.

PRECAUTIONS

General: Erythromycin is principally excreted by the liver. Caution should be exercised when erythromycin is administered to patients with impaired hepatic function. (See "Clinical Pharmacology" and "Warnings" sections).

Prolonged or repeated use of erythromycin may result in an overgrowth of nonsusceptible bacteria or fungi. If superinfection occurs, erythromycin should be discontinued and appropriate therapy instituted.

When indicated, incision and drainage or other surgical procedures should be performed in conjunction with antibiotic therapy.

Laboratory Tests: Erythromycin interferes with the fluorometric determination of urinary catecholamines.

Drug Interactions: Erythromycin use in patients who are receiving high doses of theophylline may be associated with an increase in serum theophylline levels and potential theophylline toxicity. In case of theophylline toxicity and/or elevated serum theophylline levels, the dose of theophylline should be reduced while the patient is receiving concomitant erythromycin therapy.

Concomitant administration of erythromycin and digoxin has been reported to result in elevated digoxin serum levels. There have been reports of increased anticoagulant effects when erythromycin and oral anticoagulants were used concomitantly.

Continued on next page

Abbott Laboratories—Cont.

Concurrent use of erythromycin and ergotamine or dihydro-ergotamine has been associated in some patients with acute ergot toxicity characterized by severe peripheral vasospasm and dysesthesia.

Erythromycin has been reported to decrease the clearance of triazolam and thus may increase the pharmacologic effect of triazolam.

The use of erythromycin in patients concurrently taking drugs metabolized by the cytochrome P450 system may be associated with elevations in serum erythromycin with carbamazepine, cyclosporine, hexobarbital and phenytoin. Serum concentrations of drugs metabolized by the cytochrome P450 system should be monitored closely in patients concurrently receiving erythromycin.

Troleandomycin significantly alters the metabolism of terfenadine when taken concomitantly; therefore, observe caution when erythromycin and terfenadine are used concurrently.

Patients receiving concomitant lovastatin and erythromycin should be carefully monitored; cases of rhabdomyolysis have been reported in seriously ill patients.

Carcinogenesis, Mutagenesis, Impairment of Fertility: Long-term (2-year) oral studies conducted in rats with erythromycin base did not provide evidence of tumorigenicity. Mutagenicity studies have not been conducted. There was no apparent effect on male or female fertility in rats fed erythromycin (base) at levels up to 0.25 percent of diet.

Pregnancy: Pregnancy Category B: There is no evidence of teratogenicity or any other adverse effect on reproduction in female rats fed erythromycin base (up to 0.25 percent of diet) prior to and during mating, during gestation, and through weaning of two successive litters. There are, however, no adequate and well-controlled studies in pregnant women. Because animal reproduction studies are not always predictive of human response, this drug should be used during pregnancy only if clearly needed. Erythromycin has been reported to cross the placental barrier in humans, but fetal plasma levels are generally low.

Labor and Delivery: The effect of erythromycin on labor and delivery is unknown.

Nursing Mothers: Erythromycin is excreted in breast milk, therefore, caution should be exercised when erythromycin is administered to a nursing woman.

Pediatric Use: See "Indications and Usage" and "Dosage and Administration" sections.

ADVERSE REACTIONS
The most frequent side effects of oral erythromycin preparations are gastrointestinal and are dose-related. They include nausea, vomiting, abdominal pain, diarrhea and anorexia. Symptoms of hepatic dysfunction and/or abnormal liver function test results may occur (see "Warnings" section). Pseudomembranous colitis has been rarely reported in association with erythromycin therapy.

There have been isolated reports of transient central nervous system side effects including confusion, hallucinations, seizures, and vertigo; however, a cause and effect relationship has not been established.

Occasional case reports of cardiac arrhythmias such as ventricular tachycardia have been documented in patients receiving erythromycin therapy. There have been isolated reports of other cardiovascular symptoms such as chest pain, dizziness, and palpitations; however, a cause and effect relationship has not been established.

Allergic reactions ranging from urticaria and mild skin eruptions to anaphylaxis have occurred.

There have been isolated reports of reversible hearing loss occurring chiefly in patients with renal insufficiency and in patients receiving high doses of erythromycin.

OVERDOSAGE
In case of overdosage, erythromycin should be discontinued. Overdosage should be handled with the prompt elimination of unabsorbed drug and all other appropriate measures. Erythromycin is not removed by peritoneal dialysis or hemodialysis.

DOSAGE AND ADMINISTRATION
Optimal serum levels of erythromycin are reached when ERYTHROCIN STEARATE (erythromycin stearate) is taken in the fasting state or immediately before meals.

Adults: The usual dosage is 250 mg every 6 hours; or 500 mg every 12 hours, taken in the fasting state or immediately before meals. Up to 4 g per day may be administered, depending upon the severity of the infection.

Children: Age, weight, and severity of the infection are important factors in determining the proper dosage. For the treatment of mild to moderate infections, the usual dosage is 30 to 50 mg/kg/day in 3 or 4 divided doses. When dosage is desired on a twice-a-day schedule, one-half of the total daily dose may be taken every 12 hours in the fasting state or immediately before meals. For the treatment of more severe infections the total daily dose may be doubled.

In the treatment of streptococcal infections, a therapeutic dosage of erythromycin should be administered for at least 10 days. In continuous prophylaxis of streptococcal infections in persons with a history of rheumatic heart disease, the dose is 250 mg twice a day.

For prophylaxis against bacterial endocarditis[1] in patients with congenital heart disease, or rheumatic or other acquired valvular heart disease when undergoing dental procedures or surgical procedures of the upper respiratory tract, give 1 g (20 mg/kg for children) orally $1^1/_2$ to 2 hours before the procedure, and then, 500 mg (10 mg/kg for children) orally every 6 hours for 8 doses.

For conjunctivitis of the newborn caused by *Chlamydia trachomatis:* Oral erythromycin suspension 50 mg/kg/day in 4 divided doses for at least 2 weeks.[2]

For pneumonia of infancy caused by *Chlamydia trachomatis.* Although the optimal duration of therapy has not been established, the recommended therapy is oral erythromycin suspension 50 mg/kg/day in 4 divided doses for at least 3 weeks.[2]

For urogenital infections during pregnancy due to *Chlamydia trachomatis:* Although the optimal dose and duration of therapy have not been established, the suggested treatment is erythromycin 500 mg, by mouth, 4 times a day on an empty stomach for at least 7 days. For women who cannot tolerate this regimen, a decreased dose of 250 mg, by mouth, 4 times a day should be used for at least 14 days.[2]

For adults with uncomplicated urethral, endocervical, or rectal infections caused by *Chlamydia trachomatis* in whom tetracyclines are contraindicated or not tolerated: 500 mg, by mouth, 4 times a day for at least 7 days.[2]

For treatment of primary syphilis: 30 to 40 g given in divided doses over a period of 10 to 15 days.

For treatment of acute pelvic inflammatory disease caused by *N. gonorrhoeae:* 500 mg Erythrocin Lactobionate-I.V. (erythromycin lactobionate for injection) every 6 hours for 3 days, followed by 250 mg ERYTHROCIN STEARATE every 6 hours for 7 days.

For intestinal amebiasis: Adults: 250 mg four times daily for 10 to 14 days. Children: 30 to 50 mg/kg/day in divided doses for 10 to 14 days.

For use in pertussis: Although optimal dosage and duration have not been established, doses of erythromycin utilized in reported clinical studies were 40 to 50 mg/kg/day, given in divided doses for 5 to 14 days.

For treatment of Legionnaires' Disease: Although optimal doses have not been established, doses utilized in reported clinical data were 1 to 4 g daily in divided doses.

HOW SUPPLIED
ERYTHROCIN STEARATE Filmtab Tablets (erythromycin stearate tablets, USP) are supplied as:
ERYTHROCIN STEARATE Filmtab, 250 mg
Bottles of 100 .... (NDC 0074-6346-20)
Bottles of 500 .... (NDC 0074-6346-53)
Bottles of 1000 .... (NDC 0074-6346-19)
ABBO-PAC® unit dose strip packages of
100 tablets .... (NDC 0074-6346-38)
ERYTHROCIN STEARATE Filmtab, 500 mg
Bottles of 100 .... (NDC 0074-6316-13)
Recommended storage: Store below 86°F (30°C).

REFERENCES
1. American Heart Association. 1977. Prevention of bacterial endocarditis. Circulation 56: 139A-143A.
2. CDC Sexually Transmitted Diseases Treatment Guidelines 1982.
FILMTAB—Film-sealed tablets, Abbott
Ref. 01-2538-R13
Shown in Product Identification Guide, page 303

ERYTHROMYCIN BASE FILMTAB®   ℞
[e-ri-thrō-mī'sin]
(erythromycin tablets, USP)

DESCRIPTION
Erythromycin is produced by a strain of *Streptomyces erythraeus* and belongs to the macrolide group of antibiotics. It is basic and readily forms salts with acids. The base, the stearate salt, and the esters are poorly soluble in water, and are suitable for oral administration.

ERYTHROMYCIN Base Filmtab tablets contain erythromycin, USP, in a unique, nonenteric film coating.

Inactive Ingredients: 250 mg tablet: Cellulosic polymers, corn starch, D&C Red No. 30, iron oxide, magnesium hydroxide, magnesium stearate, polyethylene glycol, propylene glycol, sodium starch glycolate, sorbic acid, sorbitan monooleate and titanium dioxide.

500 mg tablet: Cellulosic polymers, corn starch, D&C Red No. 30, magnesium hydroxide, magnesium stearate, microcrystalline cellulose, polyethylene glycol, propylene glycol, sodium starch glycolate, sorbic acid, sorbitan monooleate and titanium dioxide.

ACTIONS
Microbiology: Biochemical tests demonstrate that erythromycin inhibits protein synthesis of the pathogen without directly affecting nucleic acid synthesis. Antagonism has been demonstrated between clindamycin and erythromycin. NOTE: Many strains of *Hemophilus influenzae* are resistant to erythromycin alone, but are susceptible to erythromycin and sulfonamides together. Staphylococci resistant to erythromycin may emerge during a course of erythromycin therapy. Culture and susceptibility testing should be performed. *Disc Susceptibility Tests:* Quantitative methods that require measurement of zone diameters give the most precise estimates of antibiotic susceptibility. One recommended procedure (21 CFR section 460.1) uses erythromycin class discs for testing susceptibility; interpretations correlate zone diameters of this disc test with MIC values for erythromycin. With this procedure, a report from the laboratory of "susceptible" indicates that the infecting organism is likely to respond to therapy. A report of "resistant" indicates that the infective organism is not likely to respond to therapy. A report of "intermediate susceptibility" suggests that the organism would be susceptible if higher doses were used.

Clinical Pharmacology: Erythromycin binds to the 50 S ribosomal subunits of susceptible bacteria and suppresses protein synthesis.

Orally administered erythromycin is readily absorbed by most patients, especially on an empty stomach, but patient variation is observed. Due to its formulation and nonenteric coating, this erythromycin tablet gives reliable blood levels in the average subject; however, the levels may vary with the individual.

Erythromycin diffuses readily into most body fluids. Only low concentrations are normally achieved in the spinal fluid, but passage of the drug across the blood-brain barrier increases in meningitis. In the presence of normal hepatic function, erythromycin is concentrated in the liver and excreted in the bile; the effect of hepatic dysfunction on excretion of erythromycin by the liver into the bile is not known. Less than 5 percent of the orally administered dose of erythromycin is excreted in active form in the urine.

Erythromycin crosses the placental barrier and is excreted in breast milk.

INDICATIONS
Streptococcus pyogenes (Group A beta-hemolytic streptococcus): Upper and lower respiratory tract, skin, and soft tissue infections of mild to moderate severity.

Injectable benzathine penicillin G is considered by the American Heart Association to be the drug of choice in the treatment and prevention of streptococcal pharyngitis and in long-term prophylaxis of rheumatic fever.

When oral medication is preferred for treatment of the above conditions, penicillin G, V, or erythromycin are alternate drugs of choice.

When oral medication is given, the importance of strict adherence by the patient to the prescribed dosage regimen must be stressed. A therapeutic dose should be administered for at least 10 days.

Alpha-hemolytic streptococci (viridans group): Although no controlled clinical efficacy trials have been conducted, oral erythromycin has been suggested by the American Heart Association and American Dental Association for use in a regimen for prophylaxis against bacterial endocarditis in patients hypersensitive to penicillin who have congenital heart disease, or rheumatic or other acquired valvular heart disease when they undergo dental procedures and surgical procedures of the upper respiratory tract.[1] Erythromycin is not suitable prior to genitourinary or gastrointestinal tract surgery. NOTE: When selecting antibiotics for the prevention of bacterial endocarditis the physician or dentist should read the full joint statement of the American Heart Association and the American Dental Association.[1]

Staphylococcus aureus: Acute infections of skin and soft tissue of mild to moderate severity. Resistant organisms may emerge during treatment.

Streptococcus pneumoniae (Diplococcus pneumoniae): Upper respiratory tract infections (e.g., otitis media, pharyngitis) and lower respiratory tract infections (e.g., pneumonia) of mild to moderate degree.

Mycoplasma pneumoniae (Eaton agent, PPLO): For respiratory infections due to this organism.

Hemophilus influenzae: For upper respiratory tract infections of mild to moderate severity when used concomitantly with adequate doses of sulfonamides. (See sulfonamide labeling for appropriate prescribing information.) The concomitant use of the sulfonamides is necessary since not all strains of *Hemophilus influenzae* are susceptible to erythromycin at the concentrations of the antibiotic achieved with usual therapeutic doses.

Chlamydia trachomatis: Erythromycin is indicated for treatment of the following infections caused by *Chlamydia trachomatis:* conjunctivitis of the newborn, pneumonia of infancy and urogenital infections during pregnancy. When tetracyclines are contraindicated or not tolerated, erythromycin is indicated for the treatment of uncomplicated ure-

thral, endocervical, or rectal infections in adults due to *Chlamydia trachomatis.*[2]
Treponema pallidum: Erythromycin is an alternate choice of treatment for primary syphilis in patients allergic to the penicillins. In treatment of primary syphilis, spinal fluid examinations should be done before treatment and as part of follow-up after therapy.
Corynebacterium diphtheriae: As an adjunct to antitoxin, to prevent establishment of carriers, and to eradicate the organism in carriers.
Corynebacterium minutissimum: For the treatment of erythrasma.
Entamoeba histolytica: In the treatment of intestinal amebiasis only. Extra-enteric amebiasis requires treatment with other agents.
Listeria monocytogenes: Infections due to this organism.
Neisseria gonorrhoeae: Erythrocin® Lactobionate-I.V. (erythromycin lactobionate for injection) in conjunction with erythromycin base orally, as an alternative drug in treatment of acute pelvic inflammatory disease caused by *N. gonorrhoeae* in female patients with a history of sensitivity to penicillin. Before treatment of gonorrhea, patients who are suspected of also having syphilis should have a microscopic examination for *T. pallidum* (by immunofluorescence or darkfield) before receiving erythromycin, and monthly serologic tests for a minimum of 4 months.
Bordetella pertussis: Erythromycin is effective in eliminating the organism from the nasopharynx of infected individuals, rendering them non-infectious. Some clinical studies suggest that erythromycin may be helpful in the prophylaxis of pertussis in exposed susceptible individuals.
Legionnaires' Disease: Although no controlled clinical efficacy studies have been conducted, *in vitro* and limited preliminary clinical data suggest that erythromycin may be effective in treating Legionnaires' Disease.

CONTRAINDICATIONS

Erythromycin is contraindicated in patients with known hypersensitivity to this antibiotic.

WARNINGS

There have been reports of hepatic dysfunction with or without jaundice, occurring in patients receiving oral erythromycin products.

PRECAUTIONS

General: Erythromycin is principally excreted by the liver. Caution should be exercised when erythromycin is administered to patients with impaired hepatic function. (See "Clinical Pharmacology" and "Warnings" sections).
Prolonged or repeated use of erythromycin may result in an overgrowth of nonsusceptible bacteria or fungi. If superinfection occurs, erythromycin should be discontinued and appropriate therapy instituted.
When indicated, incision and drainage or other surgical procedures should be performed in conjunction with antibiotic therapy.
Laboratory Tests: Erythromycin interferes with the fluorometric determination of urinary catecholamines.
Drug Interactions: Erythromycin use in patients who are receiving high doses of theophylline may be associated with an increase in serum theophylline levels and potential theophylline toxicity. In case of theophylline toxicity and/or elevated serum theophylline levels, the dose of theophylline should be reduced while the patient is receiving concomitant erythromycin therapy.
Concomitant administration of erythromycin and digoxin has been reported to result in elevated digoxin serum levels.
There have been reports of increased anticoagulant effects when erythromycin and oral anticoagulants were used concomitantly.
Concurrent use of erythromycin and ergotamine or dihydroergotamine has been associated in some patients with acute ergot toxicity characterized by severe peripheral vasospasm and dysesthesia.
Erythromycin has been reported to decrease the clearance of triazolam and thus may increase the pharmacologic effect of triazolam.
The use of erythromycin in patients concurrently taking drugs metabolized by the cytochrome P450 system may be associated with elevations in serum erythromycin with carbamazepine, cyclosporine, hexobarbital and phenytoin. Serum concentrations of drugs metabolized by the cytochrome P450 system should be monitored closely in patients concurrently receiving erythromycin.
Troleandomycin significantly alters the metabolism of terfenadine when taken concomitantly; therefore, observe caution when erythromycin and terfenadine are used concurrently.
Patients receiving concomitant lovastatin and erythromycin should be carefully monitored; cases of rhabdomyolysis have been reported in seriously ill patients.
Carcinogenesis, Mutagenesis, Impairment of Fertility: Long-term (2-year) oral studies conducted in rats with erythromycin base did not provide evidence of tumorigenicity. Mutagenicity studies have not been conducted. There was no apparent effect on male or female fertility in rats fed erythromycin (base) at levels up to 0.25 percent of diet.
Pregnancy: Pregnancy Category B: There is no evidence of teratogenicity or any other adverse effect on reproduction in female rats fed erythromycin base (up to 0.25 percent of diet) prior to and during mating, during gestation, and through weaning of two successive litters. There are, however, no adequate and well-controlled studies in pregnant women. Because animal reproduction studies are not always predictive of human response, this drug should be used during pregnancy only if clearly needed. Erythromycin has been reported to cross the placental barrier in humans, but fetal plasma levels are generally low.
Labor and Delivery: The effect of erythromycin on labor and delivery is unknown.
Nursing Mothers: Erythromycin is excreted in breast milk, therefore, caution should be exercised when erythromycin is administered to a nursing woman.
Pediatric Use: See "Indications and Usage" and "Dosage and Administration" sections.

ADVERSE REACTIONS

The most frequent side effects of oral erythromycin preparations are gastrointestinal and are dose-related. They include nausea, vomiting, abdominal pain, diarrhea and anorexia. Symptoms of hepatic dysfunction and/or abnormal liver function test results may occur (see "Warnings" section).
Pseudomembranous colitis has been rarely reported in association with erythromycin therapy.
There have been isolated reports of transient central nervous system side effects including confusion, hallucinations, seizures, and vertigo; however, a cause and effect relationship has not been established.
Occasional case reports of cardiac arrhythmias such as ventricular tachycardia have been documented in patients receiving erythromycin therapy. There have been isolated reports of other cardiovascular symptoms such as chest pain, dizziness, and palpitations; however a cause and effect relationship has not been established.
Allergic reactions ranging from urticaria and mild skin eruptions to anaphylaxis have occurred.
There have been isolated reports of reversible hearing loss occurring chiefly in patients with renal insufficiency and in patients receiving high doses of erythromycin.

OVERDOSAGE

In case of overdosage, erythromycin should be discontinued. Overdosage should be handled with the prompt elimination of unabsorbed drug and all other appropriate measures.
Erythromycin is not removed by peritoneal dialysis or hemodialysis.

DOSAGE AND ADMINISTRATION

Optimum blood levels are obtained when doses are given on an empty stomach.
Adults: 250 mg every 6 hours is the usual dose; or 500 mg every 12 hours one hour before meals. Dosage may be increased up to 4 g per day according to the severity of the infection.
Children: Age, weight, and severity of the infection are important factors in determining the proper dosage. 30 to 50 mg/kg/day, in divided doses, is the usual dose. For more severe infections this dose may be doubled. If dosage is desired on a twice-a-day schedule, one-half of the total daily dose may be given every 12 hours, one hour before meals.
For treatment of streptococcal infections: a therapeutic dosage should be administered for at least 10 days. In continuous prophylaxis of streptococcal infections in persons with rheumatic heart disease history, the dose is 250 mg twice a day.
For prophylaxis against bacterial endocarditis[1] in patients with congenital heart disease, or rheumatic or other acquired valvular heart disease when undergoing dental procedures or surgical procedures of the upper respiratory tract, give 1 g (20 mg/kg for children) orally $1^1/_2$ to 2 hours before the procedure, and then, 500 mg (10 mg/kg for children) orally every 6 hours for 8 doses.
For conjunctivitis of the newborn caused by *Chlamydia trachomatis:* Oral erythromycin suspension 50 mg/kg/day in 4 divided doses for at least 2 weeks.[2]
For pneumonia of infancy caused by *Chlamydia trachomatis:* Although the optimal duration of therapy has not been established, the recommended therapy is oral erythromycin suspension 50 mg/kg/day in 4 divided doses for at least 3 weeks.[2]
For urogenital infections during pregnancy due to *Chlamydia trachomatis:* Although the optimal dose and duration of therapy have not been established, the suggested treatment is erythromycin 500 mg, by mouth, 4 times a day on an empty stomach for at least 7 days. For women who cannot tolerate this regimen, a decreased dose of 250 mg, by mouth, 4 times a day should be used for at least 14 days.[2]
For adults with uncomplicated urethral, endocervical, or rectal infections caused by *Chlamydia trachomatis* in whom tetracyclines are contraindicated or not tolerated: 500 mg, by mouth, 4 times a day for at least 7 days.[2]
For treatment of primary syphilis: 30 to 40 g given in divided doses over a period of 10 to 15 days.
For treatment of acute pelvic inflammatory disease caused by *N. gonorrhoeae:* 500 mg Erythrocin® Lactobionate-I.V. (erythromycin lactobionate for injection) every 6 hours for 3 days, followed by 250 mg erythromycin base every 6 hours for 7 days.
For intestinal amebiasis: Adults: 250 mg four times daily for 10 to 14 days. Children: 30 to 50 mg/kg/day in divided doses for 10 to 14 days.
For use in pertussis: Although optimal dosage and duration have not been established, doses of erythromycin utilized in reported clinical studies were 40 to 50 mg/kg/day, given in divided doses for 5 to 14 days.
For treatment of Legionnaires' Disease: Although optimal doses have not been established, doses utilized in reported clinical data were 1 to 4 g daily in divided doses.

HOW SUPPLIED

ERYTHROMYCIN Base Filmtab tablets (erythromycin tablets, USP) are supplied as pink, capsule-shaped tablets in two dosage strengths:
250 mg tablets:
Bottles of 100 ....(**NDC** 0074-6326-13);
Bottles of 500 ....(**NDC** 0074-6326-53);
ABBO-PAC® unit dose strip packages of
100 tablets ....(**NDC** 0074-6326-11).
500 mg tablets:
Bottles of 100 ....(**NDC** 0074-6227-13).
Recommended storage: Store below 86°F (30°C).

REFERENCES

1. American Heart Association. 1977. Prevention of bacterial endocarditis. Circulation. 56: 139A-143A.
2. CDC Sexually Transmitted Diseases Treatment Guidelines 1982.

FILMTAB—Film-sealed tablets, Abbott.
Ref. 01-2541-R3
Shown in Product Identification Guide, page 303

ERYTHROMYCIN DELAYED-RELEASE CAPSULES, USP

℞

DESCRIPTION

Erythromycin Delayed-release Capsules contain enteric-coated pellets of erythromycin base for oral administration. Erythromycin is produced by a strain of *Streptomyces erythraeus* and belongs to the macrolide group of antibiotics. It is basic and readily forms salts with acids, but it is the base which is microbiologically active. Each Erythromycin Delayed-release Capsule contains 250 milligrams of erythromycin base.
Inactive Ingredients: Cellulosic polymers, citrate ester, D&C Red No. 30, D&C Yellow No. 10, magnesium stearate and povidone. The capsule shell contains FD&C Blue No. 1, FD&C Red No. 3, gelatin, and titanium dioxide.
Erythromycin base is (3R*, 4S*, 5S*, 6R*, 7R*, 9R*, 11R*, 12R*, 13S*, 14R*)-4-[(2,6-Dideoxy-3-C-methyl-3-0-methyl-α-L-*ribo*-hexopyranosyl)oxy]-14-ethyl-7,12,13-trihydroxy-3, 5, 7, 9, 11, 13-hexamethyl-6-[[3, 4, 6-trideoxy-3-(dimethylamino)-β-D-*xylo*-hexopyranosyl]oxy]oxacyclotetradecane-2,10-dione. The structural formula is:

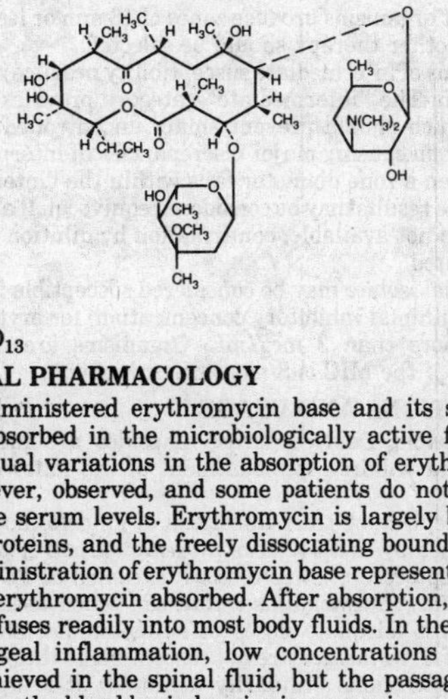

$C_{37}H_{67}NO_{13}$ MW 734

CLINICAL PHARMACOLOGY

Orally administered erythromycin base and its salts are readily absorbed in the microbiologically active form. Interindividual variations in the absorption of erythromycin are, however, observed, and some patients do not achieve acceptable serum levels. Erythromycin is largely bound to plasma proteins, and the freely dissociating bound fraction after administration of erythromycin base represents 90% of the total erythromycin absorbed. After absorption, erythromycin diffuses readily into most body fluids. In the absence of meningeal inflammation, low concentrations are normally achieved in the spinal fluid, but the passage of the drug across the blood-brain barrier increases in meningitis. Erythromycin is excreted in breast milk. The drug crosses the placental barrier but plasma levels are low.

Continued on next page

Abbott Laboratories—Cont.

In the presence of normal hepatic function, erythromycin is concentrated in the liver and is excreted in the bile; the effect of hepatic dysfunction on biliary excretion of erythromycin is not known. After oral administration, less than 5% of the administered dose can be recovered in the active form in the urine.

The enteric coating of pellets in Erythromycin Delayed-release Capsules protects the erythromycin base from inactivation by gastric acidity. Because of their small size and enteric coating, the pellets readily pass intact from the stomach to the small intestine and dissolve efficiently to allow absorption of erythromycin in a uniform manner. After administration of a single dose of a 250 mg Erythromycin Delayed-release Capsule, peak serum levels in the range of 1.13 to 1.68 mcg/mL are attained in approximately 3 hours and decline to 0.30-0.42 mcg/mL in 6 hours. Optimal conditions for stability in the presence of gastric secretion and for complete absorption are attained when Erythromycin Delayed-release Capsules are taken on an empty stomach.

Microbiology:
Erythromycin acts by inhibition of protein synthesis by binding 50 S ribosomal subunits of susceptible organisms. It does not affect nucleic acid synthesis. Antagonism has been demonstrated between clindamycin and erythromycin. Resistance to erythromycin of many strains of *Haemophilus influenzae* and some strains of staphylococci has been demonstrated. Specimens should be obtained for culture and susceptibility testing.

Erythromycin is usually active against the following organisms *in vitro* and in clinical infections:
Streptococcus pyogenes
Alpha-hemolytic streptococci (viridans group)
Staphylococcus aureus (Resistant organisms may emerge during treatment.)
Streptococcus pneumoniae
Mycoplasma pneumoniae (Eaton's Agent)
Haemophilus influenzae (Many strains are resistant to erythromycin alone, but are susceptible to erythromycin and sulfonamides together.)
Treponema pallidum
Corynebacterium diphtheriae
Corynebacterium minutissimum
Entamoeba histolytica
Listeria monocytogenes
Neisseria gonorrhoeae
Bordetella pertussis
Legionella pneumophila (agent of Legionnaires' disease)

Susceptibility Testing
Quantitative methods that require measurement of zone diameters give the most precise estimates of antibiotic susceptibility. One such standardized single-disc procedure has been recommended for use with discs to test susceptibility to erythromycin.[1] Interpretation involves correlation of the zone diameters obtained in the disc test with minimal inhibitory concentration (MIC) values for erythromycin.

Reports from the laboratory giving results of the standardized single-disc susceptibility test using a 15 mcg erythromycin disc should be interpreted according to the following criteria:

Susceptible organisms produce zones of 18 mm or greater, indicating that the tested organism is likely to respond to therapy.

Resistant organisms produce zones of 13 mm or less, indicating that other therapy should be selected.

Organisms of intermediate susceptibility produce zones of 14 to 17 mm. The "intermediate" category provides a "buffer zone" which should prevent small, uncontrolled technical factors from causing major discrepancies in interpretations; thus, when a zone diameter falls within the "intermediate" range, the results may be considered equivocal. If alternative drugs are not available, confirmation by dilution tests may be indicated.

A bacterial isolate may be considered susceptible if the MIC value[2] (minimal inhibitory concentration) for erythromycin is not more than 2 mcg/mL. Organisms are considered resistant if the MIC is 8 mcg/mL or higher.

INDICATIONS AND USAGE
Erythromycin Delayed-release Capsules are indicated in adults and children for treatment of the following conditions:

Upper respiratory tract infections of mild to moderate degree caused by *Streptococcus pyogenes* (Group A beta-hemolytic streptococci); *Streptococcus pneumoniae (Diplococcus pneumoniae)*; *Haemophilus influenzae* (when used concomitantly with adequate doses of sulfonamides, since many strains of *H. influenzae* are not susceptible to the erythromycin concentrations ordinarily achieved). (See appropriate sulfonamide labeling for prescribing information.)

Lower respiratory tract infections of mild to moderate severity caused by *Streptococcus pyogenes* (Group A beta-hemolytic streptococci); *Streptococcus pneumoniae (Diplococcus pneumoniae).*

Respiratory tract infections due to *Mycoplasma pneumoniae* (Eaton's agent).

Pertussis (whooping cough) caused by *Bordetella pertussis.* Erythromycin is effective in eliminating the organism from the nasopharynx of infected individuals, rendering them noninfectious. Some clinical studies suggest that erythromycin may be helpful in the prophylaxis of pertussis in exposed susceptible individuals.

Diphtheria—As an adjunct to antitoxin in infections due to *Corynebacterium diphtheriae*, to prevent establishment of carriers and to eradicate the organism in carriers.

Erythrasma—In the treatment of infections due to *Corynebacterium minutissimum.*

Intestinal amebiasis caused by *Entamoeba histolytica* (oral erythromycins only). Extraenteric amebiasis requires treatment with other agents.

Infections due to *Listeria monocytogenes.*

Skin and soft tissue infections of mild to moderate severity caused by *Streptococcus pyogenes* and *Staphylococcus aureus* (resistant staphylococci may emerge during treatment).

Primary syphilis caused by *Treponema pallidum.* Erythromycin (oral forms only) is an alternate choice of treatment for primary syphilis in patients allergic to the penicillins. In treatment of primary syphilis, spinal fluid should be examined before treatment and as part of the follow-up after therapy. The use of erythromycin for the treatment of *in utero* syphilis is not recommended. (See "CLINICAL PHARMACOLOGY" section.)

Erythromycins are indicated for treatment of the following infections caused by *Chlamydia trachomatis:* conjunctivitis of the newborn, pneumonia of infancy, and urogenital infections during pregnancy. When tetracyclines are contraindicated or not tolerated, erythromycin is indicated for the treatment of uncomplicated urethral, endocervical, or rectal infections in adults due to *Chlamydia trachomatis.*[3]

Legionnaires' Disease caused by *Legionella pneumophila.* Although no controlled clinical efficacy studies have been conducted, *in vitro* and limited preliminary clinical data suggest that erythromycin may be effective in treating Legionnaires' Disease.

Therapy with erythromycin should be monitored by bacteriological studies and by clinical response. (See "CLINICAL PHARMACOLOGY—Microbiology" section.)

Injectable benzathine penicillin G is considered by the American Heart Association to be the drug of choice in the treatment and prevention of streptococcal pharyngitis and in long-term prophylaxis of rheumatic fever. When oral medication is preferred for treatment of the above conditions, penicillin G, V or erythromycin are alternate drugs of choice.

Although no controlled clinical efficacy trials have been conducted, erythromycin has been suggested by the American Heart Association and the American Dental Association for use in a regimen for prophylaxis against bacterial endocarditis in patients allergic to penicillin who have congenital and/or rheumatic or other acquired valvular heart disease when they undergo dental procedures and surgical procedures of the upper respiratory tract.[3] (Erythromycin is not suitable prior to genitourinary surgery where the organisms likely to lead to bacteremia are gram-negative bacilli or the enterococcal group of streptococci).

NOTE: When selecting antibiotics for the prevention of bacterial endocarditis the physician or dentist should read the full joint 1984 statement of the American Heart Association and the American Dental Association.[3]

CONTRAINDICATION
Erythromycin is contraindicated in patients with known hypersensitivity to this antibiotic.

WARNINGS
There have been a few reports of hepatic dysfunction, with or without jaundice, occurring in patients receiving oral erythromycin products.

PRECAUTIONS
General: Erythromycin is principally excreted by the liver. Caution should be exercised when erythromycin is administered to patients with impaired hepatic function. (See "Clinical Pharmacology" and "Warnings" sections).

Prolonged or repeated use of erythromycin may result in an overgrowth of nonsusceptible bacteria or fungi. If superinfection occurs, erythromycin should be discontinued and appropriate therapy instituted.

When indicated, incision and drainage or other surgical procedures should be performed in conjunction with antibiotic therapy.

Laboratory Tests: Erythromycin interferes with the fluorometric determination of urinary catecholamines.

Drug Interactions: Erythromycin use in patients who are receiving high doses of theophylline may be associated with an increase in serum theophylline levels and potential theophylline toxicity. In case of theophylline toxicity and/or elevated serum theophylline levels, the dose of theophylline should be reduced while the patient is receiving concomitant erythromycin therapy.

Concomitant administration of erythromycin and digoxin has been reported to result in elevated digoxin serum levels.

There have been reports of increased anticoagulant effects when erythromycin and oral anticoagulants were used concomitantly.

Concurrent use of erythromycin and ergotamine or dihydroergotamine has been associated in some patients with acute ergot toxicity characterized by severe peripheral vasospasm and dysesthesia.

Erythromycin has been reported to decrease the clearance of triazolam and thus may increase the pharmacologic effect of triazolam.

The use of erythromycin in patients concurrently taking drugs metabolized by the cytochrome P450 system may be associated with elevations in serum erythromycin with carbamazepine, cyclosporine, hexobarbital and phenytoin. Serum concentrations of drugs metabolized by the cytochrome P450 system should be monitored closely in patients concurrently receiving erythromycin.

Troleandomycin significantly alters the metabolism of terfenadine when taken concomitantly; therefore, observe caution when erythromycin and terfenadine are used concurrently.

Patients receiving concomitant lovastatin and erythromycin should be carefully monitored; cases of rhabdomyolysis have been reported in seriously ill patients.

Carcinogenesis, Mutagenesis, Impairment of Fertility: Long-term (2-year) oral studies conducted in rats with erythromycin base did not provide evidence of tumorigenicity. Mutagenicity studies have not been conducted. There was no apparent effect on male or female fertility in rats fed erythromycin (base) at levels up to 0.25 percent of diet.

Pregnancy: Pregnancy Category B: There is no evidence of teratogenicity or any other adverse effect on reproduction in female rats fed erythromycin base (up to 0.25 percent of diet) prior to and during mating, during gestation, and through weaning of two successive litters. There are, however, no adequate and well-controlled studies in pregnant women. Because animal reproduction studies are not always predictive of human response, this drug should be used during pregnancy only if clearly needed. Erythromycin has been reported to cross the placental barrier in humans, but fetal plasma levels are generally low.

Labor and Delivery: The effect of erythromycin on labor and delivery is unknown.

Nursing Mothers: Erythromycin is excreted in breast milk, therefore, caution should be exercised when erythromycin is administered to a nursing woman.

Pediatric Use: See "Indications and Usage" and "Dosage and Administration" sections.

ADVERSE REACTIONS
The most frequent side effects of oral erythromycin preparations are gastrointestinal and are dose-related. They include nausea, vomiting, abdominal pain, diarrhea and anorexia. Symptoms of hepatic dysfunction and/or abnormal liver function test results may occur (see "Warnings" section). Pseudomembranous colitis has been rarely reported in association with erythromycin therapy.

There have been isolated reports of transient central nervous system side effects including confusion, hallucinations, seizures, and vertigo; however, a cause and effect relationship has not been established.

Occasional case reports of cardiac arrhythmias such as ventricular tachycardia have been documented in patients receiving erythromycin therapy. There have been isolated reports of other cardiovascular symptoms such as chest pain, dizziness, and palpitations; however, a cause and effect relationship has not been established.

Allergic reactions ranging from urticaria and mild skin eruptions to anaphylaxis have occurred.

There have been isolated reports of reversible hearing loss occurring chiefly in patients with renal insufficiency and in patients receiving high doses of erythromycin.

OVERDOSAGE
In case of overdosage, erythromycin should be discontinued. Overdosage should be handled with the prompt elimination of unabsorbed drug and all other appropriate measures. Erythromycin is not removed by peritoneal dialysis or hemodialysis.

DOSAGE AND ADMINISTRATION
Administration of a dose of Erythromycin Delayed-release Capsules in the presence of food lowers the blood levels of systemically available erythromycin. Although the blood levels obtained upon administration of enteric-coated erythromycin products in the presence of food are still above minimum inhibitory concentrations (MICs) of most organisms for which erythromycin is indicated, optimum blood levels are obtained on a fasting stomach (administration at least 1/2 hour and preferably two hours before or after a meal).

Adults: The usual dose is 250 mg every 6 hours taken one hour before meals. If twice-a-day dosage is desired, the recommended dose is 500 mg every 12 hours. Dosage may be increased up to 4 grams per day, according to the severity of

infection. Twice-a-day dosing is not recommended when doses larger than 1 gram daily are administered.

Children: Age, weight, and severity of the infection are important factors in determining the proper dosage. The usual dosage is 30 to 50 mg/kg/day, in divided doses. For the treatment of more severe infections this dosage may be doubled.

Streptococcal infections: A therapeutic dosage of oral erythromycin should be administered for at least ten days. For continuous prophylaxis against recurrences of streptococcal infections in persons with a history of rheumatic heart disease, the dose is 250 mg twice a day.

For the prevention of bacterial endocarditis in penicillin-allergic patients with valvular heart disease who are to undergo dental procedures or surgical procedures of the upper respiratory tract, the adult dose is 1 gram orally (20 mg/kg for children) one hour prior to the procedure and then 500 mg (10 mg/kg for children) orally 6 hours later.[3] (See "INDICATIONS AND USAGE" section.)

Primary syphilis: 30 to 40 g given in divided doses over a period of 10 to 15 days.

Intestinal amebiasis: 250 mg every 6 hours for 10 to 14 days for adults; 30 to 50 mg/kg/day in divided doses for 10 to 14 days for children.

Legionnaires' disease: Although optimal doses have not been established, doses utilized in reported clinical data were those recommended above (1 to 4 g daily in divided doses).

Urogenital infections during pregnancy due to *Chlamydia trachomatis:* Although the optimal dose and duration of therapy have not been established, the suggested treatment is 500 mg by mouth four times a day on an empty stomach for at least 7 days. For women who cannot tolerate this regimen, a decreased dose of 250 mg by mouth four times a day should be used for at least 14 days.[4]

For adults with uncomplicated urethral, endocervical, or rectal infections caused by *Chlamydia trachomatis,* when tetracycline is contrainidicated or not tolerated, 500 mg of erythromycin by mouth four times a day for at least 7 days.[4]

Pertussis: Although optimum dosage and duration of therapy have not been established, doses of erythromycin utilized in reported clinical studies were 40 to 50 mg/kg/day, given in divided doses for 5 to 14 days.

HOW SUPPLIED

Erythromycin Delayed-release Capsules, USP, are clear and opaque maroon capsules with pink and yellow particles containing 250 mg of erythromycin supplied in bottles of 100 (**NDC** 0074-6301-13) and 500 (**NDC** 0074-6301-53).

Storage Conditions: Protect from moisture and excessive heat. **Store below 86°F (30°C).**

REFERENCES

1. Approved Standard ASM-2 "Performance Standards for Antimicrobial Disc Susceptibility Test." National Committee for Clinical Laboratory Standards, 771 East Lancaster Avenue, Villanova, PA 19085.
2. Ericson, H.M., Sherris, J.C.: "Antibiotic Sensitivity Testing Report of an International Collaborative Study." *Acta Pathologica et Microbiologica Scandinavica,* Section B, Supp. 217, 1971.
3. American Heart Assoc. and American Dental Assoc. "Prevention of Bacterial Endocarditis," *Circulation:* Vol. 70, No. 6, December, 1984, 1123A-1127A.
4. CDC Sexually Transmitted Diseases Treatment Guidelines 1982.

Ref. 01-2563-R4

Shown in Product Identification Guide, page 303

FERO–FOLIC–500® Filmtab® Tablets ℞

[fe′ro fo-lic]

Controlled-Release Iron with Folic Acid and Vitamin C

IBERET–FOLIC–500® Filmtab® ℞

Tablets

Controlled-Release Iron with Vitamin C, and B-Complex including Folic Acid

DESCRIPTION

FERO-FOLIC-500 Filmtab is a hematinic for oral administration containing 525 mg of ferrous sulfate (equivalent to 105 mg of elemental iron) in a unique controlled-release vehicle, the Gradumet®. In addition, this product contains 800 mcg of folic acid and 500 mg of ascorbic acid present as sodium ascorbate.

Inactive Ingredients: Castor oil, cellulosic polymers, D&C Red No. 30, magnesium stearate, methyl acrylate-methyl methacrylate copolymer, pregelatinized starch (contains corn starch), polyethylene glycol, povidone, propylene glycol, talc, titanium dioxide and vanillin.

IBERET-FOLIC-500 is an Abbott hematinic containing iron in the Gradumet® controlled-release vehicle; vitamin C for enhancement of iron absorption; and the B-Complex vitamins including folic acid. The IBERET-FOLIC-500 Filmtab is for oral use.

Each Filmtab tablet provides:

*Ferrous Sulfate	525 mg
(equivalent to 105 mg of elemental iron)	
Ascorbic Acid (present as sodium ascorbate) (C)	500 mg
Niacinamide	30 mg
Calcium Pantothenate	10 mg
Thiamine Mononitrate (B_1)	6 mg
Riboflavin (B_2)	6 mg
Pyridoxine Hydrochloride (B_6)	5 mg
Folic Acid	800 mcg
Cyanocobalamin (B_{12})	25 mcg

*In controlled-release form (Gradumet)

Inactive Ingredients: Castor oil, cellulosic polymers, corn starch, D&C Red No. 7, FD&C Blue No. 1, FD&C Blue No. 2, magnesium stearate, methyl acrylate-methyl methacrylate copolymer, polyethylene glycol, povidone, propylene glycol, stearic acid, talc, titanium dioxide and vanillin.

Controlled-release of iron from the Gradumet protects against gastric side effects. The Gradumet is an inert, porous, plastic matrix which is impregnated with ferrous sulfate. Iron is leached from the Gradumet as it passes through the gastrointestinal tract, and the expended matrix is excreted harmlessly in the stool. Controlled-release iron is particularly helpful in patients who have demonstrated intolerance to oral iron preparations.

CLINICAL PHARMACOLOGY

Oral iron is absorbed most efficiently when it is administered between meals. Conventional iron preparations, however, frequently cause gastric irritation when taken on an empty stomach. Studies with iron in the Gradumet have indicated that relatively little of the iron is released in the stomach, gastric intolerance is seldom encountered, and hematologic response ranks with that obtained from plain ferrous sulfate.

Iron is found in the body principally as hemoglobin. Storage in the form of ferritin occurs in the liver, spleen, and bone marrow. Concentrations of plasma iron and the total iron-binding capacity of plasma vary greatly in different physiological conditions and disease states.

Large amounts of ascorbic acid administered orally with ferrous sulfate have been shown to enhance iron absorption. Apparently this is due to the ability of ascorbic acid to prevent the oxidation of ferrous iron to the less effectively absorbed ferric form.

Folic acid and iron are absorbed in the proximal small intestine, particularly the duodenum. Folic acid is absorbed maximally and rapidly at this site, and iron is absorbed in a descending gradient from the duodenum distally.

After absorption folic acid is rapidly converted into its metabolically active forms. Approximately two-thirds is bound to plasma protein. Half of the folic acid stored in the body is found in the liver. Folic acid is also concentrated in spinal fluid.

Except for the folates ingested in liver, yeast, and egg yolk, the percentage of absorption of food folates averages about 10%.

The B-complex vitamins in IBERET-FOLIC-500 are absorbed by the active transport process. B-complex vitamins are rapidly eliminated and therefore are not stored in the body.

Calcium pantothenate is absorbed readily from the gastrointestinal tract and distributed to all body tissues.

INDICATIONS AND USAGE

FERO-FOLIC-500 is indicated for the treatment of iron deficiency and prevention of concomitant folic acid deficiency in non-pregnant adults. FERO-FOLIC-500 is also indicated in pregnancy for the prevention and treatment of iron deficiency and to supply a maintenance dosage of folic acid.

IBERET-FOLIC-500 is indicated in non-pregnant adults for the treatment of iron deficiency and prevention of concomitant folic acid deficiency where there is an associated deficient intake or increased need for the B-complex vitamins. IBERET-FOLIC-500 is also indicated in pregnancy for the prevention and treatment of iron deficiency where there is a concomitant deficient intake or increased need for the B-complex vitamins (including folic acid).

CONTRAINDICATIONS

FERO-FOLIC-500 and IBERET-FOLIC-500 are contraindicated in patients with pernicious anemia.

FERO-FOLIC-500 and IBERET-FOLIC-500 are also contraindicated in the rare instance of hypersensitivity to folic acid.

WARNINGS

Folic acid alone is improper therapy in the treatment of pernicious anemia and other megaloblastic anemias where vitamin B_{12} is deficient.

PRECAUTIONS

Where anemia exists, its nature should be established and underlying causes determined.

FERO-FOLIC-500 and IBERET-FOLIC-500 contain 800 mcg of folic acid per tablet. Folic acid especially in doses above 0.1 mg daily may obscure pernicious anemia, in that hematologic remission may occur while neurological manifestations remain progresssive. Concomitant parenteral therapy with vitamin B_{12} may be necessary in patients with deficiency of vitamin B_{12}. Pernicious anemia is rare in women of childbearing age, and the likelihood of its occurrence along with pregnancy is reduced by the impairment of fertility associated with vitamin B_{12} deficiency.

Like other oral iron preparations, FERO-FOLIC-500 and IBERET-FOLIC-500 should be stored out of the reach of children to guard against accidental iron poisoning (see Overdosage).

Laboratory Tests: In older patients and those with conditions tending to lead to vitamin B_{12} depletion, serum B_{12} levels should be regularly assessed during treatment with FERO-FOLIC-500 or IBERET-FOLIC-500.

Drug Interactions: Absorption of iron is inhibited by *magnesium trisilicate* and *antacids containing carbonates.*

Ferrous sulfate may interfere with the absorption of *tetracyclines.*

The antiparkinsonism effects of *levodopa* may be reversed by pyridoxine.

Iron absorption is inhibited by the ingestion of eggs or milk.

Carcinogenesis: Adequate data are not available on long-term potential for carcinogenesis in animals or humans.

Pregnancy: Pregnancy Category A. Studies in pregnant women have not shown that FERO-FOLIC-500 or IBERET-FOLIC-500 increase the risk of fetal abnormalities if administered during pregnancy. If either of these drugs is used during pregnancy, the possibility of fetal harm appears remote. Because studies cannot rule out the possibility of harm, however, FERO-FOLIC-500 or IBERET-FOLIC-500 should be used during pregnancy only if clearly needed.

Nursing Mothers: Folic acid, ascorbic acid, and B-complex vitamins are excreted in breast milk.

ADVERSE REACTIONS

The likelihood of gastric intolerance to iron in the controlled-release Gradumet vehicle is remote. If such should occur, the tablet may be taken after a meal. Allergic sensitization has been reported following both oral and parenteral administration of folic acid.

OVERDOSAGE

Signs of serious toxicity may be delayed because the iron is in a controlled-release dose form. Increased capillary permeability, reduced plasma volume, increased cardiac output, and sudden cardiovascular collapse may occur in acute iron intoxication. In overdosage, efforts should be made to hasten the elimination of the Gradumet tablets ingested. An emetic should be administered as soon as possible, followed by gastric lavage if indicated. Immediately following emesis, a large dose of a saline cathartic should be used to speed passage through the intestinal tract. X-ray examination may then be considered to determine the position and number of Gradumet tablets remaining in the gastrointestinal tract.

DOSAGE AND ADMINISTRATION

FERO-FOLIC-500 is administered orally and may be taken on an empty stomach.

Adults: For treatment of iron deficiency and prevention of folic acid deficiency, the recommended dose is one tablet daily.

Pregnant Adults: For prevention and treatment of iron deficiency and to supply a maintenance dosage of folic acid, the recommended dose is one tablet daily.

IBERET-FOLIC-500 is administered orally and may be taken on an empty stomach.

Adults: For the treatment of iron deficiency and prevention of concomitant folic acid deficiency where there is an associated deficient intake or increased need for the B-complex vitamins, the recommended dose is one tablet daily.

Pregnant Adults: For the prevention and treatment of iron deficiency where there is a concomitant deficient intake or increased need for the B-complex vitamins including folic acid, the recommended dose is one tablet daily.

HOW SUPPLIED

FERO-FOLIC-500 is supplied as red Filmtab tablets in bottles of 100 (**NDC** 0074-7079-13) and 500 (**NDC** 0074-7079-53).

IBERET-FOLIC-500 is supplied as red Filmtab tablets in bottles of 60 (**NDC** 0074-7125-60).

FILMTAB—Film-sealed tablets, Abbott.

GRADUMET—Controlled-release dose form, Abbott.

Recommended storage: Store below 77°F (25°C).

Ref. 03-4410-R9

Continued on next page

Abbott Laboratories—Cont.

FERO–GRAD–500® Filmtab® tablets   OTC
[fe 'ro-grad]
CONTROLLED-RELEASE IRON, plus Vitamin C
Well-tolerated once-daily hematinic
for iron deficiency.
FERO-GRADUMET® Filmtab® tablets
For Iron Deficiency
Hematinic supplying controlled-release dose of iron

DESCRIPTION
Each Fero-Gradumet and Fero-Grad-500 tablet contains
the equivalent of 105 mg of elemental iron (525 mg of
ferrous sulfate) in a unique controlled-release vehicle, the
Gradumet®. In addition, each Fero-Grad-500 tablet contains 500 mg of vitamin C (as sodium ascorbate) to improve
iron absorption.

Inactive Ingredients: Fero-Grad-500: Castor oil, cellulosic
polymers, D&C Red No. 7, magnesium stearate,
methyl acrylate-methyl methacrylate copolymer, polyethylene glycol, povidone, pregelatinized starch (contains corn
starch), propylene glycol, talc, titanium dioxide and
vanillin.
Fero-Gradumet: Castor oil, cellulosic polymers, FD&C Red
No. 40, FD&C Yellow No. 6, magnesium stearate, methyl
acrylate-methyl methacrylate copolymer, polyethylene glycol, povidone, propylene glycol, titanium dioxide and vanillin.

WARNINGS
Close bottles tightly and keep out of reach of children. Contains iron, which can be harmful or fatal to children in large
doses. In case of accidental overdose, seek professional assistance or contact a Poison Control Center immediately.
The unit dose strip package is not intended for households
with young children.

DOSAGE AND ADMINISTRATION
Fero-Grad-500: Usual adult dose: One tablet daily, or as
directed by the physician.
Fero-Gradumet: Usual adult dose: One or two tablets daily,
or as directed by the physician.

HOW SUPPLIED
Fero-Gradumet is supplied as red tablets in bottles of 100
(NDC 0074-6852-02); Fero-Grad-500 is supplied as red tablets
in bottles of 100 (NDC 0074-7238-01) , and in Abbo-Pac unit
dose strip packages of 100 tablets (NDC 0074-7238-11).
Bottle caps are child-resistant and tamper-evident. Do not accept if
break-away ring on cap is broken or missing. Keep bottles
tightly closed. The ingredients of these products are listed in
one or more of the Medicare designated compendia.
Recommended storage: Store below 77°F (25°C).
Ref. 03-2108-8/R33 and 03-2112-8/R31

HYTRIN®   ℞
(terazosin hydrochloride)
Capsules

DESCRIPTION
HYTRIN (terazosin hydrochloride), an alpha-1-selective
adrenoceptor blocking agent, is a quinazoline derivative
represented by the following chemical name and structural
formula:
(RS)-Piperazine, 1-(4-amino-6,7-dimethoxy-2-quinazolinyl)-
4-[(tetra-hydro -2- furanyl)carbonyl]-, monohydrochloride,
dihydrate.

Terazosin hydrochloride is a white, crystalline substance,
freely soluble in water and isotonic saline and has a molecular weight of 459.93. HYTRIN capsules (terazosin hydrochloride capsules) for oral ingestion are supplied in four dosage
strengths containing terazosin hydrochloride equivalent to
1 mg, 2 mg, 5 mg, or 10 mg of terazosin.

Inactive Ingredients:
1 mg capsules: gelatin, glycerin, iron oxide, methylparaben,
mineral oil, polyethylene glycol, povidone, propylparaben,
titanium dioxide, and vanillin.
2 mg capsules: D&C yellow No. 10, gelatin, glycerin, methylparaben, mineral oil, polyethylene glycol, povidone, propylparaben, titanium dioxide, and vanillin.
5 mg capsules: D&C red No. 28, FD&C red No. 40, gelatin,
glycerin, methylparaben, mineral oil, polyethylene glycol,
povidone, propylparaben, titanium dioxide, and vanillin.

	Symptom Score (Range 0–27)			Peak Flow Rate (mL/sec)		
	N	Mean Baseline	Mean Change (%)	N	Mean Baseline	Mean Change (%)
Study 1(10 mg)[a] **Titration to fixed dose (12 wks)**						
Placebo	55	9.7	−2.3 (24)	54	10.1	+1.0 (10)
Terazosin	54	10.1	−4.5 (45)*	52	8.8	+3.0 (34)*
Study 2(2, 5, 10, 20 mg)[b] **Titration to response (24 wks)**						
Placebo	89	12.5	−3.8 (30)	88	8.8	+1.4 (16)
Terazosin	85	12.2	−5.3 (43)*	84	8.4	+2.9 (35)*
Study 3(1, 2, 5, 10 mg)[c] **Titration to response (24 wks)**						
Placebo	74	10.4	−1.1 (11)	74	8.8	+1.2 (14)
Terazosin	73	10.9	−4.6 (42)*	73	8.6	+2.6 (30)*

[a] Highest dose 10 mg shown.
[b] 23% of patients on 10 mg, 41% of patients on 20 mg.
[c] 67% of patients on 10 mg.
* Significantly (p ≤ 0.05) more improvement than placebo.

---

10 mg capsules: FD&C blue No. 1, gelatin, glycerin, methylparaben, mineral oil, polyethylene glycol, povidone, propylparaben, titanium dioxide, and vanillin.

CLINICAL PHARMACOLOGY
Pharmacodynamics:

A. Benign Prostatic Hyperplasia (BPH)
The symptoms associated with BPH are related to bladder
outlet obstruction, which is comprised of two underlying
components: a static component and a dynamic component.
The static component is a consequence of an increase in prostate size. Over time, the prostate will continue to enlarge.
However, clinical studies have demonstrated that the size of
the prostate does not correlate with the severity of BPH
symptoms or the degree of urinary obstruction. The dynamic
component is a function of an increase in smooth muscle tone
in the prostate and bladder neck, leading to constriction of
the bladder outlet. Smooth muscle tone is mediated by sympathetic nervous stimulation of alpha-l adrenoceptors,
which are abundant in the prostate, prostatic capsule and
bladder neck. The reduction in symptoms and improvement
in urine flow rates following administration of terazosin is
related to relaxation of smooth muscle produced by blockade
of alpha-l adrenoceptors in the bladder neck and prostate.
Because there are relatively few alpha-l adrenoceptors in the
bladder body, terazosin is able to reduce the bladder outlet
obstruction without affecting bladder contractility.
Terazosin has been studied in 1222 men with symptomatic
BPH. In three placebo-controlled studies, symptom evaluation and uroflowmetric measurements were performed approximately 24 hours following dosing. Symptoms were
quantified using the Boyarsky Index. The questionnaire
evaluated both obstructive (hesitancy, intermittency, terminal dribbling, impairment of size and force of stream, sensation of incomplete bladder emptying) and irritative (nocturia, daytime frequency, urgency, dysuria) symptoms by rating each of the 9 symptoms from 0-3, for a total score of 27
points. Results from these studies indicated that terazosin
statistically significantly improved symptoms and peak
urine flow rates over placebo as follows:
[See table above.]
In all three studies, both symptom scores and peak urine
flow rates showed statistically significant improvement from
baseline in patients treated with terazosin from week 2 (or
the first clinic visit) and throughout the study duration.
Analysis of the effect of terazosin on individual urinary
symptoms demonstrated that compared to placebo, terazosin
significantly improved the symptoms of hesitancy, intermittency, impairment in size and force of urinary stream, sensation of incomplete emptying, terminal dribbling, daytime
frequency and nocturia.

Global assessments of overall urinary function and symptoms were also performed by investigators who were blinded
to patient treatment assignment. In studies 1 and 3, patients
treated with terazosin had a significantly (p ≤ 0.001) greater
overall improvement compared to placebo treated patients.
In a short term study (Study 1), patients were randomized to
either 2, 5 or 10 mg of terazosin or placebo. Patients randomized to the 10 mg group achieved a statistically significant
response in both symptoms and peak flow rate compared to
placebo (Figure 1).

Figure 1
Study 1

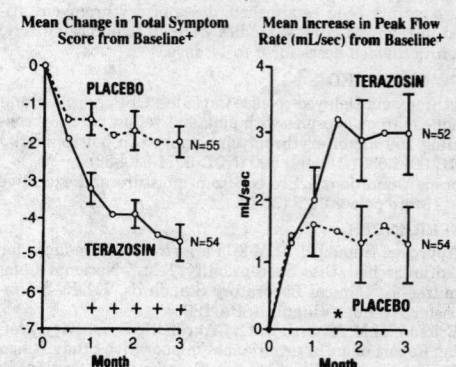

Mean Change in Total Symptom Score from Baseline+

Mean Increase in Peak Flow Rate (mL/sec) from Baseline+

†for baseline values see above table.
* p ≤ 0.05, compared to placebo group.

In a long-term, open-label, non-placebo controlled clinical
trial, 181 men were followed for 2 years and 58 of these men
were followed for 30 months. The effect of terazosin on urinary symptom scores and peak flow rates was maintained
throughout the study duration (Figures 2 and 3):
[See Figure at top of next column.]
[See second Figure at top of next column.]
In this long-term trial, both symptom scores and peak urinary flow rates showed statistically significant improvement
suggesting a relaxation of smooth muscle cells.
Although blockade of alpha-1 adrenoceptors also lowers
blood pressure in hypertensive patients with increased peripheral vascular resistance, terazosin treatment of normotensive men with BPH did not result in a clinically significant blood pressure lowering effect:
[See table below.]

Mean Changes in Blood Pressure from Baseline to Final Visit in all Double-Blind, Placebo-Controlled Studies

		Normotensive Patients DBP ≤ 90 mm Hg		Hypertensive Patients DBP > 90 mm Hg	
	Group	N	Mean Change	N	Mean Change
SBP (mm Hg)	Placebo	293	−0.1	45	−5.8
	Terazosin	519	−3.3*	65	−14.4*
DBP (mm Hg)	Placebo	293	+0.4	45	−7.1
	Terazosin	519	−2.2*	65	−15.1*

* p ≤ 0.05 vs. placebo

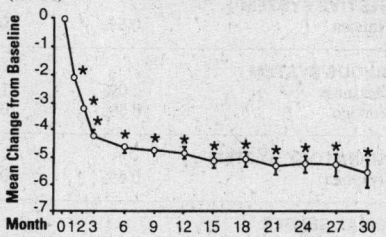

Figure 2

Mean Change in Total Symptom Score from Baseline Long-Term, Open-Label, Non-Placebo Controlled Study (N=494)

* p ≤ 0.05 vs. baseline
mean baseline = 10.7

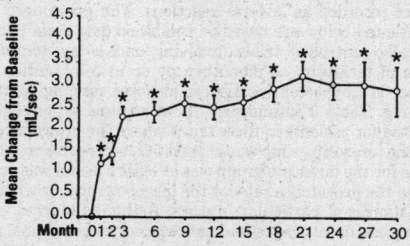

Figure 3

Mean Change in Peak Flow Rate from Baseline Long-Term, Open-Label, Non-Placebo Controlled Study (N=494)

* p ≤ 0.05 vs. baseline
mean baseline = 9.9

B. Hypertension

In animals, terazosin causes a decrease in blood pressure by decreasing total peripheral vascular resistance. The vasodilatory hypotensive action of terazosin appears to be produced mainly by blockade of alpha-1 adrenoceptors. Terazosin decreases blood pressure gradually within 15 minutes following oral administration.

Patients in clinical trials of terazosin were administered once daily (the great majority) and twice daily regimens with total doses usually in the range of 5-20 mg/day, and had mild (about 77%, diastolic pressure 95-105 mmHg) or moderate (23%, diastolic pressure 105-115 mmHg) hypertension. Because terazosin, like all alpha antagonists, can cause unusually large falls in blood pressure after the first dose or first few doses, the initial dose was 1 mg in virtually all trials, with subsequent titration to a specified fixed dose or titration to some specified blood pressure end point (usually a supine diastolic pressure of 90 mmHg).

Blood pressure responses were measured at the end of the dosing interval (usually 24 hours) and effects were shown to persist throughout the interval, with the usual supine responses 5-10 mmHg systolic and 3.5-8 mmHg diastolic greater than placebo. The responses in the standing position tended to be somewhat larger, by 1-3 mmHg, although this was not true in all studies. The magnitude of the blood pressure responses was similar to prazosin and less than hydrochlorothiazide (in a single study of hypertensive patients). In measurements 24 hours after dosing, heart rate was unchanged.

Limited measurements of peak response (2-3 hours after dosing) during chronic terazosin administration indicate that it is greater than about twice the trough (24 hour) response, suggesting some attenuation of response at 24 hours, presumably due to a fall in blood terazosin concentrations at the end of the dose interval. This explanation is not established with certainty, however, and is not consistent with the similarity of blood pressure response to once daily and twice daily dosing and with the absence of an observed dose-response relationship over a range of 5-20 mg, i.e., if blood concentrations had fallen to the point of providing less than full effect at 24 hours, a shorter dosing interval or larger dose should have led to increased response.

Further dose response and dose duration studies are being carried out. Blood pressure should be measured at the end of the dose interval; if response is not satisfactory, patients may be tried on a larger dose or twice daily dosing regimen. The latter should also be considered if possibly blood pressure-related side effects, such as dizziness, palpitations, or orthostatic complaints, are seen within a few hours after dosing. The greater blood pressure effect associated with peak plasma concentrations (first few hours after dosing) appears somewhat more position-dependent (greater in the erect position) than the effect of terazosin at 24 hours and in the erect position there is also a 6-10 beat per minute increase in heart rate in the first few hours after dosing. During the first 3 hours after dosing 12.5% of patients had a systolic pressure fall of 30 mmHg or more from supine to standing, or standing systolic pressure below 90 mmHg with a fall of at least 20 mmHg, compared to 4% of a placebo group.

There was a tendency for patients to gain weight during terazosin therapy. In placebo-controlled monotherapy trials, male and female patients receiving terazosin gained a mean of 1.7 and 2.2 pounds respectively, compared to losses of 0.2 and 1.2 pounds respectively in the placebo group. Both differences were statistically significant.

During controlled clinical trials, patients receiving terazosin monotherapy had a small but statistically significant decrease (a 3% fall) compared to placebo in total cholesterol and the combined low-density and very-low-density lipoprotein fractions. No significant changes were observed in high-density lipoprotein fraction and triglycerides compared to placebo.

Analysis of clinical laboratory data following administration of terazosin suggested the possibility of hemodilution based on decreases in hematocrit, hemoglobin, white blood cells, total protein and albumin. Decreases in hematocrit and total protein have been observed with alpha-blockade and are attributed to hemodilution.

Pharmacokinetics:

Terazosin hydrochloride administered as HYTRIN capsules is essentially completely absorbed in man. Administration of capsules immediately after meals had a minimal effect on the extent of absorption. The time to reach peak plasma concentration however, was delayed by about 40 minutes. Terazosin has been shown to undergo minimal hepatic first-pass metabolism and nearly all of the circulating dose is in the form of parent drug. The plasma levels peak about one hour after dosing, and then decline with a half-life of approximately 12 hours. In a study that evaluated the effect of age on terazosin pharmacokinetics, the mean plasma half-lives were 14.0 and 11.4 hours for the age group ≥ 70 years and the age group of 20-39 years, respectively. After oral administration the plasma clearance was decreased by 31.7% in patients 70 years of age or older compared to that in patients 20-39 years of age.

The drug is 90-94% bound to plasma proteins and binding is constant over the clinically observed concentration range. Approximately 10% of an orally administered dose is excreted as parent drug in the urine and approximately 20% is excreted in the feces. The remainder is eliminated as metabolites. Impaired renal function had no significant effect on the elimination of terazosin, and dosage adjustment of terazosin to compensate for the drug removal during hemodialysis (approximately 10%) does not appear to be necessary. Overall, approximately 40% of the administered dose is excreted in the urine and approximately 60% in the feces. The disposition of the compound in animals is qualitatively similar to that in man.

INDICATIONS AND USAGE

HYTRIN (terazosin hydrochloride) is indicated for the treatment of symptomatic benign prostatic hyperplasia (BPH). There is a rapid response, with approximately 70% of patients experiencing an increase in urinary flow and improvement in symptoms of BPH when treated with HYTRIN. The long-term effects of HYTRIN on the incidence of surgery, acute urinary obstruction or other complications of BPH are yet to be determined.

HYTRIN is also indicated for the treatment of hypertension. It can be used alone or in combination with other antihypertensive agents such as diuretics or beta-adrenergic blocking agents.

CONTRAINDICATIONS

HYTRIN capsules are contraindicated in patients known to be hypersensitive to terazosin hydrochloride.

WARNINGS

Syncope and "First-dose" Effect:

HYTRIN capsules, like other alpha-adrenergic blocking agents, can cause marked lowering of blood pressure, especially postural hypotension, and syncope in association with the first dose or first few days of therapy. A similar effect can be anticipated if therapy is interrupted for several days and then restarted. Syncope has also been reported with other alpha-adrenergic blocking agents in association with rapid dosage increases or the introduction of another antihypertensive drug. Syncope is believed to be due to an excessive postural hypotensive effect, although occasionally the syncopal episode has been preceded by a bout of severe supraventricular tachycardia with heart rates of 120-160 beats per minute. Additionally, the possibility of the contribution of hemodilution to the symptoms of postural hypotension should be considered.

To decrease the likelihood of syncope or excessive hypotension, treatment should always be initiated with a 1 mg dose of terazosin, given at bedtime. The 2 mg, 5 mg and 10 mg capsules are not indicated as initial therapy. Dosage should then be increased slowly, according to recommendations in the Dosage and Administration section and additional antihypertensive agents should be added with caution. The pa-tient should be cautioned to avoid situations, such as driving or hazardous tasks, where injury could result should syncope occur during initiation of therapy.

In early investigational studies, where increasing single doses up to 7.5 mg were given at 3 day intervals, tolerance to the first dose phenomenon did not necessarily develop and the "first-dose" effect could be observed at all doses. Syncopal episodes occurred in 3 of the 14 subjects given terazosin at doses of 2.5, 5 and 7.5 mg, which are higher than the recommended initial dose; in addition, severe orthostatic hypotension (blood pressure falling to 50/0 mmHg) was seen in two others and dizziness, tachycardia, and lightheadedness occurred in most subjects. These adverse effects all occurred within 90 minutes of dosing.

In three placebo-controlled BPH studies 1, 2, and 3 (see CLINICAL PHARMACOLOGY), the incidence of postural hypotension in the terazosin treated patients was 5.1%, 5.2%, and 3.7% respectively.

In multiple dose clinical trials involving nearly 2000 hypertensive patients treated with terazosin, syncope was reported in about 1% of patients. Syncope was not necessarily associated only with the first dose.

If syncope occurs, the patient should be placed in a recumbent position and treated supportively as necessary. There is evidence that the orthostatic effect of terazosin is greater, even in chronic use, shortly after dosing. The risk of the events is greatest during the initial seven days of treatment, but continues at all time intervals.

PRECAUTIONS

General:

Prostatic Cancer

Carcinoma of the prostate and BPH cause many of the same symptoms. These two diseases frequently co-exist. Therefore, patients thought to have BPH should be examined prior to starting HYTRIN therapy to rule out the presence of carcinoma of the prostate.

Orthostatic Hypotension

While syncope is the most severe orthostatic effect of terazosin (see Warnings), other symptoms of lowered blood pressure, such as dizziness, lightheadedness and palpitations, were more common and occurred in some 28% of patients in clinical trials of hypertension. In BPH clinical trials, 21% of the patients experienced one or more of the following: dizziness, hypotension, postural hypotension, syncope, and vertigo. Patients with occupations in which such events represent potential problems should be treated with particular caution.

Information for Patients (see Patient Package Insert):

Patients should be made aware of the possibility of syncopal and orthostatic symptoms, especially at the initiation of therapy, and to avoid driving or hazardous tasks for 12 hours after the first dose, after a dosage increase and after interruption of therapy when treatment is resumed. They should be cautioned to avoid situations where injury could result should syncope occur during initiation of terazosin therapy. They should also be advised of the need to sit or lie down when symptoms of lowered blood pressure occur, although these symptoms are not always orthostatic, and to be careful when rising from a sitting or lying position. If dizziness, lightheadedness, or palpitations are bothersome they should be reported to the physician, so that dose adjustment can be considered.

Patients should also be told that drowsiness or somnolence can occur with terazosin, requiring caution in people who must drive or operate heavy machinery.

Laboratory Tests:

Small but statistically significant decreases in hematocrit, hemoglobin, white blood cells, total protein and albumin were observed in controlled clinical trials. These laboratory findings suggested the possibility of hemodilution. Treatment with terazosin for up to 24 months had no significant effect on prostate specific antigen (PSA) levels.

Drug Interactions:

In controlled trials, terazosin has been added to diuretics, and several beta-adrenergic blockers; no unexpected interactions were observed. Terazosin has also been used in patients on a variety of concomitant therapies; while these were not formal interaction studies, no interactions were observed. Terazosin has been used concomitantly in at least 50 patients on the following drugs or drug classes: 1) analgesic/anti-inflammatory (e.g., acetaminophen, aspirin, codeine, ibuprofen, indomethacin); 2) antibiotics (e.g., erythromycin, trimethoprim and sulfamethoxazole); 3) anticholinergic/sympathomimetics (e.g., phenylephrine hydrochloride, phenylpropanolamine hydrochloride, psuedoephedrine hydrochloride); 4) antigout (e.g., allopurinol); 5) antihistamines (e.g., chlorpheniramine); 6) cardiovascular agents (e.g., atenolol, hydrochlorothiazide, methyclothiazide, propranolol); 7) corticosteroids; 8) gastrointestinal agents (e.g., antacids); 9) hypoglycemics; 10) sedatives and tranquilizers (e.g., diazepam).

Continued on next page

Abbott Laboratories—Cont.

Use with Other Drugs:
In a study (n=24) where terazosin and verapamil were administered concomitantly, terazosin's mean AUC_{0-24} increased 11% after the first verapamil dose and after 3 weeks of verapamil treatment it increased by 24% with associated increases in C_{max} (25%) and C_{min} (32%) means. Terazosin mean T_{max} decreased from 1.3 hours to 0.8 hours after 3 weeks of verapamil treatment. Statistically significant differences were not found in the verapamil level with and without terazosin. In a study (n=6) where terazosin and captopril were administered concomitantly, plasma disposition of captopril was not influenced by concomitant administration of terazosin and terazosin maximum plasma concentrations increased linearly with dose at steady-state after administration of terazosin plus captopril (see Dosage and Administration).

Carcinogenesis, Mutagenesis, Impairment of Fertility:
Terazosin was devoid of mutagenic potential when evaluated *in vivo* and *in vitro* (the Ames test, *in vivo* cytogenetics, the dominant lethal test in mice, *in vivo* Chinese hamster chromosome aberration test and V79 forward mutation assay). Terazosin, administered in the feed to rats at doses of 8, 40, and 250 mg/kg/day (70, 350, and 2100 mg/M²/day), for two years, was associated with a statistically significant increase in benign adrenal medullary tumors of male rats exposed to the 250 mg/kg dose. This dose is 175 times the maximum recommended human dose of 20 mg (12 mg/M²). Female rats were unaffected. Terazosin was not oncogenic in mice when administered in feed for 2 years at a maximum tolerated dose of 32 mg/kg/day (110 mg/M²; 9 times the maximum recommended human dose). The absence of mutagenicity in a battery of tests, of tumorigenicity of any cell type in the mouse carcinogenicity assay, of increased total tumor incidence in either species, and of proliferative adrenal lesions in female rats, suggests a male rat species-specific event. Numerous other diverse pharmacological and chemical compounds have also been associated with benign adrenal medullary tumors in male rats without supporting evidence for carcinogenicity in man.

The effect of terazosin on fertility was assessed in a standard fertility/reproductive performance study in which male and female rats were administered oral doses of 8, 30 and 120 mg/kg/day. Four of 20 male rats given 30 mg/kg (240 mg/M²; 20 times the maximum recommended human dose) and five of 19 male rats given 120 mg/kg (960 mg/M²; 80 times the maximum recommended human dose) failed to sire a litter. Testicular weights and morphology were unaffected by treatment. Vaginal smears at 30 and 120 mg/kg/day, however, appeared to contain less sperm than smears from control matings and good correlation was reported between sperm count and subsequent pregnancy.

Oral administration of terazosin for one or two years elicited a statistically significant increase in the incidence of testicular atrophy in rats exposed to 40 and 250 mg/kg/day (29 and 175 times the maximum recommended human dose), but not in rats exposed to 8 mg/kg/day (> 6 times the maximum recommended human dose). Testicular atrophy was also observed in dogs dosed with 300 mg/kg/day (> 500 times the maximum recommended human dose) for three months but not after one year when dosed with 20 mg/kg/day (38 times the maximum recommended human dose). This lesion has also been seen with Minipress®, another (marketed) selective-alpha-1 blocking agent.

Pregnancy:
Teratogenic effects: Pregnancy Category C. Terazosin was not teratogenic in either rats or rabbits when administered at oral doses up to 280 and 60 times, respectively, the maximum recommended human dose. Fetal resorptions occurred in rats dosed with 480 mg/kg/day, approximately 280 times the maximum recommended human dose. Increased fetal resorptions, decreased fetal weight and an increased number of supernumerary ribs were observed in offspring of rabbits dosed with 60 times the maximum recommended human dose. These findings (in both species) were most likely secondary to maternal toxicity. There are no adequate and well-controlled studies in pregnant women and the safety of terazosin in pregnancy has not been established. HYTRIN is not recommended during pregnancy unless the potential benefit justifies the potential risk to the mother and fetus. Nonteratogenic effects: In a peri- and post-natal development study in rats, significantly more pups died in the group dosed with 120 mg/kg/day (> 75 times the maximum recommended human dose) than in the control group during the three-week postpartum period.

Nursing Mothers:
It is not known whether terazosin is excreted in breast milk. Because many drugs are excreted in breast milk, caution should be exercised when terazosin is administered to a nursing woman.

Pediatric Use:
Safety and effectiveness in children have not been determined.

ADVERSE REACTIONS

Benign Prostatic Hyperplasia
The incidence of treatment-emergent adverse events has been ascertained from clinical trials conducted worldwide. All adverse events reported during these trials were recorded as adverse reactions. The incidence rates presented below are based on combined data from six placebo-controlled trials involving once-a-day administration of terazosin at doses ranging from 1 to 20 mg. Table 1 summarizes those adverse events reported for patients in these trials when the incidence rate in the terazosin group was at least 1% and was greater than that for the placebo group, or where the reaction is of clinical interest. Asthenia, postural hypotension, dizziness, somnolence, nasal congestion/rhinitis, and impotence were the only events that were significantly (p ≤ 0.05) more common in patients receiving terazosin than in patients receiving placebo. The incidence of urinary tract infection was significantly lower in the patients receiving terazosin than in patients receiving placebo. An analysis of the incidence rate of hypotensive adverse events (see PRECAUTIONS) adjusted for the length of drug treatment has shown that the risk of the events is greatest during the initial seven days of treatment, but continues at all time intervals.

TABLE 1
**ADVERSE REACTIONS DURING
PLACEBO-CONTROLLED TRIALS
BENIGN PROSTATIC HYPERPLASIA**

Body System	Terazosin (N=636)	Placebo (N=360)
BODY AS A WHOLE		
†Asthenia	7.4%*	3.3%
Flu Syndrome	2.4%	1.7%
Headache	4.9%	5.8%
CARDIOVASCULAR SYSTEM		
Hypotension	0.6%	0.6%
Palpitations	0.9%	1.1%
Postural Hypotension	3.9%*	0.8%
Syncope	0.6%	0.0%
DIGESTIVE SYSTEM		
Nausea	1.7%	1.1%
METABOLIC AND NUTRITIONAL DISORDERS		
Peripheral Edema	0.9%	0.3%
Weight Gain	0.5%	0.0%
NERVOUS SYSTEM		
Dizziness	9.1%*	4.2%
Somnolence	3.6%*	1.9%
Vertigo	1.4%	0.3%
RESPIRATORY SYSTEM		
Dyspnea	1.7%	0.8%
Nasal Congestion/Rhinitis	1.9%*	0.0%
SPECIAL SENSES		
Blurred Vision/Amblyopia	1.3%	0.6%
UROGENITAL SYSTEM		
Impotence	1.6%*	0.6%
Urinary Tract Infection	1.3%	3.9%*

† Includes weakness, tiredness, lassitude and fatigue.
* p ≤0.05 comparison between groups.

Additional adverse events have been reported, but these are, in general, not distinguishable from symptoms that might have occurred in the absence of exposure to terazosin. The safety profile of patients treated in the long-term open-label study was similar to that observed in the controlled studies. The adverse events were usually transient and mild or moderate in intensity, but sometimes were serious enough to interrupt treatment. In the placebo-controlled clinical trials, the rates of premature termination due to adverse events were not statistically different between the placebo and terazosin groups. The adverse events that were bothersome, as judged by their being reported as reasons for discontinuation of therapy by at least 0.5% of the terazosin group and being reported more often than in the placebo group, are shown in Table 2.

TABLE 2
**DISCONTINUATION DURING
PLACEBO-CONTROLLED TRIALS
BENIGN PROSTATIC HYPERPLASIA**

Body System	Terazosin (N=636)	Placebo (N=360)
BODY AS A WHOLE		
Fever	0.5%	0.0%
Headache	1.1%	0.8%
CARDIOVASCULAR SYSTEM		
Postural Hypotension	0.5%	0.0%
Syncope	0.5%	0.0%
DIGESTIVE SYSTEM		
Nausea	0.5%	0.3%
NERVOUS SYSTEM		
Dizziness	2.0%	1.1%
Vertigo	0.5%	0.3%
RESPIRATORY SYSTEM		
Dyspnea	0.5%	0.3%
SPECIAL SENSES		
Blurred Vision/Amblyopia	0.6%	0.0%
UROGENITAL SYSTEM		
Urinary Tract Infection	0.5%	0.3%

Hypertension
The prevalence of adverse reactions has been ascertained from clinical trials conducted primarily in the United States. All adverse experiences (events) reported during these trials were recorded as adverse reactions. The prevalence rates presented below are based on combined data from fourteen placebo-controlled trials involving once-a-day administration of terazosin, as monotherapy or in combination with other antihypertensive agents, at doses ranging from 1 to 40 mg. Table 3 summarizes those adverse events reported for patients in these trials where the prevalence rate in the terazosin group was at least 5%, where the prevalence rate for the terazosin group was at least 2% and was greater than the prevalence rate for the placebo group, or where the reaction is of particular interest. Asthenia, blurred vision, dizziness, nasal congestion, nausea, peripheral edema, palpitations and somnolence were the only symptoms that were significantly (p < 0.05) more common in patients receiving terazosin than in patients receiving placebo. Similar adverse reaction rates were observed in placebo-controlled monotherapy trials.

TABLE 3
**ADVERSE REACTIONS DURING
PLACEBO-CONTROLLED TRIALS
HYPERTENSION**

Body System	Terazosin (N=859)	Placebo (N=506)
BODY AS A WHOLE		
†Asthenia	11.3%*	4.3%
Back Pain	2.4%	1.2%
Headache	16.2%	15.8%
CARDIOVASCULAR SYSTEM		
Palpitations	4.3%*	1.2%
Postural Hypotension	1.3%	0.4%
Tachycardia	1.9%	1.2%
DIGESTIVE SYSTEM		
Nausea	4.4%*	1.4%
METABOLIC AND NUTRITIONAL DISORDERS		
Edema	0.9%	0.6%
Peripheral Edema	5.5%*	2.4%
Weight Gain	0.5%	0.2%
MUSCULOSKELETAL SYSTEM		
Pain-Extremities	3.5%	3.0%
NERVOUS SYSTEM		
Depression	0.3%	0.2%
Dizziness	19.3%*	7.5%
Libido Decreased	0.6%	0.2%
Nervousness	2.3%	1.8%
Paresthesia	2.9%	1.4%
Somnolence	5.4%*	2.6%
RESPIRATORY SYSTEM		
Dyspnea	3.1%	2.4%
Nasal Congestion	5.9%*	3.4%
Sinusitis	2.6%	1.4%
SPECIAL SENSES		
Blurred Vision	1.6%*	0.0%
UROGENITAL SYSTEM		
Impotence	1.2%	1.4%

† Includes weakness, tiredness, lassitude and fatigue.
* Statistically significant at p=0.05 level.

Additional adverse reactions have been reported, but these are, in general, not distinguishable from symptoms that might have occurred in the absence of exposure to terazosin. The following additional adverse reactions were reported by at least 1% of 1987 patients who received terazosin in controlled or open, short- or long-term clinical trials or have been reported during marketing experience: *Body as a Whole:* chest pain, facial edema, fever, abdominal pain, neck pain, shoulder pain; *Cardiovascular System:* arrhythmia, vasodilation; *Digestive System:* constipation, diarrhea, dry mouth, dyspepsia, flatulence, vomiting; *Metabolic/Nutritional Disorders:* gout; *Musculoskeletal System:* arthralgia, arthritis, joint disorder, myalgia; *Nervous System:* anxiety, insomnia; *Respiratory System:* bronchitis, cold symptoms, epistaxis, flu symptoms, increased cough, pharyngitis, rhinitis; *Skin and Appendages:* pruritus, rash, sweating; *Special Senses:* abnormal vision, conjunctivitis, tinnitus; *Urogenital System:* urinary frequency, urinary incontinence primarily reported in postmenopausal women, urinary tract infection. Post-marketing experience indicates that in rare instances patients may develop allergic reactions, including anaphylaxis, following administration of terazosin hydrochloride. There have been reports of priapism during post-marketing surveillance.

The adverse reactions were usually mild or moderate in intensity but sometimes were serious enough to interrupt treatment. The adverse reactions that were most bothersome, as judged by their being reported as reasons for discontinuation of therapy by at least 0.5% of the terazosin group and being reported more often than in the placebo group, are shown in Table 4.

TABLE 4
DISCONTINUATIONS DURING PLACEBO-CONTROLLED TRIALS
HYPERTENSION

Body System	Terazosin (N = 859)	Placebo (N = 506)
BODY AS A WHOLE		
Asthenia	1.6%	0.0%
Headache	1.3%	1.0%
CARDIOVASCULAR SYSTEM		
Palpitations	1.4%	0.2%
Postural Hypotension	0.5%	0.0%
Syncope	0.5%	0.2%
Tachycardia	0.6%	0.0%
DIGESTIVE SYSTEM		
Nausea	0.8%	0.0%
METABOLIC AND NUTRITIONAL DISORDERS		
Peripheral Edema	0.6%	0.0%
NERVOUS SYSTEM		
Dizziness	3.1%	0.4%
Paresthesia	0.8%	0.2%
Somnolence	0.6%	0.2%
RESPIRATORY SYSTEM		
Dyspnea	0.9%	0.6%
Nasal Congestion	0.6%	0.0%
SPECIAL SENSES		
Blurred Vision	0.6%	0.0%

OVERDOSAGE

Should overdosage of HYTRIN lead to hypotension, support of the cardiovascular system is of first importance. Restoration of blood pressure and normalization of heart rate may be accomplished by keeping the patient in the supine position. If this measure is inadequate, shock should first be treated with volume expanders. If necessary, vasopressors should then be used and renal function should be monitored and supported as needed. Laboratory data indicate that terazosin is 90-94% protein bound; therefore, dialysis may not be of benefit.

DOSAGE AND ADMINISTRATION

If HYTRIN administration is discontinued for several days, therapy should be reinstituted using the initial dosing regimen.

Benign Prostatic Hyperplasia:
Initial Dose:
1 mg at bedtime is the starting dose for all patients, and this dose should not be exceeded as an initial dose. Patients should be closely followed during initial administration in order to minimize the risk of severe hypotensive response.

Subsequent Doses:
The dose should be increased in a stepwise fashion to 2 mg, 5 mg, or 10 mg once daily to achieve the desired improve-

ment of symptoms and/or flow rates. Doses of 10 mg once daily are generally required for the clinical response. Therefore, treatment with 10 mg for a minimum of 4–6 weeks may be required to assess whether a beneficial response has been achieved. Some patients may not achieve a clinical response despite appropriate titration. Although some additional patients responded at a 20 mg daily dose, there was an insufficient number of patients studied to draw definitive conclusions about this dose. There are insufficient data to support the use of higher doses for those patients who show inadequate or no response to 20 mg daily. **If terazosin administration is discontinued for several days or longer, therapy should be reinstituted using the initial dosing regimen.**

Use with Other Drugs:
Caution should be observed when HYTRIN is administered concomitantly with other antihypertensive agents, especially the calcium channel blocker verapamil, to avoid the possibility of developing significant hypotension. When using HYTRIN and other antihypertensive agents concomitantly, dosage reduction and retitration of either agent may be necessary (see Precautions).

Hypertension:
The dose of HYTRIN and the dose interval (12 or 24 hours) should be adjusted according to the patient's individual blood pressure response. The following is a guide to its administration:

Initial Dose:
1 mg at bedtime is the starting dose for all patients, and this dose should not be exceeded. This initial dosing regimen should be strictly observed to minimize the potential for severe hypotensive effects.

Subsequent Doses:
The dose may be slowly increased to achieve the desired blood pressure response. The usual recommended dose range is 1 mg to 5 mg administered once a day; however, some patients may benefit from doses as high as 20 mg per day. Doses over 20 mg do not appear to provide further blood pressure effect and doses over 40 mg have not been studied. Blood pressure should be monitored at the end of the dosing interval to be sure control is maintained throughout the interval. It may also be helpful to measure blood pressure 2-3 hours after dosing to see if the maximum and minimum responses are similar, and to evaluate symptoms such as dizziness or palpitations which can result from excessive hypotensive response. If response is substantially diminished at 24 hours an increased dose or use of a twice daily regimen can be considered. **If terazosin administration is discontinued for several days or longer, therapy should be reinstituted using the initial dosing regimen.** In clinical trials, except for the initial dose, the dose was given in the morning.

Use With Other Drugs: (see above)

HOW SUPPLIED

HYTRIN capsules (terazosin hydrochloride capsules) are available in four dosage strengths:

1 mg grey capsules (imprinted with ⊟ and the Abbo-Code HH):
Bottles of 100 .... (NDC 0074-3805-13),
Abbo-Pac® unit dose strip packages
of 100 capsules .... (NDC 0074-3805-11).

2 mg yellow capsules (imprinted with ⊟ and the Abbo-Code HY):
Bottles of 100 .... (NDC 0074-3806-13),
Abbo-Pac® unit dose strip packages
of 100 capsules .... (NDC 0074-3806-11).

5 mg red capsules (imprinted with ⊟ and the Abbo-Code HK):
Bottles of 100 .... (NDC 0074-3807-13),
Abbo-Pac® unit dose strip packages
of 100 capsules .... (NDC 0074-3807-11).

10 mg blue capsules (imprinted with ⊟ and the Abbo-Code HN):
Bottles of 100 .... (NDC 0074-3808-13),
Abbo-Pac® unit dose strip packages
of 100 capsules .... (NDC 0074-3808-11).

Recommended storage: Store at controlled room temperature between 20-25 ℃ (68-77 ℉). See USP. Protect from light and moisture.
Ref. 03-4628-R2-Rev. October, 1995
ABBOTT LABORATORIES
NORTH CHICAGO, IL 60064, U.S.A.
Shown in Product Identification Guide, page 303

IBERET®–500 Filmtab® tablets   OTC
[ĭ'be-ret]
CONTROLLED-RELEASE IRON,
plus B-Complex & Vitamin C
Well-tolerated once-daily hematinic
for iron deficiency, and as a B-complex and
vitamin C supplement.
IBERET® Filmtab® tablets
Hematinic Supplying
CONTROLLED-RELEASE IRON,
Vitamin C and B-Complex Vitamins
For iron deficiency and as a vitamin C and
B-complex vitamin supplement.

DESCRIPTION

Each Iberet-500 and Iberet Filmtab tablet contains 525 mg of ferrous sulfate (equivalent to 105 mg of elemental iron) in the Gradumet® controlled-release vehicle. To enhance iron absorption, 500 mg of vitamin C has been added to each Iberet-500 Filmtab.
Each Iberet-500 Filmtab tablet contains:
Ferrous Sulfate...525 mg
  (equivalent to 105 mg of elemental iron)
Vitamin C (as Sodium Ascorbate)...............500 mg
Niacinamide...30 mg
Calcium Pantothenate....................................10 mg
Vitamin B₁ (Thiamine Mononitrate)............6 mg
Vitamin B₂ (Riboflavin)................................6 mg
Vitamin B₆ (Pyridoxine Hydrochloride).......5 mg
Vitamin B₁₂ (Cyanocobalamin).....................25 mcg
The formulation of Iberet differs from Iberet-500 only in that it contains a lesser amount of vitamin C, 150 mg per Filmtab tablet.

Inactive Ingredients:
Iberet Filmtab: Castor oil, cellulosic polymers, corn starch, FD&C Red No. 40, FD&C Yellow No. 6, magnesium stearate, methyl acrylate-methyl methacrylate copolymer, polyethylene glycol, povidone, propylene glycol, stearic acid, talc, titanium dioxide and vanillin.
Iberet-500 Filmtab: Castor oil, cellulosic polymers, corn starch, FD&C Red No. 40, FD&C Yellow No. 6, magnesium stearate, methyl acrylate-methyl methacrylate copolymer, polyethylene glycol, povidone, propylene glycol, stearic acid, talc, titanium dioxide and vanillin.

INDICATIONS

For iron deficiency and as a B-complex and vitamin C Supplement.

WARNINGS

Close bottle tightly and keep out of reach of children. These products contain iron, which can be harmful or fatal to children in large doses. In case of accidental overdose, seek professional assistance or contact a Poison Control Center immediately.
The unit dose strip package is not intended for households with young children.

DOSAGE AND ADMINISTRATION

Iberet-500 and Iberet; Usual Adult Dose: One tablet daily, or as directed by the physician.

HOW SUPPLIED

Iberet-500 is supplied as red, oval shaped tablets in bottles of 60 (NDC 0074-7235-01), and in Abbo-Pac® unit dose strip packages of 100 (NDC 0074-7235-11); Iberet is supplied as red, round tablets in bottles of 60 (NDC 0074-6863-01). Bottle caps are child-resistant and tamper-evident. Do not accept if break-away ring on cap is broken or missing. Keep bottles tightly closed.
Recommended storage: Store below 77℉ (25℃).
Ref. 03-2115-9/R27 and 03-2110-4/R34

IBERET–FOLIC–500®   ℞
Controlled-Release Iron with Vitamin C,
and B-Complex including Folic Acid
Filmtab® Tablets

See combined listing under FERO-FOLIC-500.

Continued on next page

Abbott Laboratories—Cont.

IBERET®-500 LIQUID OTC
[ī'bē-rĕt]
Hematinic Supplying Iron, Vitamin C and Vitamin B-Complex
IBERET®-LIQUID
Hematinic Supplying Iron, Vitamin C and Vitamin B-Complex

DESCRIPTION

Iberet-500 Liquid and Iberet-Liquid are hematinic preparations of ferrous sulfate, B-complex vitamins and ascorbic acid. Each teaspoonful (5 mL) of Iberet-500 Liquid provides:

Elemental Iron (as Ferrous Sulfate)	26.25 mg
Vitamin C (Ascorbic Acid)	125 mg
Niacinamide	7.5 mg
Dexpanthenol	2.5 mg
Vitamin B_1 (Thiamine Hydrochloride)	1.5 mg
Vitamin B_2 (Riboflavin)	1.5 mg
Vitamin B_6 (Pyridoxine Hydrochloride)	1.25 mg
Vitamin B_{12} (Cyanocobalamin)	6.25 mcg

In a citrus-flavored vehicle.

Iberet-Liquid has a raspberry-mint flavored vehicle; Iberet-Liquid has a smaller amount of ascorbic acid: 37.5 mg per teaspoonful. Riboflavin 5' phosphate sodium is the source of Vitamin B_2 in Iberet Liquid.

Inactive Ingredients:

Iberet-Liquid: Alcohol 1%, methylparaben, propylparaben, sorbitol, water, natural and artificial flavors.

Iberet-500 Liquid: Glycerin, methylparaben, propylene glycol, propylparaben, sodium bicarbonate, sorbitol, sucrose, water and artificial flavor.

INDICATIONS

Iberet-500 Liquid: For conditions in which iron deficiency occurs concomitantly with deficient intake or increased need for the B-complex vitamins. Iberet-Liquid: For conditions in which iron deficiency and vitamin C deficiency occur concomitantly with deficient intake or increased need for the B-complex vitamins.

WARNINGS

Close tightly and keep out of reach of children. Contains iron, which can be harmful or fatal to children in large doses. In case of accidental overdose, seek professional assistance or contact a Poison Control Center immediately.

DOSAGE AND ADMINISTRATION

Iberet-500 Liquid: Usual dosage; Adults, including pregnant females and children 4 years of age and older—2 teaspoonfuls (10 mL) twice daily, after meals; Children 1–3 years of age—1 teaspoonful (5 mL) twice daily, after meals. Otherwise as directed by the physician. Iberet-Liquid: Usual dosage: Adults, including pregnant females and children 4 years of age and older—2 teaspoonfuls (10 mL) three times daily, after meals; Children 1–3 years of age—1 teaspoonful (5 mL) three times daily, after meals. Otherwise as directed by the physician.

HOW SUPPLIED

Iberet-500 Liquid (**NDC** 0074-8422-02) and Iberet-Liquid (**NDC** 0074-7173-01) are supplied in 8 fl oz (236 mL) bottles. Bottle caps are child-resistant and provided with a tamper-evident band. Do not accept if printed band is broken or missing.

Recommended storage: Protect from temperatures above 77°F (25°C). Dispense in amber bottle only.

Ref. 02-7610-4/R23 and 02-7611-4/R20

K-LOR™ Powder ℞
[k'lor]
(Potassium Chloride for Oral Solution, USP)

DESCRIPTION

Natural fruit-flavored K-LOR (potassium chloride for oral solution, USP) is an oral potassium supplement offered in individual packets as a powder for reconstitution. Each packet of K-LOR 20 mEq powder contains potassium 20 mEq and chloride 20 mEq provided by potassium chloride 1.5 g. K-LOR powder is an electrolyte replenisher. The chemical name is potassium chloride, and the structural formula is KCl. Potassium chloride, USP, occurs as a white, granular powder or as colorless crystals. It is odorless and has a saline taste. Its solutions are neutral to litmus. It is freely soluble in water and insoluble in alcohol.

Inactive Ingredients: FD&C Yellow No. 6, maltodextrin (contains corn derivative), malic acid, saccharin, silica gel and natural flavoring.

CLINICAL PHARMACOLOGY

Potassium ion is the principal intracellular cation of most body tissues. Potassium ions participate in a number of essential physiological processes including the maintenance of intracellular tonicity, the transmission of nerve impulses, the contraction of cardiac, skeletal and smooth muscle, and the maintenance of normal renal function.

The intracellular concentration of potassium is approximately 150 to 160 mEq per liter. The normal adult plasma concentration is 3.5 to 5 mEq per liter. An active ion transport system maintains this gradient across the plasma membrane.

Potassium is a normal dietary constituent and under steady state conditions the amount of potassium absorbed from the gastrointestinal tract is equal to the amount excreted in the urine. The usual dietary intake of potassium is 50 to 100 mEq per day.

Potassium depletion will occur whenever the rate of potassium loss through renal excretion and/or loss from the gastrointestinal tract exceeds the rate of potassium intake. Such depletion usually develops as a consequence of therapy with diuretics, primary or secondary hyperaldosteronism, diabetic ketoacidosis, or inadequate replacement of potassium in patients on prolonged parenteral nutrition. Depletion can develop rapidly with severe diarrhea, especially if associated with vomiting. Potassium depletion due to these causes is usually accompanied by a concomitant loss of chloride and is manifested by hypokalemia and metabolic alkalosis. Potassium depletion may produce weakness, fatigue, disturbances of cardiac rhythm (primarily ectopic beats), prominent U-waves in the electrocardiogram, and, in advanced cases, flaccid paralysis and/or impaired ability to concentrate urine.

If potassium depletion associated with metabolic alkalosis cannot be managed by correcting the fundamental cause of the deficiency, e.g., where the patient requires long term diuretic therapy, supplemental potassium in the form of high potassium food or potassium chloride may restore normal potassium levels.

In rare circumstances, (e.g., patients with renal tubular acidosis) potassium depletion may be associated with metabolic acidosis and hyperchloremia. In such patients potassium replacement should be accomplished with potassium salts other than the chloride, such as potassium bicarbonate, potassium citrate, potassium acetate, or potassium gluconate.

INDICATIONS AND USAGE

1. For the treatment of patients with hypokalemia with or without metabolic alkalosis, in digitalis intoxication, and in patients with hypokalemic familial periodic paralysis. If hypokalemia is the result of diuretic therapy, consideration should be given to the use of a lower dose of diuretic, which may be sufficient without leading to hypokalemia.
2. For the prevention of hypokalemia in patients who would be at particular risk if hypokalemia were to develop, e.g., digitalized patients or patients with significant cardiac arrhythmias.

The use of potassium salts in patients receiving diuretics for uncomplicated essential hypertension is often unnecessary when such patients have a normal dietary pattern, and when low doses of the diuretic are used. Serum potassium should be checked periodically, however, and, if hypokalemia occurs, dietary supplementation with potassium-containing foods may be adequate to control milder cases. In more severe cases, and if dose adjustment of the diuretic is ineffective or unwarranted, supplementation with potassium salts may be indicated.

CONTRAINDICATIONS

Potassium supplements are contraindicated in patients with hyperkalemia since a further increase in serum potassium concentration in such patients can produce cardiac arrest. Hyperkalemia may complicate any of the following conditions: chronic renal failure, systemic acidosis such as diabetic acidosis, acute dehydration, extensive tissue breakdown as in severe burns, adrenal insufficiency, or the administration of a potassium-sparing diuretic, e.g., spironolactone, triamterene, or amiloride (see OVERDOSAGE).

K-LOR (potassium chloride for oral solution) is contraindicated in patients with known hypersensitivity to any ingredient in this product.

WARNINGS

Hyperkalemia: (See OVERDOSAGE)

In patients with impaired mechanisms for excreting potassium, the administration of potassium salts can produce hyperkalemia and cardiac arrest. This occurs most commonly in patients given potassium intravenously, but may also occur in patients given potassium orally. Potentially fatal hyperkalemia can develop rapidly and can be asymptomatic. The use of potassium salts in patients with chronic renal disease, or any other condition which impairs potassium excretion, requires particularly careful monitoring of the serum potassium concentration and appropriate dosage adjustment.

Interaction with Potassium-Sparing Diuretics

Hypokalemia should not be treated by the concomitant administration of potassium salts and a potassium-sparing diuretic, e.g., spironolactone, triamterene, or amiloride, since the simultaneous administration of these agents can produce severe hyperkalemia.

Interaction with Angiotensin Converting Enzyme Inhibitors

Angiotensin converting enzyme (ACE) inhibitors (e.g., captopril, enalapril) will produce some potassium retention by inhibiting aldosterone production. Potassium supplements should be given to patients receiving ACE inhibitors only with close monitoring.

Metabolic Acidosis

Hypokalemia in patients with metabolic acidosis should be treated with an alkalinizing potassium salt such as potassium bicarbonate, potassium citrate, potassium acetate or potassium gluconate.

PRECAUTIONS

General: The diagnosis of potassium depletion is ordinarily made by demonstrating hypokalemia in a patient with a clinical history suggesting some cause for potassium depletion. In interpreting the serum potassium level, the physician should bear in mind that acute alkalosis *per se* can produce hypokalemia in the absence of a deficit in total body potassium, while acute acidosis *per se* can increase the serum potassium concentration to within the normal range even in the presence of a reduced total body potassium. The treatment of potassium depletion, particularly in the presence of cardiac disease, renal disease, or acidosis, requires careful attention to acid-base balance and appropriate monitoring of serum electrolytes, the electrocardiogram, and the clinical status of the patient.

Information for Patients: Physicians should consider reminding the patient of the following:

To dilute each packet of powder in 1/2 glassful of water or other liquid and take each dose after a meal.

To take this medicine following the frequency and amount prescribed by the physician. This is especially important if the patient is also taking diuretics and/or digitalis preparations.

Laboratory Tests: When blood is drawn for analysis of plasma potassium it is important to recognize that artifactual elevations can occur after improper venipuncture technique or as a result of *in vitro* hemolysis of the sample.

Drug Interactions: Potassium-sparing diuretics, angiotensin converting enzyme inhibitors (see WARNINGS).

Carcinogenesis, Mutagenesis, Impairment of Fertility: Carcinogenicity, mutagenicity and fertility studies in animals have not been performed. Potassium is a normal dietary constituent.

Pregnancy Category C: Animal reproduction studies have not been conducted with K-LOR powder. It is unlikely that potassium supplementation that does not lead to hyperkalemia would have an adverse effect on the fetus or would affect reproductive capacity.

Nursing Mothers: The normal potassium ion content of human milk is about 13 mEq per liter. Since oral potassium becomes part of the body potassium pool, as long as body potassium is not excessive, the contribution of potassium chloride supplementation should have little or no effect on the level in human milk.

Pediatric Use: Safety and effectiveness in children have not been established.

ADVERSE REACTIONS

One of the most severe adverse effects is hyperkalemia (see CONTRAINDICATIONS, WARNINGS and OVERDOSAGE).

The most common adverse reactions to oral potassium salts are nausea, vomiting, flatulence, abdominal pain/discomfort, and diarrhea. These symptoms are due to irritation of the gastrointestinal tract and are best managed by diluting the preparation further, taking the dose with meals, or reducing the amount taken at one time.

Skin rash has been reported rarely.

OVERDOSAGE

The administration of oral potassium salts to persons with normal excretory mechanisms for potassium rarely causes serious hyperkalemia. However, if excretory mechanisms are impaired or if intravenous administration is too rapid, potentially fatal hyperkalemia can result (see CONTRAINDICATIONS and WARNINGS). It is important to recognize that hyperkalemia is usually asymptomatic and may be manifested only by an increased serum potassium concentration (6.5–8.0 mEq/L) and characteristic electrocardiographic changes (peaking of T-waves, loss of P-waves, depression of S-T segments, and prolongation of the QT intervals). Late manifestations include muscle paralysis and cardiovascular collapse from cardiac arrest (9–12 mEq/L).

Treatment measures for hyperkalemia include the following:

1. Elimination of foods and medications containing potassium and of any agents with potassium-sparing properties;
2. Intravenous administration of 300 to 500 ml/hr of 10% dextrose solution containing 10–20 units of crystalline insulin per 1,000 ml;
3. Correction of acidosis, if present, with intravenous sodium bicarbonate;
4. Use of exchange resins, hemodialysis, or peritoneal dialysis.

In treating hyperkalemia, it should be recalled that in patients who have been stabilized on digitalis, lowering the serum potassium concentration too rapidly can produce digitalis toxicity.

DOSAGE AND ADMINISTRATION

The usual dietary potassium intake by the average adult is 50 to 100 mEq per day. Potassium depletion sufficient to cause hypokalemia usually requires the loss of 200 or more mEq of potassium from the total body store.

Dosage must be adjusted to the individual needs of each patient. The dose for the prevention of hypokalemia is typically in the range of 20 mEq per day. Doses of 40–100 mEq per day or more are used for the treatment of potassium depletion. Dosage should be divided if more than 20 mEq per day is given such that no more than 20 mEq is given in a single dose. The dose should be taken after a meal.

K-LOR 20 mEq powder provides 20 mEq of potassium chloride.

Each 20 mEq (one K-LOR mEq packet) of potassium should be dissolved in at least 4 oz (approximately $^1/_2$ glassful) cold water or juice. This preparation, like other potassium supplements, must be properly diluted to avoid the possibility of gastrointestinal irritation.

HOW SUPPLIED

K-LOR 20 mEq (Potassium Chloride for Oral Solution, USP) is supplied in cartons of 30 packets (**NDC** 0074-3611-01), and cartons of 100 packets (**NDC** 0074-3611-02). Each packet contains potassium, 20 mEq, and chloride, 20 mEq, provided by potassium chloride, 1.5 g.

Recommended storage: Store below 86°F (30°C).

Caution: Federal law prohibits dispensing without prescription.

TM—Trademark

Revised: June, 1994

Ref. 13-1379-5/R25

Shown in Product Identification Guide, page 303

K-Tab® ℞

[k'tâb]

(Potassium Chloride Extended-Release Tablets, USP)

DESCRIPTION

K-TAB (potassium chloride extended-release tablets) is a solid oral dosage form of potassium chloride containing 750 mg of potassium chloride, USP, equivalent to 10 mEq of potassium in a film-coated (not enteric-coated), wax matrix tablet. This formulation is intended to slow the release of potassium so that the likelihood of a high localized concentration of potassium chloride within the gastrointestinal tract is reduced. The expended inert, porous, wax/polymer matrix is not absorbed and may be excreted intact in the stool.

K-TAB tablets are an electrolyte replenisher. The chemical name is potassium chloride, and the structural formula is KCl. Potassium chloride, USP, occurs as a white, granular powder or as colorless crystals. It is odorless and has a saline taste. Its solutions are neutral to litmus. It is freely soluble in water and insoluble in alcohol.

Inactive Ingredients

Castor oil, cellulosic polymers, colloidal silicon dioxide, D&C Yellow No. 10, magnesium stearate, paraffin, polyvinyl acetate, titanium dioxide, vanillin and vitamin E.

CLINICAL PHARMACOLOGY

Potassium ion is the principal intracellular cation of most body tissues. Potassium ions participate in a number of essential physiological processes including the maintenance of intracellular tonicity, the transmission of nerve impulses, the contraction of cardiac, skeletal, and smooth muscle, and the maintenance of normal renal function.

The intracellular concentration of potassium is approximately 150 to 160 mEq per liter. The normal adult plasma concentration is 3.5 to 5 mEq per liter. An active ion transport system maintains this gradient across the plasma membrane.

Potassium is a normal dietary constituent and under steady state conditions the amount of potassium absorbed from the gastrointestinal tract is equal to the amount excreted in the urine. The usual dietary intake of potassium is 50 to 100 mEq per day.

Potassium depletion will occur whenever the rate of potassium loss through renal excretion and/or loss from the gastrointestinal tract exceeds the rate of potassium intake. Such depletion usually develops as a consequence of therapy with diuretics, primary or secondary hyperaldosteronism, diabetic ketoacidosis, or inadequate replacement of potassium in patients on prolonged parenteral nutrition. Depletion can develop rapidly with severe diarrhea, especially if associated with vomiting. Potassium depletion due to these causes is usually accompanied by a concomitant loss of chloride and is manifested by hypokalemia and metabolic alkalosis. Potassium depletion may produce weakness, fatigue, disturbances of cardiac rhythm (primarily ectopic beats), prominent U-waves in the electrocardiogram, and in advanced cases, flaccid paralysis and/or impaired ability to concentrate urine.

If potassium depletion associated with metabolic alkalosis cannot be managed by correcting the fundamental cause of the deficiency, e.g., where the patient requires long term diuretic therapy, supplemental potassium in the form of high potassium food or potassium chloride may restore normal potassium levels.

In rare circumstances, (e.g., patients with renal tubular acidosis) potassium depletion may be associated with metabolic acidosis and hyperchloremia. In such patients potassium replacement should be accomplished with potassium salts other than the chloride, such as potassium bicarbonate, potassium citrate, potassium acetate, or potassium gluconate.

INDICATIONS AND USAGE

BECAUSE OF REPORTS OF INTESTINAL AND GASTRIC ULCERATION AND BLEEDING WITH CONTROLLED-RELEASE POTASSIUM CHLORIDE PREPARATIONS, THESE DRUGS SHOULD BE RESERVED FOR THOSE PATIENTS WHO CANNOT TOLERATE OR REFUSE TO TAKE LIQUID OR EFFERVESCENT POTASSIUM PREPARATIONS, OR FOR PATIENTS WITH WHOM THERE IS A PROBLEM OF COMPLIANCE WITH THESE PREPARATIONS.

1. For the treatment of patients with hypokalemia with or without metabolic alkalosis, in digitalis intoxication, and in patients with hypokalemic familial periodic paralysis. If hypokalemia is the result of diuretic therapy, consideration should be given to the use of a lower dose of diuretic, which may be sufficient without leading to hypokalemia.
2. For the prevention of hypokalemia in patients who would be at particular risk if hypokalemia were to develop, e.g., digitalized patients or patients with significant cardiac arrhythmias.

The use of potassium salts in patients receiving diuretics for uncomplicated essential hypertension is often unnecessary when such patients have a normal dietary pattern, and when low doses of the diuretic are used. Serum potassium should be checked periodically, however, and, if hypokalemia occurs, dietary supplementation with potassium-containing foods may be adequate to control milder cases. In more severe cases, and if dose adjustment of the diuretic is ineffective or unwarranted, supplementation with potassium salts may be indicated.

CONTRAINDICATIONS

Potassium supplements are contraindicated in patients with hyperkalemia since a further increase in serum potassium concentration in such patients can produce cardiac arrest. Hyperkalemia may complicate any of the following conditions: chronic renal failure, systemic acidosis such as diabetic acidosis, acute dehydration, extensive tissue breakdown as in severe burns, adrenal insufficiency, or the administration of potassium-sparing diuretic, e.g., spironolactone, triamterene, or amiloride. (see OVERDOSAGE).

K-TAB tablets are contraindicated in patients with known hypersensitivity to any ingredient in this product.

Controlled-release formulations of potassium chloride have produced esophageal ulceration in certain cardiac patients with esophageal compression due to an enlarged left atrium. Potassium supplementation, when indicated in such patients, should be given as a liquid preparation.

All solid dosage forms of potassium chloride are contraindicated in any patient in whom there is structural, pathological, e.g., diabetic gastroparesis, or pharmacologic (use of anticholinergic agents or other agents with anticholinergic properties at sufficient doses to exert anticholinergic effects) cause for arrest or delay in tablet passage through the gastrointestinal tract.

WARNINGS

Hyperkalemia (see OVERDOSAGE)

In patients with impaired mechanisms for excreting potassium, the administration of potassium salts can produce hyperkalemia and cardiac arrest. This occurs most commonly in patients given potassium intravenously, but may also occur in patients given potassium orally. Potentially fatal hyperkalemia can develop rapidly and can be asymptomatic. The use of potassium salts in patients with chronic renal disease, or any other condition which impairs potassium excretion, requires particularly careful monitoring of the serum potassium concentration and appropriate dosage adjustment.

Interaction with Potassium-Sparing Diuretics

Hypokalemia should not be treated by the concomitant administration of potassium salts and a potassium-sparing diuretic, e.g., spironolactone, triamterene, or amiloride, since the simultaneous administration of these agents can produce severe hyperkalemia.

Interaction with Angiotensin Converting Enzyme Inhibitors

Angiotensin converting enzyme (ACE) inhibitors (e.g., captopril, enalapril) will produce some potassium retention by inhibiting aldosterone production. Potassium supplements should be given to patients receiving ACE inhibitors only with close monitoring.

Gastrointestinal Lesions

Solid oral dosage forms of potassium chloride can produce ulcerative and/or stenotic lesions of the gastrointestinal tract. Based on spontaneous adverse reaction reports, enteric-coated preparations of potassium chloride are associated with an increased frequency of small bowel lesions (40-50 per 100,000 patient years) compared to sustained-release wax matrix formulations (less than one per 100,000 patient years). Because of the lack of extensive marketing experience with microencapsulated products, a comparison between such products and wax matrix or enteric-coated products is not available. K-TAB tablets consist of a wax matrix formulated to provide a controlled rate of release of potassium chloride and thus to minimize the possibility of a high local concentration of potassium near the gastrointestinal wall.

Prospective trials have been conducted in normal human volunteers in which the upper gastrointestinal tract was evaluated by endoscopic inspection before and after one week of solid oral potassium chloride therapy. The ability of this model to predict events occuring in usual clinical practice is unknown. Trials which approximated usual clinical practice did not reveal any clear differences between the wax matrix and microencapsulated dosage forms. In contrast, there was a higher incidence of gastric and duodenal lesions in subjects receiving a high dose of a wax matrix controlled-release formulation under conditions which did not resemble usual or recommended clinical practice, i.e., 96 mEq per day in divided doses of potassium chloride administered, to fasted patients in the presence of an anticholinergic drug to delay gastric emptying. The upper gastrointestinal lesions observed by endoscopy were asymptomatic and were not accompanied by evidence of bleeding (hemoccult testing). The relevance of these findings to the usual conditions, i.e., non-fasting, no anticholinergic agent, and smaller doses, under which controlled-release potassium chloride products are used is uncertain. Epidemiologic studies have not identified an elevated risk, compared to microencapsulated products, for upper gastrointestinal lesions in patients receiving wax matrix formulations. K-TAB tablets should be discontinued immediately and the possibility of ulceration, obstruction or perforation considered if severe vomiting, abdominal pain, distention, or gastrointestinal bleeding occurs.

Metabolic Acidosis

Hypokalemia in patients with metabolic acidosis should be treated with an alkalinizing potassium salt such as potassium bicarbonate, potassium citrate, potassium acetate, or potassium gluconate.

PRECAUTIONS

General: The diagnosis of potassium depletion is ordinarily made by demonstrating hypokalemia in a patient with a clinical history suggesting some cause for potassium depletion. In interpreting the serum potassium level, the physician should bear in mind that acute alkalosis *per se* can produce hypokalemia in the absence of a deficit in total body potassium, while acute acidosis *per se* can increase the serum potassium concentration to within the normal range even in the presence of a reduced total body potassium. The treatment of potassium depletion, particularly in the presence of cardiac disease, renal disease, or acidosis, requires careful attention to acid-base balance and appropriate monitoring of serum electrolytes, the electrocardiogram, and the clinical status of the patient.

Information for Patients: Physicians should consider reminding the patient of the following:

To take each dose with meals and with a full glass of water or other liquid.

To take this medicine following the frequency and amount prescribed by the physician. This is especially important if the patient is also taking diuretics and/or digitalis preparations.

To check with the physician if there is trouble swallowing tablets or if the tablets seem to stick in the throat.

To check with the physician at once if tarry stools or other evidence of gastrointestinal bleeding is noticed.

To take each dose without crushing, chewing or sucking the tablets.

Laboratory Tests: When blood is drawn for analysis of plasma potassium it is important to recognize that artifactual elevations can occur after improper venipuncture technique or as a result of *in vitro* hemolysis of the sample.

Drug Interactions: Potassium-sparing diuretics, angiotensin converting enzyme inhibitors (see WARNINGS).

Carcinogenesis, Mutagenesis, Impairment of Fertility: Carcinogenicity, mutagenicity and fertility studies in animals have not been performed. Potassium is a normal dietary constituent.

Pregnancy Category C: Animal reproduction studies have not been conducted with K-TAB tablets. It is unlikely that potassium supplementation that does not lead to hyperkalemia would have an adverse effect on the fetus or would affect reproductive capacity.

Continued on next page

Abbott Laboratories—Cont.

Nursing Mothers: The normal potassium ion content of human milk is about 13 mEq per liter. Since oral potassium becomes part of the body potassium pool, as long as body potassium is not excessive, the contribution of potassium chloride supplementation should have little or no effect on the level in human milk.

Pediatric Use: Safety and effectiveness in children have not been established.

ADVERSE REACTIONS

One of the most severe adverse effects is hyperkalemia (see CONTRAINDICATIONS, WARNINGS, and OVERDOSAGE). There also have been reports of upper and lower gastrointestinal conditions including obstruction, bleeding, ulceration, and perforation (see CONTRAINDICATIONS and WARNINGS).

The most common adverse reactions to oral potassium salts are nausea, vomiting, flatulence, abdominal pain/discomfort, and diarrhea. These symptoms are due to irritation of the gastrointestinal tract and are best managed by taking the dose with meals, or reducing the amount taken at one time.

Skin rash has been reported rarely.

OVERDOSAGE

The administration of oral potassium salts to persons with normal excretory mechanisms for potassium rarely causes serious hyperkalemia. However, if excretory mechanisms are impaired or if intravenous administration is too rapid, potentially fatal hyperkalemia can result (see CONTRAINDICATIONS and WARNINGS). It is important to recognize that hyperkalemia is usually asymptomatic and may be manifested only by an increased serum potassium concentration (6.5-8.0 mEq/L) and characteristic electrocardiographic changes (peaking of T-waves, loss of P-waves, depression of S-T segments, and prolongation of QT intervals). Late manifestations include muscle paralysis and cardiovascular collapse from cardiac arrest. (9-12 mEq/L).

Treatment measures for hyperkalemia include the following:

1. Elimination of foods and medications containing potassium and of any agents with potassium-sparing properties;
2. Intravenous administration of 300 to 500 mL/hr of 10% dextrose solution containing 10-20 units of crystalline insulin per 1,000 mL;
3. Correction of acidosis, if present, with intravenous sodium bicarbonate;
4. Use of exchange resins, hemodialysis, or peritoneal dialysis.

In treating hyperkalemia, it should be recalled that in patients who have been stabilized on digitalis, lowering the serum potassium concentration too rapidly can produce digitalis toxicity.

DOSAGE AND ADMINISTRATION

The usual dietary potassium intake by the average adult is 50 to 100 mEq per day. Potassium depletion sufficient to cause hypokalemia usually requires the loss of 200 or more mEq of potassium from the total body store.

Dosage must be adjusted to the individual needs of each patient.The dose for the prevention of hypokalemia is typically in the range of 20 mEq per day. Doses of 40-100 mEq per day or more are used for the treatment of potassium depletion. Dosage should be divided if more than 20 mEq per day is given such that no more than 20 mEq is given in a single dose.

K-TAB tablets provide 10 mEq of potassium chloride.

K-TAB tablets should be taken with meals and with a glass of water or other liquid. This product should not be taken on an empty stomach because of its potential for gastric irritation (see WARNINGS).

NOTE: K-TAB tablets are to be swallowed whole without crushing, chewing or sucking the tablets.

HOW SUPPLIED

K-TAB (potassium chloride extended-release tablets, USP) contains 750 mg of potassium chloride (equivalent to 10mEq). K-TAB tablets are provided as yellow, ovaloid, extended-release Filmtab® tablets in bottles of 100 (**NDC** 0074-7804-13), 1000 (**NDC** 0074-7804-19) and 5000 (**NDC** 0074-7804-59) and in ABBO-PAC® unit dose packages of 100 (**NDC** 0074-7804-11).

Recommended Storage: Store below 86°F (30°C).

CAUTION: Federal (USA) law prohibits dispensing without prescription.

Filmtab—Film-sealed tablets, Abbott

Ref. 03-4415-R14 – Rev. September, 1991

Shown in Product Identification Guide, page 303

NEMBUTAL® SODIUM CAPSULES ℞ Ⓒ II

[*nĕm-bū-tal sō-dī-um*]

(pentobarbital sodium capsules, USP)

WARNING—MAY BE HABIT FORMING

DESCRIPTION

The barbiturates are nonselective central nervous system depressants which are primarily used as sedative hypnotics. The barbiturates and their sodium salts are subject to control under the Federal Controlled Substances Act (See "Drug Abuse and Dependence" section).

Barbiturates are substituted pyrimidine derivatives in which the basic structure common to these drugs is barbituric acid, a substance which has no central nervous system (CNS) activity. CNS activity is obtained by substituting alkyl, alkenyl, or aryl groups on the pyrimidine ring. Nembutal (pentobarbital sodium) is chemically represented by sodium 5-ethyl-5-(1-methylbutyl) barbiturate.

The structural formula for pentobarbitol sodium is:

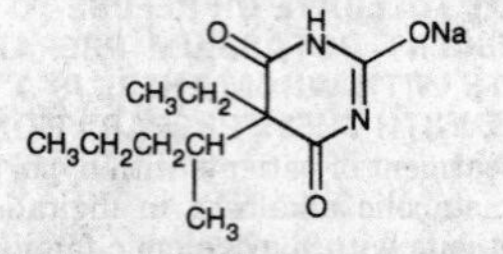

The sodium salt of pentobarbital occurs as a white, slightly bitter powder which is freely soluble in water and alcohol but practically insoluble in benzene and ether. Nembutal Sodium capsules for oral administration contain either 50 mg or 100 mg of pentobarbital sodium.

Inactive Ingredients: 50 mg Capsule: FD&C Blue No. 1, FD&C Red No. 3, FD&C Yellow No. 6, gelatin, lactose, magnesium stearate, polacrilin potassium and potassium chloride.

100 mg Capsule: colloidal silicon dioxide, corn starch, FD&C Blue No. 1, FD&C Red No. 3, FD&C Yellow No. 5 (tartrazine), FD&C Yellow No. 6, gelatin, magnesium stearate and potassium chloride.

CLINICAL PHARMACOLOGY

Barbiturates are capable of producing all levels of CNS mood alteration from excitation to mild sedation, to hypnosis, and deep coma. Overdosage can produce death. In high enough therapeutic doses, barbiturates induce anesthesia.

Barbiturates depress the sensory cortex, decrease motor activity, alter cerebellar function, and produce drowsiness, sedation, and hypnosis.

Barbiturate-induced sleep differs from physiological sleep. Sleep laboratory studies have demonstrated that barbiturates reduce the amount of time spent in the rapid eye movement (REM) phase of sleep or dreaming stage. Also, Stages III and IV sleep are decreased. Following abrupt cessation of barbiturates used regularly, patients may experience markedly increased dreaming, nightmares, and/or insomnia. Therefore, withdrawal of a single therapeutic dose over 5 or 6 days has been recommended to lessen the REM rebound and disturbed sleep which contribute to drug withdrawal syndrome (for example, decrease the dose from 3 to 2 doses a day for 1 week).

In studies, secobarbital sodium and pentobarbital sodium have been found to lose most of their effectiveness for both inducing and maintaining sleep by the end of 2 weeks of continued drug administration at fixed doses. The short-, intermediate-, and, to a lesser degree, long-acting barbiturates have been widely prescribed for treating insomnia. Although the clinical literature abounds with claims that the short-acting barbiturates are superior for producing sleep while the intermediate-acting compounds are more effective in maintaining sleep, controlled studies have failed to demonstrate these differential effects. Therefore, as sleep medications, the barbiturates are of limited value beyond short-term use.

Barbiturates have little analgesic action at subanesthetic doses. Rather, in subanesthetic doses these drugs may increase the reaction to painful stimuli. All barbiturates exhibit anticonvulsant activity in anesthetic doses. However, of the drugs in this class, only phenobarbital, mephobarbital, and metharbital have been clinically demonstrated to be effective as oral anticonvulsants in subhypnotic doses.

Barbiturates are respiratory depressants. The degree of respiratory depression is dependent upon dose. With hypnotic doses, respiratory depression produced by barbiturates is similar to that which occurs during physiologic sleep with slight decrease in blood pressure and heart rate.

Studies in laboratory animals have shown that barbiturates cause reduction in the tone and contractility of the uterus, ureters, and urinary bladder. However, concentrations of the drugs required to produce this effect in humans are not reached with sedative-hypnotic doses.

Barbiturates do not impair normal hepatic function, but have been shown to induce liver microsomal enzymes, thus increasing and/or altering the metabolism of barbiturates and other drugs. (See "Precautions—*Drug Interactions*" section).

Pharmacokinetics: Barbiturates are absorbed in varying degrees following oral, rectal, or parenteral administration. The salts are more rapidly absorbed than are the acids. The rate of absorption is increased if the sodium salt is ingested as a dilute solution or taken on an empty stomach.

The onset of action for oral or rectal administration varies from 20 to 60 minutes.

Duration of action, which is related to the rate at which the barbiturates are redistributed throughout the body, varies among persons and in the same person from time to time. In Table 1, the barbiturates are classified according to their duration of action. This classification should not be used to predict the exact duration of effect, but the grouping of drugs should be used as a guide in the selection of barbiturates.

No studies have demonstrated that the different routes of administration are equivalent with respect to bioavailability.

[See Table 1 below.]

Barbiturates are weak acids that are absorbed and rapidly distributed to all tissues and fluids with high concentrations in the brain, liver, and kidneys. Lipid solubility of the barbiturates is the dominant factor in their distribution within the body. The more lipid soluble the barbiturate, the more rapidly it penetrates all tissues of the body. Barbiturates are bound to plasma and tissue proteins to a varying degree with the degree of binding increasing directly as a function of lipid solubility.

Phenobarbital has the lowest lipid solubility, lowest plasma binding, lowest brain protein binding, the longest delay in onset of activity, and the longest duration of action. At the opposite extreme is secobarbital which has the highest lipid solubility, plasma protein binding, brain protein binding, the shortest delay in onset of activity, and the shortest duration of action. Butabarbital is classified as an intermediate barbiturate.

The plasma half-life for pentobarbital in adults is 15 to 50 hours and appears to be dose dependent.

Barbiturates are metabolized primarily by the hepatic microsomal enzyme system, and the metabolic products are excreted in the urine, and less commonly, in the feces. Approximately 25 to 50 percent of a dose of aprobarbital or phenobarbital is eliminated unchanged in the urine, whereas the amount of other barbiturates excreted unchanged in the urine is negligible. The excretion of unmetabolized barbiturate is one feature that distinguishes the long-acting category from those belonging to other categories which are almost entirely metabolized. The inactive metabolites of the barbiturates are excreted as conjugates of glucuronic acid.

INDICATIONS AND USAGE

Oral:

a. Sedatives.
b. Hypnotics, for the short-term treatment of insomnia, since they appear to lose their effectiveness for sleep induction and sleep maintenance after 2 weeks (See "Clinical Pharmacology" section).
c. Preanesthetics.

CONTRAINDICATIONS

Barbiturates are contraindicated in patients with known barbiturate sensitivity. Barbiturates are also contraindicated in patients with a history of manifest or latent porphyria.

WARNINGS

1. *Habit forming:* Barbiturates may be habit forming. Tolerance, psychological and physical dependence may occur with continued use. (See "Drug Abuse and Dependence" and "Pharmacokinetics" sections). Patients who have psychological dependence on barbiturates may increase

Table 1.—*Classification, Onset, and Duration of Action of Commonly used Barbiturates Taken Orally*

Classification	Onset of action	Duration of action
Long-acting Phenobarbital.	1 hour or longer	10 to 12 hours
Intermediate Amobarbital Butabarbital.	$^3/_4$ to 1 hour	6 to 8 hours
Short-acting Pentobarbital Secobarbital.	10 to 15 minutes	3 to 4 hours

the dosage or decrease the dosage interval without consulting a physician and may subsequently develop a physical dependence on barbiturates. To minimize the possibility of overdosage or the development of dependence, the prescribing and dispensing of sedative-hypnotic barbiturates should be limited to the amount required for the interval until the next appointment. Abrupt cessation after prolonged use in the dependent person may result in withdrawal symptoms, including delirium, convulsions, and possibly death. Barbiturates should be withdrawn gradually from any patient known to be taking excessive dosage over long periods of time. (See "Drug Abuse and Dependence" section).

2. *Acute or chronic pain:* Caution should be exercised when barbiturates are administered to patients with acute or chronic pain, because paradoxical excitement could be induced or important symptoms could be masked. However, the use of barbiturates as sedatives in the postoperative surgical period and as adjuncts to cancer chemotherapy is well established.

3. *Use in pregnancy:* Barbiturates can cause fetal damage when administered to a pregnant woman. Retrospective, case-controlled studies have suggested a connection between the maternal consumption of barbiturates and a higher than expected incidence of fetal abnormalities. Following oral or parenteral administration, barbiturates readily cross the placental barrier and are distributed throughout fetal tissues with highest concentrations found in the placenta, fetal liver, and brain.

Withdrawal symptoms occur in infants born to mothers who receive barbiturates throughout the last trimester of pregnancy. (See "Drug Abuse and Dependence" section). If this drug is used during pregnancy, or if the patient becomes pregnant while taking this drug, the patient should be apprised of the potential hazard to the fetus.

4. *Synergistic effects:* The concomitant use of alcohol or other CNS depressants may produce additive CNS depressant effects.

PRECAUTIONS

General: Barbiturates may be habit forming. Tolerance and psychological and physical dependence may occur with continuing use. (See "Drug Abuse and Dependence" section). Barbiturates should be administered with caution, if at all, to patients who are mentally depressed, have suicidal tendencies, or a history of drug abuse.

Elderly or debilitated patients may react to barbiturates with marked excitement, depression, and confusion. In some persons, barbiturates repeatedly produce excitement rather than depression.

In patients with hepatic damage, barbiturates should be administered with caution and initially in reduced doses. Barbiturates should not be administered to patients showing the premonitory signs of hepatic coma.

The 100 mg dosage strength of Nembutal Sodium capsules contains FD&C Yellow No. 5 (tartrazine) which may cause allergic-type reactions (including bronchial asthma) in certain susceptible individuals. Although the overall incidence of FD&C Yellow No. 5 (tartrazine) sensitivity in the general population is low, it is frequently seen in patients who also have aspirin hypersensitivity.

Information for the patient: Practitioners should give the following information and instructions to patients receiving barbiturates.

1. The use of barbiturates carries with it an associated risk of psychological and/or physical dependence. The patient should be warned against increasing the dose of the drug without consulting a physician.

2. Barbiturates may impair mental and/or physical abilities required for the performance of potentially hazardous tasks (e.g., driving, operating machinery, etc.).

3. Alcohol should not be consumed while taking barbiturates. Concurrent use of the barbiturates with other CNS depressants (e.g., alcohol, narcotics, tranquilizers, and antihistamines) may result in additional CNS depressant effects.

Laboratory tests: Prolonged therapy with barbiturates should be accompanied by periodic laboratory evaluation of organ systems, including hematopoietic, renal, and hepatic systems. (See "Precautions—General" and "Adverse Reactions" sections).

Drug interactions: Most reports of clinically significant drug interactions occurring with the barbiturates have involved phenobarbital. However, the application of these data to other barbiturates appears valid and warrants serial blood level determinations of the relevant drugs when there are multiple therapies.

1. *Anticoagulants:* Phenobarbital lowers the plasma levels of dicumarol (name previously used: bishydroxycoumarin) and causes a decrease in anticoagulant activity as measured by the prothrombin time. Barbiturates can induce hepatic microsomal enzymes resulting in increased metabolism and decreased anticoagulant response of oral anticoagulants (e.g., warfarin, acenocoumarol, dicumarol and phenprocoumon). Patients stabilized on anticoagulant

therapy may require dosage adjustments if barbiturates are added to or withdrawn from their dosage regimen.

2. *Corticosteroids:* Barbiturates appear to enhance the metabolism of exogenous corticosteroids probably through the induction of hepatic microsomal enzymes. Patients stabilized on corticosteroid therapy may require dosage adjustments if barbiturates are added to or withdrawn from their dosage regimen.

3. *Griseofulvin:* Phenobarbital appears to interfere with the absorption of orally administered griseofulvin, thus decreasing its blood level. The effect of the resultant decreased blood levels of griseofulvin on therapeutic response has not been established. However, it would be preferable to avoid concomitant administration of these drugs.

4. *Doxycycline:* Phenobarbital has been shown to shorten the half-life of doxycycline for as long as 2 weeks after barbiturate therapy is discontinued.

This mechanism is probably through the induction of hepatic microsomal enzymes that metabolize the antibiotic. If phenobarbital and doxycycline are administered concurrently, the clinical response to doxycycline should be monitored closely.

5. *Phenytoin, sodium valproate, valproic acid:* The effect of barbiturates on the metabolism of phenytoin appears to be variable. Some investigators report an accelerating effect, while others report no effect. Because the effect of barbiturates on the metabolism of phenytoin is not predictable, phenytoin and barbiturate blood levels should be monitored more frequently if these drugs are given concurrently. Sodium valproate and valproic acid appear to decrease barbiturate metabolism; therefore, barbiturate blood levels should be monitored and appropriate dosage adjustments made as indicated.

6. *Central nervous system depressants:* The concomitant use of other central nervous system depressants, including other sedatives or hypnotics, antihistamines, tranquilizers, or alcohol, may produce additive depressant effects.

7. *Monoamine oxidase inhibitors (MAOI):* MAOI prolong the effects of barbiturates probably because metabolism of the barbiturate is inhibited.

8. *Estradiol, estrone, progesterone and other steroidal hormones:* Pretreatment with or concurrent administration of phenobarbital may decrease the effect of estradiol by increasing its metabolism. There have been reports of patients treated with antiepileptic drugs (e.g., phenobarbital) who became pregnant while taking oral contraceptives. An alternate contraceptive method might be suggested to women taking phenobarbital.

Carcinogenesis: 1. Animal data. Phenobarbital sodium is carcinogenic in mice and rats after lifetime administration. In mice, it produced benign and malignant liver cell tumors. In rats, benign liver cell tumors were observed very late in life.

2. Human data. In a 29-year epidemiological study of 9,136 patients who were treated on an anticonvulsant protocol that included phenobarbital, results indicated a higher than normal incidence of hepatic carcinoma. Previously, some of these patients were treated with thorotrast, a drug that is known to produce hepatic carcinomas. Thus, this study did not provide sufficient evidence that phenobarbital sodium is carcinogenic in humans.

Data from one retrospective study of 235 children in which the types of barbiturates are not identified suggested an association between exposure to barbiturates prenatally and an increased incidence of brain tumor. (Gold, E., et al., "Increased Risk of Brain Tumors in Children Exposed to Barbiturates," Journal of National Cancer Institute, 61:1031–1034, 1978).

Pregnancy: 1. *Teratogenic effects.* Pregnancy Category D—See "Warnings—Use in Pregnancy" section.

2. *Nonteratogenic effects.* Reports of infants suffering from long-term barbiturate exposure in utero included the acute withdrawal syndrome of seizures and hyperirritability from birth to a delayed onset of up to 14 days. (See "Drug Abuse and Dependence" section).

Labor and delivery: Hypnotic doses of these barbiturates do not appear to significantly impair uterine activity during labor. Full anesthetic doses of barbiturates decrease the force and frequency of uterine contractions. Administration of sedative-hypnotic barbiturates to the mother during labor may result in respiratory depression in the newborn. Premature infants are particularly susceptible to the depressant effects of barbiturates. If barbiturates are used during labor and delivery, resuscitation equipment should be available. Data are currently not available to evaluate the effect of these barbiturates when forceps delivery or other intervention is necessary. Also, data are not available to determine the effect of these barbiturates on the later growth, development, and functional maturation of the child.

Nursing mothers: Caution should be exercised when a barbiturate is administered to a nursing woman since small amounts of barbiturates are excreted in the milk.

ADVERSE REACTIONS

The following adverse reactions and their incidence were compiled from surveillance of thousands of hospitalized patients. Because such patients may be less aware of certain of the milder adverse effects of barbiturates, the incidence of these reactions may be somewhat higher in fully ambulatory patients.

More than 1 in 100 patients. The most common adverse reaction estimated to occur at a rate of 1 to 3 patients per 100 is:
Nervous System: Somnolence.
Less than 1 in 100 patients. Adverse reactions estimated to occur at a rate of less than 1 in 100 patients listed below, grouped by organ system, and by decreasing order of occurrence are:
Nervous system: Agitation, confusion, hyperkinesia, ataxia, CNS depression, nightmares, nervousness, psychiatric disturbance, hallucinations, insomnia, anxiety, dizziness, thinking abnormality.
Respiratory system: Hypoventilation, apnea.
Cardiovascular system: Bradycardia, hypotension, syncope.
Digestive system: Nausea, vomiting, constipation.
Other reported reactions: Headache, injection site reactions, hypersensitivity reactions (angioedema, skin rashes, exfoliative dermatitis), fever, liver damage, megaloblastic anemia following chronic phenobarbital use.

DRUG ABUSE AND DEPENDENCE

Pentobarbital sodium capsules are subject to control by the Federal Controlled Substances Act under DEA schedule II. Barbiturates may be habit forming. Tolerance, psychological dependence, and physical dependence may occur especially following prolonged use of high doses of barbiturates. Daily administration in excess of 400 milligrams (mg) of pentobarbital or secobarbital for approximately 90 days is likely to produce some degree of physical dependence. A dosage of from 600 to 800 mg taken for at least 35 days is sufficient to produce withdrawal seizures. The average daily dose for the barbiturate addict is usually about 1.5 grams. As tolerance to barbiturates develops, the amount needed to maintain the same level of intoxication increases; tolerance to a fatal dosage, however, does not increase more than two-fold. As this occurs, the margin between an intoxicating dosage and fatal dosage becomes smaller.

Symptoms of acute intoxication with barbiturates include unsteady gait, slurred speech, and sustained nystagmus. Mental signs of chronic intoxication include confusion, poor judgment, irritability, insomnia, and somatic complaints.

Symptoms of barbiturate dependence are similar to those of chronic alcoholism. If an individual appears to be intoxicated with alcohol to a degree that is radically disproportionate to the amount of alcohol in his or her blood the use of barbiturates should be suspected. The lethal dose of a barbiturate is far less if alcohol is also ingested.

The symptoms of barbiturate withdrawal can be severe and may cause death. Minor withdrawal symptoms may appear 8 to 12 hours after the last dose of a barbiturate. These symptoms usually appear in the following order: anxiety, muscle twitching, tremor of hands and fingers, progressive weakness, dizziness, distortion in visual perception, nausea, vomiting, insomnia, and orthostatic hypotension. Major withdrawal symptoms (convulsions and delirium) may occur within 16 hours and last up to 5 days after abrupt cessation of these drugs. Intensity of withdrawal symptoms gradually declines over a period of approximately 15 days. Individuals susceptible to barbiturate abuse and dependence include alcoholics and opiate abusers, as well as other sedative-hypnotic and amphetamine abusers.

Drug dependence to barbiturates arises from repeated administration of a barbiturate or agent with barbiturate-like effect on a continuous basis, generally in amounts exceeding therapeutic dose levels. The characteristics of drug dependence to barbiturates include: (a) a strong desire or need to continue taking the drug; (b) a tendency to increase the dose; (c) a psychic dependence on the effects of the drug related to subjective and individual appreciation of those effects; and (d) a physical dependence on the effects of the drug requiring its presence for maintenance of homeostasis and resulting in a definite, characteristic, and self-limited abstinence syndrome when the drug is withdrawn.

Treatment of barbiturate dependence consists of cautious and gradual withdrawal of the drug. Barbiturate-dependent patients can be withdrawn by using a number of different withdrawal regimens. In all cases withdrawal takes an extended period of time. One method involves substituting a 30 mg dose of phenobarbital for each 100 to 200 mg dose of barbiturate that the patient has been taking. The total daily amount of phenobarbital is then administered in 3 to 4 divided doses, not to exceed 600 mg daily. Should signs of withdrawal occur on the first day of treatment, a loading dose of 100 to 200 mg of phenobarbital may be administered IM in addition to the oral dose. After stabilization on phenobarbital, the total daily dose is decreased by 30 mg a day as long as withdrawal is proceeding smoothly. A modification of this

Continued on next page

Abbott Laboratories—Cont.

Table 2.—*Concentration of Barbiturate in the Blood Versus Degree of CNS Depression*
Blood barbiturate level in ppm (μg/ml)

Barbiturate	Onset/ duration	Degree of depression in nontolerant persons*				
		1	2	3	4	5
Pentobarbital	Fast/short	≤2	0.5 to 3	10 to 15	12 to 25	15 to 40
Secobarbital	Fast/short	≤2	0.5 to 5	10 to 15	15 to 25	15 to 40
Amobarbital	Intermediate/ intermediate	≤3	2 to 10	30 to 40	30 to 60	40 to 80
Butabarbital	Intermediate/ intermediate	≤5	3 to 25	40 to 60	50 to 80	60 to 100
Phenobarbital	Slow/long	≤10	5 to 40	50 to 80	70 to 120	100 to 200

* Categories of degree of depression in nontolerant persons:
1. Under the influence and appreciably impaired for purposes of driving a motor vehicle or performing tasks requiring alertness and unimpaired judgment and reaction time.
2. Sedated, therapeutic range, calm, relaxed, and easily aroused.
3. Comatose, difficult to arouse, significant depression of respiration.
4. Compatible with death in aged or ill persons or in presence of obstructed airway, other toxic agents, or exposure to cold.
5. Usual lethal level, the upper end of the range includes those who received some supportive treatment.

regimen involves initiating treatment at the patient's regular dosage level and decreasing the daily dosage by 10 percent if tolerated by the patient.
Infants physically dependent on barbiturates may be given phenobarbital 3 to 10 mg/kg/day. After withdrawal symptoms (hyperactivity, disturbed sleep, tremors, hyperreflexia) are relieved, the dosage of phenobarbital should be gradually decreased and completely withdrawn over a 2 week period.

OVERDOSAGE

The toxic dose of barbiturates varies considerably. In general, an oral dose of 1 gram of most barbiturates produces serious poisoning in an adult. Death commonly occurs after 2 to 10 grams of ingested barbiturate. Barbiturate intoxication may be confused with alcoholism, bromide intoxication, and with various neurological disorders.
Acute overdosage with barbiturates is manifested by CNS and respiratory depression which may progress to Cheyne-Stokes respiration, areflexia, constriction of the pupils to a slight degree (though in severe poisoning they may show paralytic dilation), oliguria, tachycardia, hypotension, lowered body temperature, and coma. Typical shock syndrome (apnea, circulatory collapse, respiratory arrest, and death) may occur.
In extreme overdose, all electrical activity in the brain may cease, in which case a "flat" EEG normally equated with clinical death cannot be accepted. This effect is fully reversible unless hypoxic damage occurs. Consideration should be given to the possibility of barbiturate intoxication even in situations that appear to involve trauma.
Complications such as pneumonia, pulmonary edema, cardiac arrhythmias, congestive heart failure, and renal failure may occur. Uremia may increase CNS sensitivity to barbiturates. Differential diagnosis should include hypoglycemia, head trauma, cerebrovascular accidents, convulsive states, and diabetic coma. Blood levels from acute overdosage for some barbiturates are listed in Table 2. [See table above.]
Treatment of overdosage is mainly supportive and consists of the following:

1. Maintenance of an adequate airway, with assisted respiration and oxygen administration as necessary.
2. Monitoring of vital signs and fluid balance.
3. If the patient is conscious and has not lost the gag reflex, emesis may be induced with ipecac. Care should be taken to prevent pulmonary aspiration of vomitus. After completion of vomiting, 30 grams activated charcoal in a glass of water may be administered.
4. If emesis is contraindicated, gastric lavage may be performed with a cuffed endotracheal tube in place with the patient in the face down position. Activated charcoal may be left in the emptied stomach and a saline cathartic administered.
5. Fluid therapy and other standard treatment for shock, if needed.
6. If renal function is normal, forced diuresis may aid in the elimination of the barbiturate. Alkalinization of the urine increases renal excretion of some barbiturates, especially phenobarbital, also aprobarbital, and mephobarbital (which is metabolized to phenobarbital).
7. Although not recommended as a routine procedure, hemodialysis may be used in severe barbiturate intoxications or if the patient is anuric or in shock.
8. Patient should be rolled from side to side every 30 minutes.
9. Antibiotics should be given if pneumonia is suspected.
10. Appropriate nursing care to prevent hypostatic pneumonia, decubiti, aspiration, and other complications of patients with altered states of consciousness.

DOSAGE AND ADMINISTRATION

Adults: The usual hypnotic dose consists of 100 mg at bedtime.
Children: The preoperative dose is 2 to 6 mg/kg/24 hours (maximum 100 mg), depending on age, weight, and the desired degree of sedation.
The proper hypnotic dose for children must be judged on the basis of individual age and weight.
Dosages of barbiturates must be individualized with full knowledge of their particular characteristics and recommended rate of administration. Factors of consideration are the patient's age, weight, and condition.
Special patient population: Dosage should be reduced in the elderly or debilitated because these patients may be more sensitive to barbiturates. Dosage should be reduced for patients with impaired renal function or hepatic disease.

HOW SUPPLIED

NEMBUTAL Sodium Capsules (pentobarbital sodium capsules, USP) are supplied as follows:
50 mg transparent and orange-colored capsules in bottles of 100 (NDC 0074-3150-11)
100 mg yellow capsules in bottles of 100 (**NDC** 0074-3114-01), 500 (**NDC** 0074-3114-02) and in the Abbo-Pac® unit dose packages of 100 (**NDC** 0074-3114-21).
Recommended Storage: Store below 86°F (30°C).
Revised: March, 1992
Ref. 03-4433-R10
Shown in Product Identification Guide, page 303

NEMBUTAL® SODIUM SOLUTION Ⓒ℞

(Pentobarbital Sodium Injection, USP)
Ampuls—Vials

WARNING-MAY BE HABIT FORMING
DO NOT USE IF MATERIAL HAS PRECIPITATED

DESCRIPTION

The barbiturates are nonselective central nervous system depressants which are primarily used as sedative hypnotics and also anticonvulsants in subhypnotic doses. The barbiturates and their sodium salts are subject to control under the Federal Controlled Substances Act (See "Drug Abuse and Dependence" section).
The sodium salts of amobarbital, pentobarbital, phenobarbital, and secobarbital are available as sterile parenteral solutions.
Barbiturates are substituted pyrimidine derivatives in which the basic structure common to these drugs is barbituric acid, a substance which has no central nervous system (CNS) activity. CNS activity is obtained by substituting alkyl, alkenyl, or aryl groups on the pyrimidine ring.
NEMBUTAL Sodium Solution (pentobarbital sodium injection) is a sterile solution for intravenous or intramuscular injection. Each ml contains pentobarbital sodium 50 mg, in a vehicle of propylene glycol, 40%, alcohol, 10% and water for injection, to volume. The pH is adjusted to approximately 9.5 with hydrochloric acid and/or sodium hydroxide.
NEMBUTAL Sodium is a short-acting barbiturate, chemically designated as sodium 5-ethyl-5-(1-methylbutyl) barbiturate.
The structural formula for pentobarbital sodium is:
[See chemical structure at top of next column.]
The sodium salt occurs as a white, slightly bitter powder which is freely soluble in water and alcohol but practically insoluble in benzene and ether.

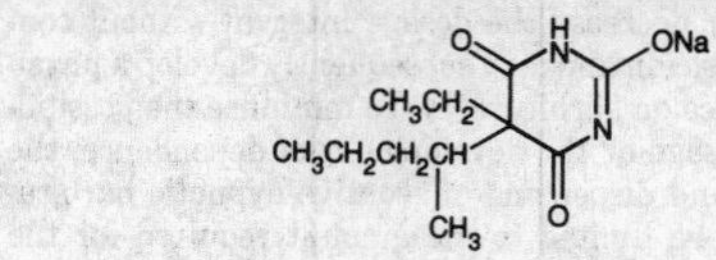

CLINICAL PHARMACOLOGY

Barbiturates are capable of producing all levels of CNS mood alteration from excitation to mild sedation, to hypnosis, and deep coma. Overdosage can produce death. In high enough therapeutic doses, barbiturates induce anesthesia.
Barbiturates depress the sensory cortex, decrease motor activity, alter cerebellar function, and produce drowsiness, sedation, and hypnosis.
Barbiturate-induced sleep differs from physiological sleep. Sleep laboratory studies have demonstrated that barbiturates reduce the amount of time spent in the rapid eye movement (REM) phase of sleep or dreaming stage. Also, Stages III and IV sleep are decreased. Following abrupt cessation of barbiturates used regularly, patients may experience markedly increased dreaming, nightmares, and/or insomnia. Therefore, withdrawal of a single therapeutic dose over 5 or 6 days has been recommended to lessen the REM rebound and disturbed sleep which contribute to drug withdrawal syndrome (for example, decrease the dose from 3 to 2 doses a day for 1 week).
In studies, secobarbital sodium and pentobarbital sodium have been found to lose most of their effectiveness for both inducing and maintaining sleep by the end of 2 weeks of continued drug administration at fixed doses. The short-, intermediate-, and, to a lesser degree, long-acting barbiturates have been widely prescribed for treating insomnia. Although the clinical literature abounds with claims that the short-acting barbiturates are superior for producing sleep while the intermediate-acting compounds are more effective in maintaining sleep, controlled studies have failed to demonstrate these differential effects. Therefore, as sleep medications, the barbiturates are of limited value beyond short-term use.
Barbiturates have little analgesic action at subanesthetic doses. Rather in subanesthetic doses these drugs may increase the reaction to painful stimuli. All barbiturates exhibit anticonvulsant activity in anesthetic doses. However, of the drugs in this class, only phenobarbital, mephobarbital, and metharbital have been clinically demonstrated to be effective as oral anticonvulsants in subhypnotic doses.
Barbiturates are respiratory depressants. The degree of respiratory depression is dependent upon dose. With hypnotic doses, respiratory depression produced by barbiturates is similar to that which occurs during physiologic sleep with slight decrease in blood pressure and heart rate.
Studies in laboratory animals have shown that barbiturates cause reduction in the tone and contractility of the uterus, ureters, and urinary bladder. However, concentration of the drugs required to produce this effect in humans are not reached with sedative-hypnotic doses.
Barbiturates do not impair normal hepatic function, but have been shown to induce liver microsomal enzymes, thus increasing and/or altering the metabolism of barbiturates and other drugs. (See "Precautions—*Drug Interactions*" section).
Pharmacokinetics: Barbiturates are absorbed in varying degrees following oral, rectal, or parenteral administration. The salts are more rapidly absorbed than are the acids.
The onset of action for oral or rectal administration varies from 20 to 60 minutes. For IM administration, the onset of action is slightly faster. Following IV administration, the onset of action ranges from almost immediately for pentobarbital sodium to 5 minutes for phenobarbital sodium. Maximal CNS depression may not occur until 15 minutes or more after IV administration for phenobarbital sodium.
Duration of action, which is related to the rate at which the barbiturates are redistributed throughout the body, varies among persons and in the same person from time to time.
No studies have demonstrated that the different routes of administration are equivalent with respect to bioavailability.
Barbiturates are weak acids that are absorbed and rapidly distributed to all tissues and fluids with high concentrations in the brain, liver, and kidneys. Lipid solubility of the barbiturates is the dominant factor in their distribution within the body. The more lipid soluble the barbiturate, the more rapidly it penetrates all tissues of the body. Barbiturates are bound to plasma and tissue proteins to a varying degree with the degree of binding increasing directly as a function of lipid solubility.
Phenobarbital has the lowest lipid solubility, lowest plasma binding, lowest brain protein binding, the longest delay in onset of activity, and the longest duration of action. At the opposite extreme is secobarbital which has the highest lipid solubility, plasma protein binding, brain protein binding, the shortest delay in onset of activity, and the shortest duration of action. Butabarbital is classified as an intermediate barbiturate.

The plasma half-life for pentobarbital in adults is 15 to 50 hours and appears to be dose dependent.

Barbiturates are metabolized primarily by the hepatic microsomal enzyme system, and the metabolic products are excreted in the urine, and less commonly, in the feces. Approximately 25 to 50 percent of a dose of aprobarbital or phenobarbital is eliminated unchanged in the urine, whereas the amount of other barbiturates excreted unchanged in the urine is negligible. The excretion of unmetabolized barbiturate is one feature that distinguishes the long-acting category from those belonging to other categories which are almost entirely metabolized. The inactive metabolities of the barbiturates are excreted as conjugates of glucuronic acid.

INDICATIONS AND USAGE
Parenteral:
a. Sedatives.
b. Hypnotics, for the short-term treatment of insomnia, since they appear to lose their effectiveness for sleep induction and sleep maintenance after 2 weeks (See "Clinical Pharmacology" section).
c. Preanesthetics.
d. Anticonvulsant, in anesthetic doses, in the emergency control of certain acute convulsive episodes, e.g., those associated with status epilepticus, cholera, eclampsia, meningitis, tetanus, and toxic reactions to strychnine or local anesthetics.

CONTRAINDICATIONS
Barbiturates are contraindicated in patients with known barbiturate sensitivity. Barbiturates are also contraindicated in patients with a history of manifest or latent porphyria.

WARNINGS
1. *Habit forming:* Barbiturates may be habit forming. Tolerance, psychological and physical dependence may occur with continued use. (See "Drug Abuse and Dependence" and "Pharmacokinetics" sections). Patients who have psychological dependence on barbiturates may increase the dosage or decrease the dosage interval without consulting a physician and may subsequently develop a physical dependence on barbiturates. To minimize the possibility of overdosage or the development of dependence, the prescribing and dispensing of sedative-hypnotic barbiturates should be limited to the amount required for the interval until the next appointment. Abrupt cessation after prolonged use in the dependent person may result in withdrawal symptoms, including delirium, convulsions, and possibly death. Barbiturates should be withdrawn gradually from any patient known to be taking excessive dosage over long periods of time. (See "Drug Abuse and Dependence" section).
2. *IV administration:* Too rapid administration may cause respiratory depression, apnea, laryngospasm, or vasodilation with fall in blood pressure.
3. *Acute or chronic pain:* Caution should be exercised when barbiturates are administered to patients with acute or chronic pain, because paradoxical excitement could be induced or important symptoms could be masked. However, the use of barbiturates as sedatives in the postoperative surgical period and as adjuncts to cancer chemotherapy is well established.
4. *Use in pregnancy:* Barbiturates can cause fetal damage when administered to a pregnant woman. Retrospective, case-controlled studies have suggested a connection between the maternal consumption of barbiturates and a higher than expected incidence of fetal abnormalities. Following oral or parenteral administration, barbiturates readily cross the placental barrier and are distributed throughout fetal tissues with highest concentrations found in the placenta, fetal liver, and brain. Fetal blood levels approach maternal blood levels following parenteral administration.

Withdrawal symptoms occur in infants born to mothers who receive barbiturates throughout the last trimester of pregnancy. (See "Drug Abuse and Dependence" section). If this drug is used during pregnancy, or if the patient becomes pregnant while taking this drug, the patient should be apprised of the potential hazard to the fetus.
5. *Synergistic effects:* The concomitant use of alcohol or other CNS depressants may produce additive CNS depressant effects.

PRECAUTIONS
General: Barbiturates may be habit forming. Tolerance and psychological and physical dependence may occur with continuing use. (See "Drug Abuse and Dependence" section). Barbiturates should be administered with caution, if at all, to patients who are mentally depressed, have suicidal tendencies, or a history of drug abuse.

Elderly or debilitated patients may react to barbiturates with marked excitement, depression, and confusion. In some persons, barbiturates repeatedly produce excitement rather than depression.

In patients with hepatic damage, barbiturates should be administered with caution and initially in reduced doses.

Barbiturates should not be administered to patients showing the premonitory signs of hepatic coma.

Parenteral solutions of barbiturates are highly alkaline. Therefore, extreme care should be taken to avoid perivascular extravasation or intra-arterial injection. Extravascular injection may cause local tissue damage with subsequent necrosis; consequences of intra-arterial injection may vary from transient pain to gangrene of the limb. Any complaint of pain in the limb warrants stopping the injection.

Information for the patient: Practitioners should give the following information and instructions to patients receiving barbiturates.
1. The use of barbiturates carries with it an associated risk of psychological and/or physical dependence. The patient should be warned against increasing the dose of the drug without consulting a physician.
2. Barbiturates may impair mental and/or physical abilities required for the performance of potentially hazardous tasks (e.g., driving, operating machinery, etc.).
3. Alcohol should not be consumed while taking barbiturates. Concurrent use of the barbiturates with other CNS depressants (e.g., alcohol, narcotics, tranquilizers, and antihistamines) may result in additional CNS depressant effects.

Laboratory tests: Prolonged therapy with barbiturates should be accompanied by periodic laboratory evaluation of organ systems, including hematopoietic, renal, and hepatic systems. (See "Precautions-*General*" and "Adverse Reactions" sections).

Drug interactions: Most reports of clinically significant drug interactions occurring with the barbiturates have involved phenobarbital. However, the application of these data to other barbiturates appears valid and warrants serial blood level determinations of the relevant drugs when there are multiple therapies.
1. *Anticoagulants:* Phenobarbital lowers the plasma levels of dicumarol (name previously used: bishydroxycoumarin) and causes a decrease in anticoagulant activity as measured by the prothrombin time. Barbiturates can induce hepatic microsomal enzymes resulting in increased metabolism and decreased anticoagulant response of oral anticoagulants (e.g., warfarin, acenocoumarol, dicumarol, and phenprocoumon). Patients stabilized on anticoagulant therapy may require dosage adjustments if barbiturates are added to or withdrawn from their dosage regimen.
2. *Corticosteroids:* Barbiturates appear to enhance the metabolism of exogenous corticosteroids probably through the induction of hepatic microsomol enzymes. Patients stabilized on corticosteroid therapy may require dosage adjustments if barbiturates are added to or withdrawn from their dosage regimen.
3. *Griseofulvin:* Phenobarbital appears to interfere with the absorption of orally administered griseofulvin, thus decreasing its blood level. The effect of the resultant decreased blood levels of griseofulvin on therapeutic response has not been established. However, it would be preferable to avoid concomitant administration of these drugs.
4. *Doxycycline:* Phenobarbital has been shown to shorten the half-life of doxycycline for as long as 2 weeks after barbiturate therapy is discontinued.

This mechanism is probably through the induction of hepatic microsomal enzymes that metabolize the antibiotic. If phenobarbital and doxycycline are administered concurrently, the clinical response to doxycycline should be monitored closely.
5. *Phenytoin, sodium valproate, valproic acid:* The effect of barbiturates on the metabolism of phenytoin appears to be variable. Some investigators report an accelerating effect, while others report no effect. Because the effect of barbiturates on the metabolism of phenytoin is not predictable, phenytoin and barbiturate blood levels should be monitored more frequently if these drugs are given concurrently. Sodium valproate and valproic acid appear to decrease barbiturate metabolism; therefore, barbiturate blood levels should be monitored and appropriate dosage adjustments made as indicated.
6. *Central nervous system depressants:* The concomitant use of other central nervous system depressants, including other sedatives or hypnotics, antihistamines, tranquilizers, or alcohol, may produce additive depressant effects.
7. *Monoamine oxidase inhibitors (MAOI):* MAOI prolong the effects of barbiturates probably because metabolism of the barbiturate is inhibited.
8. *Estradiol, estrone, progesterone and other steroidal hormones:* Pretreatment with or concurrent administration of phenobarbital may decrease the effect of estradiol by increasing its metabolism. There have been reports of patients treated with antiepileptic drugs (e.g., phenobarbital) who became pregnant while taking oral contraceptives. An alternate contraceptive method might be suggested to women taking phenobarbital.

Carcinogenesis:
1. *Animal data.* Phenobarbital sodium is carcinogenic in mice and rats after lifetime administration. In mice, it

produced benign and malignant liver cell tumors. In rats, benign liver cell tumors were observed very late in life.
2. *Human data.* In a 29-year epidemiological study of 9,136 patients who were treated on an anticonvulsant protocol that included phenobarbital, results indicated a higher than normal incidence of hepatic carcinoma. Previously, some of these patients were treated with thorotrast, a drug that is known to produce hepatic carcinomas. Thus, this study did not provide sufficient evidence that phenobarbital sodium is carcinogenic in humans.

Data from one retrospective study of 235 children in which the types of barbiturates are not identified suggested an association between exposure to barbiturates prenatally and an increased incidence of brain tumor. (Gold, E., et al., "Increased Risk of Brain Tumors in Children Exposed to Barbiturates," Journal of National Cancer Institute, 61:1031–1034, 1978).

Pregnancy: 1. *Teratogenic effects.* Pregnancy Category D—See "Warnings—Use in Pregnancy" section.

2. *Nonteratogenic effects.* Reports of infants suffering from long-term barbiturate exposure in utero included the acute withdrawal syndrome of seizures and hyperirritability from birth to a delayed onset of up to 14 days. (See "Drug Abuse and Dependence" section).

Labor and delivery: Hypnotic doses of these barbiturates do not appear to significantly impair uterine activity during labor. Full anesthetic doses of barbiturates decrease the force and frequency of uterine contractions. Administration of sedative-hypnotic barbiturates to the mother during labor may result in respiratory depression in the newborn. Premature infants are particularly susceptible to the depressant effects of barbiturates. If barbiturates are used during labor and delivery, resuscitation equipment should be available. Data are currently not available to evaluate the effect of these barbiturates when forceps delivery or other intervention is necessary. Also, data are not available to determine the effect of these barbiturates on the later growth, development, and functional maturation of the child.

Nursing mothers: Caution should be exercised when a barbiturate is administered to a nursing woman since small amounts of barbiturates are excreted in the milk.

ADVERSE REACTIONS
The following adverse reactions and their incidence were compiled from surveillance of thousands of hospitalized patients. Because such patients may be less aware of certain of the milder adverse effects of barbiturates, the incidence of these reactions may be somewhat higher in fully ambulatory patients.

More than 1 in 100 patients. The most common adverse reaction estimated to occur at a rate of 1 to 3 patients per 100 is: *Nervous System:* Somnolence.

Less than 1 in 100 patients. Adverse reactions estimated to occur at a rate of less than 1 in 100 patients listed below, grouped by organ system, and by decreasing order of occurrence are:

Nervous system: Agitation, confusion, hyperkinesia, ataxia, CNS depression, nightmares, nervousness, psychiatric disturbance, hallucinations, insomnia, anxiety, dizziness, thinking abnormality.

Respiratory system: Hypoventilation, apnea.

Cardiovascular system: Bradycardia, hypotension, syncope.

Digestive system: Nausea, vomiting, constipation.

Other reported reactions: Headache, injection site reactions, hypersensitivity reactions (angioedema, skin rashes, exfoliative dermatitis), fever, liver damage, megaloblastic anemia following chronic phenobarbital use.

DRUG ABUSE AND DEPENDENCE
Pentobarbital sodium injection is subject to control by the Federal Controlled Substances Act under DEA schedule II. Barbiturates may be habit forming. Tolerance, psychological dependence, and physical dependence may occur especially following prolonged use of high doses of barbiturates. Daily administration in excess of 400 milligrams (mg) of pentobarbital or secobarbital for approximately 90 days is likely to produce some degree of physical dependence. A dosage of from 600 to 800 mg taken for at least 35 days is sufficient to produce withdrawal seizures. The average daily dose for the barbiturate addict is usually about 1.5 grams. As tolerance to barbiturates develops, the amount needed to maintain the same level of intoxication increases; tolerance to a fatal dosage, however, does not increase more than two-fold. As this occurs, the margin between an intoxicating dosage and fatal dosage becomes smaller.

Symptoms of acute intoxication with barbiturates include unsteady gait, slurred speech, and sustained nystagmus. Mental signs of chronic intoxication include confusion, poor judgment, irritability, insomnia, and somatic complaints. Symptoms of barbiturate dependence are similar to those of chronic alcoholism. If an individual appears to be intoxicated with alcohol to a degree that is radically disproportionate to the amount of alcohol in his or her blood the use of barbitu-

Continued on next page

Abbott Laboratories—Cont.

rates should be suspected. The lethal dose of a barbiturate is far less if alcohol is also ingested.

The symptoms of barbiturate withdrawal can be severe and may cause death. Minor withdrawal symptoms may appear 8 to 12 hours after the last dose of a barbiturate. These symptoms usually appear in the following order: anxiety, muscle twitching, tremor of hands and fingers, progressive weakness, dizziness, distortion in visual perception, nausea, vomiting, insomnia, and orthostatic hypotension. Major withdrawal symptoms (convulsions and delirium) may occur within 16 hours and last up to 5 days after abrupt cessation of these drugs. Intensity of withdrawal symptoms gradually declines over a period of approximately 15 days. Individuals susceptible to barbiturate abuse and dependence include alcoholics and opiate abusers, as well as other sedative-hypnotic and amphetamine abusers.

Drug dependence to barbiturates arises from repeated administration of a barbiturate or agent with barbiturate-like effect on a continuous basis, generally in amounts exceeding therapeutic dose levels. The characteristics of drug dependence to barbiturates include: (a) a strong desire or need to continue taking the drug; (b) a tendency to increase the dose; (c) a psychic dependence on the effects of the drug related to subjective and individual appreciation of those effects; and (d) a physical dependence on the effects of the drug requiring its presence for maintenance of homeostasis and resulting in a definite, characteristic, and self-limited abstinence syndrome when the drug is withdrawn.

Treatment of barbiturate dependence consists of cautious and gradual withdrawal of the drug. Barbiturate-dependent patients can be withdrawn by using a number of different withdrawal regimens. In all cases withdrawal takes an extended period of time. One method involves substituting a 30 mg dose of phenobarbital for each 100 to 200 mg dose of barbiturate that the patient has been taking. The total daily amount of phenobarbital is then administered in 3 to 4 divided doses, not to exceed 600 mg daily. Should signs of withdrawal occur on the first day of treatment, a loading dose of 100 to 200 mg of phenobarbital may be administered IM in addition to the oral dose. After stabilization on phenobarbital, the total daily dose is decreased by 30 mg a day as long as withdrawal is proceeding smoothly. A modification of this regimen involves initiating treatment at the patient's regular dosage level and decreasing the daily dosage by 10 percent if tolerated by the patient.

Infants physically dependent on barbiturates may be given phenobarbital 3 to 10 mg/kg/day. After withdrawal symptoms (hyperactivity, disturbed sleep, tremors, hyperreflexia) are relieved, the dosage of phenobarbital should be gradually decreased and completely withdrawn over a 2-week period.

OVERDOSAGE

The toxic dose of barbiturates varies considerably. In general, an oral dose of 1 gram of most barbiturates produces serious poisoning in an adult. Death commonly occurs after 2 to 10 grams of ingested barbiturate. Barbiturate intoxication may be confused with alcoholism, bromide intoxication, and with various neurological disorders.

Acute overdosage with barbiturates is manifested by CNS and respiratory depression which may progress to Cheyne-Stokes respiration, areflexia, constriction of the pupils to a slight degree (though in severe poisoning they may show paralytic dilation), oliguria, tachycardia, hypotension, lowered body temperature, and coma. Typical shock syndrome (apnea, circulatory collapse, respiratory arrest, and death) may occur.

In extreme overdose, all electrical activity in the brain may cease, in which case a "flat" EEG normally equated with clinical death cannot be accepted. This effect is fully reversible unless hypoxic damage occurs. Consideration should be given to the possibility of barbiturate intoxication even in situations that appear to involve trauma.

Complications such as pneumonia, pulmonary edema, cardiac arrhythmias, congestive heart failure, and renal failure may occur. Uremia may increase CNS sensitivity to barbiturates. Differential diagnosis should include hypoglycemia, head trauma, cerebrovascular accidents, convulsive states, and diabetic coma. Blood levels from acute overdosage for some barbiturates are listed in Table 1. [See Table 1 in NEMBUTAL Capsules prescribing information.]

Treatment of overdosage is mainly supportive and consists of the following:

1. Maintenance of an adequate airway, with assisted respiration and oxygen administration as necessary.
2. Monitoring of vital signs and fluid balance.
3. Fluid therapy and other standard treatment for shock, if needed.
4. If renal function is normal, forced diuresis may aid in the elimination of the barbiturate. Alkalinization of the urine increases renal excretion of some barbiturates, especially phenobarbital, also aprobarbital and mephobarbital (which is metabolized to phenobarbital).
5. Although not recommended as a routine procedure, hemodialysis may be used in severe barbiturate intoxications or if the patient is anuric or in shock.
6. Patient should be rolled from side to side every 30 minutes.
7. Antibiotics should be given if pneumonia is suspected.
8. Appropriate nursing care to prevent hypostatic pneumonia, decubiti, aspiration, and other complications of patients with altered states of consciousness.

DOSAGE AND ADMINISTRATION

Dosages of barbiturates must be individualized with full knowledge of their particular characteristics and recommended rate of administration. Factors of consideration are the patient's age, weight, and condition. Parenteral routes should be used only when oral administration is impossible or impractical.

Intramuscular Administration: IM injection of the sodium salts of barbiturates should be made deeply into a large muscle, and a volume of 5 ml should not be exceeded at any one site because of possible tissue irritation. After IM injection of a hypnotic dose, the patient's vital signs should be monitored. The usual adult dosage of NEMBUTAL Sodium Solution is 150 to 200 mg as a single IM injection; the recommended pediatric dosage ranges from 2 to 6 mg/kg as a single IM injection not to exceed 100 mg.

Intravenous Administration: Nembutal Sodium Solution should not be admixed with any other medication or solution. IV injection is restricted to conditions in which other routes are not feasible, either because the patient is unconscious (as in cerebral hemorrhage, eclampsia, or status epilepticus), or because the patient resists (as in delirium), or because prompt action is imperative. Slow IV injection is essential, and patients should be carefully observed during administration. This requires that blood pressure, respiration, and cardiac function be maintained, vital signs be recorded, and equipment for resuscitation and artificial ventilation be available. The rate of IV injection should not exceed 50 mg/min for pentobarbital sodium.

There is no average intravenous dose of NEMBUTAL Sodium Solution (pentobarbital sodium injection) that can be relied on to produce similar effects in different patients. The possibility of overdose and respiratory depression is remote when the drug is injected slowly in fractional doses.

A commonly used initial dose for the 70 kg adult is 100 mg. Proportional reduction in dosage should be made for pediatric or debilitated patients. At least one minute is necessary to determine the full effect of intravenous pentobarbital. If necessary, additional small increments of the drug may be given up to a total of from 200 to 500 mg for normal adults.

Anticonvulsant use: In convulsive states, dosage of NEMBUTAL Sodium Solution should be kept to a minimum to avoid compounding the depression which may follow convulsions. The injection must be made slowly with due regard to the time required for the drug to penetrate the blood-brain barrier.

Special patient population: Dosage should be reduced in the elderly or debilitated because these patients may be more sensitive to barbiturates. Dosage should be reduced for patients with impaired renal function or hepatic disease.

Inspection: Parenteral drug products should be inspected visually for particulate matter and discoloration prior to administration, whenever solution containers permit. Solutions for injection showing evidence of precipitation should not be used.

HOW SUPPLIED

NEMBUTAL Sodium Solution (pentobarbital sodium injection, USP) is available in the following sizes: 2-ml ampul, 100 mg, in boxes of 25 (**NDC** 0074-6899-04); 20-ml multiple-dose vial, 1 g per vial (**NDC** 0074-3778-04); and 50-ml multiple-dose vial, 2.5 g per vial (**NDC** 0074-3778-05).

Each ml contains:

Pentobarbital Sodium,
derivative of barbituric acid ....50 mg
Warning—May be habit forming.
Propylene glycol ....40% v/v
Alcohol 10%
Water for Injection ....qs
(pH adjusted to approximately 9.5 with hydrochloric acid and/or sodium hydroxide.)

Exposure of pharmaceutical products to heat should be minimized. Avoid excessive heat. Protect from freezing. It is recommended that the product be stored at room temperature—86°F (30°C); however, brief exposure up to 104°F (40°C) does not adversely affect the product.

Ref. 01-2577-R5

NEMBUTAL® SODIUM SUPPOSITORIES

℃ ℞

[*nĕm-bū 'tal*]

(PENTOBARBITAL SODIUM SUPPOSITORIES)

WARNING: MAY BE HABIT FORMING

DESCRIPTION

The barbiturates are nonselective central nervous system depressants which are primarily used as sedative hypnotics. The barbiturates and their sodium salts are subject to control under the Federal Controlled Substances Act (See "Drug Abuse and Dependence" section).

Barbiturates are substituted pyrimidine derivatives in which the basic structure common to these drugs is barbituric acid, a substance which has no central nervous system (CNS) activity. CNS activity is obtained by substituting alkyl, alkenyl, or aryl groups on the pyrimidine ring. Nembutal (pentobarbital sodium) is chemically represented by sodium 5-ethyl-5-(1-methylbutyl) barbiturate.

The structural formula for pentobarbital sodium is:

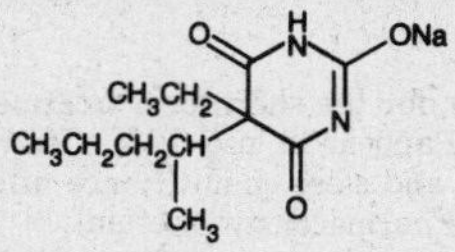

The sodium salt of pentobarbital occurs as a white, slightly bitter powder which is freely soluble in water and alcohol but practically insoluble in benzene and ether. Each rectal suppository contains either 30 mg, 60 mg, 120 mg, or 200 mg of pentobarbital sodium.

Inactive Ingredients: Semi-synthetic glycerides.

CLINICAL PHARMACOLOGY

Barbiturates are capable of producing all levels of CNS mood alteration from excitation to mild sedation, to hypnosis, and deep coma. Overdosage can produce death. In high enough therapeutic doses, barbiturates induce anesthesia.

Barbiturates depress the sensory cortex, decrease motor activity, alter cerebellar function, and produce drowsiness, sedation, and hypnosis.

Barbiturate-induced sleep differs from physiological sleep. Sleep laboratory studies have demonstrated that barbiturates reduce the amount of time spent in the rapid eye movement (REM) phase of sleep or dreaming stage. Also, Stages III and IV sleep are decreased. Following abrupt cessation of barbiturates used regularly, patients may experience markedly increased dreaming, nightmares, and/or insomnia. Therefore, withdrawal of a single therapeutic dose over 5 or 6 days has been recommended to lessen the REM rebound and disturbed sleep which contribute to drug withdrawal syndrome (for example, decrease the dose from 3 to 2 doses a day for 1 week).

In studies, secobarbital sodium and pentobarbital sodium have been found to lose most of their effectiveness for both inducing and maintaining sleep by the end of 2 weeks of continued drug administration at fixed doses. The short-, intermediate-, and, to a lesser degree, long-acting barbiturates have been widely prescribed for treating insomnia. Although the clinical literature abounds with claims that the short-acting barbiturates are superior for producing sleep while the intermediate-acting compounds are more effective in maintaining sleep, controlled studies have failed to demonstrate these differential effects. Therefore, as sleep medications, the barbiturates are of limited value beyond short-term use.

Barbiturates have little analgesic action at subanesthetic doses. Rather, in subanesthetic doses these drugs may increase the reaction to painful stimuli. All barbiturates exhibit anticonvulsant activity in anesthetic doses. However, of the drugs in this class, only phenobarbital, mephobarbital, and metharbital have been clinically demonstrated to be effective as oral anticonvulsants in subhypnotic doses.

Barbiturates are respiratory depressants. The degree of respiratory depression is dependent upon dose. With hypnotic doses, respiratory depression produced by barbiturates is similar to that which occurs during physiologic sleep with slight decrease in blood pressure and heart rate.

Studies in laboratory animals have shown that barbiturates cause reduction in the tone and contractility of the uterus, ureters, and urinary bladder. However, concentrations of the drugs required to produce this effect in humans are not reached with sedative-hypnotic doses.

Barbiturates do not impair normal hepatic function, but have been shown to induce liver microsomal enzymes, thus increasing and/or altering the metabolism of barbiturates and other drugs. (See "Precautions—*Drug Interactions*" section).

Pharmacokinetics: Barbiturates are absorbed in varying degrees following oral, rectal, or parenteral administration. The onset of action for oral or rectal administration varies from 20 to 60 minutes.

Duration of action, which is related to the rate at which the barbiturates are redistributed throughout the body, varies among persons and in the same person from time to time.

No studies have demonstrated that the different routes of administration are equivalent with respect to bioavailability.

Barbiturates are weak acids that are absorbed and rapidly distributed to all tissues and fluids with high concentrations

in the brain, liver, and kidneys. Lipid solubility of the barbiturates is the dominant factor in their distribution within the body. The more lipid soluble the barbiturate, the more rapidly it penetrates all tissues of the body. Barbiturates are bound to plasma and tissue proteins to a varying degree with the degree of binding increasing directly as a function of lipid solubility.

Phenobarbital has the lowest lipid solubility, lowest plasma binding, lowest brain protein binding, the longest delay in onset of activity, and the longest duration of action. At the opposite extreme is secobarbital which has the highest lipid solubility, plasma protein binding, brain protein binding, the shortest delay in onset of activity, and the shortest duration of action. Butabarbital is classified as an intermediate barbiturate.

The plasma half-life for phentobarbital in adults is 15 to 50 hours and appears to be dose dependent.

Barbiturates are metabolized primarily by the hepatic microsomal enzyme system, and the metabolic products are excreted in the urine, and less commonly, in the feces. Approximately 25 to 50 percent of a dose of aprobarbital or phenobarbital is eliminated unchanged in the urine, whereas the amount of other barbiturates excreted unchanged in the urine is negligible. The excretion of unmetabolized barbiturate is one feature that distinguishes the long-acting category from those belonging to other categories which are almost entirely metabolized. The inactive metabolites of the barbiturates are excreted as conjugates of glucuronic acid.

INDICATIONS AND USAGE

Rectal: Barbiturates administered rectally are absorbed from the colon and are used when oral or parenteral administration may be undesirable.
1. Sedative.
2. Hypnotic, for the short-term treatment of insomnia, since they appear to lose their effectiveness for sleep induction and sleep maintenance after 2 weeks (See "Clinical Pharmacology" section).

CONTRAINDICATIONS

Barbiturates are contraindicated in patients with known barbiturate sensitivity. Barbiturates are also contraindicated in patients with a history of manifest or latent porphyria.

WARNINGS

1. *Habit forming:* Barbiturates may be habit forming. Tolerance, psychological and physical dependence may occur with continued use. (See "Drug Abuse and Dependence" and "Pharmacokinetics" sections). Patients who have psychological dependence on barbiturates may increase the dosage or decrease the dosage interval without consulting a physician and may subsequently develop a physical dependence on barbiturates. To minimize the possibility of overdosage or the development of dependence, the prescribing and dispensing of sedative-hypnotic barbiturates should be limited to the amount required for the interval until the next appointment. Abrupt cessation after prolonged use in the dependent person may result in withdrawal symptoms, including delirium, convulsions, and possibly death. Barbiturates should be withdrawn gradually from any patient known to be taking excessive dosage over long periods of time. (See "Drug Abuse and Dependence" section).

2. *Acute or chronic pain:* Caution should be exercised when barbiturates are administered to patients with acute or chronic pain, because paradoxical excitement could be induced or important symptoms could be masked. However, the use of barbiturates as sedatives in the postoperative surgical period and as adjuncts to cancer chemotherapy is well established.

3. *Use in pregnancy:* Barbiturates can cause fetal damage when administered to a pregnant woman. Retrospective, case-controlled studies have suggested a connection between the maternal consumption of barbiturates and a higher than expected incidence of fetal abnormalities. Following oral or parenteral administration, barbiturates readily cross the placental barrier and are distributed throughout fetal tissues with highest concentrations found in the placenta, fetal liver, and brain. It is presumed that this effect will also be seen following rectal administration.

Withdrawal symptoms occur in infants born to mothers who receive barbiturates throughout the last trimester of pregnancy. (See "Drug Abuse and Dependence" section). If this drug is used during pregnancy, or if the patient becomes pregnant while taking this drug, the patient should be apprised of the potential hazard to the fetus.

4. *Synergistic effects:* The concomitant use of alcohol or other CNS depressants may produce additive CNS depressant effects.

PRECAUTIONS

General: Barbiturates may be habit forming. Tolerance and psychological and physical dependence may occur with continuing use. (See "Drug Abuse and Dependence" section). Barbiturates should be administered with caution, if at all, to patients who are mentally depressed, have suicidal tendencies, or a history of drug abuse.

Elderly or debilitated patients may react to barbiturates with marked excitement, depression, and confusion. In some persons, barbiturates repeatedly produce excitement rather than depression.

In patients with hepatic damage, barbiturates should be administered with caution and initially in reduced doses. Barbiturates should not be administered to patients showing the premonitory signs of hepatic coma.

Information for the patient: Practitioners should give the following information and instructions to patients receiving barbiturates.
1. The use of barbiturates carries with it an associated risk of psychological and/or physical dependence. The patient should be warned against increasing the dose of the drug without consulting a physician.
2. Barbiturates may impair mental and/or physical abilities required for the performance of potentially hazardous tasks (e.g., driving, operating machinery, etc.)
3. Alcohol should not be consumed while taking barbiturates. Concurrent use of the barbiturates with other CNS depressants (e.g., alcohol, narcotics, tranquilizers, and antihistamines) may result in additional CNS depressant effects.

Laboratory tests: Prolonged therapy with barbiturates should be accompanied by periodic laboratory evaluation of organ systems, including hematopoietic, renal, and hepatic systems. (See "Precautions — *General*" and "Adverse Reactions" sections).

Drug interactions: Most reports of clinically significant drug interactions occurring with the barbiturates have involved phenobarbital. However, the application of these data to other barbiturates appears valid and warrants serial blood level determinations of the relevant drugs when there are multiple therapies.
1. *Anticoagulants:* Phenobarbital lowers the plasma levels of dicumarol (name previously used: bishydroxycoumarin) and causes a decrease in anticoagulant activity as measured by the prothrombin time. Barbiturates can induce hepatic microsomal enzymes resulting in increased metabolism and decreased anticoagulant response of oral anticoagulants (e.g., warfarin, acenocoumarol, dicumarol, and phenprocoumon). Patients stabilized on anticoagulant therapy may require dosage adjustments if barbiturates are added to or withdrawn from their dosage regimen.
2. *Corticosteroids:* Barbiturates appear to enhance the metabolism of exogenous corticosteroids probably through the induction of hepatic microsomal enzymes. Patients stabilized on corticosteroid therapy may require dosage adjustments if barbiturates are added to or withdrawn from their dosage regimen.
3. *Griseofulvin:* Phenobarbital appears to interfere with the absorption of orally administered griseofulvin, thus decreasing its blood level. The effect of the resultant decreased blood levels of griseofulvin on therapeutic response has not been established. However, it would be preferable to avoid concomitant administration of these drugs.
4. *Doxycycline:* Phenobarbital has been shown to shorten the half-life of doxycycline for as long as 2 weeks after barbiturate therapy is discontinued. This mechanism is probably through the induction of hepatic microsomal enzymes that metabolize the antibiotic. If phenobarbital and doxycycline are administered concurrently, the clinical response to doxycycline should be monitored closely.
5. *Phenytoin, sodium valproate, valproic acid:* The effect of barbiturates on the metabolism of phenytoin appears to be variable. Some investigators report an accelerating effect, while others report no effect. Because the effect of barbiturates on the metabolism of phenytoin is not predictable, phenytoin and barbiturate blood levels should be monitored more frequently if these drugs are given concurrently. Sodium valproate and valproic acid appear to decrease barbiturate metabolism; therefore, barbiturate blood levels should be monitored and appropriate dosage adjustments made as indicated.
6. *Central nervous system depressants:* The concomitant use of other central nervous system depressants, including other sedatives or hypnotics, antihistamines, tranquilizers, or alcohol, may produce additive depressant effects.
7. *Monoamine oxidase inhibitors (MAOI):* MAOI prolong the effects of barbiturates probably because metabolism of the barbiturate is inhibited.
8. *Estradiol, estrone, progesterone and other steroidal hormones:* Pretreatment with or concurrent administration of phenobarbital may decrease the effect of estradiol by increasing its metabolism. There have been reports of patients treated with antiepileptic drugs (e.g., phenobarbital) who became pregnant while taking oral contraceptives. An alternate contraceptive method might be suggested to women taking phenobarbital.

Carcinogenesis:
1. Animal data. Phenobarbital sodium is carcinogenic in mice and rats after lifetime administration. In mice, it produced benign and malignant liver cell tumors. In rats, benign liver cell tumors were observed very late in life.
2. Human data. In a 29-year epidemiological study of 9,136 patients who were treated on an anticonvulsant protocol that included phenobarbital, results indicated a higher than normal incidence of hepatic carcinoma. Previously, some of these patients were treated with thorotrast, a drug that is known to produce hepatic carcinomas. Thus, this study did not provide sufficient evidence that phenobarbital sodium is carcinogenic in humans.

Data from one retrospective study of 235 children in which the types of barbiturates are not identified suggested an association between exposure to barbiturates prenatally and an increased incidence of brain tumor. (Gold, E., et al., "Increased Risk of Brain Tumors in Children Exposed to Barbiturates," Journal of National Cancer Institute, 61:1031–1034, 1978).

Pregnancy: 1. Teratogenic effects. Pregnancy Category D — See "Warnings — Use in Pregnancy" section.

2. Nonteratogenic effects. Reports of infants suffering from long-term barbiturate exposure in utero included the acute withdrawal syndrome of seizures and hyperirritability from birth to a delayed onset of up to 14 days. (See "Drug Abuse and Dependence" section).

Labor and delivery: Hypnotic doses of these barbiturates do not appear to significantly impair uterine activity during labor. Full anesthetic doses of barbiturates decrease the force and frequency of uterine contractions. Administration of sedative-hypnotic barbiturates to the mother during labor may result in respiratory depression in the newborn. Premature infants are particularly susceptible to the depressant effects of barbiturates. If barbiturates are used during labor and delivery, resuscitation equipment should be available. Data are currently not available to evaluate the effect of these barbiturates when forceps delivery or other intervention is necessary. Also, data are not available to determine the effect of these barbiturates on the later growth, development, and functional maturation of the child.

Nursing mothers: Caution should be exercised when a barbiturate is administered to a nursing woman since small amounts of barbiturates are excreted in the milk.

ADVERSE REACTIONS

The following adverse reactions and their incidence were compiled from surveillance of thousands of hospitalized patients. Because such patients may be less aware of certain of the milder adverse effects of barbiturates, the incidence of these reactions may be somewhat higher in fully ambulatory patients.

More than 1 in 100 patients. The most common adverse reaction estimated to occur at a rate of 1 to 3 patients per 100 is:
Nervous System: Somnolence.

Less than 1 in 100 patients. Adverse reactions estimated to occur at a rate of less than 1 in 100 patients listed below, grouped by organ system, and by decreasing order of occurrence are:
Nervous system: Agitation, confusion, hyperkinesia, ataxia, CNS depression, nightmares, nervousness, psychiatric disturbance, hallucinations, insomnia, anxiety, dizziness, thinking abnormality.
Respiratory system: Hypoventilation, apnea.
Cardiovascular system: Bradycardia, hypotension, syncope.
Digestive system: Nausea, vomiting, constipation.
Other reported reactions: Headache, injection site reactions, hypersensitivity reactions (angioedema, skin rashes, exfoliative dermatitis), fever, liver damage, megaloblastic anemia following chronic phenobarbital use.

DRUG ABUSE AND DEPENDENCE

Pentobarbital sodium suppositories are subject to control by the Federal Controlled Substances Act under DEA schedule III.

Barbiturates may be habit forming. Tolerance, psychological dependence, and physical dependence may occur especially following prolonged use of high doses of barbiturates. Daily administration in excess of 400 milligrams (mg) of pentobarbital or secobarbital for approximately 90 days is likely to produce some degree of physical dependence. A dosage of from 600 to 800 mg taken for at least 35 days is sufficient to produce withdrawal seizures. The average daily dose for the barbiturate addict is usually about 1.5 grams. As tolerance to barbiturates develops, the amount needed to maintain the same level of intoxication increases; tolerance to a fatal dosage, however, does not increase more than two-fold. As this occurs, the margin between an intoxicating dosage and fatal dosage becomes smaller.

Symptoms of acute intoxication with barbiturates include unsteady gait, slurred speech, and sustained nystagmus. Mental signs of chronic intoxication include confusion, poor judgment, irritability, insomnia, and somatic complaints.

Continued on next page

Abbott Laboratories—Cont.

Symptoms of barbiturate dependence are similar to those of chronic alcoholism. If an individual appears to be intoxicated with alcohol to a degree that is radically disproportionate to the amount of alcohol in his or her blood the use of barbiturates should be suspected. The lethal dose of a barbiturate is far less if alcohol is also ingested.

The symptoms of barbiturate withdrawal can be severe and may cause death. Minor withdrawal symptoms may appear 8 to 12 hours after the last dose of a barbiturate. These symptoms usually appear in the following order: anxiety, muscle twitching, tremor of hands and fingers, progressive weakness, dizziness, distortion in visual perception, nausea, vomiting, insomnia, and orthostatic hypotension. Major withdrawal symptoms (convulsions and delirium) may occur within 16 hours and last up to 5 days after abrupt cessation of these drugs. Intensity of withdrawal symptoms gradually declines over a period of approximately 15 days. Individuals susceptible to barbiturate abuse and dependence include alcoholics and opiate abusers, as well as other sedative-hypnotic and amphetamine abusers.

Drug dependence to barbiturates arises from repeated administration of a barbiturate or agent with barbiturate-like effect on a continuous basis, generally in amounts exceeding therapeutic dose levels. The characteristics of drug dependence to barbiturates include: (a) a strong desire or need to continue taking the drug; (b) a tendency to increase the dose; (c) a psychic dependence on the effects of the drug related to subjective and individual appreciation of those effects; and (d) a physical dependence on the effects of the drug requiring its presence for maintenance of homeostasis and resulting in a definite, characteristic, and self-limited abstinence syndrome when the drug is withdrawn.

Treatment of barbiturate dependence consists of cautious and gradual withdrawal of the drug. Barbiturate-dependent patients can be withdrawn by using a number of different withdrawal regimens. In all cases withdrawal takes an extended period of time. One method involves substituting a 30 mg dose of phenobarbital for each 100 to 200 mg dose of barbiturate that the patient has been taking. The total daily amount of phenobarbital is then administered in 3 to 4 divided doses, not to exceed 600 mg daily. Should signs of withdrawal occur on the first day of treatment, a loading dose of 100 to 200 mg of phenobarbital may be administered IM in addition to the oral dose. After stabilization on phenobarbital, the total daily dose is decreased by 30 mg a day as long as withdrawal is proceeding smoothly. A modification of this regimen involves initiating treatment at the patient's regular dosage level and decreasing the daily dosage by 10 percent if tolerated by the patient.

Infants physically dependent on barbiturates may be given phenobarbital 3 to 10 mg/kg/day. After withdrawal symptoms (hyperactivity, disturbed sleep, tremors, hyperreflexia) are relieved, the dosage of phenobarbital should be gradually decreased and completely withdrawn over a 2 week period.

OVERDOSAGE

The toxic dose of barbiturates varies considerably. In general, an oral dose of 1 gram of most barbiturates produces serious poisoning in an adult. Death commonly occurs after 2 to 10 grams of ingested barbiturate. Barbiturate intoxication may be confused with alcoholism, bromide intoxication, and with various neurological disorders.

Acute overdosage with barbiturates is manifested by CNS and respiratory depression which may progress to Cheyne-Stokes respiration, areflexia, constriction of the pupils to a slight degree (though in severe poisoning they may show paralytic dilation), oliguria, tachycardia, hypotension, lowered body temperature, and coma. Typical shock syndrome (apnea, circulatory collapse, respiratory arrest, and death) may occur.

In extreme overdose, all electrical activity in the brain may cease, in which case a "flat" EEG normally equated with clinical death cannot be accepted. This effect is fully reversible unless hypoxic damage occurs. Consideration should be given to the possibility of barbiturate intoxication even in situations that appear to involve trauma.

Complications such as pneumonia, pulmonary edema, cardiac arrhythmias, congestive heart failure, and renal failure may occur. Uremia may increase CNS sensitivity to barbiturates. Differential diagnosis should include hypoglycemia, head trauma, cerebrovascular accidents, convulsive states, and diabetic coma. Blood levels from acute overdosage for some barbiturates are listed in Table 1.

[See table below.]

Treatment of overdosage is mainly supportive and consists of the following:

1. Maintenance of an adequate airway, with assisted respiration and oxygen administration as necessary.
2. Monitoring of vital signs and fluid balance.
3. Fluid therapy and other standard treatment for shock, if needed.
4. If renal function is normal, forced diuresis may aid in the elimination of the barbiturate. Alkalinization of the urine increases renal excretion of some barbiturates, especially phenobarbital, also aprobarbital, and mephobarbital (which is metabolized to phenobarbital).
5. Although not recommended as a routine procedure, hemodialysis may be used in severe barbiturate intoxications or if the patient is anuric or in shock.
6. Patient should be rolled from side to side every 30 minutes.
7. Antibiotics should be given if pneumonia is suspected.
8. Appropriate nursing care to prevent hypostatic pneumonia, decubiti, aspiration, and other complications of patients with altered states of consciousness.

DOSAGE AND ADMINISTRATION

Typical hypnotic doses for adults and children are given below. These are intended only as a guide, and administration should be adjusted to the individual needs of each patient. For sedation, in children 5–14 years and in adults, reduce dose appropriately.

Adults (average to above average weight)— one 120 mg or one 200 mg suppository.

Children —

12–14 years ....one 60 mg or one
(80–110 lbs) 120 mg suppository
5–12 years ....one 60 mg suppository
(40–80 lbs)
1–4 years ....one 30 mg or one
(20–40 lbs) 60 mg suppository
2 months–1 year ....one 30 mg
(10–20 lbs) suppository

Suppositories should not be divided.

Dosages of barbiturates must be individualized with full knowledge of their particular characteristics and recommended rate of administration. Factors of consideration are the patient's age, weight, and condition.

Special patient population: Dosage should be reduced in the elderly or debilitated because these patients may be more sensitive to barbiturates. Dosage should be reduced for patients with impaired renal function or hepatic disease.

HOW SUPPLIED

NEMBUTAL Sodium Suppositories (pentobarbital sodium suppositories) are available as suppositories containing pentobarbital sodium in the amount of 30 mg (**NDC** 0074-3272-01); 60 mg (**NDC** 0074-3148-01); 120 mg (**NDC** 0074-3145-01) and 200 mg (**NDC** 0074-3164-01). Supplied in boxes of 12 suppositories.

Store in a refrigerator (36°–46°F).

Ref. 03-4514-R13

Table 1.—*Concentration of Barbiturate in the Blood Versus Degree of CNS Depression*

Blood barbiturate level in ppm (μg/ml)

Barbiturate	Onset/ duration	Degree of depression in nontolerant persons*				
		1	2	3	4	5
Pentobarbital	Fast/short	≤2	0.5 to 3	10 to 15	12 to 25	15 to 40
Secobarbital	Fast/short	≤2	0.5 to 5	10 to 15	15 to 25	15 to 40
Amobarbital	Intermediate/ intermediate	≤3	2 to 10	30 to 40	30 to 60	40 to 80
Butabarbital	Intermediate/ intermediate	≤5	3 to 25	40 to 60	50 to 80	60 to 100
Phenobarbital	Slow/long	≤10	5 to 40	50 to 80	70 to 120	100 to 200

*Categories of degree of depression in nontolerant persons:

1. Under the influence and appreciably impaired for purposes of driving a motor vehicle or performing tasks requiring alertness and unimpaired judgment and reaction time.
2. Sedated, therapeutic range, calm, relaxed, and easily aroused.
3. Comatose, difficult to arouse, significant depression of respiration.
4. Compatible with death in aged or ill persons or in presence of obstructed airway, other toxic agents, or exposure to cold.
5. Usual lethal level, the upper end of the range includes those who received some supportive treatment.

NORISODRINE® WITH CALCIUM IODIDE SYRUP ℞

[*nō-rī 'sō-drēen*]

(isoproterenol sulfate and calcium iodide)

DESCRIPTION

NORISODRINE with Calcium Iodide is a bronchodilator, expectorant in a palatable syrup.

Isoproterenol is a sympathomimetic agent which is chemically related to epinephrine. The chemical formula for isoproterenol sulfate is 1, 2-Benzenediol, 4-[1-hydroxy-2-[(1-methylethyl) amino] ethyl]-, sulfate (2:1) (salt), dihydrate and the structural formula is:

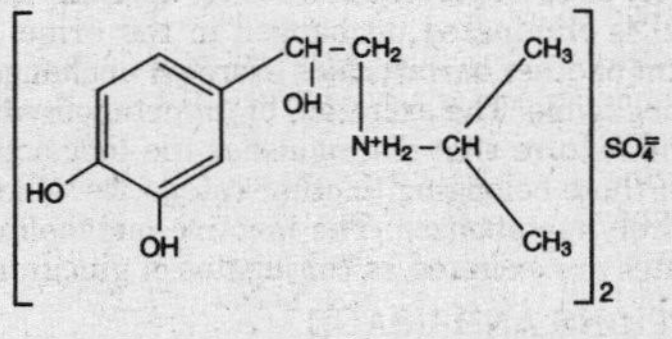

CLINICAL PHARMACOLOGY

Isoproterenol is classified as a catecholamine which acts predominantly on beta receptor sites of peripheral inhibitory and cardiac excitatory sympathetic nerves. Its primary pharmacological actions are to increase both the rate and force of cardiac contractions and to relax the smooth muscle of the bronchi, alimentary tract, and skeletal muscle vasculature. Isoproterenol can prevent or relieve bronchospasm due to drugs, as well as that due to disease. The drug lowers peripheral vascular resistance and reduces the diastolic blood pressure. Systolic pressure is unchanged or slightly increased as a consequence of increased cardiac output.

After oral administration, isoproterenol is extensively converted to its sulfate conjugate in the intestinal wall. This presystemic metabolism explains the higher doses and more variable response to isoproterenol by the oral route compared to parenteral administration. The primary excretion product found in urine is the sulfate conjugate (50 to 80% of the dose) with only minor fractions of unchanged drug (5 to 15%) and 3-O-methyl isoproterenol (15% or less).

The calorigenic effects of isoproterenol are similar to those of epinephrine. However, it causes less hyperglycemia than epinephrine. Isoproterenol can also cause central excitation. Calcium iodide is an expectorant.

INDICATIONS AND USAGE

Indicated in adults and children for the symptomatic control of bronchospasm in asthma and in allied respiratory disorders such as bronchitis and tracheobronchitis.

CONTRAINDICATIONS

This product should not be used in patients with a history of iodism, or with known hypersensitivity to iodides. It is also contraindicated in rare instances in which a patient has demonstrated hypersensitivity to isoproterenol or other sympathomimetic amines.

Use of isoproterenol is contraindicated in patients with preexisting cardiac arrhythmias because the cardiac stimulant effect may aggravate such disorders.

Long-term use of iodide-containing preparations is contraindicated during pregnancy. (See WARNINGS.)

WARNINGS

Bronchial asthma may mask the presence of cardiac asthma (pulmonary edema). A differential diagnosis should be made before instituting therapy.

Usage in Pregnancy: NORISODRINE with Calcium Iodide can cause fetal harm when administered to a pregnant woman. Maternal ingestion of large amounts of iodides during pregnancy has been associated with development of fetal goiter and resultant acute respiratory distress of the neonate. If this drug is used during pregnancy, or if the patient becomes pregnant while taking this drug, the patient should be apprised of the potential hazard to the fetus.

PRECAUTIONS

Isoproterenol should be used cautiously in patients with heart disease, hypertension, hyperthyroidism, diabetes, or unstable vasomotor systems.

Patients who must receive prolonged iodide therapy should be evaluated periodically for possible depression of thyroid function.

Drug Interactions: The concurrent administration of calcium iodide and lithium carbonate may enhance the hypothyroid and goitrogenic effects of either drug.

Concomitant use of isoproterenol and MAO inhibitors may induce acute hypertensive crisis.

Propranolol, a beta-adrenergic blocking agent, antagonizes isoproterenol.

Caution should be exercised when isoproterenol is used concomitantly with a parenteral or inhalation form of *epinephrine* or other *adrenergic agent* since the effects of these drugs are additive.

Laboratory Test Interactions: Elevated values may be obtained on thyroid function tests, and when testing for protein-bound iodine, when iodine-containing compounds have been ingested.

The use of iodides may cause false positive results when guaiac testing is performed or when testing for benzidine.

Carcinogenesis: No data is available on long-term potential for carcinogenicity in animals or humans.

Pregnancy: Pregnancy Category D. See "WARNINGS" section.

Nursing Mothers: Iodine is excreted in breast milk, therefore, caution should be exercised when NORISODRINE with Calcium Iodide is administered to a nursing woman.

ADVERSE REACTIONS

As with other sympathomimetic drugs, isoproterenol may produce undesired side effects. These effects in decreasing order of severity are cardiac arrhythmias, tachycardia, vomiting, dizziness, weakness, nausea, precordial distress and anginal-type pain, headache, palpitation, nervousness, tremor, sweating, and flushing.

Swelling of the parotid glands has been reported with prolonged use of isoproterenol. In such cases the drug should be withdrawn.

Iodism can occur with use of this drug. Symptoms of iodism include metallic taste, acneform skin lesions, mucous membrane irritation, salivary gland swelling, and gastric distress. These side effects subside quickly upon discontinuance of the iodide-containing drug. Severe and sometimes fatal skin eruptions (ioderma) occur rarely after the prolonged use of iodides.

SYMPTOMS AND TREATMENT OF OVERDOSAGE

Symptoms may include palpitation, tachycardia, restlessness, tremor, sweating, headache, dizziness, weakness, nausea, and vomiting. Blood pressure may at first be elevated slightly. Later, blood pressure may fall and the general picture of "shock" may develop.

Treatment includes general supportive measures. Sedatives may be given for restlessness.

DOSAGE AND ADMINISTRATION

The following suggestions are offered as a general guide to dosage:

Under 3 years: 1/2 teaspoonful, may be repeated every four to six hours; 3 to 10 years: 1/2 to 1 teaspoonful, may be repeated every four to six hours; over 10 years and for adults: 1 to 2 teaspoonfuls, may be repeated every four to six hours. Dosage must be adjusted to the response of the patient. Side effects may necessitate dosage reduction.

HOW SUPPLIED

Each 5 mL (teaspoonful) of NORISODRINE WITH CALCIUM IODIDE SYRUP contains 3 mg of isoproterenol sulfate and 150 mg of anhydrous calcium iodide. Norisodrine with Calcium Iodide Syrup is supplied in pint (**NDC** 0074-6953-01) bottles.

Inactive Ingredients: Alcohol 6%, ascorbic acid, caramel coloring, glycerin, liquid glucose, sucrose, water and artificial flavors forming a palatable, aromatic syrup.

Store below 77°F (25°C). Dispense in a USP tight, light-resistant glass container.

Ref. 02-7550-5/R35

NORVIR™ ℞

(ritonavir capsules)
(ritonavir oral solution)

> **WARNING**
>
> CO-ADMINISTRATION OF NORVIR WITH CERTAIN NONSEDATING ANTIHISTAMINES, SEDATIVE HYPNOTICS, OR ANTIARRHYTHMICS MAY RESULT IN POTENTIALLY SERIOUS AND/OR LIFE-THREATENING ADVERSE EVENTS DUE TO POSSIBLE EFFECTS OF NORVIR ON THE HEPATIC METABOLISM OF CERTAIN DRUGS. SEE **CONTRAINDICATIONS** AND **PRECAUTIONS** SECTIONS.

DESCRIPTION

NORVIR (ritonavir) is an inhibitor of HIV protease with activity against the Human Immunodeficiency Virus (HIV).

Ritonavir is chemically designated as 10-Hydroxy-2-methyl-5-(1-methylethyl)-1-[2-(1-methylethyl)-4-thiazolyl]-3,6-dioxo-8,11-bis(phenylmethyl)-2,4,7,12-tetraazatridecan-13-oic acid, 5-thiazolylmethyl ester, [5S-(5R*,8R*,10R*,11R*)]. Its molecular formula is $C_{37}H_{48}N_6O_5S_2$, and its molecular weight is 720.95. Ritonavir has the following structural formula:

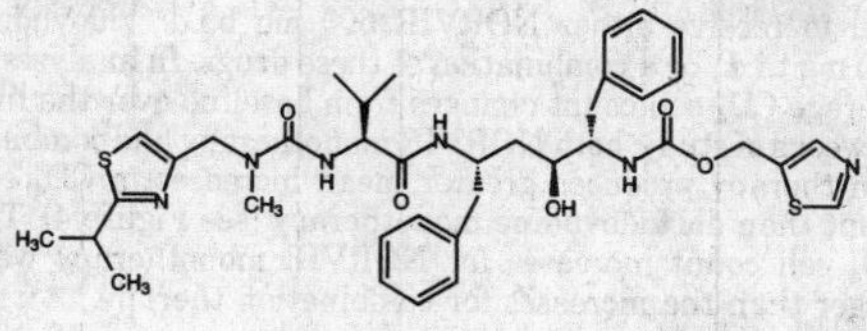

Ritonavir is a white-to-light-tan powder. Ritonavir has a bitter metallic taste. It is freely soluble in methanol and ethanol, soluble in isopropanol and practically insoluble in water.

NORVIR capsules are available for oral administration in a strength of 100 mg ritonavir with the following inactive ingredients: Caprylic/capric triglycerides, polyoxyl 35 castor oil, citric acid, gelatin, ethanol, polyglycolyzed glycerides, polysorbate 80, and propylene glycol.

NORVIR oral solution is available for oral administration as 80 mg/mL of ritonavir in a peppermint and caramel flavored vehicle. Each 8-ounce bottle contains 19.2 grams of ritonavir. NORVIR oral solution also contains ethanol, water, polyoxyl 35 castor oil, propylene glycol, anhydrous citric acid to adjust pH, saccharin sodium, peppermint oil, creamy caramel flavoring, and FD&C Yellow No. 6.

CLINICAL PHARMACOLOGY

MICROBIOLOGY

Mechanism of action: Ritonavir is a peptidomimetic inhibitor of both the HIV-1 and HIV-2 proteases. Inhibition of HIV protease renders the enzyme incapable of processing the *gag-pol* polyprotein precursor which leads to production of non-infectious immature HIV particles.

Antiviral activity *in vitro:* The activity of ritonavir was assessed *in vitro* in acutely infected lymphoblastoid cell lines and in peripheral blood lymphocytes. The concentration of drug that inhibits 50% (EC_{50}) of viral replication ranged from 3.8 to 153 nM depending upon the HIV-1 isolate and the cells employed. The average EC_{50} for low passage clinical isolates was 22 nM (n=13). In MT_4 cells, ritonavir demonstrated additive effects against HIV-1 in combination with either zidovudine (ZDV) or didanosine (ddI). Studies which measured cytotoxicity of ritonavir on several cell lines showed that > 20 μM was required to inhibit cellular growth by 50% resulting in an *in vitro* therapeutic index of at least 1000.

Resistance: HIV-1 isolates with reduced susceptibility to ritonavir have been selected *in vitro.* Genotypic analysis of these isolates showed mutations in the HIV protease gene at amino acid positions 84 (Ile to Val), 82 (Val to Phe), 71 (Ala to Val), and 46 (Met to Ile). Phenotypic (n=18) and genotypic (n=44) changes in HIV isolates from selected patients treated with ritonavir were monitored in phase I/II trials over a period of 3 to 32 weeks. Mutations associated with the HIV viral protease in isolates obtained from 41 patients appeared to occur in a stepwise and ordered fashion; in sequence, these mutations were position 82 (Val to Ala/Phe), 54 (Ile to Val), 71 (Ala to Val/Thr), and 36 (Ile to Leu), followed by combinations of mutations at an additional 5 specific amino acid positions. Of 18 patients for which both phenotypic and genotypic analysis were performed on free virus isolated from plasma, 12 showed reduced susceptibility to ritonavir *in vitro.* All 18 patients possessed one or more mutations in the viral protease gene. The 82 mutation appeared to be necessary but not sufficient to confer phenotypic resistance. Phenotypic resistance was defined as a ≥5-fold decrease in viral sensitivity *in vitro* from baseline. The clinical relevance of phenotypic and genotypic changes associated with ritonavir therapy has not been established.

Cross-resistance to other antiretrovirals: The potential for HIV cross-resistance between protease inhibitors has not been fully explored. Therefore, it is unknown what effect ritonavir therapy will have on the activity of concordantly or subsequently administered protease inhibitors. Serial HIV isolates obtained from six patients during ritonavir therapy showed a decrease in ritonavir susceptibility *in vitro* but did not demonstrate a concordant decrease in susceptibility to saquinavir *in vitro* when compared to matched baseline isolates. However, isolates from two of these patients demonstrated decreased susceptibility to indinavir *in vitro* (8-fold). Isolates from 5 patients were also tested for cross-resistance to VX-478 and nelfinavir; isolates from 2 patients had a decrease in susceptibility to nelfinavir (12 - 14-fold), and none to VX-478. Cross-resistance between ritonavir and reverse transcriptase inhibitors is unlikely because of the different enzyme targets involved. One ZDV-resistant HIV isolate tested *in vitro* retained full susceptibility to ritonavir.

Pharmacokinetics

The pharmacokinetics of ritonavir have been studied in healthy volunteers and HIV-infected patients (CD_4 ≥ 50 cells/μL). See Table 1 for ritonavir pharmacokinetic characteristics.

The absolute bioavailability of ritonavir has not been determined. After a 600 mg dose of oral solution, peak concentrations of ritonavir were achieved approximately 2 hours and 4 hours after dosing under fasting and non-fasting (514 KCal; 9% fat, 12% protein, and 79% carbohydrate) conditions, respectively. When the oral solution was given under non-fasting conditions, peak ritonavir concentrations decreased 23% and the extent of absorption decreased 7% relative to fasting conditions. Dilution of the oral solution, within one hour of administration, with 240 mL of chocolate milk, Advera® or Ensure® did not significantly affect the extent and rate of ritonavir absorption. After a single 600 mg dose under non-fasting conditions, in two separate studies, the capsule (n=21) and oral solution (n=18) formulations yielded mean ± SD areas under the plasma concentration-time curve (AUCs) of 129.5 ± 47.1 and 129.0 ± 39.3 μg•h/mL, respectively. Relative to fasting conditions, the extent of absorption of ritonavir from the capsule formulation was 15% higher when administered with a meal (771 KCal; 46% fat, 18% protein, and 37% carbohydrate).

Nearly all of the plasma radioactivity after a single oral 600 mg dose of ^{14}C-ritonavir oral solution (n=5) was attributed to unchanged ritonavir. Five ritonavir metabolites have been identified in human urine and feces. The isopropylthiazole oxidation metabolite (M-2) is the major metabolite and has antiviral activity similar to that of parent drug; however, the concentrations of this metabolite in plasma are low. Studies utilizing human liver microsomes have demonstrated that cytochrome P450 3A (CYP3A) is the major isoform involved in ritonavir metabolism, although CYP2D6 also contributes to the formation of M-2.

In a study of five subjects receiving a 600 mg dose of ^{14}C-ritonavir oral solution, 11.3 ± 2.8% of the dose was excreted into the urine, with 3.5 ± 1.8% of the dose excreted as unchanged parent drug. In that study, 86.4 ± 2.9% of the dose was excreted in the feces with 33.8 ± 10.8% of the dose excreted as unchanged parent drug. Upon multiple dosing, ritonavir accumulation is less than predicted from a single dose possibly due to a time and dose-related increase in clearance.

Table 1
Ritonavir Pharmacokinetic Characteristics

Parameter	n	Values (Mean ± SD)
C_{max} SS†	10	11.2 ± 3.6 μg/mL
C_{trough} SS†	10	3.7 ± 2.6 μg/mL
V_{β}/F‡	91	0.41 ± 0.25 L/kg
$t_{1/2}$		3 - 5 h
CL/F†	10	8.8 ± 3.2 L/h
CL/F‡	91	4.6 ± 1.6 L/h
CL_R	62	<0.1 L/h
RBC/Plasma Ratio		0.14
Percent Bound*		98 to 99%

† SS =steady state; patients taking ritonavir 600 mg q12h.
‡ Single ritonavir 600 mg dose.
* Primarily bound to human serum albumin and alpha-1 acid glycoprotein over the ritonavir concentration range of 0.01 to 30 μg/mL.

Special Populations:

Gender, Race and Age: No age-related pharmacokinetic differences have been observed in adult patients (18 to 63 years). Ritonavir pharmacokinetics have not been studied in older patients. A study of ritonavir pharmacokinetics in healthy males and females showed no statistically significant differences in the pharmacokinetics of ritonavir. Pharmacokinetic differences due to race have not been identified.

Renal Insufficiency: Ritonavir pharmacokinetics have not been studied in patients with renal insufficiency, however since renal clearance is negligible, a decrease in total body clearance is not expected in patients with renal insufficiency.

Hepatic Insufficiency: Ritonavir pharmacokinetics have not been established in subjects with hepatic insufficiency (see **PRECAUTIONS**).

Drug-Drug Interactions: Table 2 summarizes the effects on AUC and C_{max}, with 95% confidence intervals (95 CI), of co-administration of ritonavir with a variety of drugs. For information about clinical recommendations see **PRECAUTIONS-Drug Interactions.**

[See Table 2 at bottom of next page.]

INDICATIONS AND USAGE

NORVIR is indicated in combination with nucleoside analogues or as monotherapy for the treatment of HIV-infection when therapy is warranted. For patients with advanced HIV disease, this indication is based on the results from a study that showed a reduction in both mortality and AIDS-defining clinical events for patients who received NORVIR. Median duration of follow-up in this study was 6 months. The clinical benefit from NORVIR therapy for longer periods of treatment is unknown.

Continued on next page

Abbott Laboratories—Cont.

For patients with less advanced disease, this indication is based on changes in surrogate markers in studies evaluating patients who received NORVIR alone or in combination with other antiretroviral agents (see **Description of Clinical Studies**).

Description of Clinical Studies

The activity of NORVIR as monotherapy or in combination with nucleoside analogues has been evaluated in 1446 patients enrolled in two double-blind, randomized trials. NORVIR therapy in combination with zidovudine and zalcitabine was also evaluated in an open-label, non-comparative study of 32 patients. The clinical studies reported here were all conducted using ritonavir oral solution.

Advanced Patients with Prior Antiretroviral Therapy

Study 247 was a randomized, double-blind trial conducted in HIV-infected patients with at least nine months of prior antiretroviral therapy and baseline CD_4 cell counts $\leq$ 100 cells/μL. NORVIR 600 mg b.i.d. or placebo was added to each patient's baseline antiretroviral therapy regimen, which could have consisted of up to two approved antiretroviral agents. The study accrued 1090 patients, with mean baseline CD_4 cell count at study entry of 32 cells/μL. Median duration of follow-up was 6 months.

The six month cumulative incidence of clinical disease progression or death was 17% for patients randomized to NORVIR compared to 34% for patients randomized to placebo. This difference in rates was statistically significant (see Figure 1).

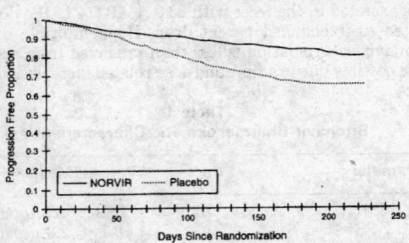

Figure 1
Time to Disease Progression or Death in Study 247

The six-month cumulative mortality was 5.8% for patients randomized to NORVIR and 10.1% for patients randomized to placebo. This difference in rates was statistically significant.

In addition, analyses of mean CD_4 cell count changes from baseline over the first 16 weeks of study for the first 211 patients enrolled (mean baseline CD_4 cell count = 29 cells/μL) showed that NORVIR was associated with larger increases in CD_4 cell counts than was placebo (see Figure 2).

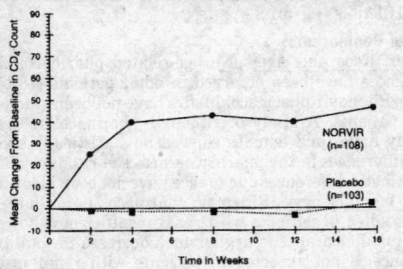

Figure 2
Mean CD₄ Count Changes (cells/μL) From Baseline In Study 247

Figure 3 summarizes the mean changes from baseline in log HIV RNA levels for Study 247.

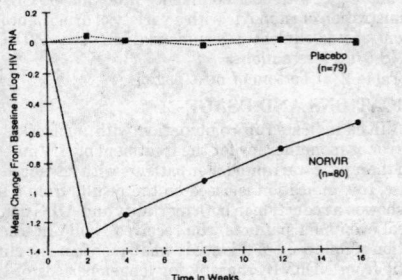

Figure 3
Mean Change From Baseline in Log HIV RNA Levels[1] in Study 247

[1] The clinical significance of changes in HIV RNA measurements has not been established.

Patients Without Prior Antiretroviral Therapy

In ongoing Study 245, 356 antiretroviral-naive HIV-infected patients (mean baseline CD_4 = 364 cells/μL) were randomized to receive either NORVIR 600 mg b.i.d., zidovudine 200 mg t.i.d., or a combination of these drugs. In analyses of average CD_4 cell count changes from baseline over the first 16 weeks of study, both NORVIR monotherapy and combination therapy produced greater mean increases in CD_4 cell count than did zidovudine monotherapy (see Figure 4). The CD_4 cell count increases for NORVIR monotherapy were larger than the increases for combination therapy.

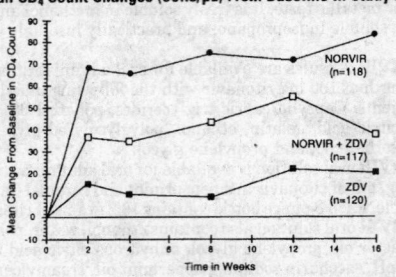

Figure 4
Mean CD₄ Count Changes (cells/μL) From Baseline In Study 245

Figure 5 summarizes the mean changes from baseline in log HIV RNA levels for Study 245.

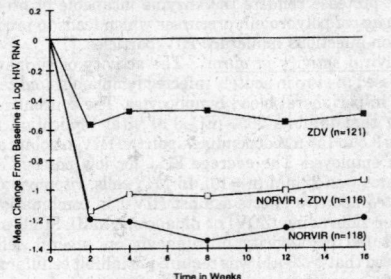

Figure 5
Mean Change From Baseline in Log HIV RNA Levels in Study 245

Combination Therapy with NORVIR, Zidovudine, and Zalcitabine in Antiretroviral-Naive Patients

In Study 208, an open-label uncontrolled trial, 32 antiretroviral-naive HIV-infected patients initially received NORVIR 600 mg b.i.d. monotherapy. Zidovudine 200 mg t.i.d. and zalcitabine 0.75 mg t.i.d. were added after 14 days of NORVIR monotherapy. Results of combination therapy for the

first 20 weeks of this study show median increases in CD_4 cell counts from baseline levels of 83 to 106 cells/μL over the treatment period. Mean decreases from baseline in HIV RNA particle levels ranged from 1.69 to 1.92 logs.

CONTRAINDICATIONS

NORVIR is contraindicated in patients with known hypersensitivity to ritonavir or any of its ingredients.

Ritonavir is expected to produce large increases in the plasma concentrations of the following drugs: amiodarone, astemizole, bepridil, bupropion, cisapride, clozapine, encainide, flecainide, meperidine, piroxicam, propafenone, propoxyphene, quinidine, rifabutin, and terfenadine. These agents have recognized risks of arrhythmias, hematologic abnormalities, seizures, or other potentially serious adverse effects. These drugs should not be co-administered with ritonavir. Ritonavir co-administration is likely to produce large increases in these highly metabolized sedatives and hypnotics: alprazolam, clorazepate, diazepam, estazolam, flurazepam, midazolam, triazolam, and zolpidem. Due to the potential for extreme sedation and respiratory depression from these agents, they should not be co-administered with ritonavir.

PRECAUTIONS

General

Ritonavir is principally metabolized by the liver. Therefore, caution should be exercised when administering this drug to patients with impaired hepatic function.

Resistance/Cross-resistance

The potential for HIV cross-resistance between protease inhibitors has not been fully explored. Therefore, it is unknown what effect ritonavir therapy will have on the activity of subsequent protease inhibitors (see **MICROBIOLOGY**).

Information For Patients

Patients should be informed that NORVIR is not a cure for HIV infection and that they may continue to acquire illnesses associated with advanced HIV infection, including opportunistic infections.

Patients should be told that the long-term effects of NORVIR are unknown at this time. They should be informed that NORVIR therapy has not been shown to reduce the risk of transmitting HIV to others through sexual contact or blood contamination.

Patients should be advised to take NORVIR with food, if possible.

Patients should be informed to take NORVIR every day as prescribed. Patients should not alter the dose or discontinue NORVIR without consulting their doctor. If a dose is missed, patients should take the next dose as soon as possible. However, if a dose is skipped, the patient should not double the next dose.

Since NORVIR interacts with some drugs when taken together, patients should be advised to report to their doctor

Table 2
Effects on AUC and C_{max} of Co-administration of Ritonavir With Other Drugs

Drug	Effect on Ritonavir				
	Ritonavir Dosage	n	AUC % (95 CI)	C_{max} % (95 CI)	
Clarithromycin 500 mg q12h 4 days	200 mg q8h 4 days	22	↑ 12% (2, 23%)	↑ 15% (2, 28%)	
Didanosine 200 mg q12h 4 days	600 mg q12h 4 days	12	↔	↔	
Fluconazole 400 mg day 1, 200 mg daily 4 days	200 mg q6h 4 days	8	↑ 12% (5, 20%)	↑ 15% (7, 22%)	
Fluoxetine 30 mg q12h 8 days	600 mg single dose	16	↑ 19% (7, 34%)	↔	
Rifampin 600 mg or 300 mg daily 10 days[2]	500 mg q12h 20 days	7,9*	↓ 35% (7, 55%)	↓ 25% (-5, 46%)	
Zidovudine 200 mg q8h 4 days	300 mg q6h 4 days	10	↔	↔	

Drug	Effect on Co-administered Drug				
	Ritonavir Dosage	n	AUC % (95 CI)	C_{max} % (95 CI)	
Clarithromycin 500 mg q12h 4 days	200 mg q8h 4 days	22	↑ 77% (56, 103%)	↑ 31% (15, 51%)	
14-OH clarithromycin metabolite			↓ 100%	↓ 99%	
Desipramine 100 mg single dose	500 mg q12h 12 days	14	↑ 145% (103, 211%)	↑ 22% (12, 35%)	
2-OH desipramine metabolite			↑ 15% (3, 26%)	↑ 67% (62, 72%)	
Didanosine 200 mg q12h 4 days	600 mg q12h 4 days	12	↓ 13% (0, 23%)	↓ 16% (5, 26%)	
Ethinyl estradiol 50 μg single dose	500 mg q12h 16 days	23	↓ 40% (31, 49%)	↓ 32% (24, 39%)	
Rifabutin 150 mg daily 16 days	500 mg q12h 10 days	5,11*	↑ 4-fold (2.8, 6.1X)	↑ 2.5-fold (1.9, 3.4X)	
25-O-desacetyl rifabutin metabolite			↑ 35-fold (25, 78X)	↑ 16-fold (14, 20X)	
Sulfamethoxazole 800 mg single dose[1]	500 mg q12h 12 days	15	↓ 20% (16, 23%)	↔	
Theophylline 3 mg/kg q8h 15 days	500 mg q12h 10 days	13,11*	↓ 43% (42, 45%)	↓ 32% (29, 34%)	
Trimethoprim 160 mg single dose[1]	500 mg q12h 12 days	15	↑ 20% (3, 43%)	↔	
Zidovudine 200 mg q8h 4 days	300 mg q6h 4 days	9	↓ 25% (15, 34%)	↓ 27% (4, 45%)	

[1] Sulfamethoxazole and trimethoprim taken as single combination tablet.
[2] Preliminary Data.
↑ Indicates increase.
↓ Indicates decrease.
↔ Indicates no change.
* Parallel group design; entries are subjects receiving combination and control regimens, respectively.

the use of any other medications, including prescription and nonprescription drugs.

Laboratory Tests

Ritonavir has been associated with alterations in triglycerides, SGOT, SGPT, GGT, CPK, and uric acid. Appropriate laboratory testing should be performed prior to initiating NORVIR therapy and at periodic intervals or if any clinical signs or symptoms occur during therapy. For comprehensive information concerning laboratory test alterations associated with nucleoside analogues, physicians should refer to the complete product information for each of these drugs.

Drug Interactions

Agents which increase CYP3A activity (e.g., phenobarbital, carbamazepine, dexamethasone, phenytoin, rifampin, and rifabutin) would be expected to increase the clearance of ritonavir resulting in decreased ritonavir plasma concentrations. Tobacco use is associated with an 18% decrease in the AUC of ritonavir.

Ritonavir can produce large increases in plasma concentrations of certain highly metabolized drugs. Ritonavir has a high affinity for several cytochrome P450 (CYP) isoforms with the following rank order: CYP3A> CYP2D6 > CYP2C9, CYP2C19 > > CYP2A6, CYP1A2, CYP2E1. There is some evidence that ritonavir may increase the activity of glucuronosyl transferases; thus, loss of therapeutic effects from directly glucuronidated agents during ritonavir therapy may signify the need for dosage alteration of these agents. A systematic review of over 200 medications prescribed to HIV-infected patients was performed to identify potential drug interactions with ritonavir. Table 3 summarizes some commonly prescribed drugs, separated by the type of metabolism and expected magnitude of interaction when co-administered with ritonavir. It is advised that concomitant use of any of these agents with ritonavir should be accompanied by therapeutic drug concentration monitoring and/or increased monitoring of therapeutic and adverse effects, especially for agents with narrow therapeutic margins (e.g., oral anticoagulants, immunosuppressants). Large dosage reductions (>50% reduction) may be required for those agents extensively metabolized by CYP3A.

The following list provides information based on studies of the co-administration of ritonavir on the pharmacokinetic properties of several commonly prescribed medications.

Clarithromycin: The mean increase in the AUC of clarithromycin in the presence of ritonavir was 77%. Clarithromycin may be administered without dosage adjustment to patients with normal renal function. However, for patients with renal impairment the following dosage adjustments should be considered. For patients with CL_{CR} 30 to 60 mL/min the dose of clarithromycin should be reduced by 50%. For patients with CL_{CR} < 30 mL/min the dose of clarithromycin should be decreased by 75%.

Desipramine: Co-administration of ritonavir resulted in a 145% mean increase in the AUC of desipramine. Dosage reduction of desipramine should be considered in patients taking the combination.

Disulfiram/Metronidazole: Ritonavir formulations contain alcohol, which can produce reactions when co-administered with disulfiram or other drugs that produce disulfiram-like reactions (e.g., metronidazole).

Oral Contraceptives: The mean AUC of ethinyl estradiol, a component in oral contraceptives, was reduced 40% during concomitant dosing with ritonavir 500 mg q12h; dosage increase or alternate contraceptive measures should be considered.

Saquinavir: Ritonavir extensively inhibits the metabolism of saquinavir resulting in greatly increased saquinavir plasma concentrations. The safety of this combination has not been established.

Theophylline: The average AUC of theophylline was reduced by 43% when co-administered with ritonavir. Increased dosage of theophylline may be required.

[See Table 3 above and on top of next page.]

Carcinogenesis and Mutagenesis

Long-term carcinogenicity studies of ritonavir in animal systems have not been completed. However, ritonavir was not mutagenic or clastogenic in a battery of in vitro and in vivo assays including bacterial reverse mutation (Ames) using S. typhimurium and E. coli, mouse lymphoma, mouse micronucleus, and chromosome aberrations in human lymphocytes.

Pregnancy, Fertility, and Reproduction

Pregnancy Category B: Ritonavir produced no effects on fertility in rats at drug exposures approximately 40% (male) and 60% (female) of that achieved with the proposed therapeutic dose. Higher dosages were not feasible due to hepatic toxicity.

No treatment-related malformations were observed when ritonavir was administered to pregnant rats or rabbits. Developmental toxicity observed in rats (early resorptions, decreased fetal body weight and ossification delays and developmental variations) occurred at a maternally toxic dosage at an exposure equivalent to approximately 30% of that achieved with the proposed therapeutic dose. A slight increase in the incidence of cryptorchidism was also noted in

Table 3
Potential Effects on Drugs Co-administered With Ritonavir

Drug Category	Representative Drugs by Potential Interaction Category				
	Large[1] ↑ AUC[2] (CYP3A)	Moderate[1] ↑ AUC[2] (CYP2D6)	Moderate[1] ↑ or ↓ AUC[2] (CYP2C9/19)	Possible ↑ AUC[2] (unknown CYP)	Possible ↓ AUC[2] (glucuronidation)
Analgesics, narcotic	Alfentanil Fentanyl	Hydrocodone Oxycodone Tramadol		Methadone	Codeine Hydromorphone Morphine
Analgesics, nonsteroidal			Diclofenac Ibuprofen Indomethacin	Nabumetone Sulindac	Ketoprofen Ketorolac Naproxen
Antiarrhythmics	Disopyramide Lidocaine	Mexiletine		Tocainide Digoxin	
Antibiotic, macrolide	Erythromycin				
Anticoagulant	R-warfarin		S-warfarin		
Anticonvulsants	Carbamazepine Clonazepam Ethosuximide		Phenytoin	Phenobarbital	Divalproex Lamotrigine
Antihistamine	Loratadine				
Antidepressants, tricyclic		Amitriptyline Clomipramine Desipramine Imipramine Maprotiline Nortriptyline		Doxepin	
Antidepressants, other	Nefazodone Sertraline Trazodone	Fluoxetine Paroxetine Venlafaxine		Fluvoxamine	
Antidiarrheal					Diphenoxylate
Antiemetics	Dronabinol Ondansetron			Prochlorperazine Promethazine	Metoclopramide
Antifungal agents				Itraconazole Ketoconazole Miconazole	
Antihypertensives			Losartan	Doxazosin Prazosin Terazosin	
Antimycobacterial	Rifampin				
Antiparasitics	Quinine		Proguanil	Albendazole Chloroquine Metronidazole Primaquine Pyrimethamine	Atovaquone
Antiulcer agents			Lansoprazole Omeprazole	Cimetidine	
β-blockers		Metoprolol Pindolol Propranolol Timolol		Acebutolol Betaxolol Penbutolol	
Calcium channel blockers	Amlodipine Diltiazem Felodipine Isradipine Nicardipine Nifedipine Nimodipine Nisoldipine Verapamil				
Cancer chemotherapeutic agents	Etoposide Paclitaxel Tamoxifen Vinblastine Vincristine			Cyclophosphamide Daunorubicin Doxorubicin	
Corticosteroids	Dexamethasone Prednisone				
Hemorrheologic agent				Pentoxifylline	
HIV protease inhibitors	Saquinavir				

Continued on next page

Abbott Laboratories—Cont.

Table 3 (continued)

Hypoglycemics		Glipizide Glyburide Tolbutamide	
Hypolipidemics	Lovastatin Pravastatin	Fluvastatin Gemfibrozil Simvastatin	Clofibrate
Immuno-suppressants	Cyclosporine Tacrolimus		
Neuroleptics		Chlorpromazine Haloperidol Perphenazine Risperidone Thioridazine	
Sedative/hypnotics			Lorazepam Oxazepam Propofol Temazepam
Stimulants		Methamphetamine	Methylphenidate

[1] Large = > 3X; Moderate = 1.5–3X.
[2] AUC = area under the plasma concentration-time curve, a measure of drug exposure.

Table 4
Percentage of Patients with Treatment-Emergent[1] Adverse Events of Moderate or Severe Intensity Occurring in ≥ 2% of Patients Receiving NORVIR

	Study 245 Naive Patients			Study 247 Advanced Patients	
Adverse Events	NORVIR +ZDV n = 116	NORVIR n = 117	ZDV n = 119	NORVIR n = 541	Placebo n = 547
Body as a Whole					
Abdominal Pain	4.3	3.4	4.2	7.0	3.1
Asthenia	27.6	9.4	10.1	14.2	5.3
Fever	1.7	0.9	1.7	4.4	2.2
Headache	7.8	5.1	7.6	6.3	4.0
Malaise	4.3	1.7	3.4	0.7	0.2
Cardiovascular					
Vasodilation	2.6	1.7	0.8	1.3	0.0
Digestive					
Anorexia	7.8	0.9	3.4	6.1	2.0
Constipation	2.6	0.0	0.8	0.0	0.4
Diarrhea	21.6	12.8	0.0	18.3	6.1
Dyspepsia	1.7	0.0	1.7	4.8	0.7
Flatulence	2.6	0.9	0.8	0.9	0.6
Local Throat Irritation	1.7	1.7	0.8	2.6	0.2
Nausea	46.6	23.1	24.4	26.2	5.7
Vomiting	22.4	12.8	12.6	15.2	2.6
Metabolic and Nutritional					
Creatine Phosphokinase Increased	1.7	3.4	3.4	0.9	0.2
Hyperlipidemia	1.7	1.7	0.0	4.1	0.0
Musculoskeletal					
Myalgia	1.7	1.7	0.8	2.2	0.9
Nervous					
Circumoral Paresthesia	5.2	2.6	0.0	5.9	0.2
Dizziness	5.2	2.6	1.7	3.3	1.1
Insomnia	3.4	2.6	0.8	1.3	0.6
Paresthesia	5.2	2.6	0.0	2.0	0.2
Peripheral Paresthesia	0.0	6.0	0.0	5.0	0.7
Somnolence	2.6	2.6	0.0	2.0	0.2
Thinking Abnormal	2.6	0.0	0.8	0.7	0.2
Respiratory					
Pharyngitis	0.9	2.6	0.0	0.4	0.4
Skin and Appendages					
Rash	0.9	0.0	0.8	2.6	0.9
Sweating	3.4	2.6	1.7	1.3	0.6
Special Senses					
Taste Perversion	15.5	10.3	7.6	5.4	1.7

[1] Includes those adverse events at least possibly related to study drug or of unknown relationship and excludes concurrent HIV conditions.

rats at an exposure approximately 22% of that achieved with the proposed therapeutic dose.

Developmental toxicity observed in rabbits (resorptions, decreased litter size and decreased fetal weights) also occurred at a maternally toxic dosage equivalent to 1.8 times the proposed therapeutic dose based on a body surface area conversion factor.

There are, however, no adequate and well-controlled studies in pregnant women. Because animal reproduction studies are not always predictive of human response, this drug should be used during pregnancy only if clearly needed.

Nursing Mothers: It is not known whether this drug is excreted in human milk. Because many drugs are excreted in human milk, caution should be exercised when ritonavir is administered to a nursing woman. However, the U.S. Public Health Service Centers for Disease Control and Prevention advises HIV-infected women not to breast-feed to avoid postnatal transmission of HIV to a child who may not be infected.

Pediatric Use
The safety and effectiveness of ritonavir in children below the age of 12 have not been established.

ADVERSE REACTIONS
The safety of NORVIR alone and in combination with nucleoside analogues was studied in 1140 patients. Table 4 lists treatment-emergent adverse events (at least possibly related and of at least moderate intensity) that occurred in 2% or greater of patients receiving NORVIR alone or in combination with nucleosides in Study 245 or Study 247. At the time of this safety assessment, the median duration of treatment in Study 245 and Study 247 was 3.7 and 2.4 months, respectively. However, safety data was collected on patients for greater than 6 months of treatment. The most frequently reported clinical adverse events, other than asthenia, among patients receiving NORVIR were gastrointestinal and neurological disturbances including nausea, diarrhea, vomiting, anorexia, abdominal pain, taste perversion, and circumoral and peripheral paresthesias. Similar adverse event profiles were reported in patients receiving ritonavir in other trials. [See Table 4 below.]

Adverse events occurring in less than 2% of patients receiving NORVIR in all phase II/phase III studies and considered at least possibly related or of unknown relationship to treatment and of at least moderate intensity are listed below by body system.

Body as a Whole: Abdomen enlarged, accidental injury, allergic reaction, back pain, cachexia, chest pain, chills, facial edema, facial pain, flu syndrome, hormone level altered, hypothermia, kidney pain, neck pain, neck rigidity, pain (unspecified), substernal chest pain, and photosensitivity reaction.

Cardiovascular System: Hemorrhage, hypotension, migraine, palpitation, peripheral vascular disorder, postural hypotension, syncope, and tachycardia.

Digestive System: Abnormal stools, bloody diarrhea, cheilitis, cholangitis, colitis, dry mouth, dysphagia, eructation, esophagitis, gastritis, gastroenteritis, gastrointestinal disorder, gastrointestinal hemorrhage, gingivitis, hepatitis, hepatomegaly, ileitis, liver damage, liver function tests abnormal, mouth ulcer, oral moniliasis, pancreatitis, periodontal abscess, rectal disorder, tenesmus, and thirst.

Endocrine System: Diabetes mellitus.

Hemic and Lymphatic System: Anemia, ecchymosis, leukopenia, lymphadenopathy, lymphocytosis, and thrombocytopenia.

Metabolic and Nutritional Disorders: Avitaminosis, dehydration, edema, glycosuria, gout, hypercholesteremia, peripheral edema, and weight loss.

Musculoskeletal System: Arthralgia, arthrosis, joint disorder, muscle cramps, muscle weakness, myositis, and twitching.

Nervous System: Abnormal dreams, abnormal gait, agitation, amnesia, anxiety, aphasia, ataxia, confusion, convulsion, depression, diplopia, emotional lability, euphoria, grand mal convulsion, hallucinations, hyperesthesia, incoordination, libido decreased, nervousness, neuralgia, neuropathy, paralysis, peripheral neuropathy, peripheral sensory neuropathy, personality disorder, tremor, urinary retention, and vertigo.

Respiratory System: Asthma, dyspnea, epistaxis, hiccup, hypoventilation, increased cough, interstitial pneumonia, lung disorder, and rhinitis.

Skin and Appendages: Acne, contact dermatitis, dry skin, eczema, folliculitis, maculopapular rash, molluscum contagiosum, pruritus, psoriasis, seborrhea, urticaria, and vesiculobullous rash.

Special Senses: Abnormal electro-oculogram, abnormal electroretinogram, abnormal vision, amblyopia/blurred vision, blepharitis, ear pain, eye pain, hearing impairment, increased cerumen, iritis, parosmia, photophobia, taste loss, tinnitus, uveitis, and visual field defect.

Urogenital System: Dysuria, hematuria, impotence, kidney calculus, kidney failure, nocturia, penis disorder, polyuria, pyelonephritis, urethritis, and urinary frequency.

Laboratory Abnormalities
Table 5 shows the percentage of patients who developed marked laboratory abnormalities.
[See Table 5 on top of next page.]

OVERDOSAGE
Acute Overdosage
Human Overdose Experience: Human experience of acute overdose with NORVIR is limited. One patient in clinical trials took NORVIR 1500 mg/day for two days. The patient reported paresthesias which resolved after the dose was decreased.

The approximate lethal dose was found to be greater than 20 times the related human dose in rats and 10 times the related human dose in mice.

Management of Overdosage
Treatment of overdose with NORVIR consists of general supportive measures including monitoring of vital signs and

Table 5
Percentage of Patients, by Study and Treatment Group, with Marked Chemistry and Hematology Laboratory Value Abnormalities

			Study 245 Naive Patients			Study 247 Advanced Patients	
Variable	Limit	NORVIR +ZDV	NORVIR		ZDV	NORVIR	Placebo
CHEMISTRY	HIGH						
Glucose	(>250 mg/dL)	2.0	–		0.9	0.4	1.1
Uric Acid	(>12 mg/dL)	–	–		–	3.6	0.2
Creatinine	(>3.6 mg/dL)	–	–		–	0.2	0.2
Potassium	(>6.0 mEq/L)	–	–		–	0.4	0.2
Chloride	(>122 mEq/L)	–	0.9		–	–	–
Total Bilirubin	(>3.6 mg/dL)	–	–		–	1.2	0.2
Alkaline Phosphatase	(>550 IU/L)	–	0.9		–	1.4	1.7
SGOT (AST)	(>180 IU/L)	2.9	6.5		1.7	3.8	4.3
SGPT (ALT)	(>215 IU/L)	3.9	5.6		2.6	6.1	2.6
GGT	(>300 IU/L)	2.0	2.8		0.9	14.7	6.7
LDH	(>1170 IU/L)	–	–		–	1.0	0.2
Triglycerides	(>1500 mg/dL)	1.0	2.8		–	10.1	0.2
Triglycerides Fasting	(>1500 mg/dL)	2.1	1.4		–	7.9	0.4
CPK	(>1000 IU/L)	7.0	7.5		7.1	8.6	4.5
Amylase	(>2 × ULN[1])	–	0.9		–	0.2	–
CHEMISTRY	LOW						
Albumin	(<2.0 g/dL)	–	–		–	0.2	0.6
Sodium	(<123 mEq/L)	–	–		–	0.2	–
Potassium	(<3.0 mEq/L)	–	0.9		–	2.0	1.1
Chloride	(<84 mEq/L)	–	0.9		–	–	0.4
Magnesium	(<1.0 mEq/L)	–	–		–	0.4	0.4
Calcium	(<6.9 mEq/L)	–	–		–	1.2	0.9
HEMATOLOGY	LOW						
Hemoglobin	(<8.0 g/dL)	–	–		–	2.8	2.4
Hematocrit	(<30%)	2.0	–		–	11.7	16.0
RBC	(<3.0 × 10^{12}/L)	1.0	–		1.7	14.9	19.7
WBC	(<2.5 × 10^9/L)	–	–		3.5	25.1	51.4
Platelet Count	(<20 × 10^9/L)	–	–		–	0.4	0.6
Neutrophils	(≤0.5 × 10^9/L)	–	–		–	4.0	6.9
HEMATOLOGY	HIGH						
WBC	(>25 × 10^9/L)	–	–		–	1.6	0.7
Neutrophils	(>20 × 10^9/L)	–	–		–	1.8	0.9
Eosinophils	(>1.0 × 10^9/L)	–	1.9		0.9	1.8	2.6
Prothrombin Time	(>1.5 × ULN[1])	1.0	–		–	1.0	1.3

[1] ULN = upper limit of the normal range.
– Indicates no events reported.

observation of the clinical status of the patient. There is no specific antidote for overdose with NORVIR. If indicated, elimination of unabsorbed drug should be achieved by emesis or gastric lavage; usual precautions should be observed to maintain the airway. Administration of activated charcoal may also be used to aid in removal of unabsorbed drug. Since ritonavir is extensively metabolized by the liver and is highly protein bound, dialysis is unlikely to be beneficial in significant removal of the drug. A Certified Poison Control Center should be consulted for up-to-date information on the management of overdose with NORVIR.

DOSAGE AND ADMINISTRATION

NORVIR is administered orally. It is recommended that NORVIR be taken with meals if possible. Patients may improve the taste of NORVIR oral solution by mixing with chocolate milk, Ensure®, or Advera® within one hour of dosing. The effects of antacids on the absorption of ritonavir have not been studied.

The recommended dosage of ritonavir is 600 mg twice daily by mouth. Some patients experience nausea upon initiation of 600 mg b.i.d. dosing; dose escalation may provide some relief: 300 mg b.i.d. for 1 day, 400 mg b.i.d. for 2 days, 500 mg b.i.d. for 1 day, and then 600 mg b.i.d. thereafter. In addition, patients initiating combination regimens with NORVIR and nucleosides may improve gastrointestinal tolerance by initiating NORVIR alone and subsequently adding nucleosides before completing two weeks of NORVIR monotherapy.

HOW SUPPLIED

NORVIR (ritonavir capsules) are white capsules imprinted with the corporate logo   , 100 mg, and the Abbo-Code PI. NORVIR is available as 100 mg capsules in the following package size:
Packages of 2 bottles
of 84 capsules each .... (NDC 0074-9492-02).

Recommended storage: Store capsules in the refrigerator between 36–46°F (2–8°C). Protect from light.
NORVIR (ritonavir oral solution) is an orange-colored liquid, supplied in amber-colored, multi-dose bottles containing 600 mg ritonavir per 7.5 mL marked dosage cup (80 mg/mL) in the following size:
240 mL bottles .... (NDC 0074-1940-63).
Recommended storage: Store NORVIR oral solution in the refrigerator between 36–46°F (2–8°C) until it is dispensed. Refrigeration of NORVIR oral solution by the patient is recommended, but not required if used within 30 days and

stored below 77°F (25°C). Product should be stored in the original container. Avoid exposure to excessive heat. Keep cap tightly closed.
Revised: May, 1996
TM - Trademark
Caution—Federal (U.S.A.) Law prohibits dispensing without prescription.
Ref. 03-4680-R2
Abbott Laboratories
North Chicago, IL 60064
Shown in Product Identification Guide, page 303

ORETIC®   ℞
[ō-re'tic]
(hydrochlorothiazide tablets, USP)

DESCRIPTION

ORETIC (hydrochlorothiazide) is a member of the benzothiadiazine (thiazide) family of drugs. It is closely related to chlorothiazide. The structural formula for hydrochlorothiazide may be represented as follows:

Clinically, hydrochlorothiazide is an orally active diuretic-antihypertensive agent.
Inactive Ingredients:
25 and 50 mg tablets: corn starch, lactose, magnesium stearate and talc.

ACTIONS

The diuretic and saluretic effects of hydrochlorothiazide result from a drug-induced inhibition of the renal tubular reabsorption of electrolytes. The excretion of sodium and chloride is greatly enhanced. Potassium excretion is also enhanced to a variable degree, as it is with the other thiazides. Although urinary excretion of bicarbonate is increased slightly, there is usually no significant change in urinary pH. Hydrochlorothiazide has a per mg natriuretic activity approximately 10 times that of the prototype thiazide, chlorothiazide. At maximal therapeutic dosages, all thiazides are approximately equal in their diuretic/natriuretic effects.

There is significant natriuresis and diuresis within two hours after administration of a single oral dose of hydrochlorothiazide. These effects reach a peak in about 6 hours and persist for about 12 hours following oral administration of a single dose.

Like other benzothiadiazines, hydrochlorothiazide also has antihypertensive properties, and may be used for this purpose either alone or to enhance the antihypertensive action of other drugs. The mechanism by which the benzothiadiazines, including hydrochlorothiazide, produce a reduction of elevated blood pressure is not known. However, sodium depletion appears to be involved.

Hydrochlorothiazide is readily absorbed from the gastrointestinal tract and is excreted unchanged by the kidneys.

INDICATIONS

ORETIC (hydrochlorothiazide) is indicated in the management of hypertension either as the sole therapeutic agent or to enhance the effect of other antihypertensive drugs in the more severe forms of hypertension.

ORETIC tablets are indicated as adjunctive therapy in edema associated with congestive heart failure, hepatic cirrhosis, and corticosteroid and estrogen therapy.

ORETIC tablets have also been found useful in edema due to various forms of renal dysfunction such as the nephrotic syndrome, acute glomerulonephritis, and chronic renal failure.

Usage in Pregnancy: The routine use of diuretics in an otherwise healthy pregnant woman is inappropriate and exposes mother and fetus to unnecessary hazard. Diuretics do not prevent development of toxemia of pregnancy, and there is no satisfactory evidence that they are useful in the treatment of developed toxemia.

Edema during pregnancy may arise from pathological causes or from the physiological and mechanical consequences of pregnancy. Thiazides are indicated in pregnancy when edema is due to pathological causes, just as they are in the absence of pregnancy (see WARNINGS). Dependent edema in pregnancy, resulting from restriction of venous return by the expanded uterus, is properly treated through elevation of the lower extremities and use of support hose; use of diuretics to lower intravascular volume in this case is illogical and unnecessary. There is hypervolemia during normal pregnancy which is harmful to neither the fetus nor the mother (in the absence of cardiovascular disease), but which is associated with edema, including generalized edema, in the majority of pregnant women. If this edema produces discomfort, increased recumbency will often provide relief. In rare instances, this edema may cause extreme discomfort which is not relieved by rest. In these cases, a short course of diuretics may provide relief and may be appropriate.

CONTRAINDICATIONS

Renal decompensation.
Hypersensitivity to this or other sulfonamide-derived drugs.

WARNINGS

Hydrochlorothiazide shares with other thiazides the propensity to deplete potassium reserves to an unpredictable degree.

Thiazides should be used with caution in patients with renal disease or significant impairment of renal function, since azotemia may be precipitated and cumulative drug effects may occur.

Thiazides should be used with caution in patients with impaired hepatic function or progressive liver disease, since minor alterations of fluid and electrolyte balance may precipitate hepatic coma.

Thiazides may be additive or potentiative of the action of other antihypertensive drugs. Potentiation occurs with ganglionic or peripheral adrenergic blocking drugs.

Sensitivity reactions may occur in patients with history of allergy or bronchial asthma.

The possibility of exacerbation or activation of systemic lupus erythematosus has been reported.

Usage in Pregnancy: Thiazides cross the placental barrier and appear in cord blood. The use of thiazides in pregnant women requires that the anticipated benefit be weighed against possible hazards to the fetus. These hazards include fetal or neonatal jaundice, thrombocytopenia, and possible other adverse reactions that have occurred in the adult.

Nursing Mothers: Thiazides appear in breast milk. If use of the drug is deemed essential, the patient should stop nursing.

PRECAUTIONS

Periodic determinations of serum electrolytes should be performed at appropriate intervals for the purpose of detecting possible electrolyte imbalances such as hyponatremia, hypochloremic alkalosis, and hypokalemia. Serum and urine electrolyte determinations are particularly important when a patient is vomiting excessively or receiving parenteral flu-

Continued on next page

Abbott Laboratories—Cont.

ids. All patients should be observed for other clinical signs of electrolyte imbalances such as dryness of mouth, thirst, weakness, lethargy, drowsiness, restlessness, muscle pains or cramps, muscular fatigue, hypotension, oliguria, tachycardia, and gastrointestinal disturbances such as nausea and vomiting.

Hypokalemia may develop with thiazides as with any other potent diuretic, especially when brisk diuresis occurs, severe cirrhosis is present, or when corticosteroids or ACTH are given concomitantly. Interference with the adequate oral intake of electrolytes will also contribute to the possible development of hypokalemia. Potassium depletion, even of a mild degree, resulting from thiazide use, may sensitize a patient to the effects of cardiac glycosides such as digitalis.

Any chloride deficit is generally mild and usually does not require specific treatment except under extraordinary circumstances (as in liver disease or renal disease). Dilutional hyponatremia may occur in edematous patients in hot weather; appropriate therapy is water restriction rather than administration of salt, except in rare instances when the hyponatremia is life threatening.

In actual salt depletion, appropriate replacement is the therapy of choice.

Hyperuricemia may occur or frank gout may be precipitated in certain patients receiving thiazide therapy.

Insulin requirements in diabetic patients may be increased, decreased, or unchanged. Latent diabetes mellitus may become manifest during thiazide administration.

Thiazide drugs may increase the responsiveness to tubocurarine.

The antihypertensive effects of the drug may be enhanced in the postsympathectomy patient.

Thiazides may decrease arterial responsiveness to norepinephrine. This diminution is not sufficient to preclude effectiveness of the pressor agent for therapeutic use.

If progressive renal impairment becomes evident as indicated by a rising-nonprotein nitrogen or blood urea nitrogen, a careful reappraisal of therapy is necessary with consideration given to withholding or discontinuing diuretic therapy.

Thiazides may decrease serum protein bound iodine levels without signs of thyroid disturbance.

Thiazides have been reported, on rare occasions, to have elevated serum calcium to hypercalcemic levels. The serum calcium levels have returned to normal when the medication has been stopped. This phenomenon may be related to the ability of the thiazide diuretics to lower the amount of calcium excreted in the urine.

ADVERSE REACTIONS

Gastrointestinal system reactions: Anorexia, gastric irritation, nausea, vomiting, cramping, diarrhea, constipation, jaundice (intrahepatic cholestatic jaundice), pancreatitis.

Central nervous system reactions: Dizziness, vertigo, paresthesias, headache, xanthopsia.

Hematologic reactions: Leukopenia, agranulocytosis, thrombocytopenia, aplastic anemia.

Dermatologic — hypersensitivity reactions: Purpura, photosensitivity, rash, urticaria, necrotizing angiitis (vasculitis) (cutaneous vasculitis).

Cardiovascular reaction: Orthostatic hypotension may occur and may be aggravated by alcohol, barbiturates, or narcotics.

Other: Hyperglycemia, glycosuria, hypercalcemia, hyperuricemia, muscle spasm, weakness, restlessness, respiratory distress including pneumonitis and pulmonary edema.

There have been isolated reports that certain nonedematous individuals developed severe fluid and electrolyte derangements after only brief exposure to normal doses of thiazide and non-thiazide diuretics. The condition is usually manifested as severe dilutional hyponatremia, hypokalemia, and hypochloremia. It has been reported to be due to inappropriately increased ADH secretion and appears to be idiosyncratic. Potassium replacement is apparently the most important therapy in the treatment of this syndrome along with removal of the offending drug.

Whenever adverse reactions are severe, treatment should be discontinued.

DOSAGE AND ADMINISTRATION

ORETIC (hydrochlorothiazide) is administered orally. Therapy should be individualized according to patient response. This therapy should be titrated to gain maximal therapeutic response as well as the minimal dose possible to maintain that therapeutic response.

For the management of edema the adult dosage ranges from 25 to 200 mg daily and may be given in single or divided doses. Usually 75 to 100 mg will produce the desired diuretic effect.

For the management of hypertension the usual initial adult dosage is 25 to 50 mg two times daily. The dosage may be increased if necessary to a maximum of 100 mg twice daily.

When therapy is prolonged or large doses are used, particular attention should be given to the patient's electrolyte status. Supplemental potassium may be required.

In the treatment of hypertension hydrochlorothiazide may be either employed alone or concurrently with other antihypertensive drugs. Combined therapy may provide adequate control of hypertension with lower dosage of the component drugs and fewer or less severe side effects. An enhanced response frequently follows its concurrent administration with Harmonyl® (deserpidine) so that dosage of both drugs may be reduced.

For treatment of moderately severe or severe hypertension, supplemental use of other more potent antihypertensive agents may be indicated.

When other antihypertensive agents are to be added to the regimen, this should be accomplished gradually. Additional potent antihypertensive agents should be given at only half the usual dose since their effect is potentiated by pretreatment with ORETIC.

OVERDOSAGE

Symptoms of overdosage include electrolyte imbalance and signs of potassium deficiency such as confusion, dizziness, muscular weakness, and gastrointestinal disturbances. General supportive measures including replacement of fluids and electrolytes may be indicated in treatment of overdosage.

HOW SUPPLIED

ORETIC (hydrochlorothiazide tablets, USP) is provided in two dosage sizes as white tablets:

25 mg tablets:
bottles of 100 (**NDC** 0074-6978-01),
bottles of 1000 (**NDC** 0074-6978-02),
Abbo-Pac® unit dose packages, 100 tablets (**NDC** 0074-6978-05).

50 mg tablets:
bottles of 100 (**NDC** 0074-6985-01),
bottles of 1000 (**NDC** 0074-6985-02),
Abbo-Pac®unit dose packages, 100 tablets (**NDC** 0074-6985-06).

Recommended Storage: Store below 86°F (30°C).

Ref. 01-2527-R7

PANHEMATIN® ℞

[*pan-hē'ma-tin*]

(HEMIN FOR INJECTION)

For I.V. Use Only

> PANHEMATIN (hemin for injection) should only be used by physicians experienced in the management of porphyrias in hospitals where the recommended clinical and laboratory diagnostic and monitoring techniques are available.
>
> PANHEMATIN therapy should be considered after an appropriate period of alternate therapy (i.e., 400 g glucose/day for 1 to 2 days). (See "WARNINGS", "PRECAUTIONS" and "DOSAGE AND ADMINISTRATION" sections.)

DESCRIPTION

PANHEMATIN (hemin for injection) is an enzyme inhibitor derived from processed red blood cells. Hemin for injection was known previously as hematin. The term hematin has been used to describe the chemical reaction product of hemin and sodium carbonate solution. Hemin is an iron containing metalloporphyrin. Chemically hemin is represented as chloro [7,12-diethenyl-3,8,13,17-tetramethyl-21H,23H-porphine-2,18-dipropanoato (2-)-N^{21},N^{22}, N^{23}, N^{24}] iron. The structural formula for hemin is:

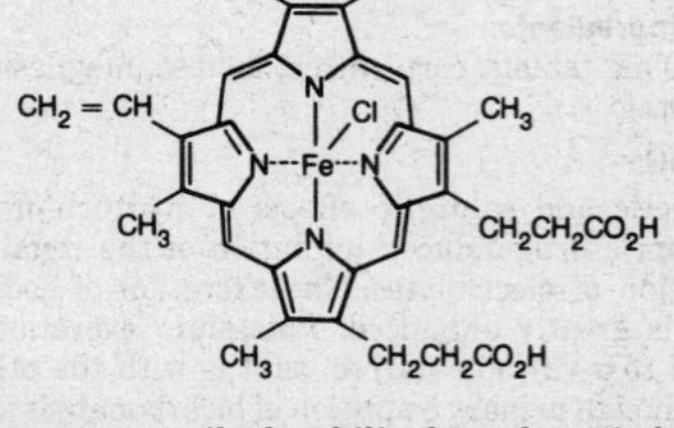

PANHEMATIN is a sterile, lyophilized powder suitable for intravenous administration after reconstitution. Each dispensing vial of PANHEMATIN contains the equivalent of 313 mg hemin, 215 mg sodium carbonate and 300 mg of sorbitol. The pH may have been adjusted with hydrochloric acid; the product contains no preservatives. When mixed as directed with Sterile Water for Injection, USP, each 43 mL provides the equivalent of approximately 301 mg hematin (7 mg/mL).

CLINICAL PHARMACOLOGY

Heme acts to limit the hepatic and/or marrow synthesis of porphyrin. This action is likely due to the inhibition of δ-aminolevulinic acid synthetase, the enzyme which limits the rate of the porphyrin/heme biosynthetic pathway. The exact mechanism by which hematin produces symptomatic improvement in patients with acute episodes of the hepatic porphyrias has not been elucidated.[1,9]

Following intravenous administration of hematin in non-jaundiced human patients, an increase in fecal urobilinogen can be observed which is roughly proportional to the amount of hematin administered. This suggests an enterohepatic pathway as at least one route of elimination. Bilirubin metabolites are also excreted in the urine following hematin injections.[2]

PANHEMATIN (hemin for injection) therapy for the acute porphyrias is not curative. After discontinuation of PANHEMATIN treatment, symptoms generally return although in some cases remission is prolonged. Some neurological symptoms have improved weeks to months after therapy although little or no response was noted at the time of treatment.

Other aspects of human pharmacokinetics have not been defined.

INDICATIONS AND USAGE

PANHEMATIN (hemin for injection) is indicated for the amelioration of recurrent attacks of acute intermittent porphyria temporally related to the menstrual cycle in susceptible women.

Manifestations such as pain, hypertension, tachycardia, abnormal mental status and mild to progressive neurologic signs may be controlled in selected patients with this disorder.

Similar findings have been reported in other patients with acute intermittent porphyria, porphyria variegata and hereditary coproporphyria. PANHEMATIN is not indicated in porphyria cutanea tarda.

CONTRAINDICATIONS

Hemin for injection is contraindicated in patients with known hypersensitivity to this drug.

WARNINGS

PANHEMATIN (hemin for injection) therapy is intended to limit the rate of porphyria/heme biosynthesis possibly by inhibiting the enzyme δ-aminolevulinic acid synthetase. For this reason, drugs such as estrogens, barbituric acid derivatives and steroid metabolites which increase the activity of δ-aminolevulinic acid synthetase should be avoided.

Also, because PANHEMATIN has exhibited transient, mild anticoagulant effects during clinical studies, concurrent anticoagulant therapy should be avoided.[9] The extent and duration of the hypocoagulable state induced by PANHEMATIN has not been established.

PRECAUTIONS

General: Clinical benefit from PANHEMATIN depends on prompt administration. Attacks of porphyria may progress to a point where irreversible neuronal damage has occurred. PANHEMATIN therapy is intended to prevent an attack from reaching the critical stage of neuronal degeneration. PANHEMATIN is not effective in repairing neuronal damage.[9]

Recommended dosage guidelines should be strictly followed. Reversible renal shutdown has been observed in a case where an excessive hematin dose (12.2 mg/kg) was administered in a single infusion. Oliguria and increased nitrogen retention occurred although the patient remained asymptomatic.[4] No worsening of renal function has been seen with administration of recommended dosages of hematin.[9]

A large arm vein or a central venous catheter should be utilized for the administration of hemin for injection to avoid the possibility of phlebitis.

Since reconstituted PANHEMATIN is not transparent, any undissolved particulate matter is difficult to see when inspected visually. Therefore, terminal filtration through a sterile 0.45 micron or smaller filter is recommended.

Tests for Diagnosis and Monitoring of Therapy: Before PANHEMATIN therapy is begun, the presence of acute porphyria must be diagnosed using the following criteria:[9]

a. Presence of clinical symptoms.

b. Positive Watson-Schwartz or Hoesch test. (A negative Watson-Schwartz or Hoesch test indicates a porphyric attack is highly unlikely. When in doubt quantitative measures of δ-aminolevulinic acid and porphobilinogen in serum or urine may aid in diagnosis.)

Urinary concentrations of the following compounds may be *monitored* during PANHEMATIN therapy. Drug effect will be

demonstrated by a decrease in one or more of the following compounds:[3–6]

ALA-δ-aminolevulinic acid
UPG-uroporphyrinogen
PBG-porphobilinogen
coproporphyrin

Carcinogenesis, Mutagenesis, Impairment of Fertility: No data are available on potential for carcinogenicity, mutagenicity or impairment of fertility in animals or humans.

Pregnancy: Teratogenic effects: Pregnancy Category C. Animal reproduction studies have not been conducted with hematin. It is also not known whether hematin can cause fetal harm when administered to a pregnant woman or can affect reproduction capacity. For this reason hemin for injection should not be given to a pregnant woman unless the expected benefits are sufficiently important to the health and welfare of the patient to outweigh the unknown hazard to the fetus.

Nursing Mothers: It is not known whether this drug is excreted in human milk. Because many drugs are excreted in human milk, caution should be exercised when hemin for injection is administered to a nursing woman.

Pediatric Use: Safety and effectiveness in children have not been established.

ADVERSE REACTIONS

Reversible renal shutdown has occurred with administration of excessive doses (See "PRECAUTIONS" section).

Phlebitis with or without leucocytosis and with or without mild pyrexia has occurred after administration of hematin through small arm veins.

There has been one report in the literature[8] of coagulopathy occurring in a patient receiving hematin therapy. This patient exhibited prolonged prothrombin time and partial thromboplastin time, thrombocytopenia, mild hypofibrinogenemia, mild elevation of fibrin split products and a 10% fall in hematocrit.

OVERDOSAGE

Reversible renal shutdown has been observed in a case where an excessive hematin dose (12.2 mg/kg) was administered in a single infusion. Treatment of this case consisted of ethacrynic acid and mannitol.[7]

DOSAGE AND ADMINISTRATION

Before administering hemin for injection, an appropriate period of alternate therapy (i.e., 400 g glucose/day for 1 to 2 days) must be considered. If improvement is unsatisfactory for the treatment of acute attacks of porphyria, an intravenous infusion of PANHEMATIN containing a dose of 1 to 4 mg/kg/day of hematin should be given over a period of 10 to 15 minutes for 3 to 14 days based on the clinical signs. In more severe cases this dose may be repeated no earlier than every 12 hours. No more than 6 mg/kg of hematin should be given in any 24-hour period.

After reconstitution each mL of PANHEMATIN contains the equivalent of approximately 7 mg of hematin. The drug may be administered directly from the vial.

Dosage Calculation Table

1 mg hematin equivalent	= 0.14 mL PANHEMATIN
2 mg hematin equivalent	= 0.28 mL PANHEMATIN
3 mg hematin equivalent	= 0.42 mL PANHEMATIN
4 mg hematin equivalent	= 0.56 mL PANHEMATIN

Since reconstituted PANHEMATIN is not transparent, any undissolved particulate matter is difficult to see when inspected visually. Therefore, terminal filtration through a sterile 0.45 micron or smaller filter is recommended.

Preparation of Solution: Reconstitute PANHEMATIN by aseptically adding 43 mL of Sterile Water for Injection, USP, to the dispensing vial. Immediately after adding diluent, the product should be shaken well for a period of 2 to 3 minutes to aid dissolution. **NOTE: Because PANHEMATIN contains no preservative and because PANHEMATIN undergoes rapid chemical decomposition in solution, it should not be reconstituted until immediately before use. After the first withdrawal from the vial, any solution remaining must be discarded.**

No drug or chemical agent should be added to a PANHEMATIN fluid admixture unless its effect on the chemical and physical stability has first been determined.

HOW SUPPLIED

PANHEMATIN (hemin for injection) is supplied as a sterile, lyophilized black powder in single dose dispensing vials (**NDC** 0074-2000-43). When mixed as directed with Sterile Water for Injection, USP, each 43 mL provides the equivalent of approximately 301 mg hematin (7 mg/mL). Store lyophilized powder in refrigerator (2–8°C) until time of use.

REFERENCES

1. Bickers, D., Treatment of the Porphyrias: Mechanisms of Action, *J Invest Dermatol* 77(1):107–113, 1981.
2. Watson, C. J., Hematin and Porphyria, editorial, *N Engl J Med* 293(12):605–607, September 18, 1975.
3. Lamon, J. M., Hematin Therapy for Acute Porphyria, *Medicine* 58(3):252–269, 1979.
4. Dhar, G. J., et al., Effects of Hematin in Hepatic Porphyria, *Ann Intern Med* 83:20–30, 1975.
5. Watson, C. J., et al., Use of Hematin in the Acute Attack of the "Inducible" Hepatic Porphyrias, *Adv Intern Med* 23:265–286, 1978.
6. McColl, K. E., et al., Treatment with Haematin in Acute Hepatic Porphyria, *Q J Med*, New Series L (198):161–174, Spring, 1981.
7. Dhar, G. J., et al., Transitory Renal Failure Following Rapid Administration of a Relatively Large Amount of Hematin in a Patient with Acute Intermittent Porphyria in Clinical Remission, *Acta Med Scand* 203:437–443, 1978.
8. Morris, D. L., et al., Coagulopathy Associated with Hematin Treatment for Acute Intermittent Porphyria, *Ann Intern Med* 95:700–701, 1981.
9. Pierach, C. A., Hematin Therapy for the Porphyric Attack, *Semin Liver Dis* 2(2):125–131, May, 1982.

Ref. 01-2388-R4

PCE® ℞
(erythromycin particles in tablets)
Dispertab® Tablets

DESCRIPTION

PCE (erythromycin particles in tablets) is an antibacterial product containing specially coated erythromycin base particles for oral administration. The coating protects the antibiotic from the inactivating effects of gastric acidity and permits efficient absorption of the antibiotic in the small intestine. PCE is available in two strengths containing either 333 mg or 500 mg of erythromycin base. PCE 500 mg tablets contain no synthetic dyes or artificial colors.

Inactive Ingredients:

PCE 333 mg tablets: Cellulosic polymers, citrate ester, colloidal silicon dioxide, D&C Red No. 30, hydrogenated vegetable oil wax, lactose, magnesium stearate, microcrystalline cellulose, povidone, propylene glycol, sodium starch glycolate, stearic acid and vanillin.

PCE 500 mg tablets: Cellulosic polymers, citrate ester, colloidal silicon dioxide, crospovidone, hydrogenated vegetable oil wax, iron oxide, microcrystalline cellulose, polyethylene glycol, povidone, propylene glycol, stearic acid, talc, titanium dioxide and vanillin.

Erythromycin is produced by a strain of *Saccaropolyspora erythraea* (formerly *Streptomyces erythraeus*) and belongs to the macrolide group of antibiotics. It is basic and readily forms salts with acids. Erythromycin is a white to off-white powder, slightly soluble in water, and soluble in alcohol, chloroform, and ether. Erythromycin is known chemically as (3R*, 4S*, 5S*, 6R*, 7R*, 9R*, 11R*, 12R*, 13S*, 14R*)-4-[(2,6-Dideoxy-3-C-methyl-3-O-methyl-α-L-*ribo*-hexopyranosyl)oxy] -14- ethyl-7,12,13-trihydroxy-3,5,7,9,11, 13-hexamethyl-6 [[3,4,6-trideoxy -3- (dimethyl-amino)-β-D-*xylo*-hexopyranosyl]oxy]oxacyclotetradecane-2,10-dione.

The structural formula is:

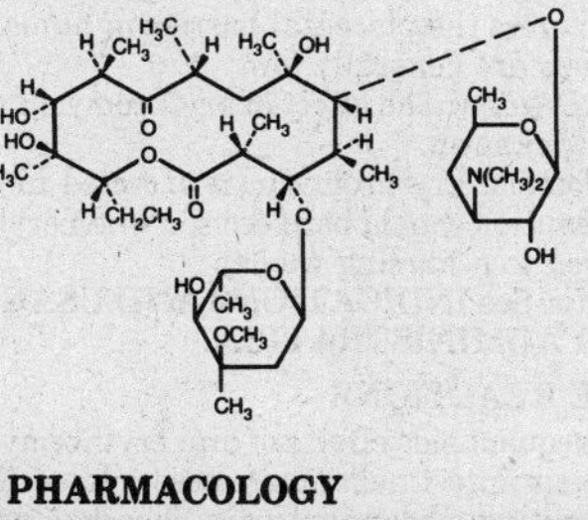

CLINICAL PHARMACOLOGY

Orally administered erythromycin base and its salts are readily absorbed in the microbiologically active form. Interindividual variations in the absorption of erythromycin are, however, observed, and some patients do not achieve optimal serum levels. Erythromycin is largely bound to plasma proteins. After absorption, erythromycin diffuses readily into most body fluids. In the absence of meningeal inflammation, low concentrations are normally achieved in the spinal fluid but the passage of the drug across the blood-brain barrier increases in meningitis. Erythromycin crosses the placental barrier and is excreted in breast milk. Erythromycin is not removed by peritoneal dialysis or hemodialysis.

In the presence of normal hepatic function, erythromycin is concentrated in the liver and is excreted in the bile; the effect of hepatic dysfunction on biliary excretion of erythromycin is not known. After oral administration, less than 5% of the administered dose can be recovered in the active form in the urine.

The erythromycin particles in PCE tablets are coated with a polymer whose dissolution is pH dependent. This coating allows for minimal release of erythromycin in acidic environments, e.g. stomach. This delivery system is designed for optimal drug release and absorption in the small intestine. In multiple-dose, steady-state studies, PCE tablets have demonstrated rapid and generally adequate drug delivery in both fasting and nonfasting conditions. However, the presence of food results in lower blood levels, and optimal blood levels are obtained when PCE tablets are given in the fasting state (at least 1/2 hour and preferably 2 hours before meals). Bioavailability data are available from Abbott Laboratories, Dept. 355.

Microbiology:

Erythromycin acts by inhibition of protein synthesis by binding 50 S ribosomal subunits of susceptible organisms. It does not affect nucleic acid synthesis. Antagonism has been demonstrated *in vitro* between erythromycin and clindamycin, lincomycin, and chloramphenicol.

Many strains of *Haemophilus influenzae* are resistant to erythromycin alone, but are susceptible to erythromycin and sulfonamides together.

Staphylococci resistant to erythromycin may emerge during a course of erythromycin therapy. Culture and susceptibility testing should be performed.

Erythromycin is usually active against the following organisms *in vitro* (prior to use, refer to INDICATIONS AND USAGE):

Gram-positive Bacteria: Staphylococcus aureus (resistant organisms may emerge during treatment),*Streptococcus pyogenes* (Group A beta-hemolytic *streptococci*), Alpha-hemolytic *streptococci* (viridans group), *Streptococcus (diplococcus) pneumoniae, Corynebacterium diphtheriae, Corynebacterium minutissimum.*

Gram-negative Bacteria: Moraxella (Branhamella) catarrhalis, Neisseria gonorrhoeae, Legionella pneumophila, Bordetella pertussis.

Mycoplasma: Mycoplasma pneumoniae, Ureaplasma urealyticum.

Other Microorganisms: Chlamydia trachomatis, Entamoeba histolytica, Treponema pallidum, Listeria monocytogenes.

Susceptibility Testing:

Quantitative methods that require measurement of zone diameters give the most precise estimates of antibiotic susceptibility. One such standardized single-disc procedure has been recommended for use with discs to test susceptibility to erythromycin.[1] Interpretation involves correlation of the zone diameters obtained in the disc test with minimal inhibitory concentration (MIC) values for erythromycin.

Reports from the laboratory giving results of the standardized single-disc susceptibility test using a 15 mcg erythromycin disc should be interpreted according to the following criteria:

Susceptible organisms produce zones of 18 mm or greater, indicating that the tested organism is likely to respond to therapy.

Resistant organisms produce zones of 13 mm or less, indicating that other therapy should be selected.

Organisms of intermediate susceptibility produce zones of 14 to 17 mm. The "intermediate" category provides a "buffer zone" which should prevent small, uncontrolled technical factors from causing major discrepancies in interpretations; thus, when a zone diameter falls within the "intermediate" range, the results may be considered equivocal. If alternative drugs are not available, confirmation by dilution tests may be indicated.

Standardized procedures require the use of control organisms. The 15 mcg erythromycin disc should give zone diameters between 22 and 30 mm for the *S. aureus* ATCC 25923 control strain.

A bacterial isolate may be considered susceptible if the MIC value[2] for erythromycin is not more than 2 mcg/mL. Organisms are considered resistant if the MIC is 8 mcg/mL or higher. The MIC of erythromycin for *S. aureus* ATCC 29213 control strain should be between 0.12 and 0.5 mcg/mL.

INDICATIONS AND USAGE

PCE tablets are indicated in the treatment of infections caused by susceptible strains of the designated microorganisms in the diseases listed below:

Upper respiratory tract infections of mild to moderate degree caused by *Streptococcus pyogenes* (Group A beta-hemolytic *streptococci*); *Streptococcus pneumoniae (Diplococcus pneumoniae); Haemophilus influenzae* (when used concomitantly with adequate doses of sulfonamides, since many strains of *H. influenzae* are not susceptible to the erythromycin concentrations ordinarily achieved). (See appropriate sulfonamide labeling for prescribing information.)

Lower respiratory tract infections of mild to moderate severity caused by *Streptococcus pyogenes* (Group A beta-hemolytic *streptococci*); *Streptococcus pneumoniae (Diplococcus pneumoniae).*

Respiratory tract infections due to *Mycoplasma pneumoniae.*

Skin and skin structure infections of mild to moderate severity caused by *Streptococcus pyogenes* and *Staphylococcus aureus* (resistant staphylococci may emerge during treatment).

Pertussis (whooping cough) caused by *Bordetella pertussis.* Erythromycin is effective in eliminating the organism from the nasopharynx of infected individuals, rendering them noninfectious. Some clinical studies suggest that erythromycin may be helpful in the prophylaxis of pertussis in exposed susceptible individuals.

Continued on next page

Abbott Laboratories—Cont.

Diphtheria—As an adjunct to antitoxin in infections due to *Corynebacterium diphtheriae* to prevent establishment of carriers and to eradicate the organism in carriers.
Erythrasma—In the treatment of infections due to *Corynebacterium minutissimum.*
Intestinal amebiasis caused by *Entamoeba histolytica* (oral erythromycins only). Extraenteric amebiasis requires treatment with other agents.
Acute pelvic inflammatory disease caused by *Neisseria gonorrhoeae:* Erythrocin® Lactobionate-I.V. (erythromycin lactobionate for injection, USP) followed by erythromycin base orally, as an alternative drug in treatment of acute pelvic inflammatory disease caused by *N. gonorrhoeae* in female patients with a history of sensitivity to penicillin. Before treatment of gonorrhea, patients who are suspected of also having syphilis should have a microscopic examination for *T. pallidum* (by immunofluorescence or darkfield) before receiving erythromycin and monthly serologic tests for a minimum of 4 months thereafter.
Erythromycins are indicated for treatment of the following infections caused by *Chlamydia trachomatis*: conjunctivitis of the newborn, pneumonia of infancy, and urogenital infections during pregnancy. When tetracyclines are contraindicated or not tolerated, erythromycin is indicated for the treatment of uncomplicated urethral, endocervical, or rectal infections in adults due to *Chlamydia trachomatis.*[3]
When tetracyclines are contraindicated or not tolerated, erythromycin is indicated for the treatment of nongonococcal urethritis caused by *Ureaplasma urealyticum.*[3]
Primary syphilis caused by *Treponema pallidum.* Erythromycin (oral forms only) is an alternative choice of treatment for primary syphilis in patients allergic to the penicillins. In treatment of primary syphilis, spinal fluid should be examined before treatment and as part of the follow-up after therapy.
Legionnaires' Disease caused by *Legionella pneumophila.* Although no controlled clinical efficacy studies have been conducted, *in vitro* and limited preliminary clinical data suggest that erythromycin may be effective in treating Legionnaires' Disease.
Prevention of Initial Attacks of Rheumatic Fever—Penicillin is considered by the American Heart Association to be the drug of choice in the prevention of initial attacks of rheumatic fever (treatment of Group A beta-hemolytic streptococcal infections of the upper respiratory tract e.g., tonsillitis, or pharyngitis).[4] Erythromycin is indicated for the treatment of penicillin-allergic patients. The therapeutic dose should be administered for ten days.
Prevention of Recurrent Attacks of Rheumatic Fever—Penicillin or sulfonamides are considered by the American Heart Association to be the drugs of choice in the prevention of recurrent attacks of rheumatic fever. In patients who are allergic to penicillin and sulfonamides, oral erythromycin is recommended by the American Heart Association in the long-term prophylaxis of streptococcal pharyngitis (for the prevention of recurrent attacks of rheumatic fever).[4]
Prevention of Bacterial Endocarditis—Although no controlled clinical efficacy trials have been conducted, oral erythromycin has been recommended by the American Heart Association for prevention of bacterial endocarditis in penicillin-allergic patients with most congenital cardiac malformations, rheumatic or other acquired valvular dysfunction, idiopathic hypertrophic subaortic stenosis (IHSS), previous history of bacterial endocarditis and mitral valve prolapse with insufficiency when they undergo dental procedures and surgical procedures of the upper respiratory tract.[5]

CONTRAINDICATIONS

Erythromycin is contraindicated in patients with known hypersensitivity to this antibiotic.
Erythromycin is contraindicated in patients taking terfenadine. (See **PRECAUTIONS**-*Drug Interactions.*)

WARNINGS

There have been reports of hepatic dysfunction with or without jaundice, occurring in patients receiving oral erythromycin products.
Rhabdomyolysis with or without renal impairment has been reported in seriously ill patients receiving erythromycin concomitantly with lovastatin. Therefore, patients receiving concomitant lovastatin and erythromycin should be monitored for creatinine kinase (CK) and serum transaminase levels. (See package insert for lovastatin.)

PRECAUTIONS

General: Erythromycin is principally excreted by the liver. Caution should be exercised when erythromycin is administered to patients with impaired hepatic function. (See **CLINICAL PHARMACOLOGY** and **WARNINGS.**)
Prolonged or repeated use of erythromycin may result in an overgrowth of nonsusceptible bacteria or fungi. If superinfection occurs, erythromycin should be discontinued and appropriate therapy instituted.
When indicated, incision and drainage or other surgical procedures should be performed in conjunction with antibiotic therapy.
Laboratory Tests: Erythromycin interferes with the fluorometric determination of urinary catecholamines.
Drug Interactions: Erythromycin use in patients who are receiving high doses of theophylline may be associated with an increase in serum theophylline levels and potential theophylline toxicity. In case of theophylline toxicity and/or elevated serum theophylline levels, the dose of theophylline should be reduced while the patient is receiving concomitant erythromycin therapy.
Concomitant administration of erythromycin and digoxin has been reported to result in elevated digoxin serum levels.
There have been reports of increased anticoagulant effects when erythromycin and oral anticoagulants were used concomitantly. Increased anticoagulation effects due to interactions of erythromycin with oral anticoagulants may be more pronounced in the elderly.
Concurrent use of erythromycin and ergotamine or dihydroergotamine has been associated in some patients with acute ergot toxicity characterized by severe peripheral vasospasm and dysesthesia.
Erythromycin has been reported to decrease the clearance of triazolam and midazolam and, thus, may increase the pharmacologic effect of these benzodiazepines.
The use of erythromycin in patients concurrently taking drugs metabolized by the cytochrome P450 system may be associated with elevations in serum levels of these drugs. There have been reports of interactions of erythromycin with carbamazepine, cyclosporine, hexobarbital, phenytoin, alfentanil, diisopyramide, lovastatin, and bromocriptine. Serum concentrations of drugs metabolized by the cytochrome P450 system should be monitored closely in patients concurrently receiving erythromycin.
Erythromycin significantly alters the metabolism of terfenadine when taken concomitantly. Rare cases of serious cardiovascular adverse events, including death, cardiac arrest, torsades de pointes, and other ventricular arrhythmias, have been observed. (See **CONTRAINDICATIONS.**)
Carcinogenesis, Mutagenesis, Impairment of Fertility: Long-term (2-year) oral studies conducted in rats with erythromycin base did not provide evidence of tumorigenicity. Mutagenicity studies have not been conducted. There was no apparent effect on male or female fertility in rats fed erythromycin (base) at levels up to 0.25 percent of diet.
Pregnancy: Pregnancy Category B: There is no evidence of teratogenicity or any other adverse effect on reproduction in female rats fed erythromycin base (up to 0.25 percent of diet) prior to and during mating, during gestation, and through weaning of two successive litters. There are, however, no adequate and well-controlled studies in pregnant women. Because animal reproduction studies are not always predictive of human response, this drug should be used during pregnancy only if clearly needed. Erythromycin has been reported to cross the placental barrier in humans, but fetal plasma levels are generally low.
Labor and Delivery: The effect of erythromycin on labor and delivery is unknown.
Nursing Mothers: Erythromycin is excreted in breast milk, therefore, caution should be exercised when erythromycin is administered to a nursing woman.
Pediatric Use: See **INDICATIONS AND USAGE** and **DOSAGE AND ADMINISTRATION.**

ADVERSE REACTIONS

The most frequent side effects of oral erythromycin preparations are gastrointestinal and are dose-related. They include nausea, vomiting, abdominal pain, diarrhea and anorexia. Symptoms of hepatic dysfunction and/or abnormal liver function test results may occur. (See **WARNINGS.**) Pseudomembranous colitis has been rarely reported in association with erythromycin therapy.
Rarely, erythromycin has been associated with the production of ventricular arrhythmias, including ventricular tachycardia and torsades de pointes, in individuals with prolonged QT interval.
Allergic reactions ranging from urticaria to anaphylaxis have occurred. Skin reactions ranging from mild eruptions to erythema multiforme, Stevens-Johnson syndrome, and toxic epidermal necrolysis have been reported rarely.
There have been isolated reports of reversible hearing loss occurring chiefly in patients with renal insufficiency and in patients receiving high doses of erythromycin.

OVERDOSAGE

In case of overdosage, erythromycin should be discontinued. Overdosage should be handled with the prompt elimination of unabsorbed drug and all other appropriate measures.
Erythromycin is not removed by peritoneal dialysis or hemodialysis.

DOSAGE AND ADMINISTRATION

In most patients, PCE tablets are well absorbed and may be dosed orally without regard to meals. However, optimal blood levels are obtained when either PCE 333 mg or PCE 500 mg tablets are given in the fasting state (at least 1/2 hour and preferably 2 hours before meals).
Adults: The usual dosage of PCE is one 333 mg tablet every 8 hours or one 500 mg tablet every 12 hours. Dosage may be increased up to 4 g per day according to the severity of the infection. However, twice-a-day dosing is not recommended when doses larger than 1 g daily are administered.
Children: Age, weight, and severity of the infection are important factors in determining the proper dosage. The usual dosage is 30 to 50 mg/kg/day, in equally divided doses. For more severe infections this dosage may be doubled but should not exceed 4 g per day.
In the treatment of Group A beta-hemolytic streptococcal infections of the upper respiratory tract (e.g., tonsillitis or pharyngitis), the therapeutic dosage of erythromycin should be administered for ten days. The American Heart Association suggests a dosage of 250 mg of erythromycin orally, twice a day in long-term prophylaxis of streptococcal upper respiratory tract infections for the prevention of recurring attacks of rheumatic fever in patients allergic to penicillin and sulfonamides.[4]
In prophylaxis against bacterial endocarditis (See **INDICATIONS AND USAGE**) the oral regimen for penicillin allergic patients is erythromycin 1 gram, 1 hour before the procedure followed by 500 mg six hours later.[5]
Conjunctivitis of the newborn caused by *Chlamydia trachomatis:*
Oral erythromycin suspension 50 mg/kg/day in 4 divided doses for at least 2 weeks.[3]
Pneumonia of infancy caused by *Chlamydia trachomatis:* Although the optimal duration of therapy has not been established, the recommended therapy is oral erythromycin suspension 50 mg/kg/day in 4 divided doses for at least 3 weeks.[3]
Urogenital infections during pregnancy due to *Chlamydia trachomatis:* Although the optimal dose and duration of therapy have not been established, the suggested treatment is 500 mg of erythromycin by mouth four times a day or two erythromycin 333 mg tablets orally every 8 hours on an empty stomach for at least 7 days. For women who cannot tolerate this regimen, a decreased dose of one erythromycin 500 mg tablet orally every 12 hours, one 333 mg tablet orally every 8 hours or 250 mg by mouth four times a day should be used for at least 14 days.[3,6]
For adults with uncomplicated urethral, endocervical, or rectal infections caused by *Chlamydia trachomatis,* when tetracycline is contraindicated or not tolerated: 500 mg of erythromycin by mouth four times a day or two 333 mg tablets orally every 8 hours for at least 7 days.[3,6]
For patients with nongonococcal urethritis caused by *Ureaplasma urealyticum* when tetracycline is contraindicated or not tolerated: 500 mg of erythromycin by mouth four times a day or two 333 mg tablets orally every 8 hours for at least 7 days.[3,6]
Primary syphilis: 30 to 40 g given in divided doses over a period of 10 to 15 days.
Acute pelvic inflammatory disease caused by N. *gonorrhoeae:* 500 mg Erythrocin Lactobionate-I.V. (erythromycin lactobionate for injection, USP) every 6 hours for 3 days, followed by 500 mg of erythromycin base orally every 12 hours, or 333 mg of erythromycin base orally every 8 hours for 7 days.
Intestinal amebiasis: Adults: 500 mg every 12 hours, 333 mg every 8 hours or 250 mg every 6 hours for 10 to 14 days. Children: 30 to 50 mg/kg/day in divided doses for 10 to 14 days.
Pertussis: Although optimal dosage and duration have not been established, doses of erythromycin utilized in reported clinical studies were 40 to 50 mg/kg/day, given in divided doses for 5 to 14 days.
Legionnaires' Disease: Although optimal dosage has not been established, doses utilized in reported clinical data were 1 to 4 g daily in divided doses.

HOW SUPPLIED

PCE (erythromycin particles in tablets) is supplied as unscored, ovaloid, Dispertab® tablets in the following strengths and packages.
333 mg, pink-speckled white (imprinted with ⓐ and PCE):
Bottles of 60 ....(**NDC** 0074-6290-60);
500 mg, white (imprinted with ⓐ and EK):
Bottles of 100 ....(**NDC** 0074-3389-13).
Recommended Storage: Store below 86°F (30°C).

REFERENCES

1. National Committee for Clinical Laboratory Standards, Approved Standard: *Performance Standards for Antimicrobial Disk Susceptibility Tests,* 3rd Edition, Vol. 4(16):M2-A3, Villanova, PA, December 1984.
2. Ericson, H.M., Sherris, J.C., Antibiotic Sensitivity Testing: Report of an International Collaborative Study, *Acta Pathologica et Microbiologica Scandinavica* Section B Suppl. 217:1-90, 1971.
3. CDC Sexually Transmitted Diseases Treatment Guidelines 1985.
4. Committee on Rheumatic Fever and Infective Endocarditis of the Council on Cardiovascular Disease of the Young:

Prevention of Rheumatic Fever, *Circulation* 70(6):1118A-1122A, December 1984.
5. Committee on Rheumatic Fever and Infective Endocarditis of the Council on Cardiovascular Disease of the Young: Prevention of Bacterial Endocarditis, *Circulation* 70(6):1123A-1127A, December 1984.
6. Data on file, Abbott Laboratories.

Revised: May, 1994
PCE 333 mg: U.S. Pat. No. 4,874,614.
PCE 500 mg: U.S. Pat. No. 4,874,614 and 5,009,897.
Ref. 03-4494-R5-Rev. May, 1994
Abbott Laboratories
North Chicago, IL 60064

Shown in Product Identification Guide, page 303

PEGANONE® ℞

[*pĕg'ă-noon*]
ETHOTOIN TABLETS, USP

DESCRIPTION

PEGANONE (ethotoin tablets, USP) is an oral antiepileptic of the hydantoin series and is chemically identified as 3-ethyl-5-phenyl-2, 4-imidazolidinedione. It is represented by the following structural formula:

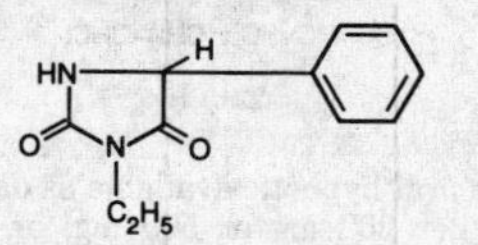

PEGANONE tablets are available in two dosage strengths of 250 mg and 500 mg respectively.

Inactive Ingredients: 250 mg and 500 mg tablets: Acacia, lactose, sodium carboxymethylcellulose, stearic acid and talc.

CLINICAL PHARMACOLOGY

PEGANONE (ethotoin tablets, USP) exerts an antiepileptic effect without causing general central nervous system depression. The mechanism of action is probably very similar to that of phenytoin. The latter drug appears to stabilize rather than to raise the normal seizure threshold, and to prevent the spread of seizure activity rather than to abolish the primary focus of seizure discharges.

In laboratory animals, the drug was found effective against electroshock convulsions, and to a lesser extent, against complex partial (psychomotor) and pentylenetetrazol-induced seizures.

In mice, the duration of antiepileptic activity was prolonged by hepatic injury but not by bilateral nephrectomy; the drug is apparently biotransformed by the liver.

Ethotoin is fairly rapidly absorbed; the extent of oral absorption is not known. The drug exhibits saturable metabolism with respect to the formation of N-deethyl and p-hydroxyl-ethotoin, the major metabolites. Where plasma concentrations are below about 8 mcg/mL, the elimination half-life of ethotoin is in the range of 3 to 9 hours. A study comparing single doses of 500 mg, 1000 mg, and 1500 mg of PEGANONE (ethotoin tablets, USP) demonstrated that ethotoin, and to a lesser extent 5-phenylhydantoin, a major metabolite, exhibits substantial nonlinear kinetics. The degree of nonlinearity with multiple dosing may be increased over that seen after a single dose, given the likelihood of plasma accumulation based on a reported elimination half-life of 6 to 9 hours and a dosing interval of 4 to 6 hours. Experience suggests that therapeutic plasma concentrations fall in the range of 15 to 50 mcg/mL; however, this range is not as extensively documented as those quoted for other antiepileptics.

INDICATIONS AND USAGE

PEGANONE (ethotoin tablets, USP) is indicated for the control of tonic-clonic (grand mal) and complex partial (psychomotor) seizures.

CONTRAINDICATIONS

PEGANONE (ethotoin tablets, USP) is contraindicated in patients with hepatic abnormalities or hematologic disorders.

WARNINGS

USAGE DURING PREGNANCY— THERE ARE MULTIPLE REPORTS IN THE CLINICAL LITERATURE WHICH INDICATE THAT THE USE OF ANTIEPILEPTIC DRUGS DURING PREGNANCY RESULTS IN AN INCREASED INCIDENCE OF BIRTH DEFECTS IN THE OFFSPRING. ALTHOUGH DATA ARE MORE EXTENSIVE WITH RESPECT TO TRIMETHADIONE, PARAMETHADIONE, PHENYTOIN, AND PHENOBARBITAL, REPORTS INDICATE A POSSIBLE SIMILAR ASSOCIATION WITH THE USE OF OTHER ANTIEPILEPTIC DRUGS. THEREFORE, ANTIEPILEPTIC DRUGS SHOULD BE ADMINISTERED TO WOMEN OF CHILDBEARING POTENTIAL ONLY IF THEY ARE CLEARLY SHOWN TO BE ESSENTIAL IN THE MANAGEMENT OF THEIR SEIZURES.

ANTIEPILEPTIC DRUGS SHOULD NOT BE DISCONTINUED IN PATIENTS IN WHOM THE DRUG IS ADMINISTERED TO PREVENT MAJOR SEIZURES BECAUSE OF THE STRONG POSSIBILITY OF PRECIPITATING STATUS EPILEPTICUS WITH ATTENDANT HYPOXIA AND RISK TO BOTH MOTHER AND THE UNBORN CHILD. CONSIDERATION SHOULD, HOWEVER, BE GIVEN TO DISCONTINUATION OF ANTIEPILEPTICS PRIOR TO AND DURING PREGNANCY WHEN THE NATURE, FREQUENCY AND SEVERITY OF THE SEIZURES DO NOT POSE A SERIOUS THREAT TO THE PATIENT. IT IS NOT, HOWEVER, KNOWN WHETHER EVEN MINOR SEIZURES CONSTITUTE SOME RISK TO THE DEVELOPING EMBRYO OR FETUS.

REPORTS HAVE SUGGESTED THAT THE MATERNAL INGESTION OF ANTIEPILEPTIC DRUGS, PARTICULARLY BARBITURATES, IS ASSOCIATED WITH A NEONATAL COAGULATION DEFECT THAT MAY CAUSE BLEEDING DURING THE EARLY (USUALLY WITHIN 24 HOURS OF BIRTH) NEONATAL PERIOD. THE POSSIBILITY OF THE OCCURRENCE OF THIS DEFECT WITH THE USE OF PEGANONE SHOULD BE KEPT IN MIND. THE DEFECT IS CHARACTERIZED BY DECREASED LEVELS OF VITAMIN K-DEPENDENT CLOTTING FACTORS, AND PROLONGATION OF EITHER THE PROTHROMBIN TIME OR THE PARTIAL THROMBOPLASTIN TIME, OR BOTH. IT HAS BEEN SUGGESTED THAT VITAMIN K BE GIVEN PROPHYLACTICALLY TO THE MOTHER ONE MONTH PRIOR TO AND DURING DELIVERY, AND TO THE INFANT, INTRAVENOUSLY, IMMEDIATELY AFTER BIRTH.

THE PHYSICIAN SHOULD WEIGH THESE CONSIDERATIONS IN TREATMENT AND COUNSELING OF EPILEPTIC WOMEN OF CHILDBEARING POTENTIAL.

PRECAUTIONS

General: Blood dyscrasias have been reported in patients receiving PEGANONE. Although the etiologic role of PEGANONE has not been definitely established, physicians should be alert for general malaise, sore throat and other symptoms indicative of possible blood dyscrasia.

There is some evidence suggesting that hydantoin-like compounds may interfere with folic acid metabolism, precipitating a megaloblastic anemia. If this should occur during gestation, folic acid therapy should be considered.

Information for Patients: Patients should be advised to report immediately such signs and symptoms as sore throat, fever, malaise, easy bruising, petechiae, epistaxis, or others that may be indicative of an infection or bleeding tendency.

Laboratory Tests: Liver function tests should be performed if clinical evidence suggests the possibility of hepatic dysfunction. Signs of liver damage are indication for withdrawal of the drug.

It is recommended that blood counts and urinalyses be performed when therapy is begun and at monthly intervals for several months thereafter. As in patients receiving other hydantoin compounds and other antiepileptic drugs, blood dyscrasias have been reported in patients receiving PEGANONE (ethotoin tablets, USP). Marked depression of the blood count is indication for withdrawal of the drug.

Drug Interactions: PEGANONE used in combination with other drugs known to adversely affect the hematopoietic system should be avoided if possible.

Considerable caution should be exercised if PEGANONE is administered concurrently with *Phenurone (phenacemide)* since paranoid symptoms have been reported during therapy with this combination.

A two-way interaction between the hydantoin antiepileptic, *phenytoin,* and the *coumarin anticoagulants* has been suggested. Presumably, phenytoin acts as a stimulator of coumarin metabolism and has been reported to cause decreased serum levels of the coumarin anticoagulants and increased prothrombin-proconvertin concentrations. Conversely, the coumarin anticoagulants have been reported to increase the serum levels and prolong the serum half-life of phenytoin by inhibiting its metabolism. Although there is no documentation of such, a similar interaction between ethotoin and the coumarin anticoagulants may occur. Caution is therefore advised when administering PEGANONE to patients receiving coumarin anticoagulants.

Carcinogenesis: No data are available on long-term potential for carcinogenicity in animals or humans.

Pregnancy: Pregnancy Category C. See "Warnings" section.

Nursing Mothers: Ethotoin is excreted in breast milk. Because of the potential for serious adverse reactions in nursing infants from ethotoin, a decision should be made whether to discontinue nursing or to discontinue the drug, taking into account the importance of the drug to the mother.

ADVERSE REACTIONS

Adverse reactions associated with PEGANONE, in decreasing order of severity, are:

Isolated cases of lymphadenopathy and systemic lupus erythematosus have been reported in patients taking hydantoin compounds, and lymphadenopathy has occurred with PEGANONE. Withdrawal of therapy has resulted in remission of the clinical and pathological findings. Therefore, if a lymphoma-like syndrome develops, the drug should be withdrawn and the patient should be closely observed for regression of signs and symptoms before treatment is resumed.

Ataxia and gum hypertrophy have occurred only rarely—usually only in patients receiving an additional hydantoin derivative. It is of interest to note that ataxia and gum hypertrophy have subsided in patients receiving other hydantoins when PEGANONE (ethotoin tablets, USP) was given as a substitute antiepileptic.

Occasionally, vomiting or nausea after ingestion of PEGANONE has been reported, but if the drug is administered after meals, the incidence of gastric distress is reduced. Other side effects have included chest pain, nystagmus, diplopia, fever, dizziness, diarrhea, headache, insomnia, fatigue, numbness and skin rash.

OVERDOSAGE

Symptoms of acute overdosage include drowsiness, visual disturbance, nausea and ataxia. Coma is possible at very high dosage.

Treatment should be begun by inducing emesis; gastric lavage may be considered as an alternative. General supportive measures will be necessary. A careful evaluation of blood-forming organs should be made following recovery.

DOSAGE AND ADMINISTRATION

PEGANONE (ethotoin tablets, USP) is administered orally in 4 to 6 divided doses daily. The drug should be taken after food, and doses should be spaced as evenly as practicable. Initial dosage should be conservative. For adults, the initial daily dose should be 1 g or less, with subsequent gradual dosage increases over a period of several days. The optimum dosage must be determined on the basis of individual response. The usual adult maintenance dose is 2 to 3 g daily. Less than 2 g daily has been found ineffective in most adults.

Pediatric dosage depends upon the age and weight of the patient. The initial dose should not exceed 750 mg daily. The usual maintenance dose in children ranges from 500 mg to 1 g daily, although occasionally 2 or (rarely) 3 g daily may be necessary.

If a patient is receiving another antiepileptic drug, it should not be discontinued when PEGANONE therapy is begun. The dosage of the other drug should be reduced gradually as that of PEGANONE is increased. PEGANONE may eventually replace the other drug or the optimal dosage of both antiepileptics may be established.

PEGANONE is compatible with all commonly employed antiepileptic medications with the possible exception of Phenurone® (phenacemide). In tonic-clonic (grand mal) seizures, use of the drug with phenobarbital may be beneficial. PEGANONE may be used in combination with drugs such as Tridione® (trimethadione) or Paradione® (paramethadione), as an adjunct in those patients with absence (petit mal) associated with tonic-clonic (grand mal).

HOW SUPPLIED

PEGANONE (ethotoin tablets, USP) grooved, white tablets are supplied in two dosage strengths: 250 mg, bottles of 100 (**NDC** 0074-6902-01); 500 mg, bottles of 100 (**NDC** 0074-6905-04).
Recommended Storage: Store below 77°F (25°C).
Ref. 01-2537-R9

PHENURONE® ℞

[*fĕn'ū-rōne*]
(PHENACEMIDE TABLETS, USP)

DESCRIPTION

PHENURONE (phenacemide) is a valuable antiepileptic drug for use in selected patients with epilepsy. Since therapy with PHENURONE involves certain risks, *physicians should thoroughly familiarize themselves with the undesirable side effects which may occur and the precautions to be observed.*

PHENURONE (phenacemide) is a substituted acetylurea derivative. Chemically PHENURONE is identified as N-(aminocarbonyl)-benzeneacetamide. The chemical structure may be represented as follows:

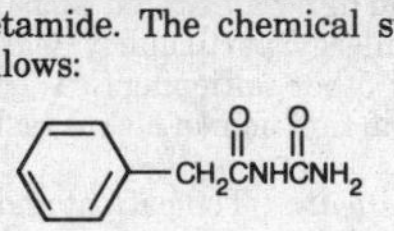

PHENURONE tablets contain 500 mg phenacemide for oral administration.

Inactive Ingredients: Corn starch, lactose and talc.

CLINICAL PHARMACOLOGY

In experimental animals, PHENURONE in doses well below those causing neurological signs, elevates the threshold for minimal electroshock convulsions and abolishes the tonic phase of maximal electroshock seizures. The drug prevents or modifies seizures induced by pentylenetetrazol or other convulsants. In comparative tests, PHENURONE was found to

Continued on next page

Abbott Laboratories—Cont.

be equal or more effective than other commonly used antiepileptics against complex partial (psychomotor) seizures which were induced in mice by low frequency stimulation of the cerebral cortex. Studies in mice have shown that Phenurone exerts a synergistic antiepileptic effect with mephenytoin, phenobarbital, or trimethadione.
Given orally to laboratory animals, Phenurone has a low acute toxicity. In mice, slight ataxia appears at 400 mg/kg and light sleep occurs at 800 mg/kg. In high doses the drug causes marked ataxia and coma, the fatal dose being in the range of 3 to 5 g/kg for mice, rats, and cats.
Phenurone is metabolized by the liver, however, further definition of human pharmacokinetics has not been determined.

INDICATIONS AND USAGE

Phenurone (phenacemide) is indicated for the control of severe epilepsy, particularly mixed forms of complex partial (psychomotor) seizures, refractory to other drugs.

CONTRAINDICATIONS

Phenurone should not be administered unless other available antiepileptics have been found to be ineffective in satisfactorily controlling seizures.

WARNINGS

Phenurone (phenacemide) can produce serious side effects as well as direct organ toxicity. As a consequence its use entails the assumption of certain risks which must be weighed against the benefit to the patient. *Ordinarily Phenurone should not be administered unless other available antiepileptics have been found to be ineffective in controlling seizures.*
Death attributable to liver damage during therapy with Phenurone has been reported. Phenurone should be used with caution in patients with a history of previous liver dysfunction. If jaundice or other signs of hepatitis appear, the drug should be discontinued.
Aplastic anemia has occurred in association with Phenurone therapy, and death from this condition has been reported. Phenurone should ordinarily not be used in patients with severe blood dyscrasias. Marked depression of the blood count is an indication for withdrawal of the drug.
Usage During Pregnancy: Phenurone can cause fetal harm when administered to a pregnant woman. There are multiple reports in the clinical literature which indicate that the use of antiepileptic drugs during pregnancy results in an increased incidence of birth defects in the offspring. Reports have also suggested that the maternal ingestion of antiepileptic drugs, particularly barbiturates, is associated with a neonatal coagulation defect that may cause bleeding during the early (usually within 24 hours of birth) neonatal period. The possibility of the occurrence of this defect with the use of Phenurone should be kept in mind. The defect is characterized by decreased levels of vitamin K-dependent clotting factors, and prolongation of either the prothrombin time or the partial thromboplastin time, or both. It has been suggested that vitamin K be given prophylactically to the mother one month prior to and during delivery, and to the infant, intravenously, immediately after birth. If this drug is used during pregnancy, or if the patient becomes pregnant while taking this drug, the patient should be apprised of the potential hazard to the fetus.

PRECAUTIONS

General: Extreme caution must be exercised in treating patients who previously have shown personality disorders. It may be advisable to hospitalize such patients during the first week of treatment. Personality changes, including attempts at suicide and the occurrence of psychoses requiring hospitalization, have been reported during therapy with Phenurone (phenacemide). Severe or exacerbated personality changes are an indication for withdrawal of the drug.
Phenurone (phenacemide) should be used with caution in patients with a history of previous liver dysfunction.
Phenurone should be administered with caution to patients with a history of allergy, particularly in association with the administration of other antiepileptics. The drug should be discontinued at the first sign of a skin rash or other allergic manifestation.
Information for Patients: The patient and his family should be aware of the possibility of personality changes so the family can watch for changes in the behavior of the patient such as decreased interest in surroundings, depression, or aggressiveness.
The patient should be told to report immediately any symptoms indicative of a developing blood dyscrasia such as malaise, sore throat, or fever.
Laboratory Tests: Liver function tests should be performed before and during therapy. Death attributable to liver damage during therapy with Phenurone has been reported. If jaundice or other signs of hepatitis appear, the drug should be discontinued.
Complete blood counts should be made before instituting Phenurone, and at monthly intervals thereafter. If no abnormality appears within 12 months, the interval between blood counts may be extended. Blood changes have been reported with leukopenia (leukocyte count of 4,000 or less per cubic millimeter of blood) as the most commonly observed effect. However, aplastic anemia has occurred in association with Phenurone therapy, and death from this condition has been reported. *The total number of each cellular element per cubic millimeter is a better index of possible blood dyscrasia than the percentage of cells.* Marked depression of the blood count is an indication for withdrawal of the drug.
Similarly, as nephritis has occasionally occurred in patients on Phenurone, the urine should be examined at regular intervals. Abnormal urinary findings are an indication for discontinuance of therapy.
Drug Interactions: Extreme caution is essential if Phenurone is administered with any other antiepileptic which is known to cause similar toxic effects.
Considerable caution should be exercised if Phenurone (phenacemide) is administered concurrently with *Peganone (ethotoin)* since paranoid symptoms have been reported during therapy with this combination.
Carcinogenesis: No data are available on long-term potential for carcinogenicity in animals or humans.
Pregnancy: Pregnancy Category D. See "Warnings" section.
Nursing Mothers: It is not known whether this drug is excreted in human milk. Because many drugs are excreted in human milk and because of the potential for serious adverse reactions in nursing infants from Phenurone, a decision should be made whether to discontinue nursing or to discontinue the drug, taking into account the importance of the drug to the mother.
Pediatric Use: Safety and effectiveness in children below the age of 5 years have not been established.

ADVERSE REACTIONS

The following adverse effects associated with Phenurone are listed by decreasing order of frequency based on data from one large clinical study[1].
Psychiatric: Psychic changes (17 in 100 patients).
Gastrointestinal: Gastrointestinal disturbances (8 in 100 patients), including anorexia (5 in 100 patients) and weight loss (less than 1 in 100 patients).
Dermatologic: Skin rash (5 in 100 patients). Stevens-Johnson Syndrome with epidermal necrolysis has been reported in one non-fatal case.
CNS: Drowsiness (4 in 100 patients), headache (2 in 100 patients), insomnia (1 in 100 patients), dizziness and paresthesias (less than 1 in 100 patients).
Hematopoietic: Blood dyscrasias (primarily leukopenia), including fatal aplastic anemia (2 in 100 patients).
Hepatic: Hepatitis, including fatalities (2 in 100 patients).
Renal: Abnormal urinary findings, including a rise in serum creatinine[2], and nephritis (1 in 100 patients or less).
Other: Fatigue, fever, muscle pain and palpitation (less than 1 in 100 patients).

OVERDOSAGE

Symptoms of acute overdosage include excitement or mania, followed by drowsiness, ataxia and coma. In one case of acute overdosage, dizziness was followed by coma which lasted nearly 24 hours. Treatment should be started by inducing emesis; gastric lavage may be considered as an alternative or adjunct. General supportive measures will be necessary. A careful evaluation of liver and kidney function, mental state, and the blood-forming organs should be made following recovery.

DOSAGE AND ADMINISTRATION

Phenurone (phenacemide) is administered orally.
Since Phenurone may produce serious toxic effects, it is strongly recommended that the dosage be held to the minimum amount necessary to achieve an adequate therapeutic effect.
For adults the usual starting dose is 1.5 g daily, administered in three divided doses of 500 mg each. After the first week, if seizures are not controlled and the drug is well tolerated, an additional 500 mg tablet may be taken upon arising. In the third week, if necessary, the dosage may be further increased by another 500 mg at bedtime. Satisfactory results have been noted in some patients on an initial dose of 250 mg three times per day. The effective total daily dose for adults usually ranges from 2 to 3 g, although some patients have required as much as 5 g daily.
For the pediatric patient from 5 to 10 years of age, approximately one-half the adult dose is recommended. It should be given at the same intervals as for adults.
Phenurone may be administered alone or in conjunction with other antiepileptics. However, extreme caution must be exercised if other antiepileptics cause toxic effects similar to Phenurone.
When Phenurone is to replace other antiepileptic medication, the latter should be withdrawn gradually as the dosage of Phenurone is increased to maintain seizure control.

HOW SUPPLIED

Phenurone (Phenacemide Tablets, USP), grooved, white, 500 mg tablets are supplied in bottles of 100 (**NDC** 0074-3971-05).

REFERENCES

1. Tyler, M. W., King, E. Q.: Phenacemide in Treatment of Epilepsy. *JAMA* 147: 17–21 (1951).
2. Richards, R.K., Bjornsson, T. D., Waterbury, L. D.: Rise in Serum and Urine Creatinine After Phenacemide. Clin. Pharmacol. Ther. 23: 430–437 (1978).

Ref. 03-4550-R11

PLACIDYL® ℞ Ⓒ

ETHCHLORVYNOL CAPSULES, USP
Oral hypnotic

DESCRIPTION

Placidyl (ethchlorvynol) is a tertiary carbinol. It is chemically designated as 1-chloro-3-ethyl-1-penten-4-yl-3-ol. Ethchlorvynol occurs as a liquid which is immiscible with water and miscible with most organic solvents. It has the following structural formula:

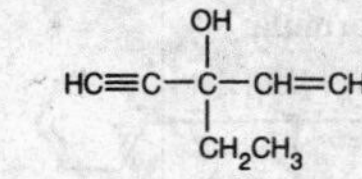
OH
HC≡C—C—CH=CHCl
CH_2CH_3

Placidyl is an oral hypnotic available as dark red capsules containing either 200 mg or 500 mg, or green capsules containing 750 mg of ethchlorvynol.
Each capsule contains the following inactive ingredients: gelatin, glycerin, iron oxide, methylparaben, polyethylene glycol, propylparaben, sorbitol and titanium dioxide. The 200 mg and 500 mg capsules also contain FD&C Red No. 40. The 750 mg capsule also contains FD&C Blue No. 1, FD&C Yellow No. 5 (tartrazine) and FD&C Yellow No. 6.

> **WARNING:** Manufactured with carbon tetrachloride, a substance which harms public health and environment by destroying ozone in the upper atmosphere.

CLINICAL PHARMACOLOGY

The usual hypnotic dose of Placidyl induces sleep within 15 minutes to one hour. The duration of the hypnotic effect is about five hours. The mechanism of action is unknown.
Placidyl is rapidly absorbed from the gastrointestinal tract with peak plasma concentrations usually occurring within two hours after a single oral fasting dose. Plasma concentrations required for hypnotic effects are unknown. The plasma half-life ($t_{1/2}$, β) of the parent compound is approximately ten to twenty hours. Studies with ^{14}C-Placidyl have demonstrated that within 24 hours, 33% of a single 500 mg dose is excreted in the urine mostly as metabolites. The major plasma and urinary metabolite is the secondary alcohol of Placidyl. The free and conjugated forms of this metabolite in the urine account for about 40% of the dose. Other minor metabolites have been identified as the primary alcohol and a secondary alcohol with an altered acetylene group. Studies with ^{14}C-Placidyl in animals indicate that the parent compound and its metabolites undergo extensive enterohepatic recirculation.
Distribution studies indicate that there is extensive tissue localization of ethchlorvynol, particularly in adipose tissue. Ethchlorvynol and/or its metabolites have also been detected in liver, kidneys, spleen, brain, bile and cerebrospinal fluid.

INDICATIONS AND USAGE

Placidyl is indicated as short-term hypnotic therapy for periods up to one week in duration for the management of insomnia. If retreatment becomes necessary, after drug-free intervals of one or more weeks, it should only be undertaken upon further evaluation of the patient.

CONTRAINDICATIONS

Placidyl is contraindicated in patients with known hypersensitivity to the drug and in patients with porphyria.

WARNINGS

PLACIDYL SHOULD BE ADMINISTERED WITH CAUTION TO MENTALLY DEPRESSED PATIENTS WITH OR WITHOUT SUICIDAL TENDENCIES. IT SHOULD ALSO BE ADMINISTERED WITH CAUTION TO THOSE WHO HAVE A PSYCHOLOGICAL POTENTIAL FOR DRUG DEPENDENCE. THE LEAST AMOUNT OF DRUG THAT IS FEASIBLE SHOULD BE PRESCRIBED FOR THESE PATIENTS.

Psychological and Physical Dependence

PROLONGED USE OF PLACIDYL MAY RESULT IN TOLERANCE AND PSYCHOLOGICAL AND PHYSICAL DEPENDENCE. PROLONGED ADMINISTRATION OF THE

DRUG IS NOT RECOMMENDED. (See "Drug Abuse and Dependence" section.)

PRECAUTIONS

General: Elderly or debilitated patients should receive the smallest effective amount of PLACIDYL (ethchlorvynol).

Caution should be exercised when treating patients with impaired hepatic or renal function.

Patients who exhibit unpredictable behavior, or paradoxical restlessness or excitement in response to barbiturates or alcohol may react in this manner to PLACIDYL.

PLACIDYL should not be used for the management of insomnia in the presence of pain unless insomnia persists after pain is controlled with analgesics.

The 750 mg dosage strength of PLACIDYL contains FD&C Yellow No. 5 (tartrazine) which may cause allergic-type reactions (including bronchial asthma) in certain susceptible individuals. Although the overall incidence of FD&C Yellow No. 5 (tartrazine) sensitivity in the general population is low, it is frequently seen in patients who also have aspirin hypersensitivity.

Information for Patients: The use of ethchlorvynol carries with it an associated risk of psychological and/or physical dependence. The patient should be warned against increasing the dose of the drug without consulting a physician.

Patients should be advised that, for the duration of the effect of PLACIDYL, mental and/or physical abilities required for the performance of potentially hazardous tasks such as the operation of dangerous machinery including motor vehicles, may be impaired.

Patients should be cautioned to avoid the concomitant use of PLACIDYL with alcohol, barbiturates, other CNS depressants, or MAO inhibitors.

Drug Interactions: The concomitant use of PLACIDYL with alcohol, barbiturates, other CNS depressants, or MAO inhibitors may produce exaggerated depressant effects.

Ethchlorvynol may cause a decreased prothrombin time response to coumarin anticoagulants; therefore, the dosage of these drugs may require adjustment when therapy with ethchlorvynol is initiated and after it is discontinued.

Transient delirium has been reported with the concomitant use of PLACIDYL and amitriptyline; therefore, PLACIDYL should be administered with caution to patients receiving tricyclic antidepressants.

Carcinogenesis: A study in mice receiving oral doses of PLACIDYL up to 7 times the maximum human daily dose for 22 to 24 months produced equivocal results. When compared to controls, a statistically significant increase in total lung tumors was found in female mice given the high dose of PLACIDYL. However, the 48% incidence is not substantially higher than the high value (39%) reported for the historical laboratory controls.

No evidence of carcinogenic potential was observed in rats given PLACIDYL at 5 to 15 times the maximum human daily dose for up to 2 years.

Usage During Pregnancy: 1. Teratogenic—Pregnancy Category C. Ethchlorvynol has been associated with a higher percentage of stillbirths and a lower survival rate of progeny among rats given 40 mg/kg/day. There are no adequate and well-controlled studies in pregnant women. Therefore, ethchlorvynol is not recommended for use during the first and second trimesters of pregnancy. Ethchlorvynol should be used during pregnancy only if the potential benefit justifies the potential risk to the fetus.

2. Non-teratogenic—Clinical experience has indicated that ethchlorvynol taken during the third trimester of pregnancy may produce CNS depression and transient withdrawal symptoms in the newborn. These symptoms resemble congenital narcotic withdrawal symptoms (See "Drug Abuse and Dependence" section).

Nursing Mothers: It is not known whether this drug is excreted in breast milk. Because many drugs are excreted in human milk and because of the potential for serious adverse reactions in nursing infants from PLACIDYL, a decision should be made whether to discontinue nursing or to discontinue the drug, taking into account the importance of the drug to the mother.

Pediatric Use: PLACIDYL is not recommended for use in children since its safety and effectiveness in the pediatric age group has not been determined.

ADVERSE REACTIONS

Adverse effects in decreasing order of severity within each of the following categories are:

Hypersensitivity: cholestatic jaundice, urticaria and rash.

Hematologic: thrombocytopenia—one case of fatal immune thrombocytopenia due to ethchlorvynol has been reported.

Gastrointestinal: vomiting, gastric upset, nausea and aftertaste.

Neurologic: dizziness and facial numbness.

Miscellaneous: blurred vision, hypotension and mild "hangover".

The following idiosyncratic responses have been reported occasionally: syncope without marked hypotension, profound muscular weakness, hysteria, marked excitement, prolonged hypnosis and mild stimulation.

Transient ataxia, and giddiness have occurred in patients in whom absorption of the drug is especially rapid. These effects can sometimes be controlled by giving PLACIDYL with food.

(See "Drug Abuse and Dependence" section for the signs and symptoms of chronic intoxication).

DRUG ABUSE AND DEPENDENCE

PLACIDYL is subject to control by the Federal Controlled Substances Act under DEA schedule IV.

Abuse: Pulmonary edema of rapid onset has resulted from the I.V. abuse of PLACIDYL (ethchlorvynol).

Dependence: Signs and symptoms of intoxication have been reported with the prolonged use of doses as low as 1 g/day. Signs and symptoms of chronic intoxication may include incoordination, tremors, ataxia, confusion, slurred speech, hyperreflexia, diplopia, and generalized muscle weakness. Toxic amblyopia, scotoma, nystagmus, and peripheral neuropathy have also been reported with prolonged use of ethchlorvynol; these symptoms are usually reversible.

Severe withdrawal symptoms similar to those seen during barbiturate and alcohol withdrawal have been reported following abrupt discontinuance of prolonged use of PLACIDYL. These symptoms may appear as late as nine days after sudden withdrawal of the drug. Signs and symptoms of PLACIDYL withdrawal may include convulsions, delirium, hallucinations, schizoid reaction, perceptual distortions, memory loss, ataxia, insomnia, slurring of speech, unusual anxiety, irritability, agitation, and tremors. Other signs and symptoms may include anorexia, nausea, vomiting, weakness, dizziness, sweating, muscle twitching, and weight loss.

Management of a patient who manifests withdrawal symptoms from PLACIDYL involves readministration of the drug to approximately the same level of chronic intoxication which existed before the abrupt discontinuance. (Phenobarbital may be substituted for PLACIDYL.) A gradual, stepwise reduction of dosage may then be made over a period of days or weeks. A phenothiazine compound may be used in addition to this regimen for those patients who exhibit psychotic symptoms during the withdrawal period. The patient undergoing withdrawal from PLACIDYL must be hospitalized or closely observed, and given general supportive care as indicated.

In one report an infant born to a mother who received 500 mg PLACIDYL at bedtime daily throughout the third trimester, exhibited withdrawal symptoms on the second day of life. The symptoms included episodic jitteriness, hyperactivity, restlessness, irritability, disturbed sleep and hunger. The neonate responded to a single oral dose of phenobarbital (3 mg/kg). The withdrawal symptoms gradually decreased and completely disappeared by the tenth day of life.

OVERDOSAGE

Acute intoxication is characterized by prolonged deep coma, severe respiratory depression, hypothermia, hypotension, and relative bradycardia. Nystagmus and pancytopenia resulting from acute PLACIDYL overdose have been reported.

Although death has occurred following the ingestion of 6 g of PLACIDYL, there have been reports of patients who have survived overdoses of 50 g and more with intensive care. Fatal blood concentrations usually range from 20 to 50 μg/mL.[1] Because large amounts of ethchlorvynol are taken up by adipose tissue, the blood concentration is an unreliable indicator of the magnitude of overdose.

Management of acute PLACIDYL intoxication is similar to that of acute barbiturate intoxication.[2] Gastric evacuation should be performed immediately. (In the unconscious patient, gastric lavage should be preceded by tracheal intubation with a cuffed tube.) Supportive care (assisted ventilation, frequent and careful monitoring of vital signs, control of blood pressure) is essential. Emphasis should be placed on pulmonary care and monitoring of blood gases. Hemoperfusion utilizing the Amberlite column technique has been reported in the literature to be the most effective method in the management of acute PLACIDYL overdose.[3] In addition, hemodialysis and peritoneal dialysis have each been reported to be of some value. (Aqueous and oil dialysates have been used. Forced diuresis with maintenance of a high urinary output has also been reported of some value.) (See "Drug Abuse and Dependence" section for the signs and symptoms of chronic intoxication.)

DOSAGE AND ADMINISTRATION

The usual adult hypnotic dose of PLACIDYL (ethchlorvynol) is 500 mg taken orally at bedtime. A dose of 750 mg may be required for patients whose sleep response to a 500 mg capsule is inadequate, or for patients being changed from barbiturates or other nonbarbiturate hypnotics. Up to 1000 mg may be given as a single bedtime dose when insomnia is unusually severe. A single supplemental dose of 200 mg may be given to reinstitute sleep in patients who may awaken after the original bedtime dose of 500 or 750 mg.

For patients whose insomnia is characterized only by untimely awakening during the early morning hours, a single dose of 200 mg taken upon awakening may be adequate for relief.

The smallest effective dose of PLACIDYL should be given to elderly or debilitated patients.

PLACIDYL should not be prescribed for periods exceeding one week. (See "Drug Abuse and Dependence" section.)

HOW SUPPLIED

PLACIDYL (ethchlorvynol capsules, USP) is supplied as:

200 mg red capsules imprinted with the ⊐ , Abbott corporate logo:

Bottles of 100 .... (**NDC** 0074-6661-08).

500 mg red capsules imprinted with the trademark PLACIDYL and 500:

Bottles of 100 .... (**NDC** 0074-6685-15).

ABBO-PAC® unit dose strip packages of 100.. (**NDC** 0074-6685-10).

750 mg green capsules imprinted with the trademark PLACIDYL and 750:

Bottles of 100 .... (**NDC** 0074-6630-01).

Recommended storage: 59°–77° F (15°–25° C).

REFERENCES

1. AMA Dept. of Drugs. *AMA Drug Evaluations*, Massachusetts: Publishing Sciences Group, Inc., 1980.
2. Khantzian, E. J., McKenna, G. J., Acute Toxic and Withdrawal Reactions Associated with Drug Use and Abuse, *Annals of Internal Medicine*, 90:361–372, 1979.
3. Lynn, R.I., et al., Resin Hemoperfusion for Treatment of Ethchlorvynol Overdose, *Annals of Internal Medicine*, 91:549–553, 1979.

Ref. 03-4566-R12

Shown in Product Identification Guide, page 303

PROSOM™ Ⓒ ℞
(estazolam tablets)

DESCRIPTION

ProSom (estazolam), a triazolobenzodiazepine derivative, is an oral hypnotic agent. Estazolam occurs as a fine, white, odorless powder that is soluble in alcohol and practically insoluble in water. The chemical name for estazolam is 8-chloro-6-phenyl-4H-s-triazolo[4,3-α][1,4]benzodiazepine. The empirical formula is $C_{16}H_{11}ClN_4$. The structural formula is represented as follows:

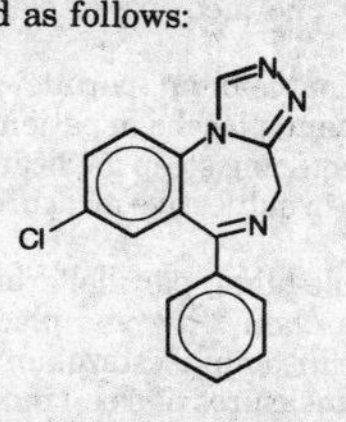

ProSom tablets are scored and contain either 1 mg or 2 mg of estazolam.

Inactive Ingredients: 1 mg tablets: corn starch, lactose, and stearic acid.

2 mg tablets: corn starch, iron oxide, lactose, and stearic acid.

CLINICAL PHARMACOLOGY

Pharmacokinetics: ProSom tablets have been found to be equivalent in absorption to an orally administered solution of estazolam. Independent of concentration, estazolam in plasma is 93% protein bound.

In healthy subjects who received up to three times the recommended dose of ProSom, peak estazolam plasma concentrations occurred within two hours after dosing (range 0.5 to 6.0 hours) and were proportional to the administered dose, suggesting linear pharmacokinetics over the dosage range tested.

The range of estimates for the mean elimination half-life of estazolam varied from 10 to 24 hours. The clearance of benzodiazepines is accelerated in smokers compared to nonsmokers, and there is evidence that this occurs with estazolam. This decrease in half-life, presumably due to enzyme induction by smoking, is consistent with other drugs with similar hepatic clearance characteristics. In all subjects and at all doses, the mean elimination half-life appeared to be independent of the dose.

In a small study (N=8) using various doses in older subjects (59 to 68 years), peak estazolam concentrations were found to be similar to those observed in younger subjects with a mean elimination half-life of 18.4 hours (range 13.5 to 34.6 hours).

Estazolam is extensively metabolized, and the metabolites are excreted primarily in the urine. Less than 5% of a 2 mg dose of estazolam is excreted unchanged in the urine, with only 4% of the dose appearing in the feces. 4′-hydroxy estazolam is the major metabolite in plasma, with concentrations approaching 12% of those of the parent eight hours after administration. While it and the lesser metabolite, 1-oxo-estazolam, have some pharmacologic activity, their low potencies and low concentrations preclude any significant contribution to the hypnotic effect of ProSom.

Continued on next page

Abbott Laboratories—Cont.

Postulated relationship between elimination rate of benzodiazepine hypnotics and their profile of common untoward effects: The type and duration of hypnotic effects and the profile of unwanted effects during administration of benzodiazepine drugs may be influenced by the biologic half-life of administered drug and any active metabolites formed. If half-lives are long, drug or metabolites may accumulate during periods of nightly administration and may be associated with impairments of cognitive and/or motor performance during waking hours; the possibility of interaction with other psychoactive drugs or alcohol will be increased. In contrast, if half-lives are short, drug and metabolites will be cleared before the next dose is ingested, and carry-over effects related to excessive sedation or CNS depression should be minimal or absent. However, during nightly use for an extended period, pharmacodynamic tolerance or adaptation to some effects of benzodiazepine hypnotics may develop. If the drug has a short elimination half-life, it is possible that a relative deficiency of the drug or its active metabolites (ie, in relationship to the receptor site) may occur at some point in the interval between each night's use. This sequence of events may account for two clinical findings reported to occur after several weeks of nightly use of rapidly eliminated benzodiazepine hypnotics, namely, increased wakefulness during the last third of the night and increased daytime anxiety in selected patients.

Controlled Trials Supporting Efficacy: In three 7-night, double-blind, parallel-group trials comparing estazolam 1 mg and/or 2 mg with placebo in adult outpatients with chronic insomnia, estazolam 2 mg was consistently superior to placebo in subjective measures of sleep induction (latency) and sleep maintenance (duration, number of awakenings, depth and quality of sleep); estazolam 1 mg was similarly superior to placebo on all measures of sleep maintenance, however, it significantly improved sleep induction in only one of two studies. In a similarly designed trial comparing estazolam 0.5 mg and 1 mg with placebo in geriatric outpatients with chronic insomnia, only the 1 mg estazolam dose was consistently superior to placebo in sleep induction (latency) and in only one measure of sleep maintenance (ie, duration of sleep).

In a single-night, double-blind, parallel-group trial comparing estazolam 2 mg and placebo in patients admitted for elective surgery and requiring sleep medications, estazolam was superior to placebo in subjective measures of sleep induction and maintenance.

In a 12-week, double-blind, parallel-group trial including a comparison of estazolam 2 mg and placebo in adult outpatients with chronic insomnia, estazolam was superior to placebo in subjective measures of sleep induction (latency) and maintenance (duration, number of awakenings, total wake time during sleep) at week 2, but produced consistent improvement over 12 weeks only for sleep duration and total wake time during sleep. Following withdrawal at week 12, rebound insomnia was seen at the first withdrawal week, but there was no difference between drug and placebo by the second withdrawal week in all parameters except latency, for which normalization did not occur until the fourth withdrawal week.

Adult outpatients with chronic insomnia were evaluated in a sleep laboratory trial comparing four doses of estazolam (0.25, 0.50, 1.0 and 2.0 mg) and placebo, each administered for 2 nights in a crossover design. The higher estazolam doses were superior to placebo in most EEG measures of sleep induction and maintenance, especially at the 2 mg dose, but only for sleep duration in subjective measures of sleep.

INDICATIONS AND USAGE

ProSom (estazolam) is indicated for the short-term management of insomnia characterized by difficulty in falling asleep, frequent nocturnal awakenings, and/or early morning awakenings. Both outpatient studies and a sleep laboratory study have shown that ProSom administered at bedtime improved sleep induction and sleep maintenance (see CLINICAL PHARMACOLOGY).

Because insomnia is often transient and intermittent, the prolonged administration of ProSom is generally neither necessary nor recommended. Since insomnia may be a symptom of several other disorders, the possibility that the complaint may be related to a condition for which there is a more specific treatment should be considered.

There is evidence to support the ability of ProSom to enhance the duration and quality of sleep for intervals up to 12 weeks (see CLINICAL PHARMACOLOGY).

CONTRAINDICATIONS

Benzodiazepines may cause fetal damage when administered during pregnancy. An increased risk of congenital malformations associated with the use of diazepam and chlordiazepoxide during the first trimester of pregnancy has been suggested in several studies. Transplacental distribution has resulted in neonatal CNS depression and also withdrawal phenomena following the ingestion of therapeutic doses of a benzodiazepine hypnotic during the last weeks of pregnancy. ProSom is contraindicated in pregnant women. If there is a likelihood of the patient becoming pregnant while receiving ProSom she should be warned of the potential risk to the fetus and instructed to discontinue the drug prior to becoming pregnant. The possibility that a woman of childbearing potential is pregnant at the time of institution of therapy should be considered.

WARNINGS

ProSom, like other benzodiazepines, has CNS depressant effects. For this reason, patients should be cautioned against engaging in hazardous occupations requiring complete mental alertness, such as operating machinery or driving a motor vehicle, after ingesting the drug, including potential impairment of the performance of such activities that may occur the day following ingestion of ProSom. Patients should also be cautioned about possible combined effects with alcohol and other CNS depressant drugs.

As with all benzodiazepines, amnesia, paradoxical reactions (eg, excitement, agitation, etc.), and other adverse behavioral effects may occur unpredictably.

There have been reports of withdrawal signs and symptoms of the type associated with withdrawal from CNS depressant drugs following the rapid decrease or the abrupt discontinuation of benzodiazepines (see DRUG ABUSE AND DEPENDENCE).

PRECAUTIONS

General: Impaired motor and/or cognitive performance attributable to the accumulation of benzodiazepines and their active metabolites following several days of repeated use at their recommended doses is a concern in certain vulnerable patients (eg, those especially sensitive to the effects of benzodiazepines or those with a reduced capacity to metabolize and eliminate them) (see DOSAGE AND ADMINISTRATION).

Elderly or debilitated patients and those with impaired renal or hepatic function should be cautioned about these risks and advised to monitor themselves for signs of excessive sedation or impaired conditions.

ProSom appears to cause dose-related respiratory depression that is ordinarily not clinically relevant at recommended doses in patients with normal respiratory function. However, patients with compromised respiratory function may be at risk and should be monitored appropriately. As a class, benzodiazepines have the capacity to depress respiratory drive; there are insufficient data available, however, to characterize their relative potency in depressing respiratory drive at clinically recommended doses.

As with other benzodiazepines, ProSom should be administered with caution to patients exhibiting signs or symptoms of depression. Suicidal tendencies may be present in such patients and protective measures may be required. Intentional overdosage is more common in this group of patients; therefore, the least amount of drug that is feasible should be prescribed for the patient at any one time.

Information for Patients: To assure the safe and effective use of ProSom, the following information and instructions should be given to patients:

1. Inform your physician about any alcohol consumption and medicine you are taking now, including drugs you may buy without a prescription. Alcohol should not be used during treatment with hypnotics.
2. Inform your physician if you are planning to become pregnant, if you are pregnant, or if you become pregnant while you are taking this medicine.
3. You should not take this medicine if you are nursing, as the drug may be excreted in breast milk.
4. Until you experience the way this medicine affects you, do not drive a car, operate potentially dangerous machinery, or engage in hazardous occupations requiring complete mental alertness after taking this medicine.
5. Since benzodiazepines may produce psychological and physical dependence, you should not increase the dose before consulting your physician. In addition, since the abrupt discontinuation of ProSom may be associated with temporary sleep disturbances, you should consult your physician before abruptly discontinuing doses of 2 mg per night or more.

Laboratory Tests: Laboratory tests are not ordinarily required in otherwise healthy patients. When treatment with ProSom is protracted, periodic blood counts, urinalyses, and blood chemistry analyses are advisable.

Drug Interactions: If ProSom is given concomitantly with other drugs acting on the central nervous system, careful consideration should be given to the pharmacology of all agents. The action of the benzodiazepines may be potentiated by anticonvulsants, antihistamines, alcohol, barbiturates, monoamine oxidase inhibitors, narcotics, phenothiazines, psychotropic medications, or other drugs that produce CNS depression. Smokers have an increased clearance of benzodiazepines as compared to nonsmokers; this was seen in studies with estazolam (see CLINICAL PHARMACOLOGY).

Carcinogenesis, Mutagenesis, Impairment of Fertility: Two-year carcinogenicity studies were conducted in mice and rats at dietary doses of 0.8, 3, and 10mg/kg/day and 0.5, 2, and 10 mg/kg/day, respectively. Evidence of tumorigenicity was not observed in either study. Incidence of hyperplastic liver nodules increased in female mice given the mid- and high-dose levels. The significance of such nodules in mice is not known at this time.

In vitro and *in vivo* mutagenicity tests including the Ames test, DNA repair in *B. subtilis, in vivo* cytogenetics in mice and rats, and the dominant lethal test in mice did not show a mutagenic potential for estazolam.

Fertility in male and female rats was not affected by doses up to 30 times the usual recommended human dose.

Pregnancy:

1. Teratogenic Effects: Pregnancy Category X (see CONTRAINDICATIONS).
2. Nonteratogenic Effects: The child born of a mother taking benzodiazepines may be at some risk for withdrawal symptoms during the postnatal period. Neonatal flaccidity has been reported in an infant born of a mother who received benzodiazepines during pregnancy.

Labor and Delivery: ProSom has no established use in labor or delivery.

Nursing Mothers: Human studies have not been conducted; however, studies in lactating rats indicate that estazolam and/or its metabolites are secreted in the milk. The use of ProSom in nursing mothers is not recommended.

Pediatric Use: Safety and effectiveness in children below the age of 18 have not been established.

Geriatric Use: Approximately 18% of individuals participating in the premarketing clinical trials of ProSom were 60 years of age or older. Overall, the adverse event profile did not differ substantively from that observed in younger individuals. Care should be exercised when prescribing benzodiazepines to small or debilitated elderly patients (see DOSAGE AND ADMINISTRATION).

ADVERSE REACTIONS

Commonly Observed: The most commonly observed adverse events associated with the use of ProSom, not seen at an equivalent incidence among placebo-treated patients were somnolence, hypokinesia, dizziness, and abnormal coordination.

Associated with Discontinuation of Treatment: Approximately 3% of 1277 patients who received ProSom in US premarketing clinical trials discontinued treatment because of an adverse clinical event. The only event commonly associated with discontinuation, accounting for 1.3% of the total, was somnolence.

Incidence in Controlled Clinical Trials: The table below enumerates adverse events that occurred at an incidence of 1% or greater among patients with insomnia who received ProSom in 7-night, placebo-controlled trials. Events reported by investigators were classified into standard dictionary (COSTART) terms to establish event frequencies. Event frequencies reported were not corrected for the occurrence of these events at baseline. The frequencies were obtained from data pooled across six studies: ProSom, N=685; placebo, N=433. The prescriber should be aware that these figures cannot be used to predict the incidence of side effects in the course of usual medical practice in which patient characteristics and other factors differ from those that prevailed in these six clinical trials. Similarly, the cited frequencies cannot be compared with figures obtained from other clinical investigators involving related drug products and uses, since each group of drug trials was conducted under a different set of conditions. However, the cited figures provide the physician with a basis of estimating the relative contribution of drug and nondrug factors to the incidence of side effects in the population studied.

INCIDENCE OF ADVERSE EXPERIENCES IN PLACEBO-CONTROLLED CLINICAL TRIALS
(Percentage of Patients Reporting)

Body System/ Adverse Event*	ProSom (N=685)	Placebo (N=433)
Body as a Whole		
Headache	16	27
Asthenia	11	8
Malaise	5	5
Lower extremity pain	3	2
Back pain	2	2
Body pain	2	2
Abdominal pain	1	2
Chest pain	1	1
Digestive System		
Nausea	4	5
Dyspepsia	2	2
Musculoskeletal System		
Stiffness	1	—
Nervous System		
Somnolence	42	27
Hypokinesia	8	4
Nervousness	8	11
Dizziness	7	3
Coordination abnormal	4	1
Hangover	3	2

Confusion	2	—
Depression	2	3
Dream abnormal	2	2
Thinking abnormal	2	1
Respiratory System		
Cold symptoms	3	5
Pharyngitis	1	2
Skin and Appendages		
Pruritus	1	—

* Events reported by at least 1% of ProSom patients.

Other Adverse Events:

During clinical trials conducted by Abbott, some of which were not placebo-controlled, ProSom was administered to approximately 1300 patients. Untoward events associated with this exposure were recorded by clinical investigators using terminology of their own choosing. To provide a meaningful estimate of the proportion of individuals experiencing adverse events, similar types of untoward events must be grouped into a smaller number of standardized event categories. In the tabulations that follow, a standard COSTART dictionary terminology has been used to classify reported adverse events. The frequencies presented, therefore, represent the proportion of the 1277 individuals exposed to ProSom who experienced an event of the type cited on at least one occasion while receiving ProSom. All reported events are included except those already listed in the previous table, those COSTART terms too general to be informative, and those events where a drug cause was remote. Events are further classified within body system categories and enumerated in order of decreasing frequency using the following definitions: frequent adverse events are defined as those occurring on one or more occasions in at least 1/100 patients; infrequent adverse events are those occurring in 1/100 to 1/1000 patients; rare events are those occurring in less than 1/1000 patients. It is important to emphasize that, although the events reported did occur during treatment with ProSom, they were not necessarily caused by it.

Body as a Whole—Infrequent: allergic reaction, chills, fever, neck pain, upper extremity pain; Rare: edema, jaw pain, swollen breast.

Cardiovascular System—Infrequent: flushing, palpitation; Rare: arrhythmia, syncope.

Digestive System—Frequent: constipation, dry mouth; Infrequent: decreased appetite, flatulence, gastritis, increased appetite, vomiting; Rare: enterocolitis, melena, ulceration of the mouth.

Endocrine System—Rare: thyroid nodule.

Hematologic and Lymphatic System— Rare: leukopenia, purpura, swollen lymph nodes.

Metabolic/Nutritional Disorders—Infrequent: thirst; Rare: increased SGOT, weight gain, weight loss.

Musculoskeletal System—Infrequent: arthritis, muscle spasm, myalgia; Rare: arthralgia.

Nervous System—Frequent: anxiety; Infrequent: agitation, amnesia, apathy, emotional lability, euphoria, hostility, paresthesia, seizure, sleep disorder, stupor, twitch; Rare: ataxia, circumoral paresthesia, decreased libido, decreased reflexes, hallucinations, neuritis, nystagmus, tremor.

Minor changes in EEG patterns, usually low-voltage fast activity, have been observed in patients during ProSom therapy or withdrawal and are of no known clinical significance.

Respiratory System—Infrequent: asthma, cough, dyspnea, rhinitis, sinusitis; Rare: epistaxis, hyperventilation, laryngitis.

Skin and Appendages—Infrequent: rash, sweating, urticaria; Rare: acne, dry skin.

Special Senses—Infrequent: abnormal vision, ear pain, eye irritation, eye pain, eye swelling, perverse taste, photophobia, tinnitus; Rare: decreased hearing, diplopia, scotomata.

Urogenital System—Infrequent: frequent urination, menstrual cramps, urinary hesitancy, urinary urgency, vaginal discharge/itching; Rare: hematuria, nocturia, oliguria, penile discharge, urinary incontinence.

Postintroduction Reports—Voluntary reports of non-US postmarketing experience with estazolam have included rare occurrences of photosensitivity and agranulocytosis. Because of the uncontrolled nature of these spontaneous reports, a causal relationship to estazolam treatment has not been determined.

DRUG ABUSE AND DEPENDENCE

Controlled Substance: ProSom tablets are a controlled substance in Schedule IV.

Abuse and Dependence: Withdrawal symptoms similar to those noted with sedatives/hypnotics and alcohol have occurred following the abrupt discontinuation of drugs in the benzodiazepine class. The symptoms can range from mild dysphoria and insomnia to a major syndrome that may include abdominal and muscle cramps, vomiting, sweating, tremors, and convulsions.

Although withdrawal symptoms are more commonly noted after the discontinuation of higher than therapeutic doses of benzodiazepines, a proportion of patients taking benzodiazepines chronically at therapeutic doses may become physically dependent on them. Available data, however, cannot provide a reliable estimate of the incidence of dependency or the relationship of the dependency to dose and duration of treatment. There is some evidence to suggest that gradual reduction of dosage will attenuate or eliminate some withdrawal phenomena. In most instances, withdrawal phenomena are relatively mild and transient; however, life-threatening events (eg, seizures, delirium, etc.) have been reported. Gradual withdrawal is the preferred course for any patient taking benzodiazepines for a prolonged period. Patients with a history of seizures, regardless of their concomitant antiseizure drug therapy, should not be withdrawn abruptly from benzodiazepines.

Individuals with a history of addiction to or abuse of drugs or alcohol should be under careful surveillance when receiving benzodiazepines because of the risk of habituation and dependence to such patients.

OVERDOSAGE

As with other benzodiazepines, experience with ProSom indicates that manifestations of overdosage include somnolence, respiratory depression, confusion, impaired coordination, slurred speech, and ultimately, coma. Patients have recovered from overdosage as high as 40 mg. As in the management of intentional overdose with any drug, the possibility should be considered that multiple agents may have been taken.

Gastric evacuation, either by the induction of emesis, lavage, or both, should be performed immediately. Maintenance of adequate ventilation is essential. General supportive care, including frequent monitoring of the vital signs and close observation of the patient, is indicated. Fluids should be administered intravenously to maintain blood pressure and encourage diuresis. The value of dialysis in treatment of benzodiazepine overdose has not been determined. The physician may wish to consider contacting a Poison Control Center for up-to-date information on the management of hypnotic drug product overdose.

Flumazenil, a specific benzodiazepine receptor antagonist, is indicated for the complete or partial reversal of the sedative effects of benzodiazepines and may be used in situations when an overdose with a benzodiazepine is known or suspected. Prior to the administration of flumazenil, necessary measures should be instituted to secure airway, ventilation, and intravenous access. Flumazenil is intended as an adjunct to, not as a substitute for, proper management of benzodiazepine overdose. Patients treated with flumazenil should be monitored for resedation, respiratory depression, and other residual benzodiazepine effects for an appropriate period after treatment. **The prescriber should be aware of a risk of seizure in association with flumazenil treatment, particularly in long-term benzodiazepine users and in cyclic antidepressant overdose.** The complete flumazenil package insert including CONTRAINDICATIONS, WARNINGS, and PRECAUTIONS should be consulted prior to use.

DOSAGE AND ADMINISTRATION

The recommended initial dose for adults is 1 mg at bedtime; however, some patients may need a 2 mg dose. In healthy elderly patients, 1 mg is also the appropriate starting dose, but increases should be initiated with particular care. In small or debilitated older patients, a starting dose of 0.5 mg, while only marginally effective in the overall elderly population, should be considered.

HOW SUPPLIED

ProSom tablets are scored tablets supplied as:

ProSom Tablets 1 mg (white)

Bottles of 100 .... (**NDC** 0074-3735-13)

ABBO-PAC® unit dose strip

packages of 100 tablets .... (**NDC** 0074-3735-11)

ProSom Tablets 2 mg (coral-colored)

Bottles of 100 .... (**NDC** 0074-3736-13)

ABBO-PAC® unit dose strip

packages of 100 tablets .... (**NDC** 0074-3736-11)

Recommended storage: Store below 86°F (30°C).

Ref. 03-4471-R5-Rev. December, 1993

Abbott Laboratories
North Chicago, IL 60064

Shown in Product Identification Guide, page 303

TRANXENE® ℂ ℞

[tran' zēen]

(clorazepate dipotassium)

T-TAB® Tablets
TRANXENE®-SD™
& TRANXENE®-SD™ HALF STRENGTH
(clorazepate dipotassium)
Tablets

DESCRIPTION

Chemically, TRANXENE (clorazepate dipotassium) is a benzodiazepine. The empirical formula is $C_{16}H_{11}ClK_2N_2O_4$; the molecular weight is 408.92; and the structural formula may be represented as follows:

[See chemical structure at top of next column.]

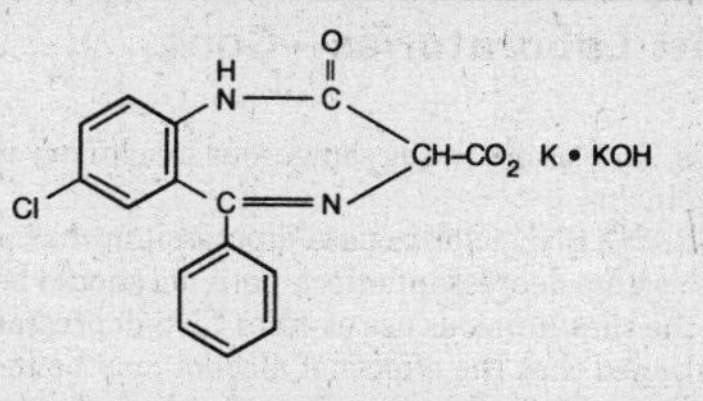

The compound occurs as a fine, light yellow, practically odorless powder. It is insoluble in the common organic solvents, but very soluble in water. Aqueous solutions are unstable, clear, light yellow, and alkaline.

TRANXENE T-TAB tablets contain either 3.75 mg, 7.5 mg or 15 mg of clorazepate dipotassium for oral administration. TRANXENE- SD and TRANXENE-SD HALF STRENGTH tablets contain 22.5 mg and 11.25 mg of clorazepate dipotassium respectively. TRANXENE-SD and TRANXENE-SD HALF STRENGTH tablets gradually release clorazepate and are designed for once-a-day administration in patients already stabilized on TRANXENE T-TAB tablets.

Inactive ingredients for TRANXENE T-TAB® Tablets: Colloidal silicon dioxide, FD&C Blue No. 2 (3.75 mg only), FD&C Yellow No. 6 (7.5 mg only), FD&C Red No. 3 (15 mg only), magnesium oxide, magnesium stearate, microcrystalline cellulose, potassium carbonate, potassium chloride, and talc.

Inactive ingredients for TRANXENE-SD and TRANXENE-SD HALF STRENGTH Tablets: Castor oil wax, FD&C Blue No. 2 (SD Half Strength, 11.25 mg only), iron oxide (SD, 22.5 mg only), lactose, magnesium oxide, magnesium stearate, potassium carbonate, potassium chloride, and talc.

CLINICAL PHARMACOLOGY

Pharmacologically, clorazepate dipotassium has the characteristics of the benzodiazepines. It has depressant effects on the central nervous system. The primary metabolite, nordiazepam, quickly appears in the blood stream. The serum half-life is about 2 days. The drug is metabolized in the liver and excreted primarily in the urine.

Studies in healthy men have shown that clorazenate dipotassium has depressant effects on the central nervous system. Prolonged administration of single daily doses as high as 120 mg was without toxic effects. Abrupt cessation of high doses was followed in some patients by nervousness, insomnia, irritability, diarrhea, muscle aches, or memory impairment.

Since orally administered clorazepate dipotassium is rapidly decarboxylated to form nordiazepam, there is essentially no circulating parent drug. Nordiazepam, the primary metabolite, quickly appears in the blood and is eliminated from the plasma with an apparent half-life of about 40 to 50 hours. Plasma levels of nordiazepam increase proportionally with TRANXENE dose and show moderate accumulation with repeated administration. The protein binding of nordiazepam in plasma is high (97-98%).

Within 10 days after oral administration of a 15 mg (50µCi) dose of ^{14}C-TRANXENE to two volunteers, 62–67% of the radioactivity was excreted in the urine and 15–19% was eliminated in the feces. Both subjects were still excreting measurable amounts of radioactivity in the urine (about 1% of the ^{14}C-dose) on day ten.

Nordiazepam is further metabolized by hydroxylation. The major urinary metabolite is conjugated oxazepam (3-hydroxynordiazepam), and smaller amounts of conjugated p-hydroxynordiazepam and nordiazepam are also found in the urine.

INDICATIONS AND USAGE

TRANXENE (clorazepate dipotassium) is indicated for the management of anxiety disorders or for the short-term relief of the symptoms of anxiety. Anxiety or tension associated with the stress of everyday life usually does not require treatment with an anxiolytic.

TRANXENE tablets are indicated as adjunctive therapy in the management of partial seizures.

The effectiveness of TRANXENE tablets in long-term management of anxiety, that is, more than 4 months, has not been assessed by systematic clinical studies. Long-term studies in epileptic patients, however, have shown continued therapeutic activity. The physician should reassess periodically the usefulness of the drug for the individual patient.

TRANXENE tablets are indicated for the symptomatic relief of acute alcohol withdrawal.

CONTRAINDICATIONS

TRANXENE tablets are contraindicated in patients with a known hypersensitivity to the drug and in those with acute narrow angle glaucoma.

WARNINGS

TRANXENE tablets are not recommended for use in depressive neuroses or in psychotic reactions.

Patients taking TRANXENE tablets should be cautioned against engaging in hazardous occupations requiring mental

Continued on next page

Abbott Laboratories—Cont.

alertness, such as operating dangerous machinery including motor vehicles.
Since TRANXENE (clorazepate dipotassium) has a central nervous system depressant effect, patients should be advised against the simultaneous use of other CNS-depressant drugs, and cautioned that the effects of alcohol may be increased.
Because of the lack of sufficient clinical experience, TRANXENE tablets are not recommended for use in patients less than 9 years of age.
Physical and Psychological Dependence:
Withdrawal symptoms (similar in character to those noted with barbiturates and alcohol) have occurred following abrupt discontinuance of clorazepate. Withdrawal symptoms associated with the abrupt discontinuation of benzodiazepines have included convulsions, delirium, tremor, abdominal and muscle cramps, vomiting, sweating, nervousness, insomnia, irritability, diarrhea, and memory impairment. The more severe withdrawal symptoms have usually been limited to those patients who had received excessive doses over an extended period of time. Generally milder withdrawal symptoms have been reported following abrupt discontinuance of benzodiazepines taken continuously at therapeutic levels for several months. Consequently, after extended therapy, abrupt discontinuation of clorazepate should generally be avoided and a gradual dosage tapering schedule followed.
Caution should be observed in patients who are considered to have a psychological potential for drug dependence.
Evidence of drug dependence has been observed in dogs and rabbits which was characterized by convulsive seizures when the drug was abruptly withdrawn or the dose was reduced; the syndrome in dogs could be abolished by administration of clorazepate.
Usage in Pregnancy: **An increased risk of congenital malformations associated with the use of minor tranquilizers (chlordiazepoxide, diazepam, and meprobamate) during the first trimester of pregnancy has been suggested in several studies. Clorazepate dipotassium, a benzodiazepine derivative, has not been studied adequately to determine whether it, too, may be associated with an increased risk of fetal abnormality. Because use of these drugs is rarely a matter of urgency, their use during this period should almost always be avoided. The possibility that a woman of childbearing potential may be pregnant at the time of institution of therapy should be considered. Patients should be advised that if they become pregnant during therapy or intend to become pregnant they should communicate with their physician about the desirability of discontinuing the drug.**
Usage during Lactation:
TRANXENE tablets should not be given to nursing mothers since it has been reported that nordiazepam is excreted in human breast milk.

PRECAUTIONS

In those patients in which a degree of depression accompanies the anxiety, suicidal tendencies may be present and protective measures may be required. The least amount of drug that is feasible should be available to the patient.
Patients taking TRANXENE tablets for prolonged periods should have blood counts and liver function tests periodically. The usual precautions in treating patients with impaired renal or hepatic function should also be observed.
In elderly or debilitated patients, the initial dose should be small, and increments should be made gradually, in accordance with the response of the patient, to preclude ataxia or excessive sedation.
Information for Patients:
To assure the safe and effective use of benzodiazepines, patients should be informed that, since benzodiazepines may produce psychological and physical dependence, it is essential that they consult with their physician before either increasing the dose or abruptly discontinuing this drug.

ADVERSE REACTIONS

The side effect most frequently reported was drowsiness. Less commonly reported (in descending order of occurrence) were: dizziness, various gastrointestinal complaints, nervousness, blurred vision, dry mouth, headache, and mental confusion. Other side effects included insomnia, transient skin rashes, fatigue, ataxia, genitourinary complaints, irritability, diplopia, depression, tremor, and slurred speech.
There have been reports of abnormal liver and kidney function tests and of decrease in hematocrit.
Decrease in systolic blood pressure has been observed.

DOSAGE AND ADMINISTRATION

For the symptomatic relief of anxiety:
TRANXENE (clorazepate dipotassium) T-TAB® tablets are administered orally in divided doses. The usual daily dose is 30 mg. The dose should be adjusted gradually within the range of 15 to 60 mg daily in accordance with the response of the patient. In elderly or debilitated patients it is advisable to initiate treatment at a daily dose of 7.5 to 15 mg.
TRANXENE tablets may also be administered in a single dose daily at bedtime; the recommended initial dose is 15 mg. After the initial dose, the response of the patient may require adjustment of subsequent dosage. Lower doses may be indicated in the elderly patient. Drowsiness may occur at the initiation of treatment and with dosage increment.
TRANXENE-SD (22.5 mg) tablets may be administered as a single dose every 24 hours. This tablet is intended as an alternate dosage form for the convenience of patients stabilized on a dose of 7.5 mg tablets three times a day. TRANXENE-SD tablets should not be used to initiate therapy.
TRANXENE-SD HALF STRENGTH (11.25 mg) tablets may be administered as a single dose every 24 hours. This tablet is intended as an alternate dosage form for the convenience of patients stabilized on a dose of 3.75 mg tablets three times a day. TRANXENE-SD HALF STRENGTH should not be used to initiate therapy.
For the symptomatic relief of acute alcohol withdrawal:
The following dosage schedule is recommended:

1st 24 hours (Day 1)	30 mg initially; followed by 30 to 60 mg in divided doses
2nd 24 hours (Day 2)	45 to 90 mg in divided doses
3rd 24 hours (Day 3)	22.5 to 45 mg in divided doses
Day 4	15 to 30 mg in divided doses

Thereafter, gradually reduce the daily dose to 7.5 to 15 mg. Discontinue drug therapy as soon as patient's condition is stable.
The maximum recommended total daily dose is 90 mg. Avoid excessive reductions in the total amount of drug administered on successive days.
As an Adjunct to Antiepileptic Drugs:
In order to minimize drowsiness, the recommended initial dosages and dosage increments should not be exceeded.
Adults: The maximum recommended initial dose in patients over 12 years old is 7.5 mg three times a day. Dosage should be increased by no more than 7.5 mg every week and should not exceed 90 mg/day.
Children (9-12 years): The maximum recommended initial dose is 7.5 mg two times a day. Dosage should be increased by no more than 7.5 mg every week and should not exceed 60 mg/day.

DRUG INTERACTIONS

If TRANXENE (clorazepate dipotassium) is to be combined with other drugs acting on the central nervous system, careful consideration should be given to the pharmacology of the agents to be employed. Animal experience indicates that clorazepate dipotassium prolongs the sleeping time after hexobarbital or after ethyl alcohol, increases the inhibitory effects of chlorpromazine, but does not exhibit monoamine oxidase inhibition. Clinical studies have shown increased sedation with concurrent hypnotic medications. The actions of the benzodiazepines may be potentiated by barbiturates, narcotics, phenothiazines, monoamine oxidase inhibitors or other antidepressants.
If TRANXENE tablets are used to treat anxiety associated with somatic disease states, careful attention must be paid to possible drug interaction with concomitant medication.
In bioavailability studies with normal subjects, the concurrent administration of antacids at therapeutic levels did not significantly influence the bioavailability of TRANXENE tablets.

OVERDOSAGE

Overdosage is usually manifested by varying degrees of CNS depression ranging from slight sedation to coma. As in the management of overdosage with any drug, it should be borne in mind that multiple agents may have been taken.
The treatment of overdosage should consist of the general measures employed in the management of overdosage of any CNS depressant. Gastric evacuation either by the induction of emesis, lavage, or both, should be performed immediately. General supportive care, including frequent monitoring of the vital signs and close observation of the patient, is indicated. Hypotension, though rarely reported, may occur with large overdoses. In such cases the use of agents such as Levophed® Bitartrate (norepinephrine bitartrate injection, USP) or Aramine® Injection (metaraminol bitartrate injection, USP) should be considered.
While reports indicate that individuals have survived overdoses of clorazepate dipotassium as high as 450 to 675 mg, these doses are not necessarily an accurate indication of the amount of drug absorbed since the time interval between ingestion and the institution of treatment was not always known. Sedation in varying degrees was the most common physiological manifestation of clorazepate dipotassium overdosage. Deep coma when it occurred was usually associated with the ingestion of other drugs in addition to clorazepate dipotassium.
Flumazenil, a specific benzodiazepine receptor antagonist, is indicated for the complete or partial reversal of the sedative effects of benzodiazepines and may be used in situations when an overdose with a benzodiazepine is known or suspected. Prior to the administration of flumazenil, necessary measures should be instituted to secure airway, ventilation, and intravenous access. Flumazenil is intended as an adjunct to, not as a substitute for, proper management of benzodiazepine overdose. Patients treated with flumazenil should be monitored for resedation, respiratory depression, and other residual benzodiazepine effects for an appropriate period after treatment. **The prescriber should be aware of a risk of seizure in association with flumazenil treatment, particularly in long-term benzodiazepine users and in cyclic antidepressant overdose.** The complete flumazenil package insert including CONTRAINDICATIONS, WARNINGS, and PRECAUTIONS should be consulted prior to use.

ANIMAL PHARMACOLOGY AND TOXICOLOGY

Studies in rats and monkeys have shown a substantial difference between doses producing tranquilizing, sedative and toxic effects. In rats, conditioned avoidance response was inhibited at an oral dose of 10 mg/kg; sedation was induced at 32 mg/kg; the LD_{50} was 1320 mg/kg. In monkeys aggressive behavior was reduced at an oral dose of 0.25 mg/kg; sedation (ataxia) was induced at 7.5 mg/kg; the LD_{50} could not be determined because of the emetic effect of large doses, but the LD_{50} exceeds 1600 mg/kg.
Twenty-four dogs were given clorazepate dipotassium orally in a 22-month toxicity study; doses up to 75 mg/kg were given. Drug-related changes occurred in the liver; weight was increased and cholestasis with minimal hepatocellular damage was found, but lobular architecture remained well preserved.
Eighteen rhesus monkeys were given oral doses of clorazepate dipotassium from 3 to 36 mg/kg daily for 52 weeks. All treated animals remained similar to control animals. Although total leucocyte count remained within normal limits it tended to fall in the female animals on the highest doses.
Examination of all organs revealed no alterations attributable to clorazepate dipotassium. There was no damage to liver function or structure.
Reproduction Studies: Standard fertility, reproduction, and teratology studies were conducted in rats and rabbits. Oral doses in rats up to 150 mg/kg and in rabbits up to 15 mg/kg produced no abnormalities in the fetuses. TRANXENE (clorazepate dipotassium) did not alter the fertility indices or reproductive capacity of adult animals. As expected, the sedative effect of high doses interfered with care of the young by their mothers (*see Usage in Pregnancy*).

HOW SUPPLIED

TRANXENE® (clorazepate dipotassium) is supplied as:
3.75 mg blue-colored, scored T-TAB® tablets:
Bottles of 100 ....(**NDC** 0074-4389-13).
Bottles of 500 ....(**NDC** 0074-4389-53).
ABBO-PAC® unit dose packages:
100 ....(**NDC** 0074-4389-11).

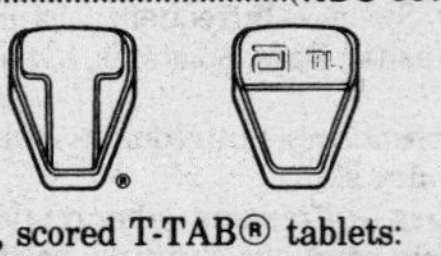

7.5 mg peach-colored, scored T-TAB® tablets:
Bottles of 100 ....(**NDC** 0074-4390-13).
Bottles of 500 ....(**NDC** 0074-4390-53).
ABBO-PAC® unit dose packages:
100 ....(**NDC** 0074-4390-11).

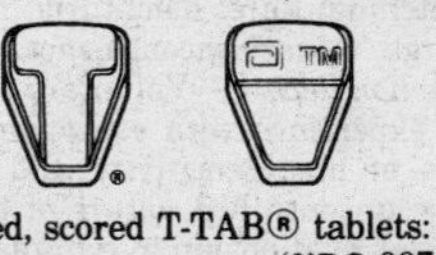

15 mg lavender-colored, scored T-TAB® tablets:
Bottles of 100 ....(**NDC** 0074-4391-13).
Bottles of 500 ....(**NDC** 0074-4391-53).
ABBO-PAC® unit dose packages:
100 ....(**NDC** 0074-4391-11).

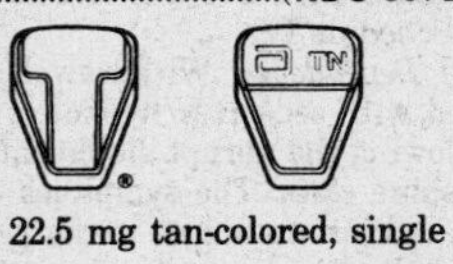

TRANXENE®-SD™ 22.5 mg tan-colored, single dose tablets:
Bottles of 100 ....(**NDC** 0074-2997-13).
TRANXENE®-SD™ HALF STRENGTH 11.25 mg blue-colored, single dose tablets:
Bottles of 100 ....(**NDC** 0074-2699-13).
T-TAB, tablet appearance and shape are trademarks of Abbott Laboratories.

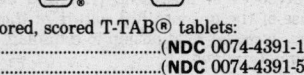

Recommended storage: Store below 77°F (25°C)
U.S. Design Pat. No. D–300,879
Ref. 03-4490-R13
Shown in Product Identification Guide, page 304

AC Laboratory
750 STIMSON AVE.
CITY OF INDUSTRY, CA 91745

Direct Inquiries to:
Yung Feng Hung
(818) 336-8889
(FAX): 818-336-1299

A C SLIM CAP   OTC

INGREDIENTS
Ma Huang 8%
Salix Alba 4:1 (White Willow Bark)
Kelp Pacific
Alfalfa Powder
Rice Flour
Sylox
Magnesium Stearate

INDICATION
A C SLIM CAP is a non habit-forming diet formula. It contains only pure, natural, hypoallergenic ingredients of the highest quality. The unique powerful synergistic blend of natural own nutrients and herbs was designed to work in your overall diet plan. A C SLIM CAP is one of the most effective and safe diet supplement products. This product is laboratory tested guaranteeing the highest standards of quality, purity, and safe potency assuring you of the finest products available. Contains no sugar, preservatives, or yeast.

DOSAGE
1–2 Capsules before meals. Take three times daily.

HOW SUPPLIED
90 / 120 Capsules Per Bottle.

CAUTION
Seek advice from a health care practitioner if you are pregnant or nursing, or if you have high blood pressure, heart or thyroid disease, diabetes, difficulty in urination due to prostate enlargement, or taking an MAO inhibitor or any other prescription drug. If nervousness, tremor, sleepiness, loss of appetite or nausea occur, reduce or discontinue use. Not intended for use by persons under age of 18.

DIA-RELIEVER   OTC
WITH ANTIOXIDANTS AND GINGKO

ACTIVE INGREDIENTS
Four Tablets Contains:

Vitamin A	20,000 I.U.
(10,000 I.U. as Beta Carotene)	
Vitamin D	600 I.U.
Vitamin K	25 mcg
Riboflavin	4 mg
Vitamin B12	12 mcg
Folate	400 mcg
Pantothenic Acid	10 mg
Iron	15 mg
Iodine	150 mcg
Zinc	15 mg
Selenium	25 mcg
Chromium	50 mcg
Vanadyl Sulfate	6.8 mg
Inositol	50 mg
Vitamin C	500 mg
Vitamin E	800 I.U.
Thiamin	4 mg
Vitamin B6	8 mg
Niacin	20 mg
Biotin	30 mcg
Calcium	80 mg
Phosphorus	20 mg
Magnesium	400 mg
Copper	2 mg
Manganese	2.5 mg
Molybdenum	2.5 mcg
Citrus Bioflavinoids	100 mg
Gingko	100 mg

INDICATION
Dia-Reliever is a unique high potency nutritional supplement which provides 100% of the USRDA for all vitamins and higher concentrations of antioxidant vitamins C, E, and A (as beta carotene.) It also supplies essential minerals and trace elements. To approximate the formula for Dia-Reliever, you would have to take;
A general-purpose multivitamin/mineral;
Antioxidant supplements of Beta Carotene, C and E;
Mineral supplements of Magnesium and Chromium, and Supplements of Citrus Bioflavinoids, Insitol, Vanadyl Sulfate, and Gingko
Many people with diabetes regularly take vitamins supplements. Now you can achieve optimum nutrition with the help of Dia-Reliever, a unique powerful formula in one convenient bottle. So Dia-Reliever is highly recommended to the people with diabetes.

DOSAGE
Four Tablets Daily

HOW SUPPLIED
90/120/ 240/ 1,000 Tablets Per Bottle

HEPLIVE   OTC

INGREDIENTS
Each Softget Capsule Contains:

Vitamin A (Palmitate)	1,200 I.U.
Vitamin E (d-Alpha Tocopherol)	10 I.U.
Vitamin C (Ascorbic Acid)	10 mg
Folic Acid	0.06 mg
Vitamin B1 (Thiamine Mononitrate)	1 mg
Vitamin B2 (Riboflavin)	1 mg
Niacinamide	10 mg
Vitamin B6 (Pyridoxine HCl)	0.5 mg
Vitamin B12 (Cobalamin)	1 mg
Biotin	3.3 mg
Pantothenia Acid	2 mg
Choline Bitartrate	21 mg
Zinc (Zinc Sulfate)	2 mg
Desiccated Liver	194.4 mg
Liver Concentrate	64.8 mg
Liver Fraction Number 2	64.8 mg
Yeast (Dried)	64.8 mg
dl-Methionine	10 mg
Inositol	10 mg

INDICATION
HEPLIVE is a balanced formulation of vitamins, minerals, lipotropic factors, and vitamin-protein supplements. It's of value as a nutritional supplement for persons who are receiving professional treatment for alcoholism, hepatic dyfunction due to hepatotoxic drugs and liver poisons, male and female infertility due to hormonal imbalance caused by hepaticdyfunction, and for nutritional supplementation after treatment.

DOSAGE
Three to Six Capsules Daily.

HOW SUPPLIED
30 / 60 / 90 / 100 / 120 / 300 / 1,000 Softgel Capsules Per Bottle.

MELATONIN   OTC
[məl″ə'tŏe-nin]

ACTIVE INGREDIENT
Melatonin .... 3 mg

DESCRIPTION & INDICATION
MELATONIN is produced by the pineal gland in the brain. It helps regulate sleep levels as a treatment for a number of conditions including: jet-lag, seasonal affective disorder (SAD), and depression.
In a volunteer study, charged by Dr. Richard J. Wurtman, professor of neurosurgery at the Massachusetts Institute of Technology, the volunteers fell asleep in five or six minutes after given a small amount of MELATONIN.
MELATONIN has also been shown to improve immunity and extend lifespan in rodents. Some research has shown that MELATONIN may improve the release of other biologically active pineal compounds through feedback communication with the pineal gland.

DOSAGE
One to Three Tablets When Needed. No More Than Three Times a Day.

HOW SUPPLIED
30 / 60 / 90 / 100 / 120 / 1,000 Tablets Per Bottle.

MELATONIN SPRAY   OTC
[məl″ə'toe-nin]
Natural Sleep Aid

MELATONIN is a hormone produced by the pineal gland, the organ which regulates the body's wake/sleep/wake cycle. The hormone is secreted in a circadian rhythm by enzymes which are activated by darkness and depressed by light. Melatonin is a safe, well tolerated supplement, which naturally augments the functioning of the pineal gland.
Melatonin Spray utilizes a new liposome delivery system which deliverys dietary ingredients in an oral spray. The patent applied for employs microscopic spheres, 1/50th the size of a human hair to speed natural absorption. This advanced method of delivery is truly efficient, there are no pills and water to wash them down.
Liposome delivery system works many times faster than conventional pills/capsules.
Melatonin Spray provides increased bio-availability of the dietary ingredients because the ingredients are immediately ready for absorption. Pills or tablets dissolve slowly in the digestive system. Melatonin Spray ingredients are just waiting to be absorbed.
A LipoCcutical multi-layered liposome system designed for sustained delivery throughout the day or night of the active ingredient.
No need to "plan" your sleep hours in advance. Melatonin Spray works within a few minutes after application.
Wide flexibility for individual use. User adjusts the number of sprays required for his/her maximum results and comfort. Tasty flavoring and breath spray.
Easy to carry - Easy to use. No need to bother with water to wash down hard to swallow pills.

HOW SUPPLIED
SIZE CONTAINER - 2 ounce spray - 49 applications @ 3 mg each.
APPLICATION - 2 sprays is equivalent to 3 mg Melatonin.
PUMP SPRAYER allows user to vary dosage according to individual needs.

Advanced Nutritional
Technology®, Inc.
6988 SIERRA CT.
DUBLIN, CA 94568

Direct Inquiries to:
(800) 624–6543
(510) 828–2128
FAX: (510) 828–6848

FORMULA 3/6/9™   OTC
(Essential Fatty Acids)

HOW SUPPLIED

	SIZE	NDC #
Formula 3/6/9 ™	30's	62617-010-01
	60's	62617-010-02

N'ODOR®   OTC
(50mg Chlorophyllin Complex)

HOW SUPPLIED

	SIZE	NDC #
N'Odor®	120's	62617-625-04

NUTR-E-SOL®   OTC
(Water Soluble Natural Vitamin E
For Maximum Absorption)

FORMULATIONS
400 I.U. Natural Vitamin E per tablespoon

PHYSIOLOGICAL CONSIDERATIONS
Advanced Nutritional Technology's Nutr-E-Sol is a high potency water soluble natural vitamin E designed for fast absorption.
Nutr-E-Sol contains a unique form of vitamin E (d-α-tocopheryl polyethylene glycol 1000 succinate or TPGS) that is absorbed directly through the intestinal wall without the use of bile for emulsification. Nutr-E-Sol is useful in raising vitamin E blood levels in diseases such as Cystic Fibrosis, Crohn's Disease, Short Bowel Syndrome, Biliary Cirrhosis and Cholestasis, where vitamin E blood levels are low.

Continued on next page

Advanced Nutritional—Cont.

Nutr-E-Sol may be taken alone or mixed with drinks. This product is tasteless and sugar-free for better compliance with the young and diabetic.

Studies indicate that Nutr-E-Sol's form of Vitamin E is absorbed better than other water-soluble vitamin E supplements, dry vitamin E supplements and emulsified forms of vitamin E.

DOSAGE
Liquid—One to three tablespoons per day.

HOW SUPPLIED

	SIZE	NDC #
Nutr-E-Sol®	8 oz.	62617-515-10
	16 oz.	62617-515-20

NUTR-EPO™   OTC
(Evening Primrose Oil)

HOW SUPPLIED

	SIZE	NDC#
NUTR-EPO™ 1300	60's	62617-035-02
NUTR-EPO™ 1000	90's	62617-030-03
NUTR-EPO™ 500	100's	62617-025-06

PEDIA-VIT® CHEWABLES   OTC
(Multi Vitamin & Minerals for Children)
(Three natural flavors)

HOW SUPPLIED

	SIZE	NDC #
Pedia-Vit® Chewables	90's	62617-115-03

PEDIA-VIT® LIQUID   OTC
(Children's Multivitamin Liquid with Iron)

HOW SUPPLIED

	SIZE	NDC #
Pedia-Vit®	8 oz.	62617-115-10

SHARKARE™   OTC
(100% pure Shark Cartilage)

HOW SUPPLIED
SHARKARE™	90's	62617-440-03

SUPER EPA®   OTC
(Eicosapentaenoic Acid and Docosahexaenoic Acid)

FORMULATION
Each softgel contains the following omega-3 fatty acid potency.
SuperEPA 2000
1000 mg
SuperEPA 1200
720 mg
SuperEPA 1000
350 mg
All strengths are cholesterol free! No Vitamin A & D or sodium are added and each product is free of toxic metals.

PHYSIOLOGICAL CONSIDERATIONS
Advanced Nutritional Technology introduces the latest development in omega-3 fatty acid therapy. All of our highly concentrated fish oils are now in their natural triglyceride form. Compared with the commonly used ethyl ester form, the natural triglyceride form is better absorbed by the body. Moreover, natural triglyceride is more stable than the free fatty acid form occasionally used—guaranteeing a product that is not rancid with peroxides.

Taken for its cardiovascular benefits, SuperEPA fish oil concentrate in its natural triglyceride form provides more omega-3 fatty acids per milligram of fish body oil in each capsule than our previous formula. Available in three strengths, you can choose the potency that best meets your dietary needs.

SuperEPA 2000 contains the highest concentration of triglyceride fish oil concentrate at 1,250 mg, providing 80% pure omega-3 fatty acids (or 1000 mg) in one capsule. At a dosage of only one or two capsules daily, this strength is the most convenient and promotes better compliance with users.

DOSAGE
SuperEPA 2000
One to two softgels daily, taken with meals.
SuperEPA 1200
One to three softgels daily, taken with meals.
SuperEPA 1000
One to six softgels daily, taken with meals

HOW SUPPLIED

	SIZE	NDC #
SuperEPA® 2000	30's	62617-050-01
	60's	62617-050-02
	90's	62617-050-03
SuperEPA® 1200	60's	62617-045-02
	90's	62617-045-03
SuperEPA® 1000	60's	62617-040-02
	90's	62617-040-03

Akorn, Inc.
100 AKORN DRIVE
ABITA SPRINGS, LA 70420

Direct Inquiries to:
Customer Service
(800) 535-7155
(504) 893-9300

OPHTHALMIC PRODUCTS

For information on Akorn ophthalmic pharmaceutical products, consult the PDR For Ophthalmology. For literature, sample material or service items, please contact Akorn, Inc. directly. (800) 535-7155

INAPSINE®   ℞
(Droperidol) Injection
FOR INTRAVENOUS OR INTRAMUSCULAR USE ONLY

DESCRIPTION
INAPSINE (droperidol) is a neuroleptic (tranquilizer) agent available in ampoules. Each milliliter contains 2.5 mg of droperidol in an aqueous solution adjusted to pH 3.4 ± 0.4 with lactic acid. Droperidol is chemically identified as 1-(1-[3-(p-fluorobenzoyl) propyl]-1,2,3,6-tetrahydro-4-pyridyl)-2-benzimidazolinone with a molecular weight of 379.43. The structural formula of INAPSINE is:

INAPSINE is a sterile, non-pyrogenic, aqueous solution for intravenous or intramuscular injection.

CLINICAL PHARMACOLOGY
INAPSINE (droperidol) produces marked tranquilization and sedation. It allays apprehension and provides a state of mental detachment and indifference while maintaining a state of reflex alertness.

INAPSINE produces an antiemetic effect as evidenced by the antagonism of apomorphine in dogs. It lowers the incidence of nausea and vomiting during surgical procedures and provides antiemetic protection in the postoperative period.

INAPSINE potentiates other CNS depressants. It produces mild alpha-adrenergic blockade, peripheral vascular dilatation and reduction of the pressor effect of epinephrine. It can produce hypotension and decreased peripheral vascular resistance and may decrease pulmonary arterial pressure (particularly if it is abnormally high). It may reduce the incidence of epinephrine-induced arrhythmias, but it does not prevent other cardiac arrhythmias.

The onset of action of single intramuscular and intravenous doses is from three to ten minutes following administration, although the peak effect may not be apparent for up to thirty minutes. The duration of the tranquilizing and sedative effects generally is two to four hours, although alteration of alertness may persist for as long as twelve hours.

INDICATIONS AND USAGE
INAPSINE (droperidol) is indicated:
- to produce tranquilization and to reduce the incidence of nausea and vomiting in surgical and diagnostic procedures.
- for premedication, induction, and as an adjunct in the maintenance of general and regional anesthesia.

- in neuroleptanalgesia in which INAPSINE is given concurrently with an opioid analgesic, such as SUBLIMAZE® (fentanyl citrate) Injection, to aid in producing tranquility and decreasing anxiety and pain.

CONTRAINDICATIONS
INAPSINE (droperidol) is contraindicated in patients with known hypersensitivity to the drug.

WARNINGS
FLUIDS AND OTHER COUNTERMEASURES TO MANAGE HYPOTENSION SHOULD BE READILY AVAILABLE.

As with other CNS depressant drugs, patients who have received INAPSINE (droperidol) should have appropriate surveillance.

It is recommended that opioids, when required, initially be used in reduced doses.

As with other neuroleptic agents, very rare reports of neuroleptic malignant syndrome (altered consciousness, muscle rigidity and autonomic instability) have occurred in patients who have received INAPSINE (droperidol).

Since it may be difficult to distinguish neuroleptic malignant syndrome from malignant hyperpyrexia in the perioperative period, prompt treatment with dantrolene should be considered if increases in temperature, heart rate or carbon dioxide production occur.

Cases of sudden death have been reported following use of droperidol at high doses (generally 25 mg or greater) in patients at risk for cardiac dysrhythmia due to anoxia, hypercarbia, severe electrolyte disturbances, or alcohol withdrawal. While these reports do not establish the cause of such death, QT prolongation after INAPSINE administration has been reported and there is at least one case of nonfatal torsade de pointes confirmed by rechallenge.

Because of these reports, INAPSINE is not recommended in the treatment of alcohol withdrawal or in other clinical situations where high doses are likely to be needed in patients at risk for dysrhythmia.

PRECAUTIONS
General: The initial dose of INAPSINE (droperidol) should be appropriately reduced in elderly, debilitated and other poor-risk patients. The effect of the initial dose should be considered in determining incremental doses.

Certain forms of conduction anesthesia, such as spinal anesthesia and some peridural anesthetics, can alter respiration by blocking intercostal nerves and can cause peripheral vasodilatation and hypotension because of sympathetic blockade. Through other mechanisms (see CLINICAL PHARMACOLOGY), INAPSINE can also alter circulation. Therefore, when INAPSINE is used to supplement these forms of anesthesia, the anesthetist should be familiar with the physiological alterations involved, and be prepared to manage them in the patients elected for these forms of anesthesia.

If hypotension occurs, the possibility of hypovolemia should be considered and managed with appropriate parenteral fluid therapy. Repositioning the patient to improve venous return to the heart should be considered when operative conditions permit. It should be noted that in spinal and peridural anesthesia, tilting the patient into a head-down position may result in a higher level of anesthesia than is desirable, as well as impair venous return to the heart. Care should be exercised in moving and positioning of patients because of a possibility of orthostatic hypotension. If volume expansion with fluids plus these other countermeasures do not correct the hypotension, then the administration of pressor agents other than epinephrine should be considered. Epinephrine may paradoxically decrease the blood pressure in patients treated with INAPSINE due to the alpha-adrenergic blocking action of INAPSINE.

Since INAPSINE may decrease pulmonary arterial pressure, this fact should be considered by those who conduct diagnostic or surgical procedures where interpretation of pulmonary arterial pressure measurements might determine final management of the patient.

Vital signs should be monitored routinely.

When the EEG is used for postoperative monitoring, it may be found that the EEG pattern returns to normal slowly.

Impaired Hepatic or Renal Function: INAPSINE should be administered with caution to patients with liver and kidney dysfunction because of the importance of these organs in the metabolism and excretion of drugs.

Pheochromocytoma: In patients with diagnosed/suspected pheochromocytoma, severe hypertension and tachycardia have been observed after the administration of INAPSINE (droperidol).

Drug Interactions: Other CNS depressant drugs (e.g. barbiturates, tranquilizers, opioids and general anesthetics) have additive or potentiating effects with INAPSINE. When patients have received such drugs, the dose of INAPSINE required will be less than usual. Following the administration of INAPSINE, the dose of other CNS depressant drugs should be reduced.

Carcinogenesis, Mutagenesis, Impairment of Fertility: No carcinogenicity studies have been carried out with INAP-

SINE. The micronucleus test in female rats revealed no mutagenic effects in single oral doses as high as 160 mg/kg. An oral study in rats (Segment I) revealed no impairment of fertility in either male or females at 0.63, 2.5 and 10 mg/kg doses (approximately 2, 9 and 36 times maximum recommended human iv/im dosage).

Pregnancy—Category C: INAPSINE administered intravenously has been shown to cause a slight increase in mortality of the newborn rat at 4.4 times the upper human dose. At 44 times the upper human dose, mortality rate was comparable to that for control animals. Following intramuscular administration, increased mortality of the offspring at 1.8 times the upper human dose is attributed to CNS depression in the dams who neglected to remove placentae from their offspring. INAPSINE has not been shown to be teratogenic in animals. There are no adequate and well-controlled studies in pregnant women. INAPSINE should be used during pregnancy only if the potential benefit justifies the potential risk to the fetus.

Labor and Delivery: There are insufficient data to support the use of INAPSINE in labor and delivery. Therefore, such use is not recommended.

Nursing Mothers: It is not known whether INAPSINE is excreted in human milk. Because many drugs are excreted in human milk, caution should be excercised when INAPSINE is administered to a nursing mother.

Pediatric Use: The safety of INAPSINE in children younger than two years of age has not been established.

ADVERSE REACTIONS

The most common somatic adverse reactions reported to occur with INAPSINE (droperidol) are mild to moderate hypotension and tachycardia, but these effects usually subside without treatment. If hypotension occurs and is severe or persists, the possibility of hypovolemia should be considered and managed with appropriate parenteral fluid therapy.

The most common behavioral adverse effects of INAPSINE (droperidol) include dysphoria, postoperative drowsiness, restlessness, hyperactivity and anxiety, which can either be the result of an inadequate dosage (lack of adequate treatment effect) or of an adverse drug reaction (part of the symptom complex of akathisia).

Care should be taken to search for extrapyramidal signs and symptoms (dystonia, akathisia, oculogyric crisis) to differentiate these different clinical conditions. When extrapyramidal symptoms are the cause, they can usually be controlled with anticholinergic agents.

Postoperative hallucinatory episodes (sometimes associated with transient periods of mental depression) have also been reported.

Other less common reported adverse reactions include anaphylaxis, dizziness, chills and/or shivering, laryngospasm, and bronchospasm.

Elevated blood pressure, with or without pre-existing hypertension, has been reported following administration of INAPSINE combined with SUBLIMAZE (fentanyl citrate) or other parenteral analgesics. This might be due to unexplained alterations in sympathetic activity following large doses; however, it is also frequently attributed to anesthetic or surgical stimulation during light anesthesia.

OVERDOSAGE

Manifestations: The manifestations of INAPSINE (droperidol) overdosage are an extension of its pharmacologic actions.

Treatment: In the presence of hypoventilation or apnea, oxygen should be administered and respiration should be assisted or controlled as indicated. A patent airway must be maintained; an oropharyngeal airway or endotracheal tube might be indicated. The patient should be carefully observed for 24 hours; body warmth and adequate fluid intake should be maintained. If hypotension occurs and is severe or persists, the possibility of hypovolemia should be considered and managed with appropriate parenteral fluid therapy. (See PRECAUTIONS).

If significant extrapyramidal reactions occur in the context of an overdose, an anticholinergic should be administered.

The intravenous LD_{50} of INAPSINE is 20–43 mg/kg in mice; 30 mg/kg in rats; 25 mg/kg in dogs and 11–13 mg/kg in rabbits. The intramuscular LD_{50} of INAPSINE is 195 mg/kg in mice; 104–110 mg/kg in rats; 97 mg/kg in rabbits and 200 mg/kg in guinea pigs.

DOSAGE AND ADMINISTRATION

Dosage should be individualized. Some of the factors to be considered in determining the dose are age, body weight, physical status, underlying pathological condition, use of other drugs, type of anesthesia to be used and the surgical procedure involved.

Vital signs should be monitored routinely.

Usual Adult Dosage

I. **Premedication**—(to be appropriately modified in the elderly, debilitated and those who have received other depressant drugs) 2.5 to 10 mg (1 to 4 mL) may be administered intramuscularly 30 to 60 minutes preoperatively.

II. **Adjunct to General Anesthesia—**
Induction—2.5 mg (1 mL) per 20 to 25 pounds may be administered (usually intravenously) along with an analgesic and/or general anesthetic. Smaller doses may be adequate. The total amount of INAPSINE (droperidol) administered should be titrated to obtain the desired effect based on the individual patient's response.
Maintenance—1.25 to 2.5 mg (0.5 to 1 mL) usually intravenously.

III. *Use without a general anesthetic in diagnostic procedures* —Administer the usual I.M. premedication 2.5 to 10 mg (1 to 4 mL) 30 to 60 minutes before the procedure. Additional 1.25 to 2.5 mg (0.5 to 1 mL) amounts of INAPSINE may be administered, usually intravenously.
NOTE: When INAPSINE is used in certain procedures, such as bronchoscopy, appropriate topical anesthesia is still necessary.

IV. *Adjunct to regional anesthesia*—2.5 to 5 mg (1 to 2 mL) may be administered intramuscularly or slowly intravenously when additional sedation is required.

Usual Children's Dosage

For children two to 12 years of age, a reduced dose as low as 1.0 to 1.5 mg (0.4 to 0.6 mL) per 20 to 25 pounds is recommended for premedication or for induction of anesthesia.

See WARNINGS and PRECAUTIONS for use of INAPSINE with other CNS depressants and in patients with altered response.

Parenteral drug products should be inspected visually for particulate matter and discoloration prior to administration, whenever solution and container permit. If such abnormalities are observed, the drug should not be administered.

HOW SUPPLIED

INAPSINE (droperidol) Injection is available as:

NDC 11098-010-01, 2.5 mg/mL, 1 mL ampoules in packages of 10

NDC 11098-010-02, 2.5 mg/mL, 2 mL ampoules in packages of 10

PROTECT FROM LIGHT. STORE AT ROOM TEMPERATURE 15°C-30°C (59°F-86°F)

AKORN MANUFACTURING, INC.
Decator, Illinois 62525
ADPAON Rev. 2/96

SUBLIMAZE® Ⓒ ℞
(fentanyl citrate)
Injection

CAUTION: Federal Law Prohibits Dispensing Without Prescription

DESCRIPTION

SUBLIMAZE (fentanyl citrate) Injection is a potent narcotic analgesic. Each milliliter of solution contains fentanyl citrate equivalent to 50 μg of fentanyl base, adjusted to pH 4.0–7.5 with sodium hydroxide. SUBLIMAZE is chemically identified as N-(1-phenethyl-4-piperidyl) propionanilide citrate (1:1) with a molecular weight of 528.60. The empirical formula is $C_{22}H_{28}N_2O \cdot C_6H_8O_7$. The structural formula of SUBLIMAZE is:

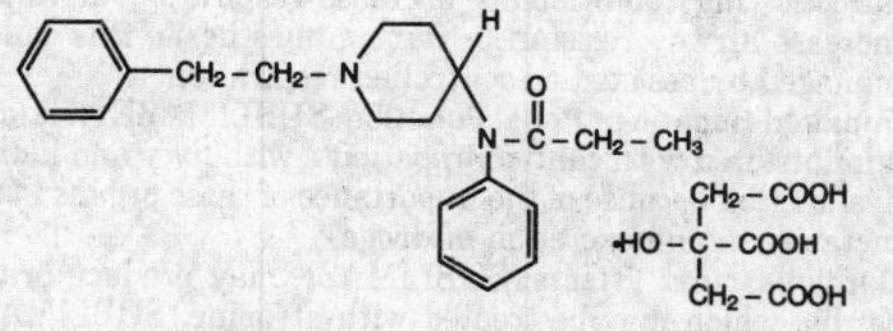

SUBLIMAZE is a sterile, non-pyrogenic, preservative free aqueous solution for intravenous or intramuscular injection.

CLINICAL PHARMACOLOGY

SUBLIMAZE (fentanyl citrate) is a narcotic analgesic. A dose of 100 μg (0.1 mg) (2.0 ml) is approximately equivalent in analgesic activity to 10 mg of morphine or 75 mg of meperidine. The principal actions of therapeutic value are analgesia and sedation. Alterations in respiratory rate and alveolar ventilation, associated with narcotic analgesics, may last longer than the analgesic effect. As the dose of narcotic is increased, the decrease in pulmonary exchange becomes greater. Large doses may produce apnea. SUBLIMAZE appears to have less emetic activity than either morphine or meperidine. Histamine assays and skin wheal testing in man indicate that clinically significant histamine release rarely occurs with SUBLIMAZE. Recent assays in man show no clinically significant histamine release in dosages up to 50 μg /kg (0.05 mg/kg) (1 ml/kg). SUBLIMAZE preserves cardiac stability, and blunts stress-related hormonal changes at higher doses.

The pharmacokinetics of SUBLIMAZE can be described as a three-compartment model, with a distribution time of 1.7 minutes, redistribution of 13 minutes and a terminal elimination half-life of 219 minutes. The volume of distribution for SUBLIMAZE is 4 L/kg.

SUBLIMAZE plasma protein binding capacity decreases with increasing ionization of the drug. Alterations in pH may affect its distribution between plasma and the central nervous system. It accumulates in skeletal muscle and fat, and is released slowly into the blood. SUBLIMAZE, which is primarily transformed in the liver, demonstrates a high first pass clearance and releases approximately 75% of an intravenous dose in urine, mostly as metabolites with less than 10% representing the unchanged drug. Approximately 9% of the dose is recovered in the feces, primarily as metabolites.

The onset of action of SUBLIMAZE is almost immediate when the drug is given intravenously; however, the maximal analgesic and respiratory depressant effect may not be noted for several minutes. The usual duration of action of the analgesic effect is 30 to 60 minutes after a single intravenous dose of up to 100 μg (0.1 mg) (2.0 ml). Following intramuscular administration, the onset of action is from seven to eight minutes, and the duration of action is one to two hours. As with longer acting narcotic analgesics, the duration of the respiratory depressant effect of SUBLIMAZE may be longer than the analgesic effect. The following observations have been reported concerning altered respiratory response to CO_2 stimulation following administration of SUBLIMAZE to man.

1. DIMINISHED SENSITIVITY TO CO_2 STIMULATION MAY PERSIST LONGER THAN DEPRESSION OF RESPIRATORY RATE. (Altered sensitivity to CO_2 stimulation has been demonstrated for up to four hours following a single dose of 600 μg (0.6 mg) (12 ml) SUBLIMAZE to healthy volunteers.) SUBLIMAZE frequently slows the respiratory rate, duration and degree of respiratory depression being dose related.
2. The peak respiratory depressant effect of a single intravenous dose of SUBLIMAZE is noted 5 to 15 minutes following injection. See also WARNINGS and PRECAUTIONS concerning respiratory depression.

INDICATIONS AND USAGE

SUBLIMAZE (fentanyl citrate) is indicated:

—for analgesic action of short duration during the anesthetic periods, premedication, induction and maintenance, and in the immediate postoperative period (recovery room) as the need arises.

—for use as a narcotic analgesic supplement in general or regional anesthesia.

—for administration with a neuroleptic such as INAPSINE® (droperidol) Injection as an anesthetic premedication, for the induction of anesthesia and as an adjunct in the maintenance of general and regional anesthesia.

—for use as an anesthetic agent with oxygen in selected high risk patients, such as those undergoing open heart surgery or certain complicated neurological or orthopedic procedures.

CONTRAINDICATIONS

SUBLIMAZE (fentanyl citrate) is contraindicated in patients with known intolerance to the drug or other opioid agonists.

WARNINGS

SUBLIMAZE (fentanyl citrate) SHOULD BE ADMINISTERED ONLY BY PERSONS SPECIFICALLY TRAINED IN THE USE OF INTRAVENOUS ANESTHETICS AND MANAGEMENT OF THE RESPIRATORY EFFECTS OF POTENT OPIOIDS.

AN OPIOID ANTAGONIST, RESUSCITATIVE AND INTUBATION EQUIPMENT AND OXYGEN SHOULD BE READILY AVAILABLE.

See also discussion of narcotic antagonists in PRECAUTIONS and OVERDOSAGE.

If SUBLIMAZE is administered with a tranquilizer such as INAPSINE (droperidol), the user should become familiar with the special properties of each drug, particularly the widely differing duration of action. In addition, when such a combination is used, fluids and other countermeasures to manage hypotension should be available.

As with other potent narcotics, the respiratory depressant effect of SUBLIMAZE may persist longer than the measured analgesic effect. The total dose of all narcotic analgesics administered should be considered by the practitioner before ordering narcotic analgesics during recovery from anesthesia. It is recommended that narcotics, when required, should be used in reduced doses initially, as low as $^1/_4$ to $^1/_3$ those usually recommended.

SUBLIMAZE may cause muscle rigidity, particularly involving the muscles of respiration. This rigidity has been reported to occur or recur infrequently in the extended postoperative period usually following high dose administration. In addition, skeletal muscle movements of various groups in the extremities, neck and external eye have been reported dur-

Continued on next page

Akorn—Cont.

ing induction of anesthesia with fentanyl; these reported movements have, on rare occasions, been strong enough to pose patient management problems. This effect is related to the dose and speed of injection and its incidence can be reduced by: 1) administration of up to 1/4 of the full paralyzing dose of a non-depolarizing neuromuscular blocking agent just prior to administration of SUBLIMAZE; 2) administration of a full paralyzing dose of a neuromuscular blocking agent following loss of eyelash reflex when SUBLIMAZE is used in anesthetic doses titrated by slow intravenous infusion; or, 3) simultaneous administration of SUBLIMAZE and a full paralyzing dose of a neuromuscular blocking agent when SUBLIMAZE is used in rapidly administered anesthetic dosages. The neuromuscular blocking agent used should be compatible with the patient's cardiovascular status.

Adequate facilities should be available for postoperative monitoring and ventilation of patients administered anesthetic doses of SUBLIMAZE. Where moderate or high doses are used (above 10 μg/kg), there must be adequate facilities for postoperative observation, and ventilation if necessary, of patients who have received SUBLIMAZE. It is essential that these facilities be fully equipped to handle all degrees of respiratory depression.

SUBLIMAZE may also produce other signs and symptoms characteristic of narcotic analgesics including euphoria, miosis, bradycardia and bronchoconstriction.

Severe and unpredictable potentiation by MAO inhibitors has been reported for other narcotic analgesics. Although this has not been reported for fentanyl, there are insufficient data to establish that this does not occur with fentanyl. Therefore, when fentanyl is administered to patients who have received MAO inhibitors within 14 days, appropriate monitoring and ready availability of vasodilators and beta-blockers for the treatment of hypertension is indicated.

Head Injuries and Increased Intracranial Pressure—SUBLIMAZE should be used with caution in patients who may be particularly susceptible to respiratory depression, such as comatose patients who may have a head injury or brain tumor. In addition, SUBLIMAZE may obscure the clinical course of patients with head injury.

PRECAUTIONS

General: The initial dose of SUBLIMAZE (fentanyl citrate) should be appropriately reduced in elderly and debilitated patients. The effect of the initial dose should be considered in determining incremental doses.

Nitrous oxide has been reported to produce cardiovascular depression when given with higher doses of SUBLIMAZE.

Certian forms of conduction anesthesia, such as spinal anesthesia and some peridural anesthetics, can alter respiration by blocking intercostal nerves. Through other mechanisms (see **CLINICAL PHARMACOLOGY**) SUBLIMAZE can also alter respiration. Therefore, when SUBLIMAZE is used to supplement these forms of anesthesia, the anesthetist should be familiar with the physiological alterations involved, and be prepared to manage them in the patients selected for these forms of anesthesia.

When a tranquilizer such as INAPSINE (droperidol) is used with SUBLIMAZE, pulmonary arterial pressure may be decreased. This fact should be considered by those who conduct diagnostic and surgical procedures where interpretation of pulmonary arterial pressure measurements might determine final management of the patient. When high dose or anesthetic dosages of SUBLIMAZE are employed, even relatively small dosages of diazepam may cause cardiovascular depression.

When SUBLIMAZE is used with a tranquilizer such as INAPSINE (droperidol), hypotension can occur. If it occurs, the possibility of hypovolemia should also be considered and managed with appropriate parenteral fluid therapy.

Repositioning the patient to improve venous return to the heart should be considered when operative conditions permit. Care should be exercised in moving and positioning of patients because of the possibility of orthostatic hypotension. If volume expansion with fluids plus other countermeasures do not correct hypotension, the administration of pressor agents other than epinephrine should be considered. Because of the alpha-adrenergic blocking action of INAPSINE (droperidol), epinephrine may paradoxically decrease the blood pressure in patients treated with INAPSINE (droperidol).

Elevated blood pressure, with and without pre-existing hypertension, has been reported following administration of SUBLIMAZE combined with INAPSINE (droperidol). This might be due to unexplained alterations in sympathetic activity following large doses; however, it is also frequently attributed to anesthetic and surgical stimulation during light anesthesia.

When INAPSINE (droperidol) is used with SUBLIMAZE and the EEG is used for postoperative monitoring, it may be found that the EEG pattern returns to normal slowly.

DOSAGE RANGE CHART

TOTAL DOSAGE

Low Dose—2 μg/kg (0.002 mg/kg) (0.04 ml/kg) SUBLIMAZE.	Moderate Dose—2–20 μg/kg (0.002–0.02 mg/kg) (0.04–0.4) ml/kg SUBLIMAZE.	High Dose—20–50 μg/kg (0.02–0.05 mg/kg) (0.4–1 ml/kg) SUBLIMAZE.
SUBLIMAZE in small doses is most useful for minor, but painful, surgical procedures. In addition to the analgesia during surgery, SUBLIMAZE may also provide some pain relief in the immediate postoperative period.	Where surgery becomes more major, a larger dose is required. With this dose, in addition to adequate analgesia, one would expect to see some abolition of the stress response. However, respiratory depression will be such that artificial ventilation during anesthesia is necessary and careful observation of ventilation postoperatively is essential.	During open heart surgery and certain more complicated neurosurgical and orthopedic procedures where surgery is more prolonged, and in the opinion of the anesthesiologist, the stress response to surgery would be detrimental to the well being of the patient, dosages of 20–50 μg/kg (0.02–0.05 mg) (0.4–1 ml) of SUBLIMAZE with nitrous oxide/oxygen have been shown to attenuate the stress response as defined by increased levels of circulating growth hormone, catecholamine, ADH and prolactin. When dosages in this range have been used during surgery, postoperative ventilation and observation are essential due to extended postoperative respiratory depression. The main objective of this technique would be to produce "stress free" anesthesia.

DOSAGE RANGE CHART

MAINTENANCE DOSAGE

Low Dose—2 μg/kg (0.002 mg/kg) (0.04 ml/kg) SUBLIMAZE.	Moderate Dose—2–20 μg/kg (0.002–0.02 mg/kg) (0.04–0.4 ml/kg) SUBLIMAZE.	High Dose—20–50 μg/kg (0.02–0.05 mg/kg) (0.4–1.0 ml/kg) SUBLIMAZE.
Additional dosages of SUBLIMAZE are infrequently needed in these minor procedures.	25 to 100 μg (0.025–0.1 mg) (0.5–2.0 ml) may be administered intravenously or intramuscularly when movement and/or changes in vital signs indicate surgical stress or lightening of analgesia.	Maintenance dosage (ranging from 25 μg (0.025 mg) (0.5 ml) to one half the initial loading dose) will be dictated by the changes in vital signs which indicate stress and lightening of analgesia. However, the additional dosage selected must be individualized especially if the anticipated remaining operative time is short.

Vital signs should be monitored routinely.

Respiratory depression caused by opioid analgesics can be reversed by opioid antagonists such as naloxone. Because the duration of respiratory depression produced by SUBLIMAZE may last longer than the duration of the opioid antagonist action, appropriate surveillance should be maintained. As with all potent opioids, profound analgesia is accompanied by respiratory depression and diminished sensitivity to CO_2 stimulation which may persist into or recur in the postoperative period. Respiratory depression secondary to chest wall rigidity has been reported in the postoperative period. Intraoperative hyperventilation may further alter postoperative response to CO_2. Appropriate postoperative monitoring should be employed to ensure that adequate spontaneous breathing is established and maintained in the absence of stimulation prior to discharging the patient from the recovery area.

Impaired Respiration: SUBLIMAZE should be used with caution in patients with chronic obstructive pulmonary disease, patients with decreased respiratory reserve, and others with potentially compromised respiration. In such patients, narcotics may additionally decrease respiratory drive and increase airway resistance. During anesthesia, this can be managed by assisted or controlled respiration.

Impaired Hepatic or Renal Function: SUBLIMAZE should be administered with caution in patients with liver and kidney dysfunction because of the importance of these organs in the metabolism and excretion of drugs.

Cardiovascular Effects: SUBLIMAZE may produce bradycardia, which may be treated with atropine. SUBLIMAZE should be used with caution in patients with cardiac bradyarrhythmias.

Drug Interactions: Other CNS depressant drugs (e.g. barbiturates, tranquilizers, narcotics and general anesthetics) will have additive or potentiating effects with SUBLIMAZE. When patients have received such drugs, the dose of SUBLIMAZE required will be less than usual. Following the administration of SUBLIMAZE, the dose of other CNS depressant drugs should be reduced.

Carcinogenesis, Mutagenesis, Impairment of Fertility: No carcinogenicity or mutagenicity studies have been conducted with SUBLIMAZE. Reproduction studies in rats revealed a significant decrease in the pregnancy rate of all experimental groups. This decrease was most pronounced in the high dosed group (1.25 mg/kg–12.5X human dose) in which one of twenty animals became pregnant.

Pregnancy—Category C: SUBLIMAZE has been shown to impair fertility and to have an embyocidal effect in rats when given in doses 0.3 times the upper human dose for a period of 12 days. No evidence of teratogenic effects have been observed after administration of SUBLIMAZE to rats. There are no adequate and well-controlled studies in pregnant women. SUBLIMAZE should be used during pregnancy only if the potential benefit justifies the potential risk to the fetus.

Labor and Delivery: There are insufficient data to support the use of SUBLIMAZE in labor and delivery. Therefore, such use is not recommended.

Nursing Mothers: It is not known whether this drug is excreted in human milk. Because many drugs are excreted in human milk, caution should be exercised when SUBLIMAZE is administered to a nursing woman.

Pediatric Use: The safety and efficacy of SUBLIMAZE in children under two years of age have not been established. Rare cases of unexplained clinically significant methemoglobinemia have been reported in premature neonates undergoing emergency anesthesia and surgery which included the combined use of fentanyl, pancuronium and atropine. A direct cause and effect relationship between the combined use of these drugs and the reported cases of methemoglobinemia has not been established.

ADVERSE REACTIONS

As with other narcotic anlagesics, the most common serious adverse reactions reported to occur with SUBLIMAZE (fentanyl citrate) are respiratory depression, apnea, rigidity, and bradycardia; if these remain untreated, respiratory arrest, circulatory depression or cardiac arrest could occur. Other adverse reactions that have been reported are hypertension, hypotension, dizziness, blurred vision, nausea, emesis, diaphoresis, pruritis, urticaria, laryngospasm and anaphylaxis. It has been reported that secondary rebound respiratory depression may occasionally occur postoperatively. Patients should be monitored for this possibility and appropriate countermeasures taken as necessary.

When a tranquilizer such as INAPSINE (droperidol) is used with SUBLIMAZE, the following adverse reactions can occur: chills and/or shivering, restlessness, and postoperative hallucinatory episodes (sometimes associated with transient periods of mental depression); extrapyramidal symptoms (dystonia, akathisia, and oculogyric crisis) have been observed up to 24 hours postoperatively. When they occur, extrapyramidal symptoms can usually be controlled with anti-parkinson agents. Postoperative drowsiness is also frequently reported following the use of INAPSINE (droperidol).

DRUG ABUSE AND DEPENDENCE

SUBLIMAZE (fentanyl citrate) is a Schedule II controlled drug substance that can produce drug dependence of the morphine type and therefore has the potential for being abused.

OVERDOSAGE

Manifestations: The manifestations of SUBLIMAZE (fentanyl citrate) overdosage are an extension of its pharmacologic actions (see CLINICAL PHARMACOLOGY) as with other

opioid analgesics. The intravenous LD_{50} of SUBLIMAZE is 3 mg/kg in rats, 1 mg/kg in cats, 14 mg/kg in dogs and 0.03 in monkeys.

Treatment: In the presence of hypoventilation or apnea, oxygen should be administered and respiration should be assisted or controlled as indicated. A patent airway must be maintained; an oropharyngeal airway or endotracheal tube might be indicated. If depressed respiration is associated with muscular rigidity, an intravenous neuromuscular blocking agent might required to facilitate assisted or controlled respiration. The patient should be carefully observed for 24 hours; body warmth and adequate fluid intake should be maintained. If hypotension occurs and is severe or persists, the possibility or hypovolemia should be considered and managed with appropriate parenteral fluid therapy. A specific narcotic antagonist such as nalorphine, levallorphan or naloxone should be available for use as indicated to manage respiratory depression. This does not preclude the use of more immediate countermeasures. The duration of respiratory depression following overdosage of SUBLIMAZE may be longer than the duration of narcotic antagonist action. Consult the package insert of the individual narcotic antagonists for details about use.

DOSAGE AND ADMINISTRATION

$$50 \ \mu g = 0.05 \ mg = 1 \ ml$$

Dosage should be individualized. Some of the factors to be considered in determining the dose are age, body weight, physical status, underlying pathological condition, use of other drugs, type of anesthesia to be used and the surgical procedure involved. Dosage should be reduced in elderly or debilitated patients (see PRECAUTIONS).
Vital signs should be monitored routinely.

I. Premedication—Premedication (to be appropriately modified in the elderly, debilitated and those who have received other depressant drugs)—50 to 100μg (0.05 to 0.1 mg) (1 to 2 ml) may be administered intramuscularly 30 to 60 minutes prior to surgery.

II. Adjunct to General Anesthesia—See Dosage Range Chart.

III. Adjunct to Regional Anesthesia-50 to 100 μg (0.05 to 0.1 mg) (1 to 2 ml) may be administered intramuscularly or slowly intravenously, over one to two minutes, when additional analgesia is required.

IV. Postoperatively (recovery room)-50 to 100 μg (0.05 to 0.1 mg) (1 to 2 ml) may be administered intramuscularly for the control of pain, tachypnea and emergence delirium. The dose may be repeated in one to two hours as needed.

Usage in Children: For induction and maintenance in children 2 to 12 years of age, a reduced dose as low as 2 to 3 μg/kg is recommended.
[See tables on top of preceding page.]

As a General Anesthetic
When attenuation of the responses to surgical stress is especially important, doses of 50 to 100 μg/kg (0.05 to 0.1 mg/kg) (1 to 2 ml/kg) may be administered with oxygen and a muscle relaxant. This technique has been reported to provide anesthesia without the use of additional anesthetic agents. In certain cases, doses up to 150 μg/kg (0.15 mg/kg) (3 ml/kg) may be necessary to produce this anesthetic effect. It has been used for open heart surgery and certain other major surgical procedures in patients for whom protection of the myocardium from excess oxygen demand is particularly indicated, and for certain complicated neurological and orthopedic procedures.
As noted above, it is essential that qualified personnel and adequate facilities be available for the management of respiratory depression.
See WARNINGS and PRECAUTIONS for use of SUBLIMAZE (fentanyl citrate) with other CNS depressants, and in patients with altered response.
Parenteral drug products should be inspected visually for particulate matter and discoloration prior to administration, whenever solution and container permit.

HOW SUPPLIED
SUBLIMAZE (fentanyl citrate) Injection is available as:
NDC 11098-030-02 50 μg/ml of fentanyl base, 2 ml ampoules in packages of 10
NDC 11098-030-05 50 μg/ml of fentanyl base, 5 ml ampoules in packages of 10
NDC 11098-030-10 50 μg/ml of fentanyl base, 10 ml ampoules in packages of 5
NDC 11098-030-20 50 μg/ml of fentanyl base, 20 ml ampoules in packages of 5
PROTECT FROM LIGHT. STORE AT CONTROLLED ROOM TEMPERATURE (59°–77°F/15°–25°C).
AKORN MANUFACTURING, INC.
Decatur, Illinois 62525

AFCA0N Rev. 2/96

Alcon Laboratories, Inc.
and its affiliates
CORPORATE HEADQUARTERS
PO BOX 6600
6201 SOUTH FREEWAY
FORT WORTH, TX 76134

Direct Inquiries to:
Sales Services
(817) 293-0450

For Medical Information Contact:
Medical Department
P.O. Box 6380
Fort Worth, TX 76115
(817) 293-0450

OPHTHALMIC PRODUCTS

For information on Alcon ophthalmic products, consult the PDR For Ophthalmology. See a complete listing of products in the Manufacturers' Index section of this book. For information, literature, samples or service items contact Alcon Sales Services.

ALOMIDE® 0.1%   ℞
(Lodoxamide Tromethamine Ophthalmic Solution)

DESCRIPTION
ALOMIDE® is a sterile ophthalmic solution containing the mast cell stabilizer lodoxamide tromethamine for topical administration to the eyes. Lodoxamide tromethamine is a white, crystalline, water-soluble powder with a molecular weight of 553.91.
Chemical Name:
N,N'-(2-chloro-5-cyano-m-phenylene)dioxamic acid tromethamine salt
Each mL of ALOMIDE® Ophthalmic Solution contains: Active: 1.78 mg lodoxamide tromethamine equivalent to 1 mg lodoxamide. **Preservative:** benzalkonium chloride 0.007%. **Inactive:** mannitol, hydroxypropyl methylcellulose 2910, sodium citrate, citric acid, edetate disodium, tyloxapol, hydrochloric acid and/or sodium hydroxide (adjust pH), and purified water.

CLINICAL PHARMACOLOGY
Lodoxamide tromethamine is a mast cell stabilizer that inhibits the *in vivo* Type 1 immediate hypersensitivity reaction. Lodoxamide therapy inhibits the increases in cutaneous vascular permeability that are associated with reagin or IgE and antigen-mediated reactions.
In vitro studies have demonstrated the ability of lodoxamide to stabilize rodent mast cells and prevent antigen-stimulated release of histamine. In addition, lodoxamide prevents the release of other mast cell inflammatory mediators (i.e., SRS-A, slow-reacting substances of anaphylaxis, also known as the peptidoleukotrienes) and inhibits eosinophil chemotaxis. Although lodoxamide's precise mechanism of action is unknown, the drug has been reported to prevent calcium influx into mast cells upon antigen stimulation.
Lodoxamide has no intrinsic vasoconstrictor, antihistaminic, cyclooxygenase inhibition, or other anti-inflammatory activity.
The disposition of ^{14}C-lodoxamide was studied in six healthy adult volunteers receiving a 3 mg (50 μCi) oral dose of lodoxamide. Urinary excretion was the major route of elimination. The elimination half-life of ^{14}C-lodoxamide was 8.5 hours in urine. In a study conducted in twelve healthy adult volunteers, topical administration of ALOMIDE® 0.1% (Lodoxamide Tromethamine Ophthalmic Solution), one drop in each eye four times per day for ten days, did not result in any measurable lodoxamide plasma levels at a detection limit of 2.5 ng/mL.

INDICATIONS AND USAGE
ALOMIDE® Ophthalmic Solution 0.1% is indicated in the treatment of the ocular disorders referred to by the terms vernal keratoconjunctivitis, vernal conjunctivitis, and vernal keratitis.

CONTRAINDICATIONS
Hypersensitivity to any component of this product.

WARNINGS
Not for injection. As with all ophthalmic preparations containing benzalkonium chloride, patients should be instructed not to wear soft contact lenses during treatment with ALOMIDE® Ophthalmic Solution.

PRECAUTIONS
General: Patients may experience a transient burning or stinging upon instillation of ALOMIDE® Ophthalmic Solution. Should these symptoms persist, the patient should be advised to contact the prescribing physician.

Carcinogenesis, Mutagenesis, Impairment of Fertility: A long-term study with lodoxamide tromethamine in rats (two-year oral administration) showed no neoplastic or tumorigenic effects at doses 100 mg/kg/day (more than 5000 times the proposed human clinical dose). No evidence of mutagenicity or genetic damage was seen in the Ames *Salmonella* Assay, Chromosomal Aberration in CHO Cells Assay, or Mouse Forward Lymphoma Assay. In the BALB/c-3T3 Cells Transformation Assay, some increase in the number of transformed foci was seen at high concentrations (greater than 4000 μg/mL). No evidence of impairment of reproductive function was shown in laboratory animal studies.
Pregnancy: Pregnancy Category B. Reproduction studies with lodoxamide tromethamine administered orally to rats and rabbits in doses of 100 mg/kg/day (more than 5000 times the proposed human clinical dose) produced no evidence of developmental toxicity. There are, however, no adequate and well-controlled studies in pregnant women. Because animal reproduction studies are not always predictive of human response, ALOMIDE® 0.1% (Lodoxamide Tromethamine Ophthalmic Solution) should be used during pregnancy only if clearly needed.
Nursing Mothers: It is not known whether lodoxamide tromethamine is excreted in human milk. Because many drugs are excreted in human milk, caution should be exercised when ALOMIDE® Ophthalmic Solution 0.1% is administered to nursing women.
Pediatric Use: Safety and effectiveness in pediatric patients below the age of 2 have not been established.

ADVERSE REACTIONS
During clinical studies of ALOMIDE® Ophthalmic Solution 0.1%, the most frequently reported ocular adverse experiences were transient burning, stinging, or discomfort upon instillation, which occurred in approximately 15% of the subjects. Other ocular events occurring in 1 to 5% of the subjects included ocular itching/pruritus, blurred vision, dry eye, tearing/discharge, hyperemia, crystalline deposits, and foreign body sensation. Events that occurred in less than 1% of the subjects included corneal erosion/ulcer, scales on lid/lash, eye pain, ocular edema/swelling, ocular warming sensation, ocular fatigue, chemosis, corneal abrasion, anterior chamber cells, keratopathy/keratitis, blepharitis, allergy, sticky sensation, and epitheliopathy.
Nonocular events reported were headache (1.5%) and (at less than 1%) heat sensation, dizziness, somnolence, nausea, stomach discomfort, sneezing, dry nose, and rash.

OVERDOSAGE
There have been no reports of ALOMIDE® 0.1% (Lodoxamide Tromethamine Ophthalmic Solution) overdose following topical ocular application. Accidental overdose of an oral preparation of 120 to 180 mg of lodoxamide resulted in a temporary sensation of warmth, profuse sweating, diarrhea, light-headedness, and a feeling of stomach distension; no permanent adverse effects were observed. Side effects reported following systemic oral administration of 0.1 mg to 10.0 mg of lodoxamide include a feeling of warmth or flushing, headache, dizziness, fatigue, sweating, nausea, loose stools, and urinary frequency/urgency. The physician may consider emesis in the event of accidental ingestion.

DOSAGE AND ADMINISTRATION
The dose for adults and children greater than two years of age is one to two drops in each affected eye four times daily for up to 3 months.

HOW SUPPLIED
ALOMIDE® Ophthalmic Solution 0.1% is supplied as follows: 10 mL in plastic ophthalmic DROP-TAINER® dispenser.

10 mL: **NDC** 0065-0345-10

STORAGE
Store at 15°C–27°C (59°F–80°F).

CAUTION
Federal (USA) law prohibits dispensing without prescription.

BETOPTIC®   ℞
(betaxolol hydrochloride)
0.5% as base
Sterile Ophthalmic Solution

DESCRIPTION
BETOPTIC® Sterile Ophthalmic Solution contains betaxolol hydrochloride, a cardioselective beta-adrenergic receptor blocking agent, in a sterile isotonic solution. Betaxolol hydrochloride is a white, crystalline powder, soluble in water, with a molecular weight of 343.89.
Chemical Name:
(±)-1-[p-[2-(Cyclopropylmethoxy)ethyl]phenoxy]-3-(isopropylamino)-2-propanol hydrochloride.

Continued on next page

Alcon Laboratories—Cont.

Each mL of BETOPTIC Ophthalmic Solution (0.5%) contains: Active: 5.6 mg betaxolol hydrochloride equivalent to betaxolol base 5 mg. Preservative: Benzalkonium Chloride 0.01%. Inactives: Edetate Disodium, Sodium Chloride, Hydrochloric Acid and/or Sodium Hydroxide (to adjust pH), and Purified Water.

CLINICAL PHARMACOLOGY

Betaxolol HCl, a cardioselective (beta-1-adrenergic) receptor blocking agent, does not have significant membrane-stabilizing (local anesthetic) activity and is devoid of intrinsic sympathomimetic action. Orally administered beta-adrenergic blocking agents reduce cardiac output in healthy subjects and patients with heart disease. In patients with severe impairment of myocardial function, beta-adrenergic receptor antagonists may inhibit the sympathetic stimulatory effect necessary to maintain adequate cardiac function.

When instilled in the eye, BETOPTIC Ophthalmic Solution has the action of reducing elevated as well as normal intraocular pressure, whether or not accompanied by glaucoma. Ophthalmic betaxolol has minimal effect on pulmonary and cardiovascular parameters.

Ophthalmic betaxolol (one drop in each eye) was compared to timolol and placebo in a three-way crossover study challenging nine patients with reactive airway disease who were selected on the basis of having at least a 15% reduction in the forced expiratory volume in one second (FEV_1) after administration of ophthalmic timolol. Betaxolol HCl had no significant effect on pulmonary function as measured by FEV_1, Forced Vital Capacity (FVC) and FEV_1/VC. Additionally, the action of isoproterenol, a beta stimulant, administered at the end of the study was not inhibited by ophthalmic betaxolol. In contrast, ophthalmic timolol significantly decreased these pulmonary functions.
[See table below.]

No evidence of cardiovascular beta-adrenergic blockade during exercise was observed with betaxolol in a double-masked, three-way crossover study in 24 normal subjects comparing ophthalmic betaxolol, timolol and placebo for effect on blood pressure and heart rate. Mean arterial blood pressure was not affected by any treatment; however, ophthalmic timolol produced a significant decrease in the mean heart rate.
[See table above.]

CLINICAL STUDIES

Optic nerve head damage and visual field loss are the result of a sustained elevated intraocular pressure and poor ocular perfusion. BETOPTIC Ophthalmic Solution has the action of reducing elevated as well as normal intraocular pressure, and the mechanism of ocular hypotensive action appears to be a reduction of aqueous production as demonstrated by tonography and aqueous fluorophotometry. The onset of action with BETOPTIC Ophthalmic Solution can generally be noted within 30 minutes and the maximal effect can usually be detected 2 hours after topical administration. A single dose provides a 12-hour reduction in intraocular pressure. Clinical observation of glaucoma patients treated with BETOPTIC Ophthalmic Solution for up to three years shows that the intraocular pressure lowering effect is well maintained.

Clinical studies show that topical BETOPTIC Ophthalmic Solution reduces mean intraocular pressure 25% from baseline. In trials using 22 mmHg as a generally accepted index of intraocular pressure control, BETOPTIC Ophthalmic Solution was effective in more than 94% of the population studied, of which 73% were treated with the beta blocker alone. In controlled, double-masked studies, the magnitude and duration of the ocular hypotensive effect of BETOPTIC Ophthalmic Solution and ophthalmic timolol solution were clinically equivalent.

BETOPTIC Ophthalmic Solution has also been used successfully in glaucoma patients who have undergone a laser trabeculoplasty and have needed additional long-term ocular hypotensive therapy.

BETOPTIC Ophthalmic Solution has been well-tolerated in glaucoma patients wearing hard or soft contact lenses and in aphakic patients.

BETOPTIC Ophthalmic Solution does not produce miosis or accommodative spasm which are frequently seen with miotic agents. The blurred vision and night blindness often associated with standard miotic therapy are not associated with BETOPTIC Ophthalmic Solution. Thus, patients with central lenticular opacities avoid the visual impairment caused by a constricted pupil.

INDICATIONS AND USAGE

BETOPTIC Ophthalmic Solution has been shown to be effective in lowering intraocular pressure and is indicated in the treatment of ocular hypertension and chronic open-angle glaucoma. It may be used alone or in combination with other anti-glaucoma drugs.

In clinical studies BETOPTIC® was safely used to lower intraocular pressure in 47 patients with both glaucoma and reactive airway disease who were followed for a mean period of 15 months. However, caution should be used in treating patients with severe reactive airway disease or a history of asthma.

CONTRAINDICATIONS

Hypersensitivity to any component of is product. BETOPTIC Ophthalmic Solution is contraindicated in patients with sinus bradycardia, greater than a first degree atrioventricular block, cardiogenic shock, or patients with overt cardiac failure.

WARNING

Topically applied beta-adrenergic blocking agents may be absorbed systemically. The same adverse reactions found with systemic administration of beta-adrenergic blocking agents may occur with topical administration. For example, severe respiratory reactions and cardiac reactions, including death due to bronchospasm in patients with asthma, and rarely death in association with cardiac failure, have been reported with topical application of beta-adrenergic blocking agents.

BETOPTIC Ophthalmic Solution has been shown to have a minor effect on heart rate and blood pressure in clinical studies. Caution should be used in treating patients with a history of cardiac failure or heart block. Treatment with BETOPTIC Ophthalmic Solution should be discontinued at the first signs of cardiac failure.

PRECAUTIONS

General: Information for Patients. Do not touch dropper tip to any surface as this may contaminate the solution.

Diabetes Mellitus. Beta-adrenergic blocking agents should be administered with caution in patients subject to spontaneous hypoglycemia or to diabetic patients (especially those with labile diabetes) who are receiving insulin or oral hypoglycemic agents. Beta-adrenergic receptor blocking agents may mask the signs and symptoms of acute hypoglycemia.

Thyrotoxicosis. Beta-adrenergic blocking agents may mask certain clinical signs (e.g., tachycardia) of hyperthyroidism. Patients suspected of developing thyrotoxicosis should be managed carefully to avoid abrupt withdrawal of beta-adrenergic blocking agents, which might precipitate a thyroid storm.

Muscle Weakness. Beta-adrenergic blockade has been reported to potentiate muscle weakness consistent with certain myasthenic symptoms (e.g., diplopia, ptosis, and generalized weakness).

Major Surgery. Consideration should be given to the gradual withdrawal of beta-adrenergic blocking agents prior to general anesthesia because of the reduced ability of the heart to respond to beta-adrenergically mediated sympathetic reflex stimuli.

Pulmonary. Caution should be exercised in the treatment of glaucoma patients with excessive restriction of pulmonary function. There have been reports of asthmatic attacks and pulmonary distress during betaxolol treatment. Although rechallenges of some such patients with ophthalmic betaxolol has not adversely affected pulmonary function test results, the possibility of adverse pulmonary effects in patients sensitive to beta blockers cannot be ruled out.

Risk from Anaphylactic Reaction: While taking beta-blockers, patients with a history of atopy or a history of severe anaphylactic reaction to a variety of allergens may be more reactive to repeated accidental, diagnostic, or therapeutic challenge with such allergens. Such patients may be unresponsive to the usual doses of epinephrine used to treat anaphylactic reactions.

Drug Interactions: Patients who are receiving a beta-adrenergic blocking agent orally and BETOPTIC Ophthalmic Solution should be observed for a potential additive effect either on the intraocular pressure or on the known systemic effects of beta blockade.

Close observation of the patient is recommended when a beta blocker is administered to patients receiving catecholamine-depleting drugs such as reserpine, because of possible additive effects and the production of hypotension and/or bradycardia.

Betaxolol is an adrenergic blocking agent; therefore, caution should be exercised in patients using concomitant adrenergic psychotropic drugs.

Ocular: In patients with angle-closure glaucoma, the immediate treatment objective is to reopen the angle by constriction of the pupil with a miotic agent. Betaxolol has little or no effect on the pupil. When BETOPTIC Ophthalmic Solution is used to reduce elevated intraocular pressure in angle-closure glaucoma, it should be used with a miotic and not alone.

Carcinogenesis, Mutagenesis, Impairment of Fertility: Lifetime studies with betaxolol HCl have been completed in mice at oral doses of 6, 20 or 60 mg/kg/day and in rats at 3, 12 or 48 mg/kg/day; betaxolol HCl demonstrated no carcinogenic effect. Higher dose levels were not tested.

In a variety of in vitro and in vivo bacterial and mammalian cell assays, betaxolol HCl was nonmutagenic.

Pregnancy: Pregnancy Category C. Reproduction, teratology, and peri- and postnatal studies have been conducted with orally administered betaxolol HCl in rats and rabbits. There was evidence of drug related postimplantation loss in

Mean Heart Rates[1]

Bruce Stress Exercise Test	TREATMENT		
Minutes	Betaxolol 1%[a]	Timolol 0.5%	Placebo
0	79.2	79.3	81.2
2	130.2	126.0	130.4
4	133.4	128.0*	134.3
6	136.4	129.2*	137.9
8	139.8	131.8*	139.4
10	140.8	131.8*	141.3

[1] Atkins, J. M. et al., Am. J. Oph. 99:173–175, Feb., 1985.
[a] Twice the clinical concentration.
* Mean pulse rate significantly lower for timolol than betaxolol or placebo ($p < 0.05$).

FEV_1 —Percent Change from Baseline[1]

	Means		
	Betaxolol 1.0%[a]	Timolol 0.5%	Placebo
Baseline	1.6	1.4	1.4
60 Minutes	2.3	−25.7*	5.8
120 Minutes	1.6	−27.4*	7.5
240 Minutes	−6.4	−26.9*	6.9
Isoproterenol[b]	36.1	−12.4*	42.8

[1] Schoene, R. B. et al., Am. J. Ophthal. 97:86, 1984.
[a] Twice the clinical concentration.
[b] Inhaled at 240 minutes; measurement at 270 minutes.
* Timolol statistically different from betaxolol and placebo ($p < 0.05$).

rabbits and rats at dose levels above 12 mg/kg and 128 mg/kg, respectively. Betaxolol HCl was not shown to be teratogenic, however, and there were no other adverse effects on reproduction at subtoxic dose levels. There are no adequate and well-controlled studies in pregnant women. BETOPTIC Ophthalmic Solution should be used during pregnancy only if the potential benefit justifies the potential risk to the fetus.

Nursing Mothers: It is not known whether betaxolol HCl is excreted in human milk. Because many drugs are excreted in human milk, caution should be exercised when BETOPTIC Ophthalmic Solution is administered to nursing women.

Pediatric Use: Safety and effectiveness in pediatric patients have not been established.

ADVERSE REACTIONS
The following adverse reactions have been reported in clinical trials with BETOPTIC Ophthalmic Solution.
Ocular: Discomfort of short duration was experienced by one in four patients, but none discontinued therapy; occasional tearing has been reported. Rare instances of decreased corneal sensitivity, erythema, itching sensation, corneal punctate staining, keratitis, anisocoria, edema, and photophobia have been reported.
Additional medical events reported with other formulations of betaxolol include blurred vision, foreign body sensation, dryness of the eyes, inflammation, discharge, ocular pain, decreased visual acuity, and crusty lashes.
Systemic: Systemic reactions following administration of BETOPTIC Ophthalmic Solution 0.5% or BETOPTIC S Ophthalmic Suspension 0.25% have been rarely reported. These include:
Cardiovascular: Bradycardia, heart block and congestive failure.
Pulmonary: Pulmonary distress characterized by dyspnea, bronchospasm, thickened bronchial secretions, asthma and respiratory failure.
Central Nervous System: Insomnia, dizziness, vertigo, headaches, depression, lethargy, and increase in signs and symptoms of myasthenia gravis.
Other: Hives, toxic epidermal necrolysis, hair loss and glossitis.

OVERDOSAGE
No information is available on overdosage of humans. The oral LD_{50} of the drug ranged from 350–920 mg/kg in mice and 860–1050 mg/kg in rats. The symptoms which might be expected with an overdose of a systemically administered beta-1-adrenergic receptor blocker agent are bradycardia, hypotension and acute cardiac failure. A topical overdose of BETOPTIC Ophthalmic Solution may be flushed from the eye(s) with warm tap water.

DOSAGE AND ADMINISTRATION
The recommended dose is one to two drops of BETOPTIC Ophthalmic Solution in the affected eye(s) twice daily. In some patients, the intraocular pressure lowering responses to BETOPTIC Ophthalmic Solution may require a few weeks to stabilize. As with any new medication, careful monitoring of patients is advised.
If the intraocular pressure of the patient is not adequately controlled on this regimen, concomitant therapy with pilocarpine and other miotics, and/or epinephrine and/or carbonic anhydrase inhibitors can be instituted.

HOW SUPPLIED
BETOPTIC Ophthalmic Solution is a sterile, isotonic, aqueous solution of betaxolol hydrochloride. Supplied as follows: 2.5, 5, 10 and 15 mL in plastic ophthalmic DROP-TAINER® dispensers.

2.5 mL: **NDC** 0065-0245-20
5 mL: **NDC** 0065-0245-05
10 mL: **NDC** 0065-0245-10
15 mL: **NDC** 0065-0245-15

STORAGE
Store at room temperature.

CAUTION
Federal (USA) law prohibits dispensing without prescription.
U.S. Patents Nos. 4,252,984; 4,311,708; 4,342,783

BETOPTIC® S   ℞
(betaxolol HCl)
0.25% as base
Sterile Ophthalmic Suspension

DESCRIPTION
BETOPTIC S Ophthalmic Suspension 0.25% contains betaxolol hydrochloride, a cardioselective beta-adrenergic receptor blocking agent, in a sterile resin suspension formulation. Betaxolol hydrochloride is a white, crystalline powder, with a molecular weight of 343.89.

Chemical Name:
(±)-1-[p-[2-(cyclopropylmethoxy)ethyl]phenoxy]-3-(isopropylamino)-2-propanol hydrochloride.
Each mL of BETOPTIC S Ophthalmic Suspension contains:
Active: betaxolol HCl 2.8 mg equivalent to 2.5 mg of betaxolol base. Preservative: benzalkonium chloride 0.01%. Inactive: Mannitol, Poly(Styrene-Divinyl Benzene) sulfonic acid, Carbomer 934P, edetate disodium, hydrochloric acid or sodium hydroxide (to adjust pH) and purified water.

CLINICAL PHARMACOLOGY
Betaxolol HCl, a cardioselective (beta-1-adrenergic) receptor blocking agent, does not have significant membrane-stabilizing (local anesthetic) activity and is devoid of intrinsic sympathomimetic action. Orally administered beta-adrenergic blocking agents reduce cardiac output in healthy subjects and patients with heart disease. In patients with severe impairment of myocardial function, beta-adrenergic receptor antagonists may inhibit the sympathetic stimulatory effect necessary to maintain adequate cardiac function.
When instilled in the eye, BETOPTIC S Ophthalmic Suspension 0.25% has the action of reducing elevated intraocular pressure, whether or not accompanied by glaucoma. Ophthalmic betaxolol has minimal effect on pulmonary and cardiovascular parameters.
Elevated IOP presents a major risk factor in glaucomatous field loss. The higher the level of IOP, the greater the likelihood of optic nerve damage and visual field loss. Betaxolol has the action of reducing elevated as well as normal intraocular pressure and the mechanism of ocular hypotensive action appears to be a reduction of aqueous production as demonstrated by tonography and aqueous fluorophotometry. The onset of action with betaxolol can generally be noted within 30 minutes and the maximal effect can usually be detected 2 hours after topical administration. A single dose provides a 12-hour reduction in intraocular pressure.
In controlled, double-masked studies, the magnitude and duration of the ocular hypotensive effect of BETOPTIC S Ophthalmic Suspension 0.25% and BETOPTIC Ophthalmic Solution 0.5% were clinically equivalent. BETOPTIC S Suspension was significantly more comfortable than BETOPTIC Solution.
Ophthalmic betaxolol solution at 1% (one drop in each eye) was compared to placebo in a crossover study challenging nine patients with reactive airway disease. Betaxolol HCl had no significant effect on pulmonary function as measured by FEV_1, Forced Vital Capacity (FVC), FEV_1/FVC and was not significantly different from placebo. The action of isoproterenol, a beta stimulant, administered at the end of the study was not inhibited by ophthalmic betaxolol.
No evidence of cardiovascular beta adrenergic-blockade during exercise was observed with betaxolol in a double-masked, crossover study in 24 normal subjects comparing ophthalmic betaxolol and placebo for effects on blood pressure and heart rate.

INDICATIONS AND USAGE
BETOPTIC S Ophthalmic Suspension 0.25% has been shown to be effective in lowering intraocular pressure and may be used in patients with chronic open-angle glaucoma and ocular hypertension. It may be used alone or in combination with other intraocular pressure lowering medications.

CONTRAINDICATIONS
Hypersensitivity to any component of this product. BETOPTIC S Ophthalmic Suspension 0.25% is contraindicated in patients with sinus bradycardia, greater than a first degree atrioventricular block, cardiogenic shock, or patients with overt cardiac failure.

WARNING
Topically applied beta-adrenergic blocking agents may be absorbed systemically. The same adverse reactions found with systemic administration of beta-adrenergic blocking agents may occur with topical administration. For example, severe respiratory reactions and cardiac reactions, including death due to bronchospasm in patients with asthma, and rarely death in association with cardiac failure, have been reported with topical application of beta-adrenergic blocking agents.
BETOPTIC S Ophthalmic Suspension 0.25% has been shown to have a minor effect on heart rate and blood pressure in clinical studies. Caution should be used in treating patients with a history of cardiac failure or heart block. Treatment with BETOPTIC S Ophthalmic Suspension 0.25% should be discontinued at the first signs of cardiac failure.

PRECAUTIONS
General:
Diabetes Mellitus. Beta-adrenergic blocking agents should be administered with caution in patients subject to spontaneous hypoglycemia or to diabetic patients (especially those with labile diabetes) who are receiving insulin or oral hypoglycemic agents. Beta-adrenergic receptor blocking agents may mask the signs and symptoms of acute hypoglycemia.
Thyrotoxicosis. Beta-adrenergic blocking agents may mask certain clinical signs (e.g., tachycardia) of hyperthyroidism. Patients suspected of developing thyrotoxicosis should be

managed carefully to avoid abrupt withdrawal of beta-adrenergic blocking agents, which might precipitate a thyroid storm.
Muscle Weakness. Beta-adrenergic blockade has been reported to potentiate muscle weakness consistent with certain myasthenic symptoms (e.g., diplopia, ptosis and generalized weakness).
Major Surgery. Consideration should be given to the gradual withdrawal of beta-adrenergic blocking agents prior to general anesthesia because of the reduced ability of the heart to respond to beta-adrenergically mediated sympathetic reflex stimuli.
Pulmonary. Caution should be exercised in the treatment of glaucoma patients with excessive restriction of pulmonary function. There have been reports of asthmatic attacks and pulmonary distress during betaxolol treatment. Although rechallenges of some such patients with ophthalmic betaxolol has not adversely affected pulmonary function test results, the possibility of adverse pulmonary effects in patients sensitive to beta blockers cannot be ruled out.
Information for Patients: Do not touch dropper tip to any surface, as this may contaminate the contents. Do not use with contact lenses in eyes.
Drug Interactions: Patients who are receiving a beta-adrenergic blocking agent orally and BETOPTIC S Ophthalmic Suspension 0.25% should be observed for a potential additive effect either on the intraocular pressure or on the known systemic effects of beta blockade.
Close observation of the patient is recommended when a beta blocker is administered to patients receiving catecholamine-depleting drugs such as reserpine, because of possible additive effects and the production of hypotension and/or bradycardia.
Betaxolol is an adrenergic blocking agent; therefore, caution should be exercised in patients using concomitant adrenergic psychotropic drugs.
Risk from anaphylactic reaction: While taking beta-blockers, patients with a history of atopy or a history of severe anaphylactic reaction to a variety of allergens may be more reactive to repeated accidental, diagnostic, or therapeutic challenge with such allergens. Such patients may be unresponsive to the usual doses of epinephrine used to treat anaphylactic reactions.
Ocular: In patients with angle-closure glaucoma, the immediate treatment objective is to reopen the angle by constriction of the pupil with a miotic agent. Betaxolol has little or no effect on the pupil. When BETOPTIC S Ophthalmic Suspension 0.25% is used to reduce elevated intraocular pressure in angle-closure glaucoma, it should be used with a miotic and not alone.
Carcinogenesis, Mutagenesis, Impairment of Fertility: Lifetime studies with betaxolol HCl have been completed in mice at oral doses of 6, 20 or 60 mg/kg/day and in rats at 3, 12 or 48 mg/kg/day; betaxolol HCl demonstrated no carcinogenic effect. Higher dose levels were not tested.
In a variety of *in vitro* and *in vivo* bacterial and mammalian cell assays, betaxolol HCl was nonmutagenic.
Pregnancy:
Pregnancy Category C. Reproduction, teratology, and peri- and postnatal studies have been conducted with orally administered betaxolol HCl in rats and rabbits. There was evidence of drug related postimplantation loss in rabbits and rats at dose levels above 12 mg/kg and 128 mg/kg, respectively. Betaxolol HCl was not shown to be teratogenic, however, and there were no other adverse effects on reproduction at subtoxic dose levels. There are no adequate and well-controlled studies in pregnant women. BETOPTIC S should be used during pregnancy only if the potential benefit justifies the potential risk to the fetus.
Nursing Mothers: It is not known whether betaxolol HCl is excreted in human milk. Because many drugs are excreted in human milk, caution should be exercised when BETOPTIC S Ophthalmic Suspension 0.25% is administered to nursing women.
Pediatric Use: Safety and effectiveness in pediatric patients not have been established.

ADVERSE REACTIONS
Ocular: In clinical trials, the most frequent event associated with the use of BETOPTIC S Ophthalmic Suspension 0.25% has been transient ocular discomfort. The following other conditions have been reported in small numbers of patients: blurred vision, corneal punctate keratitis, foreign body sensation, photophobia, tearing, itching, dryness of eyes, erythema, inflammation, discharge, ocular pain, decreased visual acuity and crusty lashes.
Additional medical events reported with other formulations of betaxolol include allergic reactions, decreased corneal sensitivity, corneal punctate staining which may appear in dendritic formations, edema and anisocoria.
Systemic: Systemic reactions following administration of BETOPTIC S Ophthalmic Suspension 0.25% or BETOPTIC Ophthalmic Solution 0.5% have been rarely reported. These include:

Continued on next page

Alcon Laboratories—Cont.

Cardiovascular: Bradycardia, heart block and congestive failure.
Pulmonary: Pulmonary distress characterized by dyspnea, bronchospasm, thickened bronchial secretions, asthma and respiratory failure.
Central Nervous System: Insomnia, dizziness, vertigo, headaches, depression, lethargy, and increase in signs and symptoms of myasthenia gravis.
Other: Hives, toxic epidermal necrolysis, hair loss, and glossitis. Perversions of taste and smell have been reported.

OVERDOSAGE

No information is available on overdosage of humans. The oral LD50 of the drug ranged from 350–920 mg/kg in mice and 860–1050 mg/kg in rats. The symptoms which might be expected with an overdose of a systemically administered beta-1-adrenergic receptor blocking agent are bradycardia, hypotension and acute cardiac failure.
A topical overdose of BETOPTIC S Ophthalmic Suspension 0.25% may be flushed from the eye(s) with warm tap water.

DOSAGE AND ADMINISTRATION

The recommended dose is one to two drops of BETOPTIC S Ophthalmic Suspension 0.25% in the affected eye(s) twice daily. In some patients, the intraocular pressure lowering responses to BETOPTIC S may require a few weeks to stabilize. As with any new medication, careful monitoring of patients is advised.
If the intraocular pressure of the patient is not adequately controlled on this regimen, concomitant therapy with pilocarpine and other miotics, and/or epinephrine and/or carbonic anhydrase inhibitors can be instituted.

HOW SUPPLIED

BETOPTIC S Ophthalmic Suspension 0.25% is supplied as follows: 2.5, 5, 10 and 15 mL in plastic ophthalmic DROP-TAINER® dispensers.

2.5 mL: **NDC** 0065-0246-20
5 mL: **NDC** 0065-0246-05
10 mL: **NDC** 0065-0246-10
15 mL: **NDC** 0065-0246-15

STORAGE

Store upright at room temperature. Shake well before using.

CAUTION

Federal (USA) Law Prohibits Dispensing Without a Prescription.
U.S. Patents Nos. 4,252,984; 4,311,708; 4,342,783; 4,911,920.

CILOXAN® ℞

(Ciprofloxacin HCl)
0.3% as base
Sterile Ophthalmic Solution

DESCRIPTION

CILOXAN® (Ciprofloxacin HCl) Ophthalmic Solution is a synthetic, sterile, multiple dose, antimicrobial for topical ophthalmic use. Ciprofloxacin is a fluoroquinolone antibacterial active against a broad spectrum of gram-positive and gram-negative ocular pathogens. It is available as the monohydrochloride monohydrate salt of 1-cyclopropyl-6-fluoro-1,4-dihydro-4-oxo-7- (1-piperazinyl)-3-quinoline-carboxylic acid. It is a faint to light yellow crystalline powder with a molecular weight of 385.8.
Ciprofloxacin differs from other quinolones in that it has a fluorine atom at the 6-position, a piperazine moiety at the 7-position, and a cyclopropyl ring at the 1-position.
Each mL of CILOXAN Ophthalmic Solution contains: Active: Ciprofloxacin HCl 3.5 mg equivalent to 3 mg base. Preservative: Benzalkonium Chloride 0.006%. Inactive: Sodium Acetate, Acetic Acid, Mannitol 4.6%, Edetate Disodium 0.05%, Hydrochloric Acid and/or Sodium Hydroxide (to adjust pH) and Purified Water. The pH is approximately 4.5 and the osmolality is approximately 300 mOsm.

CLINICAL PHARMACOLOGY

Systemic Absorption: A systemic absorbtion study was performed in which CILOXAN Ophthalmic Solution was administered in each eye every two hours while awake for two days followed by every four hours while awake for an additional 5 days. The maximum reported plasma concentration of ciprofloxacin was less than 5 ng/mL. The mean concentration was usually less than 2.5 ng/mL.
Microbiology: Ciprofloxacin has *in vitro* activity against a wide range of gram-negative and gram-positive organisms. The bactericidal action of ciprofloxacin results from interference with the enzyme DNA gyrase which is needed for the synthesis of bacterial DNA.
Ciprofloxacin has been shown to be active against most strains of the following organisms both *in vitro* and in clinical infections. (See *Indications and Usage* section).
Gram-Positive:
Staphylococcus aureus (including methicillin-susceptible and methicillin-resistant strains), *Staphylococcus epidermidis, Streptococcus pneumoniae, Streptococcus* (Viridans Group)
Gram-Negative:
Haemophilus influenzae, Pseudomonas aeruginosa, Serratia marcescens
Ciprofloxacin has been shown to be active *in vitro* against most strains of the following organisms, however, *the clinical significance of these data is unknown:*
Gram-Positive:
Enterococcus faecalis (Many strains are only moderately susceptible), *Staphylococcus haemolyticus, Staphylococcus hominis, Staphylococcus saprophyticus, Streptococcus pyogenes*
Gram-Negative:
Acinetobacter calcoaceticus subsp. anitratus, Aeromonas caviae, Aeromonas hydrophila, Brucella melitensis, Campylobacter coli, Campylobacter jejuni, Citrobacter diversus, Citrobacter freundii, Edwardsiella tarda, Enterobacter aerogenes, Enterobacter cloacae, Escherichia coli, Haemophilus ducreyi, Haemophilus parainfluenzae, Klebsiella pneumoniae, Klebsiella oxytoca, Legionella pneumophila, Moraxella (Branhamella) catarrhalis, Morganella morganii, Neisseria gonorrhoeae, Neisseria meningitidis, Pasteurella multocida, Proteus mirabilis, Proteus vulgaris, Providencia rettgeri, Providencia stuartii, Salmonella enteritidis, Salmonella typhi, Shigella sonneii, Shigella flexneri, Vibrio cholerae, Vibrio parahaemolyticus, Vibrio vulnificus, Yersinia enterocolitica
Other Organisms: *Chlamydia trachomatis* (only moderately susceptible) and *Mycobacterium tuberculosis* (only moderately susceptible).
Most strains of *Pseudomonas cepacia* and some strains of *Pseudomonas maltophilia* are resistant to ciprofloxacin as are most anaerobic bacteria, including *Bacteroides fragilis* and *Clostridium difficile.*
The minimal bactericidal concentration (MBC) generally does not exceed the minimal inhibitory concentration (MIC) by more than a factor of 2. Resistance to ciprofloxacin *in vitro* usually develops slowly (multiple-step mutation).
Ciprofloxacin does not cross-react with other antimicrobial agents such as beta-lactams or aminoglycosides; therefore, organisms resistant to these drugs may be susceptible to ciprofloxacin.
Clinical Studies:
Following therapy with CILOXAN Ophthalmic Solution, 76% of the patients with corneal ulcers and positive bacterial cultures were clinically cured and complete re-epithelialization occurred in about 92% of the ulcers.
In 3 and 7 day multicenter clinical trials, 52% of the patients with conjunctivitis and positive conjunctival cultures were clinically cured and 70–80% had all causative pathogens eradicated by the end of treatment.

INDICATIONS AND USAGE

CILOXAN Ophthalmic Solution is indicated for the treatment of infections caused by susceptible strains of the designated microorganisms in the conditions listed below:
Corneal Ulcers: *Pseudomonas aeruginosa, Serratia marcescens*, Staphylococcus aureus, Staphylococcus epidermidis, Streptococcus pneumoniae, Streptococcus* (Viridans Group)*
Conjunctivitis: *Haemophilus influenzae, Staphylococcus aureus, Staphylococcus epidermidis, Streptococcus pneumoniae*
* Efficacy for this organism was studied in fewer than 10 infections.

CONTRAINDICATIONS

A history of hypersensitivity to ciprofloxacin or any other component of the medication is a contraindication to its use. A history of hypersensitivity to other quinolones may also contraindicate the use of ciprofloxacin.

WARNINGS

NOT FOR INJECTION INTO THE EYE.
Serious and occasionally fatal hypersensitivity (anaphylactic) reactions, some following the first dose, have been reported in patients receiving systemic quinolone therapy. Some reactions were accompanied by cardiovascular collapse, loss of consciousness, tingling, pharyngeal or facial edema, dyspnea, urticaria, and itching. Only a few patients had a history of hypersensitivity reactions. Serious anaphylactic reactions require immediate emergency treatment with epinephrine and other resuscitation measures, including oxygen, intravenous fluids, intravenous antihistamines, corticosteroids, pressor amines and airway management, as clinically indicated. Remove contact lenses before using.

PRECAUTIONS

General: As with other antibacterial preparations, prolonged use of ciprofloxacin may result in overgrowth of nonsusceptible organisms, including fungi. If superinfection occurs, appropriate therapy should be initiated. Whenever clinical judgment dictates, the patient should be examined with the aid of magnification, such as slit lamp biomicroscopy and, where appropriate, fluorescein staining.
Ciprofloxacin should be discontinued at the first appearance of a skin rash or any other sign of hypersensitivity reaction.
In clinical studies of patients with bacterial corneal ulcer, a white crystalline precipitate located in the superficial portion of the corneal defect was observed in 35 (16.6%) of 210 patients. The onset of the precipitate was within 24 hours to 7 days after starting therapy. In one patient, the precipitate was immediately irrigated out upon its appearance. In 17 patients, resolution of the precipitate was seen in 1 to 8 days (seven within the first 24–72 hours), in five patients, resolution was noted in 10–13 days. In nine patients, exact resolution days were unavailable; however, at follow-up examinations, 18–44 days after onset of the event, complete resolution of the precipitate was noted. In three patients, outcome information was unavailable. The precipitate did not preclude continued use of ciprofloxacin, nor did it adversely affect the clinical course of the ulcer or visual outcome. (SEE ADVERSE REACTIONS).
Information For Patients. Do not touch dropper tip to any surface, as this may contaminate the solution.
Drug Interactions: Specific drug interaction studies have not been conducted with ophthalmic ciprofloxacin. However, the systemic administration of some quinolones has been shown to elevate plasma concentrations of theophylline, interfere with the metabolism of caffeine, enhance the effects of the oral anticoagulant, warfarin, and its derivatives and have been associated with transient elevations in serum creatinine in patients receiving cyclosporine concomitantly.
Carcinogenesis, Mutagenesis, Impairment of Fertility: Eight *in vitro* mutagenicity tests have been conducted with ciprofloxacin and the test results are listed below:
Salmonella/Microsome Test (Negative)
E. coli DNA Repair Assay (Negative)
Mouse Lymphoma Cell Forward Mutation Assay (Positive)
Chinese Hamster V_{79} Cell HGPRT Test (Negative)
Syrian Hamster Embryo Cell Transformation Assay (Negative)
Saccharomyces cerevisiae Point Mutation Assay (Negative)
Saccharomyces cerevisiae Mitotic Crossover and Gene Conversion Assay (Negative)
Rat Hepatocyte DNA Repair Assay (Positive)
Thus, two of the eight tests were positive, but the results of the following three *in vivo* test systems gave negative results:
Rat Hepatocyte DNA Repair Assay
Micronucleus Test (Mice)
Dominant Lethal Test (Mice)
Long term carcinogenicity studies in mice and rats have been completed. After daily oral dosing for up to two years, there is no evidence that ciprofloxacin had any carcinogenic or tumorigenic effects in these species.
Pregnancy—Pregnancy Category C: Reproduction studies have been performed in rats and mice at doses up to six times the usual daily human oral dose and have revealed no evidence of impaired fertility or harm to the fetus due to ciprofloxacin. In rabbits, as with most antimicrobial agents, ciprofloxacin (30 and 100 mg/kg orally) produced gastrointestinal disturbances resulting in maternal weight loss and an increased incidence of abortion. No teratogenicity was observed at either dose. After intravenous administration, at doses up to 20 mg/kg, no maternal toxicity was produced and no embryotoxicity or teratogenicity was observed. There are no adequate and well controlled studies in pregnant women. CILOXAN Ophthalmic Solution should be used during pregnancy only if the potential benefit justifies the potential risk to the fetus.
Nursing Mothers: It is not known whether topically applied ciprofloxacin is excreted in human milk; however, it is known that orally administered ciprofloxacin is excreted in the milk of lactating rats and oral ciprofloxacin has been reported in human breast milk after a single 500 mg dose. Caution should be exercised when CILOXAN Ophthalmic Solution is administered to a nursing mother.
Pediatric Use: Safety and effectiveness in pediatric patients below the age of 1 year have not been established.
Although ciprofloxacin and other quinolones cause arthropathy in immature animals after oral administration, topical ocular administration of ciprofloxacin to immature animals did not cause any arthropathy and there is no evidence that the ophthalmic dosage form has any effect on the weight bearing joints.

ADVERSE REACTIONS

The most frequently reported drug related adverse reaction was local burning or discomfort. In corneal ulcer studies with frequent administration of the drug, white crystalline precipitates were seen in approximately 17% of patients (SEE PRECAUTIONS). Other reactions occurring in less than 10% of patients included lid margin crusting, crystals/scales, foreign body sensation, itching, conjunctival hyperemia and a bad taste following instillation. Additional events occuring in less than 1% of patients included corneal staining, keratopathy/keratitis, allergic reactions, lid edema, tearing, photophobia, corneal infiltrates, nausea and decreased vision.

OVERDOSAGE

A topical overdose of CILOXAN Ophthalmic Solution may be flushed from the eye(s) with warm tap water.

DOSAGE AND ADMINISTRATION

The recommended dosage regimen for the treatment of **corneal ulcers** is: Two drops into the affected eye every 15 minutes for the first six hours and then two drops into the affected eye every 30 minutes for the remainder of the first day. On the second day, instill two drops in the affected eye hourly. On the third through the fourteenth day, place two drops in the affected eye every four hours. Treatment may be continued after 14 days if corneal re-epithelialization has not occurred.

The recommended dosage regimen for the treatment of **bacterial conjunctivitis** is: One or two drops instilled into the conjunctival sac(s) every two hours while awake for two days and one or two drops every four hours while awake for the next five days.

HOW SUPPLIED

As a sterile ophthalmic solution: 2.5 mL and 5 mL in plastic DROP-TAINER® dispensers.

2.5 mL—NDC 0065-0656-25
5 mL —NDC 0065-0656-05

STORAGE

Store at 2° to 30°C (36° to 86°F). Protect from light.

ANIMAL PHARMACOLOGY

Ciprofloxacin and related drugs have been shown to cause arthropathy in immature animals of most species tested following oral administration. However, a one-month topical ocular study using immature Beagle dogs did not demonstrate any articular lesions.

CAUTION

Federal (USA) law prohibits dispensing without prescription.

U.S. Patent No. 4,670,444

EYE-STREAM®
Sterile Eye Irrigating Solution OTC

EYE-STREAM® is a sterile and stable irrigating solution that is specially designed and packaged for use in the eye(s). Formulated as a buffered salt solution, it closely approximates normal human tear fluid.

INGREDIENTS

Each mL contains: **Tonicity Agents:** Sodium Chloride 0.64%, Potassium Chloride 0.075%, Calcium Chloride Dihydrate 0.048%, Magnesium Chloride Hexahydrate 0.03%. **Buffering Agents:** Sodium Acetate Trihydrate 0.39%, Sodium Citrate Dihydrate 0.17%. **pH Adjusters:** Sodium Hydroxide and/or Hydrochloric Acid. **Preservative:** Benzalkonium Chloride 0.013%. **Purified Water.** The pH of the solution is in the physiologic range.

INDICATIONS

> FDA APPROVED USES
> For irrigating the eye to help relieve irritation, discomfort and burning by removing loose foreign material, air pollutants (smog or pollen), or chlorinated water.

WARNINGS

If you experience eye pain, changes in vision, continued redness or irritation of the eye, or if the condition worsens or persists, consult a doctor. Obtain immediate medical treatment for all open wounds in or near the eyes. If solution changes color or becomes cloudy, do not use. To avoid contamination, do not touch tip of container to any surface. Replace cap after using. Keep this and all drugs out of the reach of children. In case of accidental ingestion, seek professional assistance or contact a Poison Control Center immediately. Not to be used as a saline solution for rinsing and soaking soft contact lenses. NOT FOR INJECTION OR INTRAOCULAR SURGERY.

DIRECTIONS

Flush the affected eye as needed, controlling the rate of flow of solution by pressure on the bottle. Please read this carton carefully and keep for future reference.

HOW SUPPLIED

In 1 fluid ounce and 4 fluid ounce plastic squeeze bottles.
1 fl. oz: NDC 0065-0530-01
4 fl. oz.: NDC 0065-0530-04

STORAGE

Store at 8°–27°C (46°–80°F).

NAPHCON® A
Eye Drops OTC
Relieves Itching & Redness

Temporary relief of the minor eye symptoms of itching and redness caused by ragweed, pollen and animal hair.

DESCRIPTION

Active: Pheniramine Maleate 0.3%, Naphazoline Hydrochloride 0.025%. **Preservative:** Benzalkonium Chloride 0.01%. **Inactive:** Sodium Chloride, Boric Acid, Sodium Borate, Edetate Disodium 0.01%, Sodium Hydroxide and/or Hydrochloric Acid (to adjust pH), Purified Water. The sterile ophthalmic solution has a pH of about 6 and a tonicity of about 270 mOsm/Kg.

DIRECTIONS

Instill 1 or 2 drops in the affected eye(s) up to 4 times daily.

WARNINGS

To avoid contamination, do not touch tip of container to any surface. Replace cap after using.
If solution changes color or becomes cloudy, do not use.
If you experience eye pain, changes in vision, continued redness or irritation of the eye, or if the condition worsens, or persists for more than 72 hours, discontinue use and consult a physician. Overuse of this product may produce increased redness of the eye.
If you are sensitive to any ingredient in this product, do not use. Do not use use this product if you have heart disease, high blood pressure, difficulty in urination due to enlargement of the prostate gland or narrow angle glaucoma unless directed by a physician.
Accidental oral ingestion in infants and children may lead to coma and marked reduction in body temperature. Before using in children under 6 years of age, consult your physician.
Keep this and all drugs out of reach of children. In case of accidental ingestion, seek professional assistance or contact a Poison Control Center immediately.
Remove contact lenses before using.
Store at 36°–80°F (2°–27°C).
Protect from light.
Use before the expiration date marked on the carton or bottle.
Keep this and all drugs out of reach of children.

TEARS NATURALE® II
Lubricant Eye Drops OTC
TEARS NATURALE FREE®
Lubricant Eye Drops

DESCRIPTION

TEARS NATURALE II is the only lubricant eye drop preserved with safe, nonsensitizing POLYQUAD 0.001%. *In vitro* studies have shown that POLYQUAD substantially avoids the damaging effects of epithelial cell toxicity possible with other tear substitute preservatives and allows epithelial cell growth. POLYQUAD has been shown to be 99% reaction-free in normal subjects and 97% reaction-free in subjects known to be preservative sensitive. TEARS NATURALE FREE is a preservative-free version of TEARS NATURALE II.

With their unique mucin like polymeric formulation, and with their natural pH, low viscosity, and isotonicity, TEARS NATURALE II and TEARS NATURALE FREE provide dry eye patients with comfort and prompt relief of dry eye symptoms.

Sterile-For Topical Eye Use Only

INGREDIENTS

TEARS NATURALE II: Each mL contains:
Active: DUASORB®, a water soluble polymeric system containing Dextran 70 0.1% and Hydroxypropyl Methylcellulose 2910 0.3%.
Preservative: POLYQUAD® (Polyquaternium-1) 0.001%. **Inactive:** Sodium Borate, Potassium Chloride, Sodium Chloride, Purified Water. May contain Hydrochloric Acid and/or Sodium Hydroxide to adjust pH.
TEARS NATURALE FREE: Each mL contains:
Active: DUASORB, a water soluble polymeric system containing Dextran 70 0.1% and Hydroxypropyl Methylcellulose 2910 0.3%.
Inactive: Sodium Borate, Potassium Chloride, Sodium Chloride, Purified Water. May contain Hydrochloric Acid and/or Sodium Hydroxide to adjust pH.

INDICATIONS

For the temporary relief of burning and irritation due to dryness of the eye and for use as a protectant against further irritation. For temporary relief of discomfort due to minor irritations of the eye or to exposure to wind or sun.

WARNINGS

Remove contact lenses before using. If you experience eye pain, changes in vision, continued redness or irritation of the eye, or if the condition worsens or persists for more than 72 hours, discontinue use and consult a doctor.
If solution changes color or becomes cloudy, do not use.
To avoid contamination, do not touch tip of container to any surface. TEARS NATURALE II: Replace cap after using. TEARS NATURALE FREE: Do not reuse. Once opened, discard. Keep this and all drugs out of the reach of children. In case of accidental ingestion, seek professional assistance or contact a Poison Control Center immediately.

DIRECTIONS

TEARS NATURALE II: Instill 1 or 2 drops in the affected eye(s) as needed. TEARS NATURALE FREE: Completely twist off tab: do not pull. Instill 1 or 2 drops in the affected eye(s) as needed.

HOW SUPPLIED

TEARS NATURALE II Lubricant Eye Drops are supplied in 15 mL and 30 mL plastic DROP-TAINER® bottles.
15 mL NDC 0065-0418-15
30 mL NDC 0065-0418-32
TEARS NATURALE FREE Lubricant Eye Drops are supplied in boxes of 32 0.02 fl. oz. single-use containers.
NDC 0065-0416-32

STORAGE

Store at room temperature.

TOBRADEX® ℞
(Tobramycin and Dexamethasone)
Sterile Ophthalmic Suspension and Ointment

DESCRIPTION

TOBRADEX® (Tobramycin and Dexamethasone) Ophthalmic Suspension and Ointment are sterile, multiple dose antibiotic and steroid combinations for topical ophthalmic use.
Tobramycin
Chemical name:
O-3-Amino-3-deoxy-α-D-glucopyranosyl-$(1 \rightarrow 4)$-O-[2,6-diamino-2,3,6-trideoxy-α-D-$ribo$-hexopyranosyl-$(1 \rightarrow 6)$]-2-deoxy-L-streptamine
Dexamethasone
Chemical Name:
9-Fluoro-11β,17,21-trihydroxy-16α-methylpregna-1,4-diene-3,20-dione
Each mL of TOBRADEX® Suspension contains: Active: Tobramycin 0.3% (3 mg) and Dexamethasone 0.1% (1 mg). Preservative: Benzalkonium Chloride 0.01%. Inactives: Tyloxapol, Edetate Disodium, Sodium Chloride, Hydroxyethyl Cellulose, Sodium Sulfate, Sulfuric Acid and/or Sodium Hydroxide (to adjust pH) and Purified Water.
Each gram of TOBRADEX® Ointment contains: Actives: Tobramycin 0.3% (3 mg) and Dexamethasone 0.1% (1 mg). Inactives: Chlorobutanol 0.5%. Inactives: Mineral Oil and White Petrolatum.

CLINICAL PHARMACOLOGY

Corticoids suppress the inflammatory response to a variety of agents and they probably delay or slow healing. Since corticoids may inhibit the body's defense mechanism against infection, a concomitant antimicrobial drug may be used when this inhibition is considered to be clinically significant. Dexamethasone is a potent corticoid.
The antibiotic component in the combination (tobramycin) is included to provide action against susceptible organisms. *In vitro* studies have demonstrated that tobramycin is active against susceptible strains of the following microorganisms:
Staphylococci, including *S. aureus* and *S. epidermidis* (coagulase-positive and coagulase-negative), including penicillin-resistant strains.
Streptococci, including some of the Group A-beta-hemolytic species, some nonhemolytic species, and some *Streptococcus pneumoniae*.
Pseudomonas aeruginosa, Escherichia coli, Klebsiella pneumoniae, Enterobacter aerogenes, Proteus mirabilis, Morganella morganii, most *Proteus vulgaris* strains, *Haemophilus influenzae* and *H. aegyptius, Moraxella lacunata, Acinetobacter calcoaceticus* and some *Neisseria* species.
Bacterial susceptibility studies demonstrate that in some cases microorganisms resistant to gentamicin remain susceptible to tobramycin.
No data are available on the extent of systemic absorption from TOBRADEX® Ophthalmic Suspension or Ointment; however, it is known that some systemic absorption can occur with ocularly applied drugs. If the maximum dose of TOBRADEX Ophthalmic Suspension is given for the first 48 hours (two drops in each eye every 2 hours) and complete systemic absorption occurs, which is highly unlikely, the daily dose of dexamethasone would be 2.4 mg. The usual physiologic replacement dose is 0.75 mg daily. If TOBRADEX Ophthalmic Suspension is given after the first 48 hours as two drops in each eye every 4 hours, the administered dose of dexamethasone would be 1.2 mg daily. The ad-

Continued on next page

Alcon Laboratories—Cont.

ministered dose for TOBRADEX Ophthalmic Ointment in both eyes four times daily would be 0.4 mg of dexamethasone daily.

INDICATIONS AND USAGE

TOBRADEX® Ophthalmic Suspension and Ointment are indicated for steroid-responsive inflammatory ocular conditions for which a corticosteroid is indicated and where superficial bacterial ocular infection or a risk of bacterial ocular infection exists.

Ocular steroids are indicated in inflammatory conditions of the palpebral and bulbar conjunctiva, cornea and anterior segment of the globe where the inherent risk of steroid use in certain infective conjunctivitides is accepted to obtain a diminution in edema and inflammation. They are also indicated in chronic anterior uveitis and corneal injury from chemical, radiation or thermal burns, or penetration of foreign bodies. The use of a combination drug with an anti-infective component is indicated where the risk of superficial ocular infection is high or where there is an expectation that potentially dangerous numbers of bacteria will be present in the eye. The particular anti-infective drug in this product is active against the following common bacterial eye pathogens: Staphylococci, including *S. aureus* and *S. epidermidis* (coagulase-positive and coagulase-negative), including penicillin-resistant strains.

Streptococci, including some of the Group A-beta-hemolytic species, some nonhemolytic species, and some *Streptococcus pneumoniae*.

Pseudomonas aeruginosa, Escherichia coli, Klebsiella pneumoniae, Enterobacter aerogenes, Proteus mirabilis, Morganella morganii, most *Proteus vulgaris* strains, *Haemophilus influenzae* and *H. aegyptius, Moraxella lacunata,* and *Acinetobacter calcoaceticus* and some *Neisseria* species.

CONTRAINDICATIONS

Epithelial herpes simplex keratitis (dendritic keratitis), vaccinia, varicella, and many other viral diseases of the cornea and conjunctiva. Mycobacterial infection of the eye. Fungal diseases of ocular structures. Hypersensitivity to a component of the medication.

WARNINGS

NOT FOR INJECTION INTO THE EYE. Sensitivity to topically applied aminoglycosides may occur in some patients. If a sensitivity reaction does occur, discontinue use.

Prolonged use of steroids may result in glaucoma, with damage to the optic nerve, defects in visual acuity and fields of vision, and posterior subcapsular cataract formation. Intraocular pressure should be routinely monitored even though it may be difficult in children and uncooperative patients. Prolonged use may suppress the host response and thus increase the hazard of secondary ocular infections. In those diseases causing thinning of the cornea or sclera, perforations have been known to occur with the use of topical steroids. In acute purulent conditions of the eye, steroids may mask infection or enhance existing infection.

PRECAUTIONS

General. The possibility of fungal infections of the cornea should be considered after long-term steroid dosing. As with other antibiotic preparations, prolonged use may result in overgrowth of nonsusceptible organisms, including fungi. If superinfection occurs, appropriate therapy should be initiated. When multiple prescriptions are required, or whenever clinical judgement dictates, the patient should be examined with the aid of magnification, such as slit lamp biomicroscopy and, where appropriate, fluorescein staining.

Cross-sensitivity to other aminoglycoside antibiotics may occur; if hypersensitivity develops with this product, discontinue use and institute appropriate therapy.

Information for Patients: Do not touch dropper or tube tip to any surface, as this may contaminate the contents.

Carcinogenesis, Mutagenesis, Impairment of Fertility. No studies have been conducted to evaluate the carcinogenic or mutagenic potential. No impairment of fertility was noted in studies of subcutaneous tobramycin in rats at doses of 50 and 100 mg/kg/day.

Pregnancy Category C. Corticosteroids have been found to be teratogenic in animal studies. Ocular administration of 0.1% dexamethasone resulted in 15.6% and 32.3% incidence of fetal anomalies in two groups of pregnant rabbits. Fetal growth retardation and increased mortality rates have been observed in rats with chronic dexamethasone therapy. Reproduction studies have been performed in rats and rabbits with tobramycin at doses up to 100 mg/kg/day parenterally and have revealed no evidence of impaired fertility or harm to the fetus. There are no adequate and well-controlled studies in pregnant women. TOBRADEX® Ophthalmic Suspension and Ointment should be used during pregnancy only if the potential benefit justifies the potential risk to the fetus.

Nursing Mothers. Systemically administered corticosteroids appear in human milk and could suppress growth, interfere with endogenous corticosteroid production, or cause

other untoward effects. It is not known whether topical administration of corticosteroids could result in sufficient systemic absorption to produce detectable quantities in human milk. Because many drugs are excreted in human milk, caution should be exercised when TOBRADEX® Ophthalmic Suspension is administered to a nursing woman.

Pediatric Use. Safety and effectiveness in pediatric patients have not been established.

ADVERSE REACTIONS

Adverse reactions have occurred with steroid/anti-infective combination drugs which can be attributed to the steroid component, the anti-infective component, or the combination. Exact incidence figures are not available. The most frequent adverse reactions to topical ocular tobramycin (TOBREX®) are hypersensitivity and localized ocular toxicity, including lid itching and swelling, and conjunctival erythema. These reactions occur in less than 4% of patients. Similar reactions may occur with the topical use of other aminoglycoside antibiotics. Other adverse reactions have not been reported; however, if topical ocular tobramycin is administered concomitantly with systemic aminoglycoside antibiotics, care should be taken to monitor the total serum concentration. The reactions due to the steroid component are: elevation of intraocular pressure (IOP) with possible development of glaucoma, and infrequent optic nerve damage; posterior subcapsular cataract formation; and delayed wound healing.

Secondary Infection. The development of secondary infection has occurred after use of combinations containing steroids and antimicrobials. Fungal infections of the cornea are particularly prone to develop coincidentally with long-term applications of steroids. The possibility of fungal invasion must be considered in any persistent corneal ulceration where steroid treatment has been used. Secondary bacterial ocular infection following suppression of host responses also occurs.

OVERDOSAGE

Clinically apparent signs and symptoms of an overdose of TOBRADEX Ophthalmic Ointment (punctate keratitis, erythema, increased lacrimation, edema and lid itching) may be similar to adverse reaction effects seen in some patients.

DOSAGE AND ADMINISTRATION

Apply a small amount (approximately 1/2 inch ribbon) into the conjunctival sac(s) up to three or four times daily.

Suspension: One or two drops instilled into the conjunctival sac(s) every four to six hours. During the initial 24 to 48 hours, the dosage may be increased to one or two drops every two (2) hours. Frequency should be decreased gradually as warranted by improvement in clinical signs. Care should be taken not to discontinue therapy prematurely. **Ointment:** Apply a small amount (approximately $^1/_2$ inch ribbon) into the conjunctival sac(s) up to three or four times daily.

How to apply TOBRADEX Ophthalmic Ointment:
1. Tilt your head back.
2. Place a finger on your cheek just under your eye and gently pull down until a "V" pocket is formed between your eyeball and your lower lid.
3. Place a small amount (about 1/2 inch) of TOBRADEX Ophthalmic Ointment in the "V" pocket. Do not let the tip of the tube touch your eye.
4. Look downward before closing your eye.

Not more than 20 mL or 8 g should be prescribed initially and the prescription should not be refilled without further evaluation as outlined in PRECAUTIONS above.

HOW SUPPLIED

Sterile ophthalmic suspension in 2.5 mL (NDC 0065-0647-25) and 5 mL (NDC 0065-0647-05) DROP-TAINER® dispensers. Sterile ophthalmic ointment in 3.5 g ophthalmic tube (NDC 0065-0648-35).

STORAGE

Store 8° to 27°C (46° to 80°F).

Store suspension upright and shake well before using.

CAUTION

Federal (USA) law prohibits dispensing without prescription.

U.S. Patent No. 5,149,694

For information on over-the-counter drugs, consult **PDR For Nonprescription Drugs**

Allergan, Inc.
2525 DUPONT DRIVE
P.O. BOX 19534
IRVINE, CA 92623-9534

Direct Inquiries to:
(714) 752-4500

OPHTHALMIC PRODUCTS

For information on Allergan, Inc. prescription, OTC, and ophthalmic products, consult the Physicians' Desk Reference For Ophthalmology. For literature, service items or sample material, contact Allergan directly. See a complete listing of products in the Manufacturers' Index section of this book.

ACULAR® ℞
(ketorolac tromethamine) 0.5%
Sterile Ophthalmic Solution

PRODUCT OVERVIEW

ACULAR® Solution is the only topical NSAID indicated for the relief of ocular itching due to seasonal allergic conjunctivitis.

ACULAR® stops the itch associated with seasonal allergic conjunctivitis due in part to its ability to inhibit prostaglandin biosynthesis.

In two double-masked, paired studies (N=241), ACULAR® Solution was found to be superior to placebo in relieving the ocular itch of seasonal allergic conjunctivitis.[1]

ACULAR® Solution is also proven safe in clinical trials, and avoids steroid-like side effects (e.g., no significant effect upon IOP).[1] There is no significant ocular toxicity reported in clinical studies to date with ACULAR® (superficial keratitis reported in 1% of patients).

The most frequently reported adverse events have been transient stinging and burning on instillation (approximately 40%). Not for use while wearing contact lenses. Caution should be used in patients with sensitivities to other NSAIDs.

ACULAR® Solution is available in 3 mL and 5 mL plastic bottles with a controlled-dropper tip.

Please see full prescribing information included.
1. Data on file, Syntex (U.S.A.) Inc.

ACULAR® , a registered trademark of Syntex (U.S.A.) Inc., is manufactured and distributed by Allergan, Inc. under license from its developer, Syntex (U.S.A.) Inc., Palo Alto, CA.

ACULAR® is marketed by Allergan, Inc.

PRESCRIBING INFORMATION

ACULAR® ℞
(ketorolac tromethamine) 0.5%
Sterile Ophthalmic Solution

DESCRIPTION

ACULAR® (ketorolac tromethamine) is a member of the pyrrolo-pyrrole group of nonsteroidal anti-inflammatory drugs (NSAIDs) for ophthalmic use. Its chemical name is (±)-5-benzoyl-2,3-dihydro-1*H*-pyrrolizine-1-carboxylic acid compound with 2-amino-2-(hydroxymethyl)-1,3-propanediol (1:1).

ACULAR® is supplied as a sterile isotonic aqueous 0.5% solution, with a pH of 7.4. ACULAR® is a racemic mixture of R-(+)- and S-(-)- ketorolac tromethamine. Ketorolac tromethamine may exist in three crystal forms. All forms are equally soluble in water. The pKa of ketorolac is 3.5. This white to off-white crystalline substance discolors on prolonged exposure to light. The molecular weight of ketorolac tromethamine is 376.41. Each mL of ACULAR® ophthalmic solution contains active: ketorolac tromethamine 0.5%; preservative: benzalkonium chloride 0.01%; inactives: edetate disodium 0.1%; octoxynol 40; sodium chloride; hydrochloric acid and/or sodium hydroxide to adjust the pH; and purified water. The osmolality of ACULAR® is 290 mOsmol/kg.

ANIMAL PHARMACOLOGY

Ketorolac tromethamine prevented the development of increased intraocular pressure induced in rabbits with topically applied arachidonic acid. Ketorolac did not inhibit rabbit lens aldose reductase *in vitro*.

Ketorolac tromethamine ophthalmic solution did not enhance the spread of ocular infections induced in rabbits with *Candida albicans, Herpes simplex* virus type one, or *Pseudomonas aeruginosa.*

CLINICAL PHARMACOLOGY

Ketorolac tromethamine is a nonsteroidal anti-inflammatory drug which, when administered systemically, has demonstrated analgesic, anti-inflammatory and anti-pyretic

activity. The mechanism of its action is thought to be due, in part, to its ability to inhibit prostaglandin biosynthesis. Ocular administration of ketorolac tromethamine reduces prostaglandin E_2 levels in aqueous humor. The mean concentration of PGE_2 was 80 pg/mL in the aqueous humor of eyes receiving vehicle and 28 pg/mL in the eyes receiving 0.5% ACULAR® ophthalmic solution. Ketorolac tromethamine given systemically does not cause pupil constriction.

Results from clinical studies indicate that ACULAR® ophthalmic solution has no significant effect upon intraocular pressure.

Two controlled clinical studies showed that ACULAR® ophthalmic solution was significantly more effective than its vehicle in relieving ocular itching caused by seasonal allergic conjunctivitis. Two drops (0.1 mL) of 0.5% ACULAR® ophthalmic solution instilled into the eyes of patients 12 hours and 1 hour prior to cataract extraction achieved measurable levels in 8 of 9 patients' eyes (mean ketorolac concentration 95 ng/mL aqueous humor, range 40 to 170 ng/mL). One drop (0.05 mL) of 0.5% ACULAR® ophthalmic solution was instilled into one eye and one drop of vehicle into the other eye tid in 26 normal subjects. Only 5 of 26 subjects had a detectable amount of ketorolac in their plasma (range 10.7 to 22.5 ng/mL) at Day 10 during topical ocular treatment. When ketorolac tromethamine 10 mg is administered systemically every 6 hours, peak plasma levels at steady state are around 960 ng/mL. ACULAR® ophthalmic solution has been safely administered in conjunction with other ophthalmic medications, such as antibiotics, beta blockers, carbonic anhydrase inhibitors, cycloplegics, and mydriatics.

INDICATIONS AND USAGE

ACULAR® ophthalmic solution is indicated for the relief of ocular itching due to seasonal allergic conjunctivitis.

CONTRAINDICATIONS

ACULAR® ophthalmic solution is contraindicated in patients while wearing soft contact lenses and in patients with previously demonstrated hypersensitivity to any of the ingredients in the formulation.

WARNINGS

There is the potential for cross-sensitivity to acetylsalicylic acid, phenylacetic acid derivatives, and other nonsteroidal anti-inflammatory agents. Therefore, caution should be used when treating individuals who have previously exhibited sensitivities to these drugs.

With some nonsteroidal anti-inflammatory drugs, there exists the potential for increased bleeding time due to interference with thrombocyte aggregation. There have been reports that ocularly applied nonsteroidal anti-inflammatory drugs may cause increased bleeding of ocular tissues (including hyphemas) in conjunction with ocular surgery.

PRECAUTIONS

General: It is recommended that ACULAR® ophthalmic solution be used with caution in patients with known bleeding tendencies or who are receiving other medications which may prolong bleeding time.

Carcinogenesis, Mutagenesis, and Impairment of Fertility: An 18-month study in mice at oral doses of ketorolac tromethamine equal to the parenteral MRHD (Maximum Recommended Human Dose) and a 24-month study in rats at oral doses 2.5 times the parenteral MRHD, showed no evidence of tumorigenicity.

Ketorolac tromethamine was not mutagenic in Ames test, unscheduled DNA synthesis and repair, and in forward mutation assays. Ketorolac did not cause chromosome breakage in the *in vivo* mouse micronucleus assay. At 1590 ug/mL (approximately 1000 times the average human plasma levels) and at higher concentrations, ketorolac tromethamine increased the incidence of chromosomal aberrations in Chinese hamster ovarian cells.

Impairment of fertility did not occur in male or female rats at oral doses of 9 mg/kg (53.1 mg/m^2) and 16 mg/kg (94.4 mg/m^2) respectively.

Pregnancy: Pregnancy Category C. Reproduction studies have been performed in rabbits, using daily oral doses at 3.6 mg/kg (42.35 mg/m^2) and in rats at 10 mg/kg (59 mg/m^2) during organogenesis. Results of these studies did not reveal evidence of teratogenicity to the fetus. Oral doses of ketorolac tromethamine at 1.5 mg/kg (8.8 mg/m^2), which was half of the human oral exposure, administered after gestation day 17 caused dystocia and higher pup mortality in rats. There are no adequate and well-controlled studies in pregnant women. Ketorolac tromethamine should be used during pregnancy only if the potential benefit justifies the potential risk to the fetus.

Nursing Mothers: Caution should be exercised when ACULAR® is administered to a nursing woman.

Pediatric Use: Safety and efficacy in pediatric patients have not been established.

ADVERSE REACTIONS

In patients with allergic conjunctivitis, the most frequent adverse events reported with the use of ACULAR® ophthalmic solution have been transient stinging and burning on instillation. These events were reported by approximately 40% of patients treated with ACULAR® ophthalmic solution. In all development studies conducted, other adverse events reported during treatment with ACULAR® include ocular irritation (3%), allergic reactions (3%), superficial ocular infections (0.5%) and superficial keratitis (1%).

DOSAGE AND ADMINISTRATION

The recommended dose of ACULAR® ophthalmic solution is one drop (0.25 mg) four times a day for relief of ocular itching due to seasonal allergic conjunctivitis. The efficacy of ACULAR® ophthalmic solution has not been established beyond one week of therapy.

HOW SUPPLIED

ACULAR® (ketorolac tromethamine) ophthalmic solution is available for topical ophthalmic administration as a 0.5% sterile solution, and is supplied in white opaque plastic bottles with a controlled dropper tip in the following sizes:
3 mL—NDC 0023-2181-03
5 mL—NDC 0023-2181-05
Store at controlled room temperature 15–30°C (59–86°F) with protection from light. CAUTION: Federal (U.S.A.) law prohibits dispensing without prescription.
U.S. Patent Nos. 4,089,969; 4,454,151; 5,110,493
ACULAR®, a registered trademark of Syntex (U.S.A.) Inc., is manufactured and distributed by Allergan, Inc. under license from its developer, Syntex (U.S.A.) Inc., Palo Alto, California, U.S.A.

ALLERGAN

©1996 Allergan, Inc.
Irvine, CA 92612

AZELEX®
(azelaic acid cream) 20%
For Dermatologic Use Only
Not for Ophthalmic Use

℞

DESCRIPTION

AZELEX® (azelaic acid cream) 20% contains azelaic acid, a naturally occurring saturated dicarboxylic acid.
Structural Formula: HOOC-(CH$_2$)$_7$-COOH. Chemical Name: 1,7-heptanedicarboxylic acid. Empirical Formula: $C_9H_{16}O_4$. Molecular Weight: 188.22.
Active Ingredient: Each gram of AZELEX® contains azelaic acid .... 0.2 gm (20% w/w).
Inactive Ingredients: cetearyl octanoate, glycerin, glyceryl stearate and cetearyl alcohol and cetyl palmitate and cocoglycerides, PEG-5 glyceryl stearate, propylene glycol and purified water. Benzoic acid is present as a preservative.

CLINICAL PHARMACOLOGY

The exact mechanism of action of azelaic acid is not known. The following *in vitro* data are available, but their clinical significance is unknown. Azelaic acid has been shown to possess antimicrobial activity against *Propionibacterium acnes* and *Staphylococcus epidermidis*. The antimicrobial action may be attributable to inhibition of microbial cellular protein synthesis.

A normalization of keratinization leading to an anticomedonal effect of azelaic acid may also contribute to its clinical activity. Electron microscopic and immunohistochemical evaluation of skin biopsies from human subjects treated with AZELEX® demonstrated a reduction in the thickness of the stratum corneum, a reduction in number and size of keratohyalin granules, and a reduction in the amount and distribution of filaggrin (a protein component of keratohyalin) in epidermal layers. This is suggestive of the ability to decrease microcomedo formation.

Pharmacokinetics: Following a single application of AZELEX® to human skin *in vitro*, azelaic acid penetrates into the stratum corneum (approximately 3 to 5% of the applied dose) and other viable skin layers (up to 10% of the dose is found in the epidermis and dermis). Negligible cutaneous metabolism occurs after topical application. Approximately 4% of the topically applied azelaic acid is systemically absorbed. Azelaic acid is mainly excreted unchanged in the urine but undergoes some β-oxidation to shorter chain dicarboxylic acids. The observed half-lives in healthy subjects are approximately 45 minutes after oral dosing and 12 hours after topical dosing, indicating percutaneous absorption rate-limited kinetics.

Azelaic acid is a dietary constituent (whole grain cereals and animal products), and can be formed endogenously from longer-chain dicarboxylic acids, metabolism of oleic acid, and ω-oxidation of monocarboxylic acids. Endogenous plasma concentration (20 to 80 ng/mL) and daily urinary excretion (4 to 28 mg) of azelaic acid are highly dependent on dietary intake. After topical treatment with AZELEX® in humans, plasma concentration and urinary excretion of azelaic acid are not significantly different from baseline levels.

INDICATIONS AND USAGE

AZELEX® is indicated for the topical treatment of mild-to-moderate inflammatory acne vulgaris.

CONTRAINDICATIONS

AZELEX® is contraindicated in individuals who have shown hypersensitivity to any of its components.

WARNINGS

AZELEX® is for dermatologic use only and not for ophthalmic use.
There have been isolated reports of hypopigmentation after use of azelaic acid. Since azelaic acid has not been well studied in patients with dark complexions, these patients should be monitored for early signs of hypopigmentation.

PRECAUTIONS

General: If sensitivity or severe irritation develop with the use of AZELEX®, treatment should be discontinued and appropriate therapy instituted.

Information for patients: Patients should be told: 1. To use AZELEX® for the full prescribed treatment period. 2. To avoid the use of occlusive dressings or wrappings. 3. To keep AZELEX® away from the mouth, eyes and other mucous membranes. If it does come in contact with the eyes, they should wash their eyes with large amounts of water and consult a physician if eye irritation persists. 4. If they have dark complexions, to report abnormal changes in skin color to their physician. 5. Due in part to the low pH of azelaic acid, temporary skin irritation (pruritus, burning, or stinging) may occur when AZELEX® is applied to broken or inflamed skin, usually at the start of treatment. However, this irritation commonly subsides if treatment is continued. If it continues, AZELEX® should be applied only once-a-day, or the treatment should be stopped until these effects have subsided. If troublesome irritation persists, use should be discontinued, and patients should consult their physician. (See ADVERSE REACTIONS.)

Carcinogenesis, mutagenesis, impairment of fertility: Azelaic acid is a human dietary component of a simple molecular structure that does not suggest carcinogenic potential, and it does not belong to a class of drugs for which there is a concern about carcinogenicity. Therefore, animal studies to evaluate carcinogenic potential with AZELEX® Cream were not deemed necessary. In a battery of tests (Ames assay, HGPRT test in Chinese hamster ovary cells, human lymphocyte test, dominant lethal assay in mice), azelaic acid was found to be nonmutagenic. Animal studies have shown no adverse effects on fertility.

Pregnancy: Teratogenic Effects: Pregnancy Category B. Embryotoxic effects were observed in Segment I and Segment II oral studies with rats receiving 2500 mg/kg/day of azelaic acid. Similar effects were observed in Segment II studies in rabbits given 150 to 500 mg/kg/day and in monkeys given 500 mg/kg/day. The doses at which these effects were noted were all within toxic dose ranges for the dams. No teratogenic effects were observed. There are, however, no adequate and well-controlled studies in pregnant women. Because animal reproduction studies are not always predictive of human response, this drug should be used during pregnancy only if clearly needed.

Nursing Mothers: Equilibrium dialysis was used to assess human milk partitioning *in vitro*. At an azelaic acid concentration of 25 µg/mL, the milk/plasma distribution coefficient was 0.7 and the milk/buffer distribution was 1.0, indicating that passage of drug into maternal milk may occur. Since less than 4% of a topically applied dose is systemically absorbed, the uptake of azelaic acid into maternal milk is not expected to cause a significant change from baseline azelaic acid levels in the milk. However, caution should be exercised when AZELEX® is administered to a nursing mother.

Pediatric Use: Safety and effectiveness in pediatric patients under 12 years of age have not been established.

ADVERSE REACTIONS

During U.S. clinical trials with AZELEX®, adverse reactions were generally mild and transient in nature. The most common adverse reactions occurring in approximately 1–5% of patients were pruritus, burning, stinging and tingling. Other adverse reactions such as erythema, dryness, rash, peeling, irritation, dermatitis, and contact dermatitis were reported in less than 1% of subjects. There is the potential for experiencing allergic reactions with use of AZELEX®.

In patients using azelaic acid formulations, the following additional adverse experiences have been reported rarely: worsening of asthma, vitiligo depigmentation, small depigmented spots, hypertrichosis, reddening (signs of keratosis pilaris), and exacerbation of recurrent herpes labialis.

DOSAGE AND ADMINISTRATION

After the skin is thoroughly washed and patted dry, a thin film of AZELEX® should be gently but thoroughly massaged into the affected areas twice daily, in the morning and evening. The hands should be washed following application. The duration of use of AZELEX® can vary from person to person and depends on the severity of the acne. Improvement of the condition occurs in the majority of patients with inflammatory lesions within four weeks.

Continued on next page

Allergan—Cont.

HOW SUPPLIED
AZELEX® is supplied in collapsible tubes in a 30 gm size: 30 g—NDC 0023-8694-30.
Note: Protect from freezing. Store between 15°-30°C (59°-86°F).
Caution: Federal (U.S.A.) law prohibits dispensing without a prescription. Distributed under license; U.S. Patent No. 4,386,104.
September 1995
ALLERGAN
Irvine, California 92612, U.S.A.

BLEPH®-10 ℞
(sulfacetamide sodium ophthalmic solution, USP) 10%

BLEPH®-10
(sulfacetamide sodium ophthalmic ointment, USP) 10%

DESCRIPTION: BLEPH®-10 (sulfacetamide sodium ophthalmic solution and ointment USP) 10% are sterile topical antibacterial agents for ophthalmic use.
Chemical Name:
N-Sulfanilylacetamide monosodium salt monohydrate.
Contains:
BLEPH®-10 solution:
Active: Sulfacetamide sodium .... 10% (100 mg/mL)
Preservative: benzalkonium chloride (0.005%)
Inactives: polyvinyl alcohol 1.4%; sodium thiosulfate; sodium phosphate dibasic; sodium phosphate monobasic; edetate disodium; polysorbate 80; hydrochloric acid and/or sodium hydroxide to adjust the pH; and purified water.
BLEPH®-10 ointment:
Active: Sulfacetamide sodium .... 10% (100 mg/g)
Preservative: phenylmercuric acetate (0.0008%)
Inactives: white petrolatum, mineral oil, and petrolatum (and) lanolin alcohol.

CLINICAL PHARMACOLOGY
Microbiology: The sulfonamides are bacteriostatic agents and the spectrum of activity is similar for all. Sulfonamides inhibit bacterial synthesis of dihydrofolic acid by preventing the condensation of the pteridine with aminobenzoic acid through competitive inhibition of the enzyme dihydropteroate synthetase. Resistant strains have altered dihydropteroate synthetase with reduced affinity for sulfonamides or produce increased quantities of aminobenzoic acid.
Topically applied sulfonamides are considered active against susceptible strains of the following common bacterial eye pathogens: *Escherichia coli, Staphylococcus aureus, Streptococcus pneumoniae, Streptococcus* (viridans group), *Haemophilus influenzae, Klebsiella* species, and *Enterobacter* species.
Topically applied sulfonamides do not provide adequate coverage against *Neisseria* species, *Serratia marcescens* and *Pseudomonas aeruginosa.* A significant percentage of staphylococcal isolates are completely resistant to sulfa drugs.

INDICATIONS AND USAGE
BLEPH®-10 solution and ointment are indicated for the treatment of conjunctivitis and other superficial ocular infections due to the following susceptible microorganisms. BLEPH®-10 solution is also indicated as an adjunctive in systemic sulfonamide therapy of trachoma:
Escherichia coli, Staphylococcus aureus, Streptococcus pneumoniae, Streptococcus (viridans group), *Haemophilus influenza, Klebsiella* species, and *Enterobacter* species.
Topically applied sulfonamides do not provide adequate coverage against *Neisseria* species, *Serratia marcescens* and *Pseudomonas aeruginosa.* A significant percentage of staphylococcal isolates are completely resistant to sulfa drugs.

CONTRAINDICATIONS
BLEPH®-10 solution and ointment are contraindicated in individuals who have a hypersensitivity to sulfonamides or to any ingredient of the preparations.

WARNINGS
FOR TOPICAL EYE USE ONLY—NOT FOR INJECTION. FATALITIES HAVE OCCURRED, ALTHOUGH RARELY, DUE TO SEVERE REACTIONS TO SULFONAMIDES INCLUDING STEVENS-JOHNSON SYNDROME, TOXIC EPIDERMAL NECROLYSIS, FULMINANT HEPATIC NECROSIS, AGRANULOCYTOSIS, APLASTIC ANEMIA AND OTHER BLOOD DYSCRASIAS. Sensitizations may recur when a sulfonamide is readministered, irrespective of the route of administration. Sensitivity reactions have been reported in individuals with no prior history of sulfonamide hypersensitivity. At the first sign of hypersensitivity, skin rash or other serious reaction, discontinue use of these preparations.

PRECAUTIONS
General: Prolonged use of topical antibacterial agents may give rise to overgrowth of nonsusceptible organisms including fungi. Bacterial resistance to sulfonamides may also develop.
The effectiveness of sulfonamides may be reduced by the para-aminobenzoic acid present in purulent exudates.
Ophthalmic ointments may retard corneal wound healing.
Sensitization may recur when a sulfonamide is readministered irrespective of the route of administration, and cross-sensitivity between different sulfonamides may occur.
At the first sign of hypersensitivity, increase in purulent discharge, or aggravation of inflammation or pain, the patient should discontinue use of the medication and consult a physician (see WARNINGS).
Information for patients: To avoid contamination, do not touch tip of container to the eye, eyelid or any surface.
Drug interactions: Sulfacetamide preparations are incompatible with silver preparations.
Carcinogenesis, Mutagenesis, Impairment of Fertility: No studies have been conducted in animals or in humans to evaluate the possibility of these effects with ocularly administered sulfacetamide. Rats appear to be especially susceptible to the goitrogenic effects of sulfonamides, and long-term oral administration of sulfonamides has resulted in thyroid malignancies in these animals.
Pregnancy: Pregnancy Category C. Animal reproduction studies have not been conducted with sulfonamide ophthalmic preparations. Kernicterus may occur in the newborn as a result of treatment of a pregnant woman at term with orally administered sulfonamides. There are no adequate and well controlled studies of sulfonamide ophthalmic preparations in pregnant women and it is not known whether topically applied sulfonamides can cause fetal harm when administered to a pregnant woman. This product should be used in pregnancy only if the potential benefit justifies the potential risk to the fetus.
Nursing mothers: Systematically administered sulfonamides are capable of producing kernicterus in infants of lactating women. Because of the potential for the development of kernicterus in neonates, a decision should be made whether to discontinue nursing or discontinue the drug taking into account the importance of the drug to the mother.
Pediatric Use: Safety and effectiveness in children below the age of two months have not been established.

ADVERSE REACTIONS
Bacterial and fungal corneal ulcers have developed during treatment with sulfonamide ophthalmic preparations.
The most frequently reported reactions are local irritation, stinging and burning. Less commonly reported reactions include non-specific conjunctivitis, conjunctival hyperemia, secondary infections and allergic reactions.
Fatalities have occurred, although rarely, due to severe reactions to sulfonamides including Stevens-Johnson syndrome, toxic epidermal necrolysis, fulminant hepatic necrosis, agranulocytosis, aplastic anemia, and other blood dyscrasias (see WARNINGS).

DOSAGE AND ADMINISTRATION
For conjunctivitis and other superficial ocular infections:
BLEPH®-10 solution:
Instill one or two drops into the conjunctival sac(s) of the affected eye(s) every two to three hours initially. Dosages may be tapered by increasing the time interval between doses as the condition responds. The usual duration of treatment is seven to ten days.
BLEPH®-10 ointment:
Apply a small amount (approximately one-half inch ribbon) into the conjunctival sac(s) of the affected eye(s) every three to four hours and at bedtime. Dosages may be tapered by increasing the time interval between doses as the condition responds. The ointment may be used as adjunct to the solution. The usual duration of treatment is seven to ten days.
For trachoma:
BLEPH®-10 solution:
Instill two drops into the conjunctival sac(s) of the affected eye(s) every two hours. Topical administration must be accompanied by systemic administration.
BLEPH®-10 (sulfacetamide sodium ophthalmic solution, USP) 10% is supplied sterile in plastic bottles in the following sizes:

2.5 mL—NDC 11980-011-03
5 mL—NDC 11980-011-05
15 mL—NDC 11980-011-15

Note: Store between 8°-25°C (46°-77°F). Protect from light. Sulfonamide solutions, on long standing, will darken in color and should be discarded.
BLEPH®-10 (sulfacetamide sodium ophthalmic ointment, USP) 10% is supplied sterile in ophthalmic ointment tubes in the following size:

3.5 g—NDC 0023-0311-04

Note: Store away from heat, 40°C (104°F)
Caution: Federal (U.S.A.) law prohibits dispensing without prescription.

BLEPHAMIDE® ℞
(sulfacetamide sodium-prednisolone acetate)

LIQUIFILM®
sterile ophthalmic suspension

DESCRIPTION
BLEPHAMIDE® LIQUIFILM® sterile ophthalmic suspension is a topical anti-inflammatory/anti-infective combination product for ophthalmic use.
Chemical Names:
Sulfacetamide sodium: N-Sulfanilylacetamide monosodium salt monohydrate.
Prednisolone acetate: 11β, 17, 21-Trihydroxypregna-1, 4-diene-3, 20-dione 21-acetate.
Contains:
Actives: sulfacetamide sodium 10.0%, prednisolone acetate (microfine suspension) 0.2%: Preservative: benzalkonium chloride: Inactives: LIQUIFILM® (polyvinyl alcohol) 1.4%: polysorbate 80; edetate disodium; sodium phosphate, dibasic; potassium phosphate, monobasic; sodium thiosulfate; hydrochloric acid and/or sodium hydroxide to adjust the pH; and purified water.

CLINICAL PHARMACOLOGY
Corticosteroids suppress the inflammatory response to a variety of agents and they probably delay or slow healing. Since corticosteroids may inhibit the body's defense mechanism against infection, a concomitant antimicrobial drug may be used when this inhibition is considered to be clinically significant in a particular case.
The anti-infective component in BLEPHAMIDE® is included to provide action against specific organisms susceptible to it. Sulfacetamide sodium is considered active against the following microorganisms: *Escherichia coli, Staphylococcus aureus, Streptococcus pneumoniae, Streptococcus* (viridans group), *Pseudomonas species, Haemophilus influenzae, Klebsiella* species, and *Enterobacter* species.
When a decision to administer both a corticosteroid and an antimicrobial is made, the administration of such drugs in combination has the advantage of greater patient compliance and convenience, with the added assurance that the appropriate dosage of both drugs is administered. When both types of drugs are in the same formulation, compatibility of ingredients is assured and the correct volume of drug is delivered and retained. The relative potency of corticosteroids depends on the molecular structure, concentration, and release from the vehicle.

INDICATIONS AND USAGE
A steroid/anti-infective combination is indicated for steroid-responsive inflammatory ocular conditions for which a corticosteroid is indicated and where bacterial infection or a risk of bacterial ocular infection exists.
Ocular steroids are indicated in inflammatory conditions of the palpebral and bulbar conjunctiva, cornea, and anterior segment of the globe where the inherent risk of steroid use in certain infective conjunctivitides is accepted to obtain a diminution in edema and inflammation. They are also indicated in chronic anterior uveitis and corneal injury from chemical, radiation, or thermal burns or penetration of foreign bodies.
The use of a combination drug with an anti-infective component is indicated where the risk of infection is high or where there is an expectation that potentially dangerous numbers of bacteria will be present in the eye.
The particular anti-infective drug in this product is active against the following common bacterial eye pathogens: *Escherichia coli, Staphylococcus aureus, Streptococcus pneumoniae, Streptococcus* (viridans group), *Pseudomonas* species, *Haemophilus influenzae, Klebsiella* species, and *Enterobacter* species. This product does not provide adequate coverage against *Neisseria* species and *Serratia marcescens.*

CONTRAINDICATIONS
BLEPHAMIDE® ophthalmic suspension is contraindicated in most viral diseases of the cornea and conjunctiva including epithelial herpes simplex keratitis (dendritic keratitis), vaccinia, and varicella, and also in mycobacterial infection of the eye and fungal diseases of ocular structures.
This product is also contraindicated in individuals with known or suspected hypersensitivity to any of the ingredients of this preparation, to other sulfonamides and to other corticosteroids. See **WARNINGS.** (Hypersensitivity to the antimicrobial component occurs at a higher rate than for other components.)

WARNINGS
NOT FOR INJECTION INTO THE EYE.
Prolonged use of corticosteroids may result in ocular hypertension/glaucoma with damage to the optic nerve, defects in

visual acuity and fields of vision, and in posterior subcapsular cataract formation.

Acute anterior uveitis may occur in susceptible individuals, primarily Blacks.

Prolonged use of BLEPHAMIDE® ophthalmic suspension may suppress the host response and thus increase the hazard of secondary ocular infections. In those diseases causing thinning of the cornea or sclera, perforation has been known to occur with the use of topical corticosteroids. In acute purulent conditions of the eye, corticosteroids may mask infection or enhance existing infection.

If the product is used for 10 days or longer, intraocular pressure should be routinely monitored even though it may be difficult in children and uncooperative patients. Corticosteroids should be used with caution in the presence of glaucoma. Intraocular pressure should be checked frequently.

A significant percentage of staphylococcal isolates are completely resistant to sulfonamides.

The use of steroids after cataract surgery may delay healing and increase the incidence of filtering blebs.

The use of ocular corticosteroids may prolong the course and may exacerbate the severity of many viral infections of the eye (including herpes simplex). Employment of corticosteroid medication in the treatment of herpes simplex requires great caution.

Topical steroids are not effective in mustard gas keratitis and Sjogren's keratoconjunctivitis.

Fatalities have occurred, although rarely, due to severe reactions to sulfonamides including Stevens-Johnson syndrome, toxic epidermal necrolysis, fulminant hepatic necrosis, agranulocytosis, aplastic anemia and other blood dyscrasias. Sensitization may recur when a sulfonamide is readministered, irrespective of the route of administration.

If signs of hypersensitivity or other serious reactions occur, discontinue use of this preparation. Cross-sensitivity among corticosteroids has been demonstrated (see **ADVERSE REACTIONS**).

PRECAUTIONS

General: The initial prescription and renewal of the medication order beyond 20 milliliters of the suspension should be made by a physician only after examination of the patient with the aid of magnification, such as slit lamp biomicroscopy and, where appropriate, fluorescein staining. If signs and symptoms fail to improve after two days, the patient should be re-evaluated.

The possibility of fungal infections of the cornea should be considered after prolonged corticosteroid dosing. Use with caution in patients with severe dry eye. Fungal cultures should be taken when appropriate.

The p-amino benzoic acid present in purulent exudates competes with sulfonamides and can reduce their effectiveness.

Information for Patients: If inflammation or pain persists longer than 48 hours or becomes aggravated, the patient should be advised to discontinue use of the medication and consult a physician (see **WARNINGS**).

This product is sterile when packaged. To prevent contamination, care should be taken to avoid touching the applicator tip to eyelids or to any other surface. The use of this bottle by more than one person may spread infection. Keep bottle tightly closed when not in use. Keep out of the reach of children.

Laboratory Tests: Eyelid cultures and tests to determine the susceptibility of organisms to sulfacetamide may be indicated if signs and symptoms persist or recur in spite of the recommended course of treatment with BLEPHAMIDE® ophthalmic suspension.

Drug Interactions: BLEPHAMIDE® ophthalmic suspension is incompatible with silver preparations. Local anesthetics related to p-amino benzoic acid may antagonize the action of the sulfonamides.

Carcinogenesis, Mutagenesis, Impairment of Fertility: Prednisolone has been reported to be noncarcinogenic. Long-term animal studies for carcinogenic potential have not been performed with sulfacetamide.

One author detected chromosomal nondisjunction in the yeast *Saccharomyces cerevisiae* following application of sulfacetamide sodium. The significance of this finding to topical ophthalmic use of sulfacetamide sodium in the human is unknown.

Mutagenic studies with prednisolone have been negative. Studies on reproduction and fertility have not been performed with sulfacetamide. A long-term chronic toxicity study in dogs showed that high oral doses of prednisolone prevented estrus. A decrease in fertility was seen in male and female rats that were mated following oral dosing with another glucocorticosteroid.

Pregnancy: Teratogenic Effects: Pregnancy Category C. Animal reproduction studies have not been conducted with sulfacetamide sodium. Prednisolone has been shown to be teratogenic in rabbits, hamsters, and mice. In mice, prednisolone has been shown to be teratogenic when given in doses 1 to 10 times the human ocular dose. Dexamethasone, hydrocortisone and prednisolone were ocularly applied to both eyes of pregnant mice five times per day on days 10 through 13 of gestation. A significant increase in the incidence of cleft pal-

ate was observed in the fetuses of the treated mice. There are no adequate well-controlled studies in pregnant women dosed with corticosteroids.

Kernicterus may be precipitated in infants by sulfonamides being given systemically during the third trimester of pregnancy. It is not known whether sulfacetamide sodium can cause fetal harm when administered to a pregnant woman or whether it can affect reproductive capacity.

BLEPHAMIDE® ophthalmic suspension should be used during pregnancy only if the potential benefit justifies the potential risk to the fetus.

Nursing Mothers: It is not known whether topical administration of corticosteroids could result in sufficient systemic absorption to produce detectable quantities in human milk. Systemically administered corticosteroids appear in human milk and could suppress growth, interfere with endogenous corticosteroid production, or cause other untoward effects. Systemically administered sulfonamides are capable of producing kernicterus in infants of lactating women. Because of the potential for serious adverse reactions in nursing infants from sulfacetamide sodium and prednisolone acetate ophthalmic suspensions, a decision should be made whether to discontinue nursing or to discontinue the medication.

Pediatric Use: Safety and effectiveness in pediatric patients below the age of six have not been established.

ADVERSE REACTIONS

Adverse reactions have occurred with corticosteroid/antibacterial combination drugs which can be attributed to the corticosteroid component, the antibacterial component, or the combination. Exact incidence figures are not available since no denominator of treated patients is available.

Reactions occurring most often from the presence of the antibacterial ingredient are allergic sensitizations. Fatalities have occurred, although rarely, due to severe reactions to sulfonamides including Stevens-Johnson syndrome, toxic epidermal necrolysis, fulminant hepatic necrosis, agranulocytosis, aplastic anemia, and other blood dyscrasias (See **WARNINGS**).

Sulfacetamide sodium may cause local irritation.

The reactions due to the corticosteroid component in decreasing order of frequency are: elevation of intraocular pressure (IOP) with possible development of glaucoma and infrequent optic nerve damage, posterior subcapsular cataract formation, and delayed wound healing.

Although systemic effects are extremely uncommon, there have been rare occurrences of systemic hypercorticoidism after use of topical steroids.

Corticosteroid-containing preparations can also cause acute anterior uveitis or perforation of the globe. Mydriasis, loss of accommodation and ptosis have occasionally been reported following local use of corticosteroids.

Secondary Infection: The development of secondary infection has occurred after use of combinations containing corticosteroids and antibacterials. Fungal and viral infections of the cornea are particularly prone to develop coincidentally with long-term applications of corticosteroid. The possibility of fungal invasion must be considered in any persistent corneal ulceration where corticosteroid treatment has been used.

Secondary bacterial ocular infection following suppression of host responses also occurs.

DOSAGE AND ADMINISTRATION

Optimal dosage is 1 drop two to four times daily, depending upon the severity of the condition.

In general, during early or acute stages of blepharitis, BLEPHAMIDE® LIQUIFILM® sterile ophthalmic suspension produces results most rapidly—and most efficiently—with instillation directly into the eye, with the excess spread on the lid (Method I). When the condition is confined to the lid, however, BLEPHAMIDE® may be applied directly to the site of the lesions (Method II).

METHOD I: In the Eye and On the Lid.
1. Wash hands carefully. Tilt head back and drop **1 drop** into the eye.
2. Close the eye and spread the excess medication present after closing the eye on the full length of the upper and lower lids.
3. Do not wipe any of the medication off the lids. It will dry completely in 4 or 5 minutes to a clear film that remains on the lids for several hours—it cannot be seen by others, nor will it interfere with vision.
4. The medication should be washed off the lids once or twice daily. **However, it should be reapplied after each washing.**

METHOD II: On the Lid.
1. Wash hands carefully. Tilt the head back and with eye closed drop 1 drop onto the lid—preferably at the corner of the eye close to the nose.
2. Spread the medication over the full length of the upper and lower lids.
3. Do not wipe away any medication—it will dry in 4 to 5 minutes to a clear, invisible film which will remain on the lids for several hours.
4. The medication should be washed off the lids once or twice a day. **However, it should be reapplied after each washing.**

Not more than 20 milliliters should be prescribed initially and the prescription should not be refilled without further evaluation as outlined in PRECAUTIONS above.

HOW SUPPLIED

BLEPHAMIDE® LIQUIFILM® is supplied in plastic dropper bottles in the following sizes:

5 mL—NDC 11980-022-05   10 mL—NDC 11980-022-10

Note: Protect from freezing. Shake well before using.
Caution: Federal (U.S.A.) law prohibits dispensing without prescription.

ALLERGAN AMERICA, Hormigueros, Puerto Rico 00660
© 1996 Allergan, Inc.

BOTOX®   ℞
(Botulinum Toxin Type A) Purified Neurotoxin Complex

DESCRIPTION

BOTOX® (Botulinum Toxin Type A) Purified Neurotoxin Complex is a sterile, vacuum-dried form of purified botulinum toxin type A, produced from a culture of the Hall strain of *Clostridium botulinum* grown in a medium containing N-Z amine and yeast extract. It is purified from the culture solution by a series of acid precipitations to a crystalline complex consisting of the active high molecular weight toxin protein and an associated hemagglutinin protein. The crystalline complex is re-dissolved in a solution containing saline and albumin and sterile filtered (0.2 microns) prior to vacuum-drying. **BOTOX®** is to be reconstituted with sterile non-preserved saline prior to intramuscular injection.

Each vial of **BOTOX®** contains 100 units (U) of *Clostridium botulinum* toxin type A, 0.5 milligrams of albumin (human), and 0.9 milligrams of sodium chloride in a sterile, vacuum-dried form without a preservative. One unit (U) corresponds to the calculated median lethal intraperitoneal dose (LD/50) in mice of the reconstituted **BOTOX®** injected.

CLINICAL PHARMACOLOGY

BOTOX® (Botulinum Toxin Type A) Purified Neurotoxin Complex blocks neuromuscular conduction by binding to receptor sites on motor nerve terminals, entering the nerve terminals, and inhibiting the release of acetylcholine. When injected intramuscularly at therapeutic doses, **BOTOX®** produces a localized chemical denervation muscle paralysis. When the muscle is chemically denervated, it atrophies and may develop extrajunctional acetylcholine receptors. There is evidence that the nerve can sprout and reinnervate the muscle, with the weakness thus being reversible.

The paralytic effect on muscles injected with **BOTOX®** Purified Neurotoxin Complex is useful in reducing the excessive, abnormal contractions associated with blepharospasm. When used for the treatment of strabismus, it is postulated that the administration of **BOTOX®** affects muscle pairs by inducing an atrophic lengthening of the injected muscle and a corresponding shortening of the muscle's antagonist. Following peri-ocular injection of **BOTOX®**, distant muscles show electrophysiologic changes but no clinical weakness or other clinical change for a period of several weeks or months, parallel to the duration of local clinical paralysis.

In one study, botulinum toxin was evaluated in 27 patients with essential blepharospasm. Twenty-six of the patients had previously undergone drug treatment utilizing benztropine mesylate, clonazepam and/or baclofen without adequate clinical results. Three of these patients then underwent muscle stripping surgery still without an adequate outcome. One patient of the 27 was previously untreated. Upon using botulinum toxin, 25 of the 27 patients reported improvement within 48 hours. One of the other patients was later controlled with a higher dosage. The remaining patient reported only mild improvement but remained functionally impaired.

In another study, 12 patients with blepharospasm were evaluated in a double-blind, placebo-controlled study. All patients receiving botulinum toxin (n=8) were improved compared with no improvements in the placebo group (n=4). The mean dystonia score improved by 72%, the self-assessment score rating improved by 61%, and a videotape evaluation rating improved by 39%. The effects of the treatment lasted a mean of 12.5 weeks.

One thousand six hundred eighty-four patients with blepharospasm evaluated in an open trial showed clinical improvement lasting an average of 12.5 weeks prior to the need for re-treatment.

Six hundred seventy-seven patients with strabismus treated with one or more injections of **BOTOX®** Purified Neurotoxin Complex were evaluated in an open trial. Fifty-five percent of these patients were improved to an alignment of 10 prism diopters or less when evaluated six months or more following injection. These results are consistent with results from additional open label trials which were conducted for this indication.

Continued on next page

Allergan—Cont.

INDICATIONS AND USAGE

BOTOX® (Botulinum Toxin Type A) Purified Neurotoxin Complex is indicated for the treatment of strabismus and blepharospasm associated with dystonia, including benign essential blepharospasm or VII nerve disorders in patients 12 years of age and above.

The efficacy of **BOTOX**® Purified Neurotoxin Complex in deviations over 50 prism diopters, in restrictive strabismus, in Duane's syndrome with lateral rectus weakness, and in secondary strabismus caused by prior surgical over-recession of the antagonist is doubtful, or multiple injections over time may be required. **BOTOX**® is ineffective in chronic paralytic strabismus except to reduce antagonist contracture in conjunction with surgical repair.

Presence of antibodies to botulinum toxin type A may reduce the effectiveness of **BOTOX**® Purified Neurotoxin Complex therapy. In clinical studies, reduction in effectiveness due to antibody production has occurred in one patient with blepharospasm receiving three doses of **BOTOX**® over a six week period totalling 92 U, and in several patients with torticollis who received multiple doses experimentally, totalling over 300 U in a one-month period. For this reason, the dose of **BOTOX**® for strabismus and blepharospasm should be kept as low as possible, in any case below 200 U in a one month period.

CONTRAINDICATIONS

BOTOX® (Botulinum Toxin Type A) Purified Neurotoxin Complex is contraindicated in individuals with known hypersensitivity to any ingredient in the formulation.

WARNINGS

The recommended dosages and frequencies of administration for **BOTOX**® Purified Neurotoxin Complex should not be exceeded. There have not been any reported instances of systemic toxicity resulting from accidental injection or oral ingestion of **BOTOX**®. Should accidental injection or oral ingestion occur, the person should be medically supervised for several days on an office or outpatient basis for signs or symptoms of systemic weakness or muscle paralysis. The entire contents of a vial is below the estimated dose for systemic toxicity in humans weighing 6 kg. or greater.

In the event of overdosage or injection into the wrong muscle, additional information may be obtained by contacting Allergan, Inc. at (800) 433-8871.

The effect of botulinum toxin may be potentiated by aminoglycoside antibiotics or any other drugs that interfere with neuromuscular transmission. Caution should be exercised when **BOTOX**® is used in patients taking any of these drugs.

PRECAUTIONS

General: The safe and effective use of **BOTOX**® (Botulinum Toxin Type A) Purified Neurotoxin Complex depends upon proper storage of the product, selection of the correct dose, and proper reconstitution and administration techniques. Physicians administering **BOTOX**® must understand the relevant neuromuscular and orbital anatomy and any alterations to the anatomy due to prior surgical procedures, and standard electromyographic techniques.

As with all biologic products, epinephrine and other precautions as necessary should be available should an anaphylactic reaction occur.

During the administration of **BOTOX**® Purified Neurotoxin Complex for the treatment of strabismus, retrobulbar hemorrhages sufficient to compromise retinal circulation have occurred from needle penetrations into the orbit. It is recommended that appropriate instruments to decompress the orbit be accessible. Ocular (globe) penetrations by needles have also occurred. An ophthalmoscope to diagnose this condition should be available.

Reduced blinking from **BOTOX**® Purified Neurotoxin Complex injection of the orbicularis muscle can lead to corneal exposure, persistent epithelial defect and corneal ulceration, especially in patients with VII nerve disorders. One case of corneal perforation in an aphakic eye requiring corneal grafting has occurred because of this effect. Careful testing of corneal sensation in eyes previously operated upon, avoidance of injection into the lower lid area to avoid ectropion, and vigorous treatment of any epithelial defect should be employed. This may require protective drops, ointment, therapeutic soft contact lenses, or closure of the eye by patching or other means.

Information for Patients: Patients with blepharospasm may have been extremely sedentary for a long time. Sedentary patients should be cautioned to resume activity slowly and carefully following the administration of **BOTOX**® Purified Neurotoxin Complex.

Drug Interactions: The effect of botulinum toxin may be potentiated by aminoglycoside antibiotics or any other drugs that interfere with neuromuscular transmission. Caution should be exercised when **BOTOX**® Purified Neurotoxin Complex is used in patients taking any of these drugs. (See Warnings).

Pregnancy: ***Pregnancy Category C:*** Animal reproduction studies have not been conducted with **BOTOX**® Purified Neurotoxin Complex. It is also not known whether **BOTOX**® can cause fetal harm when administered to a pregnant woman or can affect reproduction capacity. **BOTOX**® should be administered to pregnant women only if clearly needed.

Carcinogenesis, Mutagenesis, Impairment of Fertility: Long term studies in animals have not been performed to evaluate carcinogenic potential of **BOTOX**® Purified Neurotoxin Complex.

Nursing Mothers: It is not known whether this drug is excreted in human milk. Because many drugs are excreted in human milk, caution should be exercised when **BOTOX**® Purified Neurotoxin Complex is administered to a nursing woman.

Pediatric Use: Safety and effectiveness in children below the age of 12 have not been established.

ADVERSE REACTIONS

There have been reports of seven cases of diffuse skin rash and two cases of local swelling of the eyelid skin lasting for several days following eyelid injection.

Strabismus: Inducing paralysis in one or more extraocular muscles may produce spatial disorientation, double vision, or past-pointing. Covering the affected eye may alleviate these symptoms. Extraocular muscles adjacent to the injection site are often affected, causing ptosis or vertical deviation, especially with higher doses of **BOTOX**® (Botulinum Toxin Type A) Purified Neurotoxin Complex. The incidence rates of these side effects in 2058 adults who received 3650 injections for horizontal strabismus are listed below:

Ptosis	15.7%
Vertical deviation	16.9%

The incidence of ptosis was much less after inferior rectus injection (0.9%) and much greater after superior rectus injection (37.7%).

The incidence rates of these side effects persisting for over six months in an enlarged series of 5587 injections of horizontal muscles in 3104 patients are listed below:

Ptosis lasting over 180 days	0.3%
Vertical deviation greater than 2 prism diopters lasting over 180 days	2.1%

In these patients, the injection procedure itself caused nine scleral perforations. A vitreous hemorrhage occurred and later cleared in one case. No retinal detachment or visual loss occurred in any case. Sixteen retrobulbar hemorrhages occurred. Decompression of the orbit after five minutes was done to restore retinal circulation in one case. No eye lost vision from retrobulbar hemorrhage. Five eyes had pupillary change consistent with ciliary ganglion damage (Adies pupil).

Blepharospasm: In 1684 patients who received 4258 treatments (involving multiple injections) for blepharospasm, the incidence rates of adverse reactions per treated eye are listed below:

Ptosis	11.0%
Irritation/Tearing (includes dry eye, lagophthalmos, and photophobia)	10.0%

Ectropion, keratitis, diplopia and entropion were reported rarely (incidence less than 1%)

Ecchymosis occurs easily in the soft eyelid tissues. This can be prevented by applying pressure at the injection site immediately after the injection.

In two cases of VII nerve disorder (one case of an aphakic eye) reduced blinking from **BOTOX**® Purified Neurotoxin Complex injection of the orbicularis muscle led to serious corneal exposure, persistent epithelial defect and corneal ulceration. Perforation requiring corneal grafting occurred in one case, an aphakic eye. Avoidance of injection into the lower lid area to avoid ectropion may reduce this hazard. Vigorous treatment of any corneal epithelial defect should be employed. This may require protective drops, ointment, therapeutic soft contact lenses, or closure of the eye by patching or other means.

Two patients previously incapacitated by blepharospasm experienced cardiac collapse attributed to over-exertion within three weeks following **BOTOX**® therapy. Sedentary patients should be cautioned to resume activity slowly and carefully following the administration of **BOTOX**®.

OVERDOSAGE

In the event of overdosage or injection into the wrong muscle, additional information may be obtained by contacting Allergan, Inc. at (800) 433-8871.

DOSAGE AND ADMINISTRATION

Strabismus: **BOTOX**® (Botulinum Toxin Type A) Purified Neurotoxin Complex is intended for injection into extraocular muscles utilizing the electrical activity recorded from the tip of the injection needle as a guide to placement within the target muscle. Injection without surgical exposure or electromyographic guidance should not be attempted. Physicians should be familiar with electromyographic technique.

An injection of **BOTOX**® Purified Neurotoxin Complex is prepared by drawing into a sterile 1.0 mL tuberculin syringe an amount of the properly diluted toxin (see Dilution Table) slightly greater than the intended dose. Air bubbles in the syringe barrel are expelled and the syringe is attached to the electromyographic injection needle, preferably a 1.5 inch, 27 gauge needle. Injection volume in excess of the intended dose is expelled through the needle into an appropriate waste container to assure patency of the needle and to confirm that there is no syringe-needle leakage. A new, sterile needle and syringe should be used to enter the vial on each occasion for dilution or removal of **BOTOX**®.

To prepare the eye for **BOTOX**® Purified Neurotoxin Complex injection, it is recommended that several drops of a local anesthetic and an ocular decongestant be given several minutes prior to injection.

Note: The volume of **BOTOX**® injected for treatment of strabismus should be between 0.05 mL to 0.15 mL per muscle.

Strabismus dosage: The initial listed doses of the diluted **BOTOX**® Purified Neurotoxin Complex (see Dilution Table below) typically create paralysis of injected muscles beginning one to two days after injection and increasing in intensity during the first week. The paralysis lasts for 2–6 weeks and gradually resolves over a similar time period. Overcorrections lasting over 6 months have been rare. About one half of patients will require subsequent doses because of inadequate paralytic response of the muscle to the initial dose, or because of mechanical factors such as large deviations or restrictions, or because of the lack of binocular motor fusion to stabilize the alignment.

I. Initial doses in units (abbreviated as U). Use the lower listed doses for treatment of small deviations. Use the larger doses only for large deviations.
   A. For vertical muscles, and for horizontal strabismus of less than 20 prism diopters: 1.25 U to 2.5 U in any one muscle.
   B. For horizontal strabismus of 20 prism diopters to 50 prism diopters: 2.5 U to 5.0 U in any one muscle.
   C. For persistent VI nerve palsy of one month or longer duration: 1.25 U to 2.5 U in the medial rectus muscle.

II. Subsequent doses for residual or recurrent strabismus.
   A. It is recommended that patients be re-examined 7–14 days after each injection to assess the effect of that dose.
   B. Patients experiencing adequate paralysis of the target muscle that require subsequent injections should receive a dose comparable to the initial dose.
   C. Subsequent doses for patients experiencing incomplete paralysis of the target muscle may be increased up to twice the size of the previously administered dose.
   D. Subsequent injections should not be administered until the effects of the previous dose have dissipated as evidenced by substantial function in the injected and adjacent muscles.
   E. The maximum recommended dose as a single injection for any one muscle is 25 U.

Blepharospasm: For blepharospasm, diluted **BOTOX**® Purified Neurotoxin Complex (see Dilution Table) is injected using a sterile, 27–30 gauge needle without electromyographic guidance. 1.25 U to 2.5 U (0.05 mL to 0.1 mL volume at each site) injected into the medial and lateral pre-tarsal orbicularis oculi of the upper lid and into the lateral pre-tarsal orbicularis oculi of the lower lid is the initial recommended dose. In general, the initial effect of the injections is seen within three days and reaches a peak at one to two weeks post-treatment. Each treatment lasts approximately three months, following which the procedure can be repeated indefinitely. At repeat treatment sessions, the dose may be increased up to two-fold if the response from the initial treatment is considered insufficient—usually defined as an effect that does not last longer than two months. However there appears to be little benefit obtainable from injecting more than 5.0 U per site. Some tolerance may be found when **BOTOX**® is used in treating blepharospasm if treatments are given any more frequently than every three months, and it is rare to have the effect be permanent.

The cumulative dose of **BOTOX**® Purified Neurotoxin Complex in a 30-day period should not exceed 200 U.

DILUTION TECHNIQUE

To reconstitute lyophilized **BOTOX**® (Botulinum Toxin Type A) Purified Neurotoxin Complex, use sterile normal saline **without** a preservative; 0.9% Sodium Chloride Injection is the recommended diluent. Draw up the proper amount of diluent in the appropriate size syringe. Since **BOTOX**® is denatured by bubbling or similar violent agitation, inject the diluent into the vial gently. Discard the vial if a vacuum does not pull the diluent into the vial. Record the date and time of reconstitution on the space on the label. **BOTOX**® should be administered within 4 hours after reconstitution.

During this time period, reconstituted **BOTOX**® Purified Neurotoxin Complex should be stored in a refrigerator (2° to 8°C). Reconstituted **BOTOX**® should be clear, colorless and free of particulate matter. Parenteral drug products should be inspected visually for particulate matter and discoloration prior to administration and whenever the solution and the container permit. The use of one vial for more than one

patient is not recommended because the product and diluent do not contain a preservative.

Dilution Table

Diluent Added (0.9% Sodium Chloride Injection)	Resulting dose in Units per 0.1 mL
1.0 mL	10.0 U
2.0 mL	5.0 U
4.0 mL	2.5 U
8.0 mL	1.25 U

Note: These dilutions are calculated for an injection volume of 0.1 mL. A decrease or increase in the **BOTOX**® Purified Neurotoxin Complex dose is also possible by administering a smaller or larger injection volume—from 0.05 mL (50% decrease in dose) to 0.15 mL (50% increase in dose).

HOW SUPPLIED
Each vial contains 100 U of vacuum-dried *Clostridium botulinum* toxin type A. NDC 0023-1145-01.

CAUTION
Federal (U.S.A.) law prohibits dispensing without a prescription.

STORAGE
Store the vacuum-dried product in a freezer at or below −5°C. Administer **BOTOX**® (Botulinum Toxin Type A) Purified Neurotoxin Complex within four hours after the vial is removed from the freezer and reconstituted. During these four hours, reconstituted **BOTOX**® should be stored in a refrigerator (2° to 8°C). Reconstituted **BOTOX**® should be clear, colorless and free of particulate matter.

All vials, including expired vials, or equipment used with the drug should be disposed of carefully as is done with all medical waste.

ELIMITE® Cream
(permethrin) 5% •
℞

DESCRIPTION
ELIMITE® (permethrin) 5% Cream is a topical scabicidal agent for the treatment of infestation with *Sarcoptes scabiei* (scabies). It is available in an off-white, vanishing cream base. ELIMITE® Cream is for topical use only.

Structural Formula:

Chemical Name: The permethrin used is an approximate 1:3 mixture of the cis and trans isomers of the pyrethroid (±)-3-phenoxybenzyl 3-(2,2-dichlorovinyl)-2,2-dimethylcyclopropanecarboxylate. Permethrin has a molecular formula of $C_{21}H_{20}Cl_2O_3$ and a molecular weight of 391.29. It is a yellow to light orange-brown, low melting solid or viscous liquid.
Active Ingredient: Each gram contains permethrin 50 mg (5%).
Inactive Ingredients: Butylated hydroxytoluene, carbomer 934P, fractionated coconut oil, glycerin, glyceryl monostearate, isopropyl myristate, lanolin alcohols, mineral oil, polyoxyethylene cetyl ethers, purified water, and sodium hydroxide. Formaldehyde 1 mg (0.1%) is added as a preservative.

CLINICAL PHARMACOLOGY
Permethrin, a pyrethroid, is active against a broad range of pests including lice, ticks, fleas, mites, and other arthropods. It acts on the nerve cell membrane to disrupt the sodium channel current by which the polarization of the membrane is regulated. Delayed repolarization and paralysis of the pests are the consequences of this disturbance.

Permethrin is rapidly metabolized by ester hydrolysis to inactive metabolites which are excreted primarily in the urine. Although the amount of permethrin absorbed after a single application of the 5% cream has not been determined precisely, data from studies with ^{14}C-labeled permethrin and absorption studies of the cream applied to patients with moderate to severe scabies indicate it is 2% or less of the amount applied.

INDICATIONS AND USAGE
ELIMITE® (permethrin) 5% Cream is indicated for the treatment of infestation with *Sarcoptes scabiei* (scabies).

CONTRAINDICATIONS
ELIMITE® is contraindicated in patients with known hypersensitivity to any of its components, to any synthetic pyrethroid or pyrethrin.

WARNINGS
If hypersensitivity to ELIMITE® occurs, discontinue use.

PRECAUTIONS
General: Scabies infestation is often accompanied by pruritus, edema and erythema. Treatment with ELIMITE® may temporarily exacerbate these conditions.

Information for patients: Patients with scabies should be advised that itching, mild burning and/or stinging may occur after application of ELIMITE®. In clinical trials approximately 75% of patients treated with ELIMITE® who continued to manifest pruritus at 2 weeks had cessation by 4 weeks. If irritation persists, they should consult their physician. ELIMITE® may be very mildly irritating to the eyes. Patients should be advised to avoid contact with eyes during application and to flush with water immediately if ELIMITE® gets in the eyes.

Carcinogenesis, mutagenesis, impairment of fertility: Six carcinogenicity bioassays were evaluated with permethrin, three each in rats and mice. No tumorigenicity was seen in the rat studies. However, species-specific increases in pulmonary adenomas, a common benign tumor of mice of high spontaneous background incidence, were seen in the three mouse studies. In one of these studies there was an increased incidence of pulmonary alveolar-cell carcinomas and benign liver adenomas only in female mice when permethrin was given in their food at a concentration of 5000 ppm. Mutagenicity assays, which give useful correlative data for interpreting results from carcinogenicity bioassays in rodents, were negative. Permethrin showed no evidence of mutagenic potential in a battery of *in vitro* and *in vivo* genetic toxicity studies.

Permethrin did not have any adverse effect on reproductive function at a dose of 180 mg/kg/day orally in a three-generation rat study.

Pregnancy: *teratogenic effects:* Pregnancy Category B: Reproduction studies have been performed in mice, rats, and rabbits (200 to 400 mg/kg/day orally) and have revealed no evidence of impaired fertility or harm to the fetus due to permethrin. There are, however, no adequate and well-controlled studies in pregnant women. Because animal reproduction studies are not always predictive of human response, this drug should be used during pregnancy only if clearly needed.

Nursing mothers: It is not known whether this drug is excreted in human milk. Because many drugs are excreted in human milk and because of the evidence for tumorigenic potential of permethrin in animal studies, consideration should be given to discontinuing nursing temporarily or withholding the drug while the mother is nursing.

Pediatric use: ELIMITE® is safe and effective in pediatric patients two months of age and older. Safety and effectiveness in infants less than two months of age have not been established.

ADVERSE REACTIONS
In clinical trials, generally mild and transient burning and stinging followed application with ELIMITE® in 10% of patients and was associated with the severity of infestation. Pruritus was reported in 7% of patients at various times post-application. Erythema, numbness, tingling, and rash were reported in 1 to 2% or less of patients (see PRECAUTIONS: General).

OVERDOSAGE
No instance of accidental ingestion of ELIMITE® has been reported. If ingested, gastric lavage and general supportive measures should be employed.

DOSAGE AND ADMINISTRATION
Adults and children: Thoroughly massage ELIMITE® into the skin from the head to the soles of the feet. Scabies rarely infests the scalp of adults, although the hairline, neck, temple, and forehead may be infested in infants and geriatric patients. Usually 30 grams is sufficient for an average adult. The cream should be removed by washing (shower or bath) after 8 to 14 hours. Infants should be treated on the scalp, temple and forehead. ONE APPLICATION IS GENERALLY CURATIVE.

Patients may experience persistent pruritus after treatment. This is rarely a sign of treatment failure and is not an indication for retreatment. Demonstrable living mites after 14 days indicate that retreatment is necessary.

HOW SUPPLIED
ELIMITE® (permethrin) 5% (wt./wt.) Cream is supplied in tubes in the following size: 60 g NDC 0023-7915-60.
Note: Store at 15° to 25°C (59° to 77°F).
Caution: Federal (U.S.A.) law prohibits dispensing without prescription.
Manufactured for:
Allergan, Inc.
Irvine, CA 92612, U.S.A.
by Glaxo Wellcome Inc.
Research Triangle Park, NC 27709
© 1996 Allergan, Inc.

ERYGEL®
[är´ē-jel]
(erythromycin) 2%
Topical Gel
℞

Active Ingredient: erythromycin, USP .... 2% (20 mg/g)
Inactive Ingredients: alcohol 92% and hydroxypropyl cellulose

HOW SUPPLIED
ERYGEL® (erythromycin) 2% Topical Gel is supplied in plastic tubes in the following sizes: 30 g—NDC 0023-4312-30. 60 g—NDC 0023-4312-60; and as ERYGEL 6®, cartons of 6 —5 g tubes—NDC-0023-5147-65.
Note: FLAMMABLE. Keep away from heat and flame. Keep tube tightly closed. Store at room temperature.
© 1995 Allergan, Inc.

ERYMAX®
(Erythromycin Topical Solution USP) 2%
℞

Active Ingredient: erythromycin .... 2% (20 mg/mL).
Inactive Ingredients: SD Alcohol 40-2 with tertiary butyl alcohol and brucine sulfate (66%), propylene glycol, and citric acid.

HOW SUPPLIED
In a 2 fl oz plastic bottle with optional Dab-O-Matic applicator and a 4 fl oz plastic bottle:
2 fl oz (59 mL)—NDC 0023-0540-02
4 fl oz (118 mL)—NDC 0023-0540-04
© 1995 Allergan, Inc.

EXSEL® Lotion/Shampoo
(Selenium sulfide lotion, USP) 2.5%
℞

Active Ingredient: selenium sulfide .... 2.5% (w/v) in aqueous suspension.
Inactive Ingredients: edetate disodium; bentonite; sodium dodecylbenzene sulfonate; sodium C14-16 olefin sulfonate; glyceryl ricinoleate; dimethicone copolyol; titanium dioxide; citric acid monohydrate; sodium phosphate monobasic, monohydrate; fragrance; and purified water.

HOW SUPPLIED
EXSEL® is available in a 4 fl oz plastic bottle—NDC 0023-0817-99
© 1995 Allergan, Inc.

FLUONID®
(fluocinolone acetonide) 0.01%
Topical Solution
℞

Active Ingredient: fluocinolone acetonide 0.01%
Inactive Ingredients: propylene glycol and citric acid

HOW SUPPLIED
Topical Solution 0.01%—60 mL plastic squeeze bottles.
60 mL NDC 0023-0878-60
© 1995 Allergan, Inc.

FLUOROPLEX®
(fluorouracil)
1% Topical Cream
and
1% Topical Solution
℞

PRODUCT OVERVIEW

KEY FACTS
Effective treatment for multiple Actinic Keratoses sites.
Provides effective treatment for both clinical and subclinical lesions.
FLUOROPLEX® Cream does not contain irritating parabens or propylene glycol.

MAJOR USES
Multiple actinic keratoses.

SAFETY INFORMATION
Contraindicated in persons hypersensitive to fluorouracil or its listed ingredients.
Contraindicated in pregnancy.
Prolonged exposure to sunlight or other forms of ultraviolet irradiation may increase intensity of reaction.
Adequate long-term studies in animals to evaluate carcinogenic potential have not been conducted with fluorouracil.

Continued on next page

Allergan—Cont.

PRESCRIBING INFORMATION

FLUOROPLEX® ℞
(fluorouracil)
1% Topical Cream
and
1% Topical Solution

DESCRIPTION

FLUOROPLEX® (fluorouracil) 1% Topical Cream and 1% Topical Solution are antineoplastic/antimetabolite products for dermatological use. Fluorouracil has the empirical formula $C_4H_3FN_2O_2$ and a molecular weight of 130.08. It is sparingly soluble in water and slightly soluble in alcohol. The pH is approximately 8.5 for FLUOROPLEX® Topical Cream and 9.2 for FLUOROPLEX® Topical Solution.

Chemical Name:
2,4(1*H*, 3*H*)-Pyrimidinedione, 5-fluoro-.

FLUOROPLEX 1% Topical Cream contains:
Active Ingredient: fluorouracil .... 1.0%.
Inactive Ingredients: benzyl alcohol, emulsifying wax, mineral oil, isopropyl myristate, sodium hydroxide and purified water.

FLUOROPLEX® 1% Topical Solution contains:
Active Ingredient: fluorouracil 1.0%
Inactive Ingredients: propylene glycol, sodium hydroxide and/or hydrochloric acid to adjust the pH, and purified water

Structural Formula:

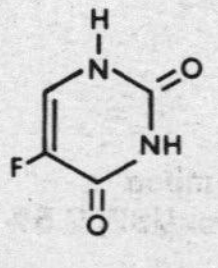

fluorouracil

CLINICAL PHARMACOLOGY

There is evidence that fluorouracil (or its metabolites) blocks the methylation reaction of deoxyuridylic acid to thymidylic acid. In this fashion, fluorouracil interferes with the synthesis of deoxyribonucleic acid (DNA) and to a lesser extent inhibits the formation of ribonucleic acid (RNA).

INDICATIONS AND USAGE

FLUOROPLEX® is indicated for the topical treatment of multiple actinic (solar) keratoses.

CONTRAINDICATIONS

Fluorouracil is contraindicated in women who are or may become pregnant. These products should not be used by patients who are allergic to any of their components.

WARNINGS

There exists the potential for a delayed hypersensitivity reaction to fluorouracil. Patch testing to prove hypersensitivity may be inconclusive.[1]

If an occlusive dressing is used, there may be an increase in the incidence of inflammatory reactions in the adjacent normal skin.

The patient should avoid prolonged exposure to sunlight or other forms of ultraviolet irradiation during treatment with FLUOROPLEX®, as the intensity of the reaction may be increased.

PRECAUTIONS

General: There is a possibility of increased absorption through ulcerated or inflamed skin.

Information for patients: The medication should be applied with care near the eyes, nose and mouth. Excessive reaction in these areas may occur due to irritation from accumulation of drug. If FLUOROPLEX® is applied with the fingers, the hands should be washed immediately afterward.

The reaction to FLUOROPLEX® in treated areas may be unsightly during therapy, and, in some cases, for several weeks following cessation of therapy.

Laboratory Tests: To rule out the presence of a frank neoplasm, a biopsy should be made of those areas failing to respond to treatment or recurring after treatment.

Carcinogenesis, mutagenesis, impairment of fertility: Adequate long-term studies in animals to evaluate carcinogenic potential have not been conducted with fluorouracil. In three *in vitro* cell transformation assays, fluorouracil produced morphological transformation of cells. Morphological transformation was also produced in one of these *in vitro* assays by a metabolite of fluorouracil and the transformed cells produced malignant tumors when injected into immunosuppressed syngeneic mice. Fluorouracil has been shown to exert mutagenic activity in the yeast cells.

Bacillus subtilis, and **Drosophila** assays. In addition, fluorouracil has produced chromosome damage at concentrations of 1.0 and 2.0 mcg/mL in an *in vitro* hamster fibroblast assay and increases in micronuclei formation in the bone marrow of mice at intraperitoneal doses within the human therapeutic dose range of 12–15 mg/kg/day. Patients receiving cumulative doses of 0.24–1.0 g of fluorouracil parenterally have shown an increase in numerical and structural chromosome aberrations in peripheral blood lymphocytes. Fluorouracil has been shown to impair fertility after parenteral administration in rats. In mice, single-dose intravenous and intraperitoneal injections of fluorouracil have been reported to kill differentiated spermatogonia and spermatocytes at a dose of 500 mg/kg and produce abnormalities in spermatids at 50 mg/kg.

Fluorouracil was negative in the dominant lethal mutation assay performed in mice.

Pregnancy: Teratogenic effects: Pregnancy Category X: Fluorouracil may cause fetal harm when administered to a pregnant woman. Fluorouracil administered parenterally has been shown to be teratogenic in mice, rats and hamsters, and embryolethal in monkeys. Fluorouracil is contraindicated in women who are or may become pregnant. If this drug is used during pregnancy, or if the patient becomes pregnant while taking this drug, the patient should be apprised of the potential hazard to the fetus.

Nursing mothers: It is not known whether this drug is excreted in human milk. Because many drugs are excreted in human milk, and because there is some systemic absorption of fluorouracil after topical administration (see **PRECAUTIONS: General**), mothers should not nurse their infants while receiving this drug.

Pediatric use: Safety and effectiveness in pediatric patients have not been established.

ADVERSE REACTIONS

Pain, pruritus, burning, irritation, inflammation, allergic contact dermatitis and telangiectasia have been reported. Occasionally, hyperpigmentation and scarring have also been reported.

OVERDOSAGE

Ordinarily, overdosage will not cause acute problems. If FLUOROPLEX® accidentally comes in contact with the eye(s), flush the eye(s) with water or normal saline. If FLUOROPLEX® is accidentally ingested, induce emesis and gastric lavage. Administer symptomatic and supportive care as needed.

DOSAGE AND ADMINISTRATION

The patient should be instructed to apply sufficient medication to cover the entire face or other affected areas.

Apply medication twice daily with non-metallic applicator or fingertips and wash hands afterwards. A treatment period of 2–6 weeks is usually required.

Increasing the frequency of application and a longer period of administration with FLUOROPLEX® may be required on areas other than the head and neck.

When FLUOROPLEX® is applied to keratotic skin, a response occurs with the following sequence: erythema, usually followed by scaling, tenderness, erosion, ulceration, necrosis and re-epithelization. When the inflammatory reaction reaches the erosion, ulceration and necrosis stages, the use of the drug should be terminated. Responses may sometimes occur in areas which appear clinically normal. These may be sites of subclinical actinic (solar) keratosis which the medication is affecting.

HOW SUPPLIED

FLUOROPLEX® (fluorouracil) 1% Topical Cream is available in 30 g tubes (NDC 0023-0812-30).

FLUOROPLEX® (fluorouracil) 1% Topical Solution is available in 30 mL plastic dropper bottles (NDC 0023-0810-30).

Note: Avoid freezing. Store at 15°–25°C (59°–77°F) in tight containers.

CAUTION: Federal (U.S.A.) law prohibits dispensing without prescription.

REFERENCE

1. Epstein E. Testing for 5-fluorouracil allergy: patch and intradermal tests. *Contact Dermatitis* 1984; 10:311.

Gris–PEG® ℞
(griseofulvin ultramicrosize)
Tablets, USP
125 mg; 250 mg

DESCRIPTION

Gris-PEG® Tablets contain ultramicrosize crystals of griseofulvin, an antibiotic derived from a species of *Penicillium*.

Each Gris-PEG® Tablet contains:
Active Ingredient: griseofulvin ultramicrosize ...... 125 mg
Inactive Ingredients: colloidal silicon dioxide, lactose, magnesium stearate; methylcellulose; methylparaben; polyethylene glycol 400 and 8000, povidone; and titanium dioxide, or
Active Ingredient: griseofulvin ultramicrosize .... 250 mg
Inactive Ingredients: colloidal silicon dioxide; magnesium stearate; methylcellulose; methylparaben; polyethylene glycol 400 and 8000; povidone; sodium lauryl sulfate; and titanium dioxide.

ACTION

Microbiology—Griseofulvin is fungistatic with *in vitro* activity against various species of *Microsporum, Epidermophyton* and *Trichophyton*. It has no effect on bacteria or other genera of fungi.

Human Pharmacology—Following oral administration, griseofulvin is deposited in the keratin precursor cells and has a greater affinity for diseased tissue. The drug is tightly bound to the new keratin which becomes highly resistant to fungal invasions.

The efficiency of gastrointestinal absorption of ultramicrocrystalline griseofulvin is approximately one and one-half times that of the conventional microsize griseofulvin. This factor permits the oral intake of two-thirds as much ultramicrocrystalline griseofulvin as the microsize form. However, there is currently no evidence that this lower dose confers any significant clinical differences with regard to safety and/or efficacy.

INDICATIONS

Gris-PEG® (griseofulvin ultramicrosize) is indicated for the treatment of the following ringworm infections; tinea corporis (ringworm of the body), tinea pedis (athlete's foot), tinea cruris (ringworm of the groin and thigh), tinea barbae (barber's itch), tinea capitis (ringworm of the scalp), and tinea unguium (onychomycosis, ringworm of the nails), when caused by one or more of the following genera of fungi: *Trichophyton rubrum, Trichophyton tonsurans, Trichophyton mentagrophytes, Trichophyton interdigitalis, Trichophyton verrucosum, Trichophyton megnini, Trichophyton gallinae, Trichophyton crateriform, Trichophyton sulphureum, Trichophyton schoenleini, Microsporum audouini, Microsporum canis, Microsporum gypseum* and *Epidermophyton floccosum.*

Note: Prior to therapy, the type of fungi responsible for the infection should be identified. The use of the drug is not justified in minor or trivial infections which will respond to topical agents alone. Griseofulvin is *not* effective in the following: bacterial infections, candidiasis (moniliasis), histoplasmosis, actinomycosis, sporotrichosis, chromoblastomycosis, coccidioidomycosis, North American blastomycosis, cryptococcosis (torulosis), tinea versicolor and nocardiosis.

CONTRAINDICATIONS

Two cases of conjoined twins have been reported since 1977 in patients taking griseofulvin during the first trimester of pregnancy. Griseofulvin should not be prescribed to pregnant patients. If the patient becomes pregnant while taking this drug, the patient should be apprised of the potential hazard to the fetus.

This drug is contraindicated in patients with porphyria or hepatocellular failure and in individuals with a history of hypersensitivity to griseofulvin.

WARNINGS

Prophylactic Usage—Safety and efficacy of griseofulvin for prophylaxis of fungal infections have not been established.

Animal Toxicology—Chronic feeding of griseofulvin, at levels ranging from 0.5%–2.5% of the diet resulted in the development of liver tumors in several strains of mice, particularly in males. Smaller particle sizes result in an enhanced effect. Lower oral dosage levels have not been tested. Subcutaneous administration of relatively small doses of griseofulvin once a week during the first three weeks of life has also been reported to induce hepatomata in mice. Thyroid tumors, mostly adenomas but some carcinomas, have been reported in male rats receiving griseofulvin at levels of 2.0%, 1.0% and 0.2% of the diet, and in female rats receiving the two higher dose levels. Although studies in other animal species have not yielded evidence of tumorigenicity, these studies were not of adequate design to form a basis for conclusion in this regard. In subacute toxicity studies, orally administered griseofulvin produced hepatocellular necrosis in mice, but this has not been seen in other species. Disturbances in porphyrin metabolism have been reported in griseofulvin-treated laboratory animals. Griseofulvin has been reported to have a colchicine-like effect on mitosis and cocarcinogenicity with methylcholanthrene in cutaneous tumor induction in laboratory animals. *Usage in Pregnancy*—See CONTRAINDICATIONS section. *Animal Reproduction Studies*—It has been reported in the literature that griseofulvin was found to be embryotoxic and teratogenic on oral administration to pregnant rats. Pups with abnormalities have been reported in the litters of a few bitches treated with griseofulvin. Suppression of spermatogenesis has been reported to occur in rats, but investigation in man failed to confirm this.

PRECAUTIONS

Patients on prolonged therapy with any potent medication should be under close observation. Periodic monitoring of organ system function, including renal, hepatic and hematopoietic, should be done. Since griseofulvin is derived from species of *Penicillium,* the possibility of cross-sensitivity with penicillin exists; however, known penicillin-sensitive patients have been treated without difficulty. Since a photosen-

sitivity reaction is occasionally associated with griseofulvin therapy, patients should be warned to avoid exposure to intense natural or artificial sunlight. Lupus erythematosus or lupus-like syndromes have been reported in patients receiving griseofulvin. Griseofulvin decreases the activity of warfarin-type anticoagulants so that patients receiving these drugs concomitantly may require dosage adjustment of the anticoagulant during and after griseofulvin therapy. Barbiturates usually depress griseofulvin activity and concomitant administration may require a dosage adjustment of the antifungal agent. There have been reports in the literature of possible interactions between griseofulvin and oral contraceptives. The effect of alcohol may be potentiated by griseofulvin, producing such effects as tachycardia and flush.

ADVERSE REACTIONS

When adverse reactions occur, they are most commonly of the hypersensitivity type such as skin rashes, urticaria, erythema multiforme, and rarely, angioneurotic edema, and may necessitate withdrawal of therapy and appropriate countermeasures. Paresthesias of the hands and feet have been reported rarely after extended therapy. Other side effects reported occasionally are oral thrush, nausea, vomiting, epigastric distress, diarrhea, headache, fatigue, dizziness, insomnia, mental confusion, and impairment of performance of routine activities. Proteinuria and leukopenia have been reported rarely. Administration of the drug should be discontinued if granulocytopenia occurs. When rare, serious reactions occur with griseofulvin, they are usually associated with high dosages, long periods of therapy, or both.

DOSAGE AND ADMINISTRATION

Accurate diagnosis of the infecting organism is essential. Identification should be made either by direct microscopic examination of a mounting of infected tissue in a solution of potassium hydroxide or by culture on an appropriate medium. Medication must be continued until the infecting organism is completely eradicated as indicated by appropriate clinical or laboratory examination. Representative treatment periods are tinea capitis, 4 to 6 weeks; tinea corporis, 2 to 4 weeks; tinea pedis, 4 to 8 weeks; tinea unguium—depending on rate of growth—fingernails, at least 4 months; toenails, at least 6 months.

General measures in regard to hygiene should be observed to control sources of infection or reinfection. Concomitant use of appropriate topical agents is usually required, particularly in treatment of tinea pedis. In some forms of athlete's foot, yeasts and bacteria may be involved as well as fungi. Griseofulvin will not eradicate the bacterial or monilial infection.

Adults: Daily administration of 375 mg (as a single dose or in divided doses) will give a satisfactory response in most patients with tinea corporis, tinea cruris, and tinea capitis. For those fungal infections more difficult to eradicate, such as tinea pedis and tinea unguium, a divided dose of 750 mg is recommended.

Pediatric Use: Approximately 3.3 mg per pound of body weight per day of ultramicrosize griseofulvin is an effective dose for most pediatric patients. On this basis, the following dosage schedule is suggested: Children weighing 35–60 pounds—125 mg to 187.5 mg daily. Children weighing over 60 pounds—187.5 mg to 375 mg daily. Children and infants 2 years of age and younger—dosage has not been established. Clinical experience with griseofulvin in children with tinea capitis indicates that a single daily dose is effective. Clinical relapse will occur if the medication is not continued until the infecting organism is eradicated.

HOW SUPPLIED

Gris-PEG® (griseofulvin ultramicrosize) Tablets, 125 mg, white, scored, elliptical-shaped, embossed "Gris-PEG" on one side and "125" on the other. Gris-PEG® (griseofulvin ultramicrosize) Tablets, 250 mg, white, scored, capsule-shaped, embossed "Gris-PEG" on one side and "250" on the other. The 125 mg strength is available in bottles of 100 (NDC 0023-0763-04). The 250 mg strength is available in bottles of 100, and 500 (NDC 0023-0773-04, and NDC 0023-0773-50 respectively). Both strengths are film-coated.

CAUTION

Federal (U.S.A.) law prohibits dispensing without prescription.

STORAGE

Store Gris-PEG® tablets at controlled room temperature 15°–30°C (59°–86°F) in tight, light-resistant containers.
Manufactured for ALLERGAN Herbert
Skin Care Division of Allergan, Inc.
Irvine, CA 92612, U.S.A.
by SANDOZ PHARMACEUTICALS CORPORATION
© 1996 Allergan, Inc.

MAXIFLOR®   ℞
(diflorasone diacetate)
Cream, USP, 0.05%
Ointment, USP, 0.05%

DESCRIPTION

MAXIFLOR Cream Contains:

Active Ingredient: 0.5 mg diflorasone diacetate, USP, in an emulsified and hydrophilic cream base.

Inactive Ingredients: Propylene glycol, stearic acid, polysorbate 60, sorbitan monostearate and monooleate, sorbic acid, citric acid and water. The corticosteroid is formulated as a solution in the vehicle using 15 percent propylene glycol to optimize drug delivery.

MAXIFLOR Ointment Contains:

Active Ingredient: 0.5 mg diflorasone diacetate, USP, in an emollient, occlusive base. *Inactive Ingredients:* Polyoxypropylene 15-stearyl ether, stearic acid, lanolin alcohol and white petrolatum.

HOW SUPPLIED

MAXIFLOR® (diflorasone diacetate) Cream, USP, 0.05% is available in collapsible tubes in the following sizes:
  30 gram NDC 0023-0766-30
  60 gram NDC 0023-0766-60
MAXIFLOR® (diflorasone diacetate) Ointment, USP, 0.05% is available in collapsible tubes in the following sizes:
  15 gram NDC 0023-0770-15
  30 gram NDC 0023-0770-30
  60 gram NDC 0023-0770-60
Manufactured for ALLERGAN Herbert
Skin Care Division of Allergan, Inc.
Irvine, California 92715, USA
by The Upjohn Company
Kalamazoo, Michigan 49001
© 1995 Allergan, Inc.

NAFTIN®   ℞
(naftifine hydrochloride) 1%
Cream

DESCRIPTION

NAFTIN® Cream, 1% contains the synthetic, broad-spectrum, antifungal agent naftifine hydrochloride.
NAFTIN® Cream, 1% is for topical use only.
Chemical Name: (E)-N-Cinnamyl-N-methyl-1-naphthalenemethyl-amine hydrochloride. Naftifine hydrochloride has an empirical formula of $C_{21}H_{21}N \cdot HCl$ and a molecular weight of 323.86.
Active Ingredient: Naftifine hydrochloride 1%
Inactive Ingredients: benzyl alcohol, cetyl alcohol, cetyl esters wax, isopropyl myristate, polysorbate 60, purified water, sodium hydroxide, sorbitan monostearate, and stearyl alcohol. Hydrochloric acid may be added to adjust pH.

CLINICAL PHARMACOLOGY

Naftifine hydrochloride is a synthetic allylamine derivative. The following *in vitro* data are available, but their clinical significance is unknown. Naftifine hydrochloride has been shown to exhibit fungicidal activity *in vitro* against a broad spectrum of organisms including *Trichophyton rubrum, Trichophyton mentagrophytes, Trichophyton tonsurans, Epidermophyton floccosum, Microsporum canis, Microsporum audouini,* and *Microsporum gypseum;* and fungistatic activity against *Candida* species, including *Candida albicans.* NAFTIN® Cream, 1% has only been shown to be clinically effective against the disease entities listed in the INDICATIONS AND USAGE section.

Although the exact mechanism of action against fungi is not known, naftifine hydrochloride appears to interfere with sterol biosynthesis by inhibiting the enzyme squalene 2,3-epoxidase. This inhibition of enzyme activity results in decreased amounts of sterols, especially ergosterol, and a corresponding accumulation of squalene in the cells.

Pharmacokinetics: *In vitro* and *in vivo* bioavailability studies have demonstrated that naftifine penetrates the stratum corneum in sufficient concentration to inhibit the growth of dermatophytes.

Following a single topical application of 1% naftifine cream to the skin of healthy subjects, systemic absorption of naftifine was approximately 6% of the applied dose. Naftifine and/or its metabolites are excreted via the urine and feces with a half-life of approximately two to three days.

INDICATIONS AND USAGE

NAFTIN® Cream, 1% is indicated for topical application in the treatment of tinea pedis, tinea cruris and tinea corporis caused by the organisms *Tricophyton rubrum, Tricophyton mentagrophytes,* and *Epidermophyton floccosum.*

CONTRAINDICATIONS

NAFTIN® Cream, 1% is contraindicated in individuals who have shown hypersensitivity to any of its components.

WARNING

NAFTIN® Cream, 1% is for topical use only and not for ophthalmic use.

PRECAUTIONS

General: NAFTIN® Cream, 1% is for external use only. If irritation or sensitivity develops with the use of NAFTIN® Cream 1%, treatment should be discontinued and appropriate therapy instituted. Diagnosis of the disease should be confirmed either by direct microscopic examination of a mounting of infected tissue in a solution of potassium hydroxide or by culture on an appropriate medium.

Information for patients: The patient should be told to:
1. Avoid the use of occlusive dressings or wrappings unless otherwise directed by the physician.
2. Keep NAFTIN® Cream, 1% away from the eyes, nose, mouth and other mucous membranes.

Carcinogenesis, mutagenesis, impairment of fertility: Long-term animal studies to evaluate the carcinogenic potential of NAFTIN® Cream, 1% have not been performed. *In vitro* and animal studies have not demonstrated any mutagenic effect or effect on fertility.

Pregnancy: Teratogenic Effects: Pregnancy Category B: Reproduction studies have been performed in rats and rabbits (via oral administration) at doses 150 times or more the topical human dose and have revealed no significant evidence of impaired fertility or harm to the fetus due to naftifine. There are, however, no adequate and well-controlled studies in pregnant women. Because animal reproduction studies are not always predictive of human response, this drug should be used during pregnancy only if clearly needed.

Nursing mothers: It is not known whether this drug is excreted in human milk. Because many drugs are excreted in human milk, caution should be exercised when NAFTIN® Cream, 1% is administered to a nursing woman.

Pediatric use: Safety and effectiveness in pediatric patients have not been established.

ADVERSE REACTIONS

During clinical trials with NAFTIN® Cream 1%, the incidence of adverse reactions was as follows: burning/stinging (6%), dryness (3%), erythema (2%), itching (2%), local irritation (2%).

DOSAGE AND ADMINISTRATION

A sufficient quantity of NAFTIN® Cream, 1% should be gently massaged into the affected and surrounding skin areas once a day. The hands should be washed after application.

If no clinical improvement is seen after four weeks of treatment with NAFTIN® Cream, 1% the patient should be reevaluated.

HOW SUPPLIED

NAFTIN® (naftifine hydrochloride) 1% Cream is supplied in collapsible tubes in the following sizes.
15 g-NDC-0023-4126-15
30 g-NDC-0023-4126-30
60 g-NDC-0023-4126-60
Note: Store below 30°C (86°F).
Caution: Federal (U.S.A.) law prohibits dispensing without prescription.
© 1996 Allergan, Inc.

NAFTIN®   ℞
(naftifine hydrochloride) 1%
Gel

DESCRIPTION

Naftin® Gel, 1% contains the synthetic, broad-spectrum, antifungal agent naftifine hydrochloride.
Naftin® Gel, 1% is for topical use only.
Chemical Name: (E)-N-Cinnamyl-N-methyl-1-naphthalenemethylamine hydrochloride. Naftifine hydrochloride has an empirical formula of $C_{21}H_{21}N \cdot HCl$ and a molecular weight of 323.86.
Contains:
Active Ingredient: Naftifine hydrochloride 1%
Inactive Ingredients: polysorbate 80, carbomer 934P, diisopropanolamine, edetate disodium, alcohol (52% v/v), and purified water.

CLINICAL PHARMACOLOGY

Naftifine hydrochloride is a synthetic allylamine derivative. The following *in vitro* data are available but their clinical significance is unknown. Naftifine hydrochloride has been shown to exhibit fungicidal activity *in vitro* against a broad spectrum of organisms including *Trichophyton rubrum, Trichophyton mentagrophytes, Trichophyton tonsurans, Epidermophyton floccosum,* and *Microsporum canis, Microsporum audouini,* and *Microsporum gypseum;* and fungistatic activity against *Candida* species including *Candida albicans.* Naftin Gel, 1% has only been shown to be clinically effective against

Continued on next page

Allergan—Cont.

the disease entities listed in the INDICATIONS AND USAGE section.

Although the exact mechanism of action against fungi is not known, naftifine hydrochloride appears to interfere with sterol biosynthesis by inhibiting the enzyme squalene 2,3-epoxidase. This inhibition of enzyme activity results in decreased amounts of sterols, especially ergosterol, and a corresponding accumulation of squalene in the cells.

Pharmacokinetics: *In vitro* and *in vivo* bioavailability studies have demonstrated that naftifine penetrates the stratum corneum in sufficient concentration to inhibit the growth of dermatophytes.

Following single topical application of ³H-labeled naftifine gel 1% to the skin of healthy subjects, up to 4.2% of the applied dose was absorbed. Naftifine and/or its metabolites are excreted via the urine and feces with a half-life of approximately two to three days.

INDICATION AND USAGE

Naftin® Gel, 1% is indicated for the topical treatment of tinea pedis, tinea cruris and tinea corporis caused by the organisms *Trichophyton rubrum*, *Trichophyton mentagrophytes*, *Trichophyton tonsurans** and *Epidermophyton floccosum.**

*Efficacy for this organism in this organ system was studied in fewer than 10 infections.

CONTRAINDICATIONS

Naftin® Gel, 1% is contraindicated in individuals who have shown hypersensitivity to any of its components.

WARNINGS

Naftin® Gel, 1% is for topical use only and not for ophthalmic use.

PRECAUTIONS

General: Naftin® Gel, 1% is for external use only. If irritation or sensitivity develop with the use of Naftin® Gel, 1%, treatment should be discontinued and appropriate therapy instituted. Diagnosis of the disease should be confirmed either by direct microscopic examination of a mounting of infected tissue in a solution of potassium hydroxide or by culture on an appropriate medium.

Information for patients:
The patient should be told to:
1. Avoid the use of occlusive dressings or wrappings unless otherwise directed by the physician.
2. Keep Naftin® Gel, 1% away from the eyes, nose, mouth and other mucous membranes.

Carcinogenesis, mutagenesis, impairment of fertility: Long-term studies to evaluate the carcinogenic potential of Naftin® Gel, 1% have not been performed. *In vitro* and animal studies have not demonstrated any mutagenic effect or effect on fertility.

Pregnancy: Teratogenic Effects: Pregnancy Category B: Reproduction studies have been performed in rats and rabbits (via oral administration) at doses 150 times or more than the topical human dose and have revealed no evidence of impaired fertility or harm to the fetus due to naftifine. There are, however, no adequate and well-controlled studies in pregnant women. Because animal reproduction studies are not always predictive of human response, this drug should be used during pregnancy only if clearly needed.

Nursing mothers: It is not known whether this drug is excreted in human milk. Because many drugs are excreted in human milk, caution should be exercised when Naftin® Gel, 1% is administered to a nursing woman.

Pediatric use: Safety and effectiveness in pediatric patients have not been established.

ADVERSE REACTIONS

During clinical trials with Naftin® Gel, 1%, the incidence of adverse reactions was as follows: burning/stinging (5.0%), itching (1.0%), erythema (0.5%), rash (0.5%), skin tenderness (0.5%).

DOSAGE AND ADMINISTRATION

A sufficient quantity of Naftin® Gel, 1% should be gently massaged into the affected and surrounding skin areas twice a day, in the morning and evening. The hands should be washed after application.

If no clinical improvement is seen after four weeks of treatment with Naftin® Gel, 1%, the patient should be reevaluated.

HOW SUPPLIED

Naftin® (naftifine hydrochloride) is supplied in collapsible tubes in the following sizes:
20 g-NDC-0023-4770-20
40 g-NDC-0023-4770-40
60 g-NDC-0023-4770-60
Note: Store at room temperature.
Caution: Federal (U.S.A.) law prohibits dispensing without prescription.
© 1996 Allergan, Inc.

OCUFLOX®   ℞
(ofloxacin ophthalmic solution)
0.3% sterile

DESCRIPTION

OCUFLOX® (ofloxacin ophthalmic solution) 0.3% is a sterile ophthalmic solution. It is a fluorinated carboxyquinolone anti-infective for topical ophthalmic use.
Structural Formula:

ofloxacin

$C_{18}H_{20}FN_3O_4$ Mol Wt 361.37

Chemical Name: (±)-9-Fluoro-2,3-dihydro-3-methyl-10-(4-methyl-1-piperazinyl)-7-oxo-7H-pyrido[1,2,3-de]-1,4 benzoxazine-6-carboxylic acid.

Contains:
Active: ofloxacin 0.3% (3 mg/mL);
Preservative: benzalkonium chloride (0.005%);
Inactives: sodium chloride and purified water. May also contain hydrochloric acid and/or sodium hydroxide to adjust pH.

OCUFLOX® solution is unbuffered and formulated with a pH of 6.4 (range—6.0 to 6.8). It has an osmolality of 300 mOsm/kg. Ofloxacin is a fluorinated 4-quinolone which differs from other fluorinated 4-quinolones in that there is a six member (pyridobenzoxazine) ring from positions 1 to 8 of the basic ring structure.

CLINICAL PHARMACOLOGY

Pharmacokinetics: Serum, urine and tear concentrations of ofloxacin were measured in 30 healthy women at various time points during a ten-day course of treatment with OCUFLOX® solution. The mean serum ofloxacin concentration ranged from 0.4 ng/mL to 1.9 ng/mL. Maximum ofloxacin concentration increased from 1.1 ng/mL on day one to 1.9 ng/mL on day 11 after QID dosing for 10½ days. Maximum serum ofloxacin concentrations after ten days of topical ophthalmic dosing were more than 1000 times lower than those reported after standard oral doses of ofloxacin. Tear ofloxacin concentrations ranged from 5.7 to 31 μg/g during the 40 minute period following the last dose on day 11. Mean tear concentration measured four hours after topical ophthalmic dosing was 9.2 μg/g.
Corneal tissue concentrations of 4.4 μg/mL were observed four hours after beginning topical ocular application of two drops of OCUFLOX® every 30 minutes. Ofloxacin was excreted in the urine primarily unmodified.
Microbiology: Ofloxacin has in vitro activity against a broad range of gram-positive and gram-negative aerobic and anaerobic bacteria. Ofloxacin is bactericidal at concentrations equal to or slightly greater than inhibitory concentrations. Ofloxacin is thought to exert a bactericidal effect on susceptible bacterial cells by inhibiting DNA gyrase, an essential bacterial enzyme which is a critical catalyst in the duplication, transcription, and repair of bacterial DNA.
Cross-resistance has been observed between ofloxacin and other fluoroquinolones. There is generally no cross-resistance between ofloxacin and other classes of antibacterial agents such as beta-lactams or aminoglycosides.
Ofloxacin has been shown to be active against most strains of the following organisms both in vitro and clinically, in conjunctival and/or corneal ulcer infections as described in the INDICATIONS AND USAGE section.
AEROBES, GRAM-POSITIVE:
 Staphylococcus aureus
 Staphylococcus epidermidis
 Streptococcus pneumoniae
AEROBES, GRAM-NEGATIVE:
 Enterobacter cloacae
 Haemophilus influenzae
 Proteus mirabilis
 Pseudomonas aeruginosa
 Serratia marcescens*
ANAEROBIC SPECIES:
 Propionibacterium acnes
*Efficacy for this organism was studied in fewer than 10 infections.
The safety and effectiveness of OCUFLOX® in treating ophthalmologic infections due to the following organisms have not been established in adequate and well-controlled clinical trials. OCUFLOX® has been shown to be active in vitro against most strains of these organisms but the clinical significance in ophthalmologic infections is unknown.

AEROBES, GRAM-POSITIVE:
 Enterococcus faecalis
 Listeria monocytogenes
 Staphylococcus capitis
 Staphylococcus hominus
 Staphylococcus simulans
 Streptococcus pyogenes
AEROBES, GRAM-NEGATIVE:
 Acinetobacter calcoaceticus var. *anitratus*
 Acinetobacter calcoaceticus var. *Iwoffii*
 Citrobacter diversus
 Citrobacter freundii
 Enterobacter aerogenes
 Enterobacter agglomerans
 Escherichia coli
 Haemophilus parainfluenzae
 Klebsiella oxytoca
 Klebsiella pneumoniae
 Moraxella (Branhamella) catarrhalis
 Moraxella lacunata
 Morganella morganii
 Neisseria gonorrhoeae
 Pseudomonas acidovorans
 Pseudomonas fluorescens
 Shigella sonnei
OTHER:
 Chlamydia trachomatis
Clinical Studies:
Conjunctivitis: In a randomized, double-masked, multicenter clinical trial, OCUFLOX® solution was superior to its vehicle after 2 days of treatment in patients with conjunctivitis and positive conjunctival cultures. Clinical outcomes for the trial demonstrated a clinical improvement rate of 86% (54/63) for the ofloxacin treated group versus 72% (48/67) for the placebo treated group after 2 days of therapy. Microbiological outcomes for the same clinical trial demonstrated an eradication rate for causative pathogens of 65% (41/63) for the ofloxacin treated group versus 25% (17/67) for the vehicle treated group after 2 days of therapy. Please note that microbiologic eradication does not always correlate with clinical outcome in anti-infective trials.
Corneal Ulcers: In a randomized, double-masked, multi-center trial of 140 subjects with positive cultures, OCUFLOX® treated subjects had an overall clinical success rate (complete re-epithelialization and no progression of the infiltrate for two consecutive visits) of 82% (61/74) compared to 80% (53/66) for the fortified antibiotic group, consisting of 1.5% tobramycin and 10% cefazolin solutions. The median time to clinical success was 11 days for the ofloxacin treated group and 10 days for the fortified treatment group.

INDICATIONS AND USAGE

OCUFLOX® solution is indicated for the treatment of infections caused by susceptible strains of the following bacteria in the conditions listed below:
CONJUNCTIVITIS:
Gram-positive bacteria:
 Staphylococcus aureus
 Staphylococcus epidermidis
 Streptococcus pneumoniae
Gram-negative bacteria:
 Enterobacter cloacae
 Haemophilus influenzae
 Proteus mirabilis
 Pseudomonas aeruginosa
CORNEAL ULCERS:
Gram-positive bacteria:
 Staphylococcus aureus
 Staphylococcus epidermidis
 Streptococcus pneumoniae
Gram-negative bacteria:
 Pseudomonas aeruginosa
 Serratia marcescens*
Anaerobic species:
 Propionibacterium acnes
*Efficacy for this organism was studied in fewer than 10 infections.

CONTRAINDICATIONS

OCUFLOX® solution is contraindicated in patients with a history of hypersensitivity to ofloxacin, to other quinolones, or to any of the components in this medication.

WARNINGS

NOT FOR INJECTION.
OCUFLOX® solution should not be injected subconjunctivally, nor should it be introduced directly into the anterior chamber of the eye.
Serious and occasionally fatal hypersensitivity (anaphylactic) reactions, some following the first dose, have been reported in patients receiving systemic quinolones, including ofloxacin. Some reactions were accompanied by cardiovascular collapse, loss of consciousness, angioedema (including laryngeal, pharyngeal or facial edema), airway obstruction, dyspnea, urticaria, and itching. A rare occurrence of Stevens-Johnson syndrome, which progressed to toxic epidermal necrolysis, has been reported in a patient who was receiving

topical ophthalmic ofloxacin. If an allergic reaction to ofloxacin occurs, discontinue the drug. Serious acute hypersensitivity reactions may require immediate emergency treatment. Oxygen and airway management, including intubation should be administered as clinically indicated.

PRECAUTIONS

General: As with other anti-infectives, prolonged use may result in overgrowth of nonsusceptible organisms, including fungi. If superinfection occurs, discontinue use and institute alternative therapy. Whenever clinical judgment dictates, the patient should be examined with the aid of magnification, such as slit lamp biomicroscopy and, where appropriate, fluorescein staining. Ofloxacin should be discontinued at the first appearance of a skin rash or any other sign of hypersensitivity reaction.

The systemic administration of quinolones, including ofloxacin, has led to lesions or erosions of the cartilage in weight-bearing joints and other signs of arthropathy in immature animals of various species. Ofloxacin, administered systemically at 10 mg/kg/day in young dogs (equivalent to 110 times the maximum recommended daily *adult ophthalmic* dose) has been associated with these types of effects.

Information for Patients: Avoid contaminating the applicator tip with material from the eye, fingers, or other source. Systemic quinolones, including ofloxacin, have been associated with hypersensitivity reactions, even following a single dose. Discontinue use immediately and contact your physician at the first sign of a rash or allergic reaction.

Drug Interactions: Specific drug interaction studies have not been conducted with OCUFLOX® ophthalmic solution. However, the systemic administration of some quinolones has been shown to elevate plasma concentrations of theophylline, interfere with the metabolism of caffeine, and enhance the effects of the oral anticoagulant warfarin and its derivatives, and has been associated with transient elevations in serum creatinine in patients receiving cyclosporine concomitantly.

Carcinogenesis, Mutagenesis, Impairment of Fertility: Long term studies to determine the carcinogenic potential of ofloxacin have not been conducted.

Ofloxacin was not mutagenic in the Ames test, in vitro and in vivo cytogenic assay, sister chromatid exchange assay (Chinese hamster and human cell lines), unscheduled DNA synthesis (UDS) assay using human fibroblasts, the dominant lethal assay, or mouse micronucleus assay. Ofloxacin was positive in the UDS test using rat hepatocyte, and in the mouse lymphoma assay.

In fertility studies in rats, ofloxacin did not affect male or female fertility or morphological or reproductive performance at oral dosing up to 360 mg/kg/day (equivalent to 4000 times the maximum recommended daily ophthalmic dose).

Pregnancy: Teratogenic Effects. Pregnancy Category C: Ofloxacin has been shown to have embryocidal effect in rats and in rabbits when given in doses of 810 mg/kg/day (equivalent to 9000 times the maximum recommended daily ophthalmic dose) and 160 mg/kg/day (equivalent to 1800 times the maximum recommended daily ophthalmic dose). These dosages resulted in decreased fetal body weight and increased fetal mortality in rats and rabbits, respectively. Minor fetal skeletal variations were reported in rats receiving doses of 810 mg/kg/day. Ofloxacin has not been shown to be teratogenic at doses as high as 810 mg/kg/day and 160 mg/kg/day when administered to pregnant rats and rabbits, respectively.

Nonteratogenic Effects: Additional studies in rats with doses up to 360 mg/kg/day during late gestation showed no adverse effect on late fetal development, labor, delivery, lactation, neonatal viability, or growth of the newborn.

There are, however, no adequate and well-controlled studies in pregnant women. OCUFLOX® solution should be used during pregnancy only if the potential benefit justifies the potential risk to the fetus.

Nursing Mothers: In nursing women a single 200 mg oral dose resulted in concentrations of ofloxacin in milk which were similar to those found in plasma. It is not known whether ofloxacin is excreted in human milk following topical ophthalmic administration. Because of the potential for serious adverse reactions from ofloxacin in nursing infants, a decision should be made whether to discontinue nursing or to discontinue the drug, taking into account the importance of the drug to the mother.

Pediatric Use: Safety and effectiveness in infants below the age of one year have not been established.

Quinolones, including ofloxacin, have been shown to cause arthropathy in immature animals after oral administration; however, topical ocular administration of ofloxacin to immature animals has not shown any arthropathy. There is no evidence that the ophthalmic dosage form of ofloxacin has any effect on weight bearing joints.

ADVERSE REACTIONS

Ophthalmic Use: The most frequently reported drug-related adverse reaction was transient ocular burning or discomfort. Other reported reactions include stinging, redness, itching,
chemical conjunctivitis/keratitis, periocular/facial edema, foreign body sensation, photophobia, blurred vision, tearing, dryness, and eye pain. Rare reports of dizziness have been received.

DOSAGE AND ADMINISTRATION

The recommended dosage regimen for the treatment of **bacterial conjunctivitis** is:

Days 1 and 2
  Instill one to two drops every two to four hours in the affected eye(s).
Days 3 through 7
  Instill one to two drops four times daily.

The recommended dosage regimen for the treatment of **bacterial corneal ulcer** is:

Days 1 and 2
  Instill one to two drops into the affected eye every 30 minutes, while awake. Awaken at approximately four and six hours after retiring and instill one to two drops.

Days 3 through 7 to 9
  Instill one to two drops hourly, while awake.
Days 7 to 9 through treatment completion
  Instill one to two drops, four times daily.

HOW SUPPLIED

OCUFLOX® (ofloxacin ophthalmic solution) 0.3% is supplied sterile in plastic dropper bottles of the following sizes:
  1 mL—NDC 11980–779–01
  5 mL—NDC 11980–779–05
  10 mL—NDC 11980–779–10
Note: Store at 15–25°C (59–77°F)
Caution: Federal (U.S.A.) law prohibits dispensing without prescription.
May 1996
Allergan America, Hormigueros, Puerto Rico 00660
Licensed from: Daiichi Pharmaceutical Co., Ltd., Tokyo, Japan and Santen Pharmaceutical Co., Ltd., Osaka, Japan
U.S. PAT. NOS. 4,382,892; 4,551,456
©1996 Allergan, Inc.   70829 10B
Shown in Product Identification Guide, page 304

PENECORT®   ℞
(hydrocortisone)
Cream, USP, 1%
Topical Solution 1%

PENECORT® Cream contains:
Active Ingredient: hydrocortisone, USP 1%
Inactive Ingredients: benzyl alcohol; petrolatum; stearyl alcohol; propylene glycol; isopropyl myristate; polyoxyl 40 stearate; carbomer 934; sodium lauryl sulfate; edetate disodium; sodium hydroxide to adjust the pH; and purified water.
PENECORT® Topical Solution contains:
Active Ingredient: hydrocortisone, USP 1%
Inactive Ingredients: SD Alcohol 40–2 with tertiary butyl alcohol and brucine sulfate (57%); propylene glycol; benzyl alcohol; and purified water.

HOW SUPPLIED
PENECORT® (hydrocortisone):
Cream, USP, 1%—30 g collapsible tubes: NDC 0023-0510-30
Topical Solution 1%—30 mL and 60 mL plastic bottles:
30 mL NDC 0023-0889-30; 60 mL NDC 0023-0889-60
© 1995 Allergan, Inc.

POLYTRIM® OPHTHALMIC SOLUTION Sterile   ℞
(TRIMETHOPRIM SULFATE AND POLYMYXIN B SULFATE)

DESCRIPTION
POLYTRIM® Ophthalmic Solution (trimethoprim sulfate and polymyxin B sulfate) is a sterile antimicrobial solution for topical ophthalmic use. Each mL contains trimethoprim sulfate equivalent to 1 mg trimethoprim and polymyxin B sulfate 10,000 units. The vehicle contains benzalkonium chloride 0.004% (added as a preservative) and the inactive ingredients sodium chloride, sodium hydroxide or sulfuric acid (added to adjust pH), and Water for Injection.
Trimethoprim sulfate, 2,4-diamino-5-(3,4,5-trimethoxy-benzyl)pyrimidine sulfate (2:1), is a white, odorless, crystalline powder with a molecular weight of 678.72.
Polymyxin B sulfate is the sulfate salt of polymyxin B_1 and B_2 which are produced by the growth of *Bacillus polymyxa* (Prazmowski) Migula (Fam. Bacillaceae). It has a potency of not less than 6,000 polymyxin B units per mg, calculated on an anhydrous basis.

CLINICAL PHARMACOLOGY

Trimethoprim is a synthetic antibacterial drug active against a wide variety of aerobic gram-positive and gram-negative ophthalmic pathogens. Trimethoprim blocks the production of tetrahydrofolic acid from dihydrofolic acid by binding to and reversibly inhibiting the enzyme dihydrofolate reductase. This binding is very much stronger for the bacterial enzyme than for the corresponding mammalian enzyme. For that reason, trimethoprim selectively interferes with bacterial biosynthesis of nucleic acids and proteins.

Polymyxin B, a cyclic lipopeptide antibiotic, is rapidly bactericidal for a variety of gram-negative organisms, especially *Pseudomonas aeruginosa*. It increases the permeability of the bacterial cell membrane by interacting with the phospholipid components of the membrane.

When used topically, trimethoprim and polymyxin B absorption through intact skin and mucous membranes is insignificant.

Blood samples were obtained from 11 human volunteers at 20 minutes, 1 hour and 3 hours following instillation in the eye of 2 drops of ophthalmic solution containing 1 mg trimethoprim and 10,000 units polymyxin B per mL. Peak serum concentrations were approximately 0.03 µg/mL trimethoprim and 1 unit/mL polymyxin B.

Microbiology: *In vitro* studies have demonstrated that the anti-infective components of POLYTRIM® are active against the following bacterial pathogens that are capable of causing external infections of the eye:
Trimethoprim: Staphylococcus aureus and *Staphylococcus epidermidis, Streptococcus pyogenes, Streptococcus faecalis, Streptococcus pneumoniae, Haemophilus influenzae, Haemophilus aegyptius, Escherichia coli, Klebsiella pneumoniae, Proteus mirabilis* (indole-negative), *Proteus vulgaris* (indole-positive), *Enterobacter aerogenes,* and *Serratia marcescens.*
Polymyxin B: Pseudomonas aeruginosa, Escherichia coli, Klebsiella pneumoniae, Enterobacter aerogenes and *Haemophilus influenzae.*

INDICATIONS AND USAGE
POLYTRIM® Ophthalmic Solution is indicated in the treatment of surface ocular bacterial infections, including acute bacterial conjunctivitis, and blepharoconjunctivitis, caused by susceptible strains of the following microorganisms: *Staphylococcus aureus, Staphylococcus epidermidis, Streptococcus pneumoniae, Streptococcus viridans, Haemophilus influenzae* and *Pseudomonas aeruginosa.* *

* Efficacy for this organism in this organ system was studied in fewer than 10 infections.

CONTRAINDICATIONS
POLYTRIM® Ophthalmic Solution is contraindicated in patients with known hypersensitivity to any of its components.

WARNINGS
NOT FOR INJECTION INTO THE EYE. If a sensitivity reaction to POLYTRIM® occurs, discontinue use. POLYTRIM® Ophthalmic Solution is not indicated for the prophylaxis or treatment of ophthalmia neonatorum.

PRECAUTIONS
General: As with other antimicrobial preparations, prolonged use may result in overgrowth of nonsusceptible organisms, including fungi. If superinfection occurs, appropriate therapy should be initiated.
Information for Patients: Avoid contaminating the applicator tip with material from the eye, fingers, or other source. This precaution is necessary if the sterility of the drops is to be maintained.
If redness, irritation, swelling or pain persists or increases, discontinue use immediately and contact your physician.
Carcinogenesis, Mutagenesis, Impairment of Fertility:
Carcinogenesis: Long-term studies in animals to evaluate carcinogenic potential have not been conducted with polymyxin B sulfate or trimethoprim.
Mutagenesis: Trimethoprim was demonstrated to be non-mutagenic in the Ames assay. In studies at two laboratories no chromosomal damage was detected in cultured Chinese hamster ovary cells at concentrations approximately 500 times human plasma levels after oral administration; at concentrations approximately 1000 times human plasma levels after oral administration in these same cells a low level of chromosomal damage was induced at one of the laboratories. Studies to evaluate mutagenic potential have not been conducted with polymyxin B sulfate.
Impairment of Fertility: Polymyxin B sulfate has been reported to impair the motility of equine sperm, but its effects on male or female fertility are unknown.
No adverse effects on fertility or general reproductive performance were observed in rats given trimethoprim in oral dosages as high as 70 mg/kg/day for males and 14 mg/kg/day for females.
Pregnancy: Teratogenic Effects: Pregnancy Category C. Animal reproduction studies have not been conducted with

Continued on next page

Allergan—Cont.

polymyxin B sulfate. It is not known whether polymyxin B sulfate can cause fetal harm when administered to a pregnant woman or can affect reproduction capacity.

Trimethoprim has been shown to be teratogenic in the rat when given in oral doses 40 times the human dose. In some rabbit studies, the overall increase in fetal loss (dead and resorbed and malformed conceptuses) was associated with oral doses 6 times the human therapeutic dose.

While there are no large well-controlled studies on the use of trimethoprim in pregnant women, Brumfitt and Pursell, in a retrospective study, reported the outcome of 186 pregnancies during which the mother received either placebo or oral trimethoprim in combination with sulfamethoxazole. The incidence of congenital abnormalities was 4.5% (3 of 66) in those who received placebo and 3.3% (4 of 120) in those receiving trimethoprim and sulfamethoxazole. There were no abnormalities in the 10 children whose mothers received the drug during the first trimester. In a separate survey, Brumfitt and Pursell also found no congenital abnormalities in 35 children whose mothers had received oral trimethoprim and sulfamethoxazole at the time of conception or shortly thereafter.

Because trimethoprim may interfere with folic acid metabolism, trimethoprim should be used during pregnancy only if the potential benefit justifies the potential risk to the fetus.

Nonteratogenic Effects: The oral administration of trimethoprim to rats at a dose of 70 mg/kg/day commencing with the last third of gestation and continuing through parturition and lactation caused no deleterious effects on gestation or pup growth and survival.

Nursing mothers: It is not known whether this drug is excreted in human milk. Because many drugs are excreted in human milk, caution should be exercised when POLYTRIM® Ophthalmic Solution is administered to a nursing woman.

Pediatric Use: Safety and effectiveness in children below the age of 2 months have not been established (see WARNINGS).

ADVERSE REACTIONS

The most frequent adverse reaction to POLYTRIM® Ophthalmic Solution is local irritation consisting of increased redness, burning, stinging, and/or itching. This may occur on instillation, within 48 hours, or at any time with extended use. There are also multiple reports of hypersensitivity reactions consisting of lid edema, itching, increased redness, tearing, and/or circumocular rash.

Photosensitivity has been reported in patients taking oral trimethoprim.

DOSAGE AND ADMINISTRATION

Adults: In mild to moderate infections, instill one drop in the affected eye(s) every three hours (maximum of 6 doses per day) for a period of 7 to 10 days.

Pediatric Use: Clinical studies have shown POLYTRIM® to be safe and effective for use in children over two months of age. The dosage regimen is the same as for adults.

HOW SUPPLIED

A sterile ophthalmic solution, each mL contains trimethoprim sulfate** equivalent to 1 mg trimethoprim and polymyxin B sulfate 10,000 units in a plastic dropper bottle of 10 mL (NDC 0023-7824-10).

Store at 15°–25°C (59°–77°F) and protect from light.

**Mfd. under U.S. Patent No. 3,956,327.

Distributed by:
ALLERGAN, INC.
Irvine, CA 92612, U.S.A.

TAC®-3 ℞
(sterile triamcinolone acetonide suspension) 3mg/mL
NOT FOR INTRAVENOUS USE
FOR INTRALESIONAL AND INTRADERMAL USE

Each mL of aqueous suspension contains: **Active Ingredient:** triamcinolone acetonide 3 mg. **Inactive Ingredients:** benzyl alcohol 0.9% as preservative; carboxymethylcellulose sodium 7.5 mg; polysorbate 80 0.4 mg; sodium chloride 2 mg; in water for injection q.s. Sodium hydroxide and/or hydrochloric acid may have been used to adjust pH.

HOW SUPPLIED

Multiple dose vials of 5 mL containing triamcinolone acetonide 3 mg/mL.
NDC 0023-0218-05.
Manufactured for ALLERGAN Herbert
Skin Care Division of Allergan, Inc.
Irvine, California 92715, U.S.A.
by
Steris Laboratories, Inc.
Phoenix, AZ 85043
©1995 Allergan, Inc.

Alpha Therapeutic Corporation
5555 VALLEY BLVD.
LOS ANGELES, CA 90032

Direct Inquiries to:
(213) 225-2221
(800) 421-0008
FAX: (213) 227-7027

For Medical Information Contact:
In Emergencies:
Jonathan Goldsmith, M.D., Medical Director
(213) 227-7210
After Hours Emergency Orders:
(800) 421-0008

ALBUTEIN® 5% ℞
Albumin (Human), USP, 5% Solution

10 bottles per case.

250mL bottle & IV set	NDC 49669-5211-1
500mL bottle & IV set	NDC 49669-5211-2

ALBUTEIN® 25% ℞
Albumin (Human), USP, 25% Solution

10 bottles per case.

20mL bottle & IV set	NDC 49669-5213-1
50mL bottle & IV set	NDC 49669-5213-2
100mL bottle & IV set	NDC 49669-5213-3

ALPHANATE™ ℞
Antihemophilic Factor, (Human)
Solvent Detergent Treated

DESCRIPTION

Alphanate™ Antihemophilic Factor (Human) Solvent Detergent Treated is a highly purified Factor VIII product for the treatment of Hemophilia A and acquired Factor VIII deficiency. It is intended for intravenous administration. The product is purified by column chromatography and utilizes a solvent detergent treatment for viral inactivation.

HOW SUPPLIED

The product is available in the following potencies:

Factor VIII Activity	Diluent	NDC Number
250 i.u.	10 mL	49669-4500-1
500 i.u.	10 mL	49669-4500-1
1000 i.u.	10 mL	49669-4500-1
1500 i.u.	10 mL	49669-4500-1

Each carton contains a single dose vial of concentrate, sterile water for injection, a vented filter spike for reconstitution, and a package insert with full prescribing information. 12 vials per case.

AlphaNine®-SD ℞
Coagulation Factor IX (Human)
Affinity Purified/Solvent Detergent Treated

AlphaNine®-SD, Coagulation Factor IX (Human) is available in 500, 1000, 1250, and 1500 assay ranges with 10 mL diluent. For intravenous administration only. Each carton and single dose vial is labeled with Factor IX dose contained; carton contains sterile diluent, transfer needle, and microaggregate filter. 12 vials per case. ASSAY RANGE 0-2000 F IX Units/Vial NDC 49669-3800-01

PLASMATEIN® 5% ℞
Plasma Protein Fraction (Human), USP, 5% Solution

10 bottles per case.

250mL bottle & IV set	NDC 49669-5721-1
500mL bottle & IV set	NDC 49669-5721-2

PROFILNINE® SD ℞
Factor IX Complex
Solvent Detergent Treated

DESCRIPTION

Profilnine® SD, Factor IX Complex, Solvent Detergent Treated is a lyophilized concentrate containing factors II, IX, and X plus low levels of factor VII. The product is available

---

in single dose vials of Factor IX for the treatment of Hemophilia B (Factor IX deficiency).

HOW SUPPLIED

The product is available in the following potencies:

Factor IX Activity	Diluent	NDC Number
500 i.u.	5 mL	49669-3200-02
1000 i.u.	10 mL	49669-3200-03
1500 i.u.	10 mL	49669-3200-03

Each individual carton contains a single dose vial of Factor IX, sterile water for injection, transfer needle, microaggregate filter, and a package insert with full prescribing information. 12 vials per case.

VENOGLOBULIN®-I ℞
Immune Globulin Intravenous (Human)

Sterile highly purified lyophilized preparation of intact, unmodified immunoglobulin. Supplies broad spectrum of IgG antibodies. Manufacturing process includes cold alcohol fractionation plus purification by PEG fractionation and DEAE Sephadex ion exchange adsorption. For intravenous administration. In 2.5g, 5.0g, and 10.0g vials with sterile diluent and transfer device. 6 vials per case.

2.5g with reconstitution kit	NDC 49669-1602-1
5.0g with reconstitution kit	NDC 49669-1603-1
10.0g with reconstitution kit and administration set	NDC 49669-1604-1

VENOGLOBULIN®-S 5% Solution ℞
Immune Globulin Intravenous (Human)
SOLVENT DETERGENT TREATED

Venoglobulin®-S 5% Solution, Solvent Detergent Treated is a sterile, highly purified solution of intact, unmodified human immunoglobulin G intended for intravenous use. IgG is isolated from large pools of human plasma using the Cohn-Oncley cold alcohol fractionation process, followed by polyethylene glycol fractionation and ion exchange chromatography. The manufacturing process includes treatment with a mixture of tri-n-butyl phosphate (TNBP) and polysorbate 80.

The process used to produce Venoglobulin®-S inactivates and/or partitions up to 13 cumulative logs of Human Immunodeficiency Virus Type 1 (HIV-1) based on *in vitro* studies. Additional solvent-detergent treatment further removes greater than 10 logs of HIV-1 and greater than 6 logs of HIV-2 as demonstrated *in vitro*, thereby providing an extra measure of safety.

Venoglobulin®-S contains all IgG antibody activities present in the donor population. The distribution of IgG subclasses corresponds to that of normal human plasma. Gamma globulin is isolated without additional chemical or enzymatic modification and the Fc portion of the molecule is maintained functionally intact. Typically IgG purity exceeds 99%.

The composition of Venoglobulin®-S is as follows:

Component	Quantity/mL
Human immunoglobulin G	50 mg
D-sorbitol	50 mg
Albumin (Human)	< 1.3 mg
Polyethylene glycol	< 100 mcg
Polysorbate 80	< 100 mcg
Tri-n-butyl phosphate	< 10 mcg

This formulation contains no preservatives. The pH of the solution ranges from 5.2 to 5.8. The osmolarity is approximately 300 mOsm/L.

10 vials per case:

50 mL	2.5g IgG	NDC 49669-1612-1
100 mL	5.0g IgG	NDC 49669-1613-1
200 mL	10.0g IgG	NDC 49669-1614-1

All sizes are packaged with a sterile I.V. administration set. Recommended storage at or below 25°C or 77°F. Do not freeze.

VENOGLOBULIN®-S 10% Solution ℞
Immune Globulin Intravenous (Human)
SOLVENT DETERGENT TREATED

DESCRIPTION

Venoglobulin®-S 10% Solution, Solvent Detergent Treated is a sterile, highly purified solution of intact, unmodified human immunoglobulin G intended for intravenous use. IgG is isolated from large pools of human plasma using the Cohn-Oncley cold alcohol fractionation process, followed by polyethylene glycol fractionation and ion exchange chromatography. The manufacturing process also includes a solvent detergent viral inactivation step.

The composition of Venoglobulin-S 10% is as follows:

Component	Quantity/mL
Human immunoglobulin G	100 mg
D-sorbitol	50 mg
Albumin (Human)	≤ 2.6 mg
Polyethylene glycol	≤ 200 mcg
Polysorbate 80	≤ 200 mcg
Tri-n-butyl phosphate	≤ 20 mcg

This formulation contains no preservatives. The pH of the solution ranges from 5.2 to 5.8. The osmolarity is approximately 330 mOsm/L.

HOW SUPPLIED

Vial size	Grams of IgG	NDC Number
50 mL	5.0 g	49669-1622-1
100 mL	10.0 g	49669-1623-1
200 mL	20.0 g	49669-1624-1

All sizes are packaged with a sterile IV administration set. 10 vials per case. Store at 2–8°C (35–46°F). Do not freeze.

EDUCATIONAL MATERIAL

Scientific publications, monographs, product literature, brochures and formulary kits available upon request.

Alpharma™
U.S Pharmaceuticals Division
Makers of Barre and NMC
Products
7205 WINDSOR BLVD.
BALTIMORE, MD 21244

For General Inquiries Contact:
Customer Service
(800) 638–9096

NDC # 0472-	PRODUCT/STRENGTH	Rx/OTC
1595	12 Hour Nasal Spray (Oxymetazoline HCl 0.05%)	OTC
1419	Acetaminophen and Codeine Phosphate Oral Soln. USP	Rx Cv
0880	Acetasol (Acetic Acid Otic Soln. USP)	Rx
0882	Acetasol HC (Hydrocortisone and Acetic Acid Otic Soln. USP)	Rx
0831	Albuterol Sulfate Inhal. Soln. 0.083%	Rx
0825	Albuterol Sulfate Syrup	Rx
0090	Aluminum Hydroxide Gel USP	OTC
0833	Amantadine HCl Syrup 50 mg/5 mL	Rx
0873	Aminophylline Oral Liquid-Dye Free 105 mg/5 mL	Rx
1417	APAP Drops (Acetaminophen 80 mg/0.8 mL)	OTC
1410	APAP Elixir-Cherry (Acetaminophen 80 mg/2.5 mL)	OTC
0647	APAP Elixir-Grape (Acetaminophen 80 mg/2.5 mL)	OTC
0016	Auroto Otic Solution (Antipyrine and Benzocaine Otic Soln. USP)	Rx
1645	Bromanate DC Cough Syrup	Rx Cv
0712	Bromanate DM	OTC
0711	Bromanate Elixir	OTC
1634	Bromanyl Cough Syrup	Rx Cv
0709	Brondelate Elixir	Rx
0933	Butabarbital Sodium Elixir USP 30 mg/5 mL	Rx CIII
0733	Cardec-DM Drops	Rx
0731	Cardec-DM Syrup	Rx
0727	Cardec-S Syrup	Rx
0036	Chlorhexidine Gluconate Oral Rinse 0.12%	Rx
0742	Chlorpromazine HCl Oral Concentrate 100 mg/mL	Rx
0514	Cimetidine Hydrochloride Oral Solution	Rx
0857	Clemastine Fumarate Syrup 0.5 mg/5 mL	Rx
0987	Clindamycin Phosphate Topical Soln. USP, 1%	Rx
0748	Codamine Pediatric Syrup	Rx CIII
0749	Codamine Syrup	Rx CIII
1358	Constulose (Lactulose Soln. USP)	Rx
0755	Cyproheptadine HCl Syrup USP 2 mg/5 mL	Rx
1517	Decofed Liquid (Pseudoephedrine HCl Syrup USP)	OTC

NDC #		
0957	Detussin Expectorant	Rx CIII
0958	Detussin Liquid	Rx CIII
0972	Dexamethasone Elixir USP 0.5 mg/5 mL	Rx
1639	Dihistine DH Elixir	OTC (See state laws) Cv
1640	Dihistine Expectorant	OTC (See state laws) Cv
0936	Diocto Liquid (Docusate Sodium Soln. USP)	OTC
0924	Diocto Syrup (Docusate Sodium Syrup USP)	OTC
0930	Diocto-C Syrup	OTC
1238	Dyphylline GG Elixir	Rx
0650	Entac Liquid	Rx
1360	Enulose (Lactulose Soln. USP)	Rx
0970	Epinephrine Mist (Epinephrine Inhalation Aerosol USP)	OTC
0977	Erythromycin Estolate Oral Susp. USP 125 mg/5 mL	Rx
0979	Erythromycin Estolate Oral Susp. USP 250 mg/5 mL	Rx
0971	Erythromycin Ethylsuccinate Oral Susp. USP 200 mg/5 mL	Rx
0974	Erythromycin Ethylsuccinate Oral Susp. USP 400 mg/5 mL	Rx
1244	Erythromycin Topical Soln. USP 2%	Rx
1469	Ferrous Sulfate Drops (15 mg iron/0.6 mL)	OTC
1465	Ferrous Sulfate Elixir (44 mg iron/5 mL)	OTC
0061	Guiatuss (Guaifenesin Syrup USP)	OTC
0012	Guiatuss AC Syrup (Sugarfree)	OTC Cv
0010	Guiatuss CF	OTC
0011	Guiatuss DAC (Sugarfree)	OTC Cv
1031	Guiatuss DM	OTC
0038	Guiatuss PE	OTC
0766	Haloperidol Oral Soln. USP 2 mg/mL	Rx
0077	Hycosin Expectorant	Rx CIII
1232	Hydramine Cough Syrup	OTC
1223	Hydramine Elixir (Alcohol Free)	OTC
1030	Hydromet Syrup	Rx CIII
0771	Hydroxyzine HCl Syrup USP 10 mg/5 mL	Rx
2430	Kaopek Suspension	OTC
0996	Lidocaine HCl Oral Topical Soln. USP 2% (Viscous)	Rx
0570	Lindane Lotion USP 1%	Rx
0572	Lindane Shampoo USP 1%	Rx
1137	Loperamide HCl Oral Soln. 1 mg/5 mL	OTC
1534	Medicated Blue Shampoo	OTC
1373	Metaproterenol Sulfate Inhalation Soln. USP 0.4%	Rx
1377	Metaproterenol Sulfate Inhalation Soln. USP 0.6%	Rx
0783	Methenamine Mandelate Oral Susp. USP 500 mg/5 mL	Rx
0454	Metoclopramide Oral Soln. USP 5 mg/5 mL	Rx
0066	Minoxidil Topical Solution 2%	OTC
0800	Multi Vit Drops with Iron	OTC
0809	Naldelate Pediatric Drops	Rx
1007	Naldelate Pediatric Syrup	Rx
0801	Naldelate Syrup	Rx
1475	Nite Time Cold Formula-Cherry Flavor	OTC
1470	Nite Time Cold Formula-Original Flavor	OTC
1245	Nucotuss Expectorant	Rx CIII
1240	Nucotuss Pediatric Expectorant	Rx Cv
1320	Nystatin Oral Suspension USP	Rx
0802	Paregoric USP	Rx CIII
1143	Phenadex Children's Cough/Cold Syrup	OTC
1142	Phenadex Pediatric Cough/Cold Drops	OTC
1015	Phenobarbital Elixir USP 20 mg/5 mL	Rx CIV
1014	Phenylephrine HCl Nasal Soln. USP, 1%	OTC
1000	Potassium Chloride Oral Soln. USP, 10% Sugar-Free	Rx
1001	Potassium Chloride Oral Soln. USP, 20% Sugar-Free	Rx
1468	Povidone Douche	OTC
1467	Povidine Surgical Scrub	OTC
1466	Povidine Topical Soln. 1%	OTC
3185	Pregnancy Test Kit	OTC
1504	Prometh Syrup Plain (Promethazine HCl Syrup USP 6.25 mg/5 mL)	Rx
1627	Prometh with Codeine Cough Syrup	Rx Cv
1628	Prometh VC Plain	Rx
1629	Prometh VC with Codeine Cough Syrup	Rx Cv
1630	Prometh with Dextromethorphan Cough Syrup	Rx
1585	Pyrinyl Lice Control Kit	OTC
1583	Pyrinyl Shampoo	OTC
1533	Selenium Sulfide Lotion USP, 2.5%	Rx
1285	Sulfatrim Pediatric Susp. (Sulfamethoxazole and Trimethoprim)	Rx
1284	Sulfatrim Susp. (Sulfamethoxazole and Trimethoprim)	Rx
1540	Theolate Liquid (Theophylline and Guaifenesin)	Rx
1444	Theophylline Elixir 80 mg/15 mL	Rx
1555	Theravite Liquid	OTC
1451	Thioridazine HCl Oral Soln. USP 100 mg/mL	Rx

1457	Thiothixene HCl Oral Soln. USP (Concentrate) 5 mg/mL	Rx
1633	Triacin-C Cough Syrup	Rx Cv
0890	Tri Vit Drops w/Fluoride 0.25 mg	Rx
0894	Tri Vit Drops w/Fluoride 0.5 mg	Rx
1040	Tussex Cough Syrup	OTC

NDC # 23317	PRODUCT/STRENGTH	Rx/OTC
805	Analgesic Balm	OTC
810	Analgesic Balm-Greaseless Muscle Rub	OTC
105	Bacitracin Zinc Ointment 500 units/g	OTC
380	Betamethasone Dipropionate Cream USP 0.05%	Rx
382	Betamethasone Dipropionate Lotion USP 0.05%	Rx
381	Betamethasone Dipropionate Ointment USP 0.05%	Rx
383	Betamethasone Dipropionate Ointment USP (Augmented), 0.05%	Rx
370	Betamethasone Valerate Cream USP 0.1%	Rx
372	Betamethasone Valerate Lotion USP 0.1%	Rx
371	Betamethasone Valerate Ointment USP 0.1%	Rx
510	Bisacodyl Suppositories	OTC
400	Clobetasol Propionate Cream 0.05%	Rx
401	Clobetasol Propionate Ointment 0.05%	Rx
402	Clobetasol Propionate Topical Solution 0.05%	Rx
710	Clotrimazole Vaginal Cream USP 1%	OTC
802	Diaper Rash Ointment	OTC
825	Dibucaine Ointment USP 1%	OTC
390	Fluocinonide Cream 0.05%	Rx
392	Fluocinonide E Cream USP 0.05%	Rx
393	Fluocinonide Topical Solution 0.05%	Rx
511	Hemorrhoidal HC Suppositories, 25 mg	Rx
320	Hydrocortisone Cream USP 0.5%	OTC
323	Hydrocortisone Acetate 0.5% Cream w/Aloe	OTC
325	Hydrocortisone 0.5% Ointment USP	OTC
321	Hydrocortisone Cream USP 1%	OTC
343	Hydrocortisone Cream USP 1%	Rx
326	Hydrocortisone Ointment USP 1%	OTC
331	Hydrocortisone Ointment USP 1%-OTC	OTC
322	Hydrocortisone Cream USP 2.5%	Rx
830	Ichthammol Ointment USP 10%	OTC
835	Ichthammol Ointment USP 20%	OTC
341	Iodochlorhydroxyquin 3% w/ Hydrocortisone 1% Cream	Rx
845	Lanolin Hydrous USP	OTC
735	Miconazole Nitrate Cream 2%	OTC
730	Miconazole Nitrate Vaginal Cream 2%	OTC
736	Miconazole Nitrate 100 mg Vaginal Suppositories	OTC
738	Miconazole Nitrate 200 mg Vaginal Suppositories	Rx
160	Nystatin Cream USP	Rx
165	Nystatin Ointment USP	Rx
150	Nystatin/Triamcinolone Acetonide Cream	Rx
155	Nystatin/Triamcinolone Acetonide Ointment	Rx
855	Povidone Iodine Ointment 10%	OTC
900	Tolnaftate Cream 1%	OTC
905	Tolnaftate Solution 1%	OTC
300	Triamcinolone Acetonide Cream USP 0.025%	Rx
301	Triamcinolone Acetonide Cream USP 0.1%	Rx
306	Triamcinolone Acetonide Ointment USP 0.1%	Rx
125	Triple Antibiotic Ointment	OTC
127	Triple Antibiotic Ointment, Plus, Maximum Strength	OTC
130	Triple Antibiotic Ointment	OTC
700	Triple Sulfa Vaginal Cream	Rx
841	Vitamin A & Vitamin D Ointment	OTC
910	White Petrolatum USP	OTC
800	Zinc Oxide Ointment USP	OTC

LINDANE LOTION USP, 1% ℞

DESCRIPTION

Lindane Lotion USP, 1% is an ectoparasiticide and ovicide effective against *Sarcoptes scabiei* (scabies). In addition to the active ingredient, lindane, it contains glycerol monostearate, cetyl alcohol, stearic acid, trolamine, carrageenan, 2-amino-2-methyl-1-propanol, methylparaben, butylparaben, perfume and water to form a non-greasy lotion. Lindane which is the highly purified gamma isomer of 1, 2, 3, 4, 5, 6, hexa-chlorocyclohexane, has the following structural formula: [See chemical structure at top of next column.]

Continued on next page

Alpharma—Cont.

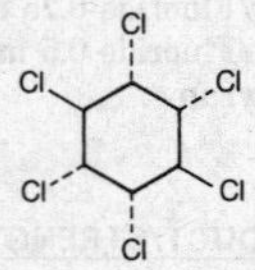

$C_6H_6Cl_6$ 290.83

CLINICAL PHARMACOLOGY

Lindane exerts its parasiticidal action by being directly absorbed into the parasites and their ova. Feldmann and Maibach[1] reported approximately 10% absorption of a lindane acetone solution applied to the forearm and left in place for 24 hours. Dale, et al[2], reported a blood level of 290 ng/mL associated with convulsions following the accidental ingestion of a lindane-containing product. Ginsburg[3] found a mean peak blood level of 28 ng/mL 6 hours after total body application of lindane lotion to scabietic infants and children. The half-life was determined to be 18 hours.

INDICATIONS AND USAGE

Because post-treatment pruritus is common and may lead to misuse, lindane lotion is indicated only for the treatment of patients infested with *Sarcoptes scabiei* (scabies) who have either failed to respond to adequate doses, or are intolerant of, other approved therapies. Reinfestation should be considered carefully before attributing the posttreatment presence of ectoparasites to a failure of response to adequate doses of other approved therapies.

CONTRAINDICATIONS

Lindane lotion is contraindicated for premature neonates because their skin may be more permeable than full term infants and their liver enzymes may not be sufficiently developed. It is also contraindicated for patients with Norwegian (crusted) scabies due to possible increased absorption. It is also contraindicated for patients with known seizure disorders and for individuals with a known sensitivity to the product or any of its components.

WARNINGS

LINDANE PENETRATES HUMAN SKIN AND HAS THE POTENTIAL FOR CNS TOXICITY (SEE CLINICAL PHARMACOLOGY SECTION). LINDANE LOTION SHOULD BE USED ACCORDING TO RECOMMENDED DOSAGE (SEE DIRECTIONS FOR USE) ESPECIALLY ON INFANTS, PREGNANT WOMEN AND NURSING MOTHERS. ANIMAL STUDIES INDICATE THAT POTENTIAL TOXIC EFFECTS OF TOPICALLY APPLIED LINDANE ARE GREATER IN THE YOUNG. SEIZURES AND, IN RARE INSTANCES, DEATHS HAVE BEEN REPORTED AFTER EXCESS DOSAGE, OVER-EXPOSURE, FREQUENT REAPPLICATIONS, AND ACCIDENTAL AND INTENTIONAL INGESTION OF LINDANE. THESE INSTANCES OF PATIENT MISUSE HAVE BEEN ASSOCIATED WITH LACK OF PATIENT UNDERSTANDING OF DIRECTIONS OF USE, PRESCRIBING OR DISPENSING EXCESSIVE QUANTITIES, AND IMPROPER REAPPLICATIONS. IN EXCEEDINGLY RARE CASES SEIZURES HAVE BEEN REPORTED WHEN USED ACCORDING TO DIRECTIONS. NO RESIDUAL EFFECTS OF LINDANE TREATMENT HAS BEEN DEMONSTRATED; THEREFORE, THIS PRODUCT SHOULD NOT BE USED TO WARD OFF A POSSIBLE INFESTATION. If accidental ingestion occurs, prompt gastric lavage is indicated. Because oils may enhance absorption, saline rather than oily cathartics should be used. Central nervous excitation can be controlled by the administration of pentobarbital, phenobarbital or diazepam.

PRECAUTIONS

General: Care should be taken to avoid contact with the eyes. If such contact occurs, eyes should be immediately flushed with water. If irritation or sensitization occurs, the patient should be advised to consult a physician.

Geriatric: Dosage may have to be reduced due to the possibility of increased absorption through elderly skin.

Information for Patients: Patient must be instructed on the proper use of the medication, especially as to amount applied and duration of use. Patient Directions for Use must accompany the product.

Laboratory Tests: No laboratory tests are needed for the proper use of this medication.

Drug Interactions: Oils may enhance absorption; therefore, simultaneous use of creams, ointments or oils should be avoided.

Carcinogenesis: Although no studies have been conducted with lindane lotion, numerous long-term feeding studies have been conducted in mice and rats to evaluate the carcinogenic potential of the technical grade of hexachlorocyclohexane (BHC) as well as the alpha, beta, gamma (lindane) and delta isomers. Both oral and topical applications have been evaluated. Nagasaki[4], Goto[5] and Hanada[6] found varying amounts of benign and malignant hepatomas associated with BHC and the alpha, delta and epsilon isomers. None reported a carcinogenic potential for lindane. Tumors were found only in the animals which had received the alpha isomer. Weisse and Herbst[7] also evaluated the carcinogenic potential of lindane in mice but could find no evidence of lindane carcinogenicity. The National Cancer Institute[8] also found no evidence of carcinogenicity.

Thorpe and Walker[9] compared beta BHC with lindane, dieldrin, DDT and hexabarbital in mice. Despite the unusually high incidence of tumors in the control group, they concluded that 600 ppm of lindane was associated with a significant increase in the incidence of hepatoma and thus, considered it a tumorigen.

Orr[10] and Kashyap, et al[11], evaluated the carcinogenic potential in mice of topically applied BHC. In neither study was there any evidence of a tumorigenic or carcinogenic potential associated with topical application of BHC.

Mutagenicity tests have been used as predictive information about the carcinogenicity of various chemical compounds. Numerous types of mutagenicity tests have been performed with lindane. The results of these tests do not indicate that lindane is mutagenic.

Pregnancy: *Teratogenic Effects:* Pregnancy Category B. Reproduction, including multigeneration studies have been performed in mice, rats, rabbits, pigs, and dogs at doses up to 10 times the human dose and have revealed no evidence of impaired fertility or harm to the fetus due to orally administered lindane. There are, however, no adequate and well-controlled studies in pregnant women. Because animal reproduction studies are not always predictive of human response, the recommended dosage should not be exceeded on pregnant women. They should be treated no more than twice during a pregnancy.

Nursing Mothers: Lindane is secreted in human milk in low concentrations. Studies conducted in the United States as well as in Europe and South America found levels of lindane in human milk ranging from 0 to 113 ppb, as the result of ingestion of foods which had been treated with lindane. There appeared to be no difference in concentrations between country and urban dwellers. Although the levels of lindane found in blood after topical application with lindane lotion make it unlikely that amounts of lindane sufficient to cause serious adverse reactions will be excreted in the milk of nursing mothers who have used lindane lotion, if there is any concern, an alternate method of feeding may be used for 4 days.

Pediatric Use: Refer to the CONTRAINDICATIONS and WARNINGS sections.

ADVERSE REACTIONS

Lindane has been reported to cause central nervous stimulation ranging from dizziness to convulsions. Cases of convulsions have been reported in connection with lindane lotion therapy. However, these incidents were almost always associated with accidental oral ingestion or misuse of the product. In exceedingly rare cases, seizures have been reported when used according to directions. Eczematous eruptions due to irritation from this product have also been reported. Incidence of these adverse reactions is relatively infrequent, occurring in less than 1 in 100,000 patients.

DRUG ABUSE AND DEPENDENCE

Lindane lotion is not subject to abuse, nor is there any dependence on the drug.

OVERDOSAGE

Overdosage or oral ingestion of lindane lotion can cause central nervous system excitation and if taken in sufficient quantities, convulsions may occur. If accidental ingestion occurs, prompt gastric lavage should be instituted. However, since oils favor absorption, saline cathartics for intestinal evacuation should be given rather than oil laxatives. If central nervous system manifestations occur, they can be antagonized by the administration of pentobarbital, phenobarbital or diazepam.

DOSAGE AND ADMINISTRATION

CAUTION: USE ONLY AS DIRECTED. DO NOT EXCEED RECOMMENDED DOSAGE.

No residual effects have been demonstrated, therefore, this product should not be used to ward off a possible infestation. However, sexual contacts should be treated simultaneously.

NOTE: PLEASE READ CAREFULLY.

DIRECTIONS FOR USE:

WARNING:

THIS PRODUCT CAN BE POISONOUS IF MISUSED. CHILDREN MUST NOT BE ALLOWED TO APPLY THIS DRUG WITHOUT DIRECT ADULT SUPERVISION. USE LOTION FOR SCABIES ONLY. APPLY ONLY ONCE. USE ONLY ENOUGH TO COVER THE BODY IN A THIN LAYER. 1 OUNCE (HALF OF A 2 OUNCE CONTAINER) SHOULD BE ALL THAT IS NEEDED FOR CHILDREN UNDER 6 YEARS OF AGE; 1 TO 2 OUNCES FOR OLDER CHILDREN AND ADULTS. DO NOT LEAVE ON FOR MORE THAN 12 HOURS. DO NOT INGEST. KEEP AWAY FROM MOUTH AND EYES. COVER INFANTS' HANDS AND FEET DURING TREATMENT TO PREVENT SUCKING AND LICKING OF LOTION. DO NOT USE IF OPEN WOUNDS, CUTS OR SORES ARE PRESENT, UNLESS DIRECTED BY YOUR PHYSICIAN.

(LOTION: SHAKE WELL)

1. APPLY THIS PREPARATION TO DRY SKIN IN A THIN LAYER AND RUB IN THOROUGHLY.
2. TRIM NAILS AND APPLY UNDER NAILS WITH TOOTHBRUSH (THROW AWAY TOOTHBRUSH AFTER USE).
3. IF A WARM BATH IS TAKEN BEFORE APPLICATION, ALLOW THE SKIN TO DRY AND COOL COMPLETELY BEFORE APPLYING THE MEDICATION.
4. A TOTAL BODY APPLICATION SHOULD BE MADE FROM THE NECK DOWN, INCLUDING SOLES OF FEET, UNLESS OTHERWISE DIRECTED BY YOUR PHYSICIAN.
5. THE LOTION SHOULD BE LEFT ON FOR 8 TO 12 HOURS (USUALLY OVERNIGHT) AND THEN REMOVED BY THOROUGH WASHING (BATH OR SHOWER).
6. AVOID UNNECESSARY CONTACT WITH YOUR SKIN IF YOU ARE APPLYING TO ANOTHER PERSON. IF TREATING MORE THAN ONE PERSON, PERSON APPLYING LOTION (ESPECIALLY PREGNANT OR NURSING WOMEN) SHOULD WEAR RUBBER GLOVES.
7. ALL RECENTLY WORN CLOTHING, UNDERWEAR AND PAJAMAS, AND USED SHEETS, PILLOW CASES, AND TOWELS SHOULD BE WASHED IN VERY HOT WATER OR DRY-CLEANED.

AFTER ONE APPLICATION, ITCHING WILL CONTINUE FOR SEVERAL WEEKS. THIS IS NORMAL AND DOES NOT REQUIRE REAPPLICATION.

IF YOU HAVE ANY QUESTIONS OR CONCERNS ABOUT YOUR CONDITION OR USE OF THE LOTION, CONTACT YOUR PHYSICIAN.

HOW SUPPLIED

Lindane Lotion USP, 1% in patient-size 2 fl oz (59 mL), pharmacy-size only pint (473 mL) and pharmacy-size only 1 gallon (3785 mL) bottles.

SHAKE WELL BEFORE USING.

Store at controlled room temperature 15°–30°C (59°–86°F).

Dispense in a tight, light-resistant container as defined in the USP, with a child-resistant closure.

CAUTION: Federal law prohibits dispensing without prescription.

REFERENCES

1. Feldmann, R.J. and Maiback, H.I., *Toxicol. Applied. Pharmacol.*, 28:126, 1974.
2. Dale, W.E., Curly, A. and Cueto, C. *Life Sci* 5:47, 1966.
3. Ginsburg, C.M., et al., *J. Pediatr.* 91:6 998–1000, 1977.
4. Nagasaki, T., Tomii, S., Mepa, T., Marugami, M. and lto. N. *Gann* (Cancer) 63(3):393, 1972.
5. Goto, M., Hattori, M., Miyagawa, T. and Enomoto, M., *Chemosphere* 6:279, 1972.
6. Hanada, M., Yatani, C., Miyaji, T., *Gann* 64:511, 1973.
7. Weisse, I., and Herbst, M., *Toxicol.* 7:233, 1977.
8. Technical Report Series, NCI-CG-TR-14, *HEW PUBLICATIONS,* No. (NIH) 77–814.
9. Thorpe, E., and Walker, A.I.T., *Food Cosmetic Toxicol.* 11:433, 1973.
10. Orr, J.W., *Nature* 162:189, 1948.
11. Kashyap, S.K. et. al., *J. Environ, Sci. Health* 14:305–318, 1979.

Manufactured by
Barre-National Inc.
Baltimore, MD 21244
an ALPHARMA USPD Company

FORM NO. 0570-02 Rev. 4/96 B1

PHARMACIST—DETACH AND GIVE TO PATIENT

LINDANE LOTION USP 1%
DIRECTIONS FOR USE

WARNING:

THIS PRODUCT CAN BE POISONOUS IF MISUSED. CHILDREN MUST NOT BE ALLOWED TO APPLY THIS DRUG WITHOUT DIRECT ADULT SUPERVISION. USE LOTION FOR SCABIES ONLY. APPLY ONLY ONCE. USE ONLY ENOUGH TO COVER THE BODY IN A THIN LAYER. 1 OUNCE (HALF OF A 2 OUNCE CONTAINER) SHOULD BE ALL THAT IS NEEDED FOR CHILDREN UNDER 6 YEARS OF AGE; 1 TO 2 OUNCES FOR OLDER CHILDREN AND ADULTS. DO NOT LEAVE ON FOR MORE THAN 12 HOURS. DO NOT INGEST. KEEP AWAY FROM MOUTH AND EYES. COVER INFANTS' HANDS AND FEET DURING TREATMENT TO PREVENT SUCKING AND LICKING OF LOTION. DO NOT USE IF OPEN WOUNDS, CUTS OR SORES ARE PRESENT, UNLESS DIRECTED BY YOUR PHYSICIAN.

(Lotion: Shake Well)

1. Apply this preparation to dry skin in a thin layer and rub in thoroughly.
2. Trim nails and apply under nails with toothbrush (throw away toothbrush after use).

3. If a warm bath is taken before application, allow the skin to dry and cool completely before applying the medication.
4. A total body application should be made from the neck down, including soles of feet, unless otherwise directed by your physician.
5. The lotion should be left on for 8 to 12 hours (usually overnight) and then removed by thorough washing (bath or shower).
6. If applying lotion to another person, wear rubber gloves, especially if you are pregnant or a nursing mother.
7. All recently worn clothing, underwear and pajamas, and used sheets, pillow cases, and towels should be washed in very hot water or dry-cleaned.

After one application, itching will continue for several weeks. This is normal and does not require reapplication.
If you have any questions or concerns about your condition or use of the lotion, contact your physician.

0570-02

LINDANE SHAMPOO, USP 1% ℞

DESCRIPTION

Lindane Shampoo, USP 1% is an ectoparasiticide and ovicide effective against *Pediculosis capitis* (head lice), *Pediculosis pubis* (crab lice) and their ova. In addition to the active ingredient, lindane, it contains trolamine lauryl sulfate, polysorbate 60, acetone and water to form a cosmetically pleasant shampoo. The pH may be adjusted with Citric Acid and/or Trolamine. Lindane, which is the highly purified gamma isomer of 1, 2, 3, 4, 5, 6, hexachlorocyclohexane, has the following structural formula:

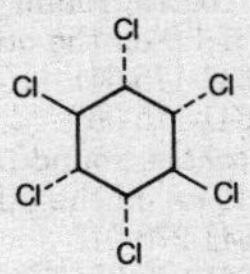

$C_6H_6Cl_6$ 290.83

CLINICAL PHARMACOLOGY

Lindane exerts its parasiticidal action by being directly absorbed into the parasites and their ova. Dale, et al[1], reported a blood level of 290 ng/mL associated with convulsions following the accidental ingestion of a lindane-containing product. Analysis of blood taken from subjects before and after the use of lindane shampoo showed a mean peak blood level of only 3 ng/mL which appeared at six hours and disappeared at eight hours after the shampoo was applied.

INDICATIONS AND USAGE

Because post-treatment pruritus is common and may lead to misuse, lindane shampoo is indicated only for the treatment of patients with pediculosis capitis (head lice) and pediculosis pubis (crab lice) who have either failed to respond to adequate doses, or are intolerant of, other approved therapies. Reinfestation should be considered carefully before attributing the posttreatment presence of ectoparasites to a failure of response to adequate doses of other approved therapies.

CONTRAINDICATIONS

Lindane shampoo is contraindicated for premature neonates because their skin may be more permeable than full term infants and their liver enzymes may not be sufficiently developed. It is also contraindicated for patients with known seizure disorders and for individuals with a known sensitivity to the product or any of its components.

WARNINGS

LINDANE PENETRATES HUMAN SKIN AND HAS THE POTENTIAL FOR CNS TOXICITY (SEE CLINICAL PHARMACOLOGY SECTION). LINDANE SHAMPOO SHOULD BE USED ACCORDING TO RECOMMENDED DOSAGE (SEE DIRECTIONS FOR USE) ESPECIALLY ON INFANTS, PREGNANT WOMEN AND NURSING MOTHERS. ANIMAL STUDIES INDICATE THAT POTENTIAL TOXIC EFFECTS OF TOPICALLY APPLIED LINDANE ARE GREATER IN THE YOUNG. SEIZURES AND, IN RARE INSTANCES, DEATHS HAVE BEEN REPORTED AFTER EXCESS DOSAGE, OVER-EXPOSURE, FREQUENT REAPPLICATIONS, AND ACCIDENTAL AND INTENTIONAL INGESTION OF LINDANE. THESE INSTANCES OF PATIENT MISUSE HAVE BEEN ASSOCIATED WITH LACK OF PATIENT UNDERSTANDING OF DIRECTIONS FOR USE, PRESCRIBING OR DISPENSING EXCESSIVE QUANTITIES, AND IMPROPER REAPPLICATIONS. IN EXCEEDINGLY RARE CASES SEIZURES HAVE BEEN REPORTED WHEN USED ACCORDING TO DIRECTIONS. NO RESIDUAL EFFECTS OF LINDANE TREATMENT HAVE BEEN DEMONSTRATED, THEREFORE, THIS PRODUCT SHOULD NOT BE USED TO WARD OFF A POSSIBLE INFESTATION.

If accidental ingestion occurs, prompt gastric lavage is indicated. Because oils may enhance absorption, saline rather than oily cathartics should be used. Central nervous excitation can be controlled by the administration of pentobarbital, phenobarbital or diazepam.

PRECAUTIONS

General: Care should be taken to avoid contact with the eyes. If such contact occurs, eyes should be immediately flushed with water. If irritation or sensitization occurs, the patient should be advised to consult a physician.

Information for Patients: Patients must be instructed on the proper use of the medication, especially as to amount applied and duration of use. Patients Directions for Use must accompany the product.

Laboratory Tests: No laboratory tests are needed for the proper use of this medication.

Drug Interactions: Oils may enhance absorption, therefore, avoid using oil treatment, or oil based hair dressings or conditioners immediately before and after applying lindane shampoo.

Carcinogenesis: Although no studies have been conducted with lindane shampoo, numerous long-term feeding studies have been conducted in mice and rats to evaluate the carcinogenic potential of the technical grade of hexachlorocyclohexane (BHC) as well as the alpha, beta, gamma (lindane) and delta isomers. Both oral and topical applications have been evaluated. Nagasaki[2], Goto[3] and Hanada[4] found varying amounts of benign and malignant hepatomas associated with BHC and the alpha, delta and epsilon isomers. None reported a carcinogenic potential for lindane. Tumors were found only in the animals which had received the alpha isomer. Weisse and Herbst[5] also evaluated the carcinogenic potential of lindane in mice but could find no evidence of lindane carcinogenicity. The National Cancer Institute[6] had also found no evidence of carcinogenicity.

Thorpe and Walker[7] compared beta BHC with lindane, dieldrin, DDT and hexabarbital in mice. Despite the unusually high incidence of tumors in the control group, they concluded that 600 ppm of lindane was associated with a significant increase in the incidence of hepatoma and thus, considered it a tumorigen.

Orr[8] and Kashyap, et al[9] evaluated the carcinogenic potential in mice of topically applied BHC. In neither study was there any evidence of a tumorigenic or carcinogenic potential associated with topical application of BHC.

Mutagenicity tests have been used as predictive information about the carcinogenicity of various chemical compounds. Numerous types of mutagenicity tests have been performed with lindane. The results of these tests do not indicate that lindane is mutagenic.

Pregnancy: *Teratogenic Effects*—Pregnancy Category B. Reproduction, including multigeneration, studies have been performed in mice, rats, rabbits, pigs, and dogs at doses up to 10 times the human dose and have revealed no evidence of impaired fertility or harm to the fetus due to orally administered lindane. There are, however, no adequate and well-controlled studies in pregnant women. Because animal reproduction studies are not always predictive of human response, the recommended dosage should not be exceeded on pregnant women. They should be treated no more than twice during a pregnancy.

Nursing Mothers: Lindane is secreted in human milk in low concentrations. Studies conducted in the United States as well as in Europe and South America found levels of lindane in human milk ranging from 0 to 113 ppb, as the result of ingestion of foods which had been treated with lindane. There appeared to be no difference in concentrations between country and urban dwellers. Although the levels of lindane found in blood after topical application with lindane shampoo make it unlikely that amounts of lindane sufficient to cause serious adverse reactions will be excreted in the milk of nursing mothers who have used lindane shampoo, if there is any concern, an alternate method of feeding may be used for 4 days.

Pediatric Use: Refer to the CONTRAINDICATIONS and WARNINGS sections.

ADVERSE REACTIONS

Lindane has been reported to cause central nervous stimulation ranging from dizziness to convulsions. Cases of convulsions have been reported in connection with lindane shampoo therapy. However, these incidents were almost always associated with accidental oral ingestion or misuse of the product. In exceedingly rare cases, seizures have been reported when used according to directions. Eczematous eruptions due to irritation from this product have also been reported. Incidence of these adverse reactions is relatively infrequent, occurring in less than 1 in 100,000 patients.

DRUG ABUSE AND DEPENDENCE

Lindane shampoo is not subject to abuse, nor is there any dependence on the drug.

OVERDOSAGE

Overdosage or oral ingestion of lindane shampoo can cause central nervous system excitation and, if taken in sufficient quantities, convulsions may occur.

If accidental ingestion occurs, prompt gastric lavage should be instituted. However, since oils favor absorption, saline cathartics for intestinal evacuation should be given rather than oil laxatives. If central nervous system manifestations occur, they can be antagonized by the administration of pentobarbital, phenobarbital or diazepam.

DOSAGE AND ADMINISTRATION

CAUTION: USE ONLY AS DIRECTED. DO NOT EXCEED RECOMMENDED DOSAGE.

No residual effects of lindane shampoo treatment have been demonstrated, therefore, this product should not be used to ward off a possible infestation. However, sexual contacts should be treated simultaneously.

NOTE: PLEASE READ CAREFULLY.

DIRECTIONS FOR USE

WARNING:

THIS PRODUCT CAN BE POISONOUS IF MISUSED. CHILDREN MUST NOT BE ALLOWED TO APPLY THIS DRUG WITHOUT DIRECT ADULT SUPERVISION. USE SHAMPOO FOR HEAD AND PUBIC LICE ONLY. DO NOT USE FOR SCABIES. USE ONLY IN AMOUNTS DIRECTED BELOW. IN NO CASE SHOULD MORE THAN 2 OUNCES BE USED BY ONE PERSON IN ONE APPLICATION. DO NOT INGEST. KEEP AWAY FROM MOUTH AND EYES. DO NOT USE IF OPEN WOUNDS, CUTS OR SORES ARE PRESENT ON SCALP OR GROIN, UNLESS DIRECTED BY YOUR PHYSICIAN.

AVOID USING OIL TREATMENTS, OIL BASED HAIR DRESSINGS OR CONDITIONERS IMMEDIATELY BEFORE AND AFTER APPLYING LINDANE SHAMPOO.

(SHAKE WELL)

1. BEFORE APPLYING LINDANE SHAMPOO, USE REGULAR SHAMPOO (WITHOUT CONDITIONERS), RINSE AND COMPLETELY DRY HAIR.
2. USE 1 OUNCE (HALF OF A 2 OUNCE BOTTLE) FOR SHORT HAIR; 1.5 OUNCES (THREE-QUARTERS OF A 2 OUNCE BOTTLE) FOR MEDIUM LENGTH HAIR; AND FULL 2 OUNCE BOTTLE FOR LONG HAIR.
3. APPLY SHAMPOO DIRECTLY TO DRY HAIR WITHOUT ADDING WATER. WORK THOROUGHLY INTO THE HAIR AND ALLOW TO REMAIN IN PLACE FOR 4 MINUTES ONLY.
4. AFTER 4 MINUTES, ADD SMALL QUANTITIES OF WATER TO HAIR UNTIL A GOOD LATHER FORMS.
5. IMMEDIATELY RINSE ALL LATHER AWAY. AVOID UNNECESSARY CONTACT OF LATHER WITH OTHER BODY SURFACES.
6. TOWEL BRISKLY AND REMOVE NITS WITH NIT COMB OR TWEEZERS.
7. AVOID UNNECESSARY CONTACT WITH YOUR SKIN IF YOU ARE APPLYING SHAMPOO TO ANOTHER PERSON. IF TREATING MORE THAN ONE PERSON, PERSON APPLYING SHAMPOO (ESPECIALLY PREGNANT AND/OR NURSING WOMEN) SHOULD WEAR RUBBER GLOVES.

RE-TREATMENT IS USUALLY NOT NECESSARY, BUT PRESENCE OF LIVING LICE IN HAIR 7 DAYS AFTER TREATMENT INDICATES THAT RE-TREATMENT MAY BE NECESSARY. DO NOT RETREAT WITHOUT THE ADVICE OF A PHYSICIAN.

HOW SUPPLIED

Lindane Shampoo, USP 1% in patient-size 2 fl oz (59 mL), pharmacy-size only pint (473 mL) and pharmacy-size only gallon (3785 mL) bottles.

SHAKE WELL BEFORE USING.

Store at controlled room temperature 15°–30°C (59°–86°F).

Dispense in a tight, light-resistant container as defined in the USP, with a child-resistant closure.

CAUTION: Federal law prohibits dispensing without prescription.

REFERENCES

1. Dale, W.E., Curly, A. and Cueto, C. *Life Sci* 5:47, 1966.
2. Nagasaki, T., Tomii, S., Mega, T., Marugami, M. and Ito, N. *Gann* (Cancer) 63(3):373, 1972.
3. Goto, M., Hattori, M., Miyagawa, T. and Enomoto, M., *Chemosphere* 6:279, 1972.
4. Hanada, M., Yatani, C., Miyaji, T., *Gann* 64:511, 1973.
5. Weisse, I., and Herbst, M., *Toxicol.* 7:233, 1977.
6. Technical Report Series, NCl-CG-TR-14, *HEW PUBLICATIONS,* No. (NIH) 77–814.
7. Thorpe, E., and Walker, A.I.T., *Food Cosmetic Toxicol. 11:433, 1973.*
8. Orr, J.W., *Nature* 162:189, 1948.
9. Kashyap, S.K. et al, *J. Environ. Sci. Health* 14:305–318, 1979.

Continued on next page

Alpharma—Cont.

Manufactured by
Barre-National Inc.
Baltimore, MD 21244
an ALPHARMA USPD Company
FORM NO. 0572-02   Rev. 4/96 B1

PHARMACIST — DETACH AND GIVE TO PATIENT

LINDANE SHAMPOO, USP 1%
A SHAMPOO
FOR THE TREATMENT OF HEAD OR PUBIC LICE
CAUTION: USE ONLY AS DIRECTED. DO NOT EXCEED
RECOMMENDED DOSE.
NOTE: PLEASE READ CAREFULLY.
DIRECTIONS FOR USE:
WARNING:
THIS PRODUCT CAN BE POISONOUS IF MISUSED. CHILDREN MUST NOT BE ALLOWED TO APPLY THIS DRUG
WITHOUT DIRECT ADULT SUPERVISION. USE SHAMPOO
FOR HEAD AND PUBIC LICE ONLY. DO NOT USE FOR
SCABIES. USE ONLY IN AMOUNTS DIRECTED BELOW. IN
NO CASE SHOULD MORE THAN 2 OUNCES BE USED BY
ONE PERSON IN ONE APPLICATION. DO NOT INGEST.
KEEP AWAY FROM MOUTH AND EYES. DO NOT USE IF
OPEN WOUNDS, CUTS OR SORES ARE PRESENT ON
SCALP OR GROIN, UNLESS DIRECTED BY YOUR PHYSICIAN.
AVOID USING OIL TREATMENTS, OIL BASED HAIR
DRESSINGS OR CONDITIONERS IMMEDIATELY BEFORE
AND AFTER APPLYING LINDANE SHAMPOO.
(SHAKE WELL)

1. BEFORE APPLYING LINDANE SHAMPOO, USE REGULAR SHAMPOO (WITHOUT CONDITIONERS), RINSE
   AND COMPLETELY DRY HAIR.
2. USE 1 OUNCE (HALF OF A 2 OUNCE BOTTLE) FOR
   SHORT HAIR; 1.5 OUNCES (THREE-QUARTERS OF A 2
   OUNCE BOTTLE) FOR MEDIUM LENGTH HAIR; AND
   FULL 2 OUNCE BOTTLE FOR LONG HAIR.
3. APPLY SHAMPOO DIRECTLY TO DRY HAIR WITHOUT ADDING WATER. WORK THOROUGHLY INTO
   THE HAIR AND ALLOW TO REMAIN IN PLACE FOR
   4 MINUTES ONLY.
4. AFTER 4 MINUTES. ADD SMALL QUANTITIES OF
   WATER TO HAIR UNTIL A GOOD LATHER FORMS.
5. IMMEDIATELY RINSE ALL LATHER AWAY. AVOID
   UNNECESSARY CONTACT OF LATHER WITH OTHER
   BODY SURFACES.
6. TOWEL BRISKLY AND REMOVE NITS WITH NIT
   COMB OR TWEEZERS.
7. AVOID UNNECESSARY CONTACT WITH YOUR SKIN
   IF YOU ARE APPLYING SHAMPOO TO ANOTHER
   PERSON. IF TREATING MORE THAN ONE PERSON,
   PERSON APPLYING SHAMPOO (ESPECIALLY PREGNANT AND/OR NURSING WOMEN) SHOULD WEAR
   RUBBER GLOVES.
RE-TREATMENT IS USUALLY NOT NECESSARY, BUT
PRESENCE OF LIVING LICE IN HAIR 7 DAYS AFTER
TREATMENT INDICATES THAT RE-TREATMENT MAY
BE NECESSARY. DO NOT RE-TREAT WITHOUT THE
ADVICE OF A PHYSICIAN.

Alra Laboratories, Inc.
**3850 CLEARVIEW CT.
GURNEE, IL 60031**

Direct Inquiries to:
Professional Services
(847) 244-9440
(800) 248-ALRA
FAX: (847) 244-9464

CHOLAC   ℞
[kō'lac]
CONSTILAC   ℞
[kŏn'stil-ac]
Lactulose Syrup, USP

Each 15 mL syrup contains:
10 g lactulose (and less than 1.6 g galactose, less than 1.2 g
lactose, 0.1 g or less of fructose); plus water and coloring.
Sodium hydroxide used to adjust pH.

HOW SUPPLIED
1 fl. oz. bottle (30 mL) (unit-dose)
  100 bottles/carton   NDC #51641-225-61
8 fl. oz. bottle (240 mL)   NDC #51641-224-68
16 fl oz. bottle (480 mL)   NDC #51641-225-76
32 fl. oz. bottle (960 mL)   NDC #51641-224-82
64 fl. oz. bottle (1920 mL)   NDC #51641-225-94
1 gal. (3785 mL)   NDC #51641-225-97

DIGOXIN TABLETS   ℞

Digoxin Tablets are available in 0.125 mg, 0.250 mg, and
0.500 mg strengths for oral administration.

HOW SUPPLIED
0.125 mg yellow, round, scored tablets debossed with Digoxin/233 and Alra logo:
Bottles of 100   NDC 51641-233-01
Bottles of 1000   NDC 51641-233-10
Bottles of 5000   NDC 51641-233-50
0.250 mg white, round, scored tablets debossed with Digoxin/234 and Alra logo:
Bottles of 100   NDC 51641-234-01
Bottles of 1000   NDC 51641-234-10
Bottles of 5000   NDC 51641-234-50
0.500 mg white, round, scored tablets debossed with Digoxin/235 and Alra logo:
Bottles of 100   NDC 51641-235-01
Bottles of 1000   NDC 51641-235-10
Bottles of 5000   NDC 51641-235-50

ERYZOLE Granules for Suspension   ℞
erythromycin ethylsuccinate and sulfisoxazole acetyl
for oral suspension USP

When reconstituted each 5mL of suspension contains:
Erythromycin Ethylsuccinate equivalent to 200mg erythromycin and Sulfisoxazole Acetyl equivalent to 600mg sulfisoxazole.

HOW SUPPLIED
Eryzole suspension is available for teaspoon dosage in bottles
of,
100 mL (NDC 51641-111-64)
150 mL (NDC 51641-111-66)
200 mL (NDC 51641-111-68)
in the form of granules to be reconstituted with water.

GELPIRIN TABLETS   OTC

Each tablet contains:
Acetaminophen .... 125 mg.
Aspirin .... 240 mg.
Caffeine .... 32 mg.
Along with two buffering agents

HOW SUPPLIED
Bottle of 100 (NDC 51641-711-01)
Bottle of 1000 (NDC 51641-711-10)

Gen–XENE®   © ℞
[jen'zēn]
Clorazepate Dipotassium Tablets

Gen–XENE Tablets are available in 3.75 mg, 7.5 mg or 15 mg
strengths for oral administration.

HOW SUPPLIED
3.75 mg gray, scored tablets debossed with ALRA and GX:
Unit dose packages of 100: NDC 51641-242-11
Bottles of 30 NDC 51641-242-03
Bottles of 100 NDC 51641-242-01
Bottles of 500 NDC 51641-242-05

7.5 mg yellow, scored tablets debossed with ALRA and GT:
Unit dose packages of 100: NDC 51641-243-11
Bottles of 30 NDC 51641-243-03
Bottles of 100 NDC 51641-243-01
Bottles of 500 NDC 51641-243-05

15 mg green, scored tablets debossed with ALRA and GN:
Unit dose packages of 100: NDC 51641-244-11
Bottles of 30 NDC 51641-244-03
Bottles of 100 NDC 51641-244-01
Bottles of 500 NDC 51641-244-05

IBU–TAB
Ibuprofen Tablets, USP

Ibuprofen Tablets are available in 200, 400, 600 and 800 mg
strengths for oral administration.

HOW SUPPLIED
IBU-TAB OTC
Ibuprofen Tablets, 200 mg (orange) film-coated, round tablets. Debossed 'ALRA' on one side and 215 on the other.

Bottles of 30   NDC 51641-215-03
Bottles of 60   NDC 51641-215-60

Bottles of 100   NDC 51641-215-01
Bottles of 250   NDC 51641-215-25
IBU-TAB ℞
Ibuprofen Tablets, 400 mg (orange) film-coated, round tablets. Debossed 'ALRA' on one side and IF 400 on the other.
Bottles of 100   NDC 51641-214-01
Bottles of 500   NDC 51641-214-05
Bottles of 1000   NDC 51641-214-10
Unit-dose packages of 100   NDC 51641-214-11
Ibuprofen Tablets, 600 mg (orange) film-coated, round tablets.
Debossed 'ALRA' on one side and IF 600 on the other.
Bottles of 100   NDC 51641-213-01
Bottles of 500   NDC 51641-213-05
Bottles of 1000   NDC 51641-213-10
Unit-dose packages of 100   NDC 51641-213-11
Ibuprofen Tablets, 800 mg (light peach) film-coated, oval
tablets. Debossed 'ALRA' on one side and IF 800 on the other.
Bottles of 100   NDC 51641-212-01
Bottles of 500   NDC 51641-212-05
Bottles of 1000   NDC 51641-212-10
Unit-dose packages of 100   NDC 51641-212-11

K+ 8   ℞
Potassium Chloride Extended-release Tablets, USP

Each K+ 8 tablet contains:
Potassium Chloride, USP .... 8 mEq (600 mg)
Equivalent to 8 mEq (312 mg) of potassium and 8 mEq
(288 mg) of chloride)

HOW SUPPLIED
8 mEq (600 mg) yellow, coated, round tablets debossed
ALRA on one side and K+8 on the other side:
Bottles of 100 (NDC 51641-175-01)
Bottles of 500 (NDC 51641-175-05)
8 mEq (600 mg) white, coated, round tablets debossed
ALRA on one side and K+8 on the other side:
Bottles of 100 (NDC 51641-275-01)
Bottles of 500 (NDC 51641-275-05)

K + 10   ℞
Potassium Chloride Extended-release Tablets, USP

Each K + 10 tablet contains:
Potassium Chloride, USP ....10 mEq (750 mg)
[Equivalent to 10 mEq (390 mg) of potassium and 10 mEq
(360 mg) of chloride]

HOW SUPPLIED
10 mEq (750 mg) yellow, coated, capsule shaped tablets
debossed ALRA on one side and K+10 on the other side.
Bottles of 100 (NDC 51641-177-01)
Bottles of 500 (NDC 51641-177-05)
Bottles of 1000 (NDC 51641-177-10)
Unit dose (100) in strips (NDC 51641-177-11)
10 mEq (750 mg) white, coated, capsule shaped tablets
debossed ALRA on one side and K+10 on the other side.
Bottles of 100 (NDC 51641-277-01)
Bottles of 500 (NDC 51641-277-05)
Bottles of 1000 (NDC 51641-277-10)

K + CARE 20 mEq   ℞
Potassium Chloride For Oral Solution, USP

Each powder packet provides:
Potassium Chloride .... 20 mEq (1.5 gm.)
[Equivalent to 20 mEq (780 mg) of potassium and 20 mEq
(720 mg) of chloride]

HOW SUPPLIED
Carton of 30 (NDC 51641-120-03) Orange flavor
Carton of 30 (NDC 51641-140-03) Fruit flavor
Carton of 100 (NDC 51641-120-01) Orange flavor
Carton of 100 (NDC 51641-140-01) Fruit flavor

K + CARE ET 25 mEq   ℞
**Potassium Bicarbonate Effervescent Tablets For Oral
Solution, USP**

Each tablet contains .... 25 mEq of Potassium
(From 2.5 Gm. of Potassium Bicarbonate)

HOW SUPPLIED
Carton of 30 (NDC 51641-135-03) Orange flavor
Carton of 30 (NDC 51641-125-03) Lime flavor
Carton of 100 (NDC 51641-135-01) Orange flavor
Carton of 100 (NDC 51641-125-01) Lime flavor

ALZA Pharmaceuticals,
A division of ALZA Corporation
950 PAGE MILL ROAD
P.O. BOX 10950
PALO ALTO, CA 94303-0802

Direct Inquiries to:
Customer Service
(800) 227-9953
FAX: (415) 962-4212

For Medical Information or Medical Emergencies Contact:
Medical Communications (for Testoderm, Progestasert, Ocusert)
(800) 634-8977
FAX: (415) 962-2488
Medical Communications (for Ethyol)
(800) 506-4959
FAX: (415) 962-2488

ETHYOL®

[a-thī-ol]
(amifostine) for Injection

℞

DESCRIPTION

ETHYOL (amifostine) is an organic thiophosphate cytoprotective agent known chemically as ethanethiol, 2-[(3-aminopropyl)amino]-, dihydrogen phosphate (ester) and has the following structural formula:

$$H_2N(CH_2)_3NH(CH_2)_2S\text{-}PO_3H_2$$

Amifostine is a white crystalline powder which is freely soluble in water. Its empirical formula is $C_5H_{15}N_2O_3PS$ and it has a molecular weight of 214.22.
ETHYOL is supplied as a sterile lyophilized powder mixture with mannitol requiring reconstitution for intravenous infusion. Each single-use 10 mL vial contains 500 mg of amifostine (anhydrous basis) and 500 mg of mannitol.

CLINICAL PHARMACOLOGY

ETHYOL (amifostine) is a prodrug that is dephosphorylated by alkaline phosphatase in tissues to a pharmacologically active free thiol metabolite that can reduce the toxic effects of cisplatin. The ability to differentially protect normal tissues is attributed to the higher capillary alkaline phosphatase activity, higher pH and better vascularity of normal tissues relative to tumor tissue, which results in a more rapid generation of the active thiol metabolite as well as a higher rate constant for uptake. The higher concentration of free thiol in normal tissues is available to bind to, and thereby detoxify, reactive metabolites of cisplatin; and also can act as a scavenger of free radicals that may be generated in tissues exposed to cisplatin. Several preclinical studies in mice and rats have demonstrated that pretreatment with ETHYOL results in protection from nephrotoxicity following administration of single and multiple doses of cisplatin.
Pharmacokinetics: Clinical pharmacokinetic studies show that ETHYOL is rapidly cleared from the plasma with a distribution half-life of <1 minute and an elimination half-life of approximately 8 minutes. Less than 10% of ETHYOL remains in the plasma 6 minutes after drug administration. ETHYOL is rapidly metabolized to an active free thiol metabolite. A disulfide metabolite is produced subsequently and is less active than the free thiol. After a 10-second bolus dose of 150 mg/m^2 of ETHYOL, renal excretion of the parent drug and its two metabolites was low during the hour following drug administration, averaging 0.69%, 2.64% and 2.22% of the administered dose for the parent, thiol and disulfide, respectively. Measurable levels of the free thiol metabolite have been found in bone marrow cells 5–8 minutes after intravenous infusion of amifostine. Pretreatment with dexamethasone or metoclopramide has no effect on ETHYOL pharmacokinetics.

Clinical Studies: A randomized controlled trial compared six cycles of cyclophosphamide 1000 mg/m^2, and cisplatin 100 mg/m^2 with or without amifostine pretreatment at 910 mg/m^2, in two successive cohorts of 121 patients with advanced ovarian cancer. In both cohorts, after multiple cycles of chemotherapy, pretreatment with ETHYOL significantly reduced the cumulative renal toxicity associated with cisplatin as assessed by the proportion of patients who had ≥40% decrease in creatinine clearance from pretreatment values, protracted elevations in serum creatinine (>1.5 mg/dL), or severe hypomagnesemia. Subgroup analyses suggested that the effect of ETHYOL was present in patients who had received nephrotoxic antibiotics, or who had pre-existing diabetes or hypertension (and thus may have been at increased risk for significant nephrotoxicity), as well as in patients who lacked these risks. Selected analyses of the effects of ETHYOL in reducing the cumulative renal toxicity of cisplatin in the randomized ovarian cancer study are provided in TABLES 1 and 2, below.

TABLE 1
Proportion of Patients with ≥40% Reduction in Calculated Creatinine Clearance*

	Amifostine + CP	CP	p-value 2-sided
All Patients	16/122 (13%)	36/120 (30%)	0.001
First Cohort	10/63	20/58	0.018
Second Cohort	6/59	16/62	0.026

*Creatinine clearance values were calculated using the Cockcroft-Gault formula. *Nephron* 1976; 16:31–41.
[See Table 2 above.]
In the randomized ovarian cancer study, ETHYOL (amifostine) had no detectable effect on the antitumor efficacy of cisplatin-cyclophosphamide chemotherapy. Objective response rates (including pathologically confirmed complete remission rates), time to progression, and survival duration were all similar in the amifostine and control study groups. The table below summarizes the principal efficacy findings of the randomized ovarian cancer study.
[See Table 3 below.]
A Phase II trial of Ethyol, 740–910 mg/m^2, and cisplatin, 120 mg/m^2, administered on day 1 and vinblastine, 5mg/m^2, administered on days 1, 8, 15 and 22 of each monthly cycle was conducted in 25 patients with Stage IV non-small cell lung cancer. This regimen was repeated until disease progression or unacceptable toxicity occurred, or a maximum of six cycles had been administered. Among 13 patients who received 4 or more cycles of this intensive cisplatin regimen, 1 had a ≥40% reduction in creatinine clearance. These results are consistent with the randomized ovarian cancer trial.

Sixteen of the 25 patients treated demonstrated a partial response to chemotherapy. With a median follow-up of 19 months, the median survival was 17 months. At one year, 64% of the patients were alive. These results indicate that ETHYOL may not adversely affect the efficacy of this chemotherapy for non-small cell lung cancer.

INDICATIONS AND USAGE

ETHYOL is indicated to reduce the cumulative renal toxicity associated with repeated administration of cisplatin in patients with advanced ovarian cancer or non-small cell lung cancer. In these settings, the clinical data do not suggest that the effectiveness of cisplatin based chemotherapy regimens is altered by ETHYOL. There are at present only limited data on the effects of ETHYOL on the efficacy of chemotherapy in other settings; therefore ETHYOL should not be administered to patients in other settings where chemotherapy can produce a significant survival benefit or cure (e.g., certain malignancies of germ cell origin), except in the context of a clinical study.

CONTRAINDICATIONS

ETHYOL is contraindicated in patients with known sensitivity to aminothiol compounds or mannitol.

WARNINGS

1. Effectiveness of the Cytotoxic Regimen
Limited data are currently available regarding the preservation of antitumor efficacy when amifostine is administered prior to cisplatin therapy in settings other than advanced ovarian cancer or non-small cell lung cancer. Although some animal data suggest interference is possible, in most tumor models the antitumor effects of chemotherapy are not altered by amifostine. The possibility of interference with the efficacy of cancer treatment would be of particular concern in those settings where chemotherapy can produce a significant survival benefit or cure. ETHYOL should therefore not be used in patients receiving chemotherapy for other malignancies in which chemotherapy can produce a significant survival benefit or cure (e.g. certain malignancies of germ cell origin), except in the context of a clinical study.
2. Hypotension
Patients who are hypotensive or in a state of dehydration should not receive ETHYOL. Patients receiving antihypertensive therapy that cannot be stopped for 24 hours preceding ETHYOL treatment also should not receive ETHYOL. Patients should be adequately hydrated prior to ETHYOL infusion and kept in a supine position during the infusion. Blood pressure should be monitored every 5 minutes during the infusion. It is important that the duration of the infusion be 15 minutes, as administration of ETHYOL as a longer infusion is associated with a higher incidence of side effects. If hypotension requiring interruption of therapy occurs, patients should be placed in the Trendelenburg position and be given and infusion of normal saline using a separate i.v. line. Guidelines for interrupting and restarting ETHYOL infusion if a decrease in systolic blood pressure should occur are provided in the DOSAGE AND ADMINISTRATION section.
3. Nausea and Vomiting
Antiemetic medication should be administered prior to and in conjunction with ETHYOL (see DOSAGE and ADMINISTRATION). When ETHYOL is administered with highly emetogenic chemotherapy, the fluid balance of the patient should be carefully monitored.
4. Hypocalcemia
Reports of clinically relevant hypocalcemia are rare, but serum calcium levels should be monitored in patients at risk of hypocalcemia, such as those with nephrotic syndrome. If necessary, calcium supplements can be administered.

TABLE 2
NCI Toxicity Grades of Serum Magnesium Levels for Each Patient's Last Cycle of Therapy

NCI-CTC Grade: (mEq/L)	0 > 1.4	1 ≤ 1.4-> 1.1	2 ≤ 1.1-> 0.8	3 ≤ 0.8-> 0.5	4 ≤ 0.5	p-value*
All Patients						
Amifostine +CP	92	13	3	0	0	0.001
CP	73	18	7	5	1	
First Cohort						
Amifostine +CP	49	10	3	0	0	0.017
CP	35	8	6	3	1	
Second Cohort						
Amifostine +CP	43	3	0	0	0	0.012
CP	38	10	1	2	0	

*Based on 2-sided Mantel-Haenszel Chi-Square statistic.

TABLE 3

	ETHYOL +CP		CP
Complete pathologic tumor response rate	21.3%		15.8%
Time to progression (months)			
Median (± 95% Cl)	15.8 (13.2, 25.1)		18.1 (12.5, 20.4)
Mean (± Std error)	19.8 (±1.04)		19.1 (±1.58)
Hazard ratio (95% Confidence Interval)		.98 (.64, 1.4)	
Survival (months)			
Median (± 95% Cl)	31.3 (28.3, 38.2)		31.8 (26.3, 39.8)
Mean (± Std error)	33.7 (±2.03)		34.3 (±2.04)
Hazard ratio (95% Confidence Interval)		.97 (.69, 1.32)	

Continued on next page

Alza—Cont.

PRECAUTIONS

GENERAL
Patients should be adequately hydrated prior to the infusion and blood pressure should be monitored during the infusion. ETHYOL should be administered as a 15-minute infusion (See DOSAGE and ADMINISTRATION).

The safety of ETHYOL administration has not been established in elderly patients, or patients with preexisting cardiovascular or cerebrovascular conditions such as ischemic heart disease, arrhythmias, congestive heart failure, or history of stroke or transient ischemic attacks. ETHYOL should be used with particular care in these and other patients in whom the common ETHYOL adverse effects of nausea/vomiting and hypotension may be more likely to have serious consequences.

Drug Interactions
There are no known drug interactions with ETHYOL. However, special consideration should be given to the administration of ETHYOL in patients receiving antihypertensive medications or other drugs that could potentiate hypotension.

Carcinogenesis, Mutagenesis and Impairment of Fertility
No long term animal studies have been performed to evaluate the carcinogenic potential of ETHYOL. ETHYOL was negative in the Ames test and in the mouse micronucleus test. The free thiol metabolite, however, was positive in the Ames test with S9 microsomal fraction in the TA1535 *Salmonella typhimurium* strain and at the TK locus in the mouse L5178Y cell assay. The metabolite was negative in the mouse micronucleus test and negative for clastogenicity in human lymphocytes.

Pregnancy
Pregnancy Category C. ETHYOL (amifostine) has been shown to be embryotoxic in rabbits at doses of 50 mg/kg, approximately sixty percent of the recommended dose in humans on a body surface area basis. There are no adequate and well-controlled studies in pregnant women. ETHYOL should be used during pregnancy only if the potential benefit justifies the potential risk to the fetus.

Nursing Mothers
No information is available on the excretion of ETHYOL or its metabolites into human milk. Because many drugs are excreted in human milk and because of the potential for adverse reactions in nursing infants, it is recommended that breast feeding be discontinued if the mother is treated with ETHYOL.

ADVERSE REACTIONS
ETHYOL produced a transient reduction in blood pressure in 62% of patients treated. The mean time of onset was 14 minutes into the 15-minute period of ETHYOL infusion, and the mean duration was 6 minutes. In some cases, the infusion had to be prematurely terminated due to a more pronounced drop in systolic blood pressure. In general, the blood pressure returned to normal within 5–15 minutes. Fewer than 3% of patients discontinued ETHYOL due to blood pressure reductions. Short term, reversible loss of consciousness has been reported rarely. Blood pressure reductions during ETHYOL administration have not been reported to cause long-term CNS, cardiovascular or renal sequelae, but clinical studies performed to date have not evaluated the safety of ETHYOL in elderly patients or patients with pre-existing cardiovascular or cerebrovascular conditions.

Hypotension that requires interruption of the ETHYOL Infusion should be treated with fluid infusion and postural management of the patient (supine or Trendelenburg position). If the blood pressure returns to normal within 5 minutes and the patient is asymptomatic, the infusion may be restarted, so that the full dose of ETHYOL can be administered.

Nausea and/or vomiting occur frequently after amifostine infusion and may be severe. In the ovarian cancer randomized study, the incidence of severe nausea/vomiting on day 1 of cyclophosphamide-cisplatin chemotherapy was 10% in patients who did not receive ETHYOL, and 19% in patients who did receive ETHYOL. Other effects which have been described during or following ETHYOL infusion are flushing/feeling of warmth, chills/feeling of coldness, dizziness, somnolence, hiccups and sneezing. These effects have not generally precluded the completion of chemotherapy.

Decrease in serum calcium concentrations is a known pharmacological effect of ETHYOL. At the recommended doses, clinically significant hypocalcemia has occurred rarely (<1%).

Allergic reactions, ranging from mild skin rashes to rigors, have occurred rarely (<1%). There has been no reported occurrence of anaphylaxis with ETHYOL.

OVERDOSAGE
In clinical trials, the maximum single dose of ETHYOL was 1300 mg/m². No information is available on single doses higher than this in adults. In the setting of a clinical trial,

children have received single ETHYOL doses of up to 2700 mg/m² with no unexpected effects. Multiple infusions (up to three) of 740–910 mg/m² doses of ETHYOL have been administered within a 24-hour period under study conditions without unexpected effects. Administration of ETHYOL at 2 and 4 hours after the initial dose has not led to increased or cumulative side effects, such as increased nausea and vomiting or hypotension. The most likely symptom of overdosage is hypotension, which should be managed by infusion of normal saline and other supportive measures, as clinically indicated.

DOSAGE AND ADMINISTRATION
In adults, the recommended starting dose of ETHYOL is 910 mg/m² administered once daily as a 15-minute i.v. infusion, starting 30 minutes prior to chemotherapy.

The 15-minute infusion is better tolerated than more extended infusions. Further reductions in infusion times have not been systematically investigated.

The infusion of ETHYOL should be interrupted if the systolic blood pressure decreases significantly from the baseline value as listed in the guideline below:

Guideline for Interrupting ETHYOL Infusion Due to Decrease in Systolic Blood Pressure

	Baseline Systolic Blood Pressure (mm Hg)				
	< 100	100–119	120–139	140–179	≥ 180
Decrease in systolic blood pressure during infusion of ETHYOL (mm Hg)	20	25	30	40	50

If the blood pressure returns to normal within 5 minutes and the patient is asymptomatic, the infusion may be restarted so that the full dose of ETHYOL may be administered. If the full dose of ETHYOL cannot be administered, the dose of ETHYOL for subsequent cycles should be 740 mg/m².

Only limited experience is available for the usage of ETHYOL in children or elderly patients (more than 70 years of age).

It is recommended that antiemetic medication, including dexamethasone 20 mg i.v. and a serotonin 5HT₃ receptor antagonist, be administered prior to and in conjunction with ETHYOL. Additional antiemetics may be required based on the chemotherapy drugs administered.

Reconstitution
ETHYOL (amifostine) for Injection is supplied as a sterile lyophilized powder mixture requiring reconstitution for intravenous infusion. Each single-use vial contains 500 mg of amifostine (anhydrous basis) and 500 mg of mannitol.

Prior to intravenous injection, ETHYOL for Injection is reconstituted with 9.5 mL of sterile Sodium Chloride Injection, USP 0.9%. The reconstituted solution (500 mg amifostine/10 mL) is chemically stable for up to 5 hours at room temperature (approximately 25°C) or up to 24 hours under refrigeration (2°C to 8°C).

ETHYOL prepared in polyvinylchloride (PVC) bags at concentrations ranging from 5 mg/mL to 40 mg/mL is chemically stable for up to 5 hours when stored at room temperature (25°C) or up to 24 hours when stored under refrigeration (2°C to 8°C).

CAUTION: Parenteral products should be inspected visually for particulate matter and discoloration prior to administration whenever solution and container permit. Do not use if cloudiness or precipitate is observed.

Incompatibilities
The compatibility of amifostine with solutions other than 0.9% Sodium Chloride for Injection, or Sodium Chloride solutions with other additives, has not been examined. The use of other solutions is not recommended.

HOW SUPPLIED
ETHYOL (amifostine) for Injection is supplied as a sterile lyophilized powder in 10 mL single-use vials (NDC 17314-3123-1). Each single-use vial contains 500 mg of amifostine (anhydrous basis) and 500 mg of mannitol. The vials are available packaged as 3 vials per carton as follows:

3 pack—3 vials per carton (NDC 17314-3123-3)

Store the lyophilized dosage form in a refrigerator (2°C to 8°C).

CAUTION: Federal (U.S.A.) law prohibits dispensing without prescription.

Manufactured by:
Ben Venue, Inc.
Bedford,
Ohio 44146

Marketed by:
Alza Pharmaceuticals
A division of Alza Corporation
Palo Alto,
California 94303

And:
U.S. Bioscience, Inc.
West Conshohocken,
Pennsylvania 19428
1-800-506-4959
©1995, U.S. Bioscience, Inc.
Revision Date 3/96   LB2005 PB
Shown in Product Identification Guide, page 304

TESTODERM® ℞
[*Tes-tō-derm*]
(Testosterone Transdermal System)
CONTROLLED DELIVERY FOR ONCE-DAILY APPLICATION

DESCRIPTION
The Testoderm® Testosterone Transdermal System is designed to release controlled amounts of testosterone, the primary circulating endogenous androgen, continuously upon application to scrotal skin.

Two sizes are available to provide nominal in vivo transdermal delivery of 4 or 6 mg testosterone for one day (patients vary in their ability to absorb testosterone transdermally, see Clinical Studies); they have a contact surface area of 40 or 60 cm² and contain 10 or 15 mg testosterone USP, respectively. The composition of the two sizes per unit area is identical. Testosterone USP is a white or creamy-white crystalline powder or crystals chemically described as 17-beta hydroxyandrost-4-en-3-one.

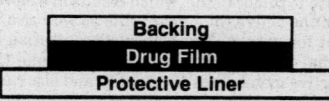

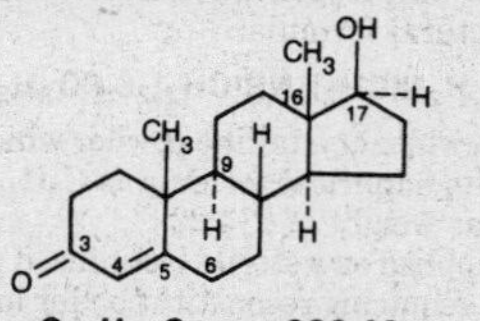

C₁₉H₂₈O₂ m.w. 288.43

Testoderm® system is composed of two layers. Proceeding from the outer surface to the film in contact with the skin, these layers are a soft flexible backing of polyethylene terephthalate and a testosterone-containing film of ethylene-vinyl acetate copolymer that contacts the skin surface and modulates the availability of the steroid. A protective liner of fluorocarbon diacrylate or silicone-coated polyester covers the drug film and must be removed before the system can be used.

Backing
Drug Film
Protective Liner

The active component of the system is testosterone. The remaining components of the system are pharmacologically inactive.

CLINICAL PHARMACOLOGY
Testoderm® releases testosterone, the primary endogenous androgenic hormone. Endogenous androgens, including testosterone and dihydrotestosterone (DHT), are responsible for the normal growth and development of the male sex organs and for maintenance of secondary sex characteristics. These effects include the growth and maturation of prostate, seminal vesicles, penis, and scrotum; the development of male hair distribution, such as facial, pubic, chest, and axillary hair; laryngeal enlargement, vocal chord thickening, alterations in body musculature, and fat distribution. DHT is necessary for the normal development of secondary sex characteristics.

Drugs in this class also cause retention of nitrogen, sodium, potassium, phosphorus, and decreased urinary excretion of calcium. Androgens have been reported to increase protein anabolism and decrease protein catabolism. Nitrogen balance is improved only when there is sufficient intake of calories and protein.

Androgens are responsible for the growth spurt of adolescence and for the eventual termination of linear growth brought about by fusion of the epiphyseal growth centers. In children, exogenous androgens accelerate linear growth rates but may cause a disproportionate advancement in bone maturation. Use over long periods may result in fusion of the epiphyseal growth centers and termination of the growth process. Androgens have been reported to stimulate the production of red blood cells by enhancing the production of erythropoietin.

During exogenous administration of androgens, endogenous testosterone release may be inhibited through feedback inhibition of pituitary luteinizing hormone (LH). At large doses of exogenous androgens, spermatogenesis may also be suppressed through feedback inhibition of pituitary follicle-stimulating hormone (FSH).

There is a lack of substantial evidence that androgens are effective in fractures, surgery, or convalescence.

Pharmacokinetics

Endogenous total testosterone serum concentrations in normal males follow a diurnal pattern. Young men and old men have slightly different patterns (Figure A). Daily application of Testoderm® approximates the natural endogenous pattern of serum testosterone of normal males. Following placement of Testoderm® on scrotal skin, the serum testosterone concentration rises to a maximum at 2 to 4 hours and returns toward baseline within approximately 2 hours after system removal. Serum levels reach a plateau at 3 to 4 weeks. Hypogonadal men using Testoderm® therapy have trough serum testosterone concentrations that are about 15% of peak levels. The testosterone levels achieved with Testoderm® therapy generally are within the range for normal men (see also Clinical Studies). The typical pattern achieved with nominal testosterone delivery of 6 mg/day from Testoderm® is shown in Figure B. Scrotal skin is at least five times more permeable to testosterone than other skin sites. Testoderm® will not produce adequate serum testosterone concentration if it is applied to nongenital skin.

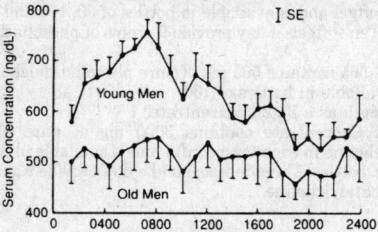

Figure A. *Hourly serum testosterone levels (mean ± SE) in normal young (n=17) and old (n=12) men. (From Bremner, 1983)*

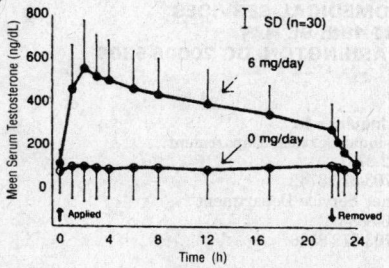

Figure B. *Serum concentration of testosterone (mean ± SD) while wearing a Testoderm® system or placebo (n=30). Systems were applied at 0 hours and removed at 22 hours.*

There is considerable variation in the half-life of testosterone as reported in the literature, ranging from 10 to 100 minutes.

Circulating testosterone is chiefly bound in the serum to sex hormone-binding globulin (SHBG) and albumin. The albumin-bound fraction of testosterone easily dissociates from albumin and is presumed to be bioactive. The portion of testosterone bound to SHBG is not considered biologically active. The amount of SHBG in the serum and the total testosterone level will determine the distribution of bioactive and nonbioactive androgen. SHBG-binding capacity is high in prepubertal children, declines during puberty and adulthood and increases again during the later decades of life.

Testosterone is a substrate for conversion to an active metabolite dihydrotestosterone (DHT).

About 90 percent of a dose of testosterone given intramuscularly is excreted in the urine as glucuronic and sulfuric acid conjugates of testosterone and its metabolites; about 6 percent of a dose is excreted in the feces, mostly in the unconjugated form. Inactivation of testosterone occurs primarily in the liver. Testosterone is metabolized to various 17-keto steroids through two different pathways, and the major active metabolites are estradiol and dihydrotestosterone (DHT). Normal concentrations of estradiol in men are 0.8 to 3.5 ng/dL. DHT concentrations in normal male serum are 30 to 85 ng/dL. DHT binds with greater affinity to SHBG than does testosterone. In reproductive tissues, DHT is further metabolized to 3-alpha and 3-beta androstanediol.

In many tissues the activity of testosterone appears to depend on reduction to dihydrotestosterone, which binds to cytosol receptor proteins. The steroid-receptor complex is transported to the nucleus where it initiates transcription and cellular changes related to androgen action.

Clinical Studies

After at least 3 weeks of Testoderm® therapy when steady state is obtained, 30 hypogonadal men treated with 6 mg/d systems for 22 hours daily achieved mean maximum serum testosterone concentrations of 593 ng/dL at 2 to 4 hours post-application. Sixty percent of the patients achieved individual maximal testosterone concentrations >500 ng/dL. The mean 24-hour steady-state AUC (area under the curve) value was 9132 ng/dL. The mean DHT serum concentrations

ranged from 134 to 162 ng/dL. Normal levels of testosterone have been maintained in patients who have worn the systems for up to six years. DHT levels also remain stable. The increase in serum testosterone concentration is proportional to the size of the system.

The variability of total testosterone concentrations among patients receiving Testoderm® treatment had a coefficient of variation from 35% to 49%. The coefficient of variation of total testosterone concentrations within individual patients was 30% to 41%. This variability is comparable to the values reported in the literature for both normal and hypogonadal men.

In two 12-week clinical studies in 72 hypogonadal men, Testoderm® therapy produced positive effects on mood and sexual behavior. By 5 weeks, 45 patients not previously treated with Testoderm® showed statistically significant increases in sexual activity. Compared to baseline, mean sexual events per week increased for sexual intercourse (0.3 to 0.8), orgasm (0.4 to 1.2), waking erections (1.0 to 3.5), and spontaneous erections (0.4 to 2.8).

Changes in nonfasting serum lipid concentrations were observed during Testoderm® therapy. By three months total cholesterol and high-density lipoprotein cholesterol decreased an average of 8% and 13%, respectively. High-density lipoprotein cholesterol remained stable thereafter. Total cholesterol continued to decrease through two years. At the end of two years, the total cholesterol/high-density lipoprotein cholesterol ratio was not different from pretreatment values.

Composite results of all studies show elevated dihydrotestosterone concentrations and a change in the ratio of testosterone to dihydrotestosterone (T/DHT) during treatment. The range in this ratio was 0.7–12.5, as compared with a ratio of 3.6–15.2 in normal untreated men. The long-term effects of the change in this ratio are not known.

Estradiol levels increased to the normal range with treatment. Sporadic elevations of estradiol above the normal range for men were observed in 3 of 72 patients and these were not associated with feminizing side effects.

INDICATIONS AND USAGE

Testoderm® is indicated for replacement therapy in males for conditions associated with a deficiency or absence of endogenous testosterone:

1. Primary hypogonadism (congenital or acquired)—testicular failure due to cryptorchidism, bilateral torsion, orchitis, vanishing testis syndrome, orchidectomy, Klinefelter's syndrome, chemotherapy, or toxic damage from alcohol or heavy metals. These men usually have low serum testosterone levels and gonadotropins (FSH, LH) above the normal range.
2. Hypogonadotropic hypogonadism (congenital or acquired) —idiopathic gonadotropin or LHRH deficiency or pituitary-hypothalamic injury from tumors, trauma, or radiation. These men have low testosterone serum levels but have gonadotropins in the normal or low range.

Testoderm® therapy has not been evaluated clinically in males under 18 years of age.

CONTRAINDICATIONS

Androgens are contraindicated in men with carcinoma of the breast or known or suspected carcinoma of the prostate.

Testoderm® therapy has not been evaluated in women and must not be used in women. Testosterone may cause fetal harm.

Testoderm® systems should not be used in patients with known hypersensitivity to any components of the system.

WARNINGS

Prolonged use of high doses of orally active 17-alpha-alkyl androgens (eg, methyltestosterone) has been associated with serious hepatic adverse effects (peliosis hepatitis, hepatic neoplasms, cholestatic hepatitis, and jaundice). Long-term therapy with testosterone enanthate, which elevates blood levels for prolonged periods, has produced multiple hepatic adenomas. Testosterone is not known to produce these adverse effects.

Geriatric patients treated with androgens may be at an increased risk for the development of prostatic hyperplasia and prostatic carcinoma (see PRECAUTIONS: Carcinogenesis, Mutagenesis, Impairment of Fertility).

Edema with or without congestive heart failure may be a serious complication in patients with preexisting cardiac, renal, or hepatic disease. In addition to discontinuation of the drug, diuretic therapy may be required.

Gynecomastia frequently develops and occasionally persists in patients being treated for hypogonadism.

PRECAUTIONS

Information for the Patient

A booklet containing instructions for use of the Testoderm® system is available.

The physician should instruct patients to report any of the following side effects of androgens:
• Too frequent or persistent erections of the penis.
• Any nausea, vomiting, changes in skin color or ankle swelling.

Virilization of female partners has been reported with use of a topical testosterone solution. Percutaneous creams leave as much as 90 mg residual testosterone on the skin. The results from one study indicated that, after removal of a Testoderm® system, the potential for transfer of testosterone to a sexual partner was 6 μg, 1/45th the daily endogenous testosterone production by the female body. Changes in body hair distribution or significant increase in acne of the female partner should be brought to the attention of a physician.

Laboratory Tests

1. Hemoglobin and hematocrit levels should be checked periodically (to detect polycythemia) in patients on long-term androgen therapy.
2. Liver function, prostatic acid phosphatase, prostatic specific antigen, cholesterol, and high-density lipoproteins should be checked periodically.

Drug Interactions

1. Anticoagulants. C-17 substituted derivatives of testosterone, such as methandrostenolone, have been reported to decrease the anticoagulant requirements of patients receiving oral anticoagulants. Patients receiving oral anticoagulant therapy require close monitoring, especially when androgens are started or stopped.
2. Oxyphenbutazone. Concurrent administration of oxyphenbutazone and androgens may result in elevated serum levels of oxyphenbutazone.
3. Insulin. In diabetic patients the metabolic effects of androgens may decrease blood glucose and, therefore, insulin requirements.

Drug/Laboratory Test Interactions

Androgens may decrease levels of thyroxin-binding globulin, resulting in decreased total T_4 serum levels and increased resin uptake of T_3 and T_4. Free thyroid hormone levels remain unchanged, however, and there is no clinical evidence of thyroid dysfunction.

Carcinogenesis, Mutagenesis, Impairment of Fertility

Animal Data. Testosterone has been tested by subcutaneous injection and implantation in mice and rats. In mice, the implant induced cervical-uterine tumors, which metastasized in some cases. There is suggestive evidence that injection of testosterone into some strains of female mice increases their susceptibility to hepatoma. Testosterone is also known to increase the number of tumors and decrease the degree of differentiation of chemically induced carcinomas of the liver in rats.

Human Data. There are rare reports of hepatocellular carcinoma in patients receiving long-term therapy with androgens in high doses. Withdrawal of the drugs did not lead to regression of the tumors in all cases.

Geriatric Use. Geriatric patients treated with androgens may be at an increased risk for the development of prostatic hyperplasia and prostatic carcinoma.

Pregnancy Category X (See Contraindications).
Teratogenic Effects. Testoderm® therapy must not be used in women.

Nursing Mothers. Testoderm® therapy must not be used in women.

Pediatric Use. Testoderm® therapy has not been evaluated clinically in males under 18 years of age.

ADVERSE REACTIONS

Adverse Reactions with the Testoderm® system

In clinical studies of 104 patients treated with Testoderm® the most common adverse effects reported were local effects. In US clinical trials, most of the 72 patients filling out a daily questionnaire reported scrotal itching, discomfort, or irritation at some time during therapy. Of all the daily questionnaire responses, 7% reported itching, 4% discomfort, and 2% irritation. All topical reactions decreased with duration of use.

The following adverse effects were reported in association with Testoderm® therapy in 104 patients using the product for up to three years; a causal relationship to Testoderm® treatment was not always determined. These effects are listed in decreasing order of occurrence with the number of patients reporting the effect in parentheses: Gynecomastia (5), acne (4), prostatitis/urinary tract infection (4), breast tenderness (3), stroke (2), memory loss (1), pupillary dilation (1), abnormal liver enzymes (1), scrotal cellulitis (1), deep vein phlebitis (1), benign prostatic hyperplasia (1), rectal mucosal lesion over prostate (1), hematuria/bladder cancer (1), papilloma on scrotum (1), and congestive heart failure (1). See CLINICAL PHARMACOLOGY, Clinical Studies subsection, regarding effects on serum lipids.

Adverse Reactions with Injection or Oral Androgen Therapy

Skin and Appendages. Hirsutism, male pattern of baldness, seborrhea, and acne.

Endocrine and Urogenital. Gynecomastia and excessive frequency and duration of penile erections. Oligospermia may occur at high dosages (see CLINICAL PHARMACOLOGY). Fluid and Electrolyte Disturbances. Retention of sodium, chloride, water, potassium, calcium, and inorganic phosphates.

Continued on next page

Alza—Cont.

Gastrointestinal. Nausea, cholestatic jaundice, alterations in liver function tests. Rare instances of hepatocellular neoplasms and peliosis hepatitis have occurred (see WARNINGS).

Hematologic. Suppression of clotting factors II, V, VII, and X, bleeding in patients on concomitant anticoagulant therapy, and polycythemia.

Nervous System. Increased or decreased libido, headache, anxiety, depression, and generalized paresthesia.

Metabolic. Increased serum cholesterol.

Miscellaneous. Rarely, anaphylactoid reactions.

DRUG ABUSE AND DEPENDENCE

Testoderm® is a Schedule III controlled substance under the Anabolic Steroids Control Act.

With oral administration, it is not possible to achieve clinically significant serum testosterone concentrations in the target organs using the testosterone in Testoderm® due to extensive first-pass metabolism. The half-life of an IM injection of testosterone is about 10 minutes.

Because scrotal skin is at least five times more permeable to testosterone than other skin sites, Testoderm® will not produce adequate serum testosterone concentrations if it is applied to nongenital skin.

OVERDOSAGE

There is one report of acute overdosage with testosterone enanthate: testosterone levels of up to 11,400 ng/dL were implicated in a cerebrovascular accident.

DOSAGE AND ADMINISTRATION

Patients should start therapy with a 6 mg/d system applied daily; if scrotal area is inadequate, a 4 mg/d system should be used. Testoderm® should be placed on clean, dry, scrotal skin. Scrotal hair should be dry-shaved for optimal skin contact. Chemical depilatories should not be used (see Patient Information). Testoderm® should be worn 22–24 hours.

After 3–4 weeks of daily system use, blood should be drawn 2–4 hours after system application for determination of serum total testosterone. Because of variability in analytical values among diagnostic laboratories, this laboratory work and later analyses for assessing the effect of the Testoderm® therapy should be performed at the same laboratory.

If patients have not achieved desired results by the end of 6–8 weeks of therapy with Testoderm®, another form of testosterone replacement therapy should be considered.

HOW SUPPLIED

Testoderm® testosterone transdermal system is a Schedule III controlled substance under the Anabolic Steroids Control Act.

Testoderm® systems are supplied as individually pouched systems, 30 per carton.

Testoderm® 4 mg/d (testosterone transdermal system) —each 40 cm² system contains 10 mg testosterone USP for nominal delivery of 4 mg for one day.*

   Carton of 30 systems .... NDC 17314-4608-3

Testoderm® 6 mg/d (testosterone transdermal system) —each 60 cm² system contains 15 mg testosterone USP for nominal delivery of 6 mg for one day.*

   Carton of 30 systems .... NDC 17314-4609-3

Store at room temperature 15–30°C

REFERENCE

Bremner WJ, Vitiello MV, Prinz PN. *Loss of Circadian Rhythmicity in Blood Testosterone Levels with Aging in Normal Men.* J Clin Endocrin Metab (1983) 56 (6): 1278-1281.

Caution: Federal law prohibits dispensing without prescription.

Manufactured by ALZA Corporation, Palo Alto, California 94304, USA

*See Clinical Studies

Edition: 6/94

PROGESTASERT EDUCATIONAL MATERIAL

All progestasert educational materials are complimentary.

Booklets—Brochures
A. Patient Information Leaflet
   (English and Spanish)
B. Clinical Evidence Brochure
C. Demonstration Kit

Videos—Audiotapes—Slides
A. Progestasert® System Insertion Technique
   Videocassette
B. Patient Audiocassette Tape
C. Instructional Slide Program

American Lecithin Company
115 HURLEY ROAD, UNIT 2B
OXFORD, CT 06478

Direct Inquiries to:
Randall E. Zigmont
(203) 262-7100
Fax: (203) 262-7101

For Medical Emergencies Contact:
In Emergencies:
Randall E. Zigmont
(203) 262-7100
Fax: (203) 262-7101

PHOSCHOL®   OTC
[fos'kol]
Phosphatidylcholine (highly purified lecithin)
Softgels and Concentrate

DESCRIPTION

PhosChol 900 contains 900 mg of pure phosphatidylcholine in each softgel.

PhosChol Concentrate contains 3000 mg of pure phosphatidylcholine in each teaspoonful.

ACTION & USES

Choline circulating in the blood after PC ingestion is taken up into all cells of the body. The brain has a unique way of ensuring that its nerve cells will receive adequate supplies of circulating choline.

A special protein molecule within the brain's capillaries traps the circulating choline, and then transports it across the blood-brain barrier, into the brain. Once in the brain, choline is incorporated into the brain's own PC, which is an essential and major part of neuronal membranes. Circulating choline transported into the brain has an additional very important function for a special group of nerve cells that make a biochemical, acetylcholine, which is released into synapses as a neurotransmitter. It provides the essential precursor used to synthesize acetylcholine. Moreover, when nerve cells are active, firing frequently and releasing large quantities of acetylcholine, their ability to make adequate amounts of the neurotransmitter requires that they receive adequate amounts of choline from the blood stream. In the absence of adequate choline, the ability of nerve cells to transmit messages to other cells across synapses is impaired and neuronal cell membranes can be depleted of PC causing cell damage. In contrast, when supplemental choline is provided, these messages can be amplified and membrane structure maintained.

PhosChol® brand of highly purified lecithin has been carefully developed to contain the highest concentration of phosphatidylcholine commercially available and can provide for the highest blood choline levels.

Figure 1.
LEVELS OF CHOLINE IN HUMAN PLASMA AFTER THE ADMINISTRATION OF 3, 6, 9, AND 18 GRAM DOSES OF LECITHIN AS PHOSCHOL

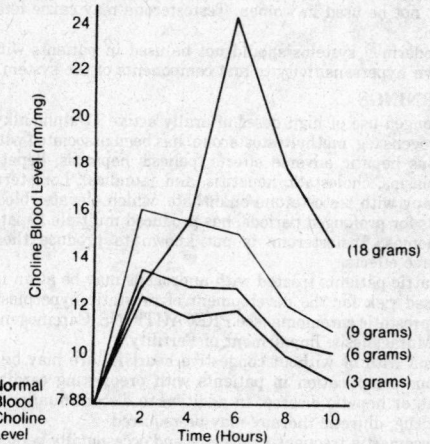

(One 9-gram dose at baseline, one 9-gram dose at 4 hours)

ADMINISTRATION

PhosChol® nutritional supplements may be recommended for two purposes:

To guard against low blood choline levels, and to restore blood choline levels in patients suffering from selected brain disorders. Amounts of PC sufficient to increase blood choline levels would help support normal cellular membrane composition and repair; they would also provide sufficient precur-

---

sor choline for the maintenance of acetylcholine biosynthesis. Taken according to these schedules, dietary supplements of PC are an aid to good health, and protect against low choline stores.

To increase blood choline by 50%, patients should take 3 grams of PhosChol before meals by noon. To double blood choline levels, patients should take 9 grams of PhosChol before meals by noon. If ingestion before meals causes intestinal distress, it is recommended that PhosChol be taken either with meals or immediately thereafter.

ADVERSE REACTIONS

No major side effects have been reported in connection with consumption of large quantities of phosphatidylcholine or commercially available (less pure) lecithin.

Minor side effects may be seen such as increased salivation, nausea and upset stomach.

HOW SUPPLIED

Two strengths as clear, amber colored, one-piece sealed softgels.

PhosChol 900 contains 900 mg of pure phosphatidylcholine in each softgel and is available in bottles of 30, 100 and 300 softgels. Ten softgels a day provide 9 grams of phosphatidylcholine.

PhosChol 565 contains 565 mg of pure phosphatidylcholine and is available in bottles of 100.

One strength as a liquid concentrate.

PhosChol Concentrate contains 3000 mg of pure phosphatidylcholine in each teaspoonful and is available in 8 oz., and 16 oz. bottles. Three teaspoonsful a day provide 9 grams of phosphatidylcholine.

American Red Cross
NATIONAL HEADQUARTERS
BIOMEDICAL SERVICES
431 18th St. N.W.
WASHINGTON, DC 20006-5306

Direct Inquiries to:
Professional Services Department
703-312-8737
FAX: 703-312-8742
Customer Service Department
800-446-8883
FAX: 703-312-8746

ANTIHEMOPHILIC FACTOR (HUMAN)   ℞
Method M
Monoclonal Purified

This product is derived from blood collected from volunteer donors by the American Red Cross Blood Services. The cost of processing, testing and packaging was paid by the American Red Cross Blood Services.

DESCRIPTION

Antihemophilic Factor (Human), Method M, is a sterile, non-pyrogenic, dried preparation of antihemophilic factor (Factor VIII, Factor VIII:C, AHF) in concentrated form with a specific activity range of 2 to 15 AHF International Units/mg of total protein. When reconstituted with the appropriate volume of diluent, it contains approximately 12.5 mg/mL Albumin (Human), 1.5 mg/mL polyethylene glycol (3350), 0.055 M histidine and 0.030 M glycine as stabilizing agents. In the absence of the added Albumin (Human), the specific activity is approximately 2,000 AHF International Units/mg of protein. It also contains, per AHF International Unit, not more than 0.1 ng mouse protein, 18 ng organic solvent [tri(n-butyl)phosphate] and 50 ng detergent (Triton X-100).

See CLINICAL PHARMACOLOGY.

Antihemophilic Factor (Human) is prepared by the Method M process from pooled human plasma by immunoaffinity chromatography utilizing a murine monoclonal antibody to Factor VIII:C, followed by an ion exchange chromatography step for further purification. Method M also includes an organic solvent [tri(n-butyl) phosphate] and detergent (Triton X-100) virus inactivation step designed to reduce the risk of transmission of hepatitis and other viral diseases. However, no procedure has been shown to be totally effective in removing viral infectivity from coagulation factor products.

Each bottle of Antihemophilic Factor (Human) is labeled with the AHF activity expressed in International Units per bottle, which is referenced to the WHO International Standard.

Antihemophilic Factor (Human) is to be administered only intravenously.

HOW SUPPLIED

Antihemophilic Factor (Human), Method M, is available as single dose bottles. Each bottle is labeled with the potency in International Units, and is packaged together with 10 mL of

Table 1

In Vitro Virus Clearance During Polygam® S/D Manufacturing

Process Step No.	Process Step Evaluated	Virus Clearance, $\log_{10}$				
		HIV-1	HIV-2	SIN	PRV	VSV
1	Fraction I + II + III Wash to Fraction I + III Supernatant	8.2*	N.D.**	5.2*	N.D.**	N.D.**
2	Fraction I + III Supernatant to Fraction I + III Filtrate	8.2*	N.D.**	4.6*	N.D.**	N.D.**
3	Fraction I + III Filtrate to Fraction II Precipitate	8.1*	N.D.**	N.A.***	N.D.**	N.D.**
4	Treatment of Resuspended Fraction II Precipitate with Solvent/Detergent Mixture	8.4*	5.7*	5.1*	4.3*	6.0*

* Minimum log reduction due to detection limit of the assay.
** Not determined.
*** Not applicable. Sindbis virus co-precipitates with Fraction II proteins.

Sterile Water for Injection, USP, a double-ended needle, and a filter needle.
NDC 52769-460-01
Manufactured by:
Baxter Healthcare Corporation
Hyland Division
Glendale, CA 91203 USA
U.S. License No. 140
Distributed by:
+ **American Red Cross**
Blood Services
Washington, DC 20006 USA
October 1992

IMMUNE GLOBULIN INTRAVENOUS ℞
(HUMAN) POLYGAM® S/D
SOLVENT/DETERGENT TREATED

This product is derived from blood collected from volunteer donors by the American Red Cross Blood Services. The cost of processing, testing and packaging was paid by the American Red Cross Blood Services.

DESCRIPTION
Immune Globulin Intravenous (Human) [IGIV], Polygam® S/D, is a solvent/detergent treated, sterile, freeze-dried preparation of highly purified immunoglobulin G (IgG) derived from large pools of human plasma. The product is manufactured by the Cohn-Oncley cold ethanol fractionation process followed by ultrafiltration and ion exchange chromatography. The manufacturing process includes treatment with an organic solvent/detergent mixture,[1,2] composed of tri(n-butyl) phosphate, octoxynol 9 and polysorbate 80.[3] The Polygam® S/D manufacturing process provides a significant viral reduction in *in vitro* studies.[3] These studies, summarized in Table 1, demonstrate virus clearance during Polygam® S/D manufacturing using infectious Human Immunodeficiency virus, Types 1 and 2 (HIV-1, HIV-2); Sindbis virus (SIN), a model virus for Hepatitis C virus; Pseudorabies virus (PRV), a model virus for lipid-enveloped DNA viruses such as Herpes; and Vesicular stomatitis virus (VSV), a model virus for lipid-enveloped RNA viruses.[3] These reductions are achieved through a combination of process chemistry, partitioning and/or inactivation during cold ethanol fractionation and the solvent/detergent treatment.[3]
[See Table 1 above.]
When reconstituted with the total volume of diluent (Sterile Water for Injection, USP) supplied, this preparation contains approximately 50 mg of protein per mL (5%), of which at least 90% is gamma globulin. The product, reconstituted to 5%, contains a physiological concentration of sodium chloride (approximately 8.5 mg/mL) and has a pH of 6.8 ± 0.4. Stabilizing agents and additional components are present in the following maximum amounts for a 5% solution: 3 mg/mL Albumin (Human), 22.5 mg/mL glycine, 20 mg/mL glucose, 2 mg/mL polyethylene glycol (PEG), 1 μg/mL tri(n-butyl) phosphate, 1μg/mL octoxynol 9, and 100 μg/mL polysorbate 80. If it is necessary to prepare a 10% (100 mg/mL) solution for infusion, half the volume of diluent should be added as described in the **DOSAGE AND ADMINISTRATION** section. In this case, the stabilizing agents and other components will be present at double the concentrations given for the 5% solution.
The manufacturing process for Immune Globulin Intravenous (Human), Polygam® S/D, isolates IgG without additional chemical or enzymatic modification and the Fc portion is maintained intact. Immune Globulin Intravenous

(Human), Polygam® S/D, contains all of the IgG antibody activities which are present in the donor population. On the average, the distribution of IgG subclasses present in this product is similar to that in normal plasma.[3] Immune Globulin Intravenous (Human), Polygam® S/D, contains only trace amounts of IgA (< 3.7 μg/mL in a 5% solution). IgM is also present in trace amounts.
Immune Globulin Intravenous (Human), Polygam® S/D, contains no preservative.

HOW SUPPLIED
Immune Globulin Intravenous (Human), Polygam® S/D, is supplied in 2.5 g, 5 g or 10 g single use bottles. Each bottle of Immune Globulin Intravenous (Human), Polygam® S/D, is furnished with a suitable volume of Sterile Water for Injection, USP, a transfer device and an administration set which contains an integral airway and a 15 micron filter.
2.5g   NDC 52769-471-72
5g   NDC 52769-471-75
10g   NDC 52769-471-80
Manufactured by:
Baxter Healthcare Corporation
Hyland Division
Glendale, CA 91203 USA
U.S. License No. 140
Distributed by:
+ **American Red Cross**
Blood Services
Washington, DC 20006 USA
February 1995

Amgen
AMGEN INC.
AMGEN CENTER
1840 DEHAVILLAND DRIVE
THOUSAND OAKS, CA 91320-1789

Direct Inquiries to:
Customer Services Department
(800) 282-6436
FAX: (800) 292-6436

For Medical Information Contact:
Professional Services Department
(800) 772-6436
FAX: (818) 865-3707
In Emergencies:
(800) 772-6436
After Hours and Weekends:
(800) 772-6436

Sales and Ordering:
Customer Services Department
(800) 282-6436
FAX: (800) 292-6436

EPOGEN® ℞
EPOETIN ALFA
For Injection

DESCRIPTION
Erythropoietin is a glycoprotein which stimulates red blood cell production. It is produced in the kidney and stimulates the division and differentiation of committed erythroid pro-

genitors in the bone marrow. EPOGEN® is the Amgen Inc. trademark for Epoetin alfa which has been selected as the proper name for recombinant human erythropoietin. EPOGEN®, a 165 amino acid glycoprotein manufactured by recombinant DNA technology, has the same biological effects as endogenous erythropoietin.[1] It has a molecular weight of 30,400 daltons and is produced by mammalian cells into which the human erythropoietin gene has been introduced. The product contains the identical amino acid sequence of isolated natural erythropoietin.
EPOGEN® is formulated as a sterile, colorless liquid in an isotonic sodium chloride/sodium citrate buffered solution for intravenous (IV) or subcutaneous (SC) administration.
Single-Dose, Preservative-Free Vial: Each 1 mL of solution contains 2,000, 3,000, 4,000 or 10,000 Units of Epoetin alfa, 2.5 mg Albumin (Human), 5.8 mg sodium citrate, 5.8 mg sodium chloride, and 0.06 mg citric acid in Water for Injection, USP (pH 6.9±0.3). This formulation contains no preservative.
Multidose, Preserved Vial: 2 mL (20,000 Units, 10,000 Units/mL). Each 1 mL of solution contains 10,000 Units of Epoetin alfa, 2.5 mg Albumin (Human), 1.3 mg sodium citrate, 8.2 mg sodium chloride, 0.11 mg citric acid, and 1% benzyl alcohol as preservative in Water for Injection, USP (pH 6.1±0.3).

CLINICAL PHARMACOLOGY
Chronic Renal Failure Patients: Endogenous production of erythropoietin is normally regulated by the level of tissue oxygenation. Hypoxia and anemia generally increase the production of erythropoietin, which in turn stimulates erythropoiesis.[2] In normal subjects, plasma erythropoietin levels range from 0.01 to 0.03 Units/mL,[2,3] and increase up to 100- to 1,000-fold during hypoxia or anemia.[2,3] In contrast, in patients with chronic renal failure (CRF), production of erythropoietin is impaired, and this erythropoietin deficiency is the primary cause of their anemia.[3,4]
Chronic renal failure is the clinical situation in which there is a progressive and usually irreversible decline in kidney function. Such patients may manifest the sequelae of renal dysfunction, including anemia, but do not necessarily require regular dialysis. Patients with end-stage renal disease (ESRD) are those patients with CRF who require regular dialysis or kidney transplantation for survival.
EPOGEN® has been shown to stimulate erythropoiesis in anemic patients with CRF, including both patients on dialysis and those who do not require regular dialysis.[4–13] The first evidence of a response to the three times weekly (T.I.W.) administration of EPOGEN® is an increase in the reticulocyte count within 10 days, followed by increases in the red cell count, hemoglobin, and hematocrit, usually within 2–6 weeks.[4,5] Because of the length of time required for erythropoiesis—several days for erythroid progenitors to mature and be released into the circulation—a clinically significant increase in hematocrit is usually not observed in less than 2 weeks and may require up to 6 weeks in some patients. Once the hematocrit reaches the suggested target range (30–36%), that level can be sustained by EPOGEN® therapy in the absence of iron deficiency and concurrent illnesses.
The rate of hematocrit increase varies between patients and is dependent upon the dose of EPOGEN®, within a therapeutic range of approximately 50–300 Units/kg T.I.W.[4] A greater biologic response is not observed at doses exceeding 300 Units/kg T.I.W.[6] Other factors affecting the rate and extent of response include availability of iron stores, the baseline hematocrit, and the presence of concurrent medical problems.
Zidovudine-treated HIV-infected Patients: Responsiveness to EPOGEN® in HIV-infected patients is dependent upon the endogenous serum erythropoietin level prior to treatment. Patients with endogenous serum erythropoietin levels ≤500 mUnits/mL, and who are receiving a dose of zidovudine ≤4,200 mg/week, may respond to EPOGEN® therapy. Patients with endogenous serum erythropoietin levels >500 mUnits/mL do not appear to respond to EPOGEN® therapy. In a series of four clinical trials involving 255 patients, 60% to 80% of HIV-infected patients treated with zidovudine had endogenous serum erythropoietin levels ≤500 mUnits/mL.
Response to EPOGEN® in zidovudine-treated HIV-infected patients is manifested by reduced transfusion requirements and increased hematocrit.
Cancer Patients on Chemotherapy: Anemia in cancer patients may be related to the disease itself or the effect of concomitantly administered chemotherapeutic agents. EPOGEN® has been shown to increase hematocrit and decrease transfusion requirements after the first month of therapy (Months 2 and 3), in anemic cancer patients undergoing chemotherapy.
A series of clinical trials enrolled 131 anemic cancer patients who were receiving cyclic cisplatin- or non cisplatin-containing chemotherapy. Endogenous baseline serum erythropoie-

Continued on next page

Amgen—Cont.

tin levels varied among patients in these trials with approximately 75% (N=83/110) having endogenous serum erythropoietin levels ≤132 mUnits/mL, and approximately 4% (N=4/110) of patients having endogenous serum erythropoietin levels >500 mUnits/mL. In general, patients with lower baseline serum erythropoietin levels responded more vigorously to EPOGEN® than patients with higher baseline erythropoietin levels. Although no specific serum erythropoietin level can be stipulated above which patients would be unlikely to respond to EPOGEN® therapy, treatment of patients with grossly elevated serum erythropoietin levels (e.g., >200 mUnits/mL) is not recommended.

Pharmacokinetics: Intravenously administered EPOGEN® is eliminated at a rate consistent with first order kinetics with a circulating half-life ranging from approximately 4 to 13 hours in patients with CRF. Within the therapeutic dose range, detectable levels of plasma erythropoietin are maintained for at least 24 hours.[7] After subcutaneous administration of EPOGEN® to patients with CRF, peak serum levels are achieved within 5–24 hours after administration and decline slowly thereafter. There is no apparent difference in half-life between patients not on dialysis whose serum creatinine levels were greater than 3, and patients maintained on dialysis.

In normal volunteers, the half-life of intravenously administered EPOGEN® is approximately 20% shorter than the half-life in CRF patients. The pharmacokinetics of EPOGEN® have not been studied in HIV-infected patients.

INDICATIONS AND USAGE

Treatment of Anemia of Chronic Renal Failure Patients: EPOGEN® is indicated in the treatment of anemia associated with chronic renal failure, including patients on dialysis (end-stage renal disease) and patients not on dialysis. EPOGEN® is indicated to elevate or maintain the red blood cell level (as manifested by the hematocrit or hemoglobin determinations) and to decrease the need for transfusions in these patients.

EPOGEN® is not intended for patients who require immediate correction of severe anemia. EPOGEN® may obviate the need for maintenance transfusions but is not a substitute for emergency transfusion.

Prior to initiation of therapy, the patient's iron stores, including transferrin saturation and serum ferritin, should be evaluated. Transferrin saturation should be at least 20% and ferritin at least 100 ng/mL. Blood pressure should be adequately controlled prior to initiation of EPOGEN® therapy, and must be closely monitored and controlled during therapy. Non-dialysis patients with symptomatic anemia considered for therapy should have a hematocrit less than 30%. All patients on EPOGEN® therapy should be regularly monitored (see "Precautions").

EPOGEN® should be administered under the guidance of a qualified physician (see "Dosage and Administration").

Treatment of Anemia in Zidovudine-treated HIV-infected Patients: EPOGEN® is indicated for the treatment of anemia related to therapy with zidovudine in HIV-infected patients. EPOGEN® is indicated to elevate or maintain the red blood cell level (as manifested by the hematocrit or hemoglobin determinations) and to decrease the need for transfusions in these patients. EPOGEN® is not indicated for the treatment of anemia in HIV-infected patients due to other factors such as iron or folate deficiencies, hemolysis or gastrointestinal bleeding, which should be managed appropriately.

EPOGEN®, at a dose of 100 Units/kg three times per week, is effective in decreasing the transfusion requirement and increasing the red blood cell level of anemic, HIV-infected patients treated with zidovudine, when the endogenous serum erythropoietin level is ≤500 mUnits/mL and when patients are receiving a dose of zidovudine ≤4,200 mg/week.

Treatment of Anemia in Cancer Patients on Chemotherapy: EPOGEN® is indicated for the treatment of anemia in patients with non-myeloid malignancies where anemia is due to the effect of concomitantly administered chemotherapy. EPOGEN® is indicated to decrease the need for transfusions in patients who will be receiving concomitant chemotherapy for a minimum of 2 months. EPOGEN® is not indicated for the treatment of anemia in cancer patients due to other factors such as iron or folate deficiencies, hemolysis or gastrointestinal bleeding which should be managed appropriately.

Clinical Experience: Response to EPOGEN®:

Chronic Renal Failure Patients: Response to EPOGEN® was consistent across all studies. In the presence of adequate iron stores (see "Pre-Therapy Iron Evaluation"), the time to reach the target hematocrit is a function of the baseline hematocrit and the rate of hematocrit rise.

The rate of increase in hematocrit is dependent upon the dose of EPOGEN® administered and individual patient variation. In clinical trials at starting doses of 50–150 Units/kg T.I.W., patients responded with an average rate of hematocrit rise of:

STARTING DOSE (T.I.W. IV)	HEMATOCRIT INCREASE POINTS/DAY	POINTS/2 WEEKS
50 Units/kg	0.11	1.5
100 Units/kg	0.18	2.5
150 Units/kg	0.25	3.5

Over this dose range, approximately 95% of all patients responded with a clinically significant increase in hematocrit, and by the end of approximately 2 months of therapy virtually all patients were transfusion-independent. Changes in the quality of life of EPOGEN®-treated patients were assessed as part of a Phase III clinical trial.[5,8] Once the target hematocrit (32–38%) was achieved, statistically significant improvements were demonstrated for most quality of life parameters measured, including energy and activity level, functional ability, sleep and eating behavior, health status, satisfaction with health, sex life, well-being, psychological effect, life satisfaction, and happiness. Patients also reported improvement in their disease symptoms. They showed a statistically significant increase in exercise capacity (VO_2max), energy, and strength with a significant reduction in aching, dizziness, anxiety, shortness of breath, muscle weakness, and leg cramps.[8,14]

Patients on Dialysis: Thirteen clinical studies were conducted, involving intravenous administration to a total of 1,010 anemic patients on dialysis for 986 patient-years of EPOGEN® therapy. In the three largest of these clinical trials, the median maintenance dose necessary to maintain the hematocrit between 30–36% was approximately 75 Units/kg (T.I.W.). In the U.S. multicenter Phase III study, approximately 65% of the patients required doses of 100 Units/kg T.I.W., or less, to maintain their hematocrit at approximately 35%. Almost 10% of patients required a dose of 25 Units/kg, or less, and approximately 10% required a dose of more than 200 Units/kg T.I.W. to maintain their hematocrit at this level.

A multicenter unit dose study was also conducted in 119 patients receiving peritoneal dialysis who self-administered EPOGEN® subcutaneously for approximately 109 patient-years of experience. Patients responded to EPOGEN® administered subcutaneously in a manner similar to patients receiving intravenous administration.[15]

Patients with CRF Not Requiring Dialysis: Four clinical trials were conducted in patients with CRF not on dialysis involving 181 EPOGEN®-treated patients for approximately 67 patient-years of experience. These patients responded to EPOGEN® therapy in a manner similar to that observed in patients on dialysis. Patients with CRF not on dialysis demonstrated a dose-dependent and sustained increase in hematocrit when EPOGEN® was administered by either an intravenous (IV) or subcutaneous (SC) route, with similar rates of rise of hematocrit when EPOGEN® was administered by either route. Moreover, EPOGEN® doses of 75–150 Units/kg per week have been shown to maintain hematocrits of 36–38% for up to 6 months. Correcting the anemia of progressive renal failure will allow patients to remain active even though their renal function continues to decrease.[16–18]

Zidovudine-treated HIV-infected Patients: EPOGEN® has been studied in four placebo-controlled trials enrolling 297 anemic (hematocrit <30%) HIV-infected (AIDS) patients receiving concomitant therapy with zidovudine (all patients were treated with Epoetin alfa manufactured by Amgen Inc.). In the subgroup of patients (89/125 EPOGEN® and 88/130 placebo) with prestudy endogenous serum erythropoietin levels ≤500 mUnits/mL (normal endogenous serum erythropoietin levels are 4–26 mUnits/mL), EPOGEN® reduced the mean cumulative number of units of blood transfused per patient by approximately 40% as compared to the placebo group.[19] Among those patients who required transfusions at baseline, 43% of EPOGEN®-treated patients versus 18% of placebo-treated patients were transfusion-independent during the second and third months of therapy. EPOGEN® therapy also resulted in significant increases in hematocrit in comparison to placebo. When examining the results according to the weekly dose of zidovudine received during Month 3 of therapy, there was a statistically significant ($p<0.003$) reduction in transfusion requirements in EPOGEN®-treated patients (N=51) compared to placebo treated patients (N=54) whose mean weekly zidovudine dose was ≤4,200 mg/week.[19] Approximately 17% of the patients with endogenous serum erythropoietin levels ≤500 mUnits/mL receiving EPOGEN® in doses from 100–200 Units/kg three times weekly (T.I.W.) achieved a hematocrit of 38% without administration of transfusions or significant reduction in zidovudine dose. In the subgroup of patients whose prestudy endogenous serum erythropoietin levels were >500 mUnits/mL, EPOGEN® therapy did not reduce transfusion requirements or increase hematocrit, compared to the corresponding responses in placebo-treated patients.

In a six month open label EPOGEN® study, patients responded with decreased transfusion requirements and sustained increases in hematocrit and hemoglobin with doses of EPOGEN® up to 300 Units/kg T.I.W.[18–20]

Responsiveness to EPOGEN® therapy may be blunted by intercurrent infectious/inflammatory episodes and by an increase in zidovudine dosage. Consequently, the dose of EPOGEN® must be titrated based on these factors to maintain the desired erythropoietic response.

Cancer Patients on Chemotherapy: EPOGEN® has been studied in a series of placebo-controlled, double-blind trials in a total of 131 anemic cancer patients. Within this group, 72 patients were treated with concomitant non cisplatin-containing chemotherapy regimens and 59 patients were treated with concomitant cisplatin-containing chemotherapy regimens. Patients were randomized to EPOGEN® 150 Units/kg or placebo subcutaneously T.I.W. for 12 weeks. EPOGEN® therapy was associated with a significantly ($p<0.008$) greater hematocrit response than in the corresponding placebo-treated patients (see TABLE).[19]

HEMATOCRIT (%): MEAN CHANGE FROM BASELINE TO FINAL VALUE*

STUDY	EPOGEN®	PLACEBO
Chemotherapy	7.6	1.3
Cisplatin	6.9	0.6

*Significantly higher in EPOGEN® patients than in placebo patients ($p<0.008$)

In the two types of chemotherapy studies (utilizing an EPOGEN® dose of 150 Units/kg T.I.W.), the mean number of units of blood transfused per patient after the first month of therapy was significantly ($p<0.02$) lower in EPOGEN®-treated patients (0.71 units in Months 2, 3) than in corresponding placebo-treated patients (1.84 units in Months 2, 3). Moreover, the proportion of patients transfused during Months 2 and 3 of therapy combined was significantly ($p<0.03$) lower in the EPOGEN®-treated patients than in the corresponding placebo-treated patients (22% versus 43%).[19]

Comparable intensity of chemotherapy in the EPOGEN® and placebo groups in the chemotherapy trials was suggested by a similar area under the neutrophil time curve in EPOGEN®- and placebo-treated patients as well as by a similar proportion of patients in EPOGEN®- and placebo-treated groups whose absolute neutrophil counts fell below 1,000 cells/μL. Available evidence suggests that patients with lymphoid and solid cancers respond equivalently to EPOGEN® therapy, and that patients with or without tumor infiltration of the bone marrow respond equivalently to EPOGEN® therapy.

CONTRAINDICATIONS

EPOGEN® is contraindicated in patients with:

1. Uncontrolled hypertension.
2. Known hypersensitivity to mammalian cell-derived products.
3. Known hypersensitivity to Albumin (Human).

WARNINGS

Chronic Renal Failure Patients

Hypertension: Patients with uncontrolled hypertension should not be treated with EPOGEN®; blood pressure should be controlled adequately before initiation of therapy. Up to 80% of patients with CRF have a history of hypertension.[21] Although there does not appear to be any direct pressor effects of EPOGEN®, blood pressure may rise during EPOGEN® therapy. During the early phase of treatment when the hematocrit is increasing, approximately 25% of patients on dialysis may require initiation of, or increases in, antihypertensive therapy. Hypertensive encephalopathy and seizures have been observed in patients with CRF treated with EPOGEN®.

Special care should be taken to closely monitor and aggressively control blood pressure in EPOGEN®-treated patients. Patients should be advised as to the importance of compliance with antihypertensive therapy and dietary restriction. If blood pressure is difficult to control by initiation of appropriate measures, the hematocrit may be reduced by decreasing or withholding the dose of EPOGEN®. A clinically significant decrease in hematocrit may not be observed for several weeks.

It is recommended that the dose of EPOGEN® be decreased if the hematocrit increase exceeds 4 points in any two-week period, because of the possible association of excessive rate of rise of hematocrit with an exacerbation of hypertension.

Seizures: Seizures have occurred in patients with CRF participating in EPOGEN® clinical trials.

In patients on dialysis, there was a higher incidence of seizures during the first 90 days of therapy (occurring in approximately 2.5% of patients) as compared with later timepoints.

Given the potential for an increased risk of seizures during the first 90 days of therapy, blood pressure and the presence of premonitory neurologic symptoms should be monitored closely. Patients should be cautioned to avoid potentially hazardous activities such as driving or operating heavy machinery during this period.

While the relationship between seizures and the rate of rise of hematocrit is uncertain, it is recommended that the dose of EPOGEN® be decreased if the hematocrit increase exceeds 4 points in any two-week period.

Thrombotic Events: During hemodialysis, patients treated with EPOGEN® may require increased anticoagulation with heparin to prevent clotting of the artificial kidney.
A relationship has not been established with statistical certainty between a rise in hematocrit and the rate of thrombotic events (including thrombosis of vascular access). In clinical trials, clotting of the vascular access (A-V shunt) has occurred at an annualized rate of about 0.25 events per patient-year on EPOGEN® therapy, a rate which appears to be no higher than that seen in untreated patients on dialysis. Overall, for patients with CRF (whether on dialysis or not), other thrombotic events (e.g., myocardial infarction, cerebrovascular accident, transient ischemic attack) have occurred in clinical trials at an annualized rate of less than 0.04 events per patient-year of EPOGEN® therapy. Patients with pre-existing vascular disease should be monitored closely. See "ADVERSE REACTIONS" for more information about thrombotic events.
Zidovudine-treated HIV-infected Patients: In contrast to CRF patients, EPOGEN® therapy has not been linked to exacerbation of hypertension, seizures, and thrombotic events in HIV-infected patients.
Miscellaneous: The multidose preserved formulation contains benzyl alcohol. Benzyl alcohol has been reported to be associated with an increased incidence of neurological and other complications in premature infants which are sometimes fatal.

PRECAUTIONS

Chronic Renal Failure Patients, Zidovudine-treated HIV-Infected Patients, and Cancer Patients on Chemotherapy

General: The parenteral administration of any biologic product should be attended by appropriate precautions in case allergic or other untoward reactions occur (see "Contraindications"). In clinical trials, while transient rashes were occasionally observed concurrently with EPOGEN® therapy, no serious allergic or anaphylactic reactions were reported. See "ADVERSE REACTIONS" for more information regarding allergic reactions.
The safety and efficacy of EPOGEN® therapy have not been established in patients with a known history of a seizure disorder or underlying hematologic disease (e.g., sickle cell anemia, myelodysplastic syndromes, or hypercoagulable disorders).
In some female patients, menses have resumed following EPOGEN® therapy; the possibility of pregnancy should be discussed and the need for contraception evaluated.
Hematology: Exacerbation of porphyria has been observed rarely in EPOGEN®-treated patients with CRF. However, EPOGEN® has not caused increased urinary excretion of porphyrin metabolites in normal volunteers, even in the presence of a rapid erythropoietic response. Nevertheless, EPOGEN® should be used with caution in patients with known porphyria.
In preclinical studies in dogs and rats, but not in monkeys, EPOGEN® therapy was associated with subclinical bone marrow fibrosis. Bone marrow fibrosis is a known complication of CRF in humans and may be related to secondary hyperparathyroidism or unknown factors. The incidence of bone marrow fibrosis was not increased in a study of patients on dialysis who were treated with EPOGEN® for 12–19 months, compared to the incidence of bone marrow fibrosis in a matched group of patients who had not been treated with EPOGEN®.
Hematocrit in CRF patients should be measured twice a week; zidovudine-treated HIV-infected, and cancer patients should have hematocrit measured once a week until hematocrit has been stabilized, and measured periodically thereafter.
Delayed or Diminished Response: If the patient fails to respond or to maintain a response to doses within the recommended dosing range, the following etiologies should be considered and evaluated:

1. Iron deficiency: Virtually all patients will eventually require supplemental iron therapy (see "Iron Evaluation").
2. Underlying infectious, inflammatory, or malignant processes.
3. Occult blood loss.
4. Underlying hematologic diseases (i.e., thalassemia, refractory anemia, or other myelodysplastic disorders).
5. Vitamin deficiencies: folic acid or vitamin B12.
6. Hemolysis.
7. Aluminum intoxication.
8. Osteitis fibrosa cystica.

Iron Evaluation: During EPOGEN® therapy, absolute or functional iron deficiency may develop. Functional iron deficiency, with normal ferritin levels but low transferrin saturation, is presumably due to the inability to mobilize iron stores rapidly enough to support increased erythropoiesis. Transferrin saturation should be at least 20% and ferritin should be at least 100 ng/mL.
Prior to and during EPOGEN® therapy, the patient's iron status, including transferrin saturation (serum iron divided by iron binding capacity) and serum ferritin, should be evaluated. Virtually all patients will eventually require supplemental iron to increase or maintain transferrin saturation to levels which will adequately support EPOGEN®-stimulated erythropoiesis.
Drug Interaction: No evidence of interaction of EPOGEN® with other drugs was observed in the course of clinical trials.
Carcinogenesis, Mutagenesis, and Impairment of Fertility: Carcinogenic potential of EPOGEN® has not been evaluated. EPOGEN® does not induce bacterial gene mutation (Ames Test), chromosomal aberrations in mammalian cells, micronuclei in mice, or gene mutation at the HGPRT locus. In female rats treated intravenously with EPOGEN®, there was a trend for slightly increased fetal wastage at doses of 100 and 500 Units/kg.
Pregnancy Category C: EPOGEN® has been shown to have adverse effects in rats when given in doses five times the human dose. There are no adequate and well-controlled studies in pregnant women. EPOGEN® should be used during pregnancy only if potential benefit justifies the potential risk to the fetus.
In studies in female rats, there were decreases in body weight gain, delays in appearance of abdominal hair, delayed eyelid opening, delayed ossification, and decreases in the number of caudal vertebrae in the F1 fetuses of the 500 Units/kg group. In female rats treated intravenously, there was a trend for slightly increased fetal wastage at doses of 100 and 500 Units/kg. EPOGEN® has not shown any adverse effect at doses as high as 500 Units/kg in pregnant rabbits (from day 6 to 18 of gestation).
Nursing Mothers: Postnatal observations of the live offspring (F1 generation) of female rats treated with EPOGEN® during gestation and lactation revealed no effect of EPOGEN® at doses of up to 500 Units/kg. There were, however, decreases in body weight gain, delays in appearance of abdominal hair, eyelid opening, and decreases in the number of caudal vertebrae in the F1 fetuses of the 500 Units/kg group. There were no EPOGEN®-related effects on the F2 generation fetuses.
It is not known whether EPOGEN® is excreted in human milk. Because many drugs are excreted in human milk, caution should be exercised when EPOGEN® is administered to a nursing woman.
Pediatric Use: The safety and effectiveness of EPOGEN® in children have not been established (see "WARNINGS").

Chronic Renal Failure Patients

Patients with CRF Not Requiring Dialysis: Blood pressure and hematocrit should be monitored no less frequently than for patients maintained on dialysis. Renal function and fluid and electrolyte balance should be closely monitored, as an improved sense of well-being may obscure the need to initiate dialysis in some patients.
Hematology: Sufficient time should be allowed to determine a patient's responsiveness to a dosage of EPOGEN® before adjusting the dose. Because of the time required for erythropoiesis and the red cell half-life, an interval of 2–6 weeks may occur between the time of a dose adjustment (initiation, increase, decrease, or discontinuation) and a significant change in hematocrit.
In order to avoid reaching the suggested target hematocrit too rapidly, or exceeding the suggested target range (hematocrit of 30–36%), the guidelines for dose and frequency of dose adjustments (see "Dosage and Administration") should be followed.
For patients who respond to EPOGEN® with a rapid increase in hematocrit (e.g., more than 4 points in any two-week period), the dose of EPOGEN® should be reduced because of the possible association of excessive rate of rise of hematocrit with an exacerbation of hypertension.
The elevated bleeding time characteristic of CRF decreases toward normal after correction of anemia in EPOGEN®-treated patients. Reduction of bleeding time also occurs after correction of anemia by transfusion.
Laboratory Monitoring: The hematocrit should be determined twice a week until it has stabilized in the suggested target range and the maintenance dose has been established. After any dose adjustment, the hematocrit should also be determined twice weekly for at least 2–6 weeks until it has been determined that the hematocrit has stabilized in response to the dose change. The hematocrit should then be monitored at regular intervals.
A complete blood count with differential and platelet count should be performed regularly. During clinical trials, modest increases were seen in platelets and white blood cell counts. While these changes were statistically significant, they were not clinically significant and the values remained within normal ranges.
In patients with CRF, serum chemistry values [including blood urea nitrogen (BUN), uric acid, creatinine, phosphorus, and potassium] should be monitored regularly. During clinical trials in patients on dialysis, modest increases were seen in BUN, creatinine, phosphorus, and potassium. In some patients with CRF not on dialysis, treated with EPOGEN®, modest increases in serum uric acid and phosphorus were observed. While changes were statistically significant, the values remained within the ranges normally seen in patients with CRF.
Diet: As the hematocrit increases and patients experience an improved sense of well-being and quality of life, the importance of compliance with dietary and dialysis prescriptions should be reinforced. In particular, hyperkalemia is not uncommon in patients with CRF. In U.S. studies in patients on dialysis, hyperkalemia has occurred at an annualized rate of approximately 0.11 episodes per patient-year of EPOGEN® therapy, often in association with poor compliance to medication, dietary and/or dialysis prescriptions.
Dialysis Management: Therapy with EPOGEN® results in an increase in hematocrit and a decrease in plasma volume which could affect dialysis efficiency. In studies to date, the resulting increase in hematocrit did not appear to adversely affect dialyzer function[9,10] or the efficiency of high-flux hemodialysis.[11] During hemodialysis, patients treated with EPOGEN® may require increased anticoagulation with heparin to prevent clotting of the artificial kidney.
Patients who are marginally dialyzed may require adjustments in their dialysis prescription. As with all patients on dialysis, the serum chemistry values [including blood urea nitrogen (BUN), creatinine, phosphorus, and potassium] in EPOGEN®-treated patients should be monitored regularly to assure the adequacy of the dialysis prescription.
Information for Patients: In those situations in which the physician determines that a home dialysis patient can safely and effectively self-administer EPOGEN®, the patient should be instructed as to the proper dosage and administration. Home dialysis patients should be referred to the full "Information for Home Dialysis Patients" section attached; it is not a disclosure of all possible effects. Patients should be informed of the signs and symptoms of allergic drug reaction and advised of appropriate actions. If home use is prescribed for a home dialysis patient, the patient should be thoroughly instructed in the importance of proper disposal and cautioned against the reuse of needles, syringes, or drug product. A puncture-resistant container for the disposal of used syringes and needles should be available to the patient. The full container should be disposed of according to the directions provided by the physician.
Renal Function: In patients with CRF not on dialysis, renal function and fluid and electrolyte balance should be closely monitored, as an improved sense of well-being may obscure the need to initiate dialysis in some patients. In patients with CRF not on dialysis, placebo-controlled studies of progression of renal dysfunction over periods of greater than one year have not been completed. In shorter term trials in patients with CRF not on dialysis, changes in creatinine and creatinine clearance were not significantly different in EPOGEN®-treated patients, compared with placebo-treated patients. Analysis of the slope of 1/serum creatinine vs. time plots in these patients indicates no significant change in the slope after the initiation of EPOGEN® therapy.

Zidovudine-treated HIV-infected Patients

Hypertension: Exacerbation of hypertension has not been observed in zidovudine-treated HIV-infected patients treated with EPOGEN®. However, EPOGEN® should be withheld in these patients if pre-existing hypertension is uncontrolled, and should not be started until blood pressure is controlled. In double-blind studies, a single seizure has been experienced by an EPOGEN®-treated patient.[19]

Cancer Patients on Chemotherapy

Hypertension: Hypertension, associated with a significant increase in hematocrit, has been noted rarely in EPOGEN®-treated cancer patients. Nevertheless, blood pressure in EPOGEN®-treated patients should be monitored carefully, particularly in patients with an underlying history of hypertension or cardiovascular disease.
Seizures: In double-blind, placebo-controlled trials, 3.2% (N=2/63) of EPOGEN®-treated patients and 2.9% (N=2/68) of placebo-treated patients had seizures. Seizures in 1.6% (N=1/63) of EPOGEN®-treated patients occurred in the context of a significant increase in blood pressure and hematocrit from baseline values. However, both EPOGEN®-treated patients also had underlying CNS pathology which may have been related to seizure activity.
Thrombotic Events: In double-blind, placebo-controlled trials, 3.2% (N=2/63) of EPOGEN®-treated patients and 11.8% (N=8/68) of placebo-treated patients had thrombotic events (e.g., pulmonary embolism, cerebrovascular accident).
Growth Factor Potential: EPOGEN® is a growth factor that primarily stimulates red cell production. However, the possibility that EPOGEN® can act as a growth factor for any tumor type, particularly myeloid malignancies, cannot be excluded.

ADVERSE REACTIONS

Chronic Renal Failure Patients

Studies analyzed to date indicate that EPOGEN® is generally well-tolerated. The adverse events reported are frequent sequelae of CRF and are not necessarily attributable to EPOGEN® therapy. In double-blind, placebo-controlled studies involving over 300 patients with CRF, the events reported in greater than 5% of EPOGEN®-treated patients during the blinded phase were:

Continued on next page

Amgen—Cont.

	Percent of Patients Reporting Event	
Event	EPOGEN®-Treated Patients (N=200)	Placebo-Treated Patients (N=135)
Hypertension	24%	19%
Headache	16%	12%
Arthralgias	11%	6%
Nausea	11%	9%
Edema	9%	10%
Fatigue	9%	14%
Diarrhea	9%	6%
Vomiting	8%	5%
Chest Pain	7%	9%
Skin Reaction (Administration Site)	7%	12%
Asthenia	7%	12%
Dizziness	7%	13%
Clotted Access	7%	2%

Significant adverse events of concern in patients with CRF treated in double-blind, placebo-controlled trials occurred in the following percent of patients during the blinded phase of the studies:

Seizure	1.1%	1.1%
CVA/TIA	0.4%	0.6%
MI	0.4%	1.1%
Death	0	1.7%

In the U.S. EPOGEN® studies in patients on dialysis (over 567 patients) the incidence (number of events per patient-year) of the most frequently reported adverse events were: hypertension (0.75), headache (0.40), tachycardia (0.31), nausea/vomiting (0.26), clotted vascular access (0.25), shortness of breath (0.14), hyperkalemia (0.11), and diarrhea (0.11). Other reported events occurred at a rate of less than 0.10 events per patient per year.

Events reported to have occurred within several hours of administration of EPOGEN® were rare, mild and transient, and included injection site stinging in dialysis patients and flu-like symptoms such as arthralgias and myalgias.

In all studies analyzed to date, EPOGEN® administration was generally well tolerated, irrespective of the route of administration.

Hypertension: Increases in blood pressure have been reported in clinical trials, often during the first 90 days of therapy. On occasion, hypertensive encephalopathy and seizures have been observed in patients with CRF treated with EPOGEN®. When data from all patients in the U.S. Phase III multicenter trial were analyzed, there was an apparent trend of more reports of hypertensive adverse events in patients on dialysis with a faster rate of rise of hematocrit (greater than 4 hematocrit points in any two-week period). However, in a double-blind, placebo-controlled trial, hypertensive adverse events were not reported at an increased rate in the EPOGEN®-treated group (150 units/kg T.I.W.) relative to the placebo group.

Seizures: There have been 47 seizures in 1,010 patients on dialysis treated with EPOGEN® in clinical trials, with an exposure of 986 patient-years for a rate of approximately 0.048 events per patient-year. However, there appeared to be a higher rate of seizures during the first 90 days of therapy (occurring in approximately 2.5% of patients) when compared to subsequent 90-day periods. The baseline incidence of seizures in the untreated dialysis population is difficult to determine; it appears to be in the range of 5–10% per patient-year.[22–24]

Thrombotic Events: In clinical trials, clotting of the vascular access has occurred at an annualized rate of about 0.25 events per patient-year on EPOGEN® therapy. Overall, for patients with CRF (whether on dialysis or not), other thrombotic events (e.g., myocardial infarction, cerebrovascular accident, transient ischemic attack) have occurred at an annualized rate of less than 0.04 events per patient-year of EPOGEN® therapy.

In over 125,000 patients treated with commercial EPOGEN®, there have been rare reports of serious or unusual thrombo-embolic events including migratory thrombophlebitis, microvascular thrombosis, pulmonary embolus, and thrombosis of the retinal artery, and temporal and renal veins. Collectively, these events have been reported in <0.0001 events per patient-year; in no case has a causal relationship been established.

Allergic Reactions: There have been no reports of serious allergic reactions or anaphylaxis associated with EPOGEN® administration during clinical trials. Skin rashes and urticaria have been observed rarely and when reported have generally been mild and transient in nature. In over 125,000 patients treated with commercial EPOGEN®, there have been rare reports of potentially serious allergic reactions including urticaria with associated

respiratory symptoms or circumoral edema (<0.0001 events per patient-year), or urticaria alone (<0.0001 events per patient-year). Most reactions occurred in situations where a causal relationship could not be established. Many of these patients resumed EPOGEN® therapy without recurrence of symptoms, some in conjunction with antihistamine pretreatment. However, symptoms recurred with rechallenge in a few instances, suggesting that allergic reactivity, although rare, may occasionally be associated with EPOGEN® therapy.

There has been no evidence for development of antibodies to erythropoietin in patients tested to date, including those receiving EPOGEN® for over 4 years. Nevertheless, if an anaphylactoid reaction occurs, EPOGEN® should be immediately discontinued and appropriate therapy initiated.

Zidovudine-treated HIV-infected Patients

Adverse events reported in clinical trials with EPOGEN® in zidovudine-treated HIV-infected patients were consistent with the progression of HIV infection. In double-blind, placebo-controlled studies of three-months duration involving approximately 300 zidovudine-treated HIV-infected patients, adverse events with an incidence of ≥10% in either EPOGEN®-treated patients or placebo-treated patients were:

	Percent of Patients Reporting Event	
Event	EPOGEN®-Treated Patients (N=144)	Placebo-Treated Patients (N=153)
Pyrexia	38%	29%
Fatigue	25%	31%
Headache	19%	14%
Cough	18%	14%
Diarrhea	16%	18%
Rash	16%	8%
Congestion, Respiratory	15%	10%
Nausea	15%	12%
Shortness of Breath	14%	13%
Asthenia	11%	14%
Skin Reaction, Medication Site	10%	7%
Dizziness	9%	10%

There were no statistically significant differences between treatment groups in the incidence of the above events.

In the 297 patients studied, EPOGEN® was not associated with significant increases in opportunistic infections or mortality.[19] In 71 patients from this group treated with EPOGEN® at 150 Units/kg T.I.W., serum p24 antigen levels did not appear to increase.[20] Preliminary data showed no enhancement of HIV replication in infected cell lines in vitro.[19]

Peripheral white blood cell and platelet counts are unchanged following EPOGEN® therapy.

Allergic Reactions: Two zidovudine-treated HIV-infected patients had urticarial reactions within 48 hours of their first exposure to study medication. One patient was treated with EPOGEN® and one was treated with placebo (EPOGEN® vehicle alone). Both patients had positive immediate skin tests against their study medication with a negative saline control. The basis for this apparent pre-existing hypersensitivity to components of the EPOGEN® formulation is unknown, but may be related to HIV-induced immunosuppression or prior exposure to blood products.

Seizures: In double-blind and open-label trials of EPOGEN® in zidovudine-treated HIV-infected patients, ten patients have experienced seizures.[19] In general, these seizures appear to be related to underlying pathology such as meningitis or cerebral neoplasms, not EPOGEN® therapy.

Cancer Patients on Chemotherapy

Adverse experiences reported in clinical trials with EPOGEN® in cancer patients were consistent with the underlying disease state. In double-blind, placebo-controlled studies of up to 3 months duration involving 131 cancer patients, adverse events with an incidence >10% in either EPOGEN®-treated or placebo-treated patients were as indicated below:

	Percent of Patients Reporting Event	
Event	EPOGEN®-Treated Patients (N=63)	Placebo-Treated Patients (N=68)
Pyrexia	29%	19%
Diarrhea	21%[a]	7%
Nausea	17%[b]	32%
Vomiting	17%	15%
Edema	17%[c]	1%
Asthenia	13%	16%
Fatigue	13%	15%
Shortness of Breath	13%	9%
Parasthesia	11%	6%
Upper Respiratory Infection	11%	4%
Dizziness	5%	12%
Trunk Pain	3%[d]	16%

a p=0.041
b p=0.069
c p=0.0016
d p=0.017

Although some statistically significant differences between EPOGEN®- and placebo-treated patients were noted, the overall safety profile of EPOGEN® appeared to be consistent with the disease process of advanced cancer. During double-blind and subsequent open-label therapy in which patients (N=72 for total EPOGEN® exposure) were treated for up to 32 weeks with doses as high as 927 Units/kg, the adverse experience profile of EPOGEN® was consistent with the progression of advanced cancer.

Based on comparable survival data and on the percentage of EPOGEN®- and placebo-treated patients who discontinued therapy due to death, disease progression, or adverse experiences (22% and 13%, respectively; p=0.25), the clinical outcome in the EPOGEN®- and placebo-treated patients appeared to be similar. Available data from animal tumor models and measurement of proliferation of solid tumor cells from clinical biopsy specimens in response to EPOGEN® suggest that EPOGEN® does not potentiate tumor growth. Nevertheless, as a growth factor, the possibility that EPOGEN® may potentiate growth of some tumors, particularly myeloid tumors, cannot be excluded. A randomized controlled Phase IV study is currently ongoing to further evaluate this issue.

The mean peripheral white blood cell count was unchanged following EPOGEN® therapy compared to the corresponding value in the placebo-treated group.

OVERDOSAGE

The maximum amount of EPOGEN® that can be safely administered in single or multiple doses has not been determined. Doses of up to 1,500 Units/kg T.I.W. for 3–4 weeks have been administered without any direct toxic effects of EPOGEN® itself.[6] Therapy with EPOGEN® can result in polycythemia if the hematocrit is not carefully monitored and the dose appropriately adjusted. If the suggested target range is exceeded, EPOGEN® may be temporarily withheld until the hematocrit returns to the suggested target range; EPOGEN® therapy may then be resumed using a lower dose (see "Dosage and Administration"). If polycythemia is of concern, phlebotomy may be indicated to decrease the hematocrit.

DOSAGE AND ADMINISTRATION

Chronic Renal Failure Patients

Starting doses of EPOGEN® over the range of 50–100 Units/kg three times weekly (T.I.W.) have been shown to be safe and effective in increasing hematocrit and eliminating transfusion dependency in patients with CRF (see "Clinical Experience"). The dose of EPOGEN® should be reduced as the hematocrit approaches 36% or increases by more than 4 points in any 2-week period. The dosage of EPOGEN® must be individualized to maintain the hematocrit within the suggested target range. At the physician's discretion, the suggested target hematocrit range may be expanded to achieve maximal patient benefit.

EPOGEN® may be given either as an intravenous (IV) or subcutaneous (SC) injection. In patients on hemodialysis, EPOGEN® usually has been administered as an IV bolus T.I.W. While the administration of EPOGEN® is independent of the dialysis procedure, EPOGEN® may be administered into the venous line at the end of the dialysis procedure to obviate the need for additional venous access. In patients with CRF not on dialysis, EPOGEN® may be given either as an IV or SC injection.

Home hemodialysis patients who have been judged competent by their physicians to self-administer EPOGEN® without medical or other supervision may give themselves either an IV or SC injection. Home peritoneal dialysis patients who have been judged competent by their physicians to self-administer EPOGEN® without medical or other supervision may give themselves a SC injection. The table below provides general therapeutic guidelines for patients with CRF:

Starting Dose:	50–100 Units/kg T.I.W.; IV or SC
Reduce Dose When:	1. Hct. approaches 36% or, 2. Hct. increases >4 points in any 2-week period
Increase Dose If:	Hct. does not increase by 5–6 points after 8 weeks of therapy, and hct. is below suggested target range.
Maintenance Dose:	Individually titrate
Suggested Target Hct. Range:	30–36%

During therapy, hematological parameters should be monitored regularly (see "Laboratory Monitoring").

Pre-Therapy Iron Evaluation: Prior to and during EPOGEN® therapy, the patient's iron stores, including transferrin saturation (serum iron divided by iron binding

capacity) and serum ferritin, should be evaluated. Transferrin saturation should be at least 20%, and ferritin should be at least 100 ng/mL. Virtually all patients will eventually require supplemental iron to increase or maintain transferrin saturation to levels that will adequately support EPOGEN®-stimulated erythropoiesis.

Dose Adjustment:
Following EPOGEN® therapy, a period of time is required for erythroid progenitors to mature and be released into circulation resulting in an eventual increase in hematocrit. Additionally, red blood cell survival time affects hematocrit and may vary due to uremia. As a result, the time required to elicit a clinically significant change in hematocrit (increase or decrease) following any dose adjustment may be 2–6 weeks.

Dose adjustment should not be made more frequently than once a month, unless clinically indicated. After any dose adjustment, the hematocrit should be determined twice weekly for at least 2–6 weeks (see "Laboratory Monitoring").
- If the hematocrit is increasing and approaching 36%, the dose should be reduced to maintain the suggested target hematocrit range. If the reduced dose does not stop the rise in hematocrit, and it exceeds 36%, doses should be temporarily withheld until the hematocrit begins to decrease, at which point therapy should be reinitiated at a lower dose.
- At any time, if the hematocrit increases by more than 4 points in a 2-week period, the dose should be immediately decreased. After the dose reduction, the hematocrit should be monitored twice weekly for 2–6 weeks, and further dose adjustments should be made as outlined in "Maintenance Dose".
- If a hematocrit increase of 5–6 points is not achieved after an 8-week period and iron stores are adequate (see "Delayed or Diminished Response"), the dose of EPOGEN® may be incrementally increased. Further increases may be made at 4–6 week intervals until the desired response is attained.

Maintenance Dose: The maintenance dose must be individualized for each patient on dialysis. In the U.S. Phase III multicenter trial in patients on hemodialysis, the median maintenance dose was 75 Units/kg T.I.W., with a range from 12.5 to 525 Units/kg T.I.W. Almost 10% of the patients required a dose of 25 Units/kg, or less, and approximately 10% of the patients required more than 200 Units/kg T.I.W. to maintain their hematocrit in the suggested target range. If the hematocrit remains below, or falls below, the suggested target range, iron stores should be re-evaluated. If the transferrin saturation is less than 20%, supplemental iron should be administered. If the transferrin saturation is greater than 20%, the dose of EPOGEN® may be increased. Such dose increases should not be made more frequently than once a month, unless clinically indicated, as the response time of the hematocrit to a dose increase can be 2–6 weeks. Hematocrit should be measured twice weekly for 2–6 weeks following dose increases. In patients with CRF not on dialysis, the maintenance dose must also be individualized. EPOGEN® doses of 75–150 Units/kg per week have been shown to maintain hematocrits of 36–38% for up to 6 months.

Delayed or Diminished Response: Over 95% of patients with CRF responded with clinically significant increases in hematocrit, and virtually all patients were transfusion-independent within approximately 2 months of initiation of EPOGEN® therapy.

If a patient fails to respond or maintain a response, other etiologies should be considered and evaluated as clinically indicated. See "PRECAUTIONS" section for discussion of delayed or diminished response.

Zidovudine-treated HIV-infected Patients
Prior to beginning EPOGEN®, it is recommended that the endogenous serum erythropoietin level be determined (prior to transfusion). Available evidence suggests that patients receiving zidovudine with endogenous serum erythropoietin levels >500 mUnits/mL are unlikely to respond to therapy with EPOGEN®.

Starting Dose: For patients with serum erythropoietin levels ≤500 mUnits/mL who are receiving a dose of zidovudine ≤4,200 mg/week, the recommended starting dose of EPOGEN® is 100 Units/kg as an intravenous or subcutaneous injection three times weekly (T.I.W.) for 8 weeks.
Increase Dose: During the dose adjustment phase of therapy, the hematocrit should be monitored weekly. If the response is not satisfactory in terms of reducing transfusion requirements or increasing hematocrit after 8 weeks of therapy, the dose of EPOGEN® can be increased by 50–100 Units/kg T.I.W. Response should be evaluated every 4–8 weeks thereafter and the dose adjusted accordingly by 50–100 Units/kg increments T.I.W. If patients have not responded satisfactorily to an EPOGEN® dose of 300 Units/kg T.I.W., it is unlikely that they will respond to higher doses of EPOGEN®.
Maintenance Dose: After attainment of the desired response (i.e., reduced transfusion requirements or increased hematocrit), the dose of EPOGEN® should be titrated to maintain the response based on factors such as variations in zidovudine dose and the presence of intercurrent infectious

or inflammatory episodes. If the hematocrit exceeds 40%, the dose should be discontinued until the hematocrit drops to 36%. The dose should be reduced by 25% when treatment is resumed and then titrated to maintain the desired hematocrit.

Cancer Patients on Chemotherapy
Baseline endogenous serum erythropoietin levels varied among patients in these trials with approximately 75% (N=83/110) having endogenous serum erythropoietin levels <132 mUnits/mL, and approximately 4% (N=4/110) of patients having endogenous serum erythropoietin levels >500 mUnits/mL. In general, patients with lower baseline serum erythropoietin levels responded more vigorously to EPOGEN® than patients with higher erythropoietin levels. Although no specific serum erythropoietin level can be stipulated above which patients would be unlikely to respond to EPOGEN® therapy, treatment of patients with grossly elevated serum erythropoietin levels (e.g., >200 mUnits/mL) is not recommended. The hematocrit should be monitored on a weekly basis in patients receiving EPOGEN® therapy until hematocrit becomes stable.

Starting Dose: The recommended starting dose of EPOGEN® is 150 Units/kg subcutaneously T.I.W.
Dose Adjustment: If the response is not satisfactory in terms of reducing transfusion requirements or increasing hematocrit after 8 weeks of therapy, the dose of EPOGEN® can be increased up to 300 Units/kg T.I.W. If patients have not responded satisfactorily to an EPOGEN® dose of 300 Units/kg T.I.W., it is unlikely that they will respond to higher doses of EPOGEN®. If the hematocrit exceeds 40%, the dose of EPOGEN® should be withheld until the hematocrit falls to 36%. The dose of EPOGEN® should be reduced by 25% when treatment is resumed and titrated to maintain the desired hematocrit. If the initial dose of EPOGEN® includes a very rapid hematocrit response (e.g., an increase of more than 4 percentage points in any 2-week period), the dose of EPOGEN® should be reduced.

PREPARATION AND ADMINISTRATION OF EPOGEN®
1. Do not shake. It is not necessary to shake EPOGEN®. Prolonged vigorous shaking may denature any glycoprotein, rendering it biologically inactive.
2. Parenteral drug products should be inspected visually for particulate matter and discoloration prior to administration. Do not use any vials exhibiting particulate matter or discoloration.
3. Using aseptic techniques, attach a sterile needle to a sterile syringe. Remove the flip top from the vial containing EPOGEN®, and wipe the septum with a disinfectant. Insert the needle into the vial, and withdraw into the syringe an appropriate volume of solution.
4. **Single-dose** 1 mL vial contains no preservative. Use one dose per vial; do not re-enter the vial. Discard unused portions.
   Multidose 2 mL vial contains preservative. Store at 2 to 8° C after initial entry and between doses. Discard 21 days after initial entry.
5. Do not dilute or administer in conjunction with other drug solutions. However, at the time of subcutaneous administration, EPOGEN® may be admixed in a syringe with bacteriostatic 0.9% sodium chloride injection, USP, with benzyl alcohol 0.9% (bacteriostatic saline) at a 1:1 ratio using aseptic technique. The benzyl alcohol in the bacteriostatic saline acts as a local anesthetic which may ameliorate subcutaneous injection site discomfort.

HOW SUPPLIED
EPOGEN®, containing Epoetin alfa, is available in the following packages:
1 mL **Single-Dose, Preservative-Free** Solution
2,000 Units/mL (NDC 55513-126-01)
3,000 Units/mL (NDC 55513-267-01)
4,000 Units/mL (NDC 55513-148-01)
10,000 Units/mL (NDC 55513-144-01)
Supplied in boxes containing 10 single-dose vials.
2 mL **Multidose, Preserved** Solution
10,000 Units/mL (NDC 55513-283-01)
Supplied in boxes containing 10 multidose vials.

STORAGE
Store at 2° to 8°C (36° to 46°F). Do not freeze or shake.

REFERENCES
1. Egrie JC, Strickland TW, Lane J, et al. (1986). "Characterization and Biological Effects of Recombinant Human Erythropoietin." *Immunobiol.* 72: 213–224.
2. Graber SE and Krantz SB (1978). "Erythropoietin and the Control of Red Cell Production." *Ann Rev Med.* 29: 51–66.
3. Eschbach JW and Adamson JW (1985). "Anemia of End-Stage Renal Disease (ESRD)." *Kidney Intl.* 28: 1–5.
4. Eschbach JW, Egrie JC, Downing MR, et al. (1987). "Correction of the Anemia of End-Stage Renal Disease with Recombinant Human Erythropoietin." *NEJM.* 316: 73–78.
5. Eschbach JW, Abdulhadi MH, Browne JK, et al. (1989). "Recombinant Human Erythropoietin in Anemic Patients with End-Stage Renal Disease." *Ann Intern Med.* 111:12.
6. Eschbach JW, Egrie JC, Downing MR, et al. (1989). "The Use of Recombinant Human Erythropoietin (r-HuEPO): Effect in End-Stage Renal Disease (ESRD)." *Prevention of Chronic Uremia* (Friedman, Beyer, DeSanto, Giordano, eds.), Field and Wood Inc., Philadelphia, PA, pp 148–155.
7. Egrie JC, Eschbach JW, McGuire T, and Adamson JW, (1988). "Pharmacokinetics of Recombinant Human Erythropoietin (r-HuEPO) Administered to Hemodialysis (HD) Patients." *Kidney Intl.* 33: 262.
8. Evans RW, Radar B, Manninen DL, et al. (1990). "The Quality of Life of Hemodialysis Recipients Treated with Recombinant Human Erythropoietin." *JAMA.* 263: 6.
9. Paganini E, Garcia J, Ellis P, et al. (1988). "Clinical Sequelae of Correction of Anemia with Recombinant Human Erythropoietin (r-HuEPO); Urea Kinetics, Dialyzer Function and Reuse." *Am J Kid Dis.* 11: 16.
10. Delano BG, Lundin AP, Golansky R, et al. (1988). "Dialyzer Urea and Creatinine Clearances Not Significantly Changed in r-HuEPO Treated Maintenance Hemodialysis (MD) Patients." *Kidney Intl.* 33: 219.
11. Stivelman J, Van Wyck D, and Ogden D (1988). "Use of Recombinant Erythropoietin (r-HuEPO) with High Flux Dialysis (HFD) Does Not Worsen Azotemia or Shorten Access Survival." *Kidney Intl.* 33: 239.
12. Lim VS, DeGowin RL, Zavala D, et al. (1989). "Recombinant Human Erythropoietin Treatment in Pre-Dialysis Patients: A Double-Blind Placebo-Controlled Trial." *Ann Int Med.* 110: 108–114.
13. Stone WJ, Graber SE, Krantz SB, et al. (1988). "Treatment of the Anemia of Pre-Dialysis Patients with Recombinant Human Erythropoietin: A Randomized, Placebo-Controlled Trial." *Am J Med Sci.* 296: 171–179.
14. Lundin AP, Akerman MJH, Chesler RM, et al. (1991). "Exercise in Hemodialysis Patients after Treatment with Recombinant Human Erythropoietin." *Nephron.* 58: 315–319.
15. Data on file, Amgen Inc.
16. Eschbach JW, Kelly MR, Galey NR, et al. (1989). "Treatment of the Anemia of Progressive Renal Failure with Recombinant Human Erythropoietin." *NEJM.* 321: 158–163.
17. The US Recombinant Human Erythropoietin Predialysis Study Group (1991). "Double-Blind, Placebo-Controlled Study of the Therapeutic Use of Recombinant Human Erythropoietin for Anemia Associated with Chronic Renal Failure in Predialysis Patients." *Am J Kid Dis.* 18(1): 50–59.
18. Danna RP, Rudnick SA, and Abels RI (1990). "Erythropoietin Therapy for the Anemia Associated with AIDS and AIDS Therapy and Cancer." *Erythropoietin in Clinical Applications—An International Perspective* (MB Garnick, ed.), Marcel Dekker, New York, NY, pp 301–324.
19. Data on file, Ortho Biologics, Inc.
20. Fischl M, Galpin JE, Levin JD, et al. (1990). "Recombinant Human Erythropoietin for Patients with AIDS Treated with Zidovudine." *NEJM.* 322: 1488–1493.
21. Kerr DN (1979). "Chronic Renal Failure." *Cecil Textbook of Medicine* (Beeson PB, McDermott W, Wyngaarden JB, eds.), W.B. Saunders, Philadelphia, PA, pp 1351–1367.
22. Raskin NH and Fishman RA (1976). "Neurologic Disorders in Renal Failure (First of Two Parts)." *NEJM.* 294: 143–148.
23. Raskin NH and Fishman RA (1976). "Neurologic Disorder in Renal Failure (Second of Two Parts)." *NEJM.* 294: 204–210.
24. Messing RO and Simon RP, (1986). "Seizures as a Manifestation of Systemic Disease." *Neurologic Clinics.* 4: 563–584.

Manufactured by:
Amgen Inc.
Amgen Center
Thousand Oaks, California 91320-1789
Issue Date 06/29/94

EPOGEN®
EPOETIN ALFA
INFORMATION FOR HOME DIALYSIS PATIENTS

EPOGEN® AND CHRONIC RENAL FAILURE
EPOGEN® (Epoetin alfa) has been prescribed for you by your doctor because you:
1. Have anemia due to your kidney disease.
2. Are able to dialyze at home.
3. Have been determined to be able to administer EPOGEN® without direct medical or other supervision.

A lack of energy or feeling of tiredness is the major symptom of anemia. Additional symptoms include shortness of breath, chest pain, and feeling cold all the time. The reason for these symptoms is that there is a lack of red blood cells. Red blood cells carry oxygen, which is important for all of the body's

Continued on next page

Amgen—Cont.

functions. When there are fewer red blood cells, the body does not get all the oxygen it needs.

Kidneys remove toxins from the blood; they also measure the amount of oxygen in the blood. If there is not enough oxygen, the kidneys will produce a hormone called erythropoietin. Erythropoietin is released into the bloodstream and travels to the bone marrow where red blood cells are made. Erythropoietin signals the bone marrow to make more oxygen-carrying red blood cells.

As the kidneys fail, they stop cleansing toxins from your body. They also make less erythropoietin than they should. Therefore, the bone marrow does not receive a strong-enough signal to make the oxygen-carrying red blood cells. Fewer red blood cells are produced so the muscles, brain, and other parts of the body do not get the oxygen they need to function properly.

EPOGEN® is a copy of human erythropoietin. EPOGEN® replaces the erythropoietin that the failed kidneys can no longer produce, and signals the bone marrow to make the oxygen-carrying red blood cells once again.

The effectiveness of EPOGEN® is measured by the increase in hematocrit (the amount of red blood cells in the blood) that results from EPOGEN® therapy. The rise in hematocrit is not immediate. It usually takes about 2 to 6 weeks before the hematocrit starts to rise. The amount of time it takes, and the dose of EPOGEN® that is needed to make the hematocrit increase, varies from patient to patient.

Most patients treated with EPOGEN® no longer need blood transfusions. However, certain medical conditions, or unexpected blood loss, may result in the need for a transfusion. In those situations where your doctor has determined that you, as a home dialysis patient, can self-administer EPOGEN®, you will receive instruction on how much EPOGEN® to use, how to inject it, how often you should inject it, and how you should dispose of the unused portions of each vial.

You will be instructed to monitor your blood pressure carefully everyday and to report any changes outside of the guidelines that your doctor has given you. When the number of red blood cells increases, your blood pressure can also increase, so your doctor may prescribe some new or additional blood pressure medication. Be sure to follow your doctor's orders. You may also be instructed to have certain laboratory tests, such as additional hematocrit or iron level measurements, done more frequently. You may be asked to report these tests to your doctor or dialysis center. Also, your doctor may prescribe additional iron for you to take. Be sure to comply with your doctor's orders.

Continue to check your access, as your doctor or nurse has shown you, to make sure it is working. Be sure to let your health care professional know right away if there is a problem.

When you receive your EPOGEN® from the dialysis center, doctor's office or home dialysis supplier, always check to see that:

1. The name EPOGEN® appears on the carton and vial label.
2. You will be able to use EPOGEN® before the expiration date stamped on the package.

EPOGEN®

EPOGEN® is produced in mammalian cells that have been genetically altered by the addition of a gene for the natural substance erythropoietin.

The EPOGEN® solution in the vial should always be clear and colorless. Do not use EPOGEN® if the contents of the vial appear discolored or cloudy, or if the vial appears to contain lumps, flakes, or particles. In addition, if the vial has been shaken vigorously, the solution may appear to be frothy and should not be used. Therefore, care should be taken not to shake the EPOGEN® vial vigorously before use.

Single-dose Vial: 2000, 3000, 4000, and 10,000 Unit vials of EPOGEN® are for single use only. Any unused portions of these vials should be discarded.

Multidose Vial: Vials of EPOGEN® marked with a white "M" on the label (10,000 Units/mL-20,000 Units in a vial) contain a preserved solution and may be entered multiple times. Multidose vials should be stored in the refrigerator between uses and thrown away 21 days after the first use. Carefully follow the instructions for "Preparing the Dose" each time you enter the multidose vial.

Follow the dialysis center's instructions on what to do with the used vials.

STORAGE

EPOGEN® should be stored in the refrigerator, but not in the freezing compartment. Do not let the vial freeze and do not leave it in direct sunlight. Do not use a vial of EPOGEN® that has been frozen or after the expiration date that is stamped on the label. If you have any questions about the safety of a vial of EPOGEN® that has been subjected to temperature extremes, be sure to check with your dialysis unit staff.

USE THE CORRECT SYRINGE

Your doctor has instructed you on how to give yourself the correct dosage of EPOGEN®. This dosage will usually be measured in Units per milliliter or cc's. It is important to use a syringe that is marked in tenths of milliliters (for example, 0.1, 0.2, etc., mL or cc). Failure to use the proper syringe can lead to a mistake in dosage, and you may receive too much or too little EPOGEN®. Too little EPOGEN® may not be effective in increasing your hematocrit, and too much EPOGEN® may lead to a hematocrit that is too high. Only use disposable syringes and needles as they do not require sterilization; they should be used once and disposed of as instructed by your doctor.

IMPORTANT: TO HELP AVOID CONTAMINATION AND POSSIBLE INFECTION, FOLLOW THESE INSTRUCTIONS EXACTLY.

PREPARING THE DOSE

1. Wash your hands thoroughly with soap and water before preparing the medication.

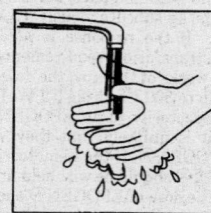

2. Check the date on the EPOGEN® vial to be sure that the drug has not expired.
3. Remove the vial of EPOGEN® from the refrigerator and allow it to reach room temperature. It is not necessary to shake EPOGEN®. Prolonged vigorous shaking may damage the product. Assemble the other supplies you will need for your injection.

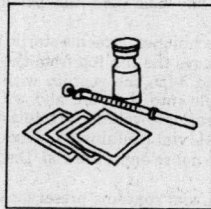

4. Hemodialysis patients should wipe off the venous port of the hemodialysis tubing with an antiseptic swab. Peritoneal dialysis patients should cleanse the skin with an antiseptic swab where the injection is to be made.

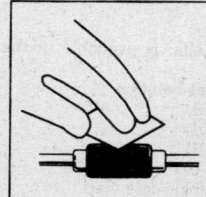
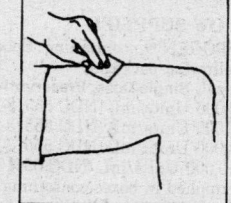

5. Flip off the red protective cap but do not remove the gray rubber stopper. Wipe the top of the gray rubber stopper with an antiseptic swab.

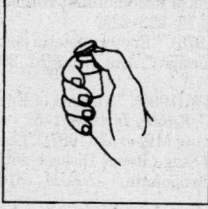
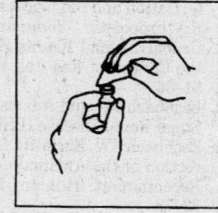

6. Using a syringe and needle designed for subcutaneous injection, draw air into the syringe by pulling back on the plunger. The amount of air should be equal to your EPOGEN® dose.

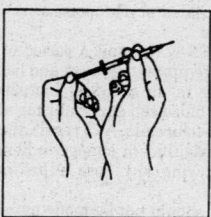

7. Carefully remove the needle cover. Put the needle through the gray rubber stopper of the EPOGEN® vial.
8. Push the plunger in to discharge air into the vial. The air injected into the vial will allow EPOGEN® to be easily withdrawn into the syringe.

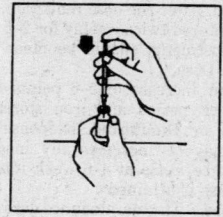

9. Turn the vial and syringe upside down in one hand. Be sure the tip of the needle is in the EPOGEN® solution. Your other hand will be free to move the plunger. Draw back on the plunger slowly to draw the correct dose of EPOGEN® into the syringe.

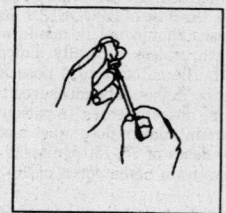

10. Check for air bubbles. The air is harmless, but too large an air bubble will reduce the EPOGEN® dose. To remove air bubbles, gently tap the syringe to move the air bubbles to the top of the syringe, then use the plunger to push the solution and the air back into the vial. Then re-measure your correct dose of EPOGEN®.
11. Double check your dose. Remove the needle from the vial. Do not lay the syringe down or allow the needle to touch anything.

INJECTING THE DOSE

Patients on home hemodialysis using the intravenous injection route:

1. Insert the needle of the syringe into the previously cleansed venous port and inject the EPOGEN®.

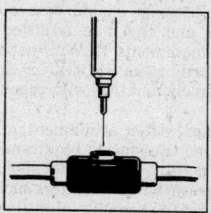

2. Remove the syringe and dispose of the whole unit. **Use the disposable syringe only once.** Dispose of syringes and needles as directed by your doctor, by following these simple steps:

- Place all used needles and syringes in a hard plastic container with a screw-on-cap, or a metal container with a plastic lid, such as a coffee can properly labeled as to content. If a metal container is used, cut a small hole in the plastic lid and tape the lid to the metal container. If a hard-plastic container is used, always screw the cap on tightly after each use. When the container is full, tape around the cap or lid, and dispose of according to your doctor's instructions.

- Do not use glass or clear plastic containers, or any container that will be recycled or returned to a store.

- Always store the container out of the reach of children.

- Please check with your doctor, nurse, or pharmacist for other suggestions. There may be special state and local laws that they will discuss with you.

Patients on home peritoneal dialysis or home hemodialysis using the subcutaneous route:

1. With one hand, stabilize the previously cleansed skin by spreading it or by pinching up a large area with your free hand.

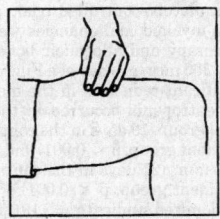

2. Hold the syringe with the other hand, as you would a pencil. Double check that the correct amount of EPOGEN® is in the syringe. Insert the needle straight into the skin (90 degree angle). Pull the plunger back slightly. If blood comes into the syringe, do not inject EPOGEN®, as the needle has entered a blood vessel; withdraw the syringe and inject at a different site. Inject the EPOGEN® by pushing the plunger all the way down.

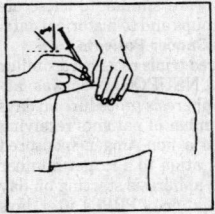 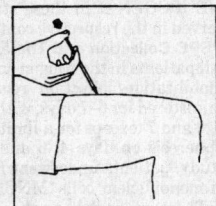

3. Hold an antiseptic swab near the needle and pull the needle straight out of the skin. Press the antiseptic swab over the injection site for several seconds.

4. **Use the disposable syringe only once.** Dispose of syringes and needles as directed by your doctor, by following these simple steps:

- Place all used needles and syringes in a hard plastic container with a screw-on-cap, or a metal container with a plastic lid, such as a coffee can properly labeled as to content. If a metal container is used, cut a small hole in the plastic lid and tape the lid to the metal container. If a hard-plastic container is used, always screw the cap on tightly after each use. When the container is full, tape around the cap or lid, and dispose of according to your doctor's instructions.

- Do not use glass or clear plastic containers, or any container that will be recycled or returned to a store.

- Always store the container out of the reach of children.

- Please check with your doctor, nurse, or pharmacist for other suggestions. There may be special state and local laws that they will discuss with you.

5. Always change the site for each injection as directed. Occasionally a problem may develop at the injection site. If you notice a lump, swelling, or bruising that doesn't go away, contact your physician. You may wish to record the site just used so that you can keep track.

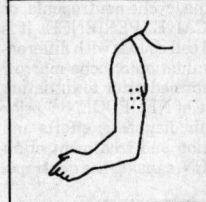 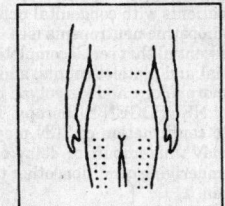

ALLERGY TO EPOGEN®
Patients occasionally experience redness, swelling, or itching at the site of injection of EPOGEN®. This may indicate an allergy to the components of EPOGEN®, or it may indicate a local reaction. If you have a local reaction, consult your doctor. A potentially more serious reaction would be a generalized allergy to EPOGEN®, which could cause a rash over the whole body, shortness of breath, wheezing, reduction in blood pressure, fast pulse, or sweating. Severe cases of generalized allergy may be life-threatening. If you think you are having a generalized allergic reaction, stop taking EPOGEN® and notify a doctor or emergency medical personnel immediately.

IMPORTANT NOTES
Since you are a home dialysis patient and your doctor allows you to self-administer EPOGEN®, please note the following:

1. Always follow the instructions of your doctor concerning dosage and administration of EPOGEN®. Do not change the dose or instructions for administration of EPOGEN® without consulting your doctor.
2. Your doctor will tell you what to do if you miss a dose of EPOGEN®. Always keep a spare syringe and needle on hand.
3. Always consult your doctor if you notice anything unusual about your condition or your use of EPOGEN®.

USAGE IN PREGNANCY
If you are pregnant or nursing a baby, consult your doctor before using EPOGEN®.
Issue date 1/19/95
Shown in Product Identification Guide, page 304

NEUPOGEN®   ℞
(Filgrastim)

DESCRIPTION
Filgrastim is a human granulocyte colony stimulating factor (G-CSF), produced by recombinant DNA technology. NEUPOGEN® is the Amgen Inc. trademark for Filgrastim, which has been selected as the name for recombinant methionyl human granulocyte colony stimulating factor (r-metHuG-CSF).

NEUPOGEN® is a 175 amino acid protein manufactured by recombinant DNA technology.[1] NEUPOGEN® is produced by *Escherichia coli (E. coli)* bacteria into which has been inserted the human granulocyte colony stimulating factor gene. NEUPOGEN® has a molecular weight of 18,800 daltons. The protein has an amino acid sequence that is identical to the natural sequence predicted from human DNA sequence analysis, except for the addition of an N- terminal methionine necessary for expression in *E. coli*. Because NEUPOGEN® is produced in *E. coli*, the product is nonglycosylated and thus differs from G-CSF isolated from a human cell.

NEUPOGEN® is a sterile, clear, colorless, preservative-free liquid for parenteral administration. Each single-use vial of NEUPOGEN® contains 300 mcg/mL of Filgrastim at a specific activity of $1.0 \pm 0.6 \times 10^8$ U/mg, (as measured by a cell mitogenesis assay). The product is formulated in a 10 mM sodium acetate buffer at pH 4.0, containing 5% mannitol, and 0.004% Tween® 80. The quantitative composition (per mL) of NEUPOGEN® is:

Filgrastim	300 mcg
Acetate	0.59 mg
Mannitol	50.0 mg
Tween® 80	0.004%
Sodium	0.035 mg
Water for Injection USP q.s. ad	1.0 mL

CLINICAL PHARMACOLOGY

Colony Stimulating Factors
Colony stimulating factors are glycoproteins which act on hematopoietic cells by binding to specific cell surface receptors and stimulating proliferation, differentiation commitment, and some end-cell functional activation.

Endogenous G-CSF is a lineage specific colony stimulating factor which is produced by monocytes, fibroblasts and endothelial cells. G-CSF regulates the production of neutrophils within the bone marrow and affects neutrophil progenitor proliferation,[2,3] differentiation[2,4] and selected end cell functional activation (including enhanced phagocytic ability,[5] priming of the cellular metabolism associated with respiratory burst,[6] antibody dependent killing,[7] and the increased expression of some functions associated with cell surface antigens.[8] G-CSF is not species specific and has been shown to have minimal direct *in vivo* or *in vitro* effects on the production of hematopoietic cell types other than the neutrophil lineage.

Pre-clinical Experience
Filgrastim was administered to monkeys, dogs, hamsters, rats, and mice as part of a pre-clinical toxicology program which included single-dose acute, repeated-dose subacute, subchronic, and chronic studies. Single-dose administration of Filgrastim by the oral, intravenous, subcutaneous, or intraperitoneal routes resulted in no significant toxicity in mice, rats, hamsters, or monkeys. Although no deaths were observed in mice, rats, or monkeys at dose levels up to 3,450 mcg/kg or in hamsters using single doses up to approximately 860 mcg/kg, deaths were observed in a subchronic (13 week) study in monkeys. In this study, evidence of neurological symptoms was seen in monkeys treated with doses of Filgrastim greater than 1,150 mcg/kg/day for up to 18 days. Deaths were seen in 5 of the 8 treated animals and were associated with 15- to 28-fold increases in peripheral leukocyte counts, and neutrophil-infiltrated hemorrhagic foci were seen in both the cerebrum and cerebellum. In contrast, no monkeys died following 13 weeks of daily intravenous administration of Filgrastim at a dose level of 115 mcg/kg. In an ensuing 52 week study, one 115 mcg/kg dose female monkey died after 18 weeks of daily IV administration of Filgrastim. Death was attributed to cardiopulmonary insufficiency.

In subacute, repeated-dose studies, changes observed were attributable to the expected pharmacological actions of Filgrastim (i.e., dose-dependent increases in white cell counts, increased circulating segmented neutrophils, and increased myeloid:erythroid ratio in bone marrow). In all species, histopathologic examination of the liver and spleen revealed evidence of ongoing extramedullary granulopoiesis; increased spleen weights were seen in all species and appeared to be dose-related. A dose-dependent increase in serum alkaline phosphatase was observed in rats, and may reflect increased activity of osteoblasts and osteoclasts. Changes in serum chemistry values were reversible following discontinuation of treatment.

In rats treated at doses of 1,150 mcg/kg/day for four weeks (5 of 32 animals) and for 13 weeks at doses of 100 mcg/kg/day (4 of 32 animals) and 500 mcg/kg/day (6 of 32 animals), articular swelling of the hind legs was observed. Some degree of hind leg dysfunction was also observed; however, symptoms reversed following cessation of dosing. In rats, osteoclasis and osteoanagenesis were found in the femur, humerus, coccyx, and hind legs (where they were accompanied by synovitis) after intravenous treatment for four weeks (115 to 1,150 mcg/kg/day), and in the sternum after intravenous treatment for 13 weeks (115 to 575 mcg/kg/day). These effects reversed to normal within 4 to 5 weeks following cessation of treatment.

In the 52-week chronic, repeated-dose studies performed in rats (intraperitoneal injection up to 57.5 mcg/kg/day), and cynomolgus monkeys (intravenous injection of up to 115 mcg/kg/day), changes observed were similar to those noted in the subacute studies. Expected pharmacological actions of Filgrastim included dose-dependent increases in white cell counts, increased circulating segmented neutrophils and alkaline phosphatase levels, and increased myeloid:erythroid ratios in the bone marrow. Decreases in platelet counts were also noted in primates. In no animals tested were hemorrhagic complications observed. Rats displayed dose-related swelling of the hind limb, accompanied by some degree of hind limb dysfunction; osteopathy was noted microscopically. Enlarged spleens (both species) and livers (monkeys), reflective of ongoing extramedullary granulopoiesis, as well as myeloid hyperplasia of the bone marrow, were observed in a dose-dependent manner.

Pharmacologic Effects of NEUPOGEN®
In Phase I studies involving 96 patients with various nonmyeloid malignancies, NEUPOGEN® administration resulted in a dose-dependent increase in circulating neutrophil

Continued on next page

Amgen—Cont.

counts over the dose range of 1–70 mcg/kg/day.[9–11] This increase in neutrophil counts was observed whether NEUPOGEN® was administered intravenously (1–70 mcg/kg twice daily),[9] subcutaneously (1–3 mcg/kg once daily),[11] or by continuous subcutaneous infusion (3–11 mcg/kg/day).[10] With discontinuation of NEUPOGEN® therapy, neutrophil counts returned to baseline, in most cases within four days. Isolated neutrophils displayed normal phagocytic (measured by zymosan-stimulated chemoluminescence) and chemotactic [measured by migration under agarose using N-formyl-methionyl-leucyl-phenylalanine (fMLP) as the chemotaxin] activity in vitro.

The absolute monocyte count was reported to increase in a dose-dependent manner in most patients receiving NEUPOGEN®, however, the percentage of monocytes in the differential count remained within the normal range. In all studies to date, absolute counts of both eosinophils and basophils did not change and were within the normal range following administration of NEUPOGEN®. Increases in lymphocyte counts following NEUPOGEN® administration have been reported in some normal subjects and cancer patients.

White blood cell differentials obtained during clinical trials have demonstrated a shift towards earlier granulocyte progenitor cells (left shift), including the appearance of promyelocytes and myeloblasts, usually during neutrophil recovery following the chemotherapy-induced nadir. In addition, Dohle bodies, increased granulocyte granulation, as well as hypersegmented neutrophils have been observed. Such changes were transient, and were not associated with clinical sequelae nor were they necessarily associated with infection.

Pharmacokinetics

Absorption and clearance of NEUPOGEN® follows first-order pharmacokinetic modeling without apparent concentration dependence. A positive linear correlation occurred between the parenteral dose and both the serum concentration and area under the concentration-time curves. Continuous intravenous infusion of 20 mcg/kg of NEUPOGEN® over 24 hours resulted in mean and median serum concentrations of approximately 48 and 56 ng/mL, respectively. Subcutaneous administration of 3.45 mcg/kg and 11.5 mcg/kg resulted in maximum serum concentrations of 4 and 49 ng/mL, respectively, within 2 to 8 hours. The volume of distribution averaged 150 mL/kg in both normal subjects and cancer patients. The elimination half-life, in both normal subjects and cancer patients, was approximately 3.5 hours. Clearance rates of NEUPOGEN® were approximately 0.5-0.7 mL/min/kg. Single parenteral doses or daily intravenous doses, over a 14 day period, resulted in comparable half-lives. The half-lives were similar for intravenous administration (231 minutes, following doses of 34.5 mcg/kg) and for subcutaneous administration (210 minutes, following NEUPOGEN® doses of 3.45 mcg/kg). Continuous 24-hour intravenous infusions of 20 mcg/kg over an 11 to 20 day period produced steady-state serum concentrations of NEUPOGEN® with no evidence of drug accumulation over the time period investigated.

INDICATIONS AND USAGE

Cancer Patients Receiving Myelosuppressive Chemotherapy

NEUPOGEN® is indicated to decrease the incidence of infection, as manifested by febrile neutropenia, in patients with non-myeloid malignancies receiving myelosuppressive anti-cancer drugs associated with a significant incidence of severe neutropenia with fever (see CLINICAL EXPERIENCE). A complete blood count and platelet count should be obtained prior to chemotherapy, and twice per week (see LABORATORY MONITORING) during NEUPOGEN® therapy to avoid leukocytosis and to monitor the neutrophil count. In Phase 3 clinical studies, NEUPOGEN® therapy was discontinued when the absolute neutrophil count (ANC) was ≥ 10,000/mm³ after the expected chemotherapy-induced nadir.

Cancer Patients Receiving Bone Marrow Transplant (BMT)

NEUPOGEN® is indicated to reduce the duration of neutropenia and neutropenia-related clinical sequelae, e.g., febrile neutropenia, in patients with non-myeloid malignancies undergoing myeloablative chemotherapy followed by marrow transplantation (see CLINICAL EXPERIENCE). It is recommended that complete blood counts and platelet counts be obtained at a minimum of three times per week (see LABORATORY MONITORING) following marrow infusion to monitor the recovery of marrow reconstitution.

Patients Undergoing Peripheral Blood Progenitor Cell (PBPC) Collection:

NEUPOGEN® is indicated for the mobilization of hematopoietic progenitor cells into the peripheral blood for collection by leukapheresis. Mobilization allows for the collection of increased numbers of progenitor cells capable of engraftment compared with collection by leukapheresis without mobilization or bone marrow harvest. After myeloablative chemotherapy, the transplantation of an increased number of progenitor cells can lead to more rapid engraftment, which may result in a decreased need for supportive care (see CLINICAL EXPERIENCE).

Patients with Severe Chronic Neutropenia (SCN)

NEUPOGEN® is indicated for chronic administration to reduce the incidence and duration of sequelae of neutropenia (e.g. fever, infections, oropharyngeal ulcers) in symptomatic patients with congenital neutropenia, cyclic neutropenia, or idiopathic neutropenia (see CLINICAL EXPERIENCE). It is essential that serial complete blood cell counts with differential and platelet counts, and an evaluation of bone marrow morphology and karyotype be performed prior to initiation of NEUPOGEN® therapy. The use of NEUPOGEN® prior to confirmation of SCN may impair diagnostic efforts and may thus impair or delay evaluation and treatment of an underlying condition, other than SCN, causing the neutropenia.

Clinical Experience: Response to NEUPOGEN®

Cancer Patients Receiving Myelosuppressive Chemotherapy

NEUPOGEN® has been shown to be safe and effective in accelerating the recovery of neutrophil counts following a variety of chemotherapy regimens. In a Phase 3 clinical trial in small cell lung cancer, patients received subcutaneous administration of NEUPOGEN® (4 to 8 mcg/kg/day, days 4–17) or placebo. In this study, the benefits of NEUPOGEN® therapy were shown to be prevention of infection as manifested by febrile neutropenia, decreased hospitalization, and decreased intravenous antibiotic usage. No difference in survival or disease progression was demonstrated.

In the Phase 3, randomized, double-blind, placebo-controlled trial conducted in patients with small cell lung cancer, patients were randomized to receive NEUPOGEN® (n = 99) or placebo (n = 111) starting on day 4, after receiving standard dose chemotherapy with cyclophosphamide, doxorubicin, and etoposide. A total of 210 patients were evaluated for efficacy and 207 evaluated for safety. Treatment with NEUPOGEN® resulted in a clinically and statistically significant reduction in the incidence of infection, as manifested by febrile neutropenia; the incidence of at least one infection over all cycles of chemotherapy was 76% (84/111) for placebo-treated patients, versus 40% (40/99) for NEUPOGEN®-treated patients (p < 0.001). The following secondary analyses were also performed. The requirements for in-patient hospitalization and antibiotic use were also significantly decreased during the first cycle of chemotherapy; incidence of hospitalization was 69% (77/111) for placebo-treated patients in cycle one, versus 52% (51/99) for NEUPOGEN®-treated patients (p = 0.032). The incidence of intravenous antibiotic usage was 60% (67/111) for placebo-treated patients in cycle one, versus 38% (38/99) for NEUPOGEN®-treated patients (p = 0.003). The incidence, severity, and duration of severe neutropenia (ANC < 500/mm³) following chemotherapy were all significantly reduced. The incidence of severe neutropenia in cycle one was 84% (83/99) for patients receiving NEUPOGEN® versus 96% (106/110) for patients receiving placebo (p = 0.004). Over all cycles, patients randomized to NEUPOGEN® had a 57% (286/500 cycles) rate of severe neutropenia versus 77% (416/543 cycles) for patients randomized to placebo. The median duration of severe neutropenia in cycle one was reduced from 6 days (range 0 to 10 days) for patients receiving placebo to 2 days (range 0 to 9 days) for patients receiving NEUPOGEN® (p < 0.001). The mean duration of neutropenia in cycle one was 5.64 ±2.27 days for patients receiving placebo versus 2.44 ±1.90 days for patients receiving NEUPOGEN®. Over all cycles, the median duration of neutropenia was 3 days for patients randomized to placebo versus 1 day for patients randomized to NEUPOGEN®. The median severity of neutropenia (as measured by ANC nadir) was 72/mm³ (range 0/mm³ –7912/mm³) in cycle one for patients receiving NEUPOGEN® versus 38/mm³ (range 0/mm³– 9520/mm³) for patients receiving placebo (p = 0.012). The mean severity of neutropenia in cycle one was 496/mm³ ±1382/mm³ for patients receiving NEUPOGEN® versus 204/mm³ ±953/mm³ for patients receiving placebo. Over all cycles, the ANC nadir for patients randomized to NEUPOGEN® was 403/mm³, versus 161/mm³ for patients randomized to placebo.

Administration of NEUPOGEN® resulted in an earlier ANC nadir following chemotherapy than was experienced by patients receiving placebo (day 10 versus day 12). NEUPOGEN® was well tolerated when given subcutaneously daily at doses of 4 to 8 mcg/kg for up to 14 consecutive days following each cycle of chemotherapy (see ADVERSE REACTIONS).

Several other Phase 1/2 studies, which did not directly measure the incidence of infection, but which did measure increases in neutrophils, support the efficacy of NEUPOGEN®. The regimens are presented to provide some background on the clinical experience with NEUPOGEN®. No claim regarding the safety or efficacy of the chemotherapy regimens is made. The effects of NEUPOGEN® on tumor growth or on the anti-tumor activity of the chemotherapy were not assessed. The doses of NEUPOGEN® used in these studies are considerably greater than those found to be effective in the Phase 3 study described above. Such Phase 1/2 studies are summarized in the following table.

[See table at top right of next page.]

Cancer Patients Receiving Bone Marrow Transplant

In two separate randomized, controlled trials, patients with Hodgkin's and non-Hodgkin's lymphoma were treated with myeloablative chemotherapy and autologous bone marrow transplantation (ABMT). In one study (n = 54), NEUPOGEN® was administered at doses of 10 or 30 mcg/kg/day; a third treatment group in this study received no NEUPOGEN®. A statistically significant reduction in the median number of days of severe neutropenia (ANC < 500/mm³) occurred in the NEUPOGEN®-treated group versus the control group [23 days in the control group, 11 days in the 10 mcg/kg/day group, and 14 days in the 30 mcg/kg/day group, (11 days in the combined treatment groups, p = 0.004)]. In the second study (n = 44, 43 patients evaluable), NEUPOGEN® was administered at doses of 10 or 20 mcg/kg/day; a third treatment group in this study received no NEUPOGEN®. A statistically significant reduction in the median number of days of severe neutropenia occurred in the NEUPOGEN®-treated group versus the control group (21.5 days in the control group and 10 days in both treatment groups, p < 0.001). The number of days of febrile neutropenia was also reduced significantly in this study [13.5 days in the control group, 5 days in the 10 mcg/kg/day group, and 5.5 days in the 20 mcg/kg/day group, (5 days in the combined treatment groups, p < 0.0001)]. Reductions in the number of days of hospitalization and antibiotic use were also seen, although these reductions were not statistically significant. There were no effects on red blood cell or platelet levels.

In a randomized, placebo-controlled trial, 70 patients with myeloid and non-myeloid malignancies were treated with myeloablative therapy and allogeneic bone marrow transplant followed by 300 mcg/m²/day of a Filgrastim product. A statistically significant reduction in the median number of days of severe neutropenia occurred in the treated group versus the control group (19 days in the control group and 15 days in the treatment group, p < 0.001) and time to recovery of ANC to ≥ 500/mm³ (21 days in the control group and 16 days in the treatment group, p < 0.001).

In three non-randomized studies (n = 119), patients received ABMT and treatment with NEUPOGEN®. One study (n = 45) involved patients with breast cancer and malignant melanoma. A second study (n = 39) involved patients with Hodgkin's disease. The third study (n = 35) involved patients with non-Hodgkin's lymphoma, acute lymphoblastic leukemia (ALL), and germ cell tumor. In these studies, the recovery of the ANC to ≥ 500/mm³ ranged from a median of 11.5 to 13 days.

None of the conditioning regimens used in the ABMT studies included radiation therapy.

While these studies were not designed to compare survival, this information was collected and evaluated. The overall survival and disease progression of patients receiving NEUPOGEN® in these studies were similar to those observed in the respective control groups and to historical data.

PBPC Collection and Therapy in Cancer Patients

All patients in the Amgen-sponsored trials received a similar mobilization/collection regimen: NEUPOGEN® was administered for 6–7 days, with an apheresis procedure on days 5, 6 and 7 (except for a limited number of patients receiving apheresis on days 4, 6 and 8). In a non-Amgen-sponsored study, patients underwent mobilization to a target number of mononuclear cells (MNC), with apheresis starting on day 5. There are no data on the mobilization of PBPCs after days 4–5 that are not confounded by leukapheresis.

Mobilization: Mobilization of PBPC was studied in 50 heavily pre-treated patients (median number of prior chemotherapy cycles = 9.5) with non-Hodgkin's lymphoma (NHL), Hodgkin's disease (HD) or acute lymphoblastic leukemia (ALL) [Amgen study 1]. CFU-GM was used as the marker for engraftable PBPC. The median CFU-GM level on each day of mobilization was determined from the data available, (CFU-GM assays were not obtained on all patients on each day of mobilization). These data are presented below.

The data from Amgen study 1 were supported by data from Amgen study 2 in which 22 pre-treated breast cancer patients (median number of prior cycles = 3) were studied. Both the CFU-GM and CD34+ cells reached a maximum on day 5 at > 10-fold over baseline and then remained elevated with leukapheresis.

[See second table on right of next page.]

In three studies of patients with prior exposure to chemotherapy, the median CFU-GM yield in the leukapheresis product ranged from 20.9 to 32.7×10⁴/kg body weight (n=105). In two of these studies where CD34+ yields in the leukapheresis product were also determined, the median CD34+ yields were 3.11 and 2.80 ×10⁶/kg respectively (n=56). In an additional study of 18 chemotherapy-naïve patients, the median CFU-GM yield was 123.4 ×10⁴/kg.

Engraftment: Engraftment following NEUPOGEN®-mobilized PBPC is summarized for 101 patients in the table below. In all studies a Cox regression model showed that the

total number of CFU-GM and/or CD34+ cells collected was a significant predictor of time to platelet recovery.

In a randomized unblinded study of patients with HD or NHL undergoing myeloablative chemotherapy (Amgen study 3), 27 patients received NEUPOGEN®-mobilized PBPC followed by NEUPOGEN® and 31 patients received ABMT followed by NEUPOGEN®. Patients randomized to the NEUPOGEN®-mobilized PBPC group compared to the ABMT group had significantly fewer days of platelet transfusions (median 6 vs. 10 days), a significantly shorter time to a sustained platelet count > 20,000/mm³ (median 16 vs. 23 days), a significantly shorter time to recovery of a sustained ANC ≥ 500/mm³ (median 11 vs. 14 days), significantly fewer days of red blood cell transfusions (median 2 vs. 3 days) and a significantly shorter duration of post-transplant hospitalization.

	Amgen-Sponsored Study 1 N=13	Amgen-Sponsored Study 2 N=22	Amgen-Sponsored Study 3 N=27	Non-Amgen-Sponsored Study N=39
Median PBPC/kg Collected:				
MNC	9.5×10⁸	9.5×10⁸	8.1×10⁸	10.3×10⁸
CD34⁺	n/a	3.1×10⁶	2.8×10⁶	6.2×10⁶
CFU-GM	63.9×10⁴	25.3×10⁴	32.6×10⁴	n/a
Days to ANC ≥ 500/mm³				
Median	9	10	11	10
Range	*8–10*	*8–15*	*9–38*	*7–40*
Day to ≥ Plt. ≥ 20,000/mm³				
Median	10	12.5	16	15.5
Range	*7–16*	*10–30*	*8–52*	*7–63*

n/a = not available

Three of the 101 patients (3%) did not achieve the criteria for engraftment as defined by a platelet count ≥ 20,000/mm³ by day 28. In clinical trials of NEUPOGEN® for the mobilization of PBPC, NEUPOGEN® was administered to patients at 5–24 mcg/kg/day after reinfusion of the collected cells until a sustainable ANC (≥500/mm³) was reached. The rate of engraftment of these cells in the absence of NEUPOGEN® post-transplantation has not been studied.

Patients with Severe Chronic Neutropenia

Severe chronic neutropenia (idiopathic, cyclic, and congenital) is characterized by a selective decrease in the number of circulating neutrophils and an enhanced susceptibility to bacterial infections.

The daily administration of NEUPOGEN® has been shown to be safe and effective in causing a sustained increase in the neutrophil count and a decrease in infectious morbidity in children and adults with the clinical syndrome of SCN.[15] In the phase 3 trial, summarized in the following table, daily treatment with NEUPOGEN® resulted in significant beneficial changes in the incidence and duration of infection, fever, antibiotic use, and oropharyngeal ulcers. In this trial, 120 patients with a median age of 12 years (range 1 to 76 years) were treated.

Overall Significant Changes in Clinical Endpoints Median Incidence[1] (events) or Duration (days) per 28-day period

	Control Patients[2]	NEUPOGEN®-treated Patients	p-value
Incidence of Infection	0.50	0.20	<0.001
Incidence of Fever	0.25	0.20	<0.001
Duration of Fever	0.63	0.20	0.005
Incidence of Oropharyngeal Ulcers	0.26	0.00	<0.001
Incidence of Antibiotic Use	0.49	0.20	<0.001

[1] Incidence values were calculated for each patient, and are defined as the total number of events experienced divided by the number of 28-day periods of exposure (on-study). Median incidence values were then reported for each patient group.

[2] Control patients were observed for a 4-month period.

The incidence for each of these five clinical parameters was lower in the NEUPOGEN® arm compared to the control arm for cohorts in each of the three major diagnostic categories. All three diagnostic groups showed favorable trends in favor of treatment. An analysis of variance showed no significant interaction between treatment and diagnosis, suggest-

Type of Malignancy	Regimen	Chemotherapy Dose	No. of Pts.	Trial Phase	NEUPOGEN® Daily Dosage[a]
Small Cell Lung Cancer	Cyclophosphamide Doxorubicin Etoposide	1 g/m²/day 50 mg/m²/day 120 mg/m²/day x 3 q 21 days	210	3	4–8 mcg/kg SC days 4–17
Small Cell Lung Cancer[11]	Ifosfamide Doxorubicin Etoposide Mesna	5 g/m²/day 50 mg/m²/day 120 mg/m²/day x 3 8 g/m²/day q 21 days	12	1/2	5.75–46 mcg/kg IV days 4–17
Urothelial Cancer[12]	Methotrexate Vinblastine Doxorubicin Cisplatin	30 mg/m²/day x 2 3 mg/m²/day x 2 30 mg/m²/day 70 mg/m²/day q 28 days	40	1/2	3.45–69 mcg/kg IV days 4–11
Various Non-Myeloid Malignancies[13]	Cyclophosphamide Etoposide Cisplatin	2.5 g/m²/day x 2 500 mg/m²/day x 3 50 mg/m²/day x 3 q 28 days	18	1/2	23–69 mcg/kg[b] IV days 8–28
Breast/Ovarian Cancer[14]	Doxorubicin[c]	75 mg/m² 100 mg/m² 125 mg/m² 150 mg/m² q 14 days	21	2	11.5 mcg/kg IV days 2–9 5.75 mcg/kg IV days 10–12
Neuroblastoma	Cyclophosphamide Doxorubicin Cisplatin	150 mg/m² x 7 35 mg/m² 90 mg/m² q 28 days (cycles 1,3,5)[d]	12	2	5.45–17.25 mcg/kg SC days 6–19

[a] NEUPOGEN® doses were those that accelerated neutrophil production. Doses which provided no additional acceleration beyond that achieved at the next lower dose are not reported.
[b] Lowest dose(s) tested in the study.
[c] Patients received doxorubicin at either 75, 100, 125, or 150 mg/m².
[d] Cycles 2,6 = cyclophosphamide 150 mg/m² x 7 and etoposide 280 mg/m² x 3
Cycle 4 = cisplatin 90 mg/m² x 1 and etoposide 280 mg/m² x 3.

	Study #1 CFU-GM/mL		Study #2 CFU-GM/mL		Study #2 CD34+ (x10⁴/mL)	
	# Samples	Median (25%, 75%)	# Samples	Median (25%, 75%)	# Samples	Median (25%, 75%)
Day 1	11	18 (13–62)	20	42 (15–151)	20	0.13 (0.02–0.66)
Day 2	7	22 (3–61)	n/a	n/a	n/a	n/a
Day 3	10	138 (39–364)	n/a	n/a	n/a	n/a
Day 4	18	365 (158–864)	18	576 (108–1819)	17	2.11 (0.58–3.93)
Day 5	36	781 (391–1608)	21	960 (72–1677)	22	3.16 (1.08–6.11)
Day 6	46	505 (199–1397)	22	756 (70–3486)	22	2.67 (1.09–4.40)
Day 7	37	333 (111–938)	22	597 (118–2009)	21	2.64 (0.78–4.22)
Day 8	15	383 (94–815)	12	51 (10–746)	12	1.61 (0.38–4.31)

Peripheral Blood Progenitor Cell Levels by Mobilization Day

n/a = not available

ing that efficacy did not differ substantially in the different diseases. Although NEUPOGEN® substantially reduced neutropenia in all patient groups, in patients with cyclic neutropenia, cycling persisted but the period of neutropenia was shortened to one day.

As a result of the lower incidence and duration of infections, there was also a lower number of episodes of hospitalization [28 hospitalizations in 62 patients in the treated group versus 44 hospitalizations in 60 patients in the control group over a 4 month period (p = 0.0034)]. Patients treated with NEUPOGEN® also reported a lower number of episodes of diarrhea, nausea, fatigue, and sore throat.

In the Phase 3 trial, untreated patients had a median ANC of 210/mm³ (range 0–1550/mm³). NEUPOGEN® therapy was adjusted to maintain the median ANC between 1,500 and 10,000/mm³. Overall, the response to NEUPOGEN® was observed in 1 to 2 weeks. The median ANC after five months of NEUPOGEN® therapy for all patients was 7,460/mm³

(range 30 to 30,880/mm³). NEUPOGEN® dosing requirements were generally higher for patients with congenital neutropenia (2.3–40 mcg/kg/day) than for patients with idiopathic (0.6–11.5 mcg/kg/day) or cyclic (0.5–6 mcg/kg/day) neutropenia.

CONTRAINDICATIONS

NEUPOGEN® is contraindicated in patients with known hypersensitivity to E. coli-derived proteins, Filgrastim, or any component of the product.

WARNINGS

Allergic-type reactions occurring on initial or subsequent treatment have been reported in < 1 in 4,000 patients treated with NEUPOGEN®. These have generally been characterized by systemic symptoms involving at least two body systems, most often skin (rash, urticaria, facial edema), respiratory (wheezing, dyspnea), and cardiovascular (hypo-

Continued on next page

Consult 1997 supplements and future editions for revisions

Amgen—Cont.

tension, tachycardia). Some reactions occurred on initial exposure. Reactions tended to occur within the first 30 minutes after administration and appeared to occur more frequently in patients receiving NEUPOGEN® intravenously. Rapid resolution of symptoms occurred in most cases after administration of antihistamines, steroids, bronchodilators, and/or epinephrine. Symptoms recurred in more than half the patients who were rechallenged.

Patients with Severe Chronic Neutropenia
The safety and efficacy of NEUPOGEN® in the treatment of neutropenia due to other hematopoietic disorders (e.g., myelodysplastic disorders or myeloid leukemia) have not been established. Care should be taken to confirm the diagnosis of SCN before initiating NEUPOGEN® therapy.

While 9 of 325 patients developed myelodysplasia or myeloid leukemia while receiving NEUPOGEN® during clinical trials, acute myeloid leukemia (AML) or abnormal cytogenetics have been reported to occur in the natural history of severe chronic neutropenia without cytokine therapy.[16] Abnormal cytogenetics have been associated with the eventual development of myeloid leukemia. The effect of NEUPOGEN® on the development of abnormal cytogenetics and the effect of continued NEUPOGEN® administration in patients with abnormal cytogenetics are unknown. If a patient with SCN develops abnormal cytogenetics, the risks and benefits of continuing NEUPOGEN® should be carefully considered (see ADVERSE REACTIONS).

PRECAUTIONS
General
Simultaneous Use with Chemotherapy and Radiation Therapy
The safety and efficacy of NEUPOGEN® given simultaneously with cytotoxic chemotherapy have not been established. Because of the potential sensitivity of rapidly dividing myeloid cells to cytotoxic chemotherapy, do not use NEUPOGEN® in the period 24 hours before through 24 hours after the administration of cytotoxic chemotherapy (see DOSAGE AND ADMINISTRATION).

The efficacy of NEUPOGEN® has not been evaluated in patients receiving chemotherapy associated with delayed myelosuppression (e.g., nitrosoureas) or with mitomycin C or with myelosuppressive doses of anti-metabolites such as 5-fluorouracil or cytosine arabinoside.

The safety and efficacy of NEUPOGEN® have not been evaluated in patients receiving concurrent radiation therapy. Simultaneous use of NEUPOGEN® with chemotherapy and radiation therapy should be avoided.

Growth Factor Potential
NEUPOGEN® is a growth factor that primarily stimulates neutrophils. However, the possibility that NEUPOGEN® can act as a growth factor for any tumor type, particularly myeloid malignancies, cannot be excluded. Therefore, because of the possibility of tumor growth, precaution should be exercised in using this drug in any malignancy with myeloid characteristics.

When NEUPOGEN® is used to mobilize PBPC, tumor cells may be released from the marrow and subsequently collected in the leukapheresis product. The effect of reinfusion of tumor cells has not been well-studied, and the limited data available are inconclusive.

Leukocytosis
Cancer Patients Receiving Myelosuppressive Chemotherapy
White blood cell counts of 100,000/mm³ or greater were observed in approximately 2% of patients receiving NEUPOGEN® at doses above 5 mcg/kg/day. There were no reports of adverse events associated with this degree of leukocytosis. In order to avoid the potential complications of excessive leukocytosis, a complete blood count (CBC) is recommended twice per week during NEUPOGEN® therapy (see LABORATORY MONITORING).

Premature Discontinuation of NEUPOGEN® Therapy
Cancer Patients Receiving Myelosuppressive Chemotherapy
A transient increase in neutrophil counts is typically seen 1 to 2 days after initiation of NEUPOGEN® therapy. However, for a sustained therapeutic response, NEUPOGEN® therapy should be continued following chemotherapy until the post nadir ANC reaches 10,000/mm³. Therefore, the premature discontinuation of NEUPOGEN® therapy, prior to the time of recovery from the expected neutrophil nadir, is generally not recommended (see DOSAGE AND ADMINISTRATION).

Other
In studies of NEUPOGEN® administration following chemotherapy, most reported side effects were consistent with those usually seen as a result of cytotoxic chemotherapy (see ADVERSE REACTIONS). Because of the potential of receiving higher doses of chemotherapy (i.e., full doses on the prescribed schedule), the patient may be at greater risk of thrombocytopenia, anemia, and non-hematologic consequences of increased chemotherapy doses (please refer to the prescribing information of the specific chemotherapy agents used). Regular monitoring of the hematocrit and platelet

count is recommended. Furthermore, care should be exercised in the administration of NEUPOGEN® in conjunction with other drugs known to lower the platelet count. In septic patients receiving NEUPOGEN®, the physician should be alert to the theoretical possibility of adult respiratory distress syndrome, due to the possible influx of neutrophils at the site of inflammation.

There have been rare reports (< 1 in 7,000 patients) of cutaneous vasculitis in patients treated with NEUPOGEN®. In most cases, the severity of cutaneous vasculitis was moderate or severe. Most of the reports involved patients with severe chronic neutropenia receiving long-term NEUPOGEN® therapy. Symptoms of vasculitis generally developed simultaneously with an increase in the ANC and abated when the ANC decreased. Many patients were able to continue NEUPOGEN® at a reduced dose.

Information for Patients
In those situations in which the physician determines that the patient can safely and effectively self-administer NEUPOGEN®, the patient should be instructed as to the proper dosage and administration. Patients should be referred to the "Information for Patients" labeling included with the Package Insert in each dispensing carton of NEUPOGEN®. This patient information, however, is not intended to be a disclosure of all known or possible effects. If home use is prescribed, patients should be thoroughly instructed in the importance of proper disposal and cautioned against the reuse of needles, syringes, or drug product. A puncture-resistant container for the disposal of used syringes and needles should be available to the patient. The full container should be disposed of according to the directions provided by the physician.

Laboratory Monitoring
Cancer Patients Receiving Myelosuppressive Chemotherapy
A CBC and platelet count should be obtained prior to chemotherapy, and at regular intervals (twice per week) during NEUPOGEN® therapy. Following cytotoxic chemotherapy, the neutrophil nadir occurred earlier during cycles when NEUPOGEN® was administered, and white blood cell differentials demonstrated a left shift, including the appearance of promyelocytes and myeloblasts. In addition, the duration of severe neutropenia was reduced, and was followed by an accelerated recovery in the neutrophil counts. Therefore, regular monitoring of white blood cell counts, particularly at the time of the recovery from the post chemotherapy nadir, is recommended in order to avoid excessive leukocytosis.

Cancer Patients Receiving Bone Marrow Transplant
Frequent complete blood counts and platelet counts are recommended (at least three times per week) following marrow transplantation.

Patients with Severe Chronic Neutropenia
During the initial four weeks of NEUPOGEN® therapy and during the two weeks following any dose adjustment, a CBC with differential and platelet count should be performed twice weekly. Once a patient is clinically stable, a CBC with differential and platelet count should be performed monthly. In clinical trials, the following laboratory results were observed.
—Cyclic fluctuations in the neutrophil counts were frequently observed in patients with congenital or idiopathic neutropenia after initiation of NEUPOGEN® therapy.
—Platelet counts were generally at the upper limits of normal prior to NEUPOGEN® therapy. With NEUPOGEN® therapy, platelet counts decreased but usually remained within normal limits (see ADVERSE REACTIONS).
—Early myeloid forms were noted in peripheral blood in most patients, including the appearance of metamyelocytes and myelocytes. Promyelocytes and myeloblasts were noted in some patients.
—Relative increases were occasionally noted in the number of circulating eosinophils and basophils. No consistent increases were observed with NEUPOGEN® therapy.
—As in other trials, increases were observed in serum uric acid, lactic dehydrogenase, and serum alkaline phosphatase.

Drug Interaction
Drug interactions between NEUPOGEN® and other drugs have not been fully evaluated. Drugs which may potentiate the release of neutrophils, such as lithium, should be used with caution.

Carcinogenesis, Mutagenesis, Impairment of Fertility
The carcinogenic potential of NEUPOGEN® has not been studied. NEUPOGEN® failed to induce bacterial gene mutations in either the presence or absence of a drug metabolizing enzyme system. NEUPOGEN® had no observed effect on the fertility of male or female rats, or on gestation at doses up to 500 mcg/kg.

Pregnancy Category C
NEUPOGEN® has been shown to have adverse effects in pregnant rabbits when given in doses 2 to 10 times the human dose. There are no adequate and well-controlled studies in pregnant women. NEUPOGEN® should be used during pregnancy only if the potential benefit justifies the potential risk to the fetus.

In rabbits, increased abortion and embryolethality were observed in animals treated with NEUPOGEN® at 80 mcg/kg/day. NEUPOGEN® administered to pregnant rabbits at doses of 80 mcg/kg/day during the period of organogenesis was associated with increased fetal resorption, genitourinary bleeding, developmental abnormalities, and decreased body weight, live births, and food consumption. External abnormalities were not observed in the fetuses of dams treated at 80 mcg/kg/day. Reproductive studies in pregnant rats have shown that NEUPOGEN® was not associated with lethal, teratogenic, or behavioral effects on fetuses when administered by daily intravenous injection during the period of organogenesis at dose levels up to 575 mcg/kg/day.

In Segment III studies in rats, offspring of dams treated at > 20 mcg/kg/day exhibited a delay in external differentiation (detachment of auricles and descent of testes) and slight growth retardation, possibly due to lower body weight of females during rearing and nursing. Offspring of dams treated at 100 mcg/kg/day exhibited decreased body weights at birth, and a slightly reduced four day survival rate.

Nursing Mothers
It is not known whether NEUPOGEN® is excreted in human milk. Because many drugs are excreted in human milk, caution should be exercised if NEUPOGEN® is administered to a nursing woman.

Pediatric Use
Serious long-term risks associated with daily administration of NEUPOGEN® have not been identified in pediatric patients (ages 4 months to 17 years) with SCN. Limited data from patients who were followed in the Phase 3 study for 1.5 years did not suggest alterations in growth and development, sexual maturation, or endocrine function.

The safety and efficacy in neonates and patients with autoimmune neutropenia of infancy have not been established. In the cancer setting, 12 pediatric patients with neuroblastoma have received up to six cycles of cyclophosphamide, cisplatin, doxorubicin, and etoposide chemotherapy concurrently with NEUPOGEN®; in this population, NEUPOGEN® was well tolerated. There was one report of palpable splenomegaly associated with NEUPOGEN® therapy, however, the only consistently reported adverse event was musculoskeletal pain, which is no different from the experience in the adult population.

ADVERSE REACTIONS
Cancer Patients Receiving Myelosuppressive Chemotherapy
In clinical trials involving over 350 patients receiving NEUPOGEN® following non-myeloablative cytotoxic chemotherapy, most adverse experiences were the sequelae of the underlying malignancy or cytotoxic chemotherapy. In all Phase 2 and 3 trials, medullary bone pain, reported in 24% of patients, was the only consistently observed adverse reaction attributed to NEUPOGEN® therapy. This bone pain was generally reported to be of mild-to-moderate severity, and could be controlled in most patients with non-narcotic analgesics; infrequently, bone pain was severe enough to require narcotic analgesics. Bone pain was reported more frequently in patients treated with higher doses (20–100 mcg/kg/day) administered intravenously, and less frequently in patients treated with lower subcutaneous doses of NEUPOGEN® (3–10 mcg/kg/day).

In the randomized, double-blind, placebo-controlled trial of NEUPOGEN® therapy following combination chemotherapy in patients (n = 207) with small cell lung cancer, the following adverse events were reported during blinded cycles of study medication (placebo or NEUPOGEN® at 4 to 8 mcg/kg/day). Events are reported as exposure adjusted since patients remained on double-blind NEUPOGEN® a median of three cycles versus one cycle for placebo.

Event	% of Blinded Cycles with Events NEUPOGEN® N = 384 patient cycles	Placebo N = 257 patient cycles
Nausea/Vomiting	57	64
Skeletal Pain	22	11
Alopecia	18	27
Diarrhea	14	23
Neutropenic Fever	13	35
Mucositis	12	20
Fever	12	11
Fatigue	11	16
Anorexia	9	11
Dyspnea	9	11
Headache	7	9
Cough	6	8
Skin Rash	6	9
Chest Pain	5	6
Generalized Weakness	4	7
Sore Throat	4	9
Stomatitis	5	10
Constipation	5	10
Pain (Unspecified)	2	7

In this study, there were no serious, life-threatening, or fatal adverse reactions attributed to NEUPOGEN® therapy. Specifically, there were no reports of flu-like symptoms, pleuritis, pericarditis, or other major systemic reactions to NEUPOGEN®.

Spontaneously reversible elevations in uric acid, lactate dehydrogenase, and alkaline phosphatase occurred in 27% to 58% of 98 patients receiving blinded NEUPOGEN® therapy following cytotoxic chemotherapy; increases were generally mild-to-moderate. Transient decreases in blood pressure (< 90/60 mmHg), which did not require clinical treatment, were reported in 7 of 176 patients in Phase 3 clinical studies following administration of NEUPOGEN®. Cardiac events (myocardial infarctions, arrhythmias) have been reported in 11 of 375 cancer patients receiving NEUPOGEN® in clinical studies; the relationship to NEUPOGEN® therapy is unknown. No evidence of interaction of NEUPOGEN® with other drugs was observed in the course of clinical trials (see PRECAUTIONS— SIMULTANEOUS USE WITH CHEMOTHERAPY AND RADIATION THERAPY).

There has been no evidence for the development of antibodies or of a blunted or diminished response to NEUPOGEN® in treated patients, including those receiving NEUPOGEN® daily for almost two years.

Cancer Patients Receiving Bone Marrow Transplant

In clinical trials, the reported adverse effects were those typically seen in patients receiving intensive chemotherapy followed by bone marrow transplantation. The most common events reported in both control and treatment groups included stomatitis and nausea and vomiting, generally of mild-to-moderate severity and were considered unrelated to NEUPOGEN®. In the randomized studies of BMT involving 167 patients who received study drug, the following events occurred more frequently in patients treated with Filgrastim than in controls: nausea (10% vs. 4%), vomiting (7% vs. 3%), hypertension (4% vs. 0%), rash (12% vs. 10%), and peritonitis (2% vs. 0%). None of these events were reported by the Investigator to be related to NEUPOGEN®. One event of erythema nodosum was reported moderate in severity and possibly related to NEUPOGEN®.

Generally, adverse events observed in non-randomized studies were similar to those seen in randomized studies, occurred in a minority of patients and were of mild-to-moderate severity. In one study (n = 45), three serious adverse events reported by the Investigator were considered possibly related to NEUPOGEN®. These included two events of renal insufficiency and one event of capillary leak syndrome. The relationship of these events to NEUPOGEN® remains unclear since they occurred in patients with culture-proven infection with clinical sepsis who were receiving potentially nephrotoxic antibacterial and antifungal therapy.

Cancer Patients Undergoing NEUPOGEN®-mobilized PBPC Collection.

In clinical trials, 126 patients received NEUPOGEN® for PBPC mobilization. In this setting, NEUPOGEN® was generally well tolerated. Adverse events related to NEUPOGEN® consisted primarily of mild-to-moderate musculoskeletal symptoms, reported in 44% of patients. These symptoms were predominantly events of medullary bone pain (33%). Headache was reported related to NEUPOGEN® in 7% of patients. Transient increases in alkaline phosphatase related to NEUPOGEN® were reported in 21% of the patients who had serum chemistries measured; most were mild-to-moderate.

All patients had increases in neutrophil counts during mobilization, consistent with the biological effects of NEUPOGEN®. Two patients had a white blood cell count > 100,000/mm^3. No sequelae were associated with any grade of leukocytosis.

Sixty-five percent of patients had mild-to-moderate anemia and 97% of patients had decreases in platelet counts; five patients (out of 126) had decreased platelet counts to < 50,000/mm^3. Anemia and thrombocytopenia have been reported to be related to leukapheresis; however, the possibility that NEUPOGEN® mobilization may contribute to anemia or thrombocytopenia has not been ruled out.

Patients with Severe Chronic Neutropenia

Mild to moderate bone pain was reported in approximately 33% of patients in clinical trials. This symptom was readily controlled with non-narcotic analgesics. Generalized musculoskeletal pain was also noted in higher frequency in patients treated with NEUPOGEN®. Palpable splenomegaly was observed in approximately 30% of patients. Abdominal or flank pain was seen infrequently and thrombocytopenia (< 50,000/mm^3) was noted in 12% of patients with palpable spleens. Fewer than 3% of all patients underwent splenectomy, and most of these had a pre-study history of splenomegaly. Fewer than 6% of patients had thrombocytopenia (< 50,000/mm^3) during NEUPOGEN® therapy, most of whom had a pre-existing history of thrombocytopenia. In most cases, thrombocytopenia was managed by NEUPOGEN® dose reduction or interruption. An additional 5% of patients had platelet counts between 50,000 to 100,000/mm^3. There were no associated serious hemorrhagic sequelae in these patients. Epistaxis was noted in 15% of patients treated with NEUPOGEN®, but was associated with thrombocytopenia in 2% of patients. Anemia was reported in approximately 10% of patients, but in most cases appeared to be related to frequent diagnostic phlebotomy, chronic illness or concomitant medications. In clinical trials, myelodysplasia or myeloid leukemia was reported to have developed during NEUPOGEN® therapy in approximately 3% of patients (9 of 325) (see WARNINGS: PATIENTS WITH SEVERE CHRONIC NEUTROPENIA). Twelve patients from a subset of 102 who had normal cytogenetic evaluations at baseline were subsequently found to have abnormalities, including monosomy 7, on routine repeat evaluation conducted after 18 to 52 months of NEUPOGEN® therapy. It is unknown whether the development of these findings is related to chronic daily NEUPOGEN® administration or reflects the natural history of SCN. Other adverse events infrequently observed and possibly related to NEUPOGEN® therapy were: injection site reaction, rash, hepatomegaly, arthralgia, osteoporosis, cutaneous vasculitis, hematuria/proteinuria, alopecia, and exacerbation of some pre-existing skin disorders (e.g., psoriasis).

OVERDOSAGE

In cancer patients receiving NEUPOGEN® as an adjunct to myelosuppressive chemotherapy, it is recommended, to avoid the potential risks of excessive leukocytosis, that NEUPOGEN® therapy be discontinued if the ANC surpasses 10,000/mm^3 after the chemotherapy-induced ANC nadir has occurred. Doses of NEUPOGEN® that increase the ANC beyond 10,000/mm^3 may not result in any additional clinical benefit.

The maximum tolerated dose of NEUPOGEN® has not been determined. Efficacy was demonstrated at doses of 4–8 mcg/kg/day in the Phase 3 study of non-myeloablative chemotherapy. Patients in the BMT studies received up to 138 mcg/kg/day without toxic effects, although there was a flattening of the dose response curve above daily doses of greater than 10 mcg/kg/day.

In NEUPOGEN® clinical trials of cancer patients receiving myelosuppressive chemotherapy, white blood cell counts > 100,000/mm^3 have been reported in less than 5% of patients, but were not associated with any reported adverse clinical effects.

In cancer patients receiving myelosuppressive chemotherapy, discontinuation of NEUPOGEN® therapy usually results in a 50% decrease in circulating neutrophils within 1 to 2 days, with a return to pretreatment levels in 1 to 7 days.

DOSAGE AND ADMINISTRATION

Cancer Patients Receiving Myelosuppressive Chemotherapy

The recommended starting dose of NEUPOGEN® is 5 mcg/kg/day, administered as a single daily injection by subcutaneous bolus injection, by short intravenous infusion (15–30 minutes), or by continuous subcutaneous or continuous intravenous infusion. A CBC and platelet count should be obtained before instituting NEUPOGEN® therapy, and monitored twice weekly during therapy. Doses may be increased in increments of 5 mcg/kg for each chemotherapy cycle, according to the duration and severity of the ANC nadir.

NEUPOGEN® should be administered no earlier than 24 hours after the administration of cytotoxic chemotherapy. NEUPOGEN® should not be administered in the period 24-hours before the administration of chemotherapy (see PRECAUTIONS). NEUPOGEN® should be administered daily for up to two weeks, until the ANC has reached 10,000/mm^3 following the expected chemotherapy-induced neutrophil nadir. The duration of NEUPOGEN® therapy needed to attenuate chemotherapy-induced neutropenia may be dependent on the myelosuppressive potential of the chemotherapy regimen employed. NEUPOGEN® therapy should be discontinued if the ANC surpasses 10,000/mm^3 after the expected chemotherapy-induced neutrophil nadir (see PRECAUTIONS). In Phase 3 trials, efficacy was observed at doses of 4 to 8 mcg/kg/day.

Cancer Patients Receiving Bone Marrow Transplant

The recommended dose of NEUPOGEN® following BMT is 10 mcg/kg/day given as an IV infusion of 4 or 24 hours, or as a continuous 24-hour subcutaneous infusion. For patients receiving bone marrow transplant, the first dose of NEUPOGEN® should be administered at least 24 hours after cytotoxic chemotherapy and at least 24 hours after bone marrow infusion.

During the period of neutrophil recovery, the daily dose of NEUPOGEN® should be titrated against the neutrophil response as follows:

Absolute Neutrophil Count	NEUPOGEN® dose adjustment
When ANC > 1,000/mm^3 for 3 consecutive days then:	Reduce to 5 mcg/kg/day (*see below)
If ANC remains > 1,000/mm^3 for 3 more consecutive days then:	Discontinue NEUPOGEN®
If ANC decreases to < 1,000/mm^3	Resume at 5 mcg/kg/day

* If ANC decreases to < 1,000/mm^3 at any time during the 5 mcg/kg/day administration, NEUPOGEN® should be increased to 10 mcg/kg/day, and the above steps should then be followed.

PBPC Collection and Therapy in Cancer Patients

The recommended dose of NEUPOGEN® for the mobilization of PBPC is 10 mcg/kg/day subcutaneously, either as a bolus or a continuous infusion. It is recommended that NEUPOGEN® be given for at least 4 days before the first leukapheresis procedure and continued until the last leukapheresis. Although the optimal duration of NEUPOGEN® administration and leukapheresis schedule have not been established, administration of NEUPOGEN® for 6–7 days with leukaphereses on days 5, 6 and 7 was found to be safe and effective (see CLINICAL EXPERIENCE: RESPONSE TO NEUPOGEN®, PBPC COLLECTION AND THERAPY IN CANCER PATIENTS for schedules used in clinical trials). Neutrophil counts should be monitored after 4 days of NEUPOGEN®, and NEUPOGEN® dose-modification should be considered for those patients who develop a white blood cell count > 100,000/mm^3.

In all clinical trials of NEUPOGEN® for the mobilization of PBPC, NEUPOGEN® was also administered after reinfusion of the collected cells (see CLINICAL EXPERIENCE).

Patients with Severe Chronic Neutropenia

NEUPOGEN® should be administered to those patients in whom a diagnosis of congenital, cyclic, or idiopathic neutropenia has been definitively confirmed. Other diseases associated with neutropenia should be ruled out.

Starting Dose:

Congenital Neutropenia: The recommended daily starting dose is 6 mcg/kg BID subcutaneously every day.

Idiopathic or Cyclic Neutropenia: The recommended daily starting dose is 5 mcg/kg as a single injection subcutaneously every day.

Dose Adjustments:

Chronic daily administration is required to maintain clinical benefit. ANC should not be used as the sole indication of efficacy. The dose should be individually adjusted based on the patients' clinical course as well as ANC. In the Phase 3 study, the target ANC was 1,500/mm^3 — 10,000/mm^3. However, patients may experience clinical benefit with ANCs below this target range. The dose should be reduced if the ANC is persistently greater than 10,000/mm^3.

Dilution

If required, NEUPOGEN® may be diluted in 5% dextrose. NEUPOGEN® diluted to concentrations between 5 and 15 mcg/mL should be protected from adsorption to plastic materials by addition of Albumin (Human) to a final concentration of 2 mg/mL. When diluted in 5% dextrose or 5% dextrose plus Albumin (Human), NEUPOGEN® is compatible with glass bottles, PVC and polyolefin IV bags, and polypropylene syringes.

Dilution of NEUPOGEN® to a final concentration of less than 5 mcg/mL is not recommended at any time. **Do not dilute with saline at any time; product may precipitate.**

Storage

NEUPOGEN® should be stored in the refrigerator at 2–8 degrees Centigrade (36–46 degrees Fahrenheit). Do not freeze. Avoid shaking. Prior to injection, NEUPOGEN® may be allowed to reach room temperature for a maximum of 24 hours. Any vial left at room temperature for greater than 24 hours should be discarded. Parenteral drug products should be inspected visually for particulate matter and discoloration prior to administration, whenever solution and container permit; if particulates or discoloration are observed, the container should not be used.

HOW SUPPLIED

NEUPOGEN®: Use only one dose per vial; do not re-enter the vial. Discard unused portions. Do not save unused drug for later administration.

Single-dose, preservative-free vials containing 300 mcg (1 mL) of Filgrastim (300 mcg/mL). Boxes of 10 (NDC 55513-347-10).

Single-dose, preservative-free vials containing 480 mcg (1.6 mL) of Filgrastim (300 mcg/mL). Boxes of 10 (NDC 55513-348-10).

NEUPOGEN® should be stored at 2-8 degrees Centigrade (36-46 degrees Fahrenheit). Do not freeze. Avoid shaking.

REFERENCES

1. Zsebo KM, Cohen AM, Murdock DC, Boone TC, Inque H, Chazin VR, Hines D, and Souza LM. Recombinant human granulocyte colony-stimulating factor: Molecular and biological characterization. *Immunobiol.* 172:175-184 (1986).
2. Welte K, Bonilla MA, Gillio AP, *et al.* Recombinant human G-CSF: Effects on hematopoiesis in normal and cyclophosphamide treated primates. *J. Exp. Med.* 165:941-948 (1987).

Continued on next page

Amgen—Cont.

3. Duhrsen U, Villeval JL, Boyd J, *et al.* Effects of recombinant human granulocyte colony-stimulating factor on hematopoietic progenitor cells in cancer patients. *Blood* 72:2074-2081 (1988).

4. Souza LM, Boone TC, Gabrilove J, *et al.* Recombinant human granulocyte colony-stimulating factor: Effects on normal and leukemic myeloid cells. *Science* 232:61-65 (1986).

5. Weisbart RH, Kacena A, Schuh A, and Golde DW. GM-CSF induces human neutrophil IgA-mediated phagocytosis by an IgA Fc receptor activation mechanism. *Nature* 332:647-648 (1988).

6. Kitagawa S, Yuo A, Souza LM, Saito M, Miura Y, and Takaku F. Recombinant human granulocyte colony-stimulating factor enhances superoxide release in human granulocytes stimulated by chemotactic peptide. *Biochem. Biophys. Res. Commun.* 144:1143 (1987).

7. Glaspy JA, Baldwin GC, Robertson PA, *et al.* Therapy for neutropenia in hairy cell leukemia with recombinant human granulocyte colony-stimulating factor. *Ann. Int. Med.* 109:789-795 (1988).

8. Yuo A, Kitagawa S, Ohsaka A, *et al.* Recombinant human granulocyte colony-stimulating factor as an activator of human granulocytes: Potentiation of responses triggered by receptor-mediated agonists and stimulation of C3bi receptor expression and adherance. *Blood* 74:2144-2149 (1989).

9. Gabrilove JL, Jakubowski A, Fain K, *et al.* Phase I study of granulocyte colony-stimulating factor in patients with transitional cell carcinoma of the urothelium. *J. Clin. Invest.* 82:1454-1461 (1988).

10. Morstyn G, Souza L, Keech J, *et al.* Effect of granulocyte colony-stimulating factor on neutropenia induced by cytotoxic chemotherapy. *Lancet* March 26:667-672 (1988).

11. Bronchud MH, Scarffe JH, Thatcher N, *et al.* Phase I/II study of recombinant human granulocyte colony-stimulating factor in patients receiving intensive chemotherapy for small cell lung cancer. *Br. J. Cancer* 56:809-813 (1987).

12. Gabrilove JL, Jakubowski A, Scher H, *et al.* Effect of granulocyte colony-stimulating factor on neutropenia and associated morbidity due to chemotherapy for transitional cell carcinoma of the urothelium. *N. Engl. J. Med.* 318:1414-1422 (1988).

13. Neidhart J, Mangalik A, Kohler W, *et al.* Granulocyte colony-stimulating factor stimulates recovery of granulocytes in patients receiving dose-intensive chemotherapy without bone-marrow transplantation. *J. Clin. Oncol.* 7:1685-1691 (1989).

14. Bronchud MH, Howell A, Crowther D, *et al.* The use of granulocyte colony-stimulating factor to increase the intensity of treatment with doxorubicin in patients with advanced breast and ovarian cancer. *Br. J. Cancer* 60:121-128 (1989).

15. Dale DC, Bonilla MA, Davis MW, *et al.* A randomized controlled phase III trial of recombinant human granulocyte colony-stimulating factor (Filgrastim) for treatment of severe chronic neutropenia. *Blood* 81:2496-2502 (1993).

16. Schroeder TM and Kurth R. Spontaneous chromosomal breakage and high incidence of leukemia in inherited disease. *Blood* 37:96-112 (1971).

Manufactured by:
Amgen Inc.   3105001
Amgen Center   Issue Date: 12/28/95
Thousand Oaks, California 91320-1789   PI Copy Rev. C

INFORMATION FOR PATIENTS

NEUPOGEN® AND CHEMOTHERAPY

Your doctor has advised you to receive chemotherapy. As your doctor has explained, chemotherapeutic drugs are used because they may help destroy rapidly growing cells, like cancer cells. However, certain normal cells in the body are affected by some chemotherapeutic drugs as well. The cells in the blood that are responsible for helping the body fight off infections are especially sensitive to these types of cancer drugs. If these infection-fighting cells, called neutrophils, fall to low levels in your blood after receiving chemotherapy, you could be more likely to get a fever and/or a serious infection. As your doctor has indicated, you must take specific precautions to avoid getting infections while you are being treated with chemotherapy.

To help speed the recovery of the infection-fighting cells after chemotherapy, and to reduce the chances of a serious infection, your doctor has prescribed NEUPOGEN® (Filgrastim). NEUPOGEN® helps to maintain adequate levels of infection-fighting cells, or neutrophils. These cells work by surrounding and destroying bacteria that may have entered the body. NEUPOGEN® works by increasing the number of neutrophils in the blood and by preventing them from falling to low levels for prolonged periods of time. You should not receive NEUPOGEN® in the period 24 hours before through 24 hours after administration of your chemotherapy. NEUPOGEN® therapy also requires that you have laboratory tests twice weekly so your doctor can monitor your white blood cell count.

You have been instructed to be alert for fever, chills, or other signs of infection while you are at home. If you experience any of these signs of infection, contact your doctor immediately. NEUPOGEN® sometimes causes bone pain. If you experience bone pain, discuss its treatment with your doctor.

NEUPOGEN® AND SEVERE CHRONIC NEUTROPENIA

Severe chronic neutropenia is a disease which results in a decrease of infection-fighting white blood cells, known as neutrophils. These cells work by surrounding and destroying bacteria that may have entered the body. When the number of infection-fighting neutrophils in the body is too low, a patient becomes more likely to develop a fever and/or a serious infection.

To help make and keep the right number of neutrophils, and to reduce the chances of a serious infection, your doctor has prescribed NEUPOGEN® (Filgrastim). NEUPOGEN® works by increasing the number of neutrophils in the blood and by preventing them from decreasing to dangerously low levels. While you are taking NEUPOGEN®, you will be required to have blood tests twice weekly during the first four weeks of therapy and for two weeks following any change in your dose, so your doctor can check your white blood cell count. Once the best dose of NEUPOGEN® has been found, your white blood cell count will be checked at least once a month as long as you are taking NEUPOGEN®. You must take your NEUPOGEN® every day.

Patients with severe chronic neutropenia are required to take NEUPOGEN® for a long period of time.

You should be alert for fever, chills, or other signs of infection while you are at home. If you have any of these or other signs of infection, you must contact your doctor immediately. NEUPOGEN® sometimes causes bone pain. If you have bone pain, discuss it with your doctor.

NEUPOGEN®

The NEUPOGEN® solution in the vial should always be clear and colorless. Do not use NEUPOGEN® if the contents of the vial appear discolored or cloudy, or if the vial appears to contain lumps, flakes, or particles. If the vial has been shaken vigorously, the solution may appear to be frothy or have bubbles at the top of the vial; this does not alter the effectiveness of NEUPOGEN®, but may decrease the amount of NEUPOGEN® that can be drawn into the syringe. Therefore, care should be taken not to shake the NEUPOGEN® vial before use. If the solution is frothy, allowing the vial to sit undisturbed for a few minutes should result in a decrease in froth or bubbles (see PREPARING THE DOSE). Vials of NEUPOGEN® are for single use. Any unused portion of a vial should be discarded.

If your doctor has told you that you can inject your own NEUPOGEN®, you will be told how much NEUPOGEN® to use, how to inject it, how often you should inject it, and how you should dispose of vials and syringes. Your treatment requires close and constant cooperation with your doctor and nurse.

When you receive your NEUPOGEN® from your doctor or pharmacist, always check to see that:
1. The name NEUPOGEN® is on the carton and vial.
2. You will be able to use NEUPOGEN® before the expiration date stamped on the package.

Storage:
NEUPOGEN® should be stored in the refrigerator, but not in the freezing compartment. Do not let the vial freeze or leave it in direct sunlight. Do not use a vial of NEUPOGEN® that has frozen or after the expiration date that is stamped on the label.

USE THE CORRECT SYRINGE

Your doctor has instructed you on how to give yourself the correct dosage of NEUPOGEN®. This dosage will usually be measured in milliliters. It is important to use a syringe that is marked in tenths of milliliters (for example, 0.1, 0.2, etc., mL). Failure to use the proper syringe can lead to a mistake in dosage, and you may receive too much or too little NEUPOGEN®. Too little NEUPOGEN® may not be effective in reducing your risk of infections, and too much NEUPOGEN® may lead to neutrophil levels that are too high.

You should only use disposable syringes and needles as they do not require sterilization; they should be used once and disposed of as instructed by your doctor.

IMPORTANT: TO HELP AVOID CONTAMINATION AND POSSIBLE INFECTION, FOLLOW THESE INSTRUCTIONS EXACTLY.

PREPARING THE DOSE

1. Wash your hands thoroughly with soap and water before preparing the medication.
2. Check the date on the NEUPOGEN® vial to be sure that the drug has not expired.

3. Remove the vial of NEUPOGEN® from the refrigerator and allow it to reach room temperature. Each NEUPOGEN® vial is designed to be used only once; do not re-enter the vial. DO NOT SHAKE. Assemble the other supplies you will need for your injection.

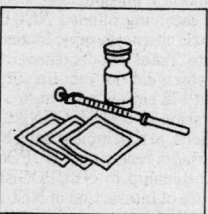

4. Cleanse the skin where the injection is to be made with an alcohol swab.

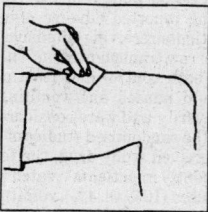

5. Flip off the protective cap but do not remove the rubber stopper. Wipe the top of the rubber stopper with an alcohol swab.

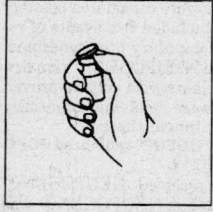
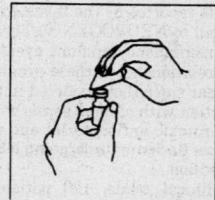

6. Using a syringe and needle designed for subcutaneous injection, draw air into the syringe by pulling back on the plunger. The amount of air should be equal to your NEUPOGEN® dose.

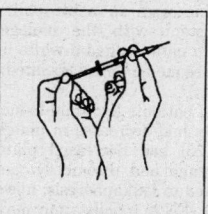

7. Carefully remove the needle cover. Put the needle through the rubber stopper of the NEUPOGEN® vial.
8. Push the plunger in to discharge air into the vial. The air injected into the vial will allow NEUPOGEN® to be easily withdrawn into the syringe.

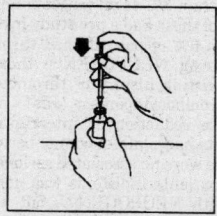

9. Turn the vial and syringe upside down in one hand. Be sure the tip of the needle is in the NEUPOGEN® solution. Your other hand will be free to move the plunger. Draw back on the plunger slowly to draw the correct dose of NEUPOGEN® into the syringe.

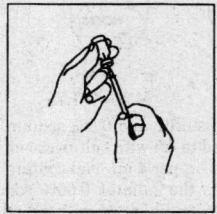

10. Check for air bubbles. The air is harmless, but too large an air bubble will reduce the NEUPOGEN® dose. To remove air bubbles, gently push the solution back into the vial and re-measure your correct dose of NEUPOGEN®.

11. Double check your dose. Remove the needle from the vial. Do not lay the syringe down or allow the needle to touch anything.

INJECTING THE DOSE

1. With one hand, stabilize the previously cleansed skin by spreading it or by pinching up a large area with your free hand.

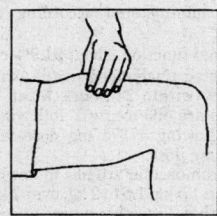

2. Hold the syringe with the other hand, as you would a pencil. Double check that the correct amount of NEUPOGEN® is in the syringe. Insert the needle straight into the skin (90 degree angle). Pull the plunger back slightly. If blood comes into the syringe, do not inject NEUPOGEN®, as the needle has entered a blood vessel; withdraw the syringe and inject at a different site. Inject the NEUPOGEN® by pushing the plunger all the way down.

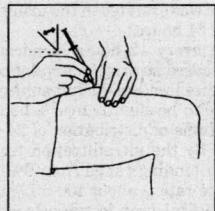 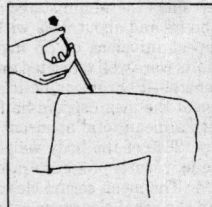

3. Hold an alcohol swab near the needle and pull the needle straight out of the skin. Press the alcohol swab over the injection site for several seconds.

4. Use the disposable syringe only once to insure sterility of the syringe and needle and to insure accuracy of the dose. Dispose of syringes and needles as directed by your physician, by following these simple steps:
   - Place all used needles and syringes in a hard plastic container with a screw-on cap, or a metal container with a plastic lid, such as a coffee can properly labeled as to content. If a metal container is used, cut a small hole in the plastic lid and tape the lid to the metal container. If a hard plastic container is used, always screw the cap on tightly after each use. When the container is full, tape around the cap or lid, and dispose of according to your doctor's instructions.
   - Do not use glass or clear plastic containers, or any container that will be recycled or returned to a store.
   - Always store the container out of the reach of children.
   - Please check with your doctor, nurse, or pharmacist for other suggestions. There may be special state and local laws that they will discuss with you.

5. Always change the site for each injection as directed by your doctor. Occasionally a problem may develop at the injection site. If you notice a lump, swelling, or bruising that doesn't go away, contact your physician.

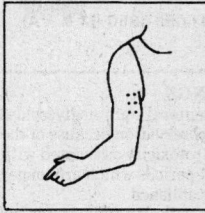 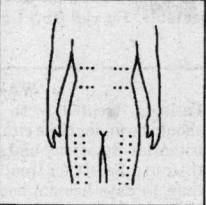

USAGE IN PREGNANCY

If you are pregnant or nursing a baby, consult your physician before using NEUPOGEN®.

ALLERGY TO NEUPOGEN®

Patients occasionally experience redness, swelling, or itching at the site of injection of NEUPOGEN®. This may indicate an allergy to the components of NEUPOGEN®, or it may indicate a local reaction. If you have a local reaction, consult your physician. A potentially more serious reaction, however, would be a generalized allergy to NEUPOGEN®, which could cause a rash over the whole body, shortness of breath, wheezing, reduction in blood pressure, fast pulse, or sweating. Severe cases of generalized allergy may be life-threatening. If you think you are having a generalized allergic reaction, stop taking NEUPOGEN® and notify a physician or emergency medical personnel immediately.

IMPORTANT NOTES

If your doctor allows you to self-administer NEUPOGEN®, please note the following:
1. Always follow the instructions of your doctor concerning the dosage and administration of NEUPOGEN®. Do not change the dose or instructions for administration of NEUPOGEN® without consulting your physician.
2. Your doctor will tell you what to do if you miss a dose of NEUPOGEN®. Always keep a spare syringe and needle on hand.
3. If you develop a fever or symptoms of infection, contact your doctor.
4. Consult your doctor if you notice anything unusual about your condition or your use of NEUPOGEN®.

Manufactured by:
Amgen Inc.   3148000
Amgen Center   Issue Date: 12/28/94
Thousand Oaks, California   PI Copy Rev. B
91320-1789   P40047D   65,000/1-95

Shown in Product Identification Guide, page 304

Apothecon
A Bristol-Myers Squibb Company
P.O. BOX 4500
PRINCETON, NJ 08543-4500

For Medical Information Contact:

Generally:
Bristol-Myers Squibb Drug Information Department
P.O. Box 4500
Princeton, NJ 08543-4500
(800) 321-1335
Adverse Drug Experiences
and Product Defects Reporting call
between 8:30 am-4:30 pm EST:
(609) 252-3737

Sales and Ordering:
Orders for Apothecon Products may be placed by:
1. Calling toll-free between 8:30 am-6:00 pm EST:
   (800) 631-5244
2. Mailing your purchase orders to:
   Apothecon
   Attn: Customer Service Department
   P.O. Box 5250
   Princeton, NJ 08543-5250
3. Faxing your purchase orders to:
   Customer Service Department
   (800) 523-2965

For listing of standard, purified, and human insulins, see Novo Nordisk Pharmaceuticals Inc.

UNILOG®
(Tablet and Capsule Identification Code)
ALPHABETICAL INDEX

Unilog Number	Product
INV 211	Amantadine Hydrochloride Capsules, USP 100 mg
BMS 37	Amoxicillin Tablets, USP (Chewable) 125 mg
BMS 38	Amoxicillin Tablets, USP (Chewable) 250 mg
INV 259	Atenolol Tablets 25 mg
INV 256	Atenolol Tablets 50 mg
INV 257	Atenolol Tablets 100 mg
BMS 5040	Atenolol Tablets 50 mg
BMS 5240	Atenolol Tablets 100 mg
INV 208	Benztropine Mesylate Tablets, USP 0.5 mg
INV 209	Benztropine Mesylate Tablets, USP 1 mg
INV 210	Benztropine Mesylate Tablets, USP 2 mg
Bristol 7271	Cefadroxil Capsules, USP 500 mg
AP 7045	Captopril Tablets, USP 12.5 mg
AP 7046	Captopril Tablets, USP 25 mg
AP 7047	Captopril Tablets, USP 50 mg
AP 7048	Captopril Tablets, USP 100 mg
7375	Cephalexin Capsules USP 250 mg
7376	Cephalexin Capsules USP 500 mg
Squibb 181	Cephalexin Capsules USP 250 mg
Squibb 239	Cephalexin Capsules USP 500 mg
INV 228	Cimetidine Tablets, USP 200 mg
INV 229	Cimetidine Tablets, USP 300 mg
INV 230	Cimetidine Tablets, USP 400 mg
INV 231	Cimetidine Tablets, USP 800 mg
Squibb W028	Cloxacillin Sodium Capsules USP 250 mg
Squibb W038	Cloxacillin Sodium Capsules USP 500 mg
7936	Cloxacillin Sodium Capsules USP 250 mg
7496	Cloxacillin Sodium Capsules USP 500 mg
INV 252	Cyclobenzaprine Hydrochloride Tablets, USP 10 mg
MJ775	Desyrel Tablets (Trazodone Hydrochloride Tablets) 50 mg
MJ776	Desyrel Tablets (Trazodone Hydrochloride Tablets) 100 mg
MJ778	Desyrel Dividose Tablets (Trazodone Hydrochloride Tablets) 150 mg
MJ796	Desyrel Dividose Tablets (Trazodone Hydrochloride Tablets) 300 mg
W048	Dicloxacillin Sodium Capsules USP 250 mg
W058	Dicloxacillin Sodium Capsules USP 500 mg
52 50	Diltiazem Hydrochloride 30 mg
55 50	Diltiazem Hydrochloride 60 mg
57 70	Diltiazem Hydrochloride 90 mg
58 50	Diltiazem Hydrochloride 120 mg
AP 0837	Doxycycline Hyclate Capsules USP 50 mg
AP 0814	Doxycycline Hyclate Capsules USP 100 mg
AP 812	Doxycycline Hyclate Tablets USP 100 mg
7892	Dynapen Capsules (Dicloxacillin Sodium Capsules USP) 125 mg
W048	Dynapen Capsules (Dicloxacillin Sodium Capsules USP) 250 mg
W058	Dynapen Capsules (Dicloxacillin Sodium Capsules USP) 500 mg
AP 025	Estradiol Tablets .5 mg
AP 026	Estradiol Tablets 1.0 mg
AP 027	Estradiol Tablets 2.0 mg
Squibb 429	Florinef Tablets (Fludrocortisone Acetate Tablets USP) 0.1 mg
INV 320	Gemfibrozil Tablets, USP 600 mg
INV 291	Glipizide Tablets, USP 5 mg
INV 292	Glipizide Tablets, USP 10 mg
INV 250	Hydroxychloroquine Sulfate Tablets, USP 200 mg
INV 246	Indapamide Tablets, USP 1.25 mg
INV 247	Indapamide Tablets, USP 2.5 mg
Bristol 3506	Kantrex Capsules (Kanamycin Sulfate Capsules) 500 mg
BL 770	Klotrix Tablets (Potassium Chloride Tablets) 10 mEq
INV 263	Metoclopramide Tablets, USP 5 mg
INV 264	Metoclopramide Tablets, USP 10 mg
W921	Metoprolol Tartrate Tablets, USP 50 mg
W933	Metoprolol Tartrate Tablets, USP 100 mg
Squibb 580	Mycostatin Oral Tablets (Nystatin Tablets USP) 500,000 u.
AP 2461	Nadolol Tablets, USP 20 mg
AP 2462	Nadolol Tablets, USP 40 mg
AP 2463	Nadolol Tablets, USP 80 mg
AP 2464	Nadolol Tablets, USP 120 mg
AP 2465	Nadolol Tablets, USP 160 mg
BL NI	Naldecon Tablets
INV 286	Naproxen Sodium Tablets, USP 275 mg
INV 287	Naproxen Sodium Tablets, USP 550 mg

Continued on next page

Apothecon—Cont.

PPP 606	**Naturetin Tablets** (Bendroflumethiazide Tablets USP) 5 mg
PPP 618	**Naturetin Tablets** (Bendroflumethazide Tablets USP) 10 mg
Squibb 611	**Niacin Tablets USP** 50 mg
Squibb 612	**Niacin Tablets USP** 100 mg
Squibb 537	**Niacin Tablets USP** 500 mg
Bristol 7977	**Oxacillin Sodium Capsules USP** 250 mg
Bristol 7982	**Oxacillin Sodium Capsules USP** 500 mg
AP 6910	**Potassium Chloride Extended Release Tablets** 10 meq
Bristol 7992	**Principen Capsules** (Ampicillin Capsules USP) 250 mg
Bristol 7993	**Principen Capsules** (Ampicillin Capsules USP) 500 mg
INV 275	**Prochlorperazine Maleate Tablets, USP** 5 mg
INV 276	**Prochlorperazine Maleate Tablets, USP** 10 mg
PPP 863	**Prolixin Tablets** (Fluphenazine Hydrochloride Tablets USP) 1 mg
PPP 864	**Prolixin Tablets** (Fluphenazine Hydrochloride Tablets USP) 2.5 mg
PPP 877	**Prolixin Tablets** (Fluphenazine Hydrochloride Tablets USP) 5 mg
PPP 956	**Prolixin Tablets** (Fluphenazine Hydrochloride Tablets USP) 10 mg
PPP 758	**Pronestyl Capsules** (Procainamide Hydrochloride Capsules USP) 250 mg
PPP 756	**Pronestyl Capsules** (Procainamide Hydrochloride Capsules USP) 375 mg
PPP 757	**Pronestyl Capsules** (Procainamide Hydrochloride Capsules USP) 500 mg
PPP 431	**Pronestyl Tablets** (Procainamide Hydrochloride Tablets USP) 250 mg
PPP 434	**Pronestyl Tablets** (Procainamide Hydrochloride Tablets USP) 375 mg
PPP 438	**Pronestyl Tablets** (Procainamide Hydrochloride Tablets USP) 500 mg
PPP 775	**Pronestyl-SR Tablets** (Procainamide Hydrochloride Tablets) 500 mg
PPP 769	**Rauzide Tablets** (Rauwolfia Serpentina with Bendroflumethiazide Tablets) 50 mg - 4 mg
138	**SMZ/TMP Tablets** (Sulfamethoxazole and Trimethoprim Tablets USP) 400 mg - 80 mg
171	**SMZ/TMP Tablets** (Sulfamethoxazole and Trimethoprim Tablets USP) 800 mg - 160 mg
Squibb 655	**Sumycin Capsules** (Tetracycline Hydrochloride Capsules USP) 250 mg
Squibb 763	**Sumycin Capsules** (Tetracycline Hydrochloride Capsules USP) 500 mg
Squibb 663	**Sumycin Tablets** (Tetracycline Hydrochloride Tablets USP) 250 mg
Squibb 603	**Sumycin Tablets** (Tetracycline Hydrochloride Tablets USP) 500 mg
Squibb 535	**Theragran Hematinic Tablets**
AP 778	**Trazodone Hydrochloride Tablets,** 150 mg
Bristol 7278	**Trimox Capsules** (Amoxicillin Capsules USP) 250 mg
Bristol 7279	**Trimox Capsules** (Amoxicillin Capsules USP) 500 mg
MJ 543	**Vasodilan Tablets** (Isoxsuprine Hydrochloride) 10 mg
MJ 544	**Vasodilan Tablets** (Isoxsuprine Hydrochloride) 20 mg
BL V1	250 mg
	Veetids Tablets (Penicillin V Potassium Tablets, USP)
BL V2	500 mg
	Veetids Tablets (Penicillin v Potassium Tablets, USP)
Squibb 113	**Velosef '250' Capsules** (Cephradine Capsules USP) 250 mg
Squibb 114	**Velosef '500' Capsules** (Cephradine Capsules USP) 500 mg

AMIKIN® ℞

[*ah-mi 'kin*]

(amikacin sulfate USP) Injectable, 500 mg vial NSN 6505-01-033-0058 (M & VA)
Injectable, 1 g vial NSN 6505-01-056-1950 (M & VA)

WARNINGS

Patients treated with parenteral aminoglycosides should be under close clinical observation because of the potential ototoxicity and nephrotoxicity associated with their use. Safety for treatment periods which are longer than 14 days has not been established.

Neurotoxicity, manifested as vestibular and permanent bilateral auditory ototoxicity, can occur in patients with preexisting renal damage and in patients with normal renal function treated at higher doses and/or for periods longer than those recommended. The risk of aminoglycoside-induced ototoxicity is greater in patients with renal damage. High frequency deafness usually occurs first and can be detected only by audiometric testing. Vertigo may occur and may be evidence of vestibular injury. Other manifestations of neurotoxicity may include numbness, skin tingling, muscle twitching and convulsions. The risk of hearing loss due to aminoglycosides increases with the degree of exposure to either high peak or high trough serum concentrations. Patients developing cochlear damage may not have symptoms during therapy to warn them of developing eighth-nerve toxicity, and total or partial irreversible bilateral deafness may occur after the drug has been discontinued. Aminoglycoside-induced ototoxicity is usually irreversible.

Aminoglycosides are potentially nephrotoxic. The risk of nephrotoxicity is greater in patients with impaired renal function and in those who receive high doses or prolonged therapy.

Neuromuscular blockade and respiratory paralysis have been reported following parenteral injection, topical instillation (as in orthopedic and abdominal irrigation or in local treatment of empyema), and following oral use of aminoglycosides. The possibility of these phenomena should be considered if aminoglycosides are administered by any route, especially in patients receiving anesthetics, neuromuscular blocking agents such as tubocurarine, succinylcholine, decamethonium, or in patients receiving massive transfusions of citrate-anticoagulated blood. If blockage occurs, calcium salts may reverse these phenomena, but mechanical respiratory assistance may be necessary.

Renal and eighth-nerve function should be closely monitored especially in patients with known or suspected renal impairment at the onset of therapy and also in those whose renal function is initially normal but who develop signs of renal dysfunction during therapy. Serum concentrations of amikacin should be monitored when feasible to assure adequate levels and to avoid potentially toxic levels and prolonged peak concentrations above 35 μg per mL. Urine should be examined for decreased specific gravity, increased excretion of proteins, and the presence of cells or casts. Blood urea nitrogen, serum creatinine, or creatinine clearance should be measured periodically. Serial audiograms should be obtained where feasible in patients old enough to be tested, particularly high risk patients. Evidence of ototoxicity (dizziness, vertigo, tinnitus, roaring in the ears, and hearing loss) or nephrotoxicity requires discontinuation of the drug or dosage adjustment.

Concurrent and/or sequential systemic, oral or topical use of other neurotoxic or nephrotoxic products, particularly bacitracin, cisplatin, amphotericin B, cephaloridine, paromomycin, viomycin, polymyxin B, colistin, vancomycin, or other aminoglycosides should be avoided. Other factors that may increase risk of toxicity are advanced age and dehydration.

The concurrent use of AMIKIN with potent diuretics (ethacrynic acid, or furosemide) should be avoided since diuretics by themselves may cause ototoxicity. In addition, when administered intravenously, diuretics may enhance aminoglycoside toxicity by altering antibiotic concentrations in serum and tissue.

DESCRIPTION

Amikacin sulfate is a semi-synthetic aminoglycoside antibiotic derived from kanamycin. It is $C_{22}H_{43}N_5O_{13} \cdot 2H_2SO_4$. D-Streptamine, *O*-3-amino-3-deoxy-α-D-glucopyranosyl-(1 → 6)-*O*-[6-amino-6-deoxy-α-D-glucopyranosyl-(1 → 4)]-N^1-(4-amino-2-hydroxy-1-oxobutyl)-2-deoxy-, (*S*)-, sulfate (1:2) (salt).

[See chemical structure at top of next column.]

The dosage form is supplied as a sterile, colorless to light straw colored solution for IM or IV use. The 100 mg per 2 mL vial contains per each mL: 50 mg amikacin (as the sulfate),

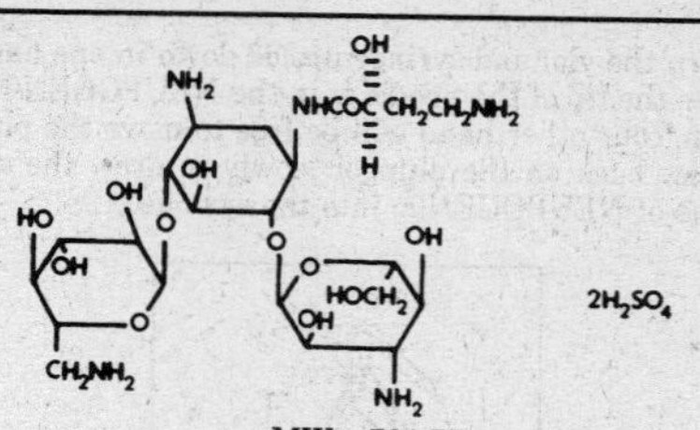

MW=781.75

0.13% sodium bisulfite and 0.5% sodium citrate dihydrate with pH adjusted to 4.5 with sulfuric acid. The 500 mg per 2 mL vial and the 1 g per 4 mL vial contain per each mL: 250 mg amikacin (as the sulfate), 0.66% sodium bisulfite and 2.5% sodium citrate dihydrate with pH adjusted to 4.5 with sulfuric acid.

Vial headspace contains nitrogen.

CLINICAL PHARMACOLOGY

Intramuscular Administration—AMIKIN is rapidly absorbed after intramuscular administration. In normal adult volunteers, average peak serum concentrations of about 12, 16, and 21 mcg are obtained 1 hour after intramuscular administration of 250 mg (3.7mg/kg), 375 mg (5 mg/kg), 500 mg (7.5 mg/kg), single doses, respectively. At 10 hours, serum levels are about 0.3 mcg/mL, 1.2 mcg/mL, and 2.1 mcg/mL, respectively.

Tolerance studies in normal volunteers reveal that amikacin is well tolerated locally following repeated intramuscular dosing, and when given at maximally recommended doses, no ototoxicity or nephrotoxicity has been reported. There is no evidence of drug accumulation with repeated dosing for 10 days when administered according to recommended doses.

With normal renal function, about 91.9% of an intramuscular dose is excreted unchanged in the urine in the first 8 hours, and 98.2% within 24 hours. Mean urine concentrations for 6 hours are 563 mcg/mL following a 250 mg dose, 697 mcg/mL following a 375 mg dose, and 832 mcg/mL following a 500 mg dose.

Preliminary intramuscular studies in newborns of different weights (less than 1.5 kg, 1.5 to 2 kg, over 2 kg) at a dose of 7.5 mg/kg revealed that, like other aminoglycosides, serum half-life values were correlated inversely with post-natal age and renal clearances of amikacin. The volume of distribution indicates that amikacin, like other aminoglycosides, remains primarily in the extracellular fluid space of neonates. Repeated dosing every 12 hours in all the above groups did not demonstrate accumulation after 5 days.

Intravenous Administration—Single doses of 500 mg (7.5 mg/kg) administered to normal adults as an infusion over a period of 30 minutes produced a mean peak serum concentration of 38 mcg/mL at the end of the infusion, and levels of 24 mcg/mL, 18 mcg/mL, and 0.75 mcg/mL at 30 minutes, 1 hour and 10 hours postinfusion, respectively. Eighty-four percent of the administered dose was excreted in the urine in 9 hours and about 94% within 24 hours.

Repeat infusions of 7.5 mg/kg every 12 hours in normal adults were well tolerated and caused no drug accumulation.

General—Pharmacokinetic studies in normal adult subjects reveal the mean serum half-life to be slightly over 2 hours with a mean total apparent volume of distribution of 24 liters (28% of the body weight). By the ultrafiltration technique, reports of serum protein binding range from 0% to 11%. The mean serum clearance rate is about 100 mL/min and the renal clearance rate is 94 mL/min in subjects with normal renal function.

Amikacin is excreted primarily by glomerular filtration. Patients with impaired renal function or diminished glomerular filtration pressure excrete the drug much more slowly (effectively prolonging the serum half-life). Therefore, renal function should be monitored carefully and dosage adjusted accordingly (see suggested dosage schedule under "**DOSAGE AND ADMINISTRATION**").

Following administration at the recommended dose, therapeutic levels are found in bone, heart, gallbladder, and lung tissue in addition to significant concentrations in urine, bile, sputum, bronchial secretions, interstitial, pleural and synovial fluids.

Spinal fluid levels in normal infants are approximately 10% to 20% of the serum concentrations and may reach 50% when the meninges are inflamed. AMIKIN has been demonstrated to cross the placental barrier and yield significant concentrations in amniotic fluid. The peak fetal serum concentration is about 16% of the peak maternal serum concentration and maternal and fetal serum half-life values are about 2 and 3.7 hours, respectively.

Microbiology

Gram-negative—Amikacin is active *in vitro* against *Pseudomonas* species, *Escherichia coli, Proteus* species (indole-positive and indole-negative), *Providencia* species, *Klebsiella-Enterobacter-Serratia* species, *Acinetobacter* (formerly *Mima-Herellea*) species, and *Citrobacter freundii.*

When strains of the above organisms are found to be resistant to other aminoglycosides, including gentamicin, tobramycin and kanamycin, many are susceptible to amikacin *in vitro*.

Gram-positive—Amikacin is active *in vitro* against penicillinase and nonpenicillinase-producing *Staphylococcus* species including methicillin-resistant strains. However, aminoglycosides in general have a low order of activity against other Gram-positive organisms; viz, *Streptococcus pyogenes,* enterococci, and *Streptococcus pneumoniae* (formerly *Diplococcus pneumoniae*).

Amikacin resists degradation by most aminoglycoside inactivating enzymes known to affect gentamicin, tobramycin, and kanamycin.

In vitro studies have shown that AMIKIN combined with a beta-lactam antibiotic acts synergistically against many clinically significant Gram-negative organisms.

Disc Susceptibility Tests—Quantitative methods that require measurement of zone diameters give the most precise estimates of antibiotic susceptibility. One such procedure[1] has been recommended for use with discs to test susceptibility to amikacin. Interpretation involves correlation of the diameters obtained in the disc test with MIC values for amikacin. When the causative organism is tested by the Kirby-Bauer method of disc susceptibility, a 30 mcg amikacin disc should give a zone of 17 mm or greater to indicate susceptibility. Zone sizes of 14 mm or less indicate resistance. Zone sizes of 15 to 16 mm indicate intermediate susceptibility. With this procedure, a report from the laboratory of "susceptible" indicates that the infecting organism is likely to respond to therapy. A report of "resistant" indicates that the infecting organism is not likely to respond to therapy. A report of "intermediate susceptibility" suggests that the organism would be susceptible if the infection is confined to tissues and fluids (e.g., urine) in which high antibiotic levels are attained.

INDICATIONS AND USAGE

AMIKIN is indicated in the short-term treatment of serious infections due to susceptible strains of Gram-negative bacteria, including *Pseudomonas* species, *Escherichia coli,* species of indole-positive and indole-negative *Proteus, Providencia* species, *Klebsiella-Enterobacter-Serratia* species, and *Acinetobacter (Mima-Herellea)* species.

Clinical studies have shown AMIKIN to be effective in bacterial septicemia (including neonatal sepsis); in serious infections of the respiratory tract, bones and joints, central nervous system (including meningitis); and skin and soft tissue; intra-abdominal infections (including peritonitis); and in burns and post-operative infections (including post-vascular surgery). Clinical studies have shown AMIKIN also to be effective in serious complicated and recurrent urinary tract infections due to these organisms. Aminoglycosides, including AMIKIN injectable, are not indicated in uncomplicated initial episodes of urinary tract infections unless the causative organisms are not susceptible to antibiotics having less potential toxicity.

Bacteriologic studies should be performed to identify causative organisms and their susceptibilities to amikacin. AMIKIN may be considered as initial therapy in suspected Gram-negative infections and therapy may be instituted before obtaining the results of susceptibility testing. Clinical trials demonstrated that AMIKIN was effective in infections caused by gentamicin and/or tobramycin-resistant strains of Gram-negative organisms, particularly *Proteus rettgeri, Providencia stuartii, Serratia marcescens, and Pseudomonas aeruginosa.* The decision to continue therapy with the drug should be based on results of the susceptibility tests, the severity of the infection, the response of the patient and the important additional considerations contained in the "WARNINGS" box above.

AMIKIN has also been shown to be effective in staphylococcal infections and may be considered as initial therapy under certain conditions in the treatment of known or suspected staphylococcal disease such as, severe infections where the causative organism may be either a Gram-negative bacterium or a staphylococcus, infections due to susceptible strains of staphylococci in patients allergic to other antibiotics, and in mixed staphylococcal/Gram-negative infections. In certain severe infections such as neonatal sepsis, concomitant therapy with a penicillin-type drug may be indicated because of the possibility of infections due to Gram-positive organisms such as streptococci or pneumococci.

CONTRAINDICATIONS

A history of hypersensitivity to amikacin is a contraindication for its use. A history of hypersensitivity or serious toxic reactions to aminoglycosides may contraindicate the use of any other aminoglycoside because of the known cross-sensitivities of patients to drugs in this class.

WARNINGS

See "WARNINGS" box above.

Aminoglycosides can cause fetal harm when administered to a pregnant woman. Aminoglycosides cross the placenta and there have been several reports of total irreversible, bilateral congenital deafness in children whose mothers received streptomycin during pregnancy. Although serious side effects to the fetus or newborns have not been reported in the treatment of pregnant women with other aminoglycosides, the potential for harm exists. Reproduction studies of amikacin have been performed in rats and mice and revealed no evidence of impaired fertility or harm to the fetus due to amikacin. There are no well controlled studies in pregnant women, but investigational experience does not include any positive evidence of adverse effects to the fetus. If this drug is used during pregnancy, or if the patient becomes pregnant while taking this drug, the patient should be apprised of the potential hazard to the fetus.

Contains sodium bisulfite, a sulfite that may cause allergic-type reactions including anaphylactic symptoms and life-threatening or less severe asthmatic episodes in certain susceptible people. The overall prevalence of sulfite sensitivity in the general population is unknown and probably low. Sulfite sensitivity is seen more frequently in asthmatic than nonasthmatic people.

PRECAUTIONS

Aminoglycosides are quickly and almost totally absorbed when they are applied topically, except to the urinary bladder, in association with surgical procedures. Irreversible deafness, renal failure, and death due to neuromuscular blockade have been reported following irrigation of both small and large surgical fields with an aminoglycoside preparation.

AMIKIN is potentially nephrotoxic, ototoxic and neurotoxic. The concurrent or serial use of other ototoxic or nephrotoxic agents should be avoided either systemically or topically because of the potential for additive effects. Increased nephrotoxicity has been reported following concomitant parenteral administration of aminoglycoside antibiotics and cephalosporins. Concomitant cephalosporins may spuriously elevate creatinine determinations.

Since AMIKIN is present in high concentrations in the renal excretory system, patients should be well hydrated to minimize chemical irritation of the renal tubules. Kidney function should be assessed by the usual methods prior to starting therapy and daily during the course of treatment.

If signs of renal irritation appear (casts, white or red cells, or albumin), hydration should be increased. A reduction in dosage (see "DOSAGE AND ADMINISTRATION") may be desirable if other evidence of renal dysfunction occurs such as decreased creatinine clearance; decreased urine specific gravity; increased BUN, creatinine, or oliguria. If azotemia increases or if a progressive decrease in urinary output occurs, treatment should be stopped.

Note: When patients are well hydrated and kidney function is normal the risk of nephrotoxic reactions with amikacin is low if the dosage recomendations (see "DOSAGE AND ADMINISTRATION") are not exceeded.

Elderly patients may have reduced renal function which may not be evident in routine screening tests such as BUN or serum creatinine. A creatinine clearance determination may be more useful. Monitoring of renal function during treatment with aminoglycosides is particularly important.

Aminoglycosides should be used with caution in patients with muscular disorders such as myasthenia gravis or parkinsonism since these drugs may aggravate muscle weakness because of their potential curare-like effect on the neuromuscular junction.

In vitro mixing of aminoglycosides with beta-lactam antibiotics (penicillin or cephalosporins) may result in a significant mutual inactivation. A reduction in serum half-life or serum level may occur when an aminoglycoside or penicillin-type drug is administered by separate routes. Inactivation of the aminoglycoside is clinically significant only in patients with severely impaired renal function. Inactivation may continue in specimens of body fluids collected for assay, resulting in inaccurate aminoglycoside readings. Such specimens should be properly handled (assayed promptly, frozen, or treated with beta-lactamase).

Cross-allergenicity among aminoglycosides has been demonstrated.

As with other antibiotics, the use of amikacin may result in overgrowth of non-susceptible organisms. If this occurs, appropriate therapy should be instituted.

Aminoglycosides should not be given concurrently with potent diuretics (See "WARNINGS" box).

Carcinogenesis, Mutagenesis, Impairment of Fertility—Long term studies in animals to evaluate carcinogenic potential have not been performed, and mutagenicity has not been studied. AMIKIN administered subcutaneously to rats at doses up to 4 times the human daily dose did not impair male or female fertility.

Pregnancy/Teratogenic Effects—Pregnancy Category D (See "WARNINGS" section).

Nursing Mothers—It is not known whether AMIKIN is excreted in human milk. Because many drugs are excreted in human milk and because of the potential for serious adverse reactions in nursing infants from AMIKIN, a decision should be made whether to discontinue nursing or to discontinue the drug, taking into account the importance of the drug to the mother.

Pediatric Use—Aminoglycosides should be used with caution in premature and neonatal infants because of the renal immaturity of these patients and the resulting prolongation of serum half-life of these drugs.

ADVERSE REACTIONS

All aminoglycosides have the potential to induce auditory, vestibular, and renal toxicity and neuromuscular blockade (see "WARNINGS" box). They occur more frequently in patients with present or past history of renal impairment, of treatment with other ototoxic or nephrotoxic drugs, and in patients treated for longer periods and/or with higher doses than recommended.

Neurotoxicity-Ototoxicity—Toxic effects on the eighth cranial nerve can result in hearing loss, loss of balance, or both. Amikacin primarily affects auditory function. Cochlear damage includes high frequency deafness and usually occurs before clinical hearing loss can be detected.

Neurotoxicity-Neuromuscular Blockage—Acute muscular paralysis and apnea can occur following treatment with aminoglycoside drugs.

Nephrotoxicity—Elevation of serum creatinine, albuminuria, presence of red and white cells, casts, azotemia, and oliguria have been reported. Renal function changes are usually reversible when the drug is discontinued.

Other—In addition to those described above, other adverse reactions which have been reported on rare occasions are skin rash, drug fever, headache, paresthesia, tremor, nausea and vomiting, eosinophilia, arthralgia, anemia, and hypotension.

OVERDOSAGE

In the event of overdosage or toxic reaction, peritoneal dialysis or hemodialysis will aid in the removal of amikacin from the blood. In the newborn infant, exchange transfusion may also be considered.

DOSAGE AND ADMINISTRATION

The patient's pretreatment body weight should be obtained for calculation of correct dosage. AMIKIN may be given intramuscularly or intravenously.

The status of renal function should be estimated by measurement of the serum creatinine concentration or calculation of the endogenous creatinine clearance rate. The blood urea nitrogen (BUN) is much less reliable for this purpose. Reassessment of renal function should be made periodically during therapy.

Whenever possible, amikacin concentrations in serum should be measured to assure adequate but not excessive levels. It is desirable to measure both peak and trough serum concentrations intermittently during therapy. Peak concentrations (30 to 90 minutes after injection) above 35 mcg per mL and trough concentrations (just prior to the next dose) above 10 mcg per mL should be avoided. Dosage should be adjusted as indicated.

Intramuscular Administration for Patients with Normal Renal Function—The recommended dosage for adults, children and older infants (see "WARNINGS" box) with normal renal function is 15 mg/kg/day divided into 2 or 3 equal doses administered at equally-divided intervals, i.e., 7.5 mg/kg q12h or 5 mg/kg q8h. Treatment of patients in the heavier weight classes should not exceed 1.5 gram per day.

When amikacin is indicated in newborns (see "WARNINGS" box), it is recommended that a loading dose of 10 mg/kg be administered initially to be followed with 7.5 mg/kg every 12 hours.

The usual duration of treatment is 7 to 10 days. It is desirable to limit the duration of treatment to short term whenever feasible. The total daily dose by all routes of administration should not exceed 15 mg/kg/day. In difficult and complicated infections where treatment beyond 10 days is considered, the use of AMIKIN should be reevaluated. If continued, amikacin serum levels, and renal, auditory, and vestibular functions should be monitored. At the recommended dosage level, uncomplicated infections due to amikacin-sensitive organisms should respond in 24 to 48 hours. If definite clinical response does not occur within 3 to 5 days, therapy should be stopped and the antibiotic susceptibility pattern of the invading organism should be rechecked. Failure of the infection to respond may be due to resistance of the organism or to the presence of septic foci requiring surgical drainage.

When AMIKIN is indicated in uncomplicated urinary tract infections, a dose of 250 mg twice daily may be used. [See table on top of next page.]

Intramuscular Administration for Patients with Impaired Renal Function—Whenever possible, serum amikacin concentrations should be monitored by appropriate assay procedures. Doses may be adjusted in patients with impaired renal function either by administering normal doses at prolonged intervals or by administering reduced doses at a fixed interval.

Both methods are based on the patient's creatinine clearance or serum creatinine values since these have been found to

Continued on next page

Apothecon—Cont.

DOSAGE GUIDELINES

ADULTS AND CHILDREN WITH NORMAL RENAL FUNCTION

Patient Weight		Dosage		
		7.5 mg/kg q 12h	OR	5mg/kg q 8h
lbs.	kg			
99	45	337.5 mg		225 mg
110	50	375 mg		250 mg
121	55	412.5 mg		275 mg
132	60	450 mg		300 mg
143	65	487.5 mg		325 mg
154	70	525 mg		350 mg
165	75	562.5 mg		375 mg
176	80	600 mg		400 mg
187	85	637.5 mg		425 mg
198	90	675 mg		450 mg
209	95	712.5 mg		475 mg
220	100	750 mg		500 mg

correlate with aminoglycoside half-lives in patients with diminished renal function. These dosage schedules must be used in conjunction with careful clinical and laboratory observations of the patient and should be modified as necessary. Neither method should be used when dialysis is being performed.

Normal Dosage at Prolonged Intervals—If the creatinine clearance rate is not available and the patient's condition is stable, a dosage interval in hours for the normal dose can be calculated by multiplying the patient's serum creatinine by 9; e.g., if the serum creatinine concentration is 2 mg/100 mL, the recommended single dose (7.5 mg/kg) should be administered every 18 hours.

Reduced Dosage at Fixed Time Intervals—When renal function is impaired and it is desirable to administer AMIKIN at a fixed time interval, dosage must be reduced. In these patients, serum AMIKIN concentrations should be measured to assure accurate administration of AMIKIN and to avoid concentrations above 35 mcg/mL. If serum assay determinations are not available and the patient's condition is stable, serum creatinine and creatinine clearance values are the most readily available indicators of the degree of renal impairment to use as a guide for dosage.

First, initiate therapy by administering a normal dose, 7.5 mg/kg, as a loading dose. This loading dose is the same as the normally recommended dose which would be calculated for a patient with a normal renal function as described above. To determine the size of maintenance doses administered every 12 hours, the loading dose should be reduced in proportion to the reduction in the patient's creatinine clearance rate:

$$\begin{array}{l} \text{Maintenance} \\ \text{Dose} \\ \text{Every 12 hours} \end{array} = \dfrac{\text{observed CC}}{\text{normal CC}} \times \begin{array}{l} \text{calculated} \\ \text{loading} \\ \text{dose in mg} \end{array}$$

(CC—creatinine clearance rate)

An alternate rough guide for determining reduced dosage at 12-hour intervals (for patients whose steady state serum creatinine values are known) is to divide the normally recommended dose by the patient's serum creatinine.

The above dosage schedules are not intended to be rigid recommendations but are provided as guides to dosage when the measurement of amikacin serum levels is not feasible.

Intravenous Administration—The individual dose, the total daily dose, and the total cumulative dose of AMIKIN are identical to the dose recommended for intramuscular administration. The solution for intravenous use is prepared by adding the contents of a 500 mg vial to 100 or 200 mL of sterile diluent such as 0.9% sodium chloride injection or 5% dextrose injection or any other compatible solutions listed below.

The solution is administered to adults over a 30 to 60 minute period. The total daily dose should not exceed 15 mg/kg/day and may be divided into either 2 or 3 equally-divided doses at equally-divided intervals.

In pediatric patients the amount of fluid used will depend on the amount of AMIKIN ordered for the patient. It should be a sufficient amount to infuse the AMIKIN over a 30 to 60 minute period. Infants should receive a 1- to 2-hour infusion.

Stability in IV Fluids—AMIKIN is stable for 24 hours at room temperature at concentrations of 0.25 and 5 mg/mL in the following solutions:

5% Dextrose Injection
5% Dextrose and 0.2% Sodium Chloride Injection
5% Dextrose and 0.45% Sodium Chloride Injection
0.9% Sodium Chloride Injection
Lactated Ringer's Injection

Normosol®M in 5% Dextrose Injection (or Plasma-Lyte 56 Injection in 5% Dextrose in Water)
Normosol®R in 5% Dextrose Injection (or Plasma-Lyte 148 Injection in 5% Dextrose in Water)

In the above solutions with AMIKIN concentrations of 0.25 and 5 mg/mL, solutions aged for 60 days at 4°C and then stored at 25°C had utility times of 24 hours.

At the same concentrations, solutions frozen and aged for 30 days at −15°C, thawed, and stored at 25°C had utility times of 24 hours.

Parenteral drug products should be inspected visually for particulate matter and discoloration prior to administration whenever the solution and container permit.

Aminoglycosides administered by any of the above routes should not be physically premixed with other drugs but should be administered separately.

Because of the potential toxicity of aminoglycosides, "fixed dosage" recommendations which are not based upon body weight are not advised. Rather, it is essential to calculate the dosage to fit the needs of each patient.

HOW SUPPLIED

AMIKIN (sterile amikacin sulfate injection, USP) is supplied in vials as a sterile nonpyrogenic colorless solution which requires no refrigeration. At times the solution may become a very pale yellow; this does not indicate a decrease in potency.

AMIKIN® (amikacin sulfate injection)
NDC 0015-3015-20 100 mg per 2 mL package of 10 vials
NDC 0015-3020-20 500 mg per 2 mL package of 10 vials
NDC 0015-3023-20 1 g per 4 mL package of 10 vials
NDC 0015-3020-21 500 mg per 2 mL in glass, disposable syringe with a rubber shielded, stainless steel needle (1 1/4″×22G), package of 10 syringes

Storage
Store at controlled room temperature 15°–30°C (59°–86°F).

REFERENCES

[1] Bauer, A. W., Kirby, W. M. M., Sherris, J. C., and Turck, M.: Antibiotic Testing by a Standardized Single Disc Method, Am. J. Clin. Pathol., 45:493, 1966; Standardized Disc Susceptibility, FEDERAL REGISTER, 37:205527–29, 1972.

Caution: Federal law prohibits dispensing without a prescription.

APOTHECON®
A Bristol-Myers Squibb Company
Princeton, NJ 08540 USA
Revised September 1993   3015DIM-17

DESYREL®   ℞
[des′ē-rel]
(trazodone HCl)

Tablets, 150 mg, bottles of 100
                              NSN 6505-01-234-4439 (M&VA)

DESCRIPTION

DESYREL (trazodone hydrochloride) is an antidepressant chemically unrelated to tricyclic, tetracyclic, or other known antidepressant agents. It is a triazolopyridine derivative designated as 2-[3-[4-(3-chlorophenyl)-1-piperazinyl] propyl]-1,2,4-triazolo[4, 3-a]pyridin-3(2H)-one hydrochloride. It is a white odorless crystalline powder which is freely soluble in water. Its molecular weight is 408.3. The empirical formula is $C_{19}H_{22}ClN_5O \cdot HCl$ and the structural formula is represented as follows:

[See chemical structure at top of next column.]

DESYREL is supplied for oral administration in 50 mg, 100 mg, 150 mg and 300 mg tablets.

DESYREL Tablets, 50 mg, contain the following inactive ingredients: dibasic calcium phosphate, castor oil, microcrystalline cellulose, ethylcellulose, FD&C Yellow No. 6 (aluminum lake), lactose, magnesium stearate, povidone, sodium starch glycolate, and starch (corn).

DESYREL Tablets, 100 mg, contain the following inactive ingredients: dibasic calcium phosphate, castor oil, microcrystalline cellulose, ethylcellulose, lactose, magnesium stearate, povidone, sodium starch glycolate, and starch (corn).

DESYREL Tablets, 150 mg, contain the following inactive ingredients: microcrystalline cellulose, FD&C Yellow No. 6 (aluminum lake), magnesium stearate, pregelatinized starch, and stearic acid.

DESYREL Tablets, 300 mg, contain the following inactive ingredients: microcrystalline cellulose, yellow ferric oxide, magnesium stearate, sodium starch glycolate, pregelatinized starch, and stearic acid.

CLINICAL PHARMACOLOGY

The mechanism of DESYREL's antidepressant action in man is not fully understood. In animals, DESYREL selectively inhibits serotonin uptake by brain synaptosomes and potentiates the behavioral changes induced by the serotonin precursor, 5-hydroxytryptophan. Cardiac conduction effects of DESYREL in the anesthetized dog are qualitatively dissimilar and quantitatively less pronounced than those seen with tricyclic antidepressants. DESYREL is not a monoamine oxidase inhibitor and, unlike amphetamine-type drugs, does not stimulate the central nervous system.

In man, DESYREL is well absorbed after oral administration without selective localization in any tissue. When DESYREL is taken shortly after ingestion of food, there may be an increase in the amount of drug absorbed, a decrease in maximum concentration, and a lengthening in the time to maximum concentration. Peak plasma levels occur approximately one hour after dosing when DESYREL is taken on an empty stomach or two hours after dosing when taken with food. Elimination of DESYREL is biphasic, consisting of an initial phase (half-life 3–6 hours) followed by a slower phase (half-life 5–9 hours), and is unaffected by the presence or absence of food. Since the clearance of DESYREL from the body is sufficiently variable, in some patients DESYREL may accumulate in the plasma.

For those patients who responded to DESYREL, one-third of the inpatients and one-half of the outpatients had a significant therapeutic response by the end of the first week of treatment. Three-fourths of all responders demonstrated a significant therapeutic effect by the end of the second week. One-fourth of responders required 2–4 weeks for a significant therapeutic response.

INDICATIONS AND USAGE

DESYREL is indicated for the treatment of depression. The efficacy of DESYREL has been demonstrated in both inpatient and outpatient settings and for depressed patients with and without prominent anxiety. The depressive illness of patients studied corresponds to the Major Depressive Episode criteria of the American Psychiatric Association's Diagnostic and Statistical Manual, III.[a]

Major Depressive Episode implies a prominent and relatively persistent (nearly every day for at least two weeks) depressed or dysphoric mood that usually interferes with daily functioning, and includes at least four of the following eight symptoms: change in appetite, change in sleep, psychomotor agitation or retardation, loss of interest in usual activities or decrease in sexual drive, increased fatigability, feelings of guilt or worthlessness, slowed thinking or impaired concentration, and suicidal ideation or attempts.

CONTRAINDICATIONS

DESYREL is contraindicated in patients hypersensitive to DESYREL.

WARNINGS

TRAZODONE HAS BEEN ASSOCIATED WITH THE OCCURRENCE OF PRIAPISM. IN MANY OF THE CASES REPORTED, SURGICAL INTERVENTION WAS REQUIRED AND, IN SOME OF THESE CASES, PERMANENT IMPAIRMENT OF ERECTILE FUNCTION OR IMPOTENCE RESULTED. MALE PATIENTS WITH PROLONGED OR INAPPROPRIATE ERECTIONS SHOULD IMMEDIATELY DISCONTINUE THE DRUG AND CONSULT THEIR PHYSICIAN.

The detumescence of priapism and drug-induced penile erections has been accomplished by both pharmacologic, e.g., the intracavernosal injection of alpha-adrenergic stimulants such as epinephrine and norepinephrine, as well as surgical procedures.[b-g]

Any pharmacologic or surgical procedure utilized in the treatment of priapism should be performed under the supervision of a urologist or a physician familiar with the procedure and should not be initiated without urologic con-

sultation if the priapism has persisted for more than 24 hours.

DESYREL (trazodone hydrochloride) is not recommended for use during the initial recovery phase of myocardial infarction.

Caution should be used when administering DESYREL to patients with cardiac disease, and such patients should be closely monitored, since antidepressant drugs (including DESYREL) have been associated with the occurrence of cardiac arrhythmias. Recent clinical studies in patients with pre-existing cardiac disease indicate that DESYREL may be arrhythmogenic in some patients in that population. Arrhythmias identified include isolated PVCs, ventricular couplets, and in two patients short episodes (3–4 beats) of ventricular tachycardia.

PRECAUTIONS

General

The possibility of suicide in seriously depressed patients is inherent in the illness and may persist until significant remission occurs. Therefore, prescriptions should be written for the smallest number of tablets consistent with good patient management.

Hypotension, including orthostatic hypotension and syncope, has been reported to occur in patients receiving DESYREL. Concomitant administration of antihypertensive therapy with DESYREL may require a reduction in the dose of the antihypertensive drug.

Little is known about the interaction between DESYREL and general anesthetics; therefore, prior to elective surgery, DESYREL should be discontinued for as long as clinically feasible.

As with all antidepressants, the use of DESYREL should be based on the consideration of the physician that the expected benefits of therapy outweigh potential risk factors.

Information for Patients

Because priapism has been reported to occur in patients receiving DESYREL, patients with prolonged or inappropriate penile erection should immediately discontinue the drug and consult with the physician (see **WARNINGS**).

Antidepressants may impair the mental and/or physical ability required for the performance of potentially hazardous tasks, such as operating an automobile or machinery; the patient should be cautioned accordingly.

DESYREL may enhance the response to alcohol, barbiturates, and other CNS depressants.

DESYREL should be given shortly after a meal or light snack. Within any individual patient, total drug absorption may be up to 20% higher when the drug is taken with food rather than on an empty stomach. The risk of dizziness/lightheadedness may increase under fasting conditions.

Laboratory Tests

Occasional low white blood cell and neutrophil counts have been noted in patients receiving DESYREL. These were not considered clinically significant and did not necessitate discontinuation of the drug; however, the drug should be discontinued in any patient whose white blood cell count or absolute neutrophil count falls below normal levels. White blood cell and differential counts are recommended for patients who develop fever and sore throat (or other signs of infection) during therapy.

Drug Interactions

Increased serum digoxin or phenytoin levels have been reported to occur in patients receiving DESYREL concurrently with either of those two drugs.

It is not known whether interactions will occur between monoamine oxidase (MAO) inhibitors and DESYREL. Due to the absence of clinical experience, if MAO inhibitors are discontinued shortly before or are to be given concomitantly with DESYREL, therapy should be initiated cautiously with gradual increase in dosage until optimum response is achieved.

Therapeutic Interactions

Concurrent administration with electroshock therapy should be avoided because of the absence of experience in this area.

There have been reports of increased and decreased prothrombin time occurring in warfarinized patients who take DESYREL.

Carcinogenesis, Mutagenesis, Impairment of Fertility

No drug- or dose-related occurrence of carcinogenesis was evident in rats receiving DESYREL in daily oral doses up to 300 mg/kg for 18 months.

Pregnancy Category C

DESYREL has been shown to cause increased fetal resorption and other adverse effects on the fetus in two studies using the rat when given at dose levels approximately 30–50 times the proposed maximum human dose. There was also an increase in congenital anomalies in one of three rabbit studies at approximately 15–50 times the maximum human dose. There are no adequate and well-controlled studies in pregnant women. DESYREL should be used during pregnancy only if the potential benefit justifies the potential risk to the fetus.

Nursing Mothers

DESYREL and/or its metabolites have been found in the milk of lactating rats, suggesting that the drug may be secreted in human milk. Caution should be exercised when DESYREL is administered to a nursing woman.

Pediatric Use

Safety and effectiveness in children below the age of 18 have not been established.

ADVERSE REACTIONS

Because the frequency of adverse drug effects is affected by diverse factors (eg, drug dose, method of detection, physician judgment, disease under treatment, etc.), a single meaningful estimate of adverse event incidence is difficult to obtain. This problem is illustrated by the variation in adverse event incidence observed and reported from the inpatients and outpatients treated with DESYREL. It is impossible to determine precisely what accounts for the differences observed.

Clinical Trial Reports

The table below is presented solely to indicate the relative frequency of adverse events reported in representative controlled clinical studies conducted to evaluate the safety and efficacy of DESYREL® (trazodone hydrochloride).

The figures cited cannot be used to predict precisely the incidence of untoward events in the course of usual medical practice where patient characteristics and other factors often differ from those which prevailed in the clinical trials. These incidence figures, also, cannot be compared with those obtained from other clinical studies involving related drug products and placebo as each group of drug trials is conducted under a different set of conditions.

[See table above.]

Occasional sinus bradycardia has occurred in long-term studies.

	Treatment-Emergent Symptom Incidence			
	Inpts.		Outpts.	
	D	P	D	P
Number of Patients	142	95	157	158
% of Patients Reporting				
Allergic				
Skin Condition/Edema	2.8	1.1	7.0	1.3
Autonomic				
Blurred Vision	6.3	4.2	14.7	3.8
Constipation	7.0	4.2	7.6	5.7
Dry Mouth	14.8	8.4	33.8	20.3
Cardiovascular				
Hypertension	2.1	1.1	1.3	*
Hypotension	7.0	1.1	3.8	0.0
Shortness of Breath	*	1.1	1.3	0.0
Syncope	2.8	2.1	4.5	1.3
Tachycardia/Palpitations	0.0	0.0	7.0	7.0
CNS				
Anger/Hostility	3.5	6.3	1.3	2.5
Confusion	4.9	0.0	5.7	7.6
Decreased Concentration	2.8	2.1	1.3	0.0
Disorientation	2.1	0.0	*	0.0
Dizziness/Lightheadedness	19.7	5.3	28.0	15.2
Drowsiness	23.9	6.3	40.8	19.6
Excitement	1.4	1.1	5.1	5.7
Fatigue	11.3	4.2	5.7	2.5
Headache	9.9	5.3	19.8	15.8
Insomnia	9.9	10.5	6.4	12.0
Impaired Memory	1.4	0.0	*	*
Nervousness	14.8	10.5	6.4	8.2
Gastrointestinal				
Abdominal/Gastric Disorder	3.5	4.2	5.7	4.4
Bad Taste in Mouth	1.4	0.0	0.0	0.0
Diarrhea	0.0	1.1	4.5	1.9
Nausea/Vomiting	9.9	1.1	12.7	9.5
Musculoskeletal				
Musculoskeletal Aches/Pains	5.6	3.2	5.1	2.5
Neurological				
Incoordination	4.9	0.0	1.9	0.0
Paresthesia	1.4	0.0	0.0	*
Tremors	2.8	1.1	5.1	3.8
Sexual Function				
Decreased Libido	*	1.1	1.3	*
Other				
Decreased Appetite	3.5	5.3	0.0	*
Eyes Red/Tired/Itching	2.8	0.0	0.0	0.0
Head Full-Heavy	2.8	0.0	0.0	0.0
Malaise	2.8	0.0	0.0	0.0
Nasal/Sinus Congestion	2.8	0.0	5.7	3.2
Nightmares/Vivid Dreams	*	1.1	5.1	5.7
Sweating/Clamminess	1.4	1.1	*	*
Tinnitus	1.4	0.0	0.0	*
Weight Gain	1.4	0.0	4.5	1.9
Weight Loss	*	3.2	5.7	2.5

*Incidence less than 1%.

D = DESYREL   P = Placebo

In addition to the relatively common (ie, greater than 1%) untoward events enumerated above, the following adverse events have been reported to occur in association with the use of DESYREL in the controlled clinical studies: akathisia, allergic reaction, anemia, chest pain, delayed urine flow, early menses, flatulence, hallucinations/delusions, hematuria, hypersalivation, hypomania, impaired speech, impotence, increased appetite, increased libido, increased urinary frequency, missed periods, muscle twitches, numbness, and retrograde ejaculation.

Postintroduction Reports:

Although the following adverse reactions have been reported in DESYREL users, the causal association has neither been confirmed nor refuted.

Voluntary reports received since market introduction include the following: abnormal dreams, agitation, alopecia, anxiety, aphasia, apnea, ataxia, breast enlargement or engorgement, cardiospams, cerebrovascular accident, chills, cholestatis, clitorism, congestive heart failure, diplopia, edema, extrapyramidal symptoms, grand mal seizures, hallucinations, hemolytic anemia, hirsutism, hyperbilirubinema, increased amylase, increased salivation, insomnia, leukocytosis, leukonychia, jaundice, lactation, liver enzyme alterations, methemoglobinemia, nausea/vomiting (most frequently), paresthesia, paranoid rection, priapism (see **WARNINGS** and **PRECAUTIONS, Information for Patients**; some patients have required surgical intervention), pruritus, psoriasis, psychosis, rash, stupor, inappropriate ADH syndrome, tardive dyskinesia, unexplained death, urinary incontinence, urinary retention, urticaria, vasodilation, vertigo, and weakness.

Continued on next page

Apothecon—Cont.

Cardiovascular system effects which have been reported include the following: conduction block, orthostatic hypotension and syncope, palpitations, bradycardia, atrial fibrillation, myocardial infarction, cardiac arrest, arrhythmia, and ventricular ectopic activity, including ventricular tachycardia (see **WARNINGS**).

OVERDOSE

Animal Oral LD_{50}

The oral LD_{50} of the drug is 610 mg/kg in mice, 486 mg/kg in rats, and 560 mg/kg in rabbits.

Signs and Symptoms

Death from overdose has occurred in patients ingesting DESYREL (trazodone hydrochloride) and other drugs concurrently (namely, alcohol; alcohol + chloral hydrate + diazepam; amobarbital; chlordiazepoxide; or meprobamate). The most severe reactions reported to have occurred with overdose of DESYREL alone have been priapism, respiratory arrest, seizures, and EKG changes. The reactions reported most frequently have been drowsiness and vomiting. Overdosage may cause an increase in incidence or severity of any of the reported adverse reactions (see **ADVERSE REACTIONS**).

Treatment

There is no specific antidote for DESYREL. Treatment should be symptomatic and supportive in the case of hypotension or excessive sedation. Any patient suspected of having taken an overdose should have the stomach emptied by gastric lavage. Forced diuresis may be useful in facilitating elimination of the drug.

DOSAGE AND ADMINISTRATION

The dosage should be initiated at a low level and increased gradually, noting the clinical response and any evidence of intolerance. Occurrence of drowsiness may require the administration of a major portion of the daily dose at bedtime or a reduction of dosage. DESYREL should be taken shortly after a meal or light snack. Symptomatic relief may be seen during the first week, with optimal antidepressant effects typically evident within two weeks. Twenty-five percent of those who respond to DESYREL require more than two weeks (up to four weeks) of drug administration.

Usual Adult Dosage

An initial dose of 150 mg/day in divided doses is suggested. The dose may be increased by 50 mg/day every three to four days. The maximum dose for outpatients usually should not exceed 400 mg/day in divided doses. Inpatients (i.e., more severely depressed patients) may be given up to but not in excess of 600 mg/day in divided doses.

Maintenance

Dosage during prolonged maintenance therapy should be kept at the lowest effective level. Once an adequate response has been achieved, dosage may be gradually reduced, with subsequent adjustment depending on therapeutic response. Although there has been no systematic evaluation of the efficacy of DESYREL beyond six weeks, it is generally recommended that a course of antidepressant drug treatment should be continued for several months.

HOW SUPPLIED

DESYREL® (trazodone hydrochloride)

Tablets, **50 mg**—round, orange/scored, film-sealed (debossed with **DESYREL** and **MJ 775**)

NDC 0087-0775-41 Bottles of 100
NDC 0087-0775-43 Bottles of 1000
NDC 0087-0775-42 Cartons of 100 Unit Doses

Tablets, **100 mg**—round, white/scored, film-sealed (debossed with **DESYREL** and **MJ 776**)

NDC 0087-0776-41 Bottles of 100
NDC 0087-0776-43 Bottles of 1000
NDC 0087-0776-42 Cartons of 100 Unit Doses

Tablets, **150 mg**—orange, in the Dividose® tablet design (debossed with **MJ** and **778** on front; "**50**," "**50**," "**50**" on reverse)

NDC 0087-0778-43 Bottles of 100
NDC 0087-0778-44 Bottles of 500

Tablets, **300 mg**—yellow, in the Dividose® tablet design (debossed with **MJ** and **796** on front; "**100**," "**100**," "**100**" on reverse)

NDC 0087-0796-41 Bottles of 100

U.S. Patent Nos. 4,215,104
4,258,027

Storage

Store at room temperature. Protect from temperatures above 104°F (40°C). Dispense in tight, light-resistant container (USP).

Caution: Federal law prohibits dispensing without prescription.

REFERENCES

a. Williams JBW, Ed: Diagnostic and Statistical Manual of Mental Disorders-III, American Psychiatric Association, May, 1980.
b. Lue TF, Physiology of erection and pathophysiology of impotence. In: Wash PC, Retik AB, Stamey TA, Vaughan ED, eds. Campbell's Urology. Sixth edition. Philadelphia: W.B. Saunders; 1992: 722–725.
c. Goldstein I, Krane RJ, Diagnosis and therapy of erectile dysfunction. In: Wash PC, Retik AB, Stamey TA, Vaughan ED, eds. Campbell's Urology. Sixth edition. Philadelphia: W.B. Saunders: 1992: 3071–3072.
d. Yealy DM, Hogya PT: Priapism. *Emerg Med Clin North Am.* 1988; 6:509–520.
e. Banos JE, Bosch F, Farre M, Drug-induced priapism. Its aetiology, incidence and treatment. *Med Toxicol Adverse Drug Exp.* 1989; 4:46–58.
f. O'Brien WM, O'Connor KP, Lynch JH. Priapism: current concepts. *Ann Emerg Med.* 1989: 980–983.
g. Bardin ED, Krieger JN. Pharmacological priapism: comparison of trazodone- and papaverine-associated cases. *Int Urol Nephrol.* 1990; 22:147–152.

Revised: October 1993 P5319-00

FLORINEF® ACETATE ℞
Fludrocortisone Acetate Tablets USP

DESCRIPTION

Florinef Acetate (Fludrocortisone Acetate Tablets USP) contains fludrocortisone acetate, a synthetic adrenocortical steroid possessing very potent mineralocorticoid properties and high glucocorticoid activity; it is used only for its mineralocorticoid effects. The chemical name for fludrocortisone acetate is 9-fluoro-11β, 17, 21-trihydroxypregn-4-ene-3,20-dione 21-acetate; its graphic formula is:

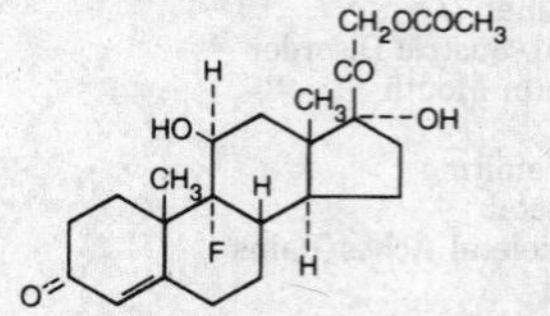

$C_{23}H_{31}FO_6$ MW422.49

Florinef Acetate is available for oral administration as scored tablets providing 0.1 mg fludrocortisone acetate per tablet. Inactive ingredients: calcium phosphate, color additive (D&C Red No. 27), corn starch, lactose, magnesium stearate, sodium benzoate, and talc.

CLINICAL PHARMACOLOGY

Corticosteroids are thought to act, at least in part, by controlling the rate of synthesis of proteins. Although there are a number of instances in which the synthesis of specific proteins is known to be induced by corticosteroids, the links between the initial actions of the hormones and the final metabolic effects have not been completely elucidated.

The physiologic action of fludrocortisone acetate is similar to that of hydrocortisone. However, the effects of fludrocotisone acetate, particularly on electrolyte balance, but also on carbohydrate metabolism, are considerably heightened and prolonged. Mineralocorticoids act on the distal tubules of the kidney to enhance the reabsorption of sodium ions from the tubular fluid into the plasma; they increase the urinary excretion of both potassium and hydrogen ions. The consequence of these three primary effects together with similar actions on cation transport in other tissues appear to account for the entire spectrum of physiological activities that are characteristic of mineralocorticoids. In small oral doses, fludrocortisone acetate produces marked sodium retention and increased urinary potassium excretion. It also causes a rise in blood pressure, apparently because of these effects on electrolyte levels.

In larger doses, fludrocortisone acetate inhibits endogenous adrenal cortical secretion, thymic activity, and pituitary corticotropin excretion; promotes the deposition of liver glycogen; and, unless protein intake is adequate, induces negative nitrogen balance.

The approximate plasma half-life of fludrocortisone (fluorohydrocortisone) is 3.5 hours or more and the biological half-life is 18 to 36 hours.

INDICATIONS AND USAGE

Florinef Acetate is indicated as partial replacement therapy for primary and secondary adrenocortical insufficiency in Addison's disease and for the treatment of salt-losing adrenogenital syndrome.

CONTRAINDICATIONS

Corticosteroids are contraindicated in patients with systemic fungal infections and in those with a history of possible or known hypersensitivity to these agents.

WARNINGS

BECAUSE OF ITS MARKED EFFECT ON SODIUM RETENTION, THE USE OF FLUDROCORTISONE ACETATE IN THE TREATMENT OF CONDITIONS OTHER THAN THOSE INDICATED HEREIN IS NOT ADVISED.

Corticosteroids may mask some signs of infection, and new infections may appear during their use. There may be decreased resistance and inability to localize infection when corticosteroids are used. If an infection occurs during fludrocortisone acetate therapy, it should be promptly controlled by suitable antimicrobial therapy.

Prolonged use of corticosteroids may produce posterior subcapsular cataracts, glaucoma with possible damage to the optic nerves, and may enhance the establishment of secondary ocular infections due to fungi or viruses.

Average and large doses of hydrocortisone or cortisone can cause elevation of blood pressure, salt and water retention, and increased excretion of potassium. These effects are less likely to occur with the synthetic derivatives except when used in large doses. However, since fludrocortisone acetate is a potent mineralocorticoid, both the dosage and salt intake should be carefully monitored in order to avoid the development of hypertension, edema, or weight gain. **Periodic checking of serum electrolyte levels is advisable during prolonged therapy; dietary salt restriction and potassium supplementation may be necessary.** All corticosteroids increase calcium excretion.

Patients should not be vaccinated against smallpox while on corticosteroid therapy. Other immunization procedures should not be undertaken in patients who are on corticosteroids, especially on high dose, because of possible hazards of neurological complications and a lack of antibody response.

The use of Florinef Acetate (Fludrocortisone Acetate Tablets USP) in patients with active tuberculosis should be restricted to those cases of fulminating or disseminated tuberculosis in which the corticosteroid is used for the management of the disease in conjunction with an appropriate antituberculous regimen. If corticosteroids are indicated in patients with latent tuberculosis or tuberculin reactivity, close observation is necessary since reactivation of the disease may occur. During prolonged corticosteroid therapy these patients should receive chemoprophylaxis.

Children who are on immunosuppressant drugs are more susceptible to infections than healthy children. Chicken pox and measles, for example, can have a more serious or even fatal course in children on immunosuppressant corticosteroids. In such children, or in adults who have not had these diseases, particular care should be taken to avoid exposure. If exposed, therapy with varicella zoster immune globulin (VZIG) or pooled intravenous immunoglobulin (IVIG), as appropriate, may be indicated. If chicken pox develops, treatment with antiviral agents may be considered.

PRECAUTIONS

General

Adverse reactions to corticosteroids may be produced by too rapid withdrawal or by continued use of large doses.

To avoid drug-induced adrenal insufficiency, supportive dosage may be required in times of stress (such as trauma, surgery, or severe illness) both during treatment with fludrocortisone acetate and for a year afterwards.

There is an enhanced corticosteroid effect in patients with hypothyroidism and in those with cirrhosis.

Corticosteroids should be used cautiously in patients with ocular herpes simplex because of possible corneal perforation.

The lowest possible dose of corticosteroid should be used to control the condition being treated. A gradual reduction in dosage should be made when possible.

Psychic derangements may appear when corticosteroids are used. These may range from euphoria, insomnia, mood swings, personality changes, and severe depression to frank psychotic manifestations. Existing emotional instability or psychotic tendencies may also be aggravated by corticosteroids.

Aspirin should be used cautiously in conjunction with corticosteroids in patients with hypoprothrombinemia.

Corticosteroids should be used with caution in patients with nonspecific ulcerative colitis if there is a probability of impending perforation, abscess, or other pyogenic infection. Corticosteroids should also be used cautiously in patients with diverticulitis, fresh intestinal anastomoses, active or latent peptic ulcer, renal insufficiency, hypertension, osteoporosis, and myasthenia gravis.

Information for Patients

The physician should advise the patient to report any medical history of heart disease, high blood pressure, or kidney or liver disease and to report current use of any medicines to determine if these medicines might interact adversely with fludrocortisone acetate (see **Drug Interactions**).

Patients who are on immunosuppressant doses of corticosteroids should be warned to avoid exposure to chicken pox or measles and, if exposed, to obtain medical advice.

The patient's understanding of his steroid-dependent status and increased dosage requirement under widely variable conditions of stress is vital. Advise the patient to carry medical identification indicating his dependence on steroid medication and, if necessary, instruct him to carry an adequate supply of medication for use in emergencies.

Stress to the patient the importance of regular follow-up visits to check his progress and the need to promptly notify

the physician of dizziness, severe or continuing headaches, swelling of feet or lower legs, or unusual weight gain.
Advise the patient to use the medicine only as directed, to take a missed dose as soon as possible, unless it is almost time for the next dose, and not to double the next dose.
Inform the patient to keep this medication and all drugs out of the reach of children.

Laboratory Tests
Patients should be monitored regularly for blood pressure determinations and serum electrolyte determinations (see **WARNINGS**).

Drug Interactions
When administered concurrently, the following drugs may interact with adrenal corticosteroids.
Amphotericin B or potassium-depleting diuretics (benzothiadiazines and related drugs, ethacrynic acid and furosemide)—enhanced hypokalemia. Check serum potassium levels at frequent intervals; use potassium supplements if necessary (see **WARNINGS**).
Digitalis glycosides—enhanced possibility of arrhythmias or digitalis toxicity associated with hypokalemia. Monitor serum potassium levels; use potassium supplements if necessary.
Oral anticoagulants—decreased prothrombin time response. Monitor prothrombin levels and adjust anticoagulant dosage accordingly.
Antidiabetic drugs (oral agents and insulin)—diminished antidiabetic effect. Monitor for symptoms of hyperglycemia; adjust dosage of antidiabetic drug upward if necessary.
Aspirin—increased ulcerogenic effect; decreased pharmacologic effect of aspirin. Rarely salicylate toxicity may occur in patients who discontinue steroids after concurrent high-dose aspirin therapy. Monitor salicylate levels or the therapeutic effect for which aspirin is given; adjust salicylate dosage accordingly if effect is altered (see **PRECAUTIONS, General**).
Barbiturates, phenytoin, or rifampin—increased metabolic clearance of fludrocortisone acetate because of the induction of hepatic enzymes. Observe the patient for possible diminished effect of steroid and increase the steroid dosage accordingly.
Anabolic steroids (particularly C-17 alkylated androgens such as oxymetholone, methandrostenolone, norethandrolone, and similar compounds)—enhanced tendency toward edema. Use caution when giving these drugs together, especially in patients with hepatic or cardiac disease.
Vaccines—neurological complications and lack of antibody response (see **WARNINGS**).
Estrogen—increased levels of corticosteroid-binding globulin, thereby increasing the bound (inactive) fraction; this effect is at least balanced by decreased metabolism of corticosteroids. When estrogen therapy is initiated, a reduction in corticosteroid dosage may be required, and increased amounts may be required when estrogen is terminated.

Drug/Laboratory Test Interactions
Corticosteroids may affect the nitrobluetetrazolium test for bacterial infection and produce false-negative results.

Carcinogenesis, Mutagenesis, Impairment of Fertility
Adequate studies have not been performed in animals to determine whether fludrocortisone acetate has carcinogenic or mutagenic activity or whether it affects fertility in males or females.

Pregnancy. Category C.
Adequate animal reproduction studies have not been conducted with fludrocortisone acetate. However, many corticosteroids have been shown to be teratogenic in laboratory animals at low doses. Teratogenicity of these agents in man has not been demonstrated. It is not known whether fludrocortisone acetate can cause fetal harm when administered to a pregnant woman or can affect reproduction capacity. Fludrocortisone acetate should be given to a pregnant woman only if clearly needed.

Pregnancy. Nonteratogenic Effects.
Infants born of mothers who have received substantial doses of fludrocortisone acetate during pregnancy should be carefully observed for signs of hypoadrenalism.
Maternal treatment with corticosteroids should be carefully documented in the infant's medical records to assist in follow up.

Nursing Mothers
Corticosteroids are found in the breast milk of lactating women receiving systemic therapy with these agents. Caution should be exercised when fludrocortisone acetate is administered to a nursing woman.

Pediatric Use
Safety and effectiveness in children have not been established.
Growth and development of infants and children on prolonged corticosteroid therapy should be carefully observed.

ADVERSE REACTIONS
Most adverse reactions are caused by the drug's mineralocorticoid activity (retention of sodium and water) and include hypertension, edema, cardiac enlargement, congestive heart failure, potassium loss, and hypokalemic alkalosis.
When fludrocortisone is used in the small dosages recommended, the glucocorticoid side effects often seen with cortisone and its derivatives are not usually a problem; however the following untoward effects should be kept in mind, particularly when fludrocortisone is used over a prolonged period of time or in conjunction with cortisone or a similar glucocorticoid.
Musculoskeletal—muscle weakness, steroid myopathy, loss of muscle mass, osteoporosis, vertebral compression fractures, aseptic necrosis of femoral and humeral heads, pathologic fracture of long bones, and spontaneous fractures.
Gastrointestinal—peptic ulcer with possible perforation and hemorrhage, pancreatitis, abdominal distention, and ulcerative esophagitis.
Dermatologic—impaired wound healing, thin fragile skin, bruising, petechiae and ecchymoses, facial erythema, increased sweating, subcutaneous fat atrophy, purpura, striae, hyperpigmentation of the skin and nails, hirsutism, acneiform eruptions, and hives and/or allergic skin rash; reactions to skin tests may be suppressed.
Neurological—convulsions, increased intracranial pressure with papilledema (pseudotumor cerebri) usually after treatment, vertigo, headache, and severe mental disturbances.
Endocrine—menstrual irregularities, development of the cushingoid state; suppression of growth in children; secondary adrenocortical and pituitary unresponsiveness, particularly in times of stress (e.g., trauma, surgery, or illness); decreased carbohydrate tolerance; manifestations of latent diabetes mellitus; and increased requirements for insulin or oral hypoglycemic agents in diabetics.
Ophthalmic—posterior subcapsular cataracts, increased intraocular pressure, glaucoma, and exophthalmos.
Metabolic—hyperglycemia, glycosuria, and negative nitrogen balance due to protein catabolism.
Other adverse reactions that may occur following the administration of a corticosteroid are necrotizing angiitis, thrombophlebitis, aggravation or masking of infections, insomnia, syncopal episodes, and anaphylactoid reactions.

OVERDOSAGE
Development of hypertension, edema, hypokalemia, excessive increase in weight, and increase in heart size are signs of overdosage of fludrocortisone acetate. When these are noted, administration of the drug should be discontinued, after which the symptoms will usually subside within several days; subsequent treatment with fludrocortisone acetate should be with a reduced dose. Muscular weakness may develop due to excessive potassium loss and can be treated by administering a potassium supplement. Regular monitoring of blood pressure and serum electrolytes can help to prevent overdosage (see **WARNINGS**).

DOSAGE AND ADMINISTRATION
Dosage depends on the severity of the disease and the response of the patient. Patients should be continually monitored for signs that indicate dosage adjustment is necessary, such as remissions or exacerbations of the disease and stress (surgery, infection, trauma) (see **WARNINGS** and **PRECAUTIONS, General**).

Addison's Disease
In Addison's disease, the combination of Florinef Acetate (Fludrocortisone Acetate Tablets USP) with a glucocorticoid such as hydrocortisone or cortisone provides substitution therapy approximating normal adrenal activity with minimal risks of unwanted effects.
The usual dose is 0.1 mg of Florinef Acetate daily, although dosage ranging from 0.1 mg three times a week to 0.2 mg daily has been employed. In the event transient hypertension develops as a consequence of therapy, the dose should be reduced to 0.05 mg daily. Florinef Acetate is preferably administered in conjunction with cortisone (10 mg to 37.5 mg daily in divided doses) or hydrocortisone (10 mg to 30 mg daily in divided doses).

Salt-Losing Adrenogenital Syndrome
The recommended dosage for treating the salt-losing adrenogenital syndrome is 0.1 mg to 0.2 mg of Florinef Acetate daily.

HOW SUPPLIED
Florinef Acetate Tablets (Fludrocortisone Acetate Tablets USP), 0.1 mg/tablet: light pink, round, biconvex, scored tablets in bottles of 100 (NDC 0003-0429-50); identification no. **429.**

Storage
Store at room temperature; avoid excessive heat.
CAUTION: Federal law prohibits dispensing without prescription.

Apothecon®
A Bristol-Myers Squibb Co.
Princeton, NJ 08540

P3345-00 Revised November 1991 P3345-00

FUNGIZONE® INTRAVENOUS ℞
Amphotericin B For Injection USP

WARNING
This drug should be used *primarily* for treatment of patients with progressive and potentially life-threatening fungal infections; it should not be used to treat noninvasive forms of fungal disease such as oral thrush, vaginal candidiasis and esophegeal candidiasis in patients with normal neutrophil counts.

DESCRIPTION
FUNGIZONE Intravenous (Amphotericin B for Injection) contains amphotericin B, an antifungal polyene antibiotic obtained from a strain of *Streptomyces nodosus.* Amphotericin B is designated chemically as [1R-(1R*,3S*,5R*,6R*,9R*, 11R*,15S*,16R*, 17R*,18S*,19E,21E,23E,25E,27E,29E,31E, 33R*,35S*,36R*,37S*)]-33-[(3-Amino-3,6-dideoxy-β-D-mannopyranosyl)-oxy]-1,3,5,6,9,11,17,37-octahydroxy-15,16, 18-trimethyl-13-oxo-14,39-dioxabicyclol[33.3.1] nonatriaconta-19,21,23,25,27,29,31-heptaene-36-carboxylic acid. Structural formula:

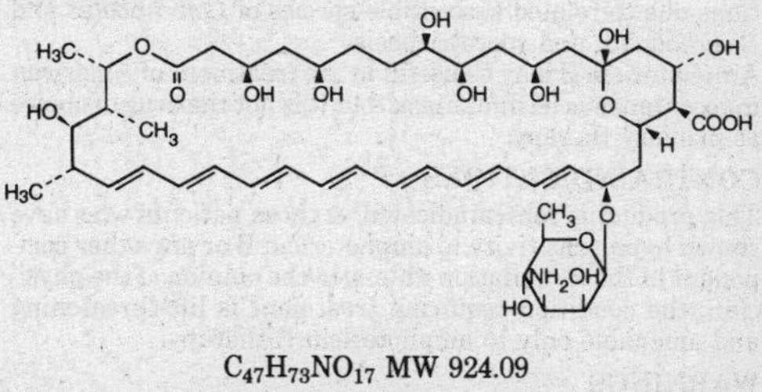

$C_{47}H_{73}NO_{17}$ MW 924.09

Each vial contains a sterile, nonpyrogenic, lyophilized cake (which may partially reduce to powder following manufacture) providing 50 mg amphotericin B and 41 mg sodium desoxycholate with 20.2 mg sodium phosphates as a buffer. Crystalline amphotericin B is insoluble in water; therefore, the antibiotic is solubilized by the addition of sodium desoxycholate to form a mixture which provides a colloidal dispersion for intravenous infusion following reconstitution.
At the time of manufacture the air in the vial is replaced by nitrogen.

CLINICAL PHARMACOLOGY
Microbiology
Amphotericin B shows a high order of *in vitro* activity against many species of fungi. *Histoplasma capsulatum, Coccidioides immitis, Candida* species, *Blastomyces dermatitidis, Rhodotorula, Cryptococcus neoformans, Sporothrix schenckii, Mucor mucedo,* and *Aspergillus fumigatus* are all inhibited by concentrations of amphotericin B ranging from 0.03 to 1.0 mcg/mL *in vitro.* While *Candida albicans* is generally quite susceptible to amphotericin B, non-*albicans* species may be less susceptible. *Pseudallescheria boydii* and *Fusarium* sp. are often resistant to amphotericin B. The antibiotic is without effect on bacteria, rickettsiae, and viruses.

Susceptibility Testing
Standardized techniques for susceptibility testing for antifungal agents have not been established and results of susceptibility studies have not been correlated with clinical outcomes.

Pharmacokinetics
Amphotericin B is fungistatic or fungicidal depending on the concentration obtained in body fluids and the susceptibility of the fungus. The drug acts by binding to sterols in the cell membrane of susceptible fungi with a resultant change in membrane permeability allowing leakage of intracellular components. Mammalian cell membranes also contain sterols and it has been suggested that the damage to human cells and fungal cells may share common mechanisms.
An initial intravenous infusion of 1 to 5 mg of amphotericin B per day, gradually increased to 0.4 to 0.6 mg/kg daily, produces peak plasma concentrations ranging from approximately 0.5 to 2 mcg/mL. Following a rapid initial fall, plasma concentrations plateau at about 0.5 mcg/mL. An elimination half-life of approximately 15 days follows an initial plasma half-life of about 24 hours. Amphotericin B circulating in plasma is highly bound (>90%) to plasma proteins and is poorly dialyzable. Approximately two thirds of concurrent plasma concentrations have been detected in fluids from inflamed pleura, peritoneum, synovium, and aqueous humor. Concentrations in the cerebrospinal fluid seldom exceed 2.5 percent of those in the plasma. Little amphotericin B penetrates into vitreous humor or normal amniotic fluid. Complete details of tissue distribution are not known.
Amphotericin B is excreted very slowly (over weeks to months) by the kidneys with two to five percent of a given

Continued on next page

Apothecon—Cont.

dose being excreted in the biologically active form. Details of possible metabolic pathways are not known. After treatment is discontinued, the drug can be detected in the urine for at least seven weeks due to the slow disappearance of the drug. The cumulative urinary output over a seven day period amounts to approximately 40 percent of the amount of drug infused.

INDICATIONS AND USAGE

FUNGIZONE Intravenous (Amphotericin B for Injection USP) should be administered primarily to patients with progressive, potentially life-threatening fungal infections. This potent drug should not be used to treat noninvasive fungal infections, such as oral thrush, vaginal candidiasis and esophageal candidiasis in patients with normal neutrophil counts.

FUNGIZONE Intravenous is specifically intended to treat potentially life-threatening fungal infections: aspergillosis, cryptococcosis (torulosis), North American blastomycosis, systemic candidiasis, coccidioidomycosis, histoplasmosis, zygomycosis including mucormycosis due to susceptible species of the genera *Absidia, Mucor* and *Rhizopus,* and infections due to related susceptible species of *Conidiobolus* and *Basidiobolus,* and sporotrichosis.

Amphotericin B may be useful in the treatment of American mucocutaneous leishmaniasis, but it is not the drug of choice as primary therapy.

CONTRAINDICATIONS

This product is contraindicated in those patients who have shown hypersensitivity to amphotericin B or any other component in the formulation unless, in the opinion of the physician, the condition requiring treatment is life-threatening and amenable only to amphotericin B therapy.

WARNINGS

Amphotericin B is frequently the only effective treatment available for potentially life-threatening fungal disease. In each case, its possible life-saving benefit must be balanced against its untoward and dangerous side effects.

PRECAUTIONS

General

Amphotericin B should be administered intravenously under close-clinical observation by medically trained personnel. It should be reserved for treatment of patients with progressive, potentially life-threatening fungal infections due to susceptible organisms (see **INDICATIONS AND USAGE**).

Acute reactions including fever, shaking chills, hypotension, anorexia, nausea, vomiting, headache, and tachypnea are common 1 to 3 hours after starting an intravenous infusion. These reactions are usually more severe with the first few doses of amphotericin B and usually diminish with subsequent doses.

Rapid intravenous infusion has been associated with hypotension, hypokalemia, arrhythmias, and shock and should, therefore, be avoided (see **DOSAGE AND ADMINISTRATION**).

Amphotericin B should be used with care in patients with reduced renal function; frequent monitoring of renal function is recommended (see **PRECAUTIONS, Laboratory Tests** and **ADVERSE REACTIONS**). In some patients hydration and sodium repletion prior to amphotericin B administration may reduce the risk of developing nephrotoxicity. Supplemental alkali medication may decrease renal tubular acidosis complications.

Since acute pulmonary reactions have been reported in patients given amphotericin B during or shortly after leukocyte tranfusions, it is advisable to temporally separate these infusions as far as possible and to monitor pulmonary function (see **PRECAUTIONS, Drug Interactions**).

Leukoencephalopathy has been reported following use of amphotericin B. Literature reports have suggested that total body irradiation may be a predisposition.

Whenever medication is interrupted for a period longer than seven days, therapy should be resumed by starting with the lowest dosage level, e.g., 0.25 mg/kg of body weight, and increased gradually as outlined under **DOSAGE AND ADMINISTRATION.**

Laboratory Tests

Renal function should be monitored frequently during amphotericin B therapy (see **ADVERSE REACTIONS**). It is also advisable to monitor on a regular basis liver function, serum electrolytes (particularly magnesium and potassium), blood counts, and hemoglobin concentrations. Laboratory test results should be used as a guide to subsequent dosage adjustments.

Drug Interactions

When administered concurrently, the following drugs may interact with amphotericin B:

Antineoplastic agents: may enhance the potential for renal toxicity, bronchospasm and hypotension. Antineoplastic agents (e.g., nitrogen mustard, etc.) should be given concomitantly only with great caution.

Corticosteroids and Corticotropin (ACTH): may potentiate amphotericin B-induced hypokalemia which may predispose the patient to cardiac dysfunction. Avoid concomitant use unless necessary to control side effects of amphotericin B. If used concomitantly, closely monitor serum electrolytes and cardiac function (see **ADVERSE REACTIONS**).

Digitalis glycosides: amphotericin B-induced hypokalemia may potentiate digitalis toxicity. Serum potassium levels and cardiac function should be closely monitored and any deficit promptly corrected.

Flucytosine: while a synergistic relationship with amphotericin B has been reported, concomitant use may increase the toxicity of flucytosine by possibly increasing its cellular uptake and/or impairing its renal excretion.

Imidazoles (e.g., ketoconazole, miconazole, clotrimazole, fluconazole, etc.): In vitro and animal studies with the combination of amphotericin B and imidazoles suggest that imidazoles may induce fungal resistance to amphotericin B. Combination therapy should be administered with caution, especially in immunocompromised patients.

Other nephrotoxic medications: agents such as aminoglycosides, cyclosporine, and pentamidine may enhance the potential for drug-induced renal toxicity, and should be used concomitantly only with great caution. Intensive monitoring of renal function is recommended in patients requiring any combination of nephrotoxic medications (see **PRECAUTIONS, Laboratory Tests**).

Skeletal muscle relaxants: amphotericin B-induced hypokalemia may enhance the curariform effect of skeletal muscle relaxants (e.g., tubocurarine). Serum potassium levels should be monitored and deficiencies corrected.

Leukocyte transfusions: acute pulmonary toxicity has been reported in patients receiving intravenous amphotericin B and leukocyte transfusions (see **PRECAUTIONS, General**).

Carcinogenesis, Mutagenesis, Impairment of Fertility

No long-term studies in animals have been performed to evaluate carcinogenic potential. There also have been no studies to determine mutagenicity or whether this medication affects fertility in males or females.

Pregnancy: Teratogenic Effects, Pregnancy Category B

Reproduction studies in animals have revealed no evidence of harm to the fetus due to amphotericin B for injection. Systemic fungal infections have been successfully treated in pregnant women with amphotericin B for injection without obvious effects to the fetus, but the number of cases reported has been small. Because animal reproduction studies are not always predictive of human response, and adequate and well-controlled studies have not been conducted in pregnant women, this drug should be used during pregnancy only if clearly indicated.

Nursing Mothers

It is not known whether amphotericin B is excreted in human milk. Because many drugs are excreted in human milk and considering the potential toxicity of amphotericin B, it is prudent to advise a nursing mother to discontinue nursing.

Pediatric Use

Safety and effectiveness in pediatric patients have not been established through adequate and well-controlled studies. Systemic fungal infections have been successfully treated in pediatric patients without reports of unusual side effects. Amphotericin B for Injection when administered to pediatric patients should be limited to the smallest dose compatible with an effective therapeutic regimen.

ADVERSE REACTIONS

Although some patients may tolerate full intravenous doses of amphotericin B without difficulty, most will exhibit some intolerance, often at less than the full therapeutic dose.

Tolerance may be improved by treatment with aspirin, antipyretics (e.g., acetaminophen), antihistamines, or antiemetics. Meperidine (25 to 50 mg IV) has been shown in some patients to decrease the duration of shaking chills and fever that may accompany the infusion of amphotericin B.

Administration of amphotericin B on alternate days may decrease anorexia and phlebitis.

Intravenous administration of small doses of adrenal corticosteroids just prior to or during the amphotericin B infusion may help decrease febrile reactions. Dosage and duration of such corticosteroid therapy should be kept to a minimum (see **PRECAUTIONS, Drug Interactions**).

Addition of heparin (1000 units per infusion), and the use of a pediatric scalp-vein needle may lessen the incidence of thrombophlebitis. Extravasation may cause chemical irritation.

The adverse reactions most commonly observed are:

General (body as a whole): fever (sometimes accompanied by shaking chills usually occurring within 15 to 20 minutes after initiation of treatment); malaise; weight loss.

Cardiopulmonary: hypotension; tachypnea.

Gastrointestinal: anorexia; nausea; vomiting; diarrhea; dyspepsia; cramping epigastric pain.

Hematologic: normochromic, normocytic anemia.

Local: pain at the injection site with or without phlebitis or thrombophlebitis.

Musculoskeletal: generalized pain, including muscle and joint pains.

Neurologic: headache.

Renal: **decreased** renal function and renal function abnormalities including: azotemia, hypokalemia, hyposthenuria, renal tubular acidosis; and nephrocalcinosis. These usually improve with interruption of therapy. However, some permanent impairment often occurs, especially in those patients receiving large amounts (over 5 g) of amphotericin B or receiving other nephrotoxic agents. In some patients hydration and sodium repletion prior to amphotericin B administration may reduce the risk of developing nephrotoxicity. Supplemental alkali medication may decrease renal tubular acidosis.

The following adverse reactions have also been reported:

General (body as a whole): flushing.

Allergic: anaphylactoid and other allergic reactions; bronchospasm; wheezing.

Cardiopulmonary: cardiac arrest; shock; cardiac failure; pulmonary edema; hypersensitivity pneumonitis; arrhythmias, including ventricular fibrillation; dyspnea; hypertension.

Dermatologic: rash, in particular maculopapular; pruritis.

Gastrointestinal: acute liver failure; hepatitis; jaundice; hemorrhagic gastroenteritis; melena.

Hematologic: agranulocytosis; coagulation defects; thrombocytopenia; leukopenia; eosinophilia; leukocytosis.

Neurologic: convulsions; hearing loss; tinnitus; transient vertigo; visual impairment; diplopia; peripheral neuropathy; encephalopathy (see **PRECAUTIONS**); other neurologic symptoms.

Renal: acute renal failure; anuria; oliguria.

Altered Laboratory Findings

Serum Electrolytes: Hypomagnesemia; hypo- and hyperkalemia; hypocalcemia.

Liver Function Tests: Elevations of AST, ALT, GGT, bilirubin, and alkaline phosphatase.

Renal Function Tests: Elevations of BUN and serum creatinine.

OVERDOSAGE

Amphotericin B overdoses can result in cardio-respiratory arrest. If an overdose is suspected, discontinue therapy and monitor the patient's clinical status (e.g., cardio-respiratory, renal, and liver function, hematologic status, serum electrolytes) and administer supportive therapy, as required. Amphotericin B is not hemodialyzable.

Prior to reinstituting therapy, the patient's condition should be stabilized (including correction of electrolyte deficiencies, etc.).

DOSAGE AND ADMINISTRATION

CAUTION: Under no circumstances should a total daily dose of 1.5 mg/kg be exceeded. Amphotericin B overdoses can result in cardio-respiratory arrest (see OVERDOSAGE).

FUNGIZONE Intravenous should be administered by *slow* intravenous infusion. Intravenous infusion should be given over a period of approximately 2 to 6 hours (depending on the dose) observing the usual precautions for intravenous therapy (see **PRECAUTIONS, General**). The recommended concentration for intravenous infusion is 0.1 mg/mL (1 mg/10 mL).

Since patient tolerance varies greatly, the dosage of amphotericin B must be individualized and adjusted according to the patient's clinical status (e.g., site and severity of infection, etiologic agent, cardio-renal function, etc.).

A single intravenous **test dose** (1 mg in 20 mL of 5% dextrose solution) administered over 20–30 minutes may be preferred. The patient's temperature, pulse, respiration, and blood pressure should be recorded every 30 minutes for 2 to 4 hours.

In patients with **good cardi-renal function** and a **well tolerated test dose,** therapy is usually initiated with a daily dose of 0.25 mg/kg of body weight. However, in those patients having **severe and rapidly progressive fungal infection,** therapy may be initiated with a daily dose of 0.3 mg/kg of body weight. In patients with **impaired cardio-renal function** or a **severe reaction to the test dose,** therapy should be initiated with smaller daily doses (i.e., 5 to 10 mg).

Depending on the patient's cardio-renal status (see **PRECAUTIONS, Laboratory Tests**), doses may gradually be increased by 5 to 10 mg per day to final daily dosage of 0.5 to 0.7 mg/kg.

There are insufficient data presently available to define total dosage requirements and duration of treatment necessary for eradication of specific mycoses. The optimal dose is unknown. Total daily dosage may range up to 1.0 mg/kg per day or up to 1.5 mg/kg when given on alternate days.

Sporotrichosis: Therapy with intravenous amphotericin B for sporotrichosis has ranged up to nine months with a total dose up to 2.5 g.

Aspergillosis: Aspergillosis has been treated with amphotericin B intravenously for a period up to eleven months with a total dose up to 3.6 g.

Rhinocerebral phycomycosis: This fulminating disease, generally occurs in association with diabetic ketoacidosis. It is, therefore, imperative that diabetic control be restored in order for treatment with FUNGIZONE Intravenous to be

successful. In contradistinction, pulmonary phycomycosis, which is more common in association with hematologic malignancies, is often an incidental finding at autopsy. A cumulative dose of at least 3 g of amphotericin B is recommended to treat rhinocerebral phycomycosis. Although a total dose of 3 to 4 g will infrequently cause lasting renal impairment, this would seem a reasonable minimum where there is clinical evidence of invasion of deep tissue. Since rhinocerebral phycomycosis usually follows a rapidly fatal course, the therapeutic approach must necessarily be more aggressive than that used in more indolent mycoses.

Preparation of Solutions

Reconstitute as follows: An initial concentrate of 5 mg amphotericin B per mL is first prepared by rapidly expressing 10 mL Sterile Water for Injection USP *without a bacteriostatic agent* directly into the lyophillized cake, using a sterile needle (minimum diameter: 20 gauge) and syringe. Shake the vial immediately until the colloidal solution is clear. The infusion solution, providing 0.1 mg amphotericin B per mL, is then obtained by further dilution (1:50) with 5% Dextrose Injection USP *of pH above 4.2.* The pH of each container of Dextrose Injection should be ascertained before use. Commercial Dextrose Injection usually has a pH above 4.2; however, if it is below 4.2, then 1 or 2 mL of buffer should be added to the Dextrose Injection before it is used to dilute the concentrated solution of amphotericin B. The recommended buffer has the following composition:

Dibasic sodium phosphate (anhydrous)	1.59 g
Monobasic sodium phosphate (anhydrous)	0.96 g
Water for Injection USP	qs 100.0 mL

The buffer should be sterilized before it is added to the Dextrose Injection, either by filtration through a bacterial retentive stone, mat, or membrane, or by autoclaving for 30 minutes at 15 lb pressure (121°C).

CAUTION: Aseptic technique must be strictly observed in all handling, since no preservative or bacteriostatic agent is present in the antibiotic or in the materials used to prepare it for administration. All entries into the vial or into the diluents must be made with a sterile needle. Do not reconstitute with saline solutions. The use of any diluent other than the ones recommended or the presence of a bacteriostatic agent (e.g., benzyl alcohol) in the diluent may cause precipitation of the antibiotic. Do not use the initial concentrate or the infusion solution if there is any evidence of precipitation or foreign matter in either one.

An in-line membrane filter may be used for intravenous infusion of amphotercin B; however, the mean pore diameter of the filter should not be less than 1.0 micron in order to assure passage of the antibiotic dispersion.

HOW SUPPLIED

FUNGIZONE Intravenous (Amphotericin B for Injection USP) Available as single vials providing 50 mg amphotericin B as a yellow to orange lyophilized cake (which may partially reduce to powder following manufacture). NDC 0003-0437-30.

Storage

Prior to reconstitution FUNGIZONE Intravenous should be stored in the refrigerator, protected against exposure to light. The concentrate (5 mg amphotericin B per mL after reconstitution with 10 mL Sterile Water for Injection USP) may be stored in the dark, at room temperature for 24 hours, or at refrigerator temperatures for one week with minimal loss of potency and clarity. Any unused material should then be discarded. Solutions prepared for intravenous infusion (0.1 mg or less amphotericin B per mL) should be used promptly after preparation and should be protected from light during administration.

CAUTION: Federal law prohibits dispensing without prescription.

Apothecon®
A Bristol-Myers Squibb Co.
Princeton, NJ 08540
J4-481B   Revised September 1993   J4-481B

K-LYTE® ℞
[k′ līt]
Effervescent Tablets

Each tablet in solution provides 25 mEq (978 mg) potassium as bicarbonate and citrate.

K-LYTE® DS ℞
Effervescent Tablets

Each tablet in solution provides 50 mEq (1955 mg) potassium as bicarbonate and citrate.

K-LYTE/CL® ℞
Effervescent Tablets

Each tablet in solution provides the equivalent of 25 mEq (1865 mg) potassium chloride.

	K-LYTE	K-LYTE DS	K-LYTE/CL	K-LYTE/CL 50
Potassium Chloride	—	—	1.5 g	2.24 g
Potassium Bicarbonate	2.5 g	2.5 g	0.5 g	2.0 g
Potassium Citrate	—	2.7 g	—	—
L-lysine Monohydrochloride	—	—	0.91 g	3.65 g
Citric Acid	2.1 g	2.1 g	0.55 g	1.0 g

K–LYTE/CL® 50 ℞
Effervescent Tablets

Each tablet in solution provides the equivalent of 50 mEq (3730 mg) potassium chloride.

Caution: Federal law prohibits dispensing without prescription.

DESCRIPTION
[See table above.]

Inactive Ingredients: All of the K-LYTE line of effervescent tablets contain docusate sodium, natural and/or artificial flavors, light mineral oil, saccharin and talc.
K-LYTE and K-LYTE DS lime tablets, and K-LYTE/Cl and K-LYTE/Cl 50 citrus tablets have D&C Yellow No. 10. K-LYTE and K-LYTE DS orange tablets and K-LYTE/Cl and K-LYTE/Cl 50 fruit punch tablets have FD&C Yellow No. 6. K-LYTE orange and lime tablets have dextrose, and K-LYTE DS orange and lime tablets have lactose.
Note: This listing of inactive ingredients is a voluntary action of Pharmaceutical Manufacturers Association members.

HOW SUPPLIED
K-LYTE® Effervescent Tablets. Each tablet in solution provides 25 mEq (978 mg) potassium.
  NDC 0087-0760-01 Lime flavor, Boxes of 30
  NDC 0087-0760-43 Lime flavor, Boxes of 100
  NDC 0087-0760-02 Lime flavor, Boxes of 250
  NDC 0087-0761-01 Orange flavor, Boxes of 30
  NDC 0087-0761-43 Orange flavor, Boxes of 100
  NDC 0087-0761-02 Orange flavor, Boxes of 250
K-LYTE® DS Effervescent Tablets. Each tablet provides 50 mEq (1955 mg) potassium.
  NDC 0087-0772-41 Lime flavor, Boxes of 30
  NDC 0087-0772-42 Lime flavor, Boxes of 100
  NDC 0087-0771-41 Orange flavor, Boxes of 30
  NDC 0087-0771-42 Orange flavor, Boxes of 100
K-LYTE/CL® Effervescent Tablets. Each tablet in solution provides the equivalent of 25 mEq (1865 mg) potassium chloride.
  NDC 0087-0766-41 Citrus flavor, Boxes of 30
  NDC 0087-0766-43 Citrus flavor, Boxes of 100
  NDC 0087-0766-42 Citrus flavor, Boxes of 250
  NDC 0087-0767-41 Fruit Punch flavor, Boxes of 30
  NDC 0087-0767-43 Fruit Punch flavor, Boxes of 100
  NDC 0087-0767-42 Fruit Punch flavor, Boxes of 250
K-LYTE/CL® 50 mEq Effervescent Tablets. Each tablet in solution provides the equivalent of 50 mEq (3730 mg) potassium chloride.
  NDC 0087-0757-41 Fruit Punch flavor, Boxes of 30
  NDC 0087-0757-42 Fruit Punch flavor, Boxes of 100
  NDC 0087-0758-41 Citrus flavor, Boxes of 30
  NDC 0087-0758-42 Citrus flavor, Boxes of 100

Store Below 86°F (30°C).

U.S. Patent No. 3,970,750

KLOTRIX® ℞
[klō′trix]
(potassium chloride)
Slow-Release Tablets 10 mEq (750 mg)

Caution: Federal law prohibits dispensing without prescription.

DESCRIPTION
KLOTRIX is a solid, oral dosage form of potassium chloride containing 750 mg of potassium chloride, USP (equivalent to 10 mEq of potassium) in a film-coated wax-matrix tablet. This formulation is intended to provide a controlled release of potassium from the matrix to minimize the likelihood of producing high, localized concentrations of potassium within the gastrointestinal tract.
KLOTRIX is an electrolyte replenisher. The chemical name is potassium chloride, and the structural formula is KCl. Potassium chloride, USP, occurs as a white, granular powder or as colorless crystals. It is odorless and has a saline taste.

Its solutions are neutral to litmus. It is freely soluble in water and insoluble in alcohol.
This product contains the following inactive ingredients: ethylcellulose, FD&C Yellow No. 6 (aluminum lake), glycerin, hydroxypropyl methylcellulose 2910, edible ink, magnesium stearate, povidone, colloidal silicon dioxide, stearic acid, and titanium dioxide.

HOW SUPPLIED
Tablets (light orange, film-coated) each containing 750 mg potassium chloride (equivalent to 10 mEq each potassium and chloride).
NDC 0087-0770-41	Bottles of 100
NDC 0087-0770-42	Bottles of 1000
NDC 0087-0770-43	Cartons of 100 individually wrapped tablets

U.S. Patent No. 4,140,756

Storage
Do not store at temperatures above 86°F (30°C).
Bristol Laboratories®
A Bristol-Myers Squibb Co.
Princeton, NJ 08543
Date of Revision August 1991

P5323-00

NYDRAZID® INJECTION ℞
Isoniazid Injection USP

CAUTION: Federal law prohibits dispensing without prescription.

> **WARNING**
> Severe and sometimes fatal hepatitis associated with isoniazid therapy may occur and may develop even after many months of treatment. This risk of developing hepatitis is age related. Approximate case rates by age are: 0 per 1,000 for persons under 20 years of age, 3 per 1,000 for persons in the 20 to 34 year age group, 12 per 1,000 for persons in the 35 to 49 year age group, 23 per 1,000 for persons in the 50 to 64 age group, and 8 per 1,000 for persons over 65 years of age. This risk of hepatitis is increased with daily consumption of alcohol. Precise data to provide a fatality rate for isoniazid-related hepatitis is not available; however, in a US Public Health Service Surveillance Study of 13,838 persons taking isoniazid, there were 8 deaths among 174 cases of hepatitis.
> Therefore, patients given isoniazid should be carefully monitored and interviewed at monthly intervals. Serum transaminase concentration becomes elevated in about 10 to 20 percent of patients, usually during the first few months of therapy but it can occur at any time. Usually enzyme levels return to normal despite continuance of drug but in some cases progressive liver dysfunction occurs. Patients should be instructed to report immediately any of the prodromal symptoms of hepatitis, such as fatigue, weakness, malaise, anorexia, nausea, or vomiting. If these symptoms appear or if signs suggestive of hepatic damage are detected, isoniazid should be discontinued promptly, since continued use of the drug in these cases has been reported to cause a more severe form of liver damage.
> Patients with tuberculosis should be given appropriate treatment with alternative drugs. If isoniazid must be reinstituted, it should be reinstituted only after symptoms and laboratory abnormalities have cleared. The drug should be restarted in a very small and gradually increasing doses and should be withdrawn immediately if there is any indication of recurrent liver involvement. Preventive treatment should be deferred in persons with acute hepatic diseases.

Continued on next page

Apothecon—Cont.

DESCRIPTION

Isoniazid is the hydrazide of isonicotinic acid. Nydrazid Injection (Isoniazid Injection) provides 100 mg isoniazid per ml with 0.25% chlorobutanol (chloral derivative) as a preservative; the pH has been adjusted to 6.0 to 7.0 with sodium hydroxide or hydrochloric acid. At the time of manufacture, the air in the container is replaced by nitrogen.

CLINICAL PHARMACOLOGY

Isoniazid acts against actively growing tubercle bacilli. Within one to two hours after oral administration, isoniazid produces peak blood levels which decline to 50 percent or less within six hours. It diffuses readily into all body fluids (cerebrospinal, pleural, and ascitic), tissues, organs, and excreta (saliva, sputum, and feces). The drug also passes through the placental barrier and into milk in concentrations comparable to those in the plasma. From 50 to 70 percent of a dose of isoniazid is excreted in the urine in 24 hours.

Isoniazid is metabolized primarily by acetylation and dehydrazination. The rate of acetylation is genetically determined. Approximately 50 percent of Blacks and Caucasians are "slow acetylators" and the rest are "rapid acetylators"; the majority of Eskimos and Orientals are "rapid acetylators."

The rate of acetylation does not significantly alter the effectiveness of isoniazid therapy when dosage is administered daily. However, slow acetylation may lead to higher blood levels of the drug and thus an increase in toxic reactions. Pyridoxine (B_6) deficiency is sometimes observed in adults with high doses of isoniazid and is considered probably due to its competition with pyridoxal phosphate for the enzyme apotryptophanase.

INDICATIONS AND USAGE

Nydrazid Injection (Isoniazid Injection) is recommended for all forms of tuberculosis in which organisms are susceptible. Intramuscular administration is intended for use whenever administration by the oral route is not possible.

Isoniazid is recommended for preventive therapy for the following groups, in order of priority:

1. Household members and other close associates of persons with recently diagnosed tuberculous disease.
2. Positive tuberculin skin test reactors with findings on the chest roentgenogram consistent with nonprogressive tuberculous disease, in whom there are neither positive bacteriologic findings nor a history of adequate chemotherapy.
3. Newly infected persons.
4. Positive tuberculin skin test reactors in the special clinical situations as follows: prolonged therapy with adrenocorticosteroids; immunosuppressive therapy; some hematologic and reticuloendothelial diseases, such as leukemia or Hodgkin's disease; diabetes mellitus; silicosis; after gastrectomy.
5. Other positive tuberculin reactors under 35 years of age. The risk of hepatitis must be weighed against the risk of tuberculosis in positive tuberculin reactors over the age of 35. However, the use of isoniazid is recommended for those with the additional risk factors listed above (1 to 4) and on an individual basis in situations where there is likelihood of serious consequences to contacts who may become infected.

CONTRAINDICATIONS

Previous isoniazid-associated hepatic injury; severe adverse reactions to isoniazid, such as drug fever, chills, and arthritis; acute liver of any etiology.

WARNINGS

See the boxed warning.

PRECAUTIONS

All drugs should be stopped and an evaluation made at the first sign of a hypersensitivity reaction. If isoniazid therapy must be reinstituted, the drug should be given only after symptoms have cleared. The drug should be restarted in very small and gradually increasing doses and should be withdrawn immediately if there is any indication of recurrent hypersensitivity reaction.

Use of isoniazid should be carefully monitored in the following:

1. Patients who are receiving phenytoin concurrently. Isoniazid may decrease the excretion of phenytoin or may enhance its effects. To avoid phenytoin intoxication, appropriate dosage adjustment of the anticonvulsant should be made.
2. Daily users of alcohol. Daily ingestion of alcohol may be associated with a higher incidence of isoniazid hepatitis.
3. Those patients with current chronic liver disease or severe renal dysfunction.

Periodic ophthalmologic examinations during isoniazid therapy are recommended when visual symptoms occur.

Usage in Pregnancy and Lactation

It has been reported that in both rats and rabbits, isoniazid may exert an embryocidal effect when administered orally during pregnancy, although no isoniazid-related congenital anomalies have been found in reproduction studies in mammalian species (mice, rats and rabbits). Isoniazid should be prescribed during pregnancy only when therapeutically necessary. The benefit of preventive therapy should be weighed against a possible risk to the fetus. Preventive treatment generally should be started after delivery because of the increased risk of tuberculosis for new mothers.

Since isoniazid is known to cross the placental barrier and to pass into maternal breast milk, neonates and breast-fed infants of isoniazid-treated mothers should be carefully observed for any evidence of adverse effects.

CARCINOGENESIS

Isoniazid has been reported to induce pulmonary tumors in a number of strains of mice.

ADVERSE REACTIONS

The most frequent reactions are those affecting the nervous system and the liver.

Nervous system: Peripheral neuropathy is the most common toxic effect. It is dose related, occurs most often in the malnourished and in those predisposed to neuritis (e.g., alcoholics and diabetics), and is usually preceded by paresthesias of the feet and hands. The incidence is higher in "slow acetylators."

Other neurotoxic effects which are uncommon with conventional doses are convulsions, toxic encephalopathy, optic neuritis and atrophy, memory impairment, and toxic psychosis.

Gastrointestinal: Nausea, vomiting, and epigastric distress.

Hepatic: Elevated serum transaminases (SGOT, SGPT), bilirubinemia, bilirubinuria, jaundice, and occasionally severe and sometimes fatal hepatitis. The common prodromal symptoms are anorexia, nausea, vomiting, fatigue, malaise, and weakness. Mild and transient elevation of serum transaminase levels occurs in 10 to 20 percent of persons taking isoniazid. The abnormality usually occurs in the first four to six months of treatment but can occur at any time during therapy. In most instances, enzyme levels return to normal without need to discontinue medication. In occasional instances, progressive liver damage occurs with accompanying symptoms. In these cases, the drug should be discontinued immediately. The frequency of progressive liver damage increases with age. It is rare in individuals under 20, but occurs in up to 2.3 percent of those over 50 years of age.

Hematologic: Agranulocytosis; hemolytic, sideroblastic, or aplastic anemia; thrombocytopenia; and eosinophilia.

Hypersensitivity: Fever, skin eruptions (morbilliform, maculopapular, purpuric, or exfoliative), lymphadenopathy, and vasculitis.

Metabolic and endocrine: Pyridoxine deficiency, pellagra, hyperglycemia, metabolic acidosis, and gynecomastia.

Miscellaneous: Rheumatic syndrome and systemic lupus erythematosus-like syndrome. Local irritation has been observed at the site of intramuscular injection.

OVERDOSAGE

Signs and Symptoms

Isoniazid overdosage produces signs and symptoms within 30 minutes to three hours after ingestion. Nausea, vomiting, dizziness, slurring of speech, blurring of vision, and visual hallucinations (including bright colors and strange designs) are among the early manifestations. With marked overdosage, respiratory distress and CNS depression, progressing rapidly from stupor to profound coma, are to be expected, along with severe, intractable seizures. Severe metabolic acidosis, acetonuria, and hyperglycemia are typical laboratory findings.

Treatment

Untreated or inadequately treated cases of gross isoniazid overdosage can terminate fatally, but good response has been reported in most patients brought under adequate treatment within the first few hours after drug ingestion. Secure the airway and establish adequate respiratory exchange. To control convulsions, administer I.V. short-acting barbiturates and I.V. pyridoxine (usually 1 mg/mg isoniazid ingested).

Obtain blood samples for immediate determination of gases, electrolytes, BUN, glucose, etc.; type and crossmatch blood in preparation for possible hemodialysis.

Rapid control of metabolic acidosis is fundamental to management. Give I.V. sodium bicarbonate at once and repeat as needed, adjusting subsequent dosage on the basis of laboratory findings (i.e., serum sodium, pH, etc.).

Forced osmotic diuresis must be started early and should be continued for some hours after clinical improvement to hasten renal clearance of the drug and help prevent relapse. Fluid intake and output should be monitored.

Hemodialysis is advised for severe cases; if this is not available, peritoneal dialysis can be used along with forced diuresis.

Along with measures based on initial and repeated determination of blood gases and other laboratory tests as needed, meticulous respiratory and other intensive care should be utilized to protect against hypoxia, hypotension, aspiration pneumonitis, etc.

Note: For preventive therapy of tuberculous infection it is recommended that physicians be familiar with the joint recommendations of the American Thoracic Society, American Lung Association, and the Center for Disease Control, as published in the American Review of Respiratory Disease, Vol. 110, No. 3, September, 1974, or CDC's Morbidity and Mortality Weekly Report, Vol. 24, No. 8, February 22, 1975.

DOSAGE AND ADMINISTRATION

Nydrazid Injection is used in conjunction with other effective antituberculous agents. If the bacilli become resistant, therapy must be changed to agents to which the bacilli are susceptible.

Usual Parenteral Dosage

For Treatment of Tuberculosis

Adults: 5 mg/kg up to 300 mg daily in a single dose.

Infants and Children: 10 to 20 mg/kg depending on severity of infection (up to 300 to 500 mg daily) in a single dose.

For Preventive Therapy

Adults: 300 mg per day in a single dose.

Infants and Children: 10 mg/kg (up to 300 mg daily) in a single dose.

Continuous administration of isoniazid for a sufficient period of time is an essential part of the regimen because relapse rates are higher if chemotherapy is stopped prematurely. In the treatment of tuberculosis, resistant organisms may multiply and their emergence during the treatment may necessitate a change in the regimen.

Concomitant administration of pyridoxine (B_6) is recommended in the malnourished and in those predisposed to neuropathy (e.g., alcoholics and diabetics).

HOW SUPPLIED

Nydrazid Injection (Isoniazid Injection USP) is available for intramuscular use in 10 mL vials providing 100 mg isoniazid per mL (NDC 0003-0643-50).

Storage

Store at room temperature.

Nydrazid Injection may crystallize at low temperatures. If this occurs, warm the vial to room temperature before use to redissolve the crystals.

APOTHECON®
A Bristol-Myers Squibb Company
Princeton, NJ 08540

J4-491   Revised October 1990   J4-491

PROLIXIN® INJECTION ℞
Fluphenazine Hydrochloride Injection USP
FOR INTRAMUSCULAR USE ONLY

PROLIXIN® ORAL CONCENTRATE ℞
Fluphenazine Hydrochloride Oral Solution USP

PROLIXIN® ELIXIR ℞
Fluphenazine Hydrochloride Elixir USP

PROLIXIN DECANOATE® ℞
Fluphenazine Decanoate Injection USP

PROLIXIN ENANTHATE® ℞
Fluphenazine Enanthate Injection USP

DESCRIPTION

PROLIXIN is a trifluoromethyl phenothiazine derivative intended for the management of schizophrenia. PROLIXIN Injection (Fluphenazine Hydrochloride Injection) is available in multiple dose vials providing 2.5 mg fluphenazine hydrochloride per mL. The preparation also includes sodium chloride for isotonicity, sodium hydroxide or hydrochloric acid to adjust the pH to 4.8–5.2, and 0.1% methylparaben and 0.01% propylparaben as preservatives. At the time of manufacture, the air in the vials is replaced by nitrogen.

PROLIXIN Oral Concentrate (Fluphenazine Hydrochloride Oral Solution) contains 5 mg fluphenazine hydrochloride per mL. Inactive ingredients: alcohol 14%, glycerin, purified water, and sodium benzoate.

PROLIXIN Elixir (Fluphenazine Hydrochloride Elixir) contains 0.5 mg fluphenazine hydrochloride per mL. Inactive ingredients: alcohol [14% (v/v)], colorant (FD&C Yellow No. 6), flavors, glycerin, polysorbate 40, purified water, sodium benzoate, and sucrose.

PROLIXIN DECANOATE is the decanoate ester of a trifluoromethyl phenothiazine derivative. It is a highly potent behavior modifier with a markedly extended duration of effect. PROLIXIN DECANOATE is available for intramuscular or subcutaneous administration, providing 25 mg fluphenazine decanoate per mL in a sesame oil vehicle with 1.2% (w/v) benzyl alcohol as a preservative. At the time of manufacture, the air in the vials is replaced by nitrogen.

PROLIXIN ENANTHATE (Fluphenazine Enanthate Injection) is an esterified trifluoromethyl phenothiazine derivative, chemically designated as 2-[4-[3-[2-(Trifluoromethyl)-

phenothiazin-10-yl]propyl]-1-piperazinyl]ethyl heptanoate. It is a highly potent behavior modifier with a markedly extended duration of effect. PROLIXIN ENANTHATE is available for intramuscular or subcutaneous administration, providing 25 mg fluphenazine enanthate per mL in a sesame oil vehicle with 1.5% (w/v) benzyl alcohol as a preservative. At the time of manufacture, the air in the vials is replaced by nitrogen.

CLINICAL PHARMACOLOGY

PROLIXIN has activity at all levels of the central nervous system as well as on multiple organ systems. The mechanism whereby its therapeutic action is exerted is unknown.

The basic effects of fluphenazine decanoate appear to be no different from those of fluphenazine hydrochloride, with the exception of duration of action. The esterification of fluphenazine markedly prolongs the drug's duration of effect without unduly attenuating its beneficial action.

The basic effects of fluphenazine enanthate appear to be no different from those of fluphenazine hydrochloride, with the exception of duration of action. The esterification of fluphenazine markedly prolongs the drug's duration of effect without unduly attenuating its beneficial action. The onset of action generally appears between 24 to 72 hours after injection, and the effects of the drug on psychotic symptoms become significant within 48 to 96 hours. Amelioration of symptoms then continues for one to three weeks or longer, with an average duration of effect of about two weeks.

Fluphenazine differs from other phenothiazine derivatives in several respects: it is more potent on a milligram basis, it has less potentiating effect on central nervous system depressants and anesthetics than do some of the phenothiazines and appears to be less sedating, and it is less likely than some of the older phenothiazines to produce hypotension (nevertheless, appropriate cautions should be observed—see sections on **PRECAUTIONS** and **ADVERSE REACTIONS**).

INDICATIONS AND USAGE

PROLIXIN is indicated in the management of manifestations of psychotic disorders.

Prolixin Decanoate (Fluphenazine Decanoate Injection) is a long-acting parenteral antipsychotic drug intended for use in the management of patients requiring prolonged parenteral neuroleptic therapy (e.g., chronic schizophrenics).

Prolixin Enanthate is a long-acting parenteral antipsychotic drug intended for use in the management of patients requiring prolonged parenteral neuroleptic therapy (e.g., chronic schizophrenics).

PROLIXIN has not been shown effective in the management of behavorial complications in patients with mental retardation.

CONTRAINDICATIONS

Phenothiazines are contraindicated in patients with suspected or established subcortical brain damage, in patients receiving large doses of hypnotics, and in comatose or severely depressed states. The presence of blood dyscrasia or liver damage precludes the use of fluphenazine decanoate, enanthate, or hydrochloride. PROLIXIN is contraindicated in patients who have shown hypersensitivity to fluphenazine; cross-sensitivity to phenothiazine derivatives may occur.

Fluphenazine decanoate and fluphenazine enanthate are not intended for use in children under 12 years of age.

Prolixin Enanthate is contraindicated in comatose or severely depressed states.

WARNINGS

Tardive Dyskinesia

Tardive dyskinesia, a syndrome consisting of potentially irreversible, involuntary, dyskinetic movements may develop in patients treated with neuroleptic (antipsychotic) drugs. Although the prevalence of the syndrome appears to be highest among the elderly, especially elderly women, it is impossible to rely upon prevalence estimates to predict, at the inception of neuroleptic treatment, which patients are likely to develop the syndrome. Whether neuroleptic drug products differ in their potential to cause tardive dyskinesia is unknown.

Both the risk of developing the syndrome and the likelihood that it will become irreversible are believed to increase as the duration of treatment and the total cumulative dose of neuroleptic drugs administered to the patient increase. However, the syndrome can develop, although much less commonly, after relatively brief treatment periods at low doses.

There is no known treatment for established cases of tardive dyskinesia, although the syndrome may remit, partially or completely, if neuroleptic treatment is withdrawn. Neuroleptic treatment, itself, however, may suppress (or partially suppress) the signs and symptoms of the syndrome and thereby may possibly mask the underlying disease process. The effect that symptomatic suppression has upon the long-term course of the syndrome is unknown.

Given these considerations, neuroleptics should be prescribed in a manner that is most likely to minimize the occurrence of tardive dyskinesia. Chronic neuroleptic treatment should generally be reserved for patients who suffer from a chronic illness that, 1) is known to respond to neuroleptic drugs, and, 2) for whom alternative, equally effective, but potentially less harmful treatments are *not* available or appropriate. In patients who do require chronic treatment, the smallest dose and the shortest duration of treatment producing a satisfactory clinical response should be sought. The need for continued treatment should be reassessed periodically.

If signs and symptoms of tardive dyskinesia appear in a patient on neuroleptics, drug discontinuation should be considered. However, some patients may require treatment despite the presence of the syndrome.

(For further information about the description of tardive dyskinesia and its clinical detection, please refer to the sections on **PRECAUTIONS, Information for Patients** and **ADVERSE REACTIONS, Tardive Dyskinesia.**)

Neuroleptic Malignant Syndrome (NMS)

A potentially fatal symptom complex sometimes referred to as Neuroleptic Malignant Syndrome (NMS) has been reported in association with antipsychotic drugs. Clinical manifestations of NMS are hyperpyrexia, muscle rigidity, altered mental status and evidence of autonomic instability (irregular pulse or blood pressure, tachycardia, diaphoresis, and cardiac dysrhythmias).

The diagnostic evaluation of patients with this syndrome is complicated. In arriving at a diagnosis, it is important to identify cases where the clinical presentation includes both serious medical illness (e.g., pneumonia, systemic infection, etc.) and untreated or inadequately treated extrapyramidal signs and symptoms (EPS). Other important considerations in the differential diagnosis include central anticholinergic toxicity, heat stroke, drug fever and primary central nervous system (CNS) pathology.

The management of NMS should include: 1) immediate discontinuation of antipsychotic drugs and other drugs not essential to concurrent therapy; 2) intensive symptomatic treatment and medical monitoring; and 3) treatment of any concomitant serious medical problems for which specific treatments are available. There is no general agreement about specific pharmacological treatment regimens for uncomplicated NMS.

If a patient requires antipsychotic drug treatment after recovery from NMS, the potential reintroduction of drug therapy should be carefully considered. The patient should be carefully monitored, since recurrences of NMS have been reported.

The use of this drug may impair the mental and physical abilities required for driving a car or operating heavy machinery.

Physicians should be alert to the possibility that severe adverse reactions may occur which require immediate medical attention.

Potentiation of the effects of alcohol may occur with the use of this drug.

Since there is no adequate experience in children who have received this drug, safety and efficacy in children have not been established.

Usage in Pregnancy

The safety for the use of this drug during pregnancy has not been established; therefore, the possible hazards should be weighed against the potential benefits when administering this drug to pregnant patients.

PRECAUTIONS

General

Because of the possibility of cross-sensitivity, fluphenazine should be used cautiously in patients who have developed cholestatic jaundice, dermatoses or other allergic reactions to phenothiazine derivatives.

Psychotic patients on large doses of a phenothiazine drug who are undergoing surgery should be watched carefully for possible hypotensive phenomena. Moreover, it should be remembered that reduced amounts of anesthetics or central nervous system depressants may be necessary.

The effects of atropine may be potentiated in some patients receiving fluphenazine because of added anticholinergic effects.

Fluphenazine should be used cautiously in patients exposed to extreme heat or phosphorus insecticides; in patients with a history of convulsive disorders, since grand mal convulsions have been known to occur; and in patients with special medical disorders, such as mitral insufficiency or other cardiovascular diseases and pheochromocytoma.

The possibility of liver damage, pigmentary retinopathy, lenticular and corneal deposits, and development of irreversible dyskinesia should be remembered when patients are on prolonged therapy.

Neuroleptic drugs elevate prolactin levels; the elevation persists during chronic administration. Tissue culture experiments indicate that approximately one-third of human breast cancers are prolactin dependent *in vitro*, a factor of potential importance if the prescription of these drugs is contemplated in a patient with a previously detected breast cancer. Although disturbances such as galactorrhea, amenorrhea, gynecomastia, and impotence have been reported, the clinical significance of elevated serum prolactin levels is unknown for most patients. An increase in mammary neoplasms has been found in rodents after chronic administration of neuroleptic drugs. Neither clinical studies nor epidemiologic studies conducted to date, however, have shown an association between chronic administration of these drugs and mammary tumorigenesis; the available evidence is considered too limited to be conclusive at this time.

Information for Patients

Given the likelihood that some patients exposed chronically to neuroleptics will develop tardive dyskinesia, it is advised that all patients in whom chronic use is contemplated be given, if possible, full information about this risk. The decision to inform patients and/or their guardians must obviously take into account the clinical circumstances and the competency of the patient to understand the information provided.

Abrupt Withdrawal

In general, phenothiazines do not produce psychic dependence; however, gastritis, nausea and vomiting, dizziness, and tremulousness have been reported following abrupt cessation of high dose therapy. Reports suggest that these symptoms can be reduced if concomitant antiparkinsonian agents are continued for several weeks after the phenothiazine is withdrawn.

Outside state hospitals or other psychiatric institutions, fluphenazine decanoate or enanthate should be administered under the direction of a physician experienced in the clinical use of psychotropic drugs, particularly phenothiazine derivatives.

Facilities should be available for periodic checking of hepatic function, renal function and the blood picture. Renal function of patients on long-term therapy should be monitored; if BUN (blood urea nitrogen) becomes abnormal, treatment should be discontinued.

As with any phenothiazine, the physician should be alert to the possible development of "silent pneumonias" in patients under treatment with fluphenazine.

ADVERSE REACTIONS

Central Nervous System: The side effects most frequently reported with phenothiazine compounds are extrapyramidal symptoms including pseudoparkinsonism, dystonia, dyskinesia, akathisia, oculogyric crises, opisthotonos, and hyperreflexia. Muscle rigidity sometimes accompanied by hyperthermia has been reported following use of fluphenazine decanoate. Most often these extrapyramidal symptoms are reversible; however, they may be persistent (see below). The frequency of such reactions is related in part to chemical structure: one can expect a higher incidence with fluphenazine decanoate or enanthate than with less potent piperazine derivatives or with straight-chain phenothiazines such as chlorpromazine. With any given phenothiazine derivative, the incidence and severity of such reactions depend more on individual patient sensitivity than on other factors, but dosage level and patient age are also determinants.

Extrapyramidal reactions may be alarming, and the patient should be forewarned and reassured. These reactions can usually be controlled by administration of antiparkinsonian drugs such as Benztropine Mesylate or intravenous Caffeine and Sodium Benzoate Injection, and by subsequent reductions in dosage.

Tardive Dyskinesia: See **WARNINGS**. The syndrome is characterized by involuntary choreoathetoid movements which variously involve the tongue, face, mouth, lips, or jaw (e.g., protrusion of the tongue, puffing of cheeks, puckering of the mouth, chewing movements), trunk and extremities. The severity of the syndrome and the degree of impairment produced vary widely.

The syndrome may become clinically recognizable either during treatment, upon dosage reduction, or upon withdrawal of treatment. Early detection of tardive dyskinesia is important. To increase the likelihood of detecting the syndrome at the earliest possible time, the dosage of neuroleptic drug should be reduced periodically (if clinically possible) and the patient observed for signs of the disorder. This maneuver is critical, since neuroleptic drugs may mask the signs of the syndrome.

Other CNS Effects: Occurrences of neuroleptic malignant syndrome (NMS) have been reported in patients on neuroleptic therapy (see **WARNINGS, Neuroleptic Malignant Syndrome**). Leukocytosis, elevated CPK, liver function abnormalities, and acute renal failure may also occur with NMS. Drowsiness or lethargy, if they occur, may necessitate a reduction in dosage; the induction of a catatonic-like state has been known to occur with dosages of fluphenazine far in excess of the recommended amounts. As with other phenothiazine compounds, reactivation or aggravation of psychotic processes may be encountered.

Phenothiazine derivatives have been known to cause, in some patients, restlessness, excitement, or bizarre dreams.

Autonomic Nervous System: Hypertension and fluctuations in blood pressure have been reported with fluphenazine.

Continued on next page

Apothecon—Cont.

Hypotension has rarely presented a problem with fluphenazine. However, patients with pheochromocytoma, cerebral vascular or renal insufficiency, or a severe cardiac reserve deficiency (such as mitral insufficiency) appear to be particularly prone to hypotensive reactions with phenothiazine compounds, and should therefore be observed closely when the drug is administered. If severe hypotension should occur, supportive measures including the use of intravenous vasopressor drugs should be instituted immediately. Levarterenol Bitartrate Injection is the most suitable drug for this purpose; *epinephrine should not be used* since phenothiazine derivatives have been found to reverse its action, resulting in a further lowering of blood pressure.

Autonomic reactions including nausea and loss of appetite, salivation, polyuria, perspiration, dry mouth, headache, and constipation may occur. Autonomic effects can usually be controlled by reducing or temporarily discontinuing dosage. In some patients, phenothiazine derivatives have caused blurred vision, glaucoma, bladder paralysis, fecal impaction, paralytic ileus, tachycardia, or nasal congestion.

Metabolic and Endocrine: Weight change, peripheral edema, abnormal lactation, gynecomastia, menstrual irregularities, false results on pregnancy tests, impotency in men and increased libido in women have all been known to occur in some patients on phenothiazine therapy.

Allergic Reactions: Skin disorders such as itching, erythema, urticaria, seborrhea, photosensitivity, eczema and even exfoliative dermatitis have been reported with phenothiazine derivatives. The possibility of anaphylactoid reactions occurring in some patients should be borne in mind.

Hematologic: Routine blood counts are advisable during therapy since blood dyscrasias including leukopenia, agranulocytosis, thrombocytopenic or nonthrombocytopenic purpura, eosinophilia, and pancytopenia have been observed with phenothiazine derivatives. Furthermore, if any soreness of the mouth, gums, or throat, or any symptoms of upper respiratory infection occur and confirmatory leukocyte count indicates cellular depression, therapy should be discontinued and other appropriate measures instituted immediately.

Hepatic: Liver damage as manifested by cholestatic jaundice may be encountered, particularly during the first months of therapy; treatment should be discontinued if this occurs. An increase in cephalin flocculation, sometimes accompanied by alterations in other liver function tests, has been reported in patients receiving fluphenazine who have had no clinical evidence of liver damage.

Others: Sudden, unexpected and unexplained deaths have been reported in hospitalized psychotic patients receiving phenothiazines. Previous brain damage or seizures may be predisposing factors; high doses should be avoided in known seizure patients. Several patients have shown sudden flareups of psychotic behavior patterns shortly before death. Autopsy findings have usually revealed acute fulminating pneumonia or pneumonitis, aspiration of gastric contents, or intramyocardial lesions.

Although this is not a general feature of fluphenazine, potentiation of central nervous system depressants (opiates, analgesics, antihistamines, barbiturates, alcohol) may occur.

The following adverse reactions have also occurred with phenothiazine derivatives: systemic lupus erythematosus-like syndrome, hypotension severe enough to cause fatal cardiac arrest, altered electrocardiographic and electroencephalographic tracings, altered cerebrospinal fluid proteins, cerebral edema, asthma, laryngeal edema and angioneurotic edema; with long-term use—skin pigmentation, and lenticular and corneal opacities.

Injections of fluphenazine decanoate or enanthate are extremely well tolerated, local tissue reactions occurring only rarely.

DOSAGE AND ADMINISTRATION

Prolixin Injection

The average well-tolerated starting dose for adult psychotic patients is 1.25 mg (0.5 mL) intramuscularly. Depending on the severity and duration of symptoms, initial total daily dosage may range from 2.5 to 10.0 mg and should be divided and given at six- to eight-hour intervals.

The smallest amount that will produce the desired results must be carefully determined for each individual, since optimal dosage levels of this potent drug vary from patient to patient. In general, the parenteral dose for fluphenazine has been found to be approximately $1/3$ to $1/2$ the oral dose. Treatment may be instituted with a *low initial dosage,* which may be increased, if necessary, until the desired clinical effects are achieved. Dosages exceeding 10.0 mg daily should be used with caution.

When symptoms are controlled, oral maintenance therapy can generally be instituted, often with single daily doses. Continued treatment, by the oral route if possible, is needed to achieve maximum therapeutic benefits; further adjust-

ments in dosage may be necessary during the course of therapy to meet the patient's requirements.

Prolixin Oral Concentrate

Depending on the severity and duration of symptoms, total daily dosage for *adult* psychotic patients may range initially from 2.5 to 10.0 mg and should be divided and given at six- to eight-hour intervals.

The smallest amount that will produce the desired results must be carefully determined for each individual, since optimal dosage levels of this potent drug vary from patient to patient. In general, the oral dose has been found to be approximately two to three times the parenteral dose of fluphenazine. Treatment is best instituted with a *low initial dosage,* which may be increased, if necessary, until the desired clinical effects are achieved. Therapeutic effect is often achieved with doses under 20 mg daily. Patients remaining severely disturbed or inadequately controlled may require upward titration of dosage. Daily doses up to 40 mg may be necessary; controlled clinical studies have not been performed to demonstrate safety of prolonged administration of such doses.

When symptoms are controlled, dosage can generally be reduced gradually to daily maintenance doses of 1.0 or 5.0 mg, often given as a single daily dose. Continued treatment is needed to achieve maximum therapeutic benefits; further adjustments in dosage may be necessary during the course of therapy to meet the patient's requirements.

For psychotic patients who have been stabilized on a fixed daily dosage of orally administered PROLIXIN (fluphenazine hydrochloride) dosage forms, conversion to the long-acting injectable PROLIXIN DECANOATE may be indicated [see package insert for PROLIXIN DECANOATE (Fluphenazine Decanoate Injection) for conversion information]. For *geriatric* patients, the suggested starting dose is 1.0 to 2.5 mg daily, adjusted according to the response of the patient. When the Oral Concentrate dosage form is to be used, the desired dose (measured by a calibrated device only) should be added to at least 60 mL (2 fl oz) of a suitable diluent *just prior to administration* to insure palatability and stability. Suggested diluents include tomato or fruit juice, milk, and uncaffeinated soft drinks. The Oral Concentrate should not be mixed with beverages containing caffeine (coffee, cola), tannics (tea), or pectinates (apple juice) because of potential incompatibility.

PROLIXIN Injection (Fluphenazine Hydrochloride Injection USP) is useful when psychotic patients are unable or unwilling to take oral therapy.

Prolixin Elixir

PROLIXIN Elixir should be inspected prior to use. Upon standing a slight wispy precipitate or globular material may develop due to the flavoring oils separating from the solution (potency is not affected). Gentle shaking redisperses the oils and the solution becomes clear. Solutions that do not clarify should not be used.

Depending on the severity and duration of symptoms, total daily dosage for *adult* psychotic patients may range initially from 2.5 to 10.0 mg and should be divided and given at six- to eight-hour intervals.

The smallest amount that will produce the desired results must be carefully determined for each individual, since optimal dosage levels of this potent drug vary from patient to patient. In general, the oral dose has been found to be approximately two to three times the parenteral dose of fluphenazine. Treatment is best instituted with a *low initial dosage,* which may be increased, if necessary, until the desired clinical effects are achieved. Therapeutic effect is often achieved with doses under 20 mg daily. Patients remaining severely disturbed or inadequately controlled may require upward titration of dosage. Daily doses up to 40 mg may be necessary; controlled clinical studies have not been performed to demonstrate safety of prolonged administration of such doses.

When symptoms are controlled, dosage can generally be reduced gradually to daily maintenance doses of 1.0 or 5.0 mg, often given as a single daily dose. Continued treatment is needed to achieve maximum therapeutic benefits; further adjustments in dosage may be necessary during the course of therapy to meet the patient's requirements.

For psychotic patients who have been stabilized on a fixed daily dosage of orally administered PROLIXIN (fluphenazine hydrochloride) dosage forms, conversion to the long-acting injectable PROLIXIN DECANOATE may be indicated [see package insert for PROLIXIN DECANOATE (Fluphenazine Decanoate Injection) for conversion information]. For *geriatric* patients, the suggested starting dose is 1.0 to 2.5 mg daily, adjusted according to the response of the patient. PROLIXIN Injection (Fluphenazine Hydrochloride Injection USP) is useful when psychotic patients are unable or unwilling to take oral therapy.

Prolixin Decanoate

Parenteral drug products should be inspected visually for particulate matter and discoloration prior to administration, whenever solution and container permit.

PROLIXIN DECANOATE (Fluphenazine Decanoate Injection) may be given intramuscularly or subcutaneously. A dry syringe and needle of at least 21 gauge should be used. Use of

a wet needle or syringe may cause the solution to become cloudy.

To begin therapy with PROLIXIN DECANOATE the following regimens are suggested:

For *most patients,* a dose of 12.5 to 25 mg (0.5 to 1 mL) may be given to initiate therapy. The onset of action generally appears between 24 and 72 hours after injection and the effects of the drug on psychotic symptoms become significant within 48 to 96 hours. Subsequent injections and the dosage interval are determined in accordance with the patient's response. When administered as maintenance therapy, a single injection may be effective in controlling schizophrenic symptoms up to four weeks or longer. The response to a single dose has been found to last as long as six weeks in a few patients on maintenance therapy.

It may be advisable that patients who have no history of taking phenothiazines should be treated initially with a shorter-acting form of fluphenazine (see **HOW SUPPLIED** section for the availability of the shorter-acting fluphenazine hydrochloride dosage forms) before administering the decanoate to determine the patient's response to fluphenazine and to establish appropriate dosage. For psychotic patients who have been stabilized on a fixed daily dosage of PROLIXIN Tablets (Fluphenazine Hydrochloride Tablets USP), PROLIXIN Elixir (Fluphenazine Hydrochloride Elixir USP), or PROLIXIN Oral Concentrate (Fluphenazine Hydrochloride Oral Solution), conversion of therapy from these short-acting oral forms to the long-acting injectable PROLIXIN DECANOATE may be indicated.

Appropriate dosage of PROLIXIN DECANOATE (Fluphenazine Decanoate Injection) should be individualized for each patient and responses carefully monitored. No precise formula can be given to convert to use of PROLIXIN DECANOATE; however, a controlled multicentered study,[*] in patients receiving oral doses from 5 to 60 mg fluphenazine hydrochloride daily, showed that 20 mg fluphenazine hydrochloride daily was equivalent to 25 mg (1 mL) PROLIXIN DECANOATE every three weeks. This represents an approximate conversion ratio of 0.5 mL (12.5 mg) of decanoate every three weeks for every 10 mg of fluphenazine hydrochloride daily.

Once conversion to PROLIXIN DECANOATE is made, careful clinical monitoring of the patient and appropriate dosage adjustment should be made at the time of each injection.

Severely agitated patients may be treated initially with a rapid-acting phenothiazine compound such as PROLIXIN Injection (Fluphenazine Hydrochloride Injection USP—see package insert accompanying that product for complete information). When acute symptoms have subsided, 25 mg (1 mL) of PROLIXIN DECANOATE may be administered; subsequent dosage is adjusted as necessary.

"Poor risk" patients (those with known hypersensitivity to phenothiazines, or with disorders that predispose to undue reactions): Therapy may be initiated cautiously with oral or parenteral fluphenazine hydrochloride (see package inserts accompanying these products for complete information). When the pharmacologic effects and an appropriate dosage are apparent, an equivalent dose of PROLIXIN DECANOATE may be administered. Subsequent dosage adjustments are made in accordance with the response of the patient.

The optimal amount of the drug and the frequency of administration must be determined for each patient, since dosage requirements have been found to vary with clinical circumstances as well as with individual response to the drug.

Dosage should not exceed 100 mg. If doses greater than 50 mg are deemed necessary, the next dose and succeeding doses should be increased cautiously in increments of 12.5 mg.

Prolixin Enanthate

PROLIXIN ENANTHATE (Fluphenazine Enanthate Injection USP) may be given intramuscularly or subcutaneously. A dry syringe and needle of at least 21 gauge should be used. Use of a wet needle or syringe may cause the solution to become cloudy.

To begin therapy with PROLIXIN ENANTHATE the following regimens are suggested:

For most patients a dose of 25 mg (1 mL) every two weeks should prove to be adequate, and therapy may be started on that basis. Subsequent adjustments in the amount and the dosage interval may be made, if necessary, in accordance with the patient's response.

It may be advisable that patients who have no history of taking phenothiazines should be treated initially with a shorter-acting form of fluphenazine before administering the enanthate to determine the patient's response to fluphenazine and to establish appropriate dosage. Since the dosage comparability of the shorter-acting forms of fluphenazine to the longer-acting enanthate is not known, special caution should be exercised when switching from the shorter-acting forms to the enanthate.

Severely agitated patients may be treated initially with a rapid-acting phenothiazine compound such as PROLIXIN Injection (Fluphenazine Hydrochloride Injection USP—see package insert accompanying that product for complete information). When acute symptoms have subsided, 25 mg (1

mL) of PROLIXIN ENANTHATE may be administered; subsequent dosage is adjusted as necessary.

"Poor risk" patients (those with known hypersensitivity to phenothiazines, or with disorders that predispose to undue reactions): Therapy may be initiated cautiously with oral or parenteral fluphenazine hydrochloride. (See package inserts accompanying these products for complete information.) When the pharmacologic effects and an appropriate dosage are apparent, an equivalent dose of PROLIXIN ENANTHATE may be administered. Subsequent dosage adjustments are made in accordance with the response of the patient.

The optimal amount of the drug and the frequency of administration must be determined for each patient, since dosage requirements have been found to vary with clinical circumstances as well as with individual response to the drug. Although in a large series of patients the optimal dose was usually 25 mg every two weeks, the amount required ranged from 12.5 to 100 mg (0.5 to 4 mL). The interval between doses ranged from one to three weeks in most instances. The response to a single dose was found to last as long as six weeks in a few patients on maintenance therapy.

Dosage should not exceed 100 mg. If doses greater than 50 mg are deemed necessary, the next dose and succeeding doses should be increased cautiously in increments of 12.5 mg.

HOW SUPPLIED

PROLIXIN INJECTION (Fluphenazine Hydrochloride Injection USP) is available in multiple dose vials as a sterile aqueous solution providing 2.5 mg fluphenazine hydrochloride per mL.

Storage
Solutions should be protected from exposure to light. Parenteral solutions may vary in color from essentially colorless to light amber. If a solution has become any darker than light amber or is discolored in any other way it should not be used. Store at room temperature; avoid freezing.

PROLIXIN ORAL CONCENTRATE (Fluphenazine Hydrochloride Oral Solution USP): 120 mL bottle with a 1 mL safety-cap dropper calibrated at 0.1 mL and in 0.2 mL increments. 5 mg fluphenazine hydrochloride per mL. NDC 0003-0801-10.

Storage
Store at room temperature; avoid freezing. Protect from light. Keep tightly closed.

PROLIXIN ELIXIR
(Fluphenazine Hydrochloride Elixir USP) 0.5 mg/mL (2.5 mg per 5 mL teaspoonful)
60 ml bottle with calibrated dropper: NDC 0003-0820-30
473 ml bottle: NDC 0003-0820-50
Storage
Store elixir at room temperature. Protect from light. Keep tightly closed. Avoid freezing.

PROLIXIN DECANOATE (Fluphenazine Decanoate Injection, USP) is available in 25 mg/mL:
1 mL Unimatic® single dose syringe
NDC 0003-0569-02
Each syringe is supplied with a 20-gauge $1^1/_2$ inch needle.
5 mL Multiple dose vial
NDC 0003-0569-15
At time of manufacture, the air in the vials is replaced by nitrogen.

PROLIXIN ENANTHATE (Fluphenazine Enanthate Injection USP) is available in vials providing 25 mg fluphenazine enanthate per mL. (NDC 0003-0824-05)

Storage
Store at room temperature; avoid freezing and excessive heat. Protect from light.

* The Initiation of Long-Term Pharmacotherapy in Schizophrenia: Dosage and Side Effect Comparisons Between Oral and Depot Fluphenazine; N.R. Schooler; Pharmakopsych. 9:159–169, 1976.

STADOL® ℞
[stā'dŏl]
(butorphanol tartrate, USP)

Full prescribing information for the above product appears under Mead Johnson Laboratories.

For information on over-the-counter drugs, consult **PDR For Nonprescription Drugs**

Arco Pharmaceuticals, Inc.
105 ORVILLE DRIVE
BOHEMIA, NY 11716

Direct Inquiries to:
Professional Service Department
(516) 567-9500

ARCO-LASE® OTC
(broad pH spectrum digestant)

COMPOSITION
Each soft, mint flavored tablet contains Trizyme*, 38 mg., and Lipase, 25 mg.
*Contains the following standardized enzymes: amylolytic 30 mg.; proteolytic 6 mg.; cellulolytic 2 mg.

ACTION AND USES
Indicated for most gastrointestinal disorders due to poor digestion: Flatulence, gas and bloating, dyspepsia, distention, fullness, heartburn, or in any condition where normal digestion is impaired by digestive insufficiencies. Arcolase provides the highest enzymatic activity, plus the protective action of the widest pH range. Thus it is effective throughout the entire G.I. tract. Requiring no enteric coating, there is assurance of a positive breakdown of its factors. This is advantageous, because quite often patients with digestive disorders cannot digest their food properly, let alone hard, or enteric coated capsules or tablets.

SIDE EFFECTS
None.

ADMINISTRATION AND DOSAGE
One tablet with or immediately following meals. Tablet may be swallowed or chewed.

SUPPLIED
Bottles of 50's. NDC 275-4040.

ARCO-LASE® PLUS ℞

COMPOSITION
Same as Arco-Lase, plus the addition of Hyoscyamine sulfate 0.10 mg., atropine sulfate 0.02 mg. and phenobarbital ⅛ gr. (Warning: may be habit forming.)

ACTION AND USES
Gastrointestinal disturbances, such as cramps, bloating, spasms, diarrhea, nausea, vomiting and peptic ulcer. The enzymes correct the digestive insufficiencies.
The antispasmodic and phenobarbital contribute to the symptomatic relief of hypermotility and nervous tension, which usually accompanies functional disturbances of the bowel.

ADMINISTRATION AND DOSAGE
One tablet following meals.

SIDE EFFECTS
May cause rapid pulse, dryness of mouth and blurred vision.

CONTRAINDICATIONS
This product is contraindicated in the presence of glaucoma or prostatic hypertrophy.

SUPPLIED
Bottles of 50's. NDC 275-45-45.

LITERATURE AVAILABLE
Yes.

MEGA-B® OTC
(super potency vitamin B complex, sugar & starch free)

COMPOSITION
Each Mega-B Tablet contains the following Mega Vitamins:
B₁ (Thiamine Mononitrate)	100 mg.
B₂ (Riboflavin)	100 mg.
B₆ (Pyridoxine Hydrochloride)	100 mg.
B₁₂ (Cyanocobalamin)	100 mcg.
Choline Bitartrate	100 mg.
Inositol	100 mg.
Niacinamide	100 mg.
Folic Acid	100 mcg.
Pantothenic Acid	100 mg.
d-Biotin	100 mcg.
Para-Aminobenzoic Acid (PABA)	100 mg.

In a base of yeast to provide the identified and unidentified B-Complex Factors.

ADVANTAGES
Each Mega-B capsule-shaped tablet provides the highest vitamin B complex available in a single dose.
Mega-B was designed for those patients who require truly Mega vitamin potencies with the convenience of minimum dosage.

INDICATIONS
Mega-B is indicated in conditions characterized by depletions or increased demand of the water-soluble B-complex vitamins. It may be useful in the nutritional management of patients during prolonged convalescence associated with major surgery. It is also indicated for stress conditions, as an adjunct to antibiotics and diuretic therapy, pre and post operative cases, liver conditions, gastrointestinal disorders interfering with intake or absorption of water-soluble vitamins, prolonged or wasting diseases, diabetes, burns, fractures, severe infections, and some psychological disorders.

WARNING
NOT INTENDED FOR TREATMENT OF PERNICIOUS ANEMIA, OR OTHER PRIMARY OR SECONDARY ANEMIAS.

DOSAGE
Usual dosage is one Mega-B tablet daily, or varied, depending on clinical needs.

SUPPLIED
Yellow capsule shaped tablets in bottles of 30, 100 and 500.

MEGADOSE™ OTC
(multiple mega-vitamin formula with minerals, sugar and starch free)

COMPOSITION
Vitamin A	25,000 USP Units
Vitamin D	1,000 USP Units
Vitamin C w/Rose Hips	250 mg.
Vitamin E	100 IU
Folic Acid	400 mcg.
Vitamin B₁	80 mg.
Vitamin B₂	80 mg.
Niacinamide	80 mg.
Vitamin B₆	80 mg.
Vitamin B₁₂	80 mcg.
Biotin	80 mcg.
Pantothenic Acid	80 mg.
Choline Bitartrate	80 mg.
Inositol	80 mg.
Para-Aminobenzoic Acid	80 mg.
Rutin	30 mg.
Citrus Bioflavonoids	30 mg.
Betaine Hydrochloride	30 mg.
Glutamic Acid	30 mg.
Hesperidin Complex	5 mg.
Iodine (from Kelp)	0.15 mg.
Calcium Gluconate*	50 mg.
Zinc Gluconate*	25 mg.
Potassium Gluconate*	10 mg.
Ferrous Gluconate*	10 mg.
Magnesium Gluconate*	7 mg.
Manganese Gluconate*	6 mg.
Copper Gluconate*	0.5 mg.

*Natural mineral chelates in a base containing natural ingredients.

DOSAGE
One tablet daily.

SUPPLIED
Capsule shaped tablets in bottles of 30, 100 and 250.

IDENTIFICATION PROBLEM?
Turn to the **Product Identification** Guide, where you'll find more than 1600 products pictured in actual size and full color.

B.F. Ascher & Company, Inc.

15501 WEST 109TH STREET
LENEXA, KS 66219-1308

Direct Inquiries to:
Product Information Department
(913) 888-1880

ANASPAZ® Tablets
[an'ah-spāz]

(l-hyoscyamine sulfate) ....0.125 mg

HOW SUPPLIED
Light yellow, compressed, scored tablets with the Ascher logo on one side and the NDC 225/295 on the other.
Bottles of 100—NDC 0225-0295-15
Bottles of 500—NDC 0225-0295-20

AYR® Saline Nasal Mist, Drops and Gel   OTC

(See PDR For Nonprescription Drugs.)

ITCH–X® Gel and Spray   OTC

(See PDR For Nonprescription Drugs.)

KWELCOF® Liquid   C III R
[kwel'cof]

Each teaspoonful (5 mL) contains:
Hydrocodone bitartrate ....5 mg
   (WARNING: May be habit-forming)
Guaifenesin ....100 mg

HOW SUPPLIED
Clear, fruit-flavored liquid which is alcohol-free, dye-free, sugar-free and corn allergen-free.
1 pint (473 mL) bottles—NDC 0225-0420-45

MOBISYL® Analgesic Creme   OTC

(See PDR For Nonprescription Drugs.)

MOBIGESIC®   OTC
Pain Reliever-Fever Reducer Tablets

(See PDR for Nonprescription Drugs.)

PEN•KERA® Creme   OTC

(See PDR For Nonprescription Drugs.)

PRETTY FEET & HANDS®   OTC
Rough Skin Remover

(See PDR For Nonprescription Drugs.)

NOTICE
Before prescribing or administering
any product described in
PHYSICIANS' DESK REFERENCE ,
check the **PDR Supplements**
for revised information.

Astra Merck Inc.

725 CHESTERBROOK BOULEVARD
WAYNE, PA 19087-5677

For Medical Information Contact:
1-800-236-9933

Adverse Drug Experiences:
1-800-236-9933

TABLETS
PLENDIL®   R
(FELODIPINE)
EXTENDED-RELEASE TABLETS

DESCRIPTION

PLENDIL* (Felodipine) is a calcium antagonist (calcium channel blocker). Felodipine is a dihydropyridine derivative that is chemically described as ± ethyl methyl 4-(2,3-dichlorophenyl)-1,4-dihydro-2,6-dimethyl-3,5-pyridinedicarboxylate. Its empirical formula is $C_{18}H_{19}Cl_2NO_4$ and its structural formula is:

Felodipine is a slightly yellowish, crystalline powder with a molecular weight of 384.26. It is insoluble in water and is freely soluble in dichloromethane and ethanol. Felodipine is a racemic mixture.
Tablets PLENDIL provide extended release of felodipine. They are available as tablets containing 2.5 mg, 5 mg or 10 mg of felodipine for oral administration. In addition to the active ingredient felodipine, the tablets contain the following inactive ingredients: Tablets PLENDIL 2.5 mg—hydroxypropyl cellulose, lactose, FD&C Blue 2, sodium stearyl fumarate, titanium dioxide, yellow iron oxide and other ingredients. Tablets PLENDIL 5 mg and 10 mg—cellulose, red and yellow oxide, lactose, polyethylene glycol, sodium stearyl fumarate, titanium dioxide and other ingredients.

---
*Registered trademark of Astra AB

CLINICAL PHARMACOLOGY

Mechanism of Action
Felodipine is a member of the dihydropyridine class of calcium channel antagonists (calcium channel blockers). It reversibly competes with nitrendipine and/or other calcium channel blockers for dihydropyridine binding sites, blocks voltage-dependent Ca^{++} currents in vascular smooth muscle and cultured rabbit atrial cells and blocks potassium-induced contracture of the rat portal vein.
In vitro studies show that the effects of felodipine on contractile processes are selective, with greater effects on vascular smooth muscle than cardiac muscle. Negative inotropic effects can be detected *in vitro*, but such effects have not been seen in intact animals.
The effect of felodipine on blood pressure is principally a consequence of a dose-related decrease of peripheral vascular resistance in man, with a modest reflex increase in heart rate (see *Cardiovascular Effects*). With the exception of a mild diuretic effect seen in several animal species and man, the effects of felodipine are accounted for by its effects on peripheral vascular resistance.
Pharmacokinetics and Metabolism
Following oral administration, felodipine is almost completely absorbed and undergoes extensive first-pass metabolism. The systemic bioavailability of PLENDIL is approximately 20 percent. Mean peak concentrations following the administration of PLENDIL are reached in 2.5 to 5 hours. Both peak plasma concentration and the area under the plasma concentration time curve (AUC) increase linearly with doses up to 20 mg. Felodipine is greater than 99 percent bound to plasma proteins.
Following intravenous administration, the plasma concentration of felodipine declined triexponentially with mean disposition half-lives of 4.8 minutes, 1.5 hours and 9.1 hours. The mean contributions of the three individual phases to the overall AUC were 15, 40 and 45 percent, respectively, in the order of increasing $t_{1/2}$.
Following oral administration of the immediate-release formulation, the plasma level of felodipine also declined polyexponentially with a mean terminal $t_{1/2}$ of 11 to 16 hours. The

mean peak and trough steady-state plasma concentrations achieved after 10 mg of the immediate-release formulation given once a day to normal volunteers, were 20 and 0.5 nmol/L, respectively. The trough plasma concentration of felodipine in most individuals was substantially below the concentration needed to effect a half-maximal decline in blood pressure (EC_{50}) [4–6 nmol/L for felodipine], thus precluding once a day dosing with the immediate-release formulation.
Following administration of a 10-mg dose of PLENDIL, the extended-release formulation, to young, healthy volunteers, mean peak and trough steady-state plasma concentrations of felodipine were 7 and 2 nmol/L, respectively. Corresponding values in hypertensive patients (mean age 64) after a 20-mg dose of PLENDIL were 23 and 7 nmol/L. Since the EC_{50} for felodipine is 4 to 6 nmol/L, a 5 to 10-mg dose of PLENDIL in some patients, and a 20-mg dose in others, would be expected to provide an antihypertensive effect that persists for 24 hours (see *Cardiovascular Effects* below and DOSAGE AND ADMINISTRATION).
The systemic plasma clearance of felodipine in young healthy subjects is about 0.8 L/min and the apparent volume of distribution is about 10 L/kg.
Following an oral or intravenous dose of ^{14}C-labeled felodipine in man, about 70 percent of the dose of radioactivity was recovered in urine and 10 percent in the feces. A negligible amount of intact felodipine is recovered in the urine and feces (< 0.5%). Six metabolites, which account for 23 percent of the oral dose, have been identified; none has significant vasodilating activity.
Following administration of PLENDIL to hypertensive patients, mean peak plasma concentrations at steady state are about 20 percent higher than after a single dose. Blood pressure response is correlated with plasma concentrations of felodipine.
The bioavailability of PLENDIL is not influenced by the presence of food in the gastrointestinal tract. In a study of six patients, the bioavailability of felodipine was increased more than two-fold when taken with doubly concentrated grapefruit juice, compared to when taken with water or orange juice. A similar finding has been seen with some other dihydropyridine calcium antagonists, but to a lesser extent than that seen with felodipine.
Age Effects: Plasma concentrations of felodipine, after a single dose and at steady state, increase with age. Mean clearance of felodipine in elderly hypertensives (mean age 74) was only 45 percent of that of young volunteers (mean age 26). At steady state mean AUC for young patients was 39 percent of that for the elderly. Data for intermediate age ranges suggest that the AUCs fall between the extremes of the young and the elderly.
Hepatic Dysfunction: In patients with hepatic disease, the clearance of felodipine was reduced to about 60 percent of that seen in normal young volunteers.
Renal impairment does not alter the plasma concentration profile of felodipine; although higher concentrations of the metabolites are present in the plasma due to decreased urinary excretion, these are inactive.
Animal studies have demonstrated that felodipine crosses the blood-brain barrier and the placenta.
Cardiovascular Effects
Following administration of PLENDIL, a reduction in blood pressure generally occurs within two to five hours. During chronic administration, substantial blood pressure control lasts for 24 hours, with trough reductions in diastolic blood pressure approximately 40–50 percent of peak reductions. The antihypertensive effect is dose-dependent and correlates with the plasma concentration of felodipine.
A reflex increase in heart rate frequently occurs during the first week of therapy; this increase attenuates over time. Heart rate increases of 5–10 beats per minute may be seen during chronic dosing. The increase is inhibited by beta-blocking agents.
The P-R interval of the ECG is not affected by felodipine when administered alone or in combination with a beta-blocking agent. Felodipine alone or in combination with a beta-blocking agent has been shown, in clinical and electrophysiologic studies, to have no significant effect on cardiac conduction (P-R, P-Q and H-V intervals).
In clinical trials in hypertensive patients without clinical evidence of left ventricular dysfunction, no symptoms suggestive of a negative inotropic effect were noted; however none would be expected in this population (see PRECAUTIONS).
Renal/Endocrine Effects
Renal vascular resistance is decreased by felodipine while glomerular filtration rate remains unchanged. Mild diuresis, natriuresis and kaliuresis have been observed during the first week of therapy. No significant effects on serum electrolytes were observed during short- and long-term therapy. In clinical trials in patients with hypertension increases in plasma noradrenaline levels have been observed.
Clinical Studies
Felodipine produces dose-related decreases in systolic and diastolic blood pressure as demonstrated in six placebo-controlled, dose response studies using either immediate-release

or extended-release dosage forms. These studies enrolled over 800 patients on active treatment, at total daily doses ranging from 2.5 to 20 mg. In those studies felodipine was administered either as monotherapy or was added to beta blockers. The results of the two studies with PLENDIL given once daily as monotherapy are shown in the table below:

MEAN REDUCTIONS IN BLOOD PRESSURE (mmHg)*
Systolic/Diastolic

Dose	N	Mean Peak Response	Mean Trough Response	Trough/ Peak Ratios (%s)
Study 1 (8 weeks)				
2.5 mg	68	9.4/4.7	2.7/2.5	29/53
5 mg	69	9.5/6.3	2.4/3.7	25/59
10 mg	67	18.0/10.8	10.0/6.0	56/56
Study 2 (4 weeks)				
10 mg	50	5.3/7.2	1.5/3.2	33/40**
20 mg	50	11.3/10.2	4.5/3.2	43/34**

* Placebo response subtracted
** Different number of patients available for peak and trough measurements

INDICATIONS AND USAGE

PLENDIL is indicated for the treatment of hypertension. PLENDIL may be used alone or concomitantly with other antihypertensive agents.

CONTRAINDICATIONS

PLENDIL is contraindicated in patients who are hypersensitive to this product.

PRECAUTIONS

General
Hypotension: Felodipine, like other calcium antagonists, may occasionally precipitate significant hypotension and rarely syncope. It may lead to reflex tachycardia which in susceptible individuals may precipitate angina pectoris. (See ADVERSE REACTIONS.)
Heart Failure: Although acute hemodynamic studies in a small number of patients with NYHA Class II or III heart failure treated with felodipine have not demonstrated negative inotropic effects, safety in patients with heart failure has not been established. Caution therefore should be exercised when using PLENDIL in patients with heart failure or compromised ventricular function, particularly in combination with a beta blocker.
Elderly Patients or Patients with Impaired Liver Function: Patients over 65 years of age or patients with impaired liver function may have elevated plasma concentrations of felodipine and may respond to lower doses of PLENDIL, therefore a starting dose of 2.5 mg once a day is recommended. These patients should have their blood pressure monitored closely during dosage adjustment of PLENDIL. (See CLINICAL PHARMACOLOGY and DOSAGE AND ADMINISTRATION.)
Peripheral Edema: Peripheral edema, generally mild and not associated with generalized fluid retention, was the most common adverse event in the clinical trials. The incidence of peripheral edema was both dose- and age-dependent. Frequency of peripheral edema ranged from about 10 percent in patients under 50 years of age taking 5 mg daily to about 30 percent in those over 60 years of age taking 20 mg daily. This adverse effect generally occurs within 2–3 weeks of the initiation of treatment.
Information for Patients
Patients should be instructed to take PLENDIL whole and not to crush or chew the tablets. They should be told that mild gingival hyperplasia (gum swelling) has been reported. Good dental hygiene decreases its incidence and severity.
NOTE: As with many other drugs, certain advice to patients being treated with PLENDIL is warranted. This information is intended to aid in the safe and effective use of this medication. It is not a disclosure of all possible adverse or intended effects.
Drug Interactions
Beta-Blocking Agents: A pharmacokinetic study of felodipine in conjunction with metoprolol demonstrated no significant effects on the pharmacokinetics of felodipine. The AUC and C_{max} of metoprolol, however, were increased approximately 31 and 38 percent, respectively. In controlled clinical trials, however, beta blockers including metoprolol were concurrently administered with felodipine and were well tolerated.
Cimetidine: In healthy subjects pharmacokinetic studies showed an approximately 50 percent increase in the area under the plasma concentration time curve (AUC) as well as the C_{max} of felodipine when given concomitantly with cimetidine. It is anticipated that a clinically significant interaction may occur in some hypertensive patients. Therefore, it is recommended that low doses of PLENDIL be used when given concomitantly with cimetidine.
Digoxin: When given concomitantly with PLENDIL the pharmacokinetics of digoxin in patients with heart failure were not significantly altered.
Anticonvulsants: In a pharmacokinetic study, maximum plasma concentrations of felodipine were considerably lower in epileptic patients on long-term anticonvulsant therapy (e.g., phenytoin, carbamazepine, or phenobarbital) than in healthy volunteers. In such patients, the mean area under the felodipine plasma concentration-time curve was also reduced to approximately six percent of that observed in healthy volunteers. Since a clinically significant interaction may be anticipated, alternative antihypertensive therapy should be considered in these patients.
Other Concomitant Therapy: In healthy subjects there were no clinically significant interactions when felodipine was given concomitantly with indomethacin or spironolactone.
Interaction with Food: See CLINICAL PHARMACOLOGY, *Pharmacokinetics and Metabolism.*
Carcinogenesis, Mutagenesis, Impairment of Fertility
In a two-year carcinogenicity study in rats fed felodipine at doses of 7.7, 23.1 or 69.3 mg/kg/day (up to 28 times* the maximum recommended human dose on a mg/m^2 basis), a dose-related increase in the incidence of benign interstitial cell tumors of the testes (Leydig cell tumors) was observed in treated male rats. These tumors were not observed in a similar study in mice at doses up to 138.6 mg/kg/day (28 times* the maximum recommended human dose on a mg/m^2 basis). Felodipine, at the doses employed in the two-year rat study, has been shown to lower testicular testosterone and to produce a corresponding increase in serum luteinizing hormone in rats. The Leydig cell tumor development is possibly secondary to these hormonal effects which have not been observed in man.
In this same rat study a dose-related increase in the incidence of focal squamous cell hyperplasia compared to control was observed in the esophageal groove of male and female rats in all dose groups. No other drug-related esophageal or gastric pathology was observed in the rats or with chronic administration in mice and dogs. The latter species, like man, has no anatomical structure comparable to the esophageal groove.
Felodipine was not carcinogenic when fed to mice at doses of up to 138.6 mg/kg/day (28 times* the maximum recommended human dose on a mg/m^2 basis) for periods of up to 80 weeks in males and 99 weeks in females.
Felodipine did not display any mutagenic activity *in vitro* in the Ames microbial mutagenicity test or in the mouse lymphoma forward mutation assay. No clastogenic potential was seen *in vivo* in the mouse micronucleus test at oral doses up to 2500 mg/kg (506 times* the maximum recommended human dose on a mg/m^2 basis) or *in vitro* in a human lymphocyte chromosome aberration assay.
A fertility study in which male and female rats were administered doses of 3.8, 9.6 or 26.9 mg/kg/day showed no significant effect of felodipine on reproductive performance.
Pregnancy
Pregnancy Category C
Teratogenic Effects: Studies in pregnant rabbits administered doses of 0.46, 1.2, 2.3 and 4.6 mg/kg/day (from 0.4 to 4 times* the maximum recommended human dose on a mg/m^2 basis) showed digital anomalies consisting of reduction in size and degree of ossification of the terminal phalanges in the fetuses. The frequency and severity of the changes appeared dose-related and were noted even at the lowest dose. These changes have been shown to occur with other members of the dihydropyridine class and are possibly a result of compromised uterine blood flow. Similar fetal anomalies were not observed in rats given felodipine.
In a teratology study in cynomolgus monkeys no reduction in the size of the terminal phalanges was observed but an abnormal position of the distal phalanges was noted in about 40 percent of the fetuses.
Nonteratogenic Effects: A prolongation of parturition with difficult labor and an increased frequency of fetal and early postnatal deaths were observed in rats administered doses of 9.6 mg/kg/day (4 times* the maximum human dose on a mg/m^2 basis) and above.
Significant enlargement of the mammary glands in excess of the normal enlargement for pregnant rabbits was found with doses greater than or equal to 1.2 mg/kg/day (equal to the maximum human dose on a mg/m^2 basis). This effect occurred only in pregnant rabbits and regressed during lactation. Similar changes in the mammary glands were not observed in rats or monkeys.
There are no adequate and well-controlled studies in pregnant women. If felodipine is used during pregnancy, or if the patient becomes pregnant while taking this drug, she should be apprised of the potential hazard to the fetus, possible digital anomalies of the infant, and the potential effects of felodipine on labor and delivery, and on the mammary glands of pregnant females.
Nursing Mothers
It is not known whether this drug is secreted in human milk and because of the potential for serious adverse reactions from felodipine in the infant, a decision should be made whether to discontinue nursing or to discontinue the drug, taking into account the importance of the drug to the mother.
Pediatric Use
Safety and effectiveness in children have not been established.

*Based on patient weight of 50 kg

ADVERSE REACTIONS

In controlled studies in the United States and overseas approximately 3000 patients were treated with felodipine as either the extended-release or the immediate-release formulation.
The most common clinical adverse events reported with PLENDIL administered as monotherapy at the recommended dosage range of 2.5 mg to 10 mg once a day were peripheral edema and headache. Peripheral edema was generally mild, but it was age- and dose-related and resulted in discontinuation of therapy in about 3 percent of the enrolled patients. Discontinuation of therapy due to any clinical adverse event occurred in about 6 percent of the patients receiving PLENDIL, principally for peripheral edema, headache, or flushing.
Adverse events that occurred with an incidence of 1.5 percent or greater at any of the recommended doses of 2.5 mg to 10 mg once a day (PLENDIL, N=861; Placebo, N=334), without regard to causality, are compared to placebo and are listed by dose in the table below. These events are reported from controlled clinical trials with patients who were randomized to a fixed dose of PLENDIL or titrated from an initial dose of 2.5 mg or 5 mg once a day. A dose of 20 mg once a day has been evaluated in some clinical studies. Although the antihypertensive effect of PLENDIL is increased at 20 mg once a day, there is a disproportionate increase in adverse events, especially those associated with vasodilatory effects (see DOSAGE and ADMINISTRATION).
[See table on top of next page.]
Adverse events that occurred in 0.5 up to 1.5 percent of patients who received PLENDIL in all controlled clinical trials at the recommended dosage range of 2.5 mg to 10 mg once a day and serious adverse events that occurred at a lower rate or events reported during marketing experience (those lower rate events are in italics) are listed below. These events are listed in order of decreasing severity within each category and the relationship of these events to administration of PLENDIL is uncertain: ***Body as a Whole:*** Chest pain, facial edema, flu-like illness; ***Cardiovascular:*** *Myocardial infarction, hypotension, syncope, angina pectoris, arrhythmia,* tachycardia, premature beats; ***Digestive:*** Abdominal pain, diarrhea, vomiting, dry mouth, flatulence, acid regurgitation; ***Hematologic:*** *Anemia;* ***Metabolic:*** ALT (SGPT) increased; ***Musculoskeletal:*** Arthralgia, back pain, leg pain, foot pain, muscle cramps, myalgia, arm pain, knee pain, hip pain; ***Nervous/Psychiatric:*** Insomnia, depression, anxiety disorders, irritability, nervousness, somnolence, decreased libido; ***Respiratory:*** Dyspnea, pharyngitis, bronchitis, influenza, sinusitis, epistaxis, respiratory infection; ***Skin:*** Contusion, erythema, urticaria; ***Special Senses:*** Visual disturbances; ***Urogenital:*** Impotence, urinary frequency, urinary urgency, dysuria, polyuria.
Gingival Hyperplasia: Gingival hyperplasia, usually mild, occurred in <0.5 percent of patients in controlled studies. This condition may be avoided or may regress with improved dental hygiene. (See PRECAUTIONS, *Information for Patients.*)
Clinical Laboratory Test Findings
Serum Electrolytes: No significant effects on serum electrolytes were observed during short- and long-term therapy (see CLINICAL PHARMACOLOGY, *Renal/Endocrine Effects*).
Serum Glucose: No significant effects on fasting serum glucose were observed in patients treated with PLENDIL in the U.S. controlled study.
Liver Enzymes: One of two episodes of elevated serum transaminases decreased once drug was discontinued in clinical studies; no follow-up was available for the other patient.

OVERDOSAGE

Oral doses of 240 mg/kg and 264 mg/kg in male and female mice, respectively and 2390 mg/kg and 2250 mg/kg in male and female rats, respectively, caused significant lethality.
In a suicide attempt, one patient took 150 mg felodipine together with 15 tablets each of atenolol and spironolactone and 20 tablets of nitrazepam. The patient's blood pressure

Continued on next page

Astra Merck—Cont.

Percent of Patients with Adverse Events in Controlled Trials*
of PLENDIL (N=861) as Monotherapy without Regard to Causality
(Incidence of discontinuations shown in parentheses)

Body System Adverse Events	Placebo N=334	2.5 mg N=255	5 mg N=581	10 mg N=408
Body as a Whole				
Peripheral Edema	3.3 (0.0)	2.0 (0.0)	8.8 (2.2)	17.4 (2.5)
Asthenia	3.3 (0.0)	3.9 (0.0)	3.3 (0.0)	2.2 (0.0)
Warm Sensation	0.0 (0.0)	0.0 (0.0)	0.9 (0.2)	1.5 (0.0)
Cardiovascular				
Palpitation	2.4 (0.0)	0.4 (0.0)	1.4 (0.3)	2.5 (0.5)
Digestive				
Nausea	1.5 (0.9)	1.2 (0.0)	1.7 (0.3)	1.0 (0.7)
Dyspepsia	1.2 (0.0)	3.9 (0.0)	0.7 (0.0)	0.5 (0.0)
Constipation	0.9 (0.0)	1.2 (0.0)	0.3 (0.0)	1.5 (0.2)
Nervous				
Headache	10.2 (0.9)	10.6 (0.4)	11.0 (1.7)	14.7 (2.0)
Dizziness	2.7 (0.3)	2.7 (0.0)	3.6 (0.5)	3.7 (0.5)
Paresthesia	1.5 (0.3)	1.6 (0.0)	1.2 (0.0)	1.2 (0.2)
Respiratory				
Upper Respiratory				
Infection	1.8 (0.0)	3.9 (0.0)	1.9 (0.0)	0.7 (0.0)
Cough	0.3 (0.0)	0.8 (0.0)	1.2 (0.0)	1.7 (0.0)
Rhinorrhea	0.0 (0.0)	1.6 (0.0)	0.2 (0.0)	0.2 (0.0)
Sneezing	0.0 (0.0)	1.6 (0.0)	0.0 (0.0)	0.0 (0.0)
Skin				
Rash	0.9 (0.0)	2.0 (0.0)	0.2 (0.0)	0.2 (0.0)
Flushing	0.9 (0.3)	3.9 (0.0)	5.3 (0.7)	6.9 (1.2)

* Patients in titration studies may have been exposed to more than one dose level of PLENDIL.

and heart rate were normal on admission to hospital; he subsequently recovered without significant sequelae. Overdosage might be expected to cause excessive peripheral vasodilation with marked hypotension and possibly bradycardia.

If severe hypotension occurs, symptomatic treatment should be instituted. The patient should be placed supine with the legs elevated. The administration of intravenous fluids may be useful to treat hypotension due to overdosage with calcium antagonists. In case of accompanying bradycardia, atropine (0.5–1 mg) should be administered intravenously. Sympathomimetic drugs may also be given if the physician feels they are warranted.

It has not been established whether felodipine can be removed from the circulation by hemodialysis.

DOSAGE AND ADMINISTRATION

The recommended starting dose is 5 mg once a day. Depending on the patient's response the dosage can be decreased to 2.5 mg or increased to 10 mg once a day. These adjustments should occur generally at intervals of not less than two weeks. The recommended dosage range is 2.5–10 mg once daily. In clinical trials, doses above 10 mg daily showed an increased blood pressure response but a large increase in the rate of peripheral edema and other vasodilatory adverse events (see ADVERSE REACTIONS). Modification of the recommended dosage is usually not required in patients with renal impairment.

PLENDIL should be swallowed whole and not crushed or chewed.

Use in the Elderly or Patients with Impaired Liver Function: Patients over 65 years of age or patients with impaired liver function, may develop higher plasma concentrations of felodipine, therefore a starting dose of 2.5 mg once a day is recommended. Dosage may be adjusted as described above. (See PRECAUTIONS.)

HOW SUPPLIED

No. 3584—Tablets PLENDIL, 2.5 mg, are sage green, round convex tablets, with code 450 on one side and PLENDIL on the other. They are supplied as follows:
NDC 61113-450-28 unit dose packages of 100
NDC 61113-450-58 unit of use bottles of 100
NDC 61113-450-31 unit of use bottles of 30.
No. 3585—Tablets PLENDIL, 5 mg, are light red-brown, round convex tablets, with code 451 on one side and PLENDIL on the other. They are supplied as follows:
NDC 61113-451-28 unit dose packages of 100
(6505-01-350-0354, 5 mg individually sealed 100's)
NDC 61113-451-58 unit of use bottles of 100
(6505-01-350-0356, 5 mg 100's)
NDC 61113-451-31 unit of use bottles of 30
(6505-01-350-0352, 5 mg 30's).
No. 3586—Tablets PLENDIL, 10 mg, are red-brown, round convex tablets, with code 452 on one side and PLENDIL on the other. They are supplied as follows:
NDC 61113-452-28 unit dose packages of 100
(6505-01-350-0353, 10 mg individually sealed 100's)

NDC 61113-452-58 unit of use bottles of 100
(6505-01-350-0355, 10 mg 100's)
NDC 61113-452-31 unit of use bottles of 30
(6505-01-350-0357, 10 mg 30's)
Storage
Store below 30°C (86°F). Keep container tightly closed. Protect from light.
Distributed by:
ASTRA MERCK
Wayne, PA 19087, USA
Manufactured by: MERCK & CO., INC., West Point, PA 19486, USA
Issued July 1995   7909008
© 1995 Astra Merck Inc.   All rights reserved.
Shown in Product Identification Guide, page 304

PRILOSEC®* 　　　　　　　　　　　　　　　℞
(OMEPRAZOLE)
DELAYED-RELEASE CAPSULES

DESCRIPTION

The active ingredient in PRILOSEC* (Omeprazole) Delayed-Release Capsules is a substituted benzimidazole, 5-methoxy-2-[[(4-methoxy-3,5-dimethyl-2-pyridinyl) methyl] sulfinyl]-1*H*-benzimidazole, a compound that inhibits gastric acid secretion. Its empirical formula is $C_{17}H_{19}N_3O_3S$, with a molecular weight of 345.42. The structural formula is:

Omeprazole is a white to off-white crystalline powder which melts with decomposition at about 155°C. It is a weak base, freely soluble in ethanol and methanol, and slightly soluble in acetone and isopropanol and very slightly soluble in water. The stability of omeprazole is a function of pH; it is rapidly degraded in acid media, but has acceptable stability under alkaline conditions.

PRILOSEC is supplied as delayed-release capsules for oral administration. Each delayed-release capsule contains either 10 mg or 20 mg of omeprazole in the form of enteric-coated granules with the following inactive ingredients: cellulose, disodium hydrogen phosphate, hydroxypropyl cellulose, hydroxypropyl methylcellulose, lactose, mannitol, sodium lauryl sulfate and other ingredients. The capsule shells have the following inactive ingredients: gelatin-NF, FD&C Blue #1, FD&C Red #40, D&C Red #28, titanium dioxide, synthetic black iron oxide, isopropanol, butyl alcohol, FD&C Blue #2, D&C Red #7 Calcium Lake, and, in addition, the 10 mg capsule shell also contains D&C Yellow #10.

*Registered trademark of AB Astra.

CLINICAL PHARMACOLOGY

Pharmacokinetics and Metabolism: Omeprazole
PRILOSEC Delayed-Release Capsules contain an enteric-coated granule formulation of omeprazole (because omeprazole is acid-labile), so that absorption of omeprazole begins only after the granules leave the stomach. Absorption is rapid, with peak plasma levels of omeprazole occurring within 0.5 to 3.5 hours. Peak plasma concentrations of omeprazole and AUC are approximately proportional to doses up to 40 mg, but because of a saturable first-pass effect, a greater than linear response in peak plasma concentration and AUC occurs with doses greater than 40 mg. Absolute bioavailability (compared to intravenous administration) is about 30–40% at doses of 20–40 mg, due in large part to presystemic metabolism. In healthy subjects the plasma half-life is 0.5 to 1 hour, and the total body clearance is 500–600 mL/min. Protein binding is approximately 95%.

The bioavailability of omeprazole increases slightly upon repeated administration of PRILOSEC Delayed-Release Capsules.

Following single dose oral administration of a buffered solution of omeprazole, little if any unchanged drug was excreted in urine. The majority of the dose (about 77%) was eliminated in urine as at least six metabolites. Two were identified as hydroxyomeprazole and the corresponding carboxylic acid. The remainder of the dose was recoverable in feces. This implies a significant biliary excretion of the metabolites of omeprazole. Three metabolites have been identified in plasma—the sulfide and sulfone derivatives of omeprazole, and hydroxyomeprazole. These metabolites have very little or no antisecretory activity.

In patients with chronic hepatic disease, the bioavailability increased to approximately 100% compared to an I.V. dose, reflecting decreased first-pass effect, and the plasma half-life of the drug increased to nearly 3 hours compared to the half-life in normals of 0.5–1 hour. Plasma clearance averaged 70 mL/min, compared to a value of 500–600 mL/min in normal subjects.

In patients with chronic renal impairment, whose creatinine clearance ranged between 10 and 62 mL/min/1.73 m², the disposition of omeprazole was very similar to that in healthy volunteers, although there was a slight increase in bioavailability. Because urinary excretion is a primary route of excretion of omeprazole metabolites, their elimination slowed in proportion to the decreased creatinine clearance.

The elimination rate of omeprazole was somewhat decreased in the elderly, and bioavailability was increased. Omeprazole was 76% bioavailable when a single 40 mg oral dose of omeprazole (buffered solution) was administered to healthy elderly volunteers, versus 58% in young volunteers given the same dose. Nearly 70% of the dose was recovered in urine as metabolites of omeprazole and no unchanged drug was detected. The plasma clearance of omeprazole was 250 mL/min (about half that of young volunteers) and its plasma half-life averaged one hour, about twice that of young healthy volunteers.

In pharmacokinetic studies of single 20 mg omeprazole doses, an increase in AUC of approximately four-fold was noted in Asian subjects compared to Caucasians. Dose adjustment, particularly where maintenance of healing of erosive esophagitis is indicated, for the hepatically impaired and Asian subjects should be considered.

Pharmacokinetics: Combination Therapy with Clarithromycin
Omeprazole 40 mg daily was given in combination with clarithromycin 500 mg every 8 hours to healthy adult male subjects. The steady state plasma concentrations of omeprazole were increased (C_{max}, AUC_{0-24}, and $T_{1/2}$ increases of 30%, 89% and 34% respectively) by the concomitant administration of clarithromyin. The observed increases in omeprazole plasma concentration were associated with the following pharmacological effects. The mean 24-hour gastric pH value was 5.2 when omeprazole was administered alone and 5.7 when coadministered with clarithromycin.

The plasma levels of clarithromycin and 14-hydroxy-clarithromycin were increased by the concomitant administration of omeprazole. For clarithromycin, the mean C_{max} was 10% greater, the mean C_{min} was 27% greater, and the mean AUC_{0-8} was 15% greater when clarithromycin was administered with omeprazole than when clarithromycin was administered alone. Similar results were seen for 14-hydroxy-clarithromycin, the mean C_{max} was 45% greater, the mean C_{min} was 57% greater, and the mean AUC_{0-8} was 45% greater. Clarithromycin concentrations in the gastric tissue and mucus were also increased by concomitant administration of omeprazole.

Clarithromycin Tissue Concentrations
2 hours after Dose[1]

Tissue	Clarithromycin	Clarithromycin + Omeprazole
Antrum	10.48±2.01 (n=5)	19.96± 4.71 (n=5)
Fundus	20.81±7.64 (n=5)	24.25± 6.37 (n=5)
Mucus	4.15±7.74 (n=4)	38.29±32.79 (n=4)

[1] Mean ± SD (µg/g)

For information on clarithromycin pharmacokinetics and microbiology, consult the clarithromycin package insert, CLINICAL PHARMACOLOGY section.

Pharmacodynamics
Mechanism of Action
Omeprazole belongs to a new class of antisecretory compounds, the substituted benzimidazoles, that do not exhibit anticholinergic or H_2 histamine antagonistic properties, but that suppress gastric acid secretion by specific inhibition of the H^+/K^+ ATPase enzyme system at the secretory surface of the gastric parietal cell. Because this enzyme system is regarded as the acid (proton) pump within the gastric mucosa, omeprazole has been characterized as a gastric acid-pump inhibitor, in that it blocks the final step of acid production. This effect is dose-related and leads to inhibition of both basal and stimulated acid secretion irrespective of the stimulus. Animal studies indicate that after rapid disappearance from plasma, omeprazole can be found within the gastric mucosa for a day or more.

Antisecretory Activity
After oral administration, the onset of the antisecretory effect of omeprazole occurs within one hour, with the maximum effect occurring within two hours. Inhibition of secretion is about 50% of maximum at 24 hours and the duration of inhibition lasts up to 72 hours. The antisecretory effect thus lasts far longer than would be expected from the very short (less than one hour) plasma half-life, apparently due to prolonged binding to the parietal H^+/K^+ ATPase enzyme. When the drug is discontinued, secretory activity returns gradually, over 3 to 5 days. The inhibitory effect of omeprazole on acid secretion increases with repeated once-daily dosing, reaching a plateau after four days.
Results from numerous studies of the antisecretory effect of multiple doses of 20 mg and 40 mg of omeprazole in normal volunteers and patients are shown below. The "max" value represents determinations at a time of maximum effect (2–6 hours after dosing), while "min" values are those 24 hours after the last dose of omeprazole.

Range of Mean Values from Multiple Studies of the Mean Antisecretory Effects of Omeprazole After Multiple Daily Dosing

Parameter % Decrease in	Omeprazole 20 mg		Omeprazole 40 mg	
	Max	Min	Max	Min
Basal Acid Output	78*	58–80	94*	80–93
Peak Acid Output	79*	50–59	88*	62–68
24-hr. Intragastric Acidity		80–97		92–94

*Single Studies

Single daily oral doses of omeprazole ranging from a dose of 10 mg to 40 mg have produced 100% inhibition of 24-hour intragastric acidity in some patients.

Enterochromaffin-like (ECL) Cell Effects
In 24-month carcinogenicity studies in rats, a dose-related significant increase in gastric carcinoid tumors and ECL cell hyperplasia was observed in both male and female animals (see PRECAUTIONS, Carcinogenesis, Mutagenesis, Impairment of Fertility). Hypergastrinemia secondary to prolonged and sustained hypochlorhydria has been postulated to be the mechanism by which ECL cell hyperplasia and gastric carcinoid tumors develop. Omeprazole may also affect other cells in the gastrointestinal tract (e.g., G cells), either directly or by inducing sustained hypochlorhydria, but this possibility has not been extensively studied.
Human gastric biopsy specimens from about 200 patients treated continuously with omeprazole for an average of over 12 months have not detected ECL cell effects of omeprazole similar to those seen in rats. Longer term data are needed to rule out the possibility of an increased risk for the development of gastric tumors in patients receiving long-term therapy with omeprazole.

Serum Gastrin Effects
In studies involving more than 200 patients, serum gastrin levels increased during the first 1 to 2 weeks of once-daily administration of therapeutic doses of omeprazole in parallel with inhibition of acid secretion. No further increase in serum gastrin occurred with continued treatment. In comparison with histamine H_2-receptor antagonists, the median increases produced by 20 mg doses of omeprazole were higher (1.3 to 3.6 fold vs. 1.1 to 1.8 fold increase). Gastrin values returned to pretreatment levels, usually within 1 to 2 weeks after discontinuation of therapy.

Other Effects
Systemic effects of omeprazole in the CNS, cardiovascular and respiratory systems have not been found to date. Ome-

prazole, given in oral doses of 30 or 40 mg for 2 to 4 weeks, had no effect on thyroid function, carbohydrate metabolism, or circulating levels of parathyroid hormone, cortisol, estradiol, testosterone, prolactin, cholecystokinin or secretin.
No effect on gastric emptying of the solid and liquid components of a test meal was demonstrated after a single dose of omeprazole 90 mg. In healthy subjects, a single I.V. dose of omeprazole (0.35 mg/kg) had no effect on intrinsic factor secretion. No systematic dose-dependent effect has been observed on basal or stimulated pepsin output in humans. However, when intragastric pH is maintained at 4.0 or above, basal pepsin output is low, and pepsin activity is decreased.
As do other agents that elevate intragastric pH, omeprazole administered for 14 days in healthy subjects produced a significant increase in the intragastric concentrations of viable bacteria. The pattern of the bacterial species was unchanged from that commonly found in saliva. All changes resolved within three days of stopping treatment.

Clinical Studies
Duodenal Ulcer Disease
Active Duodenal Ulcer: In a multicenter, double-blind, placebo-controlled study of 147 patients with endoscopically documented duodenal ulcer, the percentage of patients healed (per protocol) at 2 and 4 weeks was significantly higher with PRILOSEC 20 mg once a day than with placebo ($p \le 0.01$).

Treatment of Active Duodenal Ulcer % of Patients Healed

	PRILOSEC 20 mg a.m. (n=99)	Placebo a.m. (n=48)
Week 2	*41	13
Week 4	*75	27

*($p \le 0.01$)

Complete daytime and nighttime pain relief occurred significantly faster ($p \le 0.01$) in patients treated with PRILOSEC 20 mg than in patients treated with placebo. At the end of the study, significantly more patients who had received PRILOSEC had complete relief of daytime pain ($p \le 0.05$) and nighttime pain ($p \le 0.01$).
In a multicenter, double-blind study of 293 patients with endoscopically documented duodenal ulcer, the percentage of patients healed (per protocol) at 4 weeks was significantly higher with PRILOSEC 20 mg once a day than with ranitidine 150 mg b.i.d. ($p < 0.01$).

Treatment of Active Duodenal Ulcer % of Patients Healed

	PRILOSEC 20 mg a.m. (n=145)	Ranitidine 150 mg b.i.d. (n=148)
Week 2	42	34
Week 4	*82	63

*($p < 0.01$)

Healing occurred significantly faster in patients treated with PRILOSEC than in those treated with ranitidine 150 mg b.i.d. ($p < 0.01$).
In a foreign multinational randomized, double-blind study of 105 patients with endoscopically documented duodenal ulcer, 20 mg and 40 mg of PRILOSEC were compared to 150 mg b.i.d. of ranitidine at 2, 4 and 8 weeks. At 2 and 4 weeks both doses of PRILOSEC were statistically superior (per protocol) to ranitidine, but 40 mg was not superior to 20 mg of PRILOSEC, and at 8 weeks there was no significant difference between any of the active drugs.

Treatment of Active Duodenal Ulcer % of Patients Healed

	PRILOSEC 20 mg (n=34)	PRILOSEC 40 mg (n=36)	Ranitidine 150 mg b.i.d. (n=35)
Week 2	*83	*83	53
Week 4	*97	*100	82
Week 8	100	100	94

*($p \le 0.01$)

Duodenal Ulcer Recurrence
Four randomized double blind clinical studies in patients with *H. pylori* infection and active duodenal ulcer disease compared omeprazole plus clarithromycin to omeprazole. Two of these studies, one in the U.S., the other in the U.S. and Canada, included a clarithromycin alone arm. The dose regimen in the two multicenter U.S. studies (n=498) was PRILOSEC 40 mg q.d. plus clarithromycin 500 mg t.i.d. for 14 days followed by PRILOSEC 20 mg q.d. for 14 days; PRILOSEC 40 mg q.d. for 14 days followed by PRILOSEC 20 mg q.d. for 14 days; clarithromycin 500 mg t.i.d. for 14 days. Two foreign studies (n=369) compared PRILOSEC and clarithromycin to PRILOSEC, and did not include a clarithromycin alone arm. The dose regimen was the same as that used in the U.S. studies except for one study (M92-812b) where

PRILOSEC 40 mg q.d. was used throughout the 28 day treatment period. Endpoints studied were: eradication of *H. pylori*, duodenal ulcer healing and recurrence. *H. pylori* status was determined by histology and another bacteriological test. For a given patient, *H. pylori* was considered eradicated if at least one of these tests was negative, and none was positive.
The combination of omeprazole and clarithromycin was effective in eradicating *H. pylori*.

H. pylori Eradication Rates % of Patients Cured† [95% Confidence Interval]

	PRILOSEC + Clarithromycin	PRILOSEC	Clarithromycin
U.S. Studies			
Study M93-067	*74 [61, 85] (n=58)	0 [0, 6] (n=55)	34 [20, 50] (n=44)
Study M93-100	*64 [51, 76] (n=64)	0 [0, 6] (n=62)	38 [24, 53] (n=48)
Non U.S. Studies			
Study M92-812b	*83 [72, 91] (n=69)	1 [0, 7] (n=75)	N/A
Study M93-058	*74 [64, 83] (n=93)	4 [1, 10] (n=96)	N/A

† Evaluable patients with confirmed duodenal ulcer and *H. pylori* infection at baseline who are healed at week 4, and for whom results were available for the 4–6 week post-treatment visit are included in this analysis.
* ($p \le 0.01$) versus PRILOSEC or clarithromycin.

Ulcer healing was not significantly different when clarithromycin was added to omeprazole therapy compared to omeprazole therapy alone.
The combination of omeprazole and clarithromycin was effective in eradicating *H. pylori* and reduced duodenal ulcer recurrence.

Duodenal Ulcer Recurrence Rates by *H. pylori* Eradication Status % of Patients with Ulcer Recurrence

	H. pylori eradicated#	*H. pylori* not eradicated#
U.S. Studies†		
6 months post-treatment		
Study M93-067	*35 (n=49)	60 (n=88)
Study M93-100	*8 (n=53)	60 (n=106)
Non U.S. Studies‡		
6 months post-treatment		
Study M92-812b	*5 (n=43)	46 (n=78)
Study M93-058	*6 (n=53)	43 (n=107)
12 months post-treatment		
Study M92-812b	*5 (n=39)	68 (n=71)

H. pylori eradication status assessed at same timepoint as ulcer recurrence.
† Combined results for PRILOSEC + clarithromycin, PRILOSEC, and clarithromycin treatment arms.
‡ Combined results for PRILOSEC + clarithromycin and PRILOSEC treatment arms.
* ($p \le 0.01$) versus proportion with duodenal ulcer recurrence who were not *H. pylori* eradicated.

Gastric Ulcer
In a U.S. multicenter, double-blind, study of omeprazole 40 mg once a day, 20 mg once a day, and placebo in 520 patients with endoscopically diagnosed gastric ulcer, the following results were obtained.

Treatment of Gastric Ulcer % of Patients Healed (All Patients Treated)

	PRILOSEC 20 mg q.d. (n=202)	PRILOSEC 40 mg q.d. (n=214)	Placebo (n=104)
Week 4	47.5**	55.6**	30.8
Week 8	74.8**	82.7**,+	48.1

**($p < 0.01$) PRILOSEC 40 mg or 20 mg versus placebo
+ ($p < 0.05$) PRILOSEC 40 mg versus 20 mg

For the stratified groups of patients with ulcer size less than or equal to 1 cm, no difference in healing rates between 40 mg and 20 mg was detected at either 4 or 8 weeks. For pa-

Continued on next page

Astra Merck—Cont.

tients with ulcer size greater than 1 cm, 40 mg was significantly more effective than 20 mg at 8 weeks.

In a foreign, multinational, double-blind study of 602 patients with endoscopically diagnosed gastric ulcer, omeprazole 40 mg once a day, 20 mg once a day, and ranitidine 150 mg twice a day were evaluated.

Treatment of Gastric Ulcer
% of Patients Healed
(All Patients Healed)

	PRILOSEC 20 mg q.d. (n=200)	PRILOSEC 40 mg q.d. (n=187)	Ranitidine 150 mg b.i.d. (n=199)
Week 4	63.5	78.1**,++	56.3
Week 8	81.5	91.4**,++	78.4

**(p<0.01) PRILOSEC 40 mg versus ranitidine
++(p<0.01) PRILOSEC 40 mg versus 20 mg

Gastroesophageal Reflux Disease (GERD)
In a U.S. multicenter double-blind placebo controlled study of 20 mg or 40 mg of PRILOSEC Delayed-Release Capsules in patients with symptomatic esophagitis and endoscopically diagnosed erosive esophagitis of grade 2 or above, the percentage healing rates (per protocol) were as follows:

Week	20 mg PRILOSEC (n=83)	40 mg PRILOSEC (n=87)	Placebo (n=43)
4	39**	45**	7
8	74**	75**	14

**(p<0.01) PRILOSEC versus placebo.

In this study, the 40 mg dose was not superior to the 20 mg dose of PRILOSEC in the percentage healing rate. Other controlled clinical trials have also shown that PRILOSEC is effective in severe GERD. In comparisons with histamine H₂-receptor antagonists in patients with erosive esophagitis, grade 2 or above, PRILOSEC in a dose of 20 mg was significantly more effective than the active controls. Complete daytime and nighttime heartburn relief occurred significantly faster (p<0.01) in patients treated with PRILOSEC than in those taking placebo or histamine H₂-receptor antagonists.
Long Term Maintenance Treatment of Erosive Esophagitis
In a U.S. double-blind, randomized, multicenter, placebo controlled study, two dose regimens of PRILOSEC were studied in patients with endoscopically confirmed healed esophagitis. Results to determine maintenance of healing of erosive esophagitis are shown below.

Life Table Analysis

	PRILOSEC 20 mg q.d. (n=138)	PRILOSEC 20 mg 3 days per week (n=137)	Placebo (n=131)
Percent in endoscopic remission at 6 months	*70	34	11

*(p<0.01) PRILOSEC 20 mg q.d. versus PRILOSEC 20 mg 3 consecutive days per week or placebo.

In an international multicenter double-blind study, PRILOSEC 20 mg daily and 10 mg daily were compared to ranitidine 150 mg twice daily in patients with endoscopically confirmed healed esophagitis. The table below provides the results of this study for maintenance of healing of erosive esophagitis.

Life Table Analysis

	PRILOSEC 20 mg q.d. (n=131)	PRILOSEC 10 mg q.d. (n=133)	Ranitidine 150 mg b.i.d. (n=128)
Percent in endoscopic remission at 12 months	*77	‡58	46

*(p=0.01) PRILOSEC 20 mg q.d. versus PRILOSEC 10 mg q.d. or Ranitidine.
‡(p=0.03) PRILOSEC 10 mg q.d. versus Ranitidine.

In patients who initially had grades 3 or 4 erosive esophagitis, for maintenance after healing 20 mg daily of PRILOSEC was effective, while 10 mg did not demonstrate effectiveness.
Pathological Hypersecretory Conditions
In open studies of 136 patients with pathological hypersecretory conditions, such as Zollinger-Ellison (ZE) syndrome with or without multiple endocrine adenomas, PRILOSEC Delayed-Release Capsules significantly inhibited gastric acid secretion and controlled associated symptoms of diarrhea, anorexia, and pain. Doses ranging from 20 mg every other day to 360 mg per day maintained basal acid secretion below 10 mEq/hr in patients without prior gastric surgery, and below 5 mEq/hr in patients with prior gastric surgery.
Initial doses were titrated to the individual patient need, and adjustments were necessary with time in some patients (see

DOSAGE AND ADMINISTRATION). PRILOSEC was well tolerated at these high dose levels for prolonged periods (>5 years in some patients). In most ZE patients, serum gastrin levels were not modified by PRILOSEC. However, in some patients serum gastrin increased to levels greater than those present prior to initiation of omeprazole therapy. At least 11 patients with ZE syndrome on long-term treatment with PRILOSEC developed gastric carcinoids. These findings are believed to be a manifestation of the underlying condition, which is known to be associated with such tumors, rather than the result of the administration of PRILOSEC. (See ADVERSE REACTIONS.)

INDICATIONS AND USAGE

Duodenal Ulcer
PRILOSEC Delayed-Release Capsules are indicated for short-term treatment of active duodenal ulcer. Most patients heal within four weeks. Some patients may require an additional four weeks of therapy.

PRILOSEC Delayed-Release Capsules, in combination with clarithromycin, are also indicated for treatment of patients with *H. pylori* infection and active duodenal ulcer to eradicate *H. pylori*. Eradication of *H. pylori* has been shown to reduce the risk of duodenal ulcer recurrence (see CLINICAL PHARMACOLOGY, *Clinical Studies* and DOSAGE AND ADMINISTRATION).

In patients who fail therapy, susceptibility testing should be done. If resistance to clarithromycin is demonstrated or susceptibility testing is not possible, alternative antimicrobial therapy should be instituted. (See the clarithromycin package insert, MICROBIOLOGY section.)

Gastric Ulcer
PRILOSEC Delayed-Release Capsules are indicated for short-term treatment (4–8 weeks) of active benign gastric ulcer. (See CLINICAL PHARMACOLOGY, *Clinical Studies*, *Gastric Ulcer*).

Gastroesophageal Reflux Disease (GERD)
Erosive Esophagitis
PRILOSEC Delayed-Release Capsules are indicated for the short-term treatment (4–8 weeks) of erosive esophagitis which has been diagnosed by endoscopy (see CLINICAL PHARMACOLOGY, *Clinical Studies*).

Poorly Responsive Symptomatic GERD
PRILOSEC Delayed-Release Capsules are also indicated for the short-term treatment (4–8 weeks) of symptomatic gastroesophageal reflux disease (esophagitis) poorly responsive to customary medical treatment, usually including an adequate course of a histamine H₂-receptor antagonist.
The efficacy of PRILOSEC used for longer than 8 weeks in these patients has not been established. In the rare instance of a patient not responding to 8 weeks of treatment, it may be helpful to give up to an additional 4 weeks of treatment. If there is recurrence of erosive esophagitis or symptomatic GERD poorly responsive to customary medical treatment, additional 4–8 week courses of omeprazole may be considered.

Maintenance of Healing of Erosive Esophagitis
PRILOSEC Delayed-Release Capsules are indicated to maintain healing of erosive esophagitis.
Controlled studies do not extend beyond 12 months.

Pathological Hypersecretory Conditions
PRILOSEC Delayed-Release Capsules are indicated for the long-term treatment of pathological hypersecretory conditions (e.g., Zollinger-Ellison syndrome, multiple endocrine adenomas and systemic mastocytosis).

CONTRAINDICATIONS

Omeprazole
PRILOSEC Delayed-Release Capsules are contraindicated in patients with known hypersensitivity to any component of the formulation.

Clarithromycin
Clarithromycin is contraindicated in patients with a known hypersensitivity to any macrolide antibiotic, and in patients receiving terfenadine therapy who have pre-existing cardiac abnormalities or electrolyte disturbances. (Please refer to full prescribing information for clarithromycin before prescribing.)

WARNING:

Clarithromycin
CLARITHROMYCIN SHOULD NOT BE USED IN PREGNANT WOMEN EXCEPT IN CLINICAL CIRCUMSTANCES WHERE NO ALTERNATIVE THERAPY IS APPROPRIATE. IF PREGNANCY OCCURS WHILE TAKING CLARITHROMYCIN, THE PATIENT SHOULD BE APPRISED OF THE POTENTIAL HAZARD TO THE FETUS. (See WARNINGS in prescribing information for clarithromycin.)

PRECAUTIONS

General
Symptomatic response to therapy with omeprazole does not preclude the presence of gastric malignancy.
Atrophic gastritis has been noted occasionally in gastric corpus biopsies from patients treated long-term with omeprazole.
Information for Patients
PRILOSEC Delayed-Release Capsules should be taken before eating. Patients should be cautioned that the PRILOSEC Delayed-Release Capsule should not be opened, chewed or crushed, and should be swallowed whole.
Drug Interactions
Other
Omeprazole can prolong the elimination of diazepam, warfarin and phenytoin, drugs that are metabolized by oxidation in the liver. Although in normal subjects no interaction with theophylline or propranolol was found, there have been clinical reports of interaction with other drugs metabolized via the cytochrome P-450 system (e.g., cyclosporine, disulfiram, benzodiazepines). Patients should be monitored to determine if it is necessary to adjust the dosage of these drugs when taken concomitantly with PRILOSEC.
Because of its profound and long lasting inhibition of gastric acid secretion, it is theoretically possible that omeprazole may interfere with absorption of drugs where gastric pH is an important determinant of their bioavailability (e.g., ketoconazole, ampicillin esters, and iron salts). In the clinical trials, antacids were used concomitantly with the administration of PRILOSEC.
Combination Therapy with Clarithromycin
Co-administration of omeprazole and clarithromycin may result in increases in plasma levels of omeprazole, clarithromycin, and 14-hydroxy-clarithromycin. (See also CLINICAL PHARMACOLOGY, *Pharmacokinetics: Combination Therapy with Clarithromycin.*)
Carcinogenesis, Mutagenesis, Impairment of Fertility
In two 24-month carcinogenicity studies in rats, omeprazole at daily doses of 1.7, 3.4, 13.8, 44.0 and 140.8 mg/kg/day (approximately 4 to 352 times the human dose, based on a patient weight of 50 kg and a human dose of 20 mg) produced gastric ECL cell carcinoids in a dose-related manner in both male and female rats; the incidence of this effect was markedly higher in female rats, which had higher blood levels of omeprazole. Gastric carcinoids seldom occur in the untreated rat. In addition, ECL cell hyperplasia was present in all treated groups of both sexes. In one of these studies, female rats were treated with 13.8 mg omeprazole/kg/day (approximately 35 times the human dose) for one year, then followed for an additional year without the drug. No carcinoids were seen in these rats. An increased incidence of treatment-related ECL cell hyperplasia was observed at the end of one year (94% treated vs 10% controls). By the second year the difference between treated and control rats was much smaller (46% vs 26%) but still showed more hyperplasia in the treated group. An unusual primary malignant tumor in the stomach was seen in one rat (2%). No similar tumor was seen in male or female rats treated for two years. For this strain of rat no similar tumor has been noted historically, but a finding involving only one tumor is difficult to interpret. A 78-week mouse carcinogenicity study of omeprazole did not show increased tumor occurrence, but the study was not conclusive.
Omeprazole was not mutagenic in an *in vitro* Ames *Salmonella typhimurium* assay, an *in vitro* mouse lymphoma cell assay and an *in vivo* rat liver DNA damage assay. A mouse micronucleus test at 625 and 6250 times the human dose gave a borderline result, as did an *in vivo* bone marrow chromosome aberration test. A second mouse micronucleus study at 2000 times the human dose, but with different (suboptimal) sampling times, was negative.
In a rat fertility and general reproductive performance test, omeprazole in a dose range of 13.8 to 138.0 mg/kg/day (approximately 35 to 345 times the human dose) was not toxic or deleterious to the reproductive performance of parental animals.
Pregnancy
Omeprazole
Pregnancy Category C
Teratology studies conducted in pregnant rats at doses up to 138 mg/kg/day (approximately 345 times the human dose) and in pregnant rabbits at doses up to 69 mg/kg/day (approximately 172 times the human dose) did not disclose any evidence for a teratogenic potential of omeprazole.
In rabbits, omeprazole in a dose range of 6.9 to 69.1 mg/kg/day (approximately 17 to 172 times the human dose) produced dose-related increases in embryo-lethality, fetal resorptions and pregnancy disruptions. In rats, dose-related embryo/fetal toxicity and postnatal developmental toxicity were observed in offspring resulting from parents treated with omeprazole 13.8 to 138.0 mg/kg/day (approximately 35 to 345 times the human dose). There are no adequate or well-controlled studies in pregnant women. Sporadic reports have been received of congenital abnormalities occurring in in-

fants born to women who have received omeprazole during pregnancy. Omeprazole should be used during pregnancy only if the potential benefit justifies the potential risk to the fetus.

Clarithromycin

Pregnancy Category C. See WARNINGS (above) and full prescribing information for clarithromycin before using in pregnant women.

Nursing Mothers

It is not known whether omeprazole is excreted in human milk. In rats, omeprazole administration during late gestation and lactation at doses of 13.8 to 138 mg/kg/day (35 to 345 times the human dose) resulted in decreased weight gain in pups. Because many drugs are excreted in human milk, because of the potential for serious adverse reactions in nursing infants from omeprazole, and because of the potential for tumorigenicity shown for omeprazole in rat carcinogenicity studies, a decision should be made whether to discontinue nursing or to discontinue the drug, taking into account the importance of the drug to the mother.

Pediatric Use

Safety and effectiveness in children have not been established.

ADVERSE REACTIONS

PRILOSEC Delayed-Release Capsules were generally well tolerated during domestic and international clinical trials in 3096 patients.

In the U.S. clinical trial population of 465 patients (including duodenal ulcer, Zollinger-Ellison syndrome and resistant ulcer patients), the following adverse experiences were reported to occur in 1% or more of patients on therapy with PRILOSEC. Numbers in parentheses indicate percentages of the adverse experiences considered by investigators as possibly, probably or definitely related to the drug:

	Omeprazole (n = 465)	Placebo (n = 64)	Ranitidine (n = 195)
Headache	6.9 (2.4)	6.3	7.7 (2.6)
Diarrhea	3.0 (1.9)	3.1 (1.6)	2.1 (0.5)
Abdominal Pain	2.4 (0.4)	3.1	2.1
Nausea	2.2 (0.9)	3.1	4.1 (0.5)
URI	1.9	1.6	2.6
Dizziness	1.5 (0.6)	0.0	2.6 (1.0)
Vomiting	1.5 (0.4)	4.7	1.5 (0.5)
Rash	1.5 (1.1)	0.0	0.0
Constipation	1.1 (0.9)	0.0	0.0
Cough	1.1	0.0	1.5
Asthenia	1.1 (0.2)	1.6 (1.6)	1.5 (1.0)
Back Pain	1.1	0.0	0.5

The following adverse reactions which occurred in 1% or more of omeprazole-treated patients have been reported in international double-blind, and open-label, clinical trials in which 2,631 patients and subjects received omeprazole.

	Incidence of Adverse Experiences ≥ 1% Causal Relationship not Assessed	
	Omeprazole (n = 2631)	Placebo (n = 120)
Body as a Whole, site unspecified		
Abdominal pain	5.2	3.3
Asthenia	1.3	0.8
Digestive System		
Constipation	1.5	0.8
Diarrhea	3.7	2.5
Flatulence	2.7	5.8
Nausea	4.0	6.7
Vomiting	3.2	10.0
Acid regurgitation	1.9	3.3
Nervous System/Psychiatric		
Headache	2.9	2.5

Additional adverse experiences occurring in <1% of patients or subjects in domestic and/or international trials, or occurring since the drug was marketed, are shown below within each body system. In many instances, the relationship to PRILOSEC was unclear.

Body As a Whole: Fever, pain, fatigue, malaise, abdominal swelling

Cardiovascular: Chest pain or angina, tachycardia, bradycardia, palpitation, elevated blood pressure, peripheral edema

Gastrointestinal: Pancreatitis (some fatal), anorexia, irritable colon, flatulence, fecal discoloration, esophageal candidiasis, mucosal atrophy of the tongue, dry mouth. During treatment with omeprazole, gastric fundic gland polyps have been noted rarely. These polyps are benign and appear to be reversible when treatment is discontinued.

Gastro-duodenal carcinoids have been reported in patients with ZE syndrome on long-term treatment with PRILOSEC. This finding is believed to be a manifestation of the underlying condition, which is known to be associated with such tumors.

Hepatic: Mild and, rarely, marked elevations of liver function tests [ALT (SGPT), AST (SGOT), γ-glutamyl transpeptidase, alkaline phosphatase, and bilirubin (jaundice)]. In rare instances, overt liver disease has occurred, including hepatocellular, cholestatic, or mixed hepatitis, liver necrosis (some fatal), hepatic failure (some fatal), and hepatic encephalopathy.

Metabolic/Nutritional: Hyponatremia, hypoglycemia, weight gain

Musculoskeletal: Muscle cramps, myalgia, muscle weakness, joint pain, leg pain

Nervous System/Psychiatric: Psychic disturbances including depression, aggression, hallucinations, confusion, insomnia, nervousness, tremors, apathy, somnolence, anxiety, dream abnormalities; vertigo; paresthesia; hemifacial dysesthesia

Respiratory: Epistaxis, pharyngeal pain

Skin: Rash and, very rarely, cases of severe generalized skin reactions including toxic epidermal necrolysis (TEN; some fatal), Stevens-Johnson syndrome, and erythema multiforme (some severe); skin inflammation, urticaria, angioedema, pruritus, alopecia, dry skin, hyperhidrosis

Special Senses: Tinnitus, taste perversion

Urogenital: Interstitial nephritis (some with positive rechallenge), urinary tract infection, microscopic pyuria, urinary frequency, elevated serum creatinine, proteinuria, hematuria, glycosuria, testicular pain, gynecomastia

Hematologic: Rare instances of pancytopenia, agranulocytosis (some fatal), thrombocytopenia, neutropenia, anemia, leucocytosis, and hemolytic anemia have been reported.

The incidence of clinical adverse experiences in patients greater than 65 years of age was similar to that in patients 65 years of age or less.

Combination Therapy with Clarithromycin

In clinical trials using combination therapy with PRILOSEC and clarithromycin, no adverse experiences peculiar to this drug combination have been observed. Adverse experiences that have occurred have been limited to those that have been previously reported with omeprazole or clarithromycin.

Adverse experiences observed in controlled clinical trials using combination therapy with PRILOSEC and clarithromycin (n=346) which differed from those previously described for omeprazole alone were: Taste perversion (15%), tongue discoloration (2%), rhinitis (2%), pharyngitis (1%), and flu syndrome (1%).

For more information on clarithromycin, refer to the clarithromycin package insert, ADVERSE REACTIONS section.

OVERDOSAGE

Rare reports have been received of overdosage with omeprazole. Doses ranged from 320 mg to 900 mg (16–45 times the usual recommended clinical dose). Manifestations were variable, but included confusion, drowsiness, blurred vision, tachycardia, nausea, diaphoresis, flushing, headache, and dry mouth. Symptoms were transient, and no serious clinical outcome has been reported. No specific antidote for omeprazole overdosage is known. Omeprazole is extensively protein bound and is, therefore, not readily dialyzable. In the event of overdosage, treatment should be symptomatic and supportive.

Lethal doses of omeprazole after single oral administration are about 1500 mg/kg in mice and greater than 4000 mg/kg in rats, and about 100 mg/kg in mice and greater than 40 mg/kg in rats given single intravenous injections. Animals given these doses showed sedation, ptosis, convulsions, and decreased activity, body temperature, and respiratory rate and increased depth of respiration.

DOSAGE AND ADMINISTRATION

Duodenal Ulcer

Short-Term Treatment of Active Duodenal Ulcer: The recommended adult oral dose of PRILOSEC is 20 mg once daily. Most patients heal within four weeks. Some patients may require an additional four weeks of therapy. (See INDICATIONS AND USAGE.)

Reduction of the Risk of Duodenal Ulcer Recurrence: Combination Therapy with Clarithromycin

Days 1–14:	Days 15–28:
PRILOSEC 40 mg q.d. (in the morning) plus clarithromycin 500 mg t.i.d.	PRILOSEC 20 mg q.d.

Please refer to clarithromycin full prescribing information for CONTRAINDICATIONS and WARNING, and for information regarding dosing in the elderly and renally impaired patients (PRECAUTIONS: *General*, PRECAUTIONS: *Geriatric Use* and PRECAUTIONS: *Drug Interactions*).

Gastric Ulcer

The recommended adult oral dose is 40 mg once a day for 4–8 weeks. (See CLINICAL PHARMACOLOGY, *Clinical Studies, Gastric Ulcer,* and INDICATIONS AND USAGE, *Gastric Ulcer.)*

Erosive Esophagitis or Poorly Responsive Gastroesophageal Reflux Disease (GERD)

The recommended adult oral dose is 20 mg daily for 4 to 8 weeks (see INDICATIONS AND USAGE).

Maintenance of Healing of Erosive Esophagitis

The recommended adult oral dose is 20 mg daily. (See CLINICAL PHARMACOLOGY, *Clinical Studies.)*

Pathological Hypersecretory Conditions

The dosage of PRILOSEC in patients with pathological hypersecretory conditions varies with the individual patient. The recommended adult oral starting dose is 60 mg once a day. Doses should be adjusted to individual patient needs and should continue for as long as clinically indicated. Doses up to 120 mg t.i.d. have been administered. Daily dosages of greater than 80 mg should be administered in divided doses. Some patients with Zollinger-Ellison syndrome have been treated continuously with PRILOSEC for more than 5 years. No dosage adjustment is necessary for patients with renal impairment, hepatic dysfunction or for the elderly.

PRILOSEC Delayed-Release Capsules should be taken before eating. In the clinical trials, antacids were used concomitantly with PRILOSEC.

Patients should be cautioned that the PRILOSEC Delayed-Release Capsule should not be opened, chewed or crushed, and should be swallowed whole.

HOW SUPPLIED

No. 3426—PRILOSEC Delayed-Release Capsules, 10 mg, are opaque, hard gelatin, apricot and amethyst colored capsules, coded 606 on cap and PRILOSEC 10 on the body. They are supplied as follows:

NDC 61113-606-31 unit of use bottles of 30
NDC 61113-606-68 bottles of 100
NDC 61113-606-28 unit dose packages of 100.

No. 3440—PRILOSEC Delayed-Release Capsules, 20 mg, are opaque, hard gelatin, amethyst colored capsules, coded 742 on cap and PRILOSEC 20 on body. They are supplied as follows:

NDC 61113-742-31 unit of use bottles of 30 (6505-01-314-2716, 20 mg 30's)
NDC 61113-742-28 unit dose package of 100 (6505-01-314-2717, 20 mg individually sealed 100's)
NDC 61113-742-82 bottles of 1000.

Storage

Store PRILOSEC Delayed-Release Capsules in a tight container protected from light and moisture. Store between 15°C and 30°C (59°F and 86°F).

Distributed by:
Astra Merck
Wayne, PA 19087, USA
Manufactured by: MERCK & CO., INC.,
West Point, PA 19486, USA
Issued April 1996 7910921

© 1995 Astra Merck Inc. All rights reserved

Shown in Product Identification Guide, page 304

TABLETS
TONOCARD®
(TOCAINIDE HCl) ℞

WARNINGS

Blood Dyscrasias: Agranulocytosis, bone marrow depression, leukopenia, neutropenia, aplastic/hypoplastic anemia, thrombocytopenia and sequelae such as septicemia and septic shock have been reported in patients receiving TONOCARD. Most of these patients received TONOCARD within the recommended dosage range. Fatalities have occurred (with approximately 25 percent mortality in reported agranulocytosis cases). Since most of these events have been noted during the first 12 weeks of therapy, it is recommended that complete blood counts, including white cell, differential and platelet counts be performed, optimally, at weekly intervals for the first three months of therapy; and frequently thereafter. Complete blood counts should be performed promptly if the patient develops any signs of infection (such as fever, chills, sore throat, or stomatitis), bruising, or bleeding. If any of these hematologic disorders is identified, TONOCARD should be discontinued and appropriate treatment should be instituted if necessary. Blood counts usually return to normal within one month of discontinuation. Caution should be used in patients with pre-existing marrow failure or cytopenia of any type. (See ADVERSE REACTIONS.)

Pulmonary Fibrosis: Pulmonary fibrosis, interstitial pneumonitis, fibrosing alveolitis, pulmonary edema, and pneumonia have been reported in patients receiving TONOCARD. Many of these events occurred in patients who were seriously ill. Fatalities have been

Continued on next page

Astra Merck—Cont.

reported. The experiences are usually characterized by bilateral infiltrates on x-ray and are frequently associated with dyspnea and cough. Fever may or may not be present. Patients should be instructed to promptly report the development of any pulmonary symptoms such as exertional dyspnea, cough or wheezing. Chest x-rays are advisable at that time. If these pulmonary disorders develop, TONOCARD should be discontinued. (See ADVERSE REACTIONS.)

DESCRIPTION

TONOCARD* (Tocainide HCl) is a primary amine analog of lidocaine with antiarrhythmic properties useful in the treatment of ventricular arrhythmias. The chemical name for tocainide hydrochloride is 2-amino-*N*-(2,6-dimethylphenyl) propanamide hydrochloride. Its empirical formula is $C_{11}H_{16}N_2O{\bullet}HCl$, with a molecular weight of 228.72. The structural formula is:

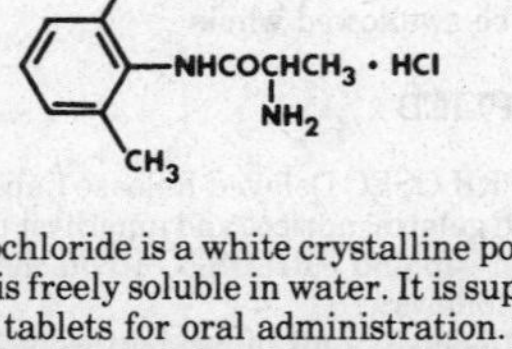

Tocainide hydrochloride is a white crystalline powder with a bitter taste and is freely soluble in water. It is supplied as 400 mg and 600 mg tablets for oral administration. Each tablet contains the following inactive ingredients: hydroxypropyl methylcellulose, iron oxide, magnesium stearate, methylcellulose, polyethylene glycol, and titanium dioxide.

*Registered trademark of Astra Pharmaceutical Products Inc.

CLINICAL PHARMACOLOGY

Action
Tocainide, like lidocaine, produces dose dependent decreases in sodium and potassium conductance, thereby decreasing the excitability of myocardial cells. In experimental animal models, the dose-related depression of sodium current is more pronounced in ischemic tissue than in normal tissue.
Electrophysiology
Tocainide is a Class I antiarrhythmic compound with electrophysiologic properties in man similar to those of lidocaine, but dissimilar from quinidine, procainamide, and disopyramide.
In studies of isolated dog Purkinje fibers, tocainide in concentrations of 1–50 mcg/mL had no significant effect on resting membrane potential, but reduced the amplitude and rate of depolarization (dv/dt) of the action potential. Tocainide decreased the effective refractory period (ERP) to a lesser extent than the action potential duration (APD) resulting in an increase in the ERP/APD ratio.
In patients with cardiac disease, TONOCARD produced no clinically significant changes in sinus nodal function, effective refractory periods, or intracardiac conduction times when studied under electrophysiologic testing procedures.
Tocainide, like lidocaine, characteristically does not prolong ventricular depolarization (QRS duration) or repolarization (QT intervals) as measured by electrocardiography. Theoretically, therefore, TONOCARD may be useful in the treatment of ventricular arrhythmias associated with a prolonged QT interval.
Patients who respond to lidocaine also respond to TONOCARD in a majority of cases. Failure to respond to lidocaine usually predicts failure to respond to TONOCARD, but there are exceptions to this.
In a controlled comparison with quinidine, 600 mg b.i.d. of TONOCARD produced a mean reduction of 42 percent in PVC count, compared to a 54 percent reduction by quinidine 300 mg every 6 hours. Among all patients entered into the study, about one-fifth of tocainide recipients and one-third of quinidine recipients had 75 percent or greater reductions in PVC count or had elimination of ventricular tachycardia.
Pharmacokinetics
Following oral administration of tocainide, peak plasma concentrations occur within 0.5 to 2 hours. The average plasma half-life in patients is approximately 15 hours. Although the effective plasma concentration may vary from patient to patient, the usual therapeutic plasma range (as defined by 50–80 percent PVC suppression) is 4–10 mcg/mL (18–45 micromole/L), expressed as tocainide hydrochloride. Tocainide is approximately 10 percent bound to plasma protein.
In contrast to lidocaine, tocainide undergoes negligible first pass hepatic degradation. Following oral administration, the bioavailability of TONOCARD approaches 100 percent. The extent of its bioavailability is unaffected by food. Tocainide has no cardioactive metabolites. Approximately 40 percent of the administered dose of tocainide is excreted unchanged in the urine. Acidification of the urine has not been shown to significantly alter tocainide excretion in the urine, but alkalinization of the urine results in a significant decrease in the percent of tocainide excreted unchanged in the urine. Animal data indicate that tocainide crosses the blood-brain barrier; however, it has less lipid solubility than lidocaine.
Hemodynamics
Cardiac catheterization studies in man utilizing intravenous tocainide infusions (0.5–0.75 mg/kg/min over 15 min) have shown that tocainide usually produces a small degree of depression of parameters of left ventricular function, such as left ventricular dP/dt, and left ventricular end diastolic pressure. There were usually no changes in cardiac output or clinical evidence of increasing congestive heart failure in the well-compensated patients studied. Small but statistically significant increases in aortic and pulmonary arterial pressures have been consistently observed and are probably related to small increases in vascular resistance. When used concomitantly with a beta-blocking drug, tocainide further reduced cardiac index and left ventricular dP/dt and further increased pulmonary wedge pressure.
No clinically significant changes in heart rate, blood pressure, or signs of myocardial depression were observed in a study of 72 post-myocardial infarction patients receiving long-term therapy with oral TONOCARD at usual doses (400 mg q8h). When tocainide was administered orally at a dose of 120 mg/kg to anesthetized dogs (14 times the initial maximum dose recommended for humans), a negative inotropic effect was observed: the rate of change of left ventricular pressure decreased by up to 29 percent of control at 3 hours after administration. This effect was not observed at lower doses (60 mg/kg). Tocainide has been used safely in patients with acute myocardial infarction and various degrees of congestive heart failure. It has, however, a small negative inotropic effect and can increase peripheral resistance slightly. It therefore should be used cautiously in patients with known heart failure, particularly if a beta blocker is given as well. (See PRECAUTIONS.)

INDICATIONS AND USAGE

TONOCARD is indicated for the treatment of documented ventricular arrhythmias, such as sustained ventricular tachycardia, that, in the judgment of the physician, are life-threatening. Because of the proarrhythmic effects of TONOCARD, as well as its potential for other serious adverse effects, (see WARNINGS), its use to treat lesser arrhythmias is not recommended. Treatment of patients with asymptomatic ventricular premature contractions should be avoided.
Initiation of treatment with TONOCARD, as with other antiarrhythmic agents used to treat life-threatening arrhythmias, should be carried out in the hospital. It is essential that each patient given TONOCARD be evaluated electrocardiographically and clinically prior to, and during, therapy with TONOCARD to determine whether the response to TONOCARD supports continued treatment.
Antiarrhythmic drugs have not been shown to enhance survival in patients with ventricular arrhythmias.

CONTRAINDICATIONS

Patients who are hypersensitive to this product or to local anesthetics of the amide type.
Patients with second or third degree atrioventricular block in the absence of an artificial ventricular pacemaker.

WARNINGS

Mortality: **In the National Heart, Lung and Blood Institute's Cardiac Arrhythmia Suppression Trial (CAST), a long-term, multi-center, randomized, double-blind study in patients with asymptomatic non-life-threatening ventricular arrhythmias who had a myocardial infarction more than six days but less than two years previously, an excessive mortality or non-fatal cardiac arrest rate (7.7%) was seen in patients treated with encainide or flecainide compared with that seen in patients assigned to carefully matched placebo-treated groups (3.0%). The average duration of treatment with encainide or flecainide in this study was ten months.**

The applicability of the CAST results to other populations (e.g., those without recent myocardial infarction) is uncertain. Considering the known proarrhythmic properties of TONOCARD (Tocainide HCl) and the lack of evidence of improved survival for any antiarrhythmic drug in patients without life-threatening arrhythmias, the use of TONOCARD as well as other antiarrhythmic agents should be reserved for patients with life-threatening ventricular arrhythmias.

Acceleration of Ventricular Rate: Acceleration of ventricular rate occurs infrequently when antiarrhythmics are administered to patients with atrial flutter or fibrillation (see ADVERSE REACTIONS).

PRECAUTIONS

General
In patients with known heart failure or minimal cardiac reserve, TONOCARD should be used with caution because of the potential for aggravating the degree of heart failure.
Caution should be used in the institution or continuation of antiarrhythmic therapy in the presence of signs of increasing depression of cardiac conductivity.
In patients with severe liver or kidney disease, the rate of drug elimination may be significantly decreased (see DOSAGE AND ADMINISTRATION).
Since antiarrhythmic drugs may be ineffective in patients with hypokalemia, the possibility of a potassium deficit should be explored and, if present, the deficit should be corrected.
Like all other oral antiarrhythmics, TONOCARD has been reported to increase arrhythmias in some patients (see ADVERSE REACTIONS).
Information for Patients
Patients should be instructed to promptly report the development of bruising or bleeding; any signs of infections such as fever, chills, sore throat, or soreness and ulcers in the mouth; any pulmonary symptoms, such as exertional dyspnea, cough, or wheezing; rash.
Laboratory Tests
As with other antiarrhythmics, abnormal liver function tests, particularly in the early stages of therapy, have been reported. Periodic monitoring of liver function should be considered. Hepatitis and jaundice have been reported in some patients.
Drug Interactions
Tocainide and lidocaine are pharmacodynamically similar. The concomitant use of these two agents may cause an increased incidence of adverse reactions, including central nervous system adverse reactions such as seizure.
Specific interaction studies with cimetidine, digoxin, metoprolol and warfarin have been conducted, no clinically significant interaction was seen with cimetidine, digoxin or warfarin; but tocainide and metoprolol had additive effects on wedge pressure and cardiac index. TONOCARD has also been used in open studies with digitalis, beta-blocking agents, other antiarrhythmic agents, anticoagulants, and diuretics, without evidence of clinically significant interactions. Nevertheless, caution should be exercised in the use of multiple drug therapy.
TONOCARD is equally effective in digitalized and non-digitalized patients. In 17 patients with refractory ventricular arrhythmias on concomitant therapy, serum digoxin levels (1.1 ± 0.4 ng/mL) remained in the expected normal range (0.5–2.5 ng/mL) during tocainide administration.
Carcinogenesis, Mutagenesis, Impairment of Fertility
The carcinogenic potential of tocainide was studied in mice using oral doses up to 300 mg/kg/day (about 6 times the maximum recommended human dose) for up to 94 weeks in males and 102 weeks in females and in rats at doses up to 200 mg/kg/day for 24 months. Tocainide did not affect the type or incidence of neoplasia in the two studies.
Tocainide did not show any mutagenic potential when evaluated *in vivo* in the micronucleus test using mice at oral doses up to 187.5 mg/kg/day (about 7 times the usual human dose). Also, no mutagenic activity was seen *in vitro* in the Ames microbial mutagen test or in the mouse lymphoma forward mutation assay.
Reproduction and fertility studies in rats showed no adverse effects on male or female fertility at oral doses up to 200 mg/kg/day (about 8 times the usual human dose).
Pregnancy
Pregnancy Category C. In a teratogenicity study in rabbits, tocainide was administered orally at doses of 25, 50, and 100 mg/kg/day (about 1 to 4 times the usual human dose). No evidence of a drug-related teratogenic effect was noted; however, these doses were maternotoxic and produced a dose-related increase in abortions and stillbirths. In a teratogenicity study in rats, an oral dose of 300 mg/kg/day (about 12 times the usual human dose) showed no evidence of treatment-related fetal malformations, but maternotoxicity and an increase in fetal resorptions were noted. An oral dose of 30 mg/kg/day (about twice the usual human dose) did not produce any adverse effects.
In reproduction studies in rats at maternotoxic oral doses of 200 and 300 mg/kg/day (about 8 and 12 times the usual human dose, respectively), dystocia, and delayed parturition occurred which was accompanied by an increase in stillbirths and decreased survival in offspring during the first week postpartum. Growth and viability of surviving offspring were not affected for the remainder of the lactation period.
There are no adequate and well-controlled studies in pregnant women. TONOCARD should be used during pregnancy

only if the potential benefit justifies the potential risk to the fetus.

Nursing Mothers
It is not known whether tocainide is secreted in human milk. Because many drugs are secreted in human milk and because of the potential for serious adverse reactions in nursing infants from TONOCARD, a decision should be made whether to discontinue nursing or to discontinue the drug, taking into account the importance of the drug to the mother.

Pediatric Use
Safety and effectiveness in children have not been established.

ADVERSE REACTIONS

TONOCARD commonly produces minor, transient, nervous system and gastrointestinal adverse reactions, but is otherwise generally well tolerated. TONOCARD has been evaluated in both short-term (n = 1,358) and long-term (n = 262) controlled studies as well as a compassionate use program. Dosages were lower in most of the controlled studies (1200 mg/day) and higher in the compassionate use program (1800 mg and more). In long-term (2–6 months) controlled studies, the most frequent adverse reactions were dizziness/vertigo (15.3 percent), nausea (14.5 percent), paresthesia (9.2 percent), and tremor (8.4 percent). These reactions were generally mild, transient, dose-related and reversible with a reduction in dosage, by taking the drug with food, or by therapy discontinuation. Tremor, when present, may be useful as a clinical indicator that the maximum dose is being approached. Adverse reactions leading to therapy discontinuation occurred in 21 percent of patients in long-term controlled trials and were usually related to the nervous system or digestive system.

Adverse reactions occurring in greater than one percent of patients from the short-term and long-term controlled studies appear in the following table:

| | Percent of Patients Controlled Studies | |
	Short-term (n = 1,358)	Long-term (n = 262)
BODY AS A WHOLE		
Tiredness/drowsiness/fatigue/ lethargy/lassitude/ sleepiness	1.6	0.8
Hot/cold feelings	0.5	1.5
CARDIOVASCULAR		
Hypotension	3.4	2.7
Bradycardia	1.8	0.4
Palpitations	1.8	0.4
Chest pain	1.6	0.4
Conduction disorders	1.5	0.0
Left ventricular failure	1.4	0.0
DIGESTIVE		
Nausea	15.2	14.5
Vomiting	8.3	4.6
Anorexia	1.2	1.9
Diarrhea/loose stools	0.0	3.8
NERVOUS SYSTEM/PSYCHIATRIC		
Dizziness/vertigo	8.0	15.3
Paresthesia	3.5	9.2
Tremor	2.9	8.4
Confusion/disorientation/ hallucinations	2.1	2.7
Headache	2.1	4.6
Nervousness	1.5	0.4
Altered mood/awareness	1.5	3.4
Incoordination/unsteadiness/ walking disturbances	1.2	0.0
Anxiety	1.1	1.5
Ataxia	0.2	3.0
SKIN		
Diaphoresis	5.1	2.3
Rash/skin lesion	0.4	8.4
SPECIAL SENSES		
Blurred vision/visual disturbances	1.3	1.5
Tinnitus/hearing loss	0.4	1.5
Nystagmus	0.0	1.1

An additional group of about 2,000 patients has been treated in a program allowing for the use of TONOCARD under compassionate use circumstances. These patients were seriously ill with the large majority on multiple drug therapy, and comparatively high doses of TONOCARD were used. Fifty-four percent of the patients continued in the program for one year or longer, and 12 percent were treated for longer than three years, with the longest duration of therapy being nine years. Adverse reactions leading to therapy discontinuation occurred in 12 percent of patients (usually central nervous system effects or rash). A tabulation of adverse reactions occurring in one percent or more of patients follows:

	Percent of Patients Compassionate Use (n = 1,927)
CARDIOVASCULAR	
Increased ventricular arrhythmias/PVCs	10.9
CHF/progression of CHF	4.0
Tachycardia	3.2
Hypotension	1.8
Conduction disorders	1.3
Bradycardia	1.0
DIGESTIVE	
Nausea	24.6
Anorexia	11.3
Vomiting	9.0
Diarrhea/loose stools	6.8
MUSCULOSKELETAL	
Arthritis/arthralgia	4.7
Myalgia	1.7
NERVOUS SYSTEM/PSYCHIATRIC	
Dizziness/vertigo	25.3
Tremor	21.6
Nervousness	11.5
Confusion/disorientation/ hallucinations	11.2
Altered mood/awareness	11.0
Ataxia	10.8
Paresthesia	9.2
SKIN	
Rash/skin lesion	12.2
Diaphoresis	8.3
Lupus	1.6
SPECIAL SENSES	
Blurred vision/vision disturbances	10.0
Nystagmus	1.1

Adverse reactions occurring in less than one percent of patients in either the controlled studies or the compassionate use program or since the drug was marketed are as follows:
Body as a Whole: Septicemia; septic shock; syncope; vasovagal episodes; edema; fever; chills; cinchonism; asthenia; malaise.
Cardiovascular: Ventricular fibrillation; extension of acute myocardial infarction; cardiogenic shock; pulmonary embolism; angina; AV block; hypertension; claudication; increased QRS duration; pleurisy/pericarditis; prolonged QT interval; right bundle branch block; cardiomegaly; sinus arrest; vasculitis; orthostatic hypotension; cold extremities.
Digestive: Hepatitis, jaundice (see PRECAUTIONS), abnormal liver function tests; pancreatitis; abdominal pain/discomfort; constipation; dysphagia; gastrointestinal symptoms (including dyspepsia); stomatitis; dry mouth; thirst.
Hematologic: Agranulocytosis; bone marrow depression; aplastic/hypoplastic anemia; hemolytic anemia; anemia; leukopenia; neutropenia; thrombocytopenia; eosinophilia.
Metabolic and Immune: Hypersensitivity Reaction (including some of the following symptoms or signs: rash, fever, joint pains, abnormal liver function tests, eosinophilia); increased ANA.
Musculoskeletal: Muscle cramps; muscle twitching/spasm; neck pain; pain radiating from neck; pressure on shoulder.
Nervous System/Psychiatric: Coma; convulsions/seizures; myasthenia gravis; depression; psychosis; psychic disturbances; agitation; decreased mental acuity; dysarthria; impaired memory; increased stuttering/slurred speech; insomnia/sleeping disturbances; local anesthesia; dream abnormalities.
Respiratory: Respiratory arrest; pulmonary edema; pulmonary fibrosis; fibrosing alveolitis; pneumonia; interstitial pneumonitis; dyspnea; hiccough; yawning.
Skin: Stevens-Johnson syndrome; exfoliative dermatitis; erythema multiforme; urticaria; alopecia; pruritus; pallor/flushed face.
Special Senses: Diplopia; earache; taste perversion/smell perversion.
Urogenital: Urinary retention; polyuria/increased diuresis.
Agranulocytosis, bone marrow depression, leukopenia, neutropenia, aplastic/hypoplastic anemia, and thrombocytopenia have been reported (0.18 percent) in patients receiving TONOCARD in controlled trials and the compassionate use program. Most of these events have been noted during the first 12 weeks of therapy. (See Box WARNINGS.)
Pulmonary fibrosis, interstitial pneumonitis, fibrosing alveolitis, pulmonary edema, and pneumonia, have been reported in patients receiving TONOCARD. The incidence of pulmonary fibrosis (including interstitial pneumonitis and fibrosing alveolitis) was 0.11 percent in controlled trials and the compassionate use program. These events usually occurred in seriously ill patients. Symptoms of these pulmo-

nary disorders and/or x-ray changes usually occurred following 3–18 weeks of therapy. Fatalities have been reported. (See Box WARNINGS.)
A number of disorders, in which a causal relationship with TONOCARD has not been established, have been reported in seriously ill patients. These include: renal failure, renal dysfunction, myocardial infarction, cerebrovascular accidents and transient ischemic attacks. These disorders may be related to the patient's underlying condition.

DRUG ABUSE AND DEPENDENCE

Drug withdrawal after chronic treatment has not shown any indication of psychological or physical dependence.

OVERDOSAGE

The initial and most important signs and symptoms of overdosage would be expected to be related to the central nervous system. Other adverse reactions, such as gastrointestinal disturbances, may follow. (See ADVERSE REACTIONS.)
Should convulsions or cardiopulmonary depression or arrest develop, the patency of the airway and adequacy of ventilation must be assured immediately. Should convulsions persist despite ventilatory therapy with oxygen, small increments of anticonvulsant agents may be given intravenously. Examples of such agents include a benzodiazepine (e.g., diazepam), an ultrashort-acting barbiturate (e.g., thiopental or thiamylal), or a short-acting barbiturate (e.g., pentobarbital or secobarbital).
The oral LD_{50} of tocainide was calculated to be about 800 mg/kg in mice, 1000 mg/kg in rats, and 230 mg/kg in guinea pigs; deaths were usually preceded by convulsions.
Studies in normal individuals to date indicate that tocainide has a hemodialysis clearance approximately equivalent to its renal clearance.

DOSAGE AND ADMINISTRATION

The dosage of TONOCARD must be individualized on the basis of antiarrhythmic response and tolerance, both of which are dose-related. Clinical and electrocardiographic evaluation (including Holter monitoring if necessary for evaluation) are needed to determine whether the desired antiarrhythmic response has been obtained and to guide titration and dose adjustment. Adverse effects appearing shortly after dosing, for example, suggest a need for dividing the dose further with a shorter dose-interval. Loss of arrhythmia control prior to the next dose suggests use of a shorter dose interval and/or a dose increase. Absence of a clear response suggests reconsideration of therapy.
The recommended initial dosage is 400 mg every 8 hours. The usual adult dosage is between 1200 and 1800 mg/day in a three dose daily divided regimen. Doses beyond 2400 mg per day have been administered infrequently. Patients who tolerate the t.i.d. regimen may be tried on a twice daily regimen with careful monitoring.
Some patients, particularly those with renal or hepatic impairment, may be adequately treated with less than 1200 mg/day.

HOW SUPPLIED

No. 3409—Tablets TONOCARD, 400 mg, are oval, yellow, scored, film-coated tablets, coded 707 on one side and TONOCARD on the other side. They are supplied as follows:
NDC 61113-707-68 bottles of 100
(6505-01-203-6240, 400 mg 100's)
NDC 61113-707-28 unit dose packages of 100.
No. 3410—Tablets TONOCARD, 600 mg, are oblong, yellow, scored, film-coated tablets, coded 709 on one side and TONOCARD on the other side. They are supplied as follows:
NDC 61113-709-68 bottles of 100
(6505-01-206-0273, 600 mg 100's)
NDC 61113-709-28 unit dose packages of 100.
Storage
Store below 40°C (104°F), preferably between 15°C and 30°C (59°F and 86°F). Store in a well-closed container.
Distributed by:
ASTRA MERCK
Wayne, PA 19087, USA
Manufactured by: MERCK & CO., INC.,
West Point, PA 19486, USA
Issued July 1995   7911313
©1995 Astra Merck Inc. All rights reserved.
Shown in Product Identification Guide, page 304

Astra USA, Inc.
50 OTIS STREET
WESTBOROUGH, MA 01581-4500

Medical Information or Medical Emergencies
Product information, adverse event reports and 24-hour emergency medical information.
Telephone: (800) 262-0460

ALBUTEROL SULFATE, USP ℞

Solution for Inhalation 0.5%*
Arm-a-Med®
(*Potency expressed as albuterol)

DESCRIPTION

Albuterol Sulfate Solution for Inhalation contains albuterol sulfate, USP, the racemic form of albuterol and a relatively selective beta$_2$-adrenergic bronchodilator (see **CLINICAL PHARMACOLOGY** section below). Albuterol sulfate has the chemical name α^1-[(*tert*-Butylamino) methyl]-4-hydroxy-*m*-xylene-α,α'-diol sulfate (2:1) (salt), and the following chemical structure:

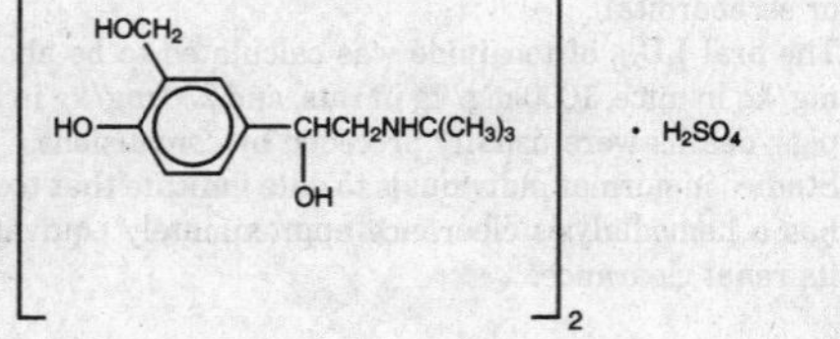

Albuterol sulfate has a molecular weight of 576.7 and the empirical formula $(C_{13}H_{21}NO_3)_2 \bullet H_2SO_4$. Albuterol sulfate is a white crystalline powder, soluble in water and slightly soluble in ethanol.

The World Health Organization's recommended name for albuterol base is salbutamol.

Albuterol Sulfate Solution for Inhalation 0.5% is in concentrated form. Dilute 0.5 mL of the solution to 3 mL with sterile normal saline solution prior to administration.

Each mL of Albuterol Sulfate Solution for Inhalation 0.5% contains 5 mg of albuterol (as 6.0 mg of albuterol sulfate) in an aqueous solution containing benzalkonium chloride; sulfuric acid is used to adjust the pH between 3 and 5. Albuterol Sulfate Solution for Inhalation 0.5% contains no sulfiting agents. It is supplied in 20 mL bottles.

Albuterol Sulfate Solution for Inhalation is a clear, colorless to light yellow solution.

CLINICAL PHARMACOLOGY

The prime action of beta-adrenergic drugs is to stimulate adenyl cyclase, the enzyme which catalyzes the formation of cyclic-3', 5'-adenosine monophosphate (cyclic AMP) from adenosine triphosphate (ATP). The cyclic AMP thus formed mediates the cellular responses. *In vitro* studies and *in vivo* pharmacologic studies have demonstrated that albuterol has a preferential effect on beta$_2$-adrenergic receptors compared with isoproterenol. While it is recognized that beta$_2$-adrenergic receptors are the predominant receptors in bronchial smooth muscle, recent data indicate that 10% to 50% of the beta receptors in the human heart may be beta$_2$ receptors. The precise function of these receptors, however, is not yet established. Albuterol has been shown in most controlled clinical trials to have more effect on the respiratory tract, in the form of bronchial smooth muscle relaxation, than isoproterenol at comparable doses while producing fewer cardiovascular effects. Controlled clinical studies and other clinical experience have shown that inhaled albuterol, like other beta-adrenergic agonist drugs, can produce a significant cardiovascular effect in some patients, as measured by pulse rate, blood pressure, symptoms, and/or ECG changes.

Albuterol is longer acting than isoproterenol in most patients by any route of administration because it is not a substrate for the cellular uptake processes for catecholamines nor for catechol-*O*-methyl transferase.

Studies in asthmatic patients have shown that less than 20% of a single alubterol dose was absorbed following either IPPB or nebulizer administration; the remaining amount was recovered from the nebulizer and apparatus and expired air. Most of the absorbed dose was recovered in the urine 24 hours after drug administration. Following a 3.0 mg dose of nebulized albuterol, the maximum albuterol plasma level at 0.5 hour was 2.1 ng/mL (range 1.4 to 3.2 ng/mL). There was a significant dose-related response in FEV_1 and peak flow rate (PFR). It has been demonstrated that following oral administration of 4 mg albuterol, the elimination half-life was 5 to 6 hours.

Animal studies show that albuterol does not pass the blood-brain barrier. Recent studies in laboratory animals (minipigs, rodents, and dogs) recorded the occurrence of cardiac arrhythmias and sudden death (with histologic evidence of myocardial necrosis) when beta-agonists and methylxanthines were administered concurrently. The significance of these findings when applied to humans is currently unknown.

In controlled clinical trials, most patients exhibited an onset of improvement in pulmonary function within 5 minutes as determined by FEV_1. FEV_1 measurements also showed that the maximum average improvement in pulmonary function usually occurred at approximately 1 hour following inhalation of 2.5 mg of albuterol by compressor-nebulizer, and remained close to peak for 2 hours. Clinically significant improvement in pulmonary function (defined as maintenance of a 15% or more increase in FEV_1 over baseline values) continued for 3 to 4 hours in most patients and in some patients continued up to 6 hours.

In repetitive dose studies, continued effectiveness was demonstrated throughout the 3-month period of treatment in some patients.

INDICATIONS AND USAGE

Albuterol Sulfate Solution for Inhalation is indicated for the relief of bronchospasm in patients with reversible obstructive airway disease and acute attacks of bronchospasm.

CONTRAINDICATIONS

Albuterol Sulfate Solution for Inhalation is contraindicated in patients with a history of hypersensitivity to any of its components.

WARNINGS

As with other inhaled beta-adrenergic agonists, Albuterol Sulfate Solution for Inhalation can produce paradoxical bronchospasm, which can be life threatening. If it occurs, the preparation should be discontinued immediately and alternative therapy instituted.

Fatalities have been reported in association with excessive use of inhaled sympathomimetic drugs and with the home use of sympathomimetic nebulizers. It is, therefore, essential that the physician instruct the patient in the need for further evaluation if his/her asthma becomes worse. In individual patients, any beta$_2$-adrenergic agonist, including albuterol inhalation solution and solution for inhalation, may have a clinically significant cardiac effect.

Immediate hypersensitivity reactions may occur after administration of alubterol as demonstrated by rare cases of urticaria, angioedema, rash, bronchospasm, and oropharyngeal edema.

PRECAUTIONS

General: Albuterol, as with all sympathomimetic amines, should be used with caution in patients with cardiovascular disorders, especially coronary insufficiency, cardiac arrhythmias and hypertension, in patients with convulsive disorders, hyperthyroidism or diabetes mellitus, and in patients who are unusually responsive to sympathomimetic amines.

Large doses of intravenous alubterol have been reported to aggravate preexisting diabetes mellitus and ketoacidosis. Additionally, beta-agonists, including albuterol, when given intravenously may cause a decrease in serum potassium, possibly through intracellular shunting. The decrease is usually transient, not requiring supplementation. The relevance of these observations to the use of Albuterol Sulfate Solution for Inhalation is unknown.

To avoid contaminating the multi-dose bottle of Albuterol Sulfate Solution for Inhalation, proper aseptic technique should be used when withdrawing and delivering the dose into the nebulizer.

Information for Patients: The action of Albuterol Sulfate Solution for Inhalation may last up to 6 hours and therefore it should not be used more frequently than recommended. Do not increase the dose or frequency of medication without medical consultation. If symptoms get worse, medical consultation should be sought promptly. While taking Albuterol Sulfate Solution for Inhalation, other anti-asthma medicines should not be used unless prescribed.

Drug stability and safety of Albuterol Sulfate Solution for Inhalation when mixed with other drugs in a nebulizer have not been established.

See illustrated **"Patient's Instructions for Use."**

Drug Interactions: Other sympathomimetic aerosol bronchodilators or epinephrine should not be used concomitantly with albuterol.

Albuterol should be administered with extreme caution to patients being treated with monoamine oxidase inhibitors or tricyclic antidepressants, since the action of albuterol on the vascular system may be potentiated.

Beta-receptor blocking agents and albuterol inhibit the effect of each other.

Since albuterol may lower serum potassium, care should be taken in patients also using other drugs which lower serum potassium as the effects may be additive.

Carcinogenesis, Mutagenesis, and Impairment of Fertility: Albuterol sulfate, like other agents in its class, caused a significant dose-related increase in the incidence of benign leiomyomas of the mesovarium in a 2-year study in the rat, at oral doses corresponding to 10, 50, and 250 times the maximum human nebulizer dose. In another study, this effect was blocked by the coadministration of propranolol. The relevance of these findings to humans is not known. An 18-month study in mice and a lifetime study in hamsters revealed no evidence of tumorigenicity. Studies with albuterol revealed no evidence of mutagenesis. Reproduction studies in rats revealed no evidence of impaired fertility.

Teratogenic Effects—Pregnancy Category C: Albuterol has been shown to be teratogenic in mice when given subcutaneously in doses corresponding to the human nebulization dose. There are no adequate and well-controlled studies in pregnant women. Albuterol should be used during pregnancy only if the potential benefit justifies the potential risk to the fetus. A reproduction study in CD-1 mice with albuterol (0.025, 0.25, and 2.5 mg/kg subcutaneously, corresponding to 0.1, 1, and 12.5 times the maximum human nebulization dose, respectively) showed cleft palate formation in 5 of 111 (4.5%) fetuses at 0.25 mg/kg and in 10 of 108 (9.3%) fetuses at 2.5 mg/kg. None were observed at 0.025 mg/kg. Cleft palate also occurred in 22 of 72 (30.5%) fetuses treated with 2.5 mg/kg isoproterenol (positive control). A reproduction study in Stride Dutch rabbits revealed cranioschisis in 7 of 19 (37%) fetuses at 50 mg/kg, corresponding to 250 times the maximum human nebulization dose. During marketing, various congenital anomalies, including cleft palate and limb defects, have been reported in the offspring of patients being treated with albuterol. Some of the mothers were taking multiple medications during their pregnancies. Because no consistent pattern of defects can be discerned, a relationship between albuterol use and congenital anomalies cannot be established.

Labor and Delivery: Oral albuterol has been shown to delay preterm labor in some reports. There are presently no well-controlled studies which demonstrate that it will stop preterm labor or prevent labor at term. Therefore, cautious use of Albuterol Sulfate Solution for Inhalation is required in pregnant patients when given for relief of bronchospasm so as to avoid interference with uterine contractibility.

Nursing Mothers: It is not known whether this drug is excreted in human milk. Because of the potential for tumorigenicity shown for alubterol in some animal studies, a decision should be made whether to discontinue nursing or to discontinue the drug, taking into account the importance of the drug to the mother.

Pediatric Use: Safety and effectiveness of albuterol inhalation solution and solution for inhalation in children below the age of 12 years have not been established.

ADVERSE REACTIONS

The results of clinical trials with Albuterol Sulfate Solution for Inhalation in 135 patients showed the following side effects which were considered probably or possibly drug related:

Central Nervous System: tremors (20%), dizziness (7%), nervousness (4%), headache (3%), insomnia (1%).
Gastrointestinal: nausea (4%), dyspepsia (1%).
Ear, Nose, and Throat: pharyngitis (<1%), nasal congestion (1%).
Cardiovascular: tachycardia (1%), hypertension (1%).
Respiratory: bronchospasm (8%), cough (4%), bronchitis (4%), wheezing (1%).

No clinically relevant laboratory abnormalities related to Albuterol Sulfate Solution for Inhalation administration were determined in these studies.

In comparing the adverse reactions reported for patients treated with Albuterol Sulfate Solution for Inhalation with those of patients treated with isoproterenol during clinical trials of 3 months, the following moderate to severe reactions, as judged by the investigators, were reported. This table does not include mild reactions.

Percent Incidence of Moderate to Severe Adverse Reactions

Reaction	Albuterol N=65	Isoproterenol N=65
Central Nervous System		
Tremors	10.7%	13.8%
Headache	3.1%	1.5%
Insomnia	3.1%	1.5%
Cardiovascular		
Hypertension	3.1%	3.1%
Arrhythmias	0%	3.0%
*Palpitation	0%	22.0%
Respiratory		
†Bronchospasm	15.4%	18.0%
Cough	3.1%	5.0%
Bronchitis	1.5%	5.0%

Wheeze	1.5%	1.5%
Sputum Increase	1.5%	1.5%
Dyspnea	1.5%	1.5%
Gastrointestinal		
Nausea	3.1%	0%
Dyspepsia	1.5%	0%
Systemic		
Malaise	1.5%	0%

* The finding of no arrhythmias and no palpitations after albuterol administration in this clinical study should not be interpreted as indicating that these adverse effects cannot occur after the administration of inhaled albuterol.

† In most cases of bronchospasm, this term was generally used to describe exacerbations in the underlying pulmonary disease.

Rare cases of urticaria, angioedema, rash, bronchospasm, and oropharyngeal edema have been reported after the use of inhaled albuterol.

OVERDOSAGE

Manifestations of overdosage may include anginal pain, hypertension, hypokalemia, and exaggeration of the pharmacological effects listed in **ADVERSE REACTIONS**.
The oral LD_{50} in rats and mice was greater than 2,000 mg/kg. The inhalational LD_{50} could not be determined.
There is insufficient evidence to determine if dialysis is beneficial for overdosage of Albuterol Sulfate Solution for Inhalation.

DOSAGE AND ADMINISTRATION

The usual dosage for adults and children 12 years and older is 2.5 mg of albuterol administration 3 to 4 times daily by nebulization. More frequent administration or higher doses are not recommended. To administer 2.5 mg of albuterol, dilute 0.5 mL of the 0.5% solution for inhalation to a total volume of 3 mL with sterile normal saline solution and administer by nebulization. The flow rate is regulated to suit the particular nebulizer so that the Albuterol Sulfate Solution for Inhalation will be delivered over approximately 5 to 15 minutes.
Drug stability and safety of Albuterol Sulfate Solution for Inhalation when mixed with other drugs in a nebulizer have not been established.
The use of Albuterol Sulfate Solution for Inhalation can be continued as medically indicated to control recurring bouts of bronchospasm. During treatment, most patients gain optimum benefit from regular use of the nebulizer solution.
If a previously effective dosage regimen fails to provide the usual relief, medical advice should be sought immediately, as this is often a sign of seriously worsening asthma which would require reassessment of therapy.

HOW SUPPLIED

Albuterol Sulfate Solution for Inhalation 0.5% is a clear, colorless to light yellow solution, and is supplied in amber glass bottles of 20 mL fill (NDC 0186-1490-01) with accompanying calibrated dropper; boxes of one.
Store between 2° and 25°C (36° and 77°F).
Manufactured for:
ASTRA®
Astra USA, Inc.
Westborough, MA 01581
Manufactured by:
Warrick Pharmaceuticals Corporation
Niles, Illinois 60714 USA

000539R01 Rev. 5/95
B-17954121

Copyright© 1994, 1995, Warrick Pharmaceuticals Corporation.
All rights reserved.

Patient's Instructions for Use

Albuterol Sulfate, USP
Solution for Inhalation 0.5%*
*Potency expressed as albuterol
Note: The Albuterol Sulfate Solution contained in the 20 mL multiple-dose bottle is concentrated and must be diluted. Read complete instructions carefully before using.

1. Draw 0.5 mL of Albuterol Sulfate Solution into the specially marked dropper that comes with each multi-dose bottle (Figure 1).

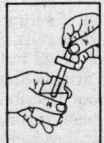

Figure 1

2. Squeeze the solution into the nebulizer reservoir through the appropriate opening (Figure 2).

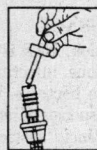

Figure 2

3. Add 2.5 mL of diluting fluid–sterile normal saline solution (as your physician has directed).

4. Gently swirl the nebulizer to mix the contents and connect it with the mouthpiece or face mask (Figure 3).

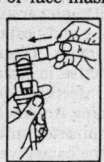

Figure 3

5. Connect the nebulizer to the compressor.

6. Sit in a comfortable, upright position; place the mouthpiece in your mouth (Figure 4) (or put on the face mask); and turn the compressor on.

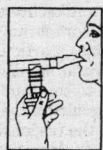

Figure 4

7. Breathe as calmly, deeply, and evenly as possible until no more mist is formed in the nebulizer chamber (about 5-15 minutes). At this point, the treatment is finished.

8. Clean the nebulizer (see manufacturer's instructions).

Note: Use only as directed by your physician. More frequent administration or higher doses are not recommended.
Drug stability and safety of Albuterol Sulfate Solution for Inhalation when mixed with other drugs in a nebulizer have not been established.
Store Albuterol Sulfate Solution for Inhalation 0.5%* between 2° and 25°C (36° and 77°F).
Pharmacist: For additional instructions, use back of this sheet.
ASTRA®
Astra USA, Inc.
Westborough, MA 01581
Rev. 5/95
Illustrations Copyright© 1993 by
Astra USA, Inc., Westborough, MA 01581
Copyright© 1994, 1995, Warrick
Pharmaceuticals Corporation, Niles, IL
60714 USA. All rights reserved.

AMIKACIN SULFATE INJECTION, USP ℞

WARNINGS

Patients treated with parenteral aminoglycosides should be under close clinical observation because of the potential ototoxicity and nephrotoxicity associated with their use. Safety for treatment periods which are longer than 14 days has not been established.
Neurotoxicity, manifested as vestibular and permanent bilateral auditory ototoxicity, can occur in patients with pre-existing renal damage and in patients with normal renal function treated at higher doses and/or for periods longer than those recommended. The risk of aminoglycoside-induced ototoxicity is greater in patients with renal damage. High frequency deafness usually occurs first and can be detected only by audiometric testing. Vertigo may occur and may be evidence of vestibular injury. Other manifestations of neurotoxicity may include numbness, skin tingling, muscle twitching and convulsions. The risk of hearing loss due to aminoglycosides increases with the degree of exposure to either high peak or high trough serum concentrations. Patients developing cochlear damage may not have symptoms during therapy to warn them of developing eighth-nerve toxicity, and total or partial irreversible bilateral deafness may occur after the drug has been discontinued. Aminoglycoside-induced ototoxicity is usually irreversible.
Aminoglycosides are potentially nephrotoxic. The risk of nephrotoxicity is greater in patients with impaired renal function and in those who receive high doses or prolonged therapy.
Neuromuscular blockade and respiratory paralysis have been reported following parenteral injection, topical instillation (as in orthopedic and abdominal irrigation or in local treatment of empyema), and following oral use of aminoglycosides. The possibility of these phenomena should be considered if aminoglycosides are administered by any route, especially in patients receiving anesthetics, neuromuscular blocking agents such as tubocurarine, succinylcholine, decamethonium, or in patients receiving massive transfusions of citrate-anticoagulated blood. If blockage occurs, calcium salts may reverse these phenomena, but mechanical respiratory assistance may be necessary.
Renal and eighth-nerve function should be closely monitored especially in patients with known or suspected renal impairment at the onset of therapy and also in those whose renal function is initially normal but who develop signs of renal dysfunction during therapy. Serum concentrations of amikacin should be monitored when feasible to assure adequate levels and to avoid potentially toxic levels and prolonged peak concentrations above 35 micrograms per mL. Urine should be examined for decreased specific gravity, increased excretion of proteins, and the presence of cells or casts. Blood urea nitrogen, serum creatinine, or creatinine clearance should be measured periodically. Serial audiograms should be obtained when feasible in patients old enough to be tested, particularly high risk patients. Evidence of ototoxicity (dizziness, vertigo, tinnitus, roaring in the ears, and hearing loss) or nephrotoxicity requires discontinuation of the drug or dosage adjustment.
Concurrent and/or sequential systemic, oral, or topical use of other neurotoxic or nephrotoxic products, particularly bacitracin, cisplatin, amphotericin B, cephaloridine, paromomycin, viomycin, polymyxin B, colistin, vancomycin, or other aminoglycosides should be avoided. Other factors that may increase the risk of toxicity are advanced age and dehydration.
The concurrent use of amikacin with potent diuretics (ethacrynic acid, or furosemide) should be avoided since diuretics by themselves may cause ototoxicity.
In addition, when administered intravenously, diuretics may enhance aminoglycoside toxicity by altering antibiotic concentrations in serum and tissue.

DESCRIPTION

Amikacin sulfate is a semi-synthetic aminoglycoside antibiotic derived from kanamycin. It is $C_{22}H_{43}N_5O_{13} \cdot 2H_2SO_4$ D-Streptamine, O-3-amino-3-deoxy-α-D-glucopyranosyl-(1->6)-O-[6-amino-6-deoxy-α-D-glucopyranosyl(1->4)]-N^1-(4-amino-2-hydroxy-1-oxobutyl)-2-deoxy-, (S)-,.sulfate (1:2)(salt). Molecular weight 781.75

Amikacin sulfate injection is a sterile, colorless to light straw colored solution available for IM or IV use. Each mL contains amikacin sulfate equivalent to 50 mg or 250 mg amikacin. The 50 mg/mL product also contains 0.13% sodium bisulfite and 0.5% sodium citrate (dihydrate) with pH adjusted to 4.5 with sulfuric acid. The 250 mg/mL product also contains 0.66% sodium bisulfite and 2.5% sodium citrate (dihydrate) with pH adjusted to 4.5 with sulfuric acid. The solutions are filled under nitrogen.

CLINICAL PHARMACOLOGY

Intramuscular Administration—Amikacin is rapidly absorbed after intramuscular administration. In normal adult volunteers, average peak serum concentrations of about 12, 16, and 21 mcg/mL are obtained 1 hour after intramuscular administration of 250 mg (3.7 mg/kg). 375 mg (5 mg/kg), 500 mg (7.5 mg/kg), single doses, respectively. At 10 hours, serum levels are about 0.3 mcg/mL, 1.2 mcg/mL, and 2.1 mcg/mL, respectively.
Tolerance studies in normal volunteers reveal that amikacin is well tolerated locally following repeated intramuscular dosing, and when given at maximally recommended doses, no ototoxicity or nephrotoxicity has been reported. There is no evidence of drug accumulation with repeated dosing for 10 days when administered according to recommended doses.

Continued on next page

Astra—Cont.

With normal renal function, about 91.9% of an intramuscular dose is excreted unchanged in the urine in the first 8 hours, and 98.2% within 24 hours. Mean urine concentrations for 6 hours are 563 mcg/mL following a 250 mg dose, 697 mcg/mL following a 375 mg dose, and 832 mcg/mL following a 500 mg dose.

Preliminary intramuscular studies in newborns of different weights (less than 1.5 kg, 1.5 to 2.0 kg, over 2.0 kg) at a dose of 7.5 mg/kg revealed that, like other aminoglycosides, serum half-life values were correlated inversely with post-natal age and renal clearances of amikacin. The volume of distribution indicates that amikacin, like other aminoglycosides, remains primarily in the extracellular fluid space of neonates. Repeated dosing every 12 hours in all the above groups did not demonstrate accumulation after 5 days.

Intravenous Administration—Single doses of 500 mg (7.5 mg/kg), administered to normal adults as an infusion over a period of 30 minutes produced a mean peak serum concentration of 38 mcg/mL at the end of the infusion, and levels of 24 mcg/mL, 18 mcg/mL, and 0.75 mcg/mL at 30 minutes. 1 hour, and 10 hours post infusion, respectively. Eighty-four percent of the administered dose was excreted in the urine in 9 hours and about 94% within 24 hours.

Repeat infusions of 7.5 mg/kg every 12 hours in normal adults were well tolerated and caused no drug accumulation.

General—Pharmacokinetic studies in normal adult subjects reveal the mean serum half-life to be slightly over 2 hours with a mean total apparent volume of distribution of 24 liters (28% of the body weight). By the ultrafiltration technique, reports of serum protein binding range from 0 to 11%. The mean serum clearance rate is about 100 mL/min and the renal clearance rate is 94 mL/min in subjects with normal renal function.

Amikacin is excreted primarily by glomerular filtration. Patients with impaired renal function or diminished glomerular filtration pressure excrete the drug much more slowly (effectively prolonging the serum half-life).

Therefore, renal function should be monitored carefully and dosage adjusted accordingly (see suggested dosage schedule under DOSAGE AND ADMINISTRATION).

Following administration at the recommended dose, therapeutic levels are found in bone, heart, gallbladder, and lung tissue in addition to significant concentrations in urine, bile, sputum, bronchial secretions, interstitial, pleural, and synovial fluids.

Spinal fluid levels in normal infants are approximately 10 to 20% of the serum concentrations and may reach 50% when the meninges are inflamed. Amikacin has been demonstrated to cross the placental barrier and yield significant concentrations in amniotic fluid. The peak fetal serum concentration is about 16% of the peak maternal serum concentration and maternal and fetal serum half-life values are about 2 and 3.7 hours, respectively.

Microbiology

Gram-negative—Amikacin is active *in vitro* against *Pseudomonas* species, *Escherichia coli, Proteus* species (indole-positive and indole-negative), *Providencia* species. *Klebsiella-Enterobacter-Serratia* species, *Acinetobacter* (formerly *Mima-Herellea*) species, and *Citrobacter freundii.*

When strains of the above organisms are found to be resistant to other aminoglycosides, including gentamicin, tobramycin and kanamycin, many are susceptible to amikacin *in vitro.*

Gram-positive—Amikacin is active *in vitro* against penicillinase and non-penicillinase-producing *Staphylococcus* species including methicillin-resistant strains. However, aminoglycosides in general have a low order of activity against other Gram-positive organisms: viz, *Streptococcus pyogenes,* enterococci, and *Streptococcus pneumoniae* (formerly *Diplococcus pneumoniae*).

Amikacin resists degradation by most aminoglycoside inactivating enzymes known to affect gentamicin, tobramycin, and kanamycin.

In vitro studies have shown that amikacin sulfate combined with a beta-lactam antibiotic acts synergistically against many clinically significant gram-negative organisms.

Disc Susceptibility Tests—Quantitative methods that require measurement of zone diameters give the most precise estimates of antibiotic susceptibility. One such procedure* has been recommended for use with discs to test susceptibility to amikacin. Interpretation involves correlation of the diameters obtained in the disc test with MIC values for amikacin. When the causative organism is tested by the Kirby-Bauer method of disc susceptibility, a 30-mcg amikacin disc should give a zone of 17 mm or greater to indicate susceptibility. Zone sizes of 14 mm or less indicate resistance. Zone sizes of 15 to 16 mm indicate intermediate susceptibility. With this procedure, a report from the laboratory of "susceptible" indicates that the infecting organism is likely to respond to therapy. A report of "resistant" indicates that the infecting organism is not likely to respond to therapy. A report of "intermediate susceptibility" suggests that the organism would be susceptible if the infection is confined to tissues and fluids (e.g., urine) in which high antibiotic levels are attained.

INDICATIONS AND USAGE

Amikacin Sulfate Injection, USP is indicated in the short-term treatment of serious infections due to susceptible strains of Gram-negative bacteria, including *Pseudomonas* species, *Escherichia coli,* species of indole-positive and indole-negative *Proteus, Providencia* species, *Klebsiella-Enterobacter-Serratia* species, and *Acinetobacter (Mima-Herellea)* species.

Clinical studies have shown Amikacin Sulfate Injection to be effective in bacterial septicemia (including neonatal sepsis); in serious infections of the respiratory tract, bones and joints, central nervous system (including meningitis) and skin and soft tissue; intra-abdominal infections (including peritonitis); and in burns and post-operative infections (including post-vascular surgery). Clinical studies have shown amikacin also to be effective in serious complicated and recurrent urinary tract infections due to these organisms. Aminoglycosides, including Amikacin Sulfate Injection, are not indicated in uncomplicated initial episodes of urinary tract infections unless the causative organisms are not susceptible to antibiotics having less potential toxicity.

Bacteriologic studies should be performed to identify causative organisms and their susceptibilities to amikacin. Amikacin may be considered as initial therapy in suspected Gram-negative infections and therapy may be instituted before obtaining the results of susceptibility testing. Clinical trials demonstrated that amikacin was effective in infections caused by gentamicin and/or tobramycin-resistant strains of Gram-negative organisms, particularly *Proteus rettgeri, Providencia stuartii, Serratia marcescens,* and *Pseudomonas aeruginosa.* The decision to continue therapy with the drug should be based on the results of the susceptiblity tests, the severity of the infection, the response of the patient and the important additional considerations contained in the WARNINGS box above.

Amikacin has also been shown to be effective in staphylococcal infections and may be considered as initial therapy under certain conditions in the treatment of known or suspected staphylococcal disease such as, severe infections where the causative organism may be either a Gram-negative bacterium or a staphylococcus, infections due to susceptible strains of staphylococci in patients allergic to other antibiotics, and in mixed staphylococcal/Gram-negative infections.

In certain severe infections such as neonatal sepsis, concomitant therapy with a penicillin-type drug may be indicated because of the possibility of infections due to Gram-positive organisms such as streptococci or pneumococci.

CONTRAINDICATIONS

A history of hypersensitivity to amikacin is a contraindication for its use. A history of hypersensitivity or serious toxic reactions to aminoglycosides may contraindicate the use of any other aminoglycoside because of the known cross-sensitivities of patients to drugs in this class.

WARNINGS

See WARNINGS box above.

Aminoglycosides can cause fetal harm when administered to a pregnant woman. Aminoglycosides cross the placenta and there have been several reports of total irreversible, bilateral congenital deafness in children whose mothers received streptomycin during pregnancy. Although serious side effects to the fetus or newborns have not been reported in the treatment of pregnant women with other aminoglycosides, the potential for harm exists. Reproduction studies of amikacin have been performed in rats and mice and revealed no evidence of impaired fertility or harm to the fetus due to amikacin. There are no well controlled studies in pregnant women, but investigational experience does not include any positive evidence of adverse effects to the fetus. If this drug is used during pregnancy, or if the patient becomes pregnant while taking this drug, the patient should be apprised of the potential hazard to the fetus.

Contains sodium bisulfite, a sulfite that may cause allergic-type reactions including anaphylactic symptoms and life-threatening or less severe asthmatic episodes in certain susceptible people. The overall prevalence of sulfite sensitivity in the general population is unknown and probably low. Sulfite sensitivity is seen more frequently in asthmatic than nonasthmatic people.

PRECAUTIONS

Aminoglycosides are quickly and almost totally absorbed when they are applied topically, except to the urinary bladder, in association with surgical procedures. Irreversible deafness, renal failure, and death due to neuromuscular blockade have been reported following irrigation of both small and large surgical fields with an aminoglycoside preparation.

Amikacin Sulfate Injection is potentially nephrotoxic, ototoxic and neurotoxic. The concurrent or serial use of other ototoxic or nephrotoxic agents should be avoided either systemically or topically because of the potential for additive effects. Increased nephrotoxicity has been reported following concomitant parenteral administration of aminoglycoside antibiotics and cephalosporins. Concomitant cephalosporins may spuriously elevate creatinine determinations.

Since amikacin is present in high concentrations in the renal excretory system, patients should be well-hydrated to minimize chemical irritation to the renal tubules.

Kidney function should be assessed by the usual methods prior to starting therapy and daily during the course of treatment.

If signs of renal irritation appear (casts, white or red cells, or albumin), hydration should be increased. A reduction in dosage (see DOSAGE AND ADMINISTRATION) may be desirable if other evidence of renal dysfunction occurs such as decreased creatinine clearance, decreased urine specific gravity, increased BUN, creatinine, or oliguria. If azotemia increases or if a progressive decrease in urinary output occurs, treatment should be stopped.

Note: When patients are well-hydrated and kidney function is normal the risk of nephrotoxic reactions with amikacin is low if the dosage recommendations (see DOSAGE AND ADMINISTRATION) are not exceeded.

Elderly patients may have reduced renal function which may not be evident in routine screening tests such as BUN or serum creatinine. A creatinine clearance determination may be more useful. Monitoring of renal function during treatment with aminoglycosides is particularly important.

Aminoglycosides should be used with caution in patients with muscular disorders such as myasthenia gravis or parkinsonism since these drugs may aggravate muscle weakness because of their potential curare-like effect on the neuromuscular junction.

In vitro mixing of aminoglycosides with beta-lactam antibiotics (penicillin or cephalosporins) may result in a significant mutual inactivation. A reduction in serum half-life or serum level may occur when an aminoglycoside or penicillin-type drug is administered by separate routes. Inactivation of the aminoglycoside is clinically significant only in patients with severely impaired renal function. Inactivation may continue in specimens of body fluids collected for assay, resulting in inaccurate aminoglycoside readings. Such specimens should be properly handled (assayed promptly, frozen, or treated with beta-lactamase).

Cross-allergenicity among aminoglycosides has been demonstrated.

As with other antibiotics, the use of amikacin may result in overgrowth of nonsusceptible organisms. If this occurs, appropriate therapy should be instituted.

Aminoglycosides should not be given concurrently with potent diuretics (see WARNINGS box).

Carcinogenesis, Mutagenesis, Impairment of Fertility—Long term studies in animals to evaluate carcinogenic potential have not been performed, and mutagenicity has not been studied. Amikacin administered subcutaneously to rats at doses up to 4 times the human daily dose did not impair male or female fertility.

Pregnancy—Category D (see WARNINGS section).

Nursing Mothers—It is not known whether amikacin is excreted in human milk. Because many drugs are excreted in human milk and because of the potential for serious adverse reactions in nursing infants from amikacin, a decision should be made whether to discontinue nursing or to discontinue the drug, taking into account the importance of the drug to the mother.

Pediatric Use—Aminoglycosides should be used with caution in premature and neonatal infants because of the renal immaturity of these patients and the resulting prolongation of serum half-life of these drugs.

ADVERSE REACTIONS

All aminoglycosides have the potential to induce auditory, vestibular, and renal toxicity and neuromuscular blockade (see WARNINGS box). They occur more frequently in patients with present or past history of renal impairment, of treatment with other ototoxic or nephrotoxic drugs, and in patients treated for longer periods and/or with higher doses than recommended.

Neurotoxicity-Ototoxicity—Toxic effects on the eighth cranial nerve can result in hearing loss, loss of balance, or both. Amikacin primarily affects auditory function. Cochlear damage includes high frequency deafness and usually occurs before clinical hearing loss can be detected.

Neurotoxicity-Neuromuscular Blockage—Acute muscular paralysis and apnea can occur following treatment with aminoglycoside drugs.

Nephrotoxicity—Elevation of serum creatinine, albuminuria, presence of red and white cells, casts, azotemia, and oliguria have been reported. Renal function changes are usually reversible when the drug is discontinued.

Other—In addition to those described above, other adverse reactions which have been reported on rare occasions are skin rash, drug fever, headache, paresthesia, tremor, nausea and vomiting, eosinophilia, arthralgia, anemia, and hypotension.

OVERDOSAGE

In the event of overdosage or toxic reaction, peritoneal dialysis or hemodialysis will aid in the removal of amikacin from the blood. In the newborn infant, exchange transfusion may also be considered.

DOSAGE AND ADMINISTRATION

The patient's pretreatment body weight should be obtained for calculation of correct dosage. Amikacin Sulfate Injection may be given intramuscularly or intravenously.
The status of renal function should be estimated by measurement of the serum creatinine concentration or calculation of the endogenous creatinine clearance rate.
The blood urea nitrogen (BUN) is much less reliable for this purpose. Reassessment of renal function should be made periodically during therapy.
Whenever possible, amikacin concentrations in serum should be measured to assure adequate but not excessive levels. It is desirable to measure both peak and trough serum concentrations intermittently during therapy. Peak concentrations (30–90 minutes after injection) above 35 micrograms per mL and trough concentrations (just prior to the next dose) above 10 micrograms per mL should be avoided. Dosage should be adjusted as indicated.
Intramuscular Administration for Patients with Normal Renal Function—The recommended dosage for adults, children and older infants (see WARNINGS box) with normal renal function is 15 mg/kg/day divided into 2 or 3 equal doses administered at equally-divided intervals, i.e., 7.5 mg/kg q12h or 5 mg/kg q8h. Treatment of patients in the heavier weight classes should not exceed 1.5 grams/day.
When amikacin is indicated in newborns (see WARNINGS box), it is recommended that a loading dose of 10 mg/kg be administered initially to be followed with 7.5 mg/kg every 12 hours.
The usual duration of treatment is 7 to 10 days. It is desirable to limit the duration of treatment to short term whenever feasible. The total daily dose by all routes of administration should not exceed 15 mg/kg/day. In difficult and complicated infections where treatment beyond 10 days is considered, the use of amikacin should be reevaluated. If continued, amikacin serum levels, and renal, auditory, and vestibular functions should be monitored. At the recommended dosage level, uncomplicated infections due to amikacin-sensitive organisms should respond in 24 to 48 hours. If definite clinical response does not occur within 3 to 5 days, therapy should be stopped and the antibiotic susceptibility pattern of the invading organism should be rechecked. Failure of the infection to respond may be due to resistance of the organism or to the presence of septic foci requiring surgical drainage.
When amikacin is indicated in uncomplicated urinary tract infections, a dose of 250 mg twice daily may be used.

DOSAGE GUIDELINES
ADULTS AND CHILDREN WITH NORMAL RENAL FUNCTION

Patient Weight		Dosage		
lbs	kg	7.5 mg/kg q12h	OR	5 mg/kg q8h
99	45	337.5 mg		225 mg
110	50	375 mg		250 mg
121	55	412.5 mg		275 mg
132	60	450 mg		300 mg
143	65	487.5 mg		325 mg
154	70	525 mg		350 mg
165	75	562.5 mg		375 mg
176	80	600 mg		400 mg
187	85	637.5 mg		425 mg
198	90	675 mg		450 mg
209	95	712.5 mg		475 mg
220	100	750 mg		500 mg

Intramuscular Administration for Patients with Impaired Renal Function—Whenever possible, serum amikacin concentrations should be monitored by appropriate assay procedures. Doses may be adjusted in patients with impaired renal function either by administering normal doses at prolonged intervals or by administering reduced doses at a fixed interval.
Both methods are based on the patient's creatinine clearance or serum creatinine values since these have been found to correlate with aminoglycoside half-lives in patients with diminished renal function. These dosage schedules must be used in conjunction with careful clinical and laboratory observations of the patient and should be modified as necessary. Neither method should be used when dialysis is being performed.
Normal Dosage at Prolonged Intervals—If the creatinine clearance rate is not available and the patient's condition is stable, a dosage interval in hours for the normal dose can be calculated by multiplying the patient's serum creatinine by 9; e.g., if the serum creatinine concentration is 2 mg/100 mL, the recommended single dose (7.5 mg/kg) should be administered every 18 hours.
Reduced Dosage at Fixed Time Intervals—When renal function is impaired and it is desirable to administer amikacin at a fixed time interval, dosage must be reduced. In these patients serum amikacin concentrations should be measured to assure accurate administration of amikacin and to avoid concentrations above 35 mcg/mL. If serum assay determinations are not available and the patient's condition is stable, serum creatinine and creatinine clearance values are the most readily availabe indicators of the degree of renal impairment to use as a guide for dosage.
First, initiate therapy by administering a normal dose, 7.5 mg/kg, as a loading dose. This loading dose is the same as the normally recommended dose which would be calculated for a patient with a normal renal function as described above.
To determine the size of maintenance doses administered every 12 hours, the loading dose should be reduced in proportion to the reduction in the patient's creatinine clearance rate:

$$\text{Maintenance Dose Every 12 Hours} = \frac{\text{observed CC in mL/min}}{\text{normal CC in mL/min}} \times \text{calculated loading dose in mg}$$

(CC-creatinine clearance rate)

An alternate rough guide for determining reduced dosage at 12 hour intervals (for patients whose steady state serum creatinine values are known) is to divide the normally recommended dose by the patient's serum creatinine.
The above dosage schedules are not intended to be rigid recommendations but are provided as guides to dosage when the measurement of amikacin serum levels is not feasible.
Intravenous Administration—The individual dose, the total daily dose, and the total cumulative dose of amikacin sulfate are identical to the dose recommended for intramuscular administration. The solution for intravenous use is prepared by adding the contents of a 500 mg vial to 100 mL or 200 mL of sterile diluent such as 0.9% sodium chloride injection or 5% dextrose injection or any of the compatible solutions listed below.
The solution is administered to adults over a 30 to 60 minute period. The total daily dose should not exceed 15 mg/kg/day and may be divided into either 2 or 3 equally-divided doses at equally-divided intervals.
In pediatric patients, the amount of fluid used will depend on the amount ordered for the patient. It should be a sufficient amount to infuse the amikacin over a 30 to 60 minute period. Infants should receive a 1 to 2 hour infusion.
Stability in IV Fluids—Amikacin sulfate is stable for 24 hours at room temperature at concentrations of 0.25 and 5 mg/mL in the following solutions:
5% Dextrose Injection
5% Dextrose and 0.2% Sodium Chloride Injection
5% Dextrose and 0.45% Sodium Chloride Injection
0.9% Sodium Chloride Injection
Lactated Ringer's Injection
Normosol®M in 5% Dextrose Injection, (or Plasma-Lyte 56 Injection in 5% Dextrose in Water)
Normosol®R in 5% Dextrose Injection, (or Plasma-Lyte 148 Injection in 5% Dextrose in Water)
In the above solutions with amikacin concentrations of 0.25 and 5 mg/mL solutions aged for 60 days at 4°C and then stored at 25°C had utility times of 24 hours.
All the same concentrations, solutions frozen and aged for 30 days at −15°C, thawed, and stored at 25°C had utility times of 24 hours.
Parenteral drug products should be inspected visually for particulate matter and discoloration prior to administration whenever the solution and container permit.
Aminoglycosides administered by any of the above routes should not be physically premixed with other drugs but should be administered separately.
Because of the potential toxicity of aminoglycosides, "fixed dosage" recommendations which are not based upon body weight are not advised. Rather it is essential to calculate the dosage to fit the needs of each patient.

HOW SUPPLIED

Amikacin Sulfate Injection, USP is supplied in vials as a colorless solution which requires no refrigeration. It is stable at room temperature for 2 years. At times the solution may become a very pale yellow; this does not indicate a decrease in potency.
Amikacin Sulfate Injection, USP is available as:

NDC 0186-1702-13	100 mg base per 2 mL vial	box of 10
NDC 0186-1703-13	500 mg base per 2 mL vial	box of 10
NDC 0186-1705-13	1 gram base per 4 mL vial	box of 10

*Bauer, A.W., Kirby, W.M.M., Sherris, J.C., and Turck, M: Antibiotic Testing by a Standardized Single Disc Method, *Am. J. Clin. Pathol.*, 45–493, 1966: Standardized Disc Susceptibility Test, FEDERAL REGISTER, 37:20527-29, 1972.

ASTRA®
Astra USA Inc., Westborough, MA 01581
021659R04 Iss. 6/94

AQUASOL A® ℞
Vitamin A Capsules, USP

DESCRIPTION

Each Vitamin A capsule, 15 mg for oral administration, contains the equivalent in activity to 15 mg of retinol or 50,000 USP Vitamin A Units. Each Vitamin A capsule, 7.5 mg, for oral administration, contains the equivalent of 7.5 mg retinol or 25,000 USP Vitamin A Units.
One USP unit is equal to 0.3 mcg of retinol or 0.6 mcg of beta-carotene. One molecule of beta-carotene yields 2 molecules of retinol, which is known as provitamin A.
Vitamin A synthetic (palmitate) is a clear, yellow to light-amber, oily liquid that has only a slight odor. It is a preisomerized vitamin A palmitate of synthetic origin. It is miscible with ether and with chloroform and is slightly soluble in alcohol.
Ordinarily fat-soluble, the vitamin A in this product has been water solubilized by special processing* to enable better absorption and utilization particularly in conditions in which absorption or utilization of fats and fat-soluble substances is impaired. The capsules also contain ethyl vanillin, FD&C Red #40, gelatin, glycerin, methylparaben, polysorbate 80, and propylparaben.

*Oil-soluble Vitamin A alcohol, water solubilized with polysorbate 80.

The structural formula of Vitamin A, retinol, is as follows:

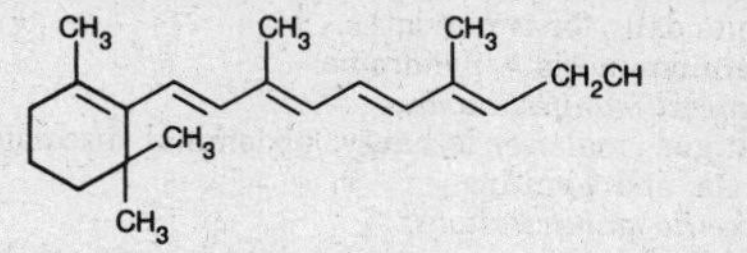

CLINICAL PHARMACOLOGY

Beta-carotene, retinol, and retinal have effective and reliable vitamin A activity. Retinal and retinol are in chemical equilibrium in the body and have equivalent antixerophthalmic activity. Retinal combines with the rod pigment, opsin, in the retina to form rhodopsin, necessary for visual dark adaptation. Vitamin A prevents retardation of growth and preserves the epithelial cells integrity. Normal adult liver storage is sufficient to satisfy two years requirements of vitamin A.
Vitamin A is readily absorbed from the gastrointestinal tract, where the biosynthesis of vitamin A from beta-carotene takes place. Vitamin A absorption requires bile salts, pancreatic lipase, and dietary fat. It is transported in the blood to the liver by the chylomicron fraction of the lymph. Vitamin A is stored in the Kupffer cells of the liver mainly as the palmitate. Normal serum vitamin A is 80–300 USP units per 100 mL (plasma range is 30–70 mcg per dL) and for carotenoids 270 to 753 USP units per 100 mL. The normal adult liver contains approximately 100 to 300 micrograms per gram, mostly as retinol palmitate.

INDICATIONS AND USAGE

Vitamin A capsules are effective for the treatment of vitamin A deficiency.

CONTRAINDICATIONS

Vitamin A is contraindicated in hypervitaminosis A; malabsorption syndrome; or when there is sensitivity to any of the ingredients of this preparation.
Usage in Pregnancy: Safety of amounts exceeding 6,000 USP units of vitamin A daily during pregnancy has not been established at this time. The use of vitamin A in excess of the recommended dietary allowance may cause fetal harm when administered to a pregnant woman.
Animal reproduction studies have shown fetal abnormalities associated with overdosage in several species. Malformations of the central nervous system, the eye, the palate, and the urogenital tract are recorded.
Vitamin A in excess of the recommended dietary allowance is contraindicated in women who are or may become pregnant. If vitamin A is used during pregnancy, or if the patient becomes pregnant while taking vitamin A, the patient should be apprised of the potential hazard to the fetus.

WARNINGS

Avoid overdosage. Keep out of the reach of children.

PRECAUTIONS

General:
Protect from light. Prolonged daily administration over 25,000 USP units of vitamin A should be under close supervision. Blood level assays are not a direct measure of liver storage. Liver storage should be adequate before discontinuing therapy. Single vitamin A deficiency is rare. Multiple vitamin deficiency is expected in any dietary deficiency.

Continued on next page

Astra—Cont.

Drug Interactions:
Women on oral contraceptives have shown a significant increase in plasma vitamin A levels.

Carcinogenesis:
There are no studies that show that administration of vitamin A will cause or prevent cancer.

Pregnancy Category X:
See CONTRAINDICATIONS section.

Nursing Mothers:
The U.S. Recommended Daily Allowance (RDA) of vitamin A (5,000 USP units) is recommended for nursing mothers.

ADVERSE REACTIONS
See OVERDOSAGE section.

OVERDOSAGE
The following amounts have been found to be toxic orally. Toxicity manifestations depended on the age, dosage size, and duration of administration.
Acute Toxicity—single dose (25,000 USP units/kg body weight)
Infant: 350,000 USP units
Adult: Over 2 million USP units
Chronic Toxicity—(4,000 USP units/kg body weight for 6 to 15 months)
Infants 3 to 6 months old: 18,500 USP units (water dispersed)/day for one to three months.
Adults: 1 million USP units daily for three days: 50,000 USP units daily for longer than 18 months: 500,000 USP units daily for two months.
Hypervitaminosis A Syndrome:
1. *General manifestations:*
Fatigue, malaise, lethargy, abdominal discomfort, anorexia, and vomiting.
2. *Specific manifestations:*
a. Skeletal: slow growth, hard tender cortical thickening over the radius and the tibia, migratory arthralgia, and premature closure of the epiphysis.
b. Central Nervous System: irritability, headache, and increased intracranial pressure as manifested by bulging fontanels, papilledema, and exophthalmos.
c. Dermatologic: fissures of the lips, drying and cracking of the skin, alopecia, scaling, massive desquamation, and increased pigmentation.
d. Systemic: hypomenorrhea, hepatosplenomegaly, jaundice, leukopenia, vitamin A plasma level over 1,200 USP units/100 mL.
The treatment of hypervitaminosis A consists of immediate withdrawal of the vitamin along with symptomatic and supportive treatment.

DOSAGE AND ADMINISTRATION
Adults and Children Over 8 years of age:
100,000 USP units daily for three days followed by 50,000 USP units daily for two weeks.
Follow-up therapy with an oral therapeutic multivitamin preparation, containing 10,000 to 20,000 USP units vitamin A for persons over 8 years old is recommended daily for two months. In malabsorption, the parenteral route must be used for an equivalent preparation.
Poor dietary habits should be corrected and an abundant and well-balanced dietary intake should be prescribed.

HOW SUPPLIED
Aquasol A capsules (vitamin A capsules USP) are available as:
NDC 0186-4301-00; 15 mg retinol (50,000 USP Units), Bottles of 100.
NDC 0186-4291-00; 7.5 mg retinol (25,000 USP Units), Bottles of 100.
These products are dark red, soft gelatin capsules.
Store at controlled room temperature, 15°–30°C (59°–86°F). Protect from light. Dispense in a tight, light-resistant container as defined in the USP.
These products are manufactured for Astra USA, Inc., by R.P. Scherer Corp., Clearwater, FL 33518.
Caution: Federal law prohibits dispensing without prescription.
Manufactured for:
Astra USA, Inc.
Westborough, MA 01581
021678R30   8/93 (30)
11164/8-93

AQUASOL A®   ℞
Parenteral
water-miscible
vitamin A Palmitate

50,000 USP Units
(15 mg retinol)/mL
with 0.5% chlorobutanol as preservative; 12% polysorbate 80, 0.1% citric acid, 0.03% butylated hydroxyanisole, 0.03%

butylated hydroxytoluene; and sodium hydroxide to adjust pH.
THIS IS A STERILE PRODUCT FOR INTRAMUSCULAR INJECTION

DESCRIPTION
AQUASOL A PARENTERAL (water-miscible vitamin A Palmitate) provides 50,000 USP Units of vitamin A per mL as retinol ($C_{20}H_{30}O$) in the form of vitamin A palmitate, a light yellow to amber oil. The structural formula of retinol is:

Ordinarily oil-soluble, the vitamin A in this product has been water solubilized by special processing* and is available in a water solution for intramuscular injection.
One USP Unit is equivalent to one international unit (IU) and to 0.3 mcg of retinol or 0.6 mcg of beta-carotene.

CLINICAL PHARMACOLOGY
Beta-carotene, retinol, and retinal have effective and reliable vitamin A activity. Retinal and retinol are in chemical equilibrium in the body and have equivalent antixerophthalmic activity. Retinal combines with the rod pigment, opsin, in the retina to form rhodopsin, necessary for visual dark adaptation. Vitamin A prevents retardation of growth and preserves the epithelial cells' integrity. Normal adult liver storage is sufficient to satisfy two years' requirements of vitamin A.
Vitamin A is readily absorbed from the gastrointestinal tract, where the biosynthesis of vitamin A from beta-carotene takes place. Vitamin A absorption requires bile salts, pancreatic lipase, and dietary fat. It is transported in the blood to the liver by the chylomicron fraction of the lymph. Vitamin A is stored in Kupffer cells of the liver mainly as the palmitate. Normal serum vitamin A is 80–300 Units per 100 mL (plasma range is 30–70 μg per dl) and for carotenoids 270–753 Units per mL. The normal adult liver contains approximately 100 to 300 micrograms per gram, mostly as retinol palmitate.

---

*Oil-soluble vitamin A water solubilized with polysorbate 80.

INDICATIONS
Vitamin A injection is effective for the treatment of vitamin A deficiency.
The parenteral administration is indicated when the oral administration is not feasible as in anorexia, nausea, vomiting, pre- and post-operative conditions, or it is not available as in the "Malabsorption Syndrome" with accompanying steatorrhea.

CONTRAINDICATIONS
The intravenous administration. Hypervitaminosis A. Sensitivity to any of the ingredients in this preparation.
Use in Pregnancy: Safety of amounts exceeding 6,000 Units of vitamin A daily during pregnancy has not been established at this time. The use of vitamin A in excess of the recommended dietary allowance may cause fetal harm when administered to a pregnant woman. Animal reproduction studies have shown fetal abnormalities associated with overdosage in several species. Malformations of the central nervous system, the eye, the palate, and the urogenital tract are recorded. Vitamin A in excess of the recommended dietary allowance is contraindicated in women who are or may become pregnant. If vitamin A is used during pregnancy, or if the patient becomes pregnant while taking vitamin A, the patient should be apprised of the potential hazard to the fetus.

WARNINGS
Avoid overdosage. Keep out of the reach of children.

PRECAUTIONS
General: Protect from light. Prolonged daily dose administration over 25,000 Units vitamin A should be under close supervision. Blood level assays are not a direct measure of liver storage. Liver storage should be adequate before discontinuing therapy. Single vitamin A deficiency is rare. Multiple vitamin deficiency is expected in any dietary deficiency.
Drug Interactions: Women on oral contraceptives have shown a significant increase in plasma vitamin A levels.
Carcinogenesis: There are no studies that show that administration of vitamin A will cause or prevent cancer.
Pregnancy Category X:
See CONTRAINDICATIONS section.
Nursing Mothers: The U.S. Recommended Daily Allowance (RDA) of vitamin A (5,000 Units) is recommended for nursing mothers.

ADVERSE REACTIONS
See OVERDOSAGE section. Anaphylactic shock and death have been reported using the intravenous route. Allergic reactions have been reported rarely with administration of Aquasol A Parenteral including one case of an anaphylactoid type reaction.

OVERDOSAGE
The following amounts have been found to be toxic orally. Toxicity manifestations depend on the age, dosage, size, and duration of administration.
Acute toxicity—single dose (25,000 Units/kg body weight)
Infant: 350,000 Units
Adult: Over 2 million Units
Chronic toxicity (4,000 Units/kg body weight for 6 to 15 months)
Infants 3 to 6 months old: 18,500 Units (water dispersed)/day for one to three months.
Adult: 1 million Units daily for three days; 50,000 Units daily for longer than 18 months; 500,000 Units daily for two months.
Hypervitaminosis A Syndrome:
1. *General manifestations:*
Fatigue, malaise, lethargy, abdominal discomfort, anorexia, and vomiting.
2. *Specific manifestations:*
a. Skeletal: slow growth, hard tender cortical thickening on the radius and tibia, migratory arthralgia and premature closure of the epiphysis.
b. Central Nervous System: irritability, headache, and increased intracranial pressure as manifested by bulging fontanels, papilledema, and exophthalmos.
c. Dermatologic: fissures of the lips, drying and cracking of the skin, alopecia, scaling, massive desquamation, and increased pigmentation.
d. Systemic: hypomenorrhea, hepatosplenomegaly, jaundice, leukopenia, vitamin A plasma level over 1,200 Units/100 mL.
The treatment of hypervitaminosis A consists of immediate withdrawal of the vitamin along with symptomatic and supportive treatment.

DOSAGE AND ADMINISTRATION
For intramuscular use.
I. Adults
100,000 Units daily for three days followed by 50,000 daily for two weeks.
II. Children 1 to 8 years old
17,500 to 35,000 Units daily for 10 days.
III. Infants
7,500 to 15,000 Units daily for 10 days.
Follow-up therapy with an oral therapeutic multi-vitamin preparation, containing 10,000 to 20,000 Units vitamin A for persons over 8 years old and 5,000 to 10,000 Units for infants and children, is recommended daily for two months. In malabsorption, the parenteral route must be used for an equivalent preparation.
Poor dietary habits should be corrected and an abundant and well-balanced dietary intake should be prescribed.

HOW SUPPLIED
Aquasol A Parenteral (water-miscible vitamin A Palmitate) is available as: NDC 0186-4239-62; 50,000 USP Units (15 mg retinol/mL); 2 mL single-dose vial, box of 10.
Store at 2°–8°C (36°–46°F). Do not freeze.
Caution: Federal law prohibits dispensing without prescription.
Manufactured by:
Centeon L.L.C.
Kankakee, IL 60901

Manufactured for:
ASTRA®
Astra USA, Inc.
Westborough, MA 01581
021646R01   Rev. 6/96

ASTRAMORPH/PF™   Ⓒ
[ās'-trä-mŏrf″]
(morphine sulfate injection, USP) Preservative-Free

DESCRIPTION
Morphine is the most important alkaloid of opium and is a phenanthrene derivative. It is available as the sulfate, having the following structural formula:

7,8-Didehydro-4,5-epoxy-17-methyl-(5α,6α)-morphinan-3,6-diol sulfate (2:1) (salt), pentahydrate

Preservative-free ASTRAMORPH/PF (Morphine Sulfate Injection, USP) is a sterile, pyrogen-free, isobaric solution free of antioxidants, preservatives or other potentially neurotoxic additives, and is intended for intravenous, epidural or intrathecal administration as a narcotic analgesic. Each milliliter contains morphine sulfate 0.5 mg or 1 mg (Warning: May Be Habit Forming) and sodium chloride 9 mg in Water for Injection. pH may be adjusted with hydrochloric acid to 2.5–6.5. Containers are sealed under nitrogen. Each container is intended for SINGLE USE ONLY. Discard any unused portion. DO NOT AUTOCLAVE.

CLINICAL PHARMACOLOGY

Morphine exerts its primary effects on the central nervous system and organs containing smooth muscle. Pharmacologic effects include analgesia, drowsiness, alteration in mood (euphoria), reduction in body temperature (at low doses), dose-related depression of respiration, interference with adrenocortical response to stress (at high doses), reduction in peripheral resistance with little or no effect on cardiac index and miosis.

Morphine, as other opioids, acts as an agonist interacting with stereo-specific and saturable binding sites/receptors in the brain, spinal cord and other tissues. These sites have been classified as μ receptors and are widely distributed throughout the central nervous system being present in highest concentration in the limbic system (frontal and temporal cortex, amygdala and hippocampus), thalamus, striatum, hypothalamus, midbrain and laminae I, II, IV and V of the dorsal horn in the spinal cord. It has been postulated that exogenously administered morphine exerts its analgesic effect, in part, by altering the central release of neurotransmitter from afferent nerves sensitive to noxious stimuli. Peripheral threshold or responsiveness to noxious stimuli is unaffected leaving monosynaptic reflexes such as the patellar or the Achilles tendon reflex intact.

Autonomic reflexes are not affected by epidural or intrathecal morphine, however morphine exerts spasmogenic effects on the gastrointestinal tract that result in decreased peristaltic activity.

Central nervous system effects of intravenously administered morphine sulfate are influenced by ability to cross the blood-brain barrier.

The delay in the onset of analgesia following epidural or intrathecal injection may be attributed to its relatively poor lipid solubility (i.e., an oil/water partition coefficient of 1.42), and its slow access to the receptor sites. The hydrophilic character of morphine may also explain its retention in the CNS and its slow release into the systemic circulation, resulting in a prolonged effect.

Nausea and vomiting may be prominent and are thought to be the result of central stimulation of the chemoreceptor trigger zone. Histamine release is common; allergic manifestations of urticaria and, rarely, anaphylaxis may occur. Bronchoconstriction may occur either as an idiosyncratic reaction or from large dosages.

Approximately one-third of intravenous morphine is bound to plasma proteins. Free morphine is rapidly redistributed in parenchymatous tissues. The major metabolic pathway is through conjugation with glucuronic acid in the liver. Elimination half-life is approximately 1.5 to 2 hours in healthy volunteers. For intravenously administered morphine, 90% is excreted in the urine within 24 hours and traces are detectable in urine up to 48 hours. About 7–10% of administered morphine eventually appears in the feces as conjugated morphine.

Peak serum levels following epidural or intrathecal administration of ASTRAMORPH/PF are reached within 30 minutes in most subjects and decline to very low levels during the next 2 to 4 hours. The onset of action occurs in 15 to 60 minutes following epidural administration or intrathecal administration; analgesia may last up to 24 hours. Due to this extended duration of action, sustained pain relief can be provided with lower daily doses (by these two routes) than are usually required with intravenous or intramuscular morphine administration.

INDICATIONS AND USAGE

Preservative-free ASTRAMORPH/PF is a systemic narcotic analgesic for administration by the intravenous, epidural or intrathecal routes. It is used for the management of pain not responsive to non-narcotic analgesics. Morphine sulfate, administered epidurally or intrathecally, provides pain relief for extended periods without attendant loss of motor, sensory or sympathetic function.

CONTRAINDICATIONS

ASTRAMORPH/PF is contraindicated in those medical conditions which would preclude the administration of opioids by the intravenous route—allergy to morphine or other opiates, acute bronchial asthma, upper airway obstruction.

Administration of morphine by the epidural or intrathecal route is contraindicated in the presence of infection at the injection site, anticoagulant therapy, bleeding diathesis, parenterally administered corticosteroids within a two week period or other concomitant drug therapy or medical condition which would contraindicate the technique of epidural or intrathecal analgesia.

WARNINGS

ASTRAMORPH/PF administration should be limited to use by those familiar with the management of respiratory depression, and in the case of epidural or intrathecal administration, familiar with the techniques and patient management problems associated with epidural or intrathecal drug administration. Because epidural administration has been associated with lessened potential for immediate or late adverse effects than intrathecal administration, the epidural route should be used whenever possible. Rapid intravenous administration may result in chest wall rigidity.

FACILITIES WHERE ASTRAMORPH/PF IS ADMINISTERED MUST BE EQUIPPED WITH RESUSCITATIVE EQUIPMENT, OXYGEN, NALOXONE INJECTION, AND OTHER RESUSCITATIVE DRUGS. WHEN THE EPIDURAL OR INTRATHECAL ROUTE OF ADMINISTRATION IS EMPLOYED, PATIENTS MUST BE OBSERVED IN A FULLY EQUIPPED AND STAFFED ENVIRONMENT FOR AT LEAST 24 HOURS.

SEVERE RESPIRATORY DEPRESSION UP TO 24 HOURS FOLLOWING EPIDURAL OR INTRATHECAL ADMINISTRATION HAS BEEN REPORTED.

Morphine sulfate may be habit forming. (**See Drug Abuse and Dependence section.**)

PRECAUTIONS

General

Preservative-free ASTRAMORPH/PF (Morphine Sulfate Injection, USP) should be administered with extreme caution in aged or debilitated patients, in the presence of increased intracranial/intraocular pressure and in patients with head injury. Pupillary changes (miosis) may obscure the course of intracranial pathology. Care is urged in patients who have a decreased respiratory reserve (e.g., emphysema, severe obesity, kyphoscoliosis).

Seizures may result from high doses. Patients with known seizure disorders should be carefully observed for evidence of morphine-induced seizure activity.

It is recommended that administration of ASTRAMORPH/PF by the epidural or intrathecal routes be limited to the lumbar area. Intrathecal use has been associated with a higher incidence of respiratory depression than epidural use.

Smooth muscle hypertonicity may result in biliary colic, difficulty in urination and possible urinary retention requiring catheterization. Consideration should be given to risks inherent in urethral catheterization, e.g., sepsis, when epidural or intrathecal administration is considered, especially in the perioperative period.

Elimination half-life may be prolonged in patients with reduced metabolic rates and with hepatic or renal dysfunction. Hence, care should be exercised in administering morphine in these conditions, particularly with repeated dosing.

Patients with reduced circulating blood volume, impaired myocardial function or on sympatholytic drugs should be observed carefully for orthostatic hypotension, particularly in transport.

Patients with chronic obstructive pulmonary disease and patients with acute asthmatic attack may develop acute respiratory failure with administration of morphine. Use in these patients should be reserved for those whose conditions require endotracheal intubation and respiratory support or control of ventilation.

Drug Interactions

Depressant effects of morphine are potentiated by either concomitant administration or in the presence of other CNS depressants such as alcohol, sedatives, antihistaminics or psychotropic drugs (e.g., MAO inhibitors, phenothiazines, butyrophenones and tricyclic antidepressants). Premedication or intra-anesthetic use of neuroleptics with morphine may increase the risk of respiratory depression.

Carcinogenesis, Mutagenesis, Impairment of Fertility

Studies of morphine sulfate in animals to evaluate the carcinogenic and mutagenic potential or the effect on fertility have not been conducted.

Pregnancy

Teratogenic effects—Pregnancy Category C

Animal reproduction studies have not been conducted with morphine sulfate. It is also not known whether morphine sulfate can cause fetal harm when administered to a pregnant woman or can affect reproduction capacity. Morphine sulfate should be given to a pregnant woman only if clearly needed.

Nonteratogenic effects

Infants born from mothers who have been taking morphine chronically may exhibit withdrawal symptoms.

Labor and Delivery

Intravenous morphine readily passes into the fetal circulation and may result in respiratory depression in the neonate. Naloxone and resuscitative equipment should be available for reversal of narcotic-induced respiratory depression in the neonate. In addition, intravenous morphine may reduce the strength, duration and frequency of uterine contraction resulting in prolonged labor.

Epidurally and intrathecally administered morphine readily passes into the fetal circulation and may result in respiratory depression of the neonate. Controlled clinical studies have shown that *epidural* administration has little or no effect on the relief of labor pain.

However, studies have suggested that in most cases 0.2 to 1 mg of morphine *intrathecally* provides adequate pain relief with little effect on the duration of first stage labor. The second stage labor, though, may be prolonged if the parturient is not encouraged to bear down. A continuous intravenous infusion of naloxone, 0.6 mg/hr, for 24 hours after intrathecal injection may be employed to reduce the incidence of potential side effects.

Nursing Mothers

Morphine is excreted in maternal milk. Effect on the nursing infant is not known.

Pediatric Use

Safety and effectiveness in children have not been established.

ADVERSE REACTIONS

The most serious side effect is respiratory depression. Because of delay in maximum CNS effect with intravenously administered drug (30 min), rapid administration may result in overdosing. Bolus administration by the epidural or intrathecal route may result in early respiratory depression due to direct venous redistribution of morphine to the respiratory centers in the brain. Late (up to 24 hours) onset of acute respiratory depression has been reported with administration by the epidural or intrathecal route and is believed to be the result of rostral spread. Reports of respiratory depression following intrathecal administration have been more frequent, but the dosage used in most of these cases has been considerably higher than that recommended. This depression may be severe and could require intervention (see Warnings and Overdosage sections). Even without clinical evidence of ventilatory inadequacy, a diminished CO_2 ventilation response may be noted for up to 22 hours following epidural or intrathecal administration.

While low doses of intravenously administered morphine have little effect on cardiovascular stability, high doses are excitatory, resulting from sympathetic hyperactivity and increase in circulating catecholamines. Excitation of the central nervous system resulting in convulsions may accompany high doses of morphine given intravenously. Dysphoric reactions may occur and toxic psychoses have been reported.

Epidural or intrathecal administration is accompanied by a high incidence of pruritus which is dose related but not confined to site of administration. Nausea and vomiting are frequently seen in patients following morphine administration. Urinary retention which may persist for 10–20 hours following single epidural or intrathecal administration has been reported in approximately 90% of males. Incidence is somewhat lower in females. Patients may require catheterization (see Precautions). Pruritus, nausea/vomiting and urinary retention frequently can be alleviated by the intravenous administration of low doses of naloxone (0.2 mg).

Tolerance and dependence to chronically administered morphine, by whatever route, is known to occur (**see Drug Abuse and Dependence section**).

Miscellaneous side effects include constipation, headache, anxiety, depression of cough reflex, interference with thermal regulation and oliguria. Evidence of histamine release such as urticaria, wheals and/or local tissue irritation may occur.

In general, side effects are amenable to reversal by narcotic antagonists. **NALOXONE HYDROCHLORIDE INJECTION AND RESUSCITATIVE EQUIPMENT SHOULD BE IMMEDIATELY AVAILABLE FOR ADMINISTRATION IN CASE OF LIFE THREATENING OR INTOLERABLE SIDE EFFECTS.**

DRUG ABUSE AND DEPENDENCE

Controlled Substance

Morphine sulfate injection is a Schedule II substance under the Drug Enforcement Administration classification.

Abuse

Morphine has recognized abuse and dependence potential.

Dependence

Cerebral and spinal receptors may develop tolerance/dependence independently, as a function of local dosage. Care must be taken to avert withdrawal in those patients who have been maintained on parenteral/oral narcotics when epidural or intrathecal administration is considered. Withdrawal may occur following chronic epidural or intrathecal administration, as well as the development of tolerance to morphine by these routes. (**See nonteratogenic effects under Pregnancy**).

OVERDOSAGE

Overdosage is characterized by respiratory depression with or without concomitant CNS depression. Since respiratory arrest may result either through direct depression of the respiratory center or as the result of hypoxia, primary atten-

Continued on next page

Astra—Cont.

tion should be given to the establishment of adequate respiratory exchange through provision of a patent airway and institution of assisted or controlled ventilation. The narcotic antagonist, naloxone hydrochloride, is a specific antidote. Naloxone hydrochloride (see package insert for full prescribing information) should be administered intravenously, simultaneously with respiratory resuscitation. *As the duration of effect of naloxone is considerably shorter than that of epidural or intrathecal morphine, repeated administration may be necessary.* Patients should be closely observed for evidence of renarcotization. *Note: Respiratory depression may be delayed in onset up to 24 hours* following epidural or intrathecal administration. In painful conditions, reversal of narcotic effect may result in acute onset of pain and release of catecholamines. Careful administration of naloxone may permit reversal of side effects without affecting analgesia. Parenteral administration of narcotics in patients receiving epidural or intrathecal morphine may result in overdosage.

DOSAGE AND ADMINISTRATION
Preservative-free ASTRAMORPH/PF (Morphine Sulfate Injection, USP) is intended for intravenous, epidural or intrathecal administration.
Intravenous Administration
Dosage
The initial dose of morphine should be 2 mg to 10 mg/70 kg of body weight. Patients under the age of 18; no information available.
Epidural Administration
ASTRAMORPH/PF SHOULD BE ADMINISTERED EPIDURALLY ONLY BY PHYSICIANS EXPERIENCED IN THE TECHNIQUES OF EPIDURAL ADMINISTRATION AND WHO ARE THOROUGHLY FAMILIAR WITH THE LABELING. IT SHOULD BE ADMINISTERED ONLY IN SETTINGS WHERE ADEQUATE PATIENT MONITORING IS POSSIBLE. RESUSCITATIVE EQUIPMENT AND A SPECIFIC ANTAGONIST (NALOXONE HYDROCHLORIDE INJECTION) SHOULD BE IMMEDIATELY AVAILABLE FOR THE MANAGEMENT OF RESPIRATORY DEPRESSION AS WELL AS COMPLICATIONS WHICH MIGHT RESULT FROM INADVERTENT INTRATHECAL OR INTRAVASCULAR INJECTION. (NOTE: INTRATHECAL DOSAGE IS USUALLY $^1/_{10}$ THAT OF EPIDURAL DOSAGE.) PATIENT MONITORING SHOULD BE CONTINUED FOR AT LEAST 24 HOURS AFTER EACH DOSE, SINCE DELAYED RESPIRATORY DEPRESSION MAY OCCUR.
Proper placement of a needle or catheter in the epidural space should be verified before ASTRAMORPH/PF is injected. Acceptable techniques for verifying proper placement include: a) aspiration to check for absence of blood or cerebrospinal fluid, or b) administration of 5 mL (3 mL in obstetric patients) of UNPRESERVED 1.5% Lidocaine and Epinephrine (1:200,000) Injection and then observe the patient for lack of tachycardia (this indicates that vascular injection has *not* been made) and lack of sudden onset of segmental anesthesia (this indicates that intrathecal injection has *not* been made).
Epidural Adult Dosage
Initial injection of 5 mg in the lumbar region may provide satisfactory pain relief for up to 24 hours. If adequate pain relief is not achieved within one hour, careful administration of incremental doses of 1 to 2 mg at intervals sufficient to assess effectiveness may be given. No more than 10 mg/24 hr should be administered.
Thoracic administration has been shown to dramatically increase the incidence of early and late respiratory depression even at doses of 1 to 2 mg.
For continuous infusion an initial dose of 2 to 4 mg/24 hours is recommended. Further doses of 1 to 2 mg may be given if pain relief is not achieved initially.
Aged or debilitated patients-Administer with extreme caution (**see Precautions section**). Doses of less than 5 mg may provide satisfactory pain relief for up to 24 hours.
Epidural Pediatric Use
No information on use in pediatric patients is available.
Intrathecal Administration

> NOTE: INTRATHECAL DOSAGE IS USUALLY $^1/_{10}$ THAT OF EPIDURAL DOSAGE.

ASTRAMORPH/PF SHOULD BE ADMINISTERED INTRATHECALLY ONLY BY PHYSICIANS EXPERIENCED IN THE TECHNIQUES OF INTRATHECAL ADMINISTRATION AND WHO ARE THOROUGHLY FAMILIAR WITH THE LABELING. IT SHOULD BE ADMINISTERED ONLY IN SETTINGS WHERE ADEQUATE PATIENT MONITORING IS POSSIBLE. RESUSCITATIVE EQUIPMENT AND A SPECIFIC ANTAGONIST (NALOXONE HYDROCHLORIDE INJECTION) SHOULD BE IMMEDIATELY AVAILABLE FOR THE MANAGEMENT OF RESPIRATORY DEPRESSION AS WELL AS COMPLICATIONS WHICH MIGHT RESULT FROM INADVERTENT

INTRAVASCULAR INJECTION. **PATIENT MONITORING SHOULD BE CONTINUED FOR AT LEAST 24 HOURS AFTER EACH DOSE, SINCE DELAYED RESPIRATORY DEPRESSION MAY OCCUR. RESPIRATORY DEPRESSION (BOTH EARLY AND LATE ONSET) HAS OCCURRED MORE FREQUENTLY FOLLOWING INTRATHECAL ADMINISTRATION.**
Intrathecal Adult Dosage
A single injection of 0.2 to 1 mg may provide satisfactory pain relief for up to 24 hours. (**CAUTION: THIS IS ONLY 0.4 TO 2 ML OF THE 0.5 MG/ML POTENCY OR 0.2 to 1 ML OF THE 1 MG/ML POTENCY OF ASTRAMORPH/PF.) DO NOT INJECT INTRATHECALLY MORE THAN 2 ML OF THE 0.5 MG/ML POTENCY OR 1 ML OF THE 1 MG/ML POTENCY. USE IN THE LUMBAR AREA ONLY IS RECOMMENDED.** Repeated intrathecal injections of ASTRAMORPH/PF are not recommended. A constant intravenous infusion of naloxone hydrochloride, 0.6 mg/hr, for 24 hours after intrathecal injection may be used to reduce the incidence of potential side effects.
Aged or debilitated patients-Administer with extreme caution (**see Precautions section**). A lower dosage is usually satisfactory.
Repeat Dosage
If pain recurs, alternative routes of administration should be considered, since experience with repeated doses of morphine by the intrathecal route is limited.
Intrathecal Pediatric Use
No information on use in pediatric patients is available.
Parenteral drug products should be inspected for particulate matter and discoloration prior to administration, whenever solution and container permit.

HOW SUPPLIED
The following strengths and container types of ASTRAMORPH/PF are available:
(0.5 mg/mL)
NDC 0186-1159-03   2 mL (1 mg) Ampule, Boxes of 10
NDC 0186-1150-02   10 mL (5 mg) Ampule, Boxes of 5
NDC 0186-1152-12   10 mL (5 mg) Single Dose Vial,
                     Boxes of 5 Astra E-Z OFF™ vial closure
(1 mg/mL)
NDC 0186-1160-03   2 mL (2 mg) Ampule, Boxes of 10
NDC 0186-1151-02   10 mL (10 mg) Ampule, Boxes of 5
NDC 0186-1153-12   10 mL (10 mg) Single Dose Vial,
                     Boxes of 5 Astra E-Z OFF™ vial closure
Storage
Protect from light. Store in carton at controlled room temperature, 15° to 30° C (59°F to 86°F) until ready to use. ASTRAMORPH/PF contains no preservative. DISCARD ANY UNUSED PORTION. DO NOT AUTOCLAVE. Do not use the Injection if darker than pale yellow or if discolored in any other way, or if it contains a precipitate.
Caution: Federal law prohibits dispensing without prescription.
021865R03   10/89 (3)

ATROPINE SULFATE ℞
[*ā'trow-peen*]
Injection, USP
0.1 mg/mL
Adult Strength

(For details of indications, dosage and administration, precautions, and adverse reactions, see circular in package.)

HOW SUPPLIED
Prefilled Syringes:
5 mL (0.5 mg) NDC 0186-0648-01
with a 21 G 15/16″ Needle
10 mL (1 mg) NDC 0186-0649-01
with a 21 G 15/16″ Needle
Solution should be stored at controlled room temperature 15°–30°C (59°–86°F).
Caution: Federal law prohibits dispensing without prescription.
                              021880R04 Rev. 9/95

BRETYLIUM TOSYLATE INJECTION ℞
For Intramuscular or Intravenous Use.

(For details of indications, dosage and administration, precautions, and adverse reactions, see circular in package.)

HOW SUPPLIED
NDC 0186-1131-04, 10 mL single dose vial, box of 1
NDC 0186-0663-01, 10 mL syringe, 21 G 15/16″ Needle, box of 1
Each unit contains 500 mg bretylium tosylate in Water for Injection, USP. The pH is adjusted when necessary, with

hydrochloric acid and/or sodium hydroxide. Sterile, nonpyrogenic.
021810R04   2/94(4)

CALCITONIN-SALMON INJECTION, SYNTHETIC ℞

DESCRIPTION
Calcitonin is a polypeptide hormone secreted by the parafollicular cells of the thyroid gland in mammals and by the ultimobranchial gland of birds and fish.
Calcitonin-salmon injection, synthetic is a synthetic polypeptide of 32 amino acids in the same linear sequence that is found in calcitonin of salmon origin. This is shown by the following graphic formula:

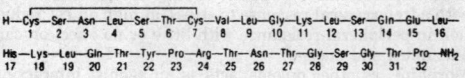

It is provided in sterile solution for subcutaneous or intramuscular injection. Each milliliter contains 200 I.U. calcitonin-salmon; 5 mg phenol (as preservative); with sodium chloride, sodium acetate, glacial acetic acid, and sodium hydroxide to adjust tonicity and pH between 3.9 and 4.5. Filled under nitrogen.
The activity of calcitonin-salmon is stated in International Units based on bioassay in comparison with the International Reference Preparation of calcitonin-salmon for Bioassay, distributed by the National Institute for Biological Standards and Control, Holly Hill, London.

HOW SUPPLIED
Calcitonin-salmon injection, synthetic is available as:
NDC 0186-1608-13; 2 mL multiple dose vial containing 200 I.U. per mL Box of 1
Store in refrigerator, between 2°-8°C (36°-46°F).
Caution: Federal law prohibits dispensing without prescription.

                         021713R01 Iss. 5/94

10% CALCIUM CHLORIDE ℞
[*cal'cium chlor'ide*]
Injection, USP
1 gram (100 mg/mL)
27.3 mg (1.4 mEq) Ca++/mL
2.04 mOsm/mL (calc.)
A Hypertonic Solution for Intravenous Injection

Caution: This solution must not be injected intramuscularly or subcutaneously.

(For details of indications, dosage and administration, precautions, and adverse reactions, see circular in package.)

HOW SUPPLIED
10% Calcium Chloride Injection, USP is supplied as follows:
NDC 0186-1166-04 10 mL single dose vials in packages of 25
NDC 0186-0651-01 10 mL prefilled syringes with 21 G 15/16″ Needle
The solution should be stored at controlled room temperature 15°–30°C (59°–86°F).
021710R03   2/95(3)

CLINDAMYCIN PHOSPHATE INJECTION, USP ℞
[*klin"dah-mī'sin*]
Sterile Solution
For Intramuscular and Intravenous Use

> **WARNING**
> Clindamycin therapy has been associated with severe colitis which may end fatally. Therefore, it should be reserved for serious infections where less toxic antimicrobial agents are inappropriate, as described in the INDICATIONS AND USAGE section. It should not be used in patients with nonbacterial infections, such as most upper respiratory tract infections. Studies indicate a toxin(s) produced by *Clostridia* is one primary cause of antibiotic-associated colitis. Cholestyramine and colestipol resins have been shown to bind the toxin *in vitro.* See WARNINGS section. The colitis is usually characterized by severe, persistent diarrhea and severe abdominal cramps and may be associated with the passage of blood and mucus. Endoscopic examination may reveal pseudomembranous colitis. Stool culture for *Clostridium difficile* and stool assay for *C. difficile* toxin may be helpful diagnostically.

When significant diarrhea occurs, the drug should be discontinued or, if necessary, continued only with close observation of the patient. Large bowel endoscopy has been recommended.

Antiperistaltic agents such as opiates and diphenoxylate with atropine may prolong and/or worsen the condition. Vancomycin has been found to be effective in the treatment of antibiotic-associated pseudomembranous colitis produced by *Clostridium difficile*. The usual adult dosage is 500 milligrams to 2 grams of vancomycin orally per day in three to four divided doses administered for 7 to 10 days. Cholestyramine or colestipol resins bind vancomycin *in vitro*. If both a resin and vancomycin are to be administered concurrently, it may be advisable to separate the time of administration of each drug.

Diarrhea, colitis, and pseudomembranous colitis have been observed to begin up to several weeks following cessation of therapy with clindamycin.

(For details of indications, dosage and administration, precautions, and adverse reactions, see circular in package.)

HOW SUPPLIED

Each mL of Clindamycin Phosphate Injection, USP contains clindamycin phosphate equivalent to 150 mg clindamycin, 0.5 mg disodium edetate and 9.45 mg benzyl alcohol as preservative. When necessary, pH is adjusted with sodium hydroxide and/or hydrochloric acid. Filled under nitrogen. Clindamycin Phosphate Injection, USP 150 mg/mL is available in the following packages:

2 mL vials	NDC 0186-1450-04 Boxes of 25
4 mL vials	NDC 0186-1451-04 Boxes of 25
6 mL vials	NDC 0186-1452-04 Boxes of 25

Also available in:
60 mL Pharmacy Bulk   NDC 0186-1453-01 Box of 1
Package
Store at controlled room temperature 15°–30°C (59°–86°F).
Caution: Federal law prohibits dispensing without prescription.

021666R04   8/92 (4)

COCAINE HYDROCHLORIDE
Topical Solution   Ⓒ II

DESCRIPTION

Each mL contains 40 mg or 100 mg cocaine HCl (Warning: May be habit forming), benzoic acid, citric acid, FD&C green #3 dye, D&C yellow #10 dye. An aqueous solution.

NOT FOR INJECTION OR OPHTHALMIC USE

NOTE (for Glass Bottle): Do not steam autoclave.
Cocaine Hydrochloride USP is a crystalline, granular, or powder substance having a saline, slightly bitter taste that numbs tongue and lips. Cocaine Hydrochloride is a local anesthetic.

CLINICAL PHARMACOLOGY

Cocaine blocks the initiation or conduction of the nerve impulse following local application, thereby effecting local anesthetic action.
Cocaine is absorbed from all sites of application, including mucous membranes and the gastrointestinal mucosa. Cocaine is degraded by plasma esterases, with the half-life in the plasma being approximately one hour.

INDICATIONS AND USAGE

Cocaine Hydrochloride Topical Solution is indicated for the introduction of local (topical) anesthesia of accessible mucous membranes of the oral, laryngeal and nasal cavities.

CONTRAINDICATIONS

Cocaine Hydrochloride is contraindicated in patients with a known history of hypersensitivity to the drug or to the components of the topical solution.

WARNINGS

RESUSCITATIVE EQUIPMENT AND DRUGS SHOULD BE IMMEDIATELY AVAILABLE WHEN ANY LOCAL ANESTHETIC IS USED.
Carcinogenesis, Mutagenesis:
Long-term studies to determine the carcinogenic and mutagenic potential of cocaine are not available.
Pregnancy: Teratogenic Effects —Pregnancy Category C:
Animal reproduction studies have not been conducted with cocaine. It is also not known whether cocaine can cause fetal harm when administered to a pregnant woman or can affect reproduction capacity. Cocaine should be given to a pregnant woman only if needed.

PRECAUTIONS

The safety and effectiveness of Cocaine Hydrochloride Topical Solution depends on proper dosage, correct technique,

adequate precautions, and readiness for emergencies. Standard textbooks should be consulted for specific techniques and precautions for various anesthetic procedures.
The lowest dosage that results in effective anesthesia should be used to avoid high plasma levels and serious adverse effects. Debilitated, elderly patients, acutely ill patients, and children should be given reduced doses commensurate with their age and physical status.
Cocaine Hydrochloride Topical Solution should be used with caution in patients with severely traumatized mucosa and sepsis in the region of the proposed application. Use with caution in persons with known drug sensitivities.

ADVERSE REACTIONS

Adverse reactions may be due to high plasma levels as a result of excessive and rapid absorption of the drug. Reactions are systemic in nature and involve the central nervous system and/or the cardiovascular system. A small number of reactions may result from hypersensitivity, idiosyncrasy or diminished tolerance on the part of the patient.
CNS reactions are excitatory and/or depressant and may be characterized by nervousness, restlessness, and excitement. Tremors and eventually clonicotonic convulsions may result. Emesis may occur. Central stimulation is followed by depression, with death resulting from respiratory failure.
Small doses of cocaine slow the heart rate, but after moderate doses, the rate is increased due to central sympathetic stimulation.
Cocaine is pyrogenic, augmenting heat production in stimulating muscular activity and causing vasoconstriction which decreases heat loss. Cocaine is known to interfere with the uptake of norepinephrine by adrenergic nerve terminals, producing sensitization to catecholamines, causing vasoconstriction and mydriasis.
Cocaine causes sloughing of the corneal epithelium, causing clouding, pitting, and occasionally ulceration of the cornea. The drug is not meant for ophthalmic use.

OVERDOSAGE

The fatal dose of cocaine has been approximated at 1.2 g, although severe toxic effects have been reported from doses as low as 20 mg.
Symptoms
The symptoms of cocaine poisoning are referable to the CNS, namely the patient becomes excited, restless, garrulous, anxious and confused. Enhanced reflexes, headache, rapid pulse, irregular respiration, chills, rise in body temperature, mydriasis, exophthalmos, nausea, vomiting and abdominal pain are noticed. In severe overdoses, delirium, Cheyne-Stokes respiration, convulsions, unconsciousness, and death from respiratory arrest result. Acute poisoning by cocaine is rapid in developing.
Treatment
The specific treatment of acute cocaine poisoning is the intravenous administration of a short-acting barbiturate or diazepam. Artificial respiration may be necessary. It is important to limit absorption of the drug. If entrance of the drug into circulation can be checked, and respiratory exchange maintained, the prognosis is favorable since cocaine is eliminated fairly rapidly.

DOSAGE AND ADMINISTRATION

The dosage varies and depends upon the area to be anesthetized, vascularity of the tissues, individual tolerance, and the technique of anesthesia. The lowest dosage needed to provide effective anesthesia should be administered. Dosages should be reduced for children and for elderly and debilitated patients. Cocaine Hydrochloride Topical Solution can be administered by means of cotton applicators or packs, instilled into a cavity, or as a spray.

HOW SUPPLIED

4% Cocaine Hydrochloride Topical Solution

NDC 0186-1790-78	4 mL Bottle	Box of 1
NDC 0186-1791-13	10 mL Multiple Dose Bottle	Box of 1

10% Cocaine Hydrochloride Topical Solution

NDC 0186-1792-78	4 mL Bottle	Box of 1
NDC 0186-1793-13	10 mL Multiple Dose Bottle	Box of 1

Store at controlled room temperature 15°–30°C (59°–86°F).
Caution: Federal law prohibits dispensing without prescription.

021661R03   Rev. 3/95

Cocaine Hydrochloride
Viscous Topical Solution   Ⓒ II Ŗ

DESCRIPTION

Each mL contains 40 mg or 100 mg cocaine HCl (Warning: May be habit forming), propylene glycol, hydroxypropylcellulose, FD&C green #3 dye. The pH is adjusted with sodium hydroxide and/or hydrochloric acid. As aqueous solution.

NOT FOR INJECTION OR OPHTHALMIC USE

NOTE (For Glass Bottle): External surface of unopened bottle may be sterilized by ethylene oxide only. Do not steam autoclave.
Cocaine Hydrochloride, USP is a crystalline, granular, or powder substance, having a saline, slightly bitter taste that numbs tongue and lips. Cocaine Hydrochloride is a local anesthetic.

HOW SUPPLIED

4% Cocaine Hydrochloride Viscous Topical Solution

NDC 0186-1794-35	4 mL Bottle	5 × 4 mL
NDC 0186-1794-45	10 mL Multiple Dose Bottle	5 × 10 mL

10% Cocaine Hydrochloride Viscous Topical Solution

NDC 0186-1795-35	4 mL Bottle	5 × 4 mL
NDC 0186-1795-45	10 mL Multiple Dose Bottle	5 × 10 mL

Store at controlled room temperature 15°–30°C (59°–86°F).
Caution: Federal law prohibits dispensing without prescription.

021690R01 Rev. 3/95

DALGAN®   Ŗ
[dăl-găn]
(dezocine)
Injection

DESCRIPTION

Dalgan (dezocine) is a synthetic opioid agonist-antagonist parenteral analgesic of the amino-tetralin series. The chemical name is (-)-[5R-(5α,11α,13S*)]-13-amino-5,6,7,8,9,10,11,12-octahydro-5-methyl-5,11-methanobenzocyclodecen-3-ol. The structural formula is:

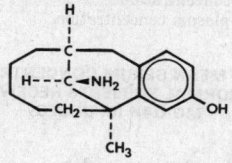

The molecular weight of the base is 245.4, and the molecular formula is $C_{16}H_{23}NO$. The n-octanol: water partition coefficient of dezocine is 1.7.
Dalgan is available in three concentrations: 5, 10, and 15 mg of dezocine per mL for intravenous or intramuscular administration. Each mL of the 5 mg strength contains 0.15 mg sodium metabisulfite and 7.236 mg lactic acid. Each mL of the 10 mg strength contains 0.15 mg sodium metabisulfite and 9.406 mg lactic acid. Each mL of the 15 mg strength contains 0.075 mg sodium metabisulfite and 11.578 mg lactic acid. Each mL of all three strengths contains 0.3 mL propylene glycol as a preservative and Water for Injection. The pH of Dalgan solutions is adjusted to 4.0 with sodium hydroxide.

CLINICAL PHARMACOLOGY

Pharmacodynamics
Dalgan (dezocine) is a strong opioid analgesic. Its analgesic potency, onset, and duration of action in the relief of postoperative pain are comparable to morphine. Pain relief in patients with postoperative pain is clinically evident when steady-state serum levels exceed 5 to 9 ng/mL. The side effects listed under ADVERSE REACTIONS were observed in patients whose average peak levels were less than 45 ng/mL. Peak analgesic effect lags peak serum levels by 20 to 60 minutes.

Table of Estimated Pharmacodynamic Parameters
Following Intramuscular Doses of Dalgan

$C(50)est^1$	5 to 9 ng/mL
$C(toxic)est^2$	45 ng/mL

1. Estimated concentration required to obtain 50% decreases in pain intensity scores in postoperative pain.
2. Estimated concentration above which side effects may be more frequent.

Pharmacokinetics (see Table and Graph)
Dalgan (dezocine) is completely and rapidly absorbed following intramuscular injection in normal volunteers, with an average peak serum concentration of 19 ng/mL (range 10 to 38 ng/mL) occurring between 10 and 90 minutes after a 10 mg intramuscular injection. Following a 10 mg intravenous infusion over 5 minutes, the average terminal half-life of dezocine is 2.4 hr (range 1.2 to 7.4 hr). The average volume of distribution (Vss) is 10.1 L/kg (range 4.7 to 20.1 L/kg), and the average total body clearance is 3.3 L/hr/kg (range 1.7 to 7.2 L/hr/kg). There is evidence of nonlinear (dose-depen-

Continued on next page

Astra—Cont.

dent) pharmacokinetics at doses above 10 mg: in a study where 5, 10, and 20 mg intravenous doses of dezocine were given (N=12), dose-proportional serum levels were observed after 5 and 10 mg injections, but the area under the serum concentration-time curve for the 20 mg dose was about 25% greater, and the total body clearance was about 20% lower, when compared to the 5 and 10 mg doses. The pharmacokinetics of dezocine following chronic administration (steady-state pharmacokinetics) have not been experimentally determined, but predicted serum levels for 5 and 15 mg intramuscular doses given every 4 hrs are presented in the graph.

Approximately two-thirds of a Dalgan dose is recovered in the urine with about 1% being excreted as unchanged dezocine and the remainder as the glucuronide conjugate. Protein binding of dezocine has not been studied.

Mean (range) Pharmacokinetic Parameters of Dezocine in Normal Volunteers

	Dose		
	5 mg (N=12)	10 mg (N=36)	20 mg (N=12)
IV			
Clearance (L/hr/kg)	3.52 (2.1–6.2)	3.33 (1.7–7.2)	2.76 (1.7–4.1)
Vss (L/kg)	10.7 (6.4–15.5)	10.1 (4.7–20.1)	8.8 (5.8–13.5)
t1/2 (hr)	1.7 (0.6–4.4)	2.4 (1.2–7.4)	2.4 (1.4–5.2)
IM		(N = 24)	
Bioavailability		100%	
Cmax[1] (ng/mL)		10–38	
tmax[2] (min)		10–90	

1. Peak plasma concentration.
2. Time-to-peak plasma concentration.

SIMULATED MEAN SERUM CONCENTRATIONS OF DEZOCINE IN NORMAL SUBJECTS RECEIVING 5 AND 15 MG Q4H IM DOSES

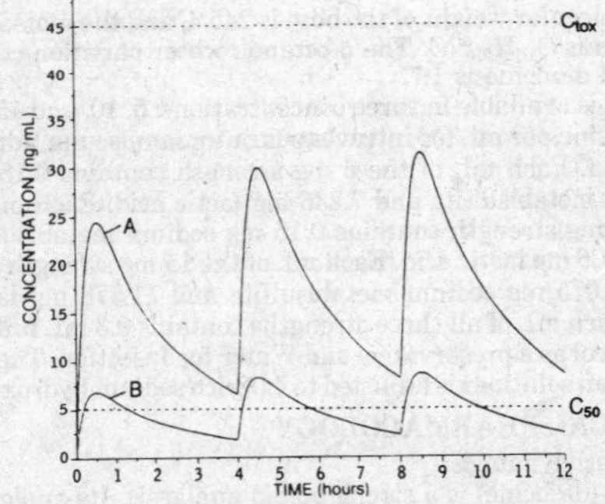

A = Dalgan 15 mg q4h
B = Dalgan 5 mg q4h
C_{tox}= Estimated concentration above which side effects may be more frequent.
C_{50}= Estimated concentration required to obtain 50% decreases in pain intensity scores in postoperative pain.

Hepatic insufficiency did not alter total body clearance in one study of 7 patients with cirrhosis. The volume of distribution and consequently the half-life, however, were increased by 30–50% relative to normal volunteers following a 10 mg intravenous dose. It is not known whether the free concentration of dezocine is altered in cirrhotic patients.

The effect of renal insufficiency on dezocine kinetics (urinary elimination) has not been studied. Because the primary elimination of dezocine is through the urine as a glucuronide, however, use in patients with renal dysfunction should be done cautiously with reduced doses.

Narcotic Antagonist Activity

Dalgan is a mixed opioid agonist-antagonist analgesic. Its opioid antagonist activity is less than that of nalorphine but greater than that of pentazocine when measured by antagonism of morphine-induced narcosis in rats.

Effect on Respiration

Dalgan and morphine produce a similar degree of respiratory depression when given in the usual analgesic doses. The effect is dose dependent and may be reversed by naloxone. As the dose of Dalgan is increased, there appears to be an upper limit to the magnitude of the respiratory depression produced by the drug in both animals and healthy human volunteers. Dalgan, like other mixed agonist-antagonist analgesics, may offer increased safety over pure agonist drugs such as morphine.

Cardiovascular Effects

Dalgan has not been found to be associated with clinically important adverse effects on cardiac performance. Dalgan has been administered to patients as a 4-minute intravenous infusion at approximately 10 times the usual recommended intravenous dose without causing significant changes in mean systemic artery pressure, mean pulmonary artery pressure, pulmonary capillary wedge pressure, cardiac output, stroke index, and left ventricular stroke work index.

Clinical Trials

Postoperative Analgesia

The analgesic efficacy of Dalgan was investigated in randomized controlled clinical trials in postoperative general surgical pain (orthopedic, gynecologic, and abdominal). The studies were primarily double-blind, single-dose, parallel trials in which Dalgan in intravenous (IV) doses of 2.5 to 10 mg (85 to 160 patients per treatment group) or intramuscular (IM) doses of 5 to 20 mg (39 to 221 patients per treatment group) was compared to 5 to 10 mg of morphine or 1 mg of IV butorphanol in patients with moderate-to-severe pain at baseline.

The onset of analgesic action was similar for Dalgan, morphine, and butorphanol, occurring within 15 minutes of IV and 30 minutes of IM administration of the drug. Dalgan in 10 mg IM doses produced analgesia similar to that produced by 10 mg of IM morphine, while 5 mg of Dalgan IV was equivalent to 1 mg of IV butorphanol.

The peak analgesic effect and duration of analgesia were comparable for both routes of administration. The time by which approximately half of the patients remedicated was dose related and independent of the route of administration. Half of the patients remedicated within 2 hours after 5 mg of Dalgan or 1 mg of butorphanol IV, 3 hours after 10 mg of Dalgan or morphine IM, and 4 hours after 15 mg of Dalgan IM.

Another measure of the effect of Dalgan was the number of patients who did not require remedication during the six hours of the trial. The percentage of patients who did not request additional medication during the trial was 21% after a single dose of 15 mg of Dalgan, 15% after 10 mg of Dalgan or morphine, and 4% after placebo.

Pain relief was proportional to the dose of Dalgan for single doses less than 20 mg. In one study with 39 to 42 patients per treatment group, comparing single doses of 20 mg or 10 mg of IM Dalgan with 10 mg of IM morphine, the patients receiving 20 mg of Dalgan did not obtain as much pain relief as that provided by 15 mg of the drug in other studies (the patients who received 10 mg of Dalgan or morphine in this study did obtain analgesia comparable to that seen in other trials). These results suggest that the maximally effective dose of Dalgan in postoperative pain may be 15 mg due to Dalgan's mixed agonist-antagonist pharmacology.

Use In Chronic Pain States:

Data on the use of Dalgan in chronic pain has been gathered in trials of burn patients (n = 16) and cancer pain (n = 88). The daily dose of Dalgan for most patients with chronic pain has ranged between 20 and 60 mg per day, although doses as large as 90 to 140 mg per day have been used in 15 patients. Dalgan has not been adequately studied in the management of chronic pain. It is not recommended for use in patients who may have developed significant tolerance to opioid drugs from long-term use because of the risk of precipitating acute withdrawal symptoms.

INDICATIONS

Dalgan is indicated for the management of pain when the use of an opioid analgesic is appropriate (see Clinical Trials).

CONTRAINDICATIONS

Dalgan should not be administered to patients who have been shown to be hypersensitive to it.

WARNINGS

Contains sodium metabisulfite, a sulfite that may cause allergic-type reactions including anaphylactic symptoms and life-threatening or less severe asthmatic episodes in certain susceptible people. The overall prevalence of sulfite sensitivity in the general population is unknown and probably low. Sulfite sensitivity is seen more frequently in asthmatic than in nonasthmatic people.

Patients Physically Dependent on Narcotics

Because of its opioid antagonist properties, Dalgan is not recommended for patients who are physically dependent on narcotics. Patients who have recently taken substantial amounts of narcotics may experience withdrawal symptoms. Because of the difficulty in assessing dependence in patients who have previously received substantial amounts of narcotic medication, caution should be used in the administration of Dalgan to such patients. To avoid precipitating an acute narcotic abstinence reaction, a sufficient period of withdrawal from opioids should be allowed before Dalgan is administered.

PRECAUTIONS

DALGAN IS A STRONG OPIOID ANALGESIC AND, LIKE ALL SUCH DRUGS, IT SHOULD BE ADMINISTERED IN CLINICAL SETTINGS WHERE RESPIRATORY DEPRESSION WILL BE PROMPTLY RECOGNIZED AND APPROPRIATELY MANAGED.

RESPIRATORY DEPRESSION INDUCED BY DALGAN CAN BE REVERSED WITH NALOXONE.

Head Injury and Increased Intracranial Pressure

Although there is no clinical experience in patients with head injury, the possible respiratory-depressant effect and the potential of strong analgesics to elevate cerebrospinal-fluid pressure (resulting from vasodilatation following CO_2 retention) may be markedly exaggerated in the presence of head injury, intracranial lesions, or a preexisting increase in intracranial pressure. Furthermore, strong analgesics can produce effects that may obscure the clinical course of patients with head injuries. In such patients, Dalgan should be used only when essential and with extreme caution.

Use in Chronic Obstructive Pulmonary Disease

Because strong opioids cause some respiratory depression, they should be administered only with caution and in low doses to patients with preexisting respiratory depression (e.g., from other medication, uremia, or severe infection), severely limited respiratory reserve, bronchial asthma, obstructive respiratory conditions, or cyanosis. Respiratory depression induced by Dalgan can be reversed by naloxone.

Use in Hepatic or Renal Disease

Dezocine undergoes extensive hepatic metabolism and renal excretion of the glucuronide metabolite (see CLINICAL PHARMACOLOGY). Administration to patients with hepatic or renal dysfunction should be cautious using reduced doses.

Use in Biliary Surgery

Although there is no evidence that Dalgan alters the tonic pressure within the common bile duct, therapeutic doses of other opioid analgesics can significantly increase pressure within the common bile duct. Therefore, Dalgan should be used with caution in such settings.

Use with Other Central Nervous System Depressants

Opioid analgesics, general anesthetics, sedatives, tranquilizers, hypnotics, or other CNS depressants (including alcohol) administered concomitantly with Dalgan may have an additive effect. When such combined therapy is contemplated, the dose of one or both agents should be reduced.

Use in Drug or Alcohol Dependence

Use of Dalgan in combination with alcohol and/or other CNS depressant drugs will result in increased risk to the patient. Dalgan should be used with caution in individuals with active drug or alcohol addiction who are not in a medically controlled environment. Self-administration of any strong opioid may increase the relapse rate in populations recovering from addiction in abstinence-based recovery programs.

Use in Ambulatory Patients

Strong opioid analgesics impair the mental or physical abilities required for the performance of potentially dangerous tasks such as driving a car or operating machinery. Patients who have been given Dalgan should not drive or operate dangerous machinery until the effects of the drug are no longer present.

Pregnancy Category C

In reproductive studies, dezocine was shown to cause a dose-related suppression of body weight and food consumption of the parenteral generation in rats receiving either intravenous or intramuscular doses. Pup body weight was suppressed in a dose-related fashion. Teratology studies conducted in mice, rats, and rabbits revealed no evidence of teratogenic effects. There are no adequate and well-controlled studies in pregnant women. Dalgan should be used during pregnancy only if the potential benefit justifies the potential risk to the fetus.

Labor and Delivery

Safety to the mother and fetus after Dalgan administration during labor is unknown. The drug should be used in labor and delivery only when the physician deems its use essential to the welfare of the mother and infant.

Nursing Mothers

The use of Dalgan in mothers nursing infants is not recommended, since it is not known whether this drug is excreted in breast milk.

Pediatric Use

Safety and efficacy in patients under the age of 18 years have not been established.

Use in the Aged

Like all strong, mixed opioid agonist-antagonist analgesics, Dalgan has the ability to depress respiration and reduce ventilatory drive to a clinically significant extent. It also has the potential to alter mental status or induce delirium in elderly patients. Dalgan has not undergone sufficient clinical testing in the geriatric population to assess its relative risk compared to other opioid analgesics, but the initial dose of all drugs of this class should be reduced in the geriatric patient and subsequent doses individualized.

ADVERSE REACTIONS

A total of 2192 patients have received Dalgan on an acute or chronic basis in the initial clinical trials of the drug. In nearly all cases, the type of incidence of side effects were those expected of a strong analgesic, and no unforeseen or unusual toxicity was reported. There is, as yet, limited information on the use of Dalgan for periods longer than 48 to 72 hours, but there was no evidence of hepatic, hematologic, or renal toxicity in 73 patients who received the drug for periods of time longer than 7 days.

The occurrence of adverse effects with Dalgan is based on data obtained from patients treated in both controlled and uncontrolled clinical trials. The adverse effects are listed below by frequency of occurrence within the body system affected.

The frequencies shown reflect the actual frequency of each adverse effect in patients who received Dalgan. There has been no attempt to correct for a placebo effect or to subtract the frequencies reported by placebo-treated patients in controlled trials.

The following adverse reactions were reported at a frequency of 1% or greater:

Reactions
Gastrointestinal System: Nausea*, vomiting*.
Nervous System: Sedation*, dizziness/vertigo.
Skin: Injection-site reactions*.
(Reactions occurring with a frequency of 1 to <3% are unmarked, while reactions occurring with a frequency of 3 to 9% are marked with an asterisk.*)

The following adverse reactions were reported with a frequency of less than 1% and are probably causally related to the administration of Dalgan:
Body as a whole: Sweating, chills, flushing, low hemoglobin, edema.
Cardiovascular system: Hypotension, heart or pulse irregularity, hypertension, chest pain, pallor, thrombophlebitis.
Gastrointestinal system: Dry mouth, constipation, diarrhea, abdominal pain/distress/disorder.
Musculoskeletal system: Cramps/aching/pain.
Nervous system: Anxiety, confusion, crying, delusions, sleep disturbance, headache, delirium, depression.
Respiratory system: Respiratory depression, respiratory symptoms, atelectasis.
Skin: Pruritus, rash, erythema.
Special senses: Diplopia, slurred speech, blurred vision.
Urogenital system: Urinary frequency, hesitancy, and retention.

The following adverse effects have been reported in less than 1% of the 2192 patients studied, and the association between these events and Dalgan administration is unknown. They are being listed to serve as alerting information for the physician.
Gastrointestinal: Increased alkaline phosphatase and SGOT.
Respiratory system: Hiccups.
Special senses: Congestion in ears, tinnitus.

There is no information available from postmarketing experience with the drug.

DRUG ABUSE AND DEPENDENCE

Dezocine has substituted for morphine in abuse-liability testing in animals. It has been identified as a narcotic in abuse-liability testing in experienced drug abusers, but has shown no evidence of abuse in clinical use during drug development. Mixed opioid agonist-antagonists of this type are generally recognized as having less potential for abuse than pure agonists such as morphine or meperidine, but all such drugs have abuse potential in certain individuals, especially those individuals with a prior history of opioid drug abuse or dependence.

Dezocine has a limited capacity to induce physical dependence in animal testing. Increasing tolerance to Dalgan or physical dependence on the drug were not seen in clinical trials.

OVERDOSAGE

Clinical Presentation
Although there have been no incidents of overdosage with Dalgan during clinical trials, and thus no human experience with the drug, overdosage with Dalgan is possible. Based on the preclinical pharmacology of dezocine, overdosage will produce acute respiratory depression, cardiovascular compromise, and delirium. The largest dose of Dalgan which has been given to nontolerant healthy volunteers without toxicity has been 30 mg/70 kg.

Treatment
The pharmacologic treatment of suspected Dalgan overdosage is intravenously administered naloxone. The respiratory and cardiac status of the patient should be evaluated constantly and appropriate supportive measures instituted, such as oxygen, intravenous fluids, vasopressors, and assisted or controlled respiration.

DOSAGE AND ADMINISTRATION

Intramuscular
Although the recommended single dose for an adult is 5 to 20 mg, the majority of patients in clinical trials received an initial dose of 10 mg. Dosage should be adjusted according to the patient's weight, age, severity of pain, physical status, and other medications that the patient may be receiving. Dalgan may be repeated every 3 to 6 hours as necessary. The recommended maximum single dose is 20 mg, with a probable upper limit of 120 mg a day based on preclinical pharmacology of the drug. There is insufficient information regarding the risk of chronic use of Dalgan to establish limits for the maximum recommended duration of treatment with the drug.

Intravenous
The recommended range for intravenous administration of Dalgan is 2.5 to 10 mg repeated every 2 to 4 hours, with most patients in clinical trials receiving an initial intravenous dose of 5 mg.

Subcutaneous
Dalgan is not recommended for subcutaneous administration. Repeated injection of Dalgan at a single site has been associated with subcutaneous inflammation, vascular irritation, and venous thrombosis in animals. The significance of this finding for patients is unknown, although injection-site reactions occurred in 4% of patients treated with Dalgan in clinical trials.

Children and Adolescents
Dalgan is not recommended for patients under 18 years of age.

HOW SUPPLIED

Dalgan® (dezocine) Injection (a clear, colorless to slightly yellow solution) is available in the following dosage strengths:
Single-Dose Vials
2 mL (1 mL Fill), 5 mg/mL, Box of 1, NDC 0186-1520-13
2 mL (1 mL Fill), 10 mg/mL, Box of 1, NDC 0186-1521-13
2 mL (1 mL Fill), 15 mg/mL, Box of 1, NDC 0186-1523-13
Multiple-Dose Vials
10 mL, 10 mg/mL, Box of 1, NDC 0186-1522-12
Syringes
2 mL (1 mL Fill), 5 mg/mL, Box of 10, NDC 0186-1529-23
2 mL (1 mL Fill), 10 mg/mL, Box of 10, NDC 0186-1524-23
2 mL (1 mL Fill), 15 mg/mL, Box of 10, NDC 0186-1525-23
For intramuscular or intravenous injection.

SAFETY AND HANDLING INSTRUCTIONS
Dalgan is supplied in sealed dosage forms and at low concentrations which pose no known risk to health-care workers. Accidental dermal exposure to Dalgan should be treated by rinsing the affected area with fresh water.

Dalgan should be stored at room temperature and protected from light. As with all parenteral products, Dalgan should be inspected visually for particulate matter and discoloration prior to administration, whenever solution and container permit. Do not use if the solution contains a precipitate.

Dalgan, like other mixed agonist-antagonist opioid analgesics, has low abuse potential in patient populations. However, strong mixed agonist-antagonist drugs have reportedly been associated with abuse and dependence in health-care providers and others with ready access to such drugs. Dalgan should be handled accordingly.

Manufactured by:
Wyeth Laboratories Inc.
Philadelphia, PA 19101
Manufactured for:
Astra USA, Inc.
Westborough, MA 01581
021575R00 (8/94)

50% DEXTROSE
[dex'trose]
Injection, USP
Concentrated Dextrose
For Intravenous
Administration

NOTE: This solution is hypertonic—see WARNINGS and PRECAUTIONS

(For details of indications, dosage and administration, precautions, and adverse reactions, see circular in package.)

HOW SUPPLIED
50% Dextrose Injection, USP is supplied as follows:
50 mL Prefilled Syringe with 19 G$^{15/16}$" needle, NDC 0186-0654-01
The solution should be stored at controlled room temperature 15°–30°C (59°–86°F).
021857R06 Rev. 10/94

DOBUTAMINE HYDROCHLORIDE INJECTION ℞

DESCRIPTION
Dobutamine Hydrochloride Injection is 1,2-benzenediol, 4-[2-[[3-(4-hydroxyphenyl)-1-methylpropyl] amino]ethyl]-, hydrochloride, (±). It is a synthetic catecholamine.

Molecular Formula: $C_{18}H_{23}NO_3 \cdot HCl$
Molecular Weight: 337.85

The clinical formulation is supplied in a sterile form for intravenous use only. Each mL contains dobutamine hydrochloride equivalent to 12.5 mg (41.5 μmol) dobutamine, 0.24 mg sodium metabisulfite (added during manufacture), and water for injection, q.s. Hydrochloric acid and/or sodium hydroxide may have been added during manufacture to adjust the pH.
Single dose vial. Discard unused portion.

HOW SUPPLIED
NDC 0186-1931-01, 20 mL single dose vial containing 250 mg dobutamine (as the hydrochloride), box of 1.
Store at controlled room temperature 15°–30°C (59°–86°F).
Caution: Federal law prohibits dispensing without prescription.
021648R03 Iss. 8/94

DOPAMINE HYDROCHLORIDE Injection, USP ℞
[do-pa-mean]

(For details of indications, dosage and administration, precautions, and adverse reactions, see circular in package.)

HOW SUPPLIED
Dopamine HCl 200 mg is supplied in the following form:
  Additive Syringe 5 mL (40 mg/mL) NDC 0186-0638-01
Dopamine HCl 400 mg is supplied in the following forms:
  Additive Syringe 5 mL (80 mg/mL) NDC 0186-0641-01
      10 mL (40 mg/mL) NDC 0186-0639-01
Dopamine HCl 800 mg is supplied in the following form:
  Additive Syringe 5 mL (160 mg/mL) NDC 0186-0642-01
Packages are color coded according to the total dosage content; 200 mg coded blue/white, 400 mg coded green/white and 800 mg coded yellow/white.
Store at controlled room temperature 15°–30°C (59°–86°F).
Protect from light.
Avoid contact with alkalies (including sodium bicarbonate), oxidizing agents, or iron salts.
NOTE: Do not use the Injection if it is darker than slightly yellow or discolored in any way.
021861R07 3/92 (7)

DOXORUBICIN HYDROCHLORIDE INJECTION, USP ℞
DOXORUBICIN HYDROCHLORIDE FOR INJECTION, USP
FOR INTRAVENOUS USE ONLY

> **WARNINGS**
> 1. Severe local tissue necrosis will occur if there is extravasation during administration (see DOSAGE AND ADMINISTRATION). Doxorubicin must not be given by the intramuscular or subcutaneous route.
> 2. Serious irreversible myocardial toxicity with delayed congestive failure often unresponsive to any cardiac supportive therapy may be encountered as total dosage approaches 550 mg/m². This toxicity may occur at lower cumulative doses in patients with prior mediastinal irradiation or on concurrent cyclophosphamide therapy.
> 3. Dosage should be reduced in patients with impaired hepatic function.
> 4. Severe myelosuppression may occur.
> 5. Doxorubicin should be administered only under the supervision of a physician who is experienced in the use of cancer chemotherapeutic agents.

DESCRIPTION
Doxorubicin is a cytotoxic anthracycline antibiotic isolated from cultures of *Streptomyces peucetius* var. *caesius*. Doxorubicin consists of a naphthacenequinone nucleus linked

Continued on next page

Astra—Cont.

through a glycosidic bond at ring atom 7 to an amino sugar, daunosamine. The structural formula is as follows:

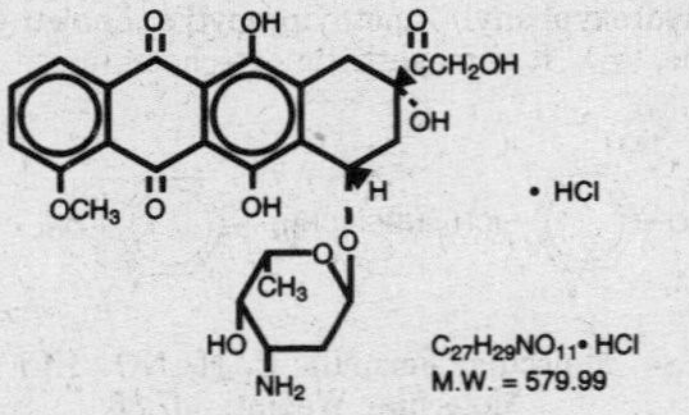
• HCl
$C_{27}H_{29}NO_{11}$• HCl
M.W. = 579.99

Doxorubicin binds to nucleic acids, presumably by specific intercalation of the planar anthracycline nucleus with the DNA double helix. The anthracycline ring is lipophilic but the saturated end of the ring system contains abundant hydroxyl groups adjacent to the amino sugar, producing a hydrophilic center. The molecule is amphoteric, containing acidic functions in the ring phenolic groups and a basic function in the sugar amino group. It binds to cell membranes as well as plasma proteins.

Doxorubicin Hydrochloride Injection, USP is a sterile, isotonic, preservative-free solution for intravenous administration. It is available in 10 mg (5 mL), 20 mg (10 mL), 50 mg (25 mL) single dose vials and 2 mg/mL (100 mL) multidose vials. Each mL contains 2 mg doxorubicin hydrochloride and the following inactive ingredients: sodium chloride 9 mg and water for injection q.s. Hydrochloric acid is used to adjust pH to a target pH of 3.0.

Doxorubicin Hydrochloride for Injection, USP, is supplied as a sterile, lyophilized powder in vials containing 10 mg, 20 mg, or 50 mg of doxorubicin hydrochloride, which, when reconstituted according to directions with a suitable diluent, produces a sterile, isotonic solution, for intravenous administration, containing 2 mg/mL of doxorubicin hydrochloride. Each vial also contains 50 mg, 100 mg, or 250 mg, respectively, of lactose monohydrate.

CLINICAL PHARMACOLOGY

Though not completely elucidated, the mechanism of action of doxorubicin is related to its ability to bind to DNA and inhibit nucleic acid synthesis. Cell culture studies have demonstrated rapid cell penetration and perinucleolar chromatin binding, rapid inhibition of mitotic activity and nucleic acid synthesis, mutagenesis and chromosomal aberrations. Animal studies have shown activity in a spectrum of experimental tumors, immunosuppression, carcinogenic properties in rodents, induction of a variety of toxic effects, including delayed and progressive cardiac toxicity, myelosuppression in all species and atrophy to testes in rats and dogs.

Pharmacokinetic studies show the intravenous administration of normal or radiolabeled doxorubicin is followed by rapid plasma clearance and significant tissue binding. Urinary excretion, as determined by fluorimetric methods, accounts for approximately 4 to 5% of the administered dose in five days. Biliary excretion represents the major excretion route, 40 to 50% of the administered dose being recovered in the bile or feces in seven days. Impairment of liver function results in slower excretion, and consequently, increased retention and accumulation in plasma and tissues. Doxorubicin does not cross the blood brain barrier.

INDICATIONS AND USAGE

Injectable doxorubicin hydrochloride has been used successfully to produce regression in disseminated neoplastic conditions such as acute lymphoblastic leukemia, acute myeloblastic leukemia, Wilms' tumor, neuroblastoma, soft tissue and bone sarcomas, breast carcinoma, ovarian carcinoma, transitional cell bladder carcinoma thyroid carcinoma, lymphomas of both Hodgkin and non-Hodgkin types, bronchogenic carcinoma in which the small cell histologic type is the most responsive compared to other cell types and gastric carcinoma.

A number of other solid tumors have also shown some responsiveness but in numbers too limited to justify specific recommendation. Studies to date have shown malignant melanoma, kidney carcinoma, large bowel carcinoma, brain tumors and metastases to the central nervous system not to be significantly responsive to doxorubicin therapy.

CONTRAINDICATIONS

Doxorubicin therapy should not be started in patients who have marked myelosuppression induced by previous treatment with other antitumor agents or by radiotherapy. Conclusive data are not available on pre-existing heart disease as a co-factor of increased risk of doxorubicin induced cardiac toxicity. Preliminary data suggest that in such cases cardiac toxicity may occur at doses lower than the recommended cumulative limit. It is therefore not recommended to start doxorubicin in such cases. Doxorubicin treatment is contraindicated in patients who received previous treatment with complete cumulative doses of doxorubicin and/or daunorubicin.

WARNINGS

Special attention must be given to the cardiac toxicity exhibited by doxorubicin. Although uncommon, acute left ventricular failure has occurred, particularly in patients who have received total dosage of the drug exceeding the currently recommended limit of 550 mg/m^2. The limit appears to be lower (400 mg/m^2) in patients who received radiotherapy to the mediastinal area or concomitant therapy with other potentially cardiotoxic agents such as cyclophosphamide. The total dose of doxorubicin administered to the individual patient should also take into account previous or concomitant therapy with related compounds such as daunorubicin. Congestive heart failure and/or cardiomyopathy may be encountered several weeks after discontinuation of doxorubicin therapy.

Cardiac failure is often not favorably affected by presently known medical or physical therapy for cardiac support. Early clinical diagnosis of drug induced heart failure appears to be essential for successful treatment with digitalis, diuretics, low salt diet and bed rest. Severe cardiac toxicity may occur precipitously without antecedent ECG changes. A baseline ECG and ECGs performed prior to each dose or course after 300 mg/m^2 cumulative dose has been given is suggested. Transient ECG changes consisting of T-wave flattening, S-T depression and arrhythmias lasting up to two weeks after a dose or course of doxorubicin are presently not considered indications for suspension of doxorubicin therapy. Doxorubicin cardiomyopathy has been reported to be associated with a persistent reduction in the voltage of the QRS wave, a prolongation of the systolic time interval and a reduction of the ejection fraction as determined by echocardiography or radionuclide angiography. None of these tests have yet been confirmed to consistently identify those individual patients that are approaching their maximally tolerated cumulative dose of doxorubicin. If test results indicate change in cardiac function associated with doxorubicin, the benefit of continued therapy must be carefully evaluated against the risk of producing irreversible cardiac damage.

Acute life-threatening arrhythmias have been reported to occur during or within a few hours after doxorubicin hydrochloride administration.

There is a high incidence of bone marrow depression, primarily of leukocytes, requiring careful hematologic monitoring. With the recommended dosage schedule, leukopenia is usually transient, reaching its nadir at 10 to 14 days after treatment with recovery usually occurring by the 21st day. White blood cell counts as low as 1000/mm^3 are to be expected during treatment with appropriate doses of doxorubicin. Red blood cell and platelet levels should also be monitored since they may also be depressed. Hematologic toxicity may require dose reduction or suspension or delay of doxorubicin therapy. Persistent severe myelosuppression may result in superinfection or hemorrhage.

Doxorubicin may potentiate the toxicity of other anticancer therapies. Exacerbation of cyclophosphamide induced hemorrhagic cystitis and enhancement of the hepatotoxicity of 6-mercaptopurine have been reported. Radiation induced toxicity to the myocardium, mucosae, skin and liver have been reported to be increased by the administration of doxorubicin.

Toxicity to recommended doses of doxorubicin hydrochloride is enhanced by hepatic impairment, therefore, prior to the individual dosing, evaluation of hepatic function is recommended using conventional clinical laboratory tests, such as SGOT, SGPT, alkaline phosphatase and bilirubin. (See DOSAGE AND ADMINISTRATION.)

Necrotizing colitis manifested by typhlitis (cecal inflammation), bloody stools and severe and sometimes fatal infections have been asociated with a combination of doxorubicin hydrochloride given by IV push daily for 3 days and cytarabine given by continuous infusion daily for 7 or more days.

On intravenous administration of doxorubicin, extravasation may occur with or without an accompanying stinging or burning sensation and even if blood returns well on aspiration of the infusion needle (see DOSAGE AND ADMINISTRATION). If any signs or symptoms of extravasation have occurred, the injection or infusion should be immediately terminated and restarted in another vein.

Doxorubicin and related compounds have also been shown to have mutagenic and carcinogenic properties when tested in experimental models.

Usage in pregnancy—Safe use of doxorubicin has not been established. Doxorubicin is embryotoxic and teratogenic in rats and embryotoxic and abortifacient in rabbits. Therefore, the benefits to the pregnant patient should be carefully weighed against the potential toxicity to fetus and embryo. The possible adverse effects on fertility in males and females in humans or experimental animals have not been adequately evaluated.

PRECAUTIONS

Initial treatment with doxorubicin requires close observation of the patient and extensive laboratory monitoring. It is recommended, therefore, that patients be hospitalized at least during the first phase of the treatment.

Like other cytotoxic drugs, doxorubicin may induce hyperuricemia secondary to rapid lysis of neoplastic cells. The clinician should monitor the patient's blood uric acid level and be prepared to use such supportive and pharmacologic measures as might be necessary to control this problem.

Doxorubicin imparts a red coloration to the urine for 1 to 2 days after administration and patients should be advised to expect this during active therapy.

Doxorubicin is not an anti-microbial agent.

ADVERSE REACTIONS

Dose limiting toxicities of therapy are myelosuppression and cardiotoxicity (see WARNINGS). Other reactions reported are:

Cutaneous—Reversible and complete alopecia occurs in most cases.

Hyperpigmentation of nailbeds and dermal creases, primarily in children, and onycholysis have been reported in a few cases. Recall of skin reaction due to prior radiotherapy has occurred with doxorubicin administration.

Gastrointestinal—Acute nausea and vomiting occurs frequently and may be severe. This may be alleviated by antiemetic therapy. Mucositis (stomatitis and esophagitis) may occur 5 to 10 days after administration. The effect may be severe leading to ulceration and represents a site of origin for severe infections. The dosage regimen consisting of administration of doxorubicin on three consecutive days results in the greater incidence and severity of mucositis. Ulceration and necrosis of the colon, especially the cecum, may occur leading to bleeding or severe infections which can be fatal. This reaction has been reported in patients with acute non-lymphocytic leukemia treated with a 3-day course of doxorubicin combined with cytarabine. Anorexia and diarrhea have been occasionally reported.

Vascular—Phlebosclerosis has been reported especially when small veins are used or a single vein is used for repeated administration. Facial flushing may occur if the injection is given too rapidly.

Local—Severe cellulitis, vesication and tissue necrosis will occur if doxorubicin is extravasated during administration. Erythematous streaking along the vein proximal to the site of the injection has been reported. (See DOSAGE AND ADMINISTRATION.)

Hypersensitivity—Fever, chills and urticaria have been reported occasionally. Anaphylaxis may occur. A case of apparent cross sensitivity to lincomycin has been reported.

Other—Conjunctivitis and lacrimation occur rarely.

OVERDOSAGE

Acute overdosage of doxorubicin enhances the toxic effects of mucositis, leukopenia and thrombopenia. Treatment of acute overdosage consists of treatment of the severely myelosuppressed patient with hospitalization, antibiotics, platelet and granulocyte transfusions and symptomatic treatment of mucositis. The 200 mg vial is packaged as a multiple dose vial and caution should be exercised to prevent inadvertent overdosage.

Chronic overdosage with cumulative doses exceeding 550 mg/m^2 increases the risk of cardiomyopathy and resultant congestive heart failure. Treatment consists of vigorous management of congestive heart failure with digitalis preparations and diuretics. The use of peripheral vasodilators has been recommended.

DOSAGE AND ADMINISTRATION

Care in the administration of doxorubicin hydrochloride will reduce the chance of perivenous infiltration. It may also decrease the chance of local reactions such as urticaria and erythematous streaking. On intravenous administration of doxorubicin, extravasation may occur with or without an accompanying stinging or burning sensation and even if blood returns well on aspiration of the infusion needle. If any signs or symptoms of extravasation have occurred, the injection or infusion should be immediately terminated and restarted in another vein. If it is known or suspected that subcutaneous extravasation has occurred, local infiltration with an injectable corticosteroid and flooding the site with normal saline has been reported to lessen the local reaction. Because of the progressive nature of extravasation reactions, the area of injection should be frequently examined and plastic surgery consultation obtained. If ulceration begins, early wide excision of the involved area should be considered.[1]

The most commonly used dosage schedule is 60 to 75 mg/m^2 as a single intravenous injection administered at 21 day intervals. The lower dose should be given to patients with inadequate marrow reserves due to old age, or prior therapy, or neoplastic marrow infiltration. An alternative dosage schedule is weekly doses of 20 mg/m^2 which has been reported to produce a lower incidence of congestive heart failure. Thirty (30) mg/m^2 on each of three successive days repeated every four weeks has also been used. Doxorubicin dosage must be reduced if the bilirubin is elevated as follows: serum bilirubin 1.2 to 3.0 mg/dL—give $^1/_2$ normal dose, > 3 mg/dL—give $^1/_4$ normal dose.

Reconstitution Directions: Doxorubicin Hydrochloride for Injection, 10 mg, 20 mg, and 50 mg vials should be reconstituted with 5mL, 10mL, and 25mL, respectively, of Sodium Chloride Injection 0.9% to give a final concentration of 2 mg/mL of doxorubicin hydrochloride. An appropriate volume of air should be withdrawn from the vial during reconstitution to avoid excessive pressure build-up. Bacteriostatic diluents are not recommended.

After adding the diluent, the vial should be shaken and the contents allowed to dissolve. The reconstituted solution is stable for 7 days at room temperature and 15 days under refrigeration 2°C to 8°C (36°F to 46°F). It should be protected from exposure to sunlight. Discard any unused solution from the 10 mg, 20 mg, and 50 mg single dose vials.

Note: Parenteral drug products should be inspected visually for particulate matter and discoloration prior to administration, whenever solution and container permit.

It is recommended that doxorubicin be slowly administered into the tubing of a freely running intravenous infusion of Sodium Chloride Injection or Dextrose Injection, 5%. The tubing should be attached to a Butterfly® needle inserted preferably into a large vein. If possible, avoid veins over joints or in extremities with compromised venous or lymphatic drainage. The rate of administration is dependent on the size of the vein and the dosage. However, the dose should be administered in not less than 3 to 5 minutes. Local erythematous streaking along the vein as well as facial flushing may be indicative of too rapid an administration. A burning or stinging sensation may be indicative of perivenous infiltration and the infusion should be immediately terminated and restarted in another vein. Perivenos infiltration may occur painlessly. Doxorubicin should not be mixed with heparin or fluorouracil since it has been reported that these drugs are incompatible to the extent that a precipitate may form. Until specific compatibility data are available, it is not recommended that doxorubicin be mixed with other drugs. Doxorubicin has been used concurrently with other approved chemotherapeutic agents. Evidence is available that in some types of neoplastic disease combination chemotherapy is superior to single agents. The benefits and risks of such therapy continue to be elucidated.

Handling and Disposal: Skin reactions associated with doxorubicin have been reported. Caution in the handling and preparation of the powder and solution must be exercised and the use of gloves is recommended. If doxorubicin powder or solution contacts the skin or mucosae, immediately wash thoroughly with soap and water.

Procedues for proper handling and disposal of anti-cancer drugs should be considered. Several guidelines on this subject have been published.[2-7] There is no general agreement that all of the procedures recommended in the guidelines are necessary or appropriate.

HOW SUPPLIED

Doxorubicin Hydrochloride Injection, USP, is supplied as a sterile, red-orange solution. Single dose vial, contains no preservatives. Discard unused portion.
NDC 0186-1532-31
10 mg vial, 2 mg/mL, 5 mL, Box of 1.
NDC 0186-1532-41
20 mg vial, 2 mg/mL, 10 mL, Box of 1.
NDC 0186-1532-61
50 mg vial, 2 mg/mL, 25 mL, Box of 1.
Store under refrigeration 2°C to 8°C (36°F to 46°F). Protect from light. Retain in carton until time of use.
Multidose vial, contains no preservatives.
NDC 0186-1532-81
200 mg vial, 2 mg/mL, 100 mL, Box of 1.
Store under refrigeration 2°C to 8°C (36°F to 46°F). Protect from light. Retain in carton until contents are used.
Doxorubicin Hydrochloride for Injection, USP, is supplied in single dose vials as a sterile red-orange lyophilized powder. The vials are packed in individual cartons.

10 mg	NDC 0186-1533-28	Box of 5
	Product No. 1530-13	
20 mg	NDC 0186-1535-28	Box of 5
	Product No. 1575-12	
50 mg	NDC 186-1534-28	Box of 1
	Product No. 1531-01	

Store unreconstituted vials at controlled room temperature 15°C to 30°C (59°F to 86°F). After reconstitution the solution is stable for 7 days at room temperature and 15 days under refrigeration 2°C to 8°C (36°F to 46°F).
Protect from light. Retain in carton until contents are used. Discard unused portion.
Caution: Federal law prohibits dispensing without prescription.

REFERENCES
1. Rudolph R, et al: Skin Ulcers Due to Adriamycin. Cancer 1976:38:1087-1094
2. Recommendations for the Safe Handling of Parenteral Antineoplastic Drugs, NIH Publication No. 83–2621. For sale by the Superintendent of Documents, U. S. Government Printing Office, Washington D. C. 20402.
3. AMA Council Report. Guidelines for Handling Parenteral Antineoplastics. JAMA, March 15, 1985.
4. National Study Commission on Cytotoxic Exposure-Recommendations for Handling Cytotoxic Agents. Available from Louis P. Jeffrey, Sc.D., Chairman, National Study Commission on Cytotoxic Exposure. Massachusetts College of Pharmacy & Allied Health Sciences, 179 Longwood Avenue, Boston, Massachusetts 02115.
5. Clinical Oncological Society of Australia: Guidelines and recommendations for safe handling of antineoplastic agents. Med J Australia 1983: 1:426-428.
6. Jones R B, et al. Safe handling of chemotherapeutic agents: A report from the Mount Sinai Medical Center. Ca-A Cancer Journal for Clinicians Sept./Oct., 1983: 258-263.
7. American Society of Hospital Pharmacists Technical Assistance Bulletin on Handling Cytotoxic and Hazardous Drugs. Am J Hosp Pharm 1990: 47:1033-1049.

MANUFACTURED FOR:
ASTRA®
Astra USA, Inc.
Westborough, MA 01581
DATE:
August 1995   021794R02
MANUFACTURED BY:
PHARMACHEMIE B.V.
Haarlem
The Netherlands   93.144.127-B

DROPERIDOL INJECTION, USP   ℞
FOR INTRAVENOUS OR INTRAMUSCULAR USE ONLY.

(For details of indications, dosage and administration, precautions, and adverse reactions, see circular in package.)

HOW SUPPLIED
Droperidol injection is available as:
Ampules, 2.5 mg/mL
2 mL, (5 mg/2 mL),   box of 10   NDC 0186-1220-03
5 mL, (12.5 mg/5 mL),   box of 10   NDC 0186-1221-03
Single Dose Vials, 2.5 mg/mL
2 mL, (5 mg/2 mL),   box of 10   NDC 0186-1226-13
5 mL, (12.5 mg/5 mL),   box of 10   NDC 0186-1227-13
Multiple Dose Vials, 2.5 mg/mL
10 mL,   box of 1   NDC 0186-1224-12

PROTECT FROM LIGHT.
Store at controlled room temperature 15°–30°C (59°–86°F).
Caution: Federal law prohibits dispensing without prescription.
021879R04   REV. (8/95)

DURANEST®   ℞
[*dur'a-nest*]
(etidocaine hydrochloride)
Injections for infiltration and nerve block

DESCRIPTION

Duranest (etidocaine HCl) Injections are sterile aqueous solutions that contain a local anesthetic agent and are administered parenterally by injection. See INDICATIONS AND USAGE for specific uses. The specific quantitative composition of each available solution is shown in Table 1. Duranest Injections contain etidocaine HCl, which is chemically designated as butanamide, N-(2,6-dimethylphenyl)-2-(ethylpropylamine)-, monohydrochloride and has the following structural formula:

Epinephrine is (-)-3, 4-Dihydroxy-α-[(methylamino) methyl] benzyl alcohol and has the following structural formula:
[See chemical structure at top of next column.]

The pK_a of etidocaine (7.74) is similar to that of lidocaine (7.86). However, etidocaine possesses a greater degree of lipid solubility and protein binding capacity than does lidocaine. Duranest Injections are sterile and, except for the 1.5% concentration, are available with or without epinephrine 1:200,000. Single dose containers of Duranest Injection without epinephrine may be reautoclaved if necessary.
See Table 1 for composition of available injections.
[See Table 1 below.]

CLINICAL PHARMACOLOGY
Mechanism of Action: Etidocaine stabilizes the neuronal membrane by inhibiting the ionic fluxes required for the initiation and conduction of impulses, thereby effecting local anesthetic action.
Onset and Duration of Action: *In vivo* animal studies have shown that etidocaine has a rapid onset (3–5 minutes) and a prolonged duration of action (5–10 hours). Based on comparative clinical studies of lidocaine and etidocaine, the anesthetic properties of etidocaine in man may be characterized as follows: Initial onset of sensory analgesia and motor blockade is rapid (usually 3–5 minutes) and similar to that produced by lidocaine. Duration of sensory analgesia is 1.5 to 2 times longer than that of lidocaine by the peridural route. The difference in analgesic duration between etidocaine and lidocaine may be even greater following peripheral nerve blockade than following central neural blockade. Duration of analgesia in excess of 9 hours is not infrequent when etidocaine is used for peripheral nerve blocks such as brachial plexus blockade. Etidocaine produces a profound degree of motor blockade and abdominal muscle relaxation when used for peridural analgesia.
Hemodynamics: Excessive blood levels may cause changes in cardiac output, total peripheral resistance, and mean arterial pressure. With central neural blockade these changes may be attributable to block of autonomic fibers, a direct depressant effect of the local anesthetic agent on various components of the cardiovascular system, and/or the beta-adrenergic receptor stimulating action of epinephrine when present. The net effect is normally a modest hypotension when the recommended dosages are not exceeded.
Pharmacokinetics and Metabolism: Information derived from diverse formulations, concentrations and usages reveals that etidocaine is completely absorbed following parenteral administration, its rate of absorption depending, for example, upon such factors as the site of administration and the presence or absence of a vasoconstrictor agent. Except for intravenous administration, the highest blood levels are obtained following intercostal nerve block and the lowest after subcutaneous administration.
The plasma binding of etidocaine is dependent on drug concentration, and the fraction bound decreases with increasing concentration. At 0.5–1.0 µg/mL, 95% is bound to plasma protein.
Etidocaine crosses the blood-brain and placental barriers, presumably by passive diffusion.
Etidocaine is metabolized rapidly by the liver, and metabolites and unchanged drug are excreted by the kidney. Biotransformation includes oxidative N-dealkylation, ring hydroxylation, cleavage of the amide linkage, and conjugation. To date, approximately 20 metabolites of etidocaine have been found in the urine. The percent of dose excreted as unchanged drug is less than 10%.
The mean elimination half-life of etidocaine following a bolus intravenous injection is about 2.5 hours. Because of the rapid rate at which etidocaine is metabolized, any condition that affects liver function may alter etidocaine kinetics. Renal dysfunction may not affect etidocaine kinetics but may increase the accumulation of metabolites.
Factors such as acidosis and the concomitant use of CNS stimulants and depressants affect the CNS levels of etidocaine required to produce overt systemic effects. In the rhe-

Table 1. Composition of Available Injections

Duranest (etidocaine HCl) Concentration %	Epinephrine Dilution (as the bitartrate)	pH	Sodium chloride (mg/mL)	Single Dose Vials/ Dental Cartridge Sodium metabisulfite (mg/mL)	Citric acid (mg/mL)
1.0	None	4.0–5.0	7.1	None	—
1.0	1:200,000	3.0–4.5	7.1	0.5	0.2
1.5	1:200,000	3.0–4.5	6.2	0.5	0.2

NOTE: pH of all solutions adjusted with sodium hydroxide and/or hydrochloric acid. Duranest dental cartridges are only available as 1.5% solution with epinephrine 1:200,000. Filled under nitrogen.

Continued on next page

Astra—Cont.

sus monkey, arterial blood levels of 4.5 µg/mL have been shown to be threshold for convulsive activity.

INDICATIONS AND USAGE

Duranest (etidocaine HCl) Injections are indicated for infiltration anesthesia, peripheral nerve blocks (e.g., brachial plexus, intercostal, retrobulbar, ulnar, inferior alveolar), and central neural block (i.e., lumbar or caudal epidural blocks).

CONTRAINDICATIONS

Etidocaine is contraindicated in patients with a known history of hypersensitivity to local anesthetics of the amide type.

WARNINGS

DURANEST INJECTIONS FOR INFILTRATION AND NERVE BLOCK SHOULD BE EMPLOYED ONLY BY CLINICIANS WHO ARE WELL VERSED IN DIAGNOSIS AND MANAGEMENT OF DOSE-RELATED TOXICITY AND OTHER ACUTE EMERGENCIES THAT MIGHT ARISE FROM THE BLOCK TO BE EMPLOYED AND THEN ONLY AFTER ENSURING THE *IMMEDIATE* AVAILABILITY OF OXYGEN, OTHER RESUSCITATIVE DRUGS, CARDIOPULMONARY EQUIPMENT, AND THE PERSONNEL NEEDED FOR PROPER MANAGEMENT OF TOXIC REACTIONS AND RELATED EMERGENCIES (see also ADVERSE REACTIONS and PRECAUTIONS). DELAY IN PROPER MANAGEMENT OF DOSE-RELATED TOXICITY, UNDERVENTILATION FROM ANY CAUSE AND/OR ALTERED SENSITIVITY MAY LEAD TO THE DEVELOPMENT OF ACIDOSIS, CARDIAC ARREST, AND POSSIBLY DEATH.

To avoid intravascular injection, aspiration should be performed before the local anesthetic solution is injected. The needle must be repositioned until no return of blood can be elicited by aspiration. Note, however, that the absence of blood in the syringe does not guarantee that intravascular injection has been avoided.

Local anesthetic solutions containing antimicrobial preservatives (e.g., methylparaben) should not be used for epidural anesthesia because the safety of these agents has not been established with regard to intrathecal injection, either intentional or accidental.

Vasopressor agents administered for the treatment of hypotension related to caudal or other epidural blocks should not be used in the presence of ergot-type oxytocic drugs, since severe persistent hypertension and even rupture of cerebral blood vessels may occur.

Duranest with epinephrine solutions contain sodium metabisulfite, a sulfite that may cause allergic-type reactions including anaphylactic symptoms and life-threatening or less severe asthmatic episodes in certain susceptible people. The overall prevalence of sulfite sensitivity in the general population is unknown and probably low. Sulfite sensitivity is seen more frequently in asthmatic than in nonasthmatic people.

PRECAUTIONS

General: The safety and effectiveness of etidocaine depend on proper dosage, correct technique, adequate precautions, and readiness for emergencies. Standard textbooks should be consulted for specific techniques and precautions for various regional anesthetic procedures. Resuscitative equipment, oxygen, and other resuscitative drugs should be available for immediate use. (See WARNINGS and ADVERSE REACTIONS.) The lowest dosage that results in effective anesthesia should be used to avoid high plasma levels and serious adverse effects. Syringe aspirations should also be performed before and during each supplemental injection when using indwelling catheter techniques. During the administration of epidural anesthesia, it is recommended that a test dose be administered initially and that the patient be monitored for central nervous system toxicity and cardiovascular toxicity, as well as for signs of unintended intrathecal administration, before proceeding. When clinical conditions permit, consideration should be given to employing local anesthetic solutions that contain epinephrine for the test dose because circulatory changes compatible with epinephrine may also serve as a warning sign of unintended intravascular injection. An intravascular injection is still possible even if aspirations for blood are negative. Repeated doses of etidocaine may cause significant increases in blood levels with each repeated dose because of slow accumulation of the drug or its metabolites. Tolerance to elevated blood levels varies with the status of the patient. Debilitated, elderly patients, acutely ill patients, and children should be given reduced doses commensurate with their age and physical condition. Etidocaine should also be used with caution in patients with severe shock or heart block.

Lumbar and caudal epidural anesthesia should be used with extreme caution in persons with the following conditions: existing neurological disease, spinal deformities, septicemia, and severe hypertension.

Local anesthetic solutions containing a vasoconstrictor should be used cautiously and in carefully circumscribed quantities in areas of the body supplied by end arteries or having otherwise compromised blood supply. Patients with peripheral vascular disease and those with hypertensive vascular disease may exhibit exaggerated vasoconstrictor response. Ischemic injury or necrosis may result. Preparations containing a vasoconstrictor should be used with caution in patients during or following the administration of potent general anesthetic agents, since cardiac arrhythmias may occur under such conditions.

Careful and constant monitoring of cardiovascular and respiratory (adequacy of ventilation) vital signs and the patient's state of consciousness should be accomplished after each local anesthetic injection. It should be kept in mind at such times that restlessness, anxiety, tinnitus, dizziness, blurred vision, tremors, depression or drowsiness may be early warning signs of central nervous system toxicity.

Since amide-type local anesthetics are metabolized by the liver, Duranest Injections should be used with caution in patients with hepatic disease.

Patients with severe hepatic disease, because of their inability to metabolize local anesthetics normally, are at greater risk of developing toxic plasma concentrations. Duranest Injection should also be used with caution in patients with impaired cardiovascular function since they may be less able to compensate for functional changes associated with the prolongation of A-V conduction produced by these drugs.

Many drugs used during the conduct of anesthesia are considered potential triggering agents for familial malignant hyperthermia. Since it is not known whether amide-type local anesthetics may trigger this reaction and since the need for supplemental general anesthesia cannot be predicted in advance, it is suggested that a standard protocol for the management of malignant hyperthermia should be available. Early unexplained signs of tachycardia, tachypnea, labile blood pressure and metabolic acidosis may precede temperature elevation. Successful outcome is dependent on early diagnosis, prompt discontinuance of the suspect triggering agent(s) and institution of treatment, including oxygen therapy, indicated supportive measures and dantrolene (consult dantrolene sodium intravenous package insert before using).

Etidocaine should be used with caution in persons with known drug sensitivities. Patients allergic to para-aminobenzoic acid derivatives (procaine, tetracaine, benzocaine, etc.) have not shown cross sensitivity to etidocaine.

Use in the Head and Neck Area: Small doses of local anesthetics injected into the head and neck area, including retrobulbar, dental and stellate ganglion blocks, may produce adverse reactions similar to systemic toxicity seen with unintentional intravascular injections of larger doses. The injection procedures require the utmost care. Confusion, convulsions, respiratory depression and/or respiratory arrest, and cardiovascular stimulation or depression have been reported. These reactions may be due to intra-arterial injection of the local anesthetic with retrograde flow to the cerebral circulation. They may also be due to puncture of the dural sheath of the optic nerve during retrobulbar block with diffusion of any local anesthetic along the subdural space to the midbrain. Patients receiving these blocks should have their circulation and respiration monitored and be constantly observed. Resuscitative equipment and personnel for treating adverse reactions should be immediately available. Dosage recommendations should not be exceeded. (See DOSAGE AND ADMINISTRATION.)

Use in Ophthalmic Surgery: When local anesthetic injections are employed for retrobulbar block, lack of corneal sensation should not be relied upon to determine whether or not the patient is ready for surgery. This is because complete lack of corneal sensation usually precedes clinically acceptable external ocular muscle akinesia.

Use in Dentistry: Because of the long duration of anesthesia, when Duranest 1.5% with epinephrine is used for dental injections, patients should be cautioned about the possibility of inadvertent trauma to tongue, lips and buccal mucosa and advised not to chew solid foods or test the anesthetized area by biting or probing.

Information for Patients: When appropriate, patients should be informed in advance that they may experience temporary loss of sensation and motor activity, usually in the lower half of the body, following proper administration of epidural anesthesia.

Clinically Significant Drug Interactions: The administration of local anesthetic solutions containing epinephrine or norepinephrine to patients receiving monoamine oxidase inhibitors, tricyclic antidepressants or phenothiazines may produce severe, prolonged hypotension or hypertension. Concurrent use of these agents should generally be avoided. In situations when concurrent therapy is necessary, careful patient monitoring is essential.

Concurrent administration of vasopressor drugs (for the treatment of hypotension related to epidural blocks) and ergot-type oxytocic drugs may cause severe, persistent hypertension or cerebrovascular accidents.

Drug Laboratory Test Interactions: The intramuscular injection of etidocaine may result in an increase in creatine phosphokinase levels. Thus, the use of this enzyme determination, without isoenzyme separation, as a diagnostic test for the presence of acute myocardial infarction may be compromised by the intramuscular injection of etidocaine.

Carcinogenesis, Mutagenesis, Impairment of Fertility: Studies of etidocaine in animals to evaluate the carcinogenic and mutagenic potential have not been conducted. Studies in rats at 1.7 times the maximum recommended human dose have revealed no impairment of fertility.

Use in Pregnancy: Teratogenic Effects. Pregnancy Category B. Reproduction studies have been performed in rats and rabbits at doses up to 1.7 times the human dose and have revealed no evidence of harm to the fetus caused by etidocaine. There are, however, no adequate and well-controlled studies in pregnant women. Animal reproduction studies are not always predictive of human response. General consideration should be given to this fact before administering etidocaine to women of childbearing potential, especially during early pregnancy when maximum organogenesis takes place.

Labor and Delivery: Local anesthetics rapidly cross the placenta and when used for epidural, paracervical, pudendal or caudal block anesthesia, can cause varying degrees of maternal, fetal and neonatal toxicity. (See CLINICAL PHARMACOLOGY—Pharmacokinetics.) The incidence and degree of toxicity depend upon the procedure performed, the type and amount of drug used, and the technique of drug administration. Adverse reactions in the parturient, fetus and neonate involve alterations of the central nervous system, peripheral vascular tone and cardiac function.

Maternal hypotension has resulted from regional anesthesia. Local anesthetics produce vasodilation by blocking sympathetic nerves. Elevating the patient's legs and positioning her on her left side will help prevent decreases in blood pressure. The fetal heart rate also should be monitored continuously and electronic fetal monitoring is highly advisable.

Epidural anesthesia may alter the forces of parturition through changes in uterine contractility or maternal expulsive efforts. Because Duranest Injection may produce profound motor block, it is not recommended for epidural anesthesia in normal delivery. Duranest Injection is, however, recommended for epidural anesthesia when caesarean section is to be performed.

The use of some local anesthetic drug products during labor and delivery may be followed by diminished muscle strength and tone for the first day or two of life. The long-term significance of these observations is unknown.

Fetal bradycardia may occur in 20 to 30 percent of patients receiving paracervical nerve block anesthesia with the amide-type local anesthetics and may be associated with fetal acidosis. Fetal heart rate should always be monitored during paracervical anesthesia. The physician should weigh the possible advantages against risks when considering paracervical block in prematurity, toxemia of pregnancy, and fetal distress. Careful adherence to recommended dosage is of the utmost importance in obstetrical paracervical block. Failure to achieve adequate analgesia with recommended doses should arouse suspicion of intravascular or fetal intracranial injection. Cases compatible with unintended fetal intracranial injection of local anesthetic solution have been reported following intended paracervical or pudendal block or both. Babies so affected present with unexplained neonatal depression at birth, which correlates with high local anesthetic serum levels, and often manifest seizures within six hours. Prompt use of supportive measures combined with forced urinary excretion of the local anesthetic has been used successfully to manage this complication. Case reports of maternal convulsions and cardiovascular collapse following use of some local anesthetics for paracervical block in early pregnancy (as anesthesia for elective abortion) suggest that systemic absorption under these circumstances may be rapid. There are inadequate data in support of safe and effective use of etidocaine for obstetrical or non-obstetrical paracervical block, therefore, such use is not recommended.

Nursing Mothers: It is not known whether this drug is excreted in human milk. Because many drugs are excreted in human milk, caution should be exercised when etidocaine is administered to a nursing woman.

Pediatric Use: No information is currently available on appropriate pediatric doses.

ADVERSE REACTIONS

Systemic: Adverse experiences following the administration of etidocaine are similar in nature to those observed with other amide local anesthetic agents. These adverse experiences are, in general, dose-related and may result from high plasma levels caused by excessive dosage, rapid absorption or unintended intravascular injection, or may result from a hypersensitivity, idiosyncrasy or diminished tolerance on the part of the patient. Serious adverse experiences are generally systemic in nature. The following types are those most commonly reported:

Central Nervous System: CNS manifestations are excitatory and/or depressant and may be characterized by lightheadedness, nervousness, apprehension, euphoria, confu-

sion, dizziness, drowsiness, tinnitus, blurred or double vision, vomiting, sensations of heat, cold or numbness, twitching, tremors, convulsions, unconsciousness, respiratory depression and arrest. The excitatory manifestations may be very brief or may not occur at all, in which case the first manifestation of toxicity may be drowsiness merging into unconsciousness and respiratory arrest.

Drowsiness following the administration of etidocaine is usually an early sign of a high blood level of the drug and may occur as a consequence of rapid absorption.

Cardiovascular System: Cardiovascular manifestations are usually depressant and are characterized by bradycardia, hypotension, and cardiovascular collapse, which may lead to cardiac arrest.

Allergic: Allergic reactions are characterized by cutaneous lesions, urticaria, edema or anaphylactoid reactions. Allergic reactions may occur as a result of sensitivity either to local anesthetic agents or to the methylparaben used as a preservative in multiple dose vials. The detection of sensitivity by skin testing is of doubtful value.

Neurologic: The incidences of adverse reactions associated with the use of local anesthetics may be related to the total dose of local anesthetic administered and are also dependent upon the particular drug used, the route of administration and the physical status of the patient.

In the practice of caudal or lumbar epidural block, occasional unintentional penetration of the subarachnoid space by the catheter may occur. Subsequent adverse effects may depend partially on the amount of drug administered subdurally. These may include spinal block of varying magnitude (including total spinal block), hypotension secondary to spinal block, loss of bladder and bowel control, and loss of perineal sensation and sexual function. Persistent motor, sensory and/or autonomic (sphincter control) deficit of some lower spinal segments with slow recovery (several months) or incomplete recovery have been reported in rare instances when caudal or lumbar epidural block has been attempted. Backache and headache have also been noted following use of these anesthetic procedures.

Other: There have been rare reports of TRISMUS in patients who have received Duranest (etidocaine HCl) for dental anesthesia. Onset of symptoms occurs within hours or days upon resolution of blockade. No correlation has been demonstrated with dosage, administration technique or dental procedure. In most patients, symptoms resolved within days to weeks, although some reports have suggested that symptoms were present for many months. Symptomatic treatment with analgesics, moist heat and physiotherapy was helpful in some cases.

OVERDOSAGE

Acute emergencies from local anesthetics are generally related to high plasma levels encountered during therapeutic use of local anesthetics or to unintended subarachnoid injection of local anesthetic solution (see ADVERSE REACTIONS, WARNINGS, and PRECAUTIONS).

Management of Local Anesthetic Emergencies: The first consideration is prevention, best accomplished by careful and constant monitoring of cardiovascular and respiratory vital signs and the patient's state of consciousness after each local anesthetic injection. At the first sign of change, oxygen should be administered.

The first step in the management of convulsions, as well as underventilation or apnea due to unintentional subarachnoid injection of drug solution, consists of immediate attention to the maintenance of a patent airway and assisted or controlled ventilation with oxygen and a delivery system capable of permitting immediate positive airway pressure by mask. Immediately after the institution of these ventilatory measures, the adequacy of the circulation should be evaluated, keeping in mind that drugs used to treat convulsions sometimes depress the circulation when administered intravenously. Should convulsions persist despite adequate respiratory support, and if the status of the circulation permits, small increments of an ultra-short acting barbiturate (such as thiopental or thiamylal) or a benzodiazepine (such as diazepam) may be administered intravenously. The clinician should be familiar, prior to use of local anesthetics, with these anticonvulsant drugs. Supportive treatment of circulatory depression may require administration of intravenous fluids and, when appropriate, a vasopressor as directed by the clinical situation (e.g., ephedrine).

Table 2. Dosage Recommendations

PROCEDURE	Duranest HCl with epinephrine 1:200,000		
	Conc. (%)	Vol. (mL)	Total Dose (mg)
Peripheral Nerve Block	1.0	5–40	50–400
Central Neural Block Lumbar Peridural			
Intraabdominal or Pelvic Surgery Lower Limb Surgery	1.0 or	10–30	100–300
Caesarean Section	1.5	10–20	150–300

PROCEDURE	Duranest HCl with epinephrine 1:200,000		
	Conc. (%)	Vol. (mL)	Total Dose (mg)
Caudal	1.0	10–30	100–300
Retrobulbar	1.0 or 1.5	2–4	20–60
Maxillary Infiltration and/or inferior Alveolar Nerve Block	1.5	1–5	15–75

If not treated immediately, both convulsions and cardiovascular depression can result in hypoxia, acidosis, bradycardia, arrhythmias and cardiac arrest. Underventilation or apnea due to unintentional subarachnoid injection of local anesthetic solution may produce these same signs and also lead to cardiac arrest if ventilatory support is not instituted. If cardiac arrest should occur, standard cardiopulmonary resuscitative measures should be instituted.

Endotracheal intubation, employing drugs and techniques familiar to the clinician, may be indicated, after initial administration of oxygen by mask, if difficulty is encountered in the maintenance of a patent airway or if prolonged ventilatory support (assisted or controlled) is indicated.

Dialysis is of negligible value in the treatment of acute overdosage with etidocaine.

The intravenous LD$_{50}$ of etidocaine HCl in female mice is 7.6 (6.6–8.5) mg/kg and the subcutaneous LD$_{50}$ is 112 (96–166) mg/kg.

DOSAGE AND ADMINISTRATION

As with all local anesthetic agents, the dose of Duranest (etidocaine HCl) Injection to be employed will depend upon the area to be anesthetized, the vascularity of the tissues, the number of neuronal segments to be blocked, the type of regional anesthetic technique, and the physical condition and tolerance of the individual patient.

The maximum dose to be employed as a single injection should be determined on the basis of the status of the patient and the type of regional anesthetic technique to be performed. Although single injections of 450 mg have been employed for regional anesthesia without adverse effects, at present it is strongly recommended that the maximal dose as a single injection should not exceed 400 mg (approximately 8.0 mg/kg or 3.6 mg/lb based on a 50 kg person) with epinephrine 1:200,000 and 300 mg (approximately 6 mg/kg or 2.7 mg/lb based on a 50 kg person) without epinephrine. Because etidocaine has been shown to disappear quite rapidly from blood, toxicity is influenced by rapidity of administration, and therefore, slow injection in vascular areas is highly recommended. Incremental doses of Duranest Injection may be repeated at 2–3 hour intervals.

Caudal and Lumbar Epidural Block: As a precaution against the adverse experiences sometimes observed following unintentional penetration of the subarachnoid space, a test dose of 2–5 mL should be administered at least 5 minutes prior to injecting the total volume required for a lumbar or caudal epidural block. The test dose should be repeated if the patient is moved in a manner that may have displaced the catheter. Epinephrine, if contained in the test dose (10–15 μg have been suggested), may serve as a warning of unintentional intravascular injection. If injected into a blood vessel, this amount of epinephrine is likely to produce a transient "epinephrine response" within 45 seconds, consisting of an increase in heart rate and systolic blood pressure, circumoral pallor, palpitations and nervousness in the unsedated patient. The sedated patient may exhibit only a pulse rate increase of 20 or more beats per minute for 15 or more seconds. Patients on beta-blockers may not manifest changes in heart rate, but blood pressure monitoring can detect an evanescent rise in systolic blood pressure. Adequate time should be allowed for onset of anesthesia after administration of each test dose. The rapid injection of a large volume of Duranest Injection through the catheter should be avoided, and when feasible, fractional doses should be administered.

In the event of the known injection of a large volume of local anesthetic solution into the subarachnoid space, after suitable resuscitation, and if the catheter is in place, consider attempting the recovery of drug by draining a moderate amount of cerebrospinal fluid (such as 10 mL) through the epidural catheter.

Use in Dentistry When used for local anesthesia in dental procedures the dosage of Duranest (etidocaine HCl) Injection depends on the physical status of the patient, the area of the oral cavity to be anesthetized, the vascularity of the oral tissues, and the technique of anesthesia. The least volume of solution that results in effective local anesthesia should be administered. For specific techniques and procedures of local anesthesia in the oral cavity, refer to standard textbooks. Dosage requirements should be determined on an individual basis. In maxillary infiltration and/or inferior alveolar nerve block, initial dosages of 1.0–5.0 mL ($1/_2$–$2^1/_2$ cartridges) of Duranest Injection 1.5% with epinephrine 1:200,000 are usually effective.

Aspiration is recommended since it reduces the possibility of intravascular injection, thereby keeping the incidence of side effects and anesthetic failures to a minimum.

The following dosage recommendations are intended as guides for the use of Duranest Injection in the average adult patient. As indicated previously, the dosage should be reduced for elderly or debilitated patients or patients with severe renal disease.

NOTE:
Parenteral drug products should be inspected visually for particulate matter and discoloration prior to administration whenever the solution and container permit. The Injection is not to be used if its color is pinkish or darker than slightly yellow or if it contains a precipitate.

[See table 2 above.]

HOW SUPPLIED
[See table below.]
021842R30   (2/93)

DYCLONE® 0.5% and 1%   ℞
Topical Solutions, USP
[díe-clone]
(dyclonine HCl)

DESCRIPTION

Dyclone (dyclonine HCl) 0.5% and 1% Topical Solutions contain a local anesthetic agent and are administered topically. See INDICATIONS for specific uses.

Dyclone 0.5% and 1% Topical Solutions contain dyclonine HCl, which is chemically designated as 4'-butoxy-3-piperidinopropiophenone HCl. Dyclonine HCl is a white crystalline powder that is sparingly soluble in water and has the following structural formula:

Dosage Form and Volume	Duranest Injection Concentration	Epinephrine Dilution (as the bitartrate)	pH	NDC Number
Single Dose Vials* 30 mL	1.0%	None	4.0–5.0	0186-0820-01
	1.0%	1:200,000	3.0–4.5	0186-0825-01
20 mL	1.5%	1:200,000	3.0–4.5	0186-0836-03
Dental Cartridge** 1.8 mL	1.5%	1:200,000	3.0–4.5	0186-0840-14

Solutions containing epinephrine should be protected from light.
*Store at controlled room temperature 15°–30°C (59°–86°F).
**Store at room temperature, approx. 25°C (77°F).

Continued on next page

Astra—Cont.

COMPOSITION OF DYCLONE 0.5% AND 1% TOPICAL SOLUTIONS

Each mL of Dyclone 0.5% Solution contains dyclonine HCl, 5 mg.
Each mL of Dyclone 1% Solution contains dyclonine HCl, 10 mg.

Both solutions also contain chlorbutanol hydrous and sodium chloride, and the pH is adjusted to 3.0–5.0 by means of hydrochloric acid.

CLINICAL PHARMACOLOGY

Dyclone Topical Solutions effect surface anesthesia when applied topically to mucous membranes. Effective anesthesia varies with different patients, but usually occurs from 2 to 10 minutes after application and persists for approximately 30 minutes.

INDICATIONS AND USAGE

Dyclone Topical Solutions are indicated for anesthetizing accessible mucous membranes (e.g., the mouth, pharynx, larynx, trachea, esophagus, and urethra) prior to various endoscopic procedures.
Dyclone 0.5% Topical Solution may also be used to block the gag reflex, to relieve the pain of oral ulcers or stomatitis and to relieve pain associated with ano-genital lesions.

CONTRAINDICATIONS

Dyclonine is contraindicated in patients known to be hypersensitive (allergic) to the local anesthetic or to other components of Dyclone Topical Solutions.

WARNINGS

IN ORDER TO MANAGE POSSIBLE ADVERSE REACTIONS, RESUSCITATIVE EQUIPMENT, OXYGEN AND OTHER RESUSCITATIVE DRUGS SHOULD BE IMMEDIATELY AVAILABLE WHENEVER LOCAL ANESTHETIC AGENTS, SUCH AS DYCLONINE, ARE ADMINISTERED TO MUCOUS MEMBRANES.
Dyclone Topical Solutions should not be injected into tissue or used in the eyes because of highly irritant properties.
Dyclone Topical Solutions should be used with extreme caution in the presence of sepsis or severely traumatized mucosa in the area of application since under such conditions there is the potential for rapid systemic absorption.

PRECAUTIONS

General: The safety and effectiveness of dyclonine depend on proper dosage, correct technique, adequate precautions, and readiness for emergencies (See WARNINGS and ADVERSE REACTIONS). The lowest dosage that results in effective anesthesia should be used to avoid high plasma levels and serious adverse effects. Repeated doses of dyclonine may cause significant increases in blood levels with each repeated dose because of slow accumulation of the drug or its metabolites. Tolerance to elevated blood levels varies with the status of the patient. Debilitated, elderly patients, acutely ill patients, and children should be given reduced doses commensurate with their age, weight and physical condition. Dyclonine should also be used with caution in patients with severe shock or heart block.
Dyclone Topical Solutions should be used with caution in persons with known drug sensitivities.
Information for Patients: When topical anesthetics are used in the mouth or throat, the patient should be aware that the production of topical anesthesia may impair swallowing and thus enhance the danger of aspiration. For this reason, food should not be ingested for 60 minutes following use of local anesthetic preparations in the mouth or throat area. This is particularly important in children because of their frequency of eating.
Numbness of the tongue or buccal mucosa may increase the danger of biting trauma. When Dyclone 0.5% Topical Solution is used to relieve the pain of oral ulcers or stomatitis which interferes with eating, patients should be warned about the risk of biting trauma before they accept this treatment; caution should be exercised in selecting food and eating. Following other uses in the mouth and throat area, food and/or chewing gum should not be used while the area is anesthetized.
Drug/Laboratory Test Interactions: Dyclone Topical Solutions should not be used in cystoscopic procedures following intravenous pyelography because an iodine precipitate occurs which interferes with visualization.
Carcinogenesis, mutagenesis, impairment of fertility: Studies of dyclonine in animals to evaluate the carcinogenic and mutagenic potential or the effect on fertility have not been conducted.
Use in Pregnancy: Teratogenic Effects:
Pregnancy Category C. Animal reproduction studies have not been conducted with dyclonine. It is also not known whether dyclonine can cause fetal harm when administered to a pregnant woman or can affect reproduction capacity. General consideration should be given to this fact before administering dyclonine to women of childbearing potential, especially during early pregnancy when maximum organogenesis takes place.
Nursing Mothers: It is not known whether this drug is excreted in human milk. Because many drugs are excreted in human milk, caution should be exercised when dyclonine is administered to a nursing woman.
Pediatric Use: Safety and effectiveness in children under the age of 12 have not been established.

ADVERSE REACTIONS

Adverse experiences following the administration of dyclonine are similar in nature to those observed with other local anesthetic agents. These adverse experiences are, in general, dose-related and may result from high plasma levels caused by excessive dosage or rapid absorption, or may result from a hypersensitivity, idiosyncrasy or diminished tolerance on the part of the patient. Serious adverse experiences are generally systemic in nature. The following types are those most commonly reported:
Central nervous system: CNS manifestations are excitatory and/or depressant and may be characterized by lightheadedness, nervousness, apprehension, euphoria, confusion, dizziness, drowsiness, tinnitus, blurred or double vision, vomiting, sensations of heat, cold or numbness, twitching, tremors, convulsions, unconsciousness, repiratory depression and arrest. The excitatory manifestations may be very brief or may not occur at all, in which case the first manifestation of toxicity may be drowsiness merging into unconsciousness and respiratory arrest.
Drowsiness following the administration of dyclonine is usually an early sign of a high blood level of the drug and may occur as a consequence of rapid absorption.
Cardiovascular system: Cardiovascular manifestations are usually depressant and are characterized by bradycardia, hypotension, and cardiovascular collapse, which may lead to cardiac arrest.
Allergic: Allergic reactions are characterized by cutaneous lesions, urticaria, edema or anaphylactoid reactions. Allergic reactions may occur as a result of sensitivity either to the local anesthetic agent or to the other ingredients used in this formulation. Allergic reactions, if they occur, should be managed by conventional means. The detection of sensitivity by skin testing is of doubtful value. Local reactions include irritation, stinging, urethritis with and without bleeding.

OVERDOSAGE

Acute emergencies from local anesthetics are generally related to high plasma levels encountered during therapeutic use of local anesthetics. (See ADVERSE REACTIONS, WARNINGS, and PRECAUTIONS).
Management of local anesthetic emergencies: The first consideration is prevention, best accomplished by careful and constant monitoring of cardiovascular and respiratory vital signs and the patient's state of consciousness after each local anesthetic administration.
The first step in the management of convulsions consists of immediate attention to the maintenance of a patent airway and assisted or controlled ventilation with oxygen and a delivery system capable of permitting immediate positive airway pressure by mask. Immediately after the institution of these ventilatory measures, the adequacy of the circulation should be evaluated, keeping in mind that drugs used to treat convulsions sometimes depress the circulation when administered intravenously. Should convulsions persist despite adequate respiratory support, and if the status of the circulation permits, small increments of an ultra-short acting barbiturate (such as thiopental or thiamylal) or a benzodiazepine (such as diazepam) may be administered intravenously. The clinician should be familiar, prior to use of local anesthetics, with these anticonvulsant drugs. Supportive treatment of circulatory depression may require administration of intravenous fluids and, when appropriate, a vasopressor as directed by the clinical situation (e.g., ephedrine).
If not treated immediately, both convulsions and cardiovascular depression can result in hypoxia, acidosis, bradycardia, arrhythmias and cardiac arrest. If cardiac arrest should occur, standard cardiopulmonary resuscitative measures should be instituted.
The median lethal dose (LD_{50}) of dyclonine HCl administered orally to female rats is 176 mg/kg and 90 mg/kg in female mice. Intraperitoneally the LD_{50} in female rats is 31 mg/kg and 43 mg/kg in female mice.

DOSAGE AND ADMINISTRATION

As with all local anesthetics, the dosage varies and depends upon the area to be anesthetized, vascularity of the tissues, individual tolerance and the technique of anesthesia. The lowest dosage needed to provide effective anesthesia should be administered.
A maximum dose of 30 mL of 1% Dyclone Topical Solution (300 mg of dyclonine HCl) may be used, although satisfactory anesthesia is usually produced within the range of 4 to 20 mL. For specific techniques and procedures refer to standard textbooks.
Although as much as 300 mg of dyclonine HCl (as a 1% solution) have been tolerated, this dosage as a 0.5% solution has not been administered primarily because satisfactory anesthesia in endoscopic procedures can usually be produced by lesser amounts. For specific techniques for endoscopic procedures refer to standard textbooks.

PROCTOLOGY

Apply pledgets of cotton or sponges moistened with the Dyclone 0.5% Solution to postoperative wounds for the relief of discomfort and pain.

GYNECOLOGY

Apply Dyclone 0.5% Solution as wet compresses or as a spray to relieve the discomfort of episiotomy or perineorrhaphy wounds.

ONCOLOGY-RADIOLOGY

Apply Dyclone 0.5% Solution as a rinse or swab to inflamed or ulcerated mucous membrane of the mouth caused by antineoplastic chemotherapy or radiation therapy. In lesions of the esophagus, 5–15 mL of the anesthetic may be swallowed to relieve pain and allow more comfortable deglutition.

OTORHINOLARYNGOLOGY

To suppress the gag reflex and to facilitate examination of the posterior pharynx or larynx, apply Dyclone 0.5% Solution as a spray or gargle.
Dyclone 0.5% Solution may be applied as a rinse or swab to relieve the discomfort of aphthous stomatitis, herpetic stomatitis, or other painful oral lesions.

DENTISTRY

Dyclone 0.5% Topical Solution is useful to suppress the gag reflex in the positioning of x-ray films, making prosthetic impressions, and doing surgical procedures in the molar areas. It is also useful as a preinjection mucous membrane anesthetic or applied to the gums prior to scaling (prophylaxis). The anesthetic can be applied as a mouthwash or gargle and the excess spit out.

HOW SUPPLIED

Sterile, in one fluid ounce bottles, DYCLONE 0.5% TOPICAL SOLUTION (NDC 0186-3001-01) and DYCLONE 1% TOPICAL SOLUTION (NDC 0186-3002-01). Keep tightly closed. Store at controlled room temperature: 15°–30°C (59°–86°F). Avoid excessive heat (temperatures above 40°C (104°F). Subject to damage by freezing.
021859R02 Rev. 8/89 (2)

EMLA® ℞

CREAM (lidocaine 2.5% and prilocaine 2.5%)

DESCRIPTION

EMLA Cream (lidocaine 2.5% and prilocaine 2.5%) is an emulsion in which the oil phase is a eutectic mixture of lidocaine and prilocaine in a ratio of 1:1 by weight. A eutectic mixture has a melting point below room temperature and therefore both local anesthetics exist as a liquid oil rather than as crystals.
Lidocaine is chemically designated as acetamide, 2-(diethylamino)-N-(2,6-dimethylphenyl), has an octanol:water partition ratio of 43 at pH 7.4, and has the following structure:

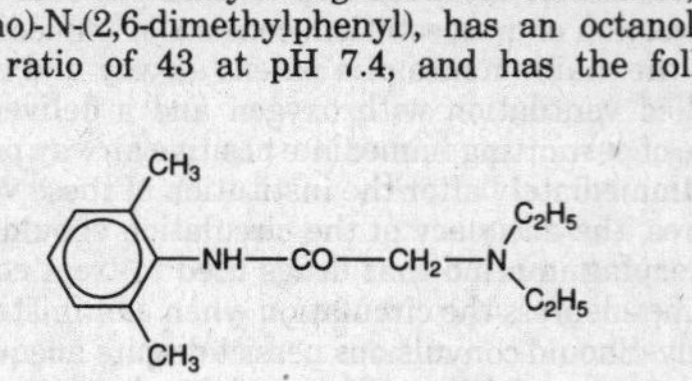

$C_{14}H_{22}N_2O$ M. W. 234.3

Prilocaine is chemically designated as propanamide, N-(2-methylphenyl)-2-(propylamino), has an octanol:water partition ratio of 25 at pH 7.4, and has the following structure:

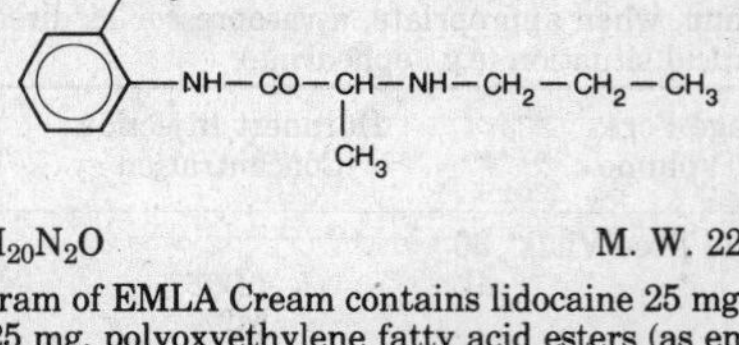

$C_{13}H_{20}N_2O$ M. W. 220.3

Each gram of EMLA Cream contains lidocaine 25 mg, prilocaine 25 mg, polyoxyethylene fatty acid esters (as emulsifiers), carboxypolymethylene (as a thickening agent), sodium hydroxide to adjust to a pH approximating 9, and purified water (about 92%) to 1 gram. EMLA Cream contains no preservative, however it passes the USP antimicrobial effectiveness test due to the pH. The specific gravity of EMLA Cream is 1.00.

CLINICAL PHARMACOLOGY

Mechanism of Action: EMLA Cream (lidocaine 2.5% and prilocaine 2.5%), applied to intact skin under occlusive dressing, provides dermal analgesia by the release of lidocaine and prilocaine from the cream into the epidermal and dermal layers of the skin and the accumulation of lidocaine and prilocaine in the vicinity of dermal pain receptors and nerve endings. Lidocaine and prilocaine are amide-type local anesthetic agents. Both lidocaine and prilocaine stabilize neuronal membranes by inhibiting the ionic fluxes required for the initiation and conduction of impulses, thereby effecting local anesthetic action.

The onset, depth and duration of dermal analgesia provided by EMLA Cream depends primarily on the duration of application. To provide sufficient analgesia for clinical procedures such as intravenous catheter placement and venipuncture, EMLA Cream should be applied under an occlusive dressing for at least 1 hour. To provide dermal analgesia for clinical procedures such as split skin graft harvesting, EMLA Cream should be applied under occlusive dressing for at least 2 hours. Satisfactory dermal analgesia is achieved 1 hour after application, reaches maximum at 2 to 3 hours, and persists for 1 to 2 hours after removal.

Dermal application of EMLA Cream may cause a transient, local blanching followed by a transient, local redness or erythema.

Pharmacokinetics: EMLA Cream is a eutectic mixture of lidocaine 2.5% and prilocaine 2.5% formulated as an oil in water emulsion. As a eutectic mixture, both anesthetics are liquid at room temperature (see DESCRIPTION) and the penetration and subsequent systemic absorption of both prilocaine and lidocaine are enhanced over that which would be seen if each component in crystalline form was applied separately as a 2.5% topical cream.

The amount of lidocaine and prilocaine systemically absorbed from EMLA Cream is directly related to both the duration of application and to the area over which it is applied. In two pharmacokinetic studies, 60 g of EMLA Cream (1.5 g lidocaine and 1.5 g prilocaine) was applied to 400 cm^2 of intact skin on the lateral thigh and then covered by an occlusive dressing. The subjects were then randomized such that one-half of the subjects had the occlusive dressing and residual cream removed after 3 hours, while the remainder left the dressing in place for 24 hours. The results from these studies are summarized below.

[See Table 1 below.]

When 60 g of EMLA was applied over 400 cm^2 for 24 hours, peak blood levels of lidocaine are approximately 1/20 the systemic toxic level. Likewise, the maximum prilocaine level is about 1/36 the toxic level. The application of EMLA Cream to broken or inflamed skin, or to 2,000 cm^2 or more of skin where more of both anesthetics are absorbed, could result in higher plasma levels that could, in susceptible individuals, produce a systemic pharmacologic response. When each drug is administered intravenously, the steady-state volume of distribution is 1.1 to 2.1 L/kg (mean 1.5, ±0.3 SD, n=13) for lidocaine and is 0.7 to 4.4 L/kg (mean 2.6, ±1.3 SD, n=13) for prilocaine. The larger distribution volume for prilocaine produces the lower plasma concentrations of prilocaine observed when equal amounts of prilocaine and lidocaine are administered. At concentrations produced by application of EMLA Cream, lidocaine is approximately 70% bound to plasma proteins, primarily alpha-1-acid glycoprotein. At much higher plasma concentrations (1 to 4 μg/mL of free base) the plasma protein binding of lidocaine is concentration dependent. Prilocaine is 55% bound to plasma proteins. Both lidocaine and prilocaine cross the placental and blood brain barrier, presumably by passive diffusion.

It is not known if lidocaine or prilocaine are metabolized in the skin. Lidocaine is metabolized rapidly by the liver to a number of metabolites including monoethylglycinexylidide (MEGX) and glycinexylidide (GX), both of which have pharmacologic activity similar to, but less potent than that of lidocaine. The metabolite, 2,6-xylidine, has unknown pharmacologic activity but is carcinogenic in rats (see Carcinogenesis subsection of PRECAUTIONS). Following intravenous administration, MEGX and GX concentrations in serum range from 11 to 36% and from 5 to 11% of lidocaine concentrations, respectively. Prilocaine is metabolized in both the liver and kidneys by amidases to various metabolites including *ortho*-toluidine and N-n-propylalanine. It is not metabolized by plasma esterases. The *ortho*-toluidine metabolite has been shown to be carcinogenic in several animal models (see Carcinogenesis subsection of PRECAUTIONS). In addition, *ortho*-toluidine can produce methemoglobinemia following systemic doses of prilocaine approximating 8 mg/kg (see ADVERSE REACTIONS). Very young patients, patients with glucose-6-phosphate deficiencies and patients taking oxidizing drugs such as antimalarials and sulfonamides are more susceptible to methemoglobinemia (see Methemoglobinemia subsection of PRECAUTIONS).

The half-life of lidocaine elimination from the plasma following IV administration is approximately 65 to 150 minutes (mean 110, ±24 SD, n=13). This half-life may be increased in cardiac or hepatic dysfunction. More than 98% of an absorbed dose of lidocaine can be recovered in the urine as metabolites or parent drug. The systemic clearance is 10 to 20 mL/min/kg (mean 13, ±3 SD, n=13). The elimination half-life of prilocaine is approximately 10 to 150 minutes (mean 70, ±48 SD, n=13). The systemic clearance is 18 to 64 mL/min/kg (mean 38, ±15 SD, n=13). Prilocaine's half-life also may be increased in hepatic or renal dysfunction since both of these organs are involved in prilocaine metabolism.

CLINICAL STUDIES

EMLA Cream application in adults prior to IV cannulation or venipuncture was studied in 200 patients in four clinical studies in Europe. Application for at least 1 hour provided significantly more dermal analgesia than placebo cream or ethyl chloride. EMLA Cream was comparable to subcutaneous lidocaine, but was less efficacious than intradermal lidocaine. Most patients found EMLA Cream treatment preferable to lidocaine infiltration or ethyl chloride spray.

EMLA Cream was compared with 0.5% lidocaine infiltration prior to skin graft harvesting in one open label study in 80 adult patients in England. Application of EMLA Cream for 2 to 5 hours provided dermal analgesia comparable to lidocaine infiltration.

EMLA Cream application in children was studied in seven non-US studies (320 patients) and one US study (100 patients). In controlled studies, application of EMLA Cream for at least 1 hour with or without presurgical medication prior to needle insertion provided significantly more pain reduction than placebo. In children under the age of seven years, EMLA Cream was less effective than in older children or adults.

EMLA Cream was compared with placebo in the laser treatment of facial port-wine stains in 72 pediatric patients (ages 5–16). EMLA Cream was effective in providing pain relief during laser treatment.

Local dermal effects associated with EMLA Cream application in these studies on intact skin included paleness, redness and edema and were transient in nature (see ADVERSE REACTIONS).

Individualization of Dose: The dose of EMLA Cream which provides effective analgesia depends on the duration of the application over the treated area.

All pharmacokinetic and clinical studies employed a thick layer of EMLA Cream (1–2 g/10 cm^2). The duration of application prior to venipuncture was 1 hour. The duration of application prior to taking split thickness skin grafts was 2 hours. Although a thinner application may be efficacious, such has not been studied and may result in less complete analgesia or a shorter duration of adequate analgesia.

The systemic absorption of lidocaine and prilocaine is a side effect of the desired local effect. The amount of drug absorbed depends on surface area and duration of application. The systemic blood levels depend on the amount absorbed and patient size (weight) and rate of systemic drug elimination. Long duration of application, large treatment area, small patients, or impaired elimination may result in high blood levels. The systemic blood levels are typically a small fraction (1/20 to 1/36) of the blood levels which produce toxicity. Table 2 which follows gives maximum recommended application areas for infants and children.

[See Table 2 at top of next column.]

TABLE 2
EMLA CREAM MAXIMUM RECOMMENDED APPLICATION AREA*
For Infants and Children
Based on Application to Intact Skin

Body Weight (kg)	Maximum Application Area (cm^2)**
up to 10 kg	100
10 to 20 kg	600
above 20 kg	2000

* These are broad guidelines for avoiding systemic toxicity in applying EMLA to patients with normal intact skin and with normal renal and hepatic function.

** For more individualized calculation of how much lidocaine and prilocaine may be absorbed, physicians can use the following estimates of lidocaine and prilocaine absorption for children and adults:

The estimated mean (±SD) absorption of lidocaine is 0.045 (±0.016) mg/cm^2/hr.

The estimated mean (±SD) absorption of prilocaine is 0.077 (±0.036) mg/cm^2/hr.

An IV antiarrhythmic dose of lidocaine is 1 mg/kg (70 mg/70 kg) and gives a blood level of about 1 μg/mL. Toxicity would be expected at blood levels above 5 μg/mL. Smaller areas of treatment are recommended in a debilitated patient, a small child or a patient with impaired elimination. Decreasing the duration of application is likely to decrease the analgesic effect.

INDICATION AND USAGE

EMLA Cream (a eutectic mixture of lidocaine 2.5% and prilocaine 2.5%) is indicated as a topical anesthetic for use on **normal intact skin** for local analgesia.

EMLA Cream is not recommended for use on mucous membranes because limited studies show much greater absorption of lidocaine and prilocaine than through intact skin. Safe dosing recommendations for use on mucous membranes cannot be made because it has not been studied adequately.

EMLA Cream is not recommended in any clinical situation in which penetration or migration beyond the tympanic membrane into the middle ear is possible because of the ototoxic effects observed in animal studies (see WARNINGS).

CONTRAINDICATIONS

EMLA Cream (lidocaine 2.5% and prilocaine 2.5%) is contraindicated in patients with a known history of sensitivity to local anesthetics of the amide type or to any other component of the product.

WARNINGS

Application of EMLA Cream to larger areas or for longer times than those recommended could result in sufficient absorption of lidocaine and prilocaine resulting in serious adverse effects (see Individualization of Dose).

Studies in laboratory animals (guinea pigs) have shown that EMLA Cream has an ototoxic effect when instilled into the middle ear. In these same studies, animals exposed to EMLA Cream in the external auditory canal only, showed no abnormality. EMLA Cream should not be used in any clinical situation in which its penetration or migration beyond the tympanic membrane into the middle ear is possible.

Methemoglobinemia: EMLA Cream should not be used in those rare patients with congenital or idiopathic methemoglobinemia and in infants under the age of twelve months who are receiving treatment with methemoglobin-inducing agents.

Very young patients or patients with glucose-6-phosphate deficiencies are more susceptible to methemoglobinemia.

Patients taking drugs associated with drug-induced methemoglobinemia such as sulfonamides, acetaminophen, acetanilid, aniline dyes, benzocaine, chloroquine, dapsone, naphthalene, nitrates and nitrites, nitrofurantoin, nitroglycerin, nitroprusside, pamaquine, para-aminosalicylic acid, phenacetin, phenobarbital, phenytoin, primaquine, quinine, are also at greater risk for developing methemoglobinemia.

A methemoglobinemia value of 28% (of total hemoglobin) developed in a three-month old male infant (5.3 kg) in clinical trials who had 5 grams of EMLA Cream under an occlusive dressing applied to the back of the hands and in the cubital regions for 5 hours. The methemoglobinemia was successfully treated with IV methylene blue. The patient was concomitantly receiving trimethoprim (16 mg/day) and sulfamethoxazole (80 mg/day) for a urinary tract infection.

PRECAUTIONS

General: Repeated doses of EMLA Cream may increase blood levels of lidocaine and prilocaine. EMLA Cream should be used with caution in patients who may be more sensitive to the systemic effects of lidocaine and prilocaine including acutely ill, debilitated, or elderly patients.

Continued on next page

TABLE 1
Absorption of Lidocaine and Prilocaine from EMLA Cream
Normal Volunteers (N=16)

EMLA (g)	Area (cm^2)	Time on (hrs)	Drug Content (mg)	Absorbed (mg)	Cmax (μg/mL)	Tmax (hr)
60	400	3	lidocaine 1500	54	0.12	4
			prilocaine 1500	92	0.07	4
60	400	24*	lidocaine 1500	243	0.28	10
			prilocaine 1500	503	0.14	10

*Maximum recommended duration of exposure is 4 hours.

Astra—Cont.

EMLA Cream coming in contact with the eye should be avoided because animal studies have demonstrated severe eye irritation. Also the loss of protective reflexes can permit corneal irritation and potential abrasion. Absorption of EMLA Cream in conjunctival tissues has not been determined. If eye contact occurs, immediately wash out the eye with water or saline and protect the eye until sensation returns.

Patients allergic to para-aminobenzoic acid derivatives (procaine, tetracaine, benzocaine, etc.) have not shown cross sensitivity to lidocaine and/or prilocaine, however, EMLA Cream should be used with caution in patients with a history of drug sensitivities, especially if the etiologic agent is uncertain.

Patients with severe hepatic disease, because of their inability to metabolize local anesthetics normally, are at greater risk of developing toxic plasma concentrations of lidocaine and prilocaine.

Information for Patients: When EMLA Cream is used, the patient should be aware that the production of dermal analgesia may be accompanied by the block of all sensations in the treated skin. For this reason, the patient should avoid inadvertent trauma to the treated area by scratching, rubbing, or exposure to extreme hot or cold temperatures until complete sensation has returned.

Drug Interactions: EMLA Cream should be used with caution in patients receiving Class I antiarrhythmic drugs (such as tocainide and mexiletine) since the toxic effects are additive and potentially synergistic.

Prilocaine may contribute to the formation of methemoglobin in patients treated with other drugs known to cause this condition (see Methemoglobinemia subsection of WARNINGS).

Carcinogenesis, Mutagenesis, Impairment of Fertility: Carcinogenesis: Metabolites of both lidocaine and prilocaine have been shown to be carcinogenic in laboratory animals. In the animal studies reported below, doses or blood levels are compared to the Single Dermal Administration (SDA) of 60 g of EMLA Cream to 400 cm^2 for 3 hours to a small person (50 kg). The typical application for one or two treatments for venipuncture sites (2.5 or 5 g) would be $1/24$ or $1/12$ of that dose in an adult or about the same mg/kg dose in an infant.

A two-year oral toxicity study of 2,6-xylidine, a metabolite of lidocaine, has shown that in both male and female rats 2,6-xylidine in daily doses of 900 mg/m^2 (60 times SDA) resulted in carcinomas and adenomas of the nasal cavity. With daily doses of 300 mg/m^2 (20 times SDA), the increase in incidence of nasal carcinomas and/or adenomas in each sex of the rat were not statistically greater than the control group. In the low dose (90 mg/m^2; 6 times SDA) and control groups, no nasal tumors were observed. A rhabdomyosarcoma, a rare tumor, was observed in the nasal cavity of both male and female rats at the high dose of 900 mg/m^2. In addition, the compound caused subcutaneous fibromas and/or fibrosarcomas in both male and female rats and neoplastic nodules of the liver in the female rats with a significantly positive trend test; pairwise comparisons using Fisher's Exact Test showed significance only at the high dose of 900 mg/m^2. The animal study was conducted at oral doses of 15, 50, and 150 mg/kg/day. The dosages have been converted to mg/m^2 for the SDA calculations above.

Chronic oral toxicity studies of *ortho*-toluidine, a metabolite of prilocaine, in mice (900 to 14,400 mg/m^2; 60 to 960 times SDA) and rats (900 to 4,800 mg/m^2; 60 to 320 times SDA) have shown that *ortho*-toluidine is a carcinogen in both species. The tumors included hepatocarcinomas/adenomas in female mice, multiple occurrences of hemangiosarcomas/hemangiomas in both sexes of mice, sarcomas of multiple organs, transitional-cell carcinomas/papillomas of urinary bladder in both sexes of rats, subcutaneous fibromas/fibrosarcomas and mesotheliomas in male rats, and mammary gland fibroadenomas/adenomas in female rats. The lowest dose tested (900 mg/m^2; 60 times SDA) was carcinogenic in both species. Thus the no-effect dose must be less than 60 times SDA. The animal studies were conducted at 150 to 2,400 mg/kg in mice and at 150 to 800 mg/kg in rats. The dosages have been converted to mg/m^2 for the SDA calculations above.

Mutagenesis: The mutagenic potential of lidocaine HCl has been tested in the Ames Salmonella/mammalian microsome test and by analysis of structural chromosome aberrations in human lymphocytes *in vitro*, and by the mouse micronucleus test *in vivo*. There was no indication in these three tests of any mutagenic effects.

The mutagenicity of 2,6-xylidine, a metabolite of lidocaine, has been studied in different tests with mixed results. The compound was found to be weakly mutagenic in the Ames test only under metabolic activation conditions. In addition, 2,6-xylidine was observed to be mutagenic at the thymidine kinase locus, with or without activation, and induced chromosome aberrations and sister chromatid exchanges at con-

centrations at which the drug precipitated out of the solution (1.2 mg/mL). No evidence of genotoxicity was found in the *in vivo* assays measuring unscheduled DNA synthesis in rat hepatocytes, chromosome damage in polychromatic erythrocytes or preferential killing of DNA repair-deficient bacteria in liver, lung, kidney, testes and blood extracts from mice. However, covalent binding studies of DNA from liver and ethmoid turbinates in rats indicate that 2,6-xylidine may be genotoxic under certain conditions *in vivo*.

Ortho-toluidine, a metabolite of prilocaine, (0.5 µg/mL) showed positive results in *Escherichia coli* DNA repair and phage-induction assays. Urine concentrates from rats treated with *ortho*-toluidine (300 mg/kg orally; 300 times SDA) were mutagenic for *Salmonella typhimurium* with metabolic activation. Several other tests on *ortho*-toluidine, including reverse mutations in five different *Salmonella typhimurium* strains with or without metabolic activation and with single strand breaks in DNA of V79 Chinese hamster cells, were negative.

Impairment of Fertility: See Use in Pregnancy.

Use in Pregnancy: Teratogenic Effects: Pregnancy Category B.

Reproduction studies with lidocaine have been performed in rats and have revealed no evidence of harm to the fetus (30 mg/kg subcutaneously; 22 times SDA). Reproduction studies with prilocaine have been performed in rats and have revealed no evidence of impaired fertility or harm to the fetus (300 mg/kg intramuscularly; 188 times SDA). There are, however, no adequate and well-controlled studies in pregnant women. Because animal reproduction studies are not always predictive of human response, EMLA Cream should be used during pregnancy only if clearly needed.

Reproduction studies have been performed in rats receiving subcutaneous administration of an aqueous mixture containing lidocaine HCl and prilocaine HCl at 1:1 (w/w). At 40 mg/kg each, a dose equivalent to 29 times SDA lidocaine and 25 times SDA prilocaine, no teratogenic, embryotoxic or fetotoxic effects were observed.

Labor and Delivery: Neither lidocaine nor prilocaine are contraindicated in labor and delivery. Should EMLA Cream be used concomitantly with other products containing lidocaine and/or prilocaine, total doses contributed by all formulations must be considered.

Nursing Mothers: Lidocaine, and probably prilocaine, are excreted in human milk. Therefore, caution should be exercised when EMLA Cream is administered to a nursing mother since the milk:plasma ratio of lidocaine is 0.4 and is not determined for prilocaine.

Pediatric Use: Controlled studies of EMLA Cream in children under the age of seven years have shown less overall benefit than in older children or adults. These results illustrate the importance of emotional and psychological support of younger children undergoing medical or surgical procedures.

EMLA Cream should be used with care in patients with conditions or therapy associated with methemoglobinemia (see Methemoglobinemia subsection of WARNINGS).

When using EMLA Cream in young children, care must be taken to insure that application of the cream is limited to the intended site (see DOSAGE AND ADMINISTRATION). Accidental ingestion may lead to dose related toxicity.

In children weighing less than 20 kg, the area and duration should be limited (see TABLE 2 in Individualization of Dose).

ADVERSE REACTIONS

Localized Reactions: During or immediately after treatment with EMLA Cream, the skin at the site of treatment may develop erythema or edema or may be the locus of abnormal sensation. Rare cases of hyperpigmentation following the use of EMLA Cream have been reported. The relationship to EMLA Cream or the underlying procedure has not been established. In clinical studies involving over 1,300 EMLA Cream-treated subjects, one or more such local reactions were noted in 56% of patients, and were generally mild and transient, resolving spontaneously within 1 or 2 hours. There were no serious reactions which were ascribed to EMLA Cream.

In patients treated with EMLA Cream, local effects observed in the trials included: paleness (pallor or blanching) 37%, redness (erythema) 30%, alterations in temperature sensations 7%, edema 6%, itching 2% and rash, less than 1%.

Allergic Reactions: Allergic and anaphylactoid reactions associated with lidocaine or prilocaine can occur. They are characterized by urticaria, angioedema, bronchospasm, and shock. If they occur they should be managed by conventional means. The detection of sensitivity by skin testing is of doubtful value.

Systemic (Dose Related) Reactions: Systemic adverse reactions following appropriate use of EMLA Cream are unlikely due to the small dose absorbed (see Pharmacokinetics subsection of CLINICAL PHARMACOLOGY). Systemic adverse effects of lidocaine and/or prilocaine are similar in nature to those observed with other amide local anesthetic agents including CNS excitation and/or depression (light-headedness, nervousness, apprehension, euphoria, confusion, dizziness, drowsiness, tinnitus, blurred or double vision, vomiting, sen-

sations of heat, cold or numbness, twitching, tremors, convulsions, unconsciousness, respiratory depression and arrest). Excitatory CNS reactions may be brief or not occur at all, in which case the first manifestation may be drowsiness merging into unconsciousness. Cardiovascular manifestations may include bradycardia, hypotension and cardiovascular collapse leading to arrest.

OVERDOSAGE

Peak blood levels following a 60 g application to 400 cm^2 for 3 hours are 0.05 to 0.16 µg/mL for lidocaine and 0.02 to 0.10 µg/mL for prilocaine. Toxic levels of lidocaine (> 5 µg/mL) and/or prilocaine (> 6 µg/mL) cause decreases in cardiac output, total peripheral resistance and mean arterial pressure. These changes may be attributable to direct depressant effects of these local anesthetic agents on the cardiovascular system. In the absence of massive topical overdose or oral ingestion, evaluation should include evaluation of other etiologies for the clinical effects or overdosage from other sources of lidocaine, prilocaine or other local anesthetics. Consult the package inserts for parenteral Xylocaine (lidocaine HCl) or Citanest (prilocaine HCl) for further information for the management of overdose.

DOSAGE AND ADMINISTRATION

A thick layer of EMLA Cream is applied to intact skin and covered with an occlusive dressing:

Minor Dermal Procedures: For minor procedures such as intravenous cannulation and venipuncture, apply 2.5 grams of EMLA Cream ($1/2$ the 5 g tube) over 20 to 25 cm^2 of skin surface for at least 1 hour. In controlled clinical trials, two sites were usually prepared in case there was a technical problem with cannulation or venipuncture at the first site.

Major Dermal Procedures: For more painful dermatological procedures involving a larger skin area such as split thickness skin graft harvesting, apply 2 grams of EMLA Cream per 10 cm^2 of skin and allow to remain in contact with the skin for at least 2 hours.

Dermal analgesia can be expected to increase for up to 3 hours under occlusive dressing and persist for 1 to 2 hours after removal of the cream. The amount of lidocaine and prilocaine absorbed during the period of application can be estimated from the information in Table 2, ** footnote, in Individualization of Dose.

A single application of EMLA Cream in a child weighing less than 10 kg should not be applied over an area larger than 100 cm^2. A single application of EMLA Cream in children weighing between 10 kg and 20 kg should not be applied over an area larger than 600 cm^2 (see Table 2 in Individualization of Dose).

When applying EMLA Cream to young children, care must be taken to maintain careful observation of the child to prevent accidental ingestion of EMLA Cream or the occlusive dressing. A secondary protective covering to prevent inadvertent disruption of the application site may be useful.

EMLA Cream should not be used in infants under the age of one month nor in infants under the age of twelve months who are receiving treatment with methemoglobin-inducing agents (see Methemoglobinemia subsection of WARNINGS).

When EMLA Cream (lidocaine 2.5% and prilocaine 2.5%) is used concomitantly with other products containing local anesthetic agents, the amount absorbed from all formulations must be considered (see Individualization of Dose). The amount absorbed in the case of EMLA Cream is determined by the area over which it is applied and the duration of application under occlusion (see Table 2, ** footnote, in Individualization of Dose).

Although the incidence of systemic adverse reactions with EMLA Cream is very low, caution should be exercised, particularly when applying it over large areas and leaving it on for longer than 2 hours. The incidence of systemic adverse reactions can be expected to be directly proportional to the area and time of exposure (see Individualization of Dose).

HOW SUPPLIED

EMLA Cream is available as the following:
NDC 0186-1515-01   5 gram tube, box of 1,
   contains 2 Tegaderm® dressings (6 cm × 7 cm)
NDC 0186-1515-03   5 gram tube, box of 5,
   contains 12 Tegaderm® dressings (6 cm × 7 cm)
NDC 0186-1516-01   30 gram tube, box of 1
NOT FOR OPHTHALMIC USE.
KEEP CONTAINER TIGHTLY CLOSED AT ALL TIMES WHEN NOT IN USE.
Store at controlled room temperature 15°–30°C (59°–86°F).
Manufactured by:
Astra Pharmaceutical Production, AB
Södertälje, Sweden
Manufactured for:
ASTRA®
Astra USA, Inc.   09-050-88-0-80
Westborough, MA 01581   000425R06   Rev. 11/95

INSTRUCTIONS FOR APPLICATION

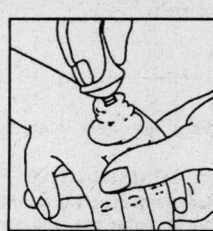

1. Apply 2.5 g of cream ($^1/_2$ the 5 g tube) per 20 to 25 cm^2 (approx. 2 in. by 2 in.) of skin in a thick layer at the site of the procedure.

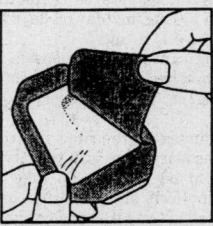

2. Take an occlusive dressing (provided with the 5 g tubes only) and remove the center cut-out piece.

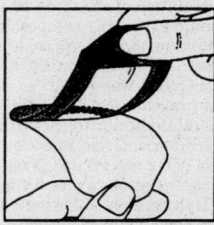

3. Peel the paper liner from the paper framed dressing.

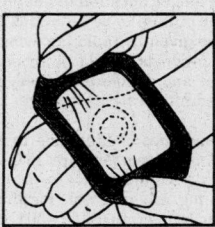

4. Cover the EMLA® Cream so that you get a thick layer underneath. Do not spread out the cream. Smooth down the dressing edges carefully and ensure it is secure to avoid leakage. (This is especially important when the patient is a child.)

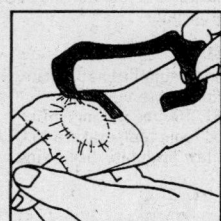

5. Remove the paper frame. The time of application can easily be marked directly on the occlusive dressing. EMLA® must be applied at least 1 hour before the start of a routine procedure and for 2 hours before the start of a painful procedure.

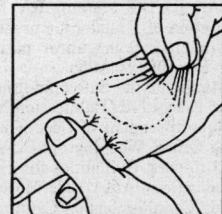

6. Remove the occlusive dressing, wipe off the EMLA® Cream, clean the entire area with an antiseptic solution and prepare the patient for the procedure. The duration of effective skin anesthesia will be at least 1 hour after removal of the occlusive dressing.

PRECAUTIONS

1. Do not apply near eyes or on open wounds.
2. Do not use in children under one month of age.
3. Keep out of reach of children.

Manufactured by:
Astra Pharmaceutical Production, AB
Södertälje, Sweden
Manufactured for:
ASTRA®
Astra USA, Inc.
Westborough, MA 01581   000425R06
Shown in Product Identification Guide, page 304

EPINEPHRINE   ℞
[ep-ē-nef'-rin]
Injection, USP
1:10,000 (0.1 mg/mL)
Adult Strength

(For details of indications, dosage and administration, precautions, and adverse reactions, see circular in package.)

HOW SUPPLIED
Epinephrine Injection, USP, 1:10,000, is supplied in 10 mL prefilled syringes with a 21 G $^{15}/_{16}''$ needle. (NDC 0186-0653-01) The solution should be stored at controlled room temperature 15°–30°C (59°–86°F) and should be protected from light by storage in the original carton until use.
021883R03   Rev. 7/91 (3)

ETOPOSIDE   ℞
INJECTION

> **WARNINGS**
> Etoposide should be administered under the supervision of a qualified physician experienced in the use of cancer chemotherapeutic agents. Severe myelosuppression with resulting infection or bleeding may occur.

DESCRIPTION
Etoposide (also commonly known as VP-16) is a semisynthetic derivative of podophyllotoxin used in the treatment of certain neoplastic diseases. It is 4'-demethylepipodophyllotoxin 9-[4,6-0-(R) ethylidene-β-D-glucopyranoside]. It is very soluble in methanol and chloroform, slightly soluble in ethanol, and sparingly soluble in water and ether. It is made more miscible with water by means of organic solvents. It has a molecular weight of 588.58 and a molecular formula of $C_{29}H_{32}O_{13}$.
Etoposide injection is available for intravenous use as 20 mg/mL (100 mg/5 mL) sterile solution in 5 mL multiple dose vials. The pH of the clear yellow solution is 3 to 4. Each mL contains 20 mg etoposide, 2 mg citric acid, 30 mg benzyl alcohol, 80 mg polysorbate 80, 650 mg polyethylene glycol 300, and 30.5 percent (v/v) alcohol. The structural formula is:

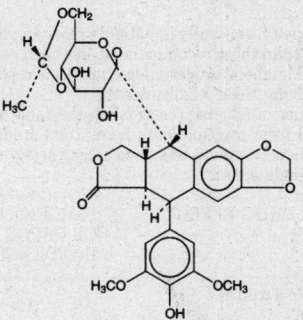

CLINICAL PHARMACOLOGY
Etoposide has been shown to cause metaphase arrest in chick fibroblasts. Its main effect, however, appears to be at the G_2 portion of the cell cycle in mammalian cells. Two different dose-dependent responses are seen. At high concentrations (10 μg/mL or more), lysis of cells entering mitosis is observed. At low concentrations (0.3 to 10 μg/mL), cells are inhibited from entering prophase. It does not interfere with microtubular assembly. The predominant macromolecular effect of etoposide appears to be DNA synthesis inhibition.
Pharmacokinetics: On intravenous administration, the disposition of etoposide is best described as a biphasic process with a distribution half-life of about 1.5 hours and terminal elimination half-life ranging from 4 to 11 hours. Total body clearance values range from 33 to 48 mL/min or 16 to 36

mL/min/m^2 and, like the terminal elimination half-life, are independent of dose over a range 100 to 600 mg/m^2. Over the same dose range, the areas under the plasma concentration vs. time curves (AUC) and the maximum plasma concentration (C_{max}) values increase linearly with dose. Etoposide does not accumulate in the plasma following daily administration of 100 mg/m^2 for 4 to 5 days.
The mean volumes of distribution at steady state fall in the range of 18 to 29 liters or 7 to 17 L/m^2. Etoposide enters the CSF poorly. Although it is detectable in CSF and intracerebral tumors, the concentrations are lower than in extracerebral tumors and in plasma. Etoposide concentrations are higher in normal lung than in lung metastases and are similar in primary tumors and normal tissues of the myometrium. *In vitro*, etoposide is highly protein bound (97%) to human plasma proteins. An inverse relationship between plasma albumin levels and etoposide renal clearance is found in children. In a study determining the effect of other therapeutic agents in the *in vitro* binding of carbon-14 labeled etoposide to human serum proteins, only phenylbutazone, sodium salicylate and aspirin displaced protein-bound etoposide at concentrations achieved *in vivo*[1].
Etoposide binding ratio correlates directly with serum albumin in patients with cancer and in normal volunteers. The unbound fraction of etoposide significantly correlated with bilirubin in a population of cancer patients[2,3].
After intravenous administration of ^{3}H-etoposide (70 to 290 mg/m^2), mean recoveries of radioactivity in the urine range from 42 to 67%, and fecal recoveries range from 0 to 16% of the dose. Less than 50% of an intravenous dose is excreted in the urine as etoposide with mean recoveries of 8 to 35% within 24 hours.
In children, approximately 55% of the dose is excreted in the urine as etoposide in 24 hours. The mean renal clearance of etoposide is 7 to 10 mL/min/m^2 or about 35% of the total body clearance over a dose range of 80 to 600 mg/m^2. Etoposide, therefore, is cleared by both renal and nonrenal processes, i.e., metabolism and biliary excretion. The effect of renal disease on plasma etoposide clearance is not known. Biliary excretion appears to be a minor route of etoposide elimination. Only 6% or less of an intravenous dose is recovered in the bile as etoposide. Metabolism accounts for most of the nonrenal clearance of etoposide. The major urinary metabolite of etoposide in adults and children is the hydroxy acid [4'-demethylepipodophyllic acid-9-[4,6-0-(R)-ethylidene-β-D-glucopyranoside)], formed by opening of the lactone ring. It is also present in human plasma, presumably as the trans isomer. Glucuronide and/or sulfate conjugates of etoposide are excreted in human urine and represent 5 to 22% of the dose.
After intravenous infusion, the C_{max} and AUC values exhibit marked intra- and inter-subject variability.
In adults, the total body clearance of etoposide is correlated with creatinine clearance, serum albumin concentration, and nonrenal clearance. In children, elevated serum SGPT levels are associated with reduced drug total body clearance. Prior use of cisplatin may also result in a decrease of etoposide total body clearance in children.

INDICATIONS AND USAGE
Etoposide Injection is indicated in the management of the following neoplasms:
Refractory Testicular Tumors—In combination therapy with other approved chemotherapeutic agents in patients with refractory testicular tumors who have already received appropriate surgical, chemotherapeutic, and radiotherapeutic therapy.
Small Cell Lung Cancer—Etoposide injection and/or capsules in combination with other approved chemotherapeutic agents as first line treatment in patients with small cell lung cancer.

CONTRAINDICATIONS
Etoposide Injection is contraindicated in patients who have demonstrated a previous hypersensitivity to it.

WARNINGS
Patients being treated with etoposide must be frequently observed for myelosuppression both during and after therapy. Dose-limiting bone marrow suppression is the most significant toxicity associated with etoposide therapy. Therefore, the following studies should be obtained at the start of therapy and prior to each subsequent dose of etoposide: platelet count, hemoglobin, white blood cell count, and differential. The occurrence of a platelet count below 50,000/mm^3 or an absolute neutrophil count below 500/mm^3 is an indication to withhold further therapy until the blood counts have sufficiently recovered.
Physicians should be aware of the possible occurrence of an anaphylactic reaction manifested by chills, fever, tachycardia, bronchospasm, dyspnea, and hypotension. (See "**ADVERSE REACTIONS**" section). Treatment is symptomatic. The infusion should be terminated immediately, followed by the administration of pressor agents, corticosteroids, antihis-

Continued on next page

Astra—Cont.

tamines, or volume expanders at the discretion of the physician.

Etoposide injection should be given only by slow intravenous infusion (usually over a 30 to 60 minute period) since hypotension has been reported as a possible side effect of rapid intravenous injection.

Pregnancy: Pregnancy "Category D". Etoposide can cause fetal harm when administered to pregnant women. Etoposide has been shown to be teratogenic in mice and rats. There are no adequate and well-controlled studies in pregnant women. If this drug is used during pregnancy, or if the patient becomes pregnant while receiving this drug, the patient should be apprised of the potential hazard to the fetus. Women of childbearing potential should be advised to avoid becoming pregnant.

Etoposide is teratogenic and embryocidal in rats and mice at doses of 1 to 3% of the recommended clinical dose based on body surface area.

In a teratology study in SPF rats, etoposide was administered intravenously at doses of 0.13, 0.4, 1.2, and 3.6 mg/kg/day on days 6 to 15 of gestation. Etoposide caused dose-related maternal toxicity, embryotoxicity, and teratogenicity at dose levels of 0.4 mg/kg/day and higher. Embryonic resorptions were 90 and 100% at the 2 highest dosages. At 0.4 and 1.2 mg/kg, fetal weights were decreased and fetal abnormalities including decreased weight, major skeletal abnormalities, exencephaly, encephalocele, and anophthalmia occurred. Even at the lowest dose tested, 0.13 mg/kg, a significant increase in retarded ossification was observed.

Etoposide administered as a single intraperitoneal, injection in Swiss-Albino mice at dosages of 1, 1.5 and 2 mg/kg on days 6, 7, or 8 of gestation caused dose-related embryotoxicity, cranial abnormalities, and major skeletal malformations.

PRECAUTIONS

General: In all instances where the use of etoposide is considered for chemotherapy, the physician must evaluate the need and usefulness of the drug against the risk of adverse reactions. Most such adverse reactions are reversible if detected early. If severe reactions occur, the drug should be reduced in dosage or discontinued and appropriate corrective measures should be taken according to the clinical judgement of the physician. Reinstitution of etoposide therapy should be carried out with caution, and with adequate consideration of the further need for the drug and alertness as to possible recurrence of toxicity.

Laboratory Tests: Periodic complete blood counts should be done during the course of etoposide treatment. They should be performed prior to therapy and at appropriate intervals during and after therapy. At least one determination should be done prior to each dose of etoposide.

Carcinogenesis, Mutagenesis, Impairment of Fertility: Carcinogenicity tests with etoposide have not been conducted in laboratory animals. Etoposide should be considered a potential carcinogen in humans. The occurence of acute leukemia with a preleukemic phase has been reported rarely in patients treated with etoposide in association with other antineo-plastic agents.

The mutagenic and genotoxic potential of etoposide has been established in mammalian cells. Etoposide caused aberrations in chromosome number and structure in embryonic murine cells and human hematopoietic cells; gene mutations in Chinese hamster ovary cells; and DNA damage by strand breakage and DNA-protein cross-links in mouse leukemia cells. Etoposide also caused a dose-related increase in sister chromatid exchanges in Chinese hamster ovary cells.

Treatment of Swiss-Albino mice with 1.5 mg/kg IP of etoposide on day 7 of gestation increased the incidence of intra-uterine death and fetal malformations as well as significantly decreased the average fetal body weight. Maternal weight gain was not affected.

Treatment of pregnant SPF rats with 1.2 mg/kg/day IV of etoposide for 10 days led to a prenatal mortality of 92%, and 50% of the implanting fetuses were abnormal.

Pregnancy: Pregnancy "Category D" (See **"WARNINGS"** section).

Nursing Mothers: It is not known whether this drug is excreted in human milk. Because many drugs are excreted in human milk and because of the potential for serious adverse reactions in nursing infants from etoposide, a decision should be made whether to discontinue nursing or to discontinue the drug, taking into account the importance of the drug to the mother.

Pediatric Use: Safety and effectiveness in pediatric patients have not been establlished.

Etoposide Injection contains polysorbate 80. In premature infants, a life-threatening syndrome consisting of liver and renal failure, pulmonary deterioration, thrombocytopenia, and ascites has been associated with an injectable vitamin E product containing polysorbate 80.

ADVERSE REACTIONS

The following data on adverse reactions are based on both oral and intravenous administration of etoposide as a single agent, using several different dose schedules for treatment of a wide variety of malignancies.

Hematologic Toxicity: Myelosuppression is dose related and dose limiting, with granulocyte nadirs occurring 7 to 14 days after drug administration and platelet nadirs occurring 9 to 16 days after drug administration. Bone marrow recovery is usually complete by day 20, and no cumulative toxicity has been reported.

The occurrence of acute leukemia with or without a preleukemic phase has been reported rarely in patients treated with etoposide in association with other antineoplastic agents.

Gastrointestinal Toxicity: Nausea and vomiting are the major gastrointestinal toxicities. The severity of such nausea and vomiting is generally mild to moderate with treatment discontinuation required in 1% of patients. Nausea and vomiting can usually be controlled with standard antiemetic therapy. Gastrointestinal toxicities are slightly more frequent after oral administration than after intravenous infusion.

Hypotension: Transient hypotension following rapid intravenous administration has been reported in 1% to 2% of patients. It has not been associated with cardiac toxicity or electrocardiographic changes. No delayed hypotension has been noted. To prevent this rare occurrence, it is recommended that etoposide be administered by slow intravenous infusion over a 30 to 60 minute period. If hypotension occurs, it usually responds to cessation of the infusion and administration of fluids or other supportive therapy as appropriate. When restarting the infusion, a slower administration rate should be used.

Allergic Reactions: Anaphylactic-like reactions characterized by chills, fever, tachycardia, bronchospasm, dyspnea, and/or hypotension have been reported to occur in 0.7% to 2% of patients receiving intravenous etoposide and in less than 1% of the patients treated with the oral capsules. These reactions have usually responded promptly to the cessation of the infusion and administration of pressor agents, corticosteroids, antihistamines, or volume expanders as appropriate; however, the reactions can be fatal. Hypertension and/or flushing have also been reported. Blood pressure usually normalizes within a few hours after cessation of the infusion. Anaphylactic-like reactions have occurred during the initial infusion of etoposide.

Facial/tongue swelling, coughing, diaphoresis, cyanosis, tightness in throat, laryngospasm, back pain, and/or loss of consciousness have sometimes occurred in association with the above reactions. In addition, an apparent hypersensitivity, associated apnea has been reported rarely.

Rash, urticaria, and/or pruritis have infrequently been reported at recommended doses. At investigational doses, a generalized pruritic erythymatous maculopapular rash, consistent with perivasculitis, has been reported.

Alopecia: Reversible alopecia, sometimes progressing to total baldness was observed in up to 66% of patients.

Other Toxicities: The following adverse reactions have been infrequently reported: aftertaste, fever, pigmentation, abdominal pain, constipation, dysphagia, transient cortical blindness, optical neuritis and a single report of radiation recall dermatitis.

Hepatic toxicity, generally in patients receiving higher doses of the drug than those recommended, has been reported with etoposide. Metabolic acidosis also has been reported in patients receiving these higher doses.

The incidence of adverse reactions in the table that follows are derived from multiple data bases from studies in 2,081 patients when etoposide was used either orally or by injection as a single agent.

ADVERSE DRUG EFFECT	PERCENT RANGE OF REPORTED INCIDENCE
Hematologic Toxicity	
Leukopenia (less than 1,000 WBC/mm³)	3-17
Leukopenia (less than 4,000 WBC/mm³)	60-91
Thrombocytopenia (less than 50,000 platelets/mm³)	1-20
Thrombocytopenia (less than 100,000 platelets/mm³)	22-41
Anemia	0-33
Gastrointestinal Toxicity	
Nausea and vomiting	31-43
Abdominal pain	0-2
Anorexia	10-13
Diarrhea	1-13
Stomatitis	1-6
Hepatic	0-3
Alopecia	8-66
Peripheral neurotoxicity	1-2
Hypotension	1-2
Allergic reactions	1-2

OVERDOSAGE

No proven antidotes have been established for etoposide overdosage.

DOSAGE AND ADMINISTRATION

Note: Plastic devices made of acrylic or ABS (a polymer composed of acrylonitrile, butadiene, and styrene) have been reported to crack and leak when used with undiluted Etoposide Injection.

The usual dose of Etoposide Injection in testicular cancer in combination with other approved chemotherapeutic agents ranges from 50 to 100 mg/m²/day on days 1 through 5 to 100 mg/m²/ day on days 1, 3, and 5.

In small cell lung cancer, the Etoposide Injection dose in combination with other approved chemotherapeutic drugs ranges from 35 mg/m²/day for 4 days to 50 mg/m²/day for 5 days.

Chemotherapy courses are repeated at 3- to 4-week intervals after adequate recovery from any toxicity.

The dosage should be modified to take into account the myelosuppressive effects of other drugs in the combination or the effects of prior X-ray therapy or chemotherapy which may have compromised bone marrow reserve.

Administration Precautions: As with other potentially toxic compounds, caution should be exercised in handling and preparing the solution of etoposide. Skin reactions associated with accidental exposure to etoposide may occur. The use of gloves is recommended. If etoposide solution contacts the skin or mucosa, immediately wash the skin or mucosa thoroughly with soap and water.

Preparation for Intravenous Administration: Etoposide Injection must be diluted prior to use with either dextrose injection 5% or sodium chloride injection 0.9%, to give a final concentration of 0.2 mg/mL to 0.4 mg/mL. If solutions are prepared at concentrations above 0.4 mg/mL, precipitation may occur. Hypotension following rapid intravenous administration has been reported, hence, it is recommended that the etoposide solution is administered over a 30 to 60 minute period. A longer duration of administration may be used if the volume of fluid to be infused is a concern. **Etoposide should not be given by rapid intravenous injection.**

Parenteral drug products should be inspected visually for particulate matter and discoloration (see "DESCRIPTION" section) prior to administration whenever solution and container permit.

Stability: Unopened vials of Etoposide Injection are stable for 24 months at room temperature 15°C–30°C (59°F–86°F). Vials diluted as recommended to a concentration of 0.2 mg/mL or 0.4 mg/mL are stable for 96 and 24 hours, respectively, at room temperature 15°C–30°C (59°F–86°F) under normal room fluorescent light in both glass and plastic containers.

Procedures for proper handling and disposal of anticancer drugs should be considered. Several guidelines on this subject have been published[4-10]. There is no general agreement that all of the procedures recommended in the guidelines are necessary or appropriate.

HOW SUPPLIED

Etoposide Injection is supplied as a sterile, clear, yellow solution, in a 5 mL multi-dose vial.

NDC 0186-1571-31, 100 mg (20 mg/mL).

Store at controlled room temperature 15°C–30°C (59°F–86°F).

Caution: Federal law prohibits dispensing without prescription.

REFERENCES

1. Gaver RC, Deeb G. The effect of other drugs on the in vitro binding of ^{14}C-etoposide to human serum proteins. Proc Am Assoc Cancer Res 1989;30:A2132.
2. Stewart CF, Pieper JA, Arbuck SG, Evans WE. Altered protein binding of etoposide in patients with cancer. Clin Pharmacol Ther 1989;45:49–55.
3. Stewart CF, Arbuck SG, Fleming RA, Evans WE. Prospective evaluation of a model for predicting etoposide plasma protein binding in cancer patients. Proc Am Assoc Cancer Res 1989;30:A958.
4. Recommendations for the Safe Handling of Parenteral Antineoplastic Drugs. NIH Publication No. 83–2621. For sale by the Superintendent of Documents, US Government Printing Office, Washington, DC 20402.
5. AMA Council Report. Guidelines for Handling Parenteral Antineoplastics. JAMA 1985 March 15.
6. National Study Commissions on Cytotoxic Exposure—Recommendations for Handling Cytotoxic Agents. Available from Louis P. Jeffrey, Sc.D., Chairman, National Study Commission on Cytotoxic Exposure, Massachusetts College of Pharmacy and Allied Health Sciences, 179 Longwood Avenue, Boston, Massachusetts 02115.

7. Clinical Oncological Society of Australia. Guidelines and Recommendations for Safe Handling of Antineoplastic Agents. Med J Australia 1983;1:426–428.

8. Jones RB, et al: Safe handling of chemotherapeutic agents: A report from the Mount Sinai Medical Center. CA—A Cancer Journal for Clinicians 1983;Sept/Oct:258–263.

9. American Society of Hospital Pharmacists Technical Assistance Bulletin on Handling Cytotoxic and Hazardous Drugs. Am J Hosp Pharm 1990;47:1033–1049.

10. OSHA Work-Practice Guidelines for Personnel Dealing with Cytotoxic (Antineoplastic) Drugs. Am J Hosp Pharm 1986;43:1193–1204.

MANUFACTURED BY
PHARMACHEMIE B.V.
Haarlem
The Netherlands
MANUFACTURED FOR
ASTRA®
Astra USA, Inc.
Westborough, MA 01581
021796R01
DATE
June, 1995
021796R01 Iss. 6/95

FENTANYL CITRATE* and DROPERIDOL Ⅽ Ⅱ ℞ INJECTION
*WARNING: May be habit forming.
FOR INTRAVENOUS OR INTRAMUSCULAR USE ONLY.

The two components of Fentanyl Citrate and Droperidol Injection, fentanyl citrate and droperidol, have different pharmacologic actions. Before administering Fentanyl Citrate and Droperidol Injection, the user should become familiar with the special properties of each drug, particularly the widely differing durations of action.

(For details of indication, dosage and administration, precautions, and adverse reactions, see circular in package.)

HOW SUPPLIED
Each mL of Fentanyl Citrate and Droperidol Injection contains fentanyl citrate (WARNING: May be habit forming) equivalent to 0.05 mg (50 mcg) of fentanyl base, droperidol 2.5 mg and lactic acid to adjust pH and is available in the following dosage forms:
Ampules
NDC 0186-1230-03, 2 mL ampule packages of 10
NDC 0186-1231-03, 5 mL ampule packages of 10
Vials
NDC 0186-1232-13, 2 mL single dose vial packages of 10
NDC 0186-1233-13, 5 mL single dose vial packages of 10
(FOR INTRAVENOUS USE BY HOSPITAL PERSONNEL SPECIFICALLY TRAINED IN THE USE OF OPIOID ANALGESICS.)
Protect from light. Store at controlled room temperature 15°–30°C (59°–86°F).
Caution: Federal law prohibits dispensing without prescription.
021881R03   Rev. 12/94

FOSCAVIR®   ℞
(foscarnet sodium) Injection

RENAL IMPAIRMENT IS THE MAJOR TOXICITY OF FOSCAVIR, AND OCCURS TO SOME DEGREE IN MOST PATIENTS. CONSEQUENTLY, CONTINUAL ASSESSMENT OF A PATIENT'S RISK AND FREQUENT MONITORING OF SERUM CREATININE WITH DOSE ADJUSTMENT FOR CHANGES IN RENAL FUNCTION ARE IMPERATIVE.
FOSCAVIR HAS BEEN SHOWN TO CAUSE ALTERATIONS IN PLASMA MINERALS AND ELECTROLYTES THAT HAVE LED TO SEIZURES. THEREFORE, PATIENTS MUST BE MONITORED FREQUENTLY FOR SUCH CHANGES AND THEIR POTENTIAL SEQUELAE.
FOSCAVIR IS INDICATED FOR USE ONLY IN THE TREATMENT OF CMV RETINITIS AND MUCOCUTANEOUS ACYCLOVIR-RESISTANT HSV INFECTIONS IN IMMUNOCOMPROMISED PATIENTS. (See INDICATIONS section.)

DESCRIPTION
FOSCAVIR is the brand name for foscarnet sodium. The chemical name of foscarnet sodium is phosphonoformic acid, trisodium salt. Foscarnet sodium is a white, crystalline powder containing 6 equivalents of water of hydration with an empirical formula of $Na_3CO_5P \bullet 6 H_2O$ and a molecular weight of 300.1. The structural formula is:

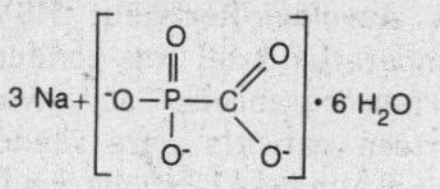

$$3\,Na+ \left[\begin{array}{c} O \\ \| \\ O-P-C \\ | \\ O- \end{array} \begin{array}{c} O \\ \| \\ \\ O- \end{array} \right] \bullet 6 H_2O$$

FOSCAVIR has the potential to chelate divalent metal ions, such as calcium and magnesium, to form stable coordination compounds. FOSCAVIR INJECTION is a sterile, isotonic aqueous solution for intravenous administration only. The solution is clear and colorless. Each milliliter of FOSCAVIR contains 24 mg of foscarnet sodium hexahydrate in Water for Injection, USP. Hydrochloric acid and/or sodium hydroxide may have been added to adjust the pH of the solution to 7.4. FOSCAVIR INJECTION contains no preservatives.

CLINICAL PHARMACOLOGY
Microbiology: *Mechanism of Action:* FOSCAVIR is an organic analogue of inorganic pyrophosphate that inhibits replication of all known herpesviruses *in vitro* including cytomegalovirus (CMV), herpes simplex virus types 1 and 2 (HSV-1, HSV-2), human herpesvirus 6 (HHV-6), Epstein-Barr virus (EBV), and varicella-zoster virus (VZV). FOSCAVIR exerts its antiviral activity by a selective inhibition at the pyrophosphate binding site on virus-specific DNA polymerases and reverse transcriptases at concentrations that do not affect cellular DNA polymerases. FOSCAVIR does not require activation (phosphorylation) by thymidine kinase or other kinases, and therefore is active *in vitro* against HSV TK deficient mutants and CMV UL97 mutants. Thus, HSV strains resistant to acyclovir or CMV strains resistant to ganciclovir may be sensitive to FOSCAVIR. However, acyclovir or ganciclovir resistant mutants with alterations in the viral DNA polymerase may be resistant to FOSCAVIR and may not respond to therapy with FOSCAVIR.

Antiviral Activity: The quantitative relationship between the *in vitro* susceptibility of human cytomegalovirus (CMV) or mucocutaneous herpes simplex virus 1 and 2 (HSV-1 and HSV-2) to FOSCAVIR and clinical response to therapy has not been clearly established in man and virus sensitivity testing has not been standardized. Sensitivity test results, expressed as the concentration of drug required to inhibit by 50% the growth of virus in cell culture (IC_{50}), vary greatly depending on the assay method used, cell type employed and the laboratory performing the test. A number of sensitive viruses and their IC_{50} values are listed below.

TABLE 1

FOSCARNET Inhibition of virus multiplication in cell culture

Virus	IC_{50} (μM)
CMV	50–800*
HSV-1, HSV-2	10–130
VZV	48–90
EBV	< 500**
HHV-6	< 67***
Ganciclovir resistant CMV	190
HSV-TK minus mutant	67
HSV-DNA polymerase mutants	5–443

* Mean = 269 μM
** 97% of viral antigen synthesis inhibited at 500 μM
*** IC_{100} = 67 μM

Clinical isolates of CMV taken from patients show different sensitivities to FOSCAVIR *in vitro*. Statistically significant decreases in positive CMV cultures from blood and urine have been demonstrated in two studies (FOS-03 and ACTG-015/915) of patients treated with FOSCAVIR. Although median time to progression of CMV retinitis was increased in patients treated with the drug, reductions in positive blood or urine cultures have not been shown to correlate with clinical efficacy in individual patients.

TABLE 2
BLOOD AND URINE CULTURE RESULTS FROM CMV RETINITIS PATIENTS*

Blood	+CMV	–CMV
Baseline	27	34
End of Induction**	1	60

Urine	+CMV	–CMV
Baseline	52	6
End of Induction**	21	37

*A combined total of 77 patients were treated with FOSCAVIR in two clinical trials (FOS-03 and ACTG-015/915). Not all patients had blood or urine cultures done and some patients had results from both cultures.
**(60 mg/kg FOSCAVIR TID for 2–3 weeks).

Drug Resistance: Strains of both HSV and CMV that are resistant to FOSCAVIR can be readily selected *in vitro* by passage of wild type virus in the presence of increasing concentrations of the drug. All FOSCAVIR resistant mutants are known to be generated through mutation in the viral DNA polymerase gene. If no clinical response to FOSCAVIR is observed, viral isolates should be tested for sensitivity to foscarnet as naturally resistant mutants may emerge under selective pressure both *in vitro* and *in vivo*. The latent state of any of the human herpesviruses is not known to be sensitive to FOSCAVIR and viral reactivation of CMV occurs after FOSCAVIR therapy is terminated. In patients treated with FOSCAVIR for mucocutaneous acyclovir-resistant HSV infections, reactivation may be with HSV sensitive to acyclovir. Therefore, in the case of a relapse, sensitivity testing of the viral isolate is advised.

Pharmacokinetics: *Protein Binding: In vitro* studies have shown that 14–17% of foscarnet is bound to plasma protein at plasma drug concentrations of 1–1000 μM.

Plasma Concentrations: The pharmacokinetics of FOSCAVIR infusions have been determined when administered as an intermittent infusion during induction therapy in AIDS patients with CMV retinitis. Observed plasma foscarnet concentrations in two studies (FOS-01 and ACTG-015 respectively) are summarized in the following table:

[See table 3 at bottom of next page.]

Clearance: Mean ($\pm SD$) plasma clearances were 130 ± 44 and 178 ± 48 mL/min in two studies in which FOSCAVIR was given by intermittent infusion (ACTG-015 and FOS-01 respectively), and 152 ± 59 and 214 ± 25 mL/min/1.73 m^2 in two studies using continuous infusion. Approximately 80–90% of IV FOSCAVIR is excreted unchanged in the urine of patients with normal renal function. Urinary excretion data suggest that both tubular secretion and glomerular filtration account for urinary elimination of foscarnet. In one study, plasma clearance was less than creatinine clearance, suggesting that FOSCAVIR may also undergo tubular reabsorption. In three studies, decreases in plasma clearance of FOSCAVIR were proportional to decreases in creatinine clearance.

Half-life: Two studies (FOS-01 and ACTG-015) in patients with initially normal renal function who were treated with intermittent infusions of FOSCAVIR showed average drug plasma half-lives of about three hours determined on days 1 or 3 of therapy. This may be an underestimate of the effective half-life of FOSCAVIR due to the limited duration of the observation period. The plasma half-life of FOSCAVIR increases with the severity of renal impairment. Half-lives of 2–8 hours have been reported in patients having estimated or measured 24-hour creatinine clearances of 44–90 mL/min. Careful monitoring of renal function and dose adjustment in patients on FOSCAVIR is imperative (see WARNINGS and DOSAGE AND ADMINISTRATION). Following the continuous infusion of FOSCAVIR for 72 hours in six HIV+ patients, plasma half-lives of 0.45 ± 0.32 and 3.3 ± 1.3 hours were determined. A terminal half-life (λ_3) of 18 ± 2.8 hours was estimated from the urinary excretion of foscarnet over 48 hours after stopping the infusion. When FOSCAVIR was administered as a continuous infusion to 13 patients with HIV infection for 8 to 21 days, plasma half-lives of 1.4 ± 0.6 and 6.8 ± 5.0 hours were determined. A terminal half-life of 87.5 ± 41.8 hours was estimated from the urinary excretion of foscarnet over six days after the last infusion; however, the renal function of these patients at the time of discontinuing the FOSCAVIR infusion was not known.

Measurements of urinary excretion are required to detect the longer terminal half-life assumed to represent release of foscarnet from bone. In animal studies (mice), 40% of an intravenous dose of FOSCAVIR is deposited in bone in young animals and 7% in adults. Postmortem data on several patients in European clinical trials provide evidence that foscarnet does accumulate in bone in humans; however, the extent to which this occurs has not been determined.

Volume of Distribution: Mean volumes of distribution at steady state range from 0.3–0.6 L/kg.

Cerebrospinal Fluid: Variable penetration of FOSCAVIR into cerebrospinal fluid has been observed. Intermittent infusion of 50 mg/kg of FOSCAVIR every 8 hours for 28 days in 9 patients produced foscarnet CSF levels 3 hours after the end of the infusion of 150–260 μM or 39–103% of plasma levels. In another 4 patients, the CSF concentrations of foscarnet were 35–69% of the plasma drug level after a dose of 230 mg/kg/day by continuous infusion for 2–13 days; however, the CSF:plasma ratio was only 13% in one patient while receiving a continuous infusion of FOSCAVIR at a rate of 274 mg/kg/day. Disease-related defects in the blood-brain barrier may be responsible for the variations seen.

Pharmacodynamics: A pharmacodynamic analysis of patient data from one U.S. clinical trial (FOS-01) revealed a relationship between cumulative exposure to foscarnet (product of plasma foscarnet concentration x time) and changes in renal function (serum creatinine) during induc-

Continued on next page

Astra—Cont.

tion. All patients had their doses adjusted according to the recommended FOSCAVIR dosing nomogram. Seventeen of 24 patients (72%) showed evidence of renal impairment (> 20% suppression from baseline estimated creatinine clearance) during induction. This occurred in 3 patients on days 5–6, in 11 patients on days 7–14 and in 3 patients after day 14. Eleven patients had at least 40% suppression from baseline estimated creatinine clearance and six patients had more than 50% suppression, demonstrating that patients vary in their degree of sensitivity to FOSCAVIR-induced renal impairment. No specific factors were identified that predicted patients at higher risk. No relationship was found between a patient's initial creatinine clearance or initial drug clearance and renal impairment. Thus initial renal function may not be predictive of a patient's potential for renal impairment induced by FOSCAVIR.

CLINICAL TRIALS

CMV Retinitis: Controlled clinical trials of FOSCAVIR have been conducted in the treatment of CMV retinitis. In most studies, treatment was begun with an induction dosage regimen of 60 mg/kg every 8 hours for the first 2–3 weeks, followed by a once-daily maintenance regimen at doses ranging from 60–120 mg/kg.

A prospective, randomized, masked, controlled clinical trial (FOS-03) was conducted in 24 patients with AIDS and CMV retinitis. All diagnoses and determinations of retinitis progression were made from retinal photographs by ophthalmologists who were masked to the patient's treatment assignment. Patients received induction treatment of FOSCAVIR, 60 mg/kg every 8 hours for 3 weeks, followed by maintenance treatment with 90 mg/kg/day until retinitis progression (appearance of a new lesion or advancement of the border of a posterior lesion greater than 750 microns in diameter). The 13 patients randomized to treatment with FOSCAVIR had a significant delay in progression of CMV retinitis compared to untreated controls. Median times to retinitis progression from study entry were 93 days (range 21– > 364) and 22 days (range 7–42), respectively, $p < 0.001$.

In another prospective clinical trial of CMV retinitis in patients with AIDS (ACTG-915), 33 patients were treated with two to three weeks of FOSCAVIR induction (60 mg/kg TID) and then randomized to two maintenance dose groups, 90 mg/kg/day and 120 mg/kg/day. Median times from study entry to retinitis progression were 96 (range 14– > 176) days and 140 (range 16– > 233) days, respectively (FDA analysis). This difference was not statistically significant. The same criteria for retinitis progression were used as described above for FOS-03.

In study ACTG 129/FGCRT SOCA study 107 patients with newly diagnosed CMV retinitis were randomized to treatment with FOSCAVIR (induction: 60 mg/kg TID for 2 weeks; maintenance: 90 mg/kg QD) and 127 were randomized to treatment with ganciclovir (induction: 5 mg/kg BID; maintenance: 5 mg/kg QD). The median time to retinitis progression in the patients treated with FOSCAVIR was 59 days (see ADVERSE REACTIONS section).

Mucocutaneous Acyclovir-Resistant HSV Infections: A prospective, comparative trial was conducted in 25 AIDS patients with mucocutaneous, acyclovir-resistant HSV infections. Fourteen patients were randomized to either FOSCAVIR (N = 8) at a dose of 40 mg/kg TID or vidarabine (N = 6) at a dose of 15 mg/kg per day; eleven patients received FOSCAVIR without being randomized. Lesions in the eight patients randomized to FOSCAVIR healed after 11 to 25 days; seven of the 11 patients non-randomly treated with FOSCAVIR healed their lesions in 10 to 30 days. Vidarabine was discontinued because of intolerance in four patients and poor therapeutic response in two patients. Five of these patients were subsequently treated with FOSCAVIR and two healed their lesions in 15 and 24 days. In a second prospective, randomized trial, forty AIDS patients and three bone marrow transplant recipients with mucocutaneous, acyclovir-resistant HSV infections were randomized to receive FOSCAVIR at a dose of either 40 mg/kg BID or 40 mg/kg TID. Fifteen of the 43 patients had healing of their lesions in 11 to 72 days with no difference in response between the two treatment groups.

INDICATIONS

CMV Retinitis: FOSCAVIR is indicated for the treatment of CMV retinitis in patients with acquired immunodeficiency syndrome (AIDS). SAFETY AND EFFICACY OF FOSCAVIR HAVE NOT BEEN ESTABLISHED FOR TREATMENT OF OTHER CMV INFECTIONS (e.g., PNEUMONITIS, GASTROENTERITIS); CONGENITAL OR NEONATAL CMV DISEASE; OR NON-IMMUNOCOMPROMISED INDIVIDUALS.

The diagnosis of CMV retinitis should be made by indirect ophthalmoscopy. Other conditions in the differential diagnosis of CMV retinitis include candidiasis, toxoplasmosis, and other diseases producing a similar retinal pattern, any of which may produce a retinal appearance similar to CMV. For this reason it is essential that the diagnosis of CMV retinitis be established by an ophthalmologist familiar with the retinal presentation of these conditions. The diagnosis of CMV retinitis may be supported by culture of CMV from urine, blood, throat, or other sites, but a negative CMV culture does not rule out CMV retinitis.

Mucocutaneous Acyclovir-Resistant HSV Infections: FOSCAVIR is indicated for the treatment of acyclovir-resistant mucocutaneous HSV infections in immunocompromised patients. SAFETY AND EFFICACY OF FOSCAVIR HAVE NOT BEEN ESTABLISHED FOR TREATMENT OF OTHER HSV INFECTIONS (e.g., RETINITIS, ENCEPHALITIS); CONGENITAL OR NEONATAL HSV DISEASE; OR HSV IN NON-IMMUNOCOMPROMISED INDIVIDUALS.

CONTRAINDICATIONS

FOSCAVIR is contraindicated in patients with clinically significant hypersensitivity to foscarnet sodium.

TABLE 3

Mean ±SD Dose mg/kg* (Infusion Time)	Day of Sampling	Mean Plasma Concentration (μM) CMAX**[range]	CMIN***[range]
FOS-01			
57±6 Q8h (1 hour)	1	573 [213–1305]	78 [< 33–139]
47±12 Q8h (1 hour)	14 or 15	579 [246–922]	110 [< 33–148]
ACTG-015			
55±6 Q8h (2 hours)	3	445 [306–720]	88 [< 33–162]
57 ±7 Q8h (2 hours)	14 or 15	517 [348–789]	105 [43–205]

* Planned dose = 60 mg/kg Q8h in both studies.

** Observed Maximum Concentration:

FOS-01:

Day 1 (N = 14): Observed 0.9–2.0 hrs after start of infusion.

Day 14/15 (N = 10): Observed 0.8–1.3 hrs after start of infusion.

ACTG-015:

Day 3 (N = 12): Observed 1.8–2.4 hrs after start of infusion.

Day 14/15 (N = 12): Observed 1.7–2.6 hrs after start of infusion.

*** Observed Minimum Concentration:

FOS-01:

Day 1 (N = 13): Observed 4–8 hrs after start of infusion. (Mean represents 5/13 observations, 8/13 < 33 μM)

Day 14/15 (N = 10): Observed 6.3–8 hrs after start of infusion. (Mean represents 9/10 observations, 1/10 < 33 μM)

ACTG-015:

Day 3 (N = 12): Observed 7.8–8.1 hrs after start of infusion. (Mean represents 9/12 observations, 3/12 < 33 μM)

Day 14/15 (N = 12): Observed 6.4–8.7 hrs after start of infusion. (Means represents 12/12 observations)

WARNINGS

Renal Impairment: THE MAJOR TOXICITY OF FOSCAVIR IS RENAL IMPAIRMENT, WHICH OCCURS TO SOME DEGREE IN MOST PATIENTS. Approximately 33% of 189 patients with AIDS and CMV retinitis who received intravenous FOSCAVIR in clinical studies developed significant impairment of renal function, manifested by a rise in serum creatinine concentration to 2.0 mg/dL or greater. FOSCAVIR must therefore be used with caution in all patients, especially those with a history of impairment of renal function. Patients vary in their sensitivity to nephrotoxicity induced by FOSCAVIR and initial renal function may not be predictive of the potential for drug induced renal impairment (see Pharmacodynamics). FOSCAVIR has not been studied in patients with baseline serum creatinine levels greater than 2.8 mg/dL or measured 24-hour creatinine clearances < 50 mL/min.

Analysis of data in one clinical trial (FOS-01) demonstrated renal impairment is most likely to become clinically evident, as assessed by increasing serum creatinine, during the second week of induction therapy at 60 mg/kg TID (see Pharmacodynamics). Renal impairment, however, may occur at any time in any patient during FOSCAVIR treatment and renal function should therefore be monitored especially carefully (see PATIENT MONITORING).

Elevations in serum creatinine are usually, but not uniformly, reversible following discontinuation or dose adjustment of FOSCAVIR. In the U.S. studies, recovery of renal function after FOSCAVIR-induced impairment usually occurred within one week of drug discontinuation. However, of 35 patients in the U.S. controlled clinical studies who experienced grade II renal impairment (serum creatinine 2–3 times the upper limit of normal), two died with renal failure within four weeks of stopping FOSCAVIR, and three others died with renal insufficiency still present less than four weeks after drug cessation.

BECAUSE OF FOSCAVIR'S POTENTIAL TO CAUSE RENAL IMPAIRMENT, DOSE ADJUSTMENT FOR DECREASED BASELINE RENAL FUNCTION AND ANY CHANGE IN RENAL FUNCTION DURING TREATMENT IS NECESSARY. In addition, it may be beneficial for adequate hydration to be established (e.g., by inducing diuresis) prior to and during FOSCAVIR administration.

Mineral and Electrolyte Imbalances: FOSCAVIR has been associated with changes in serum electrolytes including hypocalcemia (15%), hypophosphatemia (8%) and hyperphosphatemia (6%), hypomagnesemia (15%), and hypokalemia (16%). Administration of FOSCAVIR has been shown to be associated with a transient, dose-related decrease in ionized serum calcium, which may not be reflected in total serum calcium. This effect most likely is related to foscarnet's chelation of divalent metal ions such as calcium. Therefore, patients should be advised to report symptoms of low ionized calcium such as perioral tingling, numbness in the extremities and paresthesias. Physicians should be prepared to treat these as well as severe manifestations of electrolyte abnormalities such as tetany and seizures. The rate of FOSCAVIR infusion may affect the transient decrease in ionized calcium. Slowing the rate may decrease or prevent symptoms. Transient changes in calcium or other electrolytes (including magnesium, potassium or phosphate) may also contribute to a patient's risk for cardiac disturbances and seizures (see below). Therefore, particular caution is advised in patients with altered calcium or other electrolyte levels before treatment, especially those with neurologic or cardiac abnormalities and those receiving other drugs known to influence minerals and electrolytes (see PATIENT MONITORING and Drug Interactions).

Neurotoxicity and Seizures: FOSCAVIR treatment has been associated with seizures in 18/189 (10%) of AIDS patients in five controlled studies. Three patients were not taking FOSCAVIR at the time of seizure. In most cases (15/18), the patients had an active CNS condition (e.g., toxoplasmosis, HIV encephalopathy) or a history of CNS diseases. The rate of seizures did not increase with duration of treatment. Three cases were associated with overdoses of FOSCAVIR (see OVERDOSAGE).

A logistic regression analysis was performed comparing the 18 patients in these five studies who had seizures with the 161 who did not. Statistically significant ($p < 0.05$) risk factors associated with seizures were low baseline absolute neutrophil count (ANC), impaired baseline renal function, and low total serum calcium. Several cases of seizures were associated with death. However, occurrence of seizures did not always necessitate discontinuation of FOSCAVIR; ten of fifteen patients with seizures that occurred while receiving the drug continued or resumed FOSCAVIR following treatment of their underlying disease, electrolyte disturbances, and/or dose decreases. If factors predisposing a patient to seizures are present, electrolytes, including calcium and magnesium, must be monitored especially carefully (see PATIENT MONITORING).

PRECAUTIONS

General: In controlled clinical studies with FOSCAVIR, the maximum single dose administered was 120 mg/kg by intravenous infusion over 2 hours. It is likely that larger doses, or more rapid infusions, would result in increased toxicity. Care must be taken to infuse solutions containing FOSCAVIR only into veins with adequate blood flow to permit rapid dilution and distribution, and avoid local irritation (see DOSAGE AND ADMINISTRATION). Local irritation and ulcerations of penile epithelium have been reported in male patients receiving FOSCAVIR, possibly related to the presence of drug in urine. One case of vulvovaginal ulcerations in a female receiving FOSCAVIR has been reported. Adequate hydration with close attention to personal hygiene may minimize the occurrence of such events.

Hemopoietic System: Anemia has been reported in 33% of patients receiving FOSCAVIR in controlled studies. This anemia was usually manageable with transfusions and required discontinuation of FOSCAVIR in less than 1% (1/189) of patients in the studies. Granulocytopenia has been reported in 17% of patients receiving FOSCAVIR in controlled studies; however, only 1% (2/189) were terminated from these studies because of neutropenia.

Information for Patients: *CMV Retinitis:* Patients should be advised that FOSCAVIR is not a cure for CMV retinitis, and that they may continue to experience progression of retinitis during or following treatment. They should be advised to have regular ophthalmologic examinations.
Mucocutaneous Acyclovir-Resistant HSV Infections: Patients should be advised that FOSCAVIR is not a cure for HSV infections. While complete healing may occur, relapse occurs in most patients. Because relapse may be due to acyclovir-sensitive HSV, sensitivity testing of the viral isolate is advised. In addition, repeated treatment with FOSCAVIR has led to the development of resistance associated with poorer response. In the case of poor therapeutic response, sensitivity testing of the viral isolate also is advised.
General: Patients should be informed that the major toxicities of foscarnet are renal impairment, electrolyte disturbances, and seizures, and that dose modifications and possibly discontinuation may be required. The importance of close monitoring while on therapy must be emphasized. Patients should be advised of the importance of perioral tingling, numbness in the extremities or paresthesias during or after infusion as possible symptoms of electrolyte abnormalities. Should such symptoms occur, the infusion of FOSCAVIR should be stopped, appropriate laboratory samples for assessment of electrolyte concentrations obtained, and a physician consulted before resuming treatment. The rate of infusion must be no more than 1 mg/kg/minute. The potential for renal impairment may be minimized by accompanying FOSCAVIR administration with hydration adequate to establish and maintain a diuresis during dosing.

Drug Interactions: Coadministration of FOSCAVIR with other drugs could theoretically alter its antiviral activity, toxicity or pharmacokinetics.

A possible drug interaction of FOSCAVIR and intravenous pentamidine has been described. Concomitant treatment of four patients in the United Kingdom with FOSCAVIR and intravenous pentamidine may have caused hypocalcemia; one patient died with severe hypocalcemia. Toxicity associated with concomitant use of aerosolized pentamidine has not been reported.

The elimination of foscarnet may be impaired by drugs that inhibit renal tubular secretion; however, no studies have been conducted to determine whether this occurs. Nonetheless, because of foscarnet's tendency to cause renal impairment, the use of FOSCAVIR should be avoided in combination with potentially nephrotoxic drugs such as aminoglycosides, amphotericin B and intravenous pentamidine (see above) unless the potential benefits outweigh the risks to the patient.

Since FOSCAVIR decreases serum levels of ionized calcium, concurrent treatment with other drugs known to influence serum calcium levels should be used with particular caution. FOSCAVIR was used concomitantly with zidovudine in approximately one-third of patients in the U.S. studies. Although the combination was generally well tolerated, additive effects on anemia may have occurred. In one study of 24 patients (FOS-03), anemia was reported as an adverse event in 60% (3/5) of patients receiving FOSCAVIR only, 88% (7/8) of patients receiving both zidovudine and FOSCAVIR, 29% (2/7) of patients receiving only zidovudine and 25% (1/4) of patients receiving neither drug. However, no evidence of increased myelosuppression was seen with FOSCAVIR in combination with zidovudine.

Carcinogenesis, Mutagenesis, Impairment of Fertility: Carcinogenicity studies were conducted in rats and mice at oral doses of 500 mg/kg/day and 250 mg/kg/day. Oral bioavailability in unfasted rodents is <20%. No evidence of oncogenicity was reported at plasma drug levels equal to $^1/_3$ and $^1/_5$, respectively, of those in humans (at the maximum recommended human daily dose) as measured by the area-under-the-time/concentration curve (AUC).

FOSCAVIR showed genotoxic effects in the BALB/3T3 *in vitro* transformation assay at concentrations greater than 0.5 mcg/mL and an increased frequency of chromosome aberrations in the sister chromatid exchange assay at 1000 mcg/mL. A high dose of foscarnet (350 mg/kg) caused an increase in micronucleated polychromatic erythrocytes *in vivo* in mice at doses that produced exposures (Area Under Curve) comparable to that anticipated clinically.

Pregnancy: Teratogenic Effect: *Pregnancy, Category C:* FOSCAVIR did not adversely affect fertility and general reproductive performance in rats. The results of peri- and post-natal studies in rats were also negative. However, these studies used exposures that are inadequate to define the potential for impairment of fertility at human drug exposure levels.

Daily subcutaneous doses up to 75 mg/kg administered to female rats prior to and during mating, during gestation, and 21 days post-partum caused a slight increase (<5%) in the number of skeletal anomalies compared with the control group. Daily subcutaneous doses up to 75 mg/kg administered to rabbits and 150 mg/kg administered to rats during gestation caused an increase in the frequency of skeletal anomalies/variations. On the basis of estimated drug exposure (as measured by AUC), the 150 mg/kg dose in rats and 75 mg/kg dose in rabbits were approximately one-eighth (rat) and one-third (rabbit) the estimated maximal daily human exposure. These studies are inadequate to define the potential teratogenicity at levels to which women will be exposed.

There are no adequate and well controlled studies in pregnant women. Because animal reproductive studies are not always predictive of human response, FOSCAVIR should be used during pregnancy only if clearly needed.

Nursing Mothers: It is not known whether FOSCAVIR is excreted in human milk; however, in lactating rats administered 75 mg/kg, FOSCAVIR was excreted in maternal milk at concentrations three times higher than peak maternal blood concentrations. Because many drugs are excreted in human milk, caution should be exercised if FOSCAVIR is administered to a nursing woman.

Pediatric Use: The safety and effectiveness of FOSCAVIR in children have not been studied. FOSCAVIR is deposited in teeth and bone and deposition is greater in young and growing animals. FOSCAVIR has been demonstrated to adversely affect development of tooth enamel in mice and rats. The effects of this deposition on skeletal development have not been studied. Since deposition in human bone also occurs, it is likely that it does so to a greater degree in developing bone in children. Administration to children should be undertaken only after careful evaluation and only if the potential benefits for treatment outweigh the risks.

Use in the Elderly: No studies of the efficacy or safety of FOSCAVIR in persons over age 65 have been conducted. Since these individuals frequently have reduced glomerular filtration, particular attention should be paid to assessing renal function before and during FOSCAVIR administration (see DOSAGE AND ADMINISTRATION).

ADVERSE REACTIONS

In five controlled U.S. clinical trials in which 189 patients with AIDS and CMV retinitis were treated with FOSCAVIR, the most frequently reported events were the following: fever 65% (123/189), nausea 47% (88/189), anemia 33% (63/189), diarrhea 30% (57/189), abnormal renal function including acute renal failure, decreased creatinine clearance and increased serum creatinine 27% (51/189), vomiting 26% (50/189), headache 26% (49/189), and seizure 10% (18/189) (see WARNINGS and PRECAUTIONS). These incidence figures were calculated without reference to drug relationship or severity.

From the same controlled studies, adverse events categorized by investigator as "severe" were death (14%), abnormal renal function (14%), marrow suppression (10%), anemia (9%), and seizures (7%). Although death was specifically attributed to FOSCAVIR in only one case, other complications of foscarnet (i.e., renal impairment, electrolyte abnormalities, and seizures) may have contributed to patient deaths (see WARNINGS and PRECAUTIONS).

From the five U.S. controlled clinical trials of FOSCAVIR, the following list of adverse events has been compiled regardless of causal relationship to FOSCAVIR. Evaluation of these reports was difficult because of the diverse manifestations of the underlying disease and because most patients received numerous concomitant medications.

Incidence 5% or Greater

Body as a Whole: fever, fatigue, rigors, asthenia, malaise, pain, infection, sepsis, death
Central and Peripheral Nervous System: headache, paresthesia, dizziness, involuntary muscle contractions, hypoesthesia, neuropathy, seizures including grand mal seizures (see WARNINGS)
Gastrointestinal System: anorexia, nausea, diarrhea, vomiting, abdominal pain
Hematologic: anemia, granulocytopenia, leukopenia (see PRECAUTIONS)

Metabolic and Nutritional: mineral and electrolyte imbalances (see WARNINGS) including hypokalemia, hypocalcemia, hypomagnesemia, hypophosphatemia, hyperphosphatemia
Psychiatric: depression, confusion, anxiety
Respiratory System: coughing, dyspnea
Skin and Appendages: rash, increased sweating
Urinary: alterations in renal function including increased serum creatinine, decreased creatinine clearance, and abnormal renal function (see WARNINGS)
Special Senses: vision abnormalities

Incidence between 1% and 5%

Application Site: injection site pain, injection site inflammation
Body as a Whole: back pain, chest pain, edema, influenza-like symptoms, bacterial infections, moniliasis, fungal infections, abscess
Cardiovascular: hypertension, palpitations, ECG abnormalities including sinus tachycardia, first degree AV block and non-specific ST-T segment changes, hypotension, flushing, cerebrovascular disorder (see WARNINGS)
Central and Peripheral Nervous System: tremor, ataxia, dementia, stupor, generalized spasms, sensory disturbances, meningitis, aphasia, abnormal coordination, leg cramps, EEG abnormalities (see WARNINGS)
Gastrointestinal: constipation, dysphagia, dyspepsia, rectal hemorrhage, dry mouth, melena, flatulence, ulcerative stomatitis, pancreatitis
Hematologic: thrombocytopenia, platelet abnormalities, thrombosis, white blood cell abnormalities, lymphadenopathy
Liver and Biliary: abnormal A-G ratio, abnormal hepatic function, increased SGPT, increased SGOT
Metabolic and Nutritional: hyponatremia, decreased weight, increased alkaline phosphatase, increased LDH, increased BUN, acidosis, cachexia, thirst, hypercalcemia (see WARNINGS)
Musculo-Skeletal: arthralgia, myalgia
Neoplasms: lymphoma-like disorder, sarcoma
Psychiatric: insomnia, somnolence, nervousness, amnesia, agitation, aggressive reaction, hallucination
Respiratory System: pneumonia, sinusitis, pharyngitis, rhinitis, respiratory disorders, respiratory insufficiency, pulmonary infiltration, stridor, pneumothorax, hemoptysis, bronchospasm
Skin and Appendages: pruritus, skin ulceration, seborrhea, erythematous rash, maculo-papular rash, skin discoloration
Special Senses: taste perversions, eye abnormalities, eye pain, conjunctivitis
Urinary System: albuminuria, dysuria, polyuria, urethral disorder, urinary retention, urinary tract infections, acute renal failure, nocturia, facial edema

Incidence less than 1%

Body as a Whole: hypothermia, leg edema, peripheral edema, syncope, ascites, substernal chest pain, abnormal crying, malignant hyperpyrexia, herpes simplex, viral infection, toxoplasmosis
Cardiovascular: cardiomyopathy, cardiac failure, cardiac arrest, bradycardia, extrasystole, arrhythmias, atrial arrhythmias, atrial fibrillation, phlebitis, superficial thrombophlebitis of the arm, mesenteric vein thrombophlebitis
Central and Peripheral Nervous System: vertigo, coma, encephalopathy, abnormal gait, hyperesthesia, hypertonia, visual field defects, dyskinesia, extrapyramidal disorders, hemiparesis, hyperkinesia, vocal cord paralysis, paralysis, paraplegia, speech disorders, tetany, hyporeflexia, neuralgia, neuritis, peripheral neuropathy, hyperreflexia, cerebral edema, nystagmus
Endocrine: antidiuretic hormone disorders, decreased gonadotropins, gynecomastia
Gastrointestinal System: enteritis, enterocolitis, glossitis, proctitis, stomatitis, tenesmus, increased amylase, pseudomembranous colitis, gastroenteritis, oral leukoplakia, oral hemorrhage, rectal disorders, colitis, duodenal ulcer, hematemesis, paralytic ileus, esophageal ulceration, ulcerative proctitis, tongue ulceration
Hematologic: pulmonary embolism, coagulation disorders, decreased coagulation factors, epistaxis, decreased prothrombin, hypochromic anemia, pancytopenia, hemolysis, leukocytosis, cervical lymphadenopathy, lymphopenia
Special Senses: deafness, earache, tinnitus, otitis
Liver and Biliary System: cholecystitis, cholelithiasis, hepatitis, cholestatic hepatitis, hepatosplenomegaly, jaundice
Metabolic and Nutritional: dehydration, glycosuria, increased creatine phosphokinase, diabetes mellitus, abnormal glucose tolerance, hypervolemia, hypochloremia, periorbital edema, hypoproteinemia
Musculo-Skeletal System: arthrosis, synovitis, torticollis
Neoplasms: malignant lymphoma, skin hypertrophy
Psychiatric: impaired concentration, emotional lability, psychosis, suicide attempt, delirium, personality disorders, sleep disorders

Continued on next page

Astra—Cont.

Reproductive: perineal pain in women, penile inflammation

Respiratory System: bronchitis, laryngitis, respiratory depression, abnormal chest x-ray, pleural effusion, lobar pneumonia, pulmonary hemorrhage, pneumonitis

Skin and Appendages: acne, alopecia, dermatitis, anal pruritus, genital pruritus, aggravated psoriasis, psoriaform rash, skin disorders, dry skin, urticaria, verruca

Urinary System: hematuria, glomerulonephritis, micturition disorders, micturition frequency, toxic nephropathy, nephrosis, urinary incontinence, renal tubular disorders, pyelonephritis, urethral irritation, uremia

Special Senses: diplopia, blindness, retinal detachment, mydriasis, photophobia

The types and incidences of adverse events reported worldwide in post-marketing surveillance for FOSCAVIR have not been different from or greater in frequency than those observed in U.S. clinical trials. Rare events that have appeared in post-marketing surveillance include: ventricular arrhythmia, prolongation of QT interval, diabetes insipidus (usually nephrogenic), and muscle disorders including myopathy, myositis, muscle weakness and rare cases of rhabdomyolysis. Rare cases of vesiculobullous eruptions including erythema multiforme, toxic epidermal necrolysis, and Stevens-Johnson Syndrome have been reported. In most cases, patients were taking other implicated medications.

Comparative morbidity data available from the Foscarnet vs. Ganciclovir CMV Retinitis Trial (FGCRT), performed by the Studies of the Ocular Complications of AIDS (SOCA) Research Group, is found in Table 4 below.

[See table below.]

Table 4 shows selected adverse events from study ACTG 129/FGCRT SOCA study in which FOSCAVIR therapy (induction: 60 mg/kg TID for 2 weeks; maintenance: 90 mg/kg QD) was compared with ganciclovir therapy (induction: 5 mg/kg BID; maintenance: 5 mg/kg QD) for the treatment of newly diagnosed CMV retinitis. In the study 127 subjects were randomized to ganciclovir and 107 were randomized to foscarnet. Ganciclovir was associated with more decreases in absolute neutrophil counts below 500/μL than FOSCAVIR. FOSCAVIR was associated with more increases in serum creatinine levels above 260 μM than ganciclovir. In this study, the observed rate of seizures was similar in the two treatment arms.

OVERDOSAGE

In controlled clinical trials performed in the United States, overdosage with FOSCAVIR was reported in 10 out of 189 patients. All 10 patients experienced adverse events and all except one made a complete recovery. One patient died after receiving a total daily dose of 12.5 g for three days instead of the intended 10.9 g. The patient suffered a grand mal seizure and became comatose. Three days later the patient expired with the cause of death listed as respiratory/cardiac arrest. The other nine patients received doses ranging from 1.14 times to 8 times their recommended doses with an average of 4 times their recommended doses. Overall, three patients had seizures, three patients had renal function impairment, four patients had paresthesis either in limbs or periorally, and five patients had documented electrolyte disturbances primarily involving calcium and phosphate.

The pattern of adverse events associated with overdose in post-marketing surveillance is consistent wtih the symptoms previously observed during foscarnet therapy.

There is no specific antidote for FOSCAVIR overdose. Hemodialysis and hydration may be of benefit in reducing drug plasma levels in patients who receive an overdosage of FOSCAVIR, but the effectiveness of these interventions has not been evaluated. The patient should be observed for signs and symptoms of renal impairment and electrolyte imbalance. Medical treatment should be instituted if clinically warranted.

DOSAGE AND ADMINISTRATION

CAUTION—DO NOT ADMINISTER FOSCAVIR BY RAPID OR BOLUS INTRAVENOUS INJECTION. THE TOXICITY OF FOSCAVIR MAY BE INCREASED AS A RESULT OF EXCESSIVE PLASMA LEVELS. CARE SHOULD BE TAKEN TO AVOID UNINTENTIONAL OVERDOSE BY CAREFULLY CONTROLLING THE RATE OF INFUSION. THEREFORE, AN INFUSION PUMP MUST BE USED. IN SPITE OF THE USE OF AN INFUSION PUMP, OVERDOSES HAVE OCCURRED.

ADMINISTRATION

FOSCAVIR is administered by controlled intravenous infusion, either by using a central venous line or by using a peripheral vein. The standard 24 mg/mL solution may be used without dilution when using a central venous catheter for infusion. When a peripheral vein catheter is used, the 24 mg/mL solution **must** be diluted to 12 mg/mL with 5% dextrose in water or with a normal saline solution prior to administration to avoid local irritation of peripheral veins. Since the dose of FOSCAVIR is calculated on the basis of body weight, it may be desirable to remove and discard any unneeded quantity from the bottle before starting with the infusion to avoid overdosage. Dilutions and/or removals of excess quantities should be accomplished under aseptic conditions. Solutions thus prepared should be used within 24 hours of first entry into a sealed bottle.

Other drugs and supplements can be administered to a patient receiving FOSCAVIR. However, care must be taken to ensure that FOSCAVIR is only administered with normal saline or 5% dextrose solution and that no other drug or supplement is administered concurrently via the same catheter. Foscarnet has been reported to be chemically incompatible with 30% dextrose, amphotericin B, and solutions containing calcium such as Ringer's lactate and TPN. Physical incompatibility with other IV drugs has also been reported including acyclovir sodium, ganciclovir, trimetrexate glucuronate, pentamidine isethionate, vancomycin, trimethoprim/sulfamethoxazole, diazepam, midazolam, digoxin, phenytoin, leucovorin, and prochlorperazine. Because of foscarnet's chelating properties, a precipitate can potentially occur when divalent cations are administered concurrently in the same catheter.

Parenteral drug products must be inspected visually for particulate matter and discoloration prior to administration whenever the solution and container permit. Solutions that are discolored or contain particulate matter should not be used.

Accidental Exposure: Accidental skin and eye contact with foscarnet sodium solution may cause local irritation and burning sensation. If accidental contact occurs, the exposed area should be flushed with water.

DOSAGE

THE RECOMMENDED DOSAGE, FREQUENCY, OR INFUSION RATES SHOULD NOT BE EXCEEDED. ALL DOSES MUST BE INDIVIDUALIZED FOR PATIENTS' RENAL FUNCTION.

Induction Treatment: The recommended initial dose of FOSCAVIR for patients with normal renal function is 60 mg/kg (minimum one hour infusion) every eight hours for CMV retinitis patients over 2–3 weeks depending on clinical response, and 40 mg/kg (minimum one hour infusion) either every 8 or 12 hours for acyclovir-resistant HSV patients for 2–3 weeks or until healed.

An infusion pump must be used to control the rate of infusion. Adequate hydration is recommended to establish a diuresis, both prior to and during treatment to minimize renal toxicity (see WARNINGS), provided there are no clinical contraindications.

Maintenance Treatment: Following induction treatment the recommended maintenance dose of FOSCAVIR for CMV retinitis is 90 mg/kg/day to 120 mg/kg/day (individualized for renal function) given as an intravenous infusion over 2 hours. Because the superiority of the 120 mg/kg/day has not been established in controlled trials, and given the likely relationship of higher plasma foscarnet levels to toxicity, it is recommended that most patients be started on maintenance treatment with a dose of 90 mg/kg/day. Escalation to 120 mg/kg/day may be considered should early reinduction be required because of retinitis progression. Some patients who show excellent tolerance to FOSCAVIR may benefit from initiation of maintenance treatment at 120 mg/kg/day earlier in their treatment. An infusion pump must be used to control the rate of infusion with all doses. Again, hydration to establish diuresis both prior to and during treatment is recommended to minimize renal toxicity, provided there are no clinical contraindications (see WARNINGS).

Patients who experience progression of retinitis while receiving FOSCAVIR maintenance therapy may be retreated with the induction and maintenance regimens given above.

Use in Patients with Abnormal Renal Function: FOSCAVIR should be used with caution in patients with abnormal renal function because reduced plasma clearance of foscarnet will result in elevated plasma levels (see CLINICAL PHARMACOLOGY). In addition, FOSCAVIR has the potential to further impair renal function (see WARNINGS). FOSCAVIR has not been specifically studied in patients with creatinine clearances <50 mL/min or serum creatinines >2.8 mg/dL. Renal function must be monitored carefully at baseline and during induction and maintenance therapy with appropriate dose adjustments for FOSCAVIR as outlined below (see Dose Adjustment and PATIENT MONITORING). During FOSCAVIR therapy if creatinine clearance falls below the limits of the dosing nomograms (0.4 mL/min/kg), FOSCAVIR should be discontinued and the patient monitored daily until resolution of renal impairment is ensured.

Dose Adjustment: FOSCAVIR dosing must be individualized according to the patient's renal function status. Refer to TABLE 5 below for recommended doses and adjust the dose as indicated.

To use this dosing guide, actual 24-hour creatinine clearance (mL/min) must be divided by body weight (kg), or the estimated creatinine clearance in mL/min/kg can be calculated from serum creatinine (mg/dL) using the following formula (modified Cockcroft and Gault equation):

For males:

$$\frac{140 - age}{serum\ creatinine \times 72} \quad (\times\ 0.85\ for\ females)$$

TABLE 5
FOSCAVIR DOSING GUIDE
INDUCTION

CrCl (mL/min/kg)	HSV: Equivalent to 80 mg/kg/ day total (40 mg/kg Q12h)	HSV: Equivalent to 120 mg/kg/ day total (40 mg/kg Q8h)	CMV: Equivalent to 180 mg/kg/ day total (60 mg/kg Q8h)
>1.4	40 Q12h	40 Q8h	60 Q8h
>1.0–1.4	30 Q12h	30 Q8h	45 Q8h
>0.8–1.0	20 Q12h	35 Q12h	50 Q12h
>0.6–0.8	35 Q24h	25 Q12h	40 Q12h
>0.5–0.6	25 Q24h	40 Q24h	60 Q24h
≥0.4–0.5	20 Q24h	35 Q24h	50 Q24h
<0.4	Not Recommended	Not Recommended	Not Recommended

MAINTENANCE

CrCl (mL/min/kg)	CMV: Equivalent to 90 mg/kg/day (once daily)	CMV: Equivalent to 120 mg/kg/day (once daily)
>1.4	90 Q24h	120 Q24h
>1.0–1.4	70 Q24h	90 Q24h
>0.8–1.0	50 Q24h	65 Q24h
>0.6–0.8	80 Q48h	105 Q48h
>0.5–0.6	60 Q48h	80 Q48h
≥0.4–0.5	50 Q48h	65 Q48h
<0.4	Not Recommended	Not Recommended

> = greater than; ≥ = greater than or equal to; < = less than

PATIENT MONITORING

The majority of patients will experience some decrease in renal function due to FOSCAVIR administration. Therefore it is recommended that creatinine clearance, either measured or estimated using the modified Cockcroft and Gault equation based on serum creatinine, be determined at baseline, 2–3 times per week during induction therapy and at least once every one to two weeks during maintenance ther-

---

TABLE 4—SELECTED EVENTS RELATED TO MORBIDITY, ACCORDING TO TREATMENT GROUP*

EVENT	GANCICLOVIR No. of Events	GANCICLOVIR No. of Patients	GANCICLOVIR Rates†	FOSCARNET No. of Events	FOSCARNET No. of Patients	FOSCARNET Rates†
Absolute neutrophil count decreasing to <0.50 × 10⁹ per liter	63	41	1.30	31	17	0.72
Serum creatinine increasing to >260 μmol per liter	6	4	0.12	13	9	0.30
Seizure	21	13	0.37	19	13	0.37
Catheterization-related infection	49	27	1.26	51	28	1.46
Hospitalization	209	91	4.74	202	75	5.03

* Values for the treatment groups refer only to patients who completed at least one follow-up visit—i.e., 113 to 119 patients in the ganciclovir group and 93 to 100 in the foscarnet group. "Events" denotes all events observed and "patients" the number of patients with one or more of the indicated events.

† Per person-year at risk.

apy, with FOSCAVIR dose adjusted accordingly (see Dose Adjustment). More frequent monitoring may be required for some patients. It is also recommended that a 24-hour creatinine clearance be determined at baseline and periodically thereafter to ensure correct dosing (assuming verification of an adequate collection using creatinine index). FOSCAVIR should be discontinued if creatinine clearance drops below 0.4 mL/min/kg.

Due to FOSCAVIR's propensity to chelate divalent metal ions and alter levels of serum electrolytes, patients must be monitored closely for such changes. It is recommended that a schedule similar to that recommended for serum creatinine (see above) be used to monitor serum calcium, magnesium, potassium and phosphorus. Particular caution is advised in patients with decreased total serum calcium or other electrolyte levels before treatment, as well as in patients with neurologic or cardiac abnormalities, and in patients receiving other drugs known to influence serum calcium levels. Any clinically significant metabolic changes should be corrected. Also, patients who experience mild (e.g., perioral numbness or paresthesias) or severe (e.g., seizures) symptoms of electrolyte abnormalities should have serum electrolyte and mineral levels assessed as close in time to the event as possible. Careful monitoring and appropriate management of electrolytes, calcium, magnesium and creatinine are of particular importance in patients with conditions that may predispose them to seizures (see WARNINGS).

HOW SUPPLIED

FOSCAVIR (foscarnet sodium) INJECTION, 24 mg/mL for intravenous infusion, is supplied in glass bottles as follows:
NDC 0186-1906-01   500 mL bottles, cases of 12
NDC 0186-1905-01   250 mL bottles, cases of 12
FOSCAVIR INJECTION should be stored at controlled room temperature 15°–30°C (59°–86°F), and should be protected from excessive heat (above 40°C) and from freezing. FOSCAVIR INJECTION should be used only if the bottle and seal are intact, a vacuum is present, and the solution is clear and colorless.

Caution: Federal law prohibits dispensing without prescription.
Manufactured by:
Abbott Laboratories
North Chicago, IL 60064
Manufactured for:
ASTRA®
Astra USA, Inc.,
Westborough, MA 01581
000571R05
Rev. 7/96

FUROSEMIDE INJECTION, USP   ℞

[fū″rō′sĕ-mīde]
10 mg/mL

PROTECT FROM LIGHT ● DO NOT USE IF THE SOLUTION IS DISCOLORED ● STORE AT CONTROLLED ROOM TEMPERATURE
WARNING: Furosemide is a potent diuretic which, if given in excessive amounts, can lead to a profound diuresis with water and electrolyte depletion. Therefore, careful medical supervision is required, and the dose and the dose schedule have to be adjusted to each patient's needs.
(See under DOSAGE AND ADMINISTRATION.)
(For details of indications, dosage, and administration, precautions, and adverse reactions, see circular in package.)

HOW SUPPLIED

Furosemide Injection, USP, 10 mg/mL is supplied in the following forms:
Single Dose Vials
2 mL (20 mg), 25 per package, NDC 0186-1114-13
4 mL (40 mg), 25 per package, NDC 0186-1115-13
8 mL (80 mg), 25 per package, NDC 0186-1116-12
10 mL (100 mg), 25 per package, NDC 0186-1117-12
Prefilled Syringes [supplied with 21 gauge × ¹⁵/₁₆″ needle]
4 mL (40 mg), Boxes of 10 NDC 0186-0635-01
10 mL (100 mg), Boxes of 10 NDC 0186-0636-01
Store in carton to protect from light.
To insure patient safety, this needle should be handled with care and should be destroyed and discarded if damaged in any manner. If cannula is bent, no attempt should be made to straighten.
To prevent needle-stick injuries, needles should not be recapped, purposely bent, or broken by hand.
All solutions should be stored at controlled room temperature 15°–30°C (59°–86°F) and should be protected from light. Do not use if the solution is discolored.
021877R10   10/94 (10)

HYDROMORPHONE HCl INJECTION   Ⓒ

(For details of indications, dosages and administration, precautions, and adverse reactions, see circular in package.)

HOW SUPPLIED

NDC 0186-1309-01 2 mg/mL- 20 mL multiple dose vials
Storage: Store at 15°–30°C (59°–86°F). Protect from light.
021888R01   11/91 (1)

ISOETHARINE INHALATION   ℞
Solution, USP
Arm-a-Med®
0.062%, 0.125%, 0.167%,
0.2%, and 0.25%
SULFITE-FREE

DESCRIPTION

Isoetharine Inhalation Solution, USP (sulfite-free) is a sterile solution for oral inhalation packaged in plastic vials for single use. Each vial contains isoetharine hydrochloride 0.062%, 0.125%, 0.167%, 0.2% or 0.25% in a sterile aqueous solution containing Water for Injection, sodium chloride, ascorbic acid, edetate disodium and hydrochloric acid. The solution is filled under nitrogen. The solution is for use in aerosol bronchodilator therapy employing oxygen aerosolization or intermittent positive pressure breathing (IPPB). Isoetharine hydrochloride is a sympathomimetic amine and is chemically 3,4-dihydroxy-α-[1-(isopropylamino)propyl] benzyl alcohol hydrochloride, with the following structural formula:

$C_{13}H_{21}NO_3 \cdot HCl$ M.W. 275.77

CLINICAL PHARMACOLOGY

Isoetharine is a sympathomimetic amine with preferential affinity for $Beta_2$ adrenergic receptor sites of bronchial and certain arteriolar musculature and a lower order of affinity for $Beta_1$ adrenergic receptors. Its activity in symptomatic relief of bronchospasm is rapid and of relatively long duration. By relieving bronchospasm, isoetharine helps give prompt relief and significantly increases FVC, FEV_1, and FEF 25%-75%.
Recent studies in laboratory animals (minipigs, rodents and dogs) recorded the occurrence of cardiac arrhythmias and sudden death (with histologic evidence of myocardial necrosis) when beta agonists and methylxanthines were administered concurrently. The significance of these findings when applied to human usage is currently unknown.

INDICATIONS AND USAGE

Isoetharine hydrochloride is indicated for use as a bronchodilator for bronchial asthma and for reversible bronchospasm that may occur in association with bronchitis and emphysema.

CONTRAINDICATIONS

Isoetharine inhalation solution should not be administered to patients who are hypersensitive to any of its components.

WARNINGS

Not for injection.
Excessive use of an adrenergic aerosol should be discouraged as it may lose its effectiveness. Occasional patients have been reported to develop paradoxical airway resistance with repeated excessive use of an aerosol adrenergic inhalation preparation. The cause of this refractory state is unknown. It is advisable that in such instances the use of the aerosol adrenergic be discontinued immediately and alternative therapy instituted, since in the reported cases the patients did not respond to other forms of therapy until the drug was withdrawn. Cardiac arrest has been noted in several instances.
Isoetharine should not be administered along with epinephrine or other sympathomimetic amines, since these drugs are direct cardiac stimulants and may cause excessive tachycardia. They may, however, be alternated if desired.

PRECAUTIONS

General: Dosage must be carefully adjusted in patients with hyperthyroidism, hypertension, acute coronary disease, cardiac asthma, limited cardiac reserve and in individuals sensitive to sympathomimetic amines since overdosage may result in tachycardia, palpitations, nausea, headache or epinephrine-like side effects.
Drug Interactions: Isoetharine should not be administered along with epinephrine or other sympathomimetic amines, since these drugs are direct cardiac stimulants and may

cause excessive tachycardia. They may, however, be alternated if desired.
Carcinogenesis, Mutagenesis, Impairment of Fertility: Chronic toxicity studies up to twelve months in dogs with doses up to 20 mg/kg/day (equivalent to approximately 200 times the human dose based on a 70 kg individual) and chronic toxicity studies in rats with the doses up to 45 mg/kg/day (equivalent to approximately 450 times the human dose, based on a 70 kg individual) revealed no evidence of carcinogenicity due to isoetharine.
Pregnancy—Category C: Animal reproduction studies have not been conducted with isoetharine hydrochloride. It is also not known whether isoetharine hydrochloride can cause fetal harm when administered to a pregnant woman or can affect reproduction capacity, although there is no evidence of such harm or effects. Isoetharine hydrochloride should be given to a pregnant woman only if in the physician's judgment the potential benefit to the pregnant woman outweighs the risk to the fetus.
Nursing Mothers: It is not known whether this drug is excreted in human milk. Because many drugs are excreted in human milk, caution should be exercised when isoetharine hydrochloride is administered to a nursing woman.
Pediatric Use: The safety and efficacy of this product in children under the age of 12 have not been established.

ADVERSE REACTIONS

Although isoetharine hydrochloride is relatively free of toxic side effects, too frequent use may cause the following effects, as is the case with other sympathomimetic amines:
CNS Effects: headache, anxiety, tension, restlessness, insomnia, weakness, dizziness, excitement.
Cardiovascular Effects: tachycardia, palpitations, changes in blood pressure.
Gastrointestinal Effects: nausea.
Other: tremor, weakness.

OVERDOSAGE

Overdosage of isoetharine hydrochloride may produce signs and symptoms typical of excessive sympathomimetic effects, including tachycardia, palpitations, nausea, headache, blood pressure changes, anxiety, restlessness, insomnia, tremor, weakness, dizziness, and excitation. Excessive use of adrenergic aerosols may result in loss of effectiveness or severe paradoxical airway resistance. Cardiac arrest has been noted in several instances. In all cases of overdosage, the drug should be discontinued immediately and vital functions supported until the patient is stabilized. It is not known whether isoetharine hydrochloride is dialyzable.
The single dose amount of drug that may be toxic or life threatening is highly variable according to patient characteristics and drug history. The acute oral LD_{50} in mice is 1630 mg/kg of pure drug (isoetharine HCl).

DOSAGE AND ADMINISTRATION

Isoetharine hydrochloride is for oral inhalation only and can be administered by oxygen aerosolization or intermittent positive pressure breathing devices (IPPB). Usually, treatment need not be repeated more than every four hours, although in severe cases more frequent administration may be necessary.

Method of Administration	Usual Dose (1% Solution)*	Range
Oxygen aerosolization**	0.5 mL	0.25 to 0.5 mL
IPPB†	0.5 mL	0.25 to 1 mL

*The doses given are for the 1% solution which must be suitably diluted prior to administration. Below are the dose equivalents for the entire prediluted and ready-to-use product line:

Product Strength (%)	Volume (mL)	Equivalent to mL of Isoetharine HCl 1%
0.062%	4 mL	0.25 mL
0.125%	4 mL	0.5 mL
0.167%	3 mL	0.5 mL
0.2%	2.5 mL	0.5 mL
0.25%	2 mL	0.5 mL

** Administered with oxygen flow adjusted to 4 to 6 liters/minute over a period of 15 to 20 minutes.
† Usually an inspiratory flow rate of 15 liters/minute at a cycling pressure of 15 cm H_2O is recommended. It may be necessary, according to patient and type of IPPB apparatus, to adjust flow rate to 6 to 30 liters per minute, cycling pressure to 10–15 cm H_2O and further dilution according to needs of patient.

HOW SUPPLIED

Isoetharine Inhalation Solution, USP (sulfite-free) is supplied in Arm-a-Med vials. There are 5 single-use, plastic vials per pouch. There are 20 pouches per carton of 100 vials.

Continued on next page

Astra—Cont.

NDC 0186-4110-01 Isoetharine Inhalation Solution, USP, 0.062%, 4 mL vials. Total contents of 2.5 mg of isoetharine hydrochloride.
NDC 0186-4112-01 Isoetharine Inhalation Solution, USP, 0.125%, 4 mL vials. Total contents of 5 mg of isoetharine hydrochloride.
NDC 0186-4111-01 Isoetharine Inhalation Solution, USP, 0.167%, 3mL vials. Total contents of 5 mg of isoetharine hydrochloride.
NDC 0186-4113-01 Isoetharine Inhalation Solution, USP, 0.2%, 2.5 mL vials. Total contents of 5 mg of isoetharine hydrochloride.
NDC 0186-4120-01 Isoetharine Inhalation Solution, USP, 0.25%, 2 mL vials. Total contents of 5 mg of isoetharine hydrochloride.

Store at controlled room temperature, 15°–30°C (59°–86°F). PROTECT FROM LIGHT. Store vial in pouch until time of use. Do not use solution if its color is pinkish or darker than slightly yellow or if it contains a precipitate.

Caution: Federal law prohibits dispensing without prescription.

Manufactured by:
Armour Pharmaceutical Company
Kankakee, Illinois 60901
Manufactured for:
Astra USA, Inc.
Westborough, MA 01581

021637R00 Rev 1/95

LEVOTHYROXINE SODIUM, USP ℞
for Injection

DESCRIPTION

Levothyroxine Sodium, USP for Injection contains synthetic crystalline L-3,3',5,5'-tetraiodothyronine sodium salt [levothyroxine (T_4) sodium]. Synthetic T_4 is similar to that produced in the human thyroid gland. T_4 contains four iodine atoms and is formed by the coupling of two molecules of diiodotyrosine (DIT).

Levothyroxine (T_4) Sodium has an empirical formula of $C_{15}H_{10}I_4NNaO_4xH_2O$, molecular weight of 798.86 (anhydrous), and structural formula as shown:

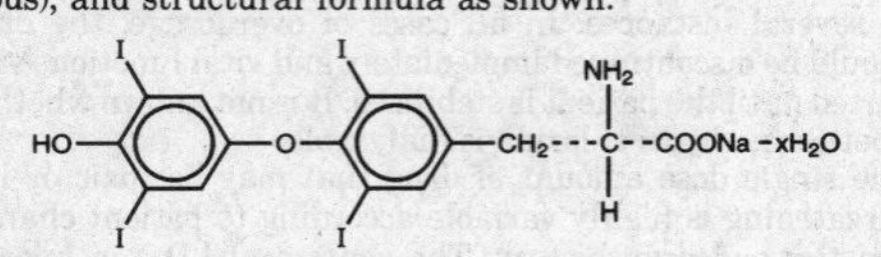

Levothyroxine Sodium, USP for Injection is a sterile, lyophilized powder. Each vial contains 200 mcg or 500 mcg Levothyroxine Sodium, 10 mg Mannitol, and 0.7 mg Tribasic Sodium Phosphate Anhydrous. pH may be adjusted with Sodium Hydroxide.

CLINICAL PHARMACOLOGY

The steps in the synthesis of thryoid hormones are controlled by throtropin (Thyroid Stimulating Hormone, TSH) secreted by the anterior pituitary. This hormone's secretion is in turn controlled by a feedback mechanism effected by the thyroid hormones themselves and by thyrotropin releasing hormone (TRH), a tripeptide of hypothalamic origin. Endogenous thyroid hormone secretion is suppressed when exogenous thyroid hormones are administered to euthyroid individuals in excess of the normal gland's secretion.

The mechanisms by which thyroid hormones exert their physiologic action are not well understood. These hormones enhance oxygen consumption by most tissues of the body and increase the basal metabolic rate and the metabolism of carbohydrates, lipids, and proteins. Thus they exert a profound influence on every organ system in the body and are of particular importance in the development of the central nervous system.

The normal thyroid gland contains approximately 200 mcg of levothyroxine (T_4) per gram of gland, and 15 mcg of triiodothyronine (T_3) per gram. The ratio of these two hormones in the circulation does not represent the ratio in the thyroid gland, since about 80 percent of peripheral triiodothyronine comes from monodeiodination of levothyroxine at the 5 position (outer ring). Peripheral monodeiodination of levothyroxine at the 5 position (inner ring) results in the formulation of reverse triiodothyronine (rT_3), which is calorigenically inactive. These facts would seem to advocate levothyroxine as the treatment of choice for the hypothyroid patient and to militate against the administration of hormone combinations which, while normalizing thyroxine levels may produce triiodothyronine levels in the thyrotoxic range.

Triiodothyronine (T_3) level is low in the fetus and newborn, in old age, in chronic caloric deprivation, hepatic cirrhosis, renal failure, surgical stress, and chronic illnesses representing what has been called the "low triiodothyronine syndrome."

PHARMACOKINETICS

More than 99 percent of circulating hormones are bound to serum proteins, including thyroxine-binding globulin (TBG), thyroxine-binding prealbumin (TBPA), and albumin (TBa), whose capacities and affinities vary for the hormones. The higher affinity of levothyroxine (T_4) for both TBG and TBPA as compared to triiodothyronine (T_3) partially explains the higher serum levels and longer half-life of the former hormone. Both protein-bound hormones exist in equilibrium with minute amounts of free hormone, the latter accounting for the metabolic activity.

Deiodination of levothyroxine (T_4) occurs at a number of sites, including liver, kidney, and other tissues. The conjugated hormone, in the form of glucuronide or sulfate, is found in the bile and gut where it may complete an enterohepatic circulation. Eighty-five percent of levothyroxine (T_4) metabolized daily is deiodinated.

INDICATIONS AND USAGE

Levothyroxine Sodium, USP for Injection is indicated:

1. As replacement or supplemental therapy in patients with hypothyroidism of any etiology, except transient hypothyroidism during the recovery phase of subacute thyroiditis. This category includes cretinism, myxedema, and ordinary hypothyroidism in patients of any age (children, adults, the elderly), or state (including pregnancy); primary hypothyroidism resulting from functional deficiency, primary atrophy, partial or total absence of thyroid gland, or the effects of surgery, radiation, or drugs, with or without the presence of goiter; and secondary (pituitary), or tertiary (hypothalamic) hypothyroidism (see **CONTRAINDICATIONS** and **PRECAUTIONS**). Levothyroxine Sodium, USP for Injection can be used intravenously whenever a rapid onset of effect is critical and either intravenously or intramuscularly in hypothyroid patients whenever the oral route is precluded for long periods of time.
2. As a pituitary TSH suppressant, in the treatment or prevention of various types of euthyroid goiters, including thyroid nodules, subacute or chronic lymphocytic thyroiditis (Hashimoto's), multinodular goiter, and in the management of thyroid cancer.
3. As a diagnostic agent in suppression tests to aid in the diagnosis of suspected mild hyperthyroidism or thyroid gland autonomy.

CONTRAINDICATIONS

Thyroid hormone preparations are generally contraindicated in patients with diagnosed but as yet uncorrected adrenal cortical insufficiency, untreated thyrotoxicosis, and apparent hypersensitivity to any of their active or extraneous constituents. There is no well documented evidence from the literature, however, of true allergic or idiosyncratic reactions to thyroid hormone.

WARNINGS

Drugs with thyroid activity, alone or together with other therapeutic agents, have been used for the treatment of obesity. In euthyroid patients, doses within the range of daily hormonal requirements are ineffective for weight reduction. Larger doses may produce serious or even life threatening manifestations of toxicity, particularly when given in association with sympathomimetic amines such as those used for their anorectic effects.

The use of thyroid hormones in the therapy of obesity, alone or combined with other drugs, is unjustified and has been shown to be ineffective. Neither is their use justified for the treatment of male or female infertility unless this condition is accompanied by hypothyroidism.

PRECAUTIONS

General: Thyroid hormones should be used with great caution in a number of circumstances where the integrity of the cardiovascular system, particularly the coronary arteries, is suspected. These include patients with angina pectoris or the elderly, who have a greater likelihood of occult cardiac disease. In these patients, therapy should be initiated with low doses, i.e., 25-50 mcg levothyroxine (T_4). When, in such patients, a euthyroid state can only be reached at the expense of an aggravation of the cardiovascular disease, thyroid hormone dosage should be reduced.

Thyroid hormone therapy in patients with concomitant diabetes mellitus or insipidus or adrenal cortical insufficiency aggravates the intensity of their symptoms. Appropriate adjustments of the various therapeutic measures directed at these concomitant endocrine diseases are required. The therapy of myxedema coma may require simultaneous administration of glucocorticoids (see **DOSAGE AND ADMINISTRATION**).

Hypothyroidism decreases and hyperthyroidism increases the sensitivity to oral anticoagulants. Prothrombin time should be closely monitored in thyroid treated patients on oral anticoagulants and dosage of the latter agents adjusted on the basis of frequent prothrombin time determinations.

In infants, excessive doses of thyroid hormone preparations may produce craniosynostosis.

Information for the Patient: Patients on thyroid hormone preparations and parents of children on thyroid therapy should be informed that:

1. Replacement therapy is to be taken essentially for life, with the exception of cases of transient hypothyroidism, usually associated with thyroiditis, and in those patients receiving a therapeutic trial of the drug.
2. They should immediately report during the course of therapy any signs or symptoms of thyroid hormone toxicity, e.g., chest pain, increased pulse rate, palpitations, excessive sweating, heat intolerance, nervousness, or any other unusual event.
3. In case of concomitant diabetes mellitus, the daily dosage of antidiabetic medication may need readjustment as thyroid hormone replacement is achieved. If thyroid medication is stopped, a downward readjustment of the dosage of insulin or oral hypoglycemic agent may be necessary to avoid hypoglycemia. At all times, close monitoring of blood or urinary glucose levels is mandatory in such patients.
4. In case of concomitant oral anticoagulant therapy, the prothrombin time should be measured frequently to determine if the dosage of oral anticoagulants is to be readjusted.
5. Partial loss of hair may be experienced by children in the first few months of thyroid therapy, but this is usually a transient phenomenon and later recovery is usually the rule.

Laboratory Tests: Treatment of patients with thyroid hormones requires the periodic assessment of thyroid status by means of appropriate laboratory tests, by full clinical evaluation, or both. The TSH suppression test can be used to test the effectiveness of any thyroid preparation bearing in mind the relative insensitivity of the infant pituitary to the negative feedback effect of thyroid hormones. Serum T_4 levels can be used to test the effectiveness of levothyroxine sodium. When the total serum T_4 is low but TSH is normal, a test specific to assess unbound (free) T_4 levels is warranted. Specific measurements of T_4 and T_3 by competitive protein binding or radioimmunoassay are not influenced by blood levels of organic or inorganic iodine and have essentially replaced older tests of thyroid hormone measurements, i.e., PBI, BEI, and T_4 by column.

Drug Interactions: *Oral Anticoagulants*—Thyroid hormones appear to increase catabolism of vitamin K-dependent clotting factors. If oral anticoagulants are also being given, compensatory increases in clotting factor synthesis are impaired. Patients stabilized on oral anticoagulants who are found to require thyroid replacement therapy should be watched very closely when thyroid is started. If a patient is truly hypothyroid, it is likely that a reduction in anticoagulant dosage will be required. No special precautions appear to be necessary when oral anticoagulant therapy is begun in a patient already stabilized on maintenance thyroid replacement therapy.

Insulin Or Oral Hypoglycemics—Initiating thyroid replacement therapy may cause increases in insulin or oral hypoglycemic requirements. The effects seen are poorly understood and depend upon a variety of factors such as dose and type of thyroid preparations and endocrine status of the patient. Patients receiving insulin or oral hypoglycemics should be closely watched during initiation of thyroid replacement therapy.

Estrogen, Oral Contraceptives—Estrogens tend to increase serum thyroxine-binding globulin (TBG). In a patient with a nonfunctioning thyroid gland who is receiving thyroid replacement therapy, free levothyroxine may be decreased when estrogens are started, thus increasing thyroid requirements. However, if the patient's thyroid gland has sufficient function, the decreased free thyroxine will result in a compensatory increase in thyroxine output by the thyroid. Therefore, patients without a functioning thyroid gland who are on thyroid replacement therapy may need to increase their thyroid dose if estrogens or estrogen-containing oral contraceptives are given.

Drug/Laboratory Test Interactions: The following drugs or moieties are known to interfere with some laboratory tests performed in patients on thyroid hormone therapy: Androgens, corticosteroids, estrogens, oral contraceptives containing estrogens, iodine-containing preparations, and the numerous preparations containing salicylates.

1. Changes in TBG concentration should be taken into consideration in the interpretation of T_4 and T_3 values. Pregnancy, estrogens, and estrogen-containing oral contraceptives increase TBG concentrations. TBG may also be increased during infectious hepatitis. Decreases in TBG concentrations are observed in nephrosis, acromegaly, and after androgen or corticosteroid therapy. Familial hyper- or hypo-thyroxine-binding-globulinemias have been described. The incidence of TBG deficiency approximates 1 in 9000. The binding of thyroxine by TBPA is inhibited by salicylates. In such cases, the unbound (free) hormone should be measured. Alternatively, an indirect measure of

free thyroxine, such as the Free Thyroxine Index (FTI) may be used.

2. Medicinal or dietary iodine interferes with all *in vivo* tests of radioiodine uptake, producing low uptakes which may not indicate a true decrease in hormone synthesis.

3. The persistence of clinical and laboratory evidence of hypothyroidism in spite of adequate dosage replacement indicates either poor patient compliance, poor absorption, or inactivity of the preparation. Intracellular resistance to thyroid hormone is quite rare, and is suggested by clinical signs and symptoms of hypothyroidism in the presence of high serum T_4 levels.

Carcinogenesis, Mutagenesis, and Impairment of Fertility: A reported association between prolonged thyroid therapy and breast cancer has not been confirmed and patients on thyroid therapy for established indications should not discontinue therapy. No confirmatory long-term studies in animals have been performed to evaluate carcinogenic potential, mutagenicity, or impairment of fertility in either males or females.

Pregnancy: Pregnancy category A. Thyroid hormones do not readily cross the placental barrier. The clinical experience to date does not indicate any adverse effect on fetuses when thyroid hormones are administered to pregnant women. On the basis of current knowledge, thyroid replacement therapy to hypothyroid women should not be discontinued during pregnancy.

Nursing Mothers: Minimal amount of thyroid hormones are excreted in human milk. Thyroid is not associated with serious adverse reactions and does not have known tumorigenic potential. While caution should be exercised when thyroid is administered to a nursing woman, adequate replacement doses of levothyroxine are generally needed to maintain normal lactation.

Pediatric Use: Pregnant mothers provide little or no thyroid hormone to the fetus. The incidence of congenital hypothyroidism is relatively high (1 in 4,000) and the hypothyroid fetus would not derive any benefit from the small amounts of hormone crossing the placental barrier. Routine determinations of serum T_4 and/or TSH is strongly advised in neonates in view of the deleterious effects of thyroid deficiency on growth and development.

Treatment should be initiated immediately upon diagnosis, and maintained for life, unless transient hypothyroidism is suspected; in which case, therapy may be interrupted for 2 to 8 weeks after the age of 3 years to reassess the condition. Cessation of therapy is justified in patients who have maintained a normal TSH during those 2 to 8 weeks.

ADVERSE REACTIONS

Adverse reactions other than those indicative of hyperthyroidism because of therapeutic overdosage, either initially or during the maintenance periods, are rare (see **OVERDOSAGE**).

OVERDOSAGE

Signs and Symptoms: Excessive doses of thyroid result in hypermetabolic state resembling in every aspect the condition of endogenous origin. The condition may be self-induced.

Treatment of Overdosage: Dosage should be reduced or therapy temporarily discontinued if signs and symptoms of overdosage appear. Treatment may be reinstated at a lower dosage. In normal individuals, normal hypothalamic-pituitary-thyroid axis function is restored in 6 to 8 weeks after thyroid suppression.

Treatment of acute massive thyroid hormone overdosage is aimed at counteracting central and peripheral effects, mainly those of increased sympathetic activity. Treatment is symptomatic and supportive. Oxygen may be administered and ventilation maintained. Cardiac glycosides may be indicated if congestive heart failure develops. Measures to control fever, hypoglycemia, or fluid loss should be instituted if needed. Antiadrenergic agents, particularly propranolol, have been used advantageously in the treatment of increased sympathetic activity. Propranolol may be administered intravenously at a dosage of 1 to 3 mg over a 10 minute period or orally, 80 to 160 mg/day, especially when no contraindications exist for its use.

DOSAGE AND ADMINISTRATION

The dosage and rate of coadministration of Levothyroxine Sodium, USP for Injection is determined by the indication and must in every case be individualized according to patient response and laboratory findings.

Hypothyroidism: Levothyroxine Sodium, USP for Injection by intravenous or intramuscular routes can be substituted for the oral dosage form when ingestion of levothyroxine sodium tablets is precluded for long periods of time. The initial parenteral dosage should be approximately one half of the previously established oral dosage of levothyroxine sodium tablets. Close observation of the patient, with individual adjustment of the dosage as needed, is recommended.

Myxedema Coma: Myxedema coma is usually precipitated in the hypothyroid patient by intercurrent illness or drugs such as sedatives and anesthetics and should be considered a medical emergency. Therapy should be directed at the correction of electrolyte disturbances and possible infection besides the administration of thyroid hormones. Corticosteroids should be administered routinely. T_4 may be administered via a nasogastric tube but the preferred route of administration is intravenous. Sodium levothyroxine (T_4) is given at a starting dose of 400 mcg (100 mcg/mL) given rapidly, and is usually well-tolerated, even in the elderly. In the presence of concomitant heart disease, the sudden administration of such large doses of L-thyroxine intravenously is clearly not without its cardiovascular risks. Under such circumstances, intravenous therapy should not be undertaken without weighing the alternative risks of the myxedema coma and the cardiovascular disease. Clinical judgement in this situation may dictate smaller intravenous doses of Levothyroxine Sodium, USP for Injection. The initial dose is followed by daily supplements of 100 to 200 mcg given intravenously. Normal T_4 levels are achieved in 24 hours followed in 3 days by threefold evaluation of T_3. Continued daily administration of lesser amounts parenterally should be maintained until the patient is fully capable of accepting a daily oral dose. A daily maintenance dose of 50 to 100 mcg parenterally should suffice to maintain the euthyroid state, once established. Oral therapy would be resumed as soon as the clinical situation has been stabilized and the patient is able to take oral medication.

TSH Suppression in Thyroid Cancer, Nodules, and Euthyroid Goiters: Exogenous thyroid hormone may produce regression of metastases from follicular and papillary carcinoma of the thyroid and is used as ancillary therapy of these conditions following surgery or radioactive iodine. Medullary carcinoma of the thyroid is usually unresponsive to this therapy. TSH should be suppressed to low or undetectable levels. Therefore, larger amounts of thyroid hormone than those used for replacement therapy are frequently required. This therapy is also used in treating nontoxic solitary nodules and multinodular goiters, and to prevent thyroid enlargement in chronic (Hashimoto's) thyroiditis.

Thyroid Suppression Therapy: Administration of thyroid hormone in doses higher than those produced physiologically by the gland results in suppression of the production of endogenous hormone. This is the basis for the thyroid suppression test and is used as an aid in the diagnosis of patients with signs of mild hyperthyroidism in whom base line laboratory tests appear normal, or to demonstrate thyroid gland autonomy in patients with Graves' ophthalmopathy. I uptake is determined before and after the administration of the exogenous hormone. A fifty percent or greater suppression of uptake indicates a normal thyroid-pituitary axis and thus rules out thyroid gland autonomy.

For adults, the average suppressive dose of levothyroxine (T_4) is 2.6 mcg/kg of body weight per day given for 7 to 10 days. These doses usually yield normal serum T_4 and T_3 levels and lack of response to TSH.

Levothyroxine sodium should be administered cautiously to patients in whom there is a strong suspicion of thyroid gland autonomy, in view of the fact that the exogenous hormone effects will be additive to the endogenous source.

HOW SUPPLIED

Levothyroxine Sodium, USP for Injection is lyophilized with 10 mg Mannitol and 0.7 mg Tribasic Sodium Phosphate Anhydrous in 10 mL vials. The pH may be adjusted with Sodium Hydroxide. It is supplied as follows:
NDC 0186-1855-01; 200 mcg per 10 mL vial
NDC 0186-1856-01; 500 mcg per 10 mL vial
Store at controlled room temperature, 15°-30°C (59°-86°F).

DIRECTIONS FOR RECONSTITUTION

Reconstitute the lyophilized levothyroxine sodium by aseptically adding 5 mL of 0.9% Sodium Chloride Injection, USP or Bacteriostatic Sodium Chloride Injection, USP with Benzyl Alcohol, only. Shake vial to insure complete mixing. Use **immediately** after reconstitution. Do not add to other intravenous fluids. Discard any unused portion.

CAUTION: Federal law prohibits dispensing without prescription.

Manufactured by:
ASTRA®
Astra USA, Inc.
Westborough, MA 01581   021669R00 Iss. 2/95

MAGNESIUM SULFATE INJECTION, USP

NDC No. 0186-	Magnesium Sulfate Heptahydrate Concentration	Container Type	Fill Volume	Magnesium per mL	Sulfate per mL
1203-04	10%	Vial	20 mL	9.9 mg	38.9 mg
1204-04	10%	Vial	50 mL	9.9 mg	38.9 mg
1209-04	50%	Vial	2 mL	49.3 mg	194.7 mg
1210-04	50%	Vial	10 mL	49.3 mg	194.7 mg
1211-04	50%	Vial	20 mL	49.3 mg	194.7 mg
0684-01	50%	Additive Syringe	5 mL	49.3 mg	194.7 mg
0685-01	50%	Additive Syringe	10 mL	49.3 mg	194.7 mg

MAGNESIUM SULFATE INJECTION, USP ℞

(For details of indications, dosages and administration, precautions, and adverse reactions, see circular in package.)

HOW SUPPLIED

[See table above.]
No preservative added. Unused portion of container should be discarded. Use only if solution is clear, and seal intact.
021874R01   2/88

MANNITOL Injection, USP 25% ℞
[*man-ĭ-tall*]

(For details of indications, dosage and administration, precautions, and adverse reactions, see circular in package.)

HOW SUPPLIED

Mannitol Injection, USP 25% is a sterile solution supplied in single dose containers as follows:
NDC 0186-1168-04: 50 mL vials, 25 vials per package
NDC 0186-0652-01: 50 mL syringes, 10 syringes per package
Caution: Federal law prohibits dispensing without prescription.
Store at controlled room temperature 15°-30°C (59°-86°F).
NOTE: Crystals may form in mannitol solutions especially if solutions are chilled. See PRECAUTIONS to dissolve the crystals.
021855R03   Rev. 1/95

MEPERIDINE HCl INJECTION, USP Ⓒ℞

WARNING: May be habit forming.
(For details of indications, dosage and administration, precautions, and adverse reactions, see circular in package.)

HOW SUPPLIED

Meperidine Hydrochloride Injection, USP is available as:
Multiple Dose Vials
NDC 0186-1283-01   100 mg/mL,   20 mL vial, box of 1
NDC 0186-1284-01   50 mg/mL,   30 mL vial, box of 1
Store at controlled room temperature 15°-30°C (59°-86°F).
021889R04   7/92 (4)

METAPROTERENOL SULFATE ℞
ARM-A-MED®
Inhalation Solution, USP
0.4% and 0.6%

DESCRIPTION

Each vial contains metaproterenol sulfate 0.4% or 0.6% in a sterile aqueous solution containing sodium chloride and edetate disodium. Sulfuric acid and/or sodium hydroxide to adjust pH to 2.8-4.0. The solution is filled under nitrogen. The solution is a bronchodilator to be administered by oral inhalation with the aid of an intermittent positive pressure breathing apparatus (IPPB).
Metaproterenol sulfate is a beta adrenergic stimulator and is chemically 1-(3,5 dihydroxyphenyl)-2-isopropylaminoethanol sulfate, a white, crystalline, racemic mixture of two optically active isomers. It differs from isoproterenol hydrochloride by having two hydroxyl groups attached at the meta positions on the benzene ring rather than one at the meta and one at the para position.
[See chemical structure at top of next column.]

Continued on next page

Astra—Cont.

metaproterenol sulfate   isoproterenol hydrochloride

CLINICAL PHARMACOLOGY

Metaproterenol is a potent beta adrenergic stimulator with a rapid onset of action. It is postulated that beta adrenergic stimulants produce many of their pharmacological effects by activation of adenyl cyclase, the enzyme which catalyzes the conversion of adenosine triphosphate to cyclic adenosine monophosphate.

Absorption, biotransformation and excretion studies following administration by inhalation have not been performed. Following oral administration in humans, an average of 40% of the drug is absorbed; it is not metabolized by catechol-O-methyltransferase but is excreted primarily as glucuronic acid conjugates.

Recent studies in laboratory animals (minipigs, rodents and dogs) recorded the occurrence of cardiac arrhythmias and sudden death (with histologic evidence of myocardial necrosis) when beta agonists and methylxanthines were administered concurrently. The significance of these findings when applied to humans is currently unknown.

INDICATIONS AND USAGE

Metaproterenol Sulfate Inhalation Solution, USP is indicated as a bronchodilator for bronchial asthma, and for reversible bronchospasm which may occur in association with bronchitis and emphysema.

Following controlled single dose studies by an intermittent positive pressure breathing apparatus (IPPB) and by hand bulb nebulizers, significant improvement (15% or greater increase in FEV_1) occurred within 5 to 30 minutes and persisted for periods varying from 2 to 6 hours.

In these studies, the longer duration of effect occurred in the studies in which the drug was administered by IPPB, i.e., 6 hours versus 2 to 3 hours when administered by hand bulb nebulizer. In these studies the doses used were 0.3 mL by IPPB and 10 inhalations by hand bulb nebulizer.

In controlled repetitive dosing studies by IPPB and by hand bulb nebulizer the onset of effect occurred within 5 to 30 minutes and duration ranged from 4 to 6 hours. In these studies the doses used were 0.3 mL b.i.d. or t.i.d. when given by IPPB, and 10 inhalations q.i.d. (no more often than q4h) when given by hand bulb nebulizer. As in the single-dose studies, effectiveness was measured as a sustained increase in FEV_1 of 15% or greater. In these repetitive dosing studies there was no apparent difference in duration between the two methods of delivery.

During other clinical tolerance studies metaproterenol was administered q.i.d. (by nebulizer) for periods of 60 and 90 days. On specified days before, during, and after these open label trials, patients were referred to a laboratory where the effects of single doses of metaproterenol and isoproterenol on pulmonary function were recorded (in a double blind crossover controlled setting). Both drugs continued to exert significant improvement in function throughout this period of treatment.

CONTRAINDICATIONS

Use in patients with cardiac arrhythmias associated with tachycardia is contraindicated.

Although rare, immediate hypersensitivity reactions can occur. Therefore, Metaproterenol Sulfate Inhalation Solution, USP is contraindicated in patients with a history of hypersensitivity to any of its components.

WARNINGS

Excessive use of adrenergic aerosols is potentially dangerous. Fatalities have been reported following excessive use of metaproterenol, as with other sympathomimetic inhalation preparations, and the exact cause is unknown. Cardiac arrest was noted in several cases.

Paradoxical bronchoconstriction with repeated excessive administration has been reported with other sympathomimetic agents.

Patients should be advised to contact their physicians in the event that they do not respond to their usual dose of sympathomimetic amine aerosol.

PRECAUTIONS

General: Because metaproterenol is a sympathomimetic drug, it should be used with great caution in patients with hypertension, coronary artery disease, congestive heart failure, hyperthyroidism or diabetes, or when there is sensitivity to sympathomimetic amines.

Information for Patients: Extreme care must be exercised with respect to the administration of additional sympatho-

mimetic agents. A sufficient interval of time should elapse prior to administration of another sympathomimetic agent.

Carcinogenesis, Mutagenesis, Impairment of Fertility: Long-term studies in mice and rats to evaluate the oral carcinogenic potential of metaproterenol sulfate have not been completed.

Studies of metaproterenol sulfate have not been conducted to determine mutagenic potential or effect on fertility.

Pregnancy: Teratogenic Effects: Pregnancy Category C. Metaproterenol has been shown to be teratogenic and embryocidal in rabbits when given orally in doses 620 times the human inhalation dose. There are no adequate and well-controlled studies in pregnant women. Metaproterenol Sulfate Inhalation Solution, USP should be used during pregnancy only if the potential benefit justifies the potential risk to the fetus.

Oral reproduction studies in mice, rats and rabbits showed no teratogenic or embryocidal effect at 50 mg/kg corresponding to 310 times the human inhalation dose. Teratogenic effects in the rabbit included skeletal abnormalities and hydrocephalus with bone separation.

Nursing Mothers: It is not known whether this drug is excreted in human milk. Because many drugs are excreted in human milk, caution should be exercised when metaproterenol sulfate is administered to a nursing woman.

Pediatric Use: Safety and effectiveness in children below the age of 12 have not been established.

ADVERSE REACTIONS

Adverse reactions are similar to those noted with other sympathomimetic agents.

The most frequent adverse reactions to metaproterenol are nervousness and tachycardia which occur in about 1 in 7 patients, tremor which occurs in about 1 in 20 patients and nausea which occurs in about 1 in 50 patients. Less frequent adverse reactions are hypertension, palpitations, vomiting and bad taste which occur in approximately 1 in 300 patients.

OVERDOSAGE

The symptoms of overdosage are those of excessive beta adrenergic stimulation listed under ADVERSE REACTIONS. These reactions usually do not require treatment other than reduction of dosage and/or frequency of administration.

DOSAGE AND ADMINISTRATION

Metaproterenol Sulfate Inhalation Solution, USP is administered by oral inhalation using an IPPB device. The usual adult dose is one vial per nebulization treatment. Each 0.4% vial is equivalent to 0.2 mL metaproterenol sulfate 5% solution diluted to 2.5 mL with normal saline. Each 0.6% vial is equivalent to 0.3 mL metaproterenol sulfate 5% solution diluted to 2.5 mL with normal saline.

Usually, treatment need not be repeated more often than every four hours to relieve acute attacks of bronchospasm. As part of a total treatment program in chronic bronchospastic pulmonary diseases, Metaproterenol Sulfate Inhalation Solution, USP may be administered three or four times a day.

As with all medications, the physician should begin therapy with the lowest effective dose and then titrate the dosage according to the individual patient's requirements.

Metaproterenol Sulfate Inhalation Solution, USP is not recommended for use in children under 12 years of age.

HOW SUPPLIED

Metaproterenol Sulfate Inhalation Solution, USP is supplied in Arm-a-Med vials and is available in pouches containing 5 single-use, plastic vials of 2.5 mL each. There are 20 pouches per carton of 100 vials.

NDC 0186-4131-01 0.4% equivalent to 0.2 mL Metaproterenol Sulfate Inhalation Solution, USP 5% diluted to 2.5 mL. Total contents of 10 mg of metaproterenol sulfate.

NDC 0186-4130-01 0.6% equivalent to 0.3 mL Metaproterenol Sulfate Inhalation Solution, USP 5% diluted to 2.5 mL. Total contents of 15 mg of metaproterenol sulfate.

DO NOT STORE ABOVE 25°C (77°F). PROTECT FROM LIGHT. Store vials in pouch until ready for use.

Do not use solution if its color is pinkish or darker than slightly yellow or if it contains a precipitate.

Caution: Federal law prohibits dispensing without prescription.

Manufactured by:
Centeon L.L.C.
Kankakee, Illinois 60901
021638R01   Rev. 4/96

MORPHINE SULFATE (Immediate Release)
Concentrated Oral Solution   ℂ ℞

(WARNING: May be habit forming.)

DESCRIPTION

Each mL of Morphine Sulfate (Immediate Release) Concentrated Oral Solution contains:

Morphine Sulfate .... 20 mg
(WARNING: May be habit forming.)
Chemically, Morphine Sulfate is Morphinan-3,6-diol,7,8-didehydro-4,5-epoxy-17-methyl-, (5α,6α)-, sulfate (2:1)(salt), pentahydrate, which can be represented by the following structural formula:

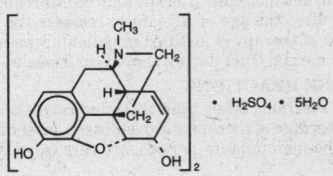

Morphine Sulfate acts as a narcotic analgesic.

HOW SUPPLIED

Morphine Sulfate (Immediate Release) Concentrated Oral Solution is available as follows:
NDC 0186-1123-85, 20 mg/mL, 120 mL bottle with calibrated dropper (box of one).
DEA Order Form Required.
Caution: Federal law prohibits dispensing without prescription.
021702R00   Iss. 3/95

MORPHINE SULFATE   ℂ ℞
Immediate Release Oral Solution

(WARNING: May be habit forming.)

DESCRIPTION

Each 5 mL of Morphine Sulfate Immediate Release Oral Solution contains:
Morphine Sulfate .... 10 mg
(WARNING: May be habit forming.)
Chemically, Morphine Sulfate is Morphinan-3,6-diol, 7,8-didehydro-4,5-epoxy-17-methyl-, (5α,6α)-, sulfate (2:1) (salt), pentahydrate, which can be represented by the following structural formula:

Morphine Sulfate acts as a narcotic analgesic.

HOW SUPPLIED

Morphine Sulfate Immediate Release Oral Solution is available as follows:
NDC 0186-1124-95, 10 mg/5 mL, 500 mL bottle
DEA Order Form Required.
Caution: Federal law prohibits dispensing without prescription.
021694R00   Iss. 3/95

MORPHINE SULFATE INJECTION, USP   ℂ ℞

WARNING—MAY BE HABIT FORMING.
FOR INTRAVENOUS USE AFTER DILUTION.
NOT FOR EPIDURAL OR INTRATHECAL USE.

DESCRIPTION

Morphine is a tertiary nitrogen base containing a phenanthrene nucleus; it has two hydroxyl groups, one phenolic and the other alcoholic (secondary). The sulfate salt occurs as white, feathery, silky crystals, cubical masses of crystals, or white, crystalline powder.

The chemical name of morphine sulfate is 7,8-didehydro-4,5α-epoxy-17-methylmorphinan-3,6α-diol sulfate (2:1) (salt), pentahydrate.

The molecular formula is $(C_{17}H_{19}NO_3)_2 \cdot H_2SO_4 \cdot 5H_2O$, and the structural formula is as follows:

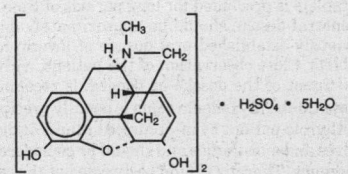

Morphine Sulfate Injection, USP, 25 mg/mL, 20 mL is a sterile solution of morphine sulfate for intravenous infusion after dilution.

Each mL contains: Morphine sulfate 25 mg, edetate disodium 0.075% and sodium bisulfite 0.1% as an antioxidant, in Water for Injection q.s.

This product contains no bacteriostat or antimicrobial agents and is intended as a single dose unit. When the dosing requirement is completed, the unused portion should be discarded in an appropriate manner.

NOTE: This product is not intended for intrathecal use, epidural use, or direct injection.

HOW SUPPLIED

Morphine Sulfate Injection, USP, 25 mg/mL is available in a single dose vial as follows:

NDC 0186-1135-51, 25 mg/mL, 20 mL vial, (box of one)
Store at controlled room temperature 15°–30°C (59°–86°F).
PROTECT FROM LIGHT.
CAUTION: Federal law prohibits dispensing without prescription.

021643R00   Iss. 9/94

MORPHINE SULFATE INJECTION, USP Ⓒ Ⅱ ℞
WARNING—MAY BE HABIT FORMING.
For Intravenous Infusion Only.
Not For Epidural Or Intrathecal Use.

DESCRIPTION

Morphine is a tertiary nitrogen base containing a phenanthrene nucleus; it has two hydroxyl groups, one phenolic and the other alcoholic (secondary). The sulfate salt occurs as white, feathery, silky crystals, cubical masses of crystals or white, crystalline powder.

The chemical name of morphine sulfate is 7,8-didehydro-4,5α-epoxy-17-methylmorphinan-3,6α-diol sulfate (2:1) (salt), pentahydrate.

The empirical formula is $(C_{17}H_{19}NO_3)_2 \cdot H_2SO_4 \cdot 5H_2O$ and the structure is as follows:

$$H_2SO_4 \cdot 5H_2O$$

M.W. 758.83

Morphine Sulfate Injection, USP, is a sterile solution of 1 mg/mL or 2 mg/mL morphine sulfate pentahydrate in Water for Injection, USP. The 1 mg/mL and 2 mg/mL solutions contain Sodium Chloride 7.6 mg; with citric acid, anhydrous 0.4 mg and sodium citrate, dihydrate 0.2 mg added as buffers. Sodium metabisulfite 0.9 mg is added as an antioxidant. May contain additional citric acid and sodium citrate for pH adjustment.

The solutions contain no bacteriostat or antimicrobial agents and are intended only as single dose units for slow intravenous use by infusion pump. When the dosing requirement is completed, the unused portion should be discarded in an appropriate manner.

HOW SUPPLIED

Morphine Sulfate Injection, USP, is available in single-dose vials as follows:

NDC 0186-1120-81 1 mg/mL, 60 mL vial (box of one)
NDC 0186-1121-81 2 mg/mL, 60 mL vial (box of one)
Store at controlled room temperature 15°–30°C (59°–86°F).
PROTECT FROM LIGHT.
NOTE: Morphine sulfate solutions may darken with age.
CAUTION: Federal law prohibits dispensing without prescription.

021691R00   Iss. 1/94

M.V.I.®-12 ℞
Multi-Vitamin Infusion
For dilution in intravenous infusions only.
M.V.I.-12
Multi-Vitamin Infusion
M.V.I.-12 Multi-Dose
PHARMACY BULK PACKAGE
NOT FOR DIRECT INFUSION
Multi-Vitamin Infusion
M.V.I.-12 UNIT VIAL
Multi-Vitamin Infusion

(For details of indications, dosage and administration, precautions, and adverse reactions, see circular in package.)

After M.V.I.-12 is diluted in an intravenous infusion, the resulting solution is ready for immediate use. Some of the vitamins in this product, particularly A and D and riboflavin, are light sensitive, and exposure to light should be minimized.

Store at 2°–8°C (36°–46°F).

HOW SUPPLIED

M.V.I.-12—NDC 0186-1199-31 Boxes of 25 and cartons of 100. Each box contains two vials—Vial 1 (5 mL) and Vial 2 (5 mL), both vials to be used for a single dose.

M.V.I.-12 Multi-Dose (PHARMACY BULK PACKAGE)—NDC 0186-1199-10 Boxes of 20 vials, 50 mL each (10 Vial 1 and 10 Vial 2). Mix contents of Vial 1 with Vial 2 to provide ten single doses.

M.V.I.-12 UNIT VIAL—NDC 0186-1199-35 Boxes of 25 two-chambered 10 mL vials.

Caution: Federal law prohibits dispensing without prescription.

Manufactured by:
Armour Pharmaceutical Company
Kankakee, Illinois 60901
Astra USA, Inc.
Westborough, MA 01581

021644R00   Rev. 11/94

M.V.I.® PEDIATRIC ℞
Multi-Vitamins for Infusion
For dilution in intravenous infusions only.

(For details of indications, dosage and administration, precautions, and adverse reactions, see circular in package.)

DISCARD ANY UNUSED PORTION.

Parenteral drug products should be inspected visually for particulate matter and discoloration prior to administration, whenever solution and container permit.

After M.V.I. Pediatric is reconstituted it should be immediately diluted into the intravenous solution. The resulting solution should be administered immediately. Some of the vitamins in this product, particularly vitamins A and D and riboflavin, are light-sensitive and exposure to light should be minimized.

HOW SUPPLIED

M.V.I Pediatric is available as:
NDC 0186-1839-35, Single Dose Vial, Boxes of 25.
NDC 0186-1839-25, Single-use, multiple dose vials (PHARMACY BULK PACKAGE), Boxes of 5.
Store at controlled room temperature, 15°–30°C (59°–86°F).
Caution: Federal law prohibits dispensing without prescription.

Manufactured by:
Armour Pharmaceutical Company
Kankakee, Illinois 60901
Astra USA, Inc.
Westborough, MA 01581

021645R00   Rev. 11/94

NALBUPHINE HCl INJECTION ℞

(For details of indications, dosage and administration, precautions, and adverse reactions, see circular in package.)

HOW SUPPLIED

Nalbuphine HCl Injection for intramuscular, subcutaneous or intravenous use is available in the following dosage forms:

Vials
10 mg/mL, 10 mL vial (box of 1),   NDC 0186-1262-12
20 mg/mL, 10 mL vial (box of 1),   NDC 0186-1266-12
Store at controlled room temperature 15°–30°C (59°–86°F).
Protect from light.

021886R04   8/90 (4)

NALOXONE HCl INJECTION, USP ℞
Narcotic Antagonist

(For details of indications, dosage and administration, precautions, and adverse reactions, see circular in package.)

HOW SUPPLIED

Naloxone HCl Injection, USP, for intravenous, intramuscular and subcutaneous administration is available as:

0.02 mg/mL		
2 mL vial,	box of 10	NDC 0186-1252-13
0.4 mg/mL		
1 mL vial,	box of 10	NDC 0186-1250-13
10 mL vial,	box of 1	NDC 0186-1254-12
1 mg/mL		
1 mL vial,	box of 10	NDC 0186-1251-13
5 mL vial,	box of 1	NDC 0186-1253-13
10 mL vial,	box of 1	NDC 0186-1255-12

Store at controlled room temperature 15°–30°C (59°–86°F).
Protect from light.

021885R07   5/93 (7)

NEOSTIGMINE METHYLSULFATE ℞
INJECTION, USP

(For details of indications, dosage and administration, precautions, and adverse reactions, see circular in package.)

HOW SUPPLIED

Neostigmine Methylsulfate Injection, USP is available in the following dosage forms:
1:1000 (1 mg/mL)—NDC 0186-1742-01
10 mL Multiple Dose Vial, box of 5
1:2000 (0.5 mg/mL)—NDC 0186-1741-01
10 mL Multiple Dose Vial, box of 5

021591R02   12/89 (2)

NESACAINE® ℞
(chloroprocaine HCl Injection, USP)
[nes′ a-caine]
NESACAINE®-MPF
(chloroprocaine HCl Injection, USP)
For Infiltration and Nerve Block.

DESCRIPTION

Nesacaine and Nesacaine-MPF Injections are sterile non pyrogenic local anesthetics. The active ingredient in Nesacaine and Nesacaine-MPF Injections is chloroprocaine HCl (benzoic acid, 4-amino-2-chloro-2-(diethylamino) ethyl ester, monohydrochloride), which is represented by the following structural formula:

$$NH_2 - \langle \rangle - COOCH_2CH_2N(C_2H_5)_2 \cdot HCl$$

[See Table 1 on bottom of next page.]

The solutions are adjusted to pH 2.7–4.0 by means of sodium hydroxide and/or hydrochloric acid. Filled under nitrogen. Nesacaine and Nesacaine-MPF Injections should not be resterilized by autoclaving.

CLINICAL PHARMACOLOGY

Chloroprocaine, like other local anesthetics, blocks the generation and the conduction of nerve impulses, presumably by increasing the threshold for electrical excitation in the nerve, by slowing the propagation of the nerve impulse and by reducing the rate of rise of the action potential. In general, the progression of anesthesia is related to the diameter, myelination and conduction velocity of affected nerve fibers. Clinically, the order of loss of nerve function is as follows: (1) pain, (2) temperature, (3) touch, (4) proprioception, and (5) skeletal muscle tone.

Systemic absorption of local anesthetics produces effects on the cardiovascular and central nervous systems. At blood concentrations achieved with normal therapeutic doses, changes in cardiac conduction, excitability, refractoriness, contractility, and peripheral vascular resistance are minimal. However, toxic blood concentrations depress cardiac conduction and excitability, which may lead to atrioventricular block and ultimately to cardiac arrest. In addition, with toxic blood concentrations myocardial contractility may be depressed and peripheral vasodilation may occur, leading to decreased cardiac output and arterial blood pressure.

Following systemic absorption, toxic blood concentrations of local anesthetics can produce central nervous system stimulation, depression, or both. Apparent central stimulation may be manifested as restlessness, tremors and shivering, which may progress to convulsions. Depression and coma may occur, possibly progressing ultimately to respiratory arrest.

However, the local anesthetics have a primary depressant effect on the medulla and on higher centers. The depressed stage may occur without a prior stage of central nervous system stimulation.

PHARMACOKINETICS

The rate of systemic absorption of local anesthetic drugs is dependent upon the total dose and concentration of drug administered, the route of administration, the vascularity of the administration site, and the presence or absence of epinephrine in the anesthetic injection. Epinephrine usually reduces the rate of absorption and plasma concentration of local anesthetics and is sometimes added to local anesthetic injections in order to prolong the duration of action.

The onset of action with chloroprocaine is rapid (usually within 6 to 12 minutes), and the duration of anesthesia, depending upon the amount used and the route of administration, may be up to 60 minutes.

Local anesthetics appear to cross the placenta by passive diffusion. However, the rate and degree of diffusion varies considerably among the different drugs as governed by: (1)

Continued on next page

Astra—Cont.

the degree of plasma protein binding, (2) the degree of ionization, and (3) the degree of lipid solubility. Fetal/maternal ratios of local anesthetics appear to be inversely related to the degree of plasma protein binding, since only the free, unbound drug is available for placental transfer. Thus, drugs with the highest protein binding capacity may have the lowest fetal/maternal ratios. The extent of placental transfer is also determined by the degree of ionization and lipid solubility of the drug. Lipid soluble, nonionized drugs readily enter the fetal blood from the maternal circulation.
Depending upon the route of administration, local anesthetics are distributed to some extent to all body tissues, with high concentrations found in highly perfused organs such as the liver, lungs, heart, and brain.
Various pharmacokinetic parameters of the local anesthetics can be significantly altered by the presence of hepatic or renal disease, addition of epinephrine, factors affecting urinary pH, renal blood flow, the route of administration, and the age of the patient. The *in vitro* plasma half-life of chloroprocaine in adults is 21 ± 2 seconds for males and 25 ± 1 seconds for females. The *in vitro* plasma half-life in neonates is 43 ± 2 seconds.
Chloroprocaine is rapidly metabolized in plasma by hydrolysis of the ester linkage by pseudocholinesterase. The hydrolysis of chloroprocaine results in the production of β-diethylaminoethanol and 2-chloro-4-aminobenzoic acid, which inhibits the action of the sulfonamides (see **PRECAUTIONS**):
The kidney is the main excretory organ for most local anesthetics and their metabolites. Urinary excretion is affected by urinary perfusion and factors affecting urinary pH.

INDICATIONS AND USAGE

Nesacaine 1% and 2% Injections, in multidose vials with methylparaben as preservative, are indicated for the production of local anesthesia by infiltration and peripheral nerve block. They are not to be used for lumbar or caudal epidural anesthesia.
Nesacaine-MPF 2% and 3% Injections, in single dose vials without preservative and without EDTA, are indicated for the production of local anesthesia by infiltration, peripheral and central nerve block, including lumbar and caudal epidural blocks.
Nesacaine and Nesacaine-MPF Injections are not to be used for subarachnoid administration.

CONTRAINDICATIONS

Nesacaine and Nesacaine-MPF Injections are contraindicated in patients hypersensitive (allergic) to drugs of the PABA ester group.
Lumbar and caudal epidural anesthesia should be used with extreme caution in persons with the following conditions: existing neurological disease, spinal deformities, septicemia, and severe hypertension.

WARNINGS

LOCAL ANESTHETICS SHOULD ONLY BE EMPLOYED BY CLINICIANS WHO ARE WELL VERSED IN DIAGNOSIS AND MANAGEMENT OF DOSE RELATED TOXICITY AND OTHER ACUTE EMERGENCIES WHICH MIGHT ARISE FROM THE BLOCK TO BE EMPLOYED, AND THEN ONLY AFTER ENSURING THE *IMMEDIATE* AVAILABILITY OF OXYGEN, OTHER RESUSCITATIVE DRUGS, CARDIOPULMONARY RESUSCITATIVE EQUIPMENT, AND THE PERSONNEL RESOURCES NEEDED FOR PROPER MANAGEMENT OF TOXIC REACTIONS AND RELATED EMERGENCIES (see also ADVERSE REACTIONS and PRECAUTIONS). DELAY IN PROPER MANAGEMENT OF DOSE RELATED TOXICITY, UNDERVENTILATION FROM ANY CAUSE AND/OR ALTERED SENSITIVITY MAY LEAD TO THE DEVELOPMENT OF ACIDOSIS, CARDIAC ARREST AND, POSSIBLY, DEATH. NESCAINE (chloroprocaine HCl Injection, USP) contains methylparaben and should not be used for lumbar or caudal epidural anesthesia because safety of this antimicrobial preservative has not been established with regard to intrathecal injection, either intentional or unintentional. NESACAINE-MPF Injection contains no preservative; discard unused injection remaining in vial after initial use
Vasopressors should not be used in the presence of ergot type oxytocic drugs, since a severe persistent hypertension may occur.
To avoid intravascular injection, aspiration should be performed before the anesthetic solution is injected. The needle must be repositioned until no blood return can be elicited. However, the absence of blood in the syringe does not guarantee that intravascular injection has been avoided.
Mixtures of local anesthetics are sometimes employed to compensate for the slower onset of one drug and the shorter duration of action of the second drug. Experiments in primates suggest that toxicity is probably additive when mixtures of local anesthetics are employed, but some experiments in rodents suggest synergism. Caution regarding toxic equivalence should be exercised when mixtures of local anesthetics are employed.

PRECAUTIONS

General

The safety and effective use of chloroprocaine depend on proper dosage, correct technique, adequate precautions and readiness for emergencies. Resuscitative equipment, oxygen and other resuscitative drugs should be available for immediate use. (See **WARNINGS** and **ADVERSE REACTIONS**.) The lowest dosage that results in effective anesthesia should be used to avoid high plasma levels and serious adverse effects. Injections should be made slowly, with frequent aspirations before and during the injection to avoid intravascular injection. Syringe aspirations should also be performed before and during each supplemental injection in continuous (intermittent) catheter techniques. During the administration of epidural anesthesia, it is recommended that a test dose be administered (3 mL of 3% or 5 mL of 2% Nesacaine-MPF Injection) initially and that the patient be monitored for central nervous system toxicity and cardiovascular toxicity, as well as for signs of unintended intrathecal administration, before proceeding. When clinical conditions permit, consideration should be given to employing a chloroprocaine solution that contains epinephrine for the test dose because circulatory changes characteristic of epinephrine may also serve as a warning sign of unintended intravascular injection. An intravascular injection is still possible even if aspirations for blood are negative. With the use of continuous catheter techniques, it is recommended that a fraction of each supplemental dose be administered as a test dose in order to verify proper location of the catheter.
Injection of repeated doses of local anesthetics may cause significant increases in plasma levels with each repeated dose due to slow accumulation of the drug or its metabolites. Tolerance to elevated blood levels varies with the physical condition of the patient. Debilitated, elderly patients, acutely ill patients, and children should be given reduced doses commensurate with their age and physical status. Local anesthetics should also be used with caution in patients with hypotension or heart block.
Careful and constant monitoring of cardiovascular and respiratory (adequacy of ventilation) vital signs and the patient's state of consciousness should be accomplished after each local anesthetic injection. It should be kept in mind at such times that restlessness, anxiety, tinnitus, dizziness, blurred vision, tremors, depression or drowsiness may be early warning signs of central nervous system toxicity.
Local anesthetic injections containing a vasoconstrictor should be used cautiously and in carefully circumscribed quantities in areas of the body supplied by end arteries or having otherwise compromised blood supply. Patients with peripheral vascular disease and those with hypertensive vascular disease may exhibit exaggerated vasoconstrictor response. Ischemic injury or necrosis may result.
Since ester-type local anesthetics are hydrolyzed by plasma cholinesterase produced by the liver, chloroprocaine should be used cautiously in patients with hepatic disease.
Local anesthetics should also be used with caution in patients with impaired cardiovascular function since they may be less able to compensate for functional changes associated with the prolongation of A-V conduction produced by these drugs.
Use in Ophthalmic Surgery: When local anesthetic injections are employed for retrobulbar block, lack of corneal sensation should not be relied upon to determine whether or not the patient is ready for surgery. This is because complete lack of corneal sensation usually precedes clinically acceptable external ocular muscle akinesia.

Information for Patients

When appropriate, patients should be informed in advance that they may experience temporary loss of sensation and motor activity, usually in the lower half of the body, following proper administration of epidural anesthesia.

Clinically Significant Drug Interactions

The administration of local anesthetic solutions containing epinephrine or norepinephrine to patients receiving monoamine oxidase inhibitors, tricyclic antidepressants or phenothiazines may produce severe, prolonged hypotension or hypertension. Concurrent use of these agents should generally be avoided. In situation when concurrent therapy is necessary, careful patient monitoring is essential.
Concurrent administration of vasopressor drugs (for the treatment of hypotension related to obstetric blocks) and ergot-type oxytocic drugs may cause severe, persistent hypertension or cerebrovascular accidents.
The para-aminobenzoic acid metabolite of chloroprocaine inhibits the action of sulfonamides. Therefore, chloroprocaine should not be used in any condition in which a sulfonamide drug is being employed.

Carcinogenesis, Mutagenesis, and Impairment of Fertility

Long-term studies in animals to evaluate carcinogenic potential and reproduction studies to evaluate mutagenesis or impairment of fertility have not been conducted with chloroprocaine.

Pregnancy: Category C

Animal reproduction studies have not been conducted with chloroprocaine. It is also not known whether chloroprocaine can cause fetal harm when administered to a pregnant woman or can affect reproduction capacity. Chloroprocaine should be given to a pregnant woman only if clearly needed. This does not preclude the use of chloroprocaine at term for the production of obstetrical anesthesia.

Labor and Delivery

Local anesthetics rapidly cross the placenta, and when used for epidural, paracervical, pudendal or caudal block anesthesia, can cause varying degrees of maternal, fetal and neonatal toxicity. (See **CLINICAL PHARMACOLOGY** and **PHARMACOKINETICS**.)
The incidence and degree of toxicity depend upon the procedure performed, the type and amount of drug used, and the technique of drug administration. Adverse reactions in the parturient, fetus and neonate involve alterations of the central nervous system, peripheral vascular tone and cardiac function.
Maternal hypotension has resulted from regional anesthesia. Local anesthetics produce vasodilation by blocking sympathetic nerves. Elevating the patient's legs and positioning her on her left side will help prevent decreases in blood pressure. The fetal heart rate also should be monitored continuously, and electronic fetal monitoring is highly advisable.
Epidural, paracervical, or pudendal anesthesia may alter the forces of parturition through changes in uterine contractility or maternal expulsive efforts. In one study, paracervical block anesthesia was associated with a decrease in the mean duration of first stage labor and facilitation of cervical dilation. However, epidural anesthesia has also been reported to prolong the second stage of labor by removing the parturient's reflex urge to bear down or by interfering with motor function. The use of obstetrical anesthesia may increase the need for forceps assistance.
The use of some local anesthetic drug products during labor and delivery may be followed by diminished muscle strength and tone for the first day or two of life. The long-term significance of these observations is unknown.
Careful adherence to recommended dosage is of the utmost importance in obstetrical paracervical block. Failure to achieve adequate analgesia with recommended doses should arouse suspicion of intravascular or fetal intracranial injection. Cases compatible with unintended fetal intracranial injection of local anesthetic injection have been reported following intended paracervical or pudendal block or both. Babies so affected present with unexplained neonatal depression at birth which correlates with high local anesthetic serum levels and usually manifest seizures within six hours. Prompt use of supportive measures combined with forced urinary excretion of the local anesthetic has been used successfully to manage this complication.
Case reports of maternal convulsions and cardiovascular collapse following use of some local anesthetics for paracervical block in early pregnancy (as anesthesia for elective abortion) suggest that systemic absorption under these circumstances may be rapid. The recommended maximum dose of each drug should not be exceeded. Injection should be made slowly and with frequent aspiration. Allow a 5-minute interval between sides.
There are no data concerning use of chloroprocaine for obstetrical paracervical block when toxemia of pregnancy is present or when fetal distress or prematurity is anticipated in advance of the block; such use is, therefore, not recommended.
The following information should be considered by clinicians who select chloroprocaine for obstetrical paracevical block anesthesia:

Table 1: Composition of Available Injections

Product Identification	Formula (mg/mL) Chloroprocaine HCl	Sodium Chloride	Disodium EDTA dihydrate	Methylparaben
Nesacaine 1%	10	6.7	0.111	1
Nesacaine 2%	20	4.7	0.111	1
Nesacaine-MPF 2%	20	4.7	—	—
Nesacaine-MPF 3%	30	3.3	—	—

1. Fetal bradycardia (generally a heart rate of less than 120 per minute for more than 2 minutes) has been noted by electronic monitoring in about 5 to 10 percent of the cases (various studies) where initial total doses of 120 mg to 400 mg of chloroprocaine were employed. The incidence of bradycardia, within this dose range, might not be dose related.
2. Fetal acidosis has not been demonstrated by blood gas monitoring around the time of bradycardia or afterwards. These data are limited and generally restricted to nontoxemic cases where fetal distress or prematurity was not anticipated in advance of the block.
3. No intract chloroprocaine and only trace quantities of a hydrolysis product, 2-chloro-4-aminobenzoic acid, have been demonstrated in umbilical cord arterial or venous plasma following properly administered paracervical block with chloroprocaine.
4. The role of drug factors and non-drug factors associated with fetal bradycardia following paracervical block are unexplained at this time.

Nursing Mothers

It is not known whether this drug is excreted in human milk. Because many drugs are excreted in human milk, caution should be exercised when chloroprocaine is administered to a nursing woman.

Pediatric Use

Guidelines for the administration of Nesacaine and Nesacaine-MPF Injections to children are presented in DOSAGE AND ADMINISTRATION.

ADVERSE REACTIONS

Systemic: The most commonly encountered acute adverse experiences that demand immediate countermeasures are related to the central nervous system and the cardiovascular system. These adverse experiences are generally dose related and may result from rapid absorption from the injection site, diminished tolerance, or from unintentional intravascular injection of the local anesthetic solution. In addition to systemic dose-related toxicity, unintentional subarachnoid injection of drug during the intended performance of caudal or lumbar epidural block or nerve blocks near the vertebral column (especially in the head and neck region) may result in under-ventilation or apnea ("Total Spinal"). Factors influencing plasma protein binding, such as acidosis, systemic diseases that alter protein production, or competition of other drugs for protein binding sites, may diminish individual tolerance. Plasma cholinesterase deficiency may also account for diminished tolerance to ester type local anesthetics.

Central Nervous System Reactions: These are characterized by excitation and/or depression. Restlessness, anxiety, dizziness, tinnitus, blurred vision or tremors may occur, possibly proceeding to convulsions. However, excitement may be transient or absent, with depression being the first manifestation of an adverse reaction. This may quickly be followed by drowsiness merging into unconsciousness and respiratory arrest.

The incidence of convulsions associated with the use of local anesthetics varies with the procedure used and the total dose administered. In a survey of studies of epidural anesthesia, overt toxicity progressing to convulsions occurred in approximately 0.1 percent of local anesthetic administrations.

Cardiovascular System Reactions: High doses, or unintended intravascular injection, may lead to high plasma levels and related depression of the myocardium, hypotension, bradycardia, ventricular arrhythmias, and, possibly, cardiac arrest.

Allergic: Allergic type reactions are rare and may occur as a result of sensitivity to the local anesthetic or to other formulation ingredients, such as the antimicrobial preservative methylparaben, contained in multiple dose vials. These reactions are characterized by signs such as urticaria, pruritis, erythema, angioneurotic edema (including laryngeal edema), tachycardia, sneezing, nausea, vomiting, dizziness, syncope, excessive sweating, elevated temperature, and possibly, anaphylactoid type symptomatology (including severe hypotension). Cross sensitivity among members of the ester-type local anesthetic group has been reported. The usefulness of screening for sensitivity has not been definitely established.

Neurologic: In the practice of caudal or lumbar epidural block, occasional unintentional penetration of the subarachnoid space by the catheter may occur (see **PRECAUTIONS**). Subsequent adverse observations may depend partially on the amount of drug administered intrathecally. These observations may include spinal block of varying magnitude (including total spinal block), hypotension secondary to spinal block, loss of bladder and bowel control, and loss of perineal sensation and sexual function. Arachnoiditis, persistent motor, sensory and/or autonomic (sphincter control) deficit of some lower spinal segments with slow recovery (several months) or incomplete recovery have been reported in rare instances. (See **DOSAGE AND ADMINISTRATION** discussion of Caudal and Lumbar Epidural Block.) Backache and headache have also been noted following lumbar epidural or caudal block.

Anesthetic Procedure	Solution Concentration %	Volume (mL)	Total Dose (mg)
Mandibular	2	2–3	40–60
Infraorbital	2	0.5–1	10–20
Brachial plexus	2	30–40	600–800
Digital (without epinephrine)	1	3–4	30–40
Pudendal	2	10 each side	400
Paracervical (see also PRECAUTIONS)	1	3 per each of 4 sites	up to 120

OVERDOSAGE

Acute emergencies from local anesthetics are generally related to high plasma levels encountered during therapeutic use of local anesthetics or to unintended subarachnoid injection of local anesthetic solution (see **ADVERSE REACTIONS, WARNINGS and PRECAUTIONS**).

In mice, the intravenous LD_{50} of chloroprocaine HCl is 97 mg/kg and the subcutaneous LD_{50} of chloroprocaine HCl is 950 mg/kg.

Management of Local Anesthetic Emergencies: The first consideration is prevention, best accomplished by careful and constant monitoring of cardiovascular and respiratory vital signs and the patient's state of consciousness after each local anesthetic injection. At the first sign of change, oxygen should be administered.

The first step in the management of convulsions, as well as underventilation or apnea due to unintentional subarachnoid injection of drug solution, consists of immediate attention to the maintenance of a patent airway and assisted or controlled ventilation with oxygen and a delivery system capable of permitting immediate positive airway pressure by mask. Immediately after the institution of these ventilatory measures, the adequacy of the circulation should be evaluated, keeping in mind that drugs used to treat convulsions sometimes depress the circulation when administered intravenously. Should convulsions persist despite adequate respiratory support, and if the status of the circulation permits, small increments of an ultra-short acting barbiturate (such as thiopental or thiamylal) or a benzodiazepine (such as diazepam) may be administered intravenously; the clinician should be familiar, prior to the use of anesthetics, with these anticonvulsant drugs. Supportive treatment of circulatory depression may require administration of intravenous fluids and, when appropriate, a vasopressor dictated by the clinical situation (such as ephedrine to enhance myocardial contractile force).

If not treated immediately, both convulsions and cardiovascular depression can result in hypoxia, acidosis, bradycardia, arrhythmias and cardiac arrest. Underventilation or apnea due to unintentional subarachnoid injection of local anesthetic solution may produce these same signs and also lead to cardiac arrest if ventilatory support is not instituted. If cardiac arrest should occur, standard cardiopulmonary resuscitative measures should be instituted. Recovery has been reported after prolonged resuscitative efforts.

Endotracheal intubation, employing drugs and techniques familiar to the clinician, may be indicated, after initial administration of oxygen by mask, if difficulty is encountered in the maintenance of a patent airway or if prolonged ventilatory support (assisted or controlled) is indicated.

DOSAGE AND ADMINISTRATION

Chloroprocaine may be administered as a single injection or continuously through an indwelling catheter. As with all local anesthetics, the dose administered varies with the anesthetic procedure, the vascularity of the tissues, the depth of anesthesia and degree of muscle relaxation required, the duration of anesthesia desired, and the physical condition of the patient. The smallest dose and concentration required to produce the desired result should be used. Dosage should be reduced for children, elderly and debilitated patients and patients with cardiac and/or liver disease. The maximum single recommended doses of chloroprocaine in adults are: without epinephrine, 11 mg/kg, not to exceed a maximum total dose of 800 mg; with epinephrine (1:200,000), 14 mg/kg, not to exceed a maximum total dose of 1000 mg. For specific techniques and procedures, refer to standard textbooks.

Caudal and Lumbar Epidural Block: In order to guard against adverse experiences sometimes noted following unintended penetration of the subarachnoid space, the following procedure modifications are recommended:

1. Use an adequate test dose (3 mL of Nesacaine-MPF 3% Injection or 5 mL of Nesacaine-MPF 2% Injection) prior to induction of complete block. This test dose should be repeated if the patient is moved in such a fashion as to have displaced the epidural catheter. Allow adequate time for onset of anesthesia following administration of each test dose.
2. Avoid the rapid injection of a large volume of local anesthetic injection through the catheter. Consider fractional doses, when feasible.
3. In the event of the known injection of a large volume of local anesthetic injection into the subarachnoid space, after suitable resuscitation and if the catheter is in place, consider attempting the recovery of drug by draining a moderate amount of cerebrospinal fluid (such as 10 mL) through the epidural catheter.

As a guide for some routine procedures, suggested doses are given below:

1. Infiltration and Peripheral Nerve Block: NESACAINE or NESACAINE-MPF (chloroprocaine HCl Injection, USP)
[See table above.]
2. Caudal and Lumbar Epidural Block: NESACAINE-MPF INJECTION. For caudal anesthesia, the initial dose is 15 to 25 mL of a 2% or 3% solution. Repeated doses may be given at 40 to 60 minute intervals.
   For lumbar epidural anesthesia, 2 to 2.5 mL per segment of a 2% or 3% solution can be used. The usual total volume of Nesacaine-MPF Injection is from 15 to 25 mL. Repeated doses 2 to 6 mL less than the original dose may be given at 40 to 50 minute intervals.

The above dosages are recommended as a guide for use in the average adult. Maximum dosages of all local anesthetics must be individualized after evaluating the size and physical condition of the patient and the rate of systemic absorption from a particular injection site.

Pediatric Dosage: It is difficult to recommend a maximum dose of any drug for children, since this varies as a function of age and weight. For children over 3 years of age who have a normal lean body mass and normal body development, the maximum dose is determined by the child's age and weight and should not exceed 11 mg/kg (5 mg/lb). For example, in a child of 5 years weighing 50 lbs (23 kg), the dose of chloroprocaine HCl without epinephrine would be 250 mg. Concentrations of 0.5–1.0% are suggested for infiltration and 1.0–1.5% for nerve block. In order to guard against systemic toxicity, the lowest effective concentration and lowest effective dose should be used at all times. Some of the lower concentrations for use in infants and smaller children are not available in pre-packaged containers; it will be necessary to dilute available concentrations with the amount of 0.9% sodium chloride injection necessary to obtain the required final concentration of chloroprocaine injection.

Preparation of Epinephrine Injections—To prepare a 1:200,000 epinephrine-chloroprocaine HCl injection, add 0.15 mL of a 1 to 1000 Epinephrine Injection USP to 30 mL of Nesacaine-MPF Injection.

Chloroprocaine is incompatible with caustic alkalis and their carbonates, soaps, silver salts, iodine and iodides.

Parenteral drug products should be inspected visually for particulate matter and discoloration prior to administration, whenever injection and container permit. As with other anesthetics having a free aromatic amino group, Nesacaine and Nesacine-MPF Injections are slightly photosensitive and may become discolored after prolonged exposure to light. It is recommended that these vials be stored in the original outer containers, protected from direct sunlight. Discolored injection should not be administered. If exposed to low temperatures, Nesacaine and Nesacaine-MPF Injections may deposit crystals of chloroprocaine HCl which will redissolve with shaking when returned to room temperature. The product should not be used if it contains undissolved (e.g., particulate) material.

HOW SUPPLIED

NESACAINE (chloroprocaine HCl Injection, USP) with preservatives is supplied as follows:

1% solution (NDC 0186-0971-66) in 30 mL multiple dose vials

2% solution (NDC 0186-0972-66) in 30 mL multiple dose vials

NESACAINE-MPF (chloroprocaine HCl Injection, USP) without preservatives and without EDTA is supplied as follows:

2% solution (NDC 0186-0991-66) in 20 mL single dose vials

3% solution (NDC 0186-0992-66) in 20 mL single dose vials

Keep from freezing. Protect from light. Store at controlled room temperature 15°–30°C (59°–86°F).

Continued on next page

Astra—Cont.

PANCURONIUM BROMIDE INJECTION ℞

> THIS DRUG SHOULD BE ADMINISTERED BY ADEQUATELY TRAINED INDIVIDUALS FAMILIAR WITH ITS ACTIONS, CHARACTERISTICS, AND HAZARDS.

HOW SUPPLIED

Pancuronium Bromide Injection is packaged in the following forms:

Vials, 1 mg/mL

NDC 0186-1322-12, 10 mL size—boxes of 5, Flip-Off vial closure

Vials, 2 mg/mL

NDC 0186-1331-13, 2 mL size—boxes of 10, Astra E-Z OFF® vial closure

NDC 0186-1334-03, 2 mL size—boxes of 10, Flip-Off vial closure

NDC 0186-1332-13, 5 mL size—boxes of 10, Astra E-Z OFF® vial closure

NDC 0186-1335-03, 5 mL size—boxes of 10, Flip-Off vial closure

Syringes, 2 mg/mL

NDC 0186-1333-23, 2 mL size—boxes of 10, 22 G, $1^1/_4''$ needle
NDC 0186-1336-23, 2 mL size—boxes of 10, Luer Hub Only
NDC 0186-0676-01, 5 mL size—box of 1, 21 G, $^{15}/_{16}''$ needle
NDC 0186-0692-01, 5 mL size—box of 1, Luer Hub Only

STORAGE

Both concentrations of Pancuronium Bromide Injection will maintain full clinical potency for six months if kept at a room temperature of 18°-22°C (65°-72°F); or for 18 months when refrigerated at 2°-8°C (36°-46°F).

Caution: Federal law prohibits dispensing without prescription.

021887R05   2/93

POLOCAINE® ℞

[pō′-lō-caine ″]

(Mepivacaine Hydrochloride Injection, USP)

POLOCAINE®-MPF (Mepivacaine Hydrochloride Injection, USP)

THESE SOLUTIONS ARE NOT INTENDED FOR SPINAL ANESTHESIA OR DENTAL USE

(For details of indications, dosages and administration, precautions, and adverse reactions, see circular in package.)

HOW SUPPLIED

POLOCAINE-MPF (Mepivacaine HCl Injection, USP) without preservatives is available as follows:

1% Single-dose vials of 30 mL (NDC 0186-0412-01)
1.5% Single-dose vials of 30 mL (NDC 0186-0418-01)
2% Single-dose vials of 20 mL (NDC 0186-0422-01)

POLOCAINE (Mepivacaine HCl Injection, USP) with preservatives is available as follows:

1% Multiple-dose vials of 50 mL (NDC 0186-0410-01)
2% Multiple-dose vials of 50 mL (NDC 0186-0420-01)

Unused portions of solutions not containing preservatives should be discarded.

Store at controlled room temperature 15°–30°C (59°–86°F).

021668R00   Issue 1/92

RHINOCORT® Nasal Inhaler ℞

(budesonide)
For Intranasal Use Only.
Shake Well Before Use.

DESCRIPTION

Budesonide, the active component of Rhinocort® Nasal Inhaler, is an anti-inflammatory glucocorticosteroid. It is designated chemically as 16α, 17α-butylidene-dioxypregna-1,4-diene-11β, 21-diol-3, 20-dione. Budesonide possesses an asymmetric carbon atom in its structure and is provided as the mixture of the two epimers, 22R and 22S. The empirical formula of budesonide is $C_{25}H_{34}O_6$ and its molecular weight is 430.5. Its structural formula is:

Budesonide is a white to off-white odorless powder that is practically insoluble in water and in heptane, sparingly soluble in ethanol, and freely soluble in chloroform. Its partition coefficient between octanol and water at pH 7.4 is 1.6×10^3. Rhinocort Nasal Inhaler is a metered-dose pressurized aerosol unit containing a suspension of micronized budesonide in a mixture of propellants, (dichlorodifluoromethane, trichloromonofluoromethane, and dichlorotetrafluoroethane) and sorbitan trioleate.

Each actuation releases 50 μg budesonide from the valve and delivers approximately 32 μg budesonide from the nasal adapter (dose to patient). Throughout the package insert 32 μg per actuation is used to calculate the dose administered. One canister provides at least 200 metered doses.

CLINICAL PHARMACOLOGY

Budesonide is a glucocorticosteroid having a potent glucocorticoid and weak mineralocorticoid activity. In standard *in vitro* and animal models, budesonide has an approximately 200 fold higher affinity for the glucocorticoid receptor and a 1000 fold higher topical anti-inflammatory potency than cortisol (rat croton oil ear edema assay). As a measure of systemic activity, budesonide is 40 times more potent than cortisol when administered subcutaneously and 25 times more potent when administered orally in the rat thymus involution assay.

The precise mechanism of glucocorticosteroid actions on allergic and nonallergic rhinitis is not known. Glucocorticosteroids have been shown to have a wide range of inhibitory activities against multiple cell types (e.g. mast cells, eosinophils, neutrophils, macrophages and lymphocytes) and mediators (e.g., histamine, eicosanoids, leukotrienes and cytokines) involved in allergic and nonallergic/irritant-mediated inflammation.

Corticoids affect the delayed (6 hour) response to an allergen challenge more than the histamine-associated immediate response (20 minute). The clinical significance of these findings is unknown.

Pharmacokinetics: The pharmacokinetics of budesonide have been studied following nasal, oral and intravenous administration. Pharmacokinetic studies were performed with doses higher than those used clinically because at clinical doses the resulting plasma levels are below the limits of detection.

The results are as follows:

[See table below.]

Only about 20% of an intranasal dose from the Rhinocort Nasal Inhaler reaches the systemic circulation.

While budesonide is well absorbed from the GI tract, the oral bioavailability of budesonide is low (~10%) primarily due to extensive first pass metabolism in the liver. After reaching the systemic circulation, plasma levels decline in a log linear manner with an apparent elimination half-life of approximately 2 hours.

Budesonide has a volume of distibution of approximately 200 L and is 88% protein bound in the plasma. Budesonide is a mixture of two epimers, 22R and 22S. In glucocorticoid receptor binding studies, the 22R form is two times as active as the 22S epimer. It is also preferentially cleared by the liver with an apparent systemic clearance of 1.4 +/− 0.3 L/min., vs. 1.0 +/− 0.2 L/min. for the 22S form. *In vitro* studies indicate that the two forms of budesonide do not interconvert.

Budesonide is rapidly and extensively metabolized in man by the liver. *In vitro* studies looking at sites of metabolism showed negligible metabolism in skin, lung, and serum. After intranasal administration of a radiolabeled dose, $^2/_3$ of the radioactivity was found in the urine and the remainder in the feces by 96 hours. The primary metabolites of budesonide in the urine following IV administration are 16α-hydroxyprednisolone (24%) and 6β-hydroxybudesonide (5%). An additional 34% of the radioactivity recovered in the urine were conjugates. No unchanged budesonide was found in the urine. These results regarding the metabolic fate of budesonide parallel results obtained in *in vitro* metabolic studies using human liver homogenates.

In vitro studies of the binding of the two primary metabolites to the glucocorticoid receptor indicate that they have less than 1% of the affinity for the receptor as the parent compound budesonide.

Pharmacodynamics: The effect of Rhinocort Nasal Inhaler at a dosage of two sprays in each nostril morning and evening (total daily dose of 256 μg) on hypothalamic-pituitary-adrenal (HPA) axis function has been evaluated in 275 adults and 61 children following short-term use (< 2 months) and in 113 adults and 116 children following longer use (6–48 months). Early morning plasma cortisol and the short cosyntropin stimulation test (30–60 minutes) were the most commonly performed assessments of HPA function.

Twenty-four hour urinary cortisol levels were determined in 50 adults (short term) and 96 children (long term). There were no statistically significant changes from baseline measurements in early morning plasma cortisol or 24-hour urinary cortisol excretion or in response to cosyntropin.

In a crossover trial using single doses of 200, 400 and 800 μg of an aqueous formulation of budesonide administered intranasally at 10 P.M., a dose-dependent decrease in urinary cortisol excretion was found between 10 P.M. and 8 A.M. the following morning. The same study has not been performed with Rhinocort Nasal Inhaler. However, in a study using the Rhinocort Nasal Inhaler administered at 10 P.M., doses four (1024 μg) and eight (2048 μg) times higher than the recommended daily dose (256 μg) were followed by a significant decrease in plasma cortisol levels at 8 A.M. the following morning (17% and 22%, respectively).

A 3 week clinical study in seasonal rhinitis, comparing Rhinocort Nasal Inhaler and orally ingested budesonide with placebo in 98 patients with allergic rhinitis due to birch pollen, demonstrated that the therapeutic effect of budesonide can be attributed to the topical effects of budesonide. Intranasally, 128 μg of budesonide applied twice daily (55 μg systemically absorbed/day) provided clinically and statistically significant evidence of efficacy, whereas 250 μg of budesonide ingested twice a day as a capsule (65 μg systemically absorbed/day) was no different from placebo in reducing nasal symptoms.

Clinical Trials: The prophylactic and therapeutic efficacy of Rhinocort Nasal Inhaler has been evaluated in 20 controlled clinical trials of seasonal or perennial rhinitis. The number of patients treated with budesonide in these studies was 50 male and 33 female patients ages 6 to 12 years old, 77 males and 62 females ages 13 to 18 years old, 185 males and 246 females ages 19 to 64 and 1 male and 2 females over 64. The patients were predominantly caucasian.

Double-blind clinical trials of two to four weeks duration have shown that, compared with placebo, Rhinocort Nasal Inhaler 128 μg b.i.d. (two sprays in each nostril morning and evening) or 256 μg q.d. (four sprays in each nostril in the morning) provides statistically significant relief of nasal symptoms such as blockage, rhinorrhea, itching, and sneezing in adults and children with seasonal allergic rhinitis or perennial allergic rhinitis. Similar improvement has also been demonstrated in adults with nonallergic perennial rhinitis.

The therapeutic effect of Rhinocort Nasal Inhaler compared with placebo has been demonstrated by rhinoscopic examinations in children and adults with seasonal or perennial allergic rhinitis and adults with nonallergic perennial rhinitis. Biopsies of the nasal mucosa of 50 adult patients after 12 months of treatment and of 10 patients after 3–5 years of therapy showed no histopathological evidence of adverse effects. The clinical significance of either of these findings is unknown.

Individualization of Dosage: It is recommended that the starting dose for all adults be 256 μg daily, as either two sprays in each nostril twice per day, morning and evening, or as four sprays in each nostril once a day in the morning. The effect should be assessed 3–7 days after initiating treatment

Route of Administration	T_{max} (hr)	C_{max}** (nmol/L)	Systemic Availability***	V_D (L)	Clearance (L/min)
	Mean* [range]				
Nasal Inhaler (N=9)	0.6 [0.3–2]	0.52 [0.24–0.88]	21 [16–27]	—	—
Oral Capsule (N=11)	1.0 [0.5–2]	0.33 [0.19–0.50]	12 [8–20]	—	—
I.V. (N=11)	—	—	100	201 [102–275]	1.2 [0.8–1.5]

* mean of the two epimers
** dose normalized to a 256 μg dose
*** % of delivered dose

and then periodically until the patient's symptoms are stable. If adequate relief of symptoms is not achieved after 3 weeks of treatment, then Rhinocort Nasal Inhaler should be discontinued.

In patients who do achieve a good result it is desirable, once the maximum benefit seems to have been achieved, to titrate an individual patient to the minimum effective dose. Because of the generally short duration of therapy for seasonal allergic rhinitis, it is usually not necessary to do this.

In patients with perennial allergic rhinitis, once adequate relief has been obtained the dose should be gradually decreased every 2–4 weeks as long as the desired clinical effect is maintained. If symptoms return, the dose may briefly be increased to the patient's starting dose and then returned to the dose the patient was on before symptoms reoccurred.

As with other aerosolized nasal glucocorticosteroids, the vehicle used to deliver the glucocorticosteroid may cause symptoms that are difficult to distinguish from the patient's rhinitis symptoms. The corticoid may suppress symptoms caused by the vehicle at higher doses but as the dose is decreased symptoms from the vehicle may emerge. If a patient needs chronic treatment and the daily dose cannot be decreased from the starting dose, it may be advisable to try alternative therapy.

INDICATIONS AND USAGE

Rhinocort Nasal Inhaler is indicated for the management of symptoms of seasonal or perennial allergic rhinitis in adults and children and nonallergic perennial rhinitis in adults.

Rhinocort Nasal Inhaler is not recommended for treatment of nonallergic rhinitis in children because adequate numbers of such children have not been studied.

CONTRAINDICATIONS

Hypersensitivity to any of the ingredients of this preparation contraindicates its use.

WARNINGS

The replacement of a systemic glucocorticosteroid with a topical glucocorticosteroid can be accompanied by signs of adrenal insufficiency, and in addition some patients may experience symptoms of withdrawal, e.g. joint and/or muscular pain, lassitude and depression. Patients previously treated for prolonged periods with systemic glucocorticosteroids and transferred to topical glucocorticosteroids should be carefully monitored for acute adrenal insufficiency in response to stress. In those patients who have asthma or other clinical conditions requiring long-term systemic glucocorticosteroid treatment, too rapid a decrease in systemic glucocorticosteroids may cause a severe exacerbation of their symptoms.

The use of Rhinocort Nasal Inhaler with alternate-day systemic prednisone could increase the likelihood of hypothalamic-pituitary-adrenal (HPA) suppression compared with a therapeutic dose of either one alone. Therefore, Rhinocort Nasal Inhaler should be used with caution in patients already receiving alternate-day prednisone treatment for any disease. In addition, the concomitant use of Rhinocort Nasal Inhaler with other inhaled glucocorticosteroids could increase the risk of signs or symptoms of hypercorticism and/or suppression of the HPA-axis.

Patients who are on drugs which suppress the immune system are more susceptible to infections than healthy individuals. Chicken pox and measles, for example, can have a more serious or even fatal course in non-immune children or adults on immunosuppressant doses of corticosteroids. In such children or adults, who have not had these diseases, particular care should be taken to avoid exposure. How the dose, route and duration of corticosteroid administration affects the risk of developing a disseminated infection is not known. The contribution of the underlying disease and/or prior corticosteroid treatment to the risk is also not known. If exposed to chicken pox, prophylaxis with varicella zoster immune globulin (VZIG) may be indicated. If exposed to measles, prophylaxis with pooled intramuscular immunoglobulin (IG) may be indicated. (See the respective package insert for complete VZIG and IG prescribing information). If chicken pox develops, treatment with antiviral agents may be considered.

PRECAUTIONS

General: Rarely, immediate hypersensitivity reactions or contact dermatitis may occur after the intranasal administration of budesonide. Rare instances of wheezing, nasal septum perforation and increased intraocular pressure have been reported following the intranasal application of aerosolized glucocorticosteroids.

Like other glucocorticosteroids, budesonide is absorbed into the circulation. Use of excessive doses of glucocorticosteroids may lead to signs or symptoms of hypercorticism, suppression of HPA function and/or suppression of growth in children or teenagers. In short term studies of the acute effect of inhaled budesonide 256 μg/day on lower leg growth (knemometry), it like other inhaled and intramuscular corticoids which have been studied showed a decrease in the rate of lower leg growth. The clinical significance of this finding is not known. In two one-year studies in 92 children taking recommended doses of Rhinocort Nasal Inhaler, height and skeletal stature were consistent with chronological age. Physicians should closely follow the growth of children taking corticoids, by any route, and weigh the benefits of corticoid therapy against the possibility of growth suppression if a child's growth appears slowed.

Although systemic effects have been minimal with recommended doses of Rhinocort Nasal Inhaler, this potential risk increases with larger doses. Therefore, larger than recommended doses of Rhinocort Nasal Inhaler should be avoided. When used at larger doses, systemic glucocorticosteroid effects such as hypercorticism and adrenal suppression may appear. If such changes occur, the dosage of Rhinocort Nasal Inhaler should be discontinued slowly, consistent with accepted procedures for discontinuing oral glucocorticosteroid therapy.

In clinical studies with budesonide administered intranasally, the development of localized infections of the nose and pharynx with Candida albicans has occurred only rarely. When such an infection develops, it may require treatment with appropriate local therapy and discontinuation of treatment with Rhinocort Nasal Inhaler. Patients using Rhinocort Nasal Inhaler over several months or longer should be examined periodically for evidence of Candida infection or other signs of adverse effects on the nasal mucosa.

Rhinocort Nasal Inhaler should be used with caution, if at all, in patients with active or quiescent tuberculous infections, untreated fungal, bacterial, or systemic viral infections, or ocular herpes simplex.

Because of the inhibitory effect of glucocorticosteroids on wound healing, patients who have experienced recent nasal septal ulcers, nasal surgery, or nasal trauma should not use a nasal glucocorticosteroid until healing has occurred.

Information for Patients: Patients being treated with Rhinocort Nasal Inhaler should receive the following information and instructions.

Patients should use Rhinocort Nasal Inhaler as prescribed. A decrease in symptoms may occur as soon as 24 hours after starting glucocorticosteroid therapy and generally can be expected to occur within a few days of initiating therapy in allergic rhinitis. The patient should contact the physician if symptoms do not improve by three weeks, or if the condition worsens. Nasal irritation and/or burning after use of the spray occur only rarely with this product. The patient should contact the physician if they occur repeatedly.

Patients who are on corticosteroids should be warned to avoid exposure to chicken pox or measles. Patients should also be advised that if they are exposed, they should consult their physician without delay.

For the proper use of this unit and to attain maximum improvement, the patient should read and follow the accompanying patient instructions carefully.

Carcinogenesis, Mutagenesis, Impairment of Fertility: Long-term studies were conducted in mice and rats using oral administration to evaluate the carcinogenic potential of budesonide.

There was no evidence of a carcinogenic effect when budesonide was administered orally for 91 weeks to mice at doses up to 200 μg/kg/day (600 μg/m^2/day).

In a 104-week carcinogenicity study in Sprague-Dawley rats (41), a statistically significant increase in the incidence of gliomas was observed in male rats receiving 50 μg/kg/day (300 μg/m^2/day) orally; no such changes were seen in male rats receiving doses of 10 and 25 μg/kg/day (60 and 150 μg/m^2/day) or in female rats at any dose. Two additional 104-week carcinogenicity studies have been performed with oral budesonide at doses of 50 μg/kg/day (300 μg/m^2/day) in male Sprague-Dawley and Fischer rats. These studies did not demonstrate an increased glioma incidence in budesonide treated animals as compared with concurrent controls or reference glucocorticosteroid treated groups (prednisolone and triamcinolone acetonide).

Compared with concurrent control male Sprague-Dawley rats there was a statistically significant increase in the incidence of hepatocellular tumors. This finding was confirmed in all three steroid groups (budesonide, prednisolone, triamcinolone acetonide) in the second study in male Sprague-Dawley rats.

The mutagenic potential of budesonide was evaluated in six different test systems; Ames Salmonella/microsome plate test, mouse micronucleus test, mouse lymphoma test, chromosome aberration test in human lymphocytes, sex-linked recessive lethal test in Drosophila melanogaster, and DNA repair analysis in rat hepatocyte culture. No mutagenic or clastogenic properties of budesonide were found in any of the tests.

The effect upon fertility and general reproductive performance was studied in rats given budesonide subcutaneously. At 20 μg/kg/day (120 μg/m^2/day) and higher dose levels, a decrease in maternal body-weight gain was observed along with a decrease in prenatal viability and viability of the young at birth and during lactation. No such effects were noted at the dose level 5 μg/kg/day (30 μg/m^2/day).

Pregnancy: Teratogenic Effects: Pregnancy Category C: As with other glucocorticoids budesonide has been shown to be teratogenic and embryocidal in rabbits and rats when given subcutaneously in doses exceeding 5 and 100 μg/kg/day (59 and 600 μg/m^2/day), respectively. In these studies budesonide at 25 μg/kg/day (295 μg/m^2/day) given to rabbits and 500 μg/kg/day (3000 μg/m^2/day) given to rats was found to produce fetal loss, decreased pup weights and skeletal abnormalities. No teratogenic or embryocidal effects have been seen in rats when budesonide was administered by inhalation at doses of 100–250 μg/kg/day (600–1500 μg/m^2/day, approximately 27–68 times the human recommended starting dose based on μg/kg/day or 4–10 times the human dose based on μg/m^2/day).

There are no adequate and well-controlled studies in pregnant women. Budesonide should be used during pregnancy only if the potential benefit justifies the potential risk to the fetus. Experience with oral glucocorticosteroids since their introduction in pharmacologic, as opposed to physiologic, doses suggests that rodents are more prone to teratogenic effects from glucocorticosteroids than humans. In addition, because there is a natural increase in glucocorticosteroid production during pregnancy, most women will require a lower exogenous glucocorticosteroid dose and many will not need glucocorticosteroid treatment during pregnancy.

Nonteratogenic Effects: Hypoadrenalism may occur in infants born of mothers receiving glucocorticosteroids during pregnancy. Such infants should be carefully observed.

Nursing Mothers: It is not known whether budesonide is excreted in human milk. Because other glucocorticosteroids are excreted in human milk, caution should be exercised when Rhinocort Nasal Inhaler is administered to nursing women.

Pediatric Use: Safety and effectiveness in children below 6 years of age have not been established. Oral glucocorticosteroids have been shown to cause growth suppression in children and teenagers with extended use. If a child or teenager on any glucocorticosteroid appears to have growth suppression, the possibility that they are particularly sensitive to this effect of glucocorticosteroids should be considered (see PRECAUTIONS).

ADVERSE REACTIONS

Adverse reaction information is derived from blinded-controlled clinical trials (see Clinical Trials), open label studies and marketing experience. In the description below, rates of rare events are derived principally from marketing experience and publications, and accurate estimates of incidence are not possible.

The incidence of common adverse reactions is based upon controlled clinical trials in 606 patients [101 girls and 145 boys (< 19 years of age) and 203 female and 157 male adults] treated with Rhinocort Nasal Inhaler 128 μg twice daily over 2–4 weeks. The most common adverse reactions were symptoms of irritation of the nasal mucous membranes. All common adverse reactions were reported with approximately the same frequency by placebo patients suggesting the possibility that the vehicle or the rhinitis itself was responsible for the symptoms. Sneezing after use of the inhaler occurred in 2% of Rhinocort treated patients and in 11% of patients using the placebo.

Systemic glucocorticosteroid side-effects were not reported during controlled clinical studies with Rhinocort Nasal Inhaler. If recommended doses are exceeded, however, or if individuals are particularly sensitive, symptoms of hypercorticism, i.e., Cushing's syndrome, could occur.

Incidence Greater than 1% (Based on controlled clinical trials):

Respiratory: nasal irritation*, pharyngitis*, cough increased*, epistaxis*.

Digestive: dry mouth, dyspepsia.

*incidence 3 to 9%; incidence of unmarked reactions 1 to 3%.

Incidence Less than 1% Causal Relationship Probable (Adverse reactions reported only in the literature or from marketing experience, and presumably rarer are *italicized*):

Respiratory: moniliasis, hoarseness, wheezing, nasal pain, *nasal septum mucosal atrophy/necrosis, nasal septum perforation.*

Special Senses: reduced sense of smell, bad taste.

Digestive: nausea.

Skin and Appendages: facial edema, rash, pruritus, *contact dermatitis,* herpes simplex.

Incidence Less than 1% Causal Relationship Unknown (Adverse reactions reported only in the literature or from marketing experience, and presumably rarer are *italicized*):

Respiratory: dyspnea.

Nervous System: nervousness.

Skin and Appendages: *alopecia.*

Musculoskeletal: myalgia, arthralgia.

OVERDOSAGE

Acute overdosage with this dosage form is unlikely since one canister of Rhinocort Nasal Inhaler only contains approximately 12.7 mg of budesonide. Chronic overdosage may result in signs/symptoms of hyerpcorticism (see WARNINGS and PRECAUTIONS).

Continued on next page

Astra—Cont.

DOSAGE AND ADMINISTRATION

Adults and children 6 years of age and older: The recommended starting dose is 256 μg daily, given as either two sprays in each nostril morning and evening or as four sprays in each nostril in the morning.

A decrease in symptoms may occur as soon as 24 hours after onset of treatment with Rhinocort Nasal Inhaler but generally it takes 3–7 days to reach maximum benefit.

If no improvement has been obtained by the third week of treatment with Rhinocort Nasal Inhaler, treatment should be discontinued.

After the desired clinical effect has been obtained, the maintenance dose should be reduced to the smallest amount necessary for control of symptoms (see Individualization of Dosage, CLINICAL PHARMACOLOGY section).

If glucocorticosteroids are discontinued when they still are needed, symptoms may not recur for several days.

At recommended doses, Rhinocort's therapeutic effects are localized to the nose, therefore, concomitant treatment may be necessary to counteract allergic eye symptoms. Doses exceeding 256 μg daily (4 sprays/nostril) are not recommended. Rhinocort Nasal Inhaler is not recommended for children below 6 years of age or for children with nonallergic perennial rhinitis because adequate numbers of these children have not been studied.

Directions for Use: Illustrated Patient's Instructions for Use accompany each package of Rhinocort Nasal Inhaler.

HOW SUPPLIED

Rhinocort Nasal Inhaler is supplied in a 7.0 g canister containing 200 metered doses provided with a metering valve and nasal adapter together with Patient's Instructions for Use. Each actuation delivers approximately 32 μg of micronized budesonide from the nasal adapter to the patient.

Caution: Federal (USA) law prohibits dispensing without prescription.

Rhinocort Nasal Inhaler should be stored between 15°C (59°F) and 30°C (86°F) with the valve downwards. Shake well before use.

Each inhaler with actuator is packaged in an aluminum foil pouch to protect the product from moisture. After opening the aluminum pouch, the product should be used within 6 months and storage in an area of high humidity should be avoided.

Contents under pressure. Do not puncture. Do not use or store near heat or open flame. Exposure to temperatures above 50°C (120°F) may cause the canister to explode.

Never throw the container into fire or an incinerator. Keep out of reach of children.

Note: The indented statement below is required by the Federal government's Clean Air Act for all products containing or manufactured with chlorofluorocarbons (CFCs).

> **WARNING:** Contains trichloromonofluoromethane, dichlorotetrafluoroethane, and dichlorodifluoromethane, substances which harm public health and environment by destroying ozone in the upper atmosphere.

A notice similar to the above WARNING has been placed in the patient information leaflet of this product pursuant to EPA regulations.

Manufactured for:
ASTRA®
Astra USA, Inc. 09-081-16-0-80
Westborough, MA 01581 000753R03 (1/95)

Patient's Instructions For Use

RHINOCORT® (budesonide)
Nasal Inhaler

Use a pair of scissors to cut the pouch open. Read the information before using Rhinocort Nasal Inhaler.

Follow the directions carefully.

1. 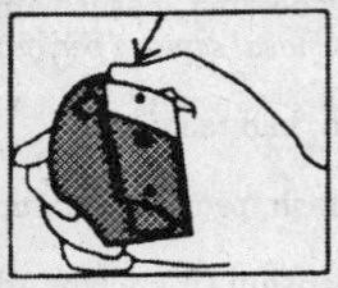
Blow your nose.
Open the nasal inhaler by pressing on the arrow and rotating until it clicks into the locked position. Shake the canister thoroughly before using.

2. 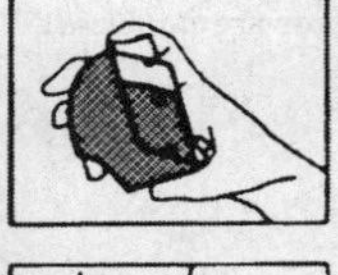
Place your thumb on the bottom of the unit while placing your index finger on the top of the canister. Wrap your fingers securely around the back.

3. 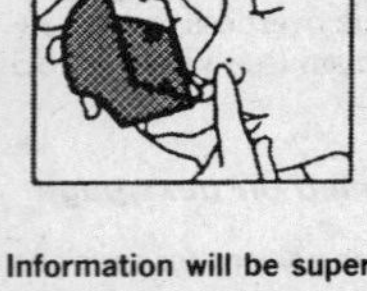
Close one nostril and insert the end of the inhaler tube into the other nostril. Hold your breath and actuate a dose by pressing straight down on the canister. For optimum results, shake the canister between sprays.

4. 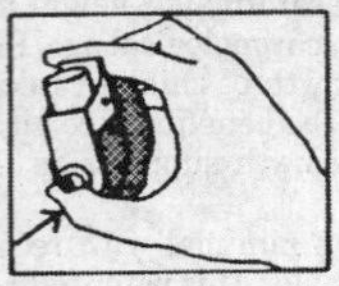
Rotate the unit closed for storage.

> **WARNING:** Contains trichloromonofluoromethane, dichlorotetrafluoroethane, and dichlorodifluoromethane, substances which harm the environment by destroying ozone in the upper atmosphere. Your physician has determined that this product is likely to help your personal health. USE THIS PRODUCT AS DIRECTED, UNLESS INSTRUCTED TO DO OTHERWISE BY YOUR PHYSICIAN. If you have any questions about alternatives, consult with your physician.

N.B.

Follow your doctor's directions and do not use Rhinocort Nasal Inhaler more often than prescribed.

Contact your doctor if you find the effect strongly reduced. Rhinocort Nasal Inhaler does not give immediate relief. Generally it will take a few days to achieve full effect. It is therefore very important that Rhinocort is used regularly.

To be used within 6 months after the aluminum pouch has been opened. After opening the pouch, avoid storage in areas of high humidity.

Cleaning:

Remove the aerosol container and wash the plastic parts regularly in warm-not hot-water with addition of mild detergent if necessary. Allow the plastic parts to dry completely and then replace the container.

Contents under pressure.

Do not puncture or throw container into incinerator. Using or storing near open flame or heating above 120°F (50°C) may cause container to burst.

Manufactured for: Astra USA, Inc., Westborough, MA 01581
000753R03 (1/95)

Shown in Product Identification Guide, page 304

SENSORCAINE® ℞

[*sén-sor-caine*]
(Bupivacaine HCl Injection, USP)
SENSORCAINE®-MPF ***(Bupivacaine HCl Injection, USP)***
SENSORCAINE® with Epinephrine ***(Bupivacaine and Epinephrine Injection, USP)*** 1:200,000 (as bitartrate)
SENSORCAINE®-MPF with Epinephrine ***(Bupivacaine and Epinephrine Injection, USP)*** 1:200,000 (as bitartrate)

DESCRIPTION

Sensorcaine® (Bupivacaine HCl) injections are sterile isotonic solutions that contain a local anesthetic agent with and without epinephrine (as bitartrate) 1:200,000 and are administered parenterally by injection. See INDICATIONS AND USAGE for specific uses. Solutions of bupivacaine HCl may be autoclaved if they do not contain epinephrine.

Sensorcaine® injections contain bupivacaine HCl which is chemically designated as 2-piperidinecarboxamide, 1-butyl-N-(2,6-dimethylphenyl)-monohydrochloride, monohydrate and has the following structure:

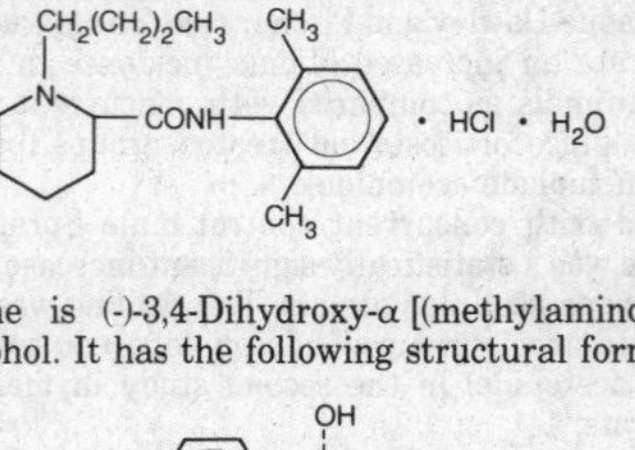

Epinephrine is (-)-3,4-Dihydroxy-α [(methylamino)methyl] benzyl alcohol. It has the following structural formula:

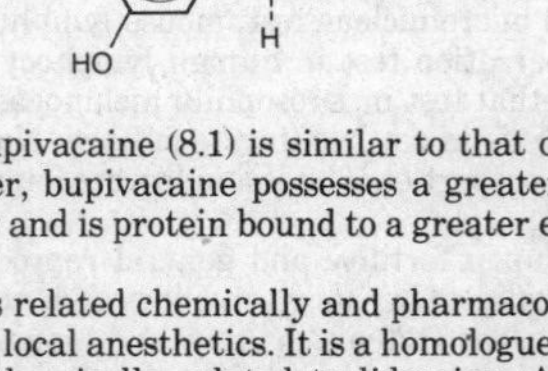

The pK_a of bupivacaine (8.1) is similar to that of lidocaine (7.86). However, bupivacaine possesses a greater degree of lipid solubility and is protein bound to a greater extent than lidocaine.

Bupivacaine is related chemically and pharmacologically to the aminoacyl local anesthetics. It is a homologue of mepivacaine and is chemically related to lidocaine. All three of these anesthetics contain an amide linkage between the aromatic nucleus and the amino or piperidine group. They differ in this respect from the procaine-type local anesthetics, which have an ester linkage.

Dosage forms listed as Sensorcaine-MPF indicates single dose solutions that are Methyl Paraben Free (MPF).

Sensorcaine-MPF is a sterile isotonic solution containing sodium chloride. Sensorcaine in multiple dose vials, each mL also contains 1 mg methylparaben as antiseptic preservative. The pH of these solutions is adjusted to between 4.0 and 6.5 with sodium hydroxide and/or hydrochloric acid.

Sensorcaine-MPF with Epinephrine 1:200,000 (as bitartrate) is a sterile isotonic solution containing sodium chloride. Each mL contains bupivacaine hydrochloride and 0.005 mg epinephrine, with 0.5 mg sodium metabisulfite as an antioxidant and 0.2 mg citric acid (anhydrous) as stabilizer. Sensorcaine with Epinephrine 1:200.000 (as bitartrate) in multiple dose vials, each mL also contains 1 mg methylparaben as antiseptic preservative. The pH of these solutions is adjusted to between 3.3 to 5.5 with sodium hydroxide and/or hydrochloric acid. Filled under nitrogen.

Note: The user should have an appreciation and awareness of the formulations and their intended uses. (See DOSAGE AND ADMINISTRATION.)

CLINICAL PHARMACOLOGY

Local anesthetics block the generation and the conduction of nerve impulses, presumably by increasing the threshold for electrical excitation in the nerve, by slowing the propagation of the nerve impulse, and by reducing the rate of rise of the action potential. In general, the progression of anesthesia is related to the diameter, myelination and conduction velocity of affected nerve fibers. Clinically, the order of loss of nerve function is as follows: (1) pain, (2) temperature, (3) touch, (4) proprioception, and (5) skeletal muscle tone.

Systemic absorption of local anesthetics produces effects on the cardiovascular and central nervous systems. At blood concentrations achieved with therapeutic doses, changes in cardiac conduction, excitability, refractoriness, contractility, and peripheral vascular resistance are minimal. However, toxic blood concentrations depress cardiac conduction and excitability, which may lead to atrioventricular block, ventricular arrhythmias and to cardiac arrest, sometimes resulting in fatalities. In addition, myocardial contractility is depressed and peripheral vasodilation occurs, leading to decreased cardiac output and arterial blood pressure. Recent clinical reports and animal research suggest that these cardiovascular changes are more likely to occur after unintended intravascular injection of bupivacaine. Therefore, incremental dosing is necessary.

Following systemic absorption, local anesthetics can produce central nervous system stimulation, depression or both. Apparent central stimulation is usually manifested as restlessness, tremors and shivering, progressing to convulsions, followed by depression and coma, progressing ultimately to respiratory arrest. However, the local anesthetics have a primary depressant effect on the medulla and on higher centers. The depressed stage may occur without a prior excited stage.

Pharmacokinetics: The rate of systemic absorption of local anesthetics is dependent upon the total dose and concentration of drug administered, the route of administration, the vascularity of the administration site, and the presence or absence of epinephrine in the anesthetic solution. A dilute concentration of epinephrine (1:200,000 or 5 μg/mL) usually reduces the rate of absorption and peak plasma concentration of bupivacaine, permitting the use of moderately larger total doses and sometimes prolonging the duration of action.

The onset of action with bupivacaine is rapid and anesthesia is long-lasting. The duration of anesthesia is significantly longer with bupivacaine than with any other commonly used local anesthetic. It has also been noted that there is a period of analgesia that persists after the return of sensation, during which time the need for potent analgesics is reduced.

Local anesthetics are bound to plasma proteins in varying degrees. Generally, the lower the plasma concentration of drug, the higher the percentage of drug bound to plasma proteins.

Local anesthetics appear to cross the placenta by passive diffusion. The rate and degree of diffusion is governed by: (1) the degree of plasma protein binding, (2) the degree of ionization, and (3) the degree of lipid solubility. Fetal/maternal ratios of local anesthetics appear to be inversely related to the degree of plasma protein binding, because only the free, unbound drug is available for placental transfer. Bupivacaine, with a high protein binding capacity (95%), has a low fetal/maternal ratio (0.2–0.4). The extent of placental transfer is also determined by the degree of ionization and lipid solubility of the drug. Lipid soluble, nonionized drugs readily enter the fetal blood from the maternal circulation.

Depending upon the route of administration, local anesthetics are distributed to some extent to all body tissues, with high concentrations found in highly perfused organs such as the liver, lungs, heart, and brain.

Pharmacokinetic studies on the plasma profile of bupivacaine after direct intravenous injection suggest a three-compartment open model. The first compartment is represented by the rapid intravascular distribution of the drug. The second compartment represents the equilibration of the drug throughout the highly perfused organs such as the brain, myocardium, lungs, kidneys, and liver. The third compartment represents an equilibration of the drug with poorly

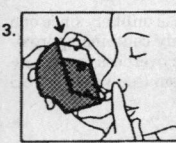

perfused tissues, such as muscle and fat. The elimination of drug from tissue depends largely upon the ability of binding sites in the circulation to carry it to the liver where it is metabolized.

After injection of Sensorcaine for caudal, epidural or peripheral nerve block in man, peak levels of bupivacaine in the blood are reached in 30 to 45 minutes, followed by a decline to insignificant levels during the next 3 to 6 hours.

Various pharmacokinetic parameters of the local anesthetics can be significantly altered by the presence of hepatic or renal disease, addition of epinephrine, factors affecting urinary pH, renal blood flow, the route of drug administration, and the age of the patient. The half-life of bupivacaine in adults is 3.5 ± 2.0 hours and in neonates 8.1 hours.

Amide-type local anesthetics such as bupivacaine are metabolized primarily in the liver via conjugation with glucuronic acid.

Patients with hepatic disease, especially those with severe hepatic disease, may be more susceptible to the potential toxicities of the amide-type local anesthetics. The major metabolite of bupivacaine is 2,6-pipecoloxylidine.

The kidney is the main excretory organ for most local anesthetics and their metabolites. Urinary excretion is affected by renal perfusion and factors affecting urinary pH. Only 5% of bupivacaine is excreted unchanged in the urine.

When administered in recommended doses and concentrations, Sensorcaine does not ordinarily produce irritation or tissue damage and does not cause methemoglobinemia.

INDICATIONS AND USAGE

Sensorcaine is indicated for the production of local or regional anesthesia or analgesia for surgery, for oral surgery procedures, for diagnostic and therapeutic procedures, and for obstetrical procedures. Only the 0.25% and 0.5% concentrations are indicated for obstetrical anesthesia. (See WARNINGS.)

Experience with non-obstetrical surgical procedures in pregnant patients is not sufficient to recommend use of the 0.75% concentration in these patients. Sensorcaine is not recommended for intravenous regional anesthesia (Bier Block). (See WARNINGS.)

The routes of administration and indicated Sensorcaine concentrations are:

local infiltration	0.25%
peripheral nerve block	0.25%, 0.5%
retrobulbar block	0.75%
sympathetic block	0.25%
lumbar epidural	0.25%, 0.5% and 0.75% (non-obstetrical)
caudal	0.25%, 0.5%
epidural test dose (see PRECAUTIONS)	

(See DOSAGE AND ADMINISTRATION for additional information.) Standard textbooks should be consulted to determine the accepted procedures and techniques for the administration of Sensorcaine.

Use only the single dose ampules and single dose vials for caudal or epidural anesthesia; the multiple dose vials contain a preservative and, therefore, should not be used for these procedures.

CONTRAINDICATIONS

Sensorcaine is contraindicated in obstetrical paracervical block anesthesia. Its use by this technique has resulted in fetal bradycardia and death.

Sensorcaine is contraindicated in patients with a known hypersensitivity to it or to any local anesthetic agent of the amide type or to other components of bupivacaine solutions.

WARNINGS

THE 0.75% CONCENTRATION OF SENSORCAINE INJECTION IS NOT RECOMMENDED FOR OBSTETRICAL ANESTHESIA. THERE HAVE BEEN REPORTS OF CARDIAC ARREST WITH DIFFICULT RESUSCITATION OR DEATH DURING USE OF BUPIVACAINE FOR EPIDURAL ANESTHESIA IN OBSTETRICAL PATIENTS. IN MOST CASES, THIS HAS FOLLOWED USE OF THE 0.75% CONCENTRATION. RESUSCITATION HAS BEEN DIFFICULT OR IMPOSSIBLE DESPITE APPARENTLY ADEQUATE PREPARATION AND APPROPRIATE MANAGEMENT. CARDIAC ARREST HAS OCCURRED AFTER CONVULSIONS RESULTING FROM SYSTEMIC TOXICITY, PRESUMABLY FOLLOWING UNINTENTIONAL INTRAVASCULAR INJECTION. THE 0.75% CONCENTRATION SHOULD BE RESERVED FOR SURGICAL PROCEDURES WHERE A HIGH DEGREE OF MUSCLE RELAXATION AND PROLONGED EFFECT ARE NECESSARY.

LOCAL ANESTHETICS SHOULD ONLY BE EMPLOYED BY CLINICIANS WHO ARE WELL VERSED IN DIAGNOSIS AND MANAGEMENT OF DOSE-RELATED TOXICITY AND OTHER ACUTE EMERGENCIES WHICH MIGHT ARISE FROM THE BLOCK TO BE EMPLOYED, AND THEN ONLY AFTER INSURING THE *IMMEDIATE* AVAILABILITY OF OXYGEN, OTHER RESUSCITATIVE DRUGS, CARDIOPULMONARY RESUSCITATIVE EQUIPMENT, AND THE PERSONNEL RESOURCES NEEDED FOR PROPER MANAGEMENT OF TOXIC REACTIONS AND RELATED EMERGENCIES. (See also ADVERSE REACTIONS, PRECAUTIONS, and OVERDOSAGE.) DELAY IN PROPER MANAGEMENT OF DOSE-RELATED TOXICITY, UNDERVENTILATION FROM ANY CAUSE AND /OR ALTERED SENSITIVITY MAY LEAD TO THE DEVELOPMENT OF ACIDOSIS, CARDIAC ARREST AND, POSSIBLY, DEATH.

Local anesthetic solutions containing antimicrobial preservatives, i.e. those supplied in multiple dose vials, should not be used for epidural or caudal anesthesia because safety has not been established with regard to intrathecal injection, either intentional or unintentional, of such preservatives.

It is essential that aspiration for blood or cerebrospinal fluid (where applicable) be done prior to injecting any local anesthetic, both the original dose and all subsequent doses, to avoid intravascular or subarachnoid injection. However, a negative aspiration does *not* ensure against an intravascular or subarachnoid injection.

Bupivacaine and Epinephrine Injection or other vasopressors should not be used concomitantly with ergot-type oxytocic drugs, because a severe persistent hypertension may occur. Likewise, solutions of bupivacaine containing a vasoconstrictor, such as epinephrine, should be used with extreme caution in patients receiving monoamine oxidase (MAO) inhibitors or antidepressants of the triptyline or imipramine types, because severe prolonged hypertension may result.

Until further experience is gained in children younger than 12 years, administration of bupivacaine in this age group is not recommended.

Reports of cardiac arrest and death have occurred with the use of bupivacaine for intravenous regional anesthesia (Bier Block). Information on safe dosages or techniques of administration of this product are lacking; therefore, bupivacaine is not recommended for use by this technique.

Prior use of chloroprocaine may interfere with subsequent use of bupivacaine. Because of this, and because safety of intercurrent use of bupivacaine and chloroprocaine has not been established, such use is not recommended.

Sensorcaine with epinephrine solutions contain sodium metabisulfite, a sulfite that may cause allergic-type reactions including anaphylactic symptoms and life-threatening or less severe asthmatic episodes in certain susceptible people. The overall prevalence of sulfite sensitivity in the general population is unknown and probably low. Sulfite sensitivity is seen more frequently in asthmatic than in nonasthmatic people.

PRECAUTIONS

General: The safety and effectiveness of local anesthetics depend on proper dosage, correct technique, adequate precautions and readiness for emergencies. Resuscitative equipment, oxygen, and other resuscitative drugs should be available for immediate use. (See WARNINGS, ADVERSE REACTIONS, and OVERDOSAGE.) During major regional nerve blocks, the patient should have I.V. fluids running via an indwelling catheter to assure a functioning intravenous pathway. The lowest dosage of local anesthetic that results in effective anesthesia should be used to avoid high plasma levels and serious adverse effects. The rapid injection of a large volume of local anesthetic solution should be avoided and fractional (incremental) doses should be used when feasible.

Epidural Anesthesia: During epidural administration of bupivacaine, concentrated solutions (0.5–0.75%) should be administered in incremental doses of 3 to 5 mL with sufficient time between doses to detect toxic manifestations of unintentional intravascular or intrathecal injection. Syringe aspirations should also be performed before and during each supplemental injection in continuous (intermittent) catheter techniques. An intravascular injection is still possible even if aspirations for blood are negative.

During the administration of epidural anesthesia, it is recommended that a test dose be administered initially and the effects monitored before the full dose is given. When using a "continuous" catheter technique, test doses should be given prior to both the original and all reinforcing doses, because plastic tubing in the epidural space can migrate into a blood vessel or through the dura. When clinical conditions permit, the test dose should contain epinephrine (10 to 15 μg have been suggested) to serve as a warning of unintentional intravascular injection. If injected into a blood vessel, this amount of epinephrine is likely to produce a transient "epinephrine response" within 45 seconds, consisting of an increase in heart rate and systolic blood pressure, circumoral pallor, palpitations and nervousness in the unsedated patient. The sedated patient may exhibit only a pulse rate increase of 20 or more beats per minute for 15 or more seconds. Therefore, following the test dose, the heart rate should be monitored for a heart rate increase. Patients on beta-blockers may not manifest changes in heart rate, but blood pressure monitoring can detect an evanescent rise in systolic blood pressure. The test dose should also contain 10 to 15 mg of Sensorcaine or an equivalent dose of a short-acting amide anesthetic such as 30 to 40 mg of lidocaine, to detect an unintentional intrathecal administration. This will be manifested within a few minutes by signs of spinal block (e.g., decreased sensation of the buttocks, paresis of the legs, or, in the sedated patient, absent knee jerk). An intravascular or subarachnoid injection is still possible even if results of the test dose are negative. The test dose itself may produce a systemic toxic reaction, high spinal or epinephrine-induced cardiovascular effects.

Injection of repeated doses of local anesthetics may cause significant increases in plasma levels with each repeated dose due to slow accumulation of the drug or its metabolites or to slow metabolic degradation. Tolerance to elevated blood levels varies with the physical condition of the patient. Debilitated, elderly patients, acutely ill patients and children should be given reduced doses commensurate with their age and physical condition. Local anesthetics should also be used with caution in patients with hypotension or heart block.

Careful and constant monitoring of cardiovascular and respiratory vital signs (adequacy of ventilation) and the patient's state of consciousness should be performed after each local anesthetic injection. It should be kept in mind at such times that restlessness, anxiety, incoherent speech, light-headedness, numbness and tingling of the mouth and lips, metallic taste, tinnitus, dizziness, blurred vision, tremors, twitching, depression, or drowsiness may be early warning signs of central nervous system toxicity.

Local anesthetic solutions containing a vasoconstrictor should be used cautiously and in carefully restricted quantities in areas of the body supplied by end arteries or having otherwise compromised blood supply such as digits, nose, external ear, penis, etc. Patients with hypertensive vascular disease may exhibit exaggerated vasoconstrictor response. Ischemic injury or necrosis may result.

Because amide-type local anesthetics such as bupivacaine are metabolized by the liver, these drugs, especially repeat doses, should be used cautiously in patients with hepatic disease. Patients with severe hepatic disease, because of their inability to metabolize local anesthetics normally, are at a greater risk of developing toxic plasma concentrations.

Local anesthetics should also be used with caution in patients with impaired cardiovascular function because they may be less able to compensate for functional changes associated with the prolongation of A-V conduction produced by these drugs.

Serious dose-related cardiac arrhythmias may occur if preparations containing a vasoconstrictor such as epinephrine are employed in patients during or following the administration of potent inhalation anesthetics. In deciding whether to use these products concurrently in the same patient, the combined action of both agents upon the myocardium, the concentration and volume of vasoconstrictor used, and the time since injection, when applicable, should be taken into account.

Many drugs used during the conduct of anesthesia are considered potential triggering agents for familial malignant hyperthermia. Because it is not known whether amide-type local anesthetics may trigger this reaction and because the need for supplemental general anesthesia cannot be predicted in advance, it is suggested that a standard protocol for management should be available. Early unexplained signs of tachycardia, tachypnea, labile blood pressure and metabolic acidosis may precede temperature elevation. Successful outcome is dependent on early diagnosis, prompt discontinuance of the suspect triggering agent(s) and prompt treatment, including oxygen therapy, dantrolene (consult dantrolene sodium intravenous package insert before using) and other supportive measures.

Use in Head and Neck Area: Small doses of local anesthetics injected into the head and neck area, including retrobulbar, dental and stellate ganglion blocks, may produce adverse reactions similar to systemic toxicity seen with unintentional intravascular injections of larger doses. The injection procedures require the utmost care. Confusion, convulsions, respiratory depression and/or respiratory arrest, and cardiovascular stimulation or depression have been reported. These reactions may be due to intraarterial injection of the local anesthetic with retrograde flow to the cerebral circulation. They also may be due to puncture of the dural sheath of the optic nerve during retrobulbar block with diffusion of any local anesthetic along the subdural space to the midbrain. Patients receiving these blocks should have their circulation and respiration monitored and be constantly observed. Resuscitative equipment and personnel for treating adverse reactions should be immediately available. Dosage recommendations should not be exceeded (See DOSAGE AND ADMINISTRATION).

Use in Ophthalmic Surgery: Clinicians who perform retrobulbar blocks should be aware that there have been reports of respiratory arrest following local anesthetic injection. Prior to retrobulbar block, as with all other regional procedures, the immediate availability of equipment, drugs, and personnel to manage respiratory arrest or depression, convulsions, and cardiac stimulation or depression should be

Continued on next page

Astra—Cont.

assured (see also WARNINGS and *Use in Head and Neck Area*, above). As with other anesthetic procedures, patients should be constantly monitored following ophthalmic blocks for signs of these adverse reactions, which may occur following relatively low total doses. A concentration of 0.75% bupivacaine is indicated for retrobulbar block; however, this concentration is not indicated for any other peripheral nerve block, including the facial nerve and not indicated for local infiltration, including the conjunctiva (see INDICATIONS and PRECAUTIONS, *General*). Mixing Sensorcaine (bupivacaine HCl) with other local anesthetics is not recommended because of insufficient data on the clinical use of such mixtures.

When Sensorcaine 0.75% is used for retrobulbar block, complete corneal anesthesia usually precedes onset of clinically acceptable external ocular muscle akinesia. Therefore, presence of akinesia rather than anesthesia alone should determine readiness of the patient for surgery.

Information for Patients: When appropriate, patients should be informed in advance that they may experience temporary loss of sensation and motor activity, usually in the lower half of the body following proper administration of caudal or lumbar epidural anesthesia. Also, when appropriate, the physician should discuss other information including adverse reactions in the Sensorcaine package insert.

Clinically Significant Drug Interactions: The administration of local anesthetic solutions containing epinephrine or norepinephrine to patients receiving monoamine oxidase inhibitors or tricyclic antidepressants may produce severe, prolonged hypertension. Concurrent use of these agents should generally be avoided. In situations in which concurrent therapy is necessary, careful patient monitoring is essential.

Concurrent administration of vasopressor drugs and of ergot-type oxytocic drugs may cause severe, persistent hypertension or cerebrovascular accidents.

Phenothiazines and butyrophenones may reduce or reverse the pressor effect of epinephrine.

Carcinogenesis, Mutagenesis, and Impairment of Fertility: Long-term studies in animals of most local anesthetics, including bupivacaine, to evaluate the carcinogenic potential have not been conducted. Mutagenic potential or the effect on fertility has not been determined. There is no evidence from human data that bupivacaine may be carcinogenic or mutagenic or that it impairs fertility.

Pregnancy Category C: Decreased pup survival in rats and embryocidal effect in rabbits have been observed when bupivacaine HCl was administered to these species in doses comparable to nine and five times, respectively, the maximum recommended daily human dose (400 mg). There are no adequate and well-controlled studies in pregnant women of the effect of bupivacaine on the developing fetus. Sensorcaine should be used during pregnancy only if the potential benefit justifies the potential risk to the fetus. This does not exclude the use of Sensorcaine (0.25% and 0.5% concentrations) at term for obstetrical anesthesia or analgesia. (See *Labor and Delivery*.)

Labor and Delivery: See Box WARNINGS regarding obstetrical use in 0.75% concentration.

Sensorcaine is contraindicated in obstetrical paracervical block anesthesia.

Local anesthetics rapidly cross the placenta, and when used for epidural, caudal or pudendal block anesthesia, can cause varying degrees of maternal, fetal and neonatal toxicity. (See *Pharmacokinetics* in CLINICAL PHARMACOLOGY.) The incidence and degree of toxicity depend upon the procedure performed, the type and amount of drug used, and the technique of drug administration. Adverse reactions in the parturient, fetus and neonate involve alterations of the central nervous system, peripheral vascular tone and cardiac function.

Maternal hypotension has resulted from regional anesthesia. Local anesthetics produce vasodilation by blocking sympathetic nerves. Elevating the patient's legs and positioning her on her left side will help prevent decreases in blood pressure. The fetal heart rate also should be monitored continuously, and electronic fetal monitoring is highly advisable.

Epidural, caudal, or pudendal anesthesia may alter the forces of parturition through changes in uterine contractility or maternal expulsive efforts. Epidural anesthesia has been reported to prolong the second stage of labor by removing the parturient's reflex urge to bear down or by interfering with motor function. The use of obstetrical anesthesia may increase the need for forceps assistance.

The use of some local anesthetic drug products during labor and delivery may be followed by diminished muscle strength and tone for the first day or two of life. This has not been reported with Sensorcaine.

It is extremely important to avoid aortocaval compression by the gravid uterus during administration of regional block to parturients. To do this, the patient must be maintained in the left lateral decubitus position or a blanket roll or sand-bag may be placed beneath the right hip and the gravid uterus displaced to the left.

Nursing Mothers: It is not known whether local anesthetic drugs are excreted in human milk. Because many drugs are excreted in human milk, caution should be exercised when local anesthetics are administered to a nursing mother.

Pediatric Use: Until further experience is gained in children younger than 12 years, administration of Sensorcaine (Bupivacaine HCl) Injection in this age group is not recommended.

ADVERSE REACTIONS

Reactions to bupivacaine are characteristic of those associated with other amide-type local anesthetics. A major cause of adverse reactions to this group of drugs may be associated with its excessive plasma levels, which may be due to overdosage, unintentional intravascular injection or slow metabolic degradation.

Systemic: The most commonly encountered acute adverse experiences that demand immediate countermeasures are related to the central nervous system and the cardiovascular system. These adverse experiences are generally dose related and due to high plasma levels which may result from overdosage, rapid absorption from the injection site, diminished tolerance or from unintentional intravascular injection of the local anesthetic solution. In addition to systemic dose-related toxicity, unintentional subarachnoid injection of drug during the intended performance of caudal or lumbar epidural block or nerve blocks near the vertebral column (especially in the head and neck region) may result in underventilation or apnea ("Total or High Spinal"). Also, hypotension due to loss of sympathetic tone and respiratory paralysis or underventilation due to cephalad extension of the motor level of anesthesia may occur. This may lead to secondary cardiac arrest if untreated. Factors influencing plasma protein binding, such as acidosis, systemic diseases that alter protein production or competition with other drugs for protein binding sites, may diminish individual tolerance.

Central Nervous System Reactions: These are characterized by excitation and/or depression. Restlessness, anxiety, dizziness, tinnitus, blurred vision or tremors may occur, possibly proceeding to convulsions. However, excitement may be transient or absent, with depression being the first manifestation of an adverse reaction. This may quickly be followed by drowsiness merging into unconsciousness and respiratory arrest. Other central nervous system effects may be nausea, vomiting, chills, and constriction of the pupils.

The incidence of convulsions associated with the use of local anesthetics varies with the procedure used and the total dose administered. In a survey of studies of epidural anesthesia, overt toxicity progressing to convulsions occurred in approximately 0.1 percent of local anesthetic administrations.

Cardiovascular System Reactions: High doses or unintentional intravascular injection may lead to high plasma levels and related depression of the myocardium, decreased cardiac output, heart block, hypotension, bradycardia, ventricular arrhythmias, including ventricular tachycardia and ventricular fibrillation, and cardiac arrest. (See WARNINGS, PRECAUTIONS, and OVERDOSAGE sections.)

Allergic: Allergic type reactions are rare and may occur as a result of sensitivity to the local anesthetic or to other formulation ingredients, such as the antimicrobial preservative methylparaben contained in multiple dose vials or sulfites in epinephrine-containing solutions (see WARNINGS). These reactions are characterized by signs such as urticaria, pruritus, erythema, angioneurotic edema (including laryngeal edema), tachycardia, sneezing, nausea, vomiting, dizziness, syncope, excessive sweating, elevated temperature, and possibly, anaphylactoid symptomatology (including severe hypotension). Cross sensitivity among members of the amide-type local anesthetic group has been reported. The usefulness of screening for sensitivity has not been definitely established.

Neurologic: The incidence of adverse neurologic reactions associated with the use of local anesthetics may be related to the total dose of local anesthetic administered and are also dependent upon the particular drug used, the route of administration and the physical status of the patient. Many of these effects may be related to local anesthetic techniques, with or without a contribution from the drug.

In the practice of caudal or lumbar epidural block, occasional unintentional penetration of the subarachnoid space by the catheter or needle may occur. Subsequent adverse effects may depend partially on the amount of drug administered intrathecally and the physiological and physical effects of a dural puncture. A high spinal is characterized by paralysis of the legs, loss of consciousness, respiratory paralysis and bradycardia.

Neurologic effects following unintentional subarachnoid administration during epidural or caudal anesthesia may include spinal block by varying magnitude (including high or total spinal block); hypotension secondary to spinal block; urinary retention; fecal and urinary incontinence; loss of perineal sensation and sexual function; persistent anesthesia, paresthesia, weakness, paralysis of the lower extremities and loss of sphincter control, all of which may have slow, incomplete or no recovery; headache; backache; septic meningitis; meningismus; slowing of labor; increased incidence of forceps delivery; or cranial nerve palsies due to traction on nerves from loss of cerebrospinal fluid.

OVERDOSAGE

Acute emergencies from local anesthetics are generally related to high plasma levels encountered during therapeutic use of local anesthetics or to unintended subarachnoid injection of local anesthetic solution. (See ADVERSE REACTIONS, WARNINGS, and PRECAUTIONS.)

Management of Local Anesthetic Emergencies: The first consideration is prevention, best accomplished by careful and constant monitoring of cardiovascular and respiratory vital signs and the patient's state of consciousness after each local anesthetic injection. At the first sign of change, oxygen should be administered.

The first step in the management of systemic toxic reactions, as well as underventilation or apnea due to unintentional subarachnoid injection of drug solution, consists of immediate attention to the establishment and maintenance of a patent airway and effective assisted or controlled ventilation with 100% oxygen with a delivery system capable of permitting immediate positive airway pressure by mask. This may prevent convulsions if they have not already occurred.

If necessary, use drugs to control the convulsions. A 50 to 100 mg bolus I.V. injection of succinylcholine will paralyze the patient without depressing the central nervous or cardiovascular systems and facilitate ventilation. A bolus I.V. dose of 5 to 10 mg of diazepam or 50 to 100 mg of thiopental will permit ventilation and counteract central nervous system stimulation, but these drugs also depress the central nervous system, respiratory and cardiac function, add to postictal depression, and may result in apnea. Intravenous barbiturates, anticonvulsant agents, or muscle relaxants should only be administered by those familiar with their use. Immediately after the institution of these ventilatory measures, the adequacy of the circulation should be evaluated. Supportive treatment of circulatory depression may require administration of intravenous fluids, and, when appropriate, a vasopressor dictated by the clinical situation (such as ephedrine or epinephrine to enhance myocardial contractile force).

If difficulty is encountered in the maintenance of a patent airway or if prolonged ventilatory support (assisted or controlled) is indicated, endotracheal intubation, employing drugs and techniques familiar to the clinician, may be indicated after initial administration of oxygen by mask.

Recent clinical data from patients experiencing local anesthetic induced convulsions demonstrated rapid development of hypoxia, hypercarbia, and acidosis with bupivacaine within a minute of the onset of convulsions. These observations suggest that oxygen consumption and carbon dioxide production are greatly increased during local anesthetic convulsions and emphasize the importance of immediate and effective ventilation with oxygen which may avoid cardiac arrest.

If not treated immediately, convulsions with simultaneous hypoxia, hypercarbia and acidosis, plus myocardial depression from the direct effects of the local anesthetic may result in cardiac arrhythmias, bradycardia, asystole, ventricular fibrillation, or cardiac arrest. Respiratory abnormalities, including apnea, may occur. Underventilation or apnea due to unintentional subarachnoid injection of local anesthetic solution may produce these same signs and also lead to cardiac arrest if ventilatory support is not instituted. If cardiac arrest should occur, a successful outcome may require prolonged resuscitative efforts.

The supine position is dangerous in pregnant women at term because of aortocaval compression by the gravid uterus. Therefore, during treatment of systemic toxicity, maternal hypotension or fetal bradycardia following regional block, the parturient should be maintained in the left lateral decubitus position if possible, or manual displacement of the uterus off the great vessels be accomplished.

The mean seizure dosage of bupivacaine in rhesus monkeys was found to be 4.4 mg/kg with mean arterial plasma concentration of 4.5 mcg/mL. The intravenous and subcutaneous LD_{50} in mice is 6 to 8 mg/kg and 38 to 54 mg/kg respectively.

DOSAGE AND ADMINISTRATION

The dose of any local anesthetic administered varies with the anesthetic procedure, the area to be anesthetized, the vascularity of the tissues, the number of neuronal segments to be blocked, the depth of anesthesia and degree of muscle relaxation required, the duration of anesthesia desired, individual tolerance, and the physical condition of the patient. The smallest dose and concentration required to produce the desired result should be administered. Dosages of Sensorcaine should be reduced for young, elderly and debilitated patients and patients with cardiac and/or liver disease. The rapid injection of a large volume of local anesthetic solution should be avoided and fractional (incremental) doses should be used when feasible.

TABLE 1. DOSAGE RECOMMENDATIONS—SENSORCAINE (Bupivacaine HCl) INJECTIONS

Type of Block	Conc.	Each Dose (mL)	(mg)	Motor Block[1]
Local Infiltration	0.25%[4]	up to max.	up to max.	—
Epidural	0.75%[2,4]	10–20	75–150	complete
	0.5%[4]	10–20	50–100	moderate to complete
	0.25%[4]	10–20	25–50	partial to moderate
Caudal	0.5%[4]	15–30	75–150	moderate to complete
	0.25%[4]	15–30	37.5–75	moderate
Peripheral Nerves	0.5%[4]	5 to max.	25 to max.	moderate to complete
	0.25%[4]	5 to max.	12.5 to max.	moderate to complete
Retrobulbar[3]	0.75%[4]	2–4	15–30	complete
Sympathetic	0.25%	20–50	50–125	—
Epidural[3] Test Dose	0.5% w/ep	2–3	10–15 (See PRECAUTIONS)	—

[1]With continuous (intermittent) techniques, repeat doses increase the degree of motor block. The first repeat dose of 0.5% may produce complete motor block. Intercostal nerve block with 0.25% may also produce complete motor block for intra-abdominal surgery.
[2]For single dose use, not for intermittent (catheter) epidural technique. Not for obstetrical anesthesia.
[3]See PRECAUTIONS.
[4]Solutions with or without epinephrine.

Sensorcaine-MPF (methylparaben free) is available in the following forms:

Single Dose Ampules:
5 mL;   0.5% with epinephrine 1:200,000
30 mL;   0.25%, 0.5% and 0.75% without epinephrine
         0.5% and 0.75% with epinephrine 1:200,000

Single Dose Vials:
10 mL; with Astra E-Z Off®   0.25%, 0.5% and 0.75% without epinephrine
   vial closure;   0.25%, 0.5% and 0.75% with epinephrine 1:200,000
30 mL;   0.25%, 0.5% and 0.75% without epinephrine
              0.25%, 0.5% and 0.75% with epinephrine 1:200,000

Sensorcaine is available in the following forms:

Multiple Dose Vial:
50 mL;   0.25% and 0.5% without epinephrine
         0.25% and 0.5% with epinephrine 1:200,000

For specific techniques and procedures, refer to standard textbooks.

In recommended doses, Sensorcaine produces complete sensory block, but the effect on motor function differs among the three concentrations.

0.25%—when used for caudal, epidural, or peripheral nerve block, produces incomplete motor block. Should be used for operations in which muscle relaxation is not important, or when another means of providing muscle relaxation is used concurrently. Onset of action may be slower than with the 0.5% or 0.75% solutions.

0.5%—provides motor blockade for caudal, epidural, or nerve block, but muscle relaxation may be inadequate for operations in which complete muscle relaxation is essential.

0.75%—produces complete motor block. Most useful for epidural block in abdominal operations requiring complete muscle relaxation, and for retrobulbar anesthesia. Not for obstetrical anesthesia.

The duration of anesthesia with Sensorcaine is such that for most indications, a single dose is sufficient.

Maximum dosage limit must be individualized in each case after evaluating the size and physical status of the patient, as well as the usual rate of systemic absorption from a particular injection site. Most experience to date is with single doses of Sensorcaine up to 225 mg with epinephrine 1:200,000 and 175 mg without epinephrine; more or less drug may be used depending on individualization of each case.

These doses may be repeated up to once every three hours. In clinical studies to date, total daily doses up to 400 mg have been reported. Until further experience is gained, this dose should not be exceeded in 24 hours. The duration of anesthetic effect may be prolonged by the addition of epinephrine.

The dosages in Table 1 have generally proved satisfactory and are recommended as a guide for use in the average adult. These dosages should be reduced for young, elderly or debilitated patients. Until further experience is gained Sensorcaine is not recommended for children younger than 12 years. Sensorcaine is contraindicated for obstetrical paracervical blocks, and is not recommended for intravenous regional anesthesia (Bier block).

Use in Epidural Anesthesia: During epidural administration of Sensorcaine, 0.5% and 0.75% solutions should be administered in incremental doses of 3 mL to 5 mL with sufficient time between doses to detect toxic manifestations of unintentional intravascular or intrathecal injection. In obstetrics, only the 0.5% and 0.25% concentrations should be used; incremental doses of 3 mL to 5 mL of the 0.5% solution not exceeding 50 mg to 100 mg at any dosing interval are recommended. Repeat doses should be preceded by a test dose containing epinephrine if not contraindicated. Use only the single dose ampules and single dose vials for caudal or epidural anesthesia; the multiple dose vials contain a preservative and therefore should not be used for these procedures.

Test dose for Caudal and Lumbar Epidural Blocks: See PRECAUTIONS.

Unused portions of solutions in single dose containers should be discarded, since this product form contains no preservatives. [See Table 1 above.]

NOTE: Parenteral drug products should be inspected visually for particulate matter and discoloration prior to administration whenever the solution and container permit. The Injection is not to be used if its color is pinkish or darker than slightly yellow or if it contains a precipitate.

HOW SUPPLIED

SOLUTIONS OF SENSORCAINE (BUPIVACAINE HYDROCHLORIDE) SHOULD NOT BE USED FOR THE PRODUCTION OF SPINAL ANESTHESIA (SUBARACHNOID BLOCK) BECAUSE OF INSUFFICIENT DATA TO SUPPORT SUCH USE. [See second table above.]

Disinfecting agents containing heavy metals, which cause release of respective ions (mercury, zinc, copper, etc.), should not be used for skin or mucous membrane disinfection since they have been related to incidents of swelling and edema. When chemical disinfection of the container surface is desired, either isopropyl alcohol (91%) or ethyl alcohol (70%) is recommended. It is recommended that chemical disinfection be accomplished by wiping the ampule or vial stopper thoroughly with cotton or gauze that has been moistened with the recommended alcohol just prior to use.

Solutions should be stored at controlled room temperature 15° to 30°C (59°–86°F).

Solutions containing epinephrine should be protected from light.

Caution: Federal law prohibits dispensing without prescription.

021680R02   Rev. 2/95

Shown in Product Identification Guide, page 304

SENSORCAINE®-MPF SPINAL   ℞
[*sén-sor-caine*]
(Bupivacaine in Dextrose Injection USP)
Bupivacaine HCl 0.75% in Dextrose 8.25% Injection
Sterile Hyperbaric Solution for Spinal Anesthesia

(For details of indications, dosages and administration, precautions, and adverse reactions, see circular in package.)

HOW SUPPLIED
NDC 0186-1026-03 2 mL ampule (15 mg bupivacaine HCl with 165 mg dextrose), boxes of 10.
Store at controlled room temperature, between 15°C and 30°C (59°F and 86°F).
021868R03   9/93 (3)

SODIUM BICARBONATE   ℞
[*so'-dĕum by-car'-bōw-nāte*]
Injection, USP

FOR CORRECTION OF METABOLIC ACIDOSIS AND OTHER CONDITIONS REQUIRING SYSTEMIC ALKALINIZATION.
(For details of indications, dosage and administration, precautions, and adverse reactions, see circular in package.)

HOW SUPPLIED
Sodium Bicarbonate Injection, USP is supplied in the following dosage forms:
[See table at bottom of page.]
Solutions should be stored at controlled room temperature 15°–30°C (59°–86°F).
021701R06   8/95

SODIUM CHLORIDE 0.9%, SODIUM CHLORIDE 0.45%, STERILE WATER FOR INHALATION   ℞
Arm-a-Vial®

INDICATIONS
For use in respiratory therapy. Contents of these vials are for use in apparatus for intermittent positive pressure-breathing (IPPB) and for tracheal lavage.

WARNING
Not for injection or in preparations to be used for injection.

DOSAGE AND ADMINISTRATION
To verify container integrity squeeze Arm-a-Vial® before use. Twist cap completely off Arm-a-Vial, invert, squeeze prescribed volume in nebulizer cup of IPPB apparatus.
Can also be used for tracheal lavage.
Internal contents sterile.
External surface of vial not sterile.
DISCARD ANY UNUSED PORTION OF THE CONTENTS OF THIS SINGLE DOSE VIAL AS WELL AS ANY UNUSED SOLUTION REMAINING IN THE NEBULIZER CUP.

HOW SUPPLIED
Single dose plastic Arm-a-Vial containing 3 mL or 5 mL solutions.
Sterile water. Non pyrogenic. Available by shelf carton of 100 × 3 mL vials (NDC 0186-4102-01) and 100 × 5 mL vials (NDC 0186-4102-03).
Sodium chloride 0.9% (normal saline-sterile). Non pyrogenic. Available by shelf carton of 100 × 3 mL vials (NDC 0186-4100-01) and 100 × 5 mL vials (NDC 0186-4100-03).
Sodium chloride 0.45% (half-normal saline-sterile). Non pyrogenic. Available by shelf carton of 100 × 3 mL vials (NDC 0186-4101-01) and 100 × 5 mL vials (NDC 0186-4101-03).
Store at controlled room temperature, 15°–30°C (59°–86°F).
021635R01   Rev. 4/96

STREPTASE®   ℞
(Streptokinase)

DESCRIPTION
Streptase®, Streptokinase, is a sterile, purified preparation of a bacterial protein elaborated by group C β-hemolytic

SODIUM BICARBONATE

NDC No. 0186-	Dosage Form	Conc. %	mg/mL (NaHCO₃)	mEq/mL (Na+)	mEq/mL (HCO₃)	mEq/Container size (mL)	mOsm
0650-01	Syringe	8.4	84	1.0	1.0	50/50	2/mL
0656-01	Syringe/ (Pediatric)	8.4	84	1.0	1.0	10/10	2/mL
0647-01	Syringe	7.5	75	0.9	0.9	44.6/50	1.79/mL
0646-01	Syringe/ (Infant)	4.2	42	0.5	0.5	5/10	1/mL
0645-01	Syringe/ (Infant)	4.2	42	0.5	0.5	2.5/5	1/mL

Continued on next page

Astra—Cont.

streptococci. It is supplied as a lyophilized white powder containing 25 mg cross-linked gelatin polypeptides, 25 mg sodium L-glutamate, sodium hydroxide to adjust pH, and 100 mg Albumin (Human) per vial or infusion bottle as stabilizers. The preparation contains no preservatives and is intended for intravenous and intracoronary administration.

CLINICAL PHARMACOLOGY

Streptase, Streptokinase, acts with plasminogen to produce an "activator complex" that converts plasminogen to the proteolytic enzyme plasmin. The $t^1/_2$ of the activator complex is about 23 minutes; the complex is inactivated, in part, by antistreptococcal antibodies. The mechanism by which dissociated streptokinase is eliminated is clearance by sites in the liver; however, no metabolites of streptokinase have been identified. Plasmin degrades fibrin clots as well as fibrinogen and other plasma proteins. Plasmin is inactivated by circulating inhibitors, such as α-2-plasmin inhibitor or α-2-macroglobulin. These inhibitors are rapidly consumed at high doses of streptokinase.

Intravenous infusion of Streptokinase is followed by increased fibrinolytic activity, which decreases plasma fibrinogen levels for 24 to 36 hours. The decrease in plasma fibrinogen is associated with decreases in plasma and blood viscosity and red blood cell aggregation. The hyperfibrinolytic effect disappears within a few hours after discontinuation, but a prolonged thrombin time may persist for up to 24 hours due to the decrease in plasma levels of fibrinogen and an increase in the amount of circulating fibrin(ogen) degradation products (FDP). Depending upon the dosage and duration of infusion of Streptokinase, the thrombin time will decrease to less than two times the normal control value within 4 hours, and return to normal by 24 hours.

Intravenous administration has been shown to reduce blood pressure and total peripheral resistance with a corresponding reduction in cardiac afterload. These expected responses were not studied with the intracoronary administration of Streptase, Streptokinase. The quantitative benefit has not been evaluated.

Variable amounts of circulating antistreptokinase antibody are present in individuals as a result of recent streptococcal infections. The recommended dosage schedule usually obviates the need for antibody titration.

Two very large, randomized, placebo-controlled studies[1,2] involving almost 30,000 patients have demonstrated that a 60-minute intravenous infusion of 1,500,000 IU of Streptokinase significantly reduces mortality following a myocardial infarction. One of these studies also evaluated concomitant oral administration of low dose aspirin (160 mg/d over one month).

In the GISSI study the reduction in mortality was time dependent. There was a 47% reduction in mortality among patients treated within one hour of the onset of chest pain, a 23% reduction among patients treated within three hours, and a 17% reduction among patients treated between three and six hours. There was also a reduction in mortality in patients treated between six and twelve hours from the onset of symptoms, but the reduction was not statistically significant.

In the ISIS-2 study the reduction in mortality was also time dependent. If Streptokinase and aspirin were administered within the first hour after symptom onset, the reduction in mortality was 44%. The reduction in the odds of death in patients treated within four hours was 53% for the combination of Streptokinase and aspirin, and 35% for Streptokinase alone. However, the reduction was still significant when treatment was started 5–24 hours after symptom onset: 33% for the combined therapy and 17% for Streptokinase alone. Overall, in the 0–24 hour time period there was a 42% reduction in the odds of death with combined treatment (Streptokinase and aspirin) versus placebo ($2p < 0.00001$) and a 25% reduction in the odds of death with Streptokinase alone versus placebo ($2p < 0.00001$).

One of eight smaller studies using a similar dosing schedule showed a statistically significant reduction in mortality. When all of these studies were pooled, the overall decrease in mortality was approximately 23%. Results from pooling several studies using different dosages with long term infusion corroborate these observations.

In addition, studies measuring left ventricular ejection fraction (LVEF) at discharge showed the mean LVEFs were 3–6 percentage points higher in the Streptokinase group than in the control group. This difference was statistically significant in some of the studies[3,4]. Furthermore, some studies reported greater improvement in LVEF among patients treated within three hours than in patients treated later.

Results from a randomized controlled trial in over 11,000 patients show that, following treatment with IV Streptokinase, there is a reduction in the number of patients with clinical congestive heart failure during the 14–21 day in-hospital period. Clinical congestive heart failure occurred in 12.8% of Streptokinase-treated patients compared with 15% of the control patients ($p = 0.001$)[1].

The rate of reocclusion of the infarct-related vessel has been reported to be approximately 15–20%. The rate of reocclusion depends on dosage, additional anticoagulant therapy and residual stenosis. When the reinfarctions were evaluated in studies involving 8800 Streptokinase-treated patients, the overall rate was 3.8% (range 2–15%). In over 8500 control patients, the rate of reinfarction was 2.4%. However, the ISIS-2 study showed that an increase in reinfarction was avoided when Streptokinase was combined with low dose aspirin. The rate of reinfarction in the combination group was 1.8% vs 1.9% in the group given aspirin alone.

Streptase, Streptokinase, administered by the intracoronary route has resulted in thrombolysis usually within one hour, and ensuing reperfusion results in improvement of cardiac function and reduction of mortality[5,6]. LVEF was increased in patients treated with Streptokinase when compared to patients treated with conventional therapy. When the initial LVEF was low, the Streptokinase-treated patients showed greater improvement than did the controls. Spontaneous reperfusion is known to occur and has been observed with angiography at various time points after infarction. Data from one study show that 73% of Streptokinase-treated patients and 47% of the placebo-allocated patients reperfused during hospitalization.

Studies with thromobolytic therapy for pulmonary embolism show no significant difference in lung perfusion scan between the thrombolysis group and the heparin group at one-year follow-up. However, measurements of pulmonary capillary blood volumes and diffusing capacities at two weeks and one year after therapy indicate that a more complete resolution of thrombotic obstruction and normalization of pulmonary physiology was achieved with thrombolytic therapy, thus preventing the long term sequelae of pulmonary hypertension and pulmonary failure[7].

The long term benefit of Streptase, Streptokinase, therapy for deep vein thrombosis (DVT) has been evaluated venographically[8]. The combined results of five randomized studies show no residual thrombotic material in 60–75% of patients treated with Streptokinase versus only 10% of those treated with heparin. Thrombolytic therapy also preserves venous valve function in a majority of cases, thus avoiding the pathologic venous changes that produce the clinical postphlebitic syndrome which occurs in 90% of the DVT patients treated with heparin.

There is a time-related decrease in effectiveness when Streptase, Streptokinase, is used in the management of peripheral arterial thromboembolism. When administered three to ten days after onset of obstruction, rates of clearance of 50–75% were reported.

INDICATIONS AND USAGE

Acute Evolving Transmural Myocardial Infarction: Streptase, Streptokinase, is indicated for use in the management of acute myocardial infarction (AMI) in adults, for the lysis of intracoronary thrombi, the improvement of ventricular function, and the reduction of mortality associated with AMI, when administered by either the intravenous or the intracoronary route, as well as for the reduction of infarct size and congestive heart failure associated with AMI when administered by the intravenous route. Earlier administration of Streptokinase is correlated with greater clinical benefit. (See CLINICAL PHARMACOLOGY.)

Pulmonary Embolism: Streptase, Streptokinase, is indicated for the lysis of objectively diagnosed (angiography or lung scan) pulmonary emboli, involving obstruction of blood flow to a lobe or multiple segments, with or without unstable hemodynamics.

Deep Vein Thrombosis: Streptase, Streptokinase, is indicated for the lysis of objectively diagnosed (preferably ascending venography), acute, extensive thrombi of the deep veins such as those involving the popliteal and more proximal vessels.

Arterial Thrombosis or Embolism: Streptase, Streptokinase, is indicated for the lysis of acute arterial thrombi and emboli. Streptokinase is not indicated for arterial emboli originating from the left side of the heart due to the risk of new embolic phenomena such as cerebral embolism.

Occlusion of Arteriovenous Cannulae: Streptase, Streptokinase, is indicated as an alternative to surgical revision for clearing totally or partially occluded arteriovenous cannulae when acceptable flow cannot be achieved.

CONTRAINDICATIONS

Because thrombolytic therapy increases the risk of bleeding, Streptase, Streptokinase, is contraindicated in the following situations:

- active internal bleeding
- recent (within 2 months) cerebrovascular accident, intracranial or intraspinal surgery (see WARNINGS)
- intracranial neoplasm
- severe uncontrolled hypertension

Streptokinase should not be administered to patients having experienced severe allergic reaction to the product.

WARNINGS

Bleeding: Following intravenous high-dose brief-duration Streptokinase therapy in acute myocardial infarction, severe bleeding complications requiring transfusion are extremely rare (0.3–0.5%), and combined therapy with low dose aspirin does not appear to increase the risk of major bleeding. The addition of aspirin to Streptokinase may cause a slight increase in the risk of minor bleeding (3.1% without aspirin vs. 3.9% with)[2].

Streptokinase will cause lysis of hemostatic fibrin deposits such as those occurring at sites of needle punctures, particularly when infused over several hours, and bleeding may occur from such sites. In order to minimize the risk of bleeding during treatment with Streptokinase, venipunctures and physical handling of the patient should be performed carefully and as infrequently as possible, and intramuscular injections must be avoided.

Should an arterial puncture be necessary during intravenous therapy, upper extremity vessels are preferable. Pressure should be applied for at least 30 minutes, a pressure dressing applied, and the puncture site checked frequently for evidence of bleeding.

In the following conditions the risks of therapy may be increased and should be weighed against the anticipated benefits.

- Recent (within 10 days) major surgery, obstetrical delivery, organ biopsy, previous puncture of noncompressible vessels
- Recent (within 10 days) serious gastrointestinal bleeding
- Recent (within 10 days) trauma including cardiopulmonary resuscitation
- Hypertension: systolic BP > 180 mm Hg and/or diastolic BP > 110 mm Hg
- High likelihood of left heart thrombus, e.g., mitral stenosis with atrial fibrillation
- Subacute bacterial endocarditis
- Hemostatic defects including those secondary to severe hepatic or renal disease
- Pregnancy
- Age > 75 years
- Cerebrovascular disease
- Diabetic hemorrhagic retinopathy
- Septic thrombophlebitis or occluded AV cannula at seriously infected site
- Any other condition in which bleeding constitutes a significant hazard or would be particularly difficult to manage because of its location.

Should serious spontaneous bleeding (not controllable by local pressure) occur, the infusion of Streptase, Streptokinase, should be terminated immediately and treatment instituted as described under ADVERSE REACTIONS.

Arrhythmias: Rapid lysis of coronary thrombi has been shown to cause reperfuson atrial or ventricular dysrhythmias requiring immediate treatment. Careful monitoring for arrhythmia is recommended during and immediately following administration of Streptase, Streptokinase, for acute myocardial infarction.

Hypotension: Hypotension, sometimes severe, not secondary to bleeding or anaphylaxis has been observed during intravenous Streptase, Streptokinase, infusion in 1% to 10% of patients. Patients should be monitored closely and, should symptomatic or alarming hypotension occur, appropriate treatment should be administered. This treatment may include a decrease in the intravenous Streptokinase infusion rate. Smaller hypotensive effects are common and have not required treatment.

Other: Non-cardiogenic pulmonary edema has been reported rarely in patients treated with Streptase, Streptokinase. The risk of this appears greatest in patients who have large myocardial infarctions and are undergoing thrombolytic therapy by the intracoronary route.

Rarely, polyneuropathy has been temporally related to the use of Streptase, Streptokinase.

Should pulmonary embolism or recurrent pulmonary embolism occur during Streptase, Streptokinase, therapy, the originally planned course of treatment should be completed in an attempt to lyse the embolus. While pulmonary embolism may occasionally occur during Streptokinase treatment, the incidence is no greater than when patients are treated with heparin alone. In addition to pulmonary embolism, embolization to other sites and rare reports of cholesterol embolization with resultant complications (such as renal failure) have been observed during Streptokinase treatment.

PRECAUTIONS

General:

Repeated Administration—Because of the increased likelihood of resistance, due to antistreptokinase antibody, Streptase, Streptokinase, may not be effective if administered between five days and twelve months of prior Streptokinase

or Anistreplase administration, or streptococcal infections, such as streptococcal pharyngitis, acute rheumatic fever, or acute glomerulonephritis secondary to a streptococcal infection.

Laboratory Tests:

Intravenous or Intracoronary Infusion for Myocardial Infarction—Intravenous administration of Streptase, Streptokinase, will cause marked decreases in plasminogen and fibrinogen and increases in thrombin time (TT), activated partial thromboplastin time (APTT), and prothrombin time (PT), which usually normalize within 12–24 hours. These changes may also occur in some patients with intracoronary administration of Streptokinase.

Intravenous Infusion for Other Indications—Before commencing thrombolytic therapy, it is desirable to obtain an activated partial thromboplastin time (APTT), a prothrombin time (PT), a thrombin time (TT), or fibrinogen levels, and a hematocrit and platelet count. If heparin has been given, it should be discontinued and the TT or APTT should be less than twice the normal control value before thrombolytic therapy is started.

During the infusion, decreases in plasminogen and fibrinogen levels and an increase in the level of FDP (the latter two causing a prolongation in the clotting times of coagulation tests) will generally confirm the existence of a lytic state. Therefore, lytic therapy can be confirmed by performing the TT, APTT, PT, or fibrinogen levels approximately 4 hours after initiation of therapy. If heparin is to be (re)instituted following the Streptase, Streptokinase, infusion, the TT or APTT should be less than twice the normal control value (see manufacturer's prescribing information for proper use of heparin).

Drug Interactions: The interaction of Streptase, Streptokinase, with other drugs has not been well studied.

Use of Anticoagulants and Antiplatelet Agents—Streptase, Streptokinase, alone or in combination with antiplatelet agents and anticoagulants, may cause bleeding complications. Therefore, careful monitoring is advised. In the treatment of acute MI, aspirin, when not otherwise contraindicated, should be administered with Streptokinase (*see below*).

Anticoagulation and Antiplatelets After Treatment for Myocardial Infarction—In the treatment of acute myocardial infarction, the use of aspirin has been shown to reduce the incidence of reinfarction and stroke. The addition of aspirin to Streptokinase causes a minimal increase in the risk of minor bleeding (3.9% vs. 3.1%), but does not appear to increase the incidence of major bleeding (see ADVERSE REACTIONS)[2]. The use of anticoagulants following administration of Streptokinase increases the risk of bleeding, but has not yet been shown to be of unequivocal clinical benefit. Therefore, whereas the use of aspirin is recommended unless otherwise contraindicated, the use of anticoagulants should be decided by the treating physician.

Anticoagulation After IV Treatment for Other Indications—Continuous intravenous infusion of heparin, without a loading dose, has been recommended following termination of Streptase, Streptokinase, infusion for treatment of pulmonary embolism or deep vein thrombosis to prevent rethrombosis. The effect of Streptokinase on thrombin time (TT) and activated partial thromboplastin time (APTT) will usually diminish within 3 to 4 hours after Streptokinase therapy, and heparin therapy without a loading dose can be initiated when the TT or the APTT is less than twice the normal control value.

Pregnancy:

Pregnancy Category C—Animal reproduction studies have not been conducted with Streptase, Streptokinase. It is also not known whether Streptokinase can cause fetal harm when administered to a pregnant woman or can affect reproduction capacity. Streptokinase should be given to a pregnant woman only if clearly needed.

Pediatric Use: Safety and effectiveness in children have not been established.

ADVERSE REACTIONS

The following adverse reactions have been associated with intravenous therapy and may also occur with intracoronary artery infusion.

Bleeding: The reported incidence of bleeding (major or minor) has varied widely depending on the indication, dose, route and duration of administration, and concomitant therapy.

Minor bleeding can be anticipated mainly at invaded or disturbed sites. If such bleeding occurs, local measures should be taken to control the bleeding.

Severe internal bleeding involving gastrointestinal, genitourinary, retroperitoneal, or intracerebral sites has occurred and has resulted in fatalities. In the treatment of acute myocardial infarction with intravenous Streptokinase, the GISSI and ISIS-2 studies reported a rate of major bleeding (requiring transfusion) of 0.3–0.5%. However, rates as high as 16% have been reported in studies which required administration of anticoagulants and invasive procedures.

Major bleed rates are difficult to determine for other dosages and patient populations because of the different dosing and

Table I
SUGGESTED DILUTIONS AND INFUSION RATES

Dosage	Vial Size (IU)	Total Solution Volume	Infusion Rate
I. **Acute Myocardial Infarction**			
A. Intravenous Infusion	1,500,000	45 mL	Infuse 45 mL within 60 min.
B. Intracoronary Infusion	250,000	125 mL	
1. 20,000 IU bolus			1. Loading Dose of 10 mL
2. 2,000 IU/minute for 60 minutes			2. Then 60 mL/hour
II. **Pulmonary Embolism, Deep Vein Thrombosis, Arterial Thrombosis or Embolism Intravenous Infusion**			
A. 1. 250,000 IU loading dose over 30 minutes	1,500,000	90 mL	1. Infuse 30 mL/hour for 30 minutes
2. 100,000 IU/hour maintenance dose			2. Infuse 6 mL per hour
B. SAME	1,500,000 infusion bottle	45 mL	1. 15 mL/hour for 30 minutes
			2. Infuse 3 mL per hour

intervals of infusions. The rates reported appear to be within the ranges reported for intravenous administration in acute myocardial infarction.

Should uncontrollable bleeding occur, Streptokinase infusion should be terminated immediately, rather than slowing the rate of administration of or reducing the dose of Streptokinase. If necessary, bleeding can be reversed and blood loss effectively managed with appropriate replacement therapy. Although the use of aminocaproic acid in humans as an antidote for Streptokinase has not been documented, it may be considered in an emergency situation.

Allergic Reactions: Fever and shivering, occuring in 1–4% of patients[1,2], are the most commonly reported allergic reactions with intravenous use of Streptase, Streptokinase, in acute myocardial infarction. Anaphylactic and anaphylactoid reactions ranging in severity from minor breathing difficulty to bronchospasm, periorbital swelling or angioneurotic edema have been observed rarely. Other milder allergic effects such as urticaria, itching, flushing, nausea, headache and musculoskeletal pain have also been observed, as have delayed hypersensitivity reactions such as vasculitis and interstitial nephritis. Anaphylactic shock is very rare, having been reported in 0–0.1% of patients[1,2,4].

Mild or moderate allergic reactions may be managed with concomitant antihistamine and/or corticosteroid therapy. Severe allergic reactions require immediate discontinuation of Streptase, Streptokinase, with adrenergic, antihistamine, and/or corticosteroid agents administered intravenously as required.

Other Adverse Reactions: Transient elevations of serum transaminases have been observed. The source of these enzyme rises and their clinical significance is not fully understood.

DOSAGE AND ADMINISTRATION

Acute Evolving Transmural Myocardial Infarction: Administer Streptokinase as soon as possible after onset of symptoms. The greatest benefit in mortality reduction was observed when Streptokinase was administered within four hours, but statistically significant benefit has been reported up to 24 hours (see CLINICAL PHARMACOLOGY).

Route	Total Dose	Dosage/Duration
Intravenous infusion	1,500,000 IU	1,500,000 IU within 60 min.
Intracoronary infusion	140,000 IU	20,000 IU by bolus followed by 2,000 IU/min. for 60 min.

Pulmonary Embolism, Deep Vein Thrombosis, Arterial Thrombosis or Embolism: Streptase, Streptokinase, treatment should be instituted as soon as possible after onset of the thrombotic event, preferably within 7 days. Any delay in instituting lytic therapy to evaluate the effect of heparin therapy decreases the potential for optimal efficacy. Since human exposure to streptococci is common, antibodies to Streptokinase are prevalent. Thus, a loading dose of Streptokinase sufficient to neutralize these antibodies is required. A dose of 250,000 IU of Streptokinase infused into a peripheral vein over 30 minutes has been found appropriate in over 90% of patients. Furthermore, if the thrombin time or any other parameter of lysis after 4 hours of therapy is not significantly different from the normal control level, discontinue Streptokinase because excessive resistance is present.

Indication	Loading Dose	IV Infusion Dosage/Duration
Pulmonary Embolism	250,000 IU/30 min.	100,000 IU/hr for 24 hr (72 hrs if concurrent DVT is suspected).
Deep Vein Thrombosis	250,000 IU/30 min.	100,000 IU/hr for 72 hr
Arterial Thrombosis or Embolism	250,000 IU/30 min.	100,000 IU/hr for 24–72 hr

Arteriovenous Cannulae Occlusion: Before using Streptase, Streptokinase, an attempt should be made to clear the cannula by careful syringe technique, using heparinized saline solution. If adequate flow is not re-established, Streptokinase may be employed. Allow the effect of any pretreatment anticoagulants to diminish. Instill 250,000 IU Streptokinase in 2 mL of solution into each occluded limb of the cannula slowly. Clamp off cannula limb(s) for 2 hours. Observe the patient closely for possible adverse effects. After treatment, aspirate contents of infused cannula limb(s), flush with saline, reconnect cannula.

Reconstitution and Dilution: The protein nature and lyophilized form of Streptase, Streptokinase, require careful reconstitution and dilution. Slight flocculation (described as thin translucent fibers) of reconstituted Streptokinase occured occasionally during clinical trials but did not interfere with the safe use of the solution. The following reconstitution and dilution procedures are recommended:

Vials and Infusion Bottles

1. Slowly add 5 mL Sodium Chloride Injection, USP or 5% Dextrose Injection, USP to the Streptase, Streptokinase, vial, directing the diluent at the side of the vacuum-packed vial rather than into the drug powder.
2. Roll and tilt the vial gently to reconstitute. Avoid shaking. (Shaking may cause foaming). (If necessary, total volume may be increased to a maximum of 500 mL in glass or 50 mL in plastic containers, and the infusion pump rate in Table 1 should be adjusted accordingly.) To facilitate setting the infusion pump rate, a total volume of 45 mL, or a multiple thereof, is recommended.
3. Withdraw the entire reconstituted contents of the vial: slowly and carefully dilute further to a total volume as recommended in Table 1. Avoid shaking and agitation on dilution.
4. When diluting the 1,500,000 IU infusion bottle (50 mL), slowly add 5 mL Sodium Chloride Injection, USP, or 5% Dextrose Injection, USP, directing it at the side of the bottle rather than into the drug powder. Roll and tilt the bottle gently to reconstitute. Avoid shaking as it may cause foaming. Add an additional 40 mL of diluent to the bottle, avoiding shaking and agitation. (Total volume = 45 mL). Administer by infusion pump at the rate indicated in Table 1.
5. Parenteral drug products should be inspected visually for particulate matter and discoloration prior to administration. (The Albumin (Human) may impart a slightly yellow color to the solution.)
6. The reconstituted solution can be filtered through a 0.8 µm or larger pore size filter.
7. Because Streptase, Streptokinase, contains no preservatives, it should be reconstituted immediately before use. The solution may be used for direct intravenous administration within eight hours following reconstitution if stored at 2–8°C (36–46°F).
8. Do not add other medication to the container of Streptase, Streptokinase.
9. Unused reconstituted drug should be discarded.
[See table 1 above.]

Continued on next page

Astra—Cont.

For Use In Arteriovenous Cannulae: Slowly reconstitute the contents of 250,000 IU Streptase, Streptokinase, vacuum-packed vial with 2 mL Sodium Chloride Injection, USP or 5% Dextrose Injection, USP.

HOW SUPPLIED

Streptase, Streptokinase, is supplied as a lyophilized white powder in 50 mL infusion bottles (1,500,000 IU) or in 6.5 mL vials with a color-coded label corresponding to the amount of purified Streptokinase in each vial as follows:

green	250,000 IU	NDC 0186-1770-01	box of 1
blue	750,000 IU	NDC 0186-1771-01	box of 1
red	1,500,000 IU	NDC 0186-1773-01	box of 1 (vials)
red	1,500,000 IU	NDC 0186-1774-01	box of 1 (infusion bottles)

Store unopened vials at controlled room temperature (15–30°C or 59–86°F).

REFERENCES

1. GISSI: Effectiveness of intravenous thrombolytic treatment in acute myocardial infarction. Lancet I: 397–402, 1986
2. ISIS-2 Collaborative Group: Randomized trial of streptokinase, oral aspirin, both, or neither among 17,187 cases of suspected acute myocardial infarction: ISIS-2. Lancet II: 349–360, 1988
3. White, H., Norris, R., Brown, M., et al: Effect of intravenous streptokinase on left ventricular function and early survival after acute myocardial infarction. N Engl J Med 317: 850–5, 1987
4. The I.S.A.M. Study Group: A prospective trial of intravenous streptokinase in acute myocardial infarction (I.S. A.M.). N Engl J Med 314: 1465–1471, 1986
5. Anderson J., Marshall, H., Bray, B., et al: A randomized trial of intracoronary streptokinase in the treatment of acute myocardial infarction. N Engl J Med 308: 1312–8, 1983
6. Kennedy, J., Ritchie, J., Davis, K., Fritz, J.: Western Washington randomized trial of intracoronary streptokinase in acute myocardial infarction. N Engl J Med 309: 1477–82, 1983
7. Sharma, G., Burleson, V., Sasahara, A.: Effect of thrombolytic therapy on pulmonary-capillary blood volume in patients with pulmonary embolism. N Engl J Med 303: 842–5, 1980
8. Arnesen, H., Heilo, A., Jakobsen, E., et al: A prospective study of streptokinase and heparin in the treatment of venous thrombosis. Acta Med Scand 203: 457–463, 1978

Manufactured by Behringwerke AG
PO Box 1140, D-35001 Marburg, Germany
US License No. 97
Distributed by Astra USA, Inc.
Westborough, MA 01581 021596R07 (Revised 10/94)

TOBRAMYCIN SULFATE INJECTION, USP ℞

WARNINGS

Patients treated with tobramycin sulfate injection and other aminoglycosides should be under close clinical observation, because these drugs have an inherent potential for causing ototoxicity and nephrotoxicity.

Neurotoxicity, manifested as both auditory and vestibular ototoxicity, can occur. The auditory changes are irreversible, are usually bilateral, and may be partial or total. Eighth-nerve impairment and nephrotoxicity may develop, primarily in patients having preexisting renal damage and in those with normal renal function to whom aminoglycosides are administered for longer periods or in higher doses than those recommended. Other manifestations of neurotoxicity may include numbness, skin tingling, muscle twitching, and convulsions. The risk of aminoglycoside-induced hearing loss increases with the degree of exposure to either high peak or high trough serum concentrations. Patients who develop cochlear damage may not have symptoms during therapy to warn them of eighth-nerve toxicity, and partial or total irreversible bilateral deafness may continue to develop after the drug has been discontinued.

Rarely, nephrotoxicity may not become apparent until the first few days after cessation of therapy. Aminoglycoside-induced nephrotoxicity usually is reversible.

Renal and eighth-nerve function should be closely monitored in patients with known or suspected renal impairment and also in those whose renal function is initially normal but who develop signs of renal dysfunction during therapy. Peak and trough serum concentrations of aminoglycosides should be monitored periodically during therapy to assure adequate levels and to avoid potentially toxic levels. Prolonged serum concentrations above 12 μg/mL should be avoided. Rising trough levels (above 2 μg/mL) may indicate tissue accumulation. Such accumulation, excessive peak concentrations, advanced age, and cumulative dose may contribute to ototoxicity and nephrotoxicity (see PRECAUTIONS). Urine should be examined for decreased specific gravity and increased excretion of protein, cells, and casts. Blood urea nitrogen, serum creatinine, and creatinine clearance should be measured periodically. When feasible, it is recommended that serial audiograms be obtained in patients old enough to be tested, particularly high-risk patients. Evidence of impairment of renal, vestibular, or auditory function requires discontinuation of the drug or dosage adjustment.

Tobramycin should be used with caution in premature and neonatal infants because of their renal immaturity and the resulting prolongation of serum half-life of the drug.

Concurrent and sequential use of other neurotoxic and/or nephrotoxic antibiotics, particularly other aminoglycosides (e.g., amikacin, streptomycin, neomycin, kanamycin, gentamicin, and paromomycin), cephaloridine, viomycin, polymyxin B, colistin, cisplatin, and vancomycin, should be avoided. Other factors that may increase patient risk are advanced age and dehydration.

Aminoglycosides should not be given concurrently with potent diuretics, such as ethacrynic acid and furosemide. Some diuretics themselves cause ototoxicity, and intravenously administered diuretics enhance aminoglycoside toxicity by altering antibiotic concentrations in serum and tissue.

Aminoglycosides can cause fetal harm when administered to a pregnant woman (see PRECAUTIONS).

For further information see PRECAUTIONS in full prescribing information.

DESCRIPTION

Tobramycin sulfate, a water-soluble antibiotic of the aminoglycoside group, is derived from the actinomycete *Streptomyces tenebrarius.* Tobramycin sulfate injection, is a clear and colorless sterile aqueous solution for parenteral administration.

Tobramycin sulfate is *O*-3-amino-3-deoxy-α-D-glucopyranosyl-(1→4)-*O*-[2,6-diamino-2,3,6-trideoxy-α-D-*ribo*-hexopyranosyl-(1→6)]-2-deoxy-L-streptamine, sulfate (2:5) (salt) and has the molecular formula $(C_{18}H_{37}N_5O_9)_2 \cdot 5H_2SO_4$. The molecular weight is 1,425.39. The structural formula for tobramycin is as follows:

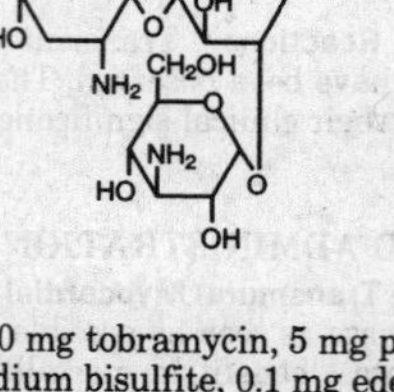

Each mL contains 40 mg tobramycin, 5 mg phenol as a preservative, 3.2 mg sodium bisulfite, 0.1 mg edetate disodium, and Water for Injection. Sulfuric acid and, if necessary, sodium hydroxide have been added to adjust the pH to 3.0–6.5. Filled under nitrogen.

HOW SUPPLIED

Tobramycin Sulfate Injection, USP is available in the following forms:

Multiple Dose Vials

NDC 0186-1783-04 80 mg*/2 mL, (40 mg*/mL) 2 mL vial—box of 25

NDC 0186-1784-01 40 mg*/mL, 30 mL—box of 1

*equivalent to tobramycin

Store at controlled room temperature 15°–30°C (59°–86°F).

Caution: Federal law prohibits dispensing without prescription.

021832R07 Rev. 2/95

TOPROL-XL® TABLETS ℞

(metoprolol succinate)
Extended Release Tablets
Tablets: 50 mg, 100 mg, and 200 mg

DESCRIPTION

Toprol-XL, metoprolol succinate, is a beta$_1$-selective (cardioselective) adrenoceptor blocking agent, for oral administration, available as extended release tablets. Toprol-XL has been formulated to provide a controlled and predictable release of metoprolol for once daily administration. The tablets comprise a multiple unit system containing metoprolol succinate in a multitude of controlled release pellets. Each pellet acts as a separate drug delivery unit and is designed to deliver metoprolol continuously over the dosage interval. The tablets contain 47.5 mg, 95 mg and 190 mg of metoprolol succinate equivalent to 50, 100 and 200 mg of metoprolol tartrate, USP, respectively. Its chemical name is (±)1-(isopropylamino) -3- [p- (2-methoxyethyl)phenoxy]-2-propanol succinate (2:1) (salt). Its structural formula is:

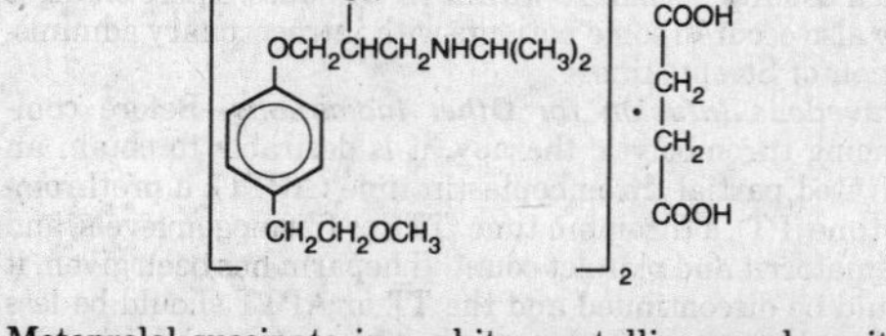

Metoprolol succinate is a white crystalline powder with a molecular weight of 652.8. It is freely soluble in water; soluble in methanol; sparingly soluble in ethanol; slightly soluble in dichloromethane and 2-propanol; practically insoluble in ethyl-acetate, acetone, diethylether and heptane. Inactive ingredients: silicon dioxide, cellulose compounds, sodium stearyl fumarate, polyethylene glycol, titanium dioxide, paraffin.

CLINICAL PHARMACOLOGY

Metoprolol is a beta$_1$-selective (cardioselective) adrenergic receptor blocking agent. This preferential effect is not absolute, however, and at higher plasma concentrations, metoprolol also inhibits beta$_2$-adrenoreceptors, chiefly located in the bronchial and vascular musculature. Metoprolol has no intrinsic sympathomimetic activity, and membrane-stabilizing activity is detectable only at plasma concentrations much greater than required for beta-blockade. Animal and human experiments indicate that metoprolol slows the sinus rate and decreases AV nodal conduction.

Clinical pharmacology studies have confirmed the beta-blocking activity of metoprolol in man, as shown by (1) reduction in heart rate and cardiac output at rest and upon exercise, (2) reduction of systolic blood pressure upon exercise, (3) inhibition of isoproterenol-induced tachycardia, and (4) reduction of reflex orthostatic tachycardia.

The relative beta$_1$-selectivity of metoprolol has been confirmed by the following: (1) In normal subjects, metoprolol is unable to reverse the beta$_2$-mediated vasodilating effects of epinephrine. This contrasts with the effect of nonselective beta-blockers, which completely reverse the vasodilating effects of epinephrine. (2) In asthmatic patients, metoprolol reduces FEV_1 and FVC significantly less than a nonselective beta-blocker, propranolol, at equivalent beta$_1$-receptor blocking doses.

In five controlled studies in normal healthy subjects, the same daily doses of Toprol-XL and immediate release metoprolol were compared in terms of the extent and duration of beta$_1$-blockade produced. Both formulations were given in a dose range equivalent to 100–400 mg of immediate release metoprolol per day. In these studies, Toprol-XL was administered once a day and immediate release metoprolol was administered once to four times a day. A sixth controlled study compared the beta$_1$-blocking effects of a 50 mg daily dose of the two formulations. In each study, beta$_1$-blockade was expressed as the percent change from baseline, in exercise heart rate following standardized submaximal exercise tolerance tests at steady state. Toprol-XL administered once a day, and immediate release metoprolol administered once to four times a day, provided comparable total beta$_1$-blockade over 24 hours (area under the beta$_1$-blockade versus time curve) in the dose range 100–400 mg. At a dosage of 50 mg once daily, Toprol-XL produced significantly higher total beta$_1$-blockade over 24 hours than immediate release metoprolol. For Toprol-XL, the percent reduction in exercise heart rate was relatively stable throughout the entire dosage interval and the level of beta$_1$-blockade increased with increasing doses from 50 to 300 mg daily. The effects at peak/trough (i.e. at 24 hours post dosing) were; 14/9, 16/10, 24/14, 27/22 and 27/20% reduction in exercise heart rate for doses of 50, 100, 200, 300 and 400 mg Toprol-XL once a day, respectively. In contrast to Toprol-XL immediate release metoprolol given at a dose of 50–100 mg once a day, produced a significantly larger peak effect on exercise tachycardia, but the effect was not evident at 24 hours. To match the peak to trough ratio obtained with Toprol-XL over the dosing range of 200 to 400 mg, a t.i.d. to q.i.d. divided dosing regimen was required for immediate release metoprolol.

The relationship between plasma metoprolol levels and reduction in exercise heart rate is independent of the pharmaceutical formulation. Using the E_{max} model, the maximal beta$_1$-blocking effect has been estimated to produce a 28.3% reduction in exercise heart rate. Beta$_1$-blocking effects in the range of 30–80% of the maximal effect (corresponding to approximately 8–23% reduction in exercise heart rate) are expected to occur at metoprolol plasma concentrations ranging from 30–540 nmol/L. The concentration-effect curve

begins reaching a plateau between 200–300 nmol/L, and higher plasma levels produce little additional beta$_1$-blocking effect. The relative beta$_1$-selectivity of metoprolol diminishes and blockade of beta$_2$-adrenoceptors increases at higher plasma concentrations.

Although beta-adrenergic receptor blockade is useful in the treatment of angina and hypertension, there are situations in which sympathetic stimulation is vital. In patients with severely damaged hearts, adequate ventricular function may depend on sympathetic drive. In the presence of AV block, beta-blockade may prevent the necessary facilitating effect of sympathetic activity on conduction. Beta$_2$-adrenergic blockade results in passive bronchial constriction by interfering with endogenous adrenergic bronchodilator activity in patients subject to bronchospasm and may also interfere with exogenous bronchodilators in such patients.

Hypertension
The mechanism of the antihypertensive effects of beta-blocking agents has not been elucidated. However, several possible mechanisms have been proposed: (1) competitive antagonism of catecholamines at peripheral (especially cardiac) adrenergic neuron sites, leading to decreased cardiac output; (2) a central effect leading to reduced sympathetic outflow to the periphery; and (3) suppression of renin activity.

In controlled clinical studies, an immediate release dosage form of metoprolol has been shown to be an effective antihypertensive agent when used alone or as concomitant therapy with thiazide-type diuretics at dosages of 100–450 mg daily. Toprol-XL, in dosages of 100 to 400 mg once daily, has been shown to possess comparable β_1-blockade as conventional metoprolol tablets administered two to four times daily. In addition, Toprol-XL administered at a dose of 50 mg once daily has been shown to lower blood pressure 24-hours post-dosing in placebo controlled studies. In controlled, comparative, clinical studies, immediate release metoprolol appeared comparable as an antihypertensive agent to propranolol, methyldopa, and thiazide-type diuretics, and affected both supine and standing blood pressure. Because of variable plasma levels attained with a given dose and lack of a consistent relationship of antihypertensive activity to drug plasma concentration, selection of proper dosage requires individual titration.

Angina Pectoris
By blocking catecholamine-induced increases in heart rate, in velocity and extent of myocardial contraction, and in blood pressure, metoprolol reduces the oxygen requirements of the heart at any given level of effort, thus making it useful in the long-term management of angina pectoris. However, in patients with heart failure, beta-adrenergic blockade may increase oxygen requirements by increasing left ventricular fiber length and end-diastolic pressure.

In controlled clinical trials, an immediate release formulation of metoprolol has been shown to be an effective antianginal agent, reducing the number of angina attacks and increasing exercise tolerance. The dosage used in these studies ranged from 100 to 400 mg daily. Toprol-XL, in dosages of 100 to 400 mg once daily, has been shown to possess comparable β_1-blockade as conventional metoprolol tablets administered two to four times daily.

Pharmacokinetics
In man, absorption of metoprolol is rapid and complete. Plasma levels following oral administration of conventional metoprolol tablets, however, approximate 50% of levels following intravenous administration, indicating about 50% first-pass metabolism. Metoprolol crosses the blood-brain barrier and has been reported in the CSF in a concentration 78% of the simultaneous plasma concentration.

Plasma levels achieved are highly variable after oral administration. Only a small fraction of the drug (about 12%) is bound to human serum albumin. Elimination is mainly by biotransformation in the liver, and the plasma half-life ranges from approximately 3 to 7 hours. Less than 5% of an oral dose of metoprolol is recovered unchanged in the urine; the rest is excreted by the kidneys as metabolites that appear to have no clinical significance. Following intravenous administration of metoprolol, the urinary recovery of unchanged drug is approximately 10%. The systemic availability and half-life of metoprolol in patients with renal failure do not differ to a clinically significant degree from those in normal subjects. Consequently, no reduction in dosage is usually needed in patients with chronic renal failure.

In comparison to conventional metoprolol, the plasma metoprolol levels following administration of Toprol-XL are characterized by lower peaks, longer time to peak and significantly lower peak to trough variation. The peak plasma levels following once daily administration of Toprol-XL average one-fourth to one-half the peak plasma levels obtained following a corresponding dose of conventional metoprolol, administered once daily or in divided doses. At steady state the average bioavailability of metoprolol following administration of Toprol-XL, across the dosage range of 50 to 400 mg once daily, was 77% relative to the corresponding single or divided doses of conventional metoprolol. Nevertheless, over the 24 hour dosing interval, β_1-blockade is comparable and dose-related (see CLINICAL PHARMACOLOGY). The bio-

availability of metoprolol shows a dose-related, although not directly proportional increase with dose and is not significantly affected by food following Toprol-XL administration.

INDICATIONS AND USAGE
Hypertension
Toprol-XL tablets are indicated for the treatment of hypertension. They may be used alone or in combination with other antihypertensive agents.

Angina Pectoris
Toprol-XL tablets are indicated in the long-term treatment of angina pectoris.

CONTRAINDICATIONS
Hypertension and Angina
Toprol-XL is contraindicated in sinus bradycardia, heart block greater than first degree, cardiogenic shock, and overt cardiac failure (see WARNINGS).

WARNINGS
Hypertension and Angina
Cardiac Failure: Sympathetic stimulation is a vital component supporting circulatory function in congestive heart failure, and beta-blockade carries the potential hazard of further depressing myocardial contractility and precipitating more severe failure. In hypertensive and angina patients who have congestive heart failure controlled by digitalis and diuretics, Toprol-XL should be administered cautiously. Both digitalis and Toprol-XL slow AV conduction.

In Patients Without a History of Cardiac Failure: Continued depression of the myocardium with beta-blocking agents over a period of time can, in some cases, lead to cardiac failure. At the first sign or symptom of impending cardiac failure, patients should be fully digitalized and/or given a diuretic. The response should be observed closely. If cardiac failure continues, despite adequate digitalization and diuretic therapy, Toprol-XL should be withdrawn.

Ischemic Heart Disease: Following abrupt cessation of therapy with certain beta-blocking agents, exacerbations of angina pectoris and, in some cases, myocardial infarction have occurred. When discontinuing chronically administered Toprol-XL, particularly in patients with ischemic heart disease, the dosage should be gradually reduced over a period of 1–2 weeks and the patient should be carefully monitored. If angina markedly worsens or acute coronary insufficiency develops, Toprol-XL administration should be reinstated promptly, at least temporarily, and other measures appropriate for the management of unstable angina should be taken. Patients should be warned against interruption or discontinuation of therapy without the physician's advice. Because coronary artery disease is common and may be unrecognized, it may be prudent not to discontinue Toprol-XL therapy abruptly even in patients treated only for hypertension.

Bronchospastic Diseases: PATIENTS WITH BRONCHOSPASTIC DISEASES SHOULD, IN GENERAL, NOT RECEIVE BETA-BLOCKERS. Because of its relative beta$_1$-selectivity, however, Toprol-XL may be used with caution in patients with bronchospastic disease who do not respond to, or cannot tolerate, other antihypertensive treatment. Since beta$_1$-selectivity is not absolute, a beta$_2$-stimulating agent should be administered concomitantly, and the lowest possible dose of Toprol-XL should be used (see DOSAGE AND ADMINISTRATION).

Major Surgery: The necessity or desirability of withdrawing beta-blocking therapy prior to major surgery is controversial; the impaired ability of the heart to respond to reflex adrenergic stimuli may augment the risks of general anesthesia and surgical procedures.
Toprol-XL like other beta-blockers, is a competitive inhibitor of beta-receptor agonists, and its effects can be reversed by administration of such agents, e.g., dobutamine or isoproterenol. However, such patients may be subject to protracted severe hypotension. Difficulty in restarting and maintaining the heart beat has also been reported with beta-blockers.

Diabetes and Hypoglycemia: Toprol-XL should be used with caution in diabetic patients if a beta-blocking agent is required. Beta-blockers may mask tachycardia occurring with hypoglycemia, but other manifestations such as dizziness and sweating may not be significantly affected.

Thyrotoxicosis: Beta-adrenergic blockade may mask certain clinical signs (e.g., tachycardia) of hyperthyroidism. Patients suspected of developing thyrotoxicosis should be managed carefully to avoid abrupt withdrawal of beta-blockade, which might precipitate a thyroid storm.

PRECAUTIONS
General
Toprol-XL should be used with caution in patients with impaired hepatic function.

Information for Patients
Patients should be advised to take Toprol-XL regularly and continuously, as directed, preferably with or immediately following meals. If a dose should be missed, the patient

should take only the next scheduled dose (without doubling it). Patients should not discontinue Toprol-XL without consulting the physician.

Patients should be advised (1) to avoid operating automobiles and machinery or engaging in other tasks requiring alertness until the patient's response to therapy with Toprol-XL has been determined; (2) to contact the physician if any difficulty in breathing occurs; (3) to inform the physician or dentist before any type of surgery that he or she is taking Toprol-XL.

Laboratory Tests
Clinical laboratory findings may include elevated levels of serum transaminase, alkaline phosphatase, and lactate dehydrogenase.

Drug Interactions
Catecholamine-depleting drugs (e.g., reserpine) may have an additive effect when given with beta-blocking agents. Patients treated with Toprol-XL plus a catecholamine depletor should therefore be closely observed for evidence of hypotension or marked bradycardia, which may produce vertigo, syncope, or postural hypotension.

Carcinogenesis, Mutagenesis, Impairment of Fertility
Long-term studies in animals have been conducted to evaluate the carcinogenic potential of metoprolol tartrate. In 2-year studies in rats at three oral dosage levels of up to 800 mg/kg/day, there was no increase in the development of spontaneously occurring benign or malignant neoplasms of any type. The only histologic changes that appeared to be drug related were an increased incidence of generally mild focal accumulation of foamy macrophages in pulmonary alveoli and a slight increase in biliary hyperplasia. In a 21-month study in Swiss albino mice at three oral dosage levels of up to 750 mg/kg/day, benign lung tumors (small adenomas) occurred more frequently in female mice receiving the highest dose than in untreated control animals. There was no increase in malignant or total (benign plus malignant) lung tumors, nor in the overall incidence of tumors or malignant tumors. This 21-month study was repeated in CD-1 mice, and no statistically or biologically significant differences were observed between treated and control mice of either sex for any type of tumor.
All mutagenicity tests performed on metoprolol tartrate (a dominant lethal study in mice, chromosome studies in somatic cells, a Salmonella/mammalian-microsome mutagenicity test, and a nucleus anomaly test in somatic interphase nuclei) and metoprolol succinate (a Salmonella/mammalian-microsome mutagenicity test) were negative.
No evidence of impaired fertility due to metoprolol tartrate was observed in a study performed in rats at doses up to 55.5 times the maximum daily human dose of 450 mg.

Pregnancy Category C
Metoprolol tartrate has been shown to increase post-implantation loss and decrease neonatal survival in rats at doses up to 55.5 times the maximum daily human dose of 450 mg. Distribution studies in mice confirm exposure of the fetus when metoprolol tartrate is administered to the pregnant animal. These studies have revealed no evidence of impaired fertility or teratogenicity. There are no adequate and well-controlled studies in pregnant women. Because animal reproduction studies are not always predictive of human response, this drug should be used during pregnancy only if clearly needed.

Nursing Mothers
Metoprolol is excreted in breast milk in very small quantities. An infant consuming 1 liter of breast milk daily would receive a dose of less than 1 mg of the drug. Caution should be exercised when Toprol-XL is administered to a nursing woman.

Pediatric Use
Safety and effectiveness in children have not been established.

Risk Of Anaphylactic Reactions
While taking beta-blockers, patients with a history of severe anaphylactic reactions to a variety of allergens may be more reactive to repeated challenge, either accidental, diagnostic or therapeutic. Such patients may be unresponsive to the usual doses of epinephrine used to treat allergic reaction.

ADVERSE REACTIONS
Hypertension and Angina
Most adverse effects have been mild and transient. The following adverse reactions have been reported for metoprolol tartrate.
Central Nervous System: Tiredness and dizziness have occurred in about 10 of 100 patients. Depression has been reported in about 5 of 100 patients. Mental confusion and short-term memory loss have been reported. Headache, somnolence, nightmares, and insomnia have also been reported.
Cardiovascular: Shortness of breath and bradycardia have occurred in approximately 3 of 100 patients. Cold extremities; arterial insufficiency, usually of the Raynaud type; palpitations; congestive heart failure; peripheral edema; syncope; chest pain; and hypotension have been reported in about 1 of 100 patients (see CONTRAINDICATIONS, WARNINGS and PRECAUTIONS).

Continued on next page

Astra—Cont.

Respiratory: Wheezing (bronchospasm) and dyspnea have been reported in about 1 of 100 patients (see WARNINGS).
Gastrointestinal: Diarrhea has occurred in about 5 of 100 patients. Nausea, dry mouth, gastric pain, constipation, flatulence, digestive tract disorders and heartburn have been reported in about 1 of 100 patients.
Hypersensitive Reactions: Pruritus or rash have occurred in about 5 of 100 patients. Worsening of psoriasis has also been reported.
Miscellaneous: Peyronie's disease has been reported in fewer than 1 of 100,000 patients. Musculoskeletal pain, blurred vision, decreased libido and tinnitus have also been reported.
There have been rare reports of reversible alopecia, agranulocytosis, and dry eyes. Discontinuation of the drug should be considered if any such reaction is not otherwise explicable. The oculomucocutaneous syndrome associated with the beta-blocker practolol has not been reported with metoprolol.

Potential Adverse Reactions
A variety of adverse reactions not listed above have been reported with other beta-adrenergic blocking agents and should be considered potential adverse reactions to Toprol-XL.
Central Nervous System: Reversible mental depression progressing to catatonia; an acute reversible syndrome characterized by disorientation for time and place, short-term memory loss, emotional lability, slightly clouded sensorium, and decreased performance on neuropsychometrics.
Cardiovascular: Intensification of AV block (see CONTRAINDICATIONS).
Hematologic: Agranulocytosis, nonthrombocytopenic purpura, thrombocytopenic purpura.
Hypersensitive Reactions: Fever combined with aching and sore throat, laryngospasm, and respiratory distress.

OVERDOSAGE

Acute Toxicity
There have been a few reports of overdosage with Toprol-XL and no specific overdosage information was obtained with this drug, with the exception of animal toxicology data. However, since Toprol-XL (metoprolol succinate salt) contains the same active moiety, metoprolol, as conventional metoprolol tablets (metoprolol tartrate salt), the recommendations on overdosage for metoprolol conventional tablets are applicable to Toprol-XL.

Signs and Symptoms
Potential signs and symptoms associated with overdosage with metoprolol are bradycardia, hypotension, bronchospasm, and cardiac failure.

Treatment
There is no specific antidote.
In general, patients with acute or recent myocardial infarction may be more hemodynamically unstable than other patients and should be treated accordingly. On the basis of the pharmacologic actions of metoprolol tartrate, the following general measures should be employed.
Elimination of the Drug: Gastric lavage should be performed.
Bradycardia: Atropine should be administered. If there is no response to vagal blockade, isoproterenol should be administered cautiously.
Hypotension: A vasopressor should be administered, e.g., levarterenol or dopamine.
Bronchospasm: A beta$_2$-stimulating agent and/or a theophylline derivative should be administered.
Cardiac Failure: A digitalis glycoside and diuretics should be administered. In shock resulting from inadequate cardiac contractility, administration of dobutamine, isoproterenol or glucagon may be considered.

DOSAGE AND ADMINISTRATION

Toprol-XL is an extended release tablet intended for once-a-day administration. When switching from immediate release metoprolol tablet to Toprol-XL, the same total daily dose of Toprol-XL should be used.
As with immediate release metoprolol, dosages of Toprol-XL should be individualized and titration may be needed in some patients.
Toprol-XL tablets are scored and can be divided; however, the whole or half tablet should be swallowed whole and not chewed or crushed.

Hypertension
The usual initial dosage is 50 to 100 mg daily in a single dose, whether used alone or added to a diuretic. The dosage may be increased at weekly (or longer) intervals until optimum blood pressure reduction is achieved. In general, the maximum effect of any given dosage level will be apparent after 1 week of therapy. Dosages above 400 mg per day have not been studied.

Angina Pectoris
The dosage of Toprol-XL should be individualized. The usual initial dosage is 100 mg daily, given in a single dose. The dosage may be gradually increased at weekly intervals until optimum clinical response has been obtained or there is a pronounced slowing of the heart rate. Dosages above 400 mg per day have not been studied. If treatment is to be discontinued, the dosage should be reduced gradually over a period of 1–2 weeks (see WARNINGS).

HOW SUPPLIED

<u>Tablets 50 mg:</u>
Contain 47.5 mg of metoprolol succinate equivalent to 50 mg of metoprolol tartrate, USP
Are white, biconvex, round, film-coated
Engraved $^{A}{}_{mo}$ on one side and scored on the other
Bottles of 100 NDC 0186-1090-05

<u>Tablets 100 mg:</u>
Contain 95 mg of metoprolol succinate equivalent to 100 mg of metoprolol tartrate, USP
Are white, biconvex, round, film-coated
Engraved $^{A}{}_{ms}$ on one side and scored on the other
Bottles of 100 NDC 0186-1092-05

<u>Tablets 200 mg:</u>
Contain 190 mg of metoprolol succinate equivalent to 200 mg of metoprolol tartrate, USP
Are white, biconvex, oval, film-coated
Engraved $^{A}{}_{my}$ and scored on one side
Bottles of 100 NDC 0186-1094-05

Store at controlled room temperature 15°-30°C (59°-86°F).
Manufactured by:
Astra Pharmaceutical Production, AB
Södertälje, Sweden
Manufactured for:
ASTRA®
Astra USA, Inc.
Westborough, MA 01581
021671R36 Rev. 4/96

Shown in Product Identification Guide, page 304

XYLOCAINE® (lidocaine hydrochloride) ℞
[*zī'lo-caine*]
Injections
XYLOCAINE® (lidocaine HCl) with Epinephrine Injections
For Infiltration and Nerve Block

DESCRIPTION

Xylocaine (lidocaine HCl) Injections are sterile, non pyrogenic aqueous solutions that contain a local anesthetic agent with or without epinephrine and are administered parenterally by injection. See INDICATIONS for specific uses.
Xylocaine solutions contain lidocaine HCl, which is chemically designated as acetamide, 2-(diethylamino)-N-(2,6-dimethylphenyl)-,monohydrochloride and has the molecular wt. 270.8. Lidocaine HCl ($C_{14}H_{22}N_2O \cdot HCl$) has the following structural formula:

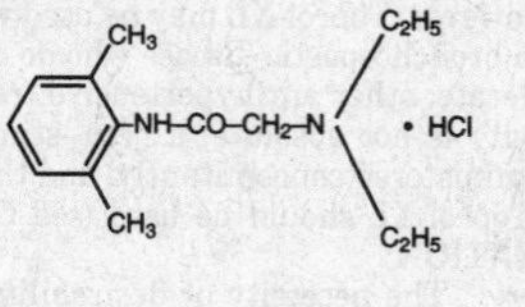

Epinephrine is (-)-3, 4-Dihydroxy-α-[(methylamino) methyl] benzyl alcohol and has the molecular wt. 183.21. Epinephrine ($C_9H_{13}NO_3$) has the following structural formula:

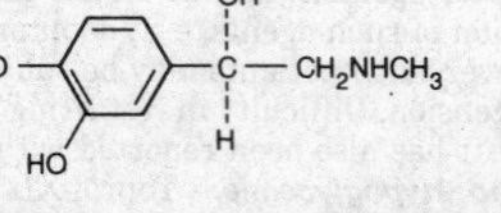

Dosage forms listed as Xylocaine-MPF indicate single dose solutions that are <u>M</u>ethyl <u>P</u>araben <u>F</u>ree (MPF).
<u>Xylocaine</u> <u>MPF</u> is a sterile, non pyrogenic, isotonic solution containing sodium chloride. <u>Xylocaine</u> in multiple dose vials, each mL also contains 1 mg methylparaben as antiseptic preservative. The pH of these solutions is adjusted to approximately 6.5 (5.0–7.0) with sodium hydroxide and/or hydrochloric acid.
<u>Xylocaine</u> <u>MPF</u> <u>with</u> <u>Epinephrine</u> is a sterile, non pyrogenic, isotonic solution containing sodium chloride. Each mL contains lidocaine hydrochloride and epinephrine, with 0.5 mg sodium metabisulfite as an antioxidant and 0.2 mg citric acid as a stabilizer. <u>Xylocaine</u> <u>with</u> <u>Epinephrine</u> in multiple dose vials, each mL also contains 1 mg methylparaben as antiseptic preservative. The pH of these solutions is adjusted to approximately 4.5 (3.3–5.5) with sodium hydroxide and/or hydrochloric acid. Filled under nitrogen.

CLINICAL PHARMACOLOGY

Mechanism of Action: Lidocaine stabilizes the neuronal membrane by inhibiting the ionic fluxes required for the initiation and conduction of impulses thereby effecting local anesthetic action.
Hemodynamics: Excessive blood levels may cause changes in cardiac output, total peripheral resistance, and mean arterial pressure. With central neural blockade these changes may be attributable to block of autonomic fibers, a direct depressant effect of the local anesthetic agent on various components of the cardiovascular system, and/or the beta-adrenergic receptor stimulating action of epinephrine when present. The net effect is normally a modest hypotension when the recommended dosages are not exceeded.
Pharmacokinetics and Metabolism: Information derived from diverse formulations, concentrations and usages reveals that lidocaine is completely absorbed following parenteral administration, its rate of absorption depending, for example, upon various factors such as the site of administration and the presence or absence of a vasoconstrictor agent. Except for intravascular administration, the highest blood levels are obtained following intercostal nerve block and the lowest after subcutaneous administration.
The plasma binding of lidocaine is dependent on drug concentration, and the fraction bound decreases with increasing concentration, At concentrations of 1 to 4 μg of free base per mL 60 to 80 percent of lidocaine is protein bound. Binding is also dependent on the plasma concentration of the alpha-1-acid glycoprotein.
Lidocaine crosses the blood-brain and placental barriers, presumably by passive diffusion.
Lidocaine is metabolized rapidly by the liver, and metabolites and unchanged drug are excreted by the kidneys. Biotransformation includes oxidative N-dealkylation, ring hydroxylation, cleavage of the amide linkage, and conjugation. N-dealkylation, a major pathway of biotransformation, yields the metabolites monoethylglycinexylidide and glycinexylidide. The pharmacological/toxicological actions of these metabolites are similar to, but less potent than, those of lidocaine. Approximately 90% of lidocaine administered is excreted in the form of various metabolites, and less than 10% is excreted unchanged. The primary metabolite in urine is a conjugate of 4-hydroxy-2, 6-dimethylaniline.
The elimination half-life of lidocaine following an intravenous bolus injection is typically 1.5 to 2.0 hours. Because of the rapid rate at which lidocaine is metabolized, any condition that affects liver function may alter lidocaine kinetics. The half-life may be prolonged two-fold or more in patients with liver dysfunction. Renal dysfunction does not affect lidocaine kinetics but may increase the accumulation of metabolites.
Factors such as acidosis and the use of CNS stimulants and depressants affect the CNS levels of lidocaine required to produce overt systemic effects. Objective adverse manifestations become increasingly apparent with increasing venous plasma levels above 6.0 μg free base per mL. In the rhesus monkey arterial blood levels of 18–21 μg/mL have been shown to be threshold for convulsive activity.

INDICATIONS AND USAGE

Xylocaine (lidocaine HCl) Injections are indicated for production of local or regional anesthesia by infiltration techniques such as percutaneous injection and intravenous regional anesthesia by peripheral nerve block techniques such as brachial plexus and intercostal and by central neural techniques such as lumbar and caudal epidural blocks, when the accepted procedures for these techniques as described in standard textbooks are observed.

CONTRAINDICATIONS

Lidocaine is contraindicated in patients with a known history of hypersensitivity to local anesthetics of the amide type.

WARNINGS

XYLOCAINE INJECTIONS FOR INFILTRATION AND NERVE BLOCK SHOULD BE EMPLOYED ONLY BY CLINICIANS WHO ARE WELL VERSED IN DIAGNOSIS AND MANAGEMENT OF DOSE-RELATED TOXICITY AND OTHER ACUTE EMERGENCIES THAT MIGHT ARISE FROM THE BLOCK TO BE EMPLOYED AND THEN ONLY AFTER ENSURING THE *IMMEDIATE* AVAILABILITY OF OXYGEN, OTHER RESUSCITATIVE DRUGS, CARDIOPULMONARY EQUIPMENT AND THE PERSONNEL NEEDED FOR PROPER MANAGEMENT OF TOXIC REACTIONS AND RELATED EMERGENCIES. (See also ADVERSE REACTIONS and PRECAUTIONS.) DELAY IN PROPER MANAGEMENT OF DOSE-RELATED TOXICITY, UNDERVENTILATION FROM ANY CAUSE AND/OR ALTERED SENSITIVITY MAY LEAD TO THE DEVELOPMENT OF ACIDOSIS, CARDIAC ARREST AND, POSSIBLY, DEATH.
To avoid intravascular injection, aspiration should be performed before the local anesthetic solution is injected. The needle must be repositioned until no return of blood can be elicited by aspiration. Note, however, that the absence of

blood in the syringe does not guarantee that intravascular injection has been avoided.

Local anesthetic solutions containing antimicrobial preservatives, (e.g., methylparaben) should not be used for epidural or spinal anesthesia because the safety of these agents has not been established with regard to intrathecal injection, either intentional or accidental.

Xylocaine with epinephrine solutions contain sodium metabisulfite, a sulfite that may cause allergic-type reactions including anaphylactic symptoms and life-threatening or less severe asthmatic episodes in certain susceptible people. The overall prevalence of sulfite sensitivity in the general population is unknown and probably low. Sulfite sensitivity is seen more frequently in asthmatic than in non-asthmatic people.

PRECAUTIONS

General: The safety and effectiveness of lidocaine depend on proper dosage, correct technique, adequate precautions, and readiness for emergencies. Standard textbooks should be consulted for specific techniques and precautions for various regional anesthetic procedures.

Resuscitative equipment, oxygen, and other resuscitative drugs should be available for immediate use. (See WARNINGS and ADVERSE REACTIONS.) The lowest dosage that results in effective anesthesia should be used to avoid high plasma levels and serious adverse effects. Syringe aspirations should also be performed before and during each supplemental injection when using indwelling catheter techniques. During the administration of epidural anesthesia, it is recommended that a test dose be administered initially and that the patient be monitored for central nervous system toxicity and cardiovascular toxicity, as well as for signs of unintended intrathecal administration, before proceeding. When clinical conditions permit, consideration should be given to employing local anesthetic solutions that contain epinephrine for the test dose because circulatory changes compatible with epinephrine may also serve as a warning sign of unintended intravascular injection. An intravascular injection is still possible even if aspirations for blood are negative. Repeated doses of lidocaine may cause significant increases in blood levels with each repeated dose because of slow accumulation of the drug or its metabolites. Tolerance to elevated blood levels varies with the status of the patient. Debilitated, elderly patients, acutely ill patients and children should be given reduced doses commensurate with their age and physical condition. Lidocaine should also be used with caution in patients with severe shock or heart block.

Lumbar and caudal epidural anesthesia should be used with extreme caution in persons with the following conditions: existing neurological disease, spinal deformities, septicemia and severe hypertension.

Local anesthetic solutions containing a vasoconstrictor should be used cautiously and in carefully circumscribed quantities in areas of the body supplied by end arteries or having otherwise compromised blood supply. Patients with peripheral vascular disease and those with hypertensive vascular disease may exhibit exaggerated vasoconstrictor response. Ischemic injury or necrosis may result. Preparations containing a vasoconstrictor should be used with caution in patients during or following the administration of potent general anesthetic agents, since cardiac arrhythmias may occur under such conditions.

Careful and constant monitoring of cardiovascular and respiratory (adequacy of ventilation) vital signs and the patient's state of consciousness should be accomplished after each local anesthetic injection. It should be kept in mind at such times that restlessness, anxiety, tinnitus, dizziness, blurred vision, tremors, depression or drowsiness may be early warning signs of central nervous system toxicity.

Since amide-type local anesthetics are metabolized by the liver, Xylocaine Injection should be used with caution in patients with hepatic disease. Patients with severe hepatic disease, because of their inability to metabolize local anesthetics normally, are at greater risk of developing toxic plasma concentrations. Xylocaine Injection should also be used with caution in patients with impaired cardiovascular function since they may be less able to compensate for functional changes associated with the prolongation of A-V conduction produced by these drugs.

Many drugs used during the conduct of anesthesia are considered potential triggering agents for familial malignant hyperthermia. Since it is not known whether amide-type local anesthetics may trigger this reaction and since the need for supplemental general anesthesia cannot be predicted in advance, it is suggested that a standard protocol for the management of malignant hyperthermia should be available. Early unexplained signs of tachycardia, tachypnea, labile blood pressure and metabolic acidosis may precede temperature elevation. Successful outcome is dependent on early diagnosis, prompt discontinuance of the suspect triggering agent(s) and institution of treatment, including oxygen therapy, indicated supportive measures and dantrolene (consult dantrolene sodium intravenous package insert before using).

Proper tourniquet technique, as described in publications and standard textbooks, is essential in the performance of intravenous regional anesthesia. Solutions containing epinephrine or other vasoconstrictors should not be used for this technique.

Lidocaine should be used with caution in persons with known drug sensitivities. Patients allergic to para-aminobenzoic acid derivatives (procaine, tetracaine, benzocaine, etc.) have not shown cross sensitivity to lidocaine.

Use in the Head and Neck Area: Small doses of local anesthetics injected into the head and neck area, including retrobulbar, dental and stellate ganglion blocks, may produce adverse reactions similar to systemic toxicity seen with unintentional intravascular injections of larger doses. Confusion, convulsions, respiratory depression and/or respiratory arrest, and cardiovascular stimulation or depression have been reported. These reactions may be due to intra-arterial injection of the local anesthetic with retrograde flow to the cerebral circulation. Patients receiving these blocks should have their circulation and respiration monitored and be constantly observed. Resuscitative equipment and personnel for treating adverse reactions should be immediately available. Dosage recommendations should not be exceeded. (See DOSAGE and ADMINISTRATION.)

Information for Patients: When appropriate, patients should be informed in advance that they may experience temporary loss of sensation and motor activity, usually in the lower half of the body, following proper administration of epidural anesthesia.

Clinically Significant Drug Interactions: The administration of local anesthetic solutions containing epinephrine or norepinephrine to patients receiving monoamine oxidase inhibitors or tricyclic antidepressants may produce severe, prolonged hypertension.

Phenothiazines and butyrophenones may reduce or reverse the pressor effect of epinephrine.

Concurrent use of these agents should generally be avoided. In situations when concurrent therapy is necessary, careful patient monitoring is essential.

Concurrent administration of vasopressor drugs (for the treatment of hypotension related to obstetric blocks) and ergot-type oxytocic drugs may cause severe, persistent hypertension or cerebrovascular accidents.

Drug/Laboratory Test Interactions: The intramuscular injection of lidocaine may result in an increase in creatine phosphokinase levels. Thus, the use of this enzyme determination, without isoenzyme separation, as a diagnostic test for the presence of acute myocardial infarction may be compromised by the intramuscular injection of lidocaine.

Carcinogenesis, Mutagenesis, Impairment of Fertility: Studies of lidocaine in animals to evaluate the carcinogenic and mutagenic potential or the effect on fertility have not been conducted.

Pregnancy: Teratogenic Effects-Pregnancy Category B. Reproduction studies have been performed in rats at doses up to 6.6 times the human dose and have revealed no evidence of harm to the fetus caused by lidocaine. There are, however, no adequate and well-controlled studies in pregnant women. Animal reproduction studies are not always predictive of human response. General consideration should be given to this fact before administering lidocaine to women of childbearing potential, especially during early pregnancy when maximum organogenesis takes place.

Labor and Delivery: Local anesthetics rapidly cross the placenta and when used for epidural, paracervical, pudendal or caudal block anesthesia, can cause varying degrees of maternal, fetal, and neonatal toxicity, (see CLINICAL PHARMACOLOGY—*Pharmacokinetics*). The potential for toxicity depends upon the procedure performed, the type and amount of drug used, and the technique of drug administration. Adverse reactions in the parturient, fetus and neonate involve alterations of the central nervous system, peripheral vascular tone and cardiac function.

Maternal hypotension has resulted from regional anesthesia. Local anesthetics produce vasodilation by blocking sympathetic nerves. Elevating the patient's legs and positioning her on her left side will help prevent decreases in blood pressure. The fetal heart rate also should be monitored continuously, and electronic fetal monitoring is highly advisable.

Epidural, spinal, paracervical, or pudendal anesthesia may alter the forces of parturition through changes in uterine contractility or maternal expulsive efforts. In one study, paracervical block anesthesia was associated with a decrease in the mean duration of first stage labor and facilitation of cervical dilation. However, spinal and epidural anesthesia have also been reported to prolong the second stage of labor by removing the parturient's reflex urge to bear down or by interfering with motor function. The use of obstetrical anesthesia may increase the need for forceps assistance.

The use of some local anesthetic drug products during labor and delivery may be followed by diminished muscle strength and tone for the first day or two of life. The long-term significance of these observations is unknown. Fetal bradycardia may occur in 20 to 30 percent of patients receiving paracervical nerve block anesthesia with the amide-type local anesthetics and may be associated with fetal acidosis. Fetal heart

rate should always be monitored during paracervical anesthesia. The physician should weigh the possible advantages against risks when considering a paracervical block in prematurity, toxemia of pregnancy, and fetal distress. Careful adherence to recommended dosage is of the utmost importance in obstetrical paracervical block. Failure to achieve adequate analgesia with recommended doses should arouse suspicion of intravascular or fetal intracranial injection. Cases compatible with unintended fetal intracranial injection of local anesthetic solution have been reported following intended paracervical or pudendal block or both. Babies so affected present with unexplained neonatal depression at birth, which correlates with high local anesthetic serum levels, and often manifest seizures within six hours. Prompt use of supportive measures combined with forced urinary excretion of the local anesthetic has been used successfully to manage this complication.

Case reports of maternal convulsions and cardiovascular collapse following use of some local anesthetics for paracervical block in early pregnancy (as anesthesia for elective abortion) suggest that systemic absorption under these circumstances may be rapid. The recommended maximum dose of each drug should not be exceeded. Injection should be made slowly and with frequent aspiration. Allow a 5-minute interval between sides.

Nursing Mothers: It is not known whether this drug is excreted in human milk. Because many drugs are excreted in human milk, caution should be exercised when lidocaine is administered to a nursing woman.

Pediatric Use: Dosages in children should be reduced, commensurate with age, body weight and physical condition. See DOSAGE AND ADMINISTRATION.

ADVERSE REACTIONS

Systemic: Adverse experiences following the administration of lidocaine are similar in nature to those observed with other amide local anesthetic agents. These adverse experiences are, in general, dose-related and may result from high plasma levels caused by excessive dosage, rapid absorption or inadvertent intravascular injection, or may result from a hypersensitivity, idiosyncrasy or diminished tolerance on the part of the patient. Serious adverse experiences are generally systemic in nature. The following types are those most commonly reported:

Central Nervous System: CNS manifestations are excitatory and/or depressant and may be characterized by lightheadedness, nervousness, apprehension, euphoria, confusion, dizziness, drowsiness, tinnitus, blurred or double vision, vomiting, sensations of heat, cold or numbness, twitching, tremors, convulsions, unconsciousness, respiratory depression and arrest. The excitatory manifestations may be very brief or may not occur at all, in which case the first manifestation of toxicity may be drowsiness merging into unconsciousness and respiratory arrest.

Drowsiness following the administration of lidocaine is usually an early sign of a high blood level of the drug and may occur as a consequence of rapid absorption.

Cardiovascular System: Cardiovascular manifestations are usually depressant and are characterized by bradycardia, hypotension, and cardiovascular collapse, which may lead to cardiac arrest.

Allergic: Allergic reactions are characterized by cutaneous lesions, urticaria, edema or anaphylactoid reactions. Allergic reactions may occur as a result of sensitivity either to local anesthetic agents or to the methylparaben used as a preservative in multiple dose vials. Allergic reactions as a result of sensitivity to lidocaine are extremely rare and, if they occur, should be managed by conventional means. The detection of sensitivity by skin testing is of doubtful value.

Neurologic: The incidences of adverse reactions associated with the use of local anesthetics may be related to the total dose of local anesthetic administered and are also dependent upon the particular drug used, the route of administration and the physical status of the patient. In a prospective review of 10,440 patients who received lidocaine for spinal anesthesia, the incidences of adverse reactions were reported to be about 3 percent each for positional headaches, hypotension and backache; 2 percent for shivering; and less than 1 percent each for peripheral nerve symptoms, nausea, respiratory inadequacy and double vision. Many of these observations may be related to local anesthetic techniques, with or without a contribution from the local anesthetic.

In the practice of caudal or lumbar epidural block, occasional unintentional penetration of the subarachnoid space by the catheter may occur. Subsequent adverse effects may depend partially on the amount of drug administered subdurally. These may include spinal block of varying magnitude (including total spinal block), hypotension secondary to spinal block, loss of bladder and bowel control, and loss of perineal sensation and sexual function. Persistent motor, sensory and/or autonomic (sphincter control) deficit of some lower spinal segments with slow recovery (several months) or incomplete recovery have been reported in rare instances when caudal or lumbar epidural block has been attempted.

Continued on next page

Astra—Cont.

Backache and headache have also been noted following use of these anesthetic procedures.

OVERDOSAGE

Acute emergencies from local anesthetics are generally related to high plasma levels encountered during therapeutic use of local anesthetics or to unintended subarachnoid injection of local anesthetic solution (see ADVERSE REACTIONS, WARNINGS, and PRECAUTIONS).

Management of Local Anesthetic Emergencies: The first consideration is prevention, best accomplished by careful and constant monitoring of cardiovascular and respiratory vital signs and the patient's state of consciousness after each local anesthetic injection. At the first sign of change, oxygen should be administered.

The first step in the management of convulsions, as well as underventilation or apnea due to unintended subarachnoid injection of drug solution, consists of immediate attention to the maintenance of a patent airway and assisted or controlled ventilation with oxygen and a delivery system capable of permitting immediate positive airway pressure by mask. Immediately after the institution of these ventilatory measures, the adequacy of the circulation should be evaluated, keeping in mind that drugs used to treat convulsions sometimes depress the circulation when administered intravenously. Should convulsions persist despite adequate repiratory support, and if the status of the circulation permits, small increments of an ultra-short acting barbiturate (such as thiopental or thiamylal) or a benzodiazepine (such as diazepam) may be administered intravenously. The clinician should be familiar, prior to the use of local anesthetics, with these anticonvulsant drugs. Supportive treatment of circulatory depression may require administration of intravenous fluids and, when appropriate, a vasopressor as directed by the clinical situation (e.g., ephedrine).

If not treated immediately, both convulsions and cardiovascular depression can result in hypoxia, acidosis, bradycardia, arrhythmias and cardiac arrest. Underventilation or apnea due to unintentional subarachnoid injection of local anesthetic solution may produce these same signs and also lead to cardiac arrest if ventilatory support is not instituted. If cardiac arrest should occur, standard cardiopulmonary resuscitative measures should be instituted.

Endotracheal intubation, employing drugs and techniques familiar to the clinician, may be indicated, after initial administration of oxygen by mask, if difficulty is encountered in the maintenance of a patent airway or if prolonged ventilatory support (assisted or controlled) is indicated.

Dialysis is of negligible value in the treatment of acute overdosage with lidocaine.

The oral LD_{50} of lidocaine HCl in non-fasted female rats is 459 (346–773) mg/kg (as the salt) and 214 (159–324) mg/kg (as the salt) in fasted female rats.

DOSAGE AND ADMINISTRATION

Table I (Recommended Dosages) summarizes the recommended volumes and concentrations of Xylocaine Injection for various types of anesthetic procedures. The dosages suggested in this table are for normal healthy adults and refer to the use of epinephrine-free solutions. When larger volumes are required, only solutions containing epinephrine should be used except in those cases where vasopressor drugs may be contraindicated.

These recommended doses serve only as a guide to the amount of anesthetic required for most routine procedures. The actual volumes and concentrations to be used depend on a number of factors such as type and extent of surgical procedure, depth of anesthesia and degree of muscular relaxation required, duration of anesthesia required, and the physical condition of the patient. In all cases the lowest concentration and smallest dose that will produce the desired result should be given. Dosages should be reduced for children and for the elderly and debilitated patients and patients with cardiac and/or liver disease.

The onset of anesthesia, the duration of anesthesia and the degree of muscular relaxation are proportional to the volume and concentration (i.e., total dose) of local anesthetic used. Thus, an increase in volume and concentration of Xylocaine Injection will decrease the onset of anesthesia, prolong the duration of anesthesia, provide a greater degree of muscular relaxation and increase the segmental spread of anesthesia. However, increasing the volume and concentration of Xylocaine Injection may result in a more profound fall in blood pressure when used in epidural anesthesia. Although the incidence of side effects with lidocaine is quite low, caution should be exercised when employing large volumes and concentrations, since the incidence of side effects is directly proportional to the total dose of local anesthetic agent injected.

For intravenous regional anesthesia, only the 50 mL single dose vial containing Xylocaine (lidocaine HCl) 0.5% Injection should be used.

Epidural Anesthesia

For epidural anesthesia, only the following dosage forms of Xylocaine Injection are recommended:

1% without epinephrine	30 mL ampules 30 mL single dose vials
1% with epinephrine 1:200,000	30 mL ampules 30 mL single dose vials
1.5% without epinephrine	20 mL ampules 20 mL single dose vials
1.5% with epinephrine 1:200,000	30 mL ampules 30 mL single dose vials
2% without epinephrine	10 mL ampules 10 mL single dose vials
2% with epinephrine 1:200,000	20 mL ampules 20 mL single dose vials

Although these solutions are intended specifically for epidural anesthesia, they may also be used for infiltration and peripheral nerve block, provided they are employed as single dose units. These solutions contain no bacteriostatic agent.

In epidural anesthesia, the dosage varies with the number of dermatomes to be anesthetized (generally 2-3 mL of the indicated concentration per dermatome).

Caudal and Lumbar Epidural Block: As a precaution against the adverse experience sometimes observed following unintentional penetration of the subarachnoid space, a test dose such as 2–3 mL of 1.5% lidocaine should be administered at least 5 minutes prior to injecting the total volume required for a lumbar or caudal epidural block. The test dose should be repeated if the patient is moved in a manner that may have displaced the catheter. Epinephine, if contained in the test dose, (10–15 μg have been suggested), may serve as a warning of unintentional intravascular injection. If injected into a blood vessel, this amount of epinephrine is likely to produce a transient "epinephrine response" within 45 seconds, consisting of an increase in heart rate and systolic blood pressure, circumoral pallor, palpitations and nervousness in the unsedated patient. The sedated patient may exhibit only a pulse rate increase of 20 or more beats per minute for 15 or more seconds. Patients on beta-blockers may not manifest changes in heart rate, but blood pressure monitoring can detect an evanescent rise in systolic blood pressure. Adequate time should be allowed for onset of anesthesia after administration of each test dose. The rapid injection of a large volume of Xylocaine Injection through the catheter should be avoided, and, when feasible, fractional doses should be administered.

In the event of the known injection of a large volume of local anesthetic solution into the subarachnoid space, after suitable resuscitation and if the catheter is in place, consider attempting the recovery of drug by draining a moderate amount of cerebrospinal fluid (such as 10 mL) through the epidural catheter.

MAXIMUM RECOMMENDED DOSAGES

Adults: For normal healthy adults, the individual maximum recommended dose of lidocaine HCl with epinephrine should not exceed 7 mg/kg (3.5 mg/lb) of body weight, and in general it is recommended that the maximum total dose not exceed 500 mg. When used without epinephrine, the maximum individual dose should not exceed 4.5 mg/kg (2 mg/lb) of body weight, and in general it is recommended that the maximum total dose does not exceed 300 mg. For continuous epidural or caudal anesthesia, the maximum recommended dosage should not be administered at intervals of less than 90 minutes. When continuous lumbar or caudal epidural anesthesia is used for non-obstetrical procedures. more drug may be administered if required to produce adequate anesthesia.

The maximum recommended dose per 90 minute period of lidocaine hydrochloride for paracervical block in obstetrical patients and non-obstetrical patients is 200 mg total. One half of the total dose is usually administered to each side. Inject slowly, five minutes between sides. (See also discussion of paracervical block in PRECAUTIONS.)

For intravenous regional anesthesia, the dose administered should not exceed 4 mg/kg in adults.

Children: It is difficult to recommend a maximum dose of any drug for children, since this varies as a function of age and weight. For children over 3 years of age who have a normal lean body mass and normal body development, the maximum dose is determined by the child's age and weight. For example, in a child of 5 years weighing 50 lbs the dose of lidocaine HCl should not exceed 75–100 mg (1.5–2 mg/lb). The use of even more dilute solutions (i.e., 0.25–0.5%) and total dosages not to exceed 3 mg/kg (1.4 mg/lb) are recommended for induction of intravenous regional anesthesia in children.

In order to guard against systemic toxicity, the lowest effective concentration and lowest effective dose should be used at all times. In some cases it will be necessary to dilute available concentrations with 0.9% sodium chloride injection in order to obtain the required final concentration.

NOTE: Parenteral drug products should be inspected visually for particulate matter and discoloration prior to administration whenever the solution and container permit. The injection is not to be used if its color is pinkish or darker than slightly yellow or if it contains a precipitate.

Table 1 Recommended Dosages

Procedure	Xylocaine (lidocaine hydrochloride) Injection (without epinephrine) Conc (%)	Vol (mL)	Total Dose (mg)
Infiltration			
Percutaneous	0.5 or 1	1–60	5–300
Intravenous regional	0.5	10–60	50–300
Peripheral Nerve Blocks, e.g.			
Brachial	1.5	15–20	225–300
Dental	2	1–5	20–100
Intercostal	1	3	30
Paravertebral	1	3–5	30–50
Pudendal (each side)	1	10	100
Paracervical			
Obstetrical analgesia (each side)	1	10	100
Sympathetic Nerve Blocks, e.g.			
Cervical (stellate ganglion)	1	5	50
Lumbar	1	5–10	50–100
Central Neural Blocks			
Epidural*			
Thoracic	1	20–30	200–300
Lumbar			
Analgesia	1	25–30	250–300
Anesthesia	1.5	15–20	225–300
	2	10–15	200–300
Caudal			
Obstetrical analgesia	1	20–30	200–300
Surgical anesthesia	1.5	15–20	225–300

* Dose determined by number of dermatomes to be anesthetized (2–3 mL/dermatome).

Xylocaine (lidocaine HCl) Concentration	Epinephrine Dilution (if present)	Xylocaine-MPF Ampules (mL) 2	5	10	20	30	Xylocaine-MPF Single Dose Vials (mL) 2	5	10	20	30	50	Xylocaine Multiple Dose Vials (mL) 10	20	50
0.5%												X			X
0.5%	1:200,000														X
1%		X	X			X	X	X	X		X		X	X	X
1%	1:100,000												X	X	X
1%	1:200,000					X		X	X		X				
1.5%					X				X	X					
1.5%	1:200,000		X			X		X	X		X				
2%		X		X			X	X	X				X	X	X
2%	1:100,000												X	X	X
2%	1:200,000				X			X	X	X					

All solutions should be stored at room temperature, approximately 25°C (77°F).

THE ABOVE SUGGESTED CONCENTRATIONS AND VOLUMES SERVE ONLY AS A GUIDE. OTHER VOLUMES AND CONCENTRATIONS MAY BE USED PROVIDED THE TOTAL MAXIMUM RECOMMENDED DOSE IS NOT EXCEEDED.

STERILIZATION, STORAGE AND TECHNICAL PROCEDURES: Disinfecting agents containing heavy metals, which cause release of respective ions (mercury, zinc, copper, etc.) should not be used for skin or mucous membrane disinfection as they have been related to incidents of swelling and edema. When chemical disinfection of multi-dose vials is desired, either isopropyl alcohol (91%) or ethyl alcohol (70%) is recommended. Many commercially available brands of rubbing alcohol, as well as solutions of ethyl alcohol not of U.S.P. grade, contain denaturants which are injurious to rubber and therefore are not to be used.

Dosage forms listed as Xylocaine-MPF indicate single dose solutions that are Methyl Paraben Free (MPF).

HOW SUPPLIED

[See table on bottom of preceding page.]

Protect from light.

021850R13   1/92 (13)

Shown in Product Identification Guide, page 304

XYLOCAINE®   ℞
[zī'lo-caine]
(lidocaine HCl Injection, USP)
FOR VENTRICULAR ARRHYTHMIAS

DESCRIPTION

Xylocaine (lidocaine HCl Injection, USP) is a sterile non pyrogenic solution of an antiarrhythmic agent administered intravenously by either direct injection or continuous infusion.

Xylocaine Injections are composed of aqueous solutions of lidocaine hydrochloride. Lidocaine HCl ($C_{14}H_{22}N_2O \cdot HCl$) is chemically designated acetamide, 2-(diethylamino)-N-(2, 6 dimethylphenyl)-, monohydrochloride.

(For details of indications, dosage and administration, precautions, and adverse reactions, see circular in package.)

HOW SUPPLIED

For direct intravenous injection, Xylocaine (lidocaine HCl Injection, USP) without preservatives is supplied in 5 mL, 50 mg and 100 mg Prefilled Syringes and in 5 mL, 100 mg Ampules.

For preparing solutions for intravenous infusions, Xylocaine, (lidocaine HCl Injection, USP) without sodium chloride or preservatives is supplied in one and two gram 25 and 50 mL Single Use Vials. Vials are available with or without presterilized transfer unit.

Solutions should be stored at controlled room temperature 15°-30°C (59°-86°F).

021679R02   8/95

4% XYLOCAINE®-MPF™ (lidocaine HCl)   ℞
[zī'lo-caine]
STERILE SOLUTION
   For transtracheal use,
   retrobulbar injection,
   and for topical application

DESCRIPTION

4% Xylocaine-MPF (lidocaine HCl) Sterile Solution (Methylparaben Free) contains a local anesthetic agent and is administered topically or by injection. See INDICATIONS for specific uses.

4% Xylocaine-MPF Sterile Solution contains lidocaine HCl, which is chemically designated as acetamide, 2-(diethylamino)-N-(2,6-dimethylphenyl)-monohydrochloride.

4% Xylocaine-MPF Sterile Solution in 5 mL ampules may be autoclaved repeatedly if necessary.

(For details of indications, dosage and administration, precautions, and adverse reactions, see circular in package.)

Composition of 4% Xylocaine-MPF Sterile Solution
Each mL contains lidocaine HCl, 40.0 mg, and sodium hydroxide and/or hydrochloric acid to adjust pH to 5.0–7.0. A sterile, aqueous solution.

HOW SUPPLIED

4% Xylocaine-MPF (lidocaine HCl) Sterile Solution, 5 mL ampule (NDC 0186-0235-03) and 5 mL prefilled sterile disposable syringe packaged in a presterilized kit containing a laryngotracheal cannula (NDC 0186-0235-72).
Store at controlled room temperature: 15°C–30°C (59°–86°F).
021562R07   8/90 (7)

XYLOCAINE® (lidocaine HCl)   ℞
[zī'lo-caine]
4% TOPICAL SOLUTION
For topical application

DESCRIPTION

Xylocaine (lidocaine HCl) 4% Topical Solution contains a local anesthetic agent and is administered topically. See INDICATIONS for specific uses.

Xylocaine 4% Topical Solution contains lidocaine HCl, which is chemically designated as acetamide, 2-(diethylamino)-N-(2,6-dimethylphenyl)-, monohydrochloride. The 50 ml screw-cap bottle should not be autoclaved, because the closure employed cannot withstand autoclaving temperatures and pressures. Composition of Xylocaine (lidocaine HCl) 4% Topical Solution: Each ml contains lidocaine HCl, 40 mg, methylparaben, and sodium hydroxide and/or hydrochloric acid to adjust pH to 6.0 - 7.0.
An aqueous solution. NOT FOR INJECTION

HOW SUPPLIED

Xylocaine (lidocaine HCl) 4% Topical Solution 50 ml screw-cap bottle, cartoned (NDC 0186-0320-01). NOT FOR INJECTION.
Store at controlled room temperature: 15°-30°C (59°-86°F).
021802R01   Rev. 7/84 (1)

1.5% XYLOCAINE®-MPF   ℞
with Dextrose 7.5%
(lidocaine HCl and dextrose Injection, USP)
   For Spinal Anesthesia
   in Obstetrics.

(For details of indications, dosage and administration, precautions, and adverse reactions, see circular in package.)

HOW SUPPLIED

Xylocaine-MPF 1.5% with Dextrose 7.5% (lidocaine HCl and dextrose Injection, USP), NDC 0186-0212-03, is supplied in 2 mL ampules in packages of 10.
Store at controlled room temperature 15°-30°C (59°-86°F).
021836R08   9/94(8)

5% XYLOCAINE®-MPF   ℞
[zī'lo-cain]
(lidocaine HCl and dextrose Injection, USP)
WITH GLUCOSE 7.5%

(For details of indications, dosage and administration, precautions, and adverse reactions, see circular in package.)

HOW SUPPLIED

Xylocaine-MPF 5% with Glucose 7.5% (lidocaine HCl and dextrose Injection, USP), NDC 0186-0225-03, is supplied in 2 mL ampules in packages of 10.
Store at controlled room temperature 15°-30°C (59°-86°F).
021564R12   Rev. 4/95

XYLOCAINE® 2% Jelly (lidocaine hydrochloride)   ℞
[zī'lo-caine]
A Topical Anesthetic
for Urological Procedures
and Lubrication
of Endotracheal Tubes

DESCRIPTION

Xylocaine (lidocaine HCl) 2% Jelly is a sterile aqueous product that contains a local anesthetic agent and is administered topically. (See INDICATIONS for specific uses.)

Xylocaine 2% Jelly contains lidocaine HCl which is chemically designated as acetamide, 2-(diethylamino)-N-(2,-6-dimethylphenyl)-, monohydrochloride.

Xylocaine 2% Jelly also contains hydroxypropylmethylcellulose, and the resulting mixture maximizes contact with mucosa and provides lubrication for instrumentation. The unused portion should be discarded after initial use. Composition of Xylocaine 2% Jelly: Each ml contains 20 mg of lidocaine HCl. The formulation also contains methylparaben, propylparaben, hydroxypropylmethylcellulose, and sodium hydroxide and/or hydrochloric acid to adjust pH to 6.0-7.0.
(For details of indications, dosage and administration, precautions, and adverse reactions, see circular in package.)

HOW SUPPLIED

Xylocaine (lidocaine HCl) 2% Jelly is supplied in the listed dosage forms. NDC 0186-0330-01, 30 mL aluminum tube, Box of 1.

A detachable applicator cone and a key for expressing the contents are included.
NDC 0186-0330-36 5 mL plastic tube, Box of 10

Store at controlled room temperature 15°-30°C (59°-86°F).
021838R14   Rev. 3/96
Shown in Product Identification Guide, page 304

5% XYLOCAINE®(lidocaine)   ℞
[zī'lo-caine]
Ointment
A Water-Soluble Topical Anesthetic Ointment

DESCRIPTION

Xylocaine (lidocaine) 5% Ointment contains a local anesthetic agent and is administered topically. See INDICATIONS for specific uses.

Xylocaine 5% Ointment contains lidocaine, which is chemically designated as acetamide, 2-(diethylamino)-N-(2,6-dimethylphenyl)-.

Composition of Xylocaine 5% Ointment
Each gram of the plain and flavored ointments contains lidocaine, 50 mg, polyethylene glycol 540 blend, polyethylene glycol 3350 and propylene glycol. The flavored ointment contains sodium saccharin, peppermint oil and spearmint oil.

(For details of indications, dosage and administration, precautions, and adverse reactions, see circular in package.)

HOW SUPPLIED

Xylocaine (lidocaine) 5% Ointment (NDC 0186-0315-21) is available in 35 gm tubes.

Xylocaine (lidocaine) 5% Ointment Flavored for application within the oral cavity, is dispensed in 3.5 gram tubes, 10 tubes per carton (NDC 0186-0350-03), and in 35-gram jars (NDC 0186-0350-01).
KEEP CONTAINER TIGHTLY CLOSED AT ALL TIMES WHEN NOT IN USE.
Store at controlled room temperature 15°-30°C (59°-86°F).
021709R13   1/94(13)

XYLOCAINE ® (lidocaine)   OTC
[zī'lo-cain]
2.5% OINTMENT

(See PDR For Nonprescription Drugs.)

XYLOCAINE® (lidocaine)   ℞
[zī'lo-caine]
10% Oral Spray
   Flavored Topical Anesthetic Aerosol
   For Use In The Oral Cavity

WARNING—CONTENTS UNDER PRESSURE

DESCRIPTION

Xylocaine (lidocaine) 10% Oral Spray contains a local anesthetic agent and is administered topically in the oral cavity. See INDICATIONS for specific uses.

Xylocaine 10% Oral Spray contains lidocaine, which is chemically designated as acetamide, 2-(diethylamino)-N-(2,6-dimethylphenyl)-.

Composition of Xylocaine (lidocaine) 10% Oral Spray:
Each actuation of the metered dose valve delivers a solution containing lidocaine, 10mg, cetylpyridinium chloride, absolute alcohol, saccharin, flavor, and polyethylene glycol.

And as propellants: trichlorofluoromethane/dichlorodifluoromethane (65%/35%).

WARNING

Contains trichlorofluoromethane and dichlorodifluoromethane, substances which harm public health and environment by destroying ozone in the upper atmosphere.
(For details of indications, dosage and administration, precautions, and adverse reactions, see circular in package.)

HOW SUPPLIED

NDC 0186-0356-01:   A 26.8 mL aerosol container provides a total amount of 3.3 g (w/w) of the active ingredient lidocaine. Each actuation of the metered dose valve delivers 10 mg of lidocaine.

Contents under pressure. Do not puncture or incinerate container. Do not expose to heat or store at temperatures above 120°F. Avoid contact with the eyes. Inhalation and swallowing should be avoided.

Keep out of the reach of children.

Use only as directed; intentional misuse by deliberately concentrating and inhaling the contents can be harmful or fatal.
STORE AT CONTROLLED ROOM TEMPERATURE 15°-30°C (59°-86°F).
Manufactured by Armstrong Laboratories, Inc., West Roxbury, MA 02132.

Continued on next page

Astra—Cont.

A flexible, disposable Cannula, 9035-05, is available in boxes of 50, to provide directed spray for easier access to oropharynx.
021731R31 11/93(31)

2% XYLOCAINE® Viscous (lidocaine hydrochloride) Solution ℞
[zī'lo-caine]
A Topical Anesthetic for the Mucous Membranes of the Mouth and Pharynx

DESCRIPTION
Xylocaine (lidocaine HCl) 2% Viscous Solution contains a local anesthetic agent and is administered topically. Xylocaine 2% Viscous Solution contains lidocaine HCl, which is chemically designated as acetamide, 2-(diethylamino)-N-(2,6-dimethylphenyl)-, monohydrochloride.
The molecular formula of lidocaine is $C_{14}H_{22}N_2O$. The molecular weight is 234.34.
(For details of indications, dosage and administration, precautions, and adverse reactions, see circular in package.)

HOW SUPPLIED
Xylocaine (lidocaine HCl) 2% Viscous Solution is available in 100 mL (NDC 0186-0360-01) and 450 mL (NDC 0186-0360-11) polyethylene squeeze bottles and in unit of use (adult dose) packages of 25 (20 mL) polyethylene bottles (NDC 0186-0361-78).
The solutions should be stored at controlled room temperature 15°–30°C (59°–86°F).
021899R02 4/94 (2)

YUTOPAR® ℞
(ritodrine hydrochloride) Injection

Caution: Federal law prohibits dispensing without prescription.

DESCRIPTION
Yutopar contains the betamimetic (beta sympathomimetic amine) ritodrine hydrochloride. Yutopar is a clear, colorless, sterile, aqueous solution; each milliliter contains either 10 mg or 15 mg of ritodrine hydrochloride, 4.35 mg of acetic acid, 2.4 mg of sodium hydroxide, 1 mg of sodium metabisulfite, and 2.9 mg of sodium chloride in Water for Injection, USP. Hydrochloric acid and/or additional sodium hydroxide is used to adjust pH. Filled under nitrogen.
FOR INTRAVENOUS USE ONLY. MUST BE DILUTED BEFORE USE. FOR DOSAGE AND ADMINISTRATION INSTRUCTIONS, SEE PRODUCT INFORMATION BELOW. DO NOT USE IF INJECTION IS DISCOLORED OR CONTAINS A PRECIPITATE.
Ritodrine hydrochloride is a white, odorless crystalline powder, freely soluble in water, with a melting point between 196° and 205°C. The chemical name of ritodrine hydrochloride is erythro-p-hydroxy-α-[1-[(p-hydroxyphenethyl)-amino]ethyl]benzyl alcohol hydrochloride and has the chemical structure:

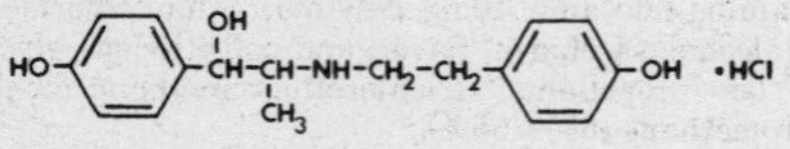

CLINICAL PHARMACOLOGY
Yutopar (ritodrine hydrochloride) is a beta-receptor agonist, which has been shown by *in vitro* and *in vivo* pharmacologic studies in animals to exert a preferential effect on the β_2 adrenergic receptors such as those in the uterine smooth muscle. Stimulation of the β_2 receptors inhibits contractility of the uterine smooth muscle.
In humans, intravenous infusions of 0.05 to 0.30 mg/min decreased the intensity and frequency of uterine contractions. These effects were antagonized by beta-blocking compounds. Intravenous administration induced an immediate dose-related elevation of heart rate with maximum mean increases between 19 and 40 beats per minute. Widening of the pulse pressure was also observed; the average increase in systolic blood pressure was 4.0 mm Hg, and the average decrease in diastolic pressure was 12.3 mm Hg.
During intravenous infusion in humans, transient elevations of blood glucose, insulin, and free fatty acids have been observed. Decreased serum potassium has also been found, but effects on other electrolytes have not been reported.
Serum kinetics in humans (non-pregnant females) of an intravenous infusion of 60 minutes duration were determined by measuring serum ritodrine levels by a radioimmunoassay technique. The distribution half-life was found to be 6 to 9 minutes, and the effective half-life 1.7 to 2.6 hours. Ninety percent of the excretion was completed within 24 hours after the dose.
Intravenous infusion at a rate of 0.15 mg/min for 1 hour yielded maximum serum levels ranging between 32 and 52 ng/mL in a group of 6 non-pregnant female volunteers.
Placental transfer was confirmed by measurement of drug concentrations in cord blood showing that ritodrine and its conjugates reach the fetal circulation.

INDICATIONS AND USAGE
Yutopar is indicated for the management of preterm labor in suitable patients.
Administered intravenously, the drug will decrease uterine activity and thus prolong gestation in the majority of such patients. Additional acute episodes may be treated by repeating the intravenous infusion. The incidence of neonatal mortality and respiratory distress syndrome increases when the normal gestation period is shortened.
Since successful inhibition of labor is more likely with early treatment, therapy with Yutopar should be instituted as soon as the diagnosis of preterm labor is established and contraindications ruled out in pregnancies of 20 or more weeks gestation. The efficacy and safety of Yutopar in advanced labor, that is, when cervical dilatation is more than 4 cm or effacement is more than 80%, have not been established.

CONTRAINDICATIONS
Yutopar is contraindicated before the 20th week of pregnancy.
Yutopar is also contraindicated in those conditions of the mother or fetus in which continuation of pregnancy is hazardous; specific contraindications include:
1. Antepartum hemorrhage which demands immediate delivery
2. Eclampsia and severe preeclampsia
3. Intrauterine fetal death
4. Chorioamnionitis
5. Maternal cardiac disease
6. Pulmonary hypertension
7. Maternal hyperthyroidism
8. Uncontrolled maternal diabetes mellitus (See PRECAUTIONS.)
9. Pre-existing maternal medical conditions that would be seriously affected by the known pharmacologic properties of a betamimetic drug; such as: hypovolemia, cardiac arrhythmias associated with tachycardia or digitalis intoxication, uncontrolled hypertension, pheochromocytoma, bronchial asthma already treated by betamimetics and/or steroids
10. Known hypersensitivity to any component of the product

WARNINGS

> Maternal pulmonary edema has been reported in patients treated with Yutopar, sometimes after delivery. It has occurred more often when patients were treated concomitantly with corticosteroids. Maternal death from this condition has been reported with or without corticosteroids given concomitantly with drugs of this class.
> Patients so treated must be closely monitored in the hospital. The patient's state of hydration should be carefully monitored; fluid overload must be avoided. (See DOSAGE AND ADMINISTRATION.) Intravenous fluid loading may be aggravated by the use of betamimetics with or without corticosteroids and may turn into manifest circulatory overloading with subsequent pulmonary edema. If pulmonary edema develops during administration, the drug should be discontinued. Edema should be managed by conventional means.

Intravenous administration of Yutopar should be supervised by persons having knowledge of the pharmacology of the drug and who are qualified to identify and manage complications of drug administration and pregnancy. Beta-adrenergic drugs increase cardiac output, and even in a normal healthy heart this added myocardial oxygen demand can sometimes lead to myocardial ischemia. Complications may include: myocardial necrosis, which may result in death; arrhythmias, including premature atrial and ventricular contractions, ventricular tachycardia, and bundle branch block; anginal pain, with or without ECG changes. Because cardiovascular responses are common and more pronounced during intravenous administration of Yutopar, cardiovascular effects, including maternal pulse rate and blood pressure and fetal heart rate, should be closely monitored. Care should be exercised for maternal signs and symptoms of pulmonary edema. A persistent high tachycardia (over 140 beats per minute) may be one of the signs of impending pulmonary edema with drugs of this class. Occult cardiac disease may be unmasked with the use of Yutopar. If the patient complains of chest pain or tightness of chest, the drug should be temporarily discontinued and an ECG should be done as soon as possible.
The drug should not be administered to patients with mild to moderate preeclampsia, hypertension, or diabetes unless the attending physician considers that the benefits clearly outweigh the risks.
Yutopar Injection contains sodium metabisulfite, a sulfite that may cause allergic-type reactions including anaphylactic symptoms and life-threatening or less severe asthmatic episodes in certain susceptible people. The overall prevalence of sulfite sensitivity in the general population is unknown and probably low. Sulfite sensitivity is seen more frequently in asthmatic than in nonasthmatic people.

PRECAUTIONS
When Yutopar is used for the management of preterm labor in a patient with premature rupture of the membranes, the benefits of delaying delivery should be balanced against the potential risks of development of chorioamnionitis.
Among low birth weight infants, approximately 9% may be growth retarded for gestational age. Therefore, Intra-Uterine Growth Retardation (IUGR) should be considered in the differential diagnosis of preterm labor; this is especially important when the gestational age is in doubt. The decision to continue or reinitiate the administration of Yutopar will depend on an assessment of fetal maturity. In addition to clinical parameters, other studies, such as sonography or amniocentesis, may be helpful in establishing the state of fetal maturity if it is in doubt.
Baseline EKG
This should be done to rule out occult maternal heart disease.
Laboratory Tests
Because intravenous administration of Yutopar has been shown to elevate plasma insulin and glucose and to decrease plasma potassium concentrations, monitoring of glucose and electrolyte levels is recommended during protracted infusions. Decrease of plasma potassium concentrations is usually transient, returning to normal within 24 hours. Special attention should be paid to biochemical variables when treating diabetic patients or those receiving potassium-depleting diuretics.
Serial hemograms may be helpful as an index of state of hydration.
Drug Interactions
Corticosteroids used concomitantly may lead to pulmonary edema. (See WARNINGS.)
Cardiovascular effects of Yutopar Injection (especially cardiac arrhythmia or hypotension) may be potentiated by concomitant use of the following drugs:
1. magnesium sulfate
2. diazoxide
3. meperidine
4. potent general anesthetic agents
Systemic hypertension may be exaggerated in the presence of parasympatholytic agents such as atropine.
The effects of other sympathomimetic amines may be potentiated when concurrently administered and these effects may be additive. A sufficient time interval should elapse prior to administration of another sympathomimetic drug.
With intravenous administration, 90% of the excretion of Yutopar is completed within 24 hours after the dose. (See CLINICAL PHARMACOLOGY.)
Beta-adrenergic blocking drugs inhibit the action of Yutopar, coadministration of these drugs should, therefore, be avoided.
With anesthetics used in surgery, the possibility that hypotensive effects may be potentiated should be considered.
Migraine Headache
Transient cerebral ischemia associated with beta sympathomimetic therapy has been reported in two patients with migraine headache.
Carcinogenesis, Mutagenesis, Impairment of Fertility
In rats given oral doses of 1, 10, and 150 mg/kg/day of ritodrine hydrochloride for 82 weeks, benign and malignant tumors were found in the various dosage groups. Since there were no important differences between untreated controls and treated groups and no dose-related trends, it was concluded that there was no evidence of tumorigenicity. The incidence (2–4%) of tumors of the type found in this study is not unusual in this species.
Reproduction studies in rats and rabbits have revealed no evidence of impaired fertility due to ritodrine hydrochloride.
Pregnancy
Teratogenic Effects
(Pregnancy Category B)
Reproduction studies were performed in rats and rabbits. The doses employed intravenously were $^1/_9$ (1 mg/kg), $^1/_3$ (3 mg/kg), and 1 (9 mg/kg) times the maximum human daily intravenous dose (but given to the animals as a bolus rather than by infusion). The oral doses, 10 and 100 mg/kg represented 5 and 50 times the maximum human daily oral maintenance dose. The results of these studies have revealed no evidence of impaired fertility or harm to the fetus due to ritodrine hydrochloride.
No adverse fetal effects were encountered when single intravenous doses of 1, 3, and 9 mg/kg/day or oral doses of 10 and 100 mg/kg/day were given to rats and rabbits on Days 6

through 15 and 6 through 18 of gestation, respectively. Intravenous doses of 1 and 8 mg/kg/day or oral doses of 10 and 100 mg/kg/day administered to the mother from Day 15 of pregnancy to Day 21 postpartum did not affect perinatal or postnatal development in rats. A slight increase in fetal weight in the rat was observed. Oral administration to both sexes did not impair fertility or reproductive performance. Lethal doses to pregnant rats did not cause immediate fetal demise. There are no adequate and well-controlled studies of Yutopar effects in pregnant women before 20 weeks gestation; therefore, this drug should not be used before the 20th week of pregnancy. Studies of Yutopar administered to pregnant women from the 20th week of gestation have not shown increased risk of fetal abnormalities. Follow-up of selected variables in a small number of children for up to 2 years has not revealed harmful effects on growth, developmental or functional maturation. Nonetheless, although clinical studies did not demonstrate a risk of permanent adverse fetal effects from Yutopar, the possibility cannot be excluded; therefore, Yutopar should be used only when clearly indicated.

Some studies indicate that infants born before 36 weeks gestation make up less than 10% of all births but account for as many as 75% of perinatal deaths and one-half of all neurologically handicapped infants. There are data available indicating that infants born at any time prior to full term may manifest a higher incidence of neurologic or other handicaps than occurs in the total population of infants born at or after full term. In delaying or preventing preterm labor, the use of Yutopar should result in an overall increase in neonatal survival. Handicapped infants who might not have otherwise survived may survive.

ADVERSE REACTIONS
The unwanted effects of Yutopar are related to its betamimetic activity and usually are controlled by suitable dosage adjustment.

Effects Associated with Intravenous Administration
Usual Effects (80–100% of patients)
Intravenous infusion of Yutopar leads almost invariably to dose-related alterations in maternal and fetal heart rates and in maternal blood pressure. During clinical studies in which the maximum infusion rate was limited to 0.35 mg/min (one patient received 0.40 mg/min), the maximum maternal and fetal heart rates averaged, respectively, 130 (range 60 to 180) and 164 (range 130 to 200) beats per minute. The maximum maternal systolic blood pressures averaged 128 mm Hg (range 96 to 162 mm Hg), an average increase of 12 mm Hg from pretreatment levels. The minimum maternal diastolic blood pressures averaged 48 mm Hg (range 0 to 76 mm Hg), an average decrease of 23 mm Hg from pretreatment levels. While the more severe effects were usually managed effectively by dosage adjustments, in less than 1% of patients, persistent maternal tachycardia or decreased diastolic blood pressure required withdrawal of the drug. A persistent high tachycardia (over 140 beats per minute) may be one of the signs of impending pulmonary edema. (See WARNINGS.)
Yutopar infusion is associated with transient elevation of blood glucose and insulin, which decreases toward normal values after 48 to 72 hours despite continued infusion. Elevation of free fatty acids and cAMP has been reported. Reduction of potassium levels should be expected; other biochemical effects have not been reported.
Frequent Effects (10–50% of patients)
Intravenous Yutopar, in about one-third of the patients, was associated with palpitation. Tremor, nausea, vomiting, headache, or erythema was observed in 10 to 15% of patients.
Occasional Effects (5–10% of patients)
Nervousness, jitteriness, restlessness, emotional upset, or anxiety was reported in 5 to 6% of patients and malaise in similar numbers.
Infrequent Effects (1–3% of patients)
Cardiac symptoms including chest pain or tightness (rarely associated with abnormalities of ECG) and arrhythmia were reported in 1 to 2% of patients. (See WARNINGS.)
Other infrequently reported maternal effects included: anaphylactic shock, rash, heart murmur, epigastric distress, ileus, bloating, constipation, diarrhea, dyspnea, hyperventilation, hemolytic icterus, glycosuria, lactic acidosis, sweating, chills, drowsiness, and weakness. Impaired liver function (i.e., increased transaminase levels and hepatitis) has also been reported infrequently (less than 1%) with the use of ritodrine and other beta sympathomimetics.
There have been cases of leukopenia and/or agranulocytosis reported in patients who have received Yutopar (ritodrine HCl) for management of preterm labor. These cases occurred in conjunction with intravenous infusion for 2 to 3 weeks or more. Leukocyte count spontaneously returned to normal after cessation of therapy in all patients. Some patients were also receiving indomethacin and magnesium sulfate as concomitant medication. At present, there has been no elucidation of the mechanism of this adverse event.
Neonatal Effects
Infrequently reported neonatal symptoms include hypoglycemia and ileus. In addition, hypocalcemia and hypotension

have been reported in neonates whose mothers were treated with other betamimetic agents.

OVERDOSAGE
The symptoms of overdosage are those of excessive beta-adrenergic stimulation including exaggeration of the known pharmacologic effects, the most prominent being tachycardia (maternal and fetal), palpitation, cardiac arrhythmia, hypotension, dyspnea, nervousness, tremor, nausea, and vomiting. When symptoms of overdose occur as a result of intravenous administration, ritodrine should be discontinued; an appropriate beta-blocking agent may be used as an antidote. Ritodrine hydrochloride is dialyzable.
Acute intravenous toxicity was studied in rats and rabbits and acute oral toxicity in mice, rats, guinea pigs, and dogs. The LD_{50} values in the most sensitive of the species used were 64 mg/kg intravenously in the nonpregnant rabbit and 540 mg/kg orally in the nonpregnant mouse. The intravenous LD_{50} value in the pregnant rat was 85 mg/kg. The amount of drug required to produce symptoms of overdose in humans is individually variable. No reports of human mortality due to overdose have been received.

DOSAGE AND ADMINISTRATION
The optimum dose of Yutopar is determined by a clinical balance of uterine response and unwanted effects.
Intravenous Therapy
Do not use intravenous Yutopar if the solution is discolored or contains any precipitate or particulate matter.
Yutopar Injection should be used promptly after preparation, but in no case after 48 hours of preparation.
Method of Administration: To minimize the risks of hypotension, the patient should be maintained in the left lateral position throughout infusion and careful attention given to her state of hydration, but fluid overload must be avoided. For appropriate control and dose titration, a controlled infusion device is recommended to adjust the rate of flow in drops/minute. An IV microdrip chamber (60 drops/mL) can provide a convenient range of infusion rates within the recommended dose range for Yutopar.
Recommended Dilution: 150 mg ritodrine hydrochloride in 500 mL fluid yielding a final concentration of 0.3 mg/mL*. Ritodrine for intravenous infusion should be diluted with 5% w/v dextrose solution. Because of the increased probability of pulmonary edema, saline diluents such as:
—0.9% w/v sodium chloride solution
—compound sodium chloride solution (Ringer's solution)
—and Hartmann's solution, should be reserved for cases where dextrose solution is medically undesirable, e.g., diabetes mellitus.
* In those cases where fluid restriction is medically desirable, a more concentrated solution may be prepared.
Intravenous therapy should be started as soon as possible after diagnosis. The usual initial dose is 0.05 mg/minute (0.17 mL/min, 10 drops/min using a microdrip chamber at the recommended dilution), to be gradually increased by 0.05 mg/min (0.17 mL/min, 10 drops/min using a microdrip chamber at the recommended dilution) every 10 minutes until the desired result is obtained, or the maternal heart rate reaches 130 beats per minute. The effective dosage usually lies between 0.15 and 0.35 mg/minute (0.50 to 1.17 mL/min, 30–70 drops/min using a microdrip chamber at the recommended dilution).
Frequent monitoring of maternal uterine contractions, heart rate, and blood pressure, and of fetal heart rate is required, with dosage individually titrated according to response. If other drugs need to be given intravenously, the use of "piggyback" or other site of intravenous administration permits the continued independent control of the rate of infusion of the Yutopar.
The infusion should generally be continued for between 12 and 24 hours after uterine contractions cease. With the recommended dilution, the maximum volume of fluid that might be administered after 12 hours at the highest dose (0.35 mg/min) will be approximately 840 mL.
The amount of IV fluids administered and the rate of administration should be monitored to avoid circulatory fluid overload (over-hydration). (See PRECAUTIONS, Laboratory Tests.)
Recurrence of unwanted preterm labor may be treated with repeated infusion of Yutopar.

HOW SUPPLIED
NDC 0186-0569-13: 5 mL vial in boxes of 10. Each vial contains 50 mg (10 mg/mL) of ritodrine hydrochloride.
NDC 0186-0599-03: 5 mL ampules in boxes of 10. Each ampule contains 50 mg (10 mg/mL) of ritodrine hydrochloride.
NDC 0186-0597-12: 10 mL vial in box of 1. Each vial contains 150 mg (15 mg/mL) of ritodrine hydrochloride.
NDC 0186-0644-01: 10 mL syringe in box of 1. Each syringe contains 150 mg (15 mg/mL) of ritodrine hydrochloride.
Store at room temperature, preferably below 86°F (30°C). Protect from excessive heat.
021843R13   Rev. 4/95

Athena Neurosciences, Inc.
800 GATEWAY BOULEVARD
SOUTH SAN FRANCISCO, CA 94080

Direct Inquiries to:
Ken Greathouse
General Manager, Athena Rx Home Pharmacy
or,
Lloyd Glenn
Director of Marketing
(415) 877-0900
FAX: (415) 877-8370

For Medical Information Contact:
In Emergencies:
(800) 578-7977
FAX: (415) 877-8370

ATAMET™   ℞
CARBIDOPA AND LEVODOPA TABLETS, USP

DESCRIPTION
When Carbidopa and Levodopa Tablets are to be given to patients who are being treated with levodopa, levodopa must be discontinued at least eight hours before therapy with this combination product is started. In order to reduce adverse reactions, it is necessary to individualize therapy. See the WARNINGS and DOSAGE AND ADMINISTRATION sections before initiating therapy.
Carbidopa, an inhibitor of aromatic amino acid decarboxylation, is a white, crystalline compound, slightly soluble in water. It is designated chemically as (—)-L-α-hydrazino-α-methyl-β-(3, 4-dihydroxybenzene) propanoic acid monohydrate.
Tablet content is expressed in terms of anhydrous carbidopa which has a molecular weight of 226.23.
Levodopa, an aromatic amino acid, is a white, crystalline compound, slightly soluble in water. It is designated chemically as (—)-L-α-amino-β-(3,4-dihydroxybenzene) propanoic acid.
Carbidopa and Levodopa is supplied as tablets in two strengths:
Carbidopa and Levodopa Tablets 25 mg/100 mg, containing 25 mg of carbidopa and 100 mg of levodopa.
Carbidopa and Levodopa Tablets 25 mg/250 mg, containing 25 mg of carbidopa and 250 mg of levodopa.
Inactive ingredients are magnesium stearate, microcrystalline cellulose, pregelatinized starch, and corn starch. Carbidopa and Levodopa Tablets 25 mg/250 mg also contain FD&C Blue 2. Carbidopa and Levodopa Tablets 25 mg/100 mg contain D&C Yellow 10 and FD&C Yellow 6.

CLINICAL PHARMACOLOGY
Current evidence indicates that symptoms of Parkinson's disease are related to depletion of dopamine in the corpus striatum. Administration of dopamine is ineffective in the treatment of Parkinson's disease apparently because it does not cross the blood-brain barrier. However, levodopa, the metabolic precursor of dopamine, does cross the blood-brain barrier, and presumably is converted to dopamine in the basal ganglia. This is thought to be the mechanism whereby levodopa relieves symptoms of Parkinson's disease.
When levodopa is administered orally it is rapidly converted to dopamine in extracerebral tissues so that only a small portion of a given dose is transported unchanged to the central nervous system. For this reason, large doses of levodopa are required for adequate therapeutic effect and these may often be attended by nausea and other adverse reactions, some of which are attributable to dopamine formed in extracerebral tissues.
Since levodopa competes with certain amino acids, the absorption of levodopa may be impaired in some patients on a high protein diet.
Carbidopa inhibits decarboxylation of peripheral levodopa. It does not cross the blood-brain barrier and does not affect the metabolism of levodopa within the central nervous system.
Since its decarboxylase inhibiting activity is limited to extracerebral tissues, administration of carbidopa with levodopa makes more levodopa available for transport to the brain. In dogs, reduced formation of dopamine in extracerebral tissues, such as the heart, provides protection against the development of dopamine-induced cardiac arrhythmias. Clinical studies tend to support the hypothesis of a similar protective effect in humans although controlled data are too limited at the present time to draw firm conclusions.
Carbidopa reduces the amount of levodopa required by about 75 percent and, when administered with levodopa, increases both plasma levels and the plasma half-life of levodopa, and

Continued on next page

Athena Neurosciences—Cont.

decreases plasma and urinary dopamine and homovanillic acid.

In clinical pharmacologic studies, simultaneous administration of carbidopa and levodopa produced greater urinary excretion of levodopa in proportion to the excretion of dopamine than administration of the two drugs at separate times.

Pyridoxine hydrochloride (vitamin B_6), in oral doses of 10 mg to 25 mg, may reverse the effects of levodopa by increasing the rate of aromatic amino acid decarboxylation. Carbidopa inhibits this action of pyridoxine.

INDICATIONS AND USAGE

Carbidopa and levodopa tablets are indicated in the treatment of the symptoms of idiopathic Parkinson's disease (paralysis agitans), postencephalitic parkinsonism, and symptomatic parkinsonism which may follow injury to the nervous system by carbon monoxide intoxication and manganese intoxication. This product is indicated in these conditions to permit the administration of lower doses of levodopa with reduced nausea and vomiting, with more rapid dosage titration, with a somewhat smoother response, and with supplemental pyridoxine (vitamin B_6).

The incidence of levodopa-induced nausea and vomiting is less with this combination product than with levodopa. In many patients this reduction in nausea and vomiting will permit more rapid dosage titration.

In some patients a somewhat smoother antiparkinsonian effect results from therapy with carbidopa and levodopa than with levodopa. However, patients with markedly irregular ("on-off") responses to levodopa have not been shown to benefit from carbidopa and levodopa therapy.

Since carbidopa prevents the reversal of levodopa effects caused by pyridoxine, carbidopa and levodopa can be given to patients receiving supplemental pyridoxine (vitamin B_6).

Although the administration of carbidopa permits control of parkinsonism and Parkinson's disease with much lower doses of levodopa, there is no conclusive evidence at present that this is beneficial other than in reducing nausea and vomiting, permitting more rapid titration, and providing a somewhat smoother response to levodopa. *Carbidopa does not decrease adverse reactions due to central effects of levodopa. By permitting more levodopa to reach the brain, particularly when nausea and vomiting is not a dose-limiting factor, certain adverse CNS effects, e.g., dyskinesias, may occur at lower dosages and sooner during therapy with carbidopa and levodopa than with levodopa.*

Certain patients who responded poorly to levodopa have improved when carbidopa and levodopa was substituted. This is most likely due to decreased peripheral decarboxylation of levodopa which results from administration of carbidopa rather than to a primary effect of carbidopa on the nervous system. Carbidopa has not been shown to enhance the intrinsic efficacy of levodopa in parkinsonian syndromes. In considering whether to give this combination product to patients already on levodopa who have nausea and /or vomiting, the practitioner should be aware that, while many patients may be expected to improve, some do not. Since one cannot predict which patients are likely to improve, this can only be determined by a trial of therapy. It should be further noted that in controlled trials comparing carbidopa and levodopa with levodopa, about half of the patients with nausea and/or vomiting on levodopa improved spontaneously despite being retained on the same dose of levodopa during the controlled portion of the trial.

CONTRAINDICATIONS

Monoamine oxidase inhibitors and carbidopa and levodopa should not be given concomitantly. These inhibitors must be discontinued at least two weeks prior to initiating therapy with this combination product.

Carbidopa and levodopa is contraindicated in patients with known hypersensitivity to this drug, and in narrow angle glaucoma.

Because levodopa may activate a malignant melanoma, it should not be used in patients with suspicious, undiagnosed skin lesions or a history of melanoma.

WARNINGS

When patients are receiving levodopa, it must be discontinued at least eight hours before therapy with this combination product is started. Carbidopa and levodopa should be substituted at a dosage that will provide approximately 25 percent of the previous levodopa dosage (see DOSAGE AND ADMINISTRATION). Patients who are taking this combination product should be instructed not to take additional levodopa unless it is prescribed by the physician.

As with levodopa, the combination product may cause involuntary movements and mental disturbances. These reactions are thought to be due to increased brain dopamine following administration of levodopa. All patients should be observed carefully for the development of depression with concomitant suicidal tendencies. Patients with past or current psychoses should be treated with caution. *Because car-*

bidopa permits more levodopa to reach the brain and, thus, more dopamine to be formed, dyskinesias may occur at lower dosages and sooner with carbidopa and levodopa than with levodopa. The occurrence of dyskinesias may require dosage reduction.

Carbidopa and levodopa should be administered cautiously to patients with severe cardiovascular or pulmonary disease, bronchial asthma, renal, hepatic or endocrine disease.

Care should be exercised in administering the combination product, as with levodopa, to patients with a history of myocardial infarction who have residual atrial, nodal, or ventricular arrhythmias. In such patients, cardiac function should be monitored with particular care during the period of initial dosage adjustment, in a facility with provisions for intensive cardiac care.

As with levodopa there is a possibility of upper gastrointestinal hemorrhage in patients with a history of peptic ulcer.

A symptom complex resembling the neuroleptic malignant syndrome including muscular rigidity, elevated body temperature, mental changes, and increased serum creatine phosphokinase has been reported when antiparkinsonian agents were withdrawn abruptly. Therefore, patients should be observed carefully when the dosage of carbidopa and levodopa is reduced abruptly or discontinued, especially if the patient is receiving neuroleptics.

Usage in Pregnancy and Lactation: Although the effects of carbidopa and levodopa on human pregnancy and lactation are unknown, both levodopa and combinations of carbidopa and levodopa have caused visceral and skeletal malformations in rabbits. Use of carbidopa and levodopa in women of childbearing potential requires that the anticipated benefits of the drug be weighed against possible hazards to mother and child. This product should not be given to nursing mothers.

Usage in Children: The safety of carbidopa and levodopa in patients under 18 years of age has not been established.

PRECAUTIONS

As with levodopa, periodic evaluations of hepatic, hematopoietic, cardiovascular, and renal function are recommended during extended therapy.

Patients with chronic wide angle glaucoma may be treated cautiously with carbidopa and levodopa provided the intraocular pressure is well controlled and the patient is monitored carefully for changes in intraocular pressure during therapy.

Laboratory Tests

Abnormalities in laboratory tests may include elevations of liver function tests such as alkaline phosphatase, SGOT (AST), SGPT (ALT), lactic dehydrogenase, and bilirubin. Abnormalities in protein-bound iodine, blood urea nitrogen and positive Coombs test have also been reported. Commonly, levels of blood urea nitrogen, creatinine, and uric acid are lower during administration of this combination product than with levodopa.

Carbidopa and levodopa may cause a false-positive reaction for urinary ketone bodies when a test tape is used for determination of ketonuria. This reaction will not be altered by boiling the urine specimen. False-negative tests may result with the use of glucose-oxidase methods of testing for glucosuria.

Drug Interactions

Caution should be exercised when the following drugs are administered concomitantly with carbidopa and levodopa.

Symptomatic postural hypotension can occur when carbidopa and levodopa is added to the treatment of a patient receiving antihypertensive drugs. Therefore, when therapy with carbidopa and levodopa is started, dosage adjustment of the antihypertensive drug may be required. For patients receiving monoamine oxidase inhibitors, see CONTRAINDICATIONS.

There have been rare reports of adverse reactions, including hypertension and dyskinesia, resulting from the concomitant use of tricyclic antidepressants and carbidopa and levodopa.

Phenothiazines and butyrophenones may reduce the therapeutic effects of levodopa. In addition, the beneficial effects of levodopa in Parkinson's disease have been reported to be reversed by phenytoin and papaverine. Patients taking these drugs with carbidopa and levodopa should be carefully observed for loss of therapeutic response.

ADVERSE REACTIONS

The most common serious adverse reactions occurring with carbidopa and levodopa are choreiform, dystonic, and other involuntary movements. Other serious adverse reactions are mental changes including paranoid ideation and psychotic episodes, depression with or without development of suicidal tendencies, and dementia. Convulsions also have occurred; however, a causal relationship with carbidopa and levodopa has not been established.

A common but less serious effect is nausea.

Less frequent adverse reactions are cardiac irregularities and/or palpitation, orthostatic hypotensive episodes, bradykinetic episodes (the "on-off" phenomenon), anorexia, vomiting, and dizziness.

Rarely, gastrointestinal bleeding, development of duodenal ulcer, hypertension, phlebitis, hemolytic and nonhemolytic anemia, thrombocytopenia, leukopenia, and agranulocytosis have occurred.

Laboratory tests which have been reported to be abnormal are alkaline phosphatase, SGOT (AST), SGPT (ALT), lactic dehydrogenase, bilirubin, blood urea nitrogen, proteinbound iodine, and Coombs test.

Other adverse reactions that have been reported with levodopa are:

Nervous System: ataxia, numbness, increased hand tremor, muscle twitching, muscle cramps, blepharospasm (which may be taken as an early sign of excess dosage, consideration of dosage reduction may be made at this time), trismus, activation of latent Horner's syndrome.

Psychiatric: confusion, sleepiness, insomnia, nightmares, hallucinations, delusions, agitation, anxiety, euphoria.

Gastrointestinal: dry mouth, bitter taste, sialorrhea, dysphagia, bruxism, hiccups, abdominal pain and distress, constipation, diarrhea, flatulence, burning sensation of tongue.

Metabolic: weight gain or loss, edema.

Integumentary: malignant melanoma (see also CONTRAINDICATIONS), flushing, increased sweating, dark sweat, skin rash, loss of hair.

Genitourinary: urinary retention, urinary incontinence, dark urine, priapism.

Special Senses: diplopia, blurred vision, dilated pupils, oculogyric crises.

Miscellaneous: weakness, faintness, fatigue, headache, hoarseness, malaise, hot flashes, sense of stimulation, bizarre breathing patterns, neuroleptic malignant syndrome.

OVERDOSAGE

Management of acute overdosage with carbidopa and levodopa is basically the same as management of acute overdosage with levodopa; however, pyridoxine is not effective in reversing the actions of this product.

General supportive measures should be employed, along with immediate gastric lavage. Intravenous fluids should be administered judiciously and an adequate airway maintained. Electrocardiographic monitoring should be instituted and the patient carefully observed for the development of arrhythmias; if required, appropriate antiarrhythmic therapy should be given. The possibility that the patient may have taken other drugs as well as carbidopa and levopoda tablets should be taken into consideration. To date, no experience has been reported with dialysis; hence, its value in overdosage is not known.

DOSAGE AND ADMINISTRATION

The optimum daily dosage of carbidopa and levodopa must be determined by careful titration in each patient. Carbidopa and.levodopa tablets are available in a 1:4 ratio of carbidopa to levodopa (25 mg/100 mg) as well as 1:10 ratio (25 mg/250 mg and 10 mg/100 mg). Tablets of the two ratios may be given separately or combined as needed to provide the optimum dosage.

Studies show that peripheral dopa decarboxylase is saturated by carbidopa at approximately 70 to 100 mg a day. Patients receiving less than this amount of carbidopa are more likely to experience nausea and vomiting.

Usual Initial Dosage

Dosage is best initiated with one tablet of carbidopa and levodopa 25 mg/100 mg three times a day. This dosage schedule provides 75 mg of carbidopa per day. Dosage may be increased by one tablet every day or every other day, as necessary, until a dosage of eight tablets of carbidopa and levodopa 25 mg/100 mg a day is reached.

If carbidopa and levodopa 10 mg/100 mg is used, dosage may be initiated with one tablet three or four times a day. However, this will not provide an adequate amount of carbidopa for many patients. Dosage may be increased by one tablet every day or every other day until a total of eight tablets (2 tablets q.i.d.) is reached.

How to Transfer Patients from Levodopa

Levodopa must be discontinued at least eight hours before starting this combination product. A daily dosage of carbidopa and levodopa should be chosen that will provide approximately 25 percent of the previous levodopa dosage. Patients who are taking less than 1500 mg of levodopa a day should be started on one tablet of carbidopa and levodopa 25 mg/100 mg three or four times a day. The suggested starting dosage for most patients taking more than 1500 mg of levodopa is one tablet of carbidopa and levodopa 25 mg/250 mg three or four times a day.

Maintenance

Therapy should be individualized and adjusted according to the desired therapeutic response. At least 70 to 100 mg of carbidopa per day should be provided. When a greater proportion of carbidopa is required, one 25 mg/100 mg tablet may be substituted for each 10 mg/100 mg tablet. When more levodopa is required, each 25 mg/250 mg tablet should be substituted for a 25 mg/100 mg tablet or a 10 mg/100 mg tablet. If necessary, the dosage of carbidopa and levodopa 25 mg/250 mg may be increased by one-half or one tablet every day or every other day to a maximum of eight tablets a day.

Experience with total daily dosages of carbidopa greater than 200 mg is limited.

Because both therapeutic and adverse responses occur more rapidly with this combination product than with levodopa alone, patients should be monitored closely during the dose adjustment period. Specifically, involuntary movements will occur more rapidly with carbidopa and levodopa than with levodopa. The occurrence of involuntary movements may require dosage reduction. Blepharospasm may be a useful early sign of excess dosage in some patients.

Current evidence indicates that other standard drugs for Parkinson's disease (except levodopa) may be continued while carbidopa and levodopa is being administered, although their dosage may have to be adjusted.

If general anesthesia is required, carbidopa and levodopa may be continued as long as the patient is permitted to take fluids and medication by mouth. If therapy is interrupted temporarily, the usual daily dosage may be administered as soon as the patient is able to take oral medication.

HOW SUPPLIED

Carbidopa and Levodopa Tablets 25 mg/100 mg NDC 59075-585-10 are available in the following form:

Mottled yellow, round, scored tablets, engraved "4"."585" on the scored side, and packaged in bottles of 100.

Carbidopa and Levodopa Tablets 25 mg/250 mg NDC 59075-587-10 are available in the following form:

Mottled blue, round, scored tablets, engraved "4"-"587" on the scored side, and packaged in bottles of 100.

Store at controlled room temperature 15°–30°C (59°–86°F). PROTECT FROM LIGHT.

Dispense in a tight, light-resistant container as defined in the USP, with a child-resistant closure (as required).

CAUTION: Federal law prohibits dispensing without prescription.

Rev. B 4/92

Manufactured by:
TEVA PHARMACEUTICAL IND. LTD.
Jerusalem, 91010, Israel
Distributed by:
ATHENA NEUROSCIENCES, Inc.
South San Francisco, CA 94080
Shown in Product Identification Guide, page 304

ATRETOL®
[ă' trĕ-tŏl]
Carbamozepine Tablets, USP 200 mg   ℞

Before prescribing Carbamazpine, the physician should be thoroughly familiar with the details of this prescribing information, particularly regarding use with other drugs, especially those which accentuate toxicity potential.

DESCRIPTION
Carbamazepine is an anticonvulsant and specific analgesic for trigeminal neuralgia, available as tablets of 200 mg for oral administration. Its chemical name is 5H-dibenz (b,f)-azepine-5-carboxamide and the structural formula is

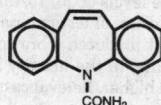

$C_{15}H_{12}N_2O$ M.W. 236.27

Carbamazepine USP is a white to off-white powder, practically insoluble in water and soluble in alcohol and in acetone.

Atretol® 200 mg tablets contain the inactive ingredients colloidal silicon dioxide, croscarmellose sodium, lactose, magnesium sterate, sodium starch glycolate and other ingredients.

CLINICAL PHARMACOLOGY
In controlled clinical trials, carbamazepine has been shown to be effective in the treatment of psychomotor and grand mal seizures, as well as trigeminal neuralgia.

It has demonstrated anticonvulsant properties in rats and mice with eletrically and chemically induced seizures. It appears to act by reducing polysynaptic responses and blocking the post-tetanic potentiation. Carbamazepine greatly reduces or abolishes pain induced by stimulation of the intraorbital nerve in cats and rats. It depresses thalamic potential and bulbar and polysynaptic reflexes, including the linguomandibular reflex in cats. Carbamazepine is chemically unrelated to other anticonvulsants or other drugs used to control the pain of trigeminal neuralgia. The mechanism of action remains unknown.

Atretol tablets are adequately absorbed after oral administration at a slower rate than a solution, thus avoiding undesirably high peak concentrations. Carbamazepine in blood is 76% bound to plasma proteins. Plasma levels of carbamazepine are variable and may range from 0.5–25 μg/mL, with no apparent relationship to the daily intake of the drug. Usual adult therapeutic levels are between 4 and 12 μg/mL. Following oral administration, serum levels peak at 4 to 5 hours. The CSF/serum ratio is 0.22, similar to the 22% unbound carbamazepine in serum. Because carbamazepine may induce its own metabolism, the half-life is also variable. Initial half-life values range from 25–65 hours, with 12–17 hours on repeated doses. Carbamazepine is metabolized in the liver. After oral administration of ^{14}C-carbamazepine, 72% of the administered radioactivity was found in the urine and 28% in the feces. This urinary radioactivity was composed largely of hydroxylated and conjugated metabolites, with only 3% of unchanged carbamazepine. Transplacental passage of carbamazepine is rapid (30 to 60 minutes), and the drug is accumulated in fetal tissues, with higher levels found in liver and kidney than in brain and in lungs.

INDICATIONS AND USAGE
Epilepsy: Atretol is indicated for use as an anticonvulsant drug. Evidence supporting efficacy or carbamazepine as an anticonvulsant was derived from active drug-controlled studies that enrolled patients with the following seizure types:
1. Partial seizures with complex symptomatology (psychomotor, temporal lobe). Patients with these seizures appear to show greater improvement than those with other types.
2. Generalized tonic-clonic seizures (grand mal).
3. Mixed seizure patterns which include the above, or other partial or generalized seizures.

Absence seizures (petit mal) do not appear to be controlled by carbamazepine (see PRECAUTIONS General).

Trigeminal Neuralgia—Atretol is indicated in the treatment of the pain associated with true trigeminal neuralgia.

Beneficial results have also been reported in glossopharyngeal neuralgia.

This drug is not a simple analgesic and should not be used for the relief of trivial aches or pains.

CONTRAINDICATIONS
Carbamazepine should not be used in patients with a history of previous bone marrow depression, hypersensitivity to the drug or known sensitivity to any of the tricyclic compounds, such as amitriptyline, desipramine, imipramine, protriptyline, nortriptyline, etc. Likewise, on theoretical grounds its use with monoamine oxidase inhibitors is not recommended. Before administration of carbamazepine, MAO inhibitors should be discontinued for a minimum of fourteen days, or longer if the clinical situation permits.

WARNINGS
Patients with a history of adverse hematologic reaction to any drug may be particularly at risk.

Severe dermatologic reactions including toxic epidermal necrolysis (Lyell's syndrome) and Stevens-Johnson syndrome, have been reported with carbamazepine. These reac-

tions have been extremely rare. However, a few fatalities have been reported.

Carbamazepine has shown mild anticholinergic activity; therefore, patients with increased intraocular pressure should be closely observed during therapy.

Because of the relationship of the drug to other tricyclic compounds, the possibility of activation of a latent psychosis and, in elderly patients, of confusion or agitation should be borne in mind.

PRECAUTIONS
General—Before initiating therapy, a detailed history and physical examination should be made.

Carbamazepine should be used with caution in patients with a mixed seizure disorder that includes atypical absence seizures, since in these patients carbamazepine has been associated with increased frequency of generalized convulsions (see INDICATIONS AND USAGE).

Therapy should be prescribed only after critical benefit-to-risk appraisal in patients with a history of cardiac, hepatic or renal damage, adverse hematologic reaction to other drugs, or interrupted courses of therapy with carbamazepine.

Information for Patients—Patients should be made aware of the early toxic signs and symptoms of a potential hematologic problem, such as fever, sore throat, ulcers in the mouth, easy bruising, petichial or purpuric hemorrhage, and should be advised to report to the physician immediately if any such signs or symptoms appear.

Since dizziness and drowsiness may occur, patients should be cautioned about the hazards of operating machinery or automobiles or engaging in other potentially dangerous tasks.

Laboratory Tests—Complete pretreatment blood counts, including platelets and possibly reticulocytes and serum iron, should be obtained as a baseline. If a patient in the course of treatment exhibits low or decreased white blood cell or plateley counts, the patient should be monitored closely. Discontinuation of the drug should be considered if any evidence of of significant bone marrow depression develops.

Baseline and periodic evaluations of liver function, particularly in patients with a history of liver disease, must be performed during treatment with this drug since liver damage may occur. The drug should be discontinued immediately in cases of aggravated liver dysfunction or active liver disease.

Baseline and periodic eye examinations, including slit-lamp, funduscopy and tonometry, are recommended since many phenothiazines and related drugs have been shown to cause eye changes.

Baseline and periodic complete urinalysis and BUN determinations are recommended for patients treated with this agent because of observed renal dysfunction.

Monitoring of blood levels (see CLINICAL PHARMACOLOGY) has increased the efficacy and safety of anticonvulsants. This monitoring may be particularly useful in cases of dramatic increase in seizure frequency and for verification of compliance. In addition, measurement of drug serum levels may aid in determining the cause of toxicity when more than one medication is being used.

Thyroid function tests have been reported to show decreased values with carbamazepine administered alone.

Hyponatremia has been reported in association with carbamazepine use, either alone or in combination with other drugs.

Drug Interactions—The simultaneous administration of phenobarbital, phenytoin, or primidone, or a combination of two, produces a marked lowering of serum levels of carbamazepine. The effect of valproic acid on carbamazepine blood levels is not clearly established, although an increase in the ratio of active 10, 11-epoxide metabolite to parent compound is a consistent finding.

The half-lives of phenytoin, warfarin, doxycycline, and theophylline were significantly shortened when administered concurrently with carbamazepine. Haloperidol and valproic acid serum levels may be reduced when the drug is administered with carbamazepine. The doses of these drugs may therefore have to be increased when carbamazepine is added to the therapeutic regimen.

Concomitant administration of carbamazepine with erythromycin, cimetidine, propoxyphene, isoniazid or calcium channel blockers has been reported to result in elevated plasma levels of carbamazepine resulting in toxicity in some cases. Also, concomitant administration of carbamazepine and lithium may increase the risk of neurotoxic side effects.

Alterations of thyroid function have been reported in combination therapy with other anticonvulsant medications.

Breakthrough bleeding has been reported among patients receiving concomitant oral contraceptives and their reliability may be adversely affected.

Carcinogenicity, Mutagenesis, Impairment of Fertility—Carbamazepine, when administered to Sprague-Dawley rats for two years in the diet at doses of 25, 75, and 250 mg/kg/day, resulted in a dose-related increase in the incidence of hepatocellular tumors in females and of benign interstitial cell adenomas in the testes of males.

Continued on next page

Athena Neurosciences—Cont.

Carbamazepine must, therefore, be considered to be carcinogenic in Sprague-Dawley rats. Bacterial and mammalian mutagenicity studies using carbamazepine produced negative results. The significance of these findings relative to the use of carbamazepine in humans is, at present, unknown.

Pregnancy Category C—Carbamazepine has been shown to have adverse effects in reproduction studies in rats when given orally in dosages 10–25 times the maximum human daily dosage of 1200 mg. In rat teratology studies, 2 of 135 offspring showed kinked ribs at 250 mg/kg and 4 of 119 offspring at 650 mg/kg showed other anomalies (cleft palate, 1; talipes, 1; anophthalmos, 2). In reproduction studies in rats, nursing offspring demonstrated a lack of weight gain and an unkempt appearance at a maternal dosage level of 200 mg/kg.

There are no adequate and well-controlled studies in pregnant women. Epidemiological data suggest that there may be an association between the use of carbamazepine during pregnancy and congenital malformations, including spina bifida. Carbamazepine should be used during pregnacy only if the potential benefit justifies the potential risk to the fetus.

Retrospective case reviews suggest that compared with monotherapy, there may be a higher prevalence of teratogenic effects associated with the use of anticonvulsants in combination therapy. Therefore, monotherapy is recommended for pregnant women.

It is important to note that anticonvulsant drugs should not be discontinued in patients in whom the drug is administered to prevent major seizures because of the strong possibility of precipitating status epilepticus with attendant hypoxia and threat to life. In individual cases where the severity and frequency of the seizure disorder are such that removal of medication does not pose a serious threat to the patient, discontinuation of the drug may be considered prior to and during pregnancy, although it cannot be said with any confidence that even minor seizures do not pose some hazard to the developing embryo or fetus.

Labor and Delivery—The effect of carbamazepine on human labor and delivery is unknown.

Nursing Mothers—During lactation, concentration of carbamazepine in milk is approximately 60% of the maternal plasma concentration.

Because of the potential for serious adverse reactions in nursing infants from carbamazepine, a decision should be made whether to discontinue nursing or to discontinue the drug, taking into account the importance of the drug to the mother.

Pediatric Use—Safety and effectiveness in children below the age of 6 years have not been established.

ADVERSE REACTIONS

If adverse reactions are of such severity that the drug must be discontinued, the physician must be aware that abrupt discontinuation of any anticonvulsant drug in a responsive epileptic patient may lead to seizures or even status epilepticus with its life-threatening hazards.

The most severe adverse reactions have been observed in the hemopoietic system (see boxed WARNING), the skin and the cardiovascular system.

The most frequently observed adverse reactions, particularly during the initial phases of therapy, are dizziness, drowsiness, unsteadiness, nausea, and vomiting. To minimize the possibility of such reactions, therapy should be initiated at the low dosage recommended.

The following additional adverse reactions have been reported:

Hemopoietic System—Aplastic anemia, agranulocytosis, pancytopenia, bone marrow depression, thrombocytopoenia, leukopenia, leukocytosis, eosinophilia, acute intermittent porphyria.

Skin—Pruritic and erythematous rashes, urticaria, toxic epidermal necrolysis (Lyell's syndrome) (see WARNINGS), Stevens-Johnson syndrome (see WARNINGS), photosensitivity reactions, alterations in skin pigmentation, exfoliative dermatitis, erythema multiforme and nodosum, purpura, aggravation of disseminated lupus erythematosus, alopecia, and diaphoresis. In certain cases, discontinuation of therapy may be necessary.

Cardiovascular System—Congestive heart failure, edema, aggravation of hypertension, hypotension, syncope and collapse, aggravation of coronary artery disease, arrhythmias and AV block, primary thrombophlebitis, recurrence of thrombophlebitis, and adenopathy or lymphadenopathy.

Some of these cardiovascular complications have resulted in fatalities. Myocardial infarction has been associated with other tricyclic compounds.

Liver—Abnormalities in liver function tests, cholestatic and hepatocellular jaundice, hepatitis.

Respiratory System—Pulmonary hypersensitivity characterized by fever, dyspnea, pneumonitis or pneumonia.

Genitourinary System—Urinary frequency, acute urinary retention, oliguria with elevated blood pressure, azotemia, renal failure, and impotence. Albuminuria, glycosuria, elevated BUN and microscopic deposits in the urine have also been reported.

Testicular atrophy occurred in rats receiving carbamazepine orally from 4 to 52 weeks at dosage levels of 50 to 400 mg/kg/day. Additionally, rats receiving carbamazepine in the diet for two years at dosage levels of 25, 75, and 250 mg/kg/day had a dose-related incidence of testicular atrophy and aspermatogenesis. In dogs, it produced a brownish discoloration, presumably a metabolite, in the urinary bladder at dosage levels of 50 mg/kg and higher. Relevance of these findings to humans is unknown.

Nervous System—Dizziness, drowsiness, disturbances of coordination, confusion, headache, fatigue, blurred vision, visual hallucinations, transient diplopia, oculomotor disturbances, nystagmus, speech disturbances, abnormal involuntary movements, peripheral neuritis and paresthesias, depression with agitation, talkativeness, tinnitus, and hyperacusis.

There have been reports of associated paralysis and other symptoms of cerebral arterial insufficiency, but the exact relationship of these reactions to the drug has not been established.

Digestive System—Nausea, vomiting, gastric distress and abdominal pain, diarrhea, constipation, anorexia, and dryness of the mouth and pharynx, including glossitis and stomatitis.

Eyes—Scattered, punctate, cortical lens opacities, as well as conjunctivitis have been reported. Although a direct casual relationship has not been established, many phenothiazines and related drugs have been shown to cause eye changes.

Musculoskeletal System—Aching joints and muscles, and leg cramps.

Metabolism—Fever and chills. Inappropriate antidiuretic hormone (ADH) secretion syndrome has been reported. Cases of frank water intoxication, with decreased serum sodium (hyponatremia) and confusion, have been reported in association with carbamazepine use (see PRECAUTIONS, Laboratory Tests).

Other—Isolated cases of a lupus erythematosus-like syndrome have been reported. There have been occasional reports of elevated levels of cholesterol, HDL cholesterol and triglycerides in patients taking anticonvulsants.

A case of aseptic meningitis, acccompanied by myoclonus and peripheral eosinophilia, has been reported in a patient taking carbamazepine in combination with other medications. The patient was successfully dechallenged, and the meningitis reappeared upon rechallenge with carbamazepine.

DRUG ABUSE AND DEPENDENCE

No evidence of abuse potential has been associated with carbamazepine, nor is there evidence of psychological or physical dependence in humans.

OVERDOSAGE

Acute toxicity—Lowest known lethal dose: adults > 60 g (39-year-old man). Highest known doses survived: adults, 30 g (31-year-old woman): children, 10 g (6-year-old boy) small children, 5 g (3-year-old girl).

Oral LD_{50} in animals (mg/kg): mice, 1100–3570; rats, 3850–4025; rabbits, 1500–2680; guinea pigs, 920.

Signs and Symptoms—The first signs and symptoms appear after 1–3 hours. Neuromuscular disturbances are the most prominent. Cardiovascular disorders are generally milder, and severe cardiac complications occur only when very high doses (> 60 g) have been ingested.

Respiration—Irregular breathing, respiratory depression.

Cardiovascular System—Tachycardia, hypertension or hypotension, shock, conduction disorders.

Nervous System and Muscles—Impairment of consciousness ranging in severity to deep coma. Convulsions, especially in small children. Motor restlessness, muscular twitching, tremor, athetoid movements, opisthotonos, ataxia, drowsiness, dizziness, mydriasis, nystagmus, adiadochokinesia, ballism, psychomotor disturbances, dysmetria. Initial hyperreflexia, followed by hyporeflexia.

Gastrointestinal Tract—Nausea, vomiting.

Kidneys and Bladder—Anuria or oliguria, urinary retention.

Laboratory Findings—Isolated instances of overdosage have included leukocytosis, reduced leukocyte count, glycosuria and acetonuria. EEG may show dysrhythmias.

Combined Poisoning—When alcohol, tricyclic antidepressants, barbiturates or hydantoins are taken at the same time, the signs and symptoms of acute poisoning with carbamazepine may be aggravated or modified.

Treatment—The prognosis in cases of severe poisoning is critically dependent upon prompt elimination of the drug, which may be achieved by inducing vomiting, irrigating the stomach and by taking appropriate steps to diminish absorption. If these measures cannot be implemented without risk on the spot, the patient should be transferred at once to a hospital, while ensuring that vital functions are safeguarded. There is no specific antidote.

Elimination of the Drug—Induction of vomiting.

Gastric lavage. Even when more than 4 hours have elapsed following ingestion of the drug, the stomach should be repeatedly irrigated, especially if the patient has also consumed alcohol.

Measures to Reduce Absorption—Activated charcoal, laxatives.

Measures to Accelerate Elimination—Forced duiresis.

Dialysis is indicated only in severe poisoning associated with renal failure. Replacement transfusion is indicated in severe poisoning in small children.

Respiratory Depression—Keep the airways free; resort, if necessary, to endotracheal intubation, artificial respiration, and administration of oxygen.

Hypotension, Shock—Keep the patient's legs raised and administer a plasma expander. If blood pressure fails to rise despite measures taken to increase plasma volume, use of vasoactive substances should be considered.

Convulsions—Diazepam or barbiturates.

Warning—Diazepam or barbiturates may aggravate respiratory depression (especially in children), hypotension, and coma. However, barbiturates should *not* be used if drugs that inhibit monoamine oxidase have also been taken by the patient either in overdosage or in recent therapy (within one week).

Surveillance—Respiration, cardiac function (ECG monitoring), blood pressure, body temperature, pupillary reflexes, and kidney and bladder function should be monitored for several days.

Treatment of Blood Count Abnormalities—If evidence of significant bone marrow depression develops, the following recommendations are suggested: (1) stop the drug, (2) perform daily CBC, platelet and reticulocyte counts, (3) do a bone marrow aspiration and trephine biopsy immediately and repeat with sufficient frequency to monitor recovery.

Specific periodic studies might be helpful as follows: (1) white cell and platelet antibodies, (2) ^{59}Fe-ferrokinetic studies, (3) peripheral blood cell typing, (4) cytogenetic studies on marrow and peripheral blood, (5) bone marrow culture studies for colony-forming units, (6) hemoglobin electrophoresis for A_2 and F hemoglobin, and (7) serum folic acid and B_{12} levels.

A fully developed aplastic anemia will require appropriate, intensive monitoring and therapy, for which specialized consultation should be sought.

DOSAGE AND ADMINISTRATION

Monitoring of blood levels has increased the efficacy and safety of anticonvulsants (see PRECAUTIONS Laboratory Tests). Dosage should be adjusted to the needs of the individual patient. A low initial daily dosage with a gradual increase is advised. As soon as adequate control is achieved, the dosage may be reduced very gradually to the minimum effective level. Tablets should be taken with meals.

Epilepsy (see INDICATIONS AND USAGE).

Adults and children over 12 years of age—Initial: 200 mg b.i.d. Increase at weekly intervals by adding up to 200 mg per day using a t.i.d. or q.i.d. regimen until the best response is obtained. Dosage should generally not exceed 1000 mg daily in children 12 to 15 years of age, and 1200 mg daily in patients above 15 years of age. Doses up to 1600 mg daily have been used in adults in rare instances. **Maintenance:** Adjust dosage to the minimum effective level, usually 800–1200 mg daily.

Children 6–12 years of age—Initital: 100 mg b.i.d. Increase at weekly intervals by adding 100 mg per day using a t.i.d. or q.i.d. regimen until the best response is obtained. Dosage should generally not exceed 1000 mg. **Maintenance:** Adjust dosage to the minimum effective level, usually 400–800 mg daily.

Combination Therapy: Atretol may be used alone or with other anticonvulsants. When added to existing anticonvulsant therapy, the drug should be added gradually while the other anticonvulsants are maintained or gradually decreased, except phenytoin, which may have to be increased, (see PRECAUTIONS, Drug Interactions and Pregnancy Category C).

Trigeminal Neuralgia (see INDICATIONS AND USAGE).

Initial: 100 mg b.i.d. on the first day for a total daily dose of 200 mg. This daily dose may be increased by up to 200 mg a day using increments of 100 mg every 12 hours only as needed to acheive freedom from pain. Do not exceed 1200 mg daily. **Maintenance:** Control of pain can be maintained in most patients with 400 mg to 800 mg daily. However, some patients may be maintained on as little as 200 mg daily, while others may require as much as 1200 mg daily. At least once every 3 months throughout the treatment period, attempts should be made to reduce the dose to the minimum effective level or even to discontinue the drug.

HOW SUPPLIED

Atretol® 200 mg (Carbamazepine Tablets, USP) is available in the following form:

Round, white, single-scored tablets, debossed "A"–"554" and are packaged in bottles of 100.
NDC 59075-554-10 (100's)
Store at controlled room temperature 15°–30°C (59°–86°F).
Protect from moisture. Store in a dry place.
Dispense in a tight container, preferably glass, as defined in the USP.
Dispense in a container labeled: Store in a dry place. Protect from moisture.
CAUTION: Federal law prohibits dispensing without prescription.

Rev. P 5/95

Manufactured by:
TEVA PHARMACEUTICAL IND. LTD.
Jerusalem, 91010, Israel
Distributed by:
ATHENA NEUROSCIENCES, INC.
South San Francisco, CA 94080

BROMOCRIPTINE MESYLATE ℞
TABLETS/CAPSULES, USP

DESCRIPTION
Bromocriptine mesylate is an ergot derivative with potent dopamine receptor agonist activity. Each bromocriptine mesylate tablet for oral administration contains $2^1/_2$ mg and each capsule contains 5 mg bromocriptine (as the mesylate). Bromocriptine mesylate is chemically designated as Ergotaman-3′, 6′, 18-trione, 2-bromo-12′-hydroxy-2′-(1-methylethyl)-5′-(2-methylpropyl)-, (5′α)-monomethanesulfonate (salt).
$2^1/_2$ mg Tablets
Active Ingredient: bromocriptine mesylate, USP
Inactive Ingredients: collodial silicon dioxide, lactose, magnesium stearate, povidone, starch, and another ingredient
5 mg Capsules
Active Ingredient: bromocriptine mesylate, USP
Inactive Ingredients: collodial silicon dioxide, gelatin, lactose, magnesium stearate, silicon dioxide, sodium lauryl sulfate, starch, titanium dioxide, and another ingredient

HOW SUPPLIED
Tablets, $2^1/_2$ mg
Round, white, scored tablets, each containing $2^1/_2$ mg bromocriptine (as the mesylate) in bottles of 100 (NDC 59075-590-10). Engraved "A" and "590" on one side and scored on reverse side.
Capsules, 5 mg
White capsules, each containing 5 mg bromocriptine (as the mesylate) in bottles of 100 (NDC 59075-591-10). Imprinted "A" on one half and "591" on other half.

Store And Dispense Below 77°F (25°C); tight, light-resistant container.
Manufactured by
Creighton Products Corporation
East Hanover, New Jersey 07936
Distributed by
Athena Neurosciences, Inc.
South San Francisco, CA 94080
Rev: March 1995

PERMAX® ℞
[pĕr′măks]
(pergolide mesylate)

DESCRIPTION
Permax® (Pergolide Mesylate) is an ergot derivative dopamine receptor agonist at both D_1 and D_2 receptor sites. Pergolide mesylate is chemically designated as 8β-[(Methylthio)methyl]-6-propylergoline monomethanesulfonate; the structural formula is as follows:

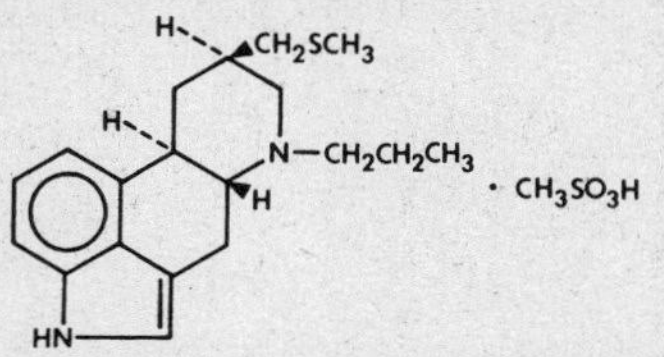

The formula weight of the base is 314.5; 1 mg of base corresponds to 3.18 μmol.
Permax is provided for oral administration in tablets containing 0.05 mg (0.159 μmol), 0.25 mg (0.795 μmol), or 1 mg (3.18 μmol) pergolide as the base. The tablets also contain croscarmellose sodium, iron oxide, lactose, magnesium stearate, and povidone. The 0.05-mg tablet also contains methionine, and the 0.25-mg tablet also contains F D & C Blue No. 2.

CLINICAL PHARMACOLOGY
Pharmacodynamic Information—Pergolide mesylate is a potent dopamine receptor agonist. Pergolide is 10 to 1,000 times more potent than bromocriptine on a milligram per milligram basis in various in vitro and in vivo test systems. Pergolide mesylate inhibits the secretion of prolactin in humans; it causes a transient rise in serum concentrations of growth hormone and a decrease in serum concentrations of luteinizing hormone. In Parkinson's disease, pergolide mesylate is believed to exert its therapeutic effect by directly stimulating postsynaptic dopamine receptors in the nigrostriatal system.
Pharmacokinetic Information (Absorption, Distribution, Metabolism, and Elimination)—Information on oral systemic bioavailability of pergolide mesylate is unavailable because of the lack of a sufficiently sensitive assay to detect the drug after the administration of a single dose. However, following oral administration of ^{14}C radiolabeled pergolide mesylate, approximately 55% of the administered radioactivity can be recovered from the urine and 5% from expired CO_2, suggesting that a significant fraction is absorbed. Nothing can be concluded about the extent of presystemic clearance, if any. Data on postabsorption distribution of pergolide are unavailable.
At least 10 metabolites have been detected, including N-despropylpergolide, pergolide sulfoxide, and pergolide sulfone. Pergolide sulfoxide and pergolide sulfone are dopamine agonists in animals. The other detected metabolites have not been identified, and it is not known whether any other metabolites are active pharmacologically.
The major route of excretion is the kidney.
Pergolide is approximately 90% bound to plasma proteins. This extent of protein binding may be important to consider when pergolide mesylate is coadministered with other drugs known to affect protein binding.

INDICATIONS AND USAGE
Permax is indicated as adjunctive treatment to levodopa/carbidopa in the management of the signs and symptoms of Parkinson's disease.
Evidence to support the efficacy of pergolide mesylate as an antiparkinsonian adjunct was obtained in a multicenter study enrolling 376 patients with mild to moderate Parkinson's disease who were intolerant to *l*-dopa/carbidopa as manifested by moderate to severe dyskinesia and/or on-off phenomena. On average, the patients evaluated had been on *l*-dopa/carbidopa for 3.9 years (range, 2 days to 16.8 years). The administration of pergolide mesylate permitted a 5% to 30% reduction in the daily dose of *l*-dopa. On average these patients treated with pergolide mesylate maintained an equivalent or better clinical status than they exhibited at baseline.

CONTRAINDICATIONS
Pergolide mesylate is contraindicated in patients who are hypersensitive to this drug or other ergot derivatives.

WARNINGS
Symptomatic Hypotension—In clinical trials, approximately 10% of patients taking pergolide mesylate with *l*-dopa versus 7% taking placebo with *l*-dopa experienced symptomatic orthostatic and/or sustained hypotension, especially during initial treatment. With gradual dosage titration, tolerance to the hypotension usually develops. It is therefore important to warn patients of the risk, to begin therapy with low doses, and to increase the dosage in carefully adjusted increments over a period of 3 to 4 weeks (*see* Dosage and Administration).
Hallucinosis—In controlled trials, pergolide mesylate with *l*-dopa caused hallucinosis in about 14% of patients as opposed to 3% taking placebo with *l*-dopa. This was of sufficient severity to cause discontinuation of treatment in about 3% of those enrolled; tolerance to this untoward effect was not observed.
Fatalities—In the placebo-controlled trial, 2 of 187 patients treated with placebo died as compared with 1 of 189 patients treated with pergolide mesylate. Of the 2,299 patients treated with pergolide mesylate in premarketing studies evaluated as of October 1988, 143 died while on the drug or shortly after discontinuing it. Because the patient population under evaluation was elderly, ill, and at high risk for death, it seems unlikely that pergolide mesylate played any role in these deaths, but the possibility that pergolide shortens survival of patients cannot be excluded with absolute certainty.
In particular, a case-by-case review of the clinical course of the patients who died failed to disclose any unique set of signs, symptoms, or laboratory results that would suggest that treatment with pergolide caused their deaths. Sixty-eight percent (68%) of the patients who died were 65 years of age or older. No death (other than a suicide) occurred within the first month of treatment; most of the patients who died had been on pergolide for years. A relative frequency of the causes of death by organ system are: Pulmonary failure/Pneumonia, 35%; Cardiovascular, 30%; Cancer, 11%; Unknown, 8.4%; Infection, 3.5%; Extrapyramidal syndrome, 3.5%; Stroke, 2.1%; Dysphagia, 2.1%; Injury, 1.4%; Suicide, 1.4%; Dehydration, 0.7%; Glomerulonephritis, 0.7%.

PRECAUTIONS
General—Caution should be exercised when administering pergolide mesylate to patients prone to cardiac dysrhythmias.
In a study comparing pergolide mesylate and placebo, patients taking pergolide mesylate were found to have significantly more episodes of atrial premature contractions (APCs) and sinus tachycardia.
The use of pergolide mesylate in patients on *l*-dopa may cause and/or exacerbate preexisting states of confusion and hallucinations (*see* Warnings) and preexisting dyskinesia. Also, the abrupt discontinuation of pergolide mesylate in patients receiving it chronically as an adjunct to *l*-dopa may precipitate the onset of hallucinations and confusion; these may occur within a span of several days. Discontinuation of pergolide should be undertaken gradually whenever possible, even if the patient is to remain on *l*-dopa.
A symptom complex resembling the neuroleptic malignant syndrome (NMS) (characterized by elevated temperature, muscular rigidity, altered consciousness, and autonomic instability), with no other obvious etiology, has been reported in association with rapid dose reduction, withdrawal of, or changes in antiparkinsonian therapy, including pergolide.
Information for Patients—Patients and their families should be informed of the common adverse consequences of the use of pergolide mesylate (*see* Adverse Reactions) and the risk of hypotension (*see* Warnings).
Patients should be advised to notify their physician if they become pregnant or intend to become pregnant during therapy.
Patients should be advised to notify their physician if they are breast-feeding an infant.
Laboratory Tests—No specific laboratory tests are deemed essential for the management of patients on Permax. Periodic routine evaluation of all patients, however, is appropriate.
Drug Interactions—Dopamine antagonists, such as the neuroleptics (phenothiazines, butyrophenones, thioxanthines) or metoclopramide, ordinarily should not be administered concurrently with Permax (a dopamine agonist); these agents may diminish the effectiveness of Permax.
Because pergolide mesylate is approximately 90% bound to plasma proteins, caution should be exercised if pergolide mesylate is coadministered with other drugs known to affect protein binding.
Carcinogenesis, Mutagenesis, and Impairment of Fertility—A 2-year carcinogenicity study was conducted in mice using dietary levels of pergolide mesylate equivalent to oral doses of 0.6, 3.7, and 36.4 mg/kg/day in males and 0.6, 4.4, and 40.8 mg/kg/day in females. A 2-year study in rats was conducted using dietary levels equivalent to oral doses of 0.04, 0.18, and 0.88 mg/kg/day in males and 0.05, 0.28, and 1.42 mg/kg/day in females. The highest doses tested in the mice and rats were approximately 340 and 12 times the maximum human oral dose administered in controlled clinical trials (6 mg/day equivalent to 0.12 mg/kg/day).
A low incidence of uterine neoplasms occurred in both rats and mice. Endometrial adenomas and carcinomas were observed in rats. Endometrial sarcomas were observed in mice. The occurrence of these neoplasms is probably attributable to the high estrogen/progesterone ratio that would occur in rodents as a result of the prolactin-inhibiting action of pergolide mesylate. The endocrine mechanisms believed to be involved in the rodents are not present in humans. However, even though there is no known correlation between uterine malignancies occurring in pergolide-treated rodents and human risk, there are no human data to substantiate this conclusion.
Pergolide mesylate was evaluated for mutagenic potential in a battery of tests that included an Ames bacterial mutation assay, a DNA repair assay in cultured rat hepatocytes, an in vitro mammalian cell-point-mutation assay in cultured L5178Y cells, and a determination of chromosome alteration in bone marrow cells of Chinese hamsters. A weak mutagenic response was noted in the mammalian cell-point-mutation assay only after metabolic activation with rat liver microsomes. No mutagenic effects were obtained in the 2 other in vitro assays and in the vivo assay. The relevance of these findings in humans is unknown.
A fertility study in male and female mice showed that fertility was maintained at 0.6 and 1.7 mg/kg/day but decreased at 5.6 mg/kg/day. Prolactin has been reported to be involved in stimulating and maintaining progesterone levels required for implantation in mice, and, therefore, the impaired fertility at the high dose may have occurred because of depressed prolactin levels.
Usage in Pregnancy—Pregnancy Category B—Reproduction studies were conducted in mice at doses of 5, 16, and 45 mg/kg/day and in rabbits at doses of 2, 6, and 16 mg/kg/day. The highest doses tested in mice and rabbits were 375 and 133 times the 6 mg/day maximum human dose administered in

Continued on next page

Athena Neurosciences—Cont.

controlled clinical trials. In these studies, there was no evidence of harm to the fetus due to pergolide mesylate. There are, however, no adequate and well-controlled studies in pregnant women. Among women who received pergolide mesylate for endocrine disorders in premarketing studies, there were 33 pregnancies that resulted in healthy babies and 6 pregnancies that resulted in congenital abnormalities (3 major, 3 minor); a causal relationship has not been established. Because human data are limited and because animal reproduction studies are not always predictive of human response, this drug should be used during pregnancy only if clearly needed.

Nursing Mothers—It is not known whether this drug is excreted in human milk. The pharmacologic action of pergolide mesylate suggests that it may interfere with lactation. Because many drugs are excreted in human milk and because of the potential for serious adverse reactions to pergolide mesylate in nursing infants, a decision should be made whether to discontinue nursing or to discontinue the drug, taking into account the importance of the drug to the mother.

Pediatric Use—Safety and effectiveness in children have not been established.

ADVERSE REACTIONS

Commonly Observed—In premarketing clinical trials, the most commonly observed adverse events associated with use of pergolide mesylate which were not seen at an equivalent incidence among placebo-treated patients were: nervous system complaints, including dyskinesia, hallucinations, somnolence, insomnia; digestive complaints, including nausea, constipation, diarrhea, dyspepsia; and respiratory system complaints, including rhinitis.

Associated With Discontinuation of Treatment—Twenty-seven percent (27%) of approximately 1,200 patients receiving pergolide mesylate for treatment of Parkinson's disease in premarketing clinical trials in the US and Canada discontinued treatment due to adverse reactions. The events most commonly causing discontinuation were related to the nervous system (15.5%), primarily hallucinations (7.8%) and confusion (1.8%).

Fatalities—See Warnings.

Incidence in Controlled Clinical Trials—The table that follows enumerates adverse events that occurred at a frequency of 1% or more among patients taking pergolide mesylate who participated in the premarketing controlled clinical trials comparing pergolide mesylate with placebo. In a double-blind, controlled study of 6 months' duration, patients with Parkinson's disease were continued on *l*-dopa/carbidopa and were randomly assigned to receive either pergolide mesylate or placebo as additional therapy.

The prescriber should be aware that these figures cannot be used to predict the incidence of side effects in the course of usual medical practice where patient characteristics and other factors differ from those which prevailed in the clinical trials. Similarly, the cited frequencies cannot be compared with figures obtained from other clinical investigations involving different treatments, uses, and investigators. The cited figures, however, do provide the prescribing physician with some basis for estimating the relative contribution of drug and nondrug factors to the side-effect incidence rate in the population studied.

[See table at right.]

Events Observed During the Premarketing Evaluation of Permax— This section reports event frequencies evaluated as of October 1988 for adverse events occurring in a group of approximately 1,800 patients who took multiple doses of pergolide mesylate. The conditions and duration of exposure to pergolide mesylate varied greatly, involving well-controlled studies as well as experience in open and uncontrolled clinical settings. In the absence of appropriate controls in some of the studies, a causal relationship between these events and treatment with pergolide mesylate cannot be determined. The following enumeration by organ system describes events in terms of their relative frequency of reporting in the data base. Events of major clinical importance are also described in the Warnings *and* Precautions sections.

The following definitions of frequency are used: frequent adverse events are defined as those occurring in at least 1/100 patients; infrequent adverse events are those occurring in 1/100 to 1/1,000 patients; rare events are those occurring in fewer than 1/1,000 patients.

Body as a Whole—*Frequent:* headache, asthenia, accidental injury, pain, abdominal pain, chest pain, back pain, flu syndrome, neck pain, fever; *Infrequent:* facial edema, chills, enlarged abdomen, malaise, neoplasm, hernia, pelvic pain, sepsis, cellulitis, moniliasis, abscess, jaw pain, hypothermia;

Incidence of Treatment-Emergent Adverse Experiences in the Placebo-Controlled Clinical Trial
Percentage of Patients Reporting Events

Body System/ Adverse Event*	Pergolide Mesylate N = 189	Placebo N = 187
Body as a Whole		
Pain	7.0	2.1
Abdominal pain	5.8	2.1
Injury, accident	5.8	7.0
Headache	5.3	6.4
Asthenia	4.2	4.8
Chest pain	3.7	2.1
Flu syndrome	3.2	2.1
Neck pain	2.7	1.6
Back pain	1.6	2.1
Surgical procedure	1.6	<1
Chills	1.1	0
Face edema	1.1	0
Infection	1.1	0
Cardiovascular		
Postural hypotension	9.0	7.0
Vasodilatation	3.2	<1
Palpitation	2.1	<1
Hypotension	2.1	<1
Syncope	2.1	1.1
Hypertension	1.6	1.1
Arrhythmia	1.1	<1
Myocardial infarction	1.1	<1
Digestive		
Nausea	24.3	12.8
Constipation	10.6	5.9
Diarrhea	6.4	2.7
Dyspepsia	6.4	2.1
Anorexia	4.8	2.7
Dry mouth	3.7	<1
Vomiting	2.7	1.6
Hemic and Lymphatic		
Anemia	1.1	<1
Metabolic and Nutritional		
Peripheral edema	7.4	4.3
Edema	1.6	0
Weight gain	1.6	0
Musculoskeletal		
Arthralgia	1.6	2.1
Bursitis	1.6	<1
Myalgia	1.1	<1
Twitching	1.1	0
Nervous System		
Dyskinesia	62.4	24.6
Dizziness	19.1	13.9
Hallucinations	13.8	3.2
Dystonia	11.6	8.0
Confusion	11.1	9.6
Somnolence	10.1	3.7
Insomnia	7.9	3.2
Anxiety	6.4	4.3
Tremor	4.2	7.5
Depression	3.2	5.4
Abnormal dreams	2.7	4.3
Personality disorder	2.1	<1
Psychosis	2.1	0
Abnormal gait	1.6	1.6
Akathisia	1.6	0
Extrapyramidal syndrome	1.6	1.1
Incoordination	1.6	<1
Paresthesia	1.6	3.2
Akinesia	1.1	1.1
Hypertonia	1.1	0
Neuralgia	1.1	<1
Speech disorder	1.1	1.6
Respiratory System		
Rhinitis	12.2	5.4
Dyspnea	4.8	1.1
Epistaxis	1.6	<1
Hiccup	1.1	0
Skin and Appendages		
Rash	3.2	2.1
Sweating	2.1	2.7
Special Senses		
Abnormal vision	5.8	5.4
Diplopia	2.1	0
Taste perversion	1.6	0
Eye disorder	1.1	0
Urogenital System		
Urinary frequency	2.7	6.4
Urinary tract infection	2.7	3.7
Hematuria	1.1	<1

*Events reported by at least 1% of patients receiving pergolide mesylate are included.

Rare: acute abdominal syndrome, LE syndrome
Cardiovascular System—*Frequent:* postural hypotension, syncope, hypertension, palpitations, vasodilatations, conges-

tive heart failure; *Infrequent:* myocardial infarction, tachycardia, heart arrest, abnormal electrocardiogram, angina pectoris, thrombophlebitis, bradycardia, ventricular ex-

trasystoles, cerebrovascular accident, ventricular tachycardia, cerebral ischemia, atrial fibrillation, varicose vein, pulmonary embolus, AV block, shock; *Rare:* vasculitis, pulmonary hypertension, pericarditis, migraine, heart block, cerebral hemorrhage

Digestive System—*Frequent:* nausea, vomiting, dyspepsia, diarrhea, constipation, dry mouth, dysphagia; *Infrequent:* flatulence, abnormal liver function tests, increased appetite, salivary gland enlargement, thirst, gastroenteritis, gastritis, periodontal abscess, intestinal obstruction, nausea and vomiting, gingivitis, esophagitis, cholelithiasis, tooth caries, hepatitis, stomach ulcer, melena, hepatomegaly, hematemesis, eructation; *Rare:* sialadenitis, peptic ulcer, pancreatitis, jaundice, glossitis, fecal incontinence, duodenitis, colitis, cholecystitis, aphthous stomatitis, esophageal ulcer

Endocrine System—*Infrequent:* hypothyroidism, adenoma, diabetes mellitus, ADH inappropriate; *Rare:* endocrine disorder, thyroid adenoma

Hemic and Lymphatic System—*Frequent:* anemia; *Infrequent:* leukopenia, lymphadenopathy, leukocytosis, thrombocytopenia, petechia, megaloblastic anemia, cyanosis; *Rare:* purpura, lymphocytosis, eosinophilia, thrombocythemia, acute lymphoblastic leukemia, polycythemia, splenomegaly

Metabolic and Nutritional System—*Frequent:* peripheral edema, weight loss, weight gain; *Infrequent:* dehydration, hypokalemia, hypoglycemia, iron deficiency anemia, hyperglycemia, gout, hypercholesteremia; *Rare:* electrolyte imbalance, cachexia, acidosis, hyperuricemia

Musculoskeletal System—*Frequent:* twitching, myalgia, arthralgia; *Infrequent:* bone pain, tenosynovitis, myositis, bone sarcoma, arthritis; *Rare:* osteoporosis, muscle atrophy, osteomyelitis

Nervous System—*Frequent:* dyskinesia, dizziness, hallucinations, confusion, somnolence, insomnia, dystonia, paresthesia, depression, anxiety, tremor, akinesia, extrapyramidal syndrome, abnormal gait, abnormal dreams, incoordination, psychosis, personality disorder, nervousness, choreoathetosis, amnesia, paranoid reaction, abnormal thinking; *Infrequent:* akathisia, neuropathy, neuralgia, hypertonia, delusions, convulsion, libido increased, euphoria, emotional lability, libido decreased, vertigo, myoclonus, coma, apathy, paralysis, neurosis, hyperkinesia, ataxia, acute brain syndrome, torticollis, meningitis, manic reaction, hypokinesia, hostility, agitation, hypotonia; *Rare:* stupor, neuritis, intracranial hypertension, hemiplegia, facial paralysis, brain edema, myelitis, hallucinations and confusion after abrupt discontinuation

Respiratory System—*Frequent:* rhinitis, dyspnea, pneumonia, pharyngitis, cough increased; *Infrequent:* epistaxis, hiccup, sinusitis, bronchitis, voice alteration, hemoptysis, asthma, lung edema, pleural effusion, laryngitis, emphysema, apnea, hyperventilation; *Rare:* pneumothorax, lung fibrosis, larynx edema, hypoxia, hypoventilation, hemothorax, carcinoma of lung

Skin and Appendages System—*Frequent:* sweating, rash; *Infrequent:* skin discoloration, pruritus, acne, skin ulcer, alopecia, dry skin, skin carcinoma, seborrhea, hirsutism, herpes simplex, eczema, fungal dermatitis, herpes zoster; *Rare:* vesiculobullous rash, subcutaneous nodule, skin nodule, skin benign neoplasm, lichenoid dermatitis

Special Senses System—*Frequent:* abnormal vision, diplopia; *Infrequent:* otitis media, conjunctivitis, tinnitus, deafness, taste perversion, ear pain, eye pain, glaucoma, eye hemorrhage, photophobia, visual field defect; *Rare:* blindness, cataract, retinal detachment, retinal vascular disorder

Urogenital System—*Frequent:* urinary tract infection, urinary frequency, urinary incontinence, hematuria, dysmenorrhea; *Infrequent:* dysuria, breast pain, menorrhagia, impotence, cystitis, urinary retention, abortion, vaginal hemorrhage, vaginitis, priapism, kidney calculus, fibrocystic breast, lactation, uterine hemorrhage, urolithiasis, salpingitis, pyuria, metrorrhagia, menopause, kidney failure, breast carcinoma, cervical carcinoma; *Rare:* amenorrhea, bladder carcinoma, breast engorgement, epididymitis, hypogonadism, leukorrhea, nephrosis, pyelonephritis, urethral pain, uricaciduria, withdrawal bleeding

Postintroduction Reports—Voluntary reports of adverse events temporally associated with pergolide that have been received since market introduction and which may have no causal relationship with the drug, include the following: neuroleptic malignant syndrome.

OVERDOSAGE

There is no clinical experience with massive overdosage. The largest overdose involved a young hospitalized adult patient who was not being treated with pergolide mesylate but who intentionally took 60 mg of the drug. He experienced vomiting, hypotension, and agitation. Another patient receiving a daily dosage of 7 mg of pergolide mesylate unintentionally took 19 mg/day for 3 days, after which his vital signs were normal but he experienced severe hallucinations. Within 36 hours of resumption of the prescribed dosage level, the hallucinations stopped. One patient unintentionally took 14 mg/day for 23 days instead of her prescribed 1.4 mg/day dosage. She experienced severe involuntary movements and tingling in her arms and legs. Another patient who inadvertently received 7 mg instead of the prescribed 0.7 mg experienced palpitations, hypotension, and ventricular extrasystoles. The highest total daily dose (prescribed for several patients with refractory Parkinson's disease) has exceeded 30 mg.

Symptoms—Animal studies indicate that the manifestations of overdosage in man might include nausea, vomiting, convulsions, decreased blood pressure, and CNS stimulation. The oral median lethal doses in mice and rats were 54 and 15 mg/kg respectively.

Treatment—To obtain up-to-date information about the treatment of overdose, a good resource is your certified Regional Poison Control Center. Telephone numbers of certified poison control centers are listed in the *Physicians' Desk Reference (PDR)*. In managing overdosage, consider the possibility of multiple drug overdoses, interaction among drugs, and unusual drug kinetics in your patient.

Management of overdosage may require supportive measures to maintain arterial blood pressure. Cardiac function should be monitored; an antiarrhythmic agent may be necessary. If signs of CNS stimulation are present, a phenothiazine or other butyrophenone neuroleptic agent may be indicated; the efficacy of such drugs in reversing the effects of overdose has not been assessed.

Protect the patient's airway and support ventilation and perfusion. Meticulously monitor and maintain, within acceptable limits, the patient's vital signs, blood gases, serum electrolytes, etc. Absorption of drugs from the gastrointestinal tract may be decreased by giving activated charcoal, which, in many cases, is more effective than emesis or lavage; consider charcoal instead of or in addition to gastric emptying. Repeated doses of charcoal over time may hasten elimination of some drugs that have been absorbed. Safeguard the patient's airway when employing gastric emptying or charcoal.

There is no experience with dialysis or hemoperfusion, and these procedures are unlikely to be of benefit.

DOSAGE AND ADMINISTRATION

Administration of Permax should be initiated with a daily dosage of 0.05 mg for the first 2 days. The dosage should then be gradually increased by 0.1 or 0.15 mg/day every third day over the next 12 days of therapy. The dosage may then be increased by 0.25 mg/day every third day until an optimal therapeutic dosage is achieved.

Permax is usually administered in divided doses 3 times per day. During dosage titration, the dosage of concurrent *l*-dopa/carbidopa may be cautiously decreased.

In clinical studies, the mean therapeutic daily dosage of Permax was 3 mg/day. The average concurrent daily dosage of *l*-dopa/carbidopa (expressed as *l*-dopa) was approximately 650 mg/day. The efficacy of Permax at doses above 5 mg/day has not been systematically evaluated.

HOW SUPPLIED

Tablets (scored):

0.05 mg, ivory, debossed with A615, (UC5336)—(RxPak* of 30) NDC 59075-615-30

0.25 mg, green, debossed with A625, (UC5337)—(RxPak of 100) NDC 59075-625-10

1 mg, pink, debossed with A630, (UC5338)—(RxPak of 100) NDC 59075-630-10

Store at controlled room temperature, 59° to 86°F (15° to 30°C).

*All RxPaks (prescription packages, Lilly) have safety closures.

Literature revised February 15, 1995

Manufactured by:
Eli Lilly & Co.
Indianapolis, IN 46285, USA

Distributed by:
Athena Neurosciences, Inc.
South San Francisco, CA 94080

Shown in Product Identification Guide, page 304

PV2274UCP

IDENTIFICATION PROBLEM?
Turn to the **Product Identification** Guide,
where you'll find more than
1600 products pictured in actual
size and full color.

Ayerst Laboratories
Division of American Home Products Corporation

See Wyeth-Ayerst Laboratories for prescription products and Whitehall-Robins for nonprescription products.

Baker Norton Pharmaceuticals, Inc.
4400 BISCAYNE BLVD.
MIAMI, FL 33137-3227

Direct Inquiries to:
(800) 347-4774
FAX: (305) 575-6298

For Medical Information Contact:
In Emergencies:
(305) 590-2254

Sales and Ordering:
(800) 735-2315
FAX: (305) 575-6444

BICITRA® ℞
[bye "si-trah]
(Brand of sodium citrate and citric acid oral solution, USP)

DESCRIPTION

BICITRA® is a stable and pleasant-tasting oral systemic alkalizer solution containing sodium citrate and citric acid in a sugar-free base. It is a nonparticulate neutralizing buffer.

BICITRA® contains in each teaspoonful (5 mL):

SODIUM CITRATE Dihydrate	500 mg (0.34 Molar)
CITRIC ACID Monohydrate	334 mg (0.32 Molar)

Each mL contains 1 mEq sodium ion and is equivalent to 1 mEq bicarbonate (HCO_3). BICITRA® also contains butylparaben, flavoring, maltitol, and sodium saccharin.

CLINICAL PHARMACOLOGY

Sodium citrate is absorbed and metabolized to sodium bicarbonate, thus acting as a systemic alkalizer. The effects are essentially those of chlorides before absorption and those of bicarbonates subsequently. Oxidation is virtually complete so that less than 5% of sodium citrate is excreted in the urine unchanged.

INDICATIONS AND USAGE

BICITRA® is an effective alkalinizing agent. It is useful in those conditions where long-term maintenance of an alkaline urine is desirable, and is of value in the alleviation of chronic metabolic acidosis, such as results from chronic renal insufficiency or the syndrome of renal tubular acidosis, especially when the administration of potassium salts is undesirable or contraindicated. BICITRA® is also useful for buffering and neutralizing gastric hydrochloric acid quickly and effectively.

BICITRA® is concentrated, and when administered after meals and before bedtime, allows one to maintain an alkaline urinary pH around the clock, usually without the necessity of a 2 A.M. dose. BICITRA® alkalinizes the urine without producing a systemic alkalosis in the recommended dosage. BICITRA® is highly palatable, pleasant tasting, and tolerable, even when administered for long periods. BICITRA® is sugar-free.

CONTRAINDICATIONS

Patients on sodium-restricted diets or with severe renal impairment. In certain situations, potassium citrate, as contained in POLYCITRA®-K, may be preferable.

PRECAUTIONS

Should be used with caution by patients with low urinary output unless under the supervision of a physician. BICITRA® should not be administered concurrently with aluminum-based antacids. Patients should be directed to dilute adequately with water and, preferably, to take each dose after meals to avoid saline laxative effect. Sodium salts should be used cautiously in patients with cardiac failure, hypertension, impaired renal function, peripheral and pulmonary edema, and toxemia of pregnancy. Periodic examinations and determinations of serum electrolytes, particularly serum bicarbonate level, should be carried out in those patients with renal disease in order to avoid these complications.

Continued on next page

Baker Norton—Cont.

ADVERSE REACTIONS

BICITRA® is generally well tolerated, without any unpleasant side effects, when given in recommended doses to patients with normal renal function and urinary output. However, as with any alkalinizing agent, caution must be used in certain patients with abnormal renal mechanisms to avoid development of alkalosis, especially in the presence of hypocalcemia.

OVERDOSAGE

Overdosage with sodium salts may cause diarrhea, nausea and vomiting, hypernoia, and convulsions.

DOSAGE AND ADMINISTRATION

BICITRA® should be taken diluted in water, followed by additional water, if desired. Palatability is enhanced if chilled before taking.

For Systemic Alkalization
Usual Adult Dose: 2 to 6 teaspoonfuls (10 to 30 mL), diluted in 1 to 3 ounces of water, after meals and at bedtime, or as directed by physician.
Usual Pediatric Dose: 1 to 3 teaspoonfuls (5 to 15 mL), diluted in 1 to 3 ounces of water, after meals and at bedtime, or as directed by physician. For children under two years of age, use is based on consultation with a physician.
As a Neutralizing Buffer: 3 teaspoonfuls (15 mL), diluted with 15 mL water, taken as a single dose, or as directed by physician.

HOW SUPPLIED

BICITRA®—is a grape flavored citrate solution supplied as:
16 fl oz. (473 mL) (NDC 0575-0225-01);
4 fl oz (118 mL) (NDC 0575-0225-04);
30 mL Unit Dose (NDC 0575-0225-30);
15 mL Unit Dose (NDC 0575-0225-15).
Keep tightly closed and protect from excessive heat or freezing.
CAUTION: Federal law prohibits dispensing without prescription.
Distributed by:
Baker Norton
Pharmaceuticals, Inc.
Miami, FL 33178-2404
Manufactured by:
H N Norton Co.
Schreveport, LA 71106-6506
L022557500
Rev. 9502   90642P

POLYCITRA® SYRUP   ℞
POLYCITRA®-LC   ℞
[polly "si-trah]
(tricitrates oral solution)

DESCRIPTION

Syrup POLYCITRA® and POLYCITRA®-LC are stable and pleasant tasting oral systemic alkalizers containing potassium citrate, sodium citrate, and citric acid. Syrup POLYCITRA® is a sugar-base preparation. POLYCITRA®-LC is a sugar-free solution, to be used by patients who desire a low-carbohydrate diet. Both products are nonalcoholic and contain identical amounts of active ingredients.

COMPOSITION

Syrup POLYCITRA® or POLYCITRA®-LC contains in each teaspoonful (5 mL):
POTASSIUM CITRATE Monohydrate .... 550 mg
SODIUM CITRATE Dihydrate .... 500 mg
CITRIC ACID Monohydrate .... 334 mg
Each mL contains 1 mEq potassium ion and 1 mEq sodium ion and is equivalent to 2 mEq bicarbonate (HCO_3).

ACTIONS

Potassium citrate and sodium citrate are absorbed and metabolized to potassium bicarbonate and sodium bicarbonate, thus acting as systemic alkalizers. The effects are essentially those of chlorides before absorption and those of bicarbonates subsequently. Oxidation is virtually complete so that less than 5% of the citrates are excreted in the urine unchanged.

INDICATIONS AND ADVANTAGES

Syrup POLYCITRA® and POLYCITRA®-LC are effective alkalinizing agents useful in those conditions where long-term maintenance of an alkaline urine is desirable, such as in patients with uric acid and cystine calculi of the urinary tract. In addition, they are valuable adjuvants when administered with uricosuric agents in gout therapy, since urates tend to crystallize out of an acid urine. They are also effective in correcting the acidosis of certain renal tubular disorders. Syrup POLYCITRA® and POLYCITRA®-LC are highly concentrated, and when administered after meals and before bedtime, allow one to maintain an alkaline urine pH

around the clock, usually without the necessity of a 2 A.M. dose. Syrup POLYCITRA® and POLYCITRA®-LC alkalinize the urine without producing a systemic alkalosis in recommended dosage. They are highly palatable, pleasant tasting, and tolerable, even when administered for long periods. Potassium citrate and sodium citrate do not neutralize the gastric juice or disturb digestion.

CONTRAINDICATIONS

Severe renal impairment with oliguria or azotemia, untreated Addison's disease, or severe myocardial damage. In certain situations, when patients are on a sodium-restricted diet, the use of potassium citrate, as contained in POLYCITRA®-K, may be preferable; or, when patients are on a potassium-restricted diet, the use of sodium citrate, as contained in BICITRA®, may be preferable.

PRECAUTIONS AND WARNINGS

Should be used with caution by patients with low urinary output or reduced glomerular filtration rates unless under the supervision of a physician. Aluminum-based antacids should be avoided in these patients. Patients should be directed to dilute adequately with water and, preferably, to take each dose after meals, to minimize the possibility of gastrointestinal injury associated with oral ingestion of potassium salt preparations and to avoid saline laxative effect. Sodium salts should be used cautiously in patients with cardiac failure, hypertension, peripheral and pulmonary edema, and toxemia of pregnancy.
Concurrent administration of potassium-containing medication, potassium-sparing diuretics, angiotensin-converting enzyme (ACE) inhibitors, or cardiac glycosides may lead to toxicity. Periodic examination and determinations of serum electrolytes, particularly serum bicarbonate level, should be carried out in those patients with renal disease in order to avoid these complications.

ADVERSE REACTIONS

Syrup POLYCITRA® and POLYCITRA®-LC, are generally well tolerated without any unpleasant side effects when given in recommended doses to patients with normal renal function and urinary output. However, as with any alkalinizing agent, caution must be used in certain patients with abnormal renal mechanisms to avoid development of hyperkalemia or alkalosis, especially in the presence of hypocalcemia. Potassium intoxication causes listlessness, weakness, mental confusion, and tingling of extremities.

DOSAGE AND ADMINISTRATION

Syrup POLYCITRA® and POLYCITRA®-LC should be taken diluted in water, followed by additional water if desired. Palatability is enhanced if chilled before taking.
Usual Adult Dose: 3 to 6 teaspoonfuls (15 to 30 mL), diluted in water, four times a day, after meals and at bedtime, or as directed by physician.
Usual Pediatric Dose: 1 to 3 teaspoonfuls (5 to 15 mL), diluted in water, four times a day, after meals and at bedtime, or as directed by physician.
Usual Dosage Range: 2 to 3 teaspoonfuls (10 to 15 mL), diluted with water, taken four times a day, will usually maintain a urine pH of 6.5–7.4. 3 to 4 teaspoonfuls (15 to 20 mL), diluted with water, taken four times a day, will usually maintain a urine pH of 7.0–7.6 throughout most of the 24 hours without unpleasant side effects. To check urine pH, HYDRION Paper (pH 6.0–8.0) or NITRAZINE Paper (pH 4.5–7.5) are available and easy to use.

OVERDOSAGE

Overdosage with sodium salts may cause diarrhea, nausea and vomiting, hypernoia, and convulsions. Overdosage with potassium salts may cause hyperkalemia and alkalosis, especially in the presence of renal disease.

HOW SUPPLIED

Syrup POLYCITRA®
16 fl oz (473 mL)
(NDC 0575-0223-01)
POLYCITRA®-LC
16 fl oz (473 mL)
(NDC 0575-0224-01)
Keep tightly closed and protect from excessive heat and freezing.
CAUTION: Federal law prohibits dispensing without prescription.
Distributed by:
Baker Norton
Pharmaceuticals, Inc.
Miami, FL 33178-2404
Manufactured by:
H N Norton Co
Schreveport, LA 71106-6506
I000431 Rev. 9412

POLYCITRA®-K CRYSTALS   ℞
[polly "si-trah- káy]
(Potassium Citrate and Citric
Acid for Oral Solution)

DESCRIPTION

POLYCITRA®-K CRYSTALS is a pleasant-tasting oral systemic alkalizer containing potassium citrate and citric acid in a sugar-free base.

COMPOSITION

POLYCITRA-K CRYSTALS® (potassium citrate and citric acid for oral solution—each unit dose packet contains:
POTASSIUM CITRATE
Monohydrate   3300 mg
CITRIC ACID
Monohydrate   1002 mg
Each unit dose packet, when reconstituted, supplies the same amount of active ingredients as is contained in 15 mL (one tablespoonful) POLYCITRA®-K Oral Solution and provides 30 mEq potassium ion and is equivalent to 30 mEq bicarbonate (HCO_3).

ACTIONS

Potassium citrate is absorbed and metabolized to potassium bicarbonate, thus acting as a systemic alkalizer. The effects are essentially those of chlorides before absorption and those of bicarbonates subsequently. Oxidation is virtually complete so that less than 5% of the potassium citrate is excreted in the urine unchanged.

INDICATIONS AND USAGE

POLYCITRA®-K CRYSTALS is an effective alkalinizing agent useful in those conditions where long-term maintenance of an alkaline urine is desirable, such as in patients with uric acid and cystine calculi of the urinary tract, especially when the administration of sodium salts is undesirable or contraindicated. In addition, it is a valuable adjuvant when administered with uricosuric agents in gout therapy, since urates tend to crystallize out of an acid urine. It is also effective in correcting the acidosis of certain renal tubular disorders where the administration of potassium citrate may be preferable. POLYCITRA®-K CRYSTALS is highly concentrated, and when administered after meals and before bedtime, allows one to maintain an alkaline urinary pH around the clock, usually without the necessity of a 2 A.M. dose. POLYCITRA®-K CRYSTALS alkalinizes the urine without producing a systemic alkalosis in recommended dosage. It is highly palatable, pleasant tasting, and tolerable even when administered for long periods. Potassium citrate does not neutralize the gastric juice or disturb digestion.

CONTRAINDICATIONS

Severe renal impairment with oliguria or azotemia, untreated Addison's disease, adynamia episodica hereditaria, acute dehydration, heat cramps, anuria, severe myocardial damage, and hyperkalemia from any cause.

WARNING

Large doses may cause hyperkalemia and alkalosis, especially in the presence of renal disease. Concurrent administration of potassium-containing medication, potassium-sparing diuretics, angiotensin-converting enzyme (ACE) inhibitors, or cardiac glycosides may lead to toxicity.

PRECAUTIONS

Should be used with caution by patients with low urinary output unless under the supervision of a physician. As with all liquids containing a high concentration of potassium, patients should be directed to dilute adequately with water to minimize the possibility of gastrointestinal injury associated with the oral ingestion of concentrated potassium salt preparations; and preferably, to take each dose after meals to avoid saline laxative effect.

ADVERSE REACTIONS

POLYCITRA-K CRYSTALS® is generally well tolerated without any unpleasant side effects when given in recommended doses to patients with normal renal function and urinary output. However, as with any alkalinizing agent, caution must be used in certain patients with abnormal renal mechanisms to avoid development of hyperkalemia or alkalosis. Potassium intoxication causes listlessness, weakness, mental confusion, tingling of extremities, and other symptoms associated with a high concentration of potassium in the serum. Periodic determinations of serum electrolytes should be carried out in those patients with renal disease in order to avoid these complications. Hyperkalemia may exhibit the following electrocardiographic abnormalities: Disappearance of the P wave, widening and slurring of QRS complex, changes of the S-T segment, tall peaked T waves, etc.

OVERDOSAGE

The administration of oral potassium salts to persons with normal excretory mechanisms for potassium rarely causes serious hyperkalemia. However, if excretory mechanisms are impaired, hyperkalemia can result (see Contraindications and Warnings). Hyperkalemia, when detected, must be

treated immediately because lethal levels can be reached in a few hours.

TREATMENT OF HYPERKALEMIA

Should hyperkalemia occur, treatment measures include the following: (1) Elimination of foods or medications containing potassium. (2) The intravenous administration of 300 to 500 mL/hr of dextrose solution (10 to 25%), containing 10 units of insulin/20 gm dextrose. (3) The use of exchange resins, hemodialysis, or peritoneal dialysis. In treating hyperkalemia, it should be recalled that in patients who have been stabilized on digitalis, too rapid a lowering of the plasma potassium concentration can produce digitalis toxicity.

DOSAGE AND ADMINISTRATION

POLYCITRA®-K CRYSTALS should be taken mixed in cool water or juice according to directions, followed by additional water, if desired.

Usual Adult Dose: POLYCITRA-K CRYSTALS®—Contents of 1 packet reconstituted with at least 6 ounces of cool water or juice, after meals and at bedtime, or as directed by physician.

Usual Pediatric Dose: POLYCITRA-K CRYSTALS® is not recommended for pediatric use. Dosage can be more easily regulated using POLYCITRA®-K Oral Solution.

Usual Dosage Range: Contents of 1 packet POLYCITRA-K CRYSTALS®, reconstituted as directed and taken four times a day, will usually maintain a urinary pH of 6.5–7.4. To check urinary pH, HYDRION Paper (pH 6.0–8.0) or NITRAZINE Paper (pH 4.5–7.5) are available and easy to use.

HOW SUPPLIED

POLYCITRA-K CRYSTALS®
—Unit Dose Packets, 100/box (NDC 0575-0221-01).
Protect from excessive heat or freezing.
CAUTION: Federal law prohibits dispensing without prescription.
POLYCITRA-K Crystals® is
Manufactured and Distributed by:
Baker Norton
Pharmaceuticals, Inc.
Miami, Florida 33178–2404
I001026   REV9502
©1995 Baker Norton Pharmaceuticals, Inc.

POLYCITRA®–K ORAL SOLUTION ℞
[polly" si-trah-ka' y]
(Potassium Citrate and Citric Acid Oral Solution, USP)

DESCRIPTION

POLYCITRA®–K is a stable and pleasant-tasting oral systemic alkalizer containing potassium citrate and citric acid in a sugar-free non-alcoholic base.

COMPOSITION

POLYCITRA®–K Oral Solution (potassium citrate and citric acid oral solution, USP) contains in each teaspoonful (5 mL):
POTASSIUM CITRATE Monohydrate .... 1100 mg
CITRIC ACID Monohydrate .... 334 mg
Each mL contains 2 mEq potassium ion and is equivalent to 2 mEq bicarbonate (HCO_3).

ACTIONS

Potassium citrate is absorbed and metabolized to potassium bicarbonate, thus acting as a systemic alkalizer. The effects are essentially those of chlorides before absorption and those of bicarbonates subsequently. Oxidation is virtually complete so that less than 5% of the potassium citrate is excreted in the urine unchanged.

INDICATIONS AND USAGE

POLYCITRA®–K Oral Solution is an effective alkalinizing agent useful in those conditions where long-term maintenance of an alkaline urine is desirable, such as in patients with uric acid and cystine calculi of the urinary tract, especially when the administration of sodium salts is undesirable or contraindicated. In addition, it is a valuable adjuvant when administered with uricosuric agents in gout therapy, since urates tend to crystallize out of an acid urine. It is also effective in correcting the acidosis of certain renal tubular disorders where the administration of potassium citrate may be preferable. POLYCITRA®–K Oral Solution is highly concentrated, and when administered after meals and before bedtime, allows one to maintain an alkaline urinary pH around the clock, usually without the necessity of a 2 A.M. dose. POLYCITRA®–K Oral Solution alkalinizes the urine without producing a systemic alkalosis in recommended dosage. It is highly palatable, pleasant tasting, and tolerable, even when administered for long periods. Potassium citrate does not neutralize the gastric juice or disturb digestion.

CONTRAINDICATIONS

Severe renal impairment with oliguria or azotemia, untreated Addison's disease, adynamia episodica hereditaria, acute dehydration, heat cramps, anuria, severe myocardial damage, and hyperkalemia from any cause.

WARNING

Large doses may cause hyperkalemia and alkalosis, especially in the presence of renal disease. Concurrent administration of potassium-containing medication, potassium-sparing diuretics, angiotensin-converting enzyme (ACE) inhibitors, or cardiac glycosides may lead to toxicity.

PRECAUTIONS

Should be used with caution by patients with low urinary output unless under the supervision of a physician. As with all liquids containing a high concentration of potassium, patients should be directed to dilute adequately with water to minimize the possibility of gastrointestinal injury associated with the oral ingestion of concentrated potassium salt preparations; and preferably, to take each dose after meals to avoid saline laxative effect.

ADVERSE REACTIONS

POLYCITRA®–K Oral Solution is generally well tolerated without any unpleasant side effects when given in recommended doses to patients with normal renal function and urinary output. However, as with any alkalinizing agent, caution must be used in certain patients with abnormal renal mechanisms to avoid development of hyperkalemia or alkalosis. Potassium intoxication causes listlessness, weakness, mental confusion, tingling of extremities, and other symptoms associated with a high concentration of potassium in the serum. Periodic determinations of serum electrolytes should be carried out in those patients with renal disease in order to avoid these complications. Hyperkalemia may exhibit the following electrocardiographic abnormalities. Disappearance of the P wave, widening and slurring of QRS complex, changes of the S-T segment, tall peaked T waves, etc.

OVERDOSAGE

The administration of oral potassium salts to persons with normal excretory mechanisms for potassium rarely causes serious hyperkalemia. However, if excretory mechanisms are impaired, hyperkalemia can result (see Contraindications and Warnings). Hyperkalemia, when detected, must be treated immediately because lethal levels can be reached in a few hours.

TREATMENT OF HYPERKALEMIA

Should hyperkalemia occur, treatment measures include the following: (1) Elimination of foods or medications containing potassium. (2) The intravenous administration of 300 to 500 mL/hr of dextrose solution (10 to 25%), containing 10 units of insulin/20 gm dextrose. (3) The use of exchange resins, hemodialysis, or peritoneal dialysis. In treating hyperkalemia, it should be recalled that in patients who have been stabilized on digitalis, too rapid a lowering of the plasma potassium concentration can produce digitalis toxicity.

DOSAGE AND ADMINISTRATION

POLYCITRA®–K Oral Solution should be taken diluted in water according to directions, followed by additional water, if desired. Palatability is enhanced if chilled before taking.
Usual Adult Dose: POLYCITRA®–K Oral Solution—3 to 6 teaspoonfuls (15 to 30 mL), diluted with 1 glass of water, after meals and at bedtime, or as directed by physician.
Usual Pediatric Dose: POLYCITRA®–K Oral Solution—1 to 3 teaspoonfuls (5 to 15 mL), diluted with ½ glass of water, after meals and at bedtime, or as directed by physician.
Usual Dosage Range: 2 to 3 teaspoonfuls (10 to 15 mL) POLYCITRA®–K Oral Solution, diluted with a glassful of water, taken four times a day. POLYCITRA®–K Oral Solution, diluted with a glassful of water, taken four times a day, will usually maintain a urinary pH of 7.0–7.6 throughout most of the 24 hours without unpleasant side effects. To check urinary pH, HYDRION Paper (pH 6.0–8.0) or NITRAZINE Paper (pH 4.5–7.5) are available and easy to use.

HOW SUPPLIED

POLYCITRA®–K ORAL SOLUTION—16 fl oz (473 mL) (NDC 0575-0222-01).
Keep tightly closed and protect from excessive heat or freezing.
CAUTION: Federal law prohibits dispensing without prescription.
POLYCITRA®–K Oral Solution is Distributed by:
Baker Norton Pharmaceuticals, Inc.
Miami, Florida 33178-2404
Manufactured by:
H N Norton Co
Shreveport, LA 71106-6506
1000432   REV9502
                                                     90442P
©1995 Baker Norton Pharmaceuticals, Inc.

PROGLYCEM® ℞
[pro-gli 'sem]
brand of diazoxide
SUSPENSION, USP
FOR ORAL ADMINISTRATION

DESCRIPTION

PROGLYCEM® (diazoxide) is a nondiuretic benzothiadiazine derivative taken orally for the management of symptomatic hypoglycemia. PROGLYCEM® **Suspension** contains 50 mg of diazoxide, USP in each milliliter and has a chocolate-mint flavor; alcohol content is approximately 7.25%.
Diazoxide has the following structural formula:

Diazoxide is 7-chloro-3-methyl-2H-1,2,4-benzothiadiazine 1,1-dioxide with the empirical formula $C_8H_7ClN_2O_2S$ and the molecular weight 230.7. It is a white powder practically insoluble to sparingly soluble in water.

CLINICAL PHARMACOLOGY

Diazoxide administered orally produces a prompt dose-related increase in blood glucose level, due primarily to an inhibition of insulin release from the pancreas, and also to an extrapancreatic effect.
The hyperglycemic effect begins within an hour and generally lasts no more than eight hours in the presence of normal renal function.
PROGLYCEM® decreases the excretion of sodium and water, resulting in fluid retention which may be clinically significant.
The hypotensive effect of diazoxide on blood pressure is usually not marked with the oral preparation. This contrasts with the intravenous preparation of diazoxide (see ADVERSE REACTIONS).
Other pharmacologic actions of PROGLYCEM® include increased pulse rate; increased serum uric acid levels due to decreased excretion; increased serum levels of free fatty acids' decreased chloride excretion; decreased para-aminohippuric acid; (PAH) clearance with no appreciable effect on glomerular filtration rate.
The concomitant administration of a benzothiazide diuretic may intensify the hyperglycemic and hyperuricemic effects of PROGLYCEM®. In the presence of hypokalemia, hyperglycemic effects are also potentiated.
PROGLYCEM®-induced hyperglycemia is reversed by the administration of insulin or tolbutamide.
The inhibition of insulin release by PROGLYCEM® is antagonized by alpha-adrenergic blocking agents.
PROGLYCEM® is extensively bound (more than 90%) to serum proteins, and is excreted in the kidneys. The plasma half-life following I.V. administration is 28 ± 8.3 hours. Limited data on oral administration revealed a half-life of 24 and 36 hours in two adults. In four children aged four months to six years, the plasma half-life varied from 9.5 to 24 hours on long-term oral administration. The half-life may be prolonged following overdosage, and in patients with impaired renal function.

INDICATIONS AND USAGE

PROGLYCEM® (ORAL DIAZOXIDE) is useful in the management of hypoglycemia due to hyperinsulinism associated with the following conditions:
Adults: Inoperable islet cell adenoma or carcinoma, or extrapancreatic malignancy.
Infants and Children: Leucine sensitivity, islet cell hyperplasia, nesidioblastosis, extrapancreatic malignancy, islet cell adenoma, or adenomatosis. PROGLYCEM® may be used preoperatively as a temporary measure, and postoperatively, if hypoglycemia persists.
PROGLYCEM® should be used only after a diagnosis of hypoglycemia due to one of the above conditions has been definitely established. When other specific medical therapy or surgical management either has been unsuccessful or is not feasible, treatment with PROGLYCEM® should be considered.

CONTRAINDICATIONS

The use of PROGLYCEM® for functional hypoglycemia is contraindicated. The drug should not be used in patients hypersensitive to diazoxide or to other thiazides unless the potential benefits outweigh the possible risks.

WARNINGS

The antidiuretic property of diazoxide may lead to significant fluid retention, which in patients with a compromised cardiac reserve, may precipitate congestive heart failure. The fluid retention will respond to conventional therapy with diuretics.

Continued on next page

Baker Norton—Cont.

It should be noted that concomitantly administered thiazides may potentiate the hyperglycemic and hyperuricemic actions of diazoxide (See DRUG INTERACTIONS and ANIMAL PHARMACOLOGY AND/OR TOXICOLOGY).

Ketoacidosis and nonketotic hyperosmolar coma have been reported in patients treated with recommended doses of PROGLYCEM® usually during intercurrent illness. Prompt recognition and treatment are essential (see OVERDOSAGE), and prolonged surveillance following the acute episode is necessary because of the long drug half-life of approximately 30 hours. The occurrence of these serious events may be reduced by careful education of patients regarding the need for monitoring the urine for sugar and ketones and for prompt reporting of abnormal findings and unusual symptoms to the physician.

Transient cataracts occur in association with hyperosmolar coma in an infant, and subsided on correction of the hyperosmolarity. Cataracts have been observed in several animals receiving daily doses of intravenous or oral diazoxide.

The development of abnormal facial features in four children treated chronically (>4 years) with PROGLYCEM® for hypoglycemia hyperinsulinism in the same clinic has been reported.

PRECAUTIONS

General: Treatment with PROGLYCEM® should be initiated under close clinical supervision, with careful monitoring of blood glucose and clinical response until the patient's condition has stabilized. This usually requires several days. If not effective in two to three weeks, the drug should be discontinued.

Prolonged treatment requires regular monitoring of the urine for sugar and ketones, especially under stress conditions, with prompt reporting of any abnormalities to the physician. Additionally, blood sugar levels should be monitored periodically by the physician to determine the need for dose adjustment.

The effects of diazoxide on the hematopoietic system and the level of serum uric acid should be kept in mind; the latter should be considered particularly in patients with hyperuricemia or a history of gout.

In some patients, higher blood levels have been observed with a oral suspension than with a capsule formulation of PROGLYCEM®. Dosage should be adjusted as necessary in individual patients if changed from one formulation to the other.

Since the plasma half-life of diazoxide is prolonged in patients with impaired renal function, a reduced dosage should be considered. Serum electrolyte levels should also be evaluated for such patients.

The antihypertensive effect of other drugs may be enhanced by PROGLYCEM®, and this should be kept in mind when administering it concomitantly with antihypertensive agents.

Because of the protein binding, administration of PROGLYCEM® with coumarin or its derivatives may require reduction in the dosage of the anticoagulant, although there has been no reported evidence of excessive anticoagulant effect. In addition, PROGLYCEM® may possibly displace bilirubin from albumin; this should be kept in mind particularly when treating newborns with increased bilirubinemia.

Information for Patients: During treatment with PROGLYCEM® the patient should be advised to consult regularly with the physician and to cooperate in the periodic monitoring of his condition by laboratory tests. In addition, the patient should be advised:

—to take the drug on a regular schedule as prescribed, not to skip doses, not to take extra doses;

—not to use this drug with other medications unless this is done with the physician's advice;

—not to allow anyone else to take this medication;

—to follow dietary instructions;

—to report promptly any adverse effects (i.e., increased urinary frequency, increased thirst, fruity breath odor);

—to report pregnancy or to discuss plans for pregnancy.

Laboratory tests: The following procedures may be especially important in patient monitoring (not necessarily inclusive); blood glucose determinations (recommended at periodic intervals in patients taking diazoxide orally for treatment of hypoglycemia, until stabilized); blood urea nitrogen (BUN) determinations and creatinine clearance determinations; hematocrit determinations; platelet count determinations; total and differential leukocyte counts; serum aspartate aminotransferase (AST) level determinations; serum uric acid level determinations; and urine testing for glucose and ketones (in patients being treated with diazoxide for hypoglycemia, semi-quantitative estimation of sugar and ketones in serum performed by the patient and reported to the physician provides frequent and relatively inexpensive monitoring of the condition).

Drug Interactions: Since diazoxide is highly bound to serum proteins, it may displace other substances which are also bound to protein, such as bilirubin or coumarin and its derivatives, resulting in higher blood levels of these substances. Concomitant administration of oral diazoxide and diphenylhydantoin may result in a loss of seizure control. These potential interactions must be considered when administering PROGLYCEM® **Suspension.**

The concomitant administration of thiazides or other commonly used diuretics may potentiate the hyperglycemic and hyperuricemic effects of diazoxide.

Drug/Laboratory Test Interactions: The hyperglycemic and hyperuricemic effects of diazoxide preclude proper assessment of these metabolic states. Increased renin secretion, IgG concentrations and decreased cortisol secretions have also been noted. Diazoxide inhibits glucagon-stimulated insulin release and causes a false-negative insulin response to glucagon.

Carcinogenesis, mutagenesis, impairment of fertility: No long-term animal dosing study has been done to evaluate the carcinogenic potential of diazoxide. No laboratory study of mutagenic potential or animal study of effects on fertility has been done.

Pregnancy Category C: Reproduction studies using the oral preparation in rats have revealed increased fetal resorptions and delayed parturition, as well as fetal skeletal anomalies; evidence of skeletal and cardiac teratogenic effects in rabbits has been noted with intravenous administration. The drug has also been demonstrated to cross the placental barrier in animals and to cause degeneration of the fetal pancreatic beta cells (See ANIMAL PHARMACOLOGY AND/OR TOXICOLOGY). Since there are no adequate data on fetal effects of this drug when given to pregnant women, safety in pregnancy has not been established. When the use of PROGLYCEM® is considered, the indications should be limited to those specified above for adults (See INDICATIONS AND USAGE), and the potential benefits to the mother must be weighed against possible harmful effects to the fetus.

Non-teratogenic Effects: Diazoxide crosses the placental barrier and appears in cord blood. When given to the mother prior to delivery of the infant, the drug may produce fetal or neonatal hyperbilirubinemia, thrombocytopenia, altered carbohydrate metabolism, and possibly other side effects that have occurred in adults.

Alopecia and hypertrichosis lanuginosa have occurred in infants whose mothers received oral diazoxide during the last 19 to 60 days of pregnancy.

Labor and delivery: Since intravenous administration of the drug during labor may cause cessation of uterine contractions, and administration of oxytocic agents may be required to reinstate labor, caution is advised in administering PROGLYCEM® at that time.

Nursing mothers: Information is not available concerning the passage of diazoxide in breast milk. Because many drugs are excreted in human milk and because of the potential for adverse reactions from diazoxide in nursing infants, a decision should be made whether to discontinue nursing or to discontinue the drug, taking into account the importance of the drug to the mother.

Pediatric use: (See INDICATIONS AND USAGE).

ADVERSE REACTIONS

Frequent and Serious: Sodium and fluid retention is most common in young infants and in adults and may precipitate congestive heart failure in patients with compromised cardiac reserve. It usually responds to diuretic therapy (See DRUG INTERACTIONS).

Infrequent but Serious: Diabetic ketoacidosis and hyperosmolar nonketotic coma may develop very rapidly. Conventional therapy with insulin and restoration of fluid and electrolyte balance is usually effective if instituted promptly. Prolonged surveillance is essential in view of the long half-life of PROGLYCEM® (See OVERDOSAGE).

Other frequent adverse reactions: Hirsutism of the lanugo type, mainly on the forehead, back and limbs, occurs most commonly in children and women and may be cosmetically unacceptable. It subsides on discontinuation of the drug.

Hyperglycemia or glycosuria may require reduction in dosage in order to avoid progression towards ketoacidosis or hyperosmolar coma.

Gastrointestinal intolerance may include anorexia, nausea, vomiting, abdominal pain, ileus, diarrhea, transient loss of taste. Tachycardia, palpitations, increased levels of serum uric acid are common.

Thrombocytopenia with or without purpura may require discontinuation of the drug. Neutropenia is transient, is not associated with increased susceptibility to infection, and ordinarily does not require discontinuation of the drug. Skin rash, headache, weakness, and malaise may also occur.

Other adverse reactions which have been observed are:

Cardiovascular: hypotension occurs occasionally, which may be augmented by thiazide diuretics given concurrently. A few cases of transient hypertension, for which no explanation is apparent, have been noted. Chest pain has been reported rarely.

Hematologic: eosinophilia; decreased hemoglobin/hematocrit; excessive bleeding, decreased IgG.

Hepato-renal: increased AST, alkaline phosphatase; azotemia, decreased creatinine clearance, reversible nephrotic syndrome, decreased urinary output, hematuria, albuminuria. Neurologic: anxiety, dizziness, insomnia, polyneuritis, paresthesia, pruritus, extrapyramidal signs. *Ophthalmologic:* transient cataracts, subconjunctival hemorrhage, ring scotoma, blurred vision, diplopia, lacrimation. *Skeletal, integumentary;* monilial dermatitis, herpes, advance in bone-age; loss of scalp hair. *Systemic:* fever, lymphadenopathy. *Other;* gout, acute pancreatitis/pancreatic necrosis, galactorrhea, enlargement of lump in breast.

OVERDOSAGE

An overdosage of PROGLYCEM® causes marked hyperglycemia which may be associated with ketoacidosis. It will respond to prompt insulin administration and restoration of fluid and electrolyte balance. Because of the drug's long half-life (approximately 30 hours), the symptoms of overdosage require prolonged surveillance for periods up to seven days until the blood sugar level stabilizes within the normal range. One investigator reported successful lowering of diazoxide blood levels by peritoneal dialysis in one patient and by hemodialysis in another.

DOSAGE AND ADMINISTRATION

Patients should be under close clinical observation when treatment with PROGLYCEM® is initiated. The clinical response and blood glucose level should be carefully monitored until the patient's condition has stabilized satisfactory; in most instances, this may be accomplished in several days. If administration of PROGLYCEM® is not effective after two or three weeks, the drug should be discontinued.

The dosage of PROGLYCEM® must be individualized based on the severity of the hypoglycemic condition and the blood glucose level and clinical response of the patient. The dosage should be adjusted until the desired clinical and laboratory effects are produced with the least amount of the drug. Special care should be taken to assure accuracy of dosage in infants and young children.

Adults and children: The usual daily dosage is 3 to 8 mg/kg, divided into two or three equal doses every 8 to 12 hours. In certain instances, patients with refractory hypoglycemia may require higher dosages. Ordinarily, an appropriate starting dosage is 3 mg/kg/day, divided into three equal doses every 8 hours. Thus an average adult would receive a starting dosage of approximately 200 mg daily.

Infants and newborns: The usual daily dosage is 8 to 15 mg/kg divided into two or three equal doses every 8 to 12 hours. An appropriate starting dosage is 10 mg/kg/day, divided into three equal doses every 8 hours.

ANIMAL PHARMACOLOGY AND/OR TOXICOLOGY

Oral diazoxide in the mouse, rat, rabbit, dog, pig, and monkey produces a rapid and transient rise in blood glucose levels. In dogs, increased blood glucose is accompanied by increased free fatty acids, lactate, and pyruvate in the serum. In mice, a marked decrease in liver glycogen and an increase in the blood urea nitrogen level occur.

In acute toxicity studies the LD$_{50}$ for oral diazoxide suspension is >5000 mg/kg in the rat, >522 mg/kg in the neonatal rat, between 1900 and 2572 mg/kg in the mouse, and 219 mg/kg in the guinea pig. Although the oral LD$_{50}$ was not determined in the dog, a dosage of up to 500 mg/kg was well tolerated.

In subacute oral toxicity studies, diazoxide at 400 mg/kg in the rat produced growth retardation, edema, increases in liver and kidney weights, and adrenal hypertrophy. Daily dosages up to 1080 mg/kg for three months produced hyperglycemia, an increase in liver weight and an increase in mortality. In dogs given oral diazoxide at approximately 40 mg/kg/day for one month, no biologically significant gross or microscopic abnormalities were observed. Cataracts, attributed to markedly disturbed carbohydrate metabolism, have been observed in a few dogs given repeated daily doses of oral or intravenous diazoxide. The lenticular changes resembled those which occur experimentally in animals with increased blood glucose levels. In chronic toxicity studies, rats given a daily dose of 200 mg/kg diazoxide for 52 weeks had a decrease in weight gain and an increase in heart, liver, adrenal and thyroid weights. Mortality in drug-treated and control groups was not different. Dogs treated with diazoxide at dosages of 50, 100, and 200 mg/kg/day for 82 weeks had higher blood glucose levels than controls. Mild bone marrow stimulation and increased pancreas weights were evident in the drug-treated dogs; several developed inguinal hernias, one had a testicular seminoma, and another had a mass near the penis. Two females had inguinal mammary swellings. The etiology of these changes was not established. There was no difference in mortality between drug-treated and control groups. In a second chronic oral toxicity study, dogs given milled diazoxide at 50, 100, and 200 mg/kg/day had anorexia and severe weight loss, causing death in a few. Hematologic, biochemical, and histologic examination did not indicate any cause of death other than inanition. After one year of treatment, there is no evidence of herniation or tissue swelling in any of the dogs.

When diazoxide was administered at high dosages concomitantly with either chlorothiazide to rats or trichlormethiazide to dogs, increased toxicity was observed. In rats, the

combination was nephrotoxic; epithelial hyperplasia was observed in the collecting tubules. In dogs, a diabetic syndrome was produced which resulted in ketosis and death. Neither of the drugs given alone produced these effects. Although the data are inconclusive, reproduction and teratology studies in several species of animals indicate that diazoxide, when administered during the critical period of embryo formation, may interfere with normal fetal development, possibly through altered glucose metabolism. Parturition was occasionally prolonged in animals treated at term. Intravenous administration of diazoxide to pregnant sheep, goats, and swine produced in the fetus an appreciable increase in blood glucose level and degeneration of the beta cells of the Islets of Langerhans. The reversibility of these effects was not studied.

HOW SUPPLIED

PROGLYCEM® Suspension, 50 mg/ml, a chocolate-mint flavored suspension; bottle of 30 ml (NDC 0575-6200-30), with dropper calibrated to deliver 10, 20, 30, 40 and 50 mg diazoxide. **Shake well before each use. Protect from light. Store in carton until contents are used. Store in light resistant container as defined in the USP. Store PROGLYCEM® Capsules and Suspension between 2° and 30°C (36° and 86°F).**

Proglycem® Suspension, Manufactured by Schering Corp. Kenilworth, New Jersey 07033
Caution: Federal (USA) Law prohibits dispensing without a prescription.
I000858
R9403

Basel Pharmaceuticals
Ciba-Geigy Corporation
556 MORRIS AVENUE
SUMMIT, NJ 07901

For Information Contact:
Consumer Affairs Department:
(800) 742-2422
Medical Services Department:
556 Morris Avenue
Summit, NJ 07901

PLEASE NOTE:
Due to the alliance between Ciba Pharmaceuticals (which includes Basel Pharmaceuticals, Ciba Pharmaceutical Company, Geigy Pharmaceuticals, and Summit Pharmaceuticals) and Geneva Pharmaceuticals, Inc, please refer to **CibaGeneva** for product information.

See CibaGeneva Pharmaceuticals for information on the following products:
Anafranil®
Tegretol®
Tegretol®-XR
See Ciba Self Medication section for information on the following product:
Habitrol®

Baxter Healthcare Corporation
Biotech Group
Hyland Division
550 NORTH BRAND BLVD.
GLENDALE, CA 91203

Direct Inquiries to:
Product Management
(800) 423-2090

For Medical Information Contact:
In Emergencies:
Edward Gomperts, M.D.
Medical Director,
Baxter Healthcare Corporation:
(818) 956-3200

ATNATIV®
Antithrombin III (Human)
Heat Treated

DESCRIPTION
ATnativ®, Antithrombin III (Human), is produced from human plasma. Antithrombin III is a glycoprotein of molecular weight 58,000 (14) and consists of 425 amino acids in a single polypeptide chain crosslinked by three disulfide bridges. Antithrombin III is identical with heparin cofactor I, a factor in plasma necessary for heparin to exert its anticoagulant effect.
ATnativ®, a sterile white powder, is intended for intravenous administration after reconstitution with Sterile Water for Injection, USP, and contains no preservative.
In addition, Antithrombin III (Human) has been heat-treated in solution at 60°C $\pm$ 0.5°C for not less than 10 hours. ATnativ® is supplied with 10 mL Sterile Water for Injection, USP. After reconstitution it contains 50 IU Antithrombin III (Human) per mL and has a pH of 6.5 to 7.5. The quantity of antithrombin III in 1 mL of normal pooled human plasma is conventionally taken as one unit. The potency assignment has been determined with a standard calibrated against a World Health Organization (WHO) Antithrombin III Reference Preparation.

HOW SUPPLIED
ATnativ®, Antithrombin III (Human), is supplied as a lyophilized powder in 50 mL infusion bottles containing 500 IU of Antithrombin III (Human). Each bottle of ATnativ® is accompanied by 10 mL Sterile Water for Injection, USP.

AUTOPLEX® T
Anti-Inhibitor Coagulant Complex, Heat Treated

DESCRIPTION
Anti-Inhibitor Coagulant Complex, Heat Treated, Autoplex® T*, is a sterile product prepared from pooled human plasma with subsequent alcohol fractionation of Cohn Fraction IV₁. It contains, in concentrated form, variable amounts of activated and precursor vitamin K-dependent clotting factors. Factors of the kinin generating system are also present. The product is standardized by its ability to correct the clotting time of Factor VIII deficient plasma or Factor VIII deficient plasma which contains inhibitors to Factor VIII.
When reconstituted, this product contains a maximum of 2 units per mL of heparin and a residual amount of polyethylene glycol (2 mg per mL, maximum). It also contains 0.02 M sodium citrate and the sodium content is 177 $\pm$ 15 milliequivalents per liter.
Laboratory testing of several lots of Anti-Inhibitor Coagulant Complex, Heat Treated, has shown the presence of Factor VIII coagulant antigent (VIII:CAg). Although anamnestic response to this antigen following administration of the product was not observed during the clinical trials, the possibility of such a response does exist.
Each lot of Anti-Inhibitor Coagulant Complex, Heat Treated, Autoplex® T, is assayed and labeled for units of Hyland Factor VIII correctional activity. Factor VIII correctional activity may not be exclusively related to the efficacious component(s). (See **Clinical Pharmacology**.)
During the manufacturing process, this product was heated for 6 days at 60°C. This heating step is designed to reduce the risk of transmission of hepatitis and other viral diseases. However, no procedure has been shown to be totally effective in removing hepatitis infectivity from Anti-Inhibitor Coagulant Complex.
Anti-Inhibitor Coagulant Complex, Heat Treated, **must be** administered intravenously.

HOW SUPPLIED
Anti-Inhibitor Coagulant Complex, Heat Treated, Autoplex® T, is furnished with a suitable volume of Sterile Water for Injection, USP; a double-ended needle; and a filter needle.

BUMINATE® 5%
Albumin (Human),
USP, 5% Solution

DESCRIPTION
Albumin (Human), 5% Solution, Buminate® 5% is a sterile, nonpyrogenic preparation of alubmin in a single dosage form for intravenous administration. Each 100 mL contains 5 g of albumin and was prepared from human venous plasma using the Cohn cold ethanol fractionation process. It has been adjusted to physiological pH with sodium bicarbonate and/or sodium hydroxide and has been stabilized with 0.004 M sodium acetyltryptophanate and 0.004 M sodium caprylate. The sodium content is 145 $\pm$ 15 mEq/L. The solution con-

tains no preservative and none of the coagulation factors found in fresh whole blood or plasma. Albumin (Human), 5% Solution, Buminate 5% is a transparent or slightly opalescent solution which may have a greenish tint or may vary from a pale straw to an amber color.
The likelihood of the presence of viable hepatitis viruses has been reduced by heating the product for 10 hours at 60°C. This procedure has been shown to be an effective method of inactivating hepatitis virus in albumin solutions even when those solutions were prepared from plasma known to be infective.[1-3]
Albumin (Human), 5% Solution, Buminate 5% contains no blood group isoagglutinins thereby permitting its administration without regard to the recipient's blood group.

HOW SUPPLIED
Albumin (Human), 5% Solution, Buminate 5% is supplied in 250 mL and 500 mL bottles.

BUMINATE® 25%
Albumin (Human),
USP, 25% Solution

DESCRIPTION
Albumin (Human), 25% Solution, Buminate® 25% is a sterile, nonpyrogenic preparation of albumin in a single dosage form for intravenous administration. Each 100 mL contains 25 g of albumin and was prepared from human venous plasma using the Cohn cold ethanol fractionation process. It has been adjusted to physiological pH with sodium bicarbonate and/or sodium hydroxide and stabilized with 0.02 M sodium acetyltryptophanate and 0.02 M sodium caprylate. The sodium content is 145 $\pm$ 15 mEq/L. This solution contains no preservative and none of the coagulation factors found in fresh whole blood or plasma. Albumin (Human), 25% Solution, Buminate 25% is a transparent or slightly opalescent solution which may have a greenish tint or may vary from a pale straw to an amber color.
The likelihood of the presence of viable hepatitis viruses has been minimized by heating the product for 10 hours at 60°C. This procedure has been shown to be an effective method of inactivating hepatitis virus in albumin solutions even when those solutions were prepared from plasma known to be infective.[1-3]

HOW SUPPLIED
Albumin (Human), 25% Solution, Buminate 25% is supplied in 20 mL, 50 mL and 100 mL bottles.

IMMUNE GLOBULIN
INTRAVENOUS (HUMAN)
GAMMAGARD® S/D
SOLVENT/DETERGENT TREATED

DESCRIPTION
Immune Globulin Intravenous (Human) [IGIV], Gammagard®S/D*, is a solvent/detergent treated, sterile, freeze-dried preparation of highly purified immunoglobulin G (IgG) derived from large pools of human plasma. The product is manufactured by the Cohn-Oncley cold ethanol fractionation process followed by ultrafiltration and ion exchange chromatography. The manufacturing process includes treatment with an organic solvent/detergent mixture,[1,2] composed of tri(n-butyl) phosphate, octoxynol 9 and polysorbate 80.[3] The Gammagard® S/D manufacturing process provides a significant viral reduction in *in vitro* studies.[3] These studies, summarized in Table 1, demonstrate virus clearance during Gammagard® S/D manufacturing using infectious Human Immunodeficiency virus, Types 1 and 2 (HIV-1, HIV-2); Sindbis virus (SIN), a model virus for Hepatitis C virus; Pseudorabies virus (PRV), a model virus for lipid-enveloped DNA viruses such as Herpes; and Vesicular stomatitis virus (VSV), a model virus for lipid-enveloped RNA viruses.[3] These reductions are achieved through a combination of process chemistry, partitioning and/or inactivation during cold ethanol fractionation and the solvent/detergent treatment.[3]
[See table 1 at bottom of next page.]
When reconstituted with the total volume of diluent (Sterile Water for Injection, USP) supplied, this preparation contains approximately 50 mg of protein per mL (5%), of which at least 90% is gamma globulin. The product, reconstituted to 5%, contains a physiological concentration of sodium chloride (approximately 8.5 mg/mL) and has a pH of 6.8 $\pm$ 0.4. Stabilizing agents and additional components are present in the following maximum amounts for a 5% solution: 3 mg/mL Albumin (Human), 22.5 mg/mL glycine, 20 mg/mL glucose, 2 mg/mL polyethylene glycol (PEG), 1 µg/mL tri(n-butyl) phosphate, 1 µg/mL octoxynol 9, and 100 µg/mL polysorbate 80. If it is necessary to prepare a 10% (100 mg/mL)

Continued on next page

Baxter Healthcare—Cont.

solution for infusion, half the volume of diluent should be added, as described in the **DOSAGE AND ADMINISTRATION** section. In this case, the stabilizing agents and other components will be present at double the concentrations given for the 5% solution.

*Manufactured under U.S. Patent No. 4,439,421.

©Copyright 1986, 1987, 1988, 1989, 1990, 1994, 1995 Baxter Healthcare Corporation. All rights reserved.

The manufacturing process for Immune Globulin Intravenous (Human), Gammagard® S/D, isolates IgG without additional chemical or enzymatic modification, and the Fc portion is maintained intact. Immune Globulin Intravenous (Human), Gammagard® S/D, contains all of the IgG antibody activities which are present in the donor population. On the average, the distribution of IgG subclasses present in this product is similar to that in normal plasma.[3] Immune Globulin Intravenous (Human), Gammagard® S/D, contains only trace amounts of IgA (< 3.7 μg/mL in a 5% solution). IgM is also present in trace amounts.

Immune Globulin Intravenous (Human), Gammagard® S/D, contains no preservative.

CLINICAL PHARMACOLOGY

Immune Globulin Intravenous (Human), Gammagard® S/D, contains a broad spectrum of IgG antibodies against bacterial and viral agents that are capable of opsonization and neutralization of microbes and toxins.

Peak levels of IgG are reached immediately after infusion of Immune Globulin Intravenous (Human), Gammagard® S/D. It has been shown that, after infusion, exogenous IgG is distributed relatively rapidly between plasma and extravascular fluid until approximately half is partitioned in the extravascular space. Therefore a rapid initial drop in serum IgG levels is to be expected.[4]

As a class, IgG survives longer *in vivo* than other serum proteins.[4,5] Studies show that the half-life of Immune Globulin Intravenous (Human), Gammagard® S/D, is approximately 37.7 ± 15 days.[3] Previous studies reported IgG half-life values of 21 to 25 days.[4,5,6] The half-life of IgG can vary considerably from person to person, however. In particular, high concentrations of IgG and hypermetabolism associated with fever and infection have been seen to coincide with a shortened half-life of IgG.[4,5,6,7]

INDICATIONS AND USAGE

Primary Immunodeficiency Diseases

Immune Globulin Intravenous (Human), Gammagard® S/D, is indicated for the treatment of primary immunodeficient states, such as: congenital agammaglobulinemias, common variable immunodeficiency, Wiskott-Aldrich syndrome, and severe combined immunodeficiencies.[6,7] This indication was supported by a clinical trial of 17 patients with primary immunodeficiency who received a total of 341 infusions. Immune Globulin Intravenous (Human), Gammagard® S/D, is especially useful when high levels or rapid elevation of circulating IgG are desired or when intramuscular injections are contraindicated (e.g., small muscle mass).

B-cell Chronic Lymphocytic Leukemia (CLL)

Immune Globulin Intravenous (Human), Gammagard® S/D, is indicated for prevention of bacterial infections in patients with hypogammaglobulinemia and/or recurrent bacterial infections associated with B-cell Chronic Lymphocytic Leukemia (CLL). In a study of 81 patients, 41 of whom were treated with Immune Globulin Intravenous (Human), Gammagard®, bacterial infections were significantly reduced in the treatment group.[8,9] In this study, the placebo group had approximately twice as many bacterial infections as the IGIV group. The median time to first bacterial infection for the IGIV group was greater than 365 days. By contrast, the time to first bacterial infection in the placebo group was 192 days. The number of viral and fungal infections, which were for the most part minor, was not statistically different between the two groups.

Idiopathic Thrombocytopenic Purpura (ITP)

When a rapid rise in platelet count is needed to prevent and/or to control bleeding in a patient with Idiopathic Thrombocytopenic Purpura, the administration of Immune Globulin Intravenous (Human), Gammagard® S/D, should be considered.

The efficacy of Immune Globulin Intravenous (Human), Gammagard®, has been demonstrated in a clinical study involving 16 patients. Of these 16 patients, 13 had chronic ITP (11 adults, 2 children), and 3 patients had acute ITP (one adult, 2 children). All 16 patients (100%) demonstrated a clinically significant rise in platelet count to a level greater than 40,000/mm^{3}following the administration of Immune Globulin Intravenous (Human), Gammagard®. Ten of the 16 patients (62.5%) exhibited a significant rise to greater than 80,000 platelets/mm^3. Of these 10 patients, 7 had chronic ITP (5 adults, 2 children), and 3 patients had acute ITP (one adult, 2 children).

The rise in platelet count to greater than 40,000/mm^3 occurred after a single 1 g/kg infusion of Gammagard® in 8 patients with chronic ITP (6 adults, 2 children), and in 2 patients with acute ITP (one adult, one child). A similar response was observed after two 1 g/kg infusions in 3 adult patients with chronic ITP, and one child with acute ITP. The remaining 2 adult patients with chronic ITP received more than two 1 g/kg infusions before achieving a platelet count greater than 40,000/mm^3. The rise in platelet count was generally rapid, occurring within 5 days. However, this rise was transient and not considered curative. Platelet count rises lasted 2 to 3 weeks, with a range of 12 days to 6 months. It should be noted that childhood ITP may resolve spontaneously without treatment.

CONTRAINDICATIONS

None known.

WARNINGS

Immune Globulin Intravenous (Human), Gammagard® S/D, should only be administered intravenously. Other routes of administration have not been evaluated.

Immediate anaphylactic and hypersensitivity reactions are a remote possibility. Epinephrine should be available for treatment of any acute anaphylactoid reactions.

Immune Globulin Intravenous (Human), Gammagard® S/D, contains only trace amounts of IgA (< 3.7 μg/mL in a 5% solution). Nonetheless, it should be given with caution to patients with antibodies to IgA or selective IgA deficiencies.[7,10]

PRECAUTIONS

An aseptic meningitis syndrome (AMS) has been reported to occur infrequently in association with Immune Globulin Intravenous (Human) (IGIV) treatment. Discontinuation of IGIV treatment has resulted in remission of AMS within several days without sequelae. The syndrome usually begins within several hours to two days following IGIV treatment. It is characterized by symptoms and signs including severe headache, nuchal rigidity, drowsiness, fever, photophobia, painful eye movements, and nausea and vomiting. Cerebrospinal fluid (CSF) studies are frequently positive with pleocytosis up to several thousand cells per cu.mm., predominantly from the granulocytic series, and elevated protein levels up to several hundred mg/dL. Patients exhibiting such symptoms and signs should receive a thorough neurological examination, including CSF studies, to rule out other causes of meningitis. AMS may occur more frequently in association with high dose (2 g/kg) IGIV treatment.

Drug Interactions

See **DOSAGE AND ADMINISTRATION** Section.

Pregnancy Category C

Animal reproduction studies have not been conducted with Immune Globulin Intravenous (Human), Gammagard® S/D. It is also not known whether Immune Globulin Intravenous (Human), Gammagard® S/D, can cause fetal harm when administered to a pregnant woman or can affect reproduction capacity. Immune Globulin Intravenous (Human), Gammagard® S/D, should be given to a pregnant woman only if clearly needed.

ADVERSE REACTIONS

In general, reported adverse reactions to Immune Globulin Intravenous (Human) Gammagard®, in patients with either congenital or acquired immunodeficiencies are similar in kind and frequency. Various minor reactions, such as headache, fatigue, chills, backache, leg cramps, lightheadedness, fever, urticaria, flushing, slight elevation of blood pressure, nausea and vomiting may occasionally occur. Slowing or stopping the infusion usually allows the symptoms to disappear promptly.

Immediate anaphylactic and hypersensitivity reactions are a remote possibility. Epinephrine should be available for treatment of any acute anaphylactoid reaction. (See **WARNINGS.**)

Primary Immunodeficiency Diseases

Twenty-one adverse reactions occurred in 341 infusions (6%), when using Immune Globulin Intravenous (Human), Gammagard® (5% solution), in a clinical trial of 17 patients with primary immunodeficiency.[11] Of the 17 patients, 12 (71%) were adults, and 5 (29%) were children (16 years or younger).

In a cross-over study comparing Gammagard® and Gammagard® S/D (5% solutions) conducted in a small number (n = 10) of primary immunodeficient patients, no unusual or unexpected adverse reactions were observed in the Gammagard® S/D group. The adverse reactions experienced in the Gammagard® S/D group were similar in frequency and nature to those observed in the control group consisting of patients receiving Gammagard®.

Gammagard®, reconstituted to a concentration of 10%, was administered intravenously at rates varying from 2–11 mL/kg/Hr. Systemic reactions occurred in 23 (10.5%) of 219 infusions. This compares with an adverse reaction incidence of 6% (only systemic reactions reported) for primary immunodeficient patients previously treated with a 5% solution at infusion rates varying between 2 and 8 mL/kg/Hr, as described above (also, see reference 11). Local pain or irritation was experienced during 35 (16%) of 219 infusions. Application of a warm compress to the infusion site alleviated local symptoms. These local reactions tended to be associated with hand vein infusions and their incidence may be reduced by infusions via the antecubital vein.

B-cell Chronic Lymphocytic Leukemia (CLL)

In the study of patients with B-cell Chronic Lymphocytic Leukemia, the incidence of adverse reactions associated with Gammagard® infusions was approximately 1.3% while that associated with placebo (normal saline) infusions was 0.6%.[9]

Idiopathic Thrombocytopenic Purpura (ITP)

During the clinical study of Gammagard® for the treatment of Idiopathic Thrombocytopenic Purpura, the only adverse reaction reported was headache which occurred in 12 of 16 patients (75%). Of these 12 patients, 11 had chronic ITP (9 adults, 2 children), and one child had acute ITP. Oral antihistamines and analgesics alleviated the symptoms and were used as pretreatment for those patients requiring additional IGIV therapy. The remaining 4 patients did not report any side effects and did not require pretreatment.

DOSAGE AND ADMINISTRATION

Primary Immunodeficiency Diseases

For patients with primary immunodeficiencies, monthly doses of at least 100 mg/kg are recommended. Initially, patients may receive 200–400 mg/kg. As there are significant differences in the half-life of IgG among patients with primary immunodeficiencies, the frequency and amount of immunoglobulin therapy may vary from patient to patient. The proper amount can be determined by monitoring clinical response. The minimum serum concentration of IgG necessary for protection has not been established.

B-cell Chronic Lymphocytic Leukemia (CLL)

For patients with hypogammaglobulinemia and/or recurrent bacterial infections due to B-cell Chronic Lymphocytic Leukemia, a dose of 400 mg/kg every 3 to 4 weeks is recommended.

Idiopathic Thrombocytopenic Purpura (ITP)

For patients with acute or chronic Idiopathic Thrombocytopenic Purpura, a dose of 1 g/kg is recommended. The need for additional doses can be determined by clinical response and platelet count. Up to three separate doses may be given on alternate days if required.

Reconstitution: Use Aseptic Technique

A. 5% Solution

1. **Note: Reconstitute immediately before use.**
2. If refrigerated, warm the Sterile Water for Injection, USP (diluent) and Immune Globulin Intravenous (Human), Gammagard® S/D (dried concentrate), to room temperature.
3. Remove caps from concentrate and diluent bottles to expose central portion of rubber stoppers.
4. Cleanse stoppers with germicidal solution.
5. Remove protective covering from the spike at one end of the transfer device (Fig. 1).
6. Place the diluent bottle on a flat surface and, while holding the bottle to prevent slipping, insert the spike of the transfer device **perpendicularly through the center** of the bottle stopper.

   Caution: Failure to use center of stopper may result in dislodging the stopper.

[See Figures 1 and 2 at top of next column.]

Press down firmly so that the transfer device fits snugly against the diluent bottle (Fig. 2). A slight twist at the end of the downward push helps ensure a snug fit.

Table 1

***In Vitro* Virus Clearance During Gammagard® S/D Manufacturing**

Process Step No.	Process Step Evaluated	Virus Clearance, $\log_{10}$ HIV-1	HIV-2	SIN	PRV	VSV
1	Fraction I + II + III Wash to Fraction I + III Supernatant	8.2*	N.D.**	5.2*	N.D.**	N.D.**
2	Fraction I + III Supernatant to Fraction I + III Filtrate	8.2*	N.D.**	4.6*	N.D.**	N.D.**
3	Fraction I + III Filtrate to Fraction II Precipitate	8.1*	N.D.**	N.A.***	N.D.**	N.D.**
4	Treatment of Resuspended Fraction II Precipitate with Solvent/Detergent Mixture	8.4*	5.7*	5.1*	4.3*	6.0*

* Minimum log reduction due to detection limit of the assay.
** Not determined.
*** Not applicable. Sindbis virus co-precipitates with Fraction II proteins.

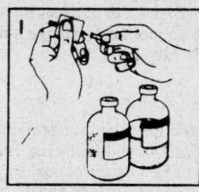 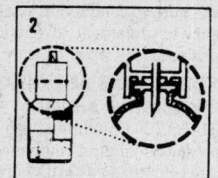

7. Remove the protective covering from the other end of the transfer device. Hold diluent bottle to prevent slipping. **Caution: Failure to use center of stopper may result in dislodging the stopper and loss of vacuum.**

Invert concentrate bottle and press firmly onto the transfer device until the concentrate bottle fits snugly against the transfer device.

8. Invert bottle/transfer device assembly (Fig. 3). Diluent will flow into the concentrate bottle. When diluent transfer is complete, remove empty diluent bottle and transfer device from concentrate bottle. Discard transfer device after single use.

9. Thoroughly wet the dried material by tilting or inverting and gently rotating the bottle (Fig. 4). **Do not shake. Avoid foaming.**

10. Repeat gentle rotation as long as undissolved product is observed.

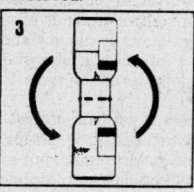 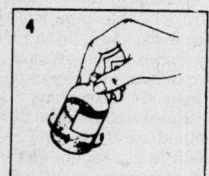

B. 10% Solution

Follow steps 1–4 as previously described in **A.**

5. To prepare a 10% solution, reconstitute with the appropriate volume of diluent by using a sterile hypodermic syringe and needle. Table 2 indicates the volume of diluent required for a 5% or 10% concentration. Using aseptic technique, draw required volume into a sterile hypodermic syringe and needle. The diluent is then injected into the concentrate bottle.

**Table 2
Required Diluent Volume**

Concentration	2.5 g bottle	5 g bottle	10 g bottle
5%	50 mL	96 mL	192 mL
10%	25 mL	48 mL	96 mL

6. Discard any unused diluent after single use.

7. Thoroughly wet the dried material by tilting or inverting and gently rotating the bottle (Fig. 4). **Do not shake. Avoid foaming.**

8. Repeat gentle rotation as long as undissolved product is observed.

Rate of Administration

It is recommended that initially a 5% solution be infused at a rate of 0.5 mL/kg/Hr. If infusion at this rate and concentration causes the patient no distress, the administration rate may be gradually increased to a maximum rate of 4 mL/kg/Hr. Patients who tolerate the 5% concentration at 4 mL/kg/Hr can be infused with the 10% concentration starting at 0.5 mL/kg/Hr. If no adverse effects occur, the rate can be increased gradually up to a maximum of 8 mL/kg/Hr.

It is recommended that antecubital veins be used especially for 10% solutions, if possible. This may reduce the likelihood of the patient experiencing discomfort at the infusion site (see **ADVERSE REACTIONS**).

A rate of administration which is too rapid may cause flushing and changes in pulse rate and blood pressure. Slowing or stopping the infusion usually allows the symptoms to disappear promptly.

Drug Interactions

Admixtures of Immune Globulin Intravenous (Human), Gammagard® S/D, with other drugs and intravenous solutions have not been evaluated. It is recommended that Immune Globulin Intravenous (Human), Gammagard® S/D, be administered separately from other drugs or medications which the patient may be receiving. The product should not be mixed with Immune Globulin Intravenous (Human) from other manufacturers.

Antibodies in immune globulin preparations may interfere with patient responses to live vaccines, such as those for measles, mumps, and rubella. The immunizing physician should be informed of recent therapy with Immune Globulin Intravenous (Human) so that appropriate precautions can be taken.

Administration

Immune Globulin Intravenous (Human), Gammagard® S/D, should be administered as soon after reconstitution as

possible. Administration should begin not more than 2 hours after reconstitution.

The reconstituted material should be at room temperature during administration.

Parenteral drug products should be inspected visually for particulate matter and discoloration prior to administration, whenever solution and container permit. Do not use if particulate matter and/or discoloration is observed.

Follow directions for use which accompany the administration set provided. If another administration set is used, ensure that the set contains a similar filter.

HOW SUPPLIED

Immune Globulin Intravenous (Human), Gammagard® S/D, is supplied in 2.5 g, 5 g or 10 g single use bottles. Each bottle of Immune Globulin Intravenous (Human), Gammagard® S/D, is furnished with a suitable volume of Sterile Water for Injection, USP, a transfer device and an administration set which contains an integral airway and a 15 micron filter.

STORAGE

Immune Globulin Intravenous (Human), Gammagard® S/D, is to be stored at a temperature not to exceed 25°C (77°F). Freezing should be avoided to prevent the diluent bottle from breaking.

REFERENCES

1. Prince AM, Horowitz B, Brotman B: Sterilisation of hepatitis and HTLV-III viruses by exposure to tri(n-butyl) phosphate and sodium cholate. **Lancet 1:**706–710, 1986
2. Horowitz B, Wiebe ME, Lippin A, et al: Inactivation of viruses in labile blood derivatives: I. Disruption of lipid enveloped viruses by tri(n-butyl) phosphate detergent combinations. **Transfusion 25:**516–522, 1985
3. Unpublished data in the files of Baxter Healthcare Corporation.
4. Waldmann TA, Storber W: Metabolism of immunoglobulins. **Prog Allergy 13:** 1–110, 1969
5. Morell A, Riesen W: Structure, function and catabolism of immunoglobulins in **Immunohemotherapy.** Nydegger UE (ed), London, Academic Press, 1981, pp 17–26
6. Stiehm ER: Standard and special human immune serum globulins as therapeutic agents. **Pediatrics 63:** 301–319, 1979
7. Buckley RH: Immunoglobulin replacement therapy: Indications and contraindications for use and variable IgG levels achieved in **Immunoglobulins: Characteristics and Use of Intravenous Preparations.** Alving BM, Finlayson JS (eds), Washington, DC, U.S. Department of Health and Human Services, 1979, pp 3–8
8. Bunch C, Chapel HM, Rai K, et al: Intravenous Immune Globulin reduces bacterial infections in Chronic Lymphocytic Leukemia: A controlled randomized clinical trial. **Blood 70 Suppl 1:** 753, 1987
9. Cooperative Group for the Study of Immunoglobulin in Chronic Lymphocytic Leukemia: Intravenous immunoglobulin for the prevention of infection in Chronic Lymphocytic Leukemia: A randomized, controlled clinical trial. **N Eng J Med 319:** 902–907, 1988
10. Burks AW, Sampson HA, Buckley RH: Anaphylactic reactions after gammaglobulin administration in patients with hypogammaglobulinemia: Detection of IgE antibodies to IgA. **N Eng J Med 314:** 560–564, 1986
11. Ochs HD, Lee ML, Fischer SH, et al: Efficacy of a New Intravenous Immunoglobulin Preparation in Primary Immunodeficient Patients. **Clinical Therapeutics 9:**512–522, 1987

BIBLIOGRAPHY

Bussel JB, Kimberly RP, Inman RD, et al: Intravenous gammaglobulin treatment of chronic idiopathic thrombocytopenic purpura. **Blood 62:** 480–486, 1983

Baxter Healthcare Corporation
Hyland Division
Glendale, CA 91203 USA
U.S. License No. 140
5771   Issued February 1995

HEMOFIL® M   ℞
Antihemophilic Factor (Human)
Method M, Monoclonal Purified

DESCRIPTION

Antihemophilic Factor (Human), Method M, Hemofil® M, is a sterile, nonpyrogenic, dried preparation of antihemophilic factor (Factor VIII, Factor VIII:C, AHF) in concentrated form with a specific activity range of 2 to 15 AHF International Units/mg of total protein. When reconstituted with the appropriate volume of diluent, it contains approximately 12.5 mg/mL Albumin (Human), 1.5 mg/mL polyethylene glycol (3350), 0.055 M histidine and 0.030 M glycine as stabilizing agents. In the absence of the added Albumin (Human), the specific activity is approximately 2,000 AHF International Units/mg of protein. It also contains, per AHF Inter-

national Unit, not more than 0.1 ng mouse protein, 18 ng organic solvent [tri(n-butyl)phosphate] and 50 ng detergent (Triton X-100) See **CLINICAL PHARMACOLOGY.**

Hemofil® M is prepared by the Method M process from pooled human plasma by immuno-affinity chromatography utilizing a murine monoclonal antibody to Factor VIII:C, followed by an ion exchange chromatography step for further purification. Method M also includes an organic solvent [tri(n-butyl)phosphate] and detergent (Triton X-100) virus inactivation step designed to reduce the risk of transmission of hepatitis and other viral diseases. However, no procedure has been shown to be totally effective in removing viral infectivity from coagulation factor products.

Each bottle of Antihemophilic Factor (Human), Hemofil® M, is labeled with the AHF activity expressed in International Units per bottle, which is referenced to the WHO International Standard.

Antihemophilic Factor (Human), Hemofil® M, is to be administered only intravenously.

HOW SUPPLIED

Antihemophilic Factor (Human), Hemofil® M, is available as single dose bottles. Each bottle is labeled with the potency in International Units, and is packaged together with 10 mL of Sterile Water for Injection, USP, a double-ended needle, and a filter needle.

PROPLEX® T   ℞
Factor IX Complex, Heat Treated

DESCRIPTION

Factor IX Complex, Heat Treated, Proplex® T*, is a sterile product prepared from normal human plasma. It contains, in concentrated form, clotting Factors II (prothrombin), VII (proconvertin), IX (PTC, antihemophilic factor B), and X (Stuart-Prower factor). Other proteins are also present in minimal amounts. The product also contains a small amount of heparin, 1.5 units or less per mL of reconstituted material as a stabilizing agent. This amount does not affect the clinical usefulness of the complex in moderate dosage.

Factor IX Complex **must** be administered intravenously.

During the manufacturing process, this product was heated for 144 hours at 60°C.

This heating step was designed to reduce the risk of transmission of hepatitis and other viral infections. No procedure has been shown to be totally effective in removing viral infectivity from Factor IX Complex.

HOW SUPPLIED

Factor IX Complex, Proplex® T, is furnished with a suitable volume of Sterile Water for Injection, USP; a double-ended needle, and a filter needle.

PROTENATE® 5%   ℞
Plasma Protein Fraction (Human),
USP, 5% Solution

DESCRIPTION

Plasma Protein Fraction (Human), Protenate® is a sterile, nonpyrogenic 5% solution of protein which has been prepared from human venous plasma using the Cohn cold ethanol fractionation method. It has been adjusted to physiological pH by the addition of sodium bicarbonate and/or sodium hydroxide and has been stabilized with 0.004 M sodium acetyltryptophanate and 0.004 M sodium caprylate. The plasma proteins consist of: albumin, not less than 83%; alpha and beta globulins, less than 17%; gamma globulin, less than 1%. Plasma Protein Fraction (Human), Protenate contains no preservative nor does it contain any of the coagulation factors of fresh whole blood or plasma. The sodium content of this product is 145 ± 15 mEq/L and the potassium content is not greater than 2 mEq/L.

Plasma Protein Fraction (Human), Protenate is a transparent or slightly opalescent solution which may vary from pale straw to amber in color.

The method of processing removes isoagglutinins and other antibodies which allows the administration of Plasma Protein Fraction (Human), Protenate without regard to the recipient's blood group. Plasma Protein Fraction (Human), Protenate is supplied in single dose bottles and must be administered intravenously.

This product has been heated for 10 hours at 60°C. This procedure has been shown to be an effective method of inactivating hepatitis virus in albumin solutions even when those solutions were prepared from plasma known to contain transmissable hepatitis virus.[1]

HOW SUPPLIED

Plasma Protein Fraction (Human), Protenate is supplied in 250 mL and 500 mL bottles.

Continued on next page

Baxter Healthcare—Cont.

Antihemophilic Factor (Recombinant) ℞

RECOMBINATE™

DESCRIPTION

Antihemophilic Factor (Recombinant), Recombinate™ is a glycoprotein synthesized by a genetically engineered Chinese Hamster Ovary (CHO) cell line. In culture the CHO cell line secretes recombinant antihemophilic factor (rAHF) into the cell culture medium. The rAHF is purified from the culture medium utilizing a series of chromatography columns. A key step in the purification process is an immunoaffinity chromatography methodology in which a purification matrix prepared by immobilization of a monoclonal antibody directed to Factor VIII is utilized to selectively isolate the rAHF in the medium. The rAHF produced has the same biological effects as Antihemophilic Factor (Human) [AHF (Human) and structurally has a similar combination of heterogeneous heavy and light chains as found in AHF (Human).

Recombinate™ is formulated as a sterile, nonpyrogenic, off-white to faint yellow, lyophilized powder preparation of concentrated recombinant AHF for intravenous injection and is available in single-dose bottles which contain nominally 250, 500 and 1000 International Units per bottle. When reconstituted with the appropriate volume of diluent, it contains the following stabilizers in maximum amounts: 12.5 mg/mL Albumin (Human), 1.5 mg/mL polyethylene glycol (3350), 180 mEq/L sodium, 55 mM histidine, 1.5 μg/AHF International Unit (IU) polysorbate-80 and 0.20 mg/mL calcium. Von Willebrand Factor (vWF) is co-expressed with the Antihemophilic Factor (Recombinant) and helps to stabilize it. The final product contains not more than 2 ng vWF/IU rAHF which will not have any clinically relevant effect in patients with von Willebrand's disease. The product contains no preservative.

Manufacturing of Recombinate™ is shared by Baxter Healthcare Corporation, Hyland Division and Genetics Institute, Inc. Genetics Institute produces Antihemophilic Factor Concentrate (Recombinant) (For Further Manufacturing Use) which is then formulated and packaged at Baxter Healthcare Corporation, Hyland Division.

Each bottle of Recombinate™ is labeled with the AHF activity expressed in IU per bottle. Biological potency is determined by an *in vitro* assay which is referenced to the World Health Organization (WHO) International Standard for Factor VIII:C Concentrate.

HOW SUPPLIED

Antihemophilic Factor (Recombinant) Recombinant™ is available in single-dose bottles which contain nominally 250, 500 and 1000 International Units per bottle. Recombinate™ is packaged with 10 mL of Sterile Water for Injection, USP, a double-ended needle, and a filter needle.

Bayer Corporation

Pharmaceutical Division
400 MORGAN LANE
WEST HAVEN, CT 06516

For Medical Information Contact:
Director, Medical Services
(800) 468-0894
(203) 937-2000

ADALAT® ℞
Capsules
(nifedipine)
For Oral Use

DESCRIPTION

ADALAT® (nifedipine) is an antianginal drug belonging to a class of pharmacological agents, the calcium channel blockers. Nifedipine is 3,5-pyridinedicarboxylic acid, 1,4-dihydro-2,6-dimethyl-4-(2-nitrophenyl)-, dimethyl ester, $C_{17}H_{18}N_2O_6$, and has the structural formula:

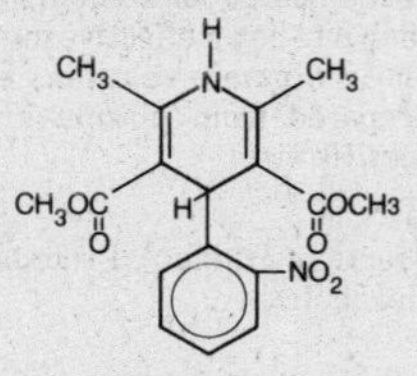

Nifedipine is a yellow crystalline substance, practically insoluble in water but soluble in ethanol. It has a molecular weight of 346.3. ADALAT® CAPSULES are formulated as soft gelatin capsules for oral administration each containing 10 mg or 20 mg of nifedipine.

Inert ingredients in the formulations are: glycerin; peppermint oil; polyethylene glycol 400; soft gelatin capsules (which contain FD&C Yellow No. 6, Red Ferric Oxide and other inert ingredients), and water. The 10 mg capsules also contain saccharin sodium.

CLINICAL PHARMACOLOGY

ADALAT® is a calcium ion influx inhibitor (slow channel blocker or calcium ion antagonist) and inhibits the transmembrane influx of calcium ions into cardiac muscle and smooth muscle. The contractile processes of cardiac muscle and vascular smooth muscle are dependent upon the movement of extracellular calcium ions into these cells through specific ion channels. ADALAT® selectively inhibits calcium ion influx across the cell membrane of cardiac muscle and vascular smooth muscle without changing serum calcium concentrations.

Mechanism of Action

The precise means by which this inhibition relieves angina has not been fully determined, but includes at least the following two mechanisms:

1) Relaxation and Prevention of Coronary Artery Spasm

ADALAT® dilates the main coronary arteries and coronary arterioles, both in normal and ischemic regions, and is a potent inhibitor of coronary artery spasm, whether spontaneous or ergonovine-induced. This property increases myocardial oxygen delivery in patients with coronary artery spasm, and is responsible for the effectiveness of ADALAT® in vasospastic (Prinzmetal's or variant) angina. Whether this effect plays any role in classical angina is not clear, but studies of exercise tolerance have not shown an increase in the maximum exercise rate-pressure product, a widely accepted measure of oxygen utilization. This suggests that, in general, relief of spasm or dilation of coronary arteries is not an important factor in classical angina.

2) Reduction of Oxygen Utilization

ADALAT® regularly reduces arterial pressure at rest and at a given level of exercise by dilating peripheral arterioles and reducing the total peripheral resistance (afterload) against which the heart works. This unloading of the heart reduces myocardial energy consumption and oxygen requirements and probably accounts for the effectiveness of ADALAT® in chronic stable angina.

Pharmacokinetics and Metabolism

ADALAT® is rapidly and fully absorbed after oral administration. The drug is detectable in serum 10 minutes after oral administration, and peak blood levels occur in approximately 30 minutes. Bioavailability is proportional to dose from 10 to 30 mg; half-life does not change significantly with dose. There is little difference in relative bioavailability when ADALAT® capsules are given orally and swallowed whole, bitten and swallowed, or bitten and held sublingually. However, biting through the capsule prior to swallowing does result in slightly earlier plasma concentrations (27 ng/mL 10 minutes after 10 mg) than if capsules are swallowed intact. It is highly bound by serum proteins. ADALAT® is extensively converted to inactive metabolites and approximately 80 percent of ADALAT® and metabolites are eliminated via the kidneys. The half-life of nifedipine in plasma is approximately two hours. Since hepatic biotransformation is the predominant route for the disposition of nifedipine, the pharmacokinetics may be altered in patients with chronic liver disease. Patients with hepatic impairment (liver cirrhosis) have a longer disposition half-life and higher bioavailability of nifedipine than healthy volunteers. The degree of serum protein binding of nifedipine is high (92–98%). Protein binding may be greatly reduced in patients with renal or hepatic impairment.

Hemodynamics

Like other slow channel blockers, ADALAT® exerts a negative inotropic effect on isolated myocardial tissue. This is rarely, if ever, seen in intact animals or man, probably because of reflex responses to its vasodilating effects. In man, ADALAT® causes decreased peripheral vascular resistance and a fall in systolic and diastolic pressure, usually modest (5–10mm Hg systolic), but sometimes larger. There is usually a small increase in heart rate, a reflex response to vasodilation. Measurements of cardiac function in patients with normal ventricular function have generally found a small increase in cardiac index without major effects on ejection fraction, left ventricular end diastolic pressure (LVEDP) or volume (LVEDV). In patients with impaired ventricular function, most acute studies have shown some increase in ejection fraction and reduction in left ventricular filling pressure.

Electrophysiologic Effects

Although like other members of its class, ADALAT® decreases sinoatrial node function and atrioventricular conduction in isolated myocardial preparations, such effects have not been seen in studies in intact animals or in man. In formal electrophysiologic studies, predominantly in patients with normal conduction system, ADALAT® has had no tendency to prolong atrioventricular conduction, prolong sinus node recovery time, or slow sinus rate.

INDICATIONS AND USAGE

I. Vasospastic Angina

ADALAT® (nifedipine) is indicated for the management of vasospastic angina confirmed by any of the following criteria: 1) classical pattern of angina at rest accompanied by ST segment elevation, 2) angina or coronary artery spasm provoked by ergonovine, or 3) angiographically demonstrated coronary artery spasm. In those patients who have had angiography, the presence of significant fixed obstructive disease is not incompatible with the diagnosis of vasospastic angina, provided that the above criteria are satisfied. ADALAT® may also be used where the clinical presentation suggests a possible vasospastic component but where vasospasm has not been confirmed, e.g., where pain has a variable threshold on exertion or when angina is refractory to nitrates and/or adequate doses of beta blockers.

II. Chronic Stable Angina (Classical Effort-Associated Angina)

ADALAT® is indicated for the management of chronic stable angina (effort-associated angina) without evidence of vasospasm in patients who remain symptomatic despite adequate dose of beta blockers and/or organic nitrates or who cannot tolerate those agents.

In chronic stable angina (effort-associated angina) ADALAT® has been effective in controlled trials of up to eight weeks duration in reducing angina frequency and increasing exercise tolerance, but confirmation of sustained effectiveness and evaluation of long term safety in these patients are incomplete.

Controlled studies in small numbers of patients suggest concomitant use of ADALAT® and beta blocking agents may be beneficial in patients with chronic stable angina, but available information is not sufficient to predict with confidence the effects of concurrent treatment, especially in patients with compromised left ventricular function or cardiac conduction abnormalities. When introducing such concomitant therapy, care must be taken to monitor blood pressure closely since severe hypotension can occur from the combined effects of the drugs (See WARNINGS).

CONTRAINDICATIONS

Known hypersensitivity reaction to ADALAT®.

WARNINGS

Excessive Hypotension

Although in most patients, the hypotensive effect of ADALAT® CAPSULES is modest and well tolerated, occasional patients have had excessive and poorly tolerated hypotension. These responses have usually occurred during initial titration or at the time of subsequent upward dosage adjustment, and may be more likely in patients on concomitant beta blockers.

Although not approved for this purpose, ADALAT® CAPSULES and other immediate-release nifedipine capsules have been used (orally and sublingually) for acute reduction of blood pressure. Several well-documented reports describe profound hypotension, myocardial infarction, and death when immediate-release nifedipine capsules were used in this way. **ADALAT® CAPSULES should not be used for acute reduction of blood pressure.**

ADALAT® CAPSULES and other immediate-release nifedipine capsules have also been used for the long-term control of essential hypertension although no properly-controlled studies have been conducted to define an appropriate dose or dose interval for such treatment. **ADALAT® CAPSULES should not be used for the control of essential hypertension.**

Several well-controlled, randomized trials studied the use of immediate-release nifedipine capsules in patients who had just sustained myocardial infarctions. In none of these trials did immediate-release nifedipine appear to provide any benefit. In some of the trials, patients who received immediate-release nifedipine had significantly worse outcomes than patients who received placebo. **ADALAT® CAPSULES should not be administered for 1 week after myocardial infarction, and it should also be avoided in the setting of acute coronary syndrome (when infarction may be imminent).**

Severe hypotension and/or increased fluid volume requirements have been reported in patients receiving ADALAT® together with a beta blocking agent who underwent coronary artery bypass surgery using high dose fentanyl anesthesia. The interaction with high dose fentanyl appears to be due to the combination of ADALAT® and a beta blocker, but the possibility that it may occur with ADALAT® alone, with low doses of fentanyl, in other surgical procedures, or with other narcotic analgesics cannot be ruled out. In ADALAT® treated patients where surgery using high dose fentanyl anesthesia is contemplated, the physician should be aware of these potential problems and, if the patient's condition permits, sufficient time (at least 36 hours) should be allowed for ADALAT® to be washed out of the body prior to surgery.

Increased Angina and/or Myocardial Infarction

Rarely, patients, particularly those who have severe obstructive coronary artery disease, have developed well docu-

mented increased frequency, duration and/or severity of angina or acute myocardial infarction on starting ADALAT® or at the time of dosage increase. The mechanism of this effect is not established.

Beta Blocker Withdrawal
Patients recently withdrawn from beta blockers may develop a withdrawal syndrome with increased angina, probably related to increased sensitivity to catecholamines. Initiation of ADALAT® treatment will not prevent this occurrence and might be expected to exacerbate it by provoking reflex catecholamine release. There have been occasional reports of increased angina in a setting of beta blocker withdrawal and ADALAT® initiation. It is important to taper beta blockers if possible, rather than stopping them abruptly before beginning ADALAT®.

Congestive Heart Failure
Rarely, patients (usually those receiving a beta blocker) have developed heart failure after beginning ADALAT®. Patients with tight aortic stenosis may be at greater risk for such an event since the unloading effect of ADALAT® would be expected to be of less benefit to these patients, owing to the fixed impedance to flow across the aortic valve.

PRECAUTIONS
General: Hypotension: Because ADALAT® decreases peripheral vascular resistance, careful monitoring of blood pressure during the initial administration and titration of ADALAT® is suggested. Close observation is especially recommended for patients already taking medications that are known to lower blood pressure (See WARNINGS).
Peripheral Edema: Mild to moderate peripheral edema, typically associated with arterial vasodilation and not due to left ventricular dysfunction, occurs in about one in ten patients treated with ADALAT® (nifedipine). This edema occurs primarily in the lower extremities and usually responds to diuretic therapy. With patients whose angina is complicated by congestive heart failure, care should be taken to differentiate this peripheral edema from the effects of increasing left ventricular dysfunction.
Laboratory Tests: Rare, usually transient, but occasionally significant elevations of enzymes such as alkaline phosphatase, CPK, LDH, SGOT, and SGPT have been noted. The relationship to ADALAT® therapy is uncertain in most cases, but probable in some. These laboratory abnormalities have rarely been associated with clinical symptoms, however, cholestasis with or without jaundice has been reported. Rare instances of allergic hepatitis have been reported. ADALAT®, like other calcium channel blockers, decreases platelet aggregation in vitro. Limited clinical studies have demonstrated a moderate but statistically significant decrease in platelet aggregation and increase in bleeding time in some ADALAT® patients. This is thought to be a function of inhibition of calcium transport across the platelet membrane. No clinical significance for these findings has been demonstrated.
Positive direct Coombs test with/without hemolytic anemia has been reported.
Although ADALAT® has been used safely in patients with renal dysfunction and has been reported to exert a beneficial effect in certain cases, rare reversible elevations in BUN and serum creatinine have been reported in patients with pre-existing chronic renal insufficiency. The relationship to ADALAT® therapy is uncertain in most cases, but probable in some.
Drug Interactions: *Beta-adrenergic blocking agents:* (See INDICATIONS and WARNINGS). Experience in over 1400 patients in a non-comparative clinical trial has shown that concomitant administration of ADALAT® and beta blocking agents is usually well tolerated, but there have been occasional literature reports suggesting that the combination may increase the likelihood of congestive heart failure, severe hypotension or exacerbation of angina.
Long acting nitrates: ADALAT® may be safely co-administered with nitrates, but there have been no controlled studies to evaluate the antianginal effectiveness of this combination.
Digitalis: Since there have been isolated reports of patients with elevated digoxin levels, and there is a possible interaction between digoxin and nifedipine, it is recommended that digoxin levels be monitored when initiating, adjusting and discontinuing nifedipine to avoid possible over- or under-digitalization.
Coumarin anticoagulants: There have been rare reports of increased prothrombin time in patients taking coumarin anticoagulants to whom ADALAT® was administered. However, the relationship to ADALAT® therapy is uncertain.
Cimetidine: A study in six healthy volunteers has shown a significant increase in peak nifedipine plasma levels (80%) and area-under-the-curve (74%) after a one week course of cimetidine at 1000 mg per day and nifedipine at 40 mg per day. Ranitidine produced smaller, non-significant increases. The effect may be mediated by the known inhibition of cimetidine on hepatic cytochrome P-450, the enzyme system probably responsible for the first-pass metabolism of nifedi-

pine. If nifedipine therapy is initiated in a patient currently receiving cimetidine, cautious titration is advised.
Quinidine: There have been rare reports of an interaction between quinidine and nifedipine (with a decreased plasma level of quinidine).
Carcinogenesis, Mutagenesis, Impairment of Fertility: Nifedipine was administered orally to rats for two years and was not shown to be carcinogenic. When given to rats prior to mating, nifedipine caused reduced fertility at a dose approximately 30 times the maximum recommended human dose. In vivo mutagenicity studies were negative.
Pregnancy: Pregnancy Category C. In rodents, rabbits, and monkeys, nifedipine has been shown to have a variety of embryotoxic, placentoxic, and fetotoxic effects, including stunted fetuses (rats, mice, and rabbits), digital anomalies (rats and rabbits), rib deformities (mice), cleft palate (mice), small placentas and underdeveloped chorionic villi (monkeys), embryonic and fetal deaths (rats, mice, and rabbits), prolonged pregnancy (rats; not evaluated in other species), and decreased neonatal survival (rats; not evaluated in other species). On a mg/kg or mg/m² basis, some of the doses associated with these various effects are higher than the maximum recommended human dose and some are lower, but all are within one order of magnitude of it.
The digital anomalies seen in nifedipine-exposed rabbit pups are strikingly similar to those seen in pups exposed to phenytoin, and these are in turn similar to the phalangeal deformities that are the most common malformation seen in human children with in utero exposure to phenytoin.
There are no adequate and well controlled studies in pregnant women. ADALAT® should be used during pregnancy only if the potential benefit justifies the potential risk to the fetus.
Nursing Mothers: Nifedipine is excreted in human milk. Therefore, a decision should be made to discontinue nursing or to discontinue the drug, taking into account the importance of the drug to the mother.

ADVERSE REACTION
In multiple-dose U.S. and foreign controlled studies in which adverse reactions were reported spontaneously, adverse effects were frequent but generally not serious and rarely required discontinuation of therapy or dosage adjustment. Most were expected consequences of the vasodilator effects of ADALAT®.

Adverse Effect	ADALAT® (%) (N=226)	Placebo (%) (N=235)
Dizziness, lightheadedness, giddiness	27	15
Flushing, heat sensation	25	8
Headache	23	20
Weakness	12	10
Nausea, heartburn	11	8
Muscle cramps, tremor	8	3
Peripheral edema	7	1
Nervousness, mood changes	7	4
Palpitation	7	5
Dyspnea, cough, wheezing	6	3
Nasal congestion, sore throat	6	8

There is also a large uncontrolled experience in over 2100 patients in the United States. Most of the patients had vasospastic or resistant angina pectoris, and about half had concomitant treatment with beta-adrenergic blocking agents. The most common adverse events were:

Incidence Approximately 10%
Cardiovascular: peripheral edema
Central Nervous System: dizziness or lightheadedness
Gastrointestinal: nausea
Systemic: headache and flushing, weakness.
Incidence Approximately 5%
Cardiovascular: transient hypotension.
Incidence 2% or Less
Cardiovascular: palpitation
Respiratory: nasal and chest congestion, shortness of breath
Gastrointestinal: diarrhea, constipation, cramps, flatulence
Musculoskeletal: inflammation, joint stiffness, muscle cramps
Central Nervous System: shakiness, nervousness, jitteriness, sleep disturbances, blurred vision, difficulties in balance
Other: dermatitis, pruritus, urticaria, fever, sweating, chills, sexual difficulties.
Incidence Approximately 0.5%
Cardiovascular: syncope. Syncopal episodes occurred mostly with initial dose and/or increase of dosage.
Incidence Less Than 0.5%
Hematologic: thrombocytopenia, anemia, leukopenia, purpura
Gastrointestinal: allergic hepatitis

Face and Throat: angioedema (mostly orpharyngeal edema with breathing difficulty in a few patients), gingival hyperplasia.
CNS: depression, paranoid syndrome
Musculoskeletal: myalgia
Special Senses: transient blindness at the peak of plasma level
Urogenital: nocturia, polyuria
Other: erythromelalgia, arthritis with ANA (+), gynecomastia, exfoliative dermatitis.
Several of these side effects appear to be dose related. Peripheral edema occurred in about one in 25 patients at doses less than 60 mg per day and in about one patient in eight at 120 mg per day or more. Transient hypotension, generally mild to moderate severity and seldom requiring discontinuation of therapy, occurred in one of 50 patients at less than 60 mg per day and in one of 20 patients at 120 mg per day or more. Very rarely, introduction of ADALAT® therapy was associated with an increase in anginal pain, possibly due to associated hypotension.
In addition, more serious adverse events were observed, not readily distinguishable from the natural history of the disease in these patients. It remains possible, however, that some or many of these events were drug related. Myocardial infarction occurred in about 4% of patients and congestive heart failure or pulmonary edema in about 2%. Ventricular arrhythmias or conduction disturbances each occurred in fewer than 0.5% of patients.
In a subgroup of over 1000 patients receiving ADALAT® with concomitant beta blocker therapy, the pattern and incidence of adverse experiences were not different from that of the entire group of ADALAT® (nifedipine) treated patients (See PRECAUTIONS).
In a subgroup of approximately 250 patients with a diagnosis of congestive heart failure as well as angina, dizziness or lightheadedness, peripheral edema, headache or flushing each occurred in one in eight patients. Hypotension occurred in about one in 20 patients. Syncope occurred in approximately one patient in 250. Myocardial infarction or symptoms of congestive heart failure each occurred in about one patient in 15. Atrial or ventricular dysrhythmias each occurred in about one patient in 150.

OVERDOSAGE
Experience with nifedipine overdosage is limited. Generally, overdosage with nifedipine leading to pronounced hypotension calls for active cardiovascular support including monitoring of cardiovascular and respiratory function, elevation of extremities, judicious use of calcium infusion, pressor agents and fluids. Clearance of nifedipine would be expected to be prolonged in patients with impaired liver function. Since nifedipine is highly protein bound, dialysis is not likely to be of any benefit; however, plasmapheresis may be beneficial.

DOSAGE AND ADMINISTRATION
The dosage of ADALAT® needed to suppress angina and that can be tolerated by the patient must be established by titration. Excessive doses can result in hypotension.
Therapy should be initiated with the 10 mg capsule. The starting dose is one 10 mg capsule, swallowed whole, 3 times/day. The usual effective dose range is 10–20 mg three times daily. Some patients, especially those with evidence of coronary artery spasm, respond only to higher doses, more frequent administration, or both. In such patients, doses of 20–30 mg three or four times daily may be effective. Doses above 120 mg daily are rarely necessary. More than 180 mg per day is not recommended.
In most cases, ADALAT® titration should proceed over a 7–14 day period so that the physician can assess the response to each dose level and monitor the blood pressure before proceeding to higher doses.
If symptoms so warrant, titration may proceed more rapidly provided that the patient is assessed frequently. Based on the patient's physical activity level, attack frequency, and sublingual nitroglycerin consumption, the dose of ADALAT® may be increased from 10 mg t.i.d. to 20 mg t.i.d. and then to 30 mg t.i.d. over a three-day period.
In hospitalized patients under close observation, the dose may be increased in 10 mg increments over four to six-hour periods as required to control pain and arrhythmias due to ischemia. A single dose should rarely exceed 30 mg.
No "rebound effect" has been observed upon discontinuation of ADALAT®. However, if discontinuation of ADALAT® is necessary, sound clinical practice suggests that the dosage should be decreased gradually with close physician supervision.
Co-Administration with Other Antianginal Drugs
Sublingual nitroglycerin may be taken as required for the control of acute manifestations of angina, particularly during ADALAT® titration. See PRECAUTIONS, Drug Interactions, for information on co-administration of ADALAT® with beta blockers or long acting nitrates.

Continued on next page

Bayer Corporation—Cont.

HOW SUPPLIED

ADALAT® soft gelatin capsules are supplied in:

Bottles of 100:	10 mg (NDC 0026-8811-51) orange
	20 mg (NDC 0026-8821-51) orange and light brown
Bottles of 300:	10 mg (NDC 0026-8811-18) orange
	20 mg (NDC 0026-8821-18) orange and light brown
Unit dose packages of 100:	10 mg (NDC 0026-8811-48) orange
	20 mg (NDC 0026-8821-48) orange and light brown

The capsules are identified as follows: 10 mg (Adalat 10), 20 mg (Adalat 20).

The capsules should be protected from light and moisture and stored at controlled room temperature 59° to 77°F (15° to 25°C). Dispense in tight, light resistant containers (USP).

Bayer Corporation
Pharmacuetical Division
400 Morgan Lane
West Haven, CT 06516

Encapsulated by
R.P. Scherer N.A., Clearwater, FL 33518

Caution: Federal (USA) law prohibits dispensing without prescription.

PD500034 3/96 BAY a 1040 6128

Shown in Product Identification Guide, page 304

ADALAT® CC ℞

(nifedipine)
Extended Release Tablets
For Oral Use

DESCRIPTION

ADALAT® CC is an extended release tablet dosage form of the calcium channel blocker nifedipine. Nifedipine is 3,5-pyridinedicarboxylic acid, 1,4-dihydro-2,6-dimethyl-4-(2-nitrophenyl)-dimethyl ester, $C_{17}H_{18}N_2O_6$, and has the structural formula:

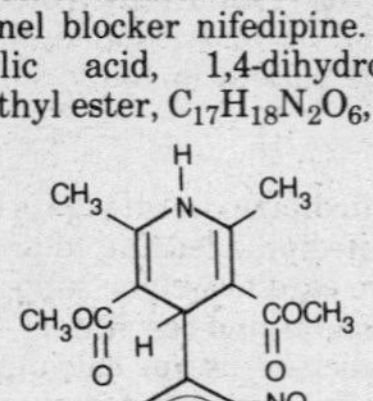

Nifedipine is a yellow crystalline substance, practically insoluble in water but soluble in ethanol. It has a molecular weight of 346.3. ADALAT CC tablets consist of an external coat and an internal core. Both contain nifedipine, the coat as a slow release formulation and the core as a fast release formulation. ADALAT CC tablets contain either 30, 60, or 90 mg of nifedipine for once-a-day oral administration.

Inert ingredients in the formulation are: hydroxypropylcellulose, lactose, corn starch, crospovidone, microcrystalline cellulose, silicon dioxide, and magnesium stearate. The inert ingredients in the film coating are: hydroxypropylmethylcellulose, polyethylene glycol, ferric oxide, and titanium dioxide.

CLINICAL PHARMACOLOGY

Nifedipine is a calcium ion influx inhibitor (slow-channel blocker or calcium ion antagonist) which inhibits the transmembrane influx of calcium ions into vascular smooth muscle and cardiac muscle. The contractile processes of vascular smooth muscle and cardiac muscle are dependent upon the movement of extracellular calcium ions into these cells through specific ion channels. Nifedipine selectively inhibits calcium ion influx across the cell membrane of vascular smooth muscle and cardiac muscle without altering serum calcium concentrations.

Mechanism of Action: The mechanism by which nifedipine reduces arterial blood pressure involves peripheral arterial vasodilatation and consequently, a reduction in peripheral vascular resistance. The increased peripheral vascular resistance that is an underlying cause of hypertension results from an increase in active tension in the vascular smooth muscle. Studies have demonstrated that the increase in active tension reflects an increase in cytosolic free calcium.

Nifedipine is a peripheral arterial vasodilator which acts directly on vascular smooth muscle. The binding of nifedipine to voltage-dependent and possibly receptor-operated channels in vascular smooth muscle results in an inhibition of calcium influx through these channels. Stores of intracellular calcium in vascular smooth muscle are limited and thus dependent upon the influx of extracellular calcium for contraction to occur. The reduction in calcium influx by nifedipine causes arterial vasodilation and decreased peripheral vascular resistance which results in reduced arterial blood pressure.

Pharmacokinetics and Metabolism: Nifedipine is completely absorbed after oral administration. The bioavailability of nifedipine as ADALAT CC relative to immediate release nifedipine is in the range of 84%–89%. After ingestion of ADALAT CC tablets under fasting conditions, plasma concentrations peak at about 2.5–5 hours with a second small peak or shoulder evident at approximately 6–12 hours post dose. The elimination half-life of nifedipine administered as ADALAT CC is approximately 7 hours in contrast to the known 2 hour elimination half-life of nifedipine administered as an immediate release capsule.

When ADALAT CC is administered as multiples of 30 mg tablets over a dose range of 30 mg to 90 mg, the area under the curve (AUC) is dose proportional; however, the peak plasma concentration for the 90 mg dose given as 3 × 30 mg is 29% greater than predicted from the 30 mg and 60 mg doses.

Two 30 mg ADALAT CC tablets may be interchanged with a 60 mg ADALAT CC tablet. Three 30 mg ADALAT CC tablets, however, result in substantially higher C_{max} values than those after a single 90 mg ADALAT CC tablet. Three 30 mg tablets should, therefore, not be considered interchangeable with a 90 mg tablet.

Once daily dosing of ADALAT CC under fasting conditions results in decreased fluctuations in the plasma concentration of nifedipine when compared to t.i.d. dosing with immediate release nifedipine capsules. The mean peak plasma concentration of nifedipine following a 90 mg ADALAT CC tablet, administered under fasting conditions, is approximately 115 ng/mL. When ADALAT CC is given immediately after a high fat meal in healthy volunteers, there is an average increase of 60% in the peak plasma nifedipine concentration, a prolongation in the time to peak concentration, but no significant change in the AUC. Plasma concentrations of nifedipine when ADALAT CC is taken after a fatty meal result in slightly lower peaks compared to the same daily dose of the immediate release formulation administered in three divided doses. This may be, in part, because ADALAT CC is less bioavailable than the immediate release formulation.

Nifedipine is extensively metabolized to highly water soluble, inactive metabolites accounting for 60% to 80% of the dose excreted in the urine. Only traces (less than 0.1% of the dose) of the unchanged form can be detected in the urine. The remainder is excreted in the feces in metabolized form, most likely as a result of biliary excretion.

No studies have been performed with ADALAT CC in patients with renal failure; however, significant alterations in the pharmacokinetics of nifedipine immediate release capsules have not been reported in patients undergoing hemodialysis or chronic ambulatory peritoneal dialysis. Since the absorption of nifedipine from ADALAT CC could be modified by renal disease, caution should be exercised in treating such patients.

Because hepatic biotransformation is the predominant route for the disposition of nifedipine, its pharmacokinetics may be altered in patients with chronic liver disease. ADALAT CC has not been studied in patients with hepatic disease; however, in patients with hepatic impairment (liver cirrhosis) nifedipine has a longer elimination half-life and higher bioavailability than in healthy volunteers.

The degree of protein binding of nifedipine is high (92%–98%). Protein binding may be greatly reduced in patients with renal or hepatic impairment.

After administration of ADALAT CC to healthy elderly men and women (age > 60 years), the mean C_{max} is 36% higher and the average plasma concentration is 70% greater than in younger patients.

Clinical Studies: ADALAT CC produced dose-related decreases in systolic and diastolic blood pressure as demonstrated in two double-blind, randomized, placebo-controlled trials in which over 350 patients were treated with ADALAT CC 30, 60 or 90mg once daily for 6 weeks. In the first study, ADALAT CC was given as monotherapy and in the second study, ADALAT CC was added to a beta-blocker in patients not controlled on a beta-blocker alone. The mean trough (24 hours post-dose) blood pressure results from these studies are shown below:

MEAN REDUCTIONS IN TROUGH SUPINE BLOOD PRESSURE (mmHg) SYSTOLIC/DIASTOLIC

STUDY 1

ADALAT CC DOSE	N	MEAN TROUGH REDUCTION*
30 MG	60	5.3/2.9
60 MG	57	8.0/4.1
90 MG	55	12.5/8.1

STUDY 2

ADALAT CC DOSE	N	MEAN TROUGH REDUCTION*
30 MG	58	7.6/3.8
60 MG	63	10.1/5.3
90 MG	62	10.2/5.8

*Placebo response subtracted.

The trough/peak ratios estimated from 24 hour blood pressure monitoring ranged from 41%–78% for diastolic and 46%–91% for systolic blood pressure.

Hemodynamics: Like other slow-channel blockers, nifedipine exerts a negative inotropic effect on isolated myocardial tissue. This is rarely, if ever, seen in intact animals or man, probably because of reflex responses to its vasodilating effects. In man, nifedipine decreases peripheral vascular resistance which leads to a fall in systolic and diastolic pressures, usually minimal in normotensive volunteers (less than 5–10 mm Hg systolic), but sometimes larger. With ADALAT CC, these decreases in blood pressure are not accompanied by any significant change in heart rate. Hemodynamic studies of the immediate release nifedipine formulation in patients with normal ventricular function have generally found a small increase in cardiac index without major effects on ejection fraction, left ventricular end-diastolic pressure (LVEDP) or volume (LVEDV). In patients with impaired ventricular function, most acute studies have shown some increase in ejection fraction and reduction in left ventricular filling pressure.

Electrophysiologic Effects: Although, like other members of its class, nifedipine causes a slight depression of sinoatrial node function and atrioventricular conduction in isolated myocardial preparations, such effects have not been seen in studies in intact animals or in man. In formal electrophysiologic studies, predominantly in patients with normal conduction systems, nifedipine administered as the immediate release capsule has had no tendency to prolong atrioventricular conduction or sinus node recovery time, or to slow sinus rate.

INDICATION AND USAGE

ADALAT CC is indicated for the treatment of hypertension. It may be used alone or in combination with other antihypertensive agents.

CONTRAINDICATIONS

Known hypersensitivity to nifedipine.

WARNINGS

Excessive Hypotension: Although in most patients the hypotensive effect of nifedipine is modest and well tolerated, occasional patients have had excessive and poorly tolerated hypotension. These responses have usually occurred during initial titration or at the time of subsequent upward dosage adjustment, and may be more likely in patients using concomitant beta-blockers.

Severe hypotension and/or increased fluid volume requirements have been reported in patients who received immediate release capsules together with a beta-blocking agent and who underwent coronary artery bypass surgery using high dose fentanyl anesthesia. The interaction with high dose fentanyl appears to be due to the combination of nifedipine and a beta-blocker, but the possibility that it may occur with nifedipine alone, with low doses of fentanyl, in other surgical procedures, or with other narcotic analgesics cannot be ruled out. In nifedipine-treated patients where surgery using high dose fentanyl anesthesia is contemplated, the physician should be aware of these potential problems and, if the patient's condition permits, sufficient time (at least 36 hours) should be allowed for nifedipine to be washed out of the body prior to surgery.

Increased Angina and/or Myocardial Infarction: Rarely, patients, particularly those who have severe obstructive coronary artery disease, have developed well documented increased frequency, duration and/or severity of angina or acute myocardial infarction upon starting nifedipine or at the time of dosage increase. The mechanism of this effect is not established.

Beta-Blocker Withdrawal: When discontinuing a beta-blocker it is important to taper its dose, if possible, rather than stopping abruptly before beginning nifedipine. Patients recently withdrawn from beta blockers may develop a withdrawal syndrome with increased angina, probably related to increased sensitivity to catecholamines. Initiation of nifedipine treatment will not prevent this occurrence and on occasion has been reported to increase it.

Congestive Heart Failure: Rarely, patients (usually while receiving a beta-blocker) have developed heart failure after beginning nifedipine. Patients with tight aortic stenosis may be at greater risk for such an event, as the unloading effect of nifedipine would be expected to be of less benefit to these patients, owing to their fixed impedance to flow across the aortic valve.

PRECAUTIONS

General—Hypotension: Because nifedipine decreases peripheral vascular resistance, careful monitoring of blood pressure during the initial administration and titration of ADALAT CC is suggested. Close observation is especially recommended for patients already taking medications that are known to lower blood pressure (See WARNINGS).

Peripheral Edema: Mild to moderate peripheral edema occurs in a dose-dependent manner with ADALAT CC. The placebo subtracted rate is approximately 8% at 30 mg, 12% at 60 mg and 19% at 90 mg daily. This edema is a localized

phenomenon, thought to be associated with vasodilation of dependent arterioles and small blood vessels and not due to left ventricular dysfunction or generalized fluid retention. With patients whose hypertension is complicated by congestive heart failure, care should be taken to differentiate this peripheral edema from the effects of increasing left ventricular dysfunction.

Information for Patients: ADALAT CC is an extended release tablet and should be swallowed whole and taken on an empty stomach. It should not be administered with food. Do not chew, divide or crush tablets.

Laboratory Tests: Rare, usually transient, but occasionally significant elevations of enzymes such as alkaline phosphatase, CPK, LDH, SGOT, and SGPT have been noted. The relationship to nifedipine therapy is uncertain in most cases, but probable in some. These laboratory abnormalities have rarely been associated with clinical symptoms; however, cholestasis with or without jaundice has been reported. A small increase (<5%) in mean alkaline phosphatase was noted in patients treated with ADALAT CC. This was an isolated finding and it rarely resulted in values which fell outside the normal range. Rare instances of allergic hepatitis have been reported with nifedipine treatment. In controlled studies, ADALAT CC did not adversely affect serum uric acid, glucose, cholesterol or potassium.

Nifedipine, like other calcium channel blockers, decreases platelet aggregation *in vitro*. Limited clinical studies have demonstrated a moderate but statistically significant decrease in platelet aggregation and increase in bleeding time in some nifedipine patients. This is thought to be a function of inhibition of calcium transport across the platelet membrane. No clinical significance for these findings has been demonstrated.

Positive direct Coombs' test with or without hemolytic anemia has been reported but a causal relationship between nifedipine administration and positivity of this laboratory test, including hemolysis, could not be determined.

Although nifedipine has been used safely in patients with renal dysfunction and has been reported to exert a beneficial effect in certain cases, rare reversible elevations in BUN and serum creatinine have been reported in patients with preexisting chronic renal insufficiency. The relationship to nifedipine therapy is uncertain in most cases but probable in some.

Drug Interactions: Beta-adrenergic blocking agents: (See WARNINGS).

ADALAT CC was well tolerated when administered in combination with a beta blocker in 187 hypertensive patients in a placebo-controlled clinical trial. However, there have been occasional literature reports suggesting that the combination of nifedipine and beta-adrenergic blocking drugs may increase the likelihood of congestive heart failure, severe hypotension, or exacerbation of angina in patients with cardiovascular disease.

Digitalis: Since there have been isolated reports of patients with elevated digoxin levels, and there is a possible interaction between digoxin and ADALAT CC, it is recommended that digoxin levels be monitored when initiating, adjusting, and discontinuing ADALAT CC to avoid possible over- or under-digitalization.

Coumarin Anticoagulants: There have been rare reports of increased prothrombin time in patients taking coumarin anticoagulants to whom nifedipine was administered. However, the relationship to nifedipine therapy is uncertain.

Quinidine: There have been rare reports of an interaction between quinidine and nifedipine (with a decreased plasma level of quinidine).

Cimetidine: Both the peak plasma level of nifedipine and the AUC may increase in the presence of cimetidine. Ranitidine produces smaller non-significant increases. This effect of cimetidine may be mediated by its known inhibition of hepatic cytochrome P-450, the enzyme system probably responsible for the first-pass metabolism of nifedipine. If nifedipine therapy is initiated in a patient currently receiving cimetidine, cautious titration is advised.

Carcinogenesis, Mutagenesis, Impairment of Fertility: Nifedipine was administered orally to rats for two years and was not shown to be carcinogenic. When given to rats prior to mating, nifedipine caused reduced fertility at a dose approximately 30 times the maximum recommended human dose. *In vivo* mutagenicity studies were negative.

Pregnancy: Pregnancy Category C. In rodents, rabbits and monkeys, nifedipine has been shown to have a variety of embryotoxic, placentotoxic and fetotoxic effects, including stunted fetuses (rats, mice and rabbits), digital anomalies (rats and rabbits), rib deformities (mice), cleft palate (mice), small placentas and underdeveloped chorionic villi (monkeys), embryonic and fetal deaths (rats, mice and rabbits), prolonged pregnancy (rats; not evaluated in other species), and decreased neonatal survival (rats; not evaluated in other species). On a mg/kg or mg/m^2 basis, some of the doses associated with these various effects are higher than the maximum recommended human dose and some are lower, but all are within an order of magnitude of it.

The digital anomalies seen in nifedipine-exposed rabbit pups are strikingly similar to those seen in pups exposed to phenytoin, and these are in turn similar to the phalangeal deformities that are the most common malformation seen in human children with *in utero* exposure to phenytoin.

There are no adequate and well-controlled studies in pregnant women. ADALAT CC should be used during pregnancy only if the potential benefit justifies the potential risk to the fetus.

Nursing Mothers: Nifedipine is excreted in human milk. Therefore, a decision should be made to discontinue nursing or to discontinue the drug, taking into account the importance of the drug to the mother.

ADVERSE EXPERIENCES

The incidence of adverse events during treatment with ADALAT CC in doses up to 90 mg daily were derived from multicenter placebo-controlled clinical trials in 370 hypertensive patients. Atenolol 50 mg once daily was used concomitantly in 187 of the 370 patients on ADALAT CC and in 64 of the 126 patients on placebo. All adverse events reported during ADALAT CC therapy were tabulated independently of their causal relationship to medication. The most common adverse event reported with ADALAT® CC was peripheral edema. This was dose related and the frequency was 18% on ADALAT CC 30 mg daily, 22% on ADALAT CC 60 mg daily and 29% on ADALAT CC 90 mg daily versus 10% on placebo.

Other common adverse events reported in the above placebo-controlled trials include:

Adverse Event	ADALAT CC (%) (n=370)	PLACEBO (%) (n=126)
Headache	19	13
Flushing/heat sensation	4	0
Dizziness	4	2
Fatigue/asthenia	4	4
Nausea	2	1
Constipation	1	0

Where the frequency of adverse events with ADALAT CC and placebo is similar, causal relationship cannot be established.

The following adverse events were reported with an incidence of 3% or less in daily doses up to 90 mg:

Body as a Whole/Systemic: chest pain, leg pain
Central Nervous System: paresthesia, vertigo
Dermatologic: rash
Gastrointestinal: constipation
Musculoskeletal: leg cramps
Respiratory: epistaxis, rhinitis
Urogenital: impotence, urinary frequency

Other adverse events reported with an incidence of less than 1.0% were:

Body as a Whole/Systemic: cellulitis, chills, facial edema, neck pain, pelvic pain, pain
Cardiovascular: atrial fibrillation, bradycardia, cardiac arrest, extrasystole, hypotension, palpitations, phlebitis, postural hypotension, tachycardia, cutaneous angiectases
Central Nervous System: anxiety, confusion, decreased libido, depression, hypertonia, insomnia, somnolence
Dermatologic: pruritus, sweating
Gastrointestinal: abdominal pain, diarrhea, dry mouth, dyspepsia, esophagitis, flatulence, gastrointestinal hemorrhage, vomiting
Hematologic: lymphadenopathy
Metabolic: gout, weight loss
Musculoskeletal: arthralgia, arthritis, myalgia
Respiratory: dyspnea, increased cough, rales, pharyngitis
Special Senses: abnormal vision, amblyopia, conjunctivitis, diplopia, tinnitus
Urogenital/Reproductive: kidney calculus, nocturia, breast engorgement

The following adverse events have been reported rarely in patients given nifedipine in other formulations: allergenic hepatitis, alopecia, anemia, arthritis with ANA (+), depression, erythromelalgia, exfoliative dermatitis, fever, gingival hyperplasia, gynecomastia, leukopenia, mood changes, muscle cramps, nervousness, paranoid syndrome, purpura, shakiness, sleep disturbances, syncope, taste perversion, thrombocytopenia, transient blindness at the peak plasma level, tremor and urticaria.

OVERDOSAGE

Experience with nifedipine overdosage is limited. Generally, overdosage with nifedipine leading to pronounced hypotension calls for active cardiovascular support including monitoring of cardiovascular and respiratory function, elevation of extremities, judicious use of calcium infusion, pressor agents and fluids. Clearance of nifedipine would be expected to be prolonged in patients with impaired liver function. Since nifedipine is highly protein bound, dialysis is not likely to be of any benefit; however, plasmapheresis may be beneficial.

There has been one reported case of massive overdosage with tablets of another extended release formulation of nifedipine. The main effects of ingestion of approximately 4800 mg of nifedipine in a young man attempting suicide as a result of cocaine-induced depression was initial dizziness, palpitations, flushing, and nervousness. Within several hours of ingestion, nausea, vomiting, and generalized edema developed. No significant hypotension was apparent at presentation, 18 hours post ingestion. Blood chemistry abnormalities consisted of a mild, transient elevation of serum creatinine, and modest elevations of LDH and CPK, but normal SGOT. Vital signs remained stable, no electrocardiographic abnormalities were noted and renal function returned to normal within 24 to 48 hours with routine supportive measures alone. No prolonged sequelae were observed.

The effect of a single 900 mg ingestion of nifedipine capsules in a depressed anginal patient on tricyclic antidepressants was loss of consciousness within 30 minutes of ingestion, and profound hypotension, which responded to calcium infusion, pressor agents, and fluid replacement. A variety of ECG abnormalities were seen in this patient with a history of bundle branch block, including sinus bradycardia and varying degrees of AV block. These dictated the prophylactic placement of a temporary ventricular pacemaker, but otherwise resolved spontaneously. Significant hyperglycemia was seen initially in this patient, but plasma glucose levels rapidly normalized without further treatment.

A young hypertensive patient with advanced renal failure ingested 280 mg of nifedipine capsules at one time, with resulting marked hypotension responding to calcium infusion and fluids. No AV conduction abnormalities, arrhythmias, or pronounced changes in heart rate were noted, nor was there any further deterioration in renal function.

DOSAGE AND ADMINISTRATION

Dosage should be adjusted according to each patient's needs. It is recommended that ADALAT CC be administered orally once daily on an empty stomach. ADALAT CC is an extended release dosage form and tablets should be swallowed whole, not bitten or divided. In general, titration should proceed over a 7–14 day period starting with 30 mg once daily. Upward titration should be based on therapeutic efficacy and safety. The usual maintenance dose is 30 mg to 60 mg once daily. Titration to doses above 90 mg daily is not recommended.

If discontinuation of ADALAT CC is necessary, sound clinical practice suggests that the dosage should be decreased gradually with close physician supervision.

Care should be taken when dispensing ADALAT CC to assure that the extended release dosage form has been prescribed.

HOW SUPPLIED

ADALAT CC extended release tablets are supplied as 30 mg, 60 mg, and 90 mg round film coated tablets. The different strengths can be identified as follows:

Strength	Color	Markings
30 mg	Pink	30 on one side and ADALAT CC on the other side
60 mg	Salmon	60 on one side and ADALAT CC on the other side
90 mg	Dark Red	90 on one side and ADALAT CC on the other side

ADALAT® CC Tablets are supplied in:

[See table at top of page.]

	Strength	NDC Code	
Bottles of 100	30 mg	0026-8841-51	Made in U.S.A.
	60 mg	0026-8851-51	Made in Germany
	90 mg	0026-8861-51	Made in Germany
Unit Dose	30 mg	0026-8841-48	Made in U.S.A.
Packages of 100	60 mg	0026-8851-48	Made in Germany
	90 mg	0026-8861-48	Made in Germany

The tablets should be protected from light and moisture and stored below 86°F (30°C). Dispense in tight, light-resistant containers.

Distributed by:
Bayer Corporation
Pharmaceutical Division
400 Morgan Lane
West Haven, CT 06516 USA
PD500025 6/95
 5387

Shown in Product Identification Guide, page 304

Continued on next page

Bayer Corporation—Cont.

BILTRICIDE® Tablets ℞
(praziquantel)

DESCRIPTION

BILTRICIDE® (praziquantel) is a trematodicide provided in tablet form for the oral treatment of schistosome infections and infections due to liver fluke.
BILTRICIDE® (praziquantel) is 2-(cyclohexylcarbonyl)-1,2,3,6,7, 11b-hexahydro-4H-pyrazino [2, 1-a] isoquinolin-4-one with the molecular formula; $C_{19}H_{24}N_2O_2$. The structural formula is as follows:

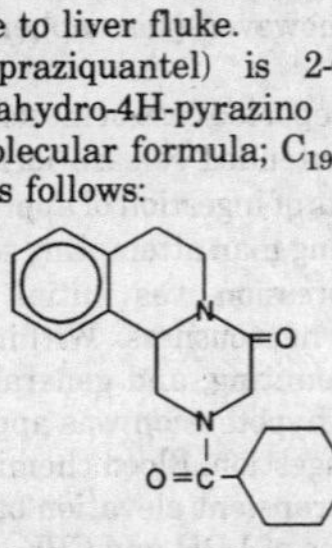

Praziquantel is a white to nearly white crystalline powder of bitter taste with a molecular weight of 312.41. The compound is stable under normal conditions and melts at 136–140°C with decomposition. The active substance is hygroscopic. Praziquantel is easily soluble in chloroform and dimethylsulfoxide, soluble in ethanol and very slightly soluble in water.
BILTRICIDE® tablets contain 600 mg of praziquantel. Inactive ingredients: corn starch, magnesium stearate, microcrystalline cellulose, povidone, sodium lauryl sulfate, polyethylene glycol, titanium dioxide and HPM cellulose.

CLINICAL PHARMACOLOGY

BILTRICIDE® induces a rapid contraction of schistosomes by a specific effect on the permeability of the cell membrane. The drug further causes vacuolization and disintegration of the schistosome tegument.
After oral administration BILTRICIDE® is rapidly absorbed (80%), subjected to a first pass effect, metabolized and eliminated by the kidneys. Maximal serum concentration is achieved 1–3 hours after dosing. The half-life of praziquantel in serum is 0.8–1.5 hours.

INDICATIONS AND USAGE

BILTRICIDE® is indicated for the treatment of infections due to: all species of schistosoma (e.g. *Schistosoma mekongi, Schistosoma japonicum, Schistosoma mansoni* and *Schistosoma hematobium),* and infections due to the liver flukes, *Clonorchis sinensis/Opisthorchis viverrini* (approval of this indication was based on studies in which the two species were not differentiated).

CONTRAINDICATIONS

BILTRICIDE® should not be given to patients who previously have shown hypersensitivity to the drug. Since parasite destruction within the eye may cause irreparable lesions, ocular cysticercosis should not be treated with this compound.

PRECAUTIONS

Information for the patient: Patients should be warned not to drive a car and not to operate machinery on the day of BILTRICIDE® treatment and the following day.
Minimal increases in liver enzymes have been reported in some patients.
When schistosomiasis or fluke infection is found to be associated with cerebral cysticercosis it is advised to hospitalize the patient for the duration of treatment.
Drug Interactions: No data are available regarding interaction of BILTRICIDE® with other drugs.
Mutagenesis, Carcinogenesis: Mutagenic effects in Salmonella tests found by one laboratory have not been confirmed in the same tested strain by other laboratories. Long term carcinogenicity studies in rats and golden hamsters did not reveal any carcinogenic effect.
Pregnancy Category B: Reproduction studies have been performed in rats and rabbits at doses up to 40 times the human dose and have revealed no evidence of impaired fertility or harm to the fetus due to BILTRICIDE® . There are, however, no adequate and well-controlled studies in pregnant women. An increase of the abortion rate was found in rats at three times the single human therapeutic dose. While animal reproduction studies are not always predictive of human response, this drug should be used during pregnancy only if clearly needed.
Nursing mothers: BILTRICIDE® appeared in the milk of nursing women at a concentration of about ¼ that of maternal serum. Women should not nurse on the day of BILTRICIDE® treatment and during the subsequent 72 hours.
Pediatric use: Safety in children under 4 years of age has not been established.

ADVERSE EFFECTS

In general BILTRICIDE® is very well tolerated. Side effects are usually mild and transient and do not require treatment. The following side effects were observed generally in order of severity: malaise, headache, dizziness, abdominal discomfort with or without nausea, rise in temperature and, rarely, urticaria. Such symptoms can, however, also result from the infection itself. Such side effects may be more frequent and/or serious in patients with a heavy worm burden. In patients with liver impairment caused by the infection, no adverse effects of BILTRICIDE® have occurred which would necessitate restriction in use.

OVERDOSAGE

In rats and mice the acute LD_{50} was about 2,500 mg/kg. No data are available in humans. In the event of overdose a fast-acting laxative should be given.

DOSAGE AND ADMINISTRATION

The dosage recommended for the treatment of schistosomiasis is: 3 × 20 mg/kg bodyweight as a one day treatment. The recommended dose for clonorchiasis and opisthorchiasis is: 3 × 25 mg/kg as a one day treatment. The tablets should be washed down unchewed with some liquid during meals. Keeping the tablets or segments thereof in the mouth can reveal a bitter taste which can promote gagging or vomiting. The interval between the individual doses should not be less than 4 and not more than 6 hours.

HOW SUPPLIED

BILTRICIDE® is supplied as a 600 mg white to orange tinged, filmcoated, oblong tablets with three scores. When broken each of the four segments contain 150 mg of active ingredient so that the dosage can be easily adjusted to the patient's bodyweight.
Segments are broken off by pressing the score (notch) with thumbnails. If ¼ of a tablet is required, this is best achieved by breaking the segment from the outer end.
BILTRICIDE® is available in bottles of 6 tablets.

	Strength	NDC	Tablet ID
Bottles of 6:	600 mg	0026-2521-06	521

Store below 86°F (30°C).
Bayer Corporation
Pharmaceutical Division
400 Morgan Lane
West Haven, CT 06516 USA
Made in Germany
Caution: Federal (USA) law prohibits dispensing without a prescription.
PD500021 5/95 EMBAY 8440 5235

Shown in Product Identification Guide, page 305

CIPRO® ℞
(ciprofloxacin hydrochloride)
TABLETS

DESCRIPTION

Cipro® (ciprofloxacin hydrochloride) is a synthetic broad spectrum antibacterial agent for oral administration. Ciprofloxacin, a fluoroquinolone, is available as the monohydrochloride monohydrate salt of 1-cyclopropyl-6-fluoro-1, 4-dihydro-4-oxo-7-(1-piperazinyl)-3-quinolinecarboxylic acid. It is a faintly yellowish to light yellow crystalline substance with a molecular weight of 385.8. Its empirical formula is $C_{17}H_{18}FN_3O_3 \cdot HCl \cdot H_2O$ and its chemical structure is as follows:

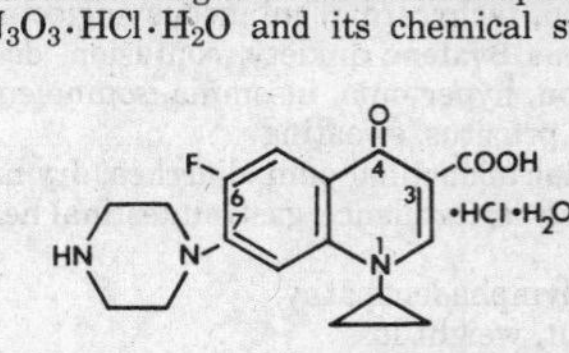

Cipro® is available in 100-mg, 250-mg, 500-mg and 750-mg (ciprofloxacin equivalent) film-coated tablets. The inactive ingredients are starch, microcrystalline cellulose, silicon dioxide, crospovidone, magnesium stearate, hydroxypropyl methylcellulose, titanium dioxide, polyethylene glycol and water. Ciprofloxacin differs from other quinolones in that it has a fluorine atom at the 6-position, a piperazine moiety at the 7-position, and a cyclopropyl ring at the 1-position.

CLINICAL PHARMACOLOGY

Cipro® tablets are rapidly and well absorbed from the gastrointestinal tract after oral administration. The absolute bioavailability is approximately 70% with no substantial loss by first pass metabolism. Ciprofloxacin maximum serum concentrations and area under the curve are shown in the chart for the 250-mg to 1000-mg dose range.

Dose (mg)	Maximum Serum Concentration (µg/mL)	Area Under Curve (AUC) (µg · hr/mL)
250	1.2	4.8
500	2.4	11.6
750	4.3	20.2
1000	5.4	30.8

Maximum serum concentrations are attained 1 to 2 hours after oral dosing. Mean concentrations 12 hours after dosing with 250, 500, or 750-mg are 0.1, 0.2, and 0.4 µg/mL, respectively. The serum elimination half-life in subjects with normal renal function is approximately 4 hours. Serum concentratrions increase proportionately with doses up to 1000-mg.
Approximately 40 to 50% of an orally administered dose is excreted in the urine as unchanged drug. After a 250-mg oral dose, urine concentrations of ciprofloxacin usually exceed 200 µg/mL during the first two hours and are approximately 30 µg/mL at 8 to 12 hours after dosing. The urinary excretion of ciprofloxacin is virtually complete within 24 hours after dosing. The renal clearance of ciprofloxacin, which is approximately 300 mL/minute, exceeds the normal glomerular filtration rate of 120 mL/minute. Thus, active tubular secretion would seem to play a significant role in its elimination. Co-administration of probenecid with ciprofloxacin results in about a 50% reduction in the ciprofloxacin renal clearance and a 50% increase in its concentration in the systemic circulation. Although bile concentrations of ciprofloxacin are several fold higher than serum concentrations after oral dosing, only a small amount of the dose administered is recovered from the bile as unchanged drug. An additional 1 to 2% of the dose is recovered from the bile in the form of metabolites. Approximately 20 to 35% of an oral dose is recovered from the feces within 5 days after dosing. This may arise from either biliary clearance or transintestinal elimination. Four metabolites have been identified in human urine which together account for approximately 15% of an oral dose. The metabolites have antimicrobial activity, but are less active than unchanged ciprofloxacin.
When Cipro® is given concomitantly with food, there is a delay in the absorption of the drug, resulting in peak concentrations that occur closer to 2 hours after dosing rather than 1 hour. The overall absorption, however, is not substantially affected. Concurrent administration of antacids containing magnesium hydroxide or aluminum hydroxide may reduce the bioavailability of ciprofloxacin by as much as 90% (See PRECAUTIONS).
Concomitant administration of ciprofloxacin with theophylline decreases the clearance of theophylline resulting in elevated serum theophylline levels and increased risk of a patient developing CNS or other adverse reactions. Ciprofloxacin also decreases caffeine clearance and inhibits the formation of paraxanthine after caffeine administration. (See PRECAUTIONS).
In patients with reduced renal function, the half-life of ciprofloxacin is slightly prolonged. Dosage adjustments may be required (See DOSAGE AND ADMINISTRATION).
In preliminary studies in patients with stable chronic liver cirrhosis, no significant changes in ciprofloxacin pharmacokinetics have been observed. The kinetics of ciprofloxacin in patients with acute hepatic insufficiency, however, have not been fully elucidated.
The binding of ciprofloxacin to serum proteins is 20 to 40% which is not likely to be high enough to cause significant protein binding interactions with other drugs.
After oral administration, ciprofloxacin is widely distributed throughout the body. Tissue concentrations often exceed serum concentrations in both men and women, particularly in genital tissue including the prostate. Ciprofloxacin is present in active form in the saliva, nasal and bronchial secretions, sputum, skin blister fluid, lymph, peritoneal fluid, bile, and prostatic secretions. Ciprofloxacin has also been detected in lung, skin, fat, muscle, cartilage, and bone. The drug diffuses into the cerebrospinal fluid (CSF); however, CSF concentrations are generally less than 10% of peak serum concentrations. Low levels of the drug have been detected in the aqueous and vitreous humors of the eye.

Microbiology: Ciprofloxacin has *in vitro* activity against a wide range of gram-negative and gram-positive organisms. The bactericidal action of ciprofloxacin results from interference with the enzyme DNA gyrase which is needed for the synthesis of bacterial DNA.
Ciprofloxacin has been shown to be active against most strains of the following microorganisms both *in vitro* and in clinical infections as described in the **INDICATIONS AND USAGE** section

Aerobic gram-positive

Enterococcus faecalis (Many strains are only moderately susceptible)	*Staphylococcus epidermidis*
Staphylococcus aureus (methicillin susceptible)	*Staphylococcus saprophyticus*
	Streptococcus pneumoniae
	Streptococcus pyogenes

Aerboic gram-negative

Campylobacter jejuni	*Proteus mirabilis*
Citrobacter diversus	*Proteus vulgaris*
Citrobacter freundii	*Providencia rettgeri*
Enterobacter cloacae	*Providencia stuartii*
Escherichia coli	*Pseudomonas aeruginosa*
Haemophilus influenzae	*Salmonella typhi*
Haemophilus parainfluenzae	*Serratia marcensens*

Klebsiella pneumoniae	*Shigella flexneri*
Morganella morganii	*Shigella sonnei*
Neisseria gonorrhoeae	

The following *in vitro* data are available, **but their clinical significance is unknown.**

Ciprofloxacin exhibits *in vitro* minimal inhibitory concentrations (MIC's) of ≤1 μg/mL against most (≥90%) strains of the following microorganisms; however, the safety and effectiveness of ciprofloxacin in treating clinical infections due to these microorganisms have not been established in adequate and well-controlled clinical trials.

Aerobic gram-positive
Staphylococcus haemolyticus
Staphylococcus hominis

Aerobic gram-negative

Acinetobacter Iwoffi	*Moraxella catarrhalis*
Aeromonas caviae	*Neisseria meningitidis*
Aeromonas hydrophila	*Pasteurella multocida*
Brucella melitensis	*Salmonella enteritidis*
Campylobacter coli	*Vibrio cholerae*
Edwardsiella tarda	*Vibrio parahaemolyticus*
Haemophilus ducreyi	*Vibrio vulnificus*
Klebsiella oxytoca	*Yersinia enterocolitica*
Legionella penumophila	

Other
Chlamydia trachomatis (moderately susceptible)
Mycobacterium tuberculosis (moderately susceptible)

Most strains of *Burkholderia cepacia* and some strains of *Stenotrophomonas maltophilia* are resistant to ciprofloxacin as are most anaerobic bacteria, including *Bacteroides fragilis* and *Clostridium difficile*.

Ciprofloxacin is slightly less active when tested at acidic pH. The inoculum size has little effect when tested *in vitro*. The minimal bactericidal concentration (MBC) generally does not exceed the minimal inhibitory concentration (MIC) by more than a factor of 2. Resistance to ciprofloxacin *in vitro* develops slowly (multiple-step mutation).

Ciprofloxacin does not cross-react with other antimicrobial agents such as beta-lactams or aminoglycosides; therefore, organisms resistant to these drugs may be susceptible to ciprofloxacin.

In vitro studies have shown that additive activity often results when ciprofloxacin is combined with other antimicrobial agents such as beta-lactams, aminoglycosides, clindamycin, or metronidazole. Synergy has been reported particularly with the combination of ciprofloxacin and a beta-lactam; antagonism is observed only rarely.

Susceptibility Tests

Diffusion Techniques: Quantitative methods are used to determine antimicrobial minimal inhibitory concentrations (MIC's). These MIC's provide estimates of the susceptibility of bacteria to antimicrobial compounds. The MIC's should be determined using a standardized procedure. Standardized procedures are based on a dilution method[1] (broth or agar) or equivalent with standardized inoculum concentrations and standardized concentrations of ciprofloxacin power. The MIC values should be interpreted according to the following criteria:

MIC (μg/mL)	Interpretation
≤1	Susceptible (S)
2	Intermediate (I)
≥4	Resistant (R)

A report of "Susceptible" indicates that the pathogen is likely to be inhibited if the antimicrobial compound in the blood reaches the concentrations usually achieveable. A report of "Intermediate" indicates that the result should be considered equivocal, and, if the microorganism is not fully susceptible to alternative, clinically feasible drugs, the test should be repeated. This category implies possible clinical applicability in body sites where the drug is physiologically concentrated or in situations where high dosage of drug can be used.. This category also provides a buffer zone which prevents small uncontrolled technical factors from causing major discrepancies in interpretation. A report of "Resistant" indicates that the pathogen is not likely to be inhibited if the antimicrobial compound in the blood reaches the concentrations usually achievable; other therapy should be selected.

Standardized susceptibility test procedures require the use of laboratory control microorganisms to control the technical aspects of the laboratory procedures. Standard ciprofloxacin powder should provide the following MIC values:

Organism		MIC (μg/mL)
E. coli	ATCC 25922	0.004–0.015
E. faecalis	ATCC 29212	0.25–2.0
P. aeruginosa	ATCC 27853	0.25–1.0
S. aureus	ATCC 29213	0.12–0.5

Diffusion Techniques: Quantitative methods that require measurement of zone diameters also provide reproducible estimates of the susceptibility of bacteria to antimicrobial compounds. One such standardized procedure[2] requires the use of standardized inoculum concentrations. This procedure uses paper disks impregnated with 5-μg ciprofloxacin to test the susceptibility of microorganisms to ciprofloxacin.

Reports from the laboratory providing results of the standardized single-disk susceptibility test with a 5-μg ciprofloxacin disk should be interpreted according to the following criteria:

Zone Diameter (mm)	Interpretation
≥21	Susceptible (S)
16–20	Intermediate (I)
≤15	Resistant (R)

Interpretation should be as stated above for results using dilution techniques. Interpretation involves correlation of the diameter obtained in the disk test with the MIC for ciprofloxacin.

As with standardized dilution techniques, diffusion methods require the use of laboratory control microorganisms that are used to control the technical aspects of the laboratory procedures. For the diffusion technique, the 5-μg ciprofloxacin disk should provide the following zone diameters in these laboratory test quality control strains:

Organism		Zone Diameter (mm)
E. coli	ATCC 25922	30–40 mm
P. aeruginosa	ATCC 27853	25–33 mm
S. aureus	ATCC 25923	22–30 mm

INDICATIONS AND USAGE

Cipro® is indicated for the treatment of infections caused by susceptible strains of the designated microorganisms in the conditions listed below. Please see DOSAGE AND ADMINISTRATION for specific recommendations.

Lower Respiratory Infections caused by *Escherichia coli, Klebsiella pneumoniae, Enterobacter cloacae, Proteus mirabilis, Pseudomonas aeruginosa, Haemophilus influenzae, Haemophilus parainfluenzae,* or *Streptococcus pneumoniae.*

NOTE: Although effective in clinical trials, ciprofloxacin is not a drug of first choice in the treatment of presumed or confirmed pneumonia secondary to *Streptococcus pneumoniae.*

Skin and Skin Structure Infections caused by *Escherichia coli, Klebsiella pneumoniae, Enterobacter cloacae, Proteus mirabilis, Proteus vulgaris, Providencia stuartii, Morganella morganii, Citrobacter freundii, Pseudomonas aeruginosa, Staphylococcus aureus,* (methicillin susceptible), *Staphylococcus epidermidis,* or *Streptococcus pyogenes.*

Bone and Joint Infections caused by *Enterobacter cloacae, Serratia marcescens,* or *Pseudomonas aeruginosa.*

Urinary Tract Infections caused by *Escherichia coli, Klebsiella pneumoniae, Enterobacter cloacae, Serratia marcescens, Proteus mirabilis, Providencia rettgeri, Morganella morganii, Citrobacter diversus, Citrobacter freundii, Pseudomonas aeruginosa, Staphylococcus epidermidis, Staphylococcus saprophyticus,* or *Enterococcus faecalis.*

Acute Uncomplicatd Cystitis in females caused by *Escherichia coli,* or *Staphylococcus saprophyticus.* (See DOSAGE AND ADMINISTRATION.)

Typhoid Fever (Enteric Fever) caused by *Salmonella typhi.*

NOTE: The efficacy of ciprofloxacin in the eradication of the chronic typhoid carrier state has not been demonstrated.

Sexually Transmitted Diseases (See WARNINGS.)

Uncomplicated cervical and urethral gonorrhea due to *Neisseria gonorrhoeae.*

Infectious Diarrhea caused by *Escherichia coli* (enterotoxigenic strains), *Campylobacter jejuni, Shigella flexneri** or *Shigella sonnei** when antibacterial therapy is indicated.

*Although treatment of infections due to this organism in this organ system demonstrated a clinically significant outcome, efficacy was studied in fewer than 10 patients.

If anaerobic organisms are suspected of contributing to the infection, appropriate therapy should be administered.

Appropriate culture and susceptibility tests should be performed before treatment in order to isolate and identify organisms causing infection and to determine their susceptibility to ciprofloxacin. Therapy with Cipro® may be initiated before results of these tests are known; once results become available appropriate therapy should be continued.

As with other drugs, some strains of *Pseudomonas aeruginosa* may develop resistance fairly rapidly during treatment with ciprofloxacin. Culture and susceptibility testing performed periodically during therapy will provide information not only on the therapeutic effect of the antimicrobial agent but also on the possible emergence of bacterial resistance.

CONTRAINDICATIONS

Cipro® (ciprofloxacin hydrochloride) is contraindicated in persons with a history of hypersensitivity to ciprofloxacin or any member of the quinolone class of antimicrobial agents.

WARNINGS

THE SAFETY AND EFFECTIVENESS OF CIPROFLOXACIN IN CHILDREN, ADOLESCENTS (LESS THAN 18 YEARS OF AGE), PREGNANT WOMEN, AND LACTATING WOMEN HAVE NOT BEEN ESTABLISHED. (SEE PRECAUTIONS—PEDIATRIC USE, PREGNANCY AND NURSING MOTHERS SUBSECTIONS.) The oral administration of ciprofloxacin caused lameness in immature dogs. Histopathological examination of the weight-bearing joints of these dogs revealed permanent lesions of the cartilage. Related quinolone-class drugs also produce erosions of cartilage of weight-bearing joints and other signs of arthropathy in immature animals of various species. (See ANIMAL PHARMACOLOGY.)

Convulsions have been reported in patients receiving ciprofloxacin. Convulsions, increased intracranial pressure, and toxic psychosis have been reported in patients receiving drugs in this class. Quinolones may also cause central nervous system (CNS) stimulation which may lead to tremors, restlessness, lightheadedness, confusion and hallucinations. If these reactions occur in patients receiving ciprofloxacin, the drug should be discontinued and appropriate measures instituted. As with all quinolones, ciprofloxacin should be used with caution in patients with known or suspected CNS disorders, such as severe cerebral arteriosclerosis, epilepsy, and other factors that predispose to seizures. (See ADVERSE REACTIONS.)

SERIOUS AND FATAL REACTIONS HAVE BEEN REPORTED IN PATIENTS RECEIVING CONCURRENT ADMINISTRATION OF CIPROFLOXACIN AND THEOPHYLLINE. These reactions have included cardiac arrest, seizure, status epilepticus and respiratory failure. Although similar serious adverse effects have been reported in patients receiving theophylline alone, the possibility that these reactions may be potentiated by ciprofloxacin cannot be eliminated. If concomitant use cannot be avoided, serum levels of theophylline should be monitored and dosage adjustments made as appropriate.

Serious and occasionally fatal hypersensitivity (anaphylactic) reactions, some following the first dose, have been reported in patients receiving quinolone therapy. Some reactions were accompanied by cardiovascular collapse, loss of consciousness, tingling, pharyngeal or facial edema, dyspnea, urticaria, and itching. Only a few patients had a history of hypersensitivity reactions. Serious anaphylactic reactions require immediate emergency treatment with epinephrine. Oxygen, intravenous steroids, and airway management, including intubation, should be administered as indicated.

Severe hypersensitivity reactions characterized by rash, fever, eosinophilia, jaundice, and hepatic necrosis with fatal outcome have also been rarely reported in patients receiving ciprofloxacin along with other drugs. The possibility that these reactions were related to ciprofloxacin cannot be excluded. Ciprofloxacin should be discontinued at the first appearance of a skin rash or any other sign of hypersensitivity.

Pseudomembranous colitis has been reported with nearly all antibacterial agents, including ciprofloxacin, and may range in severity from mild to life-threatening. Therefore, it is important to consider this diagnosis in patients who present with diarrhea subsequent to the administration of antibacterial agents.

Treatment with antibacterial agents alters the normal flora of the colon and may permit overgrowth of clostridia. Studies indicate that a toxin produced by *Clostridium difficile* is one primary cause of "antibiotic-associated colitis."

After the diagnosis of pseudomembranous colitis has been established, therapeutic measures should be initiated. Mild cases of pseudomembranous colitis usually respond to drug discontinuation alone. In moderate to severe cases, consideration should be given to management with fluids and electrolytes, protein supplementation and treatment with an antibacterial drug clinically effective against *C. difficile* colitis.

Achilles and other tendon ruptures that required surgical repair or resulted in prolonged disability have been reported with ciprofloxacin and other quinolones. Ciprofloxacin should be discontinued if the patient experiences pain, inflammation, or rupture of a tendon.

Ciprofloxacin has not been shown to be effective in the treatment of syphilis. Antimicrobial agents used in high dose for short periods of time to treat gonorrhea may mask or delay the symptoms of incubating syphilis. All patients with gonorrhea should have a serologic test for syphilis at the time of diagnosis. Patients treated with ciprofloxacin should have a follow-up serologic test for syphilis after three months.

PRECAUTIONS

General: Crystals of ciprofloxacin have been observed rarely in the urine of human subjects but more frequently in the urine of laboratory animals, which is usually alkaline. (See ANIMAL PHARMACOLOGY.) Crystalluria related to ciprofloxacin has been reported only rarely in humans because human urine is usually acidic. Alkalinity of the urine should be avoided in patients receiving ciprofloxacin. Patients should be well hydrated to prevent the formation of highly concentrated urine.

Alteration of the dosage regimen is necessary for patients with impairment of renal function. (See DOSAGE AND ADMINISTRATION.)

Continued on next page

Bayer Corporation—Cont.

Moderate to severe phototoxicity manifested as an exaggerated sunburn reaction has been observed in patients who are exposed to direct sunlight while receiving some members of the quinolone class of drugs. Excessive sunlight should be avoided. Therapy should be discontinued if phototoxicity occurs.

As with any potent drug, periodic assessment of organ system functions, including renal, hepatic, and hematopoietic function, is advisable during prolonged therapy.

Information for Patients: Patients should be advised that ciprofloxacin may be taken with or without meals. The preferred time of dosing is two hours after a meal. Patients should also be advised to drink fluids liberally and not take antacids containing magnesium, aluminum, or calcium, products containing iron, or multivitamins containing zinc. However, usual dietary intake of calcium has not been shown to alter the absorption of ciprofloxacin.

Patients should be advised that ciprofloxacin may be associated with hypersensitivity reactions, even following a single dose, and to discontinue the drug at the first sign of a skin rash or other allergic reaction.

Patients should be advised to avoid excessive sunlight or artificial ultraviolet light while receiving ciprofloxacin and to discontinue therapy if phototoxicity occurs.

Patients should be advised to discontinue treatment; rest and refrain from exercise; and inform their physician if they experience pain, inflammation, or rupture of a tendon.

Ciprofloxacin may cause dizziness and lightheadedness; therefore, patients should know how they react to this drug before they operate an automobile or machinery or engage in activities requiring mental alertness or coordination.

Patients should be advised that ciprofloxacin may increase the effects of theophylline and caffeine. There is a possibility of caffeine accumulation when products containing caffeine are consumed while taking quinolones.

Drug Interactions: As with some other quinolones, concurrent administration of ciprofloxacin with theophylline may lead to elevated serum concentrations of theophylline and prolongation of its elimination half-life. This may result in increased risk of theophylline-related adverse reactions. (See WARNINGS.) If concomitant use cannot be avoided, serum levels of theophylline should be monitored and dosage adjustments made as appropriate.

Some quinolones, including ciprofloxacin, have also been shown to interfere with the metabolism of caffeine. This may lead to reduced clearance of caffeine and a prolongation of its serum half-life.

Concurrent administration of ciprofloxacin with antacids containing magnesium, aluminum, or calcium; with sucralfate or divalent and trivalent cations such as iron may substantially interfere with the absorption of ciprofloxacin, resulting in serum and urine levels considerably lower than desired. To a lesser extent this effect is demonstrated with zinc-containing multivitamins. (See DOSAGE AND ADMINISTRATION for concurrent administration of these agents with ciprofloxacin.)

Altered serum levels of phenytoin (increased and decreased) have been reported in patients receiving concomitant ciprofloxacin.

The concomitant administration of ciprofloxacin with the sulfonylurea glyburide has, on rare occasions, resulted in severe hypoglycemia.

Some quinolones, including ciprofloxacin, have been associated with transient elevations in serum creatinine in patients receiving cyclosporine concomitantly.

Quinolones have been reported to enhance the effects of the oral anticoagulant warfarin or its derivatives. When these products are administered concomitantly, prothrombin time or other suitable coagulation tests should be closely monitored.

Probenecid interferes with renal tubular secretion of ciprofloxacin and produces an increase in the level of ciprofloxacin in the serum. This should be considered if patients are receiving both drugs concomitantly.

As with other broad spectrum antimicrobial agents, prolonged use of ciprofloxacin may result in overgrowth of non-susceptible organisms. Repeated evaluation of the patient's condition and microbial susceptibility testing is essential. If superinfection occurs during therapy, appropriate measures should be taken.

Carcinogenesis, Mutagenesis, Impairment of Fertility: Eight *in vitro* mutagenicity tests have been conducted with ciprofloxacin, and the test results are listed below:

Salmonella/Microsome Test (Negative)
E. coli DNA Repair Assay (Negative)
Mouse Lymphoma Cell Forward Mutation Assay (Positive)
Chinese Hamster V$_{79}$ Cell HGPRT Test (Negative)
Syrian Hamster Embryo Cell Transformation Assay (Negative)
Saccharomyces cerevisiae Point Mutation Assay (Negative)
Saccharomyces cerevisiae Mitotic Crossover and Gene Conversion Assay (Negative)
Rat Hepatocyte DNA Repair Assay (Positive)

Thus, 2 of the 8 tests were positive, but results of the following 3 *in vivo* test systems gave negative results:

Rat Hepatocyte DNA Repair Assay
Micronucleus Test (Mice)
Dominant Lethal Test (Mice)

Long term carcinogenicity studies in mice and rats have been completed. After daily oral dosing for up to 2 years, there was no evidence that ciprofloxacin had any carcinogenic or tumorigenic effects in these species.

Pregnancy: Teratogenic Effects. Pregnancy Category C: Reproduction studies have been performed in rats and mice at doses up to 6 times the usual daily human dose and have revealed no evidence of impaired fertility or harm to the fetus due to ciprofloxacin. In rabbits, as with most antimicrobial agents, ciprofloxacin (30 and 100 mg/kg orally) produced gastrointestinal disturbances resulting in maternal weight loss and an increased incidence of abortion. No teratogenicity was observed at either dose. After intravenous administration, at doses up to 20 mg/kg, no maternal toxicity was produced, and no embryotoxicity or teratogenicity was observed. There are, however, no adequate and well-controlled studies in pregnant women. Ciprofloxacin should be used during pregnancy only if the potential benefit justifies the potential risk to the fetus. (See WARNINGS.)

Nursing Mothers: Ciprofloxacin is excreted in human milk. Because of the potential for serious adverse reactions in infants nursing from mothers taking ciprofloxacin, a decision should be made either to discontinue nursing or to discontinue the drug, taking into account the importance of the drug to the mother.

Pediatric Use: Safety and effectiveness in children and adolescents less than 18 years of age have not been established. Ciprofloxacin causes arthropathy in juvenile animals. (See WARNINGS.)

ADVERSE REACTIONS

During clinical investigation, 2,799 patients received 2,868 courses of the drug. Adverse events that were considered likely to be drug related occurred in 7.3% of patients treated, possibly related in 9.2%, (total of 16.5% thought to be possibly or probably related to drug therapy), and remotely related in 3.0%. Ciprofloxacin was discontinued because of an adverse event in 3.5% of patients treated, primarily involving the gastrointestinal system (1.5%), skin (0.6%), and central nervous system (0.4%).

The most frequently reported events, drug related or not, were nausea (5.2%), diarrhea (2.3%), vomiting (2.0%), abdominal pain/discomfort (1.7%), headache (1.2%), restlessness (1.1%), and rash (1.1%).

Additional events that occurred in less than 1% of ciprofloxacin patients are listed below.

CARDIOVASCULAR: palpitation, atrial flutter, ventricular ectopy, syncope, hypertension, angina pectoris, myocardial infarction, cardiopulmonary arrest, cerebral thrombosis

CENTRAL NERVOUS SYSTEM: dizziness, lightheadedness, insomnia, nightmares, hallucinations, manic reaction, irritability, tremor, ataxia, convulsive seizures, lethargy, drowsiness, weakness, malaise, anorexia, phobia, depersonalization, depression, paresthesia (See above.) (See PRECAUTIONS.)

GASTROINTESTINAL: painful oral mucosa, oral candidiasis, dysphagia, intestinal perforation, gastrointestinal bleeding (See above.) Cholestatic jaundice has been reported

MUSCULOSKELETAL: arthralgia or back pain, joint stiffness, achiness, neck or chest pain, flare up of gout

RENAL/UROGENITAL: interstitial nephritis, nephritis, renal failure, polyuria, urinary retention, urethral bleeding, vaginitis, acidosis

RESPIRATORY: dyspnea, epistaxis, laryngeal or pulmonary edema, hiccough, hemoptysis, bronchospasm, pulmonary embolism

SKIN/HYPERSENSITIVITY: pruritus, urticaria, photosensitivity, flushing, fever, chills, angioedema, edema of the face, neck, lips, conjunctivae or hands, cutaneous candidiasis, hyperpigmentation, erythema nodosum (See above.)

Allergic reactions ranging from urticaria to anaphylactic reactions have been reported. (See WARNINGS).

SPECIAL SENSES: blurred vision, disturbed vision (change in color perception, overbrightness of lights), decreased visual acuity, diplopia, eye pain, tinnitus, hearing loss, bad taste.

Most of the adverse events reported were described as only mild or moderate in severity, abated soon after the drug was discontinued, and required no treatment.

In several instances nausea, vomiting, tremor, irritability, or palpitation were judged by investigators to be related to elevated serum levels of theophylline possibly as a result of drug interaction with ciprofloxacin.

In domestic clinical trials involving 214 patients receiving a single 250-mg oral dose, approximately 5% of patients reported adverse experiences without reference to drug relationship. The most common adverse experiences were vaginitis (2%), headache (1%), and vaginal pruritus (1%). Additional reactions, occurring in 0.3%–1% of patients, were abdominal discomfort, lymphadenopathy, foot pain, dizziness, and breast pain. Less than 20% of these patients had laboratory values obtained, and these results were generally consistent with the pattern noted for multi-dose therapy.

Post-Marketing Adverse Events: Additional adverse events, regardless of relationship to drug, reported from worldwide marketing experience with quinolones, including ciprofloxacin, are:

BODY AS A WHOLE: change in serum phenytoin
CARDIOVASCULAR: postural hypotension, vasculitis
CENTRAL NERVOUS SYSTEM: agitation, confusion, delirium, dysphasia, myocolonus, nystagmus, toxic psychosis
GASTROINTESTINAL: constipation, dyspepsia, flatulence, hepatic necrosis, juandice, pancreatitis, pseudomembranous colitis. (The onset of pseudomembranous colitis symptoms may occur during or after antimicrobial treatment.)
HEMIC/LYMPHATIC: agranulocytosis, hemolytic anemia, methemoglobinemia, prolongation of prothrombin time
METABOLIC/NUTRITIONAL: elevation of serum triglycerides, cholesterol, blood glucose, serum potassium
MUSCULOSKELETAL: myalgia, possible exacerbation of myasthenia gravis, tendinitis/tendon rupture
RENAL/UROGENITAL: albuminuria; candiduria, renal calculi, vaginal candidiasis
SKIN/HYPERSENSITIVITY: anaphylactic reactions, erythema multiforme/Stevens-Johnson syndrome, exfoliative dermatitis, toxic epidermal necrolysis
SPECIAL SENSES: anosmia
(See PRECAUTIONS.)

Adverse Laboratory Changes: Changes in laboratory parameters listed as adverse events without regard to drug relationship are listed below:

Hepatic—Elevations of ALT (SGPT) (1.9%), AST (SGOT) (1.7%), alkaline phosphatase (0.8%), LDH (0.4%), serum bilirubin (0.3%).

Hematologic—Eosinophilia (0.6%), leukopenia (0.4%), decreased blood platelets (0.1%), elevated blood platelets (0.1%), pancytopenia (0.1%).

Renal—Elevations of serum creatinine (1.1%), BUN (0.9%). CRYSTALLURIA, CYLINDRURIA AND HEMATURIA HAVE BEEN REPORTED.

Other changes occurring in less than 0.1% of courses were: elevation of serum gammaglutamyl transferase, elevation of serum amylase, reduction in blood glucose, elevated uric acid, decrease in hemoglobin, anemia, bleeding diathesis, increase in blood monocytes, leukocytosis.

OVERDOSAGE

In the event of acute overdosage, the stomach should be emptied by inducing vomiting or by gastric lavage. The patient should be carefully observed and given supportive treatment. Adequate hydration must be maintained. Only a small amount of ciprofloxacin (< 10%) is removed from the body after hemodialysis or peritoneal dialysis.

DOSAGE AND ADMINISTRATION

Severe/complicated urinary tract infections or urinary tract infections caused by organisms not highly susceptible to ciprofloxacin may be treated with 500-mg every 12 hours. For other mild/moderate urinary infections, the usual adult dosage is 250-mg every 12 hours.

In acute uncomplicated cystitis in females, the usual dosage is 100-mg every 12 hours. For acute uncomplicated cystitis in females, 3 days of treatment is recommended while 7 to 14 days is suggested for other mild/moderate, severe or complicated urinary tract infections.

Lower respiratory tract infections, skin and skin structure infections, and bone and joint infections may be treated with 500 mg every 12 hours. For more severe or complicated infections, a dosage of 750-mg may be given every 12 hours.

The recommended adult dosage for infectious diarrhea or typhoid fever is 500-mg every 12 hours. For the treatment of uncomplicated urethral and cervical gonococcal infections, a single 250-mg dose is recommended.

[See table at top of next page.]

The determination of dosage for any particular patient must take into consideration the severity and nature of the infection, the susceptibility of the causative organism, the integrity of the patient's host-defense mechanisms, and the status of renal function and hepatic function.

The duration of treatment depends upon the severity of infection. Generally ciprofloxacin should be continued for at least 2 days after the signs and symptoms of infection have disappeared. The usual duration is 7 to 14 days; however, for severe and complicated infections more prolonged therapy may be required. Bone and joint infections may require treatment for 4 to 6 weeks or longer. Infectious diarrhea may be treated for 5–7 days. Typhoid fever should be treated for 10 days.

DOSAGE GUIDELINES

Infection	Type or Severity	Unit Dose	Frequency	Usual Durations†
Urinary Tract	Acute Uncomplicated	100-mg	q 12 h	3 Days
	Mild/Moderate	250-mg	q 12 h	7 to 14 Days
	Severe/Complicated	500-mg	q 12 h	7 to 14 Days
Lower respiratory tract;	Mild/Moderate	500-mg	q 12 h	7 to 14 Days
Skin and Skin Structure	Severe/Complicated	750-mg	q 12 h	7 to 14 Days
Bone and Joint	Mild/Moderate	500-mg	q 12 h	≥ 4 to 6 weeks
	Severe/Complicated	750-mg	q 12 h	≥ 4 to 6 weeks
Infectious Diarrhea	Mild/Moderate/Severe	500-mg	q 12 h	5 to 7 Days
Typhoid Fever	Mild/Moderate	500-mg	q 12 h	10 Days
Urethral and Cervical Gonococcal Infections	Uncomplicated	250-mg	single dose	single dose

†Generally ciprofloxacin should be continued for at least 2 days after the signs and symptoms of infection have disappeared.

Concurrent Use With Antacids or Multivalent Cations: Concurrent administration of ciprofloxacin with sucralfate or divalent and trivalent cations such as iron or antacids containing magnesium, aluminum, or calcium may substantially interfere with the absorption of ciprofloxacin, resulting in serum and urine levels considerably lower than desired. Therefore, concurrent administration of these agents with ciprofloxacin should be avoided. However, usual dietary intake of calcium has not been shown to alter the bioavailability of ciprofloxacin. Single dose bioavailability studies have shown that antacids may be administered either 2 hours after or 6 hours before ciprofloxacin dosing without a significant decrease in bioavailability. Histamine H$_2$-receptor antagonists appear to have no significant effect on the bioavailability of ciprofloxacin.

Impaired Renal Function: Ciprofloxacin is eliminated primarily by renal excretion; however, the drug is also metabolized and partially cleared through the biliary system of the liver and through the intestine. These alternate pathways of drug elimination appear to compensate for the reduced renal excretion in patients with renal impairment. Nonetheless, some modification of dosage is recommended, particularly for patients with severe renal dysfunction. The following table provides dosage guidelines for use in patients with renal impairment; however, monitoring of serum drug levels provides the most reliable basis for dosage adjustment:

RECOMMENDED STARTING AND MAINTENANCE DOSES FOR PATIENTS WITH IMPAIRED RENAL FUNCTION

Creatinine Clearance (mL/min)	Dose
> 50	See Usual Dosage
30–50	250–500 mg q 12 h
5–29	250–500 mg q 18 h
Patients on hemodialysis or Peritoneal dialysis	250–500 mg q 24 h (after dialysis)

When only the serum creatinine concentration is known, the following formula may be used to estimate creatinine clearance.

Men: Creatinine clearance (mL/min) =

$$\frac{\text{Weight (kg)} \times (140 - \text{age})}{72 \times \text{serum creatinine (mg/dL)}}$$

Women: 0.85 × the value calculated for men.

The serum creatinine should represent a steady state of renal function.

In patients with severe infections and severe renal impairment, a unit dose of 750-mg may be administered at the intervals noted above; however, patients should be carefully monitored and the serum ciprofloxacin concentration should be measured periodically. Peak concentrations (1–2 hours after dosing) should generally range from 2 to 4 µg/mL.

For patients with changing renal function or for patients with renal impairment and hepatic insufficiency, measurement of serum concentrations of ciprofloxacin will provide additional guidance for adjusting dosage.

HOW SUPPLIED

Cipro® (ciprofloxacin hydrochloride) is available as round, slightly yellowish film-coated tablets containing 100-mg or 250-mg ciprofloxacin. The 100-mg tablet is coded with the word "Cipro" on one side and "100" on the reverse side. The 250-mg tablet is coded with the word "Cipro" on one side and "250" on the reverse side. Cipro® is also available as capsule shaped, slightly yellowish film-coated tablets containing 500-mg or 750-mg ciprofloxacin. The 500-mg tablet is coded with the word "Cipro" on one side and "500" on the reverse side. The 750-mg tablet is coded with the word "Cipro" on one side and "750" on the reverse side .Cipro® 250-mg, 500-mg, and 750-mg are available in bottles of 50's, 100's, and Unit Dose packages of 100. The 100-mg strength, is available only as Cipro® Cystitis pack containing 6 tablets for use only in female patients with acute uncomplicated cystitis.
[See table below.]

Store below 86°F (30°C).

ANIMAL PHARMACOLOGY

Ciprofloxacin and other quinolones have been shown to cause arthropathy in immature animals of most species tested. (See WARNINGS.) Damage of weight bearing joints was observed in juvenile dogs and rats. In young beagles, 100 mg/kg ciprofloxacin, given daily for 4 weeks, caused degenerative articular changes of the knee joint. At 30 mg/kg, the effect on the joint was minimal. In a subsequent study in beagles, removal of weight bearing from the joint reduced the lesions but did not totally prevent them.

Crystalluria, sometimes associated with secondary nephropathy, occurs in laboratory animals dosed with ciprofloxacin. This is primarily related to the reduced solubility of ciprofloxacin under alkaline conditions, which predominate in the urine of test animals; in man, crystalluria is rare since human urine is typically acidic. In rhesus monkeys, crystalluria without nephropathy has been noted after single oral doses as low as 5 mg/kg. After 6 months of intravenous dosing at 10 mg/kg/day, no nephropathological changes were noted; however, nephropathy was observed after dosing at 20 mg/kg/day for the same duration.

In dogs, ciprofloxacin at 3 and 10 mg/kg by rapid IV injection (15 sec.) produces pronounced hypotensive effects. These effects are considered to be related to histamine release, since they are partially antagonized by pyrilamine, an antihistamine. In rhesus monkeys, rapid IV injection also produces hypotension but the effect in this species is inconsistent and less pronounced.

In mice, concomitant administration of nonsteroidal antiinflammatory drugs such as fenbufen, phenylbutazone and indomethacin with quinolones has been reported to enhance the CNS stimulatory effect of quinolones.

Ocular toxicity seen with some related drugs has not been observed in ciprofloxacin-treated animals.

CLINICAL STUDIES

Uncomplicated Cystitis Studies

Efficacy: Two U.S. double-blind, controlled clinical studies of acute uncomplicated cystitis in women compared ciprofloxacin 100-mg BID for 3 days to ciprofloxacin 200-mg BID for 7 days or control drug. In these two studies, using strict evaluability criteria and microbiologic and clinical response criteria at the 5–9 day post-therapy follow-up, the following clinical resolution and bacterial eradication rates were obtained:

Drug Regimen	Clinical Response Resolution n (%)	Bacteriological Response By Organism (Eradication Rate)	
		E. coli n (%)	S. saprophyticus n (%)
Study 1			
Cipro 100-mg BID × 3 days	82/94 (87)	64/70 (91)	8/8 (100)
Cipro 250-mg BID × 7 days	81/86 (94)	67/69 (97)	4/4 (100)
Study 2			
Cipro 100-mg BID × 3 days	134/141 (95)	117/123 (95)	8/8 (100)
Control (3 days)	128/133 (96)	103/105 (98)	10/10 (100)

References: 1. National Committee for Clinical Laboratory Standards, Methods for Dilution Antimicrobial Susceptibility Tests for Bacteria That Grow Aerobically—Third Edition. Approved Standard NCCLS Document M7-A3, Vol. 13, No.25, NCCLS, Villanova, PA, December 1993. **2.** National Committee for Clinical Laboratory Standards, Performance Standards for Antimicrobial Disk Susceptibility Tests —Fifth Edition. Approved Standard NCCLS Document M2-A5, Vol. 13, No. 24, NCCLS, Villanova, PA, December 1993.

Bayer Corporation
Pharmaceutical Division
400 Morgan Lane
West Haven, CT 06516 USA

Caution: Federal (USA) Law prohibits dispensing without a prescription.

PZ500032   3/96   Bay o 9867   5202-2-A-U.S.-6
©1996 Bayer Corporation   6150

Shown in Product Identification Guide, page 305

CIPRO® I.V.
(ciprofloxacin)
For Intravenous Infusion

℞

DESCRIPTION

Cipro® I.V. (ciprofloxacin) is a synthetic broad-spectrum antimicrobial agent for intravenous (iv) administration. Ciprofloxacin, a fluoroquinolone, is 1-cyclopropyl-6-fluoro-1, 4-dihydro-4-oxo-7-(1-piperazinyl)-3-quinolinecarboxylic acid. Its empirical formula is $C_{17}H_{18}FN_3O_3$ and its chemical structure is:

Ciprofloxacin is a faint to light yellow crystalline powder with a molecular weight of 331.4. It is soluble in dilute (0.1N) hydrochloric acid and is practically insoluble in water and ethanol. Ciprofloxacin differs from other quinolones in that it has a fluorine atom at the 6-position, a piperazine moiety at the 7-position, and a cyclopropyl ring at the 1-position. Cipro® I.V. solutions are available as 1.0% aqueous concentrates, which are intended for dilution prior to administration, and as a 0.2% ready-for-use infusion solution in 5% Dextrose Injection. All formulas contain lactic acid as a solubilizing agent and hydrochloric acid for pH adjustment. The pH range for the 1.0% aqueous concentrates in vials is 3.3 to 3.9. The pH range for the 0.2% ready-for-use infusion solutions is 3.5 to 4.6.

The plastic container is fabricated from a specially formulated polyvinyl chloride. Solutions in contact with the plastic container can leach out certain of its chemical components in very small amounts within the expiration period, e.g., di(2-ethylhexyl) phthalate (DEHP), up to 5 parts per million. The suitability of the plastic has been confirmed in tests in animals according to USP biological tests for plastic containers as well as by tissue culture toxicity studies.

	Strength	NDC Code	Tablet Identification
Bottles of 50:	750-mg	NDC 0026-8514-50	Cipro 750
Bottles of 100:	250-mg	NDC 0026-8512-51	Cipro 250
	500-mg	NDC 0026-8513-51	Cipro 500
Unit Dose Package of 100:	250-mg	NDC 0026-8512-48	Cipro 250
	500-mg	NDC 0026-8513-48	Cipro 500
	750-mg	NDC 0026-8514-48	Cipro 750
Cystitis Package of 6:	100-mg	NDC 0026-8511-06	Cipro 100

Continued on next page

Bayer Corporation—Cont.

CLINICAL PHARMACOLOGY

Following 60-minute intravenous infusions of 200 mg and 400 mg ciprofloxacin to normal volunteers, the mean maximum serum concentrations achieved were 2.1 and 4.6 $\mu g/$mL, respectively; the concentrations at 12 hours were 0.1 and 0.2 $\mu g/$mL, respectively.

Steady-state Ciprofloxacin Serum Concentrations ($\mu g/$mL) After 60-minute IV Infusions q 12 h.

| Dose | Time after starting the infusion | | | | | |
	30 min.	1 hr	3 hr	6 hr	8 hr	12 hr
200 mg	1.7	2.1	0.6	0.3	0.2	0.1
400 mg	3.7	4.6	1.3	0.7	0.5	0.2

The pharmacokinetics of ciprofloxacin are linear over the dose range of 200 to 400 mg administered intravenously. The serum elimination half-life is approximately 5–6 hours and the total clearance is around 35 L/hr. Comparison of the pharmacokinetic parameters following the 1st and 5th iv dose on a q 12 h regimen indicates no evidence of drug accumulation.

The absolute bioavailability of oral ciprofloxacin is within a range of 70–80% with no substantial loss by first pass metabolism. An intravenous infusion of 400 mg ciprofloxacin given over 60 minutes every 12 hours has been shown to produce an area under the serum concentration time curve (AUC) equivalent to that produced by a 500 mg oral dose given every 12 hours. A 400 mg iv dose administered over 60 minutes every 12 hours results in a C_{max} similar to that observed with a 750 mg oral dose. An infusion of 200 mg ciprofloxacin given every 12 hours produces an AUC equivalent to that produced by a 250 mg oral dose given every 12 hours.

After intravenous administration, approximately 50% to 70% of the dose is excreted in the urine as unchanged drug. Following a 200 mg iv dose, concentrations in the urine usually exceed 200 $\mu g/$mL 0–2 hours after dosing and are generally greater than 15 $\mu g/$mL 8–12 hours after dosing. Following a 400 mg iv dose, urine concentrations generally exceed 400 $\mu g/$mL 0–2 hours after dosing and are usually greater than 30 $\mu g/$mL 8–12 hours after dosing. The renal clearance is approximately 22 L/hr. The urinary excretion of ciprofloxacin is virtually complete by 24 hours after dosing.

Co-administration of probenecid with ciprofloxacin results in about a 50% reduction in the ciprofloxacin renal clearance and a 50% increase in its concentration in the systemic circulation. Although bile concentrations of ciprofloxacin are severalfold higher than serum concentrations after intravenous dosing, only a small amount of the administered dose (<1%) is recovered from the bile as unchanged drug. Approximately 15% of an iv dose is recovered from the feces within 5 days after dosing.

After iv administration, three metabolites of ciprofloxacin have been identified in human urine which together account for approximately 10% of the intravenous dose.

In patients with reduced renal function, the half-life of ciprofloxacin is slightly prolonged and dosage adjustments may be required. (See DOSAGE AND ADMINISTRATION.)

In preliminary studies in patients with stable chronic liver cirrhosis, no significant changes in ciprofloxacin pharmacokinetics have been observed. However, the kinetics of ciprofloxacin in patients with acute hepatic insufficiency have not been fully elucidated.

The binding of ciprofloxacin to serum proteins is 20 to 40%.

After intravenous administration, ciprofloxacin is present in saliva, nasal and bronchial secretions, sputum, skin blister fluid, lymph, peritoneal fluid, bile and prostatic secretions. It has also been detected in the lung, skin, fat, muscle, cartilage and bone. Although the drug diffuses into cerebrospinal fluid (CSF), CSF concentrations are generally less than 10% of peak serum concentrations. Levels of the drug in the aqueous and vitreous chambers of the eye are lower than in serum.

Microbiology: Ciprofloxacin has *in vitro* activity against a wide range of gram-negative and gram-positive organisms. The bactericidal action of ciprofloxacin results from interference with the enzyme DNA gyrase which is needed for the synthesis of bacterial DNA.

Ciprofloxacin has been shown to be active against most strains of the following organisms both *in vitro* and in clinical infections. (See INDICATIONS AND USAGE section.)

Gram-positive bacteria
Enterococcus faecalis (Many strains are only moderately susceptible)
Staphylococcus aureus
Staphylococcus epidermidis
Streptococcus pneumoniae
Streptococcus pyogenes
Gram-negative bacteria
Citrobacter diversus
Citrobacter freundii
Enterobacter cloacae

Escherichia coli
Haemophilus influenzae
Haemophilus parainfluenzae
Klebsiella pneumoniae
Morganella morganii
Proteus mirabilis
Proteus vulgaris
Providencia rettgeri
Providencia stuartii
Pseudomonas aeruginosa
Serratia marcescens

Ciprofloxacin has been shown to be active *in vitro* against most strains of the following organisms; however, *the clinical significance of these data is unknown.*

Gram-positive bacteria
Staphylococcus haemolyticus
Staphylococcus hominis
Staphylococcus saprophyticus
Gram-negative bacteria
Acinetobacter calcoaceticus
Aeromonas caviae
Aeromonas hydrophila
Brucella melitensis
Campylobacter coli
Campylobacter jejuni
Edwardsiella tarda
Enterobacter aerogenes
Haemophilus ducreyi
Klebsiella oxytoca
Legionella pneumophila
Moraxella (Branhamella) catarrhalis
Neisseria gonorrhoeae
Neisseria meningitidis
Pasteurella multocida
Salmonella enteritidis
Salmonella typhi
Shigella flexneri
Shigella sonnei
Vibrio cholerae
Vibrio parahaemolyticus
Vibrio vulnificus
Yersinia enterocolitica
Other organisms
Chlamydia trachomatis (only moderately susceptible)
Mycobacterium tuberculosis (only moderately susceptible)

Most strains of *Pseudomonas cepacia* and some strains of *Pseudomonas maltophilia* are resistant to ciprofloxacin as are most anaerobic bacteria, including *Bacteroides fragilis* and *Clostridium difficile.*

Ciprofloxacin is slightly less active when tested at acidic pH. The inoculum size has little effect when tested *in vitro*. The minimum bactericidal concentration (MBC) generally does not exceed the minimum inhibitory concentration (MIC) by more than a factor of 2. Resistance to ciprofloxacin *in vitro* usually develops slowly (multiple-step mutation).

Ciprofloxacin does not cross-react with other antimicrobial agents such as beta-lactams or aminoglycosides; therefore, organisms resistant to these drugs may be susceptible to ciprofloxacin.

In vitro studies have shown that additive activity often results when ciprofloxacin is combined with other antimicrobial agents such as beta-lactams, aminoglycosides, clindamycin, or metronidazole. Synergy has been reported particularly with the combination of ciprofloxacin and a beta-lactam; antagonism is observed only rarely.

Susceptibility Tests

Diffusion Techniques: Quantitative methods that require measurement of zone diameters give the most precise estimates of antibiotic susceptibility. One such procedure recommended for use with the 5-μg ciprofloxacin disk is the National Committee for Clinical Laboratory Standards (NCCLS) approved procedure (M2-A4—Performance Standards for Antimicrobial Disc Susceptibility Tests 1990). Only a 5-μg ciprofloxacin disk should be used, and it should not be used for testing susceptibility to less active quinolones; there are no suitable surrogate disks.

Results of laboratory tests using 5-μg ciprofloxacin disks should be interpreted using the following criteria:

Zone Diameter (mm)	Interpretation
≥ 21	(S) Susceptible
16 — 20	(MS) Moderately Susceptible
≤ 15	(R) Resistant

Dilution Techniques: Broth and agar dilution methods, such as those recommended by the NCCLS (M7-A2—Methods for Dilution Antimicrobial Susceptibility Tests for Bacteria that Grow Aerobically 1990), may be used to determine the minimum inhibitory concentration (MIC) of ciprofloxacin. MIC test results should be interpreted according to the following criteria:

MIC ($\mu g/$mL)	Interpretation
≤ 1	(S) Susceptible
2	(MS) Moderately Susceptible
≥ 4	(R) Resistant

For any susceptibility test, a report of "susceptible" indicates that the pathogen is likely to be inhibited by generally achievable blood levels. A report of "resistant" indicates that the pathogen is not likely to respond. A report of "moderately susceptible" indicates that the pathogen is expected to be susceptible to ciprofloxacin if high doses are used, or if the infection is confined to tissues and fluids in which ciprofloxacin levels are attained.

The Quality Control (QC) strains should have the following assigned daily ranges for ciprofloxacin.

QC Strains	Disk Zone Diameter (mm)	MIC ($\mu g/$mL)
S. aureus (ATCC 25923)	22–30	—
S. aureus (ATCC 29213)	—	0.12–0.5
E. coli (ATCC 25922)	30–40	0.004–0.015
P. aeruginosa (ATCC 27853)	25–33	0.25–1.0
E. faecalis (ATCC 29212)	—	0.25–2.0

INDICATIONS AND USAGE

Cipro® I.V. is indicated for the treatment of infections caused by susceptible strains of the designated microorganisms in the conditions listed below when the intravenous administration offers a route of administration advantageous to the patient:

Urinary Tract Infections—mild, moderate, severe and complicated infections caused by *Escherichia coli*, (including cases with secondary bacteremia), *Klebsiella pneumoniae* subspecies *pneumoniae*, *Enterobacter cloacae*, *Serratia marcescens*, *Proteus mirabilis*, *Providencia rettgeri*, *Morganella morganii*, *Citrobacter diversus*, *Citrobacter freundii*, *Pseudomonas aeruginosa*, *Staphylococcus epidermidis*, and *Enterococcus faecalis*.

Cipro® I.V. is also indicated for the treatment of mild to moderate lower respiratory tract infections, skin and skin structure infections and bone and joint infections due to the organisms listed in each section below. In severe and complicated lower respiratory tract infections, skin and skin structure infections and bone and joint infections, safety and effectiveness of the iv formulation have not been established.

Lower Respiratory Infections—mild to moderate infections caused by *Escherichia coli*, *Klebsiella pneumoniae* subspecies *pneumoniae*, *Enterobacter cloacae*, *Proteus mirabilis*, *Pseudomonas aeruginosa*, *Haemophilus influenzae*, *Haemophilus parainfluenzae*, and *Streptococcus pneumoniae.*

Skin and Skin Structure Infections—mild to moderate infections caused by *Escherichia coli*, *Klebsiella pneumoniae* subspecies *pneumoniae*, *Enterobacter cloacae*, *Proteus mirabilis*, *Proteus vulgaris*, *Providencia stuartii*, *Morganella morganii*, *Citrobacter freundii*, *Pseudomonas aeruginosa*, *Staphylococcus aureus*, *Staphylococcus epidermidis*, and *Streptococcus pyogenes.*

Bone and Joint Infections—mild to moderate infections caused by *Enterobacter cloacae*, *Serratia marcescens*, and *Pseudomonas aeruginosa.*

If anaerobic organisms are suspected of contributing to the infection, appropriate therapy should be administered.

Appropriate culture and susceptibility tests should be performed before treatment in order to isolate and identify organisms causing infection and to determine their susceptibility to ciprofloxacin. Therapy with Cipro® I.V. may be initiated before results of these tests are known; once results become available, appropriate therapy should be continued. As with other drugs, some strains of *Pseudomonas aeruginosa* may develop resistance fairly rapidly during treatment with ciprofloxacin. Culture and susceptibility testing performed periodically during therapy will provide information not only on the therapeutic effect of the antimicrobial agent but also on the possible emergence of bacterial resistance.

CONTRAINDICATIONS

Cipro® I.V. (ciprofloxacin) is contraindicated in persons with a history of hypersensitivity to ciprofloxacin or any member of the quinolone class of antimicrobial agents.

WARNINGS

THE SAFETY AND EFFECTIVENESS OF CIPROFLOXACIN IN CHILDREN, ADOLESCENTS (LESS THAN 18 YEARS OF AGE), PREGNANT WOMEN, AND LACTATING WOMEN HAVE NOT BEEN ESTABLISHED. (SEE PRECAUTIONS—PEDIATRIC USE, PREGNANCY AND NURSING MOTHERS SUBSECTIONS.) Ciprofloxacin causes lameness in immature dogs. Histopathological examination of the weight-bearing joints of these dogs revealed permanent lesions of the cartilage. Related quinolone-class drugs also produce erosions of cartilage of weight-bearing joints and other signs of arthropathy in immature animals of various species. (See ANIMAL PHARMACOLOGY.)

Convulsions have been reported in patients receiving ciprofloxacin. Convulsions, increased intracranial pressure, and toxic psychosis have been reported in patients receiving ciprofloxacin and other drugs of this class. Quinolones may also cause central nervous system (CNS) stimulation which may lead to tremors, restlessness, lightheadedness, confusion and hallucinations. If these reactions occur in patients

receiving ciprofloxacin, the drug should be discontinued and appropriate measures instituted. As with all quinolones, ciprofloxacin should be used with caution in patients with known or suspected CNS disorders, such as severe cerebral arteriosclerosis, epilepsy, and other factors that predispose to seizures. (See ADVERSE REACTIONS.)

SERIOUS AND FATAL REACTIONS HAVE BEEN REPORTED IN PATIENTS RECEIVING CONCURRENT ADMINISTRATION OF INTRAVENOUS CIPROFLOXACIN AND THEOPHYLLINE. These reactions have included cardiac arrest, seizure, status epilepticus and respiratory failure. Although similar serious adverse events have been reported in patients receiving theophylline alone, the possibility that these reactions may be potentiated by ciprofloxacin cannot be eliminated. If concomitant use cannot be avoided, serum levels of theophylline should be monitored and dosage adjustments made as appropriate.

Serious and occasionally fatal hypersensitivity (anaphylactic) reactions, some following the first dose, have been reported in patients receiving quinolone therapy. Some reactions were accompanied by cardiovascular collapse, loss of consciousness, tingling, pharyngeal or facial edema, dyspnea, urticaria, and itching. Only a few patients had a history of hypersensitivity reactions. Serious anaphylactic reactions require immediate emergency treatment with epinephrine and other resuscitation measures, including oxygen, intravenous fluids, intravenous antihistamines, corticosteroids, pressor amines and airway management, as clinically indicated.

Severe hypersensitivity reactions characterized by rash, fever, eosinophilia, jaundice, and hepatic necrosis with fatal outcome have also been reported extremely rarely in patients receiving ciprofloxacin along with other drugs. The possibility that these reactions were related to ciprofloxacin cannot be excluded. Ciprofloxacin should be discontinued at the first appearance of a skin rash or any other sign of hypersensitivity.

Pseudomembranous colitis has been reported with nearly all antibacterial agents, including ciprofloxacin, and may range in severity from mild to life-threatening. Therefore, it is important to consider this diagnosis in patients who present with diarrhea subsequent to the administration of antibacterial agents.

Treatment with antibacterial agents alters the normal flora of the colon and may permit overgrowth of clostridia. Studies indicate that a toxin produced by *Clostridium difficile* is one primary cause of "antibiotic-associated colitis".

After the diagnosis of pseudomembranous colitis has been established, therapeutic measures should be initiated. Mild cases of pseudomembranous colitis usually respond to drug discontinuation alone. In moderate to severe cases, consideration should be given to management with fluids and electrolytes, protein supplementation and treatment with an antibacterial drug effective against *C. difficile*.

PRECAUTIONS

General: INTRAVENOUS CIPROFLOXACIN SHOULD BE ADMINISTERED BY SLOW INFUSION OVER A PERIOD OF 60 MINUTES. Local iv site reactions have been reported with the intravenous administration of ciprofloxacin. These reactions are more frequent if infusion time is 30 minutes or less or if small veins of the hand are used. (See ADVERSE REACTIONS.)

Crystals of ciprofloxacin have been observed rarely in the urine of human subjects but more frequently in the urine of laboratory animals, which is usually alkaline. (See ANIMAL PHARMACOLOGY.) Crystalluria related to ciprofloxacin has been reported only rarely in humans because human urine is usually acidic. Alkalinity of the urine should be avoided in patients receiving ciprofloxacin. Patients should be well hydrated to prevent the formation of highly concentrated urine.

Alteration of the dosage regimen is necessary for patients with impairment of renal function. (See DOSAGE AND ADMINISTRATION.)

Moderate to severe phototoxicity manifested by an exaggerated sunburn reaction has been observed in some patients who were exposed to direct sunlight while receiving some members of the quinolone class of drugs. Excessive sunlight should be avoided.

As with any potent drug, periodic assessment of organ system functions, including renal, hepatic, and hematopoietic, is advisable during prolonged therapy.

Information for Patients: Patients should be advised that ciprofloxacin may be associated with hypersensitivity reactions, even following a single dose, and to discontinue the drug at the first sign of a skin rash or other allergic reaction. Ciprofloxacin may cause dizziness and lightheadedness; therefore, patients should know how they react to this drug before they operate an automobile or machinery or engage in activities requiring mental alertness or coordination. Patients should be advised that ciprofloxacin may increase the effects of theophylline and caffeine. There is a possibility of caffeine accumulation when products containing caffeine are consumed while taking quinolones.

Drug Interactions: As with other quinolones, concurrent administration of ciprofloxacin with theophylline may lead to elevated serum concentrations of theophylline and prolongation of its elimination half-life. This may result in increased risk of theophylline-related adverse reactions. (See WARNINGS.) If concomitant use cannot be avoided, serum levels of theophylline should be monitored and dosage adjustments made as appropriate.

Some quinolones, including ciprofloxacin, have also been shown to interfere with the metabolism of caffeine. This may lead to reduced clearance of caffeine and a prolongation of its serum half-life.

Some quinolones, including ciprofloxacin, have been associated with transient elevations in serum creatinine in patients receiving cyclosporine concomitantly.

Quinolones have been reported to enhance the effects of the oral anticoagulant warfarin or its derivatives. When these products are administered concomitantly, prothrombin time or other suitable coagulation tests should be closely monitored.

Probenecid interferes with renal tubular secretion of ciprofloxacin and produces an increase in the level of ciprofloxacin in the serum. This should be considered if patients are receiving both drugs concomitantly.

As with other broad-spectrum antimicrobial agents, prolonged use of ciprofloxacin may result in overgrowth of nonsusceptible organisms. Repeated evaluation of the patient's condition and microbial susceptibility testing are essential. If superinfection occurs during therapy, appropriate measures should be taken.

Carcinogenesis, Mutagenesis, Impairment of Fertility: Eight *in vitro* mutagenicity tests have been conducted with ciprofloxacin. Test results are listed below:

Salmonella/Microsome Test (Negative)
E. coli DNA Repair Assay (Negative)
Mouse Lymphoma Cell Forward Mutation Assay (Positive)
Chinese Hamster V$_{79}$ Cell HGPRT Test (Negative)
Syrian Hamster Embryo Cell Transformation Assay (Negative)
Saccharomyces cerevisiae Point Mutation Assay (Negative)
Saccharomyces cerevisiae Mitotic Crossover and Gene Conversion Assay (Negative)
Rat Hepatocyte DNA Repair Assay (Positive)

Thus, two of the eight tests were positive, but results of the following three *in vivo* test systems gave negative results:

Rat Hepatocyte DNA Repair Assay
Micronucleus Test (Mice)
Dominant Lethal Test (Mice)

Long-term carcinogenicity studies in mice and rats have been completed. After daily oral dosing for up to 2 years, there is no evidence that ciprofloxacin has any carcinogenic or tumorigenic effects in these species.

Pregnancy: Teratogenic Effects. Pregnancy Category C: Reproduction studies have been performed in rats and mice at doses up to 6 times the usual daily human dose and have revealed no evidence of impaired fertility or harm to the fetus due to ciprofloxacin. In rabbits, ciprofloxacin (30 and 100 mg/kg orally) produced gastrointestinal disturbances resulting in maternal weight loss and an increased incidence of abortion. No teratogenicity was observed at either dose. After intravenous administration of doses up to 20 mg/kg, no maternal toxicity was produced, and no embryotoxicity or teratogenicity was observed. There are, however, no adequate and well-controlled studies in pregnant women. Ciprofloxacin should be used during pregnancy only if the potential benefit justifies the potential risk to the fetus. (See WARNINGS.)

Nursing Mothers: Ciprofloxacin is excreted in human milk. Because of the potential for serious adverse reactions in infants nursing from mothers taking ciprofloxacin, a decision should be made either to discontinue nursing or to discontinue the drug, taking into account the importance of the drug to the mother.

Pediatric Use: Safety and effectiveness in children and adolescents less than 18 years of age have not been established. Ciprofloxacin causes arthropathy in juvenile animals. (See WARNINGS.)

ADVERSE REACTIONS

The most frequently reported events, without regard to drug relationship, among patients treated with intravenous ciprofloxacin were nausea, diarrhea, central nervous system disturbance, local iv site reactions, abnormalities of liver associated enzymes (hepatic enzymes) and eosinophilia. Headache, restlessness and rash were also noted in greater than 1% of patients treated with the most common doses of ciprofloxacin.

Local iv site reactions have been reported with the intravenous administration of ciprofloxacin. These reactions are more frequent if the infusion time is 30 minutes or less. These may appear as local skin reactions which resolve rapidly upon completion of the infusion. Subsequent intravenous administration is not contraindicated unless the reactions recur or worsen.

Additional events, without regard to drug relationship or route of administration, that occurred in 1% or less of ciprofloxacin courses are listed below:

GASTROINTESTINAL: ileus; jaundice; gastrointestinal bleeding; *C. difficile* associated diarrhea; pseudomembranous colitis; pancreatitis; hepatic necrosis; intestinal perforation; dyspepsia; epigastric or abdominal pain; vomiting; constipation; oral ulceration; oral candidiasis; mouth dryness; anorexia; dysphagia; flatulence.

CENTRAL NERVOUS SYSTEM: convulsive seizures, paranoia, toxic psychosis, depression, dysphasia, phobia, depersonalization, manic reaction, unresponsiveness, ataxia, confusion, hallucinations, dizziness, lightheadedness, paresthesia, anxiety, tremor, insomnia, nightmares, weakness, drowsiness, irritability, malaise, lethargy.

SKIN/HYPERSENSITIVITY: anaphylactic reactions; erythema multiforme/Stevens-Johnson syndrome; exfoliative dermatitis; toxic epidermal necrolysis; vasculitis; angioedema; edema of the lips, face, neck, conjunctivae, hands or lower extremities; purpura; fever; chills; flushing; pruritus; urticaria; cutaneous candidiasis; vesicles; increased perspiration; hyperpigmentation; erythema nodosum; photosensitivity.

Allergic reactions ranging from urticaria to anaphylactic reactions have been reported. (See WARNINGS.)

SPECIAL SENSES: decreased visual acuity, blurred vision, disturbed vision (flashing lights, change in color perception, overbrightness of lights, diplopia), eye pain, anosmia, hearing loss, tinnitus, nystagmus, a bad taste.

MUSCULOSKELETAL: joint pain; jaw, arm or back pain; joint stiffness; neck and chest pain; achiness; flare up of gout.

RENAL/UROGENITAL: renal failure, interstitial nephritis, hemorrhagic cystitis, renal calculi, frequent urination, acidosis, urethral bleeding, polyuria, urinary retention, gynecomastia, candiduria, vaginitis. Crystalluria, cylindruria, hematuria, and albuminuria have also been reported.

CARDIOVASCULAR: cardiovascular collapse, cardiopulmonary arrest, myocardial infarction, arrhythmia, tachycardia, palpitation, cerebral thrombosis, syncope, cardiac murmur, hypertension, hypotension, angina pectoris.

RESPIRATORY: respiratory arrest, pulmonary embolism, dyspnea, pulmonary edema, respiratory distress, pleural effusion, hemoptysis, epistaxis, hiccough.

IV INFUSION SITE: thrombophlebitis, burning, pain, pruritus, paresthesia, erythema, swelling.

Also reported were agranulocytosis, prolongation of prothrombin time and possible exacerbation of myasthenia gravis.

Many of these events were described as only mild or moderate in severity, abated soon after the drug was discontinued and required no treatment.

In several instances, nausea, vomiting, tremor, irritability or palpitation were judged by investigators to be related to elevated serum levels of theophylline possibly as a result of drug interaction with ciprofloxacin.

Adverse Laboratory Changes: The most frequently reported changes in laboratory parameters with intravenous ciprofloxacin therapy, without regard to drug relationship, were:

Hepatic—Elevations of AST (SGOT), ALT (SGPT), alkaline phosphatase, LDH and serum bilirubin.

Hematologic—Elevated eosinophil and platelet counts, decreased platelet counts, hemoglobin and/or hematocrit.

Renal—Elevations of serum creatinine, BUN, uric acid.

Other—Elevations of serum creatine phosphokinase, serum theophylline (in patients receiving theophylline concomitantly), blood glucose, and triglycerides.

Other changes occurring infrequently were: decreased leukocyte count, elevated atypical lymphocyte count, immature WBCs, elevated serum calcium, elevation of serum gamma-glutamyl transpeptidase (γ GT), decreased BUN, decreased uric acid, decreased total serum protein, decreased serum albumin, decreased serum potassium, elevated serum potassium, elevated serum cholesterol.

Other changes occurring rarely during administration of ciprofloxacin were: elevation of serum amylase, decrease of blood glucose, pancytopenia, leukocytosis, elevated sedimentation rate, change in serum phenytoin, decreased prothrombin time, hemolytic anemia, and bleeding diathesis.

OVERDOSAGE

In the event of acute overdosage, the patient should be carefully observed and given supportive treatment. Adequate hydration must be maintained. Only a small amount of ciprofloxacin (< 10%) is removed from the body after hemodialysis or peritoneal dialysis.

DOSAGE AND ADMINISTRATION

The recommended adult dosage for urinary tract infections of mild to moderate severity is 200 mg every 12 hours. For severe or complicated urinary tract infections the recommended dosage is 400 mg every 12 hours.

Continued on next page

Bayer Corporation—Cont.

The recommended adult dosage for lower respiratory tract infections, skin and skin structure infections and bone and joint infections of mild to moderate severity is 400 mg every 12 hours.

The determination of dosage for any particular patient must take into consideration the severity and nature of the infection, the susceptibility of the causative organism, the integrity of the patient's host-defense mechanisms and the status of renal and hepatic function.

[See table on bottom of page.]

Cipro® I.V. should be administered by intravenous infusion over a period of 60 minutes.

The duration of treatment depends upon the severity of infection. Generally, ciprofloxacin should be continued for at least 2 days after the signs and symptoms of infection have disappeared. The usual duration is 7 to 14 days. Bone and joint infections may require treatment for 4 to 6 weeks or longer.

Ciprofloxacin hydrochloride tablets (Cipro®) for oral administration are available. Parenteral therapy may be changed to oral Cipro® tablets when the condition warrants, at the discretion of the physician. For complete dosage and administration information, see Cipro® tablet package insert.

Impaired Renal Function: The following table provides dosage guidelines for use in patients with renal impairment; however, monitoring of serum drug levels provides the most reliable basis for dosage adjustment.

RECOMMENDED STARTING AND MAINTENANCE DOSES FOR PATIENTS WITH IMPAIRED RENAL FUNCTION

Creatinine Clearance (mL/min)	Dosage
≥ 30	See usual dosage
5–29	200–400 mg q 18–24 hr

When only the serum creatinine concentration is known, the following formula may be used to estimate creatinine clearance.

Men: Creatinine clearance

$$(mL/min) = \frac{Weight\ (kg) \times (140 - age)}{72 \times serum\ creatinine\ (mg/dL)}$$

Women: 0.85 × the value calculated for men.

The serum creatinine should represent a steady state of renal function.

For patients with changing renal function or for patients with renal impairment and hepatic insufficiency, measurement of serum concentrations of ciprofloxacin will provide additional guidance for adjusting dosage.

INTRAVENOUS ADMINISTRATION

Cipro® I.V. should be administered by intravenous infusion over a period of 60 minutes. Slow infusion of a dilute solution into a large vein will minimize patient discomfort and reduce the risk of venous irritation.

Vials (Injection Concentrate): THIS PREPARATION MUST BE DILUTED BEFORE USE. The intravenous dose should be prepared by aseptically withdrawing the appropriate volume of concentrate from the vials of Cipro® I.V. This should be diluted with a suitable intravenous solution to a final concentration of 1–2 mg/mL. (See COMPATIBILITY AND STABILITY.) The resulting solution should be infused over a period of 60 minutes by direct infusion or through a Y-type intravenous infusion set which may already be in place. If this method or the "piggyback" method of administration is used, it is advisable to discontinue temporarily the administration of any other solutions during the infusion of Cipro® I.V.

Flexible Containers: Cipro® I.V. is also available as a 0.2% premixed solution in 5% dextrose in flexible containers of 100 mL or 200 mL. The solutions in flexible containers may be infused as described above.

COMPATIBILITY AND STABILITY

Ciprofloxacin injection 1% (10 mg/mL), when diluted with the following intravenous solutions to concentrations of 0.5 to 2.0 mg/mL, is stable for up to 14 days at refrigerated or room temperature storage.

0.9% Sodium Chloride Injection, USP

5% Dextrose Injection, USP

If Cipro® I.V. is to be given concomitantly with another drug, each drug should be given separately in accordance with the recommended dosage and route of administration for each drug.

HOW SUPPLIED

Cipro® I.V. (ciprofloxacin) is available as a clear, colorless to slightly yellowish solution. Cipro® I.V. is available in 200 mg and 400 mg strengths. The concentrate is supplied in vials while the premixed solution is supplied in flexible containers as follows:

CONTAINER	SIZE	STRENGTH	NDC NUMBER
Vial:	20 mL	200 mg, 1%	0026-8562-20
	40 mL	400 mg, 1%	0026-8564-64
Flexible Container:	100 mL 5% dextrose	200 mg, 0.2%	0026-8552-36
	200 mL 5% dextrose	400 mg, 0.2%	0026-8554-63

STORAGE

Vials: Store between 41–86°F (5–30°C).

Flexible Container: Store between 41–77°F (5–25°C).

Protect from light, avoid excessive heat, protect from freezing.

Ciprofloxacin is also available as Cipro® (ciprofloxacin HCl) Tablets 250, 500 and 750 mg.

ANIMAL PHARMACOLOGY

Ciprofloxacin and other quinolones have been shown to cause arthropathy in immature animals of most species tested. (See WARNINGS.) Damage of weight-bearing joints was observed in juvenile dogs and rats. In young beagles, 100 mg/kg ciprofloxacin given daily for 4 weeks caused degenerative articular changes of the knee joint. At 30 mg/kg, the effect on the joint was minimal. In a subsequent study in beagles, removal of weight-bearing from the joint reduced the lesions but did not totally prevent them.

Crystalluria, sometimes associated with secondary nephropathy, occurs in laboratory animals dosed with ciprofloxacin. This is primarily related to the reduced solubility of ciprofloxacin under alkaline conditions, which predominate in the urine of test animals; in man, crystalluria is rare since human urine is typically acidic. In rhesus monkeys, crystalluria without nephropathy has been noted after intravenous doses as low as 5 mg/kg. After 6 months of intravenous dosing at 10 mg/kg/day, no nephropathological changes were noted; however, nephropathy was observed after dosing at 20 mg/kg/day for the same duration.

In dogs, ciprofloxacin administered at 3 and 10 mg/kg by rapid intravenous injection (15 sec.) produces pronounced hypotensive effects. These effects are considered to be related to histamine release because they are partially antagonized by pyrilamine, an antihistamine. In rhesus monkeys, rapid intravenous injection also produces hypotension, but the effect in this species is inconsistent and less pronounced.

In mice, concomitant administration of nonsteroidal antiinflammatory drugs, such as fenbufen, phenylbutazone and indomethacin, with quinolones has been reported to enhance the CNS stimulatory effect of quinolones.

Ocular toxicity, seen with some related drugs, has not been observed in ciprofloxacin-treated animals.

Bayer Corporation
Pharmaceutical Division
400 Morgan Lane
West Haven, CT 06516 USA

Caution: Federal (USA) Law prohibits dispensing without a prescription.

PZ500006   2/95   BAY q 3939
5202-4-A-U.S.-3
© 1995 Bayer Corporation   4756

Shown in Product Identification Guide, page 305

CIPRO® I.V.
(ciprofloxacin)
For Intravenous Infusion

℞

PHARMACY BULK PACKAGE—NOT FOR DIRECT INFUSION

DESCRIPTION

The pharmacy bulk package is a single-entry container of a sterile preparation for parenteral use that contains many single doses. It contains ciprofloxacin as a 1% aqueous solution concentrate. The contents are intended for use in a pharmacy admixture program and are restricted to the preparation of admixtures for intravenous infusion.

Cipro® I.V. (ciprofloxacin) is a synthetic broad-spectrum antimicrobial agent for intravenous (iv) administration. Ciprofloxacin, a fluoroquinolone, is 1-cyclopropyl-6-fluoro-1, 4-dihydro-4-oxo-7-(1-piperazinyl)-3-quinolinecarboxylic acid. Its empirical formula is $C_{17}H_{18}FN_3O_3$ and its chemical structure is:

Ciprofloxacin is a faint to light yellow crystalline powder with a molecular weight of 331.4. It is soluble in dilute (0.1N) hydrochloric acid and is practically insoluble in water and ethanol. Ciprofloxacin differs from other quinolones in that it has a fluorine atom at the 6-position, a piperazine moiety at the 7-position, and a cyclopropyl ring at the 1-position. Cipro® I.V. solution is available as 1.0% aqueous concentrate, which is intended for dilution prior to administration. Ciprofloxacin solution contains lactic acid as a solubilizing agent and hydrochloric acid for pH adjustment. The pH range for the 1.0% aqueous concentrate is 3.3 to 3.9.

CLINICAL PHARMACOLOGY

Following 60-minute intravenous infusions of 200 mg and 400 mg ciprofloxacin to normal volunteers, the mean maximum serum concentrations achieved were 2.1 and 4.6 µg/mL, respectively; the concentrations at 12 hours were 0.1 and 0.2 µg/mL, respectively.

Steady-state Ciprofloxacin Serum Concentrations (µg/mL) After 60-minute IV Infusions q 12 h.

Dose	Time after starting the infusion					
	30 min.	1 hr	3 hr	6 hr	8 hr	12 hr
200 mg	1.7	2.1	0.6	0.3	0.2	0.1
400 mg	3.7	4.6	1.3	0.7	0.5	0.2

The pharmacokinetics of ciprofloxacin are linear over the dose range of 200 to 400 mg administered intravenously. The serum elimination half-life is approximately 5–6 hours and the total clearance is around 35 L/hr. Comparison of the pharmacokinetic parameters following the 1st and 5th iv dose on a q 12 h regimen indicates no evidence of drug accumulation.

The absolute bioavailability of oral ciprofloxacin is within a range of 70–80% with no substantial loss by first pass metabolism. An intravenous infusion of 400 mg ciprofloxacin given over 60 minutes every 12 hours has been shown to produce an area under the serum concentration time curve (AUC) equivalent to that produced by a 500 mg oral dose given every 12 hours. A 400 mg iv dose administered over 60 minutes every 12 hours results in a C_{max} similar to that observed with a 750 mg oral dose. An infusion of 200 mg ciprofloxacin given every 12 hours produces an AUC equivalent to that produced by a 250 mg oral dose given every 12 hours.

After intravenous administration, approximately 50% to 70% of the dose is excreted in the urine as unchanged drug. Following a 200 mg iv dose, concentrations in the urine usually exceed 200 µg/mL 0–2 hours after dosing and are generally greater than 15 µg/mL 8–12 hours after dosing. Following a 400 mg iv dose, urine concentrations generally exceed 400 µg/mL 0–2 hours after dosing and are usually greater than 30 µg/mL 8–12 hours after dosing. The renal clearance is approximately 22 L/hr. The urinary excretion of ciprofloxacin is virtually complete by 24 hours after dosing.

Co-administration of probenecid with ciprofloxacin results in about a 50% reduction in the ciprofloxacin renal clearance and a 50% increase in its concentration in the systemic circulation. Although bile concentrations of ciprofloxacin are severalfold higher than serum concentrations after intravenous dosing, only a small amount of the administered dose (<1%) is recovered from the bile as unchanged drug. Approximately 15% of an iv dose is recovered from the feces within 5 days after dosing.

		DOSAGE GUIDELINES		
Type of Infection	Type or Severity	Intravenous Unit Dose	Frequency	Daily Dose
Urinary tract	Mild/Moderate	200 mg	q 12 h	400 mg
	Severe/Complicated	400 mg	q 12 h	800 mg
Lower Respiratory tract; Skin and Skin Structure; Bone and Joint	Mild/Moderate	400 mg	q 12 h	800 mg

After iv administration, three metabolites of ciprofloxacin have been identified in human urine which together account for approximately 10% of the intravenous dose.

In patients with reduced renal function, the half-life of ciprofloxacin is slightly prolonged and dosage adjustments may be required. (See DOSAGE AND ADMINISTRATION.)

In preliminary studies in patients with stable chronic liver cirrhosis, no significant changes in ciprofloxacin pharmacokinetics have been observed. However, the kinetics of ciprofloxacin in patients with acute hepatic insufficiency have not been fully elucidated.

The binding of ciprofloxacin to serum proteins is 20 to 40%. After intravenous administration, ciprofloxacin is present in saliva, nasal and bronchial secretions, sputum, skin blister fluid, lymph, peritoneal fluid, bile and prostatic secretions. It has also been detected in the lung, skin, fat, muscle, cartilage and bone. Although the drug diffuses into cerebrospinal fluid (CSF), CSF concentrations are generally less than 10% of peak serum concentrations. Levels of the drug in the aqueous and vitreous chambers of the eye are lower than in serum.

Microbiology: Ciprofloxacin has *in vitro* activity against a wide range of gram-negative and gram-positive organisms. The bactericidal action of ciprofloxacin results from interference with the enzyme DNA gyrase which is needed for the synthesis of bacterial DNA.

Ciprofloxacin has been shown to be active against most strains of the following organisms both *in vitro* and in clinical infections. (See INDICATIONS AND USAGE section.)

Gram-positive bacteria
Enterococcus faecalis (Many strains are only moderately susceptible)
Staphylococcus aureus
Staphylococcus epidermidis
Streptococcus pneumoniae
Streptococcus pyogenes
Gram-negative bacteria

Citrobacter diversus	*Morganella morganii*
Citrobacter freundii	*Proteus mirabilis*
Enterobacter cloacae	*Proteus vulgaris*
Escherichia coli	*Providencia rettgeri*
Haemophilus influenzae	*Providencia stuartii*
Haemophilus parainfluenzae	*Pseudomonas aeruginosa*
Klebsiella pneumoniae	*Serratia marcescens*

Ciprofloxacin has been shown to be active *in vitro* against most strains of the following organisms; however, *the clinical significance of these data is unknown.*

Gram-positive bacteria
Staphylococcus haemolyticus
Staphylococcus hominis
Staphylococcus saprophyticus
Gram-negative bacteria

Acinetobacter calcoaceticus	*Neisseria gonorrhoeae*
Aeromonas caviae	*Neisseria meningitidis*
Aeromonas hydrophila	*Pasteurella multocida*
Brucella melitensis	*Salmonella enteritidis*
Campylobacter coli	*Salmonella typhi*
Campylobacter jejuni	*Shigella flexneri*
Edwardsiella tarda	*Shigella sonnei*
Enterobacter aerogenes	*Vibrio cholerae*
Haemophilus ducreyi	*Vibrio parahaemolyticus*
Klebsiella oxytoca	*Vibrio vulnificus*
Legionella pneumophila	*Yersinia enterocolitica*
Moraxella (Branhamella) catarrhalis	

Other organisms
Chlamydia trachomatis (only moderately susceptible)
Mycobacterium tuberculosis (only moderately susceptible)
Most strains of *Pseudomonas cepacia* and some strains of *Pseudomonas maltophilia* are resistant to ciprofloxacin as are most anaerobic bacteria, including *Bacteroides fragilis* and *Clostridium difficile.*

Ciprofloxacin is slightly less active when tested at acidic pH. The inoculum size has little effect when tested *in vitro.* The minimum bactericidal concentration (MBC) generally does not exceed the minimum inhibitory concentration (MIC) by more than a factor of 2. Resistance to ciprofloxacin *in vitro* usually develops slowly (multiple-step mutation).

Ciprofloxacin does not cross-react with other antimicrobial agents such as beta-lactams or aminoglycosides; therefore, organisms resistant to these drugs may be susceptible to ciprofloxacin.

In vitro studies have shown that additive activity often results when ciprofloxacin is combined with other antimicrobial agents such as beta-lactams, aminoglycosides, clindamycin, or metronidazole. Synergy has been reported particularly with the combination of ciprofloxacin and a beta-lactam; antagonism is observed only rarely.

Susceptibility Tests

Diffusion Techniques: Quantitative methods that require measurement of zone diameters give the most precise estimates of antibiotic susceptibility. One such procedure recommended for use with the 5-μg ciprofloxacin disk is the National Committee for Clinical Laboratory Standards (NCCLS) approved procedure M2-A4—Performance Standards for Antimicrobial Disc Susceptibility Tests 1990. Only

a 5-μg ciprofloxacin disk should be used, and it should not be used for testing susceptibility to less active quinolones; there are no suitable surrogate disks.

Results of laboratory tests using 5-μg ciprofloxacin disks should be interpreted using the following criteria:

Zone Diameter (mm)	Interpretation
≥ 21	(S) Susceptible
16–20	(MS) Moderately Susceptible
≤ 15	(R) Resistant

Dilution Techniques: Broth and agar dilution methods, such as those recommended by the NCCLS (M7-A2—Methods for Dilution Antimicrobial Susceptibility Tests for Bacteria that Grow Aerobically 1990), may be used to determine the minimum inhibitory concentration (MIC) of ciprofloxacin. MIC test results should be interpreted according to the following criteria:

MIC (μg/mL)	Interpretation
≤ 1	(S) Susceptible
2	(MS) Moderately Susceptible
≥ 4	(R) Resistant

For any susceptibility test, a report of "susceptible" indicates that the pathogen is likely to be inhibited by generally achievable blood levels. A report of "resistant" indicates that the pathogen is not likely to respond. A report of "moderately susceptible" indicates that the pathogen is expected to be susceptible to ciprofloxacin if high doses are used, or if the infection is confined to tissues and fluids in which high ciprofloxacin levels are attained.

The Quality Control (QC) strains should have the following assigned daily ranges for ciprofloxacin.

QC Strains	Disk Zone Diameter (mm)	MIC (μg/mL)
S. aureus (ATCC 25923)	22–30	–
S. aureus (ATCC 29213)	–	0.12–0.5
E. coli (ATCC 25922)	30–40	0.004–0.015
P. aeruginosa (ATCC 27853)	25–33	0.25–1.0
E. faecalis (ATCC 29212)	–	0.25–2.0

INDICATIONS AND USAGE

Cipro® I.V. is indicated for the treatment of infections caused by susceptible strains of the designated microorganisms in the conditions listed below when the intravenous administration offers a route of administration advantageous to the patient:

Urinary Tract Infections—mild, moderate, severe and complicated infections caused by *Escherichia coli,* (including cases with secondary bacteremia), *Klebsiella pneumoniae* subspecies *pneumoniae, Enterobacter cloacae, Serratia marcescens, Proteus mirabilis, Providencia rettgeri, Morganella morganii, Citrobacter diversus, Citrobacter freundii, Pseudomonas aeruginosa, Staphylococcus epidermidis,* and *Enterococcus faecalis.*

Cipro® I.V. is also indicated for the treatment of mild to moderate lower respiratory tract infections, skin and skin structure infections and bone and joint infections due to the organisms listed in each section below. In severe and complicated lower respiratory tract infections, skin and skin structure infections and bone and joint infections, safety and effectiveness of the iv formulation have not been established.

Lower Respiratory Infections—mild to moderate infections caused by *Escherichia coli, Klebsiella pneumoniae* subspecies *pneumoniae, Enterobacter cloacae, Proteus mirabilis, Pseudomonas aeruginosa, Haemophilus influenzae, Haemophilus parainfluenzae,* and *Streptococcus pneumoniae.*

Skin and Skin Structure Infections—mild to moderate infections caused by *Escherichia coli, Klebsiella pneumoniae* subspecies *pneumoniae, Enterobacter cloacae, Proteus mirabilis, Proteus vulgaris, Providencia stuartii, Morganella morganii, Citrobacter freundii, Pseudomonas aeruginosa, Staphylococcus aureus, Staphylococcus epidermidis,* and *Streptococcus pyogenes.*

Bone and Joint Infections—mild to moderate infections caused by *Enterobacter cloacae, Serratia marcescens,* and *Pseudomonas aeruginosa.*

If anaerobic organisms are suspected of contributing to the infection, appropriate therapy should be administered.

Appropriate culture and susceptibility tests should be performed before treatment in order to isolate and identify organisms causing infection and to determine their susceptibility to ciprofloxacin. Therapy with Cipro® I.V. may be initiated before results of these tests are known; once results become available, appropriate therapy should be continued.

As with other drugs, some strains of *Pseudomonas aeruginosa* may develop resistance fairly rapidly during treatment with ciprofloxacin. Culture and susceptibility testing performed periodically during therapy will provide information not only on the therapeutic effect of the antimicrobial agent but also on the possible emergence of bacterial resistance.

CONTRAINDICATIONS

Cipro® I.V. (ciprofloxacin) is contraindicated in persons with a history of hypersensitivity to ciprofloxacin or any member of the quinolone class of antimicrobial agents.

WARNINGS

THE SAFETY AND EFFECTIVENESS OF CIPROFLOXACIN IN CHILDREN, ADOLESCENTS (LESS THAN 18 YEARS OF AGE), PREGNANT WOMEN, AND LACTATING WOMEN HAVE NOT BEEN ESTABLISHED. (SEE PRECAUTIONS—PEDIATRIC USE, PREGNANCY AND NURSING MOTHERS SUBSECTIONS.) Ciprofloxacin causes lameness in immature dogs. Histopathological examination of the weight-bearing joints of these dogs revealed permanent lesions of the cartilage. Related quinolone-class drugs also produce erosions of cartilage of weight-bearing joints and other signs of arthropathy in immature animals of various species. (See ANIMAL PHARMACOLOGY.)

Convulsions have been reported in patients receiving ciprofloxacin. Convulsions, increased intracranial pressure, and toxic psychosis have been reported in patients receiving ciprofloxacin and other drugs of this class. Quinolones may also cause central nervous system (CNS) stimulation which may lead to tremors, restlessness, lightheadedness, confusion and hallucinations. If these reactions occur in patients receiving ciprofloxacin, the drug should be discontinued and appropriate measures instituted. As with all quinolones, ciprofloxacin should be used with caution in patients with known or suspected CNS disorders, such as severe cerebral arteriosclerosis, epilepsy, and other factors that predispose to seizures. (See ADVERSE REACTIONS.)

SERIOUS AND FATAL REACTIONS HAVE BEEN REPORTED IN PATIENTS RECEIVING CONCURRENT ADMINISTRATION OF INTRAVENOUS CIPROFLOXACIN AND THEOPHYLLINE. These reactions have included cardiac arrest, seizure, status epilepticus and respiratory failure. Although similar serious adverse events have been reported in patients receiving theophylline alone, the possibility that these reactions may be potentiated by ciprofloxacin cannot be eliminated. If concomitant use cannot be avoided, serum levels of theophylline should be monitored and dosage adjustments made as appropriate.

Serious and occasionally fatal hypersensitivity (anaphylactic) reactions, some following the first dose, have been reported in patients receiving quinolone therapy. Some reactions were accompanied by cardiovascular collapse, loss of consciousness, tingling, pharyngeal or facial edema, dyspnea, urticaria, and itching. Only a few patients had a history of hypersensitivity reactions. Serious anaphylactic reactions require immediate emergency treatment with epinephrine and other resuscitation measures, including oxygen, intravenous fluids, intravenous antihistamines, corticosteroids, pressor amines and airway management, as clinically indicated.

Severe hypersensitivity reactions characterized by rash, fever, eosinophilia, jaundice, and hepatic necrosis with fatal outcome have also been reported extremely rarely in patients receiving ciprofloxacin along with other drugs. The possibility that these reactions were related to ciprofloxacin cannot be excluded. Ciprofloxacin should be discontinued at the first appearance of a skin rash or any other sign of hypersensitivity.

Pseudomembranous colitis has been reported with nearly all antibacterial agents, including ciprofloxacin, and may range in severity from mild to life-threatening. Therefore, it is important to consider this diagnosis in patients who present with diarrhea subsequent to the administration of antibacterial agents.

Treatment with antibacterial agents alters the normal flora of the colon and may permit overgrowth of clostridia. Studies indicate that a toxin produced by *Clostridium difficile* is one primary cause of "antibiotic-associated colitis."

After the diagnosis of pseudomembranous colitis has been established, therapeutic measures should be initiated. Mild cases of pseudomembranous colitis usually respond to drug discontinuation alone. In moderate to severe cases, consideration should be given to management with fluids and electrolytes, protein supplementation and treatment with an antibacterial drug effective against *C. difficile.*

PRECAUTIONS

General: INTRAVENOUS CIPROFLOXACIN SHOULD BE ADMINISTERED BY SLOW INFUSION OVER A PERIOD OF 60 MINUTES. Local iv site reactions have been reported with the intravenous administration of ciprofloxacin. These reactions are more frequent if infusion time is 30 minutes or less or if small veins of the hand are used. (See ADVERSE REACTIONS.)

Crystals of ciprofloxacin have been observed rarely in the urine of human subjects but more frequently in the urine of laboratory animals, which is usually alkaline. (See ANIMAL PHARMACOLOGY.) Crystalluria related to ciprofloxacin has been reported only rarely in humans because human urine is usually acidic. Alkalinity of the urine should be avoided in patients receiving ciprofloxacin. Patients should be well hydrated to prevent the formation of highly concentrated urine.

Continued on next page

Bayer Corporation—Cont.

Alteration of the dosage regimen is necessary for patients with impairment of renal function. (See DOSAGE AND ADMINISTRATION.)

Moderate to severe phototoxicity manifested by an exaggerated sunburn reaction has been observed in some patients who were exposed to direct sunlight while receiving some members of the quinolone class of drugs. Excessive sunlight should be avoided.

As with any potent drug, periodic assessment of organ system functions, including renal, hepatic, and hematopoietic, is advisable during prolonged therapy.

Information for Patients: Patients should be advised that ciprofloxacin may be associated with hypersensitivity reactions, even following a single dose, and to discontinue the drug at the first sign of a skin rash or other allergic reaction. Ciprofloxacin may cause dizziness and lightheadedness; therefore, patients should know how they react to this drug before they operate an automobile or machinery or engage in activities requiring mental alertness or coordination.

Patients should be advised that ciprofloxacin may increase the effects of theophylline and caffeine. There is a possibility of caffeine accumulation when products containing caffeine are consumed while taking quinolones.

Drug Interactions: As with other quinolones, concurrent administration of ciprofloxacin with theophylline may lead to elevated serum concentrations of theophylline and prolongation of its elimination half-life. This may result in increased risk of theophylline-related adverse reactions. (See WARNINGS.) If concomitant use cannot be avoided, serum levels of theophylline should be monitored and dosage adjustments made as appropriate.

Some quinolones, including ciprofloxacin, have also been shown to interfere with the metabolism of caffeine. This may lead to reduced clearance of caffeine and a prolongation of its serum half-life.

Some quinolones, including ciprofloxacin, have been associated with transient elevations in serum creatinine in patients receiving cyclosporine concomitantly.

Quinolones have been reported to enhance the effects of the oral anticoagulant warfarin or its derivatives. When these products are administered concomitantly, prothrombin time or other suitable coagulation tests should be closely monitored.

Probenecid interferes with renal tubular secretion of ciprofloxacin and produces an increase in the level of ciprofloxacin in the serum. This should be considered if patients are receiving both drugs concomitantly.

As with other broad-spectrum antimicrobial agents, prolonged use of ciprofloxacin may result in overgrowth of non-susceptible organisms. Repeated evaluation of the patient's condition and microbial susceptibility testing are essential. If superinfection occurs during therapy, appropriate measures should be taken.

Carcinogenesis, Mutagenesis, Impairment of Fertility: Eight *in vitro* mutagenicity tests have been conducted with ciprofloxacin. Test results are listed below:

Salmonella/Microsome Test (Negative)
E. coli DNA Repair Assay (Negative)
Mouse Lymphoma Cell Forward Mutation Assay (Positive)
Chinese Hamster V_{79} Cell HGPRT Test (Negative)
Syrian Hamster Embryo Cell Transformation Assay (Negative)
Saccharomyces cerevisiae Point Mutation Assay (Negative)
Saccharomyces cerevisiae Mitotic Crossover and Gene Conversion Assay (Negative)
Rat Hepatocyte DNA Repair Assay (Positive)

Thus, two of the eight tests were positive, but results of the following three *in vivo* test systems gave negative results:

Rat Hepatocyte DNA Repair Assay
Micronucleus Test (Mice)
Dominant Lethal Test (Mice)

Long-term carcinogenicity studies in mice and rats have been completed. After daily oral dosing for up to 2 years, there is no evidence that ciprofloxacin has any carcinogenic or tumorigenic effects in these species.

Pregnancy: Teratogenic Effects. Pregnancy Category C: Reproduction studies have been performed in rats and mice at doses up to 6 times the usual daily human dose and have revealed no evidence of impaired fertility or harm to the fetus due to ciprofloxacin. In rabbits, ciprofloxacin (30

and 100 mg/kg orally) produced gastrointestinal disturbances resulting in maternal weight loss and an increased incidence of abortion. No teratogenicity was observed at either dose. After intravenous administration of doses up to 20 mg/kg, no maternal toxicity was produced, and no embryotoxicity or teratogenicity was observed. There are, however, no adequate and well-controlled studies in pregnant women. Ciprofloxacin should be used during pregnancy only if the potential benefit justifies the potential risk to the fetus. (See WARNINGS.)

Nursing Mothers: Ciprofloxacin is excreted in human milk. Because of the potential for serious adverse reactions in infants nursing from mothers taking ciprofloxacin, a decision should be made either to discontinue nursing or to discontinue the drug, taking into account the importance of the drug to the mother.

Pediatric Use: Safety and effectiveness in children and adolescents less than 18 years of age have not been established. Ciprofloxacin causes arthropathy in juvenile animals. (See WARNINGS.)

ADVERSE REACTIONS

The most frequently reported events, without regard to drug relationship, among patients treated with intravenous ciprofloxacin were nausea, diarrhea, central nervous system disturbance, local iv site reactions, abnormalities of liver associated enzymes (hepatic enzymes) and eosinophilia. Headache, restlessness and rash were also noted in greater than 1% of patients treated with the most common doses of ciprofloxacin.

Local iv site reactions have been reported with the intravenous administration of ciprofloxacin. These reactions are more frequent if the infusion time is 30 minutes or less. These may appear as local skin reactions which resolve rapidly upon completion of the infusion. Subsequent intravenous administration is not contraindicated unless the reactions recur or worsen.

Additional events, without regard to drug relationship or route of administration, that occurred in 1% or less of ciprofloxacin courses are listed below:

GASTROINTESTINAL: ileus; jaundice; gastrointestinal bleeding; *C. difficile* associated diarrhea; pseudomembranous colitis; pancreatitis; hepatic necrosis; intestinal perforation; dyspepsia; epigastric or abdominal pain; vomiting; constipation; oral ulceration; oral candidiasis; mouth dryness; anorexia; dysphagia; flatulence.

CENTRAL NERVOUS SYSTEM: convulsive seizures, paranoia, toxic psychosis, depression, dysphasia, phobia, depersonalization, manic reaction, unresponsiveness, ataxia, confusion, hallucinations, dizziness, lightheadedness, paresthesia, anxiety, tremor, insomnia, nightmares, weakness, drowsiness, irritability, malaise, lethargy.

SKIN/HYPERSENSITIVITY: anaphylactic reactions; erythema multiforme/Stevens-Johnson syndrome; exfoliative dermatitis; toxic epidermal necrolysis; vasculitis; angioedema; edema of the lips, face, neck, conjunctivae, hands or lower extremities; purpura; fever; chills; flushing; pruritus; urticaria; cutaneous candidiasis; vesicles; increased perspiration; hyperpigmentation; erythema nodosum; photosensitivity.

Allergic reactions ranging from urticaria to anaphylactic reactions have been reported. (See WARNINGS.)

SPECIAL SENSES: decreased visual acuity, blurred vision, disturbed vision (flashing lights, change in color perception, overbrightness of lights, diplopia), eye pain, anosmia, hearing loss, tinnitus, nystagmus, a bad taste.

MUSCULOSKELETAL: joint pain; jaw, arm or back pain; joint stiffness; neck and chest pain; achiness; flare up of gout.

RENAL/UROGENITAL: renal failure, interstitial nephritis, hemorrhagic cystitis, renal calculi, frequent urination, acidosis, urethral bleeding, polyuria, urinary retention, gynecomastia, candiduria, vaginitis. Crystalluria, cylindruria, hematuria, and albuminuria have also been reported.

CARDIOVASCULAR: cardiovascular collapse, cardiopulmonary arrest, myocardial infarction, arrhythmia, tachycardia, palpitation, cerebral thrombosis, syncope, cardiac murmur, hypertension, hypotension, angina pectoris.

RESPIRATORY: respiratory arrest, pulmonary embolism, dyspnea, pulmonary edema, respiratory distress, pleural effusion hemoptysis, epistaxis, hiccough.

IV INFUSION SITE: thrombophlebitis, burning, pain, pruritus, paresthesia, erythema, swelling.

Also reported were agranulocytosis, prolongation of prothrombin time and possible exacerbation of myasthenia gravis.

Many of these events were described as only mild or moderate in severity, abated soon after the drug was discontinued and required no treatment.

In several instances, nausea, vomiting, tremor, irritability or palpitation were judged by investigators to be related to elevated serum levels of theophylline possibly as a result of drug interaction with ciprofloxacin.

Adverse Laboratory Changes: The most frequently reported changes in laboratory parameters with intravenous ciprofloxacin therapy, without regard to drug relationship, were:

Hepatic	— Elevations of AST (SGOT), ALT (SGPT), alkaline phosphatase, LDH and serum billirubin.
Hematologic	— Elevated eosinophil and platelet counts, decreased platelet counts, hemoglobin and/or hematocrit.
Renal	— Elevations of serum creatinine, BUN, uric acid.
Other	— Elevations of serum creatine phosphokinase, serum theophylline (in patients receiving theophylline concomitantly), blood glucose, and triglycerides.

Other changes occurring infrequently were: decreased leukocyte count, elevated atypical lymphocyte count, immature WBCs, elevated serum calcium, elevation of serum gamma-glutamyl transpeptidase (γ GT), decreased BUN, decreased uric acid, decreased total serum protein, decreased serum albumin, decreased serum potassium, elevated serum potassium, elevated serum cholesterol.

Other changes occurring rarely during administration of ciprofloxacin were: elevation of serum amylase, decrease of blood glucose, pancytopenia, leukocytosis, elevated sedimentation rate, change in serum phenytoin, decreased prothrombin time, hemolytic anemia, and bleeding diathesis.

OVERDOSAGE

In the event of acute overdosage, the patient should be carefully observed and given supportive treatment. Adequate hydration must be maintained. Only a small amount of ciprofloxacin (< 10%) is removed from the body after hemodialysis or peritoneal dialysis.

DOSAGE AND ADMINISTRATION

The recommended adult dosage for urinary tract infections of mild to moderate severity is 200 mg every 12 hours. For severe or complicated urinary tract infections the recommended dosage is 400 mg every 12 hours.

The recommended adult dosage for lower respiratory tract infections, skin and skin structure infections and bone and joint infections of mild to moderate severity is 400 mg every 12 hours.

The determination of dosage for any particular patient must take into consideration the severity and nature of the infection, the susceptibility of the causative organism, the integrity of the patient's host-defense mechanisms and the status of renal and hepatic function.

[See table at bottom left.]

After dilution Cipro® I.V. should be administered by intravenous infusion over a period of 60 minutes.

The duration of treatment depends upon the severity of infection. Generally, ciprofloxacin should be continued for at least 2 days after the signs and symptoms of infection have disappeared. The usual duration is 7 to 14 days. Bone and joint infections may require treatment for 4 to 6 weeks or longer.

Cipro® (ciprofloxacin hydrochloride) Tablets for oral administration are available. Parenteral therapy may be changed to oral Cipro® tablets when the condition warrants, at the discretion of the physician. For complete dosage and administration information, see Cipro® tablet package insert.

Impaired Renal Function: The following table provides dosage guidelines for use in patients with renal impairment; however, monitoring of serum drug levels provides the most reliable basis for dosage adjustment.

RECOMMENDED STARTING AND MAINTENANCE DOSES FOR PATIENTS WITH IMPAIRED RENAL FUNCTION

Creatinine Clearance (mL/min)	Dosage
≥30	See usual dosage
5–29	200–400 mg q 18–24 hr

When only the serum creatinine concentration is known, the following formula may be used to estimate creatinine clearance.

Men: Creatinine clearance (mL/min) $= \dfrac{\text{Weight (kg)} \times (140 - \text{age})}{72 \times \text{serum creatinine (mg/dL)}}$

Women: 0.85 × the value calculated for men.

DOSAGE GUIDELINES

Location of Infection	Type or Severity	Intravenous Unit Dose	Frequency	Daily Dose
Urinary tract	Mild/Moderate	200 mg	q 12 h	400 mg
	Severe/Complicated	400 mg	q 12 h	800 mg
Lower Respiratory tract Skin and Skin Structure Bone and Joint	Mild/Moderate	400 mg	q 12 h	800 mg

The serum creatinine should represent a steady state of renal function.
For patients with changing renal function or for patients with renal impairment and hepatic insufficiency, measurement of serum concentrations of ciprofloxacin will provide additional guidance for adjusting dosage.

INTRAVENOUS ADMINISTRATION
After dilution Cipro® I.V. should be administered by intravenous infusion over a period of 60 minutes. Slow infusion of a dilute solution into a large vein will minimize patient discomfort and reduce the risk of venous irritation.
PHARMACY BULK PACKAGE: The pharmacy bulk package is a single-entry container of a sterile preparation for parenteral use that contains many single doses. It contains ciprofloxacin as a 1% aqueous solution concentrate. The contents are intended for use in a pharmacy admixture program and are restricted to the preparation of admixtures for intravenous infusion. **THE CLOSURE SHALL BE PENETRATED ONLY ONE TIME** with a suitable sterile transfer set or dispensing device which allows measured dispensing of the contents.
The pharmacy bulk package is to be used only in a suitable work area such as laminar flow hood or an equivalent clean air or compounding area. **THIS PREPARATION MUST BE DILUTED BEFORE USE.** The intravenous dose should be prepared by aseptically withdrawing the Cipro® I.V. concentrate from the pharmacy bulk package and diluting the appropriate volume with a suitable intravenous solution to a final concentration of 0.5–2 mg/mL (See COMPATIBILITY AND STABILITY). The resulting solution should be infused over a period of 60 minutes by direct infusion or through a Y-type intravenous set which may already be in place. If this method or the "piggyback" method of administration is used, it is advisable to discontinue the administration of any other intravenous solutions during the infusion of Cipro® I.V.

COMPATIBILITY AND STABILITY
Ciprofloxacin injection 1% (10 mg/mL), when diluted with the following intravenous solutions to concentrations of 0.5 to 2.0 mg/mL, is stable for up to 14 days at refrigerated or room temperature storage.
0.9% Sodium Chloride Injection, USP
5% Dextrose Injection, USP
If Cipro® I.V. is to be given with another drug, each drug should be given separately in accordance with the recommended dosage and route of administration for each drug.

HOW SUPPLIED
Cipro® I.V. (ciprofloxacin) is a clear, colorless to slightly yellowish solution supplied in the pharmacy bulk package as follows:

CONTAINER	SIZE	STRENGTH	NDC NUMBER
Pharmacy Bulk Package	120 mL	1200 mg, 1%	0026-8566-65

STORAGE
Store between 41–86°F (5–30°C).
Protect from light, avoid excessive heat, protect from freezing.
Cipro® I.V. (ciprofloxacin) is also available as follows:

CONTAINER	SIZE	STRENGTH	NDC NUMBER
Vial	20 mL	200 mg, 1%	0026-8562-20
	40 mL	400 mg, 1%	0026-8564-64
Flexible Container	100 mL 5% dextrose	200 mg, 0.2%	0026-8552-36
	200 mL 5% dextrose	400 mg, 0.2%	0026-8554-63

Ciprofloxacin is also available as Cipro® (ciprofloxacin HCl) Tablets 250, 500 and 750 mg.

ANIMAL PHARMACOLOGY
Ciprofloxacin and other quinolones have been shown to cause arthropathy in immature animals of most species tested. (See WARNINGS.) Damage of weight-bearing joints was observed in juvenile dogs and rats. In young beagles, 100 mg/kg ciprofloxacin given daily for 4 weeks caused degenerative articular changes of the knee joint. At 30 mg/kg, the effect on the joint was minimal. In a subsequent study in beagles, removal of weight-bearing on the joint reduced the lesions but did not totally prevent them.
Crystalluria, sometimes associated with secondary nephropathy, occurs in laboratory animals dosed with ciprofloxacin. This is primarily related to the reduced solubility of ciprofloxacin under alkaline conditions, which predominate in the urine of test animals; in man, crystalluria is rare since human urine is typically acidic. In rhesus monkeys, crystalluria without nephropathy has been noted after intravenous doses as low as 5 mg/kg. After 6 months of intravenous dosing at 10 mg/kg/day, no nephropathological changes were noted; however, nephropathy was observed after dosing at 20 mg/kg/day for the same duration.
In dogs, ciprofloxacin administered at 3 and 10 mg/kg by rapid intravenous injection (15 sec.) produces pronounced hypotensive effects. These effects are considered to be related to histamine release because they are partially antagonized by pyrilamine, an antihistamine. In rhesus monkeys, rapid intravenous injection also produces hypotension, but the effect in this species is inconsistent and less pronounced.
In mice, concomitant administration of nonsteroidal anti-inflammatory drugs, such as fenbufen, phenylbutazone and indomethacin, with quinolones has been reported to enhance the CNS stimulatory effect of quinolones.
Ocular toxicity, seen with some related drugs, has not been observed in ciprofloxacin-treated animals.

Bayer Corporation
Pharmaceutical Division
400 Morgan Lane
West Haven, CT 06516 USA

Caution: Federal (USA) Law prohibits dispensing without a prescription.

PD500015 3/95 BAY q 3939
5202-4-A-U.S.-2 5039
Shown in Product Identification Guide, page 305

DTIC-Dome® ℞
(dacarbazine)
Sterile

> **WARNING**
> It is recommended that DTIC-Dome (dacarbazine) be administered under the supervision of a qualified physician experienced in the use of cancer chemotherapeutic agents.
> 1. Hemopoietic depression is the most common toxicity with DTIC-Dome (See Warnings).
> 2. Hepatic necrosis has been reported (See Warnings).
> 3. Studies have demonstrated this agent to have a carcinogenic and teratogenic effect when used in animals.
> 4. In treatment of each patient, the physician must weigh carefully the possibility of achieving therapeutic benefit against the risk of toxicity.

DESCRIPTION
DTIC-Dome Sterile (dacarbazine) is a colorless to an ivory colored solid which is light sensitive. Each vial contains 100 mg of dacarbazine, or 200 mg of dacarbazine (the active ingredient), anhydrous citric acid and mannitol. DTIC-Dome is reconstituted and administered intravenously (pH 3–4). DTIC-Dome is an anticancer agent. Chemically, DTIC-Dome is 5-(3,3-dimethyl-1-triazeno)-imidazole-4-carboxamide (DTIC) with the following structural formula:

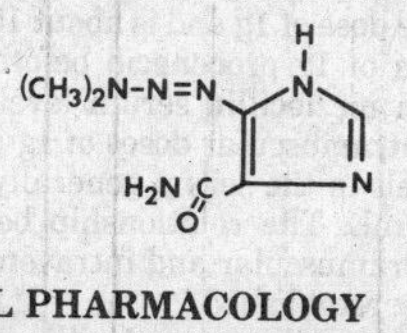

$C_6H_{10}N_6O$

CLINICAL PHARMACOLOGY
After intravenous administration of DTIC-Dome, the volume of distribution exceeds total body water content suggesting localization in some body tissue, probably the liver. Its disappearance from the plasma is biphasic with initial half-life of 19 minutes and a terminal half-life of 5 hours.[1] In a patient with renal and hepatic dysfunctions, the half-lives were lengthened to 55 minutes and 7.2 hours.[1] The average cumulative excretion of unchanged DTIC in the urine is 40% of the injected dose in 6 hours.[1] DTIC is subject to renal tubular secretion rather than glomerular filtration. At therapeutic concentrations DTIC is not appreciably bound to human plasma protein.
In man, DTIC is extensively degraded. Besides unchanged DTIC, 5-aminoimidazole -4 carboxamide (AIC) is a major metabolite of DTIC excreted in the urine. AIC is not derived endogenously but from the injected DTIC, because the administration of radioactive DTIC labeled with ^{14}C in the imidazole portion of the molecule (DTIC-2-^{14}C) gives rise to AIC-2-^{14}C.[1]
Although the exact mechanism of action of DTIC-Dome is not known, three hypotheses have been offered:
1. inhibition of DNA synthesis by acting as a purine analog
2. action as an alkylating agent
3. interaction with SH groups

INDICATIONS AND USAGE
DTIC-Dome is indicated in the treatment of metastatic malignant melanoma. In addition, DTIC-Dome is also indicated for Hodgkin's disease as a secondary-line therapy when used in combination with other effective agents.

CONTRAINDICATIONS
DTIC-Dome is contraindicated in patients who have demonstrated a hypersensitivity to it in the past.

WARNINGS
Hemopoietic depression is the most common toxicity with DTIC-Dome and involves primarily the leukocytes and platelets, although, anemia may sometimes occur. Leukopenia and thrombocytopenia may be severe enough to cause death. The possible bone marrow depression requires careful monitoring of white blood cells, red blood cells, and platelet levels. Hemopioetic toxicity may warrant temporary suspension or cessation of therapy with DTIC-Dome.
Hepatic toxicity accompanied by hepatic vein thrombosis and hepatocellular necrosis resulting in death, has been reported. The incidence of such reactions has been low; approximately 0.01% of patients treated. This toxicity has been observed mostly when DTIC-Dome has been administered concomitantly with other anti-neoplastic drugs; however, it has also been reported in some patients treated with DTIC-Dome alone.
Anaphylaxis can occur following the administration of DTIC-Dome.

PRECAUTIONS
Hospitalization is not always necessary but adequate laboratory study capability must be available. Extravasation of the drug subcutaneously during intravenous administration may result in tissue damage and severe pain. Local pain, burning sensation, and irritation at the site of injection may be relieved by locally applied hot packs.
Carcinogenicity of DTIC was studied in rats and mice. Proliferative endocardial lesions, including fibrosarcomas and sarcomas were induced by DTIC in rats. In mice, administration of DTIC resulted in the induction of angiosarcomas of the spleen.
Pregnancy Category C. DTIC-Dome has been shown to be teratogenic in rats when given in doses 20 times the human daily dose on day 12 of gestation. DTIC when administered in 10 times the human daily dose to male rats (twice weekly for 9 weeks) did not affect the male libido, although female rats mated to male rats had higher incidence of resorptions than controls. In rabbits, DTIC daily dose 7 times the human daily dose given on Days 6–15 of gestation resulted in fetal skeletal anomalies. There are no adequate and well controlled studies in pregnant women. DTIC-Dome should be used during pregnancy only if the potential benefit justifies the potential risk to the fetus.
It is not known whether this drug is excreted in human milk. Because many drugs are excreted in human milk and because of the potential for tumorigenicity shown for DTIC-Dome in animal studies, a decision should be made whether to discontinue nursing or to discontinue the drug, taking into account the importance of the drug to the mother.

ADVERSE REACTIONS
Symptoms of anorexia, nausea, and vomiting are the most frequently noted of all toxic reactions. Over 90% of patients are affected with the initial few doses. The vomiting lasts 1–12 hours and is incompletely and unpredictably palliated with phenobarbital and/or prochlorperazine. Rarely, intractable nausea and vomiting have necessitated discontinuance of therapy with DTIC-Dome. Rarely, DTIC-Dome has caused diarrhea. Some helpful suggestions include restricting the patient's oral intake of food for 4–6 hours prior to treatment. The rapid toleration of these symptoms suggests that a central nervous system mechanism may be involved, and usually these symptoms subside after the first 1 or 2 days.
There are a number of minor toxicities that are infrequently noted. Patients have experienced an influenza-like syndrome of fever to 39°C, myalgias and malaise. These symptoms occur usually after large single doses, may last for several days, and they may occur with successive treatments.
Alopecia has been noted as has facial flushing and facial paresthesia. There have been few reports of significant liver or renal function test abnormalities in man. However, these abnormalities have been observed more frequently in animal studies.
Erythematous and urticarial rashes have been observed infrequently after administration of DTIC-Dome. Rarely, photosensitivity reactions may occur.

OVERDOSAGE
Give supportive treatment and monitor blood cell counts.

DOSAGE AND ADMINISTRATION
Malignant Melanoma: The recommended dosage is 2 to 4.5mg/kg/day for 10 days. Treatment may be repeated at 4 week intervals.[2]
An alternate recommended dosage is 250mg/square meter body surface/day I.V. for 5 days. Treatment may be repeated every 3 weeks.[3,4]
Hodgkin's Disease: The recommended dosage of DTIC-Dome in the treatment of Hodgkin's Disease is 150mg/square meter body surface/day for 5 days, in combination with other effective drugs. Treatment may be repeated every 4 weeks.[5] An alternative recommended dosage is 375mg/square meter body surface on day 1, in combination with other effective drugs, to be repeated every 15 days.[6]

Continued on next page

Bayer Corporation—Cont.

DTIC-Dome (dacarbazine) 100mg/vial and 200mg/vial are reconstituted with 9.9 mL and 19.7 mL, respectively, of Sterile Water for Injection, U.S.P. The resulting solution contains 10mg/mL of dacarbazine having a pH of 3.0 to 4.0. The calculated dose of the resulting solution is drawn into a syringe and administered *only* intravenously.
The reconstituted solution may be further diluted with 5% dextrose injection, U.S.P. or sodium chloride injection, U.S.P. and administered as an intravenous infusion.
After reconstitution and prior to use, the solution in the vial may be stored at 4°C for up to 72 hours or at normal room conditions (temperature and light) for up to 8 hours. If the reconstituted solution is further diluted in 5% dextrose, injection, U.S.P. or sodium chloride injection, U.S.P., the resulting solution may be stored at 4°C for up to 24 hours or at normal room conditions for up to 8 hours.
Procedures for proper handling and disposal of anticancer drugs should be considered. Several guidelines on this subject have been published.[7–12] There is no general agreement that all of the procedures recommended in the guidelines are necessary or appropriate.

HOW SUPPLIED

10 mL vials containing 100 mg or 20 mL vials containing 200 mg of DTIC-Dome as sterile dacarbazine in boxes of 12. Store in a refrigerator 2°C to 8°C (36°F to 46°F).

REFERENCES

1. Loo, T.J., *et al.:* Mechanism of action and pharmacology studies with DTIC (NSC-45388). Cancer Treatment Reports 60: 149–152, 1976.
2. Nathanson, L., *et al.:* Characteristics of prognosis and response to an imidazole carboxamide in malignant melanoma. Clinical Pharmacology and Therapeutics 12: 955–962, 1971.
3. Costanza, M.E., *et al.:* Therapy of malignant melanoma with an imidazole carboxamide and bischloroethyl nitrosourea. Cancer 30: 1457–1461, 1972.
4. Luce, J.K., *et al.:* Clinical trials with the antitumor agent 5-(3, 3-dimethyl-1-triazeno) imidazole-4-carboxamide (NSC-45388). Cancer Chemotherapy Reports 54: 119–124, 1970.
5. Bonadonna, G., *et al.:* Combined Chemotherapy (MOPP or ABVD)—radiotherapy approach in advanced Hodgkin's disease. Cancer Treatment Reports 61: 769–777, 1977.
6. Santoro, A., and Bonadonna, G.: Prolonged disease-free survival in MOPP-resistant Hodgkin's disease after treatment with adriamycin, bleomycin, vinblastine and dacarbazine (ABVD). Cancer Chemotherapy Pharmacol. 2: 101–105, 1979.
7. Recommendations for the Safe Handling of Parenteral Antineoplastic Drugs. NIH Publication No. 83-2621. For sale by the Superintendent of Documents, U.S. Government Printing Office, Washington, D.C. 20402.
8. AMA Council Report. Guidelines for Handling Parenteral Antineoplastics. JAMA, March 15, 1985.
9. National Study Commission on Cytotoxic Exposure—Recommendations for Handling Cytotoxic Agents. Available from Louis P. Jeffrey, Sc. D., Director of Pharmacy Services, Rhode Island Hospital, 593 Eddy Street, Providence, Rhode Island 02902.
10. Clinical Oncological Society of Australia: Guidelines and recommendations for safe handling of antineoplastic agents. Med. J. Australia 1: 426–428, 1983.
11. Jones, R.B., *et al.:* Safe handling of chemotherapeutic agents: A report from the Mount Sinai Medical Center. Ca-A Cancer Journal for Clinicians Sept./Oct. 258–263, 1983.
12. American Society of Hospital Pharmacists technical assistance bulletin on handling cytotoxic drugs in hospitals. Am. J. Hosp. Pharm. 42: 131–137, 1985.

Manufactured by:
Ben Venue Laboratories
Bedford, Ohio 44146
Distributed by:
Bayer Corporation
Pharmaceutical Division
400 Morgan Lane
West Haven, CT 06516 USA
PD500002 2/95 5071

MEZLIN® ℞

Sterile mezlocillin sodium
for intravenous or intramuscular use.
BAYPEN®

DESCRIPTION

MEZLIN® (sterile mezlocillin sodium) is a semisynthetic broad spectrum penicillin antibiotic for parenteral administration. It is the monohydrate sodium salt of 6-{D-2 [3-(methyl-sulfonyl) -2- OXO- imidazolidine-1- carboxamido]-2-phenyl acetamido} penicillanic acid.

MEZLOCILLIN SERUM LEVELS IN ADULTS (mcg/mL) 2–5 MIN. IV INJECTION

DOSE	0	15 min.	30 min.	45 min.	1 hr.	2 hr.	3 hr.	4 hr.	6 hr.
4g	—	**254** (155–400)	**163** (99–260)	**122** (78–215)	**93** (67–133)	**47** (22–96)	**20** (8–45)	**9.1** (6–13)	**8.4** (5–17)

Structural Formula:

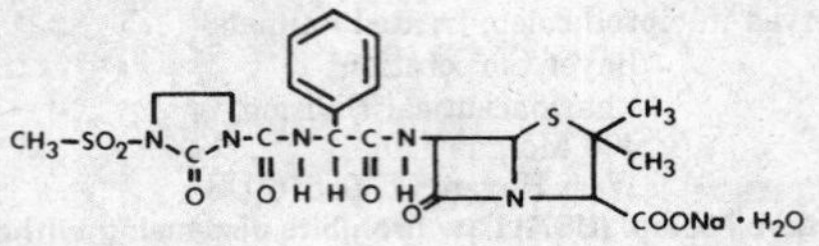

Empirical Formula:
$C_{21}H_{24}N_5O_8S_2Na \cdot H_2O$

MEZLIN® has a molecular weight of 579.6 and contains 42.6 mg (1.85 mEq) of sodium per one gram of mezlocillin activity. The dosage form is supplied as a sterile white to pale yellow crystalline powder, which is freely soluble in water. When reconstituted, solutions of MEZLIN® are clear and range from colorless to pale yellow with a pH of 4.5 to 8.0.

CLINICAL PHARMACOLOGY

Intravenous Administration. In healthy adult volunteers, mean serum levels of mezlocillin 5 minutes after a 5-minute intravenous injection of 1g, 2g, or 5g are 100, 253, or 411 mcg/mL, respectively. Serum levels, as noted below, lack dose proportionality:
[See table on top of next page.]
Fifteen minutes after a 4g intravenous injection (2–5 min.), the concentration in serum is 254 mcg/mL; 1 hour and 4 hours later levels are 93 mcg/mL and 9.1 mcg/mL, respectively:
[See table above.]
After an intravenous infusion (15 min.) of 3g, mean levels 15 minutes after dosing are 269 mcg/mL (170–280).
A 30-minute intravenous infusion of 3g produces mean peak concentrations of 263 mcg/mL; 1 hour and 4 hours later the concentrations are 57 mcg/mL and 4.4 mcg/mL, respectively:
[See second table at top of next page.]
Following intravenous infusion (2 hr.) of a 3g dose of mezlocillin every 4 hours for 7 days, mean peak serum concentrations are higher than 100 mcg/mL, and levels above 50 mcg/mL are maintained throughout dosing.
Intramuscular Administration. MEZLIN® is rapidly absorbed after intramuscular injection. In healthy volunteers, the mean peak serum concentration occurs approximately 45 minutes after a single dose of 1g and is about 15 mcg/mL. The oral administration of 1g probenecid before injection produces an increase in mezlocillin serum levels of about 50%. After repetitive intramuscular doses of 1g mezlocillin every 6 hours, peak levels in the serum generally range between 35 and 45 mcg/mL. The relationship between the pharmacokinetics of intramuscular and intravenous dosing has not yet been clearly established.
General. As with other penicillins, mezlocillin is excreted primarily by glomerular filtration and tubular secretion. The rate of elimination is dose dependent and related to the degree of renal functional impairment. In patients with normal renal function, approximately 55% of the administered dose is recovered from the urine within the first 6 hours after dosing. Two hours after an intravenous injection of 2g, concentrations of active drug in urine generally exceed 4000 mcg/mL. By 4–6 hours after injection, concentrations usually decline to a range of about 50 to 200 mcg/mL. The serum elimination half-life of mezlocillin after intravenous dosing is approximately 55 minutes.
In patients with reduced renal function, the half-life is only slightly prolonged. Dosage adjustments are usually not necessary except in patients with severe renal impairment. (See Dosage and Administration.) As with other penicillins, mezlocillin is metabolized only slightly; less than 10% of the drug excreted in the urine is in the form of the penicilloate or penilloate. The drug is readily removed from the serum by hemodialysis and, to a lesser extent, by peritoneal dialysis.
Up to 26% of a dose of mezlocillin is recovered from the bile of patients with normal liver function. Following intravenous doses of 2 to 5g, concentrations of active drug in bile generally range from 500 to 2500 mcg/mL. The biliary excretion of mezlocillin is reduced in patients with common bile duct obstruction.
Mezlocillin is not appreciably absorbed when given orally. Following parenteral administration, the apparent volume of distribution is approximately equal to the extracellular fluid volume. The drug is present in active form in the serum, urine, bile, peritoneal fluid, pleural fluid, bronchial and wound secretions, bone and other tissues. As with other penicillins, penetration into the cerebrospinal fluid (CSF) is generally poor, however higher CSF concentrations are obtained in the presence of meningeal inflammation.
Protein binding studies indicate that the degree of mezlocillin binding is low (16–42%) and depends upon testing methods and concentrations of drug studied.

Microbiology
Mezlocillin is a bactericidal antibiotic which acts by interfering with synthesis of cell wall components. It is active against a variety of gram-negative and gram-positive bacteria, including aerobic and anaerobic strains. Mezlocillin is usually active *in vitro* against most strains of the following organisms:

Gram-negative bacteria
Escherichia coli
Proteus mirabilis
Proteus vulgaris
Morganella morganii (formerly *P. morganii*)
Providencia rettgeri (formerly *Proteus rettgeri*)
Providencia stuartii
Citrobacter species*
Klebsiella species (including *K. pneumoniae*)
Enterobacter species
Shigella species*
Pseudomonas aeruginosa (and other species)
Haemophilus influenzae
Haemophilus parainfluenzae
Neisseria species
Many strains of *Serratia*, *Salmonella**, and *Acinetobacter** are also susceptible.

Gram-positive bacteria
Staphylococcus aureus (non-penicillinase producing strains)
Beta-hemolytic *streptococci* (Groups A and B)
Streptococcus pneumoniae (formerly *Diplococcus Pneumoniae*)
Streptococcus faecalis (enterococcus)

Anaerobic Organisms
Peptococcus species
Peptostreptococcus species
Clostridium species*
Bacteroides species (including *B. fragilis* group)
Fusobacterium species*
Veillonella species*
Eubacterium species*
*Mezlocillin has been shown to be active *in vitro* against these organisms, however clinical efficacy has not yet been established.
Noteworthy is mezlocillin's broadened spectrum of *in vitro* activity against important pathogenic aerobic gram-negative bacteria, including strains of *Pseudomonas, Klebsiella, Enterobacter, Serratia, Proteus, Escherichia* and *Haemophilus,* as well as *Bacteroides* and other anaerobes; and its excellent inhibitory effect against gram-positive organisms including *Streptococcus faecalis* (enterococcus). It is inactive against penicillinase-producing strains of *Staphylococcus aureus.*
In vitro studies have shown that mezlocillin combined with an aminoglycoside (e.g., gentamicin, tobramycin, amikacin, sisomicin) acts synergistically against strains of *Streptococcus faecalis* and *Pseudomonas aeruginosa.* In some instances, this combination also acts synergistically *in vitro* against other gram-negative bacteria such as *Serratia, Klebsiella* and *Acinetobacter* species.
Mezlocillin is slightly more active when tested at alkaline pH and, as with other penicillins, has reduced activity when tested *in vitro* with increasing inoculum. The minimum bactericidal concentration (MBC) generally exceeds the minimum inhibitory concentration (MIC) by a factor of 2 or 3. Resistance to mezlocillin *in vitro* develops slowly (multiple step mutation). Some strains of *Pseudomonas aeruginosa* have developed resistance fairly rapidly. Mezlocillin is not stable in the presence of penicillinase and strains of *Staphylococcus aureus* resistant to penicillin are also resistant to mezlocillin.

Susceptibility Tests
Quantitative methods that require measurement of zone diameters give good estimates of bacterial susceptibility. One such procedure* has been recommended for use with discs to test susceptibility to antimicrobials. When the causative organism is tested by the Kirby-Bauer method of disc susceptibility, a 75 mcg mezlocillin disc should give a zone of 18 mm or greater to indicate susceptibility. Zone sizes of 14 mm or less indicate resistance. Zone sizes of 15 to 17 mm indicate intermediate susceptibility. Susceptible strains of *Haemophilus* and *Neisseria* species give zones of ≥29 mm, resistant strains ≤28 mm. With this procedure, a report from the laboratory of "Susceptible" indicates that the infecting organism is likely to respond to therapy. A report of

MEZLOCILLIN SERUM LEVELS IN ADULTS (mcg/mL) 5 MIN. IV INJECTION

DOSE	0	5 min.	10 min.	20 min.	30 min.	1 hr.	2 hr.	3 hr.	4 hr.	6 hr.	8 hr.
1g	149 (132–185)	100 (64–143)	66 (47–87)	50 (31–87)	40 (22–83)	18 (8–31)	5.3 (3.3–7.7)	2.5 (1.7–3.7)	1.7 (0.7–2.8)	0.5 (0–1.2)	0.1 (0–0.2)
2g	314 (207–362)	253 (161–364)	161 (113–214)	117 (76–174)	82 (55–112)	56 (23–88)	20 (7.5–32)	11 (3.8–16)	4.4 (1.6–8.7)	1.5 (0.5–2.6)	0.6 (0.1–1.4)
5g	547 (268–854)	411 (199–597)	357 (246–456)	250 (203–353)	226 (190–333)	131 (104–193)	76 (59–104)	31 (20–40)	13 (6.4–17)	4.6 (2.1–9.4)	1.9 (1.1–3.6)

MEZLOCILLIN SERUM LEVELS IN ADULTS (mcg/mL) 30 MIN. IV INFUSION

DOSE	0	5 min.	15 min.	30 min.	45 min.	1 hr.	2 hr.	3 hr.	4 hr.	6 hr.	8 hr.
3g	263 (87–489)	170 (63–371)	141 (75–301)	109 (56–288)	79 (41–135)	57 (28–100)	26 (14–55)	12 (5.8–26)	4.4 (2.2–6.5)	1.6 (1.0–3.4)	< 1

"Resistant" indicates that the infecting organism is not likely to respond to therapy; other therapy should be selected. A report of "Intermediate Susceptibility" suggests that the organism may be susceptible if the infection is confined to tissues and fluids (e.g., urine), in which high antibiotic levels are attained. The mezlocillin disc should be used for testing susceptibility to mezlocillin. In certain conditions, it may be desirable to do additional susceptibility testing by broth or agar dilution techniques. Dilution methods, preferably the agar plate dilution procedure, are most accurate for susceptibility testing of obligate anaerobes. *Enterobacteriaceae, Pseudomonas* species and *Acinetobacter* species are considered susceptible if the MIC of mezlocillin is no greater than 64 mcg/mL and are considered resistant if the MIC is greater than 128 mcg/mL. *Haemophilus* species and *Neisseria* species are considered susceptible if the MIC of mezlocillin is less than or equal to 1 mcg/mL. Mezlocillin standard is available for broth or agar dilution studies.

*Bauer, A.W., Kirby, W.M., Sherris, J.C. and Turck, M.: Antibiotic Testing by a Standardized Single Disc Method, Am. J. Clin. Pathol., 45:493, 1966; Standardized Disc Susceptibility Test, FEDERAL REGISTER, 39:19182–19184, 1974.

INDICATIONS AND USAGE

MEZLIN® is indicated for the treatment of serious infections caused by susceptible strains of the designated microorganisms in the conditions listed below:

LOWER RESPIRATORY TRACT INFECTIONS including pneumonia and lung abscess caused by *Haemophilus influenzae, Klebsiella* species including *K. pneumoniae, Proteus mirabilis, Pseudomonas* species including *P. aeruginosa, E. coli,* and *Bacteroides* species including *B. fragilis.*

INTRA-ABDOMINAL INFECTIONS including acute cholecystitis, cholangitis, peritonitis, hepatic abscess and intra-abdominal abscess caused by susceptible *E. coli, Proteus mirabilis, Klebsiella* species, *Pseudomonas* species, *S. faecalis* (enterococcus), *Bacteroides* species, *Peptococcus* species, and *Peptostreptococcus* species.

URINARY TRACT INFECTIONS caused by susceptible *E. coli, Proteus mirabilis,* the indole positive *Proteus* species, *Morganella morganii; Klebsiella* species, *Enterobacter* species, *Serratia* species, *Pseudomonas* species, *S. faecalis* (enterococcus).

Uncomplicated gonorrhea due to susceptible *Neisseria gonorrhoeae.*

GYNECOLOGICAL INFECTIONS including endometritis, pelvic cellulitis, and pelvic inflammatory disease associated with susceptible *Neisseria gonorrhoeae, Peptococcus* species, *Peptostreptococcus* species, *Bacteroides* species, *E. coli, Proteus mirabilis, Klebsiella* species, and *Enterobacter* species.

SKIN AND SKIN STRUCTURE INFECTIONS caused by susceptible *S. faecalis* (enterococcus), *E. coli, Proteus mirabilis,* the indole positive *Proteus* species, *Proteus vulgaris,* and *Providencia rettgeri; Klebsiella* species, *Enterobacter* species, *Pseudomonas* species, *Peptococcus* species, and *Bacteroides* species.

SEPTICEMIA including bacteremia caused by susceptible *E. coli, Klebsiella* species, *Enterobacter* species, *Pseudomonas* species, *Bacteroides* species, and *Peptococcus* species.

Mezlocillin has also been shown to be effective for the treatment of infections caused by *Streptococcus* species including Group A Beta-hemolytic *Streptococcus* and *Streptococcus pneumoniae* (formerly *Diplococcus pneumoniae*) however, infections caused by these organisms are ordinarily treated with more narrow spectrum penicillins.

Appropriate culture and susceptibility tests should be performed before treatment in order to isolate and identify organisms causing infection and to determine their susceptibility to mezlocillin. Therapy with MEZLIN® may be initiated before results of these tests are known; once results become available, appropriate therapy should be continued.

Mezlocillin's broad spectrum of activity makes it particularly useful for treating mixed infections caused by susceptible strains of both gram-negative and gram-positive aerobic or anaerobic bacteria. It is not effective, however, against infections caused by penicillinase-producing *Staphylococcus aureus.*

In certain severe infections, when the causative organisms are unknown, MEZLIN® may be administered in conjunction with an aminoglycoside or a cephalosporin antibiotic as initial therapy. As soon as results of culture and susceptibility tests become available, antimicrobial therapy should be adjusted if indicated. Culture and sensitivity testing, performed periodically during therapy, will provide information on the therapeutic effect of the antimicrobial and will monitor for the possible emergence of bacterial resistance.

MEZLIN® has been used effectively in combination with an aminoglycoside antibiotic for the treatment of life-threatening infections caused by *Pseudomonas aeruginosa.* For the treatment of febrile episodes in immunosuppressed patients with granulocytopenia, MEZLIN® should be combined with an aminoglycoside or a cephalosporin antibiotic.

Prevention: The administration of MEZLIN® perioperatively (preoperatively, intraoperatively, and postoperatively) may reduce the incidence of infections in patients undergoing surgical procedures (e.g. vaginal hysterectomy and colorectal surgery) that may be classified as contaminated or potentially contaminated. Effective perioperative use for surgery depends on the time of administration. To achieve effective tissue levels, MEZLIN® should be given ½ hour to 1½ hours before surgery.

In patients undergoing Caesarean section, intraoperative (after clamping the umbilical cord) and postoperative use of MEZLIN® may reduce the incidence of certain postoperative infections. (See DOSAGE AND ADMINISTRATION section.)

For patients undergoing colorectal surgery, preoperative bowel preparation by mechanical cleansing as well as with a non-absorbable antibiotic (e.g. neomycin) is recommended. If there are signs of infection, specimens for culture should be obtained for identification of the causative organism so that appropriate therapy may be instituted.

CONTRAINDICATIONS

MEZLIN® is contraindicated in patients with a history of hypersensitivity reactions to any of the penicillins.

WARNINGS

Serious and occasionally fatal hypersensitivity (anaphylactic) reactions have occurred in patients receiving a penicillin. These reactions are more apt to occur in individuals with a history of sensitivity to multiple allergens. There have been reports of individuals with a history of penicillin hypersensitivity reactions who have experienced severe hypersensitivity reactions when treated with cephalosporin. Before therapy with mezlocillin is instituted, careful inquiry should be made to determine whether the patient has had previous hypersensitivity reactions to penicillins, cephalosporins or other drugs. Antibiotics should be used with caution in any patient who has demonstrated some form of allergy, particularly to drugs.

If an allergic reaction occurs during therapy with mezlocillin, the drug should be discontinued. SERIOUS ANAPHYLACTOID REACTIONS REQUIRE IMMEDIATE EMERGENCY TREATMENT. EPINEPHRINE, OXYGEN, INTRAVENOUS STEROIDS, AND AIRWAY MANAGEMENT, INCLUDING INTUBATION, SHOULD BE PROVIDED AS INDICATED.

PRECAUTIONS

General

Although MEZLIN® shares with other penicillins the low potential for toxicity, as with any potent drug, periodic assessment of organ system functions, including renal, hepatic and hematopoietic, is advisable during prolonged therapy. MEZLIN® has been reported rarely to cause acute interstitial nephritis.

Bleeding manifestations have occurred in some patients receiving beta-lactam antibiotics. These reactions have been associated with abnormalities of coagulation tests, such as clotting time, platelet aggregation and prothrombin time and are more likely to occur in patients with renal impairment. Although MEZLIN® has rarely been associated with clinical bleeding, the possibility of this occurring should be kept in mind, particularly in patients with severe renal impairment receiving maximum doses of the drug.

MEZLIN® has only rarely been reported to cause hypokalemia; however, the possibility of this occurring should also be kept in mind, particularly when treating patients with fluid and electrolyte imbalance. Periodic monitoring of serum potassium may be advisable in patients receiving prolonged therapy.

MEZLIN® is a monosodium salt containing only 42.6 mg (1.85 mEq) of sodium per gram of mezlocillin. This should be considered when treating patients requiring restricted salt intake.

As with any penicillin, an allergic reaction, including anaphylaxis, may occur during MEZLIN® administration, particularly in a hypersensitive individual.

As with other antibiotics, prolonged use of MEZLIN® may result in overgrowth of non-susceptible organisms. If this occurs, appropriate measures should be taken.

MEZLIN®, along with other ureidopenicillins, has been reported in one study to prolong neuromuscular blockage of vecuronium. Caution is indicated when mezlocillin is used perioperatively.

Antimicrobials used in high doses for short periods to treat gonorrhea may mask or delay the symptoms of incubating syphilis. Therefore, prior to treatment, patients with gonorrhea should also be evaluated for syphilis. Specimens for dark field examination should be obtained from any suspected primary lesion and serologic tests should be performed. Patients treated with MEZLIN® should undergo follow-up serologic tests three months after therapy.

Interactions with Drugs and Laboratory Tests

As with other penicillins, the mixing of mezlocillin with an aminoglycoside in solutions for parenteral administration can result in substantial inactivation of the aminoglycoside. Probenecid interferes with the renal tubular secretion of mezlocillin, thereby increasing serum concentrations and prolonging serum half-life of the antibiotic.

High urine concentrations of mezlocillin may produce false positive protein reactions (pseudoproteinuria) with the following methods: sulfosalicylic acid and boiling test, acetic acid test, biuret reaction, and nitric acid test. The bromphenol blue (Multi-stix®) reagent strip test has been reported to be reliable.

Pregnancy Category B

Reproduction studies have been performed in rats and mice at doses up to 2 times the human dose, and have revealed no evidence of impaired fertility or harm to the fetus, due to MEZLIN®. There are however no adequate and well-controlled studies in pregnant women. Because animal reproductive studies are not always predictive of human response, this drug should be used during pregnancy only if clearly needed. Mezlocillin crosses the placenta and is found in low concentrations in cord blood and amniotic fluid.

Nursing Mothers

Mezlocillin is detected in low concentrations in the milk of nursing mothers, therefore caution should be exercised when MEZLIN® is administered to a nursing woman.

ADVERSE REACTIONS

As with other penicillins, the following adverse reactions may occur:

Hypersensitivity reactions: skin rash, pruritus, urticaria, drug fever, acute interstitial nephritis and anaphylactic reactions.

Gastrointestinal disturbances: abnormal taste sensation, nausea, vomiting and diarrhea. If diarrhea persists, pseudomembranous colitis should be considered.

Hemic and Lymphatic Systems: thrombocytopenia, leukopenia, neutropenia, eosinophilia, reduction of hemoglobin or hematocrit, and positive Coombs' test.

Continued on next page

Bayer Corporation—Cont.

Abnormalities of hepatic and renal function tests: elevation of serum aspartate aminotransferase (SGOT), serum alanine aminotransferase (SGPT), serum alkaline phosphatase, serum bilirubin. Elevation of serum creatinine and/or BUN. Reduction in serum potassium.

Central nervous system: convulsive seizures or neuromuscular hyperirritability.

Local reactions: thrombophlebitis with intravenous administration, pain with intramuscular injection.

OVERDOSAGE

As with other penicillins, MEZLIN® in overdosage has the potential to cause neuromuscular hyperirritability or convulsive seizures. Hemodialysis, if necessary, will aid in the removal of drug from the blood.

DOSAGE AND ADMINISTRATION

MEZLIN® (sterile mezlocillin sodium) may be administered intravenously or intramuscularly. For serious infections, the intravenous route of administration should be used. Intramuscular doses should not exceed 2g per injection.

The recommended adult dosage for serious infections is 200–300 mg/kg per day given in 4 to 6 divided doses. The usual dose is 3g given every 4 hours (18g/day) or 4g given every 6 hours (16g/day). For life-threatening infections, up to 350 mg/kg per day may be administered, but the total daily dosage should ordinarily not exceed 24g.
[See first table above.]

For patients with life-threatening infections, 4g may be administered every 4 hours (24g/day).

Dosage for any individual patient must take into consideration the site and severity of infection, the susceptibility of the organisms causing infection, and the status of the patient's host defense mechanism.

The duration of therapy depends upon the severity of infection. Generally, MEZLIN® should be continued for at least 2 days after the signs and symptoms of infection have disappeared. The usual duration is 7 to 10 days; however, in difficult and complicated infections, more prolonged therapy may be required. Antibiotic therapy for Group A Beta-hemolytic streptococcal infections should be maintained for at least 10 days to reduce the risk of rheumatic fever or glomerulonephritis.

In certain deep-seated infections, involving abscess formation, appropriate surgical drainage should be performed in conjunction with antimicrobial therapy.

For acute, uncomplicated gonococcal urethritis, the usual dose is 1–2g given once intravenously or by intramuscular injection. Probenecid 1g may be given orally at the time of dosing or up to ½ -hour before. (For full prescribing information, refer to probenecid package insert.)

Prevention

To prevent postoperative infection in contaminated or potentially contaminated surgery, the following doses are recommended:

4g IV given ½ hour to 1½ hours prior to the start of surgery.

4g IV given 6 hours and 12 hours later.

Caesarean Section Patients.

The first dose of 4g is given intravenously as soon as the umbilical cord is clamped. The second and third doses of 4g should be given intravenously 4 and 8 hours, respectively, after the first dose.

Patients with Impaired Renal Function

The rate of elimination of mezlocillin is dose dependent and related to the degree of renal function impairment. After an intravenous dose of 3g, the serum half-life is approximately 1 hour in patients with creatinine clearances above 60 mL/min., 1.3 hr. in those with clearances of 30–59 mL/min., 1.6 hr. in those with clearances of 10–29 mL/min. and approximately 3.6 hr. in patients with clearances of less than 10 mL/min. Dosage adjustments of MEZLIN® are not required in patients with mild impairment of renal function. For patients with a creatinine clearance of ≤30 mL/min. (serum creatinine of approximately 3.0 mg% or greater), the following dosage guide may be used:
[See second table above.]

For life-threatening infections, 3g may be given every 6 hours to patients with creatinine clearances between 10–30 mL/min. and 2g every 6 hours to those with clearances less than 10 mL/min.

For patients with serious systemic infection undergoing hemodialysis for renal failure, 3–4g may be administered after each dialysis and then every 12 hours. Patients undergoing peritoneal dialysis may receive 3g every 12 hours.

For patients with renal failure and hepatic insufficiency, measurement of serum levels of mezlocillin will provide additional guidance for adjusting dosage.

Intravenous Administration

MEZLIN® may be administered by intermittent infusion or by direct intravenous injection.

Infusion. Each gram of mezlocillin should be reconstituted by vigorous shaking with at least 9–10 mL of Sterile Water

for Injection, 5% Dextrose Injection or 0.9% Sodium Chloride Injection. The dissolved drug should be further diluted to desired volume (50–100 mL) with an appropriate intravenous solution. (See Compatibility and Stability section.) The solution of reconstituted drug may then be administered over a period of 30 minutes by direct infusion, or through a Y-type intravenous infusion set which may already be in place. If this method or the "piggyback" method of administration is used, it is advisable to discontinue temporarily the administration of any other solutions during the infusion of MEZLIN®.

Injection. The reconstituted solution of MEZLIN® may also be injected directly into a vein or into intravenous tubing; when administered this way, the injection should be given slowly over a period of 3–5 minutes. To minimize venous irritation, the concentration of drug should not exceed 10%. When MEZLIN® is given in combination with another antimicrobial, such as an aminoglycoside, each drug should be given separately in accordance with the recommended dosage and routes of administration for each drug.

Intramuscular Administration

Each gram of mezlocillin may be reconstituted by vigorous shaking with 3–4 mL of Sterile Water for Injection or with 3–4 mL of 0.5 or 1.0% Lidocaine Hydrochloride solution (without epinephrine). (For full prescribing information, refer to lidocaine package insert.) Intramuscular doses of MEZLIN® should not exceed 2g per injection.

As with all intramuscular preparations, MEZLIN® should be injected well within the body of a relatively large muscle, such as the upper outer quadrant of the buttock (i.e., gluteus maximus); aspiration will help avoid unintentional injection into a blood vessel. Slow injection (12–15 sec.) will minimize the discomfort associated with intramuscular administration.

Infants and Children

Only limited data are available on the safety and effectiveness of MEZLIN® in the treatment of infants and children with documented serious infection. In the event a child has an infection for which MEZLIN® may be judged particularly appropriate, the following dosage guide may be used:
[See third table above.]

For infants beyond one month of age and children up to the age of 12 years, 50 mg/kg may be administered every 4 hours (300 mg/kg/day).

The drug may be infused intravenously over 30-minutes or be given by intramuscular injection.

COMPATIBILITY AND STABILITY

MEZLIN® at concentrations of 10 mg/mL and 100 mg/mL is stable (loss of potency less than 10%) in the following intravenous solutions for the time periods stated.
[See fourth table above.]

MEZLIN® at concentrations up to 250 mg/mL is stable for 24 hours at room temperature in the following diluents:

MEZLIN® DOSAGE GUIDE (ADULTS)

Condition	Daily Dosage Range	Usual Daily Dosage	Frequency and Route of Administration
Urinary tract infection (uncomplicated)	100–125 mg/kg	6–8g	1.5–2g every 6 hours IV or IM
Urinary tract infection (complicated)	150–200 mg/kg	12g	3g every 6 hours IV
Lower respiratory tract infection Intra-abdominal infection Gynecological infection Skin & skin structure infection Septicemia	225–300 mg/kg	16–18g	4g every 6 hours or 3g every 4 hours IV

MEZLIN® DOSAGE GUIDE FOR PATIENTS WITH IMPAIRED RENAL FUNCTION

Creatinine Clearance mL/min.	Urinary Tract Infection (Uncomplicated)	Urinary Tract Infection (Complicated)	Serious Systemic Infection
> 30	Usual Recommended Dosage		
10–30	1.5g every 8 hours	1.5g every 6 hours	3g every 8 hours
< 10	1.5g every 8 hours	1.5g every 8 hours	2g every 8 hours

MEZLIN® DOSAGE GUIDE (NEWBORNS)

BODY WEIGHT (gm)	AGE ≤7 DAYS	AGE >7 DAYS
≤ 2000	75 mg/kg every 12 hours (150 mg/kg/day)	75 mg/kg every 8 hours (225 mg/kg/day)
> 2000	75 mg/kg every 12 hours (150 mg/kg/day)	75 mg/kg every 6 hours (300 mg/kg/day)

STABILITY

INTRAVENOUS SOLUTION	Controlled Room Temperature	Refrigeration
Sterile Water for Injection, USP	48 hours	7 days
0.9% Sodium Chloride Injection, USP	48 hours	7 days
5% Dextrose Injection, USP	48 hours	7 days
5% Dextrose in 0.225% Sodium Chloride Injection, USP	72 hours	7 days
Lactated Ringer's Injection, USP	24 hours	7 days
5% Dextrose in Electrolyte #75 Injection	72 hours	7 days
5% Dextrose in 0.45% Sodium Chloride Injection, USP*	48 hours	48 hours
Ringer's Injection	24 hours	24 hours
10% Dextrose Injection	24 hours	24 hours
5% Fructose Injection	24 hours	24 hours

If precipitation should occur under refrigeration, the product should be warmed to 37°C for 20 minutes in a water bath and shaken well.

*This solution is stable from 10 mg/mL to 50 mg/mL under refrigeration.

Sterile Water for Injection, USP
0.9% Sodium Chloride Injection, USP
0.5% and 1.0% Lidocaine Hydrochloride solution (without epinephrine)
MEZLIN® is stable for up to 28 days when frozen at −12°C at concentrations up to 100 mg/mL in the following diluents:
Sterile Water for Injection, USP
0.9% Sodium Chloride Injection, USP or 5% Dextrose Injection, USP

HOW SUPPLIED

MEZLIN® (sterile mezlocillin sodium) is a white to pale yellow crystalline powder supplied as listed below:
MEZLIN® is available in vials, infusion bottles, pharmacy bulk packages and ADD-Vantage® vials containing mezlocillin sodium equivalent to mezlocillin, as specified:

	NDC Number
1g Vial	0026-8211-10
2g Vial	0026-8212-30
2g Infusion Bottle	0026-8212-36
3g Vial	0026-8213-35
3g Infusion Bottle	0026-8213-36
3g ADD-Vantage® Vial	0026-8213-19
4g Vial	0026-8214-35
4g Infusion Bottle	0026-8214-36
4g ADD-Vantage® Vial	0026-8214-19
20g Pharmacy Bulk Package	0026-8220-31

Unreconstituted MEZLIN® should be stored at temperatures not exceeding 86°F (30°C). The powder as well as the reconstituted solution of drug may darken slightly, depending upon storage conditions, but potency is not affected.

Bayer Corporation
Pharmaceutical Division
400 Morgan Lane
West Haven, CT 06516 USA
Made in Germany

MEZLIN®
Sterile mezlocillin sodium
BAYPEN®
℞

**PHARMACY BULK PACKAGE—
NOT FOR DIRECT INFUSION**

DESCRIPTION

A pharmacy bulk package is a container of a sterile preparation for parenteral use that contains many single doses. The contents are intended for use in a pharmacy admixture program and are restricted to the preparation of admixtures for intravenous infusion, or the filling of empty sterile syringes for intravenous injection for patients with individualized dosing requirements (see Dosage and Administration section).
MEZLIN® (sterile mezlocillin sodium) is a semisynthetic broad spectrum penicillin antibiotic for parenteral administration. It is the monohydrate sodium salt of 6-[D-2 [3-(methyl-sulfonyl) -2-OXO-imidazolidine -1- carboxamido] -2-phenyl acetamido}penicillanic acid.

Structural Formula:

CH₃—SO₂—N—C—N—C—N—C—C—... S ... CH₃ CH₃ ... N ... COONa · H₂O

Empirical Formula: $C_{21}H_{24}N_5O_8S_2Na \cdot H_2O$
MEZLIN® has a molecular weight of 579.6 and contains 42.6 mg (1.85 mEq) of sodium per one gram of mezlocillin activity. The dosage form is supplied as a sterile white to pale yellow crystalline powder, which is freely soluble in water. When reconstituted, solutions of MEZLIN® are clear and range from colorless to pale yellow with a pH of 4.5 to 8.0.

CLINICAL PHARMACOLOGY

Intravenous Administration. In healthy adult volunteers, mean serum levels of mezlocillin 5 minutes after a 5-minute intravenous injection of 1g, 2g, or 5g are 100, 253, or 411

MEZLOCILLIN SERUM LEVELS IN ADULTS (mcg/mL) 2–5 MIN. IV INJECTION

DOSE	0	15 min	30 min	45 min	1 hr	2 hr	3 hr	4 hr	6 hr
4g	—	254 (155–400)	163 (99–260)	122 (78–215)	93 (67–133)	47 (22–96)	20 (8–45)	9.1 (6–13)	8.4 (5–17)

mcg/mL, respectively. Serum levels, as noted below, lack dose proportionality:
[See table at bottom of page.]
Fifteen minutes after a 4g intravenous injection (2–5 min.), the concentration in serum is 254 mcg/mL; 1 hour and 4 hours later levels are 93 mcg/mL and 9.1 mcg/mL, respectively:
[See table above.]
After an intravenous infusion (15 min.) of 3g, mean levels 15 minutes after dosing are 269 mcg/mL (170–280).
A 30-minute intravenous infusion of 3g produces mean peak concentrations of 263 mcg/mL; 1 hour and 4 hours later the concentrations are 57 mcg/mL and 4.4 mcg/mL, respectively:
[See table at bottom of next page.]
Following intravenous infusion (2 hr.) of a 3g dose of mezlocillin every 4 hours for 7 days, mean peak serum concentrations are higher than 100 mcg/mL, and levels above 50 mcg/mL are maintained throughout dosing.
Intramuscular Administration. MEZLIN® is rapidly absorbed after intramuscular injection. In healthy volunteers, the mean peak serum concentration occurs approximately 45 minutes after a single dose of 1g and is about 15 mcg/mL. The oral administration of 1g probenecid before injection produces an increase in mezlocillin serum levels of about 50%. After repetitive intramuscular doses of 1g mezlocillin every 6 hours, peak levels in the serum generally range between 35 and 45 mcg/mL. The relationship between the pharmacokinetics of intramuscular and intravenous dosing has not yet been clearly established.
General. As with other penicillins, mezlocillin is excreted primarily by glomerular filtration and tubular secretion. The rate of elimination is dose dependent and related to the degree of renal functional impairment. In patients with normal renal function, approximately 55% of the administered dose is recovered from the urine within the first 6 hours after dosing. Two hours after an intravenous injection of 2g, concentrations of active drug in urine generally exceed 4000 mcg/mL. By 4–6 hours after injection, concentrations usually decline to a range of about 50 to 200 mcg/mL. The serum elimination half-life of mezlocillin after intravenous dosing is approximately 55 minutes.
In patients with reduced renal function, the half-life is only slightly prolonged. Dosage adjustments are usually not necessary except in patients with severe renal impairment. (See Dosage and Administration.) As with other penicillins, mezlocillin is metabolized only slightly; less than 10% of the drug excreted in the urine is in the form of the penicilloate or penilloate. The drug is readily removed from the serum by hemodialysis and, to a lesser extent, by peritoneal dialysis. Up to 26% of a dose of mezlocillin is recovered from the bile of patients with normal liver function. Following intravenous doses of 2g to 5g, concentrations of active drug in bile generally range from 500 to 2500 mcg/mL. The biliary excretion of mezlocillin is reduced in patients with common bile duct obstruction.
Mezlocillin is not appreciably absorbed when given orally. Following parenteral administration, the apparent volume of distribution is approximately equal to the extracellular fluid volume. The drug is present in active form in the serum, urine, bile, peritoneal fluid, pleural fluid, bronchial and wound secretions, bone and other tissues. As with other penicillins, penetration into the cerebrospinal fluid (CSF) is generally poor, however higher CSF concentrations are obtained in the presence of meningeal inflammation.
Protein binding studies indicate that the degree of mezlocillin binding is low (16–42%) and depends upon testing methods and concentrations of drug studied.

Microbiology

Mezlocillin is a bactericidal antibiotic which acts by interfering with synthesis of cell wall components. It is active against a variety of gram-negative and gram-positive bacteria, including aerobic and anaerobic strains. Mezlocillin is usually active in vitro against most strains of the following organisms:

Gram-negative bacteria
Escherichia coli
Proteus mirabilis
Proteus vulgaris
Morganella morganii (formerly *P. morganii*)
Providencia rettgeri (formerly *Proteus rettgeri*)
Providencia stuartii
Citrobacter species*
Klebsiella species (including *K. pneumoniae*)
Enterobacter species
Shigella species*
Pseudomonas aeruginosa (and other species)
Haemophilus influenzae
Haemophilus parainfluenzae
Neisseria species
Many strains of *Serratia, Salmonella**, and *Acinetobacter** are also susceptible.
Gram-positive bacteria
Staphylococcus aureus (non-penicillinase producing strains)
Beta-hemolytic *streptococci* (Groups A and B)
Streptococcus pneumoniae (formerly *Diplococcus pneumoniae*)
Streptococcus faecalis (enterococcus)
Anaerobic Organisms
Peptococcus species
Peptostreptococcus species
Clostridium species*
Bacteroides species (including *B. fragilis* group)
Fusobacterium species*
Veillonella species*
Eubacterium species*
*Mezlocillin has been shown to be active in vitro against these organisms, however clinical efficacy has not yet been established.
Noteworthy is mezlocillin's broadened spectrum of in vitro activity against important pathogenic aerobic gram-negative bacteria, including strains of *Pseudomonas, Klebsiella, Enterobacter, Serratia, Proteus, Escherichia* and *Haemophilus,* as well as *Bacteroides* and other anaerobes; and its excellent inhibitory effect against gram-positive organisms including *Streptococcus faecalis* (enterococcus). It is inactive against penicillinase-producing strains of *Staphylococcus aureus.*
In vitro studies have shown that mezlocillin combined with an aminoglycoside (e.g., gentamicin, tobramycin, amikacin, sisomicin) acts synergistically against strains of *Streptococcus faecalis* and *Pseudomonas aeruginosa.* In some instances, this combination also acts synergistically in vitro against other gram-negative bacteria such as *Serratia, Klebsiella* and *Acinetobacter* species.
Mezlocillin is slightly more active when tested at alkaline pH and, as with other penicillins, has reduced activity when tested in vitro with increasing inoculum. The minimum bactericidal concentration (MBC) generally exceeds the minimum inhibitory concentration (MIC) by a factor of 2 or 3. Resistance to mezlocillin in vitro develops slowly (multiple step mutation). Some strains of *Pseudomonas aeruginosa* have developed resistance fairly rapidly. Mezlocillin is not stable in the presence of penicillinase and strains of *Staphylococcus aureus* resistant to penicillin are also resistant to mezlocillin.

Susceptibility Tests

Quantitative methods that require measurement of zone diameters give good estimates of bacterial susceptibility. One such procedure* has been recommended for use with discs to test susceptibility to antimicrobials. When the causative organism is tested by the Kirby-Bauer method of disc susceptibility, a 75 mcg mezlocillin disc should give a zone of 18 mm or greater to indicate susceptibility. Zone sizes of 14 mm or less indicate resistance. Zone sizes of 15 to 17 mm indicate intermediate susceptibility. Susceptible strains of *Haemophilus* and *Neisseria* species give zones of ≥ 29 mm, resistant strains ≤ 28 mm. With this procedure, a report from the laboratory of "Susceptibile" indicates that the infecting organism is likely to respond to therapy. A report of "Resistant" indicates that the infecting organism is not

MEZLOCILLIN SERUM LEVELS IN ADULTS (mcg/mL) 5 MIN. IV INJECTION

DOSE	0	5 min	10 min	20 min	30 min	1 hr	2 hr	3 hr	4 hr	6 hr	8 hr
1g	149 (132–185)	100 (64–143)	66 (47–87)	50 (31–87)	40 (22–83)	18 (8–31)	5.3 (3.3–7.7)	2.5 (1.7–3.7)	1.7 (0.7–2.8)	0.5 (0–1.2)	0.1 (0–0.2)
2g	314 (207–362)	253 (161–364)	161 (113–214)	117 (76–174)	82 (55–112)	56 (23–88)	20 (7.5–32)	11 (3.8–16)	4.4 (1.6–8.7)	1.5 (0.5–2.6)	0.6 (0.1–1.4)
5g	547 (268–854)	411 (199–597)	357 (246–456)	250 (203–353)	226 (190–333)	131 (104–193)	76 (59–104)	31 (20–40)	13 (6.4–17)	4.6 (2.1–9.4)	1.9 (1.1–3.6)

Continued on next page

Bayer Corporation—Cont.

likely to respond to therapy; other therapy should be selected. A report of "Intermediate Susceptibility" suggests that the organism may be susceptible if the infection is confined to tissues and fluids (e.g., urine), in which high antibiotic levels are attained. The mezlocillin disc should be used for testing susceptibility to mezlocillin. In certain conditions, it may be desirable to do additional susceptibility testing by broth or agar dilution techniques. Dilution methods, preferably the agar plate dilution procedure, are most accurate for susceptibility testing of obligate anaerobes. *Enterobacteriaceae, Pseudomonas* species and *Acinetobacter* species are considered susceptible if the MIC of mezlocillin is no greater than 64 mcg/mL and are considered resistant if the MIC is greater than 128 mcg/mL. *Haemophilus* species and *Neisseria* species are considered susceptible if the MIC of mezlocillin is less than or equal to 1 mcg/mL. Mezlocillin standard is available for broth or agar dilution studies.

*Bauer, A.W., Kirby, W.M., Sherris, J.C., and Turck, M.: Antibiotic Testing by a Standardized Single Disc Method, Am. J. Clin. Pathol., 45:493, 1966; Standardized Disc Susceptibility Test, FEDERAL REGISTER, 39: 19182-19184, 1974.

INDICATIONS AND USAGE

MEZLIN® is indicated for the treatment of serious infections caused by susceptible strains of the designated microorganisms in the conditions listed below:

LOWER RESPIRATORY TRACT INFECTIONS including pneumonia and lung abscess caused by *Haemophilus influenzae, Klebsiella* species including *K. pneumoniae, Proteus mirabilis, Pseudomonas* species including *P. aeruginosa, E. coli,* and *Bacteroides* species including *B. fragilis.*

INTRA-ABDOMINAL INFECTIONS including acute cholecystitis, cholangitis, peritonitis, hepatic abscess and intraabdominal abscess caused by susceptible *E. coli, Proteus mirabilis, Klebsiella* species, *Pseudomonas* species, *S. faecalis* (enterococcus), *Bacteroides* species, *Peptococcus* species, and *Peptostreptococcus* species.

URINARY TRACT INFECTIONS caused by susceptible *E. coli, Proteus mirabilis,* the indole positive *Proteus* species, *Morganella morganii; Klebsiella* species, *Enterobacter* species, *Serratia* species, *Pseudomonas* species, *S. faecalis* (enterococcus).

Uncomplicated gonorrhea due to susceptible *Neisseria gonorrhoeae.*

GYNECOLOGICAL INFECTIONS including endometritis, pelvic cellulitis, and pelvic inflammatory disease associated with susceptible *Neisseria gonorrhoeae, Peptococcus* species, *Peptostreptococcus* species, *Bacteroides* species, *E. coli, Proteus mirabilis, Klebsiella* species, and *Enterobacter* species.

SKIN AND SKIN STRUCTURE INFECTIONS caused by susceptible *S. faecalis* (enterococcus), *E. coli, Proteus mirabilis,* the indole positive *Proteus* species, *Proteus vulgaris,* and *Providencia rettgeri; Klebsiella* species, *Enterobacter* species, *Pseudomonas* species, *Peptococcus* species, and *Bacteroides* species.

SEPTICEMIA including bacteremia caused by susceptible *E. coli, Klebsiella* species, *Enterobacter* species, *Pseudomonas* species, *Bacteroides* species, and *Peptococcus* species.

Mezlocillin has also been shown to be effective for the treatment of infections caused by *Streptococcus* species including Group A Beta-hemolytic *Streptococcus* and *Streptococcus pneumoniae* (formerly *Diplococcus pneumoniae*) however, infections caused by these organisms are ordinarily treated with more narrow spectrum penicillins.

Appropriate culture and susceptibility tests should be performed before treatment in order to isolate and identify organisms causing infection and to determine their susceptibility to mezlocillin. Therapy with MEZLIN® may be initiated before results of these tests are known; once results become available, appropriate therapy should be continued.

Mezlocillin's broad spectrum of activity makes it particularly useful for treating mixed infections caused by susceptible strains of both gram-negative and gram-positive aerobic or anaerobic bacteria. It is not effective, however, against infections caused by penicillinase-producing *Staphylococcus aureus.*

In certain severe infections, when the causative organisms are unknown, MEZLIN® may be administered in conjunction with an aminoglycoside or a cephalosporin antibiotic as initial therapy. As soon as results of culture and susceptibility tests become available, antimicrobial therapy should be adjusted if indicated. Culture and sensitivity testing, performed periodically during therapy, will provide information on the therapeutic effect of the antimicrobial and will monitor for the possible emergence of bacterial resistance. MEZLIN® has been used effectively in combination with an

MEZLIN® DOSAGE GUIDE (ADULTS)

Condition	Daily Dosage Range	Usual Daily Dosage	Frequency and Route of Administration
Urinary tract infection (uncomplicated)	100–125 mg/kg	6–8g	1.5–2g every 6 hours IV or IM
Urinary tract infection (complicated)	150–200 mg/kg	12g	3g every 6 hours IV
Lower respiratory tract infection Intra-abdominal infection Gynecological infection Skin & skin structure infection Septicemia	225–300 mg/kg	16–18g	4g every 6 hours or 3g every 4 hours IV

MEZLIN® DOSAGE GUIDE FOR PATIENTS WITH IMPAIRED RENAL FUNCTION

Creatinine Clearance mL/min.	Urinary Tract Infection (Uncomplicated)	Urinary Tract Infection (Complicated)	Serious Systemic Infection
> 30	Usual Recommended Dosage		
10–30	1.5g every 8 hours	1.5g every 6 hours	3g every 8 hours
< 10	1.5g every 8 hours	1.5g every 8 hours	2g every 8 hours

aminoglycoside antibiotic for the treatment of life-threatening infections caused by *Pseudomonas aeruginosa.* For the treatment of febrile episodes in immunosuppressed patients with granulocytopenia, MEZLIN® should be combined with an aminoglycoside or a cephalosporin antibiotic.

Prevention: The administration of MEZLIN® perioperatively (preoperatively, intraoperatively, and postoperatively) may reduce the incidence of infections in patients undergoing surgical procedures (e.g. vaginal hysterectomy and colorectal surgery) that may be classified as contaminated or potentially contaminated. Effective perioperative use for surgery depends on the time of administration. To achieve effective tissue levels, MEZLIN® should be given $1/2$ hour to $1^1/_2$ hours before surgery.

In patients undergoing Caesarean section, intraoperative (after clamping the umbilical cord) and postoperative use of MEZLIN® may reduce the incidence of certain postoperative infections. (See DOSAGE AND ADMINISTRATION section.)

For patients undergoing colorectal surgery, preoperative bowel preparation by mechanical cleansing as well as with a non-absorbable antibiotic (e.g. neomycin) is recommended. If there are signs of infection, specimens for culture should be obtained for identification of the causative organism so that appropriate therapy may be instituted.

CONTRAINDICATIONS

MEZLIN® is contraindicated in patients with a history of hypersensitivity reactions to any of the penicillins.

WARNINGS

Serious and occasionally fatal hypersensitivity (anaphylactic) reactions have occurred in patients receiving a penicillin. These reactions are more apt to occur in individuals with a history of sensitivity to multiple allergens. There have been reports of individuals with a history of penicillin hypersensitivity reactions who have experienced severe hypersensitivity reactions when treated with cephalosporin. Before therapy with mezlocillin is instituted, careful inquiry should be made to determine whether the patient has had previous hypersensitivity reactions to penicillins, cephalosporins or other drugs. Antibiotics should be used with caution in any patient who has demonstrated some form of allergy, particularly to drugs.

If an allergic reaction occurs during therapy with mezlocillin, the drug should be discontinued. SERIOUS ANAPHYLACTOID REACTIONS REQUIRE IMMEDIATE EMERGENCY TREATMENT. EPINEPHRINE, OXYGEN, INTRAVENOUS STEROIDS, AND AIRWAY MANAGEMENT, INCLUDING INTUBATION, SHOULD BE PROVIDED AS INDICATED.

PRECAUTIONS
General
Although MEZLIN® shares with other penicillins the low potential for toxicity, as with any other potent drug, periodic assessment of organ system functions, including renal, hepatic and hematopoietic, is advisable during prolonged therapy. MEZLIN® has been reported rarely to cause acute interstitial nephritis.

Bleeding manifestations have occurred in some patients receiving beta-lactam antibiotics. These reactions have been associated with abnormalities of coagulation tests, such as clotting time, platelet aggregation and prothrombin time and are more likely to occur in patients with renal impairment. Although MEZLIN® has rarely been associated with clinical bleeding, the possibility of this occurring should be kept in mind, particularly in patients with severe renal impairment receiving maximum doses of the drug.

MEZLIN® has only rarely been reported to cause hypokalemia; however, the possibility of this occurring should also be kept in mind, particularly when treating patients with fluid and electrolyte imbalance. Periodic monitoring of serum potassium may be advisable in patients receiving prolonged therapy.

MEZLIN® is a monosodium salt containing only 42.6 mg (1.85 mEq) of sodium per gram of mezlocillin. This should be considered when treating patients requiring restricted salt intake.

As with any penicillin, an allergic reaction, including anaphylaxis, may occur during MEZLIN® administration, particularly in a hypersensitive individual.

As with other antibiotics, prolonged use of MEZLIN® may result in overgrowth of non-susceptible organisms. If this occurs, appropriate measures should be taken.

MEZLIN®, along with other ureidopenicillins, has been reported in one study to prolong neuromuscular blockage of vecuronium. Caution is indicated when mezlocillin is used perioperatively.

Antimicrobials used in high doses for short periods to treat gonorrhea may mask or delay the symptoms of incubating syphilis. Therefore, prior to treatment, patients with gonorrhea should also be evaluated for syphilis. Specimens for dark field examination should be obtained from any suspected primary lesion and serologic tests should be performed. Patients treated with MEZLIN® should undergo follow-up serologic tests three months after therapy.

Interactions with Drugs and Laboratory Tests
As with other penicillins, the mixing of mezlocillin with an aminoglycoside in solutions for parenteral administration can result in substantial inactivation of the aminoglycoside. Probenecid interferes with the renal tubular secretion of mezlocillin, thereby increasing serum concentrations and prolonging serum half-life of the antibiotic.

High urine concentrations of mezlocillin may produce false positive protein reactions (pseudoproteinuria) with the following methods: sulfosalicylic acid and boiling test, acetic acid test, biuret reaction, and nitric acid test. The bromphe-

MEZLOCILLIN SERUM LEVELS IN ADULTS (mcg/mL) 30 MIN. IV INFUSION

DOSE	0	5 min	15 min	30 min	45 min	1 hr	2 hr	3 hr	4 hr	6 hr	8 hr
3g	263 (87–489)	170 (63–371)	141 (75–301)	109 (56–288)	79 (41–135)	57 (28–100)	26 (14–55)	12 (5.8–26)	4.4 (2.2–6.5)	1.6 (1.0–3.4)	< 1

nol blue (Multi-stix®) reagent strip test has been reported to be reliable.

Pregnancy Category B
Reproduction studies have been performed in rats and mice at doses up to 2 times the human dose, and have revealed no evidence of impaired fertility or harm to the fetus, due to MEZLIN®. There are however no adequate and well-controlled studies in pregnant women. Because animal reproductive studies are not always predictive of human response, this drug should be used during pregnancy only if clearly needed. Mezlocillin crosses the placenta and is found in low concentrations in cord blood and amniotic fluid.

Nursing Mothers
Mezlocillin is detected in low concentrations in the milk of nursing mothers. Therefore caution should be exercised when MEZLIN® is administered to a nursing woman.

ADVERSE REACTIONS

As with other penicillins, the following adverse reactions may occur:

Hypersensitivity reactions: skin rash, pruritus, urticaria, drug fever, acute interstitial nephritis and anaphylactic reactions.

Gastrointestinal disturbances: abnormal taste sensation, nausea, vomiting and diarrhea. If diarrhea persists, pseudomembranous colitis should be considered.

Hematologic and Lymphatic Systems: thrombocytopenia, leukopenia, neutropenia, eosinophilia, reduction of hemoglobin or hematocrit, and positive Coombs' test.

Abnormalities of hepatic and renal function tests: elevation of serum aspartate aminotransferase (SGOT), serum alanine aminotransferase (SGPT), serum alkaline phosphatase, serum bilirubin. Elevation of serum creatinine and/or BUN. Reduction in serum potassium.

Central nervous system: convulsive seizures or neuromuscular hyperirritability.

Local reactions: thrombophlebitis with intravenous administration, pain with intramuscular injection.

OVERDOSAGE

As with other penicillins, MEZLIN® in overdosage has the potential to cause neuromuscular hyperirritability or convulsive seizures. Hemodialysis, if necessary, will aid in the removal of drug from the blood.

DOSAGE AND ADMINISTRATION

MEZLIN® (sterile mezlocillin sodium) may be administered intravenously or intramuscularly. For serious infections, the intravenous route of administration should be used. Intramuscular doses should not exceed 2g per injection.

The 20g pharmacy bulk package is intended for the preparation of solutions for intravenous use. When intramuscular administration is required, the MEZLIN® vial should be used.

The recommended adult dosage for serious infections is 200–300 mg/kg per day given in 4 to 6 divided doses. The usual dose is 3g given every 4 hours (18g/day) or 4g given every 6 hours (16g/day). For life-threatening infections, up to 350 mg/kg per day may be administered, but the total daily dosage should ordinarily not exceed 24g.
[See table on top of preceding page.]
For patients with life-threatening infections, 4g may be administered every 4 hours (24g/day).
Dosage for any individual patient must take into consideration the site and severity of infection, the susceptibility of the organisms causing infection, and the status of the patient's host defense mechanism.
The duration of therapy depends upon the severity of infection. Generally, MEZLIN® should be continued for at least 2 days after the signs and symptoms of infection have disappeared. The usual duration is 7 to 10 days; however, in difficult and complicated infections, more prolonged therapy may be required. Antibiotic therapy for Group A Beta-hemolytic streptococcal infections should be maintained for at least 10 days to reduce the risk of rheumatic fever or glomerulonephritis.
In certain deep-seated infections, involving abscess formation, appropriate surgical drainage should be performed in conjunction with antimicrobial therapy.
For acute, uncomplicated gonococcal urethritis, the usual dose is 1–2g given once intravenously or by intramuscular injection. Probenecid 1g may be given orally at the time of dosing or up to ¹/₂-hour before. (For full prescribing information, refer to probenecid package insert.)

Prevention
To prevent postoperative infection in contaminated or potentially contaminated surgery, the following doses are recommended:
4g IV given ¹/₂ hour to 1¹/₂ hours prior to the start of surgery.
4g IV given 6 hours and 12 hours later.
Caesarean Section Patients.
The first dose of 4g is given intravenously as soon as the umbilical cord is clamped. The second and third doses of 4g should be given intravenously 4 and 8 hours, respectively, after the first dose.

INTRAVENOUS SOLUTION
Sterile Water for Injection, USP
0.9% Sodium Chloride Injection, USP
5% Dextrose Injection, USP
5% Dextrose in 0.225% Sodium Chloride Injection, USP
Lactated Ringer's Injection, USP
5% Dextrose in Electrolyte #75 Injection
5% Dextrose in 0.45% Sodium Chloride Injection, USP*
Ringer's Injection
10% Dextrose Injection
5% Fructose Injection

STABILITY		
Controlled Room Temperature		Refrigeration
48 hours		7 days
48 hours		7 days
48 hours		7 days
72 hours		7 days
72 hours		7 days
72 hours		7 days
48 hours		48 hours
24 hours		24 hours
24 hours		24 hours
24 hours		24 hours

If precipitation should occur under refrigeration, the product should be warmed to 37°C for 20 minutes in a water bath and shaken well.

*This solution is stable from 10 mg/mL to 50 mg/mL under refrigeration.

Patients with Impaired Renal Function
The rate of elimination of mezlocillin is dose dependent and related to the degree of renal function impairment. After an intravenous dose of 3g, the serum half-life is approximately 1 hour in patients with creatinine clearances above 60 mL/min., 1.3 hr. in those with clearances of 30–59 mL/min., 1.6 hr. in those with clearances of 10–29 mL/min. and approximately 3.6 hr. in patients with clearances of less than 10 mL/min. Dosage adjustments of MEZLIN® are not required in patients with mild impairment of renal function. For patients with a creatinine clearance of ≤30 mL/min. (serum creatinine of approximately 3.0 mg% or greater), the following dosage guide may be used:
[See second table on top of preceding page.]
For life-threatening infections, 3g may be given every 6 hours to patients with creatinine clearances between 10–30 mL/min. and 2g every 6 hours to those with clearances less than 10 mL/min.
For patients with serious systemic infection undergoing hemodialysis for renal failure, 3–4g should be administered after each dialysis and then every 12 hours. Patients undergoing peritoneal dialysis may receive 3g every 12 hours.
For patients with renal failure and hepatic insufficiency, measurement of serum levels of mezlocillin will provide additional guidance for adjusting dosage.

Directions for Proper Use of 20 gram Pharmacy Bulk Package
A pharmacy bulk package is a container of a sterile preparation for parenteral use that contains many single doses. The contents are intended for use in a pharmacy admixture program and are restricted to the preparation of admixtures for intravenous infusion, or the filling of empty sterile syringes for intravenous injection for patients with individualized dosing requirements.
THE CLOSURE SHALL BE PENETRATED ONLY ONE TIME AFTER RECONSTITUTION with a suitable sterile transfer set or dispensing device which allows measured dispensing of the contents. The pharmacy bulk package is to be used only in a suitable work area such as a laminar flow hood or an equivalent clean air compounding area.
Reconstitute by vigorous shaking with 186 mL of Sterile Water for Injection, 5% Dextrose Injection or 0.9% Sodium Chloride Injection resulting in a solution containing approximately 100 mg/mL which should be stored at controlled room temperature or under refrigeration. Within 8 hours of reconstitution, the desired dosages should be withdrawn and may be further diluted with an appropriate intravenous solution (see Compatability & Stability section).

Intravenous Administration
MEZLIN® may be administered intravenously by intermittent infusion or by direct intravenous injection.
Infusion. The dissolved drug should be further diluted to desired volume (50–100 mL) with an appropriate intravenous solution. (See Compatibility and Stability section.) The solution of reconstituted drug may then be administered over a period of 30 minutes by direct infusion, or through a Y-type intravenous infusion set which may already be in place. If this method or the "piggyback" method of administration is used, it is advisable to discontinue temporarily the administration of any other solutions during the infusion of MEZLIN®.
Injection. The reconstituted solution of MEZLIN® may also be injected directly into a vein or into intravenous tubing; when administered this way, the injection should be given slowly over a period of 3–5 minutes. To minimize venous irritation, the concentration of drug should not exceed 10%.
When MEZLIN® is given in combination with another antimicrobial, such as an aminoglycoside, each drug should be given separately in accordance with the recommended dosage and routes of administration for each drug.

Intramuscular Administration
For intramuscular administration, please refer to the Dosage and Administration section of the MEZLIN® vial package insert.

Infants and Children
Only limited data are available on the safety and effectiveness of MEZLIN® in the treatment of infants and children

with documented serious infection. In the event a child has an infection for which MEZLIN® may be judged particularly appropriate, the following dosage guide may be used:

MEZLIN DOSAGE GUIDE (NEWBORNS)

BODY WEIGHT	AGE	
(gm)	≤7 DAYS	>7 DAYS
≤2000	75 mg/kg every 12 hours (150 mg/kg/day)	75 mg/kg every 8 hours (225 mg/kg/day)
>2000	75 mg/kg every 12 hours (150 mg/kg/day)	75 mg/kg every 6 hours (300 mg/kg/day)

For infants beyond one month of age and children up to the age of 12 years, 60 mg/kg may be administered every 4 hours (300 mg/kg/day).
The drug may be infused intravenously over 30-minutes or be given by intramuscular injection.

COMPATIBILITY AND STABILITY
MEZLIN® at concentrations of 10 mg/mL and 100 mg/mL is stable (loss of potency less than 10%) in the following intravenous solutions for the time periods stated (includes time retained in pharmacy bulk package after reconstitution):
[See table on top of page.]
MEZLIN® is stable for up to 28 days when frozen at −12°C at concentrations up to 100 mg/mL in the following diluents:
Sterile Water for Injection, USP
0.9% Sodium Chloride Injection, USP or 5% Dextrose Injection, USP

HOW SUPPLIED
MEZLIN® (sterile mezlocillin sodium) is a white to pale yellow crystalline powder supplied as listed below:
MEZLIN® is available in vials, infusion bottles, pharmacy bulk packages and ADD-Vantage® vials containing mezlocillin sodium equivalent to mezlocillin, as specified:

	NDC Number
1g Vial	0026-8211-10
2g Vial	0026-8212-30
2g Infusion Bottle	0026-8212-36
3g Vial	0026-8213-35
3g Infusion Bottle	0026-8213-36
3g ADD-Vantage® Vial	0026-8213-19
4g Vial	0026-8214-35
4g Infusion Bottle	0026-8214-36
4g ADD-Vantage® Vial	0026-8214-19
20g Pharmacy Bulk Package	0026-8220-31

Unreconstituted MEZLIN® should be stored at temperatures not exceeding 86°F (30°C). The powder as well as the reconstituted solution of drug may darken slightly, depending upon storage conditions, but potency is not affected.

Bayer Corporation
Pharmaceutical Division
400 Morgan Lane
West Haven, CT 06516 USA
PD100668   BAY f 1353   5202/4/A/US/

MITHRACIN®   ℞
(plicamycin)
FOR INTRAVENOUS USE

WARNING
IT IS RECOMMENDED THAT MITHRACIN (plicamycin) BE ADMINISTERED ONLY TO HOSPITALIZED PATIENTS BY OR UNDER THE SUPERVISION OF A QUALIFIED PHYSICIAN WHO IS EXPERIENCED IN THE USE OF CANCER CHEMOTHERAPEUTIC AGENTS, BECAUSE OF THE POSSIBILITY OF SEVERE REACTIONS. FACILITIES FOR THE

Continued on next page

Bayer Corporation—Cont.

DETERMINATION OF NECESSARY LABORATORY STUDIES MUST BE AVAILABLE.

SEVERE THROMBOCYTOPENIA, A HEMORRHAGIC TENDENCY AND EVEN DEATH MAY RESULT FROM THE USE OF MITHRACIN. ALTHOUGH SEVERE TOXICITY IS MORE APT TO OCCUR IN PATIENTS WHO HAVE FAR-ADVANCED DISEASE OR ARE OTHERWISE CONSIDERED POOR RISKS FOR THERAPY, SERIOUS TOXICITY MAY ALSO OCCASIONALLY OCCUR EVEN IN PATIENTS WHO ARE IN RELATIVELY GOOD CONDITION.

IN THE TREATMENT OF EACH PATIENT, THE PHYSICIAN MUST WEIGH CAREFULLY THE POSSIBILITY OF ACHIEVING THERAPEUTIC BENEFIT VERSUS THE RISK OF TOXICITY WHICH MAY OCCUR WITH MITHRACIN THERAPY. THE FOLLOWING DATA CONCERNING THE USE OF MITHRACIN IN THE TREATMENT OF TESTICULAR TUMORS, HYPERCALCEMIC AND/OR HYPERCALCIURIC CONDITIONS ASSOCIATED WITH VARIOUS ADVANCED MALIGNANCIES, SHOULD BE THOROUGHLY REVIEWED BEFORE ADMINISTERING THIS COMPOUND.

DESCRIPTION

Mithracin (plicamycin) is a yellow crystalline compound which is produced by a microorganism, *Streptomyces plicatus.* Mithracin is available in vials as a freeze-dried, sterile preparation for intravenous administration. Each vial contains 2500 mcg (2.5 mg) of Mithracin with 100 mg of mannitol and sufficient disodium phosphate to adjust to pH 7. After reconstitution with sterile water for injection, the solution has a pH of 7. The drug is unstable in acid solutions with a pH below 4.

Mithracin is an antineoplastic agent. It has an empirical formula of $C_{52}H_{76}O_{24}$. The following structural formula has been proposed for this compound.

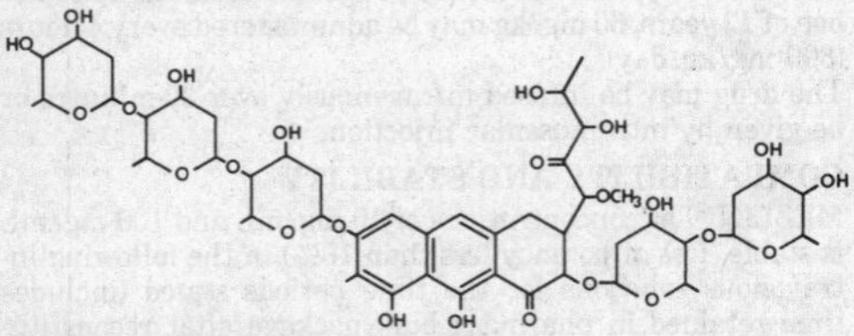

CLINICAL PHARMACOLOGY

Although the exact mechanism by which Mithracin causes tumor inhibition is not yet known, studies have indicated that this compound forms a complex with deoxyribonucleic acid (DNA) and inhibits cellular ribonucleic acid (RNA) and enzymic RNA synthesis. The binding of Mithracin to DNA in the presence of Mg^{++} (or other divalent cations) is responsible for the inhibition of DNA-dependent or DNA-directed RNA synthesis. This action presumably accounts for the biological properties of Mithracin.

Mithracin shows potent cytotoxicity against malignant cells of human origin (Hela cells) growing in tissue culture. Mithracin is lethal to Hela cells in 48 hours at concentrations as low as 0.5 micrograms per milliliter of tissue culture medium. Mithracin has shown significant anti-tumor activity against experimental leukemia in mice when administered intraperitoneally.

Plicamycin may lower serum calcium levels; the exact mechanism (or mechanisms) by which the drug exerts this effect is unknown. It appears that plicamycin may block the hypercalcemic action of pharmacologic doses of vitamin D. It has also been suggested that plicamycin may lower calcium serum levels by inhibiting the effect of parathyroid hormone upon osteoclasts. Plicamycin's inhibition of DNA-dependent RNA synthesis appears to render osteoclasts unable to fully respond to parathyroid hormone with the biosynthesis necessary for osteolysis. Decreases in serum phosphate levels and urinary calcium excretion accompany the lowering of serum calcium concentrations.

Radioautography studies[1] with ^{3}H-labeled plicamycin in C3H mice show that the greatest concentrations of the isotope are in the Kupffer cells of the liver and cells of the renal tubules. Plicamycin is rapidly cleared from the blood within the first 2 hours and excretion is also rapid. Sixty-seven percent of measured excretion occurs within 4 hours, 75% within 8 hours, and 90% is recovered in the first 24 hours after injection. There is no evidence of protein binding, nor is there any evidence of metabolism of the carbohydrate moiety of the drug to carbon dioxide and water with loss through respiration. Plicamycin crosses the blood-brain barrier; the concentration found in brain tissue is low but it persists longer than in other tissues. The experimental results in animals correlate closely with results achieved in man.[2]

INDICATIONS

Mithracin is a potent antineoplastic agent which has been shown to be useful in the treatment of carefully selected hospitalized patients with malignant tumors of the testis in whom successful treatment by surgery and/or radiation is impossible. Also, on the basis of limited clinical experience to date, it may be considered in the treatment of certain symptomatic patients with hypercalcemia and hypercalciuria associated with a variety of advanced neoplasms.

The use of Mithracin in other types of neoplastic disease is not recommended at the present time.

CONTRAINDICATIONS

Mithracin (plicamycin) is contraindicated in patients with thrombocytopenia, thrombocytopathy, coagulation disorder or an increased susceptibility to bleeding due to other causes. Mithracin should not be administered to any patient with impairment of bone marrow function.

Mithracin may cause fetal harm when administered to a pregnant woman. Mithracin is contraindicated in women who are or may become pregnant. If this drug is used during pregnancy, or if the patient becomes pregnant while taking this drug, the patient should be apprised of the potential hazard to the fetus.

PRECAUTIONS

General: Mithracin should be administered only to patients who are hospitalized and who can be observed carefully and frequently during and after therapy.

Severe thrombocytopenia, a hemorrhagic tendency and even death may result from the use of Mithracin. Although severe toxicity is more apt to occur in patients who have far-advanced disease or are otherwise considered poor risks for therapy, serious toxicity may also occasionally occur even in patients who are in relatively good condition.

Electrolyte imbalance, especially hypocalcemia, hypokalemia, and hypophosphatemia, should be corrected with appropriate electrolyte therapy prior to treatment with Mithracin.

Mithracin should be used with extreme caution in patients with significant impairment of renal or hepatic function.

Mithracin should not normally be administered to patients who are pregnant or to mothers who are breast feeding.

In the treatment of each patient, the physician must weigh carefully the possibility of achieving therapeutic benefit versus the risk of toxicity which may occur with Mithracin therapy.

Laboratory Tests: The following laboratory studies should be obtained frequently during therapy and for several days following the last dose: platelet count, prothrombin time, bleeding time. The occurrence of thrombocytopenia or a significant prolongation of prothrombin time or bleeding time is an indication for the termination of therapy.

Carcinogenesis, mutagenesis, impairment of fertility: No long-term studies in animals have been performed to evaluate the carcinogenic potential of Mithracin. Histologic evidence of inhibition of spermatogenesis was observed in a substantial number of male rats receiving doses of 0.6 mg/kg/day and above.

Pregnancy Category X: See "Contraindications" section.

Nursing Mothers: It is not known whether this drug is excreted in human milk. Because many drugs are excreted in human milk and because of the potential for serious adverse reactions in nursing infants from Mithracin, a decision should be made whether to discontinue nursing or to discontinue the drug, taking into account the importance of the drug to the mother.

ADVERSE REACTIONS

THE MOST IMPORTANT FORM OF TOXICITY ASSOCIATED WITH THE USE OF MITHRACIN CONSISTS OF A BLEEDING SYNDROME WHICH USUALLY BEGINS WITH AN EPISODE OF EPISTAXIS. This bleeding tendency may only consist of a single or several episodes of epistaxis and progress no further. However, in some cases, this hemorrhagic syndrome can start with an episode of hematemesis which may progress to more widespread hemorrhage in the gastrointestinal tract or to a more generalized bleeding tendency. This hemorrhagic diathesis is most likely due to abnormalities in multiple clotting factors.

A detailed analysis of the clinical data in 1,160 patients treated with Mithracin indicates that the hemorrhagic syndrome is dose related. With doses of 30 mcg/kg/day or less for 10 or fewer doses, the incidence of bleeding episodes has been 5.4% with an associated drug-related mortality rate of 1.6%. With doses greater than 30 mcg/kg/day and/or for more than 10 doses, a significantly larger number of bleeding episodes occurred (11.9%) and the associated drug-related mortality rate was also significantly higher (5.7%).

The most common side effects reported with the use of Mithracin consist of gastrointestinal symptoms: anorexia, nausea, vomiting, diarrhea, and stomatitis. Other less frequently reported side effects include fever, drowsiness, weakness, lethargy, malaise, headache, depression, phlebitis, facial flushing, and skin rash.

The following laboratory abnormalities have been reported during therapy with Mithracin and in most instances were reversible following cessation of treatment:

Hematologic Abnormalities: Depression of platelet count, white count, hemoglobin and prothrombin content; elevation of clotting time and bleeding time; abnormal clot retraction. Thrombocytopenia may be rapid in onset and may occur at any time during therapy or within several days following the last dose. With the occurrence of severe thrombocytopenia, the infusion of platelet concentrates of platelet-rich plasma may be helpful in elevating the platelet count.

The occurrence of leukopenia with the use of Mithracin is relatively uncommon, occurring only in approximately 6% of patients.

It has been uncommon for abnormalities in clotting time or clot retraction to be demonstrated prior to the onset of an overt bleeding episode noted in some patients treated with Mithracin. Nevertheless, the performance of these tests periodically is recommended because in a few instances, an abnormality in one of these studies may have served as a warning to terminate therapy because of impending serious toxicity.

Abnormal Liver Function Tests: Increased levels of serum glutamic oxalacetic transaminase, serum glutamic pyruvic transaminase, lactic dehydrogenase, alkaline phosphatase, serum bilirubin, ornithine carbamyl transferase, isocitric dehydrogenase, and increased retention of bromsulphalein.

Abnormal Renal Function Tests: Increased blood urea nitrogen and serum creatinine; proteinuria.

Abnormalities in Electrolyte Concentrations: Depression of serum calcium, phosphorus, and potassium.

OVERDOSAGE

Generally, adverse effects following the use of Mithracin, especially the hemorrhagic syndrome, are dose related. Therefore, following administration of an overdose, patients can be expected to experience an exaggeration of the usual adverse effects. Close monitoring of the hematologic picture, including factors involved in the clotting mechanism, hepatic and renal functions, and serum electrolytes, is necessary. No specific antidote for Mithracin is known. Management of overdosage would include general supportive measures to sustain the patient through the period of toxicity.

DOSAGE AND ADMINISTRATION

The daily dose of Mithracin is based on the patient's body weight. If a patient has abnormal fluid retention such as edema, hydrothorax or ascites, the patient's ideal weight rather than actual body weight should be used to calculate the dose.

Treatment of Testicular Tumors: In the treatment of patients with testicular tumors the recommended daily dose of Mithracin (plicamycin) is 25 to 30 mcg (0.025–0.030 mg) per kilogram of body weight. Therapy should be continued for a period of 8 to 10 days unless significant side effects or toxicity occur during therapy. A course of therapy consisting of more than 10 daily doses is not recommended. Individual daily doses should not exceed 30 mcg (0.030 mg) per kilogram of body weight.

In those patients with responsive tumors, some degree of tumor regression is usually evident within 3 or 4 weeks following the initial course of therapy. If tumor masses remain unchanged following an initial course of therapy, additional courses of therapy at monthly intervals are warranted.

When a significant tumor regression is obtained, it is suggested that additional courses of therapy be given at monthly intervals until a complete regression of tumor masses is achieved or until definite tumor progression or new tumor masses occur in spite of continued courses of therapy.

Treatment of Hypercalcemia and Hypercalciuria: Reversal of hypercalcemia and hypercalciuria can usually be achieved with Mithracin at doses considerably lower than those recommended for use in the treatment of testicular tumors. In hypercalcemia and hypercalciuria associated with advanced malignancy the recommended course of treatment with Mithracin is 25 mcg (0.025 mg) per kilogram of body weight per day for 3 or 4 days.

If the desired degree of reversal of hypercalcemia or hypercalciuria is not achieved with the initial course of therapy, additional courses of therapy may then be administered at intervals of one week or more to achieve the desired result or to maintain serum calcium and urinary calcium excretion at normal levels. It may be possible to maintain normal calcium balance with single, weekly doses or with a schedule of 2 or 3 doses per week.

NOTE: BECAUSE OF THE DRUG'S TOXICITY AND THE LIMITED CLINICAL EXPERIENCE TO DATE IN THESE INDICATIONS, THE FOLLOWING RECOMMENDATIONS SHOULD BE KEPT IN MIND BY THE PHYSICIAN.

1. **CONSIDER CASES OF HYPERCALCEMIA AND HYPERCALCIURIA NOT RESPONSIVE TO CONVENTIONAL TREATMENT.**
2. **APPLY SAME CONTRAINDICATIONS AND PRECAUTIONARY MEASURES AS IN ANTITUMOR TREATMENT.**
3. **RENAL FUNCTION SHOULD BE CAREFULLY MONITORED BEFORE, DURING, AND AFTER TREATMENT.**
4. **BENEFITS OF USE DURING PREGNANCY OR IN WOMEN OF CHILDBEARING AGE SHOULD BE WEIGHED AGAINST POTENTIAL TOXICITY TO EMBRYO OR FETUS.**

MITHRACIN

RESULTS IN 305 TESTICULAR TUMOR CASES BY TUMOR TYPE

TYPE OF TESTICULAR TUMOR	TOTAL	COMPLETE RESPONSE	PARTIAL RESPONSE	NO RESPONSE
EMBRYONAL CELL	173	26	42	105
TERATOMA	5	0	1	4
TERATOCARCINOMA	23	0	5	18
SEMINOMA	18	0	7	11
CHORIOCARCINOMA	13	1	6	6
MIXED TUMOR	73	6	19	48
TOTALS	305	33	80	192

ADMINISTRATION

By IV administration only. The appropriate daily dose of Mithracin should be diluted in one liter of 5% Dextrose Injection, USP or Sodium Chloride Injection, USP and administered by slow intravenous infusion over a period of 4 to 6 hours. Rapid direct intravenous injection of Mithracin should be avoided as it may be associated with a higher incidence and greater severity of gastrointestinal side effects. Extravasation of solutions of Mithracin may cause local irritation and cellulitis at injection sites. Should thrombophlebitis or perivascular cellulitis occur, the infusion should be terminated and reinstituted at another site. The application of moderate heat to the site of extravasation may help to disperse the compound and minimize discomfort and local tissue irritation. The use of antiemetic compounds prior to and during treatment with Mithracin may be helpful in relieving nausea and vomiting.

Procedures for proper handling and disposal of anti-cancer drugs should be considered. Several guidelines on this subject have been published.[3-8] There is no general agreement that all of the procedures recommended in the guidelines are necessary or appropriate.

HOW SUPPLIED

Mithracin is available in vials as a freeze-dried preparation for intravenous administration. Each vial contains 2500 mcg (2.5 mg) of Mithracin with 100 mg of mannitol and sufficient disodium phosphate to adjust to pH 7. These vials should be stored at refrigerator temperatures between 2°C to 8°C (36°F to 46°F).

To reconstitute, add aseptically 4.9 mL of Sterile Water for Injection to the contents of the vial and shake to dissolve. Each mL of the resulting solution will then contain 500 mcg (0.5 mg) of Mithracin. NOTE: 1 mg (milligram)=1000 mcg (micrograms). AFTER REMOVAL OF THE APPROPRIATE DOSE, THE REMAINING UNUSED SOLUTION MUST BE DISCARDED, FRESH SOLUTIONS MUST BE PREPARED IN THE ABOVE MANNER EACH DAY OF THERAPY.

ANIMAL PHARMACOLOGY AND TOXICOLOGY

In mice the average intravenous LD_{50} of Mithracin is 2,000 mcg/kg of body weight. When administered orally, it is not toxic to mice even at doses 100 times greater than the intravenous LD_{50}. In rats the average intravenous LD_{50} of Mithracin is 1,700 mcg/kg of body weight. It is not toxic to rats when administered orally at doses 17 times greater than the intravenous LD_{50}. In dogs and monkeys Mithracin is essentially non-toxic when administered intravenously for 24 days at daily doses as high as 50 and 24 mcg/kg of body weight, respectively. However, at higher doses of 100 mcg/kg/day intravenously it is lethal to dogs and monkeys. Signs of toxicity in dogs and monkeys included anorexia, vomiting, listlessness, melena, anemia, lymphopenia, elevated alkaline phosphatase, serum glutamic oxalacetic transaminase, serum glutamic pyruvic transaminase values, hypochloremia, hyponatremia, hypokalemia, hypocalcemia, and decreased prothrombin consumption. Necropsy findings consisted of necrosis of lymphoid tissue and multiple generalized hemorrhages. Mithracin (plicamycin) was only mildly irritating when injected intramuscularly in rabbits and subcutaneously in guinea pigs. Histologic evidence of inhibition of spermatogenesis was observed in a substantial number of male rats receiving doses of 0.6 mg/kg/day and above. This preclinical finding of selective drug effect constituted the scientific rationale for clinical trials in testicular tumors.

CLINICAL REPORTS

Treatment of Patients with Inoperable Testicular Tumors: In a combined series of 305 patients with inoperable testicular tumors treated with Mithracin, 33 patients (10.8%) showed a complete disappearance of tumor masses and an additional 80 patients (26.2%) responded with significant partial regression of tumor masses. The longest duration of a continuing complete response is now over 8½ years. The therapeu-

tic responses in this series of patients have been summarized by type of testicular tumor in the accompanying table. [See table above.]

Mithracin may be useful in the treatment of patients with testicular tumors which are resistant to other chemotherapeutic agents. Prior radiation therapy or prior chemotherapy did not alter the response rate with Mithracin. This suggests that there is no significant cross resistance between Mithracin and other chemotherapeutic agents.

Treatment of Patients with Hypercalcemia and Hypercalciuria: A limited number of patients with hypercalcemia (range: 12.0–25.8 mg%) and patients with hypercalciuria (range 215–492 mg/day) associated with malignant disease were treated with Mithracin. Hypercalcemia and hypercalciuria were promptly reversed in all patients. In some patients, the primary malignancy was of non-testicular origin.

REFERENCES

1. Kennedy, B.D., et al: Cancer Res. 27:1534, 1967.
2. Ransohoff, J., et al: Cancer Chemother. Rep. 49:51, 1965.
3. Recommendations for the Safe Handling of Parenteral Antineoplastic Drugs. NIH Publication No. 83-2621. For sale by the Superintendent of Documents, U.S. Government Printing Office, Washington, D.C. 20402.
4. AMA Council Report. Guidelines for Handling Parenteral Antineoplastics. JAMA, March 15, 1985.
5. National Study Commission on Cytotoxic Exposure—Recommendations for Handling Cytotoxic Agents. Available from Louis P. Jeffrey, Sc.D., Director of Pharmacy Services, Rhode Island Hospital, 593 Eddy Street, Providence, Rhode Island 02902.
6. Clinical Oncological Society of Australia: Guidelines and recommendations for safe handling of antineoplastic agents. Med J Australia 1:426–428, 1983.
7. Jones, R.B., et al: Safe handling of chemotherapeutic agents: A report from the Mount Sinai Medical Center. Ca—A Cancer Journal for Clinicians, Sept/Oct. 258–263, 1983.
8. American Society of Hospital Pharmacists technical assistance bulletin on handling cytotoxic drugs in hospitals. Am J Hosp Pharm 42:131–137, 1985.

Manufactured for
Bayer Corporation
Pharmaceutical Division
400 Morgan Lane
West Haven, CT 06516
by Ben Venue Laboratories
Bedford, Ohio 44146
PD100654—60-4178-81-4   Revised Feb. 1995

MYCELEX® ℞
(clotrimazole) TROCHE
FOR TOPICAL ORAL ADMINISTRATION

PRODUCT OVERVIEW

KEY FACTS

MYCELEX® Troche is a slow-dissolving tablet (lozenge) containing 10 mg of clotrimazole, a synthetic antifungal agent for topical use in the mouth. Clotrimazole is a broad-spectrum antifungal which exhibits fungicidal activity *in vitro* against *Candida albicans* and other species of the genus *Candida*. No single-step or multiple-step resistance to clotrimazole has developed during successive passages of *Candida albicans* in the laboratory.

MAJOR USES

MYCELEX® Troche has been proven effective in the treatment of oropharyngeal candidiasis (oral thrush) in patients over 3 years of age.

Mycelex Troches are also indicated prophylactically to reduce the incidence of oropharyngeal candidiasis in patients immunocompromised by conditions that include chemotherapy, radiotherapy, or steroid therapy utilized in the treatment of leukemia, solid tumors, or renal transplantation.

SAFETY INFORMATION

MYCELEX® Troches are contra-indicated in patients who are hypersensitive to any of its components. MYCELEX Troches are not indicated for the treatment of systemic mycoses. Since elevated SGOT levels have been reported, periodic assessment of hepatic function is advisable, particularly, in patients with pre-existing hepatic impairment.

PRESCRIBING INFORMATION

MYCELEX® ℞
(clotrimazole) TROCHE
FOR TOPICAL ORAL ADMINISTRATION

DESCRIPTION

Each Mycelex® Troche contains 10 mg clotrimazole [1-(o-chloro-α,α-diphenylbenzyl) imidazole], a synthetic antifungal agent, for topical use in the mouth.

Structural Formula:

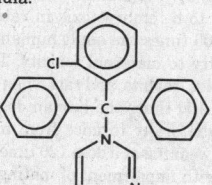

Chemical Formula:
$C_{22}H_{17}ClN_2$

The troche dosage form is a large, slowly dissolving tablet (lozenge) containing 10 mg of clotrimazole dispersed in dextrose, microcrystalline cellulose, povidone, and magnesium stearate.

CLINICAL PHARMACOLOGY

Clotrimazole is a broad-spectrum antifungal agent that inhibits the growth of pathogenic yeasts by altering the permeability of cell membranes. The action of clotrimazole is fungistatic at concentrations of drug up to 20 mcg/mL and may be fungicidal *in vitro* against *Candida albicans* and other species of the genus *Candida* at higher concentrations. No single-step or multiple-step resistance to clotrimazole has developed during successive passages of *Candida albicans* in the laboratory; however, individual organism tolerance has been observed during successive passages in the laboratory. Such *in vitro* tolerance has resolved once the organism has been removed from the antifungal environment.

After oral administration of a 10 mg clotrimazole troche to healthy volunteers, concentrations sufficient to inhibit most species of *Candida* persist in saliva for up to three hours following the approximately 30 minutes needed for a troche to dissolve. The long term persistence of drug in saliva appears to be related to the slow release of clotrimazole from the oral mucosa to which the drug is apparently bound. Repetitive dosing at three hour intervals maintains salivary levels above the minimum inhibitory concentrations of most strains of *Candida;* however, the relationship between *in vitro* susceptibility of pathogenic fungi to clotrimazole and prophylaxis or cure of infections in humans has not been established.

In another study, the mean serum concentrations were 4.98 ± 3.7 and 3.23 ± 1.4 nanograms/mL of clotrimazole at 30 and 60 minutes, respectively, after administration as a troche.

INDICATIONS AND USAGE

Mycelex® Troches are indicated for the local treatment of oropharyngeal candidiasis. The diagnosis should be confirmed by a KOH smear and/or culture prior to treatment. Mycelex Troches are also indicated prophylactically to reduce the incidence of oropharyngeal candidiasis in patients immunocompromised by conditions that include chemotherapy, radiotherapy, or steroid therapy utilized in the treatment of leukemia, solid tumors, or renal transplantation. There are no data from adequate and well-controlled trials to establish the safety and efficacy of this product for prophylactic use in patients immunocompromised by etiologies other than those listed in the previous sentence. (See DOSAGE AND ADMINISTRATION.)

CONTRAINDICATIONS

Mycelex® Troches are contraindicated in patients who are hypersensitive to any of its components.

WARNING

Mycelex® Troches are not indicated for the treatment of systemic mycoses including systemic candidiasis.

Continued on next page

Consult 1997 supplements and future editions for revisions

Bayer Corporation—Cont.

PRECAUTIONS

Abnormal liver function tests have been reported in patients treated with clotrimazole troches; elevated SGOT levels were reported in about 15% of patients in the clinical trials. In most cases the elevations were minimal and it was often impossible to distinguish effects of clotrimazole from those of other therapy and the underlying disease (malignancy in most cases). Periodic assessment of hepatic function is advisable particularly in patients with pre-existing hepatic impairment.

Since patients must be instructed to allow each troche to dissolve slowly in the mouth in order to achieve maximum effect of the medication, they must be of such an age and physical and/or mental condition to comprehend such instructions.

Carcinogenesis: An 18 month dosing study with clotrimazole in rats has not revealed any carcinogenic effect.

Usage in Pregnancy: Pregnancy Category C: Clotrimazole has been shown to be embryotoxic in rats and mice when given in doses 100 times the adult human dose (in mg/kg), possibly secondary to maternal toxicity. The drug was not teratogenic in mice, rabbits, and rats when given in doses up to 200, 180, and 100 times the human dose.

Clotrimazole given orally to mice from nine weeks before mating through weaning at a dose 120 times the human dose was associated with impairment of mating, decreased number of viable young, and decreased survival to weaning. No effects were observed at 60 times the human dose. When the drug was given to rats during a similar time period at 50 times the human dose, there was a slight decrease in the number of pups per litter and decreased pup viability.

There are no adequate and well controlled studies in pregnant women. Clotrimazole troches should be used during pregnancy only if the potential benefit justifies the potential risk to the fetus.

PEDIATRIC USE

Safety and effectiveness of clotrimazole in children below the age of 3 years have not been established; therefore, its use in such patients is not recommended.

The safety and efficacy of the prophylactic use of clotrimazole troches in children have not been established.

ADVERSE REACTIONS

Abnormal liver function tests have been reported in patients treated with clotrimazole troches; elevated SGOT levels were reported in about 15% of patients in the clinical trials (See Precautions section).

Nausea, vomiting, unpleasant mouth sensations and pruritus have also been reported with the use of the troche.

OVERDOSAGE

No data available.

DRUG ABUSE AND DEPENDENCE

No data available.

DOSAGE AND ADMINISTRATION

Mycelex® Troches are administered only as a lozenge that must be slowly dissolved in the mouth. The recommended dose is one troche five times a day for fourteen consecutive days. Only limited data are available on the safety and effectiveness of the clotrimazole troche after prolonged administration; therefore, therapy should be limited to short term use, if possible.

For prophylaxis to reduce the incidence of oropharyngeal candidiasis in patients immunocompromised by conditions that include chemotherapy, radio therapy, or steroid therapy utilized in the treatment of leukemia, solid tumors, or renal transplantation, the recommended dose is one troche three times daily for the duration of chemotherapy or until steroids are reduced to maintenance levels.

HOW SUPPLIED

Mycelex® Troches, white discoid, uncoated tablets are supplied in bottles of 70 and 140. Mycelex Troches are also available for institutional use in foil packages of 70 tablets. Each tablet will be identified with the following: Mycelex. 10

Store below 86°F (30°C).

Avoid freezing.

Bayer Corporation
Pharmaceutical Division
400 Morgan Lane
West Haven, CT 06516 USA

PD500016   BAY 5097   5041
© 1995 Bayer Corporation 3/95

Shown in Product Identification Guide, page 305

MYCELEX®-G 500 mg ℞
brand of clotrimazole
Vaginal Tablets

PRODUCT OVERVIEW

KEY FACTS

Mycelex®-G 500 mg is an effective antifungal containing 500 mg of clotrimazole (the active ingredient). Clotrimazole is a broad spectrum antifungal which exhibits fungicidal activity *in vitro* against *Candida albicans* and other species of the genus *Candida*. No single-step or multiple-step resistance to clotrimazole has developed during successive passages of *Candida albicans*.

MAJOR USES

Mycelex®-G 500 mg has proved to be clinically effective for local treatment of vulvovaginal candidiasis when one day therapy is felt warranted. In the case of severe vulvovaginal candidiasis longer antimycotic therapy such as Mycelex®-G 100 mg tablets or Mycelex®-G Cream is recommended.

SAFETY INFORMATION

Mycelex®-G 500 mg Vaginal Tablets are contraindicated in women who have shown hypersensitivity to any components of the compound. If there is a lack of response to treatment with Mycelex®-G 500 mg, appropriate microbiological studies should be performed to confirm the diagnosis and rule out other pathogens before instituting another course of antimycotic therapy. There are, however, no adequate and well-controlled studies in pregnant women during the first trimester of pregnancy.

PRESCRIBING INFORMATION

MYCELEX®-G 500 mg ℞
brand of clotrimazole
Vaginal Tablets

DESCRIPTION

Each Mycelex®-G 500 mg Vaginal Tablet contains 500 mg clotrimazole (the active ingredient) dispersed in lactose, microcrystalline cellulose, lactic acid, corn starch, crospovidone, calcium lactate, magnesium stearate, silicon dioxide and hydroxypropyl methylcellulose. Chemically, clotrimazole is [1-(o-Chloro-α, α-diphenylbenzyl) imidazole], a synthetic antifungal agent having the chemical formula $C_{22}H_{17}ClN_2$; a molecular weight of 344.84; and the following chemical structure:

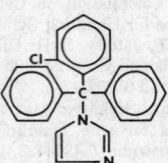

Clotrimazole is an odorless, white crystalline substance, practically insoluble in water, sparingly soluble in ether, soluble in carbon tetrachloride, and very soluble in ethanol and chloroform.

CLINICAL PHARMACOLOGY

Serum and levels in vaginal secretions of clotrimazole were measured in six healthy volunteers who had one 500 mg vaginal tablet inserted. Although serum levels of clotrimazole were higher than those in other volunteers given 100 mg and 200 mg vaginal tablets these levels did not exceed 10 nanograms/mL. It has been estimated that three to ten percent of a vaginal dose of clotrimazole may be absorbed, but the drug rapidly and efficiently degrades to microbiologically inactive metabolites. The clotrimazole concentrations remaining in vaginal secretions were still in the mg/mL range for 48 hours and in two of the six subjects at 72 hours.

The findings of high clotrimazole concentrations in vaginal secretions for up to 72 hours and low concentrations in the serum suggest that nearly all the clotrimazole given in the 500 mg vaginal tablet remains in the vagina for 48 hours, and in some cases 72 hours, in fungicidal concentrations.

Clotrimazole is a broad-spectrum antifungal agent. It has been postulated that the compound affects the permeability characteristics of the membrane allowing the leakage of essential intracellular components with a consequent inhibition of the synthesis of such macromolecules as protein, lipid, DNA, and polysaccharides.

At concentrations as low as 2–5 μg/mL, clotrimazole exhibits fungicidal activity *in vitro* against *Candida albicans* and other species of the genus *Candida*.

No single-step or multiple-step resistance to clotrimazole has developed during successive passages of *Candida albicans*.

INDICATIONS

Mycelex-G 500 mg Vaginal Tablets are indicated for the local treatment of vulvovaginal candidiasis when one day therapy is felt warranted. In the case of severe vulvovaginitis due to candidiasis, longer antimycotic therapy is recommended.

The diagnosis should be confirmed by KOH smears and/or cultures. Other pathogens commonly associated with vulvovaginitis, *Trichomonas* and *Gardnerella (Haemophilus) vaginalis*, should be ruled out by appropriate laboratory methods.

CONTRAINDICATIONS

Mycelex-G 500 mg Vaginal Tablets are contraindicated in women who have shown hypersensitivity to any components of the preparation.

WARNINGS

None.

PRECAUTIONS

If there is a lack of response to Mycelex-G 500 mg Vaginal Tablets, appropriate microbiological studies should be repeated to confirm the diagnosis and rule out other pathogens before instituting another course of antimycotic therapy.

CARCINOGENESIS

No long term studies in animals have been performed to evaluate the carcinogenic potential of Mycelex-G 500 mg Vaginal Tablets intravaginally. A long term study in rats (Wistar strains) where clotrimazole was administered orally provided no indication of carcinogenicity.

USAGE IN PREGNANCY

Pregnancy Category B: The disposition of ^{14}C-clotrimazole has been studied in humans and animals. Clotrimazole is poorly absorbed following intravaginal administration to humans, whereas it is rather well absorbed after oral administration.

In clinical trials, use of vaginally applied clotrimazole in pregnant women in their second and third trimesters has not been associated with ill effects. There are, however, no adequate and well-controlled studies in pregnant women during the first trimester of pregnancy.

Studies in pregnant rats given repeated intravaginal doses up to 100 mg/kg/day have revealed no evidence of harm to the fetus due to clotrimazole.

Repeated high oral doses of clotrimazole in rats and mice ranging from 50 to 120 mg/kg resulted in embryotoxicity (possibly secondary to maternal toxicity), impairment of mating, decreased litter size and number of viable young and decreased pup survival to weaning. However, clotrimazole was not teratogenic in mice, rabbits and rats at oral doses up to 200, 180 and 100 mg/kg, respectively. Oral absorption in the rat amounts to approximately 90% of the administered dose.

Because animal reproduction studies are not always predictive of human response, this drug should be used only if clearly indicated during the first trimester of pregnancy.

ADVERSE REACTIONS

Of 297 patients in double-blind studies with the 500 mg vaginal tablet, 3 of 149 patients treated with active drug and 3 of 148 patients treated with placebo reported complaints during therapy that were possibly drug related. In the active drug group, vomiting occurred in one patient, vaginal soreness with coitus in another, and complaints of vaginal irritation, itching, burning and dyspareunia in the third patient. In the placebo group, clitoral irritation occurred in one patient and dysuria, described as remotely related to drug, in the other. A third patient in the placebo group developed bacterial vaginitis which the investigator classed as possibly related to drug.

Eighteen (1.6%) of the 1116 patients treated with Mycelex-G in other formulations in double-blind studies reported complaints during therapy that were possibly drug-related. Mild burning occurred in six patients while other complaints such as skin rash, itching, vulval irritation, lower abdominal cramps and bloating, slight cramping, slight urinary frequency, and burning or irritation in the sexual partner, occurred rarely.

OVERDOSAGE

No data available.

DRUG ABUSE AND DEPENDENCE

Drug abuse and dependence with Mycelex-G 500 mg Vaginal Tablets has not been reported.

DOSAGE AND ADMINISTRATION

The recommended dose is one tablet inserted intravaginally one time only, preferably at bedtime. In the event of treatment failure, that is, persistence of signs and symptoms of vaginitis after five days, other pathogens commonly responsible for vaginitis should be ruled out before instituting another course of antimycotic therapy.

HOW SUPPLIED

Mycelex-G 500 mg Vaginal Tablets are white, bullet shaped, uncoated tablets, coded with Bayer on one side and 097 on the other, supplied as a single 500 mg tablet with plastic applicator and patient instructions, or in twin pack with Mycelex 1% cream 7g tube.

Store Below 86°F (30°C).

U.S. Patent Numbers 3,660,577; 3,705,172; 3,839,573; 4,457,938.

Manufactured by
Bayer Corporation
Pharmaceutical Division
400 Morgan Lane
West Haven, CT 06516
PD500010   5/95 BAY 5097
© 1995 Bayer Corporation   5213
Shown in Product Identification Guide, page 305

Study	Dose	Grade*	Number Analyzed	Patients Any Deficit Due to Spasm	Numbers With Severe Deficit
1.	20–30 mg	I–III	Nimodipine 56	13	1
			Placebo 60	16	8**
2.	60 mg	I–III	Nimodipine 31	4	2
			Placebo 39	11	10**

*Hunt and Hess Grade
**$p = 0.03$

NIMOTOP®
(nimodipine)
CAPSULES
For Oral Use

DESCRIPTION

Nimotop® (nimodipine) belongs to the class of pharmacological agents known as calcium channel blockers. Nimodipine is isopropyl (2 - methoxyethyl) 1, 4 - dihydro - 2, 6 - dimethyl - 4 - (3 - nitrophenyl) - 3, 5 - pyridine - dicarboxylate. It has a molecular weight of 418.5 and a molecular formula of $C_{21}H_{26}N_2O_7$. The structural formula is:

Nimodipine is a yellow crystalline substance, practically insoluble in water.
NIMOTOP® capsules are formulated as soft gelatin capsules for oral administration. Each liquid filled capsule contains 30 mg of nimodipine in a vehicle of glycerin, peppermint oil, purified water and polyethylene glycol 400. The soft gelatin capsule shell contains gelatin, glycerin, purified water and titanium dioxide.

CLINICAL PHARMACOLOGY

Mechanism of Action: Nimodipine is a calcium channel blocker. The contractile processes of smooth muscle cells are dependent upon calcium ions, which enter these cells during depolarization as slow ionic transmembrane currents. Nimodipine inhibits calcium ion transfer into these cells and thus inhibits contractions of vascular smooth muscle. In animal experiments, nimodipine had a greater effect on cerebral arteries than on arteries elsewhere in the body perhaps because it is highly lipophilic, allowing it to cross the blood-brain barrier; concentrations of nimodipine as high as 12.5 ng/mL have been detected in the cerebrospinal fluid of nimodipine treated subarachnoid hemorrhage (SAH) patients.
Based on animal experiments, it was hoped that nimodipine would prevent cerebral arterial spasm in SAH patients. While the clinical studies described below demonstrate a favorable effect by nimodipine on the severity of neurological deficits caused by cerebral vasospasm following SAH, there is no arteriographic evidence that the drug either prevents or relieves the spasm of these arteries. The actual mechanism of action in humans is, therefore, unknown.
Pharmacokinetics and Metabolism: In man, nimodipine is rapidly absorbed after oral administration, and peak concentrations are generally attained within one hour. The terminal elimination half-life is approximately 8 to 9 hours but earlier elimination rates are much more rapid, equivalent to a half-life of 1–2 hours; a consequence is the need for frequent (every 4 hours) dosing. There were no signs of accumulation when nimodipine was given three times a day for seven days. Nimodipine is over 95% bound to plasma proteins. The binding was concentration independent over the range of 10 ng/mL to 10 μg/mL. Nimodipine is eliminated almost exclusively in the form of metabolites and less than 1% is recovered in the urine as unchanged drug. Numerous metabolites, all of which are either inactive or considerably less active than the parent compound, have been identified. Because of a high first-pass metabolism, the bioavailability of nimodipine averages 13% after oral administration. The bioavailability is significantly increased in patients with hepatic cirrhosis, with C_{max} approximately double that in

normals which necessitates lowering the dose in this group of patients (see Dosage and Administration). In a study of 24 healthy male volunteers, administration of nimodipine capsules following a standard breakfast resulted in a 68% lower peak plasma concentration and 38% lower bioavailability relative to dosing under fasted conditions.
Clinical Trials: Nimodipine has been shown, in 4 randomized, placebo-controlled trials, to reduce the severity of neurological deficits resulting from vasospasm in patients who have had a recent subarachnoid hemorrhage (SAH). The trials used doses ranging from 20–30 mg to 90 mg every 4 hours, with drug given for 21 days in 3 studies, and for at least 18 days in the other. Three of the four trials followed patients for 3–6 months. Three of the trials studied relatively well patients, with all or most patients in Hunt and Hess Grades I–II (essentially free of focal deficits after the initial bleed); the fourth studied much sicker patients, Hunt and Hess Grades III–V. Two studies, one domestic, one French, were similar in design, with relatively unimpaired SAH patients randomized to nimodipine or placebo. In each, a judgment was made as to whether any late-developing deficit was due to spasm or other causes, and the deficits were graded. Both studies showed significantly fewer severe deficits due to spasm in the nimodipine group; the second (French) study showed fewer spasm-related deficits of all severities. No effect was seen on deficits not related to spasm.
[See table above.]
A Canadian study entered much sicker patients, who had a high rate of death and disability, and used a dose of 90 mg every 4 hours, but was otherwise similar to the first two studies. Analysis of delayed ischemic deficits, many of which result from spasm, showed a significant reduction in spasm-related deficits. Among analyzed patients (72 nimodipine, 82 placebo), there were the following outcomes.
[See table on bottom of page.]
A fourth, large, study was performed in the United Kingdom in SAH patients with all grades of severity (but about 90% were in Grades I–III). Outcomes were not defined as spasm related or not but there was a significant reduction in the overall rate of infarction and severely disabling neurological outcome at 3 months:

	Nimodipine	Placebo
Total patients	278	276
Good recovery	199*	169
Moderate disability	24	16
Severe disability	12**	31
Death	43***	60

* $p = 0.0444$—good and moderate vs severe and dead
** $p = 0.001$—severe disability
*** $p = 0.056$—death

A dose-ranging study comparing 30, 60 and 90 mg doses found a generally low rate of spasm-related neurological deficits but no significant relation of response to dose.
The effect of nimodipine on mortality is not yet clear. The large United Kingdom study showed near-significantly improved survival. The two smaller studies (domestic, French) had too few deaths to contribute to this question. The Canadian study, despite showing markedly decreased spasm-related deficits, showed overall (all patients randomized) greater 90 day mortality, 49/91 (54%) on nimodipine vs 38/97 (39%) on placebo, a significant difference. Most of the deaths appeared, in this very severely ill group (Hunt and Hess Grades III–V), to be consequences of SAH, but a drug effect cannot be ruled out. In this study 90 mg every 4 hours was the dose used, perhaps too high for the very ill population studied. The 90 mg dose is not recommended nor is treatment of Hunt and Hess Grades IV–V patients.

INDICATIONS AND USAGE

Nimotop® (nimodipine) is indicated for the improvement of neurological outcome by reducing the incidence and severity of ischemic deficits in patients with subarachnoid hemorrhage from ruptured congenital aneurysms who are in good neurological condition post-ictus (e.g., Hunt and Hess Grades I–III).

CONTRAINDICATIONS

None known.

PRECAUTIONS

General: Blood Pressure: Nimodipine has the hemodynamic effects expected of a calcium channel blocker, although they are generally not marked. In patients with subarachnoid hemorrhage given Nimotop® in clinical studies, about 5% were reported to have had lowering of the blood pressure and about 1% left the study because of this (not all could be attributed to nimodipine). Nevertheless, blood pressure should be carefully monitored during treatment with Nimotop® based on its known pharmacology and the known effects of calcium channel blockers.
Hepatic Disease: The metabolism of Nimotop® is decreased in patients with impaired hepatic function. Such patients should have their blood pressure and pulse rate monitored closely and should be given a lower dose (see Dosage and Administration).
Intestinal pseudo-obstruction and ileus have been reported rarely in patients treated with nimodipine. A causal relationship has not been established. The condition has responded to conservative management.
Laboratory Test Interactions: None known.
Drug Interaction: It is possible that the cardiovascular action of other calcium channel blockers could be enhanced by the addition of Nimotop®.
In Europe, Nimotop® was observed to occasionally intensify the effect of antihypertensive compounds taken concomitantly by patients suffering from hypertension; this phenomenon was not observed in North American clinical trials.
A study in eight healthy volunteers has shown a 50% increase in mean peak nimodipine plasma concentrations and a 90% increase in mean area under the curve, after a one-week course of cimetidine at 1,000 mg/day and nimodipine at 90 mg/day. This effect may be mediated by the known inhibition of hepatic cytochrome P-450 by cimetidine, which could decrease first-pass metabolism of nimodipine.
Carcinogenesis, Mutagenesis, Impairment of Fertility: In a two-year study, higher incidences of adenocarcinoma of the uterus and Leydig-cell adenoma of the testes were observed in rats given a diet containing 1800 ppm nimodipine (equivalent to 91 to 121 mg/kg/day nimodipine) than in placebo controls. The differences were not statistically significant, however, and the higher rates were well within historical control range for these tumors in the Wistar strain. Nimodipine was found not to be carcinogenic in a 91-week mouse study but the high dose of 1800 ppm nimodipine-in-feed (546 to 774 mg/kg/day) shortened the life expectancy of the animals. Mutagenicity studies, including the Ames, micronucleus and dominant lethal tests were negative.
Nimodipine did not impair the fertility and general reproductive performance of male and female Wistar rats following oral doses of up to 30 mg/kg/day when administered daily for more than 10 weeks in the males and 3 weeks in the females prior to mating and continued to day 7 of pregnancy. This dose in a rat is about 4 times the equivalent clinical dose of 60 mg q4h in a 50 kg patient.
Pregnancy: Pregnancy Category C. Nimodipine has been shown to have a teratogenic effect in Himalayan rabbits. Incidences of malformations and stunted fetuses were increased at oral doses of 1 and 10 mg/kg/day administered (by gavage) from day 6 through day 18 of pregnancy but not at 3.0 mg/kg/day in one of two identical rabbit studies. In the second study an increased incidence of stunted fetuses was seen at 1.0 mg/kg/day but not at higher doses. Nimodipine was embryotoxic, causing resorption and stunted growth of fetuses, in Long Evans rats at 100 mg/kg/day administered by gavage from day 6 through day 15 of pregnancy. In two other rat studies, doses of 30 mg/kg/day nimodipine administered by gavage from day 16 of gestation and continued until sacrifice (day 20 of pregnancy or day 21 post partum) were associated with higher incidences of skeletal variation,

	Delayed Ischemic Deficits (DID)		Permanent Deficits	
	Nimodipine n (%)	Placebo n (%)	Nimodipine n (%)	Placebo n (%)
DID Spasm Alone	8 (11)*	25 (31)	5 (7)*	22 (27)
DID Spasm Contributing	18 (25)	21 (26)	16 (22)	17 (21)
DID Without Spasm	7 (10)	8 (10)	6 (8)	7 (9)
No DID	39 (54)	28 (34)	45 (63)	36 (44)

*$P = 0.001$, nimodipine vs placebo

Continued on next page

Bayer Corporation—Cont.

stunted fetuses and stillbirths but no malformations. There are no adequate and well controlled studies in pregnant women to directly assess the effect on human fetuses. Nimodipine should be used during pregnancy only if the potential benefit justifies the potential risk to the fetus.

Nursing Mothers: Nimodipine and/or its metabolites have been shown to appear in rat milk at concentrations much higher than in maternal plasma. It is not known whether the drug is excreted in human milk. Because many drugs are excreted in human milk, nursing mothers are advised not to breast feed their babies when taking the drug.

Pediatric Use: Safety and effectiveness in children have not been established.

ADVERSE REACTIONS

Adverse experiences were reported by 92 of 823 patients with subarachnoid hemorrhage (11.2%) who were given nimodipine. The most frequently reported adverse experience was decreased blood pressure in 4.4% of these patients. Twenty-nine of 479 (6.1%) placebo treated patients also reported adverse experiences. The events reported with a frequency greater than 1% are displayed below by dose. [See table below.]

There were no other adverse experiences reported by the patients who were given 0.35 mg/kg q4h, 30 mg q4h or 120 mg q4h. Adverse experiences with an incidence rate of less than 1% in the 60 mg q4h dose group were: hepatitis; itching; gastrointestinal hemorrhage; thrombocytopenia; anemia; palpitations; vomiting; flushing; diaphoresis; wheezing; phenytoin toxicity; lightheadedness; dizziness; rebound vasospasm; jaundice; hypertension; hematoma.

Adverse experiences with an incidence rate less than 1% in the 90 mg q4h dose group were: itching, gastrointestinal hemorrhage; thrombocytopenia; neurological deterioration; vomiting; diaphoresis; congestive heart failure; hyponatremia; decreasing platelet count; disseminated intravascular coagulation; deep vein thrombosis.

As can be seen from the table, side effects that appear related to nimodipine use based on increased incidence with higher dose or a higher rate compared to placebo control, included decreased blood pressure, edema and headaches which are known pharmacologic actions of calcium channel blockers. It must be noted, however, that SAH is frequently accompanied by alterations in consciousness which lead to an under reporting of adverse experiences. Patients who received nimodipine in clinical trials for other indications reported flushing (2.1%), headache (4.1%) and fluid retention (0.3%), typical responses to calcium channel blockers. As a calcium channel blocker, nimodipine may have the potential to exacerbate heart failure in susceptible patients or to interfere with A-V conduction, but these events were not observed. No clinically significant effects on hematologic factors, renal or hepatic function or carbohydrate metabolism have been causally associated with oral nimodipine. Isolated cases of non-fasting elevated serum glucose levels (0.8%), elevated LDH levels (0.4%), decreased platelet counts (0.3%), elevated alkaline phosphatase levels (0.2%) and elevated SGPT levels (0.2%) have been reported rarely.

DRUG ABUSE AND DEPENDENCE

There have been no reported instances of drug abuse or dependence with Nimotop®.

OVERDOSAGE

There have been no reports of overdosage from the oral administration of Nimotop®. Symptoms of overdosage would be expected to be related to cardiovascular effects such as excessive peripheral vasodilation with marked systemic hypotension. Clinically significant hypotension due to Nimotop® overdosage may require active cardiovascular support. Norepinephrine or dopamine may be helpful in restoring blood pressure. Since Nimotop® is highly protein-bound, dialysis is not likely to be of benefit.

DOSAGE AND ADMINISTRATION

Nimotop is given orally in the form of ivory colored, soft gelatin 30 mg capsules for subarachnoid hemorrhage.

The oral dose is 60 mg (two 30 mg capsules) every 4 hours for 21 consecutive days, preferably not less than one hour before or two hours after meals. Oral Nimotop® therapy should commence within 96 hours of the subarachnoid hemorrhage. If the capsule cannot be swallowed, e.g., at the time of surgery, or if the patient is unconscious, a hole should be made in both ends of the capsule with an 18 gauge needle, and the contents of the capsule extracted into a syringe. The contents should then be emptied into the patient's *in situ* naso-gastric tube and washed down the tube with 30 mL of normal saline (0.9%).

Patients with hepatic cirrhosis have substantially reduced clearance and approximately doubled C_{max}. Dosage should be reduced to 30 mg every 4 hours, with close monitoring of blood pressure and heart rate.

HOW SUPPLIED

Each ivory colored, soft gelatin NIMOTOP® capsule is imprinted with the word Nimotop and contains 30 mg of nimodipine. The 30 mg capsules are packaged in unit dose foil pouches and supplied in cartons containing 100 capsules. The product is also available in child resistant unit dose safety pak foil pouches containing 30 capsules per carton. The capsules should be stored in the manufacturer's original foil package at a controlled room temperature of 59°F to 86°F (15°C to 30°C).

Capsules should be protected from light and freezing.

	Strength	NDC Code	Capsule Identification
Unit Dose Package of 100:	30 mg	0026-2855-48	Nimotop
Unit Dose Package of 30:	30 mg	0026-2855-70	Nimotop

Manufactured by:
Bayer Corporation
Pharmaceutical Division
400 Morgan Lane
West Haven, CT 06516

Encapsulated by:
R.P. Scherer North America
Division of R.P. Scherer Corp.
Clearwater, FL 33518

Caution: Federal (USA) law prohibits dispensing without prescription.

PD500011   3/95   BAY e 9736   5202-7-A-U.S.-4
© 1995 Bayer Corporation   4922

Shown in Product Identification Guide, page 305

Shown in Product Identification Guide, page 305

Otic DOMEBORO®
Acetic Acid 2% in
Aqueous Aluminum
Acetate Otic Solution

DESCRIPTION

Otic Domeboro® Solution contains 2% acetic acid as the active ingredient, in modified Burow's solution (water, aluminum acetate, and sodium acetate) with boric acid as a stabilizer. Otic Domeboro® solution is instilled in the external auditory canal. Acetic acid is an astringent and antimicrobial agent. The pH range is from 4.5 to 6.0.

Chemically, acetic acid is $C_2H_4O_2$ and has the following structural formula:

$$H-C-C-OH$$

Molecular weight of acetic acid is 60.05.

CLINICAL PHARMACOLOGY

Acetic acid is antibacterial and antifungal; and is effective against microorganisms (bacteria and fungi) that infect the ears of patients with acute diffuse external otitis. In *in vitro* tests, minimum lethal-time was less than 0.25 minutes when bacteria and fungi isolated from patients with otitis externa were exposed to 2% acetic acid. Quantitative absorption of acetic acid 2% from external auditory canal is not known.

INDICATIONS AND USAGE

Otic Domeboro® solution is indicated for the treatment of superficial infections of the external auditory canal caused by organisms susceptible to the action of the antimicrobial.

CONTRAINDICATIONS

Hypersensitivity to acetic acid or any of the ingredients of this product. Perforated tympanic membrane is considered a contraindication to the use of any medication in the external ear canal.

WARNINGS

Avoid use or use with caution in patients with perforated tympanic membrane (see CONTRAINDICATIONS).
NOT FOR OPHTHALMIC USE.

PRECAUTIONS

General
Care should be taken to assure that the Otic Domeboro® solution gets into the ear canal and stays in contact with the affected area long enough for the drug to act.
Discontinue promptly if sensitization or irritation occurs.
Carcinogenesis, Mutagenesis, Impairment of Fertility: No long term studies in animals have been performed to evaluate the carcinogenic potential of Otic Domeboro® solution.

ADVERSE REACTIONS

Irritation may occur.

OVERDOSAGE

No toxic effect has been reported with overdosage of Otic Domeboro® solution.

DOSAGE AND ADMINISTRATION

Patient should lie on his side with affected ear uppermost. Instill 4 to 6 drops into the external auditory canal and maintain this position for five minutes. Repeat the procedure every 2 to 3 hours.
Store below (30°C), 86°F, avoid freezing.
Otic Domeboro® Solution is a clear colorless liquid.

HOW SUPPLIED

Otic Domeboro® solution (Acetic Acid 2% in Aqueous Aluminum Acetate Otic solution) is supplied in 2 fl. oz. dropper bottle.

	NDC
2 fl. oz.	0026-4312-02

Bayer Corporation
Pharmaceutical Division
400 Morgan Lane
West Haven, CT 06516 USA
CAUTION: Federal (USA) law prohibits dispensing without prescription.
PD500003   2/95   © 1995 Bayer Corporation   4787

PRECOSE®
(acarbose tablets)

DESCRIPTION

PRECOSE® (acarbose tablets) is an oral alpha-glucosidase inhibitor for use in the management of non-insulin-dependent diabetes mellitus (NIDDM). Acarbose is an oligosaccharide which is obtained from fermentation processes of a microorganism, *Actinoplanes utahensis*, and is chemically known as O-4,6-dideoxy-4-[[(1S,4R,5S,6S)-4,5,6,-trihydroxy-3-(hydroxymethyl)-2-cyclohexen-1-yl]amino]-α-D-glucopyranosyl-(1→4)-O-α-D-glucopyranosyl-(1→4)-D-glucose. It is a white to

DOSE q4h

Number of Patients (%)

Sign/Symptom	Nimodipine 0.35 mg/kg (n = 82)	30 mg (n = 71)	60 mg (n = 494)	90 mg (n = 172)	120 mg (n = 4)	Placebo (n = 479)
Decreased Blood Pressure	1 (1.2)	0	19 (3.8)	14 (8.1)	2 (50.0)	6 (1.2)
Abnormal Liver Function Test	1 (1.2)	0	2 (0.4)	1 (0.6)	0	7 (1.5)
Edema	0	0	2 (0.4)	2 (1.2)	0	3 (0.6)
Diarrhea	0	3 (4.2)	0	3 (1.7)	0	3 (0.6)
Rash	2 (2.4)	0	3 (0.6)	2 (1.2)	0	3 (0.6)
Headache	0	1 (1.4)	6 (1.2)	0	0	1 (0.2)
Gastrointestinal Symptoms	2 (2.4)	0	0	2 (1.2)	0	0
Nausea	1 (1.2)	1 (1.4)	6 (1.2)	1 (0.6)	0	0
Dyspnea	1 (1.2)	0	0	0	0	0
EKG Abnormalities	0	1 (1.4)	0	1 (0.6)	0	0
Tachycardia	0	1 (1.4)	0	0	0	0
Bradycardia	0	0	5 (1.0)	1 (0.6)	0	0
Muscle Pain/Cramp	0	1 (1.4)	1 (0.2)	1 (0.6)	0	0
Acne	0	1 (1.4)	0	0	0	0
Depression	0	1 (1.4)	0	0	0	0

off-white powder with a molecular weight of 645.6. Acarbose is soluble in water and has a pK_a of 5.1. Its empirical formula is $C_{25}H_{43}NO_{18}$ and its chemical structure is as follows:

PRECOSE® is available as 50 mg and 100 mg tablets for oral use. The inactive ingredients are starch, microcrystalline cellulose, magnesium stearate, and colloidal silicon dioxide.

CLINICAL PHARMACOLOGY

Acarbose is a complex oligosaccharide that delays the digestion of ingested carbohydrates, thereby resulting in a smaller rise in blood glucose concentration following meals. As a consequence of plasma glucose reduction, PRECOSE® reduces levels of glycosylated hemoglobin in patients with Type II (non-insulin dependent) diabetes mellitus. Systemic nonenzymatic protein glycosylation, as reflected by levels of glycosylated hemoglobin, is a function of average blood glucose concentration over time.

Mechanism of Action: In contrast to sulfonylureas, PRECOSE® does not enhance insulin secretion. The antihyperglycemic action of acarbose results from a competitive, reversible inhibition of pancreatic alpha-amylase and membrane-bound intestinal alpha-glucoside hydrolase enzymes. Pancreatic alpha-amylase hydrolyzes complex starches to oligosaccharides in the lumen of the small intestine, while the membrane-bound intestinal alpha-glucosidases hydrolyze oligosaccharides, trisaccharides, and disaccharides to glucose and other monosaccharides in the brush border of the small intestine. In diabetic patients, this enzyme inhibition results in a delayed glucose absorption and a lowering of postprandial hyperglycemia.

Because its mechanism of action is different, the effect of PRECOSE® to enhance glycemic control is additive to that of sulfonylureas when used in combination. In addition, PRECOSE® diminishes the insulinotropic and weight-increasing effects of sulfonylureas.

Acarbose has no inhibitory activity against lactase and consequently would not be expected to induce lactose intolerance.

Pharmacokinetics:

Absorption: In a study of 6 healthy men, less than 2% of an oral dose of acarbose was absorbed as active drug, while approximately 35% of total radioactivity from a ^{14}C-labeled oral dose was absorbed. An average of 51% of an oral dose was excreted in the feces as unabsorbed drug-related radioactivity within 96 hours of ingestion. Because acarbose acts locally within the gastrointestinal tract, this low systemic bioavailability of parent compound is therapeutically desired. Following oral dosing of healthy volunteers with ^{14}C-labeled acarbose, peak plasma concentrations of radioactivity were attained 14–24 hours after dosing, while peak plasma concentrations of active drug were attained at approximately 1 hour. The delayed absorption of acarbose-related radioactivity reflects the absorption of metabolites that may be formed by either intestinal bacteria or intestinal enzymatic hydrolysis.

Metabolism: Acarbose is metabolized exclusively within the gastrointestinal tract, principally by intestinal bacteria, but also by digestive enzymes. A fraction of these metabolites (approximately 34% of the dose) was absorbed and subsequently excreted in the urine. At least 13 metabolites have been separated chromatographically from urine specimens. The major metabolites have been identified as 4-methylpyrogallol derivatives (i.e., sulfate, methyl, and glucuronide conjugates). One metabolite (formed by cleavage of a glucose molecule from acarbose) also has alpha-glucosidase inhibitory activity. This metabolite, together with the parent compound, recovered from the urine, accounts for less than 2% of the total administered dose.

Excretion: The fraction of acarbose that is absorbed as intact drug is almost completely excreted by the kidneys. When acarbose was given *intravenously*, 89% of the dose was recovered in the urine as active drug within 48 hours. In contrast, less than 2% of an *oral dose* was recovered in the urine as active (i.e., parent compound and active metabolite) drug. This is consistent with the low bioavailability of the parent drug. The plasma elimination half-life of acarbose activity is approximately 2 hours in healthy volunteers. Consequently, drug accumulation does not occur with three times a day (t.i.d.) oral dosing.

Special Populations: The mean steady-state area under the curve (AUC) and maximum concentrations of acarbose were approximately 1.5 times higher in elderly compared to young volunteers; however, these differences were not statistically significant. Patients with severe renal impairment (Clcr < 25 mL/min/1.73m²) attained about 5 times higher peak plasma

concentrations of acarbose and 6 times larger AUCs than volunteers with normal renal function. No studies of acarbose pharmacokinetic parameters according to race have been performed. In U.S. controlled clinical studies of PRECOSE® in patients with NIDDM, reductions in glycosylated hemoglobin levels were similar in whites (n = 478) and blacks (n = 167), with a trend toward a better response in hispanics (n = 132).

Drug-Drug Interactions: Studies in healthy volunteers have shown that PRECOSE® has no effect on either the pharmacokinetics or pharmacodynamics of digoxin, nifedipine, propranolol, or ranitidine. PRECOSE® did not interfere with the absorption or disposition of the sulfonylurea glyburide in diabetic patients.

CLINICAL TRIALS

Clinical Experience in Non-Insulin-Dependent Diabetes Mellitus (NIDDM) Patients on Dietary Treatment Only: Results from six controlled, fixed-dose, monotherapy studies of PRECOSE® in the treatment of NIDDM, involving 769 PRECOSE®-treated patients, were combined and a weighted average of the difference from placebo in the mean change from baseline in glycosylated hemoglobin (HbA1c) was calculated for each dose level as presented below:

Table 1

Mean Change in HbA 1c in Fixed-Dose Monotherapy Studies

Dose of PRECOSE®*	N	Change in HbA 1c %	p-Value
25 mg t.i.d.	110	-0.44	0.0307
50 mg t.i.d.	131	-0.77	0.0001
100 mg t.i.d.	244	-0.74	0.0001
200 mg t.i.d.**	231	-0.86	0.0001
300 mg t.i.d.**	53	-1.00	0.0001

* PRECOSE® was statistically significantly different from placebo at all doses. Although there were no statistically significant differences among the mean results for doses ranging from 50 to 300 mg t.i.d., some patients may derive benefit by increasing the dosage from 50 to 100 mg t.i.d.

** Although studies utilized a maximum dose of 200 or 300 mg t.i.d., the maximum recommended dose for patients ≤ 60 kg is 50 mg t.i.d.; the maximum recommended dose for patients > 60 kg is 100 mg t.i.d.

Results from these six fixed-dose, monotherapy studies were also combined to derive a weighted average of the difference from placebo in mean change from baseline for one-hour postprandial plasma glucose levels as shown in the following figure:
[See Figure 1 in next column.]

Clinical Experience in NIDDM Patients Receiving Sulfonylureas: PRECOSE® was studied as adjunctive therapy to sulfonylurea treatment in two large, placebo-controlled, double-blind, randomized studies conducted in the United States in which 540 patients were included in the efficacy analysis. In addition, PRECOSE® was studied as adjunctive therapy to sulfonylurea treatment in a third study, conducted in Canada, in which patients were stratified according to background therapy. Study 1 (Table 2) involved patients under treatment at entry with diet alone who were

Table 2

Study	Treatment	HbA 1c(%) Mean Baseline*	HbA 1c(%) Mean Change from Baseline	HbA 1c(%) Treatment Difference**	p-Value
1	Placebo	9.48	+0.05	—	—
	PRECOSE® 200† mg t.i.d.	9.19	−0.71	−0.76	0.0005
	Tolbutamide 250–1000 mg t.i.d. (mean dose 2.4 g/d)	9.28	−1.22	−1.27	0.0001
	PRECOSE® 200† mg t.i.d. + Tolbutamide 250–1000 mg t.i.d. (mean dose 1.9 g/d)	8.99	−1.73	−1.78	0.0001
2	Sulfonylurea + Placebo	9.56	+0.24	—	—
	Sulfonylurea + PRECOSE® 50–300† mg t.i.d.	9.64	−0.30	−0.54	0.0096
3	Sulfonylurea + Placebo	8.00	+0.10	—	—
	Sulfonylurea + PRECOSE® 50–200† mg t.i.d.	8.10	−0.80	−0.90	0.0020

* Normal Range: 4–6%

** The result of subtracting the placebo group average.

† Although studies utilized a maximum dose of 200 or 300 mg t.i.d., the maximum recommended dose for patients ≤ 60 kg is 50 mg t.i.d.; the maximum recommended dose for patients > 60 kg is 100 mg t.i.d.

Figure 1
Dose of PRECOSE® (t.i.d.)*

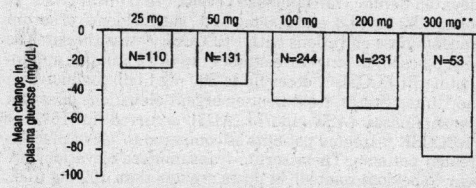

* PRECOSE® was statistically significantly different from placebo at all doses with respect to effect on one-hour postprandial plasma glucose.

** The 300 mg t.i.d. PRECOSE® regimen was superior to lower doses, but there were no statistically significant differences from 50 to 200 mg t.i.d.

subsequently randomized to four treatment groups. At the end of the study, patients in the PRECOSE® + tolbutamide group showed a mean treatment effect on glycosylated hemoglobin (HbA1c) of -1.78% and were receiving a significantly lower mean daily dose of tolbutamide than patients in the tolbutamide-alone group. Also, the efficacy in the PRECOSE® + tolbutamide group was significantly better than in the other three treatment groups. Study 2 (Table 2) involved patients taking background treatment with maximum daily doses of sulfonylureas. At the end of this study, the mean effect of the addition of PRECOSE® to maximum sulfonylurea therapy was a change in HbA1c of -0.54%. In addition, there was a significantly greater proportion of patients in the PRECOSE® + sulfonylurea group who reduced their sulfonylurea dose as compared to patients in the placebo + sulfonylurea group. In Study 3 (Table 2), the addition of PRECOSE® to a background treatment of sulfonylurea produced an additional change in mean HbA1c of -0.8%.

[See Table 2 above.]

INDICATIONS AND USAGE

PRECOSE®, as monotherapy, is indicated as an adjunct to diet to lower blood glucose in patients with non-insulin-dependent diabetes mellitus (NIDDM) whose hyperglycemia cannot be managed on diet alone. PRECOSE® may also be used in combination with a sulfonylurea when diet plus either PRECOSE® or a sulfonylurea do not result in adequate glycemic control. The effect of PRECOSE® to enhance glycemic control is additive to that of sulfonylureas when used in combination, presumably because its mechanism of action is different.

In initiating treatment for NIDDM, diet should be emphasized as the primary form of treatment. Caloric restriction and weight loss are essential in the obese diabetic patient. Proper dietary management alone may be effective in controlling blood glucose and symptoms of hyperglycemia. The importance of regular physical activity when appropriate should also be stressed. If this treatment program fails to result in adequate glycemic control, the use of PRECOSE® should be considered. The use of PRECOSE® must be viewed by both the physician and patient as a treatment in

Continued on next page

Bayer Corporation—Cont.

addition to diet, and not as a substitute for diet or as a convenient mechanism for avoiding dietary restraint.

CONTRAINDICATIONS

PRECOSE® is contraindicated in patients with known hypersensitivity to the drug and in patients with diabetic ketoacidosis or cirrhosis. PRECOSE® is also contraindicated in patients with inflammatory bowel disease, colonic ulceration, partial intestinal obstruction or in patients predisposed to intestinal obstruction. In addition, PRECOSE® is contraindicated in patients who have chronic intestinal diseases associated with marked disorders of digestion or absorption and in patients who have conditions that may deteriorate as a result of increased gas formation in the intestine.

PRECAUTIONS

General

Hypoglycemia: Because of its mechanism of action, PRECOSE® when administered alone should not cause hypoglycemia in the fasted or postprandial state. Sulfonylurea agents may cause hypoglycemia. Because PRECOSE® given in combination with a sulfonylurea will cause a further lowering of blood glucose, it may increase the hypoglycemic potential of the sulfonylurea. Oral glucose (dextrose), whose absorption is not inhibited by PRECOSE®, should be used instead of sucrose (cane sugar) in the treatment of mild to moderate hypoglycemia. Sucrose, whose hydrolysis to glucose and fructose is inhibited by PRECOSE®, is unsuitable for the rapid correction of hypoglycemia. Severe hypoglycemia. Severe hypoglycemia may require the use of either intravenous glucose infusion or glucagon injection.

Elevated Serum Transaminase Levels: In clinical trials, at doses of 50 mg t.i.d. and 100 mg t.i.d., the incidence of serum transaminase elevations with PRECOSE® was the same as with placebo. In long-term studies (up to 12 months, and including PRECOSE® doses up to 300 mg t.i.d.) conducted in the United States, treatment-emergent elevations of serum transaminases (AST and/or ALT) occurred in 15% of PRECOSE®-treated patients as compared to 7% of placebo-treated patients. These serum transaminase elevations appear to be dose related. At doses greater than 100 mg t.i.d., the incidence of serum transaminase elevations greater than three times the upper limit of normal was two to three times higher in the PRECOSE® group than in the placebo group. These elevations were asymptomatic, reversible, more common in females, and, in general, were not associated with other evidence of liver dysfunction.

In international post-marketing experience with PRECOSE® in over 500,000 patients, 19 cases of serum transaminase elevations >500 IU/L (12 of which were associated with jaundice) have been reported. Fifteen of these 19 cases received treatment with 100 mg t.i.d. or greater and 13 of 16 patients for whom weight was reported weighed <60 kg. In the 18 cases where follow-up was recorded, hepatic abnormalities improved or resolved upon discontinuation of PRECOSE®.

Loss of Control of Blood Glucose: When diabetic patients are exposed to stress such as fever, trauma, infection, or surgery, a temporary loss of control of blood glucose may occur. At such times, temporary insulin therapy may be necessary.

Information for Patients: Patients should be told to take PRECOSE® orally three times a day at the start (with the first bite) of each main meal. It is important that patients continue to adhere to dietary instructions, a regular exercise program, and regular testing of urine and/or blood glucose. PRECOSE® itself does not cause hypoglycemia even when administered to patients in the fasted state. Sulfonylurea drugs and insulin, however, can lower blood sugar levels enough to cause symptoms or sometimes life-threatening hypoglycemia. Because PRECOSE® given in combination with a sulfonylurea or insulin will cause a further lowering of blood sugar, it may increase the hypoglycemic potential of these agents. The risk of hypoglycemia, its symptoms and treatment, and conditions that predispose to its development should be well understood by patients and responsible family members. Because PRECOSE® prevents the breakdown of table sugar, patients should have a readily available source of glucose (dextrose, D-glucose) to treat symptoms of low blood sugar when taking PRECOSE® in combination with a sulfonylurea or insulin.

If side effects occur with PRECOSE®, they usually develop during the first few weeks of therapy. They are most commonly mild-to-moderate gastrointestinal effects, such as flatulence, diarrhea, or abdominal discomfort and generally diminish in frequency and intensity with time.

Laboratory Tests: Therapeutic response to PRECOSE® should be monitored by periodic blood glucose tests. Measurement of glycosylated hemoglobin levels is recommended for the monitoring of long-term glycemic control.

PRECOSE®, particularly at doses in excess of 50 mg t.i.d., may give rise to elevations of serum transaminases and, in rare instances, hyperbilirubinemia. It is recommended that serum transminase levels be checked every 3 months during the first year of treatment with PRECOSE® and periodically thereafter. If elevated transaminases are observed, a reduction in dosage or withdrawal of therapy may be indicated, particularly if the elevations persist.

Renal Impairment: Plasma concentrations of PRECOSE® in renally impaired volunteers were proportionally increased relative to the degree of renal dysfunction. Long-term clinical trials in diabetic patients with significant renal dysfunction (serum creatinine >2.0 mg/dL) have not been conducted. Therefore, treatment of these patients with PRECOSE® is not recommended.

Drug Interactions: Certain drugs tend to produce hyperglycemia and may lead to loss of blood glucose control. These drugs include the thiazides and other diuretics, corticosteroids, phenothiazines, thyroid products, estrogens, oral contraceptives, phenytoin, nicotinic acid, sympathomimetics, calcium channel-blocking drugs, and isoniazid. When such drugs are administered to a patient receiving PRECOSE®, the patient should be closely observed for loss of blood glucose control. When such drugs are withdrawn from patients receiving PRECOSE® in combination with sulfonylureas or insulin, patients should be observed closely for any evidence of hypoglycemia.

Intestinal adsorbents (e.g., charcoal) and digestive enzyme preparations containing carbohydrate-splitting enzymes (e.g., amylase, pancreatin) may reduce the effect of PRECOSE® and should not be taken concomitantly.

Carcinogenesis, Mutagenesis, and Impairment of Fertility: Nine chronic toxicity/carcinogenicity studies were conducted in three animal species (rat, hamster, dog) including two rat strains (Sprague-Dawley and Wistar).

In the first rat study, Sprague-Dawley rats received acarbose in feed at high doses (up to approximately 500 mg/kg body weight) for 104 weeks. Acarbose treatment resulted in a significant increase in the incidence of renal tumors (adenomas and adenocarcinomas) and benign Leydig cell tumors. This study was repeated with a similar outcome. Further studies were performed to separate direct carcinogenic effects of acarbose from indirect effects resulting from the carbohydrate malnutrition induced by the large doses of acarbose employed in the studies. In one study using Sprague-Dawley rats, acarbose was mixed with feed but carbohydrate deprivation was prevented by the addition of glucose to the diet. In a 26-month study of Sprague-Dawley rats, acarbose was administered by daily postprandial gavage so as to avoid the pharmacologic effects of the drug. In both of these studies, the increased incidence of renal tumors found in the original studies did not occur. Acarbose was also given in food and by postprandial gavage in two separate studies in Wistar rats. No increased incidence of renal tumors was found in either of these Wistar rat studies. In two feeding studies of hamsters, with and without glucose supplementation, there was also no evidence of carcinogenicity.

Acarbose showed no mutagenic activity when tested in six *in vitro* and three *in vivo* assays.

Fertility studies conducted in rats after oral administration produced no untoward effect on fertility or on the overall capability to reproduce.

Pregnancy:

Teratogenic Effects: Pregnancy Category B. The safety of PRECOSE® in pregnant women has not been established. Reproduction studies have been performed in rats at doses up to 480 mg/kg (corresponding to 9 times the exposure in humans, based on drug blood levels) and have revealed no evidence of impaired fertility or harm to the fetus due to acarbose. In rabbits, reduced maternal body weight gain, probably the result of the pharmacodynamic activity of high doses of acarbose in the intestines, may have been responsible for a slight increase in the number of embryonic losses. However, rabbits given 160 mg/kg acarbose (corresponding to 10 times the dose in man, based on body surface area) showed no evidence of embryotoxicity and there was no evidence of teratogenicity at a dose 32 times the dose in man (based on body surface area). There are, however, no adequate and well-controlled studies of PRECOSE® in pregnant women. Because animal reproduction studies are not always predictive of the human response, this drug should be used during pregnancy only if clearly needed. Because current information strongly suggests that abnormal blood glucose levels during pregnancy are associated with a higher incidence of congenital anomalies as well as increased neonatal morbidity and mortality, most experts recommend that insulin be used during pregnancy to maintain blood glucose levels as close to normal as possible.

Nursing Mothers: A small amount of radioactivity has been found in the milk of lactating rats after administration of radiolabeled acarbose. It is not known whether this drug is excreted in human milk. Because many drugs are excreted in human milk, PRECOSE® should not be administered to a nursing woman.

Pediatric Use: Safety and effectiveness of PRECOSE® in pediatric patients have not been established.

ADVERSE REACTIONS

Digestive Tract: Gastrointestinal symptoms are the most common reactions to PRECOSE®. In U.S. placebo-controlled trials, the incidences of abdominal pain, diarrhea, and flatulence were 21%, 33%, and 77% respectively in 1075 patients treated with PRECOSE® 50–300 mg t.i.d., whereas the corresponding incidences were 9%, 12%, and 32% in 818 placebo-treated patients. Abdominal pain and diarrhea tended to return to pretreatment levels over time, and the frequency and intensity of flatulence tended to abate with time. The increased gastrointestinal tract symptoms in patients treated with PRECOSE® is a manifestation of the mechanism of action of PRECOSE® and is related to the presence of undigested carbohydrate in the lower GI tract. Rarely, these gastrointestinal events may be severe and might be confused with paralytic ileus.

Elevated Serum Transaminase Levels: See PRECAUTIONS.

Other Abnormal Laboratory Findings: Small reductions in hematocrit occurred more often in PRECOSE®-treated patients than in placebo-treated patients but were not associated with reductions in hemoglobin. Low serum calcium and low plasma vitamin B_6 levels were associated with PRECOSE® therapy but were thought to be either spurious or of no clinical significance.

OVERDOSAGE

Unlike sulfonylureas or insulin, an overdose of PRECOSE® will not result in hypoglycemia. An overdose may result in transient increases in flatulence, diarrhea, and abdominal discomfort which shortly subside.

DOSAGE AND ADMINISTRATION

There is no fixed dosage regimen for the management of diabetes mellitus with PRECOSE® or any other pharmacologic agent. Dosage of PRECOSE® must be individualized on the basis of both effectiveness and tolerance while not exceeding the maximum recommended dose of 100 mg t.i.d. PRECOSE® should be taken three times daily at the start (with the first bite) of each main meal. PRECOSE® should be started at a low dose, with gradual dose escalation as described below, both to reduce gastrointestinal side effects and to permit identification of the minimum dose required for adequate glycemic control of the patient.

During treatment initiation and dose titration (see below), one-hour postprandial plasma glucose should be used to determine the therapeutic response to PRECOSE® and identify the minimum effective dose for the patient. Thereafter, glycosylated hemoglobin should be measured at intervals of approximately three months. The therapeutic goal should be to decrease both postprandial plasma glucose and glycosylated hemoglobin levels to normal or near normal by using the lowest effective dose of PRECOSE®, either as monotherapy or in combination with sulfonylureas.

Initial Dosage: The recommended starting dosage of PRECOSE® is 25 mg (half of a 50-mg tablet), given orally three times daily at the start (with the first bite) of each main meal.

Maintenance Dosage: Dosage of PRECOSE® should be adjusted at 4–8 week intervals based on one-hour postprandial glucose levels and on tolerance. After the initial dosage of 25 mg t.i.d., the dosage can be increased to 50 mg t.i.d. Some patients may benefit from further increasing the dosage to 100 mg t.i.d. The maintenance dose ranges from 50 mg t.i.d. to 100 mg t.i.d. However, since patients with low body weight may be at increased risk for elevated serum transaminases, only patients with body weight >60 kg should be considered for dose titration above 50 mg t.i.d. (see PRECAUTIONS). If no further reduction in postprandial glucose or glycosylated hemoglobin levels is observed with titration to 100 t.i.d., consideration should be given to lowering the dose. Once an effective and tolerated dosage is established, it should be maintained.

Maximum Dosage: The maximum recommended dose for patients ≤60 kg is 50 mg t.i.d.

The maximum recommended dose for patients >60 kg is 100 mg t.i.d.

Patients Receiving Sulfonylureas: Sulfonylurea agents may cause hypoglycemia. PRECOSE® given in combination with a sulfonylurea will cause a further lowering of blood glucose and may increase the hypoglycemic potential of the sulfonylurea. If hypoglycemia occurs, appropriate adjustments in the dosage of these agents should be made.

	Strength	NDC	Tablet Identification
Bottles of 100:	50 mg	0026-2861-51	PRECOSE 50
	100 mg	0026-2862-51	PRECOSE 100
Unit Dose	50 mg	0026-2861-48	PRECOSE 50
Packages of 100:	100 mg	0026-2862-48	PRECOSE 100

HOW SUPPLIED

PRECOSE® is available as 50 mg or 100 mg round tablets. Each tablet strength is white to yellow-tinged in color. The 50 mg tablet is scored on one side and coded with the word "PRECOSE" and "50" on the unscored side. The 100 mg tablet is unscored and is coded with the word "PRECOSE" and "100" on the same side. PRECOSE® is available in bottles of 100 and in unit dose packages of 100.

[See table on bottom of preceding page.]

Do not store above 25°C (77°F). Protect from moisture. For bottles, keep container tightly closed.

Bayer Corporation
Pharmaceutical Division
400 Morgan Lane
West Haven, CT 06516 USA
Caution: Federal law prohibits dispensing without a prescription.

PZ500036 4/96
Bay g 5421 PRECOSE® /5202/0/8/USA-1
© 1996 Bayer Corporation 6160
Shown in Product Identification Guide, page 305

TRASYLOL® ℞
(aprotinin injection)

DESCRIPTION

Trasylol® (aprotinin injection), $C_{284}H_{432}N_{84}O_{79}S_7$, is a natural proteinase inhibitor obtained from bovine lung. Aprotinin (molecular weight of 6512 daltons), consists of 58 amino acid residues that are arranged in a single polypeptide chain, cross-linked by three disulfide bridges. It is supplied as a clear, colorless, sterile isotonic solution for intravenous administration. Each milliliter contains 10,000 KIU (Kallikrein Inhibitor Units) (1.4 mg/mL) and 9 mg sodium chloride in water for injection. Hydrochloric acid and/or sodium hydroxide is used to adjust the pH to 4.5–6.5.

CLINICAL PHARMACOLOGY

Mechanism of Action: Aprotinin is a protease inhibitor with a variety of effects on the coagulation system. It inhibits plasmin and kallikrein, thus directly affecting fibrinolysis. It also inhibits the contact phase activation of coagulation which both initiates coagulation and promotes fibrinolysis. In addition to these effects on the clotting and lysis cascades in blood, aprotinin preserves the adhesive glycoproteins in the platelet membrane making them resistant to damage from the increased plasmin levels and mechanical injury that occur during cardiopulmonary bypass (CPB). The net effect is to inhibit both fibrinolysis and turnover of coagulation factors, and to decrease bleeding, although the precise mechanism of this effect is unclear.

Patients undergoing cardiac surgery with extracorporeal circulation by a heart-lung machine (cardiopulmonary bypass; CPB) develop adverse changes of their blood components, blood cells and specific coagulation proteins. These changes cause a transient hemostatic defect during the intraoperative and immediate postoperative period which may result in diffuse bleeding despite correct surgical technique. At times, this blood loss is severe enough to require multiple blood transfusions and even surgical re-exploration.

Pharmacokinetics: The studies comparing the pharmacokinetics of aprotinin in healthy volunteers, cardiac patients undergoing surgery with cardiopulmonary bypass, and women undergoing hysterectomy suggest linear pharmacokinetics over the dose range of 50,000 KIU to 2 million KIU. After intravenous (IV) injection, rapid distribution of aprotinin occurs into the total extracellular space, leading to a rapid initial decrease in plasma aprotinin concentration. Following this distribution phase, a plasma half-life of about 150 minutes is observed. At later time points, (ie, beyond 5 hours after dosing) there is a terminal elimination phase with a half-life of about 10 hours.

Average steady state intraoperative plasma concentrations were 137 KIU/mL (n = 10) after administration of the following dosage regimen: 1 million KIU IV loading dose, 1 million KIU into the pump prime volume, 250,000 KIU per hour of operation as continuous intravenous infusion (Regimen B). Average steady state intraoperative plasma concentrations were 250 KIU/mL in patients (n = 20) treated with aprotinin during cardiac surgery by administration of Regimen A (exactly double Regimen B): 2 million KIU IV loading dose, 2 million KIU into the pump prime volume, 500,000 KIU per hour of operation as continuous intravenous infusion.

Following a single IV dose of radiolabelled aprotinin, approximately 25–40% of the radioactivity is excreted in the urine over 48 hours. After a 30 minute infusion of 1 million KIU, about 2% is excreted as unchanged drug. After a larger dose of 2 million KIU infused over 30 minutes, urinary excretion of unchanged aprotinin accounts for approximately 9% of the dose. Animal studies have shown that aprotinin is accumulated primarily in the kidney. Aprotinin, after being filtered by the glomeruli, is actively reabsorbed by the proximal tubules in which it is stored in phagolysosomes. Aprotinin is slowly degraded by lysosomal enzymes. The physiological renal handling of aprotinin is similar to that of other small proteins, eg insulin.

CLINICAL TRIALS

Three placebo-controlled, double-blind studies of Trasylol® were conducted in the United States involving 523 patients undergoing repeat coronary artery bypass graft (CABG) surgery, of whom 463 were valid for efficacy analysis. The following treatments were used in the studies: Trasylol® Regimen A (2 million KIU IV loading dose, 2 million KIU into the pump prime volume, 500,000 KIU per hour of surgery as a continuous intravenous infusion); Trasylol® Regimen B (1 million KIU IV loading dose, 1 million KIU into the pump prime volume, 250,000 KIU per hour of surgery as a continuous intravenous infusion); a pump prime regimen (2 million KIU into the pump prime volume only); and a placebo regimen (normal saline).

In the three studies, fewer patients receiving Trasylol® (either Regimen A or Regimen B) required any donor blood in comparison to the placebo regimen.

[See table below.]

In these three studies there was no diminution of benefit with age. Male and female patients received benefits from Trasylol® in terms of a reduction in the average number of units of donor blood transfused. Male patients did better than female patients in terms of the percentage of patients who required any donor blood transfusions. However, the number of female patients studied was small.

A double-blind, randomized, Canadian study compared Trasylol® Regimen A (n = 28) and placebo (n = 23) in primary cardiac surgery patients (mainly CABG) requiring cardiopulmonary bypass who were treated with aspirin within 48 hours of surgery. The mean total blood loss (1209.7 mL vs. 2532.3 mL) and the mean number of units of packed red blood cells transfused (1.6 units vs. 4.3 units) were significantly less (p < 0.008) in the Trasylol® group compared to the placebo group.

In a U.S. randomized study of Trasylol® Regimen A and Regimen B versus the placebo regimen in 212 patients undergoing primary aortic and/or mitral valve replacement or repair, no benefit was found for Trasylol® in terms of the need for transfusion or the number of units of blood required.

INDICATIONS AND USAGE

Trasylol® is indicated for prophylactic use to reduce perioperative blood loss and the need for blood transfusion in patients undergoing cardiopulmonary bypass in the course of repeat coronary artery bypass graft surgery. Trasylol® is also indicated in selected cases of primary coronary artery bypass graft surgery where the risk of bleeding is especially high (impaired hemostasis, e.g., presence of aspirin or coagulopathy of other origin) or where transfusion is unavailable or unacceptable. This selected use of Trasylol® in primary CABG patients is based on the risk of renal dysfunction and on the risk of anaphylaxis (should a second procedure be needed).

REPEAT CABG PATIENTS WHO REQUIRED DONOR BLOOD

	PLACEBO REGIMEN	TRASYLOL® PUMP PRIME REGIMEN	TRASYLOL® REGIMEN B	TRASYLOL® REGIMEN A
Study 1	40/52 (77%)	Not Studied	23/49 (47%)*	22/53 (42%)*
Study 2	23/32 (72%)	Not Studied	Not Studied	7/23 (30%)*
Study 3	49/65 (75%)	49/68 (72%)	28/60 (47%)*	33/61 (54%)*

* p ≤ 0.007 compared to placebo

The number of units of donor blood required by patients was also reduced by Trasylol® Regimens A and B when compared to the placebo regimen:

UNITS OF DONOR BLOOD REQUIRED BY REPEAT CABG PATIENTS
Study 1

	PLACEBO REGIMEN	TRASYLOL® REGIMEN B	TRASYLOL® REGIMEN A
MEAN±SE	3.5±0.6	2.0±0.6**	1.8±0.6*
RANGE	0–34	0–18	0–24
MEDIAN	2	0	0

* p ≤ 0.001 compared to placebo, ANOVA on ranks
** p = 0.005 compared to placebo, ANOVA on ranks

Study 2

	PLACEBO REGIMEN	TRASYLOL® REGIMEN A
MEAN±SE	3.3±0.7	0.4±0.8*
RANGE	0–20	0–5
MEDIAN	4	0

* p = 0.0001 compared to placebo, ANOVA on ranks

Study 3

	PLACEBO REGIMEN	TRASYLOL® PUMP PRIME REGIMEN	TRASYLOL® REGIMEN B	TRASYLOL® REGIMEN A
MEAN±SE	3.4±0.5	2.5±0.3	2.3±0.8*	1.6±0.2*
RANGE	0–17	0–13	0–46	0–6
MEDIAN	3.0	2.0	0.0	1.0

* p ≤ 0.001 compared to placebo (ANOVA on ranks)

Study 2 also included 151 patients undergoing primary CABG surgery; 74 of the patients receiving Trasylol® and 67 of the patients receiving placebo were valid for efficacy analysis. Fewer patients receiving Trasylol® required any donor blood:

PRIMARY CABG PATIENTS WHO REQUIRED DONOR BLOOD
Study 2

	PLACEBO REGIMEN	TRASYLOL® REGIMEN A
	35/67 (52%)	28/74 (38%)*

* p = 0.052 compared to placebo

UNITS OF DONOR BLOOD REQUIRED BY PRIMARY CABG PATIENTS
Study 2

	PLACEBO REGIMEN	TRASYLOL® REGIMEN A
MEAN±SE	2.1±0.3	1.1±0.3*
RANGE	0–15	0–10
MEDIAN	1	0

* p = 0.0246 compared to placebo, ANOVA on ranks

Continued on next page

Bayer Corporation—Cont.

CONTRAINDICATIONS
Hypersensitivity to aprotinin.

WARNINGS
Anaphylactic reactions have been reported in less than 0.5% of patients receiving Trasylol® (including first time and re-exposures). Since Trasylol® is a foreign protein, the incidence of hypersensitivity reactions, including anaphylaxis, is considerably higher upon re-exposure. The symptoms of hypersensitivity-type reactions can range from skin eruptions, itching, dyspnea, nausea and tachycardia to fatal anaphylactic shock with circulatory failure. If hypersensitivity reactions occur during injection or infusion, administration should be stopped immediately. Emergency treatment should be initiated.

PRECAUTIONS
General: *Test Dose and Use of H₁ Antihistamine:* All patients treated with Trasylol® should first receive a test dose to assess the potential for allergic reactions. The test dose of 1 mL Trasylol® should be administered intravenously at least 10 minutes prior to the loading dose. Particular caution is necessary when administering Trasylol® (even test doses) to patients who have received aprotinin in the past because of the risk of anaphylaxis. In re-exposure cases, intravenous administration of an H₁-histamine antagonist (antihistamine) is recommended shortly before the loading dose of Trasylol®.

Loading Dose: The loading dose of Trasylol® should be given intravenously to patients in the supine position over a 20–30 minute period. Rapid intravenous administration of Trasylol® can cause a transient fall in blood pressure. (see DOSAGE AND ADMINISTRATION).

Allergic Reactions: Patients who experience any allergic reaction to the test dose of aprotinin should not receive further administration of the drug. Even after the uneventful administration of the 1 mL test dose, or without previous exposure to aprotinin, the full therapeutic dose may cause anaphylaxis. If this happens, the infusion should be stopped immediately and emergency treatment for anaphylaxis should be applied. Patients with a history of allergic reactions to drugs or other agents may be at greater risk of developing an allergic reaction.

Use of Trasylol® in patients undergoing deep hypothermic circulatory arrest: An increase in both renal failure and mortality compared to age matched historical controls has been reported in patients receiving Trasylol® while undergoing deep hypothermic circulatory arrest in connection with surgery of the aortic arch. The strength of this association is uncertain because there are no data from randomized studies to confirm or refute these findings.

Drug Interactions: Trasylol® is known to have antifibrinolytic activity and, therefore, may inhibit the effects of fibrinolytic agents.

In a study of nine patients with untreated hypertension, Trasylol® infused intravenously in a dose of 2 million KIU over two hours blocked the acute hypotensive effect of 100mg of captopril.

Trasylol®, in the presence of heparin, has been found to prolong the activated clotting time (ACT) as measured by a celite surface activation method. The kaolin activated clotting time appears to be much less affected. However, Trasylol® should not be viewed as a heparin sparing agent. (see Laboratory Monitoring of Anticoagulation During Cardiopulmonary Bypass).

Carcinogenesis, Mutagenesis, Impairment of Fertility: Long-term animal studies to evaluate the carcinogenic potential of Trasylol® or studies to determine the effect of Trasylol® on fertility have not been performed.

Results of microbial *in vitro* tests using *Salmonella typhimurium* and *Bacillus subtilis* indicate that Trasylol® is not a mutagen.

Pregnancy: Teratogenic Effects: Pregnancy Category B: Reproduction studies have been performed in rats at intravenous doses up to 200,000 KIU/kg/day for 11 days, and in rabbits at intravenous doses up to 100,000 KIU/kg/day for 13 days, 2.4 and 1.2 times the human dose on a mg/kg basis and 0.37 and 0.36 times the human mg/m² dose. They have revealed no evidence of impaired fertility or harm to the fetus due to Trasylol®. There are, however, no adequate and well-controlled studies in pregnant women. Because animal reproduction studies are not always predictive of human response, this drug should be used during pregnancy only if clearly needed.

Nursing Mother: Not applicable.

Pediatric Use: Safety and effectiveness in children have not been established.

Laboratory Monitoring of Anticoagulation during Cardiopulmonary Bypass: Trasylol® prolongs whole blood clotting time of heparinized blood as determined by a celite surface activation method. The kaolin activated clotting time appears to be much less affected. In the event of prolonged extracorporeal circulation, patients may require additional heparin, even in the presence of activated clotting time (ACT) levels that appear to represent adequate anticoagulation. Therefore, in patients on cardiopulmonary bypass (CPB) who are receiving Trasylol®, the standard system of monitoring heparinization during CPB, by keeping the celite ACT above 400–450 seconds, may lead to inadequate anticoagulation. In patients undergoing cardiopulmonary bypass with Trasylol® therapy, standard loading doses of heparin should be employed. However, additional heparin should be administered either in a fixed-dose regimen based on patient weight and duration of CPB, or on the basis of heparin levels measured by a method unaffected by Trasylol® (such as protamine titration).

ADVERSE REACTIONS
Studies analyzed to date indicate that Trasylol® is generally well tolerated. The adverse events reported are frequent sequelae of cardiac surgery and are not necessarily attributable to Trasylol® therapy. Adverse events reported, up to time of discharge from the hospital, from four double-blind, placebo-controlled studies conducted in the United States involving 886 patients undergoing cardiac surgery with cardiopulmonary bypass (Study 1—repeat CABG; Study 2—repeat and primary CABG; Study 3—repeat CABG; Study 4—primary cardiac valve replacement or repair) are listed in the following table. The table lists only those events which occurred in 2% or more of the patients treated with Trasylol® without regard to causal relationship.
[See table at left.]

In the pooled analysis of the four U.S. placebo-controlled studies, in patients undergoing cardiopulmonary bypass there was a trend toward an increased incidence of myocardial infarction in patients given Trasylol® (11% vs 8%, p=0.145). Because of the trend seen in the earlier U.S. studies (Studies 1 and 2), this issue was addressed prospectively in Study 3 (repeat CABG). In this study, the incidence rates of myocardial infarction as reported by investigators were 16%, 13%, and 7% in Trasylol® Regimen A, Regimen B, and pump prime regimens, respectively, versus 10% in the placebo regimen group. When the data were analyzed by a blinded consultant, the incidence rates for definite myocardial infarction were 12%, 15%, and 9% in the Trasylol® Regimen A, Regimen B, and pump prime regimens, respectively, versus 12% in the placebo group. The differences in the incidence rates in both analyses were not statistically significant.

In the study of patients undergoing primary or repeat CABG (Study 2), in which graft patency was evaluated by ultrafast computerized tomography (CT), a trend was seen toward an increased incidence of saphenous vein graft closure in patients who received Trasylol® Regimen A versus the placebo regimen.

Less frequent adverse events of concern, without regard to drug relationship, in cardiac surgery patients treated with Trasylol® in U.S. clinical trials were: shock (1.7%), lung edema (1.2%), phlebitis (1.0%), kidney tubular necrosis (0.9%), cerebral embolism (0.5%), liver damage (0.5%), acute kidney failure (0.5%), cerebrovascular accident (0.5%), hemolysis (0.3%), allergic reaction (0.3%).

In comparison to the placebo group, no increase in mortality in patients treated with Trasylol® was observed.

Hypersensitivity and Anaphylaxis: See WARNINGS

Laboratory Findings

Serum Creatinine: Pooled data from the four U.S. placebo-controlled studies showed a statistically significant increase in the incidence of post-operative renal dysfunction in patients treated with Trasylol®. The incidence of serum creatinine elevations ≥ 0.5 mg/dL above baseline was 21 percent in Regimen A, 18 percent in Regimen B compared to 14 percent in the placebo group (p=0.015 and p=0.495, respectively). In patients undergoing coronary artery bypass graft procedures only (Studies 1, 2, 3) the rates were 19 percent and 20 percent in the Trasylol® Regimen A and Regimen B groups and 15 percent in the placebo group (p≥0.345, versus placebo). Postoperative renal dysfunction was observed somewhat more frequently in association with primary cardiac valve procedures (30% for Trasylol® Regimen A, and 14% for Regimen B versus 8% for placebo). In the majority of instances the renal dysfunction was not severe and was reversible. A total of 4 percent of patients treated with Trasylol® Regimens A and B and 2 percent of the placebo group had a serum creatinine increase of ≥ 2 mg/dL above the preoperative value.

		Percentage of Patients Treated with Trasylol®– (N=579)	Percentage of Patients Treated with Placebo– (N=307)
	Any Event	76	73
BODY AS A WHOLE	Fever	12	8
	Infection	6	5
	Sepsis	3	2
CARDIOVASCULAR	Atrial fibrillation	24	22
	Myocardial infarction	11	8
	Heart failure	10	8
	Atrial flutter	8	5
	Hypotension	6	6
	Ventricular tachycardia	6	4
	Pericarditis	5	4
	Ventricular extrasystoles	5	4
	Arrhythmia	4	5
	Supraventricular tachycardia	4	3
	Heart arrest	3	2
	Congestive heart failure	3	1
	Peripheral edema	3	1
	Ventricular fibrillation	2	5
	Hypertension	2	4
	Atrial arrhythmia	2	3
	Tachycardia	2	5
	Surgery*	2	1
DIGESTIVE	Liver function tests abnormal	5	2
	Nausea	3	3
	Diarrhea	2	1
	Vomiting	2	1
HEMIC AND LYMPHATIC	Leukocytosis	3	2
	Thrombocytopenia	2	2
METABOLIC AND NUTRITIONAL	Creatine phosphokinase increased	5	3
	Hyperglycemia	3	2
NERVOUS	Confusion	4	3
RESPIRATORY	Lung disorder	7	7
	Pleural effusion	5	6
	Pneumonia	4	4
	Apnea	3	1
	Dyspnea	3	3
	Respiratory disorder	3	3
	Pneumothorax	3	4
	Asthma	3	2
UROGENITAL	Kidney function abnormal	5	3
	Urinary tract infection	3	4
	Kidney failure	2	1

* These surgical procedures included: rethoracotomy, pacemaker implantation, mitral valve repair, vena cava filter placement, femoral thrombectomy, and chest drainage in the Trasylol® group and pacemaker placement or revision in the placebo group.

	TEST DOSE	LOADING DOSE	"PUMP PRIME" DOSE	CONSTANT INFUSION DOSE
TRASYLOL® REGIMEN A	1 mL (1.4 mg, or 10,000 KIU)	200 mL (280 mg, or 2.0 million KIU)	200 mL (280 mg, or 2.0 million KIU)	50 mL/hr (70 mg/hr, or 500,000 KIU/hr)
TRASYLOL® REGIMEN B	1 mL (1.4 mg, or 10,000 KIU)	100 mL (140 mg, or 1.0 million KIU)	100 mL (140 mg, or 1.0 million KIU)	25 mL/hr (35 mg/hr, or 250,000 KIU/hr)

Patients with baseline elevations in serum creatinine were not at increased risk of developing postoperative renal dysfunction following Trasylol® treatment although there were mean increases in creatinine of 0.11 mg/dL after the high dose regimen (A), and of 0.09 mg/dL after the low dose regimen (B), each of which was statistically significant compared to placebo.

Serum Glucose: In the hours after cardiopulmonary bypass surgery, the serum glucose levels increased; however, the average increase in serum glucose in patients treated with the high dose regimen (61 mg/dL) was less than in the placebo treated group (78 mg/dL).

Serum Transaminases: In U.S. controlled studies, a significantly greater incidence of treatment emergent abnormal liver function tests was reported in all Trasylol® treated (Regimen A, Regimen B, and the pump prime regimen) patients (5%) compared to patients treated with the placebo regimen (2%). The percent of primary CABG patients developing an elevation of ALT (alanine amino transferase; formerly SGPT, serum glutamic pyruvic transaminase) greater than 1.8 times the upper limit of normal was not higher in the Trasylol® treated group compared to the placebo group. Among the repeat CABG patients, the percent of subjects developing an elevation of ALT of this magnitude was significantly higher in the Trasylol® treated group. This suggests an indirect effect possibly related to the risk of repeated surgery and attendant myocardial dysfunction rather than a primary drug effect. There were no differences between the Trasylol® treated and placebo groups in the incidence of elevated ALT values greater than 3.0 times the upper limit of normal.

Serum Creatine Kinase (CK): There was a trend toward an increased incidence of elevated serum creatine kinase (CK) with increased MB fractions in Trasylol® treated patients.

Partial Thromboplastin Time (PTT) and Activated Clotting Time (ACT): Significant elevations in the partial thromboplastin time (PTT) and activated clotting time (ACT) in Trasylol® treated patients are expected in the hours after surgery due to circulating concentrations of Trasylol® which are known to inhibit activation of the intrinsic clotting system by contact with a foreign surface, a method used in these tests. (See Laboratory Monitoring of Anticoagulation During Cardiopulmonary Bypass).

OVERDOSAGE

The maximum amount of Trasylol® that can be safely administered in single or multiple doses has not been determined. Doses up to 17.5 million KIU have been administered within a 24 hour period without any apparent toxicity. There is one poorly documented case, however, of a patient who received a large, but not well determined, amount of Trasylol® (in excess of 15 million KIU) in 24 hours. The patient, who had pre-existing liver dysfunction, developed hepatic and renal failure postoperatively and died. Autopsy showed hepatic necrosis and extensive renal tubular and glomerular necrosis. The relationship of these findings to Trasylol® therapy is unclear.

DOSAGE AND ADMINISTRATION

Trasylol® given prophylactically in both Regimen A and Regimen B (half Regimen A) to patients undergoing repeat CABG surgery significantly reduced the donor blood transfusion requirement relative to placebo treatment. In patients given aspirin preoperatively, while there was no difference in the number of patients requiring transfusion whether assigned to Regimen A or B, fewer units of blood and/or blood products were required by patients administered Regimen A. In high risk primary CABG surgery patients, only Regimen A was studied.

Trasylol® is supplied as a solution containing 10,000 KIU/mL, which is equal to 1.4 mg/mL. All intravenous doses of Trasylol® should be administered through a central line. **DO NOT ADMINISTER ANY OTHER DRUG USING THE SAME LINE.** Both regimens include a 1 mL test dose, a loading dose, a dose to be added to the priming fluid of the cardiopulmonary bypass circuit ("pump prime" dose), and a constant infusion dose. Regimens A and B (both incorporating a 1 mL test dose) are described in the table below:

[See table above.]

The 1 mL test dose should be administered intravenously at least 10 minutes before the loading dose. With the patient in a supine position, the loading dose is given slowly over 20–30 minutes, after induction of anesthesia but prior to sternotomy. When the loading dose is complete, it is followed by the constant infusion dose, which is continued until surgery is complete and the patient leaves the operating room. The "pump prime" dose is added to the priming fluid of the cardiopulmonary bypass circuit, by replacement of an aliquot of the priming fluid, prior to the institution of cardiopulmonary bypass. Total doses of more than 7 million KIU have not been studied in controlled trials.

Parenteral drug products should be inspected visually for particulate matter and discoloration prior to administration whenever solution and container permit. Discard any unused portion.

Renal and Hepatic Impairment: No formal studies of the pharmacokinetics of aprotinin in patients with pre-existing renal insufficiency have been conducted. However, in the placebo-controlled clinical trials conducted in the United States, patients with mildly elevated pretreatment serum creatinine levels did not have a notably higher incidence of clinically significant post-treatment elevations in serum creatinine following either Trasylol® Regimen A or Regimen B compared to administration of the placebo regimen. Changes in aprotinin pharmacokinetics with age or impaired renal function are not great enough to require any dose adjustment. No pharmacokinetic data from patients with pre-existing hepatic disease treated with Trasylol® are available.

COMPATIBILITY

Trasylol® is incompatible *in vitro* with corticosteroids, heparin, tetracyclines, and nutrient solutions containing amino acids or fat emulsion. If Trasylol® is to be given concomitantly with another drug, each drug should be administered separately through different venous lines or catheters.

HOW SUPPLIED

Size	Strength	NDC
100 mL vials	1,000,000 KIU	0026-8196-36
200 mL vials	2,000,000 KIU	0026-8197-63

STORAGE

Trasylol® should be stored between 2° and 25°C (36°–77°F). Protect from freezing.

Bayer Corporation
Pharmaceutical Division
400 Morgan Lane
West Haven, CT 06516
Made in Germany

Caution: Federal (USA) Law prohibits dispensing without a prescription.

PD500004 2/95

 4754

TRIDESILON® 0.05% ℞
(desonide cream)

DESCRIPTION

Tridesilon® Cream contains microdispersed desonide (the active ingredient) in a compatible vehicle buffered to the pH range of normal skin. Each gram of Tridesilon® Cream contains 0.5 milligrams of desonide. Tridesilon® Cream is applied topically.

Tridesilon® (desonide) is a non-fluorinated corticosteroid. Chemically, desonide is Pregna-1,4-diene-3,20-dione,11,21-dihydroxy-16,17- [(1-methylethylidene)bis(oxy)] -,(11β,16α)- with the following structural formula:

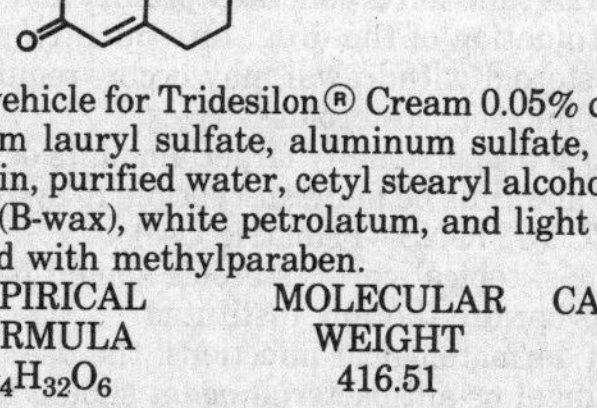

The vehicle for Tridesilon® Cream 0.05% contains glycerin, sodium lauryl sulfate, aluminum sulfate, calcium acetate, dextrin, purified water, cetyl stearyl alcohol, synthetic beeswax, (B-wax), white petrolatum, and light mineral oil. Preserved with methylparaben.

EMPIRICAL FORMULA	MOLECULAR WEIGHT	CAS REGISTRY NUMBER
$C_{24}H_{32}O_6$	416.51	638-94-8

CLINICAL PHARMACOLOGY

Topical corticosteroids share anti-inflammatory, anti-pruritic and vasoconstrictive actions.

The mechanism of anti-inflammatory activity of the topical corticosteroids is unclear. Various laboratory methods, including vasoconstrictor assays, are used to compare and predict potencies and/or clinical efficacies of the topical corticosteroids. There is some evidence to suggest that a recognizable correlation exists between vasoconstrictor potency and therapeutic efficacy in man.

Pharmacokinetics

The extent of percutaneous absorption of topical corticosteroids is determined by many factors including the vehicle, the integrity of the epidermal barrier, and the use of occlusive dressings.

Topical corticosteroids can be absorbed from normal intact skin. Inflammation and/or other disease processes in the skin increase percutaneous absorption. Occlusive dressings substantially increase the percutaneous absorption of topical corticosteroids. Thus, occlusive dressings may be a valuable therapeutic adjunct for treatment of resistant dermatoses. (See DOSAGE AND ADMINISTRATION).

Once absorbed through the skin, topical corticosteroids are handled through pharmacokinetic pathways similar to systemically administered corticosteroids. Corticosteroids are bound to plasma proteins in varying degrees. Corticosteroids are metabolized primarily in the liver and are then excreted by the kidneys. Some of the topical corticosteroids and their metabolites are also excreted into the bile.

INDICATIONS AND USAGE

Topical corticosteroids are indicated for the relief of the inflammatory and pruritic manifestations of corticosteroid-responsive dermatoses.

CONTRAINDICATIONS

Topical corticosteroids are contraindicated in those patients with a history of hypersensitivity to any of the components of the preparation.

PRECAUTIONS

General

Systemic absorption of topical corticosteroids has produced reversible hypothalamic-pituitary-adrenal (HPA) axis suppression, manifestations of Cushing's syndrome, hyperglycemia, and glucosuria in some patients.

Conditions which augment systemic absorption include the application of the more potent steroids, use over large surface areas, prolonged use, and the addition of occlusive dressings.

Therefore, patients receiving a large dose of a potent topical steroid applied to a large surface area or under an occlusive dressing should be evaluated periodically for evidence of HPA axis suppression by using the urinary free cortisol and ACTH stimulation tests. If HPA axis suppression is noted, an attempt should be made to withdraw the drug, to reduce the frequency of application, or to substitute a less potent steroid.

Recovery of HPA axis function is generally prompt and complete upon discontinuation of the drug. Infrequently, signs and symptoms of steroid withdrawal may occur, requiring supplemental systemic corticosteroids.

Children may absorb proportionally larger amounts of topical corticosteroids and thus be more susceptible to systemic toxicity. (See PRECAUTIONS—Pediatric Use).

If irritation develops, topical corticosteroids should be discontinued and appropriate therapy instituted.

In the presence of dermatological infections, the use of an appropriate antifungal or antibacterial agent should be instituted. If a favorable response does not occur promptly, the corticosteroid should be discontinued until the infection has been adequately controlled.

Information for the Patient

Patients using topical corticosteroids should receive the following information and instructions:

1. This medication is to be used as directed by the physician. It is for external use only. Avoid contact with eyes.
2. Patients should be advised not to use this medication for any disorder other than for which it was prescribed.
3. The treated skin area should not be bandaged or otherwise covered or wrapped as to be occlusive unless directed by the physician.
4. Patients should report any signs of local adverse reactions especially under occlusive dressing.
5. Parents of pediatric patients should be advised not to use tight-fitting diapers or plastic pants on a child being treated in the diaper area, as these garments may constitute occlusive dressings.

Laboratory Tests

The following tests may be helpful in evaluating the HPA axis suppression:

Urinary free cortisol test
ACTH stimulation test

Carcinogenesis, Mutagenesis, and Impairment of Fertility

Long-term animal studies have not been performed to evaluate the carcinogenic potential or the effect on fertility of topical corticosteroids.

Continued on next page

Bayer Corporation—Cont.

Studies to determine mutagenicity with prednisolone and hydrocortisone have revealed negative results.

Pregnancy Category C
Corticosteroids are generally teratogenic in laboratory animals when administered systemically at relatively low dosage levels. The more potent corticosteroids have been shown to be teratogenic after dermal application in laboratory animals. There are no adequate and well-controlled studies in pregnant women on teratogenic effects from topically applied corticosteroids. Therefore, topical corticosteroids should be used during pregnancy only if the potential benefit justifies the potential risk to the fetus. Drugs of this class should not be used extensively on pregnant patients, in large amounts, or for prolonged periods of time.

Nursing Mothers
It is not known whether topical administration of corticosteroids could result in sufficient systemic absorption to produce detectable quantities in breast milk. Systemically administered corticosteroids are secreted into breast milk in quantities *not* likely to have a deleterious effect on the infant. Nevertheless, caution should be exercised when topical corticosteroids are administered to a nursing woman.

Pediatric Use
Pediatric patients may demonstrate greater susceptibility to topical corticosteroid-induced HPA axis suppression and Cushing's syndrome than mature patients because of a larger skin surface area to body weight ratio.
Hypothalamic-pituitary-adrenal (HPA) axis suppression, Cushing's syndrome, and intracranial hypertension have been reported in children receiving topical corticosteroids. Manifestations of adrenal supression in children include linear growth retardation, delayed weight gain, low plasma cortisol levels, and absence of response to ACTH stimulation. Manifestations of intracranial hypertension include bulging fontanelles, headaches, and bilateral papilledema.
Administration of topical corticosteroids to children should be limited to the least amount compatible with an effective therapeutic regimen. Chronic corticosteroid therapy may interfere with the growth and development of children.

ADVERSE REACTIONS
The following local adverse reactions are reported infrequently with topical corticosteroids, but may occur more frequently with the use of occlusive dressings. These reactions are listed in an approximate decreasing order of occurrence:
Burning
Itching
Irritation
Dryness
Folliculitis
Hypertrichosis
Acneiform eruptions
Hypopigmentation
Perioral dermatitis
Allergic contact dermatitis
Maceration of the skin
Secondary infection
Skin atrophy
Striae
Miliaria

OVERDOSAGE
Topically applied corticosteroids can be absorbed in sufficient amounts to produce systemic effects. (See PRECAUTIONS).

DOSAGE AND ADMINISTRATION
Topical corticosteroids are generally applied to the affected area as a thin film from two to four times daily depending on the severity of the condition.
Occlusive dressings may be used for management of psoriasis or recalcitrant conditions.
If an infection develops, the use of occlusive dressings should be discontinued and appropriate antimicrobial therapy instituted.

HOW SUPPLIED
Tridesilon® (desonide) Cream 0.05% is supplied in 15 and 60 gram tubes and in 5 pound jars. It is a white semi-solid.
Store below 86°F (30°C), avoid freezing.

	NDC Number
15g	0026-5561-61
60g	0026-5561-62
5lb	0026-5561-92

Bayer Corporation
Pharmaceutical Division
400 Morgan Lane
West Haven, CT 06516 USA

CAUTION
Federal (USA) law prohibits dispensing without a prescription.
PD500007   3/95
© 1995 Bayer Corporation   5064

TRIDESILON® 0.05%   ℞
(desonide ointment)

DESCRIPTION
Tridesilon® Ointment contains microdispersed desonide (the active ingredient) in white petrolatum. Each gram of Tridesilon® Ointment contains 0.5 milligrams of desonide. Tridesilon® Ointment is applied topically.
Tridesilon® (desonide) is a non-fluorinated corticosteroid. Chemically, desonide is Pregna-1,4-diene-3,20-dione,11,21-dihydroxy-16,17- [(1-methylethylidene)bis(oxy)] -,11β, 16α)- with the following structural formula:

EMPIRICAL FORMULA	MOLECULAR WEIGHT	CAS REGISTRY NUMBER
$C_{24}H_{32}O_6$	416.51	638-94-8

CLINICAL PHARMACOLOGY
Topical corticosteroids share anti-inflammatory, anti-pruritic and vasoconstrictive actions.
The mechanism of anti-inflammatory activity of the topical corticosteroids is unclear. Various laboratory methods, including vasoconstrictor assays, are used to compare and predict potencies and/or clinical efficacies of the topical corticosteroids. There is some evidence to suggest that a recognizable correlation exists between vasoconstrictor potency and therapeutic efficacy in man.

Pharmacokinetics
The extent of percutaneous absorption of topical corticosteroids is determined by many factors including the vehicle, the integrity of the epidermal barrier, and the use of occlusive dressings.
Topical corticosteroids can be absorbed from normal intact skin. Inflammation and/or other disease processes in the skin increase percutaneous absorption. Occlusive dressings substantially increase the percutaneous absorption of topical corticosteroids. Thus, occlusive dressings may be a valuable therapeutic adjunct for treatment of resistant dermatoses. (See DOSAGE AND ADMINISTRATION).
Once absorbed through the skin, topical corticosteroids are handled through pharmacokinetic pathways similar to systemically administered corticosteroids. Corticosteroids are bound to plasma proteins in varying degrees. Corticosteroids are metabolized primarily in the liver and are then excreted by the kidneys. Some of the topical corticosteroids and their metabolites are also excreted into the bile.

INDICATIONS AND USAGE
Topical corticosteroids are indicated for the relief of the inflammatory and pruritic manifestations of corticosteroid-responsive dermatoses.

CONTRAINDICATIONS
Topical corticosteroids are contraindicated in those patients with a history of hypersensitivity to any of the components of the preparation.

PRECAUTIONS
General
Systemic absorption of topical corticosteroids has produced reversible hypothalamic-pituitary-adrenal (HPA) axis suppression, manifestations of Cushing's syndrome, hyperglycemia, and glucosuria in some patients.
Conditions which augment systemic absorption include the application of the more potent steroids, use over large surface areas, prolonged use, and the addition of occlusive dressings.
Therefore, patients receiving a large dose of a potent topical steroid applied to a large surface area or under an occlusive dressing should be evaluated periodically for evidence of HPA axis suppression by using the urinary free cortisol and ACTH stimulation tests. If HPA axis suppression is noted, an attempt should be made to withdraw the drug, to reduce the frequency of application, or to substitute a less potent steroid.
Recovery of HPA axis function is generally prompt and complete upon discontinuation of the drug. Infrequently, signs and symptoms of steroid withdrawal may occur, requiring supplemental systemic corticosteroids.
Children may absorb proportionally larger amounts of topical corticosteroids and thus be more susceptible to systemic toxicity. (See PRECAUTIONS—Pediatric Use).
If irritation develops, topical corticosteroids should be discontinued and appropriate therapy instituted.
In the presence of dermatological infections, the use of an appropriate antifungal or antibacterial agent should be instituted. If a favorable response does not occur promptly, the corticosteroid should be discontinued until the infection has been adequately controlled.

Information for the Patient
Patients using topical corticosteroids should receive the following information and instructions:
1. This medication is to be used as directed by the physician. It is for external use only. Avoid contact with the eyes.
2. Patients should be advised not to use this medication for any disorder other than for which it was prescribed.
3. The treated skin area should not be bandaged or otherwise covered or wrapped as to be occlusive unless directed by the physician.
4. Patients should report any signs of local adverse reactions especially under occlusive dressing.
5. Parents of pediatric patients should be advised not to use tight-fitting diapers or plastic pants on a child being treated in the diaper area, as these garments may constitute occlusive dressings.

Laboratory Tests
The following tests may be helpful in evaluating the HPA axis suppression:
Urinary free cortisol test
ACTH stimulation test

Carcinogenesis, Mutagenesis, and Impairment of Fertility
Long-term animal studies have not been performed to evaluate the carcinogenic potential or the effect on fertility of topical corticosteroids.
Studies to determine mutagenicity with prednisolone and hydrocortisone have revealed negative results.

Pregnancy Category C
Corticosteroids are generally teratogenic in laboratory animals when administered systemically at relatively low dosage levels. The more potent corticosteroids have been shown to be teratogenic after dermal application in laboratory animals. There are no adequate and well-controlled studies in pregnant women on teratogenic effects from topically applied corticosteroids. Therefore, topical corticosteroids should be used during pregnancy only if the potential benefit justifies the potential risk to the fetus. Drugs of this class should not be used extensively on pregnant patients, in large amounts, or for prolonged periods of time.

Nursing Mothers
It is not known whether topical administration of corticosteroids could result in sufficient systemic absorption to produce detectable quantities in breast milk. Systemically administered corticosteroids are secreted into breast milk in quantities *not* likely to have a deleterious effect on the infant. Nevertheless, caution should be exercised when topical corticosteroids are administered to a nursing woman.

Pediatric Use
Pediatric patients may demonstrate greater susceptibility to topical corticosteroid-induced HPA axis suppression and Cushing's syndrome than mature patients because of a larger skin surface area to body weight ratio.
Hypothalamic-pituitary-adrenal (HPA) axis suppression, Cushing's syndrome, and intracranial hypertension have been reported in children receiving topical corticosteroids. Manifestations of adrenal suppression in children include linear growth retardation, delayed weight gain, low plasma cortisol levels, and absence of response to ACTH stimulation. Manifestations of intracranial hypertension include bulging fontanelles, headaches, and bilateral papilledema.
Administration of topical corticosteroids to children should be limited to the least amount compatible with an effective therapeutic regimen. Chronic corticosteroid therapy may interfere with the growth and development of children.

ADVERSE REACTIONS
The following local adverse reactions are reported infrequently with topical corticosteroids, but may occur more frequently with the use of occlusive dressings. These reactions are listed in an approximate decreasing order of occurrence:
Burning
Itching
Irritation
Dryness
Folliculitis
Hypertrichosis
Acneiform eruptions
Hypopigmentation
Perioral dermatitis
Allergic contact dermatitis
Maceration of the skin
Secondary infection
Skin atrophy
Striae
Miliaria

OVERDOSAGE
Topically applied corticosteroids can be absorbed in sufficient amounts to produce systemic effects. (See PRECAUTIONS).

DOSAGE AND ADMINISTRATION
Topical corticosteroids are generally applied to the affected area as a thin film from two to four times daily depending on the severity of the condition.

Occlusive dressings may be used for the management of psoriasis or recalcitrant conditions.
If an infection develops, the use of occlusive dressings should be discontinued and appropriate antimicrobial therapy instituted.

HOW SUPPLIED

Tridesilon® (desonide) Ointment 0.05% is supplied in 15 and 60 gram tubes. It is white or faintly yellowish, transparent semisolid.

Store below 86°F (30°C). Avoid freezing.

	NDC Number
15g	0026-5591-61
60g	0026-5591-62

Bayer Corporation
Pharmaceutical Division
400 Morgan Lane
West Haven, CT 06516 USA

CAUTION: Federal (USA) law prohibits dispensing without a prescription.

PD500008 3/95
 5066

Bayer Corporation
Pharmaceutical Division
Allergy Products

400 MORGAN LANE
WEST HAVEN, CT 06516

For Medical Information Contact:
Director, Medical Services
(800) 468-0894
(203) 937-2000

ANA-KIT® ℞
ANAPHYLAXIS EMERGENCY TREATMENT KIT

DESCRIPTION

Epinephrine Injection, USP, (1:1000), contained in a sterile, 1 mL syringe, designed to deliver 2 doses of 0.3 mL each. Product is intended for subcutaneous or intramuscular use.
Each mL of Epinephrine Injection, USP, (1:1000) contains 1 mg *l*-epinephrine as the hydrochloride, 8.5 mg sodium chloride, not more than 5 mg chlorobutanol (chloral derivative) and 1.5 mg sodium bisulfite. Sealed under nitrogen.
Epinephrine is a sympathomimetic catecholamine. Its naturally occurring levo isomer, which is twenty times as active as the *d* isomer, is now obtained in pure form by separation from the synthetically produced racemate.
Chemically, epinephrine is 1-(3,4-dihydroxyphenyl)-2-(methylamino)ethanol with the following structure:

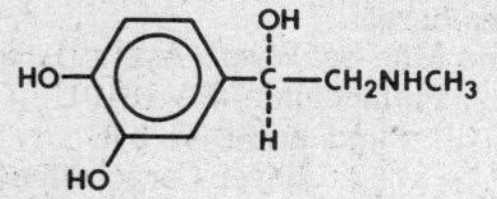

Chlo-Amine® Chlorpheniramine Maleate Tablets: 4 chewable tablets, each containing 2 mg chlorpheniramine maleate, USP, for oral administration. Contains FD&C Yellow No. 6 (Sunset Yellow) as a color additive. Chlorpheniramine maleate is an antihistamine having the chemical name γ-(4-chlorophenyl)-N,N-dimethyl-2-pyridinepropanamine, (Z)-2-butenedioate(1:1) with the following structure:

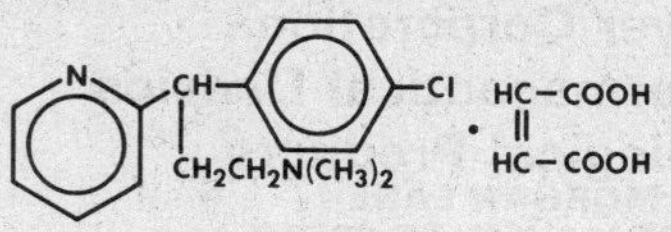

DEVICES: 2 sterile pads containing isopropyl alcohol 70% by volume. One tourniquet.

CLINICAL PHARMACOLOGY

EPINEPHRINE: The most valuable drug for the emergency treatment of severe allergic reactions is epinephrine. The vasoconstrictor effect of epinephrine on the capillary directly antagonizes the generalized vasodilation produced by histamine. Epinephrine reverses the increased permeability of dilated capillaries to plasma. The shock of severe allergic reactions is due to the loss of circulating blood volume by pooling in the dilated capillary beds and loss of plasma into the tissues. Epinephrine quickly restores circulating blood volume and blood pressure by constricting the capillary bed. The itching during episodes of hives or angioedema is promptly relieved by epinephrine. Epinephrine is a powerful relaxer of the smooth muscle of the bronchioles, stomach, intestine, pregnant uterus and urinary bladder wall. The bronchospasm, wheezing and dyspnea of the acute allergic reactions are relieved. Where abdominal cramping, defecation or involuntary urination have occurred during severe allergic attacks, epinephrine rapidly produces relief. Subcutaneously or intramuscularly administered epinephrine has a rapid onset and short duration of action. Subcutaneous administration during asthmatic attacks may produce bronchodilation within 5 to 10 minutes, and maximal effects may occur within 20 minutes.

CHLO-AMINE®: Chlo-Amine® is an effective agent in nullifying the characteristic effects of histamine and is especially valuable in the prophylaxis and relief of many allergic symptoms. It is readily absorbed from the intestinal tract and released into the tissues from the bloodstream. This action is both prompt and sustained. Elimination of the drug is such that there is a low incidence of side effects.

INDICATIONS AND USAGE

Ana-Kit® Anaphylaxis Emergency Treatment Kit is indicated for use by adult and pediatric patients under the following situations:

1. Allergic reactions including anaphylactic shock due to stinging insects (primarily of the Hymenoptera order, which includes bees, wasps, hornets, yellow jackets, bumble bees, and fire ants).
2. Severe allergic or anaphylactoid reactions due to allergy injections, exposures to pollens, dusts, molds, foods, drugs, and exercise or unknown substances (so-called idiopathic anaphylaxis).
3. Severe, life-threatening asthma attacks characterized by wheezing, dyspnea and inability to breathe.

In the sensitive patient, severe allergic reactions and anaphylactic shock may occur within minutes of the insect sting or exposure to an allergenic substance.
Symptoms may include bronchoconstriction, wheezing, sneezing, hoarseness, urticaria, angioedema, erythema, pruritis, tachycardia, thready pulse, falling blood pressure, sense of oppression or impending doom, disorientation, cramping abdominal pain, incontinance, faintness, loss of consciousness.
The Ana-Kit® is compactly designed to be carried and used by patients when severe symptoms arise, and the patient is out of reach of immediate attention by a doctor or hospital.

CONTRAINDICATIONS

EPINEPHRINE: Epinephrine must not be given intra-arterially as marked vasoconstriction may result in gangrene. **This unit is not intended for intravenous use.** Further dilution would be necessary and is not practical with this emergency syringe.
Epinephrine Injection, USP, (1:1000) must not be used if there is hypersensitivity to any of the components.
Epinephrine is contraindicated in narrow-angle glaucoma; cardiogenic, traumatic, or hemorrhagic shock; cardiac dilation; cerebral arteriosclerosis; and organic brain damage.
Epinephrine should not be used to counteract circulatory collapse or hypotension due to phenothiazines, since such agents may reverse the pressor effect of epinephrine, leading to a further lowering of blood pressure.
Epinephrine should not be administered concomitantly with other sympathomimetic agents, since the effects are additive and may be detrimental to the patient.

CHLO-AMINE®: No known contraindications.

WARNINGS

EPINEPHRINE: Overdosage or accidental intravenous administration of conventional subcutaneous doses may induce severe or fatal hypertension, or cerebrovascular hemorrhage. Fatalities may also occur from pulmonary edema resulting from peripheral constriction and cardiac stimulation. The marked pressor effects may be counteracted by use of rapidly acting vasodilators, such as the nitrites and alpha-adrenergic blockers.
Deaths have been reported in asthmatics treated with epinephrine following the use of isoproterenol or orciprenaline.
Epinephrine is the preferred treatment for serious allergic or other emergency situations even though this product contains sodium bisulfite, a sulfite that may in other products cause allergic-type reactions including anaphylactic symptoms or life-threatening or less severe asthmatic episodes in certain susceptible persons. The alternatives to using epinephrine in a life-threatening situation may not be satisfactory. The presence of a sulfite(s) in this product should not deter administration of the drug for treatment of serious allergic or other emergency situations.
Epinephrine must be administered with great caution, if at all, in patients with cardiac arrhythmias, coronary artery or organic heart disease, and hypertension. In patients with coronary insufficiency or ischemic heart disease, epinephrine may precipitate or aggravate angina pectoris as well as produce potentially fatal ventricular arrhythmias. Epinephrine should be administered only with great caution to elderly patients, those with diabetes mellitus, hyperthyroidism or psychoneurotic disorders; also to those with long-standing bronchial asthma or emphysema if such individuals may also have degenerative heart disease, and to pregnant women (see "Pregnancy").

CHLO-AMINE®: Chlorpheniramine maleate should be used with extreme caution in patients with stenosing peptic ulcer, pyloroduodenal obstruction, prostatic hypertrophy, or bladder neck obstruction. These compounds have an atropine-like action and therefore should be used with caution in patients with a history of increased intraocular pressure, cardiovascular disease, or hypertension. The asthmatic patient should take the chlorpheniramine maleate tablets with caution.

PRECAUTIONS

GENERAL: Ana-Kit® is not intended to be a substitute for medical attention or hospital care. The kit is designed to be compact and easy to carry, and to provide emergency treatment when medical care is not immediately available. Highly sensitive individuals should have the kit readily available at all times. Because of its small size it can be carried by outdoor sportsmen, golfers, gardeners, or any sensitive individual who may be exposed to stinging insects (wasps, hornets, yellow jackets, fire ants or bees) or other potentially life-threatening allergens. The drugs in the Ana-Kit®, when used as directed immediately following exposure to an allergen, may prove life-saving. Certain changes in the emergency instructions and in the kit itself may be made by the doctor according to the needs of the patient. IN ALL CASES THE PHYSICIAN SHOULD INSTRUCT THE PATIENT, AND/OR ANY OTHER PERSON WHO MIGHT BE IN A POSITION TO ADMINISTER THE EPINEPHRINE, IN THE PROPER USE OF THE SYRINGE AND THE OTHER COMPONENTS OF THIS KIT.

INFORMATION FOR PATIENTS: Complete patient information, including dosage, directions for proper administration, and precautions, can be found at the end of this package insert, as well as inside each Ana-Kit® kit.
Since epinephrine injection may produce disturbing or frightening reactions, it may be desirable to forewarn patients. Reactions commonly include an increase in pulse rate, a more forceful heartbeat, palpitations, a throbbing headache, pallor, feelings of overstimulation, anxiety, weakness, shakiness, dizziness, or nausea. Symptoms not involving an overdose generally do not indicate anything serious and usually subside rapidly with rest, quiet, and recumbency. Patients with hypertension or hyperthyroidism are prone to more severe or persistent effects, as are patients with coronary-artery disease, who may experience angina. Psychoneurotic patients may experience a worsening of symptoms. Diabetic patients may require an increased dose of insulin or other antidiabetic medication. Patients with Parkinson's disease may notice a temporary worsening of symptoms.

DRUG INTERACTIONS: Caution is indicated in patients receiving cardiac glycosides or mercurial diuretics, since these agents may sensitize the myocardium to beta-adrenergic stimulation and make cardiac arrhythmias more likely.
The effects of epinephrine may be potentiated by tricyclic antidepressants, sodium levothyroxine, and certain antihistamines, notably chlorpheniramine, tripelennamine, and diphenhydramine.
The cardiostimulating and bronchodilating effects of epinephrine are antagonized by beta-adrenergic blocking drugs, such as propranolol. The vasoconstricting and hypertensive effects are antagonized by alpha-adrenergic blocking drugs, such as phentolamine. Ergot alkaloids and phenothiazines may also reverse the pressor effects of epinephrine.
Diabetic patients receiving epinephrine may require an increased dose of insulin or oral hypoglycemic drugs.

Carcinogenesis, Mutagenesis, Impairment of Fertility: There are no data from either animal or human studies regarding the carcinogenicity or mutagenicity of epinephrine or Chlo-Amine®, and no studies have been conducted to determine their potential for the impairment of fertility.

Pregnancy: Teratogenic Effects. Pregnancy Category C—Epinephrine has been shown to be teratogenic in rats and hamsters at dose levels hundreds of times as high as the maximal human dose. Although there are no adequate or well-controlled studies in pregnant women, epinephrine crosses the placenta and its use during pregnancy may cause anoxia in the fetus. Epinephrine should be used in pregnancy only if the potential benefit justifies the potential risk to the fetus.

Pediatric Use: Administer Epinephrine or Chlo-Amine® with caution to infants and children (see "Dosage and Administration"). Syncope has occurred following the administration of epinephrine to asthmatic children.

ADVERSE REACTIONS

EPINEPHRINE: Adverse reactions include transient, moderate anxiety, apprehensiveness, restlessness, tremor, weakness, dizziness, sweating, palpitations, pallor, nausea and vomiting, headache, and respiratory difficulties. These symptoms occur in some persons receiving therapeutic doses of epinephrine, but are more likely to occur, or to occur in exaggerated form, in those with hypertension or hyperthyroidism. Excessive doses cause acute hypertension. Arrhythmias, including fatal ventricular fibrillation, have

Continued on next page

Bayer Allergy—Cont.

been reported, particularly in patients with underlying cardiac disease or those receiving certain drugs (see "Drug Interactions").

Rapid rises in blood pressure have produced cerebral hemorrhage, particularly in elderly patients with cerebrovascular disease. Angina may occur in patients with coronary-artery disease.

CHLO-AMINE®: Drowsiness, dizziness, blurred vision, dry mouth and gastrointestinal upsets may occur. Patients should not drive or operate machinery after taking the drug. Large doses produce central nervous system depression and occasionally tremors or convulsions. Reports of hematological disorders are rare.

OVERDOSAGE

EPINEPHRINE: Epinephrine is rapidly inactivated in the body, and treatment is primarily supportive. If necessary, pressor effects may be counteracted by rapidly acting vasodilators or alpha-adrenergic blocking drugs. If prolonged hypotension follows such measures, it may be necessary to administer another pressor drug, such as levarterenol.

Overdosage of epinephrine may produce extremely elevated arterial pressure, which may result in cerebrovascular hemorrhage, particularly in elderly patients.

If an epinephrine overdose induces pulmonary edema that interferes with respiration, treatment consists of a rapidly acting alpha-adrenergic blocking drug such as phentolamine and/or intermittent positive-pressure respiration.

Epinephrine overdosage can also cause transient bradycardia followed by tachycardia, and these may be accompanied by potentially fatal cardiac arrhythmias. Ventricular premature contractions may appear within one minute after injection and may be followed by multilocal ventricular tachycardia (prefibrillation rhythm). Subsidence of the ventricular effects may be followed by atrial tachycardia and occasionally by atrioventricular block. Treatment of arrhythmias consists of administration of beta-adrenergic blocking drug such as propranolol.

Overdosage sometimes also results in extreme pallor and coldness of the skin, metabolic acidosis, and kidney failure. Suitable corrective measures must be taken.

CHLO-AMINE®: Overdose symptoms may be sedation, apnea, cardiovascular collapse to stimulation, insomnia, hallucinations, tremors or convulsions. Also there may be dizziness, tinnitus, ataxia, blurred vision, hypotension, dry mouth, flushing, and abdominal symptoms.

Treatment—The patient should be induced to vomit, preferably with ipecac syrup—and large amounts of water. Prevent aspiration of vomitus. Gastric lavage may be necessary using activated charcoal and saline. Hyperosmotic cathartics such as Milk of Magnesia may hasten elimination of residual cling. Vasopressors can be used to correct hypotension. Diazepam may be used to control seizures. Hyperpyrexia can be treated with cool sponges or a hypothermic blanket.

DOSAGE AND ADMINISTRATION

Parenteral drug products should be inspected visually for particulate matter and discoloration prior to administration, whenever solution and container permit. Do not use Epinephrine Injection, USP, if it has a pinkish or darker than slightly yellow color or contains a precipitate.

The physician who prescribes the Ana-Kit® should review the package insert in detail with the patient. This review should include the proper use of the 2-dose epinephrine syringe to insure that subcutaneous or intramuscular injections are given into the deltoid region of the arm or the anteriolateral aspect of the thigh. See also the PATIENT DIRECTIONS FOR USE.

EPINEPHRINE: For subcutaneous or intramuscular injection only.

Adults and children over 12 years: 0.3 mL; 6–12 years: 0.2 mL; 2–6 years: 0.15 mL; Infants to 2 years: 0.05 to 0.1 mL. When syringe is properly set up, as directed in the Patient Instruction Sheet, a 0.3 mL dose is administered when plunger is pushed until it stops. Syringe barrel has 0.1 mL graduations so that smaller doses can be measured. (Operation of syringe is explained in the Patient Directions For Use section at the end of this package insert.)

If after 10 minutes from the first injection symptoms are not noticeably improved, administer a second dose of epinephrine from the syringe.

CHLO-AMINE®: Tablets are chewable antihistamines. Adults and children over 12 years: 4 tablets; children 6–12 years: 2 tablets; children under 6 years: 1 tablet.

HOW SUPPLIED

ANA-KIT® ANAPHYLAXIS EMERGENCY TREATMENT KIT CONTAINS:

SYRINGE: One sterile syringe containing 1 mL Epinephrine Injection, USP, (1:1000). Syringe delivers two 0.3 mL doses.

TABLETS: Four 2 mg chewable Chlo-Amine® tablets, Chlorpheniramine Maleate Tablets.

DEVICES: Two sterile pads containing 70% isopropyl alcohol (by volume) and 1 tourniquet.

PROTECT FROM LIGHT. STORE AT ROOM TEMPERATURE, APPROX. 25°C (77°F). PROTECT FROM FREEZING.

CAUTION: U.S. Federal Law Prohibits Dispensing Without Prescription.

Epinephrine Mfg. by: Wyeth-Ayerst Laboratories, Philadelphia, PA 19101

Pkgd. and Dist. by:
Bayer Corporation
Pharmaceutical Division
Spokane, WA 99207 USA

PATIENT DIRECTIONS FOR USE
ANA-KIT® Anaphylaxis Emergency Treatment Kit
(Please read entire direction sheet before an emergency arises.)

The Ana-Kit® **IS TO BE USED ONLY WHEN PRESCRIBED BY A PHYSICIAN,** for patients who are highly allergic to pollens, foods, dusts, insect stings, and drugs which may produce a life-threatening anaphylactic reaction, or have severe asthma attacks.

IN THE EVENT OF A LIFE-THREATENING SITUATION, FOLLOW THESE STEPS IMMEDIATELY TO ADMINISTER THE EPINEPHRINE.

1. Remove (pull off) blue plastic needle cover.
   Hold syringe upright and push plunger to expel air and excess epinephrine (plunger will stop).
2. Rotate rectangular plunger 1/4 turn to the right. Plunger will align with slot in barrel of syringe. Wipe injection site with alcohol swab.
3. Insert needle straight into arm or thigh as illustrated.
4. Push plunger until it stops.
   Syringe will inject a 0.3 mL dose for adults and children over 12 years.
   Children: Syringe barrel has 0.1 mL graduations so that smaller doses can be measured. Administer to infants to 2 years: 0.05 to 0.1 mL; 2–6 years: 0.15 mL; and 6–12 years: 0.2 mL.

ONCE THE INITIAL EPINEPHRINE INJECTION HAS BEEN ADMINISTERED, FOLLOW THESE ADDITIONAL STEPS.

5. CONTACT PHYSICIAN, IF POSSIBLE.
6. REMOVE STINGER if stung by insect. (Use fingernails. DO NOT push, pinch or squeeze, or further imbed the stinger into the skin as this may cause further venom to be injected.)
7. APPLY TOURNIQUET. If exposure to life-threatening agent was by injection (allergenic extract, drug) or insect sting on an arm or leg, place tourniquet between injection or sting site and body. Do not obstruct arterial blood flow with the tourniquet. (If exposure is elsewhere—neck, face, body—proceed immediately to Step 9.)
8. TIGHTEN TOURNIQUET. To tighten, pull on the end of ONE STRING. Then, at least every ten minutes, loosen the tourniquet by pulling on the small metal ring.
9. CHEW AND SWALLOW CHLO-AMINE® TABLETS. For adults and children over 12 years, take 4 tablets; children 6–12 years take 2 tablets; children under 6 years take 1 tablet. These tablets are chewable antihistamine which is generally tolerated.
10. PREPARE SYRINGE FOR A POSSIBLE SECOND INJECTION. Turn the rectangular plunger 1/4 turn to the right to line up with rectangular slot in the syringe. (A slight wiggling may aid the turning and alignment of the plunger.)
11. THE SECOND INJECTION. If after 10 minutes from the first injection symptoms are not noticeably improved, a second injection is required. Cleanse skin area with alco-

hol swab and make second injection as in STEPS 3 and 4 for the first epinephrine injection. (A small amount of epinephrine will remain in syringe after the second dose and cannot be expelled.) Note: Dispose of syringe and remaining contents if second injection is not required.

12. APPLY ICE PACKS IF AVAILABLE, AT THE SITE OF THE DRUG OR ALLERGY INJECTION, OR INSECT STING (if applicable).
13. KEEP PATIENT WARM AND AVOID EXERTION.

PRECAUTIONS

EPINEPHRINE: For subcutaneous or intramuscular injection only. **Not intended for intravenous use.**

Epinephrine Injection, USP, contains sodium bisulfite. Patients with a suspected sulfite sensitivity should consult their physician well in advance before the need to use this product becomes critical.

Epinephrine is light sensitive and should be stored in box provided. STORE AT ROOM TEMPERATURE, approximately 25°C (77°F). Protect from freezing. Any epinephrine solution in contact with the needle may cause rusting of the metal. **Do not try to force air out of the syringe until you are ready to use the epinephrine.** This may rupture the seal and allow the epinephrine solution to contact the metal promoting deterioration. **Never remove cover from needle until ready to use syringe** as this may cause needle and contents to become contaminated.

Parenteral drug products should be inspected visually for particulate matter and discoloration prior to administration, whenever solution and container permit. Do not use Epinephrine Injection, USP, if it has a pinkish or darker than slightly yellow color or contains a precipitate. Obtain replacement syringe from physician. Periodically check expiration date on syringe. If expiration date is near, re-order new syringe and discard outdated syringe after new syringe has been received.

CHLO-AMINE®: As with any drug, if you are pregnant or nursing a baby, seek the advice of a health professional before using this product.

Patients should not drive or operate machinery after taking Chlo-Amine®. Drowsiness, dizziness, blurred vision, dry mouth and gastrointestinal upsets may occur. Keep out of reach of children.

The asthmatic patient should take the chlorpheniramine maleate tablets with caution.

LIMITED WARRANTY: A number of factors beyond our control could reduce the efficacy of this product or even result in an ill effect following its use. These include storage and handling of the product after it leaves our hands, diagnosis, dosage, method of administration and biological differences in individual patients. Because of these factors, it is important that this product be stored properly and that the directions be followed carefully during use.

No warranty, express or implied, including any warranty of merchantability or fitness, is made. Representatives or the Company are not authorized to vary the terms or the contents of any printed labeling, including the package insert, for this product except by printed notice from the Company's headquarters. The prescriber and user of this product must accept the terms hereof.

Epinephrine Mfg. by: Wyeth-Ayerst Laboratories, Philadelphia, PA 19101

Pkgd. and Dist. by:
Bayer Corporation
Pharmaceutical Division
Spokane, WA 99207 USA

Hollister-Stier®
From 471103 B07 12/95   Printed in U.S.A.
Shown in Product Identification Guide, page 305

Bayer Corporation
Pharmaceutical Division
Biological Products
400 MORGAN LANE
WEST HAVEN, CT 06516

For Medical Information Contact:
Director, Medical Services
(800) 468-0894
(203) 937-2000

IMMUNE GLOBULIN INTRAVENOUS (HUMAN), 5% ℞
GAMIMUNE® N, 5%

DESCRIPTION

Immune Globulin Intravenous (Human), 5%—Gamimune® N, 5% is a sterile 4.5%–5.5% solution of human protein in 9%–11% maltose; it contains no preservative. Each milliliter (mL) contains approximately 50 mg of protein, not less than

98% of which has the electrophoretic mobility of gamma globulin. Not less than 90% of the gamma globulin is monomer. Also present are traces of IgA and of IgM. The distribution of IgG subclasses is similar to that found in normal serum. Gamimune N, 5% has a buffer capacity of 16.5 mEq/L of solution (~ 0.3 mEq/g of protein). The calculated osmolality is 309 milliosmoles per kilogram of solvent (water) and the calculated osmolarity is 278 milliosmoles per liter of solution.

The product is made by cold ethanol fractionation of large pools of human plasma. Part of the fractionation may be performed by another licensed manufacturer. The immunoglobulin is isolated from Cohn Effluent III by diafiltration and ultrafiltration. The protein has not been chemically modified other than in the adjustment of the pH of the solution to 4.0–4.5.[1] Isotonicity is achieved by the addition of maltose. The product is intended for intravenous administration.

CLINICAL PHARMACOLOGY
Primary Humoral Immunodeficiency
Gamimune N, 5% supplies a broad spectrum of opsonic and neutralizing IgG antibodies for the prevention or attenuation of a wide variety of infectious diseases. As Gamimune N, 5% is administered intravenously, essentially 100% of the infused IgG antibodies are immediately available in the recipient's circulation.[2] Studies using a modified intravenous immunoglobulin at pH 6.8 have shown that approximately 30% of the infused IgG disappeared from the circulation in the first 24 hours, due primarily to equilibration of the IgG between the plasma and the extravascular space.[2-5] A further decline to about 40% of the peak level found immediately post-infusion is to be expected during the first week.[2-5] The in vivo half-life of Gamimune N, 5% equals or exceeds the 3-week half-life reported for IgG in the literature, but individual patient variation in half-life has been observed.[2] Thus, this variable as well as the amount of immune globulin administered per dose is important in determining the frequency of administration of the drug for each individual patient.

Idiopathic Thrombocytopenic Purpura
While Gamimune N, 5% has been shown to be effective in some cases of idiopathic thrombocytopenic purpura (ITP) (see INDICATIONS AND USAGE), the mechanism of action has not been fully elucidated.

Bone Marrow Transplantation
Gamimune N, 5% has been shown to be effective in bone marrow transplant patients ≥ 20 years of age in the first 100 days posttransplant for the following: prevention of systemic and local infections, interstitial pneumonia of infectious and idiopathic etiologies and acute graft-versus-host disease (AGVHD)[6] (see INDICATIONS AND USAGE). Administration of Gamimune N, 5% to bone marrow transplant patients significantly increased IgG and IgG subclass levels while those seen in the control group fell below predicted levels. The mechanism of action of Immune Globulin Intravenous (Human), 5%—Gamimune® N, 5% in reducing the incidence of AGVHD is presently unknown.

Pediatric HIV Infection
Children infected with human immunodeficiency virus (HIV) may display defects in both cellular and humoral immunity.[7-10] As a result, some children with HIV-1 infection experience serious, potentially life-threatening recurrent bacterial infections.[11-13] In one retrospective report, among 71 HIV-infected children observed over 3.5 years, 27 (37%) experienced serious documented bacterial infections.[12] The types of bacterial and viral infections observed in HIV-infected children are similar to those seen in children with primary hypogammaglobulinemia.[14] The replacement of opsonic and neutralizing IgG antibodies has been shown to reduce serious and minor bacterial infection in HIV-infected children.[15,16]

In a randomized, double-blind, placebo-controlled, multicenter study performed between March 7, 1988 and January 15, 1991, the efficacy of Gamimune N, 5% in pediatric HIV disease to decrease the frequency of serious and minor bacterial infections and the frequency of hospitalization, and to increase the time free of serious bacterial infection was documented in children with clinical or immunologic evidence of HIV disease (see INDICATIONS AND USAGE). The primary endpoint of this study was prospectively defined as a significant reduction in the proportion of subjects who develop at least one serious bacterial infection when compared to the control group of HIV-infected children who received placebo. Serious bacterial infections were defined as laboratory-proven and clinically diagnosed (i.e., radiologically proven acute pneumonia and sinusitis) infections. The Data Safety and Monitoring Board (DSMB) recommended early termination of the study based on data presented to them from an interim analysis in December 1990 which showed that treatment with Gamimune N, 5% increased the time free from serious infections in children with CD4+counts $\geq 200/mm^3$.

General
The intravenous administration of solutions of maltose has been studied by several investigators.[17-21] Healthy subjects

tolerated the infusions well, and no adverse effects were observed at a rate of 0.25 g maltose/kg body weight per hour.[18] In safety studies conducted by Miles Inc., infusions of 10% maltose administered at 0.27–0.62 g maltose/kg per hour[21] to normal subjects produced either mild side effects (e.g., headache) or no adverse reaction.[2] Following intravenous administrations of maltose, maltose was detected in the peripheral blood; there was a dose-dependent excretion of maltose and glucose in the urine and a mild diuretic effect.[2] These alterations were well-tolerated without significant adverse effects.[2] The highest recommended infusion rate, 0.08 mL/kg body weight per minute (see DOSAGE AND ADMINISTRATION), is equivalent to 0.48 g maltose/kg body weight per hour.

The buffer capacity of Immune Globulin Intravenous (Human), 5% —Gamimune® N, 5% is 16.5 mEq/L (~ 0.33 mEq/g protein); a dose of 1000 mg/kg body weight therefore represents an acid load of 0.33 mEq/kg body weight. The total buffering capacity of whole blood in a normal individual is 45–50 mEq/L of blood, or 3.6 mEq/kg body weight.[22] Thus, the acid load delivered in the largest dose of Gamimune N, 5% would be neutralized by the buffering capacity of whole blood alone, even if the dose were infused instantaneously. (An infusion usually lasts several hours.)

In Phase I human studies, no change in arterial blood pH measurements was detected following the intravenous administration of Gamimune N, 5% at a dose of 150 mg/kg body weight;[2] following a dose of 400 mg/kg body weight in 37 patients, there were no clinically important differences in mean venous pH or bicarbonate measurements in patients who received Gamimune N, 5% compared with those who received a chemically modified intravenous immunoglobulin preparation with a pH of 6.8.[2]

In patients with limited or compromised acid-base compensatory mechanisms, consideration should be given to the effect of the additional acid load Gamimune N, 5% might present.

INDICATIONS AND USAGE
Primary Humoral Immunodeficiency
Gamimune N, 5% is efficacious in the treatment of primary immunodeficiency states in which severe impairment of antibody forming capacity has been shown, such as: congenital agammaglobulinemias, common variable immunodeficiency, Wiskott-Aldrich syndrome, x-linked immunodeficiency with hyper IgM, and severe combined immunodeficiencies.[5,23-25] Gamimune N, 5% is especially useful when high levels or rapid elevation of circulating antibodies are desired or when intramuscular injections are contraindicated.

Idiopathic Thrombocytopenic Purpura (ITP)
In clinical situations in which a rapid rise in platelet count is needed to control bleeding or to allow a patient with ITP to undergo surgery, administration of Gamimune N, 5% should be considered; in patients in whom a response is achieved, the rise of platelets is generally rapid (within 1–5 days), transient (most often lasting from several days to several weeks) and should not be considered curative. It is presently not possible to predict which patients with ITP will respond to therapy, although the increase in platelet counts in children seems to be better than that in adults. Childhood ITP may, however, respond spontaneously without treatment.

Two different dosing regimens of Gamimune N, 5% have been studied in clinical investigations: a regimen consisting of 400 mg/kg body weight daily for 5 consecutive days, and a high dose treatment regimen consisting of 1,000 mg/kg body weight administered on either 1 day or 2 consecutive days. In clinical studies of Immune Globulin Intravenous (Human), 5%—Gamimune® N, 5% five of six (83.3%) children and 12 of 16 (75%) adults with acute or chronic ITP treated with 400 mg/kg body weight for 5 consecutive days demonstrated clinically significant platelet increments of $\geq 30,000/mm^3$ over baseline. The mean platelet count in children with ITP rose from $27,800/mm^3$ at baseline to $297,000/mm^3$ (range $50,000-455,000/mm^3$) and the mean platelet count in adults with ITP rose from $27,900/mm^3$ at baseline to $124,900/mm^3$ (range $11,000-341,000/mm^3$). Two of three children with acute ITP rapidly went into complete remission.

Thirteen of 14 children (92.9%) and 26 of 29 adults (89.7%) with acute or chronic ITP treated with Gamimune N, 5% 1,000 mg/kg body weight administered on either 1 day or 2 consecutive days responded to treatment with clinically significant platelet increments of $\geq 30,000/mm^3$ over baseline. This included three of three patients with ITP that were human immunodeficiency virus (HIV) antibody positive and two of two patients with ITP that were pregnant. The mean platelet count in children with ITP treated with Gamimune N, 5% 1,000 mg/kg body weight on 1 day or 2 consecutive days rose from $44,400/mm^3$ at baseline to $285,600/mm^3$ (range $89,000-473,000/mm^3$) and the mean platelet count in adults with ITP treated with the regimen rose from $23,400/mm^3$ at baseline to $173,100/mm^3$ (range $28,000-709,000/mm^3$).

Two patients, one each with acute adult and chronic childhood ITP, entered complete remission with treatment.

Six of the 29 adult patients with ITP received Gamimune N, 5% 1,000 mg/kg on 1 day or 2 consecutive days to increase the platelet count prior to splenectomy. Mean platelet counts rose from $14,500/mm^3$ at baseline to $129,300/mm^3$ (range $51,000-242,000/mm^3$) prior to surgery.

The duration of the platelet rise following treatment of ITP with either treatment regimen of Gamimune N, 5% was variable, ranging from several days to 12 months or more. Some ITP patients have demonstrated continuing responsiveness over many months to intermittent infusions of Gamimune N, 5% 400–1,000 mg/kg body weight, administered as a single maintenance dose, at intervals as indicated by the platelet count.

Bone Marrow Transplantation (BMT)
Gamimune N, 5% should be considered for use in bone marrow transplant patients ≥ 20 years of age to decrease the risk of septicemia and other infections, interstitial pneumonia of infectious or idiopathic etiologies and acute graft-versus-host disease (AGVHD) in the first 100 days posttransplant. Gamimune N, 5% is not indicated in bone marrow transplant patients below 20 years of age. In a controlled study of 369 evaluable BMT patients (184 treated and 185 controls) who either did or did not receive Gamimune N, 5% in doses of 500 mg/kg body weight on days −7 and −2 pretransplant, then weekly through day 90 posttransplant, posttransplant complications were evaluated in the entire study group and in patients under age 20 and age 20 or older. For patients ≥ 20 years of age (128 patients in the control group and 119 patients in the treated group), there was a statistically significant reduction in interstitial pneumonia from 21% in the control group to 9% in the treated group (p=0.0032) during the first 100 days posttransplant. Also significantly reduced in this age group were: overall septicemia from 53 infections in the 128 patient control group to 26 infections in the 119 patient treated group (relative risk control treated [RR] 2.36, p=0.0025); gram-negative septicemia from 24 infections in the 128 patient control group to 9 infections in the 119 patient treated group (RR 2.53, p=0.015); gram-positive septicemia from 16 infections in the 128 patient control group to 8 infections in the 119 patient treated group (RR 2.73, p=0.046); and Grade II to IV AGVHD from an incidence of 58 of 110 in the control group to 38 of 108 in the treated group (p=0.0051).

The given p-values do not take into account multiple endpoints and subset analyses. Therefore, some of the p-values could occur by chance alone. There was no significant improvement in overall mortality in this study.

In patients below age 20, there appeared to be no benefit from treatment with Gamimune N, 5%, either in reducing the incidence of infections or the incidence of AGVHD.

Pediatric HIV Infection
Gamimune N, 5% 400 mg/kg every 28 days significantly decreased the frequency of serious and minor bacterial infections (laboratory-proven and clinically diagnosed) and the frequency of hospitalization, and increased the time free of serious bacterial infection. The effect of Gamimune N, 5% in preventing serious bacterial infections was especially apparent in preventing primary bacteremia (including Streptococcus pneumoniae bacteremia) and acute pneumonia.

In a randomized, double-blind, placebo-controlled, multicenter study, 394 HIV-infected, non-hemophilic children less than 13 years of age were randomized. Of the children randomized, 369 were included in the efficacy analysis and 376 in the safety analysis. The study population had 1) a mean age of 40 months (range 2.4–136.8 months), 2) acquired HIV primarily through vertical transmission (91%), 3) a majority (87%) of CDC Class P-2 (symptomatic), and 4) had a median CD4+count of 937 cells/mm³ (range 0–6660 cells/mm³). At the time of study entry, 14% (52 of 369) were receiving Pneumocystis carinii pneumonia (PCP) prophylaxis. During the course of the study, 51% (189 of 369) received PCP prophylaxis and 44% (164 of 369) received zidovudine (ZDV). Children with HIV-1 infection were initially stratified into two groups based upon CD4+count (< 200 cells/mm³ versus ≥ 200 cells/mm³) and CDC classification of pediatric HIV disease (history of opportunistic infections [P-2-D-1] and recurrent serious bacterial infections [P-2-D-2] versus others). Subjects received Gamimune N, 5% (400 mg/kg = 8 mL/kg) (n=185) or an equivalent volume of placebo (0.1% Albumin [Human]) (n=184) every 28 days. The mean follow-up for subjects receiving Gamimune N, 5% was 17.9 months and 17.8 months for patients on placebo.

The number of subjects who had at least one serious bacterial infection was 86 of 184 (47%) in the placebo group and 55 of 185 (30%) in the Gamimune N, 5% group (p=0.0009). All p-values reported are two-sided. Treatment with Gamimune N, 5% compared to placebo was also associated with a significant reduction in both the number of subjects with at least one laboratory-proven infection (36 of 184 vs. 18 of 185, p=0.0081), and the number of subjects with at least one clinically diagnosed infection (71 of 184 vs. 45 of 185, p=0.0036). Efficacy in patients with CD4+counts < 200/mm³ was not

Continued on next page

Bayer Biological—Cont.

established, possibly because of the small number of subjects in this category.

The 2-year treatment period defined in the protocol was truncated for some patients by the DSMB based on data from the interim analysis. Rates of serious bacterial infections per 100 patient-years were computed and analyzed to take into account both the unequal duration of treatment and follow-up, as well as recurrent infections in individual subjects. Children treated with Immune Globulin Intravenous (Human), 5%—Gamimune® N, 5% experienced a 50.5% lower frequency of laboratory-proven serious bacterial infection compared to the group treated with placebo (9.1 vs. 18.2 infections per 100 patient-years, p=0.031), a 36.0% lower frequency of clinically diagnosed serious infections (24.0 vs. 37.5 infections per 100 patient-years, p=0.013), a 40.6% reduction in total serious infections (laboratory-proven and clinically diagnosed) (33.1 vs. 55.7 infections per 100 patient-years, p=0.003), a 60% lower frequency of primary bacteremias (5.8 vs. 14.5 infections per 100 patient-years, p=0.009), a 75.6% lower frequency of *Streptococcus pneumoniae* bacteremia (1.1 vs. 4.5 bacteremias per 100 patient-years, p=0.026), a 54.3% lower frequency of clinically diagnosed pneumonia (12.7 vs. 27.8 infections per 100 patient-years, p=0.001), and a 22.5% lower frequency of minor bacterial infections (including otitis media, skin and soft tissue infections, and upper respiratory tract infections) (123.6 vs. 159.5 infections per 100 patient-years, p=0.033).

In addition to a reduced frequency of infection, children treated with Gamimune N, 5% had a 36.8% lower number of hospitalizations per 100 patient-years (72 vs. 114 per 100 patient-years, p=0.002) and a reduced number of hospital days (6.9 vs. 10.5 per patient-year, p=0.030) than patients treated with placebo. Patients treated with Gamimune N, 5% had a higher probability of remaining free of laboratory-proven infections (p=0.0093) and combined laboratory-proven and clinically diagnosed infections (p=0.0015) for 24 months than the group of children treated with placebo. At 24 months, the estimated probabilities of remaining infection-free for the Gamimune N, 5% and placebo arms were 87.8% vs. 76.1%, respectively, for laboratory-proven infections and 63.5% vs. 44.5%, respectively, for combined laboratory-proven and clinically diagnosed infections.

There was no effect of Gamimune N, 5% therapy on mortality, which was low in both treatment groups (17%), or on the frequency of opportunistic or viral infections during the period of study.

Since antibacterial prophylaxis could also account for the observed reduction in the rate of serious bacterial infections, further analysis was performed to evaluate the role of *Pneumocystis carinii* pneumonia (PCP) prophylaxis on the efficacy of Gamimune N, 5%. PCP prophylaxis consisted primarily (96%) of trimethoprim/sulfamethoxazole given 3 successive days each week. This antibiotic combination could be active against the bacteria commonly encountered in this patient population. In the subgroup of patients receiving PCP prophylaxis at study entry, treatment with Gamimune N, 5% was associated with 44.0 infections per 100 patient-years, whereas placebo recipients had 64.7 infections per 100 patient-years (p=0.047). In the subgroup of patients not receiving PCP prophylaxis at study entry, treatment with Gamimune N, 5% was associated with 22.1 infections per 100 patient-years, whereas placebo recipients had 44.9 infections per 100 patient-years on placebo (p=0.024). Thus, Gamimune N, 5% benefitted patients by reducing the rate of serious bacterial infections whether or not they were receiving PCP prophylactic treatment at study entry. However, it should be noted that the use of PCP prophylactic treatment in this study was not randomized and specific guidelines for its administration were not identified.

CONTRAINDICATIONS

Gamimune N, 5% is contraindicated in individuals who are known to have had an anaphylactic or severe systemic response to Immune Globulin (Human). Individuals with selective IgA deficiencies who have known antibody against IgA (anti-IgA antibody) should not receive Gamimune N, 5% since these patients may experience severe reactions to the IgA which may be present.[23]

WARNINGS

Gamimune N, 5% should be administered only intravenously as the intramuscular and subcutaneous routes have not been evaluated.

Gamimune N, 5% may, on rare occasions, cause a precipitous fall in blood pressure and a clinical picture of anaphylaxis, even when the patient is not known to be sensitive to immune globulin preparations. These reactions may be related to the rate of infusion. Accordingly, the infusion rate given under DOSAGE AND ADMINISTRATION should be closely followed, at least until the physician has had sufficient experience with a given patient. The patient's vital signs should be monitored continuously and careful observation made for any symptoms throughout the entire infusion.

Epinephrine should be available for the treatment of an acute anaphylactic reaction.

PRECAUTIONS
General

Any vial that has been entered should be used promptly. Partially used vials should be discarded. Do not use if turbid. Solution which has been frozen should not be used.

An aseptic meningitis syndrome (AMS) has been reported to occur infrequently in association with Immune Globulin Intravenous (Human) treatment. The syndrome usually begins within several hours to two days following Immune Globulin Intravenous (Human) treatment. It is characterized by symptoms and signs including severe headache, nuchal rigidity, drowsiness, fever, photophobia, painful eye movements, and nausea and vomiting. Cerebrospinal fluid studies are frequently positive with pleocytosis up to several thousand cells per mm³, predominantly from the granulocytic series, and elevated protein levels up to several hundred mg/dL. Patients exhibiting such symptoms and signs should receive a thorough neurological examination, including CSF studies, to rule out other causes of meningitis. AMS may occur more frequently in association with high dose (2 g/kg) Immune Globulin Intravenous (Human) treatment. Discontinuation of Immune Globulin Intravenous (Human) treatment has resulted in remission of AMS within several days without sequelae.[26–29]

Drug Interactions

Antibodies in Gamimune N, 5% may interfere with the response to live viral vaccines such as measles, mumps, and rubella. Therefore, use of such vaccines should be deferred until approximately 6 months after Gamimune N, 5% administration.

Please see DOSAGE AND ADMINISTRATION for other drug interactions.

Pregnancy Category C

Animal reproduction studies have not been conducted with Gamimune N, 5%. It is not known whether Gamimune N, 5% can cause fetal harm when administered to a pregnant woman or can affect reproduction capacity. Gamimune N, 5% should be given to a pregnant woman only if clearly needed.

ADVERSE REACTIONS
Primary Humoral Immunodeficiency

In a study of 37 patients with immunodeficiency syndromes receiving Gamimune N, 5% at a monthly dose of 400 mg/kg body weight, reactions were seen in 5.2% of the infusions of Gamimune N, 5%. Symptoms reported with Gamimune N, 5% included malaise, a feeling of faintness, fever, chills, headache, nausea, vomiting, chest tightness, dyspnea and chest, back or hip pain. In addition, mild erythema following infiltration of Gamimune N, 5% at the infusion site was reported in some cases.

Idiopathic Thrombocytopenic Purpura

In studies of Gamimune N, 5% administered at a dose of 400 mg/kg body weight in the treatment of adult and pediatric patients with ITP, systemic reactions were noted in only 4 of 154 (2.6%) infusions, and all but one occurred at rates of infusion greater than 0.04 mL/kg body weight per minute. The symptoms reported included chest tightness, a sense of tachycardia (pulse was 84 beats per minute), and a burning sensation in the head; these symptoms were all mild and transient.

In studies of Gamimune N, 5% administered at a dose of 1,000 mg/kg body weight either as a single dose or as two doses on consecutive days in the treatment of adult and pediatric patients with ITP, adverse reactions were noted in only 25 of 251 (10%) infusions. Symptoms reported included headache, nausea, fever, chills, back pain, chest tightness, and shortness of breath. In children, the high dose regimen has been well-tolerated at the highest rates of infusion. In adults, however, the frequency of adverse reactions tended to increase with infusion rates in excess of 0.06 mL/kg/min. In general, reactions reported with infusion of Immune Globulin Intravenous (Human), 5%—Gamimune® N, 5% in these studies were reported as mild or moderate, and responded to slowing of the infusion rate.

Bone Marrow Transplantation

In studies of Gamimune® N, 5% administered to 185 bone marrow transplant recipients at doses of 500 mg/kg (10 mL/kg) body weight on day −7 and day −2 pretransplant, then weekly through day 90 posttransplant, adverse reactions were noted in 12 (6.5%) of the 185 patients that received Gamimune N, 5% and in 14 (0.6%) of 2,176 infusions. All reactions reported were rate-related and classified as mild. Chills were the most common symptom reported, occurring in nine patients. The other symptoms reported included headache, flushing, fever, pruritus and slight back discomfort. All reactions resolved satisfactorily, usually without treatment or decreasing the infusion rate.

Pediatric HIV Infection

Three hundred seventy-six (376) patients, 187 treated with Gamimune N, 5% and 189 treated with placebo (0.1% Albumin [Human]), were included in the safety analysis. Adverse reactions occurred during or within 24 hours of an infusion

in 50 of 3,451 (1.4%) infusions of Gamimune N, 5% and 62 of 3,447 (1.8%) infusions of placebo. Fever was the most common adverse reaction and occurred in 30 of 105 (28.6%) patients receiving placebo and 19 of 78 (24.4%) patients treated with Gamimune N, 5%. Irritability was the second most common symptom reported, with 10 of 105 (9.5%) reports for the placebo group and 9 of 78 (11.5%) for the group treated with Gamimune N, 5%. A large number of diverse adverse reactions accounted for the remaining adverse reactions reported in both study groups. In general, the number of adverse events reported was comparable in both the placebo and Gamimune N, 5% treated groups. Three serious adverse reactions were reported. One patient experienced a hypersensitivity reaction and did not receive further Gamimune N, 5% treatment. A second patient developed tachycardia and was admitted to an intensive care unit, but later continued treatment with Gamimune N, 5%. A third patient had skin infiltration during infusion and developed a full thickness skin slough over the dorsum of the hand that required skin grafting.

General

In the studies undertaken to date, other types of reactions have not been reported with Gamimune N, 5%. It may be, however, that adverse effects will be similar to those previously reported with intravenous and intramuscular immunoglobulin administration. Potential reactions therefore, may also include anxiety, flushing, wheezing, abdominal cramps, myalgias, arthralgia, and dizziness; rash has been reported only rarely. Reactions to intravenous immunoglobulin tend to be related to the rate of infusion.

True anaphylactic reactions to Gamimune N, 5% may occur in recipients with documented prior histories of severe allergic reactions to intramuscular immunoglobulin, but some patients may tolerate cautiously administered intravenous immunoglobulin without adverse effects.[2,30] Very rarely an anaphylactoid reaction may occur in patients with no prior history of severe allergic reactions to either intramuscular or intravenous immunoglobulin.[2]

DOSAGE AND ADMINISTRATION
General

Dosages for specific indications are indicated below, but in general, it is recommended that Gamimune N, 5% be administered by itself at an initial rate of 0.01 to 0.02 mL/kg body weight per minute for 30 minutes; if well-tolerated, the rate may be **gradually** increased to a maximum of 0.08 mL/kg body weight per minute. Investigations indicate that Gamimune N, 5% is well-tolerated and less likely to produce side effects when infused at the recommended rate. If side effects occur, the rate may be reduced, or the infusion interrupted until symptoms subside. The infusion may then be resumed at the rate which is comfortable for the patient. Parenteral drug products should be inspected visually for particulate matter and discoloration prior to administration, whenever solution and container permit.

It is recommended that infusion of Immune Globulin Intravenous (Human), 5%—Gamimune® N, 5% be given by a separate line, by itself, without mixing with other intravenous fluids or medications the patient might be receiving. Gamimune N, 5% should not be mixed with Immune Globulin Intravenous (Human) from another manufacturer. Gamimune N, 5% is not compatible with saline. If dilution is required, Gamimune N, 5% may be diluted with 5% dextrose in water (D5/W). No other drug interactions or compatibilities have been evaluated.

Primary Humoral Immunodeficiency

The usual dosage of Gamimune N, 5% for prophylaxis in primary immunodeficiency syndromes is 100–200 mg/kg (2–4 mL/kg) of body weight administered approximately once a month by intravenous infusion. The dosage may be given more frequently or increased as high as 400 mg/kg (8 mL/kg) body weight, if the clinical response is inadequate, or the level of IgG achieved in the circulation is felt to be insufficient. The minimum level of IgG required for protection has not been determined.

Idiopathic Thrombocytopenic Purpura (ITP)
Induction: An increase in platelet count has been observed in children and some adults with acute or chronic ITP receiving Gamimune N, 5% 400 mg/kg body weight daily for 5 days, or alternatively, 1,000 mg/kg body weight daily for 1 day or 2 consecutive days. In the latter treatment regimen, if an adequate increase in the platelet count is observed at 24 hours, the second dose of 1,000 mg/kg body weight may be withheld. The high dose regimen (1,000 mg/kg × 1–2 days) is not recommended for individuals with expanded fluid volumes or where fluid volume may be a concern. With both treatment regimens, a response usually occurs within several days and is maintained for a variable period of time. In general, a response is seen less often in adults than in children.

Maintenance: In adults and children with ITP, if after induction therapy the platelet count falls to less than 30,000/mm³ and/or the patient manifests clinically significant bleeding, Gamimune N, 5% 400 mg/kg body weight may be given as a single infusion. If an adequate response does not result, the dose can be increased to 800–1,000 mg/kg of body

weight given as a single infusion. Maintenance infusions may be administered intermittently as clinically indicated to maintain a platelet count greater than 30,000/mm^3.

Bone Marrow Transplantation

Gamimune N, 5% should be administered in doses of 500 mg/kg (10 mL/kg) body weight beginning on days −7 and −2 pretransplant (or at the time conditioning therapy for transplantation is begun), then weekly through day 90 post-transplant. Gamimune N, 5% should be administered by itself through a Hickman line while it is in place, and thereafter through a peripheral vein. Please see DOSAGE AND ADMINISTRATION for other drug interactions.

Pediatric HIV Infection

A reduction in bacterial infections has been observed in children infected with HIV-1 receiving Gamimune N, 5% 400 mg/kg (8 mL/kg) body weight every 28 days.

HOW SUPPLIED

Immune Globulin Intravenous (Human), 5%—Gamimune® N, 5% is supplied in the following sizes:

Size	Grams Protein
10 mL	0.5
50 mL	2.5
100 mL	5.0
250 mL	12.5

STORAGE

Store at 2–8°C (36–46°F). Do not freeze. Do not use after expiration date.

CAUTION

U.S. federal law prohibits dispensing without prescription.

LIMITED WARRANTY

A number of factors beyond our control could reduce the efficacy of this product or even result in an ill effect following its use. These include improper storage and handling of the product after it leaves our hands, diagnosis, dosage, method of administration, and biological differences in individual patients. Because of these factors, it is important that this product be stored properly and that the directions be followed carefully during use.

No warranty, express or implied, including any warranty of merchantability or fitness is made. Representatives of the Company are not authorized to vary the terms or the contents of the printed labeling, including the package insert for this product, except by printed notice from the Company's headquarters. The prescriber and user of this product must accept the terms hereof.

REFERENCES

1. Tenold RA, inventor; Cutter Laboratories, assignee. Intravenously injectable immune serum globulin. U.S. Patent 4,396,608 August 2, 1983.
2. Data on file at Miles Inc.
3. Pirofsky B, Campbell SM, Montanaro A: Individual patient variations in the kinetics of intravenous immunoglobulin administration. *J Clin Immunol* 2 (2):7S–14S, 1982.
4. Pirofsky B: Intravenous immune globulin therapy in hypogammaglobulinemia. *Amer J Med* 76(3A): 53–60, 1984.
5. Pirofsky B, Anderson CJ, Bardana EJ Jr.: Therapeutic and detrimental effects of intravenous immunoglobulin therapy. In: Alving BM (ed.): *Immunoglobulins: characteristics and uses of intravenous preparations.* Washington, D.C., U.S. Government Printing Office (1980), pp 15–22.
6. Sullivan KM, Kopecky KJ, Jocom J, et al: Immunomodulatory and antimicrobial efficacy of intravenous immunoglobulin in bone marrow transplantation. *N Engl J Med* 323(11):705–12, 1990.
7. Bernstein LJ, Ochs HD, Wedgwood RJ, et al: Defective humoral immunity in pediatric acquired immune deficiency syndrome. *J Pediatr* 107(3):352–7, 1985.
8. Borkowsky W, Steele CJ, Grubman S, et al: Antibody responses to bacterial toxoids in children infected with human immunodeficiency virus. *J Pediatr* 110(4):563–6, 1987.
9. Blanche S, Le Deist F, Fischer A, et al: Longitudinal study of 18 children with perinatal LAV/HTLV III infection: attempt at prognostic evaluation. *J Pediatr* 109(6):965–70, 1986.
10. Pahwa S, Fikrig S, Menez R, et al: Pediatric acquired immunodeficiency syndrome demonstration of B-lymphocyte defects in vitro. *Diagn Immunol* 4(1):24–30, 1986.
11. Bernstein LJ, Krieger BZ, Novick B, et al: Bacterial infections in the acquired immunodeficiency syndrome of children. *Pediatr Infect Dis* 4(5):472–5, 1985.
12. Krasinski K, Borkowsky W, Bonk S, et al: Bacterial infections in human immunodeficiency virus-infected children. *Pediatr Infect Dis J* 4(5):323–8, 1988.
13. Scott GB, Buck BE, Leterman JG, et al: Acquired immunodeficiency syndrome in infants. *N Engl J Med* 310(2):76–81, 1984.
14. Mofenson LM, Willoughby A. Passive immunization. In: Pizzo PA, Wilfert CM, (eds.) *Pediatric AIDS: the challenge of HIV infection in infants, children and adolescents.* Baltimore: Williams & Wilkins (1991) pp 633–50.
15. National Institute of Child Health and Human Development Intravenous Immunoglobulin Study Group. Intravenous immune globulin for the prevention of bacterial infections in children with symptomatic human and immunodeficiency virus infection. *N Engl J Med* 325(2):73–80, 1991.
16. Mofenson LM, Moye J Jr, Bethel J, et al: Prophylactic intravenous immunoglobulin in HIV-infected children with CD4+counts of 0.20×10^9/L or more. Effect on viral, opportunistic, and bacterial infections, *JAMA* 268(4):483–88, 1992.
17. Berg G, Matzkies F: Wirkung von Maltose nach intravenöser Dauerinfusion auf den Stoffwechsel. *Z Ernährungswiss* 15:255–62, 1976.
18. Förster H, Hoos I, Boecker S: Versuche mit Probanden zur parenteralen Verwertung von Maltose. *Z Ernährungswiss* 15(3):284–93, 1976.
19. Finke C, Reinauer H: Utilization of maltose and oligosaccharides after intravenous infusion in man. *Nutr Metab* 21(Suppl 1):115–7, 1977.
20. Young EA, Drummond A, Cioletti L, et al: Metabolism of continuously infused intravenous maltose. [abstract] *Clin Res* 925(3):543A, 1977.
21. Soroff HS, Hansen LM, Sasvary D, et al: Clinical pharmacology and metabolism of maltose in normal human volunteers. *Clin Res* [abstract] 26(3):286A, 1978.
22. Guyton AC: *Textbook of Medical Physiology.* 5th ed. Philadelphia, W.B. Saunders Company, 1976, pp 499–500.
23. Buckley RH: Immunoglobulin replacement therapy: indications and contraindications for use and variable IgG levels achieved. In: Alving BM (ed.): *Immunoglobulins: characteristics and uses of intravenous preparations.* Washington, D.C., U.S. Government Printing Office (1980), pp 3–8.
24. Nolte MT, Pirofsky B, Gerritz GA, et al: Intravenous immunoglobulin therapy for antibody deficiency. *Clin Exp Immunol* 36:237–43, 1979.
25. Ochs HD: Intravenous immunoglobulin therapy of patients with primary immunodeficiency syndromes: efficacy and safety of a new modified immune globulin preparation. In: Alving BM (ed.): *Immunoglobulins: characteristics and uses of intravenous preparations.* Washington, D.C., U.S. Government Printing Office (1980), pp 9–14.
26. Sekul E, Cupler E, Dalakas M. Aseptic meningitis associated with high-dose intravenous immunoglobulin therapy: Frequency and risk factors. *Ann Int Med* 121:259–262, 1994.
27. Kato E, Shindo S, Eto Y, Hashimoto N, Yamamoto M, Sakata Y, Hiyoshi Y. Administration of Immune Globulin Associated with Aseptic Meningitis. *JAMA* 259(22):3269–3270, 1988.
28. Casteels-Van Daele M, Wijndaele L, Hunninck K, Gillis P. Intravenous immune globulin and acute aseptic meningitis. *N Engl J Med* 323(9):614–615, 1990.
29. Scribner C, Kapit R, Phillips E, Rickles N. Aseptic meningitis and intravenous immunoglobulin therapy. *Ann Intern Med* 121(4):305–306, 1994
30. Peerless AG, Stiehm ER: Intravenous gammaglobulin for reaction to intramuscular preparation. [letter] *Lancet* 2(8347):461, 1983.

Shown in Product Identification Guide, page 305

GAMIMUNE N, 10% ℞

Immune Globulin Intravenous (Human), 10%
Gamimune® N, 10%

DESCRIPTION

Immune Globulin Intravenous (Human), 10%—Gamimune® N, 10% is a sterile solution of human protein containing no preservative. Gamimune N, 10% consists of 9%–11% protein in 0.16–0.24 M glycine. Not less than 98% of the protein has the electrophoretic mobility of gamma globulin. Not less than 90% of the IgG is monomer. Also present are traces of IgA and IgM. The distribution of IgG subclasses is similar to that found in normal serum. The measured buffer capacity is 35 mEq/L and the osmolality is 274 mOsmol/kg solvent.

The product is made by cold ethanol fractionation of large pools of human plasma. Part of the fractionation may be performed by another licensed manufacturer. The immunoglobulin is isolated from Cohn effluent III by diafiltration and ultrafiltration. The protein has not been chemically modified other than in the adjustment of the pH of the solution to 4.0–4.5.[1] Isotonicity is achieved by the addition of glycine. The product is intended for intravenous administration.

CLINICAL PHARMACOLOGY

Primary Humoral Immunodeficiency

Gamimune N, 10% supplies a broad spectrum of opsonic and neutralizing IgG antibodies for the prevention or attenuation of a wide variety of infectious diseases. Since Gamimune N, 10% is administered intravenously, essentially 100% of the infused IgG antibodies are immediately available in the recipient's circulation.[2] Studies using a modified intravenous immunoglobulin at pH 6.8 have shown that approximately 30% of the infused IgG disappeared from the circulation in the first 24 hours, due primarily to equilibration of the IgG between the plasma and the extravascular space.[2–5] A further decline to about 40% of the peak level found immediately post-infusion is to be expected during the first week.[2–5] The in vivo half-life of Immune Globulin Intravenous (Human), 5%—Gamimune® N, 5% equals or exceeds the 3-week half-life reported for IgG in the literature, but individual patient variation in half-life has been observed.[2] Thus, this variable as well as the amount of immune globulin administered per dose is important in determining the frequency of administration of the drug for each individual patient. A comparative study of Gamimune N, 10% with Gamimune N, 5% (in 10% maltose) in 18 subjects demonstrated equivalent post-infusion recovery for the two preparations.

Idiopathic Thrombocytopenic Purpura

While Immune Globulin Intravenous (Human), 10%—Gaminune® N, 10% has been shown to be effective in some cases of idiopathic thrombocytopenic Purpura (ITP) (see INDICATIONS AND USAGE), the mechanism of action has not been fully elucidated.

Bone Marrow Transplantation

Clinical studies with Gamimune N, 5% have shown that it is effective in bone marrow transplant patients ≥ 20 years of age in the first 100 days posttransplant for the following: prevention of systemic and local infections, interstitial pneumonia of infectious and idiopathic etiologies and acute graft-versus-host disease (AGVHD)[6] (see INDICATIONS AND USAGE). Administration of Gamimune N, 5% to bone marrow transplant patients significantly increased IgG and IgG subclass levels while those seen in the control group fell below predicted levels. The mechanism of action of Immune Globulin Intravenous (Human), 5% — Gamimune ® N, 5% in reducing the incidence of AGVHD is presently unknown.

Pediatric HIV Infection

Children infected with human immunodeficiency virus (HIV) may display defects in both cellular and humoral immunity.[7–10] As a result, some children with HIV-1 infection experience serious, potentially life-threatening recurrent bacterial infections.[11–13] In one retrospective report, among 71 HIV-infected children observed over 3.5 years, 27 (37%) experienced serious documented bacterial infections.[12] The types of bacterial and viral infections observed in HIV-infected children are similar to those seen in children with primary hypogammaglobulinemia.[14] The replacement of opsonic and neutralizing IgG antibodies has been shown to reduce serious and minor bacterial infection in HIV-infected children.[15,16]

In a randomized, double-blind, placebo-controlled, multicenter study performed between March 7, 1988 and January 15, 1991, the efficacy of Gamimune N, 5% in pediatric HIV disease to decrease the frequency of serious and minor bacterial infections and the frequency of hospitalization, and to increase the time free of serious bacterial infection was documented in children with clinical or immunologic evidence of HIV disease (see INDICATIONS AND USAGE). The primary endpoint of this study was prospectively defined as a significant reduction in the proportion of subjects who develop at least one serious bacterial infection when compared to the control group of HIV-infected children who received placebo. Serious bacterial infections were defined as laboratory-proven and clinically diagnosed (i.e., radiologically proven acute pneumonia and sinusitis) infections. The Data Safety and Monitoring Board (DSMB) recommended early termination of the study based on data presented to them from an interim analysis in December 1990 which showed that treatment with Gamimune N, 5% increased the time free from serious infections in children with CD4+ counts ≥ 200/mm^3.

General

Glycine (aminoacetic acid) is a nonessential amino acid normally present in the body.[17] Glycine is a major ingredient in amino acid solutions employed in intravenous alimentation.[18] While toxic effects of glycine administration have been reported,[19] the doses and rates of administration were 3–4-fold greater than those for Gaminune N, 10%.

The buffer capacity of Gamimune N, 10% is 35.0 mEq/L (≃ 0.35 mEq/g protein). A dose of 1,000 mg/kg body weight therefore represents an acid load of 0.35 mEq/kg body weight. The total buffering capacity of whole blood in a normal individual is 45–50 mEq/L of blood, or 3.6 mEq/kg body weight.[20] Thus, the acid load delivered with a dose of 1000 mg/kg of Gamimune N, 10% would be neutralized by the

Continued on next page

Bayer Biological—Cont.

buffering capacity of whole blood alone, even if the dose were infused instantaneously.

In Phase I human studies comparing Gamimune N, 10% with Immune Globulin Intravenous (Human), 5%—Gamimune® N, 5% (in 10% maltose), venous blood measurements were taken following the intravenous administration of 400 mg/kg body weight in 18 patients. There were no clinically important changes in mean venous pH, bicarbonate, or base excess measurements in these patients receiving either preparation.[2]

In a similar, earlier Phase I study Gamimune N, 5% (in 10% maltose) was compared with a chemically modified 5% intravenous immunoglobulin preparation with a pH of 6.8. No clinically important changes in mean venous pH and bicarbonate measurements were detected following infusions of either preparation at doses of 400 mg/kg body weight in 37 patients.

In patients with limited or compromised acid-base compensatory mechanisms, consideration should be given to the effect of the additional acid load Gamimune N, 10% might present.

INDICATIONS AND USAGE

Primary Humoral Immunodeficiency

Gamimune N, 10% is efficacious in the treatment of primary immunodeficiency states in which severe impairment of antibody forming capacity has been shown, such as: congenital agammaglobulinemias, common variable immunodeficiency, Wiskott-Aldrich syndrome, x-linked immunodeficiency with hyper IgM, and severe combined immunodeficiencies.[5,21–23] Gamimune N, 10% is especially useful when high levels or rapid elevation of circulating antibodies are desired or when intramuscular injections are contraindicated.

Idiopathic Thrombocytopenic Purpura (ITP)

In clinical situations in which a rapid rise in platelet count is needed to control bleeding or to allow a patient with ITP to undergo surgery, administration of Gamimune N, 10% should be considered. Studies with Gamimune N, 5% demonstrate that in patients in whom a response was achieved, the rise of platelets was generally rapid (within 1–5 days), transient (most often lasting from several days to several weeks) and were not considered curative. It is presently not possible to predict which patients with ITP will respond to therapy, although the increase in platelet counts in children seems to be better than that in adults. Childhood ITP may, however, respond spontaneously without treatment.

Immune Globulin Intravenous (Human), 10%—Gamimune® N, 10% has been studied in 31 adult and pediatric subjects with ITP using a dosage of 1,000 mg/kg body weight on either 1 day or 2 consecutive days. Fourteen of 16 children (87.5%) and 9 of 10 adults with platelet follow-up (90%) responded to treatment with clinically significant platelet increments of ≥30,000/mm^3. In the 12 children with acute ITP, there was an average increase in platelet count above baseline of 274,000/mm^3 (range 33,000–529,000/mm^3).

Two different dosing regimens of Immune Globulin Intravenous (Human), 5%—Gamimune® N, 5% have been studied in clinical investigations; a regimen consisting of 400 mg/kg body weight daily for 5 consecutive days, and a high dose treatment regimen consisting of 1,000 mg/kg body weight administered on either 1 day or 2 consecutive days (these studies are summarized below).

In clinical studies of Gamimune N, 5%, five of six (83.3%) children and 12 of 16 (75%) adults with acute or chronic ITP treated with 400 mg/kg body weight for 5 consecutive days demonstrated clinically significant platelet increments of ≥30,000/mm^3 over baseline. The mean platelet count in children with ITP rose from 27,800/mm^3 at baseline to 297,000/mm^3 (range 50,000–455,000/mm^3) and the mean platelet count in adults with ITP rose from 27,900/mm^3 at baseline to 124,900/mm^3 (range 11,000–341,000/mm^3). Two of three children with acute ITP rapidly went into complete remission.

Thirteen of 14 children (92.9%) and 26 of 29 adults (89.7%) with acute or chronic ITP treated with Gamimune N, 5% 1,000 mg/kg body weight administered on either 1 day or 2 consecutive days responded to treatment with clinically significant platelet increments of ≥30,000/mm^3 over baseline. This included three of three patients with ITP that were human immunodeficiency virus (HIV) antibody positive and two of two patients with ITP that were pregnant. The mean platelet count in children with ITP treated with Gamimune N, 5% 1,000 mg/kg body weight on 1 day or 2 consecutive days rose from 44,400/mm^3 at baseline to 285,600/mm^3 (range 89,000–473,000/mm^3) and the mean platelet count in adults with ITP treated with the regimen rose from 23,400/mm^3 at baseline to 173,100/mm^3 (range 28,000–709,000/mm^3). Two patients, one each with acute adult and chronic childhood ITP, entered complete remission with treatment.

Six of the 29 adult patients with ITP received Gamimune N, 5% 1,000 mg/kg on 1 day or 2 consecutive days to increase the platelet count prior to splenectomy. Mean platelet counts rose from 14,500/mm^3 at baseline to 129,300/mm^3 (range 51,000–242,000/mm^3) prior to surgery.

The duration of the platelet rise following treatment of ITP with either treatment regimen of Gamimune N, 5% was variable, ranging from several days to 12 months or more. Some ITP patients have demonstrated continuing responsiveness over many months to intermittent infusions of Immune Globulin Intravenous (Human), 5%—Gamimune® N, 5% 400–1,000 mg/kg body weight, administered as a single maintenance dose, at intervals as indicated by the platelet count.

Bone Marrow Transplantation (BMT)

In clinical studies in bone marrow transplant patients ≥ 20 years of age, Gamimune N, 5% decreased the risk of septicemia and other infections, interstitial pneumonia of infectious or idiopathic etiologies and acute graft-versus-host disease (AGVHD) in the first 100 days posttransplant. Immune Globulin Intravenous (Human), 5% — Gamimune® N, 5% is not indicated in bone marrow transplant patients below 20 years of age. In a controlled study of 369 evaluable BMT patients (184 treated and 185 controls) who either did or did not receive Gamimune N, 5% in doses of 500 mg/kg body weight on days −7 and −2 pretransplant, then weekly through day 90 posttransplant, posttransplant complications were evaluated in the entire study group and in patients under age 20 and age 20 or older. For patients ≥ 20 years of age (128 patients in the control group and 119 patients in the treated group), there was a statistically significant reduction in interstitial pneumonia from 21% in the control group to 9% in the treated group (p=0.0032) during the first 100 days posttransplant. Also significantly reduced in this age group were: overall septicemia from 53 infections in the 128 patient control group to 26 infections in the 119 patient treated group (relative risk control:treated [RR] 2.36, p=0.0025); gram-negative septicemia from 24 infections in the 128 patient control group to 9 infections in the 119 patient treated group (RR 2.53, p=0.015); gram-positive septicemia from 16 infections in the 128 patient control group to 8 infections in the 119 patient treated group (RR 2.73, p=0.046); and Grade II to IV AGVHD from an incidence of 58 of 110 in the control group to 38 of 108 in the treated group (p=0.0051).

The given p-values do not take into account multiple endpoints and subset analyses. Therefore, some of the p-values could occur by chance alone. There was no significant improvement in overall mortality in this study.

In patients below age 20, there appeared to be no benefit from treatment with Gamimune N, 5%, either in reducing the incidence of infections or the incidence of AGVHD.

Pediatric HIV Infection

Gamimune N, 5% 400 mg/kg every 28 days significantly decreased the frequency of serious and minor bacterial infections (laboratory-proven and clinically diagnosed) and the frequency of hospitalization, and increased the time free of serious bacterial infection. The effect of Gamimune N, 5% in preventing serious bacterial infections was especially apparent in preventing primary bacteremia (including *Streptococcus pneumoniae* bacteremia) and acute pneumonia.

In a randomized, double-blind, placebo-controlled, multicenter study, 394 HIV-infected, non-hemophilic, children less than 13 years of age were randomized. Of the children randomized, 369 were included in the efficacy analysis and 376 in the safety analysis. The study population had 1) a mean age of 40 months (range 2.4–136.8 months), 2) acquired HIV primarily through vertical transmission (91%), 3) a majority (87%) of CDC Class P-2 (symptomatic), and 4) had a median CD4+ count of 937 cells/mm^3 (range 0–6660 cells/mm^3). At the time of study entry, 14% (52 of 369) were receiving *Pneumocystis carinii* pneumonia (PCP) prophylaxis. During the course of the study, 51% (189 of 369) received PCP prophylaxis and 44% (164 of 369) received zidovudine (ZDV). Children with HIV-1 infection were initially stratified into two groups based upon CD4+ count (< 200 cells/mm^3 versus ≥ 200 cells/mm^3) and CDC classification of pediatric HIV disease (history of opportunistic infections [P-2-D-1] and recurrent serious bacterial infections [P-2-D-2] versus others). Subjects received Gamimune N, 5% (400 mg/kg = 8 mL/kg) (n=185) or an equivalent volume of placebo (0.1% Albumin [Human]) (n=184) every 28 days. The mean follow-up for subjects receiving Gamimune N, 5% was 17.9 months and 17.8 months for patients on placebo.

The number of subjects who had at least one serious bacterial infection was 86 of 184 (47%) in the placebo group and 55 of 185 (30%) in the Gamimune N, 5% group (p=0.0009). All p-values reported are two-sided. Treatment with Gamimune N, 5% compared to placebo was also associated with a significant reduction in both the number of subjects with at least one laboratory-proven infection (36 of 184 vs. 18 of 185, p=0.0081), and the number of subjects with at least one clinically diagnosed infection (71 of 184 vs. 45 of 185, p=0.0036). Efficacy in patients with CD4+ counts < 200/mm^3 was not established, possibly because of the small number of subjects in this category.

The 2-year treatment period defined in the protocol was truncated for some patients by the DSMB based on data from the interim analysis. Rates of serious bacterial infections per 100 patient-years were computed and analyzed to take into account both the unequal duration of treatment and follow-up, as well as recurrent infections in individual subjects. Children treated with Immune Globulin Intravenous (Human), 5% — Gamimune® N, 5% experienced a 50.5% lower frequency of laboratory-proven serious bacterial infection compared to the group treated with placebo (9.1 vs. 18.2 infections per 100 patient-years, p=0.031), a 36.0% lower frequency of clinically diagnosed serious infections (24.0 vs. 37.5 infections per 100 patient-years, p=0.013), a 40.6% reduction in total serious infections (laboratory-proven and clinically diagnosed) (33.1 vs. 55.7 infections per 100 patient-years, p=0.003), a 60% lower frequency of primary bacteremias (5.8 vs. 14.5 infections per 100 patient-years, p=0.009), a 75.6% lower frequency of *Streptococcus pneumoniae* bacteremia (1.1 vs. 4.5 bacteremias per 100 patient-years, p=0.026), a 54.3% lower frequency of clinically diagnosed pneumonia (12.7 vs. 27.8 infections per 100 patient-years, p=0.001), and a 22.5% lower frequency of minor bacterial infections (including otitis media, skin and soft tissue infections, and upper respiratory tract infections) (123.6 vs. 159.5 infections per 100 patient-years, p=0.033).

In addition to a reduced frequency of infection, children treated with Gamimune N, 5% had a 36.8% lower number of hospitalizations per 100 patient-years (72 vs. 114 per 100 patient-years, p=0.002) and a reduced number of hospital days (6.9 vs. 10.5 per patient-year, p=0.030) than patients treated with placebo. Patients treated with Gamimune N, 5% had a higher probability of remaining free of laboratory-proven infections (p=0.0093) and combined laboratory-proven and clinically diagnosed infections (p=0.0015) for 24 months than the group of children treated with placebo. At 24 months, the estimated probabilities of remaining infection-free for the Gamimune N, 5% and placebo arms were 87.8% vs. 76.1%, respectively, for laboratory-proven infections and 63.5% vs. 44.5%, respectively, for combined laboratory-proven and clinically diagnosed infections.

There was no effect of Gamimune N, 5% therapy on mortality, which was low in both treatment groups (17%), or on the frequency of opportunistic or viral infections during the period of study.

Since antibacterial prophylaxis could also account for the observed reduction in the rate of serious bacterial infections, further analysis was performed to evaluate the role of *Pneumocystis carinii* pneumonia (PCP) prophylaxis on the efficacy of Gamimune N, 5%. PCP prophylaxis consisted primarily (96%) of trimethoprim/sulfamethoxazole given 3 successive days each week. This antibiotic combination could be active against the bacteria commonly encountered in this patient population. In the subgroup of patients receiving PCP prophylaxis at study entry, treatment with Gamimune N, 5% was associated with 44.0 infections per 100 patient-years, whereas placebo recipients had 64.7 infections per 100 patient-years (p=0.047). In the subgroup of patients not receiving PCP prophylaxis at study entry, treatment with Gamimune N, 5% was associated with 22.1 infections per 100 patient-years, whereas placebo recipients had 44.9 infections per 100 patient-years on placebo (p=0.024). Thus, Gamimune N, 5% benefitted patients by reducing the rate of serious bacterial infections whether or not they were receiving PCP prophylactic treatment at study entry. However, it should be noted that the use of PCP prophylactic treatment in this study was not randomized and specific guidelines for its administration were not identified.

CONTRAINDICATIONS

Immune Globulin Intravenous (Human), 10%—Gamimune® N, 10% is contraindicated in individuals who are known to have had an anaphylactic or severe systemic response to Immune Globulin (Human). Individuals with selective IgA deficiencies who have known antibody against IgA (anti-IgA antibody) should not receive Gamimune N, 10% since these patients may experience severe reactions to the IgA which may be present.[22]

WARNINGS

Gamimune N, 10% should be administered only intravenously as the intramuscular and subcutaneous routes have not been evaluated.

Gamimune N, 5% has, on rare occasions, caused a precipitous fall in blood pressure and a clinical picture of anaphylaxis, even when the patient is not known to be sensitive to immune globulin preparations. These reactions may be related to the rate of infusion. Accordingly, the infusion rate given under DOSAGE AND ADMINISTRATION for Gamimune N, 10% should be closely followed, at least until the physician has had sufficient experience with a given patient. The patient's vital signs should be monitored continuously and careful observation made for any symptoms throughout the entire infusion. Epinephrine should be available for the treatment of an acute anaphylactic reaction.

PRECAUTIONS

General

Any vial that has been entered should be used promptly. Partially used vials should be discarded. Do not use if turbid. Solution which has been frozen should not be used.

An aseptic meningitis syndrome (AMS) has been reported to occur infrequently in association with Immune Globulin Intravenous (Human) treatment. The syndrome usually begins within several hours to two days following Immune Globulin Intravenous (Human) treatment. It is characterized by symptoms and signs including severe headache, nuchal rigidity, drowsiness, fever, photophobia, painful eye movements, and nausea and vomiting. Cerebrospinal fluid studies are frequently positive with pleocytosis up to several thousand cells per mm^3, predominantly from the granulocytic series, and elevated protein levels up to several hundred mg/dL. Patients exhibiting such symptoms and signs should receive a thorough neurological examination, including CSF studies, to rule out other causes of meningitis. AMS may occur more frequently in association with high dose (2 g/kg) Immune Globulin Intravenous (Human) treatment. Discontinuation of Immune Globulin Intravenous (Human) treatment has resulted in remission of AMS within several days without sequelae.[24–27]

Drug Interactions

Antibodies in Gamimune N, 10% may interfere with the response to live viral vaccines such as measles, mumps and rubella. Therefore, use of such vaccines should be deferred until approximately 6 months after Gamimune N, 10% administration.

Please see DOSAGE AND ADMINISTRATION for other drug interactions.

Pregnancy Category C

Animal reproduction studies have not been conducted with Gamimune N, 10%. It is not known whether Gamimune N, 10% can cause fetal harm when administered to a pregnant woman or can affect reproduction capacity. Gamimune N, 10% should be given to a pregnant woman only if clearly needed.

ADVERSE REACTIONS

Primary Humoral Immunodeficiency

A safety study has been conducted in 20 adult and pediatric subjects with primary immunodeficiency syndrome comparing side effects of Immune Globulin Intravenous (Human), 5%—Gamimune® N, 5% with those of Immune Globulin Intravenous (Human), 10%—Gamimune® N, 10%. The incidence, nature, or severity of reactions with Gamimune N, 10% were not different from those observed with Gamimune N, 5%, and were consistent with those observed in previous studies with Gamimune N, 5%. Symptoms related to the infusion of Gamimune N, 10% were observed in 9 (3.5%) of 255 infusions. These symptoms were all mild to moderate in severity and included chills, fever, headache and emesis.

In a study of 37 patients with immunodeficiency syndromes receiving Gamimune N, 5% in a monthly dose of 400 mg/kg body weight, reactions were seen in 5.2% of the infusions. Symptoms reported included malaise, a feeling of faintness, fever, chills, headache, nausea, vomiting, chest tightness, dyspnea and chest, back or hip pain. Mild erythema following infiltration of Gamimune N, 5% at the infusion site was reported in some cases.

Idiopathic Thrombocytopenic Purpura

An investigation of Gamimune N, 10% in 31 adult and pediatric subjects with ITP encountered side effects in 17 of 119 (14.3%) infusions. The dosage in these studies was 1,000 mg/kg body weight for 1 day or 2 consecutive days. However, in the adult study, an induction dosage of 500 mg/kg body weight for 1 day or 2 consecutive days was associated with 17 of these infusions. Of those 17 infusions, three had adverse events. Overall, side effects included mild chest pain, mild and moderate emesis, moderate fever, mild or moderate headache (severe on one occasion) and a single incidence of hives, pruritus and rash. At least 17 of the 50 infusions in the pediatric study were given at rates of ≥0.1 mL/kg body weight per minute as part of a rate escalation investigation. Maximum infusion rates obtained were not limited by or interrupted due to adverse effects.

In studies of Gamimune N, 5% administered at a dose of 400 mg/kg body weight in the treatment of adult and pediatric patients with ITP, systemic reactions were noted in only 4 of 154 (2.6%) infusions, and all but one occurred at rates of infusion greater than 0.04 mL/kg body weight per minute. The symptoms reported included chest tightness, a sense of tachycardia (pulse was 84 beats per minute), and a burning sensation in the head; these symptoms were all mild and transient.

In studies of Gamimune N, 5% administered at a dose of 1,000 mg/kg body weight either as a single dose or as two doses on consecutive days in the treatment of adult and pediatric patients with ITP, adverse reactions were noted in 25 of 251 (10%) infusions. Symptoms reported included headache, nausea, fever, chills, back pain, chest tightness, and shortness of breath. In children, the high dose regimen has been well-tolerated at the highest rates of infusion. In adults, however, the frequency of adverse reactions tended to increase with infusion rates in excess of 0.06 mL/kg body weight per minute. In general, reactions reported with infusion of Immune Globulin Intravenous (Human), 5%—Gamimune® N, 5% in these studies were reported as mild or moderate, and responded to slowing of the infusion rate.

Bone Marrow Transplantation

In studies of Gamimune N, 5% administered to 185 bone marrow transplant recipients at doses of 500 mg/kg (10 mL/kg) body weight on day −7 and day −2 pretransplant, then weekly through day 90 posttransplant, adverse reactions were noted in 12 (6.5%) of the 185 patients that received Gamimune N, 5% and in 14 (0.6%) of 2,176 infusions. All reactions reported were rate-related and classified as mild. Chills were the most common symptom reported, occurring in nine patients. The other symptoms reported included headache, flushing, fever, pruritus and slight back discomfort. All reactions resolved satisfactorily, usually without treatment or decreasing the infusion rate.

Pediatric HIV Infection

Three hundred seventy-six (376) patients, 187 treated with Gamimune N, 5% and 189 treated with placebo (0.1% Albumin [Human]), were included in the safety analysis. Adverse reactions occurred during or within 24 hours of an infusion in 50 of 3,451 (1.4%) infusions of Gamimune N, 5% and 62 of 3,447 (1.8%) infusions of placebo. Fever was the most common adverse reaction and occurred in 30 of 105 (28.6%) patients receiving placebo and 19 of 78 (24.4%) patients treated with Gamimune N, 5%. Irritability was the second most common symptom reported, with 10 of 105 (9.5%) reports for the placebo group and 9 of 78 (11.5%) for the group treated with Gamimune N, 5%. A large number of diverse adverse reactions accounted for the remaining adverse reactions reported in both study groups. In general, the number of adverse events reported was comparable in both the placebo and Gamimune N, 5% treated groups. Three serious adverse reactions were reported. One patient experienced a hypersensitivity reaction and did not receive further Gamimune N, 5% treatment. A second patient developed tachycardia and was admitted to an intensive care unit, but later continued treatment with Gamimune N, 5%. A third patient had skin infiltration during infusion and developed a full thickness skin slough over the dorsum of the hand that required skin grafting.

General

In the studies undertaken to date, other types of reactions have not been reported with Gamimune N, 5% or Gamimune N, 10%. It may be, however, that adverse effects will be similar to those previously reported with intravenous and intramuscular immunoglobulin administration. Potential reactions, therefore, may also include anxiety, flushing, wheezing, abdominal cramps, myalgias, arthralgia, and dizziness; rash has been reported only rarely. Reactions to intravenous immunoglobulin tend to be related to the rate of infusion.

True anaphylactic reactions to Immune Globulin Intravenous (Human), 10%—Gamimune® N, 10% may occur in recipients with documented prior histories of severe allergic reactions to intramuscular immunoglobulin, but some patients may tolerate cautiously administered intravenous immunoglobulin without adverse effects.[2,28] Very rarely an anaphylactoid reaction may occur in patients with no prior history of severe allergic reactions to either intramuscular or intravenous immunoglobulin.[2]

DOSAGE AND ADMINISTRATION

General

Dosages for specific indications are indicated below, but in general, it is recommended that Gamimune N, 10% be infused by itself at a rate of 0.01 to 0.02 mL/kg body weight per minute for 30 minutes; if well-tolerated, the rate may be **gradually** increased to a maximum of 0.08 mL/kg body weight per minute. Investigations indicate that Gamimune N, 10% is well-tolerated and less likely to produce side effects when infused at the indicated rate. If side effects occur, the rate may be reduced, or the infusion interrupted until symptoms subside. The infusion may then be resumed at the rate which is comfortable for the patient. Parenteral drug products should be inspected visually for particulate matter and discoloration prior to administration, whenever solution and container permit.

It is recommended that infusion of Gamimune N, 10% be given by a separate line, by itself, without mixing with other intravenous fluids or medications the patient might be receiving. Gamimune N, 10% should not be mixed with Immune Globulin Intravenous (Human) from another manufacturer. Gamimune N, 10% is not compatible with saline. If dilution is required, Gamimune N, 10% may be diluted with 5% dextrose in water (D5/W). No other drug interactions or compatibilities have been evaluated.

Primary Humoral Immunodeficiency

The usual dosage of Gamimune N, 10% for prophylaxis in primary immunodeficiency syndromes is 100–200 mg/kg of body weight administered approximately once a month by intravenous infusion. The dosage may be given more frequently or increased as high as 400 mg/kg body weight, if the clinical response is inadequate, or the level of IgG achieved in the circulation is felt to be insufficient. The minimum level of IgG required for protection has not been determined.

Idiopathic Thrombocytopenic Purpura (ITP)

Induction: An increase in platelet count has been observed in children and some adults with acute or chronic ITP receiving Gamimune N, 5% 400 mg/kg body weight daily for 5 days. Alternatively, studies in adults and children with Gamimune N, 5% and Gamimune N, 10% using a dose of 1,000 mg/kg body weight daily for 1 day or 2 consecutive days have also shown increases in platelet count. In the latter treatment regimen, if an adequate increase in the platelet count is observed at 24 hours, the second dose of 1,000 mg/kg body weight may be withheld. The high dose régimen (1,000 mg/kg × 1–2 days) is not recommended for individuals with expanded fluid volumes or where fluid volume may be a concern. With both treatment regimens, a response usually occurs within several days and is maintained for a variable period of time. In general, a response is seen less often in adults than in children.

Maintenance: In adults and children with ITP, if after induction therapy the platelet count falls to less than 30,000/mm^3 and/or the patient manifests clinically significant bleeding, Immune Globulin Intravenous (Human), 10%—Gamimune® N, 10% 400 mg/kg body weight may be given as a single infusion. If an adequate response does not result, the dose can be increased to 800–1,000 mg/kg of body weight given as a single infusion. Maintenance infusions may be administered intermittently as clinically indicated to maintain a platelet count greater than 30,000/mm^3.

Bone Marrow Transplantation

A reduction in posttransplant complications has been observed in bone marrow transplant patients ≥ 20 years of age receiving Gamimune N, 5%. An equivalent dosage of Gamimune N, 10% is recommended in doses of 500 mg/kg (5 mL/kg) body weight beginning on days −7 and −2 pretransplant (or at the time conditioning therapy for transplantation is begun), then weekly through day 90 posttransplant. Gamimune N, 10% should be administered by itself through a Hickman line while it is in place, and thereafter through a peripheral vein. Please see DOSAGE AND ADMINISTRATION for other drug interactions.

Pediatric HIV Infection

A reduction in bacterial infections has been observed in children infected with HIV-1 receiving Immune Globulin Intravenous (Human), 5% — Gamimune® N, 5%. An equivalent dosage of Immune Globulin Intravenous (Human), 10% — Gamimune® N, 10% is recommended in doses of 400 mg/kg (4 mL/kg) body weight every 28 days.

HOW SUPPLIED

Gamimune N, 10% is supplied in the following sizes:

Size	Grams Protein
10 mL	1.0
50 mL	5.0
100 mL	10.0
200 mL	20.0

STORAGE

Store at 2–8°C (36–46°F). Do not freeze. Do not use after expiration date.

CAUTION

U.S. federal law prohibits dispensing without prescription.

LIMITED WARRANTY

A number of factors beyond our control could reduce the efficacy of this product or even result in an ill effect following its use. These include improper storage and handling of the product after it leaves our hands, diagnosis, dosage, method of administration, and biological differences in individual patients. Because of these factors, it is important that this product be stored properly and that the directions be followed carefully during use.

No warranty, express or implied, including any warranty of merchantability or fitness is made. Representatives of the Company are not authorized to vary the terms or the contents of the printed labeling, including the package insert for this product, except by printed notice from the Company's headquarters. The prescriber and user of this product must accept the terms hereof.

REFERENCES

1. Tenold RA, inventor; Cutter Laboratories, assignee. Intravenously injectable immune serum globulin. U.S. Patent 4,396,608, Aug. 2, 1983.
2. Data on file at Miles Inc.
3. Pirofsky B, Campbell SM, Montanaro A: Individual patient variations in the kinetics of intravenous immunoglobulin administration. *J Clin Immunol* 2(2): 7S–14S, 1982.
4. Pirofsky B: Intravenous immune globulin therapy in hypogammaglobulinemia. *Amer J Med* 76(3A): 53–60, 1984.
5. Pirofsky B, Anderson CJ, Bardana EJ Jr.: Therapeutic and detrimental effects of intravenous immunoglobulin therapy. In: Alving BM (ed.): *Immunoglobulins: characteristics and uses of intravenous preparations.* Washing-

Continued on next page

Bayer Biological—Cont.

ton, D.C., U.S. Government Printing Office, (1980), pp. 15–22.

6. Sullivan KM, Kopecky KJ, Jocom J, et al: Immunomodulatory and antimicrobial efficacy of intravenous immunoglobulin in bone marrow transplantation. *N Engl J Med* 323(11):705–12, 1990.

7. Bernstein LJ, Ochs HD, Wedgwood RJ, et al: Defective humoral immunity in pediatric acquired immune deficiency syndrome. *J Pediatr* 107(3):352–7, 1985.

8. Borkowsky W, Steele CJ, Grubman S, et al: Antibody responses to bacterial toxoids in children infected with human immunodeficiency virus. *J Pediatr* 110(4):563–6, 1987.

9. Blanche S, Le Deist F, Fischer A, et al: Longitudinal study of 18 children with perinatal LAV/HTLV III infection: attempt at prognostic evaluation. *J Pediatr* 109(6):965–70, 1986.

10. Pahwa S, Fikrig S, Menez R, et al: Pediatric acquired immunodeficiency syndrome demonstration of B-lymphocyte defects in vitro. *Diagn Immunol* 4(1):24–30, 1986.

11. Bernstein LJ, Krieger BZ, Novick B, et al: Bacterial infections in the acquired immunodeficiency syndrome of children. *Pediatr Infect Dis* 4(5):472–5, 1985.

12. Krasinski K, Borkowsky W, Bonk S, et al: Bacterial infections in human immunodeficiency virus-infected children. *Pediatr Infect Dis J* 7(5):323–8, 1988.

13. Scott GB, Buck BE, Leterman JG, et al: Acquired immunodeficiency syndrome in infants. *N Engl J Med* 310(2):76–81, 1984.

14. Mofenson LM, Willoughby A. Passive immunization. In: Pizzo PA, Wilfert CM, (eds.) *Pediatric AIDS: the challenge of HIV infection in infants, children and adolescents.* Baltimore: Williams & Wilkins (1991) pp 633–50.

15. National Institute of Child Health and Human Development Intravenous Immunoglobulin Study Group. Intravenous immune globulin for the prevention of bacterial infections in children with symptomatic human immunodeficiency virus infection. *N Engl J Med* 325(2):73–80, 1991.

16. Mofenson LM, Moye J Jr, Bethel J, et al: Prophylactic intravenous immunoglobulin in HIV-infected children with CD4+ counts of $0.20 \times 10^9/L$ or more. Effect on viral, opportunistic, and bacterial infections. *JAMA* 268(4):483–88, 1992.

17. Glycine. In: Budavari S, O'Neil MJ, Smith A, et al, eds.: *Merck Index.* 11th ed. Rahway, NJ, Merck & Co., 1989, p. 706.

18. Wretlind, A: Complete intravenous nutrition: theoretical and experimental background. *Nutr Metab* 14(Suppl):1–57, 1972.

19. Hahn RG, Stalberg HP, Gustafsson SA: Intravenous infusion of irrigating fluids containing glycine or mannitol with and without ethanol. *J Urol* 142(4): 1102–1105, 1989.

20. Guyton AC: *Textbook of Medical Physiology.* 5th ed. Philadelphia, W.B. Saunders, 1976, pp. 499–500.

21. Nolte MT, Pirofsky B, Gerritz GA, et al: Intravenous immunoglobulin therapy for antibody deficiency. *Clin Exp Immunol* 36: 237–43, 1979.

22. Buckley RH: Immunoglobulin replacement therapy: indications and contraindications for use and variable IgG levels achieved. In: Alving BM (ed): *Immunoglobulins: characteristics and uses of intravenous preparations.* Washington, D.C., U.S. Government Printing Office, (1980), pp. 3–8.

23. Ochs HD: Intravenous immunoglobulin therapy of patients with primary immunodeficiency syndromes: efficacy and safety of a new modified immune globulin preparation. In: Alving BM (ed): *Immunoglobulins: characteristics and uses of intravenous preparations.* Washington, D.C., U.S. Government Printing Office, (1980), pp. 9–14.

24. Sekul E, Cupler E, Dalakas M. Aseptic meningitis associated with high-dose intravenous immunoglobulin therapy: Frequency and risk factors. *Ann Int Med* 121:259–262, 1994.

25. Kato E, Shindo S, Eto Y, Hashimoto N, Yamamoto M, Sakata Y, Hiyoshi Y. Administration of Immune Globulin Associated with Aseptic Meningitis. *JAMA* 259(22):3269–3270, 1988.

26. Casteels-Van Daele M, Wijndaele L, Hunninck K, Gillis P. Intravenous immune globulin and acute aseptic meningitis. *N Engl J Med* 323(9):614–615, 1990.

27. Scribner C, Kapit R, Phillips E, Rickles N. Aseptic meningitis and intravenous immunoglobulin therapy. *Ann Intern Med* 121(4):305–306, 1994.

28. Peerless AG, Stiehm ER: intravenous gammaglobulin for reaction to intramuscular preparation. [letter] *Lancet* 2(8347): 461, 1983.

Shown in Product Identification Guide, page 305

HYPERAB®   ℞

[hī′per-ab ″]

Rabies Immune Globulin (Human), USP

DESCRIPTION

Rabies Immune Globulin (Human), USP—Hyperab® is a sterile solution of antirabies immunoglobulin for intramuscular administration. This product is prepared from human plasma. It is prepared by cold alcohol fractionation from the plasma of donors hyperimmunized with rabies vaccine. Hyperab is a 15%–18% solution of human protein stabilized in 0.21–0.32 M glycine. The pH of the solution has been adjusted to 6.4–7.2 with sodium carbonate. Hyperab contains the mercurial preservative sodium ethylmercurithiosalicylate (thimerosal), 80–120 μg/mL as measured by mercury assay. The product is standardized against the U.S. Standard Rabies Immune Globulin to contain an average potency value of 150 IU/mL. The U.S. unit of potency is equivalent to the International Unit (IU) for rabies antibody.

CLINICAL PHARMACOLOGY

The usefulness of prophylactic rabies antibody in preventing rabies in man when administered immediately after exposure was dramatically demonstrated in a group of persons bitten by a rabid wolf in Iran.[1,2] Similarly, beneficial results were later reported from the U.S.S.R.[3] Studies coordinated by WHO helped determine the optimal conditions under which antirabies serum of equine origin and rabies vaccine can be used in man.[4–7] These studies showed that serum can interfere to a variable extent with the active immunity induced by the vaccine, but could be minimized by booster doses of vaccine after the end of the usual dosage series. Preparation of rabies immune globulin of human origin with adequate potency was reported by Cabasso et al.[8] In carefully controlled clinical studies, this globulin was used in conjunction with rabies vaccine of duck-embryo origin (DEV).[8,9] These studies determined that a human globulin dose of 20 IU/kg of rabies antibody, given simultaneously with the first DEV dose, resulted in amply detectable levels of passive rabies antibody 24 hours after injection in all recipients. The injections produced minimal, if any, interference with the subject's endogenous antibody response to DEV.

More recently, human diploid cell rabies vaccines (HDCV) prepared from tissue culture fluids containing rabies virus have received substantial clinical evaluation in Europe and the United States.[10–16] In a study in adult volunteers, the administration of Rabies Immune Globulin (Human) did not interfere with antibody formation induced by HDCV when given in a dose of 20 IU per kilogram body weight simultaneously with the first dose of vaccine.[15]

INDICATIONS AND USAGE

Rabies vaccine and Rabies Immune Globulin (Human), USP —Hyperab® should be given to all persons suspected of exposure to rabies with one exception: persons who have been previously immunized with rabies vaccine and have a confirmed adequate rabies antibody titer should receive only vaccine. Hyperab should be administered as promptly as possible after exposure, but can be administered up to the eighth day after the first dose of vaccine is given.

Recommendations for use of passive and active immunization after exposure to an animal suspected of having rabies have been detailed by the U.S. Public Health Service Advisory Committee on Immunization Practices (ACIP).[17]

Every exposure to possible rabies infection must be individually evaluated. The following factors should be considered before specific antirabies treatment is initiated:

1. Species of Biting Animal

Carnivorous wild animals (especially skunks, foxes, coyotes, raccoons, and bobcats) and bats are the animals most commonly infected with rabies and have caused most of the indigenous cases of human rabies in the United States since 1960.[18] Unless the animal is tested and shown not to be rabid, postexposure prophylaxis should be initiated upon bite or nonbite exposure to these animals (see item 3 below). If treatment has been initiated and subsequent testing in a competent laboratory shows the exposing animal is not rabid, treatment can be discontinued.

In the United States, the likelihood that a domestic dog or cat is infected with rabies varies from region to region; hence, the need for postexposure prophylaxis also varies. However, in most of Asia and all of Africa and Latin America, the dog remains the major source of human exposure; exposures to dogs in such countries represent a special threat. Travelers to those countries should be aware that >50% of the rabies cases among humans in the United States result from exposure to dogs outside the United States.

Rodents (such as squirrels, hamsters, guinea pigs, gerbils, chipmunks, rats, and mice) and lagomorphs (including rabbits and hares) are rarely found to be infected with rabies and have not been known to cause human rabies in the United States. However, from 1971 through 1988, woodchucks accounted for 70% of the 179 cases of rabies among rodents reported to CDC.[19] In these cases, the state or local health department should be consulted before a decision is made to initiate postexposure antirabies prophylaxis.

2. Circumstances of Biting Incident

An unprovoked attack is more likely to mean that the animal is rabid. (Bites during attempts to feed or handle an apparently healthy animal may generally be regarded as provoked.)

3. Type of Exposure

Rabies is transmitted only when the virus is introduced into open cuts or wounds in skin or mucous membranes. If there has been no exposure (as described in this section), postexposure treatment is not necessary. Thus, the likelihood that rabies infection will result from exposure to a rabid animal varies with the nature and extent of the exposure. Two categories of exposure should be considered:

Bite: any penetration of the skin by teeth. Bites to the face and hands carry the highest risk, but the site of the bite should not influence the decision to begin treatment.[20] Bat-associated strains of rabies can be transmitted to humans either directly through a bat's bite or indirectly through the bite of an animal previously infected by a bat. Because some bat bites may be less severe, and therefore more difficult to recognize, than bites inflicted by larger mammalian carnivores, rabies postexposure treatment should be considered for any physical contact with bats when bite or mucous membrane contact cannot be excluded.[21]

Nonbite: scratches, abrasions, open wounds or mucous membranes contaminated with saliva or any potentially infectious material, such as brain tissue, from a rabid animal constitute nonbite exposures. If the material containing the virus is dry, the virus can be considered noninfectious. Casual contact, such as petting a rabid animal and contact with the blood, urine, or feces (e.g., guano) of a rabid animal, does not constitute an exposure and is not an indication for prophylaxis. Instances of airborne rabies have been reported rarely. Adherence to respiratory precautions will minimize the risk of airborne exposure.[22] The only documented cases of rabies from human-to-human transmission have occurred in patients who received corneas transplanted from persons who died of rabies undiagnosed at the time of death. Stringent guidelines for acceptance of donor corneas have reduced this risk. Bite and nonbite exposures from humans with rabies theoretically could transmit rabies, although no cases of rabies acquired this way have been documented.

4. Vaccination Status of Biting Animal

A properly immunized animal has only a minimal chance of developing rabies and transmitting the virus.

5. Presence of Rabies in Region

If adequate laboratory and field records indicate that there is no rabies infection in a domestic species within a given region, local health officials are justified in considering this in making recommendations on antirabies treatment following a bite by that particular species. Such officials should be consulted for current interpretations.

Rabies Postexposure Prophylaxis

The following recommendations are only a guide. In applying them, take into account the animal species involved, the circumstances of the bite or other exposure, the vaccination status of the animal, and presence of rabies in the region. Local or state public health officials should be consulted if questions arise about the need for rabies prophylaxis.

Local Treatment of Wounds: Immediate and thorough washing of all bite wounds and scratches with soap and water is perhaps the most effective measure for preventing rabies. In experimental animals, simple local wound cleansing has been shown to reduce markedly the likelihood of rabies.

Tetanus prophylaxis and measures to control bacterial infection should be given as indicated.

Active Immunization: Active immunization should be initiated as soon as possible after exposure. Many dosage schedules have been evaluated for the currently available rabies vaccines and their respective manufacturers' literature should be consulted.

Passive Immunization: A combination of active and passive immunization (vaccine and immune globulin) is considered the acceptable postexposure prophylaxis except for those persons who have been previously immunized with rabies vaccine and who have documented adequate rabies antibody titer. These individuals should receive vaccine only. For passive immunization, Rabies Immune Globulin (Human) is preferred over antirabies serum, equine.[16,17] It is recommended both for treatment of all bites by animals suspected of having rabies and for nonbite exposure inflicted by animals suspected of being rabid. Rabies Immune Globulin (Human) should be used in conjunction with rabies vaccine and can be administered through the seventh day after the first dose of vaccine is given. Beyond the seventh day, Rabies Immune Globulin (Human) is not indicated since an antibody response to cell culture vaccine is presumed to have occurred.

[See table at top of next page.]

CONTRAINDICATIONS
None known.

WARNINGS
Rabies Immune Globulin (Human), USP—Hyperab® should be given with caution to patients with a history of prior systemic allergic reactions following the administration of human immunoglobulin preparations or in patients who are known to have had an allergic response to thimerosal.

The attending physician who wishes to administer Hyperab to persons with isolated immunoglobulin A (IgA) deficiency must weigh the benefits of immunization against the potential risks of hypersensitivity reactions. Such persons have increased potential for developing antibodies to IgA and could have anaphylactic reactions to subsequent administration of blood products that contain IgA.[23]

As with all preparations administered by the intramuscular route, bleeding complications may be encountered in patients with thrombocytopenia or other bleeding disorders.

PRECAUTIONS
General
Hyperab should **not** be administered intravenously because of the potential for serious reactions. Although systemic reactions to immunoglobulin preparations are rare, epinephrine should be available for treatment of acute anaphylactoid symptoms.

Drug Interactions
Repeated doses of Rabies Immune Globulin (Human), USP—Hyperab® should not be administered once vaccine treatment has been initiated as this could prevent the full expression of active immunity expected from the rabies vaccine. Other antibodies in the Hyperab preparation may interfere with the response to live vaccines such as measles, mumps, polio or rubella. Therefore, immunization with live vaccines should not be given within 3 months after Hyperab administration.

Pregnancy Category C
Animal reproduction studies have not been conducted with Hyperab. It is also not known whether Hyperab can cause fetal harm when administered to a pregnant woman or can affect reproduction capacity. Hyperab should be given to a pregnant woman only if clearly needed.

ADVERSE REACTIONS
Soreness at the site of injection and mild temperature elevations may be observed at times. Sensitization to repeated injections has occurred occasionally in immunoglobulin-deficient patients. Angioneurotic edema, skin rash, nephrotic syndrome, and anaphylactic shock have rarely been reported after intramuscular injection, so that a causal relationship between immunoglobulin and these reactions is not clear.

DOSAGE AND ADMINISTRATION
The recommended dose for Hyperab is 20 IU/kg (0.133 mL/kg) of body weight given preferably at the time of the first vaccine dose.[8,9] It may also be given through the seventh day after the first dose of vaccine is given. If anatomically feasible, up to one-half the dose of Hyperab should be thoroughly infiltrated in the area around the wound and the rest should be administered intramuscularly in the gluteal area. Because of risk of injury to the sciatic nerve, the central region of the gluteal area MUST be avoided; only the upper, outer quadrant should be used.[24] Hyperab should never be administered in the same syringe or into the same anatomical site as vaccine.

Parenteral drug products should be inspected visually for particulate matter and discoloration prior to administration, whenever solution and container permit.

HOW SUPPLIED
Hyperab is packaged in 2 mL and 10 mL vials with an average potency value of 150 International Units per mL (IU/mL). The 2 mL vial contains a total of 300 IU which is sufficient for a child weighing 15 kg. The 10 mL vial contains a total of 1500 IU which is sufficient for an adult weighing 75 kg.

STORAGE
Hyperab should be stored under refrigeration (2°–8°C, 36°–46°F). Solution that has been frozen should not be used.

CAUTION
U.S. federal law prohibits dispensing without prescription.

LIMITED WARRANTY
A number of factors beyond our control could reduce the efficacy of this product or even result in an ill effect following its use. These include improper storage and handling of the product after it leaves our hands, diagnosis, dosage, method of administration, and biological differences in individual patients. Because of these factors, it is important that this product be stored properly and that the directions be followed carefully during use.

No warranty, express or implied, including any warranty of merchantability or fitness is made. Representatives of the Company are not authorized to vary the terms or the contents of the printed labeling, including the package insert for this product, except by printed notice from the Company's headquarters. The prescriber and user of this product must accept the terms hereof.

Rabies Postexposure Prophylaxis Guide[17]

Animal species	Condition of animal at time of attack	Treatment of exposed person [1]
Dog and cat	Healthy and available for 10 days of observation	None, unless animal develops rabies [2]
	Rabid or suspected rabid	RIGH [3] and HDCV
	Unknown (escaped)	Consult public health officials
Skunk, bat, fox, coyote raccoon, bobcat, and other carnivores; woodchuck	Regard as rabid unless geographic area is known to be free of rabies or proven negative by laboratory tests [4]	RIGH [3] and HDCV
Livestock, rodents, and lagomorphs (rabbits and hares)	Consider individually. Local and state public health officials should be consulted on questions about the need for rabies prophylaxis. In most geographical areas bites of squirrels, hamsters, guinea pigs, gerbils, chipmunks, rats, mice, other rodents, rabbits, and hares almost never call for antirabies prophylaxis.	

[1] ALL BITES AND WOUNDS SHOULD IMMEDIATELY BE THOROUGHLY CLEANSED WITH SOAP AND WATER. If antirabies treatment is indicated, both Rabies Immune Globulin (Human) [RIGH] and human diploid cell rabies vaccine (HDCV) should be given as soon as possible, REGARDLESS of the interval from exposure.

[2] During the usual holding period of 10 days, begin treatment with RIGH and vaccine (HDCV) at first sign of rabies in a dog or cat that has bitten someone. The symptomatic animal should be killed immediately and tested.

[3] If RIGH is not available, use antirabies serum, equine (ARS). Do not use more than the recommended dosage.

[4] The animal should be killed and tested as soon as possible. Holding for observation is not recommended. Discontinue vaccine if immunofluorescence test results of the animal are negative.

REFERENCES
1. Baltazard M, Bahmanyar M, Ghodssi M, et al: Essai pratique du sérum antirabique chez les mordus par loups enragés. *Bull WHO* 13:747–72, 1955.
2. Habel K, Koprowski H: Laboratory data supporting the clinical trial of antirabies serum in persons bitten by a rabid wolf. *Bull WHO* 13:773–9, 1955.
3. Selimov M, Boltucij L, Semenova E, et al: [The use of antirabies gamma globulin in subjects severely bitten by rabid wolves or other animals.] *J Hyg Epidemiol Microbiol Immunol (Praha)* 3:168–80, 1959.
4. Atanasiu P, Bahmanyar M, Baltazard M, et al: Rabies neutralizing antibody response to different schedules of serum and vaccine inoculations in non-exposed persons. *Bull WHO* 14:593–611, 1956.
5. Atanasiu P, Bahmanyar M, Baltazard M, et al: Rabies neutralizing antibody response to different schedules of serum and vaccine inoculations in non-exposed persons: Part II. *Bull WHO* 17:911–32, 1957.
6. Atanasiu P, Cannon DA, Dean DJ, et al: Rabies neutralizing antibody response to different schedules of serum and vaccine inoculations in non-exposed persons: Part 3. *Bull WHO* 25:103–14, 1961.
7. Atanasiu P, Dean DJ, Habel K, et al: Rabies neutralizing antibody response to different schedules of serum and vaccine inoculations in non-exposed persons: Part 4. *Bull WHO* 36:361–5, 1967.
8. Cabasso VJ, Loofbourow JC, Roby RE, et al: Rabies immune globulin of human origin: preparation and dosage determination in non-exposed volunteer subjects. *Bull WHO* 45:303–15, 1971.
9. Loofbourow JC, Cabasso VJ, Roby RE, et al: Rabies immune globulin (human): clinical trials and dose determination. *JAMA* 217(13): 1825–31, 1971.
10. Plotkin SA: New rabies vaccine halts disease — without severe reactions. *Mod Med* 45(20):45–8, 1977.
11. Plotkin SA, Wiktor TJ, Koprowski H, et al: Immunization schedules for the new human diploid cell vaccine against rabies. *Am J Epidemiol* 103(1):75–80, 1976.
12. Hafkin B, Hattwick MA, Smith JS, et al: A comparison of a WI-38 vaccine and duck embryo vaccine for preexposure rabies prophylaxis. *Am J Epidemiol* 107(5):439–43, 1978.
13. Kuwert EK, Marcus I, Höher PG; Neutralizing and complement-fixing antibody responses in pre- and post-exposure vaccinees to a rabies vaccine produced in human diploid cells. *J Biol Stand* 4(4):249–62, 1976.
14. Grandien M: Evaluation of tests for rabies antibody and analysis of serum responses after administration of three different types of rabies vaccines. *J Clin Microbiol* 5(3):263–7, 1977.
15. Kuwert EK, Marcus I, Werner J, et al: Postexpositionelle Schutzimpfung des Menschen gegen Tollwut mit einer neuentwickelten Gewebekulturvakzine (HDCS-Impfstoff). *Zentralbl Bakteriol [A]* 239(4):437–58, 1977.
16. Bahmanyar M, Fayaz A, Nour-Salehi S, et al: Successful protection of humans exposed to rabies infection: postexposure treatment with the new human diploid cell rabies vaccine and antirabies serum. *JAMA* 236(24):2751–4, 1976.
17. Recommendations of the Immunization Practices Advisory Committee (ACIP): Rabies prevention—United States, 1991. *MMWR* 40(RR–3):1–19, 1991.
18. Reid-Sanden FL, Dobbins JG, Smith JS, et al: Rabies surveillance in the United States during 1989. *J Am Vet Med Assoc* 197(12):1571–83, 1990.
19. Fishbein DB, Belotto AJ, Pacer RE, et al: Rabies in rodents and lagomorphs in the United States, 1971–1984: increased cases in the woodchuck (*Marmota monax*) in mid-Atlantic states. *J Wildl Dis* 22(2):151–5, 1986.
20. Hattwick MAW: Human rabies. *Public Health Rev* 3(3):229–74, 1974.
21. Epidemiologic Notes and Reports: Human Rabies—California, 1994. *MMWR* 43(25):455–457, 1994.
22. Garner JS, Simmons BP: Guideline for isolation precautions in hospitals. *Infect Control.*
23. Fudenberg HH: Sensitization to immunoglobulins and hazards of gamma globulin therapy. In: Merler E (ed.): Immunoglobulins: biologic aspects and clinical uses. Washington, DC, Nat Acad Sci, 1970, pp 211–20.
24. Recommendations of the Immunization Practices Advisory Committee (ACIP): General recommendations on immunization. *MMWR* 38(13):205–14; 219–27, 1989.

HYPERHEP®   ℞
[hī'per-hep"]
Hepatitis B Immune Globulin (Human)

DESCRIPTION
Hepatitis B Immune Globulin (Human)—HyperHep® is a sterile solution of immunoglobulin (15%-18% protein) which is prepared by cold alcohol fractionation from pooled plasma of individuals with high titers of antibody to the hepatitis B surface antigen (anti-HBs). The product is stabilized with 0.21-0.32 M glycine and is preserved with 80-120 µg/mL thimerosal (a mercury derivative), by mercury assay. The solution has a pH of 6.4-7.2 adjusted with sodium carbonate. Each vial contains anti-HBs antibody equivalent to or exceeding the potency of anti-HBs in a U.S. reference hepatitis B immune globulin (Center for Biologics Evaluation and Research, FDA). The U.S. reference has been tested against the World Health Organization standard Hepatitis B Immune Globulin and found to be equal to 217 international units (IU) per mL. HyperHep must be administered intramuscularly.

CLINICAL PHARMACOLOGY
Hepatitis B Immune Globulin (Human) provides passive immunization for individuals exposed to the hepatitis B virus (HBV) as evidenced by a reduction in the attack rate of hepatitis B following its use.[1-6] The administration of the usual recommended dose of this immune globulin generally results in a detectable level of circulating anti-HBs which persists for approximately 2 months or longer. The highest antibody (IgG) serum levels were seen in the following distribution of subjects studied:[7]

Continued on next page

Bayer Biological—Cont.

DAY	% OF SUBJECTS
3	38.9%
7	41.7%
14	11.1%
21	8.3%

Mean values for half-life were between 17.5 and 25 days, with the shortest being 5.9 days and the longest 35 days.[7]

Cases of type B hepatitis are rarely seen following exposure to HBV in persons with pre-existing anti-HBs. No confirmed instance of transmission of hepatitis B has been associated with this product.

INDICATIONS AND USAGE

Recommendations on post-exposure prophylaxis are based on available efficacy data and on the likelihood of future HBV exposure for the person requiring treatment. In all exposures, a regimen combining Hepatitis B Immune Globulin (Human) with hepatitis B vaccine will provide both short- and long-term protection, will be less costly than the two-dose Hepatitis B Immune Globulin (Human) treatment alone, and is the treatment of choice.[8]

HyperHep is indicated for post-exposure prophylaxis in the following situations:

Acute Exposure to Blood Containing HBsAg

After either parenteral exposure, e.g., by accidental "needlestick" or direct mucous membrane contact (accidental splash), or oral ingestion (pipetting accident) involving HBsAg-positive materials such as blood, plasma or serum. For inadvertent percutaneous exposure, a regimen of two doses of Hepatitis B Immune Globulin (Human), one given after exposure and one a month later, is about 75% effective in preventing hepatitis B in this setting.

Perinatal Exposure of Infants Born to HBsAg-positive Mothers

Infants born to HBsAg-positive mothers are at risk of being infected with hepatitis B virus and becoming chronic carriers.[5,8,9,10] This risk is especially great if the mother is HBeAg-positive.[11,12,13] For an infant with perinatal exposure to an HBsAg-positive and HBeAg-positive mother, a regimen combining one dose of Hepatitis B Immune Globulin (Human) at birth with the hepatitis B vaccine series started soon after birth is 85%–95% effective in preventing development of the HBV carrier state.[8,14] Regimens involving either multiple doses of Hepatitis B Immune Globulin (Human) alone or the vaccine series alone have 70%–90% efficacy, while a single dose of Hepatitis B Immune Globulin (Human) alone has only 50% efficacy.[8,15]

Sexual Exposure to an HBsAg-positive Person

Sex partners of HBsAg-positive persons are at increased risk of acquiring HBV infection. For sexual exposure to a person with acute hepatitis B, a single dose of Hepatitis B Immune Globulin (Human) is 75% effective if administered within 2 weeks of last sexual exposure.[8]

Household Exposure to Persons with Acute HBV Infection

Since infants have close contact with primary care-givers and they have a higher risk of becoming HBV carriers after acute HBV infection, prophylaxis of an infant less than 12 months of age with Hepatitis B Immune Globulin and hepatitis B vaccine is indicated if the mother or primary caregiver has acute HBV infection.[8]

Administration of Hepatitis B Immune Globulin (Human) either preceding or concomitant with the commencement of active immunization with Hepatitis B Vaccine provides for more rapid achievement of protective levels of hepatitis B antibody, than when the vaccine alone is administered.[16] Rapid achievement of protective levels of antibody to hepatitis B virus may be desirable in certain clinical situations, as in cases of accidental inoculations with contaminated medical instruments.[16] Administration of Hepatitis B Immune Globulin (Human) either 1 month preceding or at the time of commencement of a program of active vaccination with Hepatitis B Vaccine has been shown not to interfere with the active immune response to the vaccine.[16]

CONTRAINDICATIONS

None known.

WARNINGS

HyperHep should be given with caution to patients with a history of prior systemic allergic reactions following the administration of human immune globulin preparations or in patients who are known to have had an allergic response to thimerosal. Epinephrine should be available.

In patients who have severe thrombocytopenia or any coagulation disorder that would contraindicate intramuscular injections, Hepatitis B Immune Globulin (Human) should be given only if the expected benefits outweigh the risks.

PRECAUTIONS

General

Hepatitis B Immune Globulin (Human)—HyperHep® should **not** be administered intravenously because of the potential for serious reactions. Injections should be made intramuscularly, and care should be taken to draw back on the plunger of the syringe before injection in order to be certain that the needle is not in a blood vessel.

Intramuscular injections are preferably administered in the anterolateral aspects of the upper thigh and the deltoid muscle of the upper arm. The gluteal region should not be used routinely as an injection site because of the risk of injury to the sciatic nerve. An individual decision as to which muscle is injected must be made for each patient based on the volume of material to be administered. If the gluteal region is used when very large volumes are to be injected or multiple doses are necessary, the central region MUST be avoided; only the upper, outer quadrant should be used.[17]

Laboratory Tests

None required.

Drug Interactions

Although administration of Hepatitis B Immune Globulin (Human) did not interfere with measles vaccination,[18] it is not known whether Hepatitis B Immune Globulin (Human) may interfere with other live virus vaccines. Therefore, use of such vaccines should be deferred until approximately three months after Hepatitis B Immune Globulin (Human) administration. Hepatitis B Vaccine may be administered at the same time, but at a different injection site, without interfering with the immune response.[16] No interactions with other products are known.

Pregnancy Category C

Animal reproduction studies have not been conducted with HyperHep. It is also not known whether HyperHep can cause fetal harm when administered to a pregnant woman or can affect reproduction capacity. HyperHep should be given to a pregnant woman only if clearly needed.

ADVERSE REACTIONS

Local pain and tenderness at the injection site, urticaria and angioedema may occur; anaphylactic reactions, although rare, have been reported following the injection of human immune globulin preparations.[19]

OVERDOSAGE

Although no data are available, clinical experience with other immunoglobulin preparations suggests that the only manifestations would be pain and tenderness at the injection site.

DOSAGE AND ADMINISTRATION

Acute Exposure to Blood Containing HBsAg[15]

Table 1 summarizes prophylaxis for percutaneous (needle stick or bite), ocular, or mucous-membrane exposure to blood according to the source of exposure and vaccination status of the exposed person. For greatest effectiveness, passive prophylaxis with Hepatitis B Immune Globulin (Human) should be given as soon as possible after exposure (its value beyond 7 days of exposure is unclear). If Hepatitis B Immune Globulin (Human) is indicated (see Table 1 below), an injection of 0.06 mL/kg of body weight should be administered intramuscularly (see PRECAUTIONS) as soon as possible after exposure and within 24 hours, if possible. Consult Hepatitis B Vaccine package insert for dosage information regarding that product.

[See table 1 below.]

Table 1. (adapted from[20])

Recommendations for Hepatitis B Prophylaxis Following Percutaneous or Permucosal Exposure

Source	Exposed Person: Unvaccinated	Exposed Person: Vaccinated
HBsAg-Positive	1. Hepatitis B Immune Globulin (Human)×1 immediately* 2. Initiate HB Vaccine series†	1. Test exposed person for anti-HBs. 2. If inadequate antibody,‡ Hepatitis B Immune Globulin (Human) (×1) immediately plus HB Vaccine booster dose, or 2 doses of HBIG,* one as soon as possible after exposure and the second 1 month later.
Known Source (High Risk)	1. Initiate HB Vaccine series 2. Test source for HBsAg. If positive, Hepatitis B Immune Globulin (Human)×1	1. Test Source for HBsAg only if exposed is vaccine nonresponder; if source is HBsAg-positive, give Hepatitis B Immune Globulin (Human)×1 immediately plus HB Vaccine booster dose, or 2 doses of HBIG,* one as soon as possible after exposure and the second 1 month later.
Low Risk HBsAg-Positive	Initiate HB Vaccine series.	Nothing required.
Unknown Source	Initiate HB Vaccine series within 7 days of exposure.	Nothing required.

* Hepatitis B Immune Globulin (Human), dose 0.06 mL/kg IM.

† HB Vaccine dose 20 μg IM for adults; 10 μg IM for infants or children under 10 years of age. First dose within 1 week; second and third doses, 1 and 6 months later.

‡ Less than 10 sample ratio units (SRU) by radioimmunoassay (RIA), negative by enzyme immunoassay (EIA).

For persons who refuse Hepatitis B Vaccine, a second dose of Hepatitis B Immune Globulin (Human)—HyperHep® should be given 1 month after the first dose.

Prophylaxis of Infants Born to HBsAg and HBeAg Positive Mothers

Efficacy of prophylactic Hepatitis B Immune Globulin (Human) in infants at risk depends on administering Hepatitis B Immune Globulin (Human) on the day of birth. It is therefore vital that HBsAg-positive mothers be identified before delivery.

Hepatitis B Immune Globulin (Human) (0.5 mL) should be administered intramuscularly (IM) to the newborn infant after physiologic stabilization of the infant and preferably within 12 hours of birth. Hepatitis B Immune Globulin (Human) efficacy decreases markedly if treatment is delayed beyond 48 hours. Hepatitis B Vaccine should be administered IM in three doses of 0.5 mL of vaccine (10 μg) each. The first dose should be given within 7 days of birth and may be given concurrently with Hepatitis B Immune Globulin (Human) but at a separate site. The second and third doses of vaccine should be given 1 month and 6 months, respectively, after the first. If administration of the first dose of Hepatitis B Vaccine is delayed for as long as 3 months, then a 0.5 mL dose of Hepatitis B Immune Globulin (Human)—HyperHep® should be repeated at 3 months. If Hepatitis B Vaccine is refused, the 0.5 mL dose of Hepatitis B Immune Globulin (Human) should be repeated at 3 and 6 months. Hepatitis B Immune Globulin (Human) administered at birth should not interfere with oral polio and diphtheria-tetanus-pertussis vaccines administered at 2 months of age.[15]

Sexual Exposure to an HBsAg-positive Person

All susceptible persons whose sex partners have acute hepatitis B infection should receive a single dose of HBIG (0.06 mL/kg) and should begin the hepatitis B vaccine series if prophylaxis can be started within 14 days of the last sexual contact or if sexual contact with the infected person will continue (see Table 2 below). Administering the vaccine with HBIG may improve the efficacy of postexposure treatment. The vaccine has the added advantage of conferring long-lasting protection.[8]

[See table 2 at top of next page.]

Household Exposure to Persons with Acute HBV Infection

Prophylactic treatment with a 0.5 mL dose of Hepatitis B Immune Globulin (Human) and hepatitis B vaccine is indicated for infants < 12 months of age who have been exposed to a primary care-giver who has acute hepatitis B. Prophylaxis for other household contacts of persons with acute HBV infection is not indicated unless they have had identifiable blood exposure to the index patient, such as by sharing toothbrushes or razors. Such exposures should be treated like sexual exposures. If the index patient becomes an HBV carrier, all household contacts should receive hepatitis B vaccine.[8]

Hepatitis B Immune Globulin (Human) may be administered at the same time (but at a different site), or up to 1 month preceding Hepatitis B Vaccination without impairing the active immune response from Hepatitis B Vaccination.[16]

Table 2. (adapted from [21])
Recommendations for Postexposure Prophylaxis for Sexual Exposure to Hepatitis B

HBIG*		Vaccine	
Dose	Recommended timing	Dose	Recommended timing
0.06 mL/kg IM†	Single dose within 14 days of last sexual contact	1.0 mL IM†	First dose at time of HBIG* treatment¶

* HBIG = Hepatitis B Immune Globulin (Human)
† IM = intramuscularly
¶ The first dose can be administered the same time as the HBIG dose but at a different site; subsequent doses should be administered as recommended for specific vaccine.

Parenteral drug products should be inspected visually for particulate matter and discoloration prior to administration, whenever solution and container permit.
Administer intramuscularly. Do not inject intravenously.

HOW SUPPLIED

HyperHep is supplied in a 0.5 mL neonatal single dose syringe, a 1 mL and a 5 mL multiple dose vial.

STORAGE

Store at 2°–8°C (36°–46°F). Do not freeze. Do not use after expiration date.

CAUTION

U.S. federal law prohibits dispensing without prescription.

LIMITED WARRANTY

A number of factors beyond our control could reduce the efficacy of this product or even result in an ill effect following its use. These include improper storage and handling of the product after it leaves our hands, diagnosis, dosage, method of administration and biological differences in individual patients. Because of these factors, it is important that this product be stored properly and that the directions be followed carefully during use.
No warranty, express or implied, including any warranty of merchantability or fitness is made. Representatives of the Company are not authorized to vary the terms or the contents of the printed labeling, including the package insert for this product, except by printed notice from the Company's headquarters. The prescriber and user of this product must accept the terms hereof.

REFERENCES

1. Grady GF, Lee VA: Hepatitis B immune globulin—prevention of hepatitis from accidental exposure among medical personnel. *N Engl J Med* 293(21): 1067-70, 1975.
2. Seeff LB, Zimmerman HJ, Wright EC, et al: Efficacy of hepatitis B immune serum globulin after accidental exposure. *Lancet* 2(7942):939-41, 1975.
3. Krugman S, Giles JP: Viral hepatitis, type B (MS-2 strain). Further observations on natural history and prevention. *N Engl J Med* 288(15):755-60, 1973.
4. Current trends: Health status of Indochinese refugees: malaria and hepatitis B. *MMWR* 28(39):463-4; 469-70, 1979.
5. Jhaveri R, Rosenfeld W, Salazar JD, et al: High titer multiple dose therapy with HBIG in newborn infants of HBsAg positive mothers. *J Pediatr* 97(2):305-8, 1980.
6. Hoofnagle JH, Seeff LB, Bales ZB, et al: Passive-active immunity from hepatitis B immune globulin. *Ann Intern Med* 91(6):813-8, 1979.
7. Scheiermann N, Kuwert EK: Uptake and elimination of hepatitis B immunoglobulins after intramuscular application in man. *Dev Biol Stand* 54:347-55, 1983.
8. Recommendations of the Immunization Practices Advisory Committee (ACIP): Hepatitis B Virus: A Comprehensive Strategy for Eliminating Transmission in the United States Through Universal Childhood Vaccination. Appendix A: Post-exposure Prophylaxis for Hepatitis B. *MMWR* 40(RR-13):21-25, 1991.
9. Stevens CE, Beasley RP, Tsui J, et al: Vertical transmission of hepatitis B antigen in Taiwan. *N Engl J Med* 292(15):771-4, 1975.
10. Shiraki K, Yoshihara N, Kawana T, et al: Hepatitis B surface antigen and chronic hepatitis in infants born to asymptomatic carrier mothers. *Am J Dis Child* 131(6):644-7, 1977.
11. Recommendation of the Immunization Practices Advisory Committee (ACIP): Immune globulins for protection against viral hepatitis. *MMWR* 30(34):423-8; 433-5, 1981.
12. Okada K, Kamiyama I, Inomata M, et al: e antigen and anti-e in the serum of asymptomatic carrier mothers as indicators of positive and negative transmission of hepatitis B virus to their infants. *N Engl J Med* 294(14):746-9, 1976.
13. Beasley RP, Trepo C, Stevens CE, et al: The e antigen and vertical transmission of hepatitis B surface antigen. *Am J Epidemiol* 105(2):94-8, 1977.
14. Beasley RP, Hwang LY, Lee GCY, et al: Prevention of perinatally transmitted hepatitis B virus infections with hepatitis B immune globulin and hepatitis B vaccine. *Lancet* 2(8359):1099-102, 1983.
15. Recommendation of the Immunization Practices Advisory Committee (ACIP): Recommendations for protection against viral hepatitis. *MMWR* 34(22):313-35, 1985.
16. Szmuness W, Stevens CE, Olesko WR, et al: Passive-active immunisation against hepatitis B: Immunogenicity studies in adult Americans. *Lancet* 1:575-77, 1981.
17. Recommendations of the Immunization Practices Advisory Committee (ACIP): General recommendations on immunization. *MMWR* 38(13):205-14; 219-27, 1989.
18. Beasley RP, Hwang LY: Measles vaccination not interfered with by hepatitis B immune globulin. *Lancet* 1:161, 1982.
19. Ellis EF, Henney CS: Adverse reactions following administration of human gamma globulin. *J Allerg* 43(1):45-54, 1969.
20. Recommendations of the Immunization Practices Advisory Committee (ACIP): Update on Adult Immunization. Table 9. Recommendations for postexposure prophylaxis for percutaneous or permucosal exposure to hepatitis B, United States. *MMWR* 40(RR-12):70, 1991.
21. Recommendations of the Immunization Practices Advisory Committee (ACIP): Update on Adult Immunization. Table 10. Recommendations for postexposure prophylaxis for perinatal and sexual exposure to hepatitis B, United States. *MMWR* 40(RR-12):71, 1991.

HYPER-TET® ℞
[hī'per-tet"]
Tetanus Immune Globulin (Human), USP
250 Units

DESCRIPTION

Tetanus Immune Globulin (Human), USP—Hyper-Tet® is a sterile solution of tetanus hyperimmune immunoglobulin, primarily immunoglobulin G (IgG), containing 15%–18% protein, of which not less than 90% is gamma globulin. This product has been prepared from large pools of plasma obtained from individuals immunized with tetanus toxoid. Hyper-Tet is stabilized with 0.21–0.32 M glycine and contains the mercurial preservative sodium ethylmercurithiosalicylate (thimerosal), 80–120 µg per mL as measured by mercury assay. The pH is adjusted to 6.4–7.2 with sodium carbonate or acetic acid as required. The product is standardized against the U.S. Standard Antitoxin and the U.S. Control Tetanus Toxin and contains not less than 250 tetanus antitoxin units per container. Hyper-Tet must be administered intramuscularly.

CLINICAL PHARMACOLOGY

Hyper-Tet supplies passive immunity to those individuals who have low or no immunity to the toxin produced by the tetanus organism, *Clostridium tetani*. The antibodies act to neutralize the free form of the powerful exotoxin produced by this bacterium. Historically, such passive protection was provided by antitoxin derived from equine or bovine serum; however, the foreign protein in these heterologous products often produced severe allergic manifestations, even in individuals who demonstrated negative skin and/or conjunctival tests prior to administration. Estimates of the frequency of these foreign protein reactions following antitoxin of equine origin varied from 5%–30%.[1–4]

Several studies suggest the value of human tetanus antitoxin in the treatment of active tetanus.[5,6] In 1961 and 1962, Nation et al,[5] using Hyper-Tet treated 20 patients with tetanus using single doses of 3,000 to 6,000 antitoxin units in combination with other accepted clinical and nursing procedures. Six patients, all over 45 years of age, died of causes other than tetanus. The authors felt that the mortalilty rate (30%) compared favorably with their previous experience using equine antitoxin in larger doses and that the results were much better than the 60% national death rate for tetanus reported from 1951 to 1954.[7] Blake et al,[8] however, found in a data analysis of 545 cases of tetanus reported to the Centers for Disease Control from 1965 to 1971 that survival was no better with 8,000 units of human tetanus immune globulin (TIG) than with 500 units; however, an optimal dose could not be determined.

Passive immunization with Hyper-Tet may be undertaken concomitantly with active immunization using tetanus toxoid in those persons who must receive an immediate injection of tetanus antitoxin and in whom it is desirable to begin the process of active immunization. Based on the work of Rubbo,[9] McComb and Dwyer,[10] and Levine at al,[11] the physician may thus supply immediate passive protection against tetanus, and at the same time begin formation of active immunization in the injured individual which upon completion of a **full toxoid series** will preclude future need for antitoxin. Peak blood levels of IgG are obtained approximately 2 days after intramuscular injection. The half-life of IgG in the circulation of individuals with normal IgG levels is approximately 23 days.[12]

INDICATIONS AND USAGE

Tetanus Immune Globulin (Human), USP—Hyper-Tet® is indicated for prophylaxis against tetanus following injury in patients whose immunization is incomplete or uncertain (see below). It is also indicated, although evidence of effectiveness is limited, in the regimen of treatment of active cases of tetanus.[5,6,13]
The following table is a summary guide to tetanus prophylaxis in wound management:
[See table below.]

CONTRAINDICATIONS

None known.

WARNINGS

Hyper-Tet should be given with caution to patients with a history of prior systemic allergic reactions following the administration of human immunoglobulin preparations, or in patients who are known to have had an allergic response to thimerosal.
In patients who have severe thrombocytopenia or any coagulation disorder that would contraindicate intramuscular injections, Hyper-Tet should be given only if the expected benefits outweigh the risks.

PRECAUTIONS

General
Hyper-Tet should not be given intravenously. Intravenous injection of immunoglobulin intended for intramuscular use can, on occasion, cause a precipitous fall in blood pressure, and a picture not unlike anaphylaxis. Injections should only be made **intramuscularly** and care should be taken to draw back on the plunger of the syringe before injection in order to be certain that the needle is not in a blood vessel. Intramuscular injections are preferably administered in the anterolateral aspects of the upper thigh and the deltoid muscle of the upper arm. The gluteal region should not be used routinely as an injection site because of the risk of injury to the sciatic nerve. If the gluteal region is used, the central region MUST be avoided; only the upper, outer quadrant should be used.[15]

Guide to Tetanus Prophylaxis in Wound Management[14]

History of Tetanus Immunization	Clean, Minor Wounds		All Other Wounds	
(Doses)	Td*	TIG§	Td	TIG
Uncertain or less than 3	Yes	No	Yes	Yes
3 or more†	No‡	No	No£	No

* Adult type tetanus and diphtheria toxoids. If the patient is less than 7 years old, DT or DTP is given (see Dosage and Administration).
§ Tetanus Immune Globulin (Human)
† If only three doses of fluid tetanus toxoid have been received, a fourth dose of toxoid, preferably an adsorbed toxoid, should be given.
‡ Yes if more than 10 years since the last dose.
£ Yes if more than 5 years since the last dose.

Continued on next page

Bayer Biological—Cont.

Skin tests should not be done. The intradermal injection of concentrated IgG solutions often causes a localized area of inflammation which can be misinterpreted as a positive allergic reaction. In actuality, this does not represent an allergy; rather, it is localized tissue irritation. Misinterpretation of the results of such tests can lead the physician to withhold needed human antitoxin from a patient who is not actually allergic to this material. True allergic responses to human IgG given in the prescribed intramuscular manner are rare.
Although systemic reactions to human immunoglobulin preparations are rare, epinephrine should be available for treatment of acute anaphylactic reactions.

Drug Interactions
Antibodies in immunoglobulin preparations may interfere with the response to live viral vaccines such as measles, mumps, polio, and rubella. Therefore, use of such vaccines should be deferred until approximately 3 months after Tetanus Immune Globulin (Human), USP—Hyper-Tet® administration.
No interactions with other products are known.

Pregnancy Category C
Animal reproduction studies have not been conducted with Hyper-Tet. It is also not known whether Hyper-Tet can cause fetal harm when administered to a pregnant woman or can affect reproduction capacity. Hyper-Tet should be given to a pregnant woman only if clearly needed.

ADVERSE REACTIONS
Slight soreness at the site of injection and slight temperature elevation may be noted at times. Sensitization to repeated injections of human immunoglobulin is extremely rare.
In the course of routine injections of large numbers of persons with immunoglobulin there have been a few isolated occurrences of angioneurotic edema, nephrotic syndrome, and anaphylactic shock after injection.

OVERDOSAGE
Although no data are available, clinical experience with other immunoglobulin preparations suggests that the only manifestations would be pain and tenderness at the injection site.

DOSAGE AND ADMINISTRATION
Routine prophylactic dosage schedule:
Adults and children 7 years and older: Hyper-Tet, 250 units should be given by deep intramuscular injection (see PRECAUTIONS). At the same time, but in a different extremity and with a separate syringe, Tetanus and Diphtheria Toxoids Adsorbed (For Adult Use) (Td) should be administered according to the manufacturer's package insert.
Children less than 7 years old: In small children the routine prophylactic dose of Hyper-Tet may be calculated by the body weight (4.0 units/kg). However, it may be advisable to administer the entire contents of the vial or syringe of Hyper-Tet (250 units) regardless of the child's size, since theoretically the same amount of toxin will be produced in the child's body by the infecting tetanus organism as it will in an adult's body. At the same time but in a different extremity and with a different syringe, Diphtheria and Tetanus Toxoids and Pertussis Vaccine Adsorbed (DTP) or Diphtheria and Tetanus Toxoids Adsorbed (For Pediatric Use) (DT), if pertussis vaccine is contraindicated, should be administered per the manufacturer's package insert.
Note: The single injection of tetanus toxoid only initiates the series for producing active immunity in the recipient. The physician must impress upon the patient the need for further toxoid injections in 1 month and 1 year. Without such, the active immunization series is incomplete.
Current recommendations for wound management of patients definitely known to have completed a full tetanus toxoid series indicate tetanus toxoid booster only if more than 5 to 10 years have elapsed since the last dose of toxoid.[14] The prophylactic dosage schedule for these patients and for those with incomplete or uncertain immunity is shown on the table in INDICATIONS AND USAGE.
Since tetanus is actually a local infection, proper initial wound care is of paramount importance. The use of antitoxin is adjunctive to this procedure. However, in approximately 10% of recent tetanus cases, no wound or other breach in skin or mucous membrane could be implicated.[16]
Treatment of active cases of tetanus:
Standard therapy for the treatment of active tetanus including the use of Hyper-Tet must be implemented immediately. The dosage should be adjusted according to the severity of the infection.[5,6]
Parenteral drug products should be inspected visually for particulate matter and discoloration prior to administration, whenever solution and container permit. They should not be used if particulate matter and/or discoloration are present.

HOW SUPPLIED
Tetanus Immune Globulin (Human), USP—Hyper-Tet® is supplied in 250 unit prefilled disposable syringes and 250 unit vials.

STORAGE
Store at 2°-8°C (36°-46°F). Solution that has been frozen should not be used.

CAUTION
U.S. federal law prohibits dispensing without prescription.

LIMITED WARRANTY
A number of factors beyond our control could reduce the efficacy of this product or even result in an ill effect following its use. These include improper storage and handling of the product after it leaves our hands, diagnosis, dosage, method of administration, and biological differences in individual patients. Because of these factors it is important that this product be stored properly and that the directions be followed carefully during use.
No warranty, express or implied, including any warranty of merchantability or fitness is made. Representatives of the Company are not authorized to vary the terms or the contents of the printed labeling, including the package insert for this product, except by printed notice from the Company's headquarters. The prescriber and user of this product must accept the terms hereof.

REFERENCES

1. Moynihan NH: Tetanus prophylaxis and serum sensitivity tests. *Br Med J* 1:260–4, 1956.
2. Scheibel I: The uses and results of active tetanus immunization. *Bull WHO* 13:381–94, 1955.
3. Edsall G: Specific prophylaxis of tetanus. *JAMA* 171(4):417–27, 1959.
4. Bardenwerper HW: Serum neuritis from tetanus antitoxin. *JAMA* 179(10):763–6, 1962.
5. Nation NS, Pierce NF, Adler SJ, et al: Tetanus: the use of human hyperimmune globulin in treatment. *Calif Med* 98(6):305–6, 1963.
6. Ellis M: Human antitetanus serum in the treatment of tetanus. *Br Med J* 1(5338):1123–6, 1963.
7. Axnick NW, Alexander ER: Tetanus in the United States: A review of the problem. *Am J Public Health* 47(12):1493–1501, 1957.
8. Blake PA, Feldman RA, Buchanan TM, et al: Serologic therapy of tetanus in the United States, 1965–1971. *JAMA* 235(1):42–4, 1976.
9. Rubbo SD: New approaches to tetanus prophylaxis. *Lancet* 2(7461):449–53, 1966.
10. McComb JA, Dwyer RC: Passive-active immunization with tetanus immune globulin (human). *N Engl J Med* 268(16):857–62, 1963.
11. Levine L, McComb JA, Dwyer RC, et al: Active-passive tetanus immunization; choice of toxoid, dose of tetanus immune globulin and timing of injections. *N Engl J Med* 274(4);186–90, 1966.
12. Waldmann TA, Strober W, Blaese RM: Variations in the metabolism of immunoglobulins measured by turnover rates. In Merler E (ed.): Immunoglobulins: biologic aspects and clinical uses. Washington, DC, Nat Acad Sci, 1970, p 33–51.
13. McCracken GH Jr., Dowell DL, Marshall FN: Double-blind trial of equine antitoxin and human immune globulin in tetanus neonatorum. *Lancet* 1(7710):1146–9, 1971.
14. American Academy of Pediatrics, Committee on Infectious Diseases: Report ed. 20. Evanston, 1986, p. 355–9.
15. Recommendations of the Immunization Practices Advisory Committee (ACIP): General recommendations on immunization. *MMWR* 38(13): 205–14; 219–27, 1989.
16. Tetanus-Rates by year, United States, 1955–1984. Annual Summary 1984. *MMWR* 33 (54):61, 1986.

HypRho®-D Mini-Dose ℞
[hī″prō-d′]
$Rh_o(D)$ Immune Globulin (Human)

DESCRIPTION
$Rh_o(D)$ Immune Globulin (Human)—HypRho®-D Mini-Dose—is a sterile solution of immune globulin containing antibodies to $Rh_o(D)$ which is for intramuscular injection only. It is prepared from human plasma collected from carefully screened donors. It contains 15%–18% protein stabilized with 0.21–0.32 M glycine and preserved with 80–120 μg/mL thimerosal (a mercury derivative), as measured by mercury assay. The pH is adjusted with sodium carbonate.
One dose of HypRho-D Mini-Dose contains not less than one-sixth the quantity of $Rh_o(D)$ antibody contained in one standard dose of $Rh_o(D)$ Immune Globulin (Human), USP and it will suppress the immunizing potential of 2.5 mL of $Rh_o(D)$ positive packed red blood cells or the equivalent of whole blood (5 mL). The quantity of $Rh_o(D)$ antibody in HypRho-D Mini-Dose is not less than one-sixth of that contained in 1 mL of the U.S. Food and Drug Administration Reference $Rh_o(D)$ Immune Globulin (Human).

CLINICAL PHARMACOLOGY
Rh sensitization may occur in nonsensitized $Rh_o(D)$ negative women following transplacental hemorrhage resulting from spontaneous or induced abortions.[1–2] The risk of sensitization is higher in women undergoing induced abortions than in those aborting spontaneously.[1–3]
HypRho-D Mini-Dose is used to prevent the formation of anti-Rho(D) antibody in $Rh_o(D)$ negative women who are exposed to the $Rh_o(D)$ antigen at the time of spontaneous or induced abortion (up to 12 weeks' gestation).[3–5] HypRho-D Mini-Dose suppresses the stimulation of active immunity by $Rh_o(D)$ positive fetal erythrocytes that may enter the maternal circulation at the time of termination of the pregnancy.
The amount of anti-$Rh_o(D)$ in HypRho-D Mini-Dose has been shown to effectively prevent maternal isosensitization to the $Rh_o(D)$ antigens following spontaneous or induced abortion occurring up to the 12th week of gestation.[6–8] After the 12th week of gestation, a standard dose of $Rh_o(D)$ Immune Globulin (Human), USP—HypRho®-D is indicated.

INDICATIONS AND USAGE
$Rh_o(D)$ Immune Globulin (Human)—HypRho®-D Mini-Dose is recommended to prevent the isoimmunization of $Rh_o(D)$ negative women at the time of spontaneous or induced abortion of up to 12 weeks' gestation provided the following criteria are met:
1. The mother must be $Rh_o(D)$ negative and must not already be sensitized to the $Rh_o(D)$ antigen.
2. The father is not known to be $Rh_o(D)$ negative.
3. Gestation is not more than 12 weeks at termination.

Note: $Rh_o(D)$ Immune Globulin (Human) prophylaxis is not indicated if the fetus or father can be determined to be Rh negative. If the Rh status of the fetus is unknown, the fetus must be assumed to be $Rh_o(D)$ positive, and HypRho-D Mini-Dose should be administered to the mother.
FOR ABORTIONS OR MISCARRIAGES OCCURRING AFTER 12 WEEKS' GESTATION, A STANDARD DOSE OF $RH_O(D)$ IMMUNE GLOBULIN (HUMAN), USP IS INDICATED.
HypRho-D Mini-Dose should be administered within 3 hours or as soon as possible after spontaneous passage or surgical removal of the products of conception. However, if HypRho-D Mini-Dose is not given within this time period, consideration should still be given to its administration since clinical studies in male volunteers have demonstrated the effectiveness of $Rh_o(D)$ Immune Globulin (Human), USP in preventing isoimmunization as long as 72 hours after infusion of $Rh_o(D)$ positive red cells.[9]

CONTRAINDICATIONS
None known.

WARNINGS
NEVER ADMINISTER HYPRHO-D MINI-DOSE INTRAVENOUSLY. INJECT ONLY INTRAMUSCULARLY. ADMINISTER ONLY TO WOMEN POST-ABORTION OR POST-MISCARRIAGE OF UP TO 12 WEEKS' GESTATION.
HypRho-D Mini-Dose should be given with caution to patients with a history of prior systemic allergic reactions following the administration of human immune globulin preparations or in patients who are known to have had an allergic response to thimerosal.
The attending physician who wishes to administer HypRho-D Mini-Dose to persons with isolated immunoglobulin A (IgA) deficiency must weigh the benefits of immunization against the potential risks of hypersensitivity reactions. Such persons have increased potential for developing antibodies to IgA and could have anaphylactic reactions to subsequent administration of blood products that contain IgA.
As with all preparations administered by the intramuscular route, bleeding complications may be encountered in patients with thrombocytopenia or other bleeding disorders.

PRECAUTIONS
General
Although systemic reactions to immunoglobulin preparations are rare, epinephrine should be available for treatment of acute anaphylactic symptoms.

Drug Interactions
Other antibodies in the $Rh_o(D)$ Immune Globulin (Human)—HypRho®-D Mini-Dose preparation may interfere with the response to live vaccines such as measles, mumps, polio or rubella. Therefore, immunization with live vaccines should not be given within 3 months after HypRho-D Mini-Dose administration.

Pregnancy Category C
Animal reproduction studies have not been conducted with HypRho-D Mini-Dose. It is also not known whether HypRho-D Mini-Dose can cause fetal harm when administered to a pregnant woman or can affect reproduction capacity.
It should be again noted, however, that HypRho-D Mini-Dose is **not** indicated for use during pregnancy and it should be administered only post-abortion or post-miscarriage.

ADVERSE REACTIONS

Reactions to HypRho-D Mini-Dose are infrequent in Rho (D) negative individuals and consist primarily of slight soreness at the site of injection and slight temperature elevation. While sensitization to repeated injections of human globulin is extremely rare, it has occurred.

DOSAGE AND ADMINISTRATION

One syringe of HypRho-D Mini-Dose provides sufficient antibody to prevent Rh sensitization to 2.5 mL Rh_o(D) positive packed red cells or the equivalent (5 mL) of whole blood. This dose is sufficient to provide protection against maternal Rh sensitization for women undergoing spontaneous or induced abortion of up to 12 weeks' gestation.

HypRho-D Mini-Dose should be administered within 3 hours or as soon as possible following spontaneous or induced abortion. If prompt administration is not possible, HypRho-D Mini-Dose should be given within 72 hours following termination of the pregnancy.

HypRho-D Mini-Dose is administered **intramuscularly**, preferably in the anterolateral aspects of the upper thigh and the deltoid muscle of the upper arm. The gluteal region should not be used routinely as an injection site because of the risk of injury to the sciatic nerve. If the gluteal region is used, the central region must be avoided; only the upper, outer quadrant should be used.[10]

Parenteral drug products should be inspected visually for particulate matter and discoloration prior to administration, whenever solution and container permit.

HOW SUPPLIED

Each HypRho-D Mini-Dose package contains 10 single dose syringes.

STORAGE

Store at 2°-8°C (36°-46°F). Do not freeze.

CAUTION

U.S. federal law prohibits dispensing without prescription.

LIMITED WARRANTY

A number of factors beyond our control could reduce the efficacy of this product or even result in an ill effect following its use. These include improper storage and handling of the product after it leaves our hands, diagnosis, dosage, method of administration, and biological differences in individual patients. Because of these factors, it is important that this product be stored properly and that the directions be followed carefully during use.

No warranty, express or implied, including any warranty of merchantability or fitness is made. Representatives of the Company are not authorized to vary the terms or the contents of the printed labeling, including the package insert for this product, except by printed notice from the Company's headquarters. The prescriber and user of this product must accept the terms hereof.

REFERENCES

1. Queenan JT, Shah S, Kubarych SF, *et al:* Role of induced abortion in rhesus immunisation. *Lancet* 1(7704): 815–7, 1971.
2. Goldman JA, Eckerling B: Prevention of Rh immunization after abortion with anti-Rh_o(D)-immunoglobulin. *Obstet Gynecol* 40(3):366–70, 1972.
3. The selective use of Rho(D) immune globulin (RhIG). *ACOG Tech Bull* 61, 1981.
4. Prevention of Rh sensitization. *WHO Tech Rep Ser* 468, 1971.
5. Recommendation of the Public Health Service Advisory Committee on Immunization Practices: Rh immune globulin. *MMWR* 21(15):126–7, 1972.
6. Stewart FH, Burnhill MS, Bozorgi N: Reduced dose of Rh immunoglobulin following first trimester pregnancy termination. *Obstet Gynecol* 51(3):318–22, 1978.
7. McMaster conference on prevention of Rh immunization, 28-30 September, 1977. *Vox Sang* 36(1):50–64, 1979.
8. Simonovits I: Efficiency of anti-D IgG prevention after induced abortion. *Vox Sang* 26(4):361–7, 1974.
9. Freda VJ, Gorman JG, Pollack W: Prevention of Rh-hemolytic disease with Rh-immune globulin. *Am J Obstet Gynecol* 128(4):456–60, 1977.
10. Recommendations of the Immunization Practices Advisory Committee (ACIP): General recommendations on immunization. *MMWR* 38(13):205–14; 219–27, 1989.

HypRho®-D Full Dose ℞

[*hī″prō-d′*]

Rh_o(D) Immune Globulin (Human), USP

DESCRIPTION

Rh_o(D) Immune Globulin (Human), USP—HypRho®-D is a sterile solution of immune globulin containing antibodies to Rh_o(D) which is intended for intramuscular injection. This product has been prepared from large pools of human plasma. It contains 15%–18% protein stabilized with 0.21–0.32 M glycine and is preserved with 80–120 µg/mL thimerosal (a mercury derivative), as measured by mercury assay. The pH is adjusted with sodium carbonate. The potency is equal to or greater than that of the U.S. Food and Drug Administration Reference Rh_o(D) Immune Globulin. Each single dose vial or syringe contains sufficient anti-Rh_o(D) (approximately 300 µg*) to effectively suppress the immunizing potential of 15 mL of Rh_o(D) positive red blood cells.[2–4]

CLINICAL PHARMACOLOGY

HypRho-D is used to prevent isoimmunization in the Rh_o(D) negative individual exposed to Rh_o(D) positive blood as a result of a fetomaternal hemorrhage occurring during a delivery of an Rh_o(D) positive infant, abortion (either spontaneous or induced), or following amniocentesis or abdominal trauma. Similarly, immunization resulting in the production of anti-Rh_o(D) following transfusion of Rh positive red cells to an Rh_o(D) negative recipient may be prevented by administering Rh_o(D) Immune Globulin (Human), USP.[5,6]

Rh hemolytic disease of the newborn is the result of the active immunization of an Rh_o(D) negative mother by Rh_o(D) positive red cells entering the maternal circulation during a previous delivery, abortion, amniocentesis, abdominal trauma, or as a result of red cell transfusion.[7,8] HypRho-D acts by suppressing the immune response of Rh_o(D) negative individuals to Rh_o(D) positive red blood cells. The mechanism of action of HypRho-D is not fully understood.

The administration of Rh_o(D) Immune Globulin (Human), USP within 72 hours of a full-term delivery of an Rh_o(D) positive infant by an Rh_o(D) negative mother reduces the incidence of Rh isoimmunization from 12%–13% to 1%–2%.[9] The 1%–2% treatment failures are probably due to isoimmunization occurring during the latter part of pregnancy or following delivery.[10] Bowman and Pollock[11] have reported that the incidence of isoimmunization can be further reduced from approximately 1.6% to less than 0.1% by administering Rh_o(D) Immune Globulin (Human), USP in two doses, one antenatal at 28 weeks' gestation and another following delivery.

INDICATIONS AND USAGE

Pregnancy and Other Obstetric Conditions

Rh_o(D) Immune Globulin (Human), USP—HypRho®-D is recommended for the prevention of Rh hemolytic disease of the newborn by its administration to the Rh_o(D) negative mother within 72 hours after birth of an Rh_o(D) positive infant,[12] providing the following criteria are met:

1. The mother must be Rh_o(D) negative, and must not already be sensitized to the Rh_o(D) factor.
2. Her child must be Rh_o(D) positive, and should have a negative direct antiglobulin test (see PRECAUTIONS).

If HypRho-D is administered antepartum, it is essential that the mother receive another dose of HypRho-D after delivery of an Rh_o(D) positive infant.

If the father can be determined to be Rh_o(D) negative, HypRho-D need not be given.

HypRho-D should be administered within 72 hours to all nonimmunized Rh_o(D) negative women who have undergone spontaneous or induced abortion, following ruptured tubal pregnancy, amniocentesis or abdominal trauma unless the blood group of the fetus or the father is known to be Rh_o(D) negative.[7,8] If the fetal blood group cannot be determined, one must assume that it is Rh_o(D) positive,[2] and HypRho-D should be administered to the mother.

Transfusion

HypRho-D may be used to prevent isoimmunization in Rh_o(D) negative individuals who have been transfused with Rh_o(D) positive red blood cells or blood components containing red blood cells.[5,13]

CONTRAINDICATIONS

None known.

WARNINGS

NEVER ADMINISTER HYPRHO-D INTRAVENOUSLY. INJECT ONLY INTRAMUSCULARLY. NEVER ADMINISTER TO THE NEONATE.

Rh_o(D) Immune Globulin (Human), USP should be given with caution to patients with a history of prior systemic allergic reactions following the administration of human immunoglobulin preparations or to patients who are known to have had an allergic respose to thimerosal.

The attending physician who wishes to administer Rh_o(D) Immune Globulin (Human), USP to persons with isolated immunoglobulin A (IgA) deficiency must weigh the benefits of immunization against the potential risks of hypersensitivity reactions. Such persons have increased potential for developing antibodies to IgA and could have anaphylactic reactions to subsequent administration of blood products that contain IgA.

As with all preparations administered by the intramuscular route, bleeding complications may be encountered in patients with thrombocytopenia or other bleeding disorders.

PRECAUTIONS

General

A large fetomaternal hemorrhage late in pregnancy or following delivery may cause a weak mixed field positive D^u test result. If there is any doubt about the mother's Rh type, she should be given Rh_o(D) Immune Globulin (Human), USP. A screening test to detect fetal red blood cells may be helpful in such cases.

If more than 15 mL of D-positive fetal red blood cells are present in the mother's circulation, more than a single dose of Rh_o(D) Immune Globulin (Human), USP—HypRho®-D is required. Failure to recognize this may result in the administration of an inadequate dose.

Although systemic reactions to human immunoglobulin preparations are rare, epinephrine should be available for treatment of acute anaphylactic reactions.

Drug Interactions

Other antibodies in the Rh_o(D) Immune Globulin (Human), USP preparation may interfere with the response to live vaccines such as measles, mumps, polio or rubella. Therefore, immunization with live vaccines should not be given within 3 months after Rh_o(D) Immune Globulin (Human), USP administration.

Drug/Laboratory Interactions

Babies born of women given Rh_o(D) Immune Globulin (Human), USP antepartum may have a weakly positive direct antiglobulin test at birth.

Passively acquired anti-Rh_o(D) may be detected in maternal serum if antibody screening tests are performed subsequent to antepartum or postpartum administration of Rh_o(D) Immune Globulin (Human), USP.

Pregnancy Category C

Animal reproduction studies have not been conducted with HypRho-D. It is also not known whether HypRho-D can cause fetal harm when administered to a pregnant woman or can affect reproduction capacity. HypRho-D should be given to a pregnant woman only if clearly needed.

ADVERSE REACTIONS

Reactions to Rh_o(D) Immune Globulin (Human), USP are infrequent in Rh_o(D) negative individuals and consist primarily of slight soreness at the site of injection and slight temperature elevation. While sensitization to repeated injections of human immune globulin is extremely rare, it has occurred. Elevated bilirubin levels have been reported in some individuals receiving multiple doses of Rh_o(D) Immune Globulin (Human), USP following mismatched tranfusions. This is believed to be due to a relatively rapid rate of foreign red cell destruction.

DOSAGE AND ADMINISTRATION

Pregnancy and Other Obstetric Conditions

1. For postpartum prophylaxis, administer one vial or syringe of HypRho-D (300 µg*), preferably within 72 hours of delivery. Although a lesser degree of protection is afforded if Rh antibody is administered beyond the 72-hour period, HypRho-D may still be given.[7,14] Full-term deliveries can vary in their dosage requirements depending on the magnitude of the fetomaternal hemorrhage. One 300 µg* vial or syringe of HypRho-D provides sufficient antibody to prevent Rh sensitization if the volume of red blood cells that has entered the circulation is 15 mL or less.[2–4] In instances where a large (greater than 30 mL of whole blood or 15 mL red blood cells) fetomaternal hemorrhage is suspected, a fetal red cell count by an approved laboratory technique (e.g., modified Kleihauer-Betke acid elution stain technique) should be performed to determine the dosage of immune globulin required.[8,15] The red blood cell volume of the calculated fetomaternal hemorrhage is divided by 15 mL to obtain the number of vials or syringes of Rh_o(D) Immune Globulin (Human), USP—HypRho®-D for administration.[3,8,13] If more than 15 mL of red cells is suspected or if the dose calculation results in a fraction, administer the next higher whole number of vials or syringes (e.g., if 1.4, give 2 vials or syringes).
2. For antenatal prophylaxis, one 300 µg* vial or syringe of HypRho(D) is administered at approximately 28 weeks' gestation. This **must** be followed by another 300 µg* dose, preferably within 72 hours following delivery, if the infant is Rh positive.
3. Following threatened abortion at any stage of gestation with continuation of pregnancy, it is recommended that 300 µg* of HypRho-D be given. If more than 15 mL of red

Continued on next page

*A full dose of Rh_o(D) Immune Globulin (Human), USP has traditionally been referred to as a "300 µg" dose and this usage is employed here for convenience in terminology. **It should not be construed as the actual anti-D content.** Each full dose of Rh_o(D) Immune Globulin (Human), USP must contain at least as much anti-D as 1 mL of the U.S. Reference Rh_o(D) Immune Globulin. Studies performed at the FDA have shown that the U.S. Reference contains 820 international units (IU) of anti-D per mL. When the conversion factor determined for the International (WHO) Reference Preparation[1] is used, 820 IU per mL is equivalent to 164 µg per mL of anti-D.

Bayer Biological—Cont.

cells is suspected due to fetomaternal hemorrhage, the same dose modification in No. 1 above applies.

4. Following miscarriage, abortion, or termination of ectopic pregnancy at or beyond 13 weeks' gestation, it is recommended that 300 μg* of HypRho-D be given. If more than 15 mL of red blood cells is suspected due to fetomaternal hemorrhage, the same dose modification in No. 1 above applies. If pregnancy is terminated prior to 13 weeks' gestation, a single dose of HypRho®-D Mini-Dose (approximately 50 μg*) may be used instead of HypRho-D.

5. Following amniocentesis at either 15 to 18 weeks' gestation or during the third trimester, or following abdominal trauma in the second or third trimester, it is recommended that 300 μg* of HypRho-D be administered. If there is a fetomaternal hemorrhage in excess of 15 mL of red cells, the same dose modification in No. 1 applies.

If abdominal trauma, amniocentesis, or other adverse event requires the administration of HypRho-D at 13 to 18 weeks' gestation, another 300 μg* dose should be given at 26 to 28 weeks. To maintain protection throughout pregnancy, the level of passively acquired anti-Rh_o(D) should not be allowed to fall below the level required to prevent an immune response to Rh positive red cells. The half-life of IgG is 23 to 26 days. In any case, a dose of HypRho-D should be given within 72 hours after delivery if the baby is Rh positive. If delivery occurs within 3 weeks after the last dose, the postpartum dose may be withheld unless there is a fetomaternal hemorrhage in excess of 15 mL of red blood cells.[16]
*See footnote under DESCRIPTION.

Transfusion

In the case of a transfusion of Rh_o(D) positive red cells to an Rh_o(D) negative recipient, the volume of Rh positive whole blood administered is multiplied by the hematocrit of the donor unit giving the volume of red blood cells transfused. The volume of red blood cells is divided by 15 mL which provides the number of vials or syringes of HypRho-D to be administered.

If the dose calculated results in a fraction, the next higher whole number of vials or syringes should be administered (e.g., if 1.4, give 2 vials or 2 syringes). HypRho-D should be administered within 72 hours after an incompatible transfusion, but preferably as soon as possible.

Injection Procedure

DO NOT INJECT INTRAVENOUSLY. DO NOT INJECT NEONATE. Rh_o(D) Immune Globulin (Human), USP—HypRho®-D is administered **intramuscularly**, preferably in the anterolateral aspects of the upper thigh and the deltoid muscle of the upper arm. The gluteal region should not be used routinely as an injection site because of the risk of injury to the sciatic nerve. If the gluteal region is used, the central region MUST be avoided; only the upper, outer quadrant should be used.[17]

A. Single Vial or Syringe Dose
   INJECT ENTIRE CONTENTS OF THE VIAL OR SYRINGE INTO THE INDIVIDUAL INTRAMUSCULARLY.

B. Multiple Vial or Syringe Dose
   1. Calculate the number of vials or syringes of HypRho-D to be given (See Dosage section above).
   2. The total volume of HypRho-D can be given in divided doses at different sites at one time or the total dose may be divided and injected at intervals, provided the total dosage is given within 72 hours of the fetomaternal hemorrhage or transfusion. USING STERILE TECHNIQUE, INJECT THE ENTIRE CONTENTS OF THE CALCULATED NUMBER OF VIALS OR SYRINGES INTRAMUSCULARLY INTO THE PATIENT.

Parenteral drug products should be inspected visually for particulate matter and discoloration prior to administration, whenever solution and container permit.

HOW SUPPLIED

HypRho-D is available in individual and multiple-pack single dose syringes and vials.

STORAGE

Store at 2°–8°C (36°–46°F). Do not freeze.

CAUTION

U.S. federal law prohibits dispensing without prescription.

LIMITED WARRANTY

A number of factors beyond our control could reduce the efficacy of this product or even result in an ill effect following its use. These include improper storage and handling of the product after it leaves our hands, diagnosis, dosage, method of administration, and biological differences in individual patients. Because of these factors, it is important that this product be stored properly and that the directions be followed carefully during use.

No warranty, express or implied, including any warranty of merchantability or fitness is made. Representatives of the Company are not authorized to vary the terms or the contents of any printed labeling, including the package insert

for this product, except by printed notice from the Company's headquarters. The prescriber and user of this product must accept the terms hereof.

REFERENCES

1. Gunson HH, Bowell PJ, Kirkwood TBL: Collaborative study to recalibrate the International Reference Preparation of Anti-D Immunoglobulin. *J Clin Pathol* 33:249–53, 1980.
2. Rh_o(D) immune globulin (human). *Med Lett Drugs Ther* 16(1):3–4, 1974.
3. Pollack W, Ascari WQ, Kochesky RJ, et al: Studies on Rh prophylaxis I. Relationship between doses of anti-Rh and size of antigenic stimulus. *Transfusion* 11(6):333–9, 1971.
4. Unpublished data in files of Miles Inc., Cutter Biological.
5. Pollack W, Asceri WQ, Crispen JF, et al: Studies on Rh prophylaxis. II. Rh immune prophylaxis after transfusion with Rh-positive blood. *Transfusion* 11 (6):340–4, 1971.
6. Keith LG, Houser GH: Anti-Rh immune globulin after a massive transfusion accident. *Transfusion* 11(3):176, 1971.
7. The selective use of Rh_o(D) Immune Globulin (RhIG). *ACOG Tech Bull* 61, 1981.
8. Current uses of Rh_o immune globulin and detection of antibodies. *ACOG Tech Bull* 35, 1976.
9. Pollack W: Rh hemolytic disease of the newborn; its cause and prevention. *Prog Clin Biol Res* 70:185–203, 1981.
10. Bowman JM, Chown B, Lewis M, et al: Rh isoimmunization during pregnancy: antenatal prophylaxis. *Can Med Assoc J* 118(6):623–7, 1978.
11. Bowman JM, Pollock JM: Antenatal prophylaxis of Rh isommunization: 28-weeks'-gestation service program. *Can Med Assoc J* 118(6):627–30, 1978.
12. Ascari WQ, Allen AE, Baker WJ, et al: Rh_o(D) immune globulin (human): evaluation in women at risk of Rh immunization. *JAMA* 205(1): 1–4, 1968.
13. Prevention of Rh sensitization, *WHO Tech Rep Ser* 468:25, 1971.
14. Samson D, Mollison PL: Effect on primary Rh immunization of delayed administration of anti-Rh. *Immunology* 28:349–57, 175.
15. Finn R, Harper DT, Stallings, SA, et al: Transplacental hemorrhage. *Transfusion* 3(2):114–24, 1963.
16. Garraty G (ed): Hemolytic disease of the newborn. Arlington, VA, American Association of Blood Banks, 1984, p 78.
17. Recommendations of the Immunization Practices Advisory Committee (ACIP): General recommendations on immunization. *MMWR* 38(13):205–14; 219–27, 1989.

KOĀTE®-HP
[kō´ate]
Antihemophilic Factor (Human)
(Factor VIII, AHF, AHG)

℞

DESCRIPTION

Antihemophilic Factor (Human), Koāte®-HP, is a sterile, stable, purified, dried concentrate of human Antihemophilic Factor (AHF, factor VIII, AHG) which has been treated with tri-n-butyl phosphate (TNBP) and polysorbate 80 and is intended for use in therapy of classical hemophilia (hemophilia A).

Koāte-HP is purified from the cold insoluble fraction of pooled fresh-frozen plasma by modification and refinements of the methods first described by Hershgold, Pool, and Pappenhagen.[1] Koāte-HP contains purified and concentrated factor VIII. The factor VIII is 300-1000 times purified over whole plasma. Part of the fractionation may be performed by another licensed manufacturer. When reconstituted as directed, Koāte-HP contains approximately 50-150 times as much factor VIII as an equal volume of fresh plasma. The specific activity, after addition of Albumin (Human), is in the range of 9-22 IU/mg protein. Koāte-HP must be administered by the intravenous route.

Each bottle of Koāte-HP contains the labeled amount of antihemophilic factor activity in International Units (IU). One IU, as defined by the World Health Organization Standard for Blood Coagulation factor VIII, human, is approximately equal to the level of AHF found in 1.0 mL of fresh pooled human plasma. The final product when reconstituted as directed contains not more than (NMT) 5 units heparin/mL, NMT 1500 ppm polyethylene glycol (PEG), NMT 0.05 M glycine, NMT 25 ppm polysorbate 80, NMT 5 ppm tri-n-butyl phosphate (TNBP), NMT 3 mM calcium chloride, NMT 1 ppm aluminum, NMT 0.06 M histidine, and NMT 10 mg/mL Albumin (Human).

CLINICAL PHARMACOLOGY

Hemophilia A is a hereditary bleeding disorder characterized by deficient coagulant activity of the specific plasma protein clotting factor, factor VIII. In afflicted individuals, hemorrhages may occur spontaneously or after only minor

trauma. Surgery on such individuals is not feasible without first correcting the clotting abnormality. The administration of Koāte-HP provides an increase in plasma levels of factor VIII and can temporarily correct the coagulation defect in these patients.

After infusion of Koāte-HP, there is usually an instantaneous rise in the coagulant level followed by an initial rapid decrease in activity, and then a subsequent much slower rate of decrease in activity.[2–4] The early rapid phase may represent the time of equilibration with the extravascular compartment, and the second or slow phase of the survival curve presumably is the result of degradation and reflects the true biologic half-life of the infused Antihemophilic Factor (Human).[3] Studies with Koāte-HP in hemophilic patients have demonstrated a biologic half-life of approximately 9 to 14 hours.[2]

In 1984, Prince, et al[5] described the susceptibility of hepatitis B virus (HBV) and the Hutchinson strain of non-A, non-B hepatitis virus to inactivation by ether and polysorbate 80. This method is known to disrupt lipid-containing enveloped viruses. Subsequently, others[6,7] using tri-n-butyl phosphate as an alternative organic solvent to the hazardous ethyl ether in combination with a number of different detergents including polysorbate 80, sodium deoxycholate, sodium cholate, or Triton x-100, showed these forms of chemical treatment to be rapidly effective in inactivating certain lipid-enveloped viruses. These viruses included vesicular stomatitis virus (VSV), sindbis virus, and sendai virus[6] as well as, in a later study,[7] human immunodeficiency virus (HIV), HBV and non-A, non-B virus. Similar studies undertaken at Miles Inc. using TNBP and polysorbate 80 treatment of factor VIII concentrate immediately prior to a gel permeation chromatography purifying/concentrating procedure have confirmed the inactivation of VSV, visna, and sindbis viruses. Antihemophilic Factor (Human), Koāte®-HP is purified by virtue of a gel permeation chromatography step serving the dual purpose of removing the TNBP and polysorbate 80 as well as increasing the purity of the Factor VIII. Recently, concerns have been expressed concerning alterations to immune function occurring in asymptomatic hemophiliacs,[8–15] with some of the abnormalities being independent of HIV exposure. It has been suggested that the underlying mechanisms might include repeated exposure to viral agents, repeated allostimulation and/or possible contaminants in factor VIII preparations (e.g., IgG aggregates). More highly purified preparations which have minimized risks of viral transmission may therefore be desirable.[6]

INDICATIONS AND USAGE

Koāte-HP is indicated for the treatment of classical hemophilia (hemophilia A) in which there is a demonstrated deficiency of activity of the plasma clotting factor, factor VIII. Koāte-HP provides a means of temporarily replacing the missing clotting factor in order to correct or prevent bleeding episodes, or in order to perform emergency and elective surgery on hemophiliacs.

Koāte-HP has not been investigated for efficacy in the treatment of von Willebrand's disease, and hence is not approved for such usage.

CONTRAINDICATIONS

None known.

WARNINGS

This product is prepared from pooled human plasma which may contain the causative agents of hepatitis and other viral diseases. Prescribed manufacturing procedures utilized at the plasma collection centers, plasma testing laboratories, and the fractionation facilities are designed to reduce the risk of transmitting viral infection. However, the risk of viral infectivity from this product cannot be totally eliminated. The presence of hepatitis viruses should be assumed.

Individuals who receive infusions of blood or plasma products may develop signs and/or symptoms of some viral infections, particularly non-A, non-B hepatitis. It is emphasized that hepatitis B vaccination is essential for patients with hemophilia and it is recommended that this be done at birth or diagnosis.[16,17]

Fletcher et al,[18] have concluded that those who have had little exposure to blood products have a higher risk of developing hepatitis after introduction of clotting factor concentrates. For such patients, especially those with mild hemophilia, Kasper and Kipnis[19] recommend single donor products. For patients with moderate or severe hemophilia who have received numerous infusions of blood or blood products, they feel that the risk of hepatitis is small. They believe that the clotting factor concentrates have so greatly improved the management of severe hemophilia that these products should not be denied to appropriate patients. The physician and patient should consider that factor VIII concentrates may be associated with the trasmission of hepatitis and weigh the benefits of therapy accordingly.

No studies of CD4 cell count surveillance have been done in HIV seropositive patients treated exclusively with Koāte-HP; however, there have been several reports of increased rates of CD4 cell count decline in HIV seropositive hemophilia patients treated with conventionally purified FVIII concentrates compared to those treated with immunoaffinity purified products.[20–22] The clinical significance of these CD4 cell count findings remains uncertain.

PRECAUTIONS

General

1. Antihemophilic Factor (Human), Koāte-HP is intended for treatment of bleeding disorders arising from a deficiency in factor VIII. This deficiency should be proven prior to administering Koāte-HP.
2. Administer within 3 hours after reconstitution. Do not refrigerate after reconstitution.
3. Administer only by the intravenous route.
4. Filter needle should be used prior to administering.
5. Koāte-HP contains levels of blood group isoagglutinins which are not clinically significant when controlling relatively minor bleeding episodes. When large or frequently repeated doses are required, patients of blood groups A, B, or AB should be monitored by means of hematocrit for signs of progressive anemia, as well as by direct Coombs' tests.
6. Product administration and handling of the infusion set and needles must be done with caution. Percutaneous puncture with a needle contaminated with blood can transmit infectious viruses including HIV (AIDS) and hepatitis. Obtain immediate medical attention if injury occurs.

   Place needles in sharps container after single use. Discard all equipment including any reconstituted Koāte-HP product in accordance with biohazard procedures.

Pregnancy Category C

Animal reproduction studies have not been conducted with Koāte-HP. It is also not known whether Koāte-HP can cause fetal harm when administered to a pregnant woman or can affect reproduction capacity. Koāte-HP should be given to a pregnant woman only if clearly needed.

ADVERSE REACTIONS

Allergic-type reactions may result from the administration of Antihemophilic Factor (Human) preparations.[23,24]

DOSAGE AND ADMINISTRATION

Each bottle of Koāte-HP has the Antihemophilic Factor (Human) content in International Units per bottle stated on the label of the bottle. The reconstituted product must be administered intravenously by either direct syringe injection or drip infusion.

Shanbrom et al,[25] based upon studies in hemophiliacs, have suggested a linear dose-response relation with an approximate rise of 2.5% in Factor VIII activity for each unit of Antihemophilic Factor (Human) transfused per kg of body weight. Abildgaard et al,[26] in work with hemophilic children 8 months to 14 years of age, reported a response factor of 0.5 units/kg. Clinical experience with Koāte-HP has demonstrated a similar dose-response relationship.[2] The following formulas can provide a guide for dosage calculations:

Expected factor VIII increase (% of normal) =

$$\frac{\text{IU administered}}{\text{body weight (kg)} \times 0.4\ \text{IU/kg}}$$

Example:

$$\frac{840\ \text{IU}}{70\ \text{kg} \times 0.4\ \text{IU/kg}} = 30\%$$

or

IU required = body weight (kg) × desired factor VIII increase (% normal) × 0.4 IU/kg

Example: 70 kg × 0.4 IU/kg × 30% = 840 IU

All efforts should be made to follow the course of therapy with factor VIII level assays. It may be dangerous to assume any certain level has been reached unless direct evidence is obtained.

Prophylaxis of Spontaneous Hemorrhage

The level of factor VIII required to prevent spontaneous hemorrhage is approximately 5% of normal, while a level of 30% of normal is the minimum required for hemostasis following trauma and surgery.[27–29] Mild superficial or early hemorrhages may respond to a single dose of 10 IU per kg,[4,30] leading to an in vivo rise of approximately 20% in the factor VIII level. In patients with early hemarthrosis (mild pain, minimal or no swelling, erythema, warmth, and minimal or no joint limitation), if treated promptly, even smaller doses may be adequate.[30–32]

Mild Hemorrhage

In cases of mild hemorrhage, therapy need not be repeated unless there is evidence of further bleeding.

Moderate Hemorrhage and Minor Surgery

For more serious hemorrhages and for minor surgical procedures, the patient's plasma factor VIII level should be raised to 30%–50% of normal for optimum hemostasis.[30,33] This usually requires an initial dose of 15–25 IU per kg; and if further therapy is required, a maintenance dose of 10–15 IU per kg every 8–12 hours.

Severe Hemorrhage

In patients with life-threatening bleeding, or hemorrhage involving vital structures (central nervous system, retropharyngeal and retroperitoneal spaces, iliopsoas sheath), it may be desirable to raise the factor VIII level to 80%–100% of normal in order to achieve hemostasis.[30,33–35] This may be achieved with an initial Koāte-HP dose of 40–50 IU per kg and a maintenance dose of 20–25 IU per kg every 8–12 hours.

Major Surgery

For major surgical procedures, Kasper[33] recommends that a dose of Antihemophilic Factor (Human) sufficient to achieve a level of 80%–100% of normal be given an hour before the procedure. It is recommended that the factor VIII level be checked prior to going to surgery to assure the expected level is achieved. A second dose, half the size of the priming dose, should be given about 5 hours after the first dose. The factor VIII level should be maintained at a daily minimum of at least 30% for a healing period of 10–14 days, depending on the nature of the operative procedure.

The above discussion is presented as a reference and a guideline. It should be emphasized that the dosage of Antihemophilic Factor (Human), Koāte®-HP required for normalizing hemostasis must be individualized according to the needs of the patient. Factors to be considered include the weight of the patient, the severity of the deficiency, the severity of the hemorrhage, the presence of inhibitors, and the factor VIII level desired. All efforts should be made to follow the course of therapy with factor VIII level assays.

The clinical effect of Koāte-HP is the most important element in evaluating the effectiveness of treatment. It may be necessary to administer more Koāte-HP than would be estimated in order to attain satisfactory clinical results. If the calculated dose fails to attain the expected factor VIII levels, or if bleeding is not controlled after adequate calculated dosage, the presence of a factor VIII inhibitor should be suspected. Its presence should be substantiated and the inhibitor level quantitated by appropriate laboratory procedure. When an inhibitor is present, the dosage requirement for Koāte-HP is extremely variable and the dosage can be determined only by the clinical response.

Parenteral drug products should be inspected visually for particulate matter and discoloration prior to administration, whenever solution and container permit.

Reconstitution

Vacuum Transfer

1. Warm the unopened diluent and the concentrate to room temperature (NMT 37°C, 99°F).
2. After removing the plastic flip-top caps (Fig. A), aseptically cleanse the rubber stoppers of both bottles.
3. Remove the protective cover from the plastic transfer-needle cartridge with tamper-proof seal and penetrate the stopper of the diluent bottle (Fig. B).
4. Remove the remaining portion of the plastic cartridge, invert the diluent bottle and penetrate the rubber seal on the concentrate bottle (Fig. C) with the needle at an angle. Alternate method of transferring sterile water: With a sterile needle and syringe, withdraw the appropriate volume of diluent and transfer to the bottle of lyophilized concentrate.
5. The vacuum will draw the diluent into the concentrate bottle. Hold the diluent bottle at an angle to the concentrate bottle in order to direct the jet of diluent against the wall of the concentrate bottle (Fig. C). Avoid excessive foaming.
6. After removing the diluent bottle and transfer needle (Fig. D), swirl continuously until completely dissolved (Fig. E).
7. After the concentrate powder is completely dissolved, withdraw solution into the syringe through the filter needle which is supplied in the package (Fig. F). Replace the filter needle with the administration set provided and inject intravenously.
8. If the same patient is to receive more than one bottle, the contents of two bottles may be drawn into the same syringe through a separate unused filter needle before attaching the vein needle.

[See Figure at top of next column.]

Rate of Administration

The rate of administration should be adapted to the response of the individual patient, but administration of the entire dose in 5 to 10 minutes is generally well-tolerated.

HOW SUPPLIED

Antihemophilic Factor (Human), Koāte®-HP is supplied in the following single dose bottles with the total units of factor VIII activity stated on the label of each bottle. A suitable volume of Sterile Water for Injection, USP, a sterile double-ended transfer needle, a sterile filter needle, and a sterile administration set are provided.

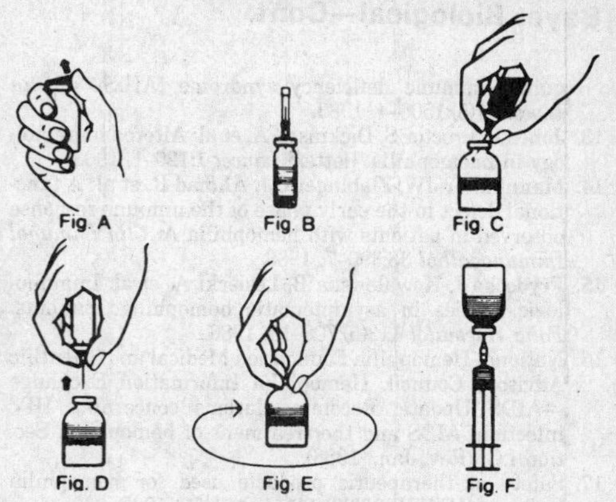
Fig. A
Fig. B
Fig. C
Fig. D
Fig. E
Fig. F

Product Code	Approximate Factor VIII Activity	Diluent
664-20	250 IU	5 mL
664-30	500 IU	5 mL
664-50	1000 IU	10 mL
664-60	1500 IU	10 mL

STORAGE

Koāte-HP should be stored under refrigeration (2°–8°C; 36°–46°F). Storage of lyophilized powder at room temperature (up to 25°C or 77°F) for 6 months, such as in home treatment situations, may be done without loss of factor VIII activity. Freezing should be avoided as breakage of the diluent bottle might occur.

CAUTION

U.S. federal law prohibits dispensing without prescription.

LIMITED WARRANTY

A number of factors beyond our control could reduce the efficacy of this product or even result in an ill effect following its use. These include improper storage and handling of the product after it leaves our hands, diagnosis, dosage, method of administration, and biological differences in individual patients. Because of these factors, it is important that this product be stored properly, that the directions be followed carefully during use, and that the risk of transmitting viruses be carefully weighed before the product is prescribed. No warranty, express or implied, including any warranty of merchantability or fitness is made. Representatives of the Company are not authorized to vary the terms or the contents of the printed labeling, including the package insert for this product, except by printed notice from the Company's headquarters. The prescriber and user of this product must accept the terms hereof.

REFERENCES

1. Hershgold EJ, Pool JG, Pappenhagen AR: The potent antihemophilic globulin concentrate derived from a cold insoluble fraction of human plasma: characterization and further data on preparation and clinical trial. *J Lab Clin Med* 67(1):23–32, 1966.
2. Unpublished data in files of Miles Inc., Cutter Biological.
3. Aronson DL: Factor VIII (antihemophilic globulin). *Semin Thromb Hemostas* 6(1):12–27, 1979.
4. Britton M, Harrison J, Abildgaard CF: Early treatment of hemophilic hemarthroses with minimal dose of new factor VIII concentrate. *J Pediatr* 85(2):245–7, 1974.
5. Prince AM, Horowitz B, Brotman B, et al: Inactivation of hepatitis B and Hutchinson strain non-A, non-B hepatitis viruses by exposure to Tween 80 and ether. *Vox Sang* 46:36–43, 1984.
6. Horowitz B, Wiebe ME, Lippin A, et al: Inactivation of viruses in labile blood derivatives. I. Distruption of lipid-enveloped viruses by tri(n-butyl) phosphate detergent combinations. *Transfusion* 25(6):516–22, 1985.
7. Piet MPJ, Chin S, Prince AM, et al: Inactivtion of viruses in plasma on treatment with tri(n-butyl) phosphate (TNBP) detergent mixtures. [abstract] *Thromb Haemost* 58(1):370, 1987.
8. Lederman MM, Ratnoff OD, Scillian JJ, et al: Impaired cell-mediated immunity in patients with classic hemophilia. *N Engl J Med* 308(2):79–83, 1983.
9. Weintrub PS, Koerper MA, Addiego JE Jr, et al: Immunologic abnormalities in patients with hemophilia A. *J Pediatr* 103(5):692–5, 1983.
10. Goldsmith JC, Moseley PL, Monick M, et al: T-lymphocyte subpopulation abnormalities in apparently healthy patients with hemophilia. *Ann Intern Med* 98:294–6, 1983.
11. Saidi P, Kim HC, Raska K Jr: T-cell subsets in hemophilia. [letter] *N Engl J Med* 308(21):1291–3, 1983.
12. Landay A, Poon MC, Abo T, et al: Immunologic studies in asymptomatic hemophilia patients: relationship to ac-

Continued on next page

Bayer Biological—Cont.

quired immune deficiency syndrome (AIDS). *J Clin Invest* 71(5):1500–4, 1983.

13. Jones P, Proctor S, Dickinson A, et al: Altered immunology in haemophilia. [letter] *Lancet* 1:120–1, 1983.
14. Mannhalter JW, Zlabinger GJ, Ahmad R, et al: A functional defect in the early phase of the immune response observed in patients with hemophilia A. *Clin Immunol Immunopathol* 38:390–7, 1986.
15. Frydecka I, Kowalewska B, Lesiecki A, et al: Immunologic studies in asymptomatic hemophiliac patients. *Folia Haematol* 113(5):708–15, 1986.
16. National Hemophilia Foundation Medical and Scientific Advisory Council. Hemophilia Information Exchange —AIDS Update: Recommendations concerning HIV infection, AIDS and the treatment of hemophilia. Section I.G. (Rev. Jan., 1988).
17. Safety of therapeutic products used for hemophilia patients. *MMWR* 37(29):441–4, 449–50, 1988.
18. Fletcher ML, Trowell JM, Craske J, et al: Non-A, non-B hepatitis after transfusion of factor VIII in infrequently treated patients. *Br Med J* 287(6407):1754–7, 1983.
19. Kasper CK, Kipnis SA: Hepatitis and clotting-factor concentrates. *JAMA* 221(5):510, 1972.
20. Madhok R, Gracie A, Lowe GDO, et al: Impaired cell mediated immunity in haemophilia in the absence of infection with human immunodeficiency virus. *Br Med J* 239(6553):978–80, 1986.
21. Goldsmith JM, Deutsche J, Tang M, et al: CD4 cells in HIV-1 infected hemophiliacs: effect of factor VIII concentrates. *Thromb Haemost* 66(4):415–9, 1991.
22. Hilgartner MW, Buckley JD, Operskalski EA, et al: Purity of factor VIII concentrates and serial CD4 counts. *Lancet* 341(8857):1373–4, 1993.
23. Eyster ME, Bowman HS, Haverstick JN: Adverse reactions to factor VIII infusions. [letter] *Ann Intern Med* 87(2):248, 1977.
24. Prager D, Djerassi I, Eyster ME, et al: Pennsylvania state-wide hemophilia program: summary of immediate reactions with the use of factor VIII and factor IX concentrate. *Blood* 53(5):1012–3, 1979.
25. Shanbrom E, Thelin GM: Experimental prophylaxis of severe hemophilia with a factor VIII concentrate. *JAMA* 208(10):1853–6, 1969.
26. Abildgaard CF, Simone JV, Corrigan JJ, et al: Treatment of hemophilia with glycine-precipitated factor VIII. *N Engl J Med* 275(9):471–5, 1966.
27. Biggs R, MacFarlane RG: Haemophilia and related conditions: a survey of 187 cases. *Br J Haematol* 4(1):1–27, 1958.
28. Langdell RD, Wagner RH, Brinkhous KM: Antihemophilic factor (AHF) levels following transfusions of blood, plasma and plasma fractions. *Proc Soc Exp Biol Med* 88(2):212–5, 1955.
29. Shulman NR, Cowan DH, Libre EP, et al: The physiologic basis for therapy of classic hemophilia (factor VIII deficiency) and related disorders. *Ann Intern Med* 67(4):856–82, 1967.
30. Abildgaard CF: Current concepts in the management of hemophilia. *Semin Hematol* 12(3):223–32, 1975.
31. Penner JA, Kelly PE: Low doses of factor VIII for hemophilia. [letter] *N Engl J Med* 297(7):401; 1977.
32. Ashenhurst JB, Langehennig PL, Seller RA: Early treatment of bleeding episodes with 10 U/kg of factor VIII. [letter] *Blood* 50(1):181–2, 1977.
33. Kasper CK: Hematologic care. In: Boone DC (ed.): Comprehensive management of hemophilia. Philadelphia, Davis, 1976, pp 3–17.
34. Edson JR: Hemophilia and related conditions. In: Conn HF (ed): Current therapy. Philadelphia, Saunders, 1980, pp 264–9.
35. Hilgartner MW; Management of hemophilia: the routine and the crises. *Drug Ther* 8(2):141–54, 1978.

Antihemophilic Factor (Recombinant) ℞
KOGENATE®

DESCRIPTION

Antihemophilic Factor (Recombinant), KOGENATE®, is a sterile, stable, purified, dried concentrate which has been manufactured by recombinant DNA technology. KOGENATE is intended for use in therapy of classical hemophilia (hemophilia A). KOGENATE is produced by Baby Hamster Kidney (BHK) cells into which the human factor VIII (FVIII) gene has been introduced.[1] KOGENATE is a highly purified glycoprotein consisting of multiple peptides including an 80 kD and various extensions of the 90 kD subunit. It has the same biological activity as FVIII derived from human plasma. In addition to the use of the classical purification methods of ion exchange chromatography and size exclusion chromatography, monoclonal antibody immunoaffinity chromatography is utilized along with other steps designed to purify recombinant factor VIII (rAHF) and remove contaminating substances. The final preparation is stabilized with Albumin (Human) and lyophilized. The concentration of KOGENATE is approximately 100 IU/mL. The product contains no preservatives.

Each vial of KOGENATE contains the labeled amount of rAHF in international units (IU). One IU, as defined by the World Health Organization standard for blood coagulation factor VIII, human, is approximately equal to the level of factor VIII activity found in 1.0 mL of fresh pooled human plasma. The final product when reconstituted as directed contains the following excipients: 10–30 mg glycine/mL, not more than (NMT) 500 μg imidazole/1000 IU, NMT 600 μg polysorbate 80/1000 IU, 2–5 mM calcium chloride, 100–130 mEq/L sodium, 100–130 mEq/L chloride and 4–10 mg Albumin (Human)/mL. KOGENATE must be administered by the intravenous route.

CLINICAL PHARMACOLOGY

The clinical trial of KOGENATE has included 168 patients, enrolled over a 55-month period. A total of 16,186 infusions have been utilized in this trial. The study was conducted in several stages.

Initial pharmacokinetic studies were conducted in 17 asymptomatic hemophilic patients, comparing pharmacokinetics of plasma-derived Antihemophilic Factor (Human) (pdAHF) and KOGENATE.[2] The mean biologic half-life of rAHF was 15.8 hours. The mean biologic half-life of pdAHF in the same individuals was 13.9 hours. A similar degree of shortening of the activated partial thromboplastin time was seen with both rAHF and pdAHF. The mean *in vivo* recovery of rAHF was similar to pdAHF, with a linear dose-response relationship. The recovery and half-life of rAHF was consistent with initial results following 13 weeks of exclusive treatment with KOGENATE. Subsequently, 826 recovery studies were conducted in 58 hemophilic patients participating in later clinical studies. Mean recovery from this group was 2.48% per IU/kg infused.

Fourteen (14) subjects from initial pharmacokinetic studies commenced home treatment with rAHF. Forty-four (44) additional subjects were then enrolled who treated themselves at home exclusively with rAHF. A total of 12,730 infusions have been administered under this portion of the study, of which 1,021 were given in clinic for recovery studies, 7,339 were given for treatment of bleeds, 4,361 were given as prophylaxis, 5 for minor surgery not requiring hospitalization, and 4 for unspecified reason.

Forty-eight (48) patients have received rAHF on 63 occasions for surgical procedures or in-hospital treatment of serious hemorrhage. Eleven (11) received rAHF for the first time in this study, while 37 were already on study or study participants under an investigation of previously untreated patients. Hemostatis has been satisfactory in all cases, with no adverse reactions.

In a study of previously untreated patients, a total of 3,254 infusions have been administered to 96 patients over a 48-month enrollment period. Hemostasis was successfully achieved in all cases.

During the analytical characterization of Antihemophilic Factor (Recombinant), KOGENATE®, analyses for carbohydrate structure revealed the presence of terminal galactose α1 3 galactose residues. Since naturally occurring antibody to this structure has been reported in humans, a trial in 18 patients was performed in which the half-life and recovery of rAHF with high levels on this carbohydrate residue was compared to that with KOGENATE, which contains low levels of this structure. As in the normal population, all patients had preexisting endogenous antibody to galactose α1 3 galactose in titers ranging from 1:320 to 1:5120 and no significant change in antibody level was noted during the study. While the mean recovery for KOGENATE in the study, 2.76%/IU/kg (N=43), was significantly different from that of rAHF with high levels of residues, 2.43%/IU/kg (N=155; p=0.0001), the recovery for rAHF with high levels of galactose $\alpha 1 \rightarrow 3$ galactose is not significantly different from the 2.48%/IU/kg recovery obtained in the larger study from the 58 patients treated with KOGENATE mentioned above. Based on these results, the galactose $\alpha 1 \rightarrow 3$ galactose residue appears to have no clinical significance.

INDICATIONS AND USAGE

KOGENATE is indicated for the treatment of classical hemophilia (hemophilia A) in which there is a demonstrated deficiency of activity of the plasma clotting factor, factor VIII. KOGENATE provides a means of temporarily replacing the missing clotting factor in order to correct or prevent bleeding episodes, or in order to perform emergency and elective surgery in hemophiliacs.

KOGENATE can also be used for treatment of hemophilia A in certain patients with inhibitors to factor VIII. In clinical studies of KOGENATE, patients who developed inhibitors on study continued to manifest a clinical response when inhibitor titers were less than 10 Bethesda Units (B.U.) per mL. When an inhibitor is present, the dosage requirement for factor VIII is variable. The dosage can be determined only by clinical response, and by monitoring of circulating factor VIII levels after treatment (see **DOSAGE AND ADMINISTRATION.)**

KOGENATE does not contain von Willebrand's factor and therefore is not indicated for the treatment of von Willebrand's disease.

CONTRAINDICATIONS

Due to the fact that Antihemophilic Factor (Recombinant) contains trace amounts of mouse protein (maximum 0.03 ng/IU rAHF) and hamster protein (maximum 0.04 ng/IU rAHF), KOGENATE should be administered with caution to individuals with previous hypersensitivity to pdAHF or known hypersensitivity to biologic preparations with trace amounts of murine or hamster proteins.

Assays to detect seroconversion to mouse and hamster protein were conducted on all patients on study. No patient has developed specific antibody titers against these proteins after commencing study, and no allergic reactions have been associated with rAHF infusions. Although no reactions were observed, patients should be warned of the theoretical possibility of a hypersensitivity reaction, and alerted to the early signs of such a reaction (e.g., hives, generalized uticaria, wheezing and hypotension). Patients should be advised to discontinue use of the product and contact their physician if such symptoms occur.

WARNINGS

None.

PRECAUTIONS

General

KOGENATE is intended for the treatment of bleeding disorders arising from a deficiency in factor VIII. This deficiency should be proven prior to administering KOGENATE.

The development of circulating neutralizing antibodies to factor VIII may occur during the treatment of patients with hemophilia A. In a study of previously untreated patients, inhibitor antibodies have developed in 17 of the 92 patients (18.5%) who have had at least one follow-up titer. The incidence of antibodies is 15/56 (26.7%) in patients with severe disease (< 2% factor VIII), 2/18 (11%) in patients with moderate disease (2–5% factor VIII) and 0/18 in patients with mild disease (> 5% factor VIII). Ten of the antibodies were high titer (> 10 Bethesda Units), three were low titer, and four were low titer and transient. Studies most closely resembling the design of the study of inhibitor development with KOGENATE have reported incidences of inhibitor formation ranging between 18.4 and 52% for patients treated with pdAHF.[3–6] The incidence of inhibitor formation in previously untreated patients treated with Antihemophilic Factor (Recombinant), KOGENATE®, appears to be consistent with that reported in the literature, however the true immunogenicity of KOGENATE is not known at present. Patients treated with rAHF should be carefully monitored for the development of antibodies to rAHF by appropriate clinical observation and laboratory tests.

Product administration and handling of the infusion set and needles must be done with caution. Percutaneous puncture with a needle contaminated with blood can transmit infectious virus including HIV (AIDS) and hepatitis. Obtain immediate medical attention if injury occurs.

Place needles in sharps container after single use. Discard all equipment including any reconstituted KOGENATE product in accordance with biohazard procedures.

Carcinogenesis, Mutagenesis, Impairment of Fertility

In vitro evaluation of the mutagenic potential of KOGENATE failed to demonstrate reverse mutation or chromosomal aberrations at doses substantially greater than the maximum expected clinical dose. *In vivo* evaluation of rAHF using doses ranging between 10 and 40 times the expected clinical maximum also indicated that KOGENATE does not possess a mutagenic potential. Long-term investigations of carcinogenic potential in animals have not been performed.

Pediatric Use

KOGENATE has been proven to be safe and efficacious in newborns and the pediatric population while under investigation as previously treated (n=21) and previously untreated patients (n=96) (see **CLINICAL PHARMACOLOGY and PRECAUTIONS**).

Pregnancy Category C

Animal reproduction studies have not been conducted with KOGENATE. It is also not known whether KOGENATE can cause fetal harm when administered to a pregnant woman or can affect reproduction capacity. KOGENATE should be given to a pregnant woman only if clearly needed.

ADVERSE REACTIONS

During the clinical studies conducted in previously treated patients, 47 out of 12,932 infusions (0.36%) were associated with 58 reported minor adverse reactions. Of these, 19 reactions were local to the injection site (e.g., burning, pruritus, erythema); and 39 were systemic complaints (dizziness, nausea, chest discomfort, sore throat, cold feet, unusual taste in mouth, and slight decrease in blood pressure). In the study with previously untreated patients, 3,254 infusions have

been associated with 11 minor adverse reactions (0.34%): two reports of erythema at the injection site, one of facial flushing related to the infusion, one report of diarrhea, two reports of nonspecific rash, two reports of fever, and three reports of emesis. No serious reactions have been reported, and all reactions have been self-limited.

DOSAGE AND ADMINISTRATION

Each bottle of KOGENATE has the rAHF content in international units per bottle stated on the label of the bottle. The reconstituted product must be administered intravenously by either direct syringe injection or drip infusion. The product must be administered within 3 hours after reconstitution.

General Approach to Treatment and Assessment of Treatment Efficacy

The dosages described below are presented as general guidance. It should be emphasized that the dosage of KOGENATE required for (hemostasis) must be individualized according to the needs of the patient, the severity of the deficiency, the severity of the hemorrhage, the presence of inhibitors, and the factor VIII level desired. It is often critical to follow the course of therapy with factor VIII level assays.

The clinical effect of KOGENATE is the most important element in evaluating the effectiveness of treatment. It may be necessary to administer more KOGENATE than would be estimated in order to attain satisfactory clinical results. If the calculated dose fails to attain the expected factor VIII levels, or if bleeding is not controlled after administration of the calculated dosage, the presence of a circulating inhibitor in the patient should be suspected. Its presence should be substantiated and the inhibitor level quantitated by appropriate laboratory tests. When an inhibitor is present, the dosage requirement for rAHF is extremely variable and the dosage can be determined only by the clinical response.

Some patients with low titer inhibitors (< 10 B.U.) can be successfully treated with factor VIII without a resultant anamnestic rise in inhibitor titer.[7] Factor VIII levels and clinical response to treatment must be assessed to insure adequate response. Use of alternative treatment products, such as Factor IX Complex concentrates, Antihemophilic Factor (Porcine) or Anti-Inhibitor Coagulant Complex, may be necessary for patients with anamnestic responses to factor VIII treatment and/or high titer inhibitors.

Calculation of Dosage

The *in vivo* percent elevation in factor VIII level can be estimated by multiplying the dose of rAHF per kilogram of body weight (IU/kg) by 2%. This method of calculation is based on clinical findings by Abildgaard *et al.*,[8] and is illustrated in the following examples.

$$\text{Expected \% factor VIII increase} = \frac{\text{\# units administered} \times 2\%/\text{IU/kg}}{\text{body weight (kg)}}$$

$$\text{Example for a 70 kg adult: } \frac{1400\ \text{IU} \times 2\%/\text{IU/kg}}{70\ \text{kg}} = 40\%$$

or

$$\text{Dosage required (IU)} = \frac{\text{body weight (kg)} \times \text{desired \% factor VIII increase}}{2\%/\text{IU/kg}}$$

$$\text{Example for a 15 kg child: } \frac{15\ \text{kg} \times 100\%}{2\%/\text{IU/kg}} = 750\ \text{IU required}$$

The dosage necessary to achieve hemostasis depends upon the type and severity of the bleeding episode, according to the following general guidelines:

Mild Hemorrhage

Mild superficial or early hemorrhages may respond to a single dose of 10 IU per kg,[9] leading to an *in vivo* rise of approximately 20% in the factor VIII level. Therapy need not be repeated unless there is evidence of further bleeding.

Moderate Hemorrhage

For more serious bleeding episodes (e.g., definite hemarthroses, known trauma), the factor VIII level should be raised to 30–50% by administering approximately 15–25 IU per kg. If further therapy is required, a repeat infusion can be given at 12–24 hours.[10]

Severe Hemorrhage

In patients with life-threatening bleeding or possible hemorrhage involving vital structures (e.g., central nervous system, retropharyngeal and retroperitoneal spaces, iliopsoas sheath), the factor VIII level should be raised to 80–100% of normal in order to achieve hemostasis. This may be achieved with an initial rAHF (Antihemophilic Factor (Recombinant). KOGENATE®) dose of 40–50 IU per kg and a maintenance dose of 20–25 IU per kg every 8–12 hours.[11,12]

Surgery

For major surgical procedures, the factor VIII level should be raised to approximately 100% by giving a preoperative dose of 50 IU/kg. The factor VIII level should be checked to assure that the expected level is achieved before the patient goes to surgery. In order to maintain hemostatic levels, repeat infusions may be necessary every 6 to 12 hours initially, and for a total of 10 to 14 days until healing is complete. The intensity of factor VIII replacement therapy required depends on the type of surgery and postoperative regimen employed. For minor surgical procedures, less intensive treatment schedules may provide adequate hemostasis.[11,12]

Prophylaxis

Factor VIII concentrates may also be administered on a regular schedule for prophylaxis of bleeding, as reported by Nilsson, *et al.*[13]

Reconstitution

Vacuum Transfer

1. Warm the unopened diluent and the concentrate to room temperature (NMT 37°C, 99°F).
2. After removing the plastic flip-top caps (Fig. A), aseptically cleanse the rubber stoppers of both bottles.
3. Remove the protective cover from the plastic transfer-needle cartridge with tamper-proof seal and penetrate the stopper of the diluent bottle (Fig. B).
4. Remove the remaining portion of the plastic cartridge, invert the diluent bottle and penetrate the rubber seal on the concentrate bottle (Fig. C) with the needle at an angle. Alternate method of transferring sterile water: With a sterile needle and syringe, withdraw the appropriate volume of diluent and transfer to the bottle of lyophilized concentrate.
5. The vacuum will draw the diluent into the concentrate bottle. Hold the diluent bottle at an angle to the concentrate bottle in order to direct the jet of diluent against the wall of the concentrate bottle (Fig. C). Avoid excessive foaming.
6. After removing the diluent bottle and transfer needle (Fig. D), swirl continuously until completely dissolved (Fig. E).
7. After the concentrate powder is completely dissolved, withdraw solution into the syringe through the filter needle which is supplied in the package (Fig. F). Replace the filter needle with the administration set provided and inject intravenously.
8. If the same patient is to receive more than one bottle, the contents of two bottles may be drawn into the same syringe through a separate unused filter needle before attaching the vein needle.

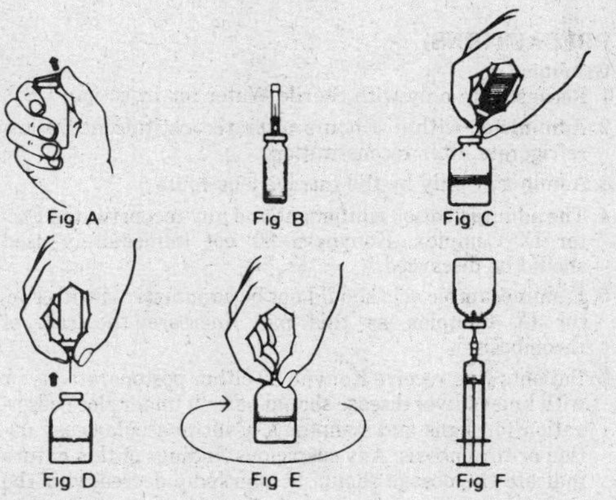
Fig A
Fig B
Fig C
Fig D
Fig E
Fig F

Rate of Administration

The rate of administration should be adapted to the response of the individual patient, but administration of the entire dose in 5 to 10 minutes or less is well-tolerated.

Parenteral drug products should be inspected visually for particulate matter and discoloration prior to administration, whenever solution and container permit.

HOW SUPPLIED

Antihemophilic Factor (Recombinant), KOGENATE®, is supplied in the following single dose bottles with the total units of factor VIII activity stated on the label of each bottle. A suitable volume of Sterile Water for Injection, USP, a sterile double-ended transfer needle, a sterile filter needle, and a sterile administration set are provided.

Product Code	Approximate Factor VIII Activity	Diluent
670-20	250 IU	2.5 mL
670-30	500 IU	5 mL
670-50	1000 IU	10 mL

STORAGE

KOGENATE should be stored under refrigeration (2–8°C; 36–46°F). Storage of lyophilized powder at room temperature (up to 25°C or 77°F) for 3 months, such as in home treatment situations, may be done without loss of factor VIII activity. Freezing should be avoided, as breakage of the diluent bottle might occur. Do not use beyond the expiration date indicated on the bottle.

CAUTION

U.S. federal law prohibits dispensing without prescription.

LIMITED WARRANTY

A number of factors beyond our control could reduce the efficacy of this product or even result in an ill effect following its use. These include improper storage and handling of the product after it leaves our hands, diagnosis, dosage, method of administration, and biological differences in individual patients. Because of these factors, it is important that this product be stored properly, and that the directions be followed carefully during use.

No warranty, express or implied, including any warranty of merchantability or fitness is made. Representatives of the Company are not authorized to vary the terms or the contents of the printed labeling, including the package insert for this product, except by printed notice from the Company's headquarters. The prescriber and user of this product must accept the terms hereof.

REFERENCES

1. Lawn RM, Vehar GA: The molecular genetics of hemophilia. *Sci Am* 254(3):48–54, 1986.
2. Schwartz RS, Abildgaard CF, Aledort LM, et al: Human recombinant DNA-derived antihemophilic factor (factor VIII) in the treatment of hemophilia A. *N Engl J Med* 323(26):1800–5, 1990.
3. Lusher JM: Viral safaety and inhibitor development associated with monoclonal antibody-purified FVIIIc. *Ann Hematol* 63(3):138–41, 1991.
4. Addiego JE Jr, Gomperts E, Liu S-L, et al: Treatment of hemophilia A with a highly purified factor VIII concentrate prepared by anti-FVIIIc immunoaffinity chromatography. *Thromb Haemost* 67(1):19–27, 1992.
5. Schwarzinger I, Pabinger I, Korninger C, et al: Incidence of inhibitors in patients with severe and moderate hemophilia A treated with factor VIII concentrates. *Am J Hematol* 24(3):241–5, 1987.
6. Ehrenforth S, Kreuz W. Scharrer I, et al: Incidence of development of factor VIII and factor IX inhibitors in hemophiliacs. *Lancet* 339(8793):594–8, 1992.
7. Kasper CK: Complications of hemophilia A treatment: factor VIII inhibitors, *Ann NY Acad Sci* 614:97–105, 1991.
8. Abildgaard CF, Simone JV, Corrigan JJ, et al: Treatment of hemophilia with glycine-precipitated Factor VIII, *N Engl J Med* 275(9):471–5, 1966.
9. Britton M, Harrison J, Abildgaard CF: Early treatment of hemophilic hemarthroses with minimal dose of new factor VIII concentrate, *J Pediatr* 85(2):245–7, 1974.
10. Abildgaard CF: Current concepts in the management of hemophilia. *Semin Hematol* 12(3):223–32, 1975.
11. Hilgartner MW: Factor replacement therapy. In: Hilgartner MW, Pochedly C, eds.: Hemophilia in the child and adult. New York, Raven Press, 1989, pp 1–26.
12. Kasper CK, Dietrich SL: Comprehensive management of haemophilia. *Clin Haematol* 14(2):489–512, 1985.
13. Nilsson IM, Berntorp E, Lofqvist T, et al: Twenty-five years' experience of prophylactic treatment in severe haemophilia A and B. *J Intern Med* 232(1):25–32, 1992.

Factor IX Complex ℞
KONŸNE® 80
Heat-Treated at 80°C

DESCRIPTION

Factor IX Complex, Konÿne® 80, heat-treated at 80°C for 72 hours, is a sterile, dried, plasma fraction comprising coagulation factors II, IX, X and low levels of factor VII.

Factor:	Nomenclature *Synonyms:*
II	prothrombin
VII	proconvertin
IX	plasma thromboplastin component, PTC, Christmas factor
X	Stuart-Prower factor

Konÿne 80 is standardized in terms of factor IX content and each vial of Konÿne 80 is labeled for factor IX. One international unit (IU) of factor IX as defined by the World Health Organization standard for blood coagulation factor IX is approximately equal to the level of factor IX found in 1.0 mL of fresh, normal plasma.

The factor IX content is approximately 50 times purified over whole plasma, and when reconstituted as directed, Konÿne 80 contains 25 times as much factor IX as an equal volume of fresh plasma. Konÿne 80, containing approximately 1000 IU of factor IX administered in 40 mL, contains the factor IX content of 1 liter of fresh plasma. Konÿne 80 must be administered intravenously.

Continued on next page

Bayer Biological—Cont.

CLINICAL PHARMACOLOGY

Factor IX Complex raises the plasma level of factor IX and restores hemostasis in patients with factor IX deficiency. In general, a level of factor IX less than 5% of normal will give rise to spontaneous hemorrhage, while levels greater than 20% of normal will lead to satisfactory hemostasis even in the face of trauma or surgery. Approximately 30% to 50% of the factor IX activity can be detected in a hemophilia B (factor IX deficiency) recipient's plasma immediately after infusion.[1,2] The biological activity of the infused factor IX disappears from the plasma with a half-life of approximately 24 hours.[2] A pharmacokinetic study in six patients found similar recoveries and half-lives for Konȳne 80 as for Konȳne®-HT. It must be noted that administration of Factor IX Complex causes an increase in blood levels of factors II, VII, IX and X.

Factors II, VII, IX and X are the vitamin K dependent coagulation factors and are synthesized in the liver. Congenital deficiencies of each of the four factors do occur and may result in a bleeding tendency. Naturally low levels of the vitamin K dependent factors may also be found in vitamin K deficiency and in severe liver disease.

This product has been heated at 80°C for 72 hours and there is no evidence of adverse effects upon the product. In a study[3] designed to assess the effectiveness of heat treatment at 68°C for 72 hours, hepatitis naive chimpanzees were inoculated with heated Antihemophilic Factor (Human) and Factor IX Complex preparations to which had been previously added non-A, non-B hepatitis Hutchinson Strain[4] to a total level of 2500 chimpanzee infectious doses (CID). The chimpanzees receiving heated preparations failed to exhibit any symptoms of non-A, non-B hepatitis. In contrast, one chimpanzee receiving Antihemophilic Factor (Human) concentrate which was not heated after the non-A, non-B inoculum was added, developed abnormally elevated alanine aminotransferase (ALT) levels beginning 10 weeks postinoculation and liver histopathology at 6 weeks. From these results, it was concluded that the heat treatment employed inactivated a known quantity of non-A, non-B hepatitis: at least 2500 CID.

Additional in vitro studies[5] on the effect of heating Factor IX Complex, Konȳne® 80, in a dried state at 80°C for 72 hours, on virus inactivation were carried out with a number of viruses, including human immunodeficiency virus (HIV), added to Factor IX Complex prior to heating. The following table shows the amount of each model virus inactivated by the process:

Virus	Starting Amount Logs*	Logs Inactivated
Vesicular Stomatitis Virus	8.0	≥7.5
Vaccinia Virus	5.75	1.0
Sindbis Virus	7.25	≥6.75
Bovine Parvovirus	4.5	3.5
Human Immunodeficiency Virus (HIV), HIV-1	4.8	≥4.3

*$\log_{10}$ $TCID_{50}$/mL (for HIV-1, $\log_{10}$ $TCID_{50}$)

INDICATIONS AND USAGE

Factor IX Complex, Konȳne® 80 is indicated for the prevention and control of bleeding caused by Factor IX deficiency due to hemophilia B.

Konȳne 80 is not indicated for use in the treatment of factor VII deficiency.

Konȳne 80 is appropriate for use in:

1. Hemophilia B (Christmas disease); demonstrated factor IX deficiency in children or adults with real or impending bleeding episodes. Spontaneous bleeding can occur even in the absence of any trauma.
2. Reversal of coumarin anticoagulant induced hemorrhage; in situations where prompt reversal is required (e.g., preceding emergency surgery, trauma, etc.), administration of fresh-frozen plasma should be initially considered as treatment; however, Konȳne 80 may be considered as a secondary approach if the risk of transmitting hepatitis is considered justifiable in the face of a life-threatening situation.[6–8]
3. Treatment of bleeding episodes in patients with hemophilia A (factor VIII deficiency) who have inhibitors to factor VIII.[9]

   In addition to coumarin anticoagulant induced deficiencies, low levels of factors II, VII, IX and X may be found in vitamin K deficiency, in patients with gut sterilization due to oral antibiotics, in patients with liver disease, and in those with nephrotic syndrome. However, Factor IX Complex, Konȳne 80® is not indicated in these situations and treatment should be aimed at correcting the primary condition.

Note: For publications on the clinical use of Konȳne®, please refer to references 1,2, 6–17.

CONTRAINDICATIONS

None known.

WARNINGS

1. Hepatitis and Viral Diseases

This product is prepared from pooled human plasma which may contain the causative agents of hepatitis and other viral diseases. Prescribed manufacturing procedures utilized at the plasma collection centers, plasma testing laboratories, and the fractionation facilities are designed to reduce the risk of transmitting viral infection. However, the risk of viral infectivity from this product cannot be totally eliminated.

Individuals who receive infusions of blood or plasma products may develop signs and/or symptoms of some viral infections, particularly non-A, non-B hepatitis.[18] It is emphasized that hepatitis B vaccination is essential for patients with hemophilia and it is recommended that this be done at birth or diagnosis.[19]

Konȳne 80 is a plasma fraction obtained from many paid donors. The presence of hepatitis viruses should be assumed and the hazard of administering Konȳne 80 should be weighed against the medical consequences of withholding it, particularly in persons with few previous transfusions of blood or blood products.

2. Thrombosis

Cases of patients developing postoperative thrombosis after treatment with Factor IX Complex have been described. Although thrombosis is a well-known risk of the postoperative period, it is found to be greater in these patients.[13–15] No other data are presently available. Until further surveys and more conclusive studies are available, Konȳne 80 is only advised for patients undergoing elective surgery where the expected beneficial effects of its use outweigh the increased risk of the possibility of thrombosis. This applies especially to those who may be predisposed to thrombosis. Do not use in cases of known liver disease where there is any suspicion of intravascular coagulation or fibrinolysis.

PRECAUTIONS

General

1. Reconstitute only with Sterile Water for Injection, USP.
2. Administer within 3 hours after reconstitution. Do not refrigerate after reconstitution.
3. Administer only by the intravenous route.
4. The administration equipment and any reconstituted Factor IX Complex, Konȳne® 80 not immediately used should be discarded.
5. E-aminocaproic acid should not be administered with Factor IX Complex as this may increase the risk of thrombosis.
6. Patients who receive Konȳne 80 either postoperatively or with known liver disease should be kept under close observation for signs and symptoms of intravascular coagulation or thrombosis. Any suspicious findings of this nature indicate the dosage should be markedly decreased if the patient's conditions are such that the treatment cannot be discontinued entirely. In the event of thrombohemorrhagic disorders occurring, reduction in dosage should be considered, and treatment with heparin may be warranted. Although this preparation does not contain heparin, it has been suggested that reconstitution with heparin in a concentration of 2–5 IU per mL may reduce the risk of development of thrombosis.[17] However, thrombosis can occur even in the presence of heparin.
7. Patients receiving Konȳne 80 for prolonged periods should be continually monitored at least for levels of factors II, IX and X. The same comments as in No. 6 above are indicated. Half-lives of factors II and X are considerably longer than the half-life of factor IX. Hence frequent repeated high-dose administration may result in build-up of factors II and X, with increasing risk of thrombotic side effects.
8. Product administration and handling of the needles must be done with caution. Percutaneous puncture with a needle contaminated with blood can transmit infectious viruses including HIV (AIDS) and hepatitis. Obtain immediate medical attention if injury occurs.

   Place needles in sharps container after single use. Discard all equipment including any reconstituted Konȳne 80 product in accordance with biohazard procedures.

Pregnancy Category C

Animal reproduction studies have not been conducted with Konȳne 80. It is also not known whether Konȳne 80 can cause fetal harm when administered to a pregnant woman or can affect reproduction capacity. Konȳne 80 should be given to a pregnant woman only if clearly needed.

ADVERSE REACTIONS

In some patients the rapid administration of Konȳne 80 can cause transient fever, chills, headache, flushing or tingling.

DOSAGE AND ADMINISTRATION

Each bottle of Konȳne 80 has the factor IX activity, in IU, stated on the bottle label. One IU is defined as the activity present in 1 mL of fresh, normal plasma. The potency is standardized in terms of factor IX content.

The amount of Konȳne 80 required for normalizing hemostasis will depend upon the patient and upon the circumstances. Sufficient Konȳne 80 should be administered to achieve and maintain a plasma level of at least 20% until hemostasis is achieved.

Levels of factor IX of 30 to 40 percent are considered effective in stopping hemorrhages.[1] Bleeds in life- or limb-threatening areas require factor IX levels of 50 to 80 percent which should be maintained at 30 to 40 percent for a few days.[1] The desired hemostatic plasma level in surgical patients for minor procedures or invasive dental surgery is between 30 and 40 percent of normal.[1] This can be achieved by a dosage not exceeding 30 to 40 units per kg body weight. In major hemorrhage, as during surgery or severe accidental trauma, plasma levels of 60 to 80 percent just prior to surgery, maintained above 30 percent for a further 5 to 7 days and then above 15 to 20 percent for 7 to 10 additional days, until healing occurs, are required.[1]

While the range of values in normal clinical practice is likely to vary depending upon differences between patients, their clinical condition and the type of assay employed, it is again stressed that high dosages, especially if frequently repeated (e.g., more than once per day) are hazardous. Such regimens can induce major thrombotic complications and hence must be avoided.

The following formulas may be used as guidelines to calculate an appropriate dose or to estimate the expected percentage increase obtained from a given dose.:

$$\text{Expected factor IX increase (in \% of normal)} = \frac{\text{IU administered} \times 1.0}{\text{body weight (in kg)}}$$

IU required = body weight (kg) × desired factor IX increase (% normal) × 1.0

Thus, in order to bring a 70 kg patient from 0% to 50% of normal, the patient would require 70 × 50 × 1.0 = 3500 IU or 50 IU/kg body weight.

Prophylaxis

The ideal treatment for proven congenital deficiency of procoagulants is prophylactic administration. For prophylaxis against hemorrhage during times of extensive physical activity, the plasma factor IX levels should be raised to 15 to 30 percent. Maintenance dosage should be adapted to the individual patient's needs. Additional Factor IX Complex, Konȳne® 80 should be administered when a patient on prophylaxis is exposed to trauma or surgery.

Maintenance Dose

Maintenance dosage should be administered according to the clinical response and the factor IX level achieved. Such dosage is usually about 10–20 IU per kg body weight per day.

Inhibitor Patients

For treatment of bleeding episodes in patients with hemophilia A (factor VIII deficiency) who have inhibitors to factor VIII, the recommended dose should be 75 IU/kg. A second dose may be administered after 12 hours if necessary.[9]

Reconstitution

Vacuum Transfer

1. Warm the unopened diluent and concentrate to room temperature (NMT 37°C, 99°F).
2. After removing the plastic flip-top caps (Fig. A) aseptically cleanse the rubber stoppers of both bottles.
3. Remove the protective cover from the plastic transfer-needle cartridge with tamper-proof seal and penetrate the stopper of the diluent bottle (Fig. B).
4. Remove the remaining portion of the plastic cartridge. Invert the diluent bottle and penetrate the rubber seal on the concentrate bottle (Fig. C) with the needle at an angle. Alternate method of transferring sterile water: With a sterile needle and syringe, withdraw the appropriate volume of diluent and transfer to the bottle of lyophilized concentrate.
5. Hold the diluent bottle at an angle to the concentrate bottle in order to direct the jet of diluent against the wall of the concentrate bottle. The vacuum will draw the diluent into the concentrate bottle. Avoid excessive foaming. Do not shake the concentrate bottle.
6. After removing the diluent bottle and transfer-needle (Fig. D), optimal reconstitution time is achieved by swirling continuously until completely dissolved (Fig. E). Reconstitution can also be achieved by very gently agitating until dissolved.

   Parenteral drug products should be inspected visually for particulate matter and discoloration prior to administration, whenever solution and container permit.
7. After the concentrate powder is completely dissolved, withdraw the Factor IX Complex, Konȳne® 80 solution into the syringe through the filter needle which is supplied

in the package (Fig. F). Replace the filter needle with an appropriate sterile injection needle, e.g., 21 gauge × 1 inch, and inject intravenously.

8. If the same patient is to receive more than one bottle of Konÿne 80, the contents of two bottles may be drawn into the same syringe through filter needles before attaching the vein needle.

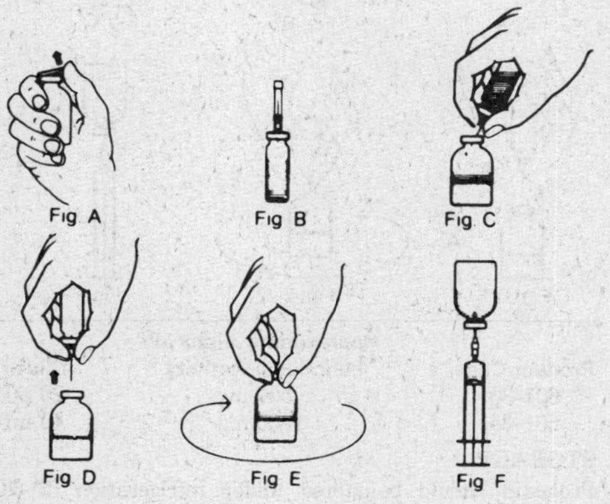

Fig A Fig B Fig C Fig D Fig E Fig F

Rate of Administration

The rate of administration should be adapted to the response of the individual patient, but is generally well-tolerated at a rate of approximately 100 IU per minute.

HOW SUPPLIED

Factor IX Complex, Konÿne® 80 is supplied in single dose bottles with the total IU of factor IX activity stated on the label of each bottle. A suitable volume of Sterile Water for Injection, USP, a sterile double-ended transfer needle, and a sterile filter needle are provided.

Product Code	Approximate Factor IX Activity	Diluent
626–20	500 IU	20 mL
626–50	1000 IU	40 mL

STORAGE

Konÿne 80 should be stored under refrigeration (2°–8°C; 36°–46°F). Freezing should be avoided as breakage of the diluent bottle might occur.

Konÿne 80 concentrate may be stored for a period of up to 1 month at temperatures not to exceed 25°C (77°F) during travel.

CAUTION

U.S. federal law prohibits dispensing without prescription.

LIMITED WARRANTY

A number of factors beyond our control could reduce the efficacy of this product or even result in an ill effect following its use. These include improper storage and handling of the product after it leaves our hands, diagnosis, dosage, method of administration, and biological differences in individual patients. Because of these factors it is important that this product be stored properly, that the directions be followed carefully during use, and that the risk of transmitting viruses be carefully weighed before the product is prescribed. No warranty, express or implied, including any warranty of merchantability or fitness is made. Representatives of the Company are not authorized to vary the terms or the contents of the printed labeling, including the package insert, for this product except by printed notice from the Company's headquarters. The prescriber and user of this product must accept the terms hereof.

REFERENCES

1. Johnson AJ, Aronson DL, Williams WJ: Preparation and clinical use of plasma and plasma fractions. In: Williams WJ (ed): *Hematology,* 4th ed, New York, McGraw-Hill, 1990, ch 170, pp 1659–1673.
2. Zauber NP, Levin J: Factor IX levels in patients with hemophilia B (Christmas disease) following transfusion with concentrates of factor IX or fresh frozen plasma (FFP). *Medicine* (Baltimore) 56(3): 213–24, 1977.
3. Mozen MM, Louie RE, Mitra G: Heat inactivation of viruses in antihemophilic factor concentrates. Abstracts, XVIth International Congress of the World Federation of Hemophilia, Rio de Janeiro, Aug. 24–28, 1984. Number 240.
4. Feinstone SM, Alter HJ, Dienes HP, et al: Non-A, non-B hepatitis in chimpanzees and marmosets. *J Infect Dis* 144(6):588–98, 1981.
5. Unpublished data in files of Miles Inc., Cutter Biological.
6. Taberner DA, Thompson JM, Poller L: Comparison of prothrombin complex concentrate and vitamin K_1 in oral anticoagulant reversal. *Br Med J* 2(6027):83–5, 1976.
7. Menache D, Roberts HR: Summary report and recommendations of the task force members and consultants. *Thromb Diath Haemorrh* 33:645–7, 1975.
8. Aronson DL: Factor IX Complex. *Semin Thromb Hemostas* 6(1):28–43, 1979.
9. Lusher JM, Shapiro SS, Palascak JE, et al: Efficacy of prothrombin-complex concentrates in hemophiliacs with antibodies to factor VIII: a multicenter therapeutic trial. *N Engl J Med* 303(8):421–5, 1980.
10. Hoag MS, Johnson FF, Robinson AJ, et al: Treatment of hemophilia B with a new clotting-factor concentrate. *N Engl J Med* 280(11):581–6, 1969.
11. Hoag MS, Johnson FF, Robinson AJ, et al: Use of plasma concentrate in congenital factor VII and IX deficiencies. *Clin Res* 17:152, 1969.
12. Breen FA Jr, Tullis JL: Prothrombin concentrates in treatment of Christmas disease and allied disorders. *JAMA* 208(10):1848–52, 1969.
13. Kasper CK: Postoperative thrombosis in hemophilia. *N Engl J Med* 289(3):160, 1973.
14. Kasper CK: Surgical operation in hemophilia B. Use of factor IX concentrate. *Calif Med* 113(1):4–8, 1970.
15. George JN, Breckenridge RT: The use of factor VIII and factor IX concentrates during surgery. *JAMA* 214(9):1673–6, 1970.
16. Gunay U, Choi HS, Maurer HS, et al: Commercial preparations of prothrombin complex. A clinical comparison. *Am J Dis Child* 126(6):775–7, 1973.
17. White GC 2d, Lundblad RL, Kingdon HS: Prothrombin complex concentrates: preparation, properties, and clinical uses. *Curr Top Hematol* 2:203–44, 1979.
18. Colombo M, Mannucci PM, Carnelli V, et al: Transmission of non-A, non-B hepatitis by heat-treated factor VIII concentrate. *Lancet* 2(8445):1–4, 1985.
19. National Hemophilia Foundation Medical and Scientific Advisory Council. Hemophilia Information Exchange—AIDS Update: Recommendations concerning AIDS and the treatment of hemophilia. HIV infection, Section I.G. (Rev. Jan., 1988).

ALPHA$_1$–PROTEINASE INHIBITOR (HUMAN) ℞

PROLASTIN®

[pro-las 'tin]

DESCRIPTION

Alpha$_1$-Proteinase Inhibitor (Human), Prolastin®, is a sterile, stable, lyophilized preparation of purified human Alpha$_1$-Proteinase Inhibitor (alpha$_1$-PI) also known as alpha$_1$-antitrypsin. Alpha$_1$-Proteinase Inhibitor (Human) is intended for use in therapy of congenital alpha$_1$-antitrypsin deficiency.

Alpha$_1$-Proteinase Inhibitor (Human) is prepared from pooled human plasma of normal donors by modification and refinements of the cold ethanol method of Cohn.[1] Part of the fractionation may be performed by another licensed manufacturer. In order to reduce the potential risk of transmission of infectious agents, Alpha$_1$-Proteinase Inhibitor (Human) has been heat-treated in solution at 60±0.5°C for not less than 10 hours. However, no procedure has been found to be totally effective in removing viral infectivity from plasma fractionation products.

The specific activity of Alpha$_1$-Proteinase Inhibitor (Human) is ≥0.35 mg functional alpha$_1$-PI/mg protein and when reconstituted as directed, the concentration of alpha$_1$-PI is ≥20 mg/mL. When reconstituted, Alpha$_1$-Proteinase Inhibitor (Human) has a pH of 6.6–7.4, a sodium content of 100–210 mEq/L, a chloride content of 60–180 mEq/L, a sodium phosphate content of 0.015–0.025 M, a polyethylene glycol content of not more than (NMT) 5 ppm, NMT 0.1% sucrose. Alpha$_1$-Proteinase Inhibitor (Human) contains small amounts of other plasma proteins including alpha$_2$-plasmin inhibitor, alpha$_1$-antichymotrypsin, C_1-esterase inhibitor, haptoglobin, antithrombin III, alpha$_1$-lipoprotein, albumin, and IgA.[1]

Each vial of Prolastin contains the labeled amount of functionally active alpha$_1$-PI in milligrams per vial (mg/vial), as determined by capacity to neutralize porcine pancreatic elastase.[1] Alpha$_1$-Proteinase Inhibitor (Human) contains no preservative and must be administered by the intravenous route.

CLINICAL PHARMACOLOGY

Alpha$_1$-antitrypsin deficiency is a chronic hereditary, usually fatal, autosomal recessive disorder in which a low concentration of alpha$_1$-PI (alpha$_1$-antitrypsin) is associated with slowly progressive, severe, panacinar emphysema that most often manifests itself in the third to fourth decades of life.[2–9] [Although the terms "Alpha$_1$-Proteinase Inhibitor" and "alpha$_1$-antitrypsin" are used interchangeably in the scientific literature, the hereditary disorder associated with a reduction in the serum level of alpha$_1$-PI is conventionally referred to as "alpha$_1$-antitrypsin deficiency" while the deficient protein is referred to as "Alpha$_1$-Proteinase Inhibitor"[10]]. The emphysema is typically worse in the lower lung zones.[4,8,9] The pathogenesis of development of emphysema in alpha$_1$-antitrypsin deficiency is not well understood at this time. It is believed, however, to be due to a chronic biochemical imbalance between elastase (an enzyme capable of degrading elastin tissues, released by inflammatory cells, primarily neutrophils, in the lower respiratory tract) and alpha$_1$-PI (the principal inhibitor of neutrophil elastase) which is deficient in alpha$_1$-antitrypsin disease.[11–15] As a result, it is believed that alveolar structures are unprotected from chronic exposure to elastase released from a chronic, low level burden of neutrophils in the lower respiratory tract, resulting in progressive degradation of elastin tissues.[11–15] The eventual outcome is the development of emphysema. Neonatal hepatitis with cholestatic jaundice appears in approximately 10% of newborns with alpha$_1$-antitrypsin deficiency.[15] In some adults, alpha$_1$-antitrypsin deficiency is complicated by cirrhosis.[15]

A large number of phenotypic variants of alpha$_1$-antitrypsin deficiency exists.[15] The most severely affected individuals are those with the PiZZ variant, typically characterized by alpha$_1$-PI serum levels <35% normal.[15] Epidemiologic studies of individuals with various phenotypes of alpha$_1$-antitrypsin deficiency have demonstrated that individuals with endogenous serum levels of alpha$_1$-PI ≤50 mg/dL (based on commercial standards) have a risk of >80% of developing emphysema over a lifetime.[3–6,8,9,16] However, individuals with endogenous alpha$_1$-PI levels >80 mg/dL, in general, do not manifest an increased risk for development of emphysema above the general population background risk.[5,15] From these observations, it is believed that the "threshold" level of alpha$_1$-PI in the serum required to provide adequate anti-elastase activity in the lung of individuals with alpha$_1$-antitrypsin deficiency is about 80 mg/dL (based on commercial standards for immunologic assay of alpha$_1$-PI).[12,15,17]

In clinical studies of Alpha$_1$-Proteinase Inhibitor (Human), Prolastin®, 23 subjects with the PiZZ variant of congenital deficiency of alpha$_1$-antitrypsin deficiency and documented destructive lung disease participated in a study of acute and/or chronic replacement therapy with Alpha$_1$-Proteinase Inhibitor (Human).[18] The mean in vivo recovery of alpha$_1$-PI was 4.2 mg (immunologic) dL per mg (functional)/kg body weight administered.[18,19] The half-life of alpha$_1$-PI in vivo was approximately 4.5 days.[18,19] Based on these observations, a program of chronic replacement therapy was developed. Nineteen of the subjects in these studies received Alpha$_1$-Proteinase Inhibitor (Human) replacement therapy, 60 mg/kg body weight, once weekly for up to 26 weeks (average 24 weeks of therapy). With this schedule of replacement therapy, blood levels of alpha$_1$-PI were maintained above 80 mg/dL (based on the commercial standards for alpha$_1$-PI immunologic assay).[18–20]. Within a few weeks of commencing this program, bronchoalveolar lavage studies demonstrated significantly increased levels of alpha$_1$-PI and functional antineutrophil elastase capacity in the epithelial lining fluid of the lower respiratory tract of the lung, as compared to levels prior to commencing the program of chronic replacement therapy with Alpha$_1$-Proteinase Inhibitor (Human).[18–20].

All 23 individuals who participated in the investigations were immunized with Hepatitis B Vaccine and received a single dose of Hepatitis B Immune Globulin (Human) on entry into the investigation. Although no other steps were taken to prevent hepatitis, neither hepatitis B nor non-A, non-B hepatitis occurred in any of the subjects.[18,19] All subjects remained seronegative for HIV antibody. None of the subjects developed any detectable antibody to alpha$_1$-PI or other serum protein.

Long-term controlled clinical trials to evaluate the effect of chronic replacement therapy with Alpha$_1$-Proteinase Inhibitor (Human), Prolastin®, on the development of or progression of emphysema in patients with congenital alpha$_1$-antitrypsin deficiency have not been performed. Estimates of the sample size required of this rare disorder and the slow progressive nature of the clinical course have been considered impediments in the ability to conduct such a trial.[21] Studies to monitor the long-term effects will continue as part of the postapproval process.

INDICATIONS AND USAGE

Congenital Alpha$_1$-Antitrypsin Deficiency

Alpha$_1$-Proteinase Inhibitor (Human) is indicated for chronic replacement therapy of individuals having congenital deficiency of alpha$_1$-PI (alpha$_1$-antitrypsin deficiency) with clinically demonstrable panacinar emphysema. Clinical and biochemical studies have demonstrated that with such therapy, it is possible to increase plasma levels of alpha$_1$-PI, and that levels of functionally active alpha$_1$-PI in the lung epithelial lining fluid are increased proportionately.[18–20] As some individuals with alpha$_1$-antitrypsin deficiency will not go on to develop panacinar emphysema, only those with early evidence of such disease should be considered for chronic replacement therapy with Alpha$_1$-Proteinase Inhibitor (Human).[22] Subjects with the PiMZ or PiMS phenotypes of alpha$_1$-antitrypsin deficiency should not be

Continued on next page

Bayer Biological—Cont.

considered for such treatment as they appear to be at small risk for panacinar emphysema.[22] Clinical data are not available as to the long-term effects derived from chronic replacement therapy of individuals with alpha$_1$-antitrypsin deficiency with Alpha$_1$-Proteinase Inhibitor (Human). Only adult subjects have received Alpha$_1$-Proteinase Inhibitor (Human) to date.

Alpha$_1$-Proteinase Inhibitor (Human) is not indicated for use in patients other than those with PiZZ, PiZ(null), or Pi(null)(null) phenotypes.

CONTRAINDICATIONS

Individuals with selective IgA deficiencies who have known antibody against IgA (anti-IgA antibody) should not receive Alpha$_1$-Proteinase Inhibitor (Human), since these patients may experience severe reactions, including anaphylaxis, to IgA which may be present.

WARNINGS

This product is prepared from pooled human plasma which may contain the causative agents of hepatitis and other viral diseases. Prescribed manufacturing procedures utilized at the plasma collection centers, plasma testing laboratories, and the fractionation facilities are designed to reduce the risk of transmitting viral infection. However, the risk of viral infectivity from this product cannot be totally eliminated.

Individuals who receive infusions of blood or plasma products may develop signs and/or symptoms of some viral infections, particularly non-A, non-B hepatitis.

Alpha$_1$-Proteinase Inhibitor (Human) has been heat-treated in solution at 60°C for 10 hours in order to reduce the potential for transmission of infectious agents.[1] No cases of hepatitis, either hepatitis B or non-A, non-B hepatitis have been recorded to date in individuals receiving Alpha$_1$-Proteinase Inhibitor (Human).[18] However, as all individuals received prophylaxis against hepatitis B, no conclusion can be drawn at this time regarding potential transmission of hepatitis B virus.

PRECAUTIONS

General

1. Administer within 3 hours after reconstitution. Do not refrigerate after reconstitution.
2. Administer only by the intravenous route.
3. As with any colloid solution there will be an increase in plasma volume following intravenous administration of Prolastin.[23] Caution should therefore be used in patients at risk for circulatory overload.
4. It is recommended that in preparation for receiving Prolastin, recipients are immunized against hepatitis B using a licensed Hepatitis B Vaccine according to the manufacturer's recommendations. Should it become necessary to treat an individual with Prolastin, and time is insufficient for adequate antibody response to vaccination, individuals should receive a single dose of Hepatitis B Immune Globulin (Human), 0.06 mL/kg body weight, intramuscularly, at the time of administration of the initial dose of Hepatitis B Vaccine.
5. Prolastin should be given alone, without mixing with other agents or diluting solutions.
6. Product administration and handling of the needles must be done with caution. Percutaneous puncture with a needle contaminated with blood can transmit infectious viruses including HIV (AIDS) and hepatitis. Obtain immediate medical attention if injury occurs.
   Place needles in sharps container after single use. Discard all equipment including any reconstituted Prolastin product in accordance with biohazard procedures.

Carcinogenesis, Mutagenesis, Impairment of Fertility

Long-term studies in animals to evaluate carcinogenesis, mutagenesis or impairment of fertility have not been conducted.

Pregnancy Category C

Animal reproduction studies have not been conducted with Prolastin. It is also not known whether Prolastin can cause fetal harm when administered to a pregnant woman or can affect reproduction capacity. Prolastin should be given to a pregnant woman only if clearly needed.

Nursing Mothers

It is not known whether Prolastin is excreted in human milk. Because many drugs are excreted in human milk, caution should be exercised when Prolastin is administered to a nursing woman.

Pediatric Use

Safety and effectiveness in the pediatric population have not been established.

ADVERSE REACTIONS

Therapeutic administration of Alpha$_1$-Proteinase Inhibitor (Human), 60 mg/kg weekly, has been demonstrated to be well-tolerated. In clinical studies, six reactions were observed with 517 infusions of Alpha$_1$-Proteinase Inhibitor (Human), or 1.16%. None of the reactions was severe.[18] The

adverse reactions reported included delayed fever (maximum temperature rise was 38.9°C, resolving spontaneously over 24 hours) occurring up to 12 hours following treatment (0.77%), light-headedness (0.19%), and dizziness (0.19%).[18] Mild transient leukocytosis and dilutional anemia several hours after infusion have also been noted.[18] Since market entry, occasional reports of other flu-like symptoms, allergic-like reactions, chills, dyspnea, rash, tachycardia, and, rarely, hypotension have also been received.

DOSAGE AND ADMINISTRATION

Each bottle of Alpha$_1$-Proteinase Inhibitor (Human) has the functional activity, as determined by inhibition of porcine pancreatic elastase,[1] stated on the label of the bottle.

The "threshold" level of alpha$_1$-PI in the serum believed to provide adequate anti-elastase activity in the lung of individuals with alpha$_1$-antitrypsin deficiency is 80 mg/dL (based on commercial standards for alpha$_1$-PI immunologic assay).[12,15,17] However, assays of alpha$_1$-PI based on commercial standards measure antigenic activity of alpha$_1$-PI whereas the labeled potency value of alpha$_1$-PI is expressed as actual functional activity, i.e., actual capacity to neutralize porcine pancreatic elastase. As functional activity may be less than antigenic activity, serum levels of alpha$_1$-PI determined using commercial immunologic assays may not accurately reflect actual functional alpha$_1$-PI levels. Therefore, although it may be helpful to monitor serum levels of alpha$_1$-PI in individuals receiving Alpha$_1$-Proteinase Inhibitor (Human), Prolastin®, using currently available commercial assays of antigenic activity, results of these assays should not be used to determine the required therapeutic dosage.

The recommended dosage of Alpha$_1$-Proteinase Inhibitor (Human) is 60 mg/kg body weight administered once weekly. This dose is intended to increase and maintain a level of functional alpha$_1$-PI in the epithelial lining of the lower respiratory tract providing adequate anti-elastase activity in the lung of individuals with alpha$_1$-antitrypsin deficiency. Alpha$_1$-Proteinase Inhibitor (Human) may be given at a rate of 0.08 mL/kg/min or greater and must be administered intravenously. The recommended dosage of 60 mg/kg takes approximately 30 minutes to infuse.

Parenteral drug products should be inspected visually for particulate matter and discoloration prior to administration, whenever solution and container permit.

Reconstitution

1. Warm the unopened diluent and concentrate to room temperature (NMT 37°C, 99°F).
2. After removing the plastic flip-top caps (Fig. A), aseptically cleanse rubber stoppers of both bottles.
3. Remove the protective cover from the plastic transfer needle cartridge with tamper-proof seal and penetrate the stopper of the diluent bottle (Fig. B).
4. Remove the remaining portion of the plastic cartridge. Invert the diluent bottle and penetrate the rubber seal on the concentrate bottle (Fig. C) with the needle at an angle.
   Alternate method of transferring sterile water: With a sterile needle and syringe, withdraw the appropriate volume of diluent and transfer to the bottle of lyophilized concentrate.
5. The vacuum will draw the diluent into the concentrate bottle. For best results, and to avoid foaming, hold the diluent bottle at an angle to the concentrate bottle in order to direct the jet of diluent against the wall of the concentrate bottle (Fig. C).
6. After removing the diluent bottle and transfer needle (Fig. D), gently swirl the concentrate bottle until the powder is completely dissolved (Fig. E).
7. Swab top of reconstituted bottle of Alpha$_1$-Proteinase Inhibitor (Human), Prolastin® again.
8. Attach the sterile filter needle provided to syringe. With filter needle in place, insert syringe into reconstituted bottle of Prolastin and withdraw Prolastin solution into syringe (Fig. F).
9. To administer Prolastin, replace filter needle with appropriate injection needle and follow procedure for I.V. administration.
10. The contents of more than one bottle of Prolastin may be drawn into the same syringe before administration. If more than one bottle of Prolastin is used, withdraw contents from bottles using aseptic technique. Place contents into an administration container (plastic minibag or glass bottle) using a syringe.* Avoid pushing an I.V. administration set spike into the product container stopper as this has been known to force the stopper into the vial, with a resulting loss of sterility.

* For a patient of average weight (about 70 kg), the volume needed will exceed the limit of one syringe.

[See Figure at top of next column.]

HOW SUPPLIED

Alpha$_1$-Proteinase Inhibitor (Human), Prolastin®, is supplied in the following single dose vials with the total alpha$_1$-PI functional activity, in milligrams, stated on the label of each vial. A suitable volume of Sterile Water for Injection, USP is provided.

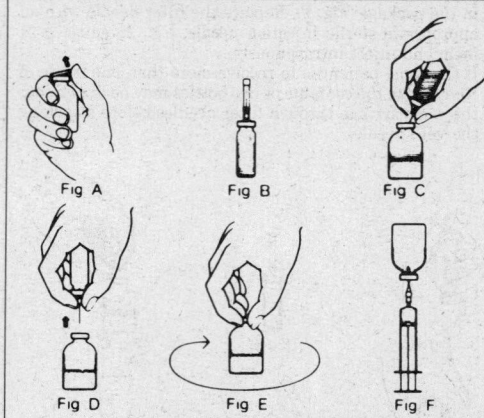

Fig A   Fig B   Fig C

Fig D   Fig E   Fig F

Product Code	Approximate Alpha$_1$-PI Functional Activity	Diluent
601-30	500 mg	20 mL
601-35	1000 mg	40 mL

STORAGE

Prolastin should be stored under refrigeration (2°–8°C; 36°–46°F). Freezing should be avoided as breakage of the diluent bottle might occur.

CAUTION

U.S. federal law prohibits dispensing without prescription.

LIMITED WARRANTY

A number of factors beyond our control could reduce the efficacy of this product or even result in an ill effect following its use. These include improper storage and handling of the product after it leaves our hands, diagnosis, dosage, method of administration, and biological differences in individual patients. Because of these factors, it is important that this product be stored properly, that the directions be followed carefully during use, and that the risk of transmitting viruses be carefully weighed before the product is prescribed. No warranty, express or implied, including any warranty of merchantability or fitness is made. Representatives of the Company are not authorized to vary the terms or the contents of the printed labeling, including the package insert for this product, except by printed notice from the Company's headquarters. The prescriber and user of this product must accept the terms hereof.

REFERENCES

1. Coan MH, Brockway WJ, Eguizabal H, et al: Preparation and properties of alpha$_1$-proteinase inhibitor concentrate from human plasma. *Vox Sang* 48(6):333–42, 1985.
2. Laurell CB, Eriksson S: The electrophoretic alpha$_1$-globulin pattern of serum in alpha$_1$-antitrypsin deficiency. *Scand J Clin Lab Invest* 15:132–40, 1963.
3. Eriksson S: Pulmonary emphysema and alpha$_1$-antitrypsin deficiency. *Acta Med Scand* 175(2):197–205, 1964.
4. Eriksson S: Studies in alpha$_1$-antitrypsin deficiency. *Acta Med Scand* Suppl 432:1–85, 1965.
5. Kueppers F, Black LF: Alpha$_1$-antitrypsin and its deficiency. *Am Rev Respir Dis* 110(2):176–94, 1974.
6. Morse JO: Alpha$_1$-antitrypsin deficiency. *N Engl J Med* 299:1045–8; 1099–105, 1978.
7. Black LF, Kueppers F: Alpha$_1$-antitrypsin deficiency in nonsmokers. *Am Rev Respir Dis* 117(3):421–8, 1978.
8. Tobin JM, Cook PJ, Hutchison DC: Alpha$_1$-antitrypsin deficiency: the clinical and physiological features of pulmonary emphysema in subjects homozygous for Pi type Z. A survey by the British Thoracic Association. *Br J Dis Chest* 77(1):14–27, 1983.
9. Larsson C. Natural history and life expectancy in severe alpha$_1$-antitrypsin deficiency, Pi Z. *Acta Med Scand* 204(5):345–51, 1978.
10. Pannell R, Johnson D, Travis J: Isolation and properties of human plasma alpha$_1$-proteinase inhibitor. *Biochemistry* 13(26):5439–45, 1974.
11. Lieberman J: Elastase, collagenase, emphysema, and alpha$_1$-antitrypsin deficiency. *Chest* 70(1):62–7, 1976.
12. Gadek JE, Fells GA, Zimmerman RL, et al: Antielastases of the human alveolar structures: implications for the protease-antiprotease theory of emphysema. *J Clin Invest* 68(4):889–98, 1981.
13. Beatty K, Bieth J, Travis J: Kinetics of association of serine proteinases with native and oxidized alpha-1-proteinase inhibitor and alpha-1-antichymotrypsin. *J Biol Chem* 255(9):3931–4, 1980.
14. Janoff A, White R, Carp H, et al: Lung injury induced by leukocytic proteases. *Am J Pathol* 97(1):111–36, 1979.
15. Gadek JE, Crystal RG: Alpha$_1$-antitrypsin deficiency. In: Stanbury JB, Wyngaarden JB, Frederickson DS, et al, eds.: *The Metabolic Basis of Inherited Disease* 5th ed. New York, McGraw-Hill, 1983, p. 1450–67.

16. Larsson C, Dirksen H, Sundstrom G, et al: Lung function studies in asymptomatic individuals with moderately (Pi SZ) and severely (Pi Z) reduced levels of alpha$_1$-antitrypsin. *Scand J Respir Dis* 57(6):267–80, 1976.
17. Gadek JE, Klein HG, Holland PV, et al: Replacement therapy of alpha$_1$-antitrypsin deficiency: reversal of protease-antiprotease imbalance within the alveolar structures of PiZ subjects. *J Clin Invest* 68(5):1158–65, 1981.
18. Data on file, Miles Inc., Cutter Biological.
19. Wewers MD, Casolaro MA, Sellers SE, et al: Replacement therapy for alpha$_1$-antitrypsin deficiency associated with emphysema. *N Engl J Med* 316(17):1055–62, 1987.
20. Wewers MD, Casolaro MA, Crystal RG: Comparison of alpha-1-antitrypsin levels and antineutrophil elastase capacity of blood and lung in a patient with the alpha-1-antitrypsin phenotype null-null before and during alpha-1-antitrypsin augmentation therapy. *Am Rev Respir Dis* 135(3):539–43, 1987.
21. Burrows B: A clinical trial of efficacy of antiproteolytic therapy: can it be done? *Am Rev Respir Dis* 127(2:2):S42–3, 1983.
22. Cohen AB: Unraveling the mysteries of alpha$_1$-antitrypsin deficiency. *N Engl J Med* 314(12):778–9, 1986.
23. Finlayson JS: Albumin products. *Semin Thromb Hemost* 6(2);85-120, 1980.

ANTITHROMBIN III (HUMAN) ℞
THROMBATE III®

DESCRIPTION
Antithrombin III (Human), THROMBATE III®, is a sterile, stable, lyophilized preparation of purified human antithrombin III.
THROMBATE III is prepared from pooled units of human plasma from normal donors by modifications and refinements of the cold ethanol method of Cohn.[1] When reconstituted, THROMBATE III has a pH of 6.0–7.5, a sodium content of 110–210 mEq/L, a chloride content of 110–210 mEq/L, an alanine content of 0.075–0.125 M and a heparin content of not more than 0.004 unit/IU AT-III. THROMBATE III contains no preservative and must be administered by the intravenous route. In addition, THROMBATE III has been heat-treated in solution at 60°C ± 0.5°C for not less than 10 hours.
Each vial of THROMBATE III contains the labeled amount of antithrombin III in international units (IU) per vial. The potency assignment has been determined with a standard calibrated against a World Health Organization (WHO) antithrombin III reference preparation.

CLINICAL PHARMACOLOGY
Antithrombin III (AT-III), an alpha$_2$-glycoprotein of molecular weight 58,000, is normally present in human plasma at a concentration of approximately 12.5 mg/dL[2,3] and is the major plasma inhibitor of thrombin.[4] Inactivation of thrombin by AT-III occurs by formation of a covalent bond resulting in an inactive 1:1 stoichiometric complex between the two, involving an interaction of the active serine of thrombin and an arginine reactive site on AT-III.[4] AT-III is also capable of inactivating other components of the coagulation cascade including factors IXa, Xa, XIa, and XIIa, as well as plasmin.[4]
The neutralization rate of serine proteases by AT-III proceeds slowly in the absence of heparin, but is greatly accelerated in the presence of heparin.[4] As the therapeutic antithrombotic effect in vivo of heparin is mediated by AT-III, heparin is ineffective in the absence or near absence of AT-III.[4–8]
The prevalence of the hereditary deficiency of AT-III is estimated to be one per 2000 to 5000 in the general population.[4,7] The pattern of inheritance is autosomal dominant. In affected individuals, spontaneous episodes of thrombosis and pulmonary embolism may be associated with AT-III levels of 40%–60% of normal.[7] These episodes usually appear after the age of 20, the risk increasing with age and in association with surgery, pregnancy and delivery. The frequency of thromboembolic events in hereditary antithrombin III (AT-III) deficiency during pregnancy has been reported to be 70%, and several studies of the beneficial use of Antithrombin III (Human) concentrates during pregnancy in women with hereditary deficiency have been reported.[9–11] In many cases, however, no precipitating factor can be identified for venous thrombosis or pulmonary embolism.[7] Greater than 85% of individuals with hereditary AT-III deficiency have had at least one thrombotic episode by the age of 50 years.[7] In about 60% of patients thrombosis is recurrent. Clinical signs of pulmonary embolism occur in 40% of affected individuals.[7] In some individuals, treatment with oral anticoagulants leads to an increase of the endogenous levels of AT-III, and treatment with oral anticoagulants may be effective in the prevention of thrombosis in such individuals.[6,7]
In clinical studies of Antithrombin III (Human), THROMBATE III® conducted in 10 asymptomatic subjects with hereditary deficiency of AT-III, the mean in vivo recovery of AT-III was 1.6% per unit per kg administered based on immunologic AT-III 1.says, and 1.4% per unit per kg administered based on functional AT-III assays.[12] The mean 50% disappearance time (the time to fall to 50% of the peak plasma level following an initial administration) was approximately 22 hours and the biologic half-life was 2.5 days based on immunologic assays and 3.8 days based on functional assays of AT-III.[12] These values are similar to the half-life for radiolabeled Antithrombin III (Human) reported in the literature of 2.8– .8 days.[13–15]
In clinical studies of THROMBATE III, none of the 13 patients with hereditary AT-III deficiency and histories of thromboembolism treated prophylactically on 16 separate occasions with THROMBATE III for high thrombotic risk situations (11 surgical procedures, 5 deliveries) developed a thrombotic complication. Heparin was also administered in 3 of the 11 surgical procedures and all 5 deliveries. Eight patients with hereditary AT-III deficiency were treated therapeutically with THROMBATE III as well as heparin for major thrombotic or thromboembolic complications, with seven patients recovering. Treatment with THROMBATE III reversed heparin resistance in two patients with hereditary AT-III deficiency being treated for thrombosis or thromboembolism.
During clinical investigation of THROMBATE III, none of 12 subjects monitored for a median of 8 months (range 2–19 months) after receiving THROMBATE III, became antibody positive to human immunodeficiency virus (HIV-1). None of 14 subjects monitored for ≥ 3 months demonstrated any evidence of hepatitis, either non-A, non-B hepatitis or hepatitis B.

INDICATIONS AND USAGE
THROMBATE III is indicated for the treatment of patients with hereditary antithrombin III deficiency in connection with surgical or obstetrical procedures or when they suffer from thromboembolism.
Subjects with AT-III deficiency should be informed about the risk of thrombosis in connection with pregnancy and surgery and about the inheritance of the disease.
The diagnosis of hereditary antithrombin III (AT-III) deficiency should be based on a clear family history of venous thrombosis as well as decreased plasma AT-III levels, and the exclusion of acquired deficiency.
AT-III in plasma may be measured by amidolytic assays using synthetic chromogenic substrates, by clotting assays, or by immunoassays. The latter does not detect all hereditary AT-III deficiencies.[16]
The AT-III level in neonates of parents with hereditary AT-III deficiency should be measured immediately after birth. (Fatal neonatal thromboembolism, such as aortic thrombi in children of women with hereditary antithrombin III deficiency, has been reported.)[17]
Plasma levels of AT-III are lower in neonates than adults, averaging approximately 60% in normal term infants.[18,19] AT-III levels in premature infants may be much lower.[18,19]
Low plasma AT-III levels, especially in a premature infant, therefore, do not necessarily indicate hereditary deficiency.
It is recommended that testing and treatment with Antithrombin III (Human), THROMBATE III® of neonates be discussed with an expert on coagulation.[11]

CONTRAINDICATIONS
None known.

WARNINGS
This product is prepared from pooled human plasma which may contain the causative agents of hepatitis and other viral diseases. Prescribed manufacturing procedures utilized at the plasma collection centers, plasma testing laboratories, and the fractionation facilities are designed to reduce the risk of transmitting viral infection. However, the risk of viral infectivity from this product cannot be totally eliminated.
Individuals who receive multiple infusions of blood or plasma products may develop signs and/or symptoms of some viral infections, particularly non-A, non-B hepatitis.
The anticoagulant effect of heparin is enhanced by concurrent treatment with THROMBATE III in patients with hereditary AT-III deficiency. Thus, in order to avoid bleeding, reduced dosage of heparin is recommended during treatment with THROMBATE III.

PRECAUTIONS
General
1. Administer within 3 hours after reconstitution. Do not refrigerate after reconstitution.
2. Administer only by the intravenous route.
3. THROMBATE III should be given alone, without mixing with other agents or diluting solutions.
4. Product administration and handling of the needles must be done with caution. Percutaneous puncture with a needle contaminated with blood can transmit infectious virus including HIV (AIDS) and hepatitis. Obtain immediate medical attention of injury occurs.
Place needles in sharps container after single use. Discard all equipment including any reconstituted THROMBATE III product in accordance with biohazard procedures.

The diagnosis of hereditary antithrombin III (AT-III) deficiency should be based on a clear family history of venous thrombosis as well as decreased plasma AT-III levels, and the exclusion of acquired deficiency.

Laboratory Tests
It is recommended that AT-III plasma levels be monitored during the treatment period. Functional levels of AT-III in plasma may be measured by amidolytic assays using chromogenic substrates or by clotting assays.

Drug Interactions
The anticoagulant effect of heparin is enhanced by concurrent treatment with THROMBATE III in patients with hereditary AT-III deficiency. Thus, in order to avoid bleeding, reduced dosage of heparin is recommended during treatment with THROMBATE III.

Pregnancy Category B
Reproduction studies have been performed in rats and rabbits at doses up to four times the human dose and have revealed no evidence of impaired fertility or harm to the fetus due to THROMBATE III. It is not known whether THROMBATE III can cause fetal harm when administered to a pregnant woman or can affect reproduction capacity. Because animal reproduction studies are not always predictive of human response, this drug should be used during pregnancy only if clearly needed.

Pediatric Use
Safety and effectiveness in the pediatric population have not been established. The AT-III level in neonates of parents with hereditary AT-III deficiency should be measured immediately after birth. (Fatal neonatal thromboembolism, such as aortic thrombi in children of women with hereditary antithrombin III deficiency, has been reported.)[17]
Plasma levels of AT-III are lower in neonates than adults, averaging approximately 60% in normal term infants.[18,19] AT-III levels in premature infants may be much lower.[18,19]
Low plasma AT-III levels, especially in a premature infant, therefore, do not necessarily indicate hereditary deficiency.
It is recommended that testing and treatment with Antithrombin III (Human), THROMBATE III® of neonates be discussed with an expert on coagulation.[11]

ADVERSE REACTIONS
In clinical studies involving THROMBATE III, adverse reactions were reported in association with 17 of the 340 infusions during the clinical studies. Included were dizziness (7), chest tightness (3), nausea (3), foul taste in mouth (3), chills (2), cramps (2), shortness of breath (1), chest pain (1), film over eye (1), light-headedness (1), bowel fullness (1), hives (1), fever (1), and oozing and hematoma formation (1). If adverse reactions are experienced, the infusion rate should be decreased, or if indicated, the infusion should be interrupted until symptoms abate.

DOSAGE AND ADMINISTRATION
Each bottle of THROMBATE III has the functional activity, in international units (IU), stated on the label of the bottle. The potency assignment has been determined with a standard calibrated against a World Health Organization antithrombin III reference preparation.
Dosage should be determined on an individual basis based on the pre-therapy plasma antithrombin III (AT-III) level, in order to increase plasma AT-III levels to the level found in normal human plasma (100%). Dosage of THROMBATE III can be calculated from the following formula:

$$\text{units required (IU)} = \frac{[\text{desired - baseline AT-III level*}] \times \text{weight (kg)}}{1.4}$$

*expressed as % normal level based on functional AT-III assay

The above formula is based on an expected incremental in vivo recovery above baseline levels for THROMBATE III of 1.4% per IU per kg administered.[12] Thus, if a 70 kg individual has a baseline AT-III level of 57%, in order to increase plasma AT-III to 120%, the initial THROMBATE III dose would be $[(120-57) \times 70]/1.4 = 3150$ IU total.
However, recovery may vary, and initially levels should be drawn at baseline and 20 minutes postinfusion. Subsequent doses can be calculated based on the recovery of the first dose. These recommendations are intended only as a guide for therapy. The exact loading dose and maintenance intervals should be individualized for each patient.
It is recommended that following an initial dose of THROMBATE III, plasma levels of AT-III be initially monitored at least every 12 hours and before the next infusion of THROMBATE III to maintain plasma AT-III levels greater than 80%. In some situations, e.g., following surgery,[20] hemorrhage or acute thrombosis, and during intravenous heparin administration,[13,21–23] the half-life of Antithrombin III (Human) has been reported to be shortened. In such conditions, plasma AT-III levels should be monitored more frequently,

Continued on next page

Bayer Biological—Cont.

and Antithrombin III (Human), THROMBATE III® administered as necessary.

When an infusion of THROMBATE III is indicated for a patient with hereditary deficiency to control an acute thrombotic episode or prevent thrombosis following surgical or obstetrical procedures, it is desirable to raise the AT-III level to normal and maintain this level for 2 to 8 days, depending on the indication for treatment, type and extent of surgery, patient's medical condition, past history and physician's judgment. Concomitant administration of heparin in each of these situations should be based on the medical judgment of the physician.

As a general recommendation, the following therapeutic program may be utilized as a starting program for treatment, modifying the program based on the actual plasma AT-III levels achieved:

a) An initial loading dose of THROMBATE III calculated to elevate the plasma AT-III level to 120%, assuming an expected rise over the baseline plasma AT-III level of 1.4% (functional activity) per IU per kg of THROMBATE III administered. Thus, if an individual has a baseline AT-III level of 57%, the initial THROMBATE III dose would be $(120-57)/1.4 = 45$ IU/kg.

b) Measure preinfusion and 20 minutes postinfusion (peak) plasma antithrombin III levels following the initial dose, plasma antithrombin III level after 12 hours, then preceding the next infusion (trough level). Subsequently measure antithrombin III levels preceding and 20 minutes after each infusion until predictable peak and trough levels have been achieved, generally between 80%–120%. Plasma levels between 80%–120% may be maintained by administration of maintenance doses of 60% of the initial loading dose, administered every 24 hours. Adjustments in the maintenance dose and/or interval between doses should be made based on actual plasma AT-III levels achieved.

The above recommendations for dosing are provided as a general guideline for therapy only. The exact loading and maintenance dosages and dosing intervals should be individualized for each subject, based on the individual clinical conditions, response to therapy, and actual plasma AT-III levels achieved. In some situations, e.g., following surgery,[20] with hemorrhage or acute thrombosis and during intravenous heparin administration,[13,21-23] in vivo survival of infused THROMBATE III has been reported to be shortened, resulting in the need to administer THROMBATE III more frequently.

THROMBATE III should be reconstituted with Sterile Water for Injection, USP and brought to room temperature prior to administration. THROMBATE III should be filtered through a sterile filter needle as supplied in the package prior to use, and should be administered within 3 hours following reconstitution. THROMBATE III may be infused over 10–20 minutes. THROMBATE III must be administered intravenously.

Parenteral drug products should be inspected visually for particulate matter and discoloration prior to administration, whenever solution and container permit.

Reconstitution

Vacuum Transfer

1. Warm the unopened diluent and the concentrate to room temperature (NMT 37℃, 99°F).
2. After removing the plastic flip-top caps (Fig. A), aseptically cleanse the rubber stoppers of both bottles.
3. Remove the protective cover from the plastic transfer needle cartridge with tamper-proof seal and penetrate the stopper of the diluent bottle (Fig. B).
4. Remove the remaining portion of the plastic cartridge, invert the diluent bottle and penetrate the rubber seal on the concentrate bottle (Fig. C) with the needle at an angle. Alternate method of transferring sterile water: With a sterile needle and syringe, withdraw the appropriate volume of diluent and transfer to the bottle of lyophilized concentrate.
5. The vacuum will draw the diluent into the concentrate bottle. Hold the diluent bottle at an angle to the concentrate bottle in order to direct the jet of diluent against the wall of the concentrate bottle (Fig. C). Avoid excessive foaming.
6. After removing the diluent bottle and transfer needle (Fig. D), swirl continuously until completely dissolved (Fig. E).
7. After the concentrate powder is completely dissolved, withdraw solution into the syringe through the filter needle which is supplied in the package (Fig. F). Replace the filter needle with an administration set (not provided) and inject intravenously.
8. If the same patient is to receive more than one bottle, the contents of two bottles may be drawn into the same syringe through a separate unused filter needle before attaching the vein needle.

Rate of Administration

The rate of administration should be adapted to the response of the individual patient, but administration of the entire dose in 10 to 20 minutes is generally well-tolerated.

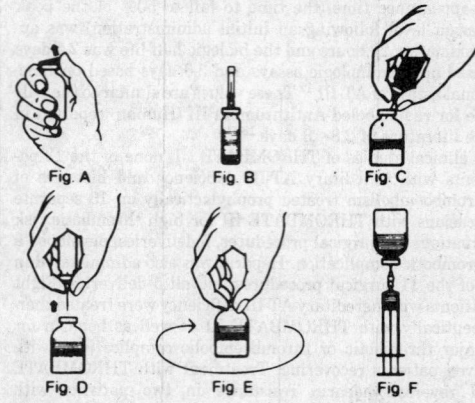

Fig. A   Fig. B   Fig. C

Fig. D   Fig E   Fig. F

HOW SUPPLIED

Antithrombin III (Human), THROMBATE III® is supplied in the following single dose vials with the potency in international units stated on the label of each vial. A suitable volume of Sterile Water for Injection, USP, a sterile double-ended transfer needle, and a sterile filter needle are provided.

Product Code	Approximate Antithrombin III Potency	Diluent
603-20	500 IU	10 mL
603-30	1000 IU	20 mL

STORAGE

Antithrombin III (Human), THROMBATE III® should be stored under refrigeration (2°–8℃; 36°–46°F). Freezing should be avoided as breakage of the diluent bottle might occur.

CAUTION

U.S. federal law prohibits dispensing without prescription.

LIMITED WARRANTY

A number of factors beyond our control could reduce the efficacy of this product or even result in an ill effect following its use. These include improper storage and handling of the product after it leaves our hands, diagnosis, dosage, method of administration, and biological differences in individual patients. Because of these factors, it is important that this product be stored properly, that the directions be followed carefully during use, and that the risk of transmitting viruses be carefully weighed before the product is prescribed. No warranty, express or implied, including any warranty of merchantability or fitness is made. Representatives of the Company are not authorized to vary the terms or the contents of the printed labeling, including the package insert for this product, except by printed notice from the Company's headquarters. The prescriber and user of this product must accept the terms hereof.

REFERENCES

1. Cohn EJ, Strong LE, Hughes WL Jr, et al: Preparation and properties of serum and plasma proteins. IV. A system for the separation into fractions of the protein and lipoprotein components of biological tissues and fluids. *J Am Chem Soc* 68(3):459–75, 1946.
2. Rosenberg RD, Bauer KA, Marcum JA: Antithrombin III "the heparin-antithrombin system." *Rev Hematol* 2:351–416, 1986.
3. Murano G, Williams L, Miller-Andersson M: Some properties of antithrombin-III and its concentration in human plasma. *Thromb Res* 18(1–2):259–62, 1980.
4. Rosenberg RD: Action and interactions of antithrombin and heparin. *N Engl J Med* 292(3):146–51, 1975.
5. Winter JH, Fenech A, Ridley W, et al: Familial antithrombin III deficiency. *Q J Med* 51(204):373–95, 1982.
6. Marciniak E, Farley CH, DeSimone PA: Familial thrombosis due to antithrombin III deficiency. *Blood* 43(2):219–31, 1974.
7. Thaler E, Lechner K: Antithrombin III deficiency and thromboembolism. *Clin Haematol* 10(2):369–90, 1981.
8. Blauhut B, Necek S, Kramar H, et al: Activity of antithrombin III and effect of heparin on coagulation in shock. *Thromb Res* 19(6):775–82, 1980.
9. Samson D, Stirling Y, Woolf L, et al: Management of planned pregnancy in a patient with congenital antithrombin III deficiency. *Br J Haematol* 56(2):243–9, 1984.
10. Brandt P: Observations during the treatment of antithrombin-III deficient women with heparin and antithrombin concentrate during pregnancy, parturition, and abortion. *Thromb Res* 22(1–2):15–24, 1981.
11. Hellgren M, Tengborn L, Abildgaard U: Pregnancy in women with congenital antithrombin III deficiency;

experience of treatment with heparin and antithrombin. *Gynecol Obstet Invest* 14(2):127–41, 1982.
12. Schwartz RS, Bauer KA, Rosenberg RD, et al: Clinical experience with antithrombin III concentrate in treatment of congenital and acquired deficiency of antithrombin. *Am J Med* 87 (Suppl 3B): 53S–60S, 1989.
13. Collen D, Schetz J, de Cock F, et al: Metabolism of antithrombin III (heparin cofactor) in man; effects of venous thrombosis and of heparin administration. *Eur J Clin Invest* 7(1):27–35, 1977.
14. Knot EAR, de Jong E, ten Cate JW, et al: Purified radiolabeled antithrombin III metabolism in three families with hereditary AT III deficiency: application of a three-compartment model. *Blood* 67(1):93–8, 1986.
15. Tengborn L, Frohm B, Nilsson LE, et al: Antithrombin III concentrate; its catabolism in health and in antithrombin III deficiency. *Scand J Clin Lab Invest* 41(5):469–77, 1981.
16. Sas G, Blasko G, Banhegyi D, et al: Abnormal antithrombin III (antithrombin III "Budapest") as a cause of familial thrombophilia. *Thromb Diath Haemorrh* 32(1):105–15, 1974.
17. Bjarke B, Herin P, Blomback M: Neonatal aortic thrombosis. A possible clinical manifestation of congenital antithrombin III deficiency. *Acta Paediatr Scand* 63:297–301, 1974.
18. Hathaway WE, Bonnar J: Perinatal coagulation, New York, Grune & Stratton, 1978, p.68.
19. Peters M, Jansen E, ten Cate JW, et al: Neonatal antithrombin III. *Br J Haematol* 58(4):579–87, 1984.
20. Mannucci PM, Boyer C, Wolf M, et al: Treatment of congenital antithrombin III deficiency with concentrates. *Br J Haematol* 50(3):531–5, 1982.
21. Marciniak E, Gockerman JP: Heparin-induced decrease in circulating antithrombin-III. *Lancet* 2(8038):581–4, 1977.
22. O'Brien JR, Etherington MD: Effect of heparin and warfarin on antithrombin III. *Lancet* 2(8050):1232, 1977.
23. Kakkar VV, Bentley PG, Scully MF, et al: Antithrombin III and heparin. *Lancet* 1(8159):103–4, 1980.

Beach Pharmaceuticals
Division of Beach Products, Inc.
5220 SOUTH MANHATTAN AVE.
TAMPA, FL 33611

Direct Inquiries to:
Richard Stephan Jenkins
(813) 839-6565
FAX (813) 837-2511

BEELITH Tablets   OTC
MAGNESIUM SUPPLEMENT
with PYRIDOXINE HCL
Each tablet supplies 362 mg (30mEq) of magnesium and 25 mg of pyridoxine HCL.

DESCRIPTION

Each tablet contains magnesium oxide 600 mg and pyridoxine hydrochloride (Vitamin B₆) 25 mg equivalent to B₆ 20 mg. Each tablet yields 362 mg of magnesium and supplies 90% of the Adult U.S. Recommended Daily Allowance (RDA) for magnesium and 1000% of the Adult RDA for vitamin B₆.

INDICATIONS

As a dietary supplement for patients with magnesium and/or Vitamin B₆ deficiencies resulting from malnutrition, alcoholism, magnesium depleting drugs, chemotheraphy and inadequate nutritional intake or absorption. Also, increases urinary magnesium levels.

DOSAGE

One tablet daily or as directed by a physician.

DRUG INTERACTION PRECAUTIONS

Do not take this product if you are presently taking a prescription drug without consulting your physician or other health professional.

WARNINGS

If you have kidney disease, take only under the supervision of a physician. Excessive dosage may cause laxation. **KEEP OUT OF THE REACH OF CHILDREN.** As with any drug, if you are pregnant or nursing a baby, seek the advice of a health professional before using this product.

HOW SUPPLIED

Golden yellow, film coated tablet with the name **BEACH** and the number **1132** printed on each tablet. Packaged in bottles of 100 (NDC 0486-1132-01) tablets.

Shown in Product Identification Guide, page 305

CITROLITH TABLETS ℞

DESCRIPTION

Each white, capsule shaped tablet contains potassium citrate, anhydrous 50 mg and sodium citrate, anhydrous 950 mg.

K-PHOS® M.F. ℞
K-PHOS® No.2 ℞

DESCRIPTION

K-PHOS® M.F.: Each tablet contains potassium acid phosphate 155 mg and sodium acid phosphate, anhydrous 350 mg. Each tablet yields approximately 125.6 mg of phosphorus, 44.5 mg of potassium or 1.1 mEq and 67 mg of sodium or 2.9 mEq. K-PHOS® No.2: Each tablet contains potassium acid phosphate 305 mg and sodium acid phosphate, anhydrous 700 mg. Each tablet yields approximately 250 mg of phosphorus, 88 mg of potassium or 2.3 mEq and 134 mg of sodium or 5.8 mEq.

Shown in Product Identification Guide, page 305

K-PHOS® NEUTRAL ℞
Supplies 250 mg of phosphorus per tablet.

DESCRIPTION

Each tablet contains 852 mg dibasic sodium phosphate anhydrous, 155 mg monobasic potassium phosphate, and 130 mg monobasic sodium phosphate monohydrate. Each tablet yields approximately 250 mg of phosphorus, 298 mg of sodium (13.0 mEq) and 45 mg of potassium (1.1 mEq).

CLINICAL PHARMACOLOGY

Phosphorus has a number of important functions in the biochemistry of the body. The bulk of the body's phosphorus is located in the bones, where it plays a key role in osteoblastic and osteoclastic activities. Enzymatically catalyzed phosphate-transfer reactions are numerous and vital in the metabolism of carbohydrate, lipid and protein, and a proper concentration of the anion is of primary importance in assuring an orderly biochemical sequence. In addition, phosphorus plays an important role in modifying steady-state tissue concentrations of calcium. Phosphate ions are important buffers of the intracellular fluid, and also play a primary role in the renal excretion of hydrogen ion.

Oral administration of inorganic phosphates increase serum phosphate levels. Phosphates lower urinary calcium levels in idiopathic hypercalciuria.

In general, in adults, about two thirds of the ingested phosphate is absorbed from the bowel, most of which is rapidly excreted into the urine.

INDICATIONS

K-PHOS® NEUTRAL increases urinary phosphate and pyrophosphate. As a phosphorus supplement, each tablet supplies 25% of the U.S. Recommended Daily Allowance (U.S.RDA) of phosphorus for adults.

CONTRAINDICATIONS

This product is contraindicated in patients with infected phosphate stones, in patients with severely impaired renal function (less than 30% of normal) and in the presence of hyperphosphatemia.

PRECAUTIONS

General: This product contains potassium and sodium and should be used with caution if regulation of these elements is desired. Occasionally, some individuals may experience a mild laxative effect during the first few days of phosphate therapy. If laxation persists to an unpleasant degree, reduce the daily dosage until this effect subsides or, if necessary, discontinue the use of this product.

Caution should be exercised when prescribing this product in the following conditions: Cardiac disease (particularly in digitalized patients); severe adrenal insufficiency (Addison's disease); acute dehydration; severe renal insufficiency; renal function impairment or chronic renal disease; extensive tissue breakdown (such as severe burns); myotonia congenita; cardiac failure; cirrhosis of the liver or severe hepatic disease; peripheral or pulmonary edema; hypernatremia; hypertension; toxemia of pregnancy; hypoparathyroidism; and acute pancreatitis. Rickets may benefit from phosphate therapy, but caution should be exercised. High serum phosphate may increase the incidence of extra-skeletal calcification.

Information for Patients: Patients with kidney stones may pass old stones when phosphate therapy is started and should be warned of this possibility. Patients should be advised to avoid the use of antacids containing aluminum, magnesium or calcium which may prevent the absorption of phosphate.

Laboratory Tests: Careful monitoring of renal function and serum electrolytes (calcium, phosphorus, potassium, sodium) may be required at periodic intervals during phosphate therapy. Other tests may be warranted in some patients, depending on conditions.

Drug Interactions: The use of antacids containing magnesium, aluminum or calcium in conjunction with phosphate preparations may bind the phosphate and prevent its absorption. Concurrent use of antihypertensives, especially diazoxide, guanethidine, hydralazine, methyldopa, or rauwolfia alkaloids; or corticosteroids, especially mineralocorticoids or corticotropin, with sodium phosphate may result in hypernatremia. Calcium-containing preparations and/or vitamin D may antagonize the effects of phosphates in the treatment of hypercalcemia. Potassium-containing medications or potassium-sparing diuretics may cause hyperkalemia. Patients should have serum potassium level determinations at periodic intervals.

Carcinogenesis, Mutagenesis, Impairment of Fertility: There have been no studies in animals or humans to evaluate the carcinogenesis, mutagenesis, or impairment of fertility for this product.

Pregnancy: Pregnancy Category C. Animal reproduction studies have not been conducted with this product. It is also not known whether this product can cause fetal harm when administered to a pregnant woman or can affect reproduction capacity. This product should be given to a pregnant woman only if clearly needed.

Nursing Mothers: It is not known whether this drug is excreted in human milk. Because many drugs are excreted in human milk, caution should be exercised when this product is administered to a nursing woman.

ADVERSE REACTIONS

Gastrointestinal upset (diarrhea, nausea, stomach pain, and vomiting) may occur with phosphate therapy. Also, bone and joint pain (possible phosphate-induced osteomalacia) could occur. The following adverse effects may be observed (primarily from sodium or potassium): headaches; dizziness; mental confusion; seizures; weakness or heaviness of legs; unusual tiredness or weakness; muscle cramps; numbness, tingling, pain, or weakness of hands or feet; numbness or tingling around lips; fast or irregular heartbeat; shortness of breath or troubled breathing; swelling of feet or lower legs; unusual weight gain; low urine output; unusual thirst.

DIRECTIONS

Adults: One or two tablets four times daily, with a full glass of water, with meals and at bedtime.

HOW SUPPLIED

White, film coated, capsule-shaped tablet with the name BEACH and number 1125 embossed on each tablet. Bottles of 100 (NDC 0486-1125-01) and 500 (NDC 0486-1125-05) tablets.

CAUTION

Federal law prohibits dispensing without prescription.

Shown in Product Identification Guide, page 305

K-PHOS® ORIGINAL (Sodium Free) ℞
(Potassium Acid Phosphate)
Urinary Acidifier
Supplies 114 mg of phosphorus per tablet.

DESCRIPTION

Each tablet contains potassium acid phosphate 500 mg. Each tablet yields approximately 114 mg of phosphorus and 144 mg of potassium or 3.7 mEq.

ACTIONS

K-PHOS® ORIGINAL (Sodium Free) is a highly effective urinary acidifier.

INDICATIONS

For use in patients with elevated urinary pH. Helps keep calcium soluble and reduces odor and rash caused by ammoniacal urine. Also, by acidifying the urine, it increases the antibacterial activity of methenamine mandelate and methenamine hippurate.

CONTRAINDICATIONS

This product is contraindicated in patients with infected phosphate stones; in patients with severely impaired renal function (less than 30% of normal) and in the presence of hyperphosphatemia and hyperkalemia.

PRECAUTIONS

General: This product contains potassium and should be used with caution if regulation of this element is desired. Occasionally, some individuals may experience a mild laxative effect during the first few days of phosphate therapy. If laxation persists to an unpleasant degree, reduce the daily dosage until this effect subsides or, if necessary, discontinue the use of this product.

Caution should be exercised when prescribing this product in the following conditions: Cardiac disease (particularly in digitalized patients); severe adrenal insufficiency (Addison's disease); acute dehydration; severe renal insufficiency or chronic renal disease; extensive tissue breakdown (such as severe burns); myotonia congenita; hypoparathyroidism; and acute pancreatitis. Rickets may benefit from phosphate therapy, but caution should be exercised. High serum phosphate levels may increase the incidence of extraskeletal calcification.

Information for Patients: Patients with kidney stones may pass old stones when phosphate therapy is started and should be warned of this possibility. Patients should be advised to avoid the use of antacids containing aluminum, calcium, or magnesium which may prevent the absorption of phosphate. To assure against gastrointestinal injury associated with oral ingestion of concentrated potassium salt preparations, patients should be instructed to dissolve tablets completely in an appropriate amount of water before taking.

Laboratory Tests: Careful monitoring of renal function and serum electrolytes (calcium, phosphorous, potassium) may be required at periodic intervals during phosphate therapy. Other tests may be warranted in some patients, depending on conditions.

Drug Interactions: The use of antacids containing magnesium, calcium, or aluminum in conjunction with phosphate preparations may bind the phosphate and prevent its absorption. Potassium-containing medications or potassium-sparing diuretics may cause hyperkalemia when used concurrently with potassium salts. Patients should have serum potassium level determinations at periodic intervals. Concurrent use of salicylates may lead to increased serum salicylate levels since excretion of salicylates is reduced in acidified urine. Serum salicylate levels should be closely monitored to avoid toxicity.

Carcincogenesis, Mutagenesis, Impairment of Fertility: There have been no studies in animals or humans to evaluate the carcinogenesis, mutagenesis, or impairment of fertility for this product.

Pregnancy: Pregnancy Category C. Animal reproduction studies have not been conducted with this product. It is also not known whether this product can cause fetal harm when administered to a pregnant woman or can affect reproduction capacity. This product should be given to a pregnant woman only if clearly needed.

Nursing Mothers: It is not known whether this drug is excreted in human milk. Because many drugs are excreted in human milk, caution should be exercised when this product is administered to a nursing woman.

ADVERSE REACTIONS

Gastrointestinal upset (diarrhea, nausea, stomach pain, and vomiting) may occur with the use of potassium phosphates. Also, bone and joint pain (possible phosphate-induced osteomalacia) could occur. The following adverse effects may be observed with potassium administration: irregular heartbeat; dizziness; mental confusion; weakness or heaviness of legs; unusual tiredness; muscle cramps; numbness, tingling, pain, or weakness in hands or feet; numbness or tingling around lips; shortness of breath or troubled breathing.

DIRECTIONS

Two tablets dissolved in 6–8 oz. of water 4 times daily with meals and at bedtime. For best results, let the tablets soak in water for 2 to 5 minutes, or more if necessary, and stir. If any tablet particles remain undissolved, they may be crushed and stirred vigorously to speed dissolution.

HOW SUPPLIED

White scored tablet with the name BEACH and the number 1111 embossed on each tablet. Bottles of 100 (NDC 0486-1111-01) and bottles of 500 (NDC 0486-1111-05) tablets.

CAUTION

Federal law prohibits dispensing without prescription.

Shown in Product Identification Guide, page 305

UROQID-Acid® No.2 Tablets ℞

DESCRIPTION

Each UROQID-Acid® No.2 tablet contains methenamine mandelate 500 mg and sodium acid phosphate, monohydrate 500 mg.

CLINICAL PHARMACOLOGY

Methenamine mandelate is rapidly absorbed and excreted in the urine. Formaldehyde is released by acid hydrolysis from methenamine with bactericidal levels rapidly reached at pH 5.0–5.5. Proportionally less formaldehyde is released as urinary pH approaches 6.0 and insufficient quantities are released above this level for therapeutic response. In acid urine, mandelic acid exerts its antibacterial action and also contributes to the acidification of the urine. Mandelic acid is excreted by both glomerular filtration and tubular excretion. In acid urine, there is equally effective antibacterial activity against both gram-positive and gram-negative or-

Continued on next page

Beach—Cont.

ganisms, since the antibacterial action of mandelic acid and formaldehyde is nonspecific. With Proteus vulgaris and urea splitting strains of Pseudomonas and Aerobacter, results may be discouraging and particular attention is required in monitoring urinary pH and overall management.

INDICATIONS AND USAGE

For the suppression or elimination of bacteriuria associated with chronic and recurrent infections of the urinary tract, including pyelitis, pyelonephritis, cystitis, and infected residual urine accompanying neurogenic bladder. When used as recommended, **UROQID-Acid®No.2** is particularly suitable for long-term therapy because of its relative safety and because resistance to the nonspecific bactericidal action of formaldehyde does not develop. Pathogens resistant to other antibacterial agents may respond because of the nonspecific effect of formaldehyde formed in an acid urine.

Prophylactic Use Rationale: Urine is a good culture medium for many urinary pathogens. Inoculation by a few organisms (relapse or reinfection) may lead to bacteriuria in susceptible individuals. Thus, the rationale of management in recurring urinary tract infection (bacteriuria) is to change the urine from a growth-supporting to a growth-inhibiting medium. There is a growing body of evidence that long-term administration of methenamine can prevent recurrence of bacteriuria in patients with chronic pyelonephritis.

Therapeutic Use Rationale: Helps to sterilize the urine and, in some situations in which underlying pathologic conditions prevent sterilization by any means, can help to suppress bacteriuria. As part of the overall management of the urinary tract infection, a thorough diagnostic evaluation should accompany the use of this product.

CONTRAINDICATIONS

UROQID-Acid®No.2 is contraindicated in patients with renal insufficiency, severe hepatic disease, severe dehydration, hyperphosphatemia, and in patients who have exhibited hypersensitivity to any components of this product.

PRECAUTIONS

General

This product should not be used as the sole therapeutic agent in acute parenchymal infections causing systemic symptoms such as chills and fever.

UROQID-Acid®No.2 contains approximately 83 mg of sodium per tablet and should be used with caution in patients on a sodium-restricted diet.

Sodium phosphates should be used with caution in the following conditions: cardiac failure; peripheral or pulmonary edema; hypernatremia; hypertension; toxemia of pregnancy; hypoparathyroidism; and acute pancreatitis. High serum phosphate levels increase the incidence of extraskeletal calcification.

Large doses of methenamine (8 grams daily for 3 to 4 weeks) have caused bladder irritation, painful and frequent micturition, albuminuria and gross hematuria. Dysuria may occur, although usually at higher than recommended doses, and can be controlled by reducing the dosage. This product contains a urinary acidifier and can cause metabolic acidosis.

Care should be taken to maintain an acidic urinary pH (below 5.5), especially when treating infections due to urea-splitting organisms such as Proteus and strains of Pseudomonas.

Drugs and/or foods which produce an alkaline urine should be restricted. Frequent urine pH tests are essential. If acidification of the urine is contraindicated or unattainable, use of this product should be discontinued.

Information For Patients: To assure an acidic pH, patients should be instructed to restrict or avoid most fruits, milk and milk products, and antacids containing sodium carbonate or bicarbonate.

Laboratory Tests: As with all urinary tract infections, the efficacy of therapy should be monitored by repeated urine cultures. During long-term therapy, careful monitoring of renal function, serum phosphorus and sodium may be required at periodic intervals.

Drug Interactions: Formaldehyde and sulfamethizole form an insoluble precipitate in acid urine and increase the risk of crystalluria; therefore, these products should not be used concurrently. Thiazide diuretics, carbonic anhydrase inhibitors, antacids, or urinary alkalinizing agents should not be used concurrently since they may cause the urine to become alkaline and reduce the effectiveness of methenamine by inhibiting its conversion to formaldehyde. Concurrent use of antihypertensives, especially diazoxide, guanethidine, hydralazine, methyldopa, or rauwolfia alkaloids; or corticosteroids, especially mineralocorticoids or corticotropin, with sodium phosphates may result in hypernatremia. Concurrent use of salicylates may lead to increased serum salicylate levels since excretion of salicylates is reduced in acidified urine. Serum salicylate levels should be closely monitored to avoid toxicity.

Laboratory Test Interactions: Formaldehyde interferes with fluorometric procedures for determination of urinary catecholamines and vanilmandelic acid (VMA) causing erroneously high results. Formaldehyde also causes falsely decreased urine estriol levels by reacting with estriol when acid hydrolysis techniques are used; estriol determinations which use enzymatic hydrolysis are unaffected by formaldehyde. Formaldehyde causes falsely elevated 17-hydroxycorticosteroid levels when the Porter-Silber method is used and falsely decreased 5-hydroxyindoleacetic acid (5HIAA) levels by inhibiting color development when nitrosonaphthol methods are used.

Carcinogenesis, Mutagenesis, Impairment Of Fertility: Long-term animal studies to evaluate the carcinogenic, mutagenic, or impairment of fertility potential of this product have not been performed.

Pregnancy: Teratogenic Effects. Pregnancy Category C. Animal reproduction studies have not been conducted with **UROQID-Acid®No.2.** It is also not known whether **UROQID-Acid®No.2** can cause fetal harm when administered to a pregnant woman or can affect reproductive capacity. Since methenamine is known to cross the placental barrier, **UROQID-Acid®No.2** should be given to a pregnant woman only if clearly needed.

Nursing Mothers: Methenamine is excreted in breast milk. Caution should be exercised when this product is administered to a nursing woman.

ADVERSE REACTIONS

Gastrointestinal disturbances (nausea, stomach upset), generalized skin rash, dysuria, painful or difficult urination may occur occasionally with the use of methenamine preparations. Microscopic and rarely, gross hematuria have also been reported.

Gastrointestinal upset (diarrhea, nausea, stomach pain, and vomiting) may occur with the use of sodium phosphates. Also, bone or joint pain (possible phosphate induced osteomalacia) could occur. The following adverse effects may be observed (primarily from sodium): headaches; dizziness; mental confusion; seizures; weakness or heaviness of legs; unusual tiredness or weakness; muscle cramps; numbness, tingling, pain, or weakness of hands or feet; numbness or tingling around lips; fast or irregular heartbeat; shortness of breath or troubled breathing; swelling of feet or lower legs; unusual weight gain; low urine output, unusual thirst.

DIRECTIONS

UROQID-Acid®No.2: Initially, 2 tablets 4 times daily. For maintenance, 2 to 4 tablets daily, in divided doses with a full glass of water.

HOW SUPPLIED

UROQID-Acid®No.2 is a yellow, film coated, capsule shaped tablet with the name **BEACH** and the number **1114** embossed on each tablet. Packaged in bottles of 100 tablets (NDC 0486-1114-01).

CAUTION

Federal law prohibits dispensing without prescription.

Shown in Product Identification Guide, page 305

Bedford Laboratories

Division of Ben Venue Laboratories
300 NORTHFIELD ROAD
BEDFORD, OH 44146

Direct Inquiries to:
Customer Service: (800) 562-4797
FAX: (216) 232-6264
Professional Services: (800) 521-5169

CERUBIDINE® ℞

[*sĭ-rew "bĭ'dēan*]
(daunorubicin HCl)
for Injection

WARNINGS

1. Cerubidine must be given into a rapidly flowing intravenous infusion. It must *never* be given by the intramuscular or subcutaneous route. Severe local tissue necrosis will occur if there is extravasation during administration.
2. Myocardial toxicity manifested in its most severe form by potentially fatal congestive heart failure may occur either during therapy or months to years after termination of therapy. The incidence of myocardial toxicity increases after a total cumulative dose exceeding 400–550 mg/m^2 in adults, 300 mg/m^2 in children more than 2 years of age, or 10 mg/kg in children less than 2 years of age.
3. Severe myelosuppression occurs when used in therapeutic doses; this may lead to infection or hemorrhage.
4. It is recommended that Cerubidine be administered only by physicians who are experienced in leukemia chemotherapy and in facilities with laboratory and supportive resources adequate to monitor drug tolerance and protect and maintain a patient compromised by drug toxicity. The physician and institution must be capable of responding rapidly and completely to severe hemorrhagic conditions and/or overwhelming infection.
5. Dosage should be reduced in patients with impaired hepatic or renal function.

DESCRIPTION

Cerubidine (daunorubicin hydrochloride) is the hydrochloride salt of an anthracycline cytotoxic antibiotic produced by a strain of *Streptomyces coeruleorubidus*. It is provided as a sterile reddish lyophilized powder in vials for intravenous administration only. Each vial contains 21.4 mg daunorubicin hydrochloride, equivalent to 20 mg daunorubicin, and 100 mg of mannitol. It is soluble in water when adequately agitated and produces a reddish solution. It has the following structural formula which may be described with the chemical name of 7-(3-amino-2,3,6-trideoxy-L-lyxohexosyloxy)-9-acetyl-7,8,9,10-tetrahydro-6,9,11-trihydroxy-4-methoxy-5, 12-naphthacenequinone hydrochloride. Its molecular formula is $C_{27}H_{29}NO_{10}HCl$ with a molecular weight of 563.99. It is a hygroscopic crystalline powder. The pH of a 5 mg/mL aqueous solution is 4.5 to 6.5.

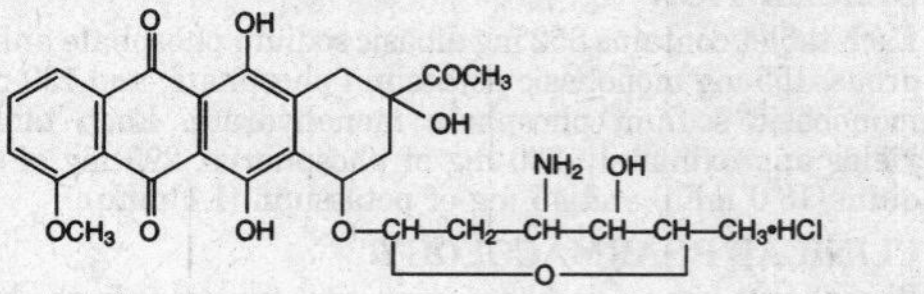

ACTION

Cerubidine inhibits the synthesis of nucleic acids; its effect on deoxyribonucleic acid is particularly rapid and marked. Cerubidine has antimitotic and cytotoxic activity although the precise mode of action is unknown. Cerubidine displays an immunosuppressive effect. It has been shown to inhibit the production of heterohemagglutinins in mice. *In vitro*, it inhibits blast-cell transformation of canine lymphocytes at 0.01 mcg/mL.

Cerubidine possesses a potent antitumor effect against a wide spectrum of animal tumors either grafted or spontaneous.

CLINICAL PHARMACOLOGY

Following intravenous injection of Cerubidine, plasma levels of daunorubicin decline rapidly, indicating rapid tissue uptake and concentration. Thereafter, plasma levels decline slowly with a half-life of 18.5 hours. By 1 hour after drug administration, the predominant plasma species is daunorubicinol, an active metabolite, which disappears with a half-life of 26.7 hours. Further metabolism via reduction cleavage of the glycosidic bond, 4-0 demethylation, and conjugation with both sulfate and glucuronide have been demonstrated. Simple glycosidic cleavage of daunorubicin or daunorubicinol is not a significant metabolic pathway in man. Twenty-five percent of an administered dose of Cerubidine is eliminated in an active form by urinary excretion and an estimated 40% by biliary excretion.

There is no evidence that Cerubidine crosses the blood-brain barrier.

In the treatment of adult acute nonlymphocytic leukemia, Cerubidine, used as a single agent, has produced complete remission rates of 40 to 50%, and in combination with cytarabine, has produced complete remission rates of 53 to 65%.

The addition of Cerubidine to the two-drug induction regimen of vincristine-prednisone in the treatment of childhood acute lymphocytic leukemia does not increase the rate of complete remission. In children receiving identical CNS prophylaxis and maintenance therapy (without consolidation), there is prolongation of complete remission duration (statistically significant, $p < 0.02$) in those children induced with the three-drug (Cerubidine-vincristine-prednisone) regimen as compared to two drugs. There is no evidence of any impact of Cerubidine on the duration of complete remission when a consolidation (intensification) phase is employed as part of a total treatment program.

In adult acute lymphocytic leukemia, in contrast to childhood acute lymphocytic leukemia, Cerubidine during induction significantly increases the rate of complete remission, but not remission duration, compared to that obtained with vincristine, prednisone, and L-asparaginase alone. The use of Cerubidine in combination with vincristine, prednisone, and L-asparaginase has produced complete remission rates of 83% in contrast to a 47% remission in patients not receiving Cerubidine.

INDICATIONS AND USAGE

Cerubidine in combination with other approved anticancer drugs is indicated for remission induction in acute nonlymphocytic leukemia (myelogenous, monocytic, erythroid) of adults and for remission induction in acute lymphocytic leukemia of children and adults.

WARNINGS

Bone Marrow: Cerubidine is a potent bone marrow suppressant. Suppression will occur in all patients given a therapeutic dose of this drug. Therapy with Cerubidine should not be started in patients with pre-existing drug-induced bone marrow suppression unless the benefit from such treatment warrants the risk. Persistent, severe myelosuppression may result in superinfection or hemorrhage.

Cardiac Effects: Special attention must be given to the potential cardiac toxicity of Cerubidine, particularly in infants and children. Pre-existing heart disease and previous therapy with doxorubicin are co-factors of increased risk of Cerubidine-induced cardiac toxicity and the benefit-to-risk ratio of Cerubidine therapy in such patients should be weighed before starting Cerubidine. In adults, at total cumulative doses less than 550 mg/m², acute congestive heart failure is seldom encountered. However, rare instances of pericarditis-myocarditis, not dose-related, have been reported.

In adults, at cumulative doses exceeding 550 mg/m², there is an increased incidence of drug-induced congestive heart failure. Based on prior clinical experience with doxorubicin, this limit appears lower, namely 400 mg/m², in patients who received radiation therapy that encompassed the heart.[1]

In infants and children, there appears to be a greater susceptibility to anthracycline-induced cardiotoxicity compared to that in adults, which is more clearly dose-related. Anthracycline therapy (including daunorubicin) in pediatric patients has been reported to produce impaired left ventricular systolic performance, reduced contractility, congestive heart failure or death. These conditions may occur months to years following cessation of chemotherapy. This appears to be dose-dependent and aggravated by thoracic irradiation. Long-term periodic evaluation of cardiac function in such patients should, thus, be performed.[2-7] In both children and adults, the total dose of Cerubidine administered should also take into account any previous or concomitant therapy with other potentially cardiotoxic agents or related compounds such as doxorubicin.

There is no absolutely reliable method of predicting the patients in whom acute congestive heart failure will develop as a result of the cardiac toxic effect of Cerubidine. However, certain changes in the electrocardiogram and a decrease in the systolic ejection fraction from pre-treatment baseline may help to recognize those patients at greatest risk to develop congestive heart failure. On the basis of the electrocardiogram, a decrease equal to or greater than 30% in limb lead QRS voltage has been associated with a significant risk of drug-induced cardiomyopathy. Therefore, an electrocardiogram and/or determination of systolic ejection fraction should be performed before each course of Cerubidine. In the event that one or the other of these predictive parameters should occur, the benefit of continued therapy must be weighed against the risk of producing cardiac damage. Early clinical diagnosis of drug-induced congestive heart failure appears to be essential for successful treatment with digitalis, diuretics, sodium restriction, and bed rest.

Evaluation of Hepatic and Renal Function: Significant hepatic or renal impairment can enhance the toxicity of the recommended doses of Cerubidine; therefore, prior to administration, evaluation of hepatic function and renal function using conventional clinical laboratory tests is recommended (See "DOSAGE AND ADMINISTRATION" Section).

Pregnancy: Cerubidine may cause fetal harm when administered to a pregnant woman because of its teratogenic potential. An increased incidence of fetal abnormalities (parieto-occipital cranioschisis, umbilical hernias, or rachischisis) and abortions was reported in rabbits. Decreases in fetal birth weight and post-delivery growth rate were observed in mice. There are no adequate and well-controlled studies in pregnant women. If this drug is used during pregnancy, or if the patient becomes pregnant while taking this drug, the patient should be apprised of the potential hazard to the fetus. Women of childbearing potential should be advised to avoid becoming pregnant.

Extravasation at Injection Site: Extravasation of Cerubidine at the site of intravenous administration can cause severe local tissue necrosis.

PRECAUTIONS

Therapy with Cerubidine requires close patient observation and frequent complete blood-count determinations. Cardiac, renal, and hepatic function should be evaluated prior to each course of treatment.

Cerubidine may induce hyperuricemia secondary to rapid lysis of leukemic cells. As a precaution, allopurinol administration is usually begun prior to initiating antileukemic therapy. Blood uric acid levels should be monitored and appropriate therapy initiated in the event that hyperuricemia develops.

Appropriate measures must be taken to control any systemic infection before beginning therapy with Cerubidine.

Cerubidine may transiently impart a red coloration to the urine after administration, and patients should be advised to expect this.

Carcinogenesis, Mutagenesis, Impairment of Fertility: Cerubidine, when injected subcutaneously into mice, causes fibrosarcomas to develop at the injection site. When administered to mice orally or intraperitoneally, no carcinogenic effect was noted after 22 months of observation.

In male dogs at a daily dose of 0.25 mg/kg administered intravenously, testicular atrophy was noted at autopsy. Histologic examination revealed total aplasia of the spermatocyte series in the seminiferous tubules with complete aspermatogenesis.

Pregnancy Category D: See "WARNINGS" Section.

ADVERSE REACTIONS

Dose-limiting toxicity includes myelosuppression and cardiotoxicity (See "WARNINGS" Section). Other reactions include:

Cutaneous: Reversible alopecia occurs in most patients.

Gastrointestinal: Acute nausea and vomiting occur but are usually mild. Antiemetic therapy may be of some help. Mucositis may occur 3 to 7 days after administration. Diarrhea has occasionally been reported.

Local: If extravasation occurs during administration, tissue necrosis can result at the site.

Acute Reactions: Rarely, anaphylactoid reaction, fever, chills, and skin rash can occur.

DOSAGE AND ADMINISTRATION

Parenteral drug products should be inspected visually for particulate matter and discoloration prior to administration, whenever solution and container permit.

Principles: In order to eradicate the leukemic cells and induce a complete remission, a profound suppression of the bone marrow is usually required. Evaluation of both the peripheral blood and bone marrow is mandatory in the formulation of appropriate treatment plans.

It is recommended that the dosage of Cerubidine be reduced in instances of hepatic or renal impairment. For example, using serum bilirubin and serum creatinine as indicators of liver and kidney function, the following dose modifications are recommended:

Serum Bilirubin	Serum Creatinine	Recommended Dose
1.2 to 3.0 mg%		³/₄ normal dose
> 3 mg%	> 3 mg%	¹/₂ normal dose

Representative Dose Schedules and Combination for the Approved Indication of Remission Induction in Adult Acute Nonlymphocytic Leukemia:

In Combination[8,9]: For patients under age 60, Cerubidine 45 mg/m²/day IV on days 1, 2, and 3 of the first course and on days 1, 2 of subsequent courses AND cytosine arabinoside 100 mg/m²/day IV infusion daily for 7 days for the first course and for 5 days for subsequent courses.

For patients 60 years of age and above, Cerubidine 30 mg/m²/day IV on days 1, 2, and 3 of the first course and on days 1, 2 of subsequent courses AND cytosine arabinoside 100 mg/m²/day IV infusion daily for 7 days for the first course and for 5 days for subsequent courses.[9] This Cerubidine dose-reduction is based on a single study and may not be appropriate if optimal supportive care is available.

The attainment of a normal-appearing bone marrow may require up to three courses of induction therapy. Evaluation of the bone marrow following recovery from the previous course of induction therapy determines whether a further course of induction treatment is required.

Representative Dose Schedule and Combination for the Approved Indication of Remission Induction in Pediatric Acute Lymphocytic Leukemia:

In Combination: Cerubidine 25 mg/m² IV on day 1 every week, vincristine 1.5 mg/m² IV on day 1 every week, prednisone 40 mg/m² PO daily. Generally, a complete remission will be obtained within four such courses of therapy; however, if after four courses the patient is in partial remission, an additional one or, if necessary, two courses may be given in an effort to obtain a complete remission.

In children less than 2 years of age or below 0.5 m² body surface area, it has been recommended that the Cerubidine dosage calculation should be based on weight (1 mg/kg) instead of body surface area.[17]

Representative Dose Schedules and Combination for the Approved Indication of Remission Induction in Adult Acute Lymphocytic Leukemia:

In Combination[10]: Cerubidine 45 mg/m²/day IV on days 1, 2, and 3 AND vincristine 2 mg IV on days 1, 8, and 15; prednisone 40 mg/m²/day PO on days 1 through 22, then tapered between days 22 to 29; L-asparaginase 500 IU/kg/day × 10 days IV on days 22 through 32.

The contents of a vial should be reconstituted with 4 mL of Sterile Water for Injection and agitated gently until the material has completely dissolved. The withdrawable vial contents provide 20 mg of daunorubicin activity, with 5 mg of daunorubicin activity per mL. The desired dose is withdrawn into a syringe containing 10 mL to 15 mL of normal saline and then injected into the tubing or sidearm in a rapidly flowing IV infusion of dextrose injection 5% or sodium chloride injection 0.9%. Cerubidine should not be administered mixed with other drugs or heparin. The reconstituted solution is stable for 24 hours at room temperature and 48 hours under refrigeration. It should be protected from exposure to sunlight.

Procedures for proper handling and disposal of anticancer drugs should be considered. Several guidelines on this subject have been published.[11-16] There is no general agreement that all of the procedures recommended in the guidelines are necessary or appropriate.

HOW SUPPLIED

Cerubidine® (daunorubicin hydrochloride) for Injection is available in butyl-rubber-stoppered vials, each containing 20 mg of base activity (21.4 mg as the hydrochloride salt) and 100 mg of mannitol, as a sterile reddish lyophilized powder. When reconstituted with 4 mL of Sterile Water for Injection, USP, each mL contains 5 mg of daunorubicin activity. Each package contains 10 vials.

NDC 55390-281-10   20 mg, single-use vials; carton of 10. Store unreconstituted powder at controlled room temperature, 15°to 30°C (59°to 86°F).

REFERENCES

1. Gilladoga AC, Manuel C, Tan CTC, et al: The cardiotoxicity of Adriamycin and daunomycin in children. *Cancer* 37:1070-1078, 1976.
2. Bleyer WA: Delayed toxicities of chemotherapy on childhood tissues. *Front Radiat Ther Onc* 16:40-54, 1982.
3. Isner JM, Ferrans VJ, Cohen SR, et al: Clinical and morphological cardiac findings after anthracycline chemotherapy. *Am J Cardiol* 51:1167-1174, 1983.
4. Rhoden WE, Jenny M, Beton DC, et al: Long term effects on left ventricular function of treatment for childhood malignancy. *Br Heart J* 66:59, 1991.
5. Steinherz LJ, Steinherz PG, Tan CTC, et al: Cardiac toxicity 4 to 20 years after completing anthracycline therapy. *JAMA* 266:1672-1677, 1991.
6. Lipshultz SE, Colan SD, Gelber RD, et al: Late cardiac effects of doxorubicin therapy for acute lymphoblastic leukemia in childhood. *N Engl J Med* 324:808-815, 1991.
7. Steinherz L, Steinherz P: Delayed cardiac toxicity from anthracycline therapy. *Pediatrician* 18:49-52, 1991.
8. Rai KR, Holland JF, Glidewell O, et al: Treatment of acute myelocytic leukemia: a study by Cancer and Leukemia Group B. *Blood* 58:1203-1212, 1981.
9. Yates J, Glidewell O, Wiernik P, et al: Cytosine arabinoside with daunorubicin or adriamycin for therapy of acute myelocytic leukemia: a CALGB study. *Blood* 60:454-462, 1982.
10. Gottlieb AJ, Weinberg V, Ellison RR, et al: Efficacy of daunorubicin in the therapy of adult acute lymphocytic leukemia: a prospective randomized trial by Cancer and Leukemia Group B. *Blood* 64:267-274, 1984.
11. Recommendations for the Safe Handling of Parenteral Antineoplastic Drugs. NIH Publication No. 83-2621. For Sale by the Superintendent of Documents, U.S. Government Printing Office, Washington, D.C. 20402.
12. AMA Council Report. Guidelines for Handling Parenteral Antineoplastics. *JAMA*, March 15, 1985.
13. National Study Commission on Cytotoxic Exposure—Recommendations for Handling Cytotoxic Agents. Available from Louis P. Jeffrey, Sc.D., Chairman, National Study Commission on Cytotoxic Exposure, Massachusetts College of Pharmacy and Allied Health Sciences, 179 Longwood Avenue, Boston, Massachusetts 02115.
14. Clinical Oncological Society of Australia: Guidelines and recommendations for safe handling of antineoplastic agents. *Med J Australia* 1:426-428, 1983.
15. Jones RB, et al: Safe handling of chemotherapeutic agents: A report from the Mount Sinai Medical Center, *Ca—A Cancer Journal for Clinicians* Sept/Oct, 258-263, 1983.
16. American Society of Hospital Pharmacists technical assistance bulletin on handling cytotoxic and hazardous drugs. *Am J Hosp Pharm* 47:1033-1049, 1990.
17. Sallan SE: Personal Communication, 1981.

MANUFACTURED BY:
Ben Venue Laboratories, Inc.
Bedford, OH 44146
MANUFACTURED FOR:
Bedford Laboratories™
Bedford, Ohio 44146
May, 1996   CRD-P00
A.H.F.S. CATEGORY 10:00

Beiersdorf Inc.
P.O. BOX 5529
NORWALK, CT 06856-5529

Direct Inquiries to:
Medical Division
(203) 853-8008

AQUAPHOR®—Original Formula   OTC
Ointment
NDC Numbers— 10356-020-01
                    10356-020-02

COMPOSITION
Petrolatum, mineral oil, mineral wax and lanolin alcohol.

ACTIONS AND USES
Aquaphor is a stable, neutral, odorless, anhydrous ointment base. It is miscible with water or aqueous solutions, forming smooth, creamy water-in-oil emulsions. In its pure form, Aquaphor is recommended for use as a topical preparation to help heal severely dry skin. Aquaphor contains no preservatives, fragrances or known irritants.

ADMINISTRATION AND DOSAGES
Use Aquaphor alone or in compounding virtually any ointment using aqueous solutions or in combination with other oil-based substances and all common topical medications. Apply Aquaphor liberally to affected area.

PRECAUTIONS
For external use only. Avoid contact with eyes. Not to be applied over third degree burns, deep or puncture wounds, infections or lacerations. If condition worsens or does not improve within 7 days, patient should consult a doctor.

HOW SUPPLIED
16 oz. jar—List No. 45585
5 lb. jar—List. No. 45586

AQUAPHOR Healing Ointment   OTC
NDC Number—10356-021-01

COMPOSITION
Petrolatum, Mineral Oil, Mineral Wax, Lanolin Alcohol, Panthenol, Bisabolol, Glycerin.

ACTIONS AND USES
Aquaphor Healing Ointment is specially formulated for healing of severely dry skin, cracked skin and minor burns. It is recommended for patients suffering from severe skin chapping and from skin disorders that result in severely dry skin. It is preservative-free, fragrance-free and hypoallergenic.[1].

ADMINISTRATION AND DOSAGE
Use Aquaphor Healing Ointment whenever a mild healing agent is needed. Apply liberally to affected dry skin areas two to three times a day. In the case of minor wounds, clean area prior to application.

PRECAUTIONS
For external use only. Avoid contact with the eyes. Not to be applied over third degree burns, deep or puncture wounds, infections or lacerations. If condition worsens or does not improve within seven days, patient should consult a physician.

HOW SUPPLIED
1.75 oz. tube—List No. 45231
1. Data on file, BDF Inc

EUCERIN®   OTC
[ū'sir-in]
Dry Skin Therapy Cleansing Bar

INDICATIONS
Use with warm water to cleanse skin.

CONTAINS
Disodium Lauryl Sulfosuccinate, Sodium Cocoyl Isethionate, Cetearyl Alcohol, Corn Starch, Glyceryl Stearate, Paraffin, Water, Titanium Dioxide, Octyldodecanol, Cyclopentadecanolide, Lanolin Alcohol, Bisabolol.

ACTIONS AND USES
Eucerin® Cleansing Bar has been specially formulated for use on sensitive skin. The formulation contains Eucerite®, a special blend of ingredients that closely resemble the natural oils of the skin, thus providing excellent moisturizing properties. This formulation is fragrance-free and non-comedo-

genic. Additionally, the pH value of Eucerin Cleansing Bar is neutral so as not to affect the skin's normal acid mantle.

DIRECTIONS
Use during shower, bath, or regular cleansing.

HOW SUPPLIED
3 oz. bar—List No. 03852

EUCERIN® Creme   OTC
[ū'sir-in]
Original Moisturizing Creme
NDC Numbers—10356-090-01
                    10356-090-05
                    10356-090-04
                    10356-090-07

INDICATIONS
Use daily to help relieve dry and very dry skin conditions.

COMPOSITION
Water, Petrolatum, Mineral Oil, Ceresin, Lanolin Alcohol, Methylchloroisothiazolinone, Methylisothiazolinone.

ACTIONS AND USES
A gentle, non-comedogenic, fragrance-free water-in-oil emulsion. Eucerin can be used for treating dry skin conditions associated with eczema, psoriasis, chapped or chafed skin, sunburn, windburn and itching associated with dryness.[1].

ADMINISTRATION AND DOSAGES
Apply freely to affected areas of the skin as often as necessary or as directed by a physician.

PRECAUTIONS
For external use only. Avoid contact with the eyes. Discontinue use if signs of irritation occur.

HOW SUPPLIED
16 oz. jar—List Number 00090
8 oz. jar—List Number 03774
4 oz. jar—List Number 03797
2 oz. tube—List Number 03868
1. Data on File.

EUCERIN®   OTC
FACIAL MOISTURIZING LOTION SPF 25
NDC Number—10356-972-01

INDICATIONS
Use daily to help relieve dry skin and provide broad spectrum sun protection.

COMPOSITION
Active Ingredients: Octyl Methoxycinnamate, Octyl Salicylate, Titanium Dioxide.
Other Ingredients: Water, Octyldodecyl Neopentanoate, Dioctyl Malate, Glycerin, Petrolatum, Zinc Oxide, Cetearyl Alcohol, DEA-Cetyl Phosphate, PEG-40 Castor Oil, Glyceryl Stearate, Sodium Hyaluronate, Lactic Acid, Lanolin Alcohol, Sodium Cetearyl Sulfate, Xanthan Gum, Methicone, Dimethicone, EDTA, Sodium Hydroxide, Methylchloroisothiazolinone, Methylisothiazolinone.

ACTIONS AND USES
Eucerin Facial Moisturizing Lotion SPF 25 is fragrance-free and non-comedogenic, with a unique sun screen (titanium dioxide) to protect skin from UVA and UVB light. It is specially formulated for dry, sensitive skin or for those undergoing therapies which irritate delicate facial skin. This light, oil-in-water formula is non-greasy and is easily absorbed into the skin.

ADMINISTRATION AND DOSAGE
Apply Eucerin Facial Moisturizing Lotion SPF 25 twice a day (especially in the morning) or as directed by a physician, to nourish and moisturize skin and protect it from harmful UVA and UVB rays.

PRECAUTIONS
For external use only. Avoid contact with eyes. Keep out of the reach of children. Discontinue use if signs of irritation occur.

HOW SUPPLIED
4 oz. bottle.—List No. 03972

EUCERIN® Lotion   OTC
[ū'sir-in]
Original Moisturizing Lotion
NDC Numbers—10356-793-01
                    10356-793-04

INDICATIONS
Use daily to help relieve dry skin.

COMPOSITION
Water, Mineral Oil, Isopropyl Myristate, PEG-40 Sorbitan Peroleate, Glyceryl Lanoleate, Sorbitol, Propylene Glycol, Cetyl Palmitate, Magnesium Sulfate, Aluminum Stearate, Lanolin Alcohol, BHT, Methylchloroisothiazolinone, Methylisothiazolinone.

ACTIONS AND USES
Eucerin Lotion is a non-comedogenic, fragrance-free, unique water-in-oil formulation that will help to alleviate and soothe dry skin, and provide long-lasting moisturization.

ADMINISTRATION AND DOSAGE
Use daily on dry skin or as directed by a physician.

PRECAUTIONS
For external use only. Avoid contact with the eyes. Discontinue use if signs of irritation occur.

HOW SUPPLIED
8 oz. bottle—List Number 3793
16 oz. bottle—List Number 3794

EUCERIN PLUS CREME   OTC
Moisturizing Alphahydroxy Creme
NDC 10356-036-01

INDICATIONS
Use daily to help relieve severely dry, flaky skin.

COMPOSITION
Water, Mineral Oil, Urea, Magnesium Stearate, Ceresin, Polyglyceryl-3 Diisostearate, Sodium Lactate, Isopropyl Palmitate, Benzyl Alcohol, Panthenol, Bisabolol, Lanolin Alcohol, Magnesium Sulfate.

CAUTION
For external use only. Avoid contact with eyes and areas where skin is inflamed or cracked. Discontinue use if signs of irritation occur. Keep out of reach of children.

ACTION AND USES
Eucerin Plus Creme is a unique alpha-hydroxy acid moisturizing creme (2.5% sodium lactate, 10% urea) that is clinically proven to help relieve severely dry, flaky skin conditions[1]. Unlike other alpha-hydroxy acid mositurizers, Eucerin Plus Creme has low irritation potential, is fragrance-free and non-comedogenic.

ADMINISTRATION AND DOSAGE
Use daily on severely dry, scaly skin or as directed by a physician.

PRECAUTIONS
Avoid contact with eyes or areas where skin is inflamed or cracked. Discontinue use if signs of irritation occur. For external use only. Keep out of reach of children.

HOW SUPPLIED
4 oz. jar—List No. 03611
1. Data on file.

EUCERIN PLUS LOTION   OTC
Alphahydroxy Moisturizing Lotion
NDC 10356-967-03
         10356-967-03

INDICATIONS
Use daily to help relieve severely dry, flaky skin.

COMPOSITION
Water, Mineral Oil, PEG-7 Hydrogenated Castor Oil, Isohexadecane, Sodium Lactate 5%, Urea 5%, Glycerin, Isopropyl Palmitate, Panthenol, Ozokerite, Magnesium Sulfate, Lanolin Alcohol, Bisabolol, Methylchloroisothiazolinone, Methylisothiazolinone.

ACTION AND USES
Eucerin Plus Lotion in a unique, patented alpha-hydroxy acid moisturizing lotion (5% Sodium Lactate, 5% Urea) that is clinically proven to help severely dry, flaky skin conditions[1]. Unlike other alpha-hydroxy acid moisturizing lotions, Eucerin Plus has low irritation potential, is fragrance free and non-comedogenic.

ADMINISTRATION AND DOSAGE
Use daily on severely dry, flaky skin or as directed by a physician.

PRECAUTIONS
Avoid contact with eyes or areas where skin is inflamed or cracked. Discontinue use if signs of irritation occur. For external use only. Keep out of reach of children.

HOW SUPPLIED
6 oz. bottle—List No. 03967
12 oz. bottle—List No.–03321
1. Data on File.

Berlex Laboratories
300 FAIRFIELD ROAD
WAYNE, NJ 07470

Direct Inquiries to:
(201) 694-4100

For Medical Information and to report drug adverse events Contact:
Department of Epidemiology and Medical Affairs
300 Fairfield Road
Wayne, NJ 07470
(800) 888-2407

Betaseron for SC Injection Only: (Medical Information Only)
15049 San Pablo Avenue
Richmond, CA 94809-0099
(800) 888-4112

Fludara for Injection Only: (Medical Information Only)
15049 San Pablo Avenue
Richmond, CA 94809-0099
(800) 888-4112

BETAPACE® ℞
[*bā′-tăh-pāce″*]
(sotalol HCl)

DESCRIPTION
BETAPACE® (sotalol hydrochloride), is an antiarrhythmic drug with Class II (beta-adrenoreceptor blocking) and Class III (cardiac action potential duration prolongation) properties. It is supplied as a light-blue, capsule-shaped tablet for oral administration. Sotalol hydrochloride is a white, crystalline solid with a molecular weight of 308.8. It is hydrophilic, soluble in water, propylene glycol and ethanol, but is only slightly soluble in chloroform. Chemically, sotalol hydrochloride is d,l-N-[4-[l-hydroxy-2-[(l-methylethyl)amino] ethyl]phenyl]methane-sulfonamide monohydrochloride. The molecular formula is $C_{12}H_{20}N_2O_3S \cdot HCl$ and is represented by the following structural formula:

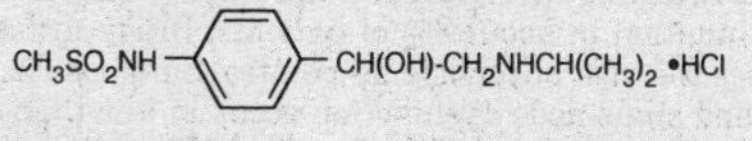
CH3SO2NH
CH(OH)-CH2NHCH(CH3)2 •HCl

BETAPACE® Tablets contain the following inactive ingredients: microcrystalline cellulose, lactose, starch, stearic acid, magnesium stearate, colloidal silicon dioxide, and FD&C blue color #2 (aluminum lake, conc.).

CLINICAL PHARMACOLOGY
Mechanism of Action: BETAPACE® (sotalol hydrochloride) has both beta-adrenoreceptor blocking (Vaughan Williams Class II) and cardiac action potential duration prolongation (Vaughan Williams Class III) antiarrhythmic properties. BETAPACE® (sotalol hydrochloride) is a racemic mixture of d- and l-sotalol. Both isomers have similar Class III antiarrhythmic effects, while the l-isomer is responsible for virtually all of the beta-blocking activity. The beta-blocking effect of sotalol is non-cardioselective, half maximal at about 80 mg/day and maximal at doses between 320 and 640 mg/day. Sotalol does not have partial agonist or membrane stabilizing activity. Although significant beta-blockade occurs at oral doses as low as 25 mg, Class III effects are seen only at daily doses of 160 mg and above.
Electrophysiology: Sotalol hydrochloride prolongs the plateau phase of the cardiac action potential in the isolated myocyte, as well as in isolated tissue preparations of ventricular or atrial muscle (Class III activity). In intact animals it slows heart rate, decreases AV nodal conduction and increases the refractory periods of atrial and ventricular muscle and conduction tissue.
In man, the Class II (beta-blockade) electrophysiological effects of BETAPACE® are manifested by increased sinus cycle length (slowed heart rate), decreased AV nodal conduction and increased AV nodal refractoriness. The Class III electrophysiological effects in man include prolongation of the atrial and ventricular monophasic action potentials, and effective refractory period prolongation of atrial muscle, ventricular muscle, and atrio-ventricular accessory pathways (where present) in both the anterograde and retrograde directions. With oral doses of 160 to 640 mg/day, the surface ECG shows dose–related mean increases of 40–100 msec in QT and 10–40 msec in QT_c. (See **WARNINGS** for description of relationship between QT_c and torsade de pointes type arrhythmias). No significant alteration in QRS interval is observed.
In a small study (n=25) of patients with implanted defibrillators treated concurrently with BETAPACE®, the average defibrillatory threshold was 6 joules (range 2–15 joules) compared to a mean of 16 joules for a non-randomized comparative group primarily receiving amiodarone.
Hemodynamics: In a study of systemic hemodynamic function measured invasively in 12 patients with a mean LV ejection fraction of 37% and ventricular tachycardia (9 sustained and 3 non-sustained), a median dose of 160 mg twice daily of BETAPACE® produced a 28% reduction in heart rate and a 24% decrease in cardiac index at 2 hours post dosing at steady-state. Concurrently, systemic vascular resistance and stroke volume showed non-significant increases of 25% and 8%, respectively. Pulmonary capillary wedge pressure increased significantly from 6.4 mmHg to 11.8 mmHg in the 11 patients who completed the study. One patient was discontinued because of worsening congestive heart failure. Mean arterial pressure, mean pulmonary artery pressure and stroke work index did not significantly change. Exercise and isoproterenol induced tachycardia are antagonized by BETAPACE®, and total peripheral resistance increases by a small amount.
In hypertensive patients, BETAPACE® (sotalol hydrochloride) produces significant reductions in both systolic and diastolic blood pressures. Although BETAPACE® (sotalol hydrochloride) is usually well-tolerated hemodynamically, caution should be exercised in patients with marginal cardiac compensation as deterioration in cardiac performance may occur. (See **WARNINGS: Congestive Heart Failure.**)
Clinical Actions: BETAPACE® (sotalol hydrochloride) has been studied in life-threatening and less severe arrhythmias. In patients with frequent premature ventricular complexes (VPC), BETAPACE® (sotalol hydrochloride) was significantly superior to placebo in reducing VPC's, paired VPCs and non-sustained ventricular tachycardia (NSVT); the response was dose-related through 640 mg/day with 80–85% of patients having at least a 75% reduction of VPCs. BETAPACE® (sotalol hydrochloride) was also superior, at the doses evaluated, to propranolol (40–80 mg TID) and similar to quinidine (200–400 mg QID) in reducing VPCs. In patients with life-threatening arrhythmias [sustained ventricular tachycardia/fibrillation (VT/VF)], BETAPACE® (sotalol hydrochloride) was studied acutely [by suppression of programmed electrical stimulation (PES) induced VT and by suppression of Holter monitor evidence of sustained VT] and, in acute responders, chronically.
In a double-blind, randomized comparison of BETAPACE® and procainamide given intravenously (total of 2 mg/kg BETAPACE® vs. 19 mg/kg of procainamide over 90 minutes), BETAPACE® suppressed PES induction in 30% of patients vs. 20% for procainamide (p=0.2).
In a randomized clinical trial [Electrophysiologic Study Versus Electrocardiographic Monitoring (ESVEM) Trial] comparing choice of antiarrhythmic therapy by PES suppression vs. Holter monitor selection (in each case followed by treadmill exercise testing) in patients with a history of sustained VT/VF who were also inducible by PES, the effectiveness acutely and chronically of BETAPACE® (sotalol hydrochloride) was compared with 6 other drugs (procainamide, quinidine, mexiletine, propafenone, imipramine and pirmenol). Overall response, limited to first randomized drug, was 39% for sotalol and 30% for the pooled other drugs. Acute response rate for first drug randomized using suppression of PES induction was 36% for BETAPACE® vs. a mean of 13% for the other drugs. Using the Holter monitoring endpoint (complete suppression of sustained VT, 90% suppression of NSVT, 80% suppression of VPC pairs, and at least 70% suppression of VPCs), BETAPACE® yielded 41% response vs. 45% for the other drugs combined. Among responders placed on long-term therapy identified acutely as effective (by either PES or Holter), BETAPACE®, when compared to the pool of other drugs, had the lowest two-year mortality (13% vs. 22%), the lowest two-year VT recurrence rate (30% vs. 60%), and the lowest withdrawal rate (38% vs. about 75–80%). The most commonly used doses of BETAPACE® (sotalol hydrochloride) in this trial were 320–480 mg/day (66% of patients), with 16% receiving 240 mg/day or less and 18% receiving 640 mg or more.
It cannot be determined, however, in the absence of a controlled comparison of BETAPACE® vs. no pharmacologic treatment (e.g., in patients with implanted defibrillators) whether BETAPACE® response causes improved survival or identifies a population with a good prognosis.
In a large double-blind, placebo controlled secondary prevention (post-infarction) trial (n=1,456), BETAPACE® (sotalol hydrochloride) was given as a non-titrated initial dose of 320 mg once daily. BETAPACE® did not produce a significant increase in survival (7.3% mortality on BETAPACE® vs 8.9% on placebo, p=0.3), but overall did not suggest an adverse effect on survival. There was, however, a suggestion of an early (i.e., first 10 days) excess mortality (3% on sotalol vs. 2% on placebo). In a second small trial (n=17 randomized to sotalol) where sotalol was administered at high doses (e.g., 320 mg twice daily) to high-risk post-infarction patients (ejection fraction <40% and either >10 VPC/hr or VT on Holter), there were 4 fatalities and 3 serious hemodynamic/electrical adverse events within two weeks of initiating sotalol.
Pharmacokinetics: In healthy subjects, the oral bioavailability of BETAPACE® (sotalol hydrochloride) is 90–100%. After oral administration, peak plasma concentrations are reached in 2.5 to 4 hours, and steady-state plasma concentrations are attained within 2–3 days (i.e., after 5–6 doses when administered twice daily). Over the dosage range 160–640 mg/day BETAPACE® (sotalol hydrochloride) displays dose proportionality with respect to plasma concentrations. Distribution occurs to a central (plasma) and to a peripheral compartment, with a mean elimination half-life of 12 hours. Dosing every 12 hours results in trough plasma concentrations which are approximately one-half of those at peak.
BETAPACE® (sotalol hydrochloride) does not bind to plasma proteins and is not metabolized. BETAPACE® (sotalol hydrochloride) shows very little intersubject variability in plasma levels. The pharmacokinetics of the d and l enantiomers of sotalol are essentially identical. BETAPACE® (sotalol hydrochloride) crosses the blood brain barrier poorly. Excretion is predominantly via the kidney in the unchanged form, and therefore lower doses are necessary in conditions of renal impairment (see **DOSAGE AND ADMINISTRATION**). Age per se does not significantly alter the pharmacokinetics of BETAPACE®, but impaired renal function in geriatric patients can increase the terminal elimination half-life, resulting in increased drug accumulation. The absorption of BETAPACE® (sotalol hydrochloride) was reduced by approximately 20% compared to fasting when it was administered with a standard meal. Since BETAPACE® (sotalol hydrochloride) is not subject to first-pass metabolism, patients with hepatic impairment show no alteration in clearance of BETAPACE®.

INDICATIONS AND USAGE
Oral BETAPACE® (sotalol hydrochloride) is indicated for the treatment of documented ventricular arrhythmias, such as sustained ventricular tachycardia, that in the judgment of the physician are life-threatening. Because of the proarrhythmic effects of BETAPACE® (See **WARNINGS**), including a 1.5 to 2% rate of torsade de pointes or new VT/VF in patients with either NSVT or supraventricular arrhythmias, its use in patients with less severe arrhythmias, even if the patients are symptomatic, is generally not recommended. Treatment of patients with asymptomatic ventricular premature contractions should be avoided.
Initiation of BETAPACE® treatment or increasing doses, as with other antiarrhythmic agents used to treat life-threatening arrhythmias, should be carried out in the hospital. The response to treatment should then be evaluated by a suitable method (e.g., PES or Holter monitoring) prior to continuing the patient on chronic therapy. Various approaches have been used to determine the response to antiarrhythmic therapy, including BETAPACE®.
In the ESVEM Trial, response by Holter monitoring was tentatively defined as 100% suppression of ventricular tachycardia, 90% suppression of non-sustained VT, 80% suppression of paired VPCs, and 75% suppression of total VPCs in patients who had at least 10 VPCs/hour at baseline; this tentative response was confirmed if VT lasting 5 or more beats was not observed during treadmill exercise testing using a standard Bruce protocol. The PES protocol utilized a maximum of three extrastimuli at three pacing cycle lengths and two right ventricular pacing sites. Response by PES was defined as prevention of induction of the following: 1) monomorphic VT lasting over 15 seconds; 2) non-sustained polymorphic VT containing more than 15 beats of monomorphic VT in patients with a history of monomorphic VT; 3) polymorphic VT or VF greater than 15 beats in patients with VF or a history of aborted sudden death without monomorphic VT; and 4) two episodes of polymorphic VT or VF of greater than 15 beats in a patient presenting with monomorphic VT. Sustained VT or NSVT producing hypotension during the final treadmill test was considered a drug failure.
In a multicenter open-label long-term study of BETAPACE® in patients with life-threatening ventricular arrhythmias which had proven refractory to other antiarrhythmic medications, response by Holter monitoring was

Continued on next page

Information on the Berlex products appearing here is based on the most current information available at the time of publication closing. Further information for these and other products may be obtained from the Medical Affairs Department, Berlex Laboratories, 300 Fairfield Road, Wayne, New Jersey 07470, 1-800-888-2407. Information on Betaseron and Fludara may be obtained from Berlex Laboratories, 15049 San Pablo Avenue, Richmond, California 94804-0016, 1-800-888-4112.

Consult 1997 supplements and future editions for revisions

Berlex Laboratories—Cont.

defined as in ESVEM. Response by PES was defined as noninducibility of sustained VT by at least double extrastimuli delivered at a pacing cycle length of 400 msec. Overall survival and arrythmia recurrence rates in this study were similar to those seen in ESVEM, although there was no comparative group to allow a definitive assessment of outcome.

Antiarrhythmic drugs have not been shown to enhance survival in patients with ventricular arrhythmias.

CONTRAINDICATIONS

BETAPACE® (sotalol hydrochloride) is contraindicated in patients with bronchial asthma, sinus bradycardia, second and third degree AV block, unless a functioning pacemaker is present, congenital or acquired long QT syndromes, cardiogenic shock, uncontrolled congestive heart failure, and previous evidence of hypersensitivity to BETAPACE®.

WARNINGS

Mortality: The National Heart, Lung, and Blood Institute's Cardiac Arrhythmia Suppression Trial I (CAST I) was a long-term, multi-center, double-blind study in patients with asymptomatic, non-life-threatening ventricular arrhythmias, 1 to 103 weeks after acute myocardial infarction. Patients in CAST I were randomized to receive placebo or individually optimized doses of encainide, flecainide, or moricizine. The Cardiac Arrhythmia Suppression Trial II (CAST II) was similar, except that the recruited patients had had their index infarction 4 to 90 days before randomization, patients with left ventricular ejection fractions greater than 40% were not admitted, and the randomized regimens were limited to placebo and moricizine.

CAST I was discontinued after an average time-on-treatment of 10 months, and CAST II was discontinued after an average time-on-treatment of 18 months. As compared to placebo treatment, all three active therapies were associated with increases in short-term (14-day) mortality, and encainide and flecainide were associated with significant increases in longer-term mortality as well. The longer-term mortality rate associated with moricizine treatment could not be statistically distinguished from that associated with placebo.

The applicability of these results to other populations (e.g., those without recent myocardial infarction) and to other than Class I antiarrhythmic agents is uncertain. BETAPACE® (sotalol hydrochloride) is devoid of Class I effects, and in a large (n=1,456) controlled trial in patients with a recent myocardial infarction, who did not necessarily have ventricular arrhythmias, BETAPACE® did not produce increased mortality at doses up to 320 mg/day (see **Clinical Actions**). On the other hand, in the large post-infarction study using a non-titrated initial dose of 320 mg once daily and in a second small randomized trial in high-risk post-infarction patients treated with high doses (320 mg BID), there have been suggestions of an excess of early sudden deaths.

Proarrhythmia: Like other antiarrhythmic agents, BETAPACE® can provoke new or worsened ventricular arrhythmias in some patients, including sustained ventricular tachycardia or ventricular fibrillation, with potentially fatal consequences. Because of its effect on cardiac repolarization (QT_c interval prolongation), torsade de pointes, a polymorphic ventricular tachycardia with prolongation of the QT interval and a shifting electrical axis is the most common form of proarrhythmia associated with BETAPACE®, occurring in about 4% of high risk (history of sustained VT/VF) patients. The risk of torsade de pointes progressively increases with prolongation of the QT interval, and is worsened also by reduction in heart rate and reduction in serum potassium (See **Electrolyte Disturbances**.)

Because of the variable temporal recurrence of arrhythmias, it is not always possible to distinguish between a new or aggravated arrhythmic event and the patient's underlying rhythm disorder. (Note, however, that torsade de pointes is usually a drug-induced arrhythmia in people with an initially normal QT_c.) Thus, the incidence of drug-related events cannot be precisely determined, so that the occurrence rates provided must be considered approximations. Note also that drug-induced arrhythmias may often not be identified, particularly if they occur long after starting the drug, due to less frequent monitoring. It is clear from the NIH-sponsored CAST (see **WARNINGS: Mortality**) that some antiarrhythmic drugs can cause increased sudden death mortality, presumably due to new arrhythmias or asystole, that do not appear early in treatment but that represent a sustained increased risk.

Overall in clinical trials with sotalol, 4.3% of 3257 patients experienced a new or worsened ventricular arrhythmia. Of this 4.3%, there was new or worsened sustained ventricular tachycardia in approximately 1% of patients and torsade de pointes in 2.4%. Additionally, in approximately 1% of patients, deaths were considered possibly drug-related; such cases, although difficult to evaluate, may have been associated with proarrhythmic events. **In patients with a history of sustained ventricular tachycardia, the incidence of torsade de pointes was 4% and worsened VT in about 1%; in patients with other, less serious, ventricular arrhythmias and supraventricular arrhythmias, the incidence of torsade de pointes was 1% and 1.4%, respectively.**

Torsade de pointes arrhythmias were dose related, as is the prolongation of QT (QT_c) interval, as shown in the table below.

Percent incidence of Torsade de Pointes and Mean QT_c Interval by Dose For Patients With Sustained VT/VF

Daily Dose (mg)	Incidence of Torsade de pointes	Mean QT_c* (msec)
80	0 (69)	463 (17)
160	0.5 (832)	467 (181)
320	1.6 (835)	473 (344)
480	4.4 (459)	483 (234)
640	3.7 (324)	490 (185)
>640	5.8 (103)	512 (62)

( ) Number of patients assessed
*Highest on-therapy value

In addition to dose and presence of sustained VT, other risk factors for torsade de pointes were gender (females had a higher incidence), excessive prolongation of the QT_c interval (see table below) and history of cardiomegaly or congestive heart failure. Patients with sustained ventricular tachycardia and a history of congestive heart failure appear to have the highest risk for serious proarrhythmia (7%). Of the patients experiencing torsade de pointes, approximately two-thirds spontaneously reverted to their baseline rhythm. The others were either converted electrically (D/C cardioversion or overdrive pacing) or treated with other drugs (see **OVERDOSAGE**). It is not possible to determine whether some sudden deaths represented episodes of torsade de pointes, but in some instances sudden death did follow a documented episode of torsade de pointes. Although BETAPACE® therapy was discontinued in most patients experiencing torsade de pointes, 17% were continued on a lower dose. Nonetheless, BETAPACE® should be used with particular caution if the QT_c is greater than 500 msec on-therapy and serious consideration should be given to reducing the dose or discontinuing therapy when the QT_c exceeds 550 msec. Due to the multiple risk-factors associated with torsade de pointes, however, caution should be exercised regardless of the QT_c interval. The table below relates the incidence of torsade de pointes to on-therapy QT_c and change in QT_c from baseline. It should be noted, however, that the highest on-therapy QT_c was in many cases the one obtained at the time of the torsade de pointes event, so that the table overstates the predictive value of a high QT_c.

[See table on bottom of page.]

Relationship Between QT_c Interval Prolongation and Torsade de Pointes

On-Therapy QT_c Interval (msec)	Incidence of Torsade de pointes
less than 500	1.3% (1787)
500–525	3.4% (236)
525–550	5.6% (125)
>550	10.8% (157)

Change in QT_c Interval From Baseline (msec)	Incidence of Torsade de pointes
less than 65	1.6% (1516)
65–80	3.2% (158)
80–100	4.1% (146)
100–130	5.2% (115)
>130	7.1% (99)

( ) Number of patients assessed

Proarrhythmic events must be anticipated not only on initiating therapy, but with every upward dose adjustment. Proarrhythmic events most often occur within 7 days of initiating therapy or of an increase in dose; 75% of serious proarrhythmias (torsade de pointes and worsened VT) occurred within 7 days of initiating BETAPACE® therapy, while 60% of such events occurred within 3 days of initiation or a dosage change. Initiating therapy at 80 mg BID with gradual upward dose titration and appropriate evaluations for efficacy (e.g., PES or Holter) and safety (e.g., QT interval, heart rate and electrolytes) prior to dose escalation, should reduce the risk of proarrhythmia. Avoiding excessive accumulation of sotalol in patients with diminished renal function, by appropriate dose reduction, should also reduce the risk of proarrhythmia (see **DOSAGE AND ADMINISTRATION**).

Congestive Heart Failure: Sympathetic stimulation is necessary in supporting circulatory function in congestive heart failure, and beta-blockade carries the potential hazard of further depressing myocardial contractility and precipitating more severe failure. In patients who have congestive heart failure controlled by digitalis and/or diuretics, BETAPACE® should be administered cautiously. Both digitalis and sotalol slow AV conduction. As with all beta-blockers, caution is advised when initiating therapy in patients with any evidence of left ventricular dysfunction. In premarketing studies, new or worsened congestive heart failure (CHF) occurred in 3.3% (n=3257) of patients and led to discontinuation in approximately 1% of patients receiving BETAPACE®. The incidence was higher in patients presenting with sustained ventricular tachycardia/fibrillation (4.6%, n=1363), or a prior history of heart failure (7.3%, n=696). Based on a life-table analysis, the one-year incidence of new or worsened CHF was 3% in patients without a prior history and 10% in patients with a prior history of CHF. NYHA Classification was also closely associated to the incidence of new or worsened heart failure while receiving BETAPACE® (1.8% in 1395 Class I patients, 4.9% in 1254 Class II patients and 6.1% in 278 Class III or IV patients).

Electrolyte Disturbances: BETAPACE® should not be used in patients with hypokalemia or hypomagnesemia prior to correction of imbalance, as these conditions can exaggerate the degree of QT prolongation, and increase the potential for torsade de pointes. Special attention should be given to electrolyte and acid-base balance in patients experiencing severe or prolonged diarrhea or patients receiving concomitant diuretic drugs.

Conduction Disturbances: Excessive prolongation of the QT interval (>550 msec) can promote serious arrhythmias and should be avoided (see **Proarrhythmias** above). Sinus bradycardia (heart rate less than 50 bpm) occurred in 13% of patients receiving BETAPACE® in clinical trials, and led to discontinuation in about 3% of patients. Bradycardia itself increases the risk of torsade de pointes. Sinus pause, sinus arrest and sinus node dysfunction occur in less than 1% of patients. The incidence of 2nd- or 3rd-degree AV block is approximately 1%.

Recent Acute MI: BETAPACE® can be used safely and effectively in the long-term treatment of life-threatening ventricular arrhythmias following a myocardial infarction. However, experience in the use of BETAPACE® to treat cardiac arrhythmias in the early phase of recovery from acute MI is limited and at least at high initial doses is not reassuring. (See **WARNINGS: Mortality**.) In the first 2 weeks post-MI caution is advised and careful dose titration is especially important, particularly in patients with markedly impaired ventricular function.

The following warnings are related to the beta-blocking activity of BETAPACE®.

Abrupt Withdrawal: Hypersensitivity to catecholamines has been observed in patients withdrawn from beta-blocker therapy. Occasional cases of exacerbation of angina pectoris, arrhythmias and, in some cases, myocardial infarction have been reported after abrupt discontinuation of beta-blocker therapy. Therefore, it is prudent when discontinuing chronically administered BETAPACE®, particularly in patients with ischemic heart disease, to carefully monitor the patient and consider the temporary use of an alternate beta-blocker if appropriate. If possible, the dosage of BETAPACE® should be gradually reduced over a period of one to two weeks. If angina or acute coronary insufficiency develops, appropriate therapy should be instituted promptly. Patients should be warned against interruption or discontinuation of therapy without the physician's advice. Because coronary artery disease is common and may be unrecognized in patients receiving BETAPACE®, abrupt discontinuation in patients with arrhythmias may unmask latent coronary insufficiency.

Non-Allergic Bronchospasm (e.g., chronic bronchitis and emphysema): **PATIENTS WITH BRONCHOSPASTIC DISEASES SHOULD IN GENERAL NOT RECEIVE BETA-BLOCKERS.** It is prudent, if BETAPACE® (sotalol hydrochloride) is

to be administered, to use the smallest effective dose, so that inhibition of bronchodilation produced by endogenous or exogenous catecholamine stimulation of $beta_2$ receptors may be minimized.

Anaphylaxis: While taking beta-blockers, patients with a history of anaphylactic reaction to a variety of allergens may have a more severe reaction on repeated challenge, either accidental, diagnostic or therapeutic. Such patients may be unresponsive to the usual doses of epinephrine used to treat the allergic reaction.

Anesthesia: The management of patients undergoing major surgery who are being treated with beta-blockers is controversial. Protracted severe hypotension and difficulty in restoring and maintaining normal cardiac rhythm after anesthesia have been reported in patients receiving beta-blockers.

Diabetes: In patients with diabetes (especially labile diabetes) or with a history of episodes of spontaneous hypoglycemia, BETAPACE® should be given with caution since beta-blockade may mask some important premonitory signs of acute hypoglycemia; e.g., tachycardia.

Sick Sinus Syndrome: BETAPACE® should be used only with extreme caution in patients with sick sinus syndrome associated with symptomatic arrhythmias, because it may cause sinus bradycardia, sinus pauses or sinus arrest.

Thyrotoxicosis: Beta-blockade may mask certain clinical signs (e.g., tachycardia) of hyperthyroidism. Patients suspected of developing thyrotoxicosis should be managed carefully to avoid abrupt withdrawal of beta-blockade which might be followed by an exacerbation of symptoms of hyperthyroidism, including thyroid storm.

PRECAUTIONS

RENAL IMPAIRMENT: BETAPACE® (sotalol hydrochloride) is mainly eliminated via the kidneys through glomerular filtration and to a small degree by tubular secretion. There is a direct relationship between renal function, as measured by serum creatinine or creatinine clearance, and the elimination rate of BETAPACE®. Guidance for dosing in conditions of renal impairment can be found under "DOSAGE AND ADMINISTRATION."

DRUG INTERACTIONS

Antiarrhythmics: Class Ia antiarrhythmic drugs, such as disopyramide, quinidine and procainamide and other Class III drugs (e.g., amiodarone) are not recommended as concomitant therapy with BETAPACE®, because of their potential to prolong refractoriness (see **WARNINGS**). There is only limited experience with the concomitant use of Class Ib or Ic antiarrhythmics. Additive Class II effects would also be anticipated with the use of other beta-blocking agents concomitantly with BETAPACE®.

Digoxin: Single and multiple doses of BETAPACE® do not substantially affect serum digoxin levels. Proarrhythmic events were more common in BETAPACE® treated patients also receiving digoxin; it is not clear whether this represents an interaction or is related to the presence of CHF, a known risk factor for proarrhythmia, in the patients receiving digoxin.

Calcium blocking drugs: BETAPACE® should be administered with caution in conjunction with calcium blocking drugs because of possible additive effects on atrioventricular conduction or ventricular function. Additionally, concomitant use of these drugs may have additive effects on blood pressure, possibly leading to hypotension.

Catecholamine-depleting agents: Concomitant use of catecholamine-depleting drugs, such as reserpine and guanethidine, with a beta-blocker may produce an excessive reduction of resting sympathetic nervous tone. Patients treated with BETAPACE® plus a catecholamine depletor should therefore be closely monitored for evidence of hypotension and or marked bradycardia which may produce syncope.

Insulin and oral antidiabetics: Hyperglycemia may occur, and the dosage of insulin or antidiabetic drugs may require adjustment. Symptoms of hypoglycemia may be masked.

Beta-2-receptor stimulants: Beta-agonists such as salbutamol, terbutaline and isoprenaline may have to be administered in increased dosages when used concomitantly with BETAPACE®.

Clonidine: Beta-blocking drugs may potentiate the rebound hypertension sometimes observed after discontinuation of clonidine; therefore, caution is advised when discontinuing clonidine in patients receiving BETAPACE®.

Other: No pharmacokinetic interactions were observed with hydrochlorothiazide or warfarin.

Drugs prolonging the QT interval: BETAPACE® should be administered with caution in conjunction with other drugs known to prolong the QT interval such as Class I antiarrhythmic agents, phenothiazines, tricyclic antidepressants, terfenadine and astemizole (see **WARNINGS**).

DRUG/Laboratory Test Interactions

The presence of sotalol in the urine may result in falsely elevated levels of urinary metanephrine when measured by fluorimetric or photometric methods. In screening patients suspected of having a pheochromocytoma and being treated with sotalol, a specific method, such as a high performance liquid chromatographic assay with solid phase extraction (e.g., J. Chromatogr. 385:241, 1987) should be employed in determining levels of catecholamines.

Carcinogenesis, Mutagenicity, Impairment of Fertility: No evidence of carcinogenic potential was observed in rats during a 24-month study at 137–275 mg/kg/day (approximately 30 times the maximum recommended human oral dose (MRHD) as mg/kg or 5 times the MRHD as mg/m^2) or in mice, during a 24-month study at 4141–7122 mg/kg/day (approximately 450–750 times the MRHD as mg/kg or 36–63 times the MRHD as mg/m^2).

Sotalol has not been evaluated in any specific assay of mutagenicity or clastogenicity.

No significant reduction in fertility occurred in rats at oral doses of 1000 mg/kg/day (approximately 100 times the MRHD as mg/kg or 9 times the MRHD as mg/m^2) prior to mating, except for a small reduction in the number of offspring per litter.

Pregnancy Category B: Reproduction studies in rats and rabbits during organogenesis at 100 and 22 times the MRHD as mg/kg (9 and 7 times the MRHD as mg/m^2), respectively, did not reveal any teratogenic potential associated with sotalol HCl. In rabbits, a high dose of sotalol HCl (160 mg/kg/day) at 16 times the MRHD as mg/kg (6 times the MRHD as mg/m^2) produced a slight increase in fetal death likely due to maternal toxicity. Eight times the maximum dose (80 mg/kg/day or 3 times the MRHD as mg/m^2) did not result in an increased incidence of fetal deaths. In rats, 1000 mg/kg/day sotalol HCl, 100 times the MRHD (18 times the MRHD as mg/m^2), increased the number of early resorptions, while at 14 times the maximum dose (2.5 times the MRHD as mg/m^2), no increase in early resorptions was noted. However, animal reproduction studies are not always predictive of human response.

Although there are no adequate and well-controlled studies in pregnant women, sotalol HCl has been shown to cross the placenta, and is found in amniotic fluid. There has been a report of subnormal birth weight with BETAPACE®. Therefore, BETAPACE® should be used during pregnancy only if the potential benefit outweighs the potential risk.

Nursing Mothers: Sotalol is excreted in the milk of laboratory animals and has been reported to be present in human milk. Because of the potential for adverse reactions in nursing infants from BETAPACE®, a decision should be made whether to discontinue nursing or to discontinue the drug, taking into account the importance of the drug to the mother.

Pediatric Use: The safety and effectiveness of BETAPACE® in children have not been established.

ADVERSE REACTIONS

During premarketing trials, 3186 patients with cardiac arrhythmias (1363 with sustained ventricular tachycardia) received oral BETAPACE®, of whom 2451 received the drug for at least two weeks. The most important adverse effects are torsade de pointes and other serious new ventricular arrhythmias (see **WARNINGS**), occurring at rates of almost 4% and 1%, respectively, in the VT/VF population. Overall, discontinuation because of unacceptable side-effects was necessary in 17% of all patients in clinical trials, and in 13% of patients treated for at least two-weeks. The most common adverse reactions leading to discontinuation of BETAPACE® are as follows: fatigue 4%, bradycardia (less than 50 bpm) 3%, dyspnea 3%, proarrhythmia 3%, asthenia 2%, and dizziness 2%.

Occasional reports of elevated serum liver enzymes have occurred with BETAPACE® therapy but no cause and effect relationship has been established. One case of peripheral neuropathy which resolved on discontinuation of BETAPACE® and recurred when the patient was rechallenged with the drug was reported in an early dose tolerance study. Elevated blood glucose levels and increased insulin requirements can occur in diabetic patients.

The following table lists as a function of dosage the most common (incidence of 2% or greater) adverse events, regardless of relationship to therapy and the percent of patients discontinued due to the event, as collected from clinical trials involving 1292 patients with sustained VT/VF.

[See table at bottom of next page.]

Potential Adverse Effects: Foreign marketing experience with sotalol hydrochloride shows an adverse experience profile similar to that described above from clinical trials. Voluntary reports since introduction include rare reports (less than one report per 10,000 patients) of: emotional lability, slightly clouded sensorium, incoordination, vertigo, paralysis, thrombocytopenia, eosinophilia, leukopenia, photosensitivity reaction, fever, pulmonary edema, hyperlipidemia, myalgia, pruritis, alopecia.

The oculomucocutaneous syndrome associated with the beta-blocker practolol has not been associated with BETAPACE® during investigational use and foreign marketing experience.

OVERDOSAGE

Intentional or accidental overdosage with BETAPACE® (sotalol hydrochloride) has rarely resulted in death.

Symptoms and Treatment of Overdosage: The most common signs to be expected are bradycardia, congestive heart failure, hypotension, bronchospasm and hypoglycemia. In cases of massive intentional overdosage (2–16 grams) of BETAPACE® the following clinical findings were seen: hypotension, bradycardia, cardiac asystole, prolongation of QT interval, torsade de pointes, ventricular tachycardia, and premature ventricular complexes. If overdosage occurs, therapy with BETAPACE® should be discontinued and the patient observed closely. Because of the lack of protein binding, hemodialysis is useful for reducing sotalol plasma concentrations. Patients should be carefully observed until QT intervals are normalized and the heart rate returns to levels > 50 bpm. In addition, if required, the following therapeutic measures are suggested:

Bradycardia or cardiac asystole: Atropine, another anticholinergic drug, a beta-adrenergic agonist or transvenous cardiac pacing.

Heart Block: (second and third degree) transvenous cardiac pacemaker.

Hypotension: (depending on associated factors) epinephrine rather than isoproterenol or norepinephrine may be useful.

Bronchospasm: Aminophylline or aerosol beta-2-receptor stimulant.

Torsade de pointes: DC cardioversion, transvenous cardiac pacing, epinephrine, magnesium sulfate.

DOSAGE AND ADMINISTRATION

As with other antiarrhythmic agents, BETAPACE® should be initiated and doses increased in a hospital with facilities for cardiac rhythm monitoring and assessment (see **INDICATIONS AND USAGE**). BETAPACE® should be administered only after appropriate clinical assessment (see **INDICATIONS AND USAGE**), and the dosage of BETAPACE® must be individualized for each patient on the basis of therapeutic response and tolerance. Proarrhythmic events can occur not only at initiation of therapy, but also with each upward dosage adjustment.

Dosage of BETAPACE® should be adjusted gradually, allowing 2–3 days between dosing increments in order to attain steady-state plasma concentrations, and to allow monitoring of QT intervals. Graded dose adjustment will help prevent the usage of doses which are higher than necessary to control the arrhythmia. The recommended initial dose is 80 mg twice daily. This dose may be increased, if necessary, after appropriate evaluation to 240 or 320 mg/day (120–160 mg twice daily). In most patients, a therapeutic response is obtained at a total daily dose of 160 to 320 mg/day, given in two or three divided doses. Some patients with life-threatening refractory ventricular arrhythmias may require doses as high as 480–640 mg/day; however, these doses should only be prescribed when the potential benefit outweighs the increased risk of adverse events, in particular proarrhythmia. Because of the long terminal elimination half-life of BETAPACE®, dosing on more than a BID regimen is usually not necessary.

DOSAGE IN RENAL IMPAIRMENT

Because sotalol is excreted predominantly in urine and its terminal elimination half-life is prolonged in conditions of renal impairment, the dosing interval (time between divided doses) of sotalol should be modified (when creatinine clearance is lower than 60 mL/min) according to the following table.

Creatinine Clearance mL/min	Dosing* Interval (hours)
> 60	12
30–59	24
10–29	36–48
< 10	Dose should be individualized

*The initial dose of 80 mg and subsequent doses should be administered at these intervals. See following paragraph for dosage escalations.

Since the terminal elimination half-life of BETAPACE® (sotalol hydrochloride) is increased in patients with renal impairment, a longer duration of dosing is required to reach steady-state. Dose escalations in renal impairment should be done after administration of at least 5–6 doses at appropriate intervals (see table above).

Extreme caution should be exercised in the use of sotalol in patients with renal failure undergoing hemodialysis. The

Continued on next page

Information on the Berlex products appearing here is based on the most current information available at the time of publication closing. Further information for these and other products may be obtained from the Medical Affairs Department, Berlex Laboratories, 300 Fairfield Road, Wayne, New Jersey 07470, 1-800-888-2407. Information on Betaseron and Fludara may be obtained from Berlex Laboratories, 15049 San Pablo Avenue, Richmond, California 94804-0016, 1-800-888-4112.

Berlex Laboratories—Cont.

half-life of sotalol is prolonged (up to 69 hours) in anuric patients. Sotalol, however, can be partly removed by dialysis with subsequent partial rebound in concentrations when dialysis is completed. Both safety (heart rate, QT interval) and efficacy (arrhythmia control) must be closely monitored.

Transfer to BETAPACE®

Before starting BETAPACE®, previous antiarrhythmic therapy should generally be withdrawn under careful monitoring for a minimum of 2–3 plasma half-lives if the patient's clinical condition permits (see **DRUG INTERACTIONS**). Treatment has been initiated in some patients receiving I.V. lidocaine without ill effect. After discontinuation of amiodarone, BETAPACE® should not be initiated until the QT interval is normalized (see **WARNINGS**).

Incidence (%) of Adverse Events and Discontinuations DAILY DOSE

Body System	160mg (n=832)	240mg (n=263)	320mg (n=835)	480mg (n=459)	640mg (n=324)	Any Dose* (n=1292)	% Patients Discontinued (n=1292)
Body as a whole							
infection	1	2	2	2	3	4	<1
fever	1	2	3	2	2	4	<1
localized pain	1	1	2	2	2	3	<1
Cardiovascular							
dyspnea	5	8	11	15	15	21	2
bradycardia	8	8	9	7	5	16	2
chest pain	4	3	10	10	14	16	<1
palpitation	3	3	8	9	12	14	<1
edema	2	2	5	3	5	8	1
ECG abnormal	4	2	4	2	2	7	1
hypotension	3	4	3	2	3	6	2
proarrhythmia	<1	<1	2	4	5	5	3
syncope	1	1	3	2	5	5	1
heart failure	2	3	2	2	2	5	1
presyncope	1	2	2	4	3	4	<1
peripheral vascular disorder	1	2	1	1	2	3	<1
cardiovascular disorder	1	<1	2	2	2	3	<1
vasodilation	1	<1	1	2	1	3	<1
AICD Discharge	<1	2	2	2	2	3	<1
hypertension	<1	1	1	1	2	2	<1
Nervous							
fatigue	5	8	12	12	13	20	2
dizziness	7	6	11	11	14	20	1
asthenia	4	5	7	8	10	13	1
light-headed	4	3	6	6	9	12	1
headache	3	2	4	4	4	8	<1
sleep problem	1	1	5	5	6	8	<1
perspiration	1	2	3	4	5	6	<1
altered consciousness	2	3	1	2	3	4	<1
depression	1	2	2	2	3	4	<1
paresthesia	1	1	2	3	2	4	<1
anxiety	2	2	2	3	2	4	<1
mood change	<1	<1	1	3	2	3	<1
appetite disorder	1	2	2	1	3	3	<1
stroke	<1	<1	1	1	<1	1	<1
Digestive							
nausea/vomiting	5	4	4	6	6	10	1
diarrhea	2	3	3	3	5	7	<1
dyspepsia	2	3	3	3	3	6	<1
abdominal pain	<1	<1	2	2	2	3	<1
colon problem	2	1	1	<1	2	3	<1
flatulence	1	<1	1	1	2	2	<1
Respiratory							
pulmonary problem	3	3	5	3	4	8	<1
upper respiratory tract problem	1	1	3	4	3	5	<1
asthma	1	<1	1	1	1	2	<1
Urogenital							
genitourinary disorder	1	0	1	1	2	3	<1
sexual dysfunction	<1	1	1	1	3	2	<1
Metabolic							
abnormal lab value	1	2	3	2	1	4	<1
weight change	1	1	1	<1	2	2	<1
Musculoskeletal							
extremity pain	2	2	4	5	3	7	<1
back pain	1	<1	2	2	2	3	<1
Skin and Appendages							
rash	2	3	2	3	4	5	<1
Hematologic							
bleeding	1	<1	1	<1	2	2	<1
Special Senses							
visual problem	1	1	2	4	5	5	<1

* Because patients are counted at each dose level tested, the Any Dose column cannot be determined by adding across the doses.

HOW SUPPLIED

BETAPACE® (sotalol hydrochloride); capsule-shaped light-blue scored tablets imprinted with the strength and "BETAPACE", are available as follows:
NDC 50419–105–10 80 mg strength, bottle of 100
NDC 50419–105–11 80 mg strength, carton of 100 unit dose
NDC 50419–109–10 120 mg strength, bottle of 100
NDC 50419–109–11 120 mg strength, carton of 100 unit dose
NDC 50419–106–10 160 mg strength, bottle of 100
NDC 50419–106–11 160 mg strength, carton of 100 unit dose
NDC 50419–107–10 240 mg strength, bottle of 100
NDC 50419–107–11 240 mg strength, carton of 100 unit dose
Store at controlled room temperature, between 15° to 30°C (59° to 86°F).
Caution: Federal law prohibits dispensing without prescription.

Manufactured for:
BERLEX Laboratories, Wayne, NJ 07470
Manufactured by:
A Bristol-Myers Company
Evansville, Indiana 47721
6063801 Rev. 4/96
Shown in Product Identification Guide, page 305

CLIMARA®
[clī-măr '-a]
(ESTRADIOL TRANSDERMAL SYSTEM)

℞

PRESCRIBING INFORMATION

> 1. ESTROGENS HAVE BEEN REPORTED TO INCREASE THE RISK OF ENDOMETRIAL CARCINOMA IN POSTMENOPAUSAL WOMEN.
> Close clinical surveillance of all women taking estrogens is important. Adequate diagnostic measures, including endometrial sampling when indicated, should be undertaken to rule out malignancy in all cases of undiagnosed persistent or recurring abnormal vaginal bleeding. There is currently no evidence that "natural" estrogens are more or less hazardous than "synthetic" estrogens at equiestrogenic doses.
> 2. ESTROGENS SHOULD NOT BE USED DURING PREGNANCY.
> Estrogen therapy during pregnancy is associated with an increased risk of congenital defects in the reproductive organs of the fetus, and possibly other birth defects. Studies of women who received diethylstilbestrol (DES) during pregnancy have shown that female offspring have an increased risk of vaginal adenosis, squamous cell dysplasia of the uterine cervix, and clear cell vaginal cancer later in life; male offspring have an increased risk of urogenital abnormalities and possibly testicular cancer later in life. The 1985 DES Task Force concluded that use of DES during pregnancy is associated with a subsequent increased risk of breast cancer in the mothers, although a causal relationship remains unproven and the observed level of excess risk is similar to that for a number of other breast cancer risk factors.
> There is no indication for estrogen therapy during pregnancy or during the immediate postpartum period. Estrogens are ineffective for the prevention or treatment of threatened or habitual abortion. Estrogens are not indicated for the prevention of postpartum breast engorgement.

DESCRIPTION

Climara®, estradiol transdermal system, is designed to release 17β-estradiol continuously upon application to intact skin. Two (12.5 and 25.0 sq cm) systems are available to provide nominal *in vivo* delivery of 0.05 or 0.1 mg respectively of estradiol per day. The period of use is 7 days. Each system has a contact surface area of either 12.5 or 25.0 sq cm, and contains 3.9 or 7.8 mg of estradiol USP respectively. The composition of the systems per unit area is identical.
Estradiol USP (17β-estradiol) is a white, crystalline powder, chemically described as estra-1,3,5(10)-triene-3,17β-diol. It has an empirical formula of $c_{18}H_{24}O_2$ and molecular weight of 272.37. The structural formula is:

The Climara® system comprises two layers. Proceeding from the visible surface toward the surface attached to the skin, these layers are (1) a translucent polyethylene film, and (2) an acrylate adhesive matrix containing estradiol USP. A protective liner (3) of siliconized or fluoropolymercoated polyester film is attached to the adhesive surface and must be removed before the system can be used.

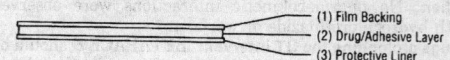

(1) Film Backing
(2) Drug/Adhesive Layer
(3) Protective Liner

The active component of the system is 17β-estradiol. The remaining components of the system (acrylate copolymer adhesive, fatty acid esters, and polyethylene backing) are pharmacologically inactive.

CLINICAL PHARMACOLOGY

The Climara® system provides systemic estrogen replacement therapy by releasing 17β-estradiol, the major estrogenic hormone secreted by the human ovary.

Estrogens are important in the development and maintenance of the female reproductive system and secondary sex characteristics. By a direct action, they cause growth and development of the uterus, fallopian tubes, and vagina. With other hormones, such as pituitary hormones and progesterone, they cause enlargement of the breasts through promotion of ductal growth, stromal development, and the accretion of fat. Estrogens are intricately involved with other hormones, especially progesterone, in the processes of the ovulatory menstrual cycle and pregnancy, and affect the release of pituitary gonadotropins. They also contribute to the shaping of the skeleton, maintenace of tone and elasticity of urogenital structures, changes in the epiphyses of the long bones that allow for the pubertal growth spurt and its termination, and pigmentation of the nipples and genitals.

Estrogens occur naturally in several forms. The primary source of estrogen in normally cycling adult women is the ovarian follicle, which secretes 70 to 500 micrograms of estradiol daily, depending on the phase of the menstrual cycle. This is converted primarily to estrone, which circulates in roughly equal proportion to estradiol, and to small amounts of estriol. After menopause, most endogenous estrogen is produced by conversion of androstenedione, secreted by the adrenal cortex, to estrone by peripheral tissues. Thus, estrone—especially in its sulfate ester form—is the most abundant circulating estrogen in postmenopausal women. Although circulating estrogens exist in a dynamic equilibrium of metabolic interconversions, estradiol is the principal intracellular human estrogen and is substantially more potent than estrone or estriol at the receptor.

Estrogen drug products act by regulating the transcription of a limited number of genes. Estrogens diffuse through cell membranes, distribute themselves throughout the cell, and bind to and activate the nuclear estrogen receptor, a DNA-binding protein which is found in estrogen-responsive tissues. The activated estrogen receptor binds to specific DNA sequences, or hormone-response elements, which enhance the transcription of adjacent genes and in turn lead to the observed effects. Estrogen receptors have been identified in tissues of the reproductive tract, breast, pituitary, hypothalamus, liver, and bone of women.

Estrogens used in therapy are well absorbed through the skin, musous membranes, and gastrointestinal tract. Administered estrogens and their esters are handled within the body essentially the same as the endogenous hormones. Metabolic conversion of estrogens occurs primarily in the liver (first pass effect), but also at local target tissue sites. Complex metabolic processes result in a dynamic equilibrium of circulating conjugated and unconjugated estrogenic forms, which are continually interconverted, especially between estrone and estradiol and between esterified and unesterified forms. Although naturally-occurring estrogens circulate in the blood largely bound to sex hormone-binding globulin and albumin, only unbound estrogens enter target tissue cells. A significant proportion of the circulating estrogen exists as sulfate conjugates, especially estrone sulfate, which serves as a circulating reservior for the formation of more active estrogenic species. A certain proportion of the estrogen is excreted into the bile and then reabsorbed from the intestine. During this enterohepatic recirculation, estrogens are desulfated and resulfated and undergo degradation through conversion to less active estrogens (estriol and other estrogens), oxidation to nonestrogenic substances (catecholestrogens, which interact with catecholamine metabolism, especially in the central nervous system), and conjugation with glucuronic acids (which are then rapidly excreted in the urine).

When given orally, naturally-occurring estrogens and their esters are extensively metabolized (first pass effect) and circulate primarily as estrone sulfate, with smaller amounts of other conjugated and unconjugated estrogenic species. This results in limited oral potency. In contrast, the skin metabolizes estradiol only to a small extent. Therefore, transdermal administration produces therapeutic serum levels of estradiol with lower circulating levels of estrone and estrone conjugates, and requires smaller total doses than does oral therapy. Because estradiol has a short half-life, transdermal administration of estradiol allows a rapid decline in blood levels after the Climara® system is removed.

PHARMACOKINETICS

Transdermal administration of estradiol is reported to produce mean serum concentrations of estradiol comparable to those produced by daily oral administration of estradiol at about 20 times the daily transdermal dose.

In a 3-week multiple-application study in 24 postmenopausal women, the 25.0 sq cm Climara® system produced average peak estradiol concentrations of approximately 100 pg/mL. Trough values at the end of each wear interval were approximately 35 pg/mL. Nearly identical serum curves were seen each week, indicating little or no accumulation of estradiol in the body. Serum estrone peak and trough levels were 60 and 40 pg/mL, respectively. Because estradiol has a short half-life (approximately 1 hour), serum concentrations of estradiol and estrone returned to preapplication levels within 6 to 24 hours after removal of the last system (to less than 17 pg/mL of estradiol and 30 pg/mL estrone.)

Linear pharmacokinetics have been demonstrated for the Climara® system. In a 1-week application study in 54 postmenopausal women, the 25.0 sq cm system produced estradiol serum level profiles and pharmacokinetic parameters that were twice as high as the 12.5 sq cm system. Statistical analyses confirmed the 2:1 dose proportionality.

On average, the Climara® 25.0 sq cm system maintained mean steady-state serum estradiol levels of approximately 70 pg/mL, and the Climara® 12.5 sq cm system maintained mean steady-state serum estradiol levels of approximately 35 pg/mL.

Table 1 summarizes the mean results from four pharmacokinetic studies. All systems were applied on the abdomen for a single 1-week period. C_{max} occurred at approximately 30 hours.

Table 1
Pharmacokinetic Summary

Surface Area (sq cm)	Delivery Rate (mg/day)	C_{max} (pg/mL)	C_{min} (pg/mL)	C_{avg} (pg/mL)
12.5	0.05	58–82	20–32	33–45
25.0	0.1	98–172	39–61	53–93

The relative standard deviation of each pharmacokinetic parameter averaged 50%, which is indicative of the considerable intersubject variability associated with transdermal drug delivery.

Two studies compared a single, 1-week application of the Climara® system with consecutive 3-day and 4-day applications of Estraderm® (a twice-a-week transdermal estradiol system). The Climara® 25.0 sq cm system was compared with the Estraderm® 20 sq cm system (see Figure 1); the Climara® 12.5 sq cm system was compared to the Estraderm® 10 sq cm system (see Figure 2). For a 1-week treatment period, both sizes of Climara® systems maintained significantly lower peak and mean steady-state levels than did the Estraderm® system; however, towards the end of each treatment period, the Climara® systems maintained similar (day 6) or higher (day 7) serum estradiol levels than did the Estraderm® system. As a result, the peak-to-end of application interval trough level fluctuations were 3- to 4-times less with the Climara® system.

Figure 1
Mean Serum Estradiol Levels for a One-Week Application of the Climara® system (25 sq cm) and Consecutive Three-Day and Four-Day Applications of the Estraderm® System (20 sq cm)

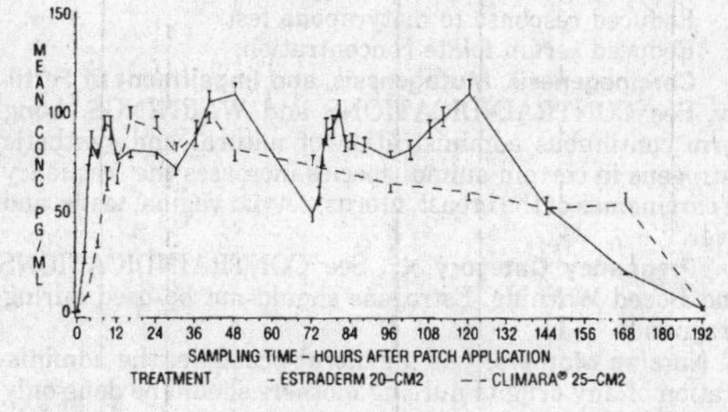

Figure 2
Mean Serum Estradiol Levels for a One-Week Application of the Climara® system (12.5 sq cm) and Consecutive Three-Day and Four-Day Applications of the Estraderm® System (10 sq cm)

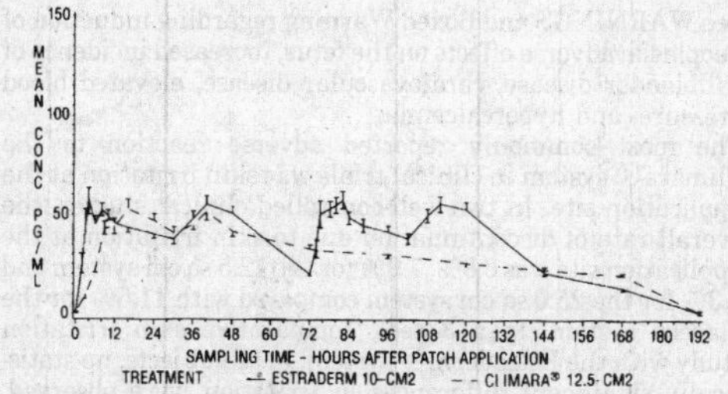

INDICATIONS AND USAGE

Climara® is indicated in the:

1. Treatment of moderate to severe vasomotor symptoms associated with the menopause. There is no adequate evidence that estrogens are effective for nervous symptoms or depression which might occur during menopause and they should not be used to treat these conditions.
2. Treatment of vulval and vaginal atrophy.
3. Treatment of hypoestrogenism due to hypogonadism, castration or primary ovarian failure.
4. Treatment of abnormal uterine bleeding due to hormonal imbalance in the absence of organic pathology and only when associated with a hypoplastic or atrophic endometrium.

CONTRAINDICATIONS

Estrogens should not be used in individuals with any of the following conditions:

1. Known or suspected pregnancy (see Boxed Warning). Estrogens may cause fetal harm when administered to a pregnant woman.
2. Undiagnosed abnormal genital bleeding.
3. Known or suspected cancer of the breast except in appropriately selected patients being treated for metastatic disease.
4. Known or suspected estrogen-dependent neoplasia.
5. Active thrombophlebitis or thromboembolic disorders.

WARNINGS

1. **Induction of malignant neoplasms.**

Endometrial cancer. The reported endometrial cancer risk among unopposed estrogen users is about 2 to 12 fold greater than in non-users, and appears dependent on duration of treatment and on estrogen dose. Most studies show no significant increased risk associated with use of estrogens for less than one year. The greatest risk appears associated with prolonged use—with increased risks of 15- to 24-fold for five to ten years or more. In three studies, persistence of risk was demonstrated for 8 to over 15 years after cessation of estrogen treatment. In one study a significant decrease in the incidence of endometrial cancer occurred six months after estrogen withdrawal. Concurrent progestin therapy may offset this risk but the overall health impact in postmenopausal women is not known (see Precautions).

Breast cancer. While the majority of studies have not shown an increased risk of breast cancer in women who have ever used estrogen replacement therapy, some have reported a moderately increased risk (relative risks of 1.3–2.0) in those taking higher doses or those taking lower doses for prolonged periods of time, especially in excess of 10 years. Other studies have not shown this relationship.

Congenital lesions with malignant potential. Estrogen therapy during pregnancy is associated with an increased risk of fetal congenital reproductive tract disorders, and possibly other birth defects. Studies of women who received DES during pregnancy have shown that female offspring have an increased risk of vaginal adenosis, squamous cell dysplasia of the uterine cervix, and clear cell vaginal cancer later in life; male offspring have an increased risk of urogenital abnormalities and possibly testicular cancer later in life. Although some of these changes are benign, others are precursors of malignancy.

2. **Gallbladder disease.** Two studies have reported a 2- to 4-fold increase in the risk of gallbladder disease requiring surgery in women receiving postmenopausal estrogens.
3. **Cardiovascular disease.** Large doses of estrogen (5 mg conjugated estrogens per day), comparable to those used to treat cancer of the prostate and breast, have been shown in a large prospective clinical trial in men to increase the risks of nonfatal myocardial infarction, pulmonary embolism, and thrombophlebitis. These risks cannot necessarily be extrapolated from men to women. However, to avoid the theoretical cardiovascular risk to women caused by high estrogen doses, the dose for estrogen replacement therapy should not exceed the lowest effective dose.
4. **Elevated blood pressure.** Occasional blood pressure increases during estrogen replacement therapy have been attributed to idiosyncratic reactions to estrogens. More often, blood pressure has remained the same or has dropped. One study showed that postmenopausal estrogen users have higher blood pressure than nonusers. Two other studies showed slightly lower blood pressure among estrogen users compared to nonusers. Postmenopausal estrogen use does not increase the risk of stroke. Nonetheless, blood pressure should be monitored at regular intervals with estrogen use. Ethinyl estradiol and conjugated estrogens have been shown to increase renin substrate. In contrast to these oral estrogens, transdermally administered estradiol has been reported not to affect renin substrate.
5. **Hypercalcemia.** Administration of estrogens may lead to severe hypercalcemia in patients with breast cancer and bone metastases. If this occurs, the drug should be stopped

Continued on next page

Information on the Berlex products appearing here is based on the most current information available at the time of publication closing. Further information for these and other products may be obtained from the Medical Affairs Department, Berlex Laboratories, 300 Fairfield Road, Wayne, New Jersey 07470, 1-800-888-2407. Information on Betaseron and Fludara may be obtained from Berlex Laboratories, 15049 San Pablo Avenue, Richmond, California 94804-0016, 1-800-888-4112.

Berlex Laboratories—Cont.

and appropriate measures taken to reduce the serum calcium level.

PRECAUTIONS

A. General

1. **Addition of a progestin.** Studies of the addition of a progestin for 10 or more days of a cycle of estrogen administration have reported a lowered incidence of endometrial hyperplasia than would be induced by estrogen treatment alone. Morphological and biochemical studies of endometria suggest that 10 to 14 days of progestin are needed to provide maximal maturation of the endometrium and to reduce the likelihood of hyperplastic changes.

There are, however, possible risks which may be associated with the use of progestins in estrogen replacement regimens. These include: (1) adverse effects on lipoprotein metabolism (lowering HDL and raising LDL) which could diminish the purported cardioprotective effect of estrogen therapy (see Precautions D.4., below); (2) impairment of glucose tolerance; and (3) possible enhancement of mitotic activity in breast epithelial tissue, although few epidemiological data are available to address this point (see Precautions below).

The choice of progestin, its dose, and its regimen may be important in minimizing these adverse effects, but these issues will require further study before they are clarified.

2. *Cardiovascular risk.* *A causal relationship between estrogen replacement therapy and reduction of cardiovascular disease in postmenopausal women has not been proven. Furthermore, the effect of added progestins on this putative benefit is not yet known.*

In recent years many published studies have suggested that there may be a cause-effect relationship between postmenopausal oral estrogen replacement therapy *without added progestins* and a decrease in cardiovascular disease in women. Although most of the observational studies which assessed this statistical association have reported a 20% to 50% reduction in coronary heart disease risk and associated mortality in estrogen takers, the following should be considered when interpreting these reports: (1) Because only one of these studies was randomized and it was too small to yield statistically significant results, all relevant studies were subject to selection bias. Thus, the apparently reduced risk of coronary artery disease cannot be attributed with certainty to estrogen replacement therapy. It may instead have been caused by life-style and medical characteristics of the women studied with the result that healthier women were selected for estrogen therapy. In general, treated women were of a higher socioeconomic and educational status, more slender, more physically active, more likely to have undergone surgical menopause, and less likely to have diabetes than the untreated women. Although some studies attempted to control for these selection factors, it is common for properly designed randomized trials to fail to confirm benefits suggested by less rigorous study designs. Thus, ongoing and future large-scale randomized trials may fail to confirm this apparent benefit. (2) Current medical practice often includes the use of concomitant progestin therapy with intact uteri (see PRECAUTIONS and WARNINGS). While the effects of added progestins on the risk of ischemic heart disease are not known, all available progestins reverse at least some of the favorable effects of estrogens on HDL and LDL levels. (3) While the effects of added progestins on the risk of breast cancer are also unknown, available epidemiological evidence suggests that progestins do not reduce, and may enhance, the moderately increased breast cancer incidence that has been reported with prolonged estrogen replacement therapy (see WARNINGS above).

Because relatively long-term use of estrogens by a woman with a uterus has been shown to induce endometrial cancer, physicians often recommend that women who are deemed candidates for hormone replacement should take progestins as well as estrogens. When considering prescribing concomitant estrogens and progestins for hormone replacement therapy, physicians and patients are advised to carefully weigh the potential benefits and risks of the added progestin. Large-scale randomized, placebo-controlled, prospective clinical trials are required to clarify these issues.

3. **Physical examination.** A complete medical and family history should be taken prior to the initiation of any estrogen therapy. The pretreatment and periodic physical examinations should include special reference to blood pressure, breasts, abdomen, and pelvic organs, and should include a Papanicolaou smear. As a general rule, estrogen should not be prescribed for longer than one year without reexamining the patient.

4. **Hypercoagulability.** Some studies have shown that women taking estrogen replacement therapy have hypercoagulability, primarily related to decreased antithrombin activity. This effect appears dose- and duration-dependent and is less pronounced than that associated with oral contraceptive use.

Also, postmenopausal women tend to have increased coagulation parameters at baseline compared to premenopausal women. There is some suggestion that low dose postmenopausal mestranol may increase the risk of thromboembolism, although the majority of studies (of primarily conjugated estrogens users) report no such increase. There is insufficient information on hypercoagulability in women who have had previous thromboembolic disease.

5. **Familial hyperlipoproteinemia.** Estrogen therapy may be associated with massive elevations of plasma triglycerides leading to pancreatitis and other complications in patients with familial defects of lipoprotein metabolism.

6. **Fluid retention.** Because estrogens may cause some degree of fluid retention, conditions which might be exacerbated by this factor, such as asthma, epilepsy, migraine, and cardiac or renal dysfunction, require careful observation.

7. **Uterine bleeding and mastodynia.** Certain patients may develop undesirable manifestations of estrogenic stimulation, such as abnormal uterine bleeding and mastodynia.

8. **Impaired liver function.** Estrogens may be poorly metabolized in patients with impaired liver function and should be administered with caution.

B. Information for the Patient. See text of Patient Package Insert after the How Supplied section.

C. Laboratory Tests. Estrogen administration should generally be guided by clinical response at the smallest dose, rather than laboratory monitoring, for relief of symptoms for those indications in which symptoms are observable.

D. Drug/Laboratory Test Interactions.

1. Accelerated prothrombin time, partial thromboplastin time, and platelet aggregation time; increased platelet count; increased factors II, VII antigen, VIII antigen, VIII coagulant activity, IX, X, XII, VII-X complex, II-VII-X complex, and betathromboglobulin; decreased levels of anti-factor Xa and antithrombin III, decreased antithrombin III activity; increased levels of fibrinogen and fibrinogen activity; increased plasminogen antigen and activity.

2. Increased thyroid-binding globulin (TBG) leading to increased circulating total thyroid hormone, as measured by protein-bound iodine (PBI), T4 levels (by column or by radioimmunoassay) or T3 levels by radioimmunoassay. T3 resin uptake is decreased, reflecting the elevated TBG. Free T4 and free T3 concentrations are unaltered.

3. Other binding proteins may be elevated in serum, i.e., corticosteroid binding globulin (CBG), sex hormone-binding globulin (SHBG), leading to increased circulating corticosteroids and sex steroids respectively. Free or biologically active hormone concentrations are unchanged. Other plasma proteins may be increased (angiotensinogen/renin substrate, alpha-1-antitrypsin, ceruloplasmin).

4. Increased plasma HDL and HDL-2 subfraction concentrations, reduced LDL cholesterol concentration, increased triglycerides levels.

5. Impaired glucose tolerance.

6. Reduced response to metyrapone test.

7. Reduced serum folate concentration.

E. Carcinogenesis, Mutagenesis, and Impairment of Fertility. See CONTRAINDICATIONS and WARNINGS. Long term continuous administration of natural and synthetic estrogens in certain animal species increases the frequency of carcinomas of the breast, uterus, cervix, vagina, testis, and liver.

F. Pregnancy Category X. See CONTRAINDICATIONS and Boxed Warning. Estrogens should not be used during pregnancy.

G. Nursing Mothers. As a general principle, the administration of any drug to nursing mothers should be done only when clearly necessary since many drugs are excreted in human milk. In addition, estrogen administration to nursing mothers has been shown to decrease the quantity and quality of the milk.

ADVERSE REACTIONS

See WARNINGS and Boxed Warning regarding induction of neoplasia, adverse effects on the fetus, increased incidence of gallbladder disease, cardiovascular disease, elevated blood pressure, and hypercalcemia.

The most commonly reported adverse reaction to the Climara® system in clinical trials was skin irritation at the application site. In two well-controlled clinical studies, the overall rate of discontinuation due to skin irritation at the application site was 6.8%; 7.9% for the 12.5 sq cm system and 5.3% for the 25.0 sq cm system compared with 11.5% for the placebo system. In a 3-week comparative skin irritation study with the Estraderm® system, in 95 subjects, no statistically significant differences in irritation were observed. Some degree of irritation at the end of week three was seen in 25% of Estraderm® and 31% of Climara® subjects. Clinically significant irritation (mild erythema associated with symptoms or moderate to severe erythema) was evident at the end of week three in 11% of Estraderm® and 9% of Climara® subjects.

The following additional adverse reactions have been reported with estrogen therapy:

1. **Genitourinary system.**

Changes in vaginal bleeding pattern and abnormal withdrawal bleeding or flow, breakthrough bleeding, spotting. Increase in size of uterine leiomyomata. Vaginal candidiasis. Change in amount of cervical secretion.

2. **Breasts.**

Tenderness, enlargement.

3. **Gastrointestinal.**

Nausea, vomiting. Abdominal cramps, bloating. Cholestatic jaundice. Increased incidence of gallbladder disease.

4. **Skin.**

Chloasma or melasma that may persist when drug is discontinued. Erythema multiforme. Erythema nodosum. Hemorrhagic eruption. Loss of scalp hair. Hirsutism.

5. **Eyes.**

Steepening of corneal curvature. Intolerance to contact lenses.

6. **Central nervous system.**

Headache, migraine, dizziness. Mental depression. Chorea.

7. **Miscellaneous.**

Increase or decrease in weight. Reduced carbohydrate tolerance. Aggravation of porphyria. Edema. Changes in libido.

OVERDOSAGE

Serious ill effects have not been reported following acute ingestion of large doses of estrogen-containing oral contraceptives by young children. Overdosage of estrogen may cause nausea and vomiting, and withdrawal bleeding may occur in females.

DOSAGE AND ADMINISTRATION

The adhesive side of the Climara® system should be placed on a clean, dry area of the abdomen. *The Climara® system should not be applied to the breasts.* The sites of application must be rotated, with an interval of at least 1 week allowed between applications to a particular site. The area selected should not be oily, damaged, or irritated. The waistline should be avoided, since tight clothing may rub and remove the system. The system should be applied immediately after opening the pouch and removing the protective liner. The system should be pressed firmly in place with the fingers for about 10 seconds, making sure there is good contact, especially around the edges. In the unlikely event that a system should fall off, a new system should be applied for the remainder of the 7-day dosing interval. Only one system should be worn at any one time during the 7-day dosing interval.

Initiation of Therapy

Two (12.5 and 25.0 sq cm) Climara® systems are available. Treatment is usually initiated with the 12.5 sq cm (0.05 mg/day) Climara® system applied to the skin once-weekly. The dose should be adjusted as necessary to control symptoms. Clinical responses (relief of symptoms) at the lowest effective dose should be the guide for establishing administration of the Climara® system, especially in women with an intact uterus. Attempts to taper or discontinue the medication should be made at 3- to 6-month intervals.

In women who are not currently taking oral estrogens, treatment with the Climara® system can be initiated at once. In women who are currently taking oral estrogen, treatment with the Climara® system can be initiated 1 week after withdrawal of oral therapy or sooner if symptoms reappear in less than 1 week.

Therapeutic Regimen

Therapy with the Climara® system is usually administered on a cyclic schedule (e.g., 3 weeks of therapy followed by 1 week without) especially in women with an intact uterus, who are not using concomitant progestin therapy.

HOW SUPPLIED

Climara® (estradiol transdermal system), 0.05 mg/day—each 12.5 sq cm system contains 3.9 mg of estradiol USP .... NDC 50419-451-04
 Individual Carton of 4 systems
 Shelf Pack Carton of 6 Individual Cartons of 4 systems
Climara® (estradiol transdermal system), 0.1 mg/day—each 25.0 sq cm system contains 7.8 mg of estradiol USP .... NDC 50419-452-04
 Individual Carton of 4 systems
 Shelf Pack Carton of 6 Individual Cartons of 4 systems
Do not store above 86°F (30°C). Do not store unpouched. Apply immediately upon removal from the protective pouch.
CAUTION: Federal law prohibits dispensing without prescription.
Manufactured for Berlex Laboratories, Wayne, NJ 07470
Manufactured by 3M Pharmaceuticals, St. Paul, MN 55144

INFORMATION FOR THE PATIENT
INTRODUCTION

The Climara® system that your doctor has prescribed for you releases small amounts of estradiol through the skin in a continuous way. Estradiol is the same hormone that your ovaries produce abundantly before menopause. The dose of estradiol you require will depend upon your individual response. The dose is adjusted by the size of the Climara® system used; the systems are available in two sizes.

This leaflet describes when and how to use estrogens, and the risks and benefits of estrogen treatment.

Estrogens have important benefits but also some risks. You must decide, with your doctor, whether the risks to you of

estrogen use are acceptable because of their benefits. If you use estrogens, check with your doctor to be sure you are using the lowest possible dose that works, and that you don't use them longer than necessary. How long you need to use estrogens will depend on the reason for use.

1. ESTROGENS INCREASE THE RISK OF CANCER OF THE UTERUS IN WOMEN WHO HAVE HAD THEIR MENOPAUSE ("CHANGE OF LIFE").
If you use any estrogen-containing drug, it is important to visit your doctor regularly and report any unusual vaginal bleeding right away. Vaginal bleeding after menopause may be a warning sign of uterine cancer. Your doctor should evaluate any unusual vaginal bleeding to find out the cause.
2. ESTROGENS SHOULD NOT BE USED DURING PREGNANCY.
Estrogens do not prevent miscarriage (spontaneous abortion) and are not needed in the days following childbirth. If you take estrogens during pregnancy, your unborn child has a greater than usual chance of having birth defects. The risk of developing these defects is small, but clearly larger than the risk in children whose mothers did not take estrogens during pregnancy. These birth defects may affect the baby's urinary system and sex organs. Daughters born to mothers who took DES (an estrogen drug) have a higher than usual chance of developing cancer of the vagina or cervix when they become teenagers or young adults. Sons may have a higher than usual chance of developing cancer of the testicles when they become teenagers or young adults.

INFORMATION ABOUT CLIMARA®

How The Climara® System Works

The Climara® system contains 17β-estradiol. When applied to the skin as directed below, the Climara® system releases 17β-estradiol, which flows through the skin into the bloodstream.

How and Where to Apply the Climara® System

Each Climara® system is individually sealed in a protective pouch. Tear open this pouch at the indentation (do not use scissors) and remove the system.

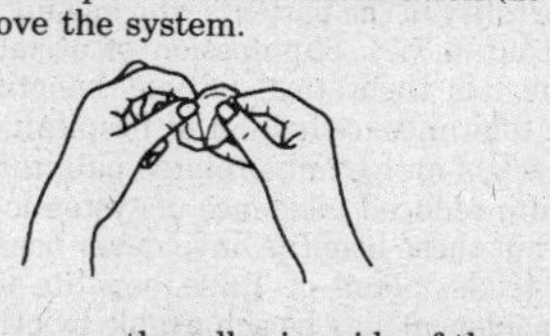

A protective liner covers the adhesive side of the system—the side that will be placed against your skin. This liner must be removed before applying the system. Remove the protective liner and discard it. Try to avoid touching the adhesive. Apply the adhesive side of the system to a clean, dry area of the skin on the abdomen. *Do not apply the Climara® system to your breasts.* The sites of application must be rotated, with an interval of at least 1 week allowed between applications to a particular site. The area selected should not be oily, damaged, or irritated. Avoid the waistline, since tight clothing may rub and remove the system. Apply the system immediately after opening the pouch and removing the protective liner. Press the system firmly in place with the fingers for about 10 seconds, making sure there is a good contact, especially around the edges.

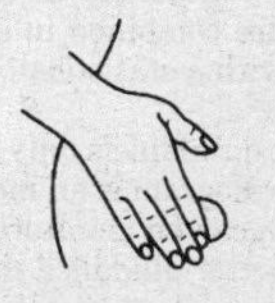

The Climara® system should be worn continuously for one week. You may wish to experiment with different locations when applying a new system, to find ones that are most comfortable for you and where clothing will not rub on the system.

When to Apply the Climara® System

The Climara® system should be changed once weekly. When changing the system, remove the used Climara® system and discard it. Any adhesive that might remain on your skin can be easily rubbed off. Then place the new Climara® system on a different skin site. (The same skin site should not be used again for at least 1 week after removal of the system). Contact with water when you are bathing, swimming, or showering will not affect the system. In the unlikely event that a system should fall off, a new system should be applied for the remainder of the 7-day dosing interval.

USES OF ESTROGEN

(Not every estrogen drug is approved for every use listed in this section. If you want to know which of these possible uses are approved for the medicine prescribed for you, ask your doctor or pharmacist to show you the professional labeling. You can also look up the specific estrogen product in a book called the "Physician's Desk Reference", which is available in many book stores and public libraries. Generic drugs carry virtually the same labeling information as their brand name versions.)

- **To reduce moderate or severe menopausal symptoms.**
  Estrogens are hormones made by the ovaries of normal women. Between ages 45 and 55, the ovaries normally stop making estrogens. This leads to a drop in body estrogen levels which causes the "change of life" or menopause (the end of monthly menstrual periods). If both ovaries are removed during an operation before natural menopause takes place, the sudden drop in estrogen levels causes "surgical menopause".
  When the estrogen levels begin dropping, some women develop very uncomfortable symptoms, such as feelings of warmth in the face, neck, and chest, or sudden intense episodes of heat and sweating ("hot flashes" or "hot flushes"). Using estrogen drugs can help the body adjust to lower estrogen levels and reduce these symptoms. Most women have only mild menopausal symptoms or none at all and do not need to use estrogen drugs for these symptoms. Others may need to take estrogens for a few months while their bodies adjust to lower estrogen levels. The majority of women do not need estrogen replacement for longer than six months for these symptoms.
- **To treat vulval and vaginal atrophy** (itching, burning, dryness in or around the vagina, difficulty or burning on urination) associated with menopause.
- **To treat certain conditions in which a young woman's ovaries do not produce enough estrogen naturally.**
- **To treat certain types of abnormal vaginal bleeding due to hormonal imbalance when your doctor has found no serious cause of the bleeding.**
- **To treat certain cancers in special situations, in men and women.**
- **To prevent thinning of bones.**
  Osteoporosis is a thinning of the bones that makes them weaker and allows them to break more easily. The bones of the spine, wrists and hips break most often in osteoporosis. Both men and women start to lose bone mass after about age 40, but women lose bone mass faster after the menopause. Using estrogens after the menopause slows down bone thinning and may prevent bones from breaking. Lifelong adequate calcium intake, either in the diet (such as dairy products) or by calcium supplements (to reach a total daily intake of 1000 milligrams per day before menopause or 1500 milligrams per day after menopause), may help to prevent osteoporosis. Regular weight-bearing exercise (like walking and running for an hour, two or three times a week) may also help to prevent osteoporosis. Before you change your calcium intake or exercise habits, it is important to discuss these lifestyle changes with your doctor to find out if they are safe for you.
  Since estrogen use has some risks, only women who are likely to develop osteoporosis should use estrogens for prevention. Women who are likely to develop osteoporosis often have the following characteristics: white or Asian race, slim, cigarette smokers, and a family history of osteoporosis in a mother, sister, or aunt. Women who have relatively early menopause, often because their ovaries were removed during an operation ("surgical menopause"), are more likely to develop osteoporosis than women whose menopause happens at the average age.

WHO SHOULD NOT USE ESTROGENS

Estrogens should not be used:

- **During pregnancy (see Boxed Warning).**
  If you think you may be pregnant, do not use any form of estrogen-containing drug. Using estrogens while you are pregnant may cause your unborn child to have birth defects. Estrogens do not prevent miscarriage.
- **If you have unusual vaginal bleeding which has not been evaluated by your doctor (see Boxed Warning).**
  Unusual vaginal bleeding can be a warning sign of cancer of the uterus, especially if it happens after menopause. Your doctor must find out the cause of the bleeding so that he or she can recommend the proper treatment. Taking estrogens without visiting your doctor can cause you serious harm if your vaginal bleeding is caused by cancer of the uterus.
- **If you have had cancer.**
  Since estrogens increase the risk of certain types of cancer, you should not use estrogens if you have ever had cancer of the breast or uterus, unless your doctor recommends that the drug may help in the cancer treatment. (For certain patients with breast or prostate cancer, estrogens may help).
- **If you have any circulation problems.**
  Estrogen drugs should not be used except in unusually special situations in which your doctor judges that you need estrogen therapy so much that the risks are acceptable. Men and women with abnormal blood clotting conditions should avoid estrogen use (see Dangers of Estrogens, below).
- **When they do not work.**
  During menopause, some women develop nervous symptoms or depression. Estrogens do not relieve these symptoms. You may have heard that taking estrogens for years after menopause will keep your skin soft and supple and keep you feeling young. There is no evidence for these claims and such long-term estrogen use may have serious risks.
- **After childbirth or when breastfeeding a baby.**
  Estrogens should not be used to try to stop the breasts from filling with milk after a baby is born. Such treatment may increase the risk of developing blood clots (see Dangers of Estrogens, below).
  If you are breastfeeding, you should avoid using any drugs because many drugs pass through to the baby in the milk. While nursing a baby, you should take drugs only on the advice of your health care provider.

DANGERS OF ESTROGENS

- **Cancer of the uterus.**
  Your risk of developing cancer of the uterus gets higher the longer you use estrogens and the larger doses you use. One study showed that after women stop taking estrogens, this higher cancer risk quickly returns to the usual level of risk (as if you had never used estrogen therapy). Three other studies showed that the cancer risk stayed high for 8 to more than 15 years after stopping estrogen treatment. Because of this risk. **IT IS IMPORTANT TO TAKE THE LOWEST DOSE THAT WORKS AND TO TAKE IT ONLY AS LONG AS YOU NEED IT.**
  Using progestin therapy together with estrogen therapy may reduce the higher risk of uterine cancer related to estrogen use (but see Other Information, below.)
  If you have had your uterus removed (total hysterectomy), there is no danger of developing cancer of the uterus.
- **Cancer of the breast.**
  Most studies have not shown a higher risk of breast cancer in women who have ever used estrogens. However, some studies have reported that breast cancer developed more often (up to twice the usual rate) in women who used estrogens for long periods of time (especially more than 10 years), or who used higher doses for shorter time periods. Regular breast examinations by a health professional and monthly self-examination are recommended for all women.
- **Gallbladder disease.**
  Women who use estrogens after menopause are more likely to develop gallbladder disease needing surgery than women who do not use estrogens.
- **Abnormal blood clotting.**
  Taking estrogens may cause changes in your blood clotting system. These changes allow the blood to clot more easily, possibly allowing clots to form in your bloodstream. If blood clots do form in your bloodstream, they can cut off the blood supply to vital organs, causing serious problems. These problems may include a stroke (by cutting off blood to the brain), a heart attack (by cutting off blood to the heart), a pulmonary embolus (by cutting off blood to the lungs), or other problems. Any of these conditions may cause death or serious long-term disability. However, most studies of low dose estrogen usage by women do not show an increased risk of these complications.

SIDE EFFECTS

In addition to the risks listed above, the following side effects have been reported with estrogen use:

—Nausea and vomiting.
—Breast tenderness or enlargement.
—Enlargement of benign tumors ("fibroids") of the uterus.
—Retention of excess fluid. This may make some conditions worsen, such as asthma, epilepsy, migraine, heart disease, or kidney disease.
—A spotty darkening of the skin, particularly on the face.

REDUCING RISK OF ESTROGEN USE

If you use estrogens, you can reduce your risks by doing these things:

- **See your doctor regularly.**
  While you are using estrogens, it is important to visit your doctor at least once a year for a check-up. If you develop vaginal bleeding while taking estrogens, you may need further evaluation. If members of your family have had breast cancer or if you have ever had breast lumps or an abnormal mammogram (breast x-ray), you may need to have more frequent breast examinations.
- **Reassess your need for estrogens.**
  You and your doctor should reevaluate whether or not you still need estrogens at least every six months.

Continued on next page

Information on the Berlex products appearing here is based on the most current information available at the time of publication closing. Further information for these and other products may be obtained from the Medical Affairs Department, Berlex Laboratories, 300 Fairfield Road, Wayne, New Jersey 07470, 1-800-888-2407. Information on Betaseron and Fludara may be obtained from Berlex Laboratories, 15049 San Pablo Avenue, Richmond, California 94804-0016, 1-800-888-4112.

Berlex Laboratories—Cont.

- **Be alert for signs of trouble.**
  If any of these warning signals (or any other unusual symptoms) happen while you are using estrogens, call your doctor immediately:
  Abnormal bleeding from the vagina (possible uterine cancer)
  Pains in the calves or chest, sudden shortness of breath, or coughing blood (possible clot in the legs, heart, or lungs)
  Severe headache or vomiting, dizziness, faintness, changes in vision or speech, weakness or numbness of an arm or leg (possible clot in the brain or eye)
  Breast lumps (possible breast cancer; ask your doctor or health professional to show you how to examine your breasts monthly)
  Yellowing of the skin or eyes (possible liver problem)
  Pain, swelling, or tenderness in the abdomen (possible gallbladder problem)

OTHER INFORMATION

1. Estrogens increase the risk of developing a condition (endometrial hyperplasia) that may lead to cancer of the lining of the uterus. Taking progestins, another hormone drug, with estrogens lowers the risk of developing this condition. Therefore, if your uterus has not been removed, your doctors may prescribe a progestin for you to take together with your estrogen.

You should know, however, that taking estrogens with progestins may have additional risks. These include:

—unhealthy effects on blood fats (especially a lowering of HDL blood cholesterol, the "good" blood fat which protects against heart disease);

—unhealthy effects on blood sugar (which might make a diabetic condition worse); and

—a possible further increase in breast cancer risk which may be associated with long-term estrogen use.

Some research has shown that estrogens taken *without* progestins may protect women against developing heart disease. However, this is not certain. The protection shown may have been caused by the characteristics of the estrogen-treated women, and not by the estrogen treatment itself. In general, treated women were slimmer, more physically active, and were less likely to have diabetes than the untreated women. These characteristics are known to protect against heart disease.

You are cautioned to discuss very carefully with your doctor or health care provider all the possible risks and benefits of long-term estrogen and progestin treatment as they affect you personally.

2. Your doctor has prescribed this drug for you and you alone. Do not give the drug to anyone else.

3. If you will be taking calcium supplements as part of the treatment to help prevent osteoporosis, check with your doctor about how much to take.

4. Keep this and all drugs out of the reach of children. In case of overdose, call your doctor, hospital or poison control center immediately.

5. This leaflet provides a summary of the most important information about estrogens. If you want more information, ask your doctor or pharmacist to show you the professional labeling. The professional labeling is also published in a book called the "Physicians' Desk Reference," which is available in book stores and public libraries. Generic drugs carry virtually the same labeling information as their brand name versions.

Do not store above 86°F (30°C). Do not store unpouched. Apply immediately upon removal from the protective pouch.

CAUTION: Federal law prohibits dispensing without prescription.

Manufactured for Berlex Laboratories, Wayne, NJ 07470
Manufactured by 3M Pharmaceuticals, St. Paul, MN 55144
©1995, Berlex Laboratories.
All Rights Reserved.
617201 January 1995
617300 January 1995
BERLEX LABORATORIES,
WAYNE, NJ 07470

Shown in Product Identification Guide, page 305

QUINAGLUTE ℞
DURA-TABS® TABLETS
[*kwĭn 'uh glōōt*]
(BRAND OF QUINIDINE GLUCONATE EXTENDED-RELEASE TABLETS, USP)

DESCRIPTION

Quinidine is an antimalarial schizonticide and an antiarrhythmic agent with Class Ia activity; it is the d-isomer of quinine, and its molecular weight is 324.43. Quinidine gluconate is the gluconate salt of quinidine; its chemical name is cinchonan-9-ol, 6'-methoxy-, (9S)-, mono-D-gluconate; its structural formula is:

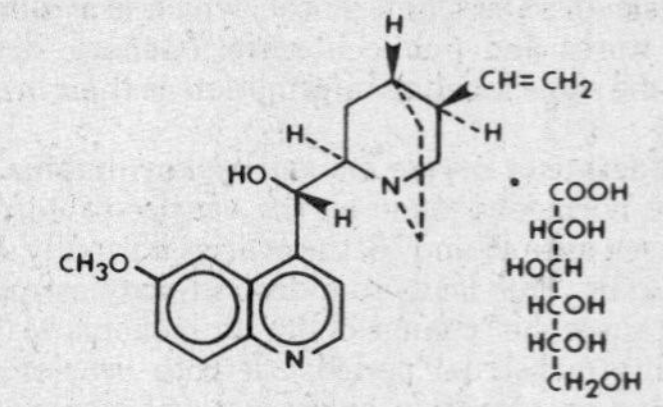

Its empirical formula is $C_{20}H_{24}N_2O_2 \cdot C_6H_{12}O_7$; and its molecular weight is 520.58, of which 62.3% is quinidine base.

Each QUINAGLUTE DURA-TABS® tablet contains 324 mg of quinidine gluconate (202 mg of quinidine base) in a matrix to provide extended-release; the inactive ingredients include confectioner's sugar, magnesium stearate, corn starch and other ingredients. Meets USP Drug Release Test 4.

CLINICAL PHARMACOLOGY

Pharmacokinetics and Metabolism:

The absolute **bioavailability** of quinidine from QUINAGLUTE® is 70–80%. Relative to a solution of quinidine sulfate, the bioavailability of quinidine from QUINAGLUTE® is reported to be 1.03. The less-than-complete bioavailability is thought to be due to first-pass elimination by the liver. Peak serum levels generally appear 3–5 hours after dosing; when the drug is taken with food, absorption is increased in both rate (27%) and extent (17%). The rate and extent of absorption of quinidine from QUINAGLUTE® are not significantly affected by the coadministration of an aluminum-hydroxide antacid.

The **volume of distribution** of quinidine is 2–3 L/kg in healthy young adults, but this may be reduced to as little as 0.5 L/kg in patients with congestive heart failure, or increased to 3–5 L/kg in patients with cirrhosis of the liver. At concentrations of 2–5 mg/L (6.5–16.2 μmol/L), the fraction of quinidine bound to plasma proteins (mainly to α_1-acid glycoprotein and to albumin) is 80–88% in adults and older children, but it is lower in pregnant women, and in infants and neonates it may be as low as 50–70%. Because α_1-acid glycoprotein levels are increased in response to stress, serum levels of total quinidine may be greatly increased in settings such as acute myocardial infarction, even though the serum content of unbound (active) drug may remain normal. Protein binding is also increased in chronic renal failure, but binding abruptly descends toward or below normal when heparin is administered for hemodialysis.

Quinidine **clearance** typically proceeds at 3–5 ml/min/kg in adults, but clearance in children may be twice or three times as rapid. The elimination half-life is 6–8 hours in adults and 3–4 hours in children. Quinidine clearance is unaffected by hepatic cirrhosis, so the increased volume of distribution seen in cirrhosis leads to a proportionate increase in the elimination half-life.

Most quinidine is eliminated hepatically via the action of cytochrome P450IIIA4; there are several different hydroxylated metabolites, and some of these have antiarrhythmic activity.

The most important of quinidine's metabolites is 3-hydroxyquinidine (3HQ), serum levels of which can approach those of quinidine in patients receiving conventional doses of QUINAGLUTE®. The volume of distribution of 3HQ appears to be larger than that of quinidine, and the elimination half-life of 3HQ is about 12 hours.

As measured by antiarrhythmic effects on animals, by QT_c prolongation in human volunteers, or by various *in vitro* techniques, 3HQ has at least half the antiarrhythmic activity of the parent compound, so it may be responsible for a substantial fraction of the effect of QUINAGLUTE® in chronic use.

When the urine pH is less than 7, about 20% of administered quinidine appears unchanged in the urine, but this fraction drops to as little as 5% when the urine is more alkaline. Renal clearance involves both glomerular filtration and active tubular secretion, moderated by (pH-dependent) tubular reabsorption. The net renal clearance is about 1 ml/min/kg in healthy adults.

When renal function is taken into account, quinidine clearance is apparently independent of patient age.

Assays of serum quinidine levels are widely available, but the results of modern assays may not be consistent with results cited in the older medical literature. The serum levels of quinidine cited in this package insert are those derived from specific assays, using either benzene extraction or (preferably) reverse-phase high-pressure liquid chromatography. In matched samples, older assays might unpredictably have given results that were as much as two or three times higher. A typical "therapeutic" concentration range is 2–6 mg/L (6.2–18.5 μmol/L).

Mechanisms of action

In patients with malaria, quinidine acts primarily as an intraerythrocytic schizonticide, with little effect upon sporozites or upon pre-erythrocytic parasites. Quinidine is gametocidal to *Plasmodium vivax* and *P. malariae*, but not to *P. falciparum*.

In cardiac muscle and in Purkinje fibers, quinidine depresses the rapid inward depolarizing sodium current, thereby slowing phase-0 depolarization and reducing the amplitude of the action potential without affecting the resting potential. In normal Purkinje fibers, it reduces the slope of phase-4 depolarization, shifting the threshold voltage upward toward zero. The result is slowed conduction and reduced automaticity in all parts of the heart, with increase of the effective refractory period relative to the duration of the action potential in the atria, ventricles, and Purkinje tissues. Quinidine also raises the fibrillation thresholds of the atria and ventricles, and it raises the ventricular defibrillation threshold as well. Quinidine's actions fall into Class Ia in the Vaughn-Williams classification.

By slowing conduction and prolonging the effective refractory period, quinidine can interrupt or prevent reentrant arrhythmias and arrhythmias due to increased automaticity, including atrial flutter, atrial fibrillation, and paroxysmal supraventricular tachycardia.

In patients with sick sinus syndrome, quinidine can cause marked sinus node depression and bradycardia. In most patients, however, use of quinidine is associated with an increase in the sinus rate.

Like other antiarrhythmic drugs with Class Ia activity, quinidine prolongs the QT interval in a dose-related fashion. This may lead to increased ventricular automaticity and polymorphic ventricular tachycardias, including *torsades de pointes* (see **Warnings**).

In addition, quinidine has anticholinergic activity, it has negative inotropic activity, and it acts peripherally as an α-adrenergic antagonist (that is, as a vasodilator).

CLINICAL EFFECTS

Maintenance of sinus rhythm after conversion from atrial fibrillation: In six clinical trials (published between 1970 and 1984) with a total of 808 patients, quinidine (418 patients) was compared to nontreatment (258 patients) or placebo (132 patients) for the maintenance of sinus rhythm after cardioversion from chronic atrial fibrillation. Quinidine was consistently more efficacious in maintaining sinus rhythm, but a meta-analysis found that mortality in the quinidine-exposed patients (2.9%) was significantly greater than mortality in the patients who had not been treated with active drug (0.8%). Suppression of atrial fibrillation with quinidine has theoretical patient benefits (e.g., improved exercise tolerance; reduction in hospitalization for cardioversion; lack of arrhythmia-related palpitations, dyspnea and chest pain; reduced incidence of systemic embolism and/or stroke), but these benefits have never been demonstrated in clinical trials. Some of these benefits (e.g., reduction in stroke incidence) may be achievable by other means (anticoagulation).

By slowing the atrial rate in atrial flutter/fibrillation, quinidine can decrease the degree of atrioventricular block and can cause an increase, sometimes marked, in the rate at which supraventricular impulses are successfully conducted by the atrioventricular node, with the resultant paradoxical increase in ventricular rate (see **Warnings**).

Non-life-threatening ventricular arrhythmias: In studies of patients with a variety of ventricular arrhythmias (mainly frequent ventricular premature beats and non-sustained ventricular tachycardia, quinidine (total n=502) has been compared with flecainide (n=141), mexiletine (n=246), propafenone (n=53), and tocainide (n=67). In each of these studies, the mortality in the quinidine group was numerically greater than the mortality in the comparator group. When the studies were combined in a meta-analysis quinidine was associated with a statistically significant threefold relative risk of death.

At therapeutic doses, quinidine's only consistent effect upon the surface electrocardiogram is an increase in the QT interval. This prolongation can be monitored as a guide to safety, and it may provide better guidance than serum drug levels (see **Warnings**).

INDICATIONS AND USAGE

Conversion of atrial fibrillation/flutter: In patients with symptomatic atrial fibrillation/flutter whose symptoms are not adequately controlled by measures that reduce the rate of ventricular response, QUINAGLUTE® is indicated as a means of restoring normal sinus rhythm. If this use of QUINAGLUTE® does not restore sinus rhythm within a reasonable time (see **Dosage and Administration**), then QUINAGLUTE® should be discontinued.

Reduction of frequency of relapse into atrial fibrillation/flutter: Chronic therapy with QUINAGLUTE® is indicated for some patients at high risk of symptomatic atrial fibrillation/flutter, generally patients who have had previous episodes of atrial fibrillation/flutter that were so frequent and poorly tolerated as to outweigh, in the judgment of the physician and the patient, the risks of prophylactic therapy with QUINAGLUTE®. The increased risk of death should specifically be considered. QUINAGLUTE® should be used only after alternative measures (e.g., use of other drugs to control the ventricular rate) have been found to be inadequate.

In patients with histories of frequent symptomatic episodes of atrial fibrillation/flutter, the goal of therapy should be an increase in the average time between episodes. In most patients, the tachyarrhythmia *will recur* during therapy, and a single recurrence should not be interpreted as therapeutic failure.

Suppression of ventricular arrhythmias: QUINAGLUTE® is also indicated for the suppression of recurrent documented ventricular arrhythmias, such as sustained ventricular tachycardia, that in the judgment of the physician are life-threatening. Because of the proarryhthmic effects of quinidine, its use with ventricular arrhythmias of lesser severity is generally not reccommended and treatment of patients with asymptomatic ventricular premature contractions should be avoided. Where possible, therapy should be guided by the results of programmed electrical stimulation and/or Holter monitoring with exercise.

Antiarrhythmic drugs (including QUINAGLUTE®) have not been shown to enhance survival in patients with ventricular arrhythmias.

CONTRAINDICATIONS

Quinidine is contraindicated in patients who are known to be allergic to it, or who have developed thrombocytopenic purpura during prior therapy with quinidine or quinine.

In the absence of a functioning artificial pacemaker, quinidine is also contraindicated in any patient whose cardiac rhythm is dependent upon a junctional or idioventricular pacemaker, including patients in complete atrioventricular block.

Quinidine is also contraindicated in patients who, like those with myasthenia gravis, might be adversely affected by an anticholinergic agent.

WARNINGS
Mortality:

> **In many trials of antiarrhythmic therapy for non-life-threatening arrhythmias, active antiarrhythmic therapy has resulted in increased mortality; the risk of active therapy is probably greatest in patients with structural heart disease.**
>
> **In the case of quinidine used to prevent or defer recurrence of atrial flutter/fibrillation, the best available data come from a meta-analysis described under** *Clinical Pharmacology/Clinical Effects* **above. In the patients studied in the trials there analyzed, the mortality associated with the use of quinidine was more than three times as great as the mortality associated with the use of placebo.**
>
> **Another meta-analysis, also described under** *Clinical Pharmacology/Clinical Effects,* **showed that in patients with various non-life-threatening ventricular arrhythmias, the mortality associated with the use of quinidine was consistently greater than that associated with the use of any of a variety of alternative antiarrhythmics.**

Proarrhythmic effects: Like many other drugs (including all other Class Ia antiarrhythmics), quinidine prolongs the QT_c interval, and this can lead to *torsades de pointes,* a life-threatening ventricular arrhythmia (see **Overdosage**). The risk of *torsades* is increased by bradycardia, hypokalemia, hypomagnesemia or high serum levels of quinidine, but it may appear in the absence of any of these risk factors. The best predictor of this arrhythmia appears to be the length of QT_c interval, and quinidine should be used with extreme care in patients who have preexisting long-QT syndromes, who have histories of *torsades de pointes* of any cause, or who have previously responded to quinidine (or other drugs that prolong ventricular repolarization) with marked lengthening of the QT_c interval. Estimation of the incidence of *torsades* in patients with therapeutic levels of quinidine is not possible from the available data.

Other ventricular arrhythmias that have been reported with quinidine include frequent extrasystoles, ventricular tachycardia, ventricular flutter, and ventricular fibrillation.

Paradoxical increase in ventricular rate in atrial flutter/fibrillation: When quinidine is administered to patients with atrial flutter/fibrillation, the desired pharmacologic reversion to sinus rhythm may (rarely) be preceded by a slowing of the atrial rate with a consequent increase in the rate of beats conducted to the ventricles. The resulting ventricular rate may be very high (greater than 200 beats per minute) and poorly tolerated. This hazard may be decreased if partial atrioventricular block is achieved prior to initiation of quinidine therapy, using conduction-reducing drugs such as digitalis, verapamil, diltiazem, or β-receptor blocking agents.

Exacerbated bradycardia in sick sinus syndrome: In patients with the sick sinus syndrome, quinidine has been associated with marked sinus node depression and bradycardia.

Pharmacokinetic considerations: Renal or hepatic dysfunction causes the elimination of quinidine to be slowed, while congestive heart failure causes a reduction in quinidine's apparent volume of distribution. Any of these conditions can lead to quinidine toxicity if dosage is not approximately reduced. In addition, interactions with coadministered drugs can alter the serum concentration and activity of quinidine, leading either to toxicity or to lack of efficacy if the dose of quinidine is not appropriately modified. (See **Precautions/Drug Interactions**.)

Vagolysis: Because quinidine opposes the atrial and A-V nodal effects of vagal stimulation, physical or pharmacological vagal maneuvers undertaken to terminate paroxysmal supraventricular tachycardia may be ineffective in patients receiving quinidine.

PRECAUTIONS
Heart block
In patients without implanted pacemakers who are at high risk of complete atrioventricular block (e.g., those with digitalis intoxication, second degree atrioventricular block, or severe intraventricular conduction defects), quinidine should be used only with caution.

Drug Interactions
Altered pharmacokinetics of quinidine: Drugs that alkalinize the urine (**carbonic-anhydrase inhibitors, sodium bicarbonate, thiazide diuretics**) reduce renal elimination of quinidine.

By pharmacokinetic mechanisms that are not well understood, quinidine levels are increased by coadministration of **amiodarone** or **cimetidine.** Very rarely, and again by mechanisms not understood, quinidine levels are decreased by coadministration of **nifedipine.**

Hepatic elimination of quinidine may be accelerated by coadministration of drugs (**phenobarbital, phenytoin, rifampin**) that include production of cytochrome P450IIIA4.

Perhaps because of competition for the P450IIIA4 metabolic pathway, quinidine levels rise when **ketaconazole** is coadministered.

Coadministration of **propranolol** usually does not affect quinidine pharmacokinetics, but in some studies the β-blocker appeared to cause increases in the peak serum levels of quinidine, decreases in quinidine's volume of distribution, and decreases in total quinidine clearance. The effects (if any) of coadministration of other β-blockers on quinidine pharmacokinetics have not been adequately studied.

Hepatic clearance of quinidine is significantly reduced during coadministration of **verapamil,** with corresponding increases in serum levels and half-life.

Altered pharmacokinetics of other drugs: Quinidine slows the elimination of **digoxin** and simultaneously reduces digoxin's apparent volume of distribution. As a result, serum digoxin levels may be as much as doubled. When quinidine and digoxin are coadministered, digoxin doses usually need to be reduced. Serum levels of **digitoxin** are also raised when quinidine is coadministered, although the effect appears to be smaller.

By a mechanism that is not understood, quinidine potentiates the anticoagulatory action of **warfarin,** and the anticoagulant dosage may need to be reduced.

Cytochrome P450IID6 is an enzyme critical to the metabolism of many drugs, notably including **mexiletine,** some **phenothiazines,** and most **polycyclic antidepressants.** Constitutional deficiency of cytochrome P450IID6 is found in less than 1% of Orientals, in about 2% of American blacks, and in about 8% of American whites. Testing with debrisoquine is sometimes used to distinguish the P450IID6-deficient "poor metabolizers" from the majority-phenotype "extensive metabolizers".

When drugs whose metabolism is P450IID6-dependent are given to poor metabolizers, the serum levels achieved are higher, sometimes much higher, than the serum levels achieved when identical doses are given to extensive metabolizers. To obtain similar clinical benefit without toxicity, doses given to poor metabolizers may need to be greatly reduced. In the case of prodrugs whose actions are actually mediated by P450IID6-produced metabolites (for example, **codeine** and **hydrocodone,** whose analgesic and antitussive effects appear to be mediated by morphine and hydromorphone, respectively), it may be possible to achieve the desired clinical benefits in poor metabolizers.

Quinidine is not metabolized by cytochrome P450IID6, but therapeutic serum levels of quinidine inhibit the action of cytochrome P450IID6, effectively converting extensive metabolizers into poor metabolizers. Caution must be exercised whenever quinidine is prescribed together with drugs metabolized by cytochrome P450IID6.

Perhaps by competing for pathways of renal clearance, coadministration of quinidine causes an increase in serum levels of **procainamide.**

Serum levels of **haloperidol** are increased when quinidine is coadministered.

Presumably because both drugs are metabolized by cytochrome P450IIIA4, coadministration of quinidine causes variable slowing of the metabolism of **nifedipine.** Interactions with other dihydropyridine calcium channel blockers have not been reported, but these agents (including **felodipine, nicardipine,** and **nimodipine**) are all dependent upon P450IIIA4 for metabolism, so similar interactions with quinidine should be anticipated.

Altered pharmacodynamics of other drugs: Quinidine's anticholinergic, vasodilating, and negative inotropic actions may be additive to those of other drugs with these effects, and antagonistic to those of drugs with cholinergic, vasoconstricting, and positive inotropic effects. For example, when quinidine and **verapamil** are coadministered in doses that are each well tolerated as monotherapy, hypotension attributable to additive peripheral α-blockade is sometimes reported.

Quinidine potentiates the actions of depolarizing (succinylcholine, decamethonium) and nondepolarizing (d-tubocurarine, pancuronium) **neuromuscular blocking agents.** These phenomena are not well understood, but they are observed in animal models as well as in humans. In addtion, *in vitro* addition of quinidine to the serum of pregnant women reduces the activity of pseudocholinesterase, an enzyme that is essential to the metabolism of succinylcholine.

Non-interactions of quinidine with other drugs: Quinidine has no clinically significant effect on the pharmacokinetics of **diltiazem, flecainide, mephenytoin, metoprolol, propafenone, propranolol, quinine, timolol,** or **tocainide.**
Conversely, the pharmacokinetics of quinidine are not significantly affected by **caffeine, ciprofloxacin, digoxin, diltiazem, felodipine, omeprazole,** or **quinine.** Quinidine's pharmacokinetics are also unaffected by cigarette smoking.

INFORMATION FOR PATIENTS
Before prescibing QUINAGLUTE® as prophylaxis against recurrence of atrial fibrillation, the physician should inform the patient of the risks and benefits to be expected (see **Clinical Pharmacology**). Discussion should include the facts.

- that the goal of therapy will be a reduction (probably not to zero) in the frequency of episodes of atrial fibrillation; and
- that reduced frequency of fibrillatory episodes may be expected, if achieved, to bring symptomatic benefit; but
- that no data are available to show that reduced frequency of fibrillatory episodes will reduce the risks of irreversible harm through stroke or death; and in fact
- that such data as are available suggest that treatment with QUINAGLUTE® is likely to increase the patient's risk of death.

Carcinogenesis, mutagenesis, impairment of fertility
Animal studies to evaluate quinidine's carcinogenic or mutagenic potential have not been performed. Similarly, there are no animal data as to quinidine's potential to impair fertility.

Pregnancy
Pregnancy Category C. Animal reproductive studies have not been conducted with quinidine. There are no adequate and well-controlled studies in pregnant women. Quinidine should be given to a pregnant woman only if clearly needed. In one neonate whose mother had received quinidine throughout her pregnancy, the serum level of quinidine was equal to that of the mother, with no apparent ill effect. The level of quinidine in amniotic fluid was about three times higher than that found in serum.

Labor and Delivery
Quinine is said to be oxytocic in humans, but there are no adequate data as to quinidine's effects (if any) on human labor and delivery.

Nursing mothers
Quinidine is present in human milk at levels slightly lower than those in maternal serum; a human infant ingesting such milk should (scaling directly by weight) be expected to develop serum quinidine levels at least an order of magnitude lower than those of the mother. On the other hand, the pharmacokinetics and pharmacodynamics of quinidine in human infants have not been adequately studied, and neonates' reduced protein binding of quinidine may increase their risk of toxicity at low total serum levels. Administration of quinidine should (if possible) be avoided in lactating women who continue to nurse.

Geriatric use
Safety and efficacy of quinidine in elderly patients have not been systematically studied.

Pediatric use
In antimalarial trials, quinidine was as safe and effective in pediatric patients as in adults. Notwithstanding the known pharmacokinetic differences between children and adults (see **Parmacokinetics and Metabolism**), children in these trials received the same doses (on a mg/kg basis) as adults. Safety and effectiveness of antiarrhythmic use in children have not been established.

Continued on next page

Information on the Berlex products appearing here is based on the most current information available at the time of publication closing. Further information for these and other products may be obtained from the Medical Affairs Department, Berlex Laboratories, 300 Fairfield Road, Wayne, New Jersey 07470, 1-800-888-2407. Information on Betaseron and Fludara may be obtained from Berlex Laboratories, 15049 San Pablo Avenue, Richmond, California 94804-0016, 1-800-888-4112.

Berlex Laboratories—Cont.

ADVERSE REACTIONS

Quinidine preparations have been used for many years, but there are only sparse data from which to estimate the incidence of various adverse reactions. The adverse reactions most frequently reported have consistently been gastrointestinal, including diarrhea, nausea, vomiting, and heartburn/esophagitis.

In the reported study that was closest in character to the predominant approved use of QUINAGLUTE®, 86 adult outpatients with atrial fibrillation were followed for six months while they received slow-release quinidine bisulfate tablets, 600 mg quinidine (approximately 400 mg of quinidine base) twice daily. The incidences of reported adverse experiences were as shown in the table below. The most serious quinidine-associated adverse reactions are described above under **Warnings.**

ADVERSE EXPERIENCES REPORTED MORE THAN ONCE IN 86 PATIENTS WITH ATRIAL FIBRILLATION

	Incidence (%)
diarrhea	21 (24%)
fever	5 (6%)
rash	5 (6%)
arrthythmia	3 (3%)
abnormal electrocardiogram	3 (3%)
nausea/vomiting	3 (3%)
dizziness	3 (3%)
headache	3 (3%)
asthenia	2 (2%)
cerebral ischemia	2 (2%)

Vomiting and diarrhea can occur as isolated reactions to therapeutic levels of quinidine, but they may also be the first signs of **cinchonism,** a syndrome that may also include tinnitus, reversible high-frequency hearing loss, deafness, vertigo, blurred vision, diplopia, photophobia, headache, confusion, and delirium. Cinchonism is most often a sign of chronic quinidine toxicity, but it may appear in sensitive patients after a single moderate dose.

A few cases of **hepatotoxicity,** including granulomatous hepatitis, have been reported in patients receiving quinidine. All of these have appeared during the first few weeks of therapy, and most (not all) have remitted once quinidine was withdrawn.

Autoimmune and inflammatory syndromes associated with quinidine therapy have included fever, urticaria, flushing, exfoliative rash, bronchospasm, psoriaform rash, pruritus and lymphadenopathy, hemolytic anemia, vasculitis, thrombocytopenic purpura, uveitis, angioedema, agranulocytosis, the sicca syndrome, arthralgia, myalgia, elevation in serum levels of skeletal-muscle enzymes, and a disorder resembling systemic lupus erythematosus, and pneumonitis.

Convulsions, apprehension, and ataxia have been reported, but it is not clear that these were not simply the results of hypotension and consequent cerebral hypoperfusion. There are many reports of syncope. Acute psychotic reactions have been reported to follow the first dose of quinidine, but these reactions appear to be extremely rare.

Other adverse reactions occasionally reported include depression, mydriasis, disturbed color perception, night blindness, scotomata, optic neurtis, visual field loss, photosensitivity, and abnormalities of pigmentation.

OVERDOSAGE

Overdoses with various oral formulations of quinidine have been well described. Death has been described after a 5-gram ingestion by a toddler, while an adolescent was reported to survive after ingesting 8 grams of quinidine.

The most important ill effects of acute quinidine overdoses are ventricular arrhythmias and hypotension. Other symptoms of overdose may include vomiting, diarrhea, tinnitus, high-frequency hearing loss, vertigo, blurred vision, diplopia, photophobia, headache, confusion and delirium.

Arrhythmias: Serum quinidine levels can be conveniently assayed and monitored, but the electrocardiographic QT_c interval is a better predictor of quinidine-induced ventricular arrhythmias.

The necessary treatment of hemodynamically unstable polymorphic ventricular tachycardia (including *torsades de pointes*) is withdrawal of treatment with quinidine and either immediate cardioversion or, if a cardiac pacemaker is in place or immediately available, immediate overdrive pacing. After pacing or cardioversion, further management must be guided by the length of the QT_c interval.

Quinidine-associated ventricular tachyarrhythmias with normal underlying QT_c intervals have not been adequately studied. Because of the theoretical possibility of QT-prolonging effects that might be additive to those of quinidine, other antiarrhythmics with Class I (disopyramide, procainamide) or Class III activities should (if possible) be avoided. Similarly, although the use of bretylium in quinidine overdose has not been reported, it is reasonable to expect that the α-blocking properties of bretylium might be additive to those of quinidine, resulting in problematic hypotension.

If the post-cardioversion QT_c interval is prolonged, then the precardioversion polymorphic ventricular tachycardia was (by definition) *torsades de pointes.* In this case, lidocaine and bretylium are unlikely to be of value, and other Class I antiarrhythmics (disopyramide, procainamide) are likely to exacerbate the situation. Factors contributing to QT_c prolongation (especially hypokalemia and hypomagnesemia) should be sought out and (if possible) aggressively corrected. Prevention of recurrent *torsades* may require sustained overdrive pacing or the cautious administration of isoproterenal (30–150 ng/kg/min).

Hypotension: Quinidine-induced hypotension that is not due to an arrhythmia is likely to be a consequence of quinidine-related α-blockade and vasorelaxation. Simple repletion of central volume (Trendelenburg positioning, saline infusion) may be sufficient therapy; other interventions reported to have been beneficial in this setting are those that increase peripheral vascular resistance, including α-agonist catecholamines (norepinephrine, metaraminol) and the Military Anti-Shock Trousers.

Treatment:

To obtain up-to-date information about the treatment of overdose, a good resource is your certified Regional Poison-Control Center. Telephone numbers of certified poison-control centers are listed in the Physicians' Desk Reference (PDR). In managing overdose, consider the possibilities of multiple-drug overdoses, drug-drug interactions, and unusual drug kinetics in your patient.

Accelerated removal: Adequate studies of orally-administered activated charcoal in human overdoses of quinidine have not been reported, but there are animal data showing significant enhancement of systemic elimination following this intervention, and there is at least one human case report in which the elimination half-life of quinidine in the serum was apparently shortened by repeated gastric lavage.

Activated charcoal should be avoided if an ileus is present; the conventional dose is 1 gram/kg administered every 2–6 hours as a slurry with 8 mL/kg of tap water.

Although renal elimination of quinidine might theoretically be accelerated by maneuvers to acidify the urine, such maneuvers are potentially hazardous and of no demonstrated benefit.

Quinidine is not usefully removed from the circulation by dialysis.

Following quinidine overdose, drugs that delay elimination of quinidine (cimetidine, carbonic-anhydrase inhibitors, thiazide diuretics) should be withdrawn unless absolutely required.

DOSAGE AND ADMINISTRATION

The dose of quinidine delivered by QUINAGLUTE DURA-TABS® tablets may be titrated by breaking a tablet in half. If tablets are crushed or chewed, their sustained-release properties will be lost.

The dosage of quinidine varies considerably depending upon the general condition and the cardiovascular state of the patient.

Conversion of atrial fibrillation/flutter to sinus rhythm

Especially in patients with known structural heart disease or other risk factors for toxicity, initiation or dose-adjustment of treatment with QUINAGLUTE® should generally be performed in a setting where facilities and personnel for monitoring and resuscitation are continuously avaliable.

Patients with symptomatic atrial fibrillation/flutter should be treated with QUINAGLUTE® only after ventricular rate control (e.g., with digitalis or β-blockers) has failed to provide satisfactory control of symptoms.

Adequate trials have not identified an optimal regimen of QUINAGLUTE® for conversion of atrial fibrillation/flutter to sinus rhythm. In one reported regimen, the patient first receives two tablets (648 mg; 403 mg of quinidine base) of QUINAGLUTE® every eight hours. If this regimen has not resulted in conversion after 3 or 4 doses, then the dose is cautiously increased. If, at any point during administration, the QRS complex widens to 130% of its pre-treatment duration; the QT_c interval widens to 130% of its pre-treatment duration and is then longer than 500 ms; P waves disappear; or the patient develops significant tachycardia, symptomatic bradycardia, or hypotension, then QUINAGLUTE® is discontinued, and other means of conversion (e.g., direct-current cardioversion) are considered.

In another regimen sometimes used, the patient receives one tablet (324 mg; 202 mg of quinidine base) every eight hours for two days; then two tablets every twelve hours for two days; and finally two tablets every eight hours for up to four days. The four-day stretch may come at one of the lower doses if, in the judgment of the physician, the lower dose is the highest one that will be tolerated. The criteria for discontinuation of treatment with QUINAGLUTE ® are the same as in the other regimen.

Reduction in the frequency of relapse into atrial fibrillation/flutter

In a patient with a history of frequent symptomatic episodes of atrial fibrillation/flutter, the goal of therapy with QUINAGLUTE® should be an increase in the average time between episodes. In most patients, the tachyarrhythmia *will recur* during therapy with QUINAGLUTE®, and a single recurrence should not be interpreted as therapeutic failure.

Especially in patients with known structural heart disease or other risk factors for toxicity, initiation or dose adjustment of treatment with QUINAGLUTE® should generally be performed in a setting where facilities and personnel for monitoring and resuscitation are continously available. Monitoring should be continued for two or three days after initiation of the regimen on which the patient will be discharged.

Therapy with QUINAGLUTE® should be begun with one tablet (324 mg; 202 mg of quinidine base) every eight or twelve hours. If this regimen is well tolerated, and if the serum quinidine level is still well within the laboratory's therapeutic range, and if the average time between arrhythmic episodes has not been satisfactorily increased, then the dose may be cautiously raised. The total daily dosage should be reduced if the QRS complex widens to 130% of its pre-treatment duration; the QT_c interval widens to 130% of its pre-treatment duration and is then longer than 500 ms; P waves disappear; or the patient develops significant tachycardia, symptomatic bradycardia, or hypotension.

Suppression of life-threatening ventricular arrhythmias

Dosing regimens for the use of quinidine gluconate in suppressing life-threatening ventricular arrhythmias have not been adequately studied. Described regimens have generally been similar to the regimen described just above for the prophylaxis of symptomatic atrial fibrillation/flutter. Where possible, therapy should be guided by the results of programmed eletrical stimulation and/or Holter monitoring with exercise.

HOW SUPPLEID

QUINAGLUTE DURA-TABS® tablets are 324 mg white to off-white, round tablets embossed with **C** in a flask design on one side and with a clock-like design on the other.

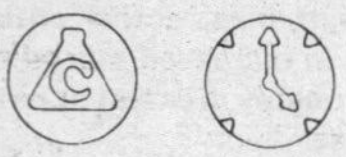

The tablets are available in bottles and unit-dose packages as follows:

bottle of 100	NDC 50419-101-10
bottle of 250	NDC 50419-101-25
bottle of 500	NDC 50419-101-50
unit-dose box of 100	NDC 50419-101-11

Store tablets at controlled room temperature (15–30°C; 59–86°F).

CAUTION: Federal (USA) law prohibits dispensing without prescription.

*Tablet designs are registered trademarks of Berlex Laboratories

BERLEX®Laboratories, Wayne, NJ 07470

Rev. 4/95 60695-1

Shown in Product Identification Guide, page 305

TRI-LEVLEN® 21 ℞

[*trī-lĕvlĕn*]

Tablets

(levonorgestrel and ethinyl estradiol tablets—triphasic regimen)

TRI–LEVLEN® 28 ℞

[*trī-lĕvlĕn*]

Tablets

(levonorgestrel and ethinyl estradiol tablets—triphasic regimen)

LEVLEN® 21 ℞

[*lĕvlĕn*]

Tablets

(levonorgestrel and ethinyl estradiol tablets)

LEVLEN® 28 ℞

[*lĕvlĕn*]

Tablets

(levonorgestrel and ethinyl estradiol tablets)

Patients should be counseled that this product does not protect against HIV infection (AIDS) and other sexually transmitted diseases.

DESCRIPTION

TRI-LEVLEN® 21 tablets

Each cycle of TRI-LEVLEN® 21 (Levonorgestrel and Ethinyl Estradiol Tablets—Triphasic Regimen) tablets consists of three different drug phases as follows: Phase 1 comprised of 6 brown film-coated tablets, each containing 0.050 mg of levonorgestrel (d(-)-13 beta-ethyl-17-alpha-ethinyl-17-beta-hydroxygon-4-en-3-one), a totally synthetic progestogen, and 0.030 mg of ethinyl estradiol (19-nor-17α-pregna-1,3,5(10)-trien-20-yne-3, 17-diol); phase 2 comprised of 5 white film-

coated tablets, each containing 0.075 mg levonorgestrel and 0.040 mg ethinyl estradiol; and, phase 3 comprised of 10 light-yellow film-coated tablets, each containing 0.125 mg levonorgestrel and 0.030 mg ethinyl estradiol. The inactive ingredients present are cellulose, iron oxides, lactose, magnesium stearate, polacrilin potassium, polyethylene glycol, titanium dioxide, and hydroxypropyl methylcellulose.

TRI-LEVLEN® 28 tablets

Each cycle of TRI-LEVLEN® 28 (Levonorgestrel and Ethinyl Estradiol Tablets—Triphasic Regimen) tablets consists of three different drug phases as follows: Phase 1 comprised of 6 brown film-coated tablets, each containing 0.050 mg of levonorgestrel (d(-)-13 beta-ethyl-17-alpha-ethinyl-17-beta-hydroxygon-4-en-3-one), a totally synthetic progestogen, and 0.030 mg of ethinyl estradiol (19-nor-17 α-pregna-1,3,5(10)-trien-20-yne-3, 17-diol); phase 2 comprised of 5 white film-coated tablets, each containing 0.075 mg levonorgestrel and 0.040 mg ethinyl estradiol; and phase 3 comprised of 10 light-yellow film-coated tablets, each containing 0.125 mg levonorgestrel and 0.030 mg ethinyl estradiol; then followed by 7 light-green film-coated inert tablets. The inactive ingredients present are cellulose, F D & C Blue 1, iron oxides, lactose, magnesium stearate, polacrilin potassium, polyethylene glycol, titanium dioxide, and hydroxypropyl methylcellulose.

LEVLEN® 21 tablets:

Each LEVLEN® 21 tablet (Levonorgestrel and Ethinyl Estradiol Tablets) contains 0.15 mg of levonorgestrel (d(-)-13 beta-ethyl-17-alpha-ethinyl-17-beta-hydroxygon-4-en-3-one), a totally synthetic progestogen, and 0.03 mg of ethinyl estradiol (19-nor-17 α-pregna-1,3,5(10)-trien-20-yne-3, 17-diol). The inactive ingredients present are cellulose, FD&C Yellow 6, lactose, magnesium stearate, and polacrillin potassium.

LEVLEN® 28 tablets:

21 light-orange LEVLEN® tablets (Levonorgestrel and Ethinyl Estradiol Tablets), each containing 0.15 mg of levonorgestrel (d(-)-13 beta-ethyl-17-alpha-ethinyl-17-beta-hydroxygon-4-en-3-one), a totally synthetic progestogen, and 0.03 mg of ethinyl estradiol (19-nor-17 α-pregna-1,3,5(10)-trien-20-yne-3, 17-diol), and 7 pink inert tablets. The inactive ingredients present are cellulose, D&C Red 30, FD&C Yellow 6, lactose, magnesium stearate, and polacrillin potassium.

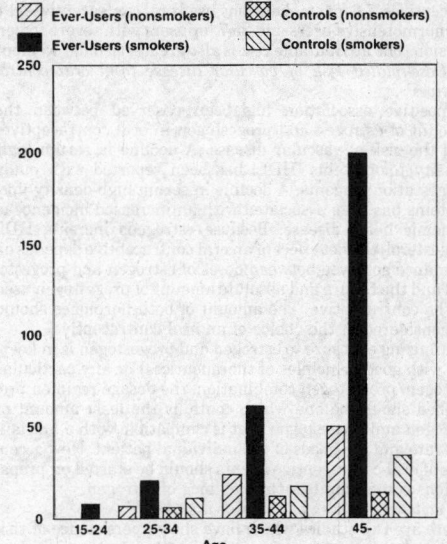

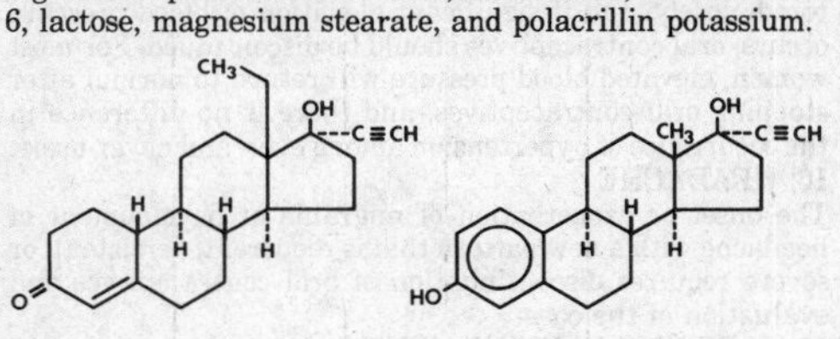

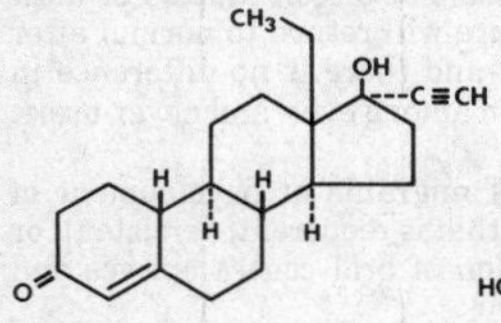

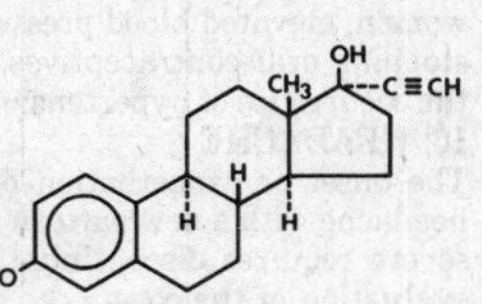

Levonorgestrel   Ethinyl Estradiol

CLINICAL PHARMACOLOGY

Combination oral contraceptives act by suppression of gonadotropins. Although the primary mechanism of this action is inhibition of ovulation, other alterations include changes in the cervical mucus (which increase the difficulty of sperm entry into the uterus) and the endometrium (which reduce the likelihood of implantation).

INDICATIONS AND USAGE

Oral contraceptives are indicated for the prevention of pregnancy in women who elect to use this product as a method of contraception.

Oral contraceptives are highly effective. Table I lists the typical accidental pregnancy rates for users of combination oral contraceptives and other methods of contraception. The efficacy of these contraceptive methods, except sterilization and the IUD, depends upon the reliability with which they are used. Correct and consistent use of methods can result in lower failure rates.

TABLE I: LOWEST EXPECTED AND TYPICAL FAILURE RATES DURING THE FIRST YEAR OF CONTINUOUS USE OF A METHOD

% of Women Experiencing an Accidental Pregnancy in the First Year of Continuous Use

Method	Lowest Expected*	Typical**
(No Contraception)	(85)	(85)
Oral contraceptives		
combined	0.1	3
progestin only	0.5	N/A***
Diaphragm with spermicidal cream or jelly	6	18
Spermicides alone (foam, and vaginal suppositories)	3	21
Vaginal Sponge		
nulliparous	6	18
multiparous	9	28
Depo-Provera (injectable progestogen)	0.3	0.3
NORPLANT® SYSTEM (implants)	0.2#	0.2#
IUD		
progesterone	2	N/A***
copper T 380A	0.8	N/A***
Condom without spermicides	2	12
Periodic abstinence	1–9	20
Female sterilization	0.2	0.4
Male sterilization	0.1	0.15

Adapted from J. Trussell et al., Table I. Studies in Family Planning, 21(1): Jan.–Feb. 1990.

* The authors' best guess of the percentage of women expected to experience an accidental pregnancy among couples who initiate a method (not necessarily for the first time) and who use it consistently and correctly during the first year if they do not stop use for any other reason.

** This term represents "typical" couples who initiate use of a method (not necessarily for the first time), who experience an accidental pregnancy during the first year if they do not stop use for any other reason.

*** N/A—Data not available.

\# This data is based on Norplant System clinical trials.

CONTRAINDICATIONS

Oral contraceptives should not be used in women with any of the following conditions:

Thrombophlebitis or thromboembolic disorders.
A past history of deep-vein thrombophlebitis or thromboembolic disorders.
Cerebral-vascular or coronary-artery disease.
Known or suspected carcinoma of the breast.
Carcinoma of the endometrium or other known or suspected estrogen-dependent neoplasia.
Undiagnosed abnormal genital bleeding.
Cholestatic jaundice of pregnancy or jaundice with prior pill use.
Hepatic adenomas or carcinomas.
Known or suspected pregnancy.

WARNINGS

> **Cigarette smoking increases the risk of serious cardiovascular side effects from oral-contraceptive use. This risk increases with age and with heavy smoking (15 or more cigarettes per day) and is quite marked in women over 35 years of age. Women who use oral contraceptives should be strongly advised not to smoke.**

The use of oral contraceptives is associated with increased risks of several serious conditions including myocardial infarction, thromboembolism, stroke, hepatic neoplasia, gallbladder disease, and hypertension, although the risk of serious morbidity or mortality is very small in healthy women without underlying risk factors. The risk of morbidity and mortality increases significantly in the presence of other underlying risk factors such as hypertension, hyperlipidemias, obesity and diabetes.

Practitioners prescribing oral contraceptives should be familiar with the following information relating to these risks. The information contained in this package insert is based principally on studies carried out in patients who used oral contraceptives with higher formulations of estrogens and progestogens than those in common use today. The effect of long-term use of the oral contraceptives with lower formulations of both estrogens and progestogens remains to be determined.

Throughout this labeling, epidemiological studies reported are of two types: retrospective or case control studies and prospective or cohort studies. Case control studies provide a measure of the relative risk of disease, namely, a ratio of the incidence of a disease among oral-contraceptive users to that among nonusers. The relative risk does not provide information on the actual clinical occurrence of a disease. Cohort studies provide a measure of attributable risk, which is the difference in the incidence of disease between oral-contraceptive users and nonusers. The attributable risk does provide information about the actual occurrence of a disease in the population. For further information, the reader is referred to a text on epidemiological methods.

1. THROMBOEMBOLIC DISORDERS AND OTHER VASCULAR PROBLEMS

a. *Myocardial Infarction*

An increased risk of myocardial infarction has been attributed to oral-contraceptive use. This risk is primarily in smokers or women with other underlying risk factors for coronary-artery disease such as hypertension, hypercholesterolemia, morbid obesity, and diabetes. The relative risk of heart attack for current oral-contraceptive users has been estimated to be two to six. The risk is very low under the age of 30.

Smoking in combination with oral-contraceptive use has been shown to contribute substantially to the incidence of myocardial infarctions in women in their mid-thirties or older with smoking accounting for the majority of excess cases. Mortality rates associated with circulatory disease have been shown to increase substantially in smokers over the age of 35 and nonsmokers over the age of 40 (Table II) among women who use oral contraceptives.

TABLE II. (Adapted from P.M. Layde and V. Beral, Lancet, 1:541–546, 1981.)

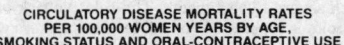

CIRCULATORY DISEASE MORTALITY RATES PER 100,000 WOMEN YEARS BY AGE, SMOKING STATUS AND ORAL-CONTRACEPTIVE USE

Ever-Users (nonsmokers)   Controls (nonsmokers)
Ever-Users (smokers)   Controls (smokers)

Oral contraceptives may compound the effects of well-known risk factors, such as hypertension, diabetes, hyperlipidemias, age and obesity. In particular, some progestogens are known to decrease HDL cholesterol and cause glucose intolerance, while estrogens may create a state of hyperinsulinism. Oral contraceptives have been shown to increase blood pressure among users (see section 9 in "WARNINGS"). Similar effects on risk factors have been associated with an increased risk of heart disease. Oral contraceptives must be used with caution in women with cardiovascular disease risk factors.

b. *Thromboembolism*

An increased risk of thromboembolic and thrombotic disease associated with the use of oral contraceptives is well established. Case control studies have found the relative risk of users compared to nonusers to be 3 for the first episode of superficial venous thrombosis, 4 to 11 for deep vein thrombosis or pulmonary embolism, and 1.5 to 6 for women with predisposing conditions for venous thromboembolic disease. Cohort studies have shown the relative risk to be somewhat lower, about 3 for new cases and about 4.5 for new cases requiring hospitalization. The risk of thromboembolic disease due to oral contraceptives is not related to length of use and disappears after pill use is stopped.

A two- to four-fold increase in relative risk of postoperative thromboembolic complications has been reported with the use of oral contraceptives. The relative risk of venous thrombosis in women who have predisposing conditions is twice that of women without such medical conditions. If feasible, oral contraceptives should be discontinued at least four weeks prior to and for two weeks after elective surgery of a type associated with an increase in risk of thromboembolism and during and following prolonged immobilization. Since the immediate post partum period is also associated with an increased risk of thromboembolism, oral contraceptives should be started no earlier than four to six weeks after delivery in women who elect not to breast-feed, or a midtrimester pregnancy termination.

c. *Cerebrovascular diseases*

Oral contraceptives have been shown to increase both the relative and attributable risks of cerebrovascular events (thrombotic and hemorrhagic strokes), although, in general, the risk is greatest among older (> 35 years), hypertensive women who also smoke. Hypertension was found to be a risk factor for both users and nonusers, for both types of strokes,

Continued on next page

Information on the Berlex products appearing here is based on the most current information available at the time of publication closing. Further information for these and other products may be obtained from the Medical Affairs Department, Berlex Laboratories, 300 Fairfield Road, Wayne, New Jersey 07470, 1-800-888-2407. Information on Betaseron and Fludara may be obtained from Berlex Laboratories, 15049 San Pablo Avenue, Richmond, California 94804-0016, 1-800-888-4112.

Berlex Laboratories—Cont.

while smoking interacted to increase the risk for hemorrhagic strokes.

In a large study, the relative risk of thrombotic strokes has been shown to range from 3 for normotensive users to 14 for users with severe hypertension. The relative risk of hemorrhagic stroke is reported to be 1.2 for nonsmokers who used oral contraceptives, 2.6 for smokers who did not use oral contraceptives, 7.6 for smokers who used oral contraceptives, 1.8 for normotensive users and 25.7 for users with severe hypertension. The attributable risk is also greater in older women.

d. *Dose-related risk of vascular disease from oral contraceptives*

A positive association has been observed between the amount of estrogen and progestogen in oral contraceptives and the risk of vascular disease. A decline in serum high-density lipoproteins (HDL) has been reported with many progestational agents. A decline in serum high-density lipoproteins has been associated with an increased incidence of ischemic heart disease. Because estrogens increase HDL cholesterol, the net effect of an oral contraceptive depends on a balance achieved between doses of estrogen and progestogen and the nature and absolute amount of progestogen used in the contraceptive. The amount of both hormones should be considered in the choice of an oral contraceptive.

Minimizing exposure to estrogen and progestogen is in keeping with good principles of therapeutics. For any particular estrogen/progestogen combination, the dosage regimen prescribed should be one which contains the least amount of estrogen and progestogen that is compatible with a low failure rate and the needs of the individual patient. New acceptors of oral-contraceptive agents should be started on preparations containing less than 50 mcg of estrogen.

e. *Persistence of risk of vascular disease*

There are two studies which have shown persistence of risk of vascular disease for ever-users of oral contraceptives. In a study in the United States, the risk of developing myocardial infarction after discontinuing oral contraceptives persists for at least 9 years for women 40–49 years who had used oral contraceptives for five or more years, but this increased risk was not demonstrated in other age groups. In another study in Great Britain, the risk of developing cerebrovascular disease persisted for at least 6 years after discontinuation of oral contraceptives, although excess risk was very small. However, both studies were performed with oral contraceptive formulations containing 50 micrograms or higher of estrogens.

2. ESTIMATES OF MORTALITY FROM CONTRACEPTIVE USE

One study gathered data from a variety of sources which have estimated the mortality rate associated with different methods of contraception at different ages (Table III). These estimates include the combined risk of death associated with contraceptive methods plus the risk attributable to pregnancy in the event of method failure. Each method of contraception has its specific benefits and risks. The study concluded that with the exception of oral-contraceptive users 35 and older who smoke and 40 and older who do not smoke, mortality associated with all methods of birth control is less than that associated with childbirth. The observation of a possible increase in risk of mortality with age for oral-contraceptive users is based on data gathered in the 1970's—but not reported until 1983. However, current clinical practice involves the use of lower estrogen dose formulations combined with careful restriction of oral-contraceptive use to women who do not have the various risk factors listed in this labeling.

Because of these changes in practice and, also, because of some limited new data which suggest that the risk of cardiovascular disease with the use of oral contraceptives may now be less than previously observed, the Fertility and Maternal Health Drugs Advisory Committee was asked to review the topic in 1989. The Committee concluded that although cardiovascular disease risks may be increased with oral-contraceptive use after age 40 in healthy nonsmoking women (even with the newer low-dose formulations), there are greater potential health risks associated with pregnancy in older women and with the alternative surgical and medical procedures which may be necessary if such women do not have access to effective and acceptable means of contraception. Therefore, the Committee recommended that the benefits of oral-contraceptive use by healthy nonsmoking women over 40 may outweigh the possible risks. Of course, older women, as all women who take oral contraceptives, should take the lowest possible dose formulation that is effective.

[See Table III below.]

3. CARCINOMA OF THE REPRODUCTIVE ORGANS

Numerous epidemiological studies have been performed on the incidence of breast, endometrial, ovarian and cervical cancer in women using oral contraceptives. The overwhelming evidence in the literature suggests that use of oral contraceptives is not associated with an increase in the risk of developing breast cancer, regardless of the age and parity of first use or with most of the marketed brands and doses. The Cancer and Steroid Hormone (CASH) study also showed no latent effect on the risk of breast cancer for at least a decade following long-term use. A few studies have shown a slightly increased relative risk of developing breast cancer, although the methodology of these studies, which included differences in examination of users and nonusers and differences in age at start of use, has been questioned.

Some studies suggest that oral-contraceptive use has been associated with an increase in the risk of cervical intraepithelial neoplasia in some populations of women. However, there continues to be controversy about the extent to which such findings may be due to differences in sexual behavior and other factors.

In spite of many studies of the relationship between oral-contraceptive use and breast and cervical cancers, a cause-and-effect relationship has not been established.

4. HEPATIC NEOPLASIA

Benign hepatic adenomas are associated with oral-contraceptive use, although the incidence of benign tumors is rare in the United States. Indirect calculations have estimated the attributable risk to be in the range of 3.3 cases/100,000 for users, a risk that increases after four or more years of use. Rupture of rare, benign, hepatic adenomas may cause death through intra-abdominal hemorrhage.

Studies from Britain have shown an increased risk of developing hepatocellular carcinoma in long-term (>8 years) oral-contraceptive users. However, these cancers are extremely rare in the U.S. and the attributable risk (the excess incidence) of liver cancers in oral-contraceptive users approaches less than one per million users.

5. OCULAR LESIONS

There have been clincial case reports of retinal thrombosis associated with the use of oral contraceptives. Oral contraceptives should be discontinued if there is unexplained partial or complete loss of vision; onset of proptosis or diplopia; papilledema; or retinal vascular lesions. Appropriate diagnostic and therapeutic measures should be undertaken immediately.

6. ORAL-CONTRACEPTIVE USE BEFORE OR DURING EARLY PREGNANCY

Extensive epidemiological studies have revealed no increased risk of birth defects in women who have used oral contraceptives prior to pregnancy. Studies also do not suggest a teratogenic effect, particularly insofar as cardiac anomalies and limb-reduction defects are concerned, when taken inadvertently during early pregnancy.

The administration of oral contraceptives to induce withdrawal bleeding should not be used as a test for pregnancy. Oral contraceptives should not be used during pregnancy to treat threatened or habitual abortion.

It is recommended that for any patient who has missed two consecutive periods, pregnancy should be ruled out before continuing oral-contraceptive use. If the patient has not adhered to the prescribed schedule, the possibility of pregnancy should be considered at the time of the first missed period. Oral-contraceptive use should be discontinued if pregnancy is confirmed.

7. GALLBLADDER DISEASE

Earlier studies have reported an increased lifetime relative risk of gallbladder surgery in users of oral contraceptives and estrogens. More recent studies, however, have shown that the relative risk of developing gallbladder disease among oral-contraceptive users may be minimal. The recent findings of minimal risk may be related to the use of oral-contraceptive formulations containing lower hormonal doses of estrogens and progestogens.

8. CARBOHYDRATE AND LIPID METABOLIC EFFECTS

Oral contraceptives have been shown to cause glucose intolerance in a significant percentage of users. Oral contraceptives containing greater than 75 micrograms of estrogens cause hyperinsulinism, while lower doses of estrogen cause less glucose intolerance. Progestogens increase insulin secretion and create insulin resistance, this effect varying with different progestational agents. However, in the nondiabetic woman, oral contraceptives appear to have no effect on fasting blood glucose. Because of these demonstrated effects, prediabetic and diabetic women should be carefully observed while taking oral contraceptives.

A small proportion of women will have persistent hypertriglyceridemia while on the pill. As discussed earlier (see "WARNINGS" 1a. and 1d.), changes in serum triglycerides and lipoprotein levels have been reported in oral-contraceptive users.

9. ELEVATED BLOOD PRESSURE

An increase in blood pressure has been reported in women taking oral contraceptives and this increase is more likely in older oral-contraceptive users and with continued use. Data from the Royal College of General Practitioners and subsequent randomized trials have shown that the incidence of hypertension increases with increasing quantities of progestogens.

Women with a history of hypertension or hypertension-related diseases, or renal disease should be encouraged to use another method of contraception. If women with hypertertension elect to use oral contraceptives, they should be monitored closely, and if significant elevation of blood pressure occurs, oral contraceptives should be discontinued. For most women, elevated blood pressure will return to normal after stopping oral contraceptives, and there is no difference in the occurrence of hypertension among ever- and never-users.

10. HEADACHE

The onset or exacerbation of migraine or development of headache with a new pattern that is recurrent, persistent, or severe requires discontinuation of oral contraceptives and evaluation of the case.

11. BLEEDING IRREGULARITIES

Breakthrough bleeding and spotting are sometimes encountered in patients on oral contraceptives, especially during the first three months of use. The type and dose of progestogen may be important. Nonhormonal causes should be considered and adequate diagnostic measures taken to rule out malignancy or pregnancy in the event of breakthrough bleeding, as in the case of any abnormal vaginal bleeding. If pathology has been excluded, time or a change to another formulation may solve the problem. In the event of amenorrhea, pregnancy should be ruled out.

Some women may encounter post-pill amenorrhea or oligomenorrhea, especially when such a condition was preexistent.

PRECAUTIONS

Patients should be counseled that this product does not protect against HIV infection (AIDS) and other sexually transmitted diseases.

1. PHYSICAL EXAMINATION AND FOLLOW UP

A complete medical history and physical examination should be taken prior to the initiation or reinstitution of oral contraceptives and at least annually during use of oral contraceptives. These physical examinations should include special reference to blood pressure, breasts, abdomen and pelvic organs, including cervical cytology, and relevant laboratory tests. In case of undiagnosed, persistent, or recurrent abnormal vaginal bleeding, appropriate diagnostic measures should be conducted to rule out malignancy. Women with a strong family history of breast cancer or who have breast nodules should be monitored with particular care.

2. LIPID DISORDERS

Women who are being treated for hyperlipidemias should be followed closely if they elect to use oral contraceptives. Some progestogens may elevate LDL levels and may render the control of hyperlipidemias more difficult. (See "WARNINGS" 1d.)

3. LIVER FUNCTION

If jaundice develops in any woman receiving such drugs, the medication should be discontinued. Steroid hormones may be poorly metabolized in patients with impaired liver function.

4. FLUID RETENTION

Oral contraceptives may cause some degree of fluid retention. They should be prescribed with caution, and only with

TABLE III—ANNUAL NUMBER OF BIRTH-RELATED OR METHOD-RELATED DEATHS ASSOCIATED WITH CONTROL OF FERTILITY PER 100,000 NONSTERILE WOMEN, BY FERTILITY-CONTROL METHOD ACCORDING TO AGE

Method of control and outcome	15–19	20–24	25–29	30–34	35–39	40–44
No fertility—control methods*	7.0	7.4	9.1	14.8	25.7	28.2
Oral contraceptives nonsmoker**	0.3	0.5	0.9	1.9	13.8	31.6
Oral contraceptives smoker**	2.2	3.4	6.6	13.5	51.1	117.2
IUD**	0.8	0.8	1.0	1.0	1.4	1.4
Condom*	1.1	1.6	0.7	0.2	0.3	0.4
Diaphragm/spermicide*	1.9	1.2	1.2	1.3	2.2	2.8
Periodic abstinence*	2.5	1.6	1.6	1.7	2.9	3.6

* Deaths are birth related
** Deaths are method related

Adapted from H.W. Ory, Family Planning Perspectives *15*:57–63, 1983.

careful monitoring, in patients with conditions which might be aggravated by fluid retention.

5. EMOTIONAL DISORDERS

Patients becoming significantly depressed while taking oral contraceptives should stop the medication and use an alternate method of contraception in an attempt to determine whether the symptom is drug related. Women with a history of depression should be carefully observed and the drug discontinued if depression recurs to a serious degree.

6. CONTACT LENSES

Contact-lens wearers who develop visual changes or changes in lens tolerance should be assessed by an ophthalmologist.

7. DRUG INTERACTIONS

Reduced efficacy and increased incidence of breakthrough bleeding and menstrual irregularities have been associated with concomitant use of rifampin. A similar assocation, though less marked, has been suggested with barbiturates, phenylbutazone, phenytoin sodium, and possibly with griseofulvin, ampicillin, and tetracyclines.

8. INTERACTIONS WITH LABORATORY TESTS

Certain endocrine- and liver-function tests and blood components may be affected by oral contraceptives:

a. Increased prothrombin and factors VII, VIII, IX, and X; decreased antithrombin 3; increased norepinephrine-induced platelet aggregability.

b. Increased thyroid-binding globulin (TBG) leading to increased circulating total thyroid hormone, as measured by protein-bound iodine (PBI), T4 by column or by radioimmunoassay. Free T3 resin uptake is decreased, reflecting the elevated TBG, free T4 concentration is unaltered.

c. Other binding proteins may be elevated in serum.

d. Sex-binding globulins are increased and result in elevated levels of total circulating sex steroids and corticoids; however, free or biologically active levels remain unchanged.

e. Triglycerides may be increased.

f. Glucose tolerance may be decreased.

g. Serum folate levels may be depressed by oral-contraceptive therapy. This may be of clinical significance if a woman becomes pregnant shortly after discontinuing oral contraceptives.

9. CARCINOGENESIS

See "WARNINGS" section.

10. PREGNANCY

Pregnancy Category X. See "CONTRAINDICATIONS" and "WARNINGS" sections.

11. NURSING MOTHERS

Small amounts of oral-contraceptive steroids have been identified in the milk of nursing mothers and a few adverse effects on the child have been reported, including jaundice and breast enlargement. In addition, oral contraceptives given in the postpartum period may interfere with lactation by decreasing the quantity and quality of breast milk. If possible, the nursing mother should be advised not to use oral contraceptives but to use other forms of contraception until she has completely weaned her child.

INFORMATION FOR THE PATIENT

See "Patient Labeling" printed below.

ADVERSE REACTIONS

An increased risk of the following serious adverse reactions has been associated with the use of oral contraceptives (see "WARNINGS" section).

Thrombophlebitis	Cerebral thrombosis
Aterial thromboembolism	Hypertension
Pulmonary embolism	Gallbladder disease
Myocardial infarction	Hepatic adenomas or benign liver tumors
Cerebral hemorrhage	

There is evidence of an association between the following conditions and the use of oral contraceptives, although additional confirmatory studies are needed:

Mesenteric thrombosis
Retinal thrombosis

The following adverse reactions have been reported in patients receiving oral contraceptives and are believed to be drug related:

Nausea
Vomiting
Gastrointestinal symptoms (such as abdominal cramps and bloating)
Breakthrough bleeding
Spotting
Change in menstrual flow
Amenorrhea
Temporary infertility after discontinuation of treatment
Edema
Melasma which may persist
Breast changes: tenderness, enlargement, and secretion
Change in weight (increase or decrease)
Change in cervical erosion and cervical secretion
Diminution in lactation when given immediately postpartum
Cholestatic jaundice
Migraine
Rash (allergic)
Mental depression
Reduced tolerance to carbohydrates
Vaginal candidiasis
Change in corneal curvature (steepening)
Intolerance to contact lenses

The following adverse reactions have been reported in users of oral contraceptives and the association has been neither confirmed nor refuted:

Congenital anomalies	Erythema nodosum
Premenstrual syndrome	Hemorrhagic eruption
Cataracts	Vaginitis
Changes in appetitie	Porphyria
Cystitis-like syndrome	Impaired renal function
Headache	Hemolytic uremic syndrome
Nervousness	Budd-Chiari syndrome
Dizziness	Acne
Hirsutism	Changes in libido
Loss of scalp hair	Colitis
Erythema multiforme	Sickle-Cell Disease
Cerebral-vascular disease with mitral valve prolapse	Optic neuritis
Lupus-like Syndromes	

OVERDOSAGE

Serious ill effects have not been reported following acute ingestion of large doses of oral contraceptives by young children. Overdosage may cause nausea, and withdrawal bleeding may occur in females.

NONCONTRACEPTIVE HEALTH BENEFITS

The following noncontraceptive health benefits related to the use of oral contraceptives are supported by epidemiological studies which largely utilized oral-contraceptive formulations containing doses exceeding 0.035 mg of ethinyl estradiol or 0.05 mg of mestranol.

Effects on menses:
- increased menstrual cycle regularity
- decreased blood loss and decreased incidence of iron deficiency anemia
- decreased incidence of dysmenorrhea

Effects related to inhibition of ovulation:
- decreased incidence of functional ovarian cysts
- decreased incidence of ectopic pregnancies

Effects from long-term use:
- decreased incidence of fibroadenomas and fibrocystic disease of the breast
- decreased incidence of acute pelvic inflammatory disease
- decreased incidence of endometrial cancer
- decreased incidence of ovarian cancer

DOSAGE AND ADMINISTRATION

TRI-LEVLEN® 21 Tablets

To achieve maximum contraceptive effectiveness, TRI-LEVLEN® 21 Tablets (levonorgestrel and ethinyl estradiol tablets—triphasic regimen) should be taken exactly as directed and at intervals not exceeding 24-hours.

TRI-LEVLEN® 21 Tablets are a three-phase preparation. The dosage of TRI-LEVLEN® 21 Tablets is **one tablet** daily for 21 consecutive days per menstrual cycle in the following order: 6 brown tablets (phase 1), followed by 5 white tablets (phase 2), and then followed by the last 10 light-yellow tablets (phase 3), according to the prescribed schedule. Tablets are then discontinued for 7 days (three weeks on, one week off).

It is recommended that TRI-LEVLEN® 21 Tablets be taken at the same time each day. During the first cycle of medication, the patient should be instructed to take one TRI-LEVLEN® 21 Tablet daily in the order of 6 brown, 5 white and, finally, 10 light-yellow tablets for twenty-one (21) consecutive days, beginning on day one (1) of her menstrual cycle. (The first day of menstruation is day one.) The tablets are then discontinued for one week (7 days). Withdrawal bleeding usually occurs within 3 days following discontinuation of TRI-LEVLEN® 21 Tablets. (If an alternate starting regimen is used [Sunday Start or postpartum], contraceptive reliance should not be placed on TRI-LEVLEN® 21 Tablets until after the first 7 consecutive days of administration. The possibility of ovulation and conception prior to initiation of medication should be considered.)

The patient begins her next and all subsequent 21-day courses of TRI-LEVLEN® 21 Tablets on the same day of the week that she began her first course, following the same schedule: 21 days on—7 days off. She begins taking her brown tablets on the 8th day after discontinuance, regardless of whether or not a menstrual period has occurred or is still in progress. Any time the next cycle of TRI-LEVLEN® 21 Tablets is started later than the 8th day, the patient should be protected by another means of contraception until she has taken a tablet daily for seven consecutive days.

If spotting or breakthrough bleeding occurs, the patient is instructed to continue on the same regimen. This type of bleeding is usually transient and without significance; however, if the bleeding is persistent or prolonged, the patient is advised to consult her physician. Although the occurrence of pregnancy is highly unlikely if TRI-LEVLEN® 21 Tablets are taken according to directions, if withdrawal bleeding does not occur, the possibility of pregnancy must be considered. If the patient has not adhered to the prescribed schedule (missed one or more tablets or started taking them on a day later than she should have), the probability of pregnancy should be considered at the time of the first missed period and appropriate diagnostic measures taken before the medication is resumed. If the patient has adhered to the prescribed regimen and misses two consecutive periods, pregnancy should be ruled out before continuing the contraceptive regimen.

The risk of pregnancy increases with each active (brown, white, or light-yellow) tablet missed. For additional patient instructions regarding missed pills, see the "WHAT TO DO IF YOU MISS PILLS" section in the DETAILED PATIENT LABELING below. If breakthrough bleeding occurs following missed active tablets, it will usually be transient and of no consequence. If the patient misses one or more light-green tablets, she is still protected against pregnancy **provided** she begins taking brown tablets again on the proper day.

In the nonlactating mother, TRI-LEVLEN® 21 Tablets may be initiated postpartum, for contraception. When the tablets are administered in the postpartum period, the increased risk of thromboembolic disease associated with the postpartum period must be considered. (See "CONTRAINDICATIONS", "WARNINGS", and "PRECAUTIONS" concerning thromboembolic disease.) It is to be noted that early resumption of ovulation may occur if Parlodel® (bromocriptine mesylate) has been used for the prevention of lactation.

TRI-LEVLEN® 28 Tablets

To achieve maximum contraceptive effectiveness, TRI-LEVLEN® 28 Tablets (levonorgestrel and ethinyl estradiol tablets—triphasic regimen) should be taken exactly as directed and at intervals not exceeding 24-hours.

TRI-LEVLEN® 28 Tablets are a three-phase preparation plus 7 inert tablets. The dosage of TRI-LEVLEN® 28 Tablets is one tablet daily for 28 consecutive days per menstrual cycle in the following order: 6 brown tablets (phase 1), followed by 5 white tablets (phase 2), followed by 10 light-yellow tablets (phase 3), plus 7 light-green inert tablets according to the prescribed schedule.

It is recommended that TRI-LEVLEN® 28 Tablets be taken at the same time each day. During the first cycle of medication, the patient should be instructed to take one TRI-LEVLEN® 28 Tablet daily in the order of 6 brown, 5 white, 10 light-yellow tablets and then 7 light-green inert tablets for twenty-eight (28) consecutive days, beginning on day one (1) of her menstrual cycle. (The first day of menstruation is day one.) Withdrawal bleeding usually occurs within 3 days following the last light-yellow tablet. (If an alternate starting regimen is used [Sunday Start or postpartum], contraceptive reliance should not be placed on TRI-LEVLEN® 28 Tablets until after the first 7 consecutive days of administration. The possibility of ovulation and conception prior to initiation of medication should be considered.)

The patient begins her next and all subsequent 28-day courses of TRI-LEVLEN® 28 Tablets on the same day of the week that she began her first course, following the same schedule. She begins taking her brown tablets on the next day after ingestion of the last light-green tablet, regardless of whether or not a menstrual period has occurred or is still in progress. Any time a subsequent cycle of TRI-LEVLEN® 28 Tablets is started later than the next day, the patient should be protected by another means of contraception until she has taken a tablet daily for seven consecutive days.

If spotting or breakthrough bleeding occurs, the patient is instructed to continue on the same regimen. This type of bleeding is usually transient and without significance; however, if the bleeding is persistent or prolonged, the patient is advised to consult her physician. Although the occurrence of pregnancy is highly unlikely if TRI-LEVLEN® 28 Tablets are taken according to directions, if withdrawal bleeding does not occur, the possibility of pregnancy must be considered. If the patient has not adhered to the prescribed schedule (missed one or more active tablets or started taking them on a day later than she should have), the probability of pregnancy should be considered at the time of the first missed period and appropriate diagnostic measures taken before the medication is resumed. If the patient has adhered to the prescribed regimen and misses two consecutive periods, pregnancy should be ruled out before continuing the contraceptive regimen.

The risk of pregnancy increases with each active (brown, white, or light-yellow) tablet missed. For additional patient instructions regarding missed pills, see the "WHAT TO DO IF YOU MISS PILLS" section in the DETAILED PATIENT

Continued on next page

Information on the Berlex products appearing here is based on the most current information available at the time of publication closing. Further information for these and other products may be obtained from the Medical Affairs Department, Berlex Laboratories, 300 Fairfield Road, Wayne, New Jersey 07470, 1-800-888-2407. Information on Betaseron and Fludara may be obtained from Berlex Laboratories, 15049 San Pablo Avenue, Richmond, California 94804-0016, 1-800-888-4112.

Berlex Laboratories—Cont.

LABELING below. If breakthrough bleeding occurs following missed active tablets, it will usually be transient and of no consequence. If the patient misses one or more light-green tablets, she is still protected against pregnancy **provided** she begins taking brown tablets again on the proper day.
In the nonlactating mother, TRI-LEVLEN® 28 Tablets may be initiated postpartum, for contraception. When the tablets are administered in the postpartum period, the increased risk of thromboembolic disease associated with the postpartum period must be considered. (See "CONTRAINDICATIONS", "WARNINGS", and "PRECAUTIONS" concerning thromboembolic disease.) It is to be noted that early resumption of ovulation may occur if Parlodel® (bromocriptine mesylate) has been used for the prevention of lactation.
LEVLEN® 21 Tablets
To achieve maximum contraceptive effectiveness, LEVLEN® 21 Tablets (levonorgestrel and ethinyl estradiol tablets) should be taken exactly as directed and at intervals not exceeding 24-hours.
The dosage of LEVLEN® 21 Tablets is **one tablet** daily for 21 consecutive days per menstrual cycle according to the prescribed schedule. Tablets are then discontinued for 7 days (three weeks on, one week off).
It is recommended that LEVLEN® 21 Tablets be taken at the same time each day. During the first cycle of medication, the patient should be instructed to take one LEVLEN® 21 Tablet daily for twenty-one (21) consecutive days, beginning on day one (1) of her menstrual cycle. (The first day of menstruation is day one.) The tablets are then discontinued for one week (7 days). Withdrawal bleeding usually occurs within 3 days following discontinuation of LEVLEN® 21 Tablets. (If an alternate starting regimen is used [Sunday Start or postpartum], contraceptive reliance should not be placed on LEVLEN® 21 Tablets until after the first 7 consecutive days of administration. The possibility of ovulation and conception prior to initiation of medication should be considered.)
The patient begins her next and all subsequent 21-day courses of LEVLEN® 21 Tablets on the same day of the week that she began her first course, following the same schedule: 21 days on—7 days off. She begins taking her light-orange tablets on the 8th day after discontinuance, regardless of whether or not a menstrual period has occurred or is still in progress. Any time the next cycle of LEVLEN® 21 Tablets is started later than the 8th day, the patient should be protected by another means of contraception until she has taken a tablet daily for seven consecutive days.
If spotting or breakthrough bleeding occurs, the patient is instructed to continue on the same regimen. This type of bleeding is usually transient and without significance; however, if the bleeding is persistent or prolonged, the patient is advised to consult her physician. Although the occurrence of pregnancy is highly unlikely if LEVLEN® 21 Tablets are taken according to directions, if withdrawal bleeding does not occur, the possibility of pregnancy must be considered. If the patient has not adhered to the prescribed schedule (missed one or more tablets or started taking them on a day later than she should have), the probability of pregnancy should be considered at the time of the first missed period and appropriate diagnostic measures taken before the medication is resumed. If the patient has adhered to the prescribed regimen and misses two consecutive periods, pregnancy should be ruled out before continuing the contraceptive regimen.
Any time the patient misses two or more tablets, she should also use another method of contraception until she has taken a tablet daily for seven consecutive days. If breakthrough bleeding occurs following missed active tablets, it usually will be transient and of no consequence. If the patient misses one or more pink tablets, she is still protected against pregnancy provided she begins taking the light-orange tablets again on the proper day.
In the nonlactating mother, LEVLEN® 21 Tablets may be initiated postpartum, for contraception. When the tablets are administered in the postpartum period, the increased risk of thromboembolic disease associated with the postpartum period must be considered. (See "CONTRAINDICATIONS", "WARNINGS", and "PRECAUTIONS" concerning thromboembolic disease.)
LEVLEN® 28 Tablets
To achieve maximum contraceptive effectiveness, LEVLEN® 28 Tablets (levonorgestrel and ethinyl estradiol tablets) should be taken exactly as directed at intervals not exceeding 24-hours.
The dosage of LEVLEN® 28 Tablets is one light-orange tablet daily for 21 consecutive days per menstrual cycle, followed by 7 pink inert tablets according to the prescribed schedule.
It is recommended that LEVLEN® 28 Tablets be taken at the same time each day. During the first cycle of medication, the patient should be instructed to take one LEVLEN® 28 Tablet daily in the order of 21 light orange and then 7 pink inert tablets for twenty-eight (28) consecutive days, beginning on day one (1) of her menstrual cycle. (The first day of menstruation is day one.) Withdrawal bleeding usually occurs within 3 days following the last light-orange tablet. (If an alternate starting regimen is used [Sunday Start or postpartum], contraceptive reliance should not be placed on LEVLEN® 28 Tablets until after the first 7 consecutive days of administration. The possibility of ovulation and conception prior to initiation of medication should be considered.)
The patient begins her next and all subsequent 28-day courses of LEVLEN® 28 Tablets on the same day of the week that she began her first course, following the same schedule. She begins taking her light-orange tablets on the next day after ingestion of the last pink tablet, regardless of whether or not a menstrual period has occurred or is still in progress. Any time a subsequent cycle of LEVLEN® 28 Tablets is started later than the next day, the patient should be protected by another means of contraception until she has taken a tablet daily for seven consecutive days.
If spotting or breakthrough bleeding occurs, the patient is instructed to continue on the same regimen. This type of bleeding is usually transient and without significance; however, if the bleeding is persistent or prolonged, the patient is advised to consult her physician. Although the occurrence of pregnancy is highly unlikely if LEVLEN® 28 Tablets are taken according to directions, if withdrawal bleeding does not occur, the possibility of pregnancy must be considered. If the patient has not adhered to the prescribed schedule (missed one or more active tablets or started taking them on a day later than she should have), the probability of pregnancy should be considered at the time of the first missed period and appropriate diagnostic measures taken before the medication is resumed. If the patient has adhered to the prescribed regimen and misses two consecutive periods, pregnancy should be ruled out before continuing the contraceptive regimen.
Any time the patient misses two or more tablets, she should also use another method of contraception until she has taken a tablet daily for seven consecutive days. If breakthrough bleeding occurs following missed active tablets, it usually will be transient and of no consequence. If the patient misses one or more pink tablets, she is still protected against pregnancy provided she begins taking the light-orange tablets again on the proper day.
In the nonlactating mother, LEVLEN® 28 Tablets may be initiated postpartum, for contraception. When the tablets are administered in the postpartum period, the increased risk of thromboembolic disease associated with the postpartum period must be considered. (See "CONTRAINDICATIONS", "WARNINGS", and "PRECAUTIONS" concerning thromboembolic disease.)

HOW SUPPLIED

TRI-LEVLEN® 21 tablets (Levonorgestrel and Ethinyl Estradiol Tablets—Triphasic Regimen), are available in packages of 3 and 6 SLIDECASE™ dispensers. Each cycle contains 21 round, film-coated tablets as follows:
NDC 50419-195, six brown tablets marked "B" on one side and "95" on the other side, each containing 0.050 mg levonorgestrel and 0.030 mg ethinyl estradiol;
NDC 50419-196, five white to off-white tablets marked "B" on one side and "96" on the other side, each containing 0.075 mg levonorgestrel and 0.040 mg ethinyl estradiol; and
NDC 50419-197, ten light-yellow tablets marked "B" on one side and "97" on the other side, each containing 0.125 mg levonorgestrel and 0.030 mg ethinyl estradiol.
In packages of:
3 SLIDECASE™ dispensers ....NDC 50419-432-03
6 SLIDECASE™ dispensers ....NDC 50419-432-06

TRI-LEVLEN® 28 tablets (Levonorgestrel and Ethinyl Estradiol Tablets—Triphasic Regimen), are available in packages of 3 and 6 SLIDECASE™ dispensers. Each cycle contains 28 round, film-coated tablets as follows:
NDC 50419-195, six brown tablets marked "B" on one side and "95" on the other side, each containing 0.050 mg levonorgestrel and 0.030 mg ethinyl estradiol;
NDC 50419-196, five white to off-white tablets marked "B" on one side and "96" on the other side, each containing 0.075 mg levonorgestrel and 0.040 mg ethinyl estradiol;
NDC 50419-197, ten light-yellow tablets marked "B" on one side and "97" on the other side, each containing 0.125 mg levonorgestrel and 0.030 mg ethinyl estradiol; and
NDC 50419-111, seven light-green inert tablets marked "B" on one side and "11" on the other side.
In packages of:
3 SLIDECASE™ dispensers ....NDC 50419-433-03
6 SLIDECASE™ dispensers ....NDC 50419-433-06

LEVLEN® 21 tablets (Levonorgestrel and Ethinyl Estradiol Tablets), are available in packages of 3 SLIDECASE™ dispensers. Each cycle contains 21 round, tablets as follows:
NDC 50419-021, 21 active, light-orange tablets marked "B" on one side and "21" on the other side, each containing 0.15 mg levonorgestrel and 0.03 mg ethinyl estradiol;
In packages of:
3 SLIDECASE™ dispensers ....NDC 50419-410-21

LEVLEN® 28 tablets (Levonorgestrel and Ethinyl Estradiol Tablets), are available in packages of 3 SLIDECASE™ dispensers. Each cycle contains 28 round tablets as follows:
NDC 50419-021, 21 active, light-orange tablets marked "B" on one side and "21" on the other side, each containing 0.15 mg levonorgestrel and 0.03 mg ethinyl estradiol;
NDC 50419-028, 7 inert pink tablets marked "B" on one side and "28" on the other side.
In packages of:
3 SLIDECASE™ dispensers ....NDC 50419-411-28

REFERENCES

References furnished upon request.

BRIEF SUMMARY PATIENT PACKAGE INSERT

This product (like all oral contraceptives) is intended to prevent pregnancy. It does not protect against HIV infection (AIDS) and other sexually transmitted diseases.
Oral contraceptives, also known as "birth control pills" or "the pill," are taken to prevent pregnancy and when taken correctly, have a failure rate of less than 1% per year when used without missing any pills. The typical failure rate of large numbers of pill users is less than 3% per year when women who miss pills are included. For most women oral contraceptives are also free of serious or unpleasant side effects. However, forgetting to take pills considerably increases the chances of pregnancy.
For the majority of women, oral contraceptives can be taken safely. But there are some women who are at high risk of developing certain serious diseases that can be life-threatening or may cause temporary or permanent disability or death. The risks associated with taking oral contraceptives increase significantly if you:

- smoke
- have high blood pressure, diabetes, high cholesterol
- have or have had clotting disorders, heart attack, stroke, angina pectoris, cancer of the breast or sex organs, jaundice or malignant or benign liver tumors

You should not take the pill if you suspect you are pregnant or have unexplained vaginal bleeding.

Cigarette smoking increases the risk of serious adverse effects on the heart and blood vessels from oral-contraceptive use. This risk increases with age and with heavy smoking (15 or more cigarettes per day) and is quite marked in women over 35 years of age. Women who use oral contraceptives are strongly advised not to smoke.

Most side effects of the pill are not serious. The most common such effects are nausea, vomiting, bleeding between menstrual periods, weight gain, breast tenderness, and difficulty wearing contact lenses. These side effects, especially nausea, and vomiting, may subside within the first three months of use.
The serious side effects of the pill occur very infrequently, especially if you are in good health and do not smoke. However, you should know that the following medical conditions have been associated with or made worse by the pill:
1. Blood clots in the legs (thrombophlebitis), lungs (pulmonary embolism), stoppage or rupture of a blood vessel in the brain (stroke), blockage of blood vessels in the heart (heart attack and angina pectoris) or other organs of the body. As mentioned above, smoking increases the risk of heart attacks and strokes and subsequent serious medical consequences.
2. Liver tumors, which may rupture and cause severe bleeding. A possible but not definite association has been found with the pill and liver cancer. However, liver cancers are extremely rare. The chance of developing liver cancer from using the pill is thus even rarer.
3. High blood pressure, although blood pressure usually returns to normal when the pill is stopped.
The symptoms associated with these serious side effects are discussed in the detailed leaflet given to you with your supply of pills. Notify your doctor or health-care provider if you notice any unusual physical disturbances while taking the pill. In addition, drugs such as rifampin, as well as some anticonvulsants and some antibiotics may decrease oral contraceptive effectiveness.
Studies to date of women taking the pill have not shown an increase in the incidence of cancer of the breast or cervix. There is, however, insufficient evidence to rule out the possibility that pills may cause such cancers.
Taking the pill provides some important noncontraceptive benefits. These include less painful menstruation, less menstrual blood loss and anemia, fewer pelvic infections, and fewer cancers of the ovary and the lining of the uterus.
Be sure to discuss any medical condition you may have with your health-care provider. Your health-care provider will take a medical and family history before prescribing oral contraceptives and will examine you.
You should be reexamined at least once a year while taking oral contraceptives. The "Detailed Patient Labeling" gives

you further information which you should read and discuss with your health-care provider.

DETAILED PATIENT LABELING

This product (like all oral contraceptives) is intended to prevent pregnancy. It does not protect against HIV infection (AIDS) and other sexually transmitted diseases.

INTRODUCTION

Any woman who considers using oral contraceptives (the "birth control pill" or the "pill") should understand the benefits and risks of using this form of birth control. This leaflet will give you much of the information you will need to make this decision and will also help you determine if you are at risk of developing any of the serious side effects of the pill. It will tell you how to use the pill properly so that it will be as effective as possible. However, this leaflet is not a replacement for a careful discussion between you and your health-care provider. You should discuss the information provided in this leaflet with him or her, both when you first start taking the pill and during your revisits. You should also follow your health-care provider's advice with regard to regular check-ups while you are on the pill.

EFFECTIVENESS OF ORAL CONTRACEPTIVES

Oral contraceptives or "birth control pills" or "the pill" are used to prevent pregnancy and are more effective than other nonsurgical methods of birth control. When they are taken correctly, the chance of becoming pregnant is less than 1% when used perfectly, without missing pills.

Typical failure rates are less than 3.0% per year. The chance of becoming pregnant increases with each missed pill during the menstrual cycle.

In comparison, typical failure rates for other nonsurgical methods of birth control during the first year of use are as follows:

Implant	<1%
Injection (Depo-Provera)	<1%
IUD	3%
Diaphragm with spermicides	18%
Spermicides alone	21%
Vaginal sponge	18%–28%
Condom alone	12%
Periodic abstinence	20%
No methods	85%

WHO SHOULD NOT TAKE ORAL CONTRACEPTIVES

> Cigarette smoking increases the risk of serious adverse effects on the heart and blood vessels from oral-contraceptive use. This risk increases with age and with heavy smoking (15 or more cigarettes per day) and is quite marked in women over 35 years of age. Women who use oral contraceptives are strongly advised not to smoke.

Some women should not use the pill. For example, you should not take the pill if you are pregnant or think you may be pregnant. You should also not use the pill if you have had any of the following conditions:

- Heart attack or stroke
- Blood clots in the legs (thrombophlebitis), lungs (pulmonary embolism), or eyes
- Blood clots in the deep veins of your legs
- Known or suspected breast cancer or cancer of the lining of the uterus, cervix or vagina
- Liver tumor (benign or cancerous)

Or, if you have any of the following:

- Chest pain (angina pectoris)
- Unexplained vaginal bleeding (until a diagnosis is reached by your doctor)
- Yellowing of the whites of the eyes or of the skin (jaundice) during pregnancy or during previous use of the pill
- Known or suspected pregnancy

Tell your health-care provider if you have ever had any of these conditions. Your health-care provider can recommend another method of birth control.

OTHER CONSIDERATIONS BEFORE TAKING ORAL CONTRACEPTIVES

Tell your health-care provider if you or any family member has ever had:

- Breast nodules, fibrocystic disease of the breast, an abnormal breast x-ray or mammogram
- Diabetes
- Elevated cholesterol or triglycerides
- High blood pressure
- Migraine or other headaches or epilepsy
- Mental depression
- Gallbladder, heart or kidney disease
- History of scanty or irregular menstrual periods

Women with any of these conditions should be checked often by their health-care provider if they choose to use oral contraceptives. Also, be sure to inform your doctor or health-care provider if you smoke or are on any medications.

ANNUAL NUMBER OF BIRTH-RELATED OR METHOD-RELATED DEATHS ASSOCIATED WITH CONTROL OF FERTILITY PER 100,000 NONSTERILE WOMEN, BY FERTILITY-CONTROL METHOD ACCORDING TO AGE

Method of control and outcome	15–19	20–24	25–29	30–34	35–39	40–44
No fertility-control methods*	7.0	7.4	9.1	14.8	25.7	28.2
Oral contraceptives nonsmoker**	0.3	0.5	0.9	1.9	13.8	31.6
Oral contraceptives smoker**	2.2	3.4	6.6	13.5	51.1	117.2
IUD**	0.8	0.8	1.0	1.0	1.4	1.4
Condom*	1.1	1.6	0.7	0.2	0.3	0.4
Diaphragm/spermicide*	1.9	1.2	1.2	1.3	2.2	2.8
Periodic abstinence*	2.5	1.6	1.6	1.7	2.9	3.6

* Deaths are birth related
** Deaths are method related

RISKS OF TAKING ORAL CONTRACEPTIVES

1. RISK OF DEVELOPING BLOOD CLOTS

Blood clots and blockage of blood vessels are the most serious side effects of taking oral contraceptives and can be fatal. In particular, a clot in the legs can cause thrombophlebitis and a clot that travels to the lungs can cause a sudden blocking of the vessel carrying blood to the lungs. Rarely, clots occur in the blood vessels of the eye and may cause blindness, double vision, or impaired vision.

If you take oral contraceptives and need elective surgery, need to stay in bed for a prolonged illness or have recently delivered a baby, you may be at risk of developing blood clots. You should consult your doctor about stopping oral contraceptives three to four weeks before surgery and not taking oral contraceptives for 2 weeks after surgery or during bed rest. You should also not take oral contraceptives soon after delivery of a baby or a midtrimester pregnancy termination. It is advisable to wait for at least 4 weeks after delivery if you are not breast-feeding. If you are breast-feeding, you should wait until you have weaned your child before using the pill. (See also the section on Breast-Feeding in "GENERAL PRECAUTIONS".)

2. HEART ATTACKS AND STROKES

Oral contraceptives may increase the tendency to develop strokes (stoppage or rupture of blood vessels in the brain) and angina pectoris and heart attacks (blockage of blood vessels in the heart). Any of these conditions can cause death or serious disability.

Smoking greatly increases the possibility of suffering heart attacks and strokes. Furthermore, smoking and the use of oral contraceptives greatly increase the chances of developing and dying of heart disease.

3. GALLBLADDER DISEASE

Oral-contraceptive users probably have a greater risk than nonusers of having gallbladder disease, although this risk may be related to pills containing high doses of estrogens.

4. LIVER TUMORS

In rare cases, oral contraceptives can cause benign but dangerous liver tumors. These benign liver tumors can rupture and cause fatal internal bleeding. In addition, a possible but not definite association has been found with the pill and liver cancers in two studies, in which a few women who developed these very rare cancers were found to have used oral contraceptives for long periods. However, liver cancers are extremely rare. The chance of developing liver cancer from using the pill is thus even rarer.

5. CANCER OF THE REPRODUCTIVE ORGANS

There is, at present, no confirmed evidence that oral contraceptives increase the risk of cancer of the reproductive organs in human studies. Several studies have found no overall increase in the risk of developing breast cancer. However, women who use oral contraceptives and have a strong family history of breast cancer or who have breast nodules or abnormal mammograms should be closely followed by their doctors.

Some studies have found an increase in the incidence of cancer of the cervix in women who use oral contraceptives. However, this finding may be related to factors other than the use of oral contraceptives.

ESTIMATED RISK OF DEATH FROM A BIRTH-CONTROL METHOD OR PREGNANCY

All methods of birth control and pregnancy are associated with a risk of developing certain diseases which may lead to disability or death. An estimate of the number of deaths associated with different methods of birth control and pregnancy has been calculated and is shown in the following table. [See table above.]

In the above table, the risk of death from any birth-control method is less than the risk of childbirth, except for oral contraceptive users over the age of 35 who smoke and pill users over the age of 40 even if they do not smoke. It can be seen in the table that for women aged 15 to 39, the risk of death was highest with pregnancy (7 to 26 deaths per 100,000 women, depending on age). Among pill users who do not smoke, the risk of death was always lower than that associated with pregnancy for any age group, except for those women over the age of 40 when the risk increases to 32 deaths per 100,000 women, compared to 28 associated with pregnancy at that

age. However, for pill users who smoke and are over the age of 35, the estimated number of deaths exceeds those for other methods of birth control. If a woman is over the age of 40 and smokes, her estimated risk of death is four times higher (117/100,000 women) than the estimated risk associated with pregnancy (28/100,000 women) in that age group. The suggestion that women over 40 who don't smoke should not take oral contraceptives is based on information from older high-dose pills and on less-selective use of pills than is practiced today. An Advisory Committee of the FDA discussed this issue in 1989 and recommended that the benefits of oral-contraceptive use by healthy, nonsmoking women over 40 years of age may outweigh the possible risks. However, all women, especially older women, are cautioned to use the lowest-dose pill that is effective.

WARNING SIGNALS

If any of these adverse effects occur while you are taking oral contraceptives, call your doctor immediately:

- Sharp chest pain, coughing of blood, or sudden shortness of breath (indicating a possible clot in the lung).
- Pain in the calf (indicating a possible clot in the leg).
- Crushing chest pain or heaviness in the chest (indicating a possible heart attack).
- Sudden severe headache or vomiting, dizziness or fainting, disturbances of vision or speech, weakness, or numbness in an arm or leg (indicating a possible stroke).
- Sudden partial or complete loss of vision (indicating a possible clot in the eye).
- Breast lumps (indicating possible breast cancer or fibrocystic disease of the breast; ask your doctor or health-care provider to show you how to examine your breasts).
- Severe pain or tenderness in the stomach area (indicating a possibly ruptured liver tumor).
- Difficulty in sleeping, weakness, lack of energy, fatigue, or change in mood (possibly indicating severe depression).
- Jaundice or a yellowing of the skin or eyeballs, accompanied frequently by fever, fatigue, loss of appetite, dark-colored urine, or light-colored bowel movements (indicating possible liver problems).

SIDE EFFECTS OF ORAL CONTRACEPTIVES

1. VAGINAL BLEEDING

Irregular vaginal bleeding or spotting may occur while you are taking the pills. Irregular bleeding may vary from slight staining between menstrual periods to breakthrough bleeding which is a flow much like a regular period. Irregular bleeding occurs most often during the first few months of oral-contraceptive use, but may also occur after you have been taking the pill for some time. Such bleeding may be temporary and usually does not indicate any serious problems. It is important to continue taking your pills on schedule. If the bleeding occurs in more than one cycle or lasts for more than a few days, talk to your doctor or health-care provider.

2. CONTACT LENSES

If you wear contact lenses and notice a change in vision or an inability to wear your lenses, contact your doctor or health-care provider.

3. FLUID RETENTION

Oral contraceptives may cause edema (fluid retention) with swelling of the fingers or ankles and may raise your blood pressure. If you experience fluid retention, contact your doctor or health-care provider.

4. MELASMA

A spotty darkening of the skin is possible, particularly of the face.

Continued on next page

Information on the Berlex products appearing here is based on the most current information available at the time of publication closing. Further information for these and other products may be obtained from the Medical Affairs Department, Berlex Laboratories, 300 Fairfield Road, Wayne, New Jersey 07470, 1-800-888-2407. Information on Betaseron and Fludara may be obtained from Berlex Laboratories, 15049 San Pablo Avenue, Richmond, California 94804-0016, 1-800-888-4112.

Berlex Laboratories—Cont.

5. OTHER SIDE EFFECTS
Other side effects include change in appetite, headache, nervousness, depression, dizziness, loss of scalp hair, rash, and vaginal infections.
If any of these side effects bother you, call your doctor or health-care provider.

GENERAL PRECAUTIONS

1. Missed periods and use of oral contraceptives before or during early pregnancy.
There may be times when you may not menstruate regularly after you have completed taking a cycle of pills. If you have taken your pills regularly and miss one menstrual period, continue taking your pills for the next cycle but be sure to inform your health-care provider before doing so. If you have not taken the pills daily as instructed and missed a menstrual period, or if you missed two consecutive menstrual periods, you may be pregnant. Check with your health-care provider immediately to determine whether you are pregnant. Do not continue to take oral contraceptives until you are sure you are not pregnant, but continue to use another method of contraception.
There is no conclusive evidence that oral contraceptive use is associated with an increase in birth defects, when taken inadvertently during early pregnancy. Previously, a few studies had reported that oral contraceptives might be associated with birth defects, but these studies have not been confirmed. Nevertheless, oral contraceptives or any other drugs should not be used during pregnancy unless clearly necessary and prescribed by your doctor. You should check with your doctor about risks to your unborn child of any medication taken during pregnancy.

2. While breast-feeding
If you are breast-feeding, consult your doctor before starting oral contraceptives. Some of the drug will be passed on to the child in the milk. A few adverse effects on the child have been reported, including yellowing of the skin (jaundice) and breast enlargement. In addition, oral contraceptives may decrease the amount and quality of your milk. If possible, do not use oral contraceptives while breast-feeding. You should use another method of contraception since breast-feeding provides only partial protection from becoming pregnant and this partial protection decreases significantly as you breast-feed for longer periods of time. You should consider starting oral contraceptives only after you have weaned your child completely.

3. Laboratory tests
If you are scheduled for any laboratory tests, tell your doctor you are taking birth-control pills. Certain blood tests may be affected by birth-control pills.

4. Drug interactions
Certain drugs may interact with birth control pills to make them less effective in preventing pregnancy or cause an increase in breakthrough bleeding. Such drugs include rifampin, drugs used for epilepsy such as barbiturates (for example, phenobarbital) and phenytoin (Dilantin is one brand of this drug), phenylbutazone (Butazolidin is one brand) and possibly certain antibiotics. You may need to use an additional method of contraception during any cycle in which you take drugs that can make oral contraceptives less effective.
This product (like all oral contraceptives) is intended to prevent pregnancy. It does not protect against transmission of HIV (AIDS) and other sexually transmitted diseases such as Chlamydia, genital herpes, genital warts, gonorrhea, hepatitis B, and Syphilis.

HOW TO TAKE THE PILL

IMPORTANT POINTS TO REMEMBER

TRI-LEVLEN® and LEVLEN® Tablets
BEFORE YOU START TAKING YOUR PILLS:
1. BE SURE TO READ THESE DIRECTIONS:
Before you start taking your pills.
Anytime you are not sure what to do.
2. THE RIGHT WAY TO TAKE THE PILL IS TO TAKE ONE PILL EVERY DAY AT THE SAME TIME.
If you miss pills you could get pregnant. This includes starting the pack late.
The more pills you miss, the more likely you are to get pregnant.
3. MANY WOMEN HAVE SPOTTING OR LIGHT BLEEDING, OR MAY FEEL SICK TO THEIR STOMACH DURING THE FIRST 1-3 PACKS OF PILLS.
If you do feel sick to your stomach, do not stop taking the pill. The problem will usually go away. If it doesn't go away, check with your doctor or clinic.
4. MISSING PILLS CAN ALSO CAUSE SPOTTING OR LIGHT BLEEDING, even when you make up these missed pills.
On the days you take 2 pills, to make up for missed pills, you could also feel a little sick to your stomach.

5. IF YOU HAVE VOMITING OR DIARRHEA, for any reason, or IF YOU TAKE SOME MEDICINES, including some antibiotics, your pills may not work as well.
Use a back-up method (such as condoms, foam, or sponge) until you check with your doctor or clinic.
6. IF YOU HAVE TROUBLE REMEMBERING TO TAKE THE PILL, talk to your doctor or clinic about how to make pill-taking easier or about using another method of birth control.
7. IF YOU HAVE ANY QUESTIONS OR ARE UNSURE ABOUT THE INFORMATION IN THIS LEAFLET, call your doctor or clinic.

BEFORE YOU START TAKING YOUR PILLS

TRI-LEVLEN® Tablets
1. DECIDE WHAT TIME OF DAY YOU WANT TO TAKE YOUR PILL.
It is important to take it at about the same time every day.
2. LOOK AT YOUR PILL PACK TO SEE IF IT HAS 21 OR 28 PILLS:
The 21-pill pack has 21 "active" (6 brown, 5 white and 10 light-yellow) pills (with hormones) to take for 3 weeks, followed by 1 week without pills.
The 28-pill pack has 21 "active" (6 brown, 5 white and 10 light yellow) pills (with hormones) to take for 3 weeks, followed by 1 week of reminder (light-green) pills (without hormones).
3. ALSO FIND:
1) where on the pack to start taking pills.
2) in what order to take the pills (follow the arrows)

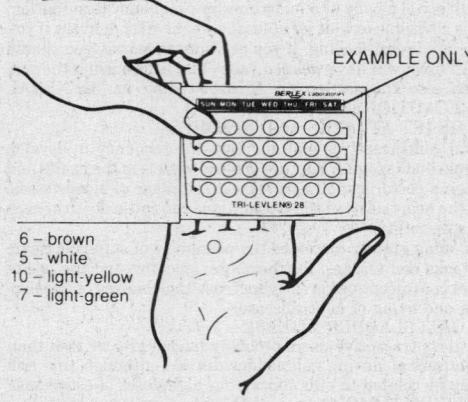

EXAMPLE ONLY

6 – brown
5 – white
10 – light-yellow
7 – light-green

4. BE SURE YOU HAVE READY AT ALL TIMES:
ANOTHER KIND OF BIRTH CONTROL (such as condoms, foam or sponge) to use as a back-up in case you miss pills.
AN EXTRA, FULL PILL PACK.

LEVLEN® Tablets
1. DECIDE WHAT TIME OF DAY YOU WANT TO TAKE YOUR PILL.
It is important to take it at about the same time every day.
2. LOOK AT YOUR PILL PACK TO SEE IF IT HAS 21 OR 28 PILLS:
The 21-pill pack has 21 "active" (light-orange) pills (with hormones) to take for 3 weeks, followed by 1 week without pills.
The 28-pill pack has 21 "active" (light-orange) pills (with hormones) to take for 3 weeks, followed by 1 week of reminder (pink) pills (without hormones).
3. ALSO FIND:
1) where on the pack to start taking pills.
2) in what order to take the pills (follow the arrows).

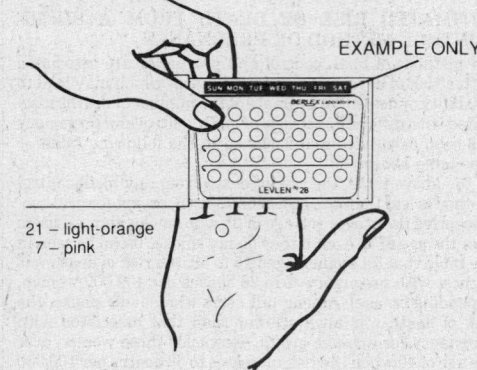

EXAMPLE ONLY

21 – light-orange
7 – pink

4. BE SURE YOU HAVE READY AT ALL TIMES:
ANOTHER KIND OF BIRTH CONTROL (such as condoms, foam or sponge) to use as a back-up in case you miss pills.
AN EXTRA, FULL PILL PACK.

WHEN TO START THE FIRST PACK OF PILLS

TRI-LEVLEN® Tablets
You have a choice for which day to start taking your first pack of pills. Decide with your doctor or clinic which is the best day for you. Pick a time of day which will be easy to remember.
DAY 1 START:
1. Take the first "active" (brown) pill of the first pack during the first 24 hours of your period.
2. You will not need to use a back-up method of birth control, since you are starting the pill at the beginning of your period.
SUNDAY START:
1. Take the first "active" (brown) pill of the first pack on the Sunday after your period starts, even if you are still bleeding. If your period begins on Sunday, start the pack that same day.
2. Use another method of birth control as a back-up method if you have sex anytime from the Sunday you start your first pack until the next Sunday (7 days). Condoms, foam, or the sponge are good back-up methods of birth control.
LEVLEN® Tablets
You have a choice for which day to start taking your first pack of pills. Decide with your doctor or clinic which is the best day for you. Pick a time of day which will be easy to remember.
DAY 1 START:
1. Take the first "active" (light-orange) pill of the first pack during the first 24 hours of your period.
2. You will not need to use a back-up method of birth control, since you are starting the pill at the beginning of your period.
SUNDAY START:
1. Take the first "active" (light-orange) pill of the first pack on the Sunday after your period starts, even if you are still bleeding. If your period begins on Sunday, start the pack that same day.
2. Use another method of birth control as a back-up method if you have sex anytime from the Sunday you start your first pack until the next Sunday (7 days). Condoms, foam, or the sponge are good back-up methods of birth control.

WHAT TO DO DURING THE MONTH

TRI-LEVLEN® and LEVLEN® Tablets
1. **TAKE ONE PILL AT THE SAME TIME EVERY DAY UNTIL THE PACK IS EMPTY.**
Do not skip pills even if you are spotting or bleeding between monthly periods or feel sick to your stomach (nausea).
Do not skip pills even if you do not have sex very often.
2. **WHEN YOU FINISH A PACK OR SWITCH YOUR BRAND OF PILLS:**
21 pills: Wait 7 days to start the next pack. You will probably have your period during that week. Be sure that no more than 7 days pass between 21-day packs.
28 pills: Start the next pack on the day after your last "reminder" pill.
Do not wait any days between packs.

WHAT TO DO IF YOU MISS PILLS

TRI-LEVLEN® Tablets
If you **MISS 1** (brown, white or light-yellow) "active" pill:
1. Take it as soon as you remember. Take the next pill at your regular time. This means you may take 2 pills in 1 day.
2. You do not need to use a back-up birth control method if you have sex.
If you **MISS 2** (brown or white) "active" pills in a row in **WEEK 1 OR WEEK 2** of your pack:
1. Take 2 pills on the day you remember and 2 pills the next day.
2. Then take 1 pill a day until you finish the pack.
3. YOU MAY BECOME PREGNANT if you have sex in the 7 days after you miss pills. You MUST use another birth control method (such as condoms, foam, or sponge) as a back-up for those 7 days.
If you **MISS 2** (light-yellow) "active" pills in a row in **THE 3rd WEEK:**
1. *If you are a Day 1 Starter:*
THROW OUT the rest of the pill pack and start a new pack that same day.
If you are a Sunday Starter:
Keep taking 1 pill every day until Sunday. On Sunday, THROW OUT the rest of the pack and start a new pack of pills that same day.

2. You may not have your period this month but this is expected. However, if you miss your period 2 months in a row, call your doctor or clinic because you might be pregnant.

3. You MAY BECOME PREGNANT if you have sex in the 7 days after you miss pills. You MUST use another birth control method (such as condoms, foam, or sponge) as a back-up for those 7 days.

If you **MISS 3 OR MORE** (brown, white or light-yellow) "active" pills in a row (during the first 3 weeks).

1. *If you are a Day 1 Starter:*
THROW OUT the rest of the pill pack and start a new pack that same day
   If you are a Sunday Starter:
Keep taking 1 pill every day until Sunday. On Sunday. THROW OUT the rest of the pack and start a new pack of pills that same day.

2. You may not have your period this month but this is expected. However, if you miss your period 2 months in a row, call your doctor or clinic because you might be pregnant.

3. You MAY BECOME PREGNANT if you have sex in the 7 days after you miss pills. You MUST use another birth control method (such as condoms, foam, or sponge) as a back-up for those 7 days.

A REMINDER FOR THOSE ON 28-DAY PACKS:

If you forget any of the 7 (light-green) "reminder" pills in Week 4:

THROW AWAY the pills you missed.

Keep taking 1 pill each day until the pack is empty.

You do not need a back-up method if you start your next pack on time.

FINALLY, IF YOU ARE STILL NOT SURE WHAT TO DO ABOUT THE PILLS YOU HAVE MISSED:

Use a BACK-UP METHOD anytime you have sex.

KEEP TAKING ONE "ACTIVE" PILL EACH DAY until you can reach your doctor or clinic.

LEVLEN® Tablets

If you **MISS 1** (light-orange) "active" pill:

1. Take it as soon as you remember. Take the next pill at your regular time. This means you may take 2 pills in 1 day.

2. You do not need to use a back-up birth control method if you have sex.

If you **MISS 2** (light-orange) "active" pills in a row in **WEEK 1 OR WEEK 2** of your pack:

1. Take 2 pills on the day you remember and 2 pills the next day.

2. Then take 1 pill a day until you finish the pack.

3. You MAY BECOME PREGNANT if you have sex in the 7 days after you miss pills. You MUST use another birth control method (such as condoms, foam, or sponge) as a back-up for those 7 days.

If you **MISS 2** (light-orange) "active" pills in a row in **THE 3rd WEEK:**

1. *If you are a Day 1 Starter:*
THROW OUT the rest of the pill pack and start a new pack that same day.
   If you are a Sunday Starter:
Keep taking 1 pill every day until Sunday. On Sunday. THROW OUT the rest of the pack and start a new pack of pills that same day.

2. You may not have your period this month but this is expected. However, if you miss your period 2 months in a row, call your doctor or clinic because you might be pregnant.

3. You MAY BECOME PREGNANT if you have sex in the 7 days after you miss pills. You MUST use another birth control method (such as condoms, foam, or sponge) as a back-up for those 7 days.

If you **MISS 3 OR MORE** (light-orange) "active" pills in a row (during the first 3 weeks).

1. *If you are a Day 1 Starter:*
THROW OUT the rest of the pill pack and start a new pack that same day.
   If you are a Sunday Starter:
Keep taking 1 pill every day until Sunday. On Sunday. THROW OUT the rest of the pack and start a new pack of pills that same day.

2. You may not have your period this month but this is expected. However, if you miss your period 2 months in a row, call your doctor or clinic because you might be pregnant.

3. You MAY BECOME PREGNANT if you have sex in the 7 days after you miss pills. You MUST use another birth control method (such as condoms, foam, or sponge) as a back-up for those 7 days.

A REMINDER FOR THOSE ON 28-DAY PACKS:

If you forget any of the 7 (pink) "reminder" pills in Week 4:

THROW AWAY the pills you missed.

Keep taking 1 pill each day until the pack is empty.

You do not need a back-up method if you start your next pack on time.

FINALLY, IF YOU ARE STILL NOT SURE WHAT TO DO ABOUT THE PILLS YOU HAVE MISSED:

Use a BACK-UP METHOD anytime you have sex.

KEEP TAKING ONE "ACTIVE" PILL EACH DAY until you can reach your doctor or clinic.

PREGNANCY DUE TO PILL FAILURE

The incidence of pill failure resulting in pregnancy is approximately less than 1.0% if taken every day as directed, but more typical failure rates are less than 3.0%. If failure does occur, the risk to the fetus is minimal.

RISKS TO THE FETUS

If you do become pregnant while using oral contraceptives, the risk to the fetus is small, and, therefore, the most pertinent, the risk to the fetus is small, on the order of no more than one per thousand. You should, however, discuss the risks to the developing child with your doctor.

PREGNANCY AFTER STOPPING THE PILL

There may be some delay in becoming pregnant after you stop using oral contraceptives, especially if you had irregular menstrual cycles before you used oral contraceptives. It may be advisable to postpone conception until you begin menstruating regularly once you have stopped taking the pill and desire pregnancy.

There does not appear to be any increase in birth defects in newborn babies when pregnancy occurs soon after stopping the pill.

OVERDOSAGE

Serious ill effects have not been reported following ingestion of large doses of oral contraceptives by young children. Overdosage may cause nausea and withdrawal bleeding in females. In case of overdosage, contact your health-care provider or pharmacist.

OTHER INFORMATION

Your health-care provider will take a medical and family history before prescribing oral contraceptives and will examine you. You should be reexamined at least once a year. Be sure to inform your health-care provider if there is a family history of any of the conditions listed previously in this leaflet. Be sure to keep all appointments with your health-care provider, because this is a time to determine if there are early signs of side effects of oral-contraceptive use.

Do not use the drug for any condition other than the one for which it was prescribed. This drug has been prescribed specifically for you; do not give it to others who may want birth-control pills.

HEALTH BENEFITS FROM ORAL CONTRACEPTIVES

In addition to preventing pregnancy, use of oral contraceptives may provide certain benefits. They are:
● Menstrual cycles may become more regular.
● Blood flow during menstruation may be lighter and less iron may be lost. Therefore, anemia due to iron deficiency is less likely to occur.
● Pain or other symptoms during menstruation may be encountered less frequently.
● Ovarian cysts may occur less frequently.
● Ectopic (tubal) pregnancy may occur less frequently.
● Noncancerous cysts or lumps in the breast may occur less frequently.
● Acute pelvic inflammatory disease may occur less frequently.
● Oral-contraceptive use may provide some protection against developing two forms of cancer: cancer of the ovaries and cancer of the lining of the uterus.

If you want more information about birth-control pills, ask your doctor or pharmacist. They have a more technical leaflet called the "Professional Labeling", which you may wish to read.

© 1993, Berlex Laboratories, All Rights Reserved.
Manufactured for:
BERLEX Laboratories, Wayne, NJ 07470
Revised Jan., 1994   60700-0
Revised Apr., 1993   60658-1
Shown in Product Identification Guide, page 305

For information on over-the-counter drugs, consult **PDR For Nonprescription Drugs**

Berlex Laboratories
**15049 SAN PABLO AVENUE
RICHMOND, CA 94804-0099**

Direct Inquiries to:
(201) 694-4100

For Medical Information and to Report Drug Adverse Events Contact:
Department of Epidemiology and Medical Affairs
300 Fairfield Road
Wayne, NJ 07470
(800) 888-2407
Betaseron for SC Injection Only:
(Medical Information Only)
15049 San Pablo Avenue
Richmond, CA 94809-0099
(800) 888-4112
Fludara For Injection Only:
(Medical Information Only)
15049 San Pablo Avenue
Richmond, CA 94809-0099
(800) 888-4112

BETASERON®
(Interferon beta-1b)   ℞

DESCRIPTION

Betaseron® (Interferon beta-1b) is a purified, sterile, lyophilized protein product produced by recombinant DNA techniques and formulated for use by injection. Interferon beta-1b is manufactured by bacterial fermentation of a strain of *Escherichia coli* that bears a genetically engineered plasmid containing the gene for human interferon beta$_{ser17}$. The native gene was obtained from human fibroblasts and altered in a way that substitutes serine for the cysteine residue found at position 17. Interferon beta-1b is a highly purified protein that has 165 amino acids and an approximate molecular weight of 18,500 daltons. It does not include the carbohydrate side chains found in the natural material.

The specific activity of Betaseron is approximately 32 million international units (IU)/mg Interferon beta-1b. Each vial contains 0.3 mg (9.6 million IU) of Interferon beta-1b. The unit measurement is derived by comparing the antiviral activity of the product to the World Health Organization (WHO) reference standard of recombinant human interferon beta. Dextrose and Albumin Human, USP (15 mg each/vial) are added as stabilizers. Prior to 1993, a different analytical standard was used to determine potency. It assigned 54 million IU to 0.3 mg Interferon beta-1b.

Lyophilized Betaseron is a sterile, white to off-white powder intended for subcutaneous injection after reconstitution with the diluent supplied (Sodium Chloride, 0.54% Solution).

CLINICAL PHARMACOLOGY

General: Interferons are a family of naturally occurring proteins, which have molecular weights ranging from 15,000 to 21,000 daltons. Three major classes of interferons have been identified: alfa, beta, and gamma. Interferon beta-1b, interferon alfa, and interferon gamma have overlapping yet distinct biologic activities.[1-5] The activities of Interferon beta-1b are species-restricted and, therefore, the most pertinent pharmacologic information on Betaseron is derived from studies of human cells in culture and in humans.

Biologic Activities: Interferon beta-1b has been shown to possess both antiviral and immunoregulatory activities. The mechanisms by which Betaseron® (Interferon beta-1b) exerts its actions in multiple sclerosis (MS) are not clearly understood. However, it is known that the biologic response-modifying properties of Interferon beta-1b are mediated through its interactions with specific cell receptors found on the surface of human cells. The binding of Interferon beta-1b to these receptors induces the expression of a number of interferon-induced gene products (e.g., 2',5'-oligoadenylate synthetase, protein kinase, and indoleamine 2,3-dioxygenase) that are believed to be the mediators of the biological actions of Interferon beta-1b.[1,3,6-10] A number of these interferon-induced products have been readily measured in the serum and cellular fractions of blood collected from patients treated with Interferon beta-1b.[11,12]

Pharmacokinetics: Because serum concentrations of Interferon beta-1b are low or not detectable following subcutane-

Continued on next page

Berlex Laboratories—Cont.

ous administration of 0.25 mg (8 million IU) or less of Betaseron, pharmacokinetic information in patients with MS receiving the recommended dose of Betaseron is not available. Following single and multiple daily subcutaneous administrations of 0.5 mg (16 million IU) Betaseron to healthy volunteers (N=12), serum Interferon beta-1b concentrations were generally below 100 IU/mL. Peak serum Interferon beta-1b concentrations occurred between 1 to 8 hours, with a mean peak serum interferon concentration of 40 IU/mL. Bioavailability, based on a total dose of 0.5 mg (16 million IU) Betaseron given as two subcutaneous injections at different sites, was approximately 50%.

After intravenous administration of Betaseron (0.006 mg [0.2 million IU] to 2.0 mg [64 million IU]), similar pharmacokinetic profiles were obtained from healthy volunteers (N=12) and from patients with diseases other than MS (N=142). In patients receiving single intravenous doses up to 2.0 mg (64 million IU), increases in serum concentrations were dose proportional. Mean serum clearance values ranged from 9.4 mL/min·kg^{-1} to 28.9 mL/min·kg^{-1} and were independent of dose. Mean terminal elimination half-life values ranged from 8.0 minutes to 4.3 hours and mean steady-state volume of distribution values ranged from 0.25 L/kg to 2.88 L/kg. Three-times-a-week intravenous dosing for 2 weeks resulted in no accumulation of Interferon beta-1b in the serum of patients. Pharmacokinetic parameters after single and multiple intravenous doses of Betaseron® (Interferon beta-1b) were comparable.

Clinical Trials: The effectiveness of Betaseron in relapsing-remitting MS was evaluated in a double-blind, multiclinic (11 sites: 4 Canadian and 7 United States), randomized, parallel, placebo-controlled clinical investigation of 2 years duration. The study enrolled MS patients, aged 18 to 50, who were ambulatory (Kurtzke expanded disability status scale [EDSS] of ≤5.5), exhibited a relapsing-remitting clinical course, met Poser's criteria[13] for clinically definite and/or laboratory supported definite MS and had experienced at least two exacerbations over 2 years preceding the trial without exacerbation in the preceding month. Patients who had received prior immunosuppressant therapy were excluded. An exacerbation was defined, per protocol, as the appearance of a new clinical sign/symptom or the clinical worsening of a previous sign/symptom (one that had been stable for at least 30 days) that persisted for a minimum of 24 hours. Patients selected for study were randomized to treatment with either placebo (N=123), 0.05 mg (1.6 million IU) of Betaseron (N=125), or 0.25 mg (8 million IU) of Betaseron (N=124) self-administered subcutaneously every other day. Outcome based on the 372 randomized patients was evaluated after 2 years.

Patients who required more than three 28-day courses of corticosteroids were removed from the study. Minor analgesics (acetaminophen, codeine), antidepressants, and oral baclofen were allowed ad libitum but chronic nonsteroidal anti-inflammatory drug (NSAID) use was not allowed.

The primary, protocol defined, outcome assessment measures were 1) frequency of exacerbations per patient and 2) proportion of exacerbation free patients. A number of secondary outcome measures were also employed as described in Table 1.

In addition to clinical measures, annual magnetic resonance imaging (MRI) was performed and quantitated for extent of disease as determined by changes in total area of lesions. In a substudy of patients (N=52) at one site, MRIs were performed every 6 weeks and quantitated for disease activity as determined by changes in size and number of lesions.

Results at the protocol designated endpoint of 2 years (see TABLE 1): In the 2-year analysis, there was a 31% reduction in annual exacerbation rate, from 1.31 in the placebo group to 0.9 in the 0.25 mg (8 million IU) group. The p-value for this difference was 0.0001. The proportion of patients free of exacerbations was 16% in the placebo group, compared with 25% in the Betaseron® (Interferon beta-1b) 0.25 mg (8 million IU) group.

Of the 372 patients randomized, 72 (19%) failed to complete 2 full years on their assigned treatments. The reasons given for withdrawal varied with treatment assignment. Excessive use of steroids accounted for 11 of the 26 placebo withdrawals, but only 2 of the 21 withdrawals from the 0.05 mg (1.6 million IU) assigned group and 1 of the 25 withdrawals from the 0.25 mg (8 million IU) assigned group. Withdrawals for adverse events attributed to study article, however, were more common among Betaseron-treated patients: 1, 5, and 10 withdrew from the placebo, 0.05 mg (1.6 million IU), and 0.25 mg (8 million IU) groups, respectively.

Over the 2-year period, there were 25 MS-related hospitalizations in the 0.25 mg (8 million IU) Betaseron® (Interferon beta-1b)-treated group compared to 48 hospitalizations in the placebo group. In comparison, non-MS hospitalizations were evenly distributed among the groups, with 16 in the 0.25 mg (8 million IU) Betaseron group and 15 in the placebo group. The average number of days of MS-related steroid use was 41 days in the 0.25 mg (8 million IU) Betaseron® (Interferon beta-1b) group and 55 days in the placebo group (p=0.004). [See table below.]

MRI data were also analyzed for patients in this study. A frequency distribution of the observed percent changes in MRI area at the end of 2 years was obtained by grouping the percentages in successive intervals of equal width. Figure 1 displays a histogram of the proportions of patients who fell into each of these intervals. The median percent change in MRI area for the 0.25 mg (8 million IU) group was −1.1% which was significantly smaller than the 16.5% observed for the placebo group (p=0.0001).

[See Figure 1 at top of next page.]

In an evaluation of frequent MRI scans (every 6 weeks) on 52 patients at one site, the percent of scans with new or expanding lesions was 29% in the placebo group and 6% in the 0.25 mg (8 million IU) treatment group (p=0.006).

MRI scanning is viewed as a useful means to visualize changes in white matter that are believed to be a reflection of the pathologic changes that, appropriately located within the central nervous system (CNS), account for some of the signs and symptoms that typify relapsing-remitting MS. The exact relationship between MRI findings and the clinical status of patients is unknown. Changes in lesion area often do not correlate with clinical exacerbations probably because many of the lesions affect so-called "silent" regions of the CNS. Moreover, it is not clear what fraction of the lesions seen on MRI become foci of irreversible demyelinization (i.e., classic white matter plaques). The prognostic significance of the MRI findings in this study has not been evaluated.

At the end of 2 years on assigned treatment, patients in the study had the option of continuing on treatment under blinded conditions. Approximately 80% of patients under each treatment accepted. Although there was a trend toward patient benefit in the Betaseron® (Interferon beta-1b) groups during the third year, particularly in the 0.25 mg (8 million IU) group, there was no statistically significant difference between the Betaseron® (Interferon beta-1b)-treated vs. placebo-treated patients in exacerbation rate, or in any of the secondary endpoints described in Table 1. As noted above, in the 2-year analysis, there was a 31% reduction in exacerbation rate in the 0.25 mg (8 million IU) group, compared with placebo. The p-value for this difference was 0.0001. In the analysis of the third year alone, the difference between treatment groups was 28%. The p-value was 0.065. The lower number of patients may account for the loss of statistical significance, and lack of direct comparability among the patient groups in this extension study make the interpretation of these results difficult. The third year MRI data did not show a trend toward additional benefit in the Betaseron arm compared with the placebo arm.

Throughout the clinical trial, serum samples from patients were monitored for the development of antibodies to Interferon beta-1b. In patients receiving 0.25 mg (8 million IU) of Betaseron (N=124) every other day in the clinical trial, 45% were found to have serum neutralizing activity at one or more of the time points tested. The relationship between antibody formation and clinical efficacy is not known.

INDICATIONS AND USAGE

Betaseron is indicated for use in ambulatory patients with relapsing-remitting multiple sclerosis to reduce the frequency of clinical exacerbations. (See **CLINICAL PHARMACOLOGY, Clinical Trials** section.) Relapsing-remitting MS is characterized by recurrent attacks of neurologic dysfunction followed by complete or incomplete recovery. The safety and efficacy of Betaseron in chronic-progressive MS has not been evaluated.

CONTRAINDICATIONS

Betaseron is contraindicated in patients with a history of hypersensitivity to natural or recombinant interferon beta, Albumin Human USP, or any other component of the formulation.

TABLE 1
2 Year Study Results
Primary and Secondary Clinical Endpoints

Efficacy Parameters	Treatment Groups			Statistical Comparisons p-value		
Primary Endpoints	Placebo	0.05 mg (1.6 mIU)	0.25 mg (8 mIU)	Placebo vs 0.05 mg (1.6 mIU)	0.05 mg (1.6 mIU) vs 0.25 mg (8 mIU)	Placebo vs 0.25 mg (8 mIU)
	(N=123)	(N=125)	(N=124)			
Annual exacerbation rate	1.31	1.14	0.90	0.005	0.113	**0.0001**
Proportion of exacerbation-free patients†	16%	18%	25%	0.609	0.288	**0.094**
Exacerbation frequency per patient 0†	20	22	29	0.151	0.077	**0.001**
1	32	31	39			
2	20	28	17			
3	15	15	14			
4	15	7	9			
≥5	21	16	8			
Secondary Endpoints††						
Median number of months to first on-study exacerbation	5	6	9	0.299	0.097	**0.010**
Rate of moderate or severe exacerbations per year	0.47	0.29	0.23	0.020	0.257	**0.001**
Mean number of moderate or severe exacerbation days per patient	44.1	33.2	19.5	0.229	0.064	**0.001**
Mean change in EDSS score‡ at endpoint	0.21	0.21	−0.07	0.995	0.108	**0.144**
Mean change in Scripps score‡‡ at endpoint	−0.53	−0.50	0.66	0.641	0.051	**0.126**
Median duration in days per exacerbation	36	33	35.5	ND	ND	**ND**
% change in mean MRI lesion area at endpoint	21.4%	9.8%	−0.9%	0.015	0.019	**0.0001**

ND - Not done

† - 14 exacerbation-free patients (0 from placebo, 6 from 0.05 mg, and 8 from 0.25 mg) dropped out of the study before completing 6 months of therapy. These patients are excluded from this analysis.

†† - Sequelae and Functional Neurologic Status, both required by protocol, were not analyzed individually but are included as a function of the EDSS.

‡ - EDSS scores range from 0–10, with higher scores reflecting greater disability.

‡‡ - Scripps neurologic rating scores range from 0–100, with smaller scores reflecting greater disability.

WARNINGS

One suicide and 4 attempted suicides were observed among 372 study patients during a 3-year period. All five patients received Betaseron® (Interferon beta-1b) (three in the 0.05 mg [1.6 million IU] group and two in the 0.25 mg [8 million IU] group). There were no attempted suicides in patients on study who did not receive Betaseron. Depression and suicide have been reported to occur in patients receiving interferon alfa, a related compound. Patients to be treated with Betaseron should be informed that depression and suicidal ideation may be a side effect of the treatment and should report these symptoms immediately to the prescribing physician. Patients exhibiting depression should be monitored closely and cessation of therapy should be considered.

PRECAUTIONS

General: Patients should be instructed in injection techniques to assure the safe self-administration of Betaseron. (See **PRECAUTIONS: Information to patients**, and **Betaseron® (Interferon beta-1b) Patient Information** sheet.)
Information to patients:
Instruction on self-injection technique and procedures. Patients should be instructed in the use of aseptic technique when administering Betaseron. Appropriate instruction for reconstitution of Betaseron and self-injection should be given including careful review of the **Betaseron® (Interferon beta-1b) Patient Information** sheet. If possible, the first injection should be performed under the supervision of an appropriately qualified health care professional.
Patients should be cautioned against the re-use of needles or syringes and instructed in safe disposal procedures. A puncture resistant container for disposal of used needles and syringes should be supplied to the patient along with instructions for safe disposal of full containers.
Eighty-five percent of patients in the controlled MS trial reported injection site reactions at one or more times during therapy. In general, these were transient and did not require discontinuation of therapy, but the nature and severity of all reported reactions should be carefully assessed. Patient understanding and use of aseptic self-injection technique and procedures should be periodically reevaluated.
Flu-like symptoms are not uncommon following initiation of therapy with Betaseron® (Interferon beta-1b). In the controlled MS clinical trial, acetaminophen was permitted for relief of fever or myalgia.
Patients should be cautioned not to change the dosage or the schedule of administration without medical consultation.
Awareness of adverse reactions. Patients should be advised about the common adverse events associated with the use of Betaseron, particularly, injection site reactions and the flu-like symptom complex (see **ADVERSE REACTIONS** section).
Patients should be cautioned to report depression or suicidal ideation (see **WARNINGS**).
Patients should be advised about the abortifacient potential of Betaseron (see **PRECAUTIONS, Pregnancy - Teratogenic effects**).
Laboratory tests: The following laboratory tests are recommended prior to initiating Betaseron therapy and at periodic intervals thereafter: hemoglobin, complete and differential white blood cell counts, platelet counts and blood chemistries including liver function tests. In the controlled MS trial, patients were monitored every 3 months. The study protocol stipulated that Betaseron therapy be discontinued in the event the absolute neutrophil count fell below 750/mm³. When the absolute neutrophil count had returned to a value greater than 750/mm³, therapy could be restarted at a 50% reduced dose. No patients were withdrawn or dose reduced for neutropenia or lymphopenia.
Similarly, if hepatic transaminase (SGOT/SGPT) levels exceeded 10 times the upper limit of normal, or if the serum bilirubin exceeded 5 times the upper limit of normal, therapy was discontinued. In each instance during the controlled MS trial, hepatic enzyme abnormalities returned to normal following discontinuation of therapy. When measurements had decreased to below these levels, therapy could be restarted at a 50% dose reduction, if clinically appropriate. Two patients were dose reduced for increased liver enzymes; one continued on treatment and one was ultimately withdrawn.
Drug interactions: Interactions between Betaseron® (Interferon beta-1b) and other drugs have not been fully evaluated. Although studies designed to examine drug interactions have not been done, it was noted that corticosteroid or ACTH treatment of relapses for periods of up to 28 days has been administered to patients (N=180) receiving Betaseron.
Betaseron administration to three cancer patients over a dose range of 0.025 mg (0.8 million IU) to 2.2 mg (71 million IU) led to a dose-dependent inhibition of antipyrine elimination.[14] The effect of alternate-day administration of 0.25 mg (8 million IU) of Betaseron on drug metabolism in MS patients is unknown.
Carcinogenesis: The carcinogenic potential of Betaseron was evaluated by studying its effect on the morphological

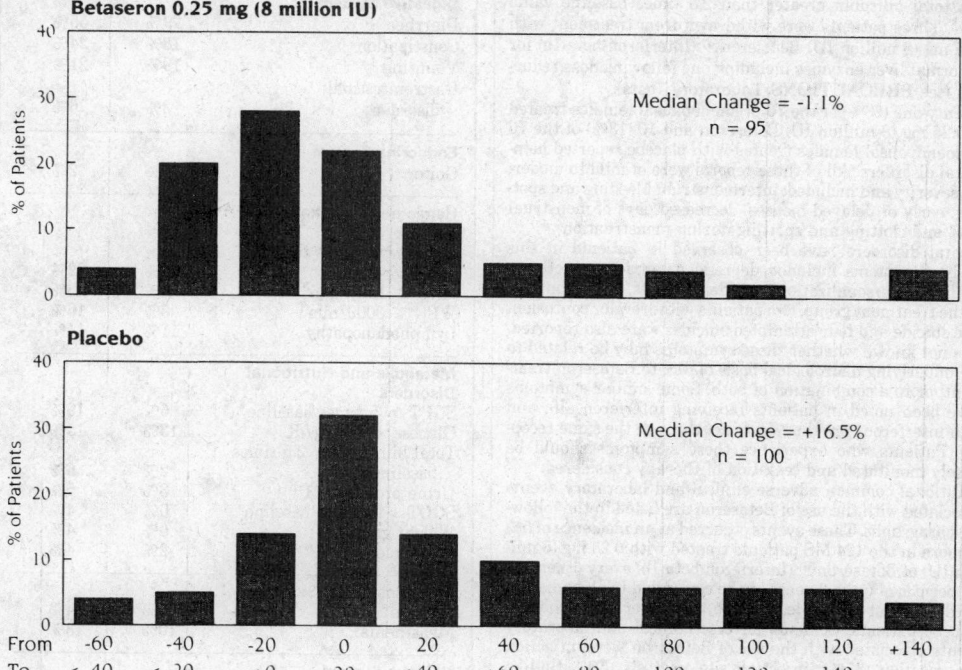

Figure 1
Distribution of Change in MRI Area

Betaseron 0.25 mg (8 million IU)

Median Change = -1.1%
n = 95

Placebo

Median Change = +16.5%
n = 100

From	-60	-40	-20	0	20	40	60	80	100	120	+140
To	< -40	< -20	< 0	< 20	< 40	< 60	< 80	< 100	< 120	< 140	

Percent Change in MRI Area

transformation of the mammalian cell line BALBc-3T3. No significant increases in transformation frequency were noted. No carcinogenicity data are available in animals or humans.
Betaseron was not mutagenic when assayed for genotoxicity in the Ames bacterial test in the presence or absence of metabolic activation.
Impairment of fertility: Studies in rhesus monkeys at doses up to .33 mg (10.7 million IU)/kg/day (32 times the recommended human dose based on body surface area comparison)* in normally cycling rhesus female monkeys had no apparent adverse effects on the menstrual cycle or on associated hormonal profiles (progesterone and estradiol) when administered over 3 consecutive menstrual cycles. The extrapolability of animal doses to human doses is not known. Effects of Betaseron on normal cycling human females are not known.
*body surface dose based on 70 kg female
Pregnancy - Teratogenic effects: Pregnancy Category C: Betaseron was not teratogenic at doses up to 0.42 mg (13.3 million IU)/kg/day in rhesus monkeys, but demonstrated a dose-related abortifacient activity when administered at doses ranging from 0.028 mg (0.89 million IU)/kg/day (2.8 times the recommended human dose based on body surface area comparison) to 0.42 mg (13.3 million IU)/kg/day (40 times the recommended human dose based on body surface area comparison). The extrapolability of animal doses to human doses is not known. Lower doses were not studied in monkeys. Spontaneous abortions while on treatment were reported in patients (N=4) who participated in the Betaseron MS clinical trial. Betaseron given to rhesus monkeys on gestation days 20 to 70 did not cause teratogenic effects, however, it is not known if teratogenic effects exist in humans. There are no adequate and well-controlled studies in pregnant women. If the patient becomes pregnant or plans to become pregnant while taking Betaseron, the patient should be apprised of the potential hazard to the fetus and it should be recommended that the patient discontinue therapy.
Nursing mothers: It is not known whether Betaseron is excreted in human milk. Because many drugs are excreted in human milk and because of the potential for serious adverse reactions in nursing infants from Betaseron, a decision should be made as to whether either to discontinue nursing or discontinue the drug, taking into account the importance of drug to the mother.
Pediatric use: Safety and efficacy in children under 18 years of age have not been established.

ADVERSE REACTIONS

Experience with Betaseron® (Interferon beta-1b) in patients with MS is limited to a total of 147 patients at the recommended dose of 0.25 mg (8 million IU) every other day or more. Consequently, adverse events that are associated with the use of Betaseron in MS patients at a low incidence may not have been observed in pre-marketing studies. Clinical experience with Betaseron in other populations (patients with cancer, HIV positive patients, etc.) provides additional data regarding adverse reactions; however, experience in non-MS populations may not be fully applicable to the MS population.
Injection site reactions (85%) and injection site necrosis (5%) occurred after administration of Betaseron. Inflammation, pain, hypersensitivity, necrosis, and non-specific reactions were significantly associated (p < 0.05) with the 0.25 mg (8 million IU) Betaseron-treated group. Only inflammation, pain, and necrosis were reported as severe events. The incidence rate for injection site reactions was calculated over the course of 3 years. This incidence rate decreased over time, with 79% of patients experiencing the event during the first 3 months of treatment compared to 47% during the last 6 months. The median time to the first occurrence of an injection site reaction was 7 days. Patients with injection site reactions reported these events 183.7 days per year. Three patients withdrew from the 0.25 mg (8 million IU) Betaseron-treated group for injection site pain.
Flu-like symptom complex was reported in 76% of the patients treated with 0.25 mg (8 million IU) Betaseron. A patient was defined as having a flu-like symptom complex if flu-like symptoms or at least two of the following symptoms were concurrently reported: fever, chills, myalgia, malaise, or sweating. Only myalgia, fever, and chills were reported as severe in more than 5% of the patients. The incidence rate for flu-like symptom complex was also calculated over the course of 3 years. The incidence rate of these events decreased over time, with 51% of patients experiencing the event during the first 3 months of treatment compared to 4% during the last 6 months. The median time to the first occurrence of flu-like symptom complex was 3 days and the median duration per patient was 10.4 days per year.
Laboratory abnormalities included absolute neutrophil count less than 1500/mm³ (18%) (no patients had absolute

Continued on next page

Information on the Berlex products appearing here is based on the most current information available at the time of publication closing. Further information for these and other products may be obtained from the Medical Affairs Department, Berlex Laboratories, 300 Fairfield Road, Wayne, New Jersey 07470, 1-800-888-2407. Information on Betaseron and Fludara may be obtained from Berlex Laboratories, 15049 San Pablo Avenue, Richmond, California 94804-0016, 1-800-888-4112.

Berlex Laboratories—Cont.

neutrophil counts less than 500/mm^3), WBC less than 3000/mm^3 (16%), SGPT greater than 5 times baseline value (19%), and total bilirubin greater than 2.5 times baseline value (6%). Three patients were withdrawn from treatment with 0.25 mg (8 million IU) Betaseron® (Interferon beta-1b) for abnormal liver enzymes including one following dose reduction (see **PRECAUTIONS, Laboratory Tests**).

Twenty-one (28%) of the 76 premenopausal females treated at 0.25 mg (8 million IU) Betaseron and 10 (13%) of the 76 premenopausal females treated with placebo reported menstrual disorders. All of these reports were of mild to moderate severity and included: intermenstrual bleeding and spotting, early or delayed menses, decreased days of menstrual flow, and clotting and spotting during menstruation.

Mental disorders have been observed in patients in this study. Symptoms included depression, anxiety, emotional lability, depersonalization, suicide attempts, confusion, etc. In the treatment group, two patients withdrew for confusion. One suicide and four attempted suicides were also reported. It is not known whether these symptoms may be related to the underlying neurological basis of MS, to Betaseron treatment, or to a combination of both. Some similar symptoms have been noted in patients receiving interferon alfa and both interferons are thought to act through the same receptor. Patients who experience these symptoms should be closely monitored and cessation of therapy considered.

Additional common adverse clinical and laboratory events associated with the use of Betaseron are listed in the following paragraphs. These events occurred at an incidence of 5% or more in the 124 MS patients treated with 0.25 mg (8 million IU) of Betaseron® (Interferon beta-1b) every other day for periods of up to 3 years in the controlled trial, and at an incidence that was at least twice that observed in the 123 placebo patients. Common adverse clinical and laboratory events associated with the use of Betaseron were: injection site reaction (85%), injection site necrosis (5%), flu-like symptoms (53%), palpitation (8%), hypertension (7%), tachycardia (6%), peripheral vascular disorders (5%), gastrointestinal disorders (6%), absolute neutrophil count < 1500/mm^3 (18%), WBC < 3000/mm^3 (16%), SGPT > 5 times baseline value (19%), total bilirubin > 2.5 times baseline value (6%), somnolence (6%), dyspnea (8%), laryngitis (6%), menstrual disorder (17%), cystitis (8%), breast pain (7%), pelvic pain (6%), and menorrhagia (6%).

A total of 277 MS patients have been treated with Betaseron in doses ranging from 0.025 mg (0.8 million IU) to 0.5 mg (16 million IU). During the first 3 years of treatment, withdrawals due to clinical adverse events or laboratory abnormalities not mentioned above included: fatigue (2%, 6 patients), cardiac arrhythmia (< 1%, 1 patient), allergic urticarial skin reaction to injections (< 1%, 1 patient), headache (< 1%, 1 patient), unspecified adverse events (< 1%, 1 patient), and "felt sick" (< 1%, 1 patient).

The table that follows enumerates adverse events and laboratory abnormalities that occurred at an incidence of 2% or more among the 124 MS patients treated with 0.25 mg (8 million IU) Betaseron every other day for periods of up to 3 years in the controlled trial and at an incidence that was at least 2% more than that observed in the 123 placebo patients. Reported adverse events have been reclassified using the standard COSTART glossary to reduce the total number of terms employed in the table. In the following table, terms so general as to be uninformative, and those events where a drug cause was remote have been excluded.

TABLE 2
Adverse Reactions and Laboratory Abnormalities

Adverse Reaction	Placebo N=123	0.25 mg (8 mIU) N=124
Body as a Whole		
Injection site reaction*	37%	85%
Headache	77%	84%
Fever*	41%	59%
Flu-like symptom complex*	56%	76%
Pain	48%	52%
Asthenia*	35%	49%
Chills*	19%	46%
Abdominal pain	24%	32%
Malaise*	3%	15%
Generalized edema	6%	8%
Pelvic pain	3%	6%
Injection site necrosis*	0%	5%
Cyst	2%	4%
Necrosis	0%	2%
Suicide attempt	0%	2%
Cardiovascular System		
Migraine	7%	12%
Palpitation*	2%	8%
Hypertension	2%	7%
Tachycardia	3%	6%
Peripheral vascular disorder	2%	5%
Hemorrhage	1%	3%
Digestive System		
Diarrhea	29%	35%
Constipation	18%	24%
Vomiting	19%	21%
Gastrointestinal disorder	3%	6%
Endocrine System		
Goiter	0%	2%
Hemic and Lymphatic System		
Lymphocytes less than 1500/mm^3	67%	82%
ANC < 1500/mm^3*	6%	18%
WBC < 3000/mm^3*	5%	16%
Lymphadenopathy	11%	14%
Metabolic and Nutritional Disorders		
SGPT > 5 times baseline*	6%	19%
Glucose < 55 mg/dL	13%	15%
Total bilirubin > 2.5 times baseline	2%	6%
Urine protein > 1+	3%	5%
SGOT > 5 times baseline*	0%	4%
Weight gain	0%	4%
Weight loss	2%	4%
Musculoskeletal System		
Myalgia*	28%	44%
Myasthenia	10%	13%
Nervous System		
Dizziness	28%	35%
Hypertonia	24%	26%
Anxiety	13%	15%
Nervousness	5%	8%
Somnolence	3%	6%
Confusion	2%	4%
Speech disorder	1%	3%
Convulsion	0%	2%
Hyperkinesia	0%	2%
Amnesia	0%	2%
Respiratory System		
Sinusitis	26%	36%
Dyspnea*	2%	8%
Laryngitis	2%	6%
Skin and Appendages		
Sweating*	11%	23%
Alopecia	2%	4%
Special Senses		
Conjunctivitis	10%	12%
Abnormal vision	4%	7%
Urogenital System		
Dysmenorrhea	11%	18%
Menstrual disorder*	8%	17%
Metrorrhagia	8%	15%
Cystitis	4%	8%
Breast pain	3%	7%
Menorrhagia	3%	6%
Urinary urgency	2%	4%
Fibrocystic breast	1%	3%
Breast neoplasm	0%	2%

* – Significantly associated with Betaseron treatment.

It should be noted that the figures cited in the table cannot be used to predict the incidence of side effects in the course of usual medical practice where patient characteristics and other factors differ from those that prevailed in the clinical trials. The cited figures do provide the prescribing physician with some basis for estimating the relative contribution of drug and nondrug factors to the side effect incidence rate in the population studied.

Other events observed during premarketing evaluation of various doses of Betaseron® (Interferon beta-1b) in 1440 patients are listed in the paragraph that follows. Because most of the events were observed in open and uncontrolled studies, the role of Betaseron® (Interferon beta-1b) in their causation cannot be reliably determined.

Body as a Whole: abscess, adenoma, anaphylactoid reaction, ascites, cellulitis, hernia, hydrocephalus, hypothermia, infection, peritonitis, photosensitivity, sarcoma, sepsis, and shock; **Cardiovascular System:** angina pectoris, arrhythmia, atrial fibrillation, cardiomegaly, cardiac arrest, cerebral hemorrhage, cerebral ischemia, endocarditis, heart failure, hypotension, myocardial infarct, pericardial effusion, postural hypotension, pulmonary embolus, spider angioma, subarachnoid hemorrhage, syncope, thrombophlebitis, thrombosis, varicose vein, vasospasm, venous pressure increased, ventricular extrasystoles, and ventricular fibrillation; **Digestive System:** aphthous stomatitis, cardiospasm, cheilitis, cholecystitis, cholelithiasis, duodenal ulcer, dry mouth, enteritis, esophagitis, fecal impaction, fecal incontinence, flatulence, gastritis, gastrointestinal hemorrhage, gingivitis, glossitis, hematemesis, hepatic neoplasia, hepatitis, hepatomegaly, ileus, increased salivation, intestinal obstruction, melena, nausea, oral leukoplakia, oral moniliasis, pancreatitis, periodontal abscess, proctitis, rectal hemorrhage, salivary gland enlargement, stomach ulcer, and tenesmus; **Endocrine System:** Cushing's Syndrome, diabetes insipidus, diabetes mellitus, hypothyroidism, and inappropriate ADH; **Hemic and Lymphatic System:** chronic lymphocytic leukemia, hemoglobin less than 9.4 g/100 mL, petechia, platelets less than 75,000/mm^3, and splenomegaly; **Metabolic and Nutritional Disorders:** alcohol intolerance, alkaline phosphatase greater than 5 times baseline value, BUN greater than 40 mg/dL, calcium greater than 11.5 mg/dL, cyanosis, edema, glucose greater than 160 mg/dL, glycosuria, hypoglycemic reaction, hypoxia, ketosis, and thirst; **Musculoskeletal System:** arthritis, arthrosis, bursitis, leg cramps, muscle atrophy, myopathy, myositis, ptosis, and tenosynovitis; **Nervous System:** abnormal gait, acute brain syndrome, agitation, apathy, aphasia, ataxia, brain edema, chronic brain syndrome, coma, delirium, delusions, dementia, depersonalization, diplopia, dystonia, encephalopathy, euphoria, facial paralysis, foot drop, hallucinations, hemiplegia, hypalgesia, hyperesthesia, incoordination, intracranial hypertension, libido decreased, manic reaction, meningitis, neuralgia, neuropathy, neurosis, nystagmus, oculogyric crisis, ophthalmoplegia, papilledema, paralysis, paranoid reaction, psychosis, reflexes decreased, stupor, subdural hematoma, torticollis, tremor, and urinary retention; **Respiratory System:** apnea, asthma, atelectasis, carcinoma of lung, hemoptysis, hiccup, hyperventilation, hypoventilation, interstitial pneumonia, lung edema, pleural effusion, pneumonia, and pneumothorax; **Skin and Appendages:** contact dermatitis, erythema nodosum, exfoliative dermatitis, furunculosis, hirsutism, leukoderma, lichenoid dermatitis, maculopapular rash, psoriasis, seborrhea, skin benign neoplasm, skin carcinoma, skin hypertrophy, skin necrosis, skin ulcer, urticaria, and vesiculobullous rash; **Special Senses:** blepharitis, blindness, deafness, dry eyes, ear pain, iritis, keratoconjunctivitis, mydriasis, otitis externa, otitis media, parosmia, photophobia, retinitis, taste loss, taste perversion, and visual field defect; **Urogenital system:** anuria, balanitis, breast engorgement, cervicitis, epididymitis, gynecomastia, hematuria, impotence, kidney calculus, kidney failure, kidney tubular disorder, leukorrhea, nephritis, nocturia, oliguria, polyuria, salpingitis, urethritis, urinary incontinence, uterine fibroids enlarged, uterine neoplasm, and vaginal hemorrhage.

DRUG ABUSE AND DEPENDENCE

No evidence or experience suggests that abuse or dependence occurs with Betaseron® (Interferon beta-1b) therapy; however, the risk of dependence has not been systematically evaluated.

DOSAGE AND ADMINISTRATION

The recommended dose of Betaseron for the treatment of ambulatory relapsing-remitting MS is 0.25 mg (8 million IU) injected subcutaneously every other day. Limited data regarding the activity of a lower dose are presented above (see **CLINICAL PHARMACOLOGY, Clinical Trials**).

Evidence of efficacy beyond 2 years is not known since the primary evidence of efficacy derives from a 2-year, double-blind, placebo-controlled clinical trial (see **CLINICAL PHARMACOLOGY, Clinical Trials**). Safety data are not available beyond the third year. Patients were discontinued from this trial due to unremitting disease progression of 6 months or greater.

To reconstitute lyophilized Betaseron® (Interferon beta-1b) for injection, use a sterile syringe and needle to inject 1.2 mL of the diluent supplied, Sodium Chloride, 0.54% Solution, into the Betaseron vial. Gently swirl the vial of Betaseron to dissolve the drug completely; do not shake. Inspect the reconstituted product visually and discard the product before use if it contains particulate matter or is discolored. After reconstitution with accompanying diluent, Betaseron vials contain 0.25 mg (8 million IU) Interferon beta-1b/mL of solution.

Withdraw 1 mL of reconstituted solution from the vial into a sterile syringe fitted with a 27-gauge needle and inject the solution subcutaneously. Sites for self-injection include arms, abdomen, hips, and thighs. A vial is suitable for single use only; unused portions should be discarded. (See **BETASERON® [Interferon beta-1b] PATIENT INFORMATION** sheet for **SELF-INJECTION PROCEDURE.**)

Stability: The reconstituted product contains no preservative. Before and after reconstitution with diluent, store at 2°

to 8°C (36° to 46°F). Product should be used within 3 hours of reconstitution.

HOW SUPPLIED

Betaseron is supplied as a lyophilized powder containing 0.3 mg (9.6 million IU) of Interferon beta-1b, 15 mg Albumin Human USP, and 15 mg dextrose, USP. Drug is packaged in a clear glass, single-use vial (3 mL capacity): a separate vial containing 2 mL of diluent (Sodium Chloride, 0.54% solution) is included for each vial of drug. Store under refrigeration, between 2° to 8°C (36° to 46°F).

NDC 50419-521-03   0.3 mg (9.6 mlU)/vial
NDC 50419-521-15   15 vials, 0.3 mg (9.6 mlU)/vial
Caution: Federal law prohibits dispensing without prescription.

REFERENCES

1. Ruzicka FJ, et al. J Biol Chem, 1987; 262: 16142–16149.
2. Uze G, et al. Cell, 1990; 60: 225–234.
3. DeMaeyer E, et al. In: Interferons and other regulatory cytokines, NY, Wiley 1988.
4. Colby CB, et al. J Immunol 1984; 133: 3091–3095.
5. Pestka S, et al. Annu Rev Biochem 1987; 56: 727–777.
6. Lengyel P, Annu Rev Biochem 1982; 51: 251–282.
7. Witt PL, et al. J Interferon Res 1990; 10: 393–402.
8. Schiller JH, et al. J Biol Resp Mod 1990; 9: 377–386.
9. Rosenblum MG, et al. J Interferon Res 1990; 10: 141–151.
10. Carlin JM, et al. J Immuno 1987; 130(7): 2414–2418.
11. Witt PL, et al. J Immunotherapy 1993; 13: 191–200.
12. Goldstein D, et al. J Natl Cancer Inst 1989; 81: 1061–1068.
13. Poser CM, et al. Ann Neurol 1983; 13(3): 227–231.
14. Blaschke TF, et al. Clinical Research 1985; 33(1): 19A.

Manufactured by:
CHIRON Corporation
Emeryville, CA 94608
U.S. License No. 1106
Distributed by:
BERLEX Laboratories
Richmond, CA 94804
©1993 Berlex Laboratories
Part Number L 1172
Revised April 1994
All rights reserved
U.S. Patent No. 4,588,585; 4,959,314; 4,737,462; 4,450,103

BETASERON® (Interferon beta-1b) PATIENT INFORMATION

Betaseron® (Interferon beta-1b) is intended for use under the guidance and supervision of a physician. Your physician or his/her delegate should instruct you in the preparation of Betaseron for administration and in the technique of self injection. Do not attempt self-administration until you are sure that you understand the requirements for mixing the product and giving an injection to yourself.

Betaseron should be used as prescribed by your physician. However, if you miss a dose, take it as soon as you remember. Your next injection, however, should be scheduled about 48 hours later. While using Betaseron, please keep in mind the following facts:

- Betaseron must be kept cold. Be sure to store it in a refrigerator before and after reconstitution. Do not freeze.
- Keep syringes and needles away from children. Do not reuse needles or syringes. Discard used syringes and needles in a syringe disposal unit as instructed by your physician.
- Women: Betaseron should not be used during pregnancy or if you are trying to become pregnant. If you wish to become pregnant while using Betaseron, discuss the matter with your doctor. While using Betaseron, women of childbearing age should use birth control measures. If you do become pregnant you should discontinue treatment and contact your doctor immediately.
- Injection site reactions are common. They include redness, pain and swelling, and discoloration. To minimize the chances for a reaction, ask your doctor to suggest a series of injection sites so that you will not have to use the same one repeatedly. Do not make an injection into skin that is tender, red, or hard.
- Flu-like symptoms are also common. They include fever, chills, sweating, fatigue, and muscle aches. Taking Betaseron at night may help lessen the impact of flu-like symptoms.
- Depression, including suicide attempts, has been reported by patients. If you experience such symptoms, contact your physician promptly.
- As with any prescription medication, side effects related to therapy can occur. Consult with your physician if you have any problems, whether or not you think they may be related to Betaseron (Interferon beta-1b).

SELF-INJECTION PROCEDURE

To mix the contents of one vial

Only the vial of diluent (liquid) that comes inside your prescription package should be used to dissolve the white cake of drug in the Betaseron vial.

1. Wash your hands thoroughly with soap and water.
2. Collect all your equipment before you begin the process. You'll need:
- vial of Diluent for Betaseron (Sodium Chloride 0.54%)
- vial of Betaseron
- 3-mL syringe with 21-gauge needle (1)
- 1-mL syringe with 27-gauge needle (1)
- alcohol wipes
- disposal unit (an opaque, puncture-resistant, sealable container for used syringes/needles)

NOTE: Be sure needle guards are on the needles tightly.
3. Remove the protective caps from both vials.
4. Use alcohol wipes to clean the tops of the vials—move in one direction and use one wipe per vial.
NOTE: Leave an alcohol wipe on top of each vial until you are ready to use it.
5. Resting your hands on a stable surface, remove the needle cover on the 3-mL syringe by pulling the cover straight off the needle.

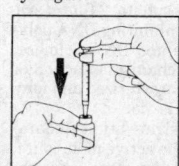

6. Pull back the plunger (on the 3-mL syringe) to the 1.2 mL mark.
NOTE: Read the labels on the vials—find the Diluent for Betaseron vial and throw away the alcohol wipe on top of it.
7. Holding the vial of Diluent for Betaseron (Interferon beta-1b) on a stable surface, slowly insert the needle straight through the stopper, into the top of the vial.

NOTE: When inserting and removing needles from vials, be sure not to touch the needles or the rubber stoppers on the vials with your hands.
If you do touch a stopper, clean it with a fresh alcohol wipe. If you touch a needle, throw away the entire syringe into the disposal unit and start over with a new syringe.
If the needle touches any surface, throw away the entire syringe into the disposal unit and start over with a new syringe.

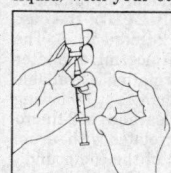

8. Push in the plunger all the way to gently inject air into the vial (leave the needle in the vial of Diluent for Betaseron).
9. Turn the vial of Diluent for Betaseron upside down.
NOTE: Keep the needle tip in the liquid.

10. Resting your hands on a stable surface, hold the vial and syringe in one hand and slowly pull back the plunger on the syringe to the 1.2 mL mark (to draw up that amount of liquid) with your other hand.
11. Keeping the vial upside down, gently tap the syringe until any air bubbles that formed rise to the top of the barrel of the syringe.
12. Carefully push in the plunger to eject ONLY THE AIR through the needle.

13. Remove the needle/syringe from the vial of Diluent for Betaseron.
NOTE: Find the Betaseron vial and throw away the alcohol wipe on top of it.
14. Holding the Betaseron vial on a stable surface, slowly insert the needle of the syringe (containing 1.2 mL of liquid) all the way through the stopper of the vial.

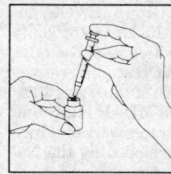

15. Push the plunger down slowly, directing the needle toward the side of the vial to allow the liquid to run down the inside wall (injecting Diluent for Betaseron (Interferon beta-1b) directly onto the cake of drug will cause excess foaming).
16. Remove the needle/syringe from the Betaseron vial.
17. Throw away the 3 mL syringe into the disposal unit.
NOTE: Double-check that you are throwing away the correct syringe into the disposal unit.

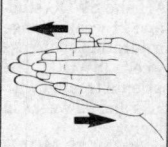

18. Roll the vial between your hands gently to completely dissolve the white cake of Betaseron (DO NOT SHAKE).
19. Look closely at the solution (it should be clear).
NOTE: If the mixture contains particles or is discolored, discard it and start again.

PREPARING THE INJECTION

1. Remove the needle guard of the 1 mL syringe and pull back the plunger to the 1 mL mark.

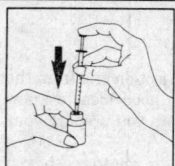

2. Insert the needle of the 1mL syringe through the stopper of the vial of Betaseron solution.
3. Gently push the plunger all the way down to inject air into the vial (leave the needle in the vial).

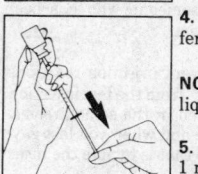

4. Turn the vial of Betaseron (Interferon beta-1b) solution upside down.
NOTE: Keep the needle tip in the liquid.
5. Pull back the plunger to withdraw 1 mL of liquid into the syringe.

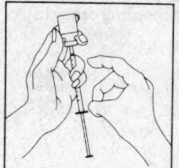

6. Hold the syringe with the needle pointing upward.
7. Tap the syringe gently until any air bubbles that formed rise to the top of the barrel of the syringe.
8. Carefully push in the plunger to eject ONLY THE AIR through the needle.

9. Remove the needle/syringe from the vial.
10. Recap the needle on the syringe.
NOTE: The injection should be administered immediately after mixing (if injection is delayed, refrigerate the solution and inject it within 3 hours). Do not freeze.
11. Throw away unused portion of the solution remaining in the vial.

GIVING THE INJECTION

Subcutaneous (under the skin) self-administration

1. Choose an injection site (see INJECTION SITES diagram); you may want to hold the syringe like a pencil or dart. Use a different site each day you inject:
- Arms (upper back portion)
- Abdomen (except around navel and waistline)
- Hips (upper, outer rear quadrant)
- Thighs (front and sides except at groin and knee)
NOTE: Do not use any areas in which you feel lumps, firm knots, depressions, pain, or discoloration; talk to your doctor or healthcare professional about anything you find.
2. Use an alcohol wipe to clean the skin at the injection site; let it air dry.
3. Throw away the wipe.

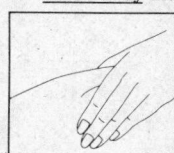

4. Uncap the needle.
5. Gently pinch the skin together around the site (to lift it up a bit).
6. Resting your wrist on the skin near the site, stick the needle straight into the skin at a 90° angle with a quick, firm motion.

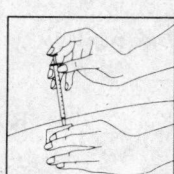

7. Inject the drug by using a slow, steady push (push the plunger all the way in until the syringe is empty).
8. Hold a swab on the injection site. Remove the needle from the skin.

9. Gently massage the injection site with a dry cotton ball or gauze.
10. Throw away the 1 mL syringe in the disposal unit.

INJECTION SITE

Picking an injection site

Betaseron (Interferon beta-1b) therapy should be injected into subcutaneous tissue (between the fat layer just under the skin and the muscles beneath). The best areas for injection are loose and soft (flabby), away from joints and nerves.

Continued on next page

Information on the Berlex products appearing here is based on the most current information available at the time of publication closing. Further information for these and other products may be obtained from the Medical Affairs Department, Berlex Laboratories, 300 Fairfield Road, Wayne, New Jersey 07470, 1-800-888-2407. Information on Betaseron and Fludara may be obtained from Berlex Laboratories, 15049 San Pablo Avenue, Richmond, California 94804-0016, 1-800-888-4112.

Berlex Laboratories—Cont.

Each therapy day you can choose an injection site from the ones identified in the diagrams. It's a good idea to know where your injection will be given before you prepare your syringe.

If there are any sites that are difficult for you to reach, you can ask your support person (or someone who has been trained to give injections) to help you.

Rotating injection sites

Changing sites each time helps prevent injection reactions: it gives the site time to "bounce back" from the last injection. Today's injection should not be given in the same areas as the last one. Keep a record of where and when you last gave yourself an injection. One way to do that is to note the injection site on a calendar.

You may use a site again after waiting 1 week. If all areas become tender, talk to the doctor about choosing other injection sites.

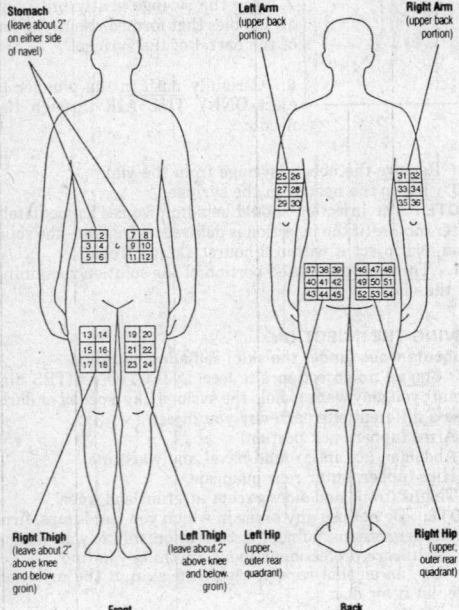

Manufactured by:
CHIRON Corporation
Emeryville, CA 94608
U.S. License No. 1106
Distributed by:
BERLEX Laboratories
Richmond, CA 94804
©1993 Berlex Laboratories
Revised April 1994
All rights reserved
Shown in Product Identification Guide, page 305

FLUDARA®   ℞
(fludarabine phosphate)
FOR INJECTION
FOR INTRAVENOUS USE ONLY

WARNING: FLUDARA FOR INJECTION should be administered under the supervision of a qualified physician experienced in the use of antineoplastic therapy. FLUDARA FOR INJECTION can severely suppress bone marrow function. When used at high doses in dose-ranging studies in patients with acute leukemia, FLUDARA FOR INJECTION was associated with severe neurologic effects, including blindness, coma, and death. This severe central nervous system toxicity occurred in 36% of patients treated with doses approximately four times greater (96 mg/m²/day for 5–7 days) than the recommended dose. Similar severe central nervous system toxicity has been rarely (≤0.2%) reported in patients treated at doses in the range of the dose recommended for chronic lymphocytic leukemia. Instances of life-threatening and sometimes fatal autoimmune hemolytic anemia have been reported to occur after one or more cycles of treatment with FLUDARA FOR INJECTION. Patients undergoing treatment with FLUDARA FOR INJECTION should be evaluated and closely monitored for hemolysis.

In a clinical investigation using FLUDARA FOR INJECTION in combination with pentostatin (deoxycoformycin) for the treatment of refractory chronic lymphocytic leukemia (CLL), there was an unacceptably high incidence of fatal pulmonary toxicity. Therefore, the use of FLUDARA FOR INJECTION in combination with pentostatin is not recommended.

DESCRIPTION

FLUDARA FOR INJECTION contains fludarabine phosphate, a fluorinated nucleotide analog of the antiviral agent vidarabine, 9-β-D-arabinofuranosyladenine (ara-A) that is relatively resistant to deamination by adenosine deaminase. Each vial of sterile lyophilized solid cake contains 50 mg of the active ingredient fludarabine phosphate, 50 mg of mannitol, and sodium hydroxide to adjust pH to 7.7. The pH range for the final product is 7.2–8.2. Reconstitution with 2 mL of Sterile Water for Injection USP results in a solution containing 25 mg/mL of fludarabine phosphate intended for intravenous administration.

The chemical name for fludarabine phosphate is 9H-Purin-6-amine, 2-fluoro-9-(5-O-phosphono-β-D-arabinofuranosyl). The molecular formula of fludarabine phosphate is $C_{10}H_{13}FN_5O_7P$ (MW 365.2) and the structure is:

$$\text{structure of fludarabine phosphate}$$

CLINICAL PHARMACOLOGY

Fludarabine phosphate is rapidly dephosphorylated to 2-fluoro-ara-A and then phosphorylated intracellularly by deoxycytidine kinase to the active triphosphate, 2-fluoro-ara-ATP. This metabolite appears to act by inhibiting DNA polymerase alpha, ribonucleotide reductase and DNA primase, thus inhibiting DNA synthesis. The mechanism of action of this antimetabolite is not completely characterized and may be multi-faceted.

Phase I studies in humans have demonstrated that fludarabine phosphate is rapidly converted to the active metabolite, 2-fluoro-ara-A, within minutes after intravenous infusion. Consequently, clinical pharmacology studies have focused on 2-fluoro-ara-A pharmacokinetics. In a study with 4 patients treated with 25 mg/m²/day for 5 days, the half-life of 2-fluoro-ara-A was approximately 10 hours. The mean total plasma clearance was 8.9 L/hr/m² and the mean volume of distribution was 98 L/m². Approximately 23% of the dose was excreted in the urine as unchanged 2-fluoro-ara-A. The mean C_{max} after the Day 1 dose was 0.57 mcg/mL and after the Day 5 dose 0.54 mcg/mL. No information is available on pharmacokinetic parameters, other than C_{max}, following the Day 5 dose of 25 mg/m². Total body clearance of 2-fluoro-ara-A has been shown to be inversely correlated with serum creatinine, suggesting renal elimination of the compound. A correlation was noted between the degree of absolute granulocyte count nadir and increased area under the concentration × time curve (AUC).

Two single-arm open-label studies of FLUDARA FOR INJECTION have been conducted in patients with CLL refractory to at least one prior standard alkylating-agent containing regimen. In a study conducted by M.D. Anderson Cancer Center (MDAH), 48 patients were treated with a dose of 22–40 mg/m² daily for 5 days every 28 days. Another study conducted by the Southwest Oncology Group (SWOG) involved 31 patients treated with a dose of 15–25 mg/m² daily for 5 days every 28 days. The overall objective response rates were 48% and 32% in the MDAH and SWOG studies, respectively. The complete response rate in both studies was 13%; the partial response rate was 35% in the MDAH study and 19% in the SWOG study. These response rates were obtained using standardized response criteria developed by the National Cancer Institute CLL Working Group[1] and were achieved in heavily pre-treated patients. The ability of FLUDARA FOR INJECTION to induce a significant rate of response in refractory patients suggests minimal cross-resistance with commonly used anti-CLL agents.

The median time to response in the MDAH and SWOG studies was 7 weeks (range of 1 to 68 weeks) and 21 weeks (range of 1 to 53 weeks) respectively. The median duration of disease control was 91 weeks (MDAH) and 65 weeks (SWOG). The median survival of all refractory CLL patients treated with FLUDARA FOR INJECTION was 43 weeks and 52 weeks in the MDAH and SWOG studies, respectively.

Rai stage improved to Stage II or better in 7 of 12 MDAH responders (58%) and in 5 of 7 SWOG responders (71%) who were Stage III or IV at baseline. In the combined studies, mean hemoglobin concentration improved from 9.0 g/dL at baseline to 11.8 g/dL at the time of response, in a subgroup of anemic patients. Similarly, average platelet count improved from 63,500/mm³ to 103,300/mm³ at the time of response in a subgroup of patients who were thrombocytopenic at baseline.

INDICATIONS AND USAGE

FLUDARA FOR INJECTION is indicated for the treatment of patients with B-cell chronic lymphocytic leukemia (CLL) who have not responded to or whose disease has progressed during treatment with at least one standard alkylating-agent containing regimen. The safety and effectiveness of FLUDARA FOR INJECTION in previously untreated or non-refractory patients with CLL have not been established.

CONTRAINDICATIONS

FLUDARA FOR INJECTION is contraindicated in those patients who are hypersensitive to this drug or its components.

WARNINGS

(See boxed warning)

There are clear dose dependent toxic effects seen with FLUDARA FOR INJECTION. Dose levels approximately 4 times greater (96 mg/m²/day for 5 to 7 days) than that recommended for CLL (25 mg/m²/day for 5 days) were associated with a syndrome characterized by delayed blindness, coma and death. Symptoms appeared from 21 to 60 days following the last dose. Thirteen of 36 patients (36%) who received FLUDARA FOR INJECTION at high doses (96 mg/m²/day for 5 to 7 days) developed this severe neurotoxicity. This syndrome has been reported rarely in patients treated with doses in the range of the recommended CLL dose of 25 mg/m²/day for 5 days every 28 days. The effect of chronic administration of FLUDARA FOR INJECTION on the central nervous system is unknown, however, patients have received the recommended dose for up to 15 courses of therapy.

Severe bone marrow suppression, notably anemia, thrombocytopenia and neutropenia, has been reported in patients treated with FLUDARA FOR INJECTION. In a Phase I study in solid tumor patients, the median time to nadir counts was 13 days (range, 3–25 days) for granulocytes and 16 days (range, 2–32) for platelets. Most patients had hematologic impairment at baseline either as a result of disease or as a result of prior myelosuppressive therapy. Cumulative myelosuppression may be seen. While chemotherapy-induced myelosuppression is often reversible, administration of FLUDARA FOR INJECTION requires careful hematologic monitoring.

Instances of life-threatening and sometimes fatal autoimmune hemolytic anemia have been reported to occur after one or more cycles of treatment with FLUDARA FOR INJECTION in patients with or without a previous history of autoimmune hemolytic anemia or a positive Coombs' test and who may or may not be in remission for their disease. Steroids may or may not be effective in controlling these hemolytic episodes. The majority of patients rechallenged with FLUDARA FOR INJECTION developed a recurrence in the hemolytic process. The mechanism(s) which predispose patients to the development of this complication has not been identified. Patients undergoing treatment with FLUDARA FOR INJECTION should be evaluated and closely monitored for hemolysis.

Transfusion related graft-versus-host disease has been observed during transfusion of non-irradiated blood in FLUDARA FOR INJECTION patients. Consideration should, therefore, be given to the use of irradiated blood products in those patients requiring transfusions while undergoing treatment with FLUDARA FOR INJECTION.

In a clinical investigation using FLUDARA FOR INJECTION in combination with pentostatin (deoxycoformycin) for the treatment of refractory chronic lymphocytic leukemia (CLL), there was an unacceptably high incidence of fatal pulmonary toxicity. Therefore, the use of FLUDARA FOR INJECTION in combination with pentostatin is not recommended.

Of the 133 CLL patients in the two trials, there were 29 fatalities during study. Approximately 50% of the fatalities were due to infection and 25% due to progressive disease.

Pregnancy Category D: FLUDARA FOR INJECTION may cause fetal harm when administered to a pregnant woman. Fludarabine phosphate was teratogenic in rats and in rabbits. Fludarabine phosphate was administered intravenously at doses of 0, 1, 10 or 30 mg/kg/day to pregnant rats on days 6 to 15 of gestation. At 10 and 30 mg/kg/day in rats, there was an increased incidence of various skeletal malformations. Fludarabine phosphate was administered intravenously at doses of 0, 1, 5 or 8 mg/kg/day to pregnant rabbits on days 6 to 15 of gestation. Dose-related teratogenic effects manifested by external deformities and skeletal malformations were observed in the rabbits at 5 and 8 mg/kg/day. Drug-related deaths or toxic effects on maternal and fetal weights were not observed. There are no adequate and well-controlled studies in pregnant women.

If FLUDARA FOR INJECTION is used during pregnancy, or if the patient becomes pregnant while taking this drug, the patient should be apprised of the potential hazard to the fe-

tus. Women of childbearing potential should be advised to avoid becoming pregnant.

PRECAUTIONS

General: FLUDARA FOR INJECTION is a potent antineoplastic agent with potentially significant toxic side effects. Patients undergoing therapy should be closely observed for signs of hematologic and nonhematologic toxicity. Periodic assessment of peripheral blood counts is recommended to detect the development of anemia, neutropenia and thrombocytopenia.

Tumor lysis syndrome associated with FLUDARA FOR INJECTION treatment has been reported in CLL patients with large tumor burdens. Since FLUDARA FOR INJECTION can induce a response as early as the first week of treatment, precautions should be taken in those patients at risk of developing this complication.

There are inadequate data on dosing of patients with renal insufficiency. FLUDARA FOR INJECTION must be administered cautiously in patients with renal insufficiency. The total body clearance of 2-fluoro-ara-A has been shown to be inversely correlated with serum creatinine, suggesting renal elimination of the compound.

Laboratory Tests: During treatment, the patient's hematologic profile (particularly neutrophils and platelets) should be monitored regularly to determine the degree of hematopoietic suppression.

Drug Interactions: The use of FLUDARA FOR INJECTION in combination with pentostatin is not recommended due to the risk of severe pulmonary toxicity (see WARNINGS section).

Carcinogenesis: No animal carcinogenicity studies with FLUDARA FOR INJECTION have been conducted.

Mutagenesis: Fludarabine phosphate has been shown to be non-mutagenic to several strains of Salmonella typhimurium, including TA-98, TA-100, TA-1535 and TA-1537. In addition, fludarabine phosphate was non-mutagenic to Chinese hamster ovary (CHO) cells at the hypoxanthine-guanine-phosphoribosyltransferase (HGPRT) locus under both activated and non-activated metabolic conditions. Fludarabine was determined to cause increased sister chromatid exchanges using an in vitro sister chromatid exchange (SCE) assay under both metabolically activated and non-activated conditions. In addition, fludarabine phosphatate has also been shown to be mutagenic as indicated by an increase in the number of micronucleated erythrocytes in the in vivo mouse micronucleus test at doses up to 1000 mg/kg.

Impairment of Fertility: Studies in mice, rats and dogs have demonstrated dose-related adverse effects on the male reproductive system. Observations consisted of a decrease in mean testicular weights in mice and rats with a trend toward decreased testicular weights in dogs and degeneration and necrosis of spermatogenic epithelium of the testes in mice, rats and dogs. The possible adverse effects on fertility in humans have not been adequately evaluated.

Pregnancy: Pregnancy Category D: (See WARNINGS section).

Nursing Mothers: It is not known whether this drug is excreted in human milk. Because many drugs are excreted in human milk and because of the potential for serious adverse reactions in nursing infants from FLUDARA FOR INJECTION, a decision should be made to discontinue nursing or discontinue the drug, taking into account the importance of the drug for the mother.

Pediatric Use: The safety and effectiveness of FLUDARA FOR INJECTION in children have not been established.

ADVERSE REACTIONS:

The most common adverse events include myelosuppression (neutropenia, thrombocytopenia and anemia), fever and chills, infection, and nausea and vomiting. Other commonly reported events include malaise, fatigue, anorexia, and weakness. Serious opportunistic infections have occurred in CLL patients treated with FLUDARA FOR INJECTION. The most frequently reported adverse events and those reactions which are more clearly related to the drug are arranged below according to body system.

Hematopoietic Systems: Hematologic events (neutropenia, thrombocytopenia, and/or anemia) were reported in the majority of CLL patients treated with FLUDARA FOR INJECTION. During FLUDARA FOR INJECTION treatment of 133 patients with CLL, the absolute neutrophil count decreased to less than 500/mm^3 in 59% of patients, hemoglobin decreased from pretreatment values by at least 2 grams percent in 60%, and platelet count decreased from pretreatment values by at least 50% in 55%. Myelosuppression may be severe and cumulative. Bone marrow fibrosis occurred in one CLL patient treated with FLUDARA FOR INJECTION. Clinically significant hemolytic anemia has been rarely reported in patients receiving FLUDARA FOR INJECTION (see WARNINGS section).

Metabolic: Tumor lysis syndrome has been reported in CLL patients treated with FLUDARA FOR INJECTION. This complication may include hyperuricemia, hyperphosphatemia, hypocalcemia, metabolic acidosis, hyperkalemia, hematuria, urate crystalluria, and renal failure. The onset of this syndrome may be heralded by flank pain and hematuria.

Nervous System: (See WARNINGS section) Objective weakness, agitation, confusion, visual disturbances, and coma have occurred in CLL patients treated with FLUDARA FOR INJECTION at the recommended dose. Peripheral neuropathy has been observed in patients treated with FLUDARA FOR INJECTION and one case of wrist-drop was reported.

Pulmonary System: Pneumonia, a frequent manifestation of infection in CLL patients, occurred in 16% and 22% of those treated with FLUDARA FOR INJECTION in the MDAH and SWOG studies, respectively. Pulmonary hypersensitivity reactions to FLUDARA FOR INJECTION characterized by dyspnea, cough and interstitial pulmonary infiltrate have been observed.

Gastrointestinal System: Gastrointestinal disturbances such as nausea and vomiting, anorexia, diarrhea, stomatitis and gastrointestinal bleeding have been reported in patients treated with FLUDARA FOR INJECTION.

Cardiovascular: Edema has been frequently reported. One patient developed a pericardial effusion possibly related to treatment with FLUDARA FOR INJECTION. No other severe cardiovascular events were considered to be drug related.

Genitourinary System: Rare cases of hemorrhagic cystitis have been reported in patients treated with FLUDARA FOR INJECTION.

Skin: Skin toxicity, consisting primarily of skin rashes, has been reported in patients treated with FLUDARA FOR INJECTION.

Data in the following table are derived from the 133 patients with CLL who received FLUDARA FOR INJECTION in the MDAH and SWOG studies.

PERCENT OF CLL PATIENTS REPORTING NON-HEMATOLOGIC ADVERSE EVENTS

ADVERSE EVENTS	MDAH (N=101)	SWOG (N=32)
ANY ADVERSE EVENT	88%	91%
BODY AS A WHOLE	72	84
FEVER	60	69
CHILLS	11	19
FATIGUE	10	38
INFECTION	33	44
PAIN	20	22
MALAISE	8	6
DIAPHORESIS	1	13
ALOPECIA	0	3
ANAPHYLAXIS	1	0
HEMORRHAGE	1	0
HYPERGLYCEMIA	1	6
DEHYDRATION	1	0
NEUROLOGICAL	21	69
WEAKNESS	9	65
PARESTHESIA	4	12
HEADACHE	3	0
VISUAL DISTURBANCE	3	15
HEARING LOSS	2	6
SLEEP DISORDER	1	3
DEPRESSION	1	0
CEREBELLAR SYNDROME	1	0
IMPAIRED MENTATION	1	0
PULMONARY	35	69
COUGH	10	44
PNEUMONIA	16	22
DYSPNEA	9	22
SINUSITIS	5	0
PHARYNGITIS	0	9
UPPER RESPIRATORY INFECTION	2	16
ALLERGIC PNEUMONITIS	0	6
EPISTAXIS	1	0
HEMOPTYSIS	1	6
BRONCHITIS	1	0
HYPOXIA	1	0
GASTROINTESTINAL	46	63
NAUSEA/VOMITING	36	31
DIARRHEA	15	13
ANOREXIA	7	34
STOMATITIS	9	0
GI BLEEDING	3	13
ESOPHAGITIS	3	0
MUCOSITIS	2	0
LIVER FAILURE	1	0
ABNORMAL LIVER FUNCTION TEST	1	3
CHOLELITHIASIS	0	3
CONSTIPATION	1	3
DYSPHAGIA	1	0
CUTANEOUS	17	18
RASH	15	15
PRURITUS	1	3
SEBORRHEA	1	0
GENITOURINARY	12	22
DYSURIA	4	3
URINARY INFECTION	2	15
HEMATURIA	2	3
RENAL FAILURE	1	0
ABNORMAL RENAL FUNCTION TEST	1	0
PROTEINURIA	1	0
HESITANCY	0	3
CARDIOVASCULAR	12	38
EDEMA	8	19
ANGINA	0	6
CONGESTIVE HEART FAILURE	0	3
ARRHYTHMIA	0	3
SUPRAVENTRICULAR TACHYCARDIA	0	3
MYOCARDIAL INFARCTION	0	3
DEEP VENOUS THROMBOSIS	1	3
PHLEBITIS	1	3
TRANSIENT ISCHEMIC ATTACK	1	0
ANEURYSM	1	0
CEREBROVASCULAR ACCIDENT	0	3
MUSCULOSKELETAL	7	16
MYALGIA	4	16
OSTEOPOROSIS	2	0
ARTHRALGIA	1	0
TUMOR LYSIS SYNDROME	1	0

More than 3000 patients received FLUDARA FOR INJECTION in studies of other leukemias, lymphomas, and other solid tumors. The spectrum of adverse effects reported in these studies was consistent with the data presented above.

OVERDOSAGE

High doses of FLUDARA FOR INJECTION (see Warnings) have been associated with an irreversible central nervous system toxicity characterized by delayed blindness, coma and death. High doses are also associated with severe thrombocytopenia and neutropenia due to bone marrow suppression. There is no known specific antidote for FLUDARA FOR INJECTION overdosage. Treatment consists of drug discontinuation and supportive therapy.

DOSAGE AND ADMINISTRATION

Usual Dose:

The recommended dose of FLUDARA FOR INJECTION is 25 mg/m^2 administered intravenously over a period of approximately 30 minutes daily for five consecutive days. Each 5 day course of treatment should commence every 28 days. Dosage may be decreased or delayed based on evidence of hematologic or nonhematologic toxicity. Physicians should consider delaying or discontinuing the drug if neurotoxicity occurs.

A number of clinical settings may predispose to increased toxicity from FLUDARA FOR INJECTION. These include advanced age, renal insufficiency, and bone marrow impairment. Such patients should be monitored closely for excessive toxicity and the dose modified accordingly.

The optimal duration of treatment has not been clearly established. It is recommended that three additional cycles of FLUDARA FOR INJECTION be administered following the achievement of a maximal response and then the drug should be discontinued.

Preparation of Solutions:

FLUDARA FOR INJECTION should be prepared for parenteral use by aseptically adding Sterile Water for Injection USP. When reconstituted with 2 mL of Sterile Water for Injection, USP, the solid cake should fully dissolve in 15 seconds or less; each mL of the resulting solution will contain 25 mg of fludarabine phosphate, 25 mg of mannitol, and sodium hydroxide to adjust the pH to 7.7. The pH range for the final product is 7.2-8.2. In clinical studies, the product has been diluted in 100 cc or 125 cc of 5% Dextrose Injection USP or 0.9% Sodium Chloride USP.

Reconstituted FLUDARA FOR INJECTION contains no antimicrobial preservative and thus should be used within 8 hours of reconstitution. Care must be taken to assure the sterility of prepared solutions. Parenteral drug products should be inspected visually for particulate matter and discoloration prior to administration.

Handling and Disposal:

Procedures for proper handling and disposal should be considered. Consideration should be given to handling and dis-

Continued on next page

Information on the Berlex products appearing here is based on the most current information available at the time of publication closing. Further information for these and other products may be obtained from the Medical Affairs Department, Berlex Laboratories, 300 Fairfield Road, Wayne, New Jersey 07470, 1-800-888-2407. Information on Betaseron and Fludara may be obtained from Berlex Laboratories, 15049 San Pablo Avenue, Richmond, California 94804-0016, 1-800-888-4112.

Berlex Laboratories—Cont.

posal according to guidelines issued for cytotoxic drugs. Several guidelines on this subject have been published.[2-8] There is no general agreement that all of the procedures recommended in the guidelines are necessary or appropriate. Caution should be exercised in the handling and preparation of FLUDARA FOR INJECTION solution. The use of latex gloves and safety glasses is recommended to avoid exposure in case of breakage of the vial or other accidental spillage. If the solution contacts the skin or mucous membranes, wash thoroughly with soap and water; rinse eyes thoroughly with plain water. Avoid exposure by inhalation or by direct contact of the skin or mucous membranes.

HOW SUPPLIED

FLUDARA FOR INJECTION is supplied as a white, lyophilized solid cake. Each vial contains 50 mg of fludarabine phosphate, 50 mg of mannitol and sodium hydroxide to adjust pH to 7.7. The pH range for the final product is 7.2-8.2. Store under refrigeration, between 2°-8°C (36°-46°F).
FLUDARA FOR INJECTION is supplied in a clear glass single dose vial (6 mL capacity) and packaged in a single dose vial carton in a shelf pack of five.
CAUTION: Federal law prohibits dispensing without prescription.
NDC 50419-511-06
Manufactured by: Ben Venue Laboratories, Bedford, OH 44146
Manufactured for: Berlex Laboratories, Richmond, CA 94804-0016
U.S. Patent Number: 4,357,324
RA 9/92
References: 1. Cheson B.D., Bennett J.M., Rai K.R. et al. Guidelines for clinical protocols for chronic lymphocytic leukemia: Recommendations of the National Cancer Institute-Sponsored Working Group. Amer J Hematol 29:152-163, 1988. **2.** Recommendations for the Safe Handling of Parenteral Antineoplastic Drugs. NIH Publication No. 83-2621. For sale by the Superintendent of Documents, U.S. Government Printing Office, Washington, D.C. 20402. **3.** AMA Council Report. Guidelines for Handling Parenteral Antineoplastics, JAMA, 1985; March 15. **4.** National Study Commission on Cytotoxic Exposure—Recommendations for Handling Cytotoxic Agents. Available from Louis P. Jeffrey, Sc.D., Chairman, National Study Commission on Cytotoxic Exposure, Massachusetts College of Pharmacy and Allied Health Sciences, 179 Longwood Avenue, Boston, Massachusetts 02115. **5.** Clinical Oncological Society of Australia: Guidelines and Recommendations for Safe Handling of Antineoplastic Agents, Med. J. Australia 1983;1:426-428. **6.** Jones, R.B. et al. Safe Handling of Chemotherapeutic Agents: A Report from the Mount Sinai Medical Center, Ca—A Cancer Journal for Clinicians 1983; Sept/Oct. 258-263. **7.** American Society of Hospital Pharmacists Technical Assistance Bulletin on Handling Cytotoxic Drugs in Hospitals, Am. J. Hosp. Pharm. 1985;42:131-137. **8.** OSHA Work-Practice Guidelines for Personnel Dealing with Cytotoxic (antineoplastic) Drugs. Am. J. Hosp. Pharm. 1986;43:1193-1204.

Shown in Product Identification Guide, page 305

Berna Products, Corp.
4216 PONCE DE LEON BLVD.
CORAL GABLES, FL 33146

Direct Inquiries to:
Michelle Moskowitz
(305) 443-2900
(800) 533-5899

For Medical Information Contact: R. Bustamante, M.D.
In Emergencies: Andres Murai, Jr
(305) 443-2900
(800) 533-5899

TE ANATOXAL BERNA™ ℞
Tetanus Toxoid Adsorbed

HOW SUPPLIED

Syringe 0.5 ml 10 ea UD (NDC: 58337-1301-2)
Vial 5 ml (NDC: 58337-1301-1)

VIVOTIF BERNA™ VACCINE ℞
Typhoid Vaccine Live Oral Ty 21a

DESCRIPTION

Vivotif Berna™ (Typhoid Vaccine Live Oral Ty 21a) is a live attenuated vaccine for oral administration. The vaccine contains the attenuated strain *Salmonella typhi* Ty 21a.
Vivotif Berna™ Vaccine is manufactured by the Swiss Serum and Vaccine Institute. The vaccine strain is grown under controlled conditions in medium containing a digest of bovine tissues, an acid digest of casein, dextrose and galactose. The bacteria are collected by centrifugation, mixed with a stabilizer containing lactose and amino acids, and lyophilized. The lyophilized bacteria are filled into gelatin capsules which are coated with an organic solution to render them resistant to dissolution in stomach acid. The enteric-coated capsules are then packaged in 4-capsule blisters for distribution. The contents of each enteric-coated capsule are shown in Table 1.

Table 1: Contents of one enteric-coated capsule of Vivotif Berna™ Vaccine

Viable *S. typhi* Ty 21a	$2 - 6 \times 10^9$ colony-forming units
Non-viable *S. typhi* Ty 21a	$5 - 50 \times 10^9$ bacterial cells
Sucrose	26 – 130 mg
Ascorbic acid	1 – 5 mg
Amino acid mixture	1.4 – 7 mg
Lactose	100 – 180 mg
Magnesium stearate	3.6 – 4.4 mg

CLINICAL PHARMACOLOGY

Salmonella typhi is the etiological agent of typhoid fever, an acute, febrile enteric disease. This vaccine will not afford protection against species of *Salmonella* other than *Salmonella typhi* or other bacteria that cause enteric disease.
There are approximately 500 cases of typhoid fever per year diagnosed in the United States (1). In 62% of these patients (statistics from 1977–1979) the disease was acquired outside of the United States while in 38% of the patients the disease was acquired within the United States (2). Of the disease acquired during foreign travel 50% of the cases were contracted in Mexico, 20% in Asian countries and 15% in India. The majority of the remaining cases were acquired in the Caribbean basin, South and Central America, North Africa, and Southern Europe (2). Typhoid fever is considered to be endemic in most areas of Central and South America, North and Central Africa, Southeast Asia and the Indian Subcontinent (3).
Of the disease acquired in the United States 23% of the cases were associated with typhoid carriers, 24% were due to food outbreaks, 23% were associated with the ingestion of contaminated food or water, 6% due to household contact with an infected person and 4% following exposure to *S. typhi* in a laboratory setting.
The majority of typhoid cases respond favorably to antibiotic therapy. However, the emergence of chloramphenicol or ampicillin-resistant strains has greatly complicated therapy. Even with appropriate antibiotic therapy there were 7 deaths among 901 acute typhoid cases reported in the United States from 1977–1979 (2). Approximately 3–5% of acute typhoid cases result in the development of a chronic carrier state (4). These non-symptomatic carriers are the natural reservoir for *S. typhi* and can serve to maintain the disease in its endemic state or to directly infect individuals (2). Eradication of the carrier state by antibiotic therapy has been unsuccessful (5).
Virulent strains of *S. typhi* upon ingestion are able to pass through the stomach acid barrier, colonize the intestinal tract, penetrate the lumen and enter the lymphatic system and bloodstream, thereby causing disease. One possible mechanism by which disease may be prevented is by evoking a local immune response in the intestinal tract. Such local immunity may be induced by oral ingestion of a live attenuated strain of *S. typhi* undergoing an aborted infection.
The ability of *S. typhi* to cause disease and to induce a protective immune response is dependent upon the bacteria possessing a complete lipopolysaccharide (6, 7). The *S. typhi* Ty 21a vaccine strain, by virtue of a reduction in enzymes essential for lipopolysaccharide biosynthesis, is restricted in its ability to produce complete lipopolysaccharide (8, 9). However, a sufficient quantity of complete lipopolysaccharide is synthesized to evoke a protective immune response. Despite low levels of lipopolysaccharide synthesis, the cells lyse before regaining a virulent phenotype due to the intracellular build-up of intermediates during lipopolysaccharide synthesis (5, 8, 9).
The efficacy of the *S. typhi* Ty 21a strain has been evaluated in a series of double-blind field trials. The first trial was performed in Alexandria, Egypt with a study population of 32,388 children aged 6 to 7 years. Three doses of vaccine, in the form of a freshly reconstituted suspension administered after ingestion of 1 g of bicarbonate, were given on alternate days. Immunization resulted in a 95% decrease in the

incidence of typhoid fever over a 3-year period of surveillance (5, 10).
A series of field trials were subsequently performed in Santiago, Chile to evaluate efficacy when the vaccine strain was administered in the form of an acid-resistant enteric-coated capsule. The initial trial involved 91,954 school-aged children, and compared 1 or 2 doses of vaccine given one week apart. After 33 months of surveillance vaccine efficacy was 21% for the single dose schedule and 54% for the 2-dose schedule (11). A further field trial was performed in Santiago, Chile involving 109,594 school-aged children (12). Three doses of enteric-coated capsules were administered either on alternate days (short immunization schedule) or 21 days apart (long immunization schedule). Following 36 months of surveillance vaccination resulted in a 67% decrease in the incidence of typhoid fever in the short immunization schedule group and a 49% reduction in the long immunization schedule group. After 48 months of surveillance the short immunization schedule resulted in a 68% decrease in typhoid fever (13). An undiminished level of protection was observed during the fifth year of surveillance. A field trial was next conducted in Santiago, Chile to determine the relative efficacy of 2, 3 and 4 doses of enteric-coated vaccine administered on alternate days to school-aged children. Relative vaccine efficacy as determined by comparison of disease incidence within the three vaccinated groups was highest for the four dose regimen. An additional field trial to determine vaccine efficacy was conducted in Plaju, Indonesia involving 22,001 individuals approximately 3 to 50 years of age. Due to logistical considerations three doses of enteric-coated capsules were administered at weekly intervals, a schedule known to provide suboptimal protection (12). After two years of surveillance vaccine efficacy for all age groups was 41%. It should be noted that vaccine efficacy was 36% for subjects 3 to 14 years of age and 60% for those 15 to 44 years of age.
At present, the precise mechanism(s) by which Vivotif Berna™ Vaccine confers protection against typhoid fever is unknown. However, it is known that immunization of adult subjects can elicit a humoral anti-*S. typhi* LPS antibody response. Taking advantage of this fact, the seroconversion rate was compared between adults living in an endemic area (Chile) and non-endemic areas (United States and Switzerland) after the ingestion of 3 doses of vaccine. Comparable seroconversion rates were seen between these groups. Other studies in North American volunteers have shown that the Ty 21a strain is capable of providing significant protection to an experimental challenge of *S. typhi*.
Because of the very low incidence of typhoid fever in United States citizens, efficacy studies are not currently feasible in this population. However, the above observations support the expectation that Vivotif Berna™ Vaccine will provide protection to recipients from non-typhoid endemic areas such as the United States.

INDICATIONS AND USAGE

Vivotif Berna™ Vaccine is indicated for immunization of adults and children greater than 6 years of age against disease caused by *Salmonella typhi*. Results from clinical studies indicate that adults and children greater than 6 years of age may be protected against typhoid fever following the oral ingestion of 4 doses of Vivotif Berna™ Vaccine. Immunization (ingestion of all 4 doses of Vivotif Berna™ Vaccine) should be completed at least 1 week prior to potential exposure to *S. typhi*.
Routine immunization against typhoid fever is not recommended in the United States of America. Selective immunization against typhoid fever is recommended under the following circumstances: 1) expected intimate exposure to a household contact with typhoid fever, 2) travelers to areas of the world with a risk of exposure to typhoid fever, and 3) workers in microbiology laboratories with expected frequent contact with *S. typhi* (14).
Not all recipients of Vivotif Berna™ Vaccine will be fully protected against typhoid fever. Travelers should take all necessary precautions to avoid contact or ingestion of potentially contaminated food or water sources. There is no evidence to support the use of typhoid vaccine to control common source outbreaks, disease following natural disasters or in persons attending rural summer camps.
Vivotif Berna™ Vaccine will not afford protection against enteric microorganisms other than *S. typhi*. An optimal booster dose has not yet been established. However, it is recommended that a booster dose consisting of 4 vaccine capsules taken on alternate days be given every 5 years under conditions of repeated or continued exposure to typhoid fever (see Dosage and Administration section).
Typhoid fever continues to be an important disease in many parts of the world. Travelers entering such areas are at risk to contracting typhoid fever following the ingestion of contaminated food or water. Parenterally administered typhoid vaccine has been shown to be effective at reducing the incidence of disease in such endemic areas. However, immunization with such vaccines is frequently accompanied by adverse reactions such as pain and/or swelling at the injection site, fever, malaise and headache.

CONTRAINDICATIONS

Hypersensitivity to any component of the vaccine or the enteric-coated capsule.

Safety of the vaccine has not been demonstrated in persons deficient in their ability to mount a humoral or cell-mediated immune response, due to either a congenital or acquired immunodeficient state including treatment with immunosuppressive or antimitotic drugs. The vaccine should not be administered to these persons regardless of benefits.

WARNINGS

Vivotif Berna™ (Typhoid Vaccine Live Oral Ty 21a) is not to be taken during an acute febrile illness or in the face of acute gastrointestinal illness. Postpone taking the vaccine if persistent diarrhea or vomiting is occurring (see general precautions).

PRECAUTIONS

General

The vaccine should not be administered to persons during an acute febrile illness or acute gastrointestinal illness. The vaccine should not be administered to individuals receiving sulfonamides and antibiotics since these agents may be active against the vaccine strain and prevent a sufficient degree of multiplication to occur in order to induce a protective immune response. The vaccine should not be administered to persons with a known hypersensitivity to any vaccine component or medium component (see description).

Information for Patients

It is essential that all 4 doses of vaccine be taken at the prescribed alternate day interval to obtain a maximal protective immune response. Vaccine potency is dependent upon storage under refrigeration [between 2°C and 8°C (35.6°F–46.4°F)]. The vaccine should be stored under refrigeration at all times. It is essential to replace unused vaccine in the refrigerator between doses. The vaccine capsule should be swallowed approximately 1 hour before a meal with a cold or lukewarm [temperature not to exceed body temperature, e.g., 37°C (98.6°F)] drink. Care should be taken not to chew the vaccine capsule. The vaccine capsule should be swallowed as soon after placing in the mouth as possible.

Carcinogenesis, Mutagenesis, Impairment of Fertility

Long-term studies in animals with Vivotif Berna™ Vaccine have not been performed to evaluate carcinogenic potential, mutagenic potential or impairment of fertility.

Pregnancy

Category C

Animal reproduction studies have not been conducted with Vivotif Berna™ Vaccine. It is not known whether Vivotif Berna™ Vaccine can cause fetal harm when administered to pregnant woman or can affect reproduction capacity. Vivotif Berna™ Vaccine should be given to pregnant woman only if clearly needed.

Nursing Mothers

There are no data to warrant the use of this product in nursing mothers. It is not known if Vivotif Berna™ Vaccine is excreted in human milk.

Pediatric Use

The safety and efficacy of Vivotif Berna™ Vaccine has not been established in children under 6 years of age. This product is therefore not recommended for use in children under 6 years of age.

ADVERSE REACTIONS

Several lots of Vivotif Berna™ Vaccine have been evaluated in several field trials both in adults and in school-aged children. Objectively monitored side-effects, e.g., abdominal pain, diarrhea, vomiting, fever, headache and skin rash, did not occur at a statistically higher frequency in the vaccinated group as compared to a placebo group (11). Post-marketing surveillance outside of the United States has found that side-effects are infrequent, transient, and resolve of their own accord. Reported adverse reactions include nausea, abdominal cramps, vomiting, skin rash or urticaria in the trunk and/or extremities.

OVERDOSAGE

Five to 8 doses of Vivotif Berna™ Vaccine containing between 3–10 × 10¹⁰ viable vaccine organisms were administered to 155 healthy adult males. This dosage was, at a minimum, 5-fold higher than the currently recommended dose. No significant reactions, e.g., vomiting, acute abdominal distress or fever, were observed. At the recommended dosage, the S. typhi Ty 21a vaccine strain is not excreted in the feces. However, clinical studies in volunteers have shown that overdosing can increase the possibility of shedding the S. typhi Ty 21a vaccine strain in the feces (15).

DOSAGE AND ADMINISTRATION

The blister containing the vaccine capsules should be inspected to ensure that the foil seal and capsules are intact. One capsule is to be swallowed approximately 1 hour before a meal with a cold or lukewarm [temperature not to exceed body temperature, e.g., 37°C (98.6°F)] drink on alternate days, e.g., days 1, 3, 5 and 7. The vaccine capsule should not be chewed and should be swallowed as soon after placing in the mouth as possible. A complete immunization schedule is the ingestion of 4 vaccine capsules as described above. Unless a complete immunization schedule is followed, an optimum immune response may not be achieved. Not all recipients of Vivotif Berna™ Vaccine will be fully protected against typhoid fever. Travelers should take all necessary precautions to avoid contact with or ingestion of potentially contaminated food or water.

Booster Use

The optimum booster schedule for Vivotif Berna™ has not been determined. Efficacy has been shown to persist for at least 5 years. Further, there is no experience with Vivotif Berna™ Vaccine as a booster in persons previously immunized with parenteral typhoid vaccine. Despite these limitations it is recommended that a booster dose consisting of four vaccine capsules taken on alternate days be given every 5 years under conditions of repeated or continued exposure to typhoid fever.

HOW SUPPLIED

A single foil blister contains 4 doses of vaccine in a single package.

STORAGE

Vivotif Berna™ Vaccine is not stable when exposed to ambient temperatures. Vivotif Berna™ Vaccine should therefore be shipped and stored between 2°C and 8°C (35.6–46.4°F). Each package of vaccine shows an expiration date. This expiration date is valid only if the product has been maintained at 2°C–8°C (35.6–46.4°F).

Vivotif Berna™ Vaccine is manufactured by Swiss Serum and Vaccine Institute Berne, Switzerland, and distributed by Berna Products Corp., Coral Gables, FL 33146.

REFERENCES

1. Centers for Disease Control. Annual summary 1980: reported morbidity and mortality in the United States. MMWR. 29: 12–17, 1981.
2. Taylor, D.N., R.A. Pollard, P.A. Blake. Typhoid in the United States and the Risk to the International Traveler. J. Infect. Dis. 148: 599–602, 1983.
3. Levine, M.M., R.E. Black, C. Lanata, and the Chilean Typhoid Committee. Precise estimation of the numbers of chronic carriers of Salmonella typhi in Santiago, Chile, an endemic area. J. Infect. Dis. 146: 724–726, 1982.
4. Ames, W.R., M. Robbins. Age and sex as factors in the development of the typhoid carrier state, and a model for estimating carrier prevalence. Am. J. Public Health 33: 221–230, 1943.
5. Germanier, R. Typhoid Fever. In, Bacterial Vaccines. R. Germanier (ed.) p. 137–165, 1984.
6. Germanier, R. Immunity in experimental salmonellosis. I. Protection induced by rough mutants of Salmonella typhimurium. Infec. Immun. 2: 309–315, 1970.
7. Germanier, R., E. Fürer. Immunity in experimental salmonellosis. II. Basis for the avirulence and protective capacity of Gal E mutants of Salmonella typhimurium. Infec. Immun. 4: 663–673, 1971.
8. Germanier, R., E. Fürer. Isolation and characterisation of Gal E mutant Ty 21a of Salmonella typhi: a candidate strain for a live, oral typhoid vaccine. J. Infect. Dis. 131: 553–558, 1975.
9. Germanier, R., E. Fürer. Characteristics of the attenuated oral vaccine strain. S. typhi Ty 21a. Develop. Biol. Standard, 53: 3–7, 1983.
10. Wahdan, M.H., C. Sérié, Y. Cerisier, S. Sallam, R. Germainer. A controlled field trial of live Salmonella typhi strain Ty 21a oral vaccine against typhoid: three-year results. J. Infect. Dis. 145: 292–296, 1982.
11. Levine, M.M., R.E. Black, C. Ferreccio, M.L. Clements, C. Lanata, J. Rooney, R. Germanier, A. Schuster, H. Rodriguez, J.M. Borgono, H. Lobos, I. Prenzel, C. Ristorio, M.E. Pinto. The efficacy of attenuated S. typhi oral vaccine strain Ty 21a evaluated in controlled field trials. In, Development of Vaccines and Drugs against Diarrhea. 11th Noble Conference, Stockholm, 1985, pp. 90–101. J. Holmgren, A. Lindberg and R. Möllby (eds.). Studentlitteratur, Lund, Sweeden, 1986.
12. Levine, M.M., C. Ferreccio, R.E. Black, R. Germanier, Chilean Typhoid Committee. Large-Scale Field Trial of Ty 21a Live Oral Typhoid Vaccine in Enteric-Coated Capsule Formulation. Lancet 1: 1049–1052, 1987.
13. Cryz, S.J., Jr., E. Fürer, M.M. Levine. Zur Wirksamkeit des oralen, attenuierten Salmonella Typhi Ty 21a Lebendimpfstoffes in kontrollierten Feldversuchen. Schweiz. Med. Wschr. 118: 467–470, 1988.
14. Report of the Committee on Infectious Diseases. Twenty-first edition, p 373–374. American Academy of Pediatrics, 141 Northwest Point Blvd., P.O. Box 927, Elk Grove Village, IL 60009-0827, 1988.
15. Gilman, R.H., R.B. Hornick, W.E. Woodward, H.L. DuPont, M.J. Snyder, M.M. Levine, J.P. Libonati. Evaluation of a UDP-Glucose-4-epimeraseless mutant of Salmonella typhi as a live oral vaccine. J. Infect. Dis. 136: 717–723, 1988.

Manufactured by:
Swiss Serum and Vaccine Institute Berne, Switzerland
U.S.-License No. 21

Distributed by:
Berna Products Corp., Coral Gables, FL 33146
Shown in Product Identification Guide, page 305

Beutlich LP Pharmaceuticals
1541 SHIELDS DRIVE
WAUKEGAN, IL 60085-8304

Direct Inquiries to:
847-473-1100
800-238-8542
FAX 847-473-1122

CEO–TWO® EVACUANT SUPPOSITORIES   OTC

NDC #0283-0763-09

COMPOSITION

Each adult rectal suppository contains sodium bicarbonate and potassium bitartrate in a water soluble polyethylene glycol base.

HOW SUPPLIED

In packages of 10, white opaque suppositories. Keep in cool, dry place.
DO NOT REFRIGERATE
(See PDR For Nonprescription Drugs)

HURRICAINE® TOPICAL ANESTHETIC   OTC

COMPOSITION

HURRICAINE contains 20% benzocaine in a flavored, water soluble polyethylene glycol base.

PACKAGING AVAILABLE

Gel
1 oz. Jar Wild Cherry NDC #0283-0871-31
1 oz. Jar Pina Colada NDC #0283-0886-31
1 oz. Jar Watermelon NDC #0283-0293-31
1/8 oz. Tube Wild Cherry NDC #0283-0871-12
1/8 oz. Tube Watermelon NDC #0283-0293-12
Liquid
1 fl. oz. Jar Wild Cherry NDC #0283-0569-31
1 fl. oz. Jar Pina Colada NDC #0283-1886-31
1/8 oz. Tube Wild Cherry NDC #0283-0569-12
.25 gm. Packet Wild Cherry NDC #0283-0569-50
.25 gm. Packet Pina Colada NDC #0283-1886-50
.25 ml Dry Handle Swab Wild Cherry NDC #0283-0693-01
Spray
2 oz. Aerosol Wild Cherry NDC #0283-679-02
Spray Kit
2 oz. Aerosol Wild Cherry NDC #0283-183-02 with 200 Disposable Extension Tubes
(See PDR For Nonprescription Drugs)

PERIDIN-C®   OTC

Vitamin-C and Bioflavonoids
(See PDR For Nonprescription Drugs)

BIOCRAFT Laboratories, Inc.

See TEVA Pharmaceuticals USA

Biogen, Inc.
14 CAMBRIDGE CENTER
CAMBRIDGE, MA 02142

Direct Inquiries to:
Customer Service (800) 456-2255
Fax (617) 679-3100

AVONEX™   ℞
[ăv′-ə-nĕx]
INTERFERON BETA-1a

DESCRIPTION

AVONEX™ (Interferon beta-1a) is produced by recombinant DNA technology. Interferon beta-1a is a 166 amino acid glycoprotein with a predicted molecular weight of approximately 22,500 daltons. It is produced by mammalian cells (Chinese Hamster Ovary cells) into which the human interferon beta gene has been introduced. The amino acid sequence of AVONEX™ is identical to that of natural human interferon beta.

Using the World Health Organization (WHO) natural interferon beta standard, Second International Standard for Interferon, Human Fibroblast (Gb-23-902-531), AVONEX™ has a specific activity of approximately 200 million international units (IU) of antiviral activity per mg; 30 mcg of AVONEX™ contains 6 million IU of antiviral activity. The activity against other standards is not known.

AVONEX™ is formulated as a sterile, white to off-white lyophilized powder for intramuscular injection after reconstitution with supplied diluent or Sterile Water for Injection, USP, preservative-free.

Each 1.0 mL (1.0 cc) of reconstituted AVONEX™ contains 30 mcg of Interferon beta-1a, 15 mg Albumin Human, USP, 5.8 mg Sodium Chloride, USP, 5.7 mg Dibasic Sodium Phosphate, USP and 1.2 mg Monobasic Sodium Phosphate, USP at a pH of approximately 7.3.

CLINICAL PHARMACOLOGY

General

Interferons are a family of naturally occurring proteins and glycoproteins that are produced by eukaryotic cells in response to viral infection and other biological inducers. Interferon beta, one member of this family, is produced by various cell types including fibroblasts and macrophages. Natural interferon beta and Interferon beta-1a are glycosylated, with each containing a single N-linked complex carbohydrate moiety. Glycosylation of other proteins is known to affect their stability, activity, biodistribution and half-life in blood. However, the effects of glycosylation of interferon beta on these properties have not been fully defined.

Biologic Activities

Interferons are cytokines that mediate antiviral, antiproliferative and immunomodulatory activities in response to viral infection and other biological inducers. Three major interferons have been distinguished: alpha, beta and gamma. Interferons alpha and beta form the Type I class of interferons, and interferon gamma is a Type II interferon. These interferons have overlapping but clearly distinct biological activities.

Interferon beta exerts its biological effects by binding to specific receptors on the surface of human cells. This binding initiates a complex cascade of intracellular events that leads to the expression of numerous interferon-induced gene products and markers. These include 2′, 5′-oligoadenylate synthetase, β_2-microglobulin and neopterin. These products have been measured in the serum and cellular fractions of blood collected from patients treated with AVONEX™ (Interferon beta-1a).

The specific interferon-induced proteins and mechanisms by which AVONEX™ exerts its effects in multiple sclerosis have not been fully defined.

Pharmacokinetics

Pharmacokinetics of AVONEX™ in multiple sclerosis patients have not been evaluated. The pharmacokinetic and pharmacodynamic profiles of AVONEX™ in healthy subjects following doses of 30 mcg through 75 mcg have been investigated. Serum levels of Interferon beta-1a as measured by antiviral activity are slightly above detectable limits following a 30 mcg intramuscular (IM) dose, and increase with higher doses.

Table 1
Mean Single Dose Pharmacokinetic
Parameters Following 60 mcg Administration

Route of Administration	AUC (IU·h/mL)	C_{max} (IU/mL)	T_{max} (Range) (h)	Elimination Half-life (h)
IM	1352	45	9.8 (3-15)	10.0
SC	478	30	7.8 (3-18)	8.6

Table 1 compares general pharmacokinetic parameters for AVONEX™ following administration of a 60 mcg dose by IM and subcutaneous (SC) routes to healthy volunteers. After an IM dose, serum levels of Interferon beta-1a typically peak between 3 and 15 hours and then decline at a rate consistent with a 10 hour elimination half-life. Serum levels of Interferon beta-1a may be sustained after IM administration due to prolonged absorption from the IM site. Systemic exposure, as determined by AUC and C_{max} values, is greater following IM than SC administration.

Biological response markers (e.g., neopterin and β_2-microglobulin) are induced by Interferon beta-1a following parenteral doses of 15 mcg through 75 mcg in healthy subjects and treated patients. Biological response marker levels increase within 12 hours of dosing and remain elevated for at least 4 days. Peak biological response marker levels are typically observed 48 hours after dosing. The relationship of serum Interferon beta-1a levels or levels of these induced biological response markers to the mechanisms by which AVONEX™ exerts its effects in multiple sclerosis is unknown.

Clinical Studies: Effects in Multiple Sclerosis

The clinical effects of AVONEX™ (Interferon beta-1a) in multiple sclerosis were studied in a randomized, multicenter, double-blind, placebo-controlled study in patients with relapsing (stable or progressive) multiple sclerosis[1]. In this study, 301 patients received either 6 million IU (30 mcg) of AVONEX™ (n=158) or placebo (n=143) by IM injection once weekly. Patients were entered into the trial over a $2^1/_2$ year period, received injections for up to 2 years, and continued to be followed until study completion. Two hundred eighty-two patients completed 1 year on study, and 172 patients completed 2 years on study. There were 144 patients treated with AVONEX™ for more than 1 year, 115 patients for more than 18 months and 82 patients for 2 years.

All patients had a definite diagnosis of multiple sclerosis of at least 1 year duration and had at least two exacerbations in the 3 years prior to study entry (or one per year if the duration of disease was less than 3 years). At entry, study participants were without exacerbation during the prior 2 months and had Kurtzke Expanded Disability Status Scale (EDSS[2]) scores ranging from 1.0 to 3.5. Patients with chronic progressive multiple sclerosis were excluded from this study.

The primary outcome assessment was time to progression in disability, measured as an increase in the EDSS of at least 1.0 point that was sustained for at least 6 months. An increase in EDSS score reflects accumulation of disability. This endpoint was used to assure that progression reflected permanent increase in disability rather than a transient effect due to an exacerbation.

Secondary outcomes included exacerbation frequency and results of magnetic resonance imaging (MRI) scans including gadolinium (Gd)-enhanced lesion number and volume and T2-weighted (proton density) lesion volume. Additional secondary endpoints included two upper limb (tested in both arms) and three lower limb function tests.

Twenty-three of the 301 patients (8%) discontinued treatment prematurely. Of these, one patient treated with placebo (1%) and six patients treated with AVONEX™ (4%) discontinued treatment due to adverse events. Thirteen of these 23 patients remained on study and were evaluated for clinical endpoints.

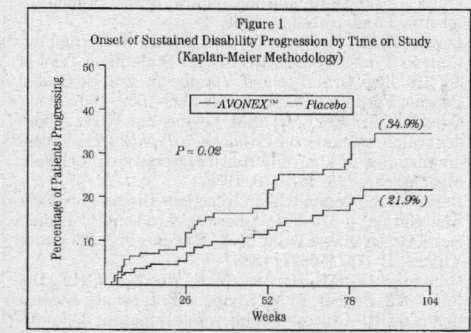

Figure 1
Onset of Sustained Disability Progression by Time on Study
(Kaplan-Meier Methodology)

Note: Disability progression represents at least a 1.0 point increase in EDSS score sustained for at least 6 months.

Time to onset of sustained progression in disability was significantly longer in patients treated with AVONEX™ than

in patients receiving placebo (p=0.02). The Kaplan-Meier plots of these data are presented in Figure 1. The Kaplan-Meier estimate of the percentage of patients progressing by the end of 2 years was 34.9% for placebo-treated patients and 21.9% for AVONEX™-treated patients, indicating a slowing of the disease process. This represents a 37% reduction in the risk of accumulating disability in the AVONEX™-treated group compared to the placebo-treated group.

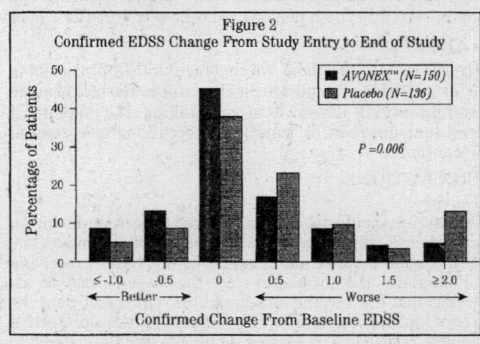

Figure 2
Confirmed EDSS Change From Study Entry to End of Study

The distribution of confirmed EDSS change from study entry (baseline) to the end of the study is shown in Figure 2. There was a statistically significant difference between treatment groups in confirmed change for patients with at least two scheduled visits (136 placebo-treated and 150 AVONEX™-treated patients; p=0.006; see Table 2). Confirmed EDSS change was calculated as the difference between the EDSS score at study entry and one of the scores determined at the last two scheduled visits. If the EDSS score at either of the last two scheduled visits showed improvement (reduction in score) the higher score was used. Otherwise, the lower score was used. Nineteen patients had one score higher and one score lower than baseline; the higher score was used. The last two scheduled visits occurred at varying time points among patients.

Table 2
Major Clinical Endpoints

Endpoint	Placebo	AVONEX™	P-Value
PRIMARY ENDPOINT:			
Time to sustained progression in disability (N: 143, 158)[1]	—See Figure 1—		0.02[2]
Percentage of patients progressing in disability at 2 years (Kaplan-Meier estimate)[1]	34.9%	21.9%	
SECONDARY ENDPOINTS:			
DISABILITY			
Mean confirmed change in EDSS from study entry to end of study (N: 136, 150)[1]	0.50	0.20	0.006[3]
EXACERBATIONS			
Number of exacerbations in subset completing 2 years (N: 87, 85)			0.03[3]
0	26%	38%	
1	30%	31%	
2	11%	18%	
3	14%	7%	
≥4	18%	7%	
Percentage of patients exacerbation-free in subset completing 2 years (N: 87, 85)	26%	38%	0.10[4]
Annual exacerbation rate (N: 143, 158)[1]	0.82	0.67	0.04[5]
MRI			
Number of Gd-enhanced lesions:			
At study entry (N: 132, 141)			
Mean (Median)	2.3 (1.0)	3.2 (1.0)	
Range	0-23	0-56	
Year 1 (N: 123, 134)			
Mean (Median)	1.6 (0)	1.0 (0)	0.02[3]
Range	0-22	0-28	
Year 2 (N: 82, 83)			
Mean (Median)	1.6 (0)	0.8 (0)	0.05[3]
Range	0-34	0-13	

T2 lesion volume:
Percentage change from
study entry to year 1
(N: 116, 123)

Median	−3.3%	−13.1%	0.02[3]

Percentage change from
study entry to year 2
(N: 83, 81)

Median	−6.5%	−13.2%	0.36[3]

Note: (N: ,) denotes the number of evaluable placebo and AVONEX™ (Interferon beta-1a) patients, respectively.
[1] *Patient data included in this analysis represent variable periods of time on study.*
[2] *Analyzed by Mantel-Cox (logrank) test.*
[3] *Analyzed by Mann-Whitney rank-sum test.*
[4] *Analyzed by Cochran-Mantel-Haenszel test.*
[5] *Analyzed by likelihood ratio test.*

The rate and frequency of exacerbations were determined as secondary outcomes. For all patients included in the study, irrespective of time on study, the annual exacerbation rate was 0.67 per year in the AVONEX™-treated group and 0.82 per year in the placebo-treated group (p=0.04).
AVONEX™ (Interferon beta-1a) treatment significantly decreased the frequency of exacerbations in the subset of patients who were enrolled in the study for at least 2 years (87 placebo-treated patients and 85 AVONEX™-treated patients; p=0.03; see Table 2).
Gd-enhanced and T2-weighted (proton density) MRI scans of the brain were obtained in most patients at baseline and at the end of 1 and 2 years of treatment. Gd-enhancing lesions seen on brain MRI scans represent areas of breakdown of the blood brain barrier thought to be secondary to inflammation. Patients treated with AVONEX™ demonstrated significantly lower Gd-enhanced lesion number after 1 and 2 years of treatment (p≤0.05; see Table 2). The volume of Gd-enhanced lesions was also analyzed, and showed similar treatment effects (p≤0.03). Percentage change in T2-weighted lesion volume from study entry to year 1 was significantly lower in AVONEX™-treated than placebo-treated patients (p=0.02). A significant difference in T2-weighted lesion volume change was not seen between study entry and year 2. The exact relationship between MRI findings and the clinical status of patients is unknown. Changes in lesion area often do not correlate with changes in disability progression. The prognostic significance of the MRI findings in this study has not been evaluated.
Of the limb function tests, only one demonstrated a statistically significant difference between treatment groups (favoring AVONEX™).
A summary of the effects of AVONEX™ on the primary and major secondary endpoints of this study is presented in Table 2.
Safety and efficacy of treatment with AVONEX™ beyond 2 years are not known.

INDICATIONS AND USAGE

AVONEX™ (Interferon beta-1a) is indicated for the treatment of relapsing forms of multiple sclerosis to slow the accumulation of physical disability and decrease the frequency of clinical exacerbations. Safety and efficacy in patients with chronic progressive multiple sclerosis have not been evaluated.

CONTRAINDICATIONS

AVONEX™ (Interferon beta-1a) is contraindicated in patients with a history of hypersensitivity to natural or recombinant interferon beta, human albumin, or any other component of the formulation.

WARNINGS

AVONEX™ (Interferon beta-1a) should be used with caution in patients with depression. Depression and suicide have been reported to occur in patients receiving other interferon compounds. Depression and suicidal ideation are known to occur at an increased frequency in the multiple sclerosis population. A relationship between occurrence of depression and/or suicidal ideation and the use of AVONEX™ has not been established. An equal incidence of depression was seen in the placebo-treated and AVONEX™-treated patients in the placebo-controlled multiple sclerosis study. Patients treated with AVONEX™ should be advised to report immediately any symptoms of depression and/or suicidal ideation to their prescribing physicians. If a patient develops depression, cessation of AVONEX™ therapy should be considered.

PRECAUTIONS

General

Caution should be exercised when administering AVONEX™ (Interferon beta-1a) to patients with pre-existing seizure disorder. In the placebo-controlled study, four patients receiving AVONEX™ experienced seizures, while no seizures occurred in the placebo group. Three of these four patients had no prior history of seizure. It is not known

whether these events were related to the effects of multiple sclerosis alone, to AVONEX™, or to a combination of both. For patients with no prior history of seizure who develop seizures during therapy with AVONEX™, an etiologic basis should be established and appropriate anti-convulsant therapy instituted prior to considering resumption of AVONEX™ treatment. The effect of AVONEX™ administration on the medical management of patients with seizure disorder is unknown.
Patients with cardiac disease, such as angina, congestive heart failure or arrhythmia, should be closely monitored for worsening of their clinical condition during initiation of therapy with AVONEX™. AVONEX™ does not have any known direct-acting cardiac toxicity; however, symptoms of flu syndrome seen with AVONEX™ therapy may prove stressful to patients with severe cardiac conditions.

Information to Patients

Patients should be informed of the most common adverse events associated with AVONEX™ administration, including symptoms associated with flu syndrome (see Adverse Reactions section and precautions in Patient Information). Symptoms of flu syndrome are most prominent at the initiation of therapy and decrease in frequency with continued treatment. In the placebo-controlled study, patients were instructed to take 650 mg acetaminophen immediately prior to injection and for an additional 24 hours after each injection to modulate acute symptoms associated with AVONEX™ administration.
Patients should be cautioned to report depression or suicidal ideation (see Warnings).
Patients should be advised about the abortifacient potential of interferon beta (see Pregnancy—Teratogenic Effects).
When a physician determines that AVONEX™ can be used outside of the physician's office, persons who will be administering AVONEX™ should receive instruction in reconstitution and injection, including the review of the injection procedures (see Dosage and Administration). If a patient is to self-administer, the physical ability of that patient to self-inject intramuscularly should be assessed. The first injection should be performed under the supervision of a qualified health care professional. A puncture-resistant container for disposal of needles and syringes should be used. Patients should be instructed in the technique and importance of proper syringe and needle disposal and be cautioned against reuse of these items.

Laboratory Tests

In addition to those laboratory tests normally required for monitoring patients with multiple sclerosis, complete blood and differential white blood cell counts, platelet counts, and blood chemistries, including liver function tests, are recommended during AVONEX™ (Interferon beta-1a) therapy. During the placebo-controlled study, these tests were performed at least every 6 months. There were no significant differences between the placebo and AVONEX™ groups in the incidence of liver enzyme elevation, leukopenia or thrombocytopenia. However, these are known to be dose-related laboratory abnormalities associated with the use of interferons. Patients with myelosuppression may require more intensive monitoring of complete blood cell counts, with differential and platelet counts.

Drug Interactions

No formal drug interaction studies have been conducted with AVONEX™. In the placebo-controlled study, corticosteroids or ACTH were administered for treatment of exacerbations in some patients concurrently receiving AVONEX™. In addition, some patients receiving AVONEX™ were also treated with anti-depressant therapy and/or oral contraceptive therapy. No unexpected adverse events were associated with these concomitant therapies.
Other interferons have been noted to reduce cytochrome P-450 oxidase-mediated drug metabolism. Formal hepatic drug metabolism studies with AVONEX™ in humans have not been conducted. Hepatic microsomes isolated from AVONEX™-treated rhesus monkeys showed no influence of AVONEX™ on hepatic P-450 enzyme metabolism activity. As with all interferon products, proper monitoring of patients is required if AVONEX™ is given in combination with myelosuppressive agents.

Carcinogenesis, Mutagenesis and Impairment of Fertility

Carcinogenesis: No carcinogenicity data for Interferon beta-1a are available in animals or humans.
Mutagenesis: Interferon beta-1a was not mutagenic when tested in the Ames bacterial test and in an *in vitro* cytogenetic assay in human lymphocytes in the presence and absence of metabolic activation. These assays are designed to detect agents that interact directly with and cause damage to cellular DNA. Interferon beta-1a is a glycosylated protein that does not directly bind to DNA.
Impairment of Fertility: No studies were conducted to evaluate the effects of interferon beta on fertility in normal women or women with multiple sclerosis. It is not known whether Interferon beta-1a can affect human reproductive capacity.
Menstrual irregularities were observed in monkeys administered interferon beta at a dose 100 times the recommended weekly human dose (based upon a body surface area compar-

ison). Anovulation and decreased serum progesterone levels were also noted transiently in some animals. These effects were reversible after discontinuation of drug.
Treatment of monkeys with interferon beta at 2 times the recommended weekly human dose (based upon a body surface area comparison) had no effects on cycle duration or ovulation.
The accuracy of extrapolating animal doses to human doses is not known. In the placebo-controlled study, 6% of patients receiving placebo and 5% of patients receiving AVONEX™ experienced menstrual disorder. If menstrual irregularities occur in humans, it is not known how long they will persist following treatment.

Pregnancy—Teratogenic Effects

Pregnancy Category C: The reproductive toxicity of AVONEX™ has not been studied in animals or humans. In pregnant monkeys given interferon beta at 100 times the recommended weekly human dose (based upon a body surface area comparison), no teratogenic or other adverse effects on fetal development were observed. Abortifacient activity was evident following 3 to 5 doses at this level. No abortifacient effects were observed in monkeys treated at 2 times the recommended weekly human dose (based upon a body surface area comparison). Although no teratogenic effects were seen in these studies, it is not known if teratogenic effects would be observed in humans. There are no adequate and well-controlled studies with interferons in pregnant women. If a woman becomes pregnant or plans to become pregnant while taking AVONEX™, she should be informed of the potential hazards to the fetus, and it should be recommended that the woman discontinue therapy.

Nursing Mothers

It is not known whether Interferon beta-1a is excreted in human milk. Because of the potential of serious adverse reactions in nursing infants, a decision should be made to either discontinue nursing or to discontinue AVONEX™.

Pediatric Use

Safety and effectiveness in pediatric patients below the age of 18 years have not been established.

ADVERSE REACTIONS

The safety data describing the use of AVONEX™ (Interferon beta-1a) in multiple sclerosis patients are based on the placebo-controlled trial in which 158 patients randomized to AVONEX™ were treated for up to 2 years (see Clinical Studies).
The five most common adverse events associated (at p ≤ 0.075) with AVONEX™ treatment were flu-like symptoms (otherwise unspecified), muscle ache, fever, chills and asthenia. The incidence of all five adverse events diminished with continued treatment.
One patient in the placebo group attempted suicide; no AVONEX™-treated patient attempted suicide. The incidence of depression was equal in the two treatment groups. However, since depression and suicide have been reported with other interferon products, AVONEX™ should be used with caution in patients with depression (see Warnings).
In the placebo-controlled study, four patients receiving AVONEX™ experienced seizures, while no seizures occurred in the placebo group. Three of these four patients had no prior history of seizure. It is not known whether these events were related to the effects of multiple sclerosis alone, to AVONEX™, or to a combination of both (see Precautions).
Table 3 enumerates adverse events and selected laboratory abnormalities that occurred at an incidence of 2% or more among the 158 multiple sclerosis patients treated with 30 mcg of AVONEX™ once weekly by IM injection. Reported adverse events have been classified using standard COSTART terms. Terms so general as to be uninformative and those events that were equal in incidence or more common in the placebo-treated patients have been excluded.

Table 3
Adverse Events and Selected Laboratory Abnormalities
in the Placebo-Controlled Study

Adverse Event	Placebo (N=143)	AVONEX™ (N=158)
Body as a Whole		
Headache	57%	67%
Flu-like symptoms (otherwise unspecified)*	40%	61%
Pain	20%	24%
Fever*	13%	23%
Asthenia	13%	21%
Chills*	7%	21%
Infection	6%	11%
Abdominal pain	6%	9%
Chest pain	4%	6%
Injection site reaction	1%	4%
Malaise	3%	4%
Injection site inflammation	0%	3%

Continued on next page

Biogen, Inc.—Cont.

Hypersensitivity reaction	0%	3%
Ovarian cyst	0%	3%
Cardiovascular System		
Syncope	2%	4%
Vasodilation	1%	4%
Digestive System		
Nausea	23%	33%
Diarrhea	10%	16%
Dyspepsia	7%	11%
Anorexia	6%	7%
Hemic and Lymphatic System		
Anemia*	3%	8%
Eosinophils ≥10%	4%	5%
HCT (%) ≤32 (females)		
or ≤37 (males)	1%	3%
Ecchymosis injection site	1%	2%
Metabolic and Nutritional Disorders		
SGOT ≥3 × ULN	1%	3%
Musculoskeletal System		
Muscle ache*	15%	34%
Arthralgia	5%	9%
Nervous System		
Sleep difficult	16%	19%
Dizziness	13%	15%
Muscle spasm	6%	7%
Suicidal tendency	1%	4%
Seizure	0%	3%
Speech disorder	0%	3%
Ataxia	0%	2%
Respiratory System		
Upper respiratory tract infection	28%	31%
Sinusitis	17%	18%
Dyspnea	3%	6%
Skin and Appendages		
Urticaria	2%	5%
Alopecia	1%	4%
Nevus	0%	3%
Herpes zoster	2%	3%
Herpes simplex	1%	2%
Special Senses		
Otitis media	5%	6%
Hearing decreased	0%	3%
Urogenital		
Vaginitis	2%	4%

*Significantly associated with AVONEX™ treatment (p ≤ 0.05).

AVONEX™ (Interferon beta-1a) has also been evaluated in 290 patients with illnesses other than multiple sclerosis. The majority of these patients were enrolled in studies to evaluate AVONEX™ treatment of chronic viral hepatitis B and C, in which the doses studied ranged from 15 mcg to 75 mcg, given SC, 3 times a week, for up to 6 months. The incidence of common adverse events in these studies was generally seen at a frequency similar to that seen in the placebo-controlled multiple sclerosis study. In these non-multiple sclerosis studies, inflammation at the site of the SC injection was seen in 52% of treated patients. In contrast, injection site inflammation was seen in 3% of multiple sclerosis patients receiving AVONEX™, 30 mcg by IM injection. Subcutaneous injections were also associated with the following local reactions: injection site necrosis, injection site atrophy, injection site edema and injection site hemorrhage. None of the above was observed in the multiple sclerosis patients participating in the placebo-controlled study.

Other events observed during premarket evaluation of AVONEX™, administered either SC or IM in all patient populations studied, are listed in the paragraph that follows. Because most of the events were observed in open and uncontrolled studies, the role of AVONEX™ in their causation cannot be reliably determined. **Body as a Whole:** abscess, ascites, cellulitis, facial edema, hernia, injection site fibrosis, injection site hypersensitivity, lipoma, neoplasm, photosensitivity reaction, sepsis, sinus headache, toothache; **Cardiovascular System:** arrhythmia, arteritis, heart arrest, hemorrhage, hypotension, palpitation, pericarditis, peripheral ischemia, peripheral vascular disorder, postural hypotension, pulmonary embolus, spider angioma, telangiectasia, vascular disorder; **Digestive System:** blood in stool, colitis, constipation, diverticulitis, dry mouth, gallbladder disorder, gastritis, gastrointestinal hemorrhage, gingivitis, gum hemorrhage, hepatoma, hepatomegaly, increased appetite, intestinal perforation, intestinal obstruction, periodontal abscess, periodontitis, proctitis, thirst, tongue disorder; **Endocrine System:** hypothyroidism; **Hemic and Lymphatic System:** coagulation time increased, ecchymosis, lymphadenopathy,

petechia; **Metabolic and Nutritional Disorders:** abnormal healing, dehydration, hypoglycemia, hypomagnesemia, hypokalemia; **Musculoskeletal System:** arthritis, bone pain, myasthenia, osteonecrosis, synovitis; **Nervous System:** abnormal gait, amnesia, Bell's Palsy, clumsiness, depersonalization, drug dependence, facial paralysis, hyperesthesia, increased libido, neurosis, psychosis; **Respiratory System:** emphysema, hemoptysis, hiccup, hyperventilation, laryngitis, pharyngeal edema, pneumonia; **Skin and Appendages:** basal cell carcinoma, blisters, cold clammy skin, contact dermatitis, erythema, furunculosis, genital pruritus, nevus, seborrhea, skin ulcer, skin discoloration; **Special Senses:** abnormal vision, conjunctivitis, earache, eye pain, labyrinthitis, vitreous floaters; **Urogenital:** breast fibroadenosis, breast mass, dysuria, epididymitis, fibrocystic change of the breast, fibroids, gynecomastia, hematuria, kidney calculus, kidney pain, leukorrhea, menopause, nocturia, pelvic inflammatory disease, penis disorder, Peyronies Disease, polyuria, postmenopausal hemorrhage, prostatic disorder, pyelonephritis, testis disorder, urethral pain, urinary urgency, urinary retention, urinary incontinence, vaginal hemorrhage.

Serum Neutralizing Activity
Throughout the placebo-controlled multiple sclerosis study, serum samples from patients were monitored for the development of Interferon beta-1a neutralizing activity. During the study, 24% of AVONEX™-treated patients were found to have serum neutralizing activity at one or more time points tested. Fifteen percent of AVONEX™-treated patients tested positive for neutralizing activity at a level at which no placebo patient tested positive. The significance of the appearance of serum neutralizing activity is unknown.

DRUG ABUSE AND DEPENDENCE
There is no evidence that abuse or dependence occurs with AVONEX™ (Interferon beta-1a) therapy. However, the risk of dependence has not been systematically evaluated.

DOSAGE AND ADMINISTRATION
The recommended dosage of AVONEX™ (Interferon beta-1a) for the treatment of relapsing forms of multiple sclerosis is 30 mcg injected intramuscularly once a week (see Figure 3).
AVONEX™ is intended for use under the guidance and supervision of a physician. Patients may self-inject only if their physician determines that it is appropriate and with medical follow-up, as necessary, after proper training in intramuscular injection technique.

FIGURE 3
RECONSTITUTION AND INJECTION
Read through entire instructions prior to starting procedure.
Wash hands prior to preparing medication and after the medication has been administered. Allow the vial of AVONEX™ (Interferon beta-1a) and the vial of diluent to reach room temperature. Reconstitute AVONEX™ using sterile technique, as discussed below.
The following supplies will be needed:
* vial of AVONEX™
* vial of diluent, single-use (Sterile Water for Injection, USP, preservative-free)
* syringe
* blue MICRO PIN®
* sterile needle
* alcohol wipes
* syringe disposal container
* adhesive bandage

Reconstitution with diluent vial
1. Remove the cap from the vial of AVONEX™ and vial of diluent, and clean the rubber stopper of each vial with an alcohol wipe.

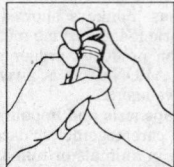

2. Remove the small protective cover from the syringe with a counterclockwise turn.

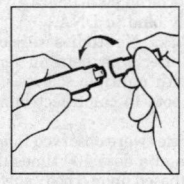

3. Attach the blue MICRO PIN® (vial access pin) to the syringe with a half turn clockwise.

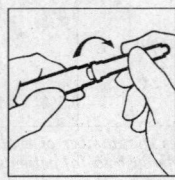

4. Remove the MICRO PIN® cover. Save for later use.

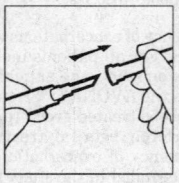

5. Pull back the syringe plunger to the 1.1 cc mark.

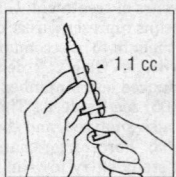

6. Push the MICRO PIN® down through the center of the rubber stopper of the diluent vial.

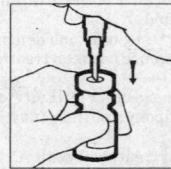

7. Inject air into the diluent vial by pushing down on the plunger until it cannot be pushed any further.
8. Turn the diluent vial and syringe upside down.
9. Keeping the MICRO PIN® in the fluid, withdraw 1.1 cc of diluent into the syringe by pulling back on the plunger.

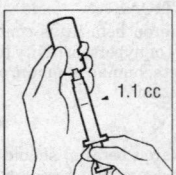

10. Tap the syringe gently to make any air bubbles rise to the top. If bubbles are present, press the plunger until the diluent is at the top of the syringe. Make sure there is still 1.1 cc of diluent in the syringe.

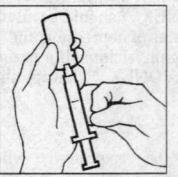

11. Pull the MICRO PIN® out of the diluent vial.
12. Insert the MICRO PIN® through the center of the rubber stopper of the vial of AVONEX™.

13. *Slowly* inject the diluent.
    CAUTION: Rapid addition of the diluent may cause foaming, making it difficult to withdraw AVONEX™.

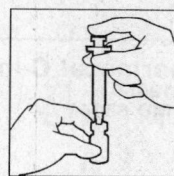

14. Without removing the syringe, *gently* swirl the vial until the white cake of AVONEX™ is dissolved. *CAUTION: DO NOT SHAKE.*

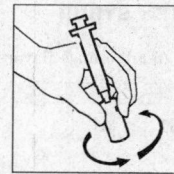

15. Check to see that all of the AVONEX™ cake is dissolved.
16. Turn the vial and syringe upside down. Slowly withdraw 1.0 cc of AVONEX™. If bubbles appear, push solution *slowly* back into the vial and withdraw the solution again.

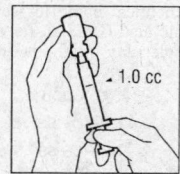

1.0 cc

17. Check the contents of the syringe. If you see areas of discoloration (other than a slightly yellow solution) or solid particles do not use the syringe. Get a new set of materials, including syringe, and start again with Step 1.
18. With the vial still upside down, tap the syringe gently to make any air bubbles rise to the top. Then press the plunger until the AVONEX™ is at the top of the syringe. Check the volume (should be 1.0 cc) and withdraw more medication if necessary. Withdraw the MICRO PIN® and syringe from the vial.
19. Replace the cover on the MICRO PIN® and remove from the syringe with a counterclockwise turn.
20. Attach a needle to the syringe with a ¹/₂ turn clockwise until the needle is secure.

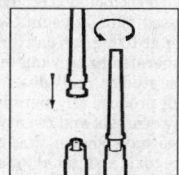

Injection

1. Use a new alcohol wipe to clean the skin at one of the recommended intramuscular injection sites. Pull the protective cover off the needle.
2. With one hand stretch the skin taut around the injection site. Hold the syringe with the other hand, making sure it is horizontal, until ready for injection. Insert the needle with a quick dart-like thrust at a 90° angle, through the skin and into the muscle. Expect to feel some resistance.

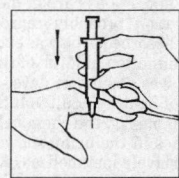

3. Once inserted, release the stretched skin and gently pull back slightly on the plunger and check for blood. If there is blood in the syringe, do not use it. Get a new set of materials, and go to Step 1 of the Reconstitution section and begin again.

4. If you do not see blood, slowly push the plunger until the syringe is empty.

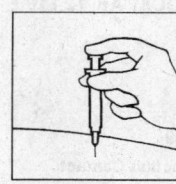

5. Hold an alcohol wipe near the needle at the injection site and pull the needle straight out. Use the wipe to apply pressure to the site for a few seconds or rub gently in a circular motion.

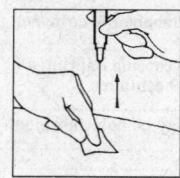

6. If there is bleeding at the site, wipe it off and, if necessary, apply an adhesive bandage.
7. Dispose of all supplies properly, including the diluent.

HOW SUPPLIED

AVONEX™ (Interferon beta-1a) is supplied as a lyophilized powder in a single-use vial containing 33 mcg (6.6 million IU) of Interferon beta-1a, 16.5 mg Albumin Human, USP, 6.4 mg Sodium Chloride, USP, 6.3 mg Dibasic Sodium Phosphate, USP, and 1.3 mg Monobasic Sodium Phosphate, USP, and is preservative-free. Diluent is supplied in a single-use vial (Sterile Water for Injection, USP, preservative-free). Reconstitute AVONEX™ with 1.1 mL (cc) of diluent and swirl gently to dissolve (approximate pH 7.3). Withdraw 1.0 mL (cc) for administration.
AVONEX™ is available in the following package configuration (NDC-59627-001-03): Package (Administration Pack) containing 4 Administration Dose Packs (each containing one vial of AVONEX™, one 10 mL (10 cc) diluent vial, two alcohol wipes, one 3 cc syringe, one Micro PIN®* vial access pin, one needle and one adhesive bandage).

Stability and Storage
Vials of AVONEX™ (Interferon beta-1a) must be stored in a 2–8°C (36–46°F) refrigerator. Should refrigeration be unavailable, AVONEX™ can be stored at 25°C (77°F) for a period of up to 30 days. DO NOT EXPOSE TO HIGH TEMPERATURES. DO NOT FREEZE. Do not use beyond the expiration date stamped on the vial. Following reconstitution, it is recommended the product be used as soon as possible within 6 hours stored at 2–8°C (36–46°F). DO NOT FREEZE.

REFERENCES

1. Jacobs LD, *et al.* Ann Neurol 1996; 39: 285-294.
2. Kurtzke JF. Neurol 1983; 33: 1444-1452.

AVONEX™ (INTERFERON BETA-1a)
Manufactured by:
BIOGEN, INC.
14 Cambridge Center
Cambridge, MA 02142 USA
©1996 Biogen, Inc. All rights reserved.
1-800-456-2255
U.S. Patent Pending
I63000-1 (5/96)
Caution: Federal law prohibits dispensing without prescription.
Micro PIN® is the trademark of B. Braun Medical Inc.

Patient Information
AVONEX™ (Interferon beta-1a) is intended for use under the guidance and supervision of a physician. If your physician recommends self-injection, you should be instructed in the preparation of AVONEX™ for administration and in the technique of self-injection. Do not attempt self-administration until you are sure that you understand the requirements for preparing the product and giving an injection to yourself.
AVONEX™ must be used as prescribed by your physician. However, if you miss a dose, take it as soon as you remember. You may resume your regular schedule, but two injections should not be administered within 2 days of each other. While using AVONEX™, please keep in mind the following facts:
● AVONEX™ (Interferon beta-1a) must be kept cold. Be sure to store it in a refrigerator before and after reconstitution. Do not freeze. If refrigeration is not available, AVONEX™ can be stored for reconstitution at 25°C (77°F) for up to 30 days. When storing outside of a refrigerator, do not allow AVONEX™ to be exposed to high temperatures as may occur in a glove compartment or on a window sill.

● For treatment of multiple sclerosis, AVONEX™ must be injected into the muscle (intramuscular injection).
● Keep syringes and needles away from children. Do not reuse needles or syringes. Discard used syringes and needles in a syringe disposal unit as instructed by your health care professional.
● Women: AVONEX™ should not be used during pregnancy or if you are trying to become pregnant. If you wish to become pregnant while using AVONEX™, discuss the matter with your doctor. While using AVONEX™, women of childbearing age should use birth control measures. If you do become pregnant you should discontinue treatment and contact your doctor immediately.
● Flu-like symptoms are common. They include fever, chills, fatigue and muscle ache. Your physician may recommend taking acetaminophen to help lessen the impact of flu-like symptoms.
● Depression has been reported by patients treated with interferon drugs. If you experience such symptoms, contact your physician promptly.
● As with any prescription medication, side effects related to therapy can occur. Consult with your physician if you have any problems, whether or not you think they may be related to AVONEX™.

Shown in Product Identification Guide, page 305

Bioglan Pharma, Inc.
**4902 EISENHOWER BOULEVARD
SUITE 150
TAMPA, FL 33634**

Direct Inquiries to:
Bioglan Pharma, Inc.
(813) 243-8833
FAX: (813) 243-8832

MICANOL®   ℞
Anthralin USP 1% Cream

DESCRIPTION
Micanol 1% (Anthralin Cream USP) is a smooth, yellow cream containing 1% anthralin USP in an aqueous cream base of glyceryl monolaurate, glyceryl monomyristate, citric acid, sodium hydroxide and purified water.
The chemical name of anthralin is 1,8-dihydroxy-9-anthrone.
The structure is:

HOW SUPPLIED
Micanol 1% (Anthralin Cream USP) is supplied in 50g tubes.
NDC 62436-401-01
Keep container tightly capped when not in use.
Avoid excessive heat.
Store at controlled room temperature 59°F–86°F (15°C–30°C).
Caution: Federal (U.S.A.) law prohibits dispensing without prescription.
Manufactured for Bioglan Pharma, Inc., Tampa, FL 33634, by Bioglan AB, Sweden
March 1996   13212051

IDENTIFICATION PROBLEM?
Turn to the **Product Identification** Guide,
where you'll find more than
1600 products pictured in actual
size and full color.

Blaine Company, Inc.
1465 JAMIKE LANE
ERLANGER, KY 41018–1039

Direct Inquiries to:
(606) 283-9437
(800) 633-9353
FAX: (606) 283-9460

For Medical Information Contact:
In Emergencies:
(606) 283-9437
(800) 633-9353
FAX: (606) 283-9460

MAG–OX 400   OTC

DESCRIPTION
Each tablet contains Magnesium Oxide 400 mg. U.S.P. (Heavy), or 241.3 mg. Elemental Magnesium (19.86 mEq.).

INDICATIONS AND USAGE
Hypomagnesemia, magnesium deficiencies and/or magnesium depletion resulting from malnutrition, restricted diet, alcoholism or magnesium depleting drugs. For increasing urinary magnesium excretion. Supplemental magnesium during pregnancy and/or as an antacid.

WARNINGS
Do not take more than 2 tablets in a 24 hour period, or use this maximum dosage for more than 2 weeks, except under the advice and supervision of a physician. Do not use this product except under the advice and supervision of a physician if you have a kidney disease. May have laxative effect. As with any drug, if you are pregnant or nursing a baby, seek professional advice before using this product. Keep this and all medicines out of children's reach.

DOSAGE
Adult dose 1 or 2 tablets daily or as directed by a physician.

HOW SUPPLIED
Bottles of 100 and 1000 and Hospital Unit Dose (UD).

URO–MAG   OTC

DESCRIPTION
Each capsule contains Magnesium Oxide 140 mg. U.S.P. (Heavy), or 84.5 mg. Elemental Magnesium (6.93 mEq.)

INDICATIONS AND USAGE
Hypomagnesemia, magnesium deficiencies and/or magnesium depletion resulting from malnutrition, restricted diet, alcoholism or magnesium depleting drugs. For increasing urinary magnesium excretion. Supplemental magnesium during pregnancy and/or as an antacid.

WARNINGS
Do not take more than 4 capsules in a 24 hour period, or use this maximum dosage for more than 2 weeks, except under the advice and supervision of a physician. Do not use this product except under the advice and supervision of a physician if you have a kidney disease. May have laxative effect. As with any drug, if you are pregnant or nursing a baby, seek professional advice before using this product. Keep this and all medicines out of children's reach.

DOSAGE
Adult dose 3–4 capsules daily or as directed by a physician.

HOW SUPPLIED
Bottles of 100 and 1000 and Hospital Unit Dose (UD).

EDUCATIONAL MATERIAL

Samples and anatomical charts available to physicians upon request.

For EMERGENCY telephone numbers, consult the **Manufacturers Index.**

Blansett Pharmacal
3304 PIKE AVENUE
N. LITTLE ROCK, AR 72118

Direct Inquiries to:
Customer Service
(501) 758-8635
FAX: (501) 758-5369

For Medical Information Contact:
In Emergencies:
Medical Information Dept
(501) 758-8635
FAX: (501) 758-5369

ANOLOR® 300   ℞
(butalbital, acetaminophen & caffeine)

Each opaque white capsule imprinted light green ANOLOR 300 and 51674-0009 contains:
Butalbital* .... 50 mg
    *(WARNING: May be habit forming)
Acetaminophen .... 325 mg
Caffeine .... 40 mg

HOW SUPPLIED
Bottles of 100

CORTANE-B OTIC   ℞
(chloroxylenol, hydrocortisone, pramoxine HCl)

Each 1 mL contains:
    Chloroxylenol .... 1 mg
    Pramoxine HCl .... 10 mg
    Hydrocortisone .... 10 mg

HOW SUPPLIED
Plastic dropper vials of 10 mL.

NALEX®-A TABLETS (Dye Free)   ℞
(Chlorpheniramine maleate, phenyltoloxamine citrate, phenylephrine HCl)

Each white timed release tablet embossed Blansett and 3 Bisect 08 contains:
    Phenylephrine HCl .... 20 mg
    Chlorpheniramine maleate .... 4 mg
    Phenyltoloxamine citrate .... 40 mg

HOW SUPPLIED
Bottles of 100

NALEX® CAPSULES   ℞
(pseudoephedrine HCl, guaifenesin)

Each opaque white-clear capsule imprinted Blansett and 30 contains:
    Pseudoephedrine HCl .... 120 mg
    In a special base providing prolonged action
    Guaifenesin .... 250 mg
    Designed for immediate release

NALEX® DH LIQUID   ©
Antitussive - Decongestant
(hydrocodone bitartrate, phenylephrine HCl & Alcohol 5%)

Each cherry flavored teaspoonful (5 mL) contains:
Hydrocodone* Bitartrate .... 1.67 mg
    *(WARNING: May be habit forming)
Phenylephrine HCl .... 5 mg
Alcohol 5%

HOW SUPPLIED
Bottles of 16 oz

NALEX® JR CAPSULES   ℞
(pseudoephedrine HCl, guaifenesin)

Each green-clear capsule imprinted Blansett and 33 contains:
Pseudoephedrine HCl .... 60 mg
    In a special base providing prolonged action
Guaifenesin .... 300 mg
    Designed for immediate release

HOW SUPPLIED
NALEX CAPSULES: Bottles of 100
NALEX JR: Bottles of 100

Bock Pharmacal Company
P.O. BOX 419056
ST. LOUIS, MO 63141

Direct Inquiries to:
telephone (314) 579-0770
FAX (314) 579-0349

BRONCHOLATE® SYRUP   ℞

Each teaspoonful (5 ml) orange flavored syrup contains:
Ephedrine HCl .... 6.25 mg
Guaifenesin .... 100.00 mg

HOW SUPPLIED
Bottles of 16 oz.

CHEMET®   ℞
SUCCIMER

DESCRIPTION
CHEMET (succimer) is an orally active, heavy metal chelating agent. The chemical name for succimer is *meso* 2, 3-dimercaptosuccinic acid (DMSA). Its empirical formula is $C_4H_6O_4S_2$ and molecular weight is 182.2. The *meso*-structural formula is:

$$\begin{array}{c} COOH \\ | \\ H-C-SH \\ | \\ H-C-SH \\ | \\ COOH \end{array}$$

Succimer is a white crystalline powder with an unpleasant, characteristic mercaptan odor and taste.
Each CHEMET opaque white capsule for oral administration, contains beads coated with 100 mg of succimer and is imprinted in black with CHEMET 100. Inactive ingredients in medicated beads are: povidone, sodium starch glycolate, starch and sucrose. Inactive ingredients in capsule are: gelatin, iron oxide, titanium dioxide and other ingredients.

CLINICAL PHARMACOLOGY
Succimer is a lead chelator; it forms water soluble chelates and, consequently, increases the urinary excretion of lead.
Preclinical Toxicology: In an ongoing six month chronic oral toxicity study in dogs, thrombocytopenia was observed in animals receiving succimer at 80 or 140 mg/kg/day after three months of dosing. Preliminary gross pathology findings in the affected dogs included ecchymoses in a number of organs. No depressed platelet counts were observed in dogs receiving succimer at 10 mg/kg/day for three months. Platelets were not enumerated in previous oral toxicity studies up to 28 days. In those studies, daily doses of succimer up to 200 mg/kg/day did not produce any significant overt toxicity in rats and dogs. However, six and twenty-eight day oral toxicity studies in dogs have shown that doses of 300 mg/kg/day or higher were toxic and lethal to some dogs. Kidney and gastrointestinal tract were the major target organs for succimer toxicity. Toxicity was manifested by anorexia, emesis, mucoid and/or bloody diarrhea, increased blood urea nitrogen concentration, increased SGPT, SGOT and alkaline phosphatase levels, renal tubular necrosis, purulent nephritis and severe gastrointestinal bleeding and ulceration. Deaths were due to renal failure.
Pharmacokinetics: In a study performed in healthy adult volunteers, after a single dose of ^{14}C-succimer at 16, 32, or 48 mg/kg, absorption was rapid but variable with peak blood radioactivity levels between one and two hours. On average, 49% of the radiolabeled dose was excreted: 39% in the feces, 9% in the urine and 1% as carbon dioxide from the lungs. Since fecal excretion probably represented non-absorbed drug, most of the absorbed drug was excreted by the kidneys. The apparent elimination half-life of the radio-labeled material in the blood was about two days.
In other studies of healthy adult volunteers receiving a single oral dose of 10 mg/kg, the chemical analysis of succimer and its metabolites in the urine showed that succimer was rapidly and extensively metabolized. Approximately 25% of the administered dose was excreted in the urine with the peak blood level and urinary excretion occurring between two and four hours. Of the total amount of drug eliminated in the urine, approximately 90% was eliminated in altered form as mixed succimer-cysteine disulfides; the remaining 10% was eliminated unchanged. The majority of mixed di-

sulfides consisted of succimer in disulfide linkages with two molecules of L-cysteine, the remaining disulfides contained one L-cysteine per succimer molecule.

Pharmacodynamics: Dose ranging studies were performed in 18 men with blood lead levels of 44–96 μg/dL. Three groups of 6 patients received either 10.0, 6.7 or 3.3 mg/kg succimer orally every 8 hours for 5 days. After five days the mean blood levels of the three groups decreased 72.5%, 58.3% and 35.5% respectively. The mean urinary lead excretions in the initial 24 hours were 28.6, 18.6 and 12.3 times the pretreatment 24 hour urinary lead excretion. As the chelatable pool was reduced during therapy, urinary lead output decreased. A mean of 19 mg of lead was excreted during a five-day course of 30 mg/kg/day succimer. Clinical symptoms, such as headache and colic and biochemical indices of lead toxicity also improved. Decrease in urinary excretion of d-aminolevulinic acid (ALA) and coproporphyrin paralleled the improvement in erythrocyte d-aminolevulinic acid dehydratase (ALA-D). Three control patients with lead poisoning of similar severity received $CaNa_2EDTA$ intravenously at a dose of 50 mg/kg/day for five days. The mean blood lead level decreased 47.4% and the mean urinary lead excretion was 21 mg in the control patients.

Effect on Essential Minerals: In the above studies succimer had no significant effect on the urinary elimination of iron, calcium or magnesium. Zinc excretion doubled during treatment. The effect of succimer on the excretion of essential minerals was small compared to that of $CaNa_2EDTA$, which can induce more than a ten-fold increase in urinary excretion of zinc and doubling of copper and iron excretion.

Efficacy: A dose ranging study was performed in 15 children aged 2 to 7 years with blood lead levels of 30–49 μg/dL and positive $CaNa_2EDTA$ lead mobilization tests. Each group of five patients received 350, 233 or 116 mg/m^2 succimer every 8 hours for 5 days. These doses corresponded to 10, 6.7 and 3.3 mg/kg. Six control patients received 1000 mg/m^2/day $CaNa_2EDTA$ intravenously for 5 days. Following therapy, the mean blood lead levels decreased 78, 63 and 42% respectively in the three groups treated with succimer. The response of the 350 mg/m^2 every 8 hours (10 mg/kg q 8 hr) group was significantly better than that of the other succimer treated groups as well as that of the control group, whose mean blood lead level fell 48%. No adverse reactions or changes in essential mineral excretion were reported in the succimer treated groups. In the $CaNa_2EDTA$ treated group, the cumulative amount of urinary lead excreted was slightly but significantly greater than in the succimer group. After $CaNa_2EDTA$, the urinary excretion of copper, zinc, iron and calcium were significantly increased.

As with other chelators, both adults and children experienced a rebound in blood lead levels after discontinuation of CHEMET. In these studies, after treatment with a dose of 350 mg/m^2 (10 mg/kg) every 8 hours for five days, the mean lead level rebounded and plateaued at 60–85% of pretreatment levels two weeks after therapy. The rebound plateau was somewhat higher with lower doses of succimer and with intravenous $CaNa_2EDTA$.

In an attempt to control rebound of blood lead levels, 19 children, ages 1–7 years, with blood lead levels of 42–67 μg/dL, were treated with 350 mg/m^2 succimer every 8 hours for five days and then divided into three groups. One group was followed for two weeks with no further therapy, the second group was treated for two weeks with 350 mg/m^2 daily, and the third with 350 mg/m^2 every 12 hours. After the initial 5 days of therapy, the mean blood lead level in all subjects declined 61%. While the untreated group and the group treated with 350 mg/m^2 daily experienced rebound during the ensuing two weeks, the group who received the 350 mg/m^2 every 12 hours experienced no such rebound during the treatment period and less rebound following cessation of therapy.

In another study, ten children, ages 21 to 72 months, with blood lead levels of 30–57 μg/dL were treated with succimer 350 mg/m^2 every eight hours for five days followed by an additional 19–22 days of therapy at a dose of 350 mg/m^2 every 12 hours. The mean blood lead levels decreased and remained stable at under 15 μg/dL during the extended dosing period.

In addition to the controlled studies, approximately 250 patients with lead poisoning have been treated with succimer either orally or parenterally in open U.S. and foreign studies with similar results reported. Succimer has been used for the treatment of lead poisoning in one patient with sickle cell anemia and in five patients with glucose-6-phosphodehydrogenase (G6PD) deficiency without adverse reactions.

Lead Encephalopathy: Three adults with lead encephalopathy have been reported in the literature to have improved with succimer therapy. However, data are not available regarding the use of succimer for the treatment of this rare and sometimes fatal complication of lead poisoning in children.

Other Heavy Metal Poisoning: No controlled clinical studies have been conducted with succimer in poisoning with other heavy metals. A limited number of patients have received succimer for mercury or arsenic poisoning. These patients showed increased urinary excretion of the heavy metal and varying degrees of symptomatic improvement.

INDICATIONS AND USAGE

CHEMET is indicated for the treatment of lead poisoning in children with blood lead levels above 45 μg/dL. CHEMET is not indicated for prophylaxis of lead poisoning in a lead-containing environment; the use of CHEMET should always be accompanied by identification and removal of the source of the lead exposure.

CONTRAINDICATIONS

CHEMET should not be administered to patients with a history of allergy to the drug.

WARNINGS

Keep out of reach of children. CHEMET is not a substitute for effective abatement of lead exposure.

Mild to moderate neutropenia has been observed in some patients receiving succimer. While a causal relationship to succimer has not been definitely established, neutropenia has been reported with other drugs in the same chemical class. A complete blood count with white blood cell differential and direct platelet counts should be obtained prior to and weekly during treatment with succimer. Therapy should either be withheld or discontinued if the absolute neutrophil count (ANC) is below 1200/μL and the patient followed closely to document recovery of the ANC to above 1500/μL or to the patient's baseline neutrophil count. There is limited experience with reexposure in patients who have developed neutropenia. Therefore, such patients should be rechallenged only if the benefit of succimer therapy clearly outweighs the potential risk of another episode of neutropenia and then only with careful patient monitoring.

Patients treated with succimer should be instructed to promptly report any signs of infection. If infection is suspected, the above laboratory tests should be conducted immediately.

PRECAUTIONS

The extent of clinical experience with CHEMET is limited. Therefore, patients should be carefully observed during treatment.

General: Elevated blood lead levels and associated symptoms may return rapidly after discontinuation of CHEMET because of redistribution of lead from bone stores to soft tissues and blood. After therapy, patients should be monitored for rebound of blood lead levels, by measuring blood lead levels at least once weekly until stable. However, the severity of lead intoxication (as measured by the initial blood lead level and the rate and degree of rebound of blood lead) should be used as a guide for more frequent blood lead monitoring.

All patients undergoing treatment should be adequately hydrated. Caution should be exercised in using CHEMET therapy in patients with compromised renal function. Limited data suggests that CHEMET is dialyzable, but that the lead chelates are not.

Transient mild elevations of serum transaminases have been observed in 6–10% of patients during the course of succimer therapy. Serum transaminases should be monitored before the start of therapy and at least weekly during therapy. Patients with a history of liver disease should be monitored closely. No data are available regarding the metabolism of succimer in patients with liver disease.

Clinical experience with repeated courses is limited. The safety of uninterrupted dosing longer than three weeks has not been established and it is not recommended.

The possibility of allergic or other mucocutaneous reactions to the drug must be borne in mind on readministration (as well as during initial courses). Patients requiring repeated courses of CHEMET should be monitored during each treatment course. One patient experienced recurrent mucocutaneous vesicular eruptions of increasing severity affecting the oral mucosa, the external urethral meatus and the perianal area on the third, fourth and fifth courses of the drug. The reaction resolved between courses and upon discontinuation of therapy.

Information for Patients: Patients should be instructed to maintain adequate fluid intake. If rash occurs, patients should consult their physician. Patients should be instructed to promptly report any indication of infection, which may be a sign of neutropenia (see WARNINGS and ADVERSE REACTIONS).

In young children unable to swallow capsules, the contents of the capsule can be administered in a small amount of food (see DOSAGE AND ADMINISTRATION).

Drug Interaction: CHEMET is not known to interact with other drugs including iron supplements; interactions have not been systematically studied. Concomitant administration of CHEMET with other chelation therapy, such as $CaNa_2EDTA$ is not recommended.

Drug/Laboratory Tests Interaction: Succimer may interfere with serum and urinary laboratory tests. *In vitro* studies have shown succimer to cause false positive results for ketones in urine using nitroprusside reagents such as Ketostix® and falsely decreased measurements of serum uric acid and CPK.

Carcinogenesis, Mutagenesis and Impairment of Fertility: CHEMET has not been tested for carcinogenic potential in long-term animal studies. CHEMET has not been tested in animals for its effect on fertility and reproductive performance in males and females. It was not mutagenic in the Ames bacterial assay and in the mammalian cell forward gene mutation assay.

Pregnancy: *Teratogenic Effects—Pregnancy Category C.* CHEMET has been shown to be teratogenic and fetotoxic in pregnant mice when given subcutaneously in a dose range of 410 to 1640 mg/kg/day during the period of organogenesis. There are no adequate and well controlled studies in pregnant women. CHEMET should be used during pregnancy only if the potential benefit justifies the potential risk to the fetus.

Nursing Mothers: It is not known whether this drug is excreted in human milk. Because many drugs and heavy metals are excreted in human milk, nursing mothers requiring CHEMET therapy should be discouraged from nursing their infants.

Pediatric Use: Refer to the INDICATIONS and DOSAGE AND ADMINISTRATION sections. There is no therapeutic experience with CHEMET in children under one year of age.

ADVERSE REACTIONS

Clinical experience with CHEMET has been limited. Consequently, the full spectrum and incidence of adverse reactions including the possibility of hypersensitivity or idiosyncratic reactions have not been determined. The most common events attributable to succimer, i.e., gastrointestinal symptoms or increases in serum transaminases, have been observed in about 10% of patients (see PRECAUTIONS). Rashes, some necessitating discontinuation of therapy, have been reported in about 4% of patients. If rash occurs, other causes (e.g. measles) should be considered before ascribing the reaction to succimer. Rechallenge with succimer may be considered if lead levels are high enough to warrant retreatment. One allergic mucocutaneous reaction has been reported on repeated administration of the drug (See PRECAUTIONS). Mild to moderate neutropenia has been observed in some patients receiving succimer (see WARNINGS). Table I presents adverse events reported with the administration of succimer for the treatment of lead and other heavy metal intoxication.

TABLE I
INCIDENCE OF ADVERSE EVENTS IN DOMESTIC STUDIES REGARDLESS OF ATTRIBUTION OR SUCCIMER DOSAGE

	Children (191)		Adults (134)	
	%	(n)	%	(n)
Digestive:	12.0	23	20.9	28
Nausea, vomiting, diarrhea, appetite loss, hemorrhoidal symptoms, loose stools, metallic taste in mouth.				
Body as a Whole:	5.2	10	15.7	21
Back pain, abdominal cramps, stomach pains, head pain, rib pain, chills, flank pain, fever, flu-like symptoms, heavy head/tired, head cold, headache, moniliasis.				
Metabolic:	4.2	8	10.4	14
Elevated SGPT, SGOT, alkaline phosphatase, elevated serum cholesterol.				
Nervous:	1.0	2	12.7	17
Drowsiness, dizziness, sensorimotor neuropathy, sleepiness, paresthesia.				
Skin and Appendages:	2.6	5	11.2	15
Papular rash, herpetic rash, rash, mucocutaneous eruptions, pruritus.				
Special Senses:	1.0	2	3.7	5
Cloudy film in eye, ears plugged, otitis media, eyes watery.				
Respiratory:	3.7	7	0.7	1
Throat sore, rhinorrhea, nasal congestion, cough.				
Urogenital:	0.0	—	3.7	5
Decreased urination, voiding difficulty, proteinuria increased.				
Cardiovascular:	0.0	—	1.8	2
Arrhythmia				
Heme/Lymphatic:	0.5*	1	1.5*	2
Mild to moderate neutropenia				
Increased platelet count, intermittent eosinophilia.				
Musculoskeletal:	0.0	—	3.0	4
Kneecap pain, leg pains.				

* Does not include neutropenia - see WARNINGS

OVERDOSAGE

Doses of 2300 mg/kg in the rat and 2400 mg/kg in the mouse produced ataxia, convulsions, labored respiration and frequently death. No case of overdosage has been reported in humans. Limited data indicate that succimer is dialyzable. In case of acute overdosage, induction of vomiting or gastric lavage followed by administration of an activated charcoal slurry and appropriate supportive therapy are recommended.

DOSAGE AND ADMINISTRATION

Start dosage at 10 mg/kg or 350 mg/m^2 every eight hours for five days. Initiation of therapy at higher doses is not recom-

Continued on next page

Bock Pharmacal—Cont.

mended. (See Table II for Dosing chart and number of capsules.) Reduce frequency of administration to 10 mg/kg or 350 mg/m^2 every 12 hours (two-thirds of initial daily dosage) for an additional two weeks of therapy. A course of treatment lasts 19 days. Repeated courses may be necessary if indicated by weekly monitoring of blood lead concentration. A minimum of two weeks between courses is recommended unless blood lead levels indicate the need for more prompt treatment.

TABLE II
CHEMET (SUCCIMER) PEDIATRIC DOSING CHART

LBS	KG	DOSE (MG)*	Number of CAPSULES*
18–35	8–15	100	1
36–55	16–23	200	2
56–75	24–34	300	3
76–100	35–44	400	4
>100	>45	500	5

*To be administered every 8 hours for 5 days, followed by dosing every 12 hours for 14 days.

In young children who cannot swallow capsules, CHEMET can be administered by separating the capsule and sprinkling the medicated beads on a small amount of soft food or putting them in a spoon and following with fruit drink. Identification of the source of lead in the child's environment and its abatement are critical to a successful therapy outcome. Chelation therapy is not a substitute for preventing further exposure to lead and should not be used to permit continued exposure to lead.
Patients who have received CaNa$_2$EDTA with or without BAL may use CHEMET for subsequent treatment after an interval of four weeks. Data on the concomitant use of CHEMET with CaNa$_2$EDTA with or without BAL are not available, and such use is not recommended.

HOW SUPPLIED
100 mg capsules in bottle of 100 (NDC 0563-0332-01)
Storage: Store between 15°C and 25°C and avoid excessive heat.
CAUTION: Federal law prohibits dispensing without prescription. Revised December, 1995.
HPG11506-01-1295BP
MANUFACTURED FOR:
bock pharmacal company
St. Louis, Mo 63141
Packaged by: Central Pharmaceuticals, Inc.
Seymour, IN 47274
©1995 Bock Pharmacal Company
All rights reserved.
Shown in Product Identification Guide, page 305

DYNABAC®
(dirithromycin tablets)   ℞

DESCRIPTION
Dynabac® (dirithromycin tablets) contain the semi-synthetic macrolide antibiotic dirithromycin for oral administration. It is a pro-drug which is converted non-enzymatically during intestinal absorption into the microbiologically active moiety erythromycylamine.
Chemically, dirithromycin is designated (9S)-9-Deoxo-11-deoxy-9, 11-[imino[(1R)-2-(2-methoxyethoxy)-ethylidene]oxy] erythromycin and has the molecular formula $C_{42}H_{78}N_2O_{14}$. Its molecular weight is 835.09. The structural formula is:

Table 1
Steady-State Tissue Concentrations of Erythromycylamine Following Two 250-mg Tablets (500 mg) of Dynabac Given Orally Once Daily

Tissue	Time After Last Dose (h)	Mean Tissue Concentration (µg/g or µg/10^7 cells)	Corresponding Mean-Plasma or Serum Concentration (µg/mL)	Tissue/Plasma (Serum) Ratio
Tonsil	14	3.47	0.17	20.4
Healthy lung	12	3.79	0.13	29.2
Pathologic/infected lung	12	3.85	0.13	29.6
Infected bronchial mucosa	12	1.70	0.13	13.1
Alveolar Macrophages	5	0.37	0.35	1.1

High tissue concentrations should not be interpreted to be quantitatively related to clinical efficacy. Erythromycylamine is concentrated in cell lysosomes, which have a low organelle pH at which drug activity is reduced.

Chemically, erythromycylamine is designated 9-(S)-9-amino-9-deoxoerythromycin and has a molecular formula of $C_{37}H_{70}N_2O_{12}$. Its molecular weight is 743.97. The structural formula is:

Dirithromycin is a basic compound. The free base is poorly soluble in water and readily soluble in polar organic solvents. Dirithromycin is hydrolyzed to erythromycylamine in acidic aqueous solutions; hydrolysis is virtually complete within 2 hours.
Dynabac tablets are enteric coated to protect the contents from gastric acid and to permit absorption of the antibiotic in the small intestine. Each enteric-coated tablet contains dirithromycin equivalent to 250 mg and the following inactive ingredients: microcrystalline cellulose, croscarmellose sodium, magnesium carbonate, magnesium stearate, sodium starch glycolate, hydroxypropyl cellulose, hydroxypropyl methylcellulose polyethylene glycol, propylene glycol, benzyl alcohol, methacrylic acid copolymer, titanium dioxide, triethyl citrate, and talc.

CLINICAL PHARMACOLOGY
Pharmacokinetics:
Absorption—Dirithromycin is rapidly absorbed and converted by nonenzymatic hydrolysis to the microbiologically active compound erythromycylamine. The absolute bioavailability of the oral formulation is approximately 10%. The pharmacokinetic parameters of erythromycylamine in plasma after single- and multiple-dose oral administration of two 250-mg Dynabac tablets once daily for 10 days in 10 fasting healthy subjects (19 to 50 years of age) were as follows: [See table below.]
Distribution—The protein binding of erythromycylamine ranges from 15% to 30%. Erythromycylamine is widely distributed throughout the body with a mean apparent volume of distribution (V_{Dss}) of 800 L (504 to 1,041 L).
Rapid distribution of erythromycylamine into tissues and high concentrations within cells result in significantly higher concentrations in tissues than in plasma or serum. There are no data available on cerebrospinal fluid penetration.
[See table above.]
Metabolism and Excretion—Erythromycylamine is primarily eliminated in the bile and undergoes little or no hepatic metabolism. Thus, the primary route of elimination is fecal/hepatic with 81% to 97% of the dose eliminated in this manner. Approximately 2% of the administered dose is eliminated through the kidney, mainly within the first 36 hours following drug administration.

The mean plasma half-life of erythromycylamine was estimated to be about 8 h (2 to 36 h), while a mean urinary terminal elimination half-life of about 44 h (16 to 65 h) and a mean apparent total body clearance of approximately 23 L/h (20 to 32 L/h) were observed in patients with normal renal function.
Food Effect on Absorption—**Dynabac tablets should be administered with food or within an hour of having eaten.** The effect of food on the bioavailability of dirithromycin was evaluated following oral administration of two 250-mg Dynabac tablets 1 or 4 hours before food and immediately after a standard breakfast. Results obtained indicated a slight increase in the absorption of erythromycylamine when dirithromycin tablets were administered after food, while a significant decrease in C_{max} (33%) and AUC (31%) occurred when administered 1 hour before food. The effects of high and low fat meals on the bioavailability of dirithromycin were also investigated. The results showed that the amount of dietary fat had little or no effect on the bioavailability of dirithromycin.
Special Populations:
Hepatic Insufficiency—In patients with mild (Child's Grade A) hepatic impairment, mean peak serum concentration, AUC, and volume of distribution increased somewhat with multiple-dose administration; however, based on the magnitude of these changes, no dosage adjustment should be necessary in patients with mildly impaired hepatic function. The pharmacokinetics of dirithromycin in patients with moderate or severe impairment in hepatic function (Child's Grade B or greater) have not been studied.
Renal Insufficiency—The mean peak plasma concentration (C_{max}) and AUC tended to increase as creatinine clearance decreased; however, based on data available to date, no dosage adjustment should be necessary in patients with impaired renal function, including dialysis patients.
Geriatric Patients—In a multiple-dose study in which 19 healthy elderly subjects (65 to 83 years of age) were given two 250-mg Dynabac tablets every day for 10 days, C_{max} and AUC tended to increase with age; however, neither C_{max} nor AUC was statistically or clinically significantly altered with age. Therefore, based on these pharmacokinetic results, no dosage adjustment should be necessary in elderly patients.
Microbiology:
Erythromycylamine, the microbiologically active product of dirithromycin hydrolysis, exerts its activity by binding to the 50S ribosomal subunits of susceptible microorganisms resulting in inhibition of protein synthesis.
Dirithromycin/Erythromycylamine has been shown to be active against most strains of the following microorganisms both *in vitro* and in clinical infections as described in the **INDICATIONS AND USAGE** section:
Gram-positive aerobes:
Staphylococcus aureus (methicillin-susceptible strains only)
Streptococcus pneumoniae
Streptococcus pyogenes
Gram-negative aerobes:
Legionella pneumophila
Moraxella catarrhalis
Other bacteria:
Mycoplasma pneumoniae
The following *in vitro* data are available, **but their clinical significance is unknown.** Dirithromycin exhibits *in vitro* minimum inhibitory concentrations (MIC's) of 2 µg/mL or less against most (≥90%) strains of the following microorganisms; however, the safety and effectiveness of Dynabac in treating clinical infections due to these microorganisms have not been established in adequate and well-controlled clinical trials.
Gram-positive aerobes:
Listeria monocytogenes
Streptococci, groups C, F, and G
Streptococcus agalactiae
Viridans group streptococci

Pharmacokinetic Parameter (n = 10 subjects)	Mean (1 S.D.) Day 1	Day 10
C_{max} (µg/mL)	0.3 (0.2)	0.4 (0.2)
T_{max} (h)	3.9 (0.9)	4.1 (1.3)
AUC_{0-24h} (µg·h/mL)	0.9 (0.7)	1.8 (1.1)

Gram-negative aerobes:
Bordetella pertussis
Anaerobic bacteria:
Propionibacterium acnes
NOTE: Microorganisms that are resistant to other macrolides are cross-resistant to dirithromycin/erythromycylamine. Enterococci and most strains of methicillin-resistant staphylococci are resistant to macrolides. In addition, due to the lack of standardized methodology and interpretive criteria, it is impossible at present to determine if strains of *Haemophilus* are susceptible or are resistant to dirithromycin/erythromycylamine.
Susceptibility Tests:
Dilution Techniques—Quantitative methods are used to determine antimicrobial minimum inhibitory concentrations (MIC's). These MIC's provide estimates of the susceptibility of bacteria to antimicrobial compounds. The MIC's should be determined using a standardized procedure. Standardized procedures are based on dilution method[1,2] (broth, agar, or microdilution) or equivalent with standardized inoculum concentrations and standardized concentrations of dirithromycin powder. The MIC values should be interpreted according to the following criteria:

MIC (μg/mL)	Interpretation
≤2	Susceptible (S)
4	Intermediate (I)
≥8	Resistant (R)

A report of "Susceptible" indicates that the pathogen is likely to be inhibited if the antimicrobial compound in blood reaches the concentrations usually achievable. A report of "Intermediate" indicates that the result should be considered equivocal, and, if the microorganism is not fully susceptible to alternative, clinically feasible drugs, the test should be repeated. This category implies possible clinical applicability in body sites where the drug is physiologically concentrated or in situations where high dosage of drug can be used. This category also provides a buffer zone which prevents small uncontrolled technical factors from causing major discrepancies in interpretation. A report of "Resistant" indicates that the pathogen is not likely to be inhibited if the antimicrobial compound in the blood reaches the concentrations usually achievable; other therapy should be selected.
Standardized susceptibility test procedures require the use of laboratory control microorganisms to control the technical aspects of the laboratory procedures. Standard dirithromycin powder should provide the following MIC values:

Microorganism	MIC (μg/mL)
S. aureus ATCC 29213	1.0 to 4.0

Diffusion Techniques—Quantitative methods that require measurement of zone diameters also provide reproducible estimates of the susceptibility of bacteria to antimicrobial compounds. One such standardized procedure[3] requires the use of standardized inoculum concentrations. This procedure uses paper disks impregnated with 15-μg dirithromycin to test the susceptibility of microorganisms to dirithromycin.
Reports from the laboratory providing results of the standard single-disk susceptibility test with a 15-μg dirithromycin disk should be interpreted according to the following criteria:

Zone diameter (mm)	Interpretation
≥19	Susceptible (S)
16 to 18	Intermediate (I)
≤15	Resistant (R)

Interpretation should be as stated above for results using dilution techniques. Interpretation involves correlation of the diameter obtained in the disk test with the MIC for dirithromycin.
As with standardized dilution techniques, diffusion methods require the use of laboratory control microorganisms that are used to control the technical aspects of the laboratory procedures. For the diffusion technique, the 15-μg dirithromycin disk should provide the following zone diameters in this laboratory test quality control strain:

Microorganism	Zone Diameter (mm)
S. aureus ATCC 25923	18 to 26

INDICATIONS AND USAGE

Dynabac (dirithromycin tablets) is indicated for the treatment of individuals age 12 years and older with mild-to-moderate infections caused by susceptible strains of the designated microorganisms in the specific conditions listed below.
Dirithromycin should not be used in patients with known, suspected, or potential bacteremias as serum levels are inadequate to provide antibacterial coverage of the blood stream.
Acute Bacterial Exacerbations of Chronic Bronchitis due to *Moraxella catarrhalis* or *Streptococcus pneumoniae.*
NOTE: Because the safety and efficacy of dirithromycin in the treatment of respiratory disease secondary to *H. influenzae* have not been demonstrated, Dynabac is NOT indicated for the empiric treatment of acute bacterial exacerbations of chronic or secondary bacterial infection of acute bronchitis. Infections known, suspected, or considered potentially to be caused by *Haemophilus* species should be treated by an antibacterial agent indicated for such treatment.
Secondary Bacterial Infection of Actue Bronchitis due to *Moraxella catarrhalis or Streptococcus pneumoniae.* (See above **NOTE.**)
Community-Acquired Pneumonia due to *Legionella pneumophila, Mycoplasma pneumoniae,* or *Streptococcus pneumoniae.*
Pharyngitis/Tonsillitis due to *Streptococcus pyogenes.*
NOTE: The usual drug of choice in the treatment and prevention of streptococcal infections and the prophylaxis of rheumatic fever is penicillin. Dynabac generally is effective in the eradication of *S. pyogenes* from the nasopharynx; however, data establishing the efficacy of Dynabac in the subsequent prevention of rheumatic fever are not available at present.
Uncomplicated Skin and Skin Structure Infections due to *Staphylococcus aureus* (methicillin-susceptible strains). (Abscesses usually require surgical drainage.)
NOTE: Because the safety and efficacy of dirithromycin in the treatment of uncomplicated skin and skin structure infections due to *S. pyogenes* have not been demonstrated, Dynabac is NOT indicated for the empiric treatment of uncomplicated skin and skin structure infections. Infections known, suspected, or potentially caused by *S. pyogenes* should be treated with an antibacterial agent indicated for such treatment.

CONTRAINDICATIONS

Dynabac is contraindicated in patients with known hypersensitivity to dirithromycin, erythromycin, or any other macrolide antibiotic.

WARNINGS

In a prospective study involving 6 healthy male volunteers, dirithromycin did not affect the metabolism of terfenadine. These six volunteers received terfenadine alone (60 mg twice daily) for 8 days, followed by terfenadine in combination with dirithromycin (500 mg once daily) for 10 days. (Both drugs were thus dosed to steady state.) The pharmacokinetics of terfenadine and its acid metabolite and the electrocardiographic QT_c interval were measured during both periods: with terfenadine alone, and with terfenadine plus dirithromycin. In five men, terfenadine levels were undetectable (<5 ng/mL) throughout the study; in one man, the C_{max} of terfenadine was 8.1 ng/mL with terfenadine alone and 7.2 ng/mL with terfenadine plus dirithromycin. The mean C_{max}, T_{max} and AUC of the acid metabolite of terfenadine were not significantly changed. The mean QT_c interval (msec) was 369 with terfenadine alone and 367 with terfenadine plus dirithromycin.
Serious cardiac dysrhythmias, some resulting in death, have occurred in patients receiving terfenadine concomitantly with other macrolide antibiotics. In addition, most macrolides are contraindicated in patients receiving terfenadine therapy who have pre-existing cardiac abnormalities (arrhythmia, bradycardia, QT_c interval prolongation, ischemic heart disease, congestive heart failure, etc.) or electrolyte disturbances. Until further use data are available, it is prudent to monitor the terfenadine levels when dirithromycin and terfenadine are coadministered. (See terfenadine package insert.)
Dirithromycin should not be used in patients with known, suspected, or potential bacteremias as serum levels are inadequate to provide antibacterial coverage of the blood stream.
Pseudomembranous colitis has been reported with nearly all antibacterial agents, including dirithromycin, and may range in severity from mild to life-threatening. Therefore, it is important to consider this diagnosis in patients who present with diarrhea subsequent to the administration of antibacterial agents.
Treatment with antibacterial agents alters the normal flora of the colon and may permit overgrowth of clostridia. Studies indicate that a toxin produced by *Clostridium difficile* is a primary cause of "antibiotic-associated colitis."
After the diagnosis of pseudomembranous colitis has been established, therapeutic measures should be initiated. Mild cases of pseudomembranous colitis usually respond to discontinuation of the drug alone. In moderate-to-severe cases, consideration should be given to management with fluids and electrolytes, protein supplementation, and treatment with an antibacterial drug clinically effective against *C. difficile* colitis.

PRECAUTIONS

Hepatic Insufficiency—Because dirithromycin/erythromycylamine is principally eliminated via the liver and because no data exist regarding the safety of administering dirithromycin to patients with Child's Grade B or greater hepatic impairment, Dynabac should be administered to such patients only when absolutely necessary. No dosage adjustment should be necessary in patients with mildly impaired hepatic function. (See **CLINICAL PHARMACOLOGY** section.)
Information to Patients—Dynabac tablets should be taken with food or within one hour of having eaten. They should not be cut, chewed, or crushed.
Drug Interactions:
Terfenadine—See **WARNINGS.**
Theophylline—Following co-administration of two 250-mg dirithromycin tablets administered once daily with 200-mg theophylline tablets administered twice daily for 10 days to 14 healthy subjects, the steady-state plasma concentration of theophylline was not significantly altered. In general, most patients treated with dirithromycin who are receiving concomitant theophylline therapy may not require empiric adjustment of theophylline dosage or monitoring of theophylline plasma concentrations. However, theophylline plasma concentrations should be monitored, with dosage adjustment as appropriate, in patients whose pulmonary disease requires maintaining a given theophylline plasma concentration for optimal pulmonary function or in patients with theophylline concentrations at the higher end of the therapeutic range.
Antacids or H_2 receptor antagonists—When dirithromycin is administered immediately following antacids or H_2-receptor antagonists, the absorption of dirithromycin is slightly enhanced.
The following drug interactions have been reported with erythromycin products. It is presently not known whether these same drug interactions occur with dirithromycin. **Until further data are available regarding the potential interaction of dirithromycin with these compounds, caution should be used during coadministration.**
Triazolam—Erythromycin has been reported to decrease the clearance of triazolam and, thus, may increase the pharmacologic effect of triazolam.
Digoxin—Concomitant administration of erythromycin and digoxin has been reported to result in elevated digoxin serum levels.
Anticoagulants—There have been reports of increased anticoagulant effects when erythromycin and oral anticoagulants were used concomitantly. Increased anticoagulation effects due to a drug interaction with erythromycin may be more pronounced in the elderly.
Ergotamine—Concurrent use of erythromycin and ergotamine or dihydroergotamine has been associated in some patients with acute ergot toxicity characterized by severe peripheral vasospasm and dysesthesia.
Other drugs—Drug interactions have been reported with concomitant administration of erythromycin and other medications, including cyclosporine, hexobarbital, carbamazepine, alfentanil, disopyramide, phenytoin, bromocriptine, valproate, astemizole, and lovastatin.
Carcinogenesis, Mutagenesis, Impairment of Fertility—Lifetime studies in animals to evaluate carcinogenic potential have not been performed with dirithromycin.
No mutagenic potential was demonstrated when dirithromycin was used in standard tests of genotoxicity, which included the following bacterial mutation tests *in vitro* and *in vivo* mammalian systems:
Bacterial Reverse-Mutation Test (Ames test)
DNA repair (UDS) in rat hepatocytes
Chinese hamster lung fibroblast (V79) test
Micronucleus test in mice
Sister-chromatid exchange—human lymphocytes
Sister-chromatid exchange—Chinese hamsters
Mouse Lymphoma Assay
In rats, fertility and reproductive performance were not affected when dirithromycin was administered at doses up to 21 times the maximum recommended human dose on a mg/m² basis.
Pregnancy: Teratogenic Effects, Pregnancy Category C—Teratology studies conducted in rats at doses up to 21 times the maximum recommended human dose on a mg/m² basis and in rabbits at doses up to 4 times the maximum recommended human dose on a mg/m² basis have revealed no evidence of impaired fertility or harm to the fetus due to dirithromycin administration. An additional teratology study in CD-1 mice demonstrated that fetal weight was significantly depressed at the 1000 mg/kg dose (8 times the maximum recommended human dose on a mg/m² basis), and there was an increased occurrence of incomplete ossification among these fetuses—a manifestation of retarded development. This decrease in ossification was also seen in rats given 1000 mg/kg/day for 2 weeks prior to mating, throughout the mating period, and throughout gestation.
There are no adequate and well-controlled studies in pregnant women. Dirithromycin should be used during pregnancy only if the potential benefit justifies the potential risk to the fetus.
Labor and Delivery—Dirithromycin has not been studied for use during labor and delivery. Treatment with dirithromycin should be given during labor and delivery only if clearly needed.
Nursing Mothers—It is not known whether either dirithromycin or erythromycylamine is excreted in human milk. It is known that dirithromycin is excreted in the milk of lactating rodents and that other drugs of this class are excreted in human milk. Because many drugs are excreted in human

Continued on next page

Bock Pharmacal—Cont.

milk, caution should be exercised when dirithromycin is administered to a nursing woman.

Pediatric Use—Safety and effectiveness in pediatric patients below the age of 12 years have not been established.

Geriatric Use—In a clinical pharmacology study, 19 healthy geriatric volunteers (65 to 83 years of age) with normal renal and hepatic function had no statistically significant differences in AUC or C_{max} when compared with 10 healthy adult volunteers (19 to 50 years of age). In clinical trials in geriatric patients who received the usual recommended adult dose (500 mg q.d. P.O.), clinical efficacy and safety were comparable with results in non-geriatric adult patients.

ADVERSE REACTIONS

Clinical Trials: In clinical trials, 3299 patients were treated with dirithromycin 500 mg q.d. P.O. for approximately 7 to 14 days. There were no deaths or permanent disabilities thought related directly to drug toxicity. Eighty-seven (2.6%) patients discontinued medication due to adverse reactions. Thirty-five (40%) of the 87 patients who discontinued therapy did so because of nausea or abdominal pain.

The following adverse clinical and laboratory reactions were reported during the dirithromycin clinical trials conducted in North America (n=1894 patients). (See Tables 2 and 3.)

Table 2
Adverse Clinical Reactions
(Incidence equal to or greater than 1%)
Clinical Trials—North America

ADVERSE REACTION	DIRITHRO-MYCIN	ERYTHRO-MYCIN
Abdominal pain	9.7%	7.5%
Headache	8.6%	8.2%
Nausea	8.3%	7.5%
Diarrhea	7.7%	7.3%
Vomiting	3.0%	2.8%
Dyspepsia	2.6%	2.1%
Dizziness/vertigo	2.3%	2.3%
Pain (non-specific)	2.2%	1.6%
Asthenia	2.0%	1.9%
Gastrointestinal disorder	1.6%	1.4%
Increased Cough	1.5%	2.6%
Flatulence	1.5%	1.5%
Rash	1.4%	2.6%
Dyspnea	1.2%	1.2%
Pruritus/Urticaria	1.2%	1.0%
Insomnia	1.0%	0.7%

Adverse reactions occurring during the clinical trials with dirithromycin with an incidence of less than 1% but greater than 0.1% included the following (listed alphabetically): Abnormal stools, allergic reaction (not further defined), amblyopia, anorexia, anxiety, constipation, dehydration, depression, dry mouth, dysmenorrhea, edema, epistaxis, eye disorder (not further defined), fever, flu syndrome, gastritis, gastroenteritis, hemoptysis, hyperventilation, malaise, mouth ulceration, myalgia, neck pain, nervousness, palpitation, paresthesia, peripheral edema, somnolence, sweating, syncope, taste perversion, thirst, tinnitus, tremor, urinary frequency vaginal moniliasis, vaginitis, vasodilatation.

Table 3
Adverse Laboratory Reactions
(Incidence equal to or greater than 1%)
Clinical Trials—North America

ADVERSE REACTION	DIRITHRO-MYCIN	ERYTHRO-MYCIN
Platelet count *increased*	3.8%	4.8%
Potassium *increased*	2.6%	0.0%
Bicarbonate *decreased*	1.4%	2.0%
CPK *increased*	1.2%	0.9%
Eosinophils *increased*	1.2%	0.6%
Seg Neutrophils *increased*	1.2%	1.3%

Adverse laboratory reactions occurring during the clinical trials with dirithromycin with an incidence of less than 1% but greater than 0.1% included the following (listed alphabetically):
Decreased:
Albumin, chloride, hematocrit, hemoglobin, seg neutrophils, phosphorus, platelet count, and total protein.
Increased:
Alkaline phosphatase, ALT, AST, bands, basophils, total bilirubin, creatinine, GGT, leukocyte count, lymphocytes, monocytes, phosphorous, and uric acid.
Macrolide-class adverse reactions—Although not observed in patients treated with dirithromycin in clinical trials, the following adverse reactions and altered laboratory test results have been reported in patients treated with macrolide antibiotics:
Bullous fixed eruptions or serious allergic reactions, including anaphylaxis, have been reported. A few cases of transient deafness have been reported with high doses of oral erythromycin. Rarely, cholestatic hepatitis has been reported. In individuals with prolonged QT intervals, erythromycin has been associated, rarely, with the production of ventricular arrhythmias, including ventricular tachycardia and torsade de pointes.

OVERDOSAGE

The toxic symptoms following an overdose of a macrolide antibiotic may include nausea, vomiting, epigastric distress, and diarrhea. Forced diuresis, peritoneal dialysis, hemodialysis, or hemoperfusion have not been established as beneficial for an overdose of dirithromycin. Hemodialysis has been shown to be ineffective in hastening the elimination of erythromycylamine from plasma in patients with chronic renal failure.

DOSAGE AND ADMINISTRATION

Dynabac (dirithromycin tablets) should be administered with food or within 1 hour of having eaten. (See CLINICAL PHARMACOLOGY, *Food Effect on Absorption*.) Dynabac tablets should not be cut, crushed, or chewed.
[See Table 4 below.]

HOW SUPPLIED

Tablets (enteric-coated) (elliptical-shaped) (white)
250 mg (UC5364)—(60s) NDC 0563-0490-60
Store at controlled room temperature, 15° to 30°C (59° to 86°F).

ANIMAL PHARMACOLOGY AND TOXICOLOGY

Cardiac and skeletal muscle lesions occurred in rats in studies up to three months by the intravenous route and in six-month studies in the rat and the dog by the oral route. While no target organ toxicity was identified in three-month oral studies, both cardiac and skeletal muscles were identified as target tissues after one-month intravenous studies in rats.

Histologic changes from oral dosing occurred only after more than four months of treatment in rats after six months in dogs. These findings were associated with high tissue-to-plasma concentration ratios of antimicrobial activity. The extensive drug uptake by tissues was reversible upon termination of treatment. Lesions in cardiac and skeletal muscle also were reversed upon termination of treatment. Dirithromycin and/or its microbiologically active metabolite appeared to accumulate in tissues with time. Despite the drug uptake in rat tissues at high multiples (approximately 14 times the anticipated clinical dose in mg/m^2), there were no lesions in this species until oral treatment was extended beyond four months.

REFERENCES

1. National Committee for Clinical Laboratory Standards. Methods for Dilution Antimicrobial Susceptibility Tests for Bacteria that Grow Aerobically—Third Edition; Approved Standard NCCLS Document M7–A3, Vol. 13, No. 25, NCCLS, Villanova, PA, December 1993
2. National Committee for Clinical Laboratory Standards. Methods for Antimicrobial Susceptibility Testing of Anaerobic Bacteria—Third Edition; Approved Standard NCCLS Document M11–A3, Vol. 13, No. 26, NCCLS, Villanova, PA, December 1993
3. National Committee for Clinical Laboratory Standards. Performance Standards for Antimicrobial Disk Susceptibility Tests—Fifth Edition; Approved Standard NCCLS Document M2–A5, Vol. 13, No. 24, NCCLS, Villanova, PA, December 1993

CAUTION

Federal (USA) law prohibits dispensing without prescription.
Literature revised April 5, 1996
Manufactured for
bock® pharmacal company
ST. LOUIS, MO 63141
by Eli Lilly and Company
Indianapolis, IN 46285, USA
PV 2592 UCP
Shown in Product Identification Guide, page 305

HEMASPAN®   OTC

Each tan colored caplet embossed bock on one side and HS bisect 33 on the other contains:
*Elemental Iron	110.0 mg
(as Ferrous Fumarate–335 mg)	
Vitamin C	200.0 mg
Docusate Sodium	20.0 mg

*In a special base to provide delayed therapeutic action.

HOW SUPPLIED

Bottles of 100.
Shown in Product Identification Guide, page 306

HISTUSSIN® D   ℂⅢ ℞
[*hĭss-tūs-ən*]

DESCRIPTION

Each 5ml teaspoonful of HISTUSSIN® D for oral use contains:
Hydrocodone Bitartrate	5 mg

(Warning: May be habit forming)
Pseudoephedrine Hydrochloride	60 mg

Antitussive-Decongestant Liquid.
Hydrocodone bitartrate is an opioid analgesic and antitussive. It occurs as fine white crystals or as crystalline powder, and is light sensitive. The chemical name is 4,5,epoxy-3-methoxy-17-methylmorphinan-6-one tartrate (1:1) hydrate (2:5). Its structural formula is shown below:

$C_{18}H_{21}NO_3 \cdot C_4H_6 \cdot 2.5H_2O$ MW 494.5

Pseudoephedrine hydrochloride is a nasal decongestant (vasoconstrictor) which occurs as fine white to off-white crystals or powder having a characteristic odor. The chemical name is α [1-(methylamino) ethyl]-benzenemethanol hydrochloride. Its chemical structure is shown below:
[See chemical structure at top of next column.]

Table 4
Recommended Dosage Schedule for Dynabac
(12 years of age and older)

Infection (Mild to Moderate Severity)	Dose	Frequency	Duration (days)
Acute Bacterial Exacerbations of Chronic Bronchitis due to *Moraxella catarrhalis* or *Streptococcus pneumoniae* **NOT FOR EMPIRIC THERAPY** (See **INDICTATIONS** and **USAGE**.)	500 mg	q day	7
Secondary Bacterial Infection of Acute Bronchitis due to *M. catarrhalis* or *S. pneumoniae* **NOT FOR EMPIRIC THERAPY** (See **INDICATIONS** and **USAGE**.)	500 mg	q day	7
Community-Acquired Pneumonia due to *Legionella pneumophila, Mycoplasma pneumoniae*, or *S. pneumoniae*	500 mg	q day	14
Pharyngitis/Tonsillitis due to *Streptococcus pyogenes*	500 mg	q day	10
Uncomplicated Skin and Skin Structure Infections due to *Staphylococcus aureus* (methicillin-susceptible) **NOT FOR EMPIRIC THERAPY** (See **INDICATIONS AND USAGE**.)	500 mg	q day	7

$C_{10}H_{15}NO \cdot HCl$ MW 201.7

CLINICAL PHARMACOLOGY

Hydrocodone is a semi-synthetic narcotic antitussive with multiple actions qualitatively similar to those of codeine. Most of these involve the central nervous system and smooth muscle. The precise mechanism of action of hydrocodone is not known; however, hydrocodone is believed to act directly on the cough center. In excessive doses, hydrocodone, like other opiates, will depress respiration. The effects of hydrocodone in therapeutic doses on the cardiovascular system are negligible. Hydrocodone can produce miosis, euphoria, physical and psychic dependence.

Following a 10 mg oral dose of hydrocodone administered to five adult male subjects, the mean peak serum concentration was 23.6 ± 5.2 ng/mL. Maximum serum levels were achieved at 1.3 ± 0.3 hours.[1] Hydrocodone exhibits a complex pattern of metabolism including O-demethylations, N-demethylation, and 6-keto reduction to the corresponding 6-α- and 6-β-hydroxy metabolites.[2]

Pseudoephedrine acts as an indirect sympathomimetic agent by stimulating sympathetic (adrenergic) nerve endings to release norepinephrine. Norepinephrine in turn stimulates alpha and beta receptors throughout the body. The action of pseudoephedrine hydrochloride is apparently more specific for the blood vessels of the upper respiratory tract and less specific for the blood vessels of the systemic circulation. The vasoconstriction produced in the respiratory tract results in the shrinking of swollen tissues in the sinuses and nasal passages. Little, if any, rebound congestion has been reported upon withdrawal of orally administered pseudoephedrine. Pseudoephedrine is rapidly and almost completely absorbed from the gastrointestinal tract. Considerable variation in elimination half-life has been observed (4.3 to 8 hours), which is attributed to individual differences in absorption, as well as excretion. Excretion rates are altered by urine pH, increasing with acidification, and decreasing with alkalization. As a result, mean half-life is approximately 3 hours at a urinary pH of 5, and increases to 16 hours at a urinary pH of 8. Approximately 43% to 96% of an administered dose is excreted unchanged in the urine; the remainder is apparently metabolized in the liver to inactive compounds by N-demethylation, parahydroxylation, and oxidative deamination.[3] The drug is distributed widely throughout body tissues and fluids including fetal tissue, breast milk, and the central nervous system.

INDICATIONS AND USAGE

For the symptomatic relief of cough accompanying upper respiratory tract congestion associated with the common cold, influenza, bronchitis and sinusitis.

CONTRAINDICATIONS

HISTUSSIN D is contraindicated in patients with severe hypertension, severe coronary artery disease, and in patients receiving MAO inhibitors.

Hypersensitivity: HISTUSSIN D is contraindicated in patients with hypersensitivity or a history of an iodiosyncratic reaction to sympathomimetic amines, phenanthrene derivatives, or to any other formula ingredients.

WARNINGS

Hydrocodone should be prescribed and administered with the same degree of caution as all oral medications containing a narcotic-analgesic. Extreme caution should be exercised in the use of hydrocodone in patients with severe respiratory impairment or patients with impaired respiratory drive.

If sympathomimetic amines are used in patients with hypertension, diabetes mellitus, ischemic heart disease, hyperthyroidism, increased intraocular pressure or prostatic hypertrophy, caution should be exercised (see CONTRAINDICATIONS). Sympathomimetic amines may produce central nervous system stimulation with convulsions or cardiovascular collapse with accompanying hypotension. DO NOT EXCEED RECOMMENDED DOSAGE.

Use in elderly: Elderly patients (60 years and older) are more likely to have adverse reactions to sympathomimetic amines. Overdosage in this age group may cause hallucinations, convulsions, CNS depression and death.

PRECAUTIONS

General: Caution should be exercised if used in patients with diabetes, hypertension, cardiovascular disease, sensitivity to ephedrine, or decreased respiratory drive (see CONTRAINDICATIONS).

Information for Patients: Hydrocodone may produce drowsiness. Persons who perform hazardous tasks requiring mental alertness or physical coordination should be cautioned accordingly. Concomitant use of hydrocodone with tranquilizers, alcohol or other depressants may produce additive depressant effects.

Do not exceed the prescribed dosage.

Drug Interactions: Hydrocodone may potentiate the effects of other narcotics, general anesthetics, tranquilizers, sedatives and hypnotics, tricyclic antidepressants, MAO inhibitors, alcohol, and other CNS depressants. Beta adrenergic blockers and MAO inhibitors potentiate the sympathomimetic effects of pseudoephedrine. Sympathomimetic amines may reduce the antihypertensive effects of methyldopa, mecamylamine, and reserpine alkaloids.

Hydrocodone-FDA Pregnancy Category C. Hydrocodone has been shown to be teratogenic in hamsters when given in doses 700 times the human dose. There are no adequate and well-controlled studies in pregnant women. HISTUSSIN D should be used during pregnancy only if the potential benefit justifies the potential risk to the fetus.

Pseudoephedrine-FDA Pregnancy Category B. Pseudoephedrine studies were conducted in rats at doses up to 150 times the human dose. No evidence of teratogenic harm to the fetus was observed. However, pseudoephedrine reduced average weight, length and rate of skeletal ossification in the animal fetus. There are, however, no adequate and well-controlled studies in pregnant women. Because animal reproduction studies are not always predictive of human response, this drug should be used during pregnancy only if clearly needed.

Nursing Mothers: Because of the potential for a serious adverse reaction from sympathomimetic amines in nursing infants, pseudoephedrine is contraindicated in nursing mothers.

ADVERSE REACTIONS

The most frequent side effects are gastrointestinal upset, nausea, drowsiness and constipation.

Individuals sensitive to pseudoephedrine may display ephedrine-like reactions such as tachycardia, palpitations, headache, dizziness or nausea. Sympathomimetic drugs have been associated with certain untoward reactions including fear, anxiety, tenseness, restlessness, tremor, weakness, pallor, respiratory difficulty, dysuria, insomnia, hallucinations, convulsions, CNS depression, arrhythmias, and cardiovascular collapse with hypotension. Patient idiosyncrasy to adrenergic agents may be mainfested by insomnia, dizziness, weakness, tremor or arrhythmias.

DRUG ABUSE AND DEPENDENCE

Controlled Substance: Hydrocodone in HISTUSSIN D mixture is controlled by the Drug Enforcement Administration. HISTUSSIN D is a Schedule III controlled substance.

Abuse: Hydrocodone is a narcotic drug related to codeine with roughly three times the abuse potential of codeine on a weight basis.

Dependence: Hydrocodone can produce drug dependence of the morphine type. Psychic dependence, physical dependence and tolerance may develop if dosage recommendations are greatly exceeded over a prolonged period of time.

Overdosage: Acute overdosage with HISTUSSIN D may produce variable clinical signs as Hydrocodone produces CNS depression and cardiovascular depression while pseudoephedrine produces CNS stimulation and variable cardiovascular effects. Hydrocodone is likely to be responsible for most of the severe reactions from overdosage. Pressor amines should be used with great caution when taking pseudoephedrine. Patients with signs of stimulation should be treated conservatively and depressant medications should be avoided if possible because of potential drug interaction with hydrocodone.

DOSAGE AND ADMINISTRATION

Adults and children over 90 lb. - 1 teaspoonful (5 ml); children 50 to 90 lb.- $^1/_2$ teaspoonful; children 25 to 50 lb.- $^1/_4$ teaspoonful. May be given four times a day as needed. May be taken with meals.

HOW SUPPLIED

HISTUSSIN D liquid is supplied as a deep red syrup with a wild cherry/black raspberry flavor. Pints NDC 0563-0864-16. **KEEP THIS AND ALL DRUGS OUT OF THE REACH OF CHILDREN. IN CASE OF ACCIDENTAL OVERDOSE, SEEK PROFESSIONAL ASSISTANCE OR CONTACT A POISON CONTROL CENTER IMMEDIATELY.**

CAUTION: Federal law prohibits dispensing without prescription.

Store at controlled room temperature.

DISPENSE IN CHILD RESISTANT CONTAINERS.

REFERENCES

1. Barnhart, J.W. & Caldwell, W.J. (1977) Gas chromatographic determination of hydrocodone in serum. *J Chromatogr*, 130;243-249.
2. Cone, E.J. & Darwin, W.D. (1978) Simultaneous determination of hydromorphone, hydrocodone and their 6alpha- and 6beta-hydroxy metabolites in urine using selected ion recording with methane chemical ionization. *Biomed Mass Spectrom*, 5, 291.
3. Kanfer, I., Dowse, R. & Vuma, V. (1993) Pharmacokinetics of oral decongestants. *Pharmacotherapy*, 13, 116S-128S, discussion 143.

HPG11795-01-0596BP
Manufactured for
bock®
pharmacal
company
ST. LOUIS, MO 63141
by Forest Pharmaceuticals, Inc.
St. Louis, MO 63045
Copyright© 1996 Bock Pharmacal Company
All rights reserved.

HISTUSSIN® HC   ℂ℟

Each 5 ml orange/pineapple flavored alcohol-free, sugar-free orange syrup contains:

Hydrocodone Bitartrate	2.5 mg
(Warning: May be habit forming.)	
Phenylephrine Hydrochloride	5.0 mg
Chlorpheniramine Maleate	2.0 mg

HOW SUPPLIED

Bottles of 16 oz.

POLY–HISTINE CS®   ℂ℟

Each 5 ml raspberry/strawberry flavored alcohol-free, red syrup contains:

Codeine Phosphate	10.0 mg
(Warning: May be habit forming.)	
Phenylpropanolamine HCl	12.5 mg
Brompheniramine Maleate	2.0 mg

HOW SUPPLIED

Bottles of 16 oz.

POLY–HISTINE ELIXIR®   ℟

Each teaspoonful (5 ml) lemon-lime flavored green elixir contains:

Phenyltoloxamine Citrate	4.0 mg
Pyrilamine Maleate	4.0 mg
Pheniramine Maleate	4.0 mg
Alcohol	4%

HOW SUPPLIED

Bottles of 16 oz.

POLY–HISTINE–D® CAPSULES   ℟

Each timed release* half red, half clear capsule with BOCK printed on both halves contains:

Phenylpropanolamine HCl	50.0 mg
Phenyltoloxamine Citrate	16.0 mg
Pyrilamine Maleate	16.0 mg
Pheniramine Maleate	16.0 mg

*In a special base to provide prolonged therapeutic action.

HOW SUPPLIED

Bottles of 100.
Shown in Product Identification Guide, page 306

POLY–HISTINE–D® ELIXIR   ℟

Each teaspoonful (5 ml) wild cherry flavored red elixir contains:

Phenylpropanolamine HCl	12.5 mg
Phenyltoloxamine Citrate	4.0 mg
Pyrilamine Maleate	4.0 mg
Pheniramine Maleate	4.0 mg
Alcohol	4%

HOW SUPPLIED

Bottles of 16 oz.

POLY–HISTINE–D® PED CAPS   ℟

Each timed release* clear capsule with BOCK printed on both halves contains:

Phenylpropanolamine HCl	25.0 mg
Phenyltoloxamine Citrate	8.0 mg
Pyrilamine Maleate	8.0 mg
Pheniramine Maleate	8.0 mg

*In a special base to provide prolonged therapeutic action.

HOW SUPPLIED

Bottles of 100.
Shown in Product Identification Guide, page 306

Continued on next page

Bock Pharmacal—Cont.

POLY–HISTINE DM® SYRUP   ℞

Each 5 ml black-raspberry flavored alcohol-free, sugar free purple syrup contains:

Dextromethorphan HBr	10.0 mg
Phenylpropanolamine HCl	12.5 mg
Brompheniramine Maleate	2.0 mg

HOW SUPPLIED
Bottles of 16 oz.

PRENATE 90®   ℞

Each white dye free oval oil- and water-soluble multivitamin/multimineral tablet embossed bock on one side and PN bisect 90 on the other side contains:

Elemental Iron	90.0 mg*
(as Ferrous Fumarate–270 mg)	
Iodine (Potassium Iodide)	150.0 mcg
Calcium (Calcium Carbonate)	250.0 mg
Copper (Cupric Oxide)	2.0 mg
Zinc (Zinc Oxide)	25.0 mg
Folic Acid	1.0 mg
Vitamin A (Acetate)	4000.0 I.U.
Vitamin D (Cholecalciferol)	400.0 I.U.
Vitamin E (Acetate)	30.0 I.U.
(as dl-alpha tocopheryl acetate)	
Vitamin C (Ascorbic Acid)	120.0 mg
Vitamin B$_1$ (Thiamine Mononitrate)	3.0 mg
Vitamin B$_2$ (Riboflavin)	3.4 mg
Vitamin B$_6$ (Pyridoxine HCl)	20.0 mg
Vitamin B$_{12}$ (Cyanocobalamin)	12.0 mcg
Niacinamide	20.0 mg
Docusate Sodium	50.0 mg

*MicroIron™ (A special base to provide delayed therapeutic action.)

HOW SUPPLIED
Bottles of 100.
Shown in Product Identification Guide, page 306

ZEPHREX® TABLETS   ℞

DESCRIPTION
ZEPHREX® is a white film coated, oval-shaped tablet with a bisect on one side and bock with 460 below the name on the other side.
Each tablet contains:

Pseudoephedrine HCl	60 mg
Guaifenesin	400 mg

HOW SUPPLIED
100's NDC 0563-2624-01
Shown in Product Identification Guide, page 306

ZEPHREX LA® TABLETS   ℞

Each timed release* orange, oval-shaped tablet embossed with bock on one side and a Z bisect LA on the other side contains:

Pseudoephedrine HCl	120.0 mg
Guaifenesin	600.0 mg

*In a special base to provide prolonged therapeutic action.

HOW SUPPLIED
Bottles of 100.
Shown in Product Identification Guide, page 306

Check the **PINK** section
to find a particular **BRAND**.

Boehringer Ingelheim Pharmaceuticals, Inc.
A subsidiary of Boehringer Ingelheim Corporation
900 RIDGEBURY ROAD
POST OFFICE BOX 368
RIDGEFIELD, CT 06877-0368

For Medical Information Contact:
(203) 791-6194

ALUPENT®   ℞
[al'u-pent]
(metaproterenol sulfate, USP)
Bronchodilator

Tablets 10 mg		BI-CODE 74
Tablets 20 mg		BI-CODE 72
Inhalation Aerosol 10 ml		BI-CODE 70
Syrup 10 mg/5 ml		BI-CODE 73
Inhalation Solution 5%		BI-CODE 71
Inhalation Solution	0.6%	BI-CODE 69
Unit-dose Vials	0.4%	BI-CODE 78

DESCRIPTION
Alupent® (metaproterenol sulfate USP) Inhalation Aerosol is a bronchodilator administered by oral inhalation. The Alupent Inhalation Aerosol containing 150 mg of metaproterenol sulfate as micronized powder is sufficient medication for 200 inhalations. Each metered dose delivers through the mouthpiece 0.65 mg of metaproterenol sulfate (each ml contains 15 mg). The inert ingredients are dichlorodifluoromethane, dichlorotetrafluoroethane and trichloromonofluoromethane as propellants, and sorbitan trioleate.
Alupent Inhalation Solution is administered by oral inhalation with the aid of a nebulizer or an intermittent positive pressure breathing apparatus (IPPB). It contains Alupent 5% in a pH-adjusted aqueous solution containing benzalkonium chloride and edetate disodium as preservatives.
Alupent Inhalation Solution Unit-dose Vial is administered by oral inhalation with the aid of an IPPB. It contains Alupent 0.4% or 0.6% in a sterile pH-adjusted aqueous solution with edetate disodium and sodium chloride.
Alupent Syrup is administered orally. Each teaspoonful (5 ml) of syrup contains metaproterenol sulfate 10 mg. The inactive ingredients are edetate disodium, FD&C Red No. 40, hydroxyethylcellulose, imitation black cherry flavor, methylparaben, propylparaben, saccharin, sorbitol solution.
Alupent Tablets are administered orally. Each tablet contains metaproterenol sulfate 10 mg or 20 mg. The inactive ingredients are colloidal silicon dioxide, cornstarch, dibasic calcium phosphate, lactose, magnesium stearate.
Chemically, Alupent is 1-(3,5 dihydroxyphenyl)-2-isopropylaminoethanol sulfate, a white crystalline, racemic mixture of two optically active isomers. It differs from isoproterenol hydrochloride by having two hydroxyl groups attached at the meta positions on the benzene ring rather than one at the meta and one at the para position.

$$\cdot H_2SO_4$$

metaproterenol sulfate (Alupent)
$(C_{11}H_{17}NO_3)_2 \cdot H_2SO_4$
Mol. Wt. 520.59

CLINICAL PHARMACOLOGY
Alupent® (metaproterenol sulfate USP) is a potent beta-adrenergic stimulator. Alupent Inhalation Aerosol and Inhalation Solution have a rapid onset of action. It is postulated that beta-adrenergic stimulants produce many of their pharmacological effects by activation of adenyl cyclase, the enzyme that catalyzes the conversion of adenosine triphosphate to cyclic adenosine monophosphate.
In vitro studies and *in vivo* pharmacologic studies have demonstrated that Alupent® (metaproterenol sulfate USP) has a preferential effect on beta-2 adrenergic receptors compared with isoproterenol. While it is recognized that beta-2 adrenergic receptors are the predominant receptors in bronchial smooth muscle, recent data indicate that there is a population of beta-2 receptors in the human heart existing in a concentration between 10–50%. The precise functions of these, however, is not yet established (see WARNINGS section).

The pharmacologic effects of beta adrenergic agonist drugs, including Alupent, are at least in part attributable to stimulation through beta adrenergic receptors of intracellular adenyl cyclase, the enzyme which catalyzes the conversion of adenosine triphosphate (ATP) to cyclic-3',5'-adenosine monophosphate (c-AMP). Increased c-AMP levels are associated with relaxation of bronchial smooth muscle and inhibition of release of mediators of immediate hypersensitivity from cells, especially from mast cells.
Pharmacokinetics: Absorption, biotransformation and excretion studies in humans following administration by inhalation have shown that approximately 3 percent of the actuated dose is absorbed intact through the lungs.
Absorption, biotransformation and excretion studies in humans following oral administration indicate that an average of less than 10% of the drug is absorbed intact; it is not metabolized by catechol-O-methyl-transferase nor converted to glucuronide conjugates but is excreted primarily as the sulfate conjugate formed in the gut. Pulmonary function tests performed after the administration of Alupent usually show improvement, e.g. an increase in one-second forced expiratory volume (FEV$_1$), maximum expiratory flow rate, peak expiratory flow rate, forced vital capacity and/or a decrease in airway resistance. The resultant decrease in airway obstruction may relieve the dyspnea associated with bronchospasm.
When administered orally or by inhalation, Alupent decreases reversible bronchospasm. Pulmonary function tests performed concomitantly usually show improvement following aerosol Alupent administration, e.g., an increase in the one-second forced expiratory volume (FEV$_1$), an increase in maximum expiratory flow rate, an increase in peak expiratory flow rate, an increase in forced vital capacity, and/or a decrease in airway resistance. The resultant decrease in airway obstruction may relieve the dyspnea associated with bronchospasm.
Controlled single- and multiple-dose studies have been performed with pulmonary function monitoring. The duration of effect of a single dose of Alupent Tablets 20 mg or Alupent Syrup (that is, the period of time during which there is a 15% or greater increase in FEV$_1$) was up to 4 hours.
Controlled single- and multiple-dose studies have been performed with pulmonary function monitoring. The duration of effect of a single dose of two to three inhalations of Alupent Inhalation Aerosol (that is, the period of time during which there is a 20% or greater increase in FEV$_1$) has varied from 1 to 5 hours.
In repetitive-dosing studies (up to q.i.d.) the duration of effect for a similar dose of Alupent Inhalation Aerosol has ranged from about 1 to 2.5 hours. Present studies are inadequate to explain the divergence in duration of the FEV$_1$ effect between single- and repetitive-dosing studies, respectively.
Following controlled single dose studies with Alupent Inhalation Solution by an intermittent positive pressure breathing apparatus (IPPB) and by hand-bulb nebulizers, significant improvement (15% or greater increase in FEV$_1$) occurred within 5 to 30 minutes and persisted for periods varying from 2 to 6 hours.
In these studies, the longer duration of effect occurred in the studies in which the drug was administered by IPPB, i.e., 6 hours, versus 2 to 3 hours when administered by hand-bulb nebulizer. In these studies, the doses used were 0.3 ml by IPPB and 10 inhalations by hand-bulb nebulizer.
In controlled repetitive-dosing studies with Alupent Inhalation Solution by IPPB and by hand-bulb nebulizer the onset of effect occurred within 5 to 30 minutes and duration ranged from 4 to 6 hours. In these studies, the doses used were 0.3 ml b.i.d. or t.i.d. when given by IPPB, and 10 inhalations q.i.d. (no more often than q4h) when given by hand-bulb nebulizer. As in the single dose studies, effectiveness was measured as a sustained increase in FEV$_1$ of 15% or greater. In these repetitive-dosing studies there was no apparent difference in duration between the two methods of delivery.
Clinical studies were conducted in which the effectiveness of Alupent Inhalation Solution was evaluated by comparison with that of isoproterenol hydrochloride over periods of two to three months. Both drugs continued to produce significant improvement in pulmonary function throughout this period of treatment.
In two well-controlled studies in children 6 to 12 years of age with acute exacerbation of asthma, 70% of patients receiving Alupent Inhalation Solution (0.1 mL to 0.2 mL) showed improvement in pulmonary function as demonstrated by a 15% increase in FEV$_1$ above baseline.
Recent studies in laboratory animals (minipigs, rodents and dogs) recorded the occurrence of cardiac arrhythmias and sudden death (with histologic evidence of myocardial necrosis) when beta agonists and methylxanthines were administered concurrently. The significance of these findings when applied to humans is currently unknown.

INDICATIONS AND USAGE
Alupent® (metaproterenol sulfate USP) is indicated as a bronchodilator for bronchial asthma and for reversible bronchospasm which may occur in association with bronchitis and emphysema. Alupent Inhalation Solution 5% is addi-

tionally indicated for the treatment of acute asthmatic attacks in children age 6 years and older.

CONTRAINDICATIONS

Use in patients with cardiac arrhythmias associated with tachycardia is contraindicated.

Although rare, immediate hypersensitivity reactions and for Alupent Inhalation Solution 5% paradoxical bronchospasm can occur. Therefore, Alupent® (metaproterenol sulfate USP) is contraindicated in patients with a history of hypersensitivity to any of its components.

WARNINGS

Excessive use of adrenergic aerosols is potentially dangerous. Fatalities have been reported following excessive use of Alupent® (metaproterenol sulfate USP) as with other sympathomimetic inhalation preparations, and the exact cause is unknown. Cardiac arrest was noted in several cases.

Alupent, like other beta adrenergic agonists, can produce a significant cardiovascular effect in some patients, as measured by pulse rate, blood pressure, symptoms and/or ECG changes. As with other beta adrenergic aerosols, Alupent can produce paradoxical bronchospasm (which can be life threatening). If it occurs, the preparation should be discontinued immediately and alternative therapy instituted.

Alupent® (metaproterenol sulfate USP) should not be used more often than prescribed. Patients should be advised to contact their physician in the event that they do not respond to their usual dose of a sympathomimetic amine aerosol.

PRECAUTIONS

General: Extreme care must be exercised with respect to the administration of additional sympathomimetic agents. Since metaproterenol is a sympathomimetic amine it should be used with caution in patients with cardiovascular disorders, including ischemic heart disease, hypertension or cardiac arrhythmias, in patients with hyperthyroidism or diabetes mellitus, and in patients who are unusually responsive to sympathomimetic amines or who have convulsive disorders. Significant changes in systolic and diastolic blood pressure could be expected to occur in some patients after use of any beta adrenergic bronchodilator.

Physicians should recognize that a single dose of nebulized Alupent® (metaproterenol sulfate USP) in the treatment of acute asthma may alleviate symptoms and improve pulmonary function temporarily but fail to completely abort an attack.

Information for Patients: Extreme care must be exercised with respect to the administration of additional sympathomimetic agents. A sufficient interval of time should elapse prior to administration of another sympathomimetic agent. Alupent Inhalation Solution 5% effects may last up to 6 hours or longer. It should not be used more often than recommended and the patient should not increase the number of inhalations or frequency of use without first consulting the physician. If symptoms of asthma get worse, adverse reactions occur, or the patient does not respond to the usual dose, the patient should be instructed to contact the physician immediately.

Alupent Tablets and Alupent Syrup should not be used more often than prescribed. If symptoms persist, patients should consult a physician promptly.

A single dose of nebulized Alupent in the treatment of an acute attack of asthma may not completely abort an attack.

Drug Interactions: Other beta adrenergic aerosol bronchodilators should not be used concomitantly with Alupent® (metaproterenol sulfate USP) because they may have additive effects. Beta adrenergic agonists should be administered with caution to patients being treated with monoamine oxidase inhibitors or tricyclic antidepressants, since the action of beta adrenergic agonists on the vascular system may be potentiated.

Carcinogenesis/Mutagenesis/Impairment of Fertility: In an 18-month study in mice, Alupent produced a significant increase in benign hepatic adenomas in males and in benign ovarian tumors in females at doses corresponding to 31 and 62 (320 and 640 for Alupent Inhalation Aerosol) times the maximum recommended dose (based on a 50 kg individual). In a 2-year study in rats, a nonsignificant incidence of benign leiomyomata of the mesovarium was noted at 62 (640 for Alupent Inhalation Aerosol) times the maximum recommended dose. The relevance of these findings to man is not known. Mutagenic studies with Alupent have not been conducted. Reproduction studies in rats revealed no evidence of impaired fertility.

Pregnancy/Teratogenic Effects

PREGNANCY CATEGORY C: Alupent has been shown to be teratogenic and embryotoxic in rabbits when given orally in doses 620 times the human inhalation dose and 100 mg/kg or 62 times the maximum recommended human oral dose. These effects included skeletal abnormalities, hydrocephalus and skull bone separation.

Embryotoxicity has also been shown in mice when given orally at doses of 50 mg/kg or 31 times the maximum recommended human oral dose. Results of other oral reproduction studies in rats (40 mg/kg) and rabbits (50 mg/kg) have not revealed any teratogenic, embryotoxic or fetotoxic effects.

There are no adequate and well-controlled studies in pregnant women. Alupent should be used during pregnancy only if the potential benefit justifies the potential risk to the fetus.

Nursing Mothers: It is not known whether Alupent is excreted in human milk; therefore, Alupent should be used during nursing only if the potential benefit justifies the possible risk to the newborn.

Pediatric Use: See **DOSAGE AND ADMINISTRATION.**

ADVERSE REACTIONS

Adverse reactions are similar to those noted with other sympathomimetic agents. Adverse reactions such as tachycardia, hypertension, palpitations, nervousness, tremor, nausea and vomiting have been reported.

The most frequent adverse reaction to Alupent® (metaproterenol sulfate USP) administered by metered-dose inhaler among 251 patients in 90-day controlled clinical trials was nervousness. This was reported in 6.8% of patients. Less frequent adverse experiences, occurring in 1–4% of patients were headache, dizziness, palpitations, gastrointestinal distress, tremor, throat irritation, nausea, vomiting, cough and asthma exacerbation. Tachycardia occurred in less than 1% of patients.

Adverse experiences associated with Alupent Inhalation Solution 5% in at least 2% of 120 patients participating in multiple-dose clinical trial of 60- and 90-day duration included nervousness (14.1%; n=17), cough (3.3%; n=4) headache (3.3%; n=4), tachycardia (2.5%; n=3) and tremor (2.5%; n=3).

Alupent Inhalation Solution 5% may be associated with a somewhat higher incidence of adverse reactions in children. In controlled clinical trials conducted in 160 pediatric patients the incidence of adverse reactions observed at the recommended doses was as follows: tachycardia, 16.6%; tremor, 33%; nausea, 14%; vomiting, 7.7%. The corresponding incidence in placebo-treated patients was: tachycardia, 7.6%; tremor, 20%; nausea, 7.7%; vomiting, 2.5%.

In two well-controlled studies in children 6 to 12 years of age with acute exacerbation of asthma, Alupent Inhalation Solution 5% was not efficacious in approximately 30% of patients, where efficacy was defined as a 15% increase in FEV_1 above baseline at two or more time points during the 1-hour testing period. In 8% of patients there was a decrease in FEV_1 of 10% or more from baseline at two or more time points during the testing period. Insufficient information exists to assess the relationship of drug administration to the decline in pulmonary function observed in these patients, but paradoxical bronchospasm is one possibility.

The most frequent adverse reactions to Alupent Inhalation Solution 0.4% and 0.6% are nervousness and tachycardia which occur in about 1 in 7 patients, tremor which occurs in about 1 in 20 patients and nausea which occurs in about 1 in 50 patients. Less frequent adverse reactions are hypertension, palpitations, vomiting and bad taste which occur in approximately 1 in 300 patients.

The following table of adverse experiences is derived from 26 controlled clinical trials with 496 patients treated with Alupent® (metaproterenol sulfate USP) Tablets:

ALUPENT® Tablets
Incidence of Adverse Events
Reported Among 496 Patients
Treated in 26 Controlled Clinical Trials

ADVERSE EXPERIENCE	Incidence Number of Patients	%
Cardiovascular		
Chest Pain	1	.2
Edema	1	.2
Hypertension	2	.4
Palpitations	19	3.8
Tachycardia	85	17.1
Central Nervous System		
Dizziness	12	2.4
Drowsiness	3	.6
Fatigue	7	1.4
Headache	35	7.0
Insomnia	9	1.8
Nervousness	100	20.2
Sensory disturbances	1	.2
Syncope	2	.4
Weakness	1	.2
Dermatological		
Diaphoresis	1	.2
Hives	1	.2
Pruritus	2	.4
Gastrointestinal		
Appetite changes	2	.4
Diarrhea	6	1.2
Gastrointestinal distress	15	3.0
Nausea	18	3.6
Vomiting	4	0.8
Musculoskeletal		
Pain	1	.2
Spasms	1	.2
Tremor	84	16.9
Ophthalmological		
Blurred vision	1	.2
Oro-Otolaryngeal		
Dry mouth/throat	2	.4
Laryngeal changes	1	.2
Bad taste	4	0.8
Respiratory		
Asthma exacerbation	10	2.0
Coughing	1	.2
Other		
Chatty	1	.2
Chills	1	.2
Clonus noted on flexing foot	1	.2
Feverish	2	.4
Flu symptoms	1	.2
Facial and finger puffiness	1	.2

The incidence of adverse events occurring in at least 1% of the 1,120 patients treated with Alupent Syrup in 44 clinical trials are tachycardia (6.1%; n=68), nervousness (4.8%; n=54), tremor (1.6%; n=18), nausea (1.3%; n=15) and headache (1.1%; n=12).

It is important to recognize that adverse reactions from beta agonist bronchodilator solutions for nebulization may occur with the use of a new container of a product in patients who have previously tolerated that same product without adverse effect. There have been reports that indicate that such patients may subsequently tolerate replacement containers of the same product without adverse effect.

OVERDOSAGE

The expected symptoms with overdosage are those of excessive beta-adrenergic stimulation and/or any of the symptoms listed under adverse reactions, e.g. angina, hypertension or hypotension, arrhythmias, nervousness, headache, tremor, dry mouth, palpitation, nausea, dizziness, fatigue, malaise and insomnia.

Treatment consists of discontinuation of metaproterenol together with appropriate symptomatic therapy.

DOSAGE AND ADMINISTRATION

If Alupent® (metaproterenol sulfate USP) is administered before or after other sympathomimetic bronchodilators, caution should be exercised with respect to possible potentiation of adrenergic effects.

Inhalation Aerosol: The usual single dose is two to three inhalations. With repetitive dosing, inhalation should usually not be repeated more often than about every three to four hours. Total dosage per day should not exceed 12 inhalations. Alupent Inhalation Aerosol is not recommended for use in children under 12 years of age.

Usually, treatment need not be repeated more often than every four hours to relieve acute attacks of bronchospasm.

As with all medications, the physician should begin therapy with the lowest effective dose and then titrate the dosage according to the individual patient's requirements.

Alupent Inhalation Solution is administered by oral inhalation with the aid of a nebulizer or an intermittent positive pressure breathing apparatus (IPPB).

Alupent Inhalation Solution may be administered three to four times a day for the treatment of reversible airways disease in adults. A single dose of nebulized Alupent in the treatment of an acute attack of asthma may not completely abort an attack.

The dosage and administration are summarized in the table below:

[See table on top of page.]

Population	Method of Administration	Usual Single Dose	Range	Dilution
Adult	Hand-bulb nebulizer	10 inhalations	5–15 inhalations	No dilution
12 years and older	IPPB or nebulizer	0.3 ml	0.2–0.3 ml	Diluted in approx. 2.5 ml saline solution or other diluent
Pediatric 6–12 years	Nebulizer	0.1 ml	0.1–0.2 ml	Diluted in saline solution to a total volume of 3 ml

Continued on next page

Boehringer Ingelheim—Cont.

Inhalation Solution 0.4% and 0.6% Unit-dose Vials: Alupent Inhalation Solution Unit-dose Vial is administered by oral inhalation using an IPPB device. The usual adult dose is one vial per nebulization treatment. Each vial of Alupent Inhalation Solution 0.4% is equivalent to 0.2 ml Alupent Inhalation Solution 5% diluted to 2.5 ml with normal saline; each vial of Alupent Inhalation Solution 0.6% is equivalent to 0.3 ml Alupent Inhalation Solution 5% diluted to 2.5 ml with normal saline.

Usually, treatment need not be repeated more often than every 4 hours to relieve acute attacks of bronchospasm. As part of a total treatment program in chronic bronchospastic pulmonary diseases, Alupent Inhalation Solution Unit-dose vials may be administered three to four times a day.

As with all medications, the physician should begin therapy with the lowest effective dose and then titrate the dosage according to the individual patient's requirements.

Alupent Inhalation Solution Unit-dose Vial is not recommended for use in children under 12 years of age.

Syrup: *Children:* Aged six to nine years or weight under 60 lbs—one teaspoonful three or four times a day. Children over nine years or weight over 60 lbs—two teaspoonfuls three or four times a day. Clinical trial experience in children under the age of 6 is limited. Of 40 children treated with Alupent Syrup for at least 1 month, daily doses of approximately 1.3 to 2.6 mg/kg were well tolerated. Adults—two teaspoonfuls three or four times a day. It is recommended that the physician titrate the dosage according to each individual patient's response to therapy.

Tablets: *Adults:* The usual dose is 20 mg three or four times a day. *Children:* Aged six to nine years or weight under 60 lbs—10 mg three or four times a day. Over nine years or weight over 60 lbs—20 mg three or four times a day. Alupent tablets are not recommended for use in children under six years at this time. It is recommended that the physician titrate the dosage according to each individual patient's response to therapy.

HOW SUPPLIED

Inhalation Aerosol: Each 200 inhalations of Alupent® (metaproterenol sulfate USP) Inhalation Aerosol contains 150 mg of metaproterenol sulfate as a micronized powder in inert propellants. Each metered dose delivers through the mouthpiece 0.65 mg metaproterenol sulfate (each ml contains 15 mg). Alupent Inhalation Aerosol with Mouthpiece (NDC 0597-0070-17), net contents 14g (10 mL).The mouthpiece is white with a clear, colorless sleeve and a blue protective cap. Alupent Inhalation Aerosol Refill (NDC 0597-0070-18), net contents 14g (10 mL).

Note: The indented statement below is required by the federal Clean Air Act for all products containing chlorofluorocarbons (CFCs), including products such as this one:

> **WARNING**
> Contains trichloromonofluoromethane (CFC-11), dichlorodifluoromethane (CFC-12) and dichlorotetrafluoroethane (CFC-114), substances which harm public health and the environment by destroying ozone in the upper atmosphere.

A notice similar to the above WARNING has been placed in the "Instructions for Use" portion of the package insert pursuant to regulations of the United States Environmental Protection Agency.

Store between 59°F (15°C) and 77°F (25°C). Avoid excessive humidity.

Inhalation Solution: Alupent Inhalation Solution is supplied as a 5% solution in bottles of 10 ml (NDC 0597-0071-75) or 30 ml (NDC 0597-0071-30) with accompanying calibrated dropper. Plastic cover on dropper should be discarded and not used to retain product. Store between 59°F (15°C) and 77°F (25°C).

Alupent Inhalation Solution Unit-dose Vial is supplied as a 0.4% (NDC 0597-0078-62) or 0.6% (NDC 0597-0069-62) clear colorless or nearly colorless solution containing 2.5 ml with 25 vials per box. Each vial is made from a low-density polyethylene resin. Store below 77°F (25°C). Protect from light. Do not use the solution if it is pinkish or darker than slightly yellow or contains a precipitate.

Syrup: Alupent is available as a cherry-flavored syrup, 10 mg per teaspoonful (5 ml) in 16 fl. oz. bottles (NDC 0597-0073-16). Store between 59°F (15°C) and 86°F (30°C). Protect from light.

Tablets: Alupent is supplied in two dosage strengths as scored round white tablets in bottles of 100. Tablets of 10 mg coded BI/74 (NDC 0597-0074-01). Tablets of 20 mg coded BI/72 (NDC 0597-0072-01). *Storage for bottles:* Store between 59°F (15°C) and 86°F (30°C). Protect from light. *Storage for blister samples:* Store between 59°F (15°C) and 77°F (25°C). Protect from light.

Caution

Federal law prohibits dispensing without prescription.

AL-PI-7/95

Shown in Product Identification Guide, page 306

ATROVENT® ℞
[*ă 'trō "vĕnt*]
(ipratropium bromide)
Inhalation Aerosol
Bronchodilator .... BI-CODE 82

PRODUCT OVERVIEW

KEY FACTS

The active ingredient in Atrovent® (ipratropium bromide) Inhalation Aerosol is ipratropium bromide. It is an anticholinergic bronchodilator classified as a synthetic quaternary ammonium compound. The bronchodilating effect of Atrovent is primarily local and site specific. It is not well absorbed systemically, resulting in a low potential for toxicity.

MAJOR USES

Atrovent Inhalation Aerosol has proved to be clinically effective for maintenance treatment of bronchospasm associated with chronic obstructive pulmonary disease, including chronic bronchitis and emphysema.

SAFETY INFORMATION

Atrovent Inhalation Aerosol is contraindicated for patients with a hypersensitivity to atropine or its derivatives or to soya lecithin or related food products such as soybean or lecithin. It is not intended for the initial treatment of acute episodes of bronchospasm where rapid response is required.

Before prescribing, please consult full prescribing information below.

PRESCRIBING INFORMATION

ATROVENT® ℞
[*ă 'trō "vĕnt*]
(ipratropium bromide)
Inhalation Aerosol
Bronchodilator

DESCRIPTION

The active ingredient in Atrovent® (ipratropium bromide) Inhalation Aerosol is ipratropium bromide. It is an anticholinergic bronchodilator chemically described as 8-azoniabicyclo(3.2.1)-octane, 3-(3-hydroxy -1- oxo-2-phenyl propoxy)-8-methyl-8-(1-methylethyl)-, bromide, monohydrate *(endo, syn)*-, (±)-; a synthetic quaternary ammonium compound, chemically related to atropine. It has the following structural formula:

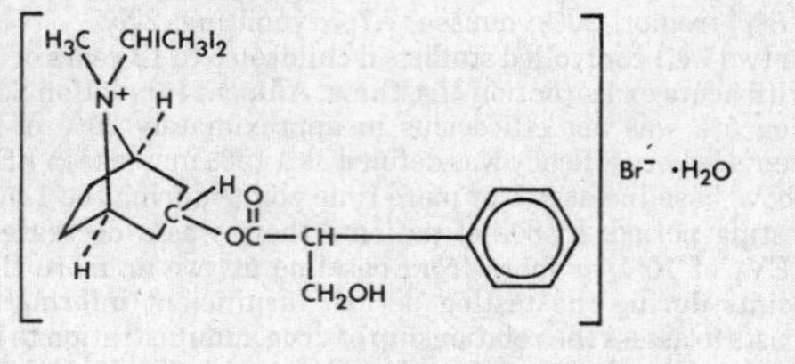

ipratropium bromide
(Atrovent)

$C_{20}H_{30}BrNO_3 \cdot H_2O$ Mol. Wt. 430.4

Ipratropium bromide is a white crystalline substance, freely soluble in water and lower alcohols but insoluble in lipophilic solvents such as ether, chloroform, and fluorocarbons.

Atrovent Inhalation Aerosol is an inhalation aerosol for oral administration. The net weight is 14 grams; it yields 200 inhalations. Each actuation of the valve delivers 18 mcg of ipratropium bromide from the mouthpiece. The inert ingredients are dichlorodifluoromethane, dichlorotetrafluoroethane, and trichloromonofluoromethane as propellants and soya lecithin.

CLINICAL PHARMACOLOGY

Atrovent® (ipratropium bromide) is an anticholinergic (parasympatholytic) agent which, based on animal studies, appears to inhibit vagally mediated reflexes by antagonizing the action of acetylcholine, the transmitter agent released from the vagus nerve. Anticholinergics prevent the increases in intracellular concentration of cyclic guanosine monophosphate (cyclic GMP) which are caused by interaction of acetylcholine with the muscarinic receptor on bronchial smooth muscle.

The bronchodilation following inhalation of Atrovent is primarily a local, site-specific effect, not a systemic one. Much of an inhaled dose is swallowed as shown by fecal excretion studies. Atrovent is not readily absorbed into the systemic circulation either from the surface of the lung or from the gastrointestinal tract as confirmed by blood level and renal excretion studies.

The half-life of elimination is about 2 hours after inhalation or intravenous administration. Autoradiographic studies in rats have shown that Atrovent does not penetrate the blood-brain barrier.

In controlled 90-day studies in patients with bronchospasm associated with chronic obstructive pulmonary disease (chronic bronchitis and emphysema) significant improvements in pulmonary function (FEV_1 and FEF_{25-75}% increases of 15% or more) occurred within 15 minutes, reached a peak in 1–2 hours, and persisted for periods of 3 to 4 hours in the majority of patients and up to 6 hours in some patients. In addition, significant increases in Forced Vital Capacity (FVC) have been demonstrated.

Controlled clinical studies have demonstrated that Atrovent (ipratropium bromide) does not alter either mucociliary clearance or the volume or viscosity of respiratory secretions. In studies without a positive control Atrovent did not alter pupil size, accommodation or visual acuity (See ADVERSE REACTIONS).

Ventilation/perfusion studies have shown no clinically significant effects on pulmonary gas exchange or arterial oxygen tension. Atrovent does not produce clinically significant changes in pulse rate or blood pressure.

INDICATIONS AND USAGE

Atrovent® (ipratropium bromide) is indicated as a bronchodilator for maintenance treatment of bronchospasm associated with chronic obstructive pulmonary disease, including chronic bronchitis and emphysema.

CONTRAINDICATIONS

Atrovent® (ipratropium bromide) is contraindicated in patients with a history of hypersensitivity to soya lecithin or related food products such as soybean and peanut. Atrovent should also not be taken by patients hypersensitive to any other components of the drug product or to atropine or its derivatives.

WARNINGS

Atrovent® (ipratropium bromide) is not indicated for the initial treatment of acute episodes of bronchospasm where rapid response is required.

PRECAUTIONS

General: Atrovent® (ipratropium bromide) should be used with caution in patients with narrow-angle glaucoma, prostatic hypertrophy or bladder-neck obstruction.

Information for Patients: Patients should be advised that temporary blurring of vision may result if the aerosol is sprayed into the eyes.

Patients should be reminded that Atrovent is not intended for occasional use, but rather, in order to be maximally effective, must be used consistently as prescribed throughout the course of therapy.

Drug Interactions: Atrovent has been used concomitantly with other drugs, including sympathomimetic bronchodilators, methylxanthines, steroids and cromolyn sodium, commonly used in the treatment of chronic obstructive pulmonary disease, without adverse drug reactions. There are no formal studies fully evaluating the interactive effects of Atrovent and these drugs with respect to effectiveness.

Carcinogenesis, Mutagenesis, Impairment of Fertility: Two-year oral carcinogenicity studies in rats and mice have revealed no carcinogenic potential at doses up to 1,250 times the maximum recommended human daily dose for Atrovent. Results of various mutagenicity studies were negative.

Fertility of male or female rats at oral doses up to approximately 10,000 times the maximum recommended human daily dose was unaffected by Atrovent administration. At doses above 18,000 times the maximum recommended human daily dose, increased resorption and decreased conception rates were observed.

Pregnancy Teratogenic Effects *PREGNANCY CATEGORY B:* Oral reproduction studies performed in mice, rats and rabbits (at doses approximately 2,000, 200,000 and 26,000 times the maximum recommended human daily dose, respectively) and inhalation reproduction studies in rats and rabbits (at doses approximately 312 and 375 times the maximum recommended human daily dose, respectively) have demonstrated no evidence of teratogenic effects as a result of Atrovent. However, no adequate or well controlled studies have been conducted in pregnant women. Because animal reproduction studies are not always predictive of human response, Atrovent® (ipratropium bromide) should be used during pregnancy only if clearly needed.

Nursing Mothers: It is not known whether Atrovent is excreted in human milk. Although lipid-insoluble quaternary bases pass into breast milk, it is unlikely that Atrovent would reach the infant to an important extent, especially when taken by aerosol. However, because many drugs are excreted in human milk, caution should be exercised when Atrovent is administered to a nursing woman.

Pediatric Use: Safety and effectiveness in the pediatric population below the age of 12 have not been established.

ADVERSE REACTIONS

Adverse reaction information concerning Atrovent® (ipratropium bromide) is derived from 90 day controlled clinical trials (N = 254), other controlled clinical trials using recommended doses of Atrovent (N = 377) and an uncontrolled study (N = 1924). Additional information is derived from the foreign post-marketing experience and the published literature.

Adverse reactions occurring in greater than one percent of patients in the 90 day controlled clinical trials appear in the following table:

	Percent of Patients	
	Ipratropium bromide	Metaproterenol sulfate
	N = 254	N = 249
Reaction		
Cardiovascular		
Palpitations	1.8	1.6
Central Nervous System		
Nervousness	3.1	6.8
Dizziness	2.4	2.8
Headache	2.4	2.0
Dermatological		
Rash	1.2	0.4
Gastrointestinal		
Nausea	2.8	1.2
Gastrointestinal distress	2.4	2.8
Vomiting	0	1.2
Musculoskeletal		
Tremor	0	2.4
Ophthalmological		
Blurred vision	1.2	0.8
Oro-Otolaryngeal		
Dry mouth	2.4	0.8
Irritation from aerosol	1.6	1.6
Respiratory		
Cough	5.9	1.2
Exacerbation of symptoms	2.4	3.6

Additional adverse reactions reported in less than one percent of the patients considered possibly due to Atrovent include urinary difficulty, fatigue, insomnia and hoarseness. The large uncontrolled, open-label study included seriously ill patients. About 7% of patients treated discontinued the program because of adverse events.

Of the 2301 patients treated in the large uncontrolled study and in clinical trials other than the 90-day studies, the most common adverse reactions reported were: dryness of the oropharynx, about 5 in 100; cough, exacerbation of symptoms and irritation from aerosol, each about 3 in 100; headache, about 2 in 100; nausea, dizziness, blurred vision/difficulty in accommodation, and drying of secretions, each about 1 in 100. Less frequently reported adverse reactions that were possibly due to Atrovent® (ipratropium bromide) include tachycardia, paresthesias, drowsiness, coordination difficulty, itching, hives, flushing, alopecia, constipation, tremor, mucosal ulcers.

Cases of precipitation or worsening of narrow-angle glaucoma, acute eye pain and hypotension have been reported. Allergic-type reactions such as skin rash, angioedema of tongue, lips and face, urticaria (including giant urticaria), laryngospasm and anaphylactic reaction have been reported, with positive rechallenge in some cases. Many of the patients had a history of allergies to other drugs and/or foods, including soybean. (See CONTRAINDICATIONS.)

OVERDOSAGE

Acute overdosage by inhalation is unlikely since Atrovent® (ipratropium bromide) is not well absorbed systemically after aerosol or oral administration. The oral LD_{50} of Atrovent ranged between 1001 and 2010 mg/kg in mice; between 1667 and more than 4000 mg/kg in rats; and between 400 and 1300 mg/kg in dogs.

DOSAGE AND ADMINISTRATION

The usual starting dose of Atrovent® (ipratropium bromide) is two inhalations (36 mcg) four times a day. Patients may take additional inhalations as required; however, the total number of inhalations should not exceed 12 in 24 hours.

HOW SUPPLIED

Atrovent® (ipratropium bromide) Inhalation Aerosol is supplied as a metered dose inhaler with a white mouthpiece which has a clear, colorless sleeve and a green protective cap. Atrovent Inhalation Aerosol with Mouthpiece (NDC 0597-0082-14), net contents 14 g. Atrovent Inhalation Aerosol Refill (NDC 0597-0082-18), net contents 14 g.

Each 14 gram vial provides sufficient medication for 200 inhalations. Each actuation delivers 18 mcg of ipratropium bromide from the mouthpiece.

Note: The indented statement below is required by the federal Clean Air Act for all products containing chlorofluorocarbons (CFCs), including products such as this one:

WARNING

Contains trichloromonofluoromethane (CFC-11), dichlorodifluoromethane (CFC-12) and dichlorotetrafluoroethane (CFC-114), substances which harm public health and the environment by destroying ozone in the upper atmosphere.

A notice similar to the above WARNING has been placed in the "Instructions for Use" portion of the package insert pursuant to regulations of the United States Environmental Protection Agency.

Store between 59°F (15°C) and 86°F (30°C). Avoid excessive humidity.

Caution
Federal law prohibits dispensing without prescription.
AT-PI-6/93
Shown in Product Identification Guide, page 306

ATROVENT® ℞
[ă′trŏ″vĕnt]
(ipratropium bromide)
Inhalation Solution .... **BI-CODE 80**

Prescribing Information

DESCRIPTION

The active ingredient in Atrovent® (ipratropium bromide) Inhalation Solution is ipratropium bromide monohydrate. It is an anticholinergic bronchodilator chemically described as 8-azoniabicyclo[3.2.1]-octane, 3-(3-hydroxy -1- oxo -2- phenyl propoxy)-8-methyl-8-(1-methylethyl)-, bromide, monohydrate *(endo, syn)*, (±); a synthetic quaternary ammonium compound, chemically related to atropine.

ipratropium bromide monohydrate (Atrovent)	$C_{20}H_{30}BrNO_3 \cdot H_2O$ Mol. Wt. 430.4

Ipratropium bromide is a white crystalline substance, freely soluble in water and lower alcohols. It is a quaternary ammonium compound and thus exists in an ionized state in aqueous solutions. It is relatively insoluble in non-polar media. Atrovent Inhalation Solution is administered by oral inhalation with the aid of a nebulizer. It contains ipratropium bromide 0.02% (anhydrous basis) in a sterile, preservative-free, isotonic saline solution, pH-adjusted 3.4 (3 to 4) with hydrochloric acid.

CLINICAL PHARMACOLOGY

Atrovent® (ipratropium bromide) is an anticholinergic (parasympatholytic) agent that, based on animal studies, appears to inhibit vagally mediated reflexes by antagonizing the action of acetylcholine, the transmitter agent released from the vagus nerve.

Anticholinergics prevent the increases in intracellular concentration of cyclic guanosine monophosphate (cyclic GMP) that are caused by interaction of acetylcholine with the muscarinic receptor on bronchial smooth muscle.

The bronchodilation following inhalation of Atrovent is primarily a local, site-specific effect, not a systemic one. Much of an administered dose is swallowed but not absorbed, as shown by fecal excretion studies. Following nebulization of a 2 mg dose, a mean 7% of the dose was absorbed into the systemic circulation either from the surface of the lung or from the gastrointestinal tract. The half-life of elimination is about 1.6 hours after intravenous administration. Ipratropium bromide is minimally (0 to 9% in vitro) bound to plasma albumin and α_1-acid glycoproteins. It is partially metabolized. Autoradiographic studies in rats have shown that Atrovent does not penetrate the blood-brain barrier. Atrovent has not been studied in patients with hepatic or renal insufficiency. It should be used with caution in those patient populations.

In controlled 12-week studies in patients with bronchospasm associated with chronic obstructive pulmonary disease (chronic bronchitis and emphysema) significant improvements in pulmonary function (FEV_1 increases of 15% or more) occurred within 15 to 30 minutes, reached a peak in 1–2 hours, and persisted for periods of 4–5 hours in the majority of patients, with about 25–38% of the patients demonstrating increases of 15% or more for at least 7–8 hours. Continued effectiveness of Atrovent Inhalation Solution was demonstrated throughout the 12-week period. In addition, significant increases in forced vital capacity (FVC) have been demonstrated. However, Atrovent did not consistently produce significant improvement in subjective symptom scores nor in quality of life scores over the 12-week duration of study.

Additional controlled 12-week studies were conducted to evaluate the safety and effectiveness of Atrovent Inhalation Solution administered concomitantly with the beta adrenergic bronchodilator solutions metaproterenol and albuterol compared with the administration of each of the beta

All Adverse Events, from a Double-blind, Parallel, 12-week Study of Patients with COPD*

	PERCENT OF PATIENTS				
	Atrovent® (500 mcg t.i.d) n=219	Alupent® (15 mg t.i.d) n=212	Atrovent®/Alupent® (500 mcg t.i.d/ 15 mg t.i.d) n=108	Albuterol (2.5 mg t.i.d) n=205	Atrovent®/Albuterol (500 mcg t.i.d/ 2.5 mg t.i.d) n=100
Body as a Whole-General Disorders					
Headache	6.4	5.2	6.5	6.3	9.0
Pain	4.1	3.3	0.9	2.9	5.0
Influenza-like symptoms	3.7	4.7	6.5	0.5	1.0
Back pain	3.2	1.9	1.9	2.4	0.0
Chest pain	3.2	4.2	5.6	2.0	1.0
Cardiovascular Disorders					
Hypertension/Hypertension Aggravated	0.9	1.9	0.9	1.5	4.0
Central & Peripheral Nervous System					
Dizziness	2.3	3.3	1.9	3.9	4.0
Insomnia	0.9	0.5	4.6	1.0	1.0
Tremor	0.9	7.1	8.3	1.0	0.0
Nervousness	0.5	4.7	6.5	1.0	1.0
Gastrointestinal System Disorders					
Mouth Dryness	3.2	0.0	1.9	2.0	3.0
Nausea	4.1	3.8	1.9	2.9	2.0
Constipation	0.9	0.0	3.7	1.0	1.0
Musculo-skeletal System Disorders					
Arthritis	0.9	1.4	0.9	0.5	3.0
Respiratory System Disorders (Lower)					
Coughing	4.6	8.0	6.5	5.4	6.0
Dyspnea	9.6	13.2	16.7	12.7	9.0
Bronchitis	14.6	24.5	15.7	16.6	20.0
Bronchospasm	2.3	2.8	4.6	5.4	5.0
Sputum Increased	1.4	1.4	4.6	3.4	0.0
Respiratory Disorder	0.0	6.1	6.5	2.0	4.0
Respiratory System Disorders (Upper)					
Upper Respiratory Tract Infection	13.2	11.3	9.3	12.2	16.0
Pharyngitis	3.7	4.2	5.6	2.9	4.0
Rhinitis	2.3	4.2	1.9	2.4	0.0
Sinusitis	2.3	2.8	0.9	5.4	4.0

* All adverse events, regardless of drug relationship, reported by three percent or more patients in the 12-week controlled clinical trials.

Continued on next page

Boehringer Ingelheim—Cont.

agonists alone. Combined therapy produced significant additional improvement in FEV_1 and FVC. On combined therapy, the median duration of 15% improvement in FEV_1 was 5–7 hours, compared with 3–4 hours in patients receiving a beta agonist alone.

INDICATIONS AND USAGE

Atrovent® (ipratropium bromide) Inhalation Solution administered either alone or with other bronchodilators, especially beta adrenergics, is indicated as a bronchodilator for maintenance treatment of bronchospasm associated with chronic obstructive pulmonary disease, including chronic bronchitis and emphysema.

CONTRAINDICATIONS

Atrovent® (ipratropium bromide) is contraindicated in known or suspected cases of hypersensitivity to ipratropium bromide, or to atropine and its derivatives.

WARNINGS

The use of Atrovent® (ipratropium bromide) Inhalation Solution as a single agent for the relief of bronchospasm in acute COPD exacerbation has not been adequately studied. Drugs with faster onset of action may be preferable as initial therapy in this situtation. Combination of Atrovent and beta agonists has not been shown to be more effective than either drug alone in reversing the bronchospasm associated with acute COPD exacerbation.

PRECAUTIONS

General: Atrovent® (ipratropium bromide) should be used with caution in patients with narrow-angle glaucoma, prostatic hypertrophy or bladder-neck obstruction.

Information for Patients: Patients should be advised that temporary blurring of vision, precipitation or worsening of narrow-angle glaucoma or eye pain may result if the solution comes into direct contact with the eyes. Use of a nebulizer with mouthpiece rather than face mask may be preferable, to reduce the likelihood of the nebulizer solution reaching the eyes. Patients should be advised that Atrovent Inhalation Solution can be mixed in the nebulizer with albuterol if used within one hour. Compatibility data are not currently available with other drugs. Patients should be reminded that Atrovent Inhalation Solution should be used consistently as prescribed throughout the course of therapy.

Drug Interactions: Atrovent has been shown to be a safe and effective bronchodilator when used in conjuction with beta adrenergic bronchodilators. Atrovent has also been used with pulmonary medications, including methylxanthines and corticosteroids, without adverse drug interactions.

Carcinogenesis, Mutagenesis, Impairment of Fertility: Two-year oral carcinogenicity studies in rats and mice have revealed no carcinogenic potential at doses up to 6 mg/kg/day of Atrovent.

Results of various mutagenicity studies (Ames test, mouse dominant lethal test, mouse micronucleus test and chromosome aberration of bone marrow in Chinese hamsters) were negative.

Fertility of male or female rats at oral doses up to 50 mg/kg/day was unaffected by Atrovent administration. At doses above 90 mg/kg, increased resorption and decreased conception rates were observed.

Pregnancy *TERATOGENIC EFFECTS*

Pregnancy Category B. Oral reproduction studies performed in mice, rats and rabbits at doses of 10, 100, and 125 mg/kg respectively, and inhalation reproduction studies in rats and rabbits at doses of 1.5 and 1.8 mg/kg (or approximately 38 and 45 times the recommended human daily dose) respectively, have demonstrated no evidence of teratogenic effects as a result of Atrovent. However, no adequate or well controlled studies have been conducted in pregnant women. Because animal reproduction studies are not always predictive of human response, Atrovent should be used during pregnancy only if clearly needed.

Nursing Mothers: It is not known whether Atrovent is excreted in human milk. Although lipid-insoluble quaternary bases pass into breast milk, it is unlikely that Atrovent® (ipratropium bromide) would reach the infant to a significant extent, especially when taken by inhalation, since Atrovent is not well absorbed systemically after inhalation or oral administration. However, because many drugs are excreted in human milk, caution should be exercised when Atrovent is administered to a nursing woman.

Pediatric Use: Safety and effectiveness in the pediatric population below the age of 12 have not been established.

ADVERSE REACTIONS

Adverse reaction information concerning Atrovent® (ipratropium bromide) Inhalation Solution is derived from 12-week active-controlled clinical trials. Additional information is derived from the foreign post-marketing experience and the published literature.

All adverse events, regardless of drug relationship, reported by three percent or more patients in the 12-week controlled clinical trials appear in the table below:

[See table on bottom of preceding page.]

Additional adverse reactions reported in less than three percent of the patients treated with Atrovent include tachycardia, palpitations, eye pain, urinary retention, urinary tract infection and urticaria. A single case of anaphylaxis thought to be possibly related to Atrovent has been reported. Cases of precipitation or worsening of narrow-angle glaucoma and acute eye pain have been reported.

Lower respiratory adverse reactions (bronchitis, dyspnea and bronchospasm) were the most common events leading to discontinuation of Atrovent therapy in the 12-week trials. Headache, mouth dryness and aggravation of COPD symptoms are more common when the total daily dose of Atrovent equals or exceeds 2,000 mcg.

OVERDOSAGE

Acute systemic overdosage by inhalation is unlikely since Atrovent® (ipratropium bromide) is not well absorbed after inhalation at up to four-fold the recommended dose, or after oral administration at up to forty-fold the recommended dose. The oral LD_{50} of Atrovent ranged between 1001 and 2010 mg/kg in mice; between 1667 and more than 4000 mg/kg in rats; and between 400 and 1300 mg/kg in dogs.

DOSAGE AND ADMINISTRATION

The usual dosage of Atrovent® (ipratropium bromide) Inhalation Solution is 500 mcg (1 Unit-Dose Vial) administered three to four times a day by oral nebulization, with doses 6 to 8 hours apart. Atrovent Inhalation Solution Unit-Dose Vials contain 500 mcg ipratropium bromide anhydrous in 2.5 ml normal saline. Atrovent Inhalation Solution can be mixed in the nebulizer with albuterol if used within one hour. Compatibility data are not currently available with other drugs.

HOW SUPPLIED

Atrovent® (ipratropium bromide) Inhalation Solution Unit Dose Vial is supplied as a 0.02% clear, colorless solution containing 2.5 ml with 25 vials per foil pouch (NDC 0597-0080-62).

Each vial is made from a low density polyethylene (LDPE) resin.

Store between 59°F (15°C) and 86°F (30°C). Protect from light. Store unused vials in the foil pouch.

ATTENTION PHARMACIST: Detach "Patient's Instructions for Use" from Package Insert and dispense with solution.

Caution

Federal law prohibits dispensing without prescription.

AS-PI 1/94

Shown in Product Identification Guide, page 306

ATTENTION PHARMACIST: Detach "Patient's Instructions for Use" from package insert and dispense it with product.

ATROVENT® ℞
(ipratropium bromide)
Nasal Spray 0.03%

Prescribing Information

DESCRIPTION

The active ingredient in ATROVENT® Nasal Spray is ipratropium bromide monohydrate. It is an anticholinergic agent chemically described as 8-azoniabicyclo (3.2.1) octane,3-(3-hydroxy-1-oxo-2-phenylpropoxy)-8-methyl-8- (1-methylethyl-), bromide, monohydrate *(endo,syn)*-, (±)- :a synthetic quaternary ammonium compound, chemically related to atropine. Its structural formula is:

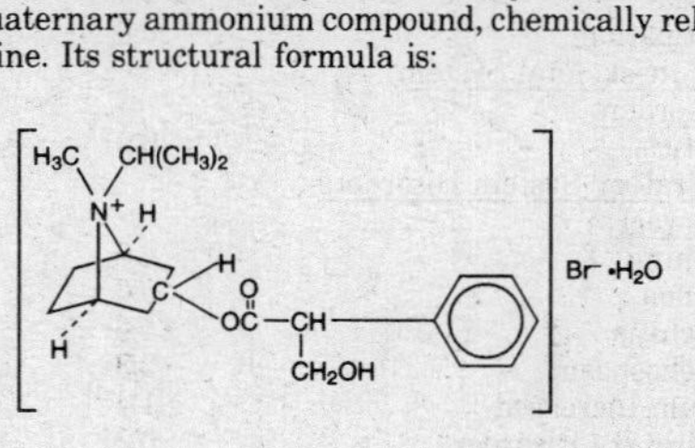

$C_{20}H_{30}BrNO_3 \bullet H_2O$
Mol. Wt. 430.4

ipratropium bromide monohydrate

Ipratropium bromide is a white to off-white, crystalline substance. It is freely soluble in lower alcohols and water, existing in an ionized state in aqueous solutions, and relatively insoluble in non-polar media.

ATROVENT® (ipratropium bromide) Nasal Spray 0.03% is intended for local administration to the nasal mucosa to control rhinorrhea in patients with perennial rhinitis. It contains 0.03% ipratropium bromide on an anhydrous basis (21 mcg/spray) in an isotonic, aqueous solution with pH adjusted to 4.7, which also contains benzalkonium chloride, edetate disodium, sodium chloride, sodium hydroxide, hydrochloric acid, and purified water.

CLINICAL PHARMACOLOGY

Mechanism of Action

Ipratropium bromide is an anticholinergic agent that inhibits vagally mediated reflexes by antagonizing the action of acetylcholine at the cholinergic receptor. In humans, ipratropium bromide has anti-secretory properties and, when applied locally, inhibits secretions from the serous and seromucous glands lining the nasal mucosa. Ipratropium bromide is a quaternary amine that minimally crosses the nasal and gastrointestinal membrane and the blood-brain barrier, resulting in a reduction of the systemic anticholinergic effects (e.g., neurologic, ophthalmic, cardiovascular and gastrointestinal effects) that are seen with tertiary anticholinergic amines.

Pharmacokinetics

Ipratropium bromide is a quaternary amine that is poorly absorbed into the systemic circulation from the nasal mucosa. Less than 20% of an 84 mcg per nostril dose is absorbed from the nasal mucosa of normal volunteers, induced-cold patients or perennial rhinitis patients, but the amount of ipratropium bromide which is systemically absorbed from nasal administration exceeds the amount of ipratropium bromide absorbed from either ATROVENT® Inhalation Solution (2% of a 500 mcg dose) or ATROVENT® Inhalation Aerosol (20% of a 36 mcg mouthpiece dose).

The half-life of elimination of ipratropium is about 1.6 hours after intravenous administration. Ipratropium bromide is minimally bound (0 to 9% *in vitro*) to plasma albumin and α_1-acid glycoprotein. It is partially metabolized to inactive ester hydrolysis products. Following intravenous administration, approximately one-half of the dose is excreted unchanged in the urine. Studies in rats have shown that ipratropium bromide does not penetrate the blood-brain barrier. The pharmacokinetics of ipratropium bromide have not been studied in patients with hepatic or renal insufficiency or in the elderly. Gender does not seem to influence the absorption or excretion of nasally administered ipratropium bromide.

Pharmacodynamic data also indicate little systemic absorption. In two single dose, pharmacokinetic trials (n = 17), solutions of up to 0.12% ipratropium bromide (336 mcg total nasal dose) did not significantly affect pupillary diameter, heart rate or systolic/diastolic blood pressure. Similarly, in an induced-cold, pharmacokinetic trial with ATROVENT® (ipratropium bromide) Nasal Spray 0.06% (84 mcg/nostril four times a day) no significant effects on pupillary diameter, heart rate or systolic/diastolic blood pressures were observed.

Controlled clinical trials demonstrated that intranasal fluorocarbon-propelled ipratropium bromide does not alter physiologic nasal functions (e.g., sense of smell, ciliary beat frequency, mucociliary clearance, or the air conditioning capacity of the nose).

Clinical Trials

The clinical trials for ATROVENT® (ipratropium bromide) Nasal Spray 0.03% were conducted in patients with nonallergic perennial rhinitis (NAPR) and in patients with allergic perennial rhinitis (APR). APR patients were those who experienced symptoms of nasal hypersecretion and nasal congestion or sneezing when exposed to specific perennial allergens (e.g., dust mites, molds) and were skin test positive to these allergens, NAPR patients were those who experienced symptoms of nasal hypersecretion and nasal congestion or sneezing throughout the year, but were skin test negative to common perennial allergens.

In four controlled, four and eight week comparisons of ATROVENT® (ipratropium bromide) Nasal Spray 0.03% (42 mcg per nostril, two or three times daily) with its vehicle, in patients with allergic or nonallergic perennial rhinitis, there was a statistically significant decrease in the severity and duration of rhinorrhea in the ATROVENT group throughout the entire study period. An effect was seen as early as the first day of therapy. There was no effect of ATROVENT® (ipratropium bromide) Nasal Spray 0.03% on degree of nasal congestion, sneezing or postnasal drip. The response to ATROVENT® (ipratropium bromide) Nasal Spray 0.03% did not appear to be affected by the type of perennial rhinitis (NAPR or APR), age or gender. No controlled clinical trials directly compared the efficacy of BID versus TID treatment.

Two nasal provocation trials in perennial rhinitis patients (n=44) using ipratropium bromide nasal spray showed a dose dependent increase in inhibition of methacholine induced nasal secretion with an onset of action within 15 minutes (time of first observation).

INDICATIONS AND USAGE

ATROVENT® (ipratropium bromide) Nasal Spray 0.03% is indicated for the symptomatic relief of rhinorrhea associated

with allergic and nonallergic perennial rhinitis in adults and children age 12 years and older. ATROVENT® (ipratropium bromide) Nasal Spray 0.03% does not relieve nasal congestion, sneezing or postnasal drip associated with allergic or nonallergic perennial rhinitis.

CONTRAINDICATIONS

ATROVENT® (ipratropium bromide) Nasal Spray 0.03% is contraindicated in patients with a history of hypersensitivity to atropine or its derivatives, or to any of the other ingredients.

WARNINGS

Immediate hypersensitivity reactions may occur after administration of ipratropium bromide, as demonstrated by rare cases of urticaria, angioedema, rash, bronchospasm and oropharyngeal edema.

PRECAUTIONS

General

ATROVENT® (ipratropium bromide) Nasal Spray 0.03% should be used with caution in patients with narrow-angle glaucoma, prostatic hypertrophy or bladder neck obstruction, particularly if they are receiving an anticholinergic by another route. Cases of precipitation or worsening of narrow-angle glaucoma and acute eye pain have been reported with direct eye contact of ipratropium bromide administered by oral inhalation.

Information for Patients

Patients should be advised that temporary blurring of vision, precipitation or worsening of narrow-angle glaucoma or eye pain may result if ATROVENT® (ipratropium bromide) Nasal Spray 0.03% comes into direct contact with the eyes. Patients should be instructed to avoid spraying ATROVENT® (ipratropium bromide) Nasal Spray 0.03% in or around their eyes. Patients who experience eye pain, blurred vision, excessive nasal dryness or episodes of nasal bleeding should be instructed to contact their doctor. Patients should be reminded to carefully read and follow the accompanying Patient's Instructions for Use.

Drug Interactions

No controlled clinical trials were conducted to investigate drug-drug interactions. ATROVENT® (ipratropium bromide) Nasal Spray 0.03% is minimally absorbed into the systemic circulation; nonetheless, there is some potential for an additive interaction with other concomitantly administered anticholinergic medications, including ATROVENT® for oral inhalation.

Carcinogenesis, Mutagenesis, Impairment of Fertility

Two-year oral carcinogenicity studies in rats and mice have revealed no carcinogenic activity at doses up to 6 mg/kg/day. This dose corresponds, in rats and mice respectively, to about 200 and 100 times the maximum recommended human daily dose (MRHD) on a mg/m^2 basis of ATROVENT® (ipratropium bromide) Nasal Spray 0.03%. Results of various mutagenicity studies (Ames test, mouse dominant lethal test, mouse micronucleus test and chromosome aberration of bone marrow in Chinese hamsters) were negative.

Fertility of male or female rats at oral doses up to 50 mg/kg/day (about 1,660 times the MRHD on a mg/m^2 basis) was unaffected by ipratropium bromide administration. At doses above 90 mg/kg/day (about 3,000 times the MRHD on a mg/m^2 basis), a decreased conception rate was observed.

Pregnancy

TERATOGENIC EFFECTS Pregnancy Category B. Oral reproduction studies were performed at doses of 10 mg/kg/day in mice, 100 mg/kg/day in rats and 125 mg/kg/day in rabbits. These doses correspond in each species respectively, to about 160, 3,000 and 8,000 times the MRHD of ATROVENT® (ipratropium bromide) Nasal Spray 0.03% in perennial rhinitis (252 mcg/day) on a mg/m^2 basis. Inhalation reproduction studies in rats and rabbits at doses of 1.5 and 1.8 mg/kg/day (about 50 and 120 times the MRHD dose on a mg/m^2 basis for each species, respectively) have demonstrated no evidence of teratogenic effects as a result of ipratropium bromide. At oral doses above 90 mg/kg/day in rats (about 3000 times the MRHD on a mg/m^2 basis) embryotoxicity was observed as increased resorption. This effect is not considered relevant to human use due to the large doses at which it was observed and the difference in route of administration. However, no adequate or well controlled studies have been conducted in pregnant women. Because animal reproduction studies are not always predictive of human response, ATROVENT® (ipratropium bromide) Nasal Spray 0.03% should be used during pregnancy only if clearly needed.

Nursing Mothers

It is known that some ipratropium bromide is systemically absorbed following nasal adminstration; however the portion which may be excreted in human milk is unknown. Although lipid-insoluble quaternary bases pass into breast milk, the minimal systemic absorption makes it unlikely that pratropium bromide would reach the infant in an amount sufficient to cause a clinical effect. However, because many drugs are excreted in human milk, caution should be exercised when ATROVENT® (ipratropium bromide) Nasal Spray 0.03% is administered to a nursing woman.

	% of Patients Reporting Events+			
	ATROVENT Nasal Spray 0.03% (n=356)		Vehicle Control (n=347)	
	Incidence %	Discontinued %	Incidence %	Discontinued %
Headache	9.8	0.6	9.2	0
Upper respiratory tract infection	9.8	1.4	7.2	1.4
Epistaxis[1]	9.0	0.3	4.6	0.3
Rhinitis*				
Nasal dryness	5.1	0	0.9	0.3
Nasal irritation[2]	2.0	0	1.7	0.6
Other nasal symptoms[3]	3.1	1.1	1.7	0.3
Pharyngitis	8.1	0.3	4.6	0
Nausea	2.2	0.3	0.9	0

1 Epistaxis reported by 7.0% of ATROVENT® patients and 2.3% of vehicle patients, blood-tinged mucus by 2.0% of ATROVENT® patients and 2.3% of vehicle patients.
2 Nasal irritation includes reports of nasal itching, nasal burning, nasal irritation and ulcerative rhinitis.
3 Other nasal symptoms include reports of nasal congestion, increased rhinorrhea, increased rhinitis, posterior nasal drip, sneezing, nasal polyps and nasal edema.
+ This table includes adverse events which occurred at an incidence of at least 2.0% in the ATROVENT® group and more frequently in the ATROVENT® group than in the vehicle group.
* All events are listed by their WHO term; rhinitis has been presented by descriptive terms for clarification.

Pediatric Use

Safety and effectiveness of ATROVENT® (ipratropium bromide) Nasal Spray 0.03% in patients below the age of 12 years have not been established.

ADVERSE REACTIONS

Adverse reaction information on ATROVENT® (ipratropium bromide) Nasal Spray 0.03% in patients with perennial rhinitis was derived from four multicenter, vehicle-controlled clinical trials involving 703 patients (356 patients on ATROVENT® and 347 patients on vehicle), and a one-year, open-label, follow-up trial. In three of the trials, patients received ATROVENT® (ipratropium bromide) Nasal Spray 0.03% three times daily, for eight weeks. In the other trial, ATROVENT® (ipratropium bromide) Nasal Spray 0.03% was given to patients two times daily for four weeks. Of the 285 patients who entered the open-label, follow-up trial, 232 were treated for 3 months, 200 for 6 months, and 159 up to one year. The majority (>86%) of patients treated for one year were maintained on 42 mcg per nostril, two or three times daily, of ATROVENT® (ipratropium bromide) Nasal Spray 0.03%.

The following table shows adverse events, and the frequency that these adverse events led to the discontinuation of treatment, reported for patients who received ATROVENT® (ipratropium bromide) Nasal Spray 0.03%, at the recommended dose of 42 mcg per nostril, or vehicle, two or three times daily for four or eight weeks. Only adverse events reported with an incidence of at least 2.0% in the ATROVENT® group and higher in the ATROVENT® group than in the vehicle group are shown.

[See table above.]

ATROVENT® (ipratropium bromide) Nasal Spray 0.03% was well tolerated by most patients. The most frequently reported nasal adverse events were transient episodes of nasal dryness or epistaxis. These adverse events were mild or moderate in nature, none was considered serious, none resulted in hospitalization and most resolved spontaneously or following a dose reduction. Treatment for nasal dryness and epistaxis was required infrequently (2% or less) and consisted of local application of pressure or a moisturizing agent (e.g., petroleum jelly or saline nasal spray). Patient discontinuation for epistaxis or nasal dryness was infrequent in both the controlled (0.3% or less) and one-year, open-label (2% or less) trials. There was no evidence of nasal rebound (i.e., a clinically significant increase in rhinorrhea, posterior nasal drip, sneezing or nasal congestion severity compared to baseline) upon discontinuation of double-blind therapy in these trials.

Adverse events reported by less than 2% of the patients receiving ATROVENT® (ipratropium bromide) Nasal Spray 0.03% during the controlled clinical trials or during the open-label follow-up trial, which are potentially related to ATROVENT®'s local effects or systemic anticholinergic effects include: dry mouth/throat, dizziness, ocular irritation, blurred vision, conjunctivitis, hoarseness, cough and taste perversion. Additional anticholinergic effects noted with other ATROVENT® dosage forms (ATROVENT® Inhalation Solution, ATROVENT® Inhalation Aerosol and ATROVENT® Nasal Spray 0.06%) include: precipitation or worsening of narrow angle glaucoma, urinary retention, prostatic disorders, tachycardia, constipation, and bowel obstruction.

There were infrequent reports of skin rash in both the controlled and uncontrolled clinical studies. Other allergic-type reactions such as angioedema of the throat, tongue, lips and face, urticaria, laryngospasm and anaphylactic reactions have been reported with other ipratropium bromide products.

No controlled trial was conducted to address the relative incidence of adverse events of BID versus TID therapy.

OVERDOSAGE

Acute overdosage by intranasal administration is unlikely since ipratropium bromide is not well absorbed systemically after intranasal or oral administration. Following administration of a 20 mg oral dose (equivalent to ingesting more than four bottles of ATROVENT® Nasal Spray 0.03%) to 10 male volunteers, no change in heart rate or blood pressure was noted. Following a 2 mg intravenous infusion over 15 minutes to the same 10 male volunteers, plasma ipratropium concentrations of 22–45 ng/mL were observed (>100 times the concentrations observed following intranasal administration). Following intravenous infusion these 10 volunteers had a mean increase of heart rate of 50 bpm and less than 20 mm Hg change in systolic or diastolic blood pressure at the time of peak ipratropium levels.

The oral LD_{50} of ipratropium bromide ranged between 1000 and 2000 mg/kg in mice (about 5,000 and 10,000 times the MRHD on a mg/m^2 basis, respectively); between 1700 and 4000 mg/kg in rats (about 9,000 and 20,000 times the MRHD on a mg/m^2 basis, respectively); and between 400 and 1300 mg/kg in dogs (about 2,000 and 7,000 times the MRHD on a mg/m^2 basis, respectively). Target organs of toxicity at repeated doses were liver, GI tract, adrenals (rat), male reproductive organs and eyes (dog).

DOSAGE AND ADMINISTRATION

The recommended dose of ATROVENT® (ipratropium bromide) Nasal Spray 0.03% is two sprays (42 mcg) per nostril two or three times daily (total dose 168 to 252 mcg/day) for the symptomatic relief of rhinorrhea associated with allergic and nonallergic perennial rhinitis in adults and children age 12 years and older. Optimum dosage varies with the response of the individual patient.

Initial pump priming requires seven actuations of the pump. If used regularly as recommended, no further priming is required. If not used for more than 24 hours, the pump will require two actuations, or if not used for more than seven days, the pump will require seven actuations to reprime.

HOW SUPPLIED

ATROVENT® (ipratropium bromide) Nasal Spray 0.03% is supplied as 30 ml of solution in a high density polyethylene (HDPE) bottle fitted with a metered nasal spray pump, a safety clip to prevent accidental discharge of the spray, and a clear plastic dust cap. The 30 ml bottle of ATROVENT® Nasal Spray is designed to deliver 345 sprays of 0.07 ml each (21 mcg ipratropium bromide), or 28 days of therapy at the maximum recommended dose (two sprays per nostril three times a day).

Store tightly closed between 59°F (15°C) and 86°F (30°C). Avoid freezing. Keep out of reach of children. Avoid spraying in or around the eyes.

Patients should be reminded to read and follow the accompanying Patient's Instructions for Use, which should be dispensed with the product.

CAUTION Federal law prohibits dispensing without prescription.

Manufactured by:
Boehringer Ingelheim
Pharmaceuticals, Inc.
Ridgefield, CT 06877
Licensed from:
Boehringer Ingelheim
International GmbH
U.S. Patent No. 4,385,048 AN.03-PI-10/95

Shown in Product Identification Guide, page 306

Continued on next page

Boehringer Ingelheim—Cont.

ATTENTION PHARMACIST: Detach "Patient's Instruction for Use" from package insert and dispense it with product.

ATROVENT® ℞
(ipratropium bromide)
Nasal Spray 0.06%

Prescribing Information

DESCRIPTION

The active ingredient in ATROVENT® Nasal Spray is ipratropium bromide monohydrate. It is an anticholinergic agent chemically described as 8-azoniabicyclo (3.2.1) octane,3-(3-hydroxy-1-oxo-2-phenylpropoxy)-8-methyl-8-(1-methylet hyl), bromide, monohydrate (*endo, syn*)-, (±)- : a synthetic quaternary ammonium compound, chemically related to atropine. Its structural formula is:

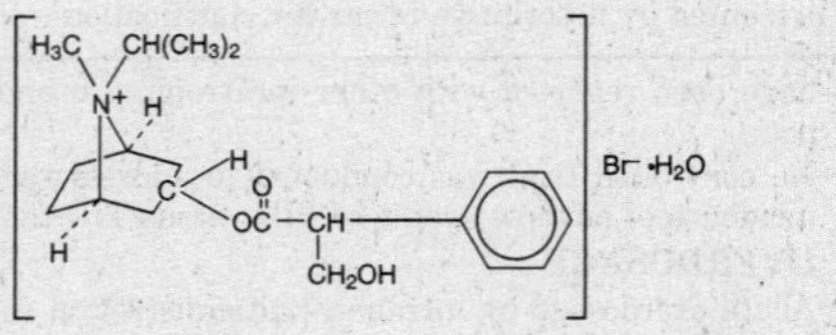

$C_{20}H_{30}BrNO_3 \bullet H_2O$
Mol. Wt. 430.4

ipratropium bromide monohydrate

Ipratropium bromide is a white to off-white, crystalline substance. It is freely soluble in lower alcohols and water, existing in an ionized state in aqueous solutions, and relatively insoluble in non-polar media.

ATROVENT® (ipratropium bromide) Nasal Spray 0.06% is intended for local administration to the nasal mucosa to control rhinorrhea in patients with the common cold. It contains 0.06% ipratropium bromide on an anhydrous basis (42 mcg/spray) in an isotonic, aqueous solution with pH adjusted to 4.7, which also contains benzalkonium chloride, edetate disodium, sodium chloride, sodium hydroxide, hydrochloric acid, and purified water.

CLINICAL PHARMACOLOGY

Mechanism of Action

Ipratropium bromide is an anticholinergic agent that inhibits vagally mediated reflexes by antagonizing the action of acetylcholine at the cholinergic receptor. In humans, ipratropium bromide has anti-secretory properties and, when applied locally, inhibits secretions from the serous and seromucous glands lining the nasal mucosa. Ipratropium bromide is a quaternary amine that minimally crosses the nasal and gastrointestinal membrane and the blood-brain barrier, resulting in a reduction of the systemic anticholinergic effects (e.g., neurologic, ophthalmic, cardiovascular and gastrointestinal effects) that are seen with tertiary anticholinergic amines.

Pharmacokinetics

Ipratropium bromide is a quaternary amine that is poorly absorbed into the systemic circulation from the nasal mucosa. Less than 20% of an 84 mcg per nostril dose is absorbed from the nasal mucosa of normal volunteers, induced-cold patients or perennial rhinitis patients, but the amount of ipratropium bromide which is systemically absorbed from nasal administration exceeds the amount of ipratropium bromide absorbed from either ATROVENT® Inhalation Solution (2% of a 500 mcg dose) or ATROVENT® Inhalation Aerosol (20% of a 36 mcg mouthpiece dose).

The half-life of elimination of ipratropium is about 1.6 hours after intravenous administration. Ipratropium bromide is minimally bound (0 to 9% *in vitro*) to plasma albumin and α_1-acid glycoprotein. It is partially metabolized to inactive ester hydrolysis products. Following intravenous administration, approximately one-half of the dose is excreted unchanged in the urine. Studies in rats have shown that ipratropium bromide does not penetrate the blood-brain barrier. The pharmacokinetics of ipratropium bromide have not been studied in patients with hepatic or renal insufficiency or in the elderly. Gender does not seem to influence the absorption or excretion of nasally administered ipratropium bromide.

Pharmacodynamic data also indicate little systemic absorption. In two single dose, pharmacokinetic trials (n = 17), solutions of up to 0.12% ipratropium bromide (336 mcg total nasal dose) did not significantly affect pupillary diameter, heart rate or systolic/diastolic blood pressure. Similarly, in an induced-cold, pharmacokinetic trial with ATROVENT® (ipratropium bromide) Nasal Spray 0.06% (84 mcg/nostril four times a day) no significant effects on pupillary diameter, heart rate or systolic/diastolic blood pressures were observed.

Controlled clinical trials demonstrated that intranasal fluorocarbon-propelled ipratropium bromide does not alter physiologic nasal functions (e.g., sense of smell, ciliary beat frequency, mucociliary clearance, or the air conditioning capacity of the nose).

Clinical Trials

The clinical trials for ATROVENT® (ipratropium bromide) Nasal Spray 0.06% were conducted in patients with rhinorrhea associated with naturally occurring common colds. In two controlled four day comparisons of ATROVENT® (ipratropium bromide) Nasal Spray 0.06% (84 mcg per nostril, administered three or four times daily; n=352) with its vehicle (n=351), there was a statistically significant reduction of rhinorrhea, as measured by both nasal discharge weight and the patients' subjective assessment of severity of rhinorrhea using a visual analog scale. These significant differences were evident within one hour following dosing. There was no effect of ATROVENT® (ipratropium bromide) Nasal Spray 0.06% on degree of nasal congestion or sneezing. The response to ATROVENT® (ipratropium bromide) Nasal Spray 0.06% did not appear to be affected by age or gender. No controlled clinical trials directly compared the efficacy of TID versus QID treatment.

INDICATIONS AND USAGE

ATROVENT® (ipratropium bromide) Nasal Spray 0.06% is indicated for the symptomatic relief of rhinorrhea associated with the common cold for adults and children age 12 years and older. ATROVENT® (ipratropium bromide) Nasal Spray 0.06% does not relieve nasal congestion or sneezing associated with the common cold.

The safety and effectiveness of the use of ATROVENT® (ipratropium bromide) Nasal Spray 0.06% beyond four days in patients with the common cold has not been established.

CONTRAINDICATIONS

ATROVENT® (ipratropium bromide) Nasal Spray 0.06% is contraindicated in patients with a history of hypersensitivity to atropine or its derivatives, or to any of the other ingredients.

WARNINGS

Immediate hypersensitivity reactions may occur after administration of ipratropium bromide, as demonstrated by rare cases of urticaria, angioedema, rash, bronchospasm and oropharyngeal edema.

PRECAUTIONS

General

ATROVENT® (ipratropium bromide) Nasal Spray 0.06% should be used with caution in patients with narrow-angle glaucoma, prostatic hypertrophy or bladder neck obstruction, particularly if they are receiving an anticholinergic by another route. Cases of precipitation or worsening of narrow-angle glaucoma and acute eye pain have been reported with direct eye contact of ipratropium bromide administered by oral inhalation.

Information for Patients

Patients should be advised that temporary blurring of vision, precipitation or worsening of narrow-angle glaucoma or eye pain may result if ATROVENT® (ipratropium bromide) Nasal Spray 0.06% comes into direct contact with the eyes. Patients should be instructed to avoid spraying ATROVENT® (ipratropium bromide) Nasal Spray 0.06% in or around the eyes. Patients who experience eye pain, blurred vision, excessive nasal dryness or episodes of nasal bleeding should be instructed to contact their doctor. Patients should be reminded to carefully read and follow the accompanying Patient's Instructions for Use.

Drug Interactions

No controlled clinical trials were conducted to investigate potential drug-drug interactions. ATROVENT® (ipratropium bromide) Nasal Spray 0.06% is minimally absorbed into the systemic circulation; nonetheless there is some potential for an additive interaction with other concomitantly administered anticholinergic medications, including ATROVENT® for oral inhalation.

Carcinogenesis, Mutagenesis, Impairment of Fertility

Two-year oral carcinogenicity studies in rats and mice have revealed no carcinogenic activity at doses up to 6 mg/kg/day. This dose corresponds, in rats and mice respectively, to about 70 and 40 times the maximum recommended human daily dose (MRHD) on a mg/m^2 basis of ATROVENT® (ipratropium bromide) Nasal Spray 0.06%. Results of various mutagenicity studies (Ames test, mouse dominant lethal test, mouse micronucleus test and chromosome aberration of bone marrow in Chinese hamsters) were negative.

Fertility of male or female rats at oral doses up to 50 mg/kg/day (about 600 times the MRHD on a mg/m^2 basis) was unaffected by ipratropium bromide administration. At doses above 90 mg/kg/day (about 1,000 times the MRHD on a mg/m^2 basis) a decreased conception rate was observed.

Pregnancy

TERATOGENIC EFFECTS Pregnancy Category B. Oral reproduction studies were performed at doses of 10 mg/kg/day in mice, 100 mg/kg/day in rats and 125 mg/kg/day in rabbits. These doses correspond, in each species respectively, to about 60, 1,200 and 3,000 times the MRHD of ATROVENT® (ipratropium bromide) Nasal Spray 0.06% in the common cold (672 mcg/day) on a mg/m^2 basis. Inhalation reproduction studies in rats and rabbits at doses of 1.5 and 1.8 mg/kg/day (about 20 and 40 times the MRHD dose on a mg/m^2 basis for each species, respectively) have demonstrated no evidence of teratogenic effects as a result of ipratropium bromide. At oral doses above 90 mg/kg/day in rats (about 1,000 times the MRHD on a mg/m^2 basis) embryotoxicity was observed as increased resorption. This effect is not considered relevant to human use due to the large doses at which it was observed and the difference in route of administration. However, no adequate or well controlled studies have been conducted in pregnant women. Because animal reproduction studies are not always predictive of human response, ATROVENT® (ipratropium bromide) Nasal spray 0.06% should be used during pregnancy only if clearly needed.

Nursing Mothers

It is known that some ipratropium bromide is systemically absorbed following nasal administration; however the portion which may be excreted in human milk is unknown. Although lipid-insoluble quaternary bases pass into breast milk, the minimal systemic absorption makes it unlikely that ipratropium bromide would reach the infant in an amount sufficient to cause a clinical effect. However, because many drugs are excreted in human milk, caution should be exercised when ATROVENT® (ipratropium bromide) Nasal Spray 0.06% is administered to a nursing woman.

Pediatric Use

Safety and effectiveness of ATROVENT® (ipratropium bromide) Nasal Spray 0.06% in patients below the age of 12 years have not been established.

ADVERSE REACTIONS

Adverse reaction information on ATROVENT® (ipratropium bromide) Nasal Spray 0.06% in patients with the common cold was derived from two multicenter, vehicle-controlled clinical trials involving 1276 patients (195 patients on ATROVENT® Nasal Spray 0.03%, 352 patients on ATROVENT® Nasal Spray 0.06%, 189 patients on ATROVENT® Nasal Spray 0.12%, 351 patients on vehicle and 189 patients receiving no treatment).

The following table shows adverse events reported for patients who received ATROVENT® (ipratropium bromide) Nasal Spray 0.06% at the recommended dose of 84 mcg per nostril, or vehicle, administered three or four times daily, where the incidence is 1% or greater in the ATROVENT® group, and higher in the ATROVENT® group than in the vehicle group.

% of Patients Reporting Events[1]

	ATROVENT® Nasal Spray 0.06% (n = 352)	Vehicle Control (n = 351)
Epistaxis[2]	8.2%	2.3%
Dry Mouth/Throat	1.4%	0.3%
Nasal Congestion	1.1%	0.0%
Nasal Dryness	4.8%	2.8%

1 This table includes adverse events for which the incidence was 1% or greater in the ATROVENT® group and higher in the ATROVENT® group than in the vehicle group

2 Epistaxis reported by 5.4% of ATROVENT® patients and 1.4% of vehicle patients, blood-tinged nasal mucus by 2.8% of ATROVENT® patients and 0.9% of vehicle patients.

ATROVENT® (ipratropium bromide) Nasal Spray 0.06% was well tolerated by most patients. The most frequently reported adverse events were transient episodes of nasal dryness or epistaxis. The majority of these adverse events (96%) were mild or moderate in nature, none was considered serious and none resulted in hospitalization. No patient required treatment for nasal dryness and only three patients (<1%) required treatment for epistaxis, which consisted of local application of pressure or a moisturizing agent (e.g., petroleum jelly). No patient receiving ATROVENT® (ipratropium bromide) Nasal Spray 0.06% was discontinued from the trial due to other nasal dryness or bleeding.

Adverse events reported by less than 1% of the patients receiving ATROVENT® (ipratropium bromide) Nasal Spray 0.06% during the controlled clinical trials which are potentially related to ATROVENT®'s local effects or systemic anticholinergic effects include: taste perversion, nasal burning, conjunctivitis, coughing, dizziness, hoarseness, palpitation, pharyngitis, tachycardia, thirst, tinnitus and blurred

vision. Additional anticholinergic effects noted with other ATROVENT® dosage forms (ATROVENT® Inhalation Solution, ATROVENT® Inhalation Aerosol and ATROVENT® Nasal Spray 0.03%) include: precipitation or worsening of narrow-angle glaucoma, urinary retention, prostate disorders, constipation and bowel obstruction.

There were no reports of allergic-type reactions in the controlled clinical trials. Allergic-type reactions such as skin rash, angioedema of the tongue, lips and face, urticaria, laryngospasm and anaphylactic reactions have been reported with other ipratropium bromide products.

No controlled trial was conducted to address the relative incidence of adverse events of TID versus QID therapy.

OVERDOSAGE

Acute overdosage by intranasal administration is unlikely since ipratropium bromide is not well absorbed systemically after intranasal or oral administration. Following administration of a 20 mg oral dose (equivalent to ingesting more than two bottles of ATROVENT® Nasal Spray 0.06%) to 10 male volunteers, no change in heart rate or blood pressure was noted. Following a 2 mg intravenous infusion over 15 minutes to the same 10 male volunteers, plasma ipratropium concentrations of 22–45 mg/mL were observed (> 100 times the concentrations observed following intranasal administration). Following intravenous infusion these 10 volunteers had a mean increase of heart rate of 50 bpm and less than 20 mm Hg change in systolic or diastolic blood pressure at the time of peak ipratropium levels.

The oral LD_{50} of ipratropium bromide ranged between 1000 and 2000 mg/kg in mice (about 2,000 and 4,000 times the MRHD on a mg/m^2 basis, respectively); between 1,700 and 4,000 mg/kg in rats (about 3,300 and 8,000 times the MRHD on a mg/m^2 basis, respectively); and between 400 and 1300 mg/kg in dogs (about 800 and 2,600 times the MRHD on a mg/m^2 basis, respectively). Target organs of toxicity at repeated doses were liver, GI tract, adrenals (rat), male reproductive organs and eyes (dog).

DOSAGE AND ADMINISTRATION

The recommended dose of ATROVENT® (ipratropium bromide) Nasal Spray 0.06% is two sprays (84 mcg) per nostril three or four times daily (total dose 504 to 672 mcg/day) for the symptomatic relief of rhinorrhea associated with the common cold in adults and children age 12 years and older. Optimum dosage varies with the response of the individual patient.

The safety and effectiveness of the use of ATROVENT® (ipratropium bromide) Nasal Spray 0.06% beyond four days in patients with the common cold have not been established.

Initial pump priming requires seven actuations of the pump. If used regularly as recommended, no further priming is required. If not used for more than 24 hours, the pump will require two actuations, or if not used for more than seven days, the pump will require seven actuations to reprime.

HOW SUPPLIED

ATROVENT® (ipratropium bromide) Nasal Spray 0.06% is supplied as 15 ml of solution in a high density polyethylene (HDPE) bottle fitted with a metered nasal spray pump, a safety clip to prevent accidental discharge of the spray, and a clear plastic dust cap. The 15 ml bottle of ATROVENT® Nasal Spray 0.06% is designed to deliver 165 sprays of 0.07 ml each (42 mcg ipratropium bromide).

Store tightly closed between 59°F (15°C) and 86°F (30°C). Avoid freezing. Keep out of reach of children. Avoid spraying in or around the eyes.

Patients should be reminded to read and follow the accompanying Patient's Instructions for Use, which should be dispensed with the product.

CAUTION Federal law prohibits dispensing without prescription.

Manufactured by:
Boehringer Ingelheim
Pharmaceuticals, Inc.
Ridgefield, CT 06877
Licensed from:
Boehringer Ingelheim
International GmbH
U.S. Patent No. 4,385,048 AN.06-PI-10/95

Shown in Product Identification Guide, page 306

CATAPRES® ℞

[kah 'tah-pres]
(clonidine hydrochloride USP)
Oral Antihypertensive
Tablets, 0.1, 0.2 and 0.3 mg
Prescribing Information

DESCRIPTION

CATAPRES (clonidine hydrochloride USP) is a centrally acting alpha-agonist hypotensive agent available as tablets for oral administration in three dosage strengths: 0.1 mg, 0.2 mg and 0.3 mg. The 0.1 mg tablet is equivalent to 0.087 mg of the free base.

The inactive ingredients are colloidal silicon dioxide, corn starch, dibasic calcium phosphate, FD&C Yellow No. 6, gelatin, glycerin, lactose, magnesium stearate, methylparaben, propylparaben. The CATAPRES 0.1 mg tablet also contains FD&C Blue No. 1 and FD&C Red No. 3.

Clonidine hydrochloride is an imidazoline derivative and exists as a mesomeric compound. The chemical name is 2-(2,6-dichlorophenylamino)-2-imidazoline hydrochloride. The following is the structural formula:

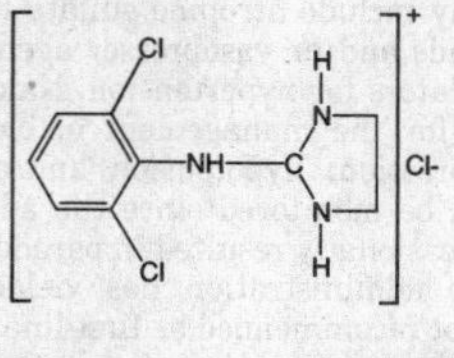

$C_9H_9Cl_2N_3 \cdot HCl$ Mol. Wt. 266.56

Clonidine hydrochloride is an odorless, bitter, white, crystalline substance soluble in water and alcohol.

CLINICAL PHARMACOLOGY

Clonidine stimulates alpha-adrenoreceptors in the brain stem. This action results in reduced sympathetic outflow from the central nervous system and in decreases in peripheral resistance, renal vascular resistance, heart rate, and blood pressure. CATAPRES (clonidine hydrochloride USP) acts relatively rapidly. The patients blood pressure declines within 30 to 60 minutes after an oral dose, the maximum decrease occurring within 2 to 4 hours. Renal blood flow and glomerular filtration rate remain essentially unchanged. Normal postural reflexes are intact; therefore, orthostatic symptoms are mild and infrequent.

Acute studies with clonidine hydrochloride in humans have demonstrated a moderate reduction (15% to 20%) of cardiac output in the supine position with no change in the peripheral resistance; at a 45° tilt there is a smaller reduction in cardiac output and a decrease of peripheral resistance. During long term therapy, cardiac output tends to return to control values, while peripheral resistance remains decreased. Slowing of the pulse rate has been observed in most patients given clonidine, but the drug does not alter normal hemodynamic response to exercise.

Tolerance to the antihypertensive effect may develop in some patients, necessitating a reevaluation of therapy.

Other studies in patients have provided evidence of a reduction in plasma renin activity and in the excretion of aldosterone and catecholamines. The exact relationship of these pharmacologic actions to the antihypertensive effect of clonidine has not been fully elucidated.

Clonidine acutely stimulates growth hormone release in both children and adults, but does not produce a chronic elevation of growth hormone with long-term use.

Pharmacokinetics: The plasma level of clonidine peaks in approximately 3 to 5 hours and the plasma half-life ranges from 12 to 16 hours. The half-life increases up to 41 hours in patients with severe impairment of renal function. Following oral administration about 40–60% of the absorbed dose is recovered in the urine as unchanged drug in 24 hours. About 50% of the absorbed dose is metabolized in the liver.

INDICATIONS AND USAGE

CATAPRES (clonidine hydrochloride USP) is indicated in the treatment of hypertension. CATAPRES may be employed alone or concomitantly with other antihypertensive agents.

CONTRAINDICATIONS

CATAPRES (clonidine hydrochloride USP) Tablets should not be used in patients with known hypersensitivity to clonidine (see PRECAUTIONS).

WARNINGS

Withdrawal Patients should be instructed not to discontinue therapy without consulting their physician. Sudden cessation of clonidine treatment has, in some cases, resulted in symptoms such as nervousness, agitation, headache, and tremor accompanied or followed by a rapid rise in blood pressure and elevated catecholamine concentrations in the plasma. The likelihood of such reactions to discontinuation of clonidine therapy appears to be greater after administration of higher doses or continuation of concomitant beta-blocker treatment and special caution is therefore advised in these situations. Rare instances of hypertensive encephalopathy, cerebrovascular accidents and death have been reported after clonidine withdrawal. When discontinuing therapy with CATAPRES®, the physician should reduce the dose gradually over 2 to 4 days to avoid withdrawal symptomatology.

An excessive rise in blood pressure following discontinuation of CATAPRES-TTS® therapy can be reversed by administration of oral clonidine hydrochloride or by intravenous phentolamine. If therapy is to be discontinued in patients receiving a beta-blocker and clonidine concurrently, the beta-blocker should be withdrawn several days before the gradual discontinuation of CATAPRES-TTS®.

"Because children commonly have gastrointestinal illnesses that lead to vomiting, they may be particularly susceptible to hypertensive episodes resulting from abrupt inability to take medication."

PRECAUTIONS

General: In patients who have developed localized contact sensitization to CATAPRES-TTS® (clonidine), continuation of CATAPRES-TTS or substitution of oral clonidine hydrochloride therapy may be associated with the development of a generalized skin rash.

In patients who develop an allergic reaction to CATAPRES-TTS, substitution of oral clonidine hydrochloride may also elicit an allergic reaction (including generalized rash, urticaria, or angioedema).

CATAPRES (clonidine hydrochloride) should be used with caution in patients with severe coronary insufficiency, conduction disturbances, recent myocardial infarction, cerebrovascular disease or chronic renal failure.

Perioperative Use: Administration of CATAPRES should be continued to within four hours of surgery and resumed as soon as possible thereafter. The blood pressure should be carefully monitored and appropriate measures instituted to control it as necessary. Blood pressure should be carefully monitored during surgery and additional measures to control blood pressure should be available if required.

Information for Patients Patients should be cautioned against interruption of CATAPRES therapy without their physician's advice.

Patients who engage in potentially hazardous activities, such as operating machinery or driving, should be advised of a possible sedative effect of clonidine. They should also be informed that this sedative effect may be increased by concomitant use of alcohol, barbiturates, or other sedating drugs.

Drug Interactions: Clonidine may potentiate the CNS-depressive effects of alcohol, barbiturates or other sedating drugs. If a patient receiving clonidine hydrochloride is also taking tricyclic antidepressants, the hypotensive effect of clonidine may be reduced, necessitating an increase in the clonidine dose.

Due to a potential for additive effects such as bradycardia and AV block, caution is warranted in patients receiving clonidine concomitantly with agents known to affect sinus node function or AV nodal conduction, e.g. digitalis, calcium channel blockers and beta-blockers.

Amitriptyline in combination with clonidine enhances the manifestation of corneal lesions in rats (see TOXICOLOGY).

Toxicology—In several studies with oral clonidine hydrochloride, a dose-dependent increase in the incidence and severity of spontaneous retinal degeneration was seen in albino rats treated for six months or longer. Tissue distribution studies in dogs and monkeys showed a concentration of clonidine in the choroid.

In view of the retinal degeneration seen in rats, eye examinations were performed during clinical trials in 908 patients before, and periodically after, the start of clonidine therapy. In 353 of these 908 patients, the eye examinations were carried out over periods of 24 months or longer. Except for some dryness of the eyes, no drug-related abnormal ophthalmological findings were recorded and, according to specialized tests such as electroretinography and macular dazzle, retinal function was unchanged.

In combination with amitriptyline, clonidine hydrochloride administration led to the development of corneal lesions in rats within 5 days.

Carcinogenesis, Mutagenesis, Impairment of Fertility: Chronic dietary administration of clonidine was not carcinogenic to rats (132 weeks) or mice (78 weeks) dosed, respectively, at up to 46 or 70 times the maximum recommended daily human dose as mg/kg (9 or 6 times the MRHD on a mg/m^2 basis). There was no evidence of genotoxicity in the Ames test for mutagenicity or mouse micronucleus test for clastogenicity.

Fertility of male or female rats was unaffected by clonidine doses as high as 150 mcg/kg (approximately 3 times the MRDHD). In a separate experiment, fertility of female rats appeared to be affected at dose levels of 500 to 2000 mcg/kg (10 to 40 times the oral MRDHD on a mg/kg basis; 2 to 8 times the MRDHD on a mg/m^2, basis).

Usage in Pregnancy: *TERATOGENIC EFFECTS Pregnancy Category C* Reproduction studies performed in rabbits at doses up to approximately 3 times the oral maximum recommended daily human dose (MRDHD) of CATAPRES (clonidine hydrochloride) produced no evidence of a teratogenic or embryotoxic potential in rabbits. In rats, however, doses as low as ⅓ the oral MRDHD ($^1/_{15}$ the MRDHD on a mg/m^2 basis) of clonidine were associated with increased resorptions in a study in which dams were treated continuously

Continued on next page

Boehringer Ingelheim—Cont.

	Programmed Delivery Clonidine *in vivo* Per Day Over 1 Week	Clonidine Content	Size	Code
Catapres-TTS®-1 (clonidine)	0.1 mg	2.5 mg	3.5 cm^2	BI-31
Catapres-TTS®-2 (clonidine)	0.2 mg	5.0 mg	7.0 cm^2	BI-32
Catapres-TTS®-3 (clonidine)	0.3 mg	7.5 mg	10.5 cm^2	BI-33

from 2 months prior to mating. Increased resorptions were not associated with treatment at the same or at higher dose levels (up to 3 times the oral MRDHD) when the dams were treated on gestation days 6–15. Increases in resorption were observed at much higher dose levels (40 times the oral MRDHD on a mg/kg basis; 4 to 8 times the MRDHD on a mg/m^2 basis) in mice and rats treated on gestation days 1–14 (lowest dose employed in the study was 500 mcg/kg).
No adequate, well-controlled studies have been conducted in pregnant women. Because animal reproduction studies are not always predictive of human response, this drug should be used during pregnancy only if clearly needed.
Nursing Mothers: As clonidine hydrochloride is excreted in human milk, caution should be exercised when CATAPRES (clonidine hydrochloride USP) is administered to a nursing woman.
Pediatric Use: Safety and effectiveness in pediatric patients below the age of twelve have not been established (See Warnings on Withdrawal).

ADVERSE REACTIONS

Most adverse effects are mild and tend to diminish with continued therapy. The most frequent (which appear to be dose-related) are dry mouth, occurring in about 40 of 100 patients; drowsiness, about 33 in 100; dizziness, about 16 in 100; constipation and sedation, each about 10 in 100.
The following less frequent adverse experiences have also been reported in patients receiving CATAPRES (clonidine hydrochloride USP), but in many cases patients were receiving concomitant medication and a causal relationship has not been established.
Body as a Whole: Weakness, about 10 in 100 patients; fatigue, about 4 in 100; headache and withdrawal syndrome each about 1 in 100. Also reported were pallor; a weakly positive Coombs' test; increased sensitivity to alcohol; and fever.
Cardiovascular: Orthostatic symptoms, about 3 in 100 patients; palpitations and tachycardia, and bradycardia, each about 5 in 1000. Syncope, Raynaud's phenomenon, congestive heart failure, and electrocardiographic abnormalities (i.e. sinus node arrest, functional bradycardia, high degree AV block and arrhythmias) have been reported rarely. Rare cases of sinus bradycardia and atrioventricular block have been reported, both with and without the use of concomitant digitalis.
Central Nervous System: Nervousness and agitation, about 3 in 100 patients, mental depression, about 1 in 100 and insomnia, about 5 in 1000. Other behavioral changes, vivid dreams or nightmares, restlessness, anxiety, visual and auditory hallucinations and delirium have rarely been reported.
Dermatological: Rash, about 1 in 100 patients; pruritus, about 7 in 1000; hives, angioneurotic edema and urticaria, about 5 in 1000; alopecia, about 2 in 1000.
Gastrointestinal: Nausea and vomiting, about 5 in 100 patients; anorexia and malaise, each about 1 in 100; mild transient abnormalities in liver function tests, about 1 in 100; hepatitis, parotitis, constipation, pseudo-obstruction, and abdominal pain, rarely.
Genitourinary: Decreased sexual activity, impotence and loss of libido, about 3 in 100 patients; nocturia, about 1 in 100; difficulty in micturition, about 2 in 1000; urinary retention, about 1 in 1000.
Hemotologic: Thrombocytopenia, rarely.
Metabolic Weight gain, about 1 in 100 patients; gynecomastia, about 1 in 1000; transient elevation of blood glucose or serum creatine phosphokinase, rarely.
Musculoskeletal—Muscle or joint pain, about 6 in 1000 and leg cramps, about 3 in 1000.
Oro-otolaryngeal: Dryness of the nasal mucosa was reported.
Ophthalmological: Dryness of the eyes, burning of the eyes and blurred vision were reported.

OVERDOSAGE

Hypertension may develop early and may be followed by hypotension, bradycardia, respiratory depression, hypothermia, drowsiness, decreased or absent reflexes, weakness, irritability and miosis. The frequency of CNS depression may be higher in children than adults. Large overdoses may result in reversible cardiac conduction defects or dysrhythmias, apnea, coma and seizures. Signs and symptoms of overdose generally occur within 30 minutes to two hours after exposure. As little as 0.1 mg of clonidine has produced signs of toxicity in children.
There is no specific antidote for clonidine overdose. Clonidine overdosage may result in the rapid development of CNS depression; therefore, induction of vomiting with ipecac syrup is not recommended. Gastric lavage may be indicated following recent and/or large ingestions. Administration of activated charcoal and/or a cathartic may be beneficial. Supportive care may include atropine sulfate for bradycardia, intravenous fluids and/or vasopressor agents for hypotension and vasodilators for hypertension. Naloxone may be a useful adjunct for the management of clonidine-induced respiratory depression, hypotension and/or coma; blood pressure should be monitored since the administration of naloxone has occasionally resulted in paradoxical hypertension. Tolazoline administration has yielded inconsistent results and is not recommended as first-line therapy. Dialysis is not likely to significantly enhance the elimination of clonidine.
The largest overdose reported to date involved a 28-year old male who ingested 100 mg of clonidine hydrochloride powder. This patient developed hypertension followed by hypotension, bradycardia, apnea, hallucinations, semicoma, and premature ventricular contractions. The patient fully recovered after intensive treatment. Plasma clonidine levels were 60 ng/ml after 1 hour, 190 ng/ml after 1.5 hours, 370 ng/ml after 2 hours, and 120 ng/ml after 5.5 and 6.5 hours. In mice and rats, the oral LD50 of clonidine is 206 and 465 mg/kg, respectively.

DOSAGE AND ADMINISTRATION

Adults: The dose of Catapres® (clonidine hydrochloride USP) must be adjusted according to the patient's individual blood pressure response. The following is a general guide to its administration.
Initial Dose: 0.1 mg tablet twice daily (morning and bedtime). Elderly patients may benefit from a lower initial dose.
Maintenance Dose: Further increments of 0.1 mg per day, may be made at weekly intervals if necessary until the desired response is achieved. Taking the larger portion of the oral daily dose at bedtime may minimize transient adjustment effects of dry mouth and drowsiness. The therapeutic doses most commonly employed have ranged from 0.2 mg to 0.6 mg per day given in divided doses. Studies have indicated that 2.4 mg is the maximum effective daily dose, but doses as high as this have rarely been employed.
Renal Impairment: Dosage must be adjusted according to the degree of impairment, and patients should be carefully monitored. Since only a minimal amount of clonidine is removed during routine hemodialysis, there is no need to give supplemental clonidine following dialysis.

HOW SUPPLIED

Catapres® (clonidine hydrochloride USP) is supplied in tablets containing 0.1 mg, 0.2 mg or 0.3 mg of clonidine hydrochloride.

[See table above.]

Store below 86°F (30°C).
Dispense in tight, light-resistant container.
Caution: Federal law prohibits dispensing without prescription.

Bottle of 1000	Unit Dose 100
NDC0597-0006-10	NDC0597-0006-61
NDC0597-0007-10	NDC0597-0007-61

Shown in Product Identification Guide, page 306

CATAPRES-TTS® ℞

(clonidine)
Transdermal Therapeutic System
Catapres-TTS -1
Catapres-TTS -2
Catapres-TTS -3
(clonidine)

Programmed delivery in vivo of 0.1, 0.2 or 0.3 mg clonidine per day, for one week.
Prescribing Information

DESCRIPTION

CATAPRES-TTS (clonidine) is a transdermal system providing continuous systemic delivery of clonidine for 7 days at an approximately constant rate. Clonidine is a centrally acting alpha-agonist hypotensive agent. It is an imidazoline derivative with the chemical name 2, 6–dichloro-N-2-imidazolidinylidenebenzenamine and has the following chemical structure:
[See chemical structure at top of next column.]
System Structure and Components: CATAPRES-TTS is a multilayered film, 0.2 mm thick, containing clonidine as the

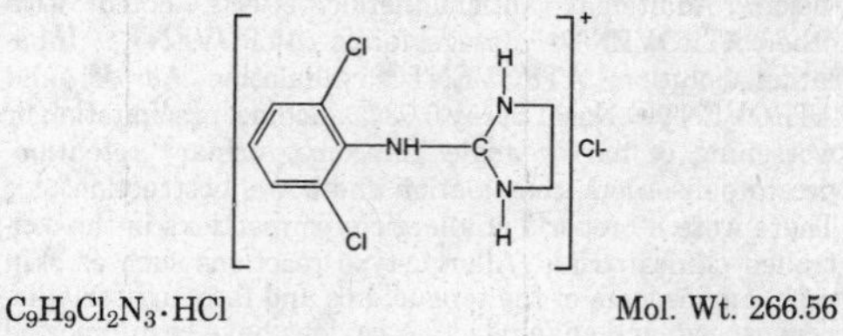

$C_9H_9Cl_2N_3 \cdot HCl$ Mol. Wt. 266.56

active agent. The system areas are 3.5 cm^2 (CATAPRES-TTS-1), 7.0 cm^2 (CATAPRES-TTS-2) and 10.5 cm^2 (CATAPRES-TTS-3) and the amount of drug released is directly proportional to the area (see Release Rate Concept). The composition per unit area is the same for all three doses. Proceeding from the visible surface towards the surface attached to the skin, there are four consecutive layers 1) a backing layer of pigmented polyester film; 2) a drug reservoir of clonidine, mineral oil, polyisobutylene, and colloidal silicon dioxide; 3) a microporous polypropylene membrane that controls the rate of delivery of clonidine from the system to the skin surface; 4) an adhesive formulation of clonidine, mineral oil, polyisobutylene, and colloidal silicon dioxide. Prior to use, a protective slit release liner of polyester that covers the adhesive layer is removed.
Corss-section of the sytsem:

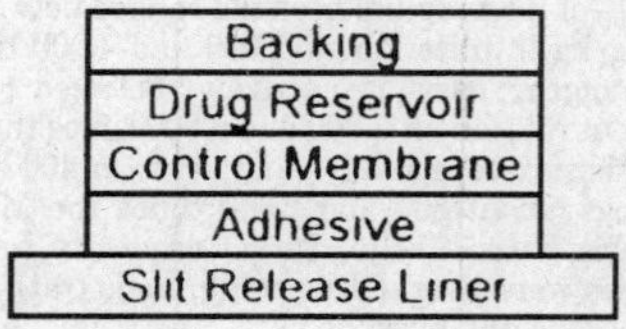

Release Rate Concept: CATAPRES-TTS is programmed to release clonidine at an approximately constant rate for 7 days. The energy for drug release is derived from the concentration gradient existing between a saturated solution of drug in the system and the much lower concentration prevailing in the skin. Clonidine flows in the direction of the lower concentration at a constant rate, limited by the rate-controlling membrane, so long as a saturated solution is maintained in the drug reservoir.
Following system application to intact skin, clonidine in the adhesive layer staurates the skin site below the system. Clonidine from the drug reservoir then begins to flow through the rate-controlling membrane and the adhesive layer of the system into the systemic circulation via the capillaries beneath the skin. Therapeutic plasma clonidine levels are achieved 2 to 3 days after initial application of CATAPRES-TTS.
The 3.5, 7.0, and 10.5 cm^2 systems deliver 0.1, 0.2, and 0.3 mg of clonidine per day, respectively. To ensure constant release of drug for 7 days, the total drug content of the system is higher than the total amount of drug delivered. Application of a new system to a fresh skin site at weekly intervals continuously maintains therapeutic plasma concentrations of clonidine. If the CATAPRES-TTS is removed and not replaced with a new system, therapeutic plasma clonidine levels will persist for about 8 hours and then decline slowly over several days. Over this time period, blood pressure returns gradually to pretreatment levels.

CLINICAL PHARMACOLOGY

Clonidine stimulates alpha-adrenoreceptors in the brain stem. This action results in reduced sympathetic outflow from the central nervous system and in decreases in peripheral resistance, renal vascular resistance, heart rate, and blood pressure. Renal blood flow and glomerular filtration rate remain essentially unchanged. Normal postural reflexes are intant; therefore, orthostatic symptoms are mild and infrequent.
Acute studies with clonidine hydrochloride in humans have demonstrated a moderate reduction (15–20%) of cardiac output in the supine position with no change in peripheral resistance, at a 45° tilt there is a smaller reduction in cardiac output and a decrease of peripheral resistance.
During long-term therapy, cardiac output tends to return to control values, while peripheral resistance remains decreased. Slowing of the pulse rate has been observed in most patients given clonidine, but the drug does not alter normal hemodynamic responses to exercise.
Tolerance to the antihypertensive effect may develop in some patients, necessitating a reevaluation of therapy.
Other studies in patients have provided evidence of a reduction in plasma renin activity and in the excretion of aldosterone and catecholamines. The exact relationship of these pharmacologic actions to the antihypertensive effect of clonidine has not been fully elucidated.

Clonidine acutely stimulates the release of growth hormone in children as well as adults but does not produce a chronic elevation of growth hormone with long-term use.

Pharmacokinetics: The plasma half-life of clonidine is 12.7 ± 7 hours. Following oral administration, about 40–60% of the absorbed dose is recovered in the urine as unchanged drug within 24 hours. The remainder of the absorbed dose is metabolized in the liver.

INDICATIONS AND USAGE

CATAPRES-TTs (clonidine) is indicated in the treatment of hypertension. It may be employed alone or concomitantly with other antihypertensive agents.

CONTRAINDICATIONS

CATAPRES-TTS (clonidine) should not be used in patients with known hypersensitivity to clonidine or to any other component of the therapeutic system.

PRECAUTIONS

General: In patients who have developed localized contact sensitization to CATAPRES-TTS (clonidine) continuation of CATAPRES-TTS or substitution of oral clonidine hydrochloride therapy may be associated with development of a generalized skin rash.

In patients who develop an allergic reaction to CATAPRES-TTS, substitution of oral clonidine hydrochloride may also elicit an allergic reaction (including generalized rash, urticaria, or angioedema).

CATAPRES-TTS should be used with caution in patients with severe coronary insufficiency, conduction distrubances, recent myocardial infarction, cerebrovascular disease, or chronic renal failure.

Withdrawal: Patients should be instructed not to discontinue therapy without consulting their physician. Sudden cessation of clonidine treatment has, in some cases, resulted in subjective symptoms such as nervousness, agitation, headache, and confusion accompanied or followed by a rapid rise in blood pressure and elevated catecholamine concentrations in the plasma. The likelihood of such reactions to discontinuation of clonidine therapy appears to be greater after administration of higher doses or continuation of concomitant beta-blocker treatment, and special caution is therefore advised in these situations. Rare instances of pulmonary edema, hypertensive encephalopathy, cerebrovascular accident and death have been reported after clonidine withdrawal.

An excessive rise in blood pressure following discontinuation of CATAPRES-TTS therapy can be reversed by administration of oral clonidine HCl or by intravenous phentolamine. If therapy is to be discontinued in patients receiving a beta-blocker and clonidine concurrently, the beta-blocker should be withdrawn several days before cessation of CATAPRES-TTS administration.

In rare instances, loss of blood pressure control has been reported in patients using CATAPRES-TTs® according to the instructions for use.

Perioperative Use: CATAPRES-TTS therapy should not be interrupted during the surgical period. Blood pressure should be carefully monitored during surgery and additional measures to control blood pressure should be available if required. Physicians considering starting CATAPRES-TTS therapy during the perioperative period must be aware that therapetic plasma clonidine levels are not achieved until 2 to 3 days after initial application of CATAPRES-TTs (see DOSAGE AND ADMINISTRATION).

Defibrillation or Cardioversion: The transdermal clonidine systems should be removed before attempting defibrillation or cardioversion because of the potential for altered electrical conductivity which may increase the risk of arcing, a phenomenon associated with the use of defibrillators.

Information for Patients: Patients should be cautioned against interruption of CATAPRES-TTS therapy without their physicians' advice.

Patients who engage in potentially hazardous activities, such as operating machinery or driving, should be advised of a possible sedative effect of clonidine. They should also be informed that this sedative effect may be increased by concomitant use of alcohol, barbiturates, or other sedating drugs.

Patients should be instructed to consult their physicians promptly about the possible need to remove the patch if they observe moderate to severe localized erythema and/or vesicle formation at the site of application or generalized skin rash.

If a patient experiences isolated, mild localized skin irritation before completing 7 days of use, the system may be removed and replaced with a new system applied to a fresh skin site.

If the system should begin to loosen from the skin after application, the patient should be instructed to place the adhesive overlay directly over the system to ensure adhesion during its 7-day use.

Used CATAPRES-TTS patches contain a substantial amount of their initial drug content which may be harmful to infants and children if accidentally applied or ingested. THEREFORE, PATIENTS SHOULD BE CAUTIONED TO KEEP BOTH USED AND UNUSED CATAPRES TTS PATCHES OUT OF REACH OF CHILDREN. After use, CATAPRES-TTS should be folded in half with the adhesive sides together and discarded away from children's reach.

Instructions for use, storage and disposal of the system are provided at the end of this monograph. These instructions also are included in each bos of Catapres-TTS.

Drug Interactions: Clonidine may potentiate the CNS-depressive effects of alcohol, barbiturates or other sedating drugs. If a patient receiving clonidine is also taking tricyclic antidepressants, the hypotensive effect of clonidine may be reduced, necessitating an increase in the clonidine dose.

Due to potential for additive effects such as bradycardia and AV block, caution is warranted in patients receiving clonidine concomitantly with agents known to affect sinus node function or AV nodal conduction e.g., digitalis, calcium channel blockers and beta-blockers.

Amitriptyline in combination with clonidine enhances the manifestation of corneal lesions in rats (See TOXICOLOGY)

Toxicology: In several studies with oral clonidine hydrochloride, a dose-dependent increase in the incidence and severity of spontaneous retinal degeneration was seen in albino rats treated for six months or longer. Tissue distribution studies in dogs and monkeys showed a concentration of clonidine in the choroid.

In view of the retinal degeneration seen in rats, eye examinations were performed during clinical trials in 908 patients before, and periodically after, the start of clonidine therapy. In 353 of these 908 patients, the eye examinations were carried out over periods of 24 months or longer. Except for some dryness of the eyes, no drug-related abnormal ophthalmological findings were recorded and, according to specialized tests such as electroretinography and macular dazzle, retinal function was unchanged.

In combination with amitriptyline, clonidine hydrochloride administration led to the development of corneal lesions in rats within 5 days.

Carcinogenesis, Mutagenesis, Impairment of Fertility: A 132-week study in rats with clonidine administered at a fixed concentration in the diet at 32–46 times the oral maximum recommended daily human dose (MRDHD) revealed no evidence of a carcinogenic potental. Mutagenicity tests were negative. Fertility of male and female rats were unaffected by clonidine doses as high as 150 mcg/kg (approximately 3 times the MRDHD). In a separate experiment, fertility of female rats appeared to be affected at dose levels of 500 to 2000 mcg/kg (10 to 40 times the oral MRDHD).

Pregnancy: *TERATOGENIC EFFECTS Pregnancy Category C* Reproduction studies performed in rabbits at doses up to approximately 3 times the oral maximum recommended daily human dose (MRDHD) of CATAPRES® (clonidine) produced no evidence of a teratogenic or embryotoxic potential in rabbits. In rats, however, doses as low as ⅓ the oral MRDHD of clonidine were associated with increased resorptions in a study in which dams were treated continuously from 2 months prior to mating. Increased resorptions were not associated with treatment at the same or at higher dose levels (up to 3 times the oral MRDHD) when the dams were treated on gestation days 6–15. Increases in resorption were observed at much higher dose levels (40 times the oral MRDHD) in rats and mice treated on gestation days 1–14 (lowest dose employed in the study was 500 mcg/kg)

No adequate, well-controlled studies have been conducted in pregnant women. Because animal reproduction studies are not always predictive of human response, this drug should be used during pregnancy only if clearly needed.

Nursing Mothers: As clonidine is excreted in human milk, caution should be exercised when CATAPRES-TTS is administered to a nursing woman.

Pediatric Use: Safety and effectiveness in children below the age of twelve have not been established.

ADVERSE REACTIONS

Clinical trial experience with Catapres-TTS Most systemic adverse effects during CATAPRES-TTS therapy have been mild and have tended to diminish with continued therapy. In a 3-month multiclinic trial of CATAPRES-TTS in 101 hypertensive patients, the systemic adverse reactions were, dry mouth (25 patients) and drowsiness (12) fatigue (6), headache (5), lethargy and sedation (3 each), insomnia, dizziness, impotence/sexual dysfunction, dry throat (2 each) and constipation, nausea, change in taste and nervousness (1 each).

In the above mentioned 3-month controlled clinical trial, as well as other uncontrolled clinical trials, the most frequent adverse reactions were **dermatological** and are described below.

In the 3-month trial, 51 of the 101 patients had localized skin reactions such as erythema (26 patients) and/or pruritus, particularly after using an adhesive overlay throughout the 7-day dosage interval. Allergic contact sensitization to Catapres-TTS was observed in 5 patients. Other skin reactions were localized vesiculation (7 patients), hyperpigmentation (5), edema (3), exoriation (3), burning (3), papules (1), throbbing (1), blanching (1), and a generalized macular rash (1).

In additional clinical experience contact dermatitis resulting in treatment discontinuation was observed in 128 of 673 patients (about 19 in 100) after a mean duration of treatment of 37 weeks. The incidence of contact dermatitis was about 34 in 100 among white women, about 18 in 100 in white men, about 14 in 100 in black women, and approximately 8 in 100 in black men. Analysis of skin reaction data showed that the risk of having to discontinue CATAPRES-TTS treatment because of contact dermatitis was greatest between treatment weeks 6 and 26, although sensitivity may develop either earlier or later in treatment.

In a large-scale clinical acceptability and safety study by 451 physicians in a total of 3539 patients, other allergic reactions were recorded for which a causal relationship to CATAPRES-TTS was not established: maculopapular rash (10 cases), urticaria (2 cases), and angioedema of the fact (2 cases), which also affected the tongue in one of the patients.

Marketing Experience with Catapres-TTS: Other adverse effects reported since the drug has been marketed are listed below by body system. In this setting, an incidence or causal relationship cannot always be accurately determined.

Body as a Whole: Fever, malaise, weakness, pallor, and discontinuation syndrome.

Cardiovascular: Congestive heart failure, cerebrovascular accident, electrocardiographic abnormalities (i.e., conduction distrubances and arrhythmias), chest pain, orthostatic symptoms, syncope, increases in blood pressure, sinus bradycardia and atrioventricular block with and without the use of concomitant digitalis, Raynaud's phenomenon, tachycardia, bradycardia, and palpitations.

Central and Peripheral Nervous System/Psychiatric: Delirium, mental depression, visual and auditory hallucinations, localized numbness, vivid dreams or nightmares, restlessness, anxiety, agitation, irritability, other behavioral changes, and drowsiness.

Dermatological: Angioneurotic edema, localized or generalized rash, hives, urticaria, contact dermatitis, pruritus, alopecia, and localized hypo or hyper pigmentation.

Gastrointestinal: Anorexia, and vomiting.

Genitourinary: Difficult micturation, loss of libido, and decreased sexual activity.

Metabolic: Gynecomastia or breast enlargement and weight gain.

Musculoskeletal: Muscle or joint pain, and leg cramps.

Ophthalmological: Blurred vision, burning of the eyes and dryness of the eyes.

Adverse Events Associated with Oral CATAPARES Therapy: In controlled trials of oral Catapres, the most common adverse reactions were dry mouth (about 40%), drowsiness (about 35%) and sedation (about 8%). The following is a list of adverse events that were reported less frequently. **Body as A Whole:** Weakness, about 10 in 100 patients; fatigue, about 4 in 100; headache and discontinuation syndrome, each about 1 in 100. Also reported were pallor; a weakly positive Coombs' test; increased sensitivity to alcohol; and fever. **Cardiovascular:** Orthostatic symptoms, about 3 in 100 patients; palpitations and tachycardia, and bradycardia, each about 5 in 1000. Syncope, raynaud's phenomenon, congestive heart failure, and electrocardiographic abnormalities (i.e., conduction distrubances and arrhythmias) have been reported rarely. Rare cases of sinus bradycardia and atrioventricular block have been reported, both with and without the use of concomitant digitalis. **Central Nervous System:** nervousness and angitation, about 3 in 100 patients; mental depression, about 1 in 100; insomnia, about 5 in 1000. Other behavioral changes, vivid dreams or nightmares, restlessness, anxiety, visual and auditory hallucinations, and delirium have been reported. **Dermatological:** Rash, about 1 in 100 patients, puritus, about 7 in 1000; hives, angioneurotic edema and urticaria, about 5 in 1000; alopecia, about 2 in 1000. **Gastrointestinal:** Nausea and vomiting, about 5 in 100 patients; anorexia and malaise, each about 1 in 100; mild transient abnormalities in liver function tests, about 1 in 100; hepatitis, parotitis and abdominal pain, rarely. **Genitourinary:** Decreased sexual activity, impotence and loss of libido, about 3 in 100 patients; nocturia, about 1 in 100; difficulty in micturition, about 2 in 1000; urinary retention, about 1 in 1000. **Hematologic:** Thrombocytopenia, rarely. **Metabolic:** Weight gain, about 1 in 100 patients; gynecomastia, about 1 in 1000; transient elevation of blood glucose or serum creatine phosphokinase, rarely. **Musculoskeletal:** muscle or joint pain, about 6 in 1000 and leg cramps, about 3 in 1000. **Oro-otolaryngeal:** dryness of the nasal mucosa was reported. **Ophthalmological:** dryness of the eyes, burning of the eyes and blurred vision was reported.

OVERDOSAGE

The signs and symptoms of clonidine overdosage may include hypotension, bradycardia, lethargy, irritability, weakness, somnolence, diminished or absent reflexes, miosis, vomiting, and hypoventilation. After large overdoses, reversible cardiac conduction defects or arrhythmias, apnea, seizures, and transient hypertension have been reported.

Continued on next page

Boehringer Ingelheim—Cont.

	Programmed Delivery Clonidine *in vivo* Per Day Over 1 Week	Clonidine Content	Size	Code
Catapres-TTS®-1 (clonidine)	0.1 mg	2.5 mg	3.5 cm^2	BI-31
Catapres-TTS®-2 (clonidine)	0.2 mg	5.0 mg	7.0 cm^2	BI-32
Catapres-TTS®-3 (clonidine)	0.3 mg	7.5 mg	10.5 cm^2	BI-33

If symptoms of overdosage occur, remove all CATAPRES-TTS systems. After their removal, the plasma clonidine levels will persist for about 8 hours, then decline slowly over a period of several days.
There is no specific antidote for clonidine. Treatment should be supportive and may include intravenous fluids as indicated, I.V. atropine sulfate for bradycardia, vasopressor agents in addition to I.V. fluids for hypotension, and vasodilators for hypertension. The alpha-blocker tolazoline has yielded inconsistent results in clonidine overdosage and is therefore not recommended as first-line treatment. The opioid antagonist naloxone may be useful as an adjunct in the management of clonidine intoxication, but cases of a paradoxical hypertensive response to this substance have been reported.
Routine hemodialysis is of limited benefit since a maximum of 5% of total body stores clonidine is removed.
Rare cases of CATAPRES-TTS overdosage due to accidental or deliberate mouthing or ingestion of the patch have been reported, many of them involving children.
In a 28-year old man who ingested 100 mg of clonidine hydrochloride powder, plasma clonidine levels were 60 ng/ml after 1 hour, 190 ng/ml after 1.5 hours, 370 ng/ml after 2 hours, and 120 ng/ml after 5.5 and 6.5 hours. This patient developed hypertension followed by hypotension, bradycardia, apnea, hallucinations, semicoma, and premature ventricular contractions. He fully recovered after intensive treatment. In mice and rats, the oral LD_{50} of clonidine is 206 and 465 mg/kg, respectively.

DOSAGE AND ADMINISTRATION

Apply CATAPRES-TTS (clonidine) once every 7 days to a hairless area of intact skin on the upper outer arm or chest. Each new application of CATAPRES-TTS should be on a different skin site from the previous location. If the system loosens during 7-day wearing, the adhesive overlay should be applied directly over the system to ensure good adhesion. There have been rare reports of the need for patch changes prior to 7 days to maintain blood pressure control.
To initiate therapy, CATAPRES-TTS dosage should be titrated according to individual therapeutic requirements, starting with CATAPRES-TTS-1. If after one or two weeks the desired reduction in blood pressure is not achieved, increase the dosage by adding another CATAPRES-TTS-1 or changing to a larger system. An increase in dosage above two CATAPRES-TTS-3 is usually not associated with additional efficacy.
When substituting CATAPRES-TTS for oral clonidine or for other antihypertensive drugs, physicians should be aware that the antihypertensive effect of CATAPRES-TTS may not commence until 2–3 days after initial application. Therefore, gradual reduction of prior drug dosage is advised. Some or all previous antihypertensive treatment may have to be continued, particularly in patients with more severe forms of hypertension.
Renal Impairment: Dosage must be adjusted according to the degree of impairment, and patients should be carefully monitored. Since only a minimal amount of clonidine is removed during routine hemodialysis, there is no need to give supplemental clonidine following dialysis.

HOW SUPPLIED

CATAPRES-TTS-1 (clonidine) and CATAPRES-TTS-2 are supplied as a 4 pouched systems and 4 adhesive overlays per carton, 3 cartons per shipper (NDC 0597-0031-12 and 0597-0032-12, respectively). CATAPRES-TTS 3 is supplied as 4 pouched systems and 4 adhesive overlays per carton (NDC 0597-0033-34). See chart below.
[See table above.]

STORAGE AND HANDLING

Store below 86° F (30° C).
CAUTION: Federal law prohibits dispensing without prescription.

Shown in Product Identification Guide, page 306

COMBIPRES® ℞

[kom 'be-pres]
Each tablet contains:
clonidine hydrochloride USP,
0.1 mg or 0.2 mg or 0.3 mg
and chlorthalidone USP, 15 mg
Oral Antihypertensive

Tablets 0.1	**BI-CODE 08**
Tablets 0.2	**BI-CODE 09**
Tablets 0.3	**BI-CODE 10**

DESCRIPTION

Combipres® is a combination of clonidine hydrochloride (a centrally acting antihypertensive agent) and chlorthalidone (a diuretic). Combipres® is available as tablets for oral administration in three dosage strengths: 0.1/15 mg, 0.2/15 mg and 0.3/15 mg of clonidine hydrochloride/chlorthalidone, respectively.
The inactive ingredients are colloidal silicon dioxide, corn starch, dibasic calcium phosphate, gelatin, glycerin, lactose, magnesium stearate, methylparaben and propylparaben. The Combipres 0.1/15 mg tablet also contains FD&C Red No. 3. The Combipres 0.2/15 mg tablet also contains FD&C Blue No. 1.
Clonidine hydrochloride:
Clonidine hydrochloride is an imidazoline derivative and exists as a mesomeric compound. The chemical name is 2-(2,6-dichlorophenylamino)-2-imidazoline hydrochloride. The following is the structural formula:

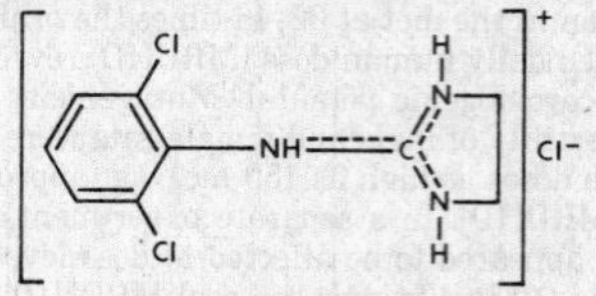

$C_9H_9Cl_2N_3 \cdot HCl$
Mol. Wt. 266.56

Clonidine hydrochloride is an odorless, bitter, white crystalline substance soluble in water and alcohol.
Chlorthalidone
Chlorthalidone is a monosulfamyl diuretic that differs chemically from thiazide diuretics in that a double ring system is incorporated in its structure. It is a racemic mixture of 2-chloro-5-(1- hydroxy-3-oxo-1-isoindolinyl) benzenesulfonamide with the following structural formula:

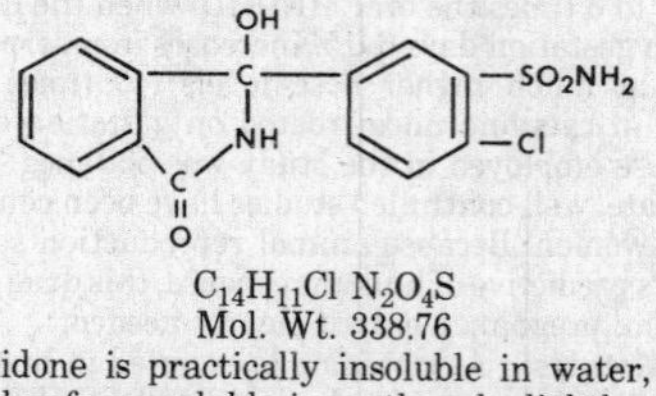

$C_{14}H_{11}Cl\ N_2O_4S$
Mol. Wt. 338.76

Chlorthalidone is practically insoluble in water, in ether and in chloroform; soluble in methanol; slightly soluble in alcohol.

CLINICAL PHARMACOLOGY

Combipres®:
Combipres produces a more pronounced antihypertensive response than occurs after either clonidine hydrochloride or chlorthalidone alone in equivalent doses.
Clonidine hydrochloride:
Clonidine hydrochloride acts relatively rapidly. The patient's blood pressure declines within 30 to 60 minutes after an oral dose, the maximum decrease occurring within 2 to 4 hours. The plasma level of clonidine hydrochloride peaks in approximately 3 to 5 hours and the plasma half-life ranges from 12 to 16 hours. The half-life increases up to 41 hours in patients with severe impairment of renal function. Following oral administration about 40–60% of the absorbed dose is recovered in the urine as unchanged drug in 24 hours. About 50% of the absorbed dose is metabolized in the liver.
Clonidine stimulates alpha-adrenoreceptors in the brain stem, resulting in reduced sympathetic outflow from the central nervous system and a decrease in peripheral resistance, renal vascular resistance, heart rate, and blood pressure. Renal blood flow and glomerular filtration rate remain essentially unchanged. Normal postural reflexes are intact and therefore orthostatic symptoms are mild and infrequent.
Acute studies with clonidine hydrochloride in humans have demonstrated a moderate reduction (15 to 20%) of cardiac output in the supine position with no change in the peripheral resistance; at a 45° tilt there is a smaller reduction in cardiac output and a decrease of peripheral resistance. During long-term therapy, cardiac output tends to return to control values, while peripheral resistance remains decreased. Slowing of the pulse rate has been observed in most patients given clonidine but the drug does not alter normal hemodynamic response to exercise.
Other studies in patients have provided evidence of a reduction in plasma renin activity and in the excretion of aldosterone and catecholamines, but the exact relationship of these pharmacologic actions to the antihypertensive effect has not been fully elucidated.
Clonidine acutely stimulates growth hormone release in both children and adults, but does not produce a chronic elevation of growth hormone with long-term use.
Tolerance may develop in some patients, necessitating a reevaluation of therapy.
Chlorthalidone:
Chlorthalidone is a long-acting oral diuretic with antihypertensive activity. Its diuretic action commences a mean of 2.6 hours after dosing and continues for up to 72 hours. The drug produces diuresis with increased excretion of sodium and chloride. The diuretic effects of chlorthalidone and the benzothiadiazine (thiazide) diuretics appear to arise from similar mechanisms and the maximal effect of chlorthalidone and the thiazides appears to be similar. The site of action appears to be the distal convoluted tubule of the nephron. The diuretic effects of chlorthalidone lead to decreased extracellular fluid volume, plasma volume, cardiac output, total exchangeable sodium, glomerular filtration rate, and renal plasma flow. Although the mechanism of action of chlorthalidone and related drugs is not wholly clear, sodium and water depletion appear to provide a basis for its antihypertensive effect. Like the thiazide diuretics, chlorthalidone produces dose-related reductions in serum potassium levels, elevations in serum uric acid and blood glucose, and it can lead to be decreased sodium and chloride levels.
The mean plasma half-life of chlorthalidone is about 40 to 60 hours. It is eliminated primarily as unchanged drug in the urine. Non-renal routes of elimination have yet to be clarified. In the blood, approximately 75% of the drug is bound to plasma proteins.

INDICATIONS AND USAGE

Combipres® (clonidine hydrochloride USP/chlorthalidone USP) is indicated in the treatment of hypertension. **This fixed combination drug is not indicated for initial therapy of hypertension. Hypertension requires therapy titrated to the individual patient. If the fixed combination represents the dosage so determined, its use may be more convenient in patient management. The treatment of hypertension is not static, but must be reevaluated as conditions in each patient warrant.**

CONTRAINDICATIONS

Anuria. Combipres® is contraindicated in patients with known hypersensitivity to chlorthalidone or other sulfonamide-derived drugs.

WARNINGS

Chlorthalidone should be used with caution in severe renal disease. In patients with renal disease, chlorthalidone or related drugs may precipitate azotemia. Cumulative effects of the drug may develop in patients with impaired renal function. Chlorthalidone should be used with caution in patients with impaired hepatic function or progressive liver disease, because minor alterations of fluid and electrolyte balance may precipitate hepatic coma.
Sensitivity reactions may occur in patients with a history of allergy or bronchial asthma. The possibility of exacerbation or activation of systemic lupus erythematosus has been reported with thiazide diuretics which are structurally related to chlorthalidone. However, systemic lupus erythematosus has not been reported following chlorthalidone administration.

PRECAUTIONS

Clonidine hydrochloride:
General In patients who have developed localized contact sensitization to Catapres-TTS® (clonidine), substitution of oral clonidine hydrochloride therapy may be associated with the development of a generalized skin rash.
In patients who develop an allergic reaction from Catapres-TTS® (clonidine) that extends beyond the local patch site (such as generalized skin rash, urticaria, or angioedema), oral clonidine hydrochloride substitution may elicit a similar reaction.
As with all antihypertensive therapy, clonidine hydrochloride should be used with caution in patients with severe coronary insufficiency, recent myocardial infarction, cerebrovascular disease or chronic renal failure.
Withdrawal Patients should be instructed not to discontinue therapy without consulting their physician. Sudden cessation of clonidine treatment has resulted in subjective symptoms such as nervousness, agitation and headache, accompanied or followed by a rapid rise in blood pressure and ele-

vated catecholamine concentrations in the plasma, but such occurrences have usually been associated with previous administration of high oral doses (exceeding 1.2 mg/day) and/or with continuation of concomitant beta-blocker therapy. Rare instances of hypertensive encephalopathy and death have been reported. When discontinuing therapy with clonidine hydrochloride, the physician should reduce the dose gradually over 2 to 4 days to avoid withdrawal symptomatology.

An excessive rise in blood pressure following clonidine hydrochloride discontinuance can be reversed by administration of oral clonidine or by intravenous phentolamine. If therapy is to be discontinued in patients receiving beta-blockers and clonidine concurrently, beta-blockers should be discontinued several days before the gradual withdrawal of clonidine hydrochloride.

Perioperative Use Administration of clonidine hydrochloride should be continued to within four hours of surgery and resumed as soon as possible thereafter. The blood pressure should be carefully monitored and appropriate measures instituted to control it as necessary.

Information for Patients Patients who engage in potentially hazardous activities, such as operating machinery or driving, should be advised of a potential sedative effect of clonidine. Patients should be cautioned against interruption of clonidine hydrochloride therapy without a physician's advice.

Drug Interactions If a patient receiving clonidine hydrochloride is also taking tricyclic antidepressants, the effect of clonidine may be reduced, thus necessitating an increase in dosage. Clonidine hydrochloride may enhance the CNS-depressive effects of alcohol, barbiturates or other sedatives. Amitriptyline in combination with clonidine enhances the manifestation of corneal lesions in rats (see OCULAR TOXICITY).

OCULAR TOXICITY

In several studies, oral clonidine hydrochloride produced a dose-dependent increase in the incidence and severity of spontaneously occurring retinal degeneration in albino rats treated for six months or longer. Tissue distribution studies in dogs and monkeys revealed that clonidine hydrochloride was concentrated in the choroid of the eye. In view of the retinal degeneration observed in rats, eye examinations were performed in 908 patients prior to the start of clonidine hydrochloride therapy, who were then examined periodically thereafter. In 353 of these 908 patients, examinations were performed for periods of 24 months or longer. Except for some dryness of the eyes, no drug-related abnormal ophthalmologic findings were recorded and clonidine hydrochloride did not alter retinal function as shown by specialized tests such as the electroretinogram and macular dazzle.

In rats, clonidine hydrochloride in combination with amitriptyline produced corneal lesions within 5 days.

Carcinogenesis, Mutagenesis, Impairment of Fertility In a 132-week (fixed concentraiton) dietary administration study in rats, clonidine hydrochloride administered at 32 to 46 times the maximum recommended daily human oral dose was unassociated with evidence of carcinogenic potential.

Fertility of male or female rats was unaffected by clonidine hydrochloride doses as high as 150 mcg/kg or about 3 times the maximum recommended daily human oral dose (MRDHD). Fertility of female rats did, however, appear to be affected (in another experiment) at dose levels of 500 to 2000 mcg/kg or 10 to 40 times the MRDHD.

Usage in Pregnancy

TERATOGENIC EFFECTS Pregnancy Category C. Reproduction studies performed in rabbits at doses up to approximately 3 times the maximum recommended daily human dose (MRDHD) of clonidine hydrochloride have revealed no evidence of teratogenic or embryotoxic potential. In rats however, doses as low as ⅓ the MRDHD were associated with increased resorptions in a study in which dams were treated continuously from 2 months prior to mating. Increased resorptions were not associated with treatment at the same or at higher dose levels (up to 3 times the MRDHD) when dams were treated days 6–15 of gestation. Increased resorptions were observed at much higher levels (40 times the MRDHD) in rats and mice treated days 1–14 of gestation (lowest dose employed in that study was 500 mcg/kg). There are, however, no adequate and well-controlled studies in pregnant women. Because animal reproduction studies are not always predictive of human response, this drug should be used during pregnancy only if clearly needed.

Nursing Mothers As clonidine hydrochloride is excreted in human milk, caution should be exercised when it is administered to a nursing woman.

Pediatric Use Safety and effectiveness in the pediatric population have not been established.

Chlorthalidone: **General**

Hypokalemia and other electrolyte abnormalities, including hyponatremia and hypochloremic alkalosis, are common in patients receiving chlorthalidone. These abnormalities are dose-related but may occur even at the lowest marketed doses of chlorthalidone. Serum electrolytes should be determined before initiating therapy and at periodic intervals during therapy. Serum and urine electrolyte determinations are particularly important when the patient is vomiting excessively or receiving parenteral fluids. All patients taking chlorthalidone should be observed for clinical signs of electrolyte imbalance, including dryness of mouth, thirst, weakness, lethargy, drowsiness, restlessness, muscle pains or cramps, muscular fatigue, hypotension, oliguria, tachycardia, palpitations and gastrointestinal disturbances, such as nausea and vomiting. Digitalis therapy may exaggerate metabolic effects of hypokalemia especially with reference to myocardial activity.

Any chloride deficit is generally mild and usually does not require specific treatment except under extraordinary circumstances (as in liver disease or renal disease). Dilutional hyponatremia may occur in edematous patients in hot weather: appropriate therapy is water restriction, rather than administration of salt, except in rare instances when the hyponatremia is life-threatening. In cases of actual salt depletion, appropriate replacement is the therapy of choice.

Uric Acid Hyperuricemia may occur or frank gout may be precipitated in certain patients receiving chlorthalidone.

Other Increases in serum glucose may occur and latent diabetes mellitus may become manifest during chlorthalidone therapy (see PRECAUTIONS Drug Interactions). Chlorthalidone and related drugs may decrease serum PBI levels without signs of thyroid disturbance.

Information for Patients Patients should inform their doctor if they have: 1) had an allergic reaction to chlorthalidone or other diuretics or have asthma 2) kidney disease 3) liver disease 4) gout 5) systemic lupus erythematosus, or 6) been taking other drugs such as cortisone, digitalis, lithium carbonate, or drugs for diabetes.

Patients should be cautioned to contact their physician if they experience any of the following symptoms of potassium loss: excess thirst, tiredness, drowsiness, restlessness, muscle pains or cramps, nausea, vomiting or increased heart rate or pulse.

Patients should also be cautioned that taking alcohol can increase the chance of dizziness occurring.

Laboratory Tests Periodic determination of serum electrolytes to detect possible electrolyte imbalance should be performed at appropriate intervals.

All patients receiving chlorthalidone should be observed for clinical signs of fluid or electrolyte imbalance: namely, hyponatremia, hypochloremic alkalosis and hypokalemia. Serum and urine electrolyte determinations are particularly important when the patient is vomiting excessively or receiving parenteral fluids.

Drug Interactions Chlorthalidone may add to or potentiate the action of other antihypertensive drugs. Insulin requirements in diabetic patients may be increased, decreased or unchanged. Higher dosage of oral hypoglycemic agents may be required. Chlorthalidone and related drugs may increase the responsiveness to tubocurarine. Chlorthalidone and related drugs may decrease arterial responsiveness to norepinephrine. This diminution is not sufficient to preclude effectiveness of the pressor agent for therapeutic use. Lithium renal clearance is reduced by chlorthalidone, increasing the risk of lithium toxicity.

Drug/Laboratory Test Interactions Chlorthalidone and related drugs may decrease serum PBI levels without signs of thyroid disturbance.

Carcinogenesis, Mutagenesis, Impairment of Fertility No information is available.

Usage in Pregnancy

TERATOGENIC EFFECTS Pregnancy Category B. Reproduction studies have been performed in the rat and the rabbit at doses up to 420 times the human dose and have revealed no evidence of harm to the fetus due to chlorthalidone. There are, however, no adequate and well-controlled studies in pregnant women. Because animal reproduction studies are not always predictive of human response, this drug should be used during pregnancy only if clearly needed.

NON-TERATOGENIC EFFECTS Thiazides cross the placental barrier and appear in cord blood. The use of chlorthalidone and related drugs in pregnant women requires that the anticipated benefits of the drug be weighed against possible hazards to the fetus. These hazards include fetal or neonatal jaundice, thrombocytopenia, and possibly other adverse reactions that have occurred in the adult.

Nursing Mothers Thiazides are excreted in human milk. Because of the potential for serious adverse reactions in nursing infants from chlorthalidone, a decision should be made whether to discontinue nursing or to discontinue the drug, taking into account the importance of the drug to the mother.

Pediatric Use Safety and effectiveness in the pediatric population have not been established.

ADVERSE REACTIONS

Combipres® is generally well tolerated. Most adverse effects are mild and tend to diminish with continued therapy. The most frequent (which appear to be dose-related) are dry mouth, occurring in about 40 to 100 patients; drowsiness, about 33 in 100; dizziness, about 16 in 100; constipation and sedation, each about 10 in 100.

In addition to the reactions listed above, certain less frequent adverse experiences, which are shown below, have also been reported in patients receiving the component drugs of Combipres® but in many cases patients were receiving concomitant medication and a causal relationship has not been established:

Clonidine hydrochloride:

Gastrointestinal Nausea and vomiting, about 5 in 100 patients; anorexia and malaise, each about 1 in 100; mild transient abnormalities in liver function tests, about 1 in 100; rare reports of hepatitis; parotitis, rarely.

Metabolic Weight gain, about 1 in 100 patients; gynecomastia, about 1 in 1000, transient elevation of blood glucose or serum creatine phosphokinase, rarely.

Central Nervous System Nervousness and agitation, about 3 in 100 patients; mental depression, about 1 in 100; headache, about 1 in 100; insomnia, about 5 in 1000. Vivid dreams or nightmares, other behavioral changes, restlessness, anxiety, visual and auditory hallucinations and delirium have been reported.

Cardiovascular Orthostatic symptoms, about 3 in 100 patients; palpitations and tachycardia, and bradycardia, each about 5 in 1000. Raynaud's phenomenon, congestive heart failure, and electrocardiographic abnormalities i.e. conduction disturbances and arrhythmias have been reported rarely. Rare cases of sinus bradycardia and atrioventricular block have been reported, both with and without the use of concomitant digitalis.

Dermatological Rash, about 1 in 100 patients; pruritus, about 7 in 1000; hives, angioneurotic edema and urticaria, about 5 in 1000, alopecia, about 2 in 1000.

Genitourinary Decreased sexual activity, impotence and loss of libido, about 3 in 100 patients; nocturia, about 1 in 100; difficulty in micturition, about 2 in 1000; urinary retention, about 1 in 1000.

Other Weakness, about 10 in 100 patients; fatigue, about 4 in 100; discontinuation syndrome, about 1 in 100; muscle or joint pain, about 6 in 1000 and cramps of the lower limbs, about 3 in 1000. Dryness, burning of the eyes, blurred vision, dryness of the nasal mucosa, pallor, weakly positive Coombs' test, increased sensitivity to alcohol and fever have been reported.

Chlorthalidone:

Gastrointestinal Anorexia, gastric irritation, nausea, vomiting, cramping, diarrhea, constipation, jaundice (intrahepatic cholestatic jaundice), pancreatitis.

Central Nervous System Dizziness, vertigo, paresthesias, headache, xanthopsia.

Hematologic Leukopenia, agranulocytosis, thrombocytopenia, aplastic anemia.

Dermatologic-Hypersensitivity Purpura, photosensitivity, rash, urticaria, necrotizing angiitis (vasculitis) (cutaneous vasculitis), Lyell's syndrome (toxic epidermal necrolysis).

Cardiovascular Orthostatic hypotension may occur and may be aggravated by alcohol, barbiturates or narcotics.

Other adverse reactions Hyperglycemia, glycosuria, hyperuricemia, muscle spasm, weakness, restlessness, impotence.

Whenever adverse reactions are moderate or severe, chlorthalidone dosage should be reduced or therapy withdrawn.

OVERDOSAGE

Clonidine hydrochloride:

The signs and symptoms of clonidine hydrochloride overdosage include hypotension, bradycardia, lethargy, irritability, weakness, somnolence, diminished or absent reflexes, miosis, vomiting and hypoventilation. With large overdoses, reversible cardiac conduction defects or arrhythmias, apnea, seizures and transient hypertension have been reported. The oral LD_{50} of clonidine in rats was 465 mg/kg, and in mice 206 mg/kg.

The general treatment of clonidine hydrochloride overdosage may include intravenous fluids as indicated. Bradycardia can be treated with intravenous atropine sulfate and hypotension with dopamine infusion in addition to intravenous fluids. Hypertension, associated with overdosage, has been treated with intravenous furosemide or diazoxide or alpha-blocking agents such as phentolamine. Tolazoline, an alpha-blocker, in intravenous doses of 10 mg at 30-minute intervals, may reverse clonidine's effects if other efforts fail. Routine hemodialysis is of limited benefit, since a maximum of 5% of circulating clonidine is removed.

In a patient who ingested 100 mg clonidine hydrochloride, plasma clonidine levels were 60 ng/ml (one hour), 190 ng/ml (1.5 hours), 370 ng/ml (two hours) and 120 ng/ml (5.5 and 6.5 hours). This patient developed hypertension followed by hypotension, bradycardia, apnea, hallucinations, semicoma, and premature ventricular contractions. The patient fully recovered after intensive treatment.

Chlorthalidone:

Symptoms of acute overdosage include nausea, weakness, dizziness and disturbances of electrolyte balance. The oral LD_{50} of the drug in the mouse and the rat is more than 25,000 mg/kg body weight. The minimum lethal dose (MLD) in humans has not been established. There is no specific antidote

Continued on next page

Boehringer Ingelheim—Cont.

but gastric lavage is recommended, followed by supportive treatment. Where necessary, this may include intravenous dextrose-saline with potassium, administered with caution.

DOSAGE AND ADMINISTRATION

The dosage must be determined by individual titration. (See INDICATIONS AND USAGE.)

Chlorthalidone is usually initiated at a dose of 25 mg once daily and may be increased to 50 mg if the response is insufficient after a suitable trial.

Clonidine hydrochloride is usually initiated at a dose of 0.1 mg twice daily. Elderly patients may benefit from a lower initial dose. Further increments of 0.1 mg/day may be made if necessary until the desired response is achieved. The therapeutic doses most commonly employed have ranged from 0.2 to 0.6 mg per day in divided doses.

One Combipres® (clonidine hydrochloride/chlorthalidone) Tablet administered once or twice daily can be used to administer a minimum of 0.1 mg clonidine hydrochloride and 15 mg chlorthalidone to a maximum of 0.6 mg clonidine hydrochloride and 30 mg chlorthalidone.

HOW SUPPLIED

Combipres® 0.1/15 mg (each tablet contains clonidine hydrochloride USP, 0.1 mg + chlorthalidone USP, 15 mg) tablets are pink, oval shaped and single scored with the marking Bl 8. Available in bottles of 100 (NDC 0597-0008-01) and 1000 (NDC 0597-0008-10).

Combipres® 0.2/15 mg (each tablet contains clonidine hydrochloride USP 0.2 mg +chlorthalidone USP, 15 mg) tablets are blue, oval shaped and single scored with the marking Bl 9. Available in bottles of 100 (NDC 0597-0009-01) and 1000 (NDC 0597-0009-10).

Combipres® 0.3/15 mg (each tablet contains clonidine hydrochloride USP, 0.3 mg + chlorthalidone USP, 15 mg) tablets are white, oval shaped and single scored with the marking Bl 10. Available in bottles of 100 (NDC 0597-0010-01).

Store below 86°F (30°C). Avoid excessive humidity.

Dispense in tight, light-resistant container.

Caution: Federal law prohibits dispensing without prescription.

CM-PI-4/91

Shown in Product Identification Guide, page 306

MEXITIL® ℞

(mexiletine hydrochloride)
Oral Antiarrhythmic
Capsules of

150 mg .... BI-CODE 66
200 mg .... BI-CODE 67
250 mg .... BI-CODE 68

DESCRIPTION

Mexitil® (mexiletine hydrochloride) is an orally active antiarrhythmic agent available as 150 mg, 200 mg and 250 mg capsules. 100 mg of mexiletine hydrochloride is equivalent to 83.31 mg of mexiletine base. It is a white to off-white crystalline powder with a slightly bitter taste, freely soluble in water and in alcohol. Mexitil® has a pKa of 9.2.

Chemically, Mexitil® is 1-methyl-2-(2,6-xylyloxy)-ethylamine hydrochloride and has the following structural formula:

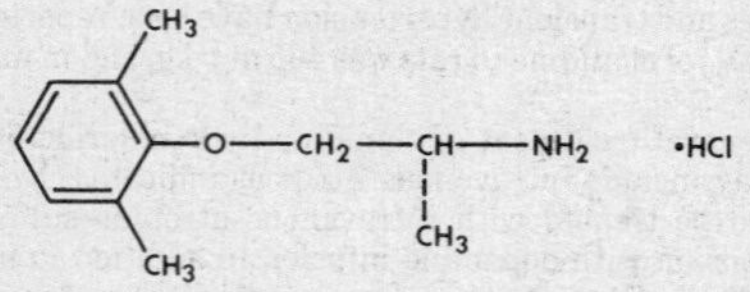

mexiletine hydrochloride (USP)

$C_{11}H_{17}NO \cdot HCl$ (MEXITIL) Mol. Wt. 215.73

Mexitil Capsules contain the following inactive ingredients: colloidal silicon dioxide, cornstarch, magnesium stearate, titanium dioxide, gelatin, FD&C Red No. 40, D&C Red No. 28, and FD&C Blue No. 1; the Mexitil 150 mg and 250 mg capsules also contain FD&C Yellow No. 10. Mexitil® capsules may contain one or more of the following components: sodium lauryl sulfate, sodium propionate, edetate calcium disodium, benzyl alcohol, carboxymethylcellulose sodium, glycerin, butylparaben, propylparaben, methylparaben, pharmaceutical glaze, ethylene glycol monoethyl ether, soya lecithin, dimethylpolysiloxane, refined shellac (food grade) and other inactive ingredients.

CLINICAL PHARMACOLOGY

Mechanism of Action Mexitil® (mexiletine hydrochloride USP) is a local anesthetic, antiarrhythmic agent, structurally similar to lidocaine, but orally active. In animal studies, Mexitil has been shown to be effective in the suppression of induced ventricular arrhythmias, including those induced by glycoside toxicity and coronary artery ligation. Mexitil®, like lidocaine, inhibits the inward sodium current, thus reducing the rate of rise of the action potential, Phase 0. Mexitil® decreased the effective refractory period (ERP) in Purkinje fibers. The decrease in ERP was of lesser magnitude than the decrease in action potential duration (APD), with a resulting increase in the ERP/APD ratio.

Electrophysiology in Man Mexiletine is a Class 1B antiarrhythmic compound with electrophysiologic properties in man similar to those of lidocaine, but dissimilar from quinidine, procainamide, and disopyramide.

In patients with normal conduction systems, Mexitil® has a minimal effect on cardiac impulse generation and propagation. In clinical trials, no development of second-degree or third-degree AV block was observed. Mexitil did not prolong ventricular depolarization (QRS duration) or repolarization (QT intervals) as measured by electrocardiography. Theoretically, therefore, Mexitil® may be useful in the treatment of ventricular arrhythmias associated with a prolonged QT interval.

In patients with pre-existing conduction defects, depression of the sinus rate, prolongation of sinus node recovery time, decreased conduction velocity and increased effective refractory period of the intraventricular conduction system have occasionally been observed.

The antiarrhythmic effect of Mexitil® has been established in controlled comparative trials against placebo, quinidine, procainamide and disopyramide. Mexitil®, at doses of 200–400 mg q8h, produced a significant reduction of ventricular premature beats, paired beats, and episodes of non-sustained ventricular tachycardia compared to placebo and was similar in effectiveness to the active agents. Among all patients entered into the studies, about 30% in each treatment group had a 70% or greater reduction in PVC count and about 40% failed to complete the three-month studies because of adverse effects. Follow-up of patients from the controlled trials has demonstrated continued effectiveness of Mexitil in long-term use.

Hemodynamics Hemodynamic studies in a limited number of patients, with normal or abnormal myocardial function, following oral administration of Mexitil, have shown small, usually not statistically significant, decreases in cardiac output and increases in systemic vascular resistance, but no significant negative inotropic effect. Blood pressure and pulse rate remain essentially unchanged. Mild depression of myocardial function, similar to that produced by lidocaine, has occasionally been observed following intravenous Mexitil therapy in patients with cardiac disease.

Pharmacokinetics Mexitil is well absorbed (~90%) from the gastrointestinal tract. Unlike lidocaine, its first-pass metabolism is low. Peak blood levels are reached in two to three hours. In normal subjects, the plasma elimination half-life of Mexitil is approximately 10–12 hours. It is 50–60% bound to plasma protein, with a volume of distribution of 5–7 liters/kg. Mexitil is metabolized in the liver. Approximately 10% is excreted unchanged by the kidney. While urinary pH does not normally have much influence on elimination, marked changes in urinary pH influence the rate of excretion: acidification accelerates excretion, while alkalinization retards it.

Several metabolites of mexiletine have shown minimal antiarrhythmic activity in animal models. The most active is the minor metabolite N-methylmexiletine, which is less than 20% as potent as mexiletine. The urinary excretion of N-methylmexiletine in man is less than 0.5%. Thus the therapeutic activity of Mexitil is due to the parent compound.

Hepatic impairment prolongs the elimination half-life of Mexitil. In eight patients with moderate to severe liver disease, the mean half-life was approximately 25 hours.

Consistent with the limited renal elimination of Mexitil, little change in the half-life has been detected in patients with reduced renal function. In eight patients with creatinine clearance less than 10 ml/min, the mean plasma elimination half-life was 15.7 hours; in seven patients with creatinine clearance between 11–40 ml/min, the mean half-life was 13.4 hours.

The absorption rate of Mexitil is reduced in clinical situations such as acute myocardial infarction in which gastric emptying time is increased. Narcotics, atropine and magnesium-aluminum hydroxide have also been reported to slow the absorption of Mexitil. Metoclopramide has been reported to accelerate absorption.

Mexiletine plasma levels of at least 0.5 mcg/ml are generally required for therapeutic response. An increase in the frequency of central nervous system adverse effects has been observed when plasma levels exceed 2.0 mcg/ml. Thus the therapeutic range is approximately 0.5 to 2.0 mcg/ml. Plasma levels within the therapeutic range can be attained with either three times daily or twice daily dosing but peak to trough differences are greater with the latter regimen, creating the possibility of adverse effects at peak and arrhythmic escape at trough. Nevertheless, some patients may be transferred successfully to the twice daily regimen (See DOSAGE AND ADMINISTRATION).

INDICATIONS AND USAGE

Mexitil® is indicated for the treatment of documented ventricular arrhythmias, such as sustained ventricular tachycardia, that, in the judgement of the physician, are life-threatening. Because of the proarrhythmic effects of Mexitil, its use with lesser arrhythmias is generally not recommended. Treatment of patients with asymptomatic ventricular premature contractions should be avoided.

Initiation of Mexitil treatment, as with other antiarrhythmic agents used to treat life-threatening arrhythmias, should be carried out in the hospital.

Antiarrhythmic drugs have not been shown to enhance survival in patients with ventricular arrhythmias.

CONTRAINDICATIONS

Mexitil® (mexiletine hydrochloride USP) is contraindicated in the presence of cardiogenic shock or pre-existing second- or third-degree AV block (if no pacemaker is present).

WARNINGS Mortality: In the National Heart, Lung and Blood Institute's Cardiac Arrhythmia Suppression Trial (CAST), a long-term, multicentered, randomized, double-blind study in patients with asymptomatic non-life-threatening ventricular arrhythmias who had a myocardial infarction more than six days but less than two years previously, an excessive mortality or non-fatal cardiac arrest rate (7.7%) was seen in patients treated with encainide or flecainide compared with that seen in patients assigned to carefully matched placebo-treated groups (3.0%). The average duration of treatment with encainide or flecainide in this study was ten months.

The applicability of the CAST results to other populations (e.g., those without recent myocardial infarction) is uncertain. Considering the known proarrhythmic properties of Mexitil and the lack of evidence of improved survival for any antiarrhythmic drug in patients without life-threatening arrhythmias, the use of Mexitil as well as other antiarrhythmic agents should be reserved for patients with life-threatening ventricular antiarrhythmia.

Acute Liver Injury In postmarketing experience abnormal liver function tests have been reported, some in the first few weeks of therapy with Mexitil® (mexiletine hydrochloride). Most of these have been observed in the setting of congestive heart failure or ischemia and their relationship to Mexitil® has not been established.

PRECAUTIONS

General If a ventricular pacemaker is operative, patients with second or third degree heart block may be treated with Mexitil® (mexiletine hydrochloride) if continuously monitored. A limited number of patients (45 of 475 in controlled clinical trials) with pre-existing first degree AV block were treated with Mexitil; none of these patients developed second or third degree AV block. Caution should be exercised when it is used in such patients or in patients with pre-existing sinus node dysfunction or intraventricular conduction abnormalities.

Like other antiarrhythmics Mexitil® (mexiletine hydrochloride) can cause worsening of arrhythmias. This has been uncommon in patients with less serious arrhythmias (frequent premature beats or non-sustained ventricular tachycardia: see ADVERSE REACTIONS), but is of greater concern in patients with life-threatening arrhythmias such as sustained ventricular tachycardia. In patients with such arrhythmias subjected to programmed electrical stimulation or to exercise provocation, 10–15% of patients had exacerbation of the arrhythmia, a rate not greater than that of other agents.

Mexitil should be used with caution in patients with hypotension and severe congestive heart failure because of the potential for aggravating these conditions.

Since Mexitil is metabolized in the liver, and hepatic impairment has been reported to prolong the elimination half-life of Mexitil, patients with liver disease should be followed carefully while receiving Mexitil. The same caution should be observed in patients with hepatic dysfunction secondary to congestive heart failure.

Concurrent drug therapy or dietary regimens which may markedly alter urinary pH should be avoided during Mexitil therapy. The minor fluctuations in urinary pH associated with normal diet do not affect the excretion of Mexitil.

SGOT Elevation and Liver Injury In three-month controlled trials, elevations of SGOT greater than three times the upper limit of normal occurred in about 1% of both mexiletine-treated and control patients. Approximately 2% of patients in the mexiletine compassionate use program had elevations of SGOT greater than or equal to three times the upper limit of normal. These elevations frequently occurred in association with identifiable clinical events and therapeutic measures such as congestive heart failure, acute myocardial infarction, blood transfusions and other medications. These

elevations were often asymptomatic and transient, usually not associated with elevated bilirubin levels and usually did not require discontinuation of therapy. Marked elevations of SGOT (>1000 U/L) were seen before death in four patients with end-stage cardiac disease (severe congestive heart failure, cardiogenic shock).

Rare instances of severe liver injury, including hepatic necrosis, have been reported in association with Mexitil treatment. It is recommended that patients in whom an abnormal liver test has occurred, or who have signs or symptoms suggesting liver dysfunction, be carefully evaluated. If persistent or worsening elevation of hepatic enzymes is detected, consideration should be given to discontinuing therapy.

Blood Dyscrasias Among 10,867 patients treated with mexiletine in the compassionate use program, marked leukopenia (neutrophils less than 1000/mm^3) or agranulocytosis were seen in 0.06%, and milder depressions of leukocytes were seen in 0.08%, and thrombocytopenia was observed in 0.16%. Many of these patients were seriously ill and receiving concomitant medications with known hematologic adverse effects. Rechallenge with mexiletine in several cases was negative. Marked leukopenia or agranulocytosis did not occur in any patient receiving Mexitil alone; five of the six cases of agranulocytosis were associated with procainamide (sustained release preparations in four) and one with vinblastine. If significant hematologic changes are observed, the patient should be carefully evaluated, and, if warranted, Mexitil should be discontinued. Blood counts usually return to normal within one month of discontinuation. (See ADVERSE REACTIONS.)

Convulsions (seizures) did not occur in Mexitil controlled clinical trials. In the compassionate use program, convulsions were reported in about 2 of 1000 patients. Twenty-eight percent of these patients discontinued therapy. Convulsions were reported in patients with and without a prior history of seizures. Mexiletine should be used with caution in patients with known seizure disorder.

Drug Interactions In a large compassionate use program Mexitil has been used concurrently with commonly employed antianginal, antihypertensive, and anticoagulant drugs without observed interactions. A variety of antiarrhythmics such as quinidine or propranolol were also added, sometimes with improved control of ventricular ectopy. When phenytoin or other hepatic enzyme inducers such as rifampin and phenobarbital have been taken concurrently with Mexitil, lowered Mexitil plasma levels have been reported. Monitoring of Mexitil plasma levels is recommended during such concurrent use to avoid ineffective therapy. In a formal study, benzodiazepines were shown not to affect Mexitil plasma concentrations. ECG intervals (PR, QRS and QT) were not affected by concurrent Mexitil and digoxin, diuretics, or propranolol.

Concurrent administration of cimetidine and Mexitil has been reported to increase, decrease, or leave unchanged Mexitil plasma levels; therefore patients should be followed carefully during concurrent therapy.

Mexitil does not alter serum digoxin levels, but magnesium-aluminum hydroxide, when used to treat gastrointestinal symptoms due to Mexitil, has been reported to lower serum digoxin levels.

Concurrent use of Mexitil and theophylline may lead to increased plasma theophylline levels. One controlled study in eight normal subjects showed a 72% mean increase (range 35–136%) in plasma theophylline levels. This increase was observed at the first test point which was the second day after starting Mexitil. Theophylline plasma levels returned to pre-Mexitil values within 48 hours after discontinuing Mexitil. If Mexitil and theophylline are to be used concurrently, theophylline blood levels should be monitored, particularly when the Mexitil dose is changed. An appropriate adjustment in theophylline dose should be considered.

Additionally, in one controlled study in five normal subjects and seven patients, the clearance of caffeine was decreased 50% following the administration of Mexitil.

Carcinogenesis, Mutagenesis and Impairment of Fertility Studies of carcinogenesis in rats (24 months) and mice (18 months) did not demonstrate any tumorigenic potential. Mexitil was found to be non-mutagenic in the Ames test. Mexitil did not impair fertility in the rat.

Pregnancy/Teratogenic Effects
PREGNANCY CATEGORY C

Reproduction studies performed with Mexitil® in rats, mice and rabbits at doses up to four times the maximum human oral dose (24 mg/kg in a 50 kg patient) revealed no evidence of teratogenicity or impaired fertility but did show an increase in fetal resorption. There are no adequate and well-controlled studies in pregnant women; this drug should be used in pregnancy only if the potential benefit justifies the potential risk to the fetus.

Nursing Mothers Mexitil appears in human milk in concentrations similar to those observed in plasma. Therefore, if the use of Mexitil is deemed essential, an alternative method of infant feeding should be considered.

Pediatric Use Safety and effectiveness in the pediatric population have not been established.

ADVERSE REACTIONS

Mexitil® (mexiletine hydrochloride) commonly produces reversible gastrointestinal and nervous system adverse reactions but is otherwise well tolerated. Mexitil has been evaluated in 483 patients in one-month and three-month controlled studies and in over 10,000 patients in a large compassionate use program. Dosages in the controlled studies ranged from 600–1200 mg/day; some patients (8%) in the

compassionate use program were treated with higher daily doses (1600–3200 mg/day). In the three-month controlled trials comparing Mexitil to quinidine, procainamide and disopyramide, the most frequent adverse reactions were upper gastrointestinal distress (41%), lightheadedness (10.5%), tremor (12.6%) and coordination difficulties (10.2%). Similar frequency and incidence were observed in the one-month placebo-controlled trial. Although these reactions were generally not serious, and were dose-related and reversible with a reduction in dosage, by taking the drug with food or antacid or by therapy discontinuation, they led to therapy discontinuation in 40% of patients in the controlled trials. A tabulation of the adverse events reported in the one-month placebo-controlled trial follows:

COMPARATIVE INCIDENCE (%) OF ADVERSE EVENTS AMONG PATIENTS TREATED WITH MEXILETINE AND PLACEBO IN THE 4-WEEK, DOUBLE-BLIND CROSSOVER TRIAL

	Mexiletine N = 53	Placebo N = 49
Cardiovascular		
Palpitations	7.5	10.2
Chest Pain	7.5	4.1
Increased Ventricular Arrhythmias/PVCs	1.9	—
Digestive		
Nausea/Vomiting/Heartburn	39.6	6.1
Central Nervous System		
Dizziness/Lightheadedness	26.4	14.3
Tremor	13.2	—
Nervousness	11.3	6.1
Coordination Difficulties	9.4	—
Changes in Sleep Habits	7.5	6.3
Paresthesias/Numbness	3.8	2.0
Weakness	1.9	4.1
Fatigue	1.9	2.0
Tinnitus	1.9	4.1
Confusion/Clouded Sensorium	1.9	2.0
Other		
Headache	7.5	6.1
Blurred Vision/Visual Disturbances	7.5	2.0
Dyspnea/Respiratory	5.7	10.2
Rash	3.8	2.0
Non-specific Edema	3.8	—

A tabulation of adverse reactions occurring in one percent or more of patients in the three-month controlled studies follows:
[See table at left.]

Less than 1%: Syncope, edema, hot flashes, hypertension, short-term memory loss, loss of consciousness, other psychological changes, diaphoresis, urinary hesitancy/retention, malaise, impotence/decreased libido, pharyngitis, congestive heart failure.

An additional group of over 10,000 patients has been treated in a program allowing administration of Mexitil® (mexiletine hydrochloride) under compassionate use circumstances. These patients were seriously ill with the large majority on multiple drug therapy. Twenty-four percent of the patients continued in the program for one year or longer. Adverse reactions leading to therapy discontinuation occurred in 15 percent of patients (usually upper gastrointestinal system or nervous system effects). In general, the more common adverse reactions were similar to those in the controlled trials. Less common adverse events possibly related to Mexitil use include:

Cardiovascular System: Syncope and hypotension, each about 6 in 1000; bradycardia, about 4 in 1000; angina/angina-like pain, about 3 in 1000; edema, atrioventricular block/conduction disturbances and hot flashes, each about 2 in 1000; atrial arrhythmias, hypertension and cardiogenic shock, each about 1 in 1000.

Central Nervous System: Short-term memory loss, about 9 in 1000 patients; hallucinations and other psychological changes, each about 3 in 1000; psychosis and convulsions/seizures, each about 2 in 1000; loss of consciousness, about 6 in 10,000.

Digestive: Dysphagia, about 2 in 1000; peptic ulcer, about 8 in 10,000; upper gastrointestinal bleeding, about 7 in 10,000; esophageal ulceration, about 1 in 10,000. Rare cases of severe hepatitis/acute hepatic necrosis.

Skin: Rare cases of exfoliative dermatitis and Stevens-Johnson Syndrome with Mexitil® (mexiletine hydrochloride) treatment have been reported.

Laboratory: Abnormal liver function tests, about 5 in 1000 patients; positive ANA and thrombocytopenia, each about 2 in 1000; leukopenia (including neutropenia and agranulocytosis), about 1 in 1000; myelofibrosis, about 2 in 10,000 patients.

COMPARATIVE INCIDENCE (%) OF ADVERSE EVENTS AMONG PATIENTS TREATED WITH MEXILETINE OR CONTROL DRUGS IN THE 12-WEEK DOUBLE-BLIND TRIALS

	Mexiletine N = 430	Quinidine N = 262	Procainamide N = 78	Disopyramide N = 69
Cardiovascular				
Palpitations	4.3	4.6	1.3	5.8
Chest Pain	2.6	3.4	1.3	2.9
Angina/Angina-like Pain	1.7	1.9	2.6	2.9
Increased Ventricular Arrhythmias/PVCs	1.0	2.7	2.6	—
Digestive				
Nausea/Vomiting/Heartburn	39.3	21.4	33.3	14.5
Diarrhea	5.2	33.2	2.6	8.7
Constipation	4.0	—	6.4	11.6
Changes in Appetite	2.6	1.9	—	—
Abdominal Pain/Cramps/Discomfort	1.2	1.5	—	1.4
Central Nervous System				
Dizziness/Lightheadedness	18.9	14.1	14.1	2.9
Tremor	13.2	2.3	3.8	1.4
Coordination Difficulties	9.7	1.1	1.3	—
Changes in Sleep Habits	7.1	2.7	11.5	8.7
Weakness	5.0	5.3	7.7	2.9
Nervousness	5.0	1.9	6.4	5.8
Fatigue	3.8	5.7	5.1	1.4
Speech Difficulties	2.6	0.4	—	—
Confusion/Clouded Sensorium	2.6	—	3.8	—
Paresthesias/Numbness	2.4	2.3	2.6	—
Tinnitus	2.4	1.5	—	—
Depression	2.4	1.1	1.3	1.4
Other				
Blurred Vision/Visual Disturbances	5.7	3.1	5.1	7.2
Headache	5.7	6.9	7.7	4.3
Rash	4.2	3.8	10.3	1.4
Dyspnea/Respiratory	3.3	3.1	5.1	2.9
Dry Mouth	2.8	1.9	5.1	14.5
Arthralgia	1.7	2.3	5.1	1.4
Fever	1.2	3.1	2.6	—

Continued on next page

Consult 1997 supplements and future editions for revisions

Boehringer Ingelheim—Cont.

Other: Diaphoresis, about 6 in 1000; altered taste, about 5 in 1000; salivary changes, hair loss and impotence/decreased libido, each about 4 in 1000; malaise, about 3 in 1000; urinary hesitancy/retention, each about 2 in 1000; hiccups, dry skin, laryngeal and pharyngeal changes and changes in oral mucous membranes, each about 1 in 1000; SLE syndrome, about 4 in 10,000.

Hematology: Blood dyscrasias were not seen in the controlled trials but did occur among the 10,867 patients treated with mexiletine in the compassionate use program (see PRECAUTIONS).

Myelofibrosis was reported in two patients in the compassionate use program: one was receiving long-term thiotepa therapy and the other had pretreatment myeloid abnormalities.

In postmarketing experience, there have been isolated, spontaneous reports of pulmonary changes including pulmonary fibrosis during Mexitil therapy with or without other drugs or diseases that are known to produce pulmonary toxicity. A causal relationship to Mexitil therapy has not been established. In addition, there have been isolated reports of exacerbation of congestive heart failure in patients with preexisting compromised ventricular function. There have been rare reports of pancreatitis associated with Mexitil® treatment.

OVERDOSAGE

Nine cases of Mexitil® (mexiletine hydrochloride) overdosage have been reported; two were fatal. In one fatality, 4400 mg of the drug was ingested. In the other death, the dose ingested was unknown. There has been a report of non-fatal ingestion of 8000 mg. Symptoms associated with overdosage include nausea, hypotension, sinus bradycardia, paresthesia, seizures, intermittent left bundle branch block and temporary asystole.

There is no specific antidote for Mexitil. Acidification of the urine, which will accelerate the excretion of mexiletine, may be useful. Treatment of overdosage should be supportive, and may include the administration of atropine if hypotension or bradycardia occurs.

DOSAGE AND ADMINISTRATION

The dosage of Mexitil® (mexiletine hydrochloride) must be individualized on the basis of response and tolerance, both of which are dose-related. Administration with food or antacid is recommended. Initiate Mexitil therapy with 200 mg every eight hours when rapid control of arrhythmia is not essential. A minimum of two to three days between dose adjustments is recommended. Dose may be adjusted in 50 or 100 mg increments up or down.

As with any antiarrhythmic drug, clinical and electrocardiographic evaluation (including Holter monitoring if necessary for evaluation) are needed to determine whether the desired antiarrhythmic effect has been obtained and to guide titration and dose adjustment.

Satisfactory control can be achieved in most patients by 200 to 300 mg given every eight hours with food or antacid. If satisfactory response has not been achieved at 300 mg q8h, and the patient tolerates Mexitil well, a dose of 400 mg q8h may be tried. As the severity of CNS side effects increases with total daily dose, the dose should not exceed 1200 mg/day.

In general, patients with renal failure will require the usual doses of Mexitil. Patients with severe liver disease, however, may require lower doses and must be monitored closely. Similarly, marked right-sided congestive heart failure can reduce hepatic metabolism and reduce the needed dose. Plasma level may also be affected by certain concomitant drugs (see PRECAUTIONS: Drug Interactions).

Loading Dose: When rapid control of ventricular arrhythmia is essential, an initial loading dose of 400 mg of Mexitil may be administered, followed by a 200 mg dose in eight hours. Onset of therapeutic effect is usually observed within 30 minutes to two hours.

Q12H Dosage Schedule: Some patients responding to Mexitil may be transferred to a 12-hour dosage schedule to improve convenience and compliance. If adequate suppression is achieved on a Mexitil dose of 300 mg or less every eight hours, the same total daily dose may be given in divided doses every 12 hours while carefully monitoring the degree of suppression of ventricular ectopy. This dose may be adjusted up to a maximum of 450 mg every 12 hours to achieve the desired response.

Transferring to Mexitil: The following dosage schedule, based on theoretical considerations rather than experimental data, is suggested for transferring patients from other Class I oral antiarrhythmic agents to Mexitil: Mexitil treatment may be initiated with a 200 mg dose, and titrated to response as described above, 6–12 hours after the last dose of quinidine sulfate, 3–6 hours after the last dose of procainamide, 6–12 hours after the last dose of disopyramide or 8–12 hours after the last dose of tocainide.

In patients in whom withdrawal of the previous antiarrhythmic agent is likely to produce life-threatening arrhythmias, hospitalization of the patient is recommended.

When transferring from lidocaine to Mexitil, the lidocaine infusion should be stopped when the first oral dose of Mexitil is administered. The infusion line should be left open until suppression of the arrhythmia appears to be satisfactorily maintained. Consideration should be given to the similarity of the adverse effects of lidocaine and Mexitil and the possibility that they may be additive.

HOW SUPPLIED

Mexitil® (mexiletine hydrochloride) is supplied in hard gelatin capsules containing 150 mg, 200 mg or 250 mg of mexiletine hydrochloride:

Mexitil® 150 mg capsules are red and caramel with the marking BI 66. Available in bottles of 100 (NDC 0597-0066-01) and individually blister-sealed unit-dose cartons of 100 (NDC 0597-0066-61).

Mexitil® 200 mg capsules are red with the marking BI 67. Available in bottles of 100 (NDC 0597-0067-01) and individually blister-sealed unit-dose cartons of 100 (NDC 0597-0067-61).

Mexitil® 250 mg capsules are red and aqua green with the marking BI 68. Available in bottles of 100 (NDC 0597-0068-01) and individually blister-sealed unit-dose cartons of 100 (NDC 0597-0068-61).

Store at room temperature 20–25°C (68–77°F).

Caution: Federal law prohibits dispensing without prescription.

ME-PI-10/93

Shown in Product Identification Guide, page 306

PERSANTINE® ℞

[per-san 'tēn]
(dipyridamole USP)

Tablets of 25 mg .... BI-CODE 17
Tablets of 50 mg .... BI-CODE 18
Tablets of 75 mg .... BI-CODE 19

DESCRIPTION

Persantine® (dipyridamole USP) is a platelet inhibitor chemically described as 2,6-bis-(diethanolamino)-4,8-dipiperidino-pyrimido-(5,4-d) pyrimidine. It has the following structural formula:

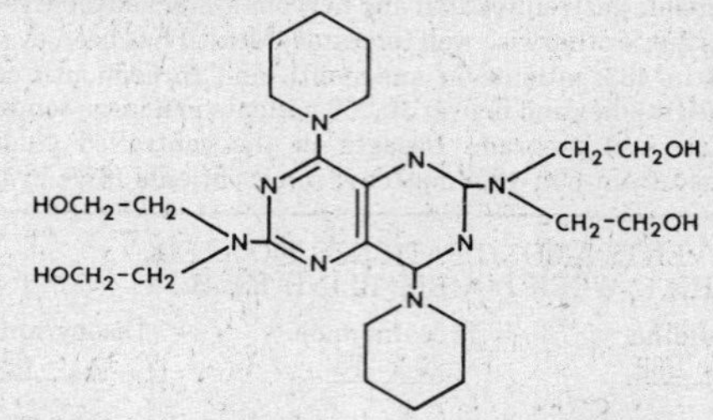

$C_{24}H_{40}N_8O_4$ Mol. Wt. 504.63

Dipyridamole is an odorless yellow crystalline powder, having a bitter taste. It is soluble in dilute acids, methanol and chloroform, and practically insoluble in water.

Persantine tablets for oral administration contain:

Active Ingredient: *TABLETS 25, 50 and 75 mg:* dipyridamole USP 25, 50 and 75 mg respectively.

Inactive Ingredients: *TABLETS 25, 50 and 75 mg:* acacia, carnauba wax, cornstarch, FD&C blue No. 1 aluminum lake, D&C yellow No. 10 aluminum lake, D&C red No. 30 aluminum lake, lactose, magnesium stearate, polyethylene glycol, povidone, shellac, sodium benzoate, sucrose, talc, titanium dioxide, white wax.

CLINICAL PHARMACOLOGY

It is believed that platelet reactivity and interaction with prosthetic cardiac valve surfaces, resulting in abnormally shortened platelet survival time, is a significant factor in thromboembolic complications occurring in connection with prosthetic heart valve replacement.

Persantine® (dipyridamole USP) has been found to lengthen abnormally shortened platelet survival time in a dose-dependent manner.

In three randomized controlled clinical trials involving 854 patients who had undergone surgical placement of a prosthetic heart valve, Persantine, in combination with warfarin, decreased the incidence of postoperative thromboembolic events by 62% to 91% compared to warfarin treatment alone. The incidence of thromboembolic events in patients receiving the combination of Persantine and warfarin ranged from 1.2% to 1.8%. In three additional studies involving 392 patients taking Persantine and coumarin-like anticoagulants, the incidence of thromboembolic events ranged from 2.3% to 6.9%.

In these trials, the coumarin anticoagulant was begun between 24 hours and 4 days postoperatively, and the Persantine was begun between 24 hours and 10 days postoperatively. The length of follow-up in these trials varied from 1 to 2 years.

Persantine does not influence prothrombin time or activity measurements when administered with warfarin.

Mechanism of Action: Persantine is a platelet adhesion inhibitor, although the mechanism of action has not been fully elucidated. The mechanism may relate to inhibition of red blood cell uptake of adenosine, itself an inhibitor of platelet reactivity, phosphodiesterase inhibition leading to increased cyclic-3', 5'-adenosine monophosphate within platelets, and inhibition of thromboxane A_2 formation, which is a potent stimulator of platelet activation.

Hemodynamics: In dogs intraduodenal doses of Persantine of 0.5 to 4.0 mg/kg produced dose-related decreases in systemic and coronary vascular resistance leading to decreases in systemic blood pressure and increases in coronary blood flow. Onset of action was in about 24 minutes and effects persisted for about 3 hours.

Similar effects were observed following IV Persantine in doses ranging from 0.025 to 2.0 mg/kg.

In man the same qualitative hemodynamic effects have been observed. However, acute intravenous administration of Persantine may worsen regional myocardial perfusion distal to partial occlusion of coronary arteries.

Pharmacokinetics and Metabolism: Following an oral dose of Persantine, the average time to peak concentration is about 75 minutes. The decline in plasma concentration following a dose of Persantine fits a two-compartment model. The alpha half-life (the initial decline following peak concentration) is approximately 40 minutes. The beta half-life (the terminal decline in plasma concentration) is approximately 10 hours. Persantine is highly bound to plasma proteins. It is metabolized in the liver where it is conjugated as a glucuronide and excreted with the bile.

INDICATIONS AND USAGE

Persantine® (dipyridamole USP) is indicated as an adjunct to coumarin anticoagulants in the prevention of postoperative thromboembolic complications of cardiac valve replacement.

CONTRAINDICATIONS

None known.

PRECAUTIONS

General: Persantine® (dipyridamole USP) should be used with caution in patients with hypotension since it can produce peripheral vasodilation.

Carcinogenesis, Mutagenesis, Impairment of Fertility: In a 111 week oral study in mice and in a 128-142 week oral study in rats, Persantine produced no significant carcinogenic effects at doses of 8, 25 and 75 mg/kg (1, 3.1 and 9.4 times the maximum recommended daily human dose). Mutagenicity testing with Persantine was negative. Reproduction studies with Persantine revealed no evidence of impaired fertility in rats at dosages up to 60 times the maximum recommended human dose. A significant reduction in number of corpora lutea with consequent reduction in implantations and live fetuses was, however, observed at 155 times the maximum recommended human dose.

Teratogenic Effects: *PREGNANCY CATEGORY B* Reproduction studies have been performed in mice at doses up to 125 mg/kg (15.6 times the maximum recommended daily human dose), rats at doses up to 1000 mg/kg (125 times the maximum recommended daily human dose) and rabbits at doses up to 40 mg/kg (5 times the maximum recommended daily human dose) and have revealed no evidence of harm to the fetus due to Persantine. There are, however, no adequate and well-controlled studies in pregnant women. Because animal reproduction studies are not always predictive of human response, this drug should be used during pregnancy only if clearly needed.

Nursing Mothers: As dipyridamole is excreted in human milk, caution should be exercised when Persantine is administered to a nursing woman.

Pediatric Use: Safety and effectiveness in the pediatric population below the age of 12 years have not been established.

ADVERSE REACTIONS

Adverse reactions at therapeutic doses are usually minimal and transient. On long-term use of Persantine® (dipyridamole USP) initial side effects usually disappear. The following reactions were reported in two heart valve replacement trials comparing Persantine and warfarin therapy to either warfarin alone or warfarin and placebo:

	Persantine/ Warfarin (N=147)	Placebo/ Warfarin (N=170)
Dizziness	13.6%	8.2%
Abdominal distress	6.1%	3.5%
Headache	2.3%	0.0
Rash	2.3%	1.1%

Other reactions from uncontrolled studies include diarrhea, vomiting, flushing and pruritus. In addition, angina pectoris has been reported rarely and there have been rare reports of liver dysfunction. On those uncommon occasions when adverse reactions have been persistent or intolerable, they have ceased on withdrawal of the medication.
When Persantine was administered concomitantly with warfarin, bleeding was no greater in frequency or severity than that observed when warfarin was administered alone.

OVERDOSAGE

Hypotension, if it occurs, is likely to be of short duration, but a vasopressor drug may be used if necessary. The oral LD_{50} in mice is 2,150 mg/kg. Single oral doses of 6,000 mg/kg in rats and 350 mg/kg in dogs were lethal. Symptoms of acute toxicity included ataxia, decreased locomotion and diarrhea in rodents and emesis, ataxia and depression in dogs. Since Persantine® (dipyridamole USP) is highly protein bound, dialysis is not likely to be of benefit.

DOSAGE AND ADMINISTRATION

Adjunctive Use in Prophylaxis of Thromboembolism after Cardiac Valve Replacement The recommended dose is 75–100 mg four times daily as an adjunct to the usual warfarin therapy. Please note that aspirin is not to be administered concomitantly with coumarin anticoagulants.

HOW SUPPLIED

Persantine® (dipyridamole USP) is available as round, orange, sugar-coated tablets of 25 mg, 50 mg and 75 mg coded BI/17, BI/18 and BI/19 respectively.
They are available in the following package sizes:

25 mg Tablets	
Bottles of 100	(NDC 0597-0017-01)
Bottles of 1000	(NDC 0597-0017-10)
Unit Dose Packages of 100	(NDC 0597-0017-61)
50 mg Tablets	
Bottles of 100	(NDC 0597-0018-01)
Bottles of 1000	(NDC 0597-0018-10)
Unit Dose Packages of 100	(NDC 0597-0018-61)
75 mg Tablets	
Bottles of 100	(NDC 0597-0019-01)
Bottles of 500	(NDC 0597-0019-05)
Unit Dose Packages of 100	(NDC 0597-0019-61)

Store below 86°F (30°C).
Caution: Federal law prohibits dispensing without prescription.

PE-PI-10/93

Shown in Product Identification Guide, page 306

PRELU–2® CIII ℞
[pra'lu (2)]
(phendimetrazine tartrate)
Timed Release Capsules .... BI-CODE 64
105 mg

DESCRIPTION

Chemical name: phendimetrazine tartrate (+) 3, 4 dimethyl-2-phenylmorpholine tartrate. Phendimetrazine tartrate is a white, odorless powder with a bitter taste. It is soluble in water, methanol and ethanol. It has a molecular weight of 341, and has the following molecular structure:

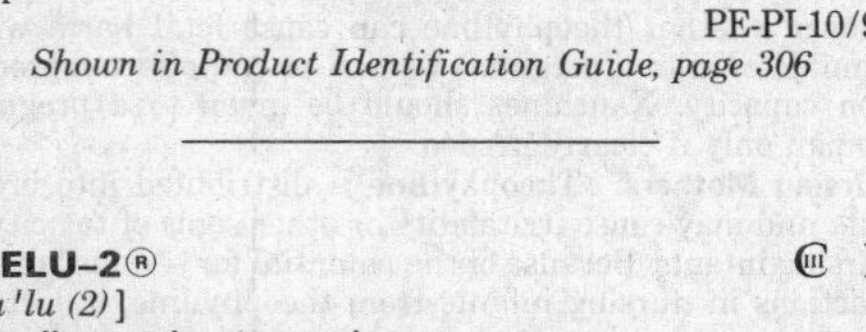

d-3, 4-dimethyl-2-phenylmorpholine tartrate

The capsule is manufactured in a special base which is designed for prolonged release.
Active Ingredient: Each timed-release capsule contains phendimetrazine tartrate 105 mg.
Inactive Ingredients: D&C Red No. 33, D&C Yellow No. 10, FD&C Blue No. 1, FD&C Yellow No. 6, gelatin, povidone, shellac, silica gel, starch, sucrose, talc, titanium dioxide.

CLINICAL PHARMACOLOGY

Phendimetrazine tartrate is a sympathomimetic amine with pharmacologic activity similar to the prototype of drugs of this class used in obesity, the amphetamines. Actions include central nervous system stimulation and elevation of blood pressure. Tachyphylaxis and tolerance have been demonstrated with all drugs of this class in which these phenomena have been looked for.
Drugs of this class used in obesity are commonly known as 'anorectics' or 'anorexigenics.' It has not been established, however, that the action of such drugs in treating obesity is primarily one of appetite suppression. Other central nervous system actions, or metabolic effects, may be involved, for example.
Adult obese subjects instructed in dietary management and treated with 'anorectic' drugs lose more weight on the average than those treated with placebo and diet, as determined in relatively short-term clinical trials.
The magnitude of increased weight loss of drug-treated patients over placebo-treated patients is only a fraction of a pound a week. The rate of weight loss is greatest in the first weeks of therapy for both drug and placebo subjects and tends to decrease in succeeding weeks. The possible origins of the increased weight loss due to the various drug effects are not established. The amount of weight loss associated with the use of an 'anorectic' drug varies from trial to trial, and the increased weight loss appears to be related in part to variables other than the drug prescribed, such as the physician-investigator, the population treated, and the diet prescribed. Studies do not permit conclusions as to the relative importance of the drug and non-drug factors on weight loss.
The natural history of obesity is measured in years, whereas the studies cited are restricted to a few weeks duration; thus, the total impact of drug-induced weight loss over that of diet alone must be considered clinically limited.
The active drug 105 mg of phendimetrazine tartrate in each capsule of this special timed release dosage form approximates the action of three 35 mg non-timed doses taken at four-hour intervals.
The major route of elimination is via the kidneys where most of the drug and metabolites are excreted. Some of the drug is metabolized to phenmetrazine and also phendimetrazine-N-oxide.
The average half-life of elimination when studied under controlled conditions is about 3.7 hours for both the timed and non-timed forms. The absorption half-life of the drug from conventional non-timed 35 mg phendimetrazine tablets is appreciably more rapid than the absorption rate of the drug from the timed release formulation.

INDICATIONS AND USAGE

Phendimetrazine tartrate is indicated in the management of exogenous obesity as a short-term adjunct (a few weeks) in a regimen of weight reduction based on caloric restriction. The limited usefulness of agents of this class (see Clinical Pharmacology) should be measured against possible risk factors inherent in their use such as those described below.

CONTRAINDICATIONS

Advanced arteriosclerosis, symptomatic cardiovascular disease, moderate to severe hypertension, hyperthyroidism, known hypersensitivity, or idiosyncrasy to the sympathomimetic amines, glaucoma.
Agitated states.
Patients with a history of drug abuse.
During or within 14 days following the administration of monoamine oxidase inhibitors (hypertensive crises may result).

WARNINGS

Tolerance to the anorectic effect usually develops within a few weeks. When this occurs, the recommended dose should not be exceeded in an attempt to increase the effect; rather, the drug should be discontinued.
Phendimetrazine tartrate may impair the ability of the patient to engage in potentially hazardous activities such as operating machinery or driving a motor vehicle; the patient should therefore be cautioned accordingly.

DRUG DEPENDENCE

Phendimetrazine tartrate is related chemically and pharmacologically to the amphetamines. Amphetamines and related stimulant drugs have been extensively abused, and the possibility of abuse of phendimetrazine tartrate should be kept in mind when evaluating the desirability of including a drug as part of a weight reduction program. Abuse of amphetamines and related drugs may be associated with intense psychological dependence and severe social dysfunction. There are reports of patients who have increased the dosage to many times that recommended. Abrupt cessation following prolonged high dosage administration results in extreme fatigue and mental depression; changes are also noted on the sleep EEG. Manifestations of chronic intoxication with anorectic drugs include severe dermatoses, marked insomnia, irritability, hyperactivity, and personality changes. The most severe manifestation of chronic intoxications is psychosis, often clinically indistinguishable from schizophrenia.
Usage in Pregnancy: The safety of phendimetrazine tartrate in pregnancy and lactation has not been established. Therefore phendimetrazine tartrate should not be taken by women who are or may become pregnant.
Pediatric Use: Phendimetrazine tartrate is not recommended for use in the pediatric population under 12 years of age.

PRECAUTIONS

Caution is to be exercised in prescribing phendimetrazine tartrate for patients with even mild hypertension.
Insulin requirements in diabetes mellitus may be altered in association with the use of phendimetrazine tartrate and the concomitant dietary regimen.
Phendimetrazine tartrate may decrease the hypotensive effect of guanethidine.
The least amount feasible should be prescribed or dispensed at one time in order to minimize the possibility of overdosage.

ADVERSE REACTIONS

Cardiovascular: Palpitation, tachycardia, elevation of blood pressure.
Central Nervous System: Overstimulation, restlessness, dizziness, insomnia, euphoria, dysphoria, tremor, headache; rarely psychotic episodes at recommended doses.
Gastrointestinal: Dryness of the mouth, unpleasant taste, diarrhea, constipation, other gastrointestinal disturbances.
Allergic: Urticaria.
Endocrine: Impotence, changes in libido.

OVERDOSAGE

Manifestations of acute overdosage with phendimetrazine tartrate include restlessness, tremor, hyperreflexia, rapid respiration, confusion, assaultiveness, hallucinations, panic states.
Fatigue and depression usually follow the central stimulation.
Cardiovascular effects include arrhythmias, hypertension or hypotension and circulatory collapse. Gastrointestinal symptoms include nausea, vomiting, diarrhea, and abdominal cramps. Fatal poisoning usually terminates in convulsions and coma. Management of acute phendimetrazine tartrate intoxication is largely symptomatic and includes lavage and sedation with a barbiturate. Experience with hemodialysis or peritoneal dialysis is inadequate to permit recommendation in this regard. Acidification of the urine increases phendimetrazine tartrate excretion. Intravenous phentolamine (Regitine) has been suggested for possible acute, severe hypertension, if this complicates phendimetrazine tartrate overdosage.

DOSAGE AND ADMINISTRATION

Since this product is a timed release dosage form, limit to one timed release capsule (105 mg phendimetrazine tartrate) in the morning.
Phendimetrazine tartrate is not recommended for use in children under 12 years of age.

HOW SUPPLIED

105 mg capsules (celery and green) in bottles of 100.
Store at controlled room temperature 15°–30°C (59°–86°F).
Federal law prohibits dispensing without prescription.

P2-PI-9/85

*Regitine® (phentolamine mesylate USP) is a registered trademark of CIBA Pharmaceutical Company.

Shown in Product Identification Guide, page 306

RESPBID® ℞
[resp 'bid]
(anhydrous theophylline, sustained release)
Tablets
250 mg .... BI-CODE 48
500 mg .... BI-CODE 49
Oral Bronchodilator

Prescribing Information

DESCRIPTION

Theophylline is a bronchodilator structurally classified as a xanthine derivative. It occurs as a white, odorless, crystalline powder having a bitter taste. Theophylline anhydrous has the chemical name, 1H-Purine-2, 6-dione, 3,7-dihydro-1,3-dimethyl-, and is represented by the following structural formula:

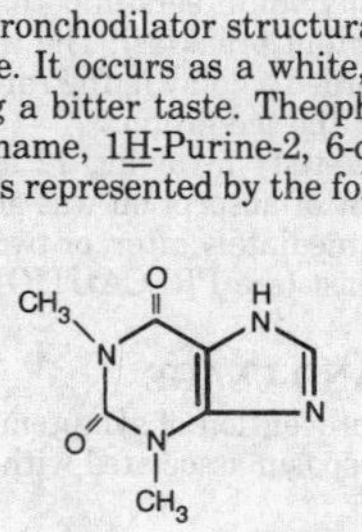

$C_7H_8N_4O_2$ Molecular Weight 180.17

Respbid® (anhydrous theophylline) Tablets contain 250 or 500 mg theophylline anhydrous, in a sustained-release formulation for oral administration. Respbid Tablets also contain: cellulose acetate phthalate, lactose, magnesium stearate.

CLINICAL PHARMACOLOGY

Theophylline directly relaxes the smooth muscle of the bronchial airways and pulmonary blood vessels, thus acting mainly as a bronchodilator and smooth muscle relaxant. It has also been demonstrated that aminophylline has a potent effect on diaphragmatic contractility in normal persons and may then be capable of reducing fatigability and thereby improve contractility in patients with chronic obstructive

Continued on next page

Boehringer Ingelheim—Cont.

airways disease. The exact mode of action remains unsettled. Although theophylline does cause inhibition of phosphodiesterase with a resultant increase in intracellular cyclic AMP, other agents similarly inhibit the enzyme producing a rise of cyclic AMP but are unassociated with any demonstrable bronchodilation. Other mechanisms proposed include an effect on translocation of intracellular calcium; prostaglandin antagonism; stimulation of catecholamines endogenously; inhibition of cyclic guanosine monophosphate metabolism and adenosine receptor antagonism. None of these mechanisms has been proved, however.

In vitro, theophylline has been shown to act synergistically with beta agonists and there are now available data which do demonstrate an additive effect *in vivo* with combined use.

Pharmacokinetics: The half-life of theophylline is influenced by a number of known variables. It may be prolonged in chronic alcoholics, particularly those with liver disease (cirrhosis or alcoholic liver disease), in patients with congestive heart failure, and in those patients taking certain other drugs (see PRECAUTIONS, Drug Interactions). Newborns and neonates have extremely slow clearance rates compared to older infants and children, i.e., those over 1 year. Older children have rapid clearance rates while most non-smoking adults have clearance rates between these two extremes. In premature neonates the decreased clearance is related to oxidative pathways that have yet to be established.

Theophylline Elimination Characteristics

	Half-Life (in Hours) Range	Half-Life (in Hours) Mean
Children	1–9	3.7
Adults	3–15	7.7

In cigarette smokers (1–2 packs/day) the mean half-life is 4–5 hours, much shorter than in non-smokers. The increase in clearance associated with smoking is presumably due to stimulation of the hepatic metabolic pathway by components of cigarette smoke. The duration of this effect after cessation of smoking is unknown but may require 6 months to 2 years before the rate approaches that of the non-smoker.

A single 500 mg dose of Respbid® (anhydrous theophylline) in 8 healthy male subjects fasted for 10 hours predose (overnight) through 4 hours postdose resulted in mean peak theophylline plasma levels of 9.1 ± 3.8 (SD) mcg/ml occurring at 5.0 ± 1.5 hours following dose administration. The extent of theophylline absorption from Respbid® (anhydrous theophylline) was complete in these subjects when compared with that from an immediate-release tablet. In another single dose study, comparable rates and extents of theophylline absorption were seen for the 250 mg Respbid Tablets in 18 healthy male subjects, fasted as above.

In a five-day multiple-dose study, 18 healthy male subjects received 250 mg Respbid Tablets in doses ranging from 375 mg to 625 mg twice daily (mean dose of 11 mg/kg per day). Subjects were allowed to take drug with milk and were permitted their normal daily meals except for fasting from 10 hours before through 4 hours after the morning dose on day 5. Following that dose, mean minimum and maximum plasma theophylline levels were 7.3 ± 2.3 mcg/ml and 10.8 ± 3.1 mcg/ml, respectively. The average percent fluctuation $[(C_{max} - C_{min}/C_{min}) \times 100]$ was 48%. The extent of theophylline absorption from Respbid averaged 94 ± 19% of that from an immediate-release liquid given four times daily.

In other studies: A single 500 mg dose of Respbid was administered to 35 healthy volunteers in both a fasting state and with a high-fat content breakfast. The resultant pharmacokinetic values recorded a delay in the rate of absorption (but not the extent) for the fed group.

In a multiple-dose study involving 12 adolescent patients, the rate and extent of absorption was similar whether the drug was taken immediately after, or two hours after, a low-fat content breakfast (see PRECAUTIONS, Drug/Food Interactions).

INDICATIONS AND USAGE

For relief and/or prevention of symptoms from asthma and reversible bronchospasm associated with chronic bronchitis and emphysema.

CONTRAINDICATIONS

Respbid® (anhydrous theophylline) Tablets are contraindicated in individuals who are hypersensitive to theophylline or any of the tablet components. It is also contraindicated in patients with active peptic ulcer disease, and in individuals with underlying seizure disorders (unless receiving appropriate anti-convulsant therapy).

WARNINGS

Serum levels above 20 mcg/ml are rarely found after appropriate administration of the recommended doses. However, in individuals in whom theophylline plasma clearance is reduced for any reason, even conventional doses may result in increased serum levels and potential toxicity. Reduced theophylline clearance has been documented in the following readily identifiable groups: 1) patients with impaired liver function; 2) patients over 55 years of age, particularly males and those with chronic lung disease; 3) those with cardiac failure from any cause; 4) patients with sustained high fever; 5) neonates and infants under 1 year of age; and 6) those patients taking certain drugs (see PRECAUTIONS, Drug Interactions). Frequently, such patients have markedly prolonged theophylline serum levels following discontinuation of the drug.

Reduction of dosage and laboratory monitoring is especially appropriate in the above individuals.

Serious side effects such as ventricular arrhythmias, convulsions or even death may appear as the first sign of toxicity without any previous warning. Less serious signs of theophylline toxicity (i.e., nausea and restlessness) may occur frequently when initiating therapy, but are usually transient; when such signs are persistent during maintenance therapy; they are often associated with serum concentrations above 20 mcg/ml. Stated differently: serious toxicity is not reliably preceded by less severe side effects. A serum concentration measurement is the only reliable method of predicting potentially life-threatening toxicity.

Many patients who require theophylline exhibit tachycardia due to their underlying disease process so that the cause/effect relationship to elevated serum theophylline concentrations may not be appreciated.

Theophylline products may cause or worsen arrhythmias and any significant change in rate and/or rhythm warrants monitoring and further investigation.

Studies in laboratory animals (minipigs, rodents, and dogs) recorded the occurrence of cardiac arrhythmias and sudden death (with histologic evidence of myocardial necrosis) when beta-agonists and methylxanthines were administered concurrently. The significance of these findings when applied to humans is currently unknown.

PRECAUTIONS

General: On the average, theophylline half-life is shorter in cigarette and marijuana smokers than in non-smokers, but smokers can have half-lives as long as non-smokers. Theophylline should not be administered concurrently with other xanthines. Use with caution in patients with hypoxemia, hypertension, or those with history of peptic ulcer. Theophylline may occasionally act as a local irritant to G.I. tract although gastrointestinal symptoms are more commonly centrally mediated and associated with serum drug concentrations over 20 mcg/ml.

Information for Patients: If nausea, vomiting, restlessness, irregular heartbeat, or convulsions occur, contact a physician immediately.

Take only the amount of drug that has been prescribed. Do not take a larger dose, or take the drug more often, or for a longer time than recommended.

Take this drug consistently with respect to food: either with meals, or fasted (at least two hours pre- or 2 hours post-meals).

Do not take other medicines, especially those for pulmonary disorders, except on the advice of a physician.

Contact your physician if pulmonary symptoms occur repeatedly, especially at the end of a dosing interval.

Avoid drinking large amounts of caffeine-containing beverages, such as coffee, tea, cocoa, or cola, or eating large quantities of chocolate while taking this medicine, since these foods increase the side effects of theophylline.

Respbid® (anhydrous theophylline) Tablets should not be chewed or crushed.

Laboratory Tests: Serum levels should be monitored periodically to determine the theophylline level associated with observed clinical response and as the method of predicting toxicity. For such measurements, the serum sample should be obtained four to six hours after administration of Respbid Tablets. It is important that the patient will not have missed or taken additional doses during the previous 48 hours and that dosing intervals will have been reasonably equally spaced. DOSAGE ADJUSTMENT BASED ON SERUM THEOPHYLLINE MEASUREMENTS WHEN THESE INSTRUCTIONS HAVE NOT BEEN FOLLOWED MAY RESULT IN RECOMMENDATIONS THAT PRESENT RISK OF TOXICITY TO THE PATIENT.

Drug Interactions: *Drug/Drug*—Toxic synergism with ephedrine has been documented and may occur with other sympathomimetic bronchodilators. In addition, the following drug interactions have been demonstrated:

Theophylline with:	
Allopurinol (high-dose)	Increased serum theophylline levels
Cimetidine	Increased serum theophylline levels
Ciprofloxacin	Increased serum theophylline levels
Erythromycin, Troleandomycin	Increased serum theophylline levels
Lithium carbonate	Increased renal excretion of lithium
Oral Contraceptives	Increased serum theophylline levels
Phenytoin	Decreased theophylline and phenytoin serum levels
Propranolol	Increased serum theophylline levels
Rifampin	Decreased serum theophylline levels

Drug/Food —Administration of a single dose of Respbid immediately after a high-fat content breakfast (8 ounces of whole milk, 2 fried eggs, 2 bacon strips, 2 ounces of hash browns and 2 slices of buttered toast, which equates to approximately 71 grams of fat and 985 calories) to 35 healthy volunteers resulted in plasma concentration levels (for the first 8 hours) of 40–60% of those noted during the fasted state and a delay in the time to peak plasma level (T-max) of 17.1 hours in contrast to the 5.1 hours observed during the fasted state.

However, when Respbid was administered on an every 12 hour schedule for 5 days, no consequential effect on absorption was noted following similar high-fat content breakfast, and the time to peak concentration averaged 5.4 hours. The rate and extent of absorption seen was similar when the drug was taken immediately after, and two hours after, a low-fat content breakfast.

The effect of other types and amounts of food, and the pharmacokinetic profile following an evening meal is not presently known.

Drug-Laboratory Test Interactions: Currently available analytical methods, including high pressure liquid chromatography and immunoassay techniques, for measuring serum theophylline levels are specific. Metabolites and other drugs generally do not affect the results. Other new analytic methods are also now in use. The physician should be aware of the laboratory method used and whether other drugs will interfere with the assay for theophylline.

Carcinogenesis, Mutagenesis, and Impairment of Fertility: Long-term carcinogenicity studies have not been performed with theophylline.

Chromosome-breaking activity was detected in human cell cultures at concentrations of theophylline up to 50 times the therapeutic serum concentration in humans. Theophylline was not mutagenic in the dominant lethal assay in male mice given theophylline intraperitoneally in doses up to 30 times the maximum daily human oral dose.

Studies to determine the effect on fertility have not been performed with theophylline.

Pregnancy: *CATEGORY C*—Animal reproduction studies have not been conducted with theophylline. It is also not known whether theophylline can cause fetal harm when administered to a pregnant woman or can affect reproduction capacity. Xanthines should be given to a pregnant woman only if clearly needed.

Nursing Mothers: Theophylline is distributed into breast milk and may cause irritability or other signs of toxicity in nursing infants. Because of the potential for serious adverse reactions in nursing infants from theophylline, a decision should be made whether to discontinue nursing or to discontinue the drug, taking into account the importance of the drug to the mother.

Pediatric Use: Respbid® (anhydrous theophylline) Tablets are not recommended for administration to the pediatric population less than six years of age.

ADVERSE REACTIONS

The following adverse reactions have been observed, but there has not been enough systematic collection of data to support an estimate of their frequency. The most consistent adverse reactions are usually due to overdosage.

1. *Gastrointestinal:* nausea, vomiting, epigastric pain, hematemesis, diarrhea.
2. *Central nervous system:* headaches, irritability, restlessness, insomnia, reflex hyperexcitability, muscle twitching, clonic and tonic generalized convulsions.
3. *Cardiovascular:* palpitation, tachycardia, extrasystoles, flushing, hypotension, circulatory failure, ventricular arrhythmias.
4. *Respiratory:* tachypnea.
5. *Renal:* potentiation of diuresis.
6. *Others:* alopecia, hyperglycemia, inappropriate ADH syndrome, rash.

OVERDOSAGE

Management: It is suggested that the management principles (consistent with the clinical status of the patient when first seen) outlined below be instituted and that simultaneous contact with a Regional Poison Control Center be established. In this way both updated information and individualization regarding required therapy may be provided.

1. When potential oral overdose is established and seizure has not occurred:

a) If patient is alert and seen within the early hours after ingestion, induction of emesis may be of value. Gastric lavage has been demonstrated to be of no value in influencing outcome in patients who present more than 1 hour after ingestion.

b) Administer a cathartic. Sorbitol solution is reported to be of value.

If serum theophylline is:		Directions:
Within desired range		Maintain dosage if tolerated. Recheck serum theophylline concentration at 6- to 12-month intervals.*
Too high	20 to 25 mcg/ml	Decrease doses by about 10% and recheck serum level after 3 days.
	25 to 30 mcg/ml	Skip the next dose and decrease subsequent doses by about 25%. Recheck serum level after 3 days.
	Over 30 mcg/ml	Skip next two doses and decrease subsequent doses by 50%. Recheck serum level after 3 days.
Too low		Increase dosage by 25% at 3 day intervals until either the desired serum concentration and/or clinical response is achieved.* The total daily dose may need to be administered at more frequent intervals if symptoms occur repeatedly at the end of the dosing interval.

The serum concentration may be rechecked at appropriate intervals, but at least at the end of any adjustment period. When the patient's condition is otherwise clinically stable, and none of the recognized factors which alter elimination are present, measurement of serum levels need be repeated only every 6 to 12 months.

*Finer adjustments in dosage may be needed for some patients.

c) Administer repeated doses of activated charcoal and monitor theophylline serum levels.
d) Prophylactic administration of phenobarbital has been shown to increase the seizure threshold in laboratory animals, and administration of this drug can be considered.

2. If patient presents with a seizure:

a) Establish an airway.
b) Administer oxygen.
c) Treat the seizure with intravenous diazepam, 0.1 to 0.3 mg/kg up to 10 mg. If seizures cannot be controlled, the use of general anesthesia should be considered.
d) Monitor vital signs, maintain blood pressure and provide adequate hydration.

3. If post-seizure coma is present:

a) Maintain airway and oxygenation.
b) If a result of oral medication, follow above recommendations to prevent absorption of the drug, but intubation and lavage will have to be performed instead of inducing emesis, and the cathartic and charcoal will need to be introduced via a large bore gastric lavage tube.
c) Continue to provide full supportive care and adequate hydration until the drug is metabolized. In general, drug metabolism is sufficiently rapid so as not to warrant dialysis. If repeated oral activated charcoal is ineffective (as noted by stable or rising serum levels) charcoal hemoperfusion may be indicated.

DOSAGE AND ADMINISTRATION

Effective use of theophylline (i.e., the concentration of drug in the serum associated with optimal benefit and minimal risk of toxicity) is considered to occur when the theophylline concentration is maintained from 10 to 20 mcg/ml. The early studies from which these levels were derived were carried out in patients immediately or shortly after recovery from acute exacerbations of their disease (some hospitalized with status asthmaticus).

Although the 20 mcg/ml level remains appropriate as a critical value (above which toxicity is more likely to occur) for safety purposes, additional data are now available which indicate that the serum theophylline concentrations required to produce maximum physiologic benefit may, in fact, fluctuate with the degree of bronchospasm present and are variable. Therefore, the physician should individualize the range appropriate to the patient's requirements, based on both symptomatic response and improvement in pulmonary function. It should be stressed that serum theophylline concentrations maintained at the upper level of the 10 to 20 mcg/ml range may be associated with potential toxicity when factors known to reduce theophylline clearance are operative (see WARNINGS).

If it is not possible to obtain serum level determinations, restriction of the daily dose (in otherwise healthy adults) to not greater than 13 mg/kg/day, to a maximum of 900 mg, in divided doses, will result in relatively few patients exceeding serum levels of 20 mcg/ml and the resultant greater risk of toxicity.

Caution should be exercised for younger children who cannot complain of minor side effects. Older adults, those with cor pulmonale, congestive heart failure, and/or liver diseases may have unusually low dosage requirements and thus may experience toxicity at the maximal dosage recommended below.

Theophylline does not distribute into fatty tissue. Dosage should be calculated on the basis of lean (ideal) body weight where mg/kg doses are presented.

Dosage guidelines are approximations only and the wide range of theophylline clearance between individuals (particularly those with concomitant disease) makes indiscriminate usage hazardous.

Respbid® (anhydrous theophylline) Tablets Should Not Be Chewed or Crushed.

Dosage Guidelines: There is information which shows that taking Respbid consistently after both high-fat and low-fat content breakfasts does not result in a decrease in peak concentration or delay in time to peak concentration that are seen when a single dose of Respbid is taken immediately after a high-fat content breakfast. Therefore, Respbid® (anhydrous theophylline) should be administered consistently with respect to food; either with meals, or fasted (at least 2 hours pre- or 2 hours post-meals). (See PRECAUTIONS, Drug/Food Interactions.)

Status asthmaticus should be considered a medical emergency and is defined as that degree of bronchospasm which is not rapidly responsive to usual doses of conventional bronchodilators. Optimal therapy for such patients frequently requires both additional medication, parenterally administered, and close monitoring, preferably in an intensive care setting.

Acute Symptoms—Respbid Tablets are not intended for patients experiencing an acute episode of bronchospasm (associated with asthma, chronic bronchitis, or emphysema). Such patients require rapid relief of symptoms and should be treated with an immediate-release theophylline preparation, an intravenous theophylline preparation or other bronchodilators, and not with controlled-release products.

Chronic Symptoms—Theophylline administration is a treatment for the management of reversible bronchospasm (asthma, chronic bronchitis and emphysema) to prevent symptoms and maintain patent airways. The appropriate dosage of theophylline can be established using an immediate-release preparation. Slow clinical titration is preferred to help assure acceptance and safety of the medication. When appropriate theophylline serum levels have been attained and clinical improvement has been maintained, the patient can usually be switched to Respbid Tablets by dividing the total daily dose of immediate-release theophylline by two and administering the appropriate Respbid Tablet every 12 hours (see conversion chart below). However, certain patients, such as the young, smokers, or some non-smoking adults are likely to metabolize theophylline rapidly and require the total daily dose administered as three equal doses at eight-hour intervals. Such patients can generally be identified as having trough serum levels lower than desired or repeatedly exhibiting symptoms near the end of a dosing interval.

If the established daily dose is:	The q 12 hr regimen is: no. tablets:	strength:
500 mg	1	Respbid 250 mg
1000 mg	1	Respbid 500 mg

Alternatively, therapy can be initiated with Respbid since it is available in dosage strengths which permit titration and adjustment of dosage as noted above. A liquid preparation should be considered for children to permit both greater ease of and more accurate dosage adjustment.

Recommended Doses for Initiating Therapy with Respbid:
Initial Dose—As an initial dose, 16 mg/kg per 24 hours or 400 mg per 24 hours (whichever is less) of Respbid® (anhydrous theophylline) Tablets in divided doses at 8– or 12–hour intervals, as appropriate (see DOSAGE AND ADMINISTRATION).

Increasing Dose—The above dosage may be increased in approximately 25% increments at three-day intervals so long as the drug is tolerated, until clinical response is satisfactory or the maximum dose as indicated in the following section is reached. The serum concentration may be checked at these intervals, but at a minimum, should be determined at the end of this adjustment period.

IT IS IMPORTANT THAT NO PATIENT BE MAINTAINED ON ANY DOSAGE THAT IS NOT TOLERATED. In instructing patients to increase dosage, they should be instructed not to take a subsequent dose if side effects occur and to resume therapy at a lower dose once adverse effects have disappeared.

Maximum Dose Where the Serum Concentration Is Not Measured:
WARNING: DO NOT ATTEMPT TO MAINTAIN ANY DOSE THAT IS NOT TOLERATED.
Do not exceed the following (or 900 mg, whichever is less):

Age 6 to under 9 years	24 mg/kg/day
Age 9 to under 12 years	20 mg/kg/day
Age 12 to under 16 years	18 mg/kg/day
Age 16 years and older	13 mg/kg/day

Measurement of Serum Theophylline Concentrations During Chronic Therapy If the above maximum doses are to be maintained or exceeded, serum theophylline measurement is essential (see PRECAUTIONS, Laboratory Tests, for guidance).

Dosage Adjustment After Serum Theophylline Measurement:
[See table at left.]

HOW SUPPLIED

Respbid® brand anhydrous theophylline is supplied as 250 mg white, round, scored sustained release tablets imprinted with "BI 48" (NDC 0597-0048-01) and 500 mg white, capsule-shaped, scored sustained-release tablets imprinted with "BI 49" (NDC 0597-0049-01) in bottles of 100.

STORE AT CONTROLLED ROOM TEMPERATURE 15°–30°C (59°–86°F).

Caution: Federal law prohibits dispensing without prescription.

RE-PI-7/91

Shown in Product Identification Guide, page 306

SERENTIL® ℞

[seh-ren 'til]
(mesoridazine besylate)

Tablets, 10 mg	**BI-CODE 20**
Tablets, 25 mg	**BI-CODE 21**
Tablets, 50 mg	**BI-CODE 22**
Tablets, 100 mg	**BI-CODE 23**
Concentrate of 25 mg/ml	**BI-CODE 25**
Ampuls of 1 ml (25 mg)	**BI-CODE 27**

Caution: Federal law prohibits dispensing without prescription.

DESCRIPTION

Serentil® (mesoridazine besylate), the besylate salt of a metabolite of thioridazine, is a phenothiazine tranquilizer that is effective in the treatment of schizophrenia, organic brain disorders, alcoholism and psychoneuroses.

Serentil is 10-[2(1-methyl-2-piperidyl) ethyl]-2- (methyl-sulfinyl)-phenothiazine [as the besylate].

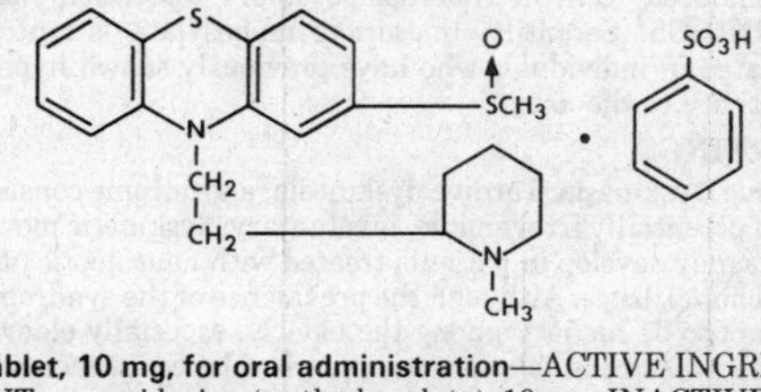

Tablet, 10 mg, for oral administration—ACTIVE INGREDIENT: mesoridazine (as the besylate), 10 mg. INACTIVE INGREDIENTS: acacia, carnauba wax, colloidal silicon dioxide, FD&C Red No. 40 aluminum lake, lactose, microcrystalline cellulose, povidone, sodium benzoate, starch, stearic acid, sucrose, synthetic black iron oxide, talc, titanium dioxide, and other ingredients.

Tablet, 25 mg, for oral administration—ACTIVE INGREDIENT: mesoridazine (as the besylate), 25 mg. INACTIVE INGREDIENTS: acacia, carnauba wax, colloidal silicon dioxide, FD&C Red No. 40 aluminum lake, lactose, microcrystalline cellulose, povidone, sodium benzoate, stearic acid, sucrose, synthetic black iron oxide, talc, titanium dioxide, and other ingredients.

Tablet, 50 mg, for oral administration—ACTIVE INGREDIENT: mesoridazine (as the besylate), 50 mg. INACTIVE INGREDIENTS: acacia, carnauba wax, colloidal silicon dioxide, FD&C Red No. 40 aluminum lake, gelatin, lactose, microcrystalline cellulose, povidone, sodium benzoate, starch, stearic acid, sucrose, synthetic black iron oxide, talc, titanium dioxide, and other ingredients.

Tablet, 100 mg, for oral administration—ACTIVE INGREDIENT: mesoridazine (as the besylate), 100 mg. INACTIVE INGREDIENTS: acacia, carnauba wax, colloidal silicon dioxide, FD&C Red No. 40 aluminum lake, gelatin, lactose, microcrystalline cellulose, povidone, sodium benzoate, starch, stearic acid, sucrose, synthetic black iron oxide, talc, titanium dioxide, and other ingredients.

Ampuls, 1 ml, for intramuscular administration—ACTIVE INGREDIENT: mesoridazine (as the besylate), 25 mg. INACTIVE INGREDIENTS: edetate disodium USP, 0.5 mg; sodium chloride USP, 7.2 mg; carbon dioxide gas (bone dry) q.s., water for injection USP, q.s. to 1 ml.

Concentrate, for oral administration—ACTIVE INGREDIENT: mesoridazine (as the besylate), 25 mg per ml. INACTIVE INGREDIENTS: alcohol, 0.61% by volume; citric acid; FD&C Red No. 40; flavors; methylparaben; propylparaben; purified water; sodium citrate, sorbitol.

Continued on next page

Boehringer Ingelheim—Cont.

ACTIONS

Based upon animal studies, Serentil® (mesoridazine besylate), as with other phenothiazines, acts indirectly on reticular formation, whereby neuronal activity into reticular formation is reduced without affecting its intrinsic ability to activate the cerebral cortex. In addition, the phenothiazines exhibit at least part of their activities through depression of hypothalamic centers. Neurochemically, the phenothiazines are thought to exert their effects by a central adrenergic blocking action.

INDICATIONS

In clinical studies Serentil® (mesoridazine besylate) has been found useful in the following disease states:

Schizophrenia: Serentil® (mesoridazine besylate) is effective in the treatment of schizophrenia. It substantially reduces the severity of emotional withdrawal, conceptual disorganization, anxiety, tension, hallucinatory behavior, suspiciousness and blunted affect in schizophrenic patients. As with other phenothiazines, patients refractory to previous medication may respond to Serentil® (mesoridazine besylate).

Behavioral Problems in Mental Deficiency and Chronic Brain Syndrome: The effect of Serentil was found to be excellent or good in the management of hyperactivity and uncooperativeness associated with mental deficiency and chronic brain syndrome.

Alcoholism—Acute and Chronic: Serentil® (mesoridazine besylate) ameliorates anxiety, tension, depression, nausea and vomiting in both acute and chronic alcoholics without producing hepatic dysfunction or hindering the functional recovery of the impaired liver.

Psychoneurotic Manifestations: Serentil® (mesoridazine besylate) reduces the symptoms of anxiety and tension, prevalent symptoms often associated with neurotic components of many disorders, and benefits personality disorders in general.

CONTRAINDICATIONS

As with other phenothiazines, Serentil® (mesoridazine besylate) is contraindicated in severe central nervous system depression or comatose states from any cause including drug-induced central nervous system depression (see WARNINGS). Serentil® (mesoridazine besylate) is contraindicated in individuals who have previously shown hypersensitivity to the drug.

WARNINGS

Tardive Dyskinesia: Tardive dyskinesia, a syndrome consisting of potentially irreversible, involuntary, dyskinetic movements may develop in patients treated with neuroleptic (antipsychotic) drugs. Although the prevalence of the syndrome appears to be highest among the elderly, especially elderly women, it is impossible to rely upon prevalence estimates to predict, at the inception of neuroleptic treatment, which patients are likely to develop the syndrome. Whether neuroleptic drug products differ in their potential to cause tardive dyskinesia is unknown.

Both the risk of developing the syndrome and the likelihood that it will become irreversible are believed to increase as the duration of treatment and the total cumulative dose of neuroleptic drugs administered to the patient increase. However, the syndrome can develop, although much less commonly, after relatively brief treatment periods at low doses. There is no known treatment for established cases of tardive dyskinesia, although the syndrome may remit, partially or completely, if neuroleptic treatment is withdrawn. Neuroleptic treatment itself, however, may suppress (or partially suppress) the signs and symptoms of the syndrome and thereby may possibly mask the underlying disease process. The effect that symptomatic suppression has upon the long-term course of the syndrome is unknown.

Given these considerations, neuroleptics should be prescribed in a manner that is most likely to minimize the occurrence of tardive dyskinesia. Chronic neuroleptic treatment should generally be reserved for patients who suffer from a chronic illness 1) that is known to respond to neuroleptic drugs, and 2) for which alternative, equally effective but potentially less harmful treatments are *not* available or appropriate. In patients who do require chronic treatment, the smallest dose and the shortest duration of treatment producing a satisfactory clinical response should be sought. The need for continued treatment should be reassessed periodically.

If signs and symptoms of tardive dyskinesia appear in a patient on neuroleptics, drug discontinuation should be considered. However, some patients may require treatment despite the presence of the syndrome.

(For further information about the description of tardive dyskinesia and its clinical detection, please refer to the sections on Information for Patients and Adverse Reactions.)

Neuroleptic Malignant Syndrome (NMS) A potentially fatal symptom complex sometimes referred to as Neuroleptic Malignant Syndrome (NMS) has been reported in association with antipsychotic drugs. Clinical manifestations of NMS are hyperpyrexia, muscle rigidity, altered mental status and evidence of autonomic instability (irregular pulse or blood pressure, tachycardia, diaphoresis, and cardiac dysrhythmias).

The diagnostic evaluation of patients with this syndrome is complicated. In arriving at a diagnosis, it is important to identify cases where the clinical presentation includes both serious medical illness (e.g., pneumonia, systemic infection, etc.) and untreated or inadequately treated extrapyramidal signs and symptoms (EPS). Other important considerations in the differential diagnosis include central anticholinergic toxicity, heat stroke, drug fever and primary central nervous system (CNS) pathology.

The management of NMS should include 1) immediate discontinuation of antipsychotic drugs and other drugs not essential to concurrent therapy, 2) intensive symptomatic treatment and medical monitoring, and 3) treatment of any concomitant serious medical problems for which specific treatments are available. There is no general agreement about specific pharmacological treatment regimens for uncomplicated NMS. If a patient requires antipsychotic drug treatment after recovery from NMS, the potential reintroduction of drug therapy should be carefully considered. The patient should be carefully monitored, since recurrences of NMS have been reported.

Where patients are participating in activities requiring complete mental alertness (e.g., driving), it is advisable to administer the phenothiazines cautiously and to increase the dosage gradually.

Central Nervous System Depressants: As in the case of other phenothiazines, Serentil® (mesoridazine besylate) is capable of potentiating central nervous system depressants (e.g., alcohol, anesthetics, barbiturates, narcotics, opiates, other psychoactive drugs, etc.) as well as atropine and phosphorus insecticides. Severe respiratory depression and respiratory arrest have been reported when a patient was given Serentil® (mesoridazine besylate) and a concomitant high dose of a barbiturate.

Usage in Pregnancy: The safety of this drug in pregnancy has not been established; hence, it should be given only when the anticipated benefits to be derived from treatment exceed the possible risks to mother and fetus.

Pediatric Use: The use of Serentil® (mesoridazine besylate USP) in the pediatric population under 12 years of age is not recommended because safe conditions for its use have not been established.

PRECAUTIONS

While ocular changes have not to date been related to Serentil® (mesoridazine besylate), one should be aware that such changes have been seen with other drugs of this class.

Because of possible hypotensive effects, reserve parenteral administration for bedfast patients or for acute ambulatory cases, and keep patient lying down for at least one-half hour after injection.

Leukopenia and/or agranulocytosis have been attributed to phenothiazine therapy. A single case of transient granulocytopenia has been associated with Serentil® (mesoridazine besylate). Since convulsive seizures have been reported, patients receiving anticonvulsant medication should be maintained on that regimen while receiving Serentil® (mesoridazine besylate).

Neuroleptic drugs elevate prolactin levels; the elevation persists during chronic administration. Tissue culture experiments indicate that approximately one-third of human breast cancers are prolactin dependent in vitro, a factor of potential importance if the prescription of these drugs is contemplated in a patient with a previously detected breast cancer. Although disturbances such as galactorrhea, amenorrhea, gynecomastia, and impotence have been reported, the clinical significance of elevated serum prolactin levels is unknown for most patients. An increase in mammary neoplasms has been found in rodents after chronic administration of neuroleptic drugs. Neither clinical studies nor epidemiologic studies conducted to date, however, have shown an association between chronic administration of these drugs and mammary tumorigenesis; the available evidence is considered too limited to be conclusive at this time.

INFORMATION FOR PATIENTS: Given the likelihood that some patients exposed chronically to neuroleptics will develop tardive dyskinesia, it is advised that all patients in whom chronic use is contemplated be given, if possible, full information about this risk.

ADVERSE REACTIONS

Drowsiness and hypotension were the most prevalent side effects encountered. Side effects tended to reach their maximum level of severity early with the exception of a few (rigidity and motoric effects) which occurred later in therapy.

With the exceptions of tremor and rigidity, adverse reactions were generally found among those patients who received relatively high doses early in treatment. Clinical data showed no tendency for the investigators to terminate treatment because of side effects.

Serentil® (mesoridazine besylate) has demonstrated a remarkably low incidence of adverse reactions when compared with other phenothiazine compounds.

Central Nervous System: Drowsiness, Parkinson's syndrome, dizziness, weakness, tremor, restlessness, ataxia, dystonia, rigidity, slurring, akathisia, and motoric reactions (opisthotonos) have been reported.

Autonomic Nervous System: Dry mouth, nausea and vomiting, fainting, stuffy nose, photophobia, constipation and blurred vision have occurred in some instances.

Genitourinary System: Inhibition of ejaculation, impotence, enuresis, and incontinence have been reported.

Skin: Itching, rash, hypertrophic papillae of the tongue and angioneurotic edema have been reported.

Cardiovascular System: Hypotension and tachycardia have been reported. EKG changes have occurred in some instances (see PHENOTHIAZINE DERIVATIVES: Cardiovascular Effects).

Phenothiazine Derivatives: It should be noted that efficacy, indications and untoward effects have varied with the different phenothiazines. The physician should be aware that the following have occurred with one or more phenothiazines and should be considered whenever one of these drugs is used:

Autonomic Reactions: Miosis, obstipation, anorexia, paralytic ileus.

Cutaneous Reactions: Erythema, exfoliative dermatitis, contact dermatitis.

Blood Dyscrasias: Agranulocytosis, leukopenia, eosinophilia, thrombocytopenia, anemia, aplastic anemia, pancytopenia.

Allergic Reactions: Fever, laryngeal edema, angioneurotic edema, asthma.

Hepatotoxicity: Jaundice, biliary stasis.

Cardiovascular Effects: Changes in the terminal portion of the electrocardiogram, including prolongation of the Q-T interval, lowering and inversion of the T wave and appearance of a wave tentatively identified as a bifid T or a U wave have been observed in some patients receiving the phenothiazine tranquilizers, including Serentil® (mesoridazine besylate). To date, these appear to be due to altered repolarization and not related to myocardial damage. They appear to be reversible. While there is no evidence at present that these changes are in any way precursors of any significant disturbance of cardiac rhythm, it should be noted that sudden and unexpected deaths apparently due to cardiac arrest have occurred in patients previously showing characteristic electrocardiographic changes while taking the drug. The use of periodic electrocardiograms has been proposed but would appear to be of questionable value as a predictive device. Hypotension, rarely resulting in cardiac arrest, has been noted.

Extrapyramidal Symptoms: Akathisia, agitation, motor restlessness, dystonic reactions, trismus, torticollis, opisthotonos, oculogyric crises, tremor, muscular rigidity, akinesia.

Tardive Dyskinesia: Chronic use of neuroleptics may be associated with the development of tardive dyskinesia. The salient features of this syndrome are described in the WARNINGS section and below.

The syndrome is characterized by involuntary choreoathetoid movements which variously involve the tongue, face, mouth, lips, or jaw (e.g., protrusion of the tongue, puffing of cheeks, puckering of the mouth, chewing movements), trunk and extremities. The severity of the syndrome and the degree of impairment produced vary widely.

The syndrome may become clinically recognizable either during treatment, upon dosage reduction, or upon withdrawal of treatment. Movements may decrease in intensity and may disappear altogether if further treatment with neuroleptics is withheld. It is generally believed that reversibility is more likely after short- rather than long-term neuroleptic exposure. Consequently, early detection of tardive dyskinesia is important. To increase the likelihood of detecting the syndrome at the earliest possible time, the dosage of neuroleptic drug should be reduced periodically (if clinically possible) and the patient observed for signs of the disorder. This maneuver is critical, for neuroleptic drugs may mask the signs of the syndrome.

Endocrine Disturbances: Menstrual irregularities, altered libido, gynecomastia, lactation, weight gain, edema. False positive pregnancy tests have been reported.

Urinary Disturbances: Retention, incontinence.

Others: Hyperpyrexia. Behavioral effects suggestive of a paradoxical reaction have been reported. These include excitement, bizarre dreams, aggravation of psychoses and toxic confusional states. More recently, a peculiar skin-eye syndrome has been recognized as a side effect following long-term treatment with phenothiazines. This reaction is marked by progressive pigmentation of areas of the skin or conjunctiva and/or accompanied by discoloration of the exposed sclera and cornea. Opacities of the anterior lens and cornea described as irregular or stellate in shape have also been reported. Systemic lupus erythematosus-like syndrome.

OVERDOSAGE

Symptoms of Acute Overdosage

—Drowsiness, confusion, disorientation, agitation, coma, death.

—Dryness of mouth, edema of glottis, laryngeal spasms, nasal congestion, blurred vision, vomiting.

—Hyperpyrexia, dilated pupils, muscle rigidity, hyperactive reflexes, areflexia.

—Stupor, and CNS depression or stimulation with convulsions followed by respiratory depression.

—Cardiac abnormalities, including QRS changes, tachycardia, hypotension, bilateral bundle branch block, ventricular fibrillation, shock, cardiac arrest and congestive heart failure. (See case descriptions below.)

Treatment of Acute Overdosage   No specific antidote is known. The drug is not dialyzable. Treatment should include:

—*General supportive* measures with *emesis* and *gastric lavage.*

—*Respiratory assistance* is apparently the most effective measure when indicated.

—The *administration of barbiturates* for control of convulsions alleviates an increase in the cardiac work load, but should be undertaken with caution to avoid potentiation of respiratory depression.

—*Intramuscular paraldehyde* or *diazepam* provides anticonvulsant activity with less respiratory depression than do the barbiturates; diazepam seems to be preferred.

—The use of *digitalis and/or physostigmine* may be considered in case of serious cardiovascular abnormalities or cardiac failure.

—Due to several cases of severe cardiotoxicity following Serentil® (mesoridazine besylate) overdose, *continuous ECG monitoring* of these patients is recommended. Two cases are described below:

Marrs-Simon P.A. et al (Cardiotoxic Manifestations of Mesoridazine Overdose. *Ann Emerg Med.* 1988;17:1074-1078) describes the management of a 20-year-old female who experienced severe cardiotoxicity following an overdose of mesoridazine. The paper also describes similar cases from the published literature.

The serum mesoridazine level in a 115-lb patient following ingestion of 4.5 g to 6.0 g of Serentil® (mesoridazine besylate) was 2.5 mcg/mL. She was comatose, hypotensive, convulsing, and had ECG changes. Twenty-four hours later, after hemoperfusion with activated charcoal, the mesoridazine blood levels fell to 1.3 mcg/mL and the patient was normotensive and responsive.

DOSAGE AND ADMINISTRATION

The dosage of Serentil® (mesoridazine besylate USP), as with most medications, should be adjusted to the needs of the individual. The lowest effective dosage should always be used. When maximum response is achieved, dosage may be reduced gradually to a maintenance level.

Schizophrenia: For most patients, regardless of severity, a starting dose of 50 mg t.i.d. is recommended. The usual optimum total daily dose range is 100-400 mg per day.

Behavioral Problems in Mental Deficiency and Chronic Brain Syndrome: For most patients a starting dose of 25 mg t.i.d. is recommended. The usual optimum total daily dose range is 75-300 mg per day.

Alcoholism: For most patients the usual starting dose is 25 mg b.i.d. The usual optimum total daily dose range is 50-200 mg per day.

Psychoneurotic Manifestations: For most patients the usual starting dose is 10 mg t.i.d. The usual optimum total daily dose range is 30-150 mg per day.

Injectable Form: In those situations in which an intramuscular form of medication is indicated, Serentil® (mesoridazine besylate) injectable is available. For most patients a starting dose of 25 mg is recommended. The dose may be repeated in 30 to 60 minutes, if necessary. The usual optimum total daily dose range is 25-200 mg per day.

HOW SUPPLIED

Tablets   10 mg (NDC 0597-0020-01), 25 mg (NDC 0597-0021-01), 50 mg (NDC 0597-0022-01), and 100 mg (NDC 0597-0023-01) mesoridazine (as the besylate). Bottles of 100.

Ampuls   1 mL [25 mg mesoridazine (as the besylate)]. Boxes of 20 (NDC 0597-0027-02).

Concentrate   Contains 25 mg mesoridazine (as the besylate) per mL, alcohol, USP, 0.61% by volume. Immediate containers: Amber glass bottles of 4 fl oz (118 mL) packaged in cartons of 12 bottles, with an accompanying dropper graduated to deliver 10 mg, 25 mg, and 50 mg of mesoridazine (as the besylate) (NDC 0597-0025-04).

STORAGE

Tablets: Below 86°F (30°C). Injection: Below 86°F (30°C); protect from light. Oral Solution: Below 77°F (25°C). Protect from light. Dispense in amber glass bottles only.

The concentrate may be diluted with distilled water, acidified tap water, orange juice or grape juice.

Each dose should be diluted just prior to administration. Preparation and storage of bulk dilutions is not recommended.

Additional information available to physicians.

PHARMACOLOGY

Pharmacological studies in laboratory animals have established that Serentil® (mesoridazine besylate USP) has a spectrum of pharmacodynamic actions typical of a major tranquilizer. In common with other tranquilizers it inhibits spontaneous motor activity in mice, prolongs thiopental and hexobarbital sleeping time in mice and produces spindles and block of arousal reaction in the EEG of rabbits. It is effective in blocking spinal reflexes in the cat and antagonizes d-amphetamine excitation and toxicity in grouped mice. It shows a moderate adrenergic blocking activity in vitro and in vivo and antagonizes 5-hydroxytryptamine in vivo. Intravenously administered, it lowers the blood pressure of anesthetized dogs. It has a weak antiacetylcholine effect in vitro. The most outstanding activity of Serentil® (mesoridazine besylate) is seen in tests developed to investigate antiemotive activity of drugs. Such tests are those in which the rat reacts to acute or chronic stress by increased defecation (emotogenic defecation) or tests in which "emotional mydriasis" is elicited in the mouse by an electric shock. In both of these tests Serentil® (mesoridazine besylate) is effective in reducing emotive reactions. Its ED_{50} in inhibiting emotogenic defecation in the rat is 0.053 mg/kg (subcutaneous administration). Serentil has a potent antiemetic action. The intravenous ED_{50} against apomorphine-induced emesis in the dog is 0.64 mg/kg. Serentil® (mesoridazine besylate), in common with other phenothiazines, demonstrates antiarrhythmic activity in anesthetized dogs.

Metabolic studies in the dog and rabbit with tritium labeled mesoridazine demonstrate that the compound is well absorbed from the gastrointestinal tract. The biological half-life of Serentil in these studies appears to be somewhere between 24 and 48 hours. Although significant urinary excretion was observed following the administration of Serentil, these studies also suggest that biliary excretion is an important excretion route for mesoridazine and/or its metabolites.

Toxicity Studies

Acute LD_{50} (mg/kg):

Route	Mouse	Rat	Rabbit	Dog
Oral	560±62.5	644±48	MLD=800	MLD=800
I.M.		509M 584 F	405	
I.V.	26±0.08	—	—	—

Chronic toxicity studies were conducted in rats and dogs. Rats were administered Serentil orally seven days per week for a period of 17 months in doses up to 160 mg/kg per day. Dogs were administered Serentil orally seven days per week for a period of 13 months. The daily dosage of the drug was increased during the period of this test such that the "top-dose" group received a daily dose of 120 mg/kg of mesoridazine for the last month of the study.

Untoward effects that occurred upon chronic administration of high dose levels included:

Rats: Reduction of food intake, slowed weight gain, morphological changes in pituitary-supported endocrine organs, and melanin-like pigment deposition in renal tissues.

Dogs: Emesis, muscle tremors, decreased food intake and death associated with aspiration of oral-gastric contents into the respiratory system.

Increased intrauterine resorptions were seen with Serentil in rats at 70 mg/kg and in rabbits at 125 mg/kg but not at 60 and 100 mg/kg, respectively. No drug-related teratology was suggested by these reproductive studies.

Local irritation from the intramuscular injection of Serentil was of the same order of magnitude as with other phenothiazines.

SR-PI-6/93

Shown in Product Identification Guide, page 306

Check the **BLUE** section
to find drugs by category.

Boehringer Mannheim Corporation

Therapeutics
101 ORCHARD RIDGE DRIVE GAITHERSBURG, MD 20878

Direct Inquiries to:
(301) 216-3900
FAX: (301) 990-3815

For Medical Information Contact:
In Emergencies:
(301) 216-3900
FAX: (301) 216-3415

DEMADEX®   ℞
[dē'-mă-dex]
torsemide tablets
torsemide injection

DESCRIPTION

DEMADEX (torsemide) is a diuretic of the pyridine-sulfonyl-urea class. Its chemical name is 1-isopropyl-3-[(4-*m*-toluidino-3-pyridyl) sulfonyl]urea and its structural formula is

Its empirical formula is $C_{16}H_{20}N_4O_3S$, its pKa is 7.1, and its molecular weight is 348.43.

DEMADEX (torsemide) is a white to off-white crystalline powder. The tablets for oral administration also contain lactose NF, crospovidone NF, povidone USP, microcrystalline cellulose NF, and magnesium stearate NF. DEMADEX (torsemide) ampuls for intravenous injection contain a sterile solution of torsemide (10 mg/mL), polyethylene glycol-400 NF, tromethamine USP, and sodium hydroxide NF (as needed to adjust pH) in water for injection USP.

CLINICAL PHARMACOLOGY

Mechanism of action: Micropuncture studies in animals have shown that DEMADEX (torsemide) acts from within the lumen of the thick ascending portion of the loop of Henle, where it inhibits the $Na^+/K^+/2Cl^-$-carrier system. Clinical pharmacology studies have confirmed this site of action in humans, and effects in other segments of the nephron have not been demonstrated. Diuretic activity thus correlates better with the rate of drug excretion in the urine than with the concentration in the blood.

DEMADEX (torsemide) increases the urinary excretion of sodium, chloride, and water, but it does not significantly alter glomerular filtration rate, renal plasma flow, or acid-base balance.

Pharmacokinetics and metabolism: The bioavailability of DEMADEX (torsemide) Tablets is approximately 80%, with little intersubject variation; the 90% confidence interval is 75% to 89%. The drug is absorbed with little first-pass metabolism, and the serum concentration reaches its peak (Cmax) within one hour after oral administration. Cmax and area under the serum concentration-time curve (AUC) after oral administration are proportional to dose over the range of 2.5 to 200 mg. Simultaneous food intake delays the time to Cmax by about 30 minutes, but overall bioavailability (AUC) and diuretic activity are unchanged. Absorption is essentially unaffected by renal or hepatic dysfunction.

The **volume of distribution** of DEMADEX (torsemide) is 12 to 15 liters in normal adults or in patients with mild to moderate renal failure or congestive heart failure. In patients with hepatic cirrhosis, the volume of distribution is approximately doubled.

In normal subjects the **elimination half-life** of DEMADEX (torsemide) is approximately 3.5 hours. DEMADEX (torsemide) is cleared from the circulation by both hepatic metabolism (approximately 80% of total clearance) and excretion into the urine (approximately 20% of total clearance in patients with normal renal function). The major metabolite in humans is the carboxylic acid derivative, which is biologically inactive. Two of the lesser metabolites possess some diuretic activity, but for practical purposes metabolism terminates the action of the drug.

Because DEMADEX (torsemide) is extensively bound to plasma protein (>99%), very little enters tubular urine via

Continued on next page

Boehringer Mannheim—Cont.

glomerular filtration. Most renal clearance of DEMADEX (torsemide) occurs via active secretion of the drug by the proximal tubules into tubular urine.

In patients with decompensated congestive heart failure, hepatic and renal clearance are both reduced, probably because of hepatic congestion and decreased renal plasma flow, respectively. The total clearance of DEMADEX (torsemide) is approximately 50% of that seen in healthy volunteers, and the plasma half-life and AUC are correspondingly increased. Because of reduced renal clearance, a smaller fraction of any given dose is delivered to the intraluminal site of action, so at any given dose there is less natriuresis in patients with congestive heart failure than in normal subjects.

In patients with renal failure, renal clearance of DEMADEX (torsemide) is markedly decreased but total plasma clearance is not significantly altered. A smaller fraction of the administered dose is delivered to the intraluminal site of action, and the natriuretic action of any given dose of diuretic is reduced. A diuretic response in renal failure may still be achieved if patients are given higher doses. The total plasma clearance and **elimination half-life** of DEMADEX (torsemide) remain normal under the conditions of impaired renal function because metabolic elimination by the liver remains intact.

In patients with hepatic cirrhosis, the volume of distribution, plasma half-life, and renal clearance are all increased, but total clearance is unchanged.

The pharmacokinetic profile of DEMADEX (torsemide) in healthy elderly subjects is similar to that in young subjects except for a decrease in renal clearance related to the decline in renal function that commonly occurs with aging. However, total plasma clearance and elimination half-life remain unchanged.

Clinical effects: The diuretic effects of DEMADEX (torsemide) begin within 10 minutes of intravenous dosing and peak within the first hour. With oral dosing, the onset of diuresis occurs within one hour and the peak effect occurs during the first or second hour. Independent of the route of administration, diuresis lasts about six to eight hours. In healthy subjects given single doses, the dose-response relationship for sodium excretion is linear over the dose range of 2.5 to 20 mg. The increase in potassium excretion is negligible after a single dose of up to 10 mg and only slight (5 to 15 mEq) after a single dose of 20 mg.

DEMADEX (torsemide) has been studied in controlled trials in patients with New York Heart Association Class II to Class IV **congestive heart failure**. Patients who received 10 to 20 mg of daily DEMADEX (torsemide) in these studies achieved significantly greater reductions in weight and edema than did patients who received placebo.

In single-dose studies in patients with **nonanuric renal failure**, high doses of DEMADEX (torsemide) (20 to 200 mg) caused marked increases in water and sodium excretion. In patients with nonanuric renal failure severe enough to require hemodialysis, chronic treatment with up to 200 mg of daily DEMADEX (torsemide) has not been shown to change steady-state fluid retention. Chronic use of any diuretic in renal disease has not been studied in adequate and well-controlled trials. When patients in a study of acute renal failure received total daily doses of 520 to 1200 mg of DEMADEX (torsemide), 19% experienced seizures. 96 total patients were treated in this study; 6/32 treated with torsemide experienced seizures, 6/32 treated with comparably high doses of furosemide experienced seizures, and 1/32 treated with placebo experienced a seizure

When given with aldosterone antagonists, DEMADEX (torsemide) also caused increases in sodium and fluid excretion in patients with edema or ascites due to **hepatic cirrhosis**. Urinary sodium excretion rate relative to the urinary excretion rate of DEMADEX (torsemide) is less in cirrhotic patients than in healthy subjects (possibly because of the hyperaldosteronism and resultant sodium retention that are characteristic of portal hypertension and ascites). However, because of the increased renal clearance of DEMADEX (torsemide) in patients with hepatic cirrhosis, these factors tend to balance each other, and the result is an overall natriuretic response that is similar to that seen in healthy subjects. Chronic use of any diuretic in hepatic disease has not been studied in adequate and well-controlled trials.

In patients with **essential hypertension**, DEMADEX (torsemide) has been shown in controlled studies to lower blood pressure when administered once a day at doses of 5 to 10 mg. The antihypertensive effect is near maximal after four to six weeks of treatment, but it may continue to increase for up to 12 weeks. Systolic and diastolic supine and standing blood pressures are all reduced. There is no significant orthostatic effect, and there is only a minimal peak-trough difference in blood-pressure reduction.

The antihypertensive effects of DEMADEX (torsemide) are, like those of other diuretics, on the average greater in black patients (a low-renin population) than in nonblack patients.

When DEMADEX (torsemide) is first administered, daily urinary sodium excretion increases for at least a week. With chronic administration, however, daily sodium loss comes into balance with dietary sodium intake. If the administration of DEMADEX (torsemide) is suddenly stopped, blood pressure returns to pretreatment levels over several days, without overshoot.

DEMADEX (torsemide) has been administered together with β-adrenergic blocking agents, ACE inhibitors, and calcium-channel blockers. Adverse drug interactions have not been observed, and special dosage adjustment has not been necessary.

INDICATIONS AND USE

DEMADEX (torsemide) is indicated for the treatment of edema associated with congestive heart failure, renal disease, or hepatic disease. Chronic use of any diuretic in renal or hepatic disease has not been studied in adequate and well-controlled trials.

DEMADEX (torsemide) Intravenous Injection is indicated when a rapid onset of diuresis is desired or when oral administration is impractical.

DEMADEX (torsemide) is indicated for the treatment of hypertension alone or in combination with other antihypertensive agents.

CONTRAINDICATIONS

DEMADEX (torsemide) is contraindicated in patients with known hypersensitivity to DEMADEX (torsemide) or to sulfonylureas.

DEMADEX (torsemide) is contraindicated in patients who are anuric.

WARNINGS

Hepatic disease with cirrhosis and ascites: DEMADEX (torsemide) should be used with caution in patients with hepatic disease with cirrhosis and ascites, since sudden alterations of fluid and electrolyte balance may precipitate hepatic coma. In these patients, diuresis with DEMADEX (torsemide) (or any other diuretic) is best initiated in the hospital. To prevent hypokalemia and metabolic alkalosis, an aldosterone antagonist or potassium-sparing drug should be used concomitantly with DEMADEX (torsemide).

Ototoxicity: Tinnitus and hearing loss (usually reversible) have been observed after rapid intravenous injection of other loop diuretics and have also been observed after oral DEMADEX (torsemide). It is not certain that these events were attributable to DEMADEX (torsemide). Ototoxicity has also been seen in animal studies when very high plasma levels of DEMADEX (torsemide) were induced. Administered intravenously, DEMADEX (torsemide) should be injected slowly over two minutes, and single doses should not exceed 200 mg.

Volume and electrolyte depletion: Patients receiving diuretics should be observed for clinical evidence of electrolyte imbalance, hypovolemia, or prerenal azotemia. Symptoms of these disturbances may include one or more of the following: dryness of the mouth, thirst, weakness, lethargy, drowsiness, restlessness, muscle pains or cramps, muscular fatigue, hypotension, oliguria, tachycardia, nausea, and vomiting. Excessive diuresis may cause dehydration, blood-volume reduction, and possibly thrombosis and embolism, especially in elderly patients. In patients who develop fluid and electrolyte imbalances, hypovolemia, or prerenal azotemia, the observed laboratory changes may include hyper- or hyponatremia, hyper- or hypochloremia, hyper- or hypokalemia, acid-base abnormalities, and increased blood urea nitrogen. If any of these occur, DEMADEX (torsemide) should be discontinued until the situation is corrected; DEMADEX (torsemide) may be restarted at a lower dose.

In controlled studies in the United States, DEMADEX (torsemide) was administered to hypertensive patients at doses of 5 mg or 10 mg daily. After six weeks at these doses, the mean decrease in serum potassium was approximately 0.1 mEq/L. The percentage of patients who had a serum potassium level below 3.5 mEq/L at any time during the studies was essentially the same in patients who received DEMADEX (torsemide) (1.5%) as in those who received placebo (3%). In patients followed for one year, there was no further change in mean serum potassium levels. In patients with congestive heart failure, hepatic cirrhosis, or renal disease treated with DEMADEX (torsemide) at doses higher than those studied in U.S. antihypertensive trials, hypokalemia was observed with greater frequency, in a dose-related manner.

In patients with cardiovascular disease, especially those receiving digitalis glycosides, diuretic-induced hypokalemia may be a risk factor for the development of arrhythmias. The risk of hypokalemia is greatest in patients with cirrhosis of the liver, in patients experiencing a brisk diuresis, in patients who are receiving inadequate oral intake of electrolytes, and in patients receiving concomitant therapy with corticosteroids or ACTH.

Periodic monitoring of serum potassium and other electrolytes is advised in patients treated with DEMADEX (torsemide).

PRECAUTIONS

Laboratory values

Potassium: See statement in Warnings.

Calcium: Single doses of DEMADEX (torsemide) increased the urinary excretion of calcium by normal subjects, but serum calcium levels were slightly increased in four- to six-week hypertension trials. In a long-term study of patients with congestive heart failure, the average one-year change in serum calcium was a decrease of 0.10 mg/dL (0.02 mmol/L). Among 426 patients treated with DEMADEX (torsemide) for an average of 11 months, hypocalcemia was not reported as an adverse event.

Magnesium: Single doses of DEMADEX (torsemide) caused healthy volunteers to increase their urinary excretion of magnesium, but serum magnesium levels were slightly increased in four- to six-week hypertension trials. In long-term hypertension studies, the average one-year change in serum magnesium was an increase of 0.03 mg/dL (0.01 mmol/L). Among 426 patients treated with DEMADEX (torsemide) for an average of 11 months, one case of hypomagnesemia (1.3 mg/dL (0.53 mmol/L)) was reported as an adverse event.

In a long-term clinical study of DEMADEX (torsemide) in patients with congestive heart failure, the estimated annual change in serum magnesium was an increase of 0.2 mg/dL (0.08 mmol/L), but these data are confounded by the fact that many of these patients received magnesium supplements. In a four-week study in which magnesium supplementation was not given, the rate of occurrence of serum magnesium levels below 1.7 mg/dL (0.70 mmol/L) was 6% and 9% in the groups receiving 5 mg and 10 mg of DEMADEX (torsemide), respectively.

Blood urea nitrogen (BUN), creatinine, and uric acid: DEMADEX (torsemide) produces small dose-related increases in each of these laboratory values. In hypertensive patients who received 10 mg of DEMADEX (torsemide) daily for six weeks, the mean increase in blood urea nitrogen was 1.8 mg/dL (0.6 mmol/L), the mean increase in serum creatinine was 0.05 mg/dL (4 μmol/L), and the mean increase in serum uric acid was 1.2 mg/dL (70 μmol/L). Little further change occurred with long-term treatment, and all changes reversed when treatment was discontinued.

Symptomatic gout has been reported in patients receiving DEMADEX (torsemide), but its incidence has been similar to that seen in patients receiving placebo.

Glucose: Hypertensive patients who received 10 mg of daily DEMADEX (torsemide) experienced a mean increase in serum glucose concentration of 5.5 mg/dL (0.3 mmol/L) after six weeks of therapy, with a further increase of 1.8 mg/dL (0.1 mmol/L) during the subsequent year. In long-term studies in diabetics, mean fasting glucose values were not significantly changed from baseline. Cases of hyperglycemia have been reported but are uncommon.

Serum lipids: In the controlled short-term hypertension studies in the United States, daily doses of 5, 10, and 20 mg of DEMADEX (torsemide) were associated with increases in total plasma cholesterol of 4, 4, and 8 mg/dL (0.10 to 0.20 mmol/L), respectively. The changes subsided during chronic therapy.

In the same short-term hypertension studies, daily doses of 5, 10, and 20 mg of DEMADEX (torsemide) were associated with mean increases in plasma triglycerides of 16, 13, and 71 mg/dL (0.15 to 0.80 mmol/L), respectively.

In long-term studies of 5 to 20 mg of DEMADEX (torsemide) daily, no clinically significant differences from baseline lipid values were observed after one year of therapy.

Other: In long-term studies in hypertensive patients, DEMADEX (torsemide) has been associated with small mean decreases in hemoglobin, hematocrit, and erythrocyte count and small mean increases in white blood cell count, platelet count, and serum alkaline phosphatase. Although statistically significant, all of these changes were medically inconsequential. No significant trends have been observed in any liver enzyme tests other than alkaline phosphatase.

DRUG INTERACTIONS

In patients with essential hypertension, DEMADEX (torsemide) has been administered together with β-blockers, ACE inhibitors, and calcium-channel blockers. In patients with congestive heart failure, DEMADEX (torsemide) has been administered together with digitalis glycosides, ACE inhibitors, and organic nitrates. None of these combined uses was associated with new or unexpected adverse events.

DEMADEX (torsemide) does not affect the protein binding of **glyburide** or of **warfarin**, the anticoagulant effect of **phenprocoumon** (a related coumarin derivative), or the pharmacokinetics of **digoxin** or **carvedilol** (a vasodilator/β-blocker). In healthy subjects, coadministration of DEMADEX (torsemide) was associated with significant reduction in the renal clearance of **spironolactone**, with corresponding increases in the AUC. However, clinical experience indicates that dosage adjustment of either agent is not required.

Because DEMADEX (torsemide) and salicylates compete for secretion by renal tubules, patients receiving high doses of **salicylates** may experience salicylate toxicity when DEMADEX (torsemide) is concomitantly administered. Also,

although possible interactions between torsemide and **nonsteroidal anti-inflammatory agents (including aspirin)** have not been studied, coadministration of these agents with another loop diuretic (furosemide) has occasionally been associated with renal dysfunction.

The natriuretic effect of DEMADEX (torsemide) (like that of many other diuretics) is partially inhibited by the concomitant administration of **indomethacin**. This effect has been demonstrated for DEMADEX (torsemide) under conditions of dietary sodium restriction (50 mEq/day) but not in the presence of normal sodium intake (150 mEq/day).

The pharmacokinetic profile and diuretic activity of DEMADEX (torsemide) are not altered by **cimetidine** or **spironolactone**. Coadministration of **digoxin** is reported to increase the area under the curve for DEMADEX (torsemide) by 50%, but dose adjustment of DEMADEX (torsemide) is not necessary.

Concomitant use of torsemide and cholestyramine has not been studied in humans but, in a study in animals, coadministration of cholestyramine decreased the absorption of orally administered DEMADEX (torsemide). If DEMADEX (torsemide) and cholestyramine are used concomitantly, simultaneous administration is not recommended.

Coadministration of **probenecid** reduces secretion of DEMADEX (torsemide) into the proximal tubule and thereby decreases the diuretic activity of DEMADEX (torsemide).

Other diuretics are known to reduce the renal clearance of **lithium**, inducing a high risk of lithium toxicity, so coadministration of lithium and diuretics should be undertaken with great caution, if at all. Coadministration of lithium and DEMADEX (torsemide) has not been studied.

Other diuretics have been reported to increase the ototoxic potential of **aminoglycoside antibiotics** and of **ethacrynic acid**, especially in the presence of impaired renal function. These potential interactions with DEMADEX (torsemide) have not been studied.

Carcinogenesis, mutagenesis, impairment of fertility

No overall increase in tumor incidence was found when DEMADEX (torsemide) was given to rats and mice throughout their lives at doses up to 9 mg/kg/day (rats) and 32 mg/kg/day (mice). On a body-weight basis, these doses are 27 to 96 times a human dose of 20 mg; on a body-surface-area basis, they are 5 to 8 times this dose. In the rat study, the high-dose female group demonstrated renal tubular injury, interstitial inflammation, and a statistically significant increase in renal adenomas and carcinomas. The tumor incidence in this group was, however, not much higher than the incidence sometimes seen in historical controls. Similar signs of chronic non-neoplastic renal injury have been reported in high-dose animal studies of other diuretics such as furosemide and hydrochlorothiazide.

No mutagenic activity was detected in any of a variety of in vivo and in vitro tests of DEMADEX (torsemide) and its major human metabolite. The tests included the Ames test in bacteria (with and without metabolic activation), tests for chromosome aberrations and sister-chromatid exchanges in human lymphocytes, tests for various nuclear anomalies in cells found in hamster and murine bone marrow, tests for unscheduled DNA synthesis in mice and rats, and others. In doses up to 25 mg/kg/day (75 times a human dose of 20 mg on a body-weight basis; 13 times this dose on a body-surface-area basis), DEMADEX (torsemide) had no adverse effect on the reproductive performance of male or female rats.

Pregnancy

Pregnancy Category B. There was no fetotoxicity or teratogenicity in rats treated with up to 5 mg/kg/day of DEMADEX (torsemide) (on a mg/kg basis, this is 15 times a human dose of 20 mg/day; on a mg/m^2 basis, the animal dose is 10 times the human dose), or in rabbits treated with 1.6 mg/kg/day (on a mg/kg basis, 5 times the human dose of 20 mg/day; on a mg/m^2 basis, 1.7 times this dose). Fetal and maternal toxicity (decrease in average body weight, increase in fetal resorption, and delayed fetal ossification) occurred in rabbits and rats given doses 4 (rabbits) and 5 (rats) times larger. Adequate and well-controlled studies have not been carried out in pregnant women. Because animal reproduction studies are not always predictive of human response, this drug should be used during pregnancy only if clearly needed.

Labor and delivery

The effect of DEMADEX (torsemide) on labor and delivery is unknown.

Nursing mothers

It is not known whether DEMADEX (torsemide) is excreted in human milk. Because many drugs are excreted in human milk, caution should be exercised when DEMADEX (torsemide) is administered to a nursing woman.

Geriatric use

Of the total number of patients who received DEMADEX (torsemide) in U.S. clinical studies, 24% were 65 or older while about 4% were 75 or older. No specific age-related differences in effectiveness or safety were observed between younger patients and elderly patients.

Pediatric use

Safety and effectiveness in children have not been established.

Administration of another loop diuretic to severely premature infants with edema due to patent ductus arteriosus and hyaline membrane disease has occasionally been associated with renal calcifications, sometimes barely visible on x-ray but sometimes in staghorn form, filling the renal pelves. Some of these calculi have been dissolved, and hypercalciuria has been reported to have decreased, when chlorothiazide has been coadministered along with the loop diuretic. In other premature neonates with hyaline membrane disease, another loop diuretic has been reported to increase the risk of persistent patent ductus arteriosus, possibly through a prostaglandin-E-mediated process. The use of DEMADEX (torsemide) in such patients has not been studied.

ADVERSE REACTIONS

At the time of approval, DEMADEX (torsemide) had been evaluated for safety in approximately 4000 subjects: over 800 of these subjects received DEMADEX (torsemide) for at least six months, and over 380 were treated for more than one year. Among these subjects were 564 who received DEMADEX (torsemide) during U.S.-based trials in which 274 other subjects received placebo.

The reported side effects of DEMADEX (torsemide) were generally transient, and there was no relationship between side effects and age, sex, race, or duration of therapy. Discontinuation of therapy due to side effects occurred in 3.5% of U.S. patients treated with DEMADEX (torsemide) and in 4.4% of patients treated with placebo. In studies conducted in the United States and Europe, discontinuation rates due to side effects were 3.0% (38/1250) with DEMADEX (torsemide) and 3.4% (13/380) with furosemide in patients with congestive heart failure, 2.0% (8/409) with DEMADEX (torsemide) and 4.8% (11/230) with furosemide in patients with renal insufficiency, and 7.6% (13/170) with DEMADEX (torsemide) and 0% (0/33) with furosemide in patients with cirrhosis.

The most common reasons for discontinuation of therapy with DEMADEX (torsemide) were (in descending order of frequency) dizziness, headache, nausea, weakness, vomiting, hyperglycemia, excessive urination, hyperuricemia, hypokalemia, excessive thirst, hypo-volemia, impotence, esophageal hemorrhage, and dyspepsia. Dropout rates for these adverse events ranged from 0.1% to 0.5%.

The side effects considered possibly or probably related to study drug that occurred in U.S. placebo-controlled trials in more than 1% of patients treated with DEMADEX (torsemide) are shown in the table below.

Reactions Possibly or Probably Drug-Related
U.S. Placebo-Controlled Studies
Incidence (Percentages of Patients)

	DEMADEX (torsemide) (N = 564)	placebo (N = 274)
headache	7.3	9.1
excessive urination	6.7	2.2
dizziness	3.2	4.0
rhinitis	2.8	2.2
asthenia	2.0	1.5
diarrhea	2.0	1.1
ECG abnormality	2.0	0.4
cough increase	2.0	1.5
constipation	1.8	0.7
nausea	1.8	0.4
arthralgia	1.8	0.7
dyspepsia	1.6	0.7
sore throat	1.6	0.7
myalgia	1.6	1.5
chest pain	1.2	0.4
insomnia	1.2	1.8
edema	1.1	1.1
nervousness	1.1	0.4

The daily doses of DEMADEX (torsemide) used in these trials ranged from 1.25 to 20 mg, with most patients receiving 5 to 10 mg; the duration of treatment ranged from one to 52 days, with a median of 41 days. Of the side effects listed in the table, only "excessive urination" occurred significantly more frequently in patients treated with DEMADEX (torsemide) than in patients treated with placebo. In the placebo-controlled hypertension studies whose design allowed side-effect rates to be attributed to dose, excessive urination was reported by 1% of patients receiving placebo, 4% of those treated with 5 mg of daily DEMADEX (torsemide), and 15% of those treated with 10 mg. The complaint of excessive urination was generally not reported as an adverse event among patients who received DEMADEX (torsemide) for cardiac, renal, or hepatic failure.

Serious adverse events reported in the clinical studies for which a drug relationship could not be excluded were atrial fibrillation, chest pain, diarrhea, digitalis intoxication, gastrointestinal hemorrhage, hyperglycemia, hyperuricemia, hypokalemia, hypotension, hypo-volemia, shunt thrombosis, rash, rectal bleeding, syncope, and ventricular tachycardia. Angioedema has been reported in a patient exposed to DEMADEX (torsemide) who was later found to be allergic to sulfa drugs.

Of the adverse reactions during placebo-controlled trials listed without taking into account assessment of relatedness to drug therapy, arthritis and various other nonspecific musculoskeletal problems were more frequently reported in association with DEMADEX (torsemide) than with placebo, even though gout was somewhat more frequently associated with placebo. These reactions did not increase in frequency or severity with the dose of DEMADEX (torsemide). One patient in the group treated with DEMADEX (torsemide) withdrew due to myalgia, and one in the placebo group withdrew due to gout.

Hypokalemia: See statement in Warnings:

OVERDOSAGE

There is no human experience with overdoses of DEMADEX (torsemide), but the signs and symptoms of overdosage can be anticipated to be those of excessive pharmacologic effect: dehydration, hypovolemia, hypotension, hyponatremia, hypokalemia, hypochloremic alkalosis, and hemoconcentration. Treatment of overdosage should consist of fluid and electrolyte replacement.

Laboratory determinations of serum levels of DEMADEX (torsemide) and its metabolites are not widely available.

No data are available to suggest physiological maneuvers (e.g., maneuvers to change the pH of the urine) that might accelerate elimination of DEMADEX (torsemide) and its metabolites. DEMADEX (torsemide) is not dialyzable, so hemodialysis will not accelerate elimination.

DOSAGE AND ADMINISTRATION

General: DEMADEX (torsemide) Tablets may be given at any time in relation to a meal, as convenient. Special dosage adjustment in the elderly is not necessary.

Because of the high bioavailablity of DEMADEX (torsemide), oral and intravenous doses are therapeutically equivalent, so patients may be switched to and from the intravenous form with no change in dose. DEMADEX (torsemide) Intravenous Injection should be administered slowly over a period of two minutes.

If DEMADEX (torsemide) is administered through an IV line, it is recommended that, as with other IV injections, the IV line be flushed with Normal Saline (Sodium Chloride Injection, USP) before and after administration. DEMADEX (torsemide) injection is formulated above pH 8.3. Flushing the line is recommended to avoid the potential for incompatibilities caused by differences in pH which could be indicated by color change, haziness or the formation of a precipitate in the solution.

Before administration, the solution of DEMADEX (torsemide) should be visually inspected for discoloration and particulate matter. If either is found, the ampul should not be used.

Congestive heart failure: The usual initial dose is 10 mg or 20 mg of once-daily oral or intravenous DEMADEX (torsemide). If the diuretic response is inadequate, the dose should be titrated upward by approximately doubling until the desired diuretic response is obtained. Single doses higher than 200 mg have not been adequately studied.

Chronic renal failure: The usual initial dose of DEMADEX (torsemide) is 20 mg of once-daily oral or intravenous DEMADEX (torsemide). If the diuretic response is inadequate, the dose should be titrated upward by approximately doubling until the desired diuretic response is obtained. Single doses higher than 200 mg have not been adequately studied.

Chronic use of any diuretic in renal disease has not been studied in adequate and well-controlled trials.

Hepatic cirrhosis: The usual initial dose is 5 mg or 10 mg of once-daily oral or intravenous DEMADEX (torsemide), administered together with an aldosterone antagonist or a potassium-sparing diuretic. If the diuretic response is inadequate, the dose should be titrated upward by approximately doubling until the desired diuretic response is obtained. Single doses higher than 40 mg have not been adequately studied.

Chronic use of any diuretic in hepatic disease has not been studied in adequate and well-controlled trials.

Hypertension: The usual initial dose is 5 mg once daily. If the 5 mg dose does not provide adequate reduction in blood pressure within four to six weeks, the dose may be increased to 10 mg once daily. If the response to 10 mg is insufficient, an additional antihypertensive agent should be added to the treatment regimen.

HOW SUPPLIED

DEMADEX (torsemide) for oral administration is available as white, scored tablets containing 5, 10, 20, or 100 mg of

Continued on next page

Boehringer Mannheim—Cont.

torsemide. The tablets are supplied in bottles and unit dose packages of 100 as follows:

dose	shape	bottle	unit dose
5 mg	oval	NDC 53169-102-01	NDC 53169-102-60
10 mg	oval	NDC 53169-103-01	NDC 53169-103-60
20 mg	oval	NDC 53169-104-01	NDC 53169-104-60
100 mg	capsule-shaped	NDC 53169-105-01	NDC 53169-105-60

Each tablet is debossed on the scored side with the Boehringer Mannheim logo and a portion (102, 103, 104, or 105) of the National Drug Code. On the opposite side, the tablet is debossed with 5, 10, 20, or 100 to indicate the dose.
DEMADEX (torsemide) for intravenous injection is supplied in clear ampuls containing 2 mL (20 mg, NDC 53169-108-80) or 5 mL (50 mg, NDC 53169-108-81) of a 10 mg/mL sterile solution.
Storage: Store all dosage forms at controlled room temperature, 15–30°C (59–86°F). Do not freeze.

Tablets manufactured by
Boehringer Mannheim GmbH, Mannheim, Germany
for
Boehringer Mannheim Corporation, Therapeutics Div., Gaithersburg, MD 20878.
Ampuls manufactured by
Sanofi Winthrop Inc. New York, NY 10016 for
Boehringer Mannheim Corporation, Therapeutics Div., Gaithersburg, MD 20878.
February 1996   0710016
Shown in Product Identification Guide, page 306

Braintree Laboratories, Inc.
P.O. BOX 850929
BRAINTREE, MA 02185-0929

Direct Inquiries to:
Harry P. Keegan, President
(617) 843-2202

For Medical Information Contact:
In Emergencies:
Jack DiPalma, M.D.
(800) 874-6756

GoLYTELY®   ℞
[go-līt'lē]
PEG–3350 and Electrolytes For Oral Solution

DESCRIPTION
A white powder in a 4 liter jug for reconstitution, containing 236 g polyethylene glycol 3350, 22.74 g sodium sulfate, 6.74 g sodium bicarbonate, 5.86 g sodium chloride, and 2.97 g potassium chloride. When dissolved in water to a volume of 4 liters, GoLYTELY is an isosmotic solution having a mildly salty taste. GoLYTELY is administered orally or via nasogastric tube.

CLINICAL PHARMACOLOGY
GoLYTELY induces a diarrhea which rapidly cleanses the bowel, usually within four hours. The osmotic activity of polyethylene glycol 3350 and the electrolyte concentration result in virtually no net absorption or excretion of ions or water. Accordingly, large volumes may be administered without significant changes in fluid or electrolyte balance.

INDICATIONS AND USAGE
GoLYTELY is indicated for bowel cleansing prior to colonoscopy and barium enema x-ray examination.

CONTRAINDICATIONS
GoLYTELY is contraindicated in patients with gastrointestinal obstruction, gastric retention, bowel perforation, toxic colitis, toxic megacolon or ileus.

WARNINGS
No additional ingredients, e.g. flavorings, should be added to the solution. GoLYTELY should be used with caution in patients with severe ulcerative colitis.

PRECAUTIONS
General: Patients with impaired gag reflex, unconscious or semiconscious patients, and patients prone to regurgitation or aspiration, should be observed during the administration of GoLYTELY, especially if it is administered via nasogastric tube. If a patient experiences severe bloating, distention or abdominal pain, administration should be slowed or temporarily discontinued until the symptoms abate. If gastrointestinal obstruction or perforation is suspected, appropriate studies should be performed to rule out these conditions before administration of GoLYTELY.

Information for patients: GoLYTELY produces a watery stool which cleanses the bowel before examination. Prepare the solution according to the instructions on the bottle. It is more palatable if chilled. For best results, no solid food should be consumed during the 3 to 4 hour period before drinking the solution, but in no case should solid foods be eaten within 2 hours of taking GoLYTELY.
Drink 240 ml (8 oz.) every 10 minutes. Rapid drinking of each portion is better than drinking small amounts continuously. The first bowel movement should occur approximately one hour after the start of GoLYTELY administration. You may experience some abdominal bloating and distention before the bowels start to move. If severe discomfort or distention occur, stop drinking temporarily or drink each portion at longer intervals until these symptoms disappear. Continue drinking until the watery stool is clear and free of solid matter. This usually requires at least 3 liters and it is best to drink all of the solution. Any unused portion should be discarded.
Drug Interactions: Oral medication administered within one hour of the start of administration of GoLYTELY may be flushed from the gastrointestinal tract and not absorbed.
Carcinogenesis, Mutagenesis, Impairment of Fertility: Carcinogenic and reproductive studies with animals have not been performed.
Pregnancy: Category C. Animal reproduction studies have not been conducted with GoLYTELY. It is also not known whether GoLYTELY can cause fetal harm when administered to a pregnant woman or can affect reproductive capacity. GoLYTELY should be given to a pregnant woman only if clearly needed.
Pediatric Use: Safety and effectiveness in children have not been established.

ADVERSE REACTIONS
Nausea, abdominal fullness and bloating are the most common adverse reactions (occurring in up to 50% of patients) to administration of GoLYTELY. Abdominal cramps, vomiting and anal irritation occur less frequently. These adverse reactions are transient and subside rapidly. Isolated cases of urticaria, rhinorrhea, dermatitis and (rarely) anaphylactic reaction have been reported which may represent allergic reactions.

DOSAGE AND ADMINISTRATION
The recommended dose for adults is 4 liters of GoLYTELY solution prior to gastrointestinal examination, as ingestion of this dose produces a satisfactory preparation in over 95% of patients. Ideally the patient should fast for approximately three or four hours prior to GoLYTELY administration, but in no case should solid food be given for at least two hours before the solution is given.
GoLYTELY is usually administered orally, but may be given via nasogastric tube to patients who are unwilling or unable to drink the solution. **Oral administration** is at a rate of 240 ml (8 oz.) every 10 minutes, until 4 liters are consumed or the rectal effluent is clear. Rapid drinking of each portion is preferred to drinking small amounts continuously. **Nasogastric tube administration** is at the rate of 20–30 ml per minute (1.2–1.8 liters per hour). The first bowel movement should occur approximately one hour after the start of GoLYTELY administration.
Various regimens have been used. One method is to schedule patients for examination in midmorning or later, allowing the patients three hours for drinking and an additional one hour period for complete bowel evacuation. Another method is to administer GoLYTELY on the evening before the examination, particularly if the patient is to have a barium enema.
Preparation of the solution: GoLYTELY solution is prepared by filling the container to the 4 liter mark with water and shaking vigorously several times to insure that the ingredients are dissolved. Dissolution is facilitated by using lukewarm water. The solution is more palatable if chilled before administration. The reconstituted solution should be refrigerated and used within 48 hours. Discard any unused portion.

HOW SUPPLIED
In powdered form, for oral administration as a solution following reconstitution. GoLYTELY® is available in a disposable jug and a packet in powdered form containing:
Disposable Jug: polyethylene glycol 3350 236 g, sodium sulfate (anhydrous) 22.74 g, sodium bicarbonate 6.74 g, sodium chloride 5.86 g, potassium chloride 2.97 g. When made up to 4 liters volume with water, the solution contains PEG 3350 17.6 mmol/L, sodium 125 mmol/L, sulfate 40 mmol/L, chloride 35 mmol/L, bicarbonate 20 mmol/L and potassium 10 mmol/L.
Packet: polyethylene glycol 3350 227.1 g, anhydrous sodium sulfate 21.5 g, sodium bicarbonate 6.36 g, sodium chloride 5.53 g, potassium chloride 2.82 g. When made up to 1 gallon volume with water, the solution contains PEG 3350 60 g/L, sodium sulfate 5.68 g/L, sodium bicarbonate 1.68 g/L, sodium chloride 1.46 g/L and potassium chloride 0.745 g/L.

CAUTION
Federal law prohibits dispensing without prescription.
STORAGE
Store in sealed container at 59°–86°F. When reconstituted, keep solution refrigerated. Use within 48 hours. Discard unused portion.
NDC 52268-0100-01
Revised 1/3/93
Distributed by Braintree Laboratories,
Braintree, MA 02185-0929
Shown in Product Identification Guide, page 306

NuLYTELY®   ℞
PEG 3350, Sodium Chloride, Sodium Bicarbonate and Potassium Chloride for Oral Solution

CHERRY FLAVOR
NuLYTELY®   ℞
PEG 3350, Sodium Chloride, Sodium Bicarbonate and Potassium Chloride for Oral Solution

DESCRIPTION
A white powder for reconstitution containing 420 g polyethylene glycol 3350, 5.72 g sodium bicarbonate, 11.2 g sodium chloride, 1.48 g potassium chloride and 2 g flavoring ingredients. When dissolved in water to a volume of 4 liters, NuLYTELY is an isosmotic solution having a pleasant cherry flavored taste. NuLYTELY is administered orally or via nasogastric tube.

CLINICAL PHARMACOLOGY
NuLYTELY induces a diarrhea which rapidly cleanses the bowel, usually within four hours. The osmotic activity of polyethylene glycol 3350 and the electrolyte concentration result in virtually no net absorption or excretion of ions or water. Accordingly, large volumes may be administered without significant changes in fluid or electrolyte balance.

INDICATIONS AND USAGE
NuLYTELY is indicated for bowel cleansing prior to colonoscopy.

CONTRAINDICATIONS
NuLYTELY is contraindicated in patients with gastrointestinal obstruction gastric retention, bowel perforation, toxic colitis or toxic megacolon.

WARNINGS
No additional ingredients, e.g. flavorings, should be added to the solution. NuLYTELY should be used with caution in patients with severe ulcerative colitis.

PRECAUTIONS
General
Patients with impaired gag reflex, unconscious, or semiconscious patients, and patients prone to regurgitation or aspiration should be observed during the administration of NuLYTELY, especially if it is administered via nasogastric tube. If a patient experiences severe bloating, distention or abdominal pain, administration should be slowed or temporarily discontinued until the symptoms abate. If gastrointestinal obstruction or perforation is suspected, appropriate studies should be performed to rule out these conditions before administration of NuLYTELY.
Information for patients: NuLYTELY produces a watery stool which cleanses the bowel before examination. Prepare the solution according to the instructions on the bottle. It is more palatable if chilled. For best results, no solid food should be consumed during the 3 to 4 hour period before drinking the solution, but in no case should solid foods be eaten within 2 hours of taking NuLYTELY.
Drink 240 ml (8 oz.) every 10 minutes. Rapid drinking of each portion is better than drinking small amounts continuously. The first bowel movement should occur approximately one hour after the start of NuLYTELY administration. You may experience some abdominal bloating and distention before the bowels start to move. If severe discomfort or distention occur, stop drinking temporarily or drink each portion at longer intervals until these symptoms disappear. Continue drinking until the watery stool is clear and free of solid matter. This usually requires at least 3 liters. Any unused portion should be discarded.
Drug Interactions: Oral medication administered within one hour of the start of administration of NuLYTELY may be flushed from the gastrointestinal tract and not absorbed.
Carcinogenesis, Mutagenesis, Impairment of Fertility: Carcinogenic and reproductive studies with animals have not been performed.
Pregnancy: Category C. Animal reproduction studies have not been conducted with NuLYTELY. It is also not known whether NuLYTELY can cause fetal harm when administered to a pregnant woman or can affect reproductive capacity. NuLYTELY should be given to a pregnant woman only if clearly needed.

Pediatric Use: Safety and effectiveness in children has not been established.

ADVERSE REACTIONS

Nausea, abdominal fullness and bloating are the most common adverse reactions (occurring in up to 50% of patients) to administration of NuLYTELY. Abdominal cramps, vomiting and anal irritation occur less frequently. These adverse reactions are transient and subside rapidly. Isolated cases of urticaria rhinorrhea and dermatitis have been reported with a related drug (GoLYTELY®) which may represent allergic reactions.

DOSAGE AND ADMINISTRATION

NuLYTELY is usually administered orally, but may be given via nasogastric tube to patients who are unwilling or unable to drink the solution. Ideally the patient should fast for approximately three or four hours prior to NuLYTELY administration, but in no case should solid food be given for at least two hours before the solution is given.

Oral administration is at a rate of 240 ml (8 oz.) every 10 minutes, until the rectal effluent is clear or 4 liters are consumed. Rapid drinking of each portion is preferred to drinking small amounts continuously. **Nasogastric tube administration** is at the rate of 20–30 ml per minute (1.2–1.8 liters per hour). The first bowel movement should occur approximately one hour after the start of NuLYTELY administration. Ingestion of 4 liters of NuLYTELY solution prior to gastrointestinal examination produces satisfactory preparation in over 95% of patients.

Various regimens have been used. One method is to schedule patients for examination in midmorning or later, allowing the patients three hours for drinking and an additional one hour period for complete bowel evacuation. Another method is to administer NuLYTELY on the evening before the examination.

Preparation of the solution: NuLYTELY solution is prepared by filling the container to the 4 liter mark with water and shaking vigorously several times to insure that the ingredients are dissolved. Dissolution is facilitated by using lukewarm water. The solution is more palatable if chilled before administration. The reconstituted solution should be refrigerated and used within 48 hours. Discard any unused portion.

HOW SUPPLIED

NuLYTELY and Cherry NuLYTELY are available in a disposable jug, in powdered form, for oral administration as a solution following reconstitution. Each jug contains:

NuLYTELY: polyethylene glycol 3350 420 g, sodium bicarbonate 5.72 g, sodium chloride 11.2 g, potassium chloride 1.48 g. When made up to 4 liters volume with water, the solution contains PEG 3350 31.3 mmol/L, sodium 65 mmol/L, chloride 53 mmol/L, bicarbonate 17 mmol/L, and potassium 5 mmol/L.

Cherry NuLYTELY: polyethylene glycol 3350 420 g, sodium bicarbonate 5.72 g, sodium chloride 11.2 g, potassium chloride 1.48 g, and flavoring ingredients, 2g. When made up to 4 liters volume with water, the solution contains PEG 3350 31.3 mmol/L, sodium 65 mmol/L, chloride 53 mmol/L, bicarbonate 17 mmol/L, and potassium 5 mmol/L.

CAUTION: Federal law prohibits dispensing without prescription.

STORAGE: Store in sealed container at 25℃. When reconstituted, keep solution refrigerated. Use within 48 hours. Discard unused portion.

NDC 52268-0301-01
Distributed by Braintree Laboratories, Inc.,
Braintree, MA 02185-0929   Revised 08/94
Shown in Product Identification Guide, page 306

PhosLo® ℞
[phos "lō"]
Calcium Acetate Tablets

DESCRIPTION

Each white round tablet (stamped "BRA 200") contains 667 mg of calcium acetate, USP (anhydrous; $Ca(CH_3COO)_2$; MW = 158.17 grams) equal to 169 mg (8.45 mEq) calcium, and 10 mg of the inert binder, polyethylene glycol 8000 NF.

CLINICAL PHARMACOLOGY

Patients with advanced renal insufficiency (creatinine clearance less than 30 ml/min) exhibit phosphate retention and some degree of hyperphosphatemia. The retention of phosphate plays a pivotal role in causing secondary hyperparathyroidism associated with osteodystrophy, and soft tissue calcification. The mechanism by which phosphate retention leads to hyperparathyroidism is not clearly delineated. Therapeutic efforts directed toward the control of hyperphosphatemia include reduction in the dietary intake of phosphate, inhibition of absorption of phosphate in the intestine with phosphate binders, and removal of phosphate from the body by more efficient methods of dialysis. The rate of removal of phosphate by dietary manipulation or by dialy-

sis is insufficient. Dialysis patients absorb 40% to 80% of dietary phosphorous. Therefore, the fraction of dietary phosphate absorbed from the diet needs to be reduced by using phopsphate binders in most renal failure patients on maintenance dialysis. Calcium acetate (PhosLo) when taken with meals, combines with dietary phosphate to form insoluble phosphate which is excreted in the feces. Maintenance of serum phosphorus below 6.0 mg/dl is generally considered as a clinically acceptable outcome of treatment with phosphate binders. PhosLo is highly soluble at neutral pH, making the calcium readily available for binding to phosphate in the proximal small intestine.

Orally administered calcium acetate from pharmaceutical dosage forms has been demonstrated to be systemically absorbed up to approximately 40% under fasting conditions and up to approximately 30% under nonfasting conditions. This range represents data from both healthy subjects and renal dialysis patients under various conditions.

INDICATIONS AND USAGE

PhosLo is indicated for the control of hyperphosphatemia in end stage renal failure and does not promote aluminum absorption.

CONTRAINDICATIONS

Patients with hypercalcemia.

WARNINGS

Patients with end stage renal failure may develop hypercalcemia when given calcium with meals. No other calcium supplements should be given concurrently with PhosLo. Progressive hypercalcemia due to overdose of PhosLo may be severe as to require emergency measures. Chronic hypercalcemia may lead to vascular calcification, and other soft-tissue calcification. The serum calcium level should be monitored twice weekly during the early dose adjustment period. **The serum calcium times phosphate (CaXP) product should not be allowed to exceed 66.** Radiographic evaluation of suspect anatomical region may be helpful in early detection of soft-tissue calcification.

PRECAUTIONS

General: Excessive dosage of PhosLo induces hypercalcemia; therefore, early in the treatment during dosage adjustment serum calcium should be determined twice weekly. Should hypercalcemia develop, the dosage should be reduced or the treatment discontinued immediately depending on the severity of hypercalcemia. PhosLo should not be given to patients on digitalis, because hypercalcemia may precipitate cardiac arrhythmias. PhosLo therapy should always be started at low dose and should not be increased without careful monitoring of serum calcium. An estimate of daily calcium intake should be made initially and the intake adjusted as needed. Serum phosphorus should also be determined periodically.

Information for the patient: The patient should be informed about compliance with dosage instructions, adherence to instructions about diet and avoidance of the use of nonprescription anatacids. Patients should be informed about the symptoms of hypercalcemia (see ADVERSE REACTIONS section).

Drug interactions: PhosLo may decrease the bioavailability of tetracyclines.

Carcinogenesis, mutagenesis, impairment of fertility: Long term animal studies have not been performed to evaluate the carcinogenic potential or effect on fertility of PhosLo.

Pregnancy: teratogenic effects: Category C. Animal reproduction studies have not been conducted with PhosLo. It is also not known whether PhosLo can cause fetal harm when administered to a pregnant woman or can affect reproduction capacity. PhosLo should be given to a pregnant woman only if clearly needed.

Pediatric use: Safety and efficacy of PhosLo have not been established.

ADVERSE REACTIONS

In clinical studies, patients have occasionally experienced nausea during PhosLo therapy. Hypercalcemia may occur during treatment with PhosLo. Mild hypercalcemia (Ca > 10.5 mg/dl) may be asymptomatic or manifest itself as constipation, anorexia, nausea and vomiting. More severe hypercalcemia (Ca > 12 mg/dl) is associated with confusion, delerium, stupor and coma. Mild hypercalcemia is easily controlled by reducing the PhosLo dose or temporarily discontinuing therapy. Severe hypercalcemia can be treated by acute hemodialysis and discontinuing PhosLo therapy. Decreasing dialysate calcium concentration could reduce the incidence and severity of PhosLo-induced hypercalcemia. The long-term effect of PhosLo on the progression of vascular or soft-tissue calcification has not been determined. Isolated cases of pruritus have been reported which may represent allergic reactions.

OVERDOSAGE

Administration of PhosLo in excess of the appropriate daily dosage can cause severe hypercalcemia (See Adverse Reactions).

DOSAGE AND ADMINISTRATION

The recommended initial dose of PhosLo for the adult dialysis patient is 2 tablets with each meal. The dosage may be increased gradually to bring serum phosphate value below 6 mg/dl, as long as hypercalcemia does not develop. Most patients require 3–4 tablets with each meal.

Store at controlled room temperature, 15°–30℃.

HOW SUPPLIED

In tablet form for oral administration. Each white round tablet contains 667 mg calcium acetate (anhydrous; $Ca(CH_3COO)_2$; MW = 158.17 equal to 169 mg (8.45 mEq) calcium and 10 mg of the inert binder, polyethylene glycol 8000.
NDC 52268-0200-01   R 5/92
Federal law prohibits dispensing without prescription.
Manufactured for Braintree Laboratories,
Braintree, MA 02185-0929
Shown in Product Identification Guide, page 306

EDUCATIONAL MATERIAL

GoLYTELY®, NuLYTELY® and Cherry Flavor NuLYTELY®

Booklets
Complimentary patient booklets are available: "Bowel Preparation Before Your Colonoscopy."

Physician Support
Lavage prescription pads and other materials are available.

PhosLo®

Brochures
Patient information booklets explaining importance of phosphate binding and PhosLo® therapy are available upon request.
Physician Support
PhosLo® prescription pads and other office/clinical materials are available.

Breckenridge Pharmaceutical, Inc.
P.O. BOX 206
BOCA RATON, FL 33429

Direct Inquiries to:
Adam P. Runsdorf
(407) 367-8512
FAX: (407) 367-8107

PRODIUM™   OTC
[prō'dē um]
(Phenazopyridine hydrochloride)
Urinary Tract Analgesic Tablets

DESCRIPTION

Each analgesic tablet contains 95 mg phenazopyridine HCl.

INDICATIONS

Phenazopyridine HCl is indicated for the temporary relief of minor pain, urgency, frequency, and burning of urination. Treatment of a urinary tract infection with phenazopyridine HCl should not exceed 2 days because there is a lack of evidence that the combined administration of phenazopyridine HCl and an antibacterial provides greater benefit than administration of the antibacterial alone after 2 days.

CONTRAINDICATIONS

Phenazopyridine HCl should not be used in patients who have previously exhibited hypersensitivity to it. Its use is also contraindicated in patients with hepatitis or renal insufficiency.

PRECAUTIONS

Do not administer to children under 12 years of age unless directed by physician. Individuals with any hepatic or renal trouble should not use this product unless directed by a physician. If symptoms persist, consult a physician. The decline in renal function associated with advanced age should be kept in mind. A yellowish tinge of the skin or sclera may indicate accumulation due to impaired renal excretion and the need to discontinue therapy.

Continued on next page

Breckenridge—Cont.

NOTE

Phenazopyridine HCl produces an orange to red color in the urine and may stain fabric. Staining of contact lenses has been reported. Phenazopyridine HCl is known to cause gastrointestinal upset in some individuals; discontinue use if symptoms occur. Taking with or following meals will reduce gastric upset.

Carcinogenesis: Long-term administration of phenazopyridine HCl has induced neoplasia in rats (large intestine) and mice (liver). Although no association between phenazopyridine HCl and human neoplasia has been reported, adequate epidemiological studies along these lines have not been conducted.

WARNING

As with any drug, if you are pregnant or nursing a baby, seek the advice of a health professional before using this product. Keep this and all medicines out of the reach of children.

DOSAGE AND ADMINISTRATION

95 mg tablets—adult dosage is two tablets 3 times a day after meals, and administration should not exceed 2 days.
Store at room temperature.

HOW SUPPLIED

Prodium™ is supplied in cartons of 30 tablets (NDC 51991-240-30) and cartons of 12 tablets (NDC 51991-240-12).

Manufactured for:
Breckenridge Pharmaceutical, Inc.
Boca Raton, FL 33429

Bristol-Myers Squibb Oncology/ Immunology Division

A Bristol-Myers Squibb Company
P.O. BOX 4500
PRINCETON, NJ 08543-4500

For Medical Information Contact:
Generally:
Bristol-Myers Squibb Drug Information Department
P.O. Box 4500
Princeton, NJ 08543-4500
(800) 426-7644
Adverse Drug Experiences
and Product Defects Reporting call
during business hours only:
(609) 252-3737

Sales and Ordering:
Orders may be placed by:
1. Calling the following toll-free number between 8:30 AM–6:00 PM EST:
 Continental U.S.: (800) 631-5244
 Alaska-Hawaii: (800) 631-5244
2. Mail orders and all inquiries should be sent to:
 Bristol-Myers Squibb Oncology Division
 Attn: Customer Service
 P.O. Box 5250
 Princeton, NJ 08543-5250
3. Faxing your purchase orders to:
 (800) 523-2965
4. Transmitting computer-to-computer on the NWDA and UCS formats through Ordernet Services use: DEA #PE0048579

BiCNU® ℞

(sterile carmustine [BCNU])

CAUTION: FEDERAL LAW PROHIBITS DISPENSING WITHOUT PRESCRIPTION.

WARNINGS

BiCNU® (sterile carmustine [BCNU]) should be administered under the supervision of a qualified physician experienced in the use of cancer chemotherapeutic agents.

Bone marrow suppression, notably thrombocytopenia and leukopenia, which may contribute to bleeding and overwhelming infections in an already compromised patient, is the most common and severe of the toxic effects of BiCNU (see "**WARNINGS**" and "**ADVERSE REACTIONS**").

Since the major toxicity is delayed bone marrow suppression, blood counts should be monitored weekly for at least 6 weeks after a dose (see "**ADVERSE REACTIONS**"). At the recommended dosage, courses of BiCNU should not be given more frequently than every 6 weeks.

The bone marrow toxicity of BiCNU is cumulative and therefore dosage adjustment must be considered on the basis of nadir blood counts from prior dose (see "Dosage Adjustment Table" under "**DOSAGE AND ADMINISTRATION**").

Pulmonary toxicity from BiCNU appears to be dose related. Patients receiving greater than 1400 mg/m^2 cumulative dose are at significantly higher risk than those receiving less. Delayed pulmonary toxicity can occur years after treatment, and can result in death, particularly in patients treated in childhood (see "**ADVERSE REACTIONS**").

DESCRIPTION

BiCNU® (sterile carmustine [BCNU]) is one of the nitrosoureas used in the treatment of certain neoplastic diseases. It is 1,3-bis (2-chloroethyl)-1-nitrosourea. It is lyophilized pale yellow flakes or congealed mass with a molecular weight of 214.06. It is highly soluble in alcohol and lipids, and poorly soluble in water. BiCNU is administered by intravenous infusion after reconstitution as recommended.

The structural formula is:

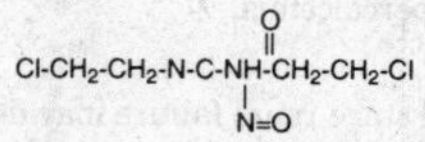

Sterile BiCNU is available in 100 mg single dose vials of lyophilized material.

CLINICAL PHARMACOLOGY

Although it is generally agreed that BiCNU alkylates DNA and RNA, it is not cross resistant with other alkylators. As with other nitrosoureas, it may also inhibit several key enzymatic processes by carbamoylation of amino acids in proteins.

Intravenously administered BiCNU is rapidly degraded, with no intact drug detectable after 15 minutes. However, in studies with C^{14} labeled drug, prolonged levels of the isotope were detected in the plasma and tissue, probably representing radioactive fragments of the parent compound.

It is thought that the antineoplastic and toxic activities of BiCNU may be due to metabolites. Approximately 60% to 70% of a total dose is excreted in the urine in 96 hours and about 10% as respiratory CO_2. The fate of the remainder is undetermined.

Because of the high lipid solubility and the relative lack of ionization at physiological pH, BiCNU crosses the blood-brain barrier quite effectively. Levels of radioactivity in the CSF are $\geq 50\%$ of those measured concurrently in plasma.

INDICATIONS AND USAGE

BiCNU is indicated as palliative therapy as a single agent or in established combination therapy with other approved chemotherapeutic agents in the following:
1. Brain tumors—glioblastoma, brainstem glioma, medulloblastoma, astrocytoma, ependymoma, and metastatic brain tumors.
2. Multiple myeloma—in combination with prednisone.
3. Hodgkin's Disease—as secondary therapy in combination with other approved drugs in patients who relapse while being treated with primary therapy, or who fail to respond to primary therapy.
4. Non-Hodgkin's lymphomas—as secondary therapy in combination with other approved drugs for patients who relapse while being treated with primary therapy, or who fail to respond to primary therapy.

CONTRAINDICATIONS

BiCNU should not be given to individuals who have demonstrated a previous hypersensitivity to it.

WARNINGS

Since the major toxicity is delayed bone marrow suppression, blood counts should be monitored weekly for at least 6 weeks after a dose (see "**ADVERSE REACTIONS**"). At the recommended dosage, courses of BiCNU should not be given more frequently than every 6 weeks.

The bone marrow toxicity of BiCNU is cumulative and therefore dosage adjustment must be considered on the basis of nadir blood counts from prior dose (See "Dosage Adjustment Table" under "**DOSAGE AND ADMINISTRATION**").

Pulmonary toxicity from BiCNU appears to be dose related. Patients receiving greater than 1400 mg/m^2 cumulative dose are at significantly higher risk than those receiving less. Additionally, delayed onset pulmonary fibrosis occurring up to 15 years after treatment has been reported in patients who received BiCNU in childhood and early adolescence (see "**ADVERSE REACTIONS**").

Long term use of nitrosoureas has been reported to be associated with the development of secondary malignancies.

Liver and renal function tests should be monitored periodically (see "**ADVERSE REACTIONS**").

BiCNU may cause fetal harm when administered to a pregnant woman. BiCNU has been shown to be embryotoxic in rats and rabbits and teratogenic in rats when given in doses equivalent to the human dose. There are no adequate and well-controlled studies in pregnant women. If this drug is used during pregnancy, or if the patient becomes pregnant while taking (receiving) this drug, the patient should be apprised of the potential hazard to the fetus. Women of childbearing potential should be advised to avoid becoming pregnant.

BiCNU has been administered through an intraarterial intracarotid route; this procedure is investigational and has been associated with ocular toxicity.

PRECAUTIONS

General: In all instances where the use of BiCNU (sterile carmustine [BCNU]) is considered for chemotherapy, the physician must evaluate the need and usefulness of the drug against the risks of toxic effects or adverse reactions. Most such adverse reactions are reversible if detected early. When such effects or reactions do occur, the drug should be reduced in dosage or discontinued and appropriate corrective measures should be taken according to the clinical judgment of the physician. Reinstitution of BiCNU therapy should be carried out with caution, and with adequate consideration of the further need for the drug and alertness as to possible recurrence of toxicity.

Laboratory Tests: Due to delayed bone marrow suppression, blood counts should be monitored weekly for at least 6 weeks after a dose.

Baseline pulmonary function studies should be conducted along with frequent pulmonary function tests during treatment. Patients with a baseline below 70% of the predicted Forced Vital Capacity (FVC) or Carbon Monoxide Diffusing Capacity (DL_{co}) are particularly at risk.

Since BiCNU may cause liver dysfunction, it is recommended that liver function tests be monitored.

Renal function tests should also be monitored periodically.

Carcinogenesis, Mutagenesis, Impairment of Fertility: BiCNU is carcinogenic in rats and mice, producing a marked increase in tumor incidence in doses approximating those employed clinically. Nitrosourea therapy does have carcinogenic potential in humans (see "**ADVERSE REACTIONS**"). BiCNU also affects fertility in male rats at doses somewhat higher than the human dose.

Pregnancy: Pregnancy "Category D". (see "**WARNINGS**").

Nursing Mothers: It is not known whether this drug is excreted in human milk. Because many drugs are excreted in human milk and because of the potential for serious adverse reactions in nursing infants from BiCNU, a decision should be made whether to discontinue nursing or to discontinue the drug, taking into account the importance of the drug to the mother.

Pediatric Use: Safety and effectiveness in children have not been established.

ADVERSE REACTIONS

Hematologic Toxicity: The most frequent and most serious toxicity of BiCNU is delayed myelosuppression. It usually occurs 4 to 6 weeks after drug administration and is dose related. Thrombocytopenia occurs at about 4 weeks postadministration and persists for 1 to 2 weeks. Leukopenia occurs at 5 to 6 weeks after a dose of BiCNU and persists for 1 to 2 weeks. Thrombocytopenia is generally more severe than leukopenia. However, both may be dose-limiting toxicities.

BiCNU may produce cumulative myelosuppression, manifested by more depressed indices or longer duration of suppression after repeated doses.

The occurrence of acute leukemia and bone marrow dysplasias have been reported in patients following long term nitrosourea therapy.

Anemia also occurs, but is less frequent and less severe than thrombocytopenia or leukopenia.

Pulmonary Toxicity: Pulmonary toxicity characterized by pulmonary infiltrates and/or fibrosis has been reported to occur from 9 days to 43 months after treatment with BiCNU and related nitrosoureas. Most of these patients were receiving prolonged therapy with total doses of BiCNU greater than 1400 mg/m^2. However, there have been reports of pulmonary fibrosis in patients receiving lower total doses. Other risk factors include past history of lung disease and duration of treatment. Cases of fatal pulmonary toxicity with BiCNU have been reported.

Additionally, delayed onset pulmonary fibrosis occurring up to 15 years after treatment has been reported in a long-term study with 17 patients who received BiCNU in childhood and early adolescence in cumulative doses ranging from 770 to 1800 mg/m^2 combined with cranial radiotherapy for intracranial tumors. Chest x-rays have demonstrated pulmonary hypoplasia with upper zone contraction. Gallium scans have been normal in all cases. Thoracic CT scans have demonstrated an unusual pattern of upper zone fibrosis. There appears to be some late reduction of pulmonary function in all long-term survivors. This form of lung fibrosis may be slowly progressive and has resulted in death in some cases. In this

long-term study, all those initially treated at less than 5 years of age died of delayed pulmonary fibrosis.

Gastrointestinal Toxicity: Nausea and vomiting after IV administration of BiCNU are noted frequently. This toxicity appears within 2 hours of dosing, usually lasting 4 to 6 hours, and is dose related. Prior administration of antiemetics is effective in diminishing and sometimes preventing this side effect.

Hepatotoxicity: A reversible type of hepatic toxicity, manifested by increased transaminase, alkaline phosphatase, and bilirubin levels, has been reported in a small percentage of patients receiving BiCNU.

Nephrotoxicity: Renal abnormalities consisting of progressive azotemia, decrease in kidney size, and renal failure have been reported in patients who received large cumulative doses after prolonged therapy with BiCNU and related nitrosoureas. Kidney damage has also been reported occasionally in patients receiving lower total doses.

Other Toxicities: Accidental contact of reconstituted BiCNU with skin has caused burning and hyperpigmentation of the affected areas.

Rapid IV infusion of BiCNU may produce intensive flushing of the skin and suffusion of the conjunctiva within 2 hours, lasting about 4 hours. It is also associated with burning at the site of injection although true thrombosis is rare. Neuroretinitis has been reported.

OVERDOSAGE

No proven antidotes have been established for BiCNU overdosage.

DOSAGE AND ADMINISTRATION

The recommended dose of BiCNU as a single agent in previously untreated patients is 150 to 200 mg/m^2 intravenously every 6 weeks. This may be given as a single dose or divided into daily injections such as 75 to 100 mg/m^2 on 2 successive days. When BiCNU is used in combination with other myelosuppressive drugs or in patients in whom bone marrow reserve is depleted, the doses should be adjusted accordingly. Doses subsequent to the initial dose should be adjusted according to the hematologic response of the patient to the preceding dose. The following schedule is suggested as a guide to dosage adjustment:

Nadir After Prior Dose		Percentage of Prior Dose to be Given
Leukocytes/mm^3	Platelets/mm^3	
>4000	>100,000	100%
3000–3999	75,000–99,999	100%
2000–2999	25,000–74,999	70%
<2000	<25,000	50%

A repeat course of BiCNU (sterile carmustine [BCNU]) should not be given until circulating blood elements have returned to acceptable levels (platelets above 100,000/mm^3, leukocytes above 4,000/mm^3), and this is usually in 6 weeks. Adequate number of neutrophils should be present on a peripheral blood smear. Blood counts should be monitored weekly and repeat courses should not be given before 6 weeks because the hematologic toxicity is delayed and cumulative.

Administration Precautions: As with other potentially toxic compounds, caution should be exercised in handling BiCNU and preparing the solution of BiCNU. Accidental contact of reconstituted BiCNU with the skin has caused transient hyperpigmentation of the affected areas. The use of gloves is recommended. If BiCNU lyophilized material or solution contacts the skin or mucosa, immediately wash the skin or mucosa thoroughly with soap and water.

The reconstituted solution should be used intravenously only and should be administered by I.V. drip. Injection of BiCNU over shorter periods of time than 1 to 2 hours may produce intense pain and burning at the site of injection.

Preparation of Intravenous Solutions: First, dissolve BiCNU with 3 mL of the supplied sterile diluent (Dehydrated Alcohol Injection, USP). Second, aseptically add 27 mL Sterile Water for Injection, USP. Each mL of resulting solution contains 3.3 mg of BiCNU in 10% ethanol, pH 5.6 to 6.0. Such solutions should be protected from light.

Reconstitution as recommended results in a clear, colorless to yellowish solution which may be further diluted with 5% Dextrose Injection, USP. Parenteral drug products should be inspected visually for particulate matter and discoloration prior to administration, whenever solution and container permit.

Important Note: The lyophilized dosage formulation contains no preservatives and is not intended as a multiple dose vial.

Stability: Unopened vials of the dry drug must be stored in a refrigerator (2℃ to 8℃). The recommended storage of unopened vials provides a stable product for 2 years. After reconstitution as recommended, BiCNU is stable for 8 hours at room temperature (25℃), protected from light.

Vials reconstituted as directed and further diluted to a concentration of 0.2 mg/mL in 5% Dextrose Injection, USP,

should be stored at room temperature, protected from light and utilized within 8 hours.

Glass containers were used for the stability data provided in this section. Only use glass containers for BiCNU administration.

Important Note: BiCNU has a low melting point (30.5° to 32.0℃ or 86.9° to 89.6°F). Exposure of the drug to this temperature or above will cause the drug to liquefy and appear as an oil film on the vials. This is a sign of decomposition and vials should be discarded. If there is a question of adequate refrigeration upon receipt of this product, immediately inspect the larger vial in each individual carton. Hold the vial to the bright light for inspection. The BiCNU will appear as a very small amount of dry flakes or dry congealed mass. If this is evident, the BiCNU is suitable for use and should be refrigerated immediately.

Procedures for proper handling and disposal of anticancer drugs should be considered. Several guidelines on this subject have been published.[1-7] There is no general agreement that all of the procedures recommended in the guidelines are necessary or appropriate.

HOW SUPPLIED

BiCNU® (sterile carmustine [BCNU]). Each package contains a vial containing 100 mg carmustine and a vial containing 3 mL sterile diluent.

NDC 0015-3012-38
Store dry powder in refrigerator (2℃ to 8℃).
For information on package sizes available refer to the current price schedule.

REFERENCES

1. Recommendations for the Safe Handling of Parenteral Antineoplastic Drugs NIH Publication No. 83-2621. For sale by the Superintendent of Documents, US Government Printing Office, Washington, DC 20402.
2. AMA Council Report Guidelines for Handling Parenteral Antineoplastics. JAMA 1985; 253 (11): 1590-1592.
3. National Study Commission on Cytotoxic Exposure-Recommendations for Handling Cytotoxic Agents. Available from Louis P. Jeffrey, ScD, Chairman, National Study Commission on Cytotoxic Exposure, Massachusetts College of Pharmacy and Allied Health Sciences, 179 Longwood Avenue, Boston, Massachusetts 02115.
4. Clinical Oncological Society of Australia. Guidelines and Recommendations for Safe Handling of Antineoplastic Agents. Med J Australia 1983; 1:426-428.
5. Jones RB, et al: Safe Handling of Chemotherapeutic Agents: A Report from the Mount Sinai Medical Center. CA–A Cancer Journal for Clinicians 1983; (Sept/Oct)258-263.
6. American Society of Hospital Pharmacists Technical Assistance Bulletin on Handling Cytotoxic and Hazardous Drugs. Am J Hosp Pharm 1990; 47:1033-1049.
7. OSHA Work-Practice Guidelines for Personnel Dealing with Cytotoxic (Antineoplastic) Drugs. Am J Hosp Pharm 1986; 43:1193-1204.

Manufactured by:
Ben Venue Laboratories, Inc., Bedford, Ohio 44146

Distributed by:

BRISTOL LABORATORIES®
ONCOLOGY PRODUCTS
A Bristol-Myers Squibb Company
Princeton, NJ 08543
U.S.A.

H1-B001-2-96   P7980-04
Latest Revised: December 1994

BLENOXANE®   ℞
(sterile bleomycin sulfate, USP)

CAUTION: FEDERAL LAW PROHIBITS DISPENSING WITHOUT PRESCRIPTION.

WARNING

It is recommended that BLENOXANE® (sterile bleomycin sulfate, USP) be administered under the supervision of a qualified physician experienced in the use of cancer chemotherapeutic agents. Appropriate management of therapy and complications is possible only when adequate diagnostic and treatment facilities are readily available.

Pulmonary fibrosis is the most severe toxicity associated with BLENOXANE. The most frequent presentation is pneumonitis occasionally progressing to pulmonary fibrosis. Its occurrence is higher in elderly patients and in those receiving greater than 400 units total dose, but pulmonary toxicity has been observed in young patients and those treated with low doses.

A severe idiosyncratic reaction consisting of hypotension, mental confusion, fever, chills, and wheezing has

been reported in approximately 1% of lymphoma patients treated with BLENOXANE.

DESCRIPTION

BLENOXANE® (sterile bleomycin sulfate, USP) is a mixture of cytotoxic glycopeptide antibiotics isolated from a strain of *Streptomyces verticillus*. It is freely soluble in water. **Note:** A unit of bleomycin is equal to the formerly used milligram activity. The term milligram activity is a misnomer and was changed to units to be more precise.

CLINICAL PHARMACOLOGY

Although the exact mechanism of action of BLENOXANE is unknown, available evidence would seem to indicate that the main mode of action is the inhibition of DNA synthesis with some evidence of lesser inhibition of RNA and protein synthesis.

In mice, high concentrations of BLENOXANE are found in the skin, lungs, kidneys, peritoneum, and lymphatics. Tumor cells of the skin and lungs have been found to have high concentrations of BLENOXANE in contrast to the low concentrations found in hematopoietic tissue. The low concentrations of BLENOXANE found in bone marrow may be related to high levels of BLENOXANE degradative enzymes found in that tissue.

In patients with normal renal function, 60 to 70% of an administered dose is recovered in the urine as active bleomycin. In patients with a creatinine clearance of >35 mL per minute, the serum or plasma terminal elimination half-life of bleomycin is approximately 115 minutes. In patients with a creatinine clearance of <35 mL per minute, the plasma or serum terminal elimination half-life increases exponentially as the creatinine clearance decreases. It was reported that patients with moderately severe renal failure excreted less than 20% of the dose in the urine. This result would suggest that severe renal impairment could lead to accumulation of the drug in blood.

Information on the dose proportionally of bleomycin is not available.

When administered intrapleurally for the treatment of malignant pleural effusion, BLENOXANE acts as a sclerosing agent.

Following intrapleural administration to a limited number of patients (n=4), the resultant bleomycin plasma concentrations suggest a systemic absorption of approximately 45%.

The safety and efficacy of BLENOXANE 60 units and tetracycline (1 gm) as treatment for malignant pleural effusion were evaluated in a multicenter, randomized trial. Patients were required to have cytologically positive pleural effusion, good performance status (0,1,2), lung re-expansion following tube thoracostomy with drainage rates of 100 mL/24 hr or less, no prior intrapleural therapy, no prior systemic BLENOXANE therapy, no chest irradiation and no recent change in systemic therapy. Overall survival did not differ between the BLENOXANE 60 units (n=44) and tetracycline (n=41) groups. Of patients evaluated within 30 days of instillation, the recurrence rate was 36% (10/28) with BLENOXANE and 67% (18/27) with tetracycline (p=0.023). Toxicity was similar between groups.

INDICATIONS & USAGE

BLENOXANE should be considered a palliative treatment. It has been shown to be useful in the management of the following neoplasms either as a single agent or in proven combinations with other approved chemotherapeutic agents:

Squamous Cell Carcinoma—Head and neck (including mouth, tongue, tonsil, nasopharynx, oropharynx, sinus, palate, lip, buccal mucosa, gingivae, epiglottis, skin, larynx), penis, cervix, and vulva. The response to BLENOXANE is poorer in patients with previously irradiated head and neck cancer.

Lymphomas—Hodgkin's Disease, non-Hodgkin's lymphoma.

Testicular Carcinoma—Embryonal cell, choriocarcinoma, and teratocarcinoma.

BLENOXANE has also been shown to be useful in the management of:

Malignant Pleural Effusion—BLENOXANE is effective as a sclerosing agent for the treatment of malignant pleural effusion and prevention of recurrent pleural effusions.

CONTRAINDICATIONS

BLENOXANE is contraindicated in patients who have demonstrated a hypersensitive or an idiosyncratic reaction to it.

WARNINGS

Patients receiving BLENOXANE must be observed carefully and frequently during and after therapy. It should be used with extreme caution in patients with significant impairment of renal function or compromised pulmonary function. Pulmonary toxicities occur in 10% of treated patients. In approximately 1%, the nonspecific pneumonitis induced by BLENOXANE progresses to pulmonary fibrosis, and death.

Continued on next page

Bristol-Myers Squibb Oncology—Cont.

Although this is age and dose related, the toxicity is unpredictable. Frequent roentgenograms are recommended.
A severe idiosyncratic reaction (similar to anaphylaxis) consisting of hypotension, mental confusion, fever, chills, and wheezing has been reported in approximately 1% of lymphoma patients treated with BLENOXANE. Since these reactions usually occur after the first or second dose, careful monitoring is essential after these doses.
Renal or hepatic toxicity, beginning as a deterioration in renal or liver function tests, have been reported, infrequently. These toxicities may occur, however, at any time after initiation of therapy.

Usage in Pregnancy

Pregnancy "Category D"—BLENOXANE (sterile bleomycin sulfate, USP) can cause fetal harm when administered to a pregnant woman. It has been shown to be teratogenic in rats. Administration of intraperitoneal doses of 1.5 mg/kg/day to rats (about 1.6 times the recommended human dose on a unit/m^2 basis) on days 6-15 of gestation caused skeletal malformations, shortened innominate artery and hydroureter. BLENOXANE is abortifacient but not teratogenic in rabbits, at intravenous doses of 1.2 mg/kg/day (about 2.4 times the recommended human dose on a unit/m^2 basis) given on gestation days 6-18.
There have been no studies in pregnant women. If BLENOXANE is used during pregnancy, or if the patient becomes pregnant while receiving this drug, the patient should be apprised of the potential hazard to the fetus. Women of childbearing potential should be advised to avoid becoming pregnant during therapy with BLENOXANE.

PRECAUTIONS

General—Bleomycin clearance may be reduced in patients with impaired renal function. No guidelines have been established for dose adjustments, but bleomycin should be used with extreme caution in patients with significant renal impairment.

Carcinogenesis, Mutagenesis, and Impairment of Fertility—The carcinogenic potential of BLENOXANE in humans is unknown. A study in F344-type male rats demonstrated an increased incidence of nodular hyperplasia after induced lung carcinogenesis by nitrosamines, followed by treatment with bleomycin. In another study where the drug was administered to rats by subcutaneous injection at 0.35mg/kg weekly (3.82 units/m^2 weekly or about 30% at the recommended human dose), necropsy findings included dose related injection site fibrosarcomas as well as various renal tumors. Bleomycin has been shown to be mutagenic both *in vitro* and *in vivo*. The effects of bleomycin on fertility have not been studied.

Pregnancy—Pregnancy "Category D". (See "**WARNINGS**" section.)

Nursing Mothers—It is not known whether the drug is excreted in human milk. Because many drugs are excreted in human milk and because of the potential for serious adverse reactions in nursing infants, it is recommended that nursing be discontinued by women receiving BLENOXANE therapy.

Pediatric Use—Safety and effectiveness of BLENOXANE in pediatric patients have not been established.

ADVERSE REACTIONS

Pulmonary—This is potentially the most serious side effect, occurring in approximately 10% of treated patients. The most frequent presentation is pneumonitis occasionally progressing to pulmonary fibrosis. Approximately 1% of patients treated have died of pulmonary fibrosis. Pulmonary toxicity is both dose and age related, being more common in patients over 70 years of age and in those receiving over 400 units total dose. This toxicity, however, is unpredictable and has been seen occasionally in young patients receiving low doses. Some published reports have suggested that the risk of pulmonary toxicity may be increased when bleomycin is used in combination with G-CSF (filgrastim) or other cytokines. However, randomized clinical studies completed to date have not demonstrated an increased risk of pulmonary complications in patients treated with bleomycin and G-CSF. Because of lack of specificity of the clinical syndrome, the identification of patients with pulmonary toxicity due to BLENOXANE has been extremely difficult. The earliest symptom associated with BLENOXANE pulmonary toxicity is dyspnea. The earliest sign is fine rales.
Radiographically, BLENOXANE-induced pneumonitis produces nonspecific patchy opacities, usually of the lower lung fields. The most common changes in pulmonary function tests are a decrease in total lung volume and a decrease in vital capacity. However, these changes are not predictive of the development of pulmonary fibrosis.
The microscopic tissue changes due to BLENOXANE toxicity include bronchiolar squamous metaplasia, reactive macrophages, atypical alveolar epithelial cells, fibrinous edema, and interstitial fibrosis. The acute stage may involve capillary changes and subsequent fibrinous exudation into alveoli producing a change similar to hyaline membrane formation and progressing to a diffuse interstitial fibrosis resembling the Hamman-Rich syndrome. These microscopic findings are nonspecific; e.g., similar changes are seen in radiation pneumonitis and pneumocystic pneumonitis.
To monitor the onset of pulmonary toxicity, roentgenograms of the chest should be taken every 1 to 2 weeks. If pulmonary changes are noted, treatment should be discontinued until it can be determined if they are drug related. Recent studies have suggested that sequential measurement of the pulmonary diffusion capacity for carbon monoxide (DL_{co}) during treatment with BLENOXANE may be an indicator of subclinical pulmonary toxicity. It is recommended that the DL_{co} be monitored monthly if it is to be employed to detect pulmonary toxicities, and thus the drug should be discontinued when the DL_{co} falls below 30 to 35% of the pretreatment value.
Because of bleomycin's sensitization of lung tissue, patients who have received bleomycin are at greater risk of developing pulmonary toxicity when oxygen is administered in surgery. While long exposure to very high oxygen concentrations is a known cause of lung damage, after bleomycin administration, lung damage can occur at lower concentrations that are usually considered safe. Suggested preventive measures are:

1. Maintain Fl O_2 at concentrations approximating that of room air (25%) during surgery and the postoperative period.
2. Monitor carefully fluid replacement, focusing more on colloid administration rather than crystalloid.

Sudden onset of an acute chest pain syndrome suggestive of pleuropericarditis has been rarely reported during BLENOXANE infusions. Although each patient must be individually evaluated, further courses of BLENOXANE do not appear to be contraindicated.
Pulmonary adverse events which may be related to the intrapleural administration of BLENOXANE have been reported only rarely.

Idiosyncratic Reactions—In approximately 1% of the lymphoma patients treated with BLENOXANE, an idiosyncratic reaction, similar to anaphylaxis clinically, has been reported. The reaction may be immediate or delayed for several hours, and usually occurs after the first or second dose. It consists of hypotension, mental confusion, fever, chills, and wheezing. Treatment is symptomatic including volume expansion, pressor agents, antihistamines, and corticosteroids.

Integument and Mucous Membranes—These are the most frequent side effects, being reported in approximately 50% of treated patients. These consist of erythema, rash, striae, vesiculation, hyperpigmentation, and tenderness of the skin. Hyperkeratosis, nail changes, alopecia, pruritus, and stomatitis have also been reported. It was necessary to discontinue BLENOXANE (sterile bleomycin sulfate, USP) therapy in 2% of treated patients because of these toxicities.
Skin toxicity is a relatively late manifestation usually developing in the 2nd and 3rd week of treatment after 150 to 200 units of BLENOXANE have been administered and appears to be related to the cumulative dose.
Intrapleural administration of BLENOXANE has occasionally been associated with local pain. Hypotension possibly requiring symptomatic treatment has been reported infrequently. Death has been very rarely reported in association with BLENOXANE pleurodesis in these very seriously ill patients.

Other—Vascular toxicities coincident with the use of BLENOXANE in combination with other antineoplastic agents have been reported rarely. The events are clinically heterogeneous and may include myocardial infarction, cerebrovascular accident, thrombotic microangiopathy (HUS) or cerebral arteritis. Various mechanisms have been proposed for these vascular complications. There are also reports of Raynaud's phenomenon occurring in patients treated with BLENOXANE in combination with vinblastine with or without cisplatin or, in a few cases, with BLENOXANE as a single agent. It is currently unknown if the cause of Raynaud's phenomenon in these cases is the disease, underlying vascular compromise, BLENOXANE, vinblastine, hypomagnesemia, or a combination of any of these factors.
Fever, chills, and vomiting were frequently reported side effects. Anorexia and weight loss are common and may persist long after termination of this medication. Pain at tumor site, phlebitis, and other local reactions were reported infrequently.

DOSAGE & ADMINISTRATION

Because of the possibility of an anaphylactoid reaction, lymphoma patients should be treated with 2 units or less for the first two doses. If no acute reaction occurs, then the regular dosage schedule may be followed.

The following dose schedule is recommended: **Squamous cell carcinoma, non-Hodgkin's lymphoma, testicular carcinoma**—0.25 to 0.50 units/kg (10 to 20 units/m^2) given intravenously, intramuscularly, or subcutaneously weekly or twice weekly.

Hodgkin's Disease—0.25 to 0.50 units/kg (10 to 20 units/m^2) given intravenously, intramuscularly, or subcutaneously weekly or twice weekly. After a 50% response, a maintenance dose of 1 unit daily or 5 units weekly intravenously or intramuscularly should be given.
Pulmonary toxicity of BLENOXANE appears to be dose related with a striking increase when the total dose is over 400 units. Total doses over 400 units should be given with great caution.

Note: When BLENOXANE is used in combination with other antineoplastic agents, pulmonary toxicities may occur at lower doses.

Improvement of Hodgkin's Disease and testicular tumors is prompt and noted within 2 weeks. If no improvement is seen by this time, improvement is unlikely. Squamous cell cancers respond more slowly, sometimes requiring as long as 3 weeks before any improvement is noted.
Malignant Pleural Effusion—60 units administered as a single dose bolus intrapleural injection.

ADMINISTRATION

BLENOXANE may be given by the intramuscular, intravenous, subcutaneous or intrapleural routes.

Intramuscular or Subcutaneous—The BLENOXANE 15 units vial should be reconstituted with 1 to 5 mL of Sterile Water for Injection, USP, Sodium Chloride for Injection, 0.9%, USP, or Bacteriostatic Water for Injection, USP. The BLENOXANE 30 units vial should be reconstituted with 2 to 10 mL of the above diluents.

Intravenous—The contents of the 15 units or 30 units vial should be dissolved in 5 mL or 10 mL, respectively of Sodium Chloride for Injection, 0.9%, USP and administered slowly over a period of 10 minutes.

Intrapleural—60 units of BLENOXANE is dissolved in 50-100 mL sodium chloride injection 0.9%, and administered through a thoracostomy tube following drainage of excess pleural fluid and confirmation of complete lung expansion. The literature suggests that successful pleurodesis is, in part, dependent upon complete drainage of the pleural fluid and reestablishment of negative intrapleural pressure prior to instillation of a sclerosing agent. Therefore, the amount of drainage from the chest tube should be as minimal as possible prior to instillation of BLENOXANE. Although there is no conclusive evidence to support this contention, it is generally accepted that chest tube drainage should be less than 100 mL in a 24 hour period prior to sclerosis. However, BLENOXANE instillation may be appropriate when drainage is between 100-300 mL under clinical conditions that necessitate sclerosis therapy. The thoracostomy tube is clamped after BLENOXANE instillation. The patient is moved from the supine to the left and right lateral positions several times during the next four hours. The clamp is then removed and suction reestablished. The amount of time the chest tube remains in place following sclerosis is dictated by the clinical situation.
The intrapleural injection of topical anesthetics or systemic narcotic analgesia is generally not required.
Parenteral drug products should be inspected visually for particulate matter and discoloration prior to administration, whenever solution and container permit.

HOW SUPPLIED

BLENOXANE® is available as follows:

NDC 0015-3010-20, 15 units per vial as sterile bleomycin sulfate, USP.

NDC 0015-3063-01, 30 units per vial as sterile bleomycin sulfate, USP.

Stability—The sterile powder is stable under refrigeration 2°C (36°F) to 8°C (46°F) and should not be used after the expiration date is reached.
BLENOXANE should not be reconstituted or diluted with D_5W or other dextrose containing diluents. When reconstituted in D_5W and analyzed by HPLC, BLENOXANE demonstrates a loss of A_2 and B_2 potency that does not occur when BLENOXANE is reconstituted in 0.9% sodium chloride.
BLENOXANE is stable for 24 hours at room temperature in Sodium Chloride.
Procedures for proper handling and disposal of anticancer drugs should be considered. Several guidelines on this subject have been published.[1-7] There is no general agreement that all of the procedures recommended in the guidelines are necessary or appropriate.

REFERENCES

1. Recommendations for the Safe Handling of Parenteral Antineoplastic Drugs. NIH Publication No. 83-2621. For sale by the Superintendent of Documents, US Government Printing Office, Washington, DC 20402.
2. AMA Council Report. Guidelines for Handling Parenteral Antineoplastics. JAMA 1985; 253(11):1590-1592.
3. National Study Commission on Cytotoxic Exposure–Recommendations for Handling Cytotoxic Agents. Available from Louis P. Jeffrey, ScD, Chairman, National Study Commission on Cytotoxic Exposure, Massachusetts College of Pharmacy and Allied Health Sciences, 179 Longwood Avenue, Boston, Massachusetts 02115.
4. Clinical Oncological Society of Australia: Guidelines and Recommendations for Safe Handling of Antineoplastic Agents. Med J Australia 1983; 1:426–428.

5. Jones RB, et al: Safe Handling of Chemotherapeutic Agents: A Report from the Mount Sinai Medical Center. CA–A Cancer Journal for Clinicians 1983; (Sept/Oct) 258–263.
6. American Society of Hospital Pharmacists Technical Assistance Bulletin on Handling Cytotoxic and Hazardous Drugs. Am J Hosp Pharm 1990; 47:1033–1049.
7. OSHA Work-Practice Guidelines for Personnel Dealing with Cytotoxic (Antineoplastic) Drugs. Am J Hosp Pharm 1986; 43:1193–1204.

Manufactured by:
Nippon Kayaku Co., Ltd.
Tokyo, Japan
Distributed by:
MeadJohnson
ONCOLOGY PRODUCTS
A Bristol-Myers Squibb Company
Princeton, NJ 08543
U.S.A.
H2-B001-3-96 P7514-01
Revised: March 1996
Shown in Product Identification Guide, page 307

CeeNU® ℞
[*cē ′nū*]
(lomustine [CCNU]) capsules

> **WARNINGS**
> CeeNU (lomustine) should be administered under the supervision of a qualified physician experienced in the use of cancer chemotherapeutic agents.
> Bone marrow suppression, notably thrombocytopenia and leukopenia, which may contribute to bleeding and overwhelming infections in an already compromised patient, is the most common and severe of the toxic effects of CeeNU (see "WARNINGS" and "ADVERSE REACTIONS").
> Since the major toxicity is delayed bone marrow suppression, blood counts should be monitored weekly for at least 6 weeks after a dose (see "ADVERSE REACTIONS"). At the recommended dosage, courses of CeeNU should not be given more frequently than every 6 weeks.
> The bone marrow toxicity of CeeNU is cumulative and therefore dosage adjustment must be considered on the basis of nadir blood counts from prior dose (see Dosage Adjustment Table under "DOSAGE AND ADMINISTRATION").

DESCRIPTION

CeeNU (lomustine) (CCNU) is one of the nitrosoureas used in the treatment of certain neoplastic diseases. It is 1- (2-chloroethyl)- 3-cyclohexyl- 1 -nitrosourea. It is a yellow powder with the empirical formula of $C_9H_{16}ClN_3O_2$ and a molecular weight of 233.71. CeeNU is soluble in 10% ethanol (0.05 mg per mL) and in absolute alcohol (70 mg per mL). CeeNU is relatively insoluble in water (<0.05 mg per mL).
It is relatively unionized at a physiological pH.
Inactive ingredients in CeeNU capsules are: magnesium stearate and mannitol.
The structural formula is:

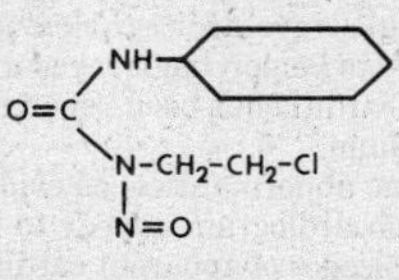

CeeNU is available in 10 mg, 40 mg and 100 mg capsules for oral administration.

CLINICAL PHARMACOLOY

Although it is generally agreed that CeeNU alkylates DNA and RNA, it is not cross resistant with other alkylators. As with other nitrosoureas, it may also inhibit several key enzymatic processes by carbamoylation of amino acids in proteins.
CeeNU may be given orally. Following oral administration of radioactive CeeNU at doses ranging from 30 mg/m^2 to 100 mg/m^2, about half of the radioactivity given was excreted in the form of degredation products within 24 hours.
The serum half-life of the metabolites ranges from 16 hours to 2 days. Tissue levels are comparable to plasma levels at 15 minutes after intravenous administration.
Because of the high lipid solubility and the relative lack of ionization at a physiological pH, CeeNU crosses the blood-brain barrier quite effectively. Levels of radioactivity in the CSF are 50% or greater than those measured concurrently in plasma.

INDICATIONS AND USAGE

CeeNU has been shown to be useful as a single agent in addition to other treatment modalities, or in established combination therapy with other approved chemotherapeutic agents in the following:
Brain tumors—both primary and metastatic, in patients who have already received appropriate surgical and/or radiotherapeutic procedures.
Hodgkin's Disease—secondary therapy in combination with other approved drugs in patients who relapse while being treated with primary therapy, or who fail to respond to primary therapy.

CONTRAINDICATIONS

CeeNU should not be given to individuals who have demonstrated a previous hypersensitivity to it.

WARNINGS

Since the major toxicity is delayed bone marrow suppression, blood counts should be monitored weekly for at least 6 weeks after a dose (see "ADVERSE REACTIONS"). At the recommended dosage, courses of CeeNU should not be given more frequently than every 6 weeks.
The bone marrow toxicity of CeeNU is cumulative and therefore dosage adjustment must be considered on the basis of nadir blood counts from prior dose (see Dosage Adjustment Table under "DOSAGE AND ADMINISTRATION").
Pulmonary toxicity from CeeNU appears to be dose related (see "ADVERSE REACTIONS").
Long term use in nitrosoureas has been reported to be possibly associated with the development of secondary malignancies.
Liver and renal function tests should be monitored periodically (see "ADVERSE REACTIONS").
Pregnancy Category D: CeeNU can cause fetal harm when administered to a pregnant woman. CeeNU is embryotoxic and teratogenic in rats and embryotoxic in rabbits at dose levels equivalent to the human dose. There are no adequate and well controlled studies in pregnant women. If this drug is used during pregnancy, or if the patient becomes pregnant while taking (receiving) this drug, the patient should be apprised of the potential hazard to the fetus. Women of childbearing potential should be advised to avoid becoming pregnant.

PRECAUTIONS

General: In all instances where the use of CeeNU is considered for chemotherapy, the physician must evaluate the need and usefulness of the drug against the risks of toxic effects or adverse reactions. Most such adverse reactions are reversible if detected early. When such effects or reactions do occur, the drug should be reduced in dosage or discontinued and appropriate corrective measures should be taken according to the clinical judgment of the physician. Reinstitution of CeeNU therapy should be carried out with caution and with adequate consideration of the further need for the drug and alertness as to possible recurrence of toxicity.
Laboratory Tests: Due to delayed bone marrow suppression, blood counts should be monitored weekly for at least 6 weeks after a dose.
Baseline pulmonary function studies should be conducted along with frequent pulmonary function tests during treatment. Patients with a baseline below 70% of the predicted Forced Vital Capacity (FVC) or Carbon Monoxide Diffusing Capacity (DL_{co}) are particularly at risk.
Since CeeNU may cause liver dysfunction, it is recommended that liver function tests be monitored periodically.
Renal function tests should also be monitored periodically.
Carcinogenesis, Mutagenesis, Impairment of Fertility: CeeNU is carcinogenic in rats and mice, producing a marked increase in tumor incidence in doses approximating those employed clinically. Nitrosourea therapy does have carcinogenic potential in humans (see "ADVERSE REACTIONS"). CeeNU also affects fertility in male rats at doses somewhat higher than the human dose.
Pregnancy: Pregnancy "Category D"—See "WARNINGS" section.
Nursing Mothers: It is not known whether this drug is excreted in human milk. Because many drugs are excreted in human milk and because of the potential for serious adverse reactions in nursing infants from CeeNU, a decision should be made whether to discontinue nursing or to discontinue the drug, taking into account the importance of the drug to the mother.
Information for the Patient: Patients receiving CeeNU should be given the following information and instructions by the physician:
1. Patients should be told that CeeNU is an anticancer drug and belongs to the group of medicines known as alkylating agents.
2. In order to provide the proper dose of CeeNU, patients should be aware that there may be two or more different types and colors of capsules in the container dispensed by the pharmacist.
3. Patients should be told that CeeNU is given as a single oral dose and will not be repeated for at least 6 weeks.
4. Patients should be told that nausea and vomiting usually last less than 24 hours, although loss of appetite may last for several days.
5. If any of the following reactions occur, notify the physician: fever, chills, sore throat, unusual bleeding or bruising, shortness of breath, dry cough, swelling of feet or lower legs, mental confusion or yellowing of eyes and skin.

ADVERSE REACTIONS

Hematologic Toxicity: The most frequent and most serious toxicity of CeeNU is delayed myelosuppression. It usually occurs 4 to 6 weeks after drug administration and is dose related. Thrombocytopenia occurs at about 4 weeks postadministration and persists for 1 to 2 weeks. Leukopenia occurs at 5 to 6 weeks after a dose of CeeNU and persists for 1 to 2 weeks. Approximately 65% of patients receiving 130 mg/m^2 develop white blood counts below 5000 wbc/mm^3. Thirty-six percent developed white blood counts below 3000 wbc/mm^3. Thrombocytopenia is generally more severe than leukopenia. However, both may be dose-limiting toxicities.
CeeNU may produce cumulative myelosuppression, manifested by more depressed indices or longer duration of suppression after repeated doses.
The occurrence of acute leukemia and bone marrow dysplasias have been reported in patients following long term nitrosourea therapy.
Anemia also occurs, but is less frequent and less severe than thrombocytopenia or leukopenia.
Pulmonary Toxicity: Pulmonary toxicity characterized by pulmonary infiltrates and/or fibrosis has been reported rarely with CeeNU. Onset of toxicity has occurred after an interval of 6 months or longer from the start of therapy with cumulative doses of CeeNU usually greater than 1100 mg/m^2. There is one report of pulmonary toxicity at a cumulative dose of only 600 mg.
Delayed onset pulmonary fibrosis occurring up to 15 years after treatment has been reported in patients who received related nitrosoureas in childhood and early adolescence combined with cranial radiotherapy for intracranial tumors.
Gastrointestinal Toxicity: Nausea and vomiting may occur 3 to 6 hours after an oral dose and usually lasts less than 24 hours. Prior administration of antiemetics is effective in diminishing and sometimes preventing this side effect. Nausea and vomiting can also be reduced if CeeNU is administered to fasting patients.
Hepatotoxicity: A reversible type of hepatic toxicity, manifested by increased transaminase, alkaline phosphatase and bilirubin levels, has been reported in a small percentage of patients receiving CeeNU.
Nephrotoxicity: Renal abnormalities consisting of progressive azotemia, decrease in kidney size and renal failure have been reported in patients who received large cumulative doses after prolonged therapy with CeeNU. Kidney damage has also been reported occasionally in patients receiving lower total doses.
Other Toxicities: Stomatitis and alopecia have been reported infrequently.
Neurological reactions such as disorientation, lethargy, ataxia, and dysarthria have been noted in some patients receiving CeeNU. However, the relationship to medication in these patients is unclear.

OVERDOSAGE

No proven antidotes have been established for CeeNU overdosage.

DOSAGE AND ADMINISTRATION

The recommended dose of CeeNU in adults and children as a single agent in previously untreated patients is 130 mg/m^2 as a single oral dose every 6 weeks. In individuals with compromised bone marrow function, the dose should be reduced to 100 mg/m^2 every 6 weeks. When CeeNU is used in combination with other myelosuppressive drugs, the doses should be adjusted accordingly.
Doses subsequent to the initial dose should be adjusted according to the hematologic response of the patient to the preceding dose. The following schedule is suggested as a guide to dosage adjustment:

Nadir After Prior Dose		Percentage of Prior Dose to be Given
Leukocytes	Platelets	
>4000	>100,000	100%
3000–3999	75,000–99,999	100%
2000–2999	25,000–74,999	70%
<2000	<25,000	50%

A repeat course of CeeNU should not be given until circulating blood elements have returned to acceptable levels (platelets above 100,000/mm^3; leukocytes above 4,000/mm^3) and this is usually in 6 weeks. Adequate number of neutrophils should be present on a peripheral blood smear. Blood counts should be monitored weekly and repeat courses

Continued on next page

Bristol-Myers Squibb Oncology—Cont.

should not be given before 6 weeks because the hematologic toxicity is delayed and cumulative.

HOW SUPPLIED

The dose pack of CeeNU (lomustine, CCNU) NDC 0015-3034-10 Capsules contains;

2—100 mg capsules (Green/Green)
2—40 mg capsules (White/Green)
2—10 mg capsules (White/White)

Stability: CeeNU Capsules are stable for the lot life indicated on package labeling when stored at room temperature in well closed containers. Avoid excessive heat (over 40°C).

Directions to the Pharmacist: The dose pack contains a total of 300 mg and will provide enough medication for titration of a single dose. The total dose prescribed by the physician can be obtained (to within 10 mg) by determining the appropriate combination of the enclosed capsule strengths. The appropriate number of capsules of each size should be placed in a single vial to which the patient information label (gummed label provided) explaining the differences in the appearance of the capsules is affixed. Each color-coded capsule is imprinted with the dose in milligrams.

A patient information sticker, to be placed on dispensing container, is enclosed.

Also available: Individual bottles of 20 capsules each.
NDC 0015-3032-20—100 mg capsules (Green/Green)
NDC 0015-3031-20—40 mg capsules (White/Green)
NDC 0015-3030-20—10 mg capsules (White/White)

Procedures for proper handling and disposal of anticancer drugs should be considered. Several guidelines on this subject have been published.[1-7] There is no general agreement that all of the procedures recommended in the guidelines are necessary or appropriate.

REFERENCES

1. Recommendations for the Safe Handling of Parenteral Antineoplastic Drugs. NIH Publication No. 83-2621. For sale by the Superintendent of Documents, U.S. Government Printing Office, Washington, D.C. 20402.
2. AMA Council Report. Guidelines for Handling Parenteral Antineoplastics. *JAMA.* 1985; 253(11):1590-1592.
3. National Study Commission on Cytotoxic Exposure—Recommendations for Handling Cytotoxic Agents. Available from Louis P. Jeffrey, Sc.D., Chairman, National Study Commission on Cytotoxic Exposure, Massachusetts College of Pharmacy and Allied Health Sciences, 179 Longwood Avenue, Boston, Massachusetts 02115.
4. Clinical Oncological Society of Australia: Guidelines and Recommendations for Safe Handling of Antineoplastic Agents. *Med J Australia.* 1983; 1:426-428.
5. Jones, R. B., et al. Safe Handling of Chemotherapeutic Agents: A report from the Mount Sinai Medical Center, *CA—A Cancer J for Clinicians.* 1983; Sept./Oct., 258-263.
6. American Society of Hospital Pharmacists Technical Assistance Bulletin on Handling Cytotoxic and Hazardous Drugs. *Am J Hosp Pharm.* 1990; 47:1033-1049.
7. OSHA Work-Practice Guidelines for Personnel Dealing with Cytotoxic (Antineoplastic) Drugs. *Am J Hosp Pharm.* 1986; 43:1193-1204.

(P6047-02)
December 1990

CYTOXAN® for Injection   ℞
[*sī-taks'an*]
(cyclophosphamide for injection, USP)
Lyophilized **CYTOXAN®** for Injection
(cyclophosphamide for injection, USP)
CYTOXAN® Tablets (cyclophosphamide tablets, USP)

DESCRIPTION

CYTOXAN for Injection is a sterile white powder blend consisting of 45 mg sodium chloride per 100 mg cyclophosphamide (anhydrous). Lyophilized CYTOXAN for Injection is a sterile white lyophilized cake or partially broken cake containing 75 mg mannitol per 100 mg cyclophosphamide (anhydrous). CYTOXAN Tablets are for oral use and contain 25 mg or 50 mg cyclophosphamide (anhydrous). Inactive ingredients in CYTOXAN tablets are acacia, FD&C Blue No. 1, D&C Yellow No. 10 Aluminum Lake, lactose, magnesium stearate, starch, stearic acid, and talc. Cyclophosphamide is a synthetic antineoplastic drug chemically related to the nitrogen mustards. Cyclophosphamide is a white crystalline powder with the molecular formula of $C_7H_{15}Cl_2N_2O_2P \cdot H_2O$ and a molecular weight of 279.1. The chemical name for cyclophosphamide is 2-[bis(2-chloroethyl)amino]tetrahydro-2H-1,3,2-oxazaphosphorine 2-oxide monohydrate. Cyclophosphamide is soluble in water, saline, or ethanol and has the following structural formula:

[See chemical structure at top of next column.]

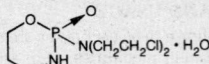

CLINICAL PHARMACOLOGY

CYTOXAN (cyclophosphamide) is biotransformed principally in the liver to active alkylating metabolites by a mixed function microsomal oxidase system. These metabolites interfere with the growth of susceptible rapidly proliferating malignant cells. The mechanism of action is thought to involve cross-linking of tumor cell DNA.

CYTOXAN is well absorbed after oral administration with a bioavailability greater than 75%. The unchanged drug has an elimination half-life of 3 to 12 hours. It is eliminated primarily in the form of metabolites, but from 5% to 25% of the dose is excreted in urine as unchanged drug. Several cytotoxic and noncytotoxic metabolites have been identified in urine and in plasma. Concentrations of metabolites reach a maximum in plasma 2 to 3 hours after an intravenous dose. Plasma protein binding of unchanged drug is low but some metabolites are bound to an extent greater than 60%. It has not been demonstrated that any single metabolite is responsible for either the therapeutic or toxic effects of cyclophosphamide. Although elevated levels of metabolites of cyclophosphamide have been observed in patients with renal failure, increased clinical toxicity in such patients has not been demonstrated.

INDICATION AND USAGE

Malignant Diseases—CYTOXAN, although effective alone in susceptible malignancies, is more frequently used concurrently or sequentially with other antineoplastic drugs.
The following malignancies are often susceptible to CYTOXAN treatment:
1. Malignant lymphomas (Stages III and IV of the Ann Arbor staging system), Hodgkin's disease, lymphocytic lymphoma (nodular or diffuse), mixed-cell type lymphoma, histiocytic lymphoma, Burkitt's lymphoma. **2.** Multiple myeloma. **3.** Leukemias: Chronic lymphocytic leukemia, chronic granulocytic leukemia (it is usually ineffective in acute blastic crisis), acute myelogenous and monocytic leukemia, acute lymphoblastic (stem-cell) leukemia in children (CYTOXAN given during remission is effective in prolonging its duration). **4.** Mycosis fungoides (advanced disease), **5.** Neuroblastoma (disseminated disease). **6.** Adenocarcinoma of the ovary. **7.** Retinoblastoma. **8.** Carcinoma of the breast.
Nonmalignant Disease: Biopsy Proven "Minimal Change" Nephrotic Syndrome in Children—CYTOXAN is useful in carefully selected cases of biopsy proven "minimal change" nephrotic syndrome in children but should not be used as primary therapy. In children whose disease fails to respond adequately to appropriate adrenocorticosteroid therapy or in whom the adrenocorticosteroid therapy produces or threatens to produce intolerable side effects. CYTOXAN may induce a remission. CYTOXAN is not indicated for the nephrotic syndrome in adults or for any other renal disease.

CONTRAINDICATIONS

Continued use of cyclophosphamide is contraindicated in patients with severely depressed bone marrow function. Cyclophosphamide is contraindicated in patients who have demonstrated a previous hypersensitivity to it. See WARNINGS and PRECAUTIONS sections.

WARNINGS

Carcinogenesis, Mutagenesis, Impairment of Fertility—Second malignancies have developed in some patients treated with cyclophosphamide used alone or in association with other antineoplastic drugs and/or modalities. Most frequently, they have been urinary bladder, myeloproliferative, or lymphoproliferative malignancies. Second malignancies most frequently were detected in patients treated for primary myeloproliferative or lymphoproliferative malignancies or nonmalignant disease in which immune processes are believed to be involved pathologically. In some cases, the second malignancy developed several years after cyclophosphamide treatment had been discontinued. In a single breast cancer trial utilizing two to four times the standard dose of cyclophosphamide, in conjunction with doxorubicin, a small number of secondary malignancies occurred within two years of beginning treatment. Urinary bladder malignancies generally have occurred in patients who previously had hemorrhagic cystitis. In patients treated with cyclophosphamide-containing regimens for a variety of solid tumors, isolated case reports of secondary malignancies have been published. One case of carcinoma of the renal pelvis was reported in a patient receiving long-term cyclophosphamide therapy for cerebral vasculitis. The possibility of cyclophosphamide-induced malignancy should be considered in any benefit-to-risk assessment for use of the drug.
Cyclophosphamide can cause fetal harm when administered to a pregnant woman and such abnormalities have been reported following cyclophosphamide therapy in pregnant women. Abnormalities were found in two infants and a 6-month-old fetus born to women treated with cyclophospha-

mide. Ectrodactylia was found in two of the three cases. Normal infants have also been born to women treated with cyclophosphamide during pregnancy, including the first trimester. If this drug is used during pregnancy, or if the patient becomes pregnant while taking (receiving) this drug, the patient should be apprised of the potential hazard to the fetus. Women of childbearing potential should be advised to avoid becoming pregnant.
Cyclophosphamide interferes with oogenesis and spermatogenesis. It may cause sterility in both sexes. Development of sterility appears to depend on the dose of cyclophosphamide, duration of therapy, and the state of gonadal function at the time of treatment. Cyclophosphamide-induced sterility may be irreversible in some patients.
Amenorrhea associated with decreased estrogen and increased gonadotropin secretion develops in a significant proportion of women treated with cyclophosphamide. Affected patients generally resume regular menses within a few months after cessation of therapy. Girls treated with cyclophosphamide during prepubescence generally develop secondary sexual characteristics normally and have regular menses. Ovarian fibrosis with apparently complete loss of germ cells after prolonged cyclophosphamide treatment in late prepubescence has been reported. Girls treated with cyclophosphamide during prepubescence subsequently have conceived.
Men treated with cyclophosphamide may develop oligospermia or azoospermia associated with increased gonadotropin but normal testosterone secretion. Sexual potency and libido are unimpaired in these patients. Boys treated with cyclophosphamide during prepubescence develop secondary sexual characteristics normally, but may have oligospermia or azoospermia and increased gonadotropin secretion. Some degree of testicular atrophy may occur. Cyclophosphamide-induced azoospermia is reversible in some patients, though the reversibility may not occur for several years after cessation of therapy. Men temporarily rendered sterile by cyclophosphamide have subsequently fathered normal children.
Urinary System—Hemorrhagic cystitis may develop in patients treated with cyclophosphamide. Rarely, this condition can be severe and even fatal. Fibrosis of the urinary bladder, sometimes extensive, also may develop with or without accompanying cystitis. Atypical urinary bladder epithelial cells may appear in the urine. These adverse effects appear to depend on the dose of cyclophosphamide and the duration of therapy. Such bladder injury is thought to be due to cyclophosphamide metabolites excreted in the urine. Forced fluid intake helps to assure an ample output of urine, necessitates frequent voiding, and reduces the time the drug remains in the bladder. This helps to prevent cystitis. Hematuria usually resolves in a few days after cyclophosphamide treatment is stopped, but it may persist. Medical and/or surgical supportive treatment may be required, rarely, to treat protracted cases of severe hemorrhagic cystitis. It is usually necessary to discontinue cyclophosphamide therapy in instances of severe hemorrhagic cystitis.
Cardiac Toxicity—Although a few instances of cardiac dysfunction have been reported following use of recommended doses of cyclophosphamide, no causal relationship has been established. Cardiotoxicity has been observed in some patients receiving high doses of cyclophosphamide ranging from 120 to 270 mg/kg administered over a period of a few days, usually as a portion of an intensive antineoplastic multidrug regimen or in conjunction with transplantation procedures. In a few instances with high doses of cyclophosphamide, severe, and sometimes fatal, congestive heart failure has occurred within a few days after the first cyclophosphamide dose. Histopathologic examination has primarily shown hemorrhagic myocarditis. Hemopericardium has occurred secondary to hemorrhagic myocarditis and myocardial necrosis. Pericarditis has been reported independent of any hemopericardium.
No residual cardiac abnormalities, as evidenced by electrocardiogram or echocardiogram appear to be present in patients surviving episodes of apparent cardiac toxicity associated with high doses of cyclophosphamide.
Cyclophosphamide has been reported to potentiate doxorubicin-induced cardiotoxicity.
Infections—Treatment with cyclophosphamide may cause significant suppression of immune responses. Serious, sometimes fatal, infections may develop in severely immunosuppressed patients. Cyclophosphamide treatment may not be indicated or should be interrupted or the dose reduced in patients who have or who develop viral, bacterial, fungal, protozoan, or helminthic infections.
Other—Rare instances of anaphylactic reaction including one death have been reported. One instance of possible cross-sensitivity with other alkylating agents has been reported.

PRECAUTIONS

General—Special attention to the possible development of toxicity should be exercised in patients being treated with cyclophosphamide if any of the following conditions are present.
1. Leukopenia. **2.** Thrombocytopenia. **3.** Tumor cell infiltration of bone marrow. **4.** Previous X-ray therapy. **5.** Previous

therapy with other cytotoxic agents. **6.** Impaired hepatic function. **7.** Impaired renal function.

Laboratory Tests—During treatment, the patient's hematologic profile (particularly neutrophils and platelets) should be monitored regularly to determine the degree of hematopoietic suppression. Urine should also be examined regularly for red cells which may precede hemorrhagic cystitis.

Drug Interactions—The rate of metabolism and the leukopenic activity of cyclophosphamide reportedly are increased by chronic administration of high doses of phenobarbital.

The physician should be alert for possible combined drug actions, desirable or undesirable, involving cyclophosphamide even though cyclophosphamide has been used successfully concurrently with other drugs, including other cytotoxic drugs.

Cyclophosphamide treatment, which causes a marked and persistent inhibition of cholinesterase activity, potentiates the effect of succinylcholine chloride.

If a patient has been treated with cyclophosphamide within 10 days of general anesthesia, the anesthesiologist should be alerted.

Adrenalectomy—Since cyclophosphamide has been reported to be more toxic in adrenalectomized dogs, adjustment of the doses of both replacement steroids and cyclophosphamide may be necessary for the adrenalectomized patient.

Wound Healing—Cyclophosphamide may interfere with normal wound healing.

Carcinogenesis, Mutagenesis, Impairment of Fertility—See WARNINGS section for information on carcinogenesis, mutagenesis, and impairment of fertility.

Pregnancy—Pregnancy Category D. See WARNINGS section.

Nursing Mothers—Cyclophosphamide is excreted in breast milk. Because of the potential for serious adverse reactions and the potential for tumorigenicity shown for cyclophosphamide in humans, a decision should be made whether to discontinue nursing or to discontinue the drug, taking into account the importance of the drug to the mother.

ADVERSE REACTIONS

Information on adverse reactions associated with the use of CYTOXAN is arranged according to body system affected or type of reaction. The adverse reactions are listed in order of decreasing incidence. The most serious adverse reactions are described in the WARNINGS section.

Reproductive System—See WARNINGS section for information on impairment of fertility.

Digestive System—Nausea and vomiting commonly occur with cyclophosphamide therapy. Anorexia and, less frequently, abdominal discomfort or pain and diarrhea may occur. There are isolated reports of hemorrhagic colitis, oral mucosal ulceration and jaundice occurring during therapy. These adverse drug effects generally remit when cyclophosphamide treatment is stopped.

Skin and Its Structures—Alopecia occurs commonly in patients treated with cyclophosphamide. The hair can be expected to grow back after treatment with the drug or even during continued drug treatment, though it may be different in texture or color. Skin rash occurs occasionally in patients receiving the drug. Pigmentation of the skin and changes in nails can occur.

Hematopoietic System—Leukopenia occurs in patients treated with cyclophosphamide, is related to the dose of drug, and can be used as a dosage guide. Leukopenia of less than 2000 cells/mm^3 develops commonly in patients treated with an initial loading dose of the drug, and less frequently in patients maintained on smaller doses. The degree of neutropenia is particularly important because it correlates with a reduction in resistance to infections. Fever has also been reported in patients with neutropenia.

Thrombocytopenia or anemia develop occasionally in patients treated with CYTOXAN. These hematologic effects usually can be reversed by reducing the drug dose or by interrupting treatment. Recovery from leukopenia usually begins in 7 to 10 days after cessation of therapy.

Urinary System—See WARNINGS section for information on cystitis and urinary bladder fibrosis.

Hemorrhagic ureteritis and renal tubular necrosis have been reported to occur in patients treated with cyclophosphamide. Such lesions usually resolve following cessation of therapy.

Infections—See WARNINGS section for information on reduced host resistance to infections.

Carcinogenesis—See WARNINGS section for information on carcinogenesis.

Respiratory System—Interstitial pulmonary fibrosis has been reported in patients receiving high doses of cyclophosphamide over a prolonged period.

Other—Rare instances of anaphylactic reaction including one death have been reported. One instance of possible cross-sensitivity with other alkylating agents has been reported.

OVERDOSAGE

No specific antidote for cyclophosphamide is known. Overdosage should be managed with supportive measures, including appropriate treatment for any concurrent infection, myelosuppression, or cardiac toxicity should it occur.

DOSAGE AND ADMINISTRATION

Treatment of Malignant Diseases: Adults and Children—When used as the only oncolytic drug therapy, the initial course of CYTOXAN for patients with no hematologic deficiency usually consists of 40 to 50 mg/kg given intravenously in divided doses over a period of 2 to 5 days. Other intravenous regimens include 10 to 15 mg/kg given every 7 to 10 days or 3 to 5 mg/kg twice weekly.

Oral CYTOXAN dosing is usually in the range of 1 to 5 mg/kg/day for both initial and maintenance dosing.

Many other regimens of intravenous and oral CYTOXAN have been reported. Dosages must be adjusted in accord with evidence of antitumor activity and/or leukopenia. The total leukocyte count is a good, objective guide for regulating dosage. Transient decreases in the total white blood cell count to 2000 cells/mm^3 (following short courses) or more persistent reduction to 3000 cells/mm^3 (with continuing therapy) are tolerated without serious risk of infection if there is no marked granulocytopenia.

When CYTOXAN is included in combined cytotoxic regimens, it may be necessary to reduce the dose of CYTOXAN as well as that of the other drugs.

CYTOXAN and its metabolites are dialyzable although there are probably quantitative differences depending upon the dialysis system being used. Patients with compromised renal function may show some measurable changes in pharmacokinetic parameters of CYTOXAN metabolism, but there is no consistent evidence indicating a need for CYTOXAN dosage modification in patients with renal function impairment.

Treatment of Nonmalignant Diseases: Biopsy Proven "Minimal Change" Nephrotic Syndrome in Children—An oral dose of 2.5 to 3 mg/kg daily for a period of 60 to 90 days is recommended. In males, the incidence of oligospermia and azoospermia increases if the duration of Cytoxan treatment exceeds 60 days. Treatment beyond 90 days increases the probability of sterility. Adrenocorticosteroid therapy may be tapered and discontinued during the course of CYTOXAN therapy. See PRECAUTIONS section concerning hematologic monitoring.

Preparation and Handling of Solutions—Parenteral drug products should be inspected visually for particulate matter and discoloration prior to administration, whenever solution and container permit.

CYTOXAN for Injection and Lyophilized CYTOXAN for Injection should be prepared for parenteral use by adding Sterile Water for Injection, USP, to the vial and shaking to dissolve. Use the quantity of diluent shown below to reconstitute the product.

Dosage Strength	Cytoxan for Injection Quantity of Diluent	Lyophilized Cytoxan for Injection Quantity of Diluent
100 mg	5 mL	5 mL
200 mg	10 mL	10 mL
500 mg	25 mL	20–25 mL
1 g	50 mL	50 mL
2 g	100 mL	80–100 mL

Solutions of CYTOXAN for Injection and Lyophilized CYTOXAN for Injection may be injected intravenously, intramuscularly, intraperitoneally, or intrapleurally or they may be infused intravenously in the following:

- Dextrose Injection, USP (5% dextrose)
- Dextrose and Sodium Chloride Injection, USP (5% dextrose and 0.9% sodium chloride)
- 5% Dextrose and Ringer's Injection
- Lactated Ringer's Injection, USP
- Sodium Chloride Injection, USP (0.45% sodium chloride)
- Sodium Lactate Injection, USP (1/6 molar sodium lactate)

Reconstituted CYTOXAN for Injection and Lyophilized CYTOXAN for Injection are chemically and physically stable for 24 hours at room temperature or for 6 days in the refrigerator; it does not contain any antimicrobial preservative and thus care must be taken to assure the sterility of prepared solutions.

The osmolarities of solutions of CYTOXAN for Injection, Lyophilized CYTOXAN for Injection, and normal saline are compared in the following table:

Lyophilized CYTOXAN for Injection	mOsm/L
4 mL diluent per 100 mg cyclophosphamide	219
5 mL diluent per 100 mg cyclophosphamide	172
CYTOXAN for Injection	352
Normal saline	287

Lyophilized CYTOXAN for Injection is slightly hypotonic while CYTOXAN for Injection is slightly hypertonic with respect to normal saline.

Extemporaneous liquid preparations of CYTOXAN for oral administration may be prepared by dissolving CYTOXAN for Injection or Lyophilized CYTOXAN for Injection in Aromatic Elixir, N.F. Such preparations should be stored under refrigeration in glass containers and used within 14 days.

HOW SUPPLIED

CYTOXAN for Injection contains 45 mg of sodium chloride per 100 mg of cyclophosphamide (anhydrous) and is supplied in vials for single dose use.

CYTOXAN for Injection (cyclophosphamide for injection, USP).

NDC 0015-0500-41 100 mg vials, carton of 12, case of 1 carton

NDC 0015-0501-41 200 mg vials, carton of 12, case of 1 carton

NDC 0015-0502-41 500 mg vials, carton of 12, case of 1 carton

NDC 0015-0505-41 1.0 g vials, carton of 6

NDC 0015-0506-41 2.0 g vials, carton of 6

Lyophilized CYTOXAN for Injection contains 75 mg mannitol per 100 mg cyclophosphamide (anhydrous) and is supplied in vials for single-dose use.

Lyophilized CYTOXAN for Injection (cyclophosphamide for injection, USP)

U.S. Patent No. 4,537,883

NDC 0015-0539-41 100 mg vials, carton of 12, case of 1 carton

NDC 0015-0546-41 200 mg vials, carton of 12, case of 1 carton

NDC 0015-0547-41 500 mg vials, carton of 12, case of 1 carton

NDC 0015-0548-41 1.0 g vials, carton of 6

NDC 0015-0549-41 2.0 g vials, carton of 6

CYTOXAN Tablets, 25 mg, and CYTOXAN Tablets, 50 mg, are white tablets with blue flecks containing 25 mg and 50 mg cyclophosphamide (anhydrous), respectively.

CYTOXAN Tablets (cyclophosphamide tablets, USP)

NDC 0015-0503-01 50 mg, bottles of 100

NDC 0015-0503-02 50 mg, bottles of 1000

NDC 0015-0503-03 50 mg, Unit Dose, cartons of 100

NDC 0015-0503-48 50 mg, Compliance Pack, cartons of 28

NDC 0015-0504-01 25 mg, bottles of 100

Storage at or below 77°F (25°C) is recommended; this product will withstand brief exposure to temperatures up to 86°F (30°C) but should be protected from temperatures above 86°F (30°C).

Procedures for proper handling and disposal of anticancer drugs should be considered. Several guidelines on this subject have been published.[1–7] There is no general agreement that all of the procedures recommended in the guidelines are necessary or appropriate.

REFERENCES

1. Recommendations for the Safe Handling of Parenteral Antineoplastic Drugs. NIH Publication No. 83-2621. For sale by the Superintendent of Documents, US Government Printing Office, Washington, DC 20402.
2. AMA Council Report, Guidelines for Handling Parenteral Antineoplastics, *JAMA.* 1985; 253(11):1590–1592.
3. National Study Commission on Cytotoxic Exposure—Recommendations for Handling Cytotoxic Agents. Available from Louis P. Jeffrey, Sc.D., Chairman, National Study Commission on Cytotoxic Exposure, Massachusetts College of Pharmacy and Allied Health Sciences, 179 Longwood Avenue, Boston, Massachusetts 02115.
4. Clinical Oncological Society of Australia. Guidelines and Recommendations for Safe Handling of Antineoplastic Agents. *Med J Australia.* 1983; 1:426–428.
5. Jones RB, et al: Safe handling of chemotherapeutic agents: A report from the Mount Sinai Medical Center. *CA—A Cancer J for Clinicians.* 1983; (Sept/Oct) 258–263.
6. American Society of Hospital Pharmacists Technical Assistance Bulletin on Handling Cytotoxic and Hazardous Drugs. *Am J Hosp Pharm.* 1990; 47:1033–1049.
7. OSHA Work-Practice Guidelines for Personnel Dealing with Cytotoxic (Antineoplastic) Drugs. *Am J Hosp Pharm.* 1986; 43:1193–1204.

(0539D1M-05)

February 1995

Shown in Product Identification Guide, page 307

ETOPOPHOS® ℞

(etoposide phosphate)

for Injection

CAUTION: FEDERAL LAW PROHIBITS DISPENSING WITHOUT A PRESCRIPTION.

WARNINGS

ETOPOPHOS® (etoposide phosphate) for Injection should be administered under the supervision of a qualified physician experienced in the use of cancer chemotherapeutic agents. Severe myelosuppression with resulting infection or bleeding may occur.

Continued on next page

Bristol-Myers Squibb Oncology—Cont.

DESCRIPTION

ETOPOPHOS® (etoposide phosphate) for Injection is an antineoplastic agent which is available for intravenous infusion as a sterile lyophile in single-dose vials containing etoposide phosphate equivalent to 100 mg etoposide, 32.7 mg sodium citrate USP and 300 mg dextran 40.
Etoposide phosphate is a water soluble ester of etoposide (commonly known as VP-16), a semi-synthetic derivative of podophyllotoxin. The water solubility of etoposide phosphate lessens the potential for precipitation following dilution and during intravenous administration.
The chemical name for etoposide phosphate is: 4'-Demethylepipodophyllotoxin 9-[4,6-O-(R)-ethylidene-β-D-glucopyranoside], 4'-(dihydrogen phosphate).
Etoposide phosphate has the following structure:

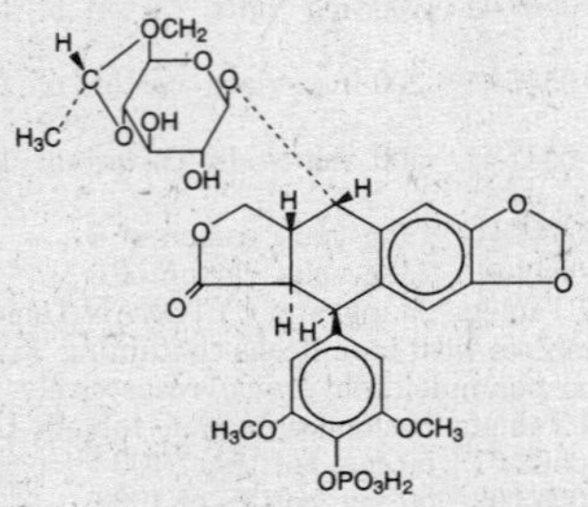

CLINICAL PHARMACOLOGY

The *in vitro* cytotoxicity observed for etoposide phosphate is significantly less than that seen with etoposide which is believed due to the necessity for conversion *in vivo* to the active moiety, etoposide, by dephosphorylation. The mechanism of action is believed to be the same as that of etoposide. Etoposide has been shown to cause metaphase arrest in chick fibroblasts. Its main effect, however, appears to be at the G_2 portion of the cell cycle in mammalian cells. Two different dose-dependent responses are seen. At high concentrations (10 μg/mL or more), lysis of cells entering mitosis is observed. At low concentrations (0.3 to 10 μg/mL), cells are inhibited from entering prophase. It does not interfere with microtubular assembly. The predominant macromolecular effect of etoposide appears to be the induction of DNA strand breaks by an interaction with DNA-topoisomerase II or the formation of free radicals.

ETOPOPHOS Bioequivalence: Following intravenous administration of ETOPOPHOS, etoposide phosphate is rapidly and completely converted to etoposide in plasma. A direct comparison of the pharmacokinetic parameters [area under the concentration time curve (AUC) and the maximum plasma concentration (CMAX)] of etoposide following intravenous administration of molar equivalent doses of ETOPOPHOS and VePesid® (etoposide) was made in two randomized cross-over studies in patients with a variety of malignancies. In the first study of 41 evaluable patients, the etoposide mean ± S.D. AUC values were 168.3 ± 48.2 μg.hr/mL and 156.7 ± 43.4 μg.hr/mL following administration of molar equivalent doses of 150 mg/m² ETOPOPHOS or VePesid with a 3.5 hour infusion time; the corresponding mean ± S.D. CMAX values were 20.0 ± 3.7 μg/mL and 19.6 ± 4.2 μg/mL, respectively. The point estimate (90% confidence interval) for the bioavailability of etoposide from ETOPOPHOS, relative to VePesid, was 107% (105%, 110%) for AUC and 103% (99%, 106%) for CMAX. In the second study of 29 evaluable patients following intravenous administration of 90, 100 and 110 mg/m² molar equivalents of ETOPOPHOS or VePesid with a 60 minute infusion time, the etoposide mean ± S.D. AUC values (normalized to the 100 mg/m² dose) were 96.1 ± 22.6 μg.hr/mL and 86.5 ± 25.8 μg.hr/mL, respectively; the corresponding mean ± S.D. CMAX values (normalized to the 100 mg/m² dose) were 20.1 ± 4.1 μg/mL and 19.0 ± 5.1 μg/mL, respectively. The point estimate (90% confidence interval) for the bioavailability of etoposide from ETOPOPHOS, relative to VePesid, was 113% (107%, 119%) for AUC and 107% (101%, 113%) for CMAX indicating bioequivalence. Results from both studies demonstrated no statistically significant differences in the AUC and CMAX parameters for etoposide when administered as ETOPOPHOS or VePesid. In addition, in the latter study, there were no statistically significant differences in the pharmacodynamic parameters (hematologic toxicity) after administration of ETOPOPHOS or VePesid. Following VePesid administration, the mean nadir values (expressed as percent decrease from baseline) for leukocytes, granulocytes, hemoglobin and thrombocytes were 67.2 ± 17.0%, 84.1 ± 14.6%, 22.6 ± 9.8% and 46.4 ± 21.9%, respectively; the corresponding values after administration of ETOPOPHOS were 67.3 ± 14.2%, 81.0 ± 16.5%, 21.4 ± 9.9% and 44.1 ± 20.7%, respectively.
Because of the similarity of pharmacokinetics and pharmacodynamics of etoposide after administration of either ETOPOPHOS or VePesid, the following information on VePesid should be considered:

VePesid Pharmacokinetics: On intravenous administration, the disposition of etoposide is best described as a biphasic process with a distribution half-life of about 1.5 hours and terminal elimination half-life ranging from 4 to 11 hours. Total body clearance values range from 33 to 48 mL/min or 16 to 36 mL/min/m² and, like the terminal elimination half-life, are independent of dose over a range 100-600 mg/m². Over the same dose range, the AUC and the CMAX values increase linearly with dose. Etoposide does not accumulate in the plasma following daily administration of 100 mg/m² for 4 to 5 days. After intravenous infusion the CMAX and AUC values exhibit marked intra- and inter-subject variability.
The mean volumes of distribution at steady state fall in the range of 18 to 29 liters or 7 to 17 L/m². Etoposide enters the CSF poorly. Although it is detectable in CSF and intracerebral tumors, the concentrations are lower than in extracerebral tumors and in plasma. Etoposide concentrations are higher in normal lung than in lung metastases and are similar in primary tumors and normal tissues of the myometrium. *In vitro*, etoposide is highly protein bound (97%) to human plasma proteins. An inverse relationship between plasma albumin levels and etoposide renal clearance is found in children. In a study determining the effect of other therapeutic agents on the *in vitro* binding of carbon-14 labeled etoposide to human serum proteins, only phenylbutazone, sodium salicylate, and aspirin displaced protein-bound etoposide at concentrations achieved *in vivo*.
Etoposide binding ratio correlates directly with serum albumin in patients with cancer and in normal volunteers. The unbound fraction of etoposide significantly correlated with bilirubin in a population of cancer patients. Data have suggested a significant inverse correlation between serum albumin concentration and free fraction of etoposide, (see "**PRECAUTIONS**").
After intravenous administration of ^{3}H-etoposide (70-290 mg/m²), mean recoveries of radioactivity in the urine range from 42 to 67%, and fecal recoveries range from 0 to 16% of the dose. Less than 50% of an intravenous dose is excreted in the urine as etoposide with mean recoveries of 8 to 35% within 24 hours.
In children, approximately 55% of the dose of VePesid (etoposide) is excreted in the urine as etoposide in 24 hours. The mean renal clearance of etoposide is 7 to 10 mL/min/m² or 35% of the total body clearance over a dose of 80 to 600 mg/m². Etoposide, therefore, is cleared by both renal and nonrenal processes, i.e., metabolism and biliary excretion. The effect of renal disease on plasma etoposide clearance is not known in children.
Biliary excretion appears to be a minor route of etoposide elimination. Only 6% or less of an intravenous dose is recovered in the bile as etoposide. Metabolism accounts for most of the nonrenal clearance of etoposide. The major urinary metabolite of etoposide in adults and children is the hydroxy acid [4'-demethylepipodophyllic acid-9-(4,6-0-(R)-ethylidene-β-D-glucopyranoside)], formed by opening of the lactone ring. It is also present in human plasma, presumably as the **trans** isomer. Glucuronide and/or sulfate conjugates of etoposide are excreted in human urine and represent 5 to 22% of the dose. In addition, O-demethylation of the dimethoxyphenol ring occurs through the CYP450 3A4 isoenzyme pathway to produce the corresponding catechol.
In adults, the total body clearance of etoposide is correlated with creatinine clearance, serum albumin concentration, and nonrenal clearance. Patients with impaired renal function receiving etoposide have exhibited reduced total body clearance, increased AUC and a lower volume of distribution at steady state, (see "**PRECAUTIONS**"). Use of cisplatin therapy is associated with reduced total body clearance. In children, elevated serum SGPT levels are associated with reduced drug total body clearance. Prior use of cisplatin may also result in a decrease of etoposide total body clearance in children.
Although some minor differences in pharmacokinetic parameters between age and gender have been observed, these differences were not considered clinically significant.

Clinical Studies: A total of 7 clinical trials with 365 patients treated (368 entered) provided the data base for the human experience summarized in this insert. Five phase I trials evaluated etoposide phosphate given on a days 1, 3 and 5 or days 1 through 5 schedule. In two trials the drug was given over 5 minutes and in three over 30 minutes. The following table summarizes the doses, schedules, infusion times and numbers of patients entered in the phase I experience.

Dose Escalation (Phase I) Trials of Etoposide Phosphate

Study	Schedule Q 21 days	Infusion Time	Dose Range (mg/m²)	Number of Patients Entered
002	Days 1–5	30 minutes	25–110	68
005	Days 1, 3, 5	30 minutes	50–175	39
006	Days 1–5	30 minutes	50–125	28
008	Days 1, 3, 5	5 minutes	50–200	36
009	Days 1–5	5 minutes	50–125	27

Two trials evaluated the pharmacokinetic equivalence of etoposide and etoposide phosphate. A phase I study (002) was expanded at the higher doses to compare the pharmacokinetic profile of etoposide following administration of etoposide or etoposide phosphate. Another, multi-institutional trial (012), was conducted at a dose of 150 mg/m² using a day 1, 3 and 5 schedule and a crossover design.
The seventh trial (011) was a randomized study in which patients with limited or extensive small cell lung cancer and no prior therapy were treated with either cisplatin plus etoposide or cisplatin plus etoposide phosphate. Patients received 20 mg/m²/day of cisplatin for 5 days and 80 mg/m²/day of etoposide or etoposide phosphate. A total of 121 patients were randomized and 120 treated (60 per group). Response rates, time to response, duration of response, time to progression, time to worsening performance status and survival were similar in the two groups whether the analysis was done for patients with limited or extensive disease or for the entire population. The following table summarizes the results regardless of disease extent.

Response to Treatment for All Patients

	Etoposide Phosphate plus Cisplatin	Etoposide plus Cisplatin	P-value
Complete Responses:	15%	15%	1.000 *
Partial Responses:	46%	43%	0.855 *
Overall Response Rate:	61%	58%	0.854 *
Median Time to Response:	48 days	46 days	0.596 **
Median Response Duration:	273 days	241 days	0.141 ***
Median Time to Progression:	211 days	213 days	0.500 ***
Median Time to Worsening:			0.472 ***
Performance Status:	210 days	149 days	0.780 ***
Median Survival:	348 days	318 days	

*Fisher's Exact test
**Wilcoxon Rank Sum test
***Logrank test

The most prominent side effects were myelosuppression and GI toxicity. Sixty-eight percent of patients treated with etoposide phosphate plus cisplatin had neutrophils less than 500/mm³ at some time during treatment as did 88% of those getting etoposide and cisplatin. Over 85% in each group had nausea and/or vomiting. No differences in the pattern or severity of side effects were observed.

INDICATION AND USAGE

ETOPOPHOS (etoposide phosphate) for Injection is indicated in the management of the following neoplasms:
Refractory Testicular Tumors: ETOPOPHOS for Injection in combination therapy with other approved chemotherapeutic agents in patients with refractory testicular tumors who have already received appropriate surgical, chemotherapeutic, and radiotherapeutic therapy.
Small Cell Lung Cancer: ETOPOPHOS for Injection in combination with other approved chemotherapeutic agents as first line treatment in patients with small cell lung cancer.

CONTRAINDICATIONS

ETOPOPHOS is contraindicated in patients who have demonstrated a previous hypersensitivity to etoposide, etoposide phosphate, or any other component of the formulations.

WARNINGS

Patients being treated with ETOPOPHOS must be frequently observed for myelosuppression both during and after therapy. Dose-limiting bone marrow suppression is the most significant toxicity associated with ETOPOPHOS therapy. Therefore, the following studies should be obtained at the start of therapy and prior to each subsequent dose of ETOPOPHOS platelet count, hemoglobin, white blood cell count, and differential. The occurrence of a platelet count below 50,000/mm³ or an absolute neutrophil count below 500/mm³ is an indication to withhold further therapy until the blood counts have sufficiently recovered. The toxicity of

rapidly infused ETOPOPHOS in patients with impaired renal or hepatic function has not been adequately evaluated. The toxicity profile of ETOPOPHOS when infused at doses >175 mg/m^2 has not been delineated.

Physicians should be aware of the possible occurrence of an anaphylactic reaction manifested by chills, fever, tachycardia, bronchospasm, dyspnea and hypotension. Higher rates of anaphylactic-like reactions have been reported in children who received infusions of etoposide at concentrations higher than those recommended. The role that concentration of infusion (or rate of infusion) plays in the development of anaphylactic-like reactions is uncertain. (See "**ADVERSE REACTIONS**" section.) Treatment is symptomatic. The infusion should be terminated immediately, followed by the administration of pressor agents, corticosteroids, antihistamines, or volume expanders at the discretion of the physician.

ETOPOPHOS can cause fetal harm when administered to a pregnant woman. Etoposide has been shown to be teratogenic in mice and rats, and it is therefore likely that ETOPOPHOS is also teratogenic.

In rats, an intravenous etoposide dose of 0.4 mg/kg/day (about 1/20th of the human dose on a mg/m^2 basis) during organogenesis caused maternal toxicity, embryotoxicity, and teratogenicity (skeletal abnormalities, exencephaly, encephalocele, and anophthalmia); higher doses of 1.2 and 3.6 mg/kg/day (about 1/7th and 1/2 of the human dose on a mg/m^2 basis) resulted in 90 and 100% embryonic resorptions. In mice, a single 1.0 mg/kg (1/16th of the human dose on a mg/m^2 basis) dose of etoposide administered intraperitoneally on days 6, 7, or 8 of gestation caused embryotoxicity, cranial abnormalities, and major skeletal malformations. An i.p. dose of 1.5 mg/kg (about 1/10th of the human dose on a mg/m^2 basis) on day 7 of gestation caused an increase in the incidence of intrauterine death and fetal malformations and a significant decrease in the average fetal body weight.

If this drug is used during pregnancy, or if the patient becomes pregnant while receiving this drug, the patient should be warned of the potential hazard to the fetus. Women of childbearing potential should be advised to avoid becoming pregnant.

ETOPOPHOS should be considered a potential carcinogen in humans. The occurrence of acute leukemia with or without a preleukemic phase has been reported in rare instances in patients treated with etoposide alone or in association with other neoplastic agents. The risk of development of a preleukemic or leukemic syndrome is unclear. Carcinogenicity tests with ETOPOPHOS have not been conducted in laboratory animals.

PRECAUTIONS

General: In all instances where the use of ETOPOPHOS is considered for chemotherapy, the physician must evaluate the need and usefulness of the drug against the risk of adverse reactions. Most such adverse reactions are reversible if detected early. If severe reactions occur, the drug should be reduced in dosage or discontinued and appropriate corrective measures should be taken according to the clinical judgement of the physician. Reinstitution of ETOPOPHOS therapy should be carried out with caution, and with adequate consideration of the further need for the drug and alertness as to possible recurrence of toxicity.

Patients with low serum albumin may be at an increased risk for etoposide associated toxicities.

Laboratory Tests: Periodic complete blood counts should be done during the course of ETOPOPHOS (etoposide phosphate) for Injection treatment. They should be performed prior to each cycle of therapy and at appropriate intervals during and after therapy.

Carcinogenesis (see "WARNINGS" section), Mutagenesis, Impairment of Fertility: ETOPOPHOS was non-mutagenic in *in vitro* Ames microbial mutagenicity assay and the *E. coli* WP2 uvrA reverse mutation assay. Since ETOPOPHOS is rapidly and completely converted to etoposide *in vivo* and etoposide has been shown to be mutagenic in Ames assay, ETOPOPHOS should be considered as a potential mutagen *in vivo*.

In rats, an oral dose of ETOPOPHOS at 86.0 mg/kg/day (about 10 times the human dose on a mg/m^2 basis) or above administered for 5 consecutive days resulted in irreversible testicular atrophy. Irreversible testicular atrophy was also present in rats treated with ETOPOPHOS intravenously for 30 days at 5.11 mg/kg/day (about 1/2 of the human dose on a mg/m^2 basis).

Pregnancy: Pregnancy "Category D." (See "**WARNINGS**" section.)

Nursing Mothers: It is not known whether this drug is excreted in human milk. Because many drugs are excreted in human milk and because of the potential for serious adverse reactions in nursing infants from ETOPOPHOS, a decision should be made whether to discontinue nursing or to discontinue the drug, taking into account the importance of the drug to the mother.

Pediatric Use: Safety and effectiveness in pediatric patients have not been established. Anaphylactic reactions have been reported in pediatric patients who received etoposide, (see "WARNINGS" section).

Drug Interactions: Caution should be exercised when administering etopophos with drugs that are known to inhibit phosphatase activities (e.g., levamisole hydrochloride). High-dose cyclosporine resulting in concentrations above 2000 ng/mL administered with oral etoposide has led to an 80% increase in etoposide exposure with a 38% decrease in total body clearance of etoposide compared to etoposide alone.

Renal Impairment: In patients with impaired renal function, the following initial dose modification should be considered based on measured creatinine clearance:

Measured Creatinine Clearance	>50 mL/min	15–50mL/min
etoposide	100% of dose	75% of dose

Subsequent etoposide dosing should be based on patient tolerance and clinical effect. Equivalent dose adjustments of ETOPOPHOS should be used.

Data are not available in patients with creatinine clearances <15 mL/min and further dose reduction should be considered in these patients.

ADVERSE REACTIONS

ETOPOPHOS has been found to be well tolerated as a single agent in clinical studies involving 206 patients with a wide variety of malignancies, and in combination with cisplatin in 60 patients with small cell lung cancer. The most frequent clinically significant adverse experiences were leukopenia and neutropenia.

The incidences of adverse experiences in the table that follows are derived from studies in which ETOPOPHOS (etoposide phosphate) for injection was administered as a single agent. A total of 98 patients received total doses at or above 450 mg/m^2 on a 5 consecutive day or day 1, 3 and 5 schedule during the first course of therapy.

Summary of Adverse Events Reports With Single Agent ETOPOPHOS Following Course 1 at Total Five Day Doses of ≥ 450 mg/m^2

		Percent of Patients
Hematologic toxicity		
Leukopenia	<4000 /mm^3	91
	<1000 /mm^3	17
Neutropenia	<2000 /mm^3	88
	<500 /mm^3	37
Thrombocytopenia	<100,000 /mm^3	23
	<50,000 /mm^3	9
Anemia	<11 g/dL	72
	<8 g/dL	19
Gastrointestinal toxicity		
Nausea and/or Vomiting		37
Anorexia		16
Mucositis		11
Constipation		8
Abdominal Pain		7
Diarrhea		6
Taste Alteration		6
Asthenia/Malaise		39
Alopecia		33
Chills and/or Fever		24
Dizziness		5
Extravasation/Phlebitis		5

Since etoposide phosphate is converted to etoposide, those adverse experiences that are associated with VePesid (etoposide) can be expected to occur with ETOPOPHOS.

Hematologic Toxicity: Myelosuppression after ETOPOPHOS administration is dose related and dose limiting with the leukocyte nadir counts occurring from day 15 to day 22 after initiation of drug therapy, granulocyte nadir counts occurring day 12-19 after initiation of drug therapy, and platelet nadirs occurring from day 10-15. Bone marrow recovery usually occurs by day 21 but may be delayed, and no cumulative toxicity has been reported. Fever and infection have also been reported in patients with neutropenia.

Gastrointestinal Toxicity: Nausea and vomiting are the major gastrointestinal toxicities. The severity of such nausea and vomiting is generally mild to moderate with treatment discontinuation required in 1% of patients. Nausea and vomiting can usually be controlled with standard antiemetic therapy.

Blood Pressure Changes: In clinical studies, one hundred fifty-one patients were treated with ETOPOPHOS (etoposide phosphate) for Injection with infusion times ranging from thirty minutes to three and one-half hours. Sixty-three patients received ETOPOPHOS as a five minute bolus infusion. Four patients experienced one or more episodes of hypertension and eight patients experienced one or more episode of hypotension, which may or may not be drug related. One episode of hypotension was reported among those patients who received a five minute bolus infusion. If clinically significant hypotension or hypertension occurs with ETOPOPHOS, appropriate supportive therapy should be initiated.

Allergic Reactions: Anaphylactic type reactions characterized by chills, rigors, tachycardia, bronchospasm, dyspnea, diaphoresis, fever, pruritus, hypertension or hypotension, loss of consciousness, nausea and vomiting have been reported to occur in 3% (7/245) of all patients treated with ETOPOPHOS. Facial flushing was reported in 2% and skin rashes in 3% of patients receiving ETOPOPHOS. These reactions have usually responded promptly to the cessation of the infusion and administration of pressor agents, corticosteroids, antihistamines, or volume expanders as appropriate; however, the reactions can be fatal. Hypertension and/or flushing have also been reported. Blood pressure usually normalized within a few hours after cessation of the initial infusion.

Anaphylactic-like reactions have occurred during the initial infusion of ETOPOPHOS, (see "**WARNINGS**" section) .Facial/tongue swelling, coughing, diaphoresis, cyanosis, tightness in throat, laryngospasm, back pain, and/or loss of consciousness have sometimes occurred in association with the above reactions. In addition, an apparent hypersensitivity-associated apnea has been reported rarely.

Rash, urticaria, and/or pruritus have infrequently been reported at recommended doses. At investigational doses, a generalized pruritic erythematous maculopapular rash, consistent with perivasculitis, has been reported.

Alopecia: Reversible alopecia, sometimes progressing to total baldness, was observed in up to 44% of patients.

Other Toxicities: The following adverse reactions have been infrequently reported: aftertaste, fever, pigmentation, abdominal pain, constipation, dysphagia, transient cortical blindness, and optic neuritis, and a single report of radiation recall dermatitis. Rarely, hepatic toxicity may be seen.

The incidences of adverse reactions in the table that follows are derived from multiple data bases from studies in 2,081 patients when VePesid (etoposide) was used either orally or by injection as a single agent.

Adverse Drug Effects Observed with Single Agent VePesid		Percent Range of Reported Incidence
Hematologic toxicity		
Leukopenia	(<1,000/mm^3)	3–17
	(<4,000/mm^3)	60–91
Thrombocytopenia	(<50,000/mm^3)	1–20
	(<100,000/mm^3)	22–41
Anemia		0–33
Gastrointestinal toxicity		
Nausea and Vomiting		31–43
Abdominal Pain		0–2
Anorexia		10–13
Diarrhea		1–13
Stomatitis		1–6
Hepatic		0–3
Alopecia		8–66
Peripheral Neurotoxicity		1–2
Hypotension		1–2
Allergic Reaction		1–2

OVERDOSAGE

No proven antidotes have been established for ETOPOPHOS (etoposide phosphate) for injection overdosage in humans. In mice, a single intravenous dose of rapidly administered ETOPOPHOS was lethal at or above 120 mg/kg (about 7 times human dose on a mg/m^2 basis) and was associated with clinical signs of neurotoxicity.

DOSAGE AND ADMINISTRATION

The usual dose of VePesid for Injection in testicular cancer in combination with other approved chemotherapeutic agents ranges from 50 to 100 mg/m^2/day on days 1 through 5 to 100 mg/m^2/day on days 1, 3, and 5. Equivalent doses of ETOPOPHOS should be used.

In small cell lung cancer, the Vepesid for Injection dose in combination with other approved chemotherapeutic drugs ranges from 35 mg/m^2/day for 4 days to 50 mg/m^2/day for 5 days. Equivalent doses of ETOPOPHOS should be used.

For recommended dosing adjustments in patients with renal impairment, see "**PRECAUTIONS**."

ETOPOPHOS solutions may be administered at infusion rates from 5 to 210 minutes. Chemotherapy courses are repeated at 3- to 4- week intervals after adequate recovery from any toxicity.

The dosage should be modified to take into account the myelosuppressive effect of other drugs in the combination or the effects prior x-ray therapy or chemotherapy which may have compromised bone marrow reserve.

Continued on next page

Bristol-Myers Squibb Oncology—Cont.

Administration Precautions: As with other potentially toxic compounds, caution should be exercised in handling and preparing the solution of ETOPOPHOS. Skin reactions associated with accidental exposure to ETOPOPHOS may occur. The use of gloves is recommended. If ETOPOPHOS solution contacts the skin or mucosa, immediately and thoroughly wash the skin with soap and water and flush the mucosa with water.

Preparation for Intravenous Administration: Prior to use, the content of each vial must be reconstituted with either 5-mL or 10-mL Sterile Water for Injection, USP; 5% Dextrose Injection, USP; 0.9% Sodium Chloride Injection, USP; Bacteriostatic Water for Injection with Benzyl Alcohol; or Bacteriostatic Sodium Chloride for Injection with Benzyl Alcohol to a concentration equivalent to 20 mg/mL or 10 mg/mL etoposide (22.7 mg/mL or 11.4 mg/mL etoposide phosphate), respectively. Following reconstitution the solution may be administered without further dilution or it can be further diluted to concentrations as low as 0.1 mg/mL etoposide with either 5% Dextrose Injection, USP or 0.9% Sodium Chloride Injection, USP.

Solutions of ETOPOPHOS (etoposide phosphate) for Injection should be prepared in an aseptic manner. Parenteral drug products should be inspected visually for particulate matter and discoloration prior to administration whenever solution and container permit.

STABILITY

Unopened vials of ETOPOPHOS for Injection are stable until the date indicated on the package when stored under refrigeration 2–8°C (36°–46°F) in the original package. When reconstituted and/or diluted as directed, ETOPOPHOS solutions can be stored in glass or plastic containers at controlled room temperature 20°–25°C (68°–77°F) or under refrigeration 2°–8°C (36°–46°F) for 24 hours. Refrigerated solutions of ETOPOPHOS should be used immediately upon return to room temperature.

HOW SUPPLIED

NDC 0015-3404-20

Individually cartoned single-dose vials with white flip-off seals containing etoposide phosphate equivalent to 100 mg etoposide.

STORAGE

Store the unopened vials under refrigeration 2–8°C (36°–46°F). Retain in original package to protect from light.

HANDLING AND DISPOSAL

Procedures for proper handling and disposal of anticancer drugs should be considered. Several guidelines on this subject have been published.[1-7] There is no general agreement that all of the procedures recommended in the guidelines are necessary or appropriate.

REFERENCES

1. Recommendations for the Safe Handling of Parenteral Antineoplastic Drugs. NIH Publication No. 83-2621. For sale by the Superintendent of Documents, US Government Printing Office, Washington, DC 20402.
2. AMA Council Report. Guidelines for Handling Parenteral Antineoplastics. JAMA 1985; 253 (11):1590-1592.
3. National Study Commission on Cytotoxic Exposure–Recommendations for Handling Cytotoxic Agents. Available from Louis P. Jeffrey, ScD, Chairman, National Study Commission on Cytotoxic Exposure, Massachusetts College of Pharmacy and Allied Health Sciences, 179 Longwood Avenue, Boston, Massachusetts 02115.
4. Clinical Oncological Society of Australia. Guidelines and Recommendations for Safe Handling of Antineoplastic Agents. Med J Australia 1983; 1:426–428.
5. Jones RB, et al. Safe Handling of Chemotherapeutic Agents: A report from the Mount Sinai Medical Center. CA–A Cancer Journal for Clinicians 1983; (Sept/Oct)258–263.
6. American Society of Hospital Pharmacists Technical Assistance Bulletin on Handling Cytotoxic and Hazardous Drugs. Am J Hosp Pharm 1990; 47:1033–1049.
7. OSHA Work-Practice Guidelines for Personnel Dealing with Cytotoxic (Antineoplastic) Drugs. Am J Hosp Pharm 1986; 43:1193–1204.

BRISTOL LABORATORIES
ONCOLOGY PRODUCTS
A Bristol-Myers Squibb Company
Princeton, NJ 08543
U.S.A.

3404DIM-01 V2-B001-5-96
51-004164-00 Issued: May 1996

Shown in Product Identification Guide, page 307

FUNGIZONE® ORAL SUSPENSION ℞

Amphotericin B Oral Suspension

CAUTION: Federal law prohibits dispensing without prescription.

DESCRIPTION

Fungizone Oral Suspension (Amphotericin B Oral Suspension) contains amphotericin B, an antifungal polyene antibiotic obtained from a strain of *Streptomyces nodosus.* Amphotericin B is designated chemically as [1R (1R*,3S*,5R*, 6R*,9R*,11R*, 15S*,16R*,17R*,18S*,19E, 21E,23E,25E,27E, 29E,31E,33R*,35S*,36R*,37S*)]-33-[(3-Amino-3,6-dideoxy-β-(D -mannopyranosyl)oxy]-1,3,5,6,9,11,17,37-octahydroxy-15, 16,18-trimethyl -13- oxo-14,39-dioxabicyclo [33.3.1] nonatriaconta-19,21,23,25,27,29,31-heptaene-36-carboxylic acid. Structural formula:

Fungizone [amphotericin B]

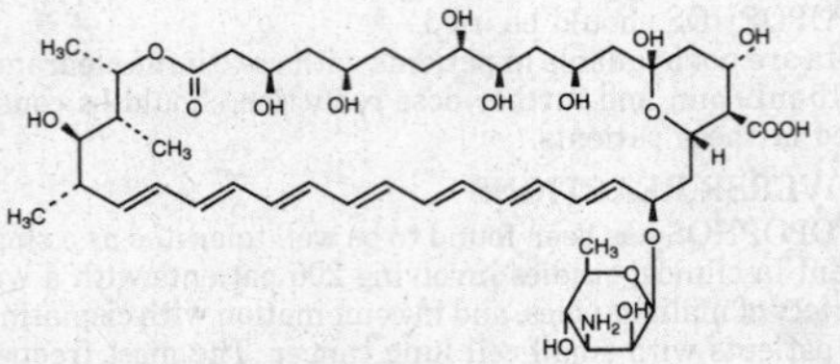

$C_{47}H_{73}NO_{17}$ MW=924.10

Fungizone Oral Suspension is a flavored aqueous suspension providing 100 mg amphotericin B per mL. Inactive ingredients: not more than 0.55 percent alcohol, carboxymethylcellulose sodium, citric acid, flavors, glycerin, methyl- and propylparaben, mono- and dibasic sodium phosphate, potassium chloride, sodium benzoate, sodium metabisulfite, and purified water.

MICROBIOLOGY

Mechanism of Action

Amphotericin B exhibits antifungal activity by binding to sterols in the cell membrane of susceptible fungi with a resultant change of membrane permeability allowing leakage of intracellular components.

Anti-Candida activity *in vitro*

Candida species are inhibited by concentrations of amphotericin B ranging from 0.03 to 2.0 μg/mL *in vitro.* While *Candida albicans* is generally quite susceptible to amphotericin B, non-*albicans* species may be less susceptible. The activity of amphotericin B is fungistatic or fungicidal depending on the concentration at the site of infection and the susceptibility of the fungal organism. However, standardized techniques for susceptibility testing of antifungal agents have not been established and results of susceptibility studies have not been correlated with clinical outcomes. The antibiotic is without effect against bacteria, rickettsiae and viruses.

Drug Resistance

Mutants with decreased susceptibility to amphotericin B have been isolated from several fungal species after serial passage *in vitro* in the presence of the drug, and from some patients receiving prolonged therapy. However, the clinical relevance of drug resistance to clinical outcome has not been established.

Drug Interaction

Antagonism between amphotericin B and imidazole derivatives, such as miconazole, and ketoconazole, which inhibit ergosterol synthesis, has been reported. However, the clinical significance of this phenomena has not been demonstrated.

CLINICAL PHARMACOLOGY

Pharmacokinetics

Amphotericin B administered as Fungizone Oral Suspension is poorly absorbed from the gastrointestinal tract. In limited studies conducted in both pediatric and adult patients administered Fungizone Oral Suspension (dose 100 mg four to six times a day), the average amphotericin B serum concentration measured by microbiological assay following at least 14 days of therapy was 0.05 μg/mL (range <0.01–0.15). Serum concentrations did not show evidence of significant antibiotic accumulation over a period of two weeks. Metabolic pathways have not been elucidated.

INDICATIONS AND USAGE

Fungizone Oral Suspension (Amphotericin B Oral Suspension) is indicated for the treatment of oral candidiasis caused by susceptible strains of *Candida albicans.*

When appropriate, it is recommended that identification of the causative pathogen be obtained by means of suitable mycologic techniques before the initiation of treatment.

CONTRAINDICATIONS

Fungizone Oral Suspension is contraindicated in patients with a history of hypersensitivity to any of its components.

PRECAUTIONS

General

Fungizone Oral Suspension is not to be used for the treatment of systemic mycoses. If a systemic mycosis is suspected or documented, appropriate therapy should be instituted. Superficial candidal lesions present in addition to the oral infection should be treated concomitantly with an appropriate topical anti-candidal preparation.

If irritation or hypersensitivity develops with Fungizone Oral Suspension, treatment should be discontinued and appropriate therapy instituted.

Information for Patients

Patients taking this medication should be provided the following information:

1. Use as directed by your physician. This medication is only for the treatment of oral candidiasis and should not be used for any other diseases or symptoms.
2. The medication works by direct contact with the oral *Candida* lesions; you should try to swish the medication around in your mouth as long as reasonably possible before swallowing.
3. If symptoms of local irritation develop, preexisting symptoms worsen, or new symptoms develop, your physician should be notified promptly.
4. Notify your physician if symptoms recur after discontinuation of medication.

Carcinogenesis, Mutagenesis, Impairment of Fertility

No long-term studies have been performed to evaluate carcinogenic or mutagenic potential of Fungizone Oral Suspension. Animal studies of Fungizone Oral Suspension have shown effects on reproduction.

Pregnancy: Category C

Fungizone Oral Suspension has been shown to cause a significantly higher incidence of stillborn fetuses when administered to pregnant rats at a dose of 200 mg/kg/day (4x the human dose, based on body surface area considerations). No signs of fetal abnormalities were observed. An increased number of deaths occurred in pregnant rabbits administered 50 mg/kg/day (2x the human dose) and 100 mg/kg/day (4x the human dose). The number of births were also reduced at those doses and one stillbirth occurred at the lower dose. No fetal abnormalities were observed. There are no adequate and well-controlled studies in pregnant women. Fungizone Oral Suspension should be used during pregnancy only if the potential benefit justifies the potential risk to the fetus.

Nursing Mothers

Though systemic absorption is poor, it is not known whether amphotericin B is excreted in human milk. Because many drugs are excreted in human milk and because of the potential for serious adverse reactions in nursing infants from Fungizone Oral Suspension, a decision should be made whether to discontinue nursing or to discontinue the drug taking into account the importance of the drug to the mother.

Pediatric Use

There has been limited study of Fungizone Oral Suspension in pediatric patients, although studies have included premature infants. Doses used have been 100 mg four times per day regardless of age. Mycological eradication of oral *Candida* in these studies has been in the range of 10 to 20%, although clinical responses are more frequent.

ADVERSE REACTIONS

Rash, gastrointestinal symptoms, including nausea, vomiting, steatorrhea, and diarrhea have been reported following administration of Fungizone Oral Suspension. Rare occurrences of urticaria, angioedema, Stevens-Johnson Syndrome and toxic epidermal necrolysis have also been reported.

DOSAGE AND ADMINISTRATION

The recommended dosage for Fungizone Oral Suspension in adults and pediatric patients is 1 mL (100 mg), four times daily. If possible, the suspension should be administered between meals to permit prolonged contact with the oral lesions.

Shake well before using. The suspension should be dropped directly on the tongue with the calibrated dropper. Patients should be directed to swish the medication in the mouth for as long as is reasonably possible before swallowing. If application by swabbing is desired, a non-absorbent swab should be used in applying medication.

The recommended duration of therapy is 2 weeks, although longer treatment may be necessary based on clinical response. Recurrence of oral candidiasis may be common depending on patient risk factors.

HOW SUPPLIED

Fungizone Oral Suspension (Amphotericin B Oral Suspension)

100 mg per mL is available in bottles of 24 mL

NDC 0087-1162-10

A dropper calibrated for 1 mL is supplied with each 24 mL bottle.

Storage

Store at controlled room temperature 15° C (59° F) to 30° C (86° F); avoid freezing. Protect from direct sunlight. Keep tightly closed.

BRISTOL-MYERS SQUIBB
Immunology
A Bristol-Myers Squibb Company
Princeton, New Jersey 08543
U.S.A.
Made in UK
Revised January 1996   51-004179-00
Shown in Product Identification Guide, page 307

HYDREA® ℞
(hydroxyurea capsules, USP)

CAUTION: FEDERAL LAW PROHIBITS DISPENSING WITHOUT PRESCRIPTION.

DESCRIPTION

HYDREA® (hydroxyurea capsules, USP) is an antineoplastic agent, available for oral use as capsules providing 500 mg hydroxyurea. Inactive ingredients: citric acid, colorants (D&C Yellow No. 10, FD&C Blue No. 1, FD&C Red 40 and D&C Red 28), gelatin, lactose, magnesium stearate, sodium phosphate, and titanium dioxide.

Hydroxyurea occurs as an essentially tasteless, white crystalline powder. Its structural formula is:

$$H_2N-\overset{\overset{\displaystyle O}{\|}}{C}-NH-OH$$

ACTIONS

Mechanism of Action—The precise mechanism by which hydroxyurea produces its cytotoxic effects cannot, at present, be described. However, the reports of various studies in tissue culture in rats and man lend support to the hypothesis that hydroxyurea causes an immediate inhibition of DNA synthesis without interfering with the synthesis of ribonucleic acid or of protein. This hypothesis explains why, under certain conditions, hydroxyurea may induce teratogenic effects.

Three mechanisms of action have been postulated for the increased effectiveness of concomitant use of hydroxyurea therapy with irradiation on squamous cell (epidermoid) carcinomas of the head and neck. *In vitro* studies utilizing Chinese hamster cells suggest that hydroxyurea (1) is lethal to normally radioresistant S-stage cells, and (2) holds other cells of the cell cycle in the G1 or pre-DNA synthesis stage where they are most susceptible to the effects of irradiation. The third mechanism of action has been theorized on the basis of *in vitro* studies of HeLa cells: it appears that hydroxyurea, by inhibition of DNA synthesis, hinders the normal repair process of cells damaged but not killed by irradiation, thereby decreasing their survival rate; RNA and protein syntheses have shown no alteration.

Absorption, Metabolism, Fate and Excretion—After oral administration in man, hydroxyurea is readily absorbed from the gastrointestinal tract. The drug reaches peak serum concentrations within 2 hours; by 24 hours the concentration in the serum is essentially zero. Approximately 80 percent of an oral or intravenous dose of 7 to 30 mg/kg may be recovered in the urine within 12 hours.

Animal Pharmacology and Toxicology—The oral LD_{50} of hydroxyurea is 7330 mg/kg in mice and 5780 mg/kg in rats, given as a single dose.

In subacute and chronic toxicity studies in the rat, the most consistent pathological findings were an apparent dose-related mild to moderate bone marrow hypoplasia as well as pulmonary congestion and mottling of the lungs. At the highest dosage levels (1260 mg/kg/day for 37 days then 2520 mg/kg/day for 40 days), testicular atrophy with absence of spermatogenesis occurred; in several animals, hepatic cell damage with fatty metamorphosis was noted. In the dog, mild to marked bone marrow depression was a consistent finding except at the lower dosage levels. Additionally, at the higher dose levels (140 to 420 mg or 140 to 1260 mg/kg/week given 3 or 7 days weekly for 12 weeks), growth retardation, slightly increased blood glucose values, and hemosiderosis of the liver or spleen were found; reversible spermatogenic arrest was noted. In the monkey, bone marrow depression, lymphoid atrophy of the spleen, and degenerative changes in the epithelium of the small and large intestines were found. At the higher, often lethal, doses (400 to 800 mg/kg/day for 7 to 15 days), hemorrhage and congestion were found in the lungs, brain, and urinary tract. Cardiovascular effects (changes in heart rate, blood pressure, orthostatic hypotension, EKG changes) and hematological changes (slight hemolysis, slight methemoglobinemia) were observed in some species of laboratory animals at doses exceeding clinical levels.

INDICATIONS AND USAGE

Significant tumor response to HYDREA has been demonstrated in melanoma, resistant chronic myelocytic leukemia, and recurrent, metastatic, or inoperable carcinoma of the ovary.

Hydroxyurea used concomitantly with irradiation therapy is intended for use in the local control of primary squamous cell (epidermoid) carcinomas of the head and neck, excluding the lip.

CONTRAINDICATIONS

Hydroxyurea is contraindicated in patients with marked bone marrow depression, i.e., leukopenia (<2500 WBC) or thrombocytopenia (<100,000), or severe anemia.

WARNINGS

Treatment with hydroxyurea should not be initiated if bone marrow function is markedly depressed (see "**CONTRAINDICATIONS**" section). Bone marrow suppression may occur, and leukopenia is generally its first and most common manifestation. Thrombocytopenia and anemia occur less often, and are seldom seen without a preceding leukopenia. However, the recovery from myelosuppression is rapid when therapy is interrupted. It should be borne in mind that bone marrow depression is more likely in patients who have previously received radiotherapy of cytotoxic cancer chemotherapeutic agents; hydroxyurea should be used cautiously in such patients.

Patients who have received irradiation therapy in the past may have an exacerbation of postirradiation erythema.

Severe anemia must be corrected with whole blood replacement before initiating therapy with hydroxyurea.

Erythrocytic abnormalities: megaloblastic erythropoiesis, which is self-limiting, is often seen early in the course of hydroxyurea therapy. The morphologic change resembles pernicious anemia, but is not related to vitamin B_{12} or folic acid deficiency. Hydroxyurea may also delay plasma iron clearance and reduce the rate of iron utilization by erythrocytes, but it does not appear to alter the red blood cell survival time.

Hydroxyurea should be used with caution in patients with marked renal dysfunction.

Elderly patients may be more sensitive to the effects of hydroxyurea, and may require a lower dose regimen.

Usage in Pregnancy—Drugs which affect DNA synthesis, such as hydroxyurea, may be potential mutagenic agents. The physician should carefully consider this possibility before administering this drug to male or female patients who may contemplate conception.

Hydroxyurea is a known teratogenic agent in animals. Therefore, hydroxyurea should not be used in women who are or may become pregnant unless in the judgment of the physician the potential benefits outweigh the possible hazards.

PRECAUTIONS

Therapy with hydroxyurea requires close supervision. The complete status of the blood, including bone marrow examination, if indicated, as well as kidney function and liver function should be determined prior to, and repeatedly during, treatment. The determination of the hemoglobin level, total leukocyte counts, and platelet counts should be performed at least once a week throughout the course of hydroxyurea therapy. If the white blood cell count decreases to less than 2500/mm³, or the platelet count to less than 100,000/mm³, therapy should be interrupted until the values rise significantly toward normal levels. Anemia, if it occurs, should be managed with whole blood replacement, without interrupting hydroxyurea therapy.

Information for Patients—Patients who take the drug by emptying the contents of the capsule into water (see **DOSAGE AND ADMINISTRATION**) should be reminded that this is a potent medication that must be handled with care. Patients must be cautioned not to allow the powder to come in contact with the skin or mucous membranes, and must be told not to inhale the powder when opening the capsules. If the powder is spilled, it should be immediately wiped up with a damp towel and disposed of, as should the empty capsules. The medication, particularly open capsules, should be kept away from children and pets.

ADVERSE REACTIONS

Adverse reactions have been primarily bone marrow depression (leukopenia, anemia, and occasionally thrombocytopenia), and less frequently gastrointestinal symptoms (stomatitis, anorexia, nausea, vomiting, diarrhea, and constipation), and dermatological reactions such as maculopapular rash, skin ulceration and facial erythema. Dysuria and alopecia occur very rarely. Large doses may produce moderate drowsiness. Neurological disturbances have occurred extremely rarely and were limited to headache, dizziness, disorientation, hallucinations, and convulsions. HYDREA (hydroxyurea capsules, USP) occasionally may cause temporary impairment of renal tubular function accompanied by elevations in serum uric acid, BUN, and creatinine levels. Abnormal BSP retention has been reported. Fever, chills, malaise, and elevation of hepatic enzymes have also been reported.

Adverse reactions observed with combined hydroxyurea and irradiation therapy are similar to those reported with the use of hydroxyurea alone. These effects primarily include bone marrow depression (anemia and leukopenia), and gastric irritation. Almost all patients receiving an adequate course of combined hydroxyurea and irradiation therapy will demonstrate concurrent leukopenia. Platelet depression (<100,000 cells/mm³) has occurred rarely and only in the presence of marked leukopenia. Gastric distress has also been reported with irradiation alone and in combination with hydroxyurea therapy.

It should be borne in mind that therapeutic doses of irradiation alone produce the same adverse reactions as hydroxyurea; combined therapy may cause an increase in the incidence and severity of these side effects.

Although inflammation of the mucous membranes at the irradiated site (mucositis) is attributed to irradiation alone, some investigators believe that the more severe cases are due to combination therapy.

The association of hydroxyurea with the development of acute pulmonary reactions consisting of diffuse pulmonary infiltrates, fever and dyspnea has been rarely reported.

DOSAGE AND ADMINISTRATION

Procedures for proper handling and disposal of antineoplastic drugs should be considered. Several guidelines on this subject have been published.[1-7] There is no general agreement that all of the procedures recommended in the guidelines are necessary or appropriate.

Because of the rarity of melanoma, resistant chronic myelocytic leukemia, carcinoma of the ovary, and carcinomas of the head and neck in children, dosage regimens have not been established.

All dosage should be based on the patient's actual or ideal weight, whichever is less.

NOTE: If the patient prefers, or is unable to swallow capsules, the contents of the capsules may be emptied into a glass of water and taken immediately. (See **PRECAUTIONS**: Information for Patients.) Some inert material used as a vehicle in the capsule may not dissolve, and may float on the surface.

SOLID TUMORS

Intermittent Therapy—80 mg/kg administered orally as a *single* dose every *third* day

Continuous Therapy—20 to 30 mg/kg administered orally as a *single* dose *daily*

The intermittent dosage schedule offers the advantage of reduced toxicity since patients on this dosage regimen have rarely required complete discontinuance of therapy because of toxicity.

Concomitant Therapy with Irradiation *Carcinoma of the head and neck*—80 mg/kg administered orally as a *single* dose every *third* day

Administration of hydroxyurea should be begun at least seven days before initiation of irradiation and continued during radiotherapy as well as indefinitely afterwards provided that the patient may be kept under adequate observation and evidences no unusual or severe reactions.

Irradiation should be given at the maximum dose considered appropriate for the particular therapeutic situation; adjustment of irradiation dosage is not usually necessary when hydroxyurea is used concomitantly.

RESISTANT CHRONIC MYELOCYTIC LEUKEMIA

Until the intermittent therapy regimen has been evaluated, CONTINUOUS therapy (20 to 30 mg/kg administered orally as a *single* dose *daily*) is recommended.

An adequate trial period for determining the antineoplastic effectiveness of hydroxyurea is six weeks of therapy. When there is regression in tumor size or arrest in tumor growth, therapy should be continued indefinitely. Therapy should be interrupted if the white blood cell count drops below 2500/mm³ or the platelet count below 100,000/mm³. In these cases, the counts should be rechecked after three days, and therapy resumed when the counts rise significantly toward normal values. Since the hematopoietic rebound is prompt, it is usually necessary to omit only a few doses. If prompt rebound has not occurred during combined HYDREA (hydroxyurea capsules, USP) and irradiation therapy, irradiation may also be interrupted. However, the need for postponement of irradiation has been rare; radiotherapy has usually been continued using the recommended dosage and technique. Anemia, if it occurs, should be corrected with whole blood replacement, without interrupting hydroxyurea therapy. Because hematopoiesis may be compromised by extensive irradiation or by other antineoplastic agents, it is recommended that hydroxyurea be administered cautiously to patients who have recently received extensive radiation therapy or chemotherapy with other cytotoxic drugs.

Pain or discomfort from inflammation of the mucous membranes at the irradiated site (mucositis) is usually controlled by measures such as topical anesthetics and orally adminis-

Continued on next page

Bristol-Myers Squibb Oncology—Cont.

tered analgesics. If the reaction is severe, hydroxyurea therapy may be temporarily interrupted; if it is extremely severe, irradiation dosage may, in addition, be temporarily postponed. However, it has rarely been necessary to terminate these therapies.
Severe gastric distress, such as nausea, vomiting, and anorexia, resulting from combined therapy may usually be controlled by temporary interruption of hydroxyurea administration; rarely has the additional interruption of irradiation been necessary.

HOW SUPPLIED

HYDREA® (hydroxyurea capsules, USP)
500 mg capsules in bottles of 100 (**NDC** 0003-0830-50).
Capsule identification number: 830.
Storage—Store at room temperature; avoid excessive heat. Keep tightly closed.

REFERENCES

1. Recommendations for the Safe Handling of Parenteral Antineoplastic Drugs. NIH Publication No. 83-2621. For sale by the Superintendent of Documents, US Government Printing Office, Washington, DC 20402.
2. AMA Council Report. Guidelines for Handling Parenteral Antineoplastics. JAMA 1985; 253(11):1590-1592.
3. National Study Commission on Cytotoxic Exposure - Recommendations for Handling Cytotoxic Agents. Available from Louis P. Jeffrey, ScD, Chairman, National Study Commission on Cytotoxic Exposure, Massachusetts College of Pharmacy and Allied Health Sciences, 179 Longwood Avenue, Boston, MA 02115.
4. Clinical Oncological Society of Australia. Guidelines and Recommendations for Safe Handling of Antineoplastic Agents. Med J Australia 1983; 1:426-428.
5. Jones RB, et al. Safe Handling of Chemotherapeutic Agents: A Report from the Mount Sinai Medical Center, CA-A Cancer Journal for Clinicians 1983; (Sept/Oct) 258-263.
6. American Society of Hospital Pharmacists Technical Assistance Bulletin on Handling Cytotoxic and Hazardous Drugs. Am J Hosp Pharm 1990; 47:1033-1049.
7. OSHA Work-Practice Guidelines for Personnel Dealing with Cytotoxic (Antineoplastic) Drugs. Am J Hosp Pharm 1986; 43:1193-1204.

BRISTOL LABORATORIES
ONCOLOGY PRODUCTS
A Bristol-Myers Squibb Company
Princeton, NJ 08543
U.S.A.
K8-B001-5-96 P9281-02
Revised: March 1996

IFEX® ℞
(sterile ifosfamide)

CAUTION: FEDERAL LAW PROHIBITS DISPENSING WITHOUT PRESCRIPTION.

> **WARNING**
> IFEX® (sterile ifosfamide) should be administered under the supervision of a qualified physician experienced in the use of cancer chemotherapeutic agents. Urotoxic side effects, especially hemorrhagic cystitis, as well as CNS toxicities such as confusion and coma have been associated with the use of IFEX. When they occur, they may require cessation of IFEX therapy. Severe myelosuppression has been reported. (See "**ADVERSE REACTIONS**" section.)

DESCRIPTION

IFEX® (sterile ifosfamide) single-dose vials for constitution and administration by intravenous infusion each contain 1 gram or 3 grams of sterile ifosfamide. Ifosfamide is a chemotherapeutic agent chemically related to the nitrogen mustards and a synthetic analog of cyclophosphamide. Ifosfamide is 3-(2-chloroethyl)-2-[(2-chloroethyl)amino]tetrahydro-2H-1,3,2-oxazaphosphorine 2-oxide. The molecular formula is $C_7H_{15}Cl_2N_2O_2P$ and its molecular weight is 261.1. Its structural formula is:

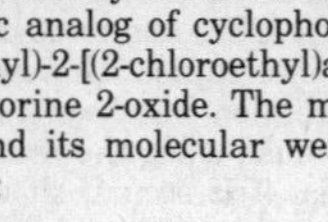

Ifosfamide is a white crystalline powder that is soluble in water.

CLINICAL PHARMACOLOGY

Ifosfamide has been shown to require metabolic activation by microsomal liver enzymes to produce biologically active metabolites. Activation occurs by hydroxylation at the ring carbon atom 4 to form the unstable intermediate 4-hydroxyifosfamide. This metabolite rapidly degrades to the stable urinary metabolite, 4-ketoifosfamide. Opening of the ring results in formation of the stable urinary metabolite, 4-carboxyifosfamide. These urinary metabolites have not been found to be cytotoxic. N, N-*bis* (2-chloroethyl)-phosphoric acid diamide (ifosphoramide) and acrolein are also found. Enzymatic oxidation of the chloroethyl side chains and subsequent dealkylation produces the major urinary metabolites, dechloroethyl ifosfamide and dechloroethyl cyclophosphamide. The alkylated metabolites of ifosfamide have been shown to interact with DNA.
In vitro incubation of DNA with activated ifosfamide has produced phosphotriesters. The treatment of intact cell nuclei may also result in the formation of DNA-DNA cross-links. DNA repair most likely occurs in G-1 and G-2 stage cells.
Pharmacokinetics: Ifosfamide exhibits dose-dependent pharmacokinetics in humans. At single doses of 3.8-5.0 g/m^2, the plasma concentrations decay biphasically and the mean terminal elimination half-life is about 15 hours. At doses of 1.6-2.4 g/m^2/day, the plasma decay is monoexponential and the terminal elimination half-life is about 7 hours. Ifosfamide is extensively metabolized in humans and the metabolic pathways appear to be saturated at high doses.
After administration of doses of 5 g/m^2 of ^{14}C-labeled ifosfamide, from 70 to 86% of the dosed radioactivity was recovered in the urine, with about 61% of the dose excreted as parent compound. At doses of 1.6-2.4 g/m^2 only 12 to 18% of the dose was excreted in the urine as unchanged drug within 72 hours.
Two different dechloroethylated derivatives of ifosfamide, 4-carboxyifosfamide, thiodiacetic acid and cysteine conjugates of chloroacetic acid have been identified as the major urinary metabolites of ifosfamide in humans and only small amounts of 4-hydroxyifosfamide and acrolein are present. Small quantities (nmole/mL) of ifosfamide mustard and 4-hydroxyifosfamide are detectable in human plasma. Metabolism of ifosfamide is required for the generation of the biologically active species and while metabolism is extensive, it is also quite variable among patients.
In a study at Indiana University, 50 fully evaluable patients with germ cell testicular cancer were treated with IFEX in combination with cisplatin and either vinblastine or etoposide after failing (47 of 50 patients) at least two prior chemotherapy regimens consisting of cisplatin/vinblastine/bleomycin, (PVB), cisplatin/vinblastine/actinomycin D/bleomycin/cyclophosphamide, (VAB6), or the combination of cisplatin and etoposide. Patients were selected for remaining cisplatin sensitivity because they had previously responded to a cisplatin containing regimen and had not progressed while on the cisplatin containing regimen or within 3 weeks of stopping it. Patients served as their own control based on the premise that long term complete responses could not be achieved by retreatment with a regimen to which they had previously responded and subsequently relapsed.
Ten of 50 fully evaluable patients were still alive 2 to 5 years after treatment. Four of the 10 long term survivors were rendered free of cancer by surgical resection after treatment with the ifosfamide regimen; median survival for the entire group of 50 fully evaluable patients was 53 weeks.

INDICATION AND USAGE

IFEX, used in combination with certain other approved antineoplastic agents, is indicated for third line chemotherapy of germ cell testicular cancer. It should ordinarily be used in combination with a prophylactic agent for hemorrhagic cystitis, such as mesna.

CONTRAINDICATIONS

Continued use of IFEX is contraindicated in patients with severely depressed bone marrow function (See "**WARNINGS**" and "**PRECAUTIONS**" sections.) IFEX is also contraindicated in patients who have demonstrated a previous hypersensitivity to it.

WARNINGS

Urinary System: Urotoxic side effects, especially hemorrhagic cystitis, have been frequently associated with the use of IFEX. It is recommended that a urinalysis should be obtained prior to each dose of IFEX (sterile ifosfamide). If microscopic hematuria (greater than 10 RBCs per high power field), is present, then subsequent administration should be withheld until complete resolution.
Further administration of IFEX should be given with vigorous oral or parenteral hydration.
Hematopoietic System: When IFEX is given in combination with other chemotherapeutic agents, severe myelosuppression is frequently observed. Close hematologic monitoring is recommended. White blood cell (WBC) count, platelet count and hemoglobin should be obtained prior to each administration and at appropriate intervals. Unless clinically essential, IFEX should not be given to patients with a WBC count below 2000/μL and/or a platelet count below 50,000/μL.
Central Nervous System: Neurologic manifestations consisting of somnolence, confusion, hallucinations and in some instances, coma, have been reported following IFEX therapy. The occurrence of these symptoms requires discontinuing IFEX therapy. The symptoms have usually been reversible and supportive therapy should be maintained until their complete resolution.
Pregnancy: Animal studies indicate that the drug is capable of causing gene mutations and chromosomal damage *in vivo*. Embryotoxic and teratogenic effects have been observed in mice, rats and rabbits at doses 0.05 to 0.075 times the human dose. Ifosfamide can cause fetal damage when administered to a pregnant woman. If IFEX is used during pregnancy, or if the patient becomes pregnant while taking this drug, the patient should be apprised of the potential hazard to the fetus.

PRECAUTIONS

General: IFEX should be given cautiously to patients with impaired renal function as well as to those with compromised bone marrow reserve, as indicated by: leukopenia, granulocytopenia, extensive bone marrow metastases, prior radiation therapy, or prior therapy with other cytotoxic agents.
Laboratory Tests: During treatment, the patient's hematologic profile (particularly neutrophils and platelets) should be monitored regularly to determine the degree of hematopoietic suppression. Urine should also be examined regularly for red cells which may precede hemorrhagic cystitis.
Drug Interactions: The physician should be alert for possible combined drug actions, desirable or undesirable, involving ifosfamide even though ifosfamide has been used successfully concurrently with other drugs, including other cytotoxic drugs.
Wound Healing: Ifosfamide may interfere with normal wound healing.
Pregnancy: Pregnancy "Category D". (See "WARNINGS" section.)
Nursing Mothers: Ifosfamide is excreted in breast milk. Because of the potential for serious adverse events and the tumorigenicity shown for ifosfamide in animal studies, a decision should be made whether to discontinue nursing or to discontinue the drug, taking into account the importance of the drug to the mother.
Carcinogenesis, Mutagenesis, Impairment of Fertility: Ifosfamide has been shown to be carcinogenic in rats, with female rats showing a significant incidence of leiomyosarcomas and mammary fibroadenomas.
The mutagenic potential of ifosfamide has been documented in bacterial systems *in vitro* and mammalian cells *in vivo. In vivo*, ifosfamide has induced mutagenic effects in mice and *Drosophila melanogaster* germ cells, and has induced a significant increase in dominant lethal mutations in male mice as well as recessive sex-linked lethal mutations in *Drosophila.*
In pregnant mice, resorptions increased and anomalies were present at day 19 after a 30 mg/m^2 dose of ifosfamide was administered on day 11 of gestation. Embryolethal effects were observed in rats following the administration of 54 mg/m^2 doses of ifosfamide from the 6th through the 15th day of gestation and embryotoxic effects were apparent after dams received 18 mg/m^2 doses over the same dosing period. Ifosfamide is embryotoxic to rabbits receiving 88 mg/m^2/day doses from the 6th through the 18th day after mating. The number of anomalies was also significantly increased over the control group.
Pediatric Use: Safety and effectiveness in pediatric patients have not been established.

ADVERSE REACTIONS

In patients receiving IFEX as a single agent, the dose-limiting toxicities are myelosuppression and urotoxicity. Dose fractionation, vigorous hydration, and a protector such as mesna can significantly reduce the incidence of hematuria, especially gross hematuria, associated with hemorrhagic cystitis. At a dose of 1.2 g/m^2 daily for 5 consecutive days, leukopenia, when it occurs, is usually mild to moderate. Other significant side effects include alopecia, nausea, vomiting, and central nervous system toxicities.

Adverse Reaction	*Incidence %
Alopecia	83
Nausea-Vomiting	58
Hematuria	46
Gross Hematuria	12
CNS Toxicity	12
Infection	8
Renal Impairment	6
Liver Dysfunction	3
Phlebitis	2
Fever	1
Allergic Reaction	<1
Anorexia	<1
Cardiotoxicity	<1
Coagulopathy	<1
Constipation	<1

Dermatitis	<1
Diarrhea	<1
Fatigue	<1
Hypertension	<1
Hypotension	<1
Malaise	<1
Polyneuropathy	<1
Pulmonary Symptoms	<1
Salivation	<1
Stomatitis	<1

*Based upon 2,070 patients from the published literature in 30 single agent studies.

Hematologic Toxicity: Myelosuppression was dose related and dose limiting. It consisted mainly of leukopenia and, to a lesser extent, thrombocytopenia. A WBC count < 3000/μL is expected in 50% of the patients treated with IFEX single agent at doses of 1.2 g/m^2 per day for 5 consecutive days. At this dose level, thrombocytopenia (platelets < 100,000/μL) occurred in about 20% of the patients. At higher dosages, leukopenia was almost universal, and at total dosages of 10-12 g/m^2/cycle, one half of the patients had a WBC count below 1000/μL and 8% of patients had platelet counts less than 50,000/μL. Myelosuppression was usually reversible and treatment can be given every 3 to 4 weeks. When IFEX is used in combination with other myelosuppressive agents, adjustments in dosing may be necessary. Patients who experience severe myelosuppression are potentially at increased risk for infection.

Digestive System: Nausea and vomiting occurred in 58% of the patients who received IFEX (sterile ifosfamide). They were usually controlled by standard antiemetic therapy. Other gastrointestinal side effects include anorexia, diarrhea, and in some cases, constipation.

Urinary System: Urotoxicity consisted of hemorrhagic cystitis, dysuria, urinary frequency and other symptoms of bladder irritation. Hematuria occurred in 6% to 92% of patients treated with IFEX. The incidence and severity of hematuria can be significantly reduced by using vigorous hydration, a fractionated dose schedule and a protector such as mesna. At daily doses of 1.2 g/m^2 for 5 consecutive days without a protector, microscopic hematuria is expected in about one half of the patients and gross hematuria in about 8% of patients.

Renal toxicity occurred in 6% of the patients treated with ifosfamide as a single agent. Clinical signs, such as elevation in BUN or serum creatinine or decrease in creatinine clearance, were usually transient. They were most likely to be related to tubular damage. One episode of renal tubular acidosis which progressed into chronic renal failure was reported. Proteinuria and acidosis also occurred in rare instances. Metabolic acidosis was reported in 31% of patients in one study when IFEX was administered at doses of 2.0 to 2.5 g/m^2/day for 4 days. Renal tubular acidosis, Fanconi syndrome and renal rickets have been reported. Close clinical monitoring of serum and urine chemistries including phosphorus, potassium, alkaline phosphatase and other appropriate laboratory studies is recommended. Appropriate replacement therapy should be administered as indicated.

Central Nervous System: CNS side effects were observed in 12% of patients treated with IFEX. Those most commonly seen were somnolence, confusion, depressive psychosis, and hallucinations. Other less frequent symptoms include dizziness, disorientation, and cranial nerve dysfunction. Seizures and coma with death were occasionally reported. The incidence of CNS toxicity may be higher in patients with altered renal function.

Other: Alopecia occurred in approximately 83% of the patients treated with IFEX as a single agent. In combination, this incidence may be as high as 100%, depending on the other agents included in the chemotherapy regimen. Increases in liver enzymes and/or bilirubin were noted in 3% of the patients. Other less frequent side effects included phlebitis, pulmonary symptoms, fever of unknown origin, allergic reactions, stomatitis, cardiotoxicity, and polyneuropathy.

OVERDOSAGE

No specific antidote for IFEX is known. Management of overdosage would include general supportive measures to sustain the patient through any period of toxicity that might occur.

DOSAGE AND ADMINISTRATION

IFEX should be administered intravenously at a dose of 1.2 g/m^2 per day for 5 consecutive days. Treatment is repeated every 3 weeks or after recovery from hematologic toxicity (Platelets ≥ 100,000/μL, WBC ≥ 4,000/μL). In order to prevent bladder toxicity, IFEX should be given with extensive hydration consisting of at least 2 liters of oral or intravenous fluid per day. A protector, such as mesna, should also be used to prevent hemorrhagic cystitis. IFEX should be administered as a slow intravenous infusion lasting a minimum of 30 minutes. Although IFEX has been administered to a small number of patients with compromised hepatic and/or renal function, studies to establish optimal dose schedules of IFEX in such patients have not been conducted.

Preparation for Intravenous Administration/Stability: Injections are prepared for parenteral use by adding *Sterile Water for Injection, USP*, or *Bacteriostatic Water for Injection, USP* (benzyl alcohol or parabens preserved), to the vial and shaking to dissolve. Use the quantity of diluent shown below to constitute the product:

Dosage Strength	Quantity of Diluent	Final Concentration
1 gram	20 mL	50 mg/mL
3 grams	60 mL	50 mg/mL

Solutions of ifosfamide may be diluted further to achieve concentrations of 0.6 to 20 mg/mL in the following fluids:

5% Dextrose Injection, USP
0.9% Sodium Chloride Injection, USP
Lactated Ringer's Injection, USP
Sterile Water for Injection, USP

Because essentially identical stability results were obtained for Sterile Water admixtures as for the other admixtures (5% Dextrose Injection, 0.9% Sodium Chloride Injection, and Lactated Ringer's Injection), the use of large volume parenteral glass bottles, Viaflex bags or PAB™ bags that contain intermediate concentrations or mixtures of excipients (eg, 2.5% Dextrose Injection, 0.45% Sodium Chloride Injection, or 5% Dextrose and 0.9% Sodium Chloride Injection) is also acceptable.

Constituted or constituted and further diluted solutions of IFEX should be refrigerated and used within 24 hours.

Parenteral drug products should be inspected visually for particulate matter and discoloration prior to administration.

HOW SUPPLIED

IFEX is only available in combination packages with the uroprotective agent MESNEX® (mesna) Injection.

IFEX® (sterile ifosfamide)/MESNEX® (mesna) Injection.

NDC 0015-3556-26 —5 × 1-gram Single Dose Vial of IFEX
—3 × 1-gram Multidose Vial of MESNEX

NDC 0015-3554-27 —10 × 1-gram Single Dose Vial of IFEX
—10 × 1-gram Multidose Vial of MESNEX

NDC 0015-3564-15 —2 × 3-gram Single Dose Vial of IFEX
—6 × 1-gram Multidose Vial of MESNEX

Store at controlled room temperature 15°C to 30°C.

Procedures for proper handling and disposal of anticancer drugs should be considered. Skin reactions associated with accidental exposure to IFEX may occur. The use of gloves is recommended. If IFEX solution contacts the skin or mucosa, immediately wash the skin thoroughly with soap and water or rinse the mucosa with copious amounts of water. Several guidelines on this subject have been published.[1-7] There is no general agreement that all of the procedures recommended in the guidelines are necessary or appropriate.

REFERENCES

1. Recommendations for the Safe Handling of Parenteral Antineoplastic Drugs. NIH Publication No. 83-2621. For sale by the Superintendent of Documents, US Government Printing Office, Washington, DC 20402.
2. AMA Council Report. Guidelines for Handling Parenteral Antineoplastics. JAMA 1985; 253 (11):1590-1592.
3. National Study Commission on Cytotoxic Exposure–Recommendations for Handling Cytotoxic Agents. Available from Louis P. Jeffrey, ScD, Chairman, National Study Commission on Cytotoxic Exposure, Massachusetts College of Pharmacy and Allied Health Sciences, 179 Longwood Avenue, Boston, Massachusetts 02115.
4. Clinical Oncological Society of Australia. Guidelines and Recommendations for Safe Handling of Antineoplastic Agents. Med J Australia 1983; 1:426–428.
5. Jones, RB, et al: Safe Handling of Chemotherapeutic Agents: A Report from the Mount Sinai Medical Center. CA-A Cancer Journal for Clinicians 1983; (Sept/Oct) 258–263.
6. American Society of Hospital Pharmacists Technical Assistance Bulletin on Handling Cytotoxic and Hazardous Drugs. Am J Hosp Pharm 1990; 47:1033–1049.
7. OSHA Work-Practice Guidelines for Personnel Dealing with Cytotoxic (Antineoplastic) Drugs. Am J Hosp Pharm 1986; 43:1193–1204.

MeadJohnson
ONCOLOGY PRODUCTS
A Bristol-Myers Squibb Company
Princeton, NJ 08543
U.S.A.

H5-B001-8-95 P7435-00
Revised: August 1995

Shown in Product Identification Guide, page 307

LYSODREN®

(mitotane tablets, USP) ℞

Caution: Federal Law Prohibits Dispensing Without Prescription.

DESCRIPTION

WARNINGS
LYSODREN® (mitotane tablets, USP) should be administered under the supervision of a qualified physician experienced in the uses of cancer chemotherapeutic agents. LYSODREN should be temporarily discontinued immediately following shock or severe trauma since adrenal suppression is its prime action. Exogenous steroids should be administered in such circumstances, since the depressed adrenal may not immediately start to secrete steroids.

LYSODREN® (mitotane tablets, USP) is an oral chemotherapeutic agent. It is best known by its trivial name, o,p'-DDD, and is chemically, 1,1-dichloro-2-(o-chlorophenyl)-2-(p-chlorophenyl) ethane. The chemical structure is shown below.

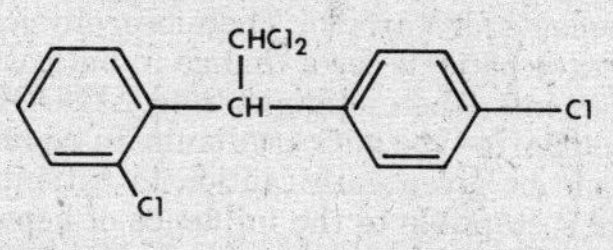

LYSODREN is a white granular solid composed of clear colorless crystals. It is tasteless and has a slight pleasant aromatic odor. It is soluble in ethanol, isoctane and carbon tetrachloride. It has a molecular weight of 320.05.

Inactive ingredients in LYSODREN tablets are: avicel, Polyethylene Glycol 3350, silicon dioxide, and starch.

LYSODREN is available as 500 mg scored tablets for oral administration.

CLINICAL PHARMACOLOGY

LYSODREN can best be described as an adrenal cytotoxic agent, although it can cause adrenal inhibition, apparently without cellular destruction. Its biochemical mechanism of action is unknown. Data are available to suggest that the drug modifies the peripheral metabolism of steroids as well as directly suppressing the adrenal cortex. The administration of LYSODREN alters the extra-adrenal metabolism of cortisol in man; leading to a reduction in measurable 17-hydroxy corticosteroids, even though plasma levels of corticosteroids do not fall. The drug apparently causes increased formation of 6-B-hydroxyl cortisol.

Data in adrenal carcinoma patients indicate that about 40% of oral LYSODREN is absorbed and approximately 10% of administered dose is recovered in the urine as water-soluble metabolite. A variable amount of metabolite (1 to 17%) is excreted in the bile and the balance is apparently stored in the tissues.

Following discontinuation of LYSODREN, the plasma terminal half life has ranged from 18 to 159 days. In most patients blood levels become undetectable after 6 to 9 weeks. Autopsy data have provided evidence that LYSODREN is found in most tissues of the body; however, fat tissues are the primary site of storage. LYSODREN is converted to a water-soluble metabolite.

No unchanged LYSODREN has been found in urine or bile.

INDICATIONS AND USAGE

LYSODREN is indicated in the treatment of inoperable adrenal cortical carcinoma of both functional and nonfunctional types.

CONTRAINDICATIONS

LYSODREN should not be given to individuals who have demonstrated a previous hypersensitivity to it.

WARNINGS

LYSODREN should be temporarily discontinued immediately following shock or severe trauma, since adrenal suppression is its prime action. Exogenous steroids should be administered in such circumstances, since the depressed adrenal may not immediately start to secrete steroids.

LYSODREN should be administered with care to patients with liver disease other than metastatic lesions from the adrenal cortex, since the metabolism of LYSODREN may be interfered with and the drug may accumulate.

All possible tumor tissues should be surgically removed from large metastatic masses before LYSODREN administration is instituted. This is necessary to minimize the possibility of infarction and hemorrhage in the tumor due to a rapid cytotoxic effect of the drug.

Long-term continuous administration of high doses of LYSODREN may lead to brain damage and impairment of function. Behavioral and neurological assessments should be made at regular intervals when continuous LYSODREN (mitotane tablets, USP) treatment exceeds 2 years.

Continued on next page

Bristol-Myers Squibb Oncology—Cont.

A substantial percentage of the patients treated show signs of adrenal insufficiency. It therefore appears necessary to watch for and institute steroid replacement in those patients. However, some investigators have recommended that steroid replacement therapy be administered concomitantly with LYSODREN. It has been shown that the metabolism of exogenous steroids is modified and consequently somewhat higher doses than normal replacement therapy may be required.

PRECAUTIONS

General: Adrenal insufficiency may develop in patients treated with LYSODREN, and adrenal steroid replacement should be considered for these patients.

Since sedation, lethargy, vertigo, and other CNS side effects can occur, ambulatory patients should be cautioned about driving, operating machinery, and other hazardous pursuits requiring mental and physical alertness.

Drug Interactions: LYSODREN has been reported to accelerate the metabolism of warfarin by the mechanism of hepatic microsomal enzyme induction, leading to an increase in dosage requirements for warfarin. Therefore, physicians should closely monitor patients for a change in anticoagulant dosage requirements when administering LYSODREN to patients on coumarin-type anticoagulants. In addition, LYSODREN should be given with caution to patients receiving other drugs susceptible to the influence of hepatic enzyme induction.

Carcinogenesis, Mutagenesis, Impairment of Fertility: The carcinogenic and mutagenic potentials of LYSODREN are unknown. However, the mechanism of action of this compound suggests that it probably has less carcinogenic potential than other cytotoxic chemotherapeutic drugs.

Pregnancy: Pregnancy "Category C". Animal reproduction studies have not been conducted with LYSODREN. It is also not known whether LYSODREN can cause fetal harm when administered to a pregnant woman or can affect reproduction capacity. LYSODREN should be given to a pregnant woman only if clearly needed.

Nursing Mothers: It is not known whether this drug is excreted in human milk. Because many drugs are excreted in human milk and because of the potential for adverse reactions in nursing infants from mitotane, a decision should be made whether to discontinue nursing or to discontinue the drug, taking into account the importance of the drug to the mother.

ADVERSE REACTIONS

A very high percentage of patients treated with LYSODREN has shown at least one type of side effect. The main types of adverse reactions consist of the following:

1. Gastrointestinal disturbances, which consist of anorexia, nausea or vomiting, and in some cases diarrhea, occur in about 80% of the patients.
2. Central nervous system side effects occur in 40% of the patients. These consist primarily of depression as manifested by lethargy and somnolence (25%), and dizziness or vertigo (15%).
3. Skin toxicity has been observed in about 15% of the cases. These skin changes consist primarily of transient skin rashes which do not seem to be dose related. In some instances, this side effect subsided while the patients were maintained on the drug without a change of dose.

Infrequently occurring side effects involve the eye (visual blurring, diplopia, lens opacity, toxic retinopathy); the genitourinary system (hematuria, hemorrhagic cystitis, and albuminuria); cardiovascular system (hypertension, orthostatic hypotension, and flushing); and some miscellaneous effects including generalized aching, hyperpyrexia, and lowered protein bound iodine (PBI).

OVERDOSAGE

No proven antidotes have been established for LYSODREN overdosage.

DOSAGE AND ADMINISTRATION

The recommended treatment schedule is to start the patient at 2 to 6 g of LYSODREN per day in divided doses, either three or four times a day. Doses are usually increased incrementally to 9 to 10 g per day. If severe side effects appear, the dose should be reduced until the maximum tolerated dose is achieved. If the patient can tolerate higher doses and improved clinical response appears possible, the dose should be increased until adverse reactions interfere. Experience has shown that the maximum tolerated dose (MTD) will vary from 2 to 16 g per day, but has usually been 9 to 10 g per day. The highest doses used in the studies to date were 18 to 19 g per day.

Treatment should be instituted in the hospital until a stable dosage regimen is achieved.

Treatment should be continued as long as clinical benefits are observed. Maintenance of clinical status or slowing of growth of metastatic lesions can be considered clinical benefits if they can clearly be shown to have occurred.

If no clinical benefits are observed after 3 months at the maximum tolerated dose, the case would generally be considered a clinical failure. However, 10% of the patients who showed a measurable response required more than 3 months at the MTD. Early diagnosis and prompt institution of treatment improve the probability of a positive clinical response. Clinical effectiveness can be shown by reduction in tumor mass; reduction in pain, weakness or anorexia; and reduction of symptoms and signs due to excessive steroid production.

A number of patients have been treated intermittently with treatment being restarted when severe symptoms have reappeared. Patients often do not respond after the third or fourth such course. Experience accumulated to date suggests that continuous treatment with the maximum possible dosage of LYSODREN (mitotane tablets, USP) is the best approach.

Procedures for proper handling and disposal of anticancer drugs should be considered. Several guidelines on this subject have been published.[1–7] There is no general agreement that all of the procedures recommended in the guidelines are necessary or appropriate.

HOW SUPPLIED

LYSODREN® (mitotane tablets, USP)

NDC 0015-3080-60–500 mg Tablets, bottle of 100

Tablets may be stored at room temperature.

REFERENCES

1. Recommendations for the Safe Handling of Parenteral Antineoplastic Drugs. NIH Publication No. 83-2621. For sale by the Superintendent of Documents, US Government Printing Office, Washington, DC 20402.
2. AMA Council Report. Guidelines for Handling Parenteral Antineoplastics. JAMA 1985; March 15.
3. National Study Commission on Cytotoxic Exposure–Recommendations for Handling Cytotoxic Agents. Available from Louis P. Jeffrey, ScD, Chairman, National Study Commission on Cytotoxic Exposure, Massachusetts College of Pharmacy and Allied Health Sciences, 179 Longwood Avenue, Boston, Massachusetts 02115.
4. Clinical Oncological Society of Australia. Guidelines and Recommendations for Safe Handling of Antineoplastic Agents. Med J Australia 1983; 1:426-428.
5. Jones, R B, et al: Safe Handling of Chemotherapeutic Agents: A Report from the Mount Sinai Medical Center. CA–A Cancer Journal for Clinicians 1983; (Sept/Oct) 258-263.
6. American Society of Hospital Pharmacists Technical Assistance Bulletin on Handling Cytotoxic Drugs in Hospitals. Am J Hosp Pharm 1985; 42:131-137.
7. OSHA Work-Practice Guidelines for Personnel Dealing with Cytotoxic (Antineoplastic) Drugs. Am J Hosp Pharm 1986; 43:1193-1204.

Manufactured by: Anabolic, Inc.
Irvine, California 92714

Distributed by:
BRISTOL LABORATORIES
ONCOLOGY PRODUCTS
A Bristol-Myers Squibb Company
Princeton, NJ 08543
U.S.A.

H6-B001-5-96 P5260-06

Revised February 1994

MEGACE® ORAL SUSPENSION ℞

[mĕg 'ace]
(megestrol acetate)

> **WARNING**
>
> THE USE OF MEGACE® (megestrol acetate) Oral Suspension IS CONTRAINDICATED IN PREGNANCY.
>
> Progestational agents have been used beginning with the first trimester of pregnancy in an attempt to prevent habitual abortion. There is no evidence that the use of a high dose progestational agent such as MEGACE Oral Suspension during any phase of pregnancy is effective for this purpose. Furthermore, in the vast majority of women, the cause of abortion is a defective ovum, which progestational agents could not be expected to influence. In addition, the use of progestational agents, with their uterine-relaxant properties, in patients with fertilized defective ova may cause a delay in spontaneous abortion.
>
> Several reports suggest an association between intrauterine exposure to progestational drugs in the first trimester of pregnancy and genital abnormalities in male and female fetuses. The risk of hypospadias, 5 to 8 per 1,000 male births in the general population, may be approximately doubled with exposure to these drugs. There are insufficient data to quantify the risk to exposed female fetuses. Because of increased genital abnormalities in male and female fetuses induced by some progestational drugs, it is prudent to avoid the use of MEGACE Oral Suspension during pregnancy.
>
> If the patient is exposed to MEGACE Oral Suspension during pregnancy or if she becomes pregnant while taking this drug, she should be apprised of the potential risks to the fetus.

DESCRIPTION

MEGACE® (megestrol acetate) Oral Suspension contains megestrol acetate, a synthetic derivative of the naturally occurring steroid hormone, progesterone. Megestrol acetate is a white, crystalline solid chemically designated as 17 α-(acetyloxy)-6-methylpregna-4,6-diene-3,20-dione. Solubility at 37°C in water is 2 μg per mL, solubility in plasma is 24 μg per mL. Its molecular weight is 384.51. The empirical formula is $C_{24}H_{32}O_4$ and the structural formula is represented as follows:

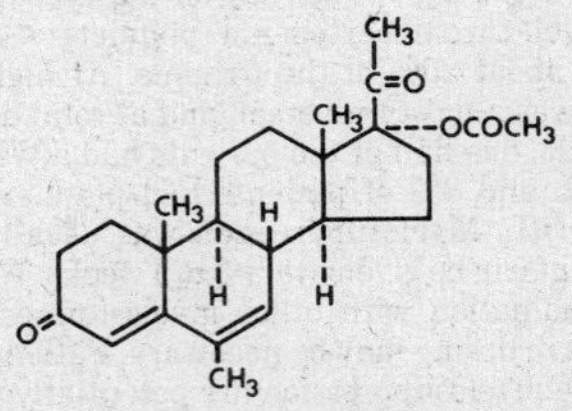

MEGACE Oral Suspension is supplied as an oral suspension containing 40 mg of micronized megestrol acetate per mL.

MEGACE Oral Suspension contains the following inactive ingredients: alcohol (max. 0.06% v/v from flavor), citric acid, lemon-lime flavor, polyethylene glycol, polysorbate 80, purified water, sodium benzoate, sodium citrate, sucrose and xanthan gum.

CLINICAL PHARMACOLOGY

Several investigators have reported on the appetite enhancing property of megestrol acetate and its possible use in cachexia. The precise mechanism by which megestrol acetate produces effects in anorexia and cachexia is unknown at the present time.

There are several analytical methods used to estimate megestrol acetate plasma concentrations, including gas chromatography-mass fragmentography (GC-MF), high pressure liquid chromatography (HPLC) and radioimmunoassay (RIA). The GC-MF and HPLC methods are specific for megestrol acetate and yield equivalent concentrations. The RIA method reacts to megestrol acetate metabolites and is, therefore, non-specific and indicates higher concentrations than the GC-MF and HPLC methods. Plasma concentrations are dependent, not only on the method used, but also on intestinal and hepatic inactivation of the drug, which may be affected by factors such as intestinal tract motility, intestinal bacteria, antibiotics administered, body weight, diet and liver function.

The major route of drug elimination in humans is urine. When radiolabeled megestrol acetate was administered to humans in doses of 4 to 90 mg, the urinary excretion within 10 days ranged from 56.5% to 78.4% (mean 66.4%) and fecal excretion ranged from 7.7% to 30.3% (mean 19.8%). The total recovered radioactivity varied between 83.1% and 94.7% (mean 86.2%). Megestrol acetate metabolites which were identified in urine constituted 5% to 8% of the dose administered. Respiratory excretion as labeled carbon dioxide and fat storage may have accounted for at least part of the radioactivity not found in urine and feces.

Plasma steady state pharmacokinetics of megestrol acetate were evaluated in 10 adult, cachectic male patients with acquired immunodeficiency syndrome (AIDS) and an involuntary weight loss greater than 10% of baseline. Patients received single oral doses of 800 mg/day of MEGACE (megestrol acetate) Oral Suspension for 21 days. Plasma concentration data obtained on day 21 were evaluated for up to 48 hours past the last dose.

Mean (±1SD) peak plasma concentration (C_{max}) of megestrol acetate was 753 (±539) ng/mL. Mean area under the concentration time-curve (AUC) was 10476 (±7788) ng × hr/mL. Median TMAX value was five hours. Seven of 10 patients gained weight in three weeks.

Additionally, 24 adult, asymptomatic HIV seropositive male subjects were dosed once daily with 750 mg of MEGACE Oral Suspension. The treatment was administered for 14 days. Mean C_{max} and AUC values 490 (±238) ng/mL and 6779 (±3048) hr × ng/mL respectively. The median TMAX value was three hours. The mean C_{min} value was 202 (±101) ng/mL. The mean %FL value was 107 (±40).

The relative bioavailability of MEGACE (megestrol acetate tablets, USP) 40 mg tablets and MEGACE Oral Suspension has not been evaluated. The effect of food on the bioavailability of MEGACE Oral Suspension has not been evaluated.

DESCRIPTION OF CLINICAL STUDIES

The clinical efficacy of MEGACE Oral Suspension was assessed in two clinical trials. One was a multicenter, random-

ized, double-blind, placebo-controlled study comparing megestrol acetate (MA) at doses of 100 mg, 400 mg, and 800 mg per day versus placebo in AIDS patients with anorexia/cachexia and significant weight loss. Of the 270 patients entered on study, 195 met all inclusion/exclusion criteria, had at least two additional post baseline weight measurements over a 12 week period or had one post baseline weight measurement but dropped out for therapeutic failure. The percent of patients gaining five or more pounds at maximum weight gain in 12 study weeks was statistically significantly greater for the 800 mg (64%) and 400 mg (57%) MA-treated groups than for the placebo group (24%). Mean weight increased from baseline to last evaluation in 12 study weeks in the 800 mg MA-treated group by 7.8 pounds, the 400 mg MA group by 4.2 pounds, the 100 mg MA group by 1.9 pounds, and decreased in the placebo group by 1.6 pounds. Mean weight changes at 4, 8 and 12 weeks for patients evaluable for efficacy in the two clinical trials are shown graphically. Changes in body composition during the 12 study weeks as measured by bioelectrical impedance analysis showed increases in non-water body weight in the MA-treated groups (See "CLINICAL STUDIES" Table). In addition, edema developed or worsened in only 3 patients.

Greater percentages of MA-treated patients in the 800 mg group (89%), the 400 mg group (68%) and the 100 mg group (72%), than in the placebo group (50%), showed an improvement in appetite at last evaluation during the 12 study weeks. A statistically significant difference was observed between the 800 mg MA-treated group and the placebo group in the change in caloric intake from baseline to time of maximum weight change. Patients were asked to assess weight change, appetite, appearance, and overall perception of well-being in 9 question survey. At maximum weight change only the 800 mg MA-treated group gave responses that were statistically significantly more favorable to all questions when compared to the placebo-treated group. A dose response was noted in the survey with positive responses correlating with higher dose for all questions.

The second trial was a multicenter, randomized, double-blind, placebo-controlled study comparing megestrol acetate 800 mg/day versus placebo in AIDS patients with anorexia/cachexia and significant weight loss. Of the 100 patients entered on study, 65 met all inclusion/exclusion criteria, had at least two additional post baseline weight measurements over a 12 week period or had one post baseline weight measurement but dropped out for therapeutic failure. Patients in the 800 mg MA-treated group had a statistically significantly larger increase in mean maximum weight change than patients in the placebo group. From baseline to study week 12, mean weight increased by 11.2 pounds in the MA-treated group and decreased 21 pounds in the placebo group. Changes in body composition as measured by bioelectrical impedance analysis showed increases in non-water weight in the MA-treated group (See "CLINICAL STUDIES" Table). No edema was reported in the MA-treated group. A greater percentage of MA-treated patients (67%) than placebo-treated patients (38%) showed an improvement in appetite at last evaluation during the 12 study weeks; this difference was statistically significant. There were no statistically significant differences between treatment groups in mean caloric change or in daily caloric intake at time to maximum weight change. In the same 9 question survey referenced in the first trial, patients' assessments of weight change, appetite, appearance, and overall perception of well-being showed increases in mean scores in MA-treated patients as compared to the placebo group.

In both trials, patients tolerated the drug well and no statistically significant differences were seen between the treatment groups with regard to laboratory abnormalities, new opportunistic infections, lymphocyte counts, T_4 counts, T_8 counts, or skin reactivity tests (See "ADVERSE REACTIONS").

CLINICAL STUDIES

[See table at right.]

Presented below are the results of mean weight changes for patients evaluable for efficacy in trials 1 and 2.

[See Figures at top of next column.]

INDICATIONS AND USAGE

MEGACE (megestrol acetate) Oral Suspension is indicated for the treatment of anorexia, cachexia, or an unexplained, significant weight loss in patients with a diagnosis of acquired immunodeficiency syndrome (AIDS).

CONTRAINDICATIONS

As a diagnostic test for pregnancy.
Known or suspected pregnancy.

WARNINGS

Megestrol acetate may cause fetal harm when administered to a pregnant woman. For animal data on fetal effects, see the "Impairment of Fertility" section under "PRECAUTIONS". There are no adequate and well-controlled studies in pregnant women. If this drug is used during pregnancy, or if the patient becomes pregnant while taking (receiving) this

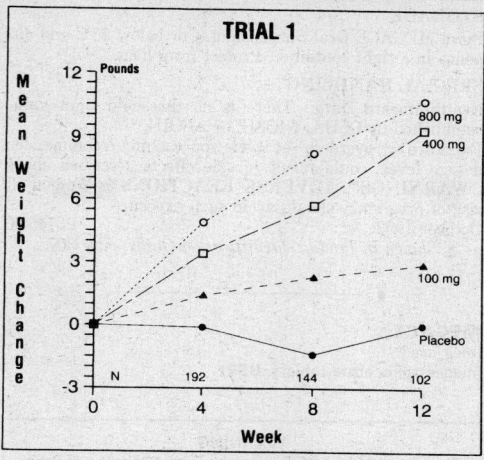

TRIAL 1

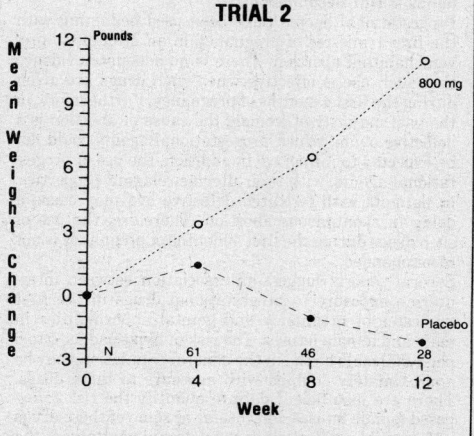

TRIAL 2

drug, the patient should be apprised of the potential hazard to the fetus. Women of childbearing potential should be advised to avoid becoming pregnant.

Megestrol acetate is not intended for prophylactic use to avoid weight loss.

See also "Carcinogenesis, Mutagenesis, and Impairment of Fertility" section under PRECAUTIONS.

PRECAUTIONS

General: Therapy with MEGACE Oral Suspension for weight loss should only be instituted after treatable causes of weight loss are sought and addressed. These treatable causes include possible malignancies, systemic infections, gastrointestinal disorders affecting absorption, endocrine disease and renal or psychiatric diseases.

Although the glucocorticoid effects of MEGACE Oral Suspension in HIV infected individuals have not been evaluated, laboratory evidence of adrenal suppression has been observed which is clinically insignificant.

Effects on HIV viral replication have not been determined. Use with caution in patients with a history of thromboembolic disease.

Information for the Patients: Patients using megestrol acetate should receive the following instructions:
1. This medication is to be used as directed by the physician.
2. Report any adverse reaction experiences while taking this medication.
3. Use contraception while taking this medication if you are a woman capable of becoming pregnant.
4. Notify your physician if you become pregnant while taking this medication.

Drug Interactions: Possible interactions of MEGACE with concomitant medications have not been investigated.

Animal Toxicology: Long-term treatment with MEGACE may increase the risk of respiratory infections. A trend toward increased frequency of respiratory infections, decreased lymphocyte counts and increased neutrophil counts was observed in a two-year chronic toxicity/carcinogenicity study of megestrol acetate conducted in rats.

Carcinogenesis, Mutagenesis, and Impairment of Fertility:
Carcinogenesis: Data on carcinogenesis were obtained from studies conducted in dogs, monkeys and rats treated with megestrol acetate at doses 53.2, 26.6 and 1.3 times *lower* than the proposed dose (13.3 mg/kg/day) for humans. No males were used in the dog and monkey studies. In female beagles, megestrol acetate (0.01, 0.1 or 0.25 mg/kg/day) administered for up to 7 years induced both benign and malignant tumors of the breast. In female monkeys, no tumors were found following 10 years of treatment with 0.01, 0.1, or 0.5 mg/kg/day megestrol acetate. Pituitary tumors were observed in female rats treated with 3.9 or 10 mg/kg/day of megestrol acetate for 2 years. The relationship of these tumors in rats and dogs to humans is unknown but should be considered in assessing the risk-to-benefit ratio when prescribing MEGACE (megestrol acetate) Oral Suspension and in surveillance of patients on therapy. Also see "WARNINGS" section.

Mutagenesis: No mutagenesis data are currently available.
Impairment of Fertility: Perinatal/postnatal (segment III) toxicity studies were performed in rats at doses (0.05–12.5mg/kg) *less* than that indicated for humans (13.3 mg/kg); in these low dose studies, the reproductive capability of male offspring of megestrol acetate-treated females was impaired. Similar results were obtained in dogs. Pregnant rats treated with megestrol acetate showed a reduction in fetal weight and number of live births, and feminization of male fetuses. No toxicity data are currently available on male reproduction (spermatogenesis).

Pregnancy: Pregnancy "Category X". (See "WARNINGS" and "Impairment of Fertility" section.) No adequate animal teratology information is available at clinically relevant doses.

Nursing Mothers: Because of the potential for adverse effects on the newborn, nursing should be discontinued if MEGACE Oral Suspension is required.

Use in HIV Infected Women: Although megestrol acetate has been used extensively in women for the treatment of endometrial and breast cancers, its use in HIV infected women has been limited.

All 10 women in the clinical trials reported breakthrough bleeding.

MEGACE (megestrol acetate) Oral Suspension Clinical Efficacy Trials

	Trial 1 Study Accrual Dates 11/88 to 12/90				Trial 2 Study Accrual Dates 5/89 to 4/91	
Megestrol Acetate, mg/day	0	100	400	800	0	800
Entered Patients	38	82	75	75	48	52
Evaluable Patients	28	61	53	53	29	36
Mean Change in Weight (lb.)						
Baseline to 12 Weeks	0.0	2.9	9.3	10.7	-2.1	11.2
% Patients ≥ 5 Pound Gain						
at Last Evaluation in 12 Weeks	21	44	57	64	28	47
Mean Changes in Body Composition*:						
Fat Body Mass (lb.)	0.0	2.2	2.9	5.5	1.5	5.7
Lean Body Mass (lb.)	-1.7	-0.3	1.5	2.5	-1.6	-0.6
Water (liters)	-1.3	-0.3	0.0	0.0	-0.1	-0.1
% Patients With Improved Appetite						
At Time of Max. Wt. Change	50	72	72	93	48	69
At Last Evaluation in 12 Wk.	50	72	68	89	38	67
Mean Change in Daily Caloric Intake: Baseline to Time of Maximum Weight Change	-107	326	308	646	30	464

* Based on bioelectrical impedance analysis determinations at last evaluation in 12 weeks

Continued on next page

Bristol-Myers Squibb Oncology—Cont.

Pediatric Use: Safety and effectiveness in children have not been established.

ADVERSE REACTIONS

Clinical Adverse Events: Adverse events which occurred in at least 5% of patients in any arm of the two clinical efficacy trials and the open trial are listed below by treatment group. All patients listed had at least one post baseline visit during the 12 study weeks. These adverse events should be considered by the physician when prescribing MEGACE (megestrol acetate) Oral Suspension.

Adverse Events
% of Patients Reporting

	Trial 1 (N=236)				Trial 2 (N=87)		Open Label Trial
Megestrol Acetate mg/day	Placebo 0	100	400	800	Placebo 0	800	1200
No. of Patients	N= 34	N= 68	N= 69	N= 65	N= 38	N= 49	N= 176
Diarrhea	15	13	8	15	8	6	10
Impotence	3	4	6	4	0	4	7
Rash	9	9	4	12	3	2	6
Flatulence	9	0	1	9	3	10	6
Hypertension	0	0	0	8	0	0	4
Asthenia	3	2	3	6	8	4	5
Insomnia	0	3	4	6	0	0	1
Nausea	9	4	0	5	3	4	5
Anemia	6	3	3	5	0	0	0
Fever	3	6	4	5	3	2	1
Libido Decreased	3	4	0	5	0	2	1
Dyspepsia	0	0	3	3	5	4	2
Hyperglycemia	3	0	6	3	0	0	3
Headache	6	10	1	3	3	0	3
Pain	6	0	0	2	5	6	4
Vomiting	9	3	0	2	3	6	4
Pneumonia	6	2	0	2	3	0	1
Urinary Freq.	0	0	1	2	5	2	1

Adverse events which occurred in 1% to 3% of all patients enrolled in the two clinical efficacy trials with at least one follow-up visit during the first 12 weeks of the study are listed below by body system. Adverse events occurring less than 1% are not included. There were no significant differences between incidence of these events in patients treated with megestrol acetate and patients treated with placebo.

Body as a Whole: abdominal pain, chest pain, infection, moniliasis and sarcoma

Cardiovascular System: cardiomyopathy and palpitation

Digestive System: constipation, dry mouth, hepatomegaly, increased salivation and oral moniliasis

Hemic and Lymphatic System: leukopenia

Metabolic and Nutritional: LDH increased, edema and peripheral edema

Nervous System: parethesia, confusion, convulsion, depression, neuropathy, hypesthesia and abnormal thinking

Respiratory System: dyspnea, cough, pharyngitis and lung disorder

Skin and Appendages: alopecia, herpes, pruritus, vesiculobulous rash, sweating and skin disorder

Special Senses: amblyopia

Urogenital System: albuminuria, urinary incontinence, urinary tract infection and gynecomastia

OVERDOSAGE

No serious unexpected side effects have resulted from studies involving MEGACE Oral Suspension administered in dosages as high as 1200 mg/day. Megestrol acetate has not been tested for dialyzability; however, due to its low solubility it is postulated that dialysis would not be an effective means of treating overdose.

DOSAGE AND ADMINISTRATION

The recommended adult initial dosage of MEGACE Oral Suspension, is 800 mg/day (20 mL/day). Shake container well before using.

In clinical trials evaluating different dose schedules, daily doses of 400 and 800 mg/day were found to be clinically effective.

A plastic dosage cup with 10 mL and 20 mL markings is provided for convenience.

HOW SUPPLIED

MEGACE® (megestrol acetate) Oral Suspension is available as a lemon-lime flavored oral suspension containing 40 mg of micronized megestrol acetate per mL

NDC 0015-0508-42 Bottles of 240 mL (8 fl. oz.)

STORAGE

Store MEGACE Oral Suspension at or below 25°C and dispense in a tight container. Protect from heat.

SPECIAL HANDLING

Health Hazard Data: There is no threshold limit value established by OSHA, NIOSH, or ACGIH.

Exposure or "overdose" at levels approaching recommended dosage levels could result in side effects described above (**"WARNINGS"**,**"ADVERSE REACTIONS"**). Women at risk of pregnancy should avoid such exposure.

October 1993 P5745-00

Shown in Product Identification Guide, page 307

MEGACE® ℞

[*mĕg'ace*]

(megestrol acetate tablets, USP)

WARNING

The Use of MEGACE During the First 4 Months of Pregnancy is Not Recommended

Progestational agents have been used beginning with the first trimester of pregnancy in an attempt to prevent habitual abortion. There is no adequate evidence that such use is effective when such drugs are given during the first 4 months of pregnancy. Furthermore, in the vast majority of women, the cause of abortion is a defective ovum, which progestational agents could not be expected to influence. In addition, the use of progestational agents, with their uterine-relaxant properties, in patients with fertilized defective ova may cause a delay in spontaneous abortion. Therefore, the use of such drugs during the first 4 months of pregnancy is not recommended.

Several reports suggest an association between intrauterine exposure to progestational drugs in the first trimester of pregnancy and genital abnormalities in male and female fetuses. The risk of hypospadias, 5 to 8 per 1,000 male births in the general population, may be approximately doubled with exposure to these drugs. There are insufficient data to quantify the risk to exposed female fetuses, but insofar as some of these drugs induce mild virilization of the external genitalia of the female fetus, and because of the increased association of hypospadias in the male fetus, it is prudent to avoid the use of these drugs during the first trimester of pregnancy.

If the patient is exposed to Megace during the first 4 months of pregnancy or if she becomes pregnant while taking this drug, she should be apprised of the potential risks to the fetus.

DESCRIPTION

Megace, megestrol acetate, is a synthetic, antineoplastic and progestational drug. Megestrol acetate is a white, crystalline solid chemically designated as 17α-acetyloxy-6-methylpregna-4, 6-diene-3, 20-dione. Solubility at 37°C in water is 2 mcg per mL, solubility in plasma is 24 mcg per mL. Its molecular weight is 384.51. The empirical formula is $C_{24}H_{32}O_4$ and the structural formula is represented as follows:

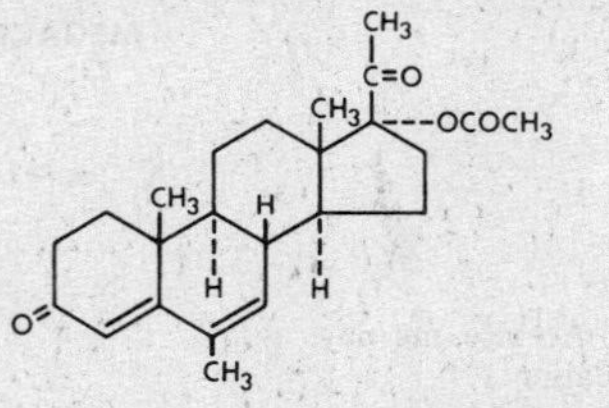

Megace is supplied as tablets for oral administration containing 20 mg and 40 mg megestrol acetate.

Megace Tablets contain the following inactive ingredients: acacia, calcium phosphate, FD&C Blue No. 1, Aluminum Lake, lactose, magnesium stearate, silicon dioxide colloidal, and starch.

CLINICAL PHARMACOLOGY

While the precise mechanism by which Megace (megestrol acetate) produces its antineoplastic effects against endometrial carcinoma is unknown at the present time, inhibition of pituitary gonadotropin production and resultant decrease in estrogen secretions may be factors. There is evidence to suggest a local effect as a result of the marked changes brought about by the direct instillation of progestational agents into the endometrial cavity. The antineoplastic action of megestrol acetate on carcinoma of the breast is effected by modifying the action of other steroid hormones and by exerting a direct cytotoxic effect on tumor cells.[1] In metastatic cancer, hormone receptors may be present in some tissues but not others. The receptor mechanism is a cyclic process whereby estrogen produced by the ovaries enters the target cell, forms a complex with cytoplasmic receptor and is transported into the cell nucleus. There it induces gene transcription and leads to the alteration of normal cell functions. Pharmacologic doses of megestrol acetate not only decrease the number of hormone-dependent human breast cancer cells but also is capable of modifying and abolishing the stimulatory effects of estrogen on these cells. It has been suggested[2] that progestins may inhibit in one of two ways: by interfering with either the stability, availability, or turnover of the estrogen receptor complex in its interaction with genes or in conjunction with the progestin receptor complex, by interacting directly with the genome to turn off specific estrogen-responsive genes.

There are several analytical methods used to estimate Megace plasma levels, including mass fragmentography, gas chromatography (GC), high pressure liquid chromatography (HPLC) and radioimmunoassay. The plasma levels by HPLC assay or radioimmunoassay methods are about one-sixth those obtained by the GC method. The plasma levels are dependent not only on the method used, but also on intestinal and hepatic inactivation of the drug, which may be affected by factors such as intestinal tract motility, intestinal bacteria, antibiotics administered, body weight, diet, and liver function.[3,4]

Metabolites account for only 5% to 8% of the administered dose and are considered negligible.[5] The major route of drug elimination in humans is the urine. When radiolabeled megestrol acetate was administered to humans in doses of 4 to 90 mg, the urinary excretion within 10 days ranged from 56.5% to 78.4% (mean 66.4%) and fecal excretion ranged from 7.7% to 30.3% (mean 19.8%). The total recovered radioactivity varied between 83.1% and 94.7% (mean 86.2%). Respiratory excretion as labeled carbon dioxide and fat storage may have accounted for at least part of the radioactivity not found in the urine and feces.

In normal male volunteers (n=23) who received 160 mg of megestrol acetate given as a 40 mg qid regimen, the oral absorption of Megace appeared to be variable. Plasma levels were assayed by a high pressure liquid chromatographic (HPLC) procedure. Peak drug levels for the first 40 mg dose ranged from 10 to 56 ng/mL (mean 27.6 ng/mL) and the times to peak concentrations ranged from 1.0 to 3.0 hours (mean 2.2 hours). Plasma elimination half-life ranged from 13.0 to 104.9 hours (mean 34.2 hours). The steady state plasma concentrations for a 40 mg qid regimen have not been established.

INDICATIONS AND USAGE

Megace (megestrol acetate) is indicated for the palliative treatment of advanced carcinoma of the breast or endometrium (ie, recurrent, inoperable, or metastatic disease). It should not be used in lieu of currently accepted procedures such as surgery, radiation, or chemotherapy.

CONTRAINDICATIONS

As a diagnostic test for pregnancy.

WARNINGS

Megestrol acetate may cause fetal harm when administered to a pregnant woman. Fertility and reproduction studies with high doses of megestrol acetate have shown a reversible feminizing effect on some male rat fetuses.[6] There are not adequate and well-controlled studies in pregnant women. If this drug is used during pregnancy, or if the patient becomes pregnant while taking (receiving) this drug, the patient should be apprised of the potential hazard to the fetus. Women of childbearing potential should be advised to avoid becoming pregnant.

The use of Megace® (megestrol acetate) in other types of neoplastic disease is not recommended.

See also "Carcinogenesis, Mutagenesis, and Impairment of Fertility" section.

PRECAUTIONS

General:

Close surveillance is indicated for any patient treated for recurrent or metastatic cancer. Use with caution in patients with a history of thrombophlebitis.

Patients should be observed for clinical evidence of adrenal cortical insufficiency when Megace is abruptly withdrawn.

Information for the Patients:

Patients using megestrol acetate should receive the following instructions.

1. This medication is to be used as directed by the physician.
2. Report any adverse reaction experiences while taking this medication.

Laboratory Tests:

Breast malignancies in which estrogen and/or progesterone receptors are positive are more likely to respond to Megace.[7,8,9]

Carcinogenesis, Mutagenesis, and Impairment of Fertility:

Administration for up to 7 years of megestrol acetate to female dogs is associated with an increased incidence of both benign and malignant tumors of the breast.[10] Comparable studies in rats and studies in monkeys are not associated

with an increased incidence of tumors. The relationship of the dog tumors to humans is unknown but should be considered in assessing the benefit-to-risk ratio when prescribing Megace and in surveillance of patients on therapy.[10,11] Also see "WARNINGS" section.

Pregnancy:
Pregnancy Category D. See "WARNINGS" section.

Nursing Mothers:
Because of the potential for adverse effects on the newborn, nursing should be discontinued if Megace is required for treatment of cancer.

Pediatric Use:
Safety and effectiveness in children have not been established.

ADVERSE REACTIONS

Weight Gain:
Weight gain is a frequent side effect of Megace.[12,13] This gain has been associated with increased appetite and is not necessarily associated with fluid retention.

Thromboembolic Phenomena:
Thromboembolic phenomena including thrombophlebitis and pulmonary embolism have been rarely reported.

Glucocorticoid Effects: The glucocorticoid effects have not been fully evaluated. Laboratory evidence of pituitary-adrenal axis abnormalities have been observed. Although the significance of these laboratory findings has not been fully established, clinically apparent adrenal insufficiency has been reported to rarely occur in patients shortly after Megace treatment was discontinued.

Other Adverse Reactions:
Nausea and vomiting, edema, breakthrough bleeding, dyspnea, tumor flare (with or without hypercalcemia), hyperglycemia, alopecia, hypertension, carpal tunnel syndrome, and rash.

OVERDOSAGE

No serious unexpected side effects have resulted from studies involving Megace (megestrol acetate) administered in dosages as high as 1600 mg/day. Oral administration of large, single doses of megestrol acetate (5 g/kg) did not produce toxic effects in mice.[6] Megestrol acetate has not been tested for dialyzability; however, due to its low solubility it is postulated that this would not be an effective means of treating overdose.

DOSAGE AND ADMINISTRATION

Breast cancer: 160 mg/day (40 mg qid)
Endometrial carcinoma: 40 to 320 mg/day in divided doses.
At least 2 months of continuous treatment is considered an adequate period for determining the efficacy of Megace (megestrol acetate).

HOW SUPPLIED

Megace® (megestrol acetate) is available as light blue, scored tablets containing 20 mg or 40 mg megestrol acetate.

NDC 0015-0595-01, 20 mg tablet	Bottles of 100
NDC 0015-0596-41, 40 mg tablet	Bottles of 100
NDC 0015-0596-45, 40 mg tablet	Bottles of 500
NDC 0015-0596-46 40 mg tablet	Bottles of 250

STORAGE

Store Megace at room temperature; protect from temperatures above 40°C (104°F).

SPECIAL HANDLING

Health Hazard Data
There is no threshold limit value established by OSHA, NIOSH, or ACGIH.
Exposure or "overdose" at levels approaching recommended dosing levels could result in side effects described above (WARNINGS, ADVERSE REACTIONS). Women at risk of pregnancy should avoid such exposure.

REFERENCES

1. Allegra JC, Kiefer SM. Mechanisms of Action of Progestational Agents. *Semin Oncol.* 1985; 12(Suppl 1):3.
2. DeSombre ER, Kuivanen PC. Progestin Modulation of Estrogen-Dependent Marker Protein Synthesis in the Endometrium. *Semin Oncol.* 1985; 12(Suppl 1):6.
3. Alexieva-Figusch J, Blankenstein MA, Hop WCJ, et al. Treatment of Metastatic Breast Cancer Patients with Different Dosages of Megestrol Acetate: Dose Relations, Metabolic and Endocrine Effects. *Eur J Cancer Clin Oncol.* 1984; 20:33–40.
4. Gaver RC, Movahhed HS, Farmen RH, Pittman KA. Liquid Chromatographic Procedure for the Quantitative Analysis of Megestrol Acetate in Human Plasma. *J Pharm Sci.* 1985; 74:664.
5. Cooper JM, Kellie AE. The Metabolism of Megestrol Acetate (17-alpha-acetoxy-6-methylpregna-4,6-diene-3,20-dione) in Women. *Steroids.* 1968;11:133.
6. David A, Edwards K, Fellowes KP, Plummer JM. Anti-Ovulatory and Other Biological Properties of Megestrol Acetate. *J Reprod Fertil.* 1963;5:331.
7. McGuire WL, Clark GM. The Prognostic Role of Progesterone Receptors in Human Breast Cancer. *Semin Oncol.* 1983;10(Suppl 4):2.
8. Horwitz KB. The Central Role of Progesterone Receptors and Progestational Agents in the Management and Treatment of Breast Cancer. *Semin Oncol.* 1988;15(Suppl 1):14.
9. Bonomi P, Johnson P, Anderson K, Wolter J, Bunting N, Strauss A, Roseman D, Shorey W, Econonou S. Primary Hormonal Therapy of Advanced Breast Cancer with Megestrol Acetate: Predictive Value of Estrogen Receptor and Progesterone Receptor Levels. *Semin Oncol.* 1985;12(1 Suppl 1):48–54.
10. Nelson LW, Weikel JH Jr., Reno FE. Mammary Nodules in Dogs during Four Years' Treatment with Megestrol Acetate or Chlormadinone Acetate. *J Natl Cancer Inst.* 1973;51:1303.
11. Owen LN, Briggs MH. Contraceptive Steroid Toxicology in the Beagle Dog and its Relevance to Human Carcinogenicity. *Curr Med Res Opin.* 1976;4:309.
12. Ansfield FJ, Kallas GJ, Singson JP. Clinical Results with Megestrol Acetate in Patients with Advanced Carcinoma of the Breast. *Surg Gynecol Obstet.* 1982;155:888.
13. Alexieva-Figusch J, van Gilse HA, Hop WCJ, *et al.* Progestin Therapy in Advanced Breast Cancer: Megestrol Acetate—An Evaluation of 160 Treated Cases. *Cancer.* 1980;46:2369.

Shown in Product Identification Guide, page 307
(P9231-03)
July 1994

MESNEX® ℞

[*mĕs-nĕx*]
(Mesna) Injection

DESCRIPTION

MESNEX Injection is a detoxifying agent to inhibit the hemorrhagic cystitis induced by ifosfamide (Ifex®). The active ingredient mesna is a synthetic sulfhydryl compound designated as sodium 2-mercaptoethanesulfonate with a molecular formula of $C_2H_5NaO_3S_2$ and a molecular weight of 164.18. Its structural formula is as follows:

$$HS\text{-}CH_2\text{-}CH_2SO_3\text{-}Na^+$$

MESNEX Injection is a sterile, nonpyrogenic aqueous solution of clear and colorless appearance in clear glass single dose ampules or multidose vials for intravenous administration. MESNEX Injection contains 100 mg/mL mesna, 0.25 mg/mL edetate disodium and sodium hydroxide for pH adjustment. MESNEX Injection multidose vials also contain 10.4 mg of benzyl alcohol as a preservative. The solution has a pH range of 6.5–8.5.

CLINICAL PHARMACOLOGY

MESNEX was developed as a prophylactic agent to prevent the hemorrhagic cystitis induced by ifosfamide. Analogous to the physiological cysteine-cystine system, following intravenous administration, mesna is rapidly oxidized to its only metabolite, mesna disulfide (dimesna). Mesna disulfide remains in the intravascular compartment and is rapidly eliminated by the kidneys.

In the kidney, the mesna disulfide is reduced to the free thiol compound, mesna, which reacts chemically with the urotoxic ifosfamide metabolites (acrolein and 4-hydroxy-ifosfamide) resulting in their detoxification. The first step in the detoxification process is the binding of mesna to 4-hydroxy-ifosfamide forming a nonurotoxic 4-sulfoethylthioifosfamide. Mesna also binds to the double bonds of acrolein and other urotoxic metabolites.

After administration of an 800 mg dose the half-lives of mesna and dimesna in the blood are 0.36 hours and 1.17 hours, respectively. Approximately 32% and 33% of the administered dose was eliminated in the urine in 24 hours as mesna and dimesna, respectively. The majority of the dose recovered was eliminated within 4 hours. Mesna has a volume of distribution of 0.652 L/kg and a plasma clearance of 1.23 L/kg/hour.

Ifosfamide has been shown to have dose-dependent pharmacokinetics in humans. At doses of 2–4 g, its terminal elimination half-life is about 7 hours. As a result, in order to maintain adequate levels of mesna in the urinary bladder during the course of elimination of the urotoxic ifosfamide metabolites, repeated doses of MESNEX are required.

Based on the pharmacokinetic profiles of mesna and ifosfamide as discussed above, MESNEX was given as bolus doses prior to ifosfamide and at 4 and 8 hours after ifosfamide administration. The hemorrhagic cystitis produced by ifosfamide is dose dependent. At a dose of 1.2 g/m² ifosfamide administered daily for 5 days, 16% to 26% of the patients who received conventional uroprophylaxis (high fluid intake, alkalinization of the urine and the administration of diuretics) developed hematuria (> 50 rbc/hpf or macrohematuria). In contrast none of the patients who received MESNEX together with this dose of ifosfamide developed hematuria.

Higher doses of ifosfamide from 2 to 4 g/m² administered for 3 to 5 days, produced hematuria in 31% to 100% of the patients. When MESNEX was administered together with these doses of ifosfamide the incidence of hematuria was less than 7%.

INDICATIONS AND USAGE

MESNEX has been shown to be effective as a prophylactic agent in reducing the incidence of ifosfamide-induced hemorrhagic cystitis.

CONTRAINDICATIONS

MESNEX is contraindicated in patients known to be hypersensitive to mesna or other thiol compounds.

WARNINGS

Allergic reactions to mesna were reported in patients with autoimmune disorders. The majority of the patients received high doses of mesna orally. The symptoms ranged from mild hypersensitivity to systemic anaphylactic reactions.

MESNEX has been developed as an agent to prevent ifosfamide-induced hemorrhagic cystitis. It will not prevent or alleviate any of the other adverse reactions or toxicities associated with ifosfamide therapy.

MESNEX does not prevent hemorrhagic cystitis in all patients. Up to 6% of patients treated with mesna have developed hematuria (> 50 rbc/hpf or WHO grade 2 and above). As a result, a morning specimen of urine should be examined for the presence of hematuria (red blood cells) each day prior to ifosfamide therapy. If hematuria develops when MESNEX is given with ifosfamide according to the recommended dosage schedule, depending on the severity of the hematuria, dosage reductions or discontinuation of ifosfamide therapy may be initiated.

In order to obtain adequate protection, MESNEX must be administered with each dose of ifosfamide as outlined in the **DOSAGE AND ADMINISTRATION** section. MESNEX is not effective in preventing hematuria due to other pathological conditions such as thrombocytopenia.

Because of the benzyl alcohol content, the multidose vial should not be used in neonates or infants and should be used with caution in older pediatric patients.

PRECAUTIONS

Laboratory Tests
A false positive test for urinary ketones may arise in patients treated with MESNEX. In this test, a red-violet color develops which, with the addition of glacial acetic acid, will return to violet.

Pediatrics
Because of the benzyl alcohol content, the multidose vial should not be used in neonates or infants and should be used with caution in older pediatric patients.

Drug Interactions
In vitro and *in vivo* animal tumor models have shown that mesna does not have any effect on the antitumor efficacy of concomitantly administered cytotoxic agents.

Carcinogenesis, Mutagenesis and Impairment of Fertility
No long term animal studies have been performed to evaluate the carcinogenic potential of mesna. The Ames **Salmonella typhimurium** test, mouse micronucleus assay and frequency of sister chromatid exchange and chromosomal aberrations in PHA-stimulated lymphocytes *in vitro* assays revealed no mutagenic activity.

Pregnancy
Pregnancy Category B. Reproduction studies in rats and rabbits with oral doses up to 1000 mg/kg have revealed no harm to the fetus due to mesna. It is not known whether MESNEX can cause fetal harm when administered to a pregnant woman or can affect reproductive capacity. MESNEX should be given to a pregnant woman only if the benefits clearly outweigh any possible risks.
Teratology studies in rats and rabbits have shown no effects.

Nursing Mothers
It is not known whether mesna or dimesna is excreted in human milk. Because many drugs are excreted in human milk and because of the potential for adverse reactions in nursing infants, from mesna, a decision should be made whether to discontinue nursing or discontinue the drug, taking into account the importance of the drug to the mother.

ADVERSE REACTIONS

Because MESNEX is used in combination with ifosfamide and other chemotherapeutic agents with documented toxicities, it is difficult to distinguish the adverse reactions which may be due to MESNEX from those caused by the concomitantly administered cytostatic agents. As a result, the adverse reaction profile of MESNEX was determined in three Phase I studies (16 subjects) utilizing intravenous and oral administration and two controlled studies in which ifosfamide and MESNEX were compared to ifosfamide and standard prophylaxis.

In Phase I studies in which IV bolus doses of 0.8 to 1.6 g/m² MESNEX were administered as single or three repeated doses to a total of 10 patients, a bad taste in the mouth (100%) and soft stools (70%) were reported. At intravenous

Continued on next page

Bristol-Myers Squibb Oncology—Cont.

and oral bolus doses of 2.4 g/m^2 which are approximately 10 times the recommended clinical doses (0.24 g/m^2) headache (50%), fatigue (33%), nausea (33%), diarrhea (83%), limb pain (50%), hypotension (17%), and allergy (17%) have also been reported in the 6 patients who participated in this study.

In controlled clinical studies, adverse reactions which can be reasonably associated with MESNEX were vomiting, diarrhea and nausea.

OVERDOSAGE

There is no known antidote for MESNEX.

DOSAGE AND ADMINISTRATION

For the prophylaxis of ifosfamide-induced hemorrhagic cystitis, MESNEX may be given on a fractionated dosing schedule of bolus intravenous injections as outlined below.

MESNEX is given as intravenous bolus injections in a dosage equal to 20% of the ifosfamide dosage (w/w) at the time of ifosfamide administration and 4 and 8 hours after each dose of ifosfamide. The total daily dose of MESNEX is 60% of the ifosfamide dose.

The recommended dosing schedule is outlined below:

	0 Hours	4 Hours	8 Hours
Ifosfamide	1.2 g/m^2	—	—
Mesnex	240 mg/m^2	240 mg/m^2	240 mg/m^2

In order to maintain adequate protection, this dosing schedule should be repeated on each day that ifosfamide is administered. When the dosage of ifosfamide is adjusted (either increased or decreased), the dose of MESNEX should be modified accordingly. When exposed to oxygen, mesna is oxidized to the disulfide, dimesna. As a result, if the ampules are used, any unused mesna remaining in the ampules after dosing should be discarded and new ampules used for each administration.

The MESNEX multidose vials may be stored and used for up to 8 days.

PREPARATION OF INTRAVENOUS SOLUTIONS/STABILITY—For I.V. administration the drug can be diluted by adding the MESNEX Injection solution to any of the following fluids obtaining final concentrations of 20 mg mesna/mL fluid:

5% Dextrose Injection, USP
5% Dextrose and 0.2% Sodium Chloride Injection, USP
5% Dextrose and 0.33% Sodium Chloride Injection, USP
5% Dextrose and 0.45% Sodium Chloride Injection, USP
0.92% Sodium Chloride Injection, USP
Lactated Ringer's Injection, USP

For example:

One mL of MESNEX (mesna) Injection multidose vial 100 mg/mL may be added to 4 mL, or one ampule of MESNEX Injection 200 mg/2 mL may be added to 8 mL of any of the solutions listed above to create a final concentration of 20 mg mesna/mL fluid.

Diluted solutions are chemically and physically stable for 24 hours at 25°C (77°F).

Mesna is not compatible with cisplatin.

Parenteral drug products should be inspected visually for particulate matter and discoloration prior to administration.

HOW SUPPLIED

MESNEX® (mesna) Injection 100 mg/mL

NDC 0015-3560-41 200 mg Single Dose Ampule,
Box of 15 Ampules of 2 mL (color-ring coding: turquoise/yellow)

NDC 0015-3563-02 1 g Multidose Vial,
Box of 1 vial of 10 mL

NDC 0015-3563-03 1 g Multidose Vial,
Box of 10 vials of 10 mL

Store at controlled room temperature 15–30°C (59°–86°F).

(P4122-00)
February 1995

Shown in Product Identification Guide, page 307

MUTAMYCIN® ℞

[*mū″-tĕ-mī′-sĭn*]
(mitomycin for injection, USP)

> **WARNING**
>
> MUTAMYCIN should be administered under the supervision of a qualified physician experienced in the use of cancer chemotherapeutic agents. Appropriate management of therapy and complications is possible only when adequate diagnostic and treatment facilities are readily available.
>
> Bone marrow suppression, notably thrombocytopenia and leukopenia, which may contribute to overwhelming infections in an already compromised patient, is the most common and severe of the toxic effects of MUTAMYCIN (see "Warnings" and "Adverse Reactions" sections).
>
> Hemolytic Uremic Syndrome (HUS) a serious complication of chemotherapy, consisting primarily of microangiopathic hemolytic anemia, thrombocytopenia, and irreversible renal failure, has been reported in patients receiving systemic MUTAMYCIN. The syndrome may occur at any time during systemic therapy with MUTAMYCIN as a single agent or in combination with other cytotoxic drugs, however, most cases occur at doses ≥ 60 mg of MUTAMYCIN. Blood product transfusion may exacerbate the symptoms associated with this syndrome.
>
> The incidence of the syndrome has not been defined.

DESCRIPTION

MUTAMYCIN (also known as mitomycin and/or mitomycin-C) is an antibiotic isolated from the broth of **Streptomyces caespitosus** which has been shown to have antitumor activity. The compound is heat stable, has a high melting point, and is freely soluble in organic solvents.

ACTION

MUTAMYCIN selectively inhibits the synthesis of deoxyribonucleic acid (DNA). The guanine and cytosine content correlates with the degree of MUTAMYCIN-induced cross-linking. At high concentrations of the drug, cellular RNA and protein synthesis are also suppressed.

In humans, MUTAMYCIN is rapidly cleared from the serum after intravenous administration. Time required to reduce the serum concentration by 50% after a 30 mg. bolus injection is 17 minutes. After injection of 30 mg., 20 mg., or 10 mg. I.V., the maximal serum concentrations were 2.4 μg./mL, 1.7 μg./mL, and 0.52 μg./mL, respectively. Clearance is effected primarily by metabolism in the liver, but metabolism occurs in other tissues as well. The rate of clearance is inversely proportional to the maximal serum concentration because, it is thought, of saturation of the degradative pathways.

Approximately 10% of a dose of MUTAMYCIN is excreted unchanged in the urine. Since metabolic pathways are saturated at relatively low doses, the percent of a dose excreted in urine increases with increasing dose. In children, excretion of intravenously administered MUTAMYCIN is similar.

Animal Toxicology—MUTAMYCIN has been found to be carcinogenic in rats and mice. At doses approximating the recommended clinical dose in man, it produces a greater than 100% increase in tumor incidence in male Sprague-Dawley rats, and a greater than 50% increase in tumor incidence in female Swiss mice.

INDICATIONS

MUTAMYCIN is not recommended as single-agent, primary therapy. It has been shown to be useful in the therapy of disseminated adenocarcinoma of the stomach or pancreas in proven combinations with other approved chemotherapeutic agents and as palliative treatment when other modalities have failed. MUTAMYCIN is not recommended to replace appropriate surgery and/or radiotherapy.

CONTRAINDICATIONS

MUTAMYCIN is contraindicated in patients who have demonstrated a hypersensitive or idiosyncratic reaction to it in the past.

MUTAMYCIN is contraindicated in patients with thrombocytopenia, coagulation disorder, or an increase in bleeding tendency due to other causes.

WARNINGS

Patients being treated with MUTAMYCIN must be observed carefully and frequently during and after therapy.

The use of MUTAMYCIN results in a high incidence of bone marrow suppression, particularly thrombocytopenia and leukopenia. Therefore, the following studies should be obtained repeatedly during therapy and for at least 8 weeks following therapy: platelet count, white blood cell count, differential, and hemoglobin. The occurrence of a platelet count below 100,000/mm^3 or a WBC below 4,000/mm^3 or a progressive decline in either is an indication to withhold further therapy until blood counts have recovered above these levels.

Patients should be advised of the potential toxicity of this drug, particularly bone marrow suppression. Deaths have been reported due to septicemia as a result of leukopenia due to the drug.

Patients receiving MUTAMYCIN should be observed for evidence of renal toxicity. MUTAMYCIN should not be given to patients with a serum creatinine greater than 1.7 mg %.

Usage in Pregnancy—Safe use of MUTAMYCIN in pregnant women has not been established. Teratological changes have been noted in animal studies. The effect of MUTAMYCIN on fertility is unknown.

PRECAUTIONS

Acute shortness of breath and severe bronchospasm have been reported following the administration of vinca alkaloids in patients who had previously or simultaneously received MUTAMYCIN. The onset of this acute respiratory distress occurred within minutes to hours after the vinca alkaloid injection. The total number of doses for each drug has varied considerably. Bronchodilators, steroids and/or oxygen have produced symptomatic relief.

A few cases of adult respiratory distress syndrome have been reported in patients receiving MUTAMYCIN in combination with other chemotherapy and maintained at FIO_2 concentrations greater than 50% perioperatively. Therefore, caution should be exercised using only enough oxygen to provide adequate arterial saturation since oxygen itself is toxic to the lungs. Careful attention should be paid to fluid balance and overhydration should be avoided.

ADVERSE REACTIONS

Bone Marrow Toxicity— This was the most common and most serious toxicity, occurring in 605 of 937 patients (64.4%). Thrombocytopenia and/or leukopenia may occur anytime within 8 weeks after onset of therapy with an average time of 4 weeks. Recovery after cessation of therapy was within 10 weeks. About 25% of the leukopenic or thrombocytopenic episodes did not recover. MUTAMYCIN produces cumulative myelosuppression.

Integument and Mucous Membrane Toxicity— This has occurred in approximately 4% of patients treated with MUTAMYCIN. Cellulitis at the injection site has been reported and is occasionally severe. Stomatitis and alopecia also occur frequently. Rashes are rarely reported. The most important dermatological problem with this drug, however, is the necrosis and consequent sloughing of tissue which results if the drug is extravasated during injection. Extravasation may occur with or without an accompanying stinging or burning sensation and even if there is adequate blood return when the injection needle is aspirated. There have been reports of delayed erythema and/or ulceration occurring either at or distant from the injection site, weeks to months after MUTAMYCIN, even when no obvious evidence of extravasation was observed during administration. Skin grafting has been required in some of the cases.

Renal Toxicity—2% of 1,281 patients demonstrated a statistically significant rise in creatinine. There appeared to be no correlation between total dose administered or duration of therapy and the degree of renal impairment.

Pulmonary Toxicity—This has occurred infrequently but can be severe and may be life threatening. Dyspnea with a nonproductive cough and radiographic evidence of pulmonary infiltrates may be indicative of MUTAMYCIN-induced pulmonary toxicity. If other etiologies are eliminated, MUTAMYCIN therapy should be discontinued. Steroids have been employed as treatment of this toxicity, but the therapeutic value has not been determined. A few cases of adult respiratory distress syndrome have been reported in patients receiving MUTAMYCIN in combination with other chemotherapy and maintained at FIO_2 concentrations greater than 50% perioperatively.

Hemolytic Uremic Syndrome (HUS)—This serious complication of chemotherapy, consisting primarily of microangiopathic hemolytic anemia (hematocrit ≤25%), thrombocytopenia (≤100,000/mm^3), and irreversible renal failure (serum creatinine ≥1.6 mg/dL) has been reported in patients receiving systemic MUTAMYCIN. Microangiopathic hemolysis with fragmented red blood cells on peripheral blood smears has occurred in 98% of patients with the syndrome. Other less frequent complications of the syndrome may include pulmonary edema (65%), neurologic abnormalities (16%), and hypertension. Exacerbation of the symptoms associated with HUS has been reported in some patients receiving blood product transfusions. A high mortality rate (52%) has been associated with this syndrome.

The syndrome may occur at any time during systemic therapy with MUTAMYCIN as a single agent or in combination with other cytotoxic drugs. Less frequently, HUS has also been reported in patients receiving combinations of cytotoxic drugs not including MUTAMYCIN. Of 83 patients studied, 72 developed the syndrome at total doses exceeding 60 mg of MUTAMYCIN. Consequently, patients receiving ≥60 mg of MUTAMYCIN should be monitored closely for unexplained anemia with fragmented cells on peripheral blood smear, thrombocytopenia, and decreased renal function.

The incidence of the syndrome has not been defined.

Therapy for the syndrome is investigational.

Cardiac Toxicity—Congestive heart failure, often treated effectively with diuretics and cardiac glycosides, has rarely been reported. Almost all patients who experienced this side effect had received prior doxorubicin therapy.

Acute Side Effects Due to MUTAMYCIN were fever, anorexia, nausea, and vomiting. They occurred in about 14% of 1,281 patients.

Other Undesirable Side Effects that have been reported during MUTAMYCIN therapy have been headache, blurring of vision, confusion, drowsiness, syncope, fatigue, edema, thrombophlebitis, hematemesis, diarrhea, and pain. These did not appear to be dose related and were not unequivocally drug related. They may have been due to the primary or metastatic disease processes.

DOSAGE AND ADMINISTRATION

MUTAMYCIN should be given intravenously only, using care to avoid extravasation of the compound. If extravasation occurs, cellulitis, ulceration, and slough may result. Each vial contains either mitomycin 5 mg and mannitol 10 mg, mitomycin 20 mg and mannitol 40 mg, or mitomycin 40 mg and mannitol 80 mg. To administer, add Sterile Water for Injection, 10 mL, 40 mL or 80 mL, respectively. Shake to dissolve. If product does not dissolve immediately, allow to stand at room temperature until solution is obtained.

After full hematological recovery (see guide to dosage adjustment) from any previous chemotherapy, the following dosage schedule may be used at 6- to 8-week intervals:

20 mg/m^2 intravenously as a single dose via a functioning intravenous catheter.

Because of cumulative myelosuppression, patients should be fully reevaluated after each course of MUTAMCYIN, and the dose reduced if the patient has experienced any toxicities. Doses greater than 20 mg/m^2 have not been shown to be more effective, and are more toxic than lower doses. The following schedule is suggested as a guide to dosage adjustment:

Nadir After Prior Dose

Leukocytes/ mm^3	Platelets/ mm^3	Percentage of Prior Dose To be Given
>4000	>100,000	100%
3000–3999	75,000–99,999	100%
2000–2999	25,000–74,999	70%
<2000	< 25,000	50%

No repeat dosage should be given until leukocyte count has returned to 4000/mm^3 and platelet count to 100,000/mm^3. When MUTAMYCIN is used in combination with other myelosuppressive agents, the doses should be adjusted accordingly. If the disease continues to progress after two courses of Mutamycin, the drug should be stopped since chances of response are minimal.

STABILITY

1. **Unreconstituted** MUTAMYCIN stored at room temperature is stable for the lot life indicated on the package. Avoid excessive heat (over 40°C).
2. **Reconstituted** with Sterile Water for Injection to a concentration of 0.5 mg. per mL, MUTAMYCIN is stable for 14 days refrigerated or 7 days at room temperature.
3. **Diluted** in various IV fluids at room temperature, to a concentration of 20 to 40 micrograms per mL:

IV Fluid	Stability
5% Dextrose Injection	3 hours
0.9% Sodium Chloride Injection	12 hours
Sodium Lactate Injection	24 hours

4. **The combination** of MUTAMYCIN (5 mg. to 15 mg.) and heparin (1,000 units to 10,000 units) in 30 mL of 0.9% Sodium Chloride Injection is stable for 48 hours at room temperature.

Procedures for proper handling and disposal of anticancer drugs should be considered. Several guidelines on this subject have been published.[1-7] There is no general agreement that all of the procedures recommended in the guidelines are necessary or appropriate.

HOW SUPPLIED

MUTAMYCIN (mitomycin for Injection, USP).
NDC 0015-3001-20—Each vial contains 5 mg. mitomycin.
NDC 0015-3002-20—Each vial contains 20 mg. mitomycin.
NDC 0015-3059-20—Each vial contains 40 mg. mitomycin.
For information on package sizes available, refer to the current price schedule.

REFERENCES

1. Recommendations for the Safe Handling of Parenteral Antineoplastic Drugs. NIH Publication No. 83-2621. For sale by the Superintendent of Documents, U.S. Government Printing Office, Washington, D.C. 20402.
2. AMA Council Report. Guidelines for Handling Parenteral Antineoplastics, *JAMA*. 1985; 253(11):1590–1592.
3. National Study Commission on Cytotoxic Exposure—Recommendations for Handling Cytotoxic Agents. Available from Louis P. Jeffrey, Sc.D., Chairman, National Study Commission on Cytotoxic Exposure, Massachusetts College of Pharmacy and Allied Health Sciences, 179 Longwood Avenue, Boston, Massachusetts 02115.
4. Clinical Oncological Society of Australia: Guidelines and Recommendations for Safe Handling of Antineoplastic Agents. *Med J Australia*. 1983; 1:426–428.
5. Jones, R. B., et. al. Safe Handling of Chemotherapeutic Agents: A Report from the Mount Sinai Medical Center, *CA—A Cancer J for Clinicians*. 1983; Sept./Oct., 258–263.
6. American Society of Hospital Pharmacists Technical Assistance Bulletin on Handling Cytotoxic and Hazardous Drugs. *Am J Hosp Pharm*. 1990; 47:1033–1049.
7. OSHA Work-Practice Guidelines for Personnel Dealing with Cytotoxic (antineoplastic) Drugs. *Am J Hosp Pharm*. 1986; 43:1193–1204.

Shown in Product Identification Guide, page 307
(3001DIM-28)
September 1992

MYCOSTATIN® PASTILLES

[mĭk'ō-stat"in]
Nystatin

℞

DESCRIPTION

Nystatin is a polyene antifungal antibiotic obtained from *Streptomyces noursei*. Structural formula:

C$_{47}$H$_{75}$NO$_{17}$ MW 926.13   CAS-1400-61-9

MYCOSTATIN (nystatin) Pastilles are round, light to dark gold-colored troches designed to dissolve slowly in the mouth. Each pastille provides 200,000 units nystatin. Inactive ingredients: anise oil, cinnamon oil, gelatin, sucrose, and other ingredients.

CLINICAL PHARMACOLOGY

Nystatin is both fungistatic and fungicidal *in vitro* against a wide variety of yeasts and yeast-like fungi. *Candida albicans* demonstrates no significant resistance to nystatin *in vitro* on repeated subculture in increasing levels of nystatin; other *Candida* species become quite resistant. Generally, resistance does not develop *in vivo*. Nystatin acts by binding to sterols in the cell membrane of susceptible fungi with a resultant change in membrane permeability allowing leakage of intracellular components. Nystatin exhibits no activity against bacteria, protozoa, trichomonads, or viruses.

Pharmacokinetics

Gastrointestinal absorption of nystatin is insignificant. Most orally administered nystatin is passed unchanged in the stool. Significant concentrations of nystatin may appear occasionally in the plasma of patients with renal insufficiency during oral therapy with conventional dosage forms. Mean nystatin concentrations in excess of those required *in vitro* to inhibit growth of clinically significant *Candida* persisted in saliva for approximately two hours after the start of oral dissolution of two nystatin pastilles (400,000 units nystatin) administered simultaneously to 12 healthy volunteers.

INDICATIONS AND USAGE

Mycostatin (nystatin) Pastilles are indicated for the treatment of candidiasis in the oral cavity.

CONTRAINDICATIONS

The pastille is contraindicated in those patients with a history of hypersensitivity to any of its components.

PRECAUTIONS

General

This medication is not to be used for the treatment of systemic mycoses.

In order to achieve maximum effect from the medication, pastilles must be allowed to dissolve slowly in the mouth; therefore, patients for whom the pastille is prescribed, including children and the elderly, must be competent to utilize the dosage form as intended.

If irritation or hypersensitivity develops with nystatin pastilles, treatment should be discontinued and appropriate therapy instituted.

Information for the Patient

Patients taking this medication should receive the following information and instructions:

1. Use as directed; the medication is not for any disorder other than for which it was prescribed.
2. Allow pastille to dissolve slowly in the mouth; **do not chew or swallow the pastille.**
3. The patient should be advised regarding replacement of any missed doses.
4. There should be no interruption or discontinuation of medication until the prescribed course of treatment is completed even though symptomatic relief may occur within a few days.
5. If symptoms of local irritation develop, the physician should be notified promptly.
6. Good oral hygiene, including proper care of dentures, is particularly important for denture wearers.

Laboratory Tests

If there is a lack of therapeutic response, appropriate microbiological studies (eg, KOH smears and/or cultures) should be repeated to confirm the diagnosis of candidiasis and rule out other pathogens before instituting another course of therapy.

Carcinogenesis, Mutagenesis, Impairment of Fertility

Studies have not been performed to evaluate carcinogenic or mutagenic potential, or possible impairment of fertility in males or females.

Pregnancy: Teratogenic Effects

Category C. Animal reproduction studies have not been conducted with nystatin pastilles. It is also not known whether nystatin pastilles can cause fetal harm when administered to a pregnant woman or can affect reproduction capacity. Nystatin pastilles should be dispensed to a pregnant woman only if clearly needed.

Pediatric Use

See PRECAUTIONS, General.

ADVERSE REACTIONS

Nystatin is generally well-tolerated by all age groups, even during prolonged use. Rarely, oral irritation or sensitization may occur. Nausea has been reported occasionally during therapy.

Large oral doses of nystatin have occasionally produced diarrhea, gastrointestinal distress, nausea and vomiting. Rash, including urticaria, has been reported rarely. Stevens-Johnson syndrome has been reported very rarely.

OVERDOSAGE

Oral doses of nystatin in excess of five million units daily have caused nausea and gastrointestinal upset. There have been no reports of serious toxic effects or superinfections (see CLINICAL PHARMACOLOGY, Pharmacokinetics).

DOSAGE AND ADMINISTRATION

Children and Adults: The recommended dose is one or two pastilles (200,000 or 400,000 units nystatin) four or five times daily for as long as 14 days if necessary. The dosage regimen should be continued for at least 48 hours after disappearance of oral symptoms.

Dosage should be discontinued if symptoms persist after the initial 14 day period of treatment (see PRECAUTIONS, Laboratory Tests).

Administration: Pastilles must be allowed to dissolve slowly in the mouth, and should not be chewed or swallowed whole.

HOW SUPPLIED

Mycostatin (nystatin) Pastilles, 200,000 units nystatin each, in packages containing 30 pleasant-tasting pastilles (NDC 0003-0543-20).

ALSO AVAILABLE

Mycostatin (Nystatin, USP) is also available as a ready-to-use oral suspension, oral tablets, vaginal tablets, and topical powder, cream, and ointment (see package inserts accompanying those products for complete information).

Storage

Refrigerate between 2° and 8°C (36° and 46°F).
Manufactured by Ernest Jackson & Co., Ltd.
Crediton, Devon, England
(P9297-01)
April 1992

PARAPLATIN®

[păr-a-plătin]
(carboplatin for injection)

℞

DESCRIPTION

PARAPLATIN® (carboplatin for injection) is supplied as a sterile lyophilized white powder available in single-dose vials containing 50 mg, 150 mg, and 450 mg of carboplatin for administration by intravenous infusion. Each vial contains equal parts by weight of carboplatin and mannitol.

Continued on next page

Bristol-Myers Squibb Oncology—Cont.

Carboplatin is a platinum coordination compound that is used as a cancer chemotherapeutic agent. The chemical name for carboplatin is platinum, diammine [1,1-cyclobutane-dicarboxylato(2-)-0,0']-, (SP-4-2), and has the following structural formula:

Carboplatin is a crystalline powder with the molecular formula of $C_6H_{12}N_2O_4Pt$ and a molecular weight of 371.25. It is soluble in water at a rate of approximately 14 mg/mL, and the pH of a 1% solution is 5–7. It is virtually insoluble in ethanol, acetone, and dimethylacetamide.

CLINICAL PHARMACOLOGY

Carboplatin, like cisplatin, produces predominantly interstrand DNA cross-links rather than DNA-protein cross-links. This effect is apparently cell-cycle nonspecific. The aquation of carboplatin, which is thought to produce the active species, occurs at a slower rate than in the case of cisplatin. Despite this difference, it appears that both carboplatin and cisplatin induce equal numbers of drug-DNA cross-links, causing equivalent lesions and biological effects. The differences in potencies for carboplatin and cisplatin appear to be directly related to the difference in aquation rates.

In patients with creatinine clearances of about 60 mL/min or greater, plasma levels of intact carboplatin decay in a biphasic manner after a 30-minute intravenous infusion of 300 to 500 mg/m² of PARAPLATIN. The initial plasma half-life (alpha) was found to be 1.1 to 2.0 hours (N=6), and the postdistribution plasma half-life (beta) was found to be 2.6 to 5.9 hours (N=6). The total body clearance, apparent volume of distribution, and mean residence time for carboplatin are 4.4 L/hour, 16 L and 3.5 hours, respectively. The Cmax values and areas under the plasma concentration vs time curves from 0 to infinity (AUC inf) increase linearly with dose, although the increase was slightly more than dose proportional. Carboplatin, therefore, exhibits linear pharmacokinetics over the dosing range studied (300–500 mg/m²).

Carboplatin is not bound to plasma proteins. No significant quantities of protein-free, ultrafilterable platinum-containing species other than carboplatin are present in plasma. However, platinum from carboplatin becomes irreversibly bound to plasma proteins and is slowly eliminated with a minimum half-life of 5 days.

The major route of elimination of carboplatin is renal excretion. Patients with creatinine clearances of approximately 60 mL/min or greater excrete 65% of the dose in the urine within 12 hours and 71% of the dose within 24 hours. All of the platinum in the 24-hour urine is present as carboplatin. Only 3% to 5% of the administered platinum is excreted in the urine between 24 and 96 hours. There are insufficient data to determine whether biliary excretion occurs.

In patients with creatinine clearances below 60 mL/min the total body and renal clearances of carboplatin decrease as the creatinine clearance decreases. PARAPLATIN dosages should therefore be reduced in these patients (see "DOSAGE AND ADMINISTRATION").

CLINICAL STUDIES

Use with cyclophosphamide for initial treatment of ovarian cancer:
In two prospectively randomized, controlled studies conducted by the National Cancer Institute of Canada, Clinical Trials Group (NCIC) and the Southwest Oncology Group (SWOG), 789 chemotherapy naive patients with advanced ovarian cancer were treated with PARAPLATIN or cisplatin, both in combination with cyclophosphamide every 28 days for six courses before surgical re-evaluation. The following results were obtained from both studies:

COMPARATIVE EFFICACY
[See table below.]

COMPARATIVE TOXICITY
The pattern of toxicity exerted by the PARAPLATIN-containing regimen was significantly different from that of the cisplatin-containing combinations. Differences between the two studies may be explained by different cisplatin dosages and by different supportive care.

The PARAPLATIN-containing regimen induced significantly more thrombocytopenia and, in one study, significantly more leukopenia and more need for transfusional support. The cisplatin-containing regimen produced significantly more anemia in one study. However, no significant differences occurred in incidences of infections and hemorrhagic episodes.

Non-hematologic toxicities (emesis, neurotoxicity, ototoxicity, renal toxicity, hypomagnesemia, and alopecia) were significantly more frequent in the cisplatin-containing arms.
[See table at top of next page.]
[See table at top of page 716.]

Use as a single agent for secondary treatment of advanced ovarian cancer:
In two prospective, randomized controlled studies in patients with advanced ovarian cancer previously treated with chemotherapy, PARAPLATIN achieved six clinical complete responses in 47 patients. The duration of these responses ranged from 45 to 71+ weeks.

INDICATIONS

Initial treatment of advanced ovarian carcinoma:
PARAPLATIN is indicated for the initial treatment of advanced ovarian carcinoma in established combination with other approved chemotherapeutic agents. One established combination regimen consists of PARAPLATIN and cyclophosphamide (Cytoxan®). Two randomized controlled studies conducted by the NCIC and SWOG with PARAPLATIN vs cisplatin, both in combination with cyclophosphamide, have demonstrated equivalent overall survival between the two groups (see "CLINICAL STUDIES" section).

There is limited statistical power to demonstrate equivalence in overall pathologic complete response rates and long-term survival (≥ 3 years) because of the small number of patients with these outcomes; the small number of patients with residual tumor < 2 cm after initial surgery also limits the statistical power to demonstrate equivalence in this subgroup.

Secondary treatment of advanced ovarian carcinoma:
PARAPLATIN is indicated for the palliative treatment of patients with ovarian carcinoma recurrent after prior chemotherapy, including patients who have been previously treated with cisplatin.

Within the group of patients previously treated with cisplatin, those who have developed progressive disease while receiving cisplatin therapy may have a decreased response rate.

CONTRAINDICATIONS

PARAPLATIN is contraindicated in patients with a history of severe allergic reactions to cisplatin or other platinum-containing compounds or mannitol.

PARAPLATIN should not be employed in patients with severe bone marrow depression or significant bleeding.

WARNINGS

Bone marrow suppression (leukopenia, neutropenia and thrombocytopenia) is dose dependent and is also the dose-limiting toxicity. Peripheral blood counts should be frequently monitored during PARAPLATIN treatment and, when appropriate, until recovery is achieved. Median nadir occurs at day 21 in patients receiving single-agent PARAPLATIN. In general, single intermittent courses of PARAPLATIN should not be repeated until leukocyte, neutrophil and platelet counts have recovered.

Since anemia is cumulative, transfusions may be needed during treatment with PARAPLATIN, particularly in patients receiving prolonged therapy.

Bone marrow suppression is increased in patients who have received prior therapy, especially regimens including cisplatin. Marrow suppression is also increased in patients with impaired kidney function. Initial PARAPLATIN dosages in these patients should be appropriately reduced (see "DOSAGE AND ADMINISTRATION") and blood counts should be carefully monitored between courses. The use of

Overview of Pivotal Trials

	NCIC	SWOG
Number of patients randomized	447	342
Median age (years)	60	62
Dose of cisplatin	75 mg/m²	100 mg/m²
Dose of carboplatin	300 mg/m²	300 mg/m²
Dose of Cytoxan	600 mg/m²	600 mg/m²
Residual tumor < 2 cm (number of patients)	39% (174/447)	14% (49/342)

Clinical Response in Measurable Disease Patients

	NCIC	SWOG
Carboplatin (number of patients)	60% (48/80)	58% (48/83)
Cisplatin (number of patients)	58% (49/85)	43% (33/76)
95% C.I. of difference (Carboplatin-Cisplatin)	(−13.9%, 18.6%)	(−2.3%, 31.1%)

Pathologic Complete Response*

	NCIC	SWOG
Carboplatin (number of patients)	11% (24/224)	10% (17/171)
Cisplatin (number of patients)	15% (33/223)	10% (17/171)
95% C.I. of difference (Carboplatin-Cisplatin)	(−10.7%, 2.5%)	(−6.9%, 6.9%)

* 114 PARAPLATIN and 109 Cisplatin patients did not undergo second-look surgery in NCIC study
 90 PARAPLATIN and 106 Cisplatin patients did not undergo second-look surgery in SWOG study

Progression-Free Survival (PFS)

	NCIC	SWOG
Median		
Carboplatin	59 weeks	49 weeks
Cisplatin	61 weeks	47 weeks
2-year PFS*		
Carboplatin	31%	21%
Cisplatin	31%	21%
95% C.I. of difference (Carboplatin-Cisplatin)	(−9.3, 8.7)	(−9.0, 9.4)
3-year PFS*		
Carboplatin	19%	8%
Cisplatin	23%	14%
95% C.I. of difference (Carboplatin-Cisplatin)	(−11.5, 4.5)	(−14.1, 0.3)
Hazard Ratio**		
95% C.I.	1.10	1.02
(Carboplatin:Cisplatin)	(0.89, 1.35)	(0.81, 1.29)

*Kaplan-Meier Estimates
 Unrelated deaths occurring in the absence of progression were counted as events (progression) in this analysis.
**Analysis adjusted for factors found to be of prognostic significance were consistent with unadjusted analysis.

Survival

	NCIC	SWOG
Median		
Carboplatin	110 weeks	86 weeks
Cisplatin	99 weeks	79 weeks
2-year Survival*		
Carboplatin	51.9%	40.2%
Cisplatin	48.4%	39.0%
95% C.I. of difference (Carboplatin-Cisplatin)	(−6.2, 13.2)	(−9.8, 12.2)
3-year Survival*		
Carboplatin	34.6%	18.3%
Cisplatin	33.1%	24.9%
95% C.I. of difference (Carboplatin-Cisplatin)	(−7.7, 10.7)	(−15.9, 2.7)
Hazard Ratio**		
95% C.I.	0.98	1.01
(Carboplatin:Cisplatin)	(0.78, 1.23)	(0.78, 1.30)

* Kaplan-Meier Estimates
** Analysis adjusted for factors found to be of prognostic significance were consistent with unadjusted analysis.

PARAPLATIN in combination with other bone marrow suppressing therapies must be carefully managed with respect to dosage and timing in order to minimize additive effects. PARAPLATIN has limited nephrotoxic potential, but concomitant treatment with aminoglycosides has resulted in increased renal and/or audiologic toxicity, and caution must be exercised when a patient receives both drugs.

PARAPLATIN can induce emesis, which can be more severe in patients previously receiving emetogenic therapy. The incidence and intensity of emesis have been reduced by using premedication with antiemetics. Although no conclusive efficacy data exist with the following schedules of PARAPLATIN, lengthening the duration of single intravenous administration to 24 hours or dividing the total dose over five consecutive daily pulse doses has resulted in reduced emesis.

Although peripheral neurotoxicity is infrequent, its incidence is increased in patients older than 65 years and in patients previously treated with cisplatin. Pre-existing cisplatin-induced neurotoxicity does not worsen in about 70% of the patients receiving PARAPLATIN as secondary treatment.

Loss of vision, which can be complete for light colors, has been reported after the use of PARAPLATIN with doses higher than those recommended in the package insert. Vision appears to recover totally or to a significant extent within weeks of stopping these high doses.

As in the case of other platinum coordination compounds, allergic reactions to PARAPLATIN have been reported. These may occur within minutes of administration and should be managed with appropriate supportive therapy.

High dosages of PARAPLATIN (more than four times the recommended dose) have resulted in severe abnormalities of liver function tests.

PARAPLATIN may cause fetal harm when administered to a pregnant woman. PARAPLATIN has been shown to be embryotoxic and teratogenic in rats. There are no adequate and well-controlled studies in pregnant women. If this drug is used during pregnancy, or if the patient becomes pregnant while receiving this drug, the patient should be apprised of the potential hazard to the fetus. Women of childbearing potential should be advised to avoid becoming pregnant.

PRECAUTIONS

General: Needles or intravenous administration sets containing aluminum parts that may come in contact with PARAPLATIN should not be used for the preparation or administration of the drug. Aluminum can react with carboplatin causing precipitate formation and loss of potency.

Drug Interactions: The renal effects of nephrotoxic compounds may be potentiated by PARAPLATIN.

Carcinogenesis, mutagenesis, impairment of fertility: The carcinogenic potential of carboplatin has not been studied, but compounds with similar mechanisms of action and mutagenicity profiles have been reported to be carcinogenic. Carboplatin has been shown to be mutagenic both **in vitro** and **in vivo**. It has also been shown to be embryotoxic and teratogenic in rats receiving the drug during organogenesis.

Pregnancy: Pregnancy "category D": (see "**WARNINGS**").

Nursing mothers: It is not known whether carboplatin is excreted in human milk. Because there is a possibility of toxicity in nursing infants secondary to PARAPLATIN treatment of the mother, it is recommended that breastfeeding be discontinued if the mother is treated with PARAPLATIN.

ADVERSE REACTIONS

For a comparison of toxicities when carboplatin or cisplatin was given in combination with cyclophosphamide, see the COMPARATIVE TOXICITY subsection of the CLINICAL STUDIES section.

[See table at top of page 717.]

In the narrative section that follows, the incidences of adverse events are based on data from 1,893 patients with various types of tumors who received PARAPLATIN as single-agent therapy.

Hematologic toxicity: Bone marrow suppression is the dose-limiting toxicity of PARAPLATIN. Thrombocytopenia with platelet counts below 50,000/mm^3 occurs in 25% of the patients (35% of pretreated ovarian cancer patients); neutropenia with granulocyte counts below 1,000/mm^3 occurs in 16% of the patients (21% of pretreated ovarian cancer patients); leukopenia with WBC counts below 2,000/mm^3 occurs in 15% of the patients (26% of pretreated ovarian cancer patients). The nadir usually occurs about day 21 in patients receiving single-agent therapy. By day 28, 90% of patients have platelet counts above 100,000/mm^3; 74% have neutrophil counts above 2,000/mm^3; 67% have leukocyte counts above 4,000/mm^3.

Marrow suppression is usually more severe in patients with impaired kidney function. Patients with poor performance status have also experienced a higher incidence of severe leukopenia and thrombocytopenia.

The hematologic effects, although usually reversible, have resulted in infectious or hemorrhagic complications in 5% of the patients treated with PARAPLATIN, with drug related death occurring in less than 1% of the patients. Fever has also been reported in patients with neutropenia.

Anemia with hemoglobin less than 11 g/dL has been observed in 71% of the patients who started therapy with a baseline above that value. The incidence of anemia increases with increasing exposure to PARAPLATIN. Transfusions have been administered to 26% of the patients treated with PARAPLATIN (44% of previously treated ovarian cancer patients).

Bone marrow depression may be more severe when PARAPLATIN is combined with other bone marrow suppressing drugs or with radiotherapy.

Gastrointestinal toxicity: Vomiting occurs in 65% of the patients (81% of previously treated ovarian cancer patients) and in about one-third of these patients it is severe. Carboplatin, as a single agent or in combination, is significantly less emetogenic than cisplatin; however, patients previously treated with emetogenic agents, especially cisplatin, appear to be more prone to vomiting. Nausea alone occurs in an additional 10%–15% of patients. Both nausea and vomiting usually cease within 24 hours of treatment and are often responsive to antiemetic measures. Although no conclusive efficacy data exist with the following schedules, prolonged administration of PARAPLATIN, either by continuous 24-hour infusion or by daily pulse doses given for 5 consecutive days, was associated with less severe vomiting than the single-dose intermittent schedule. Emesis was increased when PARAPLATIN was used in combination with other emetogenic compounds. Other gastrointestinal effects observed frequently were pain, in 17% of the patients; diarrhea, in 6%; and constipation, also in 6%.

Neurologic toxicity: Peripheral neuropathies have been observed in 4% of the patients receiving PARAPLATIN (6% of pretreated ovarian cancer patients) with mild paresthesias occurring most frequently. Carboplatin therapy produces significantly fewer and less severe neurologic side effects than does therapy with cisplatin. However, patients older than 65 years and/or previously treated with cisplatin appear to have an increased risk (10%) for peripheral neuropathies. In 70% of the patients with pre-existing cisplatin-induced peripheral neurotoxicity, there was no worsening of symptoms during therapy with PARAPLATIN. Clinical ototoxicity and other sensory abnormalities such as visual disturbances and change in taste have been reported in only 1% of the patients. Central nervous system symptoms have been reported in 5% of the patients and appear to be most often related to the use of antiemetics.

Although the overall incidence of peripheral neurologic side effects induced by PARAPLATIN is low, prolonged treatment, particularly in cisplatin pretreated patients, may result in cumulative neurotoxicity.

Nephrotoxicity: Development of abnormal renal function test results is uncommon, despite the fact that carboplatin, unlike cisplatin, has usually been administered without high-volume fluid hydration and/or forced diuresis. The incidences of abnormal renal function tests reported are 6% for serum creatinine and 14% for blood urea nitrogen (10% and 22%, respectively, in pretreated ovarian cancer patients). Most of these reported abnormalities have been mild and about one-half of them were reversible.

Creatinine clearance has proven to be the most sensitive measure of kidney function in patients receiving PARAPLATIN, and it appears to be the most useful test for correlating drug clearance and bone marrow suppression. Twenty-seven percent of the patients who had a baseline value of 60 mL/min or more demonstrated a reduction below this value during PARAPLATIN therapy.

Hepatic toxicity: The incidences of abnormal liver function tests in patients with normal baseline values were reported as follows: total bilirubin, 5%; SGOT, 15%; and alkaline phosphatase, 24%; (5%, 19%, and 37%, respectively, in pretreated ovarian cancer patients). These abnormalities have generally been mild and reversible in about one-half of the cases, although the role of metastatic tumor in the liver may complicate the assessment in many patients. In a limited series of patients receiving very high dosages of PARAPLATIN and autologous bone marrow transplantation, severe abnormalities of liver function tests were reported.

ADVERSE EXPERIENCES IN PATIENTS WITH OVARIAN CANCER
NCIC STUDY

		Paraplatin Arm Percent*	Cisplatin Arm Percent*	P-Value**
Bone Marrow				
Thrombocytopenia,	< 100,000/mm^3	70	29	< 0.001
	< 50,000/mm^3	41	6	< 0.001
Neutropenia,	< 2,000 cells/mm^3	97	96	n.s.
	< 1,000 cells/mm^3	81	79	n.s.
Leukopenia,	< 4,000 cells/mm^3	98	97	n.s.
	< 2,000 cells/mm^3	68	52	0.001
Anemia,	< 11 g/dL	91	91	n.s.
	< 8 g/dL	18	12	n.s.
Infections		14	12	n.s.
Bleeding		10	4	n.s.
Transfusions		42	31	0.018
Gastrointestinal				
Nausea and vomiting		93	98	0.010
Vomiting		84	97	< 0.001
Other GI side effects		50	62	0.013
Neurologic				
Peripheral neuropathies		16	42	< 0.001
Ototoxicity		13	33	< 0.001
Other sensory side effects		6	10	n.s.
Central neutrotoxicity		28	40	0.009
Renal				
Serum creatinine elevations		5	13	0.006
Blood urea elevations		17	31	< 0.001
Hepatic				
Bilirubin elevations		5	3	n.s.
SGOT elevations		17	13	n.s.
Alkaline phosphatase elevations		—	—	—
Electrolytes loss				
Sodium		10	20	0.005
Potassium		16	22	n.s.
Calcium		16	19	n.s.
Magnesium		63	88	< 0.001
Other side effects				
Pain		36	37	n.s.
Asthenia		40	33	n.s.
Cardiovascular		15	19	n.s.
Respiratory		8	9	n.s.
Allergic		12	9	n.s.
Genitourinary		10	10	n.s.
Alopecia+		50	62	0.017
Mucositis		10	9	n.s.

*Values are in percent of evaluable patients
**n.s. = not significant, p > 0.05
+May have been affected by cyclophosphamide dosage delivered

Continued on next page

Bristol-Myers Squibb Oncology—Cont.

Electrolyte Changes: The incidences of abnormally decreased serum electrolyte values reported were as follows: sodium, 29%; potassium, 20%; calcium, 22%; and magnesium, 29%; (47%, 28%, 31%, and 43%, respectively, in pretreated ovarian cancer patients). Electrolyte supplementation was not routinely administered concomitantly with PARAPLATIN, and these electrolyte abnormalities were rarely associated with symptoms.

Allergic reactions: Hypersensitivity to PARAPLATIN has been reported in 2% of the patients. These allergic reactions have been similar in nature and severity to those reported with other platinum-containing compounds, i.e., rash, urticaria, erythema, pruritus, and rarely bronchospasm and hypotension. These reactions have been successfully managed with standard epinephrine, corticosteroid and antihistamine therapy.

Other events: Pain and asthenia were the most frequently reported miscellaneous adverse effects; their relationship to the tumor and to anemia was likely. Alopecia was reported (3%). Cardiovascular, respiratory, genitourinary, and mucosal side effects have occurred in 6% or less of the patients. Cardiovascular events (cardiac failure, embolism, cerebrovascular accidents) were fatal in less than 1% of the patients and did not appear to be related to chemotherapy. Cancer-associated hemolytic uremic syndrome has been reported rarely.

OVERDOSAGE

There is no known antidote for PARAPLATIN overdosage. The anticipated complications of overdosage would be secondary to bone marrow suppression and/or hepatic toxicity.

DOSAGE AND ADMINISTRATION

NOTE: Aluminum reacts with carboplatin causing precipitate formation and loss of potency, therefore, needles or intravenous sets containing aluminum parts that may come in contact with the drug must not be used for the preparation or administration of PARAPLATIN.

Single agent therapy:
PARAPLATIN, as a single agent, has been shown to be effective in patients with recurrent ovarian carcinoma at a dosage of 360 mg/m² I.V. on day 1 every 4 weeks. (Alternatively see **Formula Dosing**.) In general, however, single intermittent courses of PARAPLATIN should not be repeated until the neutrophil count is at least 2,000 and the platelet count is at least 100,000.

Combination therapy with cyclophosphamide:
In the chemotherapy of advanced ovarian cancer, an effective combination for previously untreated patients consists of:
PARAPLATIN—300 mg/m² I.V. on day 1 every 4 weeks for six cycles. (Alternatively see **Formula Dosing**.)
Cyclophosphamide (Cytoxan®)—600 mg/m² I.V. on day 1 every 4 weeks for six cycles. For directions regarding the use and administration of cyclophosphamide (Cytoxan®) please refer to its package insert.
(See "CLINICAL STUDIES" section).
Intermittent courses of PARAPLATIN in combination with cyclophosphamide should not be repeated until the neutrophil count is at least 2,000 and the platelet count is at least 100,000.

Dose Adjustment Recommendations: Pretreatment platelet count and performance status are important prognostic factors for severity of myelosuppression in previously treated patients.
The suggested dose adjustments for single agent or combination therapy shown in the table below are modified from controlled trials in previously treated and untreated patients with ovarian carcinoma. Blood counts were done weekly, and the recommendations are based on the lowest post-treatment platelet or neutrophil value.

Platelets	Neutrophils	Adjusted Dose* (From Prior Course)
>100,000	>2,000	125%
50–100,000	500–2,000	No Adjustment
<50,000	<500	75%

* Percentages apply to PARAPLATIN as a single agent or to both PARAPLATIN and cyclophosphamide in combination. In the controlled studies, dosages were also adjusted at a lower level (50 to 60%) for severe myelosuppression. Escalations above 125% were not recommended for these studies.

PARAPLATIN is usually administered by an infusion lasting 15 minutes or longer. No pre- or post-treatment hydration or forced diuresis is required.

Patients with impaired kidney function: Patients with creatinine clearance values below 60 mL/min are at increased risk of severe bone marrow suppression. In renally-impaired patients who received single-agent PARAPLATIN therapy,

ADVERSE EXPERIENCES IN PATIENTS WITH OVARIAN CANCER SWOG STUDY

		Paraplatin Arm Percent*	Cisplatin Arm Percent*	P-Values**
Bone Marrow				
Thrombocytopenia,	<100,000/mm³	59	35	<0.001
	<50,000/mm³	22	11	0.006
Neutropenia,	<2,000 cells/mm³	95	97	n.s.
	<1,000 cells/mm³	84	78	n.s.
Leukopenia,	<4,000 cells/mm³	97	97	n.s.
	<2,000 cells/mm³	76	67	n.s.
Anemia,	<11 g/dL	88	87	n.s.
	<8 g/dL	8	24	<0.001
Infections		18	21	n.s.
Bleeding		6	4	n.s.
Transfusions		25	33	n.s.
Gastrointestinal				
Nausea and vomiting		94	96	n.s.
Vomiting		82	91	0.007
Other GI side effects		40	48	n.s.
Neurologic				
Peripheral neuropathies		13	28	0.001
Ototoxicity		12	30	<0.001
Other sensory side effects		4	6	n.s.
Central neurotoxicity		23	29	n.s.
Renal				
Serum creatinine elevations		7	38	<0.001
Blood urea elevations		—	—	—
Hepatic				
Bilirubin elevations		5	3	n.s.
SGOT elevations		23	16	n.s.
Alkaline phosphatase elevations		29	20	n.s.
Electrolytes loss				
Sodium		—	—	—
Potassium		—	—	—
Calcium		—	—	—
Magnesium		58	77	<0.001
Other side effects				
Pain		54	52	n.s.
Asthenia		43	46	n.s.
Cardiovascular		23	30	n.s.
Respiratory		12	11	n.s.
Allergic		10	11	n.s.
Genitourinary		11	13	n.s.
Alopecia+		43	57	0.009
Mucositis		6	11	n.s.

*Values are in percent of evaluable patients
**n.s. = not significant, p>0.05
+May have been affected by cyclophosphamide dosage delivered

the incidence of severe leukopenia, neutropenia, or thrombocytopenia has been about 25% when the dosage modifications in the table below have been used.

Baseline Creatinine Clearance	Recommended Dose on Day 1
41–59 mL/min	250 mg/m²
16–40 mL/min	200 mg/m²

The data available for patients with severely impaired kidney function (creatinine clearance below 15 mL/min) are too limited to permit a recommendation for treatment.[1,2]
These dosing recommendations apply to the initial course of treatment. Subsequent dosages should be adjusted according to the patient's tolerance based on the degree of bone marrow suppression.

Formula Dosing: Another approach for determining the initial dose of PARAPLATIN is the use of mathematical formulae, which are based on a patient's pre-existing renal function[3–4] or renal function and desired platelet nadir.[6] Renal excretion is the major route of elimination for carboplatin. (see CLINICAL PHARMACOLOGY). The use of dosing formulae, as compared to empirical dose calculation based on body surface area, allows compensation for patient variations in pretreatment renal function that might otherwise result in either underdosing (in patients with above average renal function) or overdosing (in patients with impaired renal function).
A simple formula for calculating dosage, based upon a patient's glomerular filtration rate (GFR in mL/min) and PARAPLATIN target area under the concentration versus time curve (AUC in mg/mL·min), has been proposed by Calvert[3–5]. In these studies, GFR was measured by ^{51}Cr-EDTA, which has a good correlation with creatinine clearance[7].

CALVERT FORMULA FOR CARBOPLATIN DOSING

Total Dose (mg) = (target AUC) × (GFR + 25)

Note: With the Calvert formula, the total dose of PARAPLATIN is calculated in mg, **not** mg/m².

The target AUC of 4–6 mg/mL·min using single agent PARAPLATIN appears to provide the most appropriate dose range in previously treated patients[4]. This study also showed a trend between the AUC of single agent PARAPLATIN administered to previously treated patients and the likelihood of developing toxicity[1].

	% Actual Toxicity in Previously Treated Patients	
AUC (mg/mL·min)	Gr 3 or Gr 4 Thrombocytopenia	Gr 3 or Gr 4 Leukopenia
4 to 5	16%	13%
6 to 7	33%	34%

PREPARATION OF INTRAVENOUS SOLUTIONS

Immediately before use, the content of each vial must be reconstituted with either Sterile Water for Injection, USP, 5% Dextrose in Water (D₅W), or 0.9% Sodium Chloride Injection, USP, according to the following schedule:

Vial Strength	Diluent Volume
50 mg	5 mL
150 mg	15 mL
450 mg	45 mL

These dilutions all produce a carboplatin concentration of 10 mg/mL.
PARAPLATIN can be further diluted to concentrations as low as 0.5 mg/mL with 5% Dextrose in Water (D₅W) or 0.9% Sodium Chloride Injection, USP.

STABILITY

Unopened vials of PARAPLATIN for Injection are stable for the life indicated on the package when stored at controlled room temperature 15°–30°C (59°–86°F), and protected from light.

When prepared as directed, PARAPLATIN solutions are stable for 8 hours at room temperature (25°C). Since no antibacterial preservative is contained in the formulation, it is

ADVERSE EXPERIENCES IN PATIENTS WITH OVARIAN CANCER

Bone Marrow		First Line Combination Therapy* Percent	Second Line Single Agent Therapy** Percent
Thrombocytopenia,	<100,000/mm³	66	62
	<50,000/mm³	33	35
Neutropenia,	<2,000 cells/mm³	96	67
	<1,000 cells/mm³	82	21
Leukopenia,	<4,000 cells/mm³	97	85
	<2,000 cells/mm³	71	26
Anemia,	<11 g/dL	90	90
	<8 g/dL	14	21
Infections		16	5
Bleeding		8	5
Transfusions		35	44
Gastrointestinal			
Nausea and vomiting		93	92
Vomiting		83	81
Other GI side effects		46	21
Neurologic			
Peripheral neuropathies		15	6
Ototoxicity		12	1
Other sensory side effects		5	1
Central neurotoxicity		26	5
Renal			
Serum creatinine elevations		6	10
Blood urea elevations		17	22
Hepatic			
Bilirubin elevations		5	5
SGOT elevations		20	19
Alkaline phosphatase elevations		29	37
Electrolytes loss			
Sodium		10	47
Potassium		16	28
Calcium		16	31
Magnesium		61	43
Other side effects			
Pain		44	23
Asthenia		41	11
Cardiovascular		19	6
Respiratory		10	6
Allergic		11	2
Genitourinary		10	2
Alopecia		49	2
Mucositis		8	1

* **Use with cyclophosphamide for initial treatment of ovarian cancer:** Data are based on the experience of 393 patients with ovarian cancer (regardless of baseline status) who received initial combination therapy with PARAPLATIN and cyclophosphamide in two randomized controlled studies conducted by SWOG and NCIC (see "CLINICAL STUDIES" section). Combination with cyclophosphamide as well as duration of treatment may be responsible for the differences that can be noted in the adverse experience table.

** **Single agent use for the secondary treatment of ovarian cancer:** Data are based on the experience of 553 patients with previously treated ovarian carcinoma (regardless of baseline status) who received single-agent PARAPLATIN.

recommended that PARAPLATIN solutions be discarded 8 hours after dilution.

Parenteral drug products should be inspected visually for particulate matter and discoloration prior to administration.

HOW SUPPLIED

NDC 0015-3213-30   50 mg vials, individually cartoned, shelf packs of 10 cartons, 10 shelf packs per case. (Yellow flip-off seals)

NDC 0015-3214-30   150 mg vials, individually cartoned, shelf packs of 10 cartons, 10 shelf packs per case. (Violet flip-off seals)

NDC 0015-3215-30   450 mg vials, individually cartoned, shelf packs of 6 cartons, 10 shelf packs per case. (Blue flip-off seals)

STORAGE

Store the unopened vials at controlled room temperature 15°–30°C (59°–86°F). Protect unopened vials from light. Solutions for infusion should be discarded 8 hours after preparation.

HANDLING AND DISPOSAL

Procedures for proper handling and disposal of anticancer drugs should be considered. Several guidelines on this subject have been published.[8–14] There is no general agreement that all of the procedures recommended in the guidelines are necessary or appropriate.

REFERENCES

1. Egorin, M.J., et al: Pharmacokinetics and dosage reduction of cis-diammine (1,1-cyclobutanedicarboxylato) platinum in patients with impaired renal function. *Cancer Res.* 1984; 44:5432–5438.
2. Carboplatin, Etoposide, and Bleomycin for Treatment of Stage IIC Seminoma Complicated by Acute Renal Failure. *Cancer Treatment Reports*, Vol. 71, No. 11, pp.1123–1124, November 1987.
3. Calvert AH, et al: Carboplatin dosage: Prospective evaluation of a simple formula based on renal function. *J Clin Oncol.* 1989; 7: 1748–1756.
4. Jodrell Dl, et al: Relationships between carboplatin exposure and tumor response and toxicity in patients with ovarian cancer. *J Clin Oncol.* 1992; 10:520–528.
5. Sorensen BT, et al: Dose-toxicity relationship of carboplatin in combination with cyclophosphamide in ovarian cancer patients. *Cancer Chemother Pharmacol.* 1991; 28:397–401.
6. Egorin MJ, et al: Prospective validation of a pharmacologically based dosing scheme for the cis-diamminedichloroplatinum (II) analogue diamminecyclobutanedicarboxylatoplatinum. *Cancer Res.* 1985; 45:6502–6506.
7. Daugaard G, et al: Effects of cisplatin on different measures of glomerular function in the human kidney with special emphasis on high-dose. *Cancer Chemother Pharmacol,* 1988; 21:163–167.
8. Recommendations for the Safe Handling of Parenteral Antineoplastic Drugs. NIH Publication No. 83–2621. For sale by the Superintendent of Documents, U.S. Government Printing Office, Washington, DC 20402.
9. AMA Council Report. Guidelines for Handling Parenteral Antineoplastics. *JAMA.* 1985; 253(11): 1590–1592.
10. National Study Commission on Cytotoxic Exposure—Recommendations for Handling Cytotoxic Agents. Available from Louis P. Jeffrey, ScD., Chairman, National Study Commission on Cytotoxic Exposure, Massachusetts College of Pharmacy and Allied Health Sciences, 179 Longwood Avenue, Boston, Massachusetts, 02115.
11. Clinical Oncological Society of Australia: Guidelines and Recommendations for Safe Handling of Antineoplastic Agents. *Med. J. Australia* 1983; 1:426–428.
12. Jones, R.B., et al: Safe Handling of Chemotherapeutic agents: A Report from the Mount Sinai Medical Center. *CA—A Cancer Journal for Clinicians*, 1983; (Sept/Oct) 258–263.
13. American Society of Hospital Pharmacists Technical Assistance Bulletin on Handling Cytotoxic and Hazardous Drugs. *Am. J. Hosp. Pharm.* 1990; 47:1033–1049.
14. OSHA Work-Practice Guidelines for Personnel Dealing with Cytotoxic (Antineoplastic) Drugs. *Am. J. Hosp. Pharm.* 1986; 43:1193–1204.

U.S. Patent Nos. 4,140,707
4,657,927

Shown in Product Identification Guide, page 307
(3213 DIM-08)
May 1995

PLATINOL®

[plă 'tĭ-nŏl ']
(cisplatin for injection, USP)

℞

> **WARNING**
>
> PLATINOL should be administered under the supervision of a qualified physician experienced in the use of cancer chemotherapeutic agents. Appropriate management of therapy and complications is possible only when adequate diagnostic and treatment facilities are readily available.
>
> Cumulative renal toxicity associated with PLATINOL is severe. Other major dose-related toxicities are myelosuppression, nausea, and vomiting.
>
> Ototoxicity, which may be more pronounced in children, and is manifested by tinnitus, and/or loss of high frequency hearing and occasionally deafness, is significant.
>
> *Anaphylactic-like* reactions to PLATINOL have been reported. Facial edema, bronchoconstriction, tachycardia, and hypotension may occur within minutes of PLATINOL administration. Epinephrine, corticosteroids, and antihistamines have been effectively employed to alleviate symptoms (see "**WARNINGS**" and "**ADVERSE REACTIONS**" sections).

DESCRIPTION

PLATINOL (cis-diamminedichloroplatinum) is a heavy metal complex containing a central atom of platinum surrounded by two chloride atoms and two ammonia molecules in the cis position. It is a white lyophilized powder with the molecular formula Pt $Cl_2H_6N_2$, and a molecular weight of 300.1. It is soluble in water or saline at 1 mg/mL and in dimethylformamide at 24 mg/mL. It has a melting point of 207°C.

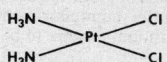

CLINICAL PHARMACOLOGY

Plasma concentrations of the parent compound, cisplatin, decay monoexponentially with a half-life of about 20 to 30 minutes following bolus administrations of 50 or 100 mg/m² doses. Monoexponential decay and plasma half-lives of about 0.5 hours are also seen following two hour or seven hour infusions of 100 mg/m². After the latter, the total-body clearances and volumes of distribution at steady-state for cisplatin are about 15 to 16 L/h/m² and 11 to 12 L/m².

Due to its unique chemical structure, the chlorine atoms of cisplatin are more subject to chemical displacement reactions by nucleophiles, such as water or sulfhydryl groups, than to enzyme-catalyzed metabolism. At physiological pH in the presence of 0.1M NaCl, the predominant molecular species are cisplatin and monohydroxymonochloro *cis*-diammine platinum (II) in nearly equal concentrations. The latter, combined with the possible direct displacement of the chlorine atoms by sulfhydryl groups of amino acids or proteins, accounts for the instability of cisplatin in biological matrices. The ratios of cisplatin to total free (ultrafilterable) platinum in the plasma vary considerably between patients and range from 0.5 to 1.1 after a dose of 100 mg/m².

Cisplatin does not undergo the instantaneous and reversible binding to plasma proteins that is characteristic of normal drug-protein binding. However, the platinum from cisplatin, but not cisplatin itself, becomes bound to several plasma proteins including albumin, transferrin, and gamma globulin. Three hours after a bolus injection and two hours after the end of a three-hour infusion, 90% of the plasma platinum is protein bound. The complexes between albumin and the

Continued on next page

Bristol-Myers Squibb Oncology—Cont.

platinum from cisplatin do not dissociate to a significant extent and are slowly eliminated with a minimum half-life of five days or more.

Following cisplatin doses of 20 to 120 mg/m², the concentrations of platinum are highest in liver, prostate, and kidney, somewhat lower in bladder, muscle, testicle, pancreas, and spleen and lowest in bowel, adrenal, heart, lung, cerebrum, and cerebellum. Platinum is present in tissues for as long as 180 days after the last administration. With the exception of intracerebral tumors, platinum concentrations in tumors are generally somewhat lower than the concentrations in the organ where the tumor is located. Different metastatic sites in the same patient may have different platinum concentrations. Hepatic metastases have the highest platinum concentrations, but these are similar to the platinum concentrations in normal liver. Maximum red blood cell concentrations of platinum are reached within 90 to 150 minutes after a 100 mg/m² dose of cisplatin and decline in a biphasic manner with a terminal half-life to 36 to 47 days.

Over a dose range of 40 to 140 mg cisplatin/m² given as a bolus injection or as infusions varying in length from 1 hour to 24 hours, from 10% to about 40% of the administered platinum is excreted in the urine in 24 hours. Over five days following administration of 40 to 100 mg/m² doses given as rapid, 2 to 3 hours, or 6 to 8 hour infusions, a mean of 35% to 51% of the dosed platinum is excreted in the urine. Similar mean urinary recoveries of platinum of about 14% to 30% of the dose are found following five daily administrations of 20, 30, or 40 mg/m² day. Only a small percentage of the administered platinum is excreted beyond 24 hours post-infusion and most of the platinum excreted in the urine in 24 hours is excreted within the first few hours. Platinum-containing species excreted in the urine are the same as those found following the incubation of cisplatin with urine from healthy subjects, except that the proportions are different.

The parent compound, cisplatin, is excreted in the urine and accounts for 13% to 17% of the dose excreted within one hour after administration of 50 mg/m². The mean renal clearance of cisplatin exceeds creatinine clearance and is 62 and 50 mL/min/m² following administration of 100 mg/m² as 2 hour or 6 to 7 hour infusions, respectively.

The renal clearance of free (ultrafilterable) platinum also exceeds the glomerular filtration rate indicating that cisplatin or other platinum-containing molecules are actively secreted by the kidneys. The renal clearance of free platinum is nonlinear and variable and is dependent on dose, urine flow rate, and individual variability in the extent of active secretion and possible tubular reabsorption.

There is a potential for accumulation of ultrafilterable platinum plasma concentrations whenever cisplatin is administered on a daily basis but not when dosed on an intermittent basis.

No significant relationships exist between the renal clearance of either free platinum or cisplatin and creatinine clearance.

Although small amounts of platinum are present in the bile and large intestine after administration of cisplatin, the fecal excretion of platinum appears to be insignificant.

INDICATIONS

PLATINOL is indicated as therapy to be employed as follows:

Metastatic Testicular Tumors—In established combination therapy with other approved chemotherapeutic agents in patients with metastatic testicular tumors who have already received appropriate surgical and/or radiotherapeutic procedures.

Metastatic Ovarian Tumors—In established combination therapy with other approved chemotherapeutic agents in patients with metastatic ovarian tumors who have already received appropriate surgical and/or radiotherapeutic procedures. An established combination consists of PLATINOL and Cytoxan® (cyclophosphamide). PLATINOL, as a single agent, is indicated as secondary therapy in patients with metastatic ovarian tumors refractory to standard chemotherapy who have not previously received PLATINOL therapy.

Advanced Bladder Cancer—PLATINOL is indicated as a single agent for patients with transitional cell bladder cancer which is no longer amenable to local treatments such as surgery and/or radiotherapy.

CONTRAINDICATIONS

PLATINOL is contraindicated in patients with preexisting renal impairment. PLATINOL should not be employed in myelosuppressed patients, or patients with hearing impairment.

PLATINOL is contraindicated in patients with a history of allergic reactions to PLATINOL or other platinum-containing compounds.

WARNINGS

PLATINOL produces cumulative nephrotoxicity which is potentiated by aminoglycoside antibiotics. The serum creati-

nine, BUN, creatinine clearance, and magnesium, sodium, potassium and calcium levels should be measured prior to initiating therapy, and prior to each subsequent course. At the recommended dosage, PLATINOL should not be given more frequently than once every 3 to 4 weeks (see "ADVERSE REACTIONS").

There are reports of severe neuropathies in patients in whom regimens are employed using higher doses of PLATINOL or greater dose frequencies than those recommended. These neuropathies may be irreversible and are seen as paresthesias in a stocking-glove distribution, areflexia, and loss of proprioception and vibratory sensation.

Loss of motor function has also been reported.

Anaphylactic-like reactions to PLATINOL have been reported. These reactions have occurred within minutes of administration to patients with prior exposure to PLATINOL, and have been alleviated by administration of epinephrine, corticosteroids, and antihistamines.

Since ototoxicity of PLATINOL is cumulative, audiometric testing should be performed prior to initiating therapy and prior to each subsequent dose of drug (see "ADVERSE REACTIONS").

PLATINOL can cause fetal harm when administered to a pregnant woman. PLATINOL is mutagenic in bacteria and produces chromosome aberrations in animal cells in tissue culture. In mice PLATINOL is teratogenic and embryotoxic. If this drug is used during pregnancy or if the patient becomes pregnant while taking this drug, the patient should be apprised of the potential hazard to the fetus. Patients should be advised to avoid becoming pregnant.

The carcinogenic effect of PLATINOL was studied in BD IX rats. PLATINOL was administered i.p. to 50 BD IX rats for 3 weeks, 3 X 1 mg/kg body weight per week. Four hundred and fifty-five days after the first application, 33 animals died, 13 of them related to malignancies: 12 leukemias and 1 renal fibrosarcoma.

The development of acute leukemia coincident with the use of PLATINOL has rarely been reported in humans. In these reports, PLATINOL was generally given in combination with other leukemogenic agents.

PRECAUTIONS

Peripheral blood counts should be monitored weekly. Liver function should be monitored periodically. Neurologic examination should also be performed regularly (see "ADVERSE REACTIONS").

Drug Interactions—Plasma levels of anticonvulsant agents may become subtherapeutic during cisplatin therapy.

In a randomized trial in advanced ovarian cancer, response duration was adversely affected when pyridoxine was used in combination with altretamine (hexamethylmelamine) and PLATINOL.[1]

Carcinogenesis, Mutagenesis, Impairment of Fertility—see "WARNINGS" section.

Pregnancy—Pregnancy "Category D". (See "WARNINGS" section.)

ADVERSE REACTIONS

Nephrotoxicity—Dose-related and cumulative renal insufficiency is the major dose-limiting toxicity of PLATINOL® (cisplatin for injection, USP). Renal toxicity has been noted in 28% to 36% of patients treated with a single dose of 50 mg/m². It is first noted during the second week after a dose and is manifested by elevations in BUN and creatinine, serum uric acid and/or a decrease in creatinine clearance. **Renal toxicity becomes more prolonged and severe with repeated courses of the drug. Renal function must return to normal before another dose of PLATINOL can be given.**

Impairment of renal function has been associated with renal tubular damage. The administration of PLATINOL using a 6- to 8-hour infusion with intravenous hydration, and mannitol has been used to reduce nephrotoxicity. However, renal toxicity still can occur after utilization of these procedures.

Ototoxicity—Ototoxicity has been observed in up to 31% of patients treated with a single dose of PLATINOL 50 mg/m², and is manifested by tinnitus and/or hearing loss in the high frequency range (4,000 to 8,000 Hz). Decreased ability to hear normal conversational tones may occur occasionally. Deafness after the initial dose of PLATINOL has been reported rarely. Ototoxic effects may be more severe in children receiving PLATINOL. Hearing loss can be unilateral or bilateral and tends to become more frequent and severe with repeated doses. Ototoxicity may be enhanced with prior or simultaneous cranial irradiation. It is unclear whether PLATINOL-induced ototoxicity is reversible. Ototoxic effects may be related to the peak plasma concentration of PLATINOL. Careful monitoring of audiometry should be performed prior to initiation of therapy and prior to subsequent doses of PLATINOL.

Vestibular toxicity has also been reported.

Ototoxicity may become more severe in patients being treated with other drugs with nephrotoxic potential.

Hematologic—Myelosuppression occurs in 25% to 30% of patients treated with PLATINOL. The nadirs in circulating platelets and leukocytes occur between days 18 to 23 (range 7.5 to 45) with most patients recovering by day 39 (range 13

to 62). Leukopenia and thrombocytopenia are more pronounced at higher doses (> 50 mg/m²). Anemia (decrease of 2 g hemoglobin/100 mL) occurs at approximately the same frequency and with the same timing as leukopenia and thrombocytopenia. Fever and infection have been reported in patients with neutropenia.

In addition to anemia secondary to myelosuppression, a Coombs' positive hemolytic anemia has been reported. In the presence of cisplatin hemolytic anemia, a further course of treatment may be accompanied by increased hemolysis and this risk should be weighed by the treating physician.

The development of acute leukemia coincident with the use of PLATINOL has rarely been reported in humans. In these reports, PLATINOL was generally given in combination with other leukemogenic agents.

Gastrointestinal—Marked nausea and vomiting occur in almost all patients treated with PLATINOL, and are occasionally so severe that the drug must be discontinued. Nausea and vomiting usually begin within 1 to 4 hours after treatment and last up to 24 hours. Various degrees of vomiting, nausea and/or anorexia may persist for up to 1 week after treatment.

Delayed nausea and vomiting (begins or persists 24 hours or more after chemotherapy) has occurred in patients attaining complete emetic control on the day of PLATINOL therapy. Diarrhea has also been reported.

OTHER TOXICITIES

Vascular toxicities coincident with the use of PLATINOL in combination with other antineoplastic agents have been reported rarely. The events are clinically heterogeneous and may include myocardial infarction, cerebrovascular accident, thrombotic microangiopathy (HUS), or cerebral arteritis. Various mechanisms have been proposed for these vascular complications. There are also reports of Raynaud's phenomenon occurring in patients treated with the combination of bleomycin, vinblastine with or without PLATINOL. It has been suggested that hypomagnesemia developing coincident with the use of PLATINOL may be an added, although not essential, factor associated with this event. However, it is currently unknown if the cause of Raynaud's phenomenon in these cases is the disease, underlying vascular compromise, bleomycin, vinblastine, hypomagnesemia, or a combination of any of these factors.

Serum Electrolyte Disturbances—Hypomagnesemia, hypocalcemia, hyponatremia, hypokalemia and hypophosphatemia have been reported to occur in patients treated with PLATINOL and are probably related to renal tubular damage. Tetany has occasionally been reported in those patients with hypocalcemia and hypomagnesemia. Generally, normal serum electrolyte levels are restored by administering supplemental electrolytes and discontinuing PLATINOL.

Inappropriate antidiuretic hormone syndrome has also been reported.

Hyperuricemia—Hyperuricemia has been reported to occur at approximately the same frequency as the increases in BUN and serum creatinine.

It is more pronounced after doses greater than 50 mg/m², and peak levels of uric acid generally occur between 3 to 5 days after the dose. Allopurinol therapy for hyperuricemia effectively reduces uric acid levels.

Neurotoxicity (see "WARNINGS" section)—Neurotoxicity, usually characterized by peripheral neuropathies, has been reported. The neuropathies usually occur after prolonged therapy (4 to 7 months); however, neurologic symptoms have been reported to occur after a single dose. Although symptoms and signs of PLATINOL neuropathy usually develop during treatment, symptoms of neuropathy may begin 3 to 8 weeks after the last dose of PLATINOL, although this is rare. PLATINOL therapy should be discontinued when the symptoms are first observed. The neuropathy, however, may progress further even after stopping treatment. Preliminary evidence suggests peripheral neuropathy may be irreversible in some patients.

Lhermitte's sign, dorsal column myelopathy, and autonomic neuropathy have also been reported.

Loss of taste and seizures have also been reported.

Muscle cramps, defined as localized, painful, involuntary skeletal muscle contractions of sudden onset and short duration, have been reported and were usually associated in patients receiving a relatively high cumulative dose of PLATINOL and with a relatively advanced symptomatic stage of peripheral neuropathy.

Ocular Toxicity—Optic neuritis, papilledema, and cerebral blindness have been reported infrequently in patients receiving standard recommended doses of PLATINOL. Improvement and/or total recovery usually occurs after discontinuing PLATINOL. Steroids with or without mannitol have been used; however, efficacy has not been established.

Blurred vision and altered color perception have been reported after the use of regimens with higher doses of PLATINOL or greater dose frequencies than those recommended in the package insert. The altered color perception manifests as a loss of color discrimination, particularly in the blue-yellow axis. The only finding on funduscopic exam is irregular retinal pigmentation of the macular area.

Anaphylactic-like Reactions—Anaphylactic-like reactions have been occasionally reported in patients previously exposed to PLATINOL. The reactions consist of facial edema, wheezing, tachycardia, and hypotension within a few minutes of drug administration. Reactions may be controlled by intravenous epinephrine with corticosteroids and/or antihistamines as indicated. Patients receiving PLATINOL should be observed carefully for possible anaphylactic-like reactions and supportive equipment and medication should be available to treat such a complication.

Hepatotoxicity—Transient elevations of liver enzymes, especially SGOT, as well as bilirubin, have been reported to be associated with PLATINOL administration at the recommended doses.

Other Events—Other toxicities reported to occur infrequently are cardiac abnormalities, hiccups, elevated serum amylase, and rash. Alopecia has also been reported.

Local soft tissue toxicity has rarely been reported following extravasation of PLATINOL. Severity of the local tissue toxicity appears to be related to the concentration of the PLATINOL solution. Infusion of solutions with a PLATINOL concentration greater than 0.5 mg/mL may result in tissue cellulitis, fibrosis, and necrosis.

OVERDOSAGE

Caution should be exercised to prevent inadvertent overdosage with PLATINOL. Acute overdosage with this drug may result in kidney failure, liver failure, deafness, ocular toxicity (including detachment of the retina), significant myelosuppression, intractable nausea and vomiting and/or neuritis. In addition, death can occur following overdosage.

No proven antidotes have been established for PLATINOL overdosage. Hemodialysis, even when initiated four hours after the overdosage, appears to have little effect on removing platinum from the body because of PATINOL's rapid and high degree of protein binding. Management of overdosage should include general supportive measures to sustain the patient through any period of toxicity that may occur.

DOSAGE AND ADMINISTRATION

Note: Needles or intravenous sets containing aluminum parts that may come in contact with PLATINOL® (cisplatin for injection, USP) should not be used for preparation or administration. Aluminum reacts with PLATINOL, causing precipitate formation and a loss of potency.

Metastatic Testicular Tumors—The usual PLATINOL dose for the treatment of testicular cancer in combination with other approved chemotherapeutic agents is 20 mg/m^2 IV daily for a 5 day cycle.

Metastatic Ovarian Tumors—The usual PLATINOL dose for the treatment of metastatic ovarian tumors in combination with Cytoxan is 75–100 mg/m^2 IV per cycle once every 4 weeks, (Day 1).[2,3]

The dose of Cytoxan when used in combination with PLATINOL is 600 mg/m^2 IV once every 4 weeks, (Day 1).[2,3]

For directions for the administration of Cytoxan refer to the Cytoxan package insert.

In combination therapy, PLATINOL and Cytoxan are administered sequentially.

As a single agent, PLATINOL should be administered at a dose of 100 mg/m^2 IV per cycle once every 4 weeks.

Advanced Bladder Cancer—PLATINOL should be administered as a single agent at a dose of 50 to 70 mg/m^2 IV per cycle once every 3 to 4 weeks depending on the extent of prior exposure to radiation therapy and/or prior chemotherapy. For heavily pretreated patients an initial dose of 50 mg/m^2 per cycle repeated every 4 weeks is recommended.

Pretreatment hydration with 1 to 2 liters of fluid infused for 8 to 12 hours prior to a PLATINOL dose is recommended. The drug is then diluted in 2 liters of 5% Dextrose in ½ or ⅓ normal saline containing 37.5 g of mannitol, and infused over a 6- to 8-hour period. If diluted solution is not to be used within 6 hours, protect solution from light. Adequate hydration and urinary output must be maintained during the following 24 hours.

A repeat course of PLATINOL should not be given until the serum creatinine is below 1.5 mg/100 mL, and/or the BUN is below 25 mg/100 mL. A repeat course should not be given until circulating blood elements are at an acceptable level (platelets $\geq$100,000/mm^3, WBC $\geq$4,000/mm^3). Subsequent doses of PLATINOL should not be given until an audiometric analysis indicates that auditory acuity is within normal limits.

As with other potentially toxic compounds, caution should be exercised in handling the powder and preparing the solution of cisplatin. Skin reactions associated with accidental exposure to cisplatin may occur. The use of gloves is recommended. If cisplatin powder or solution contacts the skin or mucosae, immediately wash the skin or mucosae thoroughly with soap and water.

PREPARATION OF INTRAVENOUS SOLUTIONS

The 10 and 50 mg vials should be reconstituted with 10 mL or 50 mL of Sterile Water for Injection, USP, respectively. Each mL of the resulting solution will contain 1 mg of PLATINOL. Reconstitution as recommended results in a clear, colorless solution.

The reconstituted solution should be used intravenously only and should be administered by IV infusion over a 6- to 8-hour period. (See "**DOSAGE AND ADMINISTRATION.**")

NOTE TO PHARMACIST: Exercise caution to prevent inadvertent PLATINOL overdosage. Please call prescriber if dose greater than 100 mg/m^2 per cycle. Aluminum and flip-off seal of vial have been imprinted with the following statement: **CALL DR. IF DOSE > 100 MG/M²/CYCLE.**

STABILITY

Unopened vials of dry powder are stable for the lot life indicated on the package when stored at room temperature (27°C).

The reconstituted solution is stable for 20 hours at room temperature (27°C). Solution removed from the amber vial should be protected from light if it is not to be used within 6 hours.

Important note: Once reconstituted, the solution should be kept at room temperature (27°C). If the reconstituted solution is refrigerated, a precipitate will form.

Procedures for proper handling and disposal of anticancer drugs should be considered. Several guidelines on this subject have been published.[4–10] There is no general agreement that all of the procedures recommended in the guidelines are necessary or appropriate.

HOW SUPPLIED

PLATINOL (cisplatin for injection, USP)

NDC 0015-3070-20—Each amber vial contains 10 mg of cisplatin.

NDC 0015-3072-20—Each amber vial contains 50 mg of cisplatin.

REFERENCES

1. Wiernik PH: Hexamethylmelamine and Low or Moderate Dose Cisplatin With or Without Pyridoxine for Treatment of Advanced Ovarian Carcinoma: A Study of the Eastern Oncology Group. Cancer Invest. 1992; 10:1–9.
2. Alberts DS, et al: Improved Therapeutic Index of Carboplatin Plus Cyclophosphamide versus Cisplatin Plus Cyclophosphamide: Final Report by the Southwest Oncology Group of a Phase III Randomized Trial in Stages III and IV Ovarian Cancer. *J Clin Oncol.* 1992; 10:706–717.
3. Swenerton K, et al: Cisplatin-Cyclophosphamide versus Carboplatin-Cyclophosphamide in Advanced Ovarian Cancer: A Randomized Phase III Study of the National Cancer Institute of Canada Clinical Trials Group. *J Clin Oncol.* 1992; 10:718–726.
4. Recommendations for the Safe Handling of Parenteral Antineoplastic Drugs. NIH Publication No. 83-2621. For sale by the Superintendent of Documents. US Government Printing Office, Washington, D.C. 20402.
5. AMA Council Report. Guidelines for Handling Parenteral Antineoplastics. *JAMA.* 1985; 253(II):1590–1592.
6. National Study Commission on Cytotoxic Exposure—Recommendations for Handling Cytotoxic Agents. Available from Louis P. Jeffrey, ScD, Chairman, National Study Commission on Cytotoxic Exposure, Massachusetts College of Pharmacy and Allied Health Sciences, 179 Longwood Avenue, Boston, Massachusetts 02115.
7. Clinical Oncological Society of Australia. Guidelines and Recommendations for Safe Handling of Antineoplastic Agents. *Med J Australia.* 1983;1:426–428.
8. Jones RB, et al: Safe Handling of Chemotherapeutic Agents: A Report from the Mount Sinai Medical Center. *CA—A Cancer Journal for Clinicians.* 1983; (Sept/Oct);258–263.
9. American Society of Hospital Pharmacists Technical Assistance Bulletin on Handling Cytotoxic and Hazardous Drugs. *Am J Hosp Pharm.* 1990;47:1033–1049.
10. OSHA Work-Practice Guidelines for Personnel Dealing with Cytotoxic (Antineoplastic) Drugs. *Am J Hosp Pharm.* 1986;43:1193–1204.

(3070 DIM-36)
December 1994

PLATINOL®-AQ ℞

[*pla-ti-nol -AQ*]
(cisplatin injection, USP)

WARNING

PLATINOL should be administered under the supervision of a qualified physician experienced in the use of cancer chemotherapeutic agents. Appropriate management of therapy and complications is possible only when adequate diagnostic and treatment facilities are readily available.

Cumulative renal toxicity associated with PLATINOL is severe. Other major dose-related toxicities are myelosuppression, nausea, and vomiting.

Ototoxicity, which may be more pronounced in children, and is manifested by tinnitus, and/or loss of high frequency hearing and occasionally deafness, is significant.

Anaphylactic-like reactions to PLATINOL have been reported. Facial edema, bronchoconstriction, tachycardia, and hypotension may occur within minutes of PLATINOL administration. Epinephrine, corticosteroids, and antihistamines have been effectively employed to alleviate symptoms (see "**WARNINGS**" and "**ADVERSE REACTIONS**" sections).

DESCRIPTION

Cisplatin (cis-diamminedichloroplatinum) is a heavy metal complex containing a central atom of platinum surrounded by two chloride atoms and two ammonia molecules in the cis position. It is a white powder with the molecular formula $PtCl_2H_6N_2$, and a molecular weight of 300.1. It is soluble in water or saline at 1 mg/mL and in dimethylformamide at 24 mg/mL. It has a melting point of 207°C. PLATINOL-AQ is a sterile aqueous solution, each mL containing 1 mg cisplatin and 9 mg sodium chloride. HCl and/or sodium hydroxide added to adjust pH.

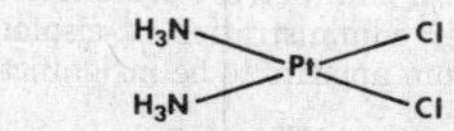

CLINICAL PHARMACOLOGY

Plasma concentrations of the parent compound, cisplatin, decay monoexponentially with a half-life of about 20 to 30 minutes following bolus administrations of 50 or 100 mg/m^2 doses. Monoexponential decay and plasma half-lives of about 0.5 hour are also seen following two hour or seven hour infusions of 100 mg/m^2. After the latter, the total-body clearances and volumes of distribution at steady-state for cisplatin are about 15 to 16 L/h/m^2 and 11 to 12 L/m^2.

Due to its unique chemical structure, the chlorine atoms of cisplatin are more subject to chemical displacement reactions by nucleophiles, such as water or sulfhydryl groups, than to enzyme-catalyzed metabolism. At physiological pH in the presence of 0.1M NaCl, the predominant molecular species are cisplatin and monohydroxymonochloro *cis*-diammine platinum (II) in nearly equal concentrations. The latter, combined with the possible direct displacement of the chlorine atoms by sulfhydryl groups of amino acids or proteins, accounts for the instability of cisplatin in biological matrices. The ratios of cisplatin to total free (ultrafilterable) platinum in the plasma vary considerably between patients and range from 0.5 to 1.1 after a dose of 100 mg/m^2.

Cisplatin does not undergo the instantaneous and reversible binding to plasma proteins that is characteristic of normal drug-protein binding. However, the platinum from cisplatin, but not cisplatin itself, becomes bound to several plasma proteins including albumin, transferrin, and gamma globulin. Three hours after a bolus injection and two hours after the end of a three-hour infusion, 90% of the plasma platinum is protein bound. The complexes between albumin and the platinum from cisplatin do not dissociate to a significant extent and are slowly eliminated with a minimum half-life of five days or more.

Following cisplatin doses of 20 to 120 mg/m^2, the concentrations of platinum are highest in liver, prostate, and kidney, somewhat lower in bladder, muscle, testicle, pancreas, and spleen and lowest in bowel, adrenal, heart, lung, cerebrum, and cerebellum. Platinum is present in tissues for as long as 180 days after the last administration. With the exception of intracerebral tumors, platinum concentrations in tumors are generally somewhat lower than the concentrations in the organ where the tumor is located. Different metastatic sites in the same patient may have different platinum concentrations. Hepatic metastases have the highest platinum concentrations, but these are similar to the platinum concentrations in normal liver. Maximum red blood cell concentrations of platinum are reached within 90 to 150 minutes after a 100 mg/m^2 dose of cisplatin and decline in a biphasic manner with a terminal half-life of 36 to 47 days.

Over a dose range of 40 to 140 mg cisplatin/m^2 given as a bolus injection or as infusions varying in length from 1 hour to 24 hours, from 10% to about 40% of the administered platinum is excreted in the urine in 24 hours. Over five days following administration of 40 to 100 mg/m^2 doses given as rapid, 2 to 3 hour, or 6 to 8 hour infusions, a mean of 35% to 51% of the dosed platinum is excreted in the urine. Similar mean urinary recoveries of platinum of about 14% to 30% of the dose are found following five daily administrations of 20, 30, or 40 mg/m^2/day. Only a small percentage of the administered platinum is excreted beyond 24 hours post-infusion and most of the platinum excreted in the urine in 24 hours is excreted within the first few hours. Platinum-containing species excreted in the urine are the same as those found

Continued on next page

Bristol-Myers Squibb Oncology—Cont.

following the incubation of cisplatin with urine from healthy subjects, except that the proportions are different.
The parent compound, cisplatin, is excreted in the urine and accounts for 13% to 17% of the dose excreted within one hour after administration of 50 mg/m^2. The mean renal clearance of cisplatin exceeds creatinine clearance and is 62 and 50 mL/min/m^2 following administration of 100 mg/m^2 as 2 hour or 6 to 7 hour infusions, respectively.
The renal clearance of free (ultrafilterable) platinum also exceeds the glomerular filtration rate indicating that cisplatin or other platinum-containing molecules are actively secreted by the kidneys. The renal clearance of free platinum is nonlinear and variable and is dependent on dose, urine flow rate, and individual variability in the extent of active secretion and possible tubular reabsorption.
There is a potential for accumulation of ultrafilterable platinum plasma concentrations whenever cisplatin is administered on a daily basis but not when dosed on an intermittent basis.
No significant relationships exist between the renal clearance of either free platinum or cisplatin and creatinine clearance.
Although small amounts of platinum are present in the bile and large intestine after administration of cisplatin, the fecal excretion of platinum appears to be insignificant.

INDICATIONS

PLATINOL is indicated as therapy to be employed as follows:
Metastatic Testicular Tumors—In established combination therapy with other approved chemotherapeutic agents in patients with metastatic testicular tumors who have already received appropriate surgical and/or radiotherapeutic procedures.
Metastatic Ovarian Tumors—In established combination therapy with other approved chemotherapeutic agents in patients with metastatic ovarian tumors who have already received appropriate surgical and/or radiotherapeutic procedures. An established combination consists of PLATINOL-AQ and Cytoxan® (cyclophosphamide). PLATINOL, as a single agent, is indicated as secondary therapy in patients with metastatic ovarian tumors refractory to standard chemotherapy who have not previously received PLATINOL therapy.
Advanced Bladder Cancer—PLATINOL is indicated as a single agent for patients with transitional cell bladder cancer which is no longer amenable to local treatments such as surgery and/or radiotherapy.

CONTRAINDICATIONS

PLATINOL is contraindicated in patients with preexisting renal impairment. PLATINOL should not be employed in myelosuppressed patients, or patients with hearing impairment.
PLATINOL is contraindicated in patients with a history of allergic reactions to PLATINOL or other platinum-containing compounds.

WARNINGS

PLATINOL produces cumulative nephrotoxicity which is potentiated by aminoglycoside antibiotics. The serum creatinine, BUN, creatinine clearance, and magnesium, sodium, potassium, and calcium levels should be measured prior to initiating therapy, and prior to each subsequent course. At the recommended dosage, PLATINOL should not be given more frequently than once every 3 to 4 weeks (see "**ADVERSE REACTIONS**").
There are reports of severe neuropathies in patients in whom regimens are employed using higher doses of PLATINOL or greater dose frequencies than those recommended. These neuropathies may be irreversible and are seen as paresthesias in a stocking-glove distribution, areflexia, and loss of proprioception and vibratory sensation.
Loss of motor function has also been reported.
Anaphylactic-like reactions to PLATINOL have been reported. These reactions have occurred within minutes of administration to patients with prior exposure to PLATINOL, and have been alleviated by administration of epinephrine, corticosteroids, and antihistamines.
Since ototoxicity of PLATINOL is cumulative, audiometric testing should be performed prior to initiating therapy and prior to each subsequent dose of drug (see "**ADVERSE REACTIONS**").
PLATINOL can cause fetal harm when administered to a pregnant woman. PLATINOL is mutagenic in bacteria and produces chromosome aberrations in animal cells in tissue culture. In mice PLATINOL is teratogenic and embryotoxic. If this drug is used during pregnancy or if the patient becomes pregnant while taking this drug, the patient should be apprised of the potential hazard to the fetus. Patients should be advised to avoid becoming pregnant.
The carcinogenic effect of PLATINOL was studied in BD IX rats. PLATINOL was administered i.p. to 50 BD IX rats for 3 weeks, 3 X 1 mg/kg body weight per week. Four hundred and fifty-five days after the first application, 33 animals died, 13 of them related to malignancies: 12 leukemias and 1 renal fibrosarcoma.
The development of acute leukemia coincident with the use of PLATINOL has rarely been reported in humans. In these reports, PLATINOL was generally given in combination with other leukemogenic agents.

PRECAUTIONS

Peripheral blood counts should be monitored weekly. Liver function should be monitored periodically. Neurologic examination should also be performed regularly (see "**ADVERSE REACTIONS**").
Drug Interactions—Plasma levels of anticonvulsant agents may become subtherapeutic during cisplatin therapy.
In a randomized trial in advanced ovarian cancer, response duration was adversely affected when pyridoxine was used in combination with altretamine (hexamethylmelamine) and PLATINOL.[1]
Carcinogenesis, Mutagenesis, Impairment of Fertility—see "**WARNINGS**" section.
Pregnancy—Pregnancy "Category D". (See "**WARNINGS**" section.)

ADVERSE REACTIONS

Nephrotoxicity—Dose-related and cumulative renal insufficiency is the major dose-limiting toxicity of PLATINOL. Renal toxicity has been noted in 28% to 36% of patients treated with a single dose of 50 mg/m^2. It is first noted during the second week after a dose and is manifested by elevations in BUN and creatinine, serum uric acid, and/or a decrease in creatinine clearance. **Renal toxicity becomes more prolonged and severe with repeated courses of the drug. Renal function must return to normal before another dose of PLATINOL can be given.**
Impairment of renal function has been associated with renal tubular damage. The administration of PLATINOL using a 6- to 8-hour infusion with intravenous hydration, and mannitol has been used to reduce nephrotoxicity. However, renal toxicity still can occur after utilization of these procedures.
Ototoxicity—Ototoxicity has been observed in up to 31% of patients treated with a single dose of PLATINOL 50 mg/m^2, and is manifested by tinnitus and/or hearing loss in the high frequency range (4,000 to 8,000 Hz). Decreased ability to hear normal conversational tones may occur occasionally. Deafness after the initial dose of PLATINOL has been reported rarely. Ototoxic effects may be more severe in children receiving PLATINOL. Hearing loss can be unilateral or bilateral and tends to become more frequent and severe with repeated doses. Ototoxicity may be enhanced with prior or simultaneous cranial irradiation. It is unclear whether PLATINOL-induced ototoxicity is reversible. Ototoxic effects may be related to the peak plasma concentration of PLATINOL. Careful monitoring of audiometry should be performed prior to initiation of therapy and prior to subsequent doses of PLATINOL.
Vestibular toxicity has also been reported.
Ototoxicity may become more severe in patients being treated with other drugs with nephrotoxic potential.
Hematologic—Myelosuppression occurs in 25% to 30% of patients treated with PLATINOL. The nadirs in circulating platelets and leukocytes occur between days 18 to 23 (range 7.5 to 45) with most patients recovering by day 39 (range 13 to 62). Leukopenia and thrombocytopenia are more pronounced at higher doses ($>$ 50 mg/m^2). Anemia (decrease of 2 g hemoglobin/100 mL) occurs at approximately the same frequency and with the same timing as leukopenia and thrombocytopenia. Fever and infection have also been reported in patients with neutropenia.
In addition to anemia secondary to myelosuppression, a Coombs' positive hemolytic anemia has been reported. In the presence of cisplatin hemolytic anemia, a further course of treatment may be accompanied by increased hemolysis and this risk should be weighed by the treating physician.
The development of acute leukemia coincident with the use of PLATINOL has rarely been reported in humans. In these reports, PLATINOL was generally given in combination with other leukemogenic agents.
Gastrointestinal—Marked nausea and vomiting occur in almost all patients treated with PLATINOL, and are occasionally so severe that the drug must be discontinued. Nausea and vomiting usually begin within 1 to 4 hours after treatment and last up to 24 hours. Various degrees of vomiting, nausea and/or anorexia may persist for up to 1 week after treatment.
Delayed nausea and vomiting (begins or persists 24 hours or more after chemotherapy) has occurred in patients attaining complete emetic control on the day of PLATINOL therapy.
Diarrhea has also been reported.

OTHER TOXICITIES

Vascular toxicities coincident with the use of PLATINOL in combination with other antineoplastic agents have been reported rarely. The events are clinically heterogeneous and may include myocardial infarction, cerebrovascular accident, thrombotic microangiopathy (HUS), or cerebral arteritis. Various mechanisms have been proposed for these vascular complications. There are also reports of Raynaud's phenomenon occurring in patients treated with the combination of bleomycin, vinblastine with or without PLATINOL. It has been suggested that hypomagnesemia developing coincident with the use of PLATINOL may be an added, although not essential, factor associated with this event. However, it is currently unknown if the cause of Raynaud's phenomenon in these cases is the disease, underlying vascular compromise, bleomycin, vinblastine, hypomagnesemia, or a combination of any of these factors.
Serum Electrolyte Disturbances—Hypomagnesemia, hypocalcemia, hyponatremia, hypokalemia and hypophosphatemia have been reported to occur in patients treated with PLATINOL and are probably related to renal tubular damage. Tetany has occasionally been reported in those patients with hypocalcemia and hypomagnesemia. Generally, normal serum electrolyte levels are restored by administering supplemental electrolytes and discontinuing PLATINOL.
Inappropriate antidiuretic hormone syndrome has also been reported.
Hyperuricemia—Hyperuricemia has been reported to occur at approximately the same frequency as the increases in BUN and serum creatinine.
It is more pronounced after doses greater than 50 mg/m^2, and peak levels of uric acid generally occur between 3 to 5 days after the dose. Allopurinol therapy for hyperuricemia effectively reduces uric acid levels.
Neurotoxicity (see "**WARNINGS**" section)—Neurotoxicity, usually characterized by peripheral neuropathies, has been reported. The neuropathies usually occur after prolonged therapy (4 to 7 months); however, neurologic symptoms have been reported to occur after a single dose. Although symptoms and signs of PLATINOL neuropathy usually develop during treatment, symptoms of neuropathy may begin 3 to 8 weeks after the last dose of PLATINOL, although this is rare. PLATINOL therapy should be discontinued when the symptoms are first observed. The neuropathy, however, may progress further even after stopping treatment. Preliminary evidence suggests peripheral neuropathy may be irreversible in some patients.
Lhermitte's sign, dorsal column myelopathy, and autonomic neuropathy have also been reported.
Loss of taste and seizures have also been reported.
Muscle cramps, defined as localized, painful, involuntary skeletal muscle contractions of sudden onset and short duration, have been reported and were usually associated in patients receiving a relatively high cumulative dose of PLATINOL and with a relatively advanced symptomatic stage of peripheral neuropathy.
Ocular Toxicity—Optic neuritis, papilledema, and cerebral blindness have been reported infrequently in patients receiving standard recommended doses of PLATINOL. Improvement and/or total recovery usually occurs after discontinuing PLATINOL. Steroids with or without mannitol have been used; however, efficacy has not been established.
Blurred vision and altered color perception have been reported after the use of regimens with higher doses of PLATINOL or greater dose frequencies than those recommended in the package insert. The altered color perception manifests as a loss of color discrimination, particularly in the blue-yellow axis. The only finding on funduscopic exam is irregular retinal pigmentation of the macular area.
Anaphylactic-like Reactions—Anaphylactic-like reactions have been occasionally reported in patients previously exposed to PLATINOL. The reactions consist of facial edema, wheezing, tachycardia, and hypotension within a few minutes of drug administration. Reactions may be controlled by intravenous epinephrine with corticosteroids, and/or antihistamines as indicated. Patients receiving PLATINOL should be observed carefully for possible anaphylactic-like reactions and supportive equipment and medication should be available to treat such a complication.
Hepatotoxicity—Transient elevations of liver enzymes, especially SGOT, as well as bilirubin, have been reported to be associated with PLATINOL administration at the recommended doses.
Other Events—Other toxicities reported to occur infrequently are cardiac abnormalities, hiccups, elevated serum amylase, and rash. Alopecia has also been reported.
Local soft tissue toxicity has rarely been reported following extravasation of PLATINOL. Severity of the local tissue toxicity appears to be related to the concentration of the PLATINOL solution. Infusion of solutions with a PLATINOL concentration greater than 0.5 mg/mL may result in tissue cellulitis, fibrosis, and necrosis.

OVERDOSAGE

Caution should be exercised to prevent inadvertent overdosage with PLATINOL. Acute overdosage with this drug may result in kidney failure, liver failure, deafness, ocular toxicity (including detachment of the retina), significant myelosuppression, intractable nausea and vomiting and/or neuritis. In addition, death can occur following overdosage.
No proven antidotes have been established for PLATINOL overdosage. Hemodialysis, even when initiated four hours after the overdosage, appears to have little effect on remov-

ing platinum from the body because of PLATINOL's rapid and high degree of protein binding. Management of overdosage should include general supportive measures to sustain the patient through any period of toxicity that may occur.

DOSAGE AND ADMINISTRATION

Note: Needles or intravenous sets containing aluminum parts that may come in contact with PLATINOL® (cisplatin injection, USP) should not be used for preparation or administration. Aluminum reacts with PLATINOL, causing precipitate formation and a loss of potency.

Metastatic Testicular Tumors—The usual PLATINOL dose for the treatment of testicular cancer in combination with other approved chemotherapeutic agents is 20 mg/m^2 IV daily for a 5 day cycle.

Metastatic Ovarian Tumors—The usual PLATINOL dose for the treatment of metastatic ovarian tumors in combination with Cytoxan is 75–100 mg/m^2 IV per cycle once every 4 weeks (Day 1).[2,3]

The dose of Cytoxan when used in combination with PLATINOL is 600 mg/m^2 IV once every 4 weeks, (Day 1).[2,3]

For directions for the administration of Cytoxan, refer to the Cytoxan package insert.

In combination therapy, PLATINOL and Cytoxan are administered sequentially.

As a single agent, PLATINOL should be administered at a dose of 100 mg/m^2 IV per cycle once every 4 weeks.

Advanced Bladder Cancer—PLATINOL should be administered as a single agent at a dose of 50 to 70 mg/m^2 IV per cycle once every 3 to 4 weeks depending on the extent of prior exposure to radiation therapy and/or prior chemotherapy. For heavily pretreated patients an initial dose of 50 mg/m^2 per cycle repeated every 4 weeks is recommended.

Pretreatment hydration with 1 to 2 liters of fluid infused for 8 to 12 hours prior to a PLATINOL dose is recommended. The drug is then diluted in 2 liters of 5% Dextrose in ½ or ⅓ normal saline containing 37.5 g of mannitol, and infused over a 6- to 8-hour period. If diluted solution is not to be used within 6 hours, protect solution from light. Do not dilute PLATINOL in just 5% Dextrose injection. Adequate hydration and urinary output must be maintained during the following 24 hours.

A repeat course of PLATINOL should not be given until the serum creatinine is below 1.5 mg/100 mL, and/or the BUN is below 25 mg/100 mL. A repeat course should not be given until circulating blood elements are at an acceptable level (platelets $\geq$ 100,000/mm^3, WBC $\geq$ 4,000/mm^3). Subsequent doses of PLATINOL should not be given until an audiometric analysis indicates that auditory acuity is within normal limits.

As with other potentially toxic compounds, caution should be exercised in handling the aqueous solution. Skin reactions associated with accidental exposure to cisplatin may occur. The use of gloves is recommended. If cisplatin solution contacts the skin or mucosae, immediately wash the skin or mucosae thoroughly with soap and water.

The aqueous solution should be used intravenously only and should be administered by IV infusion over a 6- to 8-hour period.

NOTE TO PHARMACIST: Exercise caution to prevent inadvertent PLATINOL-AQ overdosage. Please call prescriber if dose greater than 100 mg/m^2 per cycle. Aluminum and flip-off seal of vial have been imprinted with the following statement: **CALL DR. IF DOSE > 100 MG/M²/CYCLE.**

STABILITY

PLATINOL-AQ is a sterile, multidose vial without preservatives. Store at 15°C–25°C. Do not refrigerate. Protect unopened container from light.

The cisplatin remaining in the amber vial following initial entry is stable for 28 days protected from light or for seven days under fluorescent room light.

Procedures for proper handling and disposal of anticancer drugs should be considered. Several guidelines on this subject have been published.[4–10] There is no general agreement that all of the procedures recommended in the guidelines are necessary or appropriate.

HOW SUPPLIED

PLATINOL-AQ (cisplatin injection).

NDC 0015-3220-22—Each multidose vial contains 50 mg of cisplatin.

NDC 0015-3221-22—Each multidose vial contains 100 mg of cisplatin.

REFERENCES

1. Wiernik PH: Hexamethylmelamine and Low or Moderate Dose Cisplatin With or Without Pyridoxine for Treatment of Advanced Ovarian Carcinoma: A Study of the Eastern Oncology Group. Cancer Invest. 1992; 10:1–9.
2. Alberts DS, et al: Improved Therapeutic Index of Carboplatin Plus Cyclophosphamide versus Cisplatin Plus Cyclophosphamide: Final Report by the Southwest Oncology Group of a Phase III Randomized Trial in Stages III and IV Ovarian Cancer. *J Clin Oncol.* 1992; 10:706–717.
3. Swenerton K, et al: Cisplatin-Cyclophosphamide versus Carboplatin-Cyclophosphamide in Advanced Ovarian Cancer: A Randomized Phase III Study of the National Cancer Institute of Canada Clinical Trials Group. *J Clin Oncol.* 1992; 10:718–726.
4. Recommendations for the Safe Handling of Parenteral Antineoplastic Drugs. NIH Publication No. 83-2621. For sale by the Superintendent of Documents, US Government Printing Office, Washington, DC 20402.
5. AMA Council Report. Guidelines for Handling Parenteral Antineoplastics. *JAMA.* 1985; 253(11): 1590–1592.
6. National Study Commission on Cytotoxic Exposure—Recommendations for Handling Cytotoxic Agents. Available from Louis P. Jeffrey, ScD, Chairman, National Study Commission on Cytotoxic Exposure, Massachusetts College of Pharmacy and Allied Health Sciences, 179 Longwood Avenue, Boston, Massachusetts 02115.
7. Clinical Oncological Society of Australia. Guidelines and Recommendations for Safe Handling of Antineoplastic Agents. *Med J Australia.* 1983;1:426–428.
8. Jones RB, et al: Safe Handling of Chemotherapeutic Agents: A Report from the Mount Sinai Medical Center. *CA—A Cancer Journal for Clinicians.* 1983; (Sept/Oct) 258–263.
9. American Society of Hospital Pharmacists Technical Assistance Bulletin on Handling Cytotoxic and Hazardous Drugs. *Am J Hosp Pharm.* 1990;47:1033–1049.
10. OSHA Work-Practice Guidelines for Personnel Dealing with Cytotoxic (Antineoplastic) Drugs. *Am J Hosp Pharm.* 1986; 43:1193–1204.

Shown in Product Identification Guide, page 307

(3220 DIM-14)

December 1994

RUBEX® ℞

(doxorubicin hydrochloride for injection, USP)
FOR INTRAVENOUS USE ONLY

CAUTION: FEDERAL LAW PROHIBITS DISPENSING WITHOUT PRESCRIPTION.

WARNINGS

1. Severe local tissue necrosis will occur if there is extravasation during administration (see "**DOSAGE AND ADMINISTRATION**"section). Doxorubicin must not be given by the intramuscular or subcutaneous route.
2. Myocardial toxicity manifested in its most severe form by potentially fatal congestive heart failure may occur either during therapy or months to years after termination of therapy. The probability of developing impaired myocardial function based on a combined index of signs, symptoms and decline in left ventricular ejection fraction (LVEF) is estimated to be 1 to 2% at a total cumulative dose of 300 mg/m^2 of doxorubicin, 3 to 5% at a dose of 400 mg/m^2, 5 to 8% at 450 mg/m^2 and 6 to 20% at 500 mg/m^2. The risk of developing CHF increases rapidly with increasing total cumulative doses of doxorubicin in excess of 450 mg/m^2. This toxicity may occur at lower cumulative doses in patients with prior mediastinal irradiation or on concurrent cyclophosphamide therapy or with preexisting heart disease.
3. Dosage should be reduced in patients with impaired hepatic function.
4. Severe myelosuppression may occur.
5. Doxorubicin should be administered only under the supervision of a physician who is experienced in the use of cancer chemotherapeutic agents.

DESCRIPTION

Doxorubicin is a cytotoxic anthracycline antibiotic isolated from cultures of **Streptomyces peucetius** var. **caesius**. Doxorubicin consists of a naphthacenequinone nucleus linked through a glycosidic bond at ring atom 7 to an amino sugar, daunosamine. The structural formula is as follows:

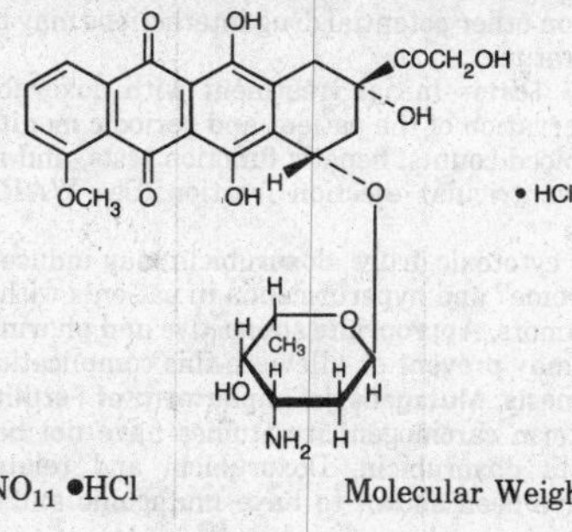

$C_{27}H_{29}NO_{11}$ •HCl Molecular Weight—579.99

Doxorubicin binds to nucleic acids, presumably by specific intercalation of the planar anthracycline nucleus with the DNA double helix. The anthracycline ring is lipophilic but the saturated end of the ring system contains abundant hydroxyl groups adjacent to the amino sugar, producing a hydrophilic center. The molecule is amphoteric, containing acidic functions in the ring phenolic groups and a basic function in the sugar amino group. It binds to cell membranes as well as plasma proteins. RUBEX® (doxorubicin hydrochloride for injection, USP) is for intravenous use only. It is available in 50 mg and 100 mg single dose vials as a lyophilized, sterile powder with added lactose (anhydrous), 250 mg and 500 mg, respectively.

CLINICAL PHARMACOLOGY

The cytotoxic effect of doxorubicin on malignant cells and its toxic effects on various organs are thought to be related to nucleotide base intercalation and cell membrane lipid binding activities of doxorubicin. Intercalation inhibits nucleotide replication and action of DNA and RNA polymerases. The interaction of doxorubicin with topoisomerase II to form DNA-cleavable complexes appears to be an important mechanism of doxorubicin cytocidal activity. Doxorubicin cellular membrane binding may effect a variety of cellular functions. Enzymatic electron reduction of doxorubicin by a variety of oxidases, reductases and dehydrogenases generate highly reactive species including the hydroxyl free radical OH®. Free radical formation has been implicated in doxorubicin cardiotoxicity by means of Cu (II) and Fe (III) reduction at the cellular level.

Animal studies have shown activity in a spectrum of experimental tumors, immunosuppression, carcinogenic properties in rodents, induction of a variety of toxic effects, including delayed and progressive cardiac toxicity, myelosuppression in all species and atrophy to testes in rats and dogs.

Pharmacokinetic studies, determined in patients with various types of tumors undergoing either single or multi-agent therapy, have shown that doxorubicin follows a multiphasic disposition after intravenous injection. The initial distributive half-life of approximately 5.0 minutes suggests rapid tissue uptake of doxorubicin, while its slow elimination from tissues is reflected by a terminal half-life of 20 to 48 hours. Steady-state distribution volumes exceed 20 to 30 L/kg and are indicative of extensive drug uptake into tissues. Plasma clearance is in the range of 8 to 20 mL/min/kg and is predominately by metabolism and biliary excretion. Approximately 40% of the dose appears in the bile in 5 days while only 5 to 12% of the drug and its metabolites appear in the urine during the same time period. Binding of doxorubicin and its major metabolite, doxorubicinol to plasma proteins is about 74 to 76% and is independent of plasma concentration of doxorubicin up to 2 μM. Enzymatic reduction at the 7 position and cleavage of the daunosamine sugar yields eglycones which are accompanied by free radical formation, the local production of which may contribute to the cardiotoxic activity of doxorubicin. Disposition of doxorubicinol (DOX-OL) in patients is formation rate limited. The terminal half-life of DOX-OL is similar to doxorubicin. The relative exposure of DOX-OL, compared to doxorubicin ranges between 0.4 to 0.6. In urine, <3% of the dose was recovered as DOX-OL over 7 days. The literature contains no information regarding gender related differences in the pharmacokinetics of doxorubicin and doxorubicinol.

In four patients dose-independent pharmacokinetics have been shown for doxorubicin in the dose range of 30 to 70 mg/m^2. Systemic clearance of doxorubicin is significantly reduced in obese women with ideal body weight greater than 130%. There was a significant reduction in clearance without any change in volume of distribution in obese patients when compared with normal patients with less than 115% ideal body weight. The clearance of doxorubicin and doxorubicinol was also reduced in patients with impaired hepatic function. Doxorubicin was excreted in the milk of one lactating patient, with peak milk concentration at 24 hours after treatment being approximately 4.4-fold greater than the corresponding plasma concentrating. Doxorubicin was detectable in the milk up to 72 hours after therapy with 70 mg/m^2 of doxorubicin given as a 15 minute intravenous infusion and 100 mg/m^2 of cisplatin as a 26 hour intravenous infusion. The peak concentration of doxorubicinol in milk at 24 hours was 0.2 μM and AUC up to 24 hours was 16.5 μM.hr while the AUC for doxorubicin was 9.9 μM.hr.

Doxorubicin does not cross the blood brain barrier.

INDICATIONS AND USAGE

Doxorubicin hydrochloride for injection, USP has been used successfully to produce regression in disseminated neoplastic conditions such as acute lymphoblastic leukemia, acute myeloblastic leukemia, Wilms' tumor, neuroblastoma, soft tissue and bone sarcomas, breast carcinoma, ovarian carcinoma, transitional cell bladder carcinoma, thyroid carcinoma, gastric carcinoma, Hodgkin's disease, malignant lymphoma and bronchogenic carcinoma in which the small cell

Continued on next page

Bristol-Myers Squibb Oncology—Cont.

histologic type is the most responsive compared to other cell types.

CONTRAINDICATIONS

Doxorubicin therapy should not be started in patients who have marked myelosuppression induced by previous treatment with other antitumor agents or by radiotherapy. Doxorubicin treatment is containdicated in patients who received previous treatment with complete cumulative doses of doxorubicin, daunorubicin, idarubicin and/or other anthracyclines and anthracenes.

WARNINGS

Special attention must be given to the cardiotoxicity induced by doxorubicin. Irreversible myocardial toxicity, manifested in its most severe form by life-threatening and potentially fatal congestive heart failure, may occur either during therapy or months to years after termination of therapy. The probability of developing impaired myocardial function, based on a combined index of signs, symptoms and decline in left ventricular ejection fraction (LVEF) is estimated to be 1 to 2% at a total cumulative dose of 300 mg/m^2 of doxorubicin, 3 to 5% at a dose of 400 mg/m^2, 5 to 8% at a dose of 450 mg/m^2 and 6 to 20% at a dose of 500 mg/m^2 given in a schedule of a bolus injection once every 3 weeks. In a retrospective review by Von Hoff *et al*, the probability of developing congestive heart failure was reported to be 5/168 (3%) at a cumulative dose of 430 mg/m^2 of doxorubicin, 8/110 (7%) at 575 mg/m^2 and 3/14 (21%) at 728 mg/m^2. The cumulative incidence of CHF was 2.2%. In a prospective study of doxorubicin in combination with cyclophosphamide, fluorouracil and/or vincristine in patients with breast cancer or small cell lung cancer, the cumulative incidence of congestive heart failure was 3 to 6%. The probability of CHF at various cumulative doses of doxorubicin was 1.5% at 300 mg/m^2, 4.9% at 400 mg/m^2, 7.7% at 450 mg/m^2 and 20.5% at 500 mg/m^2.

Cardiotoxicity may occur at lower doses in patients with prior mediastinal irradiation, concurrent cyclophosphamide therapy and advanced age. Data also suggest that pre-existing heart disease is a co-factor for increased risk of doxorubicin cardiotoxicity. In such cases, cardiac toxicity may occur at doses lower than the respective recommended cumulative dose of doxorubicin. Studies have suggested that concomitant administration of doxorubicin and calcium channel entry blockers may increase the risk of doxorubicin cardiotoxicity. The total dose of doxorubicin administered to the individual patient should also take into account previous or concomitant therapy with related compounds such as daunorubicin, idarubicin and mitoxantrone. Cardiomyopathy and/or congestive heart failure may be encountered several months or years after discontinuation of doxorubicin therapy.

The risk of congestive heart failure and other acute manifestations of doxorubicin cardiotoxicity in children may be as much or lower than in adults. Children appear to be at particular risk for developing delayed cardiac toxicity in that doxorubicin induced cardiomyopathy impairs myocardial growth as children mature, subsequently leading to possible development of congestive heart failure during early adulthood. As many as 40% of children may have subclinical cardiac dysfunction and 5 to 10% of children may develop congestive heart failure on long term follow-up. This late cardiac toxicity may be related to the dose of doxorubicin. The longer the length of follow-up the greater the increase in the detection rate.

Treatment of doxorubicin induced congestive heart failure includes the use of digitalis, diuretics, afterload reducers such as angiotensin I converting enzyme (ACE) inhibitors, low salt diet, and bed rest. Such intervention may relieve symptoms and improve the functional status of the patient.

Monitoring Cardiac Function

In adult patients severe cardiac toxicity may occur precipitously without antecedent ECG changes. Cardiomyopathy induced by anthracyclines is usually associated with very characteristic histopathologic changes on an endomyocardial biopsy (EM biopsy), and a decrease of left ventricular ejection fraction (LVEF), as measured by multi-gated radionuclide angiography (MUGA scans) and/or echocardiogram (ECHO), from pretreatment baseline values. However, it has not been demonstrated that monitoring of the ejection fraction will predict when individual patients are approaching their maximally tolerated cumulative dose of doxorubicin. Cardiac function should be carefully monitored during treatment to minimize the risk of cardiac toxicity. A baseline cardiac evaluation with an ECG, LVEF, and/or an echocardiogram (ECHO) is recommended especially in patients with risk factors for increased cardiac toxicity (pre-existing heart disease, mediastinal irradiation, or concurrent cyclophosphamide therapy). Subsequent evaluations should be obtained at a cumulative dose of doxorubicin of at least 400 mg/m^2 and periodically thereafter during the course of therapy. Children are at increased risk for developing delayed cardiotoxicity following doxorubicin administration; and, therefore, a follow-up cardiac evaluation is recommended periodically to monitor for this delayed cardiotoxicity.

In adults, a 10% decline in LVEF to below the lower limit of normal or an absolute LVEF of 45%, or a 20% decline in LVEF at any level is indicative of deterioration in cardiac function. In children, deterioration in cardiac function during or after the completion of therapy with doxorubicin is indicated by a drop in fractional shortening (FS) by an absolute value of ≥ 10 percentile units or below 29%, and a decline in LVEF of 10 percentile units or an LVEF below 55%.

In general, if test results indicate deterioration in cardiac function associated with doxorubicin, the benefit of continued therapy should be carefully evaluated against the risk of producing irreversible cardiac damage.

Acute life-threatening arrhythmias have been reported to occur during or within a few hours after doxorubicin administration.

There is a high incidence of bone marrow depression, primarily of leukocytes, requiring careful hematologic monitoring. With the recommended dose schedule, leukopenia is usually transient, reaching its nadir 10 to 14 days after treatment with recovery usually occurring by the 21st day. White blood counts as low as 1000/mm^3 are to be expected during treatment with appropriate doses of doxorubicin. Red blood cell and platelet levels should also be monitored since they may also be depressed. Hematologic toxicity may require dose reduction or suspension or delay of doxorubicin therapy. Persistent severe myelosuppression may result in superinfection or hemorrhage.

Doxorubicin may potentiate the toxicity of other anticancer therapies. Exacerbation of cyclophosphamide induced hemorrhagic cystitis and enhancement of the hepatotoxicity of 6-mercaptopurine have been reported. Radiation induced toxicity to the myocardium, mucosae, skin and liver have been reported to be increased by the administration of doxorubicin.

Since metabolism and excretion of doxorubicin occurs predominantly by the hepatobiliary route, toxicity to recommended doses of doxorubicin can be enhanced by hepatic impairment; therefore, prior to the individual dosing, evaluation of hepatic function is recommended using conventional laboratory tests such as SGOT, SGPT, alkaline phosphatase and bilirubin (see "**DOSAGE AND ADMINISTRATION**" section).

Necrotizing colitis manifested by typhlitis (cecal inflammation), bloody stools and severe and sometimes fatal infections have been associated with a combination of doxorubicin given by I.V. push daily for 3 days and cytarabine given by continuous infusion daily for 7 or more days.

On intravenous administration of doxorubicin, extravasation may occur with or without an accompanying stinging or burning sensation, even if blood returns well on aspiration of the infusion needle (see "**DOSAGE AND ADMINISTRATION**" section). If any signs or symptoms of extravasation have occurred, the injection or infusion should be immediately terminated and restarted in another vein.

Pregnancy Category D—Safe use of doxorubicin in pregnancy has not been established. Doxorubicin is embryotoxic and teratogenic in rats and embryotoxic and abortifacient in rabbits. There are no adequate and well-controlled studies in pregnant women. If doxorubicin is to be used during pregnancy, or if the patient becomes pregnant during therapy, the patient should be apprised of the potential hazard to the fetus. Women of childbearing age should be advised to avoid becoming pregnant.

PRECAUTIONS

General—Doxorubicin is not an anti-microbial agent.

Information for Patients—RUBEX® (doxorubicin hydrochloride for injection, USP) imparts a red coloration to the urine for 1 to 2 days after administration, and patients should be advised to expect this during active therapy.

Drug Interactions—Literature contain the following drug interactions with doxorubicin in humans: cyclosporine (Sandimmune) may induce coma and/or seizures, phenobarbital increases the elimination of doxorubicin, phenytoin levels may be decreased by doxorubicin, streptozocin (Zanosar) may inhibit the hepatic metabolism, and administration of live vaccines to immunosuppressed patients, including those undergoing cytotoxic chemotherapy, may be hazardous. Information on other potential drug interactions may be found in the literature.

Laboratory Tests—Initial treatment with doxorubicin requires observation of the patient and periodic monitoring of complete blood counts, hepatic function tests, and radionuclide left ventricular ejection fraction (See **WARNINGS** section).

Like other cytotoxic drugs, doxorubicin may induce "tumor lysis syndrome" and hyperuricemia in patients with rapidly growing tumors. Appropriate supportive and pharmacologic measures may prevent or alleviate this complication.

Carcinogenesis, Mutagenesis, Impairment of Fertility—Formal long-term carcinogenicity studies have not been conducted with doxorubicin. Doxorubicin and related compounds have been shown to have mutagenic and carcinogenic properties when tested in experimental models (including bacterial systems, mammalian cells in culture, and female Sprague-Dawley rats).

The possible adverse effect on fertility in males and females in humans or experimental animals have not been adequately evaluated. Testicular atrophy was observed in rats and dogs.

A variant of chemotherapy-related acute non-lymphocytic leukemia has been reported to occur infrequently a few years after multiple drug treatment of some neoplasms, which sometimes included doxorubicin. The exact role of doxorubicin has not been elucidated.

Pregnancy Category D
(See **WARNINGS** section)

Nursing Mothers: Because of the potential for serious adverse reactions in nursing infants from doxorubicin, mothers should be advised to discontinue nursing during doxorubicin therapy.

ADVERSE REACTIONS

Dose-limiting toxicities of therapy are myelosuppression and cardiotoxicity. Other reactions reported are:

Cardiotoxicity—(See **WARNINGS** section.)

Cutaneous—Reversible complete alopecia occurs in most cases. Hyperpigmentation of nailbeds and dermal creases, primarily in children, and onycholysis have been reported in a few cases. Recall of skin reaction due to prior radiotherapy has occurred with doxorubicin administration.

Gastrointestinal—Acute nausea and vomiting occurs frequently and may be severe. This may be alleviated by antiemetic therapy. Mucositis (stomatitis and esophagitis) may occur 5 to 10 days after administration. The effect may be severe leading to ulceration and represents a site of origin for severe infections. The dosage regimen consisting of administration of doxorubicin on 3 successive days results in greater incidence and severity of mucositis. Ulceration and necrosis of the colon, especially the cecum, may occur leading to bleeding or severe infections which can be fatal. This reaction has been reported in patients with acute non-lymphocytic leukemia treated with a 3-day course of doxorubicin combined with cytarabine. Anorexia and diarrhea have been occasionally reported.

Vascular—Phlebosclerosis has been reported especially when small veins are used or a single vein is used for repeated administration. Facial flushing may occur if the injection is given too rapidly.

Local—Severe cellulitis, vesication and tissue necrosis will occur if extravasation of doxorubicin occurs during administration. Erythematous streaking along the vein proximal to the site of the injection has been reported (see "**DOSAGE AND ADMINISTRATION**" section).

Hematologic—The occurrence of secondary acute myeloid leukemia with or without a preleukemic phase has been reported rarely in patients concurrently treated with doxorubicin in association with DNA-damaging antineoplastic agents. Such cases could have a short (1-3 years) latency period.

Hypersensitivity—Fever, chills and urticaria have been reported occasionally. Anaphylaxis may occur. A case of apparent cross sensitivity to lincomycin has been reported.

Other—Conjunctivitis and lacrimation occur rarely.

OVERDOSAGE

Acute overdosage with doxorubicin enhances the toxic effects of mucositis, leukopenia and thrombocytopenia. Therapy of acute overdosage consists of treatment of the severely myelosuppressed patient with hospitalization, antimicrobials, platelet transfusions and symptomatic treatment of mucositis. Use of hemopoietic growth factor (G-CSF, GM-CSF) may be considered.

The 150 mg RUBEX® (doxorubicin hydrochloride for injection, USP) and the 100 mL (2 mg/mL) RUBEX vials are packaged as multiple dose vials and caution should be exercised to prevent inadvertent over-dosage.

Cumulative dosage with doxorubicin increases the risk of cardiomyopathy and resultant congestive heart failure (See **WARNINGS** section). Treatment consists of vigorous management of congestive heart failure with digitalis preparations, diuretics, and afterload reducers such as ACE inhibitors.

DOSAGE AND ADMINISTRATION

Care in the administration of doxorubicin hydrochloride will reduce the chance of perivenous infiltration (See **WARNINGS** section). It may also decrease the chance of local reactions such as urticaria and erythematous streaking. On intravenous administration of doxorubicin, extravasation may occur with or without an accompanying stinging or burning sensation, even if blood returns well on aspiration of the infusion needle. If any signs or symptoms of extravasation have occurred, the injection or infusion should be immediately terminated and restarted in another vein. If extravasation is suspected, intermittent application of ice to the site for 15 min.,q.i.d. x 3 days may be useful. The benefit of local administration of drugs has not been clearly established. Because of the progressive nature of extravasation reactions, close observation and plastic surgery consultation is recom-

mended. Blistering, ulceration and/or persistent pain are indications for wide excision surgery, followed by split-thickness skin grafting.[1]

The most commonly used dose schedule when used as a single agent is 60 to 75 mg/m[2] as a single intravenous injection administered at 21-day intervals. The lower dosage should be given to patients with inadequate marrow reserves due to old age, or prior therapy, or neoplastic marrow infiltration. RUBEX has been used concurrently with other approved chemotherapeutic agents. Evidence is available that in some types of neoplastic disease combination chemotherapy is superior to single agents. The benefits and risks of such therapy continue to be elucidated. When used in combination with other chemotherapy drugs, the most commonly used dosage of doxorubicin is 40 to 50 mg/m[2] given as a single intravenous injection every 21 to 28 days. Doxorubicin dosage must be reduced in case of hyperbilirubinemia as follows:

Plasma bilirubin concentrate (mg/dL)	Dosage reduction (%)
1.2–3.0	50
3.1–5.0	75

Reconstitution Directions — RUBEX (doxorubicin hydrochloride for injection, USP) 50 mg and 100 mg vials should be reconstituted with 25 mL and 50 mL, respectively of Sodium Chloride Injection, USP (0.9%) to give a final concentration of 2 mg/mL of doxorubicin hydrochloride. An appropriate volume of air should be withdrawn from the vial during reconstitution to avoid excessive pressure buildup. Bacteriostatic diluents are not recommended.

After adding the diluent, the vial should be shaken and the contents allowed to dissolve. The reconstituted solution is stable for 24 hours at room temperature and 48 hours under refrigeration 2°–8°C (36°–46°F). It should be protected from exposure to sunlight and any unused solution should be discarded.

It is recommended that doxorubicin be slowly administered into the tubing of a freely running intravenous infusion of Sodium Chloride Injection, USP or 5% Dextrose Injection, USP. The tubing should be attached to a Butterfly® needle inserted preferably into a large vein. If possible, avoid veins over joints or in extremities with compromised venous or lymphatic drainage. The rate of administration is dependent on the size of the vein and the dosage. However, the dose should be administered in not less than 3 to 5 minutes. Local erythematous streaking along the vein as well as facial flushing may be indicative of too rapid an administration. A burning or stinging sensation may be indicative of perivenous infiltration and the infusion should be immediately terminated and restarted in another vein. Perivenous infiltration may occur painlessly.

Doxorubicin should not be mixed with heparin or fluorouracil since it has been reported that these drugs are incompatible to the extent that a precipitate may form. Until specific compatibility data are available, it is not recommended that doxorubicin be mixed with other drugs.

Parenteral drug products should be inspected visually for particulate matter and discoloration prior to administration, whenever solution and container permit.

Handling and Disposal — Skin reactions associated with doxorubicin have been reported. Skin accidently exposed to doxorubicin should be rinsed copiously with soap and warm water, and if the eyes are involved, standard irrigation techniques should be used immediately. The use of goggles, gloves, and protective gowns is recommended during preparation and administration of the drug.

Procedures for proper handling and disposal of anticancer drugs should be considered. Several guidelines on this subject have been published.[2-8] There is no general agreement that all of the procedures recommended in the guidelines are necessary or appropriate.

HOW SUPPLIED

RUBEX® (doxorubicin hydrochloride for injection, USP) is available as follows:

50 mg – Each single-dose vial contains 50 mg of doxorubicin HCl, USP as a sterile red-orange lyophilized powder. **NDC** 0015-3352-22
Available as one individually cartoned vial.

100 mg –Each single-dose vial contains 100 mg of doxorubicin HCl, USP as a sterile red-orange lyophilized powder. **NDC** 0015-3353-22
Available as one individually cartoned vial.

Store dry powder at controlled room temperature 15°–30°C (59°–86°F).

The reconstituted solution is stable for 24 hours at room temperature or 48 hours under refrigeration 2°-8°C (36°-46°F). Protect from exposure to sunlight. Retain in carton until time of use.

REFERENCES

1. Rudolph R, Larson DL: Etiology and Treatment of Chemotherapeutic Agent Extravasation Injuried: A Review. J Clin Oncol 1987; 5:1116-1126.

2. Recommendations for the Safe Handling of Parenteral Antineoplastic Drugs. NIH Publication No. 83-2621. For sale by the Superintendent of Documents, US Government Printing Office, Washington, DC 20402.
3. AMA Council Report. Guidelines for Handling Parenteral Antineoplastics. JAMA 1985; 253 (11): 1590-1592.
4. National Study Commission on Cytotoxic Exposure Recommendations for Handling Cytotoxic Agents. Available from Louis P. Jeffrey, ScD, Chairman, National Study Commission on Cytotoxic Exposure, Massachusetts College of Pharmacy and Allied Health Sciences, 179 Longwood Avenue, Boston, Massachusetts 02115.
5. Clinical Oncological Society of Australia. Guidelines and Recommendations for Safe Handling of Antineoplastic Agents. Med J Australia 1983; 1:426–428.
6. Jones RB, et al: Safe Handling of Chemotherapeutic Agents: A Report from the Mount Sinai Medical Center. CA-A Cancer Journal for Clinicians 1983; (Sept/Oct) 258–263.
7. American Society of Hospital Pharmacists Technical Assistance Bulletin on Handling Cytotoxic and Hazardous Drugs. Am J Hosp Pharm 1990; 47:1033–1049.
8. OSHA Work-Practice Guidelines for Personnel Dealing with Cytotoxic (Antineoplastic) Drugs. Am J Hosp Pharm 1986; 43:1193–1204.

Mead Johnson
ONCOLOGY PRODUCTS
A Bristol-Myers Squibb Company
Princeton, NJ 08543
U.S.A.
K9-B001-3-96

3351DIM-04
51-004726-00
March 1996

TAXOL® ℞
(paclitaxel) Injection

CAUTION: FEDERAL LAW PROHIBITS DISPENSING WITHOUT PRESCRIPTION.

WARNING

TAXOL® (paclitaxel) Injection should be administered under the supervision of a physician experienced in the use of cancer chemotherapeutic agents. Appropriate management of complications is possible only when adequate diagnostic and treatment facilities are readily available.

Anaphylaxis and severe hypersensitivity reactions characterized by dyspnea and hypotension requiring treatment, angioedema, and generalized urticaria have occurred in 2% of patients receiving TAXOL in clinical trials. Fatal reactions have occurred in patients despite premedication. All patients should be pretreated with corticosteriods, diphenhydramine, and H_2 antagonists. (See "**DOSAGE and ADMINISTRATION**" section.) Patients who experience severe hypersensitivity reactions to TAXOL should not be rechallenged with the drug.

TAXOL therapy should not be given to patients with baseline neutrophil counts of less than 1,500 cells/mm[3]. In order to monitor the occurrence of bone marrow suppression, primarily neutropenia, which may be severe and result in infection, it is recommended that frequent peripheral blood cell counts be performed on all patients receiving TAXOL.

DESCRIPTION

TAXOL® (paclitaxel) Injection is a clear colorless to slightly yellow viscous solution. It is supplied as a nonaqueous solution intended for dilution with a suitable parenteral fluid prior to intravenous infusion. TAXOL is available in 30 mg (5 mL) and 100 mg (16.7mL) single-dose vials. Each mL of sterile nonpyrogenic solution contains 6 mg paclitaxel, 527 mg of Cremophor® EL* (polyoxyethylated castor oil) and 49.7% (v/v) dehydrated alcohol, USP.

* Cremophor® EL is the registered trademark of BASF Aktiengesellschaft.

Paclitaxel is a natural product with antitumor activity. TAXOL (paclitaxel) is obtained via a semi-synthetic process from *Taxus baccata*. The chemical name for paclitaxel is 5β,20-Epoxy-1,2α,4,7β,10β,13α-hexahydroxytax-11-en-9-one 4,10-diacetate 2-benzoate 13-ester with (2R,3S)-N-benzoyl-3-phenylisoserine.

Paclitaxel has the following structural formula:

Paclitaxel is a white to off-white crystalline powder with the empirical formula $C_{47}H_{51}NO_{14}$ and a molecular weight of 853.9. It is highly lipophilic, insoluble in water, and melts at around 216-217°C.

CLINICAL PHARMACOLOGY

Paclitaxel is a novel antimicrotubule agent that promotes the assembly of microtubules from tubulin dimers and stabilizes microtubules by preventing depolymerization. This stability results in the inhibition of the normal dynamic reorganization of the microtubule network that is essential for vital interphase and mitotic cellular functions. In addition, paclitaxel induces abnormal arrays or "bundles" of microtubules throughout the cell cycle and multiple asters of microtubules during mitosis.

Following intravenous administration of TAXOL, paclitaxel plasma concentrations declined in a biphasic manner. The initial rapid decline represents distribution to the peripheral compartment and elimination of the drug. The later phase is due, in part, to a relatively slow efflux of paclitaxel from the peripheral compartment.

Pharmacokinetic parameters of paclitaxel following 3- and 24-hour infusions of TAXOL at dose levels of 135 and 175 mg/m[2] were determined in a Phase 3 randomized study in ovarian cancer patients and are summarized in the following table:

[See table below.]

It appeared that with the 24-hour infusion of TAXOL, a 30% increase in dose (135 mg/m[2] versus 175 mg/m[2]) increased the C_{max} by 87%, whereas the AUC (0-∞) remained proportional. However, with a 3-hour infusion, for a 30% increase in dose, the C_{max} and AUC (0-∞) were increased by 68% and 89%, respectively. The mean apparent volume of distribution at steady state, with the 24-hour infusion of TAXOL ranged from 227 to 688 L/m[2], indicating extensive extravascular distribution and/or tissue binding of paclitaxel.

The pharmacokinetics of paclitaxel were also evaluated in adult cancer patients who received single doses of 15–135 mg/m[2] given by 1-hour infusions (n=15), 30–275 mg/m[2] given by 6-hour infusions (n=36), and 200–275 mg/m[2] given by 24-hour infusions (n=54) in Phase 1 & 2 studies. Values for total body clearance and volume of distribution were consistent with the findings in the Phase 3 study.

In vitro studies of binding to human serum proteins, using paclitaxel concentrations ranging from 0.1 to 50 g/mL, indicate that between 89–98% of drug is bound; the presence of cimetidine, ranitidine, dexamethasone, or diphenhydramine did not affect protein binding of paclitaxel.

After intravenous administration of 15–275 mg/m[2] doses of TAXOL as 1, 6, 24-hour infusions, mean (SD) values for cumulative urinary recovery of unchanged drug ranged from 1.3% (0.5%) to 12.6% (16.2%) of the dose, indicating extensive non-renal clearance. In five patients administered a 225 or 250 mg/m[2] dose of radiolabeled TAXOL as a 3-hour infusion, a mean (SE) of 71% (8%) of the radioactivity was excreted in the feces in 120 hours and 14% (1%) was recovered in the urine. Total recovery of radioactivity ranged from

Summary of Non-Compartmental Pharmacokinetic Parameters
Mean (% Coefficient of Variation) Values by Single-Dose and Infusion

Dose (mg/m[2])	Infusion Duration (h)	N (patients)	C_{max} (ng/mL)	AUC (0-∞) (ng-h/mL)	T-HALF (h)	CL_T (L/h/m[2])
135	24	2	195	6300	52.7	21.7
175	24	4	365 (33)	7993 (29)	15.7 (56)	23.8 (35)
135	3	7	2170 (21)	7952 (23)	13.1 (45)	17.7 (20)
175	3	5	3650 (30)	15007 (27)	20.2 (85)	12.2 (25)

C_{max} —Maximum plasma concentration
AUC (0-∞) —Area under the plasma concentration-time curve from time 0 to infinity
CL_T —Total body clearance

Continued on next page

Bristol-Myers Squibb Oncology—Cont.

56% to 101% of the dose. Paclitaxel represented a mean of 5% of the administered radioactivity recovered in the feces, while metabolites, primary 6α-hydroxypaclitaxel, accounted for the balance. *In vitro* studies with human liver microsomes and tissue slices showed that paclitaxel was metabolized primarily to 6α-hydroxypaclitaxel by the cytochrome P450 isozyme CYP2C8; and to two minor metabolites, 3-*p*-hydroxypaclitaxel and 6α , 3'-*p*-dihydroxypaclitaxel, by CYP3A4. *In vitro*, the metabolism of paclitaxel to 6α-hydroxypaclitaxel was inhibited by a number of agents (ketoconazole, verapamil, diazepam, quinidine, dexamethasone, cyclosporin, teniposide, etoposide, and vincristine), but the concentrations used exceeded those found *in vivo* following normal therapeutic doses. Testosterone, 17α-ethinyl estrodiol, erythromycin, retinoic acid, and quercetin, a specific inhibitor of CYP2C8, also inhibited the formation of 6α-hydroxypaclitaxel *in vitro*. The pharmacokinetics of paclitaxel may also be altered *in vivo* as a result of interactions with compounds that are substrates, inducers, or inhibitors of CYP2C8 and/or CYP3A4. (See "**PRECAUTIONS: Drug Interactions**" section.) The effect of renal or hepatic dysfunction on the disposition of paclitaxel has not been investigated.

Possible interactions of paclitaxel with concomitantly administered medications have not been formally investigated.

CLINICAL STUDIES

Ovarian Carcinoma: Data from five Phase 1 and 2 clinical studies (189 patients), a multicenter, randomized Phase 3 study (407 patients), as well as an interim analysis of data from more than 300 patients enrolled in a treatment referral center program were used in support of the use of TAXOL (paclitaxel) Injection in patients who have failed initial or subsequent chemotherapy for metastatic carcinoma of the ovary. Two of the Phase 2 studies (92 patients) utilized an initial dose of 135 to 170 mg/m² in most patients (>90%) administered over 24 hours by continuous infusion. Response rates in these two studies were 22% (95% CI = 11–37%) and 30% (95% CI = 18–46%) with a total of six complete and 18 partial responses in 92 patients. The median duration of overall response in these two studies measured from the first day of treatment was 7.2 months (range: 3.5–15.8 months) and 7.5 months (range: 5.3–17.4 months), respectively. The median survival was 8.1 months (range: 0.2–36.7 months) and 15.9 months (range: 1.8–34.5+months).

The Phase 3 study had a bifactorial design and compared the efficacy and safety of TAXOL, administered at two different doses (135 or 175 mg/m²) and schedules (3- or 24-hour infusion). The overall response rate for the 407 patients was 16.2% (95% CI = 12.8–20.2%), with 6 complete and 60 partial responses. Duration of response, measured from the first day of treatment was 8.3 months (range: 3.2–21.6 months). Median time to progression was 3.7 months (range: 0.+–25.1+months). Median survival was 11.5 months (range: 0.2–26.3+ months).

Response rates, median survival and median time to progression for the 4 arms are given in the following table. The arms are listed by dose and schedule (mg·m²/hours). Comparisons between study arms should be done with caution in view of the bifactorial study design and small sample sizes per arm.

[See table below.]

Analysis were performed as planned by the study protocol, by comparing the two doses (135 or 175 mg/m²) irrespective of the schedule (3 or 24 hours) and the two schedules irrespective of dose.

Patients receiving the 175 mg/m² dose achieved a higher response rate than those receiving the 135 mg/m² dose: 18% vs. 14% (p=0.28). No difference in response rate was detected when comparing the 3-hour with the 24-hour infusion:15% vs. 17% (p=0.50). Patients receiving the 175 mg/m² dose of TAXOL had a longer time to progression than those receiving the 135 mg/m² dose: median 4.2 vs. 3.1 months (p=0.03). Time to progression was longer for patients receiving the 3-hour vs. the 24-hour infusion: 4.0

Frequency of Key Adverse Events in the Phase 3 Study

		Percent of Patients			
		175/3 (n=95)	175/24 (n=105)	135/3 (n=98)	135/24 (n=105)
● **Bone Marrow**					
– Neutropenia	<2,000/mm³	78	98	78	98
	<500/mm³	27	75	14	67
– Thrombocytopenia	<100,000/mm³	4	18	8	6
	<50,000/mm³	1	7	2	1
– Anemia	<11 g/dL	84	90	68	88
	<8 g/dL	11	12	6	10
– Infections		26	29	20	18
● **Hypersensitivity Reaction***					
– All		41	45	38	45
– Severe		2	0	2	1
● **Peripheral Neuropathy**					
– Any symptoms		63	60	55	42
– Severe symptoms		1	2	0	0
● **Mucositis**					
– Any symptoms		17	35	21	25
– Severe symptoms		0	3	0	2

* *All patients received premedication*

months vs. 3.7 months (p=0.08). No difference in survival according to dose or schedule was observed.

TAXOL remained active in patients who had developed resistance to platinum-containing therapy (defined as tumor progression while on, or tumor relapse within 6 months from completion of, platinum containing regimen) with response rates of 14% in the Phase 3 study and 31% in the Phase 1 & 2 clinical studies.

The adverse event profile in the Phase 3 study was consistent with that seen for a pooled analysis performed on 812 patients treated in ten clinical studies (see, "**ADVERSE REACTIONS**" section). For the 403 patients who received TAXOL in the Phase 3 study, the following table shows the incidence of some key adverse events by treatment arm. The arms are listed by dose and schedule (mg/m²/hours).

[See table above.]

Myelosuppression was dose and schedule related, with the schedule effect being more prominent. The development of severe hypersensitivity reactions (HSRs) was rare; 1% of the patients and 0.2% of the courses overall. There was no apparent dose or schedule effect seen for the HSRs. Additionally, peripheral neuropathy was clearly dose-related, but schedule did not appear to affect the incidence.

The results of the randomized study support the use of TAXOL at doses of 135 or 175 mg/m², administered by a 3-hour intravenous infusion. The same doses administered by 24-hour infusion were more toxic; the bifactorial study design and small sample size per arm preclude definitive conclusions regarding relative efficacy between the 4 arms of the study.

Breast Carcinoma: Data from 83 patients accrued in three phase 2 open label studies and from 471 patients enrolled in a phase 3 randomized study were available to support the use of TAXOL in patients with metastatic breast carcinoma.

Phase 2 open label studies: Two studies were conducted in 53 patients previously treated with a maximum of one prior chemotherapeutic regimen. TAXOL was administered in these 2 trials as a 24-hour infusion at initial doses of 250 mg/m² (with G-CSF support) or 200 mg/m². The response rates were 57% (95% CI: 37–75%) and 52% (95% CI: 32–72%), respectively. The third phase 2 study evaluated quality of life changes and was conducted in extensively pretreated patients who had failed anthracycline therapy and who had received a minimum of 2 chemotherapy regimens for the treatment of metastatic disease. The dose of TAXOL was 200 mg/m² as a 24-hour infusion with G-CSF support. Nine of the 30 patients analyzed achieved a partial response, for a response rate of 30% (95% CI: 15–50%).

Phase 3 randomized study: This multicenter trial was conducted in patients previously treated with one or two regimens of chemotherapy. Patients were randomized to receive TAXOL at a dose of either 175 mg/m² or 135 mg/m² given as a 3-hour infusion. In the 471 patients enrolled, 60% had symptomatic disease with impaired performance status at

study entry, and 73% had visceral metastases. These patients had failed prior chemotherapy either in the adjuvant setting (30%), the metastatic setting (39%), or both (31%). Sixty-seven percent of the patients had been previously exposed to anthracyclines and 23% of them had disease considered resistant to this class of agents.

The overall response rate for the 454 evaluable patients was 26% (95% CI: 22–30%), with 17 complete and 99 partial responses. The median duration of response, measured from the first day of treatment, was 8.1 months (range: 3.4–18.1+ months). Overall for the 471 patients, the median time to progression was 3.5 months (range: 0.03–17.1 months). Median survival was 11.7 months (range: 0–18.9 months).

Response rates, median survival and median time to progression for the 2 arms are given in the following table. The arms are listed by dose and schedule (mg·m²/hours).

Key Efficacy Parameters in the Phase 3 Study

	175/3 (n=235)	135/3 (n=236)
● **Response**		
– rate (percent)	28	22
– 95% Confidence Interval	(22–34)	(17–27)
● **Time to Progression**		
– median (months)	4.2	3.0
– 95% Confidence Interval	(3.2–4.6)	(2.5–3.8)
● **Survival**		
– median (months)	11.7	10.5
– 95% Confidence Interval	(10.0–13.8)	(9.0–12.8)

For the 458 patients who received TAXOL (paclitaxel) Injection in the Phase 3 study, the following table shows the incidence of some key adverse events by treatment arm (each arm was administered by a 3-hour infusion).

[See table at top of next page.]

Myelosuppression and peripheral neuropathy were dose related. There was one severe hypersensitivity reaction (HSR) observed at the dose of 135 mg/m².

INDICATIONS

TAXOL is indicated, after failure of first-line or subsequent chemotherapy for the treatment of metastatic carcinoma of the ovary.

TAXOL is indicated for the treatment of breast cancer after failure of combination chemotherapy for metastatic disease or relapse within 6 months of adjuvant chemotherapy. Prior therapy should have included an anthracycline unless clinically contraindicated.

CONTRAINDICATIONS

TAXOL is contraindicated in patients who have a history of hypersensitivity reactions to TAXOL or other drugs formulated in Cremophor® EL (polyoxyethylated castor oil).

TAXOL should not be used in patients with baseline neutropenia of <1,500 cells/mm³.

WARNINGS

Anaphylaxis and severe hypersensitivity reactions characterized by dyspnea and hypotension requiring treatment, angioedema, and generalized urticaria have occurred in 2% of patients receiving TAXOL in clinical trials. Fatal reactions have occurred in patients despite premedication. All patients should be pretreated with corticosteroids, diphenhydramine, and H₂ antagonists. (See "**DOSAGE and ADMINISTRATION**" section). Patients who experience severe hypersensitivity reactions to TAXOL should not be rechallenged with the drug.

Bone marrow suppression (primarily neutropenia) is dose-dependent and is the dose-limiting toxicity. Neutrophil nadirs occurred at a median of 11 days. TAXOL should not be administered to patients with baseline neutrophil counts of

Key Efficacy Parameters in the Phase 3 Study

	175/3 (n=96)	175/24 (n=106)	135/3 (n=99)	135/24 (n=106)
● **Response**				
– rate (percent)	14.6	21.7	15.2	13.2
– 95% Confidence Interval	(8.5–23.6)	(14.5–31.0)	(9.0–24.1)	(7.7–21.5)
● **Time to Progression**				
– median (months)	4.4	4.2	3.4	2.8
– 95% Confidence Interval	(3.0–5.6)	(3.5–5.1)	(2.8–4.2)	(1.9–4.0)
● **Survival**				
– median (months)	11.5	11.8	13.1	10.7
– 95% Confidence Interval	(8.4–14.4)	(8.9–14.6)	(9.1–14.6)	(8.1–13.6)

less than 1,500 cells/mm^3. Frequent monitoring of blood counts should be instituted during TAXOL treatment. Patients should not be re-treated with subsequent cycles of TAXOL until neutrophils recover to a level >1,500 cells/mm3 and platelets recover to a level >100,000 cells/mm^3. Severe conduction abnormalities have been documented in <1% of patients during TAXOL therapy and in some cases requiring pacemaker placement. If patients develop significant conduction abnormalities during TAXOL infusion, appropriate therapy should be administered and continuous cardiac monitoring should be performed during subsequent therapy with TAXOL.

TAXOL may cause fetal harm when administered to a pregnant woman. TAXOL has been shown to be embryo- and fetotoxic in rats and rabbits and to decrease fertility in rats. In these studies, TAXOL was shown to result in abortions, decreased corpora lutea, a decrease in implantations and live fetuses, and increased resorption and embryo-fetal deaths. No gross external, soft tissue or skeletal alterations occurred. There are no studies in pregnant women. If TAXOL is used during pregnancy, or if the patient becomes pregnant while receiving this drug, the patient should be apprised of the potential hazard. Women of childbearing potential should be advised to avoid becoming pregnant during therapy with TAXOL.

PRECAUTIONS

Contact of the undiluted concentrate with plasticized polyvinyl chloride (PVC) equipment or devices used to prepare solutions for infusion is not recommended. In order to minimize patient exposure to the plasticizer DEHP [di-(2-ethylhexyl)phthalate], which may be leached from PVC infusion bags or sets, diluted TAXOL solutions should preferably be stored in bottles (glass, polypropylene) or plastic bags (polypropylene, polyolefin) and administered through polyethylene-lined administration sets.

TAXOL should be administered through an in-line filter with a microporous membrane not greater than 0.22 microns. Use of filter devices such as IVEX-2® filters which incorporate short inlet and outlet PVC-coated tubing has not resulted in significant leaching of DEHP.

Drug Interaction: In a Phase I trial using escalating doses of TAXOL (110–200 mg/m^2) and cisplatin (50 or 75 mg/m^2) given as sequential infusions, myelosuppression was more profound when TAXOL was given after cisplatin than with the alternate sequence (i.e., TAXOL before cisplatin). Pharmacokinetic data from these patients demonstrated a decrease in paclitaxel clearance of approximately 33% when TAXOL was administered following cisplatin.

The metabolism of TAXOL is catalyzed by cytochrome P450 isoenzymes CYP2C8 and CYP3A4. In the absence of formal clinical drug interaction studies, caution should be exercised when administering TAXOL concomitantly with known substrates or inhibitors of the cytochrome P450 isoenzymes CYP2C8 and CYP3A4 (See "**CLINICAL PHARMACOLOGY**" section.)

Reports in the literature suggest that plasma levels of doxorubicin (and its active metabolite doxorubicinol) may be increased when paclitaxel and doxorubicin are used in combination.

Hematology: TAXOL therapy should not be administered to patients with baseline neutrophil counts of less than 1,500 cells/mm^3. In order to monitor the occurrence of myelotoxicity, it is recommended that frequent peripheral blood cell counts be performed on all patients receiving TAXOL. Patients should not be re-treated with subsequent cycles of TAXOL until neutrophils recover to a level >1,500 cells/mm^3 and platelets recover to a level >100,000 cells/mm^3. In the case of severe neutropenia (<500 cells/mm^3 for seven days or more) during a course of TAXOL therapy, a 20% reduction in dose for subsequent courses of therapy is recommended.

Hypersensitivity Reactions: Patients with a history of severe hypersensitivity reactions to products containing Cremophor® EL (e.g., cyclosporin for injection concentrate and teniposide for injection concentrate) should not be treated with TAXOL (paclitaxel) Injection. In order to avoid the occurrence of severe hypersensitivity reactions, all patients treated with TAXOL should be premedicated with corticosteroids (such as dexamethasone), diphenhydramine and H_2 antagonists (such as cimetidine or ranitidine). Minor symptoms such as flushing, skin reactions, dyspnea, hypotension or tachycardia do not require interruption of therapy. However, severe reactions, such as hypotension requiring treatment, dyspnea requiring bronchodilators, angioedema or generalized urticaria require immediate discontinuation of TAXOL and aggressive symptomatic therapy. Patients who have developed severe hypersensitivity reactions should not be rechallenged with TAXOL.

Cardiovascular: Hypotension, bradycardia, and hypertension have been observed during administration of TAXOL, but generally do not require treatment. Occasionally TAXOL infusions must be interrupted or discontinued because of initial or recurrent hypertension. Frequent vital sign monitoring, particularly during the first hour of TAXOL infusion, is recommended. Continuous cardiac monitoring is not required except for patients with serious conduction abnormalities. (See "**WARNINGS**" section.)

Frequency of Key Adverse Events in the Phase 3 Breast Carcinoma Study

		Percent of Patients	
		175 mg/m^2 (n=229)	135 mg/m^2 (n=229)
• **Bone Marrow**			
– Neutropenia*	<2,000/mm^3	90	81
	<500/mm^3	28	19
– Thrombocytopenia*	<100,000/mm^3	11	7
	<50,000/mm^3	3	2
– Anemia	<11 g/dL	55	47
	<8 g/dL	4	2
– Infections		23	15
– Febrile Neutropenia		2	2
• **Hypersensitivity Reaction****			
– All		36	31
– Severe		0	<1
• **Peripheral Neuropathy**			
– Any symptoms		70	46
– Severe symptoms		7	3
• **Mucositis**			
– Any symptoms		23	17
– Severe symptoms		3	<1

* *Based on worst course analysis*
** *All patients received premedication*

Nervous System: Although, the occurrence of peripheral neuropathy is frequent, the development of severe symptomatology is unusual and requires a dose reduction of 20% for all subsequent courses of TAXOL.

TAXOL contains dehydrated alcohol USP, 396 mg/mL; consideration should be given to possible CNS and other effects of alcohol. (See "**PRECAUTIONS: Pediatric Use**" section).

Hepatic: There is evidence that the toxicity of TAXOL is enhanced in patients with elevated liver enzymes. Caution should be exercised when administering TAXOL to patients with moderate to severe hepatic impairment and dose adjustments should be considered.

Injection Site Reaction: Injection site reactions, including reactions secondary to extravasation, were usually mild and consisted of erythema, tenderness, skin discoloration, or swelling at the injection site. These reactions have been observed more frequently with the 24-hour infusion than with the 3-hour infusion. Recurrence of skin reactions at a site of previous extravasation following administration of TAXOL at a different site, i.e., "recall", has been reported rarely. Rare reports of more severe events such as phlebitis, cellulitis, induration, skin exfoliation, necrosis and fibrosis have been received as part of the continuing surveillance of TAXOL safety. In some cases the onset of the injection site reaction either occurred during a prolonged infusion or was delayed by a week to ten days.

A specific treatment for extravasation reactions is unknown at this time. Given the possibility of extravasation, it is advisable to closely monitor the infusion site for possible infiltration during drug administration.

Carcinogenesis, Mutagenesis, Impairment of Fertility: The carcinogenic potential of TAXOL has not been studied. TAXOL has been shown to be mutagenic *in vitro* (chromosome aberrations in human lymphocytes) and *in vivo* (micronucleus test in mice) mammalian test systems, however, it did not induce mutagenicity in the Ames test or the CHO/HGPRT gene mutation assay. TAXOL at an I.V. dose of 1 mg/kg (6 mg/m^2) produced low fertility and fetal toxicity in rats. TAXOL has also been shown to be maternal and embryo-fetal toxic in rabbits receiving the drug at an I.V. dose of 3 mg/kg (33 mg/m^2) during organogenesis. (See "**WARNINGS**" section.)

Pregnancy: Pregnancy "Category D". (See "**WARNINGS**" section.)

Nursing Mothers: It is not known whether the drug is excreted in human milk. Because many drugs are excreted in human milk and because of the potential for serious adverse reactions in nursing infants, it is recommended that nursing be discontinued when receiving TAXOL therapy.

Pediatric Use: The safety and effectiveness of TAXOL in pediatric patients have not been established.

There have been reports of central nervous system (CNS) toxicity in an ongoing investigational clinical trial in pediatric patients in which TAXOL was infused intravenously over 3 hours at doses ranging from 350 mg/m^2 to 420 mg/m^2. The toxicity is most likely attributable to the high dose of the ethanol component of the TAXOL vehicle given over a short infusion time. The use of concomitant antihistamines may intensify this effect. Although a direct effect of the paclitaxel itself cannot be discounted, the high doses used in this study (over twice the recommended adult dosage) must be considered in assessing the safety of TAXOL for use in this population.

ADVERSE REACTIONS

Data in the following table are based on the experience of 812 patients (493 with ovarian carcinoma and 319 with breast carcinoma) enrolled in 10 studies. Two hundred and seventy-five patients were treated in 8 Phase 2 studies with TAXOL doses ranging from 135 to 300 mg/m^2 administered over 24 hours (in 4 of these studies, G-CSF was administered as hematopoietic support). Three hundred and one patients were treated in the randomized Phase 3 ovarian carcinoma study which compared two doses (135 or 175 mg/m^2) and two schedules (3 or 24 hours) of TAXOL. Two hundred and thirty-six patients with breast carcinoma received TAXOL (135 or 175 mg/m^2) administered over 3 hours in a controlled study.

Summary of Adverse Events in 812 Patients Receiving Taxol

		% Incidence
• **Bone Marrow**		
– Neutropenia	<2,000/mm^3	90
	<500/mm^3	52
– Leukopenia	<4,000/mm^3	90
	<1,000/mm^3	17
– Thrombocytopenia	<100,000/mm^3	20
	<50,000/mm^3	7
– Anemia	<11 g/dL	78
	<8 g/dL	16
– Infections		30
– Bleeding		14
– Red Cell Transfusions		25
– Platelet Transfusions		2
• **Hypersensitivity Reaction***		
– All		41
– Severe		2
• **Cardiovascular**		
– Vital Sign Changes**		
– Bradycardia (N=537)		3
– Hypotension (N=532)		12
– Significant Cardiovascular Events		1
• **Abnormal ECG**		
– All Pts		23
– Pts with normal baseline (N=559)		14
• **Peripheral Neuropathy**		
– Any symptoms		60
– Severe symptoms		3
• **Myalgia/Arthralgia**		
– Any symptoms		60
– Severe symptoms		8
• **Gastrointestinal**		
– Nausea and vomiting		52
– Diarrhea		38
– Mucositis		31
• **Alopecia**		87
• **Hepatic** (Pts with normal baseline and on study data)		
– Bilirubin elevations (N=765)		7
– Alkaline phosphatase elevations (N=575)		22
– AST (SGOT) elevations (N=591)		19
• **Injection Site Reaction**		13

**All patients received premedication*
** *During the first 3-hours of infusion*

None of the observed toxicities were clearly influenced by age.

The following data relate to the overall safety database of 812 patients treated in clinical studies. In addition, rare events have been reported from the postmarketing experi-

Continued on next page

Bristol-Myers Squibb Oncology—Cont.

ence or from other clinical studies. The frequency and severity of adverse events are generally similar between patients receiving TAXOL (paclitaxel) Injection for the treatment of ovarian or breast carcinoma. The frequency and severity of key adverse events for the Phase 3 ovarian and breast carcinoma studies are presented in tabular form by treatment arm in "**CLINICAL PHARMACOLOGY**", "**Clinical Studies**" section.

Hematologic: Bone marrow suppression was the major dose-limiting toxicity of TAXOL. Neutropenia, the most important hematologic toxicity, was dose and schedule dependent and was generally rapidly reversible. Among patients treated in Phase 3 ovarian study with a 3-hour infusion, neutrophil counts decline below 500 cells/mm^3 in 13% of the patients treated with a dose of 135mg/m^2 compared to 27% at a dose of 175 mg/m^2 ($p=0.05$). In the same study, severe neutropenia (<500 cells/mm^3) was more frequent with the 24-hour than with the 3-hour infusion; infusion duration had a greater impact on myelosuppression than dose. Neutropenia did not appear to increase with cumulative exposure and did not appear to be more frequent nor more severe for patients previously treated with radiation therapy.

Fever was frequent (12% of all treatment courses). Infectious episodes occurred in 30% of all patients and 9% of all courses; these episodes were fatal in 1% of all patients, and included sepsis, pneumonia and peritonitis. In the Phase 3 ovarian study, infectious episodes were reported in 19% of the patients given either 135 or 175 mg/m^2 dose by a 3 hour infusion. Urinary tract infections and upper respiratory tract infections were the most frequently reported infectious complications.

Thrombocytopenia was uncommon, and almost never severe (<50,000 cells/mm^3). Twenty percent of the patients experienced a drop in their platelet count below 100,000 cells/mm^3 at least once while on treatment; 7% had a platelet count <50,000 cells/mm^3 at the time of their worst nadir. Among the 812 patients, bleeding episodes were reported in 4% of all courses and by 14% of all patients but most of the hemorrhagic episodes were localized and the frequency of these events was unrelated to the TAXOL dose and schedule. In the Phase 3 ovarian study, bleeding episodes were reported in 10% of the patients receiving either the 135 or 175 mg/m^2 dose given by a 3-hour infusion; no patients treated with the 3-hour infusion received platelet transfusions.

Anemia (Hb <11 g/dL) was observed in 78% of all patients and was severe (Hb <8g/dL) in 16% of the cases. No consistent relationship between dose or schedule and the frequency of anemia was observed. Among all patients with normal baseline hemoglobin, 69% became anemic on study but only 7% had severe anemia. Red cell transfusions were required in 25% of all patients and in 12% of those with normal baseline hemoglobin levels.

Hypersensitivity Reactions (HSRs): All patients received premedication prior to TAXOL (See "**WARNINGS**" and "**PRECAUTIONS, Hypersensitivity Reactions**" sections). The frequency and severity of HSRs were not affected by the dose or schedule of TAXOL administration. In the Phase 3 ovarian study the 3-hour infusion was not associated with a greater increase in HSRs when compared to the 24-hour infusion. Hypersensitivity reactions were observed in 20% of all courses and in 41% of all patients. These reactions were severe in less than 2% of the patients and 1% of the courses. No severe reactions were observed after course 3 and severe symptoms occurred generally within the first hour of TAXOL infusion. The most frequent symptoms observed during these severe reactions were dyspnea, flushing, chest pain and tachycardia.

The minor hypersensitivity reactions consisted mostly of flushing (28%), rash (12%), hypotension (4%), dyspnea (2%), tachycardia (2%) and hypertension (1%). The frequency of hypersensitivity reactions remained relatively stable during the entire treatment period.

Rare reports of chills and reports of back pain in association with hypersensitivity reactions have been received as part of the continuing surveillance of TAXOL safety.

Cardiovascular: Hypotension, during the first 3-hours of infusion, occurred in 12% of all patients and 3% of all courses administered. Bradycardia, during the first 3-hours of infusion, occurred in 3% of all patients and 1% of all courses. In Phase 3 ovarian study, neither dose nor schedule had an effect on the frequency of hypotension and bradycardia. These vital sign changes most often caused no symptoms and required neither specific therapy nor treatment discontinuation. The frequency of hypotension and bradycardia were not influenced by prior anthracycline therapy.

Significant cardiovascular events possibly related to TAXOL occurred in approximately 1% of all patients. These events included syncope, rhythm abnormalities, hypertension and venous thrombosis. One of the patients with syncope treated with TAXOL at 175 mg/m^2 over 24 hours had progressive hypotension and died. The arrhythmias included asymptomatic ventricular tachycardia, bigeminy and complete AV block requiring pacemaker placement.

Electrocardiogram (ECG) abnormalities were common among patients at baseline. ECG abnormalities on study did not usually result in symptoms, were not dose-limiting, and required no intervention. ECG abnormalities were noted in 23% of all patients. Among patients with a normal ECG prior to study entry, 14% of all patients developed an abnormal tracing while on study. The most frequently reported ECG modifications were non-specific repolarization abnormalities, sinus bradycardia, sinus tachycardia and premature beats. Among patients with normal ECG at baseline, prior therapy with anthracylines did not influence the frequency of ECG abnormalities.

Cases of myocardial infarction have been reported rarely. Congestive heart failure has been reported typically in patients who have received other chemotherapy, notably anthracyclines. (See "**PRECAUTIONS**" section, "**Drug Interactions**" subsection)

Rare reports of atrial fibrillation and supraventricular tachycardia have been received as part of the continuing surveillance of TAXOL safety.

Respiratory: Rare reports of interstitial pneumonia, lung fibrosis and pulmonary embolism have been received as part of the continuing surveillance of TAXOL safety.

Neurologic: The frequency and severity of neurologic manifestations were dose-dependent, but were not influenced by infusion duration. Peripheral neuropathy was observed in 60% of all patients (3% severe) and in 52% (2% severe) of the patients without pre-existing neuropathy.

The frequency of peripheral neuropathy increased with cumulative dose. Neurologic symptoms were observed in 27% of the patients after the first course of treatment and 34–51% from course 2 to 10.

Peripheral neuropathy was the cause of TAXOL discontinuation in 1% of all patients. Sensory symptoms have usually improved or resolved within several months of TAXOL discontinuation. The incidence of neurologic symptoms did not increase in the subset of patients previously treated with cisplatin. Pre-existing neuropathies resulting from prior therapies are not a contraindication for TAXOL therapy.

Other than peripheral neuropathy, serious neurologic events following TAXOL administration have been rare (<1%) and have included grand mal seizures, syncope, ataxia and neuroencephalopathy.

Rare reports of autonomic neuropathy resulting in paralytic ileus have been received as part of the continuing surveillance of TAXOL safety. Optic nerve and/or visual disturbances (scintillating scotomata) have also been reported, particularly in patients who have received higher doses than those recommended. These effects generally have been reversible. However, rare reports in the literature of abnormal visual evoked potentials in patients have suggested persistent optic nerve damage.

Arthralgia/Myalgia: There was no consistent relationship between dose or schedule of TAXOL and the frequency or severity of arthralgia/myalgia. Sixty percent of all patients treated experienced arthralgia/myalgia; 8% experienced severe symptoms. The symptoms were usually transient, occurred two or three days after TAXOL administration, and resolved within a few days. The frequency and severity of musculoskeletal symptoms remained unchanged throughout the treatment period.

Hepatic: No relationship was observed between liver function abnormalities and either dose or schedule of TAXOL administration. Among patients with normal baseline liver function 7%, 22% and 19% had elevations in bilirubin, alkaline phosphatase and AST (SGOT), respectively. Prolonged exposure to TAXOL (paclitaxel) Injection was not associated with cumulative hepatic toxicity.

Rare reports of hepatic necrosis and hepatic encephalopathy leading to death have been received as part of the continuing surveillance of TAXOL safety.

Gastrointestinal (GI): Nausea/vomiting, diarrhea and mucositis were reported by 52%, 38% and 31% of all patients, respectively. These manifestations were usually mild to moderate. Mucositis was schedule dependent and occurred more frequently with the 24-hour than with the 3-hour infusion.

Rare reports of intestinal obstruction, intestinal perforation, pancreatitis, ischemic colitis, and dehydration have been received as part of the continuing surveillance of TAXOL safety. Rare reports of neutropenic enterocolitis (typhlitis), despite the coadministration of G-CSF, were observed in patients treated with TAXOL alone and in combination with other chemotherapeutic agents.

Injection Site Reaction: Injection site reactions, including reactions secondary to extravasation, were usually mild and consisted of erythema, tenderness, skin discoloration, or swelling at the injection site. These reactions have been observed more frequently with 24-hour infusion than with 3-hour infusion. Recurrence of skin reactions at a site of previous extravasation following administration of TAXOL at a different site, i.e., "recall", has been reported rarely.

Rare reports of more severe events such as phlebitis, cellulitis, induration, skin exfoliation, necrosis and fibrosis have been received as part of the continuing surveillance of TAXOL safety. In some cases the onset of the injection site reaction either occurred during a prolonged infusion or was delayed by a week to ten days.

A specific treatment for extravasation reactions is unknown at this time. Given the possibility of extravasation, it is advisable to closely monitor the infusion site for possible infiltration during drug administration.

Other Clinical Events: Alopecia was observed in almost all (87%) of the patients. Transient skin changes due to TAXOL related hypersensitivity reactions have been observed, but no other skin toxicities were significantly associated with TAXOL administration. Nail changes (changes in pigmentation or discoloration of nail bed) were uncommon (2%). Edema was reported in 21% of all patients (17% of those without baseline edema); only 1% had severe edema and none of these patients required treatment discontinuation. Edema was most commonly focal and disease-related. Edema was observed in 5% of all courses for patients with normal baseline and did not increase with time on study.

Rare reports of skin abnormalities related to radiation recall have been received as part of the continuing surveillance of TAXOL safety.

Rare reports of radiation pneumonitis have been rereceived in patients receiving concurrent radiotherapy.

Accidental Exposure: Upon inhalation, dyspnea, chest pain, burning eyes, sore throat and nausea have been reported. Following topical exposure, events have included tingling, burning and redness.

OVERDOSAGE

There is no known antidote for TAXOL overdosage. The primary anticipated complications of overdosage would consist of bone marrow suppression, peripheral neurotoxicity and mucositis.

DOSAGE AND ADMINISTRATION

Note: Contact of the undiluted concentrate with plasticized PVC equipment or devices used to prepare solutions for infusion is not recommended. In order to minimize patient exposure to the plasticizer DEHP [di-(2-ethylhexyl)phthalate], which may be leached from PVC infusion bags or sets, diluted TAXOL (paclitaxel) Injection solutions should be stored in bottles (glass, polypropylene) or plastic bags (polypropylene, polyolefin) and administered through polyethylene-lined administration sets.

All patients should be premedicated prior to TAXOL administration in order to prevent severe hypersensitivity reactions. Such premedication may consist of dexamethasone 20 mg PO administered approximately 12 and 6 hours before TAXOL, diphenhydramine (or its equivalent) 50 mg I.V. 30 to 60 minutes prior to TAXOL, and cimetidine (300 mg) or ranitidine (50 mg) I.V. 30 to 60 minutes before TAXOL.

In patients with carcinoma of the ovary, TAXOL has been used at several doses and schedules; however, the optimal regimen is not yet clear (see **CLINICAL PHARMACOLOGY** section). In patients previously treated with chemotherapy for ovarian cancer, the recommended regimen is TAXOL 135 mg/m^2 or 175 mg/m^2 administered intravenously over three hours every three weeks.

For patients with carcinoma of the breast, TAXOL at a dose of 175 mg/m^2 administered intravenously over 3 hours every three weeks has been shown to be effective after failure of chemotherapy for metastatic disease or relapse within 6 months of adjuvant chemotherapy.

Courses of TAXOL should not be repeated until the neutrophil count is at least 1,500 cells/mm^3 and the platelet count is at least 100,000 cells/mm^3. Patients who experience severe neutropenia (neutrophil <500 cells/mm^3 for a week or longer) or severe peripheral neuropathy during TAXOL therapy should have dosage reduced by 20% for subsequent courses of TAXOL. The incidence of neurotoxicity and the severity of neutropenia increase with dose.

Preparation and Administration Precautions: TAXOL is a cytotoxic anticancer drug and, as with other potentially toxic compounds, caution should be exercised in handling TAXOL. The use of gloves is recommended. If TAXOL solution contacts the skin, wash the skin immediately and thoroughly with soap and water. Following topical exposure, events have included tingling, burning and redness. If TAXOL contacts mucous membranes, the membranes should be flushed thoroughly with water. Upon inhalation, dyspnea, chest pain, burning eyes, sore throat, and nausea have been reported.

Given the possibility of extravasation, it is advisable to closely monitor the infusion site for possible infiltration during drug administration (See "**PRECAUTIONS: Injection Site Reaction**" section.)

Preparation for Intravenous Administration: TAXOL must be diluted prior to infusion. TAXOL should be diluted in 0.9% Sodium Chloride Injection, USP, 5% Dextrose Injection, USP, 5% Dextrose and 0.9% Sodium Chloride Injection, USP or 5% Dextrose in Ringer's Injection to a final concentration of 0.3 to 1.2 mg/mL. The solutions are physically and chemically stable for up to 27 hours at ambient temperature (approximately 25°C) and room lighting condi-

tions. Parenteral drug products should be inspected visually for particulate matter and discoloration prior to administration whenever solution and container permit.

Upon preparation, solutions may show haziness, which is attributed to the formulation vehicle. No significant losses in potency have been noted following simulated delivery of the solution through I.V. tubing containing an in-line (0.22 micron) filter.

Data collected for the presence of the extractable plasticizer DEHP [di-(2-ethylhexyl)phthalate] show that levels increase with time and concentration when dilutions are prepared in PVC containers. Consequently, the use of plasticized PVC containers and administration sets is not recommended. TAXOL solutions should be prepared and stored in glass, polypropylene, or polyolefin containers. Non-PVC containing administration sets, such as those which are polyethylene-lined, should be used.

TAXOL should be administered through an in-line filter with a microporous membrane not greater than 0.22 microns. Use of filter devices such as IVEX-2® filters which incorporate short inlet and outlet PVC-coated tubing has not resulted in significant leaching of DEHP.

The Chemo Dispensing Pin™ device or similar devices with spikes should not be used with vials of TAXOL since they can cause the stopper to collapse resulting in the loss of sterile integrity of the TAXOL solution.

Stability: Unopened vials of TAXOL are stable until the date indicated on the package when stored between 2°-25°C (36°-77°F), in the original package. Freezing does not adversely affect the product. Upon refrigeration components in the TAXOL vial may precipitate, but will redissolve upon reaching room temperature with little or no agitation. There is no impact on product quality under these circumstances. If the solution remains cloudy or if an insoluble precipitate is noted, the vial should be discarded. Solutions for infusion prepared as recommended are stable at ambient temperature (approximately 25°C) and lighting conditions for up to 27 hours.

IVEX-2® is the registered trademark of the Millipore Corporation.

Chemo Dispensing Pin™ is a trademark of B. Braun Medical Incorporated.

HOW SUPPLIED

NDC 0015-3475-27	30 mg/5 mL single-dose vial individually packaged in a carton.
NDC 0015-3476-27	100 mg/16.7 mL single-dose vial individually packaged in a carton.

Storage: Store the vials in original cartons between 2°-25°C (36°-77°F). Retain in the original package to protect from light.

Handling and Disposal: Procedures for proper handling and disposal of anticancer drugs should be considered. Several guidelines on this subject have been published[1-7]. There is no general agreement that all of the procedures recommended in the guidelines are necessary or appropriate.

REFERENCES

1. Recommendations for the Safe Handling of Parenteral Antineoplastic Drugs. NIH Publication No. 83-2621. For sale by the Superintendent of Documents, US Government Printing Office, Washington, DC 20402.
2. AMA Council Report. Guidelines for Handling Parenteral Antineoplastics. JAMA 1985; 253 (11): 1590-1592.
3. National Study Commission on Cytotoxic Exposure - Recommendations for Handling Cytotoxic Agents. Available from Louis P. Jeffrey, ScD, Chairman, National Study Commission on Cytotoxic Exposure. Massachusetts College of Pharmacy and Allied Health Sciences, 179 Longwood Avenue, Boston, Massachusetts, 02115.
4. Clinical Oncological Society of Australia. Guidelines and Recommendations for Safe Handling of Antineoplastic Agents. Med J Australia 1983; 1:426-428.
5. Jones RB, et al: Safe Handling of Chemotherapeutic Agents: A Report from the Mount Sinai Medical Center. CA-A Cancer Journal for Clinicians 1983; (Sept/Oct) 258-263.
6. American Society of Hospital Pharmacists Technical Assistance Bulletin on Handling Cytotoxic and Hazardous Drugs. Am J Hosp Pharm 1990; 47:1033-1049.
7. OSHA Work-Practice Guidelines for Personnel Dealing with Cytotoxic (Antineoplastic) Drugs. Am J Hosp Pharm 1986; 43:1193-1204.

MeadJohnson
ONCOLOGY PRODUCTS
A Bristol-Myers Squibb Company
Princeton, NJ 08543
U.S.A.

3475DIM-04
51-001978-03 Revised June 1996

Shown in Product Identification Guide, page 307

TESLAC® Ⓒ℞
(testolactone tablets, USP)

CAUTION: FEDERAL LAW PROHIBITS DISPENSING WITHOUT PRESCRIPTION.

DESCRIPTION

Teslac® (testolactone tablets, USP) is available for oral administration as tablets providing 50 mg testolactone per tablet. Testolactone is a synthetic antineoplastic agent that is structurally distinct from the androgen steroid nucleus in possessing a six-membered lactone ring in place of the usual five-membered carbocyclic D-ring. Testolactone is chemically designated as 13-hydroxy-3-oxo-13,17-secoandrosta-1,4-dien-17-oic acid δ-lactone. Graphic formula:

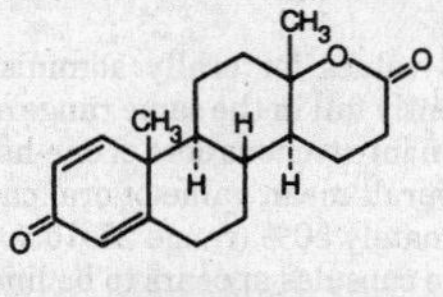

$C_{19}H_{24}O_3$ MW 300.40 CAS-968-93-4

Inactive ingredients: calcium stearate, cornstarch, gelatin, and lactose. Testolactone is a white, odorless, crystalline solid, soluble in ethanol and slightly soluble in water.

CLINICAL PHARMACOLOGY

Although the precise mechanism by which testolactone produces its clinical antineoplastic effects has not been established, its principal action is reported to be inhibition of steroid aromatase activity and consequent reduction in estrone synthesis from adrenal androstenedione, the major source of estrogen in postmenopausal women. Based on *in vitro* studies, the aromatase inhibition may be noncompetitive and irreversible. This phenomenon may account for the persistence of testolactone's effect on estrogen synthesis after drug withdrawal.

Despite some similarity to testosterone, testolactone has no *in vivo* androgenic effect. No other hormonal effects have been reported in clinical studies in patients receiving testolactone. In one study, testolactone administered orally (1000 mg/day) was reported to increase renal tubular reabsorption of calcium but to have no effect on serum calcium concentration. The mechanism of the hypocalciuric effect is unknown. No clinical effects in humans of testolactone on adrenal function have been reported; however, one study noted an increase in urinary excretion of 17-ketosteroids in most of the patients treated with 150 mg/day orally.

Testolactone is well absorbed from the gastrointestinal tract. It is metabolized to several derivatives in the liver, all of which preserve the lactone D-ring. These metabolites, as well as some unmetabolized drug, are excreted in the urine. Additional pharmacokinetic data in humans are unavailable.

For information concerning carcinogenesis, mutagenesis, pregnancy, and lactation, see the corresponding "**PRECAUTIONS**" sections.

In animals, parenteral but not oral testolactone reduced cortisone acetate induced hepatic glycogen deposits. In animal tests conducted to detect any hormonal activity for testolactone, some evidence of antiandrogenic and antiglucocorticoid activity was seen; increased growth rate in the newborn was suggested. However there was no clear manifestation of androgenic, estrogenic or antiestrogenic, progestational or antiprogestational, gonadotropin-like or antigonadotropic effects. Testolactone did not demonstrate anti-inflammatory, mineralocorticoid-like, or glucocorticoid-like properties.

INDICATIONS AND USAGE

TESLAC (testolactone tablets, USP) is recommended as adjunctive therapy in the palliative treatment of advanced or disseminated breast cancer in postmenopausal women when hormonal therapy is indicated. It may also be used in women who were diagnosed as having had disseminated breast carcinoma when premenopausal, in whom ovarian function has been subsequently terminated.

TESLAC was found to be effective in approximately 15 percent of patients with advanced or disseminated mammary cancer evaluated according to the following criteria: 1) those with a measurable decrease in size of all demonstrable tumor masses; 2) those in whom more than 50 percent of non-osseous lesions decreased in size although all bone lesions remained static; and 3) those in whom more than 50 percent of total lesions improved while the remainder were static.

CONTRAINDICATIONS

Testolactone is contraindicated in the treatment of breast cancer in men and in patients with a history of hypersensitivity to the drug.

PRECAUTIONS

Information for Patients–The physician should be consulted regarding missed doses. Notify the physician if adverse reactions occur or become more pronounced.

Laboratory Tests – Plasma calcium levels should be routinely determined in any patient receiving therapy for mammary cancer, particularly during periods of active remission of bony metastases. If hypercalcemia occurs, appropriate measures should be instituted.

Drug Interactions– When administered concurrently, testolactone may increase the effects of oral anticoagulants; monitor and adjust anticoagulant dosage accordingly.

Drug/Laboratory Test Interactions – Physiologic effects of testolactone may result in decreased estradiol concentrations with radioimmunoassays for estradiol, increased plasma calcium concentrations (See "**PRECAUTIONS, Laboratory Tests**"), and increased 24-hour urinary excretion of creatine and 17-ketosteroids.

Carcinogenesis, Mutagenesis, Impairment of Fertility – No long-term animal studies have been performed to evaluate carcinogenic potential or mutagenesis. Testolactone did not affect fertility in male or female rats.

Pregnancy: Teratogenic Effects, "Category C" – In rats, testolactone has been shown to produce increased fetal mortality, increased abnormal fetal development, and increased mortality in growing pups when given at doses 5 to 15 times the recommended human dose. In rabbits, no teratologic effects were observed at doses 2.5 to 7.5 times the recommended human dose. There are no adequate and well controlled studies in pregnant women. Testolactone is intended for use only in postmenopausal women and should not be used during pregnancy.

Nursing Mothers – It is not known whether this drug is excreted in human milk. Because many drugs are excreted in human milk, a decision should be made whether or not to discontinue nursing.

Pediatric Use–Safety and effectiveness in children have not been established.

ADVERSE REACTIONS

Certain signs and symptoms have been reported in association with the use of this drug but, in these instances, it is often impossible to determine the relationship of the underlying disease and drug administration to the reported reaction. Such reactions include maculopapular erythema, increase in blood pressure, paresthesia, aches and edema of the extremities, glossitis, anorexia and nausea and vomiting. Alopecia alone and with associated nail growth disturbance have been reported rarely; these side effects subsided without interruption of treatment.

DRUG ABUSE AND DEPENDENCE

TESLAC is classified as a controlled substance under the Anabolic Steroids Control Act of 1990 and has been assigned to Schedule III.

OVERDOSAGE

There have been no reports of acute overdosage with testolactone tablets.

DOSAGE AND ADMINISTRATION

The recommended oral dose is 250 mg qid.

In order to evaluate the response, therapy with testolactone should be continued for a minimum of three months unless there is active progression of the disease.

HOW SUPPLIED

TESLAC® (testolactone tablets, USP) **50 mg/tablet**: bottles of 100 (**NDC** 0003-0690-50). Each round, white, biconvex tablet is imprinted with the identification number 690.

Storage

Store at room temperature 25°C (77°F).

MeadJohnson
ONCOLOGY PRODUCTS
A Bristol-Myers Squibb Company
Princeton, NJ 08543
U.S.A.

K5-B001-5-96 P1-1944-00
Issued November 1994

VEPESID® ℞
(etoposide)
For Injection and Capsules

WARNINGS

VePesid (etoposide) should be administered under the supervision of a qualified physician experienced in the use of cancer chemotherapeutic agents. Severe myelosuppression with resulting infection or bleeding may occur.

DESCRIPTION

VePesid (etoposide) (also commonly known as VP-16) is a semisynthetic derivative of podophyllotoxin used in the treatment of certain neoplastic diseases. It is 4′-demethylepipodophyllotoxin 9-[4,6-0-(R)-ethylidene-β-D-glucopyranoside]. It is very soluble in methanol and chloroform,

Continued on next page

Bristol-Myers Squibb Oncology—Cont.

slightly soluble in ethanol, and sparingly soluble in water and ether. It is made more miscible with water by means of organic solvents. It has a molecular weight of 588.58 and a molecular formula of $C_{29}H_{32}O_{13}$.

VePesid may be administered either intravenously or orally. VePesid for Injection is available in 100 mg (5 mL) or 150 mg (7.5 mL), 500 mg (25 mL), or 1 gram (50 mL), sterile, multiple dose vials. The pH of the clear yellow solution is 3 to 4. Each mL contains 20 mg etoposide, 2 mg citric acid, 30 mg benzyl alcohol, 80 mg modified polysorbate 80/tween 80, 650 mg polyethylene glycol 300, and 30.5 percent (v/v) alcohol. Vial headspace contains nitrogen.

VePesid is also available as 50 mg pink capsules. Each liquid filled, soft gelatin capsule contains 50 mg of etoposide in a vehicle consisting of citric acid, glycerin, purified water, and polyethylene glycol 400. The soft gelatin capsules contain gelatin, glycerin, sorbitol, purified water and parabens (ethyl and propyl) with the following dye system: iron oxide (red) and titanium dioxide; the capsules are printed with edible ink.

The structural formula is:

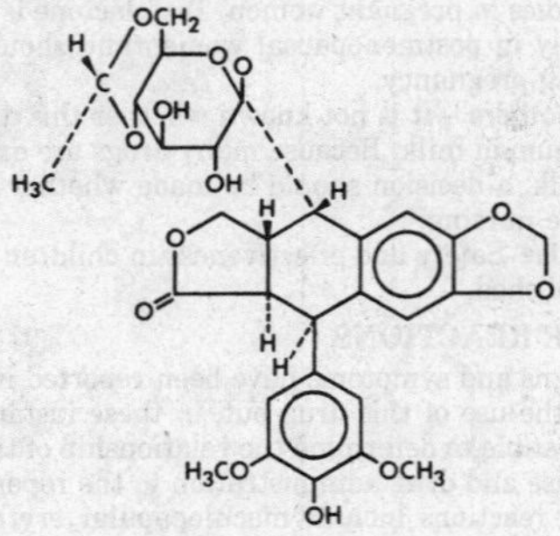

CLINICAL PHARMACOLOGY

VePesid has been shown to cause metaphase arrest in chick fibroblasts. Its main effect, however, appears to be at the G_2 portion of the cell cycle in mammalian cells. Two different dose-dependent responses are seen. At high concentrations (10 µg/mL or more), lysis of cells entering mitosis is observed. At low concentrations (0.3 to 10 µg/mL), cells are inhibited from entering prophase. It does not interfere with microtubular assembly. The predominant macromolecular effect of VePesid appears to be DNA synthesis inhibition.

Pharmacokinetics: On intravenous administration, the disposition of etoposide is best described as a biphasic process with a distribution half-life of about 1.5 hours and terminal elimination half-life ranging from 4 to 11 hours. Total body clearance values range from 33 to 48 mL/min or 16 to 36 mL/min/m^2 and, like the terminal elimination half-life, are independent of dose over a range 100–600 mg/m^2. Over the same dose range, the areas under the plasma concentration vs time curves (AUC) and the maximum plasma concentration (Cmax) values increase linearly with dose. Etoposide does not accumulate in the plasma following daily administration of 100 mg/m^2 for 4 to 5 days.

The mean volumes of distribution at steady state fall in the range of 18 to 29 liters or 7 to 17 L/m^2. Etoposide enters the CSF poorly. Although it is detectable in CSF and intracerebral tumors, the concentrations are lower than in extracerebral tumors and in plasma. Etoposide concentrations are higher in normal lung than in lung metastases and are similar in primary tumors and normal tissues of the myometrium. *In vitro,* etoposide is highly protein bound (97%) to human plasma proteins. An inverse relationship between plasma albumin levels and etoposide renal clearance is found in children. In a study determining the effect of other therapeutic agents on the *in vitro* binding of carbon-14 labeled etoposide to human serum proteins, only phenylbutazone, sodium salicylate and aspirin displaced protein-bound etoposide at concentrations achieved *in vivo.*[1]

Etoposide binding ratio correlates directly with serum albumin in patients with cancer and in normal volunteers. The unbound fraction of etoposide significantly correlated with bilirubin in a population of cancer patients.[2,3]

After intravenous administration of ^{3}H-etoposide (70–290 mg/m^2), mean recoveries of radioactivity in the urine range from 42 to 67%, and fecal recoveries range from 0 to 16% of the dose. Less than 50% of an intravenous dose is excreted in the urine as etoposide with mean recoveries of 8 to 35% within 24 hours.

In children, approximately 55% of the dose is excreted in the urine as etoposide in 24 hours. The mean renal clearance of etoposide is 7 to 10 mL/min/m^2 or about 35% of the total body clearance over a dose range of 80 to 600 mg/m^2. Etoposide, therefore, is cleared by both renal and nonrenal processes, ie, metabolism and biliary excretion. The effect of renal disease on plasma etoposide clearance is not known.

Biliary excretion appears to be a minor route of etoposide elimination. Only 6% or less of an intravenous dose is recovered in the bile as etoposide. Metabolism accounts for most of the nonrenal clearance of etoposide. The major urinary metabolite of etoposide in adults and children is the hydroxy acid [4'-demethylepipodophyllic acid-9-(4, 6-0-(R)-ethylidene-β-D-glucopyranoside)], formed by opening of the lactone ring. It is also present in human plasma, presumably as the **trans** isomer. Glucuronide and/or sulfate conjugates of etoposide are excreted in human urine and represent 5 to 22% of the dose.

After either intravenous infusion or oral capsule administration, the Cmax and AUC values exhibit marked intra- and inter-subject variability. This results in variability in the estimates of the absolute oral bioavailability of etoposide oral capsules.

Cmax and AUC values for orally administered etoposide capsules consistently fall in the same range as the Cmax and AUC values for an intravenous dose of one-half the size of the oral dose. The overall mean value of oral capsule bioavailability is approximately 50% (range 25–75%). The bioavailability of etoposide capsules appears to be linear up to a dose of at least 250 mg/m^2.

There is no evidence of a first-pass effect for etoposide. For example, no correlation exists between the absolute oral bioavailability of etoposide capsules and nonrenal clearance. No evidence exists for any other differences in etoposide metabolism and excretion after administration of oral capsules as compared to intravenous infusion.

In adults, the total body clearance of etoposide is correlated with creatinine clearance, serum albumin concentration, and nonrenal clearance. In children, elevated serum SGPT levels are associated with reduced drug total body clearance. Prior use of cisplatin may also result in a decrease of etoposide total body clearance in children.

INDICATION AND USAGE

VePesid is indicated in the management of the following neoplasms:

Refractory Testicular Tumors—VePesid for Injection in combination therapy with other approved chemotherapeutic agents in patients with refractory testicular tumors who have already received appropriate surgical, chemotherapeutic, and radiotherapeutic therapy.

Adequate data on the use of VePesid Capsules in the treatment of testicular cancer are not available.

Small Cell Lung Cancer—VePesid for Injection and/or Capsules in combination with other approved chemotherapeutic agents as first line treatment in patients with small cell lung cancer.

CONTRAINDICATIONS

VePesid is contraindicated in patients who have demonstrated a previous hypersensitivity to etoposide or any component of the formulation.

WARNINGS

Patients being treated with VePesid must be frequently observed for myelosuppression both during and after therapy. Dose-limiting bone marrow suppression is the most significant toxicity associated with VePesid therapy. Therefore, the following studies should be obtained at the start of therapy and prior to each subsequent dose of VePesid: platelet count, hemoglobin, white blood cell count and differential. The occurrence of a platelet count below 50,000/mm^3 or an absolute neutrophil count below 500/mm^3 is an indication to withhold further therapy until the blood counts have sufficiently recovered.

Physicians should be aware of the possible occurrence of an anaphylactic reaction manifested by chills, fever, tachycardia, bronchospasm, dyspnea, and hypotension. Higher rates of anaphylactic-like reactions have been reported in children who received infusions at concentrations higher than those recommended. The role that concentration of infusion (or rate of infusion) plays in the development of anaphylactic-like reactions is uncertain. (See "**ADVERSE REACTIONS**" section.) Treatment is symptomatic. The infusion should be terminated immediately, followed by the administration of pressor agents, corticosteroids, antihistamines, or volume expanders at the discretion of the physician.

For parenteral administration, VePesid should be given only by slow intravenous infusion (usually over a 30 to 60 minute period) since hypotension has been reported as a possible side effect of rapid intravenous injection.

Pregnancy: Pregnancy "Category D." VePesid can cause fetal harm when administered to a pregnant woman. VePesid has been shown to be teratogenic in mice and rats. There are no adequate and well-controlled studies in pregnant women. If this drug is used during pregnancy, or if the patient becomes pregnant while receiving this drug, the patient should be apprised of the potential hazard to the fetus. Women of childbearing potential should be advised to avoid becoming pregnant.

VePesid is teratogenic and embryocidal in rats and mice at doses of 1 to 3% of the recommended clinical dose based on body surface area.

In a teratology study in SPF rats, VePesid was administered intravenously at doses of 0.13, 0.4, 1.2, and 3.6 mg/kg/day on days 6 to 15 of gestation. VePesid caused dose-related maternal toxicity, embryotoxicity, and teratogenicity at dose levels of 0.4 mg/kg/day and higher. Embryonic resorptions were 90 and 100% at the 2 highest dosages. At 0.4 and 1.2 mg/kg, fetal weights were decreased and fetal abnormalities including decreased weight, major skeletal abnormalities, exencephaly, encephalocele, and anophthalmia occurred. Even at the lowest dose tested, 0.13 mg/kg, a significant increase in retarded ossification was observed.

VePesid administered as a single intraperitoneal, injection in Swiss-Albino mice at dosages of 1, 1.5 and 2 mg/kg on days 6, 7, or 8 of gestation caused dose-related embryotoxicity, cranial abnormalities, and major skeletal malformations.

PRECAUTIONS

General: In all instances where the use of VePesid is considered for chemotherapy, the physician must evaluate the need and usefulness of the drug against the risk of adverse reactions. Most such adverse reactions are reversible if detected early. If severe reactions occur, the drug should be reduced in dosage or discontinued and appropriate corrective measures should be taken according to the clinical judgment of the physician. Reinstitution of VePesid therapy should be carried out with caution, and with adequate consideration of the further need for the drug and alertness as to possible recurrence of toxicity.

Laboratory Tests: Periodic complete blood counts should be done during the course of VePesid treatment. They should be performed prior to therapy and at appropriate intervals during and after therapy. At least one determination should be done prior to each dose of VePesid.

Carcinogenesis, Mutagenesis, Impairment of Fertility: Carcinogenicity tests with VePesid have not been conducted in laboratory animals. VePesid should be considered a potential carcinogen in humans. The occurrence of acute leukemia with or without a preleukemic phase has been reported rarely in patients treated with VePesid in association with other antineoplastic agents.

The mutagenic and genotoxic potential of VePesid has been established in mammalian cells. VePesid caused aberrations in chromosome number and structure in embryonic murine cells and human hematopoietic cells; gene mutations in Chinese hamster ovary cells; and DNA damage by strand breakage and DNA-protein cross-links in mouse leukemia cells. VePesid also caused a dose-related increase in sister chromatid exchanges in Chinese hamster ovary cells.

Treatment of Swiss-Albino mice with 1.5 mg/kg IP of VePesid on day 7 of gestation increased the incidence of intrauterine death and fetal malformations as well as significantly decreased the average fetal body weight. Maternal weight gain was not affected.

Treatment of pregnant SPF rats with 1.2 mg/kg/day IV of VePesid for 10 days led to a prenatal mortality of 92%, and 50% of the implanting fetuses were abnormal.

Pregnancy: Pregnancy "Category D." (See "**WARNINGS**" section.)

Nursing Mothers: It is not known whether this drug is excreted in human milk. Because many drugs are excreted in human milk and because of the potential for serious adverse reactions in nursing infants from VePesid, a decision should be made whether to discontinue nursing or to discontinue the drug, taking into account the importance of the drug to the mother.

Pediatric Use: Safety and effectiveness in pediatric patients have not been established.

VePesid for Injection contains polysorbate 80. In premature infants, a life-threatening syndrome consisting of liver and renal failure, pulmonary deterioration, thrombocytopenia, and ascites has been associated with an injectable vitamin E product containing polysorbate 80. Anaphylactic reactions have been reported in pediatric patients. (See "**WARNINGS**" section).

ADVERSE REACTIONS

The following data on adverse reactions are based on both oral and intravenous administration of VePesid as a single agent, using several different dose schedules for treatment of a wide variety of malignancies.

Hematologic Toxicity: Myelosuppression is dose related and dose limiting, with granulocyte nadirs occurring 7 to 14 days after drug administration and platelet nadirs occurring 9 to 16 days after drug administration. Bone marrow recovery is usually complete by day 20, and no cumulative toxicity has been reported. Fever and infection have also been reported in patients with neutropenia.

The occurrence of acute leukemia with or without a preleukemic phase has been reported rarely in patients treated with VePesid in association with other antineoplastic agents. (See "**WARNINGS**" section).

Gastrointestinal Toxicity: Nausea and vomiting are the major gastrointestinal toxicities. The severity of such nausea and vomiting is generally mild to moderate with treatment discontinuation required in 1% of patients. Nausea and vomiting can usually be controlled with standard antie-

metic therapy. Gastrointestinal toxicities are slightly more frequent after oral administration than after intravenous infusion.

Hypotension: Transient hypotension following rapid intravenous administration has been reported in 1% to 2% of patients. It has not been associated with cardiac toxicity or electrocardiographic changes. No delayed hypotension has been noted. To prevent this rare occurrence, it is recommended that VePesid be administered by slow intravenous infusion over a 30- to 60-minute period. If hypotension occurs, it usually responds to cessation of the infusion and administration of fluids or other supportive therapy as appropriate. When restarting the infusion, a slower administration rate should be used.

Allergic Reactions: Anaphylactic-like reactions characterized by chills, fever, tachycardia, bronchospasm, dyspnea and/or hypotension have been reported to occur in 0.7% to 2% of patients receiving intravenous VePesid and in less than 1% of the patients treated with the oral capsules. These reactions have usually responded promptly to the cessation of the infusion and administration of pressor agents, corticosteroids, antihistamines, or volume expanders as appropriate; however, the reactions can be fatal. Hypertension and/or flushing have also been reported. Blood pressure usually normalizes within a few hours after cessation of the infusion. Anaphylactic-like reactions have occurred during the initial infusion of VePesid.

Facial/tongue swelling, coughing, diaphoresis, cyanosis, tightness in throat, laryngospasm, back pain and/or loss of consciousness have sometimes occurred in association with the above reactions. In addition, an apparent hypersensitivity-associated apnea has been reported rarely.

Rash, urticaria, and/or pruritus have infrequently been reported at recommended doses. At investigational doses, a generalized pruritic erythematous maculopapular rash, consistent with perivasculitis, has been reported.

Alopecia: Reversible alopecia, sometimes progressing to total baldness, was observed in up to 66% of patients.

Other Toxicities: The following adverse reactions have been infrequently reported: aftertaste, fever, pigmentation, abdominal pain, constipation, dysphagia, transient cortical blindness, and optic neuritis, and a single report of radiation recall dermatitis.

Hepatic toxicity, generally in patients receiving higher doses of the drug than those recommended, has been reported with VePesid. Metabolic acidosis has also been reported in patients receiving higher doses.

The incidences of adverse reactions in the table that follows are derived from multiple data bases from studies in 2,081 patients when VePesid was used either orally or by injection as a single agent.

ADVERSE DRUG EFFECT	PERCENT RANGE OF REPORTED INCIDENCE
Hematologic toxicity	
Leukopenia (less than 1,000 WBC/mm³)	3–17
Leukopenia (less than 4,000 WBC/mm³)	60–91
Thrombocytopenia (less than 50,000 platelets/mm³)	1–20
Thrombocytopenia (less than 100,000 platelets/mm³)	22–41
Anemia	0–33
Gastrointestinal toxicity	
Nausea and vomiting	31–43
Abdominal pain	0–2
Anorexia	10–13
Diarrhea	1–13
Stomatitis	1–6
Hepatic	0–3
Alopecia	8–66
Peripheral neurotoxicity	1–2
Hypotension	1–2
Allergic reaction	1–2

OVERDOSAGE

No proven antidotes have been established for VePesid overdosage.

DOSAGE AND ADMINISTRATION

Note: Plastic devices made of acrylic or ABS (a polymer composed of acrylonitrile, butadiene, and styrene) have been reported to crack and leak when used with underlined undiluted VePesid for Injection.

VePesid for Injection: The usual dose of VePesid for Injection in testicular cancer in combination with other approved chemotherapeutic agents ranges from 50 to 100 mg/m²/day on days 1 through 5 to 100 mg/m²/day on days 1, 3, and 5. In small cell lung cancer, the VePesid for Injection dose in combination with other approved chemotherapeutic drugs

ranges from 35 mg/m²/day for 4 days to 50 mg/m²/day for 5 days.

Chemotherapy courses are repeated at 3- to 4-week intervals after adequate recovery from any toxicity.

VePesid Capsules: In small cell lung cancer, the recommended dose of VePesid Capsules is two times the IV dose rounded to the nearest 50 mg.

The dosage, by either route, should be modified to take into account the myelosuppressive effects of other drugs in the combination or the effects of prior x-ray therapy or chemotherapy which may have compromised bone marrow reserve.

Administration Precautions: As with other potentially toxic compounds, caution should be exercised in handling and preparing the solution of VePesid. Skin reactions associated with accidental exposure to VePesid may occur. The use of gloves is recommended. If VePesid solution contacts the skin or mucosa, immediately wash the skin or mucosa thoroughly with soap and water.

Preparation for Intravenous Administration: VePesid for Injection must be diluted prior to use with either 5% Dextrose Injection, USP, or 0.9% Sodium Chloride Injection, USP, to give a final concentration of 0.2 or 0.4 mg/mL. If solutions are prepared at concentrations above 0.4 mg/mL, precipitation may occur. Hypotension following rapid intravenous administration has been reported, hence, it is recommended that the VePesid be administered over a 30- to 60-minute period. A longer duration of administration may be used if the volume of fluid to be infused is a concern. **VePesid should not be given by rapid intravenous injection.**

Parenteral drug products should be inspected visually for particulate matter and discoloration (see "**DESCRIPTION**" section) prior to administration whenever solution and container permit.

Stability: Unopened vials of VePesid for Injection are stable for 24 months at room temperature (25°C). Vials diluted as recommended to a concentration of 0.2 or 0.4 mg/mL are stable for 96 and 24 hours, respectively, at room temperature (25°C) under normal room fluorescent light in both glass and plastic containers.

VePesid Capsules must be stored under refrigeration 2°–8°C (36°–46°F). The capsules are stable for 24 months under such refrigeration conditions.

Procedures for proper handling and disposal of anticancer drugs should be considered. Several guidelines on this subject have been published[4-10]. There is no general agreement that all of the procedures recommended in the guidelines are necessary or appropriate.

HOW SUPPLIED

VePesid (etoposide) for Injection
NDC 0015-3095-20—100 mg/5 mL Sterile, Multiple Dose Vial, 10's
NDC 0015-3084-20—150 mg/7.5 mL Sterile, Multiple Dose Vial
NDC 0015-3061-20—500 mg/25 mL Sterile, Multiple Dose Vial
NDC 0015-3062-20—1 gram/50 mL Sterile, Multiple Dose Vial
VePesid (etoposide) Capsules
NDC 0015-3091-45—50 mg pink capsules with "BRISTOL 3091" printed in black in blisterpacks of 20 individually labeled blisters, each containing one capsule.
Capsules are to be stored under refrigeration 2°–8°C (36°–46°F).
DO NOT FREEZE.
Dispense in child-resistant containers.
For information on package sizes available, refer to the current price schedule.

REFERENCES

1. Gaver RC; Deeb G; "The effect of other drugs on the *in vitro* binding of 14C-etoposide to human serum proteins." *Proc Am Assoc Cancer Res.* 30:A2132, 1989.
2. Stewart CF; Pieper JA; Arbuck SG; Evans WE; "Altered protein binding of etoposide in patients with cancer." *Clin Pharmacol Ther.* 45:49–55 1989.
3. Stewart CF; Arbuck SG; Fleming RA; Evans WE; "Prospective evaluation of a model for predicting etoposide plasma protein binding in cancer patients." *Proc Am Assoc Cancer Res.* 30:A958 1989.
4. Recommendations for the Safe Handling of Parenteral Antineoplastic Drugs, NIH Publication No. 83-2621. For sale by the Superintendent of Documents, US Government Printing Office, Washington, D.C. 20402.
5. AMA Council Report. Guidelines for Handling Parenteral Antineoplastics. *JAMA.* 1985; 253 (11): 1590–1592.
6. National Study Commission on Cytotoxic Exposure—Recommendations for Handling Cytotoxic Agents. Available from Louis P. Jeffrey, Sc.D., Chairman, National Study Commission on Cytotoxic Exposure, Massachusetts College of Pharmacy and Allied Health Sciences, 179 Longwood Avenue, Boston, Massachusetts 02115.
7. Clinical Oncological Society of Australia. Guidelines and Recommendations for Safe Handling of Antineoplastic Agents. *Med J Australia.* 1983; 1:426–428.
8. Jones RB, et al; Safe handling of chemotherapeutic agents: A report from the Mount Sinai Medical Center. *CA—A Cancer Journal for Clinicians.* 1983; (Sept/Oct) 258–263.
9. American Society of Hospital Pharmacists Technical Assistance Bulletin on Handling Cytotoxic and Hazardous Drugs. *Am J Hosp Pharm.* 1990; 47:1033–1049.
10. OSHA Work-Practice Guidelines for Personnel Dealing with Cytotoxic (Antineoplastic) Drugs. *Am J Hosp Pharm.* 1986; 43:1193–1204.

(P3179-01)
June 1995
Shown in Product Identification Guide, pages 307 and 308

VUMON®
[vū 'mŏn]
**(teniposide) for Injection
Concentrate**

℞

WARNING

Vumon (teniposide) for Injection Concentrate is a cytotoxic drug, which should be administered under the supervision of a qualified physician experienced in the use of cancer chemotherapeutic agents. Appropriate management of therapy and complications is possible only when adequate treatment facilities are readily available.

Severe myelosuppression with resulting infection or bleeding may occur. Hypersensitivity reactions, including anaphylaxis-like symptoms, may occur with initial dosing or at repeated exposure to Vumon. Epinephrine, with or without corticosteroids and antihistamines has been employed to alleviate hypersensitivity reaction symptoms.

DESCRIPTION

Vumon (teniposide) for Injection Concentrate (also commonly known as VM-26), is supplied as a sterile nonpyrogenic solution in a nonaqueous medium intended for dilution with a suitable parenteral vehicle prior to intravenous infusion. Vumon is available in 50 mg (5 mL) ampules. Each mL contains 10 mg teniposide, 30 mg benzyl alcohol, 60 mg N,N-dimethylacetamide, 500 mg Cremophor® EL (polyoxyethylated castor oil)* and 42.7 percent (V/V) dehydrated alcohol. The pH of the clear solution is adjusted to approximately 5 with maleic acid.

Teniposide is a semisynthetic derivative of podophyllotoxin. The chemical name for teniposide is 4'-demethylepipodophyllotoxin 9-[4,6-0-(R)-2-thenylidene-β-D-glucopyranoside]. Teniposide differs from etoposide, another podophyllotoxin derivative, by the substitution of a thenylidene group on the glucopyranoside ring.

Teniposide has the following structural formula:

Teniposide is a white to off-white crystalline powder with the empirical formula $C_{32}H_{32}O_{13}S$ and a molecular weight of 656.66. It is a lipophilic compound with a partition coefficient value (octanol/water) of approximately 100. Teniposide is insoluble in water and ether. It is slightly soluble in methanol and very soluble in acetone and dimethylformamide.

CLINICAL PHARMACOLOGY

Teniposide is a phase-specific cytotoxic drug, acting in the late S or early G_2 phase of the cell cycle, thus preventing cells from entering mitosis.

Teniposide causes dose-dependent single- and double-stranded breaks in DNA and DNA: protein cross-links. The mechanism of action appears to be related to the inhibition of type II topoisomerase activity since teniposide does not intercalate into DNA or bind strongly to DNA. The cytotoxic effects of teniposide are related to the relative number of double-stranded DNA breaks produced in cells, which are a

Continued on next page

Bristol-Myers Squibb Oncology—Cont.

reflection of the stabilization of a topoisomerase II-DNA intermediate.

Teniposide has a broad spectrum of *in vivo* antitumor activity against murine tumors, including hematologic malignancies and various solid tumors. Notably, teniposide is active against sublines of certain murine leukemias with acquired resistance to cisplatin, doxorubicin, amsacrine, daunorubicin, mitoxantrone or vincristine.

Plasma drug levels declined biexponentially following intravenous infusion (155 mg/m^2 over 1 to 2.5 hours) of Vumon given to eight children (4–11 years old) with newly diagnosed acute lymphoblastic leukemia (ALL). The observed average pharmacokinetic parameters and associated coefficients of variation (CV%) based on a two-compartmental model analysis of the data are as follows:

[See table below.]

There appears to be some association between an increase in serum alkaline phosphatase or gamma glutamyl-transpeptidase and a decrease in plasma clearance of teniposide. Therefore, caution should be exercised if Vumon is to be administered to patients with hepatic dysfunction.

In adults, at doses of 100 to 333 mg/m^2/day, plasma levels increased linearly with dose. Drug accumulation in adult patients did not occur after daily administration of Vumon for 3 days. In pediatric patients, maximum plasma concentrations (Cmax) after infusions of 137 to 203 mg/m^2 over a period of one to two hours exceeded 40 μg/mL; by 20 to 24 hours after infusion plasma levels were generally $<2\mu g$/mL.

Renal clearance of parent teniposide accounts for about 10 percent of total body clearance. In adults, after intravenous administration of 10 mg/kg or 67 mg/m^2 of tritium-labeled teniposide, 44 percent of the radiolabel was recovered in urine (parent drug and metabolites) within 120 hours after dosing. From 4 to 12 percent of a dose is excreted in urine as parent drug. Fecal excretion of radioactivity within 72 hours after dosing accounted for 0 to 10 percent of the dose.

Mean steady-state volumes of distribution range from 8 to 44 L/m^2 for adults and 3 to 11 L/m^2 for children. The blood-brain barrier appears to limit diffusion of teniposide into the brain, although in a study in patients with brain tumors, CSF levels of teniposide were higher than CSF levels reported in other studies of patients who did not have brain tumors.

Teniposide is highly protein bound. *In vitro* plasma protein binding of teniposide is > 99 percent. The high affinity of teniposide for plasma proteins may be an important factor in limiting distribution of drug within the body. Steady state volume of distribution of the drug increases with a decrease in plasma albumin levels. Therefore, careful monitoring of children with hypoalbuminemia is indicated during therapy. Levels of teniposide in saliva, CSF and malignant ascites fluid are low relative to simultaneously measured plasma levels.

The pharmacokinetic characteristics of teniposide differ from those of etoposide, another podophyllotoxin. Teniposide is more extensively bound to plasma proteins, and its cellular uptake is greater. Teniposide also has a lower systemic clearance, a longer elimination half-life, and is excreted in the urine as parent drug to a lesser extent than etoposide.

In a study at St. Jude Children's Research Hospital (SJCRH), 9 children with acute lymphocytic leukemia (ALL) failing induction therapy with a cytarabine-containing regimen, were treated with Vumon plus cytarabine. Three of these patients were induced into complete remission with durations of remission of 30 weeks, 59 weeks, and 13 years. In another study at SJCRH, 16 children with ALL refractory to vincristine/prednisone-containing regimens were treated with Vumon plus vincristine and prednisone. Three of these patients were induced into complete remission with durations of remission of 5, 5, 37, and 73 weeks. In these two studies patients served as their own control based on the premise that long term complete remissions could not be achieved by re-treatment with drugs to which they had previously failed to respond.

INDICATIONS AND USAGE

Vumon, in combination with other approved anticancer agents, is indicated for induction therapy in patients with refractory childhood acute lymphoblastic leukemia.

Parameter	Mean	CV%
Total body clearance (mL/min/m^2)	10.3	25
Volume at steady-state (L/m^2)	3.1	30
Terminal half-life (hours)	5.0	44
Volume of central compartment (L/m^2)	1.5	36
Rate constant, central to peripheral (1/hours)	0.47	62
Rate constant, peripheral to central (1/hours)	0.42	37

CONTRAINDICATIONS

Vumon is generally contraindicated in patients who have demonstrated a previous hypersensitivity to teniposide and/or Cremophor® EL (polyoxyethylated castor oil).

WARNINGS

Vumon is a potent drug and should be used only by physicians experienced in the administration of cancer chemotherapeutic drugs. Blood counts as well as renal and hepatic function tests should be carefully monitored prior to and during therapy.

Patients being treated with Vumon (teniposide) should be observed frequently for myelosuppression both during and after therapy. Dose-limiting bone marrow suppression is the most significant toxicity associated with Vumon therapy. Therefore, the following studies should be obtained at the start of therapy and prior to each subsequent dose of Vumon: hemoglobin, white blood cell count and differential and platelet count. If necessary, repeat bone marrow examination should be performed prior to the decision to continue therapy in the setting of severe myelosuppression.

Physicians should be aware of the possible occurrence of a hypersensitivity reaction variably manifested by chills, fever, urticaria, tachycardia, bronchospasm, dyspnea, hypertension or hypotension and facial flushing. This reaction may occur with the first dose of Vumon and may be life threatening if not treated promptly with antihistamines, corticosteroids, epinephrine, intravenous fluids and other supportive measures as clinically indicated. The exact cause of these reactions is unknown. They may be due to the Cremophor® EL (polyoxyethylated castor oil) component of the vehicle or to teniposide itself[1]. Patients who have experienced prior hypersensitivity reactions to Vumon are at risk for recurrence of symptoms and should only be re-treated with Vumon if the antileukemic benefit already demonstrated clearly outweighs the risk of a probable hypersensitivity reaction for that patient. When a decision is made to re-treat a patient with Vumon in spite of an earlier hypersensitivity reaction, the patient should be pretreated with corticosteroids and antihistamines and receive careful clinical observation during and after Vumon infusion. In the clinical experience with Vumon at SJCRH and the National Cancer Institute (NCI), re-treatment of patients with prior hypersensitivity reactions has been accomplished using measures described above. To date, there is no evidence to suggest cross-sensitization between Vumon and VePesid.

One episode of sudden death, attributed to probable arrhythmia and intractable hypotension has been reported in an elderly patient receiving Vumon combination therapy for a nonleukemic malignancy. (See "ADVERSE REACTIONS" section.) Patients receiving Vumon treatment should be under continuous observation for at least the first 60 minutes following the start of the infusion and at frequent intervals thereafter. If symptoms or signs of anaphylaxis occur, the infusion should be stopped immediately, followed by the administration of epinephrine, corticosteroids, antihistamines, pressor agents, or volume expanders at the discretion of the physician. An aqueous solution of epinephrine 1:1000 and a source of oxygen should be available at the bedside.

For parenteral administration, Vumon should be given only by slow intravenous infusion (lasting at least 30- to 60-minutes) since hypotension has been reported as a possible side effect of rapid intravenous injection, perhaps due to a direct effect of Cremophor® EL[2,3]. If clinically significant hypotension develops, the Vumon infusion should be discontinued. The blood pressure usually normalizes within hours in response to cessation of the infusion and administration of fluids or other supportive therapy as appropriate. If the infusion is restarted, a slower administration rate should be used and the patient should be carefully monitored.

Acute central nervous system depression and hypotension have been observed in patients receiving investigational infusions of high-dose Vumon who were pretreated with antiemetic drugs. The depressant effects of the antiemetic agents and the alcohol content of the Vumon formulation may place patients receiving higher than recommended doses of Vumon at risk for central nervous system depression.

Pregnancy: Pregnancy "Category D."

Vumon may cause fetal harm when administered to a pregnant woman. Vumon has been shown to be teratogenic and embryotoxic in laboratory animals. In pregnant rats intravenous administration of Vumon, 0. 1–3 mg/kg (0.6–18 mg/m^2), every second day from day 6 to day 16 post coitum caused dose-related embryotoxicity and teratogenicity. Major anomalies included spinal and rib defects, deformed extremities, anophthalmia and celosomia.

There are no adequate and well-controlled studies in pregnant women. If Vumon is used during pregnancy, or if the patient becomes pregnant while receiving this drug, the patient should be apprised of the potential hazard to the fetus. Women of childbearing potential should be advised to avoid becoming pregnant during therapy with Vumon.

*Cremophor®EL is the registered trademark of BASF Aktiengesellschaft

PRECAUTIONS

General: In all instances where the use of Vumon is considered for chemotherapy, the physician must evaluate the need and usefulness of the drug against the risk of adverse reactions. Most such adverse reactions are reversible if detected early. If severe reactions occur, the drug should be reduced in dosage or discontinued and appropriate corrective measures should be taken according to the clinical judgment of the physician. Reinstitution of Vumon therapy should be carried out with caution, and with adequate consideration of the further need for the drug and alertness as to possible recurrence of toxicity.

Vumon must be administered as an intravenous infusion. Care should be taken to ensure that the intravenous catheter or needle is in the proper position and functional prior to infusion. Improper administration of Vumon may result in extravasation causing local tissue necrosis and/or thrombophlebitis. In some instances, occlusion of central venous access devices has occurred during 24-hour infusion of Vumon at a concentration of 0.1 to 0.2 mg/mL. Frequent observation during these infusions is necessary to minimize this risk[4,5].

Laboratory Tests: Periodic complete blood counts and assessments of renal and hepatic function should be done during the course of Vumon treatment. They should be performed prior to therapy and at clinically appropriate intervals during and after therapy. There should be at least one determination of hematologic status prior to therapy with Vumon.

Drug Interactions: In a study in which 34 different drugs were tested, therapeutically relevant concentrations of tolbutamide, sodium salicylate and sulfamethizole displaced protein-bound teniposide in fresh human serum to a small but significant extent. Because of the extremely high binding of teniposide to plasma proteins, these small decreases in binding could cause substantial increases in free drug levels in plasma which could result in potentiation of drug toxicity. Therefore, caution should be used in administering Vumon to patients receiving these other agents. There was no change in the plasma kinetics of teniposide when coadministered with methotrexate. However, the plasma clearance of methotrexate was slightly increased. An increase in intracellular levels of methotrexate was observed *in vitro* in the presence of teniposide.

Carcinogenesis, Mutagenesis, Impairment of Fertility: Children at SJCRH with ALL in remission who received maintenance therapy with Vumon at weekly or twice weekly doses (plus other chemotherapeutic agents), had a relative risk of developing secondary acute nonlymphocytic leukemia (ANLL) approximately 12 times that of patients treated according to other less intensive schedules[6].

A short course of Vumon for remission-induction and/or consolidation therapy was not associated with an increased risk of secondary ANLL, but the number of patients assessed was small. The potential benefit from Vumon must be weighed on a case by case basis against the potential risk of the induction of a secondary leukemia. The carcinogenicity of teniposide has not been studied in laboratory animals. Compounds with similar mechanisms of action and mutagenicity profiles have been reported to be carcinogenic and teniposide should be considered a potential carcinogen in humans. Teniposide has been shown to be mutagenic in various bacterial and mammalian genetic toxicity tests. These include positive mutagenic effects in the Ames/Salmonella and *B. subtilis* bacterial mutagenicity assays. Teniposide caused gene mutations in both Chinese hamster ovary cells and mouse lymphoma cells and DNA damage as measured by alkaline elution in human lung carcinoma derived cell lines. In addition, teniposide induced aberrations in chromosome structure in primary cultures of human lymphocytes *in vitro* and in L5178y/TK + /-mouse lymphoma cells *in vitro.* Chromosome aberrations were observed *in vivo* in the embryonic tissue of pregnant Swiss albino mice treated with teniposide. Teniposide also caused a dose-related increase in sister chromatid exchanges in Chinese hamster ovary cells and it has been shown to be embryotoxic and teratogenic in rats receiving teniposide during organogenesis. Treatment of pregnant rats IV with doses between 1.0 and 3.0 mg/kg/day on alternate days from day 6 to 16 post coitum caused retardation of embryonic development, prenatal mortality and fetal abnormalities.

Pregnancy: Pregnancy "Category D." (See "WARNINGS" section.)

Nursing Mothers: It is not known whether this drug is excreted in human milk. Because many drugs are excreted in

human milk and because of the potential for serious adverse reactions in nursing infants, a decision should be made whether to discontinue nursing or to discontinue the drug, taking into account the importance of Vumon therapy to the mother.

Patients with Down's Syndrome: Patients with both Down's Syndrome and leukemia may be especially sensitive to myelosuppressive chemotherapy. therefore, initial dosing with Vumon should be reduced in these patients. It is suggested that the first course of Vumon should be given at half the usual dose. Subsequent courses may be administered at higher dosages depending on the degree of myelosuppression and mucositis encountered in earlier courses in an individual patient.

ADVERSE REACTIONS

The table below presents the incidences of adverse reactions derived from an anlysis of data contained within literature reports of 7 studies involving 303 pediatric patients in which Vumon was administered by injection as a single agent in a variety of doses and schedules for a variety of hematologic malignancies and solid tumors. The total number of patients evaluable for a given event was not 303 since the individual studies did not address the occurrence of each event listed. Five of these 7 studies assessed Vumon activity in hematologic malignancies, such as leukemia. Thus, many of these patients had abnormal hematologic status at start of therapy with Vumon and were expected to develop significant myelosuppression as an endpoint of treatment.

Single-Agent Vumon (teniposide)
Summary of Toxicity for All Evaluable Pediatric Patients

Toxicity	Incidence in Evaluable Patients (%)
Hematologic toxicity	
Myelosuppression, nonspecified	75
Leukopenia (< 3,000 WBC/μL)	89
Neutropenia (< 2,000 ANC/μL)	95
Thrombocytopenia (< 100,000 plt/μL)	85
Anemia	88
Non-Hematologic Toxicity	
Mucositis	76
Diarrhea	33
Nausea/vomiting	29
Infection	12
Alopecia	9
Bleeding	5
Hypersensitivity reactions	5
Rash	3
Fever	3
Hypotension/Cardiovascular	2
Neurotoxicity	< 1
Hepatic dysfunction	< 1
Renal dysfunction	< 1
Metabolic abnormalities	< 1

Hematologic Toxicity: Vumon, when used with other chemotherapeutic agents for the treatment of ALL, results in severe myelosuppression. Early onset of profound myelosuppression with delayed recovery can be expected when using the doses and schedules of Vumon necessary for treatment of refractory ALL, since bone marrow hypoplasia is a desired endpoint of therapy. The occurrence of acute non-lymphocytic leukemia (ANLL), with or without a preleukemic phase, has been reported in patients treated with Vumon in combination with other antineoplastic agents. See "PRECAUTIONS" subsection "Carcinogenesis, Mutagenesis, Impairment of fertility".

Gastrointestinal Toxicity: Nausea and vomiting are the most common gastrointestinal toxicities, having occurred in 29 percent of evaluable pediatric patients. The severity of this nausea and vomiting is generally mild to moderate.

Hypotension: Transient hypotension following rapid intravenous administration has been reported in 2 percent of evaluable pediatric patients. One episode of sudden death, attributed to probable arrhythmia and intractable hypotension, has been reported in an elderly patient receiving Vumon combination therapy for a non-leukemic malignancy. No other cardiac toxicity or electrocardiographic changes have been documented. No delayed hypotension has been noted.

Allergic Reactions: Hypersensitivity reactions characterized by chills, fever, tachycardia, flushing, bronchospasm, dyspnea, and blood pressure changes (hypertension or hypotension) have been reported to occur in approximately 5 percent of evaluable pediatric patients receiving intravenous Vumon. The incidence of hypersensitivity reactions to Vumon appears to be increased in patients with brain tumors, and in patients with neuroblastoma[1].

Central Nervous System: Acute central nervous system depression and hypotension have been observed in patients receiving investigational infusions of high-dose Vumon who were pretreated with antiemetic drugs. The depressant effects of the antiemetic agents and the alcohol content of the Vumon formulation may place patients receiving higher than recommended doses of Vumon at risk for central nervous system depression.

Alopecia: Alopecia, sometimes progressing to total baldness, was observed in 9 percent of evaluable pediatric patients who received Vumon as single agent therapy. It was usually reversible.

OVERDOSAGE

There is no known antidote for Vumon overdosage. The anticipated complications of overdosage are secondary to bone marrow suppression. Treatment should consist of supportive care including blood products and antibiotics as indicated.

DOSAGE AND ADMINISTRATION

NOTE: Contact of undiluted Vumon (teniposide) for injection Concentrate with plastic equipment or devices used to prepare solutions for infusion may result in softening or cracking and possible drug product leakage. This effect has *not* been reported with *diluted solutions* of Vumon.

In order to prevent extraction of the plasticizer DEHP [di(2-ethylhexyl)phtalate], solutions of Vumon for injection Concentrate should be prepared in non-DEHP containing LVP containers such as glass or polyolefin plastic bags or containers.

Vumon solutions should be administered with non-DEHP containing IV administration sets.

In one study, childhood ALL patients failing induction therapy with a cytarabine-containing regimen were treated with the combination of Vumon 165 mg/m^2 and cytarabine 300 mg/m^2 intravenously, twice weekly for 8–9 doses. In another study, patients with childhood ALL refractory to vincristine/prednisone-containing regimens were treated with the combination of Vumon 250 mg/m^2 and vincristine 1.5 mg/m^2 intravenously, weekly for 4–8 weeks and prednisone 40 mg/m^2 orally × 28 days.

Adequate data in patients with hepatic insufficiency and/or renal insufficiency are lacking, but dose adjustments may be necessary for patients with significant renal or hepatic impairment.

Preparation and Administration Precautions: Vumon is a cytotoxic anticancer drug and as with other potentially toxic compounds, caution should be exercised in handling and preparing the solution of Vumon. Skin reactions associated with accidental exposure to Vumon may occur. The use of gloves is recommended. If Vumon solution contacts the skin, immediately wash the skin thoroughly with soap and water. If Vumon contacts mucous membranes, the membranes should be flushed thoroughly with water.

Preparation for Intravenous Administration: Vumon must be diluted with either 5 percent Dextrose Injection, USP or 0.9 percent Sodium Chloride Injection, USP, to give final teniposide concentrations of 0.1 mg/mL, 0.2 mg/mL, 0.4 mg/mL or 1.0 mg/mL. Solutions prepared in 5 percent Dextrose Injection, USP or 0.9 percent Sodium Chloride Injection, USP at teniposide concentrations of 0.1 mg/mL, 0.2 mg/mL or 0.4 mg/mL are stable at room temperature for up to 24 hours after preparation. Vumon solutions prepared at a final teniposide concentration of 1.0 mg/mL should be administered within 4 hours of preparation to reduce the potential for precipitation. **Refrigeration of Vumon solutions is not recommended.** Stability and use times are identical in glass and plastic parenteral solution containers.

Although solutions are chemically stable under the conditions indicated, precipitation of teniposide may occur at the recommended concentrations, especially if the diluted solution is subjected to more agitation than is recommended to prepare the drug solution for parenteral administration[7]. In addition, storage time prior to administration should be minimized and care should be taken to avoid contact of the diluted solution with other drugs or fluids. Parenteral drug products should be inspected visually for particulate matter and discoloration prior to administration whenever solution and container permit. **Precipitation has been reported during 24-hour infusions of Vumon diluted to teniposide concentrations of 0.1 to 0.2 mg/mL, resulting in occlusion of central venous access catheters in several patients[4,5]. Heparin solution can cause precipitation of teniposide, therefore, the administration apparatus should be flushed thoroughly with 5 percent Dextrose Injection or 0.9 percent Sodium Chloride Injection, USP before and after administration of Vumon[5].**

Hypotension has been reported following rapid intravenous administration; it is recommended that the Vumon solution be administered over at least a 30 to 60-minute period. **Vumon should not be given by rapid intravenous injection.**

In a 24-hour study under simulated conditions of actual use of the product relative to dilution strength, diluent and administration rates, dilutions at 0.1 to 1.0 mg/mL were chemically stable for at least 24 hours. Data collected for the presence of the extractable DEHP [di(2-ethylhexyl)phtalate] from PVC containers show that levels increased with time and concentration of the solutions. The data appeared similar for 0.9 percent Sodium Chloride Injection, USP, and 5 percent Dextrose Injection, USP. Consequently, the use of PVC containers is not recommended.

Similarly, the use of non-DEHP IV administration sets is recommended. Lipid administration sets or low DEHP containing nitroglycerin sets will keep patients' exposure to DEHP at low levels and are suitable for use. The diluted solutions are chemically and physically compatible with the recommended IV administration sets and LVP containers for up to 24 hours at ambient room temperature and lighting conditions. **Because of the potential for precipitation, compatibility with other drugs, infusion materials or IV pumps cannot be assured.**

Stability: Unopened ampules of Vumon (teniposide) for Injection Concentrate are stable until the date indicated on the package when stored under refrigeration (2°–8°C) in the original package. Freezing does not adversely affect the product.

HOW SUPPLIED

NDC 0015-3075-19 50 mg/5 mL sterile clear, colorless glass ampules individually packaged in a carton.

NDC 0015-3075-97 50 mg/5 mL sterile clear, colorless glass ampules individually nested in a carton tray of 10 ampules per tray.

Storage: Store the unopened ampules under refrigeration (2°–8°C). Retain in original package to protect from light.

Handling and Disposal: Procedures for proper handling and disposal of anticancer drugs should be considered. Several guidelines on this subject have been published[6–14]. There is no general agreement that all of the procedures recommended in the guidelines are necessary or appropriate.

REFERENCES

1. O'Dwyer PJ, King SA, Fortner CL and Leyland-Jones B: Hypersensitivity reactions to teniposide (VM-26): an analysis. *J Clin Oncol.* 1986; 4(8):1262–1269.
2. Lorenz W, Perlmann H-J, Schmall A, et al: Histamine release in dogs by Cremophor® EL and its derivatives. *Agents and Actions.* 1977; 7(1):63–67.
3. Lassus M, Scott D, and Leyland-Jones B: Allergic reactions associated with cremophor containing antineoplastics. *Proc Am Soc Clin Oncol* 1985; 4:268 (Abstract C-1042).
4. Strong D, Morris L: Precipitation of teniposide during infusion. *Am J Hosp Pharm* Mar 1990: Letter, 47:512,518.
5. Bogardus J, Kaplan M, Carpenter J: Precipitation of Teniposide During Infusion. *Am J Hosp Pharm;* Mar 1990: Letter, 47:518–519.
6. Pul C-H, et al: Acute Myeloid Leukemia in Children Treated with Epipodophyllotoxins for Acute Lymphoblastic Leukemia. *N Engl J Med.* 1991; 325:1682–1687.
7. Deardoff D, Schmidt C: Mixing additives in plastic LVPs. *Am J Hosp Phar.* Dec 1980: Letter, 37:1610, 1613.
8. Recommendations for the Safe Handling of Parenteral Antineoplastic Drugs. NIH Publication No. 83–2621. For sale by the Superintendent of Documents, US Government Printing office, Washington, DC 20402.
9. AMA Council Report. Guidelines for handling parenteral antineoplastics. *JAMA* 1985; 253 (11): 1590–1592.
10. National Study Commission on Cytotoxic Exposure—Recommendations for Handling Cytotoxic Agents. Available from Louis P. Jeffrey, Chairman, ScD, National Study Commission on Cytotoxic Exposure. Massachusetts College of Pharmacy and Allied Health Sciences, 179 Longwood Avenue, Boston, Massachusetts, 02115.
11. Clinical Oncological Society of Australia. Guidelines and Recommendations for Safe Handling of Antineoplastic Agents. *Med J Australia* 1983; 1:426–428.
12. Jones RB, et al: Safe handling of chemotherapeutic agents: a report from the Mount Sinai Medical Center. *CA-A Cancer Journal for Clinicians* 1983; Sept./Oct. 258–263.
13. American Society of Hospital Pharmacists Technical Assistance Bulletin on Handling Cytotoxic Drugs in Hospitals. *Am J Hosp Pharm* 1990; 47:1033–1049.
14. OSHA Work-Practice Guidelines for Personnel Dealing With Cytotoxic (Antineoplastic) drugs. *Am J Hosp Pharm* 1986; 43:1193–1204.

February 1994 P9819-02

ZERIT® ℞
(stavudine) Capsules

CAUTION: FEDERAL LAW PROHIBITS DISPENSING WITHOUT PRESCRIPTION.

WARNING

Patients receiving ZERIT® (stavudine) Capsules or any other antiretroviral therapy may continue to develop

Continued on next page

Bristol-Myers Squibb Oncology—Cont.

opportunistic infections and other complications of HIV infection, and therefore should remain under close clinical observation by physicians experienced in the treatment of patients with HIV-associated diseases.

DESCRIPTION

ZERIT® (stavudine) Capsules is the brand name for stavudine (formerly called d4T), a synthetic thymidine nucleoside analogue, active against the Human Immunodeficiency Virus (HIV). ZERIT® (stavudine) Capsules are supplied for oral administration in strengths of 15, 20, 30, and 40 mg of stavudine. Each capsule also contains inactive ingredients microcrystalline cellulose, sodium starch glycolate, lactose, and magnesium stearate. The hard gelatin shell consists of gelatin, methylparaben, propylparaben, titanium dioxide, and iron oxides.

The chemical name for stavudine is 2',3'-didehydro-3'-deoxythymidine. Stavudine has the following structural formula:

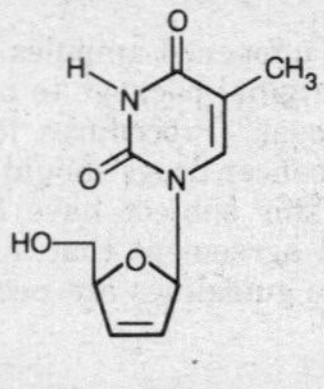

Stavudine is a white to off-white crystalline solid with the molecular formula $C_{10}H_{12}N_2O_4$ and a molecular weight of 224.2. The solubility of stavudine at 23°C is approximately 83 mg/mL in water and 30 mg/mL in propylene glycol. The n-octanol/water partition coefficient of stavudine at 23°C is 0.144.

CLINICAL PHARMACOLOGY

Mechanism of Action

Stavudine, a nucleoside analogue of thymidine, inhibits the replication of HIV in human cells *in vitro*. Stavudine is phosphorylated by cellular kinases to stavudine triphosphate which exerts antiviral activity. Stavudine triphosphate has an intracellular half-life of 3.5 hours in CEM and peripheral blood mononuclear cells. Stavudine triphosphate inhibits HIV replication by two known mechanisms: 1) it inhibits HIV reverse transcriptase by competing with the natural substrate deoxythymidine triphosphate (K1 =0.0083 to 0.032 μM); and 2) it inhibits viral DNA synthesis by causing DNA chain termination because stavudine lacks the 3'-hydroxyl group necessary for DNA elongation. In addition to the inhibitory effect on HIV reverse transcriptase, stavudine triphosphate inhibits cellular DNA polymerase beta and gamma, and markedly reduces the synthesis of mitochondrial DNA.

Microbiology

Antiviral activity *in vitro*:

The antiviral activity of stavudine has been demonstrated *in vitro* in a variety of primary and continuous cell types infected with laboratory derived and clinical isolates of HIV. However, the relationship between in vitro susceptibility of HIV to stavudine and inhibition of HIV replication in humans has not been established.

Drug resistance:

Preclinical studies: The potential for development of resistance to stavudine has been investigated *in vitro*. Selection studies performed with HIV-1 strains HXB2 and IIIb have produced isolates with reduced (7- to 30-fold) sensitivity to stavudine.

Clinical studies: Limited phenotypic and genotypic resistance studies (20 paired HIV isolates) have shown that 4- to 12-fold decreases (3/20 isolates) in stavudine susceptibility are possible; however, the genetic basis for the observed susceptibility changes has not been identified. The clinical relevance of stavudine susceptibility changes has not been established.

Five of 11 stavudine post-treatment isolates (9 of which were from patients who had previously received zidovudine) developed moderate resistance to zidovudine (9- to 176-fold) and 3 of those 11 isolates developed moderate resistance to didanosine (7- to 29-fold). The clinical relevance of these findings has not been established.

Pharmacokinetics

The pharmacokinetics of stavudine have been evaluated in 142 HIV-infected patients following administration of oral doses ranging from 0.03 to 4 mg/kg administered as single doses and as multiple doses every 6, 8, or 12 hours. Stavudine pharmacokinetics have also been evaluated in 44 HIV-infected patients after single intravenous doses ranging from 0.0625 to 1 mg/kg administered as 1-hour infusions.

Absorption and Bioavailability

Following oral administration to HIV-infected patients, stavudine was rapidly absorbed with a mean ±SD absolute bioavailability of 86.4 ±18.2% (n=25). Peak plasma concentrations (C_{max}) increased in a dose-related manner for doses (n=4 to 10 per dose level) ranging from 0.03 to 4 mg/kg and occurred ≤1 hour after dosing. Area under the plasma concentration-time curve (AUC) increased in proportion to dose after both single and multiple doses. There was no significant accumulation of stavudine with repeated administration every 6, 8, or 12 hours.

When stavudine (70 mg) was administered to 16 asymptomatic HIV-infected patients under fasting conditions, 1 hour before a standardized high-fat meal (773 Kcal, 53% fat), or immediately after the meal, systemic exposure (AUC) was similar. Mean ±SD C_{max} of stavudine was reduced from 1.44 ± 0.49 μg/mL in the fasting state to 0.75 ±0.16 μg/mL after the meal, and the median time to reach C_{max} was prolonged from 0.6 to 1.5 hours.

Distribution

Following 1-hour intravenous infusions (n=44) of stavudine doses ranging from 0.0625 to 1 mg/kg, mean ±SD volume of distribution was 58 ± 21 L, suggesting that stavudine distributes into extravascular spaces. Mean ±SD apparent volume of distribution following administration of single oral doses (n=71) ranging from 0.03 to 4 mg/kg was 66 ±22 L. Volume of distribution was independent of dose and did not correlate with body weight.

Binding of stavudine to serum proteins was negligible over the concentration range of 0.01–11.4 μg/mL. Stavudine distributes equally between red blood cells and plasma.

Metabolism

The metabolic fate of stavudine has not been elucidated in humans.

Elimination

Plasma clearance and terminal elimination half-life were independent of dose over an intravenous dosing range of 0.0625 to 1 mg/kg and an oral dosing range of 0.03 to 4 mg/kg. Following 1-hour infusions (n=44), plasma concentrations of stavudine declined in a biphasic manner with a mean ±SD terminal elimination half-life of 1.15 ± 0.35 hours. After single oral doses (n=115), the mean ±SD terminal elimination half-life was 1.44 ± 0.30 hours. Mean ±SD total body clearance, after intravenous infusion was 594 ± 164 mL/min (8.3 ± 2.3 mL/min/kg), and was independent of dose and body weight. Following single-dose oral administration (n=113), mean ±SD apparent oral clearance was independent of dose having a value of 559 ± 168 mL/min (8.03 ± 2.54 mL/min/kg). Renal elimination accounted for about 40% of the overall clearance regardless of the route of administration. The mean renal clearance was about twice the average endogenous creatinine clearance, indicating active tubular secretion in addition to glomerular filtration. Mean ±SD (n=88) cumulative urinary excretion of unchanged drug over 6 to 24 hours after administration of an oral dose was 39 ± 23% of the dose.

Special Populations

Pediatric:

(See "**PRECAUTIONS, Pediatric Use**".)

Renal Insufficiency:

Preliminary data from 14 non-HIV-infected subjects with reduced renal function and 5 subjects with normal renal function indicated that the apparent oral clearance (CL/F) of stavudine decreased as creatinine clearance (CL_{cr}) decreased (see Table 1). The terminal elimination half-life ($t^{1/2}$) was prolonged up to 8 hours. C_{max} and T_{max} were not significantly affected by reduced renal function. Based on these preliminary observations, it is recommended that ZERIT (stavudine) Capsules dosage be modified in patients with reduced creatinine clearance (see "**DOSAGE AND ADMINISTRATION**").

Table 1
Mean ±SD Pharmacokinetic Parameter Values Single 40-mg Oral Dose of ZERIT

	Creatinine Clearance		
	>50 mL/min (n=10)	26-50 mL/min (n=5)	9-25 mL/min (n=4)
CL_{cr} (mL/min)	104 ± 28	41 ± 5	15 ± 6
CL/F (mL/min)	335 ± 57	191 ± 39	106 ± 12
CL_R (mL/min)*	167 ± 65	73 ± 18	16 ± 3
$t_{1/2}$ (h)	1.7 ± 0.4	3.5 ± 2.5	4.8 ± 0.8

* CL_R=renal clearance

Hepatic Insufficiency:

Stavudine pharmacokinetics were not altered in 6 non-HIV infected patients with hepatic impairment secondary to cirrhosis (Child-Pugh classification B or C) following the administration of a single 40 mg dose.

Geriatric:

Stavudine pharmacokinetics have not been specifically investigated in patients >65 years of age.

Gender:

Stavudine pharmacokinetics have not been studied as a function of gender.

Race:

Pharmacokinetic differences due to race have not been evaluated.

INDICATIONS AND USAGE

ZERIT (stavudine) is indicated for the treatment of HIV-infected adults who have received prolonged prior zidovudine therapy.

CLINICAL STUDIES

Study AI455-019 was a multi-center, randomized, double-blind trial of ZERIT vs zidovudine for the treatment of HIV-infected adults with CD4 counts of 50 to 500 cells/mm³ who had received at least six months prior zidovudine treatment. ZERIT was administered in dosages of 40 mg BID for patients weighing ≥60 kg, and 30 mg BID for those weighing <60 kg. The zidovudine dosage was 200 mg TID.

The study enrolled 822 patients with a median baseline CD4 count of 235 cells/mm³ (range: 10 to 735 cells/mm³), and a median duration of prior zidovudine treatment of 88 weeks (range 11 to 356 weeks). Fourteen percent of subjects had AIDS at baseline, 50% had HIV-related symptoms and 36% were asymptomatic.

Table 2 gives the Kaplan-Meier estimates for the time to disease progression.

Table 2—Incidence of Disease Progression

	First AIDS–Defining Event or Death*	
	ZERIT	zidovudine
6 months	4.4%	5.7%
12 months	10.4%	14.1%
18 months	18.5%	23.3%
24 months	26.6%	31.8%

*Kaplan-Meier estimates; the overall difference between stavudine and zidovudine was not significant.

CONTRAINDICATIONS

ZERIT is contraindicated in patients with clinically significant hypersensitivity to stavudine or to any of the components contained in the formulation.

WARNINGS

The major clinical toxicity of ZERIT is peripheral neuropathy. This complication occurred in 19 and 24 percent of the 11,784 patients with advanced HIV disease who received the two dose levels of stavudine in the Parallel Track Program[1]. In patients with less advanced HIV infection in the zidovudine comparative trial, peripheral neuropathy occurred in 14 percent of ZERIT-treated patients as compared to 4 percent of zidovudine-treated patients.

[1] The parallel track program (STUDY A1455-900) Treated 12,551 HIV-infected patients with CD4 counts <300/mm³ who had failed, were intolerant of, or had contraindications to other therapies.

Patients should be monitored for the development of neuropathy that is usually characterized by numbness, tingling, or pain in the feet or hands. Stavudine-related peripheral neuropathy may resolve if therapy is withdrawn promptly. In some cases, symptoms may worsen temporarily following discontinuation of therapy. If symptoms resolve completely, resumption of treatment may be considered at a reduced dose (see "DOSAGE AND ADMINISTRATION").

Patients with a history of peripheral neuropathy are at increased risk for the development of neuropathy. If stavudine must be administered in this clinical setting, careful monitoring is essential.

PRECAUTIONS

Information for Patients

Patients should be informed that ZERIT (stavudine) Capsules is not a cure for HIV infection, and that they may continue to acquire illnesses associated with HIV infection, including opportunistic infections. Patients should be advised to remain under the care of a physician when using ZERIT.

Patients should be informed that the most common toxicity of ZERIT is peripheral neuropathy. Symptoms of peripheral neuropathy usually include tingling, burning, pain, or numbness in the hands or feet. Patients should be counseled that this toxicity occurs with greater frequency in patients with a history of peripheral neuropathy. They should be advised that these symptoms should be reported to their physicians and that dose changes may be necessary. They should also be cautioned about the use of other medications that may exacerbate peripheral neuropathy.

Patients should be informed that the long-term effects of ZERIT are unknown at this time. They should be advised that ZERIT therapy has not been shown to reduce the risk of transmission of HIV to others through sexual contact or blood contamination.

Patients should be informed that the Center for Disease Control (CDC) recommends that HIV-infected mothers not nurse newborn infants to reduce the risk of postnatal transmission of HIV infection.

Laboratory Tests
Mild to moderate increases in AST (SGOT) and ALT (SGPT) occurred commonly in clinical trials; these did not interfere with continued therapy (see "DOSAGE AND ADMINISTRATION").

Carcinogenesis, Mutagenesis, Impairment of Fertility
Long-term carcinogenicity studies of stavudine in animals have not been completed. Stavudine was not mutagenic in the Ames, E. coli reverse mutation, or the CHO/HGPRT mammalian cell forward gene mutation assays, with and without metabolic activation. Stavudine produced positive results in the in vitro human lymphocyte clastogenesis and mouse fibroblast assays, and in the in vivo mouse micronucleus test. In the in vitro assays, stavudine elevated the frequency of chromosome aberrations in human lymphocytes (concentrations of 25 to 250 μg/mL, without metabolic activation) and increased the frequency of transformed foci in mouse fibroblast cells (concentrations of 25 to 2500 μg/mL, with and without metabolic activation). In the in vivo micronucleus assay, stavudine was clastogenic in bone marrow cells following oral stavudine administration to mice at dosages of 600 to 2000 mg/kg/day for 3 days.
No evidence of impaired fertility was seen in rats with exposures (based on C_{max}) up to 216 times that observed following a clinical dosage of 1 mg/kg/day.

Pregnancy
Pregnancy "Category C". Reproduction studies have been performed in rats and rabbits with exposures (based on C_{max}) up to 399 and 183 times, respectively, of that seen at a clinical dosage of 1 mg/kg/day and have revealed no evidence of teratogenicity. The incidence in fetuses of a common skeletal variation, unossified or incomplete ossification of sternebra, was increased in rats at 399 times human exposure, while no effect was observed at 216 times human exposure. A slight post-implantation loss was noted at 216 times the human exposure with no effect noted at approximately 135 times the human exposure. An increase in early rat neonatal mortality (birth to 4 days of age) occurred at 399 times the human exposure, while survival of neonates was unaffected at approximately 135 times the human exposure. A study in rats showed that stavudine is transferred to the fetus through the placenta. The concentration in fetal tissue was approximately one-half the concentration in maternal plasma. There are no adequate and well-controlled studies in pregnant women. Because animal reproduction studies are not always predictive of human response, stavudine should be used during pregnancy only if clearly needed.

Nursing Mothers
The Center for Disease Control (CDC) recommends that HIV-infected mothers not breast feed their infants to avoid risking postnatal transmission of HIV infection. In addition, studies in which lactating rats were administered a single dose (5 or 100 mg/kg) of stavudine demonstrated that stavudine is readily excreted into breast milk. It is not known whether stavudine is excreted in human milk. Because many drugs are excreted in human milk, and because of the potential for adverse reactions from stavudine in nursing infants, mothers should be instructed not to nurse if they are receiving ZERIT.

Pediatric Use
Safety and effectiveness of ZERIT for treatment of HIV infection in pediatric patients have not been established. Limited data are available from 37 pediatric patients aged 5 months to 15 years who received ZERIT in doses ranging from 0.125 to 4.0 mg/kg/day for a median duration of 37 weeks (range 8 to 75 weeks). Serious adverse events that have been observed include AST (SGOT) and ALT (SGPT) elevations and one case of neuropathy.
Pharmacokinetics: Stavudine pharmacokinetics have been evaluated in 19 HIV-infected pediatric patients after single intravenous doses ranging from 0.125 to 2 mg/kg administered as 1-hour infusions. The pharmacokinetics of stavudine have been evaluated in 10 children (age 8 months to 4.5 years) who received stavudine oral solution and 8 children (age 6 to 15 years) who received stavudine capsules at oral doses ranging from 0.125 to 2 mg/kg administered every 12 hours.
Absorption: Stavudine was rapidly absorbed following oral administration to HIV-infected children with a mean $\pm$SD absolute bioavailability of 78.5 $\pm$ 35% and 69.2 $\pm$ 23% for capsule and solution formulations, respectively. First-dose and multiple-dose (after 12 weeks of treatment) pharmacokinetic profiles were similar, indicating no accumulation of stavudine.
Distribution: Following intravenous infusions (n=19) of stavudine at doses ranging from 0.125 to 2 mg/kg, the mean $\pm$SD volume of distribution was 13.2 $\pm$ 8.95 L (0.68 $\pm$ 0.29 L/kg), suggesting that stavudine distributes into extravascu-

lar spaces. After 12 weeks of treatment, the concentration of stavudine in cerebrospinal fluid samples collected from seven patients ranged from 0.01 to 0.12 μg/mL at times ranging from 2 to 3 hours post-dose (doses ranging from 0.125 to 1 mg/kg). The cerebrospinal fluid concentrations corresponded to 16% to 97% (mean, 55%; n=6) of the concentration in simultaneous plasma samples.
Elimination: Plasma concentrations of stavudine declined with a mean $\pm$SD terminal elimination half-life of 1.09 $\pm$ 0.28 hours following the end of a 1-hour infusion (n=19). After a single oral dose (n=18), the mean $\pm$SD terminal half-life was 0.91 $\pm$ 0.24 hours. The mean $\pm$SD total body clearance after intravenous infusion was 181.13 $\pm$ 98.36 mL/min (9.64 $\pm$ 3.10 mL/min/kg). The mean $\pm$SD apparent oral clearance after administration of solution (n=10, age <6 years) and capsule (n=8, age >6 years) formulations was 16.45 $\pm$ 4.28 and 11.01 $\pm$ 2.94 mL/min/kg, respectively.

ADVERSE REACTIONS
The major clinical toxicity of ZERIT (stavudine) Capsules is peripheral neuropathy (see "WARNINGS"). This toxicity is dose related (see Table 3). Modest elevation of hepatic transaminases was observed commonly in controlled trials.
[See Table 3 at top of next column.]

Selected adverse events that occurred in adult patients receiving ZERIT in the Phase 3 controlled comparative trial (Study AI455-019) and in the Parallel Track Program (Study AI455-900) are provided in Table 4.

[See Table 4 on top of next page.]

Table 3
Incidence of Peripheral Neuropathy Requiring Dose Modification in Controlled Clinical Trials

	%			
	Study A1455-019		Parallel Track Program	
	ZERIT (40 mg BID) (n=412)	zidovudine (200 mg TID) (n=402)	ZERIT (40 mg BID) (n=5905)	ZERIT (20 mg BID) (n=5879)
Peripheral Neuropathy[1]				
Grade 1–2	11	3	20	17
Grade 3–4	2	1	4	2
Total	13	4	24	19
Peripheral Neurologic Symptoms[2]				
Grade 1–2	38	35	5	5
Grade 3–4	<1	—	<1	1
Total	38	35	5	6

[1] Peripheral neuropathy regardless of grade leading to dose modification.
[2] Peripheral neurologic symptoms not requiring dose modification.

Table 5
Controlled Clinical Trials: Incidence of Adult Laboratory Abnormalities[a]

	%			
	Study AI455–019[b]		Parallel Track Program	
Lab Tests (units)	ZERIT (40 mg BID) (n=412)	zidovudine (200 mg TID) (n=402)	ZERIT (40 mg BID) (n=5905)	ZERIT (20 mg BID) (n=5879)
AST (SGOT) (1.25 • ≤5.0 × ULN[c])	63	49	60	59
AST (SGOT) (>5.0 × ULN)	11	10	6	6
ALT (SGPT) (1.25 • ≤5.0 × ULN)	65	46	62	62
ALT (SGPT) (>5.0 × ULN)	13	11	11	10
Bilirubin (>2.5 × ULN)	2	3	N/A[d]	N/A[d]
Anemia (<8.0 g/dL)	*	3	3	4
Neutropenia (neutrophils <750/mm^3)	5	9	12	13
Thrombocytopenia (platelets <50,000/mm^3)	3	3	4	5
Amylase (>1.4 × ULN)	14	13	N/A[d]	N/A[d]

* This abnormality was reported in fewer than 1% of patients.
a Data presented for patients for whom laboratory evaluations were performed.
b Median duration of stavudine therapy = 79 weeks; mediation duration of zidovudine therapy = 53 weeks.
c ULN = upper limit of normal.
d Collection of this data was not required per protocol.

Table 6

Creatinine Clearance (mL/min)	Recommended ZERIT Dose by Patient Weight	
	≥ 60 kg	< 60 kg
>50	40 mg every 12 hours	30 mg every 12 hours
26-50	20 mg every 12 hours	15 mg every 12 hours
10-25	20 mg every 24 hours	15 mg every 24 hours

Table 7

Product Strength	Capsule Shell Color	Markings on Capsule (in Black Ink)		Capsules per Bottle	NDC No.
15 mg	Light yellow & dark red	BMS 1964	15	60	0003–1964–01
20 mg	Light brown	BMS 1965	20	60	0003–1965–01
30 mg	Light orange & dark orange	BMS 1966	30	60	0003–1966–01
40 mg	Dark orange	BMS 1967	40	60	0003–1967–01

Continued on next page

Bristol-Myers Squibb Oncology—Cont.

Table 4
Selected Clinical Adverse Events in the Phase 3 Controlled Clinical Trials[1]

Adverse Events	Study A1455-019[2] ZERIT (40 mg BID) (n=412) %	Study A1455-019[2] zidovudine (200 mg TID) (n=402) %	Parallel Track Program ZERIT (40 mg BID) (n=5905) %	Parallel Track Program ZERIT (20 mg BID) (n=5879) %
Headache	54	49	3	4
Chills/ Fever	50	51	6	6
Diarrhea	50	43	5	5
Rash	40	35	4	4
Nausea and Vomiting	38	44	6	7
Peripheral Neurologic Symptoms[3]	38	35	5	6
Abdominal Pain	34	27	4	6
Myalgia	32	35	2	2
Insomnia	29	31	2	2
Anorexia	19	22	*	1
Peripheral Neuro-pathy[4]	14	4	24	19
Allergic Reaction	9	8	*	*
Pancrea-titis	*	*	2	2

* This event was reported in fewer than 1% of patients.
[1] Includes all clinical complaints.
[2] Median duration of stavudine therapy = 79 weeks; median duration of zidovudine therapy = 53 weeks.
[3] Peripheral neurologic symptoms not requiring dose modification.
[4] Peripheral neuropathy leading to dose modification.

Laboratory abnormalities reported in the Phase 3 controlled comparative trial (Study AI455-019) and the Parallel Track Program (Study AI455-900) are shown in Table 5.

[See Table 5 on preceding page.]

OVERDOSAGE

Experience with adults treated with 12 to 24 times the recommended daily dosage revealed no acute toxicity. Complications of chronic overdosage include peripheral neuropathy and hepatic toxicity. It is not known whether stavudine is eliminated by peritoneal dialysis or hemodialysis.

DOSAGE AND ADMINISTRATION

Adults: The interval between oral doses should be 12 hours. C_{max} was decreased by approximately 45% when stavudine was administered with food; however, the systemic availability (AUC) was unchanged (see "**CLINICAL PHARMACOLOGY**"). Thus, it appears that ZERIT (stavudine) Capsules may be taken without regard to meals. The recommended starting dose based on body weight is as follows:

40 mg twice daily for patients ≥60 kg.
30 mg twice daily for patients <60 kg.

Dosage Adjustment

Patients should be monitored for the development of peripheral neuropathy, which is usually characterized by numbness, tingling, or pain in the feet or hands. If these symptoms develop on treatment, stavudine therapy should be interrupted. Symptoms may resolve if therapy is withdrawn promptly. In some cases, symptoms may worsen temporarily following discontinuation of therapy. If symptoms resolve completely, resumption of treatment may be considered using the following dosage schedule:

20 mg twice daily for atients ≥60 kg.
15 mg twice daily for patients <60 kg.

Clinically significant elevations of hepatic transaminases should be managed in the same fashion.

Renal Impairment:

ZERIT may be administered to adult patients with impaired renal function. The following schedule is recommended:

[See Table 6 on preceding page.]

There are insufficient data to recommend a dose for patients with creatinine clearance <10 mL/min or for patients undergoing dialysis.

HOW SUPPLIED

ZERIT® (stavudine) Capsules are available in the following strengths and configurations of plastic bottles with child-resistant closures:

[See Table 7 on preceding page.]

US Patent No.: 4,978,655

Storage: ZERIT Capsules should be stored in tightly closed containers at controlled room temperature, 59° to 86°F (15° to 30°C).

BRISTOL-MEYERS SQUIBB
Immunology
Bristol-Myers Squibb Company
Princeton, NJ 08543
U.S.A.
F9-B001-4-96 P4577-02
Revised January 1996

Shown in Product Identification Guide, page 308

Bristol-Myers Products
(A Bristol-Myers Squibb Company)
345 PARK AVENUE
NEW YORK, NY 10154

Direct Inquiries to:
Products Division
Consumer Affairs Department
1350 Liberty Avenue
Hillside, NJ 07207
(800) 468-7746

Aspirin Free EXCEDRIN® OTC

COMPOSITION

Each caplet and geltab contains Acetaminophen 500 mg. and Caffeine 65 mg. Other Ingredients (caplet): Benzoic Acid, Carnauba Wax, Corn Starch, Croscarmellose Sodium, D&C Red No. 27 Lake, D&C Yellow No. 10 Lake, FD&C Blue No. 1 Lake, Hydroxypropyl Methylcellulose, Magnesium Stearate, Methylparaben, Microcrystalline Cellulose, Propylparaben, Saccharin Sodium, Simethicone Emulsion, Stearic Acid, Titanium Dioxide. May also contain: Erythorbic Acid, Mineral Oil, Polyethylene Glycol, Polysorbate 20, Polysorbate 80, Povidone, Propylene Glycol, Sorbitan Monolaurate. Other ingredients (geltab): benzoic acid, corn starch, FD&C Blue No. 1, FD&C Red No. 40, FD&C Yellow No. 6, Gelatin, Glycerin, Hydroxypropyl Methylcellulose, Magnesium Stearate, Microcrystalline Cellulose, Mineral Oil, Polysorbate 20, Povidone, Propylene Glycol, Simethicone Emulsion, Sorbitan Monolaurate, Titanium Dioxide.

INDICATIONS

For temporary relief of the pain of headache, sinusitis, colds, muscular aches, menstrual discomfort, toothaches and minor arthritis pain.

DIRECTIONS:

Adults: 2 caplets or geltabs every 6 hours while symptoms persist, not to exceed 8 caplets in 24 hours, or as directed by a doctor. Children under 12 years of age: Consult a doctor.

WARNINGS

Keep this and all other medications out of the reach of children. In case of accidental overdose, seek professional assistance or contact a poison control center immediately. Prompt medical attention is critical for adults as well as for children even if you do not notice any signs or symptoms. As with any drug, if you are pregnant or nursing a baby, seek the advice of a health professional before using this product. Do not take this product for pain for more than 10 days or for fever for more than 3 days unless directed by a doctor. If pain or fever persists or gets worse, if new symptoms occur, of if redness or swelling is present, consult a doctor because these could be signs of a serious condition. Consult a dentist promptly for toothache. If you generally consume 3 or more alcohol-containing drinks per day, you should consult your physician for advice on when and how you should take Excedrin and other pain relievers.

OVERDOSE

MUCOMYST (acetylcysteine) As An Antidote For Acetaminophen Overdose)

Acetaminophen is rapidly absorbed from the upper gastrointestinal tract with peak plasma levels occurring between 30 and 60 minutes after therapeutic doses and usually within 4 hours following an overdose. The parent compound, which is nontoxic, is extensively metabolized in the liver to form principally the sulfate and glucuronide conjugates which are also nontoxic and are rapidly excreted in the urine. A small fraction of an ingested dose is metabolized in the liver by the cytochrome P-450 mixed function oxidase enzyme system to form a reactive, potentially toxic, intermediate metabolite which preferentially conjugates with hepatic glutathione to form the nontoxic cysteine and mercapturic acid derivatives which are then excreted by the kidney. Therapeutic doses of acetaminophen do not saturate the glucuronide and sulfate conjugation pathways and do not result in the formation of sufficient reactive metabolite to deplete glutathione stores. However, following ingestion of a large overdose (150 mg/kg or greater) the glucuronide and sulfate conjugation pathways are saturated resulting in a larger fraction of the drug being metabolized via the P-450 pathway. The increased formation of reactive metabolite may deplete the hepatic stores of glutathione with subsequent binding of the metabolite to protein molecules within the hepatocyte resulting in cellular necrosis. Acetylcysteine has been shown to reduce the extent of liver injury following acetaminophen overdose. Early symptoms following a potentially hepatotoxic overdose may include: nausea, vomiting, diaphoresis and general malaise. Clinical and laboratory evidence of hepatic toxicity may not be apparent until 48 to 72 hours postingestion. In adults and adolescents, regardless of the quantity of acetaminophen reported to have been ingested, administer MUCOMYST® acetylcysteine immediately. MUCOMYST acetylcysteine therapy should be initiated and continued for a full course of therapy. Its effectiveness depends on early administration, with benefit seen principally in patients treated within 16 hours of the overdose.

If acetaminophen plasma assay capability is not available, and the estimated acetaminophen ingestion exceeds 150 mg/kg, MUCOMYST acetylcysteine therapy should be initiated and continued for a full course of therapy.

For full prescribing information, refer to the MUCOMYST package insert. Do not await the results of assays for acetaminophen level before initiating treatment with MUCOMYST acetylcysteine. The following additional procedures are recommended: The stomach should be emptied promptly by lavage or by induction of emesis with syrup of ipecac. A serum acetaminophen assay should be obtained as early as possible, but no sooner than four hours following ingestion. Liver function studies should be obtained initially and repeated at 24-hour intervals.

For additional emergency information call your regional poison center or toll-free (1-800-525-6115) to the Rocky Mountain Poison Center for assistance in diagnosis and for directions in the use of MUCOMYST acetylcysteine as an antidote.

HOW SUPPLIED

Aspirin Free EXCEDRIN® is supplied as: Coated red caplets with AFE debossed on one side

Supplied in bottles of 24's, 50's, 100's and bonus package of 125's.

All sizes packaged in child resistant closures except 100's size for caplets and 40's size for geltabs which is recommended for households without young children.

Easy to swallow red geltabs with "AF Excedrin" printed in white on one side

Supplied in bottles of 20's, 40's, 80's and bonus package of 100's.

All sizes packaged in child resistant closures except 40's which is recommended for households without young children.

Store at room temperature.

Also described in PDR For Nonprescription Drugs.

Shown in Product Identification Guide, page 306

EXCEDRIN® Extra-Strength OTC
Analgesic
[*ĕx ″cĕd ′rĭn*]

COMPOSITION

Each tablet, caplet, or geltab contains Acetaminophen 250 mg.; Aspirin 250 mg.; and Caffeine 65 mg.

Other ingredients (tablet or caplet): Benzoic Acid, FD&C Blue No. 1, Hydroxypropyl Methylcellulose, Microcrystalline Cellulose, Mineral Oil, Polysorbate 20, Povidone, Propylene Glycol, Saccharin Sodium, Simethicone Emulsion, Sorbitan Monolaurate, Stearic Acid, Titanium Dioxide. May also contain: Carnauba wax, Hydroxypropylcellulose.

Other ingredients (geltab): Benzoic Acid, D&C Yellow No. 10 Lake, Disodium EDTA, FD&C Blue No. 1 Lake, FD&C Red No. 40 Lake, Ferric Oxide, Gelatin, Glycerin, Hydroxypropyl cellulose, Hydroxypropyl Methylcellulose, Maltitol Solution, Microcrystalline Cellulose, Mineral Oil, Pepsin, Polysorbate 20, Povidone, Propylene Glycol, Propyl Gallate, Simethicon Emulsion, Sorbitan Monolaurate, Stearic Acid, Titanium Dioxide

INDICATIONS

For temporary relief of the pain of headache, sinusitis, colds, muscular aches, menstrual discomfort, toothaches and minor arthritis pain.

WARNINGS: Children and teenagers should not use this medicine for chicken pox or flu symptoms before a doctor is consulted about Reye syndrome, a rare but serious illness reported to be associated with aspirin. Keep this and all drugs out of the reach of children. In case of accidental overdose, seek professional assistance or contact a poison control center immediately. Prompt medical attention is critical for adults as well as for children even if you do not notice any signs or symptoms. As with any drug, if you are pregnant or nursing a baby, seek the advice of a health professional before using this product. **IT IS ESPECIALLY IMPORTANT NOT TO USE ASPIRIN DURING THE LAST 3 MONTHS OF PREGNANCY UNLESS SPECIFICALLY DIRECTED TO DO SO BY A DOCTOR BECAUSE IT MAY CAUSE PROBLEMS IN THE UNBORN CHILD OR COMPLICATIONS DURING DELIVERY.** Do not take this product for pain for more than 10 days or for fever for more than 3 days unless directed by a doctor. If pain or fever persists or gets worse if new symptoms occur, or if redness or swelling is present, consult a doctor because these could be signs of a serious condition. Consult a dentist promptly for toothache. Do not take this prod-

uct if you are allergic to aspirin, have asthma, have stomach problems (such as heartburn, upset stomach or stomach pain) that persist or recur, or if you have ulcers or bleeding problems, unless directed by a doctor. If ringing in the ears or loss of hearing occurs, consult a doctor before taking any more of this product. If you generally consume 3 or more alcohol-containing drinks per day, you should consult your physician for advice on when and how you should take Excedrin and other pain relievers.

DRUG INTERACTION PRECAUTION

Do not take this product if you are taking a prescription drug for anticoagulation (thinning of blood), diabetes, gout or arthritis unless directed by a doctor.

DIRECTIONS

Adults: 2 tablets or caplets with water every 6 hours while symptoms persist, not to exceed 8 tablets or caplets in 24 hours, or as directed by a doctor. Children under 12 years of age: Consult a doctor.

OVERDOSE

MUCOMYST (acetylcysteine) As An Antidote For Acetaminophen Overdose)

Acetaminophen is rapidly absorbed from the upper gastrointestinal tract with peak plasma levels occurring between 30 and 60 minutes after therapeutic doses and usually within 4 hours following an overdose. The parent compound, which is nontoxic, is extensively metabolized in the liver to form principally the sulfate and glucuronide conjugates which are also nontoxic and are rapidly excreted in the urine. A small fraction of an ingested dose is metabolized in the liver by the cytochrome P-450 mixed function oxidase enzyme system to form a reactive, potentially toxic, intermediate metabolite which preferentially conjugates with hepatic glutathione to form the nontoxic cysteine and mercapturic acid derivatives which are then excreted by the kidney. Therapeutic doses of acetaminophen do not saturate the glucuronide and sulfate conjugation pathways and do not result in the formation of sufficient reactive metabolite to deplete glutathione stores. However, following ingestion of a large overdose (150 mg/kg or greater) the glucuronide and sulfate conjugation pathways are saturated resulting in a larger fraction of the drug being metabolized via the P-450 pathway. The increased formation of reactive metabolite may deplete the hepatic stores of glutathione with subsequent binding of the metabolite to protein molecules within the hepatocyte resulting in cellular necrosis. Acetylcysteine has been shown to reduce the extent of liver injury following acetaminophen overdose. Early symptoms following a potentially hepatotoxic overdose may include: nausea, vomiting, diaphoresis and general malaise. Clinical and laboratory evidence of hepatic toxicity may not be apparent until 48 to 72 hours postingestion. In adults and adolescents, regardless of the quantity of acetaminophen reported to have been ingested, administer MUCOMYST® acetylcysteine immediately. MUCOMYST acetylcysteine therapy should be initiated and continued for a full course of therapy. Its effectiveness depends on early administration, with benefit seen principally in patients treated within 16 hours of the overdose.

If acetaminophen plasma assay capability is not available, and the estimated acetaminophen ingestion exceeds 150 mg/kg, MUCOMYST acetylcysteine therapy should be initiated and continued for a full course of therapy.

For full prescribing information, refer to the MUCOMYST package insert. Do not await the results of assays for acetaminophen level before initiating treatment with MUCOMYST acetylcysteine. The following additional procedures are recommended: The stomach should be emptied promptly by lavage or by induction of emesis with syrup of ipecac. A serum acetaminophen assay should be obtained as early as possible, but no sooner than four hours following ingestion. Liver function studies should be obtained initially and repeated at 24-hour intervals.

For additional emergency information call your regional poison center or toll-free (1-800-525-6115) to the Rocky Mountain Poison Center for assistance in diagnosis and for directions in the use of MUCOMYST acetylcysteine as an antidote.

HOW SUPPLIED

Extra Strength EXCEDRIN® is supplied as:
White circular tablet with letter "E" debossed on one side.
Supplied in bottles of 12's, 24's, 50's, 100's, 175's, metal tins of 12's.
Coated while caplets with "E" debossed on one side.
Supplied in bottles of 24's, 50's, 100's and 175's.
Excedrin Extra Strength geltabs supplied as coated green/white round tablets printed with Black "E" on one side.
Supplied in bottles of 20's, 40's, 80's and 2's.
All sizes packaged in child resistant closures except 100's for tablets, 50's for caplets which are sizes recommended for households without young children.
Also described in PDR For Nonprescription Drugs.
Shown in Product Identification Guide, page 306

EXCEDRIN P.M.®   OTC
[ĕx "cĕd 'rĭn]
Analgesic Sleeping Aid

COMPOSITION

Each tablet, caplet, or liquigel caplet contains:

	EXCEDRIN®PM Per Tablet or Caplet
Acetaminophen	500 mg.
Diphenhydramine Citrate:	38 mg.
Other Ingredients: (Tablet or Caplet)	—

Benzoic Acid
Carnauba Wax
Corn Starch
D&C Yellow No. 10 Aluminum Lake
FD&C Blue No. 1 Aluminum Lake
Hydroxypropyl Methylcellulose
Magnesium Stearate
Methylparaben, pregelatinized Starch
Propylparaben
Simethicone Emulsion
Stearic Acid
Titanium Dioxide
May Also Contain:
D&C Yellow No. 10
FD&C Blue No. 1
Polyethylene Glycol
Polysorbate 80
Propylene Glycol

	EXCEDRIN®PM Per Liquigel
Acetaminophen	500 mg.
Diphenhydramine HCL	25 mg.
Other Ingredients: (liquigel)	

D & C Red No. 33
FD&C Blue No. 1
FD&C Green No. 3
Gelatin
Glycerin
Polyethlene Glycol
Povidone
Propylene Glycol
Silicon Dioxide
Sorbitol
Titanium Dioxide
Water

INDICATIONS

For temporary relief of occasional headaches and minor aches and pains with accompanying sleeplessness.

WARNINGS

Keep this and all drugs out of the reach of children. In case of accidental overdose, seek professional assitance or contact a poison control center immediately. Prompt medical attention is critical for adults as well as for children even if you do not notice any signs or symptoms. As with any drug, if you are pregnant or nursing a baby, seek the advice of a health professional before using this product. Do not give to children under 12 years of age or use for more than 10 days unless directed by a doctor. If symptoms persist or get worse, if new ones occur, or if sleeplessness persists continuously for more than 2 weeks, consult your doctor. Insomnia may be a symptom of a serious underlying medical illness. Do not take this product, unless directed by a doctor, if you have a breathing problem such as emphysema or chronic bronchitis, or if you have glaucoma or difficulty in urination due to enlargement of the prostate gland. Avoid alcoholic beverages while taking this product. Do not take this product if you are taking sedatives or tranquilizers, without first consulting your doctor. If you generally consume 3 or more alcohol-containing drinks per day, you should consult your physician for advice on when and how you should take Excedrin PM and other pain relievers.

DIRECTIONS

Adults, 2 tablets, caplets, or liquigels at bedtime if needed or as directed by a doctor.

OVERDOSE

MUCOMYST (acetylcysteine) As An Antidote For Acetaminophen Overdose)

Acetaminophen is rapidly absorbed from the upper gastrointestinal tract with peak plasma levels occurring between 30 and 60 minutes after therapeutic doses and usually within 4 hours following an overdose. The parent compound, which is nontoxic, is extensively metabolized in the liver to form principally the sulfate and glucuronide conjugates which are also nontoxic and are rapidly excreted in the urine. A small fraction of an ingested dose is metabolized in the liver by the cytochrome P-450 mixed function oxidase enzyme system to form a reactive, potentially toxic, intermediate metabolite

---

which preferentially conjugates with hepatic glutathione to form the nontoxic cysteine and mercapturic acid derivatives which are then excreted by the kidney. Therapeutic doses of acetaminophen do not saturate the glucuronide and sulfate conjugation pathways and do not result in the formation of sufficient reactive metabolite to deplete glutathione stores. However, following ingestion of a large overdose (150 mg/kg or greater) the glucuronide and sulfate conjugation pathways are saturated resulting in a larger fraction of the drug being metabolized via the P-450 pathway. The increased formation of reactive metabolite may deplete the hepatic stores of glutathione with subsequent binding of the metabolite to protein molecules within the hepatocyte resulting in cellular necrosis. Acetylcysteine has been shown to reduce the extent of liver injury following acetaminophen overdose. Early symptoms following a potentially hepatotoxic overdose may include: nausea, vomiting, diaphoresis and general malaise. Clinical and laboratory evidence of hepatic toxicity may not be apparent until 48 to 72 hours postingestion. In adults and adolescents, regardless of the quantity of acetaminophen reported to have been ingested, administer MUCOMYST® acetylcysteine immediately. MUCOMYST acetylcysteine therapy should be initiated and continued for a full course of therapy. Its effectiveness depends on early administration, with benefit seen principally in patients treated within 16 hours of the overdose.

If acetaminophen plasma assay capability is not available, and the estimated acetaminophen ingestion exceeds 150 mg/kg, MUCOMYST acetylcysteine therapy should be initiated and continued for a full course of therapy.

For full prescribing information, refer to the MUCOMYST package insert. Do not await the results of assays for acetaminophen level before initiating treatment with MUCOMYST acetylcysteine. The following additional procedures are recommended: The stomach should be emptied promptly by lavage or by induction of emesis with syrup of ipecac. A serum acetaminophen assay should be obtained as early as possible, but no sooner than four hours following ingestion. Liver function studies should be obtained initially and repeated at 24-hour intervals.

For additional emergency information call your regional poison center or toll-free (1-800-525-6115) to the Rocky Mountain Poison Center for assistance in diagnosis and for directions in the use of MUCOMYST acetylcysteine as an antidote.

For overdose treatment information, consult a regional poison control center.

HOW SUPPLIED

EXCEDRIN P.M.® is supplied as:
Light blue circular coated tablets with "PM" debossed on one side.
Supplied in bottles of 10's, 24's, 50's and 100's.
Light blue coated caplet with "Excedrin PM" printed on one side.
Supplied in bottles of 24's, 50's, and 100's.
Light blue liquigels with "Excedrin PM" printed on one side.
Supplied in bottles of 20's and 40's.
All sizes packaged in child resistant closures except 50's tablets and caplets and 20's liquigels, which are recommended for households without young children.
Store at room temperature.
Also described in PDR For Nonprescription Drugs.

Bristol-Myers Squibb Company
P.O. BOX 4500
PRINCETON, NJ 08543-4500

For Medical Information Contact:
Generally:
Bristol-Myers Squibb Drug Information Department
P.O. Box 4500
Princeton, NJ 08543-4500
(800) 321-1335

Adverse Drug Experiences
and Product Defects Reporting call
between 8:30 AM–6:00 PM EST:
(609) 252-3737

Sales and Ordering:
Orders may be placed by:
1. Calling your purchase orders toll-free between 8:30 AM–6:00 PM EST:
(800) 631-5244
2. Mailing your purchase orders to:
Bristol-Myers Squibb U.S. Pharmaceuticals
Attn: Customer Service
P.O. Box 5250
Princeton, NJ 08543-5250
3. Faxing your purchase orders to:
(800) 523-2965
4. Transmitting computer-to-computer on the NWDA and UCS formats through Ordernet Services use: DEA# PE0048579

Continued on next page

Bristol-Myers Squibb Co.—Cont.

AZACTAM® FOR INJECTION

[a-zak'tam]
Aztreonam For Injection USP

℞

DESCRIPTION

AZACTAM (Aztreonam, Squibb) is the first member of a new class of antibiotics developed by the Squibb Institute for Medical Research and classified as monobactams. These agents were originally isolated from *Chromobacterium violaceum*. AZACTAM is a totally synthetic bactericidal antibiotic with activity against a wide spectrum of gram-negative aerobic pathogens.

The monobactams, having a unique monocyclic beta-lactam nucleus, are structurally different from other beta-lactam antibiotics (e.g., penicillins, cephalosporins, cephamycins). The sulfonic acid substituent in the 1-position of the ring activates the beta-lactam moiety; an aminothiazolyl oxime side chain in the 3-position and a methyl group in the 4-position confer the specific antibacterial spectrum and beta-lactamase stability.

Aztreonam is designated chemically as (Z)-2-[[[(2-amino-4-thiazolyl)][[(2S,3S)-2-methyl-4-oxo-1-sulfo-3-azetidinyl]carbamoyl]methylene]amino]oxy]-2-methylpropionic acid.

AZACTAM For Injection (Aztreonam For Injection) is a sterile, nonpyrogenic, sodium-free, white to yellowish-white lyophilized cake containing approximately 780 mg arginine per gram of aztreonam. Following constitution, the product is for intramuscular or intravenous use. Aqueous solutions of the product have a pH in the range of 4.5 to 7.5.

CLINICAL PHARMACOLOGY

Single 30-minute intravenous infusions of 500 mg, 1 g and 2 g doses of AZACTAM in healthy subjects produced peak serum levels of 54, 90 and 204 μg/mL, respectively, immediately after administration; at eight hours, serum levels were 1, 3 and 6 μg/mL, respectively (Figure 1). Single 3-minute intravenous injections of the same doses resulted in serum levels of 58, 125 and 242 μg/mL at five minutes following completion of injection.

Serum concentrations of aztreonam in healthy subjects following completion of single intramuscular injections of 500 mg and 1 g doses are depicted in Figure 1; maximum serum concentrations occur at about one hour. After identical single intravenous or intramuscular doses of AZACTAM, the serum concentrations of aztreonam are comparable at one hour (1.5 hours from start of intravenous infusion) with similar slopes of serum concentrations thereafter.

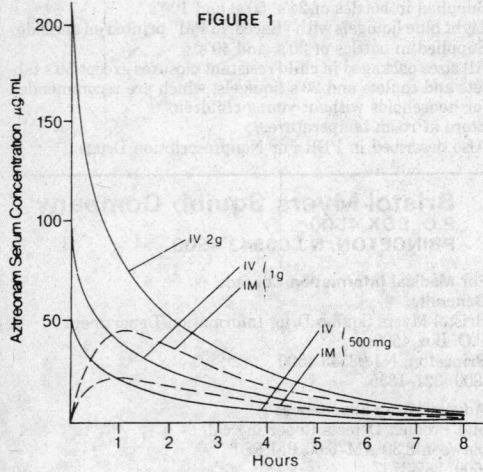

FIGURE 1

The serum levels of aztreonam following single 500 mg or 1 g (intramuscular or intravenous) or 2 g (intravenous) doses of AZACTAM (aztreonam) exceed the MIC$_{90}$ for *Neisseria* sp., *H. influenzae* and most genera of the *Enterobacteriaceae* for eight hours (for *Enterobacter* sp., the eight hour serum levels exceed the MIC for 80 percent of strains). For *Ps. aeruginosa*, a single 2 g intravenous dose produces serum levels that exceed the MIC$_{90}$ for approximately four to six hours. All of the above doses of AZACTAM result in average urine levels of aztreonam that exceed the MIC$_{90}$ for the same pathogens for up to 12 hours.

The serum half-life of aztreonam averaged 1.7 hours (1.5 to 2.0) in subjects with normal renal function, independent of the dose and route of administration. In healthy subjects, based on a 70 kg person, the serum clearance was 91 mL/min

and renal clearance was 56 mL/min; the apparent mean volume of distribution at steady-state averaged 12.6 liters, approximately equivalent to extracellular fluid volume.

In a study of healthy elderly male subjects (65 to 75 years of age), the average elimination half-life of aztreonam was slightly longer than in young healthy males.

In patients with impaired renal function, the serum half-life of aztreonam is prolonged (see DOSAGE AND ADMINISTRATION, Renal Impairment). The serum half-life of aztreonam is only slightly prolonged in patients with hepatic impairment since the liver is a minor pathway of excretion. Average urine concentrations of aztreonam were approximately 1100, 3500 and 6600 μg/mL within the first two hours following single 500 mg, 1 g and 2 g intravenous doses of AZACTAM (30-minute infusions), respectively. The range of average concentrations for aztreonam in the 8 to 12 hour urine specimens in these studies was 25 to 120 μg/mL. After intramuscular injection of single 500 mg and 1 g doses of AZACTAM, urinary levels were approximately 500 and 1200 μg/mL, respectively, within the first two hours, declining to 180 and 470 μg/mL in the six to eight hour specimens. In healthy subjects, aztreonam is excreted in the urine about equally by active tubular secretion and glomerular filtration. Approximately 60 to 70 percent of an intravenous or intramuscular dose was recovered in the urine by eight hours. Urinary excretion of a single parenteral dose was essentially complete by 12 hours after injection. About 12 percent of a single intravenous radiolabeled dose was recovered in the feces. Unchanged aztreonam and the inactive beta-lactam ring hydrolysis product of aztreonam were present in feces and urine.

Intravenous or intramuscular administration of a single 500 mg or 1 g dose of AZACTAM (aztreonam) every eight hours for seven days to healthy subjects produced no apparent accumulation of aztreonam or modification of its disposition characteristics; serum protein binding averaged 56 percent and was independent of dose. An average of about 6 percent of a 1 g intramuscular dose was excreted as a microbiologically inactive open beta-lactam ring hydrolysis product (serum half-life approximately 26 hours) of aztreonam in the zero to eight hour urine collection on the last day of multiple dosing.

Renal function was monitored in healthy subjects given aztreonam; standard tests (serum creatinine, creatinine clearance, BUN, urinalysis and total urinary protein excretion) as well as special tests (excretion of N-acetyl-β-glucosaminidase, alanine aminopeptidase and β_2-microglobulin) were used. No abnormal results were obtained.

Aztreonam achieves measurable concentrations in the following body fluids and tissues:

[See table below.]

The concentration of aztreonam in saliva at 30 minutes after a single 1 g intravenous dose (9 patients) was 0.2 μg/mL; in breast milk at two hours after a single 1 g intravenous dose (6 patients), 0.2 μg/mL, and at six hours after a single 1 g intramuscular dose (6 patients), 0.3 μg/mL; in amniotic fluid at six to eight hours after a single 1 g intravenous dose (5 pa-

tients), 2 μg/mL. The concentration of aztreonam in peritoneal fluid obtained one to six hours after multiple 2 g intravenous doses ranged between 12 and 90 μg/mL in 7 of 8 patients studied.

Aztreonam given intravenously rapidly reaches therapeutic concentrations in peritoneal dialysis fluid; conversely, aztreonam given intraperitoneally in dialysis fluid rapidly produces therapeutic serum levels.

Concomitant administration of probenecid or furosemide and AZACTAM (aztreonam) causes clinically insignificant increases in the serum levels of aztreonam. Single-dose intravenous pharmacokinetic studies have not shown any significant interaction between aztreonam and concomitantly administered gentamicin, nafcillin sodium, cephradine, clindamycin or metronidazole. No reports of disulfiram-like reactions with alcohol ingestion have been noted; this is not unexpected since aztreonam does not contain a methyl-tetrazole side chain.

The implications of the following information for predicting the occurrence of hypersensitivity reactions to AZACTAM have not been established. The number of patients included in immunologic studies is too small to draw firm conclusions with regard to clinical practice:

A study in rabbits suggests that antibodies produced in response to benzylpenicillin and to cephalothin show little cross-reactivity with aztreonam, and antibodies produced in response to aztreonam show little cross-reactivity with benzylpenicillin and cephalothin.

In a group of 22 subjects with positive skin tests to penicillin reagents, three also had positive skin tests to aztreonam. One was negative on retesting, one was confirmed as positive, and the third subject refused further evaluation. The 20 subjects with negative aztreonam skin tests were given one injection of AZACTAM 1 g IM. There were no immediate hypersensitivity reactions, but one subject later developed a localized rash that was compatible with a fixed drug eruption.

In 36 subjects receiving multiple doses of AZACTAM over a seven-day period, no IgE antibody response was detectable and only one subject demonstrated an IgG response.

Microbiology

Aztreonam exhibits potent and specific activity *in vitro* against a wide spectrum of gram-negative aerobic pathogens including *Pseudomonas aeruginosa*. The bactericidal action of aztreonam results from the inhibition of bacterial cell wall synthesis due to a high affinity of aztreonam for penicillin binding protein 3 (PBP3). Aztreonam, unlike the majority of beta-lactam antibiotics, does not induce beta-lactamase activity and its molecular structure confers a high degree of resistance to hydrolysis by beta-lactamases (i.e., penicillinases and cephalosporinases) produced by most gram-negative and gram-positive pathogens; it is therefore usually active against gram-negative aerobic organisms that are resistant to antibiotics hydrolyzed by beta-lactamases. Aztreonam maintains its antimicrobial activity over a pH range of 6 to 8 *in vitro*, as well as in the presence of human serum and under anaerobic conditions. Aztreonam is active *in vitro* and

EXTRAVASCULAR CONCENTRATIONS OF AZTREONAM AFTER A SINGLE PARENTERAL DOSE[1]

Fluid or Tissue	Dose (g)	Route	Hours Post-injection	Number of Patients	Mean Concentration (μg/mL or μg/g)
Fluids					
bile	1	IV	2	10	39
blister fluid	1	IV	1	6	20
bronchial secretion	2	IV	4	7	5
cerebrospinal fluid (inflamed meninges)	2	IV	0.9–4.3	16	3
pericardial fluid	2	IV	1	6	33
pleural fluid	2	IV	1.1–3.0	3	51
synovial fluid	2	IV	0.8–1.9	11	83
Tissues					
atrial appendage	2	IV	0.9–1.6	12	22
endometrium	2	IV	0.7–1.9	4	9
fallopian tube	2	IV	0.7–1.9	8	12
fat	2	IV	1.3–2.0	10	5
femur	2	IV	1.0–2.1	15	16
gallbladder	2	IV	0.8–1.3	4	23
kidney	2	IV	2.4–5.6	5	67
large intestine	2	IV	0.8–1.9	9	12
liver	2	IV	0.9–2.0	6	47
lung	2	IV	1.2–2.1	6	22
myometrium	2	IV	0.7–1.9	9	11
ovary	2	IV	0.7–1.9	7	13
prostate	1	IM	0.8–3.0	8	8
skeletal muscle	2	IV	0.3–0.7	6	16
skin	2	IV	0.0–1.0	8	25
sternum	2	IV	1	6	6

[1] Tissue penetration is regarded as essential to therapeutic efficacy, but specific tissue levels have not been correlated with specific therapeutic effects.

is effective in laboratory animal models and clinical infections against most strains of the following organisms, including many that are multiply-resistant to other antibiotics (i.e., certain cephalosporins, penicillins, and aminoglycosides):

Escherichia coli
Enterobacter species
Klebsiella pneumoniae and *K. oxytoca*
Proteus mirabilis
Pseudomonas aeruginosa
Serratia marcescens
Haemophilus influenzae (including ampicillin-resistant and other penicillinase-producing strains)
Citrobacter species

While *in vitro* studies have demonstrated the susceptibility to aztreonam of most strains of the following organisms, clinical efficacy for infections other than those included in the INDICATIONS AND USAGE section has not been documented:

Neisseria gonorrhoeae (including penicillinase-producing strains)
Proteus vulgaris
Morganella morganii (formerly *Proteus morganii*)
Providencia species, including *P. stuartii* and *P. rettgeri* (formerly *Proteus rettgeri*)
Pseudomonas species
Shigella species
Pasteurella multocida
Yersinia enterocolitica
Aeromonas hydrophila
Neisseria meningitidis

Aztreonam and aminoglycosides have been shown to be synergistic *in vitro* against most strains of *Ps. aeruginosa*, many strains of *Enterobacteriaceae*, and other gram-negative aerobic bacilli.

Alterations of the anaerobic intestinal flora by broad spectrum antibiotics may decrease colonization resistance, thus permitting overgrowth of potential pathogens, e.g., *Candida* and *Clostridia* species. Aztreonam has little effect on the anaerobic intestinal microflora in *in vitro* studies. *Clostridium difficile* and its cytotoxin were not found in animal models following administration of aztreonam (see ADVERSE REACTIONS, Gastrointestinal).

Susceptibility Testing

Diffusion Technique: Quantitative procedures that require measurement of zone diameters give precise estimates of microbial susceptibility to antibiotics. One such method, recommended for use with the aztreonam 30 µg disk, is the National Committee of Clinical Laboratory Standards (NCCLS) approved procedure. Only a 30 µg aztreonam disk should be used; there are no suitable surrogate disks.

Results of laboratory tests using 30 µg aztreonam disks should be interpreted using the following criteria:

Zone Diameter (mm)	Interpretation
≥ 22	(S) Susceptible
16–21	(I) Intermediate (Moderate Susceptibility)
≤ 15	(R) Resistant

Dilution Technique: Broth or agar dilution methods may be used to determine the minimal inhibitory concentration (MIC) of aztreonam.

MIC test results should be interpreted according to the concentrations of aztreonam that can be attained in serum, tissues and body fluids.

MIC (µg/mL)	Interpretation
≤ 8	(S) Susceptible
16	(I) Intermediate (Moderate Susceptibility)
≥ 32	(R) Resistant

For any susceptibility test, a report of "susceptible" indicates that the pathogen is likely to respond to AZACTAM therapy; a report of "resistant" indicates that the pathogen is not likely to respond. A report of "intermediate" (moderate susceptibility) indicates that the pathogen is expected to be susceptible to AZACTAM (aztreonam) if high dosages are used, or if the infection is confined to tissues and fluids (e.g., urine, bile) in which high aztreonam levels are attained.

The quality control cultures should have the following assigned daily ranges for aztreonam:

	Disks	Mode MIC (µg/mL)
E. coli (ATCC 25922)	28–36 mm	0.06–0.25
Ps. aeruginosa (ATCC 27853)	23–29 mm	2.0–8.0

INDICATIONS AND USAGE

Before initiating treatment with AZACTAM, appropriate specimens should be obtained for isolation of the causative organism(s) and for determination of susceptibility to aztreonam. Treatment with AZACTAM may be started empirically before results of the susceptibility testing are available; subsequently, appropriate antibiotic therapy should be continued.

AZACTAM For Injection (Aztreonam For Injection) is indicated for the treatment of the following infections caused by susceptible gram-negative microorganisms:

Urinary Tract Infections (complicated and uncomplicated), including pyelonephritis and cystitis (initial and recurrent)

caused by *Escherichia coli, Klebsiella pneumoniae, Proteus mirabilis, Pseudomonas aeruginosa, Enterobacter cloacae, Klebsiella oxytoca**, *Citrobacter* species* and *Serratia marcescens**.

Lower Respiratory Tract Infections, including pneumonia and bronchitis caused by *Escherichia coli, Klebsiella pneumoniae, Pseudomonas aeruginosa, Haemophilus influenzae, Proteus mirabilis, Enterobacter* species and *Serratia marcescens**.
Septicemia caused by *Escherichia coli, Klebsiella pneumoniae, Pseudomonas aeruginosa, Proteus mirabilis**, *Serratia marcescens** and *Enterobacter* species.

Skin and Skin-Structure Infections, including those associated with post-operative wounds, ulcers and burns caused by *Escherichia coli, Proteus mirabilis, Serratia marcescens, Enterobacter* species, *Pseudomonas aeruginosa, Klebsiella pneumoniae* and *Citrobacter* species*.

Intra-abdominal Infections, including peritonitis caused by *Escherichia coli, Klebsiella* species including *K. pneumoniae, Enterobacter* species including *E. cloacae**, *Pseudomonas aeruginosa, Citrobacter* species* including *C. freundii** and *Serratia* species* including *S. marcescens**.

Gynecologic Infections, including endometritis and pelvic cellulitis caused by *Escherichia coli, Klebsiella pneumoniae**, *Enterobacter* species* including *E. cloacae** and *Proteus mirabilis**.

---

* Efficacy for this organism in this organ system was studied in fewer than ten infections.

AZACTAM (aztreonam) is indicated for adjunctive therapy to surgery in the management of infections caused by susceptible organisms, including abscesses, infections complicating hollow viscus perforations, cutaneous infections and infections of serous surfaces. AZACTAM is effective against most of the commonly encountered gram-negative aerobic pathogens seen in general surgery.

Concurrent Therapy

Concurrent initial therapy with other antimicrobial agents and AZACTAM is recommended before the causative organism(s) is known in seriously ill patients who are also at risk of having an infection due to gram-positive aerobic pathogens. If anaerobic organisms are also suspected as etiologic agents, therapy should be initiated using an anti-anaerobic agent concurrently with AZACTAM (see DOSAGE AND ADMINISTRATION). Certain antibiotics (e.g., cefoxitin, imipenem) may induce high levels of beta-lactamase *in vitro* in some gram-negative aerobes such as *Enterobacter* and *Pseudomonas* species, resulting in antagonism to many beta-lactam antibiotics including aztreonam. These *in vitro* findings suggest that such beta-lactamase inducing antibiotics not be used concurrently with aztreonam. Following identification and susceptibility testing of the causative organism(s), appropriate antibiotic therapy should be continued.

CONTRAINDICATIONS

Aztreonam is contraindicated in patients with known allergy to this antibiotic.

WARNINGS

Careful inquiry should be made for a history of hypersensitivity reaction to any antibiotic or other drugs. Antibiotics should be given with caution to any patient who has had some form of allergy, particularly to drugs. It is recommended that patients who have had immediate hypersensitivity reactions (e.g., anaphylactic or urticarial) to penicillins and/or cephalosporins should be followed with special care. If an allergic reaction to aztreonam occurs, discontinue the drug and institute supportive treatment as appropriate (e.g., maintenance of ventilation, pressor amines, antihistamines, corticosteroids). Serious hypersensitivity reactions may require epinephrine and other emergency measures.

Pseudomembranous colitis has been reported with nearly all antibacterial agents, including aztreonam, and may range in severity from mild to life-threatening. Therefore, it is important to consider this diagnosis in patients who present with diarrhea subsequent to the administration of antibacterial agents.

Treatment with antibacterial agents alters the normal flora of the colon and may permit overgrowth of clostridia. Studies indicate that a toxin produced by *Clostridium difficile* is one primary cause of "antibiotic-associated colitis."

After the diagnosis of pseudomembranous colitis has been established, therapeutic measures should be initiated. Mild cases of pseudomembranous colitis usually respond to drug discontinuation alone. In moderate to severe cases, consideration should be given to management with fluids and electrolytes, protein supplementation, and treatment with an antibacterial drug effective against *C. difficile.*

PRECAUTIONS

General

In patients with impaired hepatic or renal function, appropriate monitoring is recommended during therapy.

If an aminoglycoside is used concurrently with aztreonam, especially if high dosages of the former are used or if therapy is prolonged, renal function should be monitored because of the potential nephrotoxicity and ototoxicity of aminoglycoside antibiotics.

The use of antibiotics may promote the overgrowth of non-susceptible organisms, including gram-positive organisms (*Staphylococcus aureus* and *Streptococcus faecalis*) and fungi. Should superinfection occur during therapy, appropriate measures should be taken.

Carcinogenesis, Mutagenesis, Impairment of Fertility

Carcinogenicity studies in animals have not been performed. Genetic toxicology studies performed *in vivo* and *in vitro* with aztreonam in several standard laboratory models revealed no evidence of mutagenic potential at the chromosomal or gene level.

Two-generation reproduction studies in rats at daily doses up to 20 times the maximum recommended human dose, prior to and during gestation and lactation, revealed no evidence of impaired fertility. There was a slightly reduced survival rate during the lactation period in the offspring of rats that received the highest dosage, but not in offspring of rats that received five times the maximum recommended human dose.

Pregnancy

Pregnancy Category B

Aztreonam crosses the placenta and enters the fetal circulation.

Studies in pregnant rats and rabbits, with daily doses up to 15 and 5 times, respectively, the maximum recommended human dose, revealed no evidence of embryo- or fetotoxicity or teratogenicity. No drug induced changes were seen in any of the maternal, fetal, or neonatal parameters that were monitored in rats receiving 15 times the maximum recommended human dose of aztreonam during late gestation and lactation.

There are no adequate and well-controlled studies in pregnant women. Because animal reproduction studies are not always predictive of human response, aztreonam should be used during pregnancy only if clearly needed.

Nursing Mothers

Aztreonam is excreted in breast milk in concentrations that are less than 1 percent of concentrations determined in simultaneously obtained maternal serum; consideration should be given to temporary discontinuation of nursing and use of formula feedings.

Pediatric Use

Safety and effectiveness have not been established in infants and children.

ADVERSE REACTIONS

Local reactions such as phlebitis/thrombophlebitis following IV administration, and discomfort/swelling at the injection site following IM administration occurred at rates of approximately 1.9 percent and 2.4 percent, respectively.

Systemic reactions (considered to be related to therapy or of uncertain etiology) occurring at an incidence of 1 to 1.3 percent include diarrhea, nausea and/or vomiting, and rash. Reactions occurring at an incidence of less than 1 percent are listed within each body system in order of decreasing severity:

Hypersensitivity—anaphylaxis, anigioedema, bronchospasm.

Hematologic—pancytopenia, neutropenia, thrombocytopenia, anemia, leukocytosis, thrombocytosis.

Gastrointestinal—abdominal cramps; rare cases of *C. difficile*-associated diarrhea, including pseudomembranous colitis, or gastrointestinal bleeding have been reported. Onset of pseudomembranous colitis symptoms may occur during or after antibiotic treatment (see WARNINGS).

Dermatologic—toxic epidermal necrolysis, purpura, erythema multiforme, exfoliative dermatitis, urticaria, petechiae, pruritus.

Cardiovascular—hypotension, transient ECG changes (ventricular bigeminy and PVC).

Respiratory—one patient experienced flushing, chest pain, and dyspnea.

Hepatobiliary—hepatitis, jaundice.

Nervous System—seizure, confusion, vertigo, paresthesia, insomnia, dizziness.

Musculoskeletal—muscular aches.

Special Senses—tinnitus, diplopia, mouth ulcer, altered taste, numb tongue, sneezing and nasal congestion, halitosis.

Other—vaginal candidiasis, vaginitis, breast tenderness.

Body as a Whole—weakness, headache, fever, malaise, diaphoresis.

Adverse Laboratory Changes

Adverse laboratory changes without regard to drug relationship that were reported during clinical trials were:

Hepatic—elevations of AST (SGOT), ALT (SGPT), and alkaline phosphatase; signs or symptoms of hepatobiliary dysfunction occurred in less than 1 percent of recipients (see above).

Hematologic—increases in prothrombin and partial thromboplastin times, eosinophilia, positive Coombs test.

Renal—increases in serum creatinine.

Continued on next page

Bristol-Myers Squibb Co.—Cont.

OVERDOSAGE
If necessary, aztreonam may be cleared from the serum by hemodialysis and/or peritoneal dialysis.

DOSAGE AND ADMINISTRATION
AZACTAM (aztreonam) For Injection may be administered intravenously or by intramuscular injection. Dosage and route of administration should be determined by susceptibility of the causative organisms, severity and site of infection, and the condition of the patient.

AZACTAM DOSAGE GUIDELINES
ADULTS

Type of Infection	Dose*	Frequency (hours)
Urinary tract infections	500 mg or 1 g	8 or 12
Moderately severe systemic infections	1 g or 2 g	8 or 12
Severe systemic or life-threatening infections	2 g	6 or 8

*Maximum recommended dose is 8 g per day.

The intravenous route is recommended for patients requiring single doses greater than 1 g or those with bacterial septicemia, localized parenchymal abscess (e.g., intra-abdominal abscess), peritonitis or other severe systemic or life-threatening infections. Because of the serious nature of infections due to *Pseudomonas aeruginosa*, dosage of 2 g every six or eight hours is recommended, at least upon initiation of therapy, in systemic infections caused by this organism.
The duration of therapy depends on the severity of infection. Generally, AZACTAM should be continued for at least 48 hours after the patient becomes asymptomatic or evidence of bacterial eradication has been obtained. Persistent infections may require treatment for several weeks. Doses smaller than those indicated should not be used.

Renal Impairment
Prolonged serum levels of aztreonam may occur in patients with transient or persistent renal insufficiency. Therefore, the dosage of AZACTAM should be halved in patients with estimated creatinine clearances between 10 and 30 mL/min/1.73 m^2 after an initial loading dose of 1 g or 2 g.
When only the serum creatinine concentration is available, the following formula (based on sex, weight, and age of the patient) may be used to approximate the creatinine clearance (Clcr). The serum creatinine should represent a steady state of renal function.

$$\text{Males:}\quad \text{Clcr} = \frac{\text{weight (kg)} \times (140 - \text{age})}{72 \times \text{serum creatinine (mg/dL)}}$$

Females: 0.85 × above value
In patients with severe renal failure (creatinine clearance less than 10 mL/min/1.73 m^2), such as those supported by hemodialysis, the usual dose of 500 mg, 1 g or 2 g should be given initially. The maintenance dose should be one-fourth of the usual initial dose given at the usual fixed interval of 6, 8 or 12 hours. For serious or life-threatening infections, in addition to the maintenance doses, one-eighth of the initial dose should be given after each hemodialysis session.

Dosage In The Elderly
Renal status is a major determinant of dosage in the elderly; these patients in particular may have diminished renal function. Serum creatinine may not be an accurate determinant of renal status. Therefore, as with all antibiotics eliminated by the kidneys, estimates of creatinine clearance should be obtained, and appropriate dosage modifications made if necessary.

Preparation Of Parenteral Solutions
General
Upon the addition of the diluent to the container, contents should be shaken **immediately** and **vigorously.** Constituted solutions are not for multiple-dose use; should the entire volume in the container not be used for a single-dose, the unused solution must be discarded.
Depending upon the concentration of aztreonam and diluent used, constituted AZACTAM (aztreonam) For Injection yields a colorless to light straw yellow solution which may develop a slight pink tint on standing (potency is not affected). Parenteral drug products should be inspected visually for particulate matter and discoloration whenever solution and container permit.

Admixtures With Other Antibiotics
Intravenous infusion solutions of AZACTAM (Aztreonam For Injection) not exceeding 2% w/v prepared with Sodium Chloride Injection USP 0.9% or Dextrose Injection USP 5%, to which clindamycin phosphate, gentamicin sulfate, tobramycin sulfate, or cefazolin sodium have been added at concentrations usually used clinically, are stable for up to 48 hours at room temperature or seven days under refrigeration. Ampicillin sodium admixtures with aztreonam in Sodium Chloride Injection USP 0.9% are stable for 24 hours at room temperature and 48 hours under refrigeration; stability in Dextrose Injection USP 5% is two hours at room temperature and eight hours under refrigeration.
Aztreonam-cloxacillin sodium and aztreonam-vancomycin hydrochloride admixtures are stable in Dianeal® 137 (Peritoneal Dialysis Solution) with 4.25% Dextrose for up to 24 hours at room temperature.
Aztreonam is incompatible with nafcillin sodium, cephradine, and metronidazole.
Other admixtures are not recommended since compatibility data are not available.

Intravenous (IV) Solutions
For Bolus Injection: The contents of an AZACTAM (aztreonam) For Injection 15 mL or 30mL capacity vial should be constituted with 6 to 10 mL Sterile Water for Injection USP.
For Infusion: Contents of the 100 mL capacity bottle should be constituted to a final concentration not exceeding 2 percent w/v (at least 50 mL of any appropriate infusion solution listed below per gram aztreonam). These solutions may be frozen immediately after constitution in the original container (see Stability below).
If the contents of a 15 mL or 30 mL capacity vial are to be transferred to an appropriate infusion solution, each gram of aztreonam should be initially constituted with at least 3 mL Sterile Water for Injection USP. Further dilution may be obtained with one of the following intravenous infusion solutions:

- Sodium Chloride Injection USP, 0.9%
- Ringer's Injection USP
- Lactated Ringer's Injection USP
- Dextrose Injection USP, 5% or 10%
- Dextrose and Sodium Chloride Injection USP, 5%:0.9%, 5%:0.45% or 5%:0.2%
- Sodium Lactate Injection USP (M/6 Sodium Lactate)
- Ionosol® B and 5% Dextrose
- Isolyte® E
- Isolyte® E with 5% Dextrose
- Isolyte® M with 5% Dextrose
- Normosol®-R
- Normosol®-R and 5% Dextrose
- Normosol®-M and 5% Dextrose
- Mannitol Injection USP, 5% or 10%
- Lactated Ringer's and 5% Dextrose Injection
- Plasma-Lyte® M and 5% Dextrose
- 10% Travert® Injection
- 10% Travert® and Electrolyte No. 1 Injection
- 10% Travert® and Electrolyte No. 2 Injection
- 10% Travert® and Electrolyte No. 3 Injection

Intramuscular (IM) Solutions
The contents of an AZACTAM (aztreonam) For Injection 15 mL or 30 mL capacity vial should be consituted with at least 3 mL of an appropriate diluent per gram aztreonam. The following diluents may be used:

- Sterile Water for Injection USP
- Bacteriostatic Water for Injection USP (with benzyl alcohol or with methyl- and propylparabens)
- Sodium Chloride Injection USP, 0.9%
- Bacteriostatic Sodium Chloride Injection USP (with benzyl alcohol)

Stability Of IV And IM Solutions
AZACTAM (aztreonam) solutions for IV infusion at concentrations not exceeding 2% w/v must be used within 48 hours following constitution if kept at controlled room temperature (59°–86°F/15°–30°C) or within seven days if refrigerated (36°–46°F/2°–8°C).
Frozen aztreonam infusion solutions may be stored for up to three months at −4°F/−20°C; frozen solutions may be thawed at controlled room temperature or by overnight refrigeration. Solutions that have been thawed and maintained at controlled room temperature or under refrigeration should be used within 24 or 72 hours after removal from the freezer, respectively. Solutions should not be refrozen.
AZACTAM solutions at concentrations exceeding 2% w/v, except those prepared with Sterile Water for Injection USP or Sodium Chloride Injection USP, should be used promptly after preparation; the two excepted solutions must be used within 48 hours if stored at controlled room temperature or within seven days if refrigerated.

Intravenous Administration
Bolus Injection: A bolus injection may be used to initiate therapy. The dose should be **slowly** injected directly into a vein, or the tubing of a suitable administration set, over a period of three to five minutes (see next paragraph regarding flushing of tubing).
Infusion: With any intermittent infusion of aztreonam and another drug with which it is not pharmaceutically compatible, the common delivery tube should be flushed before and after delivery of aztreonam with any appropriate infusion solution compatible with both drug solutions; the drugs should not be delivered simultaneously. Any AZACTAM infusion should be completed within a 20 to 60 minute period. With use of a *Y-type administration set*, careful attention should be given to the calculated volume of aztreonam solution required so that the entire dose will be infused. A *volume control administration set* may be used to deliver an initial dilution of AZACTAM (aztreonam) For Injection (see Preparation Of Parenteral Solutions, For Infusion) into a compatible infusion solution during administration; in this case, the final dilution of aztreonam should provide a concentration not exceeding 2% w/v.

Intramuscular Administration
The dose should be given by deep injection into a large muscle mass (such as the upper outer quadrant of the gluteus maximus or lateral part of the thigh). Aztreonam is well tolerated and should not be admixed with any local anesthetic agent.

HOW SUPPLIED
AZACTAM For Injection (Aztreonam For Injection)—Lyophilized
Single-dose 15 mL capacity vials:
500 mg/vial: Packages of 10 (NDC 0003-2550-10) and 25 (NDC 0003-2550-15)
1 g/vial: Packages of 10 (NDC 0003-2560-10) and 25 (NDC 0003-2560-15)
Single-dose 30 mL capacity vials:
2 g/vial: Packages of 10 (NDC 0003-2570-10) and 25 (NDC 0003-2570-15)
Single-dose 100 mL capacity intravenous infusion bottles with bail bands:
500 mg/bottle: Packages of 10 (NDC 0003-2550-20)
1 g/bottle: Packages of 10 (NDC 0003-2560-20)
2 g/bottle: Packages of 10 (NDC 0003-2570-20)

Storage
Store original packages at room temperature; avoid excessive heat.
(J4-246F)
Revised June 1994

BUSPAR® ℞
(buspirone HCl, USP)
CAUTION: FEDERAL LAW PROHIBITS DISPENSING WITHOUT PRESCRIPTION.

DESCRIPTION
BuSpar® (buspirone hydrochloride tablets, USP) is an antianxiety agent that is not chemically or pharmacologically related to the benzodiazepines, barbiturates, or other sedative/anxiolytic drugs.
Buspirone hydrochloride is a white crystalline, water soluble compound with a molecular weight of 422.0. Chemically, buspirone hydrochloride is 8-[4-[4-(2-pyrimidinyl)-1- piperazinyl]butyl]-8-azaspiro [4.5]decane-7,9- dione monohydrochloride. The empirical formula $C_{21}H_{31}N_5O_2 \cdot HCl$ is represented by the following structural formula:

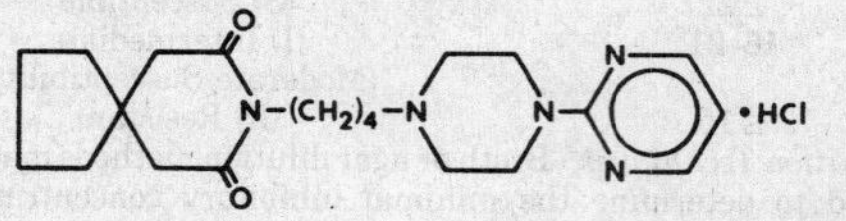

BuSpar is supplied as tablets for oral administration containing 5 mg, 10 mg, or 15 mg of buspirone hydrochloride, USP (equivalent to 4.6 mg, 9.1 mg, and 13.7 mg of buspirone free base respectively). The 15 mg tablet is provided in DIVIDOSE® tablet design. This tablet is scored so it can be either bisected or trisected. Thus, a single tablet can provide the following doses: 15 mg (entire tablet), 10 mg (two-thirds of a tablet), 7.5 mg (one-half of a tablet), or 5 mg (one-third of a tablet). BuSpar Tablets contain the following inactive ingredients: colloidal silicon dioxide, lactose, magnesium stearate, microcrystalline cellulose, and sodium starch glycolate.

CLINICAL PHARMACOLOGY
The mechanism of action of buspirone is unknown. Buspirone differs from typical benzodiazepine anxiolytics in that it does not exert anticonvulsant or muscle relaxant effects. It also lacks the prominent sedative effect that is associated with more typical anxiolytics. *In vitro* preclinical studies have shown that buspirone has a high affinity for serotonin (5-HT_{1A}) receptors. Buspirone has no significant affinity for benzodiazepine receptors and does not affect GABA binding *in vitro* or *in vivo* when tested in preclinical models.
Buspirone has moderate affinity for brain D_2-dopamine receptors. Some studies do suggest that buspirone may have indirect effects on other neurotransmitter systems.
BuSpar is rapidly absorbed in man and undergoes extensive first-pass metabolism. In a radiolabeled study, unchanged buspirone in the plasma accounted for only about 1% of the radioactivity in the plasma. Following oral administration, plasma concentrations of unchanged buspirone are very low and variable between subjects. Peak plasma levels of 1 to 6 ng/mL have been observed 40 to 90 minutes after single oral doses of 20 mg. The single-dose bioavailability of unchanged buspirone when taken as a tablet is on the average about 90% of an equivalent dose of solution, but there is large variability.

The effects of food upon the bioavailability of BuSpar have been studied in eight subjects. They were given a 20-mg dose with and without food; the area under the plasma concentration-time curve (AUC) and peak plasma concentration (C_{max}) of unchanged buspirone increased by 84% and 116% respectively, but the total amount of buspirone immunoreactive material did not change. This suggests that food may decrease the extent of presystemic clearance of buspirone, but the clinical significance of these findings is unknown.

A multiple-dose study conducted in 15 subjects suggests that buspirone has nonlinear pharmacokinetics. Thus, dose increases and repeated dosing may lead to somewhat higher blood levels of unchanged buspirone than would be predicted from results of single-dose studies.

In man, approximately 95% of buspirone is plasma protein bound, but other highly bound drugs, e.g., phenytoin, propranolol, and warfarin are not displaced by buspirone from plasma protein *in vitro*. However, *in vitro* binding studies show that buspirone does displace digoxin.

Buspirone is metabolized primarily by oxidation producing several hydroxylated derivatives and a pharmacologically active metabolite, 1-pyrimidinylpiperazine (1-PP). In animal models predictive of anxiolytic potential, 1-PP has about one quarter of the activity of buspirone, but is present in up to 20-fold greater amounts. However, this is probably not important in humans: blood samples from humans chronically exposed to BuSpar do not exhibit high levels of 1-PP; mean values are approximately 3ng/mL and the highest human blood level recorded among 108 chronically dosed patients was 17ng/mL, less than 1/200th of 1-PP levels found in animals given large doses of buspirone without signs of toxicity.

In a single-dose study using ^{14}C-labeled buspirone, 29% to 63% of the dose was excreted in the urine within 24 hours, primarily as metabolites; fecal excretion accounted for 18% to 38% of the dose. The average elimination half-life of unchanged buspirone after single doses of 10 to 40 mg is about 2 to 3 hours.

The pharmacokinetics of BuSpar in patients with hepatic or renal dysfunction has not been determined, nor has the effect of age. The effect of BuSpar on drug metabolism or concomitant drug disposition has not been investigated.

INDICATIONS AND USAGE

BuSpar is indicated for the management of anxiety disorders or the short-term relief of the symptoms of anxiety. Anxiety or tension associated with the stress of everyday life usually does not require treatment with an anxiolytic.

The efficacy of BuSpar has been demonstrated in controlled clinical trials of outpatients whose diagnosis roughly corresponds to Generalized Anxiety Disorder (GAD). Many of the patients enrolled in these studies also had coexisting depressive symptoms and BuSpar relieved anxiety in the presence of these coexisting depressive symptoms. The patients evaluated in these studies had experienced symptoms for periods of 1 month to over 1 year prior to the study, with an average symptom duration of 6 months.

Generalized Anxiety Disorder (300.02) is described in the American Psychiatric Association's Diagnostic and Statistical Manual, III[1] as follows:

Generalized, persistent anxiety (of at least 1 month continual duration), manifested by symptoms from three of the four following categories:

1. Motor tension: shakiness, jitteriness, jumpiness, trembling, tension, muscle aches, fatigability, inability to relax, eyelid twitch, furrowed brow, strained face, fidgeting, restlessness, easy startle.
2. Autonomic hyperactivity: sweating, heart pounding or racing, cold, clammy hands, dry mouth, dizziness, lightheadedness, paresthesias (tingling in hands or feet), upset stomach, hot or cold spells, frequent urination, diarrhea, discomfort in the pit of the stomach, lump in the throat, flushing, pallor, high resting pulse, and respiration rate.
3. Apprehensive expectation: anxiety, worry, fear, rumination, and anticipation of misfortune to self or others.
4. Vigilance and scanning: hyperattentiveness resulting in distractibility, difficulty in concentrating, insomnia, feeling "on edge," irritability, impatience.

The above symptoms would not be due to another mental disorder, such as a depressive disorder or schizophrenia. However,mild depressive symptoms are common in GAD.

The effectiveness of BuSpar (buspirone hydrochloride, USP) in long-term use, that is, for more than 3 to 4 weeks, has not been demonstrated in controlled trials. There is no body of evidence available that systematically addresses the appropriate duration of treatment for GAD. However, in a study of long-term use, 264 patients were treated with BuSpar for 1 year without ill effect. Therefore, the physician who elects to use BuSpar for extended periods should periodically reassess the usefulness of the drug for the individual patient.

CONTRAINDICATIONS

BuSpar is contraindicated in patients hypersensitive to buspirone hydrochloride.

WARNINGS

The administration of BuSpar to a patient taking a monoamine oxidase inhibitor (MAOI) may pose a hazard. There have been reports of the occurrence of elevated blood pressure when BuSpar has been added to a regimen including an MAOI. Therefore, it is recommended that BuSpar not be used concomitantly with an MAOI.

Because BuSpar has no established antipsychotic activity, it should not be employed in lieu of appropriate antipsychotic treatment.

PRECAUTIONS
General
Interference with cognitive and motor performance
Studies indicate that BuSpar is less sedating than other anxiolytics and that it does not produce significant functional impairment. However, its CNS effects in any individual patient may not be predictable. Therefore, patients should be cautioned about operating an automobile or using complex machinery until they are reasonably certain that buspirone treatment does not affect them adversely.

While formal studies of the interaction of BuSpar with alcohol indicate that buspirone does not increase alcohol-induced impairment in motor and mental performance, it is prudent to avoid concomitant use of alcohol and buspirone.

Potential for withdrawal reactions in sedative/hypnotic/anxiolytic drug-dependent patients
Because BuSpar does not exhibit cross-tolerance with benzodiazepines and other common sedative/hypnotic drugs, it will not block the withdrawal syndrome often seen with cessation of therapy with these drugs. Therefore, before starting therapy with BuSpar, it is advisable to withdraw patients gradually, especially patients who have been using a CNS-depressant drug chronically, from their prior treatment. Rebound or withdrawal symptoms may occur over varying time periods, depending in part on the type of drug, and its effective half-life of elimination.

The syndrome of withdrawal from sedative/hypnotic/anxiolytic drugs can appear as any combination of irritability, anxiety, agitation, insomnia, tremor, abdominal cramps, muscle cramps, vomiting, sweating, flu-like symptoms without fever, and occasionally, even as seizures.

Possible concerns related to buspirone's binding to dopamine receptors
Because buspirone can bind to central dopamine receptors, a question has been raised about its potential to cause acute and chronic changes in dopamine-mediated neurological function (e.g., dystonia, pseudo-parkinsonism, akathisia, and tardive dyskinesia). Clinical experience in controlled trials has failed to identify any significant neuroleptic-like activity; however, a syndrome of restlessness, appearing shortly after initiation of treatment, has been reported in some small fraction of buspirone-treated patients. The syndrome may be explained in several ways. For example, buspirone may increase central noradrenergic activity; alternatively, the effect may be attributable to dopaminergic effects (i.e., represent akathisia). Obviously, the question cannot be totally resolved at this point in time. Generally, long-term sequelae of any drug's use can be identified only after several years of marketing.

Information for Patients
To assure safe and effective use of BuSpar, the following information and instructions should be given to patients:
1. Inform your physician about any medications, prescription or nonprescription, alcohol, or drugs that you are now taking or plan to take during your treatment with BuSpar.
2. Inform your physician if you are pregnant, or if you are planning to become pregnant, or if you become pregnant while you are taking BuSpar.
3. Inform your physician if you are breast-feeding an infant.
4. Until you experience how this medication affects you, do not drive a car or operate potentially dangerous machinery.

Laboratory Tests
There are no specific laboratory tests recommended.

Drug Interactions
It is recommended that BuSpar (buspirone hydrochloride, USP) not be used concomitantly with MAO inhibitors (See "**WARNINGS**"). Because the effects of concomitant administration of BuSpar with most other psychotropic drugs have not been studied, the concomitant use of BuSpar with other CNS-active drugs should be approached with caution.

There is one report suggesting that the concomitant use of Desyrel® (trazodone hydrochloride) and BuSpar may have caused 3- to 6-fold elevations on SGPT (ALT) in a few patients. In a similar study, attempting to replicate this finding, no interactive effect on hepatic transaminases was identified.

In a study in normal volunteers, concomitant administration of BuSpar and haloperidol resulted in increased serum haloperidol concentrations. The clinical significance of this finding is not clear.

In vitro, buspirone does not displace tightly bound drugs like phenytoin, propranolol, and warfarin from serum proteins. However, there has been one report of prolonged prothrombin time when buspirone was added to the regimen of a patient treated with warfarin. The patient was also chronically receiving phenytoin, phenobarbital, digoxin, and Synthroid. *In vitro*, buspirone may displace less firmly bound drugs like digoxin. The clinical significance of this property is unknown.

Drug/Laboratory Test Interactions
Buspirone is not known to interfere with commonly employed clinical laboratory tests.

Carcinogenesis, Mutagenesis, Impairment of Fertility
No evidence of carcinogenic potential was observed in rats during a 24-month study at approximately 133 times the maximum recommended human oral dose; or in mice, during an 18-month study at approximately 167 times the maximum recommended human oral dose.

With or without metabolic activation, buspirone did not induce point mutations in five strains of *Salmonella typhimurium* (Ames Test) or mouse lymphoma L5178YTK$^+$ cell cultures, nor was DNA damage observed with buspirone in Wi-38 human cells. Chromosomal aberrations or abnormalities did not occur in bone marrow cells of mice given one or five daily doses of buspirone.

Pregnancy: Teratogenic Effects
Pregnancy Category B: No fertility impairment or fetal damage was observed in reproduction studies performed in rats and rabbits at buspirone doses of approximately 30 times the maximum recommended human dose. In humans, however, adequate and well-controlled studies during pregnancy have *not* been performed. Because animal reproduction studies are not always predictive of human response, this drug should be used during pregnancy only if clearly needed.

Labor and Delivery
The effect of BuSpar on labor and delivery in women is unknown. No adverse effects were noted in reproduction studies in rats.

Nursing Mothers
The extent of the excretion in human milk of buspirone or its metabolites is not known. In rats, however, buspirone and its metabolites are excreted in milk. BuSpar administration to nursing women should be avoided if clinically possible.

Pediatric Use
The safety and effectiveness of BuSpar have not been determined in individuals below 18 years of age.

Use in the Elderly
BuSpar has not been systematically evaluated in older patients; however, several hundred elderly patients have participated in clinical studies with BuSpar and no unusual adverse age-related phenomena have been identified. In 87 elderly patients for whom dosage data were available, the modal total daily dose of BuSpar was 15 mg per day, the same as that in the total sample of patients treated with BuSpar.

Use in Patients With Impaired Hepatic or Renal Function
Since BuSpar is metabolized by the liver and excreted by the kidneys, its administration to patients with severe hepatic or renal impairment cannot be recommended.

ADVERSE REACTIONS (See also "PRECAUTIONS")
Commonly Observed
The more commonly observed untoward events associated with the use of BuSpar not seen at an equivalent incidence among placebo-treated patients include dizziness, nausea, headache, nervousness, lightheadedness, and excitement.

Associated With Discontinuation of Treatment
One guide to the relative clinical importance of adverse events associated with BuSpar is provided by the frequency with which they caused drug discontinuation during clinical testing. Approximately 10% of the 2200 anxious patients who participated in the BuSpar premarketing clinical efficacy trials in anxiety disorders lasting 3 to 4 weeks discontinued treatment due to an adverse event. The more common events causing discontinuation included: central nervous system disturbances (3.4 %), primarily dizziness, insomnia, nervousness, drowsiness, and lightheaded feeling; gastrointestinal disturbances (1.2%), primarily nausea; and miscellaneous disturbances (1.1%), primarily headache and fatigue. In addition, 3.4% of patients had multiple complaints, none of which could be characterized as primary.

Incidence in Controlled Clinical Trials
The table that follows enumerates adverse events that occurred at a frequency of 1% or more among BuSpar patients who participated in 4-week, controlled trials comparing BuSpar with placebo. The frequencies were obtained from pooled data for 17 trials. The prescriber should be aware that these figures cannot be used to predict the incidence of side effects in the course of usual medical practice where patient characteristics and other factors differ from those which prevailed in the clinical trials. Similarly, the cited frequencies cannot be compared with figures obtained from other clinical investigations involving different treatments, uses, and investigators. Comparison of the cited figures, however, does provide the prescribing physician with some basis for estimating the relative contribution of drug and nondrug factors to the side-effect incidence rate in the population studied.

Continued on next page

Bristol-Myers Squibb Co.—Cont.

TREATMENT-EMERGENT ADVERSE EXPERIENCE INCIDENCE IN PLACEBO-CONTROLLED CLINICAL TRIALS*
(Percent of Patients Reporting)

Adverse Experience	BuSpar (n=477)	Placebo (n=464)
Cardiovascular		
Tachycardia/Palpitations	1	1
CNS		
Dizziness	12	3
Drowsiness	10	9
Nervousness	5	1
Insomnia	3	3
Lightheadedness	3	—
Decreased Concentration	2	2
Excitement	2	—
Anger/Hostility	2	—
Confusion	2	—
Depression	2	2
EENT		
Blurred Vision	2	—
Gastrointestinal		
Nausea	8	5
Dry Mouth	3	4
Abdominal/Gastric Distress	2	2
Diarrhea	2	—
Constipation	1	2
Vomiting	1	2
Musculoskeletal		
Musculoskeletal Aches/Pains	1	—
Neurological		
Numbness	2	—
Paresthesia	1	—
Incoordination	1	—
Tremor	1	—
Skin		
Skin Rash	1	—
Miscellaneous		
Headache	6	3
Fatigue	4	4
Weakness	2	—
Sweating/Clamminess	1	—

* Events reported by at least 1% of BuSpar (buspirone hydrochloride, USP) patients are included.
—Incidence less than 1%.

Other Events Observed During the Entire Premarketing Evaluation of BuSpar

During its premarketing assessment, BuSpar was evaluated in over 3500 subjects. This section reports event frequencies for adverse events occurring in approximately 3000 subjects from this group who took multiple doses of BuSpar in the dose range for which BuSpar is being recommended (i.e., the modal daily dose of BuSpar fell between 10 and 30 mg for 70% of the patients studied) and for whom safety data were systematically collected. The conditions and duration of exposure to BuSpar varied greatly, involving well-controlled studies as well as experience in open and uncontrolled clinical settings. As part of the total experience gained in clinical studies, various adverse events were reported. In the absence of appropriate controls in some of the studies, a causal relationship to BuSpar treatment cannot be determined. The list includes all undesirable events reasonably associated with the use of the drug.

The following enumeration by organ system describes events in terms of their relative frequency of reporting in this data base. Events of major clinical importance are also described in the "PRECAUTIONS" section.

The following definitions of frequency are used: Frequent adverse events are defined as those occurring in at least 1/100 patients. Infrequent adverse events are those occurring in 1/100 to 1/1000 patients, while rare events are those occurring in less than 1/1000 patients.

Cardiovascular
Frequent was nonspecific chest pain; infrequent were syncope, hypotension, and hypertension; rare were cerebrovascular accident, congestive heart failure, myocardial infarction, cardiomyopathy, and bradycardia.

Central Nervous System
Frequent were dream disturbances; infrequent were depersonalization, dysphoria, noise intolerance, euphoria, akathisia, fearfulness, loss of interest, dissociative reaction, hallucinations, suicidal ideation, and seizures; rare were feelings of claustrophobia, cold intolerance, stupor, and slurred speech and psychosis.

EENT
Frequent were tinnitus, sore throat, and nasal congestion; infrequent were redness and itching of the eyes, altered taste, altered smell, and conjunctivitis; rare were inner ear abnormality, eye pain, photophobia, and pressure on eyes.

Endocrine
Rare were galactorrhea and thyroid abnormality.

Gastrointestinal
Infrequent were flatulence, anorexia, increased appetite, salivation, irritable colon, and rectal bleeding; rare was burning of the tongue.

Genitourinary
Infrequent were urinary frequency, urinary hesitancy, menstrual irregularity and spotting, and dysuria; rare were amenorrhea, pelvic inflammatory disease, enuresis, and nocturia.

Musculoskeletal
Infrequent were muscle cramps, muscle spasms, rigid/stiff muscles, and arthralgias.

Neurological
Infrequent were involuntary movements and slowed reaction time; rare was muscle weakness.

Respiratory
Infrequent were hyperventilation, shortness of breath, and chest congestion; rare was epistaxis.

Sexual Function
Infrequent were decreased or increased libido; rare were delayed ejaculation and impotence.

Skin
Infrequent were edema, pruritus, flushing, easy bruising, hair loss, dry skin, facial edema, and blisters; rare were acne and thinning of nails.

Clinical Laboratory
Infrequent were increases in hepatic aminotransferases (SGOT, SGPT); rare were eosinophilia, leukopenia, and thrombocytopenia.

Miscellaneous
Infrequent were weight gain, fever, roaring sensation in the head, weight loss, and malaise; rare were alcohol abuse, bleeding disturbance, loss of voice, and hiccoughs.

POSTINTRODUCTION CLINICAL EXPERIENCE
Postmarketing experience has shown an adverse experience profile similar to that given above. Voluntary reports since introduction have included rare occurrences of allergic reactions (including urticaria), cogwheel rigidity, dystonic reactions, ataxias, extrapyramidal symptoms, dyskinesias (acute and tardive), ecchymosis, emotional lability, tunnel vision and urinary retention. Because of the uncontrolled nature of these spontaneous reports, a causal relationship to BuSpar (buspirone hydrochloride, USP) treatment has not been determined.

DRUG ABUSE AND DEPENDENCE

Controlled Substance Class
BuSpar is not a controlled substance.

Physical and Psychological Dependence
In human and animal studies, buspirone has shown no potential for abuse or diversion and there is no evidence that it causes tolerance, or either physical or psychological dependence. Human volunteers with a history of recreational drug or alcohol usage were studied in two double-blind clinical investigations. None of the subjects were able to distinguish between BuSpar and placebo. By contrast, subjects showed a statistically significant preference for methaqualone and diazepam. Studies in monkeys, mice, and rats have indicated that buspirone lacks potential for abuse.

Following chronic administration in the rat, abrupt withdrawal of buspirone did not result in the loss of body weight commonly observed with substances that cause physical dependency.

Although there is no direct evidence that BuSpar causes physical dependence or drug-seeking behavior, it is difficult to predict from experiments the extent to which a CNS-active drug will be misused, diverted, and/or abused once marketed. Consequently, physicians should carefully evaluate patients for a history of drug abuse and follow such patients closely, observing them for signs of BuSpar misuse or abuse (e.g., development of tolerance, incrementation of dose, drug-seeking behavior).

OVERDOSAGE

Signs and Symptoms
In clinical pharmacology trials, doses as high as 375 mg/day were administered to healthy male volunteers. As this dose was approached, the following symptoms were observed: nausea, vomiting, dizziness, drowsiness, miosis, and gastric distress. A few cases of overdosage have been reported, with complete recovery as the usual outcome. No deaths have been reported following overdosage with BuSpar alone. Rare cases of intentional overdosage with a fatal outcome were invariably associated with ingestion of multiple drugs and/or alcohol, and a casual relationship to buspirone could not be determined. Toxicology studies of buspirone yielded the following LD_{50} values: mice, 655 mg/kg; rats, 196 mg/kg; dogs, 586 mg/kg; and monkeys, 356 mg/kg. These dosages are 160 to 550 times the recommended human daily dose.

Recommended Overdose Treatment
General symptomatic and supportive measures should be used along with immediate gastric lavage. Respiration, pulse, and blood pressure should be monitored as in all cases of drug overdosage. No specific antidote is known to buspi-

rone, and dialyzability of buspirone has not been determined.

DOSAGE AND ADMINISTRATION
The recommended initial dose is 15 mg daily (7.5 mg b.i.d.). To achieve an optimal therapeutic response, at intervals of 2 to 3 days the dosage may be increased 5 mg per day, as needed. The maximum daily dosage should not exceed 60 mg per day. In clinical trials allowing dose titration, divided doses of 20 to 30 mg per day were commonly employed.

HOW SUPPLIED
BuSpar® (buspirone hydrochloride tablets, USP)
Tablets, 5 mg and 10 mg (white, ovoid-rectangular with score, MJ logo, strength and the name BuSpar embossed) are available in bottles of 100 and 500, and in cartons containing 100 individually packaged tablets.
5 mg tablets
NDC 0087-0818-41 Bottles of 100
NDC 0087-0818-44 Bottles of 500
NDC 0087-0818-43 Cartons of 100 unit dose
10 mg tablets
NDC 0087-0819-41 Bottles of 100
NDC 0087-0819-44 Bottles of 500
NDC 0087-0819-43 Cartons of 100 unit dose
Tablets, 15 mg white, in the DIVIDOSE® tablet design imprinted with the MJ logo, are available in bottles of 60 and 180. The 15 mg tablet is scored so that it can be either bisected or trisected. It has ID number 822 on one side and on the reverse side, the number 5 on each trisect segment.
15 mg tablets
NDC 0087-0822-32 Bottles of 60
NDC 0087-0822-33 Bottles of 180
U.S. Patent Nos. 4,182,763 and 5,015,646; (DIVIDOSE®) 4,215,104 and 4,258,027
Store at Room Temperature–Protect from temperatures greater than 86°F (30°C). Dispense in a tight, light-resistant container (USP).

REFERENCE
1. American Psychiatric Association, Ed.: Diagnostic and Statistical Manual of Mental Disorders – III, American Psychiatric Association, May 1980.
Bristol-Myers Squibb Company
Princeton, NJ 08543
U.S.A
818DIM-06   Revised April 1996
51-000648-03   D1-B001
Shown in Product Identification Guide, page 306

CAPOTEN® TABLETS   ℞
[kap'o-ten"]
Captopril Tablets

USE IN PREGNANCY
When used in pregnancy during the second and third trimesters, ACE inhibitors can cause injury and even death to the developing fetus. When pregnancy is detected, CAPOTEN should be discontinued as soon as possible. See WARNINGS: Fetal/Neonatal Morbidity and Mortality.

DESCRIPTION
CAPOTEN (captopril) is a specific competitive inhibitor of angiotensin I-converting enzyme (ACE), the enzyme responsible for the conversion of angiotensin I to angiotensin II. CAPOTEN (captopril) is designated chemically as 1-[(2S)-3-mercapto-2-methylpropionyl]-L-proline [MW 217.29] and has the following structure:

Captopril is a white to off-white crystalline powder that may have a slight sulfurous odor; it is soluble in water (approx. 160 mg/mL), methanol, and ethanol and sparingly soluble in chloroform and ethyl acetate.
CAPOTEN (captopril) is available in potencies of 12.5 mg, 25 mg, 50 mg, and 100 mg as scored tablets for oral administration. Inactive ingredients: microcrystalline cellulose, corn starch, lactose, and stearic acid.

CLINICAL PHARMACOLOGY
Mechanism of Action
The mechanism of action of CAPOTEN (captopril) has not yet been fully elucidated. Its beneficial effects in hypertension and heart failure appear to result primarily from suppression of the renin-angiotensin-aldosterone system. However, there is no consistent correlation between renin levels and response to the drug. Renin, an enzyme synthesized by the kidneys, is released into the circulation where it acts on a

plasma globulin substrate to produce angiotensin I, a relatively inactive decapeptide. Angiotensin I is then converted by angiotensin converting enzyme (ACE) to angiotensin II, a potent endogenous vasoconstrictor substance. Angiotensin II also stimulates aldosterone secretion from the adrenal cortex, thereby contributing to sodium and fluid retention.
CAPOTEN (captopril) prevents the conversion of angiotensin I to angiotensin II by inhibition of ACE, a peptidyldipeptide carboxy hydrolase. This inhibition has been demonstrated in both healthy human subjects and in animals by showing that the elevation of blood pressure caused by exogenously administered angiotensin I was attenuated or abolished by captopril. In animal studies, captopril did not alter the pressor responses to a number of other agents, including angiotensin II and norepinephrine, indicating specificity of action.
ACE is identical to "bradykininase", and CAPOTEN (captopril) may also interfere with the degradation of the vasodepressor peptide, bradykinin. Increased concentrations of bradykinin or prostaglandin E_2 may also have a role in the therapeutic effect of CAPOTEN.
Inhibition of ACE results in decreased plasma angiotensin II and increased plasma renin activity (PRA), the latter resulting from loss of negative feedback on renin release caused by reduction in angiotensin II. The reduction of angiotensin II leads to decreased aldosterone secretion, and, as a result, small increases in serum potassium may occur along with sodium and fluid loss.
The antihypertensive effects persist for a longer period of time than does demonstrable inhibition of circulating ACE. It is not known whether the ACE present in vascular endothelium is inhibited longer than the ACE in circulating blood.

Pharmacokinetics
After oral administration of therapeutic doses of CAPOTEN (captopril), rapid absorption occurs with peak blood levels at about one hour. The presence of food in the gastrointestinal tract reduces absorption by about 30 to 40 percent; captopril therefore should be given one hour before meals. Based on carbon-14 labeling, average minimal absorption is approximately 75 percent. In a 24-hour period, over 95 percent of the absorbed dose is eliminated in the urine; 40 to 50 percent is unchanged drug; most of the remainder is the disulfide dimer of captopril and captopril-cysteine disulfide.
Approximately 25 to 30 percent of the circulating drug is bound to plasma proteins. The apparent elimination half-life for total radioactivity in blood is probably less than 3 hours. An accurate determination of half-life of unchanged captopril is not, at present, possible, but it is probably less than 2 hours. In patients with renal impairment, however, retention of captopril occurs (see DOSAGE AND ADMINISTRATION).

Pharmacodynamics
Administration of CAPOTEN (captopril) results in a reduction of peripheral arterial resistance in hypertensive patients with either no change, or an increase, in cardiac output. There is an increase in renal blood flow following administration of CAPOTEN (captopril) and glomerular filtration rate is usually unchanged.
Reductions of blood pressure are usually maximal 60 to 90 minutes after oral administration of an individual dose of CAPOTEN (captopril). The duration of effect is dose related. The reduction in blood pressure may be progressive, so to achieve maximal therapeutic effects, several weeks of therapy may be required. The blood pressure lowering effects of captopril and thiazide-type diuretics are additive. In contrast, captopril and beta-blockers have a less than additive effect.
Blood pressure is lowered to about the same extent in both standing and supine positions. Orthostatic effects and tachycardia are infrequent but may occur in volume-depleted patients. Abrupt withdrawal of CAPOTEN has not been associated with a rapid increase in blood pressure.
In patients with heart failure, significantly decreased peripheral (systemic vascular) resistance and blood pressure (afterload), reduced pulmonary capillary wedge pressure (preload) and pulmonary vascular resistance, increased cardiac output, and increased exercise tolerance time (ETT) have been demonstrated. These hemodynamic and clinical effects occur after the first dose and appear to persist for the duration of therapy. Placebo controlled studies of 12 weeks duration in patients who did not respond adequately to diuretics and digitalis show no tolerance to beneficial effects on ETT; open studies, with exposure up to 18 months in some cases, also indicate that ETT benefit is maintained. Clinical improvement has been observed in some patients where acute hemodynamic effects were minimal.
The Survival and Ventricular Enlargement (SAVE) study was a multicenter, randomized, double-blind, placebo-controlled trial conducted in 2,231 patients (age 21–79 years) who survived the acute phase of a myocardial infarction and did not have active ischemia. Patients had left ventricular dysfunction (LVD), defined as a resting left ventricular ejection fraction ≤40%, but at the time of randomization were not sufficiently symptomatic to require ACE inhibitor therapy for heart failure. About half of the patients had had symptoms of heart failure in the past. Patients were given a test dose of 6.25 mg oral CAPOTEN (captopril) and were randomized within 3-16 days post-infarction to receive either CAPOTEN or placebo in addition to conventional therapy. CAPOTEN was initiated at 6.25 mg or 12.5 mg tid and after two weeks titrated to a target maintenance dose of 50 mg tid. About 80% of patients were receiving the target dose at the end of the study. Patients were followed for a minimum of two years and for up to five years, with an average follow-up of 3.5 years.
Baseline blood pressure was 113/70 mm Hg and 112/70 mm Hg for the placebo and CAPOTEN groups, respectively. Blood pressure increased slightly in both treatment groups during the study and was somewhat lower in the CAPOTEN group (119/74 vs. 125/77 mm Hg at 1 yr).
Therapy with CAPOTEN improved long-term survival and clinical outcomes compared to placebo. The risk reduction for all cause mortality was 19% (P=0.02) and for cardiovascular death was 21% (P=0.014). Captopril treated subjects had 22% (P=0.034) fewer first hospitalizations for heart failure. Compared to placebo, 22% fewer patients receiving captopril developed symptoms of overt heart failure. There was no significant difference between groups in total hospitalizations for all cause (2056 placebo; 2036 captopril).
CAPOTEN was well tolerated in the presence of other therapies such as aspirin, beta blockers, nitrates, vasodilators, calcium antagonists and diuretics.
In a multicenter, double-blind, placebo controlled trial, 409 patients, age 18–49 of either gender, with or without hypertension, with type I (juvenile type, onset before age 30) insulin-dependent diabetes mellitus, retinopahy, proteinuria ≥500 mg per day and serum creatinine ≤2.5 mg/dL, were randomized to placebo or CAPOTEN (25 mg tid) and followed for up to 4.8 years (median 3 years). To achieve blood pressure control, additional antihypertensive agents (diuretics, beta blockers, centrally acting agents, or vasodilators) were added as needed for patients in both groups.
The CAPOTEN group had a 51% reduction in risk of doubling of serum creatinine)P <0.01) and a 51% reduction in risk for the combined endpoint of end-stage renal disease (dialysis or transplantation) or death (P <0.01). CAPOTEN treatment resulted in a 30% reduction in urine protein excretion within the first 3 months (P <0.05), which was maintained throughout the trial. The CAPOTEN group had somewhat better blood pressure control than the placebo group, but the effects of CAPOTEN on renal function were greater than would be expected from the group differences in blood pressure reduction alone. CAPOTEN was well-tolerated in this patient population.
In two multicenter, double-blind, placebo controlled studies, a total of 235 normotensive patients with insulin-dependent diabetes mellitus, retinopathy and microalbuminuria (20–200 μg/min) were randomized to placebo or CAPOTEN (50 mg bid) and followed for up to 2 years. CAPOTEN delayed the progression to overt nephropathy (proteinuria ≥500 mg/day) in both studies (risk reduction 67% to 76%; P <0.05). CAPOTEN also reduced the albumin excretion rate. However, the long term clinical benefit of reducing the progression from microalbuminuria to proteinuria has not been established.
Studies in rats and cats indicate that CAPOTEN (captopril) does not cross the blood-brain barrier to any significant extent.

INDICATIONS AND USAGE

Hypertension: CAPOTEN (captopril) is indicated for the treatment of hypertension.
In using CAPOTEN, consideration should be given to the risk of neutropenia/agranulocytosis (see WARNINGS).
CAPOTEN may be used as initial therapy for patients with normal renal function, in whom the risk is relatively low. In patients with impaired renal function, particularly those with collagen vascular disease, captopril should be reserved for hypertensives who have either developed unacceptable side effects on other drugs, or have failed to respond satisfactorily to drug combinations.
CAPOTEN is effective alone and in combination with other antihypertensive agents, especially thiazide-type diuretics. The blood pressure lowering effects of captopril and thiazides are approximately additive.
Heart Failure: CAPOTEN is indicated in the treatment of congestive heart failure in combination with diuretics and digitalis. The beneficial effect of captopril in heart failure does not require the presence of digitalis, however, most controlled clinical trial experience with captopril has been in patients receiving digitalis, as well as diuretic treatment.
Left Ventricular Dysfunction After Myocardial Infarction: CAPOTEN is indicated to improve survival following myocardial infarction in clinically stable patients with left ventricular dysfunction manifested as an ejection fraction ≤40% and to reduce the incidence of overt heart failure and subsequent hospitalizations for congestive heart failure in these patients.
Diabetic Nephropathy: CAPOTEN is indicated for the treatment of diabetic nephropathy (proteinuria >500 mg/day) in patients with type I insulin-dependent diabetes mellitus and retinopathy. CAPOTEN decreases the rate of progression of renal insufficiency and development of serious adverse clinical outcomes (death or need for renal transplantation or dialysis).

CONTRAINDICATIONS

CAPOTEN is contraindicated in patients who are hypersensitive to this product or any other angiotensin-converting enzyme inhibitor (e.g., a patient who has experienced angioedema during therapy with any other ACE inhibitor).

WARNINGS

Anaphylactoid and Possibly Related Reactions
Presumably because angiotensin-converting enzyme inhibitors affect the metabolism of eicosanoids and polypeptides, including endogenous bradykinin, patients receiving ACE inhibitors (including CAPOTEN) may be subject to a variety of reactions, some of them serious.
Angioedema: Angioedema involving the extremities, face, lips, mucous membranes, tongue, glottis or larynx has been seen in patients treated with ACE inhibitors, including captopril. If angioedema involves the tongue, glottis or larynx, airway obstruction may occur and be fatal. Emergency therapy, including but not necessarily limited to, subcutaneous administration of a 1:1000 solution of epinephrine should be promptly instituted.
Swelling confined to the face, mucous membranes of the mouth, lips and extremities has usually resolved with discontinuation of captopril; some cases required medical therapy. (See PRECAUTIONS: Information for Patients and ADVERSE REACTIONS.)
Anaphylactoid reactions during desensitization: Two patients undergoing desensitizing treatment with hymenoptera venom while receiving ACE inhibitors sustained life-threatening anaphylactoid reactions. In the same patients, these reactions were avoided when ACE inhibitors were temporarily withheld, but they reappeared upon inadvertent rechallenge.
Anaphylactoid reactions during membrane exposure: Anaphylactoid reactions have been reported in patients dialyzed with high-flux membranes and treated concomitantly with an ACE inhibitor. Anaphylactoid reactions have also been reported in patients undergoing low-density lipoprotein apheresis with dextran sulfate absorption (a procedure dependent upon devices not approved in the United States.
Neutropenia/Agranulocytosis
Neutropenia (<1000/mm^3) with myeloid hypoplasia has resulted from use of captopril. About half of the neutropenic patients developed systemic or oral cavity infections or other features of the syndrome of agranulocytosis.
The risk of neutropenia is dependent on the clinical status of the patient:

In clinical trials in patients with hypertension who have normal renal function (serum creatinine less than 1.6 mg/dL and no collagen vascular disease), neutropenia has been seen in one patient out of over 8,600 exposed.

In patients with some degree of renal failure (serum creatinine at least 1.6 mg/dL) but no collagen vascular disease, the risk of neutropenia in clinical trials was about 1 per 500, a frequency over 15 times that for uncomplicated hypertension. Daily doses of captopril were relatively high in these patients, particularly in view of their diminished renal function. In foreign marketing experience in patients with renal failure, use of allopurinol concomitantly with captopril has been associated with neutropenia but this association has not appeared in U.S. reports.

In patients with collagen vascular diseases (e.g., systemic lupus erythematosus, scleroderma) and impaired renal function, neutropenia occurred in 3.7 percent of patients in clinical trials.

While none of the over 750 patients in formal clinical trials of heart failure developed neutropenia, it has occurred during the subsequent clinical experience. About half of the reported cases had serum creatinine ≥ 1.6 mg/dL and more than 75 percent were in patients also receiving procainamide. In heart failure, it appears that the same risk factors for neutropenia are present.

The neutropenia has usually been detected within three months after captopril was started. Bone marrow examinations in patients with neutropenia consistently showed myeloid hypoplasia, frequently accompanied by erythroid hypoplasia and decreased numbers of megakaryocytes (e.g., hypoplastic bone marrow and pancytopenia); anemia and thrombocytopenia were sometimes seen.
In general, neutrophils returned to normal in about two weeks after captopril was discontinued, and serious infections were limited to clinically complex patients. About 13 percent of the cases of neutropenia have ended fatally, but almost all fatalities were in patients with serious illness, having collagen vascular disease, renal failure, heart failure or immunosuppressant therapy, or a combination of these complicating factors.

Continued on next page

Bristol-Myers Squibb Co.—Cont.

Evaluation of the hypertensive or heart failure patient should always include assessment of renal function.

If captopril is used in patients with impaired renal function, white blood cell and differential counts should be evaluated prior to starting treatment and at approximately two-week intervals for about three months, then periodically.

In patients with collagen vascular disease or who are exposed to other drugs known to affect the white cells or immune response, particularly when there is impaired renal function, captopril should be used only after an assessment of benefit and risk, and then with caution.

All patients treated with captopril should be told to report any signs of infection (e.g., sore throat, fever). If infection is suspected, white cell counts should be performed without delay.

Since discontinuation of captopril and other drugs has generally led to prompt return of the white count to normal, upon confirmation of neutropenia (neutrophil count < 1000/mm³) the physician should withdraw captopril and closely follow the patient's course.

Proteinuria

Total urinary proteins greater than 1 g per day were seen in about 0.7 percent of patients receiving captopril. About 90 percent of affected patients had evidence of prior renal disease or received relatively high doses of captopril (in excess of 150 mg/day), or both. The nephrotic syndrome occurred in about one-fifth of proteinuric patients. In most cases, proteinuria subsided or cleared within six months whether or not captopril was continued. Parameters of renal function, such as BUN and creatinine, were seldom altered in the patients with proteinuria.

Hypotension

Excessive hypotension was rarely seen in hypertensive patients but is a possible consequence of captopril use in salt/volume depleted persons (such as those treated vigorously with diuretics), patients with heart failure or those patients undergoing renal dialysis. (See PRECAUTIONS: Drug Interactions.)

In heart failure, where the blood pressure was either normal or low, transient decreases in mean blood pressure greater than 20 percent were recorded in about half of the patients. This transient hypotension is more likely to occur after any of the first several doses and is usually well tolerated, producing either no symptoms or brief mild lightheadedness, although in rare instances it has been associated with arrhythmia or conduction defects. Hypotension was the reason for discontinuation of drug in 3.6 percent of patients with heart failure.

BECAUSE OF THE POTENTIAL FALL IN BLOOD PRESSURE IN THESE PATIENTS, THERAPY SHOULD BE STARTED UNDER VERY CLOSE MEDICAL SUPERVISION.
A starting dose of 6.25 or 12.5 mg tid may minimize the hypotensive effect. Patients should be followed closely for the first two weeks of treatment and whenever the dose of captopril and/or diuretic is increased. In patients with heart failure, reducing the dose of diuretic, if feasible, may minimize the fall in blood pressure.

Hypotension is not *per se* a reason to discontinue captopril. Some decrease of systemic blood pressure is a common and desirable observation upon initiation of CAPOTEN (captopril) treatment in heart failure. The magnitude of the decrease is greatest early in the course of treatment; this effect stabilizes within a week or two, and generally returns to pretreatment levels, without a decrease in therapeutic efficacy, within two months.

Fetal/Neonatal Morbidity and Mortality

ACE inhibitors can cause fetal and neonatal morbidity and death when administered to pregnant women. Several dozen cases have been reported in the world literature. When pregnancy is detected, ACE inhibitors should be discontinued as soon as possible.

The use of ACE inhibitors during the second and third trimesters of pregnancy has been associated with fetal and neonatal injury, including hypotension, neonatal skull hypoplasia, anuria, reversible or irreversible renal failure, and death. Oligohydramnios has also been reported, presumably resulting from decreased fetal renal function; oligohydramnios in this setting has been associated with fetal limb contractures, craniofacial deformation, and hypoplastic lung development. Prematurity, intrauterine growth retardation, and patent ductus arteriosus have also been reported, although it is not clear whether these occurrences were due to the ACE-inhibitor exposure.

These adverse effects do not appear to have resulted from intrauterine ACE-inhibitor exposure that has been limited to the first trimester. Mothers whose embryos and fetuses are exposed to ACE inhibitors only during the first trimester should be so informed. Nonetheless, when patients become pregnant, physicians should make every effort to discontinue the use of captopril as soon as possible.

Rarely (probably less often than once in every thousand pregnancies), no alternative to ACE inhibitors will be found.

In these rare cases, the mothers should be apprised of the potential hazards to their fetuses, and serial ultrasound examinations should be performed to assess the intraamniotic environment.

If oligohydramnios is observed, captopril should be discontinued unless it is considered life-saving for the mother. Contraction stress testing (CST), a non-stress test (NST), or biophysical profiling (BPP) may be appropriate, depending upon the week of pregnancy. Patients and physicians should be aware, however, that oligohydramnios may not appear until after the fetus has sustained irreversible injury.

Infants with histories of *in utero* exposure to ACE inhibitors should be closely observed for hypotension, oliguria, and hyperkalemia. If oliguria occurs, attention should be directed toward support of blood pressure and renal perfusion. Exchange transfusion or dialysis may be required as a means of reversing hypotension and/or substituting for disordered renal function. While captopril may be removed from the adult circulation by hemodialysis, there is inadequate data concerning the effectiveness of hemodialysis for removing it from the circulation of neonates or children. Peritoneal dialysis is not effective for removing captopril; there is no information concerning exchange transfusion for removing captopril from the general circulation.

When captopril was given to rabbits at doses about 0.8 to 70 times (on a mg/kg basis) the maximum recommended human dose, low incidences of craniofacial malformations were seen. No teratogenic effects of captopril were seen in studies of pregnant rats and hamsters. On a mg/kg basis, the doses used were up to 150 times (in hamsters) and 625 times (in rats) the maximum recommended human dose.

Hepatic Failure

Rarely, ACE inhibitors have been associated with a syndrome that starts with cholestatic jaundice and progresses to fulminant hepatic necrosis and (sometimes) death. The mechanism of this syndrome is not understood. Patients receiving ACE inhibitors who develop jaundice or marked elevations of hepatic enzymes should discontinue the ACE inhibitor and receive appropriate medical follow-up.

PRECAUTIONS

General

Impaired Renal Function

Hypertension—Some patients with renal disease, particularly those with severe renal artery stenosis, have developed increases in BUN and serum creatinine after reduction of blood pressure with captopril. Captopril dosage reduction and/or discontinuation of diuretic may be required. For some of these patients, it may not be possible to normalize blood pressure and maintain adequate renal perfusion.

Heart Failure—About 20 percent of patients develop stable elevations of BUN and serum creatinine greater than 20 percent above normal or baseline upon long-term treatment with captopril. Less than 5 percent of patients, generally those with severe preexisting renal disease, required discontinuation of treatment due to progressively increasing creatinine; subsequent improvement probably depends upon the severity of the underlying renal disease.

See CLINICAL PHARMACOLOGY, DOSAGE AND ADMINISTRATION, ADVERSE REACTIONS: Altered Laboratory Findings.

Hyperkalemia: Elevations in serum potassium have been observed in some patients treated with ACE inhibitors, including captopril. When treated with ACE inhibitors, patients at risk for the development of hyperkalemia include those with: renal insufficiency; diabetes mellitus; and those using concomitant potassium-sparing diuretics, potassium supplements or potassium-containing salt substitutes; or other drugs associated with increases in serum potassium. In a trial of type I diabetic patients with proteinuria, the incidence of withdrawal of treatment with captopril for hyperkalemia was 2% (4/207). In two trials of normotensive type I diabetic patients with microalbuminuria, no captopril group subjects had hyperkalemia (0/116). (See PRECAUTIONS: Information for Patients and Drug Interactions; ADVERSE REACTIONS: Altered Laboratory Findings.)

Cough: Presumably due to the inhibition of the degradation of endogenous bradykinin, persistent nonproductive cough has been reported with all ACE inhibitors, always resolving after discontinuation of therapy. ACE inhibitor-induced cough should be considered in the differential diagnosis of cough.

Valvular Stenosis: There is concern, on theoretical grounds, that patients with aortic stenosis might be at particular risk of decreased coronary perfusion when treated with vasodilators because they do not develop as much afterload reduction as others.

Surgery/Anesthesia: In patients undergoing major surgery or during anesthesia with agents that produce hypotension, captopril will block angiotensin II formation secondary to compensatory renin release. If hypotension occurs and is considered to be due to this mechanism, it can be corrected by volume expansion.

Hemodialysis

Recent clinical observations have shown an association of hypersensitivity-like (anaphylactoid) reactions during hemodialysis with high-flux dialysis membranes (e.g., AN69) in patients receiving ACE inhibitors. In these patients, consideration should be given to using a different type of dialysis membrane or a different class of medication. (See WARNINGS: Anaphylactoid reactions during membrane exposure).

Information for Patients

Patients should be advised to immediately report to their physician any signs or symptoms suggesting angioedema (e.g., swelling of face, eyes, lips, tongue, larynx and extremities; difficulty in swallowing or breathing; hoarseness) and to discontinue therapy. (See WARNINGS: Angioedema.)

Patients should be told to report promptly any indication of infection (e.g., sore throat, fever), which may be a sign of neutropenia, or of progressive edema which might be related to proteinuria and nephrotic syndrome.

All patients should be cautioned that excessive perspiration and dehydration may lead to an excessive fall in blood pressure because of reduction in fluid volume. Other causes of volume depletion such as vomiting or diarrhea may also lead to a fall in blood pressure; patients should be advised to consult with the physician.

Patients should be advised not to use potassium-sparing diuretics, potassium supplements or potassium-containing salt substitutes without consulting their physician. (See PRECAUTIONS: General and Drug Interactions; ADVERSE REACTIONS.)

Patients should be warned against interruption or discontinuation of medication unless instructed by the physician. Heart failure patients on captopril therapy should be cautioned against rapid increases in physical activity.

Patients should be informed that CAPOTEN (captopril) should be taken one hour before meals (see DOSAGE AND ADMINISTRATION).

Pregnancy. Female patients of childbearing age should be told about the consequences of second- and third-trimester exposure to ACE inhibitors, and they should also be told that these consequences do not appear to have resulted from intrauterine ACE-inhibitor exposure that has been limited to the first trimester. These patients should be asked to report pregnancies to their physicians as soon as possible.

Drug Interactions

Hypotension—Patients on Diuretic Therapy: Patients on diuretics and especially those in whom diuretic therapy was recently instituted, as well as those on severe dietary salt restriction or dialysis, may occasionally experience a precipitous reduction of blood pressure usually within the first hour after receiving the initial dose of captopril.

The possibility of hypotensive effects with captopril can be minimized by either discontinuing the diuretic or increasing the salt intake approximately one week prior to initiation of treatment with CAPOTEN (captopril) or initiating therapy with small doses (6.25 or 12.5 mg). Alternatively, provide medical supervision for at least one hour after the initial dose. If hypotension occurs, the patient should be placed in a supine position and, if necessary, receive an intravenous infusion of normal saline. This transient hypotensive response is not a contraindication to further doses which can be given without difficulty once the blood pressure has increased after volume expansion.

Agents Having Vasodilator Activity: Data on the effect of concomitant use of other vasodilators in patients receiving CAPOTEN for heart failure are not available; therefore, nitroglycerin or other nitrates (as used for management of angina) or other drugs having vasodilator activity should, if possible, be discontinued before starting CAPOTEN. If resumed during CAPOTEN therapy, such agents should be administered cautiously, and perhaps at lower dosage.

Agents Causing Renin Release: Captopril's effect will be augmented by antihypertensive agents that cause renin release. For example, diuretics (e.g., thiazides) may activate the renin-angiotensin-aldosterone system.

Agents Affecting Sympathetic Activity: The sympathetic nervous system may be especially important in supporting blood pressure in patients receiving captopril alone or with diuretics. Therefore, agents affecting sympathetic activity (e.g., ganglionic blocking agents or adrenergic neuron blocking agents) should be used with caution. Beta-adrenergic blocking drugs add some further antihypertensive effect to captopril, but the overall response is less than additive.

Agents Increasing Serum Potassium: Since captopril decreases aldosterone production, elevation of serum potassium may occur. Potassium-sparing diuretics such as spironolactone, triamterene, or amiloride, or potassium supplements should be given only for documented hypokalemia, and then with caution, since they may lead to a significant increase of serum potassium. Salt substitutes containing potassium should also be used with caution.

Inhibitors Of Endogenous Prostaglandin Synthesis: It has been reported that indomethacin may reduce the antihypertensive effect of captopril, especially in cases of low renin hypertension. Other nonsteroidal anti-inflammatory agents (e.g., aspirin) may also have this effect.

Lithium: Increased serum lithium levels and symptoms of lithium toxicity have been reported in patients receiving concomitant lithium and ACE inhibitor therapy. These drugs should be coadministered with caution and frequent

monitoring of serum lithium levels is recommended. If a diuretic is also used, it may increase the risk of lithium toxicity.

Drug/Laboratory Test Interaction
Captopril may cause a false-positive urine test for acetone.

Carcinogenesis, Mutagenesis and Impairment of Fertility
Two-year studies with doses of 50 to 1350 mg/kg/day in mice and rats failed to show any evidence of carcinogenic potential. The high dose in these studies is 150 times the maximum recommended human dose of 450 mg, assuming a 50-kg subject. On a body-surface-area basis, the high doses for mice and rats are 13 and 26 times the maximum recommended human dose, respectively.

Studies in rats have revealed no impairment of fertility.

Animal Toxicology
Chronic oral toxicity studies were conducted in rats (2 years), dogs (47 weeks; 1 year), mice (2 years), and monkeys (1 year). Significant drug-related toxicity included effects on hematopoiesis, renal toxicity, erosion/ulceration of the stomach, and variation of retinal blood vessels.

Reductions in hemoglobin and/or hematocrit values were seen in mice, rats, and monkeys at doses 50 to 150 times the maximum recommended human dose (MRHD) of 450 mg, assuming a 50-mg subject. On a body-surface-area basis, these doses are 5 to 25 times maximum recommended human dose (MRHD). Anemia, leukopenia, thrombocytopenia, and bone marrow suppression occurred in dogs at doses 8 to 30 times MRHD on a body-weight basis (4 to 15 times MRHD on a surface-area basis). The reductions in hemoglobin and hematocrit values in rats and mice were only significant at 1 year and returned to normal with continued dosing by the end of the study. Marked anemia was seen at all dose levels (8 to 30 times MRHD) in dogs, whereas moderate to marked leukopenia was noted only at 15 and 30 times MRHD and thrombocytopenia at 30 times MRHD. The anemia could be reversed upon discontinuation of dosing. Bone marrow suppression occurred to a varying degree, being associated only with dogs that died or were sacrificed in a moribund condition in the 1 year study. However, in the 47-week study at a dose 30 times MRHD, bone marrow suppression was found to be reversible upon continued drug administration.

Captopril caused hyperplasia of the juxtaglomerular apparatus of the kidneys in mice and rats at doses 7 to 200 times MRHD on a body-weight basis (0.6 to 35 times MRHD on a surface-area basis); in monkeys at 20 to 60 times MRHD on a body-weight basis (7 to 20 times MRHD on a surface-area basis); and in dogs at 30 times MRHD on a body-weight basis (15 times MRHD on a surface-area basis).

Gastric erosions/ulcerations were increased in incidence in male rats at 20 to 200 times MRHD on a body-weight basis (3.5 and 35 times MRHD on a surface-area basis); in dogs at 30 times MRHD on a body-weight basis (15 times on MRHD on a surface-area basis); and in monkeys at 65 times MRHD on a body-weight basis (20 times MRHD on a surface-area basis). Rabbits developed gastric and intestinal ulcers when given oral doses approximately 30 times MRHD on a body-weight basis (10 times MRHD on a surface-area basis) for only 5 to 7 days.

In the two-year rat study, irreversible and progressive variations in the caliber of retinal vessels (focal sacculations and constrictions) occurred at all dose levels (7 to 200 times MRHD) on a body-weight basis; 1 to 35 times MRHD on a surface-area basis in a dose-related fashion. The effect was first observed in the 88th week of dosing, with a progressively increased incidence thereafter, even after cessation of dosing.

Pregnancy Categories C (first trimester) and D (second and third trimesters)
See WARNINGS: Fetal/Neonatal Morbidity and Mortality.

Nursing Mothers
Concentrations of captopril in human milk are approximately one percent of those in maternal blood. Because of the potential for serious adverse reactions in nursing infants from captopril, a decision should be made whether to discontinue nursing or to discontinue the drug, taking into account the importance of CAPOTEN to the mother. (See PRECAUTIONS: Pediatric Use.)

Pediatric Use
Safety and effectiveness in children have not been established. There is limited experience reported in the literature with the use of captopril in the pediatric population; dosage, on a weight basis, was generally reported to be comparable to or less than that used in adults.

Infants, especially newborns, may be more susceptible to the adverse hemodynamic effects of captopril. Excessive, prolonged and unpredictable decreases in blood pressure and associated complications, including oliguria and seizures, have been reported.

CAPOTEN (captopril) should be used in children only if other measures for controlling blood pressure have not been effective.

ADVERSE REACTIONS
Reported incidences are based on clinical trials involving approximately 7000 patients.

Renal: About one of 100 patients developed proteinuria (see WARNINGS).

Each of the following has been reported in approximately 1 to 2 of 1000 patients and are of uncertain relationship to drug use: renal insufficiency, renal failure, nephrotic syndrome, polyuria, oliguria, and urinary frequency.

Hematologic: Neutropenia/agranulocytosis has occurred (see WARNINGS). Cases of anemia, thrombocytopenia, and pancytopenia have been reported.

Dermatologic: Rash, often with pruritus, and sometimes with fever, arthralgia, and eosinophilia, occurred in about 4 to 7 (depending on renal status and dose) of 100 patients, usually during the first four weeks of therapy. It is usually maculopapular, and rarely urticarial. The rash is usually mild and disappears within a few days of dosage reduction, short-term treatment with an antihistaminic agent, and/or discontinuing therapy; remission may occur even if captopril is continued. Pruritus, without rash, occurs in about 2 of 100 patients. Between 7 and 10 percent of patients with skin rash have shown an eosinophilia and/or positive ANA titers. A reversible associated pemphigoid-like lesion, and photosensitivity, have also been reported.

Flushing or pallor has been reported in 2 to 5 of 1000 patients.

Cardiovascular: Hypotension may occur; see WARNINGS and PRECAUTIONS [Drug Interactions] for discussion of hypotension with captopril therapy.

Tachycardia, chest pain, and palpitations have each been observed in approximately 1 of 100 patients.

Angina pectoris, myocardial infarction, Raynaud's syndrome, and congestive heart failure have each occurred in 2 to 3 of 1000 patients.

Dysgeusia: Approximately 2 to 4 (depending on renal status and dose) of 100 patients developed a diminution or loss of taste perception. Taste impairment is reversible and usually self-limited (2 to 3 months) even with continued drug administration. Weight loss may be associated with the loss of taste.

Angioedema: Angioedema involving the extremities, face, lips, mucous membranes, tongue, glottis or larynx has been reported in approximately one in 1000 patients. Angioedema involving the upper airways has caused fatal airway obstruction. (See WARNINGS: Angioedema and PRECAUTIONS: Information for Patients.)

Cough: Cough has been reported in 0.5–2% of patients treated with captopril in clinical trials (see PRECAUTIONS: General, Cough).

The following have been reported in about 0.5 to 2 percent of patients but did not appear at increased frequency compared to placebo or other treatments used in controlled trials: gastric irritation, abdominal pain, nausea, vomiting, diarrhea, anorexia, constipation, aphthous ulcers, peptic ulcer, dizziness, headache, malaise, fatigue, insomnia, dry mouth, dyspnea, alopecia, paresthesias.

Other clinical adverse effects reported since the drug was marketed are listed below by body system. In this setting, an incidence or causal relationship cannot be accurately determined.

Body as a whole: Anaphylactoid reactions (see WARNINGS: Anaphylactoid and possibly related reactions and PRECAUTIONS: Hemodialysis).

General: Asthenia, gynecomastia.

Cardiovascular: Cardiac arrest, cerebrovascular accident/insufficiency, rhythm disturbances, orthostatic hypotension, syncope.

Dermatologic: Bullous pemphigus, erythema multiforme (including Stevens-Johnson syndrome), exfoliative dermatitis.

Gastrointestinal: Pancreatitis, glossitis, dyspepsia.

Hematologic: Anemia, including aplastic and hemolytic.

Hepatobiliary: Jaundice, hepatitis, including rare cases of necrosis, cholestasis.

Metabolic: Symptomatic hyponatremia.

Musculoskeletal: Myalgia, myasthenia.

Nervous/Psychiatric: Ataxia, confusion, depression, nervousness, somnolence.

Respiratory: Bronchospasm, eosinophilic pneumonitis, rhinitis.

Special Senses: Blurred vision.

Urogenital: Impotence.

As with other ACE inhibitors, a syndrome has been reported which may include: fever, myalgia, arthralgia, interstitial nephritis, vasculitis, rash or other dermatologic manifestations, eosinophilia and an elevated ESR.

Fetal/Neonatal Morbidity and Mortality
See WARNINGS: Fetal/Neonatal Morbidity and Mortality.

Altered Laboratory Findings
Serum Electrolytes: Hyperkalemia: small increases in serum potassium, especially in patients with renal impairment (see PRECAUTIONS).

Hyponatremia: particularly in patients receiving a low sodium diet or concomitant diuretics.

BUN/Serum Creatinine: Transient elevations of BUN or serum creatinine especially in volume or salt depleted patients or those with renovascular hypertension may occur.

Rapid reduction of longstanding or markedly elevated blood pressure can result in decreases in the glomerular filtration rate and, in turn, lead to increases in BUN or serum creatinine.

Hematologic: A positive ANA has been reported.

Liver Function Tests: Elevations of liver transaminases, alkaline phosphatase, and serum bilirubin have occurred.

OVERDOSAGE
Correction of hypotension would be of primary concern. Volume expansion with an intravenous infusion of normal saline is the treatment of choice for restoration of blood pressure.

While captopril may be removed from the adult circulation by hemodialysis, there is inadequate data concerning the effectiveness of hemodialysis for removing it from the circulation of neonates or children. Peritoneal dialysis is not effective for removing captopril; there is no information concerning exchange transfusion for removing captopril from the general circulation.

DOSAGE AND ADMINISTRATION
CAPOTEN (captopril) should be taken one hour before meals. Dosage must be individualized.

Hypertension—Initiation of therapy requires consideration of recent antihypertensive drug treatment, the extent of blood pressure elevation, salt restriction, and other clinical circumstances. If possible, discontinue the patient's previous antihypertensive drug regimen for one week before starting CAPOTEN.

The initial dose of CAPOTEN (captopril) is 25 mg bid or tid. If satisfactory reduction of blood pressure has not been achieved after one or two weeks, the dose may be increased to 50 mg bid or tid. Concomitant sodium restriction may be beneficial when CAPOTEN is used alone.

The dose of CAPOTEN in hypertension usually does not exceed 50 mg tid. Therefore, if the blood pressure has not been satisfactorily controlled after one to two weeks at this dose, (and the patient is not already receiving a diuretic), a modest dose of a thiazide-type diuretic (e.g., hydrochlorothiazide, 25 mg daily), should be added. The diuretic dose may be increased at one- to two-week intervals until its highest usual antihypertensive dose is reached.

If CAPOTEN is being started in a patient already receiving a diuretic, CAPOTEN therapy should be initiated under close medical supervision (see WARNINGS and PRECAUTIONS [Drug Interactions] regarding hypotension), with dosage and titration of CAPOTEN as noted above.

If further blood pressure reduction is required, the dose of CAPOTEN may be increased to 100 mg bid or tid and then, if necessary, to 150 mg bid or tid (while continuing the diuretic). The usual dose range is 25 to 150 mg bid or tid. A maximum daily dose of 450 mg CAPOTEN should not be exceeded.

For patients with severe hypertension (e.g., accelerated or malignant hypertension), when temporary discontinuation of current antihypertensive therapy is not practical or desirable, or when prompt titration to more normotensive blood pressure levels is indicated, diuretic should be continued but other current antihypertensive medication stopped and CAPOTEN dosage promptly initiated at 25 mg bid or tid, under close medical supervision.

When necessitated by the patient's clinical condition, the daily dose of CAPOTEN may be increased every 24 hours or less under continuous medical supervision until a satisfactory blood pressure response is obtained or the maximum dose of CAPOTEN is reached. In this regimen, addition of a more potent diuretic, e.g., furosemide, may also be indicated. Beta-blockers may also be used in conjunction with CAPOTEN therapy (see PRECAUTIONS: Drug Interactions), but the effects of the two drugs are less than additive.

Heart Failure—Initiation of therapy requires consideration of recent diuretic therapy and the possibility of severe salt/volume depletion. In patients with either normal or low blood pressure, who have been vigorously treated with diuretics and who may be hyponatremic and/or hypovolemic, a starting dose of 6.25 or 12.5 mg tid may minimize the magnitude or duration of the hypotensive effect (see WARNINGS: Hypotension); for these patients, titration to the usual daily dosage can then occur within the next several days.

For most patients the usual initial daily dosage is 25 mg tid. After a dose of 50 mg tid is reached, further increases in dosage should be delayed, where possible, for at least two weeks to determine if a satisfactory response occurs. Most patients studied have had a satisfactory clinical improvement at 50 or 100 mg tid. A maximum daily dose of 450 mg of CAPOTEN (captopril) should not be exceeded.

CAPOTEN should generally be used in conjunction with a diuretic and digitalis. CAPOTEN therapy must be initiated under very close medical supervision.

Left Ventricular Dysfunction After Myocardial Infarction: The recommended dose for long-term use in patients following a myocardial infarction is a target maintenance dose of 50 mg tid.

Continued on next page

Bristol-Myers Squibb Co.—Cont.

Therapy may be initiated as early as three days following a myocardial infarction. After a single dose of 6.25 mg, CAPOTEN therapy should be initiated at 12.5 mg tid. CAPOTEN should then be increased to 25 mg tid during the next several days and to a target dose of 50 mg tid over the next several weeks as tolerated (see CLINICAL PHARMACOLOGY).

CAPOTEN may be used in patients treated with other post-myocardial infarction therapies, e.g., thrombolytics, aspirin, beta blockers.

Diabetic Nephropathy: The recommended dose of CAPOTEN for long term use to treat diabetic nephropathy is 25 mg tid.

Other antihypertensives such as diuretics, beta blockers, centrally acting agents or vasodilators may be used in conjunction with CAPOTEN if additional therapy is required to further lower blood pressure.

Dosage Adjustment in Renal Impairment—Because CAPOTEN (captopril) is excreted primarily by the kidneys, excretion rates are reduced in patients with impaired renal function. These patients will take longer to reach steady-state captopril levels and will reach higher steady-state levels for a given daily dose than patients with normal renal function. Therefore, these patients may respond to smaller or less frequent doses.

Accordingly, for patients with significant renal impairment, initial daily dosage of CAPOTEN (captopril) should be reduced, and smaller increments utilized for titration, which should be quite slow (one- to two-week intervals). After the desired therapeutic effect has been achieved, the dose should be slowly back-titrated to determine the minimal effective dose. When concomitant diuretic therapy is required, a loop diuretic (e.g., furosemide), rather than a thiazide diuretic, is preferred in patients with severe renal impairment. (See WARNINGS: Anaphylactoid reactions during membrane exposure and PRECAUTIONS: Hemodialysis.)

HOW SUPPLIED

12.5 mg tablets in bottles of 100 (NDC 0003-0450-54) and 1000 (NDC 0003-0450-75), **25 mg tablets** in bottles of 100 (NDC 0003-0452-50) and 1000 (NDC 0003-0452-75), **50 mg tablets** in bottles of 100 (NDC 0003-0482-50) and 1000 (NDC 0003-0482-75), and **100 mg tablets** in bottles of 100 (NDC 0003-0485-50). Bottles contain a desiccant-charcoal canister.

Unimatic® unit-dose packs containing 100 tablets are also available for each potency: **12.5 mg** (NDC 0003-0450-51), **25 mg** (NDC 0003-0452-51), **50 mg** (NDC 0003-0482-51), and **100 mg** (NDC 0003-0485-51).

The **12.5 mg tablet** is a biconvex oval with a partial bisect bar; the **25 mg tablet** is a biconvex rounded square with a quadrisect bar; the **50 and 100 mg tablets** are biconvex ovals with a bisect bar.

All captopril tablets are white and may exhibit a slight sulfurous odor.

Storage

Do not store above 86°F. Keep bottles tightly closed (protect from moisture).

(J4-458F)

Shown in Product Identification Guide, page 306

CAPOZIDE® 25/15 ℞
CAPOZIDE® 25/25 ℞
CAPOZIDE® 50/15 ℞
CAPOZIDE® 50/25 ℞

[kap'o-zīd"]

Captopril-Hydrochlorothiazide Tablets

USE IN PREGNANCY

When used in pregnancy during the second and third trimesters, ACE Inhibitors can cause injury and even death to the developing fetus. When pregnancy is detected, CAPOZIDE should be discontinued as soon as possible. **See WARNINGS: Captopril, Fetal/Neonatal Morbidity and Mortality.**

DESCRIPTION

CAPOZIDE (Captopril-Hydrochlorothiazide Tablets) for oral administration combines two antihypertensive agents: CAPOTEN (captopril) and hydrochlorothiazide. Captopril, the first of a new class of antihypertensive agents, is a specific competitive inhibitor of angiotensin I-converting enzyme (ACE), the enzyme responsible for the conversion of angiotensin I to angiotensin II. Hydrochlorothiazide is a benzothiadiazide (thiazide) diuretic-antihypertensive. CAPOZIDE tablets are available in four combinations of captopril with hydrochlorothiazide: 25 mg with 15 mg, 25 mg with 25 mg, 50 mg with 15 mg, and 50 mg with 25 mg. Inactive ingredients: microcrystalline cellulose, colorant (FD&C Yellow No. 6), lactose, magnesium stearate, pregelatinized starch, and stearic acid.

Captopril is designated chemically as 1-[(2S)-3-mercapto-2-methylpropionyl]-L-proline; hydrochlorothiazide is 6-Chloro-3,4-dihydro-2*H*-1, 2, 4-benzothiadiazine-7-sulfonamide 1,1-dioxide. Graphic formulas:

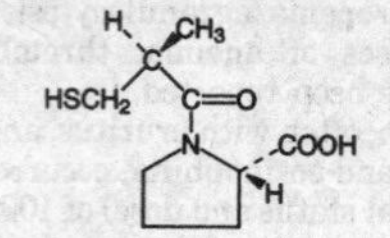

[MW 217.29]
captopril

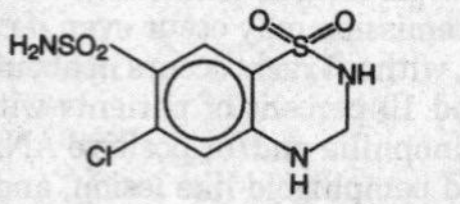

[MW 297.73]
hydrochlorothiazide

Captopril is a white to off-white crystalline powder that may have a slight sulfurous odor; it is soluble in water (approx. 160 mg/mL), methanol, and ethanol and sparingly soluble in chloroform and ethyl acetate.

Hydrochlorothiazide is a white crystalline powder slightly soluble in water but freely soluble in sodium hydroxide solution.

CLINICAL PHARMACOLOGY

Captopril

Mechanism of Action

The mechanism of action of captopril has not yet been fully elucidated. Its beneficial effects in hypertension and heart failure appear to result primarily from suppression of the renin-angiotensin-aldosterone system. However, there is no consistent correlation between renin levels and response to the drug. Renin, an enzyme synthesized by the kidneys, is released into the circulation where it acts on a plasma globulin substrate to produce angiotensin I, a relatively inactive decapeptide. Angiotensin I is then converted by angiotensin converting enzyme (ACE) to angiotensin II, a potent endogenous vasoconstrictor substance. Angiotensin II also stimulates aldosterone secretion from the adrenal cortex, thereby contributing to sodium and fluid retention.

Captopril prevents the conversion of angiotensin I to angiotensin II by inhibition of ACE, a peptidyldipeptide carboxy hydrolase. This inhibition has been demonstrated in both healthy human subjects and in animals by showing that the elevation of blood pressure caused by exogenously administered angiotensin I was attenuated or abolished by captopril. In animal studies, captopril did not alter the pressor responses to a number of other agents, including angiotensin II and norepinephrine, indicating specificity of action.

ACE is identical to "bradykininase", and captopril may also interfere with the degradation of the vasodepressor peptide, bradykinin. Increased concentrations of bradykinin or prostaglandin E_2 may also have a role in the therapeutic effect of captopril.

Inhibition of ACE results in decreased plasma angiotensin II and increased plasma renin activity (PRA), the latter resulting from loss of negative feedback on renin release caused by reduction in angiotensin II. The reduction of angiotensin II leads to decreased aldosterone secretion, and, as a result, small increases in serum potassium may occur along with sodium and fluid loss.

The antihypertensive effects persist for a longer period of time than does demonstrable inhibition of circulating ACE. It is not known whether the ACE present in vascular endothelium is inhibited longer than the ACE in circulating blood.

Pharmacokinetics

After oral administration of therapeutic doses of captopril, rapid absorption occurs with peak blood levels at about one hour. The presence of food in the gastrointestinal tract reduces absorption by about 30 to 40 percent; captopril therefore should be given one hour before meals. Based on carbon-14 labeling, average minimal absorption is approximately 75 percent. In a 24-hour period, over 95 percent of the absorbed dose is eliminated in the urine; 40 to 50 percent is unchanged drug; most of the remainder is the disulfide dimer of captopril and captopril-cysteine disulfide.

Approximately 25 to 30 percent of the circulating drug is bound to plasma proteins. The apparent elimination half-life for total radioactivity in blood is probably less than three hours. An accurate determination of half-life of unchanged captopril is not, at present, possible, but it is probably less than two hours. In patients with renal impairment, however, retention of captopril occurs (see DOSAGE AND ADMINISTRATION).

Pharmacodynamics

Administration of captopril results in a reduction of peripheral arterial resistance in hypertensive patients with either no change, or an increase, in cardiac output. There is an increase in renal blood flow following administration of captopril and glomerular filtration rate is usually unchanged. In patients with heart failure, significantly decreased peripheral (systemic vascular) resistance and blood pressure (afterload), reduced pulmonary capillary wedge pressure (preload) and pulmonary vascular resistance, increased cardiac output, and increased exercise tolerance time (ETT) have been demonstrated.

Reductions of blood pressure are usually maximal 60 to 90 minutes after oral administration of an individual dose of captopril. The duration of effect is dose related and is extended in the presence of a thiazide-type diuretic. The full effect of a given dose may not be attained for 6–8 weeks (see DOSAGE AND ADMINISTRATION). The blood pressure lowering effects of captopril and thiazide-type diuretics are additive. In contrast, captopril and beta-blockers have a less than additive effect.

Blood pressure is lowered to about the same extent in both standing and supine positions. Orthostatic effects and tachycardia are infrequent but may occur in volume-depleted patients. Abrupt withdrawal of captopril has not been associated with a rapid increase in blood pressure.

Studies in rats and cats indicate that captopril does not cross the blood-brain barrier to any significant extent.

Hydrochlorothiazide

Thiazides affect the renal tubular mechanism of electrolyte reabsorption. At maximal therapeutic dosage all thiazides are approximately equal in their diuretic potency.

Thiazides increase excretion of sodium and chloride in approximately equivalent amounts. Natriuresis causes a secondary loss of potassium and bicarbonate.

The mechanism of the antihypertensive effect of thiazides is unknown. Thiazides do not affect normal blood pressure.

The mean plasma half-life of hydrochlorothiazide in fasted individuals has been reported to be approximately 2.5 hours. Onset of diuresis occurs in two hours and the peak effect at about four hours. Its action persists for approximately six to twelve hours. Hydrochlorothiazide is eliminated rapidly by the kidney.

INDICATIONS AND USAGE

CAPOZIDE (Captopril-Hydrochlorothiazide Tablets) is indicated for the treatment of hypertension. The blood pressure lowering effects of captopril and thiazides are approximately additive.

This fixed combination drug may be used as initial therapy or substituted for previously titrated doses of the individual components.

When captopril and hydrochlorothiazide are given together it may not be necessary to administer captopril in divided doses to attain blood pressure control at trough (before the next dose). Also, with such a combination, a daily dose of 15 mg of hydrochlorothiazide may be adequate.

Treatment may, therefore, be initiated with CAPOZIDE 25 mg/15 mg once daily. Subsequent titration should be with additional doses of the components (captopril, hydrochlorothiazide) as single agents or as CAPOZIDE 50 mg/15 mg, 25 mg/25 mg, or 50 mg/25 mg (see DOSAGE AND ADMINISTRATION).

In using CAPOZIDE, consideration should be given to the risk of neutropenia/agranulocytosis (see WARNINGS).

CAPOZIDE may be used for patients with normal renal function, in whom the risk is relatively low. In patients with impaired renal function, particularly those with collagen vascular disease, CAPOZIDE should be reserved for hypertensives who have either developed unacceptable side effects on other drugs, or have failed to respond satisfactorily to other drug combinations.

CONTRAINDICATIONS

Captopril

This product is contraindicated in patients who are hypersensitive to captopril or any other angiotensin-converting enzyme inhibitor (e.g., a patient who has experienced angioedema during therapy with any other ACE inhibitor).

Hydrochlorothiazide

Hydrochlorothiazide is contraindicated in anuria. It is also contraindicated in patients who have previously demonstrated hypersensitivity to hydrochlorothiazide or other sulfonamide-derived drugs.

WARNINGS

Captopril

Anaphylactoid and Possible Related Reactions

Presumably because angiotensin-converting enzyme inhibitors affect the metabolism of eicosanoids and polypeptides, including endogenous bradykinin, patients receiving ACE inhibitors (including CAPOZIDE) may be subject to a variety of adverse reactions, some of them serious.

Angioedema: Angioedema involving the extremities, face, lips, mucous membranes, tongue, glottis or larynx has been seen in patients treated with ACE inhibitors, including captopril. If angioedema involves the tongue, glottis or larynx, airway obstruction may occur and be fatal. Emergency therapy, including but not necessarily limited to, subcutaneous

administration of a 1:1000 solution of epinephrine should be promptly instituted.
Swelling confined to the face, mucous membranes of the mouth, lips and extremities has usually resolved with discontinuation of treatment; some cases required medical therapy. (See PRECAUTIONS: Information for Patients and ADVERSE REACTIONS: Captopril.)

Anaphylactoid reactions during desensitization: Two patients undergoing desensitizing treatment with hymenoptera venom while receiving ACE inhibitors sustained life-threatening anaphylactoid reactions. In the same patients, these reactions were avoided when ACE inhibitors were temporarily withheld, but they reappeared upon inadvertent rechallenge.

Anaphylactoid reactions during membrane exposure: Anaphylactoid reactions have been reported in patients dialyzed with high-flux membranes and treated concomitantly with an ACE inhibitor. Anaphylactoid reactions have also been reported in patients undergoing low-density lipoprotein apheresis with dextran sulfate absorption (a procedure dependent upon devices not approved in the United States).

Neutropenia/Agranulocytosis
Neutropenia (<1000/mm^3) with myeloid hypoplasia has resulted from use of captopril. About half of the neutropenic patients developed systemic or oral cavity infections or other features of the syndrome of agranulocytosis.
The risk of neutropenia is dependent on the clinical status of the patient:

In clinical trials in patients with hypertension who have normal renal function (serum creatinine less than 1.6 mg/dL and no collagen vascular disease), neutropenia has been seen in one patient out of over 8,600 exposed.

In patients with some degree of renal failure (serum creatinine at least 1.6 mg/dL) but no collagen vascular disease, the risk of neutropenia in clinical trials was about 1 per 500, a frequency over 15 times that for uncomplicated hypertension. Daily doses of captopril were relatively high in these patients, particularly in view of their diminished renal function. In foreign marketing experience in patients with renal failure, use of allopurinol concomitantly with captopril has been associated with neutropenia but this association has not appeared in U.S. reports.

In patients with collagen vascular diseases (e.g., systemic lupus erythematosus, scleroderma) and impaired renal function, neutropenia occurred in 3.7 percent of patients in clinical trials.

While none of the over 750 patients in formal clinical trials of heart failure developed neutropenia, it has occurred during the subsequent clinical experience. About half of the reported cases had serum creatinine ≥1.6 mg/dL and more than 75 percent were in patients also receiving procainamide. In heart failure, it appears that the same risk factors for neutropenia are present.

The neutropenia has usually been detected within three months after captopril was started. Bone marrow examinations in patients with neutropenia consistently showed myeloid hypoplasia, frequently accompanied by erythroid hypoplasia and decreased numbers of megakaryocytes (e.g., hypoplastic bone marrow and pancytopenia); anemia and thrombocytopenia were sometimes seen.
In general, neutrophils returned to normal in about two weeks after captopril was discontinued, and serious infections were limited to clinically complex patients. About 13 percent of the cases of neutropenia have ended fatally, but almost all fatalities were in patients with serious illness, having collagen vascular disease, renal failure, heart failure or immunosuppressant therapy, or a combination of these complicating factors.

Evaluation of the hypertensive or heart failure patient should always include assessment of renal function.
If captopril is used in patients with impaired renal function, white blood cell and differential counts should be evaluated prior to starting treatment and at approximately two-week intervals for about three months, then periodically.
In patients with collagen vascular disease or who are exposed to other drugs known to affect the white cells or immune response, particularly when there is impaired renal function, captopril should be used only after an assessment of benefit and risk, and then with caution.
All patients treated with captopril should be told to report any signs of infection (e.g., sore throat, fever). If infection is suspected, white cell counts should be performed without delay.
Since discontinuation of captopril and other drugs has generally led to prompt return of the white count to normal, upon confirmation of neutropenia (neutrophil count <1000/mm^3) the physician should withdraw captopril and closely follow the patient's course.

Proteinuria
Total urinary proteins greater than 1 g per day were seen in about 0.7 percent of patients receiving captopril. About 90 percent of affected patients had evidence of prior renal disease or received relatively high doses of captopril (in excess of 150 mg/day), or both. The nephrotic syndrome occurred in about one-fifth of proteinuric patients. In most cases, proteinuria subsided or cleared within six months whether or not captopril was continued. Parameters of renal function, such as BUN and creatinine, were seldom altered in the patients with proteinuria.

Hypotension
Excessive hypotension was rarely seen in hypertensive patients but is a possible consequence of captopril use in salt/volume depleted persons (such as those treated vigorously with diuretics), patients with heart failure or those patients undergoing renal dialysis. (See PRECAUTIONS: Drug Interactions.)

Fetal/Neonatal Morbidity and Mortality
ACE inhibitors can cause fetal and neonatal morbidity and death when administerd to pregnant women. Several dozen cases have been reported in the world literature. When pregnancy is detected, ACE inhibitors should be discontinued as soon as possible.
The use of ACE inhibitors during the second and third trimesters of pregnancy has been associated with fetal and neonatal injury, including hypotension, neonatal skull hypoplasia, anuria, reversible or irreversible renal failure, and death. Oligohydramnios has also been reported, presumably resulting from decreased fetal renal function; oligohydramnios in this setting has been associated with fetal limb contractures, craniofacial deformation, and hypoplastic lung development. Prematurity, intrauterine growth retardation, and patent ductus arteriosus have also been reported, although it is not clear whether these occurrences were due to the ACE-inhibitor exposure.
These adverse effects do not appear to have resulted from intrauterine ACE-inhibitor exposure that has been limited to the first trimester. Mothers whose embryos and fetuses are exposed to ACE-inhibitors only during the first trimester should be so informed. Nonetheless, when patients become pregnant, physicians should make every effort to discontinue the use of captoril as soon as possible.
Rarely (probably less often than once in every thousand pregnancies), no alternative to ACE inhibitors will be found. In these rare cases, the mothers should be apprised of the potential hazards to their fetuses, and serial unltrasound examinations should be performed to assess the intraamniotic environment.
If oligohydramnios is observed, captopril should be discontinued unless it is considered life-saving for the mother. Contraction stress testing (CST), a non-stress test (NST), or biophysical profiling (BPP) may be appropriate, depending upon the week of pregnancy. Patients and physicians should be aware, however, that oligohydramnios may not appear until after the fetus has sustained irreversible injury.
Infants with histories of *in utero* exposure to ACE inhibitors should be closely observed for hypotension, oliguria, and hyperkalemia. If oliguria occurs, attention should be directed toward support of blood pressure and renal perfusion. Exchange transfusion or dialysis may be required as a means of reversing hypotension and/or substituting for disordered renal function. While captopril may be removed from the adult circulation by hemodialysis, there is inadequate data concerning the effectiveness of hemodialysis for removing it from the circulation of neonates or children. Peritoneal dialysis is not effective for removing captopril; there is no information concerning exchange transfusion for removing captopril from the general circulation.
When captopril was given to rabbits at doses about 0.8 to 70 times (on a mg/kg basis) the maximum recommended human dose, low incidences of craniofacial malformations were seen. No teratogenic effects of captopril were seen in studies of pregnant rats and hamsters. On a mg/kg basis, the doses used were up to 150 times (in hamsters) and 625 times (in rats) the maximum recommended human dose.

Hepatic Failure
Rarely, ACE inhibitors have been associated with a syndrome that starts with cholestatic jaundice and progresses to fulminant hepatic necrosis and (sometimes) death. The mechanism of this syndrome is not understood. Patients receiving ACE inhibitors who develop jaundice or marked elevations of hepatic enzymes should discontinue the ACE inhibitor and receive appropriate medical follow-up.

Hydrochlorothiazide
Thiazides should be used with caution in severe renal disease. In patients with renal disease, thiazides may precipitate azotemia. Cumulative effects of the drug may develop in patients with impaired renal function.
Thiazides should be used with caution in patients with impaired hepatic function or progressive liver disease, since minor alterations of fluid and electrolyte balance may precipitate hepatic coma.
Sensitivity reactions may occur in patients with or without a history of allergy or bronchial asthma.
The possibility of exacerbation or activation of systemic lupus erythematosus has been reported.
In general, lithium should not be given with diuretics (see PRECAUTIONS: Drug Interactions, Hydrochlorothiazide).

PRECAUTIONS

General
Captopril
Impaired Renal Function—Some patients with renal disease, particularly those with severe renal artery stenosis, have developed increases in BUN and serum creatinine after reduction of blood pressure with captopril. Captopril dosage reduction and/or discontinuation of diuretic may be required. For some of these patients, it may not be possible to normalize blood pressure and maintain adequate renal perfusion (see CLINICAL PHARMACOLOGY, DOSAGE AND ADMINISTRATION, ADVERSE REACTIONS: Altered Laboratory Findings).
Hyperkalemia—Elevations in serum potassium have been observed in some patients treated with ACE inhibitors, including captopril. When treated with ACE inhibitors, patients at risk for the development of hyperkalemia include those with: renal insufficiency; diabetes mellitus; and those using concomitant potassium-sparing diuretics, potassium supplements or potassium-containing salt substitutes; or other drugs associated with increases in serum potassium. (See PRECAUTIONS: Information for Patients and Drug Interactions, Captopril; ADVERSE REACTIONS: Altered Laboratory Findings.)
Cough: Presumably due to the inhibition of the degradation of endogenous bradykinin, persistent nonproductive cough has been reported with all ACE inhibitors, always resolving after discontinuation of therapy. ACE inhibitor-induced cough should be considered in the differential diagnosis of cough.
Surgery/Anesthesia—In patients undergoing major surgery or during anesthesia with agents that produce hypotension, captopril will block angiotensin II formation secondary to compensatory renin release. If hypotension occurs and is considered to be due to this mechanism, it can be corrected by volume expansion.

Hemodialysis
Recent clinical observations have shown an association of hypersensitivity-like (anaphylactoid) reactions during hemodialysis with high-flux dialysis membranes (e.g. AN69) in patients receiving ACE inhibitors as medication. In these patients, consideration should be given to using a different type of dialysis membrane or a different class of medication. (See WARNINGS: Captopril: Anaphylactoid reactions during membrane exposure.)

Hydrochlorothiazide
Periodic determination of serum electrolytes to detect possible electrolyte imbalance should be performed at appropriate intervals.
All patients receiving thiazide therapy should be observed for clinical signs of fluid or electrolyte imbalance, namely: hyponatremia, hypochloremic alkalosis, and hypokalemia. Serum and urine electrolyte determinations are particularly important when the patient is vomiting excessively or receiving parenteral fluids. Warning signs or symptoms of fluid and electrolyte imbalance may include: dryness of mouth, thirst, weakness, lethargy, drowsiness, restlessness, muscle pains or cramps, muscular fatigue, hypotension, oliguria, tachycardia, and gastrointestinal disturbances such as nausea and vomiting.
Hypokalemia may develop, especially with brisk diuresis, or when severe cirrhosis is present. Interference with adequate oral electrolyte intake will also contribute to hypokalemia. Hypokalemia can sensitize or exaggerate the response of the heart to the toxic effects of digitalis (e.g., increased ventricular irritability). Because captopril reduces the production of aldosterone, concomitant therapy with captopril reduces the diuretic-induced hypokalemia. Fewer patients may require potassium supplements and/or foods with a high potassium content (see Drug Interactions, Agents Increasing Serum Potassium).
Any chloride deficit is generally mild and usually does not require specific treatment except under extraordinary circumstances (as in liver disease or renal disease). Dilutional hyponatremia may occur in edematous patients in hot weather; appropriate therapy is water restriction, rather than administration of salt except in rare instances when the hyponatremia is life-threatening. In actual salt depletion, appropriate replacement is the therapy of choice.
Hyperuricemia may occur or frank gout may be precipitated in certain patients receiving thiazide therapy.
Latent diabetes mellitus may become manifest during thiazide administration.
The antihypertensive effect of thiazide diuretics may be enhanced in the postsympathectomy patient.
If progressive renal impairment becomes evident, as indicated by a rising nonprotein nitrogen or blood urea nitrogen (BUN), a careful reappraisal of therapy is necessary with consideration given to withholding or discontinuing diuretic therapy.
Thiazides may decrease serum PBI levels without signs of thyroid disturbance.

Continued on next page

Bristol-Myers Squibb Co.—Cont.

Calcium excretion is decreased by thiazides. Pathological changes in the parathyroid gland with hypercalcemia and hypophosphatemia have been observed in a few patients on prolonged thiazide therapy. The common complications of hyperparathyroidism such as renal lithiasis, bone resorption, and peptic ulceration have not been seen. Thiazides should be discontinued before carrying out tests for parathyroid function.

Thiazides have been shown to increase the urinary excretion of magnesium; this may result in hypomagnesemia.

Information for Patients

Patients should be advised to immediately report to their physician any signs or symptoms suggesting angioedema (e.g., swelling of face, eyes, lips, tongue, larynx and extremities; difficulty in swallowing or breathing; hoarseness) and to discontinue therapy. (See WARNINGS: Captopril: Angioedema.)

Patients should be told to report promptly any indication of infection (e.g., sore throat, fever), which may be a sign of neutropenia, or of progressive edema which might be related to proteinuria and nephrotic syndrome.

All patients should be cautioned that excessive perspiration and dehydration may lead to an excessive fall in blood pressure because of reduction in fluid volume. Other causes of volume depletion such as vomiting or diarrhea may also lead to a fall in blood pressure; patients should be advised to consult with the physician.

Patients should be advised not to use potassium-sparing diuretics, potassium supplements or potassium-containing salt substitutes without consulting their physician. (See PRECAUTIONS: General and Drug Interactions, Captopril; ADVERSE REACTIONS: Captopril.)

Patients should be warned against interruption or discontinuation of medication unless instructed by the physician.

Heart failure patients on captopril therapy should be cautioned against rapid increases in physical activity.

Patients should be informed that CAPOZIDE (Captopril-Hydrochlorothiazide Tablets) should be taken one hour before meals (see DOSAGE AND ADMINISTRATION).

Pregnancy. Female patients of childbearing age should be told about the consequences of second- and third-trimester exposure to ACE inhibitors, and they should also be told that these consequences do not appear to have resulted from intrauterine Ace-inhibitor exposure that has been limited to the first trimester. These patients should be asked to report pregnancies to their physicians as soon as possible.

Laboratory Tests

Serum electrolyte levels should be regularly monitored (see WARNINGS: Captopril and Hydrochlorothiazide; PRECAUTIONS: General, Hydrochlorothiazide).

Drug Interactions

Captopril

Hypotension—Patients on Diuretic Therapy: Patients on diuretics and especially those in whom diuretic therapy was recently instituted, as well as those on severe dietary salt restrictions or dialysis, may occasionally experience a precipitous reduction of blood pressure usually within the first hour after receiving the initial dose of captopril.

The possibility of hypotensive effects with captopril can be minimized by either discontinuing the diuretic or increasing the salt intake approximately one week prior to initiation of treatment with captopril or initiating therapy with small doses (6.25 or 12.5 mg). Alternatively, provide medical supervision for at least one hour after the initial dose. If hypotension occurs, the patient should be placed in a supine position and, if necessary, receive an intravenous infusion of normal saline. This transient hypotensive response is not a contraindication to further doses which can be given without difficulty once the blood pressure has increased after volume expansion.

Agents Having Vasodilator Activity: Data on the effect of concomitant use of other vasodilators in patients receiving captopril for heart failure are not available; therefore, nitroglycerin or other nitrates (as used for management of angina) or other drugs having vasodilator activity should, if possible, be discontinued before starting captopril. If resumed during captopril therapy, such agents should be administered cautiously, and perhaps at lower dosage.

Agents Causing Renin Release: Captopril's effect will be augmented by antihypertensive agents that cause renin release. For example, diuretics (e.g., thiazides) may activate the renin-angiotensin-aldosterone system.

Agents Affecting Sympathetic Activity: The sympathetic nervous system may be especially important in supporting blood pressure in patients receiving captopril alone or with diuretics. Therefore, agents affecting sympathetic activity (e.g., ganglionic blocking agents or adrenergic neuron blocking agents) should be used with caution. Beta-adrenergic blocking drugs add some further antihypertensive effect to captopril, but the overall response is less than additive.

Agents Increasing Serum Potassium: Since captopril decreases aldosterone production, elevation of serum potassium may occur. Potassium-sparing diuretics such as spironolactone, triamterene, or amiloride, or potassium supplements, should be given only for documented hypokalemia, and then with caution, since they may lead to a significant increase of serum potassium. Salt substitutes containing potassium should also be used with caution.

Inhibitors Of Endogenous Prostaglandin Synthesis: It has been reported that indomethacin may reduce the antihypertensive effect of captopril, especially in cases of low renin hypertension. Other nonsteroidal anti-inflammatory agents (e.g., aspirin) may also have this effect.

Lithium: Increased serum lithium levels and symptoms of lithium toxicity have been reported in patients receiving concomitant lithium and ACE inhibitor therapy. These drugs should be coadministered with caution and frequent monitoring of serum lithium levels is recommended. If a diuretic is also used, it may increase the risk of lithium toxicity (see PRECAUTIONS: Drug Interactions, Hydrochlorothiazide, Lithium).

Hydrochlorothiazide

When administered concurrently the following drugs may interact with thiazide diuretics:

Alcohol, barbiturates, or narcotics—potentiation of orthostatic hypotension may occur.

Amphotericin B, corticosteroids, or corticotropin (ACTH)—may intensify electrolyte imbalance, particularly hypokalemia. Monitor potassium levels; use potassium replacements if necessary.

Anticoagulants (oral)—dosage adjustments of anticoagulant medication may be necessary since hydrochlorothiazide may decrease their effects.

Antigout medications—dosage adjustments of antigout medication may be necessary since hydrochlorothiazide may raise the level of blood uric acid.

Other antihypertensive medications (e.g., ganglionic or peripheral adrenergic blocking agents)—dosage adjustments may be necessary since hydrochlorothiazide may potentiate their effects.

Antidiabetic drugs (oral agents and insulin)—since thiazides may elevate blood glucose levels, dosage adjustments of antidiabetic agents may be necessary.

Calcium salts—Increased serum calcium levels due to decreased excretion may occur. If calcium must be prescribed monitor serum calcium levels and adjust calcium dosage accordingly.

Cardiac glycosides—enhanced possibility of digitalis toxicity associated with hypokalemia. Monitor potassium levels (see PRECAUTIONS: Drug Interactions, Captopril).

Cholestyramine resin and colestipol HCL—may delay or decrease absorption of hydrochlorothiazide. Sulfonamide diuretics should be taken at least one hour before or four to six hours after these medications.

Diazoxide—enhanced hyperglycemic, hyperuricemic, and antihypertensive effects. Be cognizant of possible interaction; monitor blood glucose and serum uric acid levels.

Lithium—diuretic agents reduce the renal clearance of lithium and increase the risk of lithium toxicity. These drugs should be coadministered with caution and frequent monitoring of serum lithium levels is recommended (see PRECAUTIONS: Drug Interactions, Captopril, Lithium).

MAO inhibitors—dosage adjustments of one or both agents may be necessary since hypotensive effects are enhanced.

Nondepolarizing muscle relaxants, preanesthetics and anesthetics used in surgery (e.g., tubocurarine chloride and gallamine triethiodide)—effects of these agents may be potentiated; dosage adjustments may be required. Monitor and correct any fluid and electrolyte imbalances prior to surgery if feasible.

Nonsteroidal anti-inflammatory agents—in some patients, the administration of a nonsteroidal anti-inflammatory agent can reduce the diuretic, natriuretic, and antihypertensive effect of loop, potassium-sparing or thiazide diuretics. Therefore, when hydrochlorothiazide and nonsteroidal anti-inflammatory agents are used concomitantly, the patient should be observed closely to determine if the desired effect of the diuretic is obtained.

Methenamine—possible decreased effectiveness due to alkalinization of the urine.

Pressor amines (e.g., norepinephrine)—decreased arterial responsiveness, but not sufficient to preclude effectiveness of the pressor agent for therapeutic use. Use caution in patients taking both medications who undergo surgery. Administer preanesthetic and anesthetic agents in reduced dosage, and if possible, discontinue hydrochlorothiazide therapy one week prior to surgery.

Probenecid or sulfinpyrazone—increased dosage of these agents may be necessary since hydrochlorothiazide may have hyperuricemic effects.

Drug/Laboratory Test Interactions

Captopril

Captopril may cause a false-positive urine test for acetone.

Hydrochlorothiazide

Hydrochlorothiazide may cause diagnostic interference of the bentiromide test.

Carcinogenesis, Mutagenesis, Impairment of Fertility

Captopril

Two-year studies with doses of 50 to 1350 mg/kg/day in mice and rats failed to show any evidence of carcinogenic potential.

Studies in rats have revealed no impairment of fertility.

Hydrochlorothiazide

Two-year feeding studies in mice and rats conducted under the auspices of the National Toxicology Program (NTP) uncovered no evidence of a carcinogenic potential of hydrochlorothiazide in female mice (at doses of up to approximately 600 mg/kg/day) or in male and female rats (at doses of up to approximately 100 mg/kg/day). The NPT, however, found equivocal evidence for hepatocarcinogenicity in male mice.

Hydrochlorothiazide was not genotoxic in *in vitro* assays using strains TA 98, TA 100, TA 1535, TA 1537, and TA 1538 of Salmonella typhimurium (Ames assay) and in the Chinese Hamster Ovary (CHO) test for chromosomal aberrations, or in *in vivo assays using mouse germinal cell chromosomes, Chinese hamster bone marrow chromosomes, and the Drosophila* sex linked recessive lethal trait gene. Positive test results were obtained only in the *in vitro* CHO Sister Chromatid Exchange (elastogenicity) and in the Mouse Lymphoma Cell (mutagenicity) assays, using concentrations of hydrochlorothiazide from 43 to 1330 µg/mL, and in the *Aspergillus nidulans* non-disjunction assay at an unspecified concentration.

Hydrochlorothiazide has no adverse effects on the fertility of mice and rats of either sex in studies wherein these species were exposed, via their diet, to doses of up to 100 and 4 mg/kg, respectively, prior to conception and throughout gestation.

Animal Toxicology: Captopril

Chronic oral toxicity studies were conducted in rats (2 years), dogs (47 weeks; 1 year), mice (2 years), and monkeys (1 year). Significant drug-related toxicity included effects on hematopoiesis, renal toxicity, erosion/ulceration of the stomach, and variation of retinal blood vessels.

Reductions in hemoglobin and/or hematocrit values were seen in mice, rats, and monkeys at doses 50 to 150 times the maximum recommended human dose (MRHD). Anemia, leukopenia, thrombocytopenia, and bone marrow suppression occurred in dogs at doses 8 to 30 times MRHD. The reductions in hemoglobin and hematocrit values in rats and mice were only significant at 1 year and returned to normal with continued dosing by the end of the study. Marked anemia was seen at all dose levels (8 to 30 times MRHD) in dogs, whereas moderate to marked leukopenia was noted only at 15 and 30 times MRHD and thrombocytopenia at 30 times MRHD. The anemia could be reversed upon discontinuation of dosing. Bone marrow suppression occurred to a varying degree, being associated only with dogs that died or were sacrificed in a moribund condition in the 1 year study. However, in the 47-week study at a dose 30 times MRHD, bone marrow suppression was found to be reversible upon continued drug administration.

Captopril caused hyperplasia of the juxtaglomerular apparatus of the kidneys at doses 7 to 200 times the MRHD in rats and mice, at 20 to 60 times MRHD in monkeys, and at 30 times the MRHD in dogs.

Gastric erosions/ulcerations were increased in incidence at 20 and 200 times MRHD in male rats and at 30 and 65 times MRHD in dogs and monkeys, respectively. Rabbits developed gastric and intestinal ulcers when given oral doses approximately 30 times MRHD for only five to seven days.

In the two-year rat study, irreversible and progressive variations in the caliber of retinal vessels (focal sacculations and constrictions) occurred at all dose levels (7 to 200 times MRHD) in a dose-related fashion. The effect was first observed in the 88th week of dosing, with a progressively increased incidence thereafter, even after cessation of dosing.

Pregnancy Categories C (first trimester) and D (second and third trimesters)

See WARNINGS: Captopril, Fetal/Neonatal Morbidity and Mortality.

Pregnancy—Nonteratogenic Effects

Hydrochlorothiazide

Thiazides cross the placental barrier and appear in cord blood. The use of thiazides in pregnant women requires that the anticipated benefit be weighed against possible hazards to the fetus. These hazards include fetal or neonatal jaundice, thrombocytopenia, and possibly other adverse reactions which have occurred in the adult.

Nursing Mothers

Both captopril and hydrochlorothiazide are excreted in human milk. Because of the potential for serious adverse reactions in nursing infants from both drugs, a decision should be made whether to discontinue nursing or to discontinue therapy taking into account the importance of CAPOZIDE (Captopril-Hydrochlorothiazide Tablets) to the mother. (See PRECAUTIONS: Pediatric Use.)

Pediatric Use
Safety and effectiveness in children have not been established. There is limited experience reported in the literature with the use of captopril in the pediatric population; dosage, on a weight basis, was generally reported to be comparable to or less than that used in adults.
Infants, especially newborns, may be more susceptible to the adverse hemodynamic effects of captopril. Excessive, prolonged and unpredictable decreases in blood pressure and associated complications, including oliguria and seizures, have been reported.
CAPOZIDE (Captopril-Hydrochlorothiazide Tablets) should be used in children only if other measures for controlling blood pressure have not been effective.

ADVERSE REACTIONS

Captopril
Reported incidences are based on clinical trials involving approximately 7000 patients.
Renal: About one of 100 patients developed proteinuria (see WARNINGS).
Each of the following has been reported in approximately 1 to 2 of 1000 patients and are of uncertain relationship to drug use: renal insufficiency, renal failure, nephrotic syndrome, polyuria, oliguria, and urinary frequency.
Hematologic: Neutropenia/agranulocytosis has occurred (see WARNINGS). Cases of anemia, thrombocytopenia, and pancytopenia have been reported.
Dermatologic: Rash, often with pruritus, and sometimes with fever, arthralgia, and eosinophilia, occurred in about 4 to 7 (depending on renal status and dose) of 100 patients, usually during the first four weeks of therapy. It is usually maculopapular, and rarely urticarial. The rash is usually mild and disappears within a few days of dosage reduction, short-term treatment with an antihistaminic agent, and/or discontinuing therapy; remission may occur even if captopril is continued. Pruritus, without rash, occurs in about 2 of 100 patients. Between 7 and 10 percent of patients with skin rash have shown eosinophilia and/or positive ANA titers. A reversible associated pemphigoid-like lesion, and photosensitivity, have also been reported.
Flushing or pallor has been reported in 2 to 5 of 1000 patients.
Cardiovascular: Hypotension may occur; see WARNINGS and PRECAUTIONS (Drug Interactions) for discussion of hypotension with captopril therapy.
Tachycardia, chest pain, and palpitations have each been observed in approximately 1 of 100 patients.
Angina pectoris, myocardial infarction, Raynaud's syndrome, and congestive heart failure have each occurred in 2 to 3 of 1000 patients.
Dysgeusia: Approximately 2 to 4 (depending on renal status and dose) of 100 patients developed a diminution or loss of taste perception. Taste impairment is reversible and usually self-limited (2 to 3 months) even with continued drug administration. Weight loss may be associated with the loss of taste.
Angioedema: Angioedema involving the extremities, face, lips, mucous membranes, tongue, glottis or larynx has been reported in approximately one in 1000 patients. Angioedema involving the upper airways has caused fatal airway obstruction. (See WARNINGS: Captopril: Angioedema and PRECAUTIONS: Information for Patients.)
Cough: Cough has been reported in 0.5–2% of patients treated with captopril in clinical trials (see PRECAUTIONS: General, Captopril, Cough).
The following have been reported in about 0.5 to 2 percent of patients but did not appear at increased frequency compared to placebo or other treatments used in controlled trials: gastric irritation, abdominal pain, nausea, vomiting, diarrhea, anorexia, constipation, aphthous ulcers, peptic ulcer, dizziness, headache, malaise, fatigue, insomnia, dry mouth, dyspnea, alopecia, paresthesias.
Other clinical adverse effects reported since the drug was marketed are listed below by body system. In this setting, an incidence or causal relationship cannot be accurately determined.
Body as a Whole: Anaphylactoid reactions (see WARNINGS: Captopril: Anaphylactoid and possibly related reactions and PRECAUTIONS: Hemodialysis).
General: asthenia, gynecomastia.
Cardiovascular: cardiac arrest, cerebrovascular accident/insufficiency, rhythm disturbances, orthostatic hypotension, syncope.
Dermatologic: bullous pemphigus, erythema multiforme (including Stevens-Johnson syndrome), exfoliative dermatitis.
Gastrointestinal: pancreatitis, glossitis, dyspepsia.
Hematologic: anemia, including aplastic and hemolytic.
Hepatobiliary: jaundice, hepatitis, including rare cases of necrosis, cholestasis.
Metabolic: symptomatic hyponatremia.
Musculoskeletal: myalgia, myasthenia.
Nervous/Psychiatric: ataxia, confusion, depression, nervousness, somnolence.
Respiratory: bronchospasm, eosinophilic pneumonitis, rhinitis.
Special Senses: blurred vision.
Urogenital: impotence.
As with other ACE inhibitors, a syndrome has been reported which may include: fever, myalgia, arthralgia, interstitial nephritis, vasculitis, rash or other dermatologic manifestations, eosinophilia and an elevated ESR.

Fetal/Neonatal Morbidity and Mortality
See WARNINGS: Captopril, Fetal/Neonatal Morbidity and Mortality.

Hydrochlorothiazide
Gastrointestinal System: anorexia, gastric irritation, nausea, vomiting, cramping, diarrhea, constipation, jaundice (intrahepatic cholestatic jaundice), pancreatitis, and sialadenitis.
Central Nervous System: dizziness, vertigo, paresthesias, headache, and xanthopsia.
Hematologic: leukopenia, agranulocytosis, thrombocytopenia, aplastic anemia, and hemolytic anemia.
Cardiovascular: orthostatic hypotension.
Hypersensitivity: purpura, photosensitivity, rash, urticaria, necrotizing angiitis (vasculitis; cutaneous vasculitis), fever, respiratory distress including pneumonitis, and anaphylactic reactions.
Other: hyperglycemia, glycosuria, hyperuricemia, muscle spasm, weakness, restlessness, and transient blurred vision.
Whenever adverse reactions are moderate or severe, thiazide dosage should be reduced or therapy withdrawn.

Altered Laboratory Findings
Serum Electrolytes: Hyperkalemia: small increases in serum potassium, especially in patients with renal impairment (see PRECAUTIONS: Captopril).
Hyponatremia: particularly in patients receiving a low sodium diet or concomitant diuretics.
BUN/Serum Creatinine: Transient elevations of BUN or serum creatinine especially in volume or salt depleted patients or those with renovascular hypertension may occur. Rapid reduction of longstanding or markedly elevated blood pressure can result in decreases in the glomerular filtration rate and, in turn, lead to increases in BUN or serum creatinine.
Hematologic: A positive ANA has been reported.
Liver Function Tests: Elevations of liver transaminases, alkaline phosphatase, and serum bilirubin have occurred.

OVERDOSAGE

Captopril
Correction of hypotension would be of primary concern. Volume expansion with an intravenous infusion of normal saline is the treatment of choice for restoration of blood pressure.
While captopril may be removed from the adult circulation by hemodialysis, there is inadequate data concerning the effectiveness of hemodialysis for removing it from the circulation of neonates or children. Peritoneal dialysis is not effective for removing captopril; there is no information concerning exchange transfusion for removing captopril from the general circulation.

Hydrochlorothiazide
In addition to the expected diuresis, overdosage of thiazides may produce varying degrees of lethargy which may progress to coma within a few hours, with minimal depression of respiration and cardiovascular function and without evidence of serum electrolyte changes or dehydration. The mechanism of thiazide-induced CNS depression is unknown. Gastrointestinal irritation and hypermotility may occur. Transitory increase in BUN has been reported, and serum electrolyte changes may occur, especially in patients with impaired renal function.
In addition to gastric lavage and supportive therapy for stupor or coma, symptomatic treatment of gastrointestinal effects may be needed. The degree to which hydrochlorothiazide is removed by hemodialysis has not been clearly established. Measures as required to maintain hydration, electrolyte balance, respiration, and cardiovascular and renal function should be instituted.

DOSAGE AND ADMINISTRATION

DOSAGE MUST BE INDIVIDUALIZED ACCORDING TO PATIENT'S RESPONSE.
CAPOZIDE may be substituted for the previously titrated individual components.
Alternatively, therapy may be instituted with a single tablet of CAPOZIDE 25 mg/15 mg taken once daily. For patients insufficiently responsive to the initial dose, additional captopril or hydrochlorothiazide may be added as individual components or by using CAPOZIDE 50 mg/15 mg, 25 mg/25 mg or 50 mg/25 mg, or divided doses may be used.
Because the full effect of a given dose may not be attained for 6–8 weeks, dosage adjustments should generally be made at 6 week intervals, unless the clinical situation demands more rapid adjustment.
In general, daily doses of captopril should not exceed 150 mg and of hydrochlorothiazide should not exceed 50 mg.
CAPOZIDE should be taken one hour before meals.
Dosage Adjustment in Renal Impairment—Because captopril and hydrochlorothiazide are excreted primarily by the kidneys, excretion rates are reduced in patients with impaired renal function. These patients will take longer to reach steady-state captopril levels and will reach higher steady-state levels for a given daily dose than patients with normal renal function. Therefore, these patients may respond to smaller or less frequent doses of CAPOZIDE.
After the desired therapeutic effect has been achieved, the dose intervals should be increased or the total daily dose reduced until the minimal effective dose is achieved. When concomitant diuretic therapy is required in patients with severe renal impairment, a loop diuretic (e.g., furosemide), rather than a thiazide diuretic is preferred for use with captopril; therefore, for patients with severe renal dysfunction the captopril-hydrochlorothiazide combination tablet is not usually recommended. (See WARNINGS: Captopril: Anaphylactoid reactions during membrane exposure and PRECAUTIONS: Hemodialysis.)

HOW SUPPLIED

CAPOZIDE (Captopril-Hydrochlorothiazide Tablets)
25 mg captopril combined with 15 mg hydrochlorothiazide in bottles of 100 (NDC 0003-0338-50). Tablets are white with distinct orange mottling; they are biconvex rounded squares with quadrisect bars.
25 mg captopril combined with 25 mg hydrochlorothiazide in bottles of 100 (NDC 0003-0349-50). Tablets are peach-colored and may show slight mottling; they are biconvex rounded squares with quadrisect bars.
50 mg captopril combined with 15 mg hydrochlorothiazide in bottles of 100 (NDC 0003-0384-50). Tablets are white with distinct orange mottling; they are biconvex ovals with a bisect bar.
50 mg captopril combined with 25 mg hydrochlorothiazide in bottles of 100 (NDC 0003-0390-50). Tablets are peach-colored and may show slight mottling; they are biconvex ovals with a bisect bar.

STORAGE

Keep bottles tightly closed (protect from moisture); do not store above 86°F.

(5140 DIM-03)

Shown in Product Identification Guide, page 307

CEFZIL® ℞
(CEFPROZIL)
Tablets—250 mg and 500 mg
Oral Suspension—125 mg/5 mL and 250 mg/5 mL

DESCRIPTION

CEFZIL® (cefprozil) is a semi-synthetic broad-spectrum cephalosporin antibiotic.
Cefprozil is a cis and trans isomeric mixture (≥ 90% cis). The chemical name for the monohydrate is (6R, 7R)-7-[(R)-2-amino-2-(p-hydroxy-phenyl)acetamido]-8-oxo-3-propenyl-5-thia- 1-azabicyclo [4.2.0]oct-2-ene-2- carboxylic acid monohydrate, and the structural formula is:

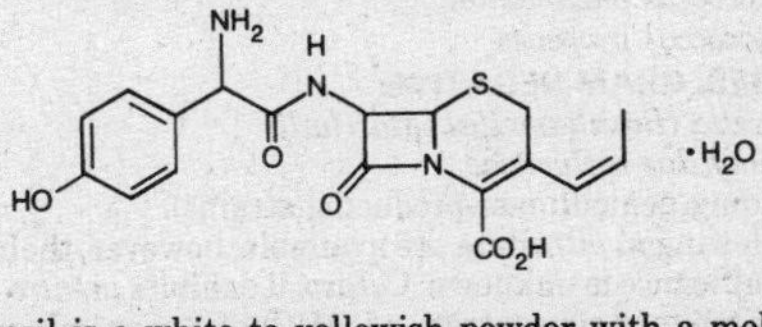

Cefprozil is a white to yellowish powder with a molecular formula for the monohydrate of $C_{18}H_{19}N_3O_5S \cdot H_20$ and a molecular weight of 407.45.
CEFZIL tablets and CEFZIL for oral suspension are intended for oral administration.
CEFZIL tablets contain cefprozil equivalent to 250 mg or 500 mg of anhydrous cefprozil. In addition, each tablet contains the following inactive ingredients: cellulose, hydroxypropyl-methylcellulose, magnesium stearate, methylcellulose, simethicone, sodium starch glycolate, polyethylene glycol, polysorbate 80, sorbic acid, and titanium dioxide. The 250 mg tablets also contain FD&C Yellow No. 6.
CEFZIL for oral suspension contains cefprozil equivalent to 125 mg or 250 mg anhydrous cefprozil per 5 mL constituted suspension. In addition, the oral suspension contains the following inactive ingredients: aspartame, cellulose, citric acid, colloidal silicone dioxide, FD&C Red No. 3, flavors (natural and artificial), glycine, polysorbate 80, simethicone, sodium benzoate, sodium carboxymethylcellulose, sodium chloride, and sucrose.

CLINICAL PHARMACOLOGY

Following oral administration of cefprozil to fasting subjects, approximately 95% of the dose was absorbed. Using the investigational capsule formulation, no food effect was ob-

Continued on next page

Bristol-Myers Squibb Co.—Cont.

served. The food effect on the tablet and on the suspension formulations has not been studied.

The pharmacokinetic data were derived from the capsule dosing; however, bioequivalence has been demonstrated for the oral solution, capsule, tablet, and suspension formulations under fasting conditions.

Average peak plasma concentrations after administration of 250 mg, 500 mg, or 1 g doses of cefprozil to fasting subjects were approximately 6.1, 10.5, and 18.3 mcg/mL respectively, and were obtained within 1.5 hours after dosing. Urinary recovery accounted for approximately 60% of the administered dose.

[See table below.]

During the first 4-hour period after drug administration, the average urine concentrations following the 250 mg, 500 mg, and 1 g doses were approximately 700 mcg/mL, 1000 mcg/mL, and 2900 mcg/mL.

Plasma protein binding is approximately 36% and is independent of concentration in the range of 2 mcg/mL to 20 mcg/mL.

The average plasma half-life in normal subjects is 1.3 hours. There was no evidence of accumulation of cefprozil in the plasma in individuals with normal renal function following multiple oral doses of up to 1000 mg every 8 hours for 10 days.

In patients with reduced renal function, the plasma half-life may be prolonged up to 5.2 hours depending on the degree of the renal dysfunction. In patients with complete absence of renal function the plasma half-life of cefprozil has been shown to be as long as 5.9 hours. The half-life is shortened during hemodialysis. Excretion pathways in patients with markedly impaired renal function have not been determined. (See PRECAUTIONS and DOSAGE AND ADMINISTRATION.)

The average AUC observed in elderly subjects (≥ 65 years of age) is approximately 35%–60% higher relative to young adults, and the average AUC in females is approximately 15%–20% higher than in males. The magnitude of these age and gender-related changes in the pharmacokinetics of cefprozil are not sufficient to necessitate dosage adjustments.

In patients with impaired hepatic function, the half-life increases to approximately 2 hours. The magnitude of the changes does not warrant a dosage adjustment for patients with impaired hepatic function.

Adequate data on CSF levels of cefprozil are not available.

MICROBIOLOGY

Cefprozil has *in vitro* activity against a broad range of gram-positive and gram-negative bacteria. The bactericidal action of cefprozil results from inhibition of cell-wall synthesis. Cefprozil has been shown to be active against most strains of the following organisms both *in vitro* and in clinical infections. (See INDICATIONS AND USAGE.)

AEROBES, GRAM-POSITIVE:

Staphylococcus aureus
(including penicillinase-producing strains)
NOTE: Cefprozil is inactive against methicillin-resistant staphylococci.
Streptococcus pneumoniae
Streptococcus pyogenes

AEROBES, GRAM-NEGATIVE:

Moraxella (Branhamella) catarrhalis
Haemophilus influenzae
(including penicillinase-producing strains)

The following *in vitro* data are available; however, their clinical significance is unknown. Cefprozil exhibits *in vitro* minimum inhibitory concentrations (MIC) of 8 mcg/mL or less against most strains of the following organisms. The safety and efficacy of cefprozil in treating infections due to these organisms have not been established in adequate and well-controlled trials.

AEROBES, GRAM-POSITIVE:

Enterococcus durans
Enterococcus faecalis
NOTE: Cefprozil is inactive against *Enterococcus faecium.*
Listeria monocytogenes
Staphylococcus epidermidis
Staphylococcus saprophyticus
Staphylococcus warneri
Streptococcus agalactiae
Streptococci (Groups C, D, F, and G)
viridans group Streptococci

AEROBES, GRAM-NEGATIVE:

Citrobacter diversus
Escherichia coli
Klebsiella pneumoniae
Neisseria gonorrhoeae
(including penicillinase-producing strains)
Proteus mirabilis
Salmonella spp.
Shigella spp.
Vibrio spp.

NOTE: Cefprozil is inactive against most strains of *Acinetobacter, Enterobacter, Morganella morganii, Proteus vulgaris, Providencia, Pseudomonas, and Serratia.*

ANAEROBES:

Bacteroides melaninogenicus
NOTE: Most strains of the *Bacteroides fragilis* group are resistant to cefprozil.
Clostridium perfringens
Clostridium difficile
Fusobacterium spp.
Peptostreptococcus spp.
Propionibacterium acnes

SUSCEPTIBILITY TESTS

Diffusion Techniques

Quantitative methods that require measurement of zone diameters give the most precise estimate of the susceptibility of bacteria to antimicrobial agents. One such standardized procedure recommended for use with the 30-mcg cefprozil disk is the National Committee for Clinical Laboratory Standards (NCCLS) approved procedure.[1] Interpretation involves correlation of the diameter obtained in the disk test with minimum inhibitory concentration (MIC) for cefprozil.

The class disk for cephalosporin susceptibility testing (the cephalothin disk) is not appropriate because of spectrum differences with cefprozil. The 30-mcg cefprozil disk should be used for all *in vitro* testing of isolates.

Reports from the laboratory giving results of the standard single-disk susceptibility test with a 30-mcg cefprozil disk should be interpreted according to the following criteria:

Zone diameter (mm)	Interpretation
≥ 18	(S) Susceptible
15–17	(MS) Moderately Susceptible
≤ 14	(R) Resistant

A report of "Susceptible" indicates that the pathogen is likely to be inhibited by generally achievable blood concentrations. A report of "Moderately Susceptible" indicates that the organism would be susceptible if high dosage is used or if the infection is confined to tissues and fluids (e.g., urine) in which high antibiotic levels are attained. A report of "Resistant" indicates that the achievable concentration of the antibiotic is unlikely to be inhibitory and other therapy should be selected.

Standardized procedures require the use of laboratory control organisms. The 30-mcg cefprozil disk should give the following zone diameters:

Organism	Zone diameter (mm)
Escherichia coli ATCC 25922	21–27
Staphylococcus aureus ATCC 25923	27–33

Dilution Techniques

Use a standardized dilution method[2] (broth, agar, microdilution) or equivalent with cefprozil powder. The MIC values obtained should be interpreted according to the following criteria:

MIC (mcg/mL)	Interpretation
≤ 8	(S) Susceptible
16	(MS) Moderately Susceptible
≥ 32	(R) Resistant

As with standard diffusion techniques, dilution techniques require the use of laboratory control organisms. Standard cefprozil powder should give the following MIC values:

Organism	MIC (mcg/mL)
Enterococcus faecalis ATCC 29212	4–16
Escherichia coli ATCC 25922	1–4
Pseudomonas aeruginosa ATCC 27853	> 32
Staphylococcus aureus ATCC 29213	0.25–1

INDICATIONS AND USAGE

CEFZIL® (cefprozil) is indicated for the treatment of patients with mild to moderate infections caused by susceptible strains of the designated microorganisms in the conditions listed below:

UPPER RESPIRATORY TRACT

Pharyngitis/Tonsillitis caused by *Streptococcus pyogenes.*

NOTE: The usual drug of choice in the treatment and prevention of streptococcal infections, including the prophylaxis of rheumatic fever, is penicillin given by the intramuscular route. Cefprozil is generally effective in the eradication of *Streptococcus pyogenes* from the nasopharynx; however, substantial data establishing the efficacy of cefprozil in the subsequent prevention of rheumatic fever are not available at present.

Otitis Media caused by *Streptococcus pneumoniae, Haemophilus influenzae,* and *Moraxella (Branhamella) catarrhalis.* (See CLINICAL STUDIES section.)

NOTE: In the treatment of otitis media due to beta-lactamase producing organisms, cefprozil had bacteriologic eradication rates somewhat lower than those observed with a product containing a specific beta-lactamase inhibitor. In considering the use of cefprozil, lower overall eradication rates should be balanced against the susceptibility patterns of the common microbes in a given geographic area and the increased potential for toxicity with products containing beta-lactamase inhibitors.

LOWER RESPIRATORY TRACT

Secondary Bacterial Infection of Acute Bronchitis and Acute Bacterial Exacerbation of Chronic Bronchitis caused by *Streptococcus pneumoniae, Haemophilus influenzae* (beta-lactamase positive and negative strains), and *Moraxella (Branhamella) catarrhalis.*

SKIN AND SKIN STRUCTURE

Uncomplicated Skin and Skin-Structure Infections caused by *Staphylococcus aureus* (including penicillinase-producing strains) and *Streptococcus pyogenes.* Abscesses usually require surgical drainage.

Culture and susceptibility testing should be performed when appropriate to determine susceptibility of the causative organism to cefprozil.

CONTRAINDICATIONS

CEFZIL is contraindicated in patients with known allergy to the cephalosporin class of antibiotics.

WARNINGS

BEFORE THERAPY WITH CEFZIL IS INSTITUTED, CAREFUL INQUIRY SHOULD BE MADE TO DETERMINE WHETHER THE PATIENT HAS HAD PREVIOUS HYPERSENSITIVITY REACTIONS TO CEFZIL, CEPHALOSPORINS, PENICILLINS, OR OTHER DRUGS. IF THIS PRODUCT IS TO BE GIVEN TO PENICILLIN-SENSITIVE PATIENTS, CAUTION SHOULD BE EXERCISED BECAUSE CROSS-SENSITIVITY AMONG BETA-LACTAM ANTIBIOTICS HAS BEEN CLEARLY DOCUMENTED AND MAY OCCUR IN UP TO 10% OF PATIENTS WITH A HISTORY OF PENICILLIN ALLERGY. IF AN ALLERGIC REACTION TO CEFZIL OCCURS, DISCONTINUE THE DRUG. SERIOUS ACUTE HYPERSENSITIVITY REACTIONS MAY REQUIRE TREATMENT WITH EPINEPHRINE AND OTHER EMERGENCY MEASURES, INCLUDING OXYGEN, INTRAVENOUS FLUIDS, INTRAVENOUS ANTIHISTAMINES, CORTICOSTEROIDS, PRESSOR AMINES, AND AIRWAY MANAGEMENT, AS CLINICALLY INDICATED.

Pseudomembranous colitis has been reported with nearly all antibacterial agents, including cefprozil, and may range in severity from mild to life-threatening. Therefore, it is important to consider this diagnosis in patients who present with diarrhea subsequent to the administration of antibacterial agents.

Treatment with antibacterial agents alters the normal flora of the colon and may permit overgrowth of clostridia. Studies indicate that a toxin produced by *Clostridium difficile* is a primary cause of "antibiotic-associated colitis."

After the diagnosis of pseudomembranous colitis has been established, appropriate therapeutic measures should be initiated. Mild cases of pseudomembranous colitis usually respond to drug discontinuation alone. In moderate to severe cases, consideration should be given to management with fluids and electrolytes, protein supplementation and treatment with an antibacterial drug clinically effective against *Clostridium difficile* colitis.

PRECAUTIONS

General

Evaluation of renal status before and during therapy is recommended, especially in seriously ill patients. In patients with known or suspected renal impairment (see DOSAGE AND ADMINISTRATION), careful clinical observation and appropriate laboratory studies should be done prior to and during therapy. The total daily dose of CEFZIL® (cefprozil) should be reduced in these patients because high and/or prolonged plasma antibiotic concentrations can occur in such individuals from usual doses. Cephalosporins, including CEFZIL, should be given with caution to patients receiving concurrent treatment with potent diuretics since these agents are suspected of adversely affecting renal function.

Prolonged use of CEFZIL may result in the overgrowth of nonsusceptible organisms. Careful observation of the patient is essential. If superinfection occurs during therapy, appropriate measures should be taken.

Dosage (mg)	Mean Plasma Cefprozil* Concentrations (mcg/mL)			8-hour Urinary Excretion (%)
	Peak appx. 1.5 hr	4 hr	8 hr	
250 mg	6.1	1.7	0.2	60%
500 mg	10.5	3.2	0.4	62%
1000 mg	18.3	8.4	1.0	54%

*Data represent mean values of 12 healthy volunteers.

Cefprozil should be prescribed with caution in individuals with a history of gastrointestinal disease, particularly colitis. Positive direct Coombs' tests have been reported during treatment with cephalosporin antibiotics.

Information for Patients
Phenylketonurics: CEFZIL (cefprozil) for oral suspension contains phenylalanine 28 mg per 5 mL (1 teaspoonful) constituted suspension for both the 125 mg/5 mL and 250 mg/5 mL dosage forms.

Drug Interactions
Nephrotoxicity has been reported following concomitant administration of aminoglycoside antibiotics and cephalosporin antibiotics. Concomitant administration of probenecid doubled the AUC for cefprozil.

Drug/Laboratory Test Interactions
Cephalosporin antibiotics may produce a false-positive reaction for glucose in the urine with copper reduction tests (Benedict's or Fehling's solution or with Clinitest®[3] tablets), but not with enzyme-based tests for glycosuria (e.g., Tes-Tape®[4]). A false-negative reaction may occur in the ferricyanide test for blood glucose. The presence of cefprozil in the blood does not interfere with the assay of plasma or urine creatinine by the alkaline picrate method.

Carcinogenesis, Mutagenesis, and Impairment of Fertility
No mutagenic potential of cefprozil was found in appropriate prokaryotic or eukaryotic cells *in vitro* or *in vivo*. No *in vivo* long-term studies have been performed to evaluate carcinogenic potential.
Reproductive studies revealed no impairment of fertility in animals.

Pregnancy: Teratogenic Effects. Pregnancy Category B
Reproduction studies have been performed in mice, rats, and rabbits at doses 14, 7, and 0.7 times the maximum daily human dose (1000 mg) based upon mg/m², and have revealed no evidence of harm to the fetus due to cefprozil. There are, however, no adequate and well-controlled studies in pregnant women. Because animal reproduction studies are not always predictive of human response, this drug should be used during pregnancy only if clearly needed.

Labor and Delivery
Cefprozil has not been studied for use during labor and delivery. Treatment should only be given if clearly needed.

Nursing Mothers
It is not known whether cefprozil is excreted in human milk. Because many drugs are excreted in human milk, caution should be exercised when CEFZIL is administered to a nursing mother.

Pediatric Use
Safety and effectiveness in pediatric patients below the age of 6 months have not been established. However, accumulation of other cephalosporin antibiotics in newborn infants (resulting from prolonged drug half-life in this age group) has been reported.

Geriatric Use
Healthy geriatric volunteers (≥ 65 years old) who received a single 1 g dose of cefprozil had 35%–60% higher AUC and 40% lower renal clearance values when compared to healthy adult volunteers 20–40 years of age. In clinical studies, when geriatric patients received the usual recommended adult doses, clinical efficacy and safety were acceptable and comparable to results in non-geriatric adult patients.

ADVERSE REACTIONS
The adverse reactions to cefprozil are similar to those observed with other orally administered cephalosporins. Cefprozil was usually well tolerated in controlled clinical trials. Approximately 2% of patients discontinued cefprozil therapy due to adverse events.
The most common adverse effects observed in patients treated with cefprozil are:
Gastrointestinal—Diarrhea (2.9%), nausea (3.5%), vomiting (1%), and abdominal pain (1%).
Hepatobiliary—Elevations of AST (SGOT) (2%), ALT (SGPT) (2%), alkaline phosphatase (0.2%), and bilirubin values (< 0.1 %). As with some penicillins and some other cephalosporin antibiotics, cholestatic jaundice has been reported rarely.
Hypersensitivity—Rash (0.9%), urticaria (0.1%). Such reactions have been reported more frequently in children than in adults. Signs and symptoms usually occur a few days after initiation of therapy and subside within a few days after cessation of therapy.
CNS—Dizziness (1%). Hyperactivity, headache, nervousness, insomnia, confusion, and somnolence have been reported rarely (<1%). All were reversible.
Hematopoietic—Decreased leukocyte count (0.2%), eosinophilia (2.3%).
Renal—Elevated BUN (0.1%), serum creatinine (0.1%).
Other—Diaper rash and superinfection (1.5%), genital pruritus and vaginitis (1.6%).
The following adverse events, regardless of established causal relationship to CEFZIL, have been rarely reported during post-marketing surveillance: anaphylaxis, colitis (including pseudomembranous colitis), erythema multiforme, fever, serum-sickness like reactions, Stevens-Johnson Syndrome and thrombocytopenia.

Population/Infection	Dosage (mg)	Duration (days)
ADULTS (13 years and older)		
UPPER RESPIRATORY TRACT		
Pharyngitis/Tonsillitis	500 q 24h	10*
LOWER RESPIRATORY TRACT		
Secondary Bacterial Infection of Acute Bronchitis and Acute Bacterial Exacerbation of Chronic Bronchitis	500 q 12h	10
SKIN AND SKIN STRUCTURE		
Uncomplicated Skin and Skin Structure Infections	250 q 12h or 500 q 24h or 500 q 12h	10
CHILDREN (2 years–12 years)		
UPPER RESPIRATORY TRACT		
Pharyngitis/Tonsillitis	7.5 mg/kg q 12h	10*
SKIN AND SKIN STRUCTURE		
Uncomplicated Skin and Skin Structure Infections	20 mg/kg q 24h	10
INFANTS & CHILDREN (6 months–12 years)		
UPPER RESPIRATORY TRACT		
Otitis Media (See INDICATIONS AND USAGE and CLINICAL STUDIES sections)	15 mg/kg q 12h	10

*In the treatment of infections due to *Streptococcus pyogenes*, CEFZIL should be administered for at least 10 days.

Cephalosporin class paragraph
In addition to the adverse reactions listed above which have been observed in patients treated with cefprozil, the following adverse reactions and altered laboratory tests have been reported for cephalosporin-class antibiotics:
Aplastic anemia, hemolytic anemia, hemorrhage, renal dysfunction, toxic epidermal necrolysis, toxic nephropathy, prolonged prothrombin time, positive Coombs' test, elevated LDH, pancytopenia, neutropenia, agranulocytosis.
Several cephalosporins have been implicated in triggering seizures, particularly in patients with renal impairment, when the dosage was not reduced. (See DOSAGE AND ADMINISTRATION and OVERDOSAGE.) If seizures associated with drug therapy occur, the drug should be discontinued. Anticonvulsant therapy can be given if clinically indicated.

OVERDOSAGE
Cefprozil is eliminated primarily by the kidneys. In case of severe overdosage, especially in patients with compromised renal function, hemodialysis will aid in the removal of cefprozil from the body.

DOSAGE AND ADMINISTRATION
CEFZIL is administered orally.
[See table above.]
Renal Impairment
Cefprozil may be administered to patients with impaired renal function. The following dosage schedule should be used.

Creatinine Clearance (mL/min)	Dosage (mg)	Dosing Interval
30–120	standard	standard
0–29*	50% of standard	standard

*Cefprozil is in part removed by hemodialysis; therefore, cefprozil should be administered after the completion of hemodialysis.

Hepatic Impairment
No dosage adjustment is necessary for patients with impaired hepatic function.

HOW SUPPLIED
CEFZIL® (cefprozil) Tablets
Each light orange film-coated tablet, imprinted with "BMS 7720 250," contains the equivalent of 250 mg anhydrous cefprozil.
Bottles of 100 Tablets NDC 0087-7720-60
Cartons of 100 Tablets NDC 0087-7720-66
(10 strips containing 10 tablets on each strip)
Each white film-coated tablet, imprinted with "BMS 7721 500," contains the equivalent of 500 mg anhydrous cefprozil.
Bottles of 50 Tablets NDC 0087-7721-50
Bottles of 100 Tablets NDC 0087-7721-60
Cartons of 100 Tablets NDC 0087-7721-66
(10 strips containing 10 tablets on each strip)
Store at controlled room temperature, 59° to 86°F (15°C to 30°C).
CEFZIL® (cefprozil) For Oral Suspension
Each 5 mL of constituted suspension contains the equivalent of 125 mg anhydrous cefprozil.
50 mL Bottle NDC 0087-7718-40
75 mL Bottle NDC 0087-7718-62
100 mL Bottle NDC 0087 7718-64

Each 5 mL of constituted suspension contains the equivalent of 250 mg anhydrous cefprozil.
50 mL Bottle NDC 0087-7719-40
75 mL Bottle NDC 0087-7719-62
100 mL Bottle NDC 0087-7719-64
All powder formulations for oral suspension contain cefprozil in a bubble-gum flavored mixture. Directions for mixing are included on the label. After mixing, store in a refrigerator, and discard unused portion after 14 days.
Store at 59° to 77°F (15° to 25°C) prior to constitution.
U.S. Patent No. 4,520,022.

CLINICAL STUDIES
Study One:
In a controlled clinical study of **acute otitis media** performed in the United States where significant rates of beta-lactamase producing organisms were found, cefprozil was compared to an oral antimicrobial agent that contained a specific beta-lactamase inhibitor. In this study, using very strict evaluability criteria and microbiologic and clinical response criteria at the 10–16 days post-therapy follow-up, the following presumptive bacterial eradication/clinical cure outcomes (i.e., clinical success) and safety results were obtained:

U.S. Acute Otitis Media Study
Cefprozil vs. beta-lactamase inhibitor-containing control drug

Efficacy: Pathogen	% of Cases with Pathogen (n = 155)	Outcome
S. pneumoniae	48.4%	cefprozil success rate 5% better than control
H. influenzae	35.5%	cefprozil success rate 17% less than control
M. catarrhalis	13.5%	cefprozil success rate 12% less than control
S. pyogenes	2.6%	cefprozil equivalent to control
Overall	100.0%	cefprozil success rate 5% less than control

Safety:
The incidence of adverse events, primarily diarrhea and rash,* were clinically and statistically significantly higher in the control arm versus the cefprozil arm.

Age Group	Cefprozil	Control
6 months–2 years	21%	41%
3–12 years	10%	19%

*The majority of these involved the diaper area in young children.

Study Two:
In a controlled clinical study of **acute otitis media** performed in Europe, cefprozil was compared to an oral antimicrobial agent that contained a specific beta-lactamase inhibitor. As expected in a European population, this study population had a lower incidence of beta-lactamase-producing organisms than usually seen in U.S. trials. In this study, using very strict evaluability criteria and microbiologic and clinical response criteria at the 10-16 days post-therapy follow-up, the following presumptive bacterial eradication/clinical cure outcomes (i.e., clinical success) were obtained:

Continued on next page

Bristol-Myers Squibb Co.—Cont.

European Acute Otitis Media Study
Cefprozil vs. beta-lactamase
inhibitor-containing control drug

Efficacy: Pathogen	% of Cases with Pathogen (n=47)	Outcome
S. pneumoniae	51.0%	cefprozil equivalent to control
H. influenzae	29.8%	cefprozil equivalent to control
M. catarrhalis	6.4%	cefprozil equivalent to control
S. pyogenes	12.8%	cefprozil equivalent to control
Overall	100.0%	cefprozil equivalent to control

Safety:
The incidence of adverse events in the cefprozil arm was comparable to the incidence of adverse events in the control arm (agent that contained a specific beta-lactamase inhibitor).

REFERENCES

1. National Committee for Clinical Laboratory Standards. *Performance Standards for Antimicrobial Disk Susceptibility Tests–Fourth Edition,* Approved Standard NCCLS Document M2-A4, Vol. 10, No. 7, NCCLS, Villanova, Pa., April, 1990.
2. National Committee for Clinical Laboratory Standards. *Methods for Dilution Antimicrobial Susceptibility Tests for Bacteria that Grow Aerobically—Second Edition.* Approved Standard NCCLS Document M7-A2, Vol. 10, No. 8, NCCLS, Villanova, Pa., April, 1990.
3. Clinitest® is a registered trademark of Miles Laboratories, Inc.
4. Tes-Tape® is a registered trademark of Eli Lilly and Company.

Revised June 1995

7718DIM-06
E2-B001-6-95

Bristol-Myers Squibb Company
Shown in Product Identification Guide, page 307

DURICEF® ℞

[dur'ĭ-sef]
(cefadroxil monohydrate, USP)

500-mg capsules, 1-g tablets, oral suspensions

DESCRIPTION

DURICEF® (cefadroxil monohydrate, USP) is a semisynthetic cephalosporin antibiotic intended for oral administration. It is a white to yellowish-white crystalline powder. It is soluble in water and it is acid-stable. It is chemically designated as 5-Thia-1-azabicyclo[4.2.0]oct-2-ene-2-carboxylic acid, 7-[[amino(4-hydroxyphenyl)acetyl]amino]-3-methyl-8-oxo-, monohydrate, [6R-[6α,7β(R*)]]-. It has the formula $C_{16}H_{17}N_3O_5S \cdot H_2O$ and the molecular weight of 381.40.
It has the following structural formula:

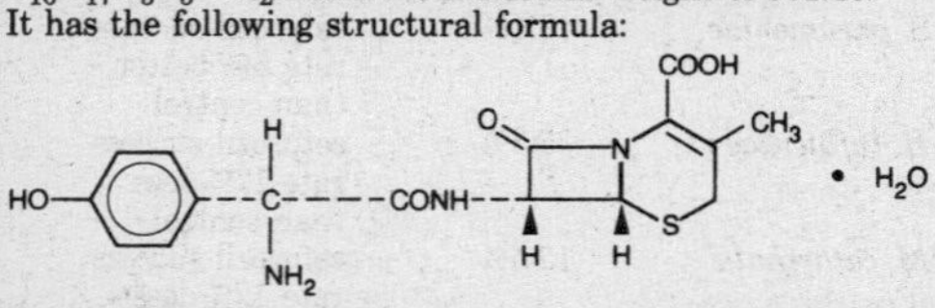

DURICEF® film-coated tablets, 1 g, contain the following inactive ingredients: microcrystalline cellulose, hydroxypropyl methylcellulose, magnesium stearate, polyethylene glycol, polysorbate 80, simethicone emulsion, and titanium dioxide.
DURICEF® for Oral Suspension contains the following inactive ingredients: FD&C Yellow No. 6, flavors (natural and artificial), polysorbate 80, sodium benzoate, sucrose, and xanthan gum.
DURICEF® capsules contain the following inactive ingredients: D&C Red No. 28, FD&C Blue No. 1, FD&C Red No. 40, gelatin, magnesium stearate, and titanium dioxide.
Clinical Pharmacology—DURICEF is rapidly absorbed after oral administration. Following single doses of 500 and 1000 mg, average peak serum concentrations were approximately 16 and 28 μg/mL, respectively. Measurable levels were present 12 hours after administration. Over 90% of the drug is excreted unchanged in the urine within 24 hours. Peak urine concentrations are approximately 1800 μg/mL during the period following a single 500-mg oral dose. Increases in dosage generally produce a proportionate increase in DURICEF urinary concentration. The urine antibiotic concentration, following a 1-g dose, was maintained well above the MIC of susceptible urinary pathogens for 20 to 22 hours.
Microbiology: *In vitro* tests demonstrate that the cephalosporins are bactericidal because of their inhibition of cell-wall synthesis. Cefadroxil has been shown to be active against the following organisms both *in vitro* and in clinical infections (see INDICATIONS AND USAGE):

Beta-hemolytic streptococci
Staphylococci, including
penicillinase-producing strains
Streptococcus (Diplococcus) pneumoniae
Escherichia coli
Proteus mirabilis
Klebsiella species
Moraxella (Branhamella) catarrhalis

Note: Most strains of *Enterococci faecalis* (formerly *Streptococcus faecalis)* and *Enterococcus faecium* (formerly *Streptococcus faecium)* are resistant to DURICEF. It is not active against most strains of *Enterobacter* species, *Morganella morganii* (formerly *Proteus morganii*), and *P. vulgaris.* It has no activity against *Pseudomonas* species and *Acinetobacter calcoaceticus* (formerly *Mima* and *Herellea* species.)
Susceptibility tests: Diffusion techniques
The use of antibiotic disk susceptibility test methods which measure zone diameter give an accurate estimation of antibiotic susceptibility. One such standard procedure[1] which has been recommended for use with disks to test susceptibility of organisms to cefadroxil uses the cephalosporin class (cephalothin) disk. Interpretation involves the correlation of the diameters obtained in the disk test with the minimum inhibitory concentration (MIC) for cefadroxil.
Reports from the laboratory giving results of the standard single-disk susceptibility test with a 30 μg cephalothin disk should be interpreted according to the following criteria:

Zone diameter (mm)	Interpretation
≥18	(S) Susceptible
15–17	(I) Intermediate
≤14	(R) Resistant

A report of "Susceptible" indicates that the pathogen is likely to be inhibited by generally achievable blood levels. A report of "Intermediate susceptibility" suggests that the organism would be susceptible if high dosage is used or if the infection is confined to tissue and fluid (eg, urine) in which high antibiotic levels are attained. A report of "Resistant" indicates that achievable concentrations of the antibiotic are unlikely to be inhibitory and other therapy should be selected.
Standardized procedures require the use of laboratory control organisms. The 30 μg cephalothin disk should give the following zone diameters:

Organism	Zone Diameter (mm)
Staphylococcus aureus ATCC 25923	29–37
Escherichia coli ATCC 25922	17–22

Dilution Techniques
When using the NCCLS agar dilution or broth dilution (including microdilution) method[2] or equivalent, a bacterial isolate may be considered susceptible if the MIC (minimum inhibitory concentration) value for cephalothin is 8 μg/mL or less. Organisms are considered resistant if the MIC is 32 μg/mL or greater. Organisms with an MIC value of less than 32 μg/mL but greater than 8 μg/mL are intermediate.
As with standard diffusion methods, dilution procedures require the use of laboratory control organisms. Standard cephalothin powder should give MIC values in the range of 0.12 μg/mL and 0.5 μg/mL for *Staphylococcus aureus* ATCC 29213. For *Escherichia coli* ATCC 25922, the MIC range should be between 4.0 μg/mL and 16.0 μg/mL. For *Streptococcus faecalis* ATCC 29212, the MIC range should be between 8.0 and 32.0 μg/mL.

INDICATIONS AND USAGE

DURICEF® (cefadroxil monohydrate, USP) is indicated for the treatment of patients with infection caused by susceptible strains of the designated organisms in the following diseases:
Urinary tract infections caused by *E. coli, P. mirabilis,* and *Klebsiella* species.
Skin and skin structure infections caused by staphylococci and/or streptococci.
Pharyngitis and tonsillitis caused by group A beta-hemolytic streptococci. (Penicillin is the usual drug of choice in the treatment and prevention of streptococcal infections, including the prophylaxis of rheumatic fever. DURICEF is generally effective in the eradication of streptococci from the nasopharynx; however, substantial data establishing the efficacy of DURICEF in the subsequent prevention of rheumatic fever are not available at present.)

Note: Culture and susceptibility tests should be initiated prior to and during therapy. Renal function studies should be performed when indicated.

CONTRAINDICATIONS

DURICEF is contraindicated in patients with known allergy to the cephalosporin group of antibiotics.

WARNINGS

BEFORE THERAPY WITH DURICEF IS INSTITUTED, CAREFUL INQUIRY SHOULD BE MADE TO DETERMINE WHETHER THE PATIENT HAS HAD PREVIOUS HYPERSENSITIVITY REACTIONS TO CEFADROXIL, CEPHALOSPORINS, PENICILLINS OR OTHER DRUGS. IF THIS PRODUCT IS TO BE GIVEN TO PENICILLIN-SENSITIVE PATIENTS, CAUTION SHOULD BE EXERCISED BECAUSE CROSS-SENSITIVITY AMONG BETA-LACTAM ANTIBIOTICS HAS BEEN CLEARLY DOCUMENTED AND MAY OCCUR IN UP TO 10% OF PATIENTS WITH A HISTORY OF PENICILLIN ALLERGY.
IF AN ALLERGIC REACTION TO DURICEF OCCURS, DISCONTINUE THE DRUG. SERIOUS ACUTE HYPERSENSITIVITY REACTIONS MAY REQUIRE TREATMENT WITH EPINEPHRINE AND OTHER EMERGENCY MEASURES, INCLUDING OXYGEN, INTRAVENOUS FLUIDS, INTRAVENOUS ANTIHISTAMINES, CORTICOSTEROIDS, PRESSOR AMINES, AND AIRWAY MANAGEMENT, AS CLINICALLY INDICATED.
Pseudomembranous colitis has been reported with nearly all antibacterial agents, including cefadroxil, and may range from mild to life-threatening. Therefore, it is important to consider this diagnosis in patients who present with diarrhea subsequent to the administration of antibacterial agents.
Treatment with antibacterial agents alters the normal flora of the colon and may permit overgrowth of clostridia. Studies indicate that a toxin produced by *Clostridium difficile* is a primary cause of "antibiotic-associated colitis".
After the diagnosis of pseudomembranous colitis has been established, therapeutic measures should be initiated. Mild cases of pseudomembranous colitis usually repond to discontinuation of the drug alone. In moderate to severe cases, consideration should be given to management with fluids and electrolytes, protein supplementation and treatment with an antibacterial drug effective against *Clostridium difficile.*

PRECAUTIONS

General: DURICEF should be used with caution in the presence of markedly impaired renal function (creatinine clearance rate of less than 50 mL/min/1.73 M^2). (See DOSAGE AND ADMINISTRATION.) In patients with known or suspected renal impairment, careful clinical observation and appropriate laboratory studies should be made prior to and during therapy.
Prolonged use of DURICEF may result in the overgrowth of nonsusceptible organisms. Careful observation of the patient is essential. If superinfection occurs during therapy, appropriate measures should be taken.
DURICEF should be prescribed with caution in individuals with history of gastrointestinal disease, particularly colitis.
Drug/Laboratory Test Interactions
Positive direct Coombs' tests have been reported during treatment with the cephalosporin antibiotics. In hematologic studies or in transfusion cross-matching procedures when antiglobulin tests are performed on the minor side or in Coombs' testing of newborns whose mothers have received cephalosporin antibiotics before parturition, it should be recognized that a positive Coombs' test may be due to the drug.
Carcinogenesis, Mutagenesis, and Impairment of Fertility: No long-term studies have been performed to determine carcinogenic potential. No genetic toxicity tests have been performed.
Pregnancy: Pregnancy Category B: Reproduction studies have been performed in mice and rats at doses up to 11 times the human dose and have revealed no evidence of impaired fertility or harm to the fetus due to cefadroxil monohydrate. There are, however, no adequate and well-controlled studies in pregnant women. Because animal reproduction studies are not always predictive of human response, this drug should be used during pregnancy only if clearly needed.
Labor and Delivery: DURICEF® (cefadroxil monohydrate, USP) has not been studied for use during labor and delivery. Treatment should only be given if clearly needed.

Child's Weight		Daily Dosage of DURICEF® Suspension		
lbs	kg	125 mg/5 mL	250 mg/5 mL	500 mg/5mL
10	4.5	1 tsp	—	
20	9.1	2 tsp	1 tsp	
30	13.6	3 tsp	1½ tsp	
40	18.2	4 tsp	2 tsp	1 tsp
50	22.7	5 tsp	2½ tsp	1¼ tsp
60	27.3	6 tsp	3 tsp	1½ tsp
70 & above	31.8+	—	—	2 tsp

Nursing Mothers: Caution should be exercised when cefadroxil monohydrate is administered to a nursing mother.
Pediatric Use: (See DOSAGE AND ADMINISTRATION).

ADVERSE REACTIONS

Gastrointestinal—Onset of pseudomembranous colitis symptoms may occur during or after antibiotic treatment (See WARNINGS). Dyspepsia, nausea and vomiting have been reported rarely. Diarrhea has also occurred.
Hypersensitivity—Allergies (in the form of rash, urticaria, angioedema, and pruritis) have been observed. These reactions usually subsided upon discontinuation of the drug. Anaphylaxis has also been reported.
Other
Other reactions have included genital pruritus, genital moniliasis, vaginitis, moderate transient neutropenia, fever, and minor elevations in serum transaminase. Agranulocytosis, thrombocytopenia, erythema multiforme, Stevens-Johnson syndrome, serum sickness, and arthralgia have been rarely reported.
In addition to the adverse reactions listed above which have been observed in patients treated with cefadroxil, the following adverse reactions and altered laboratory tests have been reported for cephalosporin-class antibiotics:
Toxic epidermal necrolysis, abdominal pain, superinfection, renal dysfunction, toxic nephropathy, hepatic dysfunction including cholestasis, aplastic anemia, hemolytic anemia, hemorrhage, prolonged prothrombin time, positive Coombs test, increased BUN, increased creatinine, elevated alkaline phosphatase, elevated aspartate aminotransferase (AST), elevated alanine aminotransferase (ALT), elevated bilirubin, elevated LDH, eosinophilia, pancytopenia, neutropenia.
Several cephalosporins have been implicated in triggering seizures, particularly in patients with renal impairment, when the dosage was not reduced (see DOSAGE AND ADMINISTRATION and OVERDOSAGE). If seizures associated with drug therapy occur, the drug should be discontinued. Anticonvulsant therapy can be given if clinically indicated.

OVERDOSAGE

A study of children under six years of age suggested that ingestion of less than 250 mg/kg of cephalosporins is not associated with significant outcomes. No action is required other than general support and observation. For amounts greater than 250 mg/kg, induce gastric emptying.
In five anuric patients. it was demonstrated that an average of 63% of a 1 g oral dose is extracted from the body during a 6–8 hour hemodialysis session.

DOSAGE AND ADMINISTRATION

DURICEF is acid-stable and may be administered orally without regard to meals. Administration with food may be helpful in diminishing potential gastrointestinal complaints occasionally associated with oral cephalosporin therapy.
Adults
Urinary Tract Infections: For uncomplicated lower urinary tract infections (ie, cystitis) the usual dosage is 1 or 2 g per day in single (q.d.) or divided doses (b.i.d.).
For all other urinary tract infections the usual dosage is 2 g per day in divided doses (b.i.d.).
Skin and Skin Structure Infections: For skin and skin structure infections the usual dosage is 1 g per day in single (q.d.) or divided doses (b.i.d.).
Pharyngitis and Tonsillitis: Treatment of group A beta-hemolytic streptococcal pharyngitis and tonsillitis—1 g per day in single (q.d.) or divided doses (b.i.d.) for 10 days.
Children
For urinary tract infections, the recommended daily dosage for children is 30 mg/kg/day in divided doses every 12 hours. For pharyngitis, tonsillitis, and impetigo, the recommended daily dosage for children is 30 mg/kg/day in a single dose or in equally divided doses every 12 hours. For other skin and skin structure infections, the recommended daily dosage is 30 mg/kg/day in equally divided doses every 12 hours. In the treatment of beta-hemolytic streptococcal infections, a therapeutic dosage of DURICEF should be administered for at least 10 days. See chart for total daily dosage for children.
[See table on bottom of preceding page.]
In patients with renal impairment, the dosage of cefadroxil monohydrate should be adjusted according to creatinine clearance rates to prevent drug accumulation. The following schedule is suggested. In adults, the initial dose is 1000 mg of DURICEF and the maintenance dose (based on the creatinine clearance rate [(mL/min/1.73 M^2]) is 500 mg at the time intervals listed below.

Creatinine Clearances	Dosage Interval
0–10 mL/min	36 hours
10–25 mL/min	24 hours
25–50 mL/min	12 hours

Patients with creatinine clearance rates over 50 mL/min may be treated as if they were patients having normal renal function.

Reconstitution Directions for Oral Suspension

Bottle Size	Reconstitution Directions
100 mL	Suspend in a total of 67 mL water. Method: Tap bottle lightly to loosen powder. Add 67 mL of water in two portions. Shake well after each addition.
75 ml	Suspend in a total of 51 mL water. Method: Tap bottle lightly to loosen powder. Add 51 mL of water in two portions. Shake well after each addition.
50 mL	Suspend in a total of 34 mL water. Method: Tap bottle lightly to loosen powder. Add 34 mL of water in two portions. Shake well after each addition.

After reconstitution, store in refrigerator. Shake well before using. Keep container tightly closed. Discard unused portion after 14 days.

HOW SUPPLIED

DURICEF® 500 mg Capsules: opaque, maroon and white hard gelatin capsules, imprinted with "PPP" and "784" on one end and with "Duricef" and "500 mg" on the other end. Capsules are supplied as follows:
NDC 0087-0784-07 Bottle of 20
NDC 0087-0784-46 Bottle of 50
NDC 0087-0784-42 Bottle of 100
NDC 0087-0784-44 10 strips of 10 individually labeled blisters with 1 capsule per blister
Store at controlled room temperature (15°–30°C).
DURICEF® 1 gram Tablets: white to off white, top bisected, oval shaped, imprinted with "PPP" on one side of the bisect and "785" on the other side of the bisect. Tablets are supplied as follows:
NDC 0087-0785-43 Bottle of 50
NDC 0087-0785-42 Bottle of 100
NDC 0087-0785-44 10 strips of 10 individually labeled blisters with 1 tablet per blister
NDC 0087-0785-45 4 packs of 10 individually labeled blisters with 1 tablet per blister
Store at controlled room temperature (15°–30°C).
DURICEF® for Oral Suspension is orange-pineapple flavored, and is supplied as follows:

125 mg/5 ml	**NDC** 0087-0786-42	50 mL Bottle
	NDC 0087-0786-41	100 mL Bottle
250 mg/5mL	**NDC** 0087-0782-42	50 mL Bottle
	NDC 0087-0782-41	100 mL Bottle
500 mg/5mL	**NDC** 0087-0783-42	50 mL Bottle
	NDC 0087-0783-05	75 mL Bottle
	NDC 0087-0783-41	100 mL Bottle

Prior to reconstitution: Store at controlled room temperature (15°–30°C).
8/91 U.S. Patent Nos. 4,160,863
4,504,657

REFERENCES

1. National Committee for Clinical Laboratory Standards, Approved Standard, *Performance Standards for Antimicrobial Disk Susceptibility Test*, 4th Edition, Vol. 10(7):M2-A4, Villanova, PA, April, 1990.
2. National Committee for Clinical Laboratory Standards, Approved Standard: *Methods for Dilution Antimicrobial Susceptibility Tests for Bacteria that Grow Aerobically*, 2nd Edition, Vol. 10(8):M7-A2, Villanova, PA, April, 1990.

Bristol-Myers Squibb Company
Princeton, NJ 08543
Made in U.S.A.
0783DIM-03
Revised October 1994

Shown in Product Identification Guide, page 307

ESTRACE® ESTRADIOL VAGINAL CREAM, USP, 0.01%) ℞
ESTRACE® ESTRADIOL TABLETS, USP)
CAUTION: FEDERAL LAW PROHIBITS DISPENSING WITHOUT PRESCRIPTION

WARNINGS

1. ESTROGENS HAVE BEEN REPORTED TO INCREASE THE RISK OF ENDOMETRIAL CARCINOMA IN POSTMENOPAUSAL WOMEN.
Close clinical surveillance of all women taking estrogens is important. Adequate diagnostic measures, including endometrial sampling when indicated, should be undertaken to rule out malignancy in all cases of undiagnosed persistent or recurring abnormal vaginal bleeding. There is no evidence that "natural" estrogens are more or less hazardous than "synthetic" estrogens at equiestrogenic doses.
2. ESTROGENS SHOULD NOT BE USED DURING PREGNANCY.
There is no indication for estrogen therapy during pregnancy or during the immediate postpartum period. Estrogens are ineffective for the prevention or treatment of threatened or habitual abortion. Estrogens are not indicated for the prevention of postpartum breast engorgement.
Estrogen therapy during pregnancy is associated with an increased risk of congenital defects in the reproductive organs of the fetus, and possibly other birth defects. Studies of women who received diethylstilbestrol (DES) during pregnancy have shown that female offspring have an increased risk of vaginal adenosis, squamous cell dysplasia of the uterine cervix, and clear cell vaginal cancer later in life; male offspring have an increased risk of urogenital abnormalities and possibly testicular cancer later in life. The 1985 DES Task Force concluded that use of DES during pregnancy is associated with a subsequent increased risk of breast cancer in the mothers, although a causal relationship remains unproven and the observed level of excess risk is similar to that for a number of other breast cancer risk factors.

DESCRIPTION

Estradiol (17β-estradiol) is a white, crystalline solid, chemically described as estra-1,3,5(10)-triene-3,17β-diol. It has an empirical formula of $C_{18}H_{24}O_2$ and molecular weight of 272.37. The structural formula is:

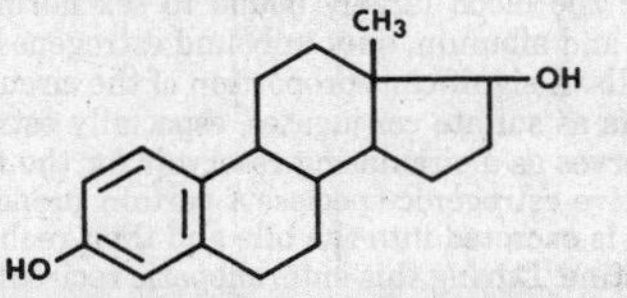

ESTRACE® (Estradiol Vaginal Cream, USP) contains 0.1 mg estradiol per gram in a nonliquefying base containing purified water, propylene glycol, stearyl alcohol, white ceresin wax, glyceryl monostearate, hydroxypropyl methylcellulose, 2208 4000 cps, sodium lauryl sulfate, methylparaben, edetate disodium and *tertiary*-butylhydroquinone.
ESTRACE® (Estradiol Tablets, USP) for oral administration contains 0.5, 1 or 2 mg of micronized estradiol per tablet.
ESTRACE Tablets, 0.5 mg, contain the following inactive ingredients: acacia, dibasic calcium phosphate, lactose, magnesium stearate, colloidal silicon dioxide, starch (corn), and talc.
ESTRACE Tablets, 1 mg, contain the following inactive ingredients: acacia, D&C Red No. 27 (aluminum lake), dibasic calcium phosphate, FD&C Blue No. 1 (aluminum lake), lactose, magnesium stearate, colloidal silicon dioxide, starch (corn), and talc.
ESTRACE Tablets, 2 mg, contain the following inactive ingredients: acacia, dibasic calcium phosphate, FD&C Blue No. 1 (aluminum lake), FD&C Yellow No. 5 (tartrazine) (aluminum lake), lactose, magnesium stearate, colloidal silicon dioxide, starch (corn), and talc.

CLINICAL PHARMACOLOGY

Estrogen drug products act by regulating the transcription of a limited number of genes. Estrogens diffuse through cell membranes, distribute themselves throughout the cell, and bind to and activate the nuclear estrogen receptor, a DNA-binding protein which is found in estrogen-responsive tissues. The activated estrogen receptor binds to specific DNA sequences, or hormone-response elements, which enhance the transcription of adjacent genes and in turn lead to the observed effects. Estrogen receptors have been identified in tissues of the reproductive tract, breast, pituitary, hypothalamus, liver, and bone of women.
Estrogens are important in the development and maintenance of the female reproductive system and secondary sex characteristics. By a direct action, they cause growth and development of the uterus, fallopian tubes, and vagina. With other hormones, such as pituitary hormones and progesterone, they cause enlargement of the breasts through promotion of ductal growth, stromal development, and the accretion of fat. Estrogens are intricately involved with other hormones, especially progesterone, in the processes of the ovulatory menstrual cycle and pregnancy, and affect the release of pituitary gonadotropins. They also contribute to the shaping of the skeleton, maintenance of tone and elasticity of urogenital structures, changes in the epiphyses of the long bones

Continued on next page

Bristol-Myers Squibb Co.—Cont.

that allow for the pubertal growth spurt and its termination, and pigmentation of the nipples and genitals.

Estrogens occur naturally in several forms. The primary source of estrogen in normally cycling adult women is the ovarian follicle, which secretes 70 to 500 micrograms of estradiol daily, depending on the phase of the menstrual cycle. This is converted primarily to estrone, which circulates in roughly equal proportion to estradiol, and to small amounts of estriol. After menopause, most endogenous estrogen is produced by conversion of androstenedione, secreted by the adrenal cortex, to estrone by peripheral tissues. Thus, estrone—especially in its sulfate ester form—is the most abundant circulating estrogen in postmenopausal women. Although circulating estrogens exist in a dynamic equilibrium of metabolic interconversions, estradiol is the principal intracellular human estrogen and is substantially more potent than estrone or estriol at the receptor.

Estrogens used in therapy are well absorbed through the skin, mucous membranes, and gastrointestinal tract. When applied for a local action, absorption is usually sufficient to cause systemic effects. When conjugated with aryl and alkyl groups for parenteral administration, the rate of absorption of oily preparations is slowed with a prolonged duration of action, such that a single intramuscular injection of estradiol valerate or estradiol cypionate is absorbed over several weeks.

Administered estrogens and their esters are handled within the body essentially the same as the endogenous hormones. Metabolic conversion of estrogens occurs primarily in the liver (first pass effect), but also at local target tissue sites. Complex metabolic processes result in a dynamic equilibrium of circulating conjugated and unconjugated estrogenic forms which are continually interconverted, especially between estrone and estradiol and between esterified and unesterified forms. Although naturally-occurring estrogens circulate in the blood largely bound to sex hormone-binding globulin and albumin, only unbound estrogens enter target tissue cells. A significant proportion of the circulating estrogen exists as sulfate conjugates, especially estrone sulfate, which serves as a circulating reservoir for the formation of more active estrogenic species. A certain proportion of the estrogen is excreted into the bile and then reabsorbed from the intestine. During this enterohepatic recirculation, estrogens are desulfated and resulfated and undergo degradation through conversion to less active estrogens (estriol and other estrogens), oxidation to nonestrogenic substances (catecholestrogens, which interact with catecholamine metabolism, especially in the central nervous system), and conjugation with glucuronic acids (which are then rapidly excreted in the urine).

When given orally, naturally-occurring estrogens and their esters are extensively metabolized (first pass effect) and circulate primarily as estrone sulfate, with smaller amounts of other conjugated and unconjugated estrogenic species. This results in limited oral potency. By contrast, synthetic estrogens, such as ethinyl estradiol and the nonsteroidal estrogens, are degraded very slowly in the liver and other tissues, which results in their high intrinsic potency. Estrogen drug products administered by non-oral routes are not subject to first-pass metabolism, but also undergo significant hepatic uptake, metabolism, and enterohepatic recycling.

INDICATIONS AND USAGE

ESTRACE® (Estradiol Vaginal Cream, USP, 0.01%) is indicated in the treatment of vulval and vaginal atrophy.

ESTRACE® (Estradiol Tablets, USP) is indicated in the:

1. Treatment of moderate to severe vasomotor symptoms associated with the menopause. There is no adequate evidence that estrogens are effective for nervous symptoms or depression which might occur during menopause and they should not be used to treat these conditions.

2. Treatment of vulval and vaginal atrophy.

3. Treatment of hypoestrogenism due to hypogonadism, castration or primary ovarian failure.

4. Treatment of breast cancer (for palliation only) in appropriately selected women and men with metastatic disease.

5. Treatment of advanced androgen-dependent carcinoma of the prostate (for palliation only).

6. Prevention of osteoporosis.

Since estrogen administration is associated with risk, selection of patients should ideally be based on prospective identification of risk factors for developing osteoporosis. Unfortunately, there is no certain way to identify those women who will develop osteoporotic fractures. Most prospective studies of efficacy for this indication have been carried out in white menopausal women, without stratification by other risk factors, and tend to show a universally salutary effect on bone. Thus, patient selection must be individualized based on the balance of risks and benefits. A more favorable risk/benefit ratio exists in a hysterectomized woman because she has no risk of endometrial cancer (see BOXED WARNINGS).

Estrogen replacement therapy reduces bone resorption and retards or halts postmenopausal bone loss. Case-control studies have shown an approximately 60 percent reduction in hip and wrist fractures in women whose estrogen replacement was begun within a few years of menopause. Studies also suggest that estrogen reduces the rate of vertebral fractures. Even when started as late as 6 years after menopause, estrogen prevents further loss of bone mass for as long as the treatment is continued. The results of a two-year, randomized, placebo-controlled, double-blind, dose-ranging study have shown that treatment with 0.5 mg estradiol daily for 23 days (of a 28 day cycle) prevents vertebral bone mass loss in postmenopausal women. When estrogen therapy is discontinued, bone mass declines at a rate comparable to the immediate postmenopausal period. There is no evidence that estrogen replacement therapy restores bone mass to premenopausal levels.

At skeletal maturity there are sex and race differences in both the total amount of bone present and its density, in favor of men and blacks. Thus, women are at higher risk than men because they start with less bone mass and, for several years following natural or induced menopause, the rate of bone mass decline is accelerated. White and Asian women are at higher risk than black women. Early menopause is one of the strongest predictors for the development of osteoporosis. In addition, other factors affecting the skeleton which are associated with osteoporosis include genetic factors (small build, family history), and endocrine factors (nulliparity, thyrotoxicosis, hyperparathyroidism, Cushing's syndrome, hyperprolactinemia, Type I diabetes), lifestyle (cigarette smoking, alcohol abuse, sedentary exercise habits) and nutrition (below average body weight, dietary calcium intake).

The mainstays of prevention and management of osteoporosis are estrogen, adequate lifetime calcium intake, and exercise. Postmenopausal women absorb dietary calcium less efficiently than premenopausal women and require an average of 1500 mg/day of elemental calcium to remain in neutral calcium balance. By comparison, premenopausal women require about 1000 mg/day and the average calcium intake in the USA is 400–600 mg/day. Therefore, when not contraindicated, calcium supplementation may be helpful.

Weight-bearing exercise and nutrition may be important adjuncts to the prevention and management of osteoporosis. Immobilization and prolonged bed rest produce rapid bone loss, while weight-bearing exercise has been shown both to reduce bone loss and to increase bone mass. The optimal type and amount of physical activity that would prevent osteoporosis have not been established, however in two studies, an hour of walking and running exercise twice or three times weekly significantly increased lumbar spine bone mass.

CONTRAINDICATIONS

Estrogens should not be used in individuals with any of the following conditions:

1. Known or suspected pregnancy (see BOXED WARNINGS). Estrogens may cause fetal harm when administered to a pregnant woman.

2. Undiagnosed abnormal genital bleeding.

3. Known or suspected cancer of the breast except in appropriately selected patients being treated for metastatic disease.

4. Known or suspected estrogen-dependent neoplasia.

5. Active thrombophlebitis or thromboembolic disorders.

WARNINGS

1. Induction of malignant neoplasms.

Endometrial cancer. The reported endometrial cancer risk among unopposed estrogen users is about 2- to 12-fold greater than in non-users, and appears dependent on duration of treatment and on estrogen dose. Most studies show no significant increased risk associated with use of estrogens for less than one year. The greatest risk appears associated with prolonged use–with increased risks of 15- to 24-fold for five to ten years or more. In three studies, persistence of risk was demonstrated for 8 to over 15 years after cessation of estrogen treatment. In one study a significant decrease in the incidence of endometrial cancer occurred six months after estrogen withdrawal. Concurrent progestin therapy may offset this risk but the overall health impact in postmenopausal women is not known (see PRECAUTIONS).

Breast Cancer. While the majority of studies have not shown an increased risk of breast cancer in women who have ever used estrogen replacement therapy, some have reported a moderately increased risk (relative risks of 1.3–2.0) in those taking higher doses or those taking lower doses for prolonged periods of time, especially in excess of 10 years. Other studies have not shown this relationship.

Congenital lesions with malignant potential. Estrogen therapy during pregnancy is associated with an increased risk of fetal congenital reproductive tract disorders, and possibly other birth defects. Studies of women who received DES during pregnancy have shown that female offspring have an increased risk of vaginal adenosis, squamous cell dysplasia of the uterine cervix, and clear cell vaginal cancer later in life; male offspring have an increased risk of urogenital abnormalities and possibly testicular cancer later in life. Although some of these changes are benign, others are precursors of malignancy.

2. Gallbladder disease. Two studies have reported a 2- to 4-fold increase in the risk of gallbladder disease requiring surgery in women receiving postmenopausal estrogens.

3. Cardiovascular disease. Large doses of estrogen (5 mg conjugated estrogens per day), comparable to those used to treat cancer of the prostate and breast, have been shown in a large prospective clinical trial in men to increase the risks of nonfatal myocardial infarction, pulmonary embolism, and thrombophlebitis. These risks cannot necessarily be extrapolated from men to women. However, to avoid the theoretical cardiovascular risk to women caused by high estrogen doses, the dose for estrogen replacement therapy should not exceed the lowest effective dose.

4. Elevated blood pressure. Occasional blood pressure increases during estrogen replacement therapy have been attributed to idiosyncratic reactions to estrogens. More often, blood pressure has remained the same or has dropped. One study showed that postmenopausal estrogen users have higher blood pressure than nonusers. Two other studies showed slightly lower blood pressure among estrogen users compared to nonusers. Postmenopausal estrogen use does not increase the risk of stroke. Nonetheless, blood pressure should be monitored at regular intervals with estrogen use.

5. Hypercalcemia. Administration of estrogens may lead to severe hypercalcemia in patients with breast cancer and bone metastases. If this occurs, the drug should be stopped and appropriate measures taken to reduce the serum calcium level.

PRECAUTIONS

A. General

1. Addition of a progestin. Studies of the addition of a progestin for seven or more days of a cycle of estrogen administration have reported a lowered incidence of endometrial hyperplasia which would otherwise be induced by estrogen treatment. Morphological and biochemical studies of endometrium suggest that 10 to 14 days of progestin are needed to provide maximal maturation of the endometrium and to eliminate any hyperplastic changes. There are possible additional risks which may be associated with the inclusion of progestins in estrogen replacement regimens. These include: (1) adverse effects on lipoprotein metabolism (lowering HDL and raising LDL) which may diminish the possible cardioprotective effect of estrogen therapy (see PRECAUTIONS D.4., below); (2) impairment of glucose tolerance; and (3) possible enhancement of mitotic activity in breast epithelial tissue (although few epidemiological data are available to address this point). The choice of progestin, its dose, and its regimen may be important in minimizing these adverse effects, but these issues remain to be clarified.

2. Physical examination. A complete medical and family history should be taken prior to the initiation of any estrogen therapy. The pretreatment and periodic physical examinations should include special reference to blood pressure, breasts, abdomen, and pelvic organs, and should include a Papanicolaou smear. As a general rule, estrogen should not be prescribed for longer than one year without reexamining the patient.

3. Hypercoagulability. Some studies have shown that women taking estrogen replacement therapy have hypercoagulability, primarily related to decreased antithrombin activity. This effect appears dose- and duration-dependent and is less pronounced than that associated with oral contraceptive use. Also, postmenopausal women tend to have increased coagulation parameters at baseline compared to pre-menopausal women. There is some suggestion that low dose postmenopausal mestranol may increase the risk of thromboembolism, although the majority of studies (of primarily conjugated estrogens users) report no such increase. There is insufficient information on hypercoagulability in women who have had previous thromboembolic disease.

4. Familial hyperlipoproteinemia. Estrogen therapy may be associated with massive elevations of plasma triglycerides leading to pancreatitis and other complications in patients with familial defects of lipoprotein metabolism.

5. Fluid retention. Because estrogens may cause some degree of fluid retention, conditions which might be exacerbated by this factor, such as asthma, epilepsy, migraine, and cardiac or renal dysfunction, require careful observation.

6. Uterine bleeding and mastodynia. Certain patients may develop undesirable manifestations of estrogenic stimulation, such as abnormal uterine bleeding and mastodynia.

7. Impaired liver function. Estrogens may be poorly metabolized in patients with impaired liver function and should be administered with caution.

ESTRACE® (Estradiol Tablets, USP), 2 mg, contain FD&C Yellow No. 5 (tartrazine) which may cause allergic-type reactions (including bronchial asthma) in certain susceptible individuals. Although the overall incidence of FD&C Yellow No. 5 (tartrazine) sensitivity in the general population is low, it is frequently seen in patients who also have aspirin hypersensitivity.

B. Information for the Patient. See text of Patient Package Insert below.

Advise patients that the number of doses per tube of ES-TRACE® (Estradiol Vaginal Cream, USP, 0.01%) will vary with dosage requirements and patient handling.

C. Laboratory Tests. Estrogen administration should generally be guided by clinical response at the smallest dose, rather than laboratory monitoring, for relief of symptoms for those indications in which symptoms are observable. For prevention of osteoporosis, however, see DOSAGE AND ADMINISTRATION section under ESTRACE® (Estradiol Tablets, USP) item 5.

D. Drug/Laboratory Test Interactions.

1. Accelerated prothrombin time, partial thromboplastin time, and platelet aggregation time; increased platelet count; increased factors II, VII antigen, VIII antigen, VIII coagulant activity, IX, X, XII, VII-X complex, II-VII-X complex, and beta-thromboglobulin; decreased levels of antifactor Xa and antithrombin III, decreased antithrombin III activity; increased levels of fibrinogen and fibrinogen activity; increased plasminogen antigen and activity.

2. Increased thyroid-binding globulin (TBG) leading to increased circulating total thyroid hormone, as measured by protein-bound iodine (PBI), T4 levels (by column or by radioimmunoassay) or T3 levels by radioimmunoassay. T3 resin uptake is decreased, reflecting the elevated TBG. Free T4 and free T3 concentrations are unaltered.

3. Other binding proteins may be elevated in serum, i.e., corticosteroid binding globulin (CBG), sex hormone-binding globulin (SHBG), leading to increased circulating corticosteroids and sex steroids, respectively. Free or biologically active hormone concentrations are unchanged. Other plasma proteins may be increased (angiotensinogen/renin substrate, alpha-1-antitrypsin, ceruloplasmin).

4. Increased plasma HDL and HDL-2 subfraction concentrations, reduced LDL cholesterol concentration, increased triglycerides levels.

5. Impaired glucose tolerance.

6. Reduced response to metyrapone test.

7. Reduced serum folate concentration.

E. Carcinogenesis, Mutagenesis, and Impairment of Fertility. Long term continuous administration of natural and synthetic estrogens in certain animal species increases the frequency of carcinomas of the breast, uterus, cervix, vagina, testis, and liver. See CONTRAINDICATIONS AND WARNINGS.

F. Pregnancy Category X. Estrogens should not be used during pregnancy. See CONTRAINDICATIONS and BOXED WARNINGS.

G. Nursing Mothers. As a general principle, the administration of any drug to nursing mothers should be done only when clearly necessary since many drugs are excreted in human milk. In addition, estrogen administration to nursing mothers has been shown to decrease the quantity and quality of the milk.

ADVERSE REACTIONS

The following additional adverse reactions have been reported with estrogen therapy (see WARNINGS regarding induction of neoplasia, adverse effects on the fetus, increased incidence of gallbladder disease, cardiovascular disease, elevated blood pressure, and hypercalcemia).

1. Genitourinary system.
Changes in vaginal bleeding pattern and abnormal withdrawal bleeding or flow; breakthrough bleeding, spotting.
Increase in size of uterine leiomyomata.
Vaginal candidiasis.
Change in amount of cervical secretion.

2. Breasts.
Tenderness, enlargement.

3. Gastrointestinal.
Nausea, vomiting.
Abdominal cramps, bloating.
Cholestatic jaundice.
Increased incidence of gallbladder disease.

4. Skin.
Chloasma or melasma which may persist when drug is discontinued.
Erythema multiforme.
Erythema nodosum.
Hemorrhagic eruption.
Loss of scalp hair.
Hirsutism.

5. Eyes.
Steepening of corneal curvature.
Intolerance to contact lenses.

6. Central Nervous System.
Headache, migraine, dizziness.
Mental depression.
Chorea.

7. Miscellaneous.
Increase or decrease in weight.
Reduced carbohydrate tolerance.
Aggravation of porphyria.

Edema.
Changes in libido.

OVERDOSAGE

Serious ill effects have not been reported following acute ingestion of large doses of estrogen-containing oral contraceptives by young children. Overdosage of estrogen may cause nausea and vomiting, and withdrawal bleeding may occur in females.

DOSAGE AND ADMINISTRATION

ESTRACE® (Estradiol Vaginal Cream, USP, 0.01%).
For treatment of vulval and vaginal atrophy associated with the menopause, the lowest dose and regimen that will control symptoms should be chosen and medication should be discontinued as promptly as possible.
Attempts to discontinue or taper medication should be made at 3-month to 6-month intervals.
Usual Dosage: The usual dosage range is 2 to 4 g (marked on the applicator) daily for one or two weeks, then gradually reduced to one half initial dosage for a similar period. A maintenance dosage of 1 g, one to three times a week, may be used after restoration of the vaginal mucosa has been achieved.
NOTE: The number of doses per tube will vary with dosage requirements and patient handling.
Patients with intact uteri should be monitored closely for signs of endometrial cancer and appropriate diagnostic measures should be taken to rule out malignancy in the event of persistent or recurring abnormal vaginal bleeding.

ESTRACE® (Estradiol Tablets, USP)

1. For treatment of moderate to severe vasomotor symptoms, vulval and vaginal atrophy associated with the menopause, the lowest dose and regimen that will control symptoms should be chosen and medication should be discontinued as promptly as possible.
Attempts to discontinue or taper medication should be made at 3-month to 6-month intervals.
The usual initial dosage range is 1 to 2 mg daily of estradiol adjusted as necessary to control presenting symptoms. The minimal effective dose for maintenance therapy should be determined by titration. Administration should be cyclic (e.g., 3 weeks on and 1 week off).

2. For treatment of female hypoestrogenism due to hypogonadism, castration, or primary ovarian failure.
Treatment is usually initiated with a dose of 1 to 2 mg daily of estradiol, adjusted as necessary to control presenting symptoms; the minimal effective dose for maintenance therapy should be determined by titration.

3. For treatment of breast cancer, for palliation only, in appropriately selected women and men with metastatic disease.
Suggested dosage is 10 mg three times daily for a period of at least three months.

4. For treatment of advanced androgen-dependent carcinoma of the prostate, for palliation only.
Suggested dosage is 1 to 2 mg three times daily. The effectiveness of therapy can be judged by phosphatase determinations as well as by symptomatic improvement of the patient.

5. For prevention of osteoporosis.
Therapy with Estrace® (Estradiol Tablets, USP) to prevent postmenopausal bone loss should be initiated as soon as possible after menopause. A daily dosage of 0.5 mg should be administered cyclically (i.e., 23 days on and 5 days off). The dosage may be adjusted if necessary to control concurrent menopausal symptoms. Discontinuation of estrogen replacement therapy may re-establish the natural rate of bone loss.

HOW SUPPLIED

ESTRACE® (Estradiol Vaginal Cream, USP, 0.01%)
NDC 0087-0754-42: Tube containing 1¹/₂oz (42.5 g) with a calibrated plastic applicator for delivery of 1,2,3, or 4 g. Store at room temperature. Protect from temperatures in excess of 40° C (104° F).
ESTRACE® (Estradiol Tablets, USP) 0.5 mg: round, white scored tablets imprinted with **021** and **MJ** on one side.
NDC 0087-0021-41   Bottles of 100
ESTRACE® (Estradiol Tablets, USP) 1 mg: round, lavender scored tablets imprinted with **755** and **MJ** on one side.
NDC 0087-0755-01   Bottles of 100
NDC 0087-0755-48   Bottles of 500
ESTRACE® (Estradiol Tablets, USP) 2 mg: round, turquoise scored tablets imprinted with **756** and **MJ** on one side.
NDC 0087-0756-01   Bottles of 100
NDC 0087-0756-48   Bottles of 500
Store at controlled room temperature 15°–30° C (59°–86° F). Dispense in a tight, light-resistant container as defined in the USP.

INFORMATION FOR THE PATIENT

INTRODUCTION

NOTE: The number of doses per tube of ESTRACE® (Estradiol Vaginal Cream, USP, 0.01%) will vary with dosage requirements and patient handling.
This leaflet describes when and how to use estrogens, and the risks and benefits of estrogen treatment.
Estrogens have important benefits but also some risks. You must decide, with your doctor, whether the risks to you of

estrogen use are acceptable because of their benefits. If you use estrogens, check with your doctor to be sure you are using the lowest possible dose that works, and that you don't use them longer than necessary. How long you need to use estrogens will depend on the reason for use.

WARNINGS

1. ESTROGENS INCREASE THE RISK OF CANCER OF THE UTERUS IN WOMEN WHO HAVE HAD THEIR MENOPAUSE ("CHANGE OF LIFE").
If you use any estrogen-containing drug, it is important to visit your doctor regularly and report any unusual vaginal bleeding right away. Vaginal bleeding after menopause may be a warning sign of uterine cancer. Your doctor should evaluate any unusual vaginal bleeding to find out the cause.

2. ESTROGENS SHOULD NOT BE USED DURING PREGNANCY.
Estrogens do not prevent miscarriage (spontaneous abortion) and are not needed in the days following childbirth. If you take estrogens during pregnancy, your unborn child has a greater than usual chance of having birth defects. The risk of developing these defects is small, but clearly larger than the risk in children whose mothers did not take estrogens during pregnancy. These birth defects may affect the baby's urinary system and sex organs. Daughters born to mothers who took DES (an estrogen drug) have a higher than usual chance of developing cancer of the vagina or cervix when they become teenagers or young adults. Sons may have a higher than usual chance of developing cancer of the testicles when they become teenagers or young adults.

USES OF ESTROGEN

(Not every estrogen drug is approved for every use listed in this section. If you want to know which of these possible uses are approved for the medicine prescribed for you, ask your doctor or pharmacist to show you the professional labeling. You can also look up the specific estrogen product in a book called the "Physicians' Desk Reference", which is available in many book stores and public libraries. Generic drugs carry virtually the same labeling information as their brand name versions.)

● **To reduce moderate or severe menopausal symptoms.** Estrogens are hormones made by the ovaries of normal women. Between ages 45 and 55, the ovaries normally stop making estrogens. This leads to a drop in body estrogen levels which causes the "change of life" or menopause (the end of monthly menstrual periods). If both ovaries are removed during an operation before natural menopause takes place, the sudden drop in estrogen levels causes "surgical menopause."
When the estrogen levels begin dropping, some women develop very uncomfortable symptoms, such as feelings of warmth in the face, neck, and chest, or sudden intense episodes of heat and sweating ("hot flashes" or "hot flushes"). Using estrogen drugs can help the body adjust to lower estrogen levels and reduce these symptoms. Most women have only mild menopausal symptoms or none at all and do not need to use estrogen drugs for these symptoms. Others may need to take estrogens for a few months while their bodies adjust to lower estrogen levels. The majority of women do not need estrogen replacement for longer than six months for these symptoms.

● **To treat vulval and vaginal atrophy** (itching, burning, dryness in or around the vagina, difficulty or burning on urination) associated with menopause.

● **To treat certain conditions in which a young woman's ovaries do not produce enough estrogen naturally.**

● **To treat certain types of abnormal vaginal bleeding due to hormonal imbalance when your doctor has found no serious cause of the bleeding.**

● **To treat certain cancers in special situations, in men and women.**

● **To prevent thinning of bones.**
Osteoporosis is a thinning of the bones that makes them weaker and allows them to break more easily. The bones of the spine, wrists and hips break most often in osteoporosis. Both men and women start to lose bone mass after about age 40, but women lose bone mass faster after the menopause. Using estrogens after the menopause slows down bone thinning and may prevent bones from breaking. Lifelong adequate calcium intake, either in the diet (such as dairy products) or by calcium supplements (to reach a total daily intake of 1000 milligrams per day before menopause or 1500 milligrams per day after menopause), may help to prevent osteoporosis. Regular weight-bearing exercise (like walking and running for an hour, two or three times a week) may also help to prevent osteoporosis. Before you change your calcium intake or exercise habits, it is important to discuss these lifestyle changes with your doctor to find out if they are safe for you.
Since estrogen use has some risks, only women who are likely to develop osteoporosis should use estrogens for prevention. Women who are likely to develop osteoporosis often

Continued on next page

Bristol-Myers Squibb Co.—Cont.

have the following characteristics: white or Asian race, slim, cigarette smokers, and a family history of osteoporosis in a mother, sister, or aunt. Women who have relatively early menopause, often because their ovaries were removed during an operation ("surgical menopause"), are more likely to develop osteoporosis than women whose menopause happens at the average age.

WHO SHOULD NOT USE ESTROGENS

Estrogens should not be used:

• **During pregnancy (see Boxed Warnings).** If you think you may be pregnant, do not use any form of estrogen-containing drug. Using estrogens while you are pregnant may cause your unborn child to have birth defects. Estrogens do not prevent miscarriage.

• **If you have unusual vaginal bleeding which has not been evaluated by your doctor (see Boxed Warnings).** Unusual vaginal bleeding can be a warning sign of cancer of the uterus, especially if it happens after menopause. Your doctor must find out the cause of the bleeding so that he or she can recommend the proper treatment. Taking estrogens without visiting your doctor can cause you serious harm if your vaginal bleeding is caused by cancer of the uterus.

• **If you have had cancer.** Since estrogens increase the risk of certain types of cancer, you should not use estrogens if you have ever had cancer of the breast or uterus, unless your doctor recommends that the drug may help in the cancer treatment. (For certain patients with breast or prostate cancer, estrogens may help.)

• **If you have any circulation problems.** Estrogen drugs should not be used except in unusually special situations in which your doctor judges that you need estrogen therapy so much that the risks are acceptable. Men and women with abnormal blood clotting conditions should avoid estrogen use (see Dangers of Estrogens, below).

• **When they do not work.** During menopause, some women develop nervous symptoms or depression. Estrogens do not relieve these symptoms. You may have heard that taking estrogens for years after menopause will keep your skin soft and supple and keep you feeling young. There is no evidence for these claims and such long-term estrogen use may have serious risks.

• **After childbirth or when breastfeeding a baby.** Estrogens should not be used to try to stop the breasts from filling with milk after a baby is born. Such treatment may increase the risk of developing blood clots (see Dangers of Estrogens, below).

If you are breastfeeding, you should avoid using any drugs because many drugs pass through to the baby in the milk. While nursing a baby, you should take drugs only on the advice of your health care provider.

DANGERS OF ESTROGENS

• **Cancer of the uterus.** Your risk of developing cancer of the uterus gets higher the longer you use estrogens and the larger doses you use. One study showed that after women stop taking estrogens, this higher cancer risk quickly returns to the usual level of risk (as if you had never used estrogen therapy). Three other studies showed that the cancer risk stayed high for 8 to more than 15 years after stopping estrogen treatment. Because of this risk, **IT IS IMPORTANT TO TAKE THE LOWEST DOSE THAT WORKS AND TO TAKE IT ONLY AS LONG AS YOU NEED IT.**

Using progestin therapy together with estrogen therapy may reduce the higher risk of uterine cancer related to estrogen use (but see Other Information, below).

If you have had your uterus removed (total hysterectomy), there is no danger of developing cancer of the uterus.

• **Cancer of the breast.** Most studies have not shown a higher risk of breast cancer in women who have ever used estrogens. However, some studies have reported that breast cancer developed more often (up to twice the usual rate) in women who used estrogens for long periods of time (especially more than 10 years), or who used higher doses for shorter time periods.

Regular breast examinations by a health professional and monthly self-examination are recommended for all women.

• **Gallbladder disease.** Women who use estrogens after menopause are more likely to develop gallbladder disease needing surgery than women who do not use estrogens.

• **Abnormal blood clotting.** Taking estrogens may cause changes in your blood clotting system. These changes allow the blood to clot more easily, possibly allowing clots to form in your bloodstream. If blood clots do form in your bloodstream, they can cut off the blood supply to vital organs, causing serious problems. These problems may include a stroke (by cutting off blood to the brain), a heart attack (by cutting off blood to the heart), a pulmonary embolus (by cutting off blood to the lungs), or other problems. Any of these conditions may cause death or serious long term disability. However, most studies of low dose estrogen usage by women do not show an increased risk of these complications.

SIDE EFFECTS

In addition to the risks listed above, the following side effects have been reported with estrogen use:

—Nausea and vomiting.

—Breast tenderness or enlargement.

—Enlargement of benign tumors ("fibroids") of the uterus.

—Retention of excess fluid. This may make some conditions worsen, such as asthma, epilepsy, migraine, heart disease, or kidney disease.

—A spotty darkening of the skin, particularly of the face.

REDUCING RISK OF ESTROGEN USE

If you use estrogens, you can reduce your risks by doing these things:

• **See your doctor regularly.** While you are using estrogens, it is important to visit your doctor at least once a year for a check-up. If you develop vaginal bleeding while taking estrogens, you may need further evaluation. If members of your family have had breast cancer or if you have ever had breast lumps or an abnormal mammogram (breast x-ray), you may need to have more frequent breast examinations.

• **Reassess your need for estrogens.** You and your doctor should reevaluate whether or not you still need estrogens at least every six months.

• **Be alert for signs of trouble.** If any of these warning signals (or any other unusual symptoms) happen while you are using estrogens, call your doctor immediately:

—Abnormal bleeding from the vagina (possible uterine cancer)

—Pains in the calves or chest, sudden shortness of breath, or coughing blood (possible clot in the legs, heart, or lungs)

—Severe headache or vomiting, dizziness, faintness, changes in vision or speech, weakness or numbness of an arm or leg (possible clot in the brain or eye)

—Breast lumps (possible breast cancer; ask your doctor or health professional to show you how to examine your breasts monthly)

—Yellowing of the skin or eyes (possible liver problem)

—Pain, swelling, or tenderness in the abdomen (possible gallbladder problem)

OTHER INFORMATION

Some doctors may choose to prescribe a progestin, a different hormonal drug, for you to take together with your estrogen treatment. Progestins lower your risk of developing endometrial hyperplasia (a possible pre-cancerous condition of the uterus) while using estrogens. Taking estrogens and progestins together may also protect you from the higher risk of uterine cancer, but this has not been clearly established. Combined use of progestin and estrogen treatment may have additional risks, however, the possible risks include unhealthy effects on blood fats (especially a lowering of HDL cholesterol, the "good" blood fat which protects against heart disease risk), unhealthy effects on blood sugar (which might worsen a diabetic condition), and a possible further increase in the breast cancer risk which may be associated with long-term estrogen use. The type of progestin drug used and its dosage schedule may be important in minimizing these effects.

Your doctor has prescribed this drug for you and you alone. Do not give the drug to anyone else.

If you will be taking calcium supplements as part of the treatment to help prevent osteoporosis, check with your doctor about how much to take.

Keep this and all drugs out of the reach of children. In case of overdose, call your doctor, hospital or poison control center immediately.

This leaflet provides a summary of the most important information about estrogens. If you want more information, ask your doctor or pharmacist to show you the professional labeling. The professional labeling is also published in a book called the "Physicians' Desk Reference", which is available in book stores and public libraries. Generic drugs carry virtually the same labeling information as their brand name versions.

Bristol-Myers Squibb Company
Princeton, New Jersey 08543
U.S.A.

P6178-01

A1-B001C-04-96 J4503C

Shown in Product Identification Guide, page 307

GLUCOPHAGE® ℞

[glü-kō-faj]

(metformin hydrochloride tablets)

DESCRIPTION

GLUCOPHAGE (metformin hydrochloride tablets) is an oral antihyperglycemic drug used in the management of non-insulin-dependent diabetes mellitus (NIDDM). Metformin hydrochloride (N,N-dimethylimidodcarbonimidic diamide hydrochloride) is not chemically or pharmacologically related to the oral sulfonylureas. The structural formula is as shown:

[See chemical structure at top of next column.]

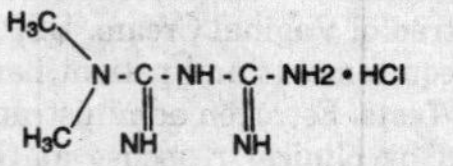

Metformin hydrochloride is a white to off-white crystalline compound with a molecular formula of $C_4H_{11}N_5 \bullet HCl$ and a molecular weight of 165.63. Metformin hydrochloride is freely soluble in water and is practically insoluble in acetone, ether or chloroform. The pK_a of metformin is 12.4. The pH of a 1% aqueous solution of metformin hydrochloride is 6.68.

GLUCOPHAGE tablets contain 500 mg and 850 mg of metformin hydrochloride. In addition, each tablet contains the following inactive ingredients: povidone, magnesium stearate and hydroxypropyl methylcellulose (hypromellose) coating.

CLINICAL PHARMACOLOGY

Antidiabetic Activity

GLUCOPHAGE is an antihyperglycemic agent which improves glucose tolerance in NIDDM subjects, lowering both basal and postprandial plasma glucose. Its pharmacologic mechanisms of action are different from those of sulfonylureas. GLUCOPHAGE decreases hepatic glucose production, decreases intestinal absorption of glucose and improves insulin sensitivity (increases peripheral glucose uptake and utilization). Unlike sulfonylureas, GLUCOPHAGE does not produce hypoglycemia in either diabetic or nondiabetic subjects (except in special circumstances, see PRECAUTIONS) and does not cause hyperinsulinemia. With metformin therapy, insulin secretion remains unchanged while fasting insulin levels and day-long plasma insulin response may actually decrease.

In a double-blind, placebo-controlled, multicenter U.S. clinical trial involving obese NIDDM patients whose hyperglycemia was not adequately controlled with dietary management alone (baseline fasting plasma glucose [FPG] of approximately 240 mg/dL), treatment with GLUCOPHAGE (up to 2.55 g/day) for 29 weeks resulted in significant mean net reduction in fasting and postprandial plasma glucose (PPG) and HbA_{1c} of 59 mg/dL, 83 mg/dL, and 1.8%, respectively, compared to placebo group (see Table 1).

Table 1. GLUCOPHAGE vs Placebo Summary of Mean Changes from Baseline* in Plasma Glucose HbA_{1c} and Body Weight, at Final Visit (29-week study)

	GLUCOPHAGE (n = 141)	Placebo (n = 145)	P–Value
FPG (mg/dL)			
Baseline	241.5	237.7	NS
Change at FINAL VISIT	−53.0	6.3	0.001**
Hemoglobin A_{1c} (%)			
Baseline	8.4	8.2	NS
Change at FINAL VISIT	−1.4	0.4	0.001**
Body Weight (lbs)			
Baseline	201.0	206.0	NS
Change at FINAL VISIT	−1.4	−2.4	NS

* All patients on diet therapy at Baseline
** Statistically significant

Monotherapy with GLUCOPHAGE may be effective in patients who have not responded to sulfonylureas or who have only a partial response to sulfonylureas or who have ceased to respond to sulfonylureas. In such patients, if adequate glycemic control is not attained with GLUCOPHAGE monotherapy, the combination of GLUCOPHAGE and a sulfonylurea may have a synergistic effect, since both agents act to improve glucose tolerance by different but complimentary mechanisms.

A 29-week, double-blind, placebo-controlled study of GLUCOPHAGE and glyburide, alone and in combination, was conducted in obese NIDDM patients who had failed to achieve adequate glycemic control while on maximum doses of glyburide (baseline FPG of approximately 250 mg/dL) (see Table 2). Patients randomized to continue on gluburide experienced worsening of glycemic control, with mean increases in FPG, PPG and HbA_{1c} of 14 mg/dL, 3 mg/dL and 0.2%, respectively. In contrast, those randomized to GLUCOPHAGE (metformin hydrochloride tablets) (up to 2.5 g/day) did not experience a deterioration in glycemic control, but rather a slight improvement, with mean reductions in FPG, PPG and HbA_{1c} of 1 mg/dL, 6 mg/dL and 0.4%, respectively. The combination of GLUCOPHAGE and glyburide was synergistic in reducing FPG, PPG and HbA_{1c} levels by 63 mg/dL, 65 mg/dL, and 1.7%, respectively. Compared to the results of glyburide treatment alone, the net differences with

combined treatment were −77 mg/dL, −68 mg/dL and −1.9%, respectively (see Table 2).

[See table at right.]

The magnitude of the decline in fasting blood glucose concentration following the institution of GLUCOPHAGE (metformin hydrochloride tablets) therapy is proportional to the level of fasting hyperglycemia. Non-insulin-dependent diabetics with higher fasting glucose concentrations will experience greater declines in plasma glucose and glycosylated hemoglobin.

GLUCOPHAGE has a modest favorable effect on serum lipids, which are often abnormal in NIDDM patients. In clinical studies, particularly when baseline levels were abnormally elevated, GLUCOPHAGE, alone or in combination with a sulfonylurea, lowered mean fasting serum triglycerides, total cholesterol and LDL cholesterol levels and had no adverse effects on other lipid levels (see Table 3).

[See table below.]

In contrast to sulfonylureas, body weight of individuals on GLUCOPHAGE tends to remain stable or may even decrease somewhat (see Table 1 and 2).

In summary, metformin-treated patients showed significant improvement in all parameters of glycemic control (FPG, PPG and HbA_{1c}), stabilization or decrease in body weight, and a tendency to improvement in the lipid profile, particularly when baseline values are abnormally elevated.

Pharmacokinetics

Absorption and Bioavailability:

The absolute bioavailability of a 500 mg metformin hydrochloride tablet given under fasting conditions is approximately 50–60%. Studies using single oral doses of metformin tablets of 500 mg and 1500 mg, and 850 mg to 2550 mg, indicate that there is a lack of dose proportionality with increasing doses, which is due to decreased absorption rather than an alteration in elimination. Food decreases the extent and slightly delays the absorption of metformin, as shown by approximately a 40% lower peak concentration and 25% lower AUC in plasma and a 35 minute prolongation of time to peak plasma concentration following administration of a single 850 mg tablet of metformin with food, compared to the same tablet strength administered fasting. The clinical relevance of these decreases is unknown.

Distribution:

The apparent volume of distribution (V/F) of metformin following single oral doses of 850 mg averaged 654 ± 358 L. Metformin is negligibly bound to plasma proteins in contrast to sulfonylureas which are more than 90% protein bound. Metformin partitions into erythrocytes, most likely as a function of time. At usual clinical doses and dosing schedules of GLUCOPHAGE (metformin hydrochloride tablets), steady state plasma concentrations of metformin are reached within 24–48 hours and are generally $< 1 \mu g/mL$. During controlled clinical trials, maximum metformin plasma levels did not exceed $5 \mu g/mL$, even at maximum doses.

Metabolism and Elimination:

Intravenous single-dose studies in normal subjects demonstrate that metformin is excreted unchanged in the urine and does not undergo hepatic metabolism (no metabolites have been identified in humans) nor biliary excretion. Renal clearance (see Table 4) is approximately 3.5 times greater than creatinine clearance which indicates that tubular secretion is the major route of metformin elimination. Following oral administration, approximately 90% of the absorbed drug is eliminated via the renal route within the first 24 hours, with a plasma elimination half-life of approximately 6.2 hours. In blood, the elimination half-life is approximately 17.6 hours, suggesting that the erythrocyte mass may be a compartment of distribution.

Table 2. Combined GLUCOPHAGE/Glyburide (Comb) vs Glyburide (Glyb) or Glucophage (GLU) Monotherapy: Summary of Mean Changes from Baseline* in Plasma Glucose, HbA$_{1c}$ and Body Weight, at Final Visit (29-week study)

	Comb (n =213)	Glyb (n =209)	GLU (n =210)	Glyb vs Comb	GLU vs Comb	GLU vs Glyb
Fasting Plasma Glucose (mg/dL)						
Baseline	250.5	247.5	253.9	NS	NS	NS
Change at FINAL VISIT	−63.5	13.7	−0.9	0.001**	0.001**	0.025**
Hemoglobin A$_{1c}$ (%)						
Baseline	8.8	8.5	8.9	NS	NS	0.007**
Change at FINAL VISIT	−1.7	0.2	−0.4	0.001**	0.001**	0.001**
Body Weight (lbs)						
Baseline	202.2	203.0	204.0	NS	NS	NS
Change at FINAL VISIT	0.9	−0.7	−8.4	0.011**	0.001**	0.001**

* All patients of glyburide, 20 mg/day, at Baseline
** Statistically significant

Special Populations:

NIDDM Subjects:

In the presence of normal renal function, there are no differences between single or multiple dose pharmacokinetics of metformin between diabetics and nondiabetics (see Table 4), nor is there any accumulation of metformin in either group at usual clinical doses.

Renal Insufficiency:

In subjects with decreased renal function (based on measured creatinine clearance), the plasma and blood half-life of metformin is prolonged and the renal clearance is decreased in proportion to the decrease in creatinine clearance (see Table 4).

Hepatic Insufficiency:

No pharmacokinetic studies have been conducted in subjects with hepatic insufficiency.

Geriatrics:

Limited data from controlled pharmacokinetic studies of metformin in healthy elderly subjects suggest that total plasma clearance is decreased, the half-life is prolonged and C_{max} is increased, compared to healthy young subjects. From these data, it appears that the change in metformin pharmacokinetics with aging is primarily accounted for by a change in renal function (see Table 4).

[See table at bottom of next page.]

Pediatrics:

No pharmacokinetic studies have been conducted in pediatric subjects.

Gender:

Metformin pharmacokinetic parameters did not differ significantly in diabetic and nondiabetic subjects when analyzed according to gender (males=19, females=16). Similarly, in controlled clinical studies in patients with NIDDM, the antihyperglycemic effect of GLUCOPHAGE (metformin hydrochloride tablets) was comparable in males and females.

Race:

No studies of metformin pharmacokinetic parameters according to race have been performed. In controlled clinical studies of GLUCOPHAGE in patients with NIDDM, the antihyperglycemic effect was comparable in whites (n=249), blacks (n=51) and hispanics (n=24).

INDICATIONS AND USE

GLUCOPHAGE (metformin hydrochloride tablets), as monotherapy, is indicated as an adjunct to diet to lower blood glucose in patients with NIDDM whose hyperglycemia cannot be satisfactorily managed on diet alone.

GLUCOPHAGE may be used concomitantly with a sulfonylurea when diet and GLUCOPHAGE or a sulfonylurea alone do not result in adequate glycemic control.

In initiating treatment for NIDDM, diet should be emphasized as the primary form of treatment. Caloric restriction and weight loss are essential in the obese diabetic patient. Proper dietary management alone may be effective in controlling the blood glucose and symptoms of hyperglycemia. Loss of blood glucose control in diet-managed patients may be transient, thus requiring only short-term pharmacologic therapy. The importance of regular physical activity should also be stressed, and cardiovascular risk factors should be identified and corrective measures taken where possible. If this treatment program fails to reduce symptoms and/or blood glucose, the use of GLUCOPHAGE alone or GLUCOPHAGE plus a sulfonylurea should be considered.

If, after a suitable trial of such treatments, glucose control still has not been achieved, consideration should be given to the use of insulin. Judgments should be based on regular clinical and laboratory evaluations.

CONTRAINDICATIONS

GLUCOPHAGE is contraindicated in patients with:

1. Renal disease or renal dysfunction (e.g., as suggested by serum creatinine levels ≥ 1.5 mg/dL [males], ≥ 1.4 mg/dL [females] or abnormal creatinine clearance) which may also result from conditions such as cardiovascular collapse (shock), acute myocardial infarction, and septicemia (see WARNINGS and PRECAUTIONS).

2. GLUCOPHAGE should be temporarily withheld in patients undergoing radiologic studies involving parenteral administration of iodinated contrast materials, because use of such products may result in acute alteration of renal function. (See also PRECAUTIONS.)

3. Known hypersensitivity to metformin hydrochloride.

4. Acute or chronic metabolic acidosis, including diabetic ketoacidosis, with or without coma. Diabetic ketoacidosis should be treated with insulin.

WARNINGS

Lactic Acidosis:

Lactic acidosis is a rare, but serious, metabolic complication that can occur due to metformin accumulation during treatment with GLUCOPHAGE; when it occurs, it is fatal in approximately 50% of cases. Lactic acidosis may also occur in association with a number of pathophysiologic conditions, including diabetes mellitus, and whenever there is significant tissue hypoperfusion and hypoxemia. Lactic acidosis is characterized by elevated blood lactate levels (> 5 mmol/L), decreased blood pH, electrolyte disturbances with an increased anion gap, and an increased lactate/pyruvate ratio. When metformin is implicated as the cause of lactic acidosis, metformin plasma levels $> 5 \mu g/mL$ are generally found.

The reported incidence of lactic acidosis in patients receiving metformin hydrochloride is very low (approximately 0.03 cases/1,000 patient-years, with approximately 0.015 fatal cases/1,000 patient-years). Reported cases have occurred primarily in diabetic patients with significant renal insufficiency, including both intrinsic renal disease and renal hypoperfusion, often in the setting of multiple concomitant medical/surgical problems and multiple concomitant medications. The risk of lactic acidosis increases with the degree of renal dysfunction and the patient's age. The risk of lactic acidosis may, therefore, be significantly decreased by regular monitoring of renal function in patients taking GLUCOPHAGE and by the use of the mini-

Table 3. Summary of Mean Percent Reduction of Major Serum Lipid Variables at Final Visit (29-week study)

	Glucophage vs. Placebo (% Change from Baseline)		Combined Glucophage/Glyburide vs. Monotherapy (% Change from Baseline)		
	Glucophage (n =141)	Placebo (n =145)	Glucophage (n =210)	Glucophage/ Glyburide (n =213)	Glyburide (n =209)
Total Cholesterol	−5%*	1%	− 2%	−4%**	1%
Total Triglycerides	−16%	1%	− 3%**	−8%**	4%
LDL-Cholesterol	−8%*	1%	− 4%**	−6%**	3%
HDL-Cholesterol	2%	−1%	5%	3%	1%

* <0.05 vs. Placebo
** <0.05 vs. Glyburide

Continued on next page

Bristol-Myers Squibb Co.—Cont.

mum effective dose of GLUCOPHAGE. In addition, GLUCOPHAGE should be promptly withheld in the presence of any condition associated with hypoxemia or dehydration. Because impaired hepatic function may significantly limit the ability to clear lactate, GLUCOPHAGE (metformin hydrochloride tablets) should generally be avoided in patients with clinical or laboratory evidence of hepatic disease. Patients should be cautioned against excessive alcohol intake, either acute or chronic, when taking GLUCOPHAGE (metformin hydrochloride tablets), since alcohol potentiates the effects of metformin hydrochloride on lactate metabolism. In addition, GLUCOPHAGE should be temporarily discontinued prior to any intravascular radiocontrast study for any surgical procedure (see also PRECAUTIONS).

The onset of lactic acidosis often is subtle, and accompanied only by nonspecific symptoms such as malaise, myalgias, respiratory distress, increasing somnolence and nonspecific abdominal distress. There may be associated hypothermia, hypotension and resistant bradyarrhythmias with more marked acidosis. The patient and the patient's physician must be aware of the possible importance of such symptoms and the patient should be instructed to notify the physician immediately if they occur (see also PRECAUTIONS). GLUCOPHAGE should be withdrawn until the situation is clarified. Serum electrolytes, ketones, blood glucose and, if indicated, blood pH, lactate levels and even blood metformin levels may be useful. Once a patient is stabilized on any dose level of GLUCOPHAGE, gastrointestinal symptoms, which are common during initiation of therapy, are unlikely to be drug related. Later occurrence of gastrointestinal symptoms could be due to lactic acidosis or other serious disease.

Levels of fasting venous plasma lactate above the upper limit of normal but less than 5 mmol/L in patients taking GLUCOPHAGE do not necessarily indicate impending lactic acidosis and may be explainable by other mechanisms, such as poorly controlled diabetes or obesity, vigorous physical activity or technical problems in sample handling. (See also PRECAUTIONS.)

Lactic acidosis should be suspected in any diabetic patient with metabolic acidosis lacking evidence of ketoacidosis (ketonuria and ketonemia).

Lactic acidosis is a medical emergency that must be treated in a hospital setting. In a patient with lactic acidosis who is taking GLUCOPHAGE, the drug should be discontinued immediately and general supportive measures promptly instituted. Because metformin hydrochloride is dialyzable (with a clearance of up to 170 mL/min under good hemodynamic conditions), prompt hemodialysis is recommended to correct the acidosis and remove the accumulated metformin. Such management often results in prompt reversal of symptoms and recovery. (See also CONTRAINDICATIONS and PRECAUTIONS).

SPECIAL WARNING ON INCREASED RISK OF CARDIOVASCULAR MORTALITY:

The administration of oral antidiabetic drugs has been reported to be associated with increased cardiovascular mortality as compared to treatment with diet alone or diet plus insulin. This warning is based on the study conducted by the University Group Diabetes Program (UGDP), a long-term prospective clinical trial designed to evaluate the effectiveness of glucose-lowering drugs in preventing or delaying vascular complications in patients with non-insulin-dependent diabetes. The study involved 1027 patients who were randomly assigned to one of five treatment groups (*Diabetes*, 19 (Suppl.2):747–830, 1970; ***Diabetes*,** 24 (Suppl.1):65–184, 1975).

The UGDP reported that patients treated for 5 to 8 years with diet plus a fixed dose of tolbutamide (1.5 g per day) or diet plus a fixed dose of phenformin (100 mg per day), had a rate of cardiovascular mortality approximately 2.5 times that of patients treated with diet alone, resulting in discontinuation of both these treatments in the UGDP study. Total mortality was increased in both the tolbutamide- and phenformin-treated groups and this increase was statistically significant in the phenformin-treated group. Despite controversy regarding the interpretation of these results, the findings of the UGDP study provide an adequate basis for this warning. The patient should be informed of the potential risks and benefits of GLUCOPHAGE and alternative modes of therapy.

Although only one drug in the sulfonylurea category (tolbutamide) and one in the biguanide category (phenformin) were included in this study, it is prudent from a safety standpoint to consider that this warning may also apply to other related oral antidiabetic drugs, in view of the similarities in mode of action and chemical structure among the drugs in each category.

PRECAUTIONS

General:

Monitoring of renal function—GLUCOPHAGE is known to be substantially excreted by the kidney, and the risk of metformin accumulation and lactic acidosis increases with the degree of impairment of renal function. Thus, patients with serum creatinine levels above the upper limit of normal for their age should not receive GLUCOPHAGE. In patients with advanced age, GLUCOPHAGE should be carefully titrated to establish the minimum dose for adequate glycemic effect, because aging is associated with reduced renal function. In elderly patients, renal function should be monitored regularly and, generally, GLUCOPHAGE should not be titrated to the maximum dose (see DOSAGE AND ADMINISTRATION).

Before initiation of GLUCOPHAGE therapy and at least annually thereafter, renal function should be assessed and verified as normal. In patients in whom development of renal dysfunction is anticipated, renal function should be assessed more frequently and GLUCOPHAGE discontinued if evidence of renal impairment is present.

Use of concomitant medications that may affect renal function or metformin disposition—Concomitant medication(s) that may affect renal function or result in significant hemodynamic change or may interfere with the disposition of GLUCOPHAGE, such as cationic drugs that are eliminated by renal tubular secretion (See Drug Interactions), should be used with caution.

Radiologic studies involving the use of iodinated contrast materials (for example, intravenous urogram, intravenous cholangiography, angiography, and scans with contrast materials)—Parenteral contrast studies with iodinated materials can lead to acute renal failure and have been associated with lactic acidosis in patients receiving GLUCOPHAGE (see CONTRAINDICATIONS). Therefore, in patients in whom any such study is planned, GLUCOPHAGE should be withheld for at least 48 hours prior to, and 48 hours subsequent to, the procedure and reinstituted only after renal function has been re-evaluated and found to be normal.

Hypoxic states—Cardiovascular collapse (shock) from whatever cause, acute congestive heart failure, acute myocardial infarction and other conditions characterized by hypoxemia have been associated with lactic acidosis and may also cause prerenal azotemia. When such events occur in patients on GLUCOPHAGE therapy, the drug should be promptly discontinued.

Surgical procedures—GLUCOPHAGE therapy should be temporarily suspended for any surgical procedure (except minor procedures not associated with restricted intake of food and fluids) and should not be restarted until the patient's oral intake has resumed and renal function has been evaluated as normal.

Alcohol intake—Alcohol is known to potentiate the effect of metformin on lactate metabolism. Patients, therefore, should be warned against excessive alcohol intake, acute or chronic, while receiving GLUCOPHAGE.

Impaired hepatic function—Since impaired hepatic function has been asociated with some cases of lactic acidosis, GLUCOPHAGE should generally be avoided in patients with clinical or laboratory evidence of hepatic disease.

Vitamin B_{12} levels—A decrease to subnormal levels of previously normal serum vitamin B_{12} levels, without clinical manifestations, is observed in approximately 7% of patients receiving GLUCOPHAGE in controlled clinical trials of 29 weeks duration. Such decrease, possibly due to interference with B_{12} absorption from the B_{12}-intrinsic factor complex, is, however, very rarely associated with anemia and appears to be rapidly reversible with discontinuation of GLUCOPHAGE (metformin hydrochloride tablets) or vitamin B_{12} supplementation. Measurement of hematologic parameters on an annual basis is advised in patients on GLUCOPHAGE and any apparent abnormalities should be appropriately investigated and managed (see Laboratory Tests).

Certain individuals (those with inadequate vitamin B_{12} or calcium intake or absorption) appear to be predisposed to developing subnormal vitamin B_{12} levels. In these patients, routine serum vitamin B_{12} measurements at two- to three-year intervals may be useful.

Change in clinical status of previously controlled diabetic—A diabetic patient previously well controlled on GLUCOPHAGE who develops laboratory abnormalities or clinical illness (especially vague and poorly defined illness) should be evaluated promptly for evidence of ketoacidosis or lactic acidosis. Evaluation should include serum electrolytes and ketones, blood glucose and, if indicated, blood pH, lactate, pyruvate and metformin levels. If acidosis of either form occurs, GLUCOPHAGE must be stopped immediately and other appropriate corrective measures initiated (see also WARNINGS).

Hypoglycemia—Hypoglycemia does not occur in patients receiving GLUCOPHAGE alone under usual circumstances of use, but could occur when caloric intake is deficient, when strenuous exercise is not compensated by caloric supplementation, or during concomitant use with other glucose-lowering agents (such as sulfonylureas) or ethanol.

Elderly, debilitated or malnourished patients, and those with adrenal or pituitary insufficiency or alcohol intoxication are particularly susceptible to hypoglycemic effects. Hypoglycemia may be difficult to recognize in the elderly, and in people who are taking beta-adrenergic blocking drugs.

Loss of control of blood glucose—When a patient stabilized on any diabetic regimen is exposed to stress such as fever, trauma, infection, or surgery, a temporary loss of glycemic control may occur. At such times, it may be necessary to withhold GLUCOPHAGE and temporarily administer insulin. GLUCOPHAGE may be reinstituted after the acute episode is resolved.

The effectiveness of oral antidiabetic drugs in lowering blood glucose to a targeted level decreases in many patients over a period of time. This phenomenon, which may be due to progression of the underlying disease or to diminished responsiveness to the drug, is known as secondary failure, to distinguish it from primary failure in which the drug is ineffective during initial therapy. Should secondary failure occur with GLUCOPHAGE or sulfonylurea monotherapy, combined therapy with GLUCOPHAGE (metformin hydrochloride tablets) and sulfonylurea may result in a response. Should secondary failure occur with combined GLUCOPHAGE/sulfonylurea therapy, it may be necessary to initiate insulin therapy.

Information for Patients:

Patients should be informed of the potential risks and advantages of GLUCOPHAGE and of alternative modes of therapy. They should also be informed about the importance of adherence to dietary instructions, of a regular exercise pro-

Table 4. Select Mean (±S.D.) Metformin Pharmacokinetic Parameters Following Single or Multiple Oral Doses of GLUCOPHAGE

Subject Groups: GLUCOPHAGE dose[a] (number of subjects)	C_{max}[b] (μg/mL)	t_{max}[c] (hrs)	**Renal Clearance (mL/min)**
Healthy, nondiabetic adults:			
500 mg SD[d] (24)	1.03 (±0.33)	2.75 (±0.81)	600 (±132)
850 mg SD (74)[e]	1.60 (±0.38)	2.64 (±0.82)	552 (±139)
850 mg t.i.d. for 19 doses[f] (9)	2.01 (±0.42)	1.79 (±0.94)	642 (±173)
Adults with NIDDM:			
850 mg SD (23)	1.48 (±0.5)	3.32 (±1.08)	491 (±138)
850 mg t.i.d. for 19 doses[f] (9)	1.90 (±0.62)	2.01 (±1.22)	550 (±160)
Elderly[g], healthy nondiabetic adults:			
850 mg SD (12)	2.45 (±0.70)	2.71 (±1.05)	412 (±98)
Renal-impaired adults: 850 mg SD			
Mild (CL_{cr}[h] 61–90 mL/min) (5)	1.86 (±0.52)	3.20 (±0.45)	384 (±122)
Moderate (CL_{cr} 31–60 mL/min) (4)	4.12 (±1.83)	3.75 (±0.50)	108 (±57)
Severe (CL_{cr} 10–30 mL/min) (6)	3.93 (±0.92)	4.01 (±1.10)	130 (±90)

[a]–All doses given fasting except the first 18 doses of the multiple dose studies;
[b]–Peak plasma concentration;
[c]–Time to peak plasma concentration;
[d]–SD=single dose;
[e]–Combined results (average means) of five studies: mean age 32 years (range 23–59 yrs).
[f]–Kinetic study done following dose 19, given fasting.
[g]–Elderly subjects, mean age 71 years (range 65–81 years).
[h]–CL_{cr}=creatinine clearance normalized to body surface area of 1.73 m^2.

gram, and of regular testing of blood glucose, glycosylated hemoglobin, renal function and hematologic parameters. The risks of lactic acidosis, its symptoms, and conditions that predispose to its development, as noted in the WARNINGS and PRECAUTIONS sections should be explained to patients. Patients should be advised to discontinue GLUCO-PHAGE immediately and to promptly notify their health practitioner if unexplained hyperventilation, myalgia, malaise, unusual somnolence or other nonspecific symptoms occur. Once a patient is stabilized on any dose level of GLUCOPHAGE, gastrointestinal symptoms, which are common during initiation of therapy, are unlikely to be drug related. Later occurrence of gastrointestinal symptoms could be due to lactic acidosis or other serious disease.

Patients should be counselled against excessive alcohol intake, either acute or chronic, while receiving GLUCO-PHAGE.

GLUCOPHAGE alone does not usually cause hypoglycemia, although it may occur when GLUCOPHAGE is used in conjunction with oral sulfonylureas. When initiating combination therapy, the risks of hypoglycemia, its symptoms and treatment, and conditions that predispose to its development should be explained to patients.

(See Patient Labeling Printed Below)

Laboratory Tests:
Response to all diabetic therapies should be monitored by periodic measurements of fasting blood glucose and glycosylated hemoglobin levels, with a goal of decreasing these levels toward the normal range. During initial dose titration, fasting glucose can be used to determine the therapeutic response. Thereafter, both glucose and glycosylated hemoglobin should be monitored. Measurements of glycosylated hemoglobin may be especially useful for evaluating long-term control (see also DOSAGE AND ADMINISTRATION). Initial and periodic monitoring of hematologic parameters (e.g., hemoglobin/hematocrit and red blood cell indices) and renal function (serum creatinine) should be performed, at least on an annual basis. While megaloblastic anemia has rarely been seen with GLUCOPHAGE (metformin hydrochloride tablets) therapy, if this is suspected, vitamin B_{12} deficiency should be excluded.

Drug Interactions:
Glyburide: In a single-dose interaction study in NIDDM subjects, co-administration of metformin and glyburide did not result in any changes in either metformin pharmacokinetics or pharmacodynamics. Decreases in glyburide AUC and C_{max} were observed, but were highly variable. The single-dose nature of this study and the lack of correlation between glyburide blood levels and pharmacodynamic effects, makes the clinical significance of this interaction uncertain (see DOSAGE AND ADMINISTRATION, Concomitant Glucophage and Oral Sulfonylurea Therapy).

Furosemide: A single-dose, metformin-furosemide drug interaction study in healthy subjects demonstrated that pharmacokinetic parameters of both compounds were affected by co-administration. Furosemide increased the metformin plasma and blood C_{max} by 22% and blood AUC by 15%, without any significant change in metformin renal clearance. When administered with metformin, the C_{max} and AUC of furosemide were 31% and 12% smaller, respectively, than when administered alone, and the terminal half-life was decreased by 32%, without any significant change in furosemide renal clearance. No information is available about the interaction of metformin and furosemide when co-administered chronically.

Nifedipine: A single-dose, metformin-nifedipine drug interaction study in normal healthy volunteers demonstrated that co-administration of nifedipine increased plasma metformin C_{max} and AUC by 20% and 9%, respectively, and increased the amount excreted in the urine. T_{max} and half-life were unaffected. Nifedipine appears to enhance the absorption metformin. Metformin had minimal effects on nifedipine.

Cationic Drugs: Cationic drugs (e.g., amiloride, digoxin, morphine, procainamide, quinidine, quinine, ranitidine, triamterene, trimethoprim, and vancomycin) that are eliminated by renal tubular secretion theoretically have the potential for interaction with metformin by competing for common renal tubular transport systems. Such interaction between metformin and oral cimetidine has been observed in normal healthy volunteers in both single- and multiple-dose, metformin-cimetidine drug interaction studies, with a 60% increase in peak metformin plasma and whole blood concentrations and a 40% increase in plasma and whole blood metformin AUC. There was no change in elimination half-life in the single-dose study. Metformin had no effect on cimetidine pharmacokinetics. Although such interactions remain theoretical (except for cimetidine), careful patient monitoring and dose adjustment of GLUCOPHAGE and/or the interfering drug is recommended in patients who are taking cationic medications that are excreted via the proximal renal tubular secretory system.

Other: Certain drugs tend to produce hyperglycemia and may lead to loss of glycemic control. These drugs include thiazide and other diuretics, corticosteroids, phenothiazines, thyroid products, estrogens, oral contraceptives, phenytoin,

nicotinic acid, sympathomimetics, calcium channel blocking drugs, and isoniazid. When such drugs are administered to a patient receiving GLUCOPHAGE, the patient should be closely observed to maintain adequate glycemic control.

In healthy volunteers, the pharmacokinetics of metformin and propranolol and metformin and Ibuprofen were not affected when co-administered in single-dose interaction studies.

Metformin is negligibly bound to plasma proteins and is, therefore, less likely to interact with highly protein-bound drugs such as salicylates, sulfonamides, chloramphenicol, and probenecid, as compared to the sulfonylureas, which are extensively bound to serum proteins.

Carcinogenesis, Mutagenesis, Impairment of Fertility:
Long-term carcinogenicity studies have been performed in rats (dosing duration of 104 weeks) and mice (dosing duration of 91 weeks) at doses up to and including 900 mg/kg/day and 1500 mg/kg/day, respectively. These doses are both approximately three times the maximum recommended human daily dose on a body surface area basis. No evidence of carcinogenicity with metformin was found in either male or female mice. Similarly, there was no tumorigenic potential observed with metformin in male rats. However, an increased incidence of benign stromal uterine polyps was seen in female rats treated with 900 mg/kg/day.

No evidence of a mutagenic potential to metformin was found in the Ames test (*S. typhimurium*), gene mutation test (mouse lymphoma cells), chromosomal aberrations test (human lymphocytes), or *in-vivo* micronuclei formation test (mouse bone marrow).

Fertility of male or female rats was unaffected by metformin administration at doses as high as 600 mg/kg/day, or approximately two times the maximum recommended human daily dose on a body surface area basis.

Pregnancy:
Teratogenic effects:
Pregnancy Category B. Safety in pregnant women has not been established. Metformin was not teratogenic in rats and rabbits at doses up to 600 mg/kg/day, or about two times the maximum recommended human daily dose on a body surface area basis. Determination of fetal concentrations demonstrated a partial placental barrier to metformin. Because animal reproduction studies are not always predictive of human response, any decision to use this drug should be balanced against the benefits and risks.

Because recent information suggests that abnormal blood glucose levels during pregnancy are associated with a higher incidence of congenital abnormalities, there is a consensus among experts that insulin be used during pregnancy to maintain blood glucose levels as close to normal as possible.

Nursing Mothers:
Studies in lactating rats show that metformin is excreted into milk and reaches levels comparable to those in plasma. Similar studies have not been conducted in nursing mothers, but caution should be exercised in such patients, and a decision should be made whether to discontinue nursing or to discontinue the drug, taking into account the importance of the drug to the mother.

Pediatric Use:
Safety and effectiveness in children have not been established. Studies in maturity-onset diabetes of the young (MODY) have not been conducted.

Geriatric Use:
Controlled clinical studies of GLUCOPHAGE (metformin hydrochloride tablets) did not include sufficient numbers of elderly patients to determine whether they respond differently from younger patients, although other reported clinical experience has not identified differences in responses between the elderly and younger patients. GLUCOPHAGE is known to be substantially excreted by the kidney and because the risk of serious adverse reactions to the drug is greater in patients with impaired renal function, it should only be used in patients with normal renal function (see CONTRAINDICATIONS, CLINICAL PHARMACOLOGY, Pharmacokinetics). Because aging is associated with reduced renal function, GLUCOPHAGE should be used with caution as age increases. Care should be taken in dose selection and should be based on careful and regular monitoring of renal function. Generally, elderly patients should not be titrated to the maximum dose of GLUCOPHAGE (see also DOSAGE AND ADMINISTRATION).

ADVERSE REACTIONS
Lactic Acidosis: See WARNINGS, PRECAUTIONS and OVERDOSAGE Sections.
Gastrointestinal Reactions: Gastrointestinal symptoms (diarrhea, nausea, vomiting, abdominal bloating, flatulence, and anorexia) are the most common reactions to GLUCO-PHAGE and are approximately 30% more frequent in patients on GLUCOPHAGE monotherapy than in placebo-treated patients, particularly during initiation of GLUCO-PHAGE therapy. These symptoms are generally transient and resolve spontaneously during continued treatment. Occasionally, temporary dose reduction may be useful. In controlled trials, GLUCOPHAGE was discontinued due to gastrointestinal reactions in approximately 4% of patients.

Because gastrointestinal symptoms during therapy initiation appear to be dose-related, they may be decreased by gradual dose escalation and by having patients take GLUCO-PHAGE (metformin hydrochloride tablets) with meals (see DOSAGE and ADMINISTRATION).

Because significant diarrhea and/or vomiting may cause dehydration and prerenal azotemia, under such circumstances, GLUCOPHAGE should be temporarily discontinued.

For patients who have been stabilized on GLUCOPHAGE, nonspecific gastrointestinal symptoms should not be attributed to therapy unless intercurrent illness or lactic acidosis have been excluded.

Special Senses: During initiation of GLUCOPHAGE therapy, approximately 3% of patients may complain of an unpleasant or metallic taste, which usually resolves spontaneously.

Dermatologic Reactions: The incidence of rash/dermatitis in controlled clinical trials was comparable to placebo for GLUCOPHAGE monotherapy and to sulfonylurea for GLUCOPHAGE/sulfonylurea therapy.

Hematologic: (See also PRECAUTIONS). During controlled clinical trials of 29 weeks duration, approximately 9% of patients on GLUCOPHAGE monotherapy and 6% of patients on GLUCOPHAGE/sulfonylurea therapy developed asymptomatic subnormal serum vitamin B_{12} levels; serum folic acid levels did not decrease significantly. However, only five cases of megaloblastic anemia have been reported with metformin administration (none during U.S. clinical studies) and no increased incidence of neuropathy has been observed. Therefore, serum B_{12} levels should be appropriately monitored or periodic parenteral B_{12} supplementation considered.

DRUG ABUSE AND DEPENDENCE
GLUCOPHAGE possesses no pharmacodynamic properties, either primary or secondary, which could be expected to result in abuse as a recreational drug or addiction.

OVERDOSAGE
Hypoglycemia has not been seen with ingestion of up to 85 grams of GLUCOPHAGE, although lactic acidosis has occurred in such circumstances (see WARNINGS). Metformin is dialyzable with a clearance of up to 170 mL/min under good hemodynamic conditions. Therefore, hemodialysis may be useful for removal of accumulated drug from patients in whom metformin overdosage is suspected.

DOSAGE AND ADMINISTRATION
There is no fixed dosage regimen for the management of hyperglycemia in diabetes mellitus with GLUCOPHAGE or any other pharmacologic agent. Dosage of GLUCOPHAGE must be individualized on the basis of both effectiveness and tolerance, while not exceeding the maximum recommended daily dose of 2550 mg. GLUCOPHAGE should be given in divided doses with meals and should be started at a low dose, with gradual dose escalation, as described below, both to reduce gastrointestinal side effects and to permit identification of the minimum dose required for adequate glycemic control of the patient.

During treatment initiation and dose titration (see below, USUAL STARTING DOSE), fasting plasma glucose should be used to determine the therapeutic response to GLUCO-PHAGE and identify the minimum effective dose for the patient. Thereafter, glycosylated hemoglobin should be measured at intervals of approximately three months. **The therapeutic goal should be to decrease both fasting plasma glucose and glycosylated hemoglobin levels to normal or near normal by using the lowest effective dose of GLUCOPHAGE, either when used as monotherapy or in combination with sulfonylurea.**

Monitoring of blood glucose and glycosylated hemoglobin will also permit detection of primary failure, i.e., inadequate lowering of blood glucose at the maximum recommended dose of medication, and secondary failure, i.e., loss of an adequate blood glucose lowering response after an initial period of effectiveness.

Short-term administration of GLUCOPHAGE (metformin hydrochloride tablets) may be sufficient during periods of transient loss of control in patients usually well-controlled on diet alone.

Usual Starting Dose:
In general, clinically significant responses are not seen at doses below 1500 mg per day. However, a lower recommended starting dose and gradually increased dosage is advised to minimize gastrointestinal symptoms.

GLUCOPHAGE 500 mg Tablets:
The usual starting dose of GLUCOPHAGE 500 mg tablets is one tablet b.i.d., given with the morning and evening meals. Dosage increases should be made in increments of one tablet every week, given in divided doses, up to a maximum of 2500 mg per day. GLUCOPHAGE can be administered twice a day up to 2000 mg per day (e.g., 1000 mg b.i.d. with morning and evening meals). If a 2500 mg daily dose is required, it may be better tolerated given t.i.d. with meals.

Continued on next page

Bristol-Myers Squibb Co.—Cont.

GLUCOPHAGE 850 mg Tablets:
The usual starting dose of GLUCOPHAGE 850 mg tablets is one tablet daily, given with the morning meal. Dosage increases should be made in increments of one tablet every OTHER week, given in divided doses, up to a maximum of 2550 mg per day. The usual maintenance dose is 850 mg b.i.d. with the morning and evening meals. When necessary, patients may be given 850 mg t.i.d. with meals.

Transfer from Other Antidiabetic Therapy:
When transferring patients from standard oral hypoglycemic agents other than chlorpropamide to GLUCOPHAGE, no transition period generally is necessary. While transferring patients from chlorpropamide, care should be exercised during the first two weeks because of the prolonged retention of chlorpropamide in the body, leading to overlapping drug effects and possible hypoglycemia.

Concomitant GLUCOPHAGE and Oral Sulfonylurea Therapy:
If patients have not responded to four weeks of the maximum dose of GLUCOPHAGE monotherapy, consideration should be given to gradual addition of an oral sulfonylurea while continuing GLUCOPHAGE at the maximum dose, even if prior primary or secondary failure to a sulfonylurea has occurred. Clinical and pharmacokinetic drug-drug interaction data are currently available only for metformin plus glyburide (glibenclamide). Published clinical information exists for the use of metformin with either chlorpropamide, tolbutamide or glipizide. No published clinical information exists regarding concomitant use of metformin with acetohexamide or tolazamide.
With concomitant GLUCOPHAGE and sulfonylurea therapy, the desired control of blood glucose may be obtained by adjusting the dose of each drug. However, attempts should be made to identify the minimum effective dose of each drug to achieve this goal. With concomitant GLUCOPHAGE and sulfonylurea therapy, the risk of hypoglycemia associated with sulfonylurea therapy continues and may be increased. Appropriate precautions should be taken. (See Package Insert of the respective sulfonylurea).
If patients have not satisfactorily responded to one to three months of concomitant therapy with the maximum dose of GLUCOPHAGE and the maximum dose of an oral sulfonylurea, institution of insulin therapy and discontinuation of these oral agents should be considered.

Specific Patient Populations:
GLUCOPHAGE is not recommended for use in pregnancy or for use in children.
The initial and maintenance dosing of GLUCOPHAGE should be conservative in patients with advanced age, due to the potential for decreased renal function in this population. Any dosage adjustment should be based on a careful assessment of renal function. Generally, elderly patients should not be titrated to the maximum dose of GLUCOPHAGE.
In debilitated or malnourished patients, the dosing should also be conservative and based on a careful assessment of renal function.

HOW SUPPLIED

GLUCOPHAGE® (brand of metformin hydrochloride tablets) is supplied as white, unscored, film-coated, cylindrical, biconvex tablets, available in the following strengths:

500 mg	Bottles of 100	NDC 0087-6060-05
850 mg	Bottles of 100	NDC 0087-6070-05

Tablets are debossed with the letters "GL" and either "500" or "850" to indicate strength.

Storage
Store between 15°–30°C (59°–86°F).

PATIENT INFORMATION ABOUT GLUCOPHAGE® (metformin hydrochloride tablets) 500 mg and 850 mg

WARNING: A small number of people who have taken Glucophage have developed a serious condition called lactic acidosis. Properly functioning kidneys are needed to help prevent lactic acidosis. Most people with kidney problems should not take Glucophage. (See Question Nos. 7–11)

Q1. Why do I need to take GLUCOPHAGE?
Your doctor has prescribed GLUCOPHAGE (GLUE-coe-fahj) to treat your type II diabetes. This is also known as non-insulin-dependent diabetes mellitus (NIDDM).

Q2. What is type II diabetes?
People with diabetes are not able to make enough insulin and/or respond normally to the insulin their body does make. When this happens, sugar (glucose) builds up in the blood. This can lead to serious medical problems including kidney damage, amputations and blindness. Diabetes is also closely linked to heart disease. The main goal of treating diabetes is to lower your blood sugar to a normal level.

Q3. How is type II diabetes usually controlled?
High blood sugar can be lowered by diet and exercise, by a number of oral medications and by insulin injections. Before taking GLUCOPHAGE you should first try to control your diabetes by exercise and weight loss. Even if you are taking GLUCOPHAGE, you should still exercise and follow the diet recommended for your diabetes.

Q4. Does GLUCOPHAGE work differently from other glucose-control medications?
Yes it does. Until GLUCOPHAGE was introduced, all the available oral glucose-control medications were from the same chemical group called sulfonylureas. These drugs lower blood sugar primarily by causing more of the body's own insulin to be released. GLUCOPHAGE (metformin hydrochloride tablets) lowers the amount of sugar in your blood by helping your body respond better to its own insulin. GLUCOPHAGE does not cause your body to produce more insulin. Therefore, GLUCOPHAGE rarely causes hypoglycemia (low blood sugar) and it doesn't usually cause weight gain.

Q5. What happens if my blood sugar is still too high?
When blood sugar cannot be lowered enough by either GLUCOPHAGE (metformin hydrochloride tablets) or a sulfonylurea, the two medications may be effective taken together. However, if you are unable to maintain your blood sugar with diet, exercise and glucose-control medication taken orally, then your doctor may prescribe injectable insulin to control your diabetes.

Q6. Can GLUCOPHAGE cause side effects?
GLUCOPHAGE, like all blood-sugar lowering medications, can cause side effects in some patients. Most of these side effects are minor and will go away after you've taken GLUCOPHAGE for a while. However, there are also serious, but rare side effects related to GLUCOPHAGE (see below).

Q7. What kind of side effects can GLUCOPHAGE cause?
If side effects occur, they usually occur during the first few weeks in therapy. They are normally minor ones such as diarrhea, nausea and upset stomach. Taking your GLUCOPHAGE with meals can help reduce these side effects.
Although these side effects are likely to go away, call your doctor if you have severe discomfort or if these effects last for more than a few weeks. Some patients may need to have their dose lowered or stop taking GLUCOPHAGE, either temporarily or permanently. Although these problems occur in up to one-third of patients when they first start taking GLUCOPHAGE, you should tell your doctor if the problems come back or start later on during the therapy.
About three out of one hundred people report having a temporary unpleasant or metallic taste when they start taking GLUCOPHAGE.

Q8. Are there any serious side effects that GLUCOPHAGE can cause?
GLUCOPHAGE rarely causes serious side effects. The most serious side effect that GLUCOPHAGE can cause is called lactic acidosis.

Q9. What is lactic acidosis and can it happen to me?
Lacitic acidosis is caused by a buildup of lactic acid in the blood. Lactic acidosis associated with GLUCOPHAGE is rare and has occurred mostly in people whose kidneys were not working normally. Lactic acidosis has been reported in about one in 33,000 patients taking GLUCOPHAGE over the course of a year. Although rare, if lactic acidosis does occur, it can be fatal in up to half the cases.
It is also important for your liver to be working normally when you take GLUCOPHAGE. Your liver helps remove lactic acid from your bloodstream.
Your doctor will monitor your diabetes and may perform blood tests on you from time to time to make sure your kidneys and your liver are functioning normally.
There is no evidence that GLUCOPHAGE causes harm to the kidneys or liver.

Q10. Are there other risk factors for lactic acidosis?
Your risk of developing lactic acidosis from taking GLUCOPHAGE is very low as long as your kidneys and liver are healthy. However, some factors can increase your risk because they can affect kidney and liver function. You should not take GLUCOPHAGE if:

- You have chronic kidney or liver problems
- You drink alcohol excessively (all the time or short-term "binge" drinking)
- You are seriously dehydrated (have lost a large amount of body fluids)
- You are going to have certain x-ray procedures with injectable contrast agents
- You are going to have surgery
- You develop a serious condition such as a heart attack, severe infection, or a stroke.

Q11. What are the symptoms of lactic acidosis?
Some of the symptoms include: feeling very weak, tired or uncomfortable; unusual muscle pain, trouble breathing, unusual or unexpected stomach discomfort, feeling cold, feeling dizzy or lightheaded, or suddenly developing slow or irregular heartbeat.
If you notice these symptoms, or if your medical condition has suddenly changed, stop taking GLUCOPHAGE and call your doctor right away. Lactic acidosis is a medical emergency that must be treated in a hospital.

Q12. What does my doctor need to know to decrease my risk of lactic acidosis?
Tell your doctor if you have an illness that results in severe vomiting, diarrhea and/or fever, or if your intake of fluids is significantly reduced. These situations can lead to severe dehydration, and it may be necessary to stop taking GLUCOPHAGE temporarily.
You should let your doctor know if you are going to have any surgery or specialized x-ray procedures that require injection of contrast agents. GLUCOPHAGE therapy will need to be stopped temporarily in such instances.

Q13. Can I take GLUCOPHAGE with other medications?
Remind your doctor that you are taking GLUCOPHAGE when any new drug is prescribed or a change is made in how you take a drug already prescribed. GLUCOPHAGE may interfere with the way some drugs work and some drugs may interfere with the action of GLUCOPHAGE.

Q14. What if I become pregnant while taking GLUCOPHAGE?
Tell your doctor if you plan to become pregnant or have become pregnant. As with other oral glucose-control medications, you should not take GLUCOPHAGE during pregnancy.
Usually your doctor will prescribe insulin while you are pregnant. As with all medications, you and your doctor should discuss the use of GLUCOPHAGE if you are nursing a child.

Q15. Are there other risks associated with GLUCOPHAGE?
There is some evidence that any oral diabetes drug may increase the risk of heart problems. Experts are not sure what the real risk for heart problems, if any, from taking oral diabetes medicine.

Q16. How do I take GLUCOPHAGE?
Your doctor will tell you how many GLUCOPHAGE tablets to take and how often. This should also be printed on the label of your prescription. You will probably be started on a low dose of GLUCOPHAGE and your dosage will be increased gradually until your blood sugar is controlled.

Q17. Where can I get more information about GLUCOPHAGE?
This leaflet is a summary of the most important information about GLUCOPHAGE. If you have any questions or problems, you should talk to your doctor or other healthcare provider about type II diabetes as well as GLUCOPHAGE and its side effects. There is also a leaflet (package insert) written for health professionals that your pharmacist can let you read.
Glucophage is a registered trademark of LIPHA s.a.
Licensed to Bristol-Myers Squibb Company.
(P8330-00) (Issued 2/95)

Shown in Product Identification Guide, page 307

MAXIPIME® ℞

(Cefepime Hydrochloride) for Injection
For Intravenous or Intramuscular Use

Caution: Federal law prohibits dispensing without prescription

DESCRIPTION

Cefepime hydrochloride is a semi-synthetic, broad spectrum, cephalosporin antibiotic for parenteral administration. The chemical name is 1-[[(6R,7R)-7-[2- (2- amino-4-thiazolyl)-glyoxylamido]-2-carboxy-8-oxo-5-thia-1- azabicyclo[4.2.0]oct-2-en-3-yl]methyl]-1-methylpyrrolidinium chloride, 7^2-(Z)- (*O*-methyloxime), monohydrochloride, monohydrate, which corresponds to the following structural formula:

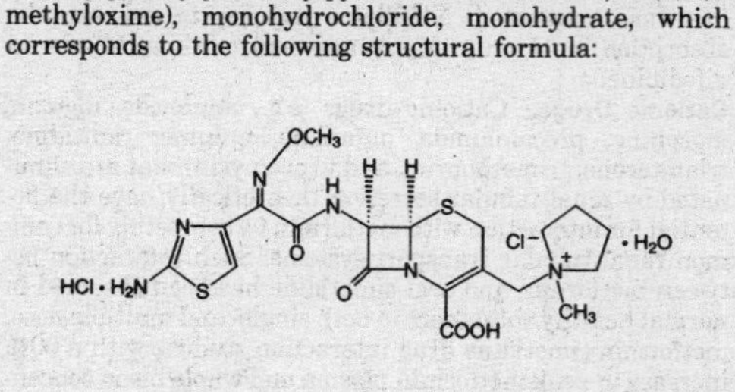

Cefepime hydrochloride is a white to pale yellow powder with a molecular formula of $C_{19}H_{25}ClN_6O_5S_2 \cdot HCl \cdot H_2O$ and a molecular weight of 571.5. It is highly soluble in water. MAXIPIME® (cefepime hydrochloride) for Injection, is supplied for intramuscular or intravenous administration in strengths equivalent to 500 mg, 1 g and 2 g of cefepime. (See **DOSAGE AND ADMINISTRATION**.) MAXIPIME is a sterile, dry mixture of cefepime hydrochloride and L-arginine. The L-arginine, at an approximate concentration of 725 mg/g of cefepime, is added to control the pH of the constituted solution at 4.0-6.0. Freshly constituted solutions of MAXIPIME will range in color from colorless to amber.

CLINICAL PHARMACOLOGY

Pharmacokinetics

The average plasma concentrations of cefepime observed in healthy adult male volunteers (n=9) at various times following single 30-minute infusions (IV) of cefepime 500 mg, 1 g, and 2 g are summarized in Table 1. Elimination of cefepime is principally via renal excretion with an average ($\pm$SD) half-life of 2.0 ($\pm$0.3) hours and total body clearance of 120.0 ($\pm$8.0) mL/min in healthy volunteers. Cefepime pharmacokinetics are linear over the range 250 mg to 2 g. There is no evidence of accumulation in healthy adult male volunteers (n=7) receiving clinically relevant doses for a period of 9 days.

Absorption

The average plasma concentrations of cefepime and its derived pharmacokinetic parameters after intravenous administration are portrayed in Table 1.

TABLE 1

Average Plasma Concentrations in µg/mL of Cefepime and Derived Pharmacokinetic Parameters ($\pm$SD), Intravenous Administration

		Maxipime	
Parameter	500 mg IV	1 g IV	2 g IV
0.5 hr	38.2	78.7	163.1
1.0 hr	21.6	44.5	85.8
2.0 hr	11.6	24.3	44.8
4.0 hr	5.0	10.5	19.2
8.0 hr	1.4	2.4	3.9
12.0 hr	0.2	0.6	1.1
C_{max}, µg/mL	39.1 (3.5)	81.7 (5.1)	163.9 (25.3)
AUC, hr·µg/mL	70.8 (6.7)	148.5 (15.1)	284.8 (30.6)
Number of subjects (male)	9	9	9

Following intramuscular (IM) administration, cefepime is completely absorbed. The average plasma concentrations of cefepime at various times following a single IM injection are summarized in Table 2. The pharmacokinetics of cefepime are linear over the range of 500 mg to 2 g IM and do not vary with respect to treatment duration.

TABLE 2

Average Plasma Concentrations in µg/mL of Cefepime and Derived Pharmacokinetic Parameters ($\pm$SD), Intramuscular Administration

		Maxipime (cefepime hydrochloride)	
Parameter	500 mg IM	1 g IM	2 g IM
0.5 hr	8.2	14.8	36.1
1.0 hr	12.5	25.9	49.9
2.0 hr	12.0	26.3	51.3
4.0 hr	6.9	16.0	31.5
8.0 hr	1.9	4.5	8.7
12.0 hr	0.7	1.4	2.3
C_{max}, µg/mL	13.9 (3.4)	29.6 (4.4)	57.5 (9.5)
T_{max}, hr	1.4 (0.9)	1.6 (0.4)	1.5 (0.4)
AUC, hr·µg/mL	60.0 (8.0)	137.0 (11.0)	262.0 (23.0)
Number of subjects (male)	6	6	12

Distribution

The average steady state volume of distribution of cefepime is 18.0 ($\pm$2.0)L. The serum protein binding of cefepime is approximately 20% and is independent of its concentration in serum.

Cefepime is excreted in human milk. A nursing infant consuming approximately 1000 mL of human milk per day would receive approximately 0.5 mg of cefepime per day. (See **PRECAUTIONS, Nursing Mothers.**)

Concentrations of cefepime achieved in specific tissues and body fluids are listed in Table 3.

TABLE 3

Average Concentrations of Cefepime in Specific Body Fluids (µg/mL) or Tissues (µg/g)

Tissue or Fluid	Dose/ Route	# of Patients	Average Time of Sample Post-Dose (hr)	Average Concentration
Blister Fluid	2 gIV	6	1.5	81.4 µg/mL
Bronchial Mucosa	2 g IV	20	4.8	24.1 µg/g
Sputum	2 g IV	5	4.0	7.4 µg/g
Urine	500 mg IV	8	0–4	292 µg/mL
	1 g IV	12	0–4	926 µg/mL
	2 g IV	12	0–4	3120 µg/mL

Data suggest that cefepime does cross the inflamed blood-brain barrier. **The clinical relevance of these data are uncertain at this time.**

Metabolism and Excretion

Cefepime is metabolized to N-methylpyrrolidine (NMP) which is rapidly converted to the N-oxide (NMP-N-oxide). Urinary recovery of unchanged cefepime accounts for approximately 85% of the administered dose. Less than 1% of the administered dose is recovered from urine as NMP, 6.8% as NMP-N-oxide, and 2.5% as an epimer of cefepime. Because renal excretion is a significant pathway of elimination, patients with renal dysfunction and patients undergoing hemodialysis require dosage adjustment. (see **DOSAGE AND ADMINISTRATION.**)

Special Populations

Geriatric patients: Cefepime pharmacokinetics have been investigated in elderly (65 years of age and older) men (n=12) and women (n=12) whose creatinine clearance was 74.0 ($\pm$15.0) mL/min. There appeared to be a decrease in cefepime total body clearance as a function of creatinine clearance. Therefore, dosage administration of cefepime in the elderly should be adjusted as appropriate if the patient's creatinine clearance is 60 mL/min or less. (See **DOSAGE AND ADMINISTRATION.**)

Renal Insufficiency: Cefepime pharmacokinetics have been investigated in patients with various degrees of renal insufficiency (n=30). The average half-life in patients requiring hemodialysis was 13.5 ($\pm$2.7) hours and in patients requiring continuous peritoneal dialysis was 19.0 ($\pm$2.0) hours. Cefepime total body clearance decreased proportionally with creatinine clearance in patients with abnormal renal function, which serves as the basis for dosage adjustment recommendations in this group of patients. (See **DOSAGE AND ADMINISTRATION.**)

Hepatic Insufficiency: The pharmacokinetics of cefepime were unaltered in patients with impaired hepatic function who received a single 1 g dose (n=11).

Microbiology

Cefepime is a bactericidal agent that acts by inhibition of bacterial cell wall synthesis. Cefepime has a broad spectrum of in vitro activity that encompasses a wide range of gram-positive and gram-negative bacteria. Cefepime has a low affinity for chromosomally-encoded beta-lactamases. Cefepime is highly resistant to hydrolysis by most beta-lactamases and exhibits rapid penetration into gram-negative bacterial cells. Within bacterial cells, the molecular targets of cefepime are the penicillin binding proteins (PBP).

Cefepime has also been shown to be active against most strains of the following microorganisms, both in vitro **and in clinical infections as described in the INDICATIONS AND USAGE section.**

Aerobic Gram-Negative Microorganisms:

Enterobacter spp.
Escherichia coli
Klebsiella pneumoniae
Proteus mirabilis

Pseudomonas aeruginosa

Aerobic Gram-Positive Microorganisms:

Staphylococcus aureus (methicillin-susceptible strains only)
Streptococcus pneumoniae
Streptococcus pyogenes (Lancefield's Group A streptococci)

The following in vitro data are available; **but their clinical significance is unknown.** Cefepime has been shown to have in vitro activity against most strains of the following microorganisms; however, the safety and effectiveness of cefepime in treating clinical infections due to these microorganisms have not been established in adequate and well-controlled trials.

Aerobic Gram-Positive Microorganisms:

Staphylococcus epidermidis (methicillin-susceptible strains only)
Staphylococcus saprophyticus
Streptococcus agalactiae (Lancefield's Group B streptococci)

NOTE: Most strains of enterococci, *e.g. Enterococcus faecalis,* and methicillin-resistant staphylococci are resistant to cefepime.

Aerobic Gram-Negative Microorganisms:

Acinetobacter calcoaceticus subsp. lwoffi
Citrobacter diversus
Citrobacter freundii
Enterobacter agglomerans
Haemophilus influenzae (including beta-lactamase producing strains)
Hafnia alvei
Klebsiella oxytoca
Moraxella (Branhamella) catarrhalis (including beta-lactamase producing strains)
Morganella morganii
Proteus vulgaris
Providencia rettgeri

Providencia stuartii
Serratia marcescens

NOTE: Cefepime is inactive against many strains of *Stenotrophomonas* (formerly *Xanthomonas maltophilia* and *Pseudomonas maltophilia*).

Anaerobic Microorganisms:

NOTE: Cefepime is inactive against most strains of *Clostridium difficile.*

Susceptibility Tests

Dilution Techniques:

Quantitative methods are used to determine antimicrobial minimum inhibitory concentrations (MIC's). These MIC's provide estimates of the susceptibility of bacteria to antimicrobial compounds. The MIC's should be determined using a standardized procedure. Standardized procedures are based on a dilution method[1] (broth or agar) or equivalent with standardized inoculum concentrations and standardized concentrations of cefepime powder. The MIC values should be interpreted according to the following criteria:

TABLE 4

Average Plasma Concentrations in µg/mL of Cefepime and Derived Pharmacokinetic Parameters ($\pm$SD), Intramuscular Administration

	MIC (µg/mL)		
Microorganism	Suscept-ible (S)	Intermed-iate (I)	Resist-ant (R)
Microorganisms other than *Haemophilus* spp.* and *S. pneumoniae**	≤8	16	≥32
Haemophilus spp.*	≤2	–*	–*
*Streptococcus pneumoniae**	≤0.5	1	≥2

*NOTE: Isolates from these species should be tested for susceptibility using specialized dilution testing methods.[1] Also, strains of *Haemophilus* spp. with MIC's greater than 2 µg/mL should be considered equivocal and should be further evaluated.

A report of "Susceptible" indicates that the pathogen is likely to be inhibited if the antimicrobial compound in the blood reaches the concentrations usually achievable. A report of "Intermediate" indicates that the result should be considered equivocal, and, if the microorganism is not fully susceptible to alternative, clinically feasible drugs, the test should be repeated. This category implies possible clinical applicability in body sites where the drug is physiologically concentrated or in situations where high dosage of drug can be used. This category also provides a buffer zone which prevents small uncontrolled technical factors from causing major discrepancies in interpretation. A report of "Resistant" indicates that the pathogen is not likely to be inhibited if the antimicrobial compound in the blood reaches the concentrations usually achievable; other therapy should be selected. Standardized susceptibility test procedures require the use of laboratory control microorganisms to control the technical aspects of the laboratory procedures. Laboratory control microorganisms are specific strains of microbiological assay organisms with intrinsic biological properties relating to resistance mechanisms and their genetic expression within bacteria; the specific strains are not clinically significant in their current microbiological status. Standard cefepime powder should provide the following MIC values (Table 5) when tested against the designated quality control strains:

TABLE 5

Microorganism	ATCC	MIC (µg/mL)
Escherichia coli	25922	0.015–0.06
Staphylococcus aureus	29213	1–4
Pseudomonas aeruginosa	27853	1–4
Haemophilus influenzae	49247	0.5–2
Streptococcus pneumoniae	49619	0.06–0.25

Diffusion techniques:

Quantitative methods that require measurement of zone diameters also provide reproducible estimates of the susceptibility of bacteria to antimicrobial compounds. One such standardized procedure[2] requires the use of standardized inoculum concentrations. This procedure uses paper disks impregnated with 30 µg of cefepime to test the susceptibility of microorganisms to cefepime. Interpretation is identical to that stated above for results using dilution techniques.

Reports from the laboratory providing results of the standard single-disk susceptibility test with a 30-µg cefepime disk should be interpreted according to the following criteria:

Continued on next page

Bristol-Myers Squibb Co.—Cont.

TABLE 6

Microorganism	Zone Diameter (mm) Suscept-ible (S)	Intermed-iate (I)	Resist-ant (R)
Microorganisms other than *Haemophilus* spp.* and *S. pneumoniae**	≥18	15–17	≤14
Haemophilus spp.*	≥26	—*	—*

*NOTE: Isolates from these species should be tested for susceptibility using specialized diffusion testing methods[2]. Isolates of *Haemophilus* spp. with zones smaller than 26 mm should be considered equivocal and should be further evaluated. Isolates of *S. pneumoniae* should be tested against a 1 μg oxacillin disk; isolates with oxacillin zone sizes larger than or equal to 20 mm may be considered susceptible to cefepime.

As with standardized dilution techniques, diffusion methods require the use of laboratory control microorganisms to control the technical aspects of the laboratory procedures. Laboratory control microorganisms are specific strains of microbiological assay organisms with intrinsic biological properties relating to resistance mechanisms and their genetic expression within bacteria; the specific strains are not clinically significant in their current microbiological status. For the diffusion technique, the 30-μg cefepime disk should provide the following zone diameters in these laboratory test quality control strains (Table 7):

TABLE 7

Microorganism	ATCC	Zone Size Range (mm)
Escherichia coli	25922	29–35
Staphylococcus aureus	25923	23–29
Pseudomonas aeruginosa	27853	24–30
Haemophilus influenzae	49247	25–31

INDICATIONS AND USAGE

MAXIPIME is indicated in the treatment of the following infections when caused by susceptible strains of the designated microorganisms:

Uncomplicated and Complicated Urinary Tract Infections (including pyelonephritis) caused by *Escherichia coli* or *Klebsiella pneumoniae,* when the infection is severe, or caused by *Escherichia coli, Klebsiella pneumoniae,* or *Proteus mirabilis,* when the infection is mild to moderate, including cases associated with concurrent bacteremia with these microorganisms.

Uncomplicated Skin and Skin Structure Infections caused by *Staphylococcus aureus* (methicillin-susceptible strains only) or *Streptococcus pyogenes.*

Pneumonia (moderate to severe) caused by *Streptococcus pneumoniae,* including cases associated with concurrent bacteremia, *Pseudomonas aeruginosa, Klebsiella pneumoniae,* or *Enterobacter* species.

Culture and susceptibility studies should be performed where appropriate to determine the susceptibility of the causative microorganism(s) to cefepime.

Therapy with MAXIPIME may be instituted before results of susceptibility studies are known; however, once these results become available, the antibiotic treatment should be adjusted accordingly.

CONTRAINDICATIONS

MAXIPIME is contraindicated in patients who have shown immediate hypersensitivity reactions to cefepime or the cephalosporin class of antibiotics, penicillins or other beta-lactam antibiotics.

WARNINGS

BEFORE THERAPY WITH MAXIPIME (CEFEPIME HYDROCHLORIDE) FOR INJECTION IS INSTITUTED, CAREFUL INQUIRY SHOULD BE MADE TO DETERMINE WHETHER THE PATIENT HAS HAD PREVIOUS IMMEDIATE HYPERSENSITIVITY REACTIONS TO CEFEPIME, CEPHALOSPORINS, PENICILLINS, OR OTHER DRUGS. IF THIS PRODUCT IS TO BE GIVEN TO PENICILLIN-SENSITIVE PATIENTS, CAUTION SHOULD BE EXERCISED BECAUSE CROSS-HYPERSENSITIVITY AMONG BETA-LACTAM ANTIBIOTICS HAS BEEN CLEARLY DOCUMENTED AND MAY OCCUR IN UP TO 10% OF PATIENTS WITH A HISTORY OF PENICILLIN ALLERGY. IF AN ALLERGIC REACTION TO MAXIPIME OCCURS, DISCONTINUE THE DRUG. SERIOUS ACUTE HYPERSENSITIVITY REACTIONS MAY REQUIRE TREATMENT WITH EPINEPHRINE AND OTHER EMERGENCY MEASURES INCLUDING OXYGEN, CORTICOSTEROIDS, INTRAVENOUS FLUIDS, INTRAVENOUS ANTIHISTAMINES, PRESSOR AMINES, AND AIRWAY MANAGEMENT, AS CLINICALLY INDICATED.

Pseudomembranous colitis has been reported with nearly all antibacterial agents, including MAXIPIME, and may range in severity from mild to life-threatening. Therefore, it is important to consider this diagnosis in patients who present with diarrhea subsequent to the administration of antibacterial agents.

Treatment with antibacterial agents alters the normal flora of the colon and may permit overgrowth clostridia. Studies indicate that a toxin produced by *Clostridium difficile* is a primary cause of "antibiotic-associated colitis".

After the diagnosis of pseudomenbranous colitis has been established, therapeutic measures should be initiated. Mild cases of pseudomembranous colitis usually respond to drug discontinuation alone. In moderate-to-severe cases, consideration should be given to management with fluids and electrolytes, protein supplementation, and treatment with an antibacterial drug clinically effective against *Clostridium difficile* colitis.

PRECAUTIONS

General

As with other antimicrobials, prolonged use of MAXIPIME may result in overgrowth of nonsusceptible microorganisms. Repeated evaluation of the patient's condition is essential. Should superinfection occur during therapy, appropriate measures should be taken.

Many cephalosporins, including cefepime, have been associated with a fall in prothrombin activity. Those at risk include patients with renal or hepatic impairment, or poor nutritional state, as well as patients receiving a protracted course of antimicrobial therapy. Prothrombin time should be monitored in patients at risk, and exogenous vitamin K administered as indicated.

Positive direct Coombs' tests have been reported during treatment with MAXIPIME. In hematologic studies or in transfusion cross-matching procedures when antiglobulin tests are performed on the minor side or in Coombs' testing of newborns whose mothers have received cephalosporin antibiotics before parturition, it should be recognized that a positive Coombs' test may be due to the drug.

MAXIPIME should be prescribed with caution in individuals with a history of gastrointestinal disease, particularly colitis.

Arginine has been shown to alter glucose metabolism and elevate serum potassium transiently when administered at 50 times the amount provided by the maximum recommended human dose of MAXIPIME. The effect of lower doses is not presently known.

Drug Interactions

Renal function should be monitored carefully if high doses of aminoglycosides are to be administered with MAXIPIME because of the increased potential of nephrotoxicity and ototoxicity of aminoglycoside antibiotics. Nephrotoxicity has been reported following concomitant administration of other cephalosporins with potent diuretics such as furosemide.

Drug/Laboratory Test Interactions

The administration of cefepime may result in a false-positive reaction for glucose in the urine when using Clinitest® tablets. It is recommended that glucose tests based on enzymatic glucose oxidase reactions (such as Clinistix® or Tes-Tape®) be used.

Carcinogenesis, Mutagenesis, and Impairment of Fertility

No long-term animal carcinogenicity studies have been conducted with cefepime. A battery of *in vivo* and *in vitro* genetic toxicity tests, including the Ames Salmonella reverse mutation assay, CHO/HGPRT mammalian cell forward gene mutation assay, chromosomal aberration and sister chromatid exchange assays in human lymphocytes, CHO fibroblast clastogenesis assay, and cytogenetic and micronucleus assays in mice were conducted. The overall conclusion of these tests indicated no definitive evidence of genotoxic potential. No untoward effects on fertility or reproduction have been observed in rats, mice, and rabbits when cefepime is administered subcutaneously at 1 to 4 times the recommended maximum human dose calculated on a mg/m^2/day basis.

Usage in Pregnancy—Teratogenic effects—Pregnancy Category B

Cefepime was not teratogenic or embryocidal when administered during the period of organogenesis to rats at doses up to 1000 mg/kg/day (4 times the recommended maximum human dose calculated on a mg/m^2/day basis) or to mice at doses up to 1200 mg/kg/day (2 times the recommended maximum human dose calculated on a mg/m^2/day basis) or to rabbits at a dose level of 100 mg/kg/day (approximately equal to the recommended maximum daily human dose calculated on a mg/m^2/day basis).

There are, however, no adequate and well-controlled studies of cefepime use in pregnant women. Because animal reproduction studies are not always predictive of human response, this drug should be used during pregnancy only if clearly needed.

Nursing Mothers

Cefepime is excreted in human breast milk in very low concentrations [0.5μg/mL]. Caution should be exercised when cefepime is administered to a nursing woman.

Labor and Delivery

Cefepime has not been studied for use during labor and delivery. Treatment should only be given if clearly indicated.

Pediatric Use

The safety and efficacy of MAXIPIME (cefepime hydrochloride) in pediatric patients below the age of 12 years have not been established. This product is intended for use in patients 12 years of age and older.

Geriatric Use

In clinical studies, when geriatric patients received the usual recommended adult dose, clinical efficacy and safety were comparable to clinical efficacy and safety in non-geriatric adult patients.

In elderly patients, dosage and administration of cefepime should be adjusted in the presence of renal insufficiency. (see **DOSAGE and ADMINISTRATION.**)

ADVERSE REACTIONS

Clinical Trials:

In clinical trials using multiple doses of cefepime, 4,137 patients were treated with the recommended dosages of cefepime (500 mg to 2 g IV q 12h). There were no deaths or permanent disabilities thought related to drug toxicity. Sixty-four (1.5%) patients discontinued medication due to adverse events thought by the investigators to be possibly, probably, or almost certainly related to drug toxicity. Thirty-three (51%) of these 64 patients who discontinued therapy did so because of rash. The percentage of cefepime-treated patients who discontinued study drug because of drug-related adverse events was very similar at daily doses of 500 mg, 1 g and 2 g q 12h (0.8%, 1.1%, and 2.0%, respectively). However, the incidence of discontinuation due to rash increased with the higher recommended doses.

The following adverse events were thought to be probably related to cefepime during evaluation of the drug in clinical trials conducted in North America (n=3,125 cefepime-treated patients).

TABLE 8

ADVERSE CLINICAL REACTIONS CEFEPIME MULTIPLE-DOSE DOSING REGIMENS CLINICAL TRIALS—NORTH AMERICA

INCIDENCE EQUAL TO OR GREATER THAN 1%	Local reactions (3.0%), including phlebitis (1.3%), pain and/or inflammation (0.6%)*; rash (1.1%)
INCIDENCE LESS THAN 1% BUT GREATER THAN 0.1%	Colitis (including pseudomembranous colitis), diarrhea, fever, headache, nausea, oral moniliasis, pruritus, urticaria, vaginitis, vomiting

*local reactions, irrespective of relationship to cefepime in those patients who received intravenous infusion (n=3,048).

The following adverse laboratory changes, irrespective of relationship to therapy with cefepime, were seen during clinical trials conducted in North America.

TABLE 9

ADVERSE LABORATORY CHANGES CEFEPIME MULTIPLE-DOSE DOSING REGIMENS CLINICAL TRIALS—NORTH AMERICA

INCIDENCE EQUAL TO OR GREATER THAN 1%	Positive Coombs' test (without hemolysis) (16.2%); decreased phosphorous (2.8%); increased ALT/SGPT (2.8%), AST/SGOT (2.4%), eosinophils (1.7%); abnormal PTT (1.6%), PT (1.4%)
INCIDENCE LESS THAN 1% BUT GREATER THAN 0.1%	Increased alkaline phosphatase, BUN, calcium, creatinine, phosphorous, potassium, total bilirubin; decreased calcium*, hematocrit, neutrophils, platelets, WBC

*Hypocalcemia was more common among elderly patients. Clinical consequences from changes in either calcium or phosphorous were not reported.

In Postmarketing Experience:

In addition to the events reported during North American clinical trials with cefepime, the following adverse experiences have been reported from foreign sources during worldwide postmarketing experience:

Encephalopathy has been reported in renally impaired patients treated with unadjusted dosing regimens of cefepime. Several cephalosporins have been implicated in triggering seizures, particularly in patients with renal impairment when the dosage was not reduced. (see **DOSAGE AND AD-**

TABLE 13
CEFEPIME ADMIXTURE STABILITY

MAXIPIME Concentration	Admixture and Concentration	IV Infusion Solutions	Stability Time for RT/L (20°–25°C)	Refrigeration (2°–8°C)
40 mg/mL	Amikacin 6 mg/mL	NS or D5W	24 hours	7 days
40 mg/mL	Ampicillin 1 mg/mL	D5W	8 hours	8 hours
40 mg/mL	Ampicillin 10 mg/mL	D5W	2 hours	8 hours
40 mg/mL	Ampicillin 1 mg/mL	NS	24 hours	48 hours
40 mg/mL	Ampicillin 10 mg/mL	NS	8 hours	48 hours
4 mg/mL	Ampicillin 40 mg/mL	NS	8 hours	8 hours
4–40 mg/mL	Clindamycin Phosphate 0.25-6 mg/mL	NS or D5W	24 hours	7 days
4 mg/mL	Heparin 10–50 units/mL	NS or D5W	24 hours	7 days
4 mg/mL	Potassium Chloride 10–40 mEq/L	NS or D5W	24 hours	7 days
4 mg/mL	Theophylline 0.8 mg/mL	D5W	24 hours	7 days
1–4 mg/mL	na	Aminosyn® II 4.25% with electrolytes and calcium	8 hours	3 days
0.125–0.25 mg/mL	na	Inpersol® with 4.25% dextrose	24 hours	7 days

NS = 0.9% Sodium Chloride Injection
D5W = 5% Dextrose Injection
na = not applicable
RT/L = Ambient room temperature and light

MINISTRATION and OVERDOSAGE.) If seizures associated with drug therapy occur, the drug should be discontinued. Anticonvulsant therapy can be given if clinically indicated.

Cephalosporin—class adverse reactions:
In addition to the adverse reactions listed above that have been observed in patients treated with cefepime, the following adverse reactions and altered laboratory tests have been reported for cephalosporin-class antibiotics:
Stevens-Johnson syndrome, erythema multiforme, toxic epidermal necrolysis, renal dysfunction, toxic nephropathy, aplastic anemia, hemolytic anemia, hemorrhage and hepatic dysfunction including cholestasis, pancytopenia.

OVERDOSAGE
In clinical trials, MAXIPIME (cefepime hydrochloride) overdosage occurred in a patient with renal failure (creatinine clearance <11 mL/min) who received 2 g q 24h for seven days. The patient exhibited seizures, encephalopathy, and neuromuscular excitability. Patients who receive an overdose should be carefully observed and given supportive treatment. In the presence of renal insufficiency, hemodialysis, not peritoneal dialysis, is recommended to aid in the removal of cefepime from the body.

DOSAGE AND ADMINISTRATION
The recommended adult dosages and routes of administration are outlined in the following table. MAXIPIME should be administered intravenously over approximately 30 minutes.

TABLE 10
Recommended Dosage Schedule for MAXIPIME

Site and Type of Infection	Dose	Frequency	Duration (days)
Mild to Moderate Uncomplicated or Complicated Urinary Tract Infections, including pyelonephritis, due to *E. coli*, *K. pneumoniae*, or *P. mirabilis*.*	0.5-1g IV/IM**	q12h	7–10
Severe Uncomplicated or Complicated Urinary Tract Infections, including pyelonephritis, due to *E. coli* or *K. pneumoniae*.*	2 g IV	q12h	10
Moderate to Severe Pneumonia due to *S. pneumoniae**, *Pseudomonas*			

aeruginosa, *Klebsiella pneumoniae*, or *Enterobacter* species.	1-2 g IV	q12h	10
Moderate to Severe Uncomplicated Skin and Skin Structure Infections due to *S. aureus* or *S. pyogenes*.	2 g IV	q12h	10

*including cases associated with concurrent bacteremia.
**IM route of administration is indicated only for mild to moderate, uncomplicated or complicated UTI's due to *E. coli* when the IM route is considered to be a more appropriate route of drug administration.

Impaired Hepatic Function—No adjustment is necessary for patients with impaired hepatic function.
Impaired Renal Function—In patients with impaired renal function (creatinine clearance <60mL/min), the dose of MAXIPIME should be adjusted to compensate for the slower rate of renal elimination. The recommended initial dose of MAXIPIME should be the same as in patients with normal renal function. The recommended maintenance doses of MAXIPIME in patients with renal insufficiency are presented in Table 11.

TABLE 11

Recommended Maintenance Schedule in Patients with Renal Impairment Relative to Normal Recommended Dosing Schedule

Creatinine Clearance (mL/min)	Recommended Maintenance Schedule		
>60 Normal recommended dosing schedule	500 mg q12h	1 g q12h	2 g q12h
30–60	500 mg q24h	1 g q24h	2 g q24h
11–29	500 mg q24h	500 mg q24h	1 g q24h
≤10	250 mg q24h	250 mg q24h	500 mg q24h

When only serum creatinine is available, the following formula (Cockcroft and Gault equation)[3] may be used to estimate creatinine clearance. The serum creatinine should represent a steady state of renal function:

Males: Creatinine Clearance (mL/min)

$$= \frac{\text{Weight (kg)} \times (140 - \text{age})}{72 \times \text{serum creatinine (mg/dL)}}$$

Females: 0.85 × above value

In patients undergoing hemodialysis, approximately 68% of the total amount of cefepime present in the body at the start of dialysis will be removed during a 3-hour dialysis period. A repeat dose, equivalent to the initial dose, should be given at the completion of each dialysis session.
In patients undergoing continuous ambulatory peritoneal dialysis, MAXIPIME may be administered at normally recommended doses at a dosage interval of every 48 hours.

Administration:
For Intravenous Infusion, constitute the 1 g or 2 g piggyback (100 mL) bottle with 50 or 100 mL of a compatible IV fluid listed in the **Compatibility and Stability** subsection. Alternatively, constitute the 500 mg, 1 g, or 2 g vial, and add an appropriate quantity of the resulting solution to an IV container with one of the compatible IV fluids. **THE RESULTING SOLUTION SHOULD BE ADMINISTERED OVER APPROXIMATELY 30 MINUTES.**
Intermittent IV infusion with a Y-type administration set can be accomplished with compatible solutions. However, during infusion of a solution containing cefepime, it is desirable to discontinue the other solution.
ADD-Vantage® vials are to be constituted only with 50 or 100 mL of 5% Dextrose Injection or 0.9% Sodium Chloride Injection in Abbott ADD-Vantage® flexible diluent containers. (see ADD-Vantage® Vial Instructions for Use.)
Intramuscular Administration: For IM administration, MAXIPIME (cefepime hydrochloride) should be constituted with one of the following diluents: Sterile Water for Injection, 0.9% Sodium Chloride, 5% Dextrose Injection, 0.5% or 1.0% Lidocaine Hydrochloride, or Bacteriostatic Water for Injection with Parabens or Benzyl Alcohol (Refer to Table 12).
Preparation of MAXIPIME solutions is summarized in Table 12:

TABLE 12
PREPARATION OF SOLUTIONS OF MAXIPIME

Single Dose Vials for Intravenous/Intramuscular Administration	Amount of Diluent to be added (mL)	Approximate Available Volume (mL)	Approximate Cefepime Concentration (mg/mL)
Cefepime vial content			
500 mg (iv)	5.0	5.6	100
500 mg (im)	1.3	1.8	280
1 g (iv)	10.0	11.3	100
1 g (im)	2.4	3.6	280
2 g (iv)	10.0	12.5	160
Piggyback (100 mL)			
1 g bottle	50	50	20
1 g bottle	100	100	10
2 g bottle	50	50	40
2 g bottle	100	100	20
ADD-Vantage®			
1 g vial	50	50	20
1 g vial	100	100	10

Compatibility and Stability:
Intravenous: MAXIPIME is compatible at concentrations between 1 and 40 mg/mL with the following IV infusion fluids: 0.9% Sodium Chloride Injection, 5% and 10% Dextrose Injection, M/6 Sodium Lactate Injection, 5% Dextrose and 0.9% Sodium Chloride Injection, Lactated Ringers and 5% Dextrose Injection, Normosol-R®, and Normosol-M® in 5% Dextrose Injection. These solutions may be stored up to 24 hours at controlled room temperature 20°–25° (68°–77°F) or 7 days in a refrigerator 2°–8°C (36°–46°F). MAXIPIME in ADD-Vantage® vials is stable at concentrations of 10–20 mg/mL in 5% Dextrose Injection or 0.9% Sodium Chloride Injection for 24 hours at controlled room temperature 20°–25°C or 7 days in a refrigerator 2°–8°C.
MAXIPIME admixture compatibility information is summarized in Table 13.
[See table above.]
Solutions of MAXIPIME, like those of most beta-lactam antibiotics, should not be added to solutions of ampicillin at a concentration greater than 40 mg/mL, and should not be added to metronidazole, vancomycin, gentamicin, tobramycin, netilmicin sulfate or aminophylline because of potential interaction. However, if concurrent therapy with MAXIPIME is indicated, each of these antibiotics can be administered separately.
Intramuscular: MAXIPIME (cefepime hydrochloride) constituted as directed is stable for 24 hours at controlled room temperature 20°–25 °C (68°–77°F) or for 7 days in a refrigerator 2°–8°C (36°–46°F) with the following diluents: Sterile Water for Injection, 0.9% Sodium Chloride Injection, 5% Dextrose Injection, Bacteriostatic Water for Injection with

Continued on next page

Bristol-Myers Squibb Co.—Cont.

Parabens or Benzyl Alcohol, or 0.5% or 1% Lidocaine Hydrochloride.

NOTE: PARENTERAL DRUGS SHOULD BE INSPECTED VISUALLY FOR PARTICULATE MATTER BEFORE ADMINISTRATION.

As with other cephalosporins, the color of MAXIPIME powder, as well as its solutions, tend to darken depending on storage conditions; however, when stored as recommended, the product potency is not adversely affected.

HOW SUPPLIED

MAXIPIME® (cefepime hydrochloride) for Injection is supplied as follows:

NDC 0003-7731-99   500 mg*   15 mL vial (tray of 10)
NDC 0003-7732-95   1 g*   Piggyback bottle 100 mL (tray of 10)
NDC 0003-7732-89   1 g*   ADD-Vantage® vial (tray of 10)
NDC 0003-7732-99   1 g*   15 mL vial (tray of 10)
NDC 0003-7733-95   2 g*   Piggyback bottle 100 mL (tray of 10)
NDC 0003-7733-99   2 g*   20 mL vial (tray of 10)
    *Based on cefepime activity

Storage

MAXIPIME IN THE DRY STATE SHOULD BE STORED BETWEEN 2°–25°C (36°–77°F) AND PROTECTED FROM LIGHT.
U.S. Patent No. 4,406,899; 4,910,301; 4,994,451 and 5,244,891

REFERENCES

(1) National Committee for Clinical Laboratory Standards. *Methods for Dilution Antimicrobial Susceptibility Tests for Bacteria that Grow Aerobically*—Third Edition. Approved Standard NCCLS Document M7-A3, Vol. 13, No. 25, NCCLS, Villanova, PA, December, 1993.
(2) National Committee for Clinical Laboratory Standards. *Performance Standards for Antimicrobial Disk Susceptibility Tests*—Fifth Edition. Approved Standard NCCLS Document M2-A5, Vol. 13, No. 24, NCCLS, Villanova, PA, December, 1993.
(3) Cockcroft DW, Gault MH. Prediction of creatinine clearance from serum creatinine. *Nephron*. 1976; 16:31-41.

ADD-Vantage® is a registered trademark of Abbott Laboratories
Normosol-R® is a registered trademark of Abbott Laboratories
Normosol-M® is a registered trademark of Abbott Laboratories
Aminosyn® is a registered trademark of Abbott Laboratories
Inpersol® is a registered trademark of Abbott Laboratories
Clinitest® and Clinistix® are registered trademarks of Ames Division, Miles Laboratories, Inc.
Tes-Tape® is a registered trademark of Eli Lilly and Company

Issued: January, 1996   7733DIM-02
E4-B001-1-96   51-004476-00
Shown in Product Identification Guide, page 307

MONOPRIL®
Fosinopril Sodium Tablets

℞

CAUTION: Federal law prohibits dispensing without prescription.

> **USE IN PREGNANCY**
>
> When used in pregnancy during the second and third trimesters, ACE inhibitors can cause injury and even death to the developing fetus. When pregnancy is detected, MONOPRIL should be discontinued as soon as possible. See **WARNINGS: Fetal/Neonatal Morbidity and Mortality.**

DESCRIPTION

MONOPRIL (Fosinopril Sodium) is the sodium salt of fosinopril, the ester prodrug of an angiotensin converting enzyme (ACE) inhibitor, fosinoprilat. It contains a phosphinate group capable of specific binding to the active site of angiotensin converting enzyme. Fosinopril sodium is designated chemically as: L-proline, 4-cyclohexyl-1-[[[2-methyl-1-(1-oxopropoxy) propoxy] (4-phenylbutyl) phosphinyl]acetyl]-, sodium salt,*trans*-.

Fosinopril sodium is a white to off-white crystalline powder. It is soluble in water (100 mg/mL), methanol, and ethanol and slightly soluble in hexane.

Its empiric formula is $C_{30}H_{45}NNaO_7P$, and its molecular weight is 585.65.

MONOPRIL is available for oral administration as 10 mg, 20 mg, and 40 mg tablets. Inactive ingredients include: lactose, microcrystalline cellulose, crospovidone, povidone, and sodium stearyl fumarate.

CLINICAL PHARMACOLOGY
Mechanism of Action

In animals and humans, fosinopril sodium is hydrolyzed by esterases to the pharmacologically active form, fosinoprilat, a specific competitive inhibitor of angiotensin converting enzyme (ACE).

ACE is a peptidyl dipeptidase that catalyzes the conversion of angiotensin I to the vasoconstrictor substance, angiotensin II. Angiotensin II also stimulates aldosterone secretion by the adrenal cortex. Inhibition of ACE results in decreased plasma angiotensin II, which leads to decreased vasopressor activity and to decreased aldosterone secretion. The latter decrease may result in a small increase of serum potassium.

In 647 hypertensive patients treated with fosinopril alone for an average of 29 weeks, mean increases in serum potassium of 0.1 mEq/L were observed. Similar increases were observed among all patients treated with fosinopril, including those receiving concomitant diuretic therapy. Removal of angiotensin II negative feedback on renin secretion leads to increased plasma renin activity.

ACE is identical to kininase, an enzyme that degrades bradykinin. Whether increased levels of bradykinin, a potent vasodepressor peptide, play a role in the therapeutic effects of MONOPRIL remains to be elucidated.

While the mechanism through which MONOPRIL lowers blood pressure is believed to be primarily suppression of the renin-angiotensin-aldosterone system, MONOPRIL has an antihypertensive effect even in patients with low-renin hypertension. Although MONOPRIL was antihypertensive in all races studied, black hypertensive patients (usually a low-renin hypertensive population) had a smaller average response to ACE inhibitor monotherapy than non-black patients.

In patients with heart failure, the beneficial effects of MONOPRIL are thought to result primarily from suppression of the renin-angiotensin-aldosterone system; inhibition of the angiotensin-converting enzyme produces decreases in both preload and afterload.

Pharmacokinetics and Metabolism

Following oral administration, fosinopril (the prodrug) is absorbed slowly. The absolute absorption of fosinopril averaged 36% of an oral dose. The primary site of absorption is the proximal small intestine (duodenum/jejunum). While the rate of absorption may be slowed by the presence of food in the gastrointestinal tract, the extent of absorption of fosinopril is essentially unaffected.

Fosinoprilat is highly protein-bound (approximately 99.4%), has a relatively small volume of distribution, and has negligible binding to cellular components in blood. After single and multiple oral doses, plasma levels, areas under plasma concentration-time curves (AUCs) and peak concentrations (Cmaxs) are directly proportional to the dose of fosinopril. Times to peak concentrations are independent of dose and are achieved in approximately 3 hours.

After an oral dose of radiolabeled fosinopril, 75% of radioactivity in plasma was present as active fosinoprilat, 20–30% as a glucuronide conjugate of fosinoprilat, and 1–5% as a *p*-hydroxy metabolite of fosinoprilat. Since fosinoprilat is not biotransformed after intravenous administration, fosinopril, not fosinoprilat, appears to be the precursor for the glucuronide and *p*-hydroxy metabolites. In rats, the *p*-hydroxy metabolite of fosinoprilat is as potent an inhibitor of ACE as fosinoprilat; the glucuronide conjugate is devoid of ACE inhibitory activity.

After intravenous administration, fosinoprilat was eliminated approximately equally by the liver and kidney. After oral administration of radiolabeled fosinopril, approximately half of the absorbed dose is excreted in the urine and the remainder is excreted in the feces. In two studies involving healthy subjects, the mean body clearance of intravenous fosinoprilat was between 26 and 39 mL/min.

In healthy subjects, the terminal elimination half-life ($t^1/_2$) of an intravenous dose of radiolabeled fosinoprilat is approximately 12 hours. In hypertensive patients with normal renal and hepatic function, who received repeated doses of fosinopril, the effective $t^1/_2$ for accumulation of fosinoprilat averaged 11.5 hours. In patients with heart failure, the effective $t^1/_2$ was 14 hours.

In patients with mild to severe renal insufficiency (creatinine clearance 10–80 mL/min/1.73m²), the clearance of fosinoprilat does not differ appreciably from normal, because of the large contribution of hepatobiliary elimination. In patients with end-stage renal disease (creatinine clearance < 10 mL/min/1.73m²), the total body clearance of fosinoprilat is approximately one-half of that in patients with normal renal function. (See DOSAGE AND ADMINISTRATION.)

Fosinopril is not well dialyzed. Clearance of fosinoprilat by hemodialysis and peritoneal dialysis averages 2% and 7%, respectively, of urea clearances.

In patients with hepatic insufficiency (alcoholic or biliary cirrhosis), the extent of hydrolysis of fosinopril is not appreciably reduced, although the rate of hydrolysis may be slowed; the apparent total body clearance of fosinoprilat is approximately one-half of that in patients with normal hepatic function.

In elderly (male) subjects (65–74 years old) with clinically normal renal and hepatic function, there appear to be no significant differences in pharmacokinetic parameters for fosinoprilat compared to those of younger subjects (20–35 years old).

Fosinoprilat was found to cross the placenta of pregnant animals.

Studies in animals indicate that fosinopril and fosinoprilat do not cross the blood-brain barrier.

Pharmacodynamics and Clinical Effects

Serum ACE activity was inhibited by ≥ 90% at 2 to 12 hours after single doses of 10 to 40 mg of fosinopril. At 24 hours, serum ACE activity remained suppressed by 85%, 93%, and 93% in the 10, 20, and 40 mg dose groups, respectively.

Hypertension

Administration of MONOPRIL (Fosinopril Sodium) to patients with mild to moderate hypertension results in a reduction of both supine and standing blood pressure to about the same extent with no compensatory tachycardia. Symptomatic postural hypotension is infrequent, although it can occur in patients who are salt- and/or volume-depleted (see WARNINGS.) Use of MONOPRIL in combination with thiazide diuretics gives a blood pressure-lowering effect greater than that seen with either agent alone.

Following oral administration of single doses of 10–40 mg, MONOPRIL lowered blood pressure within one hour, with peak reductions achieved 2–6 hours after dosing. The antihypertensive effect of a single dose persisted for 24 hours. Following four weeks of monotherapy in placebo-controlled trials in patients with mild to moderate hypertension, once daily doses of 20–80 mg lowered supine or seated systolic and diastolic blood pressures 24 hours after dosing by an average of 8–9/6–7 mmHg more than placebo. The trough effect was about 50–60% of the peak diastolic response and about 80% of the peak systolic response.

In most trials, the antihypertensive effect of MONOPRIL increased during the first several weeks of repeated measurements. The antihypertensive effect of MONOPRIL has been shown to continue during long-term therapy for at least 2 years. Abrupt withdrawal of MONOPRIL has not resulted in a rapid increase in blood pressure.

Limited experience in controlled and uncontrolled trials combining fosinopril with a calcium channel blocker or a loop diuretic has indicated no unusual drug-drug interactions. Other ACE inhibitors have had less than additive effects with beta-adrenergic blockers, presumably because both drugs lower blood pressure by inhibiting parts of the renin-angiotensin system.

ACE inhibitors are generally less effective in blacks than in non-blacks. The effectiveness of MONOPRIL was not influenced by age, sex, or weight.

In hemodynamic studies in hypertensive patients, after three months of therapy, responses (changes in BP, heart rate, cardiac index, and PVR) to various stimuli (e.g., isometric exercise, 45° head-up tilt, and mental challenge) were unchanged compared to baseline, suggesting that MONOPRIL does not affect the activity of the sympathetic nervous system. Reduction in systemic blood pressure appears to have been mediated by a decrease in peripheral vascular resistance without reflex cardiac effects. Similarly, renal, splanchnic, cerebral, and skeletal muscle blood flow were unchanged compared to baseline, as was glomerular filtration rate.

Heart Failure

In a randomized, double-blind, placebo-controlled trial, 179 patients with heart failure, all receiving diuretics and some receiving digoxin, were administered single doses of 1, 20 or 40 mg of MONOPRIL or placebo. Doses of 20 and 40 mg of MONOPRIL resulted in acute decreases in pulmonary capillary wedge pressure (preload) and mean arterial blood pressure and systemic vascular resistance (afterload). One hundred fifty-five of these patients were re-randomized to once daily therapy with MONOPRIL (1, 20, or 40 mg) for an additional 10 weeks. Hemodynamic measurements made 24 hours after dosing showed (relative to baseline) continued reduction in pulmonary capillary wedge pressure, mean arterial blood pressure, right atrial pressure and an increase in cardiac index and stroke volume for the 20 and 40 mg dose groups. No tachyphylaxis was seen.

MONOPRIL was studied in 3 double-blind, placebo-controlled, 12–24 week trials including a total of 734 patients with heart failure, with MONOPRIL doses from 10 to 40 mg daily. Concomitant therapy in 2 of these 3 trials included diuretics and digitalis; in the third trial patients were receiving only diuretics. All 3 trials showed statistically significant benefits of MONOPRIL therapy, compared to placebo, in one or more of the following: exercise tolerance (one study), symptoms of dyspnea, orthopnea and paroxysmal nocturnal dyspnea (2 studies), NYHA classification (2 studies), hospitalization for heart failure (2 studies), study withdrawals for worsening heart failure (2 studies), and/or need for supplemental diuretics (2 studies). Favorable effects were maintained for up to two years. Effects of MONOPRIL on long-

term mortality in heart failure have not been evaluated. The once daily dosage (differing from the once or twice daily dosage for hypertension) for the treatment of heart failure is a consequence of being the only dosage regimen used during clinical trial development and may not represent a known optimum dosage schedule.

INDICATIONS AND USAGE

MONOPRIL is indicated for the treatment of hypertension. It may be used alone or in combination with thiazide diuretics.

MONOPRIL is indicated in the management of heart failure as adjunctive therapy when added to conventional therapy including diuretics with or without digitalis (see DOSAGE AND ADMINISTRATION).

In using MONOPRIL (Fosinopril Sodium), consideration should be given to the fact that another angiotensin converting enzyme inhibitor, captopril, has caused agranulocytosis, particularly in patients with renal impairment or collagenvascular disease. Available data are insufficient to show that MONOPRIL does not have a similar risk (see WARNINGS).

CONTRAINDICATIONS

MONOPRIL is contraindicated in patients who are hypersensitive to this product or to any other angiotensin converting enzyme inhibitor (e.g., a patient who has experienced angioedema with any other ACE inhibitor therapy).

WARNINGS

Anaphylactoid and Possibly Related Reactions

Presumably because angiotensin-converting enzyme inhibitors affect the metabolism of eicosanoids and polypeptides, including endogenous bradykinin, patients receiving ACE inhibitors (including MONOPRIL) may be subject to a variety of adverse reactions, some of them serious.

Angioedema: Angioedema involving the extremities, face, lips, mucous membranes, tongue, glottis or larynx has been reported in patients treated with ACE inhibitors. If angioedema involves the tongue, glottis or larynx, airway obstruction may occur and be fatal. If laryngeal stridor or angioedema of the face, lips, mucous membranes, tongue, glottis or extremities occurs, treatment with MONOPRIL should be discontinued and appropriate therapy instituted immediately. **Where there is involvement of the tongue, glottis, or larynx, likely to cause airway obstruction, appropriate therapy, e.g., subcutaneous epinephrine solution 1:1000 (0.3 mL to 0.5 mL) should be promptly administered** (See PRECAUTIONS: Information for Patients and ADVERSE REACTIONS).

Anaphylactoid reactions during desensitization: Two patients undergoing desensitizing treatment with hymenoptera venom while receiving ACE inhibitors sustained lifethreatening anaphylactoid reactions. In the same patients, these reactions were avoided when ACE inhibitors were temporarily withheld, but they reappeared upon inadvertent rechallenge.

Anaphylactoid reactions during membrane exposure: Anaphylactoid reactions have been reported in patients dialyzed with high-flux membranes and treated concomitantly with an ACE inhibitor. Anaphylactoid reactions have also been reported in patients undergoing low-density lipoprotein apheresis with dextran sulfate absorption (a procedure dependent upon devices not approved in the United States).

Hypotension

MONOPRIL can cause symptomatic hypotension. Like other ACE inhibitors, fosinopril has been only rarely associated with hypotension in uncomplicated hypertensive patients. Symptomatic hypotension is most likely to occur in patients who have been volume- and/or salt-depleted as a result of prolonged diuretic therapy, dietary salt restriction, dialysis, diarrhea, or vomiting. Volume and/or salt depletion should be corrected before initiating therapy with MONOPRIL.

In patients with heart failure, with or without associated renal insufficiency, ACE inhibitor therapy may cause excessive hypotension, which may be associated with oliguria or azotemia and, rarely, with acute renal failure and death. In such patients, MONOPRIL therapy should be started under close medical supervision; they should be followed closely for the first 2 weeks of treatment and whenever the dose of fosinopril or diuretic is increased. Consideration should be given to reducing the diuretic dose in patients with normal or low blood pressure who have been treated vigorously with diuretics or who are hyponatremic.

If hypotension occurs, the patient should be placed in a supine position, and, if necessary, treated with intravenous infusion of physiological saline. MONOPRIL treatment usually can be continued following restoration of blood pressure and volume.

Neutropenia/Agranulocytosis

Another angiotensin converting enzyme inhibitor, captopril, has been shown to cause agranulocytosis and bone marrow depression, rarely in uncomplicated patients, but more frequently in patients with renal impairment, especially if they also have a collagen-vascular disease such as systemic lupus erythematosus or scleroderma. Available data from clinical trials of fosinopril are insufficient to show that fosinopril does not cause agranulocytosis at similar rates. Monitoring

of white blood cell counts should be considered in patients with collagen-vascular disease, especially if the disease is associated with impaired renal function.

Fetal/Neonatal Morbidity and Mortality

ACE inhibitors can cause fetal and neonatal morbidity and death when administered to pregnant women. Several dozen cases have been reported in the world literature. When pregnancy is detected, ACE inhibitors should be discontinued as soon as possible.

The use of ACE inhibitors during the second and third trimesters of pregnancy has been associated with fetal and neonatal injury, including hypotension, neonatal skull hypoplasia, anuria, reversible or irreversible renal failure, and death. Oligohydramnios has also been reported, presumably resulting from decreased fetal renal function; oligohydramnios in this setting has been associated with fetal limb contractures, craniofacial deformation, and hypoplastic lung development. Prematurity, intrauterine growth retardation, and patent ductus arteriosus have also been reported, although it is not clear whether these occurrences were due to the ACE-inhibitor exposure.

These adverse effects do not appear to have resulted from intrauterine ACE-inhibitor exposure that has been limited to the first trimester. Mothers whose embryos and fetuses are exposed to ACE inhibitors only during the first trimester should be so informed. Nonetheless, when patients become pregnant, physicians should make every effort to discontinue the use of fosinopril as soon as possible.

Rarely (probably less often than once in every thousand pregnancies), no alternative to ACE inhibitors will be found. In these rare cases, the mothers should be apprised of the potential hazards to their fetuses, and serial ultrasound examinations should be performed to assess the intraamniotic environment.

If oligohydramnios is observed, fosinopril should be discontinued unless it is considered life-saving for the mother. Contraction stress testing (CST), a non-stress test (NST), or biophysical profiling (BPP) may be appropriate, depending upon the week of pregnancy. Patients and physicians should be aware, however, that oligohydramnios may not appear until after the fetus has sustained irreversible injury.

Infants with histories of *in utero* exposure to ACE inhibitors should be closely observed for hypotension, oliguria, and hyperkalemia. If oliguria occurs, attention should be directed toward support of blood pressure and renal perfusion. Exchange transfusion or dialysis may be required as a means of reversing hypotension and/or substituting for disordered renal function. Fosinopril is poorly dialyzed from the circulation of adults by hemodialysis and peritoneal dialysis. There is no experience with any procedure for removing fosinopril from the neonatal circulation.

When fosinopril was given to pregnant rats at doses about 80 to 250 times (on a mg/kg basis) the maximum recommended human dose, three similar orofacial malformations and one fetus with *situs inversus* were observed among the offspring. No teratogenic effects of fosinopril were seen in studies in pregnant rabbits at doses up to 25 times (on a mg/kg basis) the maximum recommended human dose.

Hepatic Failure

Rarely, ACE Inhibitors have been associated with a syndrome that starts with cholestatic jaundice and progresses to fulminant hepatic necrosis and (sometimes) death. The mechanism of this syndrome is not understood. Patients receiving ACE inhibitors who develop jaundice or marked elevations of hepatic enzymes should discontinue the ACE inhibitor and receive appropriate medical follow-up.

PRECAUTIONS

General

Impaired Renal Function: As a consequence of inhibiting the renin-angiotensin-aldosterone system, changes in renal function may be anticipated in susceptible individuals. In patients with severe congestive heart failure whose renal function may depend on the activity of the renin-angiotensin-aldosterone system, treatment with angiotensin converting enzyme inhibitors, including MONOPRIL (Fosinopril Sodium), may be associated with oliguria and/or progressive azotemia and (rarely) with acute renal failure and/or death. In hypertensive patients with renal artery stenosis in a solitary kidney or bilateral renal artery stenosis, increases in blood urea nitrogen and serum creatinine may occur. Experience with another angiotensin converting enzyme inhibitor suggests that these increases are usually reversible upon discontinuation of ACE inhibitor and/or diuretic therapy. In such patients, renal function should be monitored during the first few weeks of therapy. Some hypertensive patients with no apparent pre-existing renal vascular disease have developed increases in blood urea nitrogen and serum creatinine, usually minor and transient, especially when MONOPRIL has been given concomitantly with a diuretic. This is more likely to occur in patients with pre-existing renal impairment. Dosage reduction of MONOPRIL and/or discontinuation of the diuretic may be required.

Evaluation of patients with hypertension or heart failure should always include assessment of renal function (see DOSAGE AND ADMINISTRATION).

Impaired renal function decreases total clearance of fosinoprilat and approximately doubles AUC. In general, no adjustment of dosing is needed. However, patients with heart failure and severely reduced renal function may be more sensitive to the hemodynamic effects (e.g., hypotension) of ACE inhibition (see CLINICAL PHARMACOLOGY).

Hyperkalemia: In clinical trials, hyperkalemia (serum potassium greater than 10% above the upper limit of normal) has occurred in approximately 2.6% of hypertensive patients receiving MONOPRIL. In most cases, these were isolated values which resolved despite continued therapy. In clinical trials, 0.1% of patients (two patients) were discontinued from therapy due to an elevated serum potassium. Risk factors for the development of hyperkalemia include renal insufficiency, diabetes mellitus, and the concomitant use of potassium-sparing diuretics, potassium supplements, and/or potassium-containing salt substitutes, which should be used cautiously, if at all, with MONOPRIL (see PRECAUTIONS: Drug Interactions).

Cough: Presumably due to the inhibition of the degradation of endogenous bradykinin, persistent nonproductive cough has been reported with all ACE inhibitors, always resolving after discontinuation of therapy. ACE inhibitor-induced cough should be considered in the differential diagnosis of cough.

Impaired Liver Function: Since fosinopril is primarily metabolized by hepatic and gut wall esterases to its active moiety, fosinoprilat, patients with impaired liver function could develop elevated plasma levels of unchanged fosinopril. In a study in patients with alcoholic or biliary cirrhosis, the extent of hydrolysis was unaffected, although the rate was slowed. In these patients, the apparent total body clearance of fosinoprilat was decreased and the plasma AUC approximately doubled.

Surgery/Anesthesia: In patients undergoing surgery or during anesthesia with agents that produce hypotension, fosinopril will block the angiotensin II formation that could otherwise occur secondary to compensatory renin release. Hypotension that occurs as a result of this mechanism can be corrected by volume expansion.

Hemodialysis

Recent clinical observations have shown an association of hypersensitivity-like (anaphylactoid) reactions during hemodialysis with high-flux dialysis membranes (e.g., AN69) in patients receiving ACE inhibitors as medication. In these patients, consideration should be given to using a different type of dialysis membrane or a different class of medication. (See WARNINGS: Anaphylactoid reactions during membrane exposure.)

Information for Patients

Angioedema: Angioedema, including laryngeal edema, can occur with treatment with ACE inhibitors, especially following the first dose. Patients should be advised to immediately report to their physician any signs or symptoms suggesting angioedema (e.g., swelling of face, eyes, lips, tongue, larynx, mucous membranes, and extremities; difficulty in swallowing or breathing; hoarseness) and to discontinue therapy. (See WARNINGS: Angioedema and ADVERSE REACTIONS).

Symptomatic Hypotension: Patients should be cautioned that light-headedness can occur, especially during the first days of therapy, and it should be reported to a physician. Patients should be told that if syncope occurs, MONOPRIL (Fosinopril Sodium) should be discontinued until the physician has been consulted.

All patients should be cautioned that inadequate fluid intake or excessive perspiration, diarrhea, or vomiting can lead to an excessive fall in blood pressure, with the same consequences of lightheadedness and possible syncope.

Hyperkalemia: Patients should be told not to use potassium supplements or salt substitutes containing potassium without consulting the physician.

Neutropenia: Patients should be told to promptly report any indication of infection (e.g., sore throat, fever), which could be a sign of neutropenia.

Pregnancy: Female patients of childbearing age should be told about the consequences of second- and third-trimester exposure to ACE inhibitors, and they should also be told that these consequences do not appear to have resulted from intrauterine ACE-inhibitor exposure that has been limited to the first trimester. These patients should be asked to report pregnancies to their physicians as soon as possible.

Drug Interactions

With diuretics: Patients on diuretics, especially those with intravascular volume depletion, may occasionally experience an excessive reduction of blood pressure after initiation of therapy with MONOPRIL. The possibility of hypotensive effects with MONOPRIL can be minimized by either discontinuing the diuretic or increasing salt intake prior to initiation of treatment with MONOPRIL. If this is not possible, the starting dose should be reduced and the patient should be observed closely for several hours following an initial dose

Continued on next page

Bristol-Myers Squibb Co.—Cont.

and until blood pressure has stabilized (see DOSAGE AND ADMINISTRATION).

With potassium supplements and potassium-sparing diuretics: MONOPRIL can attenuate potassium loss caused by thiazide diuretics. Potassium-sparing diuretics (spironolactone, amiloride, triamterene, and others) or potassium supplements can increase the risk of hyperkalemia. Therefore, if concomitant use of such agents is indicated, they should be given with caution, and the patient's serum potassium should be monitored frequently.

With lithium: Increased serum lithium levels and symptoms of lithium toxicity have been reported in patients receiving ACE inhibitors during therapy with lithium. These drugs should be coadministered with caution, and frequent monitoring of serum lithium levels is recommended. If a diuretic is also used, the risk of lithium toxicity may be increased.

With antacids: In a clinical pharmacology study, coadministration of an antacid (aluminum, hydroxide, magnesium hydroxide, and simethicone) with fosinopril reduced serum levels and urinary excretion of fosinoprilat as compared with fosinopril administrated alone, suggesting that antacids may impair absorption of fosinopril.Therefore, if concomitant administration of these agents is indicated, dosing should be separated by 2 hours.

Other: Neither MONOPRIL nor its metabolites have been found to interact with food. In separate single or multiple dose pharmacokinetic interaction studies with chlorthalidone, nifedipine, propranolol, hydrochlorothiazide, cimetidine, metoclopramide, propantheline, digoxin, and warfarin, the bioavailability of fosinoprilat was not altered by coadministration of fosinopril with any one of these drugs. In a study with concomitant administration of aspirin and MONOPRIL the bioavailability of unbound fosinoprilat was not altered.

In a pharmacokinetic interaction study with warfarin, bioavailability parameters, the degree of protein binding, and the anticoagulant effect (measured by prothrombin time) of warfarin were not significantly changed.

Drug/Laboratory Test Interaction
Fosinopril may cause a false low measurement of serum digoxin levels with the Digi-Tab® RIA Kit for Digoxin. Other kits, such as the Coat-A-Count® RIA Kit, may be used.

Carcinogenesis, Mutagenesis, and Impairment of Fertility
No evidence of a carcinogenic effect was found when fosinopril was given in the diet to mice and rats for up to 24 months at doses up to 400 mg/kg/day. On a body weight basis, the highest dose in mice and rats is about 250 times the maximum human dose of 80 mg, assuming a 50 kg subject. On a body surface area basis, in mice, this dose is 20 times the maximum human dose; in rats, this dose is 40 times the maximum human dose. Male rats given the highest dose level had a slightly higher incidence of mesentery/omentum lipomas.

Neither fosinopril nor the active fosinoprilat was mutagenic in the Ames microbial mutagen test, the mouse lymphoma forward mutation assay, or a mitotic gene conversion assay. Fosinopril was also not genotoxic in a mouse micronucleus test *in vivo* and a mouse bone marrow cytogenetic assay *in vivo*.

In the Chinese hamster ovary cell cytogenetic assay, fosinopril increased the frequency of chromosomal aberrations when tested without metabolic activation at a concentration that was toxic to the cells. However, there was no increase in chromosomal aberrations at lower drug concentrations without metabolic activation or at any concentration with metabolic activation.

There were no adverse reproductive effects in male and female rats treated with 15 or 60 mg/kg daily. On a body weight basis, the high dose of 60 mg/kg is about 38 times the maximum recommended human dose. On a body surface area basis, this dose is 6 times the maximum recommended human dose. There was no effect on pairing time prior to mating in rats until a daily dose of 240 mg/kg, a toxic dose, was given; at this dose, a slight increase in pairing time was observed. On a body weight basis, this dose is 150 times the maximum recommended human dose. On a body surface area basis, this dose is 24 times the maximum recommended human dose.

Pregnancy Categories C (first trimester) and D (second and third trimesters)
See WARNINGS: Fetal/Neonatal Morbidity and Mortality.
Nursing Mothers
Ingestion of 20 mg daily for three days resulted in detectable levels of fosinoprilat in breast milk. MONOPRIL (Fosinopril Sodium) should not be administered to nursing mothers.
Geriatric Use
Of the total number of patients who received fosinopril in US clinical studies of MONOPRIL, 13% were 65 and older while 1.3% were 75 and older. No overall differences in effectiveness or safety were observed between these patients and younger patients, and other reported clinical experience has

not identified differences in response between the elderly and younger patients, but greater sensitivity of some older individuals cannot be ruled out.

In a pharmacokinetic study comparing elderly (65–74 years old) and non-elderly (20–35 years old) healthy volunteers, there were no differences between the groups in peak fosinoprilat levels or area under the plasma concentration time curve (AUC).
Pediatric Use
Safety and effectiveness in pediatric patients have not been established.

ADVERSE REACTIONS

MONOPRIL has been evaluated for safety in more than 2100 individuals in hypertension and heart failure trials, including approximately 530 patients treated for a year or more. Generally adverse events were mild and transient, and their frequency was not prominently related to dose within the recommended daily dosage range.

Hypertension
In placebo-controlled clinical trials (688 MONOPRIL-treated patients), the usual duration of therapy was two to three months. Discontinuations due to any clinical or laboratory adverse event were 4.1 and 1.1 percent in MONOPRIL-treated and placebo-treated patients, respectively. The most frequent reasons (0.4 to 0.9%) were headache, elevated transaminases, fatigue, cough (see PRECAUTIONS: General, Cough), diarrhea, and nausea and vomiting.

During clinical trials with any MONOPRIL regimen, the incidence of adverse events in the elderly (≥ 65 years old) was similar to that seen in younger patients.

Clinical adverse events probably or possibly related or of uncertain relationship to therapy, occurring in at least 1% of patients treated with MONOPRIL alone and at least as frequent on MONOPRIL as on placebo in placebo-controlled clinical trials are shown in the table below.

Clinical Adverse Events in Placebo-Controlled Trials (Hypertension)

	MONOPRIL (N = 688) Incidence (Discontinuation)	Placebo (N = 184) Incidence (Discontinuation)
Cough	2.2 (0.4)	0.0 (0.0)
Dizziness	1.6 (0.0)	0.0 (0.0)
Nausea/Vomiting	1.2 (0.4)	0.5 (0.0)

The following events were also seen at > 1% on MONOPRIL but occurred in the placebo group at a greater rate: headache, diarrhea, fatigue, and sexual dysfunction. Other clinical events probably or possibly related, or of uncertain relationship to therapy occurring in 0.2 to 1.0% of patients (except as noted) treated with MONOPRIL in controlled or uncontrolled clinical trials (N=1479) and less frequent, clinically significant events include (listed by body system):
General: Chest pain, edema, weakness, excessive sweating.
Cardiovascular: Angina/myocardial infarction, cerebrovascular accident, hypertensive crisis, rhythm disturbances, palpitations, hypotension, syncope, flushing, claudication. Orthostatic hypotension occurred in 1.4% of patients treated with fosinopril monotherapy. Hypotension or orthostatic hypotension was a cause for discontinuation of therapy in 0.1% of patients.
Dermatologic: Urticaria, rash, photosensitivity, pruritis.
Endocrine/Metabolic: Gout, decreased libido.
Gastrointestinal: Pancreatitis, hepatitis, dysphagia, abdominal distention, abdominal pain, flatulence, constipation, heartburn, appetite/weight change, dry mouth.
Hematologic: Lymphadenopathy.
Immunologic: Angioedema. (See WARNINGS: Angioedema).
Musculoskeletal: Arthralgia, musculoskeletal pain, myalgia/muscle cramp.
Nervous/Psychiatric: Memory disturbance, tremor, confusion, mood change, paresthesia, sleep disturbance, drowsiness, vertigo.
Respiratory: Bronchospasm, pharyngitis, sinusitis/rhinitis, laryngitis/hoarseness, epistaxis. A symptom-complex of cough, bronchospasm, and eosinophilia has been observed in two patients treated with fosinopril.
Special Senses: Tinnitus, vision disturbance, taste disturbance, eye irritation.
Urogenital: Renal insufficiency, urinary frequency.
Heart Failure
In placebo-controlled clinical trials (361 MONOPRIL-treated patients), the usual duration of therapy was 3–6 months. Discontinuations due to any clinical or laboratory adverse event, except for heart failure, were 8.0% and 7.5% in MONOPRIL-treated and placebo-treated patients, respectively. The most frequent reason for discontinuation of MONOPRIL was angina pectoris (1.1%). Significant hypotension after the first dose of MONOPRIL occurred in 14/590 (2.4%) of patients; 5/590 (0.8%) patients discontinued due to first dose hypotension.

Clinical adverse events probably or possibly related or of uncertain relationship to therapy, occurring in at least 1% of patients treated with MONOPRIL and at least as common as the placebo group, in placebo-controlled trials are shown in the table below.

Clinical Adverse Events in Placebo-Controlled Trials (Heart Failure)

	MONOPRIL (N = 361) Incidence (Discontinuation)	Placebo (N = 373) Incidence (Discontinuation)
Dizziness	11.9 (0.6)	5.4 (0.3)
Cough	9.7 (0.8)	5.1 (0.0)
Hypotension	4.4 (0.8)	0.8 (0.0)
Musculoskeletal Pain	3.3 (0.0)	2.7 (0.0)
Nausea/Vomiting	2.2 (0.6)	1.6 (0.3)
Diarrhea	2.2 (0.0)	1.3 (0.0)
Chest Pain (non-cardiac)	2.2 (0.0)	1.6 (0.0)
Upper Respiratory Infection	2.2 (0.0)	1.3 (0.0)
Orthostatic Hypotension	1.9 (0.0)	0.8 (0.0)
Subjective Cardiac Rhythm Disturbance	1.4 (0.6)	0.8 (0.3)
Weakness	1.4 (0.3)	0.5 (0.0)

The following events also occurred at a rate of 1% or more on MONOPRIL (Fosinopril Sodium) but occurred on placebo more often: fatigue, dyspnea, headache, rash, abdominal pain, muscle cramp, angina pectoris, edema, and insomnia. The incidence of adverse events in the elderly (≥ 65 years old) was similar to that seen in younger patients.

Other clinical events probably or possibly related, or of uncertain relationship to therapy occurring in 0.4 to 1.0% of patients (except as noted) treated with MONOPRIL in controlled clinical trials (N=516) and less frequent, clinically significant events include (listed by body system):
General: Fever, influenza, weight gain, hyperhidrosis, sensation of cold, fall, pain.
Cardiovascular: Sudden death, cardiorespiratory arrest, shock (0.2%), atrial rhythm disturbance, cardiac rhythm disturbances, non anginal chest pain, edema lower extremity, hypertension, syncope, conduction disorder, bradycardia, tachycardia.
Dermatologic: Pruritus.
Endocrine/Metabolic: Gout, sexual dysfunction.
Gastrointestinal: Hepatomegaly, abdominal distension, decreased appetite, dry mouth, constipation, flatulence.
Immunologic: Angioedema. (0.2%).
Musculoskeletal: Muscle ache, swelling of an extremity, weakness of an extremity.
Nervous/Psychiatric: Cerebral infarction, TIA, depression, numbness, paresthesia, vertigo, behavior change, tremor.
Respiratory: Abnormal vocalization, rhinitis, sinus abnormality, tracheobronchitis, abnormal breathing, pleuritic chest pain.
Special Senses: Visual disturbance, taste disturbance.
Urogenital: Abnormal urination, kidney pain.
Fetal/Neonatal Morbidity and Mortality
See WARNINGS: Fetal/Neonatal Morbidity and Mortality.
Potential Adverse Effects Reported with ACE Inhibitors
Body as a whole: Anaphylactoid reactions (see WARNINGS: Anaphylactoid and possible related reactions and PRECAUTIONS: Hemodialysis).

Other medically important adverse effects reported with ACE inhibitors include: Cardiac arrest; eosinophilic pneumonitis; neutropenia/agranulocytosis, pancytopenia, anemia (including hemolytic and aplastic), thrombocytopenia; acute renal failure; hepatic failure, jaundice (hepatocellular or cholestatic); symptomatic hyponatremia; bullous pemphigus, exfoliative dermatitis; a syndrome which may include: arthralgia/arthritis, vasculitis, serositis, myalgia, fever, rash or other dermatologic manifestations, a positive ANA, leukocytosis, eosinophilia, or an elevated ESR.
Laboratory Test Abnormalities
Serum Electrolytes: Hyperkalemia, (see PRECAUTIONS); hyponatremia, (see PRECAUTIONS: Drug Interactions, With diuretics).
BUN/Serum Creatinine: Elevations, usually transient and minor, of BUN or serum creatinine have been observed. In placebo-controlled clinical trials, there were no significant differences in the number of patients experiencing increases in serum creatinine (outside the normal range or 1.33 times the pre-treatment value) between the fosinopril and placebo treatment groups. Rapid reduction of longstanding or markedly elevated blood pressure by any antihypertensive therapy can result in decreases in the glomerular filtration rate and, in turn, lead to increases in BUN or serum creatinine. (See PRECAUTIONS: General.)
Hematology: In controlled trials, a mean *hemoglobin* decrease of 0.1 g/dL was observed in fosinopril-treated patients. In individual patients decreases in hemoglobin or

hematocrit were usually transient, small, and not associated with symptoms. No patient was discontinued from therapy due to the development of anemia. *Other:* Neutropenia (see WARNINGS), leukopenia and eosinophilia.

Liver Function Tests: Elevations of transaminases, LDH, alkaline phosphatase and serum bilirubin have been reported. Fosinopril therapy was discontinued because of serum transaminase elevations in 0.7% of patients. In the majority of cases, the abnormalities were either present at baseline or were associated with other etiologic factors. In those cases which were possibly related to fosinopril therapy, the elevations were generally mild and transient and resolved after discontinuation of therapy.

OVERDOSAGE

Oral doses of fosinopril at 2600 mg/kg in rats were associated with significant lethality. Human overdoses of fosinopril have not been reported, but the most common manifestations of human fosinopril overdosage is likely to be hypotension.

Laboratory determinations of serum levels of fosinoprilat and its metabolites are not widely available, and such determinations have, in any event, no established role in the management of fosinopril overdose. No data are available to suggest physiological maneuvers (e.g., maneuvers to change the pH of the urine) that might accelerate elimination of fosinopril and its metabolites. Fosinoprilat is poorly removed from the body by both hemodialysis and peritoneal dialysis.

Angiotensin II could presumably serve as a specific antagonist-antidote in the setting of fosinopril overdose, but angiotensin II is essentially unavailable outside of scattered research facilities. Because the hypotensive effect of fosinopril is achieved through vasodilation and effective hypovolemia, it is reasonable to treat fosinopril overdose by infusion of normal saline solution.

DOSAGE AND ADMINISTRATION

Hypertension

The recommended initial dose of MONOPRIL (Fosinopril Sodium) is 10 mg once a day, both as monotherapy and when the drug is added to a diuretic. Dosage should then be adjusted according to blood pressure response at peak (2–6 hours) and trough (about 24 hours after dosing) blood levels. The usual dosage range needed to maintain a response at trough is 20–40 mg but some patients appear to have a further response to 80 mg. In some patients treated with once daily dosing, the antihypertensive effect may diminish toward the end of the dosing interval. If trough response is inadequate, dividing the daily dose should be considered. If blood pressure is not adequately controlled with MONOPRIL alone, a diuretic may be added.

Concomitant administration of MONOPRIL with potassium supplements, potassium salt substitutes, or potassium-sparing diuretics can lead to increases of serum potassium (see PRECAUTIONS).

In patients who are currently being treated with a diuretic, symptomatic hypotension occasionally can occur following the initial dose of MONOPRIL. To reduce the likelihood of hypotension, the diuretic should, if possible, be discontinued two to three days prior to beginning therapy with MONOPRIL (see WARNINGS). Then, if blood pressure is not controlled with MONOPRIL alone, diuretic therapy should be resumed. If diuretic therapy cannot be discontinued, an initial dose of 10 mg of MONOPRIL should be used with careful medical supervision for several hours and until blood pressure has stabilized. (See WARNINGS; PRECAUTIONS: Information for Patients and Drug Interactions.)

Since concomitant administration of MONOPRIL with potassium supplements, or potassium-containing salt substitutes or potassium-sparing diuretics may lead to increases in serum potassium, they should be used with caution (see PRECAUTIONS).

Heart Failure

Digitalis is not required for MONOPRIL to manifest improvements in exercise tolerance and symptoms. Most placebo-controlled clinical trial experience has been with both digitalis and diuretics present as background therapy.

The usual starting dose of MONOPRIL should be 10 mg once daily. Following the initial dose of MONOPRIL, the patient should be observed under medical supervision for at least two hours for the presence of hypotension or orthostasis and, if present, until blood pressure stabilizes. An initial dose of 5 mg is preferred in heart failure patients with moderate to severe renal failure or those who have been vigorously diuresed.

Dosage should be increased, over a several week period, to a dose that is maximal and tolerated but not exceeding 40 mg once daily. The usual effective dosage range is 20 to 40 mg once daily.

The appearance of hypotension, orthostasis, or azotemia early in dose titration should not preclude further careful dose titration. Consideration should be given to reducing the dose of concomitant diuretic.

For Hypertensive or Heart Failure Patients With Renal Impairment: In patients with impaired renal function, the total body clearance of fosinoprilat is approximately 50% slower than in patients with normal renal function. Since hepatobiliary elimination partially compensates for diminished renal elimination, the total body clearance of fosinoprilat does not differ appreciably with any degree of renal insufficiency (creatinine clearances <80 mL/min/1.73m^2), including end-stage renal failure (creatinine clearance <10 mL/min/1.73m^2). This relative constancy of body clearance of active fosinoprilat, resulting from the dual route of elimination, permits use of the usual dose in patients with any degree of renal impairment. (See WARNINGS: Anaphylactoid reactions during membrane exposure and PRECAUTIONS: Hemodialysis).

HOW SUPPLIED

10 mg tablets: White to off-white, biconvex flat-end diamond shaped, compressed partially scored tablets with unilog number **158** and **MJ** on one side and **m** on the other. They are supplied in bottles of 30 (NDC 0087-0158-22), bottles of 90 (NDC 0087-0158-46) and 1000 (NDC 0087-0158-85). Bottles contain a desiccant canister.

20 mg tablets: White to off-white, oval shaped, compressed tablets with unilog number **609** and **MJ** on one side and **m** on the other. They are supplied in bottles of 30 (NDC 0087-0609-41), bottles of 90 (NDC 0087-0609-42) and 1000 (NDC 0087-0609-85). Bottles contain a desiccant canister.

40 mg tablets: White to off-white, biconvex hexagonal shaped, compressed tablets with unilog number **1202** and **MJ** on one side and **m** on the other. They are supplied in bottles of 30 (NDC 0087-1202-12), bottles of 90 (NDC 0087-1202-13) and 1000 (NDC 0087-1202-51). Bottles contain a desiccant canister.

UNIMATIC® unit-dose packs containing 100 tablets are also available for each potency: **10 mg** (NDC 0087-0158-45), **20 mg** (NDC 0087-0609-45) and **40 mg** (NDC 0087-1202-45).

STORAGE

Store between 15°C (59°F) and 30°C (86°F). Avoid prolonged exposure to temperatures above 30°C (86°F). Keep bottles tightly closed (protect from moisture).

J4-502F

F4-B001-11-95 Revised: November 1995

Bristol-Myers Squibb Company

Shown in Product Identification Guide, page 307

OVCON® 35 ℞
OVCON® 50 (NORETHINDRONE AND ETHINYL ESTRADIOL TABLETS, USP)

CAUTION: FEDERAL LAW PROHIBITS DISPENSING WITHOUT PRESCRIPTION

21- and 28-DAY REGIMENS

Patients should be counseled that this product does not protect against HIV infection (AIDS) and other sexually transmitted diseases.

DESCRIPTION

21-Day OVCON 35 provides a regimen for oral contraception derived from 21 tablets composed of norethindrone and ethinyl estradiol. The chemical name for norethindrone is 17-hydroxy-19-nor-17α-pregn-4-en-20-yn-3-one and for ethinyl estradiol the chemical name is 19-nor-17α-pregna-1,3,5 (10)-trien-20-yne-3,17-diol.

28-Day OVCON® 35 and OVCON® 50 (norethindrone and ethinyl estradiol tablets, USP) provide a continuous regimen for oral contraception derived from 21 tablets composed of norethindrone and ethinyl estradiol to be followed by 7 green tablets of inert ingredients. The structural formulas are:

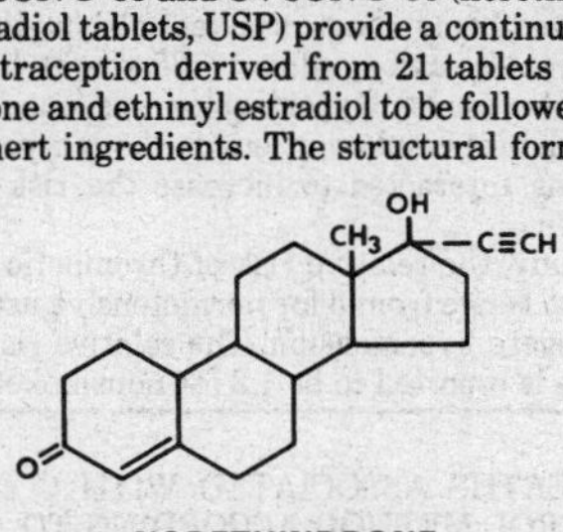

NORETHINDRONE

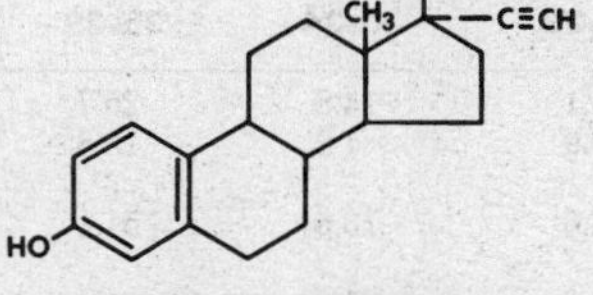

ETHINYL ESTRADIOL

The active OVCON 35 tablets contain 0.4 mg norethindrone and 0.035 mg ethinyl estradiol. The active OVCON 50 tablets contain 1 mg norethindrone and 0.05 mg ethinyl estradiol. The green tablets contain inert ingredients.

OVCON 35, 21-Day contains the following inactive ingredients: dibasic calcium phosphate, FD&C Yellow No. 6 (aluminum lake), lactose, magnesium stearate, povidone, and sodium starch glycolate.

OVCON 35, 28-Day contains the following inactive ingredients: acacia, dibasic calcium phosphate, D&C Yellow No. 10 (aluminum lake), FD&C Blue No. 1 (aluminum lake), FD&C Yellow No. 6 (aluminum lake), lactose, magnesium stearate, povidone, sodium starch glycolate, starch (corn), and talc.

OVCON 50, 28-Day contains the following inactive ingredients: acacia, dibasic calcium phosphate, D&C Yellow No. 10 (aluminum lake), FD&C Blue No.1 (aluminum lake), FD&C Yellow No. 6 (aluminum lake), lactose, magnesium stearate, povidone, sodium starch glycolate, starch (corn), and talc.

CLINICAL PHARMACOLOGY

Combination oral contraceptives act by suppression of gonadotropins. Although the primary mechanism of this action is inhibition of ovulation, other alterations include changes in the cervical mucus (which increase the difficulty of sperm entry into the uterus) and the endometrium (which reduce the likelihood of implantation).

INDICATIONS AND USAGE

Oral contraceptives are indicated for the prevention of pregnancy in women who elect to use this product as a method of contraception.

Oral contraceptives are highly effective. Table 1 lists the typical accidental pregnancy rates for users of combination oral contraceptives and other methods of contraception. The efficacy of these contraceptive methods, except sterilization, depends upon the reliability with which they are used. Correct and consistent use of methods can result in lower failure rates.

TABLE 1
LOWEST EXPECTED AND TYPICAL FAILURE RATES DURING THE FIRST YEAR OF CONTINUOUS USE OF A METHOD
% of Women Experiencing an Accidental Pregnancy in the First Year of Continuous Use

Method	Lowest Expected*	Typical**
(No contraception)	(85)	(85)
Oral contraceptives		
combined	0.1	3***
progestin only	0.5	3***
Diaphragm with spermicidal cream or jelly	6	18
Spermicides alone (foam, creams, jellies and vaginal suppositories)	3	21
Vaginal sponge		
nulliparous	6	18
multiparous	9	28
IUD	0.8–2.0	3#
Condom without spermicides	2	12
Periodic abstinence (all methods)	1–9	20
Injectible progestogen	0.3–0.4	0.3–0.4
Implants		
6 capsules	0.04	0.04
2 rods	0.03	0.03
Female sterilization	0.2	0.4
Male sterilization	0.1	0.15

Reproduced with permission of the Population Council from J. Trussell, et al: Contraceptive failure in the United States: An update. Studies in Family Planning, 21 (1), January–February 1990.

* The authors' best guess of the percentage of women expected to experience an accidental pregnancy among couples who initiate a method (not necessarily for the first time) and who use it consistently and correctly during the first year if they do not stop for any reason other than pregnancy.

** This term represents "typical" couples who initiate use of a method (not necessarily for the first time), who experience an accidental pregnancy during the first year if they do not stop use for any reason other than pregnancy.

*** Combined typical rate for both combined and progestin only.

\# Combined typical rate for both medicated and non-medicated IUD.

CONTRAINDICATIONS

Oral contraceptives should not be used in women who currently have the following conditions:

- Thrombophlebitis or thromboembolic disorders
- A past history of deep vein thrombophlebitis or thromboembolic disorders
- Cerebrovascular or coronary artery disease
- Known or suspected carcinoma of the breast
- Carcinoma of the endometrium or other known or suspected estrogen-dependent neoplasia

Continued on next page

Bristol-Myers Squibb Co.—Cont.

- Undiagnosed abnormal genital bleeding
- Cholestatic jaundice of pregnancy or jaundice with prior pill use
- Hepatic adenomas or carcinomas
- Known or suspected pregnancy

WARNINGS

Cigarette smoking increases the risk of serious cardiovascular side effects from oral contraceptive use. This risk increases with age and with heavy smoking (15 or more cigarettes per day) and is quite marked in women over 35 years of age. Women who use oral contraceptives should be strongly advised not to smoke.

The use of oral contraceptives is associated with increased risk of several serious conditions including myocardial infarction, thromboembolism, stroke, hepatic neoplasia, and gallbladder disease, although the risk of serious morbidity or mortality is very small in healthy women without underlying risk factors. The risk of morbidity and mortality increases significantly in the presence of other underlying risk factors such as hypertension, hyperlipidemias, obesity and diabetes.

Practitioners prescribing oral contraceptives should be familiar with the following information relating to these risks.

The information contained in this package insert is principally based on studies carried out in patients who used oral contraceptives with higher formulations of estrogens and progestogens than those in common use today. The effect of long-term use of the oral contraceptives with lower formulations of both estrogens and progestogens remains to be determined.

Throughout this labeling, epidemiological studies reported are of two types: retrospective or case control studies and prospective or cohort studies. Case control studies provide a measure of the relative risk of a disease, namely, a *ratio* of the incidence of a disease among oral contraceptive users to that among nonusers. The relative risk does not provide information on the actual clinical occurrence of a disease. Cohort studies provide a measure of attributable risk, which is the *difference* in the incidence of disease between oral contraceptive users and nonusers. The attributable risk does provide information about the actual occurrence of a disease in the population. *For further information, the reader is referred to a text on epidemiological methods.

*Adapted from Stadel BB: Oral contraceptives and cardiovascular disease. *N Engl J Med*, 1981;305:612–618, 672–677; with author's permission.

1. THROMBOEMBOLIC DISORDERS AND OTHER VASCULAR PROBLEMS

The physician should be alert to the earliest manifestations of thromboembolic thrombotic disorders as discussed below. Should any of these occur or be suspected the drug should be discontinued immediately.

a. Myocardial Infarction

An increased risk of myocardial infarction has been attributed to oral contraceptive use. This risk is primarily in smokers or women with other underlying risk factors for coronary artery disease such as hypertension, hypercholesterolemia, morbid obesity, and diabetes. The relative risk of heart attack for current oral contraceptive users has been estimated to be two to six. The risk is very low under the age of 30.

Smoking in combination with oral contraceptive use has been shown to contribute substantially to the incidence of myocardial infarctions in women in their mid-thirties or older, with smoking accounting for the majority of excess cases. Mortality rates associated with circulatory disease have been shown to increase substantially in smokers over the age of 35 and nonsmokers over the age of 40 (Figure 1) among women who use oral contraceptives.

FIGURE 1
CIRCULATORY DISEASE MORTALITY RATES PER 100,000 WOMAN-YEARS BY AGE, SMOKING STATUS AND ORAL CONTRACEPTIVE USE

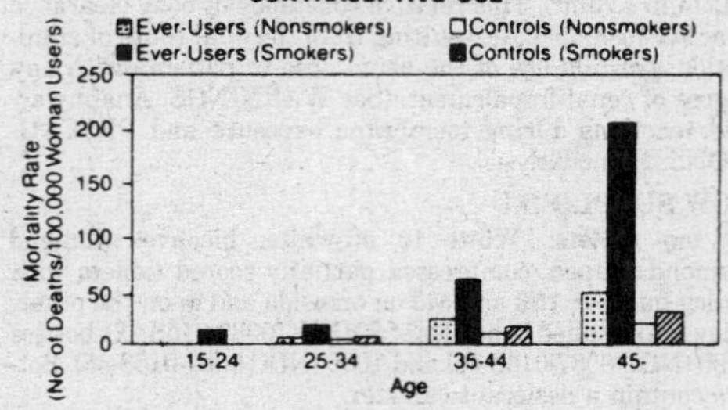

Layde PM, Beral V: Further analyses of mortality in oral contraceptive users: Royal College of General Practitioners' oral contraception study. (Table 5) *Lancet* 1981;1:541–546.

Oral contraceptives may compound the effects of well-known risk factors, such as hypertension, diabetes, hyperlipidemias, age, and obesity. In particular, some progestogens are known to decrease HDL cholesterol and cause glucose intolerance, while estrogens may create a state of hyperinsulinism. Oral contraceptives have been shown to increase blood pressure among users (see section 9 in Warnings). Such increases in risk factors have been associated with an increased risk of heart disease and the risk increases with the number of risk factors present. Oral contraceptives must be used with caution in women with cardiovascular disease risk factors.

b. Thromboembolism

An increased risk of thromboembolic and thrombotic disease associated with the use of oral contraceptives is well established. Case control studies have found the relative risk of users compared to nonusers to be 3 for the first episode of superficial venous thrombosis, 4 to 11 for deep vein thrombosis or pulmonary embolism, and 1.5 to 6 for women with predisposing conditions for venous thromboembolic disease. Cohort studies have shown the relative risk to be somewhat lower, about 3 for new cases and about 4.5 for new cases requiring hospitalization. The risk of thromboembolic disease due to oral contraceptives is not related to length of use and disappears after pill use is stopped.

A two- to four-fold increase in relative risk of postoperative thromboembolic complications has been reported with the use of oral contraceptives. The relative risk of venous thrombosis in women who have predisposing conditions is twice that of women without such medical conditions. If feasible, oral contraceptives should be discontinued at least four weeks prior to and for two weeks after elective surgery of a type associated with an increase in risk of thromboembolism and during and following prolonged immobilization. Since the immediate postpartum period is also associated with an increased risk of thromboembolism, oral contraceptives should be started no earlier than four to six weeks after delivery in women who elect not to breastfeed.

c. Cerebrovascular diseases

Oral contraceptives have been shown to increase both the relative and attributable risk of cerebrovascular events (thrombotic and hemorrhagic strokes); although, in general, the risk is greatest among older (> 35 years), hypertensive women who also smoke. Hypertension was found to be a risk factor for both users and nonusers, for both types of strokes, while smoking interacted to increase the risk for hemorrhagic strokes.

In a large study, the relative risk of thrombotic strokes has been shown to range from 3 for normotensive users to 14 for users with severe hypertension. The relative risk of hemorrhagic stroke is reported to be 1.2 for nonsmokers who used oral contraceptives, 2.6 for smokers who did not use oral contraceptives, 7.6 for smokers who used oral contraceptives, 1.8 for normotensive users and 25.7 for users with severe hypertension. The attributable risk is also greater in older women.

d. Dose-related risk of vascular disease from oral contraceptives

A positive association has been observed between the amount of estrogen and progestogen in oral contraceptives and the risk of vascular disease. A decline in serum high density lipoproteins (HDL) has been reported with many progestational agents. A decline in serum high density lipoproteins has been associated with an increased incidence of ischemic heart disease. Because estrogens increase HDL cholesterol, the net effect of an oral contraceptive depends on a balance achieved between doses of estrogen and progestogen and the nature and absolute amount of progestogens used in the contraceptive. The amount of both hormones should be considered in the choice of an oral contraceptive.

Minimizing exposure to estrogen and progestogen is in keeping with good principles of therapeutics. For any particular estrogen/progestogen combination, the dosage regimen prescribed should be one which contains the least amount of estrogen and progestogen that is compatible with a low failure rate and the needs of the individual patient. New acceptors of oral contraceptive agents should be started on preparations containing 0.05 mg or less of estrogen.

e. Persistence of risk

There are two studies which have shown persistence of risk of vascular disease for ever-users of oral contraceptives. In a study in the United States, the risk of developing myocardial infarction after discontinuing oral contraceptives persists for at least 9 years for women 40–49 years old who had used oral contraceptives for 5 or more years, but this increased risk was not demonstrated in other age groups. In another study in Great Britain, the risk of developing cerebrovascular disease persisted for at least 6 years after discontinuation of oral contraceptives, although excess risk was very small. However, both studies were performed with oral contraceptive formulations containing 50 micrograms or higher of estrogens.

2. ESTIMATES OF MORTALITY FROM CONTRACEPTIVE USE

One study gathered data from a variety of sources which have estimated the mortality rate associated with different methods of contraception at different ages (Table 2).

[See table below.]

These estimates include the combined risk of death associated with contraceptive methods plus the risk attributable to pregnancy in the event of method failure. Each method of contraception has its specific benefits and risk. The study concluded that with the exception of oral contraceptive users 35 and older who smoke and 40 and older who do not smoke, mortality associated with all methods of birth control is low and below that associated with childbirth.

The observation of a possible increase in risk of mortality with age for oral contraceptive users is based on data gathered in the 1970s—but not reported until 1983. However, current clinical practice involves the use of lower estrogen dose formulations combined with careful restriction of oral contraceptive use to women who do not have the various risk factors listed in this labeling.

Because of these changes in practice and, also, because of some limited new data which suggest that the risk of cardiovascular disease with the use of oral contraceptives may now be less than previously observed (Porter JB, Hunter J, Jick H, et al. Oral contraceptives and nonfatal vascular disease. *Obstet Gynecol* 1985;66:1–4 and Porter JB, Jick H, Walker AM. Mortality among oral contraceptive users. *Obstet Gynecol* 1987;70:29–32), the Fertility and Maternal Health Drugs Advisory Committee was asked to review the topic in 1989. The Committee concluded that although cardiovascular disease risk may be increased with oral contraceptive use after age 40 in healthy nonsmoking women (even with the newer low-dose formulations), there are greater potential health risks associated with pregnancy in older women and with the alternative surgical and medical procedures which may be necessary if such women do not have access to effective and acceptable means of contraception.

Therefore, the Committee recommended that the benefits of oral contraceptive use by healthy nonsmoking women over 40 may outweigh the possible risks. Of course, older women, as all women who take oral contraceptives, should take the lowest possible dose formulation that is effective.

3. CARCINOMA OF THE REPRODUCTIVE ORGANS

Numerous epidemiological studies have been performed on the incidence of breast, endometrial, ovarian, and cervical cancer in women using oral contraceptives. The overwhelming evidence in the literature suggests that use of oral contraceptives is not associated with an increase in the risk of developing breast cancer, regardless of the age and parity of first use or with most of the marketed brands and doses. The Cancer and Steroid Hormone (CASH) study also showed no latent effect on the risk of breast cancer for at least a decade following long-term use. A few studies have shown a slightly increased relative risk of developing breast cancer, although the methodology of these studies, which included differences

TABLE 2
ANNUAL NUMBER OF BIRTH-RELATED OR METHOD-RELATED DEATHS ASSOCIATED WITH CONTROL OF FERTILITY PER 100,000 NON-STERILE WOMEN, BY FERTILITY CONTROL METHOD ACCORDING TO AGE

Method of control and outcome	AGE 15–19	20–24	25–29	30–34	35–39	40–44
No fertility control methods*	7.0	7.4	9.1	14.8	25.7	28.2
Oral contraceptives nonsmoker**	0.3	0.5	0.9	1.9	13.8	31.6
Oral contraceptives smoker**	2.2	3.4	6.6	13.5	51.1	117.2
IUD**	0.8	0.8	1.0	1.0	1.4	1.4
Condom*	1.1	1.6	0.7	0.2	0.3	0.4
Diaphragm/spermicide*	1.9	1.2	1.2	1.3	2.2	2.8
Periodic abstinence*	2.5	1.6	1.6	1.7	2.9	3.6

* Deaths are birth related
** Deaths are method related

Ory HW: Mortality associated with fertility and fertility control:1983. *Fam Plann Perspect* 1983;15:50–56.

in examination of users and nonusers and differences in age at start of use, has been questioned.
Some studies suggest that oral contraceptive use has been associated with an increase in the risk of cervical intraepithelial neoplasia in some populations of women.
However, there continues to be controversy about the extent to which such findings may be due to differences in sexual behavior and other factors.
In spite of many studies of the relationship between oral contraceptive use and breast cancer and cervical cancers, a cause-and-effect relationship has not been established.

4. HEPATIC NEOPLASIA

Benign hepatic adenomas are associated with oral contraceptive use, although their occurrence is rare in the United States. Indirect calculations have estimated the attributable risk to be in the range of 3.3 cases/100,000 for users, a risk that increases after four or more years of use. Rupture of hepatic adenomas may cause death through intra-abdominal hemorrhage.
Studies from Britain have shown an increased risk of developing hepatocellular carcinoma in long-term (> 8 years) oral contraceptive users. However, these cancers are extremely rare in the U.S. and the attributable risk (the excess incidence) of liver cancers in oral contraceptive users approaches less than one per million users.

5. OCULAR LESIONS

There have been clinical case reports of retinal thrombosis associated with the use of oral contraceptives. Oral contraceptives should be discontinued if there is unexplained partial or complete loss of vision; onset of proptosis or diplopia; papilledema; or retinal vascular lesions. Appropriate diagnostic and therapeutic measures should be undertaken immediately.

6. ORAL CONTRACEPTIVE USE BEFORE OR DURING EARLY PREGNANCY

Extensive epidemiological studies have revealed no increased risk of birth defects in women who have used oral contraceptives prior to pregnancy. Studies also do not suggest a teratogenic effect, particularly in so far as cardiac anomalies and limb reduction defects are concerned, when taken inadvertently during early pregnancy.
The administration of oral contraceptives to induce withdrawal bleeding should not be used as a test for pregnancy. Oral contraceptives should not be used during pregnancy to treat threatened or habitual abortion.
It is recommended that for any patient who has missed two consecutive periods, pregnancy should be ruled out before continuing oral contraceptive use. If the patient has not adhered to the prescribed schedule, the possibility of pregnancy should be considered at the time of the first missed period. Oral contraceptive use should be discontinued if pregnancy is confirmed.

7. GALLBLADDER DISEASE

Earlier studies have reported an increased lifetime relative risk of gallbladder surgery in users of oral contraceptives and estrogens. More recent studies, however, have shown that the relative risk of developing gallbladder disease among oral contraceptive users may be minimal.
The recent findings of minimal risk may be related to the use of oral contraceptive formulations containing lower hormonal doses of estrogens and progestogens.

8. CARBOHYDRATE AND LIPID METABOLIC EFFECTS

Oral contraceptives have been shown to cause glucose intolerance in a significant percentage of users. Oral contraceptives containing greater than 75 micrograms of estrogens cause hyperinsulinism, while lower doses of estrogen cause less glucose intolerance. Progestogens increase insulin secretion and create insulin resistance, this effect varying with different progestational agents.
However, in the nondiabetic woman, oral contraceptives appear to have no effect on fasting blood glucose. Because of these demonstrated effects, prediabetic and diabetic women should be carefully observed while taking oral contraceptives.
A small proportion of women will have persistent hypertriglyceridemia while on the pill. As discussed earlier (see Warnings 1.a. and 1.d.), changes in serum trigylcerides and lipoprotein levels have been reported in oral contraceptive users.

9. ELEVATED BLOOD PRESSURE

An increase in blood pressure has been reported in women taking oral contraceptives and this increase is more likely in older oral contraceptive users and with continued use. Data from the Royal College of General Practitioners and subsequent randomized trials have shown that the incidence of hypertension increases with increasing concentrations of progestogens.
Women with a history of hypertension or hypertension-related diseases, or renal disease should be encouraged to use another method of contraception. If women elect to use oral contraceptives, they should be monitored closely and if significant elevation of blood pressure occurs, oral contraceptives should be discontinued. For most women, elevated blood pressure will return to normal after stopping oral contraceptives, and there is no difference in the occurrence of hypertension among ever- and never-users.

10. HEADACHE

The onset or exacerbation of migraine or development of headache with a new pattern which is recurrent, persistent, or severe requires discontinuation of oral contraceptives and evaluation of the cause.

11. BLEEDING IRREGULARITIES

Breakthrough bleeding and spotting are sometimes encountered in patients on oral contraceptives, especially during the first three months of use. Nonhormonal causes should be considered and adequate diagnostic measures taken to rule out malignancy or pregnancy in the event of breakthrough bleeding, as in the case of any abnormal vaginal bleeding. If pathology has been excluded, time or a change to another formulation may solve the problem. In the event of amenorrhea, pregnancy should be ruled out.
Women with a history of oligomenorrhea or secondary amenorrhea or young women without regular cycles prior to taking oral contraceptives may again have irregular bleeding or amenorrhea after discontinuation of oral contraceptives.

PRECAUTIONS

1. SEXUALLY-TRANSMITTED DISEASES

Patients should be counseled that this product does not protect against HIV infection (AIDS) and other sexually transmitted diseases.

2. PHYSICAL EXAMINATION AND FOLLOW-UP

It is good medical practice for all women to have annual history and physical examinations, including women using oral contraceptives. The physical examination, however, may be deferred until after initiation of oral contraceptives if requested by the woman and judged appropriate by the clinician. The physical examination should include special reference to blood pressure, breasts, abdomen, and pelvic organs, including cervical cytology, and relevant laboratory tests. In case of undiagnosed, persistent, or recurrent abnormal vaginal bleeding, appropriate measures should be conducted to rule out malignancy. Women with a strong family history of breast cancer or who have breast nodules should be monitored with particular care.

3. LIPID DISORDERS

Women who are being treated for hyperlipidemias should be followed closely if they elect to use oral contraceptives. Some progestogens may elevate LDL levels and may render the control of hyperlipidemias more difficult.

4. LIVER FUNCTION

If jaundice develops in any woman receiving such drugs, the medication should be discontinued. Steroid hormones may be poorly metabolized in patients with impaired liver function.

5. FLUID RETENTION

Oral contraceptives may cause some degree of fluid retention. They should be prescribed with caution, and only with careful monitoring, in patients with conditions which might be aggravated by fluid retention.

6. EMOTIONAL DISORDERS

Women with a history of depression should be carefully observed and the drug discontinued if depression recurs to a serious degree.
Patients becoming significantly depressed while taking oral contraceptives should stop the medication and use an alternate method of contraception in an attempt to determine whether the symptom is drug related.

7. CONTACT LENSES

Contact lens wearers who develop visual changes or changes in lens tolerance should be assessed by an ophthalmologist.

8. DRUG INTERACTIONS

Reduced efficacy and increased incidence of breakthrough bleeding and menstrual irregularities have been associated with concomitant use of rifampin. A similar association, though less marked, has been suggested with barbiturates, phenylbutazone, phenytoin sodium, and possibly with griseofulvin, ampicillin, and tetracyclines.

9. INTERACTIONS WITH LABORATORY TESTS

Certain endocrine and liver function tests and blood components may be affected by oral contraceptives:
a. Increased prothrombin and factors VII, VIII, IX, and X; decreased antithrombin 3; increased norepinephrine-induced platelet aggregability.
b. Increased thyroid-binding globulin (TBG) leading to increased circulating total thyroid hormone, as measured by protein-bound iodine (PBI), T4 by column or by radioimmunoassay. Free T3 resin uptake is decreased, reflecting the elevated TBG, free T4 concentration is unaltered.
c. Other binding proteins may be elevated in serum.
d. Sex-binding globulins are increased and result in elevated levels of total circulating sex steroids and corticoids; however, free or biologically active levels remain unchanged.
e. Triglycerides may be increased.
f. Glucose tolerance may be decreased.
g. Serum folate levels may be depressed by oral contraceptive therapy. This may be of clinical significance if a woman becomes pregnant shortly after discontinuing oral contraceptives.

10. CARCINOGENESIS

See **WARNINGS** section.

11. PREGNANCY

Pregnancy Category X. See **CONTRAINDICATIONS** and **WARNINGS** sections.

12. NURSING MOTHERS

Small amounts of oral contraceptive steroids have been identified in the milk of nursing mothers and a few adverse effects on the child have been reported, including jaundice and breast enlargement. In addition, oral contraceptives given in the postpartum period may interfere with lactation by decreasing the quantity and quality of breast milk. If possible, the nursing mother should be advised not to use oral contraceptives but to use other forms of contraception until she has completely weaned her child.

13. VOMITING AND/OR DIARRHEA

Although a cause-and-effect relationship has not been clearly established, several cases of oral contraceptive failure have been reported in association with vomiting and/or diarrhea. If significant gastrointestinal disturbance occurs in any woman receiving contraceptive steroids, the use of a back-up method of contraception for the remainder of that cycle is recommended.

INFORMATION FOR THE PATIENT

See Patient Labeling Printed Below

ADVERSE REACTIONS

An increased risk of the following serious adverse reactions has been associated with the use of oral contraceptives (see **WARNINGS** section):

- Thrombophlebitis
- Arterial thromboembolism
- Pulmonary embolism
- Myocardial infarction
- Cerebral hemorrhage
- Cerebral thrombosis
- Hypertension
- Gallbladder disease
- Hepatic adenomas or benign liver tumors

There is evidence of an association between the following conditions and the use of oral contraceptives, although additional confirmatory studies are needed:

- Mesenteric thrombosis
- Retinal thrombosis

The following adverse reactions have been reported in patients receiving oral contraceptives and are believed to be drug related:

- Nausea
- Vomiting
- Gastrointestinal symptoms (such as abdominal cramps and bloating)
- Breakthrough bleeding
- Spotting
- Change in menstrual flow
- Amenorrhea
- Temporary infertility after discontinuation of treatment
- Edema
- Melasma which may persist
- Breast changes: tenderness, enlargement, and secretion
- Change in weight (increase or decrease)
- Change in cervical ectropion and secretion
- Possible diminution in lactation when given immediately postpartum
- Cholestatic jaundice
- Migraine
- Rash (allergic)
- Mental depression
- Reduced tolerance to carbohydrates
- Vaginal candidiasis
- Change in corneal curvature (steepening)
- Intolerance to contact lenses

The following adverse reactions have been reported in users of oral contraceptives, and the association has been neither confirmed nor refuted:

- Premenstrual syndrome
- Cataracts
- Changes in appetite
- Cystitis-like syndrome
- Headache
- Nervousness
- Dizziness
- Hirsutism
- Loss of scalp hair
- Erythema multiforme
- Erythema nodosum
- Hemorrhagic eruption
- Vaginitis
- Porphyria
- Impaired renal function
- Hemolytic uremic syndrome
- Budd-Chiari syndrome
- Acne
- Changes in libido
- Colitis

Continued on next page

Bristol-Myers Squibb Co.—Cont.

OVERDOSAGE

Serious ill effects have not been reported following acute ingestion of large doses of oral contraceptives by young children. Overdosage may cause nausea, and withdrawal bleeding may occur in females.

NONCONTRACEPTIVE HEALTH EFFECTS

The following noncontraceptive health benefits related to the use of oral contraceptives are supported by epidemiological studies which largely utilized oral contraceptive formulations containing estrogen doses exceeding 0.035 mg of ethinyl estradiol or 0.05 mg of mestranol.

Effects on menses:
- Increased menstrual cycle regularity
- Decreased blood loss and decreased incidence of iron deficiency anemia
- Decreased incidence of dysmenorrhea

Effects related to inhibition of ovulation:
- Decreased incidence of functional ovarian cysts
- Decreased incidence of ectopic pregnancies

Effects from long-term use:
- Decreased incidence of fibroadenomas and fibrocystic disease of the breast
- Decreased incidence of acute pelvic inflammatory disease
- Decreased incidence of endometrial cancer
- Decreased incidence of ovarian cancer

DOSAGE AND ADMINISTRATION

The following is a summary of the instructions given to the patient in the "HOW TO TAKE THE PILL" section of the DETAILED PATIENT PACKAGE INSERT.

The patient is given instructions in five (5) categories.

1. IMPORTANT POINTS TO REMEMBER: The patient is told (a) that she should take one pill every day at the same time, (b) many women have spotting or light bleeding or gastric distress during the first one to three cycles, (c) missing pills can also cause spotting or light bleeding, (d) she should use a back-up method for contraception if she has vomiting or diarrhea or takes some concomitant medications, and/or if she has trouble remembering the pill, (e) if she has any other questions, she should consult her physician.

2. BEFORE SHE STARTS TAKING HER PILLS: She should decide what time of day she wishes to take the pill, check whether her pill pack has 21 or 28 pills, and note the order in which she should take the pills (diagrammatic drawings of the pill pack are included in the patient insert).

3. WHEN SHE SHOULD START THE FIRST PACK: The Day-One start is listed as the first choice and the Sunday start (the Sunday after her period starts) is given as the second choice. If she uses the Sunday start she should use a back-up method in the first cycle if she has intercourse before she has taken seven pills.

4. WHAT TO DO DURING THE CYCLE: The patient is advised to take one pill at the same time every day until the pack is empty. If she is on a 21 day regimen, she should wait seven days to start the next pack. If she is on the 28 day regimen, she should start the next pack the day after the last inactive tablet and not wait any days between packs.

5. WHAT TO DO IF SHE MISSED A PILL OR PILLS: The patient is given instructions about what she should do if she misses one, two or more than two pills at varying times in her cycle for both the Day-One and the Sunday start. The patient is warned that she may become pregnant if she has unprotected intercourse in the seven days after missing pills. To avoid this, she must use another birth control method such as condom, foam, or sponge in these seven days.

HOW SUPPLIED

OVCON® 35 (norethindrone and ethinyl estradiol tablets, USP) is available in 21- and 28-day regimens. Each package contains 21 round, peach tablets of 0.4 mg norethindrone and 0.035 mg ethinyl estradiol, imprinted with **MJ** on one side and **583** on the other. Each round, green tablet in the 28-day regimen contains inert ingredients and is imprinted with **MJ** on one side and **850** on the other.

OVCON 35, 21-Day
NDC 0087-0583-42 Carton of 6 compacts
OVCON 35, 28-Day
NDC 0087-0578-41 Carton of 6 compacts
OVCON® 50 (norethindrone and ethinyl estradiol tablets, USP) is available in 28-day regimens. Each package contains 21 round, yellow tablets of 1.0 mg norethindrone and 0.05 mg ethinyl estradiol, imprinted with **MJ** on one side and **584** on the other. Each round, green tablet in the 28-day regimen contains inert ingredients and is imprinted with **MJ** on one side and **850** on the other.

OVCON 50, 28-Day
NDC 0087-0579-41 Carton of 6 compacts
Store below 30°C (86°F)
References are available upon request.

PATIENT PACKAGE INSERT BRIEF SUMMARY

This product (like all oral contraceptives) is intended to prevent pregnancy. It does not protect against HIV infection (AIDS) and other sexually transmitted diseases.

Oral contraceptives, also known as "birth control pills" or "the pill," are taken to prevent pregnancy and when taken correctly, have a failure rate of about 1% per year when used without missing any pills. The typical failure rate of large numbers of pill users is less than 3% per year when women who miss pills are included.

Oral contraceptive use is associated with certain serious diseases that can be life-threatening or may cause temporary or permanent disability. The risks associated with taking oral contraceptives increase significantly if you:
- Smoke
- Have high blood pressure, diabetes, high cholesterol
- Have or have had clotting disorders, heart attack, stroke, angina pectoris, cancer of the breast or sex organs, jaundice or malignant or benign liver tumors.

You should not take the pill if you suspect you are pregnant or have unexplained vaginal bleeding.

> **Cigarette smoking increases the risk of serious cardiovascular side effects from oral contraceptive use. This risk increases with age and with heavy smoking (15 or more cigarettes per day) and is quite marked in women over 35 years of age. Women who use oral contraceptives should not smoke.**

Most side effects of the pill are not serious. The most common such effects are nausea, vomiting, bleeding between menstrual periods, weight gain, breast tenderness, and difficulty wearing contact lenses. These side effects, especially nausea and vomiting, may subside within the first three months of use.

The serious side effects of the pill occur very infrequently, especially if you are in good health and are young. However, you should know that the following medical conditions have been associated with or made worse by the pill:

1. Blood clots in the legs (thrombophlebitis), lungs (pulmonary embolism), stoppage or rupture of a blood vessel in the brain (stroke), blockage of blood vessels in the heart (heart attack or angina pectoris), or other organs of the body. As mentioned above, smoking increases the risk of heart attacks and strokes and subsequent serious medical consequences.

2. Liver tumors, which may rupture and cause severe bleeding. A possible but not definite association has been found with the pill and liver cancer. However, liver cancers are extremely rare. The chance of developing liver cancer from using the pill is thus even rarer.

3. High blood pressure, although blood pressure usually returns to normal when the pill is stopped.

The symptoms associated with these serious side effects are discussed in the detailed leaflet given to you with your supply of pills. Notify your doctor or health care provider if you notice any unusual physical disturbances while taking the pill. In addition, drugs such as rifampin, as well as some anticonvulsants and some antibiotics may decrease oral contraceptive effectiveness.

Studies to date of women taking the pill have not shown an increase in the incidence of cancer of the breast or cervix. There is, however, insufficient evidence to rule out the possibility that the pill may cause such cancers.

Taking the pill provides some important noncontraceptive effects. These include less painful menstruation, less menstrual blood loss and anemia, fewer pelvic infections, and fewer cancers of the ovary and the lining of the uterus.

Be sure to discuss any medical condition you may have with your health care provider. Your health care provider will take a medical and family history before prescribing oral contraceptives and will examine you. The physical examination may be delayed to another time if you request it and the health care provider believes that it is a good medical practice to postpone it. You should be reexamined at least once a year while taking oral contraceptives. The detailed patient information booklet gives you further information which you should read and discuss with your health care professional.

DOSAGE AND ADMINISTRATION

HOW TO TAKE THE PILL

The instructions given in the DETAILED PATIENT PACKAGE INSERT are also given in the **BRIEF SUMMARY** included inside each compact. In the event the patient may read only the brief summary, these instructions include the directions on starting the first pack on Day-One (first choice) of her period and the Sunday start (Sunday after period starts). The patient is advised that, if she used the Sunday start, she should use a back-up method in the first cycle if she has intercourse before she has taken seven pills. The patient is also instructed as to what she should do if she misses a pill or pills. The patient is warned that she may become pregnant if she misses a pill or pills and that she should use a back-up method of birth control in the event she has inter-

course any time during the seven day period following the missed pill or pills.

A diagrammatic drawing of the specific pill pack is included in the **BRIEF SUMMARY**.

PATIENT PACKAGE INSERT

This product (like all oral contraceptives) is intended to prevent pregnancy. It does not protect against HIV infection (AIDS) and other sexually transmitted diseases.

INTRODUCTION

Any woman who considers using oral contraceptives (the birth control pill or the pill) should understand the benefits and risks of using this form of birth control.

Although the oral contraceptives have important advantages over other methods of contraception, they have certain risks that no other method has and some of these risks may continue after you have stopped using the oral contraceptive. This booklet will give you much of the information you will need to make this decision and will also help you determine if you are at risk of developing any of the serious side effects of the pill. It will tell you how to use the pill properly so that it will be as effective as possible. However, this booklet is not a replacement for a careful discussion between you and your health care professional. You should discuss the information provided in this booklet with him or her, both when you first start taking the pill and during your revisits. You should also follow your health care professional's advice with regard to regular check-ups while you are on the pill.

EFFECTIVENESS OF ORAL CONTRACEPTIVES

Oral contraceptives or "birth control pills" or "the pill" are used to prevent pregnancy and are more effective than other nonsurgical methods of birth control. The chance of becoming pregnant is less than 1% (1 pregnancy per 100 women per year of use) when the pills are used correctly and no pills are missed. Typical failure rates are actually 3% per year. The chance of becoming pregnant increases with each missed pill during a menstrual cycle.

In comparison, typical accidental pregnancy rates for other nonsurgical methods of birth control during the first year of use are as follows:

IUD: 3%
Diaphragm with spermicides: 18%
Spermicides alone: 21%
Vaginal sponge: 18% to 28%
Condom alone: 12%
Periodic abstinence: 20%
Injectible progestogen: 0.3% to 0.4%
Implants: 0.03% to 0.04%
No methods: 85%

WHO SHOULD NOT TAKE ORAL CONTRACEPTIVES

> **Cigarette smoking increases the risk of serious cardiovascular side effects from oral contraceptive use. This risk increases with age and with heavy smoking (15 or more cigarettes per day) and is quite marked in women over 35 years of age. Women who use oral contraceptives should not smoke.**

Some women should not use the pill. For example, you should not take the pill if you are pregnant or think you may be pregnant. You should also not use the pill if you have or have ever had any of the following conditions:
- A history of heart attack or stroke
- Blood clots in the legs (thrombophlebitis), lungs (pulmonary embolism), or eyes
- A history of blood clots in the deep veins of your legs
- Chest pain (angina pectoris)
- Known or suspected breast cancer or cancer of the lining of the uterus
- Unexplained vaginal bleeding (until a diagnosis is reached by your doctor)
- Yellowing of the whites of the eyes or of the skin (jaundice) during pregnancy or during previous use of the pill
- Liver tumor (benign or cancerous)

Tell you health care professional if you have ever had any of these conditions. Your health care professional can recommend a safer method of birth control.

OTHER CONSIDERATIONS BEFORE TAKING ORAL CONTRACEPTIVES

Tell your health care professional if you have:
- Breast nodules, fibrocystic disease of the breast or an abnormal breast x-ray or mammogram
- Diabetes
- Elevated cholesterol or triglycerides
- High blood pressure
- Migraine or other headaches or epilepsy
- Mental depression
- Gallbladder, heart, or kidney disease
- History of scanty or irregular menstrual periods

Women with any of these conditions should be checked often by their health care professional if they choose to use oral contraceptives.

Also, be sure to inform your doctor or health care professional if you smoke or are on any medications.

RISKS OF TAKING ORAL CONTRACEPTIVES

1. Risk of developing blood clots.

Blood clots and blockage of blood vessels are the most serious side effects of taking oral contraceptives. In particular, a clot in the legs can cause thrombophlebitis and a clot that travels to the lungs can cause a sudden blockage of the vessel carrying blood to the lungs. Either of these can cause death or disability. Rarely, clots occur in the blood vessels of the eye and may cause blindness, double vision, or impaired vision.

If you take oral contraceptives and need elective surgery, need to stay in bed for a prolonged illness, or have recently delivered a baby, you may be at risk of developing blood clots. You should consult your doctor about stopping oral contraceptives three to four weeks before surgery and not taking oral contraceptives for two weeks after surgery or during bed rest. You should also not take oral contraceptives soon after delivery of a baby. It is advisable to wait for at least four weeks after delivery if you are not breastfeeding. If you are breastfeeding see the section on Breastfeeding in **GENERAL PRECAUTIONS.**

2. Heart attacks and strokes

Oral contraceptives may increase the tendency of developing strokes (stoppage or rupture of blood vessels in the brain) and angina pectoris and heart attacks (blockage of blood vessels in the heart). Any of these conditions can cause death or disability.

Smoking greatly increases the possibility of suffering heart attacks and strokes. Furthermore, smoking and the use of oral contraceptives greatly increase the chances of developing and dying of heart disease.

3. Gallbladder disease

Oral contraceptive users probably have a greater risk than nonusers of having gallbladder disease, although this risk may be related to pills containing high doses of estrogens.

4. Liver tumors

In rare cases, oral contraceptives can cause benign but dangerous liver tumors. These benign liver tumors can rupture and cause fatal internal bleeding. In addition, a possible, but not definite, association has been found with the pill and liver cancers in two studies, in which a few women who developed these very rare cancers were found to have used oral contraceptives for long periods. However, liver cancers in general are extremely rare and the chance of developing liver cancer from using the pill is thus even rarer.

5. Cancer of the reproductive organs

There is, at present, no confirmed evidence that oral contraceptives increase the risk of cancer of the reproductive organs and breasts in human studies. Several studies have found no overall increase in the risk of developing breast cancer. However, women who use oral contraceptives and have a strong family history of breast cancer, or who have breast nodules or abnormal mammograms, should be closely followed by their doctors.

Some studies have found an increase in the incidence of cancer of the cervix in women who use oral contraceptives. However, this finding may be related to factors other than the use of oral contraceptives.

ESTIMATED RISK OF DEATH FROM A BIRTH CONTROL METHOD OR PREGNANCY

All methods of birth control and pregnancy are associated with a risk of developing certain diseases which may lead to disability or death. An estimate of the number of deaths associated with different methods of birth control and pregnancy has been calculated and is shown in the following table. [See table above.]

It can be seen in the table that for women aged 15 to 39, the risk of death was highest with pregnancy (7–26 deaths per 100,000 women, depending on age). Among pill users who do not smoke, the risk of death was always lower than that associated with pregnancy for any age group, although over the age of 40, the risk increases to 32 deaths per 100,000 women, compared to 28 associated with pregnancy at that age. However, for pill users who smoke and are over the age of 35, the estimated number of deaths exceeds those for other methods of birth control. If a woman is over the age of 40 and smokes, her estimated risk of death is four times higher (117/100,000 women) than the estimated risk associated with pregnancy (28/100,000 women) in that age group.

The suggestion that women over 40 who don't smoke should not take oral contraceptives is based on information from older high-dose pills and on less selective use of pills than is practiced today. An Advisory Committee of the FDA discussed this issue in 1989 and recommended that the benefits of oral contraceptive use by healthy, nonsmoking women over 40 years of age may outweigh the possible risks. However, all women, especially older women, are cautioned to use the lowest dose pill that is effective.

In the above table, the risk of death from any birth control method is less than the risk of childbirth, except for oral contraceptive users over the age of 35 who smoke and pill users over the age of 40 even if they do not smoke.

You should discuss this information with your health care professional.

ANNUAL NUMBER OF BIRTH-RELATED OR METHOD-RELATED DEATHS ASSOCIATED WITH CONTROL OF FERTILITY PER 100,000 NON-STERILE WOMEN, BY FERTILITY CONTROL METHOD ACCORDING TO AGE

Method of control and outcome	AGE					
	15–19	20–24	25–29	30–34	35–39	40–44
No fertility control methods*	7.0	7.4	9.1	14.8	25.7	28.2
Oral contraceptives nonsmoker**	0.3	0.5	0.9	1.9	13.8	31.6
Oral contraceptives smoker**	2.2	3.4	6.6	13.5	51.1	117.2
IUD**	0.8	0.8	1.0	1.0	1.4	1.4
Condom*	1.1	1.6	0.7	0.2	0.3	0.4
Diaphragm/spermicide*	1.9	1.2	1.2	1.3	2.2	2.8
Periodic abstinence*	2.5	1.6	1.6	1.7	2.9	3.6

* Deaths are birth related
** Deaths are method related

WARNING SIGNALS

If any of these adverse conditions occur while you are taking oral contraceptives, call your doctor immediately.

- Sharp chest pain, coughing of blood, or sudden shortness of breath (indicating a possible clot in the lung)
- Pain in the calf (indicating a possible clot in the leg)
- Crushing chest pain or heaviness in the chest (indicating a possible heart attack)
- Sudden severe headache or vomiting, dizziness or fainting, disturbances of vision or speech, weakness, or numbness in an arm or leg (indicating a possible stroke)
- Sudden partial or complete loss of vision (indicating a possible clot in the eye)
- Breast lumps (indicating possible breast cancer or fibrocystic disease of the breast; ask your doctor or health care professional to show you how to examine your breasts)
- Severe pain or tenderness in the stomach area (indicating a possibly ruptured liver tumor)
- Difficulty in sleeping, weakness, lack of energy, fatigue, or change in mood (possibly indicating severe depression)
- Jaundice or a yellowing of the skin or eyeballs, accompanied frequently by fever, fatigue, loss of appetite, dark-colored urine, or light-colored bowel movements (indicating possible liver problems)
- Abnormal vaginal bleeding (See **SIDE EFFECTS OF ORAL CONTRACEPTIVES,** 1. Vaginal bleeding, below).

SIDE EFFECTS OF ORAL CONTRACEPTIVES

In addition to the risks and more serious side effects discussed above (See **RISKS OF TAKING ORAL CONTRACEPTIVES, ESTIMATED RISK OF DEATH FROM A BIRTH CONTROL METHOD OR PREGNANCY** and **WARNING SIGNALS** sections, above), the following may also occur:

1. Vaginal bleeding

Irregular vaginal bleeding or spotting may occur while you are taking the pills. Irregular bleeding may vary from slight staining between menstrual periods to breakthrough bleeding which is a flow much like a regular period. Irregular bleeding occurs most often during the first few months of oral contraceptive use, but may also occur after you have been taking the pill for some time. Such bleeding may be temporary and usually does not indicate any serious problems. It is important to continue taking your pills on schedule. If the bleeding occurs in more than one cycle or lasts for more than a few days, talk to your doctor or health care professional.

2. Gastrointestinal effects

The most frequent, unpleasant side effects are nausea and vomiting, stomach cramps, bloating, and a change in appetite.

3. Contact lenses

If you wear contact lenses and notice a change in vision or an inability to wear your lenses, contact your doctor or health care professional.

4. Fluid retention

Oral contraceptives may cause edema (fluid retention) with swelling of the fingers or ankles and may raise your blood pressure. If you experience fluid retention, contact your doctor or health care professional.

5. Melasma

A spotty darkening of the skin is possible, particularly of the face.

6. Other side effects

Other side effects may include change in appetite, headache, nervousness, depression, dizziness, loss of scalp hair, rash, and vaginal infections.

If any of these side effects bother you, call your doctor or health care professional.

GENERAL PRECAUTIONS

1. Missed periods and use of oral contraceptives before or during early pregnancy

There may be times when you may not menstruate regularly after you have completed taking a cycle of pills. If you have taken your pills regularly and miss one menstrual period, continue taking your pills for the next cycle but be sure to inform your health care professional before doing so. If you have not taken the pills daily as instructed and missed a menstrual period, or if you missed two consecutive menstrual periods, you may be pregnant. Check with your health care professional immediately to determine whether you are pregnant. Do not continue to take oral contraceptives until you are sure you are not pregnant, but continue to use another method of contraception.

There is no conclusive evidence that oral contraceptive use is associated with an increase in birth defects, when taken inadvertently during early pregnancy. Previously, a few studies had reported that oral contraceptives might be associated with birth defects, but these studies have not been confirmed. Nevertheless, oral contraceptives or any other drugs should not be used during pregnancy unless clearly necessary and prescribed by your doctor. You should check with your doctor about risks to your unborn child of any medication taken during pregnancy.

2. While breastfeeding

If you are breastfeeding, consult your doctor before starting oral contraceptives. Some of the drug will be passed on to the child in the milk. A few adverse effects on the child have been reported, including yellowing of the skin (jaundice) and breast enlargement. In addition, oral contraceptives may decrease the amount and quality of your milk. If possible, do not use oral contraceptives while breastfeeding. You should use another method of contraception since breastfeeding provides only partial protection from becoming pregnant and this partial protection decreases significantly as you breastfeed for longer periods of time. You should consider starting oral contraceptives only after you have weaned your child completely.

3. Laboratory tests

If you are scheduled for any laboratory tests, tell your doctor you are taking birth control pills. Certain blood tests may be affected by birth control pills.

4. Drug interactions

Certain drugs may interact with birth control pills to make them less effective in preventing pregnancy or cause an increase in breakthrough bleeding. Such drugs include rifampin, drugs used for epilepsy such as barbiturates (for example, phenobarbital) and phenytoin (Dilantin is one brand of this drug), phenylbutazone (Butazolidin is one brand) and possibly ampicillin and tetracyclines (several brand names). You may need to use an additional method of contraception when you take drugs which can make oral contraceptives less effective.

HOW TO TAKE THE PILL

IMPORTANT POINTS TO REMEMBER

SEXUALLY-TRANSMITTED DISEASES

This product (like all oral contraceptives) is intended to prevent pregnancy. It does not protect against transmission of HIV (AIDS) and other sexually transmitted diseases such as chlamydia, genital herpes, genital warts, gonorrhea, hepatitis B, and syphilis.

BEFORE YOU START TAKING YOUR PILLS

1. BE SURE TO READ THESE DIRECTIONS:
Before you start taking your pills.
Anytime you are not sure what to do.

2. THE RIGHT WAY TO TAKE THE PILL IS TO TAKE ONE PILL EVERY DAY AT THE SAME TIME.
If you miss pills you could get pregnant. This includes starting the pack late. The more pills you miss, the more likely you are to get pregnant.

3. MANY WOMEN HAVE SPOTTING OR LIGHT BLEEDING, OR MAY FEEL SICK TO THEIR STOMACH DURING THE FIRST 1–3 PACKS OF PILLS.
If you do feel sick to your stomach, do not stop taking the pill. The problem will usually go away. If it doesn't go away, check with your doctor or clinic.

4. MISSING PILLS CAN ALSO CAUSE SPOTTING OR LIGHT BLEEDING, even when you make up these missed pills.

Continued on next page

Bristol-Myers Squibb Co.—Cont.

On the days you take 2 pills to make up for missed pills, you could also feel a little sick to you stomach.

5. IF YOU HAVE VOMITING OR DIARRHEA, for any reason, or IF YOU TAKE SOME MEDICINES, including some antibiotics, your pills may not work as well.

Use a back-up method (such as condoms, foam, or sponge) until you check with your doctor or clinic.

6. IF YOU HAVE TROUBLE REMEMBERING TO TAKE THE PILL, talk to your doctor or clinic about how to make pill-taking easier or about using another method of birth control.

7. IF YOU HAVE ANY QUESTIONS OR ARE UNSURE ABOUT THE INFORMATION IN THIS LEAFLET, call your doctor or clinic.

BEFORE YOU START TAKING YOUR PILLS

1. DECIDE WHAT TIME OF DAY YOU WANT TO TAKE YOUR PILL.

It is important to take it at about the same time every day.

2. LOOK AT YOUR PILL PACK TO SEE IF IT HAS 21 OR 28 PILLS:

The 21-pill pack has 21 "active" peach pills (with hormones) to take for 3 weeks, followed by 1 week without pills.

The 28-pill pack has 21 "active" peach or yellow pills (with hormones) to take for 3 weeks, followed by 1 week of reminder green pills (without hormones).

Ovcon® 35
(Norethindrone and Ethinyl Estradiol Tablets, USP)

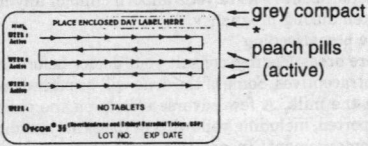

21-pill pack

Each of the 21 peach pills contains norethindrone (0.4 mg) and ethinyl estradiol (0.035 mg).

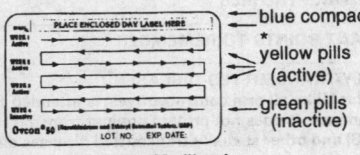

28-pill pack

Each of the 21 peach pills contains norethindrone (0.4 mg) and ethinyl estradiol (0.035 mg). Each green pill in the 28-day regimen contains inert ingredients.

Ovcon® 50
(Norethindrone and Ethinyl Estradiol Tablets, USP)

28-pill pack

Each of the 21 yellow pills contains norethindrone (1 mg) and ethinyl estradiol (0.05 mg). Each green pill in the 28-day regimen contains inert ingredients.

*For use of day labels, see WHEN TO START THE FIRST PACK OF PILLS below.

3. BE SURE YOU HAVE READY AT ALL TIMES:
ANOTHER KIND OF BIRTH CONTROL (such as condoms, foam, or sponge) to use as a back-up in case you miss pills.
AN EXTRA, FULL PILL PACK.

WHEN TO START THE FIRST PACK OF PILLS

You have a choice of which day to start taking your first pack of pills. Decide with your doctor or clinic which is the best day for you. Once you have decided which day you will begin taking your pills, immediately do the following: remove the Brief Summary from inside the compact and look for the day label sheet attached; peel the label from the sheet which has the start day printed on the left hand side; affix the label to the blister card in the designated location. Take your pill

daily in the order indicated by the arrows on the blister card. Pick a time of day which will be easy to remember..

DAY 1 START:

1. Take the first "active" peach or yellow pill of the first pack during the first 24 hours of your period.

2. You will not need to use a back-up method of birth control, since you are starting the pill at the beginning of your period.

SUNDAY START:

1. Take the first "active" peach or yellow pill of the first pack on the Sunday after your period starts, even if you are still bleeding. If your period begins on Sunday, start the pack that same day.

2. Use another method of birth control as a back-up method if you have sex anytime from the Sunday you start your first pack until the next Sunday (7 days). Condoms, foam, or the sponge are good back-up methods of birth control.

WHAT TO DO DURING THE MONTH

1. TAKE ONE PILL AT THE SAME TIME EVERY DAY UNTIL THE PACK IS EMPTY.

Do not skip pills even if you are spotting or bleeding between monthly periods or feel sick to your stomach (nausea).

Do not skip pills even if you do not have sex very often.

2. WHEN YOU FINISH A PACK OR SWITCH YOUR BRAND OF PILLS:

21 pills: Wait 7 days to start the next pack. You will probably have your period during that week. Be sure that no more than 7 days pass between the 21-day packs.

28 pills: Start the next pack on the day after your last "reminder" pill. Do not wait any days between packs.

WHAT TO DO IF YOU MISS PILLS

If you MISS 1 peach or yellow "active" pill:

1. Take it as soon as you remember. Take the next pill at your regular time. This means you may take 2 pills in 1 day.

2. You do not need to use a back-up birth control method if you have sex.

If you MISS 2 peach or yellow "active" pills in a row in WEEK 1 or WEEK 2 of your pack:

1. Take 2 pills on the day you remember and 2 pills the next day.

2. Then take 1 pill a day until you finish the pack.

3. You MAY BECOME PREGNANT if you have sex in the 7 days after you miss pills. You MUST use another birth control method (such as condoms, foam, or sponge) as a back-up for those 7 days.

If you MISS 2 peach or yellow "active" pills in a row in THE 3rd WEEK:

1. If you are a DAY 1 Starter:

THROW OUT the rest of the pill pack and start a new pack that same day.

If you are a Sunday Starter:

Keep taking 1 pill every day until Sunday.

On Sunday, THROW OUT the rest of the pack and start a new pack of pills that same day.

2. You may not have your period this month but this is expected. However, if you miss your period 2 months in a row, call your doctor or clinic because you might be pregnant.

3. You MAY BECOME PREGNANT if you have sex in the 7 days after you miss pills. You MUST use another birth control method (such as condoms, foam, or sponge) as a back-up for those 7 days.

If you MISS 3 OR MORE peach or yellow "active" pills in a row (during the first 3 weeks):

1. If you are a DAY 1 Starter:

THROW OUT the rest of the pill pack and start a new pack that same day.

If you are a Sunday Starter:

Keep taking 1 pill every day until Sunday.

On Sunday, THROW OUT the rest of the pack and start a new pack of pills that same day.

2. You may not have your period this month but this is expected. However, if you miss your period 2 months in a row, call your doctor or clinic because you might be pregnant.

3. You MAY BECOME PREGNANT if you have sex in the 7 days after you miss pills. You MUST use another birth control method (such as condoms, foam, or sponge) as a back-up for those 7 days.

A REMINDER FOR THOSE ON 28-DAY PACKS: If you forget any of the 7 green "reminder" pills in Week 4:
THROW AWAY the pills you missed.

Keep taking 1 pill each day until the pack is empty.

You do not need a back-up method.

FINALLY, IF YOU ARE STILL NOT SURE WHAT TO DO ABOUT THE PILLS YOU HAVE MISSED:

Use a BACK-UP METHOD anytime you have sex.

KEEP TAKING ONE "ACTIVE" PILL EACH DAY until you can reach your doctor or clinic.

GENERAL

1. Pregnancy due to pill failure

The incidence of pill failure resulting in pregnancy is approximately 1% (i.e., one pregnancy per 100 women per year) if taken every day as directed, but more typical failure rates

are about 3%. If failure does occur, the risk to the fetus is minimal.

2. Pregnancy after stopping the pill

There may be some delay in becoming pregnant after you stop using oral contraceptives, especially if you had irregular menstrual cycles before you used oral contraceptives. It may be advisable to postpone conception until you begin menstruating regularly once you have stopped taking the pill and desire pregnancy.

There does not appear to be any increase in birth defects in newborn babies when pregnancy occurs soon after stopping the pill.

3. Other

a. Overdosage

Serious ill effects have not been reported following ingestion of large doses of oral contraceptives by young children. Overdosage may cause nausea and withdrawal bleeding in females. In case of overdosage, contact your poison control center, health care professional, or nearest emergency room. KEEP THIS DRUG AND ALL DRUGS OUT OF THE REACH OF CHILDREN.

b. General medical information

Your health care professional will take a medical and family history before prescribing oral contraceptives and will examine you. The physical examination may be delayed to another time if you request it and the health care provider believes that it is a good medical practice to postpone it. You should be reexamined at least once a year. Be sure to inform your health care professional if there is a family history of any of the conditions listed previously in this leaflet. Be sure to keep all appointments with your health care professional, because this is a time to determine if there are early signs of side effects of oral contraceptive use.

Do not use the drug for any condition other than the one for which it was prescribed. This drug has been prescribed specifically for you; do not give it to others who may want birth control pills.

NONCONTRACEPTIVE EFFECTS OF ORAL CONTRACEPTIVES

In addition to preventing pregnancy, use of oral contraceptives may provide certain benefits. They are:

- Menstrual cycles may become more regular
- Blood flow during menstruation may be lighter and less iron may be lost. Therefore, anemia due to iron deficiency is less likely to occur
- Pain or other symptoms during menstruation may be encountered less frequently
- Ectopic (tubal) pregnancy may occur less frequently
- Noncancerous cysts or lumps in the breast may occur less frequently
- Acute pelvic inflammatory disease may occur less frequently
- Oral contraceptive use may provide some protection against developing two forms of cancer: cancer of the ovaries and cancer of the lining of the uterus.

If you want more information about birth control pills, ask your doctor or pharmacist. They have a more technical leaflet called the Professional Labeling, which you may wish to read.

Bristol-Myers Squibb Company
Revised August 1995

P6962-00
A3-B001-8-95

Shown in Product Identification Guide, page 307

PRAVACHOL® ℞
Pravastatin Sodium Tablets

DESCRIPTION

PRAVACHOL (pravastatin sodium) is one of a new class of lipid-lowering compounds, the HMG-CoA reductase inhibitors, which reduce cholesterol biosynthesis. These agents are competitive inhibitors of 3-hydroxy-3-methylglutaryl-coenzyme A (HMG-CoA) reductase, the enzyme catalyzing the early rate-limiting step in cholesterol biosynthesis, conversion of HMG-CoA to mevalonate.

Pravastatin sodium is designated chemically as 1-Naphthalene-heptanoic acid, 1,2,6,7,8,8a-hexahydro-β,δ,6-trihydroxy-2-methyl-8-(2-methyl-1-oxobutoxy)-, monosodium salt, [1S-[1α(βS*,δS*), 2α, 6α, 8β(R*), 8aα]]-.

Pravastatin sodium is an odorless, white to off-white, fine or crystalline powder. It is a relatively polar hydrophilic compound with a partition coefficient (octanol/water) of 0.59 at a pH of 7.0. It is soluble in methanol and water (> 300 mg/mL), slightly soluble in isopropanol, and practically insoluble in acetone, acetonitrile, chloroform, and ether.

PRAVACHOL is available for oral administration as 10 mg, 20 mg and 40 mg tablets. Inactive ingredients include: croscarmellose sodium, lactose, magnesium oxide, magnesium stearate, microcrystalline cellulose, and povidone. The 10 mg tablet also contains Red Ferric Oxide, the 20 mg tablet also contains Yellow Ferric Oxide, and the 40 mg tablet also contains Green Lake Blend (mixture of D&C Yellow No. 10-Aluminum Lake and FD&C Blue No. 1-Aluminum Lake).

CLINICAL PHARMACOLOGY

Cholesterol and triglycerides in the bloodstream circulate as part of lipoprotein complexes. These complexes can be separated by density ultracentrifugation into high (HDL), intermediate (IDL), low (LDL), and very low (VLDL) density lipoprotein fractions. Triglycerides (TG) and cholesterol synthesized in the liver are incorporated into very low density lipoproteins (VLDLs) and released into the plasma for delivery to peripheral tissues. In a series of subsequent steps, VLDLs are transformed into intermediate density lipoproteins (IDLs), and cholesterol-rich low density lipoproteins (LDLs). High density lipoproteins (HDLs), containing apolipoprotein A, are hypothesized to participate in the reverse transport of cholesterol from tissues back to the liver.

PRAVACHOL produces its lipid-lowering effect in two ways. First, as a consequence of its reversible inhibition of HMG-CoA reductase activity, it effects modest reductions in intracellular pools of cholesterol. This results in an increase in the number of LDL-receptors on cell surfaces and enhanced receptor-mediated catabolism and clearance of circulating LDL. Second, pravastatin inhibits LDL production by inhibiting hepatic synthesis of VLDL, the LDL precursor.

Clinical and pathologic studies have shown that elevated levels of total cholesterol (Total-C), low density lipoprotein cholesterol (LDL-C), and apolipoprotein B (a membrane transport complex for LDL) promote human atherosclerosis. Similarly, decreased levels of HDL-cholesterol (HDL-C) and its transport complex, apolipoprotein A, are associated with the development of atherosclerosis. Epidemiologic investigations have established that cardiovascular morbidity and mortality vary directly with the level of Total-C and LDL-C and inversely with the level of HDL-C. In multicenter clinical trials, those pharmacologic and/or non-pharmacologic interventions that simultaneously lowered LDL-C and increased HDL-C reduced the rate of cardiovascular events (both fatal and non-fatal myocardial infarctions). In both normal volunteers and patients with hypercholesterolemia, treatment with PRAVACHOL reduced Total-C, LDL-C, and apolipoprotein B. PRAVACHOL also modestly reduced VLDL-C and TG while producing increases of variable magnitude in HDL-C and apolipoprotein A. The effects of pravastatin on Lp (a), fibrinogen, and certain other independent biochemical risk markers for coronary heart disease are unknown. Although pravastatin is relatively more hydrophilic than other HMG-CoA reductase inhibitors, the effect of relative hydrophilicity, if any, on either efficacy or safety has not been established.

In the Pravastatin Primary Prevention Study (West of Scotland Coronary Prevention Study—WOS), the effect of improving lipoprotein levels with PRAVACHOL on fatal and non-fatal coronary heart diseases (CHD) was assessed in 6595 men, without a previous myocardial infarction, and with LDL-C levels between 156-254 mg/dl (4-6.7 mmol/l). The patients were followed for a median of 4.8 years. In this randomized, double-blind, placebo-controlled study, PRAVACHOL reduced the risk of a first coronary event [either CHD death or non-fatal myocardial infarction (MI)] by 31% [7.9% vs 5.5%, placebo vs PRAVACHOL, p=0.0001: 248 events in the placebo group (CHD death=44, non-fatal MI=204) vs 174 event in the PRAVACHOL group (CHD death=31, non-fatal MI=143)]. PRAVACHOL also decreased the risk for undergoing myocardial revascularization procedures (coronary artery bypass graft surgery or coronary angioplasty) by 37% (2.5% vs 1.7%, p=0.009) and coronary angiography by 31% (4.2% vs 2.8%, p=0.007). Cardiovascular deaths were decreased by 32% (2.3% vs 1.6%, p=0.03), and there was no increase in death from non-cardiovascular causes.

Pharmacokinetics/Metabolism

PRAVACHOL is administered orally in the active form. In clinical pharmacology studies in man, pravastatin is rapidly absorbed, with peak plasma levels of parent compound attained 1 to 1.5 hours following ingestion. Based on urinary recovery of radiolabeled drug, the average oral absorption of pravastatin is 34% and absolute bioavailability is 17%. While the presence of food in the gastrointestinal tract reduces systemic bioavailability, the lipid-lowering effects of the drug are similar whether taken with, or 1 hour prior to, meals.

Pravastatin undergoes extensive first-pass extraction in the liver (extraction ratio 0.66), which is its primary site of action, and the primary site of cholesterol synthesis and of LDL-C clearance. In vitro studies demonstrated that pravastatin is transported into hepatocytes with substantially less uptake into other cells. In view of pravastatin's apparently extensive first-pass hepatic metabolism, plasma levels may not necessarily correlate perfectly with lipid-lowering efficacy. Pravastatin plasma concentrations [including: area under the concentration-time curve (AUC), peak (Cmax), and steady-state minimum (Cmin)] are directly proportional to administered dose. Systemic bioavailability of pravastatin administered following a bedtime dose was decreased 60% compared to that following an AM dose. Despite this decrease in systemic bioavailability, the efficacy of pravastatin administered once daily in the evening, although not statistically significant, was marginally more effective than that after a morning dose. This finding of lower systemic bioavailability suggests greater hepatic extraction of the drug following the evening dose. Steady-state AUCs, Cmax and Cmin plasma concentrations showed no evidence of pravastatin accumulation following once or twice daily administration of PRAVACHOL (pravastatin sodium) tablets. Approximately 50% of the circulating drug is bound to plasma proteins. Following single dose administration of ^{14}C-pravastatin, the elimination half-life ($t^1/_2$) for total radioactivity (pravastatin plus metabolites) in humans is 77 hours.

Pravastatin, like other HMG-CoA reductase inhibitors, has variable bioavailability. The coefficient of variation, based on between-subject variability, was 50% to 60% for AUC. Approximately 20% of a radiolabeled oral dose is excreted in urine and 70% in the feces. After intravenous administration of radiolabeled pravastatin to normal volunteers, approximately 47% of total body clearance was via renal excretion and 53% by non-renal routes (i.e., biliary excretion and biotransformation). Since there are dual routes of elimination, the potential exists both for compensatory excretion by the alternate route as well as for accumulation of drug and/or metabolites in patients with renal or hepatic insufficiency.

In a study comparing the kinetics of pravastatin in patients with biopsy confirmed cirrhosis (N=7) and normal subjects (N=7), the mean AUC varied 18-fold in cirrhotic patients and 5-fold in healthy subjects. Similarly, the peak pravastatin values varied 47-fold for cirrhotic patients compared to 6-fold for healthy subjects.

Biotransformation pathways elucidated for pravastatin include: (a) isomerization to 6-epi pravastatin and the 3α-hydroxyisomer of pravastatin (SQ 31,906), (b) enzymatic ring hydroxylation to SQ 31,945, (c) ω-1 oxidation of the ester side chain, (d) β-oxidation of the carboxy side chain, (e) ring oxidation followed by aromatization, (f) oxidation of a hydroxyl group to a keto group, and (g) conjugation. The major degradation product is the 3α-hydroxy isomeric metabolite, which has one-tenth to one-fortieth the HMG-CoA reductase inhibitory activity of the parent compound.

Clinical Studies

PRAVACHOL is highly effective in reducing Total-C and LDL-C in patients with heterozygous familial, presumed familial combined, and non-familial (non-FH) forms of primary hypercholesterolemia. A therapeutic response is seen within 1 week, and the maximum response usually is achieved within 4 weeks. This response is maintained during extended periods of therapy. In addition, PRAVACHOL is effective in reducing the risk of acute coronary events in hypercholesterolemic patients with and without previous myocardial infarction.

A single daily dose administered in the evening (the recommended dosing) is as effective as the same total daily dose given twice a day. Once daily administration in the evening appears to be marginally more effective than once daily administration in the morning, perhaps because hepatic cholesterol is synthesized mainly at night. In multicenter, double-blind, placebo-controlled studies of patients with primary hypercholesterolemia, treatment with pravastatin in daily doses ranging from 10 mg to 40 mg consistently and significantly decreased Total-C, LDL-C, and Total-C/HDL-C and LDL-C/HDL-C ratios; modestly decreased VLDL-C and plasma TG levels; and produced increases in HDL-C of variable magnitude.

Primary Hypercholesterolemia Study Dose Response of PRAVACHOL* Once Daily Administration At Bedtime

Dose	Total-C	LDL-C	HDL-C	TG
10 mg	−16%	−22%	+7%	−15%
20 mg	−24%	−32%	+2%	−11%
40 mg	−25%	−34%	+12%	−24%

* Mean percent change from baseline after 8 weeks

In another clinical trial, patients treated with pravastatin in combination with cholestyramine (70% of patients were taking cholestyramine 20 or 24 g per day) had reductions equal to or greater than 50% in LDL-C. Furthermore, pravastatin attenuated cholestyramine-induced increases in TG levels (which are themselves of uncertain clinical significance).

Prevention of Coronary Heart Disease

In the Pravastatin Primary Prevention Study (West of Scotland Coronary Prevention Study—WOS[1], the effect of PRAVACHOL on fatal and non-fatal coronary heart disease (CHD) was assessed in 6595 men 45-64 years of age, without a previous MI, and with LDL-C levels between 156-254 mg/dl (4-6.7 mmol/l). In this randomized, double-blind, placebo-controlled study, patients were treated with standard care, including dietary advice, and either PRAVACHOL 40 mg daily (N=3302) or placebo (N=3293) and followed for a median duration of 4.8 years.

PRAVACHOL significantly reduced the rate of first coronary events (either CHD death or non-fatal MI) by 31% [248 events in the placebo group (CHD death=44, non-fatal MI=204) vs 174 events in the PRAVACHOL group (CHD death=31, non-fatal MI=143), p=0.0001 (see figure below)]. The risk reduction with PRAVACHOL was similar and significant throughout the entire range of baseline LDL cholesterol levels. This reduction was also similar and significant across the age range studied with a 40% risk reduction for patients younger than 55 years and a 27% risk reduction for patients 55 years and older. The Pravastatin Primary Prevention Study included only men and therefore it is not clear to what extent these data can be extrapolated to a similar population of female patients.

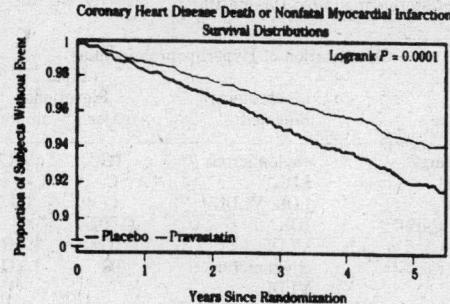

Coronary Heart Disease Death or Nonfatal Myocardial Infarction Survival Distributions

PRAVACHOL also significantly decreased the risk for undergoing myocardial revascularization procedures (coronary artery bypass graft surgery or coronary angioplasty) by 37% (80 vs 51 patients, p=0.009) and coronary angiography by 31% (128 vs 90, p=0.007). Cardiovascular deaths were decreased by 32% (73 vs 50, p=0.03), and there was no increase in death from non-cardiovascular causes.

Atherosclerosis and Myocardial Infarction

In the Pravastatin Limitation of Atherosclerosis in the Coronary Arteries (PLAC I)[2] study, the effect of pravastatin therapy on coronary atherosclerosis was assessed by coronary angiography in patients with coronary disease and moderate hypercholesterolemia (baseline LDL-C range =130-190 mg/dL). In this double-blind, multicenter, controlled clinical trial angiograms were evaluated at baseline and at three years in 264 patients. Although the difference between pravastatin and placebo for the primary endpoint (per-patient change in mean coronary artery diameter) and one of two secondary endpoints (change in percent lumen diameter stenosis) did not reach statistical significance, for the secondary endpoint of change in minimum lumen diameter, statistically significant slowing of disease was seen in the pravastatin treatment group (p=0.02).

In the Regression Growth Evaluation Statin Study (REGRESS)[3], the effect of pravastatin on coronary atherosclerosis was assessed by coronary angiography in 885 patients with angina pectoris, angiographically documented coronary artery disease and hypercholesterolemia (baseline total cholesterol range =160-310 mg/dL). In this double-blind, multicenter, controlled clinical trial, angiograms were evaluated at baseline and at two years in 653 patients (323 treated with pravastatin). Progression of coronary atherosclerosis was significantly slowed in the pravastatin group as assessed by changes in mean segment diameter (p=0.037) and minimum obstruction diameter (p=0.001).

Analysis of pooled events from PLAC I, the Pravastatin, Lipids and Atherosclerosis in the Carotids (PLAC II)[4], REGRESS, and the Kuopio Atherosclerosis Prevention Study (KAPS)[5] (combined N=1,891) showed that treatment with pravastatin was associated with a significant reduction in the composite event rate of fatal and nonfatal myocardial infarction (46 events or 6.4% for placebo versus 21 events or 2.4% for pravastatin, p=0.001). The predominant effect of pravastatin was to reduce the rate of nonfatal myocardial infarction.

INDICATIONS AND USAGE

Therapy with lipid-altering agents should be considered a component of multiple risk factor intervention in those individuals at increased risk for atherosclerotic vascular disease due to hypercholesterolemia. Lipid-altering agents should be used in addition to diet restricted in saturated fat and cholesterol when the response to diet and other nonpharmacological measures alone has been inadequate (see NCEP Guidelines below).

Primary Prevention of Coronary Events

In hypercholesterolemic patients without clinically evident coronary heart disease. PRAVACHOL (pravastatin sodium) is indicated to:

—Reduce the risk of myocardial infarction

—Reduce the risk of undergoing myocardial revascularization procedures

Reduce the risk of cardiovascular mortality with no increase in death from non-cardiovascular causes.

Continued on next page

Bristol-Myers Squibb Co.—Cont.

Atherosclerosis
In hypercholesterolemic patients with clinically evident coronary artery disease, including prior MI, PRAVACHOL (pravastatin sodium) is indicated to:
—Slow the progression of coronary atherosclerosis
—Reduce the risk of acute coronary events

Hypercholesterolemia
PRAVACHOL is indicated for the reduction of elevated total and LDL-cholesterol levels in patients with primary hypercholesterolemia (Type IIa and IIb)[6].

Classification of Hyperlipoproteinemias

Type	Lipoproteins Elevated	Lipid Elevations major	minor
I (rare)	chylomicrons	TG	↑→C
IIa	LDL	C	—
IIb	LDL, VLDL	C	TG
III (rare)	IDL	C/TG	—
IV	VLDL	TG	↑→C
V (rare)	chylomicrons, VLDL	TG	↑→C

C = cholesterol, TG = triglycerides,
LDL = low density lipoprotein,
VLDL = very low density lipoprotein,
IDL = intermediate density lipoprotein.

(For a discussion of efficacy results, see **CLINICAL PHARMACOLOGY: Clinical Studies**).

Prior to initiating therapy with pravastatin, secondary causes for hypercholesterolemia (e.g., poorly controlled diabetes mellitus, hypothyroidism, nephrotic syndrome, dysproteinemias, obstructive liver disease, other drug therapy, alcoholism) should be excluded, and a lipid profile performed to measure Total-C, HDL-C, and TG. For patients with triglycerides (TG) <400 mg/dL (<4.5 mmol/L), LDL-C can be estimated using the following equation:

$$\text{LDL-C} = \text{Total-C} - \text{HDL-C} - \tfrac{1}{5}\,\text{TG}$$

For TG levels >400 mg/dL (>4.5 mmol/L), this equation is less accurate and LDL-C concentrations should be determined by ultracentrifugation. In many hypertriglyceridemic patients, LDL-C may be low or normal despite elevated Total-C. In such cases, HMG-CoA reductase inhibitors are not indicated.

Lipid determinations should be performed at intervals of no less than four weeks and dosage adjusted according to the patient's response to therapy.

The National Cholesterol Education Program's Treatment Guidelines are summarized below:

Definite Atherosclerotic Disease*	Two or More Other Risk Factors**	LDL-Cholesterol mg/dL (mmol/L) Initiation Level	Goal
NO	NO	≥190 (≥4.9)	<160 (<4.1)
NO	YES	≥160 (≥4.1)	<130 (<3.4)
YES	YES or NO	≥130 (≥3.4)	≤100 (≤2.6)

* Coronary heart disease or peripheral vascular disease (including symptomatic carotid artery disease).

**Other risk factors for coronary heart disease (CHD) include: age (males: ≥45 years; females: ≥55 years or premature menopause without estrogen replacement therapy); family history of premature CHD; current cigarette smoking; hypertension; confirmed HDL-C <35 mg/dL (<0.91 mmol/L); and diabetes mellitus. Subtract one risk factor if HDL-C is ≥60 mg/dL (≥1.6 mmol/L).

Since the goal of treatment is lower LDL-C, the NCEP recommends that LDL-C levels be used to initiate and assess treatment response. Only if LDL-C levels are not available should the Total-C be used to monitor therapy.

As with other lipid-lowering therapy, PRAVACHOL (pravastatin sodium) is not indicated when hypercholesterolemia is due to hyperalphalipoproteinemia (elevated HDL-C). The efficacy of pravastatin has not been evaluated in patients with combined elevated Total-C and hypertriglyceridemia [>500 mg/dL (>5.7 mmol/L)]or in patients with elevated intermediate density lipoproteins as their primary lipid abnormality.

CONTRAINDICATIONS
Hypersensitivity to any component of this medication.
Active liver disease or unexplained, persistent elevations in liver function tests (see **WARNINGS**).

Pregnancy and lactation. Atherosclerosis is a chronic process and discontinuation of lipid-lowering drugs during pregnancy should have little impact on the outcome of long-term therapy of primary hypercholesterolemia. Cholesterol and other products of cholesterol biosynthesis are essential components for fetal development (including synthesis of steroids and cell membranes). Since HMG-CoA reductase inhibitors decrease cholesterol synthesis and possibly the synthesis of other biologically active substances derived from cholesterol, they may cause fetal harm when administered to pregnant women. Therefore, HMG-CoA reductase inhibitors are contraindicated during pregnancy and in nursing mothers. **Pravastatin should be administered to women of childbearing age only when such patients are highly unlikely to conceive and have been informed of the potential hazards.** If the patient becomes pregnant while taking this class of drug, therapy should be discontinued and the patient apprised of the potential hazard to the fetus.

WARNINGS
Liver Enzymes
HMG-CoA reductase inhibitors, like some other lipid-lowering therapies, have been associated with biochemical abnormalities of liver function. Increases of serum transaminase (ALT, AST) values to more than 3 times the upper limit of normal occurring on 2 or more (not necessarily sequential) occasions have been reported in 1.3% of patients treated with pravastatin in the US over an average period of 18 months. These abnormalities were not associated with cholestasis and did not appear to be related to treatment duration. In those patients in whom these abnormalities were believed to be related to pravastatin and who were discontinued from therapy, the transaminase levels usually fell slowly to pretreatment levels. These biochemical findings are usually asymptomatic although worldwide experience indicates that anorexia, weakness, and/or abdominal pain may also be present in rare patients.

It is recommended that liver function tests be performed before the initiation of treatment, at 6 and 12 weeks after initiation of therapy or elevation in dose, and periodically thereafter (e.g., semiannually). Patients who develop increased transaminase levels should be monitored with a second liver function evaluation to confirm the finding and be followed thereafter with frequent liver function tests until the abnormality(ies) return to normal. Should an increase in AST or ALT of three times the upper limit of normal or greater persist, withdrawal of pravastatin therapy is recommended.

Active liver disease or unexplained transaminase elevations are contraindications to the use of pravastatin (see **CONTRAINDICATIONS**). Caution should be exercised when pravastatin is administered to patients with a history of liver disease or heavy alcohol ingestion (see **CLINICAL PHARMACOLOGY: Pharmacokinetics/Metabolism**). Such patients should be closely monitored, started at the lower end of the recommended dosing range, and titrated to the desired therapeutic effect.

Skeletal Muscle
Rare cases of rhabdomyolysis with acute renal failure secondary to myoglobinuria have been reported with pravastatin and other drugs in this class. Uncomplicated myalgia has also been reported in pravastatin-treated patients (see **ADVERSE REACTIONS**). Myopathy, defined as muscle aching or muscle weakness in conjunction with increases in creatine phosphokinase (CPK) values to greater than 10 times the upper normal limit, was rare (<0.1%) in pravastatin clinical trials. Myopathy should be considered in any patient with diffuse myalgias, muscle tenderness or weakness, and/or marked elevation of CPK. Patients should be advised to report promptly unexplained muscle pain, tenderness or weakness, particularly if accompanied by malaise or fever. **Pravastatin therapy should be discontinued if markedly elevated CPK levels occur or myopathy is diagnosed or suspected. Pravastatin therapy should also be temporarily withheld in any patient experiencing an acute or serious condition predisposing to the development of renal failure secondary to rhabdomyolysis, e.g., sepsis; hypotension; major surgery; trauma; severe metabolic, endocrine, or electrolyte disorders; or uncontrolled epilepsy.**

The risk of myopathy during treatment with another HMG-CoA reductase inhibitor is increased with concurrent therapy with either erythromycin, cyclosporine, niacin, or fibrates. However, neither myopathy nor significant increases in CPK levels have been observed in three reports involving a total of 100 post-transplant patients (24 renal and 76 cardiac) treated for up to two years concurrently with pravastatin 10–40 mg and cyclosporine. Some of these patients also received other concomitant immunosuppressive therapies. In one single-dose study, pravastatin levels were found to be increased in cardiac transplant patients receiving cyclosporine. Further, in clinical trials involving small numbers of patients who were treated concurrently with pravastatin and niacin, there were no reports of myopathy. Also, myopathy was not reported in a trial of combination pravastatin (40 mg/day) and gemfibrozil (1200 mg/day), although 4 of 75 patients on the combination showed marked CPK elevations versus one of 73 patients receiving placebo. There was a trend toward more frequent CPK elevations and patient withdrawals due to musculoskeletal symptoms in the group receiving combined treatment as compared with the groups receiving placebo, gemfibrozil, or pravastatin monotherapy (see **PRECAUTIONS: Drug Interactions**). **The use of fibrates alone may occasionally be associated with myopathy. The combined use of pravastatin and fibrates should be avoided unless the benefit of further alterations in lipid levels is likely to outweigh the increased risk of this drug combination.**

PRECAUTIONS
General
Pravastatin may elevate creatinine phosphokinase and transaminase levels (see **ADVERSE REACTIONS**). This should be considered in the differential diagnosis of chest pain in a patient on therapy with pravastatin.

Homozygous Familial Hypercholesterolemia. Pravastatin has not been evaluated in patients with rare homozygous familial hypercholesterolemia. In this group of patients, it has been reported that HMG-CoA reductase inhibitors are less effective because the patients lack functional LDL receptors.

Renal Insufficiency. A single 20 mg oral dose of pravastatin was administered to 24 patients with varying degrees of renal impairment (as determined by creatinine clearance). No effect was observed on the pharmacokinetics of pravastatin or its 3α-hydroxy isomeric metabolite (SQ 31,906). A small increase was seen in mean AUC values and half-life ($t^1/_2$) for the inactive enzymatic ring hydroxylation metabolite (SQ 31,945). Given this small sample size, the dosage administered, and the degree of individual variability, patients with renal impairment who are receiving pravastatin should be closely monitored.

Information for Patients
Patients should be advised to report promptly unexplained muscle pain, tenderness or weakness, particularly if accompanied by malaise or fever.

Drug Interactions
Immunosuppressive Drugs, Gemfibrozil, Niacin (Nicotinic Acid), Erythromycin: See **WARNINGS: Skeletal Muscle**.

Antipyrine: Since concomitant administration of pravastatin had no effect on the clearance of antipyrine, interactions with other drugs metabolized via the same hepatic cytochrome isozymes are not expected.

Cholestyramine/Colestipol: Concomitant administration resulted in an approximately 40 to 50% decrease in the mean AUC of pravastatin. However, when pravastatin was administered 1 hour before or 4 hours after cholestyramine or 1 hour before colestipol and a standard meal, there was no clinically significant decrease in bioavailability or therapeutic effect. (See **DOSAGE AND ADMINISTRATION: Concomitant Therapy.**)

Warfarin: In a study involving 10 healthy male subjects given pravastatin and warfarin concomitantly for 6 days, bioavailability parameters at steady state for pravastatin (parent compound) were not altered. Pravastatin did not alter the plasma protein-binding of warfarin. Concomitant dosing did increase the AUC and Cmax of warfarin but did not produce any changes in its anticoagulant action (i.e., no increase was seen in mean prothrombin time after 6 days of concomitant therapy). However, bleeding and extreme prolongation of prothrombin time has been reported with another drug in this class. Patients receiving warfarin-type anticoagulants should have their prothrombin times closely monitored when pravastatin is initiated or the dosage of pravastatin is changed.

Cimetidine: The $AUC_{0\text{–}12hr}$ for pravastatin when given with cimetidine was not significantly different from the AUC for pravastatin when given alone. A significant difference was observed between the AUC's for pravastatin when given with cimetidine compared to when administered with antacid.

Digoxin: In a crossover trial involving 18 healthy male subjects given pravastatin and digoxin concurrently for 9 days, the bioavailability parameters of digoxin were not affected. The AUC of pravastatin tended to increase, but the overall bioavailability of pravastatin plus its metabolites SQ 31,906 and SQ 31,945 was not altered.

Cyclosporine: Some investigators have measured cyclosporine levels in patients on pravastatin, and to date, these results indicate no clinically meaningful elevations in cyclosporine levels. In one single-dose study, pravastatin levels were found to be increased in cardiac transplant patients receiving cyclosporine.

Gemfibrozil: In a crossover study in 20 healthy male volunteers given concomitant single doses of pravastatin and gemfibrozil, there was a significant decrease in urinary excretion and protein binding of pravastatin. In addition, there was a significant increase in AUC, Cmax, and Tmax for the pravastatin metabolite SQ 31,906. Combination therapy with pravastatin and gemfibrozil is generally not recommended.

In interaction studies with aspirin, antacids (1 hour prior to PRAVACHOL (pravastatin sodium)), *cimetidine, nicotinic acid, or probucol,* no statistically significant differences in

bioavailability were seen when PRAVACHOL was administered.

Other Drugs: During clinical trials, no noticeable drug interactions were reported when PRAVACHOL was added to: diuretics, antihypertensives, digitalis, ACE inhibitors, calcium channel blockers, beta-blockers, or nitroglycerin.

Endocrine Function

HMG-CoA reductase inhibitors interfere with cholesterol synthesis and lower circulating cholesterol levels and, as such, might theoretically blunt adrenal or gonadal steroid hormone production. Results of clinical trials with pravastatin in males and post-menopausal females were inconsistent with regard to possible effects of the drug on basal steroid hormone levels. In a study of 21 males, the mean testosterone response to human chorionic gonadotropin was significantly reduced (p < 0.004) after 16 weeks of treatment with 40 mg of pravastatin. However, the percentage of patients showing a ≥50% rise in plasma testosterone after human chorionic gonadotropin stimulation did not change significantly after therapy in these patients. The effects of HMG-CoA reductase inhibitors on spermatogenesis and fertility have not been studied in adequate numbers of patients. The effects, if any, of pravastatin on the pituitary-gonadal axis in pre-menopausal females are unknown. Patients treated with pravastatin who display clinical evidence of endocrine dysfunction should be evaluated appropriately. Caution should also be exercised if an HMG-CoA reductase inhibitor or other agent used to lower cholesterol levels is administered to patients also receiving other drugs (e.g., ketoconazole, spironolactone, cimetidine) that may diminish the levels or activity of steroid hormones.

CNS Toxicity

CNS vascular lesions, characterized by perivascular hemorrhage and edema and mononuclear cell infiltration of perivascular spaces, were seen in dogs treated with pravastatin at a dose of 25 mg/kg/day, a dose that produced a plasma drug level about 50 times higher than the mean drug level in humans taking 40 mg/day. Similar CNS vascular lesions have been observed with several other drugs in this class. A chemically similar drug in this class produced optic nerve degeneration (Wallerian degeneration of retinogeniculate fibers) in clinically normal dogs in a dose-dependent fashion starting at 60 mg/kg/day, a dose that produced mean plasma levels about 30 times higher than the mean drug level in humans taking the highest recommended dose (as measured by total enzyme inhibitory activity). This same drug also produced vestibulocochlear Wallerian-like degeneration and retinal ganglion cell chromatolysis in dogs treated for 14 weeks at 180 mg/kg/day, a dose which resulted in a mean plasma drug level similar to that seen with the 60 mg/kg/day dose.

Carcinogenesis, Mutagenesis, Impairment of Fertility

In a 2-year study in rats fed pravastatin at doses of 10, 30, or 100 mg/kg body weight, there was an increased incidence of hepatocellular carcinomas in males at the highest dose (p < 0.01). Although rats were given up to 125 times the human dose (HD) on a mg/kg body weight basis, serum drug levels were only 6 to 10 times higher than those measured in humans given 40 mg pravastatin as measured by AUC.

The oral administration of 10, 30, or 100 mg/kg (producing plasma drug levels approximately 0.5 to 5.0 times human drug levels at 40 mg) of pravastatin to mice for 22 months resulted in a statistically significant increase in the incidence of malignant lymphomas in treated females when all treatment groups were pooled and compared to controls (p < 0.05). The incidence was not dose-related and male mice were not affected.

A chemically similar drug in this class was administered to mice for 72 weeks at 25, 100, and 400 mg/kg body weight, which resulted in mean serum drug levels approximately 3, 15, and 33 times higher than the mean human serum drug concentration (as total inhibitory activity) after a 40 mg oral dose. Liver carcinomas were significantly increased in high-dose females and mid- and high-dose males, with a maximum incidence of 90 percent in males. The incidence of adenomas of the liver was significantly increased in mid- and high-dose females. Drug treatment also significantly increased the incidence of lung adenomas in mid- and high-dose males and females. Adenomas of the eye Harderian gland (a gland of the eye of rodents) were significantly higher in high-dose mice than in controls.

No evidence of mutagenicity was observed in vitro, with or without rat-liver metabolic activation, in the following studies: microbial mutagen tests, using mutant strains of *Salmonella typhimurium or Escherichia coli;* a forward mutation assay in L5178Y TK +/− mouse lymphoma cells; a chromosomal aberration test in hamster cells; and a gene conversion assay using *Saccharomyces cerevisiae.* In addition, there was no evidence of mutagenicity in either a dominant lethal test in mice or a micronucleus test in mice.

In a study in rats, with daily doses up to 500 mg/kg, pravastatin did not produce any adverse effects on fertility or general reproductive performance. However, in a study with another HMG-CoA reductase inhibitor, there was decreased fertility in male rats treated for 34 weeks at 25 mg/kg body weight, although this effect was not observed in a subsequent

fertility study when this same dose was administered for 11 weeks (the entire cycle of spermatogenesis, including epididymal maturation). In rats treated with this same reductase inhibitor at 180 mg/kg/day, seminiferous tubule degeneration (necrosis and loss of spermatogenic epithelium) was observed. Although not seen with pravastatin, two similar drugs in this class caused drug-related testicular atrophy, decreased spermatogenesis, spermatocytic degeneration, and giant cell formation in dogs. The clinical significance of these findings is unclear.

Pregnancy
Pregnancy Category X
See CONTRAINDICATIONS.

Safety in pregnant women has not been established. Pravastatin was not teratogenic in rats at doses up to 1000 mg/kg daily or in rabbits at doses of up to 50 mg/kg daily. These doses resulted in 20 × (rabbit) or 240 × (rat) the human exposure based on surface area (mg/meter2). However, in studies with another HMG-CoA reductase inhibitor, skeletal malformations were observed in rats and mice. There has been one report of severe congenital bony deformity, tracheo-esophageal fistula, and anal atresia (Vater association) in a baby born to a woman who took another HMG-CoA reductase inhibitor with dextroamphetamine sulfate during the first trimester of pregnancy. PRAVACHOL (pravastatin sodium) should be administered to women of child-bearing potential only when such patients are highly unlikely to conceive and have been informed of the potential hazards. If the woman becomes pregnant while taking PRAVACHOL, it should be discontinued and the patient advised again as to the potential hazards to the fetus.

Nursing Mothers

A small amount of pravastatin is excreted in human breast milk. Because of the potential for serious adverse reactions in nursing infants, women taking PRAVACHOL (pravastatin sodium) should not nurse (see **CONTRAINDICATIONS**).

Pediatric Use

Safety and effectiveness in individuals less than 18 years old have not been established. Hence, treatment in patients less than 18 years old is not recommended at this time.

ADVERSE REACTIONS

Pravastatin is generally well tolerated; adverse reactions have usually been mild and transient. In 4-month long placebo-controlled trials, 1.7% of pravastatin-treated patients and 1.2% of placebo-treated patients were discontinued from treatment because of adverse experiences attributed to study drug therapy; this difference was not statistically significant. In long-term studies, the most common reasons for discontinuation were asymptomatic serum transaminase increases and mild, non-specific gastrointestinal complaints. During clinical trials the overall incidence of adverse events in the elderly was not different from the incidence observed in younger patients.

Body System/ Event	All Events		Events Attributed to Study Drug	
	Pravastatin (N = 900) %	Placebo (N = 411) %	Pravastatin (N = 900) %	Placebo (N = 411) %
Cardiovascular				
Cardiac Chest Pain	4.0	3.4	0.1	0.0
Dermatologic				
Rash	4.0*	1.1	1.3	0.9
Gastrointestinal				
Nausea/Vomiting	7.3	7.1	2.9	3.4
Diarrhea	6.2	5.6	2.0	1.9
Abdominal Pain	5.4	6.9	2.0	3.9
Constipation	4.0	7.1	2.4	5.1
Flatulence	3.3	3.6	2.7	3.4
Heartburn	2.9	1.9	2.0	0.7
General				
Fatigue	3.8	3.4	1.9	1.0
Chest Pain	3.7	1.9	0.3	0.2
Influenza	2.4*	0.7	0.0	0.0
Musculoskeletal				
Localized Pain	10.0	9.0	1.4	1.5
Myalgia	2.7	1.0	0.6	0.0
Nervous System				
Headache	6.2	3.9	1.7*	0.2
Dizziness	3.3	3.2	1.0	0.5
Renal/Genitourinary				
Urinary Abnormality	2.4	2.9	0.7	1.2
Respiratory				
Common Cold	7.0	6.3	0.0	0.0
Rhinitis	4.0	4.1	0.1	0.0
Cough	2.6	1.7	0.1	0.0

*Statistically significantly different from placebo.

Adverse Clinical Events

All adverse clinical events (regardless of attribution) reported in more than 2% of pravastatin-treated patients in the placebo-controlled trials are identified in the table below; also shown are the percentages of patients in whom these medical events were believed to be related or possibly related to the drug:
[See table above.]

In the Pravastatin Primary Prevention Study (West of Scotland Coronary Prevention Study) (see **CLINICAL PHARMACOLOGY: Clinical Studies**) involving 6595 patients treated with PRAVACHOL (pravastatin sodium) (N=3302) or placebo (n=3293) the adverse event profile in the pravastatin group was comparable to that of the placebo group over the median 4.8 years of the study.

The following effects have been reported with drugs in this class; not all the effects listed below have necessarily been associated with pravastatin therapy:

Skeletal: myopathy, rhabdomyolysis, arthralgia.

Neurological: dysfunction of certain cranial nerves (including alteration of taste, impairment of extra-ocular movement, facial paresis), tremor, vertigo, memory loss, paresthesia, peripheral neuropathy, peripheral nerve palsy, anxiety, insomnia, depression.

Hypersensitivity Reactions: An apparent hypersensitivity syndrome has been reported rarely which has included one or more of the following features: anaphylaxis, angioedema, lupus erythematous-like syndrome, polymyalgia rheumatica, dermatomyositis, vasculitis, purpura, thrombocytopenia, leukopenia, hemolytic anemia, positive ANA, ESR increase, eosinophilia, arthritis, arthralgia, urticaria, asthenia, photosensitivity, fever, chills, flushing, malaise, dyspnea, toxic epidermal necrolysis, erythema multiforme, including Stevens-Johnson syndrome.

Gastrointestinal: pancreatitis, hepatitis, including chronic active hepatitis, cholestatic jaundice, fatty change in liver, and, rarely, cirrhosis, fulminant hepatic necrosis, and hepatoma; anorexia, vomiting.

Skin: alopecia, pruritus. A variety of skin changes (e.g., nodules, discoloration, dryness of skin/mucous membranes, changes to hair/nails) have been reported.

Reproductive: gynecomastia, loss of libido, erectile dysfunction.

Eye: progression of cataracts (lens opacities), ophthalmoplegia.

Laboratory Abnormalities: elevated transaminases, alkaline phosphatase, and bilirubin; thyroid function abnormalities.

Laboratory Test Abnormalities

Increases in serum transaminase (ALT, AST) values and CPK have been observed (see **WARNINGS**).

Transient, asymptomatic eosinophilia has been reported. Eosinophil counts usually returned to normal despite contin-

Continued on next page

Bristol-Myers Squibb Co.—Cont.

ued therapy. Anemia, thrombocytopenia, and leukopenia have been reported with HMG-CoA reductase inhibitors.

Concomitant Therapy

Pravastatin has been administered concurrently with cholestyramine, colestipol, nicotinic acid, probucol and gemfibrozil. Preliminary data suggest that the addition of either probucol or gemfibrozil to therapy with lovastatin or pravastatin is **not** associated with greater reduction in LDL-cholesterol than that achieved with lovastatin or pravastatin alone. No adverse reactions unique to the combination or in addition to those previously reported for each drug alone have been reported. Myopathy and rhabdomyolysis (with or without acute renal failure) have been reported when another HMG-CoA reductase inhibitor was used in combination with immunosuppressive drugs, gemfibrozil, erythromycin, or lipid-lowering doses of nicotinic acid. Concomitant therapy with HMG-CoA reductase inhibitors and these agents is generally not recommended. (See **WARNINGS: Skeletal Muscle** and **PRECAUTIONS: Drug Interactions**.)

OVERDOSAGE

To date, there are two reported cases of overdosage with pravastatin, both of which were asymptomatic and not associated with clinical laboratory abnormalities. If an overdose occurs, it should be treated symptomatically and supportive measures should be instituted as required.

DOSAGE AND ADMINISTRATION

The patient should be placed on a standard cholesterol-lowering diet before receiving PRAVACHOL (pravastatin sodium) and should continue on this diet during treatment with PRAVACHOL (see NCEP Treatment Guidelines for details on dietary therapy).

The recommended starting dose is 10 or 20 mg once daily at bedtime. In primary hypercholesterolemic patients with a history of significant renal or hepatic dysfunction, and in the elderly, a starting dose of 10 mg daily at bedtime is recommended. PRAVACHOL may be taken without regard to meals.

Since the maximal effect of a given dose is seen within 4 weeks, periodic lipid determinations should be performed at this time and dosage adjusted according to the patient's response to therapy and established treatment guidelines. The recommended dosage range is generally 10 to 40 mg administered once a day at bedtime. In the elderly, maximum reductions in LDL-cholesterol may be achieved with daily doses of 20 mg or less.

In patients taking immunosuppressive drugs such as cyclosporine (see **WARNINGS: Skeletal Muscle**) concomitantly with pravastatin, therapy should begin with 10 mg of pravastatin once-a-day at bedtime and titration to higher doses should be done with caution. Most patients treated with this combination received a maximum pravastatin dose of 20 mg/day.

Concomitant Therapy

The lipid-lowering effects of PRAVACHOL on total and LDL cholesterol are enhanced when combined with a bile-acid-binding resin. When administering a bile-acid-binding resin (e.g., cholestyramine, colestipol) and pravastatin, PRAVACHOL should be given either 1 hour or more before or at least 4 hours following the resin. (See also **ADVERSE REACTIONS: Concomitant Therapy**.)

HOW SUPPLIED

10 mg tablets: Pink to peach, rounded, rectangular-shaped, biconvex with a P embossed on one side and PRAVACHOL 10 engraved on the opposite side. They are supplied in bottles of 90 (NDC 0003-5154-05). Bottles contain a desiccant canister.

20 mg tablets: Yellow, rounded, rectangular-shaped, biconvex with a P embossed on one side and PRAVACHOL 20 engraved on the opposite side. They are supplied in bottles of 90 (NDC 0003-5178-05) and bottles of 1000 (NDC 0003-5178-75). Bottles contain a desiccant canister.

40 mg tablets: Green, rounded, rectangular-shaped, biconvex with a P embossed on one side and PRAVACHOL 40 engraved on the opposite side. They are supplied in bottles of 90 (NDC 0003-5194-10). Bottles contain a desiccant canister. Unimatic® unit-dose packs containing 100 tablets are also available for each potency: **10 mg** (NDC 0003-5154-06), **20 mg** (NDC 0003-5178-06) and **40 mg** (NDC 0003-5194-11).

Storage

Do not store above 86°F (30°C). Keep tightly closed (protect from moisture). Protect from light.

REFERENCES

[1] Shepherd J, et al. Prevention of coronary heart disease with pravastatin in men with hypercholesterolemia. *N Engl J Med* 1995; 333:1301–7.
[2] Pitt B, et al. Design and recruitment in the United States of a multicenter quantitative angiographic trial of pravastatin to limit atherosclerosis in the coronary arteries (PLAC I). *Am J Cardiol* 72:31, 1983.
[3] Jukema JW, et al. Effects of Lipid Lowering by Pravastatin on Progression and Regression of Coronary Artery Disease

in Symptomatic Man With Normal to Moderately Elevated Serum Cholesterol Levels. The Regression Growth Evaluation Statin Study (REGRESS). *Circulation* 1995; 91:2528–2540.
[4] Crouse JR, et al. Pravastatin, lipids, and atherosclerosis in the carotid arteries: design features of a clinical trial with carotid atherosclerosis outcome, *Controlled Clinical Trials* 13:495, 1992.
[5] Salonen R, et al. Kuopio Atherosclerosis Prevention Study (KAPS). A population-based primary preventive trial of the effect of LDL lowering on antherosclerotic progression in carotid and femoral arteries. Research Institute of Public Health, University of Kuopio, Finland. *Circulation* 92:1758, 1995.
[6] Frederickson classification: Type IIa-elevation of LDL; Type IIb-elevation of LDL and VLDL. Type III (familial dysbetalipoproteinemia)—elevation of IDL. Frederickson, DS, Fat transport in lipoproteins—an integrated approach to mechanism and disorders. *N Engl J Med* 276:34, 1967.

CAUTION: Federal (USA) law prohibits dispensing without prescription.
Revised July 1996
D3-B001-7-96   J4-538D
Bristol-Myers Squibb Company
Princeton, NJ 08543
Shown in Product Identification Guide, page 307

QUESTRAN® POWDER
QUESTRAN® LIGHT
(Cholestyramine for Oral Suspension, USP)   ℞

CAUTION: FEDERAL LAW PROHIBITS DISPENSING WITHOUT PRESCRIPTION

DESCRIPTION

QUESTRAN (Cholestyramine for Oral Suspension, USP), the chloride salt of a basic anion exchange resin, a cholesterol lowering agent, is intended for oral administration. Cholestyramine resin is quite hydrophilic, but insoluble in water. The cholestyramine resin in QUESTRAN is not absorbed from the digestive tract. Nine grams of QUESTRAN POWDER contain 4 grams of anhydrous cholestyramine resin. Five grams of QUESTRAN LIGHT contain 4 grams of anhydrous cholestyramine resin.

QUESTRAN Powder contains the following inactive ingredients: acacia, citric acid, D&C Yellow No. 10, FD&C Yellow No. 6, flavor (natural and artificial), polysorbate 80, propylene glycol alginate, and sucrose (421 mg/g powder). QUESTRAN LIGHT contains the following inactive ingredients: aspartame, citric acid, D&C Yellow No. 10, FD&C Red No. 40, flavor (natural and artificial), propylene glycol alginate, colloidal silicon dioxide, sucrose (144 mg/g powder), and xanthan gum.

ACTIONS/CLINICAL PHARMACOLOGY

Cholesterol is probably the sole precursor of bile acids. During normal digestion, bile acids are secreted into the intestines. A major portion of the bile acids is absorbed from the intestinal tract and returned to the liver via the enterohepatic circulation. Only very small amounts of bile acids are found in normal serum.

QUESTRAN resin adsorbs and combines with the bile acids in the intestine to form an insoluble complex which is excreted in the feces. This results in a partial removal of bile acids from the enterohepatic circulation by preventing their absorption.

The increased fecal loss of bile acids due to QUESTRAN administration leads to an increased oxidation of cholesterol to bile acids, a decrease in beta lipoprotein or low density lipoprotein plasma levels and a decrease in serum cholesterol levels. Although in man, QUESTRAN produces an increase in hepatic synthesis of cholesterol, plasma cholesterol levels fall.

In patients with partial biliary obstruction, the reduction of serum bile acid levels by QUESTRAN reduces excess bile acids deposited in the dermal tissue with resultant decrease in pruritus.

Clinical Studies

In a large, placebo-controlled, multi-clinic study, LRC-CPPT[1], hypercholesterolemic subjects treated with QUESTRAN had mean reductions in total and low-density lipoprotein cholesterol (LDL-C) which exceeded those for diet and placebo treatment by 7.2% and 10.4%, respectively. Over the seven-year study period the QUESTRAN group experienced a 19% reduction (relative to the incidence in the placebo group) in the combined rate of coronary heart disease death plus non-fatal myocardial infarction (cumulative incidences of 7% QUESTRAN and 8.6% placebo). The subjects included in the study were men aged 35-59 with serum cholesterol levels above 265 mg/dL and no previous history of heart disease. It is not clear to what extent these findings can be ex-

trapolated to females and other segments of the hypercholesterolemic population. (See also **PRECAUTIONS: Carcinogenesis, Mutagenesis, and Impairment of Fertility.**)

Two controlled clinical trials have examined the effects of QUESTRAN monotherapy upon coronary atherosclerotic lesions using coronary arteriography. In the NHLBI Type II Coronary Intervention Trial[2], 116 patients (80% male) with coronary artery disease (CAD) documented by arteriography were randomized to QUESTRAN or placebo for five years of treatment. Final study arteriography revealed progression of coronary artery disease in 49% of placebo patients compared to 32% of the QUESTRAN (Cholestyramine for Oral Suspension, USP) group (p <0.05).

In the St. Thomas Atherosclerosis Regression Study (STARS)[3], 90 hypercholesterolemic men with CAD were randomized in three blinded treatments: usual care, lipid-lowering diet, and lipid-lowering diet plus QUESTRAN. After 36 months, follow-up coronary arteriography revealed progression of disease in 46% of usual care patients, 15% of patients on lipid-lowering diet and 12% of those receiving diet plus QUESTRAN (p <0.02). The mean absolute width of coronary segments decreased in the usual care group, increased slightly (0.003 mm) in the diet group and increased by 0.103 mm in the diet plus QUESTRAN group (p <0.05). Thus in these randomized controlled clinical trials using coronary arteriography, QUESTRAN monotherapy has been demonstrated to slow progression[2,3] and promote regression[3] of atherosclerotic lesions in the coronary arteries of patients with coronary artery disease.

The effect of intensive lipid-lowering therapy on coronary atherosclerosis has been assessed by arteriography in hyperlipidemic patients. In these randomized, controlled clinical trials, patients were treated for two to four years by either conventional measures (diet, placebo, or in some cases low dose resin), or intensive combination therapy using diet plus colestipol (an anion exchange resin with a mechanism of action and an effect on serum lipids similar to that of QUESTRAN and QUESTRAN LIGHT) plus either nicotinic acid or lovastatin. When compared to conventional measures, intensive lipid-lowering combination therapy significantly reduced the frequency of progression and increased the frequency of regression of coronary atherosclerotic lesions in patients with or at risk for coronary artery disease.

INDICATIONS AND USAGE

1.) QUESTRAN (Cholestyramine for Oral Suspension, USP) is indicated as adjunctive therapy to diet for the reduction of elevated serum cholesterol in patients with primary hypercholesterolemia (elevated low density lipoprotein [LDL] cholesterol) who do not respond adequately to diet. QUESTRAN may be useful to lower LDL cholesterol in patients who also have hypertriglyceridemia, but it is not indicated where hypertriglyceridemia is the abnormality of most concern.

Therapy with lipid-altering agents should be a component of multiple risk factor intervention in those individuals at significantly increased risk for atherosclerotic vascular disease due to hypercholesterolemia. Treatment should begin and continue with dietary therapy specific for the type of hyperlipoproteinemia determined prior to initiation of drug therapy. Excess body weight may be an important factor and caloric restriction for weight normalization should be addressed prior to drug therapy in the overweight.

Prior to initiating therapy with QUESTRAN, secondary causes of hypercholesterolemia (e.g., poorly controlled diabetes mellitus, hypothyroidism, nephrotic syndrome, dysproteinemias, obstructive liver disease, other drug therapy, alcoholism), should be excluded, and a lipid profile performed to assess Total cholesterol, HDL-C, and triglycerides (TG). For individuals with TG less than 400 mg/dl (<4.5 mmol/L), LDL-C can be estimated using the following equation:

$$LDL\text{-}C = \text{Total cholesterol} - [(TG/5) + HDL\text{-}C]$$

For TG levels >400 mg/dl, this equation is less accurate and LDL-C concentration should be determined by ultracentrifugation. In hypertriglyceridemic patients, LDL-C may be low or normal despite elevated Total-C. In such cases QUESTRAN may not be indicated.

Serum cholesterol and triglyceride levels should be determined periodically based on NCEP guidelines to confirm initial and adequate long-term response. A favorable trend in cholesterol reduction should occur during the first month of QUESTRAN therapy. The therapy should be continued to sustain cholesterol reduction. If adequate cholesterol reduction is not attained, increasing the dosage of QUESTRAN or adding other lipid-lowering agents in combination with QUESTRAN should be considered.

Since the goal of treatment is to lower LDL-C, the NCEP[4] recommends that LDL-C levels be used to initiate and assess treatment response. If LDL-C levels are not available then Total-C alone may be used to monitor long-term therapy. A lipoprotein analysis (including LDL-C determination) should be carried out once a year. The NCEP treatment guidelines are summarized below.

Definite Atherosclerotic Disease*	Two or More Other Risk Factors**	LDL-Cholesterol mg/dl (mmol/L) Initiation Level	Goal
NO	NO	≥190 (≥4.9)	<160 (<4.1)
NO	YES	≥160 (≥4.1)	<130 (<3.4)
YES	YES or NO	≥130 (≥3.4)	≤100 (≤2.6)

* Coronary heart disease or peripheral vascular disease (including symptomatic carotid artery disease).

**Other risk factors for coronary heart disease (CHD) include: age (males: ≥45 years; females: ≥55 years or premature menopause without estrogen replacement therapy); family history of premature CHD; current cigarette smoking; hypertension; confirmed HDL-C <35 mg/dl (<0.91 mmol/L); and diabetes mellitus. Subtract one risk factor if HDL-C is ≥60 mg/dl (≥1.6 mmol/L).

QUESTRAN (Cholestyramine for Oral Suspension, USP) monotherapy has been demonstrated to retard the rate of progression[2,3] and increase the rate of regression[3] of coronary atherosclerosis.

2.) QUESTRAN is indicated for the relief of pruritus associated with partial biliary obstruction. QUESTRAN has been shown to have a variable effect on serum cholesterol in these patients. Patients with primary biliary cirrhosis may exhibit an elevated cholesterol as part of their disease.

CONTRAINDICATIONS

QUESTRAN is contraindicated in patients with complete biliary obstruction where bile is not secreted into the intestine and in those individuals who have shown hypersensitivity to any of its components.

WARNING: PHENYLKETONURICS: QUESTRAN LIGHT CONTAINS 16.8 mg PHENYLALANINE PER 5-GRAM DOSE.

PRECAUTIONS

General

Chronic use of QUESTRAN may be associated with increased bleeding tendency due to hypoprothrombinemia associated with Vitamin K deficiency. This will usually respond promptly to parenteral Vitamin K_1 and recurrences can be prevented by oral administration of Vitamin K_1. Reduction of serum or red cell folate has been reported over long term administration of QUESTRAN. Supplementation with folic acid should be considered in these cases.

There is a possibility that prolonged use of QUESTRAN, since it is a chloride form of anion exchange resin, may produce hyperchloremic acidosis. This would especially be true in younger and smaller patients where the relative dosage may be higher. Caution should also be exercised in patients with renal insufficiency or volume depletion, and in patients receiving concomitant spironolactone.

QUESTRAN may produce or worsen pre-existing constipation. The dosage should be increased gradually in patient to minimize the risk of developing fecal impaction. In patients with pre-existing constipation, the starting dose should be 1 packet or 1 scoop once daily for 5–7 days, increasing to twice daily with monitoring of constipation and of serum lipoproteins, at least twice, 4–6 weeks apart. Increased fluid intake and fiber intake should be encouraged to alleviate constipation and a stool softener may occasionally be indicated if the initial dose is well tolerated, the dose may be increased as needed by one dose/day (at monthly intervals) with periodic monitoring of serum lipoproteins. If constipation worsens or the desired therapeutic response is not achieved at one to six doses/day, combination therapy or alternate therapy should be considered. Particular effort should be made to avoid constipation in patients with symptomatic coronary artery disease. Constipation associated with QUESTRAN may aggravate hemorrhoids.

Information for Patients

Inform your physician if you are pregnant or plan to become pregnant or are breastfeeding. Drink plenty of fluids and mix each 9-gram dose of QUESTRAN Powder in at least 2 to 6 ounces of fluid or 5-gram dose of QUESTRAN LIGHT in at least 2–3 ounces of fluid before taking. Sipping or holding the resin suspension in the mouth for prolonged periods may lead to changes in the surface of the teeth resulting in discoloration, erosion of enamel or decay; good oral hygiene should be maintained.

Laboratory Tests

Serum cholesterol levels should be determined frequently during the first few months of therapy and periodically thereafter. Serum triglyceride levels should be measured periodically to detect whether significant changes have occurred.

The LRC-CPPT showed a dose-related increase in serum triglycerides of 10.7%–17.1% in the cholestyramine-treated group, compared with an increase of 7.9%–11.7% in the placebo group. Based on the mean values and adjusting for the placebo group, the cholestyramine-treated group showed an increase of 5% over pre-entry levels the first year of the study and an increase of 4.3% the seventh year.

Drug Interactions

QUESTRAN (Cholestyramine for Oral Suspension, USP) may delay or reduce the absorption of concomitant oral medication such as phenylbutazone, warfarin, thiazide diuretics (acidic), or propranolol (basic), as well as tetracycline, penicillin G, phenobarbital, thyroid and thyroxine preparations, estrogens and progestins, and digitalis. Interference with the absorption of oral phosphate supplements has been observed with another positively-charged bile acid sequestrant. QUESTRAN may interfere with the pharmacokinetics of drugs that undergo enterohepatic circulation. The discontinuance of QUESTRAN could pose a hazard to health if a potentially toxic drug such as digitalis has been titrated to a maintenance level while the patient was taking QUESTRAN.

Because cholestyramine binds bile acids, QUESTRAN may interfere with normal fat digestion and absorption and thus may prevent absorption of fat soluble vitamins such as A, D, E, and K. When QUESTRAN is given for long periods of time, concomitant supplementation with water-miscible (or parenteral) forms of fat-soluble vitamins should be considered.

SINCE QUESTRAN MAY BIND OTHER DRUGS GIVEN CONCURRENTLY, IT IS RECOMMENDED THAT PATIENTS TAKE OTHER DRUGS AT LEAST ONE HOUR <u>BEFORE</u> OR 4 TO 6 HOURS <u>AFTER</u> QUESTRAN (OR AT AS GREAT AN INTERVAL AS POSSIBLE) TO AVOID IMPEDING THEIR ABSORPTION.

Carcinogenesis, Mutagenesis, and Impairment of Fertility

In studies conducted in rats in which cholestyramine resin was used as a tool to investigate the role of various intestinal factors, such as fat, bile salts, and microbial flora, in the development of intestinal tumors induced by potent carcinogens, the incidence of such tumors was observed to be greater in cholestyramine resin-treated rats than in control rats.

The relevance of this laboratory observation from studies in rats to the clinical use of QUESTRAN is not known. In the LRC-CPPT study referred to above, the total incidence of fatal and nonfatal neoplasms was similar in both treatment groups. When the many different categories of tumors are examined, various alimentary system cancers were somewhat more prevalent in the cholestyramine group. The small numbers and the multiple categories prevent conclusions from being drawn. However, in view of the fact that cholestyramine resin is confined to the GI tract and not absorbed, and in light of the animal experiments referred to above, a six-year post-trial follow-up of the LRC-CPPT[5] patient population has been completed (a total of 13.4 years of in-trial plus post-trial follow-up) and revealed no significant difference in the incidence of cause-specific mortality or cancer morbidity between cholestyramine and placebo treated patients.

Pregnancy

Pregnancy Category C

There are no adequate and well controlled studies in pregnant women. The use of QUESTRAN in pregnancy or lactation or by women of childbearing age requires that the potential benefits of drug therapy be weighed against the possible hazards to the mother and child. QUESTRAN (Cholestyramine for Oral Suspension, USP) is not absorbed systemically, however, it is known to interfere with absorption of fat-soluble vitamins; accordingly, regular prenatal supplementation may not be adequate (see PRECAUTIONS: Drug Interactions).

Nursing Mothers

Caution should be exercised when QUESTRAN is administered to a nursing mother. The possible lack of proper vitamin absorption described in the "Pregnancy" section may have an effect on nursing infants.

Pediatric Use

As experience in the pediatric population is limited, a practical dosage schedule has not been established.

In calculating pediatric dosages, 44.4 mg of anhydrous cholestyramine resin are contained in 100 mg of QUESTRAN Powder and 80 mg of anhydrous cholestyramine are contained in 100 mg of QUESTRAN LIGHT.

The effects of long-term administration, as well as its effect in maintaining lowered cholesterol levels in pediatric patients, are unknown.

ADVERSE REACTIONS

The most common adverse reaction is constipation. When used as a cholesterol-lowering agent predisposing factors for most complaints of constipation are high dose and increased age (more than 60 years old). Most instances of constipation are mild, transient, and controlled with conventional therapy. Some patients require a temporary decrease in dosage or discontinuation of therapy.

Less Frequent Adverse Reactions: Abdominal discomfort and/or pain, flatulence, nausea, vomiting, diarrhea, eructation, anorexia, and steatorrhea, bleeding tendencies due to hypoprothrombinemia (Vitamin K deficiency) as well as Vitamin A (one case of night blindness reported) and D deficiences, hyperchloremic acidosis in children, osteoporosis, rash and irritation of the skin, tongue and perianal area. One ten-month-old baby with biliary atresia had an impaction presumed to be due to QUESTRAN after three days administration of 9 grams daily. She developed acute intestinal sepsis and died.

Occasional calcified material has been observed in the biliary tree, including calcification of the gallbladder, in patients to whom QUESTRAN has been given. However, this may be a manifestation of the liver disease and not drug related.

One patient experienced biliary colic on each of three occasions on which he took QUESTRAN. One patient diagnosed as acute abdominal symptom complex was found to have a "pasty mass" in the transverse colon on x-ray.

Other events (not necessarily drug related) reported in patients taking QUESTRAN include:

Gastrointestinal—GI-rectal bleeding, black stools, hemorrhoidal bleeding, bleeding from known duodenal ulcer, dysphagia, hiccups, ulcer attack, sour taste, pancreatitis, rectal pain, diverticulitis.

Laboratory test changes—Liver function abnormalities.

Hematologic—Prolonged prothrombin time, ecchymosis, anemia.

Hypersensitivity—Urticaria, asthma, wheezing, shortness of breath.

Musculoskeletal—Backache, muscle and joint pains, arthritis.

Neurologic—Headache, anxiety, vertigo, dizziness, fatigue, tinnitus, syncope, drowsiness, femoral nerve pain, paresthesia.

Eye—Uveitis.

Renal—Hematuria, dysuria, burnt odor to urine, diuresis.

Miscellaneous—Weight loss, weight gain, increased libido, swollen glands, edema, dental bleeding, dental caries, erosion of tooth enamel, tooth discoloration.

OVERDOSAGE

Overdosage with QUESTRAN has been reported in a patient taking 150% of the maximum recommended daily dosage for a period of several weeks. No ill effects were reported. Should an overdosage occur, the chief potential harm would be obstruction of the gastrointestinal tract. The location of such potential obstruction, the degree of obstruction, and the presence or absence of normal gut motility would determine treatment.

DOSAGE AND ADMINISTRATION

The recommended starting adult dose for QUESTRAN Powder is one packet or one level scoopful (9 grams of QUESTRAN contains 4 grams of anhydrous cholestyramine resin) once or twice a day. The recommended starting adult dose for QUESTRAN LIGHT is one packet or one level scoopful (5 grams of QUESTRAN LIGHT contains 4 grams of anhydrous cholestyramine resin) once or twice a day. The recommended maintenance dose for QUESTRAN Powder and QUESTRAN LIGHT is 2 to 4 packets or scoopfuls daily (8–16 grams anhydrous cholestyramine resin) divided into two doses. It is recommended that increases in dose be gradual with periodic assessment of lipid/lipoprotein levels at intervals of not less than 4 weeks. The maximum recommended daily dose is six packets or scoopfuls of QUESTRAN (24 grams of anhydrous cholestyramine resin). The suggested time of administration is at mealtime but may be modified to avoid interference with absorption of other medications. Although the recommended dosing schedule is twice daily, QUESTRAN may be administered in 1-6 doses per day.

QUESTRAN should not be taken in its dry form. Always mix QUESTRAN with water or other fluids before ingesting. See Preparation Instructions.

Concomitant Therapy

Preliminary evidence suggests that the lipid-lowering effects of QUESTRAN on total and LDL-cholesterol are enhanced when combined with a HMG-CoA reductase inhibitor, e.g., pravastatin, lovastatin, simvastatin, and fluvastatin. Additive effects on LDL-cholesterol are also seen with combined nicotinic acid/QUESTRAN therapy. See the Drug Interactions subsection of the PRECAUTIONS section for recommendations on administering concomitant therapy.

Preparation

The color of QUESTRAN may vary somewhat from batch to batch but this variation does not affect the performance of the product. Place the contents of one single-dose packet or one level scoopful of QUESTRAN in a glass or cup. Add at least 2 to 6 ounces of water or the beverage of your choice. Stir to a uniform consistency.

QUESTRAN may also be mixed with highly fluid soups or pulpy fruits with a high moisture content such as applesauce or crushed pineapple.

HOW SUPPLIED

QUESTRAN Powder (Cholestyramine for Oral Suspension, USP) is available in cartons of sixty 9-gram packets and in

Continued on next page

Bristol-Myers Squibb Co.—Cont.

cans containing 378 grams. Nine grams of QUESTRAN Powder contain 4 grams of anhydrous cholestyramine resin.

NDC 0087-0580-11   **Cartons of 60 packets**
NCE 0087-0580-05   **Cans, 378 g**

QUESTRAN LIGHT is available in cartons of sixty 5-gram packets and in cans containing 210 grams. Five grams of QUESTRAN LIGHT contain 4 grams of anhydrous cholestyramine resin.

NDC 0087-0589-01   **210 g cans, 42 doses**
NCE 0087-0589-03   **Cartons of 60, 5 g packets**

Store at room temperature.

REFERENCES

1. The Lipid Research Clinics Coronary Primary Prevention Trial Results: (I) Reduction in Incidence of Coronary Heart Disease; (II) The Relationship of Reduction in Incidence of Coronary Heart Disease to Cholesterol Lowering. *JAMA* 1984;251:351-374.
2. Brensike JF, Levy RI, Kelsey SF, et al. Effects of therapy with cholestyramine on progression of coronary arteriosclerosis: results of the NHLBI type II coronary intervention study: *Circulation* 1984;69:313-24.
3. Walts, GF, Lewis B, Brunt HNH, Lewis ES, et al. Effects on coronary artery disease of lipid lowering diet, or diet plus cholestyramine, in the St Thomas Atherosclerosis Regression Study (STARS). *Lancet* 1992;339:563-69.
4. National Cholesterol Education Program. Second Report of the Expert Panel on Detection, Evaluation, and Treatment of High Blood Cholesterol in Adults (Adult Treatment Panel II). *Circulation.* 1994 Mar;89(3):1333-445
5. The Lipid Research Clinics Investigators. The Lipid Research Clinics Coronary Primary Prevention Trial Results of 6 Years of Post-Trial Follow-up. *Arch Intern Med.* 1992:152:1399-1410.

Revised September 1995
58903DIM-8
51-000895-1

Shown in Product Identification Guide, page 307

SERZONE®   ℞
(nefazodone hydrochloride) Tablets

DESCRIPTION

SERZONE (nefazodone hydrochloride) is an antidepressant for oral administration with a chemical structure unrelated to selective serotonin reuptake inhibitors, tricyclics, tetracyclics, or monoamine oxidase inhibitors (MAOI).

Nefazodone hydrochloride is a synthetically derived phenylpiperazine antidepressant. The chemical name for nefazodone hydrochloride is 2-[3-[4-(3-chlorophenyl)-1-piperazinyl]propyl]-5-ethyl-2,4-dihydro-4-(2-phenoxyethyl)-3H-1,2,4-triazol-3-one monohydrochloride. The molecular formula is $C_{25}H_{32}ClN_5O_2 \bullet HCl$, which corresponds to a molecular weight of 506.5.

Nefazodone hydrochloride is a nonhygroscopic, white crystalline solid. It is freely soluble in chloroform, soluble in propylene glycol, and slightly soluble in polyethylene glycol and water.

SERZONE is supplied as hexagonal tablets containing 100 mg, 150 mg, 200 mg, or 250 mg of nefazodone hydrochloride and the following inactive ingredients: microcrystalline cellulose, povidone, sodium starch glycolate, colloidal silicon dioxide, magnesium stearate, and iron oxides (red and/or yellow) as colorants.

CLINICAL PHARMACOLOGY

Pharmacodynamics

The mechanism of action of nefazodone, as with other antidepressants, is unknown.

Preclinical studies have shown that nefazodone inhibits neuronal uptake of serotonin and norepinephrine.

Nefazodone occupies central 5-HT$_2$ receptors at nanomolar concentrations, and acts as an antagonist at this receptor. Nefazodone was shown to antagonize alpha$_1$-adrenergic receptors, a property which may be associated with postural hypotension. *In vitro* binding studies showed that nefazodone had no significant affinity for the following receptors: alpha$_2$ and beta adrenergic, 5-HT$_{1A}$, cholinergic, dopaminergic, or benzodiazepine.

Pharmacokinetics

Nefazodone hydrochloride is rapidly and completely absorbed but is subject to extensive metabolism, so that its absolute bioavailability is low, about 20%, and variable. Peak plasma concentrations occur at about one hour and the half-life of nefazodone is 2–4 hours.

Both nefazodone and its pharmacologically similar metabolite, hydroxynefazodone, exhibit nonlinear kinetics for both dose and time, with AUC and C_{max} increasing more than proportionally with dose increases and more than expected upon multiple dosing over time, compared to single dosing. For example, in a multiple-dose study involving BID dosing with 50, 100, and 200 mg, the AUC for nefazodone and hydroxynefazodone increased by about 4-fold with an increase

in dose from 200 to 400 mg per day; C_{max} increased by about 3-fold with the same dose increase. In a multiple-dose study involving BID dosing with 25, 50, 100, and 150 mg, the accumulation ratios for nefazodone and hydroxynefazodone AUC, after 5 days of BID dosing relative to the first dose, ranged from approximately 3 to 4 at the lower doses (50–100 mg/day) and from 5 to 7 at the higher doses (200–300 mg/day); there were also approximately 2- to 4-fold increases in C_{max} after 5 days of BID dosing relative to the first dose, suggesting extensive and greater than predicted accumulation of nefazodone and its hydroxy metabolite with multiple dosing. Steady-state plasma nefazodone and metabolite concentrations are attained within 4 to 5 days of initiation of BID dosing or upon dose increase or decrease.

Nefazodone is extensively metabolized after oral administration by n-dealkylation and aliphatic and aromatic hydroxylation, and less than 1% of administered nefazodone is excreted unchanged in urine. Attempts to characterize three metabolites identified in plasma, hydroxynefazodone (HO-NEF), meta-chlorophenylpiperazine (mCPP), and a triazoledione metabolite, have been carried out. The AUC (expressed as a multiple of the AUC for nefazodone dosed at 100 mg BID) and elimination half-lives for these three metabolites were as follows:

AUC Multiples and T$^{1/2}$ for Three Metabolites of Nefazodone (100 mg BID)		
Metabolite	AUC Multiple	T$^{1/2}$
HO-NEF	0.4	1.5–4 hrs
mCPP	0.07	4–8 hrs
Triazole-dione	4.0	18 hrs

HO-NEF possesses a pharmacological profile qualitatively and quantitatively similar to that of nefazodone. mCPP has some similarities to nefazodone, but also has agonist activity at some serotonergic receptor subtypes. The pharmacological profile of the triazole-dione metabolite has not yet been well characterized. In addition to the above compounds, several other metabolites were present in plasma but have not been tested for pharmacological activity.

After oral administration of radiolabelled nefazodone, the mean half-life of total label ranged between 11 and 24 hours. Approximately 55% of the administered radioactivity was detected in urine and about 20–30% in feces.

Distribution—Nefazodone is widely distributed in body tissues, including the central nervous system (CNS). In humans the volume of distribution of nefazodone ranges from 0.22 to 0.87 l/kg.

Protein Binding—At concentrations of 25–2500 ng/mL nefazodone is extensively (>99%) bound to human plasma proteins *in vitro*. While nefazodone did not alter the *in vitro* protein binding of chlorpromazine, desipramine, diazepam, diphenylhydantoin, lidocaine, prazosin, propranolol, verapamil, or warfarin, it is unknown whether or not displacement of either nefazodone or other drugs occurs *in vivo*. There was a 5% decrease in the protein binding of haloperidol; this is probably of no clinical significance.

Effect of Food—Food delays the absorption of nefazodone and decreases the bioavailability of nefazodone by approximately 20%.

Renal Disease—In studies involving 29 renally-impaired patients, renal impairment (creatinine clearances ranging from 7 to 60 mL/min/1.73m^2) had no effect on steady-state nefazodone plasma concentrations.

Liver Disease—In a multiple-dose study of patients with liver cirrhosis, the AUC values for nefazodone and HO-NEF at steady state were approximately 25% greater than those observed in normal volunteers.

Age/Gender Effects—After single doses of 300 mg to younger and older patients, C_{max} and AUC for nefazodone and hydroxynefazodone were up to twice as high in the older patients. With multiple doses, however, differences were much smaller, 10–20%. A similar result was seen for gender, with a higher C_{max} and AUC in women after single doses but no difference after multiple doses.

Treatment with SERZONE should be initiated at half the usual dose in elderly patients, especially women (see **DOSAGE AND ADMINISTRATION** Section), but the therapeutic dose range is similar in younger and older patients.

Clinical Trials Supporting the Effectiveness Claim

The efficacy of SERZONE (nefazodone hydrochloride) as a treatment for depression was established in two placebo-controlled, short-term trials in outpatients meeting DSM-III or DSM-IIIR criteria for major depression. One was a 6-week dose-titration study comparing SERZONE in two dose ranges (up to 300 mg/day and up to 600 mg/day [mean modal dose for this group was about 400 mg/day], on a BID schedule) and placebo. The other was an 8-week dose-titration study comparing SERZONE (up to 600 mg/day; mean modal dose was 375 mg/day), imipramine (up to 300 mg/day), and placebo, all on a BID schedule. Overall, these studies demonstrated SERZONE, at doses titrated up to 600 mg/day, to be

superior to placebo on at least three of the following four measures: 17-Item Hamilton Depression Rating Scale or HDRS (total score), Hamilton Depressed Mood item, CGI Severity score, and CGI Improvement score. Significant differences were also found for certain factors of the HDRS (e.g., anxiety factor, sleep disturbance factor, and retardation factor). Two other 6–8 week placebo- and imipramine-controlled studies in depressed outpatients provided additional support for the superiority of nefazodone (titrated up to 500 or 600 mg/day; mean modal doses of 462 mg/day and 363 mg/day) over placebo.

There were no efficacy studies focusing specifically on the elderly or on men and women separately. Overall, approximately two-thirds of patients in these trials were women, and an analysis of the effects of gender on outcome did not suggest any differential responsiveness on the basis of sex. There were too few elderly patients in these trials to reveal possible age-related differences in response.

INDICATIONS AND USAGE

SERZONE (nefazodone hydrochloride) is indicated for the treatment of depression.

The efficacy of SERZONE in the treatment of depression was established in 6–8 week controlled trials of outpatients whose diagnoses corresponded most closely to the DSM-III or DSM-IIIR category of major depressive disorder (see **CLINICAL PHARMACOLOGY** Section).

A major depressive episode implies a prominent and relatively persistent depressed or dysphoric mood that usually interferes with daily functioning (nearly every day for at least 2 weeks). It must include either depressed mood or loss of interest or pleasure and at least 5 of the following 9 symptoms: depressed mood, loss of interest in usual activities, significant change in weight and/or appetite, insomnia or hypersomnia, psychomotor agitation or retardation, increased fatigue, feelings of guilt or worthlessness, slowed thinking or impaired concentration, a suicide attempt or suicidal ideation.

The antidepressant effectiveness of SERZONE in hospitalized depressed patients has not been adequately studied.

The effectiveness of SERZONE in long-term use, that is, for more than 6 to 8 weeks, has not been systematically evaluated in controlled trials. Therefore, the physician who elects to use SERZONE for extended periods should periodically re-evaluate the long-term usefulness of the drug for the individual patient.

CONTRAINDICATIONS

Coadministration of terfenadine, astemizole or cisapride with SERZONE (nefazodone hydrochloride) is contraindicated (see **WARNINGS** and **PRECAUTIONS** Sections).

SERZONE is contraindicated in patients with known hypersensitivity to nefazodone or other phenylpiperazine antidepressants.

WARNINGS

Potential for Interaction with Monoamine Oxidase Inhibitors

In patients receiving antidepressants with pharmacological properties similar to nefazodone in combination with a monoamine oxidase inhibitor (MAOI), there have been reports of serious, sometimes fatal, reactions. For a selective serotonin reuptake inhibitor, these reactions have included hyperthermia, rigidity, myoclonus, autonomic instability with possible rapid fluctuations of vital signs, and mental status changes that include extreme agitation progressing to delirium and coma. These reactions have also been reported in patients who have recently discontinued that drug and have been started on a MAOI. Some cases presented with features resembling neuroleptic malignant syndrome. Severe hyperthermia and seizures, sometimes fatal, have been reported in association with the combined use of tricyclic antidepressants and MAOIs. These reactions have also been reported in patients who have recently discontinued these drugs and have been started on an MAOI. Although the effects of combined use of nefazodone and MAOI have not been evaluated in humans or animals, because nefazodone is an inhibitor of both serotonin and norepinephrine reuptake, it is recommended that nefazodone not be used in combination with an MAOI, or within 14 days of discontinuing treatment with an MAOI. At least 1 week should be allowed after stopping nefazodone before starting a MAOI.

Interaction with Triazolobenzodiazepines

Interaction studies of nefazodone with two triazolobenzodiazepines, i.e., triazolam and alprazolam, metabolized by cytochrome P$_{450}$IIIA$_4$, have revealed substantial and clinically important increases in plasma concentrations of these compounds when administered concomitantly with nefazodone.

Triazolam

When a single oral 0.25-mg dose of triazolam was coadministered with nefazodone (200 mg BID) at steady state, triazolam half-life and AUC increased 4-fold and peak concentrations increased 1.7-fold. Nefazodone plasma concentrations were unaffected by triazolam. ***Coadministration of nefazodone potentiated the effects of triazolam on psychomotor***

performance tests. If triazolam is coadministered with SER-ZONE, a 75% reduction in the initial triazolam dosage is recommended. For many patients, e.g., the elderly, it is recommended that triazolam not be used in combination with nefazodone. No dosage adjustment is required for SER-ZONE.

Alprazolam

When alprazolam (1 mg BID) and nefazodone (200 mg BID) were coadministered, steady-state peak concentrations, AUC and half-life values for alprazolam increased by approximately 2-fold. Nefazodone plasma concentrations were unaffected by alprazolam. If alprazolam is coadministered with SERZONE, a 50% reduction in the initial alprazolam dosage is recommended. No dosage adjustment is required for SERZONE.

Potential Terfenadine, Astemizole, and Cisapride Interactions

Terfenadine, astemizole, and cisapride are all metabolized by the cytochrome $P_{450}IIIA_4$ isozyme, and it has been demonstrated that ketoconazole, erythromycin, and other inhibitors of $IIIA_4$ can block the metabolism of these drugs, resulting in increased plasma concentrations of parent drug. Increased plasma concentrations of terfenadine, astemizole, and cisapride are associated with QT prolongation and with rare cases of serious cardiovascular adverse events, including death, due principally to ventricular tachycardia of the torsades de pointes type. Nefazodone has been shown *in vitro* to be an inhibitor of $IIIA_4$. Consequently, it is recommended that nefazodone not be used in combination with either terfenadine, astemizole, or cisapride (see CONTRAINDICATIONS and PRECAUTIONS Sections).

PRECAUTIONS

General

Postural Hypotension

A pooled analysis of the vital signs monitored during placebo-controlled premarketing studies revealed that 5.1% of nefazodone patients compared to 2.5% of placebo patients (p ≤ 0.01) met criteria for a potentially important decrease in blood pressure at some time during treatment (systolic blood pressure ≤ 90 mmHg *and* a change from baseline of ≥ 20 mmHg). While there was no difference in the proportion of nefazodone and placebo patients having adverse events characterized as 'syncope' (nefazodone, 0.2%; placebo, 0.3%), the rates for adverse events characterized as 'postural hypotension' were as follows: nefazodone (2.8%), tricyclic antidepressants (10.9%), SSRI (1.1%), and placebo (0.8%). Thus, the prescriber should be aware that there is some risk of postural hypotension in association with nefazodone use. SERZONE should be used with caution in patients with known cardiovascular or cerebrovascular disease that could be exacerbated by hypotension (history of myocardial infarction, angina, or ischemic stroke) and conditions that would predispose patients to hypotension (dehydration, hypovolemia, and treatment with antihypertensive medication).

Activation of Mania/Hypomania

During premarketing testing, hypomania or mania occurred in 0.3% of nefazodone-treated unipolar patients, compared to 0.3% of tricyclic- and 0.4% of placebo-treated patients. In patients classified as bipolar the rate of manic episodes was 1.6% for nefazodone, 5.1% for the combined tricyclic-treated groups, and 0% for placebo-treated patients. Activation of mania/hypomania is a known risk in a small proportion of patients with major affective disorder treated with other marketed antidepressants. As with all antidepressants, SERZONE (nefazodone hydrochloride) should be used cautiously in patients with a history of mania.

Suicide

The possibility of a suicide attempt is inherent in depression and may persist until significant remission occurs. Close supervision of high risk patients should accompany initial drug therapy. Prescriptions for SERZONE should be written for the smallest quantity of tablets consistent with good patient management in order to reduce the risk of overdose.

Seizures

During premarketing testing, a recurrence of a petit mal seizure was observed in a patient receiving nefazodone who had a history of such seizures. One nonstudy participant took 2000–3000 mg of nefazodone with methocarbamol and alcohol; this person reportedly experienced a convulsion (type not documented).

Priapism

While priapism did not occur during premarketing experience with nefazodone, priapism has been reported with a structurally related drug, trazodone. If patients present with prolonged or inappropriate erections, they should discontinue therapy immediately and consult their physicians. If the condition persists for more than 24 hours, a urologist should be consulted to determine appropriate management.

Use in Patients with Concomitant Illness

SERZONE has not been evaluated or used to any appreciable extent in patients with a recent history of myocardial infarction or unstable heart disease. Patients with these diagnoses were systematically excluded from clinical studies during the product's premarketing testing. Evaluation of electrocardiograms of 1153 patients who received nefazodone in 6- to

8-week, double-blind, placebo-controlled trials did not indicate that nefazodone is associated with the development of clinically important ECG abnormalities. However, sinus bradycardia, defined as heart rate ≤ 50 bpm and a decrease of at least 15 bpm from baseline, was observed in 1.5% of nefazodone-treated patients compared to 0.4% of placebo-treated patients (p ≤ 0.05). Because patients with a recent history of myocardial infarction or unstable heart disease were excluded from clinical trials, such patients should be treated with caution.

In patients with cirrhosis of the liver, the AUC values of nefazodone and HO-NEF were increased by approximately 25%.

Information for Patients

Physicians are advised to discuss the following issues with patients for whom they prescribe SERZONE.

Time to Response/Continuation

As with all antidepressants, several weeks on treatment may be required to obtain the full antidepressant effect. Once improvement is noted, it is important for patients to continue drug treatment as directed by their physician.

Interference With Cognitive and Motor Performance

Since any psychoactive drug may impair judgment, thinking, or motor skills, patients should be cautioned about operating hazardous machinery, including automobiles, until they are reasonably certain that SERZONE therapy does not adversely affect their ability to engage in such activities.

Pregnancy

Patients should be advised to notify their physician if they become pregnant or intend to become pregnant during therapy.

Nursing

Patients should be advised to notify their physician if they are breast-feeding an infant (see **PRECAUTIONS** Section, **Nursing Mothers** Subsection).

Concomitant Medication

Patients should be advised to inform their physicians if they are taking, or plan to take, any prescription or over-the-counter drugs, since there is a potential for interactions. Significant caution is indicated if SERZONE is to be used in combination with either Halcion or Xanax, and concomitant use with Seldane, Hismanal, or Propulsid is contraindicated (see **CONTRAINDICATIONS** and **WARNINGS** Sections).

Alcohol

Patients should be advised to avoid alcohol while taking SERZONE.

Allergic Reactions

Patients should be advised to notify their physician if they develop a rash, hives, or a related allergic phenomenon.

Laboratory Tests

There are no specific laboratory tests recommended.

Drug Interactions

Drugs Highly Bound to Plasma Protein

Because nefazodone is highly bound to plasma protein (see **CLINICAL PHARMACOLOGY** Section, **Pharmacokinetics** Subsection), administration of SERZONE to a patient taking another drug that is highly protein bound may cause increased free concentrations of the other drug, potentially resulting in adverse events. Conversely, adverse effects could result from displacement of nefazodone by other highly bound drugs.

CNS Active Drugs

Monoamine Oxidase Inhibitors—See **WARNINGS** Section

Haloperidol—When a single oral 5-mg dose of haloperidol was coadministered with nefazodone (200 mg BID) at steady state, haloperidol apparent clearance decreased by 35% with no significant increase in peak haloperidol plasma concentrations or time of peak. This change is of unknown clinical significance. Pharmacodynamic effects of haloperidol were generally not altered significantly. There were no changes in the pharmacokinetic parameters for nefazodone. Dosage adjustment of haloperidol may be necessary when coadministered with nefazodone.

Lorazepam—When lorazepam (2 mg BID) and nefazodone (200 mg BID) were coadministered to steady state, there was no change in any pharmacokinetic parameter for either drug compared to each drug administered alone. Therefore, dosage adjustment is not necessary for either drug when coadministered.

Triazolam/Alprazolam—See **WARNINGS** Section

• Alcohol—Although nefazodone did not potentiate the cognitive and psychomotor effects of alcohol in experiments with normal subjects, the concomitant use of SERZONE and alcohol in depressed patients is not advised.

General Anesthetics—Little is known about the potential for interaction between nefazodone and general anesthetics; therefore, prior to elective surgery, SERZONE should be discontinued for as long as clinically feasible.

Other CNS Active Drugs—The use of nefazodone in combination with other CNS-active drugs has not been systematically evaluated. Consequently, caution is advised if concomitant administration of SERZONE and such drugs is required.

Cimetidine

When nefazodone (200 mg BID) and cimetidine (300 mg QID) were coadministered for one week, no change in the steady-

state pharmacokinetics of either nefazodone or cimetidine was observed compared to each dosed alone. Therefore, dosage adjustment is not necessary for either drug when coadministered.

Cardiovascular Active Drugs

Digoxin—When nefazodone (200 mg BID) and digoxin (0.2 mg QD) were coadministered for 9 days to healthy male volunteers (n =18) who were phenotyped as $P_{450}IID_6$ extensive metabolizers, C_{max}, C_{min}, and AUC of digoxin were increased by 29%, 27%, and 15%, respectively. Digoxin had no effects on the pharmacokinetics of nefazodone and its active metabolites. Because of the narrow therapeutic index of digoxin, caution should be exercised when nefazodone and digoxin are coadministered; plasma level monitoring for digoxin is recommended.

Propranolol—The coadministration of nefazodone (200 mg BID) and propranolol (40 mg BID) for 5.5 days to healthy male volunteers (n =18), including 3 poor and 15 extensive $P_{450}IID_6$ metabolizers, resulted in 30% and 14% reductions in C_{max} and AUC of propranolol, respectively, and a 14% reduction in C_{max} for the metabolite, 4-hydroxypropranolol. The kinetics of nefazodone, hydroxynefazodone, and triazoledione were not affected by coadministration of propranolol. However, C_{max}, C_{min}, and AUC of m-chlorophenylpiperazine were increased by 23%, 54%, and 28%, respectively. No change in initial dose of either drug is necessary and dose adjustments should be made on the basis of clinical response.

Pharmacokinetics of Nefazodone in 'Poor Metabolizers' and Potential Interaction with Drugs That Inhibit and/or are Metabolized by Cytochrome P450 Isozymes

$IIIA_4$ Isozyme—Nefazodone has been shown *in vitro* to be an inhibitor of cytochrome $P_{450}IIIA_4$. This is consistent with the interaction observed between nefazodone and the benzodiazepines triazolam and alprazolam, drugs metabolized by this isozyme. Consequently, caution is indicated in the combined use of nefazodone with any drugs known to be metabolized by the $IIIA_4$ isozyme. In particular, the combined use of nefazodone with terfenadine, astemizole, or cisapride is contraindicated (see **CONTRAINDICATIONS** and **WARNINGS** Sections).

IID_6 Isozyme—A subset (3% to 10%) of the population has reduced activity of the drug-metabolizing enzyme cytochrome $P_{450}IID_6$. Such individuals are referred to commonly as "poor metabolizers" of drugs such as debrisoquin, dextromethorphan, and the tricyclic antidepressants. The pharmacokinetics of nefazodone and its major metabolites are not altered in these "poor metabolizers." Plasma concentrations of one minor metabolite (mCPP) are increased in this population; the adjustment of SERZONE dosage is not required when administered to "poor metabolizers." Nefazodone and its metabolites have been shown *in vitro* to be extremely weak inhibitors of $P_{450}IID_6$. Thus, it is not likely that nefazodone will decrease the metabolic clearance of drugs metabolized by this isozyme.

IA_2 Isozyme—Nefazodone and its metabolites have been shown *in vitro* not to inhibit cytochrome $P_{450}IA_2$. Thus, metabolic interactions between nefazodone and drugs metabolized by this isozyme are unlikely.

Electro-Convulsive Therapy (ECT)

There are no clinical studies of the combined use of ECT and nefazodone.

Carcinogenesis, Mutagenesis, Impairment of Fertility

Carcinogenesis

There is no evidence of carcinogenicity with nefazodone. The dietary administration of nefazodone to rats and mice for 2 years at daily doses of up to 200 mg/kg and 800 mg/kg, respectively, which are approximately 3 and 6 times, respectively, the maximum human daily dose on a mg/m^2 basis, produced no increase in tumors.

Mutagenesis

Nefazodone has been shown to have no genotoxic effects based on the following assays: bacterial mutation assays, a DNA repair assay in cultured rat hepatocytes, a mammalian mutation assay in Chinese hamster ovary cells, an *in vivo* cytogenetics assay in rat bone marrow cells, and a rat dominant lethal study.

Impairment of Fertility

A fertility study in rats showed a slight decrease in fertility at 200 mg/kg/day (approximately three times the maximum human daily dose on a mg/m^2 basis) but not at 100 mg/kg/day (approximately 1.5 times the maximum human daily dose on a mg/m^2 basis).

Pregnancy

Teratogenic Effects—Pregnancy Category C

Reproduction studies have been performed in pregnant rabbits and rats at daily doses up to 200 and 300 mg/kg, respectively (approximately 6 and 5 times, respectively, the maximum human daily dose on a mg/m^2 basis). No malformations were observed in the offspring as a result of nefazodone treatment. However, increased early pup mortality was seen in rats at a dose approximately five times the maximum human dose, and decreased pup weights were seen at this and lower doses, when dosing began during pregnancy and con-

Continued on next page

Bristol-Myers Squibb Co.—Cont.

tinued until weaning. The cause of these deaths is not known. The no-effect dose for rat pup mortality was 1.3 times the human dose on a mg/m^2 basis. There are no adequate and well-controlled studies in pregnant women. Nefazodone should be used during pregnancy only if the potential benefit justifies the potential risk to the fetus.

Labor and Delivery
The effect of SERZONE on labor and delivery in humans is unknown.

Nursing Mothers
It is not known whether SERZONE or its metabolites are excreted in human milk. Because many drugs are excreted in human milk, caution should be exercised when SERZONE is administered to a nursing woman.

Pediatric Use
Safety and effectiveness in individuals below 18 years of age have not been established.

Geriatric Use
Over 500 elderly (≥ 65 years) individuals participated in clinical studies with nefazodone. No unusual adverse age-related phenomena were identified in this cohort of elderly patients treated with nefazodone. Due to the increased systemic exposure to nefazodone seen in single dose studies in elderly patients (see **CLINICAL PHARMACOLOGY** Section, **Pharmacokinetics** Subsection), treatment should be initiated at half the usual dose, but titration upward should take place over the same range as in younger patients (see **DOSAGE AND ADMINISTRATION** Section). The usual precautions should be observed in elderly patients who have concomitant medical illnesses or who are receiving concomitant drugs.

ADVERSE REACTIONS

Associated with Discontinuation of Treatment
Approximately 16% of the 3496 patients who received SERZONE (nefazodone hydrochloride) in worldwide premarketing clinical trials discontinued treatment due to an adverse experience. The more common ($\geq 1\%$) events in clinical trials associated with discontinuation and considered to be drug related (i.e., those events associated with dropout at a rate approximately twice or greater for SERZONE compared to placebo) included: nausea (3.5%), dizziness (1.9%), insomnia (1.5%), asthenia (1.3%), and agitation (1.2%).

Incidence in Controlled Trials
Commonly Observed Adverse Events in Controlled Clinical Trials:

The most commonly observed adverse events associated with the use of SERZONE (incidence of 5% or greater) and not seen at an equivalent incidence among placebo-treated patients (i.e., significantly higher incidence for SERZONE compared to placebo, $p \leq 0.05$), derived from the table below, were: somnolence, dry mouth, nausea, dizziness, constipation, asthenia, lightheadedness, blurred vision, confusion, and abnormal vision.

Adverse Events Occurring at an Incidence of 1% or More Among SERZONE-Treated Patients:

The table that follows enumerates adverse events that occurred at an incidence of 1% or more, and were more frequent than in the placebo group, among SERZONE-treated patients who participated in short-term (6- to 8-week) placebo-controlled trials in which patients were dosed with SERZONE to ranges of 300 to 600 mg/day. This table shows the percentage of patients in each group who had at least one episode of an event at some time during their treatment. Reported adverse events were classified using a standard COSTART-based Dictionary terminology.

The prescriber should be aware that these figures cannot be used to predict the incidence of side effects in the course of usual medical practice where patient characteristics and other factors differ from those which prevailed in the clinical trials. Similarly, the cited frequencies cannot be compared with figures obtained from other clinical investigations involving different treatments, uses, and investigators. The cited figures, however, do provide the prescribing physician with some basis for estimating the relative contribution of drug and nondrug factors to the side-effect incidence rate in the population studied.

[See first table above.]

Dose Dependency of Adverse Events
The table that follows enumerates adverse events that were more frequent in the SERZONE dose range of 300 to 600 mg/day than in the SERZONE dose range of up to 300 mg/day. This table shows only those adverse events for which there was a statistically significant difference (p ≤ 0.05) in incidence between the SERZONE dose ranges as well as a difference between the high dose range and placebo.

[See second table above.]

Treatment-Emergent Adverse Experience Incidence in 6- to 8-Week Placebo-Controlled Clinical Trials[1] SERZONE 300 to 600 mg/day Dose Range

Body System	Preferred Term	SERZONE (n = 393)	Placebo (n = 394)
Body as a Whole	Headache	36%	33%
	Asthenia	11%	5%
	Infection	8%	6%
	Flu syndrome	3%	2%
	Chills	2%	1%
	Fever	2%	1%
	Neck Rigidity	1%	0
Cardiovascular	Postural hypotension	4%	1%
	Hypotension	2%	1%
Dermatological	Pruritus	2%	1%
	Rash	2%	1%
Gastrointestinal	Dry mouth	25%	13%
	Nausea	22%	12%
	Constipation	14%	8%
	Dyspepsia	9%	7%
	Diarrhea	8%	7%
	Increased appetite	5%	3%
	Nausea & Vomiting	2%	1%
Metabolic	Peripheral edema	3%	2%
	Thirst	1%	<1%
Musculoskeletal	Arthralgia	1%	<1%
Nervous	Somnolence	25%	14%
	Dizziness	17%	5%
	Insomnia	11%	9%
	Lightheadedness	10%	3%
	Confusion	7%	2%
	Memory impairment	4%	2%
	Paresthesia	4%	2%
	Vasodilatation[2]	4%	2%
	Abnormal dreams	3%	2%
	Concentration decreased	3%	1%
	Ataxia	2%	0
	Incoordination	2%	1%
	Psychomotor retardation	2%	1%
	Tremor	2%	1%
	Hypertonia	1%	0
	Libido decreased	1%	<1%
Respiratory	Pharyngitis	6%	5%
	Cough increased	3%	1%
Special Senses	Blurred vision	9%	3%
	Abnormal vision[3]	7%	1%
	Tinnitus	2%	1%
	Taste perversion	2%	1%
	Visual field defect	2%	0
Urogenital	Urinary frequency	2%	1%
	Urinary tract infection	2%	1%
	Urinary retention	2%	1%
	Vaginitis[4]	2%	1%
	Breast pain[4]	1%	<1%

[1] Events reported by at least 1% of patients treated with SERZONE and more frequent than the placebo group are included; incidence is rounded to the nearest 1% (<1% indicates an incidence less than 0.5%). Events for which the SERZONE incidence was equal to or less than placebo are not listed in the table, but included the following: abdominal pain, pain, back pain, accidental injury, chest pain, neck pain, palpitation, migraine, sweating, flatulence, vomiting, anorexia, tooth disorder, weight gain, edema, myalgia, cramp, agitation, anxiety, depression, hypesthesia, CNS stimulation, dysphoria, emotional lability, sinusitis, rhinitis, dysmenorrhea[4], dysuria.
[2] Vasodilatation—flushing, feeling warm.
[3] Abnormal vision—scotoma, visual trails.
[4] Incidence adjusted for gender.

Dose Dependency of Adverse Events in Placebo-Controlled Trials[1]

Body System	Preferred Term	SERZONE 300–600 mg/day (n = 209)	SERZONE ≤ 300 mg/day (n = 211)	Placebo (n = 212)
Gastrointestinal	Nausea	23%	14%	12%
	Constipation	17%	10%	9%
Nervous	Somnolence	28%	16%	13%
	Dizziness	22%	11%	4%
	Confusion	8%	2%	1%
Special Senses	Abnormal vision	10%	0	2%
	Blurred vision	9%	3%	2%
	Tinnitus	3%	0	1%

[1] Events for which there was a statistically significant difference (p ≤ 0.05) between the nefazodone dose groups.

Vital Sign Changes

(See **PRECAUTIONS** Section, *Postural Hypotension* Subsection)

Weight Changes

In a pooled analysis of placebo-controlled premarketing studies, there were no differences between nefazodone and placebo groups in the proportions of patients meeting criteria for potentially important increases or decreases in body weight (a change of $\geq 7\%$).

Laboratory Changes
Of the serum chemistry, serum hematology, and urinalysis parameters monitored during placebo-controlled premarketing studies with nefazodone, a pooled analysis revealed a statistical trend between nefazodone and placebo for hematocrit, i.e., 2.8% of nefazodone patients met criteria for a potentially important decrease in hematocrit ($\leq 37\%$ male or $\leq 32\%$ female) compared to 1.5% of placebo patients (0.05 <p ≤ 0.10). Decreases in hematocrit, presumably dilutional, have been reported with many other drugs that block $alpha_1$-adrenergic receptors. There was no apparent clinical signifi-

cance of the observed changes in the few patients meeting these criteria.

ECG Changes

Of the ECG parameters monitored during placebo-controlled premarketing studies with nefazodone, a pooled analysis revealed a statistically significant difference between nefazodone and placebo for sinus bradycardia, i.e., 1.5% of nefazodone patients met criteria for a potentially important decrease in heart rate (≤ 50 bpm and a decrease of ≥ 15 bpm) compared to 0.4% of placebo patients ($p < 0.05$). There was no obvious clinical significance of the observed changes in the few patients meeting these criteria.

Other Events Observed During the Premarketing Evaluation of SERZONE

During its premarketing assessment, multiple doses of SERZONE were administered to 3496 patients in clinical studies, including more than 250 patients treated for at least one year. The conditions and duration of exposure to SERZONE varied greatly, and included (in overlapping categories) open and double-blind studies, uncontrolled and controlled studies, inpatient and outpatient studies, fixed-dose and titration studies. Untoward events associated with this exposure were recorded by clinical investigators using terminology of their own choosing. Consequently, it is not possible to provide a meaningful estimate of the proportion of individuals experiencing adverse events without first grouping similar types of untoward events into a smaller number of standardized event categories.

In the tabulations that follow, reported adverse events were classified using a standard COSTART-based Dictionary terminology. The frequencies presented, therefore, represent the proportion of the 3496 patients exposed to multiple doses of SERZONE who experienced an event of the type cited on at least one occasion while receiving SERZONE. All reported events are included except those already listed in the Treatment-Emergent Adverse Experience Incidence table, those events listed in other safety-related sections of this insert, those adverse experiences subsumed under COSTART terms that are either overly general or excessively specific so as to be uninformative, those events for which a drug cause was very remote, and those events which were not serious and occurred in fewer than two patients.

It is important to emphasize that, although the events reported occurred during treatment with SERZONE, they were not necessarily caused by it.

Events are further categorized by body system and listed in order of decreasing frequency according to the following definitions: frequent adverse events are those occurring on one or more occasions in at least 1/100 patients (only those not already listed in the tabulated results from placebo-controlled trials appear in this listing); infrequent adverse events are those occurring in 1/100 to 1/1000 patients; rare events are those occurring in fewer than 1/1000 patients.

Body as a whole—Infrequent: allergic reaction, malaise, photosensitivity reaction, face edema, hangover effect, abdomen enlarged, hernia, pelvic pain, and halitosis. Rare: cellulitis.

Cardiovascular system—Infrequent: tachycardia, hypertension, syncope, ventricular extrasystoles, and angina pectoris. Rare: AV block, congestive heart failure, hemorrhage, pallor, and varicose vein.

Dermatological system—Infrequent: dry skin, acne, alopecia, urticaria, maculopapular rash, vesiculobullous rash, and eczema.

Gastrointestinal system—Frequent: gastroenteritis. *Infrequent:* eructation, periodontal abscess, abnormal liver function tests, gingivitis, colitis, gastritis, mouth ulceration, stomatitis, esophagitis, peptic ulcer, and rectal hemorrhage. *Rare:* glossitis, hepatitis, dysphagia, gastrointestinal hemorrhage, oral moniliasis, and ulcerative colitis.

Hemic and lymphatic system—Infrequent: ecchymosis, anemia, leukopenia, and lymphadenopathy.

Metabolic and nutritional system—Infrequent: weight loss, gout, dehydration, lactic dehydrogenase increased, SGOT increased, and SGPT increased. *Rare*: hypercholesteremia and hypoglycemia.

Musculoskeletal system—Infrequent: arthritis, tenosynovitis, muscle stiffness, and bursitis. *Rare*: tendinous contracture.

Nervous system—Infrequent: vertigo, twitching, depersonalization, hallucinations, suicide attempt, apathy, euphoria, hostility, suicidal thoughts, abnormal gait, thinking abnormal, attention decreased, derealization, neuralgia, paranoid reaction, dysarthria, increased libido, suicide, and myoclonus. *Rare*: hyperkinesia, increased salivation, cerebrovascular accident, hyperesthesia, hypotonia, ptosis, and neuroleptic malignant syndrome.

Respiratory system—Frequent: dyspnea and bronchitis. *Infrequent:* asthma, pneumonia, laryngitis, voice alteration, epistaxis, hiccup. *Rare*: hyperventilation and yawn.

Special senses—Frequent: eye pain. *Infrequent*: dry eye, ear pain, abnormality of accommodation, diplopia, conjunctivitis, mydriasis, keratoconjunctivitis, hyperacusis, and photophobia. *Rare*: deafness, glaucoma, night blindness, and taste loss.

Urogenital system—Frequent: impotence.[a] *Infrequent:* cystitis, urinary urgency, metrorrhagia[a], amenorrhea[a], polyuria, vaginal hemorrhage[a], breast enlargement[a], menorrhagia[a], urinary incontinence, abnormal ejaculation[a], hematuria, nocturia, and kidney calculus. *Rare:* uterine fibroids enlarged[a], uterine hemorrhage[a], anorgasmia, and oliguria.

[a]Adjusted for gender.

DRUG ABUSE AND DEPENDENCE

Controlled Substance Class

SERZONE (nefazodone hydrochloride) is not a controlled substance.

Physical and Psychological Dependence

In animal studies, nefazodone did not act as a reinforcer for intravenous self-administration in monkeys trained to self-administer cocaine, suggesting no abuse liability. In a controlled study of abuse liability in human subjects, nefazodone showed no potential for abuse.

Nefazodone has not been systematically studied in humans for its potential for tolerance, physical dependence, or withdrawal. While the premarketing clinical experience with nefazodone did not reveal any tendency for a withdrawal syndrome or any drug-seeking behavior, it is not possible to predict on the basis of this limited experience the extent to which a CNS-active drug will be misused, diverted, and/or abused once marketed. Consequently, physicians should carefully evaluate patients for a history of drug abuse and follow such patients closely, observing them for signs of misuse or abuse of SERZONE (e.g., development of tolerance, dose escalation, drug-seeking behavior).

OVERDOSAGE

Human Experience

There is very limited experience with nefazodone overdose. In premarketing clinical studies, there were seven reports of nefazodone overdose alone or in combination with other pharmacological agents. The amount of nefazodone ingested ranged from 1000 mg to 11,200 mg. Commonly reported symptoms from overdose of nefazodone included nausea, vomiting, and somnolence. One nonstudy participant took 2000–3000 mg of nefazodone with methocarbamol and alcohol; this person reportedly experienced a convulsion (type not documented). None of the patients died.

Overdose Management

Overdosage may cause an increase in incidence or severity of any of the reported adverse reactions (see **ADVERSE REACTIONS** Section).

There is no specific antidote for SERZONE (nefazodone hydrochloride). Treatment should be symptomatic and supportive in the case of hypotension or excessive sedation. Any patient suspected of having taken an overdose should have the stomach emptied by gastric lavage.

In managing overdosage, consider the possibility of multiple drug involvement. The physician should consider contacting a poison control center on the treatment of any overdose.

DOSAGE AND ADMINISTRATION

Initial Treatment

The recommended starting dose for SERZONE (nefazodone hydrochloride) is 200 mg/day, administered in two divided doses (BID). In the controlled clinical trials establishing the antidepressant efficacy of SERZONE, the effective dose range was generally 300 to 600 mg/day. Consequently, most patients, depending on tolerability and the need for further clinical effect, should have dose increased. Dose increases should occur in increments of 100 mg/day to 200 mg/day, again on a BID schedule, at intervals of no less than 1 week. As with all antidepressants, several weeks on treatment may be required to obtain a full antidepressant response.

Dosage for Elderly or Debilitated Patients

The recommended initial dose for elderly or debilitated patients is 100 mg/day on a BID schedule. These patients often have reduced nefazodone clearance and/or increased sensitivity to the side effects of CNS-active drugs. It may also be appropriate to modify the rate of subsequent dose titration. As steady-state plasma levels do not change with age, the final target dose based on a careful assessment of the patient's clinical response may be similar in healthy younger and older patients.

Maintenance/Continuation/Extended Treatment

There is no body of evidence available from controlled trials to indicate how long the depressed patient should be treated with SERZONE. It is generally agreed, however, that pharmacological treatment for acute episodes of depression should continue for up to six months or longer. Whether the dose of antidepressant needed to induce remission is identical to the dose needed to maintain euthymia is unknown. Although there are no efficacy data that specifically address maintenance antidepressant treatment with SERZONE, the safety of nefazodone in long-term use is supported by data from both double-blind and open-label trials involving more than 250 patients treated for at least one year.

Switching Patients to or from a Monoamine Oxidase Inhibitor

At least 14 days should elapse between discontinuation of an MAOI and initiation of therapy with SERZONE. In addition, at least 7 days should be allowed after stopping SERZONE before starting an MAOI.

HOW SUPPLIED

SERZONE® (nefazodone hydrochloride) tablets are hexagonal tablets imprinted with BMS and the strength (i.e., 100 mg) on one side and the identification code number on the other. The 100 mg and 150 mg tablets are bisect scored on both tablet faces. The 200 mg and 250 mg tablets are unscored.

NDC CODE	*DESCRIPTION*
NDC 0087-0032-31	100 mg white tablet, bottle of 60
NDC 0087-0032-44	100 mg white tablet, blister pack of 100
NDC 0087-0039-31	150 mg peach tablet, bottle of 60
NDC 0087-0039-01	150 mg peach tablet, blister pack of 100
NDC 0087-0033-31	200 mg light yellow tablet, bottle of 60
NDC 0087-0033-44	200 mg light yellow tablet, blister pack of 100
NDC 0087-0041-31	250 mg white tablet, bottle of 60

Store at room temperature, below 40°C (104°F) and dispense in a tight container.

Based on P4460-01

Bristol-Myers Squibb Company

D5-B001-10-95

Shown in Product Identification Guide, page 307

STADOL® ℞

[*stā'-dōl*]

(butorphanol tartrate) Injectable

STADOL® NS™ ℞

(butorphanol tartrate)

Nasal Spray

DESCRIPTION

Butorphanol tartrate is a synthetically derived opioid agonist-antagonist analgesic of the phenanthrene series. The chemical name is (-)-17-(cyclobutylmethyl) morphinan-3,14-diol [S-(R*,R*)] -2,3- dihydroxybutanedioate (1:1) (salt). The molecular formula is $C_{21}H_{29}NO_2 . C_4H_6O_6$, which corresponds to a molecular weight of 477.55 and the following structural formula:

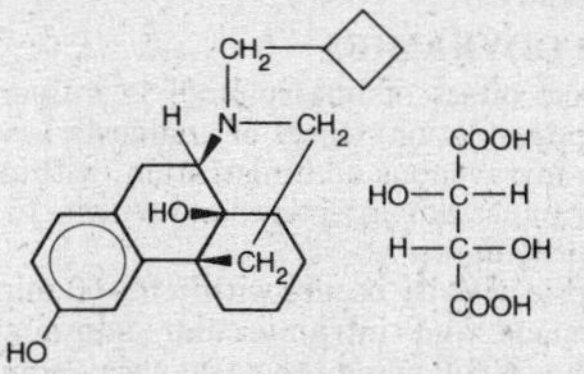

Butorphanol tartrate is a white crystalline substance. The dose is expressed as the tartrate salt. One milligram of the salt is equivalent to 0.68 mg of the free base. The n-octanol/aqueous buffer partition coefficient of butorphanol is 180:1 at pH 7.5.

STADOL® (butorphanol tartrate) Injectable is a sterile, parenteral, aqueous solution of butorphanol tartrate for intravenous or intramuscular administration. In addition to 1 or 2 mg of butorphanol tartrate, each mL of solution contains 3.3 mg of citric acid, 6.4 mg of sodium citrate, and 6.4 mg sodium chloride, and 0.1 mg benzethonium chloride (in multiple dose vial only) as a preservative.

STADOL® NS™ (butorphanol tartrate) Nasal Spray is an aqueous solution of butorphanol tartrate for administration as a metered spray to the nasal mucosa. Each bottle of STADOL NS contains 2.5 mL of a 10 mg/mL solution of butorphanol tartrate with sodium chloride, citric acid, and benzethonium chloride in purified water with sodium hydroxide and/or hydrochloric acid added to adjust the pH to 5.0. The pump reservoir must be fully primed (see PATIENT INSTRUCTIONS) prior to initial use. After initial priming each metered spray delivers an average of 1.0 mg of butorphanol tartrate and the 2.5 mL bottle will deliver an average of 14–15 doses of STADOL NS. If not used for 48 hours or longer, the unit must be re-primed (see PATIENT INSTRUCTIONS). With intermittent use requiring repriming before each dose, the 2.5 mL bottle will deliver an average of 8–10 doses of STADOL NS depending on how much repriming is necessary.

CLINICAL PHARMACOLOGY

GENERAL PHARMACOLOGY AND MECHANISM OF ACTION

Butorphanol and its major metabolites are agonists at k-opioid receptors and mixed agonist-antagonists at μ-opioid receptors.

Continued on next page

Bristol-Myers Squibb Co.—Cont.

Its interactions with these receptors in the central nervous system apparently mediate most of its pharmacologic effects, including analgesia.

In addition to analgesia, CNS effects include depression of spontaneous respiratory activity and cough, stimulation of the emetic center, miosis and sedation. Effects possibly mediated by non-CNS mechanisms include alteration in cardiovascular resistance and capacitance, bronchomotor tone, gastrointestinal secretory and motor activity and bladder sphincter activity.

In an animal model, the dose of the butorphanol tartrate required to antagonize morphine analgesia by 50% was similar to that for nalorphine, less than that for pentazocine and more than that for naloxone.

The pharmacological activity of butorphanol metabolites has not been studied in humans; in animal studies, butorphanol metabolites have demonstrated some analgesic activity.

In human studies of butorphanol (see CLINICAL TRIALS), sedation is commonly noted at doses of 0.5 mg or more. Narcosis is produced by 10–12 mg doses of butorphanol administered over 10–15 minutes intravenously.

Butorphanol, like other mixed agonist-antagonists with a high affinity for the kappa receptor, may produce unpleasant psychotomimetic effects in some individuals.

Nausea and/or vomiting may be produced by doses of 1 mg or more administered by any route.

In human studies involving individuals without significant respiratory dysfunction, 2 mg of butorphanol IV and 10 mg of morphine sulfate IV depressed respiration to a comparable degree. At higher doses, the magnitude of respiratory depression with butorphanol is not appreciably increased; however, the duration of respiratory depression is longer. Respiratory depression noted after administration of butorphanol to humans by any route is reversed by treatment with naloxone, a specific opioid antagonist (see Treatment in OVERDOSAGE).

Butorphanol tartrate demonstrates antitussive effects in animals at doses less than those required for analgesia.

Hemodynamic changes noted during cardiac catheterization in patients receiving single 0.025 mg/kg intravenous doses of butorphanol have included increases in pulmonary artery pressure, wedge pressure and vascular resistance, increases in left ventricular end diastolic pressure and in systemic arterial pressure.

PHARMACODYNAMICS

The analgesic effect of butorphanol is influenced by the route of administration. Onset of analgesia is within a few minutes for intravenous administration, within 10–15 minutes for intramuscular injection, and within 15 minutes for the nasal spray doses.

Peak analgesic activity occurs within 30–60 minutes following intravenous and intramuscular administration and within 1–2 hours following the nasal spray administration. The duration of analgesia varies depending on the pain model as well as the route of administration, but is generally 3–4 hours with IM and IV doses as defined by the time 50% of

patients required remedication. In postoperative studies, the duration of analgesia with IV or IM butorphanol was similar to morphine, meperidine and pentazocine when administered in the same fashion at equipotent doses (see CLINICAL TRIALS). Compared to the injectable form and other drugs in this class, STADOL NS (butorphanol tartrate) Nasal Spray has a longer duration of action (4–5 hours) (see CLINICAL TRIALS).

PHARMACOKINETICS

STADOL (butorphanol tartrate) Injectable is rapidly absorbed after IM injection and peak plasma levels are reached in 20–40 minutes.

After nasal administration, mean peak blood levels of 0.9–1.04 ng/mL occur at 30–60 minutes after a 1 mg dose (see Table 1). The absolute bioavailability of STADOL NS is 60–70% and is unchanged in patients with allergic rhinitis. In patients using a nasal vasoconstrictor (oxymetazoline) the fraction of the dose absorbed was unchanged, but the rate of absorption was slowed. The peak plasma concentrations were approximately half those achieved in the absence of the vasoconstrictor.

Following its initial absorption/distribution phase, the single dose pharmacokinetics of butorphanol by the intravenous, intramuscular, and nasal routes of administration are similar (see Figure 1).

Figure 1 — Butorphanol Plasma Levels After IV, IM and Nasal Spray Administration of 2 mg Dose

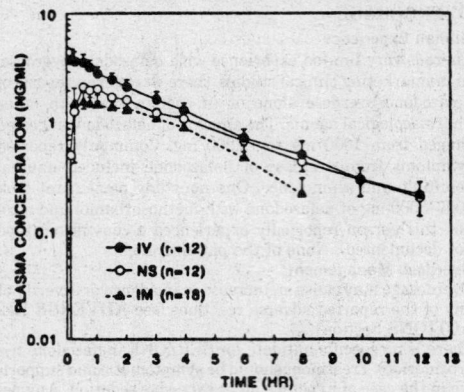

Serum protein binding is independent of concentration over the range achieved in clinical practice (up to 7 ng/mL) with a bound fraction of approximately 80%.

The volume of distribution of butorphanol varies from 305–901 liters and total body clearance from 52–154 liters/hr (see Table 1).

[See table below.]

Dose proportionality for STADOL NS (butorphanol tartrate) Nasal Spray has been determined at steady state in doses up to 4 mg at 6 hour intervals. Steady state is achieved within 2 days. The mean peak plasma concentration at steady state was 1.8-fold (maximal 3-fold) following a single dose.

The drug is transported across the blood brain and placental barriers and into human milk (see Labor and Delivery and Nursing Mothers).

Butorphanol is extensively metabolized in the liver. Metabolism is qualitatively and quantitatively similar following intravenous, intramuscular, or nasal administration. Oral bioavailability is only 5–17% because of extensive first pass metabolism of butorphanol.

The major metabolite of butorphanol is hydroxybutorphanol, while norbutorphanol is produced in small amounts. Both have been detected in plasma following administration of butorphanol. Preliminary evidence suggests the elimination half-life of hydroxybutorphanol may be greater than that of its parent.

Elimination occurs by urine and fecal excretion. When ^{3}H labelled butorphanol is administered to normal subjects, most (70–80%) of the dose is recovered in the urine, while approximately 15% is recovered in the feces.

About 5% of the dose is recovered in the urine as butorphanol. Forty-nine percent is eliminated in the urine as hydroxybutorphanol. Less than 5% is excreted in the urine as norbutorphanol (see also CLINICAL PHARMACOLOGY above).

Butorphanol pharmacokinetics in the elderly differ from younger patients (see Table 1). The mean absolute bioavailability of STADOL NS (butorphanol tartrate) Nasal Spray in elderly women (48%) was less than that in elderly men (75%), young men (68%) or young women (70%). Elimination of half-life is increased in the elderly (6.6 hours as opposed to 4.7 hours in younger subjects).

In renally impaired patients with creatinine clearances < 30 mL/min the elimination half-life is approximately doubled and the total body clearance was reduced about half (10.5 hours [clearance 150 L/h] as compared to 5.8 hours [clearance 260 L/h] in normals). No effect was observed on Cmax or Tmax after a single dose.

For further recommendations refer to statements on use in Geriatric Patients, Renal Disease, Hepatic Disease, and statement on Drug Interactions in the PRECAUTIONS, and INDIVIDUALIZATION OF DOSAGE sections below.

CLINICAL TRIALS

The effectiveness of opioid analgesics varies in different pain syndromes. Studies with STADOL (butorphanol tartrate) Injectable have been performed in postoperative (primarily abdominal and orthopedic) pain and pain during labor and delivery, as preoperative and preanesthetic medication, and as a supplement to balanced anesthesia (see below).

Studies with STADOL NS have been performed in postoperative (general, orthopedic, oral, cesarean section) pain, in post-episiotomy pain, in pain of musculoskeletal origin, and in migraine headache pain (see below).

Use in the Management of Pain

Postoperative Analgesia

The analgesic efficacy of STADOL Injectable in postoperative pain was investigated in several double-blind active-controlled studies involving 958 butorphanol-treated patients. The following doses were found to have approximately equivalent analgesic effect: 2 mg butorphanol, 10 mg morphine, 40 mg pentazocine and 80 mg meperidine.

After intravenous administration of STADOL Injectable, onset and peak analgesic effect occurred by the time of first observation (30 minutes). After intramuscular administration, pain relief onset occurred at 30 minutes or less, and peak effect occurred between 30 minutes and one hour. The duration of action of STADOL Injectable was 3–4 hours when defined as the time necessary for pain intensity to return to pretreatment level or the time to retreatment.

The analgesic efficacy of STADOL NS was evaluated (approximately 35 patients per treatment group) in a general and orthopedic surgery trial. Single doses of STADOL NS (1 or 2 mg) and IM meperidine (37.5 or 75 mg) were compared. Analgesia provided by 1 and 2 mg doses of STADOL NS was similar to 37.5 or 75 mg meperidine, respectively, with onset of analgesia within 15 minutes and peak analgesic effect within 1 hour. The median duration of pain relief was 2.5 hours with 1 mg STADOL NS, (butorphanol tartrate) Nasal Spray, 3.5 hours with 2 mg STADOL NS and 3.3 hours with either dose of meperidine.

In a postcesarean section trial, STADOL NS administered to 35 patients as two 1 mg doses 60 minutes apart was compared with a single 2 mg dose of STADOL NS or a single 2 mg IV dose of STADOL (butorphanol tartrate) Injectable (37 patients each). Onset of analgesia was within 15 minutes for all STADOL regimens. Peak analgesic effects of 2 mg intravenous STADOL Injectable and STADOL NS were similar in magnitude. The duration of pain relief provided by both 2 mg STADOL NS regimens was approximately 4.5 hours and was greater than intravenous STADOL Injectable (2.6 h).

Migraine Headache Pain

The analgesic efficacy of two 1 mg doses one hour apart of STADOL NS in migraine headache pain was compared with a single dose of 10 mg IM methadone (31 and 32 patients respectively). Significant onset of analgesia occurred within 15 minutes for both STADOL NS and IM methadone. Peak an-

Table 1 — Mean Pharmacokinetic Parameters of Butorphanol in Young and Elderly Subjects[a]

Parameters	Intravenous		Nasal	
	Young	Elderly	Young	Elderly
Tmax[b] (hr)			0.62 (0.32)[e] (0.15–1.50)[g]	1.03 (0.74) (0.25–3.00)
Cmax[c] (ng/mL)			1.04 (0.40) (0.35–1.97)	0.90 (0.57) (0.10–2.68)
AUC (inf)[d] (hr.ng/mL)	7.24 (1.57) (4.40–9.77)	8.71 (2.02) (4.76–13.03)	4.93 (1.24) (2.16–7.27)	5.24 (2.27) (0.30–10.34)
Half-life (hr)	4.56 (1.67) (2.06–8.70)	5.61 (1.36) (3.25–8.79)	4.74 (1.57) (2.89–8.79)	6.56 (1.51) (3.75–9.17)
Absolute Bioavailability (%)			69 (16) (44–113)	61 (25) (3–121)
Volume of Distribution[f] (L)	487 (155) (305–901)	552 (124) (305–737)		
Total body Clearance (L/hr)	99 (23) (70–154)	82 (21) (52–143)		

a) Young subjects (n=24) are from 20 to 40 years old and elderly (n=24) are greater than 65 years of age.
b) Time to peak plasma concentration.
c) Peak plasma concentration normalized to 1 mg dose.
d) Area under the plasma concentration-time curve after a 1 mg dose.
e) Mean (1 S.D.)
f) Derived from IV data.
g) (range of observed values)

algesic effect occurred at 2 hours for STADOL NS and 1.5 hours for methadone. The median duration of pain relief was 6 hours with STADOL NS and 4 hours with methadone as judged by the time when approximately half of the patients remedicated.

In two other trials in patients with migraine headache pain, a 2 mg initial dose of STADOL NS followed by an additional 1 mg dose 1 hr later (76 patients) was compared with either 75 mg IM meperidine (24 patients) or placebo (72 patients). Onset, peak activity and duration were similar with both active treatments; however, the incidence of adverse experiences (nausea, vomiting, dizziness) was higher in these two trials with the 2 mg initial dose of STADOL NS than in the trial with the 1 mg initial dose.

Preanesthetic Medication
STADOL Injectable (2 mg and 4 mg) and meperidine (80 mg) were studied for use as preanesthetic medication in hospitalized surgical patients. Patients received a single intramuscular dose of either STADOL Injectable or meperidine approximately 90 minutes prior to anesthesia. The anesthesia regimen included barbiturate induction, followed by nitrous oxide and oxygen with halothane or enflurane, with or without a muscle relaxant.

Anesthetic preparation was rated as satisfactory in all 42 STADOL Injectable patients regardless of the type of surgery.

Balanced Anesthesia
STADOL Injectable administered intravenously (mean dose 2 mg) was compared to intravenous morphine sulfate (mean dose 10 mg) as premedication shortly before thiopental induction, followed by balanced anesthesia in 50 ASA Class 1 and 2 patients. Anesthesia was then maintained by repeated intravenous doses, averaging 4.6 mg STADOL Injectable and 22.8 mg morphine per patient.

Anesthetic induction and maintenance were generally rated as satisfactory with both STADOL Injectable (25 patients) and morphine (25 patients) regardless of the type of surgery performed. Emergence from anesthesia was comparable with both agents.

Labor (see PRECAUTIONS)
The analgesic efficacy of intravenous STADOL (butorphanol tartrate) Injectable was studied in pain during labor. In a total of 145 patients STADOL Injectable (1 mg and 2 mg) was as effective as 40 mg and 80 mg of meperidine (144 patients) in the relief of pain in labor with no effect on the duration or progress of labor. Both drugs readily crossed the placenta and entered fetal circulation. The condition of the infants in these studies, determined by Apgar scores at 1 and 5 minutes (8 or above) and time to sustained respiration, showed that STADOL Injectable had the same effects on the infants as meperidine.

In these studies neurobehavioral testing in infants exposed to STADOL Injectable at a mean of 18.6 hours after delivery, showed no significant differences between treatment groups.

INDIVIDUALIZATION OF DOSAGE
The usual starting doses of butorphanol are: 1 mg repeated every 3–4 hours IV; 2 mg repeated every 3–4 hours IM; and 1 mg followed by 1 mg in 60–90 minutes nasally repeated every 3–4 hours (see DOSAGE AND ADMINISTRATION). Use of butorphanol in geriatric patients, patients with renal impairment, patients with hepatic impairment, and during labor requires extra caution (see below and the appropriate sections in PRECAUTIONS).

STADOL Injectable
For pain relief the recommended initial dosage regimen of STADOL Injectable is 1 mg IV or 2 mg IM with repeated doses every three to four hours, as necessary. This dosage regimen is likely to be effective for the majority of patients. Dosage adjustments of STADOL Injectable should be based on observations of its beneficial and adverse effects. The initial dose in the elderly and in patients with renal or hepatic impairment should generally be half the recommended adult dose (0.5 mg IV and 1.0 mg IM). Repeat doses in these patients should be determined by the patient's response rather than at fixed intervals but will generally be no less than 6 hours (see PRECAUTIONS).

The usual preoperative dose is 2 mg IM given 60–90 minutes before surgery or 2 mg IV shortly before induction. This is approximately equivalent in sedative effect to 10 mg morphine or 80 mg of meperidine. This single preoperative dose should be individualized based on age, body weight, physical status, underlying pathological condition, use of other drugs, type of anesthesia to be used and the surgical procedure involved.

During maintenance in balanced anesthesia the usual incremental dose of STADOL Injectable is 0.5 to 1.0 mg IV. The incremental dose may be higher, up to 0.06 mg/kg (4 mg/70 kg), depending on previous sedative, analgesic, and hypnotic drugs administered. The total dose of STADOL Injectable will vary; however, patients seldom require less than 4 mg or more than 12.5 mg (approximately 0.06 to 0.18 mg/kg).

As with other opioids of this class, STADOL Injectable may not provide adequate intraoperative analgesia in every patient or under all conditions. A failure to achieve successful analgesia during balanced anesthesia is commonly reflected

by increases in general sympathetic tone. Consequently, if blood pressure or heart rate continue to rise, consideration should be given to adding a potent volatile liquid inhalation anesthetic or another intravenous medication.

In labor, the recommended initial dose of STADOL Injectable is 1 or 2 mg IM or IV in mothers with fetuses of 37 weeks gestation or beyond and without signs of fetal distress. Dosage adjustments of STADOL Injectable in labor should be based on initial response with consideration given to concomitant analgesic or sedative drugs and the expected time of delivery. A dose should not be repeated in less than four hours nor administered less than four hours prior to the anticipated delivery (see PRECAUTIONS).

STADOL NS (butorphanol tartrate) Nasal Spray
Since STADOL NS does not require an injection, it allows the physician to initiate therapy with a low dose and repeat the dose if needed.

The usual recommended dose for initial nasal administration is 1 mg (1 spray in **one** nostril). If adequate pain relief is not achieved within 60–90 minutes, an additional 1 mg dose may be given.

The initial dose sequence outlined above may be repeated in 3–4 hours as required.

For the management of severe pain, an initial dose of 2 mg (1 spray in **each** nostril) may be used in patients who will be able to remain recumbent in the event drowsiness or dizziness occur. In such patients additional doses should not be given for 3–4 hours. The incidence of adverse events is higher with an initial 2 mg dose (see CLINICAL TRIALS).

The initial dose sequence in elderly patients and patients with renal or hepatic impairment should be limited to 1 mg followed by 1 mg in 90–120 minutes. The repeat dose sequence in these patients should be determined by the patients response rather than at fixed times but will generally be no less than at 6 hour intervals (see PRECAUTIONS).

INDICATIONS AND USAGE
STADOL (butorphanol tartrate) Injectable and STADOL NS (butorphanol tartrate) Nasal Spray are indicated for the management of pain when the use of an opioid analgesic is appropriate.

STADOL Injectable is also indicated as a preoperative or preanesthetic medication, as a supplement to balanced anesthesia, and for the relief of pain during labor.

CONTRAINDICATIONS
STADOL Injectable and STADOL NS are contraindicated in patients hypersensitive to butorphanol tartrate or the preservative benzethonium chloride in STADOL NS or STADOL Injectable in the multi-dose vial.

WARNINGS
PATIENTS DEPENDENT ON NARCOTICS
Because of its opioid antagonist properties, butorphanol is not recommended for use in patients dependent on narcotics. Such patients should have an adequate period of withdrawal from opioid drugs prior to beginning butorphanol therapy. In patients taking opioid analgesics chronically, butorphanol has precipitated withdrawal symptoms such as anxiety, agitation, mood changes, hallucinations, dysphoria, weakness and diarrhea.

Because of the difficulty in assessing opioid tolerance in patients who have recently received repeated doses of narcotic analgesic medication, caution should be used in the administration of butorphanol to such patients.

PRECAUTIONS
GENERAL
Hypotension associated with syncope during the first hour of dosing with STADOL NS (butorphanol tartrate) Nasal Spray has been reported rarely, particularly in patients with past history of similar reactions to opioid analgesics. Therefore, patients should be advised to avoid activities with potential risks.

HEAD INJURY AND INCREASED INTRACRANIAL PRESSURE
As with other opioids, the use of butorphanol in patients with head injury may be associated with carbon dioxide retention and secondary elevation of cerebrospinal fluid pressure, drug-induced miosis, and alterations in mental state that would obscure the interpretation of the clinical course of patients with head injuries. In such patients, butorphanol should be used only if the benefits of use outweigh the potential risks.

DISORDERS OF RESPIRATORY FUNCTION OR CONTROL
Butorphanol may produce respiratory depression, especially in patients receiving other CNS active agents, or patients suffering from CNS diseases or respiratory impairment.

HEPATIC AND RENAL DISEASE
In patients with severe hepatic or renal disease the initial dosage interval for STADOL (butorphanol tartrate) Injectable and STADOL NS should be increased to 6–8 hours until the response has been well characterized. Subsequent doses should be determined by patient response rather than being scheduled at fixed intervals (see INDIVIDUALIZATION OF DOSAGE).

CARDIOVASCULAR EFFECTS
Because butorphanol may increase the work of the heart, especially the pulmonary circuit (see CLINICAL PHARMACOLOGY), the use of butorphanol in patients with acute myocardial infarction, ventricular dysfunction, or coronary insufficiency should be limited to those situations where the benefits clearly outweigh the risk.

Severe hypertension has been reported rarely during butorphanol therapy. In such cases, butorphanol should be discontinued and the hypertension treated with antihypertensive drugs. In patients who are not opioid dependent, naloxone has also been reported to be effective.

INFORMATION FOR PATIENTS
1. Opioid analgesics impair the mental or physical abilities required for the performance of potentially dangerous tasks such as driving a car or operating machinery. Patients who have taken butorphanol should not drive or operate dangerous machinery for at least one hour and until the effects of the drug are no longer present.

2. Alcohol should not be consumed while using butorphanol. Concurrent use of butorphanol with drugs that affect the central nervous system (e.g., alcohol, barbiturates, tranquilizers, and antihistamines) may result in increased central nervous system depressant effects such as drowsiness, dizziness and impaired mental function.

3. Patients should be instructed on the proper use of STADOL NS (see PATIENT INSTRUCTIONS).

DRUG INTERACTIONS
Concurrent use of butorphanol with central nervous system depressants (e.g., alcohol, barbiturates, tranquilizers, and antihistamines) may result in increased central nervous system depressant effects. When used concurrently with such drugs, the dose of butorphanol should be the smallest effective dose and the frequency of dosing reduced as much as possible when administered concomitantly with drugs that potentiate the action of opioids.

In healthy volunteers, the pharmacokinetics of a 1 mg dose of butorphanol administered as STADOL NS were not affected by the co-administration of a single 6 mg subcutaneous dose of sumatriptan.

The pharmacokinetics of a 1 mg dose of butorphanol administered as STADOL NS were not affected by the co-administration of cimetidine (300 mg QID). Conversely, the administration of STADOL NS (1 mg butorphanol QID) did not alter the pharmacokinetics of a 300 mg dose of cimetidine.

It is not known if the effects of butorphanol are altered by other concomitant medications that affect hepatic metabolism of drugs (erythromycin, theophylline, etc.), but physicians should be alert to the possibility that a smaller initial dose and longer intervals between doses may be needed.

The fraction of STADOL NS (butorphanol tartrate) Nasal Spray absorbed is unaffected by the concomitant administration of a nasal vasoconstrictor (oxymetazoline), but the rate of absorption is decreased. Therefore, a slower onset can be anticipated if STADOL NS is administered concomitantly with, or immediately following, a nasal vasoconstrictor.

No information is available about the use of butorphanol concurrently with MAO inhibitors.

USE IN AMBULATORY PATIENTS
Opioid analgesics impair the mental or physical abilities required for the performance of potentially dangerous tasks such as driving a car or operating machinery. Patients who have taken butorphanol should not drive or operate dangerous machinery for at least one hour and until the effects of the drug are no longer present.

Alcohol should not be consumed while using butorphanol. Concurrent use of butorphanol with central nervous system depressants (e.g., alcohol, barbiturates, tranquilizers, and antihistamines) may result in increased central nervous system depressant effects.

Patients should be instructed on the proper use of STADOL NS (see PATIENT INSTRUCTIONS).

CARCINOGENESIS, MUTAGENESIS, IMPAIRMENT OF FERTILITY
Two year carcinogenicity studies were conducted in mice and rats given butorphanol tartrate in the diet at 5, 15 and 60 mg/kg/day (up to 200 times the maximum recommended human dose on a mg/kg basis, or up to 16 times (mice) or 39 times (rats) on a mg/m² basis. There was no evidence of carcinogenicity in either species in these studies.

Butorphanol was not genotoxic in *S. typhimurium* or *E. coli* assays or in unscheduled DNA synthesis and repair assays conducted in cultured human fibroblast cells.

Rats treated orally with 160 mg/kg/day (944 mg/sq.m.) had a reduced pregnancy rate. However, a similar effect was not observed with a 2.5 mg/kg/day (14.75 mg/sq.m.) subcutaneous dose.

PREGNANCY
Pregnancy Category C
Reproduction studies in mice, rats and rabbits during organogenesis did not reveal any teratogenic potential to butorphanol. However, pregnant rats treated subcutaneously with butorphanol at 1 mg/kg (5.9 mg/sq.m.) had a higher

Continued on next page

Bristol-Myers Squibb Co.—Cont.

frequency of stillbirths than controls. Butorphanol at 30 mg/kg/oral (5.1 mg/sq.m.) and 60 mg/kg/oral (10.2 mg/sq.m.) also showed higher incidences of post-implantation loss in rabbits.

There are no adequate and well-controlled studies of STADOL (butorphanol tartrate) in pregnant women before 37 weeks gestation. STADOL should be used during pregnancy only if the potential benefit justifies the potential risk to the infant.

LABOR AND DELIVERY

Although there have been rare reports of infant respiratory distress/apnea following the administration of STADOL (butorphanol tartrate) Injectable during labor, this adverse effect was not attributed to STADOL Injectable as used during controlled clinical trials. The reports of respiratory distress/apnea have been associated with administration of a dose within two hours of delivery, use of multiple doses, use with additional analgesic or sedative drugs, or use in preterm pregnancies.

In a study of 119 patients, the administration of 1 mg of IV STADOL Injectable during labor was associated with transient (10–90 minutes) sinusoidal fetal heart rate patterns, but was not associated with adverse neonatal outcomes. In the presence of an abnormal fetal heart rate pattern, STADOL Injectable should be used with caution.

STADOL NS (butorphanol tartrate) Nasal Spray is not recommended during labor or delivery because there is no clinical experience with its use in this setting.

NURSING MOTHERS

Butorphanol has been detected in milk following administration of STADOL (butorphanol tartrate) Injectable to nursing mothers. The amount an infant would receive is probably clinically insignificant (estimated 4 microgram/liter of milk in a mother receiving 2 mg IM four times a day).

Although there is no clinical experience with the use of STADOL NS in nursing mothers, it should be assumed that butorphanol will appear in the milk in similar amounts following the nasal route of administration.

PEDIATRIC USE

Butorphanol is not recommended for use in patients below 18 years of age because safety and efficacy have not been established in this population.

GERIATRIC USE

The initial dose of STADOL Injectable recommended for elderly patients is half the usual dose at twice the usual interval. Subsequent doses and intervals should be based on the patient response (see INDIVIDUALIZATION OF DOSAGE).

Initially a 1 mg dose of STADOL NS should generally be used in geriatric patients and 90–120 minutes should elapse before deciding whether a second 1 mg dose is needed (see INDIVIDUALIZATION OF DOSAGE).

Due to changes in clearance, the mean half-life of butorphanol is increased by 25% (to over 6 hours) in patients over the age of 65. Elderly patients may be more sensitive to its side effects. Results from a long-term clinical safety trial suggest that elderly patients may be less tolerant of dizziness due to STADOL NS than younger patients.

ADVERSE REACTIONS

A total of 2446 patients were studied in butorphanol clinical trials. Approximately half received STADOL Injectable with the remainder receiving STADOL NS. In nearly all cases the type and incidence of side effects with butorphanol by any route were those commonly observed with opioid analgesics. The adverse experiences described below are based on data from short- and long-term clinical trials in patients receiving butorphanol by any route and from post-marketing experience with STADOL Injectable. There has been no attempt to correct for placebo effect or to subtract the frequencies reported by placebo treated patients in controlled trials.

The most frequently reported adverse experiences across all clinical trials with STADOL Injectable and STADOL NS were somnolence (43%), dizziness (19%), nausea and/or vomiting (13%). In long-term trials with STADOL NS (butorphanol tartrate) Nasal Spray only, nasal congestion (13%) and insomnia (11%) were frequently reported.

The following adverse experiences were reported at a frequency of 1% or greater, and were considered to be probably related to the use of butorphanol:

BODY AS A WHOLE: asthenia/lethargy*, headache*, sensation of heat

CARDIOVASCULAR: VASODILATION*, PALPITATIONS

DIGESTIVE: ANOREXIA*, CONSTIPATION*, dry mouth*, nausea and/or vomiting (13%), stomach pain

NERVOUS: anxiety, confusion*, dizziness (19%), euphoria, floating feeling, INSOMNIA (11%), nervousness, paresthesia, somnolence (43%), TREMOR

RESPIRATORY: BRONCHITIS, COUGH, DYSPNEA*, EPISTAXIS*, NASAL CONGESTION (13%), NASAL IRRITATION*, PHARYNGITIS*, RHINITIS*, SINUS CONGESTION*, SINUSITIS, UPPER RESPIRATORY INFECTION*

SKIN AND APPENDAGES: sweating/clammy*, pruritus
SPECIAL SENSES: blurred vision, EAR PAIN, TINNITUS*, UNPLEASANT TASTE* (also seen in short-term trials with STADOL® NS™ [butorphanol tartrate] Nasal Spray).

(Reactions occurring with a frequency of 3–9% are marked with an asterisk.* Reactions reported predominantly from long-term trials with STADOL NS are CAPITALIZED.)
The following adverse experiences were reported with a frequency of less than 1%, in clinical trials or from post-marketing experience, and were considered to be probably related to the use of butorphanol.

BODY AS A WHOLE: *excessive drug effect associated with transient difficulty speaking and/or executing purposeful movements.*

CARDIOVASCULAR: hypotension, syncope.

NERVOUS: abnormal dreams, agitation, *drug dependence,* dysphoria, hallucinations, hostility

SKIN AND APPENDAGES: rash/hives

UROGENITAL: impaired urination

(Reactions reported only from post-marketing experience are *italicized.*)
The following infrequent additional adverse experiences were reported in a frequency of less than 1% of the patients studied in short-term STADOL NS trials and from post-marketing experiences under circumstances where the association between these events and butorphanol administration is unknown. They are being listed as alerting information for the physician.

BODY AS A WHOLE: chest pain, edema
CARDIOVASCULAR: hypertension, tachycardia
NERVOUS: *convulsion, delusion,* depression
RESPIRATORY: *apnea,* shallow breathing
(Reactions reported only from post-marketing experience are *italicized.*)

DRUG ABUSE AND DEPENDENCE

Although the mixed agonist-antagonist opioid analgesics, as a class, have lower abuse potential than morphine, all such drugs can be and have been reported to be abused.

Chronic use of STADOL (butorphanol tartrate) Injectable has been reported to result in mild withdrawal syndromes, and reports of overuse and self-reported addiction have been received.

Among 161 patients who used STADOL NS for 2 months or longer approximately 3% had behavioral symptoms suggestive of possible abuse. Approximately 1% of these patients reported significant overuse. Symptoms such as anxiety, agitation, and diarrhea were observed. Symptoms suggestive of opioid withdrawal occurred in 2 patients who stopped the drug abruptly after using 16 mg a day or more for longer than 3 months.

Special care should be exercised in administering butorphanol to emotionally unstable patients and to those with a history of drug misuse. When long-term therapy is necessary, such patients should be closely supervised.

OVERDOSAGE

CLINICAL MANIFESTATIONS

The clinical manifestations of overdose are those of opioid drugs, the most serious of which are hypoventilation, cardiovascular insufficiency and/or coma.

Overdose can occur due to accidental or intentional misuse of butorphanol, especially in young children who may gain access to the drug in the home.

TREATMENT

The management of suspected butorphanol overdosage includes maintenance of adequate ventilation, peripheral perfusion, normal body temperature, and protection of the airway. Patients should be under continuous observation with adequate serial measures of mental state, responsiveness and vital signs. Oxygen and ventilatory assistance should be available with continual monitoring by pulse oximetry if indicated. In the presence of coma, placement of an artificial airway may be required. An adequate intravenous portal should be maintained to facilitate treatment of hypotension associated with vasodilation.

The use of a specific opioid antagonist such as naloxone should be considered. As the duration of butorphanol action usually exceeds the duration of action of naloxone, repeated dosing with naloxone may be required.

DOSAGE AND ADMINISTRATION

Factors to be considered in determining the dose are age, body weight, physical status, underlying pathological condition, use of other drugs, type of anesthesia to be used, and surgical procedure involved. Use in the elderly, patients with hepatic or renal disease or in labor requires extra caution (see PRECAUTIONS and INDIVIDUALIZATION OF DOSAGE). The following doses are for patients who do not have impaired hepatic or renal function and who are not on CNS active agents.

USE FOR PAIN

Intravenous: The usual recommended single dose for IV administration is 1 mg repeated every three to four hours as necessary. The effective dosage range, depending on the se-

verity of pain, is 0.5 to 2 mg repeated every three to four hours.

Intramuscular: The usual recommended single dose for IM administration is 2 mg in patients who will be able to remain recumbent, in the event drowsiness or dizziness occurs. This may be repeated every three to four hours, as necessary. The effective dosage range depending on the severity of pain is 1 to 4 mg repeated every three to four hours. There are insufficient clinical data to recommend single doses above 4 mg.

NASAL SPRAY: The usual recommended dose for initial nasal administration is 1 mg (1 spray in **one** nostril). Adherence to this dose reduces the incidence of drowsiness and dizziness. If adequate pain relief is not achieved within 60–90 minutes, an additional 1 mg dose may be given.

The initial two dose sequence outlined above may be repeated in 3–4 hours as needed.

Depending on the severity of the pain, an initial dose of 2 mg (1 spray in **each** nostril) may be used in patients who will be able to remain recumbent in the event drowsiness or dizziness occur. In such patients single additional 2 mg doses should not be given for 3–4 hours.

USE AS PREOPERATIVE/PREANESTHETIC MEDICATION

The preoperative medication dosage of STADOL (butorphanol tartrate) Injectable should be individualized (see INDIVIDUALIZATION OF DOSAGE). The usual adult dose is 2 mg IM, administered 60–90 minutes before surgery. This is approximately equivalent in sedative effect to 10 mg morphine or 80 mg meperidine.

USE IN BALANCED ANESTHESIA

The usual dose of STADOL Injectable is 2 mg IV shortly before induction and/or 0.5 to 1.0 mg IV in increments during anesthesia. The increment may be higher, up to 0.06 mg/kg (4 mg/70 kg), depending on previous sedative, analgesic, and hypnotic drugs administered. The total dose of STADOL Injectable will vary; however, patients seldom require less than 4 mg or more than 12.5 mg (approximately 0.06 to 0.18 mg/kg).

The use of STADOL NS (butorphanol tartrate) Nasal Spray is not recommended, because it has not been studied in induction or maintenance of anesthesia.

LABOR

In patients at full term in early labor a 1–2 mg dose of Stadol Injectable IV or IM may be administered and repeated after 4 hours. Alternative analgesia should be used for pain associated with delivery or if delivery is expected to occur within 4 hours.

If concomitant use of STADOL with drugs that may potentiate its effects is deemed necessary (see Drug Interactions in PRECAUTIONS section) the lowest effective dose should be employed.

The use of STADOL NS is not recommended as it has not been studied in labor.

SAFETY AND HANDLING

STADOL Injectable is supplied in sealed delivery systems that have a low risk of accidental exposure to health care workers. Ordinary care should be taken to avoid aerosol generation while preparing a syringe for use. Following skin contact, rinsing with cool water is recommended.

STADOL NS is an open delivery system with increased risk of exposure to health care workers.

In the priming process, a certain amount of butorphanol may be aerosolized; therefore, the pump sprayer should be aimed away from the patient or other people or animals.

The unit should be disposed of by unscrewing the cap, rinsing the bottle, and placing the parts in a waste container.

HOW SUPPLIED

STADOL (butorphanol tartrate) Injectable for IM or IV use is available as follows:
NDC 0015-5644-20—2 mg per mL, 2-mL vial
NDC 0015-5645-20—1 mg per mL, 1-mL vial
NDC 0015-5646-20—2 mg per mL, 1-mL vial
NDC 0015-5648-20—2 mg per mL, 10-mL multi-dose vial
STADOL NS (butorphanol tartrate) Nasal Spray is supplied in a child-resistant prescription vial containing a metered-dose spray pump with protective clip and dust cover, a bottle of nasal spray solution, and a patient instruction leaflet. On average, one bottle will deliver 14–15 doses if no repriming is necessary.
NDC 0087-5650-41—10 mg per mL, 2.5-mL bottle.

PHARMACIST ASSEMBLY INSTRUCTIONS FOR STADOL NS (BUTORPHANOL TARTRATE) NASAL SPRAY

The pharmacist will assemble STADOL NS (butorphanol tartrate) Nasal Spray prior to dispensing to the patient, according to the following instructions:
1. Open the child-resistant prescription vial and remove the spray pump and solution bottle.
2. Assemble STADOL NS by first unscrewing the white cap from the solution bottle and screwing the pump unit tightly onto the bottle. Make sure the clear cover is on the pump unit.
3. Return the STADOL NS bottle to the child-resistant prescription vial for dispensing to the patient.

Storage Conditions
Store below 86°F (30°C). Parenteral drug products should be inspected visually for particulate matter and discoloration prior to administration, whenever solution and container permit.
CAUTION: FEDERAL LAW PROHIBITS DISPENSING WITHOUT PRESCRIPTION
Bristol-Myers Squibb Company
APOTHECON®
A Bristol-Myers Squibb Company
Princeton, New Jersey 08543 USA   P5993-01
STADOL NS also promoted by Cephalon, Inc.
Shown in Product Identification Guide, page 307

VAGISTAT®-1   ℞
vaginal ointment
(tioconazole 6.5%)

DESCRIPTION
Tioconazole,   1-[2-[(2-chloro-3-thienyl)methoxy]-2(2,4-dichlorophenyl)ethyl]-1H-imidazole, is a topical antifungal agent. Its chemical formula is $C_{16}H_{13}Cl_3N_2OS$ with a molecular weight of 387.7. The structural formula is given below:

VAGISTAT-1 (tioconazole 6.5%) is formulated in a base of white, soft paraffin and aluminum magnesium silicate with butylated hydroxyanisole (BHA) added as a preservative. Each applicator-full of VAGISTAT-1 provides approximately 4.6 grams of ointment containing 300 mg of tioconazole.

CLINICAL PHARMACOLOGY
Tioconazole is a broad-spectrum antifungal agent that inhibits the growth of human pathogenic yeasts. Tioconazole exhibits fungicidal activity *in vitro* against *Candida albicans,* other species of the genus *Candida,* and against *Torulopsis glabrata.*
Pharmacokinetics: Systemic absorption of tioconazole after a single intravaginal application of VAGISTAT-1 in nonpregnant patients is negligible.

INDICATIONS AND USAGE
VAGISTAT-1 is indicated for the local treatment of vulvovaginal candidiasis (moniliasis). As VAGISTAT-1 has been shown to be effective only for candidal vulvovaginitis, the diagnosis should be confirmed by KOH smears and/or cultures. Other pathogens commonly associated with vulvovaginitis should be ruled out by appropriate methods.
Studies have shown that women taking oral contraceptives have a cure rate similar to those not taking such agents when treated with VAGISTAT-1.
Safety and effectiveness in pregnant and diabetic patients have not been established (see Precautions).

CONTRAINDICATIONS
VAGISTAT-1 is contraindicated in individuals who have been shown to be sensitive to imidazole antifungal agents or to other components of the ointment.

PRECAUTIONS
General: VAGISTAT-1 is intended for intravaginal administration only. Applicators should be opened just prior to administration to prevent contamination. Administration of VAGISTAT-1 just prior to bedtime may be preferred. The VAGISTAT-1 ointment base may interact with rubber or latex products such as condoms or vaginal contraceptive diaphragms; therefore, use of such products within 72 hours following treatment is not recommended.
If clinical symptoms persist, appropriate microbiological tests should be repeated to rule out other pathogens and to confirm the diagnosis.
Information for Patients: The VAGISTAT-1 ointment base may interact with rubber or latex products such as condoms or vaginal contraceptive diaphragms; therefore, use of such products within 72 hours following treatment is not recommended.
Carcinogenesis: No long-term studies in animals have been performed to evaluate the carcinogenic potential of tioconazole.
Mutagenesis: Tioconazole did not demonstrate mutagenic activity at the levels examined in tests at either the chromosomal or subchromosomal level.
Impairment of Fertility: No impairment of fertility was seen in male rats administered tioconazole hydrochloride in oral doses up to 150 mg/kg/day. However, there was evidence of preimplantation loss in female rats at oral dose levels above 35 mg/kg/day.

Pregnancy—Pregnancy Category C: Tioconazole hydrochloride had no adverse effects on fetal viability or growth when administered orally to pregnant rats at doses of 55, 110, and 165 mg/kg/day during the period of organogenesis. A drug-related increase in the incidence of dilated ureters, hydroureters, and hydronephrosis observed in the fetuses of this study was transient and no longer evident in pups raised to 21 days of age. These effects did not occur following intravaginal administration of approximately 10 mg/kg/day in a 2% cream. There was no evidence of major structural anomalies. No embryotoxic or teratogenic effects were observed in rabbits receiving oral dose levels as high as 165 mg/kg/day or daily intravaginal application of approximately 2–3 mg/kg in a 2% tioconazole cream during organogenesis. Tioconazole hydrochloride, like other azole antimycotic agents, causes dystocia in rats when treatment is extended through parturition. Associated effects in rats include prolongation of pregnancy, *in utero* deaths, and impaired pup survival. The "no-effect" level for this phenomenon is 20 mg/kg/day orally and approximately 9 mg/kg/day intravaginally. No effect on parturition occurred in rabbits at 50 mg/kg/day orally.
There are no adequate and well-controlled studies in pregnant women. VAGISTAT-1 (tioconazole 6.5%) should be used during pregnancy only if the potential benefit justifies the potential risk to the fetus.
Nursing Mothers: It is not known whether this drug is excreted in human milk. Because many drugs are excreted in human milk, nursing should be temporarily discontinued while VAGISTAT-1 is administered.
Pediatric Use: Safety and effectiveness in children have not been established.

ADVERSE REACTIONS
The incidence of adverse reactions to VAGISTAT-1 is based on clinical trials involving 1000 patients. Burning and itching were the most frequent side effects occurring in approximately 6% and 5% of the patients, respectively. In most instances these did not interfere with the course of therapy. There were occasional reports (less than 1%) of other side effects including irritation, discharge, vulvar edema and swelling, vaginal pain, dysuria, nocturia, dyspareunia, dryness of vaginal secretions, desquamation, and burning sensation.

DOSAGE AND ADMINISTRATION
VAGISTAT-1 (tioconazole 6.5%) has been found to be effective as a single-dose treatment for vulvovaginal candidiasis. Using the prefilled applicator, insert one applicator-full intravaginally. Administration of VAGISTAT-1 just prior to bedtime may be preferred.

HOW SUPPLIED
VAGISTAT-1 is supplied in a ready-to-use, prefilled, single-dose vaginal applicator (NDC 0087-0657-40). Each applicator-full will deliver approximately 4.6 grams of VAGISTAT-1 containing 65 mg of tioconazole per gram of ointment.

Storage
Store at controlled room temperature 15°–30° C (59°–86° F).
WARNING: Manufactured with 1,1,1-tri-chloroethane, a substance which harms public health and environment by destroying ozone in the upper atmosphere.

Manufactured in Canada for Bristol-Myers Squibb Company Princeton, NJ 08543 by Pfizer Canada, Inc.
Arnprior, Ontario, Canada   P9518-05

BTG Pharmaceuticals
70 WOOD AVENUE SOUTH
ISELIN, NJ 08830

For Medical Information or Emergencies Contact:
(800) 741-2698

For Customer Service and Ordering:
(800) 741-2698
FAX: (800) 741-2696

DELATESTRYL®   ℞
Testosterone Enanthate Injection USP

DESCRIPTION
DELATESTRYL (Testosterone Enanthate Injection) provides testosterone enanthate, a derivative of the primary endogenous androgen testosterone, for intramuscular administration. In their active form, androgens have a 17-beta-hydroxy group. Esterification of the 17-beta-hydroxy group increases the duration of action of testosterone; hydrolysis to free testosterone occurs *in vivo.* Each mL of sterile, colorless to pale yellow solution provides 200 mg testosterone enan-

thate in sesame oil with 5 mg chlorobutanol (chloral derivative) as a preservative.

HOW SUPPLIED
DELATESTRYL (Testosterone Enanthate Injection USP) is available in 1 mL (200 mg/mL) Unimatic single dose syringes (NDC 54396-328-16). Each syringe is supplied with a sterile disposable 20-gauge. 1½-inch needle. DELATESTRYL is also available in 5 mL (200 mg/mL) multiple dose vials (NDC 54396-328-40).

Storage
DELATESTRYL (Testosterone Enanthate Injection USP) should be stored at room temperature. Warming and rotating the syringe unit or vial between the palms of the hands will redissolve any crystals that may have formed during storage at low temperatures.

Manufactured for
BTG Pharmaceuticals
Iselin, NJ 08830
by: Bristol-Myers Squibb
Princeton, NJ 08543

J4-484C   Issued October 1995

OXANDRIN®   ⒸⒾⒾⒾ ℞
(Oxandrolone Tablets)

DESCRIPTION
Oxandrin® oral tablets contain 2.5 mg of the anabolic steroid oxandrolone. Oxandrolone is 17β-hydroxy-17α-methyl-2-oxa-5α-androstan-3-one with the following structural formula:

Inactive ingredients include corn starch, lactose, magnesium stearate, and hydroxypropyl methylcellulose.

CLINICAL PHARMACOLOGY
Anabolic steroids are synthetic derivatives of testosterone. Certain clinical effects and adverse reactions demonstrate the androgenic properties of this class of drugs. Complete dissociation of anabolic and androgenic effects has not been achieved. The actions of anabolic steroids are therefore similar to those of male sex hormones with the possibility of causing serious disturbances of growth and sexual development if given to young children. Anabolic steroids suppress the gonadotropic functions of the pituitary and may exert a direct effect upon the testes.
During exogenous administration of anabolic androgens, endogenous testosterone release is inhibited through inhibition of pituitary luteinizing hormone (LH). At large doses, spermatogenesis may be suppressed through feedback inhibition of pituitary follicle-stimulating hormone (FSH).
Anabolic steroids have been reported to increase low-density lipoproteins and decrease high-density lipoproteins. These levels revert to normal on discontinuation of treatment.

INDICATIONS AND USAGE
Oxandrin is indicated as adjunctive therapy to promote weight gain after weight loss following extensive surgery, chronic infections, or severe trauma, and in some patients who without definite pathophysiologic reasons fail to gain or to maintain normal weight, to offset the protein catabolism associated with prolonged administration of corticosteroids, and for the relief of the bone pain frequently accompanying osteoporosis (See DOSAGE AND ADMINISTRATION).

DRUG ABUSE AND DEPENDENCE
Oxandrin is classified as a controlled substance under the Anabolic Steroids Control Act of 1990 and has been assigned to Schedule III (non-narcotic).

CONTRAINDICATIONS
1. Known or suspected carcinoma of the prostate or the male breast.
2. Carcinoma of the breast in females with hypercalcemia (androgenic anabolic steroids may stimulate osteolytic bone resorption).
3. Pregnancy, because of possible masculinization of the fetus. Oxandrin has been shown to cause embryotoxicity, fetotoxicity, infertility, and masculinization of female animal offspring when given in doses 9 times the human dose.
4. Nephrosis, the nephrotic phase of nephritis.
5. Hypercalcemia.

Continued on next page

BTG Pharmaceuticals—Cont.

WARNINGS

PELIOSIS HEPATIS, A CONDITION IN WHICH LIVER AND SOMETIMES SPLENIC TISSUE IS REPLACED WITH BLOOD-FILLED CYSTS, HAS BEEN REPORTED IN PATIENTS RECEIVING ANDROGENIC ANABOLIC STEROID THERAPY. THESE CYSTS ARE SOMETIMES PRESENT WITH MINIMAL HEPATIC DYSFUNCTION, BUT AT OTHER TIMES THEY HAVE BEEN ASSOCIATED WITH LIVER FAILURE. THEY ARE OFTEN NOT RECOGNIZED UNTIL LIFE-THREATENING LIVER FAILURE OR INTRA-ABDOMINAL HEMORRHAGE DEVELOPS. WITHDRAWAL OF DRUG USUALLY RESULTS IN COMPLETE DISAPPEARANCE OF LESIONS.

LIVER CELL TUMORS ARE ALSO REPORTED. MOST OFTEN THESE TUMORS ARE BENIGN AND ANDROGEN-DEPENDENT, BUT FATAL MALIGNANT TUMORS HAVE BEEN REPORTED. WITHDRAWAL OF DRUG OFTEN RESULTS IN REGRESSION OR CESSATION OF PROGRESSION OF THE TUMOR. HOWEVER, HEPATIC TUMORS ASSOCIATED WITH ANDROGENS OR ANABOLIC STEROIDS ARE MUCH MORE VASCULAR THAN OTHER HEPATIC TUMORS AND MAY BE SILENT UNTIL LIFE-THREATENING INTRAABDOMINAL HEMORRHAGE DEVELOPS. BLOOD LIPID CHANGES THAT ARE KNOWN TO BE ASSOCIATED WITH INCREASED RISK OF ATHEROSCLEROSIS ARE SEEN IN PATIENTS TREATED WITH ANDROGENS OR ANABOLIC STEROIDS. THESE CHANGES INCLUDE DECREASED HIGH-DENSITY LIPOPROTEINS AND SOMETIMES INCREASED LOW-DENSITY LIPOPROTEINS. THE CHANGES MAY BE VERY MARKED AND COULD HAVE A SERIOUS IMPACT ON THE RISK OF ATHEROSCLEROSIS AND CORONARY ARTERY DISEASE.

Cholestatic hepatitis and jaundice may occur with 17-alpha-alkylated androgens at a relatively low dose. If cholestatic hepatitis with jaundice appears or if liver function tests become abnormal, Oxandrin should be discontinued and the etiology should be determined. Drug-induced jaundice is reversible when the medication is discontinued.

In patients with breast cancer, anabolic steroid therapy may cause hypercalcemia by stimulating osteolysis. Oxandrin therapy should be discontinued if hypercalcemia occurs.

Edema with or without congestive heart failure may be a serious complication in patients with preexisting cardiac, renal, or hepatic disease. Concomitant administration of adrenal cortical steroid or ACTH may increase the edema.

In children, androgen therapy may accelerate bone maturation without producing compensatory gain in linear growth. This adverse effect results in compromised adult height. The younger the child, the greater the risk of compromising final mature height. The effect on bone maturation should be monitored by assessing bone age of the left wrist and hand every 6 months (See **PRECAUTIONS: Laboratory tests**).

Geriatric patients treated with androgenic anabolic steroids may be at an increased risk for the development of prostatic hypertrophy and prostatic carcinoma.

ANABOLIC STEROIDS HAVE NOT BEEN SHOWN TO ENHANCE ATHLETIC ABILITY.

PRECAUTIONS

General:
Women should be observed for signs of virilization (deepening of the voice, hirsutism, acne, clitoromegaly). Discontinuation of drug therapy at the time of evidence of mild virilism is necessary to prevent irreversible virilization. Some virilizing changes in women are irreversible even after prompt discontinuation of therapy and are not prevented by concomitant use of estrogens. Menstrual irregularities may also occur.

Anabolic steroids may cause suppression of clotting factors II, V, VII, and X, and an increase in prothombin time.

Information for patients:
The physician should instruct patients to report any of the following side effects of androgens:

Males: Too frequent or persistent erections of the penis, appearance or aggravation of acne.

Females: Hoarseness, acne, changes in menstrual periods, or more facial hair.

All patients: Nausea, vomiting, changes in skin color, or ankle swelling.

Laboratory tests:
Women with disseminated breast carcinoma should have frequent determination of urine and serum calcium levels during the course of therapy (See **WARNINGS**).

Because of the hepatotoxicity associated with the use of 17-alpha-alkylated androgens, liver function tests should be obtained periodically.

Periodic (every 6 months) x-ray examinations of bone age should be made during treatment of children to determine the rate of bone maturation and the effects of androgen therapy on the epiphyseal centers.

Serum lipids and high-density lipoprotein cholesterol determinations should be done periodically as androgenic anabolic steroids have been reported to increase low-density lipoproteins. Serum cholesterol levels may increase during therapy. Therefore, caution is required when administering these agents to patients with a history of myocardial infarction or coronary artery disease. Serial determinations of serum cholesterol should be made and therapy adjusted accordingly.

Hemoglobin and hematocrit should be checked periodically for polycythemia in patients who are receiving high doses of anabolic steroids.

Drug Interactions
Anticoagulants:
Anabolic steroids may increase sensitivity to oral anticoagulants. Dosage of the anticoagulant may have to be decreased in order to maintain desired prothrombin time. Patients receiving oral anticoagulant therapy require close monitoring, especially when anabolic steroids are started or stopped.

Oral hypoglycemic agents:
Oxandrin may inhibit the metabolism of oral hypoglycemic agents.

Adrenal steroids or ACTH:
In patients with edema, concomitant administration with adrenal cortical steroids or ACTH may increase the edema.

Drug/Laboratory test interactions:
Anabolic steroids may decrease levels of thyroxine-binding globulin, resulting in decreased total T_4 serum levels and increased resin uptake of T_3 and T_4. Free thyroid hormone levels remain unchanged. In addition, a decrease in PBI and radioactive iodine uptake may occur.

Carcinogenesis, mutagenesis, impairment of fertility
Animal data:
Oxandrin has not been tested in laboratory animals for carcinogenic or mutagenic effects. In 2-year chronic oral rat studies, a dose-related reduction of spermatogenesis and decreased organ weights (testes, prostate, seminal vesicles, ovaries, uterus, adrenals, and pituitary) were shown.

Human data:
Liver cell tumors have been reported in patients receiving long-term therapy with androgenic anabolic steroids in high doses (See **WARNINGS**). Withdrawal of the drugs did not lead to regression of the tumors in all cases.

Geriatric patients treated with androgenic anabolic steroids may be at an increased risk for the development of prostatic hypertrophy and prostatic carcinoma.

Pregnancy:
Teratogenic effects—Pregnancy Category X (See **CONTRAINDICATIONS**).

Nursing mothers:
It is not known whether anabolic steroids are excreted in human milk. Because of the potential for serious adverse reactions in nursing infants from Oxandrin, a decision should be made whether to discontinue nursing or to discontinue the drug, taking into account the importance of the drug to the mother.

Pediatric use:
Anabolic agents may accelerate epiphyseal maturation more rapidly than linear growth in children and the effect may continue for 6 months after the drug has been stopped. Therefore, therapy should be monitored by x-ray studies at 6-month intervals in order to avoid the risk of compromising adult height. Androgenic anabolic steroid therapy should be used very cautiously in children and only by specialists who are aware of the effects on bone maturation (See **WARNINGS**).

ADVERSE REACTIONS

The following adverse reactions have been associated with use of anabolic steroids:

Hepatic: Cholestatic jaundice with, rarely, hepatic necrosis and death. Hepatocellular neoplasms and peliosis hepatis with long-term therapy (See **WARNINGS**). Reversible changes in liver function tests also occur including increased bromsulfophthalein (BSP) rentention, and increases in serum bilirubin, aspartate aminotransferase (AST, SGOT) and alkaline phosphatase.

In *males:*

Prepubertal: Phallic enlargement and increased frequency or persistence of erections.

Postpubertal: Inhibition of testicular function, testicular atrophy and oligospermia, impotence, chronic priapism, epididymitis, and bladder irritability.

In *females:*
Clitoral enlargement, menstrualirregularities.

CNS: Habituation, excitation, insomnia, depression, and changes in libido.

Hematologic: Bleeding in patients on concomitant anticoagulant therapy.

Breast: Gynecomastia.

Larynx: Deepening of the voice in females.

Hair: Hirsutism and male pattern baldness in females.

Skin: Acne (especially in females and prepubertal males).

Skeletal: Premature closure of epiphyses in children (See **PRECAUTIONS: Pediatric use**).

Fluid and electrolytes: Edema, retention of serum electrolytes (sodium, chloride, potassium, phosphate, calcium).

Metabolic/Endocrine: Decreased glucose tolerance (See **PRECAUTIONS: Laboratory tests**), increased creatinine excretion, increased serum levels of creatinine phosphokinase (CPK). Masculinization of the fetus. Inhibition of gonadotropin secretion.

OVERDOSAGE

No symptoms or signs associated with overdosage have been reported. It is possible that sodium and water retention may occur.

The oral LD_{50} of Oxandrin in mice and dogs is greater than 5,000 mg/kg. No specific antidote is known, but gastric lavage may be used.

DOSAGE AND ADMINISTRATION

Therapy with anabolic steroids is adjunctive to and not a replacement for conventional therapy. The duration of therapy with Oxandrin will depend on the response of the patient and the possible appearance of adverse reactions. Therapy should be intermittent.

Adults: The *usual adult* dosage of Oxandrin is one 2.5-mg tablet two to four times daily. However, the response of individuals to anabolic steroids varies, and a daily dosage of as little as 2.5 mg or as much as 20 mg may be required to achieve the desired response. A course of therapy of 2 to 4 weeks in usually adequate. This may be repeated intermittently as indicated.

Children: For children the total daily dosage of Oxandrin is ≤0.1 mg per kilogram body weight or ≤0.045 mg per pound of body weight. This may be repeated intermittently as indicated.

HOW SUPPLIED

Oxandrin 2.5 mg tablets are oval, white, and scored with BTG on one side and "11" on each side of the scoreline on the other side; bottles of 100 (NDC 54396-111-11).

Caution: Federal law prohibits dispensing without prescription.

Manufactured for
BTG Pharmaceuticals
by:
G.D. Searle & Co.
Chicago, IL 60680

Address medical inquires to:
BTG Pharmaceuticals
Medical Affairs
70 Wood Avenue South
Iselin, NJ 08830

Revised, May 1996
BTG PHARMACEUTICALS
©1995, BTG Pharmaceuticals
BTG PHARMACEUTICALS

Oxandrin®
(Oxandrolone) tablets   Ⓒ

J.R. Carlson Laboratories, Inc.
15 COLLEGE DR.
ARLINGTON HEIGHTS, IL 60004-1985

Direct Inquiries to:
Customer Service
(847) 255-1600
FAX: (847) 255-1605

For Medical Information Contact:
In Emergencies:
Customer Service
(847) 255-1600
FAX: (847) 255-1605

ACES®   OTC

DESCRIPTION

ACES provides four natural antioxidant nutrients.

Two Soft Gels Contain:		% U.S. RDA
Beta-Carotene (Pro-Vitamin A)	10,000 IU	200%
Vitamin C (Calcium Ascorbate)	1000 mg	1667%
Vitamin E (d-Alpha Tocopherol)	400 IU	1333%
Selenium (L-selenomethionine)	100 mcg	*

RDA: Recommended Daily Allowance—Adults
*U.S. RDA not determined

The nutrients in ACES are: Beta Carotene—(Pro-vitamin A) derived from tiny sea plants or algae (*D. salina*) grown in the fresh ocean waters off southern Australia; Vitamin C provided as the gentle, buffered calcium ascorbate; Vitamin E 100% natural-source from soy, the most biologically active form; And Selenium—organically bound with the essential nutrient methionine to promote assimilation.
Suggested Use: For dietary supplementation, take two soft gels daily, preferably at mealtime.
Corn-free. Wheat-free. Milk-free. Sugar-free. Yeast-free. Preservative-free. Soft Gel Contents: Nutrients listed above, soybean oil, vegetable stearin, lecithin, beeswax. Soft Gel Shell: Beef gelatin, glycerin, water, carob.

HOW SUPPLIED

In bottles of 50, 90, 200, and 360.
Also available as *ACES ® plus ZINC*.

CO-Q10 OTC

As a key component of the electron transport chain, Co-Enzyme Q-10 plays an important role in the production of ATP energy. Carlson Co-Q10 is in opaque soft-gels, which protect against degradation by heat, light, and air. Natural Vitamin E is added to protect freshness and potency. Available in 10 mg, 30 mg, 50 mg, 100 mg strengths.

HOW SUPPLIED

Bottles of 30, 50, 60, 90, 100, 120, 240, 300, 360.

E-GEMS® OTC

DESCRIPTION

100% natural-source vitamin E (d-alpha tocopheryl acetate) soft gels. Available in 8 strengths: 30 IU, 100 IU, 200 IU, 400 IU, 600 IU, 800 IU, 1000 IU, 1200 IU.

HOW SUPPLIED

Supplied in a variety of bottle sizes.

Carnrick Laboratories, Inc.
65 HORSE HILL ROAD
CEDAR KNOLLS, NJ 07927

Direct Inquiries to:
(201) 267-2670
FAX: (201) 267-2728

For Medical Information Contact:
Medical Director
(201) 267-2670
FAX: (201) 267-2728

AMEN® ℞
[*ā 'men '*]
(medroxyprogesterone acetate tablets USP 10 mg)

CAUTION

Federal Law Prohibits Dispensing Without Prescription

WARNING

THE USE OF AMEN® (MEDROXYPROGESTERONE ACETATE) DURING THE FIRST FOUR MONTHS OF PREGNANCY IS NOT RECOMMENDED.
Progestational agents have been used beginning with the first trimester of pregnancy in an attempt to prevent habitual abortion. There is no adequate evidence that such use is effective when such drugs are given during the first four months of pregnancy. Furthermore, in the vast majority of women, the cause of abortion is a defective ovum, which progestational agents could not be expected to influence. In addition, the use of progestational agents, with their uterine-relaxant properties, in patients with fertilized defective ova may cause a delay in spontaneous abortion. Therefore, the use of such drugs during the first four months of pregnancy is not recommended.
Several reports suggest an association between intrauterine exposure to progestational drugs in the first trimester of pregnancy and genital abnormalities in male and female fetuses. The risk of hypospadias, 5 to 8 per 1,000 male births in the general population, may be approximately doubled with exposure to these drugs. There are insufficient data to quantify the risk to exposed female fetuses, but insofar as some of these drugs induce mild virilization of the external genitalia of the female fetus, and because of the increased association of hypospadias in the male fetus, it is prudent to avoid the use of these drugs during the first trimester of pregnancy.
If the patient is exposed to AMEN® Tablets (medroxyprogesterone acetate) during the first four months of pregnancy or if she becomes pregnant while taking this drug, she should be apprised of the potential risks to the fetus.

DESCRIPTION

AMEN® tablets contain medroxyprogesterone acetate, which is a derivative of progesterone. It is a white to off-white, odorless crystalline powder, stable in air, melting between 200° and 210°C. It is freely soluble in chloroform, soluble in acetone and in dioxane, sparingly soluble in alcohol and in methanol, slightly soluble in ether, and insoluble in water.
The chemical name for medroxyprogesterone acetate is pregn-4-ene-3,20-dione, 17-(acetyloxy)-6-methyl-, (6α)- with molecular formula $C_{24}H_{34}O_4$ and a molecular weight of 386.53. The structural formula is:

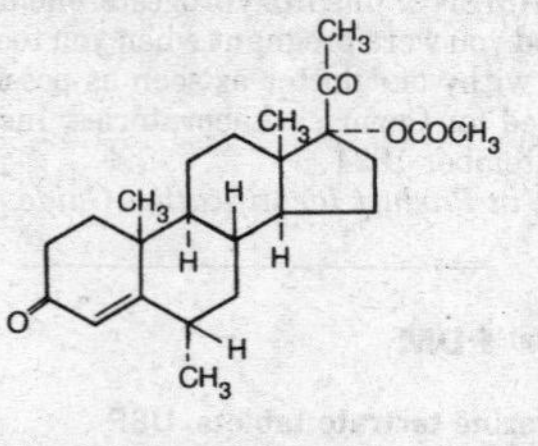

Each AMEN tablet for oral administration contains 10 mg of medroxyprogesterone acetate.
AMEN tablets contain Anhydrous Lactose, Colloidal Silicon Dioxide, Magnesium Stearate, Microcrystalline Cellulose, D&C Yellow #10, FD&C Blue #1, FD&C Red #40, and FD&C Yellow #6 as color additives.

CLINICAL PHARMACOLOGY

Medroxyprogesterone acetate administered orally or parenterally in the recommended doses to women with adequate endogenous estrogen, transforms proliferative into secretory endometrium. Androgenic and anabolic effects have been noted, but the drug is apparently devoid of significant estrogenic activity. While parenterally administered medroxyprogesterone acetate inhibits gonadotropin production, which in turn prevents follicular maturation and ovulation, available data indicate that this does not occur when the usually recommended oral dosage is given as single daily doses.

INDICATIONS AND USAGE

Secondary amenorrhea; abnormal uterine bleeding due to hormonal imbalance in the absence of organic pathology, such as fibroids or uterine cancer.

CONTRAINDICATIONS

1. Thrombophlebitis, thromboembolic disorders, cerebral apoplexy or patients with a past history of these conditions. **2.** Liver dysfunction or disease. **3.** Known or suspected malignancy of breast or genital organs. **4.** Undiagnosed vaginal bleeding. **5.** Missed abortion. **6.** As a diagnostic test for pregnancy. **7.** Known sensitivity to AMEN (medroxyprogesterone acetate tablets).

WARNINGS

1. The physician should be alert to the earliest manifestations of thrombotic disorders (thrombophlebitis, cerebrovascular disorders, pulmonary embolism, and retinal thrombosis). Should any of these occur or be suspected, the drug should be discontinued immediately.
2. Beagle dogs treated with medroxyprogesterone acetate developed mammary nodules, some of which were malignant. Although nodules occasionally appeared in control animals, they were intermittent in nature, whereas the nodules in the drug treated animals were larger, more numerous, persistent, and there were some breast malignancies with metastases. Their significance with respect to humans has not been established.
3. Discontinue medication pending examination if there is sudden partial or complete loss of vision, or if there is a sudden onset of proptosis, diplopia or migraine. If examination reveals papilledema, or retinal vascular lesions, medication should be withdrawn.
4. Detectable amounts of progestin have been identified in the milk of mothers receiving the drug. The effect of this on the nursing infant has not been determined.
5. Usage in pregnancy is not recommended (See WARNING Box).
6. Retrospective studies of morbidity and mortality in Great Britain and studies of morbidity in the United States have shown a statistically significant association between thrombophlebitis, pulmonary embolism, and cerebral thrombosis and embolism and the use of oral contraceptives.[1–4] The estimate of the relative risk of thromboembolism in the study by Vessey and Doll[3] was about sevenfold, while Sartwell and associates[4] in the United States found a relative risk of 4.4, meaning that the users are several times as likely to undergo thromboembolic disease without evident cause as nonusers. The American study also indicated that the risk did not persist after discontinuation of administration, and that it was not enhanced by long continued administration. The American study was not designed to evaluate a difference between products.

PRECAUTIONS

1. The pretreatment physical examination should include special reference to breast and pelvic organs, as well as Papanicolaou smear.
2. Because progestogens may cause some degree of fluid retention, conditions which might be influenced by this factor, such as epilepsy, migraine, asthma, cardiac or renal dysfunction require careful observation.
3. In cases of breakthrough bleeding, as in all cases of irregular bleeding per vaginum, nonfunctional causes should be borne in mind. In cases of undiagnosed vaginal bleeding adequate diagnostic measures are indicated.
4. Patients who have a history of psychic depression should be carefully observed and the drug discontinued if the depression recurs to a serious degree.
5. Any possible influence of prolonged progestin therapy on pituitary, ovarian, adrenal, hepatic or uterine functions awaits further study.
6. A decrease in glucose tolerance has been observed in a small percentage of patients on estrogen-progestin combination drugs. The mechanism of this decrease is obscure. For this reason, diabetic patients should be carefully observed while receiving progestin therapy.
7. The age of the patient constitutes no absolute limiting factor although treatment with progestins may mask the onset of the climacteric.
8. The pathologist should be advised of progestin therapy when relevant specimens are submitted.
9. Because of the occasional occurrence of thromobotic disorders, (thrombophlebitis, pulmonary embolism, retinal thrombosis, and cerebrovascular disorders) in patients taking estrogen-progestin combinations and since the mechanism is obscure, the physician should be alert to the earliest manifestation of these disorders.
10. Studies of the addition of a progestin product to an estrogen replacement regimen for seven or more days of a cycle of estrogen administration have reported a lowered incidence of endometrial hyperplasia. Morphological and biochemical studies of endometrium suggest that 10–13 days of a progestin are needed to provide maximal maturation of the endometrium and to eliminate any hyperplastic changes. Whether this will provide protection from endometrial carcinoma has not been clearly established. There are possible additional risks which may be associated with the inclusion of progestin in estrogen replacement regimens. The potential risks include adverse effects on carbohydrate and lipid metabolism. The dosage used may be important in minimizing these adverse effects.
11. Aminoglutethimide administered concomitantly with AMEN may significantly depress the bioavailability of AMEN.

Carcinogenesis, Mutagenesis, Impairment of Fertility.
Long-term intramuscular administration of medroxyprogesterone acetate has been shown to produce mammary tumors in beagle dogs (see WARNINGS). There was no evidence of a carcinogenic effect associated with the oral administration of medroxyprogesterone acetate to rats and mice. Medroxyprogesterone acetate was not mutagenic in a battery of *in vitro* or *in vivo* genetic toxicity assays.
Medroxyprogesterone acetate at high doses is an antifertility drug and high doses would be expected to impair fertility until the cessation of treatment.

Information for the Patient
See Patient Information at end of insert.

ADVERSE REACTIONS

Pregnancy—(See WARNING Box for possible adverse effects on the fetus).
Breast—Breast tenderness or galactorrhea has been reported rarely.
Skin—Sensitivity reactions consisting of urticaria, pruritus, edema and generalized rash have occured in an occasional patient. Acne, alopecia and hirsutism have been reported in a few cases.
Thromboembolic Phenomena—Thromboembolic phenomena including thrombophlebitis and pulmonary embolism have been reported.
The following adverse reactions have been observed in women taking progestins including medroxyprogesterone acetate tablets: breakthrough bleeding; spotting; change in menstrual flow; amenorrhea; edema; change in weight (increase or decrease); changes in cervical erosion and cervical secretions; cholestatic jaundice; anaphylactoid reactions and

Continued on next page

Carnrick Laboratories—Cont.

anaphylaxis; rash (allergic) with and without pruritus; mental depression; pyrexia; insomnia; nausea; somnolence.
A statistically significant association has been demonstrated between use of estrogen-progestin combination drugs and the following serious adverse reactions: thrombophlebitis, pulmonary embolism and cerebral thrombosis and embolism. For this reason patients on progestin therapy should be carefully observed.
Although available evidence is suggestive of an association, such a relationship has been neither confirmed nor refuted for the following serious adverse reactions: neuro-ocular lesions, eg. retinal thrombosis and optic neuritis.
The following adverse reactions have been observed in patients receiving estrogen-progestin combination drugs: rise in blood pressure in susceptible individuals; premenstrual-like syndrome; changes in libido; changes in appetite; cystitis-like syndrome; headache; nervousness; fatigue; backache; hirsutism; loss of scalp hair; erythema multiforme; erythema nodosum; hemorrhagic eruption; itching; dizziness.
In view of these observations, patients on progestin therapy should be carefully observed.
The following laboratory results may be altered by the use of estrogen-progestin combination drugs:
Increased sulfobromophthalein retention and other hepatic function tests.
Coagulation tests: increase in prothrombin factors VII, VIII, IX and X.
Metyrapone test.
Pregnanediol determination.
Thyroid function: increase in PBI, and butanol extractable protein bound iodine and decrease in T^3 uptake values.

DOSAGE AND ADMINISTRATION

Secondary Amenorrhea—AMEN® (medroxyprogesterone acetate tablets) may be given in dosages of 5 to 10 mg daily for from 5 to 10 days. A dose for inducing an optimum secretory transformation of an endometrium that has been adequately primed with either endogenous or exogenous estrogen is 10 mg of AMEN daily for 10 days. In cases of seconary amenorrhea, therapy may be started at any time. Progestin withdrawal bleeding usually occurs within three to seven days after discontinuing AMEN® therapy.
Abnormal Uterine Bleeding Due to Hormonal Imbalance in the Absence of Organic Pathology—Beginning on the calculated 16th or 21st day of the menstrual cycle, 5 to 10 mg of medroxyprogesterone acetate may be given daily for from 5 to 10 days. To produce an optimum secretory transformation of an endometrium that has been adequately primed with either endogenous or exogenous estrogen, 10 mg of medroxyprogesterone acetate daily for 10 days beginning on the 16th day of the cycle is suggested. Progestin withdrawal bleeding usually occurs within three to seven days after discontinuing therapy with AMEN®. Patients with a past history of recurrent episodes of abnormal uterine bleeding may benefit from planned menstrual cycling with AMEN®.

HOW SUPPLIED

Two-layered peach and white scored tablet with "C" on one side and "AMEN" on the other. AMEN® tablets containing 10 mg of medroxyprogesterone acetate USP are available in bottles of 50 (NDC 0086-0049-05), 100 (NDC 0086-0049-10) and 1000 (NDC 0086-0049-90).
Store at controlled room temperature 15°–30°C (59°–86°F).

REFERENCES

1. Royal College of General Practitioners: Oral contraception and thromboembolic disease. J Coll Gen Prac *13*:267–279, 1967.
2. Inman WHW, Vessey MP: Investigation of deaths from pulmonary, coronary, and cerebral thrombosis and embolism in women of child-bearing age. Br Med J *2*:193–199, 1968.
3. Vessey MP, Doll R: Investigation of relation between use of oral contraceptives and thromboembolic disease. A further report. Br Med J *2*:651–657, 1969.
4. Sartwell PE, Masi AT, Arthes FG, et al: Thromboembolism and oral contraceptives: An epidemiological case-control study. Am J Epidemiol *90*:365–380, 1969.

The text of the patient insert for progesterone and progesterone-like drugs is set forth below.

PATIENT INFORMATION: AMEN Tablets contain medroxyprogesterone acetate, a progesterone. The information below is that which the U.S. Food and Drug Administration requires be provided for all patients taking progesterones. The information below relates only to the risk to the unborn child associated with use of progesterone during pregnancy. For further information on the use, side effects and other risks associated with this product, ask your doctor.

WARNING FOR WOMEN

Progesterone or progesterone-like drugs have been used to prevent miscarriage in the first few months of pregnancy. No adequate evidence is available to show that they are effective for this purpose. Furthermore, most cases of early miscarriage are due to causes which could not be helped by these drugs.
There is an increased risk of minor birth defects in children whose mothers take this drug during the first 4 months of pregnancy. Several reports suggest an association between mothers who take these drugs in the first trimester of pregnancy and genital abnormalities in male and female babies. The risk to the male baby is the possibility of being born with a condition in which the opening of the penis is on the underside rather than the tip of the penis (hypospadias). Hypospadias occurs in about 5 to 8 per 1,000 male births and is about doubled with exposure to these drugs. There is not enough information to quantify the risk to exposed female fetuses, but enlargement of the clitoris and fusion of the labia may occur, although rarely.
Therefore, since drugs of this type may induce mild masculinization of the external genitalia of the female fetus, as well as hypospadias in the male fetus, it is wise to avoid using the drug during the first trimester of pregnancy.
These drugs have been used as a test for pregnancy but such use is no longer considered safe because of possible damage to a developing baby. Also, more rapid methods for testing for pregnancy are now available.
If you take AMEN® (medroxyprogesterone acetate tablets) and later find you were pregnant when you took it, be sure to discuss this with your doctor as soon as possible.
Manufactured for Carnrick Laboratories, Inc.
Revised September 1994

Shown in Product Identification Guide, page 308

BONTRIL® PDM Ⓒ III

[*bŏn'tril*]
(phendimetrazine tartrate tablets, USP 35 mg)

HOW SUPPLIED

Three layered green, white and yellow tablet with 8648 on the scored side and the letter "C" on the other. Bontril® PDM tablets containing 35 mg of phendimetrazine tartrate are available in bottles of 100 (NDC 0086-0048-10) and 1,000 (NDC 0086-0048-90).

CAUTION

Federal law prohibits dispensing without prescription.
See product insert for complete information.
Manufactured for Carnrick Laboratories, Inc.

Shown in Product Identification Guide, page 308

BONTRIL® SLOW-RELEASE Ⓒ III

[*bŏn'tril*]
(brand of phendimetrazine tartrate slow-release capsules 105 mg)

DESCRIPTION

Phendimetrazine tartrate, as the dextro isomer, has the chemical name of (+)-3,4-Dimethyl-2-phenylmorpholine Tartrate.
The structural formula is as follows:

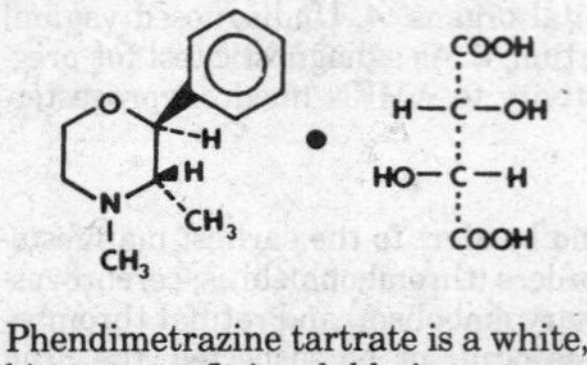

M.W. 341

Phendimetrazine tartrate is a white, odorless powder with a bitter taste. It is soluble in water, methanol and ethanol. Bontril Slow-Release capsules contain FD&C Yellow No. 6 as a color additive.

ACTIONS

Phendimetrazine tartrate is a sympathomimetic amine with pharmacological activity similar to the prototype drugs of this class used in obesity, the amphetamines. Actions include central nervous system stimulation and elevation of blood pressure. Tachyphylaxis and tolerance have been demonstrated with all drugs of this class in which these phenomena have been looked for.
Drugs of this class used in obesity are commonly known as "anorectics" or "anorexigenics". It has not been established, however, that the action of such drugs in treating obesity is primarily one of appetite suppression. Other central nervous system actions or metabolic effects may be involved.
Adult obese subjects instructed in dietary management and treated with anorectic drugs lose more weight on the average than those treated with placebo and diet, as determined in relatively short term clinical trials.
The magnitude of increased weight loss of drug-treated patients over placebo-treated patients is only a fraction of a pound a week. The rate of weight loss is greatest in the first weeks of therapy for both drug and placebo subjects and tends to decrease in succeeding weeks. The possible origin of the increased weight loss due to the various drug effects is not established. The amount of weight loss associated with the use of an anorectic drug varies from trial to trial, and the increased weight loss appears to be related in part to variables other than the drug prescribed, such as the physician investigator, the population treated, and the diet prescribed. Studies do not permit conclusions as to the relative importance of the drug and non-drug factors on weight loss.
The natural history of obesity is measured in years, whereas the studies cited are restricted to a few weeks duration; thus, the total impact of drug-induced weight loss over that of diet alone must be considered clinically limited.
The active drug 105 mg of phendimetrazine tartrate in each capsule of this special slow-release dosage form approximates the action of three 35 mg non-time release doses taken at 4 hours intervals.
The major route of elimination is via the kidneys where most of the drug and metabolites are excreted. Some of the drug is metabolized to phenmetrazine and also phendimetrazine-N-oxide.
The average half-life of elimination when studied under controlled conditions is about 1.9 hours for the non-time and 9.8 hours for the slow-release dosage form. The absorption half-life of the drug from conventional non-time 35 mg phendimetrazine tablets is approximately the same. These data indicate that the slow-release product has a similar onset of action to the conventional non-time-release product and, in addition, has a prolonged therapeutic effect.

INDICATIONS

Phendimetrazine tartrate is indicated in the management of exogenous obesity as a short term adjunct (a few weeks) in a regimen of weight reduction based on caloric restriction. The limited usefulness of agents of this class (see ACTIONS) should be measured against possible risk factors inherent in their use such as those described below.

CONTRAINDICATIONS

Advanced arteriosclerosis, symptomatic cardiovascular disease, moderate and severe hypertension, hyperthyroidism, known hypersensitivity, or idiosyncrasy to the sympathomimetic amines, glaucoma. Agitated states. Patients with a history of drug abuse. Use in patients taking other CNS stimulants including monoamine oxidase inhibitors.

WARNINGS

Tolerance to the anorectic effect usually develops within a few weeks. When this occurs, the recommended dose should not be exceeded in an attempt to increase the effect; rather, the drug should be discontinued.
Use of phendimetrazine within 14 days following the administration of monoamine oxidase inhibitors may result in a hypertensive crisis.
Abrupt cessation of administration following prolonged high dosage results in extreme fatigue and depression. Because of the effect on the central nervous system phendimetrazine tartrate may impair the ability of the patient to engage in potentially hazardous activities such as operating machinery or driving a motor vehicle; the patient should therefore be cautioned accordingly.

PRECAUTIONS

Caution is to be exercised in prescribing phendimetrazine for patients with even mild hypertension.
Insulin requirements in diabetes mellitus may be altered in association with the use of phendimetrazine and the concomitant dietary regimen.
Phendimetrazine may decrease the hypotensive effect of guanethidine.
The least amount feasible should be prescribed or dispensed at one time in order to minimize the possibility of overdosage.
Usage in Pregnancy: Safe use in pregnancy has not been established. Until more information is available, phendimetrazine tartrate should not be taken by women who are or may become pregnant unless, in the opinion of the physician, the potential benefits outweigh the possible hazards.
Usage in Children: Phendimetrazine tartrate is not recommended for use in children under 12 years of age.

ADVERSE REACTIONS

Cardiovascular: Palpitation, tachycardia, elevation of blood pressure.
Central Nervous System: Overstimulation, restlessness, dizziness, insomnia, tremor, headache; rarely psychotic episodes at recommended doses, agitation, flushing, sweating, blurring of vision.
Gastrointestinal: Dryness of the mouth, diarrhea, constipation, nausea, stomach pain.
Genitourinary: Changes in libido, urinary frequency, dysuria.

DRUG ABUSE AND DEPENDENCE

Controlled Substance: Phendimetrazine is a Schedule III controlled substance.
Dependence: Phendimetrazine Tartrate is related chemically and pharmacologically to the amphetamines. Amphet-

amines and related stimulant drugs have been extensively abused, and the possibility of abuse of phendimetrazine should be kept in mind when evaluating the desirability of including a drug as part of a weight reduction program. Abuse of amphetamines and related drugs may be associated with intense psychological dependence and severe social dysfunction. There are reports of patients who have increased the dosage to many times that recommended. Abrupt cessation following prolonged high dosage administration results in extreme fatigue and mental depression; changes are also noted on the sleep EEG. Manifestations of chronic intoxication with anorectic drugs include severe dermatoses, marked insomnia, irritability, hyperactivity and personality changes. The most severe manifestation of chronic intoxications is psychosis, often clinically indistinguishable from schizophrenia.

OVERDOSAGE

Manifestations of acute overdosage may include restlessness, tremor, hyperreflexia, rapid respiration, confusion, assaultiveness, hallucinations, panic states.

Fatigue and depression usually follow the central stimulation.

Cardiovascular effects include arrhythmias, hypertension, or hypotension and circulatory collapse. Gastrointestinal symptoms include nausea, vomiting, diarrhea, and abdominal cramps. Poisoning may result in convulsions, coma, and death.

Management of acute intoxication is largely symptomatic and includes lavage and sedation with a barbiturate. Experience with hemodialysis or peritoneal dialysis is inadequate to permit recommendation in this regard.

Acidification of the urine increases phendimetrazine tartrate excretion.

Intravenous phentolamine (Regitine) has been suggested for possible acute, severe hypertension, if this complicates overdosage.

DOSAGE AND ADMINISTRATION

One Slow-Release Capsule (105 mg) in the morning, taken 30-60 minutes before the morning meal.

Phendimetrazine Tartrate is not recommended for use in children under twelve years of age.

HOW SUPPLIED

Phendimetrazine Slow-Release Capsules, 105 mg is supplied in bottles of 100 opaque green and clear yellow capsules, imprinted with the letter "C" and 8647. NDC # 0086-0047-10. Store at controlled room temperature, 15°- 30°C(59°-86°F). The most recent revision of this labeling is Nov. 1990.

CAUTION

Federal law prohibits dispensing without prescription.
Manufactured for Carnrick Laboratories, Inc.
Shown in Product Identification Guide, page 308

CAPITAL® AND CODEINE SUSPENSION

(acetaminophen and codeine phosphate oral suspension)

HOW SUPPLIED

CAPITAL® AND CODEINE SUSPENSION contains 120 mg of acetaminophen and 12 mg of codeine phosphate/5 mL and is given orally. CAPITAL® AND CODEINE SUSPENSION is a fruit punch-flavored pink suspension available in 16 fluid oz. (473 mL) bottles, NDC 0086-0046-16.
SHAKE WELL BEFORE USING
Store at controlled room temperature 15°-30°C (59°-86°F). Dispense in tight, light-resistant glass container and label "Shake Well Before Using."

CAUTION

Federal law prohibits dispensing without prescription.
See product insert for complete information.
Manufactured for Carnrick Laboratories, Inc.
Shown in Product Identification Guide, page 308

EXGEST® LA

(phenylpropanolamine hydrochloride/guaifenesin)

DESCRIPTION

Each EXGEST® LA white, blue-speckled, oval, scored, long-acting tablet for oral administration contains:
phenylpropanolamine hydrochloride .... 75 mg
guaifenesin .... 400 mg
in a special base to provide a prolonged therapeutic effect. This product contains ingredients of the following therapeutic classes: decongestant and expectorant.
Phenylpropanolamine hydrochloride is a decongestant having the chemical name, benzenemethanol, α-(l-aminoethyl)-, hydrochloride (R*, S*), (±), with the following structure:
[See chemical structure at top of next column.]

Guaifenesin is an expectorant having the chemical name, 1,2-propanediol, 3-(2-methoxyphenoxy)-, with the following structure:

CLINICAL PHARMACOLOGY

Phenylpropanolamine hydrochloride is an α-adrenergic receptor agonist (sympathomimetic) which produces vasoconstriction by stimulating α-receptors within the mucosa of the respiratory tract. Clinically, phenylpropanolamine shrinks swollen mucous membranes, reduces tissue hyperemia, edema, and nasal congestion, and increases nasal airway patency. Guaifenesin promotes lower respiratory tract drainage by thinning bronchial secretions, lubricates irritated respiratory tract membranes through increased mucous flow, and facilitates removal of viscous, inspissated mucus. As a result, sinus and bronchial drainage is improved, and dry, nonproductive coughs become more productive and less frequent.

INDICATIONS AND USAGE

EXGEST® LA is indicated for the symptomatic relief of sinusitis, bronchitis, pharyngitis, and coryza when these conditions are associated with nasal congestion and viscous mucus in the lower respiratory tract.

CONTRAINDICATIONS

EXGEST® LA is contraindicated in individuals with known hypersensitivity to sympathomimetics, severe hypertension, or in patients receiving monoamine oxidase inhibitors.

WARNINGS

Sympathomimetic amines should be used with caution in patients with hypertension, diabetes mellitus, heart disease, peripheral vascular disease, increased intraocular pressure, hyperthyroidism, or prostatic hypertrophy.

PRECAUTIONS

Information for Patients: Do not crush or chew EXGEST® LA tablets prior to swallowing.
Drug Interactions: EXGEST® LA should not be used in patients taking monoamine oxidase inhibitors or other sympathomimetics.
Drug/Laboratory Test Interactions: Guaifenesin has been reported to interfere with clinical laboratory determinations of urinary 5-hydroxyindoleacetic acid (5-HIAA) and urinary vanillylmandelic acid (VMA).
Pregnancy: Pregnancy Category C. Animal reproduction studies have not been conducted with EXGEST® LA. It is also not known whether EXGEST® LA can cause fetal harm when administered to a pregnant woman or can affect reproduction capacity. EXGEST® LA should not be given to a pregnant woman, unless clearly needed.
Nursing Mothers: It is not known whether the drugs in EXGEST® LA are excreted in human milk. Because many drugs are excreted in human milk and because of the potential for serious adverse reactions in nursing infants, a decision should be made whether to discontinue nursing or to discontinue the product, taking into account the importance of the drug to the mother.
Pediatric Use: Safety and effectivness of EXGEST® LA tablets in children below the age of 6 have not been established.

ADVERSE REACTIONS

Possible adverse reactions include nervousness, insomnia, restlessness, headache, nausea, or gastric irritation. These reactions seldom, if ever, require discontinuation of therapy. Urinary retention may occur in patients with prostatic hypertrophy.

OVERDOSAGE

The treatment of overdosage should provide symptomatic and supportive care. If the amount ingested is considered dangerous or excessive, induce vomiting with ipecac syrup unless the patient is convulsing, comatose, or has lost the gag reflex, in which case perform gastric lavage using a large-bore tube. If indicated, follow with activated charcoal and a saline cathartic. Since the effects of EXGEST® LA may last up to 12 hours, treatment should be continued for at least that length of time.

DOSAGE AND ADMINISTRATION

Adults and children 12 years of age and older—one tablet twice daily (every 12 hours); **children 6 to under 12 years** —one-half (½) tablet twice daily (every 12 hours). EXGEST® LA is not recommended for children under 6 years of age. Tablets may be broken in half for ease of administration without affecting release of medication but should not be crushed or chewed prior to swallowing.

HOW SUPPLIED

EXGEST® LA is available as a white, blue-speckled, oval, scored, long-acting tablet for oral administration. It is inscribed with "8673" on the scored side and "C" on the other. Each long-acting tablet contains phenylpropanolamine hydrochloride 75 mg and guaifenesin 400 mg. Supplied in bottles of 100 tablets (NDC 0086-0063-10) and in bottles of 500 tablets (NDC 0086-0063-50).
Store at controlled room temperature, 15°-30°C (59°-86°F.)

CAUTION

Federal law prohibits dispensing without prescription.
Manufactured for Carnrick Laboratories, Inc.
7/95
Shown in Product Identification Guide, page 308

HYDROCET® CAPSULES
(HYDROCODONE BITARTRATE AND ACETAMINOPHEN CAPSULES)

CAUTION Federal law prohibits dispensing without prescription.

DESCRIPTION

Hydrocodone bitartrate and acetaminophen is supplied in capsule form for oral administration.
Hydrocodone bitartrate is an opioid analgesic and antitussive and occurs as fine, white crystals or as a crystalline powder. It is affected by light. The chemical name is 4,5α-epoxy-3 methoxy-17-methylmorphinan-6-one tartrate (1:1) hydrate (2:5). It has the following structural formula:

$$C_{18}H_{21}NO_3 \cdot C_4H_6O_6 \cdot 2\frac{1}{2}\ H_2O \qquad MW = 494.50$$

Acetaminophen, 4'-hydroxyacetanilide, a slightly bitter, white, odorless, crystalline powder, is a non-opiate, non-salicylate analgesic and antipyretic. It has the following structural formula:

$$C_8H_9NO_2 \qquad MW = 151.16$$

Each Hydrocet® Capsule contains:
Hydrocodone Bitartrate*, USP .... 5 mg
*(WARNING: MAY BE HABIT FORMING)
Acetaminophen, USP .... 500 mg
In addition, each imprinted capsule contains the following inactive ingredients: Deionized Water, Ethylene Glycol Monoethyl Ether, FD&C Blue #1, Lecithin, Pharmaceutical Glaze (Modified), Simethicone, Sodium Propionate, and Titanium Dioxide.

CLINICAL PHARMACOLOGY

Hydrocodone is a semisynthetic narcotic analgesic and antitussive with multiple actions qualitatively similar to those of codeine. Most of these involve the central nervous system and smooth muscle. The precise mechanism of action of hydrocodone and other opiates is not known, although it is believed to relate to the existence of opiate receptors in the central nervous system. In addition to analgesia, narcotics may produce drowsiness, changes in mood and mental clouding.

The analgesic action of acetaminophen involves peripheral influences, but the specific mechanism is as yet undetermined. Antipyretic activity is mediated through hypothalamic heat regulating centers. Acetaminophen inhibits prostaglandin synthetase. Therapeutic doses of acetaminophen have negligible effects on the cardiovascular or respiratory systems; however, toxic doses may cause circulatory failure and rapid, shallow breathing.
Pharmacokinetics: The behavior of the individual components is described below.
Hydrocodone: Following a 10 mg oral dose of hydrocodone administered to five adult male subjects, the mean peak concentration was 23.6 ± 5.2 ng/mL. Maximum serum levels were achieved at 1.3 ± 0.3 hours and the half-life was determined to be 3.8 ± 0.3 hours. Hydrocodone exhibits a complex pattern of metabolism including O-demethylation, N-demethylation and 6-keto reduction to the corresponding 6-α-and 6-β-hydroxymetabolites.

Continued on next page

Carnrick Laboratories—Cont.

See OVERDOSAGE for toxicity information.

Acetaminophen: Acetaminophen is rapidly absorbed from the gastrointestinal tract and is distributed throughout most body tissues. The plasma half-life is 1.25 to 3 hours, but may be increased by liver damage and following overdosage. Elimination of acetaminophen is principally by liver metabolism (conjugation) and subsequent renal excretion of metabolites. Approximately 85% of an oral dose appears in the urine within 24 hours of administration, most as the glucuronide conjugate, with small amounts of other conjugates and unchanged drug.

See OVERDOSAGE for toxicity information.

INDICATIONS AND USAGE

Hydrocet® Capsules (Hydrocodone bitartrate and acetaminophen) are indicated for the relief of moderate to moderately severe pain.

CONTRAINDICATIONS

This product should not be administered to patients who have previously exhibited hypersensitivity to hydrocodone or acetaminophen.

WARNINGS

Respiratory Depression: At high doses or in sensitive patients, hydrocodone may produce dose-related respiratory depression by acting directly on the brain stem respiratory center. Hydrocodone also affects the center that controls respiratory rhythm, and may produce irregular and periodic breathing.

Head Injury and Increased Intracranial Pressure: The respiratory depressant effects of narcotics and their capacity to elevate cerebrospinal fluid pressure may be markedly exaggerated in the presence of head injury, other intracranial lesions or a preexisting increase in intracranial pressure. Furthermore, narcotics produce adverse reactions which may obscure the clinical course of patients with head injuries.

Acute Abdominal Conditions: The administration of narcotics may obscure the diagnosis or clinical course of patients with acute abdominal conditions.

PRECAUTIONS

General: Special Risk Patients: As with any narcotic analgesic agent, Hydrocet® Capsules (hydrocodone bitartrate and acetaminophen) should be used with caution in elderly or debilitated patients, and those with severe impairment of hepatic or renal function, hypothyroidism, Addison's disease, prostatic hypertrophy or urethral stricture. The usual precautions should be observed and the possibility of respiratory depression should be kept in mind.

Cough reflex: Hydrocodone suppresses the cough reflex; as with all narcotics, caution should be exercised when Hydrocet® Capsules (hydrocodone bitartrate and acetaminophen) are used postoperatively and in patients with pulmonary disease.

Information for Patients: Hydrocodone, like all narcotics, may impair mental and/or physical abilities required for the performance of potentially hazardous tasks such as driving a car or operating machinery; patients should be cautioned accordingly.

Alcohol and other CNS depressants may produce an additive CNS depression, when taken with this combination product, and should be avoided.

Hydrocodone may be habit-forming. Patients should take the drug only for as long as it is prescribed, in the amounts prescribed, and no more frequently than prescribed.

Laboratory Tests: In patients with severe hepatic or renal disease, effects of therapy should be monitored with serial liver and/or renal function tests.

Drug Interactions: Patients receiving narcotics, antihistamines, antipsychotics, antianxiety agents, or other CNS depressants (including alcohol) concomitantly with Hydrocet® Capsules (hydrocodone bitartrate and acetaminophen) may exhibit an additive CNS depression. When combined therapy is contemplated, the dose of one or both agents should be reduced.

The use of MAO inhibitors or tricyclic antidepressants with hydrocodone preparations may increase the effect of either the antidepressant or hydrocodone.

Drug/Laboratory Test Interactions: Acetaminophen may produce false-positive test results for urinary 5-hydroxyindoleacetic acid.

Carcinogenesis, Mutagenesis, Impairment of Fertility: No adequate studies have been conducted in animals to determine whether hydrocodone or acetaminophen have a potential for carcinogenesis, mutagenesis, or impairment of fertility.

Pregnancy:
Teratogenic Effects: Pregnancy Category C: There are no adequate and well-controlled studies in pregnant women. Hydrocet® Capsules (hydrocodone bitartrate and acetaminophen) should be used during pregnancy only if the potential benefit justifies the potential risk to the fetus.

Nonteratogenic Effects: Babies born to mothers who have been taking opioids regularly prior to delivery will be physically dependent. The withdrawal signs include irritability and excessive crying, tremors, hyperactive reflexes, increased respiratory rate, increased stools, sneezing, yawning, vomiting and fever. The intensity of the syndrome does not always correlate with the duration of maternal opioid use or dose. There is no consensus on the best method of managing withdrawal.

Labor and Delivery: As with all narcotics, administration of this product to the mother shortly before delivery may result in some degree of respiratory depression in the newborn, especially if higher doses are used.

Nursing Mothers: Acetaminophen is excreted in breast milk in small amounts, but the significance of its effects on nursing infants is not known. It is not known whether hydrocodone is excreted in human milk. Because many drugs are excreted in human milk and because of the potential for serious adverse reactions in nursing infants from hydrocodone and acetaminophen, a decision should be made whether to discontinue nursing or to discontinue the drug, taking into account the importance of the drug to the mother.

Pediatric Use: Safety and effectiveness in pediatric patients have not been established.

ADVERSE REACTIONS

The most frequently reported adverse reactions are lightheadedness, dizziness, sedation, nausea and vomiting. These effects seem to be more prominent in ambulatory than in non-ambulatory patients, and some of these adverse reactions may be alleviated if the patient lies down.

Other adverse reactions include:

Central Nervous System: Drowsiness, mental clouding, lethargy, impairment of mental and physical performance, anxiety, fear, dysphoria, psychic dependence, mood changes.

Gastrointestinal System: Prolonged administration of Hydrocet® Capsules (hydrocodone bitartrate and acetaminophin) may produce constipation.

Genitourinary System: Ureteral spasm, spasm of vesical sphincters and urinary retention have been reported with opiates.

Respiratory Depression: Hydrocodone bitartrate may produce dose-related respiratory depression by acting directly on brain stem respiratory centers (see OVERDOSAGE).

Dermatological: Skin rash, pruritis.

The following adverse drug events may be borne in mind as potential effects of acetaminophen: allergic reactions, rash, thrombocytopenia, agranulocytosis.

Potential effects of high dosage are listed in the OVERDOSAGE section.

DRUG ABUSE AND DEPENDENCE

Controlled Substance: Hydrocet® Capsules (hydrocodone bitartrate and acetaminophen) are classified as a Schedule III controlled substance.

Abuse and Dependence: Psychic dependence, physical dependence, and tolerance may develop upon repeated administration of narcotics; therefore, this product should be prescribed and administered with caution. However, psychic dependence is unlikely to develop when Hydrocet® Capsules (hydrocodone bitartrate and acetaminophen) are used for a short time for the treatment of pain.

Physical dependence, the condition in which continued administration of the drug is required to prevent the appearance of a withdrawal syndrome, assumes clinically significant proportions only after several weeks of continued narcotic use, although some mild degree of physical dependence may develop after a few days of narcotic therapy. Tolerance, in which increasingly large doses are required in order to produce the same degree of analgesia, is manifested initially by a shortened duration of analgesic effect, and subsequently by decreases in the intensity of analgesia. The rate of development of tolerance varies among patients.

OVERDOSAGE

Following an acute overdosage, toxicity may result from hydrocodone or acetaminophen.

Signs and Symptoms:

Hydrocodone: Serious ovedose with hydrocodone is characterized by respiratory depression (a decrease in respiratory rate and/or tidal volume, Cheyne-Stokes respiration, cyanosis) extreme somnolence progressing to stupor or coma, skeletal muscle flaccidity, cold and clammy skin, and sometimes bradycardia and hypotension. In severe overdosage, apnea, circulatory collapse, cardiac arrest and death may occur.

Acetaminophen: In acetaminophen overdosage; dose-dependent, potentially fatal hepatic necrosis is the most serious adverse effect. Renal tubular necrosis, hypoglycemic coma and thrombocytopenia may also occur.

Early symptoms following a potentially hepatotoxic overdose may include: nausea, vomiting, diaphoresis and general malaise. Clinical and laboratory evidence of hepatic toxicity may not be apparent until 48 to 72 hours post-ingestion.

In adults, hepatic toxicity has rarely been reported with acute overdoses of less than 10 grams or fatalities with less than 15 grams.

Treatment: A single or multiple overdose with hydrocodone and acetaminophen is a potentially lethal polydrug overdose, and consultation with a regional poison control center is recommended.

Immediate treatment includes support of cardiorespiratory function and measures to reduce drug absorption. Vomiting should be induced mechanically, or with syrup of ipecac, if the patient is alert (adequate pharyngeal and laryngeal reflexes). Oral activated charcoal (1g/kg) should follow gastric emptying. The first dose should be accompanied by an appropriate cathartic. If repeated doses are used, the cathartic might be included with alternate doses as required. Hypotension is usually hypovolemic and should respond to fluids. Vasopressors and other supportive measures should be employed as indicated. A cuffed endo-tracheal tube should be inserted before gastric lavage of the unconscious patient and, when necessary, to provide assisted respiration.

Meticulous attention should be given to maintaining adequate pulmonary ventilation. In severe cases of intoxication, peritoneal dialysis, or preferably hemodialysis may be considered. if hypoprothrombinemia occurs due to acetaminophen overdose, vitamin K should be administered intravenously.

Naloxone, a narcotic antagonist, can reverse respiratory depression and coma associated with opioid overdose. Naloxone hydrochloride 0.4 mg to 2 mg is given parenterally. Since the duration of action of hydrocodone may exceed that of the naloxone, the patient should be kept under continuous surveillance and repeated doses of the antagonist should be administered as needed to maintain adequate respiration. A narcotic antagonist should not be administered in the absence of clinically significant respiratory or cardiovascular depression.

If the dose of acetaminophen may have exceeded 140 mg/kg, acetylcysteine should be administered as early as possible. Serum acetaminophen levels should be obtained, since levels four or more hours following ingestion help predict acetaminophen toxicity. Do not await acetaminophen assay results before initiating treatment. Hepatic enzymes should be obtained initially, and repeated at 24-hour intervals. Methemoglobinemia over 30% should be treated with methylene blue by slow intravenous administration.

The toxic dose for adults for acetaminophen is 10 g.

DOSAGE AND ADMINISTRATION

Dosage should be adjusted according to severity of pain and response of the patient. However, it should be kept in mind that tolerance to hydrocodone can develop with continued use and that the incidence of untoward effects is dose related.

The usual adult dosage is one or two capsules every four to six hours as needed for pain. The total daily dosage should not exceed 8 capsules.

HOW SUPPLIED

Blue and white, opaque capsules imprinted with the letter "C" and 8657.

Each capsule contains Hydrocodone Bitartrate*, USP 5 mg *(WARNING: MAY BE HABIT FORMING.) and Acetaminophen, USP 500 mg. Keep in tight, light resistant containers. Supplied in bottles of 100 capsules NDC 0086-0057-10.

Store at controlled room temperature, 15°–30°C (59°–86°F). The most recent revision of this labeling is February 1995.

Manufactured for:

Carnrick Laboratories, Inc.
Shown in Product Identification Guide, page 308

MIDRIN® ℞

[*mid 'rin*]

CAUTION

Federal law prohibits dispensing without prescription.

DESCRIPTION

Each red capsule with pink band contains Isometheptene Mucate 65 mg., Dichloralphenazone 100 mg., and Acetaminophen 325 mg.

Isometheptene Mucate is a white crystalline powder having a characteristic aromatic odor and bitter taste. It is an unsaturated aliphatic amine with sympathomimetic properties. Dichloralphenazone is a white, microcrystalline powder, with slight odor and tastes saline at first, becoming acrid. It is a mild sedative.

Acetaminophen, a non-salicylate, occurs as a white, odorless, crystalline powder possessing a slightly bitter taste.

Midrin capsules contain FD&C Yellow No. 6 as a color additive.

ACTIONS

Isometheptene Mucate, a sympathomimetic amine, acts by constricting dilated cranial and cerebral arterioles, thus reducing the stimuli that lead to vascular headaches. Dichloralphenazone, a mild sedative, reduces the patient's emotional reaction to the pain of both vascular and tension headaches. Acetaminophen raises the threshold to painful

stimuli, thus exerting an analgesic effect against all types of headaches.

INDICATIONS

For relief of tension and vascular headaches.*

---

*Based on a review of this drug (isometheptene mucate) by the National Academy of Sciences-National Research Council and/or other information, FDA has classified the other indication as "possibly" effective in the treatment of migraine headache.
Final classification of the less-than-effective indication requires further investigation.

CONTRAINDICATIONS

Midrin is contraindicated in glaucoma and/or severe cases of renal disease, hypertension, organic heart disease, hepatic disease and in those patients who are on monoamine-oxidase (MAO) inhibitor therapy.

PRECAUTIONS

Caution should be observed in hypertension, peripheral vascular disease and after recent cardiovascular attacks.

ADVERSE REACTIONS

Transient dizziness and skin rash may appear in hypersensitive patients. This can usually be eliminated by reducing the dose.

DOSAGE AND ADMINISTRATION

FOR RELIEF OF MIGRAINE HEADACHE: The usual adult dosage is two capsules at once, followed by one capsule every hour until relieved, up to 5 capsules within a twelve hour period.

FOR RELIEF OF TENSION HEADACHE: The usual adult dosage is one or two capsules every four hours up to 8 capsules a day.

HOW SUPPLIED

Red capsules imprinted with pink band, the letter "C" and 86120. Bottles of 50 capsules, NDC 0086-0120-05. Bottles of 100 capsules, NDC 0086-0120-10. Store at controlled room temperature 15–30°C (59–86°F) in a dry place.
The most recent revision of this labeling is Nov. 1988.
Manufactured for Carnrick Laboratories, Inc.
Shown in Product Identification Guide, page 308

MOTOFEN®

Tablets
(difenoxin hydrochloride with atropine sulfate)
antidiarrheal

DESCRIPTION

Each five-sided dye free MOTOFEN tablet contains:
Difenoxin (as the hydrochloride) .... 1.0 mg
Warning—May be habit forming.
Atropine sulfate .... 0.025 mg
Difenoxin hydrochloride, 1-(3-cyano-3,3-diphenylpropyl)-4-phenyl-4-piperidinecarboxylic acid monohydrochloride, is an orally administered antidiarrheal agent which is chemically related to the narcotic meperidine.
The structural formula is:

Difenoxin Hydrochloride

Atropine sulfate is present to discourage deliberate overdosage.
Atropine sulfate, an anticholinergic, is endo ($\pm$)-α-(hydroxymethyl) benzeneacetic acid 8-methyl-8-azabicyclo[3.2.1] oct-3-yl ester sulfate (2:1) (salt) monohydrate and has the following structural formula:

Atropine Sulfate

Inactive ingredients: calcium stearate, cellulose, lactose, corn starch.

CLINICAL PHARMACOLOGY

Animal studies have shown that difenoxin hydrochloride manifests its antidiarrheal effect by slowing intestinal motility. The mechanism of action is by a local effect on the gastrointestinal wall.
Difenoxin is the principal active metabolite of diphenoxylate.
Following oral administration of MOTOFEN, difenoxin is rapidly and extensively absorbed. Mean peak plasma levels of approximately 160 ng/mL occurred within 40 to 60 minutes in most patients following an oral dose of 2mg. Plasma levels decline to less than 10% of their peak values within 24 hours and to less than 1% of their peak values within 72 hours. This decline parallels the appearance of difenoxin and its metabolites in the urine. Difenoxin is metabolized to an inactive hydroxylated metabolite. Both the drug and its metabolites are excreted, mainly as conjugates, in urine and feces.

INDICATIONS AND USAGE

MOTOFEN (difenoxin hydrochloride with atropine sulfate) is indicated as adjunctive therapy in the management of acute nonspecific diarrhea and acute exacerbations of chronic functional diarrhea.

CONTRAINDICATIONS

MOTOFEN is contraindicated in patients with diarrhea associated with organisms that penetrate the intestinal mucosa (toxigenic *E. coli*, *Salmonella* species, *Shigella*) and pseudomembranous colitis associated with broad spectrum antibiotics. Antiperistaltic agents should not be used in these conditions because they may prolong and/or worsen diarrhea.
MOTOFEN is *contraindicated in children under 2 years of age* because of the decreased margin of safety of drugs in this class in younger age groups.
MOTOFEN is contraindicated in patients with a known hypersensitivity to difenoxin, atropine, or any of the inactive ingredients, and in patients who are jaundiced.

WARNINGS

MOTOFEN IS *NOT* AN INNOCUOUS DRUG AND DOSAGE RECOMMENDATIONS SHOULD BE STRICTLY ADHERED TO. MOTOFEN IS NOT RECOMMENDED FOR CHILDREN UNDER 2 YEARS OF AGE. OVERDOSAGE MAY RESULT IN SEVERE RESPIRATORY DEPRESSION AND COMA, POSSIBLY LEADING TO PERMANENT BRAIN DAMAGE OR DEATH (SEE *OVERDOSAGE*). THEREFORE, KEEP THIS MEDICATION OUT OF THE REACH OF CHILDREN.
FLUID AND ELECTROLYTE BALANCE—THE USE OF MOTOFEN DOES NOT PRECLUDE THE ADMINISTRATION OF APPROPRIATE FLUID AND ELECTROLYTE THERAPY. DEHYDRATION, PARTICULARLY IN CHILDREN, MAY FURTHER INFLUENCE THE VARIABILITY OF RESPONSE TO MOTOFEN AND MAY PREDISPOSE TO DELAYED DIFENOXIN INTOXICATION. DRUG-INDUCED INHIBITION OF PERISTALSIS MAY RESULT IN FLUID RETENTION IN THE COLON, AND THIS MAY FURTHER AGGRAVATE DEHYDRATION AND ELECTROLYTE IMBALANCE.
IF SEVERE DEHYDRATION OR ELECTROLYTE IMBALANCE IS MANIFESTED, MOTOFEN SHOULD BE WITHHELD UNTIL APPROPRIATE CORRECTIVE THERAPY HAS BEEN INITIATED.
Ulcerative Colitis—In some patients with acute ulcerative colitis, agents which inhibit intestinal motility or delay intestinal transit time have been reported to induce toxic megacolon. Consequently, patients with acute ulcerative colitis should be carefully observed and MOTOFEN therapy should be discontinued promptly if abdominal distention occurs or if other untoward symptoms develop.
Liver and Kidney Disease—MOTOFEN (difenoxin hydrochloride with atropine sulfate) should be used with extreme caution in patients with advanced hepatorenal disease and in all patients with abnormal liver function tests since hepatic coma may be precipitated.
Atropine—A subtherapeutic dose of atropine has been added to difenoxin hydrochloride to discourage deliberate overdosage. Usage of MOTOFEN in recommended doses is not likely to cause prominent anticholinergic side effects, but MOTOFEN should be avoided in patients in whom anticholinergic drugs are contraindicated. The warnings and precautions for use of anticholinergic agents should be observed. In children, signs of atropinism may occur even with recommended doses of MOTOFEN, particularly in patients with Down's Syndrome.

PRECAUTIONS

Information for Patients

CAUTION PATIENTS TO ADHERE STRICTLY TO RECOMMENDED DOSAGE SCHEDULES. THE MEDICATION SHOULD BE KEPT OUT OF REACH OF CHILDREN SINCE ACCIDENTAL OVERDOSAGE MAY RESULT IN SEVERE, EVEN FATAL, RESPIRATORY DEPRESSION. MOTOFEN may produce drowsiness or dizziness. The patient should be cautioned regarding activities requiring men-

tal alertness, such as driving or operating dangerous machinery.

Drug Interactions

Since the chemical structure of difenoxin hydrochloride is similar to meperidine hydrochloride, the concurrent use of MOTOFEN with monoamine oxidase inhibitors may, in theory, precipitate a hypertensive crisis.
MOTOFEN may potentiate the action of barbiturates, tranquilizers, narcotics, and alcohol. When these medications are used concomitantly with MOTOFEN, the patient should be closely monitored.
Diphenoxylate hydrochloride, from which the principal active metabolite difenoxin is derived, was found to inhibit the hepatic microsomal enzyme system at a dose of 2 mg/kg/day in studies conducted with male rats. Therefore, difenoxin has the potential to prolong the biological half-lives of drugs for which the rate of elimination is dependent on the microsomal drug metabolizing enzyme system.

Carcinogenesis, Mutagenesis, Impairment of Fertility

No evidence of carcinogenesis was found in a long-term study of difenoxin hydrochloride/atropine in the rat. In this 104 week study, rats received dietary doses of 0, 1.25, 2.5, or 5 mg/kg/day difenoxin/atropine (20:1 ratio).
No experiments have been conducted to determine the mutagenic potential of MOTOFEN. MOTOFEN did not significantly impair fertility in rats.

Pregnancy/Teratogenic Effects

Pregnancy Category C. Reproduction studies in rats and rabbits with doses at 31 and 61 times the human therapeutic dose respectively, on a mg/kg basis, demonstrated no evidence of teratogenesis due to MOTOFEN (difenoxin hydrochloride with atropine sulfate).
Pregnant rats receiving oral doses of difenoxin hydrochloride/atropine 20 times the maximum human dose had an increase in delivery time as well as a significant increase in the percent of stillbirths.
Neonatal survival in rats was also reduced with most deaths occurring within four days of delivery.
There are no well controlled studies in pregnant women. MOTOFEN should be used during pregnancy only if the potential benefit justifies the potential risk to the fetus.

Nursing Mothers

Because of the potential for serious adverse reactions in nursing infants from MOTOFEN, a decision should be made whether to discontinue nursing or to discontinue the drug, taking into account the importance of the drug to the mother.

Pediatric Use

SAFETY AND EFFECTIVENESS IN CHILDREN BELOW THE AGE OF 12 HAVE NOT BEEN ESTABLISHED. MOTOFEN IS CONTRAINDICATED IN CHILDREN UNDER 2 YEARS OF AGE. See OVERDOSAGE section for information on hazards from accidental poisoning in children.

ADVERSE REACTIONS

In view of the small amount of atropine present (0.025 mg/tablet), effects such as dryness of the skin and mucous membranes, flushing, hyperthermia, tachycardia and urinary retention are very unlikely to occur, except perhaps in children.
Many of the adverse effects reported during clinical investigation of MOTOFEN are difficult to distinguish from symptoms associated with the diarrheal syndrome. However, the following events were reported at the stated frequencies:
Gastrointestinal: Nausea, 1 in 15 patients; vomiting, 1 in 30 patients; dry mouth, 1 in 30 patients; epigastric distress, 1 in 100 patients; and constipation, 1 in 300 patients.
Central Nervous System: Dizziness and light-headedness, 1 in 20 patients; drowsiness, 1 in 25 patients; and headache, 1 in 40 patients; tiredness, nervousness, insomnia and confusion ranged from 1 in 200 to 1 in 600 patients.
Other less frequent reactions: Burning eyes and blurred vision occurred in a few cases.
The following adverse reactions have been reported in patients receiving chemically-related drugs: numbness of extremities, euphoria, depression, sedation, anaphylaxis, angioneurotic edema, urticaria, swelling of the gums, pruritus, toxic megacolon, paralytic ileus, pancreatitis, and anorexia.
THIS MEDICATION SHOULD BE KEPT IN A CHILD-RESISTANT CONTAINER AND OUT OF THE REACH OF CHILDREN SINCE AN OVERDOSAGE MAY RESULT IN SEVERE RESPIRATORY DEPRESSION AND COMA, POSSIBLY LEADING TO PERMANENT BRAIN DAMAGE OR DEATH.

DRUG ABUSE AND DEPENDENCE

MOTOFEN (difenoxin hydrochloride with atropine sulfate) tablets are a Schedule IV controlled substance.
Addiction to (dependence on) difenoxin hydrochloride is theoretically possible at high dosage. Therefore, the recommended dosage should not be exceeded. Because of the structural and pharmacological similarities of difenoxin hydrochloride to drugs with a definite addiction potential, MOTOFEN should be administered with considerable cau-

Continued on next page

Carnrick Laboratories—Cont.

tion to patients who are receiving addicting drugs, to individuals known to be addiction prone, or to those in whom histories suggest may increase the dosage on their own initiative.

OVERDOSAGE

Diagnosis and Treatment

In the event of overdosage (initial signs may include dryness of the skin and mucous membranes, flushing, hyperthermia and tachycardia followed by lethargy or coma, hypotonic reflexes, nystagmus, pinpoint pupils and respiratory depression) gastric lavage, establishment of a patent airway and possibly mechanically assisted respiration are advised.

The narcotic antagonist naloxone may be used in the treatment of respiratory depression caused by narcotic analgesics or pharmacologically related compounds such as MOTOFEN tablets. When naloxone is administered intravenously, the onset of action is generally apparent within two minutes. Naloxone may also be administered subcutaneously or intramuscularly providing a slightly less rapid onset of action but a more prolonged effect.

To counteract respiratory depression caused by MOTOFEN overdosage, the following dosage schedule for naloxone should be followed:

Adult Dosage: The usual initial adult dose of naloxone is 0.4 mg (one mL) administered intravenously. If respiratory function does not adequately improve after the initial dose, the same IV dose may be repeated at two-to-three minute intervals.

Children: The usual adult dose of naloxone for children is 0.01 mg/kg of body weight administered intravenously and repeated at two-to-three minute intervals if necessary.

Since the duration of action of difenoxin hydrochloride is longer than that of naloxone, improvement of respiration following administration may be followed by recurrent respiratory depression. Consequently, continuous observation is necessary until the effect of difenoxin hydrochloride on respiration (which effect may persist for many hours) has passed. Supplemental intramuscular doses of naloxone may be utilized to produce a longer lasting effect. TREAT ALL POSSIBLE MOTOFEN OVERDOSAGES AS SERIOUS AND MAINTAIN MEDICAL OBSERVATION FOR AT LEAST 48 HOURS, PREFERABLY UNDER CONTINUOUS HOSPITAL CARE.

Although signs of overdosage and respiratory depression may not be evident soon after ingestion of difenoxin hydrochloride, respiratory depression may occur from 12 to 30 hours later.

DOSAGE AND ADMINISTRATION

The recommended starting dose of MOTOFEN tablets in adults is 2 tablets (2 mg), then 1 tablet (1 mg) after each loose stool or 1 tablet (1 mg) every 3 to 4 hours as needed, but the total dosage during any 24-hour treatment period should not exceed 8 tablets (8 mg). In the treatment of diarrhea, if clinical improvement is not observed in 48 hours, continued administration of this type medication is not recommended. For acute diarrheas and acute exacerbations of functional diarrhea, treatment beyond 48 hours is usually not necessary.

Studies in children below the age of 12 have been inadequate to evaluate the safety and effectiveness of MOTOFEN in this age group. MOTOFEN is contraindicated in children under 2 years of age.

HOW SUPPLIED

MOTOFEN® is available as a white, dye-free, five-sided, scored tablet with "8674" on the scored side and "C" on the other. Each tablet contains 1.0 mg difenoxin (as the hydrochloride salt) and 0.025 mg atropine sulfate. Supplied in bottles of 100 tablets (NDC 0086-0074-10) and in bottles of 50 tablets (NDC 0086-0074-05).

Store at controlled room temperature, 15°–30°C (59°–86°F).

CAUTION: FEDERAL LAW PROHIBITS DISPENSING WITHOUT PRESCRIPTION

Manufactured for: Carnrick Laboratories, Inc.

12/91

Shown in Product Identification Guide, page 308

NOLAHIST® OTC

[nō 'lă-hist]

(phenindamine tartrate)

ANTIHISTAMINE

Alcohol-free

Allergy Tablets

DESCRIPTION

Each dye-free, alcohol-free NOLAHIST® tablet contains:

Phenindamine Tartrate .... 25 mg

INDICATIONS

Temporarily relieves runny nose, sneezing, itching of the nose or throat, and itchy, watery eyes due to hay fever or other upper respiratory allergies or allergic rhinitis.

WARNINGS

May cause excitability especially in children. Do not take this product if you have a breathing problem such as emphysema or chronic bronchitis, or if you have glaucoma or difficulty in urination due to enlargement of the prostate gland, unless directed by a doctor. May cause drowsiness; alcohol, sedatives, and tranquilizers may increase the drowsiness effect. Avoid alcoholic beverages while taking this product. Do not take this product if you are taking sedatives or tranquilizers without first consulting your doctor. Use caution when driving a motor vehicle or operating machinery. May cause nervousness and insomnia in some individuals. As with any drug, if you are pregnant or nursing a baby, seek the advice of a health professional before using this product. Keep this and all medication out of the reach of children. In case of accidental overdose, seek professional assistance or contact a Poison Control Center immediately.

DIRECTIONS

Adults and children 12 years of age and over: oral dosage is one tablet every 4 to 6 hours, not to exceed six tablets in 24 hours, or as directed by a doctor. Children 6 to under 12 years of age: oral dosage is one-half tablet every 4 to 6 hours, not to exceed 3 tablets in 24 hours, or as directed by a doctor. Children under 6 years of age: consult a doctor.

TAMPER-RESISTANT PACKAGE FEATURE

Bottle of 100—If printed outer wrap on carton is broken or removed, do not purchase. Blisters—Tablets are individually sealed with Nolahist® identifying copy on the back. If seal is broken, do not use.

HOW SUPPLIED

White, capsule-shaped, scored tablet inscribed with 8652 on one side and C logo on the other side in bottles of 100 (NDC 0086-0052-10) and 7 boxes of 24 blisters (NDC 0086-0052-24). Each tablet contains phenindamine tartrate 25 mg. Store at 15°–30°C (59°–86°F) and keep tightly closed away from light.

Manufactured for Carnrick Laboratories, Inc. 6/96

Shown in Product Identification Guide, page 308

NOLAMINE® ℞

[nō 'lă-mēn ']

DESCRIPTION

Each timed-release tablet contains:

Phenindamine tartrate .... 24 mg

Chlorpheniramine maleate .... 4 mg

Phenylpropanolamine hydrochloride .... 50 mg

Formulated to provide 8 to
12 hours of continuous relief.

CAUTION

Federal law prohibits dispensing without prescription.

INDICATIONS

As a nasal decongestant associated with the common cold, sinusitis, hay fever and other allergies.

CONTRAINDICATIONS

Hypersensitivity to any of the components. Contraindicated in concurrent MAO inhibitor therapy.

SIDE EFFECTS

Nervousness, insomnia, tremors, dizziness and drowsiness may occur occasionally.

PRECAUTIONS

Antihistamines may cause drowsiness and should be used with caution in patients who operate motor vehicles or dangerous machinery. Use with caution in patients with hypertension, cardiovascular disease, diabetes or hyperthyroidism. This product should be used with caution in patients with prostatic hypertrophy or glaucoma.

DOSAGE

Usual adult dose: Orally, one tablet every 8 hours. In mild cases, one tablet every 10 to 12 hours.

WARNING: Keep this and all medication out of the reach of children.

HOW SUPPLIED

Pink, timed release tablets coded C 86204 in bottles of 100 (NDC 0086-0204-10) and 250 (NDC 0086-0204-25). Store at controlled room temperature, 15°–30°C (59°–86°F) and keep away from light.

Manufactured for Carnrick Laboratories, Inc. 6/90

Shown in Product Identification Guide, page 308

PHRENILIN® ℞

[fren 'ĭ-lin]

(Butalbital* 50 mg and Acetaminophen 325 mg Tablet)

and

PHRENILIN® FORTE ℞

(Butalbital* 50 mg and Acetaminophen 650 mg Capsule)

*****(WARNING—May be habit forming)**

DESCRIPTION

PHRENILIN®: Each PHRENILIN® tablet, for oral administration, contains Butalbital*, USP 50 mg *(WARNING—May be habit forming), Acetaminophen, USP 325 mg.

In addition each PHRENILIN Tablet contains the following inactive ingredients: alginic acid, cornstarch, D&C Red No. 27—Aluminum Lake, FD&C Blue No. 1—Aluminum Lake, gelatin, magnesium stearate, microcrystalline cellulose and pregelatinized starch.

PHRENILIN® FORTE: Each PHRENILIN® FORTE capsule, for oral administration, contains Butalbital*, USP 50 mg *(WARNING—May be habit forming), Acetaminophen, USP 650 mg.

In addition each PHRENILIN FORTE capsule may also contain the following inactive ingredients: benzyl alcohol, butylparaben, D&C Red No. 28, D&C Red No. 33, edetate calcium disodium, FD&C Blue No. 1, FD&C Red No. 40, gelatin, methylparaben, propylparaben, silicon dioxide, sodium lauryl sulfate, sodium propionate and titanium dioxide.

Butalbital (5-allyl-5-isobutylbarbituric acid), a slightly bitter, white, odorless, crystalline powder, is a short to intermediate-acting barbiturate. It has the following structural formula:

$C_{11}H_{16}N_2O_3$ MW = 224.26

Acetaminophen, (4'-hydroxyacetanilide), a slightly bitter, white, odorless, crystalline powder, is a non-opiate, non-salicylate analgesic and antipyretic. It has the following structural formula:

$C_8H_9NO_2$ MW = 151.16

CLINICAL PHARMACOLOGY

This combination drug product is intended as a treatment for tension headache.

It consists of a fixed combination of butalbital and acetaminophen. The role each component plays in the relief of the complex of symptoms known as tension headache is incompletely understood.

Pharmacokinetics: The behavior of the individual components is described below.

Butalbital: Butalbital is well absorbed from the gastrointestinal tract and is expected to distribute to most tissues in the body. Barbiturates in general may appear in breast milk and readily cross the placental barrier. They are bound to plasma and tissue proteins to a varying degree and binding increases directly as a function of lipid solubility.

Elimination of butalbital is primarily via the kidney (59% to 88% of the dose) as unchanged drug or metabolites. The plasma half-life is about 35 hours. Urinary excretion products include parent drug (about 3.6% of the dose), 5-isobutyl-5-(2,3-dihydroxypropyl) barbituric acid (about 24% of the dose), 5-allyl-5(3-hydroxy-2- methyl-1-propyl) barbituric acid (about 4.8% of the dose), products with the barbituric acid ring hydrolyzed with excretion of urea (about 14% of the dose), as well as unidentified materials. Of the material excreted in the urine, 32% is conjugated.

See OVERDOSAGE for toxicity information.

Acetaminophen: Acetaminophen is rapidly absorbed from the gastrointestinal tract and is distributed throughout most body tissues. The plasma half-life is 1.25 to 3 hours, but may be increased by liver damage and following overdosage. Elimination of acetaminophen is principally by liver metabolism (conjugation) and subsequent renal excretion of metabolites. Approximately 85% of an oral dose appears in the urine within 24 hours of administration, most as the glucuronide conjugate, with small amounts of other conjugates and unchanged drug.

See OVERDOSAGE for toxicity information.

INDICATIONS AND USAGE

PHRENILIN tablets & PHRENILIN FORTE capsules are indicated for the relief of the symptom complex of tension (or muscle contraction) headache.

Evidence supporting the efficacy and safety of this combination product in the treatment of multiple recurrent head-

aches is unavailable. Caution in this regard is required because butalbital is habit-forming and potentially abusable.

CONTRAINDICATIONS

This product is contraindicated under the following conditions:

- Hypersensitivity or intolerance to any component of this product.
- Patients with porphyria.

WARNINGS

Butalbital is habit-forming and potentially abusable. Consequently, the extended use of this product is not recommended.

PRECAUTIONS

General: PHRENILIN tablets & PHRENILIN FORTE capsules (Butalbital and Acetaminophen) should be prescribed with caution in certain special-risk patients, such as the elderly or debilitated, and those with severe impairment of renal or hepatic function, or acute abdominal conditions.

Information for Patients: This product may impair mental and/or physical abilities required for the performance of potentially hazardous tasks such as driving a car or operating machinery. Such tasks should be avoided while taking this product.

Alcohol and other CNS depressants may produce an additive CNS depression, when taken with this combination product, and should be avoided.

Butalbital may be habit-forming. Patients should take the drug only for as long as it is prescribed, in the amounts prescribed, and no more frequently than prescribed.

Laboratory Tests: In patients with severe hepatic or renal disease, effects of therapy should be monitored with serial liver and/or renal function tests.

Drug Interactions: The CNS effects of butalbital may be enhanced by monoamine oxidase (MAO) inhibitors.

Butalbital and acetaminophen may enhance the effects of: other narcotic analgesics, alcohol, general anesthetics, tranquilizers such as chlordiazepoxide, sedative-hypnotics, or other CNS depressants, causing increased CNS depression.

Drug/Laboratory Test Interactions: Acetaminophen may produce false-positive test results for urinary 5-hydroxyindoleacetic acid.

Carcinogenesis, Mutagenesis, Impairment of Fertility: No adequate studies have been conducted in animals to determine whether acetaminophen or butalbital have a potential for carcinogenesis, mutagenesis or impairment of fertility.

Pregnancy: *Teratogenic Effects:* Pregnancy Category C: Animal reproduction studies have not been conducted with this combination product. It is also not known whether butalbital and acetaminophen can cause fetal harm when administered to a pregnant woman or can affect reproduction capacity. These products should be given to a pregnant woman only when clearly needed.

Nonteratogenic Effects: Withdrawal seizures were reported in a two-day-old male infant whose mother had taken a butalbital-containing drug during the last two months of pregnancy. Butalbital was found in the infant's serum. The infant was given phenobarbital 5 mg/kg, which was tapered without further seizure or other withdrawal symptoms.

Nursing Mothers: Barbiturates and acetaminophen are excreted in breast milk in small amounts, but the significance of their effects on nursing infants is not known. Because of potential for serious adverse reactions in nursing infants from butalbital and acetaminophen, a decision should be made whether to discontinue nursing or to discontinue the drug, taking into account the importance of the drug to the mother.

Pediatric Use: Safety and effectiveness in children below the age of 12 have not been established.

ADVERSE REACTIONS

Frequently Observed: The most frequently reported adverse reactions are drowsiness, lightheadedness, dizziness, sedation, shortness of breath, nausea, vomiting, abdominal pain, and intoxicated feeling.

Infrequently Observed: All adverse events tabulated below are classified as infrequent.

Central Nervous: headache, shaky feeling, tingling, agitation, fainting, fatigue, heavy eyelids, high energy, hot spells, numbness, sluggishness, seizure. Mental confusion, excitement or depression can also occur due to intolerance, particularly in elderly or debilitated patients, or due to overdosage of butalbital.

Autonomic Nervous: dry mouth, hyperhidrosis.

Gastrointestinal: difficulty swallowing, heartburn, flatulence, constipation.

Cardiovascular: tachycardia.

Musculoskeletal: leg pain, muscle fatigue.

Genitourinary: diuresis.

Miscellaneous: pruritus, fever, earache, nasal congestion, tinnitus, euphoria, allergic reactions.

Several cases of dermatological reactions, including toxic epidermal necrolysis and erythema multiforme, have been reported.

The following adverse drug events may be borne in mind as potential effects of the components of this product. Potential effects of high dosage are listed in the OVERDOSAGE section.

Acetaminophen: allergic reactions, rash, thrombocytopenia, agranulocytosis.

DRUG ABUSE AND DEPENDENCE

Abuse and Dependence: Butalbital: *Barbiturates may be habit-forming:* Tolerance, psychological dependence, and physical dependence may occur especially following prolonged use of high doses of barbiturates. The average daily dose for the barbiturate addict is usually about 1500 mg. As tolerance to barbiturates develops, the amount needed to maintain the same level of intoxication increases; tolerance to a fatal dosage, however, does not increase more than twofold. As this occurs, the margin between an intoxication dosage and fatal dosage becomes smaller. The lethal dose of a barbiturate is far less if alcohol is also ingested. Major withdrawal symptoms (convulsions and delirium) may occur within 16 hours and last up to 5 days after abrupt cessation of these drugs. Intensity of withdrawal symptoms gradually declines over a period of approximately 15 days. Treatment of barbiturate dependence consists of cautious and gradual withdrawal of the drug. Barbiturate-dependent patients can be withdrawn by using a number of different withdrawal regimens. One method involves initiating treatment at the patient's regular dosage level and gradually decreasing the daily dosage as tolerated by the patient.

OVERDOSAGE

Following an acute overdosage of butalbital and acetaminophen, toxicity may result from the barbiturate or acetaminophen.

Signs and Symptoms: Toxicity from barbiturate poisoning include drowsiness, confusion, and coma; respiratory depression; hypotension; and hypovolemic shock.

In acetaminophen overdosage: dose-dependent, potentially fatal hepatic necrosis is the most serious adverse effect. Renal tubular necroses, hypoglycemic coma and thrombocytopenia may also occur. Early symptoms following a potentially hepatotoxic overdose may include: nausea, vomiting, diaphoresis and general malaise. Clinical and laboratory evidence of hepatic toxicity may not be apparent until 48 to 72 hours post-ingestion. In adults hepatic toxicity has rarely been reported with acute overdoses of less than 10 grams, or fatalities with less than 15 grams.

Treatment: A single or multiple overdose with these combination products is a potentially lethal polydrug overdose, and consultation with a regional poison control center is recommended.

Immediate treatment includes support of cardiorespiratory function and measures to reduce drug absorption. Vomiting should be induced mechanically, or with syrup of ipecac, if the patient is alert (adequate pharyngeal and laryngeal reflexes). Oral activated charcoal (1 g/kg) should follow gastric emptying. The first dose should be accompanied by an appropriate cathartic. If repeated doses are used, the cathartic might be included with alternate doses as required. Hypotension is usually hypovolemic and should respond to fluids. Pressors should be avoided. A cuffed endotracheal tube should be inserted before gastric lavage of the unconscious patient and, when necessary, to provide assisted respiration. If renal function is normal, forced diuresis may aid in the elimination of the barbiturate. Alkalinization of the urine increases renal excretion of some barbiturates, especially phenobarbital.

Meticulous attention should be given to maintaining adequate pulmonary ventilation. In severe cases of intoxication, peritoneal dialysis, or preferably hemodialysis may be considered. If hypoprothrombinemia occurs due to acetaminophen overdose, vitamin K should be administered intravenously.

If the dose of acetaminophen may have exceeded 140 mg/kg, acetylcysteine should be administered as early as possible. Serum acetaminophen levels should be obtained, since levels four or more hours following ingestion help predict acetaminophen toxicity. Do not await acetaminophen assay results before initiating treatment. Hepatic enzymes should be obtained initially, and repeated at 24-hour intervals.

Methemoglobinemia over 30% should be treated with methylene blue by slow intravenous administration.

Toxic Doses (for adults):

PHRENILIN tablets (Butalbital 50 mg and Acetaminophen 325 mg tablets)

Butalbital: toxic dose 1 g (20 tablets)

Acetaminophen: toxic dose 10 g (30 tablets)

PHRENILIN FORTE capsules (Butalbital 50 mg and Acetaminophen 650 mg capsules)

Butalbital: toxic dose 1 g (20 capsules)

Acetaminophen: toxic dose 10 g (15 capsules)

DOSAGE AND ADMINISTRATION

PHRENILIN®: Oral: One or two tablets every four hours. Total daily dosage should not exceed 6 tablets.

PHRENILIN® FORTE: Oral: One capsule every four hours. Total daily dosage should not exceed 6 capsules.

Extended and repeated use of these products is not recommended because of the potential for physical dependence.

HOW SUPPLIED

PHRENILIN®: Pale violet scored tablets with the letter C on one side and 8650 on the other, in bottles of 100 (NDC 0086-0050-10). Each tablet contains butalbital, USP 50 mg (WARNING: May be habit forming) and acetaminophen, USP 325 mg.

PHRENILIN® FORTE: Amethyst, opaque capsules imprinted with the letter C and 8656, in bottles of 100 (NDC 0086-0056-10). Each capsule contains butalbital, USP 50 mg (WARNING: May be habit forming) and acetaminophen USP 650 mg.

Store PHRENILIN® and PHRENILIN® FORTE (Butalbital and Acetaminophen) at controlled room temperature, 15°–30°C (59°–86°F). Dispense in a tight container as defined in the USP.

Caution: Federal Law Prohibits Dispensing Without Prescription

The most recent revision of this labeling is June 1993.

Manufactured for Carnrick Laboratories, Inc.

Shown in Product Identification Guide, page 308

PROPAGEST®   OTC
(Phenylpropanolamine HCl)
Alcohol-free
NASAL DECONGESTANT TABLETS

DESCRIPTION

Each alcohol-free tablet contains:
Phenylpropanolamine HCl .... 25 mg

INDICATIONS

For the temporary relief of nasal congestion associated with the common cold, sinusitis, hay fever or other upper respiratory allergies.

DOSAGE

Adult oral dosage is one tablet every 4 hours not to exceed 6 tablets in 24 hours. Children 6 to under 12 years oral dosage is one-half tablet every 4 hours not to exceed 3 tablets in 24 hours. For children under 6 years, there is no recommended dosage except under the advice and supervision of a doctor.

WARNINGS

Do not exceed recommended dosage because at higher doses nervousness, dizziness, sleeplessness, rapid pulse or high blood pressure may occur.

Do not take this product for more than 7 days. If symptoms do not improve or are accompanied by fever, consult a doctor.

Do not take this product if you have heart disease, high blood pressure, thyroid disease, glaucoma, diabetes, or difficulty in urination due to enlargement of the prostate gland unless directed by a doctor.

As with any drug, if you are pregnant or nursing a baby, seek the advice of a health professional before using this product.

Keep this and all medication out of the reach of children.

In case of accidental overdose, seek professional assistance or contact a Poison Control Center immediately.

Drug Interaction Precaution: Do not take this product if you are presently taking a prescription drug for high blood pressure or depression, without first consulting your doctor. Do not take this product concurrently with other medication except on the advice of a doctor.

TAMPER-RESISTANT PACKAGE FEATURE:

Bottle of 100—If printed outer wrap on carton is broken or removed, do not purchase.

HOW SUPPLIED

White, oval, scored tablets inscribed with 8651 on one side and "C" logo on the other, containing 25 mg phenylpropanolamine HCl in bottles of 100. (NDC 0086-0051-10). Keep tightly closed, away from light and store at room temperature.   1/96

Manufactured for Carnrick Laboratories, Inc.

Shown in Product Identification Guide, page 308

SALFLEX®   ℞
(salsalate tablets USP)

DESCRIPTION

SALFLEX (salsalate) is a nonsteroidal anti-inflammatory agent for oral administration. Chemically, salsalate (salicylsalicylic acid or 2-hydroxy-benzoic acid, 2-carboxyphenyl ester) is a dimer of salicylic acid; its structural formula is shown below.

Chemical Structure:

[See chemical structure at top of next column.]

Each round, white, dye-free, film-coated SALFLEX tablet contains 500 mg salsalate.

Continued on next page

Carnrick Laboratories—Cont.

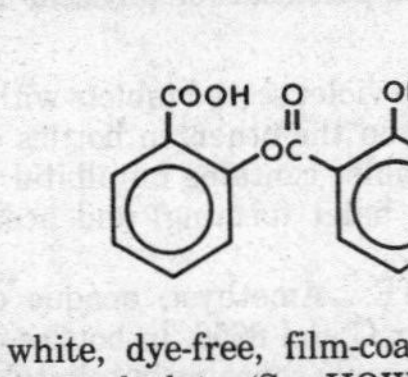

Each oval, white, dye-free, film-coated SALFLEX tablet contains 750 mg salsalate. (See HOW SUPPLIED.)

CLINICAL PHARMACOLOGY

Salsalate is insoluble in acid gastric fluids (<0.1 mg/ml at pH 1.0), but readily soluble in the small intestine where it is partially hydrolyzed to two molecules of salicylic acid. A significant portion of the parent compound is absorbed unchanged and undergoes rapid esterase hydrolysis in the body; its half-life is about one hour. About 13% is excreted through the kidneys as a glucuronide conjugate of the parent compound, the remainder as salicylic acid and its metabolites. Thus, the amount of salicylic acid available from SALFLEX (salsalate) is about 15% less than from aspirin, when the two drugs are administered on a salicylic acid molar equivalent basis (3.6 g salsalate/5 g aspirin). Salicylic acid biotransformation is saturated at anti-inflammatory doses of salsalate. Such capacity-limited biotransformation results in an increase in the half-life of salicylic acid from 3.5 to 16 or more hours. Thus, dosing with SALFLEX twice a day will satisfactorily maintain blood levels within the desired therapeutic range (10 to 30 mg/100 ml) throughout the 12-hour intervals. Therapeutic blood levels continue for up to 16 hours after the last dose. The parent compound does not show capacity-limited biotransformation, nor does it accumulate in the plasma on multiple dosing. Food slows the absorption of all salicylates including salsalate.

The mode of anti-inflammatory action of salsalate and other nonsteroidal anti-inflammatory drugs is not fully defined. Although salicylic acid (the primary metabolite of salsalate) is a weak inhibitor of prostaglandin synthesis **in vitro,** salsalate appears to selectively inhibit prostaglandin synthesis **in vivo,**[1] providing anti-inflammatory activity equivalent to aspirin[2] and indomethacin.[3] Unlike aspirin, salsalate does not inhibit platelet aggregation.[4]

The usefulness of salicylic acid, the active **in vivo** product of salsalate, in the treatment of arthritic disorders has been established.[5,6] In contrast to aspirin, salsalate causes no greater fecal gastrointestinal blood loss than placebo.[7]

INDICATIONS AND USAGE

SALFLEX (salsalate) is indicated for relief of the signs and symptoms of rheumatoid arthritis, osteoarthritis and related rheumatic disorders.

CONTRAINDICATIONS

SALFLEX is contraindicated in patients hypersensitive to salsalate.

WARNINGS

Reye Syndrome may develop in individuals who have chicken pox, influenza, or flu symptoms. Some studies suggest possible association between the development of Reye Syndrome and the use of medicines containing salicylate or aspirin. SALFLEX contains a salicylate and therefore is not recommended for use in patients with chicken pox, influenza or flu symptoms. See PRECAUTIONS.

PRECAUTIONS

General Precautions: Patients on treatment with SALFLEX should be warned not to take other salicylates so as to avoid potentially toxic concentrations. Great care should be exercised when SALFLEX is prescribed in the presence of chronic renal insufficiency or peptic ulcer disease. Protein binding of salicylic acid can be influenced by nutritional status, competitive binding of other drugs, and fluctuations in serum proteins caused by disease (rheumatoid arthritis, etc.). Although cross reactivity, including bronchospasm, has been reported occasionally with non-acetylated salicylates, including salsalate, in aspirin-sensitive patients,[8,9] salsalate is less likely than aspirin to induce asthma in such patients.[10]

Laboratory Tests: Plasma salicylic acid concentrations should be periodically monitored during long-term treatment with SALFLEX to aid maintenance of therapeutically effective levels: 10 to 30 mg/100 ml. Toxic manifestations are not usually seen until plasma concentrations exceed 30 mg/100 ml (see OVERDOSAGE). Urinary pH should also be regularly monitored: sudden acidification, as from pH 6.5 to 5.5, can double the plasma level, resulting in toxicity.

Drug Interactions: Salicylates antagonize the uricosuric action of drugs used to treat gout. ASPIRIN AND OTHER SALICYLATE DRUGS WILL BE ADDITIVE TO SALFLEX (salsalate) AND MAY INCREASE PLASMA CONCENTRATIONS OF SALICYLIC ACID TO TOXIC LEVELS. Drugs and foods that raise urine pH will increase renal clearance and urinary excretion of salicylic acid, thus lowering plasma levels; acidifying drugs or foods will decrease urinary excretion and increase plasma levels. Salicylates given concomitantly with anticoagulant drugs may predispose to systemic bleeding. Salicylates may enhance the hypoglycemic effect of oral antidiabetic drugs of the sulfonylurea class. Salicylate competes with a number of drugs for protein binding sites, notably penicillin, thiopental, thyroxine, triiodothyronine, phenytoin, sulfinpyrazone, naproxen, warfarin, methotrexate, and possibly corticosteroids.

Drug/Laboratory Test Interactions: Salicylate competes with thyroid hormone for binding to plasma proteins, which may be reflected in a depressed plasma T_4 value in some patients: thyroid function and basal metabolism are unaffected.

Carcinogenesis: No long-term animal studies have been performed with salsalate to evaluate its carcinogenic potential.

Use in Pregnancy: Pregnancy Category C: Salsalate and salicylic acid have been shown to be teratogenic and embryocidal in rats when given in doses 4 to 5 times the usual human dose. These effects were not observed at doses twice as great as the usual human dose. There are no adequate and well-controlled studies in pregnant women. SALFLEX should be used during pregnancy only if the potential benefit justifies the potential risk to the fetus.

Labor and Delivery: There exist no adequate and well-controlled studies in pregnant women. Although adverse effects on mother or infant have not been reported with salsalate use during labor, caution is advised when anti-inflammatory dosage is involved. However, other salicylates have been associated with prolonged gestation and labor, maternal and neonatal bleeding sequelae, potentiation of narcotic and barbiturate effects (respiratory or cardiac arrest in the mother), delivery problems and stillbirth.

Nursing Mothers: It is not known whether salsalate per se is excreted in human milk; salicylic acid, the primary metabolite of salsalate, has been shown to appear in human milk in concentrations approximating the maternal blood level. Thus the infant of a mother on SALFLEX therapy might ingest in mother's milk 30 to 80% as much salicylate per kg body weight as the mother is taking. Accordingly, caution should be exercised when SALFLEX (salsalate) is administered to a nursing woman.

Pediatric Use: Safety and effectiveness of SALFLEX use in children have not been established. (See WARNINGS section.)

ADVERSE REACTIONS

In two well-controlled clinical trials, the following reversible adverse experiences characteristic of salicylates were most commonly reported with salsalate (n=280 pts; listed in descending order of frequency): tinnitus, nausea, hearing impairment, rash, and vertigo. These common symptoms of salicylates, i.e., tinnitus or reversible hearing impairment, are often used as a guide to therapy.

Although cause-and-effect relationships have not been established, spontaneous reports over a ten-year period have included the following additional medically significant adverse experiences: abdominal pain, abnormal hepatic function, anaphylactic shock, angioedema, bronchospasm, decreased creatinine clearance, diarrhea, G.I. bleeding, hepatitis, hypotension, nephritis and urticaria.

DRUG ABUSE AND DEPENDENCE

Drug abuse and dependence have not been reported with salsalate.

OVERDOSAGE

Death has followed ingestion of 10 to 30 g of salicylates in adults, but much larger amounts have been ingested without fatal outcome.

Symptoms: The usual symptoms of salicylism—tinnitus, vertigo, headache, confusion, drowsiness, sweating, hyperventilation, vomiting and diarrhea—will occur. More severe intoxication will lead to disruption of electrolyte balance and blood pH, and hyperthermia and dehydration.

Treatment: Further absorption of salsalate from the G.I. tract should be prevented by emesis (syrup of ipecac) and, if necessary, by gastric lavage.

Fluid and electrolyte imbalance should be corrected by the administration of appropriate I.V. therapy. Adequate renal function should be maintained. Hemodialysis or peritoneal dialysis may be required in extreme cases.

DOSAGE AND ADMINISTRATION

Adults: The usual dosage is 3000 mg daily, given in divided doses as follows:

1) two doses of two 750 mg tablets;
2) two doses of three 500 mg tablets; or
3) three doses of two 500 mg tablets.

Some patients, e.g., the elderly, may require a lower dosage to achieve therapeutic blood concentrations and to avoid the more common side effects such as auditory.

Alleviation of symptoms is gradual, and full benefit may not be evident for 3 to 4 days, when plasma salicylate levels have achieved steady state. There is no evidence for development of tissue tolerance (tachyphylaxis), but salicylate therapy may induce increased activity of metabolizing liver enzymes, causing a greater rate of salicyluric acid production and excretion, with a resultant increase in dosage requirement for maintenance of therapeutic serum salicylate levels.

Children: Dosage recommendations and indications for SALFLEX use in children have not been established.

HOW SUPPLIED

SALFLEX 500 mg tablets:

Each round, white, dye-free, film-coated SALFLEX tablet is inscribed with 8671 on one side and "C" on the other. Each tablet contains 500 mg salsalate and is available in bottles of 100 tablets (NDC 0086-0071-10).

SALFLEX 750 mg tablets:

Each oval, white, dye-free, film-coated SALFLEX tablet is inscribed with 8672 on the scored side and "C" on the other. Each tablet contains 750 mg salsalate and is available in bottles of 100 tablets (NDC 0086-0072-10) and 500 tablets (NDC 0086-0072-50).

Store at controlled room temperature, 15°–30°C (59°–86°F).

Dispense in a tight container as defined in the USP.

CAUTION: Federal law prohibits dispensing without prescription.

REFERENCES

1. Morris HG, Sherman NA, McQuain C., et al: Effects of Salsalate (Nonacetylated) Salicylate and Aspirin on Serum Prostaglandins in Humans. Ther. Drug Monit. 7:435-438, 1985.
2. April PA, Curran NJ, Ekholm BP, et al: Multicenter Comparative Study of Salsalate (SSA) vs Aspirin (ASA) in Rheumatoid Arthritis (RA), Arthritis Rheumatism **30**(4 supplement):S93, 1987.
3. Deodhar SD, McLeod MM, Dick WC, et al: A Short-Term Comparative Trial of Salsalate and Indomethacin in Rheumatoid Arthritis. Curr. Med. Res. Opin. **5**:185–188, 1977.
4. Estes D, Kaplan K: Lack of Platelet Effect With the Aspirin Analog, Salsalate, Arthritis and Rheumatism, **23**:1303–1307, 1980.
5. Dick C, Dick PH, Nuki G, et al: Effect of Anti-inflammatory Drug Therapy on Clearance of ^{133}Xe from Knee Joints of Patients with Rheumatoid Arthritis. British Med. J. **3**:278–280, 1969.
6. Dick WC, Grayson MF, Woodburn A, et al: Indices of Inflammatory Activity. Ann. of the Rheum. Dis. **29**:643–648, 1970.
7. Cohen, A: Fecal Blood Loss and Plasma Salicylate Study of Salicylsalicylic Acid and Aspirin. J. Clin. Pharmacol. **19**:242–247, 1979.
8. Chudwin DS, Strub M, Golden HE, et al: Sensitivity to Non-Acetylated Salicylates in a Patient with Asthma, Nasal Polyps, and Rheumatoid Arthritis. Annals of Allergy **57**:133–134, 1986.
9. Spector SL, Wangaard CH, Farr RS: Aspirin and Concomitant Idiosyncrasies in Adult Asthmatic Patients. J. Allergy Clin. Immunol. **64**:500–506, 1979.
10. Stevenson DD, Schrank PJ, Hougham AJ, et al: Salsalate Cross Sensitivity in Aspirin-Sensitive Asthmatics. J. Allergy Clin. Immunol. **81**:181, 1988.

June 1993

Shown in Product Identification Guide, page 308

SINULIN® OTC

Alcohol-free

Analgesic • Antihistamine • Decongestant

DESCRIPTION

SINULIN contains acetaminophen, an analgesic and antipyretic that relieves pain, sinus headache and reduces fever; phenylpropanolamine HCl, a decongestant that promotes nasal drainage and relieves sinus pressure; and chlorpheniramine maleate, an antihistamine that helps control allergic symptoms.

ACTIVE INGREDIENTS

Each alcohol-free tablet contains: acetaminophen 650 mg. (650 mg. is a nonstandard strength of acetaminophen per tablet compared to the established standard of 325 mg. acetaminophen per tablet), chlorpheniramine maleate 4 mg., phenylpropanolamine HCl 25 mg.

INDICATIONS

For the temporary relief of nasal and sinus congestion, runny nose, sneezing, itching of the nose or throat, itchy watery eyes, headache and fever associated with the common cold, sinusitis, hay fever or other upper respiratory allergies.

WARNINGS

Sinulin tablets contain FD&C Yellow No. 6 as a color additive. Do not exceed recommended dosage because severe liver damage may occur and at higher doses, nervousness, dizziness, sleeplessness, rapid pulse or high blood pressure may occur. Adults should not take this product for more than 7 days. Children 6 to under 12 years of age should not take this product for more than 5 days. If fever persists for more than 3 days, or recurs, consult a doctor. If symptoms persist,

do not improve, or new ones occur, consult a doctor. Do not take this product if you have high blood pressure; heart disease; diabetes; thyroid disease; glaucoma; a breathing problem such as emphysema or chronic bronchitis, asthma, chronic pulmonary disease, shortness of breath or difficulty in breathing; or difficulty in urination due to enlargement of the prostate gland, or if you are presently taking a prescription drug for high blood pressure or depression, unless directed by a doctor. May cause drowsiness; alcohol, sedatives and tranquilizers may increase the drowsiness effect. Avoid alcoholic beverages while taking this product. Do not take this product if you are taking sedatives or tranquilizers, without first consulting your doctor. Use caution when driving a motor vehicle or operating machinery. May cause excitability especially in children. If a rare sensitivity reaction occurs, discontinue use and consult a doctor. As with any drug, if you are pregnant or nursing a baby, seek the advice of a health professional before using this product. Keep this and all medication out of the reach of children. In case of accidental overdose, seek professional assistance or contact a Poison Control Center immediately.

DRUG INTERACTION PRECAUTION

Do not take this product if you are presently taking a prescription drug for high blood pressure or depression, or if you are taking a sedative or tranquilizer, without first consulting your doctor. Do not take this product concurrently with other medication except on the advise of a doctor.

DIRECTIONS

Adults: oral dosage is one tablet every 4 to 6 hours, or as directed by a doctor. Do not exceed 6 tablets in 24 hours.
Children 6 to under 12 years of age: oral dosage is one-half tablet every 4 to 6 hours, or as directed by a doctor. Do not exceed 3 tablets in 24 hours.
Children under 6 years of age: do not use unless directed by a doctor.

TAMPER-RESISTANT PACKAGE FEATURE

Bottles of 20's & 100's—If printed outer wrap on carton is broken or removed, do not purchase. Blisters—Tablets are individually sealed with Sinulin® identifying copy on the back. If seal is broken, do not use.

HOW SUPPLIED

Peach color, scored tablets inscribed with 8666 on one side and C logo on the other. Bottles of 20 (NDC 0086-0066-02), 7 boxes of 24 blisters (NDC 0086-0066-24), and Bottles of 100 (NDC 0086-0066-10). Store at controlled room temperature (59°–86°F). 9/95
Manufactured for Carnrick Laboratories, Inc.
Shown in Product Identification Guide, page 308

SKELAXIN® ℞
brand of metaxalone

CAUTION

Federal law prohibits dispensing without prescription.

DESCRIPTION

Each pale rose, scored tablet contains: metaxalone, 400 mg.
Skelaxin (metaxalone) has the following chemical structure and name:
5-[(3,4-dimethylphenoxy)methyl]-2 oxazolidinone

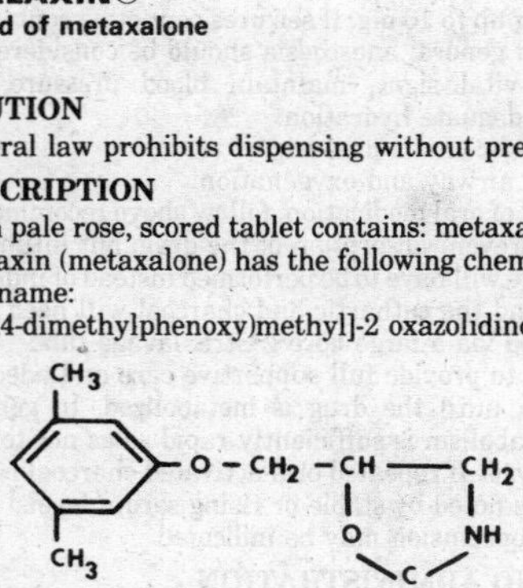

ACTIONS

The mechanism of action of metaxalone in humans has not been established, but may be due to general central nervous system depression. It has no direct action on the contractile mechanism of striated muscle, the motor end plate or the nerve fiber.

INDICATIONS

Skelaxin (metaxalone) is indicated as an adjunct to rest, physical therapy, and other measures for the relief of discomforts associated with acute, painful musculoskeletal conditions. The mode of action of this drug has not been clearly identified, but may be related to its sedative properties. Metaxalone does not directly relax tense skeletal muscles in man.

CONTRAINDICATIONS

Metaxalone is contraindicated in individuals who have shown hypersensitivity to the drug. Metaxalone should not be administered to patients with a known tendency to drug-induced, hemolytic, or other anemias. It is contraindicated in patients with significantly impaired renal or hepatic function.

PRECAUTIONS

Elevation in cephalin flocculation tests without concurrent changes in other liver function parameters have been noted. Hence, it is recommended that metaxalone be administered with great care to patients with pre-existing liver damage and that serial liver function studies be performed as required.
False-positive Benedict's tests, due to an unknown reducing substance, have been noted. A glucose-specific test will differentiate findings.
Pregnancy: Reproduction studies have been performed in rats and have revealed no evidence of impaired fertility or harm to the fetus due to metaxalone. Reactions reports from marketing experience have not revealed evidence of fetal injury, but such experience cannot exclude the possibility of infrequent or subtle damage to the human fetus. Safe use of metaxalone has not been established with regard to possible adverse effects upon fetal development. Therefore, metaxalone tablets should not be used in women who are or may become pregnant and particularly during early pregnancy unless in the judgment of the physician the potential benefits outweigh the possbile hazards.
Nursing Mothers: It is not known whether this drug is secreted in human milk. As a general rule, nursing should not be undertaken while a patient is on a drug since many drugs are excreted in human milk.
Pediatric Use: Safety and effectiveness in children 12 years of age and below have not been established.

ADVERSE REACTIONS

The most frequent reactions to metaxalone include nausea, vomiting, gastrointestinal upset, drowsiness, dizziness, headache, and nervousness or "irritability." Other adverse reactions are: hypersensitivity reaction, characterized by a light rash with or without pruritus; leukopenia; hemolytic anemia; jaundice.

DOSAGE

The recommended dose for adults and children over 12 years of age is two tablets (800 mg) three to four times a day.

MANAGEMENT OF OVERDOSAGE

Gastric lavage and supportive therapy as indicated. (When determining the LD_{50} in rats and mice, progressive sedation, hypnosis and finally respiratory failure were noted as the dosage increased. In dogs, no LD_{50} could be determined as the higher doses produced an emetic action in 15 to 30 minutes). No documented case of major toxicity has been reported.

HOW SUPPLIED

Skelaxin (metaxalone) is available as a 400 mg. pale rose tablet, inscribed with 8662 on the scored side and "C" on the other. Available in bottles of 100 (NDC 0086-0062-10) and in bottles of 500 (NDC 0086-0062-50).
Store at Controlled Room Temperature, between 15°C and 30°C (59°F and 86°F).
8/90
Manufactured for Carnrick Laboratories, Inc.
Shown in Product Identification Guide, page 308

THEO-X™ ℞
(Theophylline Extended-Release Tablets)

DESCRIPTION

Theophylline is a bronchodilator structurally classified as a xanthine derivative. It occurs as a white, odorless, crystalline powder having a bitter taste. Theophylline anhydrous has the chemical name 1*H*-Purine-2, 6-dione, 3,7-dihydro-1, 3-dimethyl-, and is represented by the following structural formula:

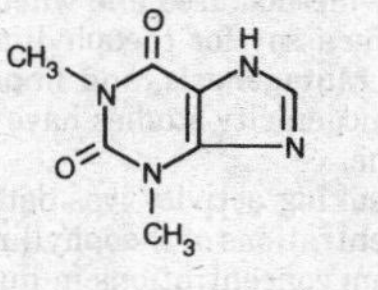

$C_7H_8N_4O_2$ 180.17

This product allows a 12-hour dosing interval for a majority of patients and a 24-hour dosing interval for selected patients (see DOSAGE AND ADMINISTRATION section for description of appropriate patient populations).
This product is available as extended-release tablets intended for oral administration, containing 100 mg, 200 mg, or 300 mg of theophylline anhydrous. Also contains Povidone, USP, Hydroxypropyl Methylcellulose, USP, Lactose Anhydrous, NF, and Magnesium Stearate, NF.

CLINICAL PHARMACOLOGY

Theophylline directly relaxes the smooth muscle of the bronchial airways and pulmonary blood vessels, thus acting mainly as a bronchodilator and smooth muscle relaxant. It has also been demonstrated that aminophylline has a potent effect on diaphragmatic contractility in normal persons and may then be capable of reducing fatigability and thereby improve contractility in patients with chronic obstructive airways disease. The exact mode of action remains unsettled. Although theophylline does cause inhibition of phosphodiesterase with a resultant increase in intracellular cyclic AMP, other agents similarly inhibit the enzyme, producing a rise of cyclic AMP, but are unassociated with any demonstrable bronchodilation. Other mechanisms proposed include an effect on translocation of intracellular calcium, prostaglandin antagonism, stimulation of catecholamines endogenously; inhibition of cyclic guanosine monophosphate metabolism, and adenosine receptor antagonism. None of these mechanisms has been proved, however.
In vitro, theophylline has been shown to act synergistically with beta agonists, and there are now available data which demonstrate an additive effect *in vivo* with combined use.
Pharmacokinetics: The half-life of theophylline is influenced by a number of known variables. It may be prolonged in chronic alcoholics, particularly those with liver disease (cirrhosis or alcoholic liver disease), in patients with congestive heart failure, and in those patients taking certain other drugs (see **PRECAUTIONS, Drug interactions**).
Newborns and neonates have extremely slow clearance rates compared to older infants and children, ie, those over 1 year. Older children have rapid clearance rates while most nonsmoking adults have clearance rates between these two extremes. In premature neonates the decreased clearance is related to oxidative pathways that have yet to be established.

Theophylline Elimination Characteristics
Theophylline

	Half-Life (in hours) Range	Mean
Children	1–9	3.7
Adults	3–15	7.7

In cigarette smokers (1–2 packs/day) the mean half-life is 4–5 hours, much shorter than in nonsmokers. The increase in clearance associated with smoking is presumably due to stimulation of the hepatic metabolic pathway by components of cigarette smoke. The duration of this effect after cessation of smoking is unknown but may require 6 months to 2 years before the rate approaches that of the nonsmoker.

Single-Dose Study:

A single-dose crossover study was conducted in twelve healthy male volunteers to compare pharmacokinetic parameters when theophylline extended-release tablets were administered with and without food. Subjects were fasted overnight and received a single 300 mg tablet early the following morning.
When dosing was done under fed conditions, the subjects received a standard breakfast consisting of 2 fried eggs, 2 strips of bacon, 4 oz. hash brown potatoes, 1 slice of toast with a pat of butter, and 8 oz. whole milk 15 minutes pre-dosing. No food was allowed for five hours post-dosing then a standard lunch was served; at ten hours post-dosing a standard supper was served. Mean peak theophylline serum levels for the two treatments were 3.7 mcg/mL (fasting) and 4.4 mcg/mL (with food). The time of peak serum level varied from subject to subject, occurring from 4 to 14 hours after dosing. However, 92% of the subjects had serum levels at least 75% of the maximum value at 4 to 8 hours after dosing, during each phase.
Thus, blood samples taken 4 to 8 hours post-dosing should reference the peak serum level for most patients. The mean T_{max} was 6.2 hours (fasting) and 8.7 hours (with food). The respective AUC (0- inf.) for these treatments were 73.3 mcg × hr/mL and 82.2 mcg × hr/mL, respectively.

Multiple-Dose Study:
(300 mg)

A multiple-dose, steady-state study was conducted under fed conditions. Three high fat content meals were served at 6:30 a.m., 12 noon and 6:30 p.m. Nineteen normal subjects were dosed as 300 mg every 12 hours (7 p.m. and 7 a.m.) for eight doses. Dosing began one-half hour after the evening meal with the test dose occurring one-half hour after breakfast. At steady-state, the mean peak concentration was 8.8 mcg/mL and the mean trough concentration was 5.9 mcg/mL.
The time of peak concentration (T_{max}) was 6.2 hours. The average percent fraction of fluctuation $[(C_{max}- C_{min}/C_{min}) \times 100]$ was 49% for this formulation and dosing regimen.
The subjects used for this study exhibited a mean half-life of 8.3 hours (range 5.2–12.2) and a mean clearance of 3.5 L/hour (range 2.3–5.6) as determined in a separate single-dose clearance study using 500 mg of immediate release theophylline, prior to this multiple-dose study.

(200 mg)

A multiple-dose steady-state study was conducted in sixteen normal subjects, with one 200 mg tablet given every 12 hours

Continued on next page

Carnrick Laboratories—Cont.

for eight doses. Three high fat content meals were served at 6:30 a.m., 12 noon and 6:30 p.m. Dosing began one-half hour after the evening meal with the test dose occurring one-half hour after breakfast. At steady-state following the eighth dose, the mean C_{max} was 5.1 mcg/mL and the mean C_{min} was 3.7 mcg/mL. The mean time to peak concentration was 6.2 hours. The average percent fraction of fluctuation was 39%. The subjects used for this study exhibited a mean half-life of 8.7 hours (range 5.0–14.6) and a mean clearance of 3.6 L/hour (range 2.2–6.1).

(100 mg)

A multiple-dose steady-state study was conducted in sixteen normal subjects, with three 100 mg tablets given every 12 hours for eight doses. Three high fat content meals were served at 6:30 a.m., 12 noon and 6:30 p.m. Dosing began one-half hour after the evening meal with the test dose occurring one-half hour after breakfast. At steady-state following the eighth dose, the mean C_{max} was 8.1 mcg/mL and the mean C_{min} was 5.6 mcg/mL. The mean time to peak concentration was 6.2 hours. The average percent fraction of fluctuation was 45%.

The subjects used for this study were the same as those used in the previously cited 200 mg study.

Once-a-Day Dosing:

A multiple-dose, steady-state study was conducted under fed conditions with once-a-day dosing. Fed conditions were the same as those previously cited. Sixteen subjects were dosed as 2×300 mg tablets every morning at 8 a.m. for five doses. At steady-state, the mean C_{max} was 11.7 mcg/mL, and the mean C_{min} was 3.4 mcg/mL. The average percent fraction of fluctuation was 244%. The mean t_{max} was 8.7 hours. The subjects used in the above study exhibited a mean half-life of 7.9 hours (range 5.3–13.4) and a mean clearance of 3.8 L/hour (range 2.3–5.7).

INDICATIONS AND USAGE

For relief and/or prevention of symptoms from asthma and reversible bronchospasm associated with chronic bronchitis and emphysema.

CONTRAINDICATIONS

This product is contraindicated in individuals who have shown hypersensitivity to its components. It is also contraindicated in patients with active peptic ulcer disease, and in individuals with underlying seizure disorders (unless receiving appropriate anticonvulsant medication).

WARNINGS

Serum levels above 20 mcg/mL are rarely found after appropriate administration of the recommended doses. However, in individuals in whom theophylline plasma clearance is reduced *for any reason*, even conventional doses may result in increased serum levels and potential toxicity. Reduced theophylline clearance has been documented in the following readily identifiable groups: 1) patients with impaired renal or liver function; 2) patients over 55 years of age; particularly males and those with chronic lung disease; 3) those with cardiac failure from any cause; 4) patients with sustained high fever; 5) neonates and infants under 1 year of age; and 6) those patients taking certain drugs (see **PRECAUTIONS, Drug Interactions**). Frequently, such patients have markedly prolonged theophylline serum levels following discontinuation of the drug.

Reduction of dosage and laboratory monitoring are especially appropriate in the above individuals.

Serious side effects such as ventricular arrhythmias, convulsions, or even death may appear as the first sign of theophylline toxicity without any previous warning. Less serious signs of theophylline toxicity (ie, nausea and restlessness) may occur frequently when initiating therapy, but are usually transient; when such signs are persistent during maintenance therapy, they are often associated with serum concentrations above 20 mcg/mL.

Stated differently, *serious toxicity is not reliably preceded by less severe side-effects.* A serum concentration measurement is the only reliable method of predicting potentially life-threatening toxicity.

Many patients who require theophylline may exhibit tachycardia due to their underlying disease process so that the cause/effect relationship to elevated serum theophylline concentrations may not be appreciated.

Theophylline products may cause or worsen arrhythmias and any significant change in rate and/or rhythm warrants monitoring and further investigation.

Studies in laboratory animals (minipigs, rodents, and dogs) recorded the occurrence of cardiac arrhythmias and sudden death (with histologic evidence of myocardial necrosis) when beta-agonists and methylxanthines were administered concurrently. The significance of these findings when applied to humans is currently unknown.

PRECAUTIONS

THEO-X TABLETS SHOULD NOT BE CHEWED OR CRUSHED.

General: On the average, theophylline half-life is shorter in cigarette and marijuana smokers than in non-smokers, but smokers can have half-lives as long as non-smokers. Theophylline should not be administered concurrently with other xanthines. Use with caution in patients with hypoxemia, hypertension, or those with history of peptic ulcer. Theophylline may occasionally act as a local irritant to the G.I. tract although gastrointestinal symptoms are more commonly centrally mediated and associated with serum drug concentrations over 20 mcg/mL.

Information for Patients: The importance of taking only the prescribed dose and time interval between doses should be reinforced. THEO-X Extended-Release Tablets should not be chewed or crushed. When dosing THEO-X on a once daily (q24h) basis, tablets should be taken whole and not split. The patient should alert the physician if symptoms occur repeatedly, especially near the end of a dosing interval.

Laboratory Tests: Serum levels should be monitored periodically to determine the theophylline level associated with observed clinical response and as the method of predicting toxicity. For such measurements, the serum sample should be obtained at the time of peak concentration, under steady-state conditions at approximately 6 hours after administration for this sustained-release product. It is important that the patient will not have missed or taken additional doses during the previous 48 hours and that dosing intervals will have been reasonably equally spaced. DOSAGE ADJUSTMENT BASED ON SERUM THEOPHYLLINE MEASUREMENTS WHEN THESE INSTRUCTIONS HAVE NOT BEEN FOLLOWED MAY RESULT IN RECOMMENDATIONS THAT PRESENT RISK OF TOXICITY TO THE PATIENT.

Drug Interactions:

Drug-Drug: Toxic synergism with ephedrine has been documented and may occur with some other sympathomimetic bronchodilators. In addition, the following drug interactions have been demonstrated:

Theophylline with:

Allopurinol (high-dose)	Increased serum theophylline levels
Cimetidine	Increased serum theophylline levels
Ciprofloxacin	Increased serum theophylline levels
Erythromycin, Troleandomycin	Increased serum theophylline levels
Lithium carbonate	Increased renal excretion of lithium
Oral contraceptives	Increased serum theophylline levels
Phenytoin	Decreased theophylline and pheyntoin serum levels
Propranolol	Increased serum theophylline levels
Rifampin	Decreased serum theophylline levels

Drug-Food: Taking THEO-X Extended-Release Tablets immediately after ingesting a high fat content meal (45 g fat, 55 g carbohydrates, 28 g protein, 789 calories) may result in a somewhat higher C_{max} and delayed T_{max}, and a somewhat greater extent of absorption when compared to taking in the fasting state. The influence of the type and amount of other foods, as well as the time interval between drug and food, has not been studied.

Drug-Laboratory Tests Interactions: Currently available analytical methods, including high pressure liquid chromatography and immunoassay techniques, for measuring serum theophylline levels are specific. Metabolites and other drugs generally do not affect the results. Other new analytic methods are also now in use. The physician should be aware of the laboratory method used and whether other drugs will interfere with the assay for theophylline.

Carcinogenesis, Mutagenesis, and Impairment of Fertility: Long-term carcinogenicity studies have not been performed with theophylline.

Chromosome-breaking activity was detected in human cell cultures at concentrations of theophylline up to 50 times the therapeutic serum concentrations in humans. Theophylline was not mutagenic in the dominant lethal assay in male mice given theophylline intraperitoneally in doses up to 30 times the maximum daily human oral dose.

Studies to determine the effect on fertility have not been performed with theophylline.

Pregnancy: Category C—Animal reproduction studies have not been conducted with theophylline. It is also not known whether theophylline can cause fetal harm when administered to a pregnant woman or can affect reproduction capacity. Xanthines should be given to a pregnant woman only if clearly needed.

Nursing Mothers: Theophylline is distributed into breast milk and may cause irritability or other signs of toxicity in nursing infants. Because of the potential for serious adverse

reactions in nursing infants from theophylline, a decision should be made whether to discontinue nursing or to discontinue the drug, taking into account the importance of the drug to the mother.

Pediatric Use: Safety and effectiveness of THEO-X Extended-Release Tablets administered:

1. Every 24 hours in children under 12 years of age, have not been established.
2. Every 12 hours in children under 6 years of age, have not been established.

ADVERSE REACTIONS

The following adverse reactions have been observed, but there has not been enough systematic collection of data to support an estimate of their frequency. The most consistent adverse reactions are usually due to overdosage.

1. *Gastrointestinal:* nausea, vomiting, epigastric pain, hematemesis, diarrhea.
2. *Central nervous system:* headaches, irritability, restlessness, insomnia, reflex hyperexcitability, muscle twitching, clonic and tonic generalized convulsions.
3. *Cardiovascular:* palpitation, tachycardia, extrasystoles, flushing, hypotension, circulatory failure, ventricular arrhythmias.
4. *Respiratory:* tachypnea.
5. *Renal:* potentiation of diuresis.
6. *Others:* alopecia, hyperglycemia, inappropriate ADH syndrome, rash.

OVERDOSAGE

Management: It is suggested that the management principles (consistent with the clinical status of the patient when first seen) outlined below be instituted and that simultaneous contact with a Regional Poison Control Center be established. In this way both updated information and individualization regarding required therapy may be provided.

1. When potential oral overdose is established and seizure has not occurred:
   a. If patient is alert and seen within the early hours after ingestion, induction of emesis may be of value. Gastric lavage has been demonstrated to be of no value in influencing outcome in patients who present more than 1 hour after ingestion.
   b. Administer a cathartic. Sorbitol solution is reported to be of value.
   c. Administer repeated doses of activated charcoal and monitor theophylline serum levels.
   d. Prophylactic administration of phenobarbital has been shown to increase the seizure threshold in laboratory animals and administration of this drug can be considered.
2. If patient presents with a seizure:
   a. Establish an airway.
   b. Administer oxygen.
   c. Treat the seizure with intravenous diazepam, 0.1 to 0.3 mg/kg up to 10 mg. If seizures cannot be controlled, the use of general anesthesia should be considered.
   d. Monitor vital signs, maintain blood pressure, and provide adequate hydration.
3. If postseizure coma is present:
   a. Maintain airway and oxygenation.
   b. If a result of oral medication, follow above recommendations to prevent absorption of the drug, but intubation and lavage will have to be performed instead of inducing emesis, and the cathartic and charcoal will need to be introduced via a large bore gastric lavage tube.
   c. Continue to provide full supportive care and adequate hydration until the drug is metabolized. In general, drug metabolism is sufficiently rapid so as not to warrant dialysis. If repeated oral activated charcoal is ineffective (as noted by stable or rising serum levels) charcoal hemoperfusion may be indicated.

DOSAGE AND ADMINISTRATION

Taking THEO-X Extended-Release Tablets immediately after a high-fat content meal may result in a somewhat higher C_{max} and delayed T_{max}, and somewhat greater extent of absorption. However, the differences are usually not great and this product may normally be administered without regard to meals.

Effective use of theophylline (ie, the concentration of drug in the serum associated with optimal benefit and minimal risk of toxicity) is considered to occur when the theophylline concentration is maintained from 10 to 20 mcg/mL. The early studies from which these levels were derived were carried out in patients immediately or shortly after recovery from acute exacerbations of their disease (some hospitalized with status asthmaticus).

Although the 20 mcg/mL level remains appropriate as a critical value (above which toxicity is more likely to occur) for safety purposes, additional data are now available which indicate that the serum theophylline concentrations required to produce maximum physiologic benefit may, in fact, fluctuate with the degree of bronchospasm present and are variable. Therefore, the physician should individualize the range appropriate to the patient's requirements, based on both symptomatic response and improvement in pulmonary

function. It should be stressed that serum theophylline concentrations maintained at the upper level of the 10 to 20 mcg/mL range may be associated with potential toxicity when factors known to reduce theophylline clearance are operative. (See **WARNINGS**).

If it is not possible to obtain serum level determinations, restriction of the daily dose (in otherwise healthy adults) to not greater than 13 mg/kg/day, to a maximum of 900 mg in divided doses will result in relatively few patients exceeding serum levels of 20 mcg/mL and the resultant greater risk of toxicity.

Caution should be exercised for younger children who cannot complain of minor side-effects. Older adults, those with cor pulmonale, congestive heart failure, and/or liver disease may have unusually low dosage requirements, and thus, may experience toxicity at the maximal dosage recommended below.

Theophylline does not distribute into fatty tissue. Dosage should be calculated on the basis of lean (ideal) body weight were mg/kg doses are presented.

THEO-X (Theophylline Extended-Release Tablets) are recommended for chronic or long-term management and prevention of symptoms, and not for use in treating acute symptoms of asthma and reversible bronchospasm.

Dosage Guidelines:
WARNING: DO NOT ATTEMPT TO MAINTAIN ANY DOSE THAT IS NOT TOLERATED.
Dosage guidelines are approximations only and the wide range of theophylline clearance between individuals (particularly those with concomitant disease) makes indiscriminate usage hazardous.

I. Acute Symptoms:
NOTE: Status asthmaticus should be considered a medical emergency and is defined as that degree of bronchospasm that is not rapidly responsive to usual doses of conventional bronchodilators. Optimal therapy for such patients frequently requires both **additional medication** parenterally administered, and **close monitoring**, preferably in an intensive care setting.
THEO-X (Theophylline Extended-Release Tablets) are not intended for patients experiencing an acute episode of bronchospasm (associated with asthma, chronic bronchitis, or emphysema). Such patients require rapid relief of symptoms and should be treated with an immediate-release or intravenous theophylline preparation (or other bronchodilators) and not with extended-release products.

II. Chronic Therapy:
A. Initiating Therapy with an Immediate-Release Product:
It is recommended that the appropriate dosage be established using an immediate-release preparation. A dosage form which allows small incremental doses is desirable for initiating therapy. A liquid preparation should be considered for children to permit easier and more accurate dosage adjustment. Slow clinical titration is generally preferred to help aassure acceptance and safety of the medication and to allow the patient to develop tolerance to transient caffeine-like side-effects. Then, if the total 24-hour dose can be given by use of the available strengths of this product, the patient can usually be switched to THEO-X Extended-Release Tablets giving one-half of the daily dose at 12 hour intervals or one-third daily dose at 8-hour intervals. Patients who metabolize theophylline rapidly, such as the young, smokers and some non-smoking adults, are the most likely candidates for dosing at 8-hour intervals. Such patients can generally be identified as having trough serum concentrations lower than desired or repeatedly exhibiting symptoms near the end of a dosing interval.

B. Initiating Therapy with THEO-X (Theophylline Extended-Release Tablets):
Alternatively, therapy can be initiated with THEO-X (Theophylline Extended-Release Tablets) since it is available in dosage forms/strengths which permit titration and adjustment of dosage as outlined in the following dosing guidelines. It is recommended that for children under 25 kg proper dosage be established with a liquid preparation to permit titration in small increments.
Initial Dose:
16 mg/kg/24 hours or 400 mg/24 hours (whichever is less) of theophylline in divided doses at 12 hours intervals.
Increasing Dose:
The above dosage may be increased in approximately 25 percent increments at 3 day intervals so long as the drug is tolerated. Following each adjustment, if the clinical response is satisfactory and serum levels can be measured, then such measurements should be obtained, then that dosage level should be maintained. Dosage increases may be made in this manner until the maximum dose indicated in section III below is reached.
It is important that no patient be maintained on any dosage that is not tolerated. When instructing patients to increase dosage according to the schedule above, they should be told not to take a subsequent dose if apparent side effects occur and to resume therapy at a lower dose once adverse effects have disappeared.

Titration and Adjustment and Chronic Maintenance:
If the desired response is not achieved with the above AVERAGE INITIAL DOSE recommendations, there are no adverse reactions and the serum theophylline level cannot be measured, dosage adjustment should proceed by increasing the dose in approximately 25% increments at three-day intervals. Following each adjustment, if the clinical response is satisfactory, then the dosage level should be maintained. DOSAGE increases may be made in this manner up to the following.

III. Maximum Dose of Theophylline Where the Serum Concentration is not Measured:
WARNING: DO NOT ATTEMPT TO MAINTAIN ANY DOSE THAT IS NOT TOLERATED.
Not to exceed the following: (or 900 mg, whichever is less)

Age 6 to under 9 years	24 mg/kg/day
Age 9 to under 12 years	20 mg/kg/day
Age 12 to under 16 Years	18 mg/kg/day
Age 16 years and older	13 mg/kg/day

IV. Measurement of Serum Theophylline Concentrations During Chronic Therapy:
If the above maximum doses are to be maintained or exceeded, serum theophylline measurement is essential (see **PRECAUTIONS, Laboratory Tests,** for guidance).
V. Final Adjustment of Dosage:
Dosage adjustment after serum theophylline measurement:

If serum theophylline is:		Directions:
Within desired range		Maintain dosage if tolerated.
Too high	20 to 25 mcg/mL	Decrease doses by about 10% and recheck serum level after 3 days.
	25 to 30 mcg/mL	Skip the next dose and decrease subsequent doses by about 25%. Recheck serum level after 3 days.
	Over 30 mcg/mL	Skip the next 2 doses and decrease subsequent doses by 50%. Recheck serum level after 3 days.
Too low		Increase dosage by 25% at 3-day intervals until either the desired serum concentration and/or clinical response is achieved. The total daily dose may need to be administered at more frequent intervals if symptoms occur repeatedly at the end of a dosing interval.

The serum concentration may be rechecked at appropriate intervals, but at least at the end of any adjustment period. When the patient's condition is otherwise clinically stable and none of the recognized factors which alter elimination are present, measurement of serum levels need be repeated only every 6 to 12 months.
DOSAGE ADJUSTMENT BASED ON SERUM THEOPHYLLINE CONCENTRATION MEASUREMENTS WHEN THESE INSTRUCTIONS HAVE NOT BEEN FOLLOWED MAY RESULT IN RECOMMENDATIONS THAT PRESENT RISK OF TOXICITY TO THE PATIENT.
Once-Daily Dosing: The slow absorption rate of this preparation may allow once-daily administration in adult non-smokers with appropriate total body clearance and other patients with low dosage requirements. Once-daily dosing should be considered only after the patient has been gradually and satisfactorily titrated to therapeutic levels with q12h dosing. Once-daily dosing should be based on twice the q12h dose and should be initiated at the end of the last q12h dosing interval. The trough concentration (C_{min}) obtained following conversion to once-daily dosing may be lower (especially in high clearance patients) and the peak concentration (C_{max}) may be higher (especially in low clearance patients) than that obtained with q12h dosing. If symptoms recur, or signs of toxicity appear during the once-daily dosing interval, dosing on the q12h basis should be reinstituted.
It is essential that serum theophylline concentrations be monitored before and after transfer to once-daily dosing. Food and posture, along with changes associated with circadian rhythm, may influence the rate of absorpiton and/or clearance rates of theophylline from extended-release dosage forms administered at night. The exact relationship of these and other factors to nightime serum concentrations and the clinical significance of such findings require additional study. Therefore, it is not recommended that THEO-X, when used as a once-a-day product, be administered at night.

HOW SUPPLIED
THEO-X (Theophylline Extended-Release Tablets) for oral administration is available as:
100 mg—White, dye-free, round, bisected, extended-release tablets inscribed with "C" on one side and "8631" on the

scored side. Supplied in bottles of 100 (NDC 0086-0031-10) and 500 (NDC 0086-0031-50).
200 mg—White, dye-free, oval-shaped, bisected, extended-release tablets inscribed with "C" on one side and "8632" on the scored side. Supplied in bottles of 100 (NDC 0086-0032-10), 500 (NDC 0086-0032-50) and 1,000 (NDC 0086-0032-90).
300 mg—White, dye-free, capsule-shaped, bisected, extended-release tablets inscribed with "C" on one side and "8633" on the scored side. Supplied in bottles of 100 (NDC 0086-0033-10), 500 (NDC 0086-0033-50) and 1,000 (NDC 0086-0033-90).
Dispense in a well-closed container as defined in the USP.
Store at controlled room temperature 15°–30°C (59°–86°F).
CAUTION: Federal law prohibits dispensing without prescription.

Issued 6/93
Shown in Product Identification Guide, page 308

Centeon
1020 FIRST AVENUE
KING OF PRUSSIA, PA 19406-1310

Direct Inquiries to:
(610) 878-4000

Sales and Ordering:
Customer Support Center
1020 First Avenue
King of Prussia, PA 19406-1310
(800) 683-1288
FAX: (610) 878-4888

ALBUMINAR®-5
[al-byōō'mĭn-är]
Albumin (Human) U.S.P. 5%

℞

DESCRIPTION
Albumin (Human) 5%, ALBUMINAR®-5 is a sterile solution of albumin obtained from large pools of adult human venous plasma by low temperature controlled fractionation according to the Cohn process. It is heated at 60°C for 10 hours and stabilized with 0.004 M sodium acetyltryptophanate and 0.004 M sodium caprylate.
Each 50 mL bottle of 5% solution contains 2.5 grams of albumin in normal saline. Each 250 mL bottle of 5% solution contains 12.5 grams of albumin in normal saline. Each 500 mL bottle of 5% solution contains 25 grams of albumin in normal saline. Each 1000 mL bottle of 5% solution contains 50 grams of albumin in normal saline. The 5% solution is osmotically equivalent with citrated plasma. The pH of the solution is adjusted to 6.9 ± 0.5 with sodium bicarbonate, sodium hydroxide, or acetic acid. Approximate concentrations of significant electrolytes per liter are: Sodium 130–160 mEq; and Potassium—n.m.t. 1 mEq. The solution contains no preservative. This product has been prepared in accordance with the requirements established by the Food and Drug Administration and is in compliance with the standards of the United States Pharmacopeia.
Albumin (Human) 5%, ALBUMINAR®-5, is to be administered by the intravenous route.

CLINICAL PHARMACOLOGY
Albumin (Human) 5%, ALBUMINAR®-5, being active osmotically, is useful in regulating the volume of circulating blood. It is a valuable therapeutic aid for the treatment of conditions that will be benefited by its marked osmotic effect. When the circulating blood volume has been depleted, the hemodilution following albumin administration persists for many hours. In individuals with normal blood volume, it usually lasts only a few hours.
Albumin (Human), unlike whole blood or plasma, is considered free of the danger of viral hepatitis because it is heated at 60 °C for 10 hours. It is convenient to use since no cross-matching is required and the absence of cellular elements removes the danger of sensitization with repeated infusions.

INDICATIONS AND USAGE
Shock—Albumin (Human) 5% is indicated in the emergency treatment of shock due to burns, trauma, operations and infections, in the treatment of severe injuries, and in other similar conditions where the restoration of blood volume is urgent. The primary function is maintenance of colloid osmotic pressure. If there has been considerable loss of red blood cells, transfusion with whole blood is indicated.
Burns—Albumin (Human) 5% is indicated in conjunction with adequate infusions of crystalloid to counteract hemoconcentration and the loss of protein, electrolytes and water that usually follow severe burns. Because of changes in per-

Continued on next page

Centeon—Cont.

meability, little administered albumin is likely to be retained intravenously in the first 12 hours after a major burn. However, an optimum regimen for the use of colloid, electrolytes and water in the treatment of burns has not been established.

Hypoproteinemia—Albumin (Human) 5%, ALBUMINAR®-5 may be used in acutely hypoproteinemic patients, provided sodium restriction is not a problem.

CONTRAINDICATIONS

Albumin (Human) 5%, ALBUMINAR®-5 is contraindicated in patients with severe anemia or cardiac failure and in patients with a history of allergic reactions to human albumin.

WARNINGS

Do not use if the solution is turbid or if there is a sediment in the bottle. Since the product contains no antimicrobial preservative, do not begin administration more than 4 hours after the container has been entered. Destroy unused portions to prevent the possibility of subsequent use of a solution that may have become contaminated.

PRECAUTIONS

GENERAL—Administration of large quantities of albumin should be supplemented with red blood cells or replaced by whole blood to combat the relative anemia which would follow such use. The quick response of blood pressure, which may follow the rapid administration of albumin, necessitates careful observation of the injured patient to detect bleeding points which failed to bleed at lower blood pressure. Albumin (Human) 5%, ALBUMINAR®-5 should be administered with caution to patients with low cardiac reserve or with no albumin deficiency because a rapid increase in plasma volume may cause circulatory embarrassment or pulmonary edema.

PREGNANCY CATEGORY C—Animal reproduction studies have not been conducted with Albumin (Human) 5%, ALBUMINAR®-5. It is also not known whether ALBUMINAR®-5 can cause fetal harm when administered to a pregnant woman or can affect reproduction capacity. ALBUMINAR®-5 should be given to a pregnant woman only if clearly needed.

ADVERSE REACTIONS

The incidence of untoward reactions to Albumin (Human) 5% is low although nausea, vomiting, increased salivation, chills and febrile reactions occasionally may occur. Urticaria and skin rash have been reported following administration of albumin.

DOSAGE AND ADMINISTRATION

Albumin (Human) 5%, ALBUMINAR®-5 may be given intravenously without further dilution. This concentration is approximately isotonic and iso-osmotic with citrated plasma. Albumin (Human) in this concentration provides additional fluid for plasma volume expansion. Therefore, when it is administered to patients with normal blood volume, the rate of infusion should be slow enough to prevent too rapid expansion of plasma volume.

In the treatment of shock in an adult patient an initial dose of 500 mL of the 5% albumin solution is given as rapidly as tolerated. If response within 30 minutes is inadequate, an additional 500 mL of 5% albumin solution may be given. The 50 mL dosage form would be appropriate for pediatric use, with a dose of 10-20 mL per Kg of body weight infused intravenously at a rate up to 5-10 mL per minute. Therapy should be guided by the clinical response, blood pressure and an assessment of relative anemia. If more than 1000 mL are given, or if hemorrhage has occurred, the administration of Whole Blood or Red Blood Cells may be desirable.

In severe burns, immediate therapy should include large volumes of crystalloid with lesser amounts of 5% albumin solution to maintain an adequate plasma volume. After the first 24 hours, the ratio of albumin to crystalloid may be increased to establish and maintain a plasma albumin level of about 2.5 g/100 mL or a total serum protein level of about 5.2 g/100 mL. However, an optimal regimen for the use of colloids, electrolytes and water after severe burns has not been established.

The infusion of Albumin (Human) as a nutrient in the treatment of chronic hypoproteinemia is not recommended. In acute hypoproteinemia 5% albumin may be used in replacing the protein lost in hypoproteinemic conditions. However, if edema is present or if large amounts of albumin are lost, Albumin (Human) 25% is preferred because of the greater amount of protein in the concentrated solution.

Parenteral drug products should be inspected visually for particulate matter and discoloration prior to administration, whenever solution and container permit.

HOW SUPPLIED

Albumin (Human) 5%, ALBUMINAR®-5 is supplied as a 5% solution in:

NDC 0053-7670-06 50 mL bottles containing 2.5 grams of albumin,

NDC 0053-7670-01 250 mL bottles containing 12.5 grams of albumin,

NDC 0053-7670-02 500 mL bottles containing 25.0 grams of albumin,

NDC 0053-7670-03 1000 mL bottles containing 50.0 grams of albumin.

Store at controlled room temperature—between 15°-30°C (59°-86°F).

CAUTION: FEDERAL (U.S.A.) LAW PROHIBITS DISPENSING WITHOUT PRESCRIPTION.

REFERENCES

1. Finlayson, J.S.: Albumin Products. Seminars in Thrombosis and Hemostasis 6:85–120, 1980.
2. Tullis, J.L.: Albumin. JAMA 237: 355–360 and 460–463, 1977.
3. Rudolph, A.M.: *Pediatrics.* 18th ED., p. 1839, Appleton and Lange, 1987.

Revised: May, 1996 (2/93) IBM 12602

Centeon L.L.C.
Kankakee, Illinois 60901, U.S.A.
U.S. Government License No. 149

ALBUMINAR®-25 ℞

[*ăl-byōō'mĭn-är"*]

Albumin (Human) U.S.P. 25%

DESCRIPTION

Albumin (Human) 25%, ALBUMINAR®-25 is a sterile aqueous solution of albumin obtained from large pools of adult human plasma by low temperature controlled fractionation according to the Cohn process. It is stabilized with 0.02 M sodium acetyltryptophanate and 0.02 M sodium caprylate and pasteurized at 60°C for 10 hours.

Albumin (Human) 25%, ALBUMINAR®-25 is a solution containing in each 100 mL, 25 grams of serum albumin, osmotically equivalent to 500 mL of normal human plasma. The pH of the solution is adjusted with sodium bicarbonate, sodium hydroxide, or acetic acid. Approximate concentrations of significant electrolytes per liter are: sodium 130–160 mEq; and potassium—n.m.t. 1 mEq. The solution contains no preservative. This product has been prepared in accordance with the requirements established by the Food and Drug Administration and is in compliance with the standards of the United States Pharmacopeia.

Albumin (Human) 25%, ALBUMINAR®-25 is to be administered by the intravenous route.

CLINICAL PHARMACOLOGY

ALBUMINAR®-25 is active osmotically and is therefore important in regulating the volume of circulating blood. When injected intravenously, 50 mL of 25% albumin draws approximately 175 mL of additional fluid into the circulation within 15 minutes, except in the presence of marked dehydration. This extra fluid reduces hemoconcentration and blood viscosity. The degree of volume expansion is dependent on the initial blood volume. When the circulating blood volume has been depleted, the hemodilution following albumin administration persists for many hours. In individuals with normal blood volume, it usually lasts only a few hours.

Albumin, unlike whole blood or plasma, is considered free of the danger of homologous serum hepatitis. Albumin (Human) 25%, ALBUMINAR®-25 may be given in conjunction with other parenteral fluids—such as saline, glucose or sodium lactate. It is convenient to use since no crossmatching is required and the absence of cellular elements removes the danger of sensitization with repeated infusions.

INDICATIONS AND USAGE

Shock—Albumin is indicated in the emergency treatment of shock and in other similar conditions where the restoration of blood volume is urgent. If there has been considerable loss of red blood cells, transfusion with whole blood is indicated.

Burns—Albumin or Albumin in either normal saline or glucose is indicated to prevent marked hemoconcentration and to maintain appropriate electrolyte balance.

Hypoproteinemia with or without edema—Albumin is indicated in those clinical situations usually associated with a low concentration of plasma protein and a resulting decreased circulating blood volume. Although diuresis may occur soon after albumin administration has been instituted, best results are obtained if albumin is continued until the normal serum protein level is regained.

CONTRAINDICATIONS

Albumin (Human) 25%, ALBUMINAR®-25 may be contraindicated in patients with severe anemia or cardiac failure.

WARNING

Do not use if the solution is turbid. Since this product contains no antimicrobial preservative, do not begin administration more than 4 hours after the container has been entered.

PRECAUTIONS

General

If dehydration is present additional fluids must accompany or follow the administration of albumin. Administration of large quantities of albumin should be supplemented with or replaced by whole blood to combat the relative anemia which would follow such use. The quick response of blood pressure which may follow the rapid administration of concentrated albumin necessitates careful observation of the injured patient to detect bleeding points which failed to bleed at lower blood pressure. Albumin (Human) 25% should be administered with caution to patients with low cardiac reserve or with no albumin deficiency because a rapid increase in plasma volume may cause circulatory embarrassment or pulmonary edema. In cases of hypertension, a slower rate of administration is desired—200 mL of albumin solution may be mixed with 300 mL of 10% glucose solution and administered at a rate of 10 grams of albumin (100 mL) per hour.

Pregnancy Category C

Animal reproduction studies have not been conducted with Albumin (Human) 25%, ALBUMINAR®-25. It is also not known whether ALBUMINAR®-25 can cause fetal harm when administered to a pregnant woman or can affect reproduction capacity. ALBUMINAR®-25 should be given to a pregnant woman only if clearly needed.

ADVERSE REACTIONS

The incidence of untoward reactions to Albumin (Human) 25% is low although nausea, vomiting, increased salivation and febrile reactions occasionally may occur.

DOSAGE AND ADMINISTRATION

Albumin (Human) 25%, ALBUMINAR®-25 may be given intravenously without dilution or it may be diluted with normal saline or 5% glucose before administration. Two hundred mL per liter gives a solution which is approximately isotonic and iso-osmotic with citrated plasma.

When undiluted albumin solution is administered in patients with normal blood volume, the rate of infusion should be slow enough (1 mL per minute) to prevent too rapid expansion of plasma volume.

In the treatment of shock the amount of albumin and duration of therapy must be based on the responsiveness of the patient as indicated by blood pressure, degree of pulmonary congestion, and hematocrit. The initial dose may be followed by additional albumin within 15–30 minutes if the response is deemed inadequate. If there is continued loss of protein, it also may be desirable to give whole blood and/or other blood fractions.

In the treatment of burns an optimal regimen involving use of albumin, crystalloids, electrolytes and water has not been established. Suggested therapy during the first 24 hours includes administration of large volumes of crystalloid solution to maintain an adequate plasma volume. Continuation of therapy beyond 24 hours usually requires more albumin and less crystalloid solution to prevent marked hemoconcentration and maintain electrolyte balance.

Duration of treatment varies depending upon the extent of protein loss through renal excretion, denuded areas of skin and decreased albumin synthesis. Attempts to raise the albumin level above 4.0 g/100 mL may only result in an increased rate of catabolism.

In the treatment of hypoproteinemia, 200 to 300 mL of 25% albumin may be required to reduce edema and to bring serum protein values to normal. Since such patients usually have approximately normal blood volume, doses of more than 100 mL of 25% albumin should not be given faster than 100 mL in 30 to 45 minutes to avoid circulatory embarrassment. If slower administration is desired, 200 mL of 25% albumin may be mixed with 300 mL of 10% glucose solution and administered by continuous drip at a rate of 100 mL of this glucose solution an hour.

Parenteral drug products should be inspected visually for particulate matter and discoloration prior to administration, whenever solution and container permit.

HOW SUPPLIED

Albumin (Human), ALBUMINAR®-25 is supplied as a 25% solution in:

NDC 0053-7680-01 20 mL vials containing 5.0 grams of albumin

NDC 0053-7680-02 50 mL vials containing 12.5 grams of albumin

NDC 0053-7680-03 100 mL vials containing 25.0 grams of albumin

Store at controlled room temperature—between 15°-30°C (59°-86°F).
Caution: Federal (U.S.A.) law prohibits dispensing without prescription

Revised: May, 1996 (10/90) IBM 12522

Centeon L.L.C.
Kankakee, Illinois 60901, U.S.A.
U.S. Government License 149

Antihemophilic Factor (Recombinant) ℞
BIOCLATE™
[*Bī′·ō·clāte*]

DESCRIPTION

Antihemophilic Factor (Recombinant), Bioclate™ is a glycoprotein synthesized by a genetically engineered Chinese Hamster Ovary (CHO) cell line. In culture the CHO cell line secretes recombinant antihemophilic factor (rAHF) into the cell culture medium. The rAHF is purified from the culture medium utilizing a series of chromatography columns. A key step in the purification process is an immunoaffinity chromatography methodology in which a purification matrix prepared by immobilization of a monoclonal antibody directed to factor VIII is utilized to selectively isolate the rAHF in the medium. The rAHF produced has the same biological effects as Antihemophilic Factor (Human) [AHF (Human)] and structurally has a similar combination of heterogeneous heavy and light chains as found in AHF (Human).

Bioclate™ is formulated as a sterile, nonpyrogenic, off-white to faint yellow, lyophilized powder preparation of concentrated recombinant AHF for intravenous injection and is available in single-dose bottles which contain nominally 250, 500 and 1000 International Units per bottle. When reconstituted with the appropriate volume of diluent, it contains the following stabilizers in maximum amounts: 12.5 mg/mL Albumin (Human), 1.5 mg/mL polyethylene glycol (3350), 180 mEq/L sodium, 55 mM histidine, 1.5 μg/AHF International Unit (IU) polysorbate-80 and 0.20 mg/mL calcium. Von Willebrand Factor (vWF) is coexpressed with the Antihemophilic Factor (Recombinant) and helps to stabilize it. The final product contains not more than 2 ng vWF/IU rAHF which will not have any clinically relevant effect in patients with von Willebrand's disease. The product contains no preservative.

Manufacturing of Bioclate™ is shared by Baxter Healthcare Corporation, Hyland Division and Genetics Institute, Inc. Genetics Institute produces Antihemophilic Factor Concentrate (Recombinant) (For Further Manufacturing Use) which is then formulated and packaged at Baxter Healthcare Corporation, Hyland Division.

Each bottle of Bioclate™ is labeled with the AHF activity expressed in IU per bottle. Biological potency is determined by an *in vitro* assay which is referenced to the World Health Organization (WHO) International Standard for Factor VIII:C Concentrate.

CLINICAL PHARMACOLOGY

AHF is the specific clotting factor deficient in patients with hemophilia A (classical hemophilia). Hemophilia A is a genetic bleeding disorder characterized by hemorrhages which may occur spontaneously or after minor trauma. The administration of Bioclate™ provides an increase in plasma levels of AHF and can temporarily correct the coagulation defect in these patients.

Pharmacokinetic studies on sixty-six (66) patients revealed the circulating mean half-life for rAHF to be 14.4 ± 4.9 hours, which was not statistically significantly different from plasma-derived Antihemophilic Factor (Human), Hemofil®M, (pdAHF), which had a mean half-life of 14.0 ± 3.9 hours (n = 59). Mean highest *in vivo* recovery in plasma was also similar at 2.18 ± 0.72 (n = 19) IU/dL per IU/kg body weight compared to the mean highest recovery point above the pre-infusion baseline for Hemofil®M of 1.97 ± 0.66 (n = 57) IU/dL per IU/kg.

The clinical study of rAHF in previously treated patients (individuals with hemophilia A who had been treated with plasma derived AHF) was based on observations made on a study group of 67 patients. These individuals received 18,451 to 1,110,111 IU over the 58.2 month study period in 13,394 infusions for a total of 21,437,195 IU rAHF.

These patients were successfully treated for bleeding episodes on a demand basis and also for the prevention of bleeds (prophylaxis). Spontaneous bleeding episodes successfully managed include hemarthroses, soft tissue and muscle bleeds. Management of hemostatis was also evaluated in surgeries. A total of 24 procedures on 13 patients were performed during this study. These included minor (*e.g.* tooth extraction) and major (*e.g.* bilateral osteotomies, thoracotomy and liver transplant) procedures. Hemostasis was maintained perioperatively and postoperatively with individualized AHF replacement.

A study of rAHF in previously untreated patients was also performed. The study group comprised seventy-nine (79) patients of whom seventy-five (75) had received at least one infusion of rAHF. In total this cohort has been given 1,054 infusions totalling 437,126 IU rAHF. Hemostasis was appropriately managed in spontaneous bleeding episodes, intracranial hemorrhage and surgical procedures.

INDICATIONS AND USAGE

The use of Antihemophilic Factor (Recombinant), Bioclate™ is indicated in hemophilia A (classical hemophilia) for the prevention and control of hemorrhagic episodes.[1] Bioclate™ is also indicated in the perioperative management of patients with hemophilia A (classical hemophilia).

Bioclate™ can be of significant therapeutic value in patients with acquired AHF inhibitors not exceeding 10 Bethesda Units per mL.[2] In clinical studies with Bioclate™, patients with inhibitors who were entered into the previously treated patient trial and those previously untreated children who have developed inhibitor activity on study, showed clinical hemostatic response when the titer of inhibitor was less than 10 Bethesda Units per mL. However, in such uses, the dosage of Bioclate™ should be controlled by frequent laboratory determinations of circulating AHF levels.

Bioclate™ is not indicated in von Willebrand's disease.

CONTRAINDICATIONS

Known hypersensitivity to mouse, hamster or bovine protein may be a contraindication to the use of Antihemophilic Factor (Recombinant) (see **PRECAUTIONS**).

WARNINGS

None.

PRECAUTIONS

General

Identification of the clotting defect as a Factor VIII deficiency is essential before the administration of Antihemophilic Factor (Recombinant), Bioclate™ is initiated. No benefit may be expected from this product in treating other deficiencies.

The formation of neutralizing antibodies, inhibitors, to factor VIII is a known complication in the management of individuals with hemophilia A. The reported prevalence of these antibodies in patients receiving plasma derived AHF is 10-20%[3,4,5,6,7,10,11,12]. These inhibitors are invariably IgG immunoglobulins, the factor VIII procoagulant inhibitory activity of which is expressed as Bethesda Units (B.U.) per mL of plasma or serum[3,4,5,6,7]. Over the investigational period, none of the 65 previously treated individuals, without an inhibitor at entry into the study, developed an inhibitor. In the previously untreated patient group there were 66 patients with factor VIII levels less than or equal to 2% who were tested for inhibitor after treatment with Bioclate™ rAHF. Of this group 12 individuals developed detectable inhibitor and of these, 3 patients showed a titer greater than 10 B.U. The true immunogenicity of Antihemophilic Factor (Recombinam). Bioclate™ is uncertain at this time. Patients treated with rAHF should be carefully monitored for the development of antibodies to rAHF by appropriate clinical observations and laboratory tests.

Formation of Antibodies to Mouse, Hamster or Bovine Protein

As Antihemophilic Factor (Recombinant), Bioclate™ contains trace amounts of mouse protein (maximum of 0.1 ng/IU rAHF), hamster protein (maximum of 1 ng CHO protein/IU rAHF), and bovine protein maximum of 1 ng BSA/IU rAHF), the remote possibility exists that patients treated with this product may develop hypersensitivity to these non-human mammalian proteins.

Information for Patients

Although allergic type hypersensitivity reactions were not observed in any patient receiving Bioclate™ on study, such reactions are theoretically possible. Patients should be informed of the early signs of hypersensitivity reactions including hives, generalized urticaria, tightness of the chest, wheezing, hypotension, and anaphylaxis. Patients should be advised to discontinue use of the product and contact their physician if these symptoms occur.

Laboratory Tests

Although dosage can be estimated by the calculations which follow, it is strongly recommended that whenever possible, appropriate laboratory tests be performed on the patient's plasma at suitable intervals to assure that adequate AHF levels have been reached and are maintained.

If the patient's plasma AHF fails to reach expected levels or if bleeding is not controlled after adequate dosage, the presence of inhibitor should be suspected. By performing appropriate laboratory procedures, the presence of an inhibitor can be demonstrated and quantified in terms of AHF International Units neutralized by each mL of plasma or by the total estimated plasma volume. If the inhibitor is present at levels less than 10 Bethesda Units per mL, administration of additional AHF may neutralize the inhibitor. Thereafter the administration of additional AHF International Units should elicit the predicted response. The control of AHF levels by laboratory assay is necessary in this situation.

Inhibitor titers above 10 Bethesda Units per mL may make hemostasis control with AHF either impossible or impractical because of the very large dose required. In addition, the inhibitor titer may rise following AHF infusion because of an anamnestic response to the AHF antigen.

Carcinogenesis, Mutagenesis, Impairment of Fertility

Bioclate™ was tested for mutagenicity at doses considerably exceeding plasma concentrations of rAHF *in vitro* and at doses up to ten times the expected maximum clinical dose *in vivo*, and did not cause reverse mutations, chromosomal aberrations, or an increase in micronuclei in bone marrow polychromatic erythrocytes. Long term studies in animals have not been performed to evaluate carcinogenic potential.

Pediatric Use

Bioclate™ is appropriate for use in children of all ages, including the newborn. Safety and efficacy studies have been performed in both previously treated (n = 23) and previously untreated (n = 75) children. (See **CLINICAL PHARMACOLOGY** and **PRECAUTIONS**).

Pregnancy

Pregnancy Category C. Animal reproduction studies have not been conducted with Antihemophilic Factor (Recombinant). It is not known whether Antihemophilic Factor (Recombinant) can cause fetal harm when administered to a pregnant woman or can affect reproductive capacity. Antihemophilic Factor (Recombinant) should be given to a pregnant woman only if clearly needed.

ADVERSE REACTIONS

During the clinical studies conducted in the previously treated patient group, there were 13 infusion related minor adverse reactions reported out of 13,394 infusions (0.097%). One patient experienced flushing and nausea during his first infusion which abated on decreasing the infusion rate. A second patient experienced mild fatigue during and following one infusion and the third patient had a series of eleven nose bleeds with a periodicity associated with the infusions.

The protein in greatest concentration in Antihemophilic Factor (Recombinant) Bioclate™ is Albumin (Human). Reactions associated with intravenous administration of albumin are extremely rare, although nausea, fever, chills or urticaria have been reported. Other allergic reactions could theoretically be encountered in the use of this Antihemophilic Factor preparation. See **Information for Patients.**

DOSAGE AND ADMINISTRATION

Each bottle of Bioclate™ is labeled with the AHF activity expressed in IU per bottle. This potency assignment is referenced to the World Health Organization International Standard for Factor VIII:C Concentrate. The high purity of Bioclate™ has been thought to influence the difficulty of producing an accurate potency measurement *in vitro*. Experiments have shown that, to achieve accurate activity levels, such a potency assay should be conducted using plastic test tubes and pipets as well as substrate containing normal levels of von Willebrand Factor.

The expected *in vivo* peak increase in AHF level expressed as IU/dL of plasma or % (percent) of normal can be estimated by multiplying the dose administered per kg body weight (IU/kg) by two. This calculation is based on the clinical findings of Abildgaard *el al*[8] and is supported by the data generated by 419 clinical pharmacokinetic studies with rAHF in 67 patients over time. This pharmacokinetic data demonstrated a peak recovery point above the pre-infusion baseline of approximately 2.0 IU/dL per IU/kg body weight.

Example (Assuming patient's baseline AHF level is at < 1%):

(1) A dose of 1750 IU AHF administered to a 70 kg patient, *i.e.* 25 IU/kg (1750/70), should be expected to cause a peak postinfusion AHF increase of 25 × 2 = 50 IU/dL (50% of normal).

(2) A peak level of 70% is required in a 40 kg child. In this situation the dose would be 70/2 × 40 = 1400 IU.

Physician supervision of the dosage is required. The following dosage schedule may be used as a guide.

[See table on top of next page.]

The careful control of the substitution therapy is especially important in cases of major surgery or life threatening hemorrhages.

Although dosage can be estimated by the calculations above, it is strongly recommended that whenever possible, appropriate laboratory tests including serial AHF assays be performed on the patient's plasma at suitable intervals to assure that adequate AHF levels have been reached and are maintained.

Other dosage regimens have been proposed such as that of Schimpf, *et al*, which describes continuous maintenance therapy.[9]

Reconstitution: Use Aseptic Technique

1. Bring Antihemophilic Factor (Recombinant). Bioclate™, (dry concentrate) and Sterile Water for Injection, USP, (diluent) to room temperature.
2. Remove caps from concentrate and diluent bottles to expose central portion of rubber stoppers.
3. Cleanse stoppers with germicidal solution and allow to dry prior to use.
4. Remove protective covering from one end of double-ended needle and insert exposed needle through diluent stopper.
5. Remove protective covering from other end of double-ended needle. Invert diluent bottle over the upright Bioclate™ bottle, then rapidly insert free end of the needle through the Bioclate™ bottle stopper at its center. The vacuum in the bottle will draw in the diluent.
6. Disconnect the two bottles by removing needle from diluent bottle stopper, then remove needle from Bioclate™ bottle. Swirl gently until all material is dissolved. Be sure

Continued on next page

Centeon—Cont.

Hemorrhage

Degree of hemorrhage	Required peak post-infusion AHF activity in the blood (as % of normal or IU/dL plasma)	Frequency of infusion
Early hemarthrosis or muscle bleed or oral bleed	20–40	Begin infusion every 12 to 24 hours for one–three days until the bleeding episode as indicated by pain is resolved or healing is achieved.
More extensive hemarthrosis, muscle bleed, or hematoma	30–60	Repeat infusion every 12 to 24 hours for usually three days or more until pain and disability are resolved.
Life threatening bleeds such as head injury, throat bleed, severe abdominal pain	60–100	Repeat infusion every 8 to 24 hours until threat is resolved.

Surgery

Type of operation		
Minor surgery, including tooth extraction	60–80	A single infusion plus oral antifibrinolytic therapy within one hour is sufficient in approximately 70% of cases.
Major Surgery	80–100 (pre- and post-operative)	Repeat infusion every 8 to 24 hours depending on state of healing.

that Bioclate™ is completely dissolved, otherwise active material will be removed by the filter.

NOTE: Do not refrigerate after reconstitution. See **Administration.**

Administration: Use Aseptic Technique

Administer at room temperature. Bioclate™ should be administered not more than 3 hours after reconstitution.

Intravenous Syringe Injection

Parenteral drug products should be inspected for particulate matter and discoloration prior to administration, whenever solution and container permit. A colorless to faint yellow appearance is acceptable for Antihemophilic Factor (Recombinant), Bioclate™.

Plastic syringes are recommended for use with this product since proteins such as AHF tend to stick to the ground-glass surface of all-glass syringes.

1. Attach filter needle to a disposable syringe and draw back plunger to admit air into syringe.
2. Insert needle into reconstituted Bioclate™.
3. Inject air into bottle and then withdraw the reconstituted material into the syringe.
4. Remove and discard the filter needle from the syringe; attach a suitable needle and inject intravenously as instructed under **Rate of Administration.**
5. If a patient is to receive more than one bottle of Bioclate™, the contents of multiple bottles may be drawn into the same syringe by drawing up each bottle through a separate unused filter needle. This practice lessens the loss of Bioclate™. Please note, filter needles are intended to filter the contents of a single bottle of Bioclate™ only.

Rate of Administration

Preparations of Bioclate™ can be administered at a rate of up to 10 mL per minute with no significant reactions. The pulse rate should be determined before and during administration of Bioclate™. Should a significant increase in pulse rate occur, reducing the rate of administration or temporarily halting the injection usually allows the symptoms to disappear promptly.

HOW SUPPLIED

Antihemophilic Factor (Recombinant), Bioclate™ is available in single-dose bottles which contain nominally 250, 500 and 1000 International Units per bottle. Bioclate™ is packaged with 10 mL of Sterile Water for Injection, USP, a double-ended needle, and a filter needle.

STORAGE

Bioclate™ can be stored under refrigeration [2–8°C (36–46°F)] or at room temperature, not to exceed 30°C (86°F). Avoid freezing to prevent damage to the diluent bottle. Do not use beyond the expiration date printed on the bottle.

REFERENCES

1. White GC, McMillan CW, Kingdon HS, *et al:* Use of recombinant antihemophilic factor in the treatment of two patients with classic hemophilia. **New Eng J Med** 320:166–170, 1989
2. Kessler CM: An Introduction to Factor VIII Inhibitors: The Detection and Quantitation. **Am. J Med 91 (Suppl 5A):** 1S-5S, 1991
3. Schwarzinger I, Pabinger I, Korninger C, Haschke F, Kundi M, Niessner H, Lechner K: Incidence of inhibitors in patients with severe and moderate hemophilia A treated with factor VIII concentrates. **Am J Hematology** 24:241–245, 1987
4. Penner JA, Kelly PE: Management of patients with factor VIII or IX inhibitors. **Sem Thromb Hemostasis** 1:386–399, 1975
5. Ehrenforth S, Kreuz W, Scharrer I, *et al:* Incidence of development of factor VIII and factor IX inhibitors in haemophiliacs. **Lancet 339:**594–598, 1992
6. McMillan CW, Shapiro SS, Whitehurst D, *et al:* The natural history of factor VIII inhibitors in patients with hemophilia A: a national cooperative study. II. Observations on the initial development of factor VIII:C inhibitors. **Blood 71:**344–348, 1988
7. Addiego JE Jr., Gomperts E, Liu S, *et al:* Treatment of hemophilia A with a highly purified factor VIII concentrate prepared by Anti-FVIIIc immunoaffinity chromatography. **Thrombosis and Haemostasis 67:**19–27, 1992
8. Abildgaard CF, Simone JV, Corrigan JJ, *et al:* Treatment of hemophilia with glycine-precipitated Factor VIII. **New Eng J Med 275:**471–475, 1966
9. Schimpf K, Rothmann P, Zimmermann K: Factor VIII dosis in prophylaxis of hemophilia A; A further controlled study, in **Proc Xlth Cong W.F.H.** Kyoto, Japan, Academic Press, 1976, pp 363–366
10. Gil FM: The Natural History of Factor VIII Inhibitors in Patients With Hemophilia A. Hoyer LW (ed), Factor VIII Inhibitors, **N.Y., AR Liss,** 1984, pp 19–29
11. Rasi V, Ikkala E: Haemophiliacs with factor VIII inhibitors in Finland: prevalence, incidence and outcome. **Br J Haematol 76:**369–371, 1990
12. Lusher, JM, Salzman PM: Viral Safety and Inhibitor Development Associated With Factor VIIIC Ultra-Purified From Plasma in Hemophiliacs Previously Unexposed to Factor VIIIC Concentrates. **Seminars in Hematology 27:**1–7, 1990

Manufactured by:

Baxter Healthcare Corporation
Hyland Division
Glendale, CA 91203 USA
U.S. License No. 140

Distributed by:

Centeon L.L.C.
Kankakee, Illinois 60901 USA

IMMUNE GLOBULIN INTRAVENOUS (HUMAN) GAMMAR®-P I.V.

$[găm' är]$

℞

DESCRIPTION

Immune Globulin Intravenous (Human), Gammar®-P I.V., is a sterile, lyophilized preparation of intact, unmodified, immunoglobulin, primarily IgG, stabilized with Albumin (Human) and sucrose. The distribution of IgG sub-classes is similar to that present in normal human plasma. It is prepared by cold alcohol fractionation of pooled plasma and is not chemically altered or enzymatically degraded. When reconstituted with the appropriate volume of Sterile Water for Injection USP, Gammar®-P I.V. contains 5% IgG, 3% Albumin (Human), 5% sucrose, and 0.5% sodium chloride. The pH of the solution has been adjusted to 6.8 ± 0.4 with citric acid and/or sodium carbonate. Gammar®-P I.V. contains no preservative. This product is intended for intravenous administration.

The heat treatment step employed in the manufacture of Immune Globulin Intravenous (Human), Gammar®-P I.V., pasteurization at 60 °C for 10 hours in aqueous solution form with stabilizers, has been validated in a series of *in vitro* experiments for its capacity to inactivate Human Immunodeficiency Virus (HIV) and the following model viruses: Sindbis, Vesicular Stomatitis (VSV), Bovine Viral Diarrhea Virus (BVD), Vaccinia, Pseudorabies and Murine Encephalomyocarditis (EMC), a non-lipid enveloped model virus. HIV was reduced by 6.0 and 5.4 $\log_{10}$ to an undetectable level after 0.5 hours of heating in two independent experiments. For each of the model viruses studied, two independent experiments were also conducted with the following results: Sindbis was reduced by 7.5 and 7.9 $\log_{10}$ to an undetectable level after two hours of heating, VSV was reduced by 6.8 and 7.2 $\log_{10}$ to an undetectable level after 0.5 hours of heating, BVD, a model for hepatitis C virus, was reduced by 6.4 and 6.5 $\log_{10}$ to an undetectable level after four hours of heating, Vaccinia was reduced by 5.6 and 5.6 $\log_{10}$ to an undetectable level after two hours of heating, Pseudorabies was reduced by 4.9 and 3.6 $\log_{10}$ to an undetectable level after six hours of heating and EMC, a non-lipid enveloped model virus, was reduced by 4.5 and 4.8 $\log_{10}$ after ten hours of heating.[1]

The viral reduction capacity of the purification procedures used in the manufacture of Immune Globulin Intravenous (Human), Gammar®-P I.V., exclusive of heat treatment, were also studied in a series of *in vitro* experiments using HIV and the model virus EMC, a non-lipid enveloped virus. EMC was reduced by 4.9 $\log_{10}$ and 3.4 $\log_{10}$ by two, independent purification steps which are conducted before and after heat treatment, respectively. HIV was reduced by at least 6.7 $\log_{10}$ by the processing steps employed to isolate Cohn Fraction II from pooled plasma during the initial purification of Gammar®-P I.V. The total viral reduction capacity for HIV and EMC attributable to the Gammar®-P I.V. manufacturing procedure, inclusive of both the heat treatment protocol and the fractionation steps studied, is, therefore, $\geq 12.1 \log_{10}$ for HIV and $\geq 12.8 \log_{10}$ for EMC.[1]

CLINICAL PHARMACOLOGY

The half-life of Immune Globulin Intravenous (Human), Gammar®-P I.V., was evaluated in a double blind clinical study in which it was compared to Gammar® I.V. The mean half-life of Gammar®-P I.V. in nine patients was determined to be approximately 40 days and was not statistically different from the mean half-life of 34 days found for Gammar® I.V. in seven patients; however, the half-life of IgG can vary considerably from patient to patient.[1]

Immune Globulin Intravenous (Human), Gammar®-P I.V., is a native, nonchemically modified IgG fractionated from pooled human donor plasma. The distribution of IgG subclasses $(IgG_1, IgG_2, IgG_3, IgG_4)$ is similar to that present in Cohn Fraction II. Since the IgG concentrate is prepared from a large pool of at least 1000 donors, it represents the expected diversity of antibodies in that population. In a study of an unheated version of this product, Gammar® I.V., it was found that Gammar® I.V. provided a broad range of antibodies, capable of opsonization and neutralization of microbes and toxins, against bacterial and viral antigens for prevention or attenuation of infectious diseases.[2] In *in vitro* testing, Gammar®-P I.V. has been shown to provide equivalent levels of a broad range of antibodies when compared to Gammar® I.V.[1]

Albumin (Human) and sucrose are added to the formulation in order to provide adequate stabilization of the IgG molecules and the reconstituted product. Because sucrose, when given intravenously, is excreted unchanged in the urine, Immune Globulin Intravenous (Human), Gammar®-P I.V., may be given to diabetics without compensatory changes in insulin dosage regimen.[3]

INDICATIONS AND USAGE

Gammar®-P I.V. is indicated for patients with primary defective antibody synthesis such as agammaglobulinemia or hypogammaglobulinemia, who are at increased risk of infection. When high levels or rapid elevation of circulating gamma globulins are desired, intravenous administration is more desirable than intramuscular therapy.

CONTRAINDICATIONS

Gammar®-P I.V. is contraindicated in individuals with a history of anaphylactic or severe systemic response to immune globulin intramuscular or intravenous preparations or in individuals with a history of allergic reactions to human albumin.

Immune Globulin Intravenous (Human), Gammar®-P I.V., should not be given to persons with isolated immunoglobulin A (IgA) deficiency. Such persons have the potential for devel-

oping antibodies to IgA and could have anaphylactic reactions to subsequent administration of blood products that contain IgA.[4]

WARNINGS

If anaphylactic or severe anaphylactoid reactions occur, discontinue infusion immediately. Epinephrine should be available for the treatment of any acute anaphylactoid reactions.

Patients with agammaglobulinemia or extreme hypogammaglobulinemia who have never received immunoglobulin substitution therapy before or who have not received immunoglobulin therapy within the preceding 8 weeks may be at risk of developing inflammatory reactions upon the infusion of human immunoglobulins. These reactions are manifested by a rise in temperature, chills, nausea and vomiting, and appear to be related to the rate of infusion.

Infusion rates and the patient's clinical state should be monitored closely during infusion. (See **Administration** section under **DOSAGE AND ADMINISTRATION**)

PRECAUTIONS

GENERAL – Epinephrine should be available for treatment of acute allergic reactions.

See **DOSAGE AND ADMINISTRATION** section for product compatibility information.

DRUG INTERACTIONS—It is reported that antibodies in immune globulin preparations may interfere with the response by pediatric patients to live viral vaccines such as measles, mumps and rubella. Immunizing physicians should be informed of recent therapy with Immune Globulin Intravenous (Human) so that appropriate precautions may be taken.

PREGNANCY CATEGORY C – Animal reproduction studies have not been performed with Immune Globulin Intravenous (Human), Gammar®-P I.V. It is also not known whether Immune Globulin Intravenous (Human), Gammar®-P.I.V. can cause fetal harm when administered to a pregnant woman or can affect reproduction capacity. Gammar®-P I.V. should be given to a pregnant woman only if clearly needed.

ASEPTIC MENINGITIS SYNDROME—An aseptic meningitis syndrome (AMS) has been reported to occur infrequently in association with Immune Globulin Intravenous (Human) (IGIV) treatment. The syndrome usually begins within several hours to two days following IGIV treatment. It is characterized by symptoms and signs including severe headache, nuchal rigidity, drowsiness, fever, photophobia, painful eye movements, and nausea and vomiting. Cerebrospinal fluid (CSF) studies are frequently positive with pleocytosis up to several thousand cells per cubic millimeter, predominantly from the granulocytic series, and elevated protein levels up to several hundred mg/dl. Patients exhibiting such symptoms and signs should receive a thorough neurological examination, including CSF studies, to rule out other causes of meningitis. AMS may occur more frequently in association with high dose (2 g/kg) IGIV treatment. Discontinuation of IGIV treatment has resulted in remission of AMS within several days without sequelae.[5-8]

ACUTE RENAL FAILURE—Recently, there have been several reports in the literature of patients who experienced acute renal failure after receiving Immune Globulin Intravenous (Human), particularly in patients with compromised renal function.[9]

ADVERSE REACTIONS

Potential reactions for all Immune Globulin Intravenous (Human) products are often related to infusion rate and may include: nausea, vomiting, abdominal cramps, chills, pyrexia, chest tightness, palpitations, tachycardia, blood pressure changes, edema, flushing, diaphoresis, acute renal failure, rash, erythema, pruritus, cyanosis, dizziness, headache, backache or other body aches, anxiety, wheezing (and other respiratory events), myalgia, shaking, fatigue, malaise and arthralgia, usually beginning within one hour of the start of the infusion.

A double blind study comparing Gammar® I.V. and Gammar®-P I.V. as replacement therapy was conducted in 19 patients (108 infusions) with primary defective antibody synthesis, such as common variable or X-linked hypogammaglobulinemia. The types of infusion related adverse reactions noted were similar in frequency and nature. For the ten patients receiving only Gammar®-P I.V. (56 infusions), all of the infusion related adverse reactions were characterized as mild and of short duration. These included the following most frequent reactions: Chills 8.9% (5/56), Headache 5.4% (3/56), and Pain: Back/Neck 3.6% (2/56). The overall incidence of infusions associated with an adverse reaction was 16% (9/56 infusions) for Gammar®-P I.V. which compared favorably to the overall incidence of infusions associated with an adverse reaction for Gammar® I.V (25%; 13/52 infusions).[1]

True anaphylactic reactions may occur in patients with a history of prior systemic allergic reactions or seizure following administration of human immunoglobulin preparations. Very rarely an anaphylactoid reaction may occur in patients with no prior history of severe allergic reactions to human immunoglobulin preparations. Patients previously sensitized to certain antigens, most commonly IgA, may be at risk of immediate anaphylactoid and hypersensitivity reactions.[4] Epinephrine should be available for the treatment of any acute anaphylactoid reaction. (See **WARNINGS and CONTRAINDICATIONS**)

Infusion rates and clinical state should be monitored closely during infusion. If an adverse reaction occurs, the infusion rate should be reduced or the infusion stopped until the symptoms have subsided. (See **DOSAGE AND ADMINISTRATION**)

DOSAGE AND ADMINISTRATION

The usual dose of Immune Globulin Intravenous (Human), Gammar®–P I.V., is directed toward restoration of the immune deficient patient's circulating IgG level to near-normal levels. Use of 200-400 mg/kg body weight every three to four weeks is recommended although some patients may require 600 mg/kg every three to four weeks. An initial loading dose of at least 200 mg/kg at more frequent intervals, proceeding to 200-600 mg/kg at three week intervals once a therapeutic plasma level has been established can be used. However, treatment must be individualized for each patient due to variation among patients in catabolic rate of IgG.

PRODUCT COMPATIBILITY – It is recommended that Immune Globulin Intravenous (Human), Gammar®–P I.V., be administered by a separate infusion line without admixture with other drugs or medications which the patient may be receiving. However, based upon compatibility studies, Gammar®–P I.V. may be infused sequentially into a primary I.V. line containing either 0.9% sodium chloride injection or 5% dextrose injection or flushed with 0.9% sodium chloride injection or 5% dextrose injection. **Do not mix Immune Globulin Intravenous (Human) products of differing formulations.** If several doses of Immune Globulin Intravenous (Human), Gammar®–P I.V. are to be administered, several reconstituted vials of identical formulation and diluent may be pooled, using proper aseptic technique. As described under **Reconstitution**, below, do not shake or cause excessive foaming. Swirl gently to mix. Filtration is acceptable but not required; pore sizes of greater than or equal to 15 microns will be less likely to slow infusion.

Reconstitution

Directions must be followed exactly.

Caution: The double-end, vented transfer spike included in this package is constructed with a plastic piercing pin (identified by the clear guard and having a double orifice) and a plastic needle (identified by the green guard and having a single orifice). The plastic piercing pin should be inserted into the diluent vial and the plastic needle into the product vial, as described below. Reference should be made to the diagram below.

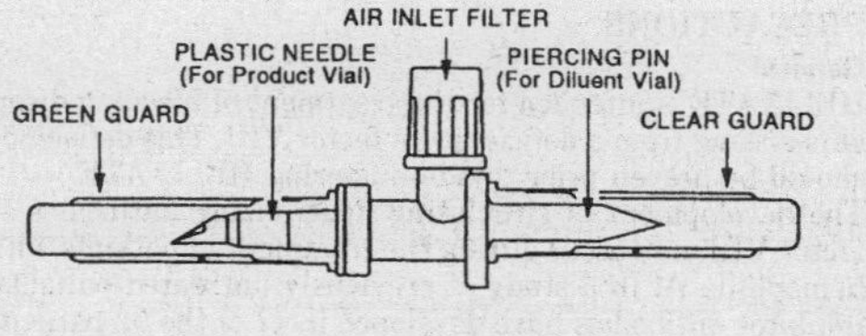

1) Bring diluent and lyophilized product vials to room temperature prior to reconstitution.
2) Remove plastic flip-off caps from both vials.
3) Treat rubber stoppers with antiseptic solution and allow to dry.
4) Remove the **clear** guard from the plastic piercing pin (with double orifice). Insert plastic piercing pin of the transfer spike into the upright **diluent** vial first.
5) Remove the **green** guard from the plastic needle (with single orifice). Invert the diluent vial with the attached transfer spike and insert plastic needle into the upright **product** vial.
6) The vacuum in the product vial will pull the diluent into the product vial. As soon as all diluent has been transferred the transfer spike will automatically admit filtered air to the product. An additional venting of the product vial after diluent addition is not necessary. Withdraw and discard transfer spike.
7) **Do not shake product vial.** Solubilize the product by continuous, gentle swirling in an upright position. Avoid the formation of foam.

   NOTE: If product cake is badly broken prior to addition of diluent, allow product vial to remain undisturbed for 2–3 minutes after addition of diluent **before** gently swirling to mix product.
8) Examine solution. Any small particles will dissolve with gentle swirling of vial. The solution should be clear and ready to administer in less than 20 minutes.
9) Product contains no preservative. Use within 3 hours of reconstitution.

   NOTE: If several doses of Immune Globulin Intravenous (Human), Gammar®–P I.V., are to be pooled aseptically for administration, avoid excessive formation of foam in the pooling container and gently swirl the pooling container to mix. DO NOT SHAKE THE POOLING CONTAINER.

Administration

CAUTION: When entering the product stopper with an IV set spike for administration, care should be taken to follow the path made by the plastic needle of the transfer spike (see **Reconstitution**).

Immune Globulin Intravenous (Human), Gammar®–P I.V., is to be administereds by intravenous infusion. The infusion should begin at a rate of 0.01 mL/kg/minute, increasing to 0.02 mL/kg/minute after 15 to 30 minutes. Most patients tolerate a gradual increase to 0.03–0.06 mL/kg/minute. For the average 70 kg person this is equivalent to 2 to 4 mL/minute. If adverse reactions develop, slowing the infusion rate will usually eliminate the reaction. Discard any unused solution.

Parenteral drug products should be inspected visually for particulate matter and discoloration prior to administration whenever solution and container permit.

HOW SUPPLIED

Individual Vial Packages

Immune Globulin Intravenous (Human), Gammar®–P I.V., is supplied in single dose vials, with diluent and sterile, vented transfer spike for reconstitution. The 10 g dosage form package also contains an administration set. The following dosage forms are available:

	Product	Diluent
NDC0053–7486–01	1.0 g immune globulin/vial	20 mL
NDC0053–7486–02	2.5 g immune globulin/vial	50 mL
NDC0053–7486–05	5.0 g immune globulin/vial	100 mL
NDC0053–7486–10	10.0 g immune globulin/vial	200 mL

Bulk Package

Immune Globulin Intravenous (Human), Gammar®–P I.V., 5.0 g immune globulin/vial is supplied in a bulk pack (NDC 0053–7486–06) of six (6) single dose vials. Each single dose vial should be reconstituted with 100 mL Sterile Water for Injection, U.S.P. (not supplied).

STORAGE

When stored at temperatures not exceeding 25°C (77°F), Immune Globulin Intravenous (Human), Gammar®–P I.V., is stable for the period indicated by the expiration date on its label. Avoid freezing which may damage container for the diluent.

CAUTION: FEDERAL (U.S.A.) LAW PROHIBITS DISPENSING WITHOUT PRESCRIPTION.

REFERENCES: 1. Data on File: Centeon L.L.C. **2.** Steele RW, Augustine RA, Tannenbaum AS, Marmer DJ. Intravenous Immune Globulin for Hypogammaglobulinaemia: A Comparison of Opsonizing Capacity in Recipient Sera. *Clin. Immunol. Immunopathol.* 1985; 34:275–283. **3.** Martindale. *The Extra Pharmacopoeia* 27th ed. Edited by Wade A. London: The Pharmaceutical Press. 1979; 65. **4.** Fudenberg HH. Sensitization to Immunoglobulins and Hazards of Gamma Globulin Therapy. *Immunoglobulins, Biologic Aspects and Clinical Uses.* 1970; 211–220. Edited by Merler E. National Academy of Sciences, Washington, D.C. **5.** Sekul EA, Cupler EJ, Dalakas MC. Aseptic Meningitis Associated with High Dose Intravenous Immunoglobulin Therapy: Frequency and Risk Factors. *Ann Int Med* 1994; 121:4, 259–262. **6.** Kato E, Shindo S, Eto Y, et al. Administration of Immune Globulin Associated with Aseptic Meningitis. *JAMA* 1988; 259:3269–3271. **7.** Casteels-Van Daele M, Wijndaele L, Hunninck K, Gillis P, Ziekenhuis V. Intravenous Immune Globulin and Acute Aseptic Meningitis. *N Engl J Med* 1990; 323:614–615. **8.** Scribner C, Kapit R, Phillips E, Rickels N. Aseptic Meningitis and Intravenous Immunoglobulin Therapy. *Ann Int Med* 1994; 121:305–306. **9.** Tan E, et al. Acute Renal Failure Resulting from Intravenous Immunoglobulin Therapy. *Arch Neurol.* 1993; 50(2):137–139.

BIBLIOGRAPHY: Polley MJ, Fischetti VA, Landaburu PH. Native Intravenous IgG Exhibits Greater Biological Activity than Modified IgG. From the *XX Cong. Int. Soc. of Hematology;* 1984.

Revised: May 1996 (9/95) IBM 12173
Centeon L.L.C.
Kankakee, Illinois 60901, U.S.A.
U.S. Government License No. 149

Antihemophilic Factor (Recombinant) ℞
HELIXATE®
[*hē"lĭxāté*]

DESCRIPTION

Antihemophilic Factor (Recombinant), HELIXATE® is a sterile, stable, purified, non-pyrogenic dried concentrate which has been manufactured by recombinant DNA technology. HELIXATE is intended for use in therapy of classical

Continued on next page

Centeon—Cont.

hemophilia (hemophilia A). HELIXATE is produced by Baby Hamster Kidney (BHK) cells into which the human factor VIII (FVIII) gene has been introduced.[1] HELIXATE is a highly purified glycoprotein consisting of multiple peptides including an 80 kD and various extensions of the 90 kD subunit. It has the same biological activity as FVIII derived from human plasma. In addition to the use of the classical purification methods of ion exchange chromatography and size exclusion chromatography, monoclonal antibody immunoaffinity chromatography is utilized along with other steps designed to purify recombinant factor VIII (rAHF) and remove contaminating substances. The final preparation is stabilized with Albumin (Human) and lyophilized. The concentration of HELIXATE is approximately 100 IU/mL. The product contains no preservatives.

Each vial of HELIXATE contains the labeled amount of rAHF in international units (IU). One IU, as defined by the World Health Organization standard for blood coagulation factor VIII, human, is approximately equal to the level of factor VIII activity found in 1.0 mL of fresh pooled human plasma. The final product when reconstituted as directed contains the following excipients: 10–30 mg glycine/mL, not more than (NMT) 500 μg imidazole/1000 IU, NMT 600 μg polysorbate 80/1000 IU, 2–5 mM calcium chloride, 100–130 mEq/L sodium, 100–130 mEq/L chloride and 4–10 mg Albumin (Human)/mL. HELIXATE must be administered by the intravenous route.

CLINICAL PHARMACOLOGY

The clinical trial of HELIXATE has included 168 patients, enrolled over a 55 month period. A total of 16,186 infusions have been utilized in this trial. The study was conducted in several stages.

Initial pharmacokinetic studies were conducted in 17 asymptomatic hemophilic patients, comparing pharmacokinetics of plasma-derived Antihemophilic Factor (Human) (pdAHF) and HELIXATE.[2] The mean biologic half-life of rAHF was 15.8 hours. The mean biologic half-life of pdAHF in the same individuals was 13.9 hours. A similar degree of shortening of the activated partial thromboplastin time was seen with both rAHF and pdAHF. The mean in vivo recovery of rAHF was similar to pdAHF, with a linear dose-response relationship. The recovery and half-life of rAHF was consistent with initial results following 13 weeks of exclusive treatment with HELIXATE. Subsequently, 826 recovery studies were conducted in 58 hemophilic patients participating in later clinical studies. Mean recovery from this group was 2.48% per IU/kg infused.

Fourteen (14) subjects from initial pharmacokinetic studies commenced home treatment with rAHF. Forty-four (44) additional subjects were then enrolled who treated themselves at home exclusively with rAHF. A total of 12,730 infusions have been administered under this portion of the study, of which 1,021 were given in clinic for recovery studies, 7,339 were given for treatment of bleeds, 4,361 were given as prophylaxis, 5 for minor surgery not requiring hospitalization, and 4 for unspecified reason.

Forty-eight (48) patients have received rAHF on 63 occasions for surgical procedures or in-hospital treatment of serious hemorrhage. Eleven (11) received rAHF for the first time in this study, while 37 were already on study or study participants under an investigation of previously untreated patients. Hemostasis has been satisfactory in all cases, with no adverse reactions.

In a study of previously untreated patients, a total of 3,254 infusions have been administered to 96 patients over a 48-month enrollment period. Hemostasis was successfully achieved in all cases.

During the analytical characterization of Antihemophilic Factor (Recombinant), HELIXATE®, analyses for carbohydrate structure revealed the presence of terminal galactose $\alpha 1 \rightarrow 3$ galactose residues. Since naturally occurring antibody to this structure has been reported in humans, a trial in 18 patients was performed in which the half-life and recovery of rAHF with high levels of this carbohydrate residue was compared to that with HELIXATE, which contains low levels of this stucture. As in the normal population, all patients had preexisting endogenous antibody to galactose $\alpha 1 \rightarrow 3$ galactose in liters ranging from 1:320 to 1:5120 and no significant change in antibody level was noted during the study. While the mean recovery for HELIXATE in the study, 2.76%/IU/kg (N=43), was significantly different from that of rAHF with high levels of residues, 2.43%/IU/kg (N=155; p=0.0001), the recovery for rAHF with high levels of galactose $\alpha 1 \rightarrow 3$ galactose is not significantly different from the 2.48%/IU/kg recovery obtained in the larger study from the 58 patients treated with HELIXATE mentioned above. Based on these results, the galactose $\alpha 1 \rightarrow 3$ galactose residue appears to have no clinical significance.

INDICATIONS AND USAGE

HELIXATE is indicated for the treatment of classical hemophilia (hemophilia A) in which there is a demonstrated deficiency of activity of the plasma clotting factor, factor VIII. HELIXATE provides a means of temporarily replacing the missing clotting factor in order to correct or prevent bleeding episodes, or in order to perform emergency and elective surgery in hemophiliacs.

HELIXATE can also be used for treatment of hemophilia A in certain patients with inhibitors to factor VIII. In clinical studies of HELIXATE, patients who developed inhibitors on study continued to manifest a clinical response when inhibitor titers were less than 10 Bethesda Units (B.U.) per mL. When an inhibitor is present, the dosage requirement for factor VIII is variable. The dosage can be determined only by clinical response, and by monitoring of circulating factor VIII levels after treatment (see **DOSAGE AND ADMINISTRATION**).

HELIXATE does not contain von Willebrand's factor and therefore is not indicated for the treatment of von Willebrand's disease.

CONTRAINDICATIONS

Due to the fact that Antihemophilic Factor (Recombinant) contains trace amounts of mouse protein (maximum 0.03 ng/IU rAHF) and hamster protein (maximum 0.04 ng/IU rAHF), HELIXATE should be administered with caution to individuals with previous hypersensitivity to pdAHF or known hypersensitivity to biologic preparations with trace amounts of murine or hamster proteins.

Assays to detect seroconversion to mouse and hamster protein were conducted on all patients on study. No patient has developed specific antibody titers against these proteins after commencing study, and no allergic reactions have been associated with rAHF infusions. Although no reactions were observed, patients should be warned of the theoretical possibility of a hypersensitivity reaction, and alerted to the early signs of such a reaction (e.g., hives, generalized urticaria, wheezing and hypotension). Patients should be advised to discontinue use of the product and contact their physician if such symptoms occur.

WARNINGS

None.

PRECAUTIONS

General

HELIXATE is intended for the treatment of bleeding disorders arising from a deficiency in factor VIII. This deficiency should be proven prior to administering HELIXATE.

The development of circulating neutralizing antibodies to factor VIII may occur during the treatment of patients with hemophilia A. In a study of previously untreated patients, inhibitor antibodies have developed in 17 of the 92 patients (18.5%) who have had at least one follow-up titer. The incidence of antibodies is 15/56 (26.7%) in patients with severe disease (<2% factor VIII), 2/18 (11%) in patients with moderate disease (2–5% factor VIII) and 0/18 in patients with mild disease (>5% factor VIII). Ten of the antibodies were high titer (>10 Bethesda Units), three were low titer, and four were low titer and transient. Studies most closely resembling the design of the study of inhibitor development with Antihemophilic Factor (Recombinant) HELIXATE® have reported incidences of inhibitor formation ranging between 18.4 and 52% for patients treated with pdAHF.[3-6] The incidence of inhibitor formation in previously untreated patients treated with HELIXATE appears to be consistent with that reported in the literature, however the true immunogenicity of HELIXATE is not known at present. Patients treated with rAHF should be carefully monitored for the development of antibodies to rAHF by appropriate clinical observation and laboratory tests. Product administration and handling of the infusion set and needles must be done with caution. Percutaneous puncture with a needle contaminated with blood can transmit infectious virus including HIV (AIDS) and hepatitis. Obtain immediate medical attention if injury occurs. Place needles in sharps container after single use. Discard all equipment including any reconstituted HELIXATE product in accordance with biohazard procedures.

Carcinogenesis, Mutagenesis, Impairment of Fertility

In vitro evaluation of the mutagenic potential of HELIXATE failed to demonstrate reverse mutation or chromosomal aberrations at doses substantially greater than the maximum expected clinical dose. In vivo evaluation of rAHF using doses ranging between 10 and 40 times the expected clinical maximum also indicated that HELIXATE does not possess a mutagenic potential. Long-term investigations of carcinogenic potential in animals have not been performed.

Pediatric Use

HELIXATE has been proven to be safe and efficacious in newborns and children while under investigation as previously treated (n=21) and previously untreated patients (n=96) (see **CLINICAL PHARMACOLOGY** and **PRECAUTIONS**).

Pregnancy Category C

Animal reproduction studies have not been conducted with HELIXATE. It is also not known whether HELIXATE can cause fetal harm when administered to a pregnant woman or can affect reproduction capacity. HELIXATE should be given to a pregnant woman only if clearly needed.

ADVERSE REACTIONS

During the clinical studies conducted in previously treated patients, 47 out of 12,932 infusions (0.36%) were associated with 58 reported minor adverse reactions. Of these, 19 reactions were local to the injection site (e.g., burning, pruritus, erythema); and 39 were systemic complaints (dizziness, nausea, chest discomfort, sore throat, cold feet, unusual taste in mouth, and slight decrease in blood pressure). In the study with previously untreated patients, 3,254 infusions have been associated with 11 minor adverse reactions (0.34%): two reports of erythema at the injection site, one of facial flushing related to the infusion, one report of diarrhea, two reports of nonspecific rash, two reports of fever, and three reports of emesis. No serious reactions have been reported, and all reactions have been self-limited.

DOSAGE AND ADMINISTRATION

Each bottle of HELIXATE has the rAHF content in international units per bottle stated on the label of the bottle. The reconstituted product must be administered intravenously by either direct syringe injection or drip infusion. The product must be administered within 3 hours after reconstitution.

General Approach to Treatment and Assessment of Treatment Efficacy

The dosages described below are presented as general guidance. It should be emphasized that the dosage of HELIXATE required for hemostasis must be individualized according to the needs of the patient, the severity of the deficiency, the severity of the hemorrhage, the presence of inhibitors, and the factor VIII level desired. It is often critical to follow the course of therapy with factor VIII level assays.

The clinical effect of HELIXATE is the most important element in evaluating the effectiveness of treatment. It may be necessary to administer more HELIXATE than would be estimated in order to attain satisfactory clinical results. If the calculated dose fails to attain the expected factor VIII levels, or if bleeding is not controlled after administration of the calculated dosage, the presence of a circulating inhibitor in the patient should be suspected. Its presence should be substantiated and the inhibitor level quantitated by appropriate laboratory tests. When an inhibitor is present, the dosage requirement for rAHF is extremely variable and the dosage can be determined only by the clinical response.

Some patients with low titer inhibitors (<10 B.U.) can be successfully treated with factor VIII without a resultant anamnestic rise in inhibitor titer.[7] Factor VIII levels and clinical response to treatment must be assessed to insure adequate response. Use of alternative treatment products, such as Factor IX Complex concentrates, Antihemophilic Factor (Porcine) or Anti-Inhibitor Coagulant Complex, may be necessary for patients with anamnestic responses to factor VIII treatment and/or high titer inhibitors.

Calculation of Dosage

The in vivo percent elevation in factor VIII level can be estimated by multiplying the dose of rAHF per kilogram of body weight (IU/kg) by 2%. This method of calculation is based on clinical findings by Abildgaard et al,[8] and is illustrated in the following examples:

[See table at left.]

$$\text{Expected \% factor VIII increase} = \frac{\text{\# units administered} \times 2\%/\text{IU/kg}}{\text{body weight (kg)}}$$

$$\text{Example for a 70 kg adult:} = \frac{1400 \text{ IU} \times 2\%/\text{IU/kg}}{70 \text{ kg}} = 40\%$$

or

$$\text{Dosage required (IU)} = \frac{\text{body weight (kg)} \times \text{desired \% factor VIII increase}}{2\%/\text{IU/kg}}$$

$$\text{Example for a 15 kg child:} = \frac{15 \text{ kg} \times 100\%}{2\%/\text{IU/kg}} = 750 \text{ IU required}$$

The dosage necessary to achieve hemostasis depends upon the type and severity of the bleeding episode, according to the following general guidelines:

Mild Hemorrhage

Mild superficial or early hemorrhages may respond to a single dose of 10 IU per kg,[9] leading to an in vivo rise of approximately 20% in the factor VIII level. Therapy need not be repeated unless there is evidence of further bleeding.

Moderate Hemorrhage

For more serious bleeding episodes (e.g., definite hemarthroses, known trauma), the factor VIII level should be raised to 30–50% by administering approximately 15–25 IU per kg. If further therapy is required, a repeat infusion can be given at 12–24 hours.[10]

Severe Hemorrhage

In patients with life-threatening bleeding or possible hemorrhage involving vital structures (e.g., central nervous system, retropharyngeal and retroperitoneal spaces, iliopsoas sheath), the factor VIII level should be raised to 80–100% of normal in order to achieve hemostasis. This may be achieved with an initial rAHF (Antihemophilic Factor (Recombinant), HELIXATE®) dose of 40–50 IU per kg and a maintenance dose of 20–25 IU per kg every 8–12 hours.[11,12]

Surgery

For major surgical procedures, the factor VIII level should be raised to approximately 100% by giving a preoperative dose of 50 IU/kg. The factor VIII level should be checked to assure that the expected level is achieved before the patient goes to surgery. In order to maintain hemostatic levels, repeat infusions may be necessary every 6 to 12 hours initially, and for a total of 10 to 14 days until healing is complete. The intensity of factor VIII replacement therapy required depends on the type of surgery and postoperative regimen employed. For minor surgical procedures, less intensive treatment schedules may provide adequate hemostasis.[11,12]

Prophylaxis

Factor VIII concentrates may also be administered on a regular schedule for prophylaxis of bleeding, as reported by Nilsson, et al.[13]

Reconstitution

Vacuum Transfer

1. Warm the unopened diluent and the concentrate to room temperature (NMT 37°C, 99°F).
2. After removing the plastic flip-top caps (Fig. A), aseptically cleanse the rubber stoppers of both bottles.
3. Remove the protective cover from the plastic transfer needle cartridge with tamper-proof seal and penetrate the stopper of the diluent bottle (Fig. B).
4. Remove the remaining portion of the plastic cartridge, invert the diluent bottle and penetrate the rubber seal on the concentrate bottle (Fig. C) with the needle at an angle.
   Alternate method of transferring sterile water: With a sterile needle and syringe, withdraw the appropriate volume of diluent and transfer to the bottle of lyophilized concentrate.
5. The vacuum will draw the diluent into the concentrate bottle. Hold the diluent bottle at an angle to the concentrate bottle in order to direct the jet of diluent against the wall of the concentrate bottle (Fig. C). Avoid excessive foaming.
6. After removing the diluent bottle and transfer needle (Fig. D). swirl continuously until completely dissolved (Fig. E).
7. After the concentrate powder is completely dissolved, withdraw solution into the syringe through the filter needle which is supplied in the package (Fig. F). Replace the filter needle with the administration set provided and inject intravenously.
8. If the same patient is to receive more than one bottle, the contents of two bottles may be drawn into the same syringe through a separate unused filter needle before attaching the vein needle.

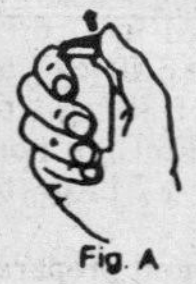

Fig. A

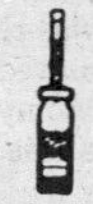

Fig. B

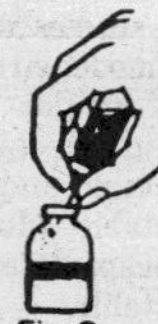

Fig. C

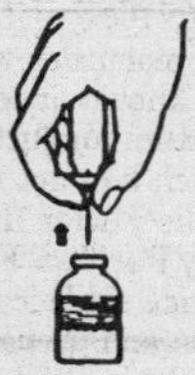

Fig. D

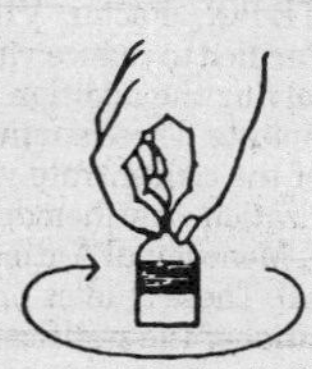

Fig. E

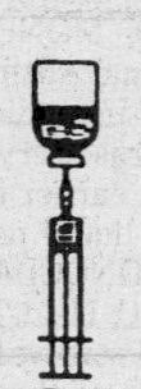

Fig. F

Rate of Administration

The rate of administration should be adapted to the response of the individual patient, but administration of the entire dose in 5 to 10 minutes or less is well tolerated.

Parenteral drug products should be inspected visually for particulate matter and discoloration prior to administration, whenever solution and container permit.

HOW SUPPLIED

Antihemophilic Factor (Recombinant), HELIXATE® is supplied in the following single use bottles with the total units of factor VIII activity stated on the label of each bottle. A suitable volume of Sterile Water for Injection, USP, a sterile double-ended transfer needle, a sterile filter needle, and a sterile administration set are provided.

Product Code	Approximate Factor VIII Activity	Diluent
NDC 0053-8120-01	250 IU	2.5 mL
NDC 0053-8120-02	500 IU	5 mL
NDC 0053-8120-04	1000 IU	10 mL

STORAGE

HELIXATE should be stored under refrigeration (2–8°C; 36–46°F). Storage of lyophilized powder at room temperature (up to 25°C or 77°F) for 3 months, such as in home treatment situations, may be done without loss of factor VIII activity. Freezing should be avoided, as breakage of the diluent bottle might occur. Do not use beyond the expiration date indicated on the bottle.

CAUTION

U.S. federal law prohibits dispensing without prescription.

LIMITED WARRANTY

A number of factors beyond our control could reduce the efficacy of this product or even result in an ill effect following its use. These include improper storage and handling of the product after it leaves our hands, diagnosis, dosage, method of administration, and biological differences in individual patients. Because of these factors, it is important that this product be stored properly, and that the directions be followed carefully during use.

No warranty, express or implied, including any warranty of merchantability or fitness is made. Representatives of the Company are not authorized to vary the terms or the contents of the printed labeling, including the package insert for this product, except by printed notice from the Company's headquarters. The prescriber and user of this product must accept the terms hereof.

REFERENCES

1. Lawn RM, Vehar GA: The molecular genetics of hemophilia. *Sci Am* 254(3): 48–54, 1986.
2. Schwartz RS, Abildgaard CF, Aledort LM, et al: Human recombinant DNA-derived antihemophilic factor (factor VIII) in the treatment of hemophilia A. *N Engl J Med* 323(26):1800–5, 1990.
3. Lusher JM: Viral safety and inhibitor development associated with monoclonal antibody-purified FVIIIc. *Ann Hematol* 63(3):138–41, 1991.
4. Addiego JE Jr, Gomperts E, Liu S-L, et al: Treatment of hemophilia A with a highly purified factor VIII concentrate prepared by anti-FVIIIc immunoaffinity chromatography. *Thromb Haemost* 67(1):19–27, 1992.
5. Schwarzinger I, Pabinger I, Korninger C, et al: Incidence of inhibitors in patients with severe and moderate hemophilia A treated with factor VIII concentrates. *Am J Hematol* 24(3):241–5, 1987.
6. Ehrenforth S, Kreuz W, Scharrer I, et al: Incidence of development of factor VIII and factor IX inhibitors in hemophiliacs. *Lancet* 339(8793):594–8, 1992.
7. Kasper CK: Complications of hemophilia A treatment: factor VIII inhibitors. *Ann NY Acad Sci* 614:97–105, 1991.
8. Abildgaard CF, Simone JV, Corrigan JJ, et al: Treatment of hemophilia with glycine-precipitated Factor VIII. *N Engl J Med* 275(9):471–5, 1966.
9. Britton M, Harrison J, Abildgaard CF: Early treatment of hemophilic hemarthroses with minimal dose of new factor VIII concentrate. *J Pediatr* 85(2):245–7, 1974.
10. Abildgaard CF: Current concepts in the management of hemophilia. *Semin Hematol* 12(3):223–32, 1975.
11. Hilgartner MW: Factor replacement therapy. In: Hilgartner MW, Pochedly C, eds.: Hemophilia in the child and adult. New York, Raven Press, 1989, pp 1–26.
12. Kasper CK, Dietrich SL: Comprehensive management of haemophilia. *Clin Haematol* 14(2):489–512, 1985.
13. Nilsson IM, Berntorp E, Lofqvist T, et al: Twenty-five years' experience of prophylactic treatment in severe haemophilia A and B. *J Intern Med* 232(1):25–32, 1992.

14–7670–214 (Rev. June 1996)

Manufactured by:
Bayer Corporation
Pharmaceutical Division
Elkhart, IN 46515, USA
U.S. License No. 8
Canadian License No. 24

Distributed by:
Centeon L.L.C.
Kankakee, Illinois 60901, USA

HUMATE-P™ ℞

[*hyōō'māt*]

Antihemophilic Factor (Human), Dried Pasteurized

DESCRIPTION

Antihemophilic Factor (Human), Pasteurized, Humate-P™ is a stable, purified, sterile, lyophilized concentrate of Antihemophilic Factor (Human) (Factor VIII, AHF) to be administered by the intravenous route in the treatment of patients with classical hemophilia (hemophilia A).

Humate-P™ is purified from the cold insoluble fraction of pooled human fresh-frozen plasma and contains highly purified and concentrated Antihemophilic Factor (Human). Humate-P™ has a high degree of purity with a low amount of non-factor VIII proteins and contains no fibrinogen (as detected by the Clauss method). Humate-P™ has a higher AHF potency than cryoprecipitate preparations. Each bottle of Humate-P™ contains the labeled amount of antihemophilic activity in international units. The Unit (IU) is defined by an international standard established by the World Health Organization: one AHF international unit is approximately equal to the level of AHF found in 1.0 mL of fresh-pooled human plasma.

Each 100 IU of Antihemophilic Factor (Human) contains 60 to 100 mg of glycine, 14 to 28 mg of sodium citrate, 8 to 16 mg of sodium chloride, 16 to 24 mg of albumin (human), 4 to 20 mg of other proteins and 20 to 44 mg of total proteins.

This product is prepared from pooled human plasma collected in the United States. Humate-P™ may also be prepared from source material supplied by other U.S. licensed manufacturers.

Antihemophilic Factor (Human), Pasteurized, Humate-P™ is pasteurized by a new procedure: heating to 60°C for 10 hours in aqueous solution form.[1] This procedure has been shown to inactivate several DNA viruses (cytomegalovirus, herpes, and hepatitis B) and RNA viruses (rubella, mumps, measles, and poliomyelitis). However, no procedure has been shown to be totally effective in removing hepatitis infectivity from Antihemophilic Factor (Human) (See Clinical Pharmacology and Warnings).

Humate-P™ contains anti-A and anti-B blood group isoagglutinins (see PRECAUTIONS).

CLINICAL PHARMACOLOGY

After I.V. injection in humans, there is a rapid increase in plasma Antihemophilic Factor followed by a rapid decrease in activity (time of equilibration with the extravascular compartment) and a subsequent slower rate of decrease in activity (biological half-life). Studies with Humate-P™ in hemophilic patients have demonstrated a mean initial half-disappearance time of 8 hours and a mean half-life of 12 hours.

Tests of infectivity on chimpanzees have confirmed the realiability of this pasteurization method in eliminating the risk of transmission of hepatitis B virus. Two chimpanzee studies were used to evaluate the efficacy of the pasteurization process in inactivating hepatitis B virus. In studies of six and nine months duration, cryoprecipitate was infected with hepatitis B virus to give a concentration of 3000 infectious units/mL. All chimpanzees injected with either cryoprecipitate or non-pasteurized Antihemophilic Factor (Human) developed hepatitis B markers (HbsAg, Anti-Hbs, Anti-Hbc). All chimpanzees injected with the pasteurized Antihemophilic Factor (Human) product consistently remained serologically negative.

The pasteurization process used in the manufacture of this product has demonstrated *in vitro* inactivation of a number of infectious agents, including HIV, Epstein-Barr virus, cytomegalovirus, herpes simplex virus, rubella virus, measles virus, mumps virus, and poliomyelitis virus. *In vivo* experiments have demonstrated inactivation of hepatitis B virus and at least one type of nonA, nonB-hepatitis virus. Furthermore, clinical studies using this product have indicated an absence of transmission of HIV, hepatitis B virus, and nonA, nonB-hepatitis.

Clinical evidence confirms the hepatitis B safety of the pasteurization procedure. Of the 34 patients who had serological follow-up for hepatitis B markers, none had developed seroconversion of the antibodies, Anti-Hbs or Anti-Hbc caused by the administration of Antihemophilic Factor (Human), Pasteurized, Humate-P.™[2]

A total of 24 lots of Humate-P™ were administered to a cohort of 16 patients who had not previously received any blood products. The study showed no elevation in ALT levels over observation periods ranging from 2 months to 12 months.

In a retrospective study of 56 patients all have remained negative for the presence of HIV-1 antibody for time periods ranging from 2 months to 5 years from initial administration of product.

Continued on next page

Centeon—Cont.

INDICATIONS AND USAGE

The usage of Humate-P™ is indicated in hemophilia A (classical hemophilia) for the prevention and control of hemorrhagic episodes. Antihemophilic Factor (Human) is not indicated in von Willebrands disease.

CONTRAINDICATIONS

None known.

WARNINGS

This product is prepared from pooled human plasma which may contain the causative agents of hepatitis and other viral diseases. Prescribed manufacturing procedures utilized at the plasma collection centers, plasma testing laboratories, and the fractionation facilities are designed to reduce the risk of transmitting viral infection. However, the risk of viral infectivity from this product cannot be totally eliminated. Accordingly, the benefits and risks of treatment with this concentrate should be carefully assessed prior to use. Individuals who receive infusions of blood or plasma products may develop signs and/or symptoms of some viral infections, particularly nonA, nonB hepatitis.

PRECAUTIONS

It is important to determine that the coagulation disorder is caused by factor VIII deficiency, since no benefit in treating other deficiencies can be expected.

This Antihemophilic Factor (Human), Pasteurized, Humate-P™ preparation contains blood group isoagglutinins (anti-A and anti-B). When large or frequently repeated doses are needed, as when inhibitors are present or when pre- and post-surgical care is involved, patients of blood groups A, B and AB should be monitored for signs of intravascular hemolysis and decreasing hematocrit values. In the event of severe hemolysis, type-specific cryoprecipitate can be given instead. Hemolytic anemia, when present, may be corrected by the administration of compatible Group O Red Blood Cells (Human).

Other precautions are as follows:

- The filter needle should only be used to transfer solution from the preparation vial to a syringe or infusion bottle or bag. The filter needle must not be used for injection.
- The administration equipment and any unused Antihemophilic Factor (Human), Pasteurized, Humate-P™ should be discarded.

Pregnancy Category C.

Animal reproduction studies have not been conducted with Antihemophilic Factor (Human). It is also not known whether Antihemophilic Factor (Human) can cause fetal harm when administered to a pregnant woman or can affect reproduction capacity. Antihemophilic Factor (Human) should be given to a pregnant woman only if clearly needed.

ADVERSE REACTIONS

Antihemophilic Factor (Human), Pasteurized, Humate-P,™ is usually tolerated without reaction. Rare cases of allergic reaction and rise in temperature have been observed.

DOSAGE AND ADMINISTRATION

Humate-P™ is for intravenous administration only. Although dosage must be individualized according to the needs of the patient (weight, severity of hemorrhage, presence of inhibitors), the following general dosages are suggested:

1. OVERT BLEEDING—Initially 15 units per kg of body weight followed by 8 units per kg every 8 hours for the first 24 hours and the same dose every 12 hours for 3 or 4 days.
2. MUSCLE HEMORRHAGES—
   a. Minor hemorrhages in extremities or non-vital areas: 8 units per kg once a day for 2 or 3 days.
   b. Massive hemorrhages in non-vital areas: 8 units per kg by infusion at 12 hour intervals for 2 days and then one a day for 2 more days.
   c. Hemorrhages near vital organs (neck, throat, subperitoneal), 15 units per kg initially, then 8 units per kg every 8 hours.
   After 2 days the dose may be reduced by one-half.
3. JOINT HEMORRHAGES—The usual dose is 8 units per kg every 8 hours for 1 day; then every 12 hours for 1 or 2 days. However, recent experience suggests that a substantially lower dose, 5–8 units per kg given once, may be sufficient for most hemorrhages. If aspiration is carried out, 8 units per kg are given just prior to aspiration; 8 hours later and again on the following day.
4. SURGERY—Dosages of 26 to 30 units per kg body weight prior to surgery are recommended. After surgery, 15 units per kg every 8 hours should be administered. Close laboratory control to maintain the blood AHF at the level deemed appropriate for the surgical procedure is recommended for at least 10 days postoperatively. As a general rule, 1 unit of AHF activity per kg will increase the circulating AHF level by 2%. Adequacy of treatment must be judged by the clinical effects—thus the dosage may vary with individual cases.

Reconstitution

1. Warm both diluent and Antihemophilic Factor (Human), Pasteurized, Humate-P™ in unopened vials to room temperature [not above 37℃ (98°F)].
2. Remove caps from both vials to expose central portions of the rubber stoppers.
3. Treat surface of rubber stoppers with antiseptic solution and allow to dry.
4. Using aseptic technique, pierce the double needle of the blue transfer set into the diluent vial. Remove the protective cap and insert the exposed (longer) needle into the upright Antihemophilic Factor (Human), Pasteurized, Humate-P™ vial. The diluent will be transferred into the Humate-P™ by vacuum.
5. Remove the diluent vial, then the transfer set, from the Humate-P™ vial.
6. Gently rotate the vial. DO NOT SHAKE VIAL. Vigorous shaking will prolong the reconstitution time. Continue swirling until the powder is dissolved and the solution is ready for administration. To assure product sterility, Humate-P™ should be administered within three hours after reconstitution.
7. Parenteral drug products should be inspected visually for particulate matter and discoloration prior to administration, whenever solution and container permit.

Administration

INTRAVENOUS INJECTION

Plastic disposable syringes are recommended with Antihemophilic Factor (Human), Pasteurized, Humate-P™ solution. The ground glass surface of all-glass syringes tend to stick with solutions of this type.

1. Open the package containing the disposable filter. Attach the filter to a sterile disposable syringe and take the filter out of the package.
2. Remove the protective cap and—without touching the tip of the filter—insert the disposable filter into the stopper of the Humate-P™ vial; inject air.
3. Draw up the solution slowly (when using several syringes leave the filter in the vial). Discard the filter.
4. Slowly inject the solution (maximally 4 mL/minute) intravenously with an infusion kit or with a suitable injection needle.
   Aspiration of blood into the filled syringe must be avoided.

HOW SUPPLIED

Antihemophilic Factor (Human), Pasteurized, Humate-P,™ is supplied in a single dose vial with a vial of diluent and sterile needles for reconstitution and withdrawal. I.U. activity is stated on the carton and label of each vial.

STORAGE

When stored at refrigerator temperature, 2°–8℃ (36°–46°F), Antihemophilic Factor (Human), Pasteurized, Humate-P™ is stable for the period indicated by the expiration date on its label. Within this period, Humate-P™ may be stored at room termperature not to exceed 30℃ (86°F), for up to 6 months. Avoid freezing, which may damage container for the diluent.

CAUTION: FEDERAL (U.S.A.) LAW PROHIBITS DISPENSING WITHOUT PRESCRIPTION.

REFERENCES

1. Heimburger N, Schwinn H, Gratz P, et al: Factor VIII Concentrate—highly purified and heated in solution. Arzneim Forsch 31(1):619-22, 1981.
2. Experimental and clinical studies of a new pasteurized antihemophilic factor concentrate. In press.
3. Abildgaard CF, Simone JV, Corrigan JJ, et al: Treatment of hemophilia with glycine-precipitated factor VIII. New Engl J Med 275: 471–475, 1966.
4. Hilgartner MW: Current Therapy, in Hilgartner MW (ed): Hemophilia in children. Littelton, MA, Publishing Sciences Group Inc., 1976, p 158.
5. Schimpf K, Rothman P, Zimmermann K: Factor VIII dosis in prophylaxis of hemophilia A; A further controlled study, Proc XIth Cong. W.F.H. Tokyo, Academia Press, 1976, p 363.
Revised: May, 1996 (7/91)   IBM 12684
Manufactured by:
Behringwerke AG
Marburg/Lahn, Germany
U.S. License No. 97
Distributed by:
Centeon L.L.C.
Kankakee, Illinois 60901, U.S.A.

**Antihemophilic Factor (Human)
MONOCLATE-P®**   ℞
[mŏn 'ō-clāte ″]
**Factor VIII:C Pasteurized
Monoclonal Antibody Purified**

DESCRIPTION

Antihemophilic Factor (Human), MONOCLATE-P®, Factor VIII:C Pasteurized, Monoclonal Antibody Purified is a sterile, stable, lyophilized concentrate of Factor VIII:C with reduced amounts of vWf:Ag and purified of extraneous plasma-derived protein by use of affinity chromatography. A murine monoclonal antibody to vWf:Ag is used as an affinity ligand to first isolate the Factor VIII Complex. Factor VIII:C is then dissociated from vWf:Ag, recovered, formulated and provided as a sterile lyophilized powder.[1,2,3] The concentrate as formulated contains Albumin (Human) as a stabilizer, resulting in a concentrate with a specific activity between 5 and 10 units/mg of total protein. In the absence of this added Albumin (Human) stabilizer, specific activity has been determined to exceed 3000 units/mg of protein.[4] MONOCLATE-P® has been prepared from pooled human plasma and is intended for use in therapy of classical hemophilia (Hemophilia A).

This concentrate has been pasteurized by heating at 60℃ for 10 hours in aqueous solution form during its manufacture in order to further reduce the risk of viral transmission.[5] However, no procedure has been shown to be totally effective in removing viral infectivity from coagulant factor concentrates. (See CLINICAL PHARMACOLOGY and WARNINGS)

MONOCLATE-P® is a highly purified preparation of Factor VIII:C. When stored as directed, it will maintain its labeled potency for the period indicated on the container and package labels.[8,9]

Upon reconstitution, a clear, colorless solution is obtained, containing 50 to 150 times as much Factor VIII:C as does an equal volume of plasma.

Each vial contains the labeled amount of antihemophilic factor (AHF) activity as expressed in terms of International Units of antihemophilic activity. One unit of antihemophilic activity is equivalent to that quantity of AHF present in one mL of normal human plasma. When reconstituted as recommended, the resulting solution contains approximately 300 to 450 millimoles of sodium ions per liter and has 2 to 3 times the tonicity of saline. It contains approximately 2–5 millimoles of calcium ions per liter, contributed as calcium chloride, approximately 1 to 2% Albumin (Human), 0.8% mannitol, and 1.2 mM histidine. The pH is adjusted with hydrochloric acid and/or sodium hydroxide. MONOCLATE-P® also contains trace amounts (≤50 ng per 100 I.U. of AHF) of the murine monoclonal antibody used in its purification (see CLINICAL PHARAMCOLOGY).

MONOCLATE-P® is to be administered only intravenously.

CLINICAL PHARMACOLOGY

Factor VIII:C is the coagulant portion of the Factor VIII complex circulating in plasma. It is noncovalently associated with the von Willebrand protein responsible for von Willebrand factor activity. These two proteins have distinct biochemical and immunological properties and are under separate genetic control. Factor VIII:C acts as a cofactor for Factor IX to activate Factor X in the intrinsic pathway of blood coagulation.[6] Hemophilia A, an hereditary disorder of blood coagulation due to decreased levels of Factor VIII:C, results in profuse bleeding into joints, muscles or internal organs as a result of a trauma. Antihemophilic Factor (Human), MONOCLATE-P®, Factor VIII:C Pasteurized, Monoclonal Antibody Purified provides an increase in plasma levels of AHF, thereby enabling temporary correction of Hemophilia A bleeding.

Clinical evaluation of MONOCLATE-P®, Factor VIII:C Pasteurized, Monoclonal Antibody Purified concentrate for its half-life characteristics in hemophilic patients showed it to be comparable to other commercially available Antihemophilic Factor (Human) concentrates. The mean half-life obtained from six patients was 17.5 hours with a mean recovery of 1.9 Units/dl rise/U/kg.

The pasteurization process used in the manufacture of this concentrate has demonstrated *in vitro* inactivation of human immunodeficiency virus (HIV) and several model viruses. In two separate studies, HIV was reduced by ≥7.0 $\log_{10}$ to an undetectable level and by 10.5 $\log_{10}$, respectively. In addition to HIV, studies were also performed using three lipid containing model viruses and one non-lipid, encapsulated model virus. Vesicular stomatitis (VSV) was reduced by ≥6.79 $\log_{10}$ to undetectable, Sindbis was reduced by ≥6.48 $\log_{10}$ to undetectable and Vaccinia was reduced by ≥5.36 $\log_{10}$ to undetectable. Murine encephalomyocarditis (EMC), a non-lipid, encapsulated model virus, was reduced by ≥7.1 $\log_{10}$ to undetectable.

Evidence of the capability of the purification and preparative steps used in the production of Antihemophilic Factor (Human), MONOCLATE-P®, Factor VIII:C Pasteurized, Monoclonal Antibody Purified to reduce viral bioburden was obtained in studies involving the addition of known quantities of virus to cryoprecipitate. These studies were conducted using an earlier form of the concentrate which had not undergone liquid pasteurization (Antihemophilic Factor (Human), MONOCLATE®, Monoclonal Antibody Purified, Factor VIII:C, Heat-Treated). These studies provide evidence of the viral removal potential of the purification and preparative steps of the manufacturing process (exclusive of heat treatment) which are common to both concentrates. In one

study, the viruses used were human immunodeficiency virus (HIV), sindbis virus, vesicular stomatitis virus (VSV) and pseudorabies virus (PsRV). A comparison of the cumulative mean reductions for all viruses tested with the individual values obtained in each experiment indicates that the combined effects of the manufacturing steps, which purify the Factor VIII:C and prepare the concentrate in a final sterile container as a lyophilized powder, contribute viral reduction capabilities of approximately 5 to 6 logs. In a separate study, aluminum hydroxide treatment followed by antibody affinity chromatography reduced vaccinia virus infectivity by 4.81 logs. These studies indicate that the purification and preparative steps of the manufacturing process are capable of providing a non-specific, viral reduction of approximately 5 to 6 logs, independent of the pasteurization process.

MONOCLATE-P® contains trace amounts of mouse protein[7] (≤50 ng per 100 I.U. of AHF). In a study using an earlier form of the concentrate which had not undergone pasteurization (MONOCLATE®), a number of patients seronegative for Anti-HIV-1 were monitored to determine whether they would develop antibody or experience adverse reactions as a result of repeated exposure. These patients were treated on multiple occasions. Pre-study serum measurements of 27 patients for human anti-mouse IgG showed that, prior to treatment, 6 of them had either detectable antibody to mouse proteins or cross-reactive proteins. These patients continued to demonstrate similar or lower antibody levels during the study. Of the remaining 21 patients, 6 were shown to have low antibody levels on one or more occasions. In no case was observance of low antibody level associated with an anamnestic response or with any clinical adverse reaction. Patients were observed for time periods ranging from 2 to 30 months.

INDICATIONS AND USAGE

Antihemophilic Factor (Human), MONOCLATE-P®, Factor VIII:C Pasteurized, Monoclonal Antibody Purified is indicated for treatment of classical hemophilia (Hemophilia A). Affected individuals frequently require therapy following minor accidents. Surgery, when required in such individuals, must be preceded by temporary corrections of the clotting abnormality. Presurgical correction of severe AHF deficiency can be accomplished with a small volume of MONOCLATE-P®.

MONOCLATE-P® is not effective in controlling the bleeding of patients with von Willebrand's disease.

CONTRAINDICATIONS

Known hypersensitivity to mouse protein is a contraindication to Antihemophilic Factor (Human), MONOCLATE-P®, Factor VIII:C Pasteurized, Monoclonal Antibody Purified.

WARNINGS

This product is prepared from pooled human plasma which may contain the causative agents of hepatitis and other viral diseases. Prescribed manufacturing procedures utilized at the plasma collection centers, plasma testing laboratories, and the fractionation facilities are designed to reduce the risk of transmitting viral infection. However, the risk of viral infectivity from this product cannot be totally eliminated. Accordingly, the benefits and risks of treatment with this concentrate should be carefully assessed prior to use. Individuals who receive infusions of blood or plasma products may develop signs and/or symptoms of some viral infections, particularly nonA, nonB hepatitis.

PRECAUTIONS

General—Most Antihemophilic Factor (Human) concentrates contain naturally occurring blood group specific antibodies. However, the processing of MONOCLATE-P® significantly reduces the presence of blood group specific antibodies in the final product. Nevertheless, when large or frequently repeated doses of product are needed, patients should be monitored by means of hematocrit and direct Coombs tests for signs of progressive anemia.

Formation of Antibodies to Mouse Protein—Although no hypersensitivity reactions have been observed, because MONOCLATE-P® contains trace amounts of mouse protein (≤50 ng per 100 I.U. of AHF), the possibility exists that patients treated with MONOCLATE-P® may develop hypersensitivity to the mouse proteins.

Information for Patients—Patients should be informed of the early signs of hypersensitivity reactions including hives, generalized urticaria, tightness of the chest, wheezing, hypotension, and anaphylaxis, and should be advised to discontinue use of the concentrate and contact their physician if these symptoms occur.

Pregnancy Category C—Animal reproduction studies have not been conducted with Antihemophilic Factor (Human), MONOCLATE-P®, Factor VIII:C Pasteurized, Monoclonal Antibody Purified. It is also not known whether MONOCLATE-P® can cause fetal harm when administered to a pregnant woman or can affect reproduction capacity. MONOCLATE-P® should be given to a pregnant woman only if clearly needed.

ADVERSE REACTIONS

Products of this type are known to cause allergic reactions, mild chills, nausea or stinging at the infusion site.

DOSAGE AND ADMINISTRATION

Antihemophilic Factor (Human), MONOCLATE-P®, Factor VIII:C Pasteurized, Monoclonal Antibody Purified is for intravenous administration only. As a general rule 1 unit of AHF activity per kg will increase the circulating AHF level by 2%.[10] The following formula provides a guide for dosage calculations:

Number of AHF I.U. Required	=	Body weight (in kg)	×	desired Factor VIII increase (% normal)	×	0.5[10]

Although dosage must be individualized according to the needs of the patient (weight, severity of hemorrhage, presence of inhibitors), the following general dosages are suggested.[11]

1. MILD HEMORRHAGES—Minor hemorrhagic episodes will generally subside with a single infusion if a level of 30% or more is attained.
2. MODERATE HEMORRHAGE AND MINOR SURGERY—For more serious hemorrhages and minor surgical procedures, the patient's Factor VIII level should be raised to 30–50% of normal, which usually requires an initial dose of 15–25 I.U. per kg. If further therapy is required a maintenance dose is 10–15 I.U. per kg every 8–12 hours.
3. SEVERE HEMORRHAGE—In hemorrhages near vital organs (neck, throat, subperitoneal) it may be desirable to raise the Factor VIII level to 80–100% of normal which can be achieved with an initial dose of 40–50 I.U. per kg and a maintenance dose of 20–25 I.U. per kg every 8–12 hours.
4. MAJOR SURGERY—For surgical procedures a dose of AHF sufficient to achieve a level 80–100% of normal should be given an hour prior to surgery. A second dose, half the size of the priming dose, should be given five hours after the first dose. Factor VIII levels should be maintained at a daily minimum of at least 30% for a period of 10–14 days postoperatively. Close laboratory control to maintain AHF plasma levels deemed appropriate to maintain hemostasis is recommended.

Reconstitution

1. Warm both the diluent and Antihemophilic Factor (Human), MONOCLATE-P®, Factor VIII:C Pasteurized, Monoclonal Antibody Purified in unopened vials to room temperature [not above 37°C (98°F)].
2. Remove the caps from both vials to expose the central portions of the rubber stoppers.
3. Treat the surface of the rubber stoppers with antiseptic solution and allow them to dry.
4. Using aseptic technique, insert one end of the double-end needle into the rubber stopper of the diluent vial. Invert the diluent vial and insert the other end of the double-end needle into the rubber stopper of the MONOCLATE-P® vial. Direct the diluent, which will be drawn in by vacuum, over the entire surface of the MONOCLATE-P® cake. (In order to assure transfer of all the diluent, adjust the position of the tip of the needle in the diluent vial to the inside edge of the diluent stopper.) Rotate the vial to ensure complete wetting of the cake during the transfer process.
5. Remove the diluent vial to release the vacuum, then remove the double-end needle, from the MONOCLATE-P® vial.
6. Gently swirl the vial until the powder is dissolved and the solution is ready for administration. The concentrate routinely and easily reconstitutes within one minute. To assure sterility, MONOCLATE-P® should be administered within three hours after reconstitution.
7. Parenteral drug preparations should be inspected visually for particulate matter and discoloration prior to administration, whenever solution and container permit.

Administration

CAUTION: This kit contains two devices, a stainless steel 5 micron filter needle, individually labeled as a 5 micron filter needle and contained in a separate blister pack, and an all plastic 5 micron vented filter spike which is supplied with the four-item administration components blister pack, either of which may be used to withdraw the reconstituted product for administration. The withdrawal directions specific for each of these alternate devices must be followed exactly for whichever device is chosen for use as described below. Product loss or inability to withdraw product will result if the improper instructions are followed.

A. Administration using the Stainless Steel Filter Needle for Withdrawal (This item is individually packaged in a separate, labeled blister pack.)

Intravenous Injection

Plastic disposable syringes are recommended with Antihemophilic Factor (Human), MONOCLATE-P®, Factor VIII:C Pasteurized, Monoclonal Antibody Purified solution. The ground glass surface of all-glass syringes tend to stick with solutions of this type.

1. Using aseptic technique, attach the filter needle to a sterile disposable syringe.
2. Draw air into the syringe equal to or greater than the contents of the vial.
3. Insert the filter needle into the stopper of the MONOCLATE-P® vial, invert the vial, position the filter needle above the level of the liquid and inject all of the air into the vial.
4. Pull the filter needle back down below the level of the liquid until the tip is at the inside edge of the stopper.
5. Withdraw the reconstituted solution into the syringe being careful to always keep the tip of the needle below the level of the liquid.
   CAUTION: Failure to inject air into the vial, or allowing air to pass through the filter needle while filling the syringe with reconstituted solution, may cause the needle to clog.
6. Discard the filter needle. Perform venipuncture using the enclosed winged needle with microbore tubing. Attach the syringe to the luer end of the tubing.
   CAUTION: Use of other winged needles without microbore tubing, although compatible with the concentrate, will result in a larger retention of solution within the winged infusion set.
7. **Administer solution intravenously at a rate (approximately 2 mL/minute) comfortable to the patient.**

B. Administration using the all plastic Vented Filter Spike for Withdrawal (This spike is supplied in the four-item Administration Components pack.)

Intravenous Injection

Plastic disposable syringes are recommended with Antihemophilic Factor (Human), MONOCLATE-P®, Factor VIII:C Pasteurized, Monoclonal Antibody Purified solution. The ground glass surface of all-glass syringes tend to stick with solutions of this type.

1. Using aseptic technique, attach the vented filter spike to a sterile disposable syringe.
   CAUTION: DO NOT INJECT AIR INTO THE MONOCLATE-P® VIAL. The self-venting feature of the vented filter spike precludes the need to inject air in order to facilitate withdrawal of the reconstituted solution. The injection of air could cause partial product loss through the vent filter.
   CAUTION: The use of other, non-vented filter needles or spikes without the proper procedure may result in an air lock and prevent the complete transfer of the concentrate.
2. Insert the vented filter spike into the stopper of the MONOCLATE-P® vial, invert the vial, and position the filter spike so that the orifice is at the inside edge of the stopper.
3. Withdraw the reconstituted solution into the syringe.
4. Discard the filter spike. Perform venipuncture using the enclosed winged needle with microbore tubing. Attach the syringe to the luer end of the tubing.
   CAUTION: Use of other winged needles without microbore tubing, although compatible with the concentrate, will result in a larger retention of solution within the winged infusion set.
5. **Administer solution intravenously at a rate (approximately 2 mL/minute) comfortable to the patient.**

STORAGE

When stored at refrigerator temperature, 2°–8°C (36°–46°F), Antihemophilic Factor (Human), MONOCLATE-P®, Factor VIII:C Pasteurized, Monoclonal Antibody Purified, is stable for the period indicated by the expiration date on its label. Within this period, MONOCLATE-P® may be stored at room temperature not to exceed 30°C (86°F), for up to 6 months.

Avoid freezing which may damage container for the diluent.

HOW SUPPLIED

MONOCLATE-P® is supplied in a single dose vial with diluent, double-ended needle for reconstitution, vented filter spike for withdrawal, filter needle for withdrawal, winged infusion set and alcohol swabs. I.U. activity is stated on the label of each vial.

CAUTION: FEDERAL (U.S.A.) LAW PROHIBITS DISPENSING WITHOUT PRESCRIPTION.

REFERENCES

1. W. Terry, A. Schreiber, C. Tarr, M. Hrinda, W. Curry, and F. Feldman, "Human Factor VIII:C Produced Using Monoclonal Antibodies," in *Research in Clinic and Laboratory*, Vol. XVI, (#1), 202 (1986) from the XVIIth International Congress of the World Federation of Hemophilia.
2. A.B. Schreiber, "The Preclinical Characterization of Monoclate Factor VIII C Antihemophilic Factor Human," *Semin Hematol* 25 (2 Suppl. 1), 1988, pp. 27–32.
3. E. Berntorp and I.M. Nilsson, "Biochemical Properties of Human Factor VIII C Monoclate Purified Using Monoclonal Antibody to VWF," *Thromb Res* O (Suppl.7), 1987, p. 60, from the Satellite Symposia of the XIth Inter-

Continued on next page

Centeon—Cont.

national Congress on Thrombosis and Haemostasis, Brussels, Belgium, July 11, 1987.
4. S. Chandra, C.C. Huang, R.L. Weeks, K. Beatty and F. Feldman, "Purity of a Factor VIII:C Preparation (Monoclate) Manufactured by Monoclonal Immunoaffinity Chromatography Technique," from the XVIII International Congress of the World Federation of Hemophilia, May 1988.
5. B. Spire, D. Dormont, F. Barre-Sinousii, L. Montagnier, and J.C. Chermann, "Inactivation of Lymphadenopathy Associated Virus by Heat, Gamma Rays, and Ultraviolet Light," *Lancet*, Jan. 26, 1985, p.188.
6. L.W. Hoyer, "The Factor VIII Complex: Structure and Function," *Blood* 58 (1981), p.1.
7. F. Feldman, S. Chandra, R. Kleszynski, C.C. Huang and R.L. Weeks, "Measurement of Murine Protein Levels in Monoclonal Antibody Purified Coagulation Factor," from the XVIII International Congress of the World Federation of Hemophilia, May 1988.
8. F. Feldman, R. Kleszynski, L. Ho, R. Kling, S. Chandra and C.C. Huang, "Validation of Coagulation Test Methods for Evaluation of Monoclate (Factor VIII:C) Potencies," from the XVIII International Congress of the World Federation of Hemophilia, May 1988.
9. S. Chandra, C.C. Huang, L. Ho, R. Kling, R.L. Weeks and F. Feldman, "Studies on the Stability of Factor VIII:C (Monoclate) in Lyophilized and Solution Form," from the XVIII International Congress of the World Federation of Hemophilia, May 1988.
10. C.F. Abilgaard, J.V. Simone, J.J. Corrigan, et al., "Treatment of Hemophilia with Glycine—Precipitated Factor VIII," *New Eng J Med*, 275 (1966), p.471.
11. C.K. Kasper, "Hematologic Care," *Comprehensive Management of Hemophilia*, ed. Boone, D.C., Philadelphia, F.A. Davis Co., (1976) pp. 2–20.

BIBLIOGRAPHY

Hershman, R.J., Naconti, S.B., and Shulman, N.R., "Prophylactic Treatment of Factor VIII Deficiency." *Blood* 35 (1970), p. 189.

Kasper, C. K., Dietrich, S. I. and Rapaport, S.K. "Hemophilia Prophylaxis in Factor VIII Concentrate." *Arch. Int. Med.* 125 (1970), p. 1004.

Biggs, R., ed. "The Treatment of Hemophilia A and B and von Willebrands Disease." Oxford: Blackwell, 1978.

Fulcher, C.A., Zimmerman, T.S., "Characterization of the Human Factor VIII Procoagulant Protein With a Heterologous Precipitating Antibody." *Proc. Natl. Acad. Sci.* 79 (1982), pp. 1648–1652.

Levine, P.H., "Factor VIII C Purified from Plasma Via Monoclonal Antibodies Human Studies." *Semin Hematol* 25 (2 Suppl. 1), 1988, pp. 38–41.

Revised: May, 1996 (1/93) IBM 12810

Centeon L.L.C.
Kankakee, Illinois 60901, U.S.A.
U.S. Government License No. 149
U.S. Patent No. Re. 32,011
U.S. Patent No. 4,876,241

COAGULATION FACTOR IX (HUMAN) MONONINE® ℞
[*mŏn ′ō nīn*]
Monoclonal Antibody Purified

DESCRIPTION

Coagulation Factor IX (Human), Mononine,® is a sterile, stable, lyophilized concentrate of Factor IX prepared from pooled human plasma and is intended for use in therapy of Factor IX deficiency, known as Hemophilia B or Christmas disease. Coagulation Factor IX (Human), Mononine,® is purified of extraneous plasma-derived proteins, including Factors II, VII and X, by use of immunoaffinity chromatography. A murine monoclonal antibody to Factor IX is used as an affinity ligand to isolate Factor IX from the source material. Factor IX is then dissociated from the monoclonal antibody, recovered, purified further, formulated and provided as a sterile, lyophilized powder. The immunoaffinity protocol utilized results in a highly pure Factor IX preparation. It shows predominantly a single component by SDS polyacrylamide electrophoretic evaluation and has a specific activity of not less than 150 Factor IX units per mg total protein. This concentrate has been processed by monoclonal antibody immunoaffinity chromatography during its manufacture which has been shown to be capable of reducing the risk of viral transmission. Additionally, a chemical treatment protocol and an ultrafiltration step used in its manufacture have also been shown to be capable of significant viral reductions. However, no procedure has been shown to be totally effective in removing viral infectivity from coagulation factor concentrates (See CLINICAL PHARMACOLOGY and WARNINGS).

Mononine® is a highly purified preparation of Factor IX. When stored as directed, it will maintain its labeled potency for the period indicated on the container and package labels. Each vial contains the labeled amount of Factor IX activity expressed in International Units (I.U.). One I.U. represents the activity of Factor IX present in 1 mL of normal, pooled plasma. When reconstituted as recommended, the resulting solution is a clear, colorless, isotonic preparation of neutral pH, containing approximately 100 times the Factor IX potency found in an equal volume of plasma. Each mL of the reconstituted concentrate contains approximately 100 I.U. of Factor IX and non-detectable levels of Factors II, VII and X (<0.0025 units per Factor IX unit using standard coagulation assays). It also contains histidine (approx. 10mM), sodium chloride (approx. 0.066M) and mannitol (approximately 3%). Hydrochloric acid and/or sodium hydroxide may have been used to adjust pH. Mononine® also contains trace amounts (≤ 50 ng mouse protein/100 Factor IX activity units) of the murine monoclonal antibody used in its purification (See CLINICAL PHARMACOLOGY).

Mononine® is to be administered only intravenously.

CLINICAL PHARMACOLOGY

Hemophilia B, or Christmas disease, is an X-linked recessively inherited disorder of blood coagulation characterized by insufficient or abnormal synthesis of the clotting protein Factor IX. Factor IX is a vitamin K-dependent coagulation factor which is synthesized in the liver. Factor IX is activated by Factor XIa in the intrinsic coagulation pathway. Activated Factor IX (IXa), in combination with Factor VIII:C, activates Factor X to Xa, resulting ultimately in the conversion of prothrombin to thrombin and the formation of a fibrin clot. The infusion of exogenous Factor IX to replace the deficiency present in Hemophilia B temporarily restores hemostasis. Depending upon the patient's level of biologically active Factor IX, clinical symptoms range from moderate skin bruising or excessive hemorrhage after trauma or surgery to spontaneous hemorrhage into joints, muscles or internal organs including the brain. Severe or recurring hemorrhages can produce death, organ dysfunction or orthopedic deformity.

Infusion of Factor IX Complex concentrates which contain varying but significant amounts of the other liver-dependent blood coagulation proteins, Factors II, VII and X, into patients with Hemophilia B results in Factor IX recoveries ranging from approximately 0.57–1.1 IU/dL rise per IU/Kg body weight infused with plasma half-lives for Factor IX ranging from approximately 23 hours to 31 hours.[1,2]

Infusion of Coagulation Factor IX (Human), Mononine,® into ten patients with severe or moderate Hemophilia B has shown a mean recovery of 0.67 IU/dL rise per IU/Kg body weight infused and a mean half-life 22.6 hours.[3] After six months of experience with repeated infusions performed on the nine patients who remained in the study, it was shown that the half-life and recovery was maintained at a level comparable to that found with the initial infusion. The six-month data showed a mean recovery of 0.68 IU/dL rise per IU/Kg body weight infused and a mean half-life of 25.3 hours.[3] The data show no statistically significant differences between the initial and six-month values.

The manufacturing procedure for Coagulation Factor IX (Human), Mononine,® includes multiple processing steps which have been designed to reduce the risk of viral transmission. Validation studies of the monoclonal antibody (MAb) immunoaffinity chromatography/chemical treatment steps and an ultrafiltration step used in the production of Mononine® document the viral reduction capacity of the processes employed. These studies were conducted using the Human Immunodeficiency Virus (HIV) and four model viruses representing a broad range of viral characteristics, i.e., Sindbis, Vaccinia, Vesicular Stomatitis (VSV) and Murine Encephalomyocarditis (EMC), a non-lipid encapsulated model virus. The results of these validation studies (see table below) document an HIV viral reduction capacity of $\geq 11.56 \log_{10}$ and a viral reduction capacity of $10.24 \log_{10}$ for Sindbis, $11.64 \log_{10}$ for EMC, $\geq 14.23 \log_{10}$ for VSV, and $\geq 10.90 \log_{10}$ for Vaccinia.

[See table below.]

The viral safety of Coagulation Factor IX (Human), Mononine,® is being studied in clinical trials of two cohorts of hemophilia B patients previously unexposed to blood or blood products. One cohort of patients includes those with moderate to severe Factor IX deficiency requiring chronic replacement therapy and the second cohort of patients includes those with a mild deficiency requiring Factor IX replacement for surgical procedures. These patients are being followed for serum ALT levels as well as for a range of viral serologies. Available serum ALT data, representing 22 patients, 13 of whom were followed for 6–15 months and 9 of whom were followed for less than 6 months, and available serology results, representing 19 patients, have continued to show no evidence of transmission of hepatitis or HIV. Although these studies are ongoing, these preliminary results show no evidence of viral transmission resulting from the infusion of Mononine® (See WARNINGS).

Coagulation Factor IX (Human), Mononine,® contains trace amounts of the murine monoclonal antibody used in its purification (≤ 50 ng mouse protein per 100 Factor IX activity units). Using another murine monoclonal antibody purified concentrate, Antihemophilic Factor (Human), Monoclate,® Factor VIII:C, Heat Treated, also containing trace amounts of murine protein (≤ 50 ng per 100 AHF activity units), a number of patients seronegative for Anti-HIV-1 were monitored to determine whether they would develop antibody to mouse protein or experience adverse reactions as a result of repeated exposure. Pre-study serum measurements of 27 patients for human anti-mouse lgG showed that, prior to treatment, 6 of them had either detectable antibody to mouse proteins or cross-reactive proteins. These patients continued to demonstrate similar or lower antibody levels during the study. Of the remaining 21 patients, 6 were shown to have low antibody levels on one or more occasions. In no case was observance of low antibody level associated with an anamnestic response or with any clinical adverse reaction. Patients were observed for time periods ranging from 2 to 30 months.

In similar clinical studies with Mononine,® a cohort of nine Anti-HIV seropositive hemophilia B patients were administered Mononine® for periods of 15–24 months. No appreciable increases in levels of lgG, lgM or lgE Human Anti-Mouse Antibodies (HAMA) were observed when compared to pre-study levels.

In clinical studies of Coagulation Factor IX (Human), Mononine,® patients were monitored for evidence of disseminated intravascular coagulation. In six patients evaluated after infusion, fibrinogen levels and platelet counts were unchanged, and fibrin degradation products did not appear.[3]

In further clinical evaluations of Coagulation Factor IX (Human), Mononine,® in a crossover study with a Factor IX Complex concentrate, Mononine® was not associated with the formation of prothrombin activation fragment (F_{1+2}) whereas the Factor IX Complex was.[3,4] Prothrombin activation fragment (F_{1+2}) is indicative of activation of prothrombin.

INDICATIONS AND USAGE

Coagulation Factor IX (Human), Mononine,® is indicated for the prevention and control of bleeding in Factor IX deficiency, also known as Hemophilia B or Christmas disease.

Mononine® is not indicated in the treatment or prophylaxis of Hemophilia A patients with inhibitors to Factor VIII.

Coagulation Factor IX (Human), Mononine,® contains non-detectable levels of Factors II, VII and X (<0.0025 units per Factor IX unit using standard coagulation assays) and is, therefore, not indicated for replacement therapy of these clotting factors.

Mononine® is also not indicated in the treatment or reversal of coumarin-induced anticoagulation or in a hemorrhagic

Summary of Virus Reduction Studies
($\log_{10}$ Reduction)

Processing Step	HIV	Sindbis	EMC	VSV	Vaccinia
MAb Chromatography	*	2.76	3.89	≥7.18**	≥3.60
Sodium Thiocyanate Chemical Treatment	≥4.16	0	0	**	0
Ultrafiltration	≥7.4	7.48	7.75	7.05	≥7.30
Total $\log_{10}$ Reduction	≥11.56	10.24	11.64	≥14.23	≥10.90

* MAb Chromatography not studied
** Results are for combined MAb chromatography/sodium thiocyanate step.

state caused by hepatitis-induced lack of production of liver dependent coagulation factors.

CONTRAINDICATIONS

Known hypersensitivity to mouse protein is a contraindication to Coagulation Factor IX (Human), Mononine.®

WARNINGS

This product is prepared from pooled human plasma which may contain the causative agents of hepatitis and other viral diseases. Prescribed manufacturing procedures utilized at the plasma collection centers, plasma testing laboratories, and the fractionation facilities are designed to reduce the risk of transmitting viral infection. However, the risk of viral infectivity from this product cannot be totally eliminated. Accordingly, the benefits and risks of treatment with this concentrate should be carefully assessed prior to use. Individuals who receive infusions of blood or plasma products may develop signs and/or symptoms of some viral infections, particularly nonA, nonB hepatitis.

Since the use of Factor IX Complex concentrates has historically been associated with the development of thromboembolic complications, the use of Factor IX-containing products may be potentially hazardous in patients with signs of fibrinolysis and in patients with disseminated intravascular coagulation (DIC).

PRECAUTIONS

The administration of Factor IX Complex concentrates, containing Factors II, VII, IX and X, has been associated with the development of thromboembolic complications. Although Coagulation Factor IX (Human), Mononine,® contains highly purified Factor IX, the potential risk of thrombosis or disseminated intravascular coagulation observed with the use of other products containing Factor IX should be recognized. Patients given Mononine® should be observed closely for signs or symptoms of intravascular coagulation or thrombosis. Because of the potential risk of thromboembolic complications, caution should be exercised when administering this concentrate to patients with liver disease, to patients post-operatively, to neonates, or to patients at risk of thromboembolic phenomena or disseminated intravascular coagulation.[5,6] In each of these situations, the potential benefit of treatment with Mononine® should be weighed against the risk of these complications.

Coagulation Factor IX (Human), Mononine,® should be administered intravenously at a rate that will permit observation of the patient for any immediate reaction. Rates of infusion of up to 225 units per minute have been regularly tolerated with no adverse reactions. If any reaction takes place that is thought to be related to the administration of Mononine,® the rate of infusion should be decreased or the infusion stopped, as dictated by the response of the patient.

During the course of treatment, determination of daily Factor IX levels is advised to guide the dose to be administered and the frequency of repeated infusions. Individual patients may vary in their response to Mononine,® achieving different levels of *in vivo* recovery and demonstrating different half-lives.

The use of high doses of Factor IX Complex concentrates has been reported to be associated with instances of myocardial infarction, disseminated intravascular coagulation, venous thrombosis and pulmonary embolism. Generally a Factor IX level of 25% to 50% is considered adequate for hemostasis, including major hemorrhages and surgery. Attempting to maintain Factor IX levels of >75% to 100% during treatment is not recommended. To achieve Factor IX levels that will remain above 25% between once a day administrations, each daily dose should attempt to raise the level to 50–60%. (See DOSAGE AND ADMINISTRATION.)

No data are available regarding the use of -amino caproic acid following an initial infusion of Mononine® for the prevention or treatment of oral bleeding following trauma or dental procedures such as extractions.

Formation of Antibodies to Mouse Protein—Although no hypersensitivity reactions have been observed, because Mononine® contains trace amounts of mouse protein (≤50 ng per 100 Factor IX activity units), the possibility exists that patients treated with Mononine® may develop hypersensitivity to the mouse protein.

$$\text{Number of Factor IX I.U. required} = \text{Body Weight (in Kg)} \times \text{desired Factor IX increase (\% normal)} \times 1.0\ \text{unit/Kg}$$

Information For Patients

Patients should be informed of the early signs of hypersensitivity reactions including hives, generalized urticaria, tightness of the chest, wheezing, hypotension, and anaphylaxis, and should be advised to discontinue use of the concentrate and contact their physician if these symptoms occur.

Pregnancy Category C

Animal reproduction studies have not been conducted with Coagulation Factor IX (Human), Mononine.® It is also not known whether Mononine® can cause fetal harm when administered to a pregnant woman or can affect reproduction capacity. Mononine® should be given to a pregnant woman only if clearly needed.

ADVERSE REACTIONS

As with the administration of any product intravenously, the following reactions may be observed following administration: headache, fever, chills, flushing, nausea, vomiting, tingling, lethargy, hives, stinging or burning at the infusion site or other manifestations of allergic reactions.

There is a potential risk of thromboembolic episodes following the administration of Mononine.® (See WARNINGS and PRECAUTIONS.)

The patient should be monitored closely during the infusion of Mononine® to observe for the development of any reaction. If any reaction takes place that is thought to be related to the administration of Mononine,® the rate of infusion should be decreased or the infusion stopped, as dictated by the response of the patient.

DOSAGE AND ADMINISTRATION

Coagulation Factor IX (Human), Mononine,® is intended for intravenous administration only. It should be reconstituted with the volume of Sterile Water for Injection, USP supplied with the lot, and administered within three hours of reconstitution. Do not refrigerate after reconstitution. After administration, any unused solution and the administration equipment should be discarded.

As a general rule, 1 unit of Factor IX activity per Kg can be expected to increase the circulating level of Factor IX by 1% of normal. The following formula provides a guide to dosage calculations:

[See table above.]

The amount of Coagulation Factor IX (Human), Mononine,® to be infused, as well as the frequency of infusions, will vary with each patient and with the clinical situation.[7,8]

As a general rule, the level of Factor IX required for treatment of different conditions is as follows:

[See table below.]

Recovery of the loading dose varies from patient to patient. Doses administered should be titrated to the patient's response.

In the presence of an inhibitor to Factor IX, higher doses of Mononine® might be necessary to overcome the inhibitor (see PRECAUTIONS). No data on the treatment of patients with inhibitors to Factor IX with Mononine® are available.

For information on rate of administration, see Rate of Administration, below.

Reconstitution

1. Warm both the diluent and Coagulation Factor IX (Human), Mononine,® in unopened vials to room temperature [not above 37°C (98°F)].
2. Remove the caps from both vials to expose the central portions of the rubber stoppers.
3. Treat the surface of the rubber stoppers with antiseptic solution and allow them to dry.
4. Using aseptic technique, insert one end of the double-end needle into the rubber stopper of the diluent vial. Invert the diluent vial and insert the other end of the double-end needle into the rubber stopper of the Mononine® vial. Direct the diluent, which will be drawn in by vacuum, over the entire surface of the Mononine® cake. (In order to assure transfer of all the diluent, adjust the position of the tip of the needle in the diluent vial to the inside edge of the diluent stopper.) Rotate the vial to ensure complete wetting of the cake during the transfer process.
5. Remove the diluent vial to release the vacuum, then remove the double-end needle from the Mononine® vial.
6. Gently swirl the vial until the powder is dissolved and the solution is ready for administration. The concentrate routinely and easily reconstitutes within one minute. To assure sterility, Mononine® should be administered within three hours after reconstitution.
7. Product should be filtered prior to use as described under Administration. Parenteral drug preparations should be inspected visually for particulate matter and discoloration prior to administration, whenever solution and container permit.

Administration

Intravenous Injection

Plastic disposable syringes are recommended with Coagulation Factor IX (Human), Mononine,® solution. The ground glass surface of all-glass syringes tend to stick with solutions of this type. Please note, this concentrate is supplied with a SELF-VENTING filter spike.

1. Using aseptic technique, attach the vented filter spike to a sterile disposable syringe.
   CAUTION: The use of other, non-vented filter needles or spikes without the proper procedure may result in an air lock and prevent the complete transfer of the concentrate.
   CAUTION: DO NOT INJECT AIR INTO THE MONONINE™ VIAL. The self-venting feature of the vented filter spike precludes the need to inject air in order to facilitate withdrawal of the reconstituted solution. The injection of air could cause partial product loss through the vent filter.
2. Insert the vented filter spike into the stopper of the Mononine® vial, invert the vial, and position the filter spike so that the orifice is at the inside edge of the stopper.
3. Withdraw the reconstituted solution into the syringe.
4. Discard the filter spike. Perform venipuncture using the enclosed winged needle with microbore tubing. Attach the syringe to the luer end of the tubing.
   CAUTION: Use of other winged needles without microbore tubing, although compatible with the concentrate, will result in a larger retention of solution within the winged infusion set.

Rate of Administration

The rate of administration should be determined by the response and comfort of the patient; intravenous dosage administration rates of up to 225 units/minute have been regularly tolerated without incident. When reconstituted as directed, i.e., to approximately 100 units/mL, Mononine® should be administered at a rate of approximately 2.0 mL per minute.

STORAGE

When stored at refrigerator temperature, 2°–8°C (36°–46°F), Coagulation Factor IX (Human), Mononine,® is stable for the period indicated by the expiration date on its label. Within this period, Mononine® may be stored at room temperature not to exceed 30°C (86°F), for up to one month. Avoid freezing which may damage container for the diluent.

HOW SUPPLIED

Mononine® is supplied in a single dose vial with diluent, double-ended needle for reconstitution, vented filter spike for withdrawal, winged infusion set and alcohol swabs. Factor IX activity in I.U. is stated on the label of each vial.

CAUTION: FEDERAL (U.S.A.) LAW PROHIBITS DISPENSING WITHOUT PRESCRIPTION.

	Minor Spontaneous Hemorrhage, Prophylaxis	Major Trauma or Surgery
Desired levels of Factor IX for Hemostasis	15–25%	25–50%
Initial loading dose to achieve desired level	up to 20–30 units/kg	up to 75 units/kg
Frequency of dosing	once; repeated in 24 hours if necessary	every 18–30 hours, depending on $T_{1/2}$ and measured Factor IX levels
Duration of treatment	once; repeated if necessary	up to ten days, depending upon nature of insult

REFERENCES

1. Zauber NP, Levin J: Factor IX levels in patients with hemophilia B (Christmas disease) following transfusion with concentrates of Factor IX or fresh frozen plasma (FFP). *Medicine* (Baltimore) 56(3): 213–24, 1977.
2. Smith KJ, Thompson AR: Labeled Factor IX Kinetics in Patients with Hemophilia-B. *Blood* 58(3): 625–629, 1981.
3. Kim HC, McMillan CW, White GC, Bergman GE, Horton MW, Saidi P: Purified Factor IX Using Monoclonal Immunoaffinity Technique: Clinical Trials in Hemophilia B and Comparison to Prothrombin Complex Concentrates. *Blood* 79, No. 3: pp 568–575, 1992.
4. Kim HC, Matts L, Eisele J, Czachur M, Saidi P: Monoclonal Antibody Purified Factor IX—Comparative Thrombogenicity to Prothrombin Complex Concentrate. Seminars in Hematology, Vol. 28, No. 3, Suppl. 6, July, 1991, pp. 15–20.
5. Aledort LM: Factor IX and Thrombosis. *Scand. J. Haematology* Suppl. 30:40, 1977.
6. Cederbaum AI, Blatt PM, Roberts HR: Intravascular coagulation with use of human prothrombin complex concentrates. *Ann. Intern. Med.* 84: 683–687, 1976.
7. Kasper CK, Dietrich SL: Comprehensive Management of Hemophilia. *Clin. Haematol.* 14(2): 489–512, 1985.

Continued on next page

Centeon—Cont.

8. Johnson AJ, Aronson DL, Williams WJ: Preparation and clinical use of plasma and plasma fractions. Chap. 167 in *Hematology* 3rd Edition, Williams WJ, Beutler E, Erslev AJ, Lichtman MA (Eds.), McGraw Hill Book Co, New York: pp 1563–1583, 1983.

Revised: May, 1996 (10/94)   IBM 12835
Centeon L.L.C.
Kankakee, Illinois 60901, U.S.A.
U.S. License No. 149
U.S. Patent No. 5,055,557

PLASMA–PLEX®

[*plāz'ma-plĕks*]
Plasma Protein Fraction (Human) U.S.P.
5% Solution Heat-Treated

DESCRIPTION

Plasma Protein Fraction (Human) 5%—Plasma-Plex® is a sterile solution of protein consisting of Albumin and Globulin derived from human venous plasma. Each 100 mL contains 5.0 g selected plasma proteins. The plasma proteins, as determined by electrophoresis, are at least 83% Albumin and no more than 17% Globulins; no more than 1% of the proteins are Gamma Globulins. The solution is iso-osmotic with normal human plasma. Approximate concentrations of significant electrolytes are: Sodium 130–160 mEq per liter; and Potassium not more than 2mEq per liter.

Plasma-Plex® is stabilized with 0.004 molar Sodium Acetyltryptophanate and 0.004 molar Sodium Caprylate, and contains no preservative. It is heat treated at 60°C. for 10 hours. This product has been prepared in accordance with the requirements established by the Food and Drug Administration and is in compliance with the standards of the United States Pharmacopeia.

Plasma Protein Fraction (Human) 5%—Plasma-Plex® is to be administered by the intravenous route.

CLINICAL PHARMACOLOGY

Plasma Protein Fraction (Human) is effective in the maintenance of a normal blood volume but has not been proved effective in the maintenance of oncotic pressure. When the circulating blood volume has been depleted, the hemodilution following albumin administration persists for many hours. In individuals with normal blood volume, it usually lasts only a few hours.

Unlike whole blood plasma, Plasma Protein Fraction (Human) 5%—Plasma-Plex® is considered free of the danger of homologous serum hepatitis. No cross-matching is required and the absence of cellular elements removes the risk of sensitization with repeated infusions.

INDICATIONS AND USAGE

Shock: Plasma-Plex® is indicated in the emergency treatment of shock due to burns, trauma, surgery, infections, in the treatment of injuries of such severity that shock, although not immediately present, is likely to ensue, and in other similar conditions where the restoration of blood volume is urgent. It supplies additional fluid for adequate plasma volume expansion in dehydrated patients. Blood transfusion may be indicated if there has been considerable loss of red blood cells.

Burns: Plasma-Plex® is indicated to prevent marked hemoconcentration and to maintain appropriate electrolyte balance.

Hypoproteinemia: Plasma Protein Fraction (Human) 5%—Plasma-Plex® may be used in hypoproteinemic patients, providing sodium restriction is not a problem. If sodium restriction is imperative, the use of 25% Albumin (Human) is recommended.

CONTRAINDICATIONS

Plasma-Plex® may be contraindicated in patients with severe anemia or cardiac failure. Do not use in patients on cardiopulmonary bypass.

WARNINGS

Do not use if the solution is turbid, or if there is a sediment in the bottle. Since the product contains no preservative, do not begin administration more than 4 hours after opening the bottle. Unused portions should be discarded.

PRECAUTIONS

General

Administration of large quantities of Plasma-Plex® should be supplemented with or replaced by whole blood to combat the relative anemia which would follow such use. Rapid infusion (greater than 10 mL/minute) may produce hypotension. Blood pressure should be monitored during use and infusion slowed or ceased if sudden hypotension occurs.

When used to reverse shock or hypotension, careful observation of the patient is necessary to detect bleeding points which failed to bleed at lower pressure.

Dehydrated patients require administration of additional fluids to replace fluid withdrawn from tissues by osmotic action of Plasma-Plex.®

Administer with caution to patients with low cardiac reserve or with no albumin deficiency because a rapid increase in plasma volume may cause circulatory embarrassment or pulmonary edema.

This product cannot be used for correction of defects of the coagulation mechanism. Administration should be by intravenous route only.

Pregnancy Category C

Animal reproduction studies have not been conducted with Plasma Protein Fraction (Human) 5%—Plasma-Plex.® It is also not known whether Plasma-Plex® can cause fetal harm when administered to a pregnant woman or can affect reproduction capacity. Plasma-Plex® should be given to a pregnant woman only if clearly needed.

ADVERSE REACTIONS

Incidence of untoward reactions is low. Nausea may occur, but should be evaluated with respect to the nature of the present illness. Hypotension, particularly following rapid infusion or intraarterial administration to patients on cardiopulmonary bypass.

DOSAGE AND ADMINISTRATION

Plasma Protein Fraction (Human) 5%—Plasma-Plex® is given intravenously without further dilution. This concentration is iso-osmotic with normal human plasma. When it is administered to patients with normal blood volume, the rate of infusion should be slow enough (1 mL per minute) to present too rapid expansion of plasma volume.

Treatment of Shock: Dosage is based almost entirely on the nature of the individual case and the response to therapy. The usual minimum effective dose is 250–500 mL.

The rate of administration for the emergency treatment of shock in adults is dependent on the response to therapy and the flow should be adjusted as the patient improves. Administration rates of 10 mL per minute should not be exceeded.

In infants and small children, Plasma-Plex® has been found to be very useful in the initial therapy of shock due to dehydration and infection. A dose of 15 mL per pound of body weight infused intravenously at a rate up to 5 to 10 mL per minute for the treatment of acute shock states in infants is desirable. As with any plasma expander the rate should be adjusted or slowed according to the clinical response and rising blood pressure.

Treatment of Burns: The dosage is dependent on the extent and severity of the burn. An optimal regimen for use of Plasma Protein Fraction (Human), crystalloids, electrolytes and water in the treatment of burns has not been established.

Treatment of Hypoproteinemia: The adult dose of Plasma Protein Fraction (Human) 5%—Plasma-Plex® is 1000 to 1500 mL daily to yield 50 to 75 g of plasma protein. Since blood volume in these patients may be normal, doses of more than 500 mL should not be given faster than 500 mL in 30 to 45 minutes to avoid circulatory embarrassment. If slower administration is desired, 1000 mL may be given by continuous drip at a rate of 100 mL per hour. If sodium restriction is imperative, 25% Albumin (Human) is recommended.

Parenteral drug products should be inspected visually for particulate matter and discoloration prior to administration whenever solution and container permit.

HOW SUPPLIED

Plasma Protein Fraction (Human) 5%—Plasma-Plex® is supplied as a 5% solution in:

NDC 0053-7753-03 50 mL bottles containing 2.5 g of selected plasma proteins.

NDC 0053-7753-01 250 mL bottles containing 12.5 g of selected plasma proteins.

NDC 0053-7753-02 500 mL bottles containing 25.0 g of selected plasma proteins.

Store at controlled room temperature—between 15°–30°C (59°–86°F). Do not allow to freeze.

Caution: Federal (U.S.A.) law prohibits dispensing without prescription.

BIBLIOGRAPHY

1. Bertrand, J.J.; Feichtmeir, T.V.; Kolomeyer, N.; Beatty, J.O.; Murphy, P.L.; Waldschmidt, W.D.; and McLean, E.B.; Clinical Investigations with a Heat-Treated Plasma Protein Fraction, Vox. Sang. 4:385–402, 1959.
2. Cock, T.C.; Binger, C.M.; and Dennis, J.L.; A New Plasma Substitute for Pediatric Therapy, Calif. Med. 89:257, 1958.
3. Hink, J.H. Jr.; Hidalgo, J.; Seeberg, V.P.; and Johnson, F.F.; Preparation and Properties of a Heat-Treated Human Plasma Protein Fraction, Vox Sanguinis 2:174, 1957.
4. Bland, J.H.; Laver, M.B.; and Lowenstein, E.; Vasodilator Effect of Commercial 5% Plasma Protein Fraction Solutions, JAMA 224:1721–1724, 1973.

Revised: May, 1996 (8/90)   IBM 12761
Centeon L.L.C.
Kankakee, Illinois 60901, U.S.A.
U.S. Government License No. 149

STIMATE®

[*stĭ-māte*]
(desmopressin acetate)
Nasal Spray, 1.5 mg/mL

DESCRIPTION

Stimate® (desmopressin acetate) is a synthetic analogue of the natural pituitary hormone 8-arginine vasopressin (ADH), an antidiuretic hormone affecting renal water conservation. Stimate® Nasal Spray contains 1.5 mg/mL desmopressin acetate in a pH-adjusted aqueous solution with chlorobutanol and sodium chloride as inactive ingredients. Stimate® Nasal Spray's compression pump delivers 0.1 mL (150 μg) of solution per spray. It is chemically defined as follows:

Mol. Wt. 1183.32

$$\text{Empirical formula: } C_{46}H_{64}N_{14}O_{12}S_2 \cdot C_2H_4O_2 \cdot 3H_2O$$

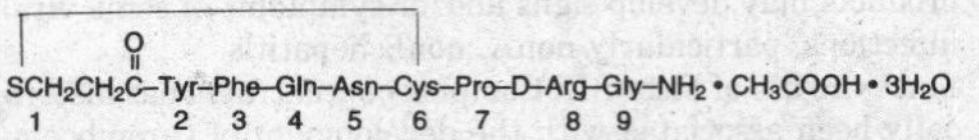

$$SCH_2CH_2C-Tyr-Phe-Gln-Asn-Cys-Pro-D-Arg-Gly-NH_2 \cdot CH_3COOH \cdot 3H_2O$$
$$1 \quad\quad 2 \quad 3 \quad 4 \quad 5 \quad 6 \quad 7 \quad 8 \quad 9$$

1-(3-Mercaptopropionic acid)-8-D-arginine vasopressin monoacetate (salt) trihydrate. Stimate® Nasal Spray is provided as an aqueous solution for intranasal use.

Each mL contains:

Desmopressin acetate	1.5 mg
Chlorobutanol	5.0 mg
Sodium Chloride	9.0 mg
Hydrochloric acid to adjust pH to approximately 4	

CLINICAL PHARMACOLOGY

Stimate® Nasal Spray contains as active substance, 1-(3-mercaptopropionic acid)-8-D-arginine vasopressin, which is a synthetic analogue of the natural hormone arginine vasopressin. One spray or 0.1 mL (150 μg) of Stimate® Nasal Spray solution has an antidiuretic activity of about 600 IU. Desmopressin acetate has been shown to be more potent than arginine vasopressin in increasing plasma levels of Factor VIII activity in patients with hemophilia and von Willebrand's disease Type I.

Dose-response studies were performed in healthy persons using doses of 150 to 450 μg, administered as one to three sprays. The response to Stimate® Nasal Spray is dose-related, with maximal plasma levels of 150 to 250 percent of initial concentrations achieved for both Factor VIII and von Willebrand factor [1]. The increase is rapid and evident within 30 minutes, reaching a maximum at about 1.5 hours [1].

The percentage increase of Factor VIII and von Willebrand factor levels in patients with mild hemophilia A and von Willebrand's disease was not notably different from that observed in normal healthy individuals when treated with 300 μg of Stimate® Nasal Spray [1–4]. In patients with von Willebrand's disease, levels of Factor VIII coagulant activity and von Willebrand factor antigen remained greater than 30 U/dL for 8 hours after a 300 μg dose of Stimate® Nasal Spray [7]. After 300 μg of Stimate® Nasal Spray, the percentage increase of Factor VIII and von Willebrand factor levels in patients with mild hemophilia A and von Willebrand's disease was less than observed after 0.3 μg/kg of intravenous desmopressin acetate [2–4].

Plasminogen activator activity increases rapidly after intravenous desmopressin acetate infusion, but there has been no clinically significant fibrinolysis in patients treated with desmopressin acetate.

The effect of repeated intravenous desmopressin acetate administration when doses were given every 12 to 24 hours has generally shown a diminution of the Factor VIII activity increase noted after a single dose. It is possible to reproduce the initial response in some patients after an interval of one week, but other patients may require as long as 6 weeks [2,4,6].

The half-life of Stimate® Nasal Spray was between 3.3 and 3.5 hours, over the range of intranasal doses, 150 to 450 μg [1]. Plasma concentrations of Stimate® Nasal Spray were maximal approximately 40 to 45 minutes after dosing [1]. The bioavailability of Stimate® Nasal Spray when administered by the intranasal route as a 1.5 mg/mL solution is between 3.3 and 4.1 percent [1].

The change in structure of arginine vasopressin to desmopressin acetate has resulted in a decreased vasopressor action and decreased actions on visceral smooth muscle relative to the enhanced antidiuretic activity, so that clinically effective antidiuretic doses are usually below threshold levels for effects on vascular or visceral smooth muscle.

INDICATIONS AND USAGE

Before the initial therapeutic administration of Stimate® Nasal Spray, the physician should establish that the patient shows an appropriate change in the coagulation profile following a test dose of intranasal administration of Stimate® Nasal Spray [2–4].

Desmopressin acetate is also available as a solution for injection (DDAVP® Injection) when the intranasal route may be compromised. These situations include nasal congestion and

blockage, nasal discharge, atrophy of nasal mucosa, and severe atrophic rhinitis. Intranasal delivery may also be inappropriate where there is an impaired level of consciousness.

Hemophilia A

Stimate® Nasal Spray is indicated for patients with hemophilia A with Factor VIII coagulant activity levels greater than 5%.

Desmopressin acetate will also stop bleeding in patients with hemophilia A with episodes of spontaneous or trauma-induced injuries such as hemarthroses, intramuscular hematomas or mucosal bleeding [2,3].

In the outpatient setting during two clinical trials where patients recorded bleeding episodes, **Stimate® Nasal Spray** provided effective hemostasis 100% of the time in 2 of the 5 patients. For those patients not responding in 100% of bleeding occasions, 45% (14 of 31) of bleeding episodes were effectively controlled with **Stimate® Nasal Spray**.

Desmopressin acetate is not indicated for the treatment of hemophilia A with Factor VIII coagulant activity levels equal to or less than 5%, or for the treatment of hemophilia B, or in patients who have Factor VIII antibodies.

von Willebrand's Disease (Type I)

Stimate® Nasal Spray is indicated for patients with mild to moderate classic von Willebrand's disease (Type I) with Factor VIII levels greater than 5%.

Desmopressin acetate will also stop bleeding in mild to moderate von Willebrand's disease patients with episodes of spontaneous or trauma-induced injuries such as hemarthroses, intramuscular hematomas, mucosal bleeding or menorrhagia [2,3].

In the outpatient setting during two clinical trials where patients recorded bleeding episodes, **Stimate® Nasal Spray** provided effective hemostasis 100% of the time in 75% of the patients (n=16). For those patients not responding in 100% of bleeding occasions, 78% (64 of 82) of bleeding episodes were effectively controlled with **Stimate® Nasal Spray**.

Patients may respond in a variable fashion depending on the type of molecular defect they have. Bleeding time and Factor VIII coagulant activity, ristocetin cofactor activity, and von Willebrand factor antigen should be checked after initial administration of **Stimate® Nasal Spray** to ensure that adequate levels have been achieved.

Stimate® Nasal Spray is not indicated for the treatment of severe classic von Willebrand's disease (Type I) and when there is evidence of an abnormal molecular form of Factor VIII antigen. See WARNING.

CONTRAINDICATION

Stimate® Nasal Spray is contraindicated in individuals with known hypersensitivity to desmopressin acetate or to any of the components of **Stimate® Nasal Spray**.

WARNINGS

For intranasal use only.

Patients who do not have need of antidiuretic hormone for its antidiuretic effect, in particular those who are young or elderly, should be cautioned to ingest only enough fluid to satisfy thirst, in order to decrease the potential occurrence of water intoxication and hyponatremia.

Fluid intake should be adjusted downward, particularly in very young and elderly patients, in order to decrease the potential occurrence of water intoxication and hyponatremia [1]. Particular attention should be paid to the possibility of the rare occurrence of an extreme decrease in plasma osmolality that may result in seizures which could lead to coma.

Stimate® Nasal Spray should not be used to treat patients with Type IIB von Willebrand's disease since platelet aggregation may be induced.

PRECAUTIONS

General

Desmopressin acetate has infrequently produced changes in blood pressure causing either a slight elevation in blood pressure or a transient fall in blood pressure and a compensatory increase in heart rate. The drug should be used with caution in patients with coronary artery insufficiency and/or hypertensive cardiovascular disease.

Stimate® Nasal Spray should be used with caution in patients with conditions associated with fluid and electrolyte imbalance, such as cystic fibrosis, because these patients are prone to hyponatremia.

There have been rare reports of thrombotic events (thrombosis [9], acute cerebrovascular thrombosis, acute myocardial infarction) following desmopressin acetate injection in patients predisposed to thrombus formation. No causality has been determined; however, the drug should be used with caution in these patients.

Severe allergic reactions have been reported rarely [2, 11-13]. Fatal anaphylaxis has been reported in one patient who received intravenous DDAVP® (desmopressin acetate). It is not known whether antibodies to desmopressin acetate are produced after repeated administration.

Since **Stimate® Nasal Spray** is used intranasally, changes in the nasal mucosa such as scarring, edema, or other disease may cause erratic, unreliable absorption in which case **Stimate® Nasal Spray** should be discontinued until the na-

sal problems resolve. For such situations, DDAVP® Injection should be considered.

Information for Patients: Patients should be informed that the bottle accurately delivers 25 doses of 150 μg each. Any solution remaining after 25 doses should be discarded since the amount delivered thereafter may be substantially less than 150 μg of drug. No attempt should be made to transfer remaining solution to another bottle. Patients should be instructed to read accompanying directions on use of the spray pump carefully before use.

Patients should also be advised that if bleeding is not controlled, the physician should be contacted [2,3].

Hemophilia A

Laboratory tests for assessing patient status include levels of Factor VIII coagulant. Factor VIII antigen and Factor VIII ristocetin cofactor (von Willebrand factor) as well as activated partial thromboplastin time. Factor VIII coagulant activity should be determined before giving **Stimate® Nasal Spray** for hemostasis. If Factor VIII coagulant activity is present at less than 5% of normal, **Stimate® Nasal Spray** should not be relied on.

von Willebrand's Disease

Laboratory tests for assessing patient status include levels of Factor VIII coagulant activity, Factor VIII ristocetin cofactor activity, and Factor VIII von Willebrand factor antigen. The skin bleeding time may be helpful in following these patients.

Drug Interactions

Although the pressor activity of desmopressin acetate is very low, its use with other pressor agents should be done only with careful patient monitoring.

DDAVP® Injection has been used with epsilon aminocaproic acid without adverse effects.

Carcinogenicity, Mutagenicity, Impairment of Fertility: There have been no long-term studies in animals to assess the carcinogenic, mutagenic or impairment of fertility potential of **Stimate® Nasal Spray**.

Pregnancy Category B: Reproduction studies performed in rats and rabbits by the subcutaneous route at doses up to 10 μg/kg/day have revealed no evidence of harm to the fetus due to desmopressin acetate. This dose is equivalent to 10 times (for Factor VIII stimulation) or 38 times (for diabetes insipidus) the systemic human dose based on a mg/M^2 surface area.

There are no adequate and well-controlled studies in pregnant women. Several publications of desmopressin acetate's use in the management of diabetes insipidus during pregnancy are available; these include a few anecdotal reports of congenital anomalies and low birth weight babies. However, no causal connection between these events and desmopressin acetate has been established. A 15-year, Swedish epidemiologic study of the use of desmopressin acetate in pregnant women with diabetes insipidus found the rate of birth defects to be no greater than that in the general population. As opposed to preparations containing natural hormones, desmopressin acetate in antidiuretic doses has no uterotonic action and the physician will have to weigh the therapeutic advantages against the possible risks in each case.

Nursing Mothers: There have been no controlled studies in nursing mothers. A single study in postpartum women demonstrated a marked change in plasma, but little if any change in assayable DDAVP in breast milk following an intranasal dose of 10 μg. It is not known whether this drug is excreted in human milk. Because many drugs are excreted in human milk, caution should be exercised when **Stimate® Nasal Spray** is administered to a nursing woman.

Pediatric Use: Use in infants and children will require careful fluid intake restriction to prevent possible hyponatremia and water intoxication. **Stimate® Nasal Spray** should not be used in infants younger than 11 months in the treatment of hemophilia A or von Willebrand's disease; safety and effectiveness in children between 11 months and 12 years of age has been demonstrated [2-4].

ADVERSE REACTIONS

Infrequently, DDAVP® Injection has produced transient headache, nausea, mild abdominal cramps and vulval pain. These symptoms disappeared with reduction in dosage. Occasional facial flushing has been reported with the administration of DDAVP® Injection. Infrequently, high doses of intranasal DDAVP® have produced transient headache and nausea. Nasal congestion, rhinitis and flushing have also been reported occasionally along with mild abdominal cramps. These symptoms disappeared with reduction in dosage. Nosebleed, sore throat, cough and upper respiratory infections have also been reported.

In addition to those listed above, the following have also been reported in clinical trials with **Stimate® Nasal Spray**: Somnolence, dizziness, itchy or light-sensitive eyes, insomnia, chills, warm feeling, pain, chest pain, palpitations, tachycardia, dyspepsia, edema, vomiting, agitation and balanitis [1-4].

DDAVP® Injection (desmopressin acetate) has infrequently produced changes in blood pressure causing either a slight elevation or a transient fall and a compensatory increase in

heart rate. Severe allergic reactions including anaphylaxis have been reported rarely with DDAVP® Injection.

See WARNING for the possibility of water intoxication, hyponatremia and coma [10].

OVERDOSAGE

See ADVERSE REACTIONS above. In cases of overdosage, the dosage should be reduced, frequency of administration decreased, or the drug withdrawn according to the severity of the condition.

There is no known specific antidote for desmopressin acetate or **Stimate® Nasal Spray**.

An oral LD$_{50}$ has not been established. An intravenous dose of 2 mg/kg in mice demonstrated no effect.

DOSAGE AND ADMINISTRATION

Hemophilia A and von Willebrand's Disease (Type I)

Stimate® Nasal Spray is administered by nasal insufflation, one spray per nostril, to provide a total dose of 300 μg. In patients weighing less than 50 kg, 150 μg administered as a single spray provided the expected effect on Factor VIII coagulant activity, Factor VIII ristocetin cofactor activity and skin bleeding time [3,4]. If **Stimate® Nasal Spray** is used preoperatively, it should be administered 2 hours prior to the scheduled procedure [5,8].

The necessity for repeat administration of **Stimate® Nasal Spray** or use of any blood products for hemostasis should be determined by laboratory response as well as the clinical condition of the patient. The tendency toward tachyphylaxis (lessening of response) with repeated administration given more frequently than every 48 hours should be considered in treating each patient.

The nasal spray pump can only deliver doses of 0.1 mL (150 μg) or multiples of 0.1 mL. If doses other than these are required, DDAVP® Injection may be used.

The spray pump must be primed prior to the first use. To prime pump, press down 4 times. The bottle should be discarded after 25 doses since the amount delivered thereafter per spray may be substantially less than 150 μg of drug.

HOW SUPPLIED

A 2.5 mL bottle with spray pump capable of delivering 25 doses of 150 μg (NDC 0053-2453-00).

KEEP REFRIGERATED AT 2°–8°C (36°–46°F). When traveling, product will maintain stability for up to 3 weeks when stored at room temperature, 22°C (72°F).

Caution: Federal (U.S.A.) law prohibits dispensing without prescription.

REFERENCES

1. RHÔNE-POULENC RORER STUDY RG-83884-141: An Open-Label Pharmacokinetic Comparison of Desmopressin Acetate Administration by Intranasal (1.5 mg/mL) and Intravenous Routes: A Dose-Proportionality Trial.
2. RHÔNE-POULENC RORER STUDY RG-83884-142: Nasal Spray Desmopressin (DDAVP): A simple Technique for Treatment of Mild Hemophillia A and von Willebrand's disease.
3. RHÔNE-POULENC RORER STUDY RG-83884-143: Intranasal Desmopressin (DDAVP) by spray in Mild Hemophilia A and von Willebrand's disease Type I.
4. RHÔNE-POULENC RORER STUDY RG-83884-144: Evaluation of Intranasal Spray DDAVP in Patients with Mild or Moderate Hemophilia A or von Willebrand's disease: Inpatient Trial.
5. Chistolini A, Dragoni F, Ferrari A, La Verde G, Arcieri R, Mohamud AE and Mazzucconi MG: Intranasal DDAVP: Biological and clinical evaluation in mild Factor VIII deficiency. Haemostasis, 21:273–277, 1991.
6. Lethagen S, Harris AS, Sjörin E and Nilsson IM: Intranasal and intravenous administration of desmopressin: Effect on FVIII/vWF, pharmacokinetics and reproducibility. Thromb. Haemost., 58:1033-1036, 1987.
7. Lethagen S, Harris AS and Nilsson IM: Intranasal desmopressin (DDAVP) by spray in mild hemophilia A and von Willebrand's disease type I. Blut, 60: 187–191, 1990.
8. Rose EH and Aledort LM: Nasal spray desmopressin (DDAVP) for mild hemophilia A and von Willebrand's disease. Ann. Int. Med., 114:563–568, 1991.
9. Viron B, Michel C, Serrato T and Verdy E: Risque thrombogène du D.D.A.V.P. dans L'insuffisance rénale chronique (Thrombogenic risk of DDAVP in chronic renal failure). Néphrologie, 8:225, 1987.
10. RHÔNE-POULENC RORER PHARMACEUTICALS INC. ADVERSE REACTION REPORT No. 01-003827; Coma, grand mal seizure, etc.
11. RHÔNE-POULENC RORER PHARMACEUTICALS INC. ADVERSE REACTION REPORT No. 01-000657; Anaphylaxis, etc.
12. RHÔNE-POULENC RORER PHARMACEUTICALS INC. ADVERSE REACTION REPORT No. 01-001182; Anaphylactoid reaction.
13. RHÔNE-POULENC RORER PHARMACEUTICALS INC. ADVERSE REACTION REPORT No. US-870671; Erythema, rash.

Continued on next page

Centeon—Cont.

Revised: May, 1996 (3/95)   IBM 23790
Manufactured for
CENTEON L.L.C.
KING OF PRUSSIA, PA 19406-1310
By Ferring Pharmaceuticals, Malmö, Sweden

EDUCATIONAL MATERIAL

Monoclate-P® Factor VIII:C
Mononine® Factor IX
Watercise Video
Flexercise Video
Raising a Child with Hemophilia Book
Family Guide to Hemophilia B Book
My Blood Doesn't Have Muscles Book
Family First: Hemophilia Kit
  A Guide for Parents of Infants with Hemophilia
  A Guide for Parents of School Age Children with
  Hemophilia
  A Guide for Young Adults with Hemophilia
Stimate® (desmopressin acetate) Nasal Spray, 1.5 mg/mL
Diane Dino's Dilemma Book
Patient Q & A Brochure
Understanding Mild To Moderate von Willebrand's Disease
Bioclate™
Patient Q & A Brochure
Helixate®
Patient Q & A Brochure
Gamma®-P I.V.
Immunoglobulin Therapy: Your Questions Answered
Brochure
*Available to physicians and pharmacists—contact Centeon
Corporate Headquarters.*

Center Laboratories
Division of EM Industries, Inc.
35 CHANNEL DRIVE
PORT WASHINGTON, NY 11050

Direct Inquiries to:
Customer Services
(800) 223-6837

For Medical Information Contact:
In Emergencies:
Technical Services
(516) 767-1800

EPIPEN®/EPIPEN® JR.   ℞
Epinephrine Auto-Injectors

**Brief summary: Before prescribing, please consult package
insert.**

DESCRIPTION
The EpiPen Auto-Injectors contain 2 mL Epinephrine Injection for emergency intramuscular use. Each EpiPen Auto-Injector delivers a single dose of 0.3 mg epinephrine from Epinephrine Injection, USP, 1:1000 (0.3 mL) in a sterile solution. Each EpiPen Jr. Auto-Injector delivers a single dose of 0.15 mg epinephrine from Epinephrine Injection, USP, 1:2000 (0.3 mL) in a sterile solution. Each 0.3 mL also contains 1.8 mg sodium chloride, 0.5 mg sodium metabisulfite, hydrochloric acid to adjust pH, and water for injection. The pH range is 2.5–5.0.

CLINICAL PHARMACOLOGY
Epinephrine is a sympathomimetic drug, acting on both alpha and beta receptors. It is the drug of choice for the emergency treatment of severe allergic reactions (Type I) to insect stings or bites, foods, drugs, and other allergens. It can also be used in the treatment of idiopathic or exercise-induced anaphylaxis. Epinephrine when given subcutaneously or intramuscularly has a rapid onset and short duration of action.

INDICATIONS AND USAGE
Epinephrine is indicated in the emergency treatment of allergic reactions (anaphylaxis) to insect stings or bites, foods, drugs and other allergens as well as idiopathic or exercise-induced anaphylaxis. The EpiPen Auto-Injector is intended for immediate self-administration by a person with a history of an anaphylactic reaction. Such reactions may occur within minutes after exposure and consist of flushing, apprehension, syncope, tachycardia, thready or unobtainable

pulse associated with a fall in blood pressure, convulsions, vomiting, diarrhea and abdominal cramps, involuntary voiding, wheezing, dyspnea due to laryngeal spasm, pruritis, rashes, urticaria or angioedema. The EpiPen is designed as emergency supportive therapy only and is not a replacement or substitute for immediate medical or hospital care.

CONTRAINDICATIONS
There are no absolute contraindications to the use of epinephrine in a life-threatening situation.

WARNINGS
Epinephrine is light sensitive and should be stored in the tube provided. Store at room temperature (15°–30°C/59°–86°F). Do not refrigerate. Before using, check to make sure solution in Auto-Injector is not discolored.
Replace the Auto-Injector if the solution is discolored or contains a precipitate. Avoid possible inadvertent intravascular administration. Select an appropriate injection site such as the thigh. DO NOT INJECT INTO BUTTOCK. Large doses or accidental intravenous injection of epinephrine may result in cerebral hemorrhage due to sharp rise in blood pressure. DO NOT INJECT INTRAVENOUSLY. Rapid acting vasodilators can counteract the marked pressor effects of epinephrine.
Epinephrine is the preferred treatment for serious allergic or other emergency situations even though this product contains sodium metabisulfite, a sulfite that may in other products cause allergic-type reactions including anaphylactic symptoms or life-threatening or less severe asthmatic episodes in certain susceptible persons. The alternatives to using epinephrine in a life-threatening situation may not be satisfactory. The presence of a sulfite in this product should not deter administration of the drug for treatment of serious allergic or other emergency situations.

PRECAUTIONS
Epinephrine is ordinarily administered with extreme caution to patients who have heart disease. Use of epinephrine with drugs that may sensitize the heart to arrhythmias, e.g., digitalis, mercurial diuretics, or quinidine, ordinarily is not recommended. Anginal pain may be induced by epinephrine in patients with coronary insufficiency. The effects of epinephrine may be potentiated by tricyclic antidepressants and monoamine oxidase inhibitors. Hyperthyroid individuals, individuals with cardiovascular disease, hypertension, or diabetes, elderly individuals, pregnant women, and children under 30 kg (66 lbs.) body weight may be theoretically at greater risk of developing adverse reactions after epinephrine administration. Despite these concerns, epinephrine is essential for the treatment of anaphylaxis. Therefore, patients with these conditions, and/or any other person who might be in a position to administer EpiPen or EpiPen Jr. to a patient experiencing anaphylaxis should be carefully instructed in regard to the circumstances under which this lifesaving medication should be used.

CARCINOGENESIS, MUTAGENESIS, IMPAIRMENT OF FERTILITY
Studies of epinephrine in animals to evaluate the carcinogenic and mutagenic potential or the effect on fertility have not been conducted.

USAGE IN PREGNANCY
Pregnancy Category C: Epinephrine has been shown to be teratogenic in rats when given in doses about 25 times the human dose. There are no adequate and well-controlled studies in pregnant women. Epinephrine should be used during pregnancy only if the potential benefit justifies the potential risk to the fetus.

PEDIATRIC USE
Epinephrine may be given safely to children at a dosage appropriate to body weight (see Dosage and Administration).

ADVERSE REACTIONS
Side effects of epinephrine may include palpitations, tachycardia, sweating, nausea and vomiting, respiratory difficulty, pallor, dizziness, weakness, tremor, headache, apprehension, nervousness and anxiety.
Cardiac arrhythmias may follow administration of epinephrine.

OVERDOSAGE
Overdosage or inadvertent intravascular injection of epinephrine may cause cerebral hemorrhage resulting from a sharp rise in blood pressure. Fatalities may also result from pulmonary edema because of peripheral vascular constriction together with cardiac stimulation.

DOSAGE AND ADMINISTRATION
Usual epinephrine adult dose for allergic emergencies is 0.3 mg. For pediatric use, the appropriate dosage may be 0.15 or 0.30 mg depending upon the body weight of the patient. However, the prescribing physician has the option of prescribing more or less than these amounts, based on careful assessment of each individual patient and recognizing the life-threatening nature of the reactions for which this drug is being prescribed. With severe persistant anaphylaxis, repeat injections with an additional EpiPen may be necessary.

HOW SUPPLIED
EpiPen and EpiPen Jr. Auto-Injectors are available singly or in packages of twelve.
EPIPEN® NDC 0268-0301-01
EPIPEN® JR NDC 0268-0302-01

CAUTION
Federal (U.S.A.) law prohibits dispensing without a prescription.

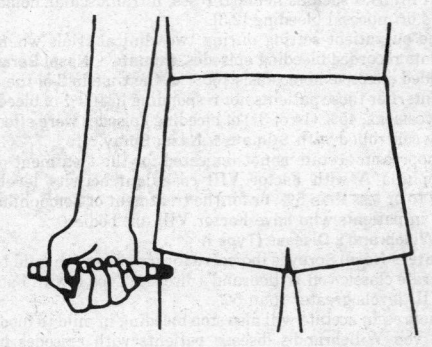

Issued: April 1988

Central Pharmaceuticals, Inc.
120 EAST THIRD STREET
SEYMOUR, IN 47274

Direct Inquiries to:
Schwarz Pharma
Drug Safety and Information
P.O. Box 2038
Milwaukee, WI 53201
(800) 558–5114

AZDŌNE® TABLETS   Ⓒ ℞
[ăz'dōn]

DESCRIPTION
Each tablet contains:
  Hydrocodone* Bitartrate .... 5 mg
    *(WARNING—May be habit forming)
  Aspirin .... 500 mg
Hydrocodone bitartrate is an opioid analgesic and antitussive and occurs as fine, white crystals or as a crystalline powder. It is affected by light. The chemical name is: 4,5α-epoxy-3-methoxy-17-methylmorphinan-6-one tartrate (1:1) hydrate (2:5).
Aspirin, salicylic acid acetate, is a non-opiate salicylate analgesic, anti-inflammatory, and antipyretic which occurs as a white, crystalline tabular or needle-like powder and is odorless or has a faint odor.
Inactive Ingredients: Corn Starch, D&C Red #7 (Calcium Lake), Sodium Starch Glycolate, and Stearic Acid.

HOW SUPPLIED
Flat, truncated oval, bisected mottled pink tablet containing 5 mg Hydrocodone Bitartrate (WARNING: May be habit forming) and 500 mg of Aspirin. Each tablet is debossed with the Central logo on one side and the number 21 and the score on the other side.
Bottles of 100 tablets—NDC 0131-2821-37
Bottles of 1000 tablets—NDC 0131-2821-43
  Shown in Product Identification Guide, page 308

CODICLEAR® DH SYRUP   Ⓒ ℞
[kō'dĭ-klēr"]

DESCRIPTION
A clear, colorless, sweet-tasting syrup for oral administration, which is alcohol-free, dye-free. sugar-free and contains no parabens.
Each teaspoonful (5 mL) contains:
Hydrocodone* bitartrate .... 5 mg
*(Warning—May be habit forming)
Guaifenesin .... 100 mg
This product contains ingredients of the following therapeutic classes: antitussive and expectorant.

CAUTION

Federal law prohibits dispensing without prescription.

INACTIVE INGREDIENTS

Benzoic Acid, Citric Acid, Flavors, Glycerin, Polyethylene Glycol, Povidone, Propylene Glycol, Purified Water, Saccharin Sodium, Sodium Citrate and Sorbitol.

CLINICAL PHARMACOLOGY

Hydrocodone bitartrate is a potent antitussive which causes suppression of the cough reflex by a direct action on the cough center. Hydrocodone is approximately three times as potent as codeine on a weight basis, and has a higher addiction potential. Guaifenesin is used as an expectorant. It is thought to increase mucous flow in the lung by stimulation of gastric mucosal reflexes.

INDICATIONS

For the temporary relief of dry, non-productive cough associated with upper and lower respiratory tract congestion.

CONTRAINDICATIONS

Hypersensitivity to hydrocodone or guaifenesin. Hydrocodone is contraindicated in the presence of increased intracranial pressure and whenever ventilatory function is depressed.

WARNINGS

Hydrocodone can produce drug dependence and therefore has the potential for being abused. Codiclear DH should be prescribed and administered with the degree of caution appropriate for this type product.

PRECAUTIONS

General: The hydrocodone in this product may exhibit additive effects with other CNS depressants, including alcohol. Respiratory depression can be a real hazard so caution should be used, especially in patients with chronic obstructive pulmonary disease.

Information for Patients: The hydrocodone may cause drowsiness and ambulatory patients who operate machinery or motor vehicles should be cautioned accordingly.

Drug Interactions: Patients receiving other narcotic analgesics, general anesthetics, phenothiazines, other tranquilizers, sedative hypnotics or other CNS depressants (including alcohol) concomitantly with hydrocodone may exhibit an additive CNS depression. When such combined therapy is contemplated the dose of one or both agents should be reduced. (See WARNINGS.)

Laboratory Interactions: The metabolite of guaifenesin has been found to produce an apparent increase in urinary 5-hydroxyindoleacetic acid, and guaifenesin therefore may interfere with the interpretation of this test for the diagnosis of carcinoid syndrome. Guaifenesin administration should be discontinued 24 hours prior to the collection of urine specimens for the determination of 5-hydroxyindoleacetic acid.

Usage in Pregnancy: Pregnancy Category C. Hydrocodone has been shown to be teratogenic in hamsters when given in doses 700 times the human dose. There are no adequate and well-controlled studies in pregnant women. CODICLEAR DH Syrup should be used during pregnancy only if the potential benefit justifies the potential risk to the fetus.

ADVERSE REACTIONS

Adverse reactions include drowsiness, lassitude, nausea, giddiness, constipation, respiratory depression and addiction.

DRUG ABUSE AND DEPENDENCE

This product is a Schedule III Controlled Sustance. Because of the hydrocodone content, some abuse might be expected. Psychic dependence, physical dependence and tolerance may develop upon repeated administration. It should be prescribed and administered with the degree of caution appropriate for this type product.

OVERDOSAGE

Symptoms of overdosage include respiratory depression, extreme somnolence progressing to stupor or coma, skeletal muscle flaccidity, cold and clammy skin and other symptoms common with narcotic overdosage.

Primary treatment consists of insuring adequate respiration through provision of a patent airway and the institution of assisted or controlled ventilation. Naloxone hydrochloride should be administered in small intravenous doses (consult specific product labeling before use). In addition, oxygen, intravenous fluids, vasopressors and other supportive measures should be employed as indicated. Gastric emptying may be useful in removing unabsorbed drug. Activated charcoal may also be of benefit.

DOSAGE AND ADMINISTRATION

Usual Adult Dose—One teaspoonful (5 mL) after meals and at bedtime, not less than 4 hours apart (not to exceed 6 teaspoonsful in a 24 hour period.) Treatment should be initiated with one teaspoonful and subsequent doses, up to a maximum single dose of 3 teaspoonsful, adjusted if required. Usual Children's Dose—Over 12 years: Initial dose 1 teaspoonful; maximum single dose, 2 teaspoonsful. 6–12 years:

Initial dose ½ teaspoonful: maximum single dose, 1 teaspoonful.

HOW SUPPLIED

Bottles of 4 fl oz—NDC 0131-5134-64
Bottles of one pint—NDC 0131-5134-70

CODIMAL® DH   ⓒ ℞
[kō'di-mahl"]

DESCRIPTION

Each teaspoonful (5 mL) of CODIMAL DH contains: Hydrocodone Bitartrate 1.66 mg. (Warning—May be habit forming); Phenylephrine Hydrochloride 5 mg.; Pyrilamine Maleate 8.33 mg. Alcohol-Free.

HOW SUPPLIED

Codimal DH (Red Syrup)
4oz—NDC# 0131-5129-64
Pint—NDC# 0131-5129-70
Gallon—NDC# 0131-5129-72

CODIMAL® DM   OTC
[kō' di-mahl"]

DESCRIPTION

Each teaspoonful (5 mL) of CODIMAL® DM contains: Dextromethorphan hydrobromide 10 mg.; Phenylephrine hydrochloride 5 mg; Pyrilamine maleate 8.33 mg.; Alcohol-Free, Dye-Free, Sugar-Free, Paraben-Free.

HOW SUPPLIED

Codimal® DM (Clear Syrup)
4 oz-NDC # 0131-5131-64
Pint-NDC# 0131-5131-70
Gallon-NDC# 0131-5131-72
For full information see product labeling.

CODIMAL®-L.A. CAPSULES   ℞
[kō'di-mahl"]

DESCRIPTION

Each Extended-Release Capsule contains:
Chlorpheniramine maleate .... 8 mg
Pseudoephedrine
  hydrochloride .... 120 mg
in a specially prepared base to provide prolonged action.

HOW SUPPLIED

No. 1 clear body, red cap printed with white Central logo and 40, filled with red, white, and blue beads.
Bottle of 100 Capsules-NDC 0131-4213-37
Bottle of 1000 Capsules-NDC 0131-4213-43
Shown in Product Identification Guide, page 308

CODIMAL®–L.A. HALF CAPSULES   ℞

DESCRIPTION

Each Extended-Release Capsule contains:
Chlorpheniramine Maleate .... 4 mg
Pseudoephedrine Hydrochloride .... 60 mg
in a specially prepared base to provide prolonged action.

HOW SUPPLIED

Codimal®-L.A. Half capsules are clear, colorless capsules with red, white and blue beads. Black printing on capsule indicates Central on cap and 60/4 on the body.
Bottle of 100 Capsules
NDC 0131-4501-37
Shown in Product Identification Guide, page 308

CODIMAL® PH   OTC
[kō' di-mahl"]

DESCRIPTION

Each teaspoonful (5 mL) of CODIMAL® PH contains: Codeine Phosphate 10 mg. (Warning-May be habit forming); Phenylephrine Hydrochloride 5 mg.; Pyrilamine Maleate 8.33 mg. Alcohol-Free

HOW SUPPLIED

Codimal® PH (Red Syrup)
4 oz-NDC# 0131-5038-64
Pint-NDC# 0131-5038-70
Gallon-NDC# 0131-5038-72

CO-GESIC®   ⓒ ℞
TABLETS
(Hydrocodone Bitartrate and Acetaminophen Tablets)

DESCRIPTION

Each CO-GESIC® Tablet contains:
Hydrocodone Bitartrate* .... 5 mg
*WARNING: May be habit forming.
Acetaminophen... 500 mg

HOW SUPPLIED

CO-GESIC® [Hydrocodone Bitartrate 5 mg (Warning: May be habit forming) and Acetaminophen 500 mg] Tablets are oval-shaped, white, scored compressed tablets debossed with 500 and 5 separated by bisect on one side and Central logo on the other.
Bottle of 100 tablets: NDC 0131-2104-37
Bottle of 500 tablets: NDC 0131-2104-41
Shown in Product Identification Guide, page 308

GUAIMAX-D®   ℞
[guī'-max"]

DESCRIPTION

Each GUAIMAX-D® white to off-white uncoated, scored, extended-release tablet for oral administration contains:
Pseudoephedrine
  Hydrochloride .... 120 mg
  Guaifenesin .... 600 mg
in a special base to provide a prolonged therapeutic effect. Dye-free.
This product contains ingredients of the following therapeutic classes: nasal decongestant and expectorant.
Pseudoephedrine hydrochloride is a nasal decongestant having the chemical name, benzenemethanol, $\alpha[1$-(methylamino) ethyl]-, $[S-(R^*,R^*)]$-, hydrochloride, with the following structure:

$C_{10}H_{15}NO \cdot HCl$ M.W. 201.70

Guaifenesin is an expectorant having the chemical name, 1, 2-propanediol, 3-(2-methoxyphenoxy)-, with the following structure:

$C_{10}H_{14}O_4$ M.W. 198.22

Inactive Ingredients: Each tablet contains Flavor, Magnesium Stearate, Microcrystalline Cellulose, Talc and other ingredients.

CLINICAL PHARMACOLOGY

Pseudoephedrine hydrochloride is an α-adrenergic receptor agonist (sympathomimetic) which produces vasoconstriction by stimulating α-receptors within the mucosa of the respiratory tract. Clinically, pseudoephedrine shrinks swollen mucous membranes, reduces tissue hyperemia, edema, and nasal congestion, and increases nasal airway patency. Guaifenesin promotes lower respiratory tract drainage by thinning bronchial secretions, lubricates irritated respiratory tract membranes through increased mucus flow, and facilitates removal of viscous, inspissated mucus. As a result of these drugs, sinus and bronchial drainage is improved, and dry, nonproductive coughs become more productive and less frequent.

INDICATIONS AND USAGE

GUAIMAX-D® tablets are indicated for the relief of nasal congestion due to the common cold, hay fever or other upper respiratory allergies, and nasal congestion associated with sinusitis; to promote nasal or sinus drainage; for the symptomatic relief of respiratory conditions characterized by dry nonproductive cough and in the presence of tenacious mucus and/or mucous plugs in the respiratory tract.

CONTRAINDICATIONS

GUAIMAX-D® tablets are contraindicated in patients with a known hypersensitivity to any of its ingredients, in nursing mothers, or in patients with severe hypertension, severe coronary artery disease, prostatic hypertrophy, or in patients on MAO inhibitor therapy.

WARNINGS

Sympathomimetic amines should be used with caution in patients with hypertension, diabetes mellitus, heart disease,

Continued on next page

Central—Cont.

peripheral vascular disease, increased intraocular pressure, hyperthyroidism, or prostatic hypertrophy.

PRECAUTIONS

General: Hypertensive patients should use GUAIMAX-D® tablets only with medical advice, as they may experience a change in blood pressure due to added vasoconstriction.

Information for Patients: Persistent cough may indicate a serious condition. If cough persists for more than one week, tends to recur, or is accompanied by a high fever, rash, or persistent headache, consult a physician.

Drug Interactions: MAO inhibitors and beta adrenergic blockers increase effects of sympathomimetics. Sympathomimetics may reduce the antihypertensive effects of methyldopa, guanethidine, mecamylamine, reserpine and veratrum alkaloids.

Drug/Laboratory Test Interactions: Guaifenesin has been reported to interfere with clinical laboratory determinations of urinary 5-hydroxyindoleacetic acid (5-HIAA) and urinary vanillylmandelic acid (VMA).

Pregnancy: Pregnancy Category C. Animal reproduction studies have not been conducted with GUAIMAX-D® tablets. It is also not known whether GUAIMAX-D® tablets can cause fetal harm when administered to a pregnant woman or can affect reproduction capacity. GUAIMAX-D® tablets should be given to a pregnant woman only if clearly needed.

Nursing Mothers: GUAIMAX-D® tablets are contraindicated in the nursing mother because of the higher than usual risks to infants from sympathomimetic agents.

Usage in Elderly: Patients 60 years and older are more likely to experience adverse reactions to sympathomimetics. Overdose may cause hallucinations, convulsions, CNS depression and death. Demonstrate safe use of a short-acting sympathomimetic before use of a sustained action formulation in elderly patients.

Pediatric Use: Safety and effectiveness of GUAIMAX-D® tablets in pediatric patients below the age of 6 have not been established.

ADVERSE REACTIONS

Gastrointestinal: nausea and vomiting.

Central Nervous System: nervousness, dizziness, sleeplessness, lightheadedness, tremor, hallucinations, convulsions, CNS depression, fear, anxiety, headache, increased irritability or excitement.

Cardiovascular: palpitations, tachycardia, cardiovascular collapse and death.

General: weakness.

Respiratory: respiratory difficulties.

OVERDOSAGE

Symptoms: Overdosage may cause hallucinations, convulsions, CNS depression, cardiovascular collapse and death.

Treatment: Treatment of overdosage should provide symptomatic care. If the amount ingested is considered dangerous or excessive, induce vomiting with ipecac syrup unless the patient is convulsing, comatose, or has lost the gag reflex, in which case, perform gastric lavage using a large-bore tube. If indicated, follow with activated charcoal and a saline cathartic. Since the effects of GUAIMAX-D® tablets may last up to 12 hours, treatment should be continued for at least that length of time.

DOSAGE AND ADMINISTRATION

Adults and pediatric patients 12 years of age and older: one tablet twice daily (every 12 hours). Pediatric patients 6 to under 12 years: one-half ($^1/_2$) tablet twice daily (every 12 hours). GUAIMAX-D® tablets are not recommended for pediatric patients under 6 years of age. Tablets may be broken in half for ease of administration without affecting release of medication but should not be crushed or chewed prior to swallowing.

HOW SUPPLIED

GUAIMAX-D® tablets are uncoated white to off-white, debossed with the product name on one side and scored on the other with 131 on the left side and 2055 on the right side.

Bottles of 100 NDC 0131-2055-37

Shown in Product Identification Guide, page 308

MONO-GESIC® TABLETS ℞

[mon″o-je′zik]

(salsalate)

DESCRIPTION

Each oval, pink film-coated tablet contains:

Salsalate.. 750 mg

Mono-Gesic® (Salsalate Tablets, USP) is a non-steroidal anti-inflammatory agent for oral administration. Chemically, salsalate (salicylsalicylic acid or 2-hydroxy-benzoic acid 2-carboxyphenyl ester) is a dimer of salicylic acid. It is represented by the following formula:

[See structure at top of next column.]

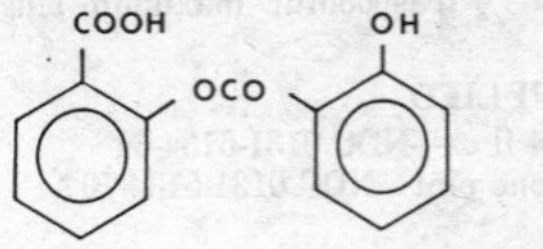

$C_{14}H_{10}O_5$ M.W. 258.2

The ingredient in this product is of the following classes: non-steroidal anti-inflammatory agent and analgesic.

Inactive Ingredients: Castor Oil, D&C Red #30 Lake, Hydroxypropyl Cellulose, Hydroxypropyl Methylcellulose, Microcrystalline Cellulose, Pharmaceutical Glaze, Polyethylene Glycol, Povidone, Propylene Glycol, Sodium Lauryl Sulfate, Sodium Starch Glycolate, Stearic Acid, Titanium Dioxide.

CLINICAL PHARMACOLOGY

Mono-Gesic® is insoluble in acid gastric fluids (< 0.1 mg/mL at pH 1.0), but readily soluble in the small intestine where it is partially hydrolyzed to two molecules of salicylic acid. A significant portion of the parent compound is absorbed unchanged and undergoes rapid esterase hydrolysis in the body; its half-life is about one hour. About 13% is excreted through the kidneys as a glucuronide conjugate of the parent compound, the remainder as salicylic acid and its metabolites. Thus, the amount of salicylic acid available from Mono-Gesic® is about 15% less than from aspirin, when the two drugs are administered on a salicylic acid molar equivalent basis (3.6 g salsalate/5 g aspirin). Salicylic acid biotransformation is saturated at anti-inflammatory doses of Mono-Gesic®. Such capacity-limited biotransformation results in an increase in the half-life of salicylic acid from 3.5 to 16 or more hours. Thus, dosing with Mono-Gesic® twice a day will satisfactorily maintain blood levels within the desired therapeutic range (10 to 30 mg/100 mL) throughout the 12-hour intervals. Therapeutic blood levels continue for up to 16 hours after the last dose. The parent compound does not show capacity-limited biotransformation, nor does it accumulate in the plasma on multiple dosing. Food slows the absorption of all salicylates including Mono-Gesic®.

The mode of anti-inflammatory action of Mono-Gesic® and other nonsteroidal anti-inflammatory drugs is not fully defined. Although salicylic acid (the primary metabolite of Mono-Gesic®) is a weak inhibitor of prostaglandin synthesis *in vitro*, Mono-Gesic® appears to selectively inhibit prostaglandin synthesis *in vivo*; providing anti-inflammatory activity equivalent to aspirin and indomethacin. Unlike aspirin, Mono-Gesic® does not inhibit platelet aggregation.

The usefulness of salicylic acid, the active *in vivo* product of Mono-Gesic®, in the treatment of arthritic disorders has been established. In contrast to aspirin, Mono-Gesic® causes no greater fecal gastrointestinal blood loss than placebo.

INDICATIONS AND USAGE

Mono-Gesic® is indicated for the temporary relief of symptoms of rheumatoid arthritis, osteoarthritis and related rheumatic disorders.

CONTRAINDICATIONS

Hypersensitivity to salsalate.

WARNINGS

Drugs of this class, salicylates, have been reported to be associated with the development of Reye Syndrome in children and teenagers with chicken pox, influenza, and influenza-like infections.

PRECAUTIONS

General: To avoid potentially toxic concentrations, the plasma salicylic acid levels should be monitored to maintain the therapeutically effective levels of 10 to 30 mg/100 mL. Changes in urinary pH can have significant effects on the plasma level of salicylic acid. Acidification can result in an increase in the plasma level resulting in toxicity while an increase in urinary pH will increase renal clearance and urinary excretion of salicylic acid, thus lowering plasma levels.

Information for Patients: Patients on long-term treatment should be warned not to take other salicylates. They should also be warned that if symptoms of overdosage, such as tinnitus, vertigo, headache, confusion, drowsiness, sweating, hyperventilation, vomiting or diarrhea appear, the drug should be stopped and physician notified.

Drug Interactions: Salicylates antagonize the uricosuric action of drugs used to treat gout. Salicylates will be additive to Mono-Gesic® and could increase plasma concentrations to toxic levels. Drugs and foods that raise urine pH will increase renal clearance and urinary excretion of salicylic acid, thus lowering plasma levels; acidifying drugs or foods will decrease urinary excretion and increase plasma levels. Salicylates may competitively displace anticoagulant drugs from plasma protein binding sites and thereby predispose to systemic bleeding. Salicylates may enhance the hypoglycemic effect of oral antidiabetic drugs of the sulfonylurea class. Salicylate competes with a number of drugs for protein binding sites, notably penicillin, thiopental, thyroxine, triiodothyronine, phenytoin, sulfinpyrazone, naproxen, warfarin, methotrexate, and possibly corticosteroids.

Drug/Laboratory Test Interactions: Salicylate competes with thyroid hormone for binding to plasma proteins, which may be reflected in a depressed plasma T_4 value in some patients; thyroid function and basal metabolism are unaffected.

Carcinogenesis: No long-term animal studies have been performed with Mono-Gesic® to evaluate its carcinogenic potential; however, several such studies using aspirin and other salicylates have failed to demonstrate any association of these agents with cancerous cell changes.

Use in Pregnancy: Pregnancy Category C: Salsalate and salicylic acid have been shown to be teratogenic and embryocidal in rats when given in doses four to five times the usual human dose. These effects were not observed at doses twice as great as the usual human dose. There are no adequate and well-controlled studies in pregnant women. Mono-Gesic® should be used during pregnancy only if the potential benefit justifies the potential risk to the fetus.

Labor and Delivery: There are no adequate and well-controlled studies in pregnant women. Although adverse effects on mother or infant have not been reported with Mono-Gesic® used during labor, caution is advised when anti-inflammatory dosage is involved. However, other salicylates have been associated with prolonged gestation and labor, maternal and neonatal bleeding sequelae, potentiation of narcotic and barbiturate effects (respiratory or cardiac arrest in the mother), delivery problems and stillbirth.

Nursing Mothers: It is not known whether salsalate per se is excreted in human milk; salicylic acid, the primary metabolite of Mono-Gesic®, has been shown to appear in human milk in concentrations approximating the maternal blood level. Thus the infant of a mother on Mono-Gesic® therapy might ingest in mother's milk 30 to 80 percent as much salicylate per kg body weight as the mother is taking. Accordingly, caution should be exercised when Mono-Gesic® is administered to a nursing woman.

Pediatric Use: Safety and effectiveness in pediatric patients have not been established.

ADVERSE REACTIONS

Adverse reactions are usually the result of overdosage and may include tinnitus and temporary hearing loss, vertigo, headache, confusion, drowsiness, sweating, hyperventilation, vomiting and diarrhea.

DRUG ABUSE AND DEPENDENCE

Drug abuse and dependence have not been reported with Mono-Gesic®.

OVERDOSAGE

IN ALL CASES OF SUSPECTED OVERDOSE, IMMEDIATELY CALL YOUR REGIONAL POISON CENTER and/or SEEK PROFESSIONAL ASSISTANCE. No deaths after overdosage have been reported for Mono-Gesic®. Death has followed ingestion of 10 to 30 g of other salicylates in adults, but much larger amounts have been ingested without fatal outcome.

Signs and Symptoms: The usual symptoms of salicylism (tinnitus, vertigo, headache, confusion, drowsiness, sweating, hyperventilation, vomiting and diarrhea) will occur. More severe intoxication will lead to disruption of electrolyte balance and blood pH, hyperthermia and dehydration.

Treatment: Further absorption of Mono-Gesic® from the G.I. tract should be prevented by emesis (syrup of ipecac) and, if necessary, by gastric lavage.

Fluid and electrolyte imbalance should be corrected by the administration of appropriate I.V. therapy. Adequate renal function should be maintained. Hemodialysis or peritoneal dialysis may be required in extreme cases.

DOSAGE AND ADMINISTRATION

Dosage should be adjusted according to the severity of the disease and the response of the patient. Response will be gradual and full benefits may not be evident for three to four days when plasma salicylate levels have achieved steady state.

The usual dosage is 3,000 mg daily, given in divided doses, such as two tablets twice daily or one tablet four times daily.

HOW SUPPLIED

MONO-GESIC® 750 mg tablets:

An oval, pink, film-coated tablet debossed with Central logo on one side and 750 bisect mg on the other side.

Bottles of 100 tablets—NDC 0131-2164-37

Bottles of 500 tablets—NDC 0131-2164-41

Shown in Product Identification Guide, page 308

NIFEREX® TABLETS/ELIXIR   OTC
[ni'fer"ex]
NIFEREX® with VITAMIN C TABLETS
(polysaccharide-iron complex, as cell-contracted akaganéite)

DESCRIPTION
NIFEREX is a highly water-soluble complex of iron and a low molecular weight polysaccharide. Each NIFEREX Film Coated Tablet and each NIFEREX with Vitamin C Chewable Tablet contains 50 mg elemental iron. In addition, each NIFEREX with Vitamin C tablet contains Ascorbic acid, U.S.P., 100 mg. and Sodium ascorbate, 168.75 mg. Each 5 mL (teaspoonful) NIFEREX Elixir contains 100 mg elemental iron, alcohol 10% (dye-free, sugar free).

ACTION AND USES
NIFEREX is an easily assimilated source of iron for treatment of uncomplicated iron deficiency anemia. Because NIFEREX is a polysaccharide bound iron complex, it is relatively nontoxic and there are relatively few, if any, of the gastrointestinal side effects associated with iron therapy, thus permitting full therapeutic dosage (150 to 300 mg elemental iron daily) in a single dose if desirable. There is no staining of teeth and no metallic aftertaste.

INDICATIONS
For treatment of uncomplicated iron deficiency anemia.

CONTRAINDICATIONS
In patients with hemochromatosis and hemosiderosis, and in those with a known hypersensitivity to any of the ingredients.

DOSAGE AND ADMINISTRATION
ADULTS: One or two NIFEREX or NIFEREX with Vitamin C Tablets twice daily, or one to two teaspoonfuls NIFEREX Elixir daily or as directed by a physician. CHILDREN 6 to 12 years of age: One or two NIFEREX or one NIFEREX with Vitamin C Tablet daily, or one teaspoonful NIFEREX Elixir daily or as directed by a physician, Children 2 to 6 years of age: $^1/_2$ teaspoonful NIFEREX Elixir daily or as directed by a physician.

HOW SUPPLIED
Niferex Elixir (dark brown liquid)
Bottles of 8 ounces—NDC 0131-5066-68
Niferex Tablets (round, brown film-coated)
Bottles of 100—NDC 0131-2200-37
Niferex with Vitamin C Tablets (round, brown, compressed, chewable tablet imprinted with Central logo)
Bottles of 50—NDC 0131-2202-34

NIFEREX®-150 CAPSULES   OTC
[ni'fer"ex]
(polysaccharide-iron complex, as cell-contracted akaganéite)

DESCRIPTION
NIFEREX is a highly water-soluble complex of iron and a low molecular weight polysaccharide. Each bead-filled NIFEREX-150 Capsule contains 150 mg elemental iron as polysaccharide-iron complex, as cell-contracted akaganéite.

ACTIONS AND USES
NIFEREX is an easily assimilated source of iron for treatment of uncomplicated iron deficiency anemia. Because NIFEREX is a polysaccharide bound iron complex, it is relatively nontoxic and there are relatively few, if any, of the gastrointestinal side effects associated with iron therapy, thus permitting full therapeutic dosage (150 to 300 mg elemental iron daily) in a single dose if desirable. There is no staining of teeth and no metallic aftertaste.

INDICATIONS
For treatment of uncomplicated iron deficiency anemia.

CONTRAINDICATIONS
In patients with hemochromatosis and hemosiderosis, and in those with a known hypersensitivity to any of the ingredients.

DOSAGE AND ADMINISTRATION
ADULTS: One or two NIFEREX-150 Capsules daily.

HOW SUPPLIED
Niferex-150 Capsules (Opaque orange cap, clear colorless body printed with white Central logo and 4220, filled with brown beads.)
Bottles of 100-NDC 0131-4220-37
Bottles of 1000-NDC 0131-4220-43
Shown in Product Identification Guide, page 308

NIFEREX®-150 FORTE CAPSULES   Rx
[ni'fer"ex for'ta]

DESCRIPTION
Each capsule Niferex®-150 Forte contains:
Iron (Elemental) .... 150 mg
  (polysaccharide-iron complex, as cell-contracted akaganéite)
Folic Acid .... 1 mg
Vitamin B$_{12}$ .... 25 mcg

PRECAUTION
Folic acid, especially in doses above 0.1 mg–0.4 mg daily, may obscure pernicious anemia, in that hematologic remission may occur while neurological manifestations remain progressive.

DOSAGE AND ADMINISTRATION
Adults—one capsule or one teaspoonful of elixir daily or as prescribed by a physician.

HOW SUPPLIED
Niferex-150 Forte Capsules (Opaque red cap, clear colorless body printed with Central logo and 4330, filled with brown beads)
Bottle of 100—NDC 0131-4330-37
Bottle of 1000—NDC 0131-4330-43
Shown in Product Identification Guide, page 308

NIFEREX®—PN TABLETS   Rx
[ni'fer"ex]

DESCRIPTION
Each film-coated tablet contains:
Iron (Elemental) .... 60 mg
  (polysaccharide-iron complex, as cell-contracted akaganéite)
Folic acid .... 1 mg
Ascorbic acid .... 50 mg
  (as sodium ascorbate)
Cyanocobalamin (Vitamin B$_{12}$) .... 3 mcg
Vitamin A .... 4000 IU
Vitamin D .... 400 IU
Thiamine mononitrate .... 3 mg
Riboflavin .... 3 mg
Pyridoxine hydrochloride .... 2 mg
Niacinamide .... 10 mg
Calcium (as calcium carbonate) .... 125 mg
Zinc (as zinc sulfate monohydrate) .... 18 mg
This product contains ingredients of the following therapeutic classes: vitamins and minerals.

INACTIVE INGREDIENTS
Castor Oil, FD&C Blue #1 Lake, Gelatin, Hydrogenated Vegetable Oil, Hydroxypropyl Cellulose, Hydroxypropyl Methylcellulose, Magnesium Stearate, Microcrystalline Cellulose, Pharmaceutical Glaze, Polyethylene Glycol, Povidone, Propylene Glycol, Starch and Titanium Dioxide.

CLINICAL PHARMACOLOGY
This product is formulated to meet the needs of the pregnant or lactating patient with special consideration given to adequate amounts of the hematopoietic factors, iron, folic acid and cyanocobalamin. Calcium (phosphorus-free) is also included in the formula to help supply the increased requirements of this mineral. The 60 mg of elemental iron is available in the form of Niferex® (polysaccharide-iron complex, as cell-contracted akaganéite). This form of iron is especially useful in the pregnant patient because, although it is absorbed as well as ferrous sulfate, it does not produce the gastrointestinal irritation commonly associated with iron salts. In addition, folic acid and cyanocobalamin in therapeutic amounts are included to prevent or treat the significant number of pregnant patients who develop megaloblastic anemia of pregnancy.

INDICATIONS AND USAGE
For the prevention and/or treatment of dietary vitamin and mineral deficiencies associated with pregnancy and lactation.

CONTRAINDICATIONS
Hypersensitivity to any of the ingredients.

WARNINGS
Folic acid alone is improper therapy in the treatment of pernicious anemia and other megaloblastic anemias where vitamin B$_{12}$ is deficient.

PRECAUTIONS
Folic acid, especially in doses above 0.1 mg–0.4 mg daily may obscure pernicious anemia, in that hematologic remission may occur while neurological manifestations remain progressive.

ADVERSE REACTIONS
Allergic sensitization has been reported following both oral and parenteral administration of folic acid.

DOSAGE AND ADMINISTRATION
One tablet daily or as prescribed by a physician.

HOW SUPPLIED
(Oval, blue film coated tablet debossed with 131/05)
Bottles of 100 tablets—NDC 0131-2209-37
Bottles of 1000 tablets—NDC 0131-2209-43
Shown in Product Identification Guide, page 308

NIFEREX®-PN FORTE TABLETS   Rx

DESCRIPTION
Each tablet contains:
Iron (Elemental) .... 60 mg
  (polysaccharide-iron complex, as cell-contracted akaganéite)
Vitamin A acetate .... 5000 IU
Vitamin D .... 400 IU
Vitamin E .... 30 IU
  (as dl-alpha-tocopheryl acetate)
Vitamin C (ascorbic acid) .... 80 mg
Folic acid .... 1 mg
Thiamine (vitamin B$_1$) .... 3 mg
  (as thiamine mononitrate)
Riboflavin (vitamin B$_2$) .... 3.4 mg
Vitamin B$_6$ (as pyridoxine hydrochloride) .... 4 mg
Niacinamide .... 20 mg
Vitamin B$_{12}$ (Cyanocobalamin) .... 12 mcg
Calcium (as calcium carbonate) .... 250 mg
Iodine (as potassium iodide) .... 0.2 mg
Magnesium (as magnesium oxide) .... 10 mg
Copper (as cupric oxide) .... 2 mg
Zinc (as zinc sulfate) .... 25 mg
Dye-Free

HOW SUPPLIED
Capsule shaped, white film coated tablet debossed with Central on one side and 1 bisect O on the other.
Bottles of 100 Tablets—NDC 0131-2309-37
Shown in Product Identification Guide, page 308

PEDIAPAP™   OTC
Acetaminophen Oral Solution, USP

DESCRIPTION
Each teaspoonful (5 mL) of PEDIAPAP contains: Acetaminophen 160 mg. Alcohol-free, Dye-free, Sugar-free.

HOW SUPPLIED
PEDIAPAP™
4 oz—NDC# 0131-5080-64

PREDNICEN®–M 21-Pak   Rx
[pred"ni-sen']
(Prednisone Tablets, USP)

DESCRIPTION
Each white film-coated tablet debossed with 131/07 contains:
Prednisone .... 5 mg

HOW SUPPLIED
Unit Pack 21 x 5 mg.—NDC # 0131-2228-81

THEOCLEAR®–80 Syrup   Rx
[the'ō-klēr"]
(theophylline syrup)

DESCRIPTION
THEOCLEAR-80: Each 15 mL (1 tablespoonful) contains 80 mg Theophylline Anhydrous as the active ingredient. Other ingredients are Benzoic Acid, Citric Acid, Flavor, Glycerin, Propylene Glycol, Saccharin Sodium, Sorbitol, Tartaric Acid and Purified Water. This formulation provides an alcohol-free, dye-free, and sugar-free vehicle containing no corn allergens.

HOW SUPPLIED
Theoclear-80 Syrup (Clear, colorless liquid with an anise odor)
One Pint—NDC 0131-5098-70
One Gallon—NDC 0131-5098-72

Cetylite Industries, Inc.
9051 RIVER ROAD
P.O. BOX 90006
PENNSAUKEN, NJ 08110-0700

Direct Inquiries to:
Mr. Stanley L. Wachman, President
(609) 665-6111
(800) 257-7740
FAX: (609) 665-5408

CETACAINE®
[set 'a-cane "]
TOPICAL ANESTHETIC

℞

ACTIVE INGREDIENTS
Benzocaine 14.0%
Butyl Aminobenzoate 2.0%
Tetracaine Hydrochloride 2.0%

CONTAINS
Benzalkonium Chloride 0.5%
Cetyl Dimethyl Ethyl
    Ammonium Bromide 0.005%
In a bland water soluble base.

ACTION
Cetacaine produces anesthesia rapidly in approximately 30 seconds.

INDICATIONS
Cetacaine is a topical anesthetic indicated for the production of anesthesia of accessible mucous membrane.
Cetacaine Spray is indicated for use to control pain or gagging. Cetacaine in all forms is indicated for use to control pain.

DOSAGE AND ADMINISTRATION
Cetacaine Spray should be applied for approximately one second or less for normal anesthesia. Only limited quantity of Cetacaine is required for anesthesia. Spray in excess of two seconds is contraindicated. Average expulsion rate of residue from spray, at normal temperatures, is 200 mg. per second. Tissue need not be dried prior to application of Cetacaine. Cetacaine should be applied directly to the site where pain control is required.
Cetacaine Liquid or Cetacaine Ointment may be applied with a cotton pledget or directly to tissue. Cotton pledget should not be held in position for extended periods of time, since local reactions to benzoate topical anesthetics are related to the length of time of application.

ADVERSE REACTION
Systemic reactions to Cetacaine have not been reported. Localized allergic reactions may occur after prolonged or repeated use. Dehydration of the epithelium or an escharotic effect may result from prolonged contact. Allergic reactions are known to occur in some patients with preparations containing benzocaine.
Usage in Pregnancy: Safe use of Cetacaine has not been established with respect to possible adverse effects upon fetal development. Therefore Cetacaine should not be used during early pregnancy, unless in the judgment of a physician the potential benefits outweigh the unknown hazards.
Routine precaution for the use of any topical anesthetic should be observed when Cetacaine is used.

CONTRAINDICATIONS
Cetacaine is not for injection.
Do not use on the eyes.
To avoid excessive systemic absorption, Cetacaine should not be applied to large areas of denuded or inflamed tissue.
Cetacaine should not be administered to patients who are hypersensitive to any of its ingredients.
Individual dosage of tetracaine hydrochloride in excess of 20 mg. is contraindicated. Cetacaine should not be used under dentures or cotton rolls, as retention of the active ingredients under a denture or cotton roll could possibly cause an escharotic effect.
Jetco-Spray® Cannula
The autoclavable, stainless steel Jetco cannula for Cetacaine Spray is specially designed for accessibility and application of Cetacaine, at the required site of pain control.
The Jetco cannula is supplied in various lengths and shapes.
The Jetco cannula is inserted firmly onto the protruding plastic tubing on each bottle of Cetacaine Spray.
The Jetco cannula may be removed and re-inserted as many times as required for cleansing or sterilization.

PACKAGING AVAILABLE
Cetacaine Spray 56 g. including propellant.
Cetacaine Liquid 56 g.
Cetacaine Hospital Gel 29 g Tube.
Cetacaine Ointment 37 g Jar.

CAUTION
Federal law prohibits dispensing Cetacaine without prescription.
Made in U.S.A.   (Rev. 7/93)

Chattem, Inc.
1715 WEST 38TH STREET
CHATTANOOGA, TN 37409

Direct Inquiries to:
Gary Galante
(423) 821-4571, Ext. 336

HERPECIN-L® Cold Sore Lip Balm Stick   OTC
[her "puh-sin-el "]

PRODUCT OVERVIEW
KEY FACTS
HERPECIN-L Lip Balm Stick is a convenient, easy-to-use treatment for perioral *herpes simplex* [HSV-1] infections. It has sunscreens for an SPF of 15.

MAJOR USES
HERPECIN-L not only treats cold sores, sun and fever blisters, but with prophylactic use, its sunscreens also protect to help prevent them. Users report early use at the *prodromal* stages of an attack will often abort the lesions and prevent or lessen scabbing. Prescribe: Apply "early, liberally and often".

SAFETY INFORMATION
For topical use only. A rare sensitivity may occur.

PRESCRIBING INFORMATION
HERPECIN-L® Cold Sore Lip Balm   OTC
COMPOSITION
A soothing, emollient, lip balm incorporating allantoin, the sunscreen, Padimate O, in a balanced, slightly acidic lipid base that includes petrolatum and titanium dioxide at a cosmetically acceptable level. (Has no caines, antibiotics, phenol or camphor.) (NDC 38083-777-31)

ACTIONS AND USES
HERPECIN-L relieves dryness and chapping by providing a lipid barrier to help restore normal moisture balance to the lips. Skin protectants help to soften the crusts and scabs of "cold sores". The sunscreen is effective in 290-320 AU range while titanium dioxide, though at low levels, helps to screen, block, reflect the sun's rays and help prevent sun-induced *herpes labialis*. Used as directed, SPF is 15.

ADMINISTRATION
(1) Recurrent *"cold sores, sun and fever blisters "*: Simply put, use **soon, liberally** and **often**. Frequent sufferers report that with *prophylactic* use (BID/PRN), attacks are fewer and less severe. Most recurrent *herpes labialis* patients are aware of the prodromal symptoms: tingling, itching, burning. At this stage, or if the lesion has already developed, HERPECIN-L should be applied liberally every hour, or as often as is convenient. (2) *Outdoor protection:* Apply before and during sun exposure, after swimming and again at bedtime (h.s.). (3) *Dry, chapped lips:* Apply as needed.

ADVERSE REACTIONS
If sensitive to any of the ingredients, discontinue use.

CONTRAINDICATIONS
None. Sunscreens are not recommended for children under 2 years.

HOW SUPPLIED
2.8 gm. swivel tubes.

SAMPLES AVAILABLE
Yes. (Please request on professional letterhead or Rx pad.)

For information on over-the-counter drugs,
consult **PDR For Nonprescription Drugs**

Chiron Therapeutics
4560 HORTON STREET
EMERYVILLE, CA 94608-2997

For Medical Information Contact:
Generally:
Professional Services (6:00 AM to 5:00 PM PST):
(800) CHIRON-8
(800) 244-7668
FAX: (510) 601-3435
In Emergencies:
(6:00 AM to 5:00 PM PST):
(800) CHIRON-8
(800) 244-7668
After Hours and Weekend Emergencies:
(415) 885-8777

Sales and Ordering:
(800) CHIRON-8
(800) 244-7668
FAX: (510) 601-3434

PROLEUKIN®
[prō-lū '-kin]
Aldesleukin
For Injection

℞

> **WARNINGS**
> PROLEUKIN® (aldesleukin) for injection should be administered only in a hospital setting under the supervision of a qualified physician experienced in the use of anti-cancer agents. An intensive care facility and specialists skilled in cardiopulmonary or intensive care medicine must be available.
> PROLEUKIN administration has been associated with capillary leak syndrome (CLS). CLS results in hypotension and reduced organ perfusion which may be severe and can result in death.
> Therapy with PROLEUKIN should be restricted to patients with normal cardiac and pulmonary functions as defined by thallium stress testing and formal pulmonary function testing. Extreme caution should be used in patients with normal thallium stress tests and pulmonary function tests who have a history of prior cardiac or pulmonary disease.
> PROLEUKIN administration should be held in patients developing moderate to severe lethargy or somnolence; continued administration may result in coma.

DESCRIPTION
PROLEUKIN® (aldesleukin) for injection, a human recombinant interleukin-2 product, is a highly purified protein with a molecular weight of approximately 15,300 daltons. The chemical name is des-alanyl-1, serine-125 human interleukin-2. PROLEUKIN, a lymphokine, is produced by recombinant DNA technology using a genetically engineered *E. coli* strain containing an analog of the human interleukin-2 gene. Genetic engineering techniques were used to modify the human IL-2 gene, and the resulting expression clone encodes a modified human interleukin-2. This recombinant form differs from native interleukin-2 in the following ways: a) PROLEUKIN is not glycosylated because it is derived from *E. coli*. ; b) The molecule has no N-terminal alanine; the codon for this amino acid was deleted during the genetic engineering procedure; c) The molecule has serine substituted for cysteine at amino acid position 125; this was accomplished by site specific manipulation during the genetic engineering procedure; and d) the aggregation state of PROLEUKIN is likely to be different from that of native interleukin-2.
Biological activities tested *in vitro* for the native non-recombinant molecule have been reproduced with PROLEUKIN.[1,2]
PROLEUKIN is supplied as a sterile, white to off-white, lyophilized cake in single-use vials intended for intravenous (IV) administration. When reconstituted with 1.2 mL Sterile Water for Injection, USP, each mL contains 18 million IU (1.1 mg) PROLEUKIN, 50 mg mannitol, and 0.18 mg sodium dodecyl sulfate, buffered with approximately 0.17 mg monobasic and 0.89 mg dibasic sodium phosphate to a pH of 7.5 (range 7.2 to 7.8). The manufacturing process for PROLEUKIN involves fermentation in a defined medium containing tetracycline hydrochloride. The presence of the antibiotic is not detectable in the final product. PROLEUKIN contains no preservatives in the final product. PROLEUKIN biological potency is determined by a lymphocyte proliferation bioassay and is expressed in International Units (IU) as established by the World Health Organization 1ST International Standard for interleukin-2 (human). The relationship between potency and protein mass is as follows:
18 million (18×10^6) IU PROLEUKIN® = 1.1 mg protein

CLINICAL PHARMACOLOGY

PROLEUKIN® (aldesleukin) has been shown to possess the biological activity of human native interleukin-2.[1,2] *In vitro* studies performed on human cell lines demonstrate the immunoregulatory properties of PROLEUKIN, including: a) enhancement of lymphocyte mitogenesis and stimulation of long-term growth of human interleukin-2 dependent cell lines; b) enhancement of lymphocyte cytotoxicity; c) induction of killer cell [lymphokine-activated (LAK) and natural (NK)] activity; and d) induction of interferon-gamma production.

The *in vivo* administration of PROLEUKIN in select murine tumor models and in the clinic produces multiple immunological effects in a dose-dependent manner. These effects include activation of cellular immunity with profound lymphocytosis, eosinophilia, and thrombocytopenia, and the production of cytokines including tumor necrosis factor, IL-1, and gamma interferon.[3] *In vivo* experiments in murine tumor models have shown inhibition of tumor growth.[4] The exact mechanism by which PROLEUKIN mediates its antitumor activity in animals and humans is unknown.

Pharmacokinetics: PROLEUKIN exists as biologically active, non-covalently bound microaggregates with an average size of 27 recombinant interleukin-2 molecules. The solubilizing agent, sodium dodecyl sulfate, may have an effect on the kinetic properties of this product. The pharmacokinetic profile of PROLEUKIN is characterized by high plasma concentrations following a short IV infusion, rapid distribution to extravascular, extracellular space and elimination from the body by metabolism in the kidneys with little or no bioactive protein excreted in the urine.

Studies of IV PROLEUKIN in sheep and humans indicate that approximately 30% of the administered dose initially distributes to the plasma.

This is consistent with studies in rats that demonstrate a rapid (<1 minute) and preferential uptake of approximately 70% of an administered dose into the liver, kidney, and lung.

The serum half-life ($T^1/_2$) curves of PROLEUKIN remaining in the plasma are derived from studies done in 52 cancer patients following a 5-minute IV infusion.[5] These patients were shown to have a distribution and elimination $T^1/_2$ of 13 and 85 minutes, respectively.

The relatively rapid clearance rate of PROLEUKIN has led to dosage schedules characterized by frequent, short infusions. Observed serum levels are proportional to the dose of PROLEUKIN.

Following the initial rapid organ distribution described above, the primary route of clearance of circulating PROLEUKIN is the kidney. In humans and animals, PROLEUKIN is cleared from the circulation by both glomerular filtration and peritubular extraction in the kidney.[6–8] This dual mechanism for delivery of PROLEUKIN to the proximal tubule may account for the preservation of clearance in patients with rising serum creatinine values. Greater than 80% of the amount of PROLEUKIN distributed to plasma, cleared from the circulation and presented to the kidney is metabolized to amino acids in the cells lining the proximal convoluted tubules. In humans, the mean clearance rate in cancer patients is 268 mL/min.

Immunogenicity: Fifty-seven of 77 renal cancer patients (74%) treated with the every 8-hour PROLEUKIN regimen developed low titers of non-neutralizing anti-interleukin-2 antibodies. Neutralizing antibodies were not detected in this group of patients but have been detected in 1/106 (<1%) patients treated with IV PROLEUKIN using a wide variety of schedules and doses. The clinical significance of anti-interleukin-2 antibodies is unknown.

Clinical Experience: Two hundred and fifty-five patients with metastatic renal cell cancer were treated with single agent PROLEUKIN. Treatment was given by the every 8-hour regimen in seven clinical studies conducted at 21 institutions. To be eligible for study, patients were required to have bidimensionally measurable disease; Eastern Cooperative Oncology Group (ECOG) Performance Status (PS) of 0 or 1 (see Table I); and normal organ function, including normal cardiac stress test and pulmonary function tests. Patients with brain metastases, active infections, organ allografts, and diseases requiring steroid treatment were excluded. In addition, it was noted that 218 of the 255 (85%) patients had undergone nephrectomy prior to treatment with PROLEUKIN.

TABLE I
PERFORMANCE STATUS SCALE

Performance Status Equivalent: ECOG*	Karnofsky	Performance Status Definitions
0	100	Asymptomatic
1	80-90	Symptomatic: fully ambulatory
2	60-70	Symptomatic; in bed less than 50% of day
3	40-50	Symptomatic: in bed more than 50% of day
4	20-30	Bedridden

Zubrod, CG, et al. *J Chron Dis* 11:7-33, 1960

PROLEUKIN was given by 15-minute IV infusion every 8 hours for up to 5 days (maximum of 14 doses). No treatment was given on days 6 to 14 and then dosing was repeated for up to 5 days on days 15 to 19 (maximum of 14 doses). These two cycles constituted one course of therapy. All patients were treated with 28 doses or until dose-limiting toxicity occurred requiring ICU-level support. Patients received a median of 20 of 28 scheduled doses of PROLEUKIN. Doses were held for specific toxicities (See "**DOSAGE AND ADMINISTRATION**" Section, "**Dose Modification**" Subsection). A variety of serious adverse events were encountered including: hypotension; oliguria/anuria; mental status changes including coma; pulmonary congestion and dyspnea; GI bleeding; respiratory failure leading to intubation; ventricular arrhythmias; myocardial ischemia and/or infarction; ileus or intestinal perforation; renal failure requiring dialysis; gangrene; seizures; sepsis and death (See "**ADVERSE REACTIONS**" Section).

Due to the toxicities encountered during the clinical trials, investigators used the following concomitant medications. Acetaminophen and indomethacin were started immediately prior to PROLEUKIN to reduce fever. Renal function was particularly monitored because indomethacin may cause synergistic nephrotoxicity. Meperidine was added to control the rigors associated with fever. Ranitidine or cimetidine were given for prophylaxis of gastrointestinal irritation and bleeding. Antiemetics and antidiarrheals were used as needed to treat other gastrointestinal side effects. These medications were discontinued 12 hours after the last dose of PROLEUKIN. Hydroxyzine or diphenhydramine was used to control symptoms from pruritic rashes and continued until resolution of pruritus. **NOTE: Prior to the use of any product mentioned in this paragraph, the physician should refer to the package insert for the respective product.**

For the 255 patients in the PROLEUKIN database, objective response was seen in 15% or 37 patients with nine (4%) complete and 28 (11%) partial responders. The 95% confidence interval for response was 11 to 20%. Onset of tumor regression has been observed as early as 4 weeks after completion of the first course of treatment, and tumor regression may continue for up to 12 months after the start of treatment. Durable responses were achieved with a median duration of objective (partial or complete) response by Kaplan-Meier projection of 23.2 months (1 to 50 months). The median duration of objective partial response was 18.8 months. The proportion of responding patients who will have response durations of 12 months or greater is projected to be 85% for all responders and 79% for patients with partial responses (Kaplan-Meier).

Complete Responders	Partial Responders	Response Rate	Onset of Response	Median Duration of Response
9 (4%)	28 (11%)	15%	1 to 12 mos.	23.2 months (range 1-50)

Response was observed in both lung and non-lung sites (e.g., liver, lymph node, renal bed recurrences, soft tissue). Patients with individual bulky lesions (> 5 × 5 cm), as well as large cumulative tumor burden (>25 cm² tumor area) achieved durable responses.

An analysis of prognostic factors showed that performance status as defined by the ECOG (see Table I) was a significant predictor of response. PS 0 patients had an 18% overall rate of objective response, which included all nine complete response patients and 21 of 28 partial response patients. PS 1 patients had a lower rate of response (9%), all of which were partial responses. In this group it was notable that six of the seven responders had resolution of tumor-related symptoms and improved performance status to PS 0. All seven patients were fully functional and four of the seven returned to work, suggesting that responses among the PS 1 patients were clinically meaningful as well (see Table II).

In addition, the frequency of toxicity was related to the performance status. As a group, PS 0 patients, when compared with PS 1 patients, had lower rates of adverse events with fewer on-study deaths (4% vs. 6%), less frequent intubations (8% vs. 25%), gangrene (0% vs. 6%), coma (1% vs. 6%), GI bleeding (4% vs. 8%), and sepsis (6% vs. 18%). These differences in toxicity are reflected in the shorter mean time to hospital discharge for PS 0 patients (2 vs. 3 days), as well as the smaller percentage of PS 0 patients experiencing a delayed (> 7 days) discharge from the hospital (8% vs. 19%).

[See Table I above.]

[See Table II below.]

TABLE II
PROLEUKIN RESPONSE ANALYZED BY ECOG* PERFORMANCE STATUS (PS)

Pre-Treatment ECOG PS	No. of Patients Treated (n=255)	Response CR	Response PR	Patients Responding	On-Study Death Rate
0	166	9	21	18%	4%
1	80	0	7	9%	6%
≥2	9	0	0	0%	0%

* Eastern Cooperative Oncology Group

INDICATIONS AND USAGE

PROLEUKIN® (aldesleukin) is indicated for the treatment of adults (≥ 18 years of age) with metastatic renal cell carcinoma.

Careful patient selection is mandatory prior to the administration of PROLEUKIN. See "**CONTRAINDICATIONS**", "**WARNINGS**" and "**PRECAUTIONS**" Sections regarding patient screening, including recommended cardiac and pulmonary function tests and laboratory tests.

Evaluation of clinical studies to date reveals that patients with more favorable ECOG performance status (ECOG PS 0) at treatment initiation respond better to PROLEUKIN, with a higher response rate and lower toxicity (See "**CLINICAL PHARMACOLOGY**" Section, "**Clinical Experience**" Subsection). Therefore, selection of patients for treatment should include assessment of performance status, as described in Table 1.

Experience in patients with PS >1 is extremely limited.

CONTRAINDICATIONS

PROLEUKIN® (aldesleukin) is contraindicated in patients with a known history of hypersensitivity to interleukin-2 or any component of the PROLEUKIN formulation.

Patients with an abnormal thallium stress test or pulmonary function tests are excluded from treatment with PROLEUKIN. Patients with organ allografts should be excluded as well. In addition, retreatment with PROLEUKIN is contraindicated in patients who experienced the following toxicities while receiving an earlier course of therapy:

- Sustained ventricular tachycardia (≥5 beats)
- Cardiac rhythm disturbances not controlled or unresponsive to management
- Recurrent chest pain with ECG changes, consistent with angina or myocardial infarction
- Intubation required >72 hours
- Pericardial tamponade
- Renal dysfunction requiring dialysis >72 hours
- Coma or toxic psychosis lasting >48 hours
- Repetitive or difficult to control seizures
- Bowel ischemia/perforation
- GI bleeding requiring surgery

WARNINGS

See boxed "**WARNINGS**"

PROLEUKIN® (aldesleukin) administration has been associated with capillary leak syndrome (CLS) which results from extravasation of plasma proteins and fluid into the extravascular space and loss of vascular tone. CLS results in hypotension and reduced organ perfusion which may be severe and can result in death. The CLS may be associated with cardiac arrhythmias (supraventricular and ventricular), angina, myocardial infarction, respiratory insufficiency requiring intubation, gastrointestinal bleeding or infarction, renal insufficiency, and mental status changes.

Because of the severe adverse events which generally accompany PROLEUKIN therapy at the recommended dosages, thorough clinical evaluation should be performed to exclude from treatment patients with significant cardiac, pulmonary, renal, hepatic, or CNS impairment.

Should adverse events occur, which require dose modification, dosage should be withheld rather than reduced (See "**DOSAGE AND ADMINISTRATION**" Section, "**Dose Modification**" Subsection).

PROLEUKIN may exacerbate pre-existing autoimmune disease. Because not all patients who develop interleukin-2-associated autoimmune phenomena have a pre-existing

Continued on next page

Chiron Therapeutics—Cont.

history of autoimmune disease, awareness and close monitoring for thyroid abnormalities or other potentially autoimmune phenomena is warranted. Two patients with quiescent Crohn's disease had activation of their disease following treatment with PROLEUKIN, and both required surgical intervention.

PROLEUKIN may exacerbate disease symptoms in patients with clinically unrecognized or untreated CNS metastases. All patients should have thorough evaluation and treatment of CNS metastases prior to receiving PROLEUKIN therapy. They should be neurologically stable with a negative CT scan. In addition, extreme caution should be exercised in treating patients with a history of seizure disorder because PROLEUKIN may cause seizures.

Intensive PROLEUKIN treatment is associated with impaired neutrophil function (reduced chemotaxis) and with an increased risk of disseminated infection, including sepsis and bacterial endocarditis, in treated patients. Consequently, pre-existing bacterial infections should be adequately treated prior to initiation of PROLEUKIN therapy. Additionally, all patients with indwelling central lines should receive antibiotic prophylaxis effective against *S. aureus*.[9–11] Antibiotic prophylaxis which has been associated with a reduced incidence of staphylococcal infections in PROLEUKIN studies includes the use of oxacillin, nafcillin, ciprofloxacin, or vancomycin. Disseminated infections acquired in the course of PROLEUKIN treatment are a major contributor to treatment morbidity and use of antibiotic prophylaxis and aggressive treatment of suspected and documented infections may reduce the morbidity of PROLEUKIN treatment. **NOTE: Prior to the use of any product mentioned in this paragraph, the physician should refer to the package insert for the respective product.**

PRECAUTIONS

General: Patients should have normal cardiac, pulmonary, hepatic, and CNS function at the start of therapy. Patients who have had a nephrectomy are still eligible for treatment if they have serum creatinine levels $\leq$ 1.5 mg/dL.

Adverse events are frequent, often serious, and sometimes fatal.

Capillary leak syndrome (CLS) begins immediately after PROLEUKIN® (aldesleukin) treatment starts and is marked by increased capillary permeability to protein and fluids and reduced vascular tone. In most patients, this results in a concomitant drop in mean arterial blood pressure within 2 to 12 hours after the start of treatment. With continued therapy, clinically significant hypotension (defined as systolic blood pressure below 90 mm Hg or a 20 mm Hg drop from baseline systolic pressure), and hypoperfusion will occur. In addition, extravasation of protein and fluids into the extravascular space will lead to edema formation and creation of effusions.

Medical management of CLS begins with careful monitoring of the patient's fluid and organ perfusion status. This is achieved by frequent determination of blood pressure and pulse, and by monitoring organ function, which includes assessment of mental status and urine output. Hypovolemia is assessed by catheterization and central pressure monitoring.

Flexibility in fluid and pressor management is essential for maintaining organ perfusion and blood pressure. Consequently, extreme caution should be used in treating patients with fixed requirements for large volumes of fluid (e.g., patients with hypercalcemia).

Patients with hypovolemia are managed by administering IV fluids, either colloids or crystalloids. IV fluids are usually given when the central venous pressure (CVP) is below 3 to 4 mm H_2O. Correction of hypovolemia may require large volumes of IV fluids, but caution is required because unrestrained fluid administration may exacerbate problems associated with edema formation or effusions.

With extravascular fluid accumulation, edema is common, and some patients may develop ascites or pleural effusions. Management of these events depends on a careful balancing of the effects of fluid shifts so that neither the consequences of hypovolemia (e.g., impaired organ perfusion) nor the consequences of fluid accumulations (e.g., pulmonary edema) exceeds the patient's tolerance.

Clinical experience has shown that early administration of dopamine (1 to 5 μg/kg/min) to patients manifesting capillary leak syndrome, before the onset of hypotension, can help to maintain organ perfusion particularly to the kidney and thus preserve urine output. Weight and urine output should be carefully monitored. If organ perfusion and blood pressure are not sustained by dopamine therapy, clinical investigators have increased the dose of dopamine to 6 to 10 μg/kg/min or have added phenylephrine hydrochloride (1 to 5 μg/kg/min) to low dose dopamine (See **"CLINICAL PHARMACOLOGY"** Section, **"Clinical Experience"** Subsection). Prolonged use of pressors, either in combination or as individual agents, at relatively high doses, may be associated with cardiac rhythm disturbances. **NOTE: Prior to the use of any product mentioned in this paragraph, the physician should refer to the package insert for the respective product.**

Failure to maintain organ perfusion, demonstrated by altered mental status, reduced urine output, a fall in the systolic blood pressure below 90 mm Hg or onset of cardiac arrhythmias, should lead to holding the subsequent doses until recovery of organ perfusion and a return of systolic blood pressure above 90 mm Hg are observed (See **"DOSAGE AND ADMINISTRATION"** Section, **"Dose Modification"** Subsection).

Recovery from CLS begins soon after cessation of PROLEUKIN therapy. Usually, within a few hours, the blood pressure rises, organ perfusion is restored and resorption of extravasated fluid and protein begins. If there has been excessive weight gain or edema formation, particularly if associated with shortness of breath from pulmonary congestion, use of diuretics, once blood pressure has normalized, has been shown to hasten recovery.

Oxygen is given to the patient if pulmonary function monitoring confirms that P_aO_2 is decreased.

PROLEUKIN administration may cause anemia and/or thrombocytopenia. Packed red blood cell transfusions have been given both for relief of anemia and to insure maximal oxygen-carrying capacity. Platelet transfusions have been given to resolve absolute thrombocytopenia and to reduce the risk of GI bleeding. In addition, leukopenia and neutropenia are observed.

PROLEUKIN administration results in fever, chills, rigors, pruritus, and gastrointestinal side effects in most patients treated at recommended doses. These side effects have been aggressively managed as described in the **"CLINICAL PHARMACOLOGY"** Section, **"Clinical Experience"** Subsection.

Renal and hepatic function are impaired during PROLEUKIN treatment. Use of concomitant medications known to be nephrotoxic or hepatotoxic may further increase toxicity to the kidney or liver. In addition, reduced kidney and liver function secondary to PROLEUKIN treatment may delay elimination of concomitant medications and increase the risk of adverse events from those drugs.

Patients may experience mental status changes including irritability, confusion, or depression while receiving PROLEUKIN. These mental status changes may be indicators of bacteremia or early bacterial sepsis. Mental status changes due solely to PROLEUKIN are generally reversible when drug administration is discontinued. However, alterations in mental status may progress for several days before recovery begins.

Impairment of thyroid function has been reported following PROLEUKIN treatment. A small number of these patients required thyroid replacement therapy. This impairment of thyroid function may be a manifestation of autoimmunity.

PROLEUKIN enhancement of cellular immune function may increase the risk of allograft rejection in transplant patients.

Laboratory Tests: The following clinical evaluations are recommended for all patients, prior to beginning treatment and then daily during drug administration.

- Standard hematologic tests—including CBC, differential, and platelet counts
- Blood chemistries—including electrolytes, renal and hepatic function tests
- Chest x-rays

All patients should have baseline pulmonary function tests with arterial blood gases. Adequate pulmonary function should be documented (FEV_1 >2 liters or $\geq$75% of predicted for height and age) prior to initiating therapy. All patients should be screened with a stress thallium study. Normal ejection fraction and unimpaired wall motion should be documented. If a thallium stress test suggests minor wall motion abnormalities of questionable significance, a stress echocardiogram to document normal wall motion may be useful to exclude significant coronary artery disease.

Daily monitoring during therapy with PROLEUKIN should include vital signs (temperature, pulse, blood pressure, and respiration rate) and weight. In a patient with a decreased blood pressure, especially less than 90 mm Hg, constant cardiac monitoring for rhythm should be conducted. If an abnormal complex or rhythm is seen, an ECG should be performed. Vital signs in these hypotensive patients should be taken hourly and central venous pressure (CVP) checked.

During treatment, pulmonary function should be monitored on a regular basis by clinical examination, assessment of vital signs and pulse oximetry. Patients with dyspnea or clinical signs of respiratory impairment (tachypnea or rales) should be further assessed with arterial blood gas determination. These tests are to be repeated as often as clinically indicated.

Cardiac function is assessed daily by clinical examination and assessment of vital signs. Patients with signs or symptoms of chest pain, murmurs, gallops, irregular rhythm or palpitations should be further assessed with an ECG examination and CPK evaluation. If there is evidence of cardiac ischemia or congestive heart failure, a repeat thallium study should be done.

Drug Interactions: PROLEUKIN may affect central nervous function. Therefore, interactions could occur following concomitant administration of psychotropic drugs (e.g., narcotics, analgesics, antiemetics, sedatives, tranquilizers).

Concurrent administration of drugs possessing nephrotoxic (e.g., aminoglycosides, indomethacin), myelotoxic (e.g., cytotoxic chemotherapy), cardiotoxic (e.g., doxorubicin), or hepatotoxic (e.g., methotrexate, asparaginase) effects with PROLEUKIN may increase toxicity in these organ systems. The safety and efficacy of PROLEUKIN in combination with chemotherapies have not been established.

Although glucocorticoids have been shown to reduce PROLEUKIN-induced side effects including fever, renal insufficiency, hyperbilirubinemia, confusion, and dyspnea,[12] concomitant administration of these agents with PROLEUKIN may reduce the antitumor effectiveness of PROLEUKIN and thus should be avoided.

Beta-blockers and other antihypertensives may potentiate the hypotension seen with PROLEUKIN.

Delayed adverse reactions to iodinated contrast media: A review of the literature revealed that 12.6% (range 11–28%) of 501 patients treated with various interleukin-2-containing regimens who were subsequently administered radiographic iodinated contrast media experienced acute, atypical adverse reactions. The onset of symptoms usually occurred within hours (most commonly 1 to 4 hours) following the administration of contrast media. These reactions include fever, chills, nausea, vomiting, pruritus, rash, diarrhea, hypotension, edema, and oliguria. Some clinicians have noted that these reactions resemble the immediate side effects caused by interleukin-2 administration; however, the cause of contrast reactions after interleukin-2 therapy is unknown. Most events were reported to occur when contrast media was given within 4 weeks after the last dose of interleukin-2. These events were also reported to occur when contrast media was given several months after interleukin-2 treatment.[13]

Carcinogenesis, Mutagenesis, Impairment of Fertility: There have been no studies conducted assessing the carcinogenic or mutagenic potential of PROLEUKIN.

There have been no studies conducted assessing the effect of PROLEUKIN on fertility. It is recommended that this drug not be administered to fertile persons of either sex not practicing effective contraception.

Pregnancy: *Pregnancy Category C.* Animal reproduction studies have not been conducted with PROLEUKIN. It is also not known whether PROLEUKIN can cause fetal harm when administered to a pregnant woman or can affect reproduction capacity. In view of the known adverse effects of PROLEUKIN, it should only be given to a pregnant woman with extreme caution, weighing the potential benefit with the risks associated with therapy.

Nursing Mothers: It is not known whether this drug is excreted in human milk. Because many drugs are excreted in human milk and because of the potential for serious adverse reactions in nursing infants from PROLEUKIN, a decision should be made whether to discontinue nursing or to discontinue the drug, taking into account the importance of the drug to the mother.

Pediatric Use: Safety and effectiveness in children under 18 years of age have not been established.

ADVERSE REACTIONS

The rate of drug-related deaths in the 255 metastatic renal cell carcinoma patients on study who received single-agent PROLEUKIN® (aldesleukin) was 4% (11/255).

Frequency and severity of adverse reactions to PROLEUKIN have generally been shown to be dose-related and schedule-dependent. Most adverse reactions are self-limiting and are usually, but not invariably, reversible within 2 or 3 days of discontinuation of therapy.

Examples of adverse reactions with permanent sequelae include: myocardial infarction, bowel perforation/infarction, and gangrene.

The most frequently reported serious adverse reactions include hypotension, renal dysfunction with oliguria/anuria, dyspnea or pulmonary congestion, and mental status changes (i.e., lethargy, somnolence, confusion, and agitation). Other serious toxicities have included myocardial ischemia, myocarditis, gangrene, respiratory failure leading to intubation, GI bleeding requiring surgery, intestinal perforation/ileus, coma, seizure, sepsis and renal impairment requiring dialysis. The incidence of these events has been higher in PS 1 patients than in PS 0 patients (See **"CLINICAL PHARMACOLOGY"** Section, **"Clinical Experience"** Subsection).

The following data on adverse reactions are based on 373 patients (255 with renal cell cancer and 118 with other tumors) treated with the recommended every 8-hour 15-minute infusion dosing regimen. These patients had metastatic or recurrent carcinoma and were enrolled in investigational trials in the United States.

Organ systems in which reactions occurred in a significant number of the patients treated are found in the following table:

[See table at top of next page.]

Other serious adverse events were derived from trials involving more than 1,800 patients treated with PROLEUKIN-based regimens using a variety of doses and schedules. These events each occurred with a frequency of <1% and included: liver or renal failure resulting in death; duodenal ulceration; fatal intestinal perforation; bowel necrosis; fatal cardiac arrest, myocarditis, and supraventricular tachycardia; permanent or transient blindness secondary to optic neuritis; fatal malignant hyperthermia; pulmonary edema resulting in death; respiratory arrest; fatal respiratory failure; fatal stroke; transient ischemic attack; meningitis; cerebral edema; pericarditis; allergic interstitial nephritis; tracheoesophageal fistula; fatal pulmonary emboli; severe depression leading to suicide.

Exacerbation of pre-existing autoimmune disease (Crohn's Disease and Thyroid Disease, see "WARNINGS" Section) and delayed adverse reactions to iodinated contrast media (see "PRECAUTIONS" Section) have also been reported. In clinical investigations, persistent but non-progressive vitiligo has been observed in malignant melanoma patients treated with interleukin-2.

OVERDOSAGE

Side effects following the use of PROLEUKIN® (aldesleukin) are dose-related. Administration of more than the recommended dose has been associated with a more rapid onset of expected dose-limiting toxicities. Adverse reactions generally will reverse when the drug is stopped, particularly because its serum half-life is short (See "CLINICAL PHARMACOLOGY" Section, "Pharmacokinetics" Subsection). Any continuing symptoms should be treated supportively. Life-threatening toxicities have been ameliorated by the intravenous administration of dexamethasone,[12] which may result in loss of therapeutic effect from PROLEUKIN. **NOTE: Prior to the use of dexamethasone, the physician should refer to the package insert for this product.**

DOSAGE AND ADMINISTRATION

PROLEUKIN® (aldesleukin) for injection should be administered by a 15-minute IV infusion every 8 hours. Before initiating treatment, carefully review the "INDICATIONS AND USAGE", "CONTRAINDICATIONS", "WARNINGS", "PRECAUTIONS", and "ADVERSE REACTIONS" Sections, particularly regarding patient selection, possible serious adverse events, patient monitoring, and withholding dosage.

The following schedule has been used to treat adult patients with metastatic renal cell carcinoma. Each course of treatment consists of two 5-day treatment cycles separated by a rest period.

600,000 IU/kg (0.037 mg/kg) dose administered every 8 hours by a 15-minute IV infusion for a total of 14 doses. Following 9 days of rest, the schedule is repeated for another 14 doses, for a maximum of 28 doses per course. During clinical trials, doses were frequently held for toxicity (See "Dose Modification" Subsection). Patients treated with this schedule received a median of 20 of the 28 doses during the first course of therapy.

Retreatment: Patients should be evaluated for response approximately 4 weeks after completion of a course of therapy and again immediately prior to the scheduled start of the next treatment course. Additional courses of treatment may be given to patients only if there is some tumor shrinkage following the last course, and retreatment is not contraindicated (See "CONTRAINDICATIONS" Section). Each treatment course should be separated by a rest period of at least 7 weeks from the date of hospital discharge. Tumors have continued to regress up to 12 months following the initiation of PROLEUKIN therapy.

Dose Modification: Dose modification for toxicity should be accomplished by holding or interrupting a dose rather than reducing the dose to be given. Decisions to stop, hold, or restart PROLEUKIN therapy must be made after a global assessment of the patient. With this in mind, the following guidelines should be used:

Treatment with PROLEUKIN should be permanently discontinued for:

Organ System	Permanently discontinue treatment for the following toxicities
Cardiovascular	Sustained ventricular tachycardia (≥ 5 beats) Cardiac rhythm disturbances not controlled or unresponsive to management Recurrent chest pain with ECG changes, documented angina, or myocardial infarction Pericardial tamponade
Pulmonary	Intubation required > 72 hours
Renal	Renal dysfunction requiring dialysis > 72 hours
Central Nervous System	Coma or toxic psychosis lasting > 48 hours. Repetitive or difficult to control seizures

TABLE III
Incidence of Adverse Events

Events by Body System	% of Patients	Events by Body System	% of Patients
Cardiovascular		**Gastrointestinal**	
Hypotension	85	Nausea and Vomiting	87
(requiring pressors)	71	Diarrhea	76
Sinus Tachycardia	70	Stomatitis	32
Arrhythmias	22	Anorexia	27
Atrial	8	GI Bleeding	13
Supraventricular	5	(requiring surgery)	2
Ventricular	3	Dyspepsia	7
Junctional	1	Constipation	5
Bradycardia	7	Intestinal Perforation/Ileus	2
Premature Ventricular Contractions	5	Pancreatitis	<1
Premature Atrial Contractions	4	**Neurologic**	
Myocardial Ischemia	3	Mental Status Changes	73
Myocardial Infarction	2	Dizziness	17
Cardiac Arrest	2	Sensory Dysfunction	10
Congestive Heart Failure	1	Special Sensory Disorders	
Myocarditis	1	(vision, speech, taste)	7
Stroke	1	Syncope	3
Gangrene	1	Motor Dysfunction	2
Pericardial Effusion	1	Coma	1
Endocarditis	1	Seizure (grand mal)	1
Thrombosis	1		
Pulmonary		**Renal**	
Pulmonary Congestion	54	Oliguria/Anuria	76
Dyspnea	52	BUN Elevation	63
Pulmonary Edema	10	Serum Creatinine Elevation	61
Respiratory Failure		Proteinuria	12
(leading to intubation)	9	Hematuria	9
Tachypnea	8	Dysuria	3
Pleural Effusion	7	Renal Impairment Requiring Dialysis	2
Wheezing	6	Urinary Retention	1
Apnea	1	Urinary Frequency	1
Pneumothorax	1	**Dermatologic**	
Hemoptysis	1	Pruritus	48
Hepatic		Erythema	41
Elevated Bilirubin	64	Rash	26
Elevated Transaminase	56	Dry Skin	15
Elevated Alkaline Phosphatase	56	Exfoliative Dermatitis	14
Jaundice	11	Purpura/Petechiae	4
Ascites	4	Urticaria	2
Hepatomegaly	1	Alopecia	1
Hematologic		**Musculoskeletal**	
Anemia	77	Arthralgia	6
Thrombocytopenia	64	Myalgia	6
Leukopenia	34	Arthritis	1
Coagulation Disorders	10	Muscle Spasm	1
Leukocytosis	9	**Endocrine**	
Eosinophilia	6	Hypothyroidism	<1
Abnormal Laboratory Findings		**General**	
Hypomagnesemia	16	Fever and/or Chills	89
Acidosis	16	Pain (all sites)	54
Hypocalcemia	15	Abdominal	15
Hypophosphatemia	11	Chest	12
Hypokalemia	9	Back	9
Hyperuricemia	9	Fatigue/Weakness/Malaise	53
Hypoalbuminemia	8	Edema	47
Hypoproteinemia	7	Infection	23
Hyponatremia	4	(including urinary tract, injection site, catheter tip, phlebitis, sepsis)	
Hyperkalemia	4	Weight Gain (≥ 10%)	23
Alkalosis	4	Headache	12
Hypoglycemia	2	Weight Loss (≥ 10%)	5
Hyperglycemia	2	Conjunctivitis	4
Hypocholesterolemia	1	Injection Site Reactions	3
Hypercalcemia	1	Allergic Reactions (non-anaphylactic)	1
Hypernatremia	1		
Hyperphosphatemia	1		

Gastrointestinal	Bowel ischemia/perforation/GI bleeding requiring surgery

[See table at top of next page.]

Reconstitution and Dilution Directions:
Reconstitution and dilution procedures other than those recommended may alter the delivery and/or pharmacology of PROLEUKIN and thus should be avoided.

1. PROLEUKIN (aldesleukin) is a sterile, white to off-white, preservative-free, lyophilized powder suitable for IV infusion upon reconstitution and dilution. **EACH VIAL CONTAINS 22 MILLION IU (1.3 MG) OF PROLEUKIN AND SHOULD BE RECONSTITUTED ASEPTICALLY WITH 1.2 ML OF STERILE WATER FOR INJECTION, USP. WHEN RECONSTITUTED AS DIRECTED, EACH ML CONTAINS 18 MILLION IU (1.1 MG) OF PROLEUKIN.** The resulting solution should be a clear, colorless to slightly yellow liquid. The vial is for single-use only and any unused portion should be discarded.

2. During reconstitution, the Sterile Water for Injection, USP should be directed at the side of the vial and the contents gently swirled to avoid excess foaming. **DO NOT SHAKE.**

3. The dose of PROLEUKIN, reconstituted in Sterile Water for Injection, USP (without preservative) should be diluted aseptically in 50 mL of 5% Dextrose Injection, USP and infused over a 15-minute period. Although glass bottles and plastic (polyvinyl chloride) bags have been used in clinical trials with comparable results, it is recommended that plastic bags be used as the dilution container since experimental studies suggest that use of plastic containers results in more consistent drug delivery. In-line filters should not be used when administering PROLEUKIN.

4. Before and after reconstitution and dilution, store in a refrigerator at 2° to 8°C (36° to 46°F). Do not freeze. Administer PROLEUKIN within 48 hours of reconstitution. The solution should be brought to room temperature prior to infusion in the patient.

5. Reconstitution or dilution with Bacteriostatic Water for Injection, USP, or 0.9% Sodium Chloride Injection, USP should be avoided because of increased aggregation. Animal studies have shown that dilution with albumin can alter the pharmacology of PROLEUKIN. PROLEUKIN should not be mixed with other drugs.

Continued on next page

Chiron Therapeutics—Cont.

Doses should be held and restarted according to the following:

Organ System	Hold dose for	Subsequent doses may be given if
Cardiovascular	Atrial fibrillation, supraventricular tachycardia, or bradycardia that requires treatment or is recurrent or persistent	Patient is asymptomatic with full recovery to normal sinus rhythm.
	Systolic BP <90 mm Hg with increasing requirements for pressors	Systolic BP ≥90 mm Hg and stable or improving requirements for pressors
	Any ECG change consistent with MI or ischemia with or without chest pain; suspicion of cardiac ischemia	Patient is asymptomatic, MI has been ruled out, clinical suspicion of angina is low
Pulmonary	O₂ saturation <94% on room air or <90% with 2 liters O₂ by nasal prongs	O₂ saturation ≥94% on room air or ≥90% with 2 liters O₂ by nasal prongs
Central Nervous System	Mental status changes, including moderate confusion or agitation	Mental status changes completely resolved
Systemic	Sepsis syndrome, patient is clinically unstable	Sepsis syndrome has resolved, patient is clinically stable, infection is under treatment
Renal	Serum creatinine ≥4.5 mg/dL or a serum creatinine of 4 mg/dL in the presence of severe volume overload, acidosis, or hyperkalemia	Serum creatinine <4 mg/dL and fluid and electrolyte status is stable
	Persistent oliguria, urine output of ≤10 mL/hour for 16 to 24 hours with rising serum creatinine	Urine output >10 mL/hour with a decrease of serum creatinine ≥1.5 mg/dL or normalization of serum creatinine
Hepatic	Signs of hepatic failure including encephalopathy, increasing ascites, liver pain, hypoglycemia	All signs of hepatic failure have resolved*
Gastrointestinal	Stool guaiac repeatedly >3–4+	Stool guaiac negative
Skin	Bullous dermatitis or marked worsening of pre-existing skin condition (avoid topical steroid therapy)	Resolution of all signs of bullous dermatitis

*Discontinue all further treatment for that course. Consider starting a new course of treatment at least 7 weeks after cessation of adverse event and hospital discharge.

6. Parenteral drug products should be inspected visually for particulate matter and discoloration prior to administration, whenever solution and container permit.

HOW SUPPLIED
PROLEUKIN® (aldesleukin) for injection is supplied in individually-boxed single-use vials. Each vial contains 22 × 10⁶ IU of PROLEUKIN. Discard unused portion.
NDC 53905-991-01 Individually-boxed single-use vial Store vials of lyophilized PROLEUKIN in a refrigerator at 2° to 8°C (36° to 46°F).
Reconstituted or diluted PROLEUKIN is stable for up to 48 hours at refrigerated and room temperatures, 2° to 25°C (36° to 77°F). However, since this product contains no preservative, the reconstituted and diluted solutions should be stored in the refrigerator.
Do not use beyond the expiration date printed on the vial.
Note: This product contains no preservative.
CAUTION: Federal law (USA) prohibits dispensing without a prescription.

REFERENCES
1. Doyle MV, Lee MT, Fong S. Comparison of the biological activities of human recombinant interleukin-2₁₂₅ and native interleukin-2. *J Biol Response Mod* 1985; **4**:96–109.
2. Ralph P, Nakoinz I, Doyle M, et al. Human B and T lymphocyte stimulating properties of interleukin-2 (IL-2) muteins. In: *Immune Regulation by Characterized Polypeptides.* Alan R. Liss, Inc. **1987**:453–62.
3. Winkelhake JL and Gauny SS. Human recombinant interleukin-2 as an experimental therapeutic. *Pharmacol Rev* 1990: **42**:1–28.
4. Rosenberg SA, Mule JJ, Spiess PJ, et al. Regression of established pulmonary metastases and subcutaneous tumor mediated by the systemic administration of high-dose recombinant interleukin-2. *J Exp Med* 1985; **161**:1169–88.
5. Konrad MW, Hemstreet G, Hersh EM, et al. Pharmacokinetics of recombinant interleukin-2 in humans. *Cancer Res* 1990; **50**:2009–17.
6. Donohue JH and Rosenberg SA. The fate of interleukin-2 after *in vivo* administration. *J Immunol* 1983; **130**:2203–8.
7. Koths K, Halenbeck R. Pharmacokinetic studies on ³⁵S-labeled recombinant interleukin-2 in mice. In: Sorg C and Schimpl A, eds. *Cellular and Molecular Biology of Lymphokines.* Academic Press: Orlando, Fl, **1985**:779.
8. Moyer BR, Young JD, Bauer RJ, et al. Renal mechanisms for the clearance of recombinant human IL-2 in the rat. *Pharmaceutical Res* 1990: **7**:S284 (abstract).
9. Bock SN, Lee RE, Fisher B, et al. A prospective randomized trial evaluating prophylactic antibiotics to prevent triple-lumen catheter-related sepsis in patients treated with immunotherapy. *J Clin Oncol* 1990; **8**:161–69.
10. Hartman LC, Urba, WJ, Steis RG, et al. Use of prophylactic antibiotics for prevention of intravascular catheter-related infections in interleukin-2-treated patients. *J Natl Cancer Inst* 1989; **81**:1190–93.
11. Snydman DR, Sullivan B, Gill M, et al. Nosocomial sepsis associated with interleukin-2. *Ann Intern Med* 1990; **112**:102–07.
12. Mier JW, Vachino G, Klempner MS, et al. Inhibition of interleukin-2-induced tumor necrosis factor release by dexamethasone: Prevention of an acquired neutrophil chemotaxis defect and differential suppression of interleukin-2-associated side effects. *Blood* 1990; **76**:1933–40.
13. Choyke PL, Miller DL, Lotze MT, et al. Delayed reactions to contrast media after interleukin-2 immunotherapy. *Radiology* 1992; **183**:111–114.

MANUFACTURED BY:
Chiron Corporation
Emeryville, CA 94608
U.S. License No. 1106
U.S. Patent Nos.
RE 33653; 4,530,787; 4,569,790; 4,604,377; 4,853,332; 4,748,234; 4,572,798; 4,959,314
© 1994 Chiron Corporation
DISTRIBUTED BY:
Chiron Therapeutics
Emeryville, CA 94608
Z0-P-03

CibaGeneva Pharmaceuticals

Ciba-Geigy Corporation
556 MORRIS AVENUE
SUMMIT, NJ 07901
(for branded products)

Geneva Pharmaceuticals, Inc.
2655 WEST MIDWAY BOULEVARD
PO BOX 446
BROOMFIELD, CO 80038-0446
(for branded generic products)

For Information Contact:
Consumer Affairs Department:
(800) 742-2422
Medical Services Department
556 Morris Avenue
Summit, NJ 07901
(for branded products)

For Information Contact:
Customer Support Department
(800) 525-8747
(303) 466-2400
FAX (303) 469-6467
(for branded generic products)

To provide a convenient and accurate means of identifying CibaGeneva solid dosage form products, a code number has been imprinted on all tablets and capsules. To help you quickly identify a CibaGeneva tablet or capsule by its code number, an alphabetical listing of products (with corresponding codes and identification numbers) has been compiled below.

CibaGeneva Product Identification Number	ALPHABETICAL LISTING	National Drug Code Number
	Actigall® ursodiol	
153	CAPSULES, 300 mg (white and pink, hard gelatin)	
	100's	57267-153-30
	Anafranil® clomipramine HCl	
115	CAPSULES, 25 mg (ivory/melon yellow)	
		58887-115-30
116	CAPSULES, 50 mg (ivory/aqua blue)	
		58887-116-30
117	CAPSULES, 75 mg (ivory/yellow)	
		58887-117-30
	Anturane® sulfinpyrazone USP	
41	TABLETS (white, single-scored) each containing 100 mg sulfinpyrazone USP	
	100's	0083-0041-30
168	CAPSULES (green) each containing 200 mg sulfinpyrazone USP	
	100's	0083-0168-30
	Apresazide® hydralazine HCl and hydrochlorothiazide	
139	CAPSULES 25/25 (light blue and white opaque), each containing 25 mg hydralazine HCl and 25 mg hydrochlorothiazide	
	100's	0083-0139-30
149	CAPSULES 50/50 (pink and white opaque), each containing 50 mg hydralazine HCl and 50 mg hydrochlorothiazide	
	100's	0083-0149-30
159	CAPSULES 100/50 (pink flesh and white opaque), each containing 100 mg hydralazine HCl and 50 mg hydrochlorothiazide	
	100's	0083-0159-30
	Apresoline® hydrochloride hydralazine hydrochloride USP	
37	TABLETS, 10 mg (pale yellow, dry coated)	
	100's	0083-0037-30
39	TABLETS, 25 mg (deep blue, dry-coated)	
	100's	0083-0039-30
73	TABLETS, 50 mg (light blue, dry-coated)	
	100's	0083-0073-30
101	TABLETS, 100 mg (peach, dry-coated)	
	100's	0083-0101-30
72	**Brethine® Tablets** terbutaline sulfate USP	2.5 mg
	Oval, white, scored tablets	
	100's	0028-0072-01
	1000's	0028-0072-10
	100's Unit Dose Pkg.	0028-0072-61
	Gy-Pak® 100's	
	One Unit (12 ×100)	0028-0072-65
105	**Brethine® Tablets** terbutaline sulfate USP	5 mg
	Round, scored, white tablets	
	100's	0028-0105-01
	1000's	0028-0105-10
	100's Unit Dose Pkg.	0028-0105-61
	Gy-Pak® 100's	
	One unit (12 ×100)	0028-0105-65
151	**Cataflam® Tablets** diclofenac potassium	50 mg
	Light brown, round, biconvex	
	100's	0028-0151-01
	100's Unit Dose Pkg.	0028-0151-61
	Cytadren® aminoglutethamide USP	
24	TABLETS-250 mg (white, round, scored into quarters)	
	100's	0083-0024-30
	Esidrix® hydrochlorothiazide USP	
22	TABLETS, 25 mg (pink, scored)	
	100's	0083-0022-30
46	TABLETS, 50 mg (yellow, scored)	
	100's	0083-0046-30
	Esimil®	
47	TABLETS (white, scored), each containing 10 mg guanethidine monosulfate USP and 25 mg hydrochlorothiazide USP	
	100's	0083-0047-30
	Estraderm® 0.05 mg estradiol transdermal system	

2310 Package of 6 Patient Calendar Packs 0083-2310-62
(8 systems per Patient Calendar Pack)
Package of 1 Patient Calendar Pack 0083-2310-24
(24 systems per Patient Calendar Pack)

Estraderm® 0.1 mg
estradiol transdermal system
2320 Package of 6 Patient Calendar Packs 0083-2320-62
(8 systems per Patient Calendar Pack)
Package of 1 Patient Calendar Pack 0083-2320-24
(24 systems per Patient Calendar Pack)

Ismelin® sulfate
guanethidine monosulfate
49 TABLETS, 10 mg (pale yellow, scored)
100's 0083-0049-30
103 TABLETS, 25 mg (white, scored)
100's 0083-0103-30

108 **Lamprene® Capsules**
clofazimine 50 mg
Brown, spherical capsules
100's 0028-0108-01

23 **Lioresal® Tablets**
baclofen 10 mg
White, oval, scored tablets
100's 0028-0023-01
100's Unit Dose Pkg. 0028-0023-61

33 **Lioresal® Tablets**
baclofen 20 mg
White, capsule shaped, scored tablets
100's 0028-0033-01
100's Unit Dose Pkg. 0028-0033-61

51 **Lopressor® Tablets**
metoprolol tartrate 50 mg
Light red, capsule-shaped, scored tablets
100's 0028-0051-01
1000's 0028-0051-10
100's Unit Dose Pkg. 0028-0051-61
Gy-Pak® 100's
One Unit (12 ×100) 0028-0051-65

71 **Lopressor® Tablets**
metoprolol tartrate 100 mg
Light blue, capsule-shaped, scored tablets
100's 0028-0071-01
1000's 0028-0071-10
100's Unit Dose Pkg. 0028-0071-61
Gy-Pak® 60's
One Unit (12 ×60) 0028-0071-73
Gy-Pak® 100's
One Unit (12 ×100) 0028-0071-65

Lopressor HCT®
metoprolol tartrate and hydrochlorothiazide
35 TABLETS, 50/25 mg (white and blue, capsule-shaped, scored)
100's 0028-0035-01
53 TABLETS, 100/25 mg (white and pink, capsule-shaped, scored)
100's 0028-0053-01
73 TABLETS, 100/50 mg (white and yellow, capsule-shaped, scored)
100's 0028-0073-01

Lotensin®
benazepril hydrochloride
59 TABLETS, 5 mg (round, light yellow, coated)
100's 0083-0059-30
Accu-Pak® 100's 0083-0059-32
63 TABLETS, 10 mg (round, dark yellow, coated)
100's 0083-0063-30
Accu-Pak® 100's 0083-0063-32
79 TABLETS, 20 mg (round, tan, coated)
100's 0083-0079-30
Accu-Pak® 100's 0083-0079-32
94 TABLETS, 40 mg (round, dark rose, coated)
100's 0083-0094-30
Accu-Pak® 100's 0083-0094-32

Lotensin HCT®
benazepril HCl and hydrochlorothiazide USP
57 TABLETS, 5 mg/6.25 mg (white, oblong, scored)
100's 0083-0057-30
Accu-Pak® 100's 0083-0057-32
72 TABLETS, 10 mg/12.5 mg (light pink, oblong, scored)
100's 0083-0072-30
Accu-Pak® 100's 0083-0072-32
74 TABLETS, 20 mg/12.5 mg (grayish-violet, oblong, scored)
100's 0083-0074-30
Accu-Pak® 100's 0083-0074-32
75 TABLETS, 20 mg/25 mg (red, oblong, scored)
100's 0083-0075-30
Accu-Pak® 100's 0083-0075-32

Lotrel®
amlodipine and benazepril hydrochloride combination capsules

Transderm-Nitro®
nitroglycerin

Code	Transderm-Nitro System*	Total Nitroglycerin in System	System Size	National Drug Code Number	Carton Size
902	0.1 mg/hr	12.5 mg	5 cm^2	57267-902-26	30 Systems
				57267-902-42	**30 Systems
				57267-902-30	**100 Systems
905	0.2 mg/hr	25 mg	10 cm^2	57267-905-26	30 Systems
				57267-905-42	**30 Systems
				57267-905-30	**100 Systems
910	0.4 mg/hr	50 mg	20 cm^2	57267-910-26	30 Systems
				57267-910-42	**30 Systems
				57267-910-30	**100 Systems
915	0.6 mg/hr	75 mg	30 cm^2	57267-915-26	30 Systems
				57267-915-42	**30 Systems
				57267-915-30	**100 Systems
920	0.8 mg/hr	100 mg	40 cm^2	57267-920-26	30 Systems
				57267-920-42	**30 Systems

**Institutional Pack

* Rated release in vivo. Release rates were formerly described in terms of drug delivered per 24 hours. In these terms, the supplied Transderm-Nitro systems would be rated at 2.5 mg/24 hr (0.1 mg/hr), 5 mg/24 hr (0.2 mg/hr), 10 mg/24 hr (0.4 mg/hr), 15 mg/24 hr (0.6 mg/hr), and 20 mg/24 hr (0.8 mg/hr).

2255 CAPSULES, 2.5/10 mg (white with 2 gold bands) 0083-2255-30
2260 CAPSULES, 5/10 mg (light brown with 2 white bands) 0083-2260-30
2265 CAPSULES, 5/20 mg (pink with 2 white bands) 0083-2265-30

Ludiomil®
maprotiline hydrochloride USP
110 TABLETS, 25 mg (oval, dark orange, coated)
100's 0083-0110-30
Accu-Pak® 100's 0083-0110-32
26 TABLETS, 50 mg (round, dark orange, coated)
100's 0083-0026-30
135 TABLETS, 75 mg (oval, white, coated)
100's 0083-0135-30

111 **PBZ® Tablets**
tripelennamine hydrochloride USP 25 mg
Round, white, scored tablets
100's 0028-0111-01

117 **PBZ® Tablets**
tripelennamine hydrochloride USP 50 mg
Round, white, scored tablets
100's 0028-0117-01

48 **PBZ-SR® Tablets**
tripelennamine hydrochloride 100 mg
Lavender-colored tablets
100's 0028-0048-01

Rimactane®
rifampin USP
154 CAPSULES, 300 mg (opaque scarlet and caramel)
30's 0083-0154-26
60's 0083-0154-29
100's 0083-0154-30

Ritalin® hydrochloride Ⓒ II
methylphenidate hydrochloride USP
07 TABLETS, 5 mg (yellow)
100's 0083-0007-30
03 TABLETS, 10 mg (pale green, scored)
100's 0083-0003-30
34 TABLETS, 20 mg (pale yellow, scored)
100's 0083-0034-30

Ritalin-SR® Ⓒ II
methylphenidate hydrochloride sustained-release tablets
16 TABLETS, 20 mg (round, white, scored)
100's 0083-0016-30

Ser-Ap-Es®
71 TABLETS (light salmon pink, dry-coated), each containing 0.1 mg reserpine, 25 mg hydralazine hydrochloride and 15 mg hydrochlorothiazide
100's 0083-0071-30
1000's 0083-0071-40

Slow-K®
potassium chloride USP
165 TABLETS (round, buff-colored, sugar-coated), each containing 8 mEq (600 mg) potassium chloride
100's 57267-165-30
1000's 57267-165-40
Consumer Pack 100's 57267-165-65

Tegretol®
carbamazepine
52 TABLETS, 100 mg (round, red-speckled, pink)
0083-0052-30
27 TABLETS, 200 mg (capsule-shaped, pink)
0083-0027-30
7019 SUSPENSION, 100 mg/5 ml (tsp) (yellow-orange, citrus-vanilla flavored)
0083-0019-76

Tegretol®-XR
carbamazepine extended-release tablets
61 TABLETS, 100 mg (round, yellow, coated)
0083-0061-30
62 TABLETS, 200 mg (round, pink, coated)
0083-0062-30
60 TABLETS, 400 mg (round, brown, coated)
0083-0060-30

32 **Tofranil® Tablets**
imipramine hydrochloride USP 10 mg
Triangular, coral-colored, coated tablets
100's 0028-0032-01

136 **Tofranil® Tablets**
imipramine hydrochloride USP 50 mg
Coral-colored (white Geigy imprint) coated tablets
100's 0028-0136-01
1000's 0028-0136-10
Gy-Pak® 100's
One unit (12 ×100) 0028-0136-65

140 **Tofranil® Tablets**
imipramine hydrochloride USP 25 mg
Coral-colored (black Geigy imprint) coated tablets
100's 0028-0140-01
1000's 0028-0140-10
Gy-Pak® 100's
One unit (12 ×100) 0028-0140-65

40 **Tofranil-PM® Capsules**
imipramine pamoate 100 mg
Dark yellow/coral-colored capsules
30's 0028-0040-26
100's 0028-0040-01

45 **Tofranil-PM® Capsules**
imipramine pamoate 125 mg
Light yellow/coral-colored capsules
30's 0028-0045-26
100's 0028-0045-01

20 **Tofranil-PM® Capsules**
imipramine pamoate 75 mg
Coral-colored capsules
30's 0028-0020-26
100's 0028-0020-01

22 **Tofranil-PM® Capsules**
imipramine pamoate 150 mg
Coral-colored capsules
30's 0028-0022-26
100's 0028-0022-01

[See table above.]

Vivelle™ 0.0375 mg
estradiol transdermal system
232562 Package of 6 Patient Calendar Packs 0083-2325-62
(8 Systems per Patient Calendar Pack)
232525 Package of 1 Patient Calendar Pack 0083-2325-25
(24 systems per Patient Calendar Pack)

Vivelle™ 0.05 mg
estradiol transdermal system
232662 Package of 6 Patient Calendar Packs 0083-2326-62
(8 systems per Patient Calendar Pack)
232625 Package of 1 Patient Calendar Pack 0083-2326-25
(24 systems per Patient Calendar Pack)

Vivelle™ 0.075 mg
estradiol transdermal system
232762 Package of 6 Patient Calendar Packs 0083-2327-62
(8 systems per Patient Calendar Pack)

Continued on next page

CibaGeneva—Cont.

232725 Package of 1 Patient Calendar Pack 0083-2327-25
(24 systems per Patient Calendar Pack)

Vivelle™ 0.1 mg
estradiol transdermal system

232862 Package of 6 Patient Calendar Packs 0083-2328-62
(8 systems per Patient Calendar Pack)

232825 Package of 1 Patient Calendar Pack 0083-2328-25
(24 systems per Patient Calendar Pack)

162 **Voltaren® Tablets**
diclofenac sodium 50 mg
Light brown, biconvex, triangular-shaped

60's	0028-0262-60
100's	0028-0262-01
1000's	0028-0262-10
100's Unit Dose Pkg.	0028-0262-61

164 **Voltaren® Tablets**
diclofenac sodium 75 mg
Light pink, biconvex, triangular-shaped

60's	0028-0264-60
100's	0028-0264-01
1000's	0028-0264-10
100's Unit Dose Pkg.	0028-0264-61

58 **Voltaren® Tablets**
diclofenac sodium 25 mg
Yellow, biconvex, triangular-shaped

60's	0028-0258-60
100's	0028-0258-01
100's Unit Dose Pkg.	0028-0258-61

205 **Voltaren®-XR Tablets**
diclofenac sodium 100 mg
Light pink, coated, round, biconvex

100's	0028-0205-01
100's Unit Dose Pkg.	0028-0205-61

ACTIGALL® ℞
ursodiol USP
Capsules

SPECIAL NOTE

Gallbladder stone dissolution with Actigall treatment requires months of therapy. Complete dissolution does not occur in all patients and recurrence of stones within 5 years has been observed in up to 50% of patients who do dissolve their stones on bile acid therapy. Patients should be carefully selected for therapy with ursodiol, and alternative therapies should be considered.

DESCRIPTION

Actigall is a bile acid available as 300-mg capsules suitable for oral administration.

Actigall is ursodiol USP (ursodeoxycholic acid), a naturally occurring bile acid found in small quantities in normal human bile and in larger quantities in the biles of certain species of bears. It is a bitter-tasting, white powder freely soluble in ethanol, methanol, and glacial acetic acid; sparingly soluble in chloroform; slightly soluble in ether; and practically insoluble in water. The chemical name for ursodiol is 3α,7β-dihydroxy-5β-cholan-24-oic acid ($C_{24}H_{40}O_4$). Ursodiol USP has a molecular weight of 392.56.

Inactive Ingredients. Gelatin, iron oxide, magnesium stearate, colloidal silicon dioxide, starch, and titanium dioxide.

CLINICAL PHARMACOLOGY

About 90% of a therapeutic dose of Actigall is absorbed in the small bowel after oral administration. After absorption, ursodiol enters the portal vein and undergoes efficient extraction from portal blood by the liver (i.e., there is a large "first-pass" effect) where it is conjugated with either glycine or taurine and is then secreted into the hepatic bile ducts. Ursodiol in bile is concentrated in the gallbladder and expelled into the duodenum in gallbladder bile via the cystic and common ducts by gallbladder contractions provoked by physiologic responses to eating. Only small quantities of ursodiol appear in the systemic circulation and very small amounts are excreted into urine. The sites of the drug's therapeutic actions are in the liver, bile, and gut lumen.

Beyond conjugation, ursodiol is not altered or catabolized appreciably by the liver or intestinal mucosa. A small proportion of orally administered drug undergoes bacterial degradation with each cycle of enterohepatic circulation. Ursodiol can be both oxidized and reduced at the 7-carbon, yielding either 7-keto-lithocholic acid or lithocholic acid, respectively. Further, there is some bacterially catalyzed deconjugation of glyco- and tauro- ursodeoxycholic acid in the small bowel. Free ursodiol, 7-keto-lithocholic acid, and lithocholic acid are relatively insoluble in aqueous media and larger proportions of these compounds are lost from the distal gut into the feces. Reabsorbed free ursodiol is reconjugated by the liver. Eighty percent of lithocholic acid formed in the small bowel is excreted in the feces, but the 20% that is absorbed is sulfated at the 3-hydroxyl group in the liver to relatively insoluble lithocholyl conjugates which are excreted into bile and lost in feces. Absorbed 7-keto-lithocholic acid is stereospecifically reduced in the liver to chenodiol.

Lithocholic acid causes cholestatic liver injury and can cause death from liver failure in certain species unable to form sulfate conjugates. Lithocholic acid is formed by 7-dehydroxylation of the dihydroxy bile acids (ursodiol and chenodiol) in the gut lumen. The 7-dehydroxylation reaction appears to be alpha-specific, i.e., chenodiol is more efficiently 7-dehydroxylated than ursodiol and, for equimolar doses of ursodiol and chenodiol, levels of lithocholic acid appearing in bile are lower with the former. Man has the capacity to sulfate lithocholic acid. Although liver injury has not been associated with ursodiol therapy, a reduced capacity to sulfate may exist in some individuals, but such a deficiency has not yet been clearly demonstrated.

Pharmacodynamics

Ursodiol suppresses hepatic synthesis and secretion of cholesterol, and also inhibits intestinal absorption of cholesterol. It appears to have little inhibitory effect on synthesis and secretion into bile of endogenous bile acids, and does not appear to affect secretion of phospholipids into bile.

With repeated dosing, bile ursodeoxycholic acid concentrations reach a steady state in about 3 weeks. Although insoluble in aqueous media, cholesterol can be solubilized in at least two different ways in the presence of dihydroxy bile acids. In addition to solubilizing cholesterol in micelles, ursodiol acts by an apparently unique mechanism to cause dispersion of cholesterol as liquid crystals in aqueous media. Thus, even though administration of high doses (e.g., 15–18 mg/kg/day) does not result in a concentration of ursodiol higher than 60% of the total bile acid pool, ursodiol-rich bile effectively solubilizes cholesterol. The overall effect of ursodiol is to increase the concentration level at which saturation of cholesterol occurs.

The various actions of ursodiol combine to change the bile of patients with gallstones from cholesterol-precipitating to cholesterol-solubilizing, thus resulting in bile conducive to cholesterol stone dissolution.

After ursodiol dosing is stopped, the concentration of the bile acid in bile falls exponentially, declining to about 5%–10% of its steady-state level in about 1 week.

Clinical Results

Gallstone Dissolution

On the basis of clinical trial results in a total of 868 patients with radiolucent gallstones treated in 8 studies (three in the U.S. involving 282 patients, one in the U.K. involving 130 patients, and four in Italy involving 456 patients) for periods ranging from 6–78 months with Actigall doses ranging from about 5 to 20 mg/kg/day, an Actigall dose of about 8–10 mg/kg/day appeared to be the best dose. With an Actigall dose of about 10 mg/kg/day, complete stone dissolution can be anticipated in about 30% of unselected patients with uncalcified gallstones <20 mm in maximal diameter treated for up to 2 years. Patients with calcified gallstones prior to treatment, or patients who develop stone calcification or gallbladder nonvisualization on treatment, and patients with stones >20 mm in maximal diameter rarely dissolve their stones. The chance of gallstone dissolution is increased up to 50% in patients with floating or floatable stones (i.e., those with high cholesterol content), and is inversely related to stone size for those <20 mm in maximal diameter. Complete dissolution was observed in 81% of patients with stones up to 5 mm in diameter. Age, sex, weight, degree of obesity, and serum cholesterol level are not related to the chance of stone dissolution with Actigall.

A nonvisualizing gallbladder by oral cholecystogram prior to the initiation of therapy is not a contraindication to Actigall therapy (the group of patients with nonvisualizing gallbladders in the Actigall studies had complete stone dissolution rates similar to the group of patients with visualizing gallbladders). However, gallbladder nonvisualization developing during ursodiol treatment predicts failure of complete stone dissolution and in such cases therapy should be discontinued.

Partial stone dissolution occurring within 6 months of beginning therapy with Actigall appears to be associated with a >70% chance of eventual complete stone dissolution with further treatment; partial dissolution observed within 1 year of starting therapy indicates a 40% probability of complete dissolution.

Stone recurrence after dissolution with Actigall therapy was seen within 2 years in 8/27 (30%) of patients in the U.K. studies. Of 16 patients in the U.K. study whose stones had previously dissolved on chenodiol but later recurred, 11 had complete dissolution on Actigall. Stone recurrence has been observed in up to 50% of patients within 5 years of complete stone dissolution on ursodiol therapy. Serial ultrasonographic examinations should be obtained to monitor for recurrence of stones, bearing in mind that radiolucency of the stones should be established before another course of Actigall is instituted. A prophylactic dose of Actigall has not been established.

Gallstone Prevention

Two placebo-controlled, multicenter, double-blind, randomized, parallel group trials in a total of 1316 obese patients were undertaken to evaluate Actigall in the prevention of gallstone formation in obese patients undergoing rapid weight loss. The first trial consisted of 1004 obese patients with a body mass index (BMI) ≥38 who underwent weight loss induced by means of a very low calorie diet for a period of 16 weeks. An intent-to-treat analysis of this trial showed that gallstone formation occurred in 23% of the placebo group, while those patients on 300, 600, or 1200 mg/day of Actigall experienced a 6%, 3%, and 2% incidence of gallstone formation, respectively. The mean weight loss for this 16-week trial was 47 lb for the placebo group, and 47, 48, and 50 lb for the 300, 600, and 1200 mg/day Actigall groups, respectively.

The second trial consisted of 312 obese patients (BMI ≥40) who underwent rapid weight loss through gastric bypass surgery. The trial drug treatment period was for 6 months following this surgery. Results of this trial showed that gallstone formation occurred in 23% of the placebo group, while those patients on 300, 600, or 1200 mg/day of Actigall experienced a 9%, 1%, and 5% incidence of gallstone formation, respectively. The mean weight loss for this 6-month trial was 64 lb for the placebo group, and 67, 74, and 72 lb for the 300, 600, and 1200 mg/day Actigall groups, respectively.

ALTERNATIVE THERAPIES

Watchful Waiting

Watchful waiting has the advantage that no therapy may ever be required. For patients with silent or minimally symptomatic stones, the rate of development of moderate-to-severe symptoms or gallstone complications is estimated to be between 2% and 6% per year, leading to a cumulative rate of 7% to 27% in 5 years. Presumably the rate is higher for patients already having symptoms.

Cholecystectomy

For patients with symptomatic gallstones, surgery offers the advantage of immediate and permanent stone removal, but carries a high risk in some patients. About 5% of cholecystectomized patients have residual symptoms or retained common duct stones. The spectrum of surgical risk varies as a function of age and the presence of disease other than cholelithiasis.

Mortality Rates for Cholecystectomy in the U.S.
(National Halothane Study, JAMA 1966; 197:775-8)
27,600 Cholecystectomies (Smoothed Rates)
Deaths/1000 Operations***

Low Risk Patients*	Age (Yrs)	Cholecystectomy	Cholecystectomy +Common Duct Exploration
Women	0–49	.54	2.13
	50–69	2.80	10.10
Men	0–49	1.04	4.12
	50–69	5.41	19.23
High Risk Patients**			
Women	0–49	12.66	47.62
	50–69	17.24	58.82
Men	0–49	24.39	90.91
	50–69	33.33	111.11

* In good health or with moderate systemic disease.
** With severe or extreme systemic disease.
*** Includes both elective and emergency surgery.

Women in good health or who have only moderate systemic disease and are under 49 years of age have the lowest surgical mortality rate (0.054); men in all categories have a surgical mortality rate twice that of women. Common duct exploration quadruples the rates in all categories. The rates rise with each decade of life and increase tenfold or more in all categories with severe or extreme systemic disease.

INDICATIONS AND USAGE

1. Actigall is indicated for patients with radiolucent, noncalcified gallbladder stones <20 mm in greatest diameter in whom elective cholecystectomy would be undertaken except for the presence of increased surgical risk due to systemic disease, advanced age, idiosyncratic reaction to general anesthesia, or for those patients who refuse surgery. Safety of use of Actigall beyond 24 months is not established.
2. Actigall is indicated for the prevention of gallstone formation in obese patients experiencing rapid weight loss.

CONTRAINDICATIONS

1. Actigall will not dissolve calcified cholesterol stones, radiopaque stones, or radiolucent bile pigment stones. Hence, patients with such stones are not candidates for Actigall therapy.
2. Patients with compelling reasons for cholecystectomy including unremitting acute cholecystitis, cholangitis, biliary obstruction, gallstone pancreatitis, or biliary-gastrointestinal fistula are not candidates for Actigall therapy.
3. Allergy to bile acids.

PRECAUTIONS

Liver Tests
Ursodiol therapy has not been associated with liver damage. Lithocholic acid, a naturally occurring bile acid, is known to be a liver-toxic metabolite. This bile acid is formed in the gut from ursodiol less efficiently and in smaller amounts than that seen from chenodiol. Lithocholic acid is detoxified in the liver by sulfation and, although man appears to be an efficient sulfater, it is possible that some patients may have a congenital or acquired deficiency in sulfation, thereby predisposing them to lithocholate-induced liver damage. Abnormalities in liver enzymes have not been associated with Actigall therapy and, in fact, Actigall has been shown to decrease liver enzyme levels in liver disease. However, patients given Actigall should have SGOT (AST) and SGPT (ALT) measured at the initiation of therapy and thereafter as indicated by the particular clinical circumstances.

Drug Interactions
Bile acid sequestering agents such as cholestyramine and colestipol may interfere with the action of Actigall by reducing its absorption.

Aluminum-based antacids have been shown to adsorb bile acids in vitro and may be expected to interfere with Actigall in the same manner as the bile acid sequestering agents. Estrogens, oral contraceptives, and clofibrate (and perhaps other lipid-lowering drugs) increase hepatic cholesterol secretion, and encourage cholesterol gallstone formation and hence may counteract the effectiveness of Actigall.

Carcinogenesis, Mutagenesis, Impairment of Fertility
Ursodeoxycholic acid was tested in 2-year oral carcinogenicity studies in CD-1 mice and Sprague-Dawley rats at daily doses of 50, 250, and 1000 mg/kg/day. It was not tumorigenic in mice. In the rat study, it produced statistically significant dose-related increased incidences of pheochromocytomas of adrenal medulla in males (p=0.014, Peto trend test) and females (p=0.004, Peto trend test.) A 78-week rat study employing intrarectal instillation of lithocholic acid and taurodeoxycholic acid, metabolites of ursodiol and chenodiol, has been conducted. These bile acids alone did not produce any tumors. A tumor-promoting effect of both metabolites was observed when they were coadministered with a carcinogenic agent. Results of epidemiologic studies suggest that bile acids might be involved in the pathogenesis of human colon cancer in patients who had undergone a cholecystectomy, but direct evidence is lacking. Ursodiol is not mutagenic in the Ames test. Dietary administration of lithocholic acid to chickens is reported to cause hepatic adenomatous hyperplasia.

Pregnancy Category B
Reproduction studies have been performed in rats and rabbits with ursodiol doses up to 200-fold the therapeutic dose and have revealed no evidence of impaired fertility or harm to the fetus at doses of 20- to 100-fold the human dose in rats and at 5-fold the human dose (highest dose tested) in rabbits. Studies employing 100- to 200-fold the human dose in rats have shown some reduction in fertility rate and litter size. There have been no adequate and well-controlled studies of the use of ursodiol in pregnant women, but inadvertent exposure of 4 women to therapeutic doses of the drug in the first trimester of pregnancy during the Actigall trials led to no evidence of effects on the fetus or newborn baby.

Although it seems unlikely, the possibility that ursodiol can cause fetal harm cannot be ruled out; hence, the drug is not recommended for use during pregnancy.

Nursing Mothers
It is not known whether ursodiol is excreted in human milk. Because many drugs are excreted in human milk, caution should be exercised when Actigall is administered to a nursing mother.

Pediatric Use
The safety and effectiveness of Actigall in pediatric patients have not been established.

ADVERSE REACTIONS
The nature and frequency of adverse experiences were similar across all groups.

The following tables provide comprehensive listings of the adverse experiences reported that occurred with a 5% incidence level:

GALLSTONE DISSOLUTION

	Ursodiol 8-10 mg/kg/day (N=155)		Placebo (N=159)	
	N	(%)	N	(%)
Body as a Whole				
Allergy	8	(5.2)	7	(4.4)
Chest Pain	5	(3.2)	10	(6.3)
Fatigue	7	(4.5)	8	(5.0)
Infection Viral	30	(19.4)	41	(25.8)
Digestive System				
Abdominal Pain	67	(43.2)	70	(44.0)
Cholecystitis	8	(5.2)	7	(4.4)
Constipation	15	(9.7)	14	(8.8)
Diarrhea	42	(27.1)	34	(21.4)
Dyspepsia	26	(16.8)	18	(11.3)
Flatulence	12	(7.7)	12	(7.5)
Gastrointestinal Disorder	6	(3.9)	8	(5.0)
Nausea	22	(14.2)	27	(17.0)
Vomiting	15	(9.7)	11	(6.9)
Musculoskeletal System				
Arthralgia	12	(7.7)	24	(15.1)
Arthritis	9	(5.8)	4	(2.5)
Back Pain	11	(7.1)	18	(11.3)
Myalgia	9	(5.8)	9	(5.7)
Nervous System				
Headache	28	(18.1)	34	(21.4)
Insomnia	3	(1.9)	8	(5.0)
Respiratory System				
Bronchitis	10	(6.5)	6	(3.8)
Coughing	11	(7.1)	7	(4.4)
Pharyngitis	13	(8.4)	5	(3.1)
Rhinitis	8	(5.2)	11	(6.9)
Sinusitis	17	(11.0)	18	(11.3)
Upper Respiratory Tract Infection	24	(15.5)	21	(13.2)
Urogenital System				
Urinary Tract Infection	10	(6.5)	7	(4.4)

GALLSTONE PREVENTION

	Actigall 600 mg (N=322)		Placebo (N=325)	
	N	(%)	N	(%)
Body as a Whole				
Fatigue	25	(7.8)	33	(10.2)
Infection Viral	29	(9.0)	29	(8.9)
Influenza-like Symptoms	21	(6.5)	19	(5.8)
Digestive System				
Abdominal Pain	20	(6.2)	39	(12.0)
Constipation	85	(26.4)	72	(22.2)
Diarrhea	81	(25.2)	68	(20.9)
Flatulence	15	(4.7)	24	(7.4)
Nausea	56	(17.4)	43	(13.2)
Vomiting	44	(13.7)	44	(13.5)
Musculoskeletal System				
Back Pain	38	(11.8)	21	(6.5)
Musculoskeletal Pain	19	(5.9)	15	(4.6)
Nervous System				
Dizziness	53	(16.5)	42	(12.9)
Headache	80	(24.8)	78	(24.0)
Respiratory System				
Pharyngitis	10	(3.1)	19	(5.8)
Sinusitis	17	(5.3)	18	(5.5)
Upper Respiratory Tract Infection	40	(12.4)	35	(10.8)
Skin and Appendages				
Alopecia	17	(5.3)	8	(2.5)
Urogenital System				
Dysmenorrhea	18	(5.6)	19	(5.8)

OVERDOSAGE
Neither accidental nor intentional overdosing with Actigall has been reported. Doses of Actigall in the range of 16–20 mg/kg/day have been tolerated for 6–37 months without symptoms by 7 patients. The LD$_{50}$ for ursodiol in rats is over 5000 mg/kg given over 7–10 days and over 7500 mg/kg for mice. The most likely manifestation of severe overdose with Actigall would probably be diarrhea, which should be treated symptomatically.

DOSAGE AND ADMINISTRATION

Gallstone Dissolution
The recommended dose for Actigall treatment of radiolucent gallbladder stones is 8–10 mg/kg/day given in 2 or 3 divided doses.

Ultrasound images of the gallbladder should be obtained at 6-month intervals for the first year of Actigall therapy to monitor gallstone response. If gallstones appear to have dissolved, Actigall therapy should be continued and dissolution confirmed on a repeat ultrasound examination within 1 to 3 months. Most patients who eventually achieve complete stone dissolution will show partial or complete dissolution at the first on-treatment reevaluation. If partial stone dissolution is not seen by 12 months of Actigall therapy, the likelihood of success is greatly reduced.

Gallstone Prevention
The recommended dosage of Actigall for gallstone prevention in patients undergoing rapid weight loss is 600 mg/day (300 mg b.i.d.).

HOW SUPPLIED
Capsules 300 mg—opaque, white, pink (imprinted Actigall 300 mg)

Bottles of 100 ....NDC 57267-153-30

Samples, when available, are identified by the word SAMPLE appearing on each capsule.

Caution: Federal law prohibits dispensing without prescription.

Do not store above 86°F (30°C).

Dispense in tight container (USP).

C96-39 (Rev. 4/96)

Dist. by:
Ciba-Geigy Corporation
Pharmaceuticals Division
Summit, New Jersey 07901

Shown in Product Identification Guide, page 308

ANAFRANIL®   ℞
clomipramine hydrochloride
Capsules

DESCRIPTION
Anafranil, clomipramine hydrochloride, is an antiobsessional drug that belongs to the class (dibenzazepine) of pharmacologic agents known as tricyclic antidepressants. Anafranil is available as capsules of 25, 50, and 75 mg for oral administration.

Clomipramine hydrochloride is 3-chloro-5-[3-(dimethylamino)propyl]-10,11-dihydro-5H-dibenz[b,f]azepine monohydrochloride.

Clomipramine hydrochloride is a white to off-white crystalline powder. It is freely soluble in water, in methanol, and in methylene chloride, and insoluble in ethyl ether and in hexane. Its molecular weight is 351.3.

Inactive Ingredients. D&C Red No. 33 (25-mg capsules only), D&C Yellow No. 10, FD&C Blue No. 1 (50-mg capsules only), FD&C Yellow No. 6, gelatin, magnesium stearate, methylparaben, propylparaben, silicon dioxide, sodium lauryl sulfate, starch, and titanium dioxide.

CLINICAL PHARMACOLOGY

Pharmacodynamics
Clomipramine (CMI) is presumed to influence obsessive and compulsive behaviors through its effects on serotonergic neuronal transmission. The actual neurochemical mechanism is unknown, but CMI's capacity to inhibit the reuptake of serotonin (5-HT) is thought to be important.

Pharmacokinetics
Absorption/Bioavailability: CMI from Anafranil capsules is as bioavailable as CMI from a solution. The bioavailability of CMI from capsules is not significantly affected by food. In a dose proportionality study involving multiple CMI doses, steady-state plasma concentrations (C_{SS}) and area-under-plasma-concentration-time curves (AUC) of CMI and CMI's major active metabolite, desmethylclomipramine (DMI), were not proportional to dose over the ranges evaluated, i.e., between 25–100 mg/day and between 25–150 mg/day, although C_{SS} and AUC are approximately linearly related to dose between 100–150 mg/day. The relationship between dose and CMI/DMI concentrations at higher daily doses has not been systematically assessed, but if there is significant dose dependency at doses above 150 mg/day, there is the potential for dramatically higher C_{SS} and AUC even for patients dosed within the recommended range. This may pose a potential risk to some patients (see WARNINGS and PRECAUTIONS, Drug Interactions).

After a single 50-mg oral dose, maximum plasma concentrations of CMI occur within 2-6 hours (mean, 4.7 hr) and range from 56 ng/ml to 154 ng/ml (mean, 92 ng/ml). After multiple daily doses of 150 mg of Anafranil, steady-state maximum plasma concentrations range from 94 ng/ml to 339 ng/ml (mean, 218 ng/ml) for CMI and from 134 ng/ml to 532 ng/ml (mean, 274 ng/ml) for DMI. No pharmacokinetic information is available for doses ranging from 150 mg/day to 250 mg/day, the maximum recommended daily dose.

Distribution: CMI distributes into cerebrospinal fluid (CSF) and brain and into breast milk. DMI also distributes into CSF, with a mean CSF/plasma ratio of 2.6. The protein binding of CMI is approximately 97%, principally to albumin, and is independent of CMI concentration. The interaction between CMI and other highly protein-bound drugs has not been fully evaluated, but may be important (see PRECAUTIONS, Drug Interactions).

Metabolism: CMI is extensively biotransformed to DMI and other metabolites and their glucuronide conjugates. DMI is pharmacologically active, but its effects on OCD behaviors are unknown. These metabolites are excreted in urine and feces, following biliary elimination. After a 25-mg radiolabeled dose of CMI in two subjects, 60% and 51%, respectively, of the dose were recovered in the urine and 32% and 24%, respectively, in feces. In the same study, the com-

Continued on next page

CibaGeneva—Cont.

bined urinary recoveries of CMI and DMI were only about 0.8–1.3% of the dose administered. CMI does not induce drug-metabolizing enzymes, as measured by antipyrine half-life.

Elimination: Evidence that the C_{SS} and AUC for CMI and DMI may increase disproportionately with increasing oral doses suggests that the metabolism of CMI and DMI may be capacity limited. This fact must be considered in assessing the estimates of the pharmacokinetic parameters presented below, as these were obtained in individuals exposed to doses of 150 mg. If the pharmacokinetics of CMI and DMI are nonlinear at doses above 150 mg, their elimination half-lives may be considerably lengthened at doses near the upper end of the recommended dosing range (i.e., 200 mg/day to 250 mg/day). Consequently, CMI and DMI may accumulate, and this accumulation may increase the incidence of any dose- or plasma-concentration-dependent adverse reactions, in particular seizures (see WARNINGS).

After a 150-mg dose, the half-life of CMI ranges from 19 hours to 37 hours (mean, 32 hr) and that of DMI ranges from 54 hours to 77 hours (mean, 69 hr). Steady-state levels after multiple dosing are typically reached within 7–14 days for CMI. Plasma concentrations of the metabolite exceed the parent drug on multiple dosing. After multiple dosing with 150 mg/day, the accumulation factor for CMI is approximately 2.5 and for DMI is 4.6. Importantly, it may take two weeks or longer to achieve this extent of accumulation at constant dosing because of the relatively long elimination half-lives of CMI and DMI (see DOSAGE AND ADMINISTRATION). The effects of hepatic and renal impairment on the disposition of Anafranil have not been determined.

Interactions: Coadministration of haloperidol with CMI increases plasma concentrations of CMI. Coadministration of CMI with phenobarbital increases plasma concentrations of phenobarbital (see PRECAUTIONS, Drug Interactions). Younger subjects (18–40 years of age) tolerated CMI better and had significantly lower steady-state plasma concentrations, compared with subjects over 65 years of age. Children under 15 years of age had significantly lower plasma concentration/dose ratios, compared with adults. Plasma concentrations of CMI were significantly lower in smokers than in nonsmokers.

INDICATIONS AND USAGE

Anafranil is indicated for the treatment of obsessions and compulsions in patients with Obsessive-Compulsive Disorder (OCD). The obsessions or compulsions must cause marked distress, be time-consuming, or significantly interfere with social or occupational functioning, in order to meet the DSM-III-R (circa 1989) diagnosis of OCD.

Obsessions are recurrent, persistent ideas, thoughts, images, or impulses that are ego-dystonic. Compulsions are repetitive, purposeful, and intentional behaviors performed in response to an obsession or in a stereotyped fashion, and are recognized by the person as excessive or unreasonable.

The effectiveness of Anafranil for the treatment of OCD was demonstrated in multicenter, placebo-controlled, parallel-group studies, including two 10-week studies in adults and one 8-week study in children and adolescents 10–17 years of age. Patients in all studies had moderate-to-severe OCD (DSM-III), with mean baseline ratings on the Yale-Brown Obsessive Compulsive Scale (YBOCS) ranging from 26 to 28 and a mean baseline rating of 10 on the NIMH Clinical Global Obsessive Compulsive Scale (NIMH-OC). Patients taking CMI experienced a mean reduction of approximately 10 on the YBOCS, representing an average improvement on this scale of 35% to 42% among adults and 37% among children and adolescents. CMI-treated patients experienced a 3.5 unit decrement on the NIMH-OC. Patients on placebo showed no important clinical response on either scale. The maximum dose was 250 mg/day for most adults and 3 mg/kg/day (up to 200 mg) for all children and adolescents. The effectiveness of Anafranil for long-term use (i.e., for more than 10 weeks) has not been systematically evaluated in placebo-controlled trials. The physician who elects to use Anafranil for extended periods should periodically reevaluate the long-term usefulness of the drug for the individual patient (see DOSAGE AND ADMINISTRATION).

CONTRAINDICATIONS

Anafranil is contraindicated in patients with a history of hypersensitivity to Anafranil or other tricyclic antidepressants.

Anafranil should not be given in combination, or within 14 days before or after treatment, with a monoamine oxidase (MAO) inhibitor. Hyperpyretic crisis, seizures, coma, and death have been reported in patients receiving such combinations.

Anafranil is contraindicated during the acute recovery period after a myocardial infarction.

WARNINGS

Seizures

During premarket evaluation, seizure was identified as the most significant risk of Anafranil use.

The observed cumulative incidence of seizures among patients exposed to Anafranil at doses up to 300 mg/day was 0.64% at 90 days, 1.12% at 180 days, and 1.45% at 365 days. The cumulative rates correct the crude rate of 0.7% (25 of 3519 patients) for the variable duration of exposure in clinical trials.

Although dose appears to be a predictor of seizure, there is a confounding of dose and duration of exposure, making it difficult to assess independently the effect of either factor alone. The ability to predict the occurrence of seizures in subjects exposed to doses of CMI greater than 250 mg is limited, given that the plasma concentration of CMI may be dose-dependent and may vary among subjects given the same dose. Nevertheless, prescribers are advised to limit the daily dose to a maximum of 250 mg in adults and 3 mg/kg (or 200 mg) in children and adolescents (see DOSAGE AND ADMINISTRATION).

Caution should be used in administering Anafranil to patients with a history of seizures or other predisposing factors, e.g., brain damage of varying etiology, alcoholism, and concomitant use with other drugs that lower the seizure threshold.

Rare reports of fatalities in association with seizures have been reported by foreign post-marketing surveillance, but not in U.S. clinical trials. In some of these cases, Anafranil had been administered with other epileptogenic agents; in others, the patients involved had possibly predisposing medical conditions. Thus a causal association between Anafranil treatment and these fatalities has not been established.

Physicians should discuss with patients the risk of taking Anafranil while engaging in activities in which sudden loss of consciousness could result in serious injury to the patient or others, e.g., the operation of complex machinery, driving, swimming, climbing.

PRECAUTIONS

General

Suicide: Since depression is a commonly associated feature of OCD, the risk of suicide must be considered. Prescriptions for Anafranil should be written for the smallest quantity of capsules consistent with good patient management, in order to reduce the risk of overdose.

Cardiovascular Effects: Modest orthostatic decreases in blood pressure and modest tachycardia were each seen in approximately 20% of patients taking Anafranil in clinical trials; but patients were frequently asymptomatic. Among approximately 1400 patients treated with CMI in the premarketing experience who had ECGs, 1.5% developed abnormalities during treatment, compared with 3.1% of patients receiving active control drugs and 0.7% of patients receiving placebo. The most common ECG changes were PVCs, ST-T wave changes, and intraventricular conduction abnormalities. These changes were rarely associated with significant clinical symptoms. Nevertheless, caution is necessary in treating patients with known cardiovascular disease, and gradual dose titration is recommended.

Psychosis, Confusion, And Other Neuropsychiatric Phenomena: Patients treated with Anafranil have been reported to show a variety of neuropsychiatric signs and symptoms including delusions, hallucinations, psychotic episodes, confusion, and paranoia. Because of the uncontrolled nature of many of the studies, it is impossible to provide a precise estimate of the extent of risk imposed by treatment with Anafranil. As with tricyclic antidepressants to which it is closely related, Anafranil may precipitate an acute psychotic episode in patients with unrecognized schizophrenia.

Mania/Hypomania: During premarketing testing of Anafranil in patients with affective disorder, hypomania or mania was precipitated in several patients. Activation of mania or hypomania has also been reported in a small proportion of patients with affective disorder treated with marketed tricyclic antidepressants, which are closely related to Anafranil.

Hepatic Changes: During premarketing testing, Anafranil was occasionally associated with elevations in SGOT and SGPT (pooled incidence of approximately 1% and 3%, respectively) of potential clinical importance (i.e., values greater than 3 times the upper limit of normal). In the vast majority of instances, these enzyme increases were not associated with other clinical findings suggestive of hepatic injury; moreover, none were jaundiced. Rare reports of more severe liver injury, some fatal, have been recorded in foreign postmarketing experience. Caution is indicated in treating patients with known liver disease, and periodic monitoring of hepatic enzyme levels is recommended in such patients.

Hematologic Changes: Although no instances of severe hematologic toxicity were seen in the premarketing experience with Anafranil, there have been postmarketing reports of leukopenia, agranulocytosis, thrombocytopenia, anemia, and pancytopenia in association with Anafranil use. As is

the case with tricyclic antidepressants to which Anafranil is closely related, leukocyte and differential blood counts should be obtained in patients who develop fever and sore throat during treatment with Anafranil.

Central Nervous System: More than 30 cases of hyperthermia have been recorded by nondomestic postmarketing surveillance systems. Most cases occurred when Anafranil was used in combination with other drugs. When Anafranil and a neuroleptic were used concomitantly, the cases were sometimes considered to be examples of a neuroleptic malignant syndrome.

Sexual Dysfunction: The rate of sexual dysfunction in male patients with OCD who were treated with Anafranil in the premarketing experience was markedly increased compared with placebo controls (i.e., 42% experienced ejaculatory failure and 20% experienced impotence, compared with 2.0% and 2.6%, respectively, in the placebo group). Approximately 85% of males with sexual dysfunction chose to continue treatment.

Weight Changes: In controlled studies of OCD, weight gain was reported in 18% of patients receiving Anafranil, compared with 1% of patients receiving placebo. In these studies, 28% of patients receiving Anafranil had a weight gain of at least 7% of their initial body weight, compared with 4% of patients receiving placebo. Several patients had weight gains in excess of 25% of their initial body weight. Conversely, 5% of patients receiving Anafranil and 1% receiving placebo had weight losses of at least 7% of their initial body weight.

Electroconvulsive Therapy: As with closely related tricyclic antidepressants, concurrent administration of Anafranil with electroconvulsive therapy may increase the risks; such treatment should be limited to those patients for whom it is essential, since there is limited clinical experience.

Surgery: Prior to elective surgery with general anesthetics, therapy with Anafranil should be discontinued for as long as is clinically feasible, and the anesthetist should be advised.

Use in Concomitant Illness: As with closely related tricyclic antidepressants, Anafranil should be used with caution in the following:

(1) Hyperthyroid patients or patients receiving thyroid medication, because of the possibility of cardiac toxicity;
(2) Patients with increased intraocular pressure, a history of narrow-angle glaucoma, or urinary retention, because of the anticholinergic properties of the drug;
(3) Patients with tumors of the adrenal medulla (e.g., pheochromocytoma, neuroblastoma) in whom the drug may provoke hypertensive crises;
(4) Patients with significantly impaired renal function.

Withdrawal Symptoms: A variety of withdrawal symptoms have been reported in association with abrupt discontinuation of Anafranil, including dizziness, nausea, vomiting, headache, malaise, sleep disturbance, hyperthermia, and irritability. In addition, such patients may experience a worsening of psychiatric status. While the withdrawal effects of Anafranil have not been systematically evaluated in controlled trials, they are well known with closely related tricyclic antidepressants, and it is recommended that the dosage be tapered gradually and the patient monitored carefully during discontinuation (see DRUG ABUSE AND DEPENDENCE).

Information for Patients

Physicians are advised to discuss the following issues with patients for whom they prescribe Anafranil:

(1) The risk of seizure (see WARNINGS);
(2) The relatively high incidence of sexual dysfunction among males (see Sexual Dysfunction);
(3) Since Anafranil may impair the mental and/or physical abilities required for the performance of complex tasks, and since Anafranil is associated with a risk of seizures, patients should be cautioned about the performance of complex and hazardous tasks (see WARNINGS);
(4) Patients should be cautioned about using alcohol, barbiturates, or other CNS depressants concurrently, since Anafranil may exaggerate their response to these drugs;
(5) Patients should notify their physician if they become pregnant or intend to become pregnant during therapy;
(6) Patients should notify their physician if they are breastfeeding.

Drug Interactions

The risks of using Anafranil in combination with other drugs have not been systematically evaluated. Given the primary CNS effects of Anafranil, caution is advised in using it concomitantly with other CNS-active drugs (see Information for Patients). Anafranil should *not* be used with MAO inhibitors (see CONTRAINDICATIONS).

Close supervision and careful adjustment of dosage are required when Anafranil is administered with anticholinergic or sympathomimetic drugs.

Several tricyclic antidepressants have been reported to block the pharmacologic effects of guanethidine, clonidine, or similar agents, and such an effect may be anticipated with CMI because of its structural similarity to other tricyclic antidepressants.

The plasma concentration of CMI has been reported to be increased by the concomitant administration of haloperidol;

plasma levels of several closely related tricyclic antidepressants have been reported to be increased by the concomitant administration of methylphenidate or hepatic enzyme inhibitors (e.g., cimetidine, fluoxetine) and decreased by the concomitant administration of hepatic enzyme inducers (e.g., barbiturates, phenytoin), and such an effect may be anticipated with CMI as well. Administration of CMI has been reported to increase the plasma levels of phenobarbital, if given concomitantly (see CLINICAL PHARMACOLOGY, Interactions).

Drugs Metabolized by P450 2D6: The biochemical activity of the drug metabolizing isozyme cytochrome P450 2D6 (debrisoquin hydroxylase) is reduced in a subset of the Caucasian population (about 7%–10% of Caucasians are so-called "poor metabolizers"); reliable estimates of the prevalence of reduced P450 2D6 isozyme activity among Asian, African and other populations are not yet available. Poor metabolizers have higher than expected plasma concentrations of tricyclic antidepressants (TCAs) when given usual doses. Depending on the fraction of drug metabolized by P450 2D6, the increase in plasma concentration may be small, or quite large (8 fold increase in plasma AUC of the TCA). In addition, certain drugs inhibit the activity of this isozyme and make normal metabolizers resemble poor metabolizers. An individual who is stable on a given dose of TCA may become abruptly toxic when given one of these inhibiting drugs as concomitant therapy. The drugs that inhibit cytochrome P450 2D6 include some that are not metabolized by the enzyme (quinidine; cimetidine) and many that are substrates for P450 2D6 (many other antidepressants, phenothiazines, and the Type 1C antiarrhythmics propafenone and flecainide). While all the selective serotonin reuptake inhibitors (SSRIs), e.g., fluoxetine, sertraline, and paroxetine, inhibit P450 2D6, they may vary in the extent of inhibition. The extent to which SSRI-TCA interactions may pose clinical problems will depend on the degree of inhibition and the pharmacokinetics of the SSRI involved. Nevertheless, caution is indicated in the co-administration of TCAs with any of the SSRIs and also in switching from one class to the other. Of particular importance, sufficient time must elapse before initiating TCA treatment in a patient being withdrawn from fluoxetine, given the long half-life of the parent and active metabolite (at least 5 weeks may be necessary). Concomitant use of tricyclic antidepressants with drugs that can inhibit cytochrome P450 2D6 may require lower doses than usually prescribed for either the tricyclic antidepressant or the other drug. Furthermore, whenever one of these drugs is withdrawn from co-therapy, an increased dose of tricyclic antidepressant may be required. It is desirable to monitor TCA plasma levels whenever a TCA is going to be co-administered with another drug known to be an inhibitor of P450 2D6. Because Anafranil is highly bound to serum protein, the administration of Anafranil to patients taking other drugs that are highly bound to protein (e.g., warfarin, digoxin) may cause an increase in plasma concentrations of these drugs, potentially resulting in adverse effects. Conversely, adverse effects may result from displacement of protein-bound Anafranil by other highly bound drugs (see CLINICAL PHARMACOLOGY, Distribution).

Carcinogenesis, Mutagenesis, Impairment of Fertility
In a 2-year bioassay, no clear evidence of carcinogenicity was found in rats given doses 20 times the maximum daily human dose. Three out of 235 treated rats had a rare tumor (hemangioendothelioma); it is unknown if these neoplasms are compound related.
In reproduction studies, no effects on fertility were found in rats given doses approximately 5 times the maximum daily human dose.

Pregnancy Category C
No teratogenic effects were observed in studies performed in rats and mice at doses up to 20 times the maximum daily human dose. Slight nonspecific fetotoxic effects were seen in the offspring of pregnant mice given doses 10 times the maximum daily human dose. Slight nonspecific embryotoxicity was observed in rats given doses 5–10 times the maximum daily human dose.
There are no adequate or well-controlled studies in pregnant women. Withdrawal symptoms, including jitteriness, tremor, and seizures, have been reported in neonates whose mothers had taken Anafranil until delivery. Anafranil should be used during pregnancy only if the potential benefit justifies the potential risk to the fetus.

Nursing Mothers
Anafranil has been found in human milk. Because of the potential for adverse reactions, a decision should be made whether to discontinue nursing or to discontinue the drug, taking into account the importance of the drug to the mother.

Pediatric Use
In a controlled clinical trial in children and adolescents (10–17 years of age), 46 outpatients received Anafranil for up to 8 weeks. In addition, 150 adolescent patients have received Anafranil in open-label protocols for periods of several months to several years. Of the 196 adolescents studied, 50 were 13 years of age or less and 146 were 14–17 years of age. While the adverse reaction profile in this age group (see AD-

Incidence of Treatment-Emergent Adverse Experience in Placebo-Controlled Clinical Trials (Percentage of Patients Reporting Event)

Body System/ Adverse Event*	Adults Anafranil (N=322)	Adults Placebo (N=319)	Children and Adolescents Anafranil (N=46)	Children and Adolescents Placebo (N=44)
Nervous System				
Somnolence	54	16	46	11
Tremor	54	2	33	2
Dizziness	54	14	41	14
Headache	52	41	28	34
Insomnia	25	15	11	7
Libido change	21	3	—	—
Nervousness	18	2	4	2
Myoclonus	13	—	2	—
Increased appetite	11	2	—	2
Paresthesia	9	3	2	2
Memory impairment	9	1	7	2
Anxiety	9	4	—	—
Twitching	7	1	4	5
Impaired concentration	5	2	—	—
Depression	5	1	—	—
Hypertonia	4	1	2	—
Sleep disorder	4	—	9	5
Psychosomatic disorder	3	—	—	—
Yawning	3	—	—	—
Confusion	3	—	2	—
Speech disorder	3	—	—	—
Abnormal dreaming	3	—	—	2
Agitation	3	—	—	—
Migraine	3	—	—	—
Depersonalization	2	—	—	—
Irritability	2	2	2	—
Emotional lability	2	—	—	2
Panic reaction	1	—	2	—
Aggressive reaction	—	—	2	—
Paresis	—	—	2	—
Skin and Appendages				
Increased sweating	29	3	9	—
Rash	8	1	4	2
Pruritis	6	—	2	2
Dermatitis	2	—	—	2
Acne	2	2	—	5
Dry skin	2	—	—	5
Urticaria	1	—	—	—
Abnormal skin odor	—	—	2	—
Digestive System				
Dry mouth	84	17	63	16
Constipation	47	11	22	9
Nausea	33	14	9	11
Dyspepsia	22	10	13	2
Diarrhea	13	9	7	5
Anorexia	12	—	22	—
Abdominal pain	11	9	13	16
Vomiting	7	2	7	—
Flatulence	6	3	—	2
Tooth disorder	5	—	—	—
Gastrointestinal disorder	2	—	—	2
Dysphagia	2	—	—	—
Esophagitis	1	—	—	—
Eructation	—	—	2	2
Ulcerative stomatitis	—	—	2	—
Body as a Whole				
Fatigue	39	18	35	9
Weight increase	18	1	2	—
Flushing	8	—	7	—
Hot flushes	5	—	2	—
Chest pain	4	4	7	—
Fever	4	—	2	7
Allergy	3	3	7	5
Pain	3	2	4	2
Local edema	2	4	—	—
Chills	2	1	—	—
Weight decrease	—	—	7	—
Otitis media	—	—	4	5
Asthenia	—	—	2	—
Halitosis	—	—	2	—
Cardiovascular System				
Postural hypotension	6	—	4	—
Palpitation	4	2	2	—
Tachycardia	4	—	2	—
Syncope	—	—	2	—
Respiratory System				
Pharyngitis	14	9	—	5
Rhinitis	12	10	7	9
Sinusitis	6	4	2	5
Coughing	6	6	4	5
Bronchospasm	2	—	7	2
Epistaxis	2	—	—	2
Dyspnea	—	—	2	—
Laryngitis	—	1	2	—

Continued on next page

CibaGeneva—Cont.

Incidence of Treatment-Emergent Adverse Experience in Placebo-Controlled Clinical Trials (Percentage of Patients Reporting Event)

Body System/ Adverse Event*	Adults		Children and Adolescents	
	Anafranil (N=322)	Placebo (N=319)	Anafranil (N=46)	Placebo (N=44)
Urogenital System				
Male and Female Patients Combined				
Micturition disorder	14	2	4	2
Urinary tract infection	6	1	—	—
Micturition frequency	5	3	—	—
Urinary retention	2	—	7	—
Dysuria	2	2	—	—
Cystitis	2	—	—	—
Female Patients Only	(N=182)	(N=167)	(N=10)	(N=21)
Dysmenorrhea	12	14	10	10
Lactation (nonpuerperal)	4	—	—	—
Menstrual disorder	4	2	—	—
Vaginitis	2	—	—	—
Leukorrhea	2	—	—	—
Breast enlargement	2	—	—	—
Breast pain	1	—	—	—
Amenorrhea	1	—	—	—
Male Patients Only	(N=140)	(N=152)	(N=36)	(N=23)
Ejaculation failure	42	2	6	—
Impotence	20	3	—	—
Special Senses				
Abnormal vision	18	4	7	2
Taste perversion	8	—	4	—
Tinnitus	6	—	4	—
Abnormal lacrimation	3	2	—	—
Mydriasis	2	—	—	—
Conjunctivitis	1	—	—	—
Anisocoria	—	—	2	—
Blepharospasm	—	—	2	—
Ocular allergy	—	—	2	—
Vestibular disorder	—	—	2	2
Musculoskeletal				
Myalgia	13	9	—	—
Back pain	6	6	—	—
Arthralgia	3	5	—	—
Muscle weakness	1	—	2	—
Hemic and Lymphatic				
Purpura	3	—	—	—
Anemia	—	—	2	2
Metabolic and Nutritional				
Thirst	2	2	—	2

*Events reported by at least 1% of Anafranil patients are included.

VERSE REACTIONS) is similar to that in adults, it is unknown what, if any, effects long-term treatment with Anafranil may have on the growth and development of children.

The safety and effectiveness in pediatric patients below the age of 10 have not been established. Therefore, specific recommendations cannot be made for the use of Anafranil in children under the age of 10.

Use in Elderly

Anafranil has not been systematically studied in older patients; but 152 patients at least 60 years of age participating in U.S. clinical trials received Anafranil for periods of several months to several years. No unusual age-related adverse events have been identified in this elderly population, but these data are insufficient to rule out possible age-related differences, particularly in elderly patients who have concomitant systemic illnesses or who are receiving other drugs concomitantly.

ADVERSE REACTIONS

Commonly Observed

The most commonly observed adverse events associated with the use of Anafranil and not seen at an equivalent incidence among placebo-treated patients were gastrointestinal complaints, including dry mouth, constipation, nausea, dyspepsia, and anorexia; nervous system complaints, including somnolence, tremor, dizziness, nervousness, and myoclonus; genitourinary complaints, including changed libido, ejaculatory failure, impotence, and micturition disorder; and other miscellaneous complaints, including fatigue, sweating, increased appetite, weight gain, and visual changes.

Leading to Discontinuation of Treatment

Approximately 20% of 3616 patients who received Anafranil in U.S. premarketing clinical trials discontinued treatment because of an adverse event. Approximately one-half of the patients who discontinued (9% of the total) had multiple complaints, none of which could be classified as primary. Where a primary reason for discontinuation could be identified, most patients discontinued because of nervous system complaints (5.4%), primarily somnolence. The second-most-frequent reason for discontinuation was digestive system complaints (1.3%), primarily vomiting and nausea.

Incidence in Controlled Clinical Trials

The following table enumerates adverse events that occurred at an incidence of 1% or greater among patients with OCD who received Anafranil in adult or pediatric placebo-controlled clinical trials. The frequencies were obtained from pooled data of clinical trials involving either adults receiving Anafranil (N=322) or placebo (N=319) or children treated with Anafranil (N=46) or placebo (N=44). The prescriber should be aware that these figures cannot be used to predict the incidence of side effects in the course of usual medical practice, in which patient characteristics and other factors differ from those that prevailed in the clinical trials. Similarly, the cited frequencies cannot be compared with figures obtained from other clinical investigations involving different treatments, uses, and investigators. The cited figures, however, provide the physician with a basis for estimating the relative contribution of drug and nondrug factors to the incidence of side effects in the populations studied.

[See table on preceding page.]

[See table above.]

Other Events Observed During the Premarketing Evaluation of Anafranil

During clinical testing in the U.S., multiple doses of Anafranil were administered to approximately 3600 subjects. Untoward events associated with this exposure were recorded by clinical investigators using terminology of their own choosing. Consequently, it is not possible to provide a meaningful estimate of the proportion of individuals experiencing adverse events without first grouping similar types of untoward events into a smaller number of standardized event categories.

In the tabulations that follow, a modified World Health Organization dictionary of terminology has been used to classify reported adverse events. The frequencies presented, therefore, represent the proportion of the 3525 individuals exposed to Anafranil who experienced an event of the type cited on at least one occasion while receiving Anafranil. All events are included except those already listed in the previous table, those reported in terms so general as to be uninformative, and those in which an association with the drug was remote. It is important to emphasize that although the events reported occurred during treatment with Anafranil, they were not necessarily caused by it.

Events are further categorized by body system and listed in order of decreasing frequency according to the following definitions: frequent adverse events are those occurring on one or more occasions in at least 1/100 patients; infrequent adverse events are those occurring in 1/100 to 1/1000 patients; rare events are those occurring in less than 1/1000 patients.

Body as a Whole: *Infrequent*—general edema, increased susceptibility to infection, malaise. *Rare*—dependent edema, withdrawal syndrome.

Cardiovascular System: *Infrequent*—abnormal ECG, arrhythmia, bradycardia, cardiac arrest, extrasystoles, pallor. *Rare*—aneurysm, atrial flutter, bundle branch block, cardiac failure, cerebral hemorrhage, heart block, myocardial infarction, myocardial ischemia, peripheral ischemia, thrombophlebitis, vasospasm, ventricular tachycardia.

Digestive System: *Infrequent*—abnormal hepatic function, blood in stool, colitis, duodenitis, gastric ulcer, gastritis, gastroesophageal reflux, gingivitis, glossitis, hemorrhoids, hepatitis, increased saliva, irritable bowel syndrome, peptic ulcer, rectal hemorrhage, tongue ulceration, tooth caries. *Rare*—cheilitis, chronic enteritis, discolored feces, gastric dilatation, gingival bleeding, hiccup, intestinal obstruction, oral/pharyngeal edema, paralytic ileus, salivary gland enlargement.

Endocrine System: *Infrequent*—hypothyroidism. *Rare*—goiter, gynecomastia, hyperthyroidism.

Hemic and Lymphatic System: *Infrequent*—lymphadenopathy. *Rare*—leukemoid reaction, lymphoma-like disorder, marrow depression.

Metabolic and Nutritional Disorder: *Infrequent*—dehydration, diabetes mellitus, gout, hypercholesterolemia, hyperglycemia, hyperuricemia, hypokalemia. *Rare*—fat intolerance, glycosuria.

Musculoskeletal System: *Infrequent*—arthrosis. *Rare*—dystonia, exostosis, lupus erythematosus rash, bruising, myopathy, myositis, polyarteritis nodosa, torticollis.

Nervous System: *Frequent*—abnormal thinking, vertigo. *Infrequent*—abnormal coordination, abnormal EEG, abnormal gait, apathy, ataxia, coma, convulsions, delirium, delusion, dyskinesia, dysphonia, encephalopathy, euphoria, extrapyramidal disorder, hallucinations, hostility, hyperkinesia, hypnagogic hallucinations, hypokinesia, leg cramps, manic reaction, neuralgia, paranoia, phobic disorder, psychosis, sensory disturbance, somnambulism, stimulation, suicidal ideation, suicide attempt, teeth-grinding. *Rare*—anticholinergic syndrome, aphasia, apraxia, catalepsy, cholinergic syndrome, choreoathetosis, generalized spasm, hemiparesis, hyperesthesia, hyperreflexia, hypoesthesia, illusion, impaired impulse control, indecisiveness, mutism, neuropathy, nystagmus, oculogyric crisis, oculomotor nerve paralysis, schizophrenic reaction, stupor, suicide.

Respiratory System: *Infrequent*—bronchitis, hyperventilation, increased sputum, pneumonia. *Rare*—cyanosis, hemoptysis, hypoventilation, laryngismus.

Skin and Appendages: *Infrequent*—alopecia, cellulitis, cyst, eczema, erythematous rash, genital pruritus, maculopapular rash, photosensitivity reaction, psoriasis, pustular rash, skin discoloration. *Rare*—chloasma, folliculitis, hypertrichosis, piloerection, seborrhea, skin hypertrophy, skin ulceration.

Special Senses: *Infrequent*—abnormal accommodation, deafness, diplopia, earache, eye pain, foreign body sensation, hyperacusis, parosmia, photophobia, scleritis, taste loss. *Rare*—blepharitis, chromatopsia, conjunctival hemorrhage, exophthalmos, glaucoma, keratitis, labyrinth disorder, night blindness, retinal disorder, strabismus, visual field defect.

Urogenital System: *Infrequent*—endometriosis, epididymitis, hematuria, nocturia, oliguria, ovarian cyst, perineal pain, polyuria, prostatic disorder, renal calculus, renal pain, urethral disorder, urinary incontinence, uterine hemorrhage, vaginal hemorrhage. *Rare*—albuminuria, anorgasmy, breast engorgement, breast fibroadenosis, cervical dysplasia, endometrial hyperplasia, premature ejaculation, pyelonephritis, pyuria, renal cyst, uterine inflammation, vulvar disorder.

DRUG ABUSE AND DEPENDENCE

Anafranil has not been systematically studied in animals or humans for its potential for abuse, tolerance, or physical dependence. While a variety of withdrawal symptoms have been described in association with Anafranil discontinuation (see PRECAUTIONS, Withdrawal Symptoms), there is no evidence for drug-seeking behavior, except for a single report of potential Anafranil abuse by a patient with a history of dependence on codeine, benzodiazepines, and multiple psychoactive drugs. The patient received Anafranil for depression and panic attacks and appeared to become dependent after hospital discharge.

Despite the lack of evidence suggesting an abuse liability for Anafranil in foreign marketing, it is not possible to predict the extent to which Anafranil might be misused or abused once marketed in the U.S. Consequently, physicians should carefully evaluate patients for a history of drug abuse and follow such patients closely.

OVERDOSAGE

Deaths may occur from overdosage with this class of drugs. Multiple drug ingestion (including alcohol) is common in deliberate tricyclic overdose. As the management is complex and changing, it is recommended that the physician contact a poison control center for current information on treatment. Signs and symptoms of toxicity develop rapidly after tricyclic overdose. Therefore, hospital monitoring is required as soon as possible.

Human Experience

In U.S. clinical trials, 2 deaths occurred in 12 reported cases of acute overdosage with Anafranil either alone or in combination with other drugs. One death involved a patient suspected of ingesting a dose of 7000 mg. The second death involved a patient suspected of ingesting a dose of 5750 mg. The 10 nonfatal cases involved doses of up to 5000 mg, accompanied by plasma levels of up to 1010 ng/ml. All 10 patients completely recovered. Among reports from other countries of Anafranil overdose, the lowest dose associated with a fatality was 750 mg. Based upon postmarketing reports in the United Kingdom, CMI's lethality in overdose is considered to be similar to that reported for closely related tricyclic compounds marketed as antidepressants.

Manifestations

Signs and symptoms vary in severity depending upon factors such as the amount of drug absorbed, the age of the patient, and the time elapsed since drug ingestion. Critical manifestations of overdose include cardiac dysrhythmias, severe hypotension, convulsions, and CNS depression including coma. Changes in the electrocardiogram, particularly in QRS axis or width, are clinically significant indicators of tricyclic toxicity. Other CNS manifestations may include drowsiness, stupor, ataxia, restlessness, agitation, delirium, severe perspiration, hyperactive reflexes, muscle rigidity, and athetoid and choreiform movements. Cardiac abnormalities may include tachycardia, signs of congestive heart failure, and in very rare cases, cardiac arrest. Respiratory depression, cyanosis, shock, vomiting, hyperpyrexia, mydriasis, and oliguria or anuria may also be present.

Management

Obtain an ECG and immediately initiate cardiac monitoring. Protect the patient's airway, establish an intravenous line, and initiate gastric decontamination. A minimum of 6 hours of observation with cardiac monitoring and observation for signs of CNS or respiratory depression, hypotension, cardiac dysrhythmias and/or conduction blocks, and seizures is necessary. If signs of toxicity occur at any time during this period, extended monitoring is required. There are case reports of patients succumbing to fatal dysrhythmias late after overdose; these patients had clinical evidence of significant poisoning prior to death and most received inadequate gastrointestinal decontamination. Monitoring of plasma drug levels should not guide management of the patient.

Gastrointestinal Decontamination: All patients suspected of tricyclic overdose should receive gastrointestinal decontamination. This should include large volume gastric lavage followed by activated charcoal. If consciousness is impaired, the airway should be secured prior to lavage. Emesis is contraindicated.

Cardiovascular: A maximal limb-lead QRS duration of ≥ 0.10 seconds may be the best indication of the severity of the overdose. Serum alkalinization, to a pH of 7.45 to 7.55, using intravenous sodium bicarbonate and hyperventilation (as needed) should be instituted for patients with dysrhythmias and/or QRS widening. A pH >7.60 or a Pco_2 <20 mmHg is undesirable. Dysrhythmias unresponsive to sodium bicarbonate therapy/hyperventilation may respond to lidocaine, bretylium, or phenytoin. Type 1A and 1C antiarrhythmics are generally contraindicated (e.g., quinidine, disopyramide, and procainamide).

In rare instances, hemoperfusion may be beneficial in acute refractory cardiovascular instability in patients with acute toxicity. However, hemodialysis, peritoneal dialysis, exchange transfusions, and forced diuresis generally have been reported as ineffective in tricyclic poisoning.

CNS: In patients with CNS depression, early intubation is advised because of the potential for abrupt deterioration. Seizures should be controlled with benzodiazepines, or if these are ineffective, other anticonvulsants (e.g., phenobarbital, phenytoin). Physostigmine is not recommended except to treat life-threatening symptoms that have been unresponsive to other therapies, and then only in consultation with a poison control center.

Psychiatric Follow-up: Since overdosage is often deliberate, patients may attempt suicide by other means during the recovery phase.

Psychiatric referral may be appropriate.

Pediatric Management: The principles of management of child and adult overdosages are similar. It is strongly recommended that the physician contact the local poison control center for specific pediatric treatment.

DOSAGE AND ADMINISTRATION

The treatment regimens described below are based on those used in controlled clinical trials of Anafranil in 520 adults, and 91 children and adolescents with OCD. During initial titration, Anafranil should be given in divided doses with meals to reduce gastrointestinal side effects. The goal of this initial titration phase is to minimize side effects by permitting tolerance to side effects to develop or allowing the patient time to adapt if tolerance does not develop.

Because both CMI and its active metabolite, DMI, have long elimination half-lives, the prescriber should take into consideration the fact that steady-state plasma levels may not be achieved until 2–3 weeks after dosage change (see CLINICAL PHARMACOLOGY). Therefore, after initial titration, it may be appropriate to wait 2–3 weeks between further dosage adjustments.

Initial Treatment/Dose Adjustment (Adults)

Treatment with Anafranil should be initiated at a dosage of 25 mg daily and gradually increased, as tolerated, to approximately 100 mg during the first 2 weeks. During initial titration, Anafranil should be given in divided doses with meals to reduce gastrointestinal side effects. Thereafter, the dosage may be increased gradually over the next several weeks, up to a maximum of 250 mg daily. After titration, the total daily dose may be given once daily at bedtime to minimize daytime sedation.

Initial Treatment/Dose Adjustment (Children and Adolescents)

As with adults, the starting dose is 25 mg daily and should be gradually increased (also given in divided doses with meals to reduce gastrointestinal side effects) during the first 2 weeks, as tolerated, up to a daily maximum of 3 mg/kg or 100 mg, whichever is smaller. Thereafter, the dosage may be increased gradually over the next several weeks up to a daily maximum of 3 mg/kg or 200 mg, whichever is smaller (see PRECAUTIONS, Pediatric Use). As with adults, after titration, the total daily dose may be given once daily at bedtime to minimize daytime sedation.

Maintenance/Continuation Treatment (Adults, Children, and Adolescents)

While there are no systematic studies that answer the question of how long to continue Anafranil, OCD is a chronic condition and it is reasonable to consider continuation for a responding patient. Although the efficacy of Anafranil after 10 weeks has not been documented in controlled trials, patients have been continued in therapy under double-blind conditions for up to 1 year without loss of benefit. However, dosage adjustments should be made to maintain the patient on the lowest effective dosage, and patients should be periodically reassessed to determine the need for treatment. During maintenance, the total daily dose may be given once daily at bedtime.

HOW SUPPLIED

Capsules 25 mg—ivory/melon yellow (imprinted ANAFRANIL 25 mg)
Bottles of 100 .... NDC 58887-115-30
Unit Dose (blister pack)
Box of 100 (strips of 10) .... NDC 58887-115-32

Capsules 50 mg—ivory/aqua blue (imprinted ANAFRANIL 50 mg)
Bottles of 100 .... NDC 58887-116-30
Unit Dose (blister pack)
Box of 100 (strips of 10) .... NDC 58887-116-32

Capsules 75 mg—ivory/yellow (imprinted ANAFRANIL 75 mg)
Bottles of 100 .... NDC 58887-117-30
Unit Dose (blister pack)
Box of 100 (strips of 10) .... NDC 58887-117-32

Samples, when available, are identified by the word *SAMPLE* appearing on each capsule.

Do not store above 86°F (30°C). Protect from moisture.

Dispense in tight container (USP).

ANIMAL TOXICOLOGY

Testicular and lung changes commonly associated with tricyclic compounds have been observed with Anafranil. In 1- and 2-year studies in rats, changes in the testes (atrophy, aspermatogenesis, and calcification) and drug-induced phospholipidosis in the lungs were observed at doses 4 times the maximum daily human dose. Testicular atrophy was also observed in a 1-year oral toxicity study in dogs at 10 times the maximum daily human dose.

C96-11 (Rev. 2/96)

Ciba-Geigy Corporation
Pharmaceuticals Division
Summit, New Jersey 07901

Shown in Product Identification Guide, page 308

ANTURANE®

℞

[ann 'too-rain]
sulfinpyrazone USP
Tablets, Capsules

DESCRIPTION

Anturane, sulfinpyrazone USP, is a uricosuric agent available as 100-mg tablets and 200-mg capsules for oral administration. Its chemical name is 1,2-diphenyl-4-[2-(phenylsulfinyl)ethyl]-3,5-pyrazolidinedione.

Sulfinpyrazone USP is a white to off-white powder practically insoluble in water and in solvent hexane, soluble in alcohol and in acetone, and sparingly soluble in dilute alkali. Its molecular weight is 404.48.

Inactive Ingredients. Anturane tablets: Colloidal silicon dioxide, gelatin, lactose, magnesium stearate, cornstarch, stearic acid, and talc.

Anturane capsules: D&C Red No. 33, D&C Yellow No. 10, FD&C Blue No. 1, gelatin, lactose, magnesium stearate, methylparaben, propylparaben, silicon dioxide, sodium lauryl sulfate, cornstarch, stearic acid, talc, and titanium dioxide.

CLINICAL PHARMACOLOGY

Its pharmacologic activity is the potentiation of the urinary excretion of uric acid. It is useful for reducing the blood urate levels in patients with chronic tophaceous gout and acute intermittent gout, and for promoting the resorption of tophi.

INDICATIONS

Anturane is indicated for the treatment of:

1. Chronic gouty arthritis
2. Intermittent gouty arthritis

CONTRAINDICATIONS

Patients with an active peptic ulcer or symptoms of gastrointestinal inflammation or ulceration should not receive the drug.

The drug is contraindicated in patients with a history or the presence of:

1. Hypersensitivity to phenylbutazone or other pyrazoles
2. Blood dyscrasias

WARNINGS

Studies on the teratogenicity of pyrazole compounds in animals have yielded inconclusive results. Up to the present time, however, there have been no reported cases of human congenital malformation proved to be due to the use of the drug.

It is suggested that Anturane be used with caution in pregnant women, weighing the potential risks against the possible benefits.

PRECAUTIONS

As with all pyrazole compounds, patients receiving Anturane should be kept under close medical supervision and periodic blood counts are recommended. It may be administered with care to patients with a history of healed peptic ulcer.

Recent reports have indicated that Anturane potentiates the action of certain sulfonamides, such as sulfadiazine and sulfisoxazole. In addition, other pyrazole compounds (phenylbutazone) have been observed to potentiate the hypoglycemic sulfonylurea agents, as well as insulin. In view of these observations, it is suggested that Anturane be used with caution in conjunction with sulfa drugs, the sulfonylurea hypoglycemic agents and insulin.

Because Anturane is a potent uricosuric agent, it may precipitate urolithiasis and renal colic, especially in the initial stages of therapy. For this reason, an adequate fluid intake and alkalinization of the urine are recommended. In cases with significant renal impairment, periodic assessment of renal function is indicated. Occasional cases of renal failure have been reported; but a cause-and-effect relationship has not always been clearly established.

Salicylates antagonize the uricosuric action of Anturane and for this reason their concomitant use is contraindicated in gouty arthritis.

Anturane may accentuate the action of coumarin-type anticoagulants and further depress prothrombin activity when these medications are employed simultaneously.

Continued on next page

CibaGeneva—Cont.

Pediatric Use
Safety and effectiveness in pediatric patients have not been established.

NOTE
Anturane has minimal anti-inflammatory effect and is not intended for the relief of an acute attack of gout.
In the initial stages of therapy, because of the marked ability of Anturane to mobilize urates, acute attacks of gouty arthritis may be precipitated.

ADVERSE REACTIONS
The most frequently reported adverse reactions with Anturane have been upper gastrointestinal disturbances. In these patients it is advisable to administer the drug with food, milk, or antacids. Despite this precaution, Anturane may aggravate or reactivate peptic ulcer.
Rash has been reported. In most instances, this reaction did not necessitate discontinuance of therapy. In general, Anturane has not been observed to affect electrolyte balance.
Blood dyscrasias (anemia, leukopenia, agranulocytosis, thrombocytopenia and aplastic anemia) have rarely been reported. There has also been a published report associating Anturane, administered concomitantly with other drugs including colchicine, with leukemia following long-term treatment of patients with gout. However, the circumstances involved in the two cases reported are such that a cause-and-effect relationship to Anturane has not been clearly established.

OVERDOSAGE
Symptoms: Nausea, vomiting, diarrhea, epigastric pain, ataxia, labored respiration, convulsions, coma. Possible symptoms, seen after overdosage with other pyrazolone derivatives: anemia, jaundice, ulceration.
Treatment: No specific antidote. Induce emesis; gastric lavage; supportive treatment (intravenous glucose infusions, analeptics).

DOSAGE AND ADMINISTRATION
Initial: 200–400 mg daily in two divided doses, with meals or milk, gradually increasing when necessary to full maintenance dosage in one week.
Maintenance: 400 mg daily, given in two divided doses, as above. This dosage may be increased to 800 mg daily, if necessary, and may sometimes be reduced to as low as 200 mg daily after the blood urate level has been controlled. Treatment should be continued without interruption even in the presence of acute exacerbations, which can be concomitantly treated with phenylbutazone or colchicine. Patients previously controlled with other uricosuric therapy may be transferred to Anturane at full maintenance dosage.

HOW SUPPLIED
Tablets 100 mg—round, white, scored (imprinted CIBA 41)
  Bottles of 100 ....NDC 0083-0041-30
Capsules 200 mg—green (imprinted Anturane 200 CIBA 168)
  Bottles of 100 ....NDC 0083-0168-30
Do not store above 86°F (30°C).
Dispense in tight container (USP).

C96-18 (Rev. 4/96)
Shown in Product Identification Guide, page 309

APRESAZIDE® ℞
[a-press 'a-zyde]
hydralazine hydrochloride and
hydrochlorothiazide
Capsules

WARNING
This fixed-combination drug is not indicated for initial therapy of hypertension. Hypertension requires therapy titrated to the individual patient. If the fixed combination represents the dosage so determined, its use may be more convenient in patient management. The treatment of hypertension is not static but must be reevaluated as conditions in each patient warrant.

DESCRIPTION
Apresazide, hydralazine hydrochloride and hydrochlorothiazide, is an antihypertensive-diuretic combination available as capsules for oral administration. Apresazide capsules of 25/25 contain 25 mg of hydralazine hydrochloride USP and 25 mg of hydrochlorothiazide USP; capsules of 50/50 contain 50 mg of hydralazine hydrochloride USP and 50 mg of hydrochlorothiazide USP; and capsules of 100/50 contain 100 mg of hydralazine hydrochloride USP and 50 mg of hydrochlorothiazide USP.

Hydralazine hydrochloride is 1-hydrazinophthalazine monohydrochloride.
Hydralazine hydrochloride USP is a white to off-white, odorless crystalline powder. It is soluble in water, slightly soluble in alcohol, and very slightly soluble in ether. It melts at about 275°C, with decomposition, and has a molecular weight of 196.64.
Hydrochlorothiazide is 6-chloro-3,4-dihydro-2*H*-1,2,4-benzothiadiazine-7-sulfonamide 1,1-dioxide.
Hydrochlorothiazide USP is a white, or practically white, practically odorless crystalline powder. It is freely soluble in sodium hydroxide solution, in *n*-butylamine, and in dimethylformamide; sparingly soluble in methanol; slightly soluble in water; and insoluble in ether, in chloroform, and in dilute mineral acids. Its molecular weight is 297.73.
Inactive Ingredients: D&C Red No. 28 (25/25 and 50/50 capsules only); D&C Red No. 33 and D&C Yellow No. 10 (100/50 capsules only); FD&C Blue No. 1 (25/25 and 50/50 capsules only); FD&C Red No. 40 (50/50 capsules only); gelatin; magnesium stearate; methylparaben; propylparaben; silicon dioxide; sodium lauryl sulfate; starch; and titanium dioxide.

CLINICAL PHARMACOLOGY
Hydralazine
Although the precise mechanism of action of hydralazine is not fully understood, the major effects are on the cardiovascular system. Hydralazine apparently lowers blood pressure by exerting a peripheral vasodilating effect through a direct relaxation of vascular smooth muscle. Hydralazine, by altering cellular calcium metabolism, interferes with the calcium movements within the vascular smooth muscle that are responsible for initiating or maintaining the contractile state. The peripheral vasodilating effect of hydralazine results in decreased arterial blood pressure (diastolic more than systolic); decreased peripheral vascular resistance; and an increased heart rate, stroke volume, and cardiac output. The preferential dilatation of arterioles, as compared to veins, minimizes postural hypotension and promotes the increase in cardiac output. Hydralazine usually increases renin activity in plasma, presumably as a result of increased secretion of renin by the renal juxtaglomerular cells in response to reflex sympathetic discharge. This increase in renin activity leads to the production of angiotensin II, which then causes stimulation of aldosterone and consequent sodium reabsorption. Hydralazine also maintains or increases renal and cerebral blood flow.
Hydrochlorothiazide
Thiazides affect the renal tubular mechanism of electrolyte reabsorption. At maximal therapeutic dosage, all thiazides are approximately equal in their diuretic potency. Thiazides increase excretion of sodium and chloride in approximately equivalent amounts. Natriuresis causes a secondary loss of potassium.
The mechanism of the antihypertensive effect of thiazides is unknown. Thiazides do not affect normal blood pressure.
Pharmacokinetics
Hydralazine. Hydralazine is rapidly absorbed after oral administration, and peak plasma levels are reached at 1–2 hours. Plasma levels decline with a half-life of 3–7 hours. Binding to human plasma protein is 87%. Plasma levels of hydralazine vary widely among individuals. Hydralazine is subject to polymorphic acetylation; slow acetylators generally have higher plasma levels of hydralazine and require lower doses to maintain control of blood pressure. Hydralazine undergoes extensive hepatic metabolism; it is excreted mainly in the form of metabolites in the urine.
Administration of hydralazine with food results in higher levels of the drug in plasma.
Hydrochlorothiazide. Onset of action of thiazides occurs in 2 hours and the peak effect at about 4 hours. The action persists for approximately 6–12 hours. Hydrochlorothiazide is rapidly absorbed, as indicated by peak concentrations 1–2.5 hours after oral administration. Plasma levels of the drug are proportional to dose; the concentration in whole blood is 1.6–1.8 times higher than in plasma. Thiazides are eliminated rapidly by the kidney. After oral administration of 25- to 100-mg doses, 72–97% of the dose is excreted in the urine, indicating dose-independent absorption. Hydrochlorothiazide is eliminated from plasma in a biphasic fashion with a terminal half-life of 10–17 hours. Plasma protein binding is 67.9%. Plasma clearance is 15.9–30.0 L/hr; volume of distribution is 3.6–7.8 L/kg.
Gastrointestinal absorption of hydrochlorothiazide is enhanced when administered with food. Absorption is decreased in patients with congestive heart failure, and the pharmacokinetics are considerably different in these patients.

INDICATIONS AND USAGE
Hypertension (see boxed **WARNING**).

CONTRAINDICATIONS
Hydralazine
Hypersensitivity to hydralazine; coronary artery disease; mitral valvular rheumatic heart disease.

Hydrochlorothiazide
Anuria; hypersensitivity to this or other sulfonamide-derived drugs.

WARNINGS
Hydralazine
In a few patients hydralazine may produce a clinical picture simulating systemic lupus erythematosus including glomerulonephritis. In such patients hydralazine should be discontinued unless the benefit-to-risk determination requires continued antihypertensive therapy with this drug. Signs and symptoms usually regress when the drug is discontinued, but residua have been detected many years later. Long-term treatment with steroids may be necessary. (See **PRECAUTIONS, Laboratory Tests.**)
Hydrochlorothiazide
Thiazides should be used with caution in patients with severe renal disease. In patients with renal disease, thiazides may precipitate azotemia. Cumulative effects of the drug may develop in patients with impaired renal function.
Thiazides should be used with caution in patients with impaired hepatic function or progressive liver disease, since minor alterations of fluid and electrolyte imbalance may precipitate hepatic coma.
Thiazides may add to or potentiate the action of other antihypertensive drugs. Potentiation occurs with ganglionic or peripheral adrenergic blocking drugs.
Sensitivity reactions are more likely to occur in patients with a history of allergy or bronchial asthma.
The possibility of exacerbation or activation of systemic lupus erythematosus has been reported.

PRECAUTIONS
General
Hydralazine. Myocardial stimulation produced by hydralazine can cause anginal attacks and ECG changes indicative of myocardial ischemia. The drug has been implicated in the production of myocardial infarction. It must, therefore, be used with caution in patients with suspected coronary artery disease.
The "hyperdynamic" circulation caused by hydralazine may accentuate specific cardiovascular inadequacies. For example, hydralazine may increase pulmonary artery pressure in patients with mitral valvular disease. The drug may reduce the pressor responses to epinephrine. Postural hypotension may result from hydralazine but is less common than with ganglionic blocking agents. It should be used with caution in patients with cerebral vascular accidents.
In hypertensive patients with normal kidneys who are treated with hydralazine, there is evidence of increased renal blood flow and a maintenance of glomerular filtration rate. In some instances where control values were below normal, improved renal function has been noted after administration of hydralazine. However, as with any antihypertensive agent, hydralazine should be used with caution in patients with advanced renal damage.
Peripheral neuritis, evidenced by paresthesia, numbness, and tingling, has been observed. Published evidence suggests that hydralazine has an antipyridoxine effect and that pyridoxine should be added to the regimen if symptoms develop.
Hydrochlorothiazide. All patients receiving thiazide therapy should be observed for clinical signs of fluid or electrolyte imbalance, namely hyponatremia, hypochloremic alkalosis, and hypokalemia (see **Laboratory Tests** and **Drug/Drug Interactions**). Warning signs are dryness of mouth, thirst, weakness, lethargy, drowsiness, restlessness, muscle pains or cramps, muscular fatigue, hypotension, oliguria, tachycardia, and gastrointestinal disturbance, such as nausea or vomiting.
Hypokalemia may develop, especially in cases of brisk diuresis or severe cirrhosis.
Interference with adequate oral intake of electrolytes will also contribute to hypokalemia. Hypokalemia may be avoided or treated by the use of potassium supplements or foods with a high potassium content.
Any chloride deficit is generally mild and usually does not require specific treatment, except under extraordinary circumstances (as in liver disease or renal disease). Dilutional hyponatremia may occur in edematous patients in hot weather; appropriate therapy is water restriction, rather than administration of salt, except in rare instances when the hyponatremia is life-threatening. In cases of actual salt depletion, appropriate replacement is the therapy of choice.
Hyperuricemia may occur or frank gout may be precipitated in certain patients receiving thiazide therapy.
Latent diabetes may become manifest during thiazide administration (see **Drug/Drug Interactions**).
The antihypertensive effects of the drug may be enhanced in the postsympathectomy patient.
If progressive renal impairment becomes evident, withholding or discontinuing diuretic therapy should be considered.
Calcium excretion is decreased by thiazides. Pathological changes in the parathyroid gland with hypercalcemia and hypophosphatemia have been observed in a few patients on prolonged thiazide therapy. The common complications of

hyperparathyroidism, such as renal lithiasis, bone resorption, and peptic ulceration, have not been seen.
Thiazide diuretics have been shown to increase the urinary excretion of magnesium; this may result in hypomagnesemia.

Information for Patients
Patients should be informed of possible side effects and advised to take the medication regularly and continuously as directed.

Laboratory Tests
Hydralazine. Complete blood counts and antinuclear antibody titer determinations are indicated before and periodically during prolonged therapy with hydralazine even though the patient is asymptomatic. These studies are also indicated if the patient develops arthralgia, fever, chest pain, continued malaise, or other unexplained signs or symptoms.
A positive antinuclear antibody titer requires that the physician carefully weigh the implications of the test results against the benefits to be derived from antihypertensive therapy with a combination drug containing hydralazine.
Blood dyscrasias, consisting of reduction in hemoglobin and red cell count, leukopenia, agranulocytosis, and purpura, have been reported. If such abnormalities develop, therapy should be discontinued.
Hydrochlorothiazide. Initial and periodic determinations of serum electrolytes to detect possible electrolyte imbalance should be performed at appropriate intervals.
Serum and urine electrolyte determinations are particularly important when the patient is vomiting excessively or receiving parenteral fluids.

Drug/Drug Interactions
Hydralazine. MAO inhibitors should be used with caution in patients receiving hydralazine.
When other potent parenteral antihypertensive drugs, such as diazoxide, are used in combination with hydralazine, patients should be continously observed for several hours for any excessive fall in blood pressure. Profound hypotensive episodes may occur when diazoxide injections and hydralazine are used concomitantly.
Hydrochlorothiazide. Hypokalemia can sensitize or exaggerate the response of the heart to the toxic effects of digitalis (e.g., increased ventricular irritability).
Hypokalemia may develop during concomitant use of steroids or ACTH.
Insulin requirements in diabetic patients may be increased, decreased, or unchanged.
Thiazides may decrease arterial responsiveness to norepinephrine, but not enough to preclude effectiveness of the pressor agent for therapeutic use.
Thiazides may increase the responsiveness to tubocurarine.
Lithium renal clearance is reduced by thiazides, increasing the risk of lithium toxicity.
There have been rare reports in the literature of hemolytic anemia occurring with the concomitant use of hydrochlorothiazide and methyldopa.
Concurrent administration of some nonsteroidal anti-inflammatory agents may reduce the diuretic, natriuretic and antihypertensive effects of thiazide diuretics.
Cholestyramine and colestipol resins: Absorption of hydrochlorothiazide is impaired in the presence of anionic exchange resins. Single doses of either cholestyramine or colestipol resins bind the hydrochlorothiazide and reduce its absorption from the gastrointestinal tract by up to 85% and 43%, respectively.

Drug/Laboratory Test Interactions
Thiazides may decrease serum levels of protein-bound iodine without signs of thyroid disturbance. Apresazide should be discontinued before tests for parathyroid function are made (See **General, *Hydrochlorothiazide,*** Calcium excretion).

Carcinogenesis, Mutagenesis, Impairment of Fertility
Carcinogenicity, mutagenicity, and fertility studies in animals have not been conducted with Apresazide.
Hydralazine. In a lifetime study in Swiss albino mice, there was a statistically significant increase in the incidence of lung tumors (adenomas and adenocarcinomas) of both male and female mice given hydralazine continuously in their drinking water at a dosage of about 250 mg/kg per day (about 80 times the maximum recommended human dose). In a 2-year carcinogenicity study of rats given hydralazine by gavage at dosages of 15, 30, and 60 mg/kg per day (approximately 5 to 20 times the recommended human daily dose), microscopic examination of the liver revealed a small, but statistically significant, increase in benign neoplastic nodules in male and female rats from the high-dose group and in female rats from the intermediate-dose group. Benign interstitial cell tumors of the testes were also significantly increased in male rats from the high-dose group. The tumors observed are common in aged rats, and a significantly increased incidence was not observed until 18 months of treatment. Hydralazine was shown to be mutagenic in bacterial systems (Gene Mutation and DNA Repair) and in one of two rat and one rabbit hepatocyte in vitro DNA repair studies. Additional in vivo and in vitro studies using lymphoma cells, germinal cells, and fibroblasts from mice, bone marrow cells from Chinese hamsters, and fibroblasts from human cell lines did not demonstrate any mutagenic potential for hydralazine.
The extent to which these findings indicate a risk to man is uncertain. While long-term clinical observation has not suggested that human cancer is associated with hydralazine use, epidemiologic studies have so far been insufficient to arrive at any conclusions.
Fertility studies in animals have not been conducted with hydralazine.
Hydrochlorothiazide. Two-year feeding studies in mice and rats conducted under the auspices of the National Toxicology Program (NTP) uncovered no evidence of a carcinogenic potential of hydrochlorothiazide in female mice (at doses of up to approximately 600 mg/kg/day) or in male and female rats (at doses of up to approximately 100 mg/kg/day). The NTP, however, found equivocal evidence for hepatocarcinogenicity in male mice.
Hydrochlorothiazide was not genotoxic in in vitro assays using strains TA 98, TA 100, TA 1535, TA 1537, and TA 1538 of *Salmonella typhimurium* (Ames assay) and in the Chinese Hamster Ovary (CHO) test for chromosomal aberrations, or in in vivo assays using mouse germinal cell chromosomes, Chinese hamster bone marrow chromosomes, and the *Drosophila* sex-linked recessive lethal trait gene. Positive test results were obtained only in the in vitro CHO Sister Chromatid Exchange (clastogenicity) and in the Mouse Lymphoma Cell (mutagenicity) assays, using concentrations of hydrochlorothiazide from 43 to 1300 μg/mL, and in the *Aspergillus nidulans* nondisjunction assay at an unspecified concentration.
Hydrochlorothiazide had no adverse effects on the fertility of mice and rats of either sex in studies wherein these species were exposed, via their diet, to doses of up to 100 and 4 mg/kg/day, respectively, prior to mating, and throughout gestation.

Pregnancy: Teratogenic Effects. Pregnancy Category C
Animal reproduction studies have not been conducted with Apresazide.
Hydralazine. Animal studies indicate that hydralazine is teratogenic in mice at 20–30 times the maximum daily human dose of 200–300 mg and possibly in rabbits at 10–15 times the maximum daily human dose, but that it is nonteratogenic in rats. Teratogenic effects observed were cleft palate and malformations of facial and cranial bones.
Hydrochlorothiazide. Studies in which hydrochlorothiazide was orally administered to pregnant mice and rats during their respective periods of major organogenesis at doses up to 3000 and 1000 mg/kg/day, respectively, provided no evidence of harm to the fetus. There are, however, no adequate and well-controlled studies of Apresazide in pregnant women. Because animal reproduction studies are not always predictive of human response, this combination drug should be used during pregnancy only if clearly needed.

Nonteratogenic Effects. *Hydrochlorothiazide.* There are no adequate and well-controlled studies of Apresazide in pregnant women. However, thiazides cross the placental barrier and appear in cord blood, and there is a risk of fetal or neonatal jaundice, thrombocytopenia, and possibly other adverse reactions that have occurred in adults.

Nursing Mothers
It is not known whether hydralazine is excreted in human milk. Thiazides are excreted in human milk. Because of the potential for serious adverse reactions in nursing infants, a decision should be made whether to discontinue nursing or to discontinue the drug, taking into account the importance of the drug to the mother.

Pediatric Use
Safety and effectiveness of the combination drug in pediatric patients have not been established.

ADVERSE REACTIONS
Adverse reactions are usually reversible upon reduction of dosage or discontinuation of Apresazide. Whenever adverse reactions are moderate or severe, it may be necessary to discontinue the drug.

Hydralazine
The following adverse reactions have been observed, but there has not been enough systematic collection of data to support an estimate of their frequency.

Common
Headache, anorexia, nausea, vomiting, diarrhea, palpitations, tachycardia, angina pectoris.

Less Frequent
Digestive: Constipation, paralytic ileus.
Cardiovascular: Hypotension, paradoxical pressor response, edema.
Respiratory: Dyspnea.
Neurologic: Peripheral neuritis, evidenced by paresthesia, numbness, and tingling; dizziness; tremors; muscle cramps; psychotic reactions characterized by depression, disorientation, or anxiety.
Genitourinary: Difficulty in urination.
Hematologic: Blood dyscrasias, consisting of reduction in hemoglobin and red cell count, leukopenia, agranulocytosis, purpura; lymphadenopathy; splenomegaly.
Hypersensitive Reactions: Rash, urticaria, pruritus, fever, chills, arthralgia, eosinophilia, and, rarely, hepatitis.
Other: Nasal congestion, flushing, lacrimation, conjunctivitis.

Hydrochlorothiazide
The following adverse reactions have been observed, but there has not been enough systematic collection of data to support an estimate of their frequency. Consequently the reactions are categorized by organ systems and are listed in decreasing order of severity and not frequency.
Digestive: Pancreatitis, jaundice (intrahepatic cholestatic), sialadenitis, vomiting, diarrhea, cramping, nausea, gastric irritation, constipation, anorexia.
Cardiovascular: Orthostatic hypotension (may be potentiated by alcohol, barbiturates, or narcotics).
Neurologic: Vertigo, dizziness, transient blurred vision, headache, paresthesia, xanthopsia, weakness, restlessness.
Musculoskeletal: Muscle spasm.
Hematologic: Aplastic anemia, agranulocytosis, leukopenia, thrombocytopenia.
Metabolic: Hyperglycemia, glycosuria, hyperuricemia.
Hypersensitive Reactions: Necrotizing angiitis, Stevens-Johnson syndrome, respiratory distress including pneumonitis and pulmonary edema, purpura, urticaria, rash, photosensitivity.

OVERDOSAGE
Acute Toxicity
Oral LD_{50}'s in rats (mg/kg): hydralazine, 173 and 187; hydrochlorothiazide, 2750.

Signs and Symptoms
Hydralazine. Signs and symptoms of overdosage include hypotension, tachycardia, headache, and generalized skin flushing.
Complications can include myocardial ischemia and subsequent myocardial infarction, cardiac arrhythmia, and profound shock.
Hydrochlorothiazide. The most prominent feature of poisoning is acute loss of fluid and electrolytes.
Cardiovascular: Tachycardia, hypotension, shock.
Neuromuscular: Weakness, confusion, dizziness, cramps of the calf muscles, paresthesia, fatigue, impairment of consciousness.
Digestive: Nausea, vomiting, thirst.
Renal: Polyuria, oliguria, or anuria (due to hemoconcentration).
Laboratory Findings: Hypokalemia, hyponatremia, hypochloremia, alkalosis; increased BUN (especially in patients with renal insufficiency).
Combined Poisoning: Signs and symptoms may be aggravated or modified by concomitant intake of antihypertensive medication, barbiturates, curare, digitalis (hypokalemia), corticosteroids, narcotics, or alcohol.

Treatment
There is no specific antidote.
The gastric contents should be evacuated, taking adequate precautions against aspiration and for protection of the airway. An activated charcoal slurry may be instilled if conditions permit. Dialysis may not be effective for elimination of Apresazide because of its plasma protein binding (see **CLINICAL PHARMACOLOGY**).
These manipulations may have to be omitted or carried out after cardiovascular status has been stabilized, since they might precipitate cardiac arrhythmias or increase the depth of shock.
Support of the cardiovascular system is of primary importance in suspected hydralazine overdosage. Shock should be treated with plasma expanders. The patient's legs should be kept raised and lost fluid and electrolytes (potassium, sodium) should be replaced. If possible, vasopressors should not be given, but if a vasopressor is required, care should be taken not to precipitate or aggravate cardiac arrhythmia. Tachycardia responds to beta blockers. Digitalization may be necessary, and renal function should be monitored and supported as required.

DOSAGE AND ADMINISTRATION
Dosage should be determined by individual titration (see boxed **WARNING**).
The usual dosage is one Apresazide capsule twice daily, the strength depending upon individual requirement following titration. For maintenance, the dosage should be adjusted to the lowest effective level.
When necessary, other antihypertensive agents such as sympathetic inhibitors may be added gradually in reduced dosages, and the effects should be watched carefully.

HOW SUPPLIED
Capsules 25/25—light blue and white opaque (imprinted APRESAZIDE® 25/25 CIBA 139)
25 mg of hydralazine hydrochloride and 25 mg of hydrochlorothiazide
Bottles of 100 .... NDC 0083-0139-30

Continued on next page

CibaGeneva—Cont.

Capsules 50/50—pink and white opaque (imprinted APRESAZIDE® 50/50 CIBA 149)

50 mg of hydralazine hydrochloride and 50 mg of hydrochlorothiazide

Bottles of 100 .... NDC 0083-0149-30

Capsules 100/50—flesh pink and white opaque (imprinted APRESAZIDE® 100/50 CIBA 159)

100 mg of hydralazine hydrochloride and 50 mg of hydrochlorothiazide

Bottles of 100 .... NDC 0083-0159-30

Samples, when available, are identified by the word *SAMPLE* appearing on each capsule.
Do not store above 86°F (30°C).
Dispense in tight, light-resistant container (USP).

C96-15 (Rev. 3/96)

Shown in Product Identification Guide, page 309

APRESOLINE® hydrochloride ℞

[a-press 'oh-leen]
hydralazine hydrochloride USP
Tablets

DESCRIPTION

Apresoline, hydralazine hydrochloride USP, is an antihypertensive, available as 10-, 25-, 50-, and 100-mg tablets for oral administration. Its chemical name is 1-hydrazinophthalazine monohydrochloride.
Hydralazine hydrochloride USP is a white to off-white, odorless crystalline powder. It is soluble in water, slightly soluble in alcohol, and very slightly soluble in ether. It melts at about 275°C, with decomposition, and has a molecular weight of 196.64.
Inactive Ingredients: Acacia, D&C Yellow No. 10 (10-mg tablets), FD&C Blue No. 1 (25-mg and 50-mg tablets), FD&C Yellow No. 5 and FD&C Yellow No. 6 (100-mg tablets), lactose, magnesium stearate, mannitol, polyethylene glycol, sodium starch glycolate, starch and stearic acid.

CLINICAL PHARMACOLOGY

Although the precise mechanism of action of hydralazine is not fully understood, the major effects are on the cardiovascular system. Hydralazine apparently lowers blood pressure by exerting a peripheral vasodilating effect through a direct relaxation of vascular smooth muscle. Hydralazine, by altering cellular calcium metabolism, interferes with the calcium movements within the vascular smooth muscle that are responsible for initiating or maintaining the contractile state.
The peripheral vasodilating effect of hydralazine results in decreased arterial blood pressure (diastolic more than systolic); decreased peripheral vascular resistance; and an increased heart rate, stroke volume, and cardiac output. The preferential dilatation of arterioles, as compared to veins, minimizes postural hypotension and promotes the increase in cardiac output. Hydralazine usually increases renin activity in plasma, presumably as a result of increased secretion of renin by the renal juxtaglomerular cells in response to reflex sympathetic discharge. This increase in renin activity leads to the production of angiotensin II, which then causes stimulation of aldosterone and consequent sodium reabsorption. Hydralazine also maintains or increases renal and cerebral blood flow.
Hydralazine is rapidly absorbed after oral administration, and peak plasma levels are reached at 1–2 hours. Plasma levels of apparent hydralazine decline with a half-life of 3–7 hours. Binding to human plasma protein is 87%. Plasma levels of hydralazine vary widely among individuals. Hydralazine is subject to polymorphic acetylation; slow acetylators generally have higher plasma levels of hydralazine and require lower doses to maintain control of blood pressure. Hydralazine undergoes extensive hepatic metabolism; it is excreted mainly in the form of metabolites in the urine.

INDICATIONS AND USAGE

Essential hypertension, alone or as an adjunct.

CONTRAINDICATIONS

Hypersensitivity to hydralazine; coronary artery disease; mitral valvular rheumatic heart disease.

WARNINGS

In a few patients hydralazine may produce a clinical picture simulating systemic lupus erythematosus including glomerulonephritis. In such patients hydralazine should be discontinued unless the benefit-to-risk determination requires continued antihypertensive therapy with this drug. Symptoms and signs usually regress when the drug is discontinued but residua have been detected many years later. Long-term treatment with steroids may be necessary. (See **PRECAUTIONS, Laboratory Tests.**)

PRECAUTIONS

General: Myocardial stimulation produced by Apresoline can cause anginal attacks and ECG changes of myocardial ischemia. The drug has been implicated in the production of myocardial infarction. It must, therefore, be used with caution in patients with suspected coronary artery disease.
The "hyperdynamic" circulation caused by Apresoline may accentuate specific cardiovascular inadequacies. For example, Apresoline may increase pulmonary artery pressure in patients with mitral valvular disease. The drug may reduce the pressor responses to epinephrine. Postural hypotension may result from Apresoline but is less common than with ganglionic blocking agents. It should be used with caution in patients with cerebral vascular accidents.
In hypertensive patients wiith normal kidneys who are treated with Apresoline, there is evidence of increased renal blood flow and a maintenance of glomerular filtration rate. In some instances where control values were below normal, improved renal function has been noted after administration of Apresoline. However, as with any antihypertensive agent, Apresoline should be used with caution in patients with advanced renal damage.
Peripheral neuritis, evidenced by paresthesia, numbness, and tingling, has been observed. Published evidence suggests an antipyridoxine effect, and that pyridoxine should be added to the regimen if symptoms develop.
The Apresoline tablets (100 mg) contain FD&C Yellow No. 5 (tartrazine), which may cause allergic-type reactions (including bronchial asthma) in certain susceptible individuals. Although the overall incidence of FD&C Yellow No. 5 (tartrazine) sensitivity in the general population is low, it is frequently seen in patients who are also hypersensitive to aspirin.
Information for Patients: Patients should be informed of possible side effects and advised to take the medication regularly and continuously as directed.
Laboratory Tests: Complete blood counts and antinuclear antibody titer determinations are indicated before and periodically during prolonged therapy with hydralazine even though the patient is asymptomatic. These studies are also indicated if the patient develops arthralgia, fever, chest pain, continued malaise, or other unexplained signs or symptoms.
A positive antinuclear antibody titer requires that the physician carefully weigh the implications of the test results against the benefits to be derived from antihypertensive therapy with hydralazine.
Blood dyscrasias, consisting of reduction in hemoglobin and red cell count, leukopenia, agranulocytosis, and purpura, have been reported. If such abnormalities develop, therapy should be discontinued.
Drug/Drug Interactions: MAO inhibitors should be used with caution in patients receiving hydralazine.
When other potent parenteral antihypertensive drugs, such as diazoxide, are used in combination with hydralazine, patients should be continuously observed for several hours for any excessive fall in blood pressure. Profound hypotensive episodes may occur when diazoxide injection and Apresoline are used concomitantly.
Drug/Food Interactions: Administration of hydralazine with food results in higher plasma levels.
Carcinogensis, Mutagenesis, Impairment of Fertility: In a lifetime study in Swiss albino mice, there was a statistically significant increase in the incidence of lung tumors (adenomas and adenocarcinomas) of both male and female mice given hydralazine continuously in their drinking water at a dosage of about 250 mg/kg per day (about 80 times the maximum recommended human dose). In a 2-year carcinogenicity study of rats given hydralazine by gavage at dose levels of 15, 30, and 60 mg/kg/day (approximately 5 to 20 times the recommended human daily dosage), microscopic examination of the liver revealed a small, but statistically significant, increase in benign neoplastic nodules in male and female rats from the high-dose group and in female rats from the intermediate-dose group. Benign interstitial cell tumors of the testes were also significantly increased in male rats from the high-dose group. The tumors observed are common in aged rats and a significantly increased incidence was not observed until 18 months of treatment. Hydralazine was shown to be mutagenic in bacterial systems (Gene Mutation and DNA Repair) and in one of two rat and one rabbit hepatocyte *in vitro* DNA repair studies. Additional *in vivo* and *in vitro* studies using lymphoma cells, germinal cells, and fibroblasts from mice, bone marrow cells from chinese hamsters and fibroblasts from human cell lines did not demonstrate any mutagenic potential for hydralazine.
The extent to which these findings indicate a risk to man is uncertain. While long-term clinical observation has not suggested that human cancer is associated with hydralazine use, epidemiologic studies have so far been insufficient to arrive at any conclusions.
Pregnancy Category C: Animal studies indicate that hydralazine is teratogenic in mice at 20–30 times the maximum daily human dose of 200–300 mg and possibly in rabbits at 10–15 times the maximum daily human dose, but that it is nonteratogenic in rats. Teratogenic effects observed were cleft palate and malformations of facial and cranial bones. There are no adequate and well-controlled studies in pregnant women. Although clinical experience does not include any positive evidence of adverse effects on the human fetus, hydralazine should be used during pregnancy only if the expected benefit justifies the potential risk to the fetus.
Nursing Mothers: Hydralazine has been shown to be excreted in breast milk.
Pediatric Use: Safety and effectiveness in pediatric patients have not been established in controlled clinical trials, although there is experience with the use of Apresoline in these patients. The usual recommended oral starting dosage is 0.75 mg/kg of body weight daily in four divided doses. Dosage may be increased gradually over the next 3–4 weeks to a maximum of 7.5 mg/kg or 200 mg daily.

ADVERSE REACTIONS

Adverse reactions with Apresoline are usually reversible when dosage is reduced. However, in some cases it may be necessary to discontinue the drug.
The following adverse reactions have been observed, but there has not been enough systematic collection of data to support an estimate of their frequency.
Common: Headache, anorexia, nausea, vomiting, diarrhea, palpitations, tachycardia, angina pectoris.
Less Frequent: *Digestive:* constipation, paralytic ileus.
Cardiovascular: hypotension, paradoxical pressor response, edema.
Respiratory: dyspnea.
Neurologic: peripheral neuritis, evidenced by paresthesia, numbness, and tingling; dizziness; tremors; muscle cramps; psychotic reactions characterized by depression, disorientation, or anxiety.
Genitourinary: difficulty in urination.
Hematologic: blood dyscrasias, consisting of reduction in hemoglobin and red cell count, leukopenia, agranulocytosis, purpura; lymphadenopathy; splenomegaly.
Hypersensitive Reactions: rash, urticaria, pruritus, fever, chills, arthralgia, eosinophilia, and, rarely, hepatitis.
Other: nasal congestion, flushing, lacrimation, conjunctivitis.

OVERDOSAGE

Acute Toxicity: No deaths due to acute poisoning have been reported.
Highest known dose survived: adults, 10 g orally.
Oral LD_{50} in rats: 173 and 187 mg/kg.
Signs and Symptoms: Signs and symptoms of overdosage include hypotension, tachycardia, headache, and generalized skin flushing.
Complications can include myocardial ischemia and subsequent myocardial infarction, cardiac arrhythmia, and profound shock.
Treatment: There is no specific antidote.
The gastric contents should be evacuated, taking adequate precautions against aspiration and for protection of the airway. An activated charcoal slurry may be instilled if conditions permit. These manipulations may have to be omitted or carried out after cardiovascular status has been stabilized, since they might precipitate cardiac arrhythmias or increase the depth of shock.
Support of the cardiovascular system is of primary importance. Shock should be treated with plasma expanders. If possible, vasopressors should not be given, but if a vasopressor is required, care should be taken not to precipitate or aggravate cardiac arrhythmia. Tachycardia responds to beta blockers. Digitalization may be necessary, and renal function should be monitored and supported as required.
No experience has been reported with extracorporeal or peritoneal dialysis.

DOSAGE AND ADMINISTRATION

Initiate therapy in gradually increasing dosages; adjust according to individual response. Start with 10 mg four times daily for the first 2–4 days, increase to 25 mg four times daily for the balance of the first week. For the second and subsequent weeks, increase dosage to 50 mg four times daily. For maintenance, adjust dosage to the lowest effective levels.
The incidence of toxic reactions, particularly the L.E. cell syndrome, is high in the group of patients receiving large doses of Apresoline.
In a few resistant patients, up to 300 mg of Apresoline daily may be required for a significant antihypertensive effect. In such cases, a lower dosage of Apresoline combined with a thiazide and/or reserpine or a beta blocker may be considered. However, when combining therapy, individual titration is essential to ensure the lowest possible therapeutic dose of each drug.

HOW SUPPLIED

Tablets 10 mg—round, pale yellow, dry-coated (imprinted CIBA 37)

Bottles of 100—NDC 0083-0037-30

Tablets 25 mg—round, deep blue, dry-coated (imprinted CIBA 39)

Bottles of 100—NDC 0083-0039-30

Tablets 50 mg—round, light blue, dry-coated (imprinted CIBA 73)

Bottles of 100—NDC 0083-0073-30

Tablets 100 mg—round, peach, dry-coated (imprinted CIBA 101)

Bottles of 100—NDC 0083-0101-30

Samples, when available, are identified by the word *SAMPLE* appearing on each tablet.

Do not store above 86°F (30°C).

Dispense in tight, light-resistant container (USP).

C95-14 (Rev. 5/95)

Shown in Product Identification Guide, page 309

AREDIA® ℞

pamidronate disodium for injection
For Intravenous Infusion

Prescribing Information

DESCRIPTION

Aredia, pamidronate disodium, (APD), is a bone-resorption inhibitor available in 30-mg, 60-mg, or 90-mg vials for intravenous administration. Each 30-mg, 60-mg, and 90-mg vial contains, respectively, 30 mg, 60 mg, and 90 mg of sterile, lyophilized pamidronate disodium and 470 mg, 400 mg, and 375 mg of mannitol, USP. The pH of a 1% solution of pamidronate disodium in distilled water is approximately 8.3. Aredia, a member of the group of chemical compounds known as bisphosphonates, is an analog of pyrophosphate. Pamidronate disodium is designated chemically as phosphonic acid (3-amino-1-hydroxypropylidene) bis-, disodium salt, pentahydrate, (APD).

Pamidronate disodium is a white-to-practically-white powder. It is soluble in water and in 2N sodium hydroxide, sparingly soluble in 0.1N hydrochloric acid and in 0.1N acetic acid, and practically insoluble in organic solvents. Its molecular formula is $C_3H_9NO_7P_2Na_2 \cdot 5H_2O$ and its molecular weight is 369.1.

Inactive Ingredients. Mannitol, USP, and phosphoric acid (for adjustment to pH 6.5 prior to lyophilization).

CLINICAL PHARMACOLOGY

The principal pharmacologic action of Aredia is inhibition of bone resorption. Although the mechanism of antiresorptive action is not completely understood, several factors are thought to contribute to this action. Aredia adsorbs to calcium phosphate (hydroxyapatite) crystals in bone and may directly block dissolution of this mineral component of bone. In vitro studies also suggest that inhibition of osteoclast activity contributes to inhibition of bone resorption. In animal studies, at doses recommended for the treatment of hypercalcemia, Aredia inhibits bone resorption apparently without inhibiting bone formation and mineralization. Of relevance to the treatment of hypercalcemia of malignancy is the finding that Aredia inhibits the accelerated bone resorption that results from osteoclast hyperactivity induced by various tumors in animal studies.

Pharmacokinetics

Distribution

Body retention of pamidronate was calculated to be 54 ± 14% of the dose over 120 hours (Table 1).

Metabolism

Pamidronate is not metabolized and is exclusively eliminated by renal excretion.

Excretion

After administration of 30, 60, and 90 mg of Aredia over 4 and 24 hours, an overall mean ± SD of 46 ± 14% of the drug was excreted unchanged in the urine within 120 hours. Cumulative urinary excretion was linearly related to dose. The mean ± SD elimination half-life is 28 ± 7 hours. Total and renal clearances of pamidronate were 110 ± 52 mL/min and 50 ± 27 mL/min, respectively. The rate of elimination from bone has not been determined.

Special Populations

There are no data available on the effects of age, gender, or race on the pharmacokinetics of pamidronate.

Pediatric

Pamidronate is not labeled for use in the pediatric population.

Renal Insufficiency

The pharmacokinetics of pamidronate were studied in cancer patients (n=19) with normal and varying degrees of renal impairment. Each patient received a single 90-mg dose of Aredia infused over 4 hours. The renal clearance of pamidronate in patients was found to closely correlate with creatinine clearance (see Figure 1). A trend toward a lower percentage of drug excreted unchanged in urine was observed in renally impaired patients. Adverse experiences noted were not found to be related to changes in renal clearance of pamidronate. Given the recommended dose, 90 mg infused over 4 hours, excessive accumulation of pamidronate in renally impaired patients is not anticipated if Aredia is administered on a monthly basis.

Figure 1: Pamidronate renal clearance as a function of creatinine clearance in patients with normal and impaired renal function. The lines are the mean prediction line and 95% confidence intervals.

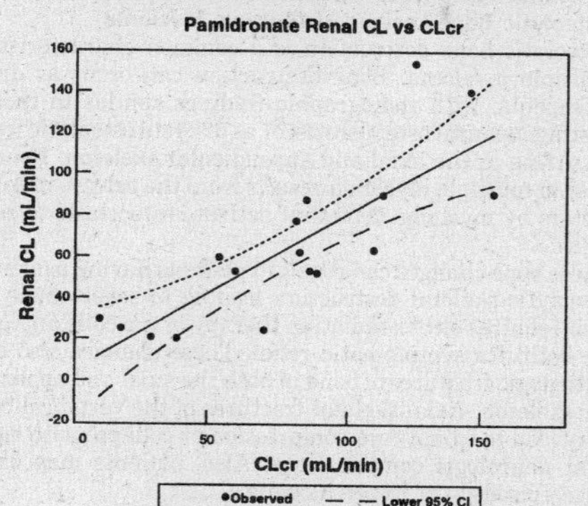
Pamidronate Renal CL vs CLcr
Renal CL (mL/min)
CLcr (mL/min)
•Observed
Predicted
Lower 95% CI
Upper 95% CI

Hepatic Insufficiency

There are no human pharmacokinetic data for Aredia in patients who have hepatic insufficiency.

Drug-Drug Interactions

There are no human pharmacokinetic data for drug interactions with Aredia.

[See table below.]

After intravenous administration of radiolabeled pamidronate in rats, approximately 50%–60% of the compound was rapidly adsorbed by bone and slowly eliminated from the body by the kidneys. In rats given 10 mg/kg bolus injections of radiolabeled Aredia, approximately 30% of the compound was found in the liver shortly after administration and was then redistributed to bone or eliminated by the kidneys over 24-48 hours. Studies in rats injected with radiolabeled Aredia showed that the compound was rapidly cleared from the circulation and taken up mainly by bones, liver, spleen, teeth, and tracheal cartilage. Radioactivity was eliminated from most soft tissues within 1–4 days; was detectable in liver and spleen for 1 and 3 months, respectively; and remained high in bones, trachea, and teeth for 6 months after dosing. Bone uptake occurred preferentially in areas of high bone turnover. The terminal phase of elimination half-life in bone was estimated to be approximately 300 days.

Pharmacodynamics

Serum phosphate levels have been noted to decrease after administration of Aredia, presumably because of decreased release of phosphate from bone and increased renal excretion as parathyroid hormone levels, which are usually suppressed in hypercalcemia associated with malignancy, return toward normal. Phosphate therapy was administered in 30% of the patients in response to a decrease in serum phosphate levels. Phosphate levels usually returned toward normal within 7–10 days.

Urinary calcium/creatinine and urinary hydroxyproline/creatinine ratios decrease and usually return to within or below normal after treatment with Aredia. These changes occur within the first week after treatment, as do decreases in serum calcium levels, and are consistent with an antiresorptive pharmacologic action.

Hypercalcemia of Malignancy

Osteoclastic hyperactivity resulting in excessive bone resorption is the underlying pathophysiologic derangement in metastatic bone disease and hypercalcemia of malignancy. Excessive release of calcium into the blood as bone is resorbed results in polyuria and gastrointestinal disturbances, with progressive dehydration and decreasing glomerular filtration rate. This, in turn, results in increased renal resorption of calcium, setting up a cycle of worsening systemic hypercalcemia. Correction of excessive bone resorption and adequate fluid administration to correct volume deficits are therefore essential to the management of hypercalcemia.

Most cases of hypercalcemia associated with malignancy occur in patients who have breast cancer; squamous-cell tumors of the lung or head and neck; renal-cell carcinoma; and certain hematologic malignancies, such as multiple myeloma and some types of lymphomas. A few less-common malignancies, including vasoactive intestinal-peptide-producing tumors and cholangiocarcinoma, have a high incidence of hypercalcemia as a metabolic complication. Patients who have hypercalcemia of malignancy can generally be divided into two groups, according to the pathophysiologic mechanism involved.

In humoral hypercalcemia, osteoclasts are activated and bone resorption is stimulated by factors such as parathyroid-hormone-related protein, which are elaborated by the tumor and circulate systemically.

Humoral hypercalcemia usually occurs in squamous-cell malignancies of the lung or head and neck or in genitourinary tumors such as renal-cell carcinoma or ovarian cancer. Skeletal metastases may be absent or minimal in these patients.

Extensive invasion of bone by tumor cells can also result in hypercalcemia due to local tumor products that stimulate bone resorption by osteoclasts. Tumors commonly associated with locally mediated hypercalcemia include breast cancer and multiple myeloma.

Total serum calcium levels in patients who have hypercalcemia of malignancy may not reflect the severity of hypercalcemia, since concomitant hypoalbuminemia is commonly present. Ideally, ionized calcium levels should be used to diagnose and follow hypercalcemic conditions; however, these are not commonly or rapidly available in many clinical situations. Therefore, adjustment of the total serum calcium value for differences in albumin levels is often used in place of measurement of ionized calcium; several nomograms are in use for this type of calculation (see DOSAGE AND ADMINISTRATION).

Clinical Trials

In one double-blind clinical trial, 52 patients who had hypercalcemia of malignancy were enrolled to receive 30 mg, 60 mg, or 90 mg of Aredia as a single 24-hour intravenous infusion if their corrected serum calcium levels were ≥12.0 mg/dL after 48 hours of saline hydration.

The mean baseline-corrected serum calcium for the 30-mg, 60-mg and 90-mg groups were 13.8 mg/dL, 13.8 mg/dL and 13.3 mg/dL, respectively.

The majority of patients (64%) had decreases in albumin-corrected serum calcium levels by 24 hours after initiation of treatment. Mean-corrected serum calcium levels at days 2-7 after initiation of treatment with Aredia were significantly reduced from baseline in all three dosage groups. As a result, by 7 days after initiation of treatment with Aredia, 40%, 61%, and 100% of the patients receiving 30 mg, 60 mg, and 90 mg of Aredia, respectively, had normal-corrected serum calcium levels. Many patients (33%-53%) in the 60-mg and 90-mg dosage groups continued to have normal-corrected serum calcium levels, or a partial response (≥15% decrease of corrected serum calcium from baseline), at day 14.

In a second double-blind, controlled clinical trial, 65 cancer patients who had corrected serum calcium levels of ≥12.0 mg/dL after at least 24 hours of saline hydration were randomized to receive either 60 mg of Aredia as a single 24-hour intravenous infusion or 7.5 mg/kg of Didronel (etidronate disodium) as a 2-hour intravenous infusion daily for 3 days. Thirty patients were randomized to receive Aredia and 35 to receive Didronel.

The mean baseline-corrected serum calcium for the Aredia 60 mg and Didronel groups were 14.6 mg/dL and 13.8 mg/dL, respectively.

By day 7, 70% of the patients in the Aredia group and 41% of the patients in the Didronel group had normal-corrected serum calcium levels ($P < 0.05$). When partial responders (≥15% decrease of serum calcium from baseline) were also included, the response rates were 97% for the Aredia group and 65% for the Didronel group ($P < 0.01$). Mean-corrected serum calcium for the Aredia and Didronel groups decreased from baseline values to 10.4 and 11.2 mg/dL, respectively, on day 7. At day 14, 43% of patients in the Aredia group and 18% of patients in the Didronel group still had normal-corrected serum calcium levels, or maintenance of a partial response. For responders in the Aredia and Didronel groups, the median duration of response was similar (7 and 5 days, respectively). The time course of effect on corrected serum calcium is summarized in the following table.

Continued on next page

Table 1
Mean (SD, CV%) Pamidronate Pharmacokinetic Parameters in Cancer Patients
(n=6 for each group)

Dose (Infusion rate)	Maximum Concentration (ug/mL)	Percent of dose excreted in urine	Total Clearance (mL/min)	Renal Clearance (mL/min)
30 mg (4 hrs)	0.73 (0.14, 19.1%)	43.9 (14.0, 31.9%)	136 (44, 32.4%)	58 (27, 46.5%)
60 mg (4 hrs)	1.44 (0.57, 39.6%)	47.4 (47.4, 54.4%)	88 (56, 63.6%)	42 (28, 66.7%)
90 mg (4 hrs)	2.61 (0.74, 28.3%)	45.3 (25.8, 56.9%)	103 (37, 35.9%)	44 (16, 36.4%)
90 mg (24 hrs)	1.38 (1.97, 142.7%)	47.5 (10.2, 21.5%)	101 (58, 57.4%)	52 (42, 80.8%)

CibaGeneva—Cont.

Change in Corrected Serum Calcium by Time from Initiation of Treatment

Time (hr)	Mean Change from Baseline in Corrected Serum Calcium (mg/dL)		
	Aredia	Didronel	p Value[1]
Baseline	14.6	13.8	
24	−0.3	−0.5	
48	−1.5	−1.1	
72	−2.6	−2.0	
96	−3.5	−2.0	<0.01
168	−4.1	−2.5	<0.01

[1] Comparison between treatment groups

In a third multicenter, randomized, parallel double-blind trial, a group of 69 cancer patients with hypercalcemia was enrolled to receive 60 mg of Aredia as a 4- or 24-hour infusion, which was compared to a saline treatment group. Patients who had a corrected serum calcium level of ≥12.0 mg/dL after 24 hours of saline hydration were eligible for this trial.

The mean baseline-corrected serum calcium levels for Aredia 60-mg 4-hour infusion, Aredia 60-mg 24-hour infusion, and saline infusion were 14.2 mg/dL, 13.7 mg/dL, and 13.7 mg/dL, respectively.

By day 7 after initiation of treatment, 78%, 61%, and 22% of the patients had normal-corrected serum calcium levels for the 60-mg 4-hour infusion, 60-mg 24 hour infusion, and saline infusion, respectively. At day 14, 39% of the patients in the Aredia 60-mg 4-hour infusion group and 26% of the patients in the Aredia 60-mg 24-hour infusion group had normal-corrected serum calcium levels or maintenance of a partial response.

For responders, the median duration of complete responses was 4 days and 6.5 days for Aredia 60-mg 4-hour infusion and Aredia 60-mg 24-hour infusion, respectively.

In all three trials, patients treated with Aredia had similar response rates in the presence or absence of bone metastases. Concomitant administration of furosemide did not affect response rates.

Thirty-two patients who had recurrent or refractory hypercalcemia of malignancy were given a second course of 60 mg of Aredia over a 4- or 24-hour period. Of these, 41% showed a complete response and 16% showed a partial response to the retreatment, and these responders had about a 3-mg/dL fall in mean-corrected serum calcium levels 7 days after retreatment.

Unlike Aredia 60 mg, the drug has not been investigated in a controlled clinical trial employing a 90-mg dose infused over a 4-hour period.

Paget's Disease

Paget's disease of bone (osteitis deformans) is an idiopathic disease characterized by chronic, focal areas of bone destruction complicated by concurrent excessive bone repair, affecting one or more bones. These changes result in thickened but weakened bones that may fracture or bend under stress. Signs and symptoms may be bone pain, deformity, fractures, neurological disorders resulting from cranial and spinal nerve entrapment and from spinal cord and brain stem compression, increased cardiac output to the involved bone, increased serum alkaline phosphatase levels (reflecting increased bone formation) and/or urine hydroxyproline excretion (reflecting increased bone resorption).

Clinical Trials

In one double-blind clinical trial, 64 patients with moderate to severe Paget's disease of bone were enrolled to receive 5 mg, 15 mg, or 30 mg of Aredia as a single 4-hour infusion on 3 consecutive days, for total doses of 15 mg, 45 mg, and 90 mg of Aredia.

The mean baseline serum alkaline phosphatase levels were 1409 U/L, 983 U/L, and 1085 U/L, and the mean baseline urine hydroxyproline/creatinine ratios were 0.25, 0.19, and 0.19 for the 15-mg, 45-mg, and 90-mg groups, respectively.

The effects of Aredia on serum alkaline phosphatase (SAP) and urine hydroxyproline/creatinine ratios (UOHP/C) are summarized in the following table:

Percent of Patients With Significant % Decreases in SAP and UOHP/C

% Decrease	SAP			UOHP/C		
	15 mg	45 mg	90 mg	15 mg	45 mg	90 mg
≥50	26	33	60	15	47	72
≥30	40	65	83	35	57	85

The median maximum percent decreases from baseline in serum alkaline phosphatase and urine hydroxyproline/creatinine ratios were 25%, 41%, and 57%, and 25%, 47%, and 61% for the 15-mg, 45-mg, and 90-mg groups, respectively. The median time to response (≥50% decrease) for serum alkaline phosphatase was approximately 1 month for the 90-mg group, and the response duration ranged from 1 to 372 days.

No statistically significant differences between treatment groups, or statistically significant changes from baseline were observed for the bone pain response, mobility, and global evaluation in the 45-mg and 90-mg groups. Improvement in radiologic lesions occurred in some patients in the 90-mg group.

Twenty-five patients who had Paget's disease were retreated with 90 mg of Aredia. Of these, 44% had a ≥50% decrease in serum alkaline phosphatase from baseline after treatment, and 39% had a ≥50% decrease in urine hydroxyproline/creatinine ratio from baseline after treatment.

Osteolytic Bone Lesions of Multiple Myeloma

Osteolytic bone destruction is a common characteristic of multiple myeloma. Bone destruction can occur as diffuse osteopenia, with radiographic findings similar to those of postmenopausal osteoporosis, or as discrete osteolytic lesions occurring in the axial and appendicular skeleton. Bone disease in multiple myeloma results from the release of soluble factors by myeloma cells that activate osteoclasts to resorb bone.

These bone changes can result in patients having evidence of osteolytic skeletal destruction leading to severe bone pain that requires either radiation therapy or narcotic analgesics (or both) for symptomatic relief. These changes also cause pathologic fractures of bone in both the axial and appendicular skeleton. Axial skeletal fractures of the vertebral bodies may lead to spinal cord compression or collapse with significant neurologic complications. Also, patients may experience episode(s) of hypercalcemia.

Clinical Trials

In a double-blind, randomized, placebo-controlled trial, 392 patients with advanced multiple myeloma were enrolled to receive Aredia or placebo in addition to their underlying antimyeloma therapy to determine the effect of Aredia on the occurrence of skeletal-related events (SRE's).

SRE's were defined as episodes of pathologic fractures, radiation therapy to bone, surgery to bone, and spinal cord compression. Patients received either 90 mg of Aredia or placebo as a monthly 4-hour intravenous infusion for 9 months. Of the 392 patients, 377 were evaluable for efficacy (196 Aredia, 181 placebo). The proportion of patients developing any SRE was significantly smaller in the Aredia group (24% vs 41%, P<0.001), and the mean skeletal morbidity rate (#SRE/year) was significantly greater for placebo than for Aredia patients (2.1 vs 1.1, P<.02). The times to the first SRE occurrence, pathologic fracture, and radiation to bone were significantly longer in the Aredia group (P=.001, .006, and .046, respectively). Moreover, fewer-Aredia patients suffered any pathologic fracture (17% vs 30%, P=.004) or needed radiation to bone (14% vs 22%, P=.049).

In addition, decreases in pain scores from baseline occurred at the last measurement for those Aredia patients with pain at baseline (P=.026) but not in the placebo group. At the last measurement, a worsening from baseline was observed in the placebo group for the Spitzer quality of life variable (P<.001) and ECOG performance status (P<.011) while there was no significant deterioration from baseline in these parameters observed in Aredia-treated patients.*

*The statistical significance of analyses of these secondary endpoints of pain, quality of life, and performance status may be overestimated since numerous analyses were performed.

INDICATIONS AND USAGE

Hypercalcemia of Malignancy

Aredia, in conjunction with adequate hydration, is indicated for the treatment of moderate or severe hypercalcemia associated with malignancy, with or without bone metastases. Patients who have either epidermoid or non-epidermoid tumors respond to treatment with Aredia. Vigorous saline hydration, an integral part of hypercalcemia therapy, should be initiated promptly and an attempt should be made to restore the urine output to about 2 L/day throughout treatment. Mild or asymptomatic hypercalcemia may be treated with conservative measures (i.e., saline hydration, with or without loop diuretics). Patients should be hydrated adequately throughout the treatment, but overhydration, especially in those patients who have cardiac failure, must be avoided. Diuretic therapy should not be employed prior to correction of hypovolemia. The safety and efficacy of Aredia in the treatment of hypercalcemia associated with hyperparathyroidism or with other non-tumor-related conditions has not been established.

Paget's Disease

Aredia is indicated for the treatment of patients with moderate to severe Paget's disease of bone. The effectiveness of Aredia was demonstrated primarily in patients with serum alkaline phosphatase ≥3 times the upper limit of normal. Aredia therapy in patients with Paget's disease has been effective in reducing serum alkaline phosphatase and urinary hydroxyproline levels by ≥50% in at least 50% of patients, and by ≥30% in at least 80% of patients. Aredia therapy has also been effective in reducing these biochemical markers in patients with Paget's disease who failed to respond, or no longer responded to other treatments.

Osteolytic Bone Lesions of Multiple Myeloma

Aredia is indicated, in conjunction with standard antimyeloma chemotherapy, for the treatment of patients with osteolytic bone lesions of multiple myeloma.

CONTRAINDICATIONS

Aredia is contraindicated in patients with clinically significant hypersensitivity to Aredia or other bisphosphonates.

WARNINGS

In both rats and dogs, nephropathy has been associated with intravenous (bolus and infusion) administration of Aredia.

Two 7-day intravenous infusion studies were conducted in the dog wherein Aredia was given for 1, 4, or 24 hours at doses of 1–20 mg/kg for up to 7 days. In the first study, the compound was well tolerated at 3 mg/kg (1.7 × highest recommended human dose [HRHD] for a single intravenous infusion) when administered for 4 or 24 hours, but renal findings such as elevated BUN and creatinine levels and renal tubular necrosis occurred when 3 mg/kg was infused for 1 hour and at doses of ≥10 mg/kg. In the second study, slight renal tubular necrosis was observed in 1 male at 1 mg/kg when infused for 4 hours. Additional findings included elevated BUN levels in several treated animals and renal tubular dilation and/or inflammation at ≥1 mg/kg after each infusion time.

Aredia was given to rats at doses of 2, 6, and 20 mg/kg and to dogs at doses of 2, 4, 6, and 20 mg/kg as a 1-hour infusion, once a week, for 3 months followed by a 1-month recovery period. In rats, nephrotoxicity was observed at ≥6 mg/kg and included increased BUN and creatinine levels and tubular degeneration and necrosis. These findings were still present at 20 mg/kg at the end of the recovery period. In dogs, moribundity/death and renal toxicity occurred at 20 mg/kg as did kidney findings of elevated BUN and creatinine levels at ≥6 mg/kg and renal tubular degeneration at ≥4 mg/kg. The kidney changes were partially reversible at 6 mg/kg. In both studies, the dose level that produced no adverse renal effects was considered to be 2 mg/kg (1.1 × HRHD for a single intravenous infusion).

Patients who receive an intravenous infusion of Aredia should have periodic evaluations of standard laboratory and clinical parameters of renal function.

Studies conducted in young rats have reported the disruption of dental dentine formation following single- and multi-dose administration of bisphosphonates. The clinical significance of these findings is unknown.

PRECAUTIONS

General

Standard hypercalcemia-related metabolic parameters, such as serum levels of calcium, phosphate, magnesium, and potassium should be carefully monitored following initiation of therapy with Aredia. Cases of asymptomatic hypophosphatemia (12%), hypokalemia (7%), hypomagnesemia (11%), and hypocalcemia (5%–12%), were reported in Aredia-treated patients. Rare cases of symptomatic hypocalcemia (including tetany) have been reported in association with Aredia therapy. If hypocalcemia occurs, short-term calcium therapy may be necessary. In Paget's disease of bone, 17% of patients treated with 90 mg of Aredia showed serum calcium levels below 8 mg/dL.

Aredia has not been tested in patients who have class Dc renal impairment (creatinine >5.0 mg/dL), and in few multiple myeloma patients with serum creatinine ≥3.0 mg/dL. (See also CLINICAL PHARMACOLOGY, Pharmacokinetics.) Clinical judgment should determine whether the potential benefit outweighs the potential risk in such patients.

Laboratory Tests

Serum calcium, electrolytes, phosphate, magnesium and creatinine, and CBC, differential, and hematocrit/hemoglobin must be closely monitored in patients treated with Aredia. Patients who have preexisting anemia, leukopenia, or thrombocytopenia should be monitored carefully in the first 2 weeks following treatment.

Drug Interactions

Concomitant administration of a loop diuretic had no effect on the calcium-lowering action of Aredia.

Carcinogenesis, Mutagenesis, Impairment of Fertility

In a 104-week carcinogenicity study (daily oral administration) in rats, there was a positive dose response relationship for benign adrenal pheochromocytoma in males (p <0.00001). Although this condition was also observed in females, the incidence was not statistically significant. When the dose calculations were adjusted to account for the limited oral bioavailability of Aredia in rats, the lowest daily dose associated with adrenal pheochromocytoma was similar to the intended clinical dose. Adrenal pheochromocytoma was also observed in low numbers in the control animals and is considered a relatively common spontaneous neoplasm in the rat. Aredia (daily oral administration) was not carcinogenic in an 80-week study in mice.

Aredia was nonmutagenic in six mutagenicity assays: Ames test, *Salmonella* and *Escherichia*/liver-microsome test, nu-

cleus-anomaly test, sister-chromatid-exchange study, point-mutation test, and micronucleus test in the rat.

In rats, decreased fertility occurred in first-generation offspring of parents who had received 150 mg/kg of Aredia orally; however, this occurred only when animals were mated with members of the same dose group. Aredia has not been administered intravenously in such a study.

Pregnancy Category C

There are no adequate and well-controlled studies in pregnant women.

Bolus intravenous studies conducted in rats and rabbits determined that Aredia produces maternal toxicity and embryo/fetal effects when given during organogenesis at doses of 0.6 to 8.3 times the highest recommended human dose for a single intravenous infusion. As it has been shown that Aredia can cross the placenta in rats and has produced marked maternal and nonteratogenic embryo/fetal effects in rats and rabbits, it should not be given to women during pregnancy.

Nursing Mothers

It is not known whether Aredia is excreted in human milk. Because many drugs are excreted in human milk, caution should be exercised when Aredia is administered to a nursing woman.

Pediatric Use

Safety and effectiveness of Aredia in pediatric patients have not been established.

ADVERSE REACTIONS

Hypercalcemia of Malignancy

Transient mild elevation of temperature by at least 1°C was noted 24 to 48 hours after administration of Aredia in 34% of patients in clinical trials. In the saline trial, 18% of patients had a temperature elevation of at least 1°C 24 to 48 hours after treatment.

Drug-related local soft-tissue symptoms (redness, swelling or induration and pain on palpation) at the site of catheter insertion were most common (18%) in patients treated with 90 mg of Aredia. When all on-therapy events are considered, that rate rises to 41%. Symptomatic treatment resulted in rapid resolution in all patients.

Rare cases of uveitis, iritis, scleritis, and episcleritis have been reported, including one case of scleritis, and one case of uveitis upon separate rechallenges.

Four of 128 patients (3%) who received Aredia during the three U.S. controlled hypercalcemia clinical studies were reported to have had seizures, 2 of whom had preexisting seizure disorders. None of the seizures were considered to be drug-related by the investigators. However, a possible relationship between the drug and the occurrence of seizures cannot be ruled out. It should be noted that in the saline arm 1 patient (4%) had a seizure.

At least 15% of patients treated with Aredia for hypercalcemia of malignancy also experienced the following adverse events during a clinical trial:

General: Fluid overload, generalized pain
Cardiovascular: Hypertension
Gastrointestinal: Abdominal pain, anorexia, constipation, nausea, vomiting
Genitourinary: Urinary tract infection
Musculoskeletal: Bone pain
Laboratory abnormality: Anemia, hypokalemia, hypomagnesemia, hypophosphatemia

Many of these adverse experiences may have been related to the underlying disease state.

The following table lists the adverse experiences considered to be treatment-related during comparative, controlled U.S. trials.

[See table above.]

Paget's Disease

Transient mild elevation of temperature >1°C above pretreatment baseline was noted within 48 hours after completion of treatment in 21% of the patients treated with 90 mg of Aredia in clinical trials.

Drug-related musculoskeletal pain and nervous system symptoms (dizziness, headache, paresthesia, increased sweating) were more common in patients with Paget's disease treated with 90 mg of Aredia than in patients with hypercalcemia of malignancy treated with the same dose.

Adverse experiences considered to be related to trial drug, which occurred in at least 5% of patients with Paget's disease treated with 90 mg of Aredia in two U.S. clinical trials, were fever, nausea, back pain, and bone pain.

At least 10% of all Aredia-treated patients with Paget's disease also experienced the following adverse experiences during clinical trials:

Cardiovascular: Hypertension
Musculoskeletal: Arthrosis, bone pain
Nervous system: Headache

Most of these adverse experiences may have been related to the underlying disease state.

Osteolytic Bone Lesions of Multiple Myeloma

The most commonly reported (> 15%) adverse experiences occurred with similar frequencies in the Aredia and placebo treatment groups, and most of these adverse experiences may have been related to the underlying disease state or antimyeloma therapy.

Treatment-Related Adverse Experiences Reported in Three U.S. Controlled Clinical Trials					
Percent of Patients					
	Aredia			Didronel	Saline
	60 mg over 4 hr n=23	60 mg over 24 hr n=73	90 mg over 24 hr n=17	7.5 mg/kg × 3 days n=35	n=23
General					
Edema	0	1	0	0	0
Fatigue	0	0	12	0	0
Fever	26	19	18	9	0
Fluid overload	0	0	0	6	0
Infusion-site reaction	0	4	18	0	0
Moniliasis	0	0	6	0	0
Rigors	0	0	0	0	4
Gastrointestinal					
Abdominal pain	0	1	0	0	0
Anorexia	4	1	12	0	0
Constipation	4	0	6	3	0
Diarrhea	0	1	0	0	0
Dyspepsia	4	0	0	0	0
Gastrointestinal hemorrhage	0	0	6	0	0
Nausea	4	0	18	6	0
Stomatitis	0	1	0	3	0
Vomiting	4	0	0	0	0
Respiratory					
Dyspnea	0	0	0	3	0
Rales	0	0	6	0	0
Rhinitis	0	0	6	0	0
Upper respiratory infection	0	3	0	0	0
CNS					
Anxiety	0	0	0	0	4
Convulsions	0	0	0	3	0
Insomnia	0	1	0	0	0
Nervousness	0	0	0	0	4
Psychosis	4	0	0	0	0
Somnolence	0	1	6	0	0
Taste perversion	0	0	0	3	0
Cardiovascular					
Atrial fibrillation	0	0	6	0	4
Atrial flutter	0	1	0	0	0
Cardiac failure	0	1	0	0	0
Hypertension	0	0	6	0	4
Syncope	0	0	6	0	0
Tachycardia	0	0	6	0	4
Endocrine					
Hypothyroidism	0	0	6	0	0
Hemic and Lymphatic					
Anemia	0	0	6	0	0
Leukopenia	4	0	0	0	0
Neutropenia	0	1	0	0	0
Thrombocytopenia	0	1	0	0	0
Musculoskeletal					
Myalgia	0	1	0	0	0
Urogenital					
Uremia	4	0	0	0	0
Laboratory Abnormalities					
Hypocalcemia	0	1	12	0	0
Hypokalemia	4	4	18	0	0
Hypomagnesemia	4	10	12	3	4
Hypophosphatemia	0	9	18	3	0
Abnormal liver function	0	0	0	3	0

Commonly Reported Adverse Experiences In One U.S. Controlled Clinical Trial

	Aredia %	Placebo %
Fever	31.5	27.0
Anemia*	29.6	31.7
Nausea	26.6	31.2
Fatigue	22.7	21.2
Upper Respiratory Infection	23.2	19.6
Diarrhea	19.2	19.6
Constipation	18.2	20.1
Headache	17.7	16.4
Coughing	15.9	15.8
Dyspnea	16.4	14.8

*Severe anemia (whether or not trial-drug-related) was reported in 10.8% and 5.8% of the patients treated with Aredia and placebo, respectively.

Toxicities commonly associated with chemotherapy, including cytopenia, infection, nausea and vomiting, and cachexia,

were not more frequent or severe in Aredia patients than in placebo patients. Mineral and electrolyte disturbances, including hypocalcemia, were reported rarely and in similar percentages of Aredia-treated patients compared with those in the placebo group. The reported frequencies of hypocalcemia, hypokalemia, hypophosphatemia, and hypomagnesemia for Aredia-treated patients were 3.4%, 5.9%, 1.5%, and 3.4%, respectively, and for placebo-treated patients were 0.5%, 8.5%, 0.5%, and 4.2%, respectively. In previous hypercalcemia of malignancy trials, patients treated with Aredia (60 or 90 mg over 24 hours) developed electrolyte abnormalities more frequently (see ADVERSE REACTIONS, Hypercalcemia of Malignancy).

Arthralgias and myalgias were reported slightly more frequently in the Aredia group than in the placebo group (6.4% and 14.8% vs 3.7% and 9.5%, respectively).

One Aredia-treated patient experienced allergic reactions (of moderate severity) characterized by swollen and itchy eyes, runny nose, and scratchy throat within 24 hours after the sixth infusion.

Continued on next page

Consult 1997 supplements and future editions for revisions

CibaGeneva—Cont.

OVERDOSAGE

There have been several cases of drug maladministration of intravenous Aredia in hypercalcemia patients with total doses of 225 mg to 300 mg given over $2^1/_2$ to 4 days. All of these patients survived, but they experienced hypocalcemia that required intravenous and/or oral administration of calcium.

In addition, one obese woman (95 kg) who was treated with 285 mg of Aredia/day for 3 days, experienced high fever (39.5°C), hypotension (from 170/90 mmHg to 90/60 mmHg), and transient taste perversion, noted about 6 hours after the first infusion. The fever and hypotension were rapidly corrected with steroids.

If overdosage occurs, symptomatic hypocalcemia could also result; such patients should be treated with short-term intravenous calcium.

DOSAGE AND ADMINISTRATION

Hypercalcemia of Malignancy

Consideration should be given to the severity of as well as the symptoms of hypercalcemia. Vigorous saline hydration alone may be sufficient for treating mild, asymptomatic hypercalcemia. Overhydration should be avoided in patients who have potential for cardiac failure. In hypercalcemia associated with hematologic malignancies, the use of glucocorticoid therapy may be helpful.

Moderate Hypercalcemia

The recommended dose of Aredia in moderate hypercalcemia (corrected serum calcium* of approximately 12–13.5 mg/dL) is 60 to 90 mg. The 60-mg dose is given as an initial, SINGLE-DOSE, intravenous infusion over at least 4 hours. The 90-mg dose must be given by an initial, SINGLE-DOSE, intravenous infusion over 24 hours.

Severe Hypercalcemia

The recommended dose of Aredia in severe hypercalcemia (corrected serum calcium* > 13.5 mg/dL) is 90 mg. The 90-mg dose must be given by an initial, SINGLE-DOSE, intravenous infusion over 24 hours.

*** Albumin-corrected serum calcium (CCa, mg/dL) = serum calcium, mg/dL + 0.8 (4.0-serum albumin, g/dL).**

Retreatment

A limited number of patients have received more than one treatment with Aredia for hypercalcemia. Retreatment with Aredia, in patients who show complete or partial response initially, may be carried out if serum calcium does not return to normal or remain normal after initial treatment. **It is recommended that a minimum of 7 days elapse before retreatment, to allow for full response to the initial dose.** The dose and manner of retreatment is identical to that of the initial therapy.

Paget's Disease

The recommended dose of Aredia in patients with moderate to severe Paget's disease of bone is 30 mg daily, administered as a 4-hour infusion on 3 consecutive days for a total dose of 90 mg.

Retreatment

A limited number of patients with Paget's disease have received more than one treatment of Aredia in clinical trials. When clinically indicated, patients should be retreated at the dose of initial therapy.

Osteolytic Bone Lesions of Multiple Myeloma

The recommended dose of Aredia in patients with osteolytic bone lesions of multiple myeloma is 90 mg administered as a 4-hour infusion given on a monthly basis. Aredia has been given frequently with dexamethasone, prednisone, prednisolone, cyclophosphamide, melphalan, vincristine, interferon alfa, carmustine, and infrequently with etoposide, cisplatin, mitoxantrone, cytarabine, solumedrol, idarubicin, thiotepa, and carboplatin.

Patients with marked Bence-Jones proteinuria and dehydration should receive adequate hydration prior to Aredia infusion.

Limited information is available on the use of Aredia in multiple myeloma patients with a serum creatinine ≥3.0 mg/dL.

There is little data on the safety or efficacy of Aredia given beyond a duration of 9 months.

Preparation of Solution

Reconstitution

Aredia is reconstituted by adding 10 mL of Sterile Water for Injection, USP, to each vial, resulting in a solution of 30 mg/10 mL, 60 mg/10 mL, or 90 mg/10 mL. The pH of the reconstituted solution is 6.0–7.4. The drug should be completely dissolved before the solution is withdrawn.

Hyercalcemia of Malignancy

The daily dose must be administered as an intravenous infusion over at least 4 hours for the 60-mg dose, and over 24 hours for the 90-mg dose. The recommended dose should be diluted in 1000 mL of sterile 0.45% or 0.9% Sodium Chloride, USP, or 5% Dextrose Injection, USP. This infusion solution is stable for up to 24 hours at room temperature.

Paget's Disease

The recommended dose of 30 mg should be diluted in 500 mL of sterile 0.45% or 0.9% Sodium Chloride, USP, or 5% Dextrose Injection, USP, and administered over a 4-hour period for 3 consecutive days.

Osteolytic Bone Lesions of Multiple Myeloma

The recommended dose of 90 mg should be diluted with 500 mL of sterile 0.45% or 0.9% Sodium Chloride, USP, or 5% Dextrose Injection, USP, and administered over a 4–hour period on a monthly basis.

Aredia must not be mixed with calcium-containing infusion solutions, such as Ringer's solution, and should be given in a single intravenous solution and line separate from all other drugs.

Note: **Parenteral drug products should be inspected visually for particulate matter and discoloration prior to administration, whenever solution and container permit.**

Aredia reconstituted with Sterile Water for Injection may be stored under refrigeration at 36°–46°F (2°–8°C) for up to 24 hours.

HOW SUPPLIED

Vials—30 mg—each contains 30 mg of sterile, lyophilized pamidronate disodium and 470 mg of mannitol, USP.

Carton of 4 vials .... NDC 0083-2601-04

Vials—60 mg—each contains 60 mg of sterile, lyophilized pamidronate disodium and 400 mg of mannitol, USP.

Carton of 1 vial .... NDC 0083-2606-01

Vials—90 mg—each contains 90 mg of sterile, lyophilized pamidronate disodium and 375 mg of mannitol, USP.

Carton of 1 vial .... NDC 0083-2609-01

Do not store above 86°F (30°C).

Caution: Federal law prohibits dispensing without prescription.

C95-38 (Rev. 8/95)

Dist. by:
Ciba-Geigy Corporation
Pharmaceuticals Division
Summit, New Jersey 07901

BRETHAIRE® ℞

[*breth-air'*]

terbutaline sulfate inhalation aerosol
Bronchodilator Aerosol
For Oral Inhalation Only

DESCRIPTION

Brethaire is a bronchodilator aerosol for oral inhalation. The active ingredient of Brethaire is terbutaline sulfate USP, (±)-α-[(*tert*-butylamino) methyl]-3,5-dihydroxybenzylalcohol sulfate (2:1) (salt), a beta-adrenergic agonist. The empirical formula is $(C_{12}H_{19}NO_3)_2 \cdot H_2SO_4$.

Terbutaline sulfate USP is a white to gray-white crystalline powder. It is odorless or has a faint odor of acetic acid. It is soluble in water and in 0.1N hydrochloric acid, slightly soluble in methanol, and insoluble in chloroform. Its molecular weight is 548.65.

Brethaire is a metered-dose dispenser containing micronized terbutaline sulfate in a suspension of the following composition:

	7.5-ml (10.5-g) Canister
terbutaline sulfate USP	0.075 g
sorbitan trioleate	0.105 g
trichloromonofluoromethane NF	2.58 g
dichlorotetrafluoroethane NF	2.58 g
dichlorodifluoromethane NF	5.16 g

Each actuation delivers 0.20 mg of terbutaline sulfate from the mouthpiece (0.25 mg valve delivery). Each canister provides at least 300 inhalations.

CLINICAL PHARMACOLOGY

Brethaire is a beta-adrenergic-receptor agonist that has been shown by in vitro and in vivo studies in animals to exert a preferential effect on $beta_2$-adrenergic receptors. While it is recognized that $beta_2$-adrenergic receptors are the predominant receptors in bronchial smooth muscle, recent data indicate that there is a population of $beta_2$-receptors in the human heart existing in a concentration between 10–50%. The precise function of these, however, is not yet established (see PRECAUTIONS). Controlled clinical studies in patients who were administered Brethaire have not revealed a preferential $beta_2$-adrenergic effect.

The pharmacologic effects of beta-adrenergic agonists, including Brethaire, are at least in part attributable to stimulation through beta-adrenergic receptors of intracellular adenyl cyclase, the enzyme which catalyzes the conversion of adenosine triphosphate (ATP) to cyclic 3'5'- adenosine monophosphate (cAMP). Increased cAMP levels are associated with relaxation of bronchial smooth muscle and inhibition of release of mediators of immediate hypersensitivity from cells, especially from mast cells.

Terbutaline sulfate by inhaler has been shown in controlled clinical studies to relieve bronchospasm associated with chronic obstructive pulmonary disease such as asthma, chronic bronchitis, and emphysema. This action was manifested by a clinically significant improvement in pulmonary function as demonstrated by an increase in FEV_1 of 15% or more in some patients. Terbutaline sulfate by inhaler also produced clinically significant increases in peak expiratory flow rate and instantaneous flow rates at 75, 50, and 25% of vital capacity. There were also clinically significant reductions in functional residual capacity, residual volume, and airway resistance in some patients. Clinically significant improvement in pulmonary function occurred within 5 to 30 minutes in most patients after administration of the drug. The response was well established by 5 minutes and the maximal effect usually occurred between 1 and 2 hours in most patients. Significant bronchodilator activity has been observed to persist for 3 to 4 hours after dosing in many patients in 3-month repetitive-dose studies. With continued administration of Brethaire, the duration of effectiveness decreases in most patients.

Recent studies in laboratory animals (minipigs, rodents, and dogs), recorded the occurrence of cardiac arrhythmias and sudden death (with histologic evidence of myocardial necrosis) when beta agonists and methylxanthines were administered concurrently. The significance of these findings when applied to humans is currently unknown.

INDICATIONS AND USAGE

Brethaire is indicated for the relief of bronchospasm in patients with reversible obstructive airway disease.

In controlled clinical trials the onset of improvement in pulmonary function was within 5 to 30 minutes. These studies also showed that maximum improvement in pulmonary function occurred at 120 minutes following two inhalations of Brethaire and that clinically significant improvement (i.e., 15% increase in FEV_1/predicted FEV_1) generally continued for 3 to 4 hours in most patients. In some studies there was a significant decrease in improvement of pulmonary function noted with continued administration of terbutaline sulfate aerosol. Continued effectiveness of Brethaire was demonstrated over a 14-week period in some patients in these clinical trials. Some patients with asthma, in single-dose studies only, have shown a therapeutic response that was still apparent at 6 hours.

CONTRAINDICATIONS

Brethaire is contraindicated in patients with a history of hypersensitivity to any of its components.

WARNINGS

As with other adrenergic aerosols, the potential for paradoxical bronchospasm (which can be life-threatening) should be kept in mind. If it occurs, the preparation should be discontinued immediately and alternative therapy instituted.

Fatalities have been reported in association with excessive use of inhaled sympathomimetic drugs. The exact cause of death is unknown. As with other beta-adrenergic aerosols, Brethaire should not be used in excess. Controlled clinical studies and other clinical experience have shown that Brethaire, like other inhaled beta-adrenergic agonists, can produce a significant cardiovascular effect in some patients, as measured by pulse rate, blood pressure, symptoms, and/or ECG changes.

There have been rare reports of seizures in patients receiving terbutaline; seizures did not recur in these patients after the drug was discontinued.

The contents of Brethaire are under pressure. Do not puncture the container. Do not use or store it near heat or open flame. Exposure to temperatures above 120°F may cause bursting. Never throw the container into a fire or incinerator. Keep it out of children's reach.

PRECAUTIONS

General

Terbutaline sulfate is a sympathomimetic amine and, as such, should be used with caution in patients with cardiovascular disorders, including coronary insufficiency and hypertension, in patients with hyperthyroidism or diabetes mellitus, and in patients who are unusually responsive to sympathomimetic amines.

Immediate hypersensitivity reactions and exacerbation of bronchospasm have been reported after terbutaline administration.

Large doses of intravenous terbutaline sulfate have been reported to aggravate preexisting diabetes and ketoacidosis.

Terbutaline sulfate should not be used for tocolysis.

Although there have been no reports concerning the use of aerosol terbutaline sulfate during labor and delivery, it has been reported that high doses of terbutaline sulfate administered intravenously inhibit uterine contractions. Although this effect is extremely unlikely as a consequence of aerosol use, it should be kept in mind.

Information for Patients

The action of Brethaire may last up to 6 hours, and therefore, it should not be used more frequently than recommended.

Patients should not increase the number or frequency of doses without consulting the physician. If symptoms get worse, patients should consult their physician promptly.

While taking Brethaire, patients should not take other

inhaled medicines that have not been prescribed by the physician.
See illustrated Instructions for Patients.

Drug Interactions

Other sympathomimetic aerosol bronchodilators or epinephrine should not be used concomitantly with terbutaline sulfate. Terbutaline sulfate should be administered with caution to patients being treated with monoamine oxidase inhibitors or tricyclic antidepressants, since the action of terbutaline sulfate on the vascular system may be potentiated.
Beta-receptor-blocking agents and terbutaline sulfate inhibit the effect of each other.

Carcinogenesis, Mutagenesis, Impairment of Fertility

A 2-year oral carcinogenesis bioassay of terbutaline sulfate (50, 500, 1000, and 2000 mg/kg, corresponding to 1042, 10,417, 20,833, and 41,667 times the recommended daily adult dose) in Sprague-Dawley rats revealed drug-related changes in the female genital system. Female rats showed drug-related increases in leiomyomas of the mesovarium: 3 (5%) at 50 mg/kg, 17 (28%) at 500 mg/kg, 21 (35%) at 1000 mg/kg, and 23 (38%) at 2000 mg/kg, which were significant at the three highest levels. None occurred in female controls. The incidence of ovarian cysts was significantly elevated at all dose levels except 2000 mg/kg, and hyperplasia of the mesovarium was increased significantly at 500 and 2000 mg/kg.
A 21-month oral (feeding) study of terbutaline sulfate (5, 50, and 200 mg/kg, corresponding to 104, 1042, and 4167 times the recommended daily adult dose) in the mouse revealed no evidence of carcinogenicity.
Studies of terbutaline sulfate have not been conducted to determine mutagenic potential.
A Segment 1 oral reproduction study of terbutaline sulfate (up to 50 mg/kg corresponding to 1042 times the maximum clinical dose) in the rat revealed no adverse effects on fertility.

Pregnancy Category B

Reproduction studies have been performed in rats and rabbits at doses up to 1042 times the human dose and have revealed no evidence of impaired fertility or harm to the fetus due to terbutaline sulfate. There are, however, no adequate and well-controlled studies in pregnant women. Because animal reproduction studies are not always predictive of human response, this drug should be used during pregnancy only if clearly needed. For use in labor and delivery, see PRECAUTIONS, General.

Nursing Mothers

It is not known whether this drug is excreted in human milk. Because many drugs are excreted in human milk, caution should be exercised when terbutaline sulfate is administered to a nursing woman.

Pediatric Use

Safety and effectiveness in pediatric patients below the age of 12 years have not been established.

ADVERSE REACTIONS

The adverse reactions of terbutaline sulfate are similar to those of other sympathomimetic agents. A 14-week double-blind study compared terbutaline sulfate and isoproterenol aerosols in 259 asthmatic patients. The results of this study showed that the incidence of cardiovascular effects was as follows: palpitations, none with terbutaline and fewer than 5 per 100 with isoproterenol; tachycardia, about 3 per 100 with terbutaline and about 2 per 100 with isoproterenol; and increased blood pressure, fewer than 1 per 100 with terbutaline and about 2 per 100 with isoproterenol. In the same study, both drugs caused headache and nausea or digestive disorder in fewer than 10 patients per 100, tremor or nervousness in fewer than 5 patients per 100, and drowsiness in fewer than 5 patients per 100. About 4% of patients receiving terbutaline and about 1% of patients receiving isoproterenol had dysrhythmias. In addition, terbutaline sulfate, like other sympathomimetic agents, can cause adverse reactions such as angina, dyspnea and wheezing, vomiting, vertigo, central stimulation, insomnia, unusual taste, and drying or irritation of the oropharynx. Significantly more patients experienced dyspnea or wheezing, or both, after terbutaline than after isoproterenol administration. ECG changes such as sinus pause, atrial premature beats, AV block, ventricular premature beats, ST-T-wave depression, T-wave inversion, sinus bradycardia, and atrial escape beat with aberrant conduction were described after terbutaline administration. ECG changes were similar in frequency after isoproterenol administration.

OVERDOSAGE

Overdosage experience is limited. Excessive adrenergic-receptor stimulation may augment the signs and symptoms listed under ADVERSE REACTIONS and may be accompanied by other adrenergic effects. In the case of terbutaline overdosage, the patient should be treated symptomatically for the sympathomimetic overdosage with careful consideration given to the appropriateness of any chosen therapy and to the possible effect on the patient's underlying disease state.

DOSAGE AND ADMINISTRATION

The usual dosage for adults and children 12 years and older is two inhalations separated by a 60-second interval, repeated every 4 to 6 hours. Dosing should not be repeated more often than every 4 to 6 hours. The use of Brethaire can be continued as medically indicated to control recurring bouts of bronchospasm. During this time most patients gain optimal benefit from regular use of the inhaler. Safe usage for periods extending over several years has been documented.
If a previously effective dosage regimen fails to provide the usual relief, medical advice should be sought immediately, as this is often a sign of seriously worsening asthma, which would require reassessment of therapy.

HOW SUPPLIED

Brethaire contains 75 mg of terbutaline sulfate as a micronized powder in an inert propellant. This is sufficient medication for at least 300 actuations. Each actuation delivers approximately 0.20 mg of terbutaline sulfate from the mouthpiece (0.25 mg valve delivery).
Brethaire canister with mouthpiece, 7.5 ml (10.5 g)
....NDC 0028-5557-88
Each canister is supplied with a white plastic mouthpiece with a yellow-colored cap.
Brethaire canister refill without mouthpiece, 7.5 ml (10.5 g)
....NDC 0028-5557-87
Canister is for use with Brethaire inhalation aerosol mouthpiece only. The mouthpiece should not be used with other aerosol medications.
Store between 59°–86°F(15°–30°C).
Avoid spraying in eyes.
Dispense with enclosed instructions for use.
Note: The indented statement below is required by the Federal Government's Clean Air Act for all products containing or manufactured with chlorofluorocarbons (CFC's).

WARNING

> Contains trichloromonofluoromethane, dichlorotetrafluorethane and dichlorodifluoromethane, substances which harm public health and environment by destroying ozone in the upper atmosphere.

A notice similar to the above **WARNING** has been placed in the patient information leaflet of this product pursuant to EPA regulations.
Federal law prohibits dispensing without a prescription.
C95-50 (Rev. 11/95)

Dist. by:
Geigy Pharmaceuticals
Ciba-Geigy Corporation
Ardsley, New York 10502

BRETHAIRE® ℞
terbutaline sulfate inhalation aerosol

Instructions For Patients

Before using your BRETHAIRE inhaler, read complete instructions carefully.

1. **SHAKE THE INHALER WELL** immediately before each use. Then remove the cap from the mouthpiece. Test spray into the air before using for the first time and when the aerosol has not been used for a prolonged period. Inspect mouthpiece for possible foreign objects before each subsequent use.
2. **BREATHE OUT FULLY,** expelling as much air from your lungs as possible. Place the mouthpiece fully into the mouth holding the inhaler as shown in Figure 1 and closing the lips around it.

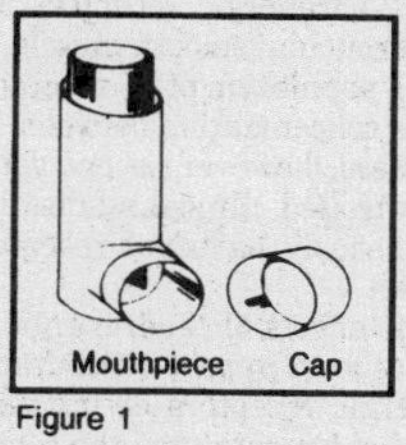

Figure 1

3. **WHILE BREATHING IN DEEPLY, FULLY DEPRESS THE TOP OF THE METAL CANISTER** with your index finger (see Figure 2).

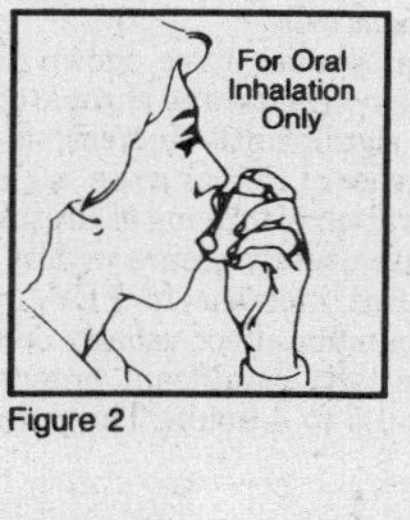

Figure 2

4. **HOLD YOUR BREATH AS LONG AS POSSIBLE.** Before breathing out, remove the inhaler from your mouth and release your finger from the canister.
5. Wait one minute and SHAKE the inhaler again. Repeat steps two through four for a second inhalation if prescribed by your doctor.
6. Replace cap after each use.
7. **CLEANSE THE INHALER THOROUGHLY AND FREQUENTLY.** Remove the metal canister and cleanse the plastic case and cap by rinsing thoroughly in warm running water at least once a day. After thoroughly drying the plastic case and cap, gently replace the canister into the case with a twisting motion and replace the cap.

DOSAGE: Use only as directed by your doctor.
WARNINGS: The action of BRETHAIRE inhaler may last up to six hours and therefore it should not be used more frequently than recommended. Do not increase the number or frequency of doses without consulting your physician. If symptoms do not improve, or get worse, consult your physician immediately. While taking BRETHAIRE inhaler, other inhaled medicines should be used only as prescribed by your physician.
Contents Under Pressure. Do not puncture.
Do not use or store near heat or open flame. Exposure to temperatures above 120°F may cause bursting.
Never throw container into fire or incinerator.
Keep out of reach of children.
Store between 59°–86°F (15°–30°C).
Canister is for use with Brethaire inhalation aerosol mouthpiece only. The mouthpiece should not be used with other aerosol medications.
Avoid spraying in eyes.
Note: The indented statement below is required by the Federal Government's Clean Air Act for all products containing or manufactured with chlorofluorocarbons (CFC's).
This product contains trichloromonofluoromethane, dichlorotetrafluoroethane and dichlorodifluoromethane, substances which harm public health and environment by destroying ozone in the upper atmosphere.
Your physician has determined that this product is likely to help your personal health. USE THIS PRODUCT AS DIRECTED, UNLESS INSTRUCTED TO DO OTHERWISE BY YOUR PHYSICIAN. If you have any questions about alternatives, consult with your physician.
C95-49 (Rev.11/95)

Dist. by:
Ciba-Geigy Corporation
Pharmaceuticals Division
Summit, NJ 07901
Shown in Product Identification Guide, page 309

BRETHINE® ℞
[breth-een ']
terbutaline sulfate tablets USP
Tablets of 5 mg
Tablets of 2.5 mg

DESCRIPTION

Brethine, terbutaline sulfate USP, is a bronchodilator available as tablets of 2.5 mg (2.05 mg of the free base) and 5 mg (4.1 mg of the free base) for oral administration. Terbutaline sulfate is ±-α-[(*tert*-Butylamino)methyl]-3,5-dihydroxybenzyl alcohol sulfate (2:1) (salt).
Terbutaline sulfate USP is a white to gray-white crystalline powder. It is odorless or has a faint odor of acetic acid. It is soluble in water and in 0.1N hydrochloric acid, slightly soluble in methanol, and insoluble in chloroform. Its molecular weight is 548.65.
Inactive Ingredients. Cellulose compounds, lactose, magnesium stearate, povidone, and starch.

ACTIONS

Brethine is a β-adrenergic receptor agonist which has been shown by *in vitro* and *in vivo* pharmacological studies in animals to exert a preferential effect on β_2-adrenergic receptors such as those located in bronchial smooth muscle. Controlled clinical studies in patients who were administered the drug orally have revealed proportionally greater changes in pulmonary function parameters than in heart rate or blood pressure. While this *suggests* a relative preference for the β_2 receptor in man, the usual cardiovascular effects commonly associated with sympathomimetic agents were also observed with Brethine.
Brethine has been shown in controlled clinical studies to relieve bronchospasm in chronic obstructive pulmonary disease.
This action is manifested by a clinically significant increase in pulmonary function as demonstrated by an increase of 15% or more in FEV_1 and in $FEF_{25\text{-}75\%}$. Following administration of Brethine tablets, a measurable change in flow rate is usually observed in 30 minutes, and a clinically significant improvement in pulmonary function occurs at 60–120 min-

Continued on next page

CibaGeneva—Cont.

utes. The maximum effect usually occurs within 120-180 minutes. Brethine also produces a clinically significant decrease in airway and pulmonary resistance which persists for at least four hours or longer. Significant bronchodilator action, as measured by various pulmonary function determinations (airway resistance, $FEF_{25\text{-}75\%}$, or PEFR), has been demonstrated in some studies for periods up to eight hours. Clinical studies were conducted in which the effectiveness of Brethine was evaluated in comparison with ephedrine over periods up to three months. Both drugs continued to produce significant improvement in pulmonary function throughout this period of treatment.

INDICATIONS

Brethine is indicated as a bronchodilator for bronchial asthma and for reversible bronchospasm which may occur in association with bronchitis and emphysema.

CONTRAINDICATIONS

Brethine is contraindicated when there is known hypersensitivity to sympathomimetic amines.

WARNINGS

There have been rare reports of seizures in patients receiving terbutaline; seizures did not recur in these patients after the drug was discontinued.

Controlled clinical studies and other clinical experience have shown that Brethine, like other β-adrenergic agonists, can produce a significant cardiovascular effect in some patients, as measured by pulse rate, blood pressure, symptoms, and/or ECG changes.

Usage in Pregnancy: Animal reproductive studies have been negative with respect to adverse effects on fetal development. The safe use of Brethine has not, however, been established in human pregnancy. As with any medication, the use of the drug in pregnancy, lactation, or women of childbearing potential requires that the expected therapeutic benefit of the drug be weighed against its possible hazards to the mother or child.

Usage in Pediatrics: Brethine tablets are not presently recommended for children below the age of 12 years due to insufficient clinical data in this pediatric group.

PRECAUTIONS

Brethine should be used with caution in patients with diabetes, hypertension, hyperthyroidism, and a history of seizures. Large doses of intravenous terbutaline sulfate have been reported to aggravate preexisting diabetes and ketoacidosis.

As with other sympathomimetic bronchodilator agents, Brethine should be administered cautiously to cardiac patients, especially those with associated arrhythmias.

The concomitant use of Brethine with other sympathomimetic agents is not recommended, since their combined effect on the cardiovascular system may be deleterious to the patient. However, this does not preclude the use of an aerosol bronchodilator of the adrenergic stimulant type for the relief of an acute bronchospasm in patients receiving chronic oral Brethine therapy.

Terbutaline sulfate should not be used for tocolysis. Serious adverse reactions may occur after administration of terbutaline sulfate to women in labor. In the mother, these include increased heart rate, transient hyperglycemia, hypokalemia, cardiac arrhythmias, pulmonary edema, and myocardial ischemia. Increased fetal heart rate and neonatal hypoglycemia may occur as a result of maternal administration.

Immediate hypersensitivity reactions and exacerbation of bronchospasm have been reported after terbutaline administration.

PEDIATRIC USE

Safety and effectiveness in pediatric patients below the age of 12 years have not been established.

ADVERSE REACTIONS

Commonly observed side effects include nervousness and tremor. Other reported reactions include headache, increased heart rate, palpitations, drowsiness, nausea, vomiting, sweating, and muscle cramps. These reactions are generally transient in nature and usually do not require treatment. The frequency of these side effects appears to diminish with continued therapy. In general, all the side effects observed are characteristic of those commonly seen with sympathomimetic amines.

There have been rare reports of elevations in liver enzymes and of hypersensitivity vasculitis.

DOSAGE AND ADMINISTRATION

The usual oral dose of Brethine for adults is 5 mg administered at approximately six-hour intervals, three times daily, during the hours the patient is usually awake. If side effects are particularly disturbing, the dose may be reduced to 2.5 mg three times daily, and still provide a clinically significant improvement in pulmonary function. A dose of 2.5 mg, three times daily, also is recommended for children in the 12- to 15-year group. Brethine is not recommended at present for use in children below the age of 12 years. In adults, a total dose of 15 mg should not be exceeded in a 24-hour period. In children, a total dose of 7.5 mg should not be exceeded in a 24-hour period.

OVERDOSAGE

Overdosage experience is limited. Excessive beta-adrenergic receptor stimulation may augment the signs or symptoms listed under **ADVERSE REACTIONS** and they may be accompanied by other adrenergic effects. Treat the alert patient who has taken excessive oral medication by emptying the stomach by means of induced emesis, followed by gastric lavage. In the unconscious patient, secure the airway with a cuffed endotracheal tube before beginning lavage (do not induce emesis). Instillation of activated charcoal slurry may help reduce absorption of terbutaline sulfate. Maintain adequate respiratory exchange. Provide cardiac and respiratory support as needed. Continue observation until symptom-free.

HOW SUPPLIED

Tablets 2.5 mg—oval, white, scored (imprinted Geigy 72)
Bottles of 100 .... NDC 0028-0072-01
Bottles of 1000 .... NDC 0028-0072-10
Gy-Pak®—One Unit
12 bottles—100 tablets each .... NDC 0028-0072-65
Unit Dose (blister pack)
Box of 100 (strips of 10) .... NDC 0028-0072-61
Tablets 5 mg—round, white, scored (imprinted Geigy 105)
Bottles of 100 .... NDC 0028-0105-01
Bottles of 1000 .... NDC 0028-0105-10
Gy-Pak®—one Unit
12 bottles—100 tablets each .... NDC 0028-0105-65
Unit Dose (blister pack)
Box of 100 (strips of 10) .... NDC 0028-0105-61

Store at controlled room temperature 59°-86°F (15°-30°C).
Dispense in tight, light-resistant container (USP).

C95-48 (Rev. 11/95)

Shown in Product Identification Guide, page 309

BRETHINE® ℞

[breth-een′]
terbutaline sulfate Injection USP
Ampuls
A sterile aqueous solution for subcutaneous injection.

DESCRIPTION

Brethine, terbutaline sulfate injection USP, is a β-adrenergic agonist bronchodilator available as a sterile, nonpyrogenic, aqueous solution in ampuls, for subcutaneous administration. Each milliliter of solution contains 1 mg of terbutaline sulfate USP (0.82 mg of the free base); sodium chloride ACS, for isotonicity; and hydrochloric acid ACS, for adjustment to a target pH of 4. Terbutaline sulfate is (±)-α-[(*tert*-butylamino)methyl]-3,5-dihydroxybenzyl alcohol sulfate (2:1) (salt). The empirical formula is $(C_{12}H_{19}NO_3)_2 \cdot H_2SO_4$.

Terbutaline sulfate USP is a white to gray-white crystalline powder. It is odorless or has a faint odor of acetic acid. It is soluble in water and in 0.1N hydrochloric acid, slightly soluble in methanol, and insoluble in chloroform. Its molecular weight is 548.65.

CLINICAL PHARMACOLOGY

Brethine is a β-adrenergic receptor agonist. In vitro and in vivo studies in animals have shown that Brethine exerts a preferential effect on β_2-adrenergic receptors. While it is recognized that β_2-adrenergic receptors are the predominant receptors in bronchial smooth muscle, recent data indicate that there is a population of β_2-receptors in the human heart, existing in a concentration between 10–50%. The precise function of these, however, is not yet established (see WARNINGS). Controlled clinical studies in patients given Brethine subcutaneously have not revealed a preferential β_2-adrenergic effect.

The pharmacologic effects of β-adrenergic agonists, including Brethine, are at least in part attributable to stimulation through β-adrenergic receptors of intracellular adenylcyclase, the enzyme which catalyzes the conversion of adenosine triphosphate (ATP) to cyclic 3′, 5′-adenosine monophosphate (cAMP). Increased cAMP levels are associated with relaxation of bronchial smooth muscle and inhibition of release of mediators of immediate hypersensitivity from cells, especially from mast cells.

Controlled clinical studies have shown that Brethine relieves bronchospasm in acute and chronic obstructive pulmonary disease by significantly increasing pulmonary flow rates (e.g., an increase of 15% or more in FEV_1). After subcutaneous administration of 0.25 mg of Brethine, a measurable change in flow rate usually occurs within 5 minutes, and a clinically significant increase in FEV_1 occurs within 15 minutes. The maximum effect usually occurs within 30–60 minutes, and clinically significant bronchodilator activity may continue for 1.5 to 4 hours. The duration of clinically significant improvement is comparable to that observed with equimilligram doses of epinephrine.

Recent studies in laboratory animals (minipigs, rodents, and dogs) recorded the occurrence of cardiac arrhythmias and sudden death (with histological evidence of necrosis) when β-agonists and methylxanthines were administered concurrently. The significance of these findings when applied to humans is currently unknown.

Pharmacokinetics

After subcutaneous administration of 0.25 mg of terbutaline sulfate to two male subjects, peak terbutaline serum concentrations of 5.2 and 5.3 ng/ml were observed at about 20 minutes after dosing. Further studies are needed to confirm these results.

Elimination half-life of the drug in 10 of 14 patients was approximately 2.9 hr after subcutaneous administration, but longer elimination half-lives (between 6–14 hr) were found in the other 4 patients. About 90% of the drug was excreted in the urine at 96 hr after subcutaneous administration, with about 60% of this being unchanged drug. It appears that the sulfate conjugate is a major metabolite of terbutaline and urinary excretion is the primary route of elimination.

INDICATIONS AND USAGE

Brethine is indicated for the prevention and reversal of bronchospasm in patients with bronchial asthma and reversible bronchospasm associated with bronchitis and emphysema.

CONTRAINDICATIONS

Brethine is contraindicated in patients known to be hypersensitive to sympathomimetic amines or any component of this drug product.

WARNINGS

There have been rare reports of seizures in patients receiving terbutaline; seizures did not recur in these patients after the drug was discontinued.

Controlled clinical studies and other clinical experience have shown that Brethine, like other β-adrenergic agonists, can produce a significant cardiovascular effect in some patients, as measured by pulse rate, blood pressure, symptoms, and/or ECG changes.

PRECAUTIONS

General

Since Brethine is a sympathomimetic amine, it should be used with caution in patients with cardiovascular disorders, including ischemic heart disease, hypertension, and cardiac arrhythmias; in patients with hyperthyroidism or diabetes mellitus; and in patients who are unusually responsive to sympathomimetic amines or who have convulsive disorders. Significant changes in systolic and diastolic blood pressure can be expected to occur in some patients after use of any β-adrenergic bronchodilator.

Immediate hypersensitivity reactions and exacerbations of bronchospasm have been reported after terbutaline administration.

Terbutaline sulfate should not be used for tocolysis.

Drug Interactions

The concomitant use of Brethine with other sympathomimetic agents is not recommended, since the combined effect on the cardiovascular system may be deleterious to the patient.

β-adrenergic agonists should be administered with caution to patients being treated with monoamine oxidase inhibitors or tricyclic antidepressants, since the action of β-adrenergic agonists on the vascular system may be potentiated.

Carcinogenesis, Mutagenesis, Impairment of Fertility

In a 2-year oral study in the rat, terbutaline sulfate caused a significant dose-related increase in the incidence of benign leiomyomas of the mesovarium at doses corresponding to 5,000, 50,000, 100,000, and 200,000 times the maximum recommended human subcutaneous dose (0.01 mg/kg). The relevance of these findings to humans is not known. An 18-month oral study in mice revealed no evidence of tumorigenicity at doses up to 200 mg/kg (20,000 times the maximum recommended human subcutaneous dose). Mutagenicity studies have not been performed. A reproduction study in rats at oral doses up to 5000 times the maximum subcutaneous dose (0.01 mg/kg) revealed no evidence of impaired fertility.

Pregnancy Category B

Reproduction studies performed in mice, rats, or rabbits at doses up to 1500 times the subcutaneous maximum daily human dose of 0.01 mg/kg have revealed no evidence of impaired fertility or harm to the fetus due to Brethine. Increased levels of maternal and fetal blood glucose have been observed after intravenous administration of terbutaline to near-term pregnant baboons at doses up to 4 times the maximum recommended human subcutaneous dose.

There are, however, no adequate and well-controlled studies in pregnant women. Because animal reproduction studies are not always predictive of human response, this drug should be used during pregnancy only if clearly needed. Administration of the drug under these conditions requires careful benefit-to-risk determination.

Percent Incidence of Adverse Reactions

	Terbutaline		Epinephrine	
	0.25 mg N=77	0.5 mg N=205	0.25 mg N=153	0.5 mg N=61
Reaction				
Central Nervous System				
Tremors	7.8%	38.0%	16.3%	18.0%
Nervousness	16.9%	30.7%	8.5%	31.1%
Dizziness	1.3%	10.2%	7.8%	3.3%
Headache	7.8%	8.8%	3.3%	9.8%
Drowsiness	11.7%	9.8%	14.4%	8.2%
Cardiovascular				
Palpitations	7.8%	22.9%	7.8%	29.5%
Tachycardia	1.3%	1.5%	2.6%	0.0%
Respiratory				
Dyspnea	0.0%	2.0%	2.0%	0.0%
Chest Discomfort	1.3%	1.5%	2.6%	0.0%
Gastrointestinal				
Nausea/Vomiting	1.3%	3.9%	1.3%	11.5%
Systemic				
Weakness	1.3%	0.5%	2.6%	1.6%
Flushed Feeling	0.0%	2.4%	1.3%	0.0%
Sweating	0.0%	2.4%	0.0%	0.0%
Pain at Injection Site	2.6%	0.5%	2.6%	1.6%

Note: Some patients received more than one dosage strength of terbutaline sulfate and epinephrine. In addition, there were reports of anxiety, muscle cramps, and dry mouth (<0.5%).

Labor and Delivery
Terbutaline sulfate should not be used for tocolysis. Serious adverse reactions may occur after administration of terbutaline sulfate to women in labor. In the mother, these include increased heart rate, transient hyperglycemia, hypokalemia, cardiac arrhythmias, pulmonary edema, and myocardial ischemia. Increased fetal heart rate and neonatal hypoglycemia may occur as a result of maternal administration.

Nursing Mothers
It is not known whether this drug is excreted in human milk. Therefore, Brethine should be used during nursing only if the potential benefit justifies the possible risk to the newborn.

Pediatric Use
Brethine is not recommended for pediatric patients under the age of 12 years because of insufficient clinical data to establish safety and effectiveness.

ADVERSE REACTIONS
Adverse reactions observed with Brethine are similar to those commonly seen with other sympathomimetic agents. All these reactions are transient in nature and usually do not require treatment.
The following table compares adverse reactions seen in patients treated with terbutaline sulfate injection (0.25 mg and 0.5 mg) with those seen in patients treated with epinephrine injection (0.25 mg and 0.5 mg), during eight double-blind crossover studies involving a total of 214 patients.
[See table above.]
There have been rare reports of elevations of liver enzymes and of hypersensitivity vasculitis with terbutaline administration.

OVERDOSAGE
Acute Toxicity
Intravenous LD_{50}'s (mg/kg): rats, 61.5; mice, 48.4. Oral LD_{50} in rats is > 5000 mg/kg.
Signs and Symptoms
Excessive β-adrenergic receptor stimulation may augment the signs and symptoms listed under ADVERSE REACTIONS.
Treatment
There is no specific antidote. Treatment consists of discontinuation of Brethine along with the institution of appropriate symptomatic therapy.

DOSAGE AND ADMINISTRATION
Ampuls should be used only for subcutaneous administration and not intravenous infusion. Sterility and accurate dosing cannot be assured if the ampuls are not used in accordance with DOSAGE AND ADMINISTRATION.
The usual subcutaneous dose of Brethine is 0.25 mg injected into the lateral deltoid area. If significant clinical improvement does not occur within 15–30 minutes, a second dose of 0.25 mg may be administered. If the patient then fails to respond within another 15–30 minutes, other therapeutic measures should be considered. The total dose within 4 hours should not exceed 0.5 mg.
Note: Parenteral drug products should be inspected visually for particulate matter and discoloration prior to administration, whenever solution and container permit.

HOW SUPPLIED
Ampuls 1 mg/ml—The drug is supplied at a volume of 1 ml contained in a 2 ml clear glass ampul. Each ampul contains 1 mg of Brethine per 1 ml of solution; 0.25 ml of solution will provide the usual clinical dose of 0.25 mg. Ampuls are expiration-dated.

Box of 10 ampuls ....NDC 0028-7507-23
Box of 100 ampuls ....NDC 0028-7507-01
Keep at controlled room temperature 59°–86°F (15°–30°C).
Protect from light by storing ampuls in original carton until dispensed. Do not use if solution is discolored.

C95-51 (Rev. 12/95)
Shown in Product Identification Guide, page 309

CATAFLAM® ℞
diclofenac potassium
Immediate-Release Tablets

VOLTAREN® ℞
diclofenac sodium
Delayed-Release (enteric-coated) Tablets

VOLTAREN®-XR ℞
diclofenac sodium
Extended-Release Tablets

Prescribing Information

DESCRIPTION
Diclofenac, as the sodium or potassium salt, is a benzeneacetic acid derivative, designated chemically as 2-[(2,6-dichlorophenyl)amino] benzeneacetic acid, monosodium or monopotassium salt.
Diclofenac, as the sodium or potassium salt, is a faintly yellowish white to light beige, virtually odorless, slightly hygroscopic crystalline powder. Molecular weights of the sodium and potassium salts are 318.14 and 334.25, respectively. It is freely soluble in methanol, soluble in ethanol, and practically insoluble in chloroform and in dilute acid. Diclofenac sodium is sparingly soluble in water while diclofenac potassium is soluble in water. The n-octanol/water partition coefficient is, for both diclofenac salts, 13.4 at pH 7.4 and 1545 at pH 5.2. Both salts have a single dissociation constant (pKa) of 4.0 ± 0.2 at 25° C in water.
Diclofenac potassium is available as **Cataflam Immediate-Release Tablets** of 50 mg for oral administration.
CATAFLAM Inactive Ingredients: Calcium phosphate, colloidal silicon dioxide, iron oxides, magnesium stearate, microcrystalline cellulose, polyethylene glycol, povidone, sodium starch glycolate, starch, sucrose, talc, titanium dioxide.
Diclofenac sodium is available as **VOLTAREN Delayed-Release (enteric-coated) Tablets** of 25 mg, 50 mg, and 75 mg for oral administration, and **VOLTAREN-XR Extended-Release Tablets** of 100 mg.
VOLTAREN Inactive Ingredients: Hydroxypropyl methylcellulose, iron oxide, lactose, magnesium stearate, methacrylic acid copolymer, microcrystalline cellulose, polyethylene glycol, povidone, propylene glycol, sodium hydroxide, sodium starch glycolate, talc, titanium dioxide, D&C Yellow No. 10 Aluminum Lake (25-mg tablet only), FD&C Blue No. 1 Aluminum Lake (50-mg tablet only).
VOLTAREN-XR Inactive Ingredients: Cetyl alcohol, hydroxypropyl methylcellulose, iron oxide, magnesium stearate, polyethylene glycol, polysorbate, povidone, silicon dioxide, sucrose, talc, titanium dioxide.

CLINICAL PHARMACOLOGY
Pharmacodynamics
Diclofenac, the anion in Cataflam, Voltaren, and Voltaren-XR, is a nonsteroidal anti-inflammatory drug (NSAID). In pharmacologic studies, diclofenac has shown anti-inflammatory, analgesic, and antipyretic activity. As with other NSAIDs, its mode of action is not known; its ability to inhibit prostaglandin synthesis, however, may be involved in its anti-inflammatory activity, as well as contribute to its efficacy in relieving pain related to inflammation and primary dysmenorrhea. With regard to its analgesic effect, diclofenac is not a narcotic.

Pharmacokinetics
Cataflam Immediate-Release Tablets, Voltaren Delayed-Release Tablets, and Voltaren-XR Extended-Release Tablets, contain the same therapeutic moiety, diclofenac. They differ in the cationic portion of the salt (see DESCRIPTION), as well as in their release characteristics. Cataflam Immediate-Release Tablets are formulated to release diclofenac in the stomach. Voltaren Delayed-Release (enteric-coated) Tablets are in a pharmaceutical formulation that resists dissolution in the low pH of gastric fluid but allows a rapid release of drug in the higher pH-environment of the duodenum. Conversely, Voltaren-XR Extended-Release Tablets are formulated to release drug over a prolonged period. The primary pharmacokinetic difference between the three products is the pattern of drug release and absorption, as described below and shown in Table 1.

Table 1
Mean (% CV) Pharmacokinetics of Diclofenac Following Single Oral Doses of CATAFLAM, VOLTAREN Delayed-Release, and VOLTAREN-XR

Drug	Dose (mg)	AUC (ng·hr/mL)	C_{max} (ng/mL)	T_{max} (hr)
Cataflam	50	1309 (21.7%)	1312 (44.1%)	1.00 (74.6%)
Voltaren	50	1429 (38.4%)	1417 (22.4%)	2.22 (49.8%)
Voltaren-XR	100	2079 (33.7%)	417 (40.7%)	5.25 (28.3%)

For this reason, separate sections are provided below to describe the different absorption profiles of Cataflam Immediate-Release Tablets, Voltaren Delayed-Release Tablets, and Voltaren-XR Extended-Release Tablets.

Absorption
Under fasting condition, diclofenac is completely absorbed from the gastrointestinal tract. However, due to first-pass metabolism, only about 50% of the absorbed dose is systemically available.
Cataflam Immediate-Release Tablets: In some fasting volunteers, measurable plasma levels are observed within 10 minutes of dosing with Cataflam. Peak plasma levels are achieved in approximately 1 hour in fasting normal volunteers, with a range from 0.33 to 2 hours.
The extent of diclofenac absorption is not significantly affected when Cataflam is taken with food. However, the rate of absorption is reduced by food, as indicated by a delay in T_{max} and decrease in C_{max} values by approximately 30%. After repeated oral administration of Cataflam 50 mg t.i.d. no accumulation of diclofenac in plasma occurred.
Voltaren Delayed-Release Tablets: Peak plasma levels are achieved in 2 hours in fasting normal volunteers, with a range from 1 to 4 hours. The area-under-the-plasma-concentration curve (AUC) is dose-proportional within the range of 25 mg to 150 mg. Peak plasma levels are less than dose-proportional and are approximately 1.0, 1.5, and 2.0 μg/mL for 25-mg, 50-mg, and 75-mg doses, respectively. It should be noted that the administration of several individual Voltaren tablets may not yield equivalent results in peak concentration as the administration of one tablet of a higher strength. This is probably due to the staggered gastric emptying of tablets into the duodenum. After repeated oral administration of Voltaren 50 mg b.i.d., diclofenac did not accumulate in plasma.
When Voltaren is taken with food, there is usually a delay in the onset of absorption of 1 to 4.5 hours, with delays as long as 10 hours in some patients, and a reduction in peak plasma levels of approximately 40%. The extent of absorption of diclofenac, however, is not significantly affected by food intake.
Voltaren-XR Extended-Release Tablets: The extent of diclofenac absorption from the extended-release tablet is not significantly affected when the drug is taken with food, however, food significantly altered the absorption pattern as indicated by a delay of 1 to 2 hours in T_{max} and a two-fold increase in C_{max} values. The plasma profile of the extended-release tablet, under fasting conditions, was characterized by multiple peaks and high intersubject variability in blood profiles. In contrast, the plasma profile for the extended-release tablets under fed conditions showed a more consistent absorption pattern with a single peak usually occurring between 5 and 6 hours after the meal.

Distribution
Plasma concentrations of diclofenac decline from peak levels in a biexponential fashion, with the terminal phase having a half-life of approximately 2 hours. Clearance and volume of distribution are about 350 mL/min and 550 mL/kg, respec-

Continued on next page

CibaGeneva—Cont.

tively. More than 99% of diclofenac is reversibly bound to human plasma albumin.

As with other NSAIDs, diclofenac diffuses into and out of the synovial fluid. Diffusion into the joint occurs when plasma levels are higher than those in the synovial fluid, after which the process reverses and synovial fluid levels are higher than plasma levels. It is not known whether diffusion into the joint plays a role in the effectiveness of diclofenac.

Metabolism and Elimination

Diclofenac is eliminated through metabolism and subsequent urinary and biliary excretion of the glucuronide and the sulfate conjugates of the metabolites. Approximately 65% of the dose is excreted in the urine, and approximately 35% in the bile.

Conjugates of unchanged diclofenac account for 5%–10% of the dose excreted in the urine and for less than 5% excreted in the bile. Little or no unchanged unconjugated drug is excreted. Conjugates of the principal metabolite account for 20%–30% of the dose excreted in the urine and for 10%–20% of the dose excreted in the bile. Conjugates of three other metabolites together account for 10%–20% of the dose excreted in the urine and for small amounts excreted in the bile. The elimination half-life values for these metabolites are shorter than those for the parent drug. Urinary excretion of an additional metabolite (half-life 80 hours) accounts for only 1.4% of the oral dose. The degree of accumulation of diclofenac metabolites is unknown. Some of the metabolites may have activity.

Special Populations

A 4-week study, comparing plasma level profiles of diclofenac (Voltaren 50 mg b.i.d.) in younger (26–46 years) versus older (66–81 years) adults, did not show differences between age groups (10 patients per age group).

Geriatric Population: An 8-day study, comparing the kinetics of diclofenac (100 mg Voltaren-XR q.d.) in osteoarthritis patients older than 65 years versus younger than 65 years showed no significant differences between the two groups with respect to peak plasma levels, time to peak levels, or AUC.

Patients with Renal and/or Hepatic Impairment: To date, no differences in the pharmacokinetics of diclofenac have been detected in studies of patients with renal (50 mg intravenously) or hepatic impairment (100-mg oral solution). In patients with renal impairment (N=5, creatinine clearance 3 to 42 mL/min), AUC values and elimination rates were comparable to those in healthy subjects. In patients with biopsy-confirmed cirrhosis or chronic active hepatitis (variably elevated transaminases and mildly elevated bilirubins, N=10), diclofenac concentrations and urinary elimination values were comparable to those in healthy subjects.

Clinical Studies

Cataflam Immediate-Release Tablets in Analgesia/Primary Dysmenorrhea: The analgesic efficacy of Cataflam was demonstrated in trials of patients with postoperative pain (following gynecologic, oral, and orthopedic surgery), osteoarthritis of the knee, and primary dysmenorrhea. The effectiveness of Cataflam in studies of pain or primary dysmenorrhea showed that onset of analgesia began, in some patients, as soon as 30 minutes, and relief of pain lasted as long as 8 hours, following single 50-mg or 100-mg doses. Duration of pain relief was judged by the time at which approximately half of the patients need remedication. The onset and duration of pain relief for either the 50-mg or 100-mg dose was essentially the same, whether patients had moderate or severe pain at baseline.

Cataflam was studied in single-dose and multiple-dose pain trials. The pain models in single-dose studies were post-dental extraction and post-gynecologic surgery: the efficacy of the 50-mg dose (N=258) and the 100-mg dose (N=255) was comparable to aspirin 650 mg in onset of pain relief, but generally provided a longer duration of analgesia than aspirin. The pain models for multiple-dose trials were post-orthopedic surgery pain as well as pain associated with primary dysmenorrhea: the efficacy of the 50-mg dose (N=101) and the 100-mg dose (N=442), followed by 50 mg every 8 hours, was comparable to naproxen sodium 550 mg followed by 275 mg every 8 hours. In one study of chronic pain, in patients with osteoarthritis (N=196), Cataflam 50 mg t.i.d. was comparable in efficacy to ibuprofen 800 mg t.i.d. and Voltaren Delayed-Release Tablets 50 mg t.i.d.

Voltaren Delayed-Release Tablets in Osteoarthritis: Voltaren was evaluated for the management of the signs and symptoms of osteoarthritis of the hip or knee in a total of 633 patients treated for up to 3 months in placebo- and active-controlled clinical trials against aspirin (N=449), and naproxen (N=92). Voltaren was given both in variable (100–150 mg/day) and fixed (150 mg/day) dosing schedules in either b.i.d. or t.i.d. dosing regimens. In these trials, Voltaren was found to be comparable to 2400 to 3600 mg/day of aspirin or 500 mg/day of naproxen. Voltaren was effective when administered as either b.i.d. or t.i.d. dosing regimens.

Voltaren Delayed-Release Tablets in Rheumatoid Arthritis: Voltaren was evaluated for managing the signs and symptoms of rheumatoid arthritis in a total of 468 patients treated for up to 3 months in placebo- and active-controlled clinical trials against aspirin (N=290), and ibuprofen (N=74). Voltaren was given in a fixed (150 or 200 mg/day) dosing schedule as either b.i.d. or t.i.d. dosing regimens. Voltaren was found to be comparable to 3600 to 4800 mg/day of aspirin, and 2400 mg/day of ibuprofen. Voltaren was used b.i.d. or t.i.d., administering 150 mg/day in most trials, but 50 mg q.i.d. (200 mg/day) was also studied.

Voltaren Delayed-Release Tablets in Ankylosing Spondylitis: Voltaren was evaluated for the management of the signs and symptoms of ankylosing spondylitis in a total of 132 patients in one active-controlled clinical trial against indomethacin (N=130). Both Voltaren and indomethacin patients were started on 25 mg t.i.d. and were permitted to increase the dose 25 mg/day each week to a maximum dose of 125 mg/day. Voltaren 75–125 mg/day was found to be comparable to indomethacin 75–125 mg/day.

Voltaren-XR Extended-Release Tablets in Osteoarthritis: The use of Voltaren-XR Tablets in controlling the signs and symptoms of osteoarthritis was assessed in two double-blind, controlled trials in which 742 patients participated and 517 patients were treated for 3 months. In one active- and placebo-controlled study, Voltaren-XR Tablets at doses of 100 mg q.d. were comparable to Voltaren Delayed-Release Tablets 50 mg b.i.d. in patients whose osteoarthritis symptoms were stabilized after 2 weeks of treatment with Voltaren Delayed-Release Tablets 75 mg b.i.d. In another study, Voltaren-XR Tablets at doses of 100 mg q.d. and 100 mg b.i.d. were compared to Voltaren Delayed-Release Tablets 50 mg q.i.d. Voltaren-XR Tablets 100 mg b.i.d. were comparable to Voltaren Delayed-Release Tablets 50 mg q.i.d. With the Voltaren-XR Tablet formulation, although there was a trend toward greater efficacy at doses of 200 mg daily than 100 mg daily, there was also an increase in side effects when 200 mg of Voltaren-XR Tablets were administered to patients with osteoarthritis.

Voltaren-XR Extended-Release Tablets in Rheumatoid Arthritis: The use of Voltaren-XR Tablets in controlling the signs and symptoms of rheumatoid arthritis was assessed in two double-blind, controlled trials in which 704 patients participated and 441 patients were treated for 3 months. In one active- and placebo-controlled study, Voltaren-XR Tablets 100 mg q.d. were comparable to Voltaren Delayed-Release Tablets 50 mg b.i.d. in patients whose rheumatoid arthritis symptoms were stabilized after 2 weeks' treatment of Voltaren Delayed-Release Tablets 75 mg b.i.d. In another study, Voltaren-XR Tablets at doses of 100 mg q.d. and 100 mg b.i.d. were compared to Voltaren Delayed-Release Tablets 50 mg q.i.d.; Voltaren-XR Tablets 100 mg b.i.d. were comparable to Voltaren Delayed-Release Tablets 50 mg q.i.d. There was a trend toward greater efficacy with doses of 200 mg daily as compared to 100 mg daily of Voltaren-XR Tablets. There was also an increase in side effects when 200 mg of Voltaren-XR Tablets were administered to patients with rheumatoid arthritis.

Special Studies *(The clinical significance of the findings outlined below is unknown.)*

G.I. Blood Loss/Endoscopy Data: G.I. blood loss and endoscopy studies were performed with Voltaren Delayed-Release (enteric-coated) Tablets that, unlike Immediate-Release Tablets, do not dissolve in the stomach where the endoscopic lesions are primarily seen; Cataflam Immediate-Release Tablets have not been similarly studied. A repeat-dose endoscopy study, in patients with rheumatoid arthritis or osteoarthritis treated with Voltaren Delayed-Release Tablets 75 mg b.i.d. (N=101), or naproxen (immediate-release tablets) 500 mg b.i.d. (N=103) for 3 months, resulted in a significantly smaller number of patients with an increase in endoscopy score from baseline and a significantly lower mean endoscopy score after treatment in the Voltaren-treated patients. Two repeat-dose endoscopic studies, in normal volunteers showed that daily doses of Voltaren Delayed-Release Tablets 75 or 100 mg (N=6 and N=14, respectively) for 1 week caused fewer gastric lesions, and those that did occur had lower scores than those observed following daily 500-mg doses of naproxen (immediate-release tablets). In healthy subjects, the daily administration of 150 mg of Voltaren (N=8) for 3 weeks resulted in a mean fecal blood loss less than that observed with 3.0 g of aspirin daily (N=8). In four repeat-dose studies, mean fecal blood loss with 150 mg of Voltaren was also less than that observed with 750 mg of naproxen (N=8 and N=6) or 150 mg of indomethacin (N=8 and N=6).

INDIVIDUALIZATION OF DOSAGE

Diclofenac, like other NSAIDs, shows interindividual differences in both pharmacokinetics and clinical response (pharmacodynamics). Consequently, the recommended strategy for initiating therapy is to use a starting dose likely to be effective for the majority of patients and to adjust dosage thereafter based on observation of diclofenac's beneficial and adverse effects.

In patients weighing less than 60 kg (132 lb), or where the severity of the disease, concomitant medication, or other diseases warrant, the maximum recommended total daily dose of Cataflam, Voltaren, or Voltaren-XR should be reduced. Experience with other NSAIDs has shown that starting therapy with maximum doses in patients at increased risk due to renal or hepatic disease, low body weight (<60 kg), advanced age, a known ulcer diathesis, or known sensitivity to NSAID effects, is likely to increase frequency of adverse reactions and is not recommended (see PRECAUTIONS).

Osteoarthritis/Rheumatoid Arthritis/Ankylosing Spondylitis: The usual starting dose of Cataflam Immediate-Release Tablets or Voltaren Delayed-Release for patients with osteoarthritis, is 100 to 150 mg/day, using a b.i.d. or t.i.d. dosing regimen. For patients with osteoarthritis, the ususal starting dose of Voltaren-XR Extended-Release Tablets is 100 mg q.d. In two variable-dose clinical trials in osteoarthritis using Voltaren Delayed-Release Tablets, of 266 patients started on 100 mg/day, 176 chose to increase the dose to 150 mg/day. Dosages above 200 mg/day have not been studied in patients with osteoarthritis.

For most patients with rheumatoid arthritis, the usual starting dose of Cataflam Immediate-Release Tablets or Voltaren Delayed-Release Tablets is 150 mg/day, using a b.i.d. or t.i.d. dosing regimen. The usual starting dose of Voltaren-XR Extended-Release Tablets is 100 mg q.d. Patients requiring more relief of pain and inflammation may increase the dose to 200 mg/day. In clinical trials, patients receiving 200 mg/day were less likely to drop from the trial due to lack of efficacy than patients receiving 150 mg/day as Voltaren Delayed-Release Tablets or 100 mg/day as Voltaren-XR Extended-Release Tablets. Dosages above 225 mg/day are not recommended in patients with rheumatoid arthritis because of increased risk of adverse events.

The recommended dose of Voltaren Delayed-Release Tablets for patients with ankylosing spondylitis is 100 to 125 mg/day, using a q.i.d. dosing regimen (see DOSAGE AND ADMINISTRATION regarding the 125 mg/day dosing regimen). In a variable-dose clinical trial, of 132 patients started on 75 mg/day, 122 chose to increase the dose to 125 mg/day. Dosages above 125 mg/day have not been studied in patients with ankylosing spondylitis.

Analgesia/Primary Dysmenorrhea: Because of earlier absorption of diclofenac from Cataflam Immediate-Release Tablets, it is the formulation indicated for management of pain and primary dysmenorrhea when prompt onset of pain relief is desired. The results of clinical trials suggest an initial Cataflam dose of 50 mg for pain or for primary dysmenorrhea, followed by doses of 50 mg every 8 hours, as needed. With experience, some patients with recurring pain, such as dysmenorrhea, may find that an initial dose of 100 mg of Cataflam, followed by 50-mg doses, will provide better relief. After the first day, when the maximum recommended dose may be 200 mg, the total daily dose should generally not exceed 150 mg.

INDICATIONS AND USAGE

Cataflam Immediate-Release Tablets and Voltaren Delayed-Release Tablets are indicated for the acute and chronic treatment of signs and symptoms of osteoarthritis and rheumatoid arthritis. Voltaren-XR Extended-Release Tablets are indicated for chronic therapy of osteoarthritis and rheumatoid arthritis. In addition, Cataflam Immediate-Release Tablets and Voltaren Delayed-Release Tablets are indicated for the treatment of ankylosing spondylitis. Only Cataflam is indicated for the management of pain and primary dysmenorrhea, when prompt pain relief is desired, because it is formulated to provide earlier plasma concentrations of diclofenac (see CLINICAL PHARMACOLOGY, Pharmacokinetics and Clinical Studies).

CONTRAINDICATIONS

Diclofenac in all formulations, Cataflam, Voltaren, and Voltaren-XR, is contraindicated in patients with known hypersensitivity to diclofenac and diclofenac-containing products. Diclofenac should not be given to patients who have experienced asthma, urticaria, or other allergic-type reactions after taking aspirin or other NSAIDs. Severe, rarely fatal, anaphylactic-like reactions to diclofenac have been reported in such patients (see WARNINGS—Anaphylactoid Reactions, and PRECAUTIONS—Preexisting Asthma).

WARNINGS

Gastrointestinal Effects

Peptic ulceration and gastrointestinal bleeding have been reported in patients receiving diclofenac. Physicians and patients should therefore remain alert for ulceration and bleeding in patients treated chronically with diclofenac even in the absence of previous G.I. tract symptoms. It is recommended that patients be maintained on the lowest dose of diclofenac possible, consistent with achieving a satisfactory therapeutic response.

Risk of G.I. Ulcerations, Bleeding, and Perforation with NSAID Therapy: Serious gastrointestinal toxicity such as bleeding, ulceration, and perforation can occur at any time, with or without warning symptoms, in patients treated

chronically with NSAID therapy. Although minor upper gastrointestinal problems, such as dyspepsia, are common, usually developing early in therapy, physicians should remain alert for ulceration and bleeding in patients treated chronically with NSAIDs even in the absence of previous G.I. tract symptoms. In patients observed in clinical trials of several months to 2 years' duration, symptomatic upper G.I. ulcers, gross bleeding, or perforation appear to occur in approximately 1% of patients for 3–6 months, and in about 2%–4% of patients treated for 1 year. Physicians should inform patients about the signs and/or symptoms of serious G.I. toxicity and what steps to take if they occur.

Studies to date have not identified any subset of patients not at risk of developing peptic ulceration and bleeding. Except for a prior history of serious G.I. events and other risk factors known to be associated with peptic ulcer disease, such as alcoholism, smoking, etc., no risk factors (e.g., age, sex) have been associated with increased risk. Elderly or debilitated patients seem to tolerate ulceration or bleeding less well than other individuals, and most spontaneous reports of fatal G.I. events are in this population. Studies to date are inconclusive concerning the relative risk of various NSAIDs in causing such reactions. High doses of any NSAID probably carry a greater risk of these reactions, although controlled clinical trials showing this do not exist in most cases. In considering the use of relatively large doses (within the recommended dosage range), sufficient benefit should be anticipated to offset the potential increased risk of G.I. toxicity.

Hepatic Effects
Elevations of one or more liver tests may occur during diclofenac therapy. These laboratory abnormalities may progress, may remain unchanged, or may be transient with continued therapy. Borderline elevations (i.e., less than 3 times the ULN [=the Upper Limit of the Normal range]), or greater elevations of transaminases occurred in about 15% of diclofenac-treated patients. Of the hepatic enzymes, ALT (SGPT) is the one recommended for the monitoring of liver injury.

In clinical trials, meaningful elevations (i.e., more than 3 times the ULN) of AST (SGOT) (ALT was not measured in all studies) occurred in about 2% of approximately 5700 patients at some time during Voltaren treatment. In a large, open, controlled trial, meaningful elevations of ALT and/or AST occurred in about 4% of 3700 patients treated for 2–6 months, including marked elevations (i.e., more than 8 times the ULN) in about 1% of the 3700 patients. In that open-label study, a higher incidence of borderline (less than 3 times the ULN), moderate (3–8 times the ULN), and marked (>8 times the ULN) elevations of ALT or AST was observed in patients receiving diclofenac when compared to other NSAIDs. Transaminase elevations were seen more frequently in patients with osteoarthritis than in those with rheumatoid arthritis (see ADVERSE REACTIONS).

In addition to enzyme elevations seen in clinical trials, postmarketing surveillance has found rare cases of severe hepatic reactions, including liver necrosis, jaundice, and fulminant fatal hepatitis with and without jaundice. Some of these rare reported cases underwent liver transplantation. Physicians should measure transaminases periodically in patients receiving long-term therapy with diclofenac, because severe hepatotoxicity may develop without a prodrome of distinguishing symptoms. The optimum times for making the first and subsequent transaminase measurements are not known. In the largest U.S. trial (open-label) that involved 3700 patients monitored first at 8 weeks and 1200 patients monitored again at 24 weeks, almost all meaningful elevations in transaminases were detected before patients became symptomatic. In 42 of the 51 patients in all trials who developed marked transaminase elevations, abnormal tests occurred during the first 2 months of therapy with diclofenac. Postmarketing experience has shown severe hepatic reactions can occur at any time during treatment with diclofenac. Cases of drug-induced hepatotoxicity have been reported in the first month, and in some cases, the first two months of therapy. Based on these experiences, transaminases should be monitored within 4 to 8 weeks after initiating treatment with diclofenac (see PRECAUTIONS—Laboratory Tests). As with other NSAIDs, if abnormal liver tests persist or worsen, if clinical signs and/or symptoms consistent with liver disease develop, or if systemic manifestations occur (e.g., eosinophilia, rash, etc.), diclofenac should be discontinued immediately.

To minimize the possibility that hepatic injury will become severe between transaminase measurements, physicians should inform patients of the warning signs and symptoms of hepatotoxicity (e.g., nausea, fatigue, lethargy, pruritus, jaundice, right upper quadrant tenderness, and "flu-like" symptoms), and the appropriate action patients should take if these signs and symptoms appear.

Anaphylactoid Reactions
As with other NSAIDs, anaphylactoid reactions may occur in patients without prior exposure to diclofenac. Diclofenac should not be given to patients with the aspirin triad. The triad typically occurs in asthmatic patients who experience rhinitis with or without nasal polyps, or who exhibit severe,

potentially fatal bronchospasm after taking aspirin or other nonsteroidal anti-inflammatory drugs. Fatal reactions have been reported in such patients (see CONTRAINDICATIONS, and PRECAUTIONS—Preexisting Asthma). Emergency help should be sought in cases where an anaphylactoid reaction occurs.

Advanced Renal Disease
In cases with advanced kidney disease, treatment with diclofenac, as with other NSAIDs, should only be initiated with close monitoring of the patient's kidney functions (see PRECAUTIONS—Renal Effects).

Pregnancy
In late pregnancy, diclofenac should, as with other NSAIDs, be avoided because it will cause premature closure of the ductus arteriosus (see PRECAUTIONS—Pregnancy, *Teratogenic Effects, Pregnancy Category B*, and Labor and Delivery).

PRECAUTIONS
General
Cataflam Immediate-Release Tablets, Voltaren Delayed-Release Tablets, and Voltaren-XR Extended-Release Tablets should not be used concomitantly with other diclofenac-containing products since they also circulate in plasma as the diclofenac anion.

Fluid Retention and Edema: Fluid retention and edema have been observed in some patients taking diclofenac. Therefore, as with other NSAIDs, diclofenac should be used with caution in patients with a history of cardiac decompensation, hypertension, or other conditions predisposing to fluid retention.

Hematologic Effects: Anemia is sometimes seen in patients receiving diclofenac or other NSAIDs. This may be due to fluid retention, G.I. blood loss, or an incompletely described effect upon erythropoiesis.

Renal Effects: As a class, NSAIDs have been associated with renal papillary necrosis and other abnormal renal pathology in long-term administration to animals. In oral diclofenac studies in animals, some evidence of renal toxicity was noted. Isolated incidents of papillary necrosis were observed in a few animals at high doses (20–120 mg/kg) in several baboon subacute studies. In patients treated with diclofenac, rare cases of interstitial nephritis and papillary necrosis have been reported (see ADVERSE REACTIONS). A second form of renal toxicity, generally associated with NSAIDs, is seen in patients with conditions leading to a reduction in renal blood flow or blood volume, where renal prostaglandins have a supportive role in the maintenance of renal perfusion. In these patients, administration of an NSAID results in a dose-dependent decrease in prostaglandin synthesis and, secondarily, in a reduction of renal blood flow, which may precipitate overt renal failure. Patients at greatest risk of this reaction are those with impaired renal function, heart failure, liver dysfunction, those taking diuretics, and the elderly. Discontinuation of NSAID therapy is typically followed by recovery to the pretreatment state. Cases of significant renal failure in patients receiving diclofenac have been reported from marketing experience, but were not observed in over 4000 patients in clinical trials during which serum creatinine and BUN values were followed serially. There were only 11 patients (0.3%) whose serum creatinine and concurrent serum BUN values were greater than 2.0 mg/dL and 40 mg/dL, respectively, while on diclofenac (mean rise in the 11 patients: creatinine 2.3 mg/dL and BUN 28.4 mg/dL).

Since diclofenac metabolites are eliminated primarily by the kidneys, patients with significantly impaired renal function should be more closely monitored than subjects with normal renal function.

Porphyria: The use of diclofenac in patients with hepatic porphyria should be avoided. To date, 1 patient has been described in whom diclofenac probably triggered a clinical attack of porphyria. The postulated mechanism, demonstrated in rats, for causing such attacks by diclofenac, as well as some other NSAIDs, is through stimulation of the porphyrin precursor delta-aminolevulinic acid (ALA).

Aseptic Meningitis: As with other NSAIDs, aseptic meningitis with fever and coma has been observed on rare occasions in patients on diclofenac therapy. Although it is probably more likely to occur in patients with systemic lupus erythematosus and related connective tissue diseases, it has been reported in patients who do not have an underlying chronic disease. If signs or symptoms of meningitis develop in a patient on diclofenac, the possibility of its being related to diclofenac should be considered.

Preexisting Asthma: About 10% of patients with asthma may have aspirin-sensitive asthma. The use of aspirin in patients with aspirin-sensitive asthma has been associated with severe bronchospasm which can be fatal. Since cross-reactivity, including bronchospasm, between aspirin and other nonsteroidal anti-inflammatory drugs has been reported in such aspirin-sensitive patients, diclofenac should not be administered to patients with this form of aspirin sensitivity and should be used with caution in all patients with preexisting asthma.

Other Precautions: The pharmacologic activity of diclofenac may reduce fever and inflammation, thus diminish-

ing their utility as diagnostic signs in detecting underlying conditions.

In order to avoid exacerbation of manifestations of adrenal insufficiency, patients who have been on prolonged corticosteroid treatment should have their therapy tapered slowly rather than discontinued abruptly when diclofenac is added to the treatment program.

Blurred and/or diminished vision, scotomata, and/or changes in color vision have been reported. If a patient develops such complaints while receiving diclofenac, the drug should be discontinued and the patient should have an ophthalmologic examination which includes central visual fields and color vision testing.

Information for Patients
Diclofenac, like other drugs of its class, is not free of side effects. The side effects of these drugs can cause discomfort and, rarely, more serious side effects, such as gastrointestinal bleeding, and more rarely. liver toxicity (see WARNINGS, Hepatic Effects), which may result in hospitalization and even fatal outcomes.

NSAIDs are often essential agents in the management of arthritis and have a major role in the management of pain, but they also may be commonly employed for conditions that are less serious.

Physicians may wish to discuss with their patients the potential risks (see WARNINGS, PRECAUTIONS, and ADVERSE REACTIONS) and likely benefits of NSAID treatment, particularly when the drugs are used for less serious conditions where treatment without NSAIDs may represent an acceptable alternative to both the patient and physician.

Because serious G.I. tract ulceration and bleeding can occur without warning symptoms, physicians should follow chronically treated patients for the signs and symptoms of ulceration and bleeding and should inform them of the importance of this follow-up (see WARNINGS, Gastrointestinal Effects, *Risk of G.I. Ulcerations, Bleeding, and Perforation with NSAID Therapy*). If diclofenac is used chronically, patients should also be instructed to report any signs and symptoms that might be due to hepatotoxicity of diclofenac; these symptoms may become evident between visits when periodic liver laboratory tests are performed (see WARNINGS, Hepatic Effects, and PRECAUTIONS—Laboratory Tests).

Laboratory Tests
Hepatic Effects: Transaminases and other hepatic enzymes should be monitored in patients treated with NSAIDs. For patients on diclofenac therapy, it is recommended that a determination be made within 4 weeks of initiating therapy and at intervals thereafter. If clinical signs and symptoms consistent with liver disease develop, or if systemic manifestations occur (e.g. eosinophilia, rash, etc.) and abnormal liver tests are detected, persist or worsen, diclofenac should be discontinued immediately.

Hematologic Effects: Patients on long-term treatment with NSAIDs, including diclofenac, should have their hemoglobin or hematocrit checked periodically for signs or symptoms of anemia. Appropriate measures should be taken in case such signs of anemia occur.

Drug Interactions
Aspirin: Concomitant administration of diclofenac and aspirin is not recommended because diclofenac is displaced from its binding sites during the concomitant administration of aspirin, resulting in lower plasma concentrations, peak plasma levels, and AUC values.

Anticoagulants: While studies have not shown diclofenac to interact with anticoagulants of the warfarin type, caution should be exercised, nonetheless, since interactions have been seen with other NSAIDs. Because prostaglandins play an important role in hemostasis, and NSAIDs affect platelet function as well, concurrent therapy with all NSAIDs, including diclofenac, and warfarin requires close monitoring of patients to be certain that no change in their anticoagulant dosage is required.

Digoxin, Methotrexate, Cyclosporine: Diclofenac, like other NSAIDs, may affect renal prostaglandins and increase the toxicity of certain drugs. Ingestion of diclofenac may increase serum concentrations of digoxin and methotrexate and increase cyclosporine's nephrotoxicity. Patients who begin taking diclofenac or who increase their diclofenac dose or any other NSAID while taking digoxin, methotrexate, or cyclosporine may develop toxicity characteristics for these drugs. They should be observed closely, particularly if renal function is impaired. In the case of digoxin, serum levels should be monitored.

Lithium: Diclofenac decreases lithium renal clearance and increases lithium plasma levels. In patients taking diclofenac and lithium concomitantly, lithium toxicity may develop.

Oral Hypoglycemics: Diclofenac does not alter glucose metabolism in normal subjects nor does it alter the effects of oral hypoglycemic agents. There are rare reports, however, from marketing experiences, of changes in effects of insulin or oral hypoglycemic agents in the presence of diclofenac that necessitated changes in the doses of such agents. Both

Continued on next page

CibaGeneva—Cont.

hypo- and hyperglycemic effects have been reported. A direct causal relationship has not been established, but physicians should consider the possibility that diclofenac may alter a diabetic patient's response to insulin or oral hypoglycemic agents.

Diuretics: Diclofenac and other NSAIDs can inhibit the activity of diuretics. Concomitant treatment with potassium-sparing diuretics may be associated with increased serum potassium levels.

Other Drugs: In small groups of patients (7–10/interaction study), the concomitant administration of azathioprine, gold, chloroquine, D-penicillamine, prednisolone, doxycycline, or digitoxin did not significantly affect the peak levels and AUC values of diclofenac. Phenobarbital toxicity has been reported to have occurred in a patient on chronic phenobarbital treatment following the initiation of diclofenac therapy.

Protein Binding

In vitro, diclofenac interferes minimally or not at all with the protein binding of salicylic acid (20% decrease in binding), tolbutamide, prednisolone (10% decrease in binding), or warfarin. Benzylpenicillin, ampicillin, oxacillin, chlortetracycline, doxycycline, cephalothin, erythromycin, and sulfamethoxazole have no influence *in vitro* on the protein binding of diclofenac in human serum.

Drug/Laboratory Test Interactions

Effect on Blood Coagulation: Diclofenac increases platelet aggregaton time but does not affect bleeding time, plasma thrombin clotting time, plasma fibrinogen, or factors V and VII to XII. Statistically significant changes in prothrombin and partial thromboplastin times have been reported in normal volunteers. The mean changes were observed to be less than 1 second in both instances, however, and are unlikely to be clinically important. Diclofenac is a prostaglandin synthetase inhibitor, however, and all drugs that inhibit prostaglandin synthesis interfere with platelet function to some degree; therefore, patients who may be adversely affected by such an action should be carefully observed.

Carcinogenesis, Mutagenesis, Impairment of Fertility

Long-term carcinogenicity studies in rats given diclofenac sodium up to 2 mg/kg/day (or 12 mg/m^2/day, approximately the human dose) have revealed no significant increases in tumor incidence. There was a slight increase in benign mammary fibroadenomas in mid-dose-treated (0.5 mg/kg/day or 3 mg/m^2/day) female rats (high-dose females had excessive mortality), but the increase was not significant for this common rat tumor. A 2-year carcinogenicity study conducted in mice employing diclofenac sodium at doses up to 0.3 mg/kg/day (0.9 mg/m^2/day) in males and 1 mg/kg/day (3 mg/m^2/day) in females did not reveal any oncogenic potential. Diclofenac sodium did not show mutagenic activity in *in vitro* point mutation assays in mammalian (mouse lymphoma) and microbial (yeast, Ames) test systems and was nonmutagenic in several mammalian *in vitro* and *in vivo* tests, including dominant lethal and male germinal epithelial chromosomal studies in mice, and nucleus anomaly and chromosomal aberration studies in Chinese hamsters. Diclofenac sodium administered to male and female rats at 4 mg/kg/day (24 mg/m^2/day) did not affect fertility.

Pregnancy, *Teratogenic Effects, Pregnancy Category B*

Reproduction studies have been performed in mice given diclofenac sodium (up to 20 mg/kg/day or 60 mg/m^2/day) and in rats and rabbits given diclofenac sodium (up to 10 mg/kg/day or 60 mg/m^2/day for rats, and 80 mg/m^2/day for rabbits), and have revealed no evidence of teratogenicity despite the induction of maternal toxicity and fetal toxicity. In rats, maternally toxic doses were associated with dystocia, prolonged gestation, reduced fetal weights and growth, and reduced fetal survival. Diclofenac has been shown to cross the placental barrier in mice and rats. There are, however, no adequate and well-controlled studies in pregnant women. Because animal reproduction studies are not always predictive of human response, this drug should not be used during pregnancy unless the benefits to the mother justify the potential risk to the fetus. Because of the risk to the fetus resulting in premature closure of the ductus arteriosus, diclofenac should be avoided in late pregnancy.

Labor and Delivery

The effects of diclofenac on labor and delivery in pregnant women are unknown. Because of the known effects of prostaglandin-inhibiting drugs on the fetal cardiovascular system (closure of ductus arteriosus), use of diclofenac during late pregnancy should be avoided and, as with other nonsteroidal anti-inflammatory drugs, it is possible that diclofenac may inhibit uterine contractions and delay parturition.

Nursing Mothers

Because of the potential for serious adverse reactions in nursing infants from diclofenac, a decision should be made whether to discontinue nursing or to discontinue the drug, taking into account the importance of the drug to the mother.

Pediatric Use

Safety and effectiveness of diclofenac in pediatric patients have not been established.

Geriatric Use

Of the more than 6000 patients treated with diclofenac in U.S. trials, 31% were older than 65 years of age. No overall difference was observed between efficacy, adverse event, or pharmacokinetic profiles of older and younger patients. As with any NSAID, the elderly are likely to tolerate adverse reactions less well than younger patients.

ADVERSE REACTIONS

Adverse reaction information is derived from blinded, controlled, and open-label clinical trials, as well as worldwide marketing experience. In the description below, rates of more common events represent clinical study results; rarer events are derived principally from marketing experience and publications, and accurate rate estimates are generally not possible.

In 718 patients treated for shorter periods, i.e., 2 weeks or less, with Cataflam Immediate-Release Tablets, adverse reactions were reported one-half to one-tenth as frequently as by patients treated for longer periods. In a 6-month, double-blind trial comparing Cataflam Immediate-Release Tablets (N=196) versus Voltaren Delayed-Release Tablets (N=197) verus ibuprofen (N=197), adverse reactions were similar in nature and frequency. In controlled clinical trials, the incidence of adverse reactions for Voltaren Delayed-Release Tablets and Voltaren-XR Extended-Release Tablets at comparable doses were similar.

The incidence of common adverse reactions (greater than 1%) is based upon controlled clinical trials in 1543 patients treated up to 13 weeks with Voltaren Delayed-Release Tablets. By far the most common adverse effects were gastrointestinal symptoms, most of them minor, occurring in about 20%, and leading to discontinuation in about 3%, of patients. Peptic ulcer or G.I. bleeding occurred in clinical trials in 0.6% (95% confidence interval: 0.2% to 1%) of approximately 1800 patients during their first 3 months of diclofenac treatment and in 1.6% (95% confidence interval: 0.8% to 2.4%) of approximately 800 patients followed for 1 year.

Gastrointestinal symptoms were followed in frequency by central nervous system side effects such as headache (7%) and dizziness (3%).

Meaningful (exceeding 3 times the Upper Limit of Normal) elevations of ALT (SGPT) or AST (SGOT) occurred at an overall rate of approximately 2% during the first 2 months of Voltaren treatment. Unlike aspirin-related elevations, which occur more frequently in patients with rheumatoid arthritis, these elevations were more frequently observed in patients with osteoarthritis (2.6%) than in patients with rheumatoid arthritis (0.7%). Marked elevations (exceeding 8 times the ULN) were seen in 1% of patients treated for 2–6 months (see WARNINGS, Hepatic Effects).

The following adverse reactions were reported in patients treated with disclofenac:

Incidence Greater Than 1%—Causal Relationship Probable:

(All derived from clinical trials.)

*Incidence, 3% to 9% (incidence of unmarked reactions is 1%–3%).

Body as a Whole: Abdominal pain or cramps,* headache,* fluid retention, abdominal distention.

Digestive: Diarrhea,* indigestion,* nausea,* constipation,* flatulence, liver test abnormalities,* PUB, i.e., peptic ulcer, with or without bleeding and/or perforation, or bleeding without ulcer (see above and also WARNINGS).

Nervous System: Dizziness.

Skin and Appendages: Rash, pruritus.

Special Senses: Tinnitus.

Incidence Less Than 1%—Causal Relationship Probable:

(Adverse reactions reported only in worldwide marketing experience or in the literature, not seen in clinical trials, are considered rare and are *italicized.*)

Body as a Whole: Malaise, swelling of lips and tongue, photosensitivity, *anaphylaxis,* anaphylactoid reactions.

Cardiovascular: Hypertension, congestive heart failure.

Digestive: Vomiting, jaundice, melena, *esophageal lesions,* aphthous stomatitis, dry mouth and mucous membranes, bloody diarrhea, hepatitis, *hepatic necrosis, cirrhosis, hepatorenal syndrome,* appetite change, pancreatitis with or without concomitant hepatitis, *colitis.*

Hemic and Lymphatic: Hemoglobin decrease, leukopenia, thrombocytopenia, *eosinophilia, hemolytic anemia, aplastic anemia, agranulocytosis,* purpura, *allergic purpura.*

Metabolic and Nutritional Disorders: Azotemia.

Nervous System: Insomnia, drowsiness, depression, diplopia, anxiety, irritability, *aseptic meningitis, convulsions.*

Respiratory: Epistaxis, asthma, laryngeal edema.

Skin and Appendages: Alopecia, urticaria, eczema, dermatitis, *bullous eruption, erythemia multiforme major,* angioedema, *Stevens-Johnson syndrome.*

Special Senses: Blurred vision, taste disorder, reversible and irreversible hearing loss, scotoma.

Urogenital: *Nephrotic syndrome,* proteinuria, *oliguria, interstitial nephritis, papillary necrosis, acute renal failure.*

Incidence Less Than 1%—Causal Relationship Unknown:

(The following reactions have been reported in patients taking diclofenac under circumstances that do not permit a clear attribution of the reaction to diclofenac. These reactions are being included as alerting information to physicians. Adverse reactions reported only in worldwide marketing experience or in the literature, not seen in clinical trials, are considered rare and are *italicized.*)

Body as a Whole: Chest pain.

Cardiovascular: Palpitations, *flushing,* tachycardia, premature ventricular contractions, myocardial infarction, *hypotension.*

Digestive: *Intestinal perforation.*

Hemic and Lymphatic: *Bruising.*

Metabolic and Nutritional Disorders: Hypoglycemia, *weight loss.*

Nervous System: Paresthesia, memory disturbance, nightmares, tremor, tic, *abnormal coordination, disorientation, psychotic reaction.*

Respiratory: Dyspnea, hyperventilation, edema of pharynx.

Skin and Appendages: Excess perspiration, *exfoliative dermatitis.*

Special Senses: Vitreous floaters, night blindness, amblyopia.

Urogenital: Urinary frequency, nocturia, hematuria, impotence, vaginal bleeding.

OVERDOSAGE

Worldwide reports of overdosage with diclofenac cover 66 cases. In approximately one-half of these reports of overdosage, concomitant medications were also taken. The highest dose of diclofenac was 5.0 g in a 17-year-old male who suffered loss of consciousness, increased intracranial pressure, aspiration pneumonitis, and died 2 days after overdose. The next highest doses of diclofenac were 4.0 g and 3.75 g. The 24-year-old female who took 4.0 g and the 28- and 42-year-old females, each of whom took 3.75 g, did not develop any clinically significant signs or symptoms. However, there was a report of a 17-year-old female who experienced vomiting and drowsiness after an overdose of 2.37 g of diclofenac.

Animal LD_{50} values show a wide range of susceptibilities to acute overdosage, with primates being more resistant to acute toxicity than rodents (LD_{50} in mg/kg—rats, 55; dogs, 500; monkeys, 3200).

In case of acute overdosage, it is recommended that the stomach be emptied by vomiting or lavage. Forced diuresis may theoretically be beneficial because the drug is excreted in the urine. The effect of dialysis or hemoperfusion in the elimination of diclofenac (99% protein-bound: see CLINICAL PHARMACOLOGY) remains unproven. In addition to supportive measures, the use of oral activated charcoal may help to reduce the absorption of diclofenac.

DOSAGE AND ADMINISTRATION

Diclofenac may be administered as 50-mg Cataflam Immediate-Release Tablets, as 25-mg, 50-mg, and 75-mg Voltaren Delayed-Release Tablets, or as 100-mg Voltaren-XR Extended-Release Tablets. Cataflam Immediate-Release Tablets is the formulation indicated for management of acute pain and primary dysmenorrhea when prompt onset of pain relief is desired because of earlier absorption of diclofenac. For the same reason, Voltaren-XR is not indicated for the management of acute painful conditions and should be used as chronic therapy in patients with osteoarthritis and rheumatoid arthritis.

The dosage of diclofenac should be individualized to the lowest effective dose to minimize adverse effects (see INDIVIDUALIZATION OF DOSAGE).

Osteoarthritis: The recommended dosage is 100 to 150 mg/day: Cataflam or Voltaren Delayed-Release 50 mg b.i.d. or t.i.d; or Voltaren Delayed-Release 75 mg b.i.d. The recommended dosage for chronic therapy with Voltaren-XR is 100 mg q.d. Dosages of Voltaren-XR Extended Release Tablets of 200 mg daily are not recommended for patients with osteoarthritis. Dosages above 200 mg/day have not been studied in patients with osteoarthritis.

Rheumatoid Arthritis: The recommended dosage is 100 to 200 mg/day: Cataflam or Voltaren Delayed-Release 50 mg t.i.d. or q.i.d.; or Voltaren Delayed-Release 75 mg b.i.d. The recommended dosage for chronic therapy with Voltaren-XR is 100 mg q.d. In the rare patient where Voltaren-XR 100 mg/day is unsatisfactory, the dose may be increased to 100 mg b.i.d. if the benefits outweigh the clinical risks. Dosages above 225 mg/day are not recommended in patients with rheumatoid arthritis.

Ankylosing Spondylitis: The recommended dosage is 100 to 125 mg/day: Voltaren 25 mg q.i.d. with an extra 25-mg dose at bedtime if necessary. Dosages above 125 mg/day have not been studied in patients with ankylosing spondylitis.

Analgesia and Primary Dysmenorrhea: The recommended starting dose of Cataflam Immediate-Release Tablets is 50 mg t.i.d. With experience, physicians may find that in some patients an initial dose of 100 mg of Cataflam, followed by 50-mg doses, will provide better relief. After the first day,

when the maximum recommended dose may be 200 mg, the total daily dose should generally not exceed 150 mg.

HOW SUPPLIED

Cataflam Tablets
50 mg—light brown, round, biconvex (imprinted CATAFLAM on one side and 50 on the other side)

Bottles of 100 .... NDC 0028-0151-01
Unit Dose (blister pack)
Box of 100 (strips of 10) .... NDC 0028-0151-61

Voltaren *Delayed-Release* Tablets
25 mg—yellow, biconvex, triangular-shaped (imprinted VOLTAREN 25 on one side)

Bottles of 60 .... NDC 0028-0258-60
Bottles of 100 .... NDC 0028-0258-01
Unit Dose (blister pack)
Box of 100 (strips of 10) .... NDC 0028-0258-61

50 mg—light brown, biconvex, triangular-shaped (imprinted VOLTAREN 50 on one side)

Bottles of 60 .... NDC 0028-0262-60
Bottles of 100 .... NDC 0028-0262-01
Bottles of 1000 .... NDC 0028-0262-10
Unit Dose (blister pack)
Box of 100 (strips of 10) .... NDC 0028-0262-61

75 mg—light pink, biconvex, triangular-shaped (imprinted VOLTAREN 75 on one side)

Bottles of 60 .... NDC 0028-0264-60
Bottles of 100 .... NDC 0028-0264-01
Bottles of 1000 .... NDC 0028-0264-10
Unit Dose (blister pack)
Box of 100 (strips of 10) .... NDC 0028-0264-61

Voltaren-XR *Extended-Release* Tablets
100 mg—light pink, coated, round, biconvex, with beveled edges (imprinted Voltaren-XR on one side and 100 on the other side)

Bottles of 100 .... NDC 0028-0205-01
Unit Dose (blister pack)
Box of 100 (strips of 10) .... NDC 0028-0205-61

Do not store above 86°F (30°C). Protect from moisture. Dispense in *tight* container (USP).

C96-10 (Rev. 2/96)

Dist. by:
Ciba-Geigy Corporation
Pharmaceuticals Division
Ardsley, New York 10502
Shown in Product Identification Guide, page 309

CYTADREN® Tablets   ℞
[*sight 'a-dren*]
aminoglutethimide tablets USP

DESCRIPTION

Cytadren, aminoglutethimide tablets USP, is an inhibitor of adrenocortical steroid synthesis, available as 250-mg tablets for oral administration. Its chemical name is 3-(4-aminophenyl)-3-ethyl-2, 6-piperidinedione.

Aminoglutethimide USP is a fine, white or creamy white, crystalline powder. It is very slightly soluble in water, and readily soluble in most organic solvents. It forms water-soluble salts with strong acids. Its molecular weight is 232.28.

Inactive Ingredients. Cellulose compounds, colloidal silicon dioxide, starch, stearic acid, and talc.

CLINICAL PHARMACOLOGY

Cytadren inhibits the enzymatic conversion of cholesterol to Δ^5-pregnenolone, resulting in a decrease in the production of adrenal glucocorticoids, mineralocorticoids, estrogens, and androgens.

Cytadren blocks several other steps in steroid synthesis, including the C-11, C-18, and C-21 hydroxylations and the hydroxylations required for the aromatization of androgens to estrogens, mediated through the binding of Cytadren to cytochrome P-450 complexes.

A decrease in adrenal secretion of cortisol is followed by an increased secretion of pituitary adrenocorticotropic hormone (ACTH), which will overcome the blockade of adrenocortical steroid synthesis by Cytadren. The compensatory increase in ACTH secretion can be suppressed by the simultaneous administration of hydrocortisone. Since Cytadren increases the rate of metabolism of dexamethasone but not that of hydrocortisone, the latter is preferred as the adrenal glucocorticoid replacement.

Although Cytadren inhibits the synthesis of thyroxine by the thyroid gland, the compensatory increase in thyroid-stimulating hormone (TSH) is frequently of sufficient magnitude to overcome the inhibition of thyroid synthesis due to Cytadren. In spite of an increase in TSH, Cytadren has not been associated with increased prolactin secretion.

Note: Cytadren was marketed previously as an anticonvulsant but was withdrawn from marketing for that indication in 1966 because of the effects on the adrenal gland.

Pharmacokinetics
Cytadren is rapidly and completely absorbed after oral administration. In 6 healthy male volunteers, maximum plasma levels of Cytadren averaged 5.9 μg/ml at a median of 1.5 hours after ingestion of two 250-mg tablets. The bioavailability of tablets is equivalent to equal doses given as a solution. After ingestion of a single oral dose, 34–54% is excreted in the urine as unchanged drug during the first 48 hours, and an additional fraction as the N-acetyl derivative.

The half-life of Cytadren in normal volunteers given single oral doses averaged 12.5 ± 1.6 hours.

Upon withdrawal of therapy with Cytadren, the ability of the adrenal glands to synthesize steroid returns, usually within 72 hours.

INDICATIONS AND USAGE

Cytadren is indicated for the suppression of adrenal function in selected patients with Cushing's syndrome. Morning levels of plasma cortisol in patients with adrenal carcinoma and ectopic ACTH-producing tumors were reduced on the average to about one half of the pretreatment levels, and in patients with adrenal hyperplasia to about two thirds of the pretreatment levels, during 1–3 months of therapy with Cytadren. Data available from the few patients with adrenal adenoma suggest similar reductions in plasma cortisol levels. Measurements of plasma cortisol showed reductions to at least 50% of baseline or to normal levels in one third or more of the patients studied, depending on diagnostic groups and time of measurement.

Because Cytadren does not affect the underlying disease process, it is used primarily as an interim measure until more definitive therapy such as surgery can be undertaken or in cases where such therapy is not appropriate. Only small numbers of patients have been treated for longer than 3 months. A decreased effect or "escape phenomenon" seems to occur more frequently in patients with pituitary-dependent Cushing's syndrome, probably because of increasing ACTH levels in response to decreasing glucocorticoid levels. Cytadren should be used only in those patients who are responsive to treatment.

CONTRAINDICATIONS

Cytadren is contraindicated in those patients with serious forms, and/or severe manifestations, of hypersensitivity to glutethimide or aminoglutethimide.

WARNINGS

Cytadren may cause adrenocortical hypofunction, especially under conditions of stress, such as surgery, trauma, or acute illness. Patients should be carefully monitored and given hydrocortisone and mineralocorticoid supplements as indicated. Dexamethasone should not be used. (See **PRECAUTIONS, Drug Interactions.**)

Cytadren also may suppress aldosterone production by the adrenal cortex and may cause orthostatic or persistent hypotension. The blood pressure should be monitored in all patients at appropriate intervals. Patients should be advised of the possible occurrence of weakness and dizziness as symptoms of hypotension, and of measures to be taken should they occur.

The effects of Cytadren may be potentiated if it is taken in combination with alcohol.

Cytadren can cause fetal harm when administered to a pregnant woman. In the earlier experience with the drug in about 5000 patients, two cases of pseudohermaphroditism were reported in female infants whose mothers were treated with Cytadren and concomitant anticonvulsants. Normal pregnancies have also occurred in patients treated with Cytadren.

When administered to rats at doses ½ and 1¼ times the maximum daily human dose, Cytadren caused a decrease in fetal implantation, an increase in fetal deaths, and a variety of teratogenic effects. The compound also caused pseudohermaphroditism in rats treated with approximately 3 times the maximum daily human dose. If this drug must be used during pregnancy, or if the patient becomes pregnant while taking the drug, the patient should be apprised of the potential hazard to the fetus.

PRECAUTIONS

General
This drug should be administered only by physicians familiar with its use and hazards. Therapy should be initiated in a hospital. (See **DOSAGE AND ADMINISTRATION.**)

Information for Patients
Patients should be warned that drowsiness may occur and that they should not drive, operate potentially dangerous machinery, or engage in other activities that may become hazardous because of decreased alertness.

Patients should also be warned of the possibility of hypotension and its symptoms (see **WARNINGS**).

Laboratory Tests
Hypothyroidism may occur in association with Cytadren; hence, appropriate clinical observations should be made and laboratory studies of thyroid function performed as indicated. Supplementary thyroid hormone may be required.

Hematologic abnormalities in patients receiving Cytadren have been reported (see **ADVERSE REACTIONS**). Therefore, baseline hematologic studies should be performed, followed by periodic hematologic evaluation.

Since elevations in SGOT, alkaline phosphatase, and bilirubin have been reported, appropriate clinical observations and regular laboratory studies should be performed before and during therapy.

Serum electrolyte levels should be determined periodically.

Drug Interactions
Cytadren accelerates the metabolism of dexamethasone; therefore, if glucocorticoid replacement is needed, hydrocortisone should be prescribed.

Aminoglutethimide diminishes the effect of coumarin and warfarin.

Carcinogenesis, Mutagenesis, Impairment of Fertility
A 2-year carcinogenicity study of Cytadren conducted in rats at doses of 10–60 mg/kg/day (approximately 0.04 to 0.2 times the maximum daily therapeutic dose based on surface area, mg/m²) revealed a highly statistically dose-related trend in the incidence of benign and malignant neoplasms of the adrenal cortex and thyroid follicular cells in both sexes. A borderline statistically significant increase (0.05 level) in ovarian tubular adenomas was observed at 60 mg/kg/day. Urinary bladder papillomas also showed a statistically significant dose-related trend in males.

Cytadren affects fertility in female rats (see **WARNINGS**). The relevance of these findings to humans is not known.

Pregnancy Category D
See **WARNINGS**.

Nursing Mothers
It is not known whether this drug is excreted in human milk. Because many drugs are excreted in human milk and because of the potential for serious adverse reactions in nursing infants from Cytadren, a decision should be made whether to discontinue nursing or to discontinue the drug, taking into account the importance of the drug to the mother.

Pediatric Use
Safety and effectiveness in pediatric patients have not been established (see **CLINICAL STUDIES IN CHILDREN**).

ADVERSE REACTIONS

Untoward effects have been reported in about 2 out of 3 patients with Cushing's syndrome who were treated for 4 or more weeks with Cytadren as the only adrenocortical suppressant.

The most frequent and reversible side effects were drowsiness (approximately 1 in 3 patients), morbilliform skin rash (1 in 6 patients), nausea and anorexia (each approximately 1 in 8 patients), and dizziness (about 1 in 20 patients). The dizziness was possibly caused by lowered vascular resistance or orthostasis. These reactions often disappear spontaneously with continued therapy.

Other Effects Observed
Hematologic: Single instances of neutropenia, leukopenia (patient received concomitant *o,p* '-DDD), pancytopenia (patient received concomitant 5-fluorouracil), and agranulocytosis occurred in 4 of 27 patients with Cushing's syndrome caused by adrenal carcinoma who were treated for at least 4 weeks. In 1 patient with adrenal hyperplasia, hemoglobin levels and hematocrit decreased during the course of treatment with Cytadren. From the earlier experience with the drug used as an anticonvulsant in 1,214 patients, transient leukopenia was the only hematologic effect and was reported once; Coombs'-negative hemolytic anemia also occurred once. In approximately 300 patients with nonadrenal malignancy, 1 in 25 showed some degree of anemia, and 1 in 150 developed pancytopenia during treatment with Cytadren.

Endocrine: Adrenal insufficiency occurred in about 1 in 30 patients with Cushing's syndrome who were treated with Cytadren for 4 or more weeks. This insufficiency tended to involve glucocorticoids as well as mineralocorticoids. Hypothyroidism is occasionally associated with thyroid enlargement and may be detected or confirmed by measuring plasma levels of the thyroid hormone. Masculinization and hirsutism have occasionally occurred in females, as has precocious sexual development in males.

Central Nervous System: Headache was reported in about 1 in 20 patients.

Cardiovascular: Hypotension, occasionally orthostatic, occurred in 1 in 30 patients receiving Cytadren. Tachycardia occurred in 1 in 40 patients.

Gastrointestinal and Liver: Vomiting occurred in 1 in 30 patients. Isolated instances of abnormal findings on liver function tests were reported. Suspected hepatotoxicity occurred in less than 1 in 1000 patients.

Skin: In addition to rash (1 in 6 patients, and often reversible with continued therapy), pruritus was reported in 1 in 20 patients. These may be allergic or hypersensitive reactions. Urticaria has occurred rarely.

Miscellaneous: Fever was reported in several patients who were treated with Cytadren for less than 4 weeks; some of these patients also received other drugs. Myalgia occurred in 1 in 30 patients.

Pulmonary hypersensitivity, including allergic alveolitis and interstitial alveolar infiltrates, has occurred rarely.

Continued on next page

CibaGeneva—Cont.

OVERDOSAGE

Acute Toxicity

No deaths due to overdosage with Cytadren have been reported.

The highest known doses that have been survived are 7 g (33-year-old woman), 7.5-10 g (16-year-old girl), and 10 g (10-year-old boy).

Oral LD_{50}'s (mg/kg): rats, 1800; dogs, > 100. Intravenous LD_{50}'s (mg/kg): rats, 156; dogs > 100.

Signs and Symptoms

An acute overdose with Cytadren may reduce the production of steroids in the adrenal cortex to a degree that is clinically relevant. The following manifestations may be expected:

Respiratory Function: Respiratory depression, hypoventilation.

Cardiovascular System: Hypotension, hypovolemic shock due to dehydration.

Central Nervous System/Muscles: Somnolence, lethargy, coma, ataxia, dizziness, fatigue. (Extreme weakness has been reported with divided doses of 3 g daily.)

Gastrointestinal System: Nausea, vomiting.

Renal Function: Loss of sodium and water.

Laboratory Findings: Hyponatremia, hypochloremia, hyperkalemia, hypoglycemia.

The signs and symptoms of acute overdosage with Cytadren may be aggravated or modified if alcohol, hypnotics, tranquilizers, or tricyclic antidepressants have been taken at the same time.

Treatment

Symptomatic treatment of overdosage is recommended.

Since aminoglutethimide and glutethimide are chemically related, measures that have been used in successfully removing glutethimide from the body might be useful in removing aminoglutethimide.

Gastric lavage and unspecified supportive treatment have been employed. Full consciousness following deep coma was regained 40 hours or less after ingestion of 3 or 4 g without lavage. No evidence of hematologic, renal, or hepatic effects was subsequently found.

Close monitoring should be provided, and appropriate measures taken to support vital functions, if necessary.

If deficiency of circulating glucocorticoid develops, an intravenous infusion of a soluble hydrocortisone preparation (100 mg of hydrocortisone sodium succinate in 500 ml of isotonic sodium chloride solution) and 50 ml of 40% glucose solution should be given within 3 hours. After the initial infusion is completed, an intravenous administration of hydrocortisone, 10 mg per hour, should be continued until the patient is able to take oral cortisone.

If hypovolemia or hypotension occurs, an intravenous administration of norepinephrine, 10 mg, in 500 ml of isotonic sodium chloride should be administered according to the patient's needs and response. After rehydration, 500 ml of plasma or blood should be given for maintenance of sufficient circulatory volume.

Dialysis may be considered in severe intoxication.

DOSAGE AND ADMINISTRATION

Adults

Treatment should be instituted in a hospital until a stable dosage regimen is achieved. Therapy should be initiated with 250 mg orally four times daily, preferably at 6-hour intervals. Adrenocortical response should be followed by careful monitoring of plasma cortisol levels until the desired level of suppression is achieved. If the level of cortisol suppression is inadequate, the dosage may be increased in increments of 250 mg daily at intervals of 1–2 weeks to a total daily dose of 2 g. Dose reduction or temporary discontinuation of therapy may be required in the event of adverse effects, including extreme drowsiness, severe skin rash, or excessively low cortisol levels. If a skin rash persists for longer than 5–8 days or becomes severe, the drug should be discontinued. It may be possible to reinstate therapy at a lower dosage following the disappearance of a mild or moderate rash. Mineralocorticoid replacement (e.g., fludrocortisone) may be necessary. If glucocorticoid replacement therapy is needed, 20–30 mg of hydrocortisone orally in the morning will replace endogenous secretion.

HOW SUPPLIED

Tablets 250 mg — white, round, scored into quarters (imprinted CIBA 24)

Bottles of 100 ....NDC 0083-0024-30

Protect from light.

Dispense in tight, light-resistant container (USP).

Do not store above 86°F (30°C).

CLINICAL STUDIES IN CHILDREN

Clinical investigations included 9 patients aged 2½ to 16 years; 4 of these were aged 10 or less. Seven of the patients received other therapies (drugs or irradiation) either with Cytadren or within a short period before initiation of therapy with Cytadren. Diagnoses included 5 patients with adre-

nal carcinoma, 3 with adrenal hyperplasia, and 1 with ectopic ACTH-producing tumor. Duration of treatment ranged from 3 days to 6½ months. Dosages ranged from 0.375 g to 1.5 g daily. In general, smaller doses were used for younger patients; for example, a 2½-year-old received 0.5–0.75 g daily, a 3½-year-old received 0.5 g daily, and all others over 10 years of age received 0.75–1.5 g daily. Results are difficult to evaluate because of the concomitant therapy, duration of therapy, or inadequate laboratory documentation. Most patients did show decreases in plasma or urinary steroids at some time during treatment, but these may have been due to other therapeutic modalities or their combinations.

C96-19 (Rev. 4/96)

Shown in Product Identification Guide, page 309

DESFERAL®

[des'fer-all]

deferoxamine mesylate USP

Vials

℞

DESCRIPTION

Desferal, deferoxamine mesylate USP, is an iron-chelating agent, available in vials for intramuscular, subcutaneous, and intravenous administration. Each vial contains 500 mg of deferoxamine mesylate USP in sterile, lyophilized form. Deferoxamine mesylate is N-[5-[3-[(5-aminopentyl)-hydroxycarbamoyl]propionamido]-pentyl]-3-[[5-(N-hydroxy-acetamido)pentyl]carbamoyl] propionohydroxamic acid monomethanesulfonate (salt).

Deferoxamine mesylate USP is a white to off-white powder. It is freely soluble in water and slightly soluble in methanol. Its molecular weight is 656.79.

CLINICAL PHARMACOLOGY

Desferal chelates iron by forming a stable complex that prevents the iron from entering into further chemical reactions. It readily chelates iron from ferritin and hemosiderin but not readily from transferrin; it does not combine with the iron from cytochromes and hemoglobin. Desferal does not cause any demonstrable increase in the excretion of electrolytes or trace metals. Theoretically, 100 parts by weight of Desferal is capable of binding approximately 8.5 parts by weight of ferric iron.

Desferal is metabolized principally by plasma enzymes, but the pathways have not yet been defined. The chelate is readily soluble in water and passes easily through the kidney, giving the urine a characteristic reddish color. Some is also excreted in the feces via the bile.

INDICATIONS AND USAGE

Desferal is indicated for the treatment of acute iron intoxication and of chronic iron overload due to transfusion-dependent anemias.

Acute Iron Intoxication

Desferal is an adjunct to, and not a substitute for, standard measures used in treating acute iron intoxication, which may include the following: induction of emesis with syrup of ipecac; gastric lavage; suction and maintenance of a clear airway; control of shock with intravenous fluids, blood, oxygen, and vasopressors; and correction of acidosis.

Chronic Iron Overload

Desferal can promote iron excretion in patients with secondary iron overload from multiple transfusions (as may occur in the treatment of some chronic anemias, including thalassemia). Long-term therapy with Desferal slows accumulation of hepatic iron and retards or eliminates progression of hepatic fibrosis.

Iron mobilization with Desferal is relatively poor in patients under the age of 3 years with relatively little iron overload. The drug should ordinarily not be given to such patients unless significant iron mobilization (e.g., 1 mg or more of iron per day) can be demonstrated.

Desferal is not indicated for the treatment of primary hemochromatosis, since phlebotomy is the method of choice for removing excess iron in this disorder.

CONTRAINDICATIONS

Desferal is contraindicated in patients with severe renal disease or anuria, since the drug and the iron chelate are excreted primarily by the kidney.

WARNINGS

Ocular and auditory disturbances have been reported when Desferal was administered over prolonged periods of time, at high doses, or in patients with low ferritin levels. The ocular disturbances observed have been blurring of vision; cataracts after prolonged administration in chronic iron overload; decreased visual acuity including visual loss; impaired peripheral, color, and night vision; and retinal pigmentary abnormalities. The auditory abnormalities reported have been tinnitus and hearing loss including high frequency sensorineural hearing loss. In most cases, both ocular and auditory disturbances were reversible upon immediate cessation of treatment. Slit-lamp examinations performed in patients

treated with Desferal for acute iron intoxication have not revealed cataracts.

Visual acuity tests, slit-lamp examinations, funduscopy and audiometry are recommended periodically in patients treated for prolonged periods of time. Toxicity is more likely to be reversed if symptoms or test abnormalities are detected early.

PRECAUTIONS

General

Flushing of the skin, urticaria, hypotension, and shock have occurred in a few patients when Desferal was administered by rapid intravenous injection. THEREFORE, DESFERAL SHOULD BE GIVEN INTRAMUSCULARLY OR BY SLOW SUBCUTANEOUS OR INTRAVENOUS INFUSION.

Iron overload increases susceptibility of patients to Yersinia enterocolitica infections. In some rare cases, treatment with Desferal has enhanced this susceptibility, resulting in generalized infections by providing this bacteria with a siderophore otherwise missing. In such cases, Desferal treatment should be discontinued until the infection is resolved.

In patients undergoing hemodialysis while receiving Desferal, there have been rare reports of fungal infections (i.e., mucormycosis) that have sometimes been fatal; however, a causal relationship to the drug has not been established.

Information for Patients

Patients should be informed that occasionally their urine may show a reddish discoloration.

Carcinogenesis, Mutagenesis, Impairment of Fertility

Long-term carcinogenicity studies in animals have not been performed with Desferal.

Cytotoxicity may occur, since Desferal has been shown to inhibit DNA synthesis *in vitro*.

Pregnancy Category C

Delayed ossification in mice and skeletal anomalies in rabbits were observed after Desferal was administered in daily doses up to 4.5 times the maximum daily human dose. No adverse effects were observed in similar studies in rats.

There are no adequate and well-controlled studies in pregnant women. Desferal should be used during pregnancy only if the potential benefit justifies the potential risk to the fetus.

Nursing Mothers

It is not known whether this drug is excreted in human milk. Because many drugs are excreted in human milk, caution should be exercised when Desferal is administered to a nursing woman.

Pediatric Use

Safety and effectiveness in children under the age of 3 years have not been established (see INDICATIONS AND USAGE).

ADVERSE REACTIONS

The following adverse reactions have been observed, but there are not enough data to support an estimate of their frequency.

Skin: Localized irritation and pain, swelling and induration, pruritus, erythema, wheal formation.

Hypersensitive Reactions: Generalized erythema (rash), urticaria, anaphylactic reaction.

Cardiovascular: Tachycardia, hypotension, shock.

Digestive: Abdominal discomfort, diarrhea.

Special Senses: Ocular and auditory disturbances (see WARNINGS).

Other: Dysuria, leg cramps, fever.

OVERDOSAGE

Acute Toxicity

Intravenous LD_{50}'s (mg/kg): mice, 287; rats, 329.

Signs and Symptoms

Since Desferal is available only for parenteral administration, acute poisoning is unlikely to occur. However, tachycardia, hypotension, and gastrointestinal symptoms have occasionally developed in patients who received overdoses of Desferal.

Treatment

There is no specific antidote.

Signs and symptoms of overdosage may be eliminated by reducing the dosage.

Desferal is readily dialyzable.

DOSAGE AND ADMINISTRATION

Acute Iron Intoxication

Intramuscular Administration

This route is preferred and should be used for ALL PATIENTS NOT IN SHOCK.

Dosage. A dose of 1.0 g should be administered initially. This may be followed by 500 mg (one vial) every 4 hours for two doses. Depending upon the clinical response, subsequent doses of 500 mg may be administered every 4–12 hours. The total amount administered should not exceed 6.0 g in 24 hours.

Preparation of Solution. Desferal is dissolved by adding 2 ml of Sterile Water for Injection to each vial, resulting in a solution of 250 mg/ml. The drug should be completely dis-

solved before the solution is withdrawn. Desferal is then administered intramuscularly. See *NOTE* below.

Intravenous Administration

THIS ROUTE SHOULD BE USED ONLY FOR PATIENTS IN A STATE OF CARDIOVASCULAR COLLAPSE AND THEN ONLY BY SLOW INFUSION. THE RATE OF INFUSION SHOULD NOT EXCEED 15 MG/KG PER HOUR.

Dosage: An initial dose of 1.0 g should be administered at a rate NOT TO EXCEED 15 mg/kg per hour. This may be followed by 500 mg every 4 hours for two doses. Depending upon the clinical response, subsequent doses of 500 mg may be administered every 4–12 hours. The total amount administered should not exceed 6.0 g in 24 hours.

As soon as the clinical condition of the patient permits, intravenous administration should be discontinued and the drug should be administered intramuscularly.

Preparation of Solution. Desferal is dissolved by adding 2 ml of Sterile Water for Injection to each vial, resulting in a solution of 250 mg/ml. The drug should be completely dissolved before the solution is withdrawn. The solution is then added to physiologic saline, glucose in water, or Ringer's lactate solution and administered at a rate NOT TO EXCEED 15 mg/kg per hour. See *NOTE* below.

Chronic Iron Overload

The more effective of the following routes of administration must be chosen on an individual basis for each patient.

Intramuscular Administration

A daily dose of 0.5–1.0 g should be administered intramuscularly. In addition, 2.0 g should be administered intravenously with each unit of blood transfused; however, Desferal should be administered separately from the blood. The rate of intravenous infusion must not exceed 15 mg/kg per hour.

Subcutaneous Administration

A daily dose of 1.0–2.0 g (20–40 mg/kg per day) should be administered over 8–24 hours, utilizing a small portable pump capable of providing continuous mini-infusion. The duration of infusion must be individualized. In some patients, as much iron will be excreted after a short infusion of 8–12 hours as with the same dose given over 24 hours.

Preparation of Solution for Subcutaneous or Intramuscular Administration. Desferal is dissolved by adding 2.0 ml of Sterile Water for Injection to each vial, resulting in a solution of 250 mg/ml. The drug should be completely dissolved before the solution is withdrawn into the syringe to be used for administration. See *NOTE* below.

NOTE: Parenteral drug products should be inspected visually for particulate matter and discoloration prior to administration, whenever solution and container permit.

Desferal reconstituted with Sterile Water for Injection may be stored under sterile conditions and protected from light at room temperature for not longer than 1 week. Do not refrigerate reconstituted solution.

Reconstituting Desferal in solvents or under conditions other than indicated may result in precipitation. Turbid solutions should not be used.

HOW SUPPLIED

Vials —each containing 500 mg of sterile, lyophilized deferoxamine mesylate

Cartons of 4 vials ....NDC 0083-3801-04

Do not store above 77°F (25°C).

C94-10 (Rev. 5/94)

Dist. by:
Ciba-Geigy Corporation
Pharmaceuticals Division
Summit, New Jersey 07901

ESIDRIX®
[ess'a-dricks]
hydrochlorothiazide USP
Tablets

℞

DESCRIPTION

Esidrix, hydrochlorothiazide USP, is a diuretic and antihypertensive available as 25-mg and 50-mg tablets for oral administration. Its chemical name is 6-chloro-3,4-dihydro-2*H*-1,2,4-benzothiadiazine-7-sulfonamide 1,1-dioxide.

Hydrochlorothiazide USP is a white, or practically white, practically odorless, crystalline powder. It is slightly soluble in water, freely soluble in sodium hydroxide solution, in *n*-butylamine and in dimethylformamide, sparingly soluble in methanol, and insoluble in ether, in chloroform, and in dilute mineral acids. Its molecular weight is 297.73.

Inactive Ingredients: Colloidal silicon dioxide, D&C Yellow No. 10 (50-mg tablets), FD&C Red No. 40 and FD&C Yellow No. 6 (25-mg tablets), lactose, starch, stearic acid, and sucrose.

CLINICAL PHARMACOLOGY

Thiazides affect the renal tubular mechanism of electrolyte reabsorption. At maximal therapeutic dosage all thiazides are approximately equal in their diuretic potency. Thiazides increase excretion of sodium and chloride in approximately

equivalent amounts. Natriuresis causes a secondary loss of potassium.

The mechanism of the antihypertensive effect of thiazides is unknown. Thiazides do not affect normal blood pressure. Onset of action of thiazides occurs in 2 hours and the peak effect at about 4 hours. Its action persists for approximately 6 to 12 hours. Thiazides are eliminated rapidly by the kidney.

INDICATIONS AND USAGE

Hypertension

In the management of hypertension either as the sole therapeutic agent or to enhance the effect of other antihypertensive drugs in the more severe forms of hypertension.

Edema

As adjunctive therapy in edema associated with congestive heart failure, hepatic cirrhosis, and corticosteroid and estrogen therapy.

Esidrix has also been found useful in edema due to various forms of renal dysfunction, such as the nephrotic syndrome, acute glomerulonephritis, and chronic renal failure.

Usage in Pregnancy: The routine use of diuretics in an otherwise healthy woman is inappropriate and exposes mother and fetus to unnecessary hazard. Diuretics do not prevent development of toxemia of pregnancy, and there is no satisfactory evidence that they are useful in the treatment of developed toxemia.

Edema during pregnancy may arise from pathological causes or from the physiologic and mechanical consequences of pregnancy. Thiazides are indicated in pregnancy when edema is due to pathologic causes, just as they are in the absence of pregnancy (however, see **PRECAUTIONS, Pregnancy**). Dependent edema in pregnancy, resulting from restriction of venous return by the expanded uterus, is properly treated through elevation of the lower extremities and use of support hose; use of diuretics to lower intravascular volume in this case is illogical and unnecessary. There is hypervolemia during normal pregnancy which is not harmful to either the fetus or the mother (in the absence of cardiovascular disease) but which is associated with edema, including generalized edema, in the majority of pregnant women. If this edema produces discomfort, increased recumbency will often provide relief. In rare instances, this edema may cause extreme discomfort which is not relieved by rest. In these cases, a short course of diuretics may provide relief and may be appropriate.

CONTRAINDICATIONS

Anuria; hypersensitivity to this or other sulfonamide-derived drugs.

WARNINGS

Use with caution in severe renal disease. In patients with renal disease, thiazides may precipitate azotemia. Cumulative effects of the drug may develop in patients with impaired renal function.

Thiazides should be used with caution in patients with impaired hepatic function or progressive liver disease, since minor alterations of fluid and electrolyte imbalance may precipitate hepatic coma.

Thiazides may add to or potentiate the action of other antihypertensive drugs. Potentiation occurs with ganglionic or peripheral adrenergic blocking drugs.

Sensitivity reactions are more likely to occur in patients with a history of allergy or bronchial asthma.

The possibility of exacerbation or activation of systemic lupus erythematosus has been reported.

PRECAUTIONS

General

All patients receiving thiazide therapy should be observed for clinical signs of fluid or electrolyte imbalance: namely, hyponatremia, hypochloremic alkalosis, and hypokalemia (see **Laboratory Tests** and **Drug/Drug Interactions**). Warning signs are dryness of mouth, thirst, weakness, lethargy, drowsiness, restlessness, muscle pains or cramps, muscular fatigue, hypotension, oliguria, tachycardia, and gastrointestinal disturbance such as nausea or vomiting.

Hypokalemia may develop, especially with brisk diuresis or when severe cirrhosis is present.

Interference with adequate oral intake of electrolytes will also contribute to hypokalemia. Hypokalemia may be avoided or treated by use of potassium supplements or foods with a high potassium content.

Any chloride deficit is generally mild and usually does not require specific treatment except under extraordinary circumstances (as in liver disease or renal disease). Dilutional hyponatremia may occur in edematous patients in hot weather; appropriate therapy is water restriction rather than administration of salt, except in rare instances when the hyponatremia is life-threatening. In actual salt depletion, appropriate replacement is the therapy of choice.

Hyperuricemia may occur or frank gout may be precipitated in certain patients receiving thiazide therapy.

Latent diabetes may become manifest during thiazide administration (see **Drug/Drug Interactions**).

The antihypertensive effects of the drug may be enhanced in the postsympathectomy patient.

If progressive renal impairment becomes evident, withholding or discontinuing diuretic therapy should be considered. Calcium excretion is decreased by thiazides. Pathological changes in the parathyroid gland with hypercalcemia and hypophosphatemia have been observed in a few patients on prolonged thiazide therapy. The common complications of hyperparathyroidism such as renal lithiasis, bone resorption, and peptic ulceration have not been seen.

Thiazide diuretics have been shown to increase the urinary excretion of magnesium; this may result in hypomagnesemia.

Information for Patients

Patients should be informed of possible side effects and advised to take the medication regularly and continuously as directed.

Laboratory Tests

Initial and periodic determinations of serum electrolytes to detect possible electrolyte imbalance should be performed at appropriate intervals.

Serum and urine electrolyte determinations are particularly important when the patient is vomiting excessively or receiving parenteral fluids.

Drug/Drug Interactions

Hypokalemia can sensitize or exaggerate the response of the heart to the toxic effects of digitalis (e.g., increased ventricular irritability).

Hypokalemia may develop during concomitant use of steroids or ACTH.

Insulin requirements in diabetic patients may be increased, decreased, or unchanged.

Thiazides may decrease arterial responsiveness to norepinephrine. This diminution is not sufficient to preclude effectiveness of the pressor agent for therapeutic use.

Thiazide drugs may increase the responsiveness to tubocurarine.

Lithium renal clearance is reduced by thiazides, increasing the risk of lithium toxicity.

There have been rare reports in the literature of hemolytic anemia occurring with the concomitant use of hydrochlorothiazide and methyldopa.

Concurrent administration of some nonsteroidal anti-inflammatory agents may reduce the diuretic, natriuretic and antihypertensive effects of thiazide diuretics.

Cholestyramine and colestipol resins: Absorption of hydrochlorothiazide is impaired in the presence of anionic exchange resins. Single doses of either cholestyramine or colestipol resins bind the hydrochlorothiazide and reduce its absorption from the gastrointestinal tract by up to 85% and 43%, respectively.

Drug/Laboratory Test Interactions

Thiazides may decrease serum PBI levels without signs of thyroid disturbance.

Thiazides should be discontinued before carrying out tests for parathyroid function (see **PRECAUTIONS, General,** calcium excretion).

Carcinogenesis, Mutagenesis, Impairment of Fertility

Two-year feeding studies in mice and rats conducted under the auspices of the National Toxicology Program (NTP) uncovered no evidence of a carcinogenic potential of hydrochlorothiazide in female mice (at doses of up to approximately 600 mg/kg/day) or in male and female rats (at doses of up to approximately 100 mg/kg/day). The NTP, however, found equivocal evidence for hepatocarcinogenicity in male mice. Hydrochlorothiazide was not genotoxic in in vitro assays using strains TA 98, TA 100, TA 1535, TA 1537, and TA 1538 of *Salmonella typhimurium* (Ames assay) and in the Chinese Hamster Ovary (CHO) test for chromosomal aberrations, or in in vivo assays using mouse germinal cell chromosomes, Chinese hamster bone marrow chromosomes, and the *Drosophilia* sex-linked recessive lethal trait gene. Positive test results were obtained only in the in vitro CHO Sister Chromatid Exchange (clastogenicity) and in the Mouse Lymphoma Cell (mutagenicity) assays, using concentrations of hydrochlorothiazide from 43 to 1300 μg/mL, and in the *Aspergillus nidulans* nondisjunction assay at an unspecified concentration.

Hydrochlorothiazide had no adverse effect on the fertility of mice and rats of either sex in studies wherein these species were exposed, via their diet, to doses of up to 100 and 4 mg/kg/day, respectively, prior to mating and throughout gestation.

Pregnancy: Teratogenic Effects. Pregnancy Category B

Studies in which hydrochlorothiazide was orally administered to pregnant mice and rats during their respective periods of major organogenesis at doses up to 3000 and 1000 mg/kg/day, respectively, provided no evidence of harm to the fetus. There are however, no adequate and well-controlled studies in pregnant women. Because animal reproduction studies are not always predictive of human response, this drug should be used during pregnancy only if clearly needed.

Nonteratogenic Effects. Thiazides cross the placental barrier and appear in cord blood. There is a risk of fetal or neo-

Continued on next page

CibaGeneva—Cont.

natal jaundice, thrombocytopenia, and possibly other adverse reactions that have occurred in adults.

Nursing Mothers

Thiazides are excreted in breast milk. Because of the potential for serious adverse reactions in nursing infants, a decision should be made whether to discontinue nursing or to discontinue Esidrix, taking into account the importance of the drug to the mother.

Pediatric Use

Safety and effectiveness in pediatric patients have not been established.

ADVERSE REACTIONS

Adverse reactions are usually reversible upon reduction of dosage or discontinuation of Esidrix. Whenever adverse reactions are moderate or severe, it may be necessary to discontinue the drug.

The following adverse reactions have been observed, but there has not been enough systematic collection of data to support an estimate of their frequency. Consequently the reactions are categorized by organ systems and are listed in decreasing order of severity and not frequency.

Digestive: Pancreatitis, jaundice (intrahepatic cholestatic), sialadenitis, vomiting, diarrhea, cramping, nausea, gastric irritation, constipation, anorexia.

Cardiovascular: Orthostatic hypotension (may be potentiated by alcohol, barbiturates, or narcotics).

Neurologic: Vertigo, dizziness, transient blurred vision, headache, paresthesia, xanthopsia, weakness, restlessness.

Musculoskeletal: Muscle spasm.

Hematologic: Aplastic anemia, agranulocytosis, leukopenia, thrombocytopenia.

Metabolic: Hyperglycemia, glycosuria, hyperuricemia.

Hypersensitive Reactions: Necrotizing angiitis, Stevens-Johnson syndrome, respiratory distress including pneumonitis and pulmonary edema, purpura, urticaria, rash, photosensitivity.

OVERDOSAGE

Acute Toxicity

No deaths due to acute poisoning with Esidrix have been reported.

Highest known doses ingested: children, 500 mg (14-year-old girl); young children, 125 mg ($2^{1}/_{2}$-year-old child).

Oral LD_{50} in rats: > 2750 mg/kg.

Signs and Symptoms

The most prominent feature of poisoning with Esidrix is acute loss of fluid and electrolytes.

Cardiovascular: Tachycardia, hypotension, shock.

Neuromuscular: Weakness, confusion, dizziness, cramps of the calf muscles, paresthesia, fatigue, impairment of consciousness.

Gastrointestinal: Nausea, vomiting, thirst.

Renal: Polyuria, oliguria or anuria (due to hemoconcentration).

Laboratory findings: Hypokalemia, hyponatremia, hypochloremia, alkalosis, increased BUN (especially in patients with renal insufficiency).

Combined poisoning: Signs and symptoms may be aggravated or modified by concomitant intake of antihypertensive medication, barbiturates, curare, digitalis (hypokalemia), corticosteroids, narcotics, or alcohol.

Treatment

There is no specific antidote.

Elimination of the drug: Induction of vomiting, gastric lavage.

Measures to reduce absorption: Activated charcoal.

Hypotension, shock: The patient's legs should be kept raised, and lost fluid and electrolytes (potassium, sodium) should be replaced.

Surveillance: Fluid and electrolyte balance (especially serum potassium) and renal function should be monitored until conditions become normal.

DOSAGE AND ADMINISTRATION

Therapy should be individualized according to patient response. Dosage should be titrated to gain maximal therapeutic response as well as the minimal dose possible to maintain that therapeutic response.

ADULTS

Hypertension

To Initiate Therapy: Usual dosage is 50–100 mg daily. May be given as a single dose every morning.

Maintenance: After a week dosage may be adjusted downward to as little as 25 mg a day, or upward. Rarely patients may require up to 200 mg daily in divided doses.

Combined Therapy: When necessary, other antihypertensive agents may be added cautiously. Since this drug potentiates the antihypertensive effect of other agents, such additions should be gradual. Dosages of ganglionic blockers in particular should be halved initially.

Edema

To Initiate Diuresis: 25 to 200 mg daily for several days, or until dry weight is attained.

Maintenance: 25 to 100 mg daily or intermittently depending on the patient's response. A few refractory patients may require up to 200 mg daily.

INFANTS AND CHILDREN

The usual pediatric dosage is administered twice daily. The total daily dosage for infants up to 2 years of age: 12.5 to 37.5 mg; for children 2 to 12 years of age: 37.5 to 100 mg. Dosages should be based on body weight at the rate of 1 mg per pound, but infants below 6 months of age may require 1.5 mg per pound.

HOW SUPPLIED

Tablets 25 mg—round, pink, scored (imprinted CIBA 22)
    Bottles of 100 .... NDC 0083-0022-30
Tablets 50 mg—round, yellow, scored (imprinted CIBA 46)
    Bottles of 100 .... NDC 0083-0046-30
Do not store above 86°F (30°C)
Dispense in tight, light-resistant container (USP).

C96-27 (Rev. 3/96)

Shown in Product Identification Guide, page 309

ESIMIL®

[ess 'a-mill]
guanethidine monosulfate USP 10 mg
hydrochlorothiazide USP 25 mg
Combination Tablets

℞

> ### WARNING
> This fixed-combination drug is not indicated for initial therapy of hypertension. Hypertension requires therapy titrated to the individual patient. If the fixed combination represents the dosage so determined, its use may be more convenient in patient management. The treatment of hypertension is not static but must be reevaluated as conditions in each patient warrant.

DESCRIPTION

Esimil is an antihypertensive-diuretic combination, available as tablets for oral administration. Each tablet contains Ismelin (guanethidine monosulfate USP), 10 mg, and Esidrix (hydrochlorothiazide USP), 25 mg.

Guanethidine monosulfate is [2-(hexahydro-1(2H)-azocinyl) ethyl]guanidine sulfate 1:1.

Guanethidine monosulfate USP is a white to off-white crystalline powder with a molecular weight of 296.38. It is very soluble in water, sparingly soluble in alcohol and practically insoluble in chloroform.

Hydrochlorothiazide is 6-chloro-3,4-dihydro-2H-1,2,4-benzothiadiazine-7-sulfonamide 1,1-dioxide.

Hydrochlorothiazide USP is a white, or practically white, practically odorless crystalline powder. It is slightly soluble in water; freely soluble in sodium hydroxide solution, in *n*-butylamine, and in dimethylformamide; sparingly soluble in methanol; and insoluble in ether, in chloroform, and in dilute mineral acids. Its molecular weight is 297.73.

Inactive Ingredients: Colloidal silicon dioxide, lactose, starch, stearic acid, and sucrose.

CLINICAL PHARMACOLOGY

Guanethidine

Guanethidine acts at the sympathetic neuroeffector junction by inhibiting or interfering with the release and/or distribution of the chemical mediator (presumably the catecholamine norepinephrine), rather than acting at the effector cell by inhibiting the association of the transmitter with its receptors. In contrast to ganglionic blocking agents, guanethidine suppresses equally the responses mediated by alpha- and beta-adrenergic receptors but does not produce parasympathetic blockade. Since sympathetic blockade results in modest decreases in peripheral resistance and cardiac output, guanethidine lowers blood pressure in the supine position. It further reduces blood pressure by decreasing the degree of vasoconstriction that normally results from reflex sympathetic nervous activity upon assumption of the upright posture, thus reducing venous return and cardiac output more. The inhibition of sympathetic venoconstrictive mechanisms results in venous pooling of blood. Therefore, the effect of guanethidine is especially pronounced when the patient is standing. Both the systolic and diastolic pressures are reduced.

Other actions at the sympathetic nerve terminal include depletion of norepinephrine. Once it gains access to the neuron, guanethidine accumulates within the intraneuronal storage vesicles and causes depletion of norepinephrine stores within the nerve terminal. Prolonged oral administration of guanethidine produces a denervation sensitivity of the neuroeffector junction, probably resulting from the chronic reduction in norepinephrine released by the sympathetic nerve endings. Systemic responses to catecholamines released from the adrenal medulla are not prevented and may even be augmented as a result of this denervation sensitivity. A paradoxical hypertensive crisis may occur if guan-

ethidine is given to patients with pheochromocytoma or if norepinephrine is given to a patient receiving the drug. Due to its poor lipid solubility, guanethidine does not readily cross the blood-brain barrier. In contrast to most neural blocking agents, guanethidine does not appear to suppress plasma renin activity in many patients.

Pharmacokinetics

The pharmacokinetics of guanethidine are complex. The amount of drug in plasma and in urine is linearly related to dose, although large differences occur between individuals because of variation in absorption and metabolism. Adrenergic blockade occurs with a minimum concentration in plasma of 8 ng/ml; this concentration is achieved in different individuals with doses of 10–50 mg per day at steady state. Guanethidine is eliminated slowly because of extensive tissue binding. After chronic oral administration, the initial phase of elimination with a half-life of 1.5 days is followed by a second phase of elimination with a half-life of 4–8 days. The renal clearance of guanethidine is 56 ml/min. Guanethidine is converted by the liver to three metabolites, which are excreted in the urine. The metabolites are pharmacologically less active than guanethidine.

Hydrochlorothiazide

Thiazides affect the renal tubular mechanism of electrolyte reabsorption. At maximal therapeutic dosage, all thiazides are approximately equal in their diuretic potency. Thiazides increase excretion of sodium and chloride in approximately equivalent amounts. Natriuresis causes a secondary loss of potassium.

The mechanism of the antihypertensive effect of thiazides is unknown. Thiazides do not affect normal blood pressure.

Pharmacokinetics

The onset of action of thiazides occurs in 2 hours, and the peak effect at about 4 hours. The action persists for approximately 6–12 hours. Hydrochlorothiazide is rapidly absorbed, as indicated by peak plasma concentrations 1–2.5 hours after oral administration. Plasma levels of the drug are proportional to dose; the concentration in whole blood is 1.6–1.8 times higher than in plasma. Thiazides are eliminated rapidly by the kidney. After oral administration of 25- to 100-mg doses of hydrochlorothiazide, 72–97% of the dose is excreted in the urine, indicating dose-independent absorption. Hydrochlorothiazide is eliminated from plasma in a biphasic fashion with a terminal half-life of 10–17 hours. Plasma protein binding is 67.9%. Plasma clearance is 15.9–30.0 L/hr; volume of distribution is 3.6–7.8 L/kg.

Gastrointestinal absorption of hydrochlorothiazide is enhanced when administered with food. Absorption is decreased in patients with congestive heart failure, and the pharmacokinetics are considerably different in these patients.

INDICATIONS AND USAGE

Esimil is indicated for the treatment of hypertension (see boxed **WARNING**).

CONTRAINDICATIONS

Guanethidine

Known or suspected pheochromocytoma; hypersensitivity; frank congestive heart failure not due to hypertension; use of monoamine oxidase (MAO) inhibitors.

Hydrochlorothiazide

Anuria; hypersensitivity to this or other sulfonamide-derived drugs.

WARNINGS

Guanethidine and hydrochlorothiazide are potent drugs, and their use can lead to disturbing and serious clinical problems. Physicians should be familiar with both drugs and their combination before prescribing, and patients should be warned not to deviate from instructions.

Guanethidine

> Orthostatic hypotension can occur frequently, and patients should be properly instructed about this potential hazard. Fainting spells may occur unless the patient is forewarned to sit or lie down with the onset of dizziness or weakness. Postural hypotension is most marked in the morning and is accentuated by hot weather, alcohol, or exercise. Dizziness or weakness may be particularly bothersome during the initial period of dosage adjustment and with postural changes, such as arising in the morning. The potential occurrence of these symptoms may require alteration of previous daily activity. The patient should be cautioned to avoid sudden or prolonged standing or exercise while taking the drug.

Inhibition of ejaculation has been reported in animals (see **PRECAUTIONS, Carcinogenesis, Mutagenesis, Impairment of Fertility**) as well as in men given guanethidine. This effect, which results from the sympathetic blockade caused by the drug's action, is reversible after guanethidine has been discontinued for several weeks. The drug does not cause parasympathetic blockade, and erectile potency is usually retained during administration of guanethidine. The possible occurrence of inhibition of ejaculation should be kept in

mind when considering the use of guanethidine in men of reproductive age.
If possible, therapy should be withdrawn 2 weeks prior to surgery to reduce the possibility of vascular collapse and cardiac arrest during anesthesia. If emergency surgery is indicated, preanesthetic and anesthetic agents should be administered cautiously in reduced dosage. Oxygen, atropine, vasopressors, and adequate solutions for volume replacement should be ready for immediate use to counteract vascular collapse in the surgical patient. Vasopressors should be used only with extreme caution, since guanethidine augments responsiveness to exogenously administered norepinephrine and vasopressors; specifically, blood pressure may rise and cardiac arrhythmias may be produced.

Hydrochlorothiazide

Thiazides should be used with caution in patients with severe renal disease. In patients with renal disease, thiazides may precipitate azotemia. Cumulative effects of the drug may develop in patients with impaired renal function.
Thiazides should be used with caution in patients with impaired hepatic function or progressive liver disease, since minor alterations of fluid and electrolyte imbalance may precipitate hepatic coma.
Thiazides may add to or potentiate the action of other antihypertensive drugs. Potentiation occurs with ganglionic or peripheral adrenergic blocking drugs.
Sensitivity reactions are more likely to occur in patients with a history of allergy or bronchial asthma.
The possibility of exacerbation of activation of systemic lupus erythematosus has been reported.

PRECAUTIONS

General

Guanethidine. Dosage requirements may be reduced in the presence of fever.
Special care should be exercised when treating patients with a history of bronchial asthma; asthmatic patients are more apt to be hypersensitive to catecholamine depletion, and their condition may be aggravated.
The effects of guanethidine are cumulative over long periods; initial doses should be small and increased gradually in small increments.
Guanethidine should be used very cautiously in hypertensive patients with: renal disease and nitrogen retention or rising BUN levels, since decreased blood pressure may further compromise renal function; coronary insufficiency or recent myocardial infarction; and cerebrovascular disease, especially with encephalopathy.
Guanethidine should not be given to patients with severe cardiac failure except with extreme caution, since guanethidine may interfere with the compensatory role of the adrenergic system in producing circulatory adjustment in patients with congestive heart failure.
Patients with incipient cardiac decompensation should be watched for weight gain or edema.
Guanethidine should be used cautiously in patients with a history of peptic ulcer or other chronic disorders that may be aggravated by a relative increase in parasympathetic tone.
Hydrochlorothiazide. All patients receiving thiazide therapy should be observed for clinical signs of fluid or electrolyte imbalance, namely hyponatremia, hypochloremic alkalosis, and hypokalemia (see **Laboratory Tests** and **Drug/Drug Interactions**). Warning signs are dryness of mouth, thirst, weakness, lethargy, drowsiness, restlessness, muscle pains or cramps, muscular fatigue, hypotension, oliguria, tachycardia, and gastrointestinal disturbance, such as nausea or vomiting.
Thiazide diuretics have been shown to increase the urinary excretion of magnesium; this may result in hypomagnesemia.
Hypokalemia may develop, especially in cases of brisk diuresis or severe cirrhosis.
Interference with adequate oral intake of electrolytes will also contribute to hypokalemia. Hypokalemia may be avoided or treated by use of potassium supplements or foods with a high potassium content.
Any chloride deficit is generally mild and usually does not require specific treatment, except under extraordinary circumstances (as in liver disease or renal disease). Dilutional hyponatremia may occur in edematous patients in hot weather; appropriate therapy is water restriction, rather than administration of salt, except in rare instances when the hyponatremia is life-threatening. In cases of actual salt depletion, appropriate replacement is the therapy of choice.
Hyperuricemia may occur or frank gout may be precipitated in certain patients receiving thiazide therapy.
Latent diabetes may become manifest during thiazide administration (see **Drug/Drug Interactions**).
The antihypertensive effects of the drug may be enhanced in the postsympathectomy patient.
If progressive renal impairment becomes evident, withholding or discontinuing diuretic therapy should be considered.
Calcium excretion is decreased by thiazides. Pathological changes in the parathyroid gland with hypercalcemia and hypophosphatemia have been observed in a few patients on prolonged thiazide therapy. The common complications of hyperparathyroidism, such as renal lithiasis, bone resorption, and peptic ulceration, have not been seen.

Information for Patients

The patient should be advised to take this medication exactly as directed. If the patient misses a dose, he or she should be told to take only the next scheduled dose (without doubling it).
The patient should be advised to avoid sudden or prolonged standing or exercise and to arise slowly, especially in the morning, to reduce the orthostatic hypotensive effects of dizziness, lightheadedness, or fainting.
The patient should be cautioned about ingesting alcohol, since it aggravates the orthostatic hypotensive effects of guanethidine.
Male patients should be advised that guanethidine may interfere with ejaculation.

Laboratory Tests

Hydrochlorothiazide. Initial and periodic determinations of serum electrolytes to detect possible electrolyte imbalance should be performed at appropriate intervals.
Serum and urine electrolyte determinations are particularly important when the patient is vomiting excessively or receiving parenteral fluids.

Drug/Drug Interactions

Guanethidine. Concurrent use of guanethidine and rauwolfia derivatives may cause excessive postural hypotension, bradycardia, and mental depression.
Both digitalis and guanethidine slow the heart rate.
Amphetamine-like compounds, stimulants (e.g., ephedrine, methylphenidate), tricyclic antidepressants (e.g., amitriptyline, imipramine, desipramine) and other psychopharmacologic agents (e.g., phenothiazines and related compounds), as well as oral contraceptives, may reduce the hypotensive effect of guanethidine.
MAO inhibitors should be discontinued for at least 1 week before starting therapy with guanethidine.
Hydrochlorothiazide. Hypokalemia can sensitize or exaggerate the response of the heart to the toxic effects of digitalis (e.g., increased ventricular irritability).
Hypokalemia may develop during concomitant use of steroids or ACTH.
Insulin requirements in diabetic patients may be increased, decreased, or unchanged.
Thiazides may decrease arterial responsiveness to norepinephrine, but not enough to preclude effectiveness of the pressor agent for therapeutic use.
Thiazides may increase the responsiveness to tubocurarine.
Lithium renal clearance is reduced by thiazides, increasing the risk of lithium toxicity.
There have been rare reports in the literature of hemolytic anemia occurring with the concomitant use of hydrochlorothiazide and methyldopa.
Concurrent administration of some nonsteroidal anti-inflammatory agents may reduce the diuretic, natriuretic and antihypertensive effects of thiazide diuretics.
Cholestyramine and colestipol resins: Absorption of hydrochlorothiazide is impaired in the presence of anionic exchange resins. Single doses of either cholestyramine or colestipol resins bind the hydrochlorothiazide and reduce its absorption from the gastrointestinal tract by up to 85% and 43%, respectively.

Drug/Laboratory Test Interactions

Thiazides may decrease serum levels of protein-bound iodine without signs of thyroid disturbance. Esimil should be discontinued before tests for parathyroid function are made (see **General, Hydrochlorothiazide,** Calcium excretion).

Carcinogenesis, Mutagenesis, Impairment of Fertility

Long-term carcinogenicity studies in animals have not been conducted with Esimil. Fertility was not impaired in rats receiving at least 4 times the average daily human dose of Esimil.
Guanethidine: While inhibition of sperm passage and accumulation of sperm debris have been reported in rats and rabbits after several weeks of administration of guanethidine, 5 or 10 mg/kg per day, subcutaneously or intraperitoneally, recovery of ejaculatory function and fertility has been demonstrated in rats given guanethidine intramuscularly, 25 mg/kg per day, for 8 weeks. Inhibition of ejaculation has also been reported in men (see **WARNINGS** and **ADVERSE REACTIONS**). This effect, which is attributable to the sympathetic blockade caused by the drug, is reversible several weeks after discontinuance of the drug.
Hydrochlorothiazide: Two-year feeding studies in mice and rats conducted under the auspices of the National Toxicology Program (NTP) uncovered no evidence of a carcinogenic potential of hydrochlorothiazide in female mice (at doses of up to approximately 600 mg/kg/day) or in male and female rats (at doses of up to approximately 100 mg/kg/day). The NTP, however, found equivocal evidence for hepatocarcinogenicity in male mice.
Hydrochlorothiazide was not genotoxic in in vitro assays using strains TA 98, TA 100, TA 1535, TA 1537, and TA 1538 of *Salmonella typhimurium* (Ames assay) and in the Chinese Hamster Ovary (CHO) test for chromosomal aberrations, or in in vivo assays using mouse germinal cell chromosomes, Chinese hamster bone marrow chromosomes, and the *Drosophila* sex-linked recessive lethal trait gene. Positive test results were obtained only in the in vitro CHO Sister Chromatid Exchange (clastogenicity) and in the Mouse Lymphoma Cell (mutagenicity) assays, using concentrations of hydrochlorothiazide from 43 to 1300 μg/mL, and in the *Aspergillus nidulans* nondisjunction assay at an unspecified concentration.
Hydrochlorothiazide had no adverse effects on the fertility of mice and rats of either sex in studies wherein these species were exposed, via their diet, to doses of up to 100 and 4 mg/kg/day, respectively, prior to mating and throughout gestation.

Pregnancy: Teratogenic Effects. Pregnancy Category B

A reproduction study performed in rats receiving at least 150 times the average daily human dose of Esimil has revealed no evidence of harm to the fetus due to this drug.
There are no adequate and well-controlled studies of Esimil in pregnant women. Because animal reproduction studies are not always predictive of human response, this drug should be used during pregnancy only if clearly needed.
Guanethidine. The effects of guanethidine on teratogenesis have not been studied in animals.
Hydrochlorothiazide. Studies in which hydrochlorothiazide was orally administered to pregnant mice and rats during their respective periods of major organogenesis at doses up to 3000 and 1000 mg/kg/day, respectively, provided no evidence of harm to the fetus.
Nonteratogenic Effects. *Hydrochlorothiazide.* Thiazides cross the placental barrier and appear in cord blood, and there is a risk of fetal or neonatal jaundice, thrombocytopenia, and possibly other adverse reactions that have occurred in adults.

Nursing Mothers

Guanethidine is excreted in breast milk in very small quantity. Thiazides are also excreted in breast milk. Because of the potential for serious adverse reactions in nursing infants, a decision should be made whether to discontinue nursing or to discontinue Esimil, taking into account the importance of the drug to the mother.

Pediatric Use

Safety and effectiveness of the combination drug in pediatric patients have not been established.

ADVERSE REACTIONS

Whenever adverse reactions are moderate or severe, it may be necessary to reduce the dosage of Esimil, discontinuing the drug, or administer the individual active components, reducing the dosage of either guanethidine or hydrochlorothiazide.
The following adverse reactions have been observed, but there are not enough data to support an estimate of their frequency. Consequently the reactions are categorized by organ system and are listed in decreasing order of severity and not frequency.

Guanethidine

Digestive: Diarrhea, which may be severe at times and necessitate discontinuance of medication; vomiting; nausea; increased bowel movements; dry mouth; parotid tenderness.
Cardiovascular: Chest pains (angina); bradycardia; a tendency toward fluid retention and edema with occasional development of congestive heart failure.
Respiratory: Dyspnea; asthma in susceptible individuals; nasal congestion.
Neurologic: Syncope resulting from either postural or exertional hypotension; dizziness; blurred vision; muscle tremor; ptosis of the lids; mental depression; chest paresthesias; weakness; lassitude; fatigue.
Muscular: Myalgia.
Genitourinary: Rise in BUN; urinary incontinence; inhibition of ejaculation; nocturia.
Metabolic: Weight gain.
Skin and Appendages: Dermatitis; scalp hair loss.
Although a causal relationship has not been established, a few instances of blood dyscrasias (anemia, thrombocytopenia, and leukopenia) and of priapism or impotence have been reported.

Hydrochlorothiazide

Digestive: Pancreatitis, jaundice (intrahepatic cholestatic), sialadenitis, vomiting, diarrhea, cramping, nausea, gastric irritation, constipation, anorexia.
Cardiovascular: Orthostatic hypotension (may be potentiated by alcohol, barbiturates, or narcotics).
Neurologic: Vertigo, dizziness, transient blurred vision, headache, paresthesia, xanthopsia, weakness, restlessness.
Musculoskeletal: Muscle spasm.
Hematologic: Aplastic anemia, agranulocytosis, leukopenia, thrombocytopenia.
Metabolic: Hyperglycemia, glycosuria, hyperuricemia.
Hypersensitive Reactions: Necrotizing angiitis, Stevens-Johnson syndrome, respiratory distress including pneumonitis and pulmonary edema, purpura, urticaria, rash, photosensitivity.

Continued on next page

CibaGeneva—Cont.

OVERDOSAGE

Acute Toxicity

No deaths due to acute poisoning with Esimil have been reported.

Oral LD_{50}'s in rats (mg/kg): guanethidine, 1262; hydrochlorothiazide, 2750.

Signs and Symptoms

Guanethidine. Postural hypotension (with dizziness, blurred vision, and possibly syncope when standing), shock, and bradycardia are most likely to occur; diarrhea (possibly severe), nausea, and vomiting may also occur. Unconsciousness is unlikely if adequate blood pressure and cerebral perfusion can be maintained by placing the patient in the supine position and by administering other treatment as required.

Hydrochlorothiazide. The most prominent feature of poisoning is acute loss of fluid and electrolytes.

Cardiovascular: Tachycardia, hypotension, shock.

Neuromuscular: Weakness, confusion, dizziness, cramps of the calf muscles, paresthesia, fatigue, impairment of consciousness.

Digestive: Nausea, vomiting, thirst.

Renal: Polyuria, oliguria, or anuria (due to hemoconcentration).

Laboratory Findings: Hypokalemia, hyponatremia, hypochloremia, alkalosis, increased BUN (especially in patients with renal insufficiency).

Combined Poisoning: Signs and symptoms may be aggravated or modified by concomitant intake of antihypertensive medication, barbiturates, digitalis (hypokalemia), corticosteroids, narcotics, or alcohol.

Treatment

There is no specific antidote.

The stomach contents should be evacuated. An activated charcoal slurry should be instilled and laxatives given, if conditions permit.

If hypotension or shock occurs, the patient's legs should be kept raised, and lost fluid and electrolytes (potassium, sodium) should be replaced. Renal function should be monitored until conditions become normal.

In sinus bradycardia, atropine should be administered.

In previously normotensive patients, treatment has consisted essentially of restoring blood pressure and heart rate to normal by keeping the patient in the supine position. Normal homeostatic control usually returns gradually over a 72-hour period in these patients.

In previously hypertensive patients, particularly those with impaired cardiac reserve or other cardiovascular-renal disease, intensive treatment may be required to support vital functions and to control cardiac irregularities that might be present. The supine position must be maintained; if vasopressors are required, they must be used with extreme caution, since guanethidine may increase responsiveness, causing a rise in blood pressure and development of cardiac arrhythmias.

Diarrhea, if severe or persistent, should be treated with anticholinergic agents to reduce intestinal hypermotility, and hydration and electrolyte balance should be maintained.

Since guanethidine is excreted slowly, cardiovascular and renal function should be monitored for a few days.

DOSAGE AND ADMINISTRATION

Dosage should be determined by titration of individual components (see boxed WARNING). Once the patient has successfully been given titrated doses of the individual components, Esimil may be substituted if the titrated doses are the same as those in the fixed combination.

When combined with other antihypertensive agents, doses of hydrochlorothiazide in excess of 50 mg should be avoided. Therefore, since each Esimil tablet contains 25 mg of hydrochlorothiazide, the daily dosage of this fixed combination should not exceed two tablets. If further blood pressure control is indicated, additional doses of guanethidine or other nondiuretic antihypertensive agents should be considered. Before using any guanethidine-containing product, at least 1 week should elapse after MAO inhibitors (see CONTRAINDICATIONS) or ganglionic blockers have been discontinued.

HOW SUPPLIED

Tablets —round, white, scored (imprinted CIBA 47)

    10 mg of guanethidine monosulfate

    25 mg of hydrochlorothiazide

    Bottles of 100 ....NDC 0083-0047-30

Do not store above 86°F (30°C).

Dispense in tight container (USP)   C96-16 (Rev. 3/96)

Shown in Product Identification Guide, page 309

ESTRADERM® ℞
estradiol transdermal system
Continuous delivery for twice-weekly application

Prescribing Information

> **1. ESTROGENS HAVE BEEN REPORTED TO INCREASE THE RISK OF ENDOMETRIAL CARCINOMA IN POSTMENOPAUSAL WOMEN.**
>
> Close clinical surveillance of all women taking estrogens is important. Adequate diagnostic measures, including endometrial sampling when indicated, should be undertaken to rule out malignancy in all cases of undiagnosed persistent or recurring abnormal vaginal bleeding. There is no evidence that "natural" estrogens are more or less hazardous than "synthetic" estrogens at equiestrogenic doses.
>
> **2. ESTROGENS SHOULD NOT BE USED DURING PREGNANCY.**
>
> Estrogen therapy during pregnancy is associated with an increased risk of congenital defects in the reproductive organs of the fetus, and possibly other birth defects. Studies of women who received diethylstilbestrol (DES) during pregnancy have shown that female offspring have an increased risk of vaginal adenosis, squamous cell dysplasia of the uterine cervix, and clear cell vaginal cancer later in life; male offspring have an increased risk of urogenital abnormalities and possible testicular cancer later in life. The 1985 DES Task Force concluded that use of DES during pregnancy is associated with a subsequent increased risk of breast cancer in the mothers, although a causal relationship remains unproven and the observed level of excess risk is similar to that for a number of other breast cancer risk factors.
>
> There is no indication for estrogen therapy during pregnancy.
>
> Estrogens are ineffective for the prevention or treatment of threatened or habitual abortion. Estrogens are not indicated for the prevention of postpartum breast engorgement.

DESCRIPTION

Estraderm, estradiol transdermal system, is designed to release 17β-estradiol through a rate-limiting membrane continuously upon application to intact skin.

Two systems are available to provide nominal in vivo delivery of 0.05 or 0.1 mg of estradiol per day via skin of average permeability (interindividual variation in skin permeability is approximately 20%). Each corresponding system having an active surface area of 10 or 20 cm² contains 4 or 8 mg of estradiol USP and 0.3 or 0.6 mL of alcohol USP, respectively. The composition of the systems per unit area is identical. Estradiol USP (17β-estradiol) is a white, crystalline powder, chemically described as estra-1,3,5(10)-triene-3, 17β-diol.

The Estraderm system comprises four layers. Proceeding from the visible surface toward the surface attached to the skin, these layers are (1) a transparent polyester film, (2) a drug reservoir of estradiol USP and alcohol USP gelled with hydroxypropyl cellulose, and (3) an ethylene-vinyl acetate copolymer membrane, and (4) an adhesive formulation of light mineral oil and polyisobutylene. A protective liner (5) of siliconized polyethylene terephthalate film is attached to the adhesive surface and must be removed before the system can be used.

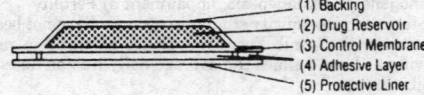

- (1) Backing
- (2) Drug Reservoir
- (3) Control Membrane
- (4) Adhesive Layer
- (5) Protective Liner

The active component of the system is estradiol. The remaining components of the system are pharmacologically inactive. Alcohol is also released from the system during use.

CLINICAL PHARMACOLOGY

The Estraderm system releases estradiol, the major estrogenic hormone secreted by the human ovary. Although circulating estrogens exist in a dynamic equilibrium of metabolic interconversions, estradiol is the principal intracellular human estrogen and is substantially more potent than estrone or estriol at the receptor level.

Estraderm provides systemic estrogen replacement therapy. Estrogen receptors have been identified in tissues of the reproductive tract, breast, pituitary, hypothalamus, liver, and in the bone of women. Among numerous effects, estradiol is largely responsible for the development and maintenance of the female reproductive system and of secondary sexual characteristics. By a direct action, it causes growth and development of the vagina, uterus, and fallopian tubes. With other hormones, such as pituitary hormones and progesterone, they cause enlargement of the breasts through promotion of ductal growth, stromal development, and the accretion of fat. Estrogens contribute to the shaping of the skeleton, to the maintenance of tone and elasticity of urogenital

---

structures, to changes in the epiphyses of the long bones that allow for the pubertal growth spurt and its termination, to the growth of axillary and pubic hair, and to the pigmentation of the nipples and genitals.

Estrogens are intricately involved with other hormones, especially progesterone, in the processes of the ovulatory menstrual cycle and pregnancy and affect the release of pituitary gonadotropins.

Loss of ovarian estradiol secretion after menopause can result in instability of thermoregulation, causing hot flushes associated with sleep disturbance and excessive sweating, and urogenital atrophy, causing dyspareunia and urinary incontinence. Estradiol replacement therapy alleviates many of these symptoms of estradiol deficiency in the menopausal woman.

Transdermal administration produces therapeutic serum levels of estradiol with lower circulating levels of estrone and estrone conjugates, and requires smaller total doses than does oral therapy. Because estradiol has a short half-life (~1 hour), transdermal administration of estradiol allows a rapid decline in blood levels after an Estraderm system is removed, e.g., in a cycling regimen.

In a study using transdermally administered estradiol, 0.1 mg daily, plasma levels increased by 66 pg/mL, resulting in an average plasma level of 73 pg/mL. There were no significant increases in the concentration of renin substrate or other hepatic proteins (sex hormone-binding globulin, thyroxine-binding globulin, and corticosteroid-binding globulin).

Pharmacokinetics

Administration of Estraderm produces mean serum concentrations of estradiol comparable to those produced by a daily oral administration of estradiol at about 20 times the daily transdermal dose. In single-application studies in 14 postmenopausal women using Estraderm systems that provided 0.05 and 0.1 mg of exogenous estradiol per day, these systems produced increased blood levels within 4 hours and maintained respective mean serum estradiol concentrations of 32 and 67 pg/mL above baseline over the application period. At the same time, increases in estrone serum concentration averaged only 9 and 27 pg/mL above baseline, respectively. Serum concentrations of estradiol and estrone returned to preapplication levels within 24 hours after removal of the system. The estimated daily urinary output of estradiol conjugates increased 5 to 10 times the baseline values and returned to near baseline within 2 days after removal of the system.

By comparison, estradiol (2 mg/day) administered orally to postmenopausal women resulted in increases in mean serum concentration of 59 pg/mL of estradiol and 302 pg/mL of estrone above baseline on the third consecutive day of dosing. Urinary output of estradiol conjugates after oral administration increased to about 100 times the baseline values and did not approach baseline until 7–8 days after the last dose.

In a 3-week multiple-application study of 14 postmenopausal women in which Estraderm 0.05 was applied twice weekly, the mean increments in steady-state serum concentration were 30 pg/mL for estradiol and 12 pg/mL for estrone. Urinary output of estradiol conjugates returned to baseline within 3 days after removal of the last (6th) system, indicating little or no estrogen accumulation in the body.

INDICATIONS AND USAGE

Estraderm® (estradiol transdermal system) is indicated in the following:

1. Treatment of moderate-to-severe vasomotor symptoms associated with menopause. There is no adequate evidence that estrogens are effective for nervous symptoms or depression that might occur during menopause, and they should not be used to treat these conditions.
2. Treatment of atrophic vaginitis and kraurosis vulvae.
3. Treatment of atrophic urethritis.
4. Treatment of hypoestrogenism due to hypogonadism, castration, or primary ovarian failure.
5. Prevention of osteoporosis (loss of bone mass). The mainstays of prevention and management of osteoporosis are estrogen, an adequate lifetime calcium intake, and exercise. Estrogen replacement therapy is the most effective single modality for the prevention of postmenopausal osteoporosis in women. Estrogen replacement therapy reduces bone resorption and retards or halts postmenopausal bone loss. Case-controlled studies have shown an approximately 60% reduction in hip and wrist fractures in women whose estrogen replacement was begun within a few years of menopause. Studies also suggest that estrogen reduces the rate of vertebral fractures. Even when started as late as 6 years after menopause, estrogen prevents further loss of bone mass for as long as treatment is continued. When estrogen therapy is discontinued, bone mass declines at a rate comparable to the immediate postmenopausal period. A well-controlled, double-blind, prospective trial conducted at the Mayo Clinic has demonstrated that treatment with Estraderm prevents bone loss in postmenopausal women at a dosage of 0.05 mg/day.

Treatment with Estraderm 0.05 mg showed full maintenance of bone density with a slight (0.8%), but not significant, increase. Placebo treatment resulted in a significant loss of more than 6% below baseline vertebral bone mass. Patients using either Estraderm 0.1 or 0.05 mg had significantly greater bone densities than those using placebo. Women are at higher risk than men because they have less bone mass, and for several years following natural or induced menopause, the rate of bone mass decline is accelerated. Early menopause is one of the strongest predictors for the development of osteoporosis. In addition, other factors affecting the skeleton that are associated with osteoporosis include race (white and Asian women are at higher risk than black women); genetic factors (small build, family history); endocrine factors (nulliparity, thyrotoxicosis, hyperparathyroidism, Cushing's syndrome, hyperprolactinemia, Type I diabetes); life-style (cigarette smoking, alcohol abuse, sedentary habits); and nutrition (below-average body weight, dietary calcium intake). Calcium deficiency has been implicated in the pathogenesis of the disease. Therefore, when not contraindicated, it is recommended that postmenopausal women receive calcium supplementation.

Immobilization and prolonged bed rest produce rapid bone loss, while weight-bearing exercise has been shown both to reduce bone loss and to increase bone mass. The optimal type and amount of physical activity that would prevent osteoporosis have not been established.

CONTRAINDICATIONS

Patients with known hypersensitivity to any of the components of the therapeutic system should not use Estraderm. Estrogens should not be used in women with any of the following conditions:

1. Known or suspected pregnancy (see Boxed Warning). Estrogen may cause fetal harm when administered to a pregnant woman.
2. Known or suspected cancer of the breast.
3. Known or suspected estrogen-dependent neoplasia.
4. Undiagnosed abnormal genital bleeding.
5. Active thrombophlebitis or thromboembolic disorders.

WARNINGS

1. *Induction of malignant neoplasms.* Some studies have suggested a possible increased incidence of breast cancer in those women taking estrogen therapy at higher doses or for prolonged periods of time. The majority of studies, however, have not shown an association with the usual doses used for estrogen replacement therapy. Women on this therapy should have regular breast examinations and should be instructed in breast self-examination. The reported endometrial cancer risk among unopposed estrogen users is about 2- to 12-fold greater than in nonusers and appears dependent on duration of treatment and on estrogen dose. Most studies show no significant increased risk associated with use of estrogens for less than 1 year. The greatest risk appears associated with prolonged use with increased risks of 15- to 24-fold for 5 to 10 years or more. In three studies, persistence of risk was demonstrated for 8 to over 15 years after cessation of estrogen treatment. In one study, a significant decrease in the incidence of endometrial cancer occurred 6 months after estrogen withdrawal. Concurrent progestin therapy may offset this risk, but the overall health impact in postmenopausal women is not known (see PRECAUTIONS).

Estrogen therapy during pregnancy is associated with an increased risk of fetal congenital reproductive tract disorders. In female offspring, there is an increased risk of vaginal adenosis, squamous cell dysplasia of the cervix, and clear cell vaginal cancer later in life; in males, urogenital and possibly testicular abnormalities. Although some of these changes are benign, it is not known whether they are precursors of malignancy.

2. *Gallbladder disease.* Two studies have reported a 2- to 4-fold increase in the risk of surgically confirmed gallbladder disease in postmenopausal women receiving oral estrogen replacement therapy, similar to the 2-fold increase previously noted in users of oral contraceptives.

3. *Cardiovascular disease.* Large doses of oral estrogen (5 mg conjugated estrogens per day), comparable to those used to treat cancer of the prostate and breast, have been shown in a large prospective clinical trial in men to increase the risk of nonfatal myocardial infarction, pulmonary embolism, and thrombophlebitis. It cannot necessarily be extrapolated from men to women. However, to avoid the theoretical cardiovascular risk to women caused by high estrogen doses, the dose for estrogen replacement therapy should not exceed the lowest effective dose.

4. *Elevated blood pressure.* Occasional blood pressure increases during postmenopausal estrogen replacement therapy have been attributed to idiosyncratic reactions to estrogens. More often, blood pressure has remained the same or has dropped. Postmenopausal estrogen use does not increase the risk of stroke; nonetheless, blood pressure should be monitored at regular intervals with estrogen use, especially if high doses are used. Ethinyl estradiol and conjugated estrogens have been shown to increase renin substrate. In con-

trast to these oral estrogens, transdermally administered estradiol does not affect renin substrate.

5. *Hypercalcemia.* Administration of estrogen may lead to severe hypercalcemia in patients with breast cancer and bone metastases. If this occurs, the drug should be stopped and appropriate measures taken to reduce the serum calcium levels.

PRECAUTIONS

General

1. *Addition of a progestin.* Studies of the addition of a progestin for 10 or more days of a cycle of estrogen administration have reported a lowered incidence of endometrial hyperplasia than would be induced by estrogen treatment alone. Morphologic and biochemical studies of endometria suggest that 10 to 14 days of progestin are needed to provide maximal maturation of the endometrium and to reduce the likelihood of hyperplastic changes. There are possible additional risks that may be associated with the use of progestins in estrogen replacement regimens. These include (1) adverse effects on lipoprotein metabolism (lowering HDL and raising LDL), which could diminish the purported cardioprotective effect of estrogen therapy (see PRECAUTIONS, below); (2) impairment of glucose tolerance; and (3) possible enhancement of mitotic activity in breast epipthelial tissue, although few epidemiologic data are available to address this point (see PRECAUTIONS, below). The choice of progestin, its dose, and its regimen may be important in minimizing these adverse effects, but these issues will require further study before they are clarified.

2. *Cardiovascular risk.* A causal relationship between estrogen replacement therapy and reduction of cardiovascular disease in postmenopausal women has not been proven. Furthermore, the effect of added progestins on this putative benefit is not yet known.

In recent years, many published studies have suggested that there may be a cause-effect relationship between postmenopausal oral estrogen replacement therapy *without added progestins* and a decrease in cardiovascular disease in women. Although most of the observational studies that assessed this statistical association have reported a 20% to 50% reduction in coronary heart disease risk and associated mortality in estrogen takers, the following should be considered when interpreting these reports:

1. Because only one of these studies was randomized and it was too small to yield statistically significant results, all relevant studies were subject to selection bias. The apparently reduced risk of coronary artery disease cannot be attributed with certainty to estrogen replacement therapy. It may instead have been caused by life-style and medical characteristics of the women studied with the possibility that healthier women were selected for estrogen therapy. Thus, ongoing and future large-scale randomized trials may fail to confirm this apparent benefit.

2. Current medical practice often includes the use of concomitant progestin therapy in women with intact uteri (see PRECAUTIONS and WARNINGS). While the effects of added progestins on the risk of ischemic heart disease are not known, all available progestins reverse at least some of the favorable effects of estrogens on HDL and LDL levels.

3. While the effects of added progestins on the risk of breast cancer are also unknown, available epidemiological evidence suggests that progestins do not reduce, and may enhance, the moderately increased breast cancer incidence that has been reported with prolonged estrogen replacement therapy (see WARNINGS, above).

Because relatively long-term use of estrogens by women with uteri has been shown to induce endometrial cancer, physicians often recommend that women who are deemed candidates for hormone replacement should take progestins as well as estrogens. When considering prescribing concomitant estrogens and progestins for hormone replacement therapy, physicians and patients are advised to carefully weigh the potential benefits and risks of the added progestin. Large-scale, randomized, placebo-controlled, prospective clinical trials are required to clarify these issues.

3. *Physical examination.* A complete medical and family history should be taken prior to the initiation of any estrogen therapy. The pretreatment and periodic physical examinations should include special reference to blood pressure, breasts, abdomen, and pelvic organs and should include a Papanicolaou smear. As a general rule, estrogen should not be prescribed for longer than 1 year without another physical examination being performed.

4. *Hypercoagulability.* Some studies have shown that women taking estrogen replacement therapy have hypercoagulability, primarily related to decreased antithrombin activity. This effect appears dose- and duration-dependent and is less pronounced than that associated with oral contraceptive use. Also, postmenopausal women tend to have increased coagulation parameters at baseline compared to premenopausal women. There is some suggestion that low-dose postmenopausal mestranol may increase the risk of thromboembolism, although the majority of studies (primarily of users of conjugated estrogens) report no such increase. There is in-

sufficient information on hypercoagulability in women who have had previous thromboembolic disease. Women on estrogen replacement therapy have not been reported to have an increased risk of thrombophlebitis and/or thromboembolic disease. However, there is insufficient information regarding women who have had previous thromboembolic disease.

5. *Familial hyperlipoproteinemia.* Estrogen therapy may be associated with massive elevations of plasma triglycerides, leading to pancreatitis and other complications in patients with familial defects of lipoprotein metabolism.

6. *Fluid retention.* Because estrogens may cause some degree of fluid retention, conditions that might be influenced by this factor, such as asthma, epilepsy, migraine, and cardiac or renal dysfunction, require careful observation.

7. *Uterine bleeding and mastodynia.* Certain patients may develop undesirable manifestations of estrogenic stimulation, such as abnormal uterine bleeding and mastodynia.

8. *Impaired liver function.* Estrogens may be poorly metabolized in patients with impaired liver function and should be administered with caution.

Information for the Patient

See text of Patient Package Insert, which appears after the HOW SUPPLIED section.

Laboratory Tests

Estrogen administration should generally be guided by clinical response at the smallest dose, rather than laboratory monitoring, for relief of symptoms for those indications in which symptoms are observable. For prevention and treatment of osteoporosis, however, see DOSAGE AND ADMINISTRATION. Tests used to measure adequacy of estrogen replacement therapy include serum estrone and estradiol levels and suppression of serum gonadotropin levels.

Drug/Laboratory Test Interactions

Some of these drug/laboratory test interactions have been observed only with estrogen-progestin combinations (oral contraceptives):

1. Accelerated prothrombin time, partial thromboplastin time, and platelet aggregation time; increased platelet count; increased factors II, VII antigen, VIII antigen, VIII coagulant activity, IX, X, XII, VII-X complex, II-VII-X complex, and beta-thromboglobulin; decreased levels of antifactor Xa and antithrombin III; decreased antithrombin III activity; increased levels of fibrinogen and fibrinogen activity; increased plasminogen antigen and activity.

2. Increased thyroid-binding globulin (TBG) leading to increased circulating total thyroid hormone, as measured by T_4 levels determined either by column or by radioimmunoassay. Free T_3 resin uptake is decreased, reflecting the elevated TBG; free T_4 and free T_3 concentrations are unaltered.

3. Other binding proteins may be elevated in serum, i.e., corticosteroid-binding globulin (CBG), sex hormone-binding globulin (SHBG), leading to increased circulating corticosteroids and sex steroids respectively. Free or biologically active hormone concentrations are unchanged. Other plasma proteins may be increased (angiotensinogen/renin substrate, alpha-1–antitrypsin, ceruloplasmin).

4. Increased plasma HDL and HDL-2 subfraction concentrations, reduced LDL cholesterol concentration, increased triglyceride levels.

5. Impaired glucose tolerance.

6. Reduced response to metyrapone test.

7. Reduced serum folate concentration.

Carcinogenesis, Mutagenesis, Impairment of Fertility

Long-term, continuous administration of natural and synthetic estrogens in certain animal species increases the frequency of carcinomas of the breast, cervix, vagina, testis, and liver (see CONTRAINDICATIONS and WARNINGS).

Pregnancy Category X

Estrogens should not be used during pregnancy (see CONTRAINDICATIONS and Boxed Warning).

Nursing Mothers

As a general principle, the administration of any drug to nursing mothers should be done only when clearly necessary since many drugs are excreted in human milk.

ADVERSE REACTIONS

(See WARNINGS regarding induction of neoplasia, adverse effects on the fetus, gallbladder disease, cardiovascular disease, elevated blood pressure, and hypercalcemia.)

The most commonly reported adverse reaction to Estraderm in clinical trials was redness and irritation at the application site. This occurred in about 17% of the women treated and caused approximately 2% to discontinue therapy. Reports of rash have been rare. There have also been rare reports of severe systemic allergic reactions.

The following additional adverse reactions have been reported with estrogen therapy:

1. *Genitourinary system.* Changes in vaginal bleeding pattern and abnormal withdrawal bleeding or flow; breakthrough bleeding; spotting; increase in size of uterine leiomyomata; vaginal candidiasis; change in amount of cervical secretion.

Continued on next page

CibaGeneva—Cont.

2. *Breasts.* Tenderness, enlargement.
3. *Gastrointestinal.* Nausea, vomiting; abdominal cramps, bloating; cholestatic jaundice; gallbladder disease.
4. *Skin.* Chloasma or melasma that may persist when drug is discontinued; erythema multiforme; erythema nodosum; hemorrhagic eruption; loss of scalp hair; hirsutism.
5. *Eyes.* Steepening of corneal curvature; intolerance to contact lenses.
6. *CNS.* Headache, migraine, dizziness; mental depression; chorea.
7. *Miscellaneous.* Increase or decrease in weight; reduced carbohydrate tolerance; aggravation of porphyria; edema; changes in libido.

ACUTE OVERDOSAGE

Serious ill effects have not been reported following acute ingestion of large doses of estrogen-containing oral contraceptives by young children. Overdosage of estrogen may cause nausea and vomiting, and withdrawl beeding may occur in females.

DOSAGE AND ADMINISTRATION

The adhesive side of the Estraderm system should be placed on a clean, dry area of the skin on the trunk of the body (including the buttocks and abdomen). The site selected should be one that is not exposed to sunlight. *Estraderm should not be applied to the breasts.* The Estraderm system should be replaced twice weekly. The sites of application must be rotated, with an interval of at least 1 week allowed between applications to a particular site. The area selected should not be oily, damaged, or irritated. The waistline should be avoided, since tight clothing may rub the system off. The system should be applied immediately after opening the pouch and removing the protective liner. The system should be pressed firmly in place with the palm of the hand for about 10 seconds, making sure there is good contact, especially around the edges. In the unlikely event that a system should fall off, the same system may be reapplied. If necessary, a new system may be applied. In either case, the original treatment schedule should be continued.

Initiation of Therapy

Estraderm is currently available in two dosage forms—0.05 mg and 0.1 mg. For treatment of moderate-to-severe vasomotor symptoms, atrophic vaginitis, and atrophic urethritis associated with menopause, initiate therapy with Estraderm 0.05 applied to the skin twice weekly. The lowest dose that will control symptoms should be chosen, and medication should be discontinued as promptly as possible. Attempts to discontinue or taper medication given only for these menopausal symptoms should be made at 3-month to 6-month intervals.

Prophylactic therapy with Estraderm to prevent postmenopausal bone loss should be initiated with the 0.05 mg/day dosage as soon as possible after menopause. The dosage may be adjusted if necessary. Discontinuation of estrogen replacement therapy may reestablish bone loss at a rate comparable to the immediate postmenopausal period.

In women not currently taking oral estrogens, treatment with Estraderm may be initiated at once. In women who are currently taking oral estrogen, treatment with Estraderm should be initiated 1 week after withdrawal of oral hormone replacement therapy, or sooner if menopausal symptoms reappear in less than 1 week.

Therapeutic Regimen

Estraderm therapy may be given continuously in patients who do not have an intact uterus. In those patients with an intact uterus, Estraderm may be given on a cyclic schedule (e.g., 3 weeks on drug followed by 1 week off drug).

HOW SUPPLIED

Estraderm estradiol transdermal system 0.05 mg/day—each 10 cm^2 system contains 4 mg of estradiol USP for nominal* delivery of 0.05 mg of estradiol per day.

Patient Calendar Pack
of 8 Systems .... NDC 0083-2310-08
Carton of 6 Patient Calendar Packs
of 8 Systems .... NDC 0083-2310-62
Carton of 1 Patient Calendar Pack
of 24 Systems .... NDC 0083-2310-24

Estraderm estradiol transdermal system 0.1 mg/day—each 20 cm^2 system contains 8 mg of estradiol USP for nominal* delivery of 0.1 mg of estradiol per day.

Patient Calendar Pack
of 8 Systems .... NDC 0083-2320-08
Carton of 6 Patient Calendar Packs
of 8 Systems .... NDC 0083-2320-62
Carton of 1 Patient Calendar Pack
of 24 Systems .... NDC 0083-2320-24

*See DESCRIPTION.
Do not store above 86°F (30°C).
Do not store unpouched. Apply immediately upon removal from the protective pouch.

C95-43 (Rev. 10/95)

Information for the Patient

ESTRADERM® ℞

Generic name: estradiol transdermal system pronounced ess-tra-DYE-all

1. ESTROGENS INCREASE THE RISK OF CANCER OF THE UTERUS IN WOMEN WHO HAVE HAD THEIR MENOPAUSE ("CHANGE OF LIFE").
If you use any estrogen-containing drug, it is important to visit your doctor regularly and report any unusual vaginal bleeding right away. Vaginal bleeding after menopause may be a warning sign of uterine cancer. Your doctor should evaluate any unusual vaginal bleeding to find out the cause.
2. ESTROGENS SHOULD NOT BE USED DURING PREGNANCY.
Estrogens do not prevent miscarriage (spontaneous abortion) and are not needed in the days following childbirth. If you take estrogens during pregnancy, your unborn child has a greater than usual chance of having birth defects. The risk of developing these defects is small, but clearly larger than the risk in children whose mothers did not take estrogens during pregnancy. These birth defects may affect the baby's urinary system and sex organs. Daughters born to mothers who took DES (an estrogen drug) have a higher than usual chance of developing cancer of the vagina or cervix when they become teenagers or young adults. Sons may have a higher than usual chance of developing cancer of the testicles when they become teenagers or young adults.

INTRODUCTION

Your doctor has prescribed Estraderm for the treatment of your menopausal symptoms and/or to prevent osteoporosis. During menopause, production of estrogen hormones by your body decreases well below the amounts normally produced during your fertile years. In many women, this decrease in estrogen production causes uncomfortable symptoms, most noticeably, hot flushes and sleep disturbance. Estrogens can be given to reduce or eliminate these symptoms and/or to prevent osteoporosis.

The Estraderm system that your doctor has prescribed for you releases small amounts of estradiol through the skin in a continuous way. Estradiol is the same hormone that your ovaries produce abundantly before menopause. Your doctor will prescribe the lowest dose you require, depending upon your individual response. The dose is adjusted by the size of the Estraderm system used; the systems are available in two sizes. The length of treatment will depend on the reason for use.

INFORMATION ABOUT ESTRADERM

How Estraderm Works

Estraderm contains estradiol. When applied to the skin as directed below, the Estraderm system releases estradiol, which flows through the skin into the bloodstream.

How and Where to Apply Estraderm

Each Estraderm system is individually sealed in a protective pouch. Tear open this pouch at the indentation (do not use scissors) and remove the system. Bubbles in the system are normal.

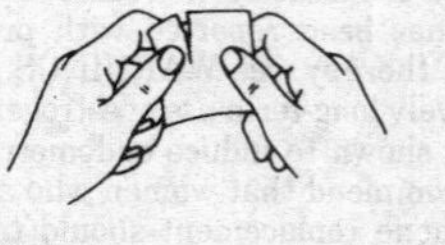

A stiff protective liner covers the adhesive side of the system—the side that will be placed against your skin. This liner must be removed before applying the system. Slide the protective liner sideways between your thumb and index finger. Then hold the system at one edge. Remove the protective liner and discard it. Try to avoid touching the adhesive.

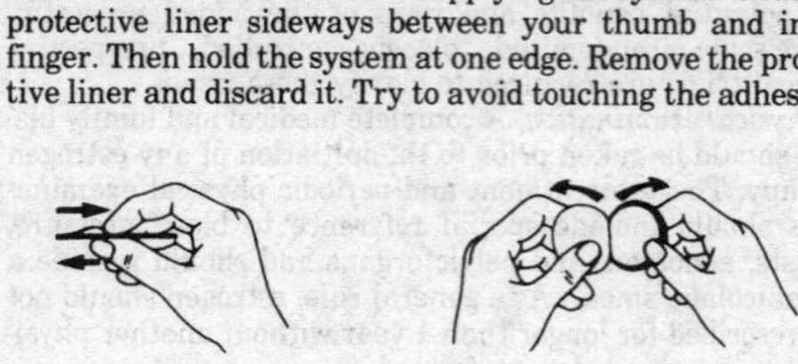

Apply the adhesive side of the system to a clean, dry area of the skin on the trunk of the body (including the buttocks and abdomen).

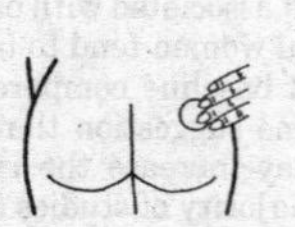

The site selected should be one that is not exposed to sunlight. Some women may find that it is more comfortable to wear Estraderm on the buttocks. *Do not apply Estraderm to your breasts.* The sites of application must be rotated, with an interval of at least 1 week allowed between applications to a particular site. The area selected should not be oily, damaged, or irritated. Avoid the waistline, since tight clothing may rub the system off. Apply the system immediately after opening the pouch and removing the protective liner. Press the system firmly in place with the palm of your hand for about 10 seconds, making sure there is good contact, especially around the edges.

The Estraderm system should be worn continuously until it is time to replace it with a new system. You may wish to experiment with different locations when applying a new system, to find ones that are most comfortable for you and where clothing will not rub on the system.

When to Apply Estraderm

The Estraderm system should be replaced twice weekly. Your Estraderm package contains a calendar checklist on the back to help you remember a schedule. Mark the 2-day schedule you plan to follow. Always change the system on the 2 days of the week you have marked.

When changing the system, remove the used Estraderm and discard it. Any adhesive that might remain on your skin can be easily rubbed off. Then place the new Estraderm on a different skin site. (The same skin site should not be used again for at least 1 week after removal of the system.)

Please note: Contact with water when you are bathing, swimming, or showering will not affect the system. In the unlikely event that a system should fall off, put this same system back on and continue to follow your original treatment schedule. If necessary, you may apply a new system but continue to follow your original schedule.

Benefits of Treatment With Estraderm

Regular use of Estraderm twice weekly offers relief of moderate-to-severe symptoms of menopause and has been shown to help prevent osteoporosis, which is a thinning of the bones that makes them more fragile. In the years following the menopause, unless estrogen therapy is taken regularly, your bones can rapidly lose strength, possibly leading to osteoporosis and bone fractures. Estraderm may prevent this bone loss and the development of osteoporosis and may help you to avoid fractures of your spine ("dowager's hump"), wrist, and hip later in life.

Small quantities of the naturally occurring hormone estradiol are absorbed through the skin from the Estraderm system, ensuring a continuous supply of circulating hormone in the body.

There is no medical evidence that the use of any estrogen during menopause will keep you feeling young, keep your skin soft, or relieve nervousness.

USES OF ESTROGEN

To reduce moderate-to-severe menopausal symptoms. Estrogens are hormones produced by the ovaries. The decrease in the amount of estrogen that occurs in all women, usually between ages 45 and 55, causes the menopause. Sometimes the ovaries are removed by an operation, causing "surgical menopause." When the amount of estrogen begins to decrease, some women develop very uncomfortable symptoms, such as feelings of warmth in the face, neck, and chest or sudden intense episodes of heat and sweating ("hot flashes"). The use of drugs containing estrogens can help the body adjust to lower estrogen levels.

Some women have only mild menopausal symptoms, or none at all, and do not need estrogen therapy for these particular symptoms. Other women may need estrogens for a few months while their bodies adjust to lower estrogen levels. For the treatment of menopausal symptoms only, most women need estrogen replacement therapy for no longer than 6 months. The prevention of osteoporosis may require longer-term therapy.

To prevent osteoporosis (brittle bones). After age 40, and especially after menopause, women begin to lose bone more rapidly, and some women develop osteoporosis. This thinning of the bones makes the bones weaker and more likely to break, often leading to fractures of the spine, hip, and wrist. Taking estrogens after the menopause slows down or halts bone loss and may prevent bones from breaking. Rapid loss of bone may begin soon after estrogen therapy is discontinued. Eating foods that are high in calcium (such as milk products) or taking calcium supplements and certain types of exercise may also help prevent osteoporosis. Before you change your calcium intake or exercise habits, it is important to discuss these life-style changes with your doctor to find out if they are safe for you. Since estrogen use is associated with some risk, its use in the prevention of osteoporosis should be confined to women who appear to be susceptible to this condition. The following characteristics are often present in women who are likely to develop osteoporosis: early menopause; white or Asian race; a family history of osteoporosis in a mother, sister, or aunt; slight build; cigarette smoking; alcohol abuse; or sedentary life-style.

Women who had their menopause by the surgical removal of their ovaries at a relatively young age may be good candidates for Estraderm therapy to help prevent osteoporosis.

To treat atrophic vaginitis (itching, burning, dryness in or around the vagina) *and atrophic urethritis* (which may cause difficulty or burning on urination).

WHEN ESTROGENS SHOULD NOT BE USED

During pregnancy. Although the possibility is fairly small, there is a greater risk of having a child born with a birth defect if you take estrogens during pregnancy. A male child may have an increased risk of developing abnormalities of the urinary system and sex organs. A female child may have an increased risk of developing cancer of the vagina or cervix in her teens or twenties. Estrogen is not effective in preventing miscarriage (abortion). In addition, estrogen should not be used after childbirth to prevent the breast from filling with milk, or while breast-feeding.

If you have undiagnosed vaginal bleeding. Unusual vaginal bleeding can be a warning sign of uterine cancer, especially if it happens after menopause. Your doctor must find out the proper treatment, if any. Taking estrogens without visiting your doctor can cause you serious harm if your vaginal bleeding is caused by cancer of the uterus.

If you have any circulation problems. Estrogen therapy should be used only after consultation with your doctor and only in recommended doses. Patients with a tendency for abnormal blood clotting should avoid estrogen use (see DANGERS OF ESTROGENS).

If you have had cancer. Since estrogens increase the risk of certain cancers, you should not take estrogens if you have ever had cancer of the breast or uterus.

When they are ineffective. Sometimes women experience nervous symptoms or depression during menopause. There is no evidence that estrogens are effective for such symptoms. You may have heard that taking estrogens for long periods (years) after menopause will keep your skin soft and supple and keep you feeling young. There is no evidence for these claims, and such long-term treatment may carry serious risks.

DANGERS OF ESTROGENS

Cancer of the uterus. The risk of cancer of the uterus increases the longer estrogens are used and when larger doses are taken. One study showed that when estrogens are discontinued, this increased risk of cancer seems to fall off quickly. Three other studies showed that the risk for uterine cancer stayed high for 8 to more than 15 years after stopping estrogen treatment. Because of this risk, *it is important to take the lowest dose of estrogen that will control your symptoms and to take it only as long as you need it.* Using progestin therapy together with estrogen therapy may reduce the higher risk of uterine cancer related to estrogen use (see OTHER INFORMATION).

If you have had your uterus removed (total hysterectomy), there is no danger of developing cancer of the uterus.

Cancer of the breast. The majority of studies have shown no association between the usual doses used for estrogen replacement therapy and breast cancer. Some studies have suggested a possible increased incidence of breast cancer in those women taking estrogens for prolonged periods of time and especially if higher doses are used.

Regular breast examinations by a health professional and monthly self-examination are recommended for women receiving estrogen therapy, as they are for all women.

Gallbladder disease. Women who use estrogens after menopause are more likely to develop gallbladder disease needing surgery than women who do not use estrogens.

Abnormal blood clotting. Taking estrogens may increase the risk of blood clots. These clots can cause a stroke, heart attack, or pulmonary embolus, any of which may be fatal. However, most studies of low-dose estrogen usage by women do not show an increased risk of these complications.

SIDE EFFECTS

In addition to the risks listed above, the following side effects have been reported with estrogen use:

● Nausea and vomiting.
● Breast tenderness or enlargement.
● Enlargement of benign tumors of the uterus.
● Retention of excess fluid. This may make some conditions worsen, such as asthma, epilepsy, migraine, heart disease, or kidney disease.
● A spotty darkening of the skin, particularly on the face.
● Skin irritation, redness, or rash may occur at the site of Estraderm application.

REDUCING RISK OF ESTROGEN USE

If you decide to take estrogen replacement therapy, you can reduce your risks by carefully monitoring your treatment.

See your doctor regularly. While you are taking estrogens, it is important that you visit your doctor at least once a year for a physical examination. If members of your family have had breast cancer or if you have ever had breast nodules or an abnormal mammogram (breast x-ray), you may need to have more frequent breast examinations.

Reevaluate your need for estrogens. You and your doctor should reevaluate your need for estrogens at least every 6 months.

Be alert for signs of trouble. Report these or any other unusual side effects to your doctor immediately:

● Abnormal bleeding from the vagina.
● Pains in the calves or chest, a sudden shortness of breath,

or coughing blood (indicating possible clots in the legs, heart, or lungs).
● Severe headache, dizziness, faintness, or changes in vision, indicating possible clots in the brain or eye.
● Breast lumps.
● Yellowing of the skin.
● Pain, swelling, or tenderness in the abdomen.
● Skin irritation, redness, or rash.

OTHER INFORMATION

If your uterus has not been removed, your doctor may choose to prescribe a progestin, a different hormonal drug, to be used in association with estrogen treatment. Progestins lower the risk of developing endometrial hyperplasia, a possible precancerous condition of the uterine lining, which may occur while using estrogens. There are possible additional risks that may be associated with the inclusion of a progestin in estrogen treatment. The possible risks include unfavorable effects on blood fats and sugars, as well as a possible further increase in breast cancer risk that may be associated with long-term estrogen use.

Some research has suggested that estrogens taken *without progestins* may protect women against developing heart disease. However, this effect of estrogens is not certain.

You are cautioned to discuss very carefully with your doctor or health care provider all the possible risks and benefits of long-term estrogen and progestin treatment, as they affect you personally.

Your doctor has prescribed this drug for you and you alone. Do not give the drug to anyone else.

If you will be taking calcium supplements as part of the treatment to help prevent osteoporosis, check with your doctor about the amounts recommended.

Keep this and all other drugs out of the reach of children. In case of overdose, remove the Estraderm system and call your doctor, hospital, or poison control center immediately.

This leaflet provides the most important information about estrogens. If you want to read more, ask your doctor or pharmacist to let you read the professional labeling.

C95-44 (Rev. 10/95)
C95-43/C95-44 (Rev. 10/95)

Ciba-Geigy Corporation
Pharmaceuticals Division
Summit, New Jersey 07901

Shown in Product Identification Guide, page 309

ISMELIN® sulfate   ℞
[*iz'mel-lin*]
guanethidine monosulfate USP
Tablets

DESCRIPTION

Ismelin, guanethidine monosulfate USP, is an antihypertensive, available as tablets of 10 mg and 25 mg for oral administration. Each 10-mg and 25-mg tablet contains guanethidine monosulfate USP equivalent to 10 mg and 25 mg of guanethidine sulfate, USP. Its chemical name is [2-(hexahydro-1(2*H*)-azocinyl)ethyl]guanidine sulfate 1:1.

Guanethidine monosulfate USP is a white to off-white crystalline powder with a molecular weight of 296.38. It is very soluble in water, sparingly soluble in alcohol, and practically insoluble in chloroform.

Inactive ingredients: Calcium stearate, colloidal silicon dioxide, D&C Yellow No. 10 (10-mg tablets), lactose, starch, stearic acid, and sucrose.

CLINICAL PHARMACOLOGY

Ismelin acts at the sympathetic neuroeffector junction by inhibiting or interfering with the release and/or distribution of the chemical mediator (presumably the catecholamine norepinephrine), rather than acting at the effector cell by inhibiting the association of the transmitter with its receptors. In contrast to ganglionic blocking agents, Ismelin suppresses equally the responses mediated by alpha- and beta-adrenergic receptors but does not produce parasympathetic blockade. Since sympathetic blockade results in modest decreases in peripheral resistance and cardiac output, Ismelin lowers blood pressure in the supine position. It further reduces blood pressure by decreasing the degree of vasoconstriction that normally results from reflex sympathetic nervous activity upon assumption of the upright posture, thus reducing venous return and cardiac output more. The inhibition of sympathetic venoconstrictive mechanisms results in venous pooling of blood. Therefore, the effect of Ismelin is especially pronounced when the patient is standing. Both the systolic and diastolic pressures are reduced.

Other actions at the sympathetic nerve terminal include depletion of norepinephrine. Once it gains access to the neuron, Ismelin accumulates within the intraneuronal storage vesicles and causes depletion of norepinephrine stores within the nerve terminal. Prolonged oral administration of Ismelin produces a denervation sensitivity of the neuroeffector junction, probably resulting from the chronic reduction in norepinephrine released by the sympathetic nerve endings. Systemic responses to catecholamines released from

the adrenal medulla are not prevented and may even be augmented as a result of this denervation sensitivity. A paradoxical hypertensive crisis may occur if Ismelin is given to patients with pheochromocytoma or if norepinephrine is given to a patient receiving the drug.

Due to its poor lipid solubility, Ismelin does not readily cross the blood-brain barrier. In contrast to most neural blocking agents, Ismelin does not appear to suppress plasma renin activity in many patients.

Pharmacokinetics

The pharmacokinetics of Ismelin are complex. The amount of drug in plasma and in urine is linearly related to dose, although large differences occur between individuals because of variation in absorption and metabolism. Adrenergic blockade occurs with a minimum concentration in plasma of 8 ng/ml; this concentration is achieved in different individuals with dosages of 10–50 mg/day at steady state. Ismelin is eliminated slowly because of extensive tissue binding. After chronic oral administration, the initial phase of elimination with a half-life of 1.5 days is followed by a second phase of elimination with a half-life of 4–8 days. The renal clearance of Ismelin is 56 ml/min. Ismelin is converted by the liver to three metabolites, which are excreted in the urine. The metabolites are pharmacologically less active than Ismelin.

INDICATIONS AND USAGE

Ismelin is indicated for the treatment of moderate and severe hypertension, either alone or as an adjunct, and for the treatment of renal hypertension, including that secondary to pyelonephritis, renal amyloidosis, and renal artery stenosis.

CONTRAINDICATIONS

Known or suspected pheochromocytoma; hypersensitivity; frank congestive heart failure not due to hypertension; use of monoamine oxidase (MAO) inhibitors.

WARNINGS

Ismelin is a potent drug and its use can lead to disturbing and serious clinical problems. Before prescribing, physicians should familiarize themselves with the details of its use and warn patients not to deviate from instructions.

> Orthostatic hypotension can occur frequently, and patients should be properly instructed about this potential hazard. Fainting spells may occur unless the patient is forewarned to sit or lie down with the onset of dizziness or weakness. Postural hypotension is most marked in the morning and is accentuated by hot weather, alcohol, or exercise. Dizziness or weakness may be particularly bothersome during the initial period of dosage adjustment and with postural changes, such as arising in the morning. The potential occurrence of these symptoms may require alteration of previous daily activity. The patient should be cautioned to avoid sudden or prolonged standing or exercise while taking the drug.

Inhibition of ejaculation has been reported in animals (see PRECAUTIONS, Carcinogenesis, Mutagenesis, Impairment of Fertility) as well as in men given Ismelin. This effect, which results from the sympathetic blockade caused by the drug's action, is reversible after Ismelin has been discontinued for several weeks. The drug does not cause parasympathetic blockade, and erectile potency is usually retained during administration of Ismelin. The possible occurrence of inhibition of ejaculation should be kept in mind when considering the use of guanethidine in men of reproductive age. If possible, therapy should be withdrawn 2 weeks prior to surgery to reduce the possibility of vascular collapse and cardiac arrest during anesthesia. If emergency surgery is indicated, preanesthetic and anesthetic agents should be administered cautiously in reduced dosage. Oxygen, atropine, vasopressors, and adequate solutions for volume replacement should be ready for immediate use to counteract vascular collapse in the surgical patient. Vasopressors should be used only with extreme caution, since Ismelin augments responsiveness to exogenously administered norepinephrine and vasopressors; specifically, blood pressure may rise and cardiac arrhythmias may be produced.

PRECAUTIONS

General

Dosage requirements may be reduced in the presence of fever.

Special care should be exercised when treating patients with a history of bronchial asthma; asthmatic patients are more apt to be hypersensitive to catecholamine depletion, and their condition may be aggravated.

The effects of Ismelin are cumulative over long periods; initial doses should be small and increased gradually in small increments.

Ismelin should be used very cautiously in hypertensive patients with renal disease and nitrogen retention or rising BUN levels, since decreased blood pressure may further compromise renal function, coronary insufficiency or recent

Continued on next page

CibaGeneva—Cont.

myocardial infarction, and cerebrovascular disease, especially with encephalopathy.
Ismelin should not be given to patients with severe cardiac failure except with extreme caution, since Ismelin may interfere with the compensatory role of the adrenergic system in producing circulatory adjustment in patients with congestive heart failure.
Patients with incipient cardiac decompensation should be watched for weight gain or edema, which may be averted by the concomitant administration of a thiazide.
Ismelin should be used cautiously in patients with a history of peptic ulcer or other chronic disorders that may be aggravated by a relative increase in parasympathetic tone.

Information for Patients
The patient should be advised to take Ismelin exactly as directed. If the patient misses a dose, he or she should be told to take only the next scheduled dose (without doubling it).
The patient should be advised to avoid sudden or prolonged standing or exercise and to arise slowly, especially in the morning, to reduce the orthostatic hypotensive effects of dizziness, lightheadedness, or fainting.
The patient should be cautioned about ingesting alcohol, since it aggravates the orthostatic hypotensive effects of Ismelin.
Male patients should be advised that guanethidine may interfere with ejaculation.

Drug Interactions
Concurrent use of Ismelin and rauwolfia derivatives may cause excessive postural hypotension, bradycardia, and mental depression.
Both digitalis and Ismelin slow the heart rate.
Thiazide diuretics enhance the antihypertensive action of Ismelin (see **DOSAGE AND ADMINISTRATION**).
Amphetamine-like compounds, stimulants (e.g., ephedrine, methylphenidate), tricylic antidepressants (e.g., amitriptyline, imipramine, desipramine) and other psychopharmacologic agents (e.g., phenothiazines and related compounds), as well as oral contraceptives, may reduce the hypotensive effect of Ismelin.
MAO inhibitors should be discontinued for at least 1 week before starting therapy with Ismelin.

Carcinogenesis, Mutagenesis, Impairment of Fertility
Long-term carcinogenicity studies in animals have not been conducted with Ismelin.
While inhibition of sperm passage and accumulation of sperm debris have been reported in rats and rabbits after several weeks of administration of Ismelin, 5 or 10 mg/kg per day, subcutaneously or intraperitoneally, recovery of ejaculatory function and fertility has been demonstrated in rats given Ismelin intramuscularly, 25 mg/kg per day, for 8 weeks. Inhibition of ejaculation has also been reported in men (see **WARNINGS** and **ADVERSE REACTIONS**). This effect, which is attributable to the sympathetic blockade caused by the drug, is reversible several weeks after discontinuance of the drug.

Pregnancy Category C
Animal reproduction studies have not been conducted with Ismelin. It is also not known whether Ismelin can cause fetal harm when administered to a pregnant woman or can affect reproduction capacity. Ismelin should be given to a pregnant woman only if clearly needed.

Nursing Mothers
Ismelin is excreted in breast milk in very small quantity. Caution should be exercised when Ismelin is administered to a nursing woman.

Pediatric Use
Safety and effectiveness in pediatric patients have not been established.

ADVERSE REACTIONS
The following adverse reactions have been observed, but there are not enough data to support an estimate of their frequency. Consequently the reactions are categorized by organ system and are listed in decreasing order of severity and not frequency.
Digestive: Diarrhea, which may be severe at times and necessitate discontinuance of medication; vomiting, nausea, increased bowel movements; dry mouth, parotid tenderness.
Cardiovascular: Chest pains (angina); bradycardia; a tendency toward fluid retention and edema with occasional development of congestive heart failure.
Respiratory: Dyspnea; asthma in susceptible individuals; nasal congestion.
Neurologic: Syncope resulting from either postural or exertional hypotension; dizziness; blurred vision; muscle tremor; ptosis of the lids; mental depression; chest paresthesias; weakness; lassitude; fatigue.
Muscular: Myalgia.
Genitourinary: Rise in BUN; urinary incontinence; inhibition of ejaculation; nocturia.
Metabolic: Weight gain.
Skin and Appendages: Dermatitis; scalp hair loss.
Although a causal relationship has not been established, a few instances of blood dyscrasia (anemia, thrombocytopenia, and leukopenia) and of priapism or impotence have been reported.

OVERDOSAGE
Acute Toxicity
No deaths due to acute poisoning have been reported.
Oral LD_{50} in rats: 1262 mg/kg.

Signs and Symptoms
Postural hypotension (with dizziness, blurred vision, and possibly syncope when standing), shock, and bradycardia are most likely to occur, diarrhea (possibly severe), nausea and vomiting may also occur. Unconsciousness is unlikely if adequate blood pressure and cerebral perfusion can be maintained by placing the patient in the supine position and by administering other treatment as required.

Treatment
There is no specific antidote.
Treatment should consist of gastric lavage. An activated charcoal slurry should be instilled and laxatives given, if conditions permit.
In sinus bradycardia, atropine should be administered.
In previously normotensive patients, treatment has consisted essentially of restoring blood pressure and heart rate to normal by keeping the patient in the supine position. Normal homeostatic control usually returns gradually over a 72-hour period in these patients.
In previously hypertensive patients, particularly those with impaired cardiac reserve or other cardiovascular-renal disease, intensive treatment may be required to support vital functions and to control cardiac irregularities that might be present. The supine position must be maintained; if vasopressors are required, they must be used with extreme caution, since Ismelin may increase responsiveness, causing a rise in blood pressure and development of cardiac arrhythmias.
Diarrhea, if severe or persistent, should be treated with anticholinergic agents to reduce intestinal hypermotility; hydration and electrolyte balance should be maintained.
Since Ismelin is excreted slowly, cardiovascular and renal function should be monitored for a few days.

DOSAGE AND ADMINISTRATION
Better control may be obtained, especially in the initial phases of treatment, if the patient can have his blood pressure recorded regularly at home.

Ambulatory Patients
Initial doses should be small (10 mg) and increased gradually, depending upon the patient's response. Ismelin has a long duration of action; therefore, dosage increases should not be made more often than every 5–7 days, unless the patient is hospitalized.
Blood pressure should be measured in the supine position, after standing for 10 minutes, and immediately after exercise if feasible. Dosage may be increased only if there has been no decrease in the standing blood pressure from previous levels. The average daily dose is 25–50 mg; only one dose a day is usually required.

Dosage Chart for Ambulatory Patients

Visits (Intervals of 5–7 Days)	*Daily Dose*
Visit 1 (Patient may be started on 10-mg tablets)	10 mg
Visit 2	20 mg
Visit 3 (Patient may be changed to 25-mg tablets whenever convenient)	30 mg (three 10-mg tablets) or 37.5 mg (one and one-half 25-mg tablets)
Visit 4	50 mg
Visit 5 and subsequent	Dosage may be increased by 12.5 mg or 25 mg if necessary.

The dosage should be reduced in any of the following situations: (1) normal supine pressure (2) excessive orthostatic fall in pressure (3) severe diarrhea.

Hospitalized Patients
Initial oral dose is 25–50 mg, increased by 25 mg or 50 mg daily or every other day, as indicated. This higher dosage is possible because hospitalized patients can be watched carefully. Unless absolutely impossible, the standing blood pressure should be measured regularly. Patients should not be discharged from the hospital until the effect of the drug on the standing blood pressure is known. Patients should be told about the possibility of orthostatic hypotension and warned not to get out of bed without help during the period of dosage adjustment.

Combination Therapy
Ismelin may be added gradually to thiazides and/or hydralazine. Thiazide diuretics enhance the effectiveness of Ismelin and may reduce the incidence of edema. When thiazide diuretics are added to the regimen in patients taking Ismelin, it is usually necessary to reduce the dosage of Ismelin. After control is established, the dosage of all drugs should be reduced to the lowest effective level.
Note: When Ismelin is replacing MAO inhibitors, at least 1 week should elapse before commencing treatment with Ismelin (see **CONTRAINDICATIONS**). If ganglionic blockers have not been discontinued before Ismelin is started, they should be gradually withdrawn to prevent a spiking blood pressure response during the transfer period.

HOW SUPPLIED
Tablets 10 mg—round, pale yellow, scored (imprinted CIBA 49)
Bottles of 100 ....NDC 0083-0049-30
Tablets 25 mg—round, white, scored (imprinted CIBA 103)
Bottles of 100 ....NDC 0083-0103-30
Do not store above 86°F (30°C).
Dispense in tight container (USP).

C96-14 (Rev. 3/96)

Shown in Product Identification Guide, page 309

LAMPRENE® ℞
clofazimine
Capsules

DESCRIPTION
Lamprene, clofazimine, is an antileprosy agent available as capsules for oral administration. Each capsule contains 50 mg of micronized clofazimine suspended in an oil-wax base. Clofazimine is a substituted iminophenazine bright-red dye. Its chemical name is 3-(*p*-chloroanilino)-10-(*p*-chlorophenyl)-2, 10-dihydro-2-isopropyliminophenazine.
Clofazimine is a reddish-brown powder. It is readily soluble in benzene; soluble in chloroform; poorly soluble in acetone and in ethyl acetate; sparingly soluble in methanol and in ethanol; and virtually insoluble in water. Its molecular weight is 473.4.
Inactive Ingredients. Beeswax, butylated hydroxytoluene, citric acid, ethyl vanillin, gelatin, glycerin, iron oxide, lecithin, p-methoxy acetophenone, parabens, plant oils, propylene glycol.

CLINICAL PHARMACOLOGY
Lamprene exerts a slow bactericidal effect on *Mycobacterium leprae* (Hansen's bacillus). Lamprene inhibits mycobacterial growth and binds preferentially to mycobacterial DNA. Lamprene also exerts anti-inflammatory properties in controlling erythema nodosum leprosum reactions. However, its precise mechanisms of action are unknown.

Pharmacokinetics
Lamprene has a variable absorption rate in leprosy patients, ranging from 45–62% after oral administration. The average serum concentrations in leprosy patients treated with 100 mg and 300 mg daily were 0.7 μg/ml and 1.0 μg/ml, respectively. After ingestion of a single dose of 300 mg, elimination of unchanged Lamprene and its metabolites in a 24-hour urine collection was negligible. Lamprene is retained in the human body for a long time. The half-life of Lamprene following repeated oral doses is estimated to be at least 70 days. Part of the ingested drug recovered from the feces may represent excretion via the bile. A small amount is also eliminated in the sputum, sebum, and sweat.
Lamprene is highly lipophilic and tends to be deposited predominantly in fatty tissue and in cells of the reticuloendothelial system. It is taken up by macrophages throughout the body. In autopsies performed on leprosy patients, clofazimine crystals were found predominantly in the mesenteric lymph nodes, adrenals, subcutaneous fat, liver, bile, gall bladder, spleen, small intestine, muscles, bones, and skin.

Microbiology
Measurement of the minimum inhibitory concentration (MIC) of Lamprene against leprosy bacilli *in vitro* is not yet feasible. In the mouse footpad system, the multiplication of *M. leprae* is inhibited by introducing 0.0001–0.001% Lamprene in the diet. Although bacterial killing may begin shortly after starting the drug, it cannot be measured in biopsy tissues taken from patients for mouse footpad studies until approximately 50 days after the start of therapy.
Lamprene does not show cross-resistance with dapsone or rifampin.
The following *in vitro* data are available, but their clinical significance is unknown. Lamprene has been shown *in vitro* to inhibit *M. avium* and *M. bovis* at concentrations of approximately 0.1–1.0 μg/ml. The MIC for *M. avium-intracellulare* isolated from patients with acquired immuno-deficiency syndrome (AIDS) ranged from 1.0 to 5.0 μg/ml. With a few exceptions, microorganisms other than mycobacteria are not inhibited by Lamprene.

INDICATIONS AND USAGE
Lamprene is indicated in the treatment of lepromatous leprosy, including dapsone-resistant lepromatous leprosy and lepromatous leprosy complicated by erythema nodosum leprosum. Lamprene has not been demonstrated to be effective in the treatment of other leprosy-associated inflammatory reactions.

Combination drug therapy has been recommended for initial treatment of multibacillary leprosy to prevent the development of drug resistance.

CONTRAINDICATIONS

There are no known contraindications.

WARNINGS

Severe abdominal symptoms (see below) have necessitated exploratory laparotomies in some patients receiving Lamprene. Rare reports have included splenic infarction, bowel obstruction, and gastrointestinal bleeding. There have also been reports of death following severe abdominal symptoms. Autopsies have revealed crystalline deposits of clofazimine in various tissues including the intestinal mucosa, liver, spleen, and mesenteric lymph nodes.

Lamprene should be used with caution in patients who have gastrointestinal problems such as abdominal pain and diarrhea. Dosages of Lamprene of more than 100 mg daily should be given for as short a period as possible and only under close medical supervision. If a patient complains of colicky or burning pain in the abdomen, nausea, vomiting, or diarrhea, the dose should be reduced, and, if necessary, the interval between doses should be increased, or the drug should be discontinued.

PRECAUTIONS

General

Physicians should be aware that skin discoloration due to Lamprene may result in depression. Two suicides have been reported in patients receiving Lamprene. For skin dryness and ichthyosis, oil can be applied to the skin.

Information for Patients

Patients should be warned that Lamprene may cause a discoloration of the skin from red to brownish black, as well as discoloration of the conjunctivae, lacrimal fluid, sweat, sputum, urine, and feces. Patients should be advised that skin discoloration, although reversible, may take several months or years to disappear after the conclusion of therapy with Lamprene.

Patients should be told to take Lamprene with meals.

Drug Interactions

Preliminary data which suggest that dapsone may inhibit the anti-inflammatory activity of Lamprene have not been confirmed. If leprosy-associated inflammatory reactions develop in patients being treated with dapsone and clofazimine, it is still advisable to continue treatment with both drugs.

Carcinogenesis, Mutagenesis, Impairment of Fertility

Long-term carcinogenicity studies in animals have not been conducted with Lamprene. Results of mutagenicity studies (Ames test) were negative. There was some evidence of impaired fertility in one study in rats treated at a dose 25 times the usual human dose; the number of offspring was reduced and there was a lower proportion of implantations.

Pregnancy Category C

Lamprene was not teratogenic in laboratory animals at dose levels equivalent to 8 times (rabbit) and 25 times (rat) the usual human daily dose. However, there was evidence of fetotoxicity in the mouse at 12-25 times the human dose, i.e., retardation of fetal skull ossification, increased incidence of abortions and stillbirths, and impaired neonatal survival. The skin and fatty tissue of offspring became discolored approximately 3 days after birth, which was attributed to the presence of Lamprene in the maternal milk.

It has been found that Lamprene crosses the human placenta. The skin of infants born to women who had received the drug during pregnancy was found to be deeply pigmented at birth. No evidence of teratogenicity was found in these infants. There are no adequate and well-controlled studies in pregnant women. Lamprene should be used during pregnancy only if the potential benefit justifies the risk to the fetus.

Nursing Mothers

Lamprene is excreted in the milk of nursing mothers. Lamprene should not be administered to a nursing woman unless clearly indicated.

Pediatric Use

Safety and effectiveness in pediatric patients have not been established. Several cases of pediatric patients treated with Lamprene have been reported in the literature.

ADVERSE REACTIONS

In general, Lamprene is well tolerated when administered in dosages no greater than 100 mg daily. The most consistent adverse reactions are usually dose related and are usually reversible when Lamprene is discontinued.

Adverse Reactions Occuring in More Than 1% of Patients
Skin: Pigmentation from pink to brownish-black in 75–100% of the patients within a few weeks of treatment; ichthyosis and dryness (8–28%); rash and pruritus (1–5%).
Gastrointestinal: Abdominal and epigastric pain, diarrhea, nausea, vomiting, gastrointestinal intolerance (40–50%).
Ocular: Conjunctival and corneal pigmentation due to clofazimine crystal deposits; dryness; burning; itching; irritation.

Other: Discoloration of urine, feces, sputum, sweat; elevated blood sugar; elevated ESR.

Adverse Reactions Occurring in Less Than 1% of Patients
Skin: Phototoxicity, erythroderma, acneiform eruptions, monilial cheilosis.
Gastrointestinal: Bowel obstruction (see WARNINGS), gastrointestinal bleeding (see WARNINGS), anorexia, constipation, weight loss, hepatitis, jaundice, eosinophilic enteritis, enlarged liver.
Ocular: Diminished vision.
Nervous: Dizziness, drowsiness, fatigue, headache, giddiness, neuralgia, taste disorder.
Psychiatric: Depression secondary to skin discoloration; two suicides have been reported.
Laboratory: Elevated levels of albumin, serum bilirubin, and AST (SGOT); eosinophilia; hypokalemia.
Other: Splenic infarction (see WARNINGS), thromboembolism, anemia, cystitis, bone pain, edema, fever, lymphadenopathy, vascular pain.

OVERDOSAGE

No specific data are available on the treatment of overdosage with Lamprene. However, in case of overdose, the stomach should be emptied by inducing vomiting or by gastric lavage, and supportive symptomatic treatment should be employed.

DOSAGE AND ADMINISTRATION

Lamprene should be taken with meals.

Lamprene should be used preferably in combination with one or more other antileprosy agents to prevent the emergence of drug resistance.

For the treatment of proven dapsone-resistant leprosy, Lamprene should be given at a dosage of 100 mg daily in combination with one or more other antileprosy drugs for 3 years, followed by monotherapy with 100 mg of Lamprene daily. Clinical improvement usually can be detected between the first and third months of treatment and is usually clearly evident by the sixth month.

For dapsone-sensitive multibacillary leprosy, a combination therapy with two other antileprosy drugs is recommended. The triple-drug regimen should be given for at least 2 years and continued, if possible, until negative skin smears are obtained. At this time, monotherapy with an appropriate antileprosy drug can be instituted.

The treatment of erythema nodosum leprosum reactions depends on the severity of symptoms. In general, the basic antileprosy treatment should be continued, and if nerve injury or skin ulceration is threatened, corticosteriods should be given. Where prolonged corticosteroid therapy becomes necessary, Lamprene administered at dosages of 100 mg to 200 mg daily for up to 3 months may be useful in eliminating or reducing corticosteroid requirements. Dosages above 200 mg daily are not recommended, and the dosage should be tapered to 100 mg daily as quickly as possible after the reactive episode is controlled. The patient must remain under medical surveillance.

For advice about combination drug regimens, contact the USPHS Gillis W. Long Hansen's Disease Center, Carville, LA (504-642-7771).

HOW SUPPLIED

Capsules 50 mg—brown, spherical
Bottles of 100 ....NDC 0028-0108-01
Store below 30°C (86°F). Protect from moisture.
Dispense in tight container (USP).

C95-53 (Rev. 11/95)

Dist. by:
Ciba-Geigy Corporation
Pharmaceuticals Division
Summit, NJ 07901
Shown in Product Identification Guide, page 309

LIORESAL®	Tablets	℞
[lye-oar'eh-sal]		
baclofen USP	10 mg	
Muscle Relaxant, Antispastic	20 mg	℞

DESCRIPTION

Lioresal, baclofen USP, is a muscle relaxant and antispastic, available as 10-mg and 20-mg tablets for oral administration. Its chemical name is 4-amino-3-(4-chlorophenyl)-butanoic acid.

Baclofen USP is a white to off-white, odorless or practically odorless crystalline powder, with a molecular weight of 213.66. It is slightly soluble in water, very slightly soluble in methanol, and insoluble in chloroform.

Inactive Ingredients. Cellulose compounds, magnesium stearate, povidone, and starch.

ACTIONS

The precise mechanism of action of Lioresal is not fully known. Lioresal is capable of inhibiting both monosynaptic and polysynaptic reflexes at the spinal level, possibly by hyperpolarization of afferent terminals, although actions at supraspinal sites may also occur and contribute to its clinical

effect. Although Lioresal is an analog of the putative inhibitory neurotransmitter gamma-aminobutyric acid (GABA), there is no conclusive evidence that actions on GABA systems are involved in the production of its clinical effects. In studies with animals, Lioresal has been shown to have general CNS depressant properties as indicated by the production of sedation with tolerance, somnolence, ataxia, and respiratory and cardiovascular depression. Lioresal is rapidly and extensively absorbed and eliminated. Absorption may be dose-dependent, being reduced with increasing doses. Lioresal is excreted primarily by the kidney in unchanged form and there is relatively large intersubject variation in absorption and/or elimination.

INDICATIONS

Lioresal is useful for the alleviation of signs and symptoms of spasticity resulting from multiple sclerosis, particularly for the relief of flexor spasms and concomitant pain, clonus, and muscular rigidity.

Patients should have reversible spasticity so that Lioresal treatment will aid in restoring residual function.

Lioresal may also be of some value in patients with spinal cord injuries and other spinal cord diseases.

Lioresal is not indicated in the treatment of skeletal muscle spasm resulting from rheumatic disorders.

The efficacy of Lioresal in stroke, cerebral palsy, and Parkinson's disease has not been established and, therefore, it is not recommended for these conditions.

CONTRAINDICATIONS

Hypersensitivity to baclofen.

WARNINGS

a. *Abrupt Drug Withdrawal:* Hallucinations and seizures have occurred on abrupt withdrawal of Lioresal. Therefore, except for serious adverse reactions, the dose should be reduced slowly when the drug is discontinued.

b. *Impaired Renal Function:* Because Lioresal is primarily excreted unchanged through the kidneys, it should be given with caution, and it may be necessary to reduce the dosage.

c. *Stroke:* Lioresal has not significantly benefited patients with stroke. These patients have also shown poor tolerability to the drug.

d. *Pregnancy:* Lioresal has been shown to increase the incidence of omphaloceles (ventral hernias) in fetuses of rats given approximately 13 times the maximum dose recommended for human use, at a dose which caused significant reductions in food intake and weight gain in dams. This abnormality was not seen in mice or rabbits. There was also an increased incidence of incomplete sternebral ossification in fetuses of rats given approximately 13 times the maximum recommended human dose, and an increased incidence of unossified phalangeal nuclei of forelimbs and hindlimbs in fetuses of rabbits given approximately 7 times the maximum recommended human dose. In mice, no teratogenic effects were observed, although reductions in mean fetal weight with consequent delays in skeletal ossification were present when dams were given 17 or 34 times the human daily dose. There are no studies in pregnant women. Lioresal should be used during pregnancy only if the benefit clearly justifies the potential risk to the fetus.

PRECAUTIONS

Because of the possibility of sedation, patients should be cautioned regarding the operation of automobiles or other dangerous machinery, and activities made hazardous by decreased alertness. Patients should also be cautioned that the central nervous system effects of Lioresal may be additive to those of alcohol and other CNS depressants.

Lioresal should be used with caution where spasticity is utilized to sustain upright posture and balance in locomotion or whenever spasticity is utilized to obtain increased function. In patients with epilepsy, the clinical state and electroencephalogram should be monitored at regular intervals, since deterioration in seizure control and EEG have been reported occasionally in patients taking Lioresal.

It is not known whether this drug is excreted in human milk. As a general rule, nursing should not be undertaken while a patient is on a drug since many drugs are excreted in human milk.

A dose-related increase in incidence of ovarian cysts and a less marked increase in enlarged and/or hemorrhagic adrenal glands was observed in female rats treated chronically with Lioresal.

Ovarian cysts have been found by palpation in about 4% of the multiple sclerosis patients that were treated with Lioresal for up to one year. In most cases these cysts disappeared spontaneously while patients continued to receive the drug. Ovarian cysts are estimated to occur spontaneously in approximately 1% to 5% of the normal female population.

Pediatric Use

Safety and effectiveness in pediatric patients below the age of 12 years have not been established.

Continued on next page

CibaGeneva—Cont.

ADVERSE REACTIONS

The most common is transient drowsiness (10–63%). In one controlled study of 175 patients, transient drowsiness was observed in 63% of those receiving Lioresal compared to 36% of those in the placebo group. Other common adverse reactions are dizziness (5–15%), weakness (5–15%) and fatigue (2–4%). Others reported:

Neuropsychiatric: Confusion (1–11%), headache (4–8%), insomnia (2–7%); and, rarely, euphoria, excitement, depression, hallucinations, paresthesia, muscle pain, tinnitus, slurred speech, coordination disorder, tremor, rigidity, dystonia, ataxia, blurred vision, nystagmus, strabismus, miosis, mydriasis, diplopia, dysarthria, epileptic seizure.

Cardiovascular: Hypotension (0–9%). Rare instances of dyspnea, palpitation, chest pain, syncope.

Gastrointestinal: Nausea (4–12%), constipation (2–6%); and, rarely, dry mouth, anorexia, taste disorder, abdominal pain, vomiting, diarrhea, and positive test for occult blood in stool.

Genitourinary: Urinary frequency (2–6%); and, rarely, enuresis, urinary retention, dysuria, impotence, inability to ejaculate, nocturia, hematuria.

Other: Instances of rash, pruritus, ankle edema, excessive perspiration, weight gain, nasal congestion.

Some of the CNS and genitourinary symptoms may be related to the underlying disease rather than to drug therapy. The following laboratory tests have been found to be abnormal in a few patients receiving Lioresal: increased SGOT, elevated alkaline phosphatase, and elevation of blood sugar.

OVERDOSAGE

Signs and Symptoms: Vomiting, muscular hypotonia, drowsiness, accommodation disorders, coma, respiratory depression, and seizures.

Treatment: In the alert patient, empty the stomach promptly by induced emesis followed by lavage. In the obtunded patient, secure the airway with a cuffed endotracheal tube before beginning lavage (do not induce emesis). Maintain adequate respiratory exchange, do not use respiratory stimulants.

DOSAGE AND ADMINISTRATION

The determination of optimal dosage requires individual titration. Start therapy at a low dosage and increase gradually until optimum effect is achieved (usually between 40–80 mg daily).

The following dosage titration schedule is suggested:

5 mg t.i.d. for 3 days
10 mg t.i.d. for 3 days
15 mg t.i.d. for 3 days
20 mg t.i.d. for 3 days

Thereafter additional increases may be necessary but the total daily dose should not exceed a maximum of 80 mg daily (20 mg q.i.d.).

The lowest dose compatible with an optimal response is recommended. If benefits are not evident after a reasonable trial period, patients should be slowly withdrawn from the drug (see **WARNINGS** *Abrupt Drug Withdrawal*).

HOW SUPPLIED

Tablets 10 mg —oval, white, scored (imprinted Lioresal on one side and 10 twice on the scored side)

Bottles of 100 ....NDC 0028-0023-01
Unit Dose (blister pack)
Box of 100 (strips of 10) ....NDC 0028-0023-61

Tablets 20 mg —capsule-shaped, white, scored (imprinted Lioresal on one side and 20 twice on the scored side)

Bottles of 100 ....NDC 0028-0033-01
Unit Dose (blister pack)
Box of 100 (strips of 10) ....NDC 0028-0033-61

Samples, when available, are identified by the word *Sample* appearing on each tablet.

Do not store above 86°F (30°C).

Dispense in tight container (USP).

C96-37 (Rev 3/96)

Shown in Product Identification Guide, page 309

LOPRESSOR®   ℞
metoprolol tartrate tablets, USP
metoprolol tartrate injection, USP

DESCRIPTION

Lopressor, metoprolol tartrate, is a selective beta$_1$-adrenoreceptor blocking agent, available as 50- and 100-mg tablets for oral administration and in 5-ml ampuls for intravenous administration. Each ampul contains a sterile solution of metoprolol tartrate USP, 5 mg, and sodium chloride USP, 45 mg. Metoprolol tartrate is 1-(isopropylamino)-3-[*p* -(2-methoxyethyl) phenoxy]-2-propanol (2:1) *dextro* -tartrate salt.

Metoprolol tartrate is a white, practically odorless, crystalline powder with a molecular weight of 684.82. It is very soluble in water; freely soluble in methylene chloride, in chloroform, and in alcohol; slightly soluble in acetone; and insoluble in ether.

Inactive Ingredients: Tablets contain cellulose compounds, colloidal silicon dioxide, D&C Red No. 30 aluminum lake (50-mg tablets), FD&C Blue No. 2 aluminum lake (100-mg tablets), lactose, magnesium stearate, polyethylene glycol, propylene glycol, povidone, sodium starch glycolate, talc, and titanium dioxide.

CLINICAL PHARMACOLOGY

Lopressor is a beta-adrenergic receptor blocking agent. In vitro and in vivo animal studies have shown that it has a preferential effect on beta$_1$ adrenoreceptors, chiefly located in cardiac muscle. This preferential effect is not absolute, however, and at higher doses, Lopressor also inhibits beta$_2$ adrenoreceptors, chiefly located in the bronchial and vascular musculature.

Clinical pharmacology studies have confirmed the beta-blocking activity of metoprolol in man, as shown by (1) reduction in heart rate and cardiac output at rest and upon exercise, (2) reduction of systolic blood pressure upon exercise, (3) inhibition of isoproterenol-induced tachycardia, and (4) reduction of reflex orthostatic tachycardia.

Relative beta$_1$ selectivity has been confirmed by the following: (1) In normal subjects, Lopressor is unable to reverse the beta$_2$-mediated vasodilating effects of epinephrine. This contrasts with the effect of nonselective (beta$_1$ plus beta$_2$) beta blockers, which completely reverse the vasodilating effects of epinephrine. (2) In asthmatic patients, Lopressor reduces FEV$_1$ and FVC significantly less than a nonselective beta blocker, propranolol, at equivalent beta$_1$-receptor blocking doses.

Lopressor has no intrinsic sympathomimetic activity, and membrane-stabilizing activity is detectable only at doses much greater than required for beta blockade. Lopressor crosses the blood-brain barrier and has been reported in the CSF in a concentration 78% of the simultaneous plasma concentration. Animal and human experiments indicate that Lopressor slows the sinus rate and decreases AV nodal conduction.

In controlled clinical studies, Lopressor has been shown to be an effective antihypertensive agent when used alone or as concomitant therapy with thiazide-type diuretics, at dosages of 100–450 mg daily. In controlled, comparative, clinical studies, Lopressor has been shown to be as effective an antihypertensive agent as propranolol, methyldopa, and thiazide-type diuretics, and to be equally effective in supine and standing positions.

The mechanism of the antihypertensive effects of beta-blocking agents has not been elucidated. However, several possible mechanisms have been proposed: (1) competitive antagonism of catecholamines at peripheral (especially cardiac) adrenergic neuron sites, leading to decreased cardiac output; (2) a central effect leading to reduced sympathetic outflow to the periphery; and (3) suppression of renin activity.

By blocking catecholamine-induced increases in heart rate, in velocity and extent of myocardial contraction, and in blood pressure, Lopressor reduces the oxygen requirements of the heart at any given level of effort, thus making it useful in the long-term management of angina pectoris. However, in patients with heart failure, beta-adrenergic blockade may increase oxygen requirements by increasing left ventricular fiber length and end-diastolic pressure.

Although beta-adrenergic receptor blockade is useful in the treatment of angina and hypertension, there are situations in which sympathetic stimulation is vital. In patients with severely damaged hearts, adequate ventricular function may depend on sympathetic drive. In the presence of AV block, beta blockade may prevent the necessary facilitating effect of sympathetic activity on conduction. Beta$_2$-adrenergic blockade results in passive bronchial constriction by interfering with endogenous adrenergic bronchodilator activity in patients subject to bronchospasm and may also interfere with exogenous bronchodilators in such patients.

In controlled clinical trials, Lopressor, administered two or four times daily, has been shown to be an effective antianginal agent, reducing the number of angina attacks and increasing exercise tolerance. The dosage used in these studies ranged from 100 to 400 mg daily. A controlled, comparative, clinical trial showed that Lopressor was indistinguishable from propranolol in the treatment of angina pectoris.

In a large (1,395 patients randomized), double-blind, placebo-controlled clinical study, Lopressor was shown to reduce 3-month mortality by 36% in patients with suspected or definite myocardial infarction.

Patients were randomized and treated as soon as possible after their arrival in the hospital, once their clinical condition had stabilized and their hemodynamic status had been carefully evaluated. Subjects were ineligible if they had hypotension, bradycardia, peripheral signs of shock, and/or more than minimal basal rales as signs of congestive heart failure. Initial treatment consisted of intravenous followed by oral administration of Lopressor or placebo, given in a coronary care or comparable unit. Oral maintenance therapy with Lopressor or placebo was then continued for 3 months. After this double-blind period, all patients were given Lopressor and followed up to 1 year.

The median delay from the onset of symptoms to the initiation of therapy was 8 hours in both the Lopressor and placebo treatment groups. Among patients treated with Lopressor, there were comparable reductions in 3-month mortality for those treated early (≤ 8 hours) and those in whom treatment was started later. Significant reductions in the incidence of ventricular fibrillation and in chest pain following initial intravenous therapy were also observed with Lopressor and were independent of the interval between onset of symptoms and initiation of therapy.

The precise mechanism of action of Lopressor in patients with suspected or definite myocardial infarction is not known.

In this study, patients treated with metoprolol received the drug both very early (intravenously) and during a subsequent 3-month period, while placebo patients received no beta-blocker treatment for this period. The study thus was able to show a benefit from the overall metoprolol regimen but cannot separate the benefit of very early intravenous treatment from the benefit of later beta-blocker therapy. Nonetheless, because the overall regimen showed a clear beneficial effect on survival without evidence of an early adverse effect on survival, one acceptable dosage regimen is the precise regimen used in the trial. Because the specific benefit of very early treatment remains to be defined however, it is also reasonable to administer the drug orally to patients at a later time as is recommended for certain other beta blockers.

Pharmacokinetics

In man, absorption of Lopressor is rapid and complete. Plasma levels following oral administration, however, approximate 50% of levels following intravenous administration, indicating about 50% first-pass metabolism.

Plasma levels achieved are highly variable after oral administration. Only a small fraction of the drug (about 12%) is bound to human serum albumin. Elimination is mainly by biotransformation in the liver, and the plasma half-life ranges from approximately 3 to 7 hours. Less than 5% of an oral dose of Lopressor is recovered unchanged in the urine; the rest is excreted by the kidneys as metabolites that appear to have no clinical significance. The systemic availability and half-life of Lopressor in patients with renal failure do not differ to a clinically significant degree from those in normal subjects. Consequently, no reduction in dosage is usually needed in patients with chronic renal failure.

Significant beta-blocking effect (as measured by reduction of exercise heart rate) occurs within 1 hour after oral administration, and its duration is dose-related. For example, a 50% reduction of the maximum registered effect after single oral doses of 20, 50, and 100 mg occurred at 3.3, 5.0, and 6.4 hours, respectively, in normal subjects. After repeated oral dosages of 100 mg twice daily, a significant reduction in exercise systolic blood pressure was evident at 12 hours.

Following intravenous administration of Lopressor, the urinary recovery of unchanged drug is approximately 10%. When the drug was infused over a 10-minute period, in normal volunteers, maximum beta blockade was achieved at approximately 20 minutes. Doses of 5 mg and 15 mg yielded a maximal reduction in exercise-induced heart rate of approximately 10% and 15%, respectively. The effect on exercise heart rate decreased linearly with time at the same rate for both doses, and disappeared at approximately 5 hours and 8 hours for the 5-mg and 15-mg doses, respectively.

Equivalent maximal beta-blocking effect is achieved with oral and intravenous doses in the ratio of approximately 2.5:1.

There is a linear relationship between the log of plasma levels and reduction of exercise heart rate. However, antihypertensive activity does not appear to be related to plasma levels. Because of variable plasma levels attained with a given dose and lack of a consistent relationship of antihypertensive activity to dose, selection of proper dosage requires individual titration.

In several studies of patients with acute myocardial infarction, intravenous followed by oral administration of Lopressor caused a reduction in heart rate, systolic blood pressure, and cardiac output. Stroke volume, diastolic blood pressure, and pulmonary artery end diastolic pressure remained unchanged.

In patients with angina pectoris, plasma concentration measured at 1 hour is linearly related to the oral dose within the range of 50 to 400 mg. Exercise heart rate and systolic blood pressure are reduced in relation to the logarithm of the oral dose of metoprolol. The increase in exercise capacity and the reduction in left ventricular ischemia are also significantly related to the logarithm of the oral dose.

INDICATIONS AND USAGE

Hypertension

Lopressor tablets are indicated for the treatment of hypertension. They may be used alone or in combination with other antihypertensive agents.

Angina Pectoris
Lopressor is indicated in the long-term treatment of angina pectoris.

Myocardial Infarction
Lopressor ampuls and tablets are indicated in the treatment of hemodynamically stable patients with definite or suspected acute myocardial infarction to reduce cardiovascular mortality. Treatment with intravenous Lopressor can be initiated as soon as the patient's clinical condition allows (see **DOSAGE AND ADMINISTRATION, CONTRAINDICATIONS, and WARNINGS**). Alternatively, treatment can begin within 3 to 10 days of the acute event (see **DOSAGE AND ADMINISTRATION**).

CONTRAINDICATIONS

Hypertension and Angina
Lopressor is contraindicated in sinus bradycardia, heart block greater than first degree, cardiogenic shock, and overt cardiac failure (see **WARNINGS**).

Myocardial Infarction
Lopressor is contraindicated in patients with a heart rate < 45 beats/min; second- and third-degree heart block; significant first-degree heart block (P-R interval $\geq$ 0.24 sec); systolic blood pressure < 100 mmHg; or moderate-to-severe cardiac failure (see **WARNINGS**).

WARNINGS

Hypertension and Angina
Cardiac Failure: Sympathetic stimulation is a vital component supporting circulatory function in congestive heart failure, and beta blockade carries the potential hazard of further depressing myocardial contractility and precipitating more severe failure. In hypertensive and angina patients who have congestive heart failure controlled by digitalis and diuretics, Lopressor should be administered cautiously. Both digitalis and Lopressor slow AV conduction.
In Patients Without a History of Cardiac Failure: Continued depression of the myocardium with beta-blocking agents over a period of time can, in some cases, lead to cardiac failure. At the first sign or symptom of impending cardiac failure, patients should be fully digitalized and/or given a diuretic. The response should be observed closely. If cardiac failure continues, despite adequate digitalization and diuretic therapy, Lopressor should be withdrawn.

Ischemic Heart Disease: Following abrupt cessation of therapy with certain beta-blocking agents, exacerbations of angina pectoris and, in some cases, myocardial infarction have occurred. When discontinuing chronically administered Lopressor, particularly in patients with ischemic heart disease, the dosage should be gradually reduced over a period of 1–2 weeks and the patient should be carefully monitored. If angina markedly worsens or acute coronary insufficiency develops, Lopressor administration should be reinstated promptly, at least temporarily, and other measures appropriate for the management of unstable angina should be taken. Patients should be warned against interruption or discontinuation of therapy without the physician's advice. Because coronary artery disease is common and may be unrecognized, it may be prudent not to discontinue Lopressor therapy abruptly even in patients treated only for hypertension.

Bronchospastic Diseases: PATIENTS WITH BRONCHOSPASTIC DISEASES SHOULD, IN GENERAL, NOT RECEIVE BETA-BLOCKERS. Because of its relative beta₁ selectivity, however, Lopressor may be used with caution in patients with bronchospastic disease who do not respond to, or cannot tolerate, other antihypertensive treatment. Since beta₁ selectivity is not absolute, a beta₂-stimulating agent should be administered concomitantly, and the lowest possible dose of Lopressor should be used. In these circumstances it would be prudent initially to administer Lopressor in smaller doses three times daily, instead of larger doses two times daily, to avoid the higher plasma levels associated with the longer dosing interval. (See **DOSAGE AND ADMINISTRATION**.)
Major Surgery: The necessity or desirability of withdrawing beta-blocking therapy prior to major surgery is controversial; the impaired ability of the heart to respond to reflex adrenergic stimuli may augment the risks of general anesthesia and surgical procedures.
Lopressor, like other beta blockers, is a competitive inhibitor of beta-receptor agonists, and its effects can be reversed by administration of such agents, e.g., dobutamine or isoproterenol. However, such patients may be subject to protracted severe hypotension. Difficulty in restarting and maintaining the heart beat has also been reported with beta blockers.
Diabetes and Hypoglycemia: Lopressor should be used with caution in diabetic patients if a beta-blocking agent is required. Beta blockers may mask tachycardia occurring with hypoglycemia, but other manifestations such as dizziness and sweating may not be significantly affected.
Thyrotoxicosis: Beta-adrenergic blockade may mask certain clinical signs (e.g., tachycardia) of hyperthyroidism. Patients suspected of developing thyrotoxicosis should be

managed carefully to avoid abrupt withdrawal of beta blockade, which might precipitate a thyroid storm.

Myocardial Infarction
Cardiac Failure: Sympathetic stimulation is a vital component supporting circulatory function, and beta blockade carries the potential hazard of depressing myocardial contractility and precipitating or exacerbating minimal cardiac failure.
During treatment with Lopressor, the hemodynamic status of the patient should be carefully monitored. If heart failure occurs or persists despite appropriate treatment, Lopressor should be discontinued.
Bradycardia: Lopressor produces a decrease in sinus heart rate in most patients; this decrease is greatest among patients with high initial heart rates and least among patients with low initial heart rates. Acute myocardial infarction (particularly inferior infarction) may in itself produce significant lowering of the sinus rate. If the sinus rate decreases to < 40 beats/min, particularly if associated with evidence of lowered cardiac output, atropine (0.25–0.5 mg) should be administered intravenously. If treatment with atropine is not successful, Lopressor should be discontinued, and cautious administration of isoproterenol or installation of a cardiac pacemaker should be considered.
AV Block: Lopressor slows AV conduction and may produce significant first- (P-R interval $\geq$0.26 sec), second-, or third-degree heart block. Acute myocardial infarction also produces heart block.
If heart block occurs, Lopressor should be discontinued and atropine (0.25–0.5 mg) should be administered intravenously. If treatment with atropine is not successful, cautious administration of isoproterenol or installation of a cardiac pacemaker should be considered.
Hypotension: If hypotension (systolic blood pressure $\leq$ 90 mmHg) occurs, Lopressor should be discontinued, and the hemodynamic status of the patient and the extent of myocardial damage carefully assessed. Invasive monitoring of central venous, pulmonary capillary wedge, and arterial pressures may be required. Appropriate therapy with fluids, positive inotropic agents, balloon counterpulsation, or other treatment modalities should be instituted. If hypotension is associated with sinus bradycardia or AV block, treatment should be directed at reversing these (see above).
Bronchospastic Diseases: PATIENTS WITH BRONCHOSPASTIC DISEASES SHOULD, IN GENERAL, NOT RECEIVE BETA BLOCKERS. Because of its relative beta₁ selectivity, Lopressor may be used with extreme caution in patients with bronchospastic disease. Because it is unknown to what extent beta₂-stimulating agents may exacerbate myocardial ischemia and the extent of infarction, these agents should *not* be used prophylactically. If bronchospasm not related to congestive heart failure occurs, Lopressor should be discontinued. A theophylline derivative or a beta₂ agonist may be administered cautiously, depending on the clinical condition of the patient. Both theophylline derivatives and beta₂ agonists may produce serious cardiac arrhythmias.

PRECAUTIONS

General
Lopressor should be used with caution in patients with impaired hepatic function.

Information for Patients
Patients should be advised to take Lopressor regularly and continuously, as directed, with or immediately following meals. If a dose should be missed, the patient should take only the next scheduled dose (without doubling it). Patients should not discontinue Lopressor without consulting the physician.
Patients should be advised (1) to avoid operating automobiles and machinery or engaging in other tasks requiring alertness until the patient's response to therapy with Lopressor has been determined; (2) to contact the physician if any difficulty in breathing occurs; (3) to inform the physician or dentist before any type of surgery that he or she is taking Lopressor.

Laboratory Tests
Clinical laboratory findings may include elevated levels of serum transaminase, alkaline phosphatase, and lactate dehydrogenase.

Drug Interactions
Catecholamine-depleting drugs (e.g., reserpine) may have an additive effect when given with beta-blocking agents. Patients treated with Lopressor plus a catecholamine depletor should therefore be closely observed for evidence of hypotension or marked bradycardia, which may produce vertigo, syncope, or postural hypotension.
Risk of Anaphylactic Reaction. While taking beta-blockers, patients with a history of severe anaphylactic reaction to a variety of allergens may be more reactive to repeated challenge, either accidental, diagnostic, or therapeutic. Such patients may be unresponsive to the usual doses of epinephrine used to treat allergic reactions.

Carcinogenesis, Mutagenesis, Impairment of Fertility
Long-term studies in animals have been conducted to evaluate carcinogenic potential. In 2-year studies in rats at three oral dosage levels of up to 800 mg/kg per day, there was no

increase in the development of spontaneously occurring benign or malignant neoplasms of any type. The only histologic changes that appeared to be drug related were an increased incidence of generally mild focal accumulation of foamy macrophages in pulmonary alveoli and a slight increase in biliary hyperplasia. In a 21-month study in Swiss albino mice at three oral dosage levels of up to 750 mg/kg per day, benign lung tumors (small adenomas) occurred more frequently in female mice receiving the highest dose than in untreated control animals. There was no increase in malignant or total (benign plus malignant) lung tumors, nor in the overall incidence of tumors or malignant tumors. This 21-month study was repeated in CD-1 mice, and no statistically or biologically significant differences were observed between treated and control mice of either sex for any type of tumor.
All mutagenicity tests performed (a dominant lethal study in mice, chromosome studies in somatic cells, a Salmonella/mammalian-microsome mutagenicity test, and a nucleus anomaly test in somatic interphase nuclei) were negative.
No evidence of impaired fertility due to Lopressor was observed in a study performed in rats at doses up to 55.5 times the maximum daily human dose of 450 mg.

Pregnancy Category C
Lopressor has been shown to increase postimplantation loss and decrease neonatal survival in rats at doses up to 55.5 times the maximum daily human dose of 450 mg. Distribution studies in mice confirm exposure of the fetus when Lopressor is administered to the pregnant animal. These studies have revealed no evidence of impaired fertility or teratogenicity. There are no adequate and well-controlled studies in pregnant women. Because animal reproduction studies are not always predictive of human response, this drug should be used during pregnancy only if clearly needed.

Nursing Mothers
Lopressor is excreted in breast milk in very small quantity. An infant consuming 1 liter of breast milk daily would receive a dose of less than 1 mg of the drug. Caution should be exercised when Lopressor is administered to a nursing woman.

Pediatric Use
Safety and effectiveness in pediatric patients have not been established.

ADVERSE REACTIONS

Hypertension and Angina
Most adverse effects have been mild and transient.
Central Nervous System: Tiredness and dizziness have occurred in about 10 of 100 patients. Depression has been reported in about 5 of 100 patients. Mental confusion and short-term memory loss have been reported. Headache, nightmares, and insomnia have also been reported.
Cardiovascular: Shortness of breath and bradycardia have occurred in approximately 3 of 100 patients. Cold extremities; arterial insufficiency, usually of the Raynaud type; palpitations; congestive heart failure; peripheral edema; and hypotension have been reported in about 1 of 100 patients. (See **CONTRAINDICATIONS, WARNINGS, and PRECAUTIONS**.)
Respiratory: Wheezing (bronchospasm) and dyspnea have been reported in about 1 of 100 patients (see **WARNINGS**).
Gastrointestinal: Diarrhea has occurred in about 5 of 100 patients. Nausea, dry mouth, gastric pain, constipation, flatulence, and heartburn have been reported in about 1 of 100 patients.
Hypersensitive Reactions: Pruritus or rash have occurred in about 5 of 100 patients. Worsening of psoriasis has also been reported.
Miscellaneous: Peyronie's disease has been reported in fewer than 1 of 100,000 patients. Musculoskeletal pain, blurred vision, and tinnitus have also been reported.
There have been rare reports of reversible alopecia, agranulocytosis, and dry eyes. Discontinuation of the drug should be considered if any such reaction is not otherwise explicable. The oculomucocutaneous syndrome associated with the beta blocker practolol has not been reported with Lopressor.

Myocardial Infarction
Central Nervous System: Tiredness has been reported in about 1 of 100 patients. Vertigo, sleep disturbances, hallucinations, headache, dizziness, visual disturbances, confusion, and reduced libido have also been reported, but a drug relationship is not clear.
Cardiovascular: In the randomized comparison of Lopressor and placebo described in the **CLINICAL PHARMACOLOGY** section, the following adverse reactions were reported:

	Lopressor	Placebo
Hypotension (systolic BP < 90 mmHg)	27.4%	23.2%
Bradycardia (heart rate < 40 beats/min)	15.9%	6.7%
Second- or third-degree heart block	4.7%	4.7%
First-degree heart block (P-R $\geq$ 0.26 sec)	5.3%	1.9%
Heart failure	27.5%	29.6%

Continued on next page

CibaGeneva—Cont.

Respiratory: Dyspnea of pulmonary origin has been reported in fewer than 1 of 100 patients.
Gastrointestinal: Nausea and abdominal pain have been reported in fewer than 1 of 100 patients.
Dermatologic: Rash and worsened psoriasis have been reported, but a drug relationship is not clear.
Miscellaneous: Unstable diabetes and claudication have been reported, but a drug relationship is not clear.

Potential Adverse Reactions

A variety of adverse reactions not listed above have been reported with other beta-adrenergic blocking agents and should be considered potential adverse reactions to Lopressor.
Central Nervous System: Reversible mental depression progressing to catatonia; an acute reversible syndrome characterized by disorientation for time and place, short-term memory loss, emotional lability, slightly clouded sensorium, and decreased performance on neuropsychometrics.
Cardiovascular: Intensification of AV block (See **CONTRAINDICATIONS**).
Hematologic: Agranulocytosis, nonthrombocytopenic purpura, thrombocytopenic purpura.
Hypersensitive Reactions: Fever combined with aching and sore throat, laryngospasm, and respiratory distress.

OVERDOSAGE

Acute Toxicity

Several cases of overdosage have been reported, some leading to death.
Oral LD_{50}'s (mg/kg): mice, 1158–2460; rats, 3090–4670.

Signs and Symptoms

Potential signs and symptoms associated with overdosage with Lopressor are bradycardia, hypotension, bronchospasm, and cardiac failure.

Treatment

There is no specific antidote.
In general, patients with acute or recent myocardial infarction may be more hemodynamically unstable than other patients and should be treated accordingly (see **WARNINGS**, Myocardial Infarction).
On the basis of the pharmacologic actions of Lopressor, the following general measures should be employed:
Elimination of the Drug: Gastric lavage should be performed.
Bradycardia: Atropine should be administered. If there is no response to vagal blockade, isoproterenol should be administered cautiously.
Hypotension: A vasopressor should be administered, e.g., levarterenol or dopamine.
Bronchospasm: A $beta_2$-stimulating agent and/or a theophylline derivative should be administered.
Cardiac Failure: A digitalis glycoside and diuretic should be administered. In shock resulting from inadequate cardiac contractility, administration of dobutamine, isoproterenol, or glucagon may be considered.

DOSAGE AND ADMINISTRATION

Hypertension

The dosage of Lopressor should be individualized. Lopressor should be taken with or immediately following meals.
The usual initial dosage is 100 mg daily in single or divided doses, whether used alone or added to a diuretic. The dosage may be increased at weekly (or longer) intervals until optimum blood pressure reduction is achieved. In general, the maximum effect of any given dosage level will be apparent after 1 week of therapy. The effective dosage range is 100 to 450 mg per day. Dosages above 450 mg per day have not been studied. While once-daily dosing is effective and can maintain a reduction in blood pressure throughout the day, lower doses (especially 100 mg) may not maintain a full effect at the end of the 24-hour period, and larger or more frequent daily doses may be required. This can be evaluated by measuring blood pressure near the end of the dosing interval to determine whether satisfactory control is being maintained throughout the day. $Beta_1$ selectivity diminishes as the dose of Lopressor is increased.

Angina Pectoris

The dosage of Lopressor should be individualized. Lopressor should be taken with or immediately following meals.
The usual initial dosage is 100 mg daily, given in two divided doses. The dosage may be gradually increased at weekly intervals until optimum clinical response has been obtained or there is pronounced slowing of the heart rate. The effective dosage range is 100 to 400 mg per day. Dosages above 400 mg per day have not been studied. If treatment is to be discontinued, the dosage should be reduced gradually over a period of 1–2 weeks. (See **WARNINGS**.)

Myocardial Infarction

Early Treatment: During the early phase of definite or suspected acute myocardial infarction, treatment with Lopressor can be initiated as soon as possible after the patient's arrival in the hospital. Such treatment should be initiated in a coronary care or similar unit immediately after the patient's hemodynamic condition has stabilized.

Treatment in this early phase should begin with the intravenous administration of three bolus injections of 5 mg of Lopressor each; the injections should be given at approximately 2-minute intervals. During the intravenous administration of Lopressor, blood pressure, heart rate, and electrocardiogram should be carefully monitored.
In patients who tolerate the full intravenous dose (15 mg), Lopressor tablets, 50 mg every 6 hours, should be initiated 15 minutes after the last intravenous dose and continued for 48 hours. Thereafter, patients should receive a maintenance dosage of 100 mg twice daily (see *Late Treatment* below). Patients who appear not to tolerate the full intravenous dose should be started on Lopressor tablets either 25 mg or 50 mg every 6 hours (depending on the degree of intolerance) 15 minutes after the last intravenous dose or as soon as their clinical condition allows. In patients with severe intolerance, treatment with Lopressor should be discontinued (see **WARNINGS**).
Late Treatment: Patients with contraindications to treatment during the early phase of suspected or definite myocardial infarction, patients who appear not to tolerate the full early treatment, and patients in whom the physician wishes to delay therapy for any other reason should be started on Lopressor tablets, 100 mg twice daily, as soon as their clinical condition allows. Therapy should be continued for at least 3 months. Although the efficacy of Lopressor beyond 3 months has not been conclusively established, data from studies with other beta blockers suggest that treatment should be continued for 1–3 years.

Note: **Parenteral drug products should be inspected visually for particulate matter and discoloration prior to administration, whenever solution and container permit.**

HOW SUPPLIED

Metoprolol tartrate tablets, USP
Tablets 50 mg—capsule-shaped, biconvex, pink, scored (imprinted GEIGY on one side and 51 twice on the scored side)

Bottles of 100	NDC 0028-0051-01
Bottles of 1000	NDC 0028-0051-10
Gy-Pak®—One Unit	
12 bottles—60 tablets each	NDC 0028-0051-73
12 bottles—100 tablets each	NDC 0028-0051-65
Unit Dose (blister pack)	
Box of 100 (strips of 10)	NDC 0028-0051-61

Tablets 100 mg—capsule-shaped, biconvex, light blue, scored (imprinted GEIGY on one side and 71 twice on the scored side)

Bottles of 100	NDC 0028-0071-01
Bottles of 1000	NDC 0028-0071-10
Gy-Pak®—One Unit	
12 bottles—60 tablets each	NDC 0028-0071-73
12 bottles—100 tablets each	NDC 0028-0071-65
Unit Dose (blister pack)	
Box of 100 (strips of 10)	NDC 0028-0071-61

Samples, when available, are identified by the word *SAMPLE* appearing on each tablet.
Store between 59°-86°F (15°-30°C). Protect from moisture.
Dispense in tight, light-resistant container (USP).
Metoprolol tartrate injection, USP
Ampuls 5 ml—each containing 5 mg of metoprolol tartrate

Tray of 4 packs of 3 ampuls	NDC 0028-4201-33

Do not store above 86°F (30°C). Protect from light.

C96–12 (Rev. 3/96)

Shown in Product Identification Guide, page 309

LOPRESSOR HCT®   ℞
metoprolol tartrate USP and hydrochlorothiazide USP
50/25 Tablets
100/25 Tablets
100/50 Tablets
Beta Blocker/Diuretic Antihypertensive

Prescribing Information

DESCRIPTION

Lopressor HCT has the antihypertensive effect of Lopressor®, metoprolol tartrate, a selective $beta_1$-adrenoreceptor blocking agent, and the antihypertensive and diuretic actions of hydrochlorothiazide. It is available as tablets for oral administration. The 50/25 tablets contain 50 mg of metoprolol tartrate USP and 25 mg of hydrochlorothiazide USP; the 100/25 tablets contain 100 mg of metoprolol tartrate USP and 25 mg of hydrochlorothiazide USP; and the 100/50 tablets contain 100 mg of metoprolol tartrate USP and 50 mg of hydrochlorothiazide USP.
Metoprolol tartrate USP is $(\pm)$-1-Isopropylamino-3-[p-(2-methoxyethyl)phenoxy]-2-propanol 2:1 *dextro*-tartrate salt.
Metoprolol tartrate USP is a white, crystalline powder. It is very soluble in water; freely soluble in methylene chloride, in chloroform, and in alcohol; slightly soluble in acetone; and insoluble in ether. Its molecular weight is 684.82.

Hydrochlorothiazide is 6-chloro-3,4-dihydro-2H-1,2,4-benzothiadiazine-7-sulfonamide, 1,1-dioxide.
Hydrochlorothiazide USP is a white, or practically white, practically odorless, crystalline powder. It is freely soluble in sodium hydroxide solution, in n-butylamine, and in dimethylformamide; sparingly soluble in methanol; slightly soluble in water; and insoluble in ether, in chloroform, and in dilute mineral acids. Its molecular weight is 297.73.
Inactive Ingredients: Cellulose compounds, colloidal silicon dioxide, D&C Yellow No. 10 (100/50-mg tablets), FD&C Blue No. 1 (50/25-mg tablets), FD&C Red No. 40 and FD&C Yellow No. 6 (100/25-mg tablets), lactose, magnesium stearate, povidone, sodium starch glycolate, starch, stearic acid, and sucrose.

CLINICAL PHARMACOLOGY

Lopressor

Lopressor is a beta-adrenergic receptor blocking agent. *In vitro* and *in vivo* animal studies have shown that it has a preferential effect on $beta_1$ adrenoreceptors, chiefly located in cardiac muscle. This preferential effect is not absolute, however, and at higher doses, Lopressor also inhibits $beta_2$ adrenoreceptors, chiefly located in the bronchial and vascular musculature.
Clinical pharmacology studies have confirmed the beta-blocking activity of metoprolol in man, as shown by (1) reduction in heart rate and cardiac output at rest and upon exercise, (2) reduction of systolic blood pressure upon exercise, (3) inhibition of isoproterenol-induced tachycardia, and (4) reduction of reflex orthostatic tachycardia.
Relative $beta_1$ selectivity has been confirmed by the following: (1) in normal subjects, Lopressor is unable to reverse the $beta_2$-mediated vasodilating effects of epinephrine. This contrasts with the effect of nonselective ($beta_1$ plus $beta_2$) beta blockers, which completely reverse the vasodilating effects of epinephrine. (2) In asthmatic patients, Lopressor reduces FEV_1 and FVC significantly less than a nonselective beta blocker, propranolol at equivalent $beta_1$-receptor blocking doses.
Lopressor has no intrinsic sympathomimetic activity and only weak membrane-stabilizing activity. Lopressor crosses the blood-brain barrier and has been reported in the CSF in a concentration 78% of the simultaneous plasma concentration. Animal and human experiments indicate that Lopressor slows the sinus rate and decreases AV nodal conduction.
In controlled clinical studies, Lopressor has been shown to be an effective antihypertensive agent when used alone or as concomitant therapy with thiazide-type diuretics, at dosages of 100–450 mg daily. In controlled, comparative, clinical studies, Lopressor has been shown to be as effective an antihypertensive agent as propranolol, methyldopa, and thiazide-type diuretics, and to be equally effective in supine and standing positions.
The mechanism of the antihypertensive effects of beta-blocking agents has not been elucidated. However, several possible mechanisms have been proposed: (1) competitive antagonism of catecholamines at peripheral (especially cardiac) adrenergic neuron sites, leading to decreased cardiac output; (2) a central effect leading to reduced sympathetic outflow to the periphery; and (3) suppression of renin activity.
In man, absorption of Lopressor is rapid and complete. Plasma levels following oral administration, however, approximate 50% of levels following intravenous administration, indicating about 50% first-pass metabolism. Plasma levels achieved are highly variable after oral administration. Only a small fraction of the drug (about 12%) is bound to human serum albumin. Elimination is mainly by biotransformation in the liver, and the plasma half-life ranges from approximately 3 to 7 hours. Less than 5% of an oral dose of Lopressor is recovered unchanged in the urine; the rest is excreted by the kidneys as metabolites that appear to have no clinical significance. The systemic availability and half-life of Lopressor in patients with renal failure do not differ to a clinically significant degree from those in normal subjects. Consequently, no reduction in dosage is usually needed in patients with chronic renal failure.
Significant beta-blocking effect (as measured by reduction of exercise heart rate) occurs within 1 hour after oral administration, and its duration is dose-related. For example, a 50% reduction of the maximum registered effect after single oral doses of 20, 50, and 100 mg occurred at 3.3, 5.0, and 6.4 hours, respectively, in normal subjects. After repeated oral dosages of 100 mg twice daily, a significant reduction in exercise systolic blood pressure was evident at 12 hours.
There is a linear relationship between the log of plasma levels and reduction of exercise heart rate. However, antihypertensive activity does not appear to be related to plasma levels. Because of variable plasma levels attained with a given dose and lack of a consistent relationship of antihypertensive activity to dose, selection of proper dosage requires individual titration.

Hydrochlorothiazide

Thiazides affect the renal tubular mechanism of electrolyte reabsorption. At maximal therapeutic dosage, all thiazides

are approximately equal in their diuretic potency. Thiazides increase excretion of sodium and chloride in approximately equivalent amounts. Natriuresis causes a secondary loss of potassium.

The mechanism of the antihypertensive effect of thiazides is unknown. Thiazides do not affect normal blood pressure.

The onset of action of thiazides occurs in 2 hours and the peak effect at about 4 hours. The action persists for approximately 6–12 hours. Hydrochlorothiazide is rapidly absorbed, as indicated by peak plasma concentrations 1–2.5 hours after oral administration. Plasma levels of the drug are proportional to dose; the concentration in whole blood is 1.6–1.8 times higher than in plasma. Thiazides are eliminated rapidly by the kidney. After oral administration of 25- to 100-mg doses, 72–97% of the dose is excreted in the urine, indicating dose-independent absorption. Hydrochlorothiazide is eliminated from plasma in a biphasic fashion with a terminal half-life of 10–17 hours. Plasma protein binding is 67.9%. Plasma clearance is 15.9–30.0 L/hr; volume of distribution is 3.6–7.8 L/kg.

Gastrointestinal absorption of hydrochlorothiazide is enhanced when administered with food. Absorption is decreased in patients with congestive heart failure, and the pharmacokinetics are considerably different in these patients.

INDICATIONS AND USAGE

Lopressor HCT is indicated for the management of hypertension.

This fixed-combination drug is not indicated for initial therapy of hypertension. If the fixed combination represents the dose titrated to the individual patient's needs, therapy with the fixed combination may be more convenient than with the separate components.

CONTRAINDICATIONS

Lopressor

Lopressor is contraindicated in sinus bradycardia, heart block greater than first degree, cardiogenic shock, and overt cardiac failure (see **WARNINGS**).

Hydrochlorothiazide

Hydrochlorothiazide is contraindicated in patients with anuria or hypersensitivity to this or other sulfonamide-derived drugs (see **WARNINGS**).

WARNINGS

Lopressor

Cardiac Failure. Sympathetic stimulation is a vital component supporting circulatory function in congestive heart failure, and beta blockade carries the potential hazard of further depressing myocardial contractility and precipitating more severe failure. In hypertensive patients who have congestive heart failure controlled by digitalis and diuretics, Lopressor should be administered cautiously. Both digitalis and Lopressor slow AV conduction.

In Patients Without a History of Cardiac Failure. Continued depression of the myocardium with beta-blocking agents over a period of time can, in some cases, lead to cardiac failure. At the first sign or symptom of impending cardiac failure, patients should be fully digitalized and/or given a diuretic. The response should be observed closely. If cardiac failure continues, despite adequate digitalization and diuretic therapy, Lopressor should be withdrawn.

Ischemic Heart Disease. Following abrupt cessation of therapy with certain beta-blocking agents, exacerbations of angina pectoris and, in some cases, myocardial infarction have been reported. Even in the absence of overt angina pectoris, when discontinuing therapy, Lopressor should not be withdrawn abruptly, and patients should be cautioned against interruption of therapy without the physician's advice (see **PRECAUTIONS**, Information for Patients).

Bronchospastic Diseases. **PATIENTS WITH BRONCHOSPASTIC DISEASES SHOULD, IN GENERAL, NOT RECEIVE BETA BLOCKERS. Because of its relative $beta_1$ selectivity, however, Lopressor may be used with caution in patients with bronchospastic disease who do not respond to, or cannot tolerate, other antihypertensive treatment. Since $beta_1$ selectivity is not absolute, a $beta_2$-stimulating agent should be administered concomitantly, and the lowest possible dose of Lopressor should be used. In these circumstances it would be prudent initially to administer Lopressor in smaller doses three times daily, instead of larger doses two times daily, to avoid the higher plasma levels associated with the longer dosing interval. (See DOSAGE AND ADMINISTRATION.)**

Major Surgery. The necessity or desirability of withdrawing beta-blocking therapy prior to major surgery is controversial; the impaired ability of the heart to respond to reflex adrenergic stimuli may augment the risks of general anesthesia and surgical procedures.

Lopressor, like other beta blockers, is a competitive inhibitor of beta-receptor agonists, and its effects can be reversed by administration of such agents, e.g., dobutamine or isoproterenol. However, such patients may be subject to protracted severe hypotension. Difficulty in restarting and maintaining the heart beat has also been reported with beta blockers.

Diabetes and Hypoglycemia. Lopressor should be used with caution in diabetic patients if a beta-blocking agent is required. Beta blockers may mask tachycardia occurring with hypoglycemia, but other manifestations such as dizziness and sweating may not be significantly affected. Selective beta blockers do not potentiate insulin-induced hypoglycemia and, unlike nonselective beta blockers, do not delay recovery of blood glucose to normal levels.

Thyrotoxicosis. Beta-adrenergic blockade may mask certain clinical signs (e.g., tachycardia) or hyperthyroidism. Patients suspected of developing thyrotoxicosis should be managed carefully to avoid abrupt withdrawal of beta blockade, which might precipitate a thyroid storm.

Hydrochlorothiazide

Thiazides should be used with caution in patients with severe renal disease. In patients with renal disease, thiazides may precipitate azotemia. Cumulative effects of the drug may develop in patients with impaired renal function.

Thiazides should be used with caution in patients with impaired hepatic function or progressive liver disease, since minor alterations of fluid and electrolyte imbalance may precipitate hepatic coma.

Thiazides may add to or potentiate the action of other antihypertensive drugs. Potentiation occurs with ganglionic or peripheral adrenergic blocking drugs.

Sensitivity reactions are more likely to occur in patients with a history of allergy or bronchial asthma.

The possibility of exacerbation or activation of systemic lupus erythematosus has been reported.

PRECAUTIONS

General

Lopressor. Lopressor should be used with caution in patients with impaired hepatic function.

Hydrochlorothiazide. All patients receiving thiazide therapy should be observed for clinical signs of fluid or electrolyte imbalance, namely hyponatremia, hypochloremic alkalosis, and hypokalemia (see Laboratory Tests and Drug/Drug Interactions). Warning signs are dryness of mouth, thirst, weakness, lethargy, drowsiness, restlessness, muscle pains or cramps, muscular fatigue, hypotension, oliguria, tachycardia, and gastrointestinal disturbance, such as nausea or vomiting.

Hypokalemia may develop, especially in cases of brisk diuresis or severe cirrhosis.

Interference with adequate oral intake of electrolytes will also contribute to hypokalemia. Hypokalemia may be avoided or treated by the use of potassium supplements or foods with a high potassium content.

Any chloride deficit is generally mild and usually does not require specific treatment, except under extraordinary circumstances (as in liver disease or renal disease). Dilutional hyponatremia may occur in edematous patients in hot weather; appropriate therapy is water restriction, rather than administration of salt, except in rare instances when the hyponatremia is life-threatening. In cases of actual salt depletion, appropriate replacement is the therapy of choice.

Hyperuricemia may occur or frank gout may be precipitated in certain patients receiving thiazide therapy.

Latent diabetes may become manifest during thiazide administration (see Drug/Drug Interactions).

The antihypertensive effects of the drug may be enhanced in the postsympathectomy patient.

If progressive renal impairment becomes evident, withholding or discontinuing diuretic therapy should be considered.

Calcium excretion is decreased by thiazides. Pathological changes in the parathyroid gland with hypercalcemia and hypophosphatemia have been observed in a few patients on prolonged thiazide therapy. The common complications of hyperparathyroidism, such as renal lithiasis, bone resorption, and peptic ulceration, have not been seen.

Thiazide diuretics have been shown to increase the urinary excretion of magnesium; this may result in hypomagnesmia.

Information for Patients

Patients should be advised to take Lopressor HCT regularly and continuously, as directed, with or immediately following meals. If a dose should be missed, the patient should take only the next scheduled dose (without doubling it). Patients should not discontinue Lopressor HCT without consulting the physician.

Patients should be advised (1) to avoid operating automobiles and machinery or engaging in other tasks requiring alertness until the patient's response to therapy with Lopressor has been determined; (2) to contact the physician if any difficulty in breathing occurs; (3) to inform the physician or dentist before any type of surgery that he or she is taking Lopressor HCT.

Laboratory Tests

Lopressor. Clinical laboratory findings may include elevated levels of serum transaminase, alkaline phosphatase, and lactate dehydrogenase.

Hydrochlorothiazide. Initial and periodic determinations of serum electrolytes to detect possible electrolyte imbalance should be performed at appropriate intervals.

Serum and urine electrolyte determinations are particularly important when the patient is vomiting excessively or receiving parenteral fluids.

Drug/Drug Interactions

Lopressor. Catecholamine-depleting drugs (e.g., reserpine) may have an additive effect when given with beta-blocking agents. Patients treated with Lopressor plus a catecholamine depletor should therefore be closely observed for evidence of hypotension or marked bradycardia, which may produce vertigo, syncope, or postural hypotension.

Risk of Anaphylactic Reaction. While taking beta-blockers, patients with a history of severe anaphylactic reaction to a variety of allergens may be more reactive to repeated challenge, either accidental, diagnostic, or therapeutic. Such patients may be unresponsive to the usual doses of epinephrine used to treat allergic reaction.

Hydrochlorothiazide. Hypokalemia can sensitize or exaggerate the response of the heart to the toxic effects of digitalis (e.g., increased ventricular irritability).

Hypokalemia may develop during concomitant use of steroids or ACTH.

Insulin requirements in diabetic patients may be increased, decreased, or unchanged.

Thiazides may decrease arterial responsiveness to norepinephrine, but not enough to preclude effectiveness of the pressor agent for therapeutic use.

Thiazides may increase the responsiveness to tubocurarine.

Lithium renal clearance is reduced by thiazides, increasing the risk of lithium toxicity.

There have been rare reports in the literature of hemolytic anemia occurring with the concomitant use of hydrochlorothiazide and methyldopa.

Concurrent administration of some nonsteroidal anti-inflammatory agents may reduce the diuretic, natriuretic and antihypertensive effects of thiazide diuretics.

Cholestyramine and colestipol resins: Absorption of hydrochlorothiazide is impaired in the presence of anionic exchange resins. Single doses of either cholestyramine or colestipol resins bind the hydrochlorothiazide and reduce its absorption from the gastrointestinal tract by up to 85% and 43%, respectively.

Drug/Laboratory Test Interactions

Hydrochlorothiazide. Thiazides may decrease serum levels of protein-bound iodine without signs of thyroid disturbance. Thiazides should be discontinued before tests for parathyroid function are made. (See General, *Hydrochlorothiazide,* Calcium excretion.)

Carcinogenesis, Mutagenesis, Impairment of Fertility

Lopressor HCT. Carcinogenicity and mutagenicity studies have not been conducted with Lopressor HCT. Lopressor HCT produced no evidence of impaired fertility in male or female rats administered gavaged doses up to 200/50 mg/kg (100/50 times the maximum recommended daily human dose) prior to mating and throughout gestation and rearing of young.

Lopressor. Long-term studies in animals have been conducted to evaluate carcinogenic potential. In a 2-year study in rats at three oral dosage levels of up to 800 mg/kg per day, there was no increase in the development of spontaneously occurring benign or malignant neoplasms of any type. The only histologic changes that appeared to be drug related were an increased incidence of generally mild focal accumulation of foamy macrophages in pulmonary alveoli and a slight increase in biliary hyperplasia. In a 21-month study in Swiss albino mice at three oral dosage levels of up to 750 mg/kg per day, benign lung tumors (small adenomas) occurred more frequently in female mice receiving the highest dose than in untreated control animals. There was no increase in malignant or total (benign plus malignant) lung tumors, nor in the overall incidence of tumors or malignant tumors. This 21-month study was repeated in CD-1 mice, and no statistically or biologically significant differences were observed between treated and control mice of either sex for any type of tumor.

All mutagenicity tests performed (a dominant lethal study in mice, chromosome studies in somatic cells, a *Salmonella*/mammalian-microsome mutagenicity test, and a nucleus anomaly test in somatic interphase nuclei) were negative.

No evidence of impaired fertility due to Lopressor was observed in a study performed in rats at doses up to 55.5 times the maximum daily human dose of 450 mg.

Hydrochlorothiazide. Two-year feeding studies in mice and rats conducted under the auspices of the National Toxicology Program (NTP) uncovered no evidence of a carcinogenic potential of hydrochlorothiazide in female mice (at doses up to approximately 600 mg/kg/day) or in male and female rats (at doses up to approximately 100 mg/kg/day). The NTP, however, found equivocal evidence for hepatocarcinogenicity in male mice.

Hydrochlorothiazide was not genotoxic in in vitro assays using strains TA 98, TA 100, TA 1535, TA 1537, and TA 1538 of *Salmonella typhimurium* (Ames assay) and in the Chinese Hamster Ovary (CHO) test for chromosomal aberrations, or in in vivo assays using mouse germinal cell chromosomes, Chinese hamster bone marrow chromosomes, and the *Drosophila* sex-linked recessive lethal trait gene. Positive test

Continued on next page

CibaGeneva—Cont.

results were obtained only in the in vitro CHO Sister Chromatid Exchange (clastogenicity) and in the Mouse Lymphoma Cell (mutagenicity) assays, using concentrations of hydrochlorothiazide from 43 to 1300 μg/mL, and in the *Aspergillus nidulans* nondisjunction assay at an unspecified concentration.

Hydrochlorothiazide had no adverse effects on the fertility of mice and rats of either sex in studies wherein these species were exposed, via their diet, to doses of up to 100 and 4 mg/kg/day, respectively, prior to mating and throughout gestation.

Pregnancy: Teratogenic Effects. Pregnancy Category C

Lopressor HCT. No evidence of adverse effects on pregnancy or the fetus were observed in rats when dams were administered gavaged doses up to 200/50 mg/kg of Lopressor HCT (100/50 times the maximum recommended daily human dose) during the period of organogenesis. Increased postimplantation loss and decreased postnatal survival were observed with these doses when administered later in pregnancy (gestation days 15–21). In rabbits, increased fetal loss was observed with oral doses of 25/6.25 mg/kg of Lopressor HCT (12/6 times the maximum recommended daily human dose), but not with lower doses. There are no adequate and well-controlled studies of Lopressor HCT in pregnant women. Lopressor HCT should be used during pregnancy only if the potential benefit justifies the potential risk to the fetus.

Lopressor. Lopressor has been shown to increase postimplantation loss and decrease neonatal survival in rats at doses up to 55.5 times the maximum daily human dose of 450 mg. Distribution studies in mice confirm exposure of the fetus when Lopressor is administered to the pregnant animal. These studies have revealed no evidence of teratogenicity.

Hydrochlorothiazide. Studies in which hydrochlorothiazide was orally administered to pregnant mice and rats during their respective periods of major organogenesis at doses up to 3000 and 1000 mg/kg/day, respectively, provided no evidence of harm to the fetus.

Nonteratogenic Effects

Hydrochlorothiazide. Thiazides cross the placental barrier and appear in cord blood, and there is a risk of fetal or neonatal jaundice, thrombocytopenia, and possibly other adverse reactions that have occurred in adults.

Nursing Mothers

Lopressor is excreted in breast milk in very small quantity. An infant consuming 1 liter of breast milk daily would receive a dose of metoprolol of less than 1 mg. Thiazides are also excreted in breast milk. If the use of Lopressor HCT is deemed essential, the patient should stop nursing.

Pediatric Use

Safety and effectiveness in pediatric patients have not been established.

ADVERSE REACTIONS

Lopressor HCT

The following adverse reactions were reported in controlled clinical studies of the combination of Lopressor and hydrochlorothiazide.

Body as a Whole: Fatigue or lethargy and flu syndrome have each been reported in about 10 in 100 patients.

Nervous System: Dizziness or vertigo, drowsiness or somnolence, and headache have each occurred in about 10 in 100 patients. Nightmare has occurred in 1 in 100 patients.

Cardiovascular: Bradycardia has occurred in about 6 in 100 patients. Decreased exercise tolerance and dyspnea have each occurred in about 1 of 100 patients.

Digestive: Diarrhea, digestive disorder, dry mouth, nausea or vomiting, and constipation have each occurred in about 1 in 100 patients.

Metabolic and Nutritional: Hypokalemia has occurred in fewer than 10 in 100 patients. Edema, gout, and anorexia have each occurred in 1 in 100 patients.

Special Senses: Blurred vision, tinnitus, and earache have each been reported in 1 in 100 patients.

Skin: Sweating and purpura have each occurred in 1 in 100 patients.

Urogenital: Impotence has occurred in 1 in 100 patients.

Musculoskeletal: Muscle pain has occurred in 1 in 100 patients.

Lopressor

Most adverse effects have been mild and transient.

Central Nervous System: Tiredness and dizziness have occurred in about 10 of 100 patients. Depression has been reported in about 5 of 100 patients. Mental confusion and short-term memory loss have been reported. Headache, nightmares, and insomnia have also been reported, but a drug relationship is not clear.

Cardiovascular: Shortness of breath and bradycardia have occurred in approximately 3 of 100 patients. Cold extremities; arterial insufficiency, usually of the Raynaud type; palpitations; and congestive heart failure have been reported. (See **CONTRAINDICATIONS, WARNINGS,** and **PRECAUTIONS**).

Respiratory: Wheezing (bronchospasm) has been reported in fewer than 1 of 100 patients (see **WARNINGS**).

Gastrointestinal: Diarrhea has occurred in about 5 of 100 patients. Nausea, gastric pain, constipation, flatulence, and heartburn have been reported in 1 of 100, or fewer, patients.

Hypersensitive Reactions: Pruritus has occurred in fewer than 1 of 100 patients. Rash has been reported.

Miscellaneous: Peyronie's disease has been reported in fewer than 1 of 100,000 patients. Alopecia has been reported. The oculomucocutaneous syndrome associated with the beta blocker practolol has not been reported with Lopressor.

Potential Adverse Reactions

A variety of adverse reactions not listed above have been reported with other beta-adrenergic blocking agents and should be considered potential adverse reactions to Lopressor.

Central Nervous System: Reversible mental depression progressing to catatonia; visual disturbances; hallucinations; an acute reversible syndrome characterized by disorientation for time and place, short-term memory loss, emotional lability, slightly clouded sensorium, and decreased performance on neuropsychometrics.

Cardiovascular: Intensification of AV block (see **CONTRAINDICATIONS**).

Hematologic: Agranulocytosis, nonthrombocytopenic purpura, thrombocytopenic purpura.

Hypersensitive Reactions: Fever combined with aching and sore throat, laryngospasm, and respiratory distress.

Hydrochlorothiazide

The following adverse reactions have been observed, but there has not been enough systematic collection of data to support an estimate of their frequency. Consequently the reactions are categorized by organ systems and are listed in decreasing order of severity and not frequency.

Digestive: Pancreatitis, jaundice (intrahepatic cholestatic), sialadenitis, vomiting, diarrhea, cramping, nausea, gastric irritation, constipation, anorexia.

Cardiovascular: Orthostatic hypotension (may be potentiated by alcohol, barbiturates, or narcotics).

Neurologic: Vertigo, dizziness, transient blurred vision, headache, paresthesia, xanthopsia, weakness, restlessness.

Musculoskeletal: Muscle spasm.

Hematologic: Aplastic anemia, agranulocytosis, leukopenia, thrombocytopenia.

Metabolic: Hyperglycemia, glycosuria, hyperuricemia.

Hypersensitive Reactions: Necrotizing angiitis, Stevens-Johnson syndrome, respiratory distress including pneumonitis and pulmonary edema, purpura, urticaria, rash, photosensitivity.

OVERDOSAGE

Acute Toxicity

Several cases of overdosage with Lopressor have been reported, some leading to death. No deaths have been reported with hydrochlorothiazide.

Oral LD_{50}'s (mg/kg): mice, 1158 (Lopressor); rats, 3090 (Lopressor), 2750 (hydrochlorothiazide).

Signs and Symptoms

Lopressor. Potential signs and symptoms associated with overdosage with Lopressor are bradycardia, hypotension, bronchospasm, and cardiac failure.

Hydrochlorothiazide. The most prominent feature of poisoning is acute loss of fluid and electrolytes.

Cardiovascular: Tachycardia, hypotension, shock.

Neuromuscular: Weakness, confusion, dizziness, cramps of the calf muscles, paresthesia, fatigue, impairment of consciousness.

Digestive: Nausea, vomiting, thirst.

Renal: Polyuria, oliguria, or anuria (due to hemoconcentration).

Laboratory Findings: Hypokalemia, hyponatremia, hypochloremia, alkalosis; increased BUN (especially in patients with renal insufficiency).

Combined Poisoning: Signs and symptoms may be aggravated or modified by concomitant intake of antihypertensive medication, barbiturates, curare, digitalis (hypokalemia), corticosteroids, narcotics, or alcohol.

Treatment

There is no specific antidote.

On the basis of the pharmacologic actions of Lopressor and hydrochlorothiazide, the following general measures should be employed:

Elimination of the Drug: Inducement of vomiting, gastric lavage, and activated charcoal.

Bradycardia: Atropine should be administered. If there is no response to vagal blockade, isoproterenol should be administered cautiously.

Hypotension: The patient's legs should be elevated, and lost fluid and electrolytes (potassium, sodium) should be replaced. A vasopressor should be administered, e.g., levarterenol or dopamine.

Bronchospasm: A $beta_2$-stimulating agent and/or a theophylline derivative should be administered.

Cardiac Failure: A digitalis glycoside and diuretic should be administered. In shock resulting from inadequate cardiac contractility, administration of dobutamine, isoproterenol, or glucagon may be considered.

Surveillance: Fluid and electrolyte balance (especially serum potassium) and renal function should be monitored until conditions become normal.

DOSAGE AND ADMINISTRATION

Dosage should be determined by individual titration (see **INDICATIONS AND USAGE**).

Hydrochlorothiazide is usually given at a dosage of 25 to 100 mg per day. The usual initial dosage of Lopressor is 100 mg daily in single or divided doses. Dosage may be increased gradually until optimum blood pressure control is achieved. The effective dosage range is 100 to 450 mg per day. While once-daily dosing is effective and can maintain a reduction in blood pressure throughout the day, lower doses (especially 100 mg) may not maintain a full effect at the end of the 24-hour period, and larger or more frequent daily doses may be required. This can be evaluated by measuring blood pressure near the end of the dosing interval to determine whether satisfactory control is being maintained thhroughout the day. $Beta_1$ selectivity diminishes as dosage of Lopressor is increased.

The following dosage schedule may be used to administer from 100 to 200 mg of Lopressor per day and from 25 to 50 mg of hydrochlorothiazide per day:

Lopressor HCT	***Dosage***
Tablets of 50/25	2 tablets per day in single or divided doses
Tablets of 100/25	1 to 2 tablets per day in single or divided doses
Tablets of 100/50	1 tablet per day in single or divided doses

Dosing regimens that exceed 50 mg of hydrochlorothiazide per day are not recommended. When necessary, another antihypertensive agent may be added gradually, beginning with 50% of the usual recommended starting dose to avoid an excessive fall in blood pressure.

HOW SUPPLIED

Tablets 50/25—capsule-shaped, white and blue, scored (imprinted Geigy on one side and 35 twice on the scored side) 50 mg of metoprolol tartrate and 25 mg of hydrochlorothiazide

Bottles of 100 .... NDC 0028-0035-01

Tablets 100/25—capsule-shaped, white and pink, scored (imprinted Geigy on one side and 53 twice on the scored side) 100 mg of metoprolol tartrate and 25 mg of hydrochlorothiazide

Bottles of 100 .... NDC 0028-0053-01

Tablets 100/50—capsule-shaped, white and yellow, scored (imprinted Geigy on one side and 73 twice on the scored side) 100 mg of metoprolol tartrate and 50 mg of hydrochlorothiazide

Bottles of 100 .... NDC 0028-0073-01

Samples, when available, are identified by the word *Sample* appearing on each tablet.

Store between 59°–86°F (15°–30°C). Protect from moisture.

Dispense in tight, light-resistant container (USP).

C96-28 (Rev. 3/96)

Shown in Product Identification Guide, page 309

LOTENSIN® ℞

benazepril hydrochloride
Tablets

Prescribing Information

Use in Pregnancy
When used in pregnancy during the second and third trimesters, ACE inhibitors can cause injury and even death to the developing fetus. When pregnancy is detected, Lotensin should be discontinued as soon as possible. See **WARNINGS, Fetal/Neonatal Morbidity and Mortality.**

DESCRIPTION

Benazepril hydrochloride is a white to off-white crystalline powder, soluble (> 100 mg/mL) in water, in ethanol, and in methanol. Benazepril's chemical name is 3-[[1-(ethoxy-carbonyl)-3-phenyl-(1S)-propyl]amino]-2,3,4,5-tetrahydro-2-oxo-1*H*-1-(3S)-benzazepine-1-acetic acid monohydrochloride.

Its empirical formula is $C_{24}H_{28}N_2O_5 \cdot HCl$, and its molecular weight is 460.96.

Benazeprilat, the active metabolite of benazepril, is a non-sulfhydryl angiotensin-converting enzyme inhibitor. Benazepril is converted to benazeprilat by hepatic cleavage of the ester group.

Lotensin is supplied as tablets containing 5 mg, 10 mg, 20 mg, and 40 mg of benazepril for oral administration. The inactive ingredients are cellulose compounds, colloidal silicon dioxide, crospovidone, hydrogenated castor oil (5-mg, 10-mg, and 20-mg tablets), iron oxides, lactose, magnesium stea-

rate (40-mg tablets), polysorbate 80, propylene glycol (5-mg and 40-mg tablets), starch, talc, and titanium dioxide.

CLINICAL PHARMACOLOGY

Mechanism of Action

Benazepril and benazeprilat inhibit angiotensin-converting enzyme (ACE) in human subjects and animals. ACE is a peptidyl dipeptidase that catalyzes the conversion of angiotensin I to the vasoconstrictor substance, angiotensin II. Angiotensin II also stimulates aldosterone secretion by the adrenal cortex.

Inhibition of ACE results in decreased plasma angiotensin II, which leads to decreased vasopressor activity and to decreased aldosterone secretion. The latter decrease may result in a small increase of serum potassium. Hypertensive patients treated with Lotensin alone for up to 52 weeks had elevations of serum potassium of up to 0.2 mEq/L. Similar patients treated with Lotensin and hydrochlorothiazide for up to 24 weeks had no consistent changes in their serum potassium (see PRECAUTIONS).

Removal of angiotensin II negative feedback on renin secretion leads to increased plasma renin activity. In animal studies, benazepril had no inhibitory effect on the vasopressor response to angiotensin II and did not interfere with the hemodynamic effects of the autonomic neurotransmitters acetylcholine, epinephrine, and norepinephrine.

ACE is identical to kininase, an enzyme that degrades bradykinin. Whether increased levels of bradykinin, a potent vasodepressor peptide, play a role in the therapeutic effects of Lotensin remains to be elucidated.

While the mechanism through which benazepril lowers blood pressure is believed to be primarily suppression of the renin-angiotensin-aldosterone system, benazepril has an antihypertensive effect even in patients with low-renin hypertension. (see INDICATIONS AND USAGE).

Pharmacokinetics and Metabolism

Following oral administration of Lotensin, peak plasma concentrations of benazepril are reached within 0.5-1.0 hours. The extent of absorption is at least 37% as determined by urinary recovery and is not significantly influenced by the presence of food in the GI tract.

Cleavage of the ester group (primarily in the liver) converts benazepril to its active metabolite, benazeprilat. Peak plasma concentrations of benazeprilat are reached 1-2 hours after drug intake in the fasting state and 2-4 hours after drug intake in the nonfasting state. The serum protein binding of benazepril is about 96.7% and that of benazeprilat about 95.3%, as measured by equilibrium dialysis; on the basis of in vitro studies, the degree of protein binding should be unaffected by age, hepatic dysfunction, or concentration (over the concentration range of 0.24-23.6 μmol/L).

Benazepril is almost completely metabolized to benazeprilat, which has much greater ACE inhibitory activity than benazepril, and to the glucuronide conjugates of benazepril and benazeprilat. Only trace amounts of an administered dose of Lotensin can be recovered in the urine as unchanged benazepril, while about 20% of the dose is excreted as benazeprilat, 4% as benazepril glucuronide, and 8% as benazeprilat glucuronide.

The kinetics of benazepril are approximately dose-proportional within the dosage range of 10-80 mg.

The effective half-life of accumulation of benazeprilat following multiple dosing of benazepril hydrochloride is 10-11 hours. Thus, steady-state concentrations of benazeprilat should be reached after 2 or 3 doses of benazepril hydrochloride given once daily.

The kinetics did not change, and there was no significant accumulation during chronic administration (28 days) of once-daily doses between 5 mg and 20 mg. Accumulation ratios based on AUC and urinary recovery of benazeprilat were 1.19 and 1.27, respectively.

When dialysis was started two hours after ingestion of 10 mg of benazepril, approximately 6% of benazeprilat was removed in 4 hours of dialysis. The parent compound, benazepril, was not detected in the dialysate.

The disposition of benazepril and benazeprilat in patients with mild-to-moderate renal insufficiency (creatinine clearance > 30 mL/min) is similar to that in patients with normal renal function. In patients with creatinine clearance ≤30 mL/min, peak benazeprilat levels and the initial (alpha phase) half-life increase, and time to steady state may be delayed (see DOSAGE AND ADMINISTRATION).

Benazepril and benazeprilat are cleared predominantly by renal excretion in healthy subjects with normal renal function. Nonrenal (i.e., biliary) excretion accounts for approximately 11%-12% of benazeprilat excretion in healthy subjects. In patients with renal failure, biliary clearance may compensate to an extent for deficient renal clearance.

In patients with hepatic dysfunction due to cirrhosis, levels of benazeprilat are essentially unaltered. The pharmacokinetics of benazepril and benazeprilat do not appear to be influenced by age.

In studies in rats given ^{14}C-benazepril, benazepril and its metabolites crossed the blood-brain barrier only to an extremely low extent. Multiple doses of benazepril did not result in accumulation in any tissue except the lung, where, as

with other ACE inhibitors in similar studies, there was a slight increase in concentration due to slow elimination in that organ.

Some placental passage occurred when the drug was administered to pregnant rats.

Pharmacodynamics

Single and multiple doses of 10 mg or more of Lotensin cause inhibition of plasma ACE activity by at least 80%-90% for at least 24 hours after dosing. Pressor responses to exogenous angiotensin I were inhibited by 60%-90% (up to 4 hours post-dose) at the 10-mg dose.

Administration of Lotensin to patients with mild-to-moderate hypertension results in a reduction of both supine and standing blood pressure to about the same extent with no compensatory tachycardia. Symptomatic postural hypotension is infrequent, although it can occur in patients who are salt- and/or volume-depleted (see WARNINGS).

In single-dose studies, Lotensin lowered blood pressure within 1 hour, with peak reductions achieved 2-4 hours after dosing. The antihypertensive effect of a single dose persisted for 24 hours. In multiple-dose studies, once-daily doses of 20-80 mg decreased seated pressure (systolic/diastolic) 24 hours after dosing by about 6-12/4-7 mmHg. The trough values represent reductions of about 50% of that seen at peak.

Four dose-response studies using once-daily dosing were conducted in 470 mild-to-moderate hypertensive patients not using diuretics. The minimal effective once-daily dose of Lotensin was 10 mg; but further falls in blood pressure, especially at morning trough, were seen with higher doses in the studied dosing range (10-80 mg). In studies comparing the same daily dose of Lotensin given as a single morning dose or as a twice-daily dose, blood pressure reductions at the time of morning trough blood levels were greater with the divided regimen.

During chronic therapy, the maximum reduction in blood pressure with any dose is generally achieved after 1-2 weeks. The antihypertensive effects of Lotensin have continued during therapy for at least two years. Abrupt withdrawal of Lotensin has not been associated with a rapid increase in blood pressure.

In patients with mild-to-moderate hypertension, Lotensin 10-20 mg was similar in effectiveness to captopril, hydrochlorothiazide, nifedipine SR, and propranolol.

The antihypertensive effects of Lotensin were not appreciably different in patients receiving high- or low-sodium diets. In hemodynamic studies in dogs, blood pressure reduction was accompanied by a reduction in peripheral arterial resistance, with an increase in cardiac output and renal blood flow and little or no change in heart rate. In normal human volunteers, single doses of benazepril caused an increase in renal blood flow but had no effect on glomerular filtration rate.

Use of Lotensin in combination with thiazide diuretics gives a blood-pressure-lowering effect greater than that seen with either agent alone. By blocking the renin-angiotensin-aldosterone axis, administration of Lotensin tends to reduce the potassium loss associated with the diuretic.

INDICATIONS AND USAGE

Lotensin is indicated for the treatment of hypertension. It may be used alone or in combination with thiazide diuretics. In using Lotensin, consideration should be given to the fact that another angiotensin-converting enzyme inhibitor, captopril, has caused agranulocytosis, particularly in patients with renal impairment or collagen-vascular disease. Available data are insufficient to show that Lotensin does not have a similar risk (see WARNINGS).

Black patients receiving ACE-inhibitor monotherapy have been reported to have a higher incidence of angioedema compared to nonblacks. It should also be noted that in controlled clinical trials ACE inhibitors have an effect on blood pressure that is less in black patients than in nonblacks.

CONTRAINDICATIONS

Lotensin is contraindicated in patients who are hypersensitive to this product or to any other ACE inhibitor.

WARNINGS

Anaphylactoid and Possibly Related Reactions

Presumably because angiotensin-converting enzyme inhibitors affect the metabolism of eicosanoids and polypeptides, including endogenous bradykinin, patients receiving ACE inhibitors (including Lotensin) may be subject to a variety of adverse reactions, some of them serious.

Angioedema: Angioedema of the face, extremities, lips, tongue, glottis, and larynx has been reported in patients treated with angiotensin-converting enzyme inhibitors. In U.S. clinical trials, symptoms consistent with angioedema were seen in none of the subjects who received placebo and in about 0.5% of the subjects who received Lotensin. Angioedema associated with laryngeal edema can be fatal. If laryngeal stridor or angioedema of the face, tongue, or glottis occurs, treatment with Lotensin should be discontinued and appropriate therapy instituted immediately. **Where there is involvement of the tongue, glottis, or larynx, likely to cause airway obstruction, appropriate therapy, e.g., subcutaneous**

epinephrine injection 1:1000 (0.3 mL to 0.5 mL) should be promptly administered (see ADVERSE REACTIONS).

Anaphylactoid Reactions During Desensitization: Two patients undergoing desensitizing treatment with hymenoptera venom while receiving ACE inhibitors sustained life-threatening anaphylactoid reactions. In the same patients, these reactions were avoided when ACE inhibitors were temporarily withheld, but they reappeared upon inadvertent rechallenge.

Anaphylactoid Reactions During Membrane Exposure: Anaphylactoid reactions have been reported in patients dialyzed with high-flux membranes and treated concomitantly with an ACE inhibitor. Anaphylactoid reactions have also been reported in patients undergoing low-density lipoprotein apheresis with dextran sulfate absorption (a procedure dependent upon devices not approved in the United States).

Hypotension

Lotensin can cause symptomatic hypotension. Like other ACE inhibitors, benazepril has been only rarely associated with hypotension in uncomplicated hypertensive patients. Symptomatic hypotension is most likely to occur in patients who have been volume- and/or salt-depleted as a result of prolonged diuretic therapy, dietary salt restriction, dialysis, diarrhea, or vomiting. Volume- and/or salt-depletion should be corrected before initiating therapy with Lotensin.

In patients with congestive heart failure, with or without associated renal insufficiency, ACE inhibitor therapy may cause excessive hypotension, which may be associated with oliguria or azotemia and, rarely, with acute renal failure and death. In such patients, Lotensin therapy should be started under close medical supervision; they should be followed closely for the first 2 weeks of treatment and whenever the dose of benazepril or diuretic is increased.

If hypotension occurs, the patient should be placed in a supine position, and, if necessary, treated with intravenous infusion of physiological saline. Lotensin treatment usually can be continued following restoration of blood pressure and volume.

Neutropenia/Agranulocytosis

Another angiotensin-converting enzyme inhibitor, captopril, has been shown to cause agranulocytosis and bone marrow depression, rarely in uncomplicated patients, but more frequently in patients with renal impairment, especially if they also have a collagen-vascular disease such as systemic lupus erythematosus or scleroderma. Available data from clinical trials of benazepril are insufficient to show that benazepril does not cause agranulocytosis at similar rates. Monitoring of white blood cell counts should be considered in patients with collagen-vascular disease, especially if the disease is associated with impaired renal function.

Fetal/Neonatal Morbidity and Mortality

ACE inhibitors can cause fetal and neonatal morbidity and death when administered to pregnant women. Several dozen cases have been reported in the world literature. When pregnancy is detected, ACE inhibitors should be discontinued as soon as possible.

The use of ACE inhibitors during the second and third trimesters of pregnancy has been associated with fetal and neonatal injury, including hypotension, neonatal skull hypoplasia, anuria, reversible or irreversible renal failure, and death. Oligohydramnios has also been reported, presumably resulting from decreased fetal renal function; oligohydramnios in this setting has been associated with fetal limb contractures, craniofacial deformation, and hypoplastic lung development. Prematurity, intrauterine growth retardation, and patent ductus arteriosus have also been reported, although it is not clear whether these occurrences were due to the ACE inhibitor exposure.

These adverse effects do not appear to have resulted from intrauterine ACE inhibitor exposure that has been limited to the first trimester. Mothers whose embryos and fetuses are exposed to ACE inhibitors only during the first trimester should be so informed. Nonetheless, when patients become pregnant, physicians should make every effort to discontinue the use of benazepril as soon as possible.

Rarely (probably less often than once in every thousand pregnancies), no alternative to ACE inhibitors will be found. In these rare cases, the mothers should be apprised of the potential hazards to their fetuses, and serial ultrasound examinations should be performed to assess the intraamniotic environment.

If oligohydramnios is observed, benazepril should be discontinued unless it is considered life-saving for the mother. Contraction stress testing (CST), a nonstress test (NST), or biophysical profiling (BPP) may be appropriate, depending upon the week of pregnancy. Patients and physicians should be aware, however, that oligohydramnios may not appear until after the fetus has sustained irreversible injury.

Infants with histories of in utero exposure to ACE inhibitors should be closely observed for hypotension, oliguria, and hyperkalemia. If oliguria occurs, attention should be directed toward support of blood pressure and renal perfusion. Exchange transfusion or dialysis may be required as means

Continued on next page

CibaGeneva—Cont.

of reversing hypotension and/or substituting for disordered renal function. Benazepril, which crosses the placenta, can theoretically be removed from the neonatal circulation by these means; there are occasional reports of benefit from these maneuvers with another ACE inhibitor, but experience is limited.

No teratogenic effects of Lotensin were seen in studies of pregnant rats, mice, and rabbits. On a mg/m^2 basis, the doses used in these studies were 60 times (in rats), 9 times (in mice), and more than 0.8 times (in rabbits) the maximum recommended human dose (assuming a 50-kg woman). On a mg/kg basis these multiples are 300 times (in rats), 90 times (in mice) and more than 3 times (in rabbits) the maximum recommended human dose.

Hepatic Failure

Rarely, ACE inhibitors have been associated with a syndrome that starts with cholestatic jaundice and progresses to fulminant hepatic necrosis and (sometimes) death. The mechanism of this syndrome is not understood. Patients receiving ACE inhibitors who develop jaundice or marked elevations of hepatic enzymes should discontinue the ACE inhibitor and receive appropriate medical follow-up.

PRECAUTIONS

General

Impaired Renal Function: As a consequence of inhibiting the renin-angiotensin-aldosterone system, changes in renal function may be anticipated in susceptible individuals. In patients with severe congestive heart failure whose renal function may depend on the activity of the renin-angiotensin-aldosterone system, treatment with angiotensin-converting enzyme inhibitors, including Lotensin, may be associated with oliguria and/or progressive azotemia and (rarely) with acute renal failure and/or death. In a small study of hypertensive patients with renal artery stenosis in a solitary kidney or bilateral renal artery stenosis, treatment with Lotensin was associated with increases in blood urea nitrogen and serum creatinine; these increases were reversible upon discontinuation of Lotensin or diuretic therapy, or both. When such patients are treated with ACE inhibitors, renal function should be monitored during the first few weeks of therapy. Some hypertensive patients with no apparent preexisting renal vascular disease have developed increases in blood urea nitrogen and serum creatinine, usually minor and transient, especially when Lotensin has been given concomitantly with a diuretic. This is more likely to occur in patients with preexisting renal impairment. Dosage reduction of Lotensin and/or discontinuation of the diuretic may be required. **Evaluation of the hypertensive patient should always include assessment of renal function (see DOSAGE AND ADMINISTRATION).**

Hyperkalemia: In clinical trials, hyperkalemia (serum potassium at least 0.5 mEq/L greater than the upper limit of normal) occurred in approximately 1% of hypertensive patients receiving Lotensin. In most cases, these were isolated values which resolved despite continued therapy. Risk factors for the development of hyperkalemia include renal insufficiency, diabetes mellitus, and the concomitant use of potassium-sparing diuretics, potassium supplements, and/or potassium-containing salt substitutes, which should be used cautiously, if at all, with Lotensin (see Drug Interactions).

Cough: Presumably due to the inhibition of the degradation of endogenous bradykinin, persistent nonproductive cough has been reported with all ACE inhibitors, always resolving after discontinuation of therapy. ACE inhibitor-induced cough should be considered in the differential diagnosis of cough.

Impaired Liver Function: In patients with hepatic dysfunction due to cirrhosis, levels of benazeprilat are essentially unaltered. (See WARNINGS, Hepatic Failure.)

Surgery/Anesthesia: In patients undergoing surgery or during anesthesia with agents that produce hypotension, benazepril will block the angiotensin II formation that could otherwise occur secondary to compensatory renin release. Hypotension that occurs as a result of this mechanism can be corrected by volume expansion.

Information for Patients

Pregnancy: Female patients of childbearing age should be told about the consequences of second- and third-trimester exposure to ACE inhibitors, and they should also be told that these consequences do not appear to have resulted from intrauterine ACE inhibitor exposure that has been limited to the first trimester. These patients should be asked to report pregnancies to their physicians as soon as possible.

Angioedema: Angioedema, including laryngeal edema, can occur at any time with treatment with ACE inhibitors. Patients should be so advised and told to report immediately any signs or symptoms suggesting angioedema (swelling of face, eyes, lips, or tongue, or difficulty in breathing) and to take no more drug until they have consulted with the prescribing physician.

Symptomatic Hypotension: Patients should be cautioned that lightheadedness can occur, especially during the first days of therapy, and it should be reported to the prescribing physician. Patients should be told that if syncope occurs, Lotensin should be discontinued until the prescribing physician has been consulted.

All patients should be cautioned that inadequate fluid intake or excessive perspiration, diarrhea, or vomiting can lead to an excessive fall in blood pressure, with the same consequences of lightheadedness and possible syncope.

Hyperkalemia: Thrombocytopenia. Patients should be told not to use potassium supplements or salt substitutes containing potassium without consulting the prescribing physician.

Neutropenia: Patients should be told to promptly report any indication of infection (e.g., sore throat, fever), which could be a sign of neutropenia.

Drug Interactions

Diuretics: Patients on diuretics, especially those in whom diuretic therapy was recently instituted, may occasionally experience an excessive reduction of blood pressure after initiation of therapy with Lotensin. The possibility of hypotensive effects with Lotensin can be minimized by either discontinuing the diuretic or increasing the salt intake prior to initiation of treatment with Lotensin. If this is not possible, the starting dose should be reduced (see DOSAGE AND ADMINISTRATION).

Potassium Supplements and Potassium-Sparing Diuretics: Lotensin can attenuate potassium loss caused by thiazide diuretics. Potassium-sparing diuretics (spironolactone, amiloride, triamterene, and others) or potassium supplements can increase the risk of hyperkalemia. Therefore, if concomitant use of such agents is indicated, they should be given with caution, and the patient's serum potassium should be monitored frequently.

Oral Anticoagulants: Interaction studies with warfarin and acenocoumarol failed to identify any clinically important effects on the serum concentrations or clinical effects of these anticoagulants.

Lithium: Increased serum lithium levels and symptoms of lithium toxicity have been reported in patients receiving ACE inhibitors during therapy with lithium. These drugs should be coadministered with caution, and frequent monitoring of serum lithium levels is recommended. If a diuretic is also used, the risk of lithium toxicity may be increased.

Other: No clinically important pharmacokinetic interactions occurred when Lotensin was administered concomitantly with hydrochlorothiazide, chlorthalidone, furosemide, digoxin, propranolol, atenolol, naproxen, or cimetidine.

Lotensin has been used concomitantly with beta-adrenergic-blocking agents, calcium-channel-blocking agents, diuretics, digoxin, and hydralazine, without evidence of clinically important adverse interactions. Benazepril, like other ACE inhibitors, has had less than additive effects with beta-adrenergic blockers, presumably because both drugs lower blood pressure by inhibiting parts of the renin-angiotensin system.

Carcinogenesis, Mutagenesis, Impairment of Fertility

No evidence of carcinogenicity was found when benazepril was administered to rats and mice for up to two years at doses of up to 150 mg/kg/day. When compared on the basis of body weights, this dose is 110 times the maximum recommended human dose. When compared on the basis of body surface areas, this dose is 18 and 9 times (rats and mice, respectively) the maximum recommended human dose (calculations assume a patient weight of 60 kg). No mutagenic activity was detected in the Ames test in bacteria (with or without metabolic activation), in an in vitro test for forward mutations in cultured mammalian cells, or in a nucleus anomaly test. In doses of 50–500 mg/kg/day (6–60 times the maximum recommended human dose based on mg/m^2 comparison and 37–375 times the maximum recommended human dose based on a mg/kg comparison), Lotensin had no adverse effect on the reproductive performance of male and female rats.

Pregnancy Categories C (first trimester) and D (second and third trimesters)

See WARNINGS, Fetal/Neonatal Morbidity and Mortality.

Nursing Mothers

Minimal amounts of unchanged benazepril and of benazeprilat are excreted into the breast milk of lactating women treated with benazepril. A newborn child ingesting entirely breast milk would receive less than 0.1% of the mg/kg maternal dose of benazepril and benazeprilat.

Geriatric Use

Of the total number of patients who received benazepril in U.S. clinical studies of Lotensin, 18% were 65 or older while 2% were 75 or older. No overall differences in effectiveness or safety were observed between these patients and younger patients, and other reported clinical experience has not identified differences in responses between the elderly and younger patients, but greater sensitivity of some older individuals cannot be ruled out.

Pediatric Use

Safety and effectiveness in pediatric patients have not been established.

ADVERSE REACTIONS

Lotensin has been evaluated for safety in over 6000 patients with hypertension; over 700 of these patients were treated for at least one year. The overall incidence of reported adverse events was comparable in Lotensin and placebo patients.

The reported side effects were generally mild and transient, and there was no relation between side effects and age, duration of therapy, or total dosage within the range of 2 to 80 mg. Discontinuation of therapy because of a side effect was required in approximately 5% of U.S. patients treated with Lotensin and in 3% of patients treated with placebo.

The most common reasons for discontinuation were headache (0.6%) and cough (0.5%). (See PRECAUTIONS, Cough).

The side effects considered possibly or probably related to study drug that occurred in U.S. placebo-controlled trials in more than 1% of patients treated with Lotensin are shown below.

PATIENTS IN U.S. PLACEBO-CONTROLLED STUDIES

	LOTENSIN (N=964)		PLACEBO (N=496)	
	N	%	N	%
Headache	60	6.2	21	4.2
Dizziness	35	3.6	12	2.4
Fatigue	23	2.4	11	2.2
Somnolence	15	1.6	2	0.4
Postural Dizziness	14	1.5	1	0.2
Nausea	13	1.3	5	1.0
Cough	12	1.2	5	1.0

Other adverse experiences reported in controlled clinical trials (in less than 1% of benazepril patients), and rarer events seen in postmarketing experience, include the following (in some, a causal relationship to drug use is uncertain):

Cardiovascular: Symptomatic hypotension was seen in 0.3% of patients, postural hypotension in 0.4%, and syncope in 0.1%; these reactions led to discontinuation of therapy in 4 patients who had received benazepril monotherapy and in 9 patients who had received benazepril with hydrochlorothiazide (see PRECAUTIONS and WARNINGS). Other reports include angina pectoris, palpitations, and peripheral edema.

Renal: Of hypertensive patients with no apparent preexisting renal disease, about 2% have sustained increases in serum creatinine to at least 150% of their baseline values while receiving Lotensin, but most of these increases have disappeared despite continuing treatment. A much smaller fraction of these patients (less than 0.1%) developed simultaneous (usually transient) increases in blood urea nitrogen and serum creatinine.

Fetal/Neonatal Morbidity and Mortality: See WARNINGS, Fetal/Neonatal Morbidity and Mortality.

Angioedema: Angioedema has been reported in patients receiving ACE inhibitors. During clinical trials in hypertensive patients with benazepril, 0.5% of patients experienced edema of the lips or face without other manifestations of angioedema. Angioedema associated with laryngeal edema and/or shock may be fatal. If angioedema of the face, extremities, lips, tongue, or glottis and/or larynx occurs, treatment with Lotensin should be discontinued and appropriate therapy instituted immediately (see WARNINGS).

Dermatologic: Stevens-Johnson syndrome, apparent hypersensitivity reactions (manifested by dermatitis, pruritus, or rash), photosensitivity, and flushing. There have been rare reports of pemphigus in patients receiving ACE inhibitors.

Gastrointestinal: Pancreatitis, constipation, gastritis, vomiting, and melena.

Hematologic: Thrombocytopenia. There have been rare reports of hemolytic anemia in patients receiving ACE inhibitors.

Neurologic and Psychiatric: Anxiety, decreased libido, hypertonia, insomnia, nervousness, and paresthesia.

Other: Arthralgia, arthritis, asthenia, asthma, bronchitis, dyspnea, impotence, infection, myalgia, sinusitis, sweating, and urinary tract infection.

Clinical Laboratory Test Findings

Creatinine and Blood Urea Nitrogen: Of hypertensive patients with no apparent preexisting renal disease, about 2% have sustained increases in serum creatinine to at least 150% of their baseline values while receiving Lotensin, but most of these increases have disappeared despite continuing treatment. A much smaller fraction of these patients (less than 0.1%) developed simultaneous (usually transient) increases in blood urea nitrogen and serum creatinine. None of these increases required discontinuation of treatment. Increases in these laboratory values are more likely to occur in patients with renal insufficiency or those pretreated with a diuretic and, based on experience with other ACE inhibitors, would be expected to be especially likely in patients with renal artery stenosis (see PRECAUTIONS, General).

Potassium: Since benazepril decreases aldosterone secretion, elevation of serum potassium can occur. Potassium supplements and potassium-sparing diuretics should be given with caution, and the patient's serum potassium should be monitored frequently (see PRECAUTIONS).

Dose	Tablet Color	Bottle of 100	Accu-Pak® of 100
5 mg	light yellow	NDC 0083-0059-30	NDC 0083-0059-32
10 mg	dark yellow	NDC 0083-0063-30	NDC 0083-0063-32
20 mg	tan	NDC 0083-0079-30	NDC 0083-0079-32
40 mg	dark rose	NDC 0083-0094-30	NDC 0083-0094-32

Hemoglobin: Decreases in hemoglobin (a low value and a decrease of 5 g/dL) were rare, occurring in only 1 of 2014 patients receiving Lotensin alone and in 1 of 1357 patients receiving Lotensin plus a diuretic. No U.S. patients discontinued treatment because of decreases in hemoglobin.

Other (causal relationships unknown): Clinically important changes in standard laboratory tests were rarely associated with Lotensin administration. Elevations of uric acid, blood glucose, serum bilirubin, and liver enzymes (see WARNINGS) have been reported, as have scattered incidents of hyponatremia, electrocardiographic changes, leukopenia, eosinophilia, and proteinuria. In U.S. trials, less than 0.5% of patients discontinued treatment because of laboratory abnormalities.

OVERDOSAGE

Single oral doses of 3 g/kg benazepril were associated with significant lethality in mice. Rats, however, tolerated single oral doses of up to 6 g/kg. Reduced activity was seen at 1 g/kg in mice and at 5 g/kg in rats. Human overdoses of benazepril have not been reported, but the most common manifestation of human benazepril overdosage is likely to be hypotension. Laboratory determinations of serum levels of benazepril and its metabolites are not widely available, and such determinations have, in any event, no established role in the management of benazepril overdose.

No data are available to suggest physiological maneuvers (e.g., maneuvers to change the pH of the urine) that might accelerate elimination of benazepril and its metabolites. Benazepril is only slightly dialyzable, but dialysis might be considered in overdosed patients with severely impaired renal function (see WARNINGS).

Angiotensin II could presumably serve as a specific antagonist-antidote in the setting of benazepril overdose, but angiotensin II is essentially unavailable outside of scattered research facilities. Because the hypotensive effect of benazepril is achieved through vasodilation and effective hypovolemia, it is reasonable to treat benazepril overdose by infusion of normal saline solution.

DOSAGE AND ADMINISTRATION

The recommended initial dose for patients not receiving a diuretic is 10 mg once-a-day. The usual maintenance dosage range is 20–40 mg per day administered as a single dose or in two equally divided doses. A dose of 80 mg gives an increased response, but experience with this dose is limited. The divided regimen was more effective in controlling trough (predosing) blood pressure than the same dose given as a once-daily regimen. Dosage adjustment should be based on measurement of peak (2–6 hours after dosing) and trough responses. If a once-daily regimen does not give adequate trough response, an increase in dosage or divided administration should be considered. If blood pressure is not controlled with Lotensin alone, a diuretic can be added.

Total daily doses above 80 mg have not been evaluated.

Concomitant administration of Lotensin with potassium supplements, potassium salt substitutes, or potassium-sparing diuretics can lead to increases of serum potassium (see PRECAUTIONS).

In patients who are currently being treated with a diuretic, symptomatic hypotension occasionally can occur following the initial dose of Lotensin. To reduce the likelihood of hypotension, the diuretic should, if possible, be discontinued two to three days prior to beginning therapy with Lotensin (see WARNINGS). Then, if blood pressure is not controlled with Lotensin alone, diuretic therapy should be resumed. If the diuretic cannot be discontinued, an initial dose of 5 mg Lotensin should be used to avoid excessive hypotension.

Dosage Adjustment in Renal Impairment

For patients with a creatinine clearance <30 mL/min/1.73 m^2 (serum creatinine >3 mg/dL), the recommended initial dose is 5 mg Lotensin once daily. Dosage may be titrated upward until blood pressure is controlled or to a maximum total daily dose of 40 mg (see WARNINGS).

HOW SUPPLIED

Lotensin is available in tablets of 5 mg, 10 mg, 20 mg, and 40 mg, packaged with a desiccant in bottles of 100 tablets. Lotensin is also supplied in blister packages (1 tablet/blister), in Accu-Pak® Unit Dose boxes containing 10 strips of 10 blisters each.

Each tablet is imprinted with LOTENSIN on one side and the tablet strength ("5", "10", "20", or "40") on the other. Samples, when available, are identified by the word *SAMPLE* on each tablet.

The National Drug Codes for the various packages are: [See table above]

Storage: Do not store above 86°F (30°C). Protect from moisture.

Dispense in tight container (USP).

C95-41 (Rev. 10/95)

Dist. by:
Ciba-Geigy Corporation
Pharmaceuticals Division
Summit, New Jersey 07901
Shown in Product Identification Guide, page 309

LOTENSIN HCT® ℞
benazepril hydrochloride and hydrochlorothiazide USP
Combination Tablets
5 mg/6.25 mg
10 mg/12.5 mg
20 mg/12.5mg
20 mg/25 mg

Prescribing Information

> **USE IN PREGNANCY**
> When used in pregnancy during the second and third trimesters, ACE inhibitors can cause injury and even death to the developing fetus. When pregnancy is detected, Lotensin HCT should be discontinued as soon as possible. See **WARNINGS, Fetal/Neonatal Morbidity and Mortality.**

DESCRIPTION

Benazepril hydrochloride is a white to off-white crystalline powder, soluble (>100 mg/mL) in water, in ethanol, and in methanol. Benazepril hydrochloride's chemical name is 3-[[1-(ethoxycarbonyl)-3-phenyl-(1S)-propyl]amino]-2,3,4,5-tetrahydro-2-oxo-1H-1-(3S)-benzazepine-1-acetic acid monohydrochloride.

Its empirical formula is $C_{24}H_{28}N_2O_5 \cdot HCl$, and its molecular weight is 460.96.

Benazeprilat, the active metabolite of benazepril, is a nonsulfhydryl angiotensin-converting enzyme inhibitor. Benazepril is converted to benazeprilat by hepatic cleavage of the ester group.

Hydrochlorothiazide USP is a white, or practically white, practically odorless, crystalline powder. It is slightly soluble in water; freely soluble in sodium hydroxide solution, in *n*-butylamine, and in dimethylformamide; sparingly soluble in methanol; and insoluble in ether, in chloroform, and in dilute mineral acids. Hydrochlorothiazide's chemical name is 6-chloro-3,4-dihydro -2H-1,2,4- benzothiadiazine-7-sulfonamide 1,1-dioxide.

Its empirical formula is $C_7H_8ClN_3O_4S_2$, and its molecular weight is 297.73. Hydrochlorothiazide is a thiazide diuretic. Lotensin HCT is a combination of benazepril hydrochloride and hydrochlorothiazide USP. The tablets are formulated for oral administration with a combination of 5, 10, or 20 mg of benazapril hydrochloride and 6.25, 12.5, or 25 mg of hydrochlorothiazide USP. The inactive ingredients of the tablets are cellulose compounds, crospovidone, hydrogenated castor oil, iron oxides (10/12.5-mg, 20/12.5-mg, and 20/25 mg tablets), lactose, polyethylene glycol, talc, and titanium dioxide.

CLINICAL PHARMACOLOGY

Mechanism of Action

Benazepril and benazeprilat inhibit angiotensin-converting enzyme (ACE) in human subjects and in animals. ACE is a peptidyl dipeptidase that catalyzes the conversion of angiotensin I to the vasoconstrictor substance, angiotensin II. Angiotensin II also stimulates aldosterone secretion by the adrenal cortex.

Inhibition of ACE results in decreased plasma angiotensin II, which leads to decreased vasopressor activity and to decreased aldosterone secretion. The latter decrease may result in a small increase of serum potassium. Hypertensive patients treated with benazepril alone for up to 52 weeks had elevations of serum potassium of up to 0.2 mEq/L. Similar patients treated with benazepril and hydrochlorothiazide for up to 24 weeks had no consistent changes in their serum potassium (see PRECAUTIONS).

Removal of angiotensin II negative feedback on renin secretion leads to increased plasma renin activity. In animal studies, benazepril had no inhibitory effect on the vasopressor response to angiotensin II and did not interfere with the hemodynamic effects of the autonomic neurotransmitters acetylcholine, epinephrine, and norepinephrine.

ACE is identical to kininase, an enzyme that degrades bradykinin. Whether increased levels of bradykinin, a potent vasodepressor peptide, play a role in the therapeutic effects of Lotensin HCT remains to be elucidated.

While the mechanism through which benazepril lowers blood pressure is believed to be primarily suppression of the renin-angiotensin-aldosterone system, benazepril has an antihypertensive effect even in patients with low-renin hypertension.

Hydrochlorothiazide is a thiazide diuretic. Thiazides affect the renal tubular mechanisms of electrolyte reabsorption, directly increasing excretion of sodium and chloride in approximately equivalent amounts. Indirectly, the diuretic action of hydrochlorothiazide reduces plasma volume, with consequent increases in plasma renin activity, increases in aldosterone secretion, increases in urinary potassium loss, and decreases in serum potassium. The renin-aldosterone link is mediated by angiotensin, so coadministration of an ACE inhibitor tends to reverse the potassium loss associated with these diuretics.

The mechanism of the antihypertensive effect of thiazides is unknown.

Pharmacokinetics and Metabolism

Following oral administration of Lotensin HCT, peak plasma concentrations of benazepril are reached within 0.5–1.0 hours. As determined by urinary recovery, the extent of absorption is at least 37%. The absorption of hydrochlorothiazide is somewhat slower (1–2.5 hours) and somewhat more complete (50%–80%). In fasting subjects, the rate and extent of absorption of benazepril and hydrochlorothiazide from Lotensin HCT are not different, respectively, from the rate and extent of absorption of benazepril and hydrochlorothiazide from immediate-release monotherapy formulations.

The absorption of benazepril from Lotensin® tablets is not influenced by the presence of food in the gastrointestinal tract, but possible effects of food upon absorption of either component from Lotensin HCT tablets have not been studied. The reported studies of food effects on hydrochlorothiazide absorption have been inconclusive. The absorption of hydrochlorothiazide is increased by agents that reduce gastrointestinal motility, but it is reported to be reduced by 50% in patients with congestive heart failure.

Cleavage of the ester group (primarily in the liver) converts benazepril to its active metabolite, benazeprilat. Peak plasma concentrations of benazeprilat are reached 1–2 hours after drug intake in the fasting state and 2–4 hours after drug intake in the nonfasting state. The serum protein binding of benazepril is about 96.7% and that of benazeprilat about 95.3%, as measured by equilibrium dialysis; on the basis of in vitro studies, the degree of protein binding should be unaffected by age, hepatic dysfunction, or—over the concentration range of 0.24–23.6 μmol/L—concentration.

Hydrochlorothiazide is not metabolized. Its apparent volume of distribution is 3.6–7.8 L/kg, and its measured plasma protein binding is 67.9%. The drug also accumulates in red blood cells, so that whole blood levels are 1.6–1.8 times those measured in plasma.

In studies of rats given ^{14}C-benazepril, benazepril and its metabolites crossed the blood-brain barrier only to an extremely low extent. Multiple doses of benazepril did not result in accumulation in any tissue except the lung, where, as with other ACE inhibitors in similar studies, there was a slight increase in concentration due to slow elimination in that organ.

Some placental passage occurred when benazepril was administered to pregnant rats. In humans, hydrochlorothiazide crosses the placenta freely, and levels in umbilical-cord blood are similar to those in the maternal circulation.

Benazepril is almost completely metabolized to benazeprilat, which has much greater ACE inhibitory activity than benazepril, and to the glucuronide conjugates of benazepril and benazeprilat. Only trace amounts of an administered dose of benazepril can be recovered unchanged in the urine; about 20% of the dose is excreted as benazeprilat, 4% as benazepril glucuronide, and 8% as benazeprilat glucuronide. In patients with hepatic dysfunction due to cirrhosis, levels of benazeprilat are essentially unaltered. Similarly, the pharmacokinetics of benazepril and benazeprilat do not appear to be influenced by age.

The kinetics of benazepril are dose-proportional within the dosage range of 5–20 mg. Small deviations from dose proportionality were observed when the broader range of 2–80 mg was studied, possibly due to the saturable binding of the compound to ACE.

The effective half-life of accumulation of benazeprilat following multiple dosing of benazepril hydrochloride is 10–11 hours. Thus, steady-state concentrations of benazeprilat should be reached after 2 or 3 doses of benazepril hydrochloride given once daily.

During chronic administration (28 days) of once-daily doses of benazepril between 5 mg and 20 mg, the kinetics did not change, and there was no significant accumulation. Accumulation ratios based on AUC and urinary recovery of benazeprilat were 1.19 and 1.27, respectively.

When dialysis was started 2 hours after ingestion of 10 mg of benazepril, approximately 6% of benazeprilat was removed in 4 hours of dialysis. The parent compound, benazepril, was not detected in the dialysate.

Benazepril and benazeprilat are cleared predominantly by renal excretion in healthy subjects with normal renal func-

Continued on next page

CibaGeneva—Cont.

tion. Nonrenal (i.e., biliary) excretion accounts for approximately 11%–12% of benazeprilat excretion in healthy subjects. In patients with renal failure, biliary clearance may compensate to an extent for deficient renal clearance.
The disposition of benazepril and benazeprilat in patients with mild-to-moderate renal insufficiency (creatinine clearance > 30 mL/min) is similar to that in patients with normal renal function. In patients with creatinine clearance ≤30 mL/min, peak benazeprilat levels and the initial (alpha phase) half-life increase, and time to steady state may be delayed (see DOSAGE AND ADMINISTRATION).
Thiazide diuretics are eliminated by the kidney, with a terminal half-life of 5–15 hours. In a study of patients with impaired renal function (mean creatinine clearance of 19 mL/min), the half-life of hydrochlorothiazide elimination was lengthened to 21 hours.

Pharmacodynamics

Single and multiple doses of 10 mg or more of **benazepril** cause inhibition of plasma ACE activity by at least 80%–90% for at least 24 hours after dosing. For up to 4 hours after a 10-mg dose, pressor responses to exogenous angiotensin I were inhibited by 60%–90%.
Administration of benazepril to patients with mild-to-moderate hypertension results in a reduction of both supine and standing blood pressure to about the same extent, with no compensatory tachycardia. Symptomatic postural hypotension is infrequent, although it can occur in patients who are salt and/or volume depleted (see WARNINGS, Hypotension).
In single-dose studies, benazepril lowered blood pressure within 1 hour, with peak reductions achieved 2–4 hours after dosing. The antihypertensive effect of a single dose persisted for 24 hours. In multiple-dose studies, once-daily doses of 20–80 mg decreased seated pressure (systolic/diastolic) 24 hours after dosing by about 6–12/4–7 mmHg. The reductions at trough are about 50% of those seen at peak.
Four dose-response studies of benazepril monotherapy using once-daily dosing were conducted in 470 mild-to-moderate hypertensive patients not using diuretics. The minimal effective once-daily dose of benazepril was 10 mg; further falls in blood pressure, especially at morning trough, were seen with higher doses in the studied dosing range (10–80 mg). In studies comparing the same daily dose of benazepril given as a single morning dose or as a twice-daily dose, blood pressure reductions at the time of morning trough blood levels were greater with the divided regimen.
During chronic therapy with benazepril, the maximum reduction in blood pressure with any given dose is generally achieved after 1–2 weeks. The antihypertensive effects of benazepril have continued during therapy for at least 2 years. Abrupt withdrawal of benazepril has not been associated with a rapid increase in blood pressure.
In patients with mild-to-moderate hypertension, total daily doses of Lotensin 20–40 mg were similar in effectiveness to total daily doses of captopril 50–100 mg, hydrochlorothiazide 25–50 mg, nifedipine SR 40–80 mg, and propranolol 80–160 mg.
The antihypertensive effects of benazepril were not appreciably different in patients receiving high- or low-sodium diets.
In hemodynamic studies in dogs, blood pressure reduction was accompanied by a reduction in peripheral arterial resistance, with an increase in cardiac output and renal blood flow and little or no change in heart rate. In normal human volunteers, single doses of benazepril caused an increase in renal blood flow but had no effect on glomerular filtration rate.
In clinical trials of **benazepril/hydrochlorothiazide** using benazepril doses of 5–20 mg and hydrochlorothiazide doses of 6.25–25 mg, the antihypertensive effects were sustained for at least 24 hours, and they increased with increasing dose of either component. Although benazepril monotherapy is somewhat less effective in blacks than in nonblacks, the efficacy of combination therapy appears to be independent of race.
By blocking the renin-angiotensin-aldosterone axis, administration of benazepril tends to reduce the potassium loss associated with the diuretic. In clinical trials of Lotensin HCT, the average change in serum potassium was near zero in subjects who received 5/6.25 mg or 20/12.5 mg, but the average subject who received 10/12.5 mg or 20/25 mg experienced a mild reduction in serum potassium, similar to that experienced by the average subject receiving the same dose of hydrochlorothiazide monotherapy.

INDICATIONS AND USAGE

Lotensin HCT is indicated for the treatment of hypertension. **This fixed combination drug is not indicated for the initial therapy of hypertension (see DOSAGE AND ADMINISTRATION).**
In using Lotensin HCT, consideration should be given to the fact that another angiotensin-converting enzyme inhibitor, captopril, has caused agranulocytosis, particularly in patients with renal impairment or collagen-vascular disease. Available data are insufficient to show that benazepril does not have a similar risk (see WARNINGS, Neutropenia/Agranulocytosis).
Black patients receiving ACE inhibitors have been reported to have a higher incidence of angioedema compared to nonblacks.

CONTRAINDICATIONS

Lotensin HCT is contraindicated in patients who are anuric. Lotensin HCT is also contraindicated in patients who are hypersensitive to benazepril, to any other ACE inhibitor, to hydrochlorothiazide, or to other sulfonamide-derived drugs. Hypersensitivity reactions are more likely to occur in patients with a history of allergy or bronchial asthma.

WARNINGS

Anaphylactoid and Possibly Related Reactions

Presumably because angiotensin-converting enzyme inhibitors affect the metabolism of eicosanoids and polypeptides, including endogenous bradykinin, patients receiving ACE inhibitors (including Lotensin HCT) may be subject to a variety of adverse reactions, some of them serious.
Angioedema: Angioedema of the face, extremities, lips, tongue, glottis, and larynx has been reported in patients treated with angiotensin-converting enzyme inhibitors. In U.S. clinical trials, symptoms consistent with angioedema were seen in none of the subjects who received placebo and in about 0.5% of the subjects who received benazepril. Angioedema associated with laryngeal edema can be fatal. If laryngeal stridor or angioedema of the face, tongue, or glottis occurs, treatment with Lotensin HCT should be discontinued and appropriate therapy instituted immediately. *When involvement of the tongue, glottis, or larynx appears likely to cause airway obstruction, appropriate therapy, e.g., subcutaneous epinephrine injection 1:1000 (0.3–0.5 mL) should be promptly administered* (see PRECAUTIONS and ADVERSE REACTIONS).
Anaphylactoid Reactions During Desensitization: Two patients undergoing desensitizing treatment with hymenoptera venom while receiving ACE inhibitors sustained life-threatening anaphylactoid reactions. In the same patients, these reactions were avoided when ACE inhibitors were temporarily withheld, but they reappeared upon inadvertent rechallenge.
Anaphylactoid Reactions During Membrane Exposure: Anaphylactoid reactions have been reported in patients dialyzed with high-flux membranes and treated concomitantly with an ACE inhibitor. Anaphylactoid reactions have also been reported in patients undergoing low-density lipoprotein apheresis with dextran sulfate absorption.

Hypotension

Lotensin HCT can cause symptomatic hypotension. Like other ACE inhibitors, benazepril has been only rarely associated with hypotension in uncomplicated hypertensive patients. Symptomatic hypotension is most likely to occur in patients who have been volume and/or salt depleted as a result of prolonged diuretic therapy, dietary salt restriction, dialysis, diarrhea, or vomiting. Volume and/or salt depletion should be corrected before initiating therapy with Lotensin HCT.
Lotensin HCT should be used cautiously in patients receiving concomitant therapy with other antihypertensives. The thiazide component of Lotensin HCT may potentiate the action of other antihypertensive drugs, especially ganglionic or peripheral adrenergic-blocking drugs. The antihypertensive effects of the thiazide component may also be enhanced in the postsympathectomy patient.
In patients with congestive heart failure, with or without associated renal insufficiency, ACE inhibitor therapy may cause excessive hypotension, which may be associated with oliguria, azotemia, and (rarely) with acute renal failure and death. In such patients, Lotensin HCT therapy should be started under close medical supervision; they should be followed closely for the first 2 weeks of treatment and whenever the dose of benazepril or diuretic is increased.
If hypotension occurs, the patient should be placed in a supine position, and, if necessary, treated with intravenous infusion of physiological saline. Lotensin HCT treatment usually can be continued following restoration of blood pressure and volume.

Impaired Renal Function

Lotensin HCT should be used with caution in patients with severe renal disease. Thiazides may precipitate azotemia in such patients, and the effects of repeated dosing may be cumulative.
When the renin-angiotensin-aldosterone system is inhibited by benazepril, changes in renal function may be anticipated in susceptible individuals. In patients with **severe congestive heart failure,** whose renal function may depend on the activity of the renin-angiotensin-aldosterone system, treatment with angiotensin-converting enzyme inhibitors (including benazepril) may be associated with oliguria and/or progressive azotemia and (rarely) with acute renal failure and/or death.
In a small study of hypertensive patients with **unilateral or bilateral renal artery stenosis,** treatment with benazepril was associated with increases in blood urea nitrogen and serum creatinine; these increases were reversible upon discontinuation of benazepril therapy, concomitant diuretic therapy, or both. When such patients are treated with Lotensin HCT, renal function should be monitored during the first few weeks of therapy.
Some benazepril-treated hypertensive patients with **no apparent preexisting renal vascular disease** have developed increases in blood urea nitrogen and serum creatinine, usually minor and transient, especially when benazepril has been given concomitantly with a diuretic. Dosage reduction of Lotensin HCT may be required. **Evaluation of the hypertensive patient should always include assessment of renal function** (see DOSAGE AND ADMINISTRATION).

Neutropenia/Agranulocytosis

Another angiotensin-converting enzyme inhibitor, captopril, has been shown to cause agranulocytosis and bone marrow depression, rarely in uncomplicated patients (incidence probably less than once per 10,000 exposures) but more frequently (incidence possibly as great as once per 1000 exposures) in patients with renal impairment, especially those who also have collagen-vascular diseases such as systemic lupus erythematosus or scleroderma. Available data from clinical trials of benazepril are insuffıcent to show that benazepril does not cause agranulocytosis at similar rates. Monitoring of white blood cell counts should be considered in patients with collagen-vascular disease, especially if the disease is associated with impaired renal function.

Fetal/Neonatal Morbidity and Mortality

ACE inhibitors can cause fetal and neonatal morbidity and death when administered to pregnant women. Several dozen cases have been reported in the world literature. When pregnancy is detected, Lotensin HCT should be discontinued as soon as possible.
The use of ACE inhibitors during the second and third trimesters of pregnancy has been associated with fetal and neonatal injury, including hypotension, neonatal skull hypoplasia, anuria, reversible or irreversible renal failure, and death. Oligohydramnios has also been reported, presumably resulting from decreased fetal renal function; oligohydramnios in this setting has been associated with fetal limb contractures, craniofacial deformation, and hypoplastic lung development. Prematurity, intrauterine growth retardation, and patent ductus arteriosus have also been reported, although it is not clear whether these occurrences were due to the ACE inhibitor exposure.
These adverse effects do not appear to have resulted from intrauterine ACE inhibitor exposure that has been limited to the first trimester. Mothers whose embryos and fetuses are exposed to ACE inhibitors only during the first trimester should be so informed. Nonetheless, when patients become pregnant, physicians should make every effort to discontinue the use of benazepril as soon as possible.
Rarely (probably less often than once in every thousand pregnancies), no alternative to ACE inhibitors will be found. In these rare cases, the mothers should be apprised of the potential hazards to their fetuses, and serial ultrasound examinations should be performed to assess the intraamniotic environment.
If oligohydramnios is observed, benazepril should be discontinued unless it is considered life-saving for the mother. Contraction stress testing (CST), a nonstress test (NST), or biophysical profiling (BPP) may be appropriate, depending upon the week of pregnancy. Patients and physicians should be aware, however, that oligohydramnios may not appear until after the fetus has sustained irreversible injury.
Infants with histories of in utero exposure to ACE inhibitors should be closely observed for hypotension, oliguria, and hyperkalemia. If oliguria occurs, attention should be directed toward support of blood pressure and renal perfusion. Exchange transfusion or peritoneal dialysis may be required as means of reversing hypotension and/or substituting for disordered renal function. Benazepril, which crosses the placenta, can theoretically be removed from the neonatal circulation by these means; there are occasional reports of benefit from these maneuvers, but experience is limited.
Intrauterine exposure to thiazide diuretics is associated with fetal or neonatal jaundice, thrombocytopenia, and possibly other adverse reactions that have occurred in adults.
No teratogenic effects were seen when benazepril and hydrochlorothiazide were administered to pregnant rats at a dose ratio of 4:5. On a mg/kg basis, the doses used were up to 167 times the maximum recommended human dose. Similarly, no teratogenic effects were seen when benazepril and hydrochlorothiazide were administered to pregnant mice at total doses up to 160 mg/kg/day, with benazepril:hydrochlorothiazide ratios of 15:1. When hydrochlorothiazide was orally administered without benazepril to pregnant mice and rats during their respective periods of major organogenesis, at doses up to 3000 and 1000 mg/kg/day respectively, there was no evidence of harm to the fetus. Similarly, no teratogenic effects of benazepril were seen in studies of pregnant rats, mice, and rabbits; on a mg/kg basis, the doses used in these studies were 300 times (in rats), 90 times (in mice), and more

than 3 times (in rabbits) the maximum recommended human dose.

Hepatic Failure

Rarely, ACE inhibitors have been associated with a syndrome that starts with cholestatic jaundice and progresses to fulminant hepatic necrosis and (sometimes) death. The mechanism of this syndrome is not understood. Patients receiving ACE inhibitors who develop jaundice or marked elevations of hepatic enzymes should discontinue the ACE inhibitor and receive appropriate medical follow-up.

Impaired Hepatic Function

Lotensin HCT should be used with caution in patients with impaired hepatic function or progressive liver disease, since minor alterations of fluid and electrolyte balance may precipitate hepatic coma (see Hepatic Failure, above). In patients with hepatic dysfunction due to cirrhosis, levels of benazeprilat are essentially unaltered. No formal pharmacokinetic studies have been carried out in hypertensive patients with impaired liver function.

Systemic Lupus Erythematosus

Thiazide diuretics have been reported to cause exacerbation or activation of systemic lupus erythematosus.

PRECAUTIONS

General

Derangements of Serum Electrolytes: In clinical trials of benazepril monotherapy, hyperkalemia (serum potassium at least 0.5 mEq/L greater than the upper limit of normal) occurred in approximately 1% of hypertensive patients receiving benazepril. In most cases, these were isolated values which resolved despite continued therapy. Risk factors for the development of hyperkalemia included renal insufficiency, diabetes mellitus, and the concomitant use of potassium-sparing diuretics, potassium supplements, and/or potassium-containing salt substitutes.

Conversely, treatment with thiazide diuretics has been associated with hypokalemia, hyponatremia, and hypochloremic alkalosis. These disturbances have sometimes been manifest as one or more of dryness of mouth, thirst, weakness, lethargy, drowsiness, restlessness, muscle pains or cramps, muscular fatigue, hypotension, oliguria, tachycardia, nausea, and vomiting. Hypokalemia can also sensitize or exaggerate the response of the heart to the toxic effects of digitalis. The risk of hypokalemia is greatest in patients with cirrhosis of the liver, in patients experiencing a brisk diuresis, in patients who are receiving inadequate oral intake of electrolytes, and in patients receiving concomitant therapy with corticosteroids or ACTH.

The opposite effects of benazepril and hydrochlorothiazide on serum potassium will approximately balance each other in many patients, so that no net effect upon serum potassium will be seen. In other patients, one or the other effect may be dominant. Initial and periodic determinations of serum electrolytes to detect possible electrolyte imbalance should be performed at appropriate intervals.

Chloride deficits are generally mild and require specific treatment only under extraordinary circumstances (e.g., in liver disease or renal disease). Dilutional hyponatremia may occur in edematous patients; appropriate therapy is water restriction rather than administration of salt, except in rare instances when the hyponatremia is life-threatening. In actual salt depletion, appropriate replacement is the therapy of choice.

Calcium excretion is decreased by thiazides. In a few patients on prolonged thiazide therapy, pathological changes in the parathyroid gland have been observed, with hypercalcemia and hypophosphatemia. More serious complications of hyperparathyroidism (renal lithiasis, bone resorption, and peptic ulceration) have not been seen.

Thiazides increase the urinary excretion of magnesium, and hypomagnesemia may result.

Other Metabolic Disturbances: Thiazide diuretics tend to reduce glucose tolerance and to raise serum levels of cholesterol, triglycerides, and uric acid. These effects are usually minor, but frank gout or overt diabetes may be precipitated in susceptible patients.

Cough: Presumably due to the inhibition of the degradation of endogenous bradykinin, persistent nonproductive cough has been reported with all ACE inhibitors, always resolving after discontinuation of therapy. ACE inhibitor-induced cough should be considered in the differential diagnosis of cough.

Surgery/Anesthesia: In patients undergoing surgery or during anesthesia with agents that produce hypotension, benazepril will block the angiotensin II formation that could otherwise occur secondary to compensatory renin release. Hypotension that occurs as a result of this mechanism can be corrected by volume expansion.

Information for Patients

Angioedema: Angioedema, including laryngeal edema, can occur at any time with treatment with ACE inhibitors. A patient receiving Lotensin HCT should be told to report immediately any signs or symptoms suggesting angioedema (swelling of face, eyes, lips, or tongue, or difficulty in breathing) and to take no more drug until after consulting with the prescribing physician.

Pregnancy: Female patients of childbearing age should be told about the consequences of second- and third-trimester exposure to ACE inhibitors, and they should also be told that these consequences do not appear to have resulted from intrauterine ACE-inhibitor exposure that has been limited to the first trimester. These patients should be asked to report pregnancies to their physicians as soon as possible.

Symptomatic Hypotension: A patient receiving Lotensin HCT should be cautioned that lightheadedness can occur, especially during the first days of therapy, and that it should be reported to the prescribing physician. The patient should be told that if syncope occurs, Lotensin HCT should be discontinued until the physician has been consulted.

All patients should be cautioned that inadequate fluid intake, excessive perspiration, diarrhea, or vomiting can lead to an excessive fall in blood pressure, with the same consequences of lightheadedness and possible syncope.

Hyperkalemia: A patient receiving Lotensin HCT should be told not to use potassium supplements or salt substitutes containing potassium without consulting the prescribing physician.

Neutropenia: Patients should be told to promptly report any indication of infection (e.g., sore throat, fever), which could be a sign of neutropenia.

Laboratory Tests

The hydrochlorothiazide component of Lotensin HCT may decrease serum PBI levels without signs of thyroid disturbance.

Therapy with Lotensin HCT should be interrupted for a few days before carrying out tests of parathyroid function.

Drug Interactions

Potassium Supplements and Potassium-Sparing Diuretics: As noted above (Derangements of Serum Electrolytes), the net effect of Lotensin HCT may be to elevate a patient's serum potassium, to reduce it, or to leave it unchanged. Potassium-sparing diuretics (spironolactone, amiloride, triamterene, and others) or potassium supplements can increase the risk of hyperkalemia. If concomitant use of such agents is indicated, they should be given with caution, and the patient's serum potassium should be monitored frequently.

Lithium: Increased serum lithium levels and symptoms of lithium toxicity have been reported in patients receiving ACE inhibitors during therapy with lithium. Because renal clearance of lithium is reduced by thiazides, the risk of lithium toxicity is presumably raised further when, as in therapy with Lotensin HCT, a thiazide diuretic is coadministered with the ACE inhibitor. Lotensin HCT and lithium should be coadministered with caution, and frequent monitoring of serum lithium levels is recommended.

Other: Benazepril has been used concomitantly with beta-adrenergic-blocking agents, calcium-blocking agents, cimetidine, diuretics, digoxin, hydralazine, and naproxen without evidence of clinically important adverse interactions. Other ACE inhibitors have had less than additive effects with beta-adrenergic blockers, presumably because drugs of both classes lower blood pressure by inhibiting parts of the renin-angiotensin system.

Interaction studies with warfarin and acenocoumarol have failed to identify any clinically important effects of benazepril on the serum concentrations or clinical effects of these anticoagulants.

Insulin requirements in diabetic patients may be increased, decreased, or unchanged.

Thiazides may decrease arterial responsiveness to norepinephrine, but not enough to preclude effectiveness of the pressor agent for therapeutic use.

Thiazides may increase the responsiveness to tubocurarine.

The diuretic, natriuretic, and antihypertensive effects of thiazide diuretics may be reduced by concurrent administration of nonsteroidal anti-inflammatory agents.

Cholestyramine and colestipol resins: Absorption of hydrochlorothiazide is impaired in the presence of anionic exchange resins. Single doses of either cholestyramine or colestipol resins bind the hydrochlorothiazide and reduce its absorption from the gastrointestinal tract by up to 85% and 43%, respectively.

Carcinogenesis, Mutagenesis, Impairment of Fertility

No evidence of carcinogenicity was found when **benazepril** was given to rats and mice for 104 weeks at doses up to 150 mg/kg/day. On a body-weight basis, this dose is over 100 times the maximum recommended human dose; on a body-surface-area basis, this dose is 18 times (rats) and 9 times (mice) the maximum recommended human dose. No mutagenic activity was detected in the Ames test in bacteria (with or without metabolic activation), in an in vitro test for forward mutations in cultured mammalian cells, or in a nucleus anomaly test. At doses of 50–500 mg/kg/day (38–375 times the maximum recommended human dose on a body-weight basis; 6–61 times the maximum recommended dose on a body-surface-area basis), benazepril had no adverse effect on the reproductive performance of male and female rats.

Under the auspices of the National Toxicology Program, rats and mice received **hydrochlorothiazide** in their feed for two years, at doses up to 600 mg/kg/day in mice and up to 100 mg/kg/day in rats. These studies uncovered no evidence of a carcinogenic potential of hydrochlorothiazide in rats or female mice, but there was equivocal evidence of hepatocarcinogenicity in male mice. Hydrochlorothiazide was not genotoxic in in vitro assays using strains TA 98, TA 100, TA 1535, TA 1537, and TA 1538 of *Salmonella typhimurium* (the Ames test); in the Chinese Hamster Ovary (CHO) test for chromosomal aberrations; or in in vivo assays using mouse germinal cell chromosomes, Chinese hamster bone marrow chromosomes; and the *Drosophila* sex-linked recessive lethal trait gene. Positive test results were obtained in the in vitro CHO Sister Chromatid Exchange (clastogenicity) test and in the Mouse Lymphoma Cell (mutagenicity) assays, using concentrations of hydrochlorothiazide of 43–1300 μg/mL. Positive test results were also obtained in the *Aspergillus nidulans* nondisjunction assay, using an unspecified concentration of hydrochlorothiazide.

Hydrochlorothiazide had no adverse effects on the fertility of mice and rats of either sex in studies wherein these species were exposed, via their diets, to doses up to 100 and 4 mg/kg/day, respectively, prior to mating and throughout gestation.

Pregnancy

Pregnancy Categories C (first trimester) and D (second and third trimesters): See WARNINGS, Fetal/Neonatal Morbidity and Mortality.

Nursing Mothers

Minimal amounts of unchanged benazepril and of benazeprilat are excreted into the breast milk of lactating women treated with benazepril, so that a newborn child ingesting nothing but breast milk would receive less than 0.1% of the maternal doses of benazepril and benazeprilat. Thiazides, on the other hand, are definitely excreted into breast milk. Because of the potential for serious adverse reactions in nursing infants from hydrochlorothiazide and the unknown effects of benazepril in infants, a decision should be made whether to discontinue nursing or to discontinue Lotensin HCT, taking into account the importance of the drug to the mother.

Geriatric Use

Of the total number of patients who received Lotensin HCT in U.S. clinical studies of Lotensin HCT, 19% were 65 or older while about 1.5% were 75 or older. Overall differences in effectiveness or safety were not observed between these patients and younger patients, and other reported clinical experience has not identified differences in responses between the elderly and younger patients, but greater sensitivity of some older individuals cannot be ruled out.

Pediatric Use

Safety and effectiveness in pediatric patients have not been established.

ADVERSE REACTIONS

Lotensin HCT has been evaluated for safety in over 2500 patients with hypertension; over 500 of these patients were treated for at least 6 months, and over 200 were treated for more than 1 year.

The reported side effects were generally mild and transient, and there was no relationship between side effects and age, sex, race, or duration of therapy. Discontinuation of therapy due to side effects was required in approximately 7% of U.S. patients treated with Lotensin HCT and in 4% of patients treated with placebo.

The most common reasons for discontinuation of therapy with Lotensin HCT in U.S. studies were cough (1.0%; see PRECAUTIONS), "dizziness" (1.0%), headache (0.6%), and fatigue (0.6%).

The side effects considered possibly or probably related to study drug that occurred in U.S. placebo-controlled trials in more than 1% of patients treated with Lotensin HCT are shown in the table below.

Reactions Possibly or Probably Drug Related
Patients in U.S. Placebo-Controlled Studies

	LOTENSIN HCT N=655		Placebo N=235	
	N	%	N	%
"Dizziness"	41	6.3	8	3.4
Fatigue	34	5.2	6	2.6
Postural Dizziness	23	3.5	1	0.4
Headache	20	3.1	10	4.3
Cough	14	2.1	3	1.3
Hypertonia	10	1.5	3	1.3
Vertigo	10	1.5	2	0.9
Nausea	9	1.4	2	0.9
Impotence	8	1.2	0	0.0
Somnolence	8	1.2	1	0.4

Other side effects considered possibly or probably related to study drug that occurred in U.S. placebo-controlled trials in 0.3% to 1.0% of patients treated with Lotensin HCT were the following:

Continued on next page

CibaGeneva—Cont.

Angioedema: Edema of the lips or face without other manifestations of angioedema (0.3%). See WARNINGS, Angioedema.

Cardiovascular: Hypotension (seen in 0.6% of patients), postural hypotension (0.3%), palpitations, and flushing.

Gastrointestinal: Vomiting, diarrhea, dyspepsia, anorexia, and constipation.

Neurologic and Psychiatric: Insomnia, nervousness, paresthesia, libido decrease, dry mouth, taste perversion, and tinnitus.

Dermatologic: Rash and sweating.

Other: Gout, urinary frequency, arthralgia, myalgia, asthenia, and pain (including chest pain and abdominal pain).

Other adverse experiences reported in 0.3% or more of Lotensin HCT patients in U.S. controlled clinical trials, and rarer events seen in postmarketing experience, were the following; asterisked entries occurred in more than 1% of patients (in some, a causal relationship to Lotensin HCT is uncertain).

Angioedema: Edema of the lips or face without other manifestations of angioedema. See WARNINGS, Angioedema.

Cardiovascular: Syncope, peripheral vascular disorder, and tachycardia.

Body as a Whole: Infection, back pain,* flu syndrome,* fever, chills, and neck pain.

Dermatologic: Photosensitivity and pruritus. There have been rare reports of pemphigus in patients receiving ACE inhibitors.

Gastrointestinal: Gastroenteritis, flatulence, and tooth disorder. There have been rare reports of pancreatitis in patients receiving ACE inhibitors.

Hematologic: There have been rare reports of hemolytic anemia in patients receiving ACE inhibitors.

Neurologic and Psychiatric: Hypesthesia, abnormal vision, abnormal dreams, and retinal disorder.

Respiratory: Upper respiratory infection,* epistaxis, bronchitis, rhinitis,* sinusitis,* and voice alteration.

Other: Conjunctivitis, arthritis, urinary tract infection, and urinary frequency.*

Fetal/Neonatal Morbidity and Mortality: See WARNINGS, Fetal/Neonatal Morbidity and Mortality.

Monotherapy with **benazepril** has been evaluated for safety in over 6000 patients. In clinical trials, the observed adverse reactions to benazepril were similar to those seen in trials of Lotensin HCT. In postmarketing experience with benazepril, there have been rare reports of Stevens-Johnson syndrome and thrombocytopenia.

Hydrochlorothiazide has been extensively prescribed for many years, but there has not been enough systematic collection of data to support an estimate of the frequency of the observed adverse reactions. Within organ-system groups, the reported reactions are listed here in decreasing order of severity, without regard to frequency.

Cardiovascular: Orthostatic hypotension (may be potentiated by alcohol, barbiturates, or narcotics).

Digestive: Pancreatitis, jaundice (intrahepatic cholestatic) (see WARNINGS), sialadenitis, vomiting, diarrhea, cramping, nausea, gastric irritation, constipation, and anorexia.

Neurologic: Vertigo, lightheadedness, transient blurred vision, headache, paresthesia, xanthopsia, weakness, and restlessness.

Musculoskeletal: Muscle spasm.

Hematologic: Aplastic anemia, agranulocytosis, leukopenia, and thrombocytopenia.

Metabolic: Hyperglycemia, glycosuria, and hyperuricemia.

Hypersensitivity: Necrotizing angiitis, Stevens-Johnson syndrome, respiratory distress (including pneumonitis and pulmonary edema), purpura, urticaria, rash, and photosensitivity.

Clinical Laboratory Test Findings

Serum Electrolytes: See PRECAUTIONS.

Creatinine: Minor reversible increases in serum creatinine were observed in patients with essential hypertension treated with Lotensin HCT. Such increases occurred most frequently in patients with renal artery stenosis (see PRECAUTIONS).

PBI and Tests of Parathyroid Function: See PRECAUTIONS.

Other (Causal Relationships Unknown): Other clinically important changes in standard laboratory tests were rarely associated with Lotensin HCT administration. Elevations in blood urea nitrogen, uric acid, glucose, SGOT, and SGPT (see WARNINGS) have been reported. In the somewhat larger patient population exposed to benazepril monotherapy in U.S. trials, the same abnormalities were reported, together with scattered accounts of hyponatremia, melena, electrocardiographic changes, leukopenia, eosinophilia, and proteinuria.

OVERDOSAGE

No specific information is available on the treatment of overdosage with Lotensin HCT; treatment should be symptomatic and supportive. Therapy with Lotensin HCT should be discontinued, and the patient should be observed. Dehydration electrolyte imbalance, and hypotension should be treated by established procedures.

Single oral doses of 1 g/kg of benazepril caused reduced activity in mice, and doses of 3 g/kg were associated with significant lethality. Reduction of activity in rats was not seen until they had received doses of 5 g/kg, and doses of 6 g/kg were not lethal. In single-dose studies of hydrochlorothiazide, most rats survived doses up to 2.75 g/kg.

Data from human overdoses of benazepril are scanty, but the most common manifestation of human benazepril overdosage is likely to be hypotension. In human hydrochlorothiazide overdose, the most common signs and symptoms observed have been those of dehydration and electrolyte depletion (hypokalemia, hypochloremia, hyponatremia). If digitalis has also been administered, hypokalemia may accentuate cardiac arrhythmias.

Laboratory determinations of serum levels of benazepril and its metabolites are not widely available, and such determinations have, in any event, no established role in the management of benazepril overdose.

No data are available to suggest physiological maneuvers (e.g., maneuvers to change the pH of the urine) that might accelerate elimination of benazepril and its metabolites. Benazeprilat is only slightly dialyzable, but dialysis might be considered in overdosed patients with severely impaired renal function (see WARNINGS).

Angiotensin II could presumably serve as a specific antagonist-antidote in the setting of benazepril overdose, but angiotensin II is essentially unavailable outside of scattered research facilities. Because the hypotensive effect of benazepril is achieved through vasodilation and effective hypovolemia, it is reasonable to treat benazepril overdose by infusion of normal saline solution.

DOSAGE AND ADMINISTRATION

Benazepril is an effective treatment of hypertension in once-daily doses of 10–80 mg, while hydrochlorothiazide is effective in doses of 25–100 mg. In clinical trials of benazepril/hydrochlorothiazide combination therapy using benazepril doses of 5–20 mg and hydrochlorothiazide doses of 6.25–25 mg, the antihypertensive effects increased with increasing dose of either component.

The side effects (see WARNINGS) of benazepril are generally rare and apparently independent of dose; those of hydrochlorothiazide are a mixture of dose-dependent phenomena (primarily hypokalemia) and dose-independent phenomena (e.g., pancreatitis), the former much more common than the latter. Therapy with any combination of benazepril and hydrochlorothiazide will be associated with both sets of dose-independent side effects, but regimens in which benazepril is combined with low doses of hydrochlorothiazide produce minimal effects on serum potassium. In clinical trials of Lotensin HCT, the average change in serum potassium was near zero in subjects who received 5/6.25 mg or 20/12.5 mg, but the average subject who received 10/12.5 mg or 20/25 mg experienced a mild reduction in serum potassium, similar to that experienced by the average subject receiving the same dose of hydrochlorothiazide monotherapy.

To minimize dose-independent side effects, it is usually appropriate to begin combination therapy only after a patient has failed to achieve the desired effect with monotherapy.

Dose Titration Guided by Clinical Effect: A patient whose blood pressure is not adequately controlled with benazepril monotherapy may be switched to Lotensin HCT 10/12.5 or Lotensin HCT 20/12.5. Further increases of either or both components could depend on clinical response. The hydrochlorothiazide dose should generally not be increased until 2–3 weeks have elapsed. Patients whose blood pressures are adequately controlled with 25 mg of daily hydrochlorothiazide, but who experience significant potassium loss with this regimen, may achieve similar blood-pressure control without electrolyte disturbance if they are switched to Lotensin HCT 5/6.25.

Replacement Therapy: The combination may be substituted for the titrated individual components.

Use in Renal Impairment: Regimens of therapy with Lotensin HCT need not take account of renal function as long as the patient's creatinine clearance is >30 mL/min/1.73m² (serum creatinine roughly ≤3 mg/dL or 265 μmol/L). In patients with more severe renal impairment, loop diuretics are preferred to thiazides, so Lotensin HCT is not recommended (see WARNINGS).

HOW SUPPLIED

Lotensin HCT is available in tablets of four different strengths:

Benazepril	Hydrochlorothiazide	Tablet Color
5 mg	6.25 mg	white
10 mg	12.50 mg	light pink
20 mg	12.50 mg	grayish-violet
20 mg	25.00 mg	red

Tablets of each strength are supplied in bottles that contain a desiccant and 100 tablets.

The National Drug Codes for the various packages are

Dose	Bottle of 100
5/6.25	NDC 0083-0057-30
10/12.5	NDC 0083-0072-30
20/12.5	NDC 0083-0074-30
20/25	NDC 0083-0075-30

Tablets are oblong and scored, with "Lotensin HCT" on one side and a portion of the NDC code ("57," "72," "74," or "75") on the other. Samples, when available, are identified by the word SAMPLE on each tablet.

Storage: Do not store above 86°F (30°C). Protect from moisture and light. Dispense in tight, light-resistant container (USP).

C96-35 (Rev. 3/96)

Dist. by:
Ciba-Geigy Corporation
Pharmaceuticals Division
Summit, New Jersey 07901

Shown in Product Identification Guide, page 309

LOTREL® ℞
amlodipine and benazepril hydrochloride
Combination Capsules

2.5 mg/10 mg
5 mg/10 mg
5mg/20 mg

Prescribing Information

> **USE IN PREGNANCY**
> When used in pregnancy during the second and third trimesters, ACE inhibitors can cause injury and even death to the developing fetus.
> When pregnancy is detected, Lotrel should be discontinued as soon as possible. See WARNINGS, Fetal/Neonatal Morbidity and Mortality.

DESCRIPTION

Benazepril hydrochloride is a white to off-white crystalline powder, soluble (>100 mg/mL) in water, in ethanol, and in methanol. Benazepril hydrochloride's chemical name is 3-[[1-(ethoxycarbonyl)-3-phenyl- (1S) -propyl]amino]-2,3,4,5-tetrahydro-2-oxo-1H-1-(3S)-benzazepine-1-acetic acid monohydrochloride.

Its empirical formula is $C_{24}H_{28}N_2O_5 \cdot HCl$, and its molecular weight is 460.96.

Benazeprilat, the active metabolite of benazepril, is a non-sulfhydryl angiotensin-converting enzyme (ACE) inhibitor. Benazepril is converted to benazeprilat by hepatic cleavage of the ester group.

Amlodipine besylate is a white crystalline powder, slightly soluble in water and sparingly soluble in ethanol. Its chemical name is (R,S) 3-ethyl-5-methyl-2-(2-aminoethoxymethyl)-4-(2-chlorophenyl)-1,4-dihydro-6-methyl -3,5- pyridinedicarboxylate benzenesulfonate.

Its empirical formula is $C_{20}H_{25} ClN_2O_5 \cdot C_6H_6O_3S$, and its molecular weight is 567.1.

Amlodipine besylate is the besylate salt of amlodipine, a dihydropyridine calcium channel blocker.

Lotrel is a combination of amlodipine besylate and benazepril hydrochloride. The capsules are formulated for oral administration with a combination of amlodipine besylate equivalent to 2.5 mg or 5 mg of amlodipine and 10 mg or 20 mg of benazepril hydrochloride. The inactive ingredients of the capsules are calcium phosphate, cellulose compounds, colloidal silicon dioxide, crospovidone, gelatin, hydrogenated castor oil, iron oxides, lactose, magnesium stearate, polysorbate 80, silicon dioxide, sodium lauryl sulfate, sodium starch glycolate, starch, talc, and titanium dioxide.

CLINICAL PHARMACOLOGY

Mechanism of Action

Benazepril and benazeprilat inhibit angiotensin-converting enzyme (ACE) in human subjects and in animals. ACE is a peptidyl dipeptidase that catalyzes the conversion of angiotensin I to the vasoconstrictor substance angiotensin II. Angiotensin II also stimulates aldosterone secretion by the adrenal cortex.

Inhibition of ACE results in decreased plasma angiotensin II, which leads to decreased vasopressor activity and to decreased aldosterone secretion. The latter decrease may result in a small increase of serum potassium. Hypertensive patients treated with benazepril and amlodipine for up to 56 weeks had elevations of serum potassium up to 0.2 mEq/L (see PRECAUTIONS).

Removal of angiotensin II negative feedback on renin secretion leads to increased plasma renin activity. In animal studies, benazepril had no inhibitory effect on the vasopressor response to angiotensin II and did not interfere with the hemodynamic effects of the autonomic neurotransmitters acetylcholine, epinephrine, and norepinephrine.

ACE is identical to kininase, an enzyme that degrades bradykinin. Whether increased levels of bradykinin, a potent

vasodepressor peptide, play a role in the therapeutic effects of Lotrel remains to be elucidated.
While the mechanism through which benazepril lowers blood pressure is believed to be primarily suppression of the renin-angiotensin-aldosterone system, benazepril has an antihypertensive effect even in patients with low-renin hypertension.
Amlodipine is a dihydropyridine calcium antagonist (calcium ion antagonist or slow channel blocker) that inhibits the transmembrane influx of calcium ions into vascular smooth muscle and cardiac muscle. Experimental data suggest that amlodipine binds to both dihydropyridine and nondihydropyridine binding sites. The contractile processes of cardiac muscle and vascular smooth muscle are dependent upon the movement of extracellular calcium ions into these cells through specific ion channels. Amlodipine inhibits calcium ion influx across cell membranes selectively, with a greater effect on vascular smooth muscle cells than on cardiac muscle cells. Negative inotropic effects can be detected in vitro but such effects have not been seen in intact animals at therapeutic doses. Serum calcium concentration is not affected by amlodipine. Within the physiologic pH range, amlodipine is an ionized compound (pKa=8.6), and its kinetic interaction with the calcium channel receptor is characterized by a gradual rate of association and dissociation with the receptor binding site, resulting in a gradual onset of effect.
Amlodipine is a peripheral arterial vasodilator that acts directly on vascular smooth muscle to cause a reduction in peripheral vascular resistance and reduction in blood pressure.

Pharmacokinetics and Metabolism

The rate and extent of absorption of benazepril and amlodipine from Lotrel are not significantly different, respectively, from the rate and extent of absorption of benazepril and amlodipine from individual tablet formulations. Absorption from the individual tablets is not influenced by the presence of food in the gastrointestinal tract; food effects on absorption from Lotrel have not been studied.
Following oral administration of Lotrel, peak plasma concentrations of benazepril are reached in 0.5–2 hours. Cleavage of the ester group (primarily in the liver) converts benazepril to its active metabolite, benazeprilat, which reaches peak plasma concentrations in 1.5–4 hours. The extent of absorption of benazepril is at least 37%.
Peak plasma concentrations of amlodipine are reached 6–12 hours after administration of Lotrel; the extent of absorption is 64%–90%.
The apparent volumes of **distribution** of amlodipine and benazeprilat are about 21 L/kg and 0.7 L/kg, respectively. Approximately 93% of circulating amlodipine is bound to plasma proteins, and the bound fraction of benazeprilat is slightly higher. On the basis of in vitro studies, benazeprilat's degree of protein binding should be unaffected by age, by hepatic dysfunction, or—over the therapeutic concentration range—by concentration.
Benazeprilat has much greater ACE-inhibitory activity than benazepril, and the **metabolism** of benazepril to benazeprilat is almost complete. Only trace amounts of an administered dose of benazepril can be recovered unchanged in the urine; about 20% of the dose is excreted as benazeprilat, 8% as benazeprilat glucuronide, and 4% as benazepril glucuronide.
Amlodipine is extensively metabolized in the liver, with 10% of the parent compound and 60% of the metabolites excreted in the urine. In patients with hepatic dysfunction, decreased clearance of amlodipine may increase the area under the plasma-concentration curve by 40%–60%, and dosage reduction may be required (see DOSAGE AND ADMINISTRATION). In patients with renal impairment, the pharmacokinetics of amlodipine are essentially unaffected.
Benazeprilat's effective **elimination** half-life is 10–11 hours, while that of amlodipine is about 2 days, so steady-state levels of the two components are achieved after about a week of once-daily dosing. The clearance of benazeprilat from the plasma is primarily renal, but biliary excretion accounts for 11%–12% of benazepril elimination in normal subjects. In patients with severe renal insufficiency (creatinine clearance less than 30 mL/min), peak benazeprilat levels and the time to steady state may be increased (see DOSAGE AND ADMINISTRATION). In patients with hepatic impairment, on the other hand, the pharmacokinetics of benazeprilat are essentially unaffected.
Although the pharmacokinetics of benazepril and benazeprilat are unaffected by **age**, clearance of amlodipine is decreased in the elderly, with resulting increases of 35%–70% in peak plasma levels, elimination half-life, and area under the plasma-concentration curve. Dose adjustment may be required.

Pharmacodynamics

Single and multiple doses of 10 mg or more of **benazepril** cause inhibition of plasma ACE activity by at least 80%–90% for at least 24 hours after dosing. For up to 4 hours after a 10-mg dose, pressor responses to exogenous angiotensin I were inhibited by 60%–90%.
Administration of benazepril to patients with mild-to-moderate hypertension results in a reduction of both supine and standing blood pressure to about the same extent, with no compensatory tachycardia. Symptomatic postural hypotension is infrequent, although it can occur in patients who are salt and/or volume depleted (see WARNINGS, Hypotension).
The antihypertensive effects of benazepril were not appreciably different in patients receiving high- or low-sodium diets.
In normal human volunteers, single doses of benazepril caused an increase in renal blood flow but had no effect on glomerular filtration rate.
Following administration of therapeutic doses to patients with hypertension, **amlodipine** produces vasodilation resulting in a reduction of supine and standing blood pressures. These decreases in blood pressure are not accompanied by a significant change in heart rate or plasma catecholamine levels with chronic dosing. Plasma concentrations correlate with effect in both young and elderly patients.
As with other calcium channel blockers, hemodynamic measurements of cardiac function at rest and during exercise (or pacing) in patients with normal ventricular function treated with amlodipine have generally demonstrated a small increase in cardiac index without significant influence on dP/dt or on left ventricular and diastolic pressure or volume. In hemodynamic studies, amlodipine has not been associated with a negative inotropic effect when administered in the therapeutic dose range to intact animals and humans, even when coadministered with beta blockers to humans.
Amlodipine does not change sinoatrial (SA) nodal function or atrioventricular (AV) conduction in intact animals or humans. In clinical studies in which amlodipine was administered in combination with beta blockers to patients with either hypertension or angina, no adverse effects on electrocardiographic parameters were observed.
Over 700 patients received Lotrel once daily in five double-blind, placebo-controlled studies. Lotrel lowered blood pressure within 1 hour, with peak reductions achieved 2–8 hours after dosing. The antihypertensive effect of a single dose persisted for 24 hours.
Once-daily doses of benazepril/amlodipine using benazepril doses of 10–20 mg and amlodipine doses of 2.5–5 mg decreased seated pressure (systolic/diastolic) 24 hours after dosing by about 10–25/6–13 mmHg.
Combination therapy was effective in blacks and nonblacks. Both components contributed to the antihypertensive efficacy in nonblacks, but virtually all of the antihypertensive effect in blacks could be attributed to the amlodipine component. Among nonblack patients in placebo-controlled trials comparing Lotrel to the individual components, the blood pressure lowering effects of the combination were shown to be additive and in some cases synergistic.
During chronic therapy with Lotrel, the maximum reduction in blood pressure with any given dose is generally achieved after 1–2 weeks. The antihypertensive effects of Lotrel have continued during therapy for at least 1 year. Abrupt withdrawal of Lotrel has not been associated with a rapid increase in blood pressure.

INDICATIONS AND USAGE

Lotrel is indicated for the treatment of hypertension.
This fixed combination drug is not indicated for the initial therapy of hypertension (see DOSAGE AND ADMINISTRATION).
In using Lotrel, consideration should be given to the fact that an ACE inhibitor, captopril, has caused agranulocytosis, particularly in patients with renal impairment or collagen-vascular disease. Available data are insufficient to show that benazepril does not have a similar risk (see WARNINGS, Neutropenia/Agranulocytosis).
Black patients receiving ACE inhibitors have been reported to have a higher incidence of angioedema compared to nonblacks.

CONTRAINDICATIONS

Lotrel is contraindicated in patients who are hypersensitive to benazepril, to any other ACE inhibitor, or to amlodipine.

WARNINGS

Anaphylactoid and Possibly Related Reactions

Presumably because angiotensin-converting enzyme inhibitors affect the metabolism of eicosanoids and polypeptides, including endogenous bradykinin, patients receiving ACE inhibitors (including Lotrel) may be subject to a variety of adverse reactions, some of them serious. These reactions usually occur after one of the first few doses of the ACE inhibitor, but they sometimes do not appear until after months of therapy.
Angioedema: Angioedema of the face, extremities, lips, tongue, glottis, and larynx has been reported in patients treated with ACE inhibitors. In U.S. clinical trials, symptoms consistent with angioedema were seen in none of the subjects who received placebo and in about 0.5% of the subjects who received benazepril. Angioedema associated with laryngeal edema can be fatal. If laryngeal stridor or angioedema of the face, tongue, or glottis occurs, treatment with Lotrel should be discontinued and appropriate therapy instituted immediately. *When involvement of the tongue, glottis, or larynx appears likely to cause airway obstruction, appropriate therapy, e.g., subcutaneous epinephrine injection 1:1000 (0.3–0.5 mL), should be promptly administered (see ADVERSE REACTIONS).*
Anaphylactoid Reactions During Desensitization: Two patients undergoing desensitizing treatment with hymenoptera venom while receiving ACE inhibitors sustained life-threatening anaphylactoid reactions. In the same patients, these reactions were avoided when ACE inhibitors were temporarily withheld, but they reappeared upon inadvertent rechallenge.
Anaphylactoid Reactions During Membrane Exposure: Anaphylactoid reactions have been reported in patients dialyzed with high-flux membranes and treated concomitantly with an ACE inhibitor. Anaphylactoid reactions have also been reported in patients undergoing low-density lipoprotein apheresis with dextran sulfate absorption.
Increased Angina and/or Myocardial Infarction: Rarely, patients, particularly those with severe obstructive coronary artery disease, have developed documented increased frequency, duration, and/or severity of angina or acute myocardial infarction on starting calcium channel blocker therapy or at the time of dosage increase. The mechanism of this effect has not been elucidated.

Hypotension

Lotrel can cause symptomatic hypotension. Like other ACE inhibitors, benazepril has been only rarely associated with hypotension in uncomplicated hypertensive patients. Symptomatic hypotension is most likely to occur in patients who have been volume and/or salt depleted as a result of prolonged diuretic therapy, dietary salt restriction, dialysis, diarrhea, or vomiting. Volume and/or salt depletion should be corrected before initiating therapy with Lotrel.
Since the vasodilation induced by amlodipine is gradual in onset, acute hypotension has rarely been reported after oral administration of amlodipine. Nonetheless, caution should be exercised when administering Lotrel as with any other peripheral vasodilator, particularly in patients with severe aortic stenosis.
In patients with congestive heart failure, with or without associated renal insufficiency, ACE inhibitor therapy may cause excessive hypotension, which may be associated with oliguria, azotemia, and (rarely) with acute renal failure and death. In such patients, Lotrel therapy should be started under close medical supervision; they should be followed closely for the first 2 weeks of treatment and whenever the dose of the benazepril component is increased or a diuretic is added or its dose increased.
If hypotension occurs, the patient should be placed in a supine position, and if necessary, treated with intravenous infusion of physiologic saline. Lotrel treatment usually can be continued following restoration of blood pressure and volume.

Neutropenia/Agranulocytosis

Another ACE inhibitor, captopril, has been shown to cause agranulocytosis and bone marrow depression, rarely in uncomplicated patients (incidence probably less than once per 10,000 exposures) but more frequently (incidence possibly as great as once per 1000 exposures) in patients with renal impairment, especially those who also have collagen-vascular diseases such as systemic lupus erythematosis or scleroderma. Available data from clinical trials of benazepril are insufficient to show that benazepril does not cause agranulocytosis at similar rates. Monitoring of white blood cell counts should be considered in patients with collagen-vascular disease, especially if the disease is associated with impaired renal function.

Fetal/Neonatal Morbidity and Mortality

ACE inhibitors can cause fetal and neonatal morbidity and death when administered to pregnant women. Several dozen cases have been reported in the world literature. When pregnancy is detected, Lotrel should be discontinued as soon as possible.
The use of ACE inhibitors during the second and third trimesters of pregnancy has been associated with fetal and neonatal injury, including hypotension, neonatal skull hypoplasia, anuria, reversible or irreversible renal failure, and death. Oligohydramnios has also been reported, presumably resulting from decreased fetal renal function; oligohydramnios in this setting has been associated with fetal limb contractures, craniofacial deformation, and hypoplastic lung development. Prematurity, intrauterine growth retardation, and patent ductus arteriosus have also been reported, although it is not clear whether these occurrences were due to the ACE inhibitor exposure.
These adverse effects do not appear to have resulted from intrauterine ACE inhibitor exposure that has been limited to the first trimester. Mothers whose embryos and fetuses are exposed to ACE inhibitors only during the first trimester should be so informed. Nonetheless, when patients become pregnant, physicians should make every effort to discontinue the use of benazepril as soon as possible.

Continued on next page

CibaGeneva—Cont.

Rarely (probably less often than once in every thousand pregnancies), no alternative to ACE inhibitors will be found. In these rare cases, the mothers should be apprised of the potential hazards to their fetuses, and serial ultrasound examinations should be performed to assess the intraamniotic environment.

If oligohydramnios is observed, benazepril should be discontinued unless it is considered life-saving for the mother. Contraction stress testing (CST), a nonstress test (NST), or biophysical profiling (BPP) may be appropriate, depending upon the week of pregnancy. Patients and physicians should be aware, however, that oligohydramnios may not appear until after the fetus has sustained irreversible injury.

Infants with histories of in utero exposure to ACE inhibitors should be closely observed for hypotension, oliguria, and hyperkalemia. If oliguria occurs, attention should be directed toward support of blood pressure and renal perfusion. Exchange transfusion or peritoneal dialysis may be required as means of reversing hypotension and/or substituting for disordered renal function. Benazepril, which crosses the placenta, can theoretically be removed from the neonatal circulation by these means; there are occasional reports of benefit from these maneuvers, but experience is limited.

Lotrel has not been adequately studied in pregnant women. When rats received benazepril:amlodipine at doses ranging from 5:2.5 to 50:25 mg/kg/day, dystocia was observed with increasing dose-related incidence at all doses tested. On a mg/m^2 basis, the 2.5 mg/kg/day dose of amlodipine is 3.6 times the amlodipine dose delivered when the maximum recommended dose of Lotrel is given to a 50-kg woman. Similarly, the 5 mg/kg/day dose of benazepril is approximately 2 times the benazepril dose delivered when the maximum recommended dose of Lotrel is given to a 50-kg woman.

No teratogenic effects were seen when benazepril and amlodipine were administered in combination to pregnant rats or rabbits. Rats received dose ratios up to 50:25 mg/kg/day (benazepril:amlodipine) (24 times the maximum recommended human dose on a mg/m^2 basis, assuming a 50-kg woman). Rabbits received doses up to 1.5:0.75 (benazepril:amlodipine) mg/kg/day; on a mg/m^2 basis, this is 0.97 times the size of a maximum recommended dose of Lotrel given to a 50-kg woman.

Similar results were seen in animal studies involving benazepril alone and amlodipine alone.

Hepatic Failure

Rarely, ACE inhibitors have been associated with a syndrome that starts with cholestatic jaundice and progresses to fulminant hepatic necrosis and (sometimes) death. The mechanism of this syndrome is not understood. Patients receiving ACE inhibitors who develop jaundice or marked elevations of hepatic enzymes should discontinue the ACE inhibitor and receive appropriate medical follow-up.

PRECAUTIONS

General

Impaired Renal Function: Lotrel should be used with caution in patients with severe renal disease.

When the renin-angiotensin-aldosterone system is inhibited by benazepril, changes in renal function may be anticipated in susceptible individuals. In patients with **severe congestive heart failure**, whose renal function may depend on the activity of the renin-angiotensin-aldosterone system, treatment with ACE inhibitors (including benazepril) may be associated with oliguria and/or progressive azotemia and (rarely) with acute renal failure and/or death.

In a small study of hypertensive patients with **unilateral or bilateral renal artery stenosis**, treatment with benazepril was associated with increases in blood urea nitrogen and serum creatinine; these increases were reversible upon discontinuation of benazepril therapy, concomitant diuretic therapy, or both. When such patients are treated with Lotrel, renal function should be monitored during the first few weeks of therapy.

Some benazepril-treated hypertensive patients with **no apparent preexisting renal vascular disease** have developed increases in blood urea nitrogen and serum creatinine, usually minor and transient, especially when benazepril has been given concomitantly with a diuretic. Dosage reduction of Lotrel may be required. **Evaluation of the hypertensive patient should always include assessment of renal function** (see DOSAGE AND ADMINISTRATION).

Hyperkalemia: In U.S. placebo-controlled trials of Lotrel, hyperkalemia (serum potassium at least 0.5 mEq/L greater than the upper limit of normal) not present at baseline occurred in approximately 1.5% of hypertensive patients receiving Lotrel. Increases in serum potassium were generally reversible. Risk factors for the development of hyperkalemia include renal insufficiency, diabetes mellitus, and the concomitant use of potassium-sparing diuretics, potassium supplements, and/or potassium-containing salt substitutes.

Patients With Congestive Heart Failure: Although hemodynamic studies and a controlled trial in patients with NYHA Class II-III heart failure have shown that amlodipine did not lead to clinical deterioration as measured by exercise tolerance, left ventricular ejection fraction, and clinical symptomatology, studies have not been performed in patients with NYHA Class IV heart failure. In general, all calcium channel blockers should be used with caution in patients with heart failure.

Patients With Hepatic Failure: In patients with hepatic dysfunction due to cirrhosis, levels of benazeprilat are essentially unaltered. However, since amlodipine is extensively metabolized by the liver and the plasma elimination half-life ($t_{1/2}$) is 56 hours in patients with impaired hepatic function, caution should be exercised when administering Lotrel to patients with severe hepatic impairment (see also WARNINGS).

Cough: Presumably due to the inhibition of the degradation of endogenous bradykinin, persistent nonproductive cough has been reported with all ACE inhibitors, always resolving after discontinuation of therapy. ACE inhibitor-induced cough should be considered in the differential diagnosis of cough.

Surgery/Anesthesia: In patients undergoing surgery or during anesthesia with agents that produce hypotension, benazepril will block the angiotensin II formation that could otherwise occur secondary to compensatory renin release. Hypotension that occurs as a result of this mechanism can be corrected by volume expansion.

Drug Interactions

Diuretics: Patients on diuretics, especially those in whom diuretic therapy was recently instituted, may occasionally experience an excessive reduction of blood pressure after initiation of therapy with Lotrel. The possibility of hypotensive effects with Lotrel can be minimized by either discontinuing the diuretic or increasing the salt intake prior to initiation of treatment with Lotrel.

Potassium Supplements and Potassium-Sparing Diuretics: Benazepril can attenuate potassium loss caused by thiazide diuretics. Potassium-sparing diuretics (spironolactone, amiloride, triamterene, and others) or potassium supplements can increase the risk of hyperkalemia. If concomitant use of such agents is indicated, they should be given with caution, and the patient's serum potassium should be monitored frequently.

Lithium: Increased serum lithium levels and symptoms of lithium toxicity have been reported in patients receiving ACE inhibitors during therapy with lithium. Lotrel and lithium should be coadministered with caution, and frequent monitoring of serum lithium levels is recommended.

Other: Benazepril has been used concomitantly with oral anticoagulants, beta-adrenergic-blocking agents, calcium-blocking agents, cimetidine, diuretics, digoxin, hydralazine, and naproxen without evidence of clinically important adverse interactions.

In clinical trials, amlodipine has been safely administered with thiazide diuretics, beta blockers, ACE inhibitors, long-acting nitrates, sublingual nitroglycerin, digoxin, warfarin, nonsteroidal anti-inflammatory drugs, antibiotics, and oral hypoglycemic drugs.

In vitro data in human plasma indicate that amlodipine has no effect on the protein binding of drugs tested (digoxin, phenytoin, warfarin, and indomethacin). Special studies have indicated that the coadministration of amlodipine with digoxin did not change serum digoxin levels or digoxin renal clearance in normal volunteers; that coadministration with cimetidine did not alter the pharmacokinetics of amlodipine; and that coadministration with warfarin did not change the warfarin-induced prothrombin response time.

Carcinogenesis, Mutagenesis, Impairment of Fertility

No evidence of carcinogenicity was found when **benazepril** was given, via dietary administration, to rats and mice for 104 weeks at doses up to 150 mg/kg/day. On a body-weight basis, this dose is over 100 times the maximum recommended human dose; on a body-surface-area basis, this dose is 18 times (rats) and 9 times (mice) the maximum recommended human dose. No mutagenic activity was detected in the Ames test in bacteria, in an in vitro test for forward mutations in cultured mammalian cells, or in a nucleus anomaly test. At doses of 50–500 mg/kg/day (38–375 times the maximum recommended human dose on a body-weight basis; 6–61 times the maximum recommended dose on a body-surface-area basis), benazepril had no adverse effect on the reproductive performance of male and female rats.

Rats and mice treated with amlodipine in the diet for 2 years, at concentrations calculated to provide daily dosage levels of 0.5, 1.25, and 2.5 mg/kg/day, showed no evidence of carcinogenicity. For mice, but not for rats, the highest dose was close to the maximum tolerated dose. On a mg/m^2 basis, this dose given to mice was approximately equal to the maximum recommended clinical dose. On the same basis, the same dose given to rats was approximately twice the maximum recommended clinical dose.

Mutagenicity studies with amlodipine revealed no drug-related effects at either the gene or chromosome levels.

There was no effect on the fertility of rats treated with amlodipine (males for 64 days and females for 14 days prior to mating) at doses up to 10 mg/kg/day (8 times the maximum recommended human dose of 10 mg on a mg/m^2 basis, assuming a 50-kg person).

No adverse effects on fertility occurred when the benazepril:amlodipine combination was given orally to rats of either sex at dose ratios up to 15:7.5 mg/kg/day (benazepril:amlodipine), prior to mating and throughout gestation.

Pregnancy

Pregnancy Categories C (first trimester) and D (second and third trimesters): See WARNINGS, Fetal/Neonatal Morbidity and Mortality.

Nursing Mothers

Minimal amounts of unchanged benazepril and of benazeprilat are excreted into the breast milk of lactating women treated with benazepril, so that a newborn child ingesting nothing but breast milk would receive less than 0.1% of the maternal doses of benazepril and benazeprilat.

It is not known whether amlodipine is excreted in human milk. In the absence of this information, it is recommended that nursing be discontinued while Lotrel is administered.

Geriatric Use

Of the total number of patients who received Lotrel in U.S. clinical studies of Lotrel, 19% were 65 or older while about 2% were 75 or older. Overall differences in effectiveness or safety were not observed between these patients and younger patients. Clinical experience has not identified differences in responses between the elderly and younger patients, but greater sensitivity of some older individuals cannot be ruled out.

Pediatric Use

Safety and effectiveness in pediatric patients have not been established.

ADVERSE REACTIONS

Lotrel has been evaluated for safety in over 1600 patients with hypertension; over 500 of these patients were treated for at least 6 months, and over 400 were treated for more than 1 year.

The reported side effects were generally mild and transient, and there was no relationship between side effects and age, sex, race, or duration of therapy. Discontinuation of therapy due to side effects was required in approximately 4% of patients treated with Lotrel and in 3% of patients treated with placebo.

The most common reasons for discontinuation of therapy with Lotrel in U.S. studies were cough and edema.*

The side effects considered possibly or probably related to study drug that occurred in U.S. placebo-controlled trials in more than 1% of patients treated with Lotrel are shown in the table below.

PERCENT INCIDENCE IN U.S. PLACEBO-CONTROLLED TRIALS

	Benazepril/ Amlodipine N=760	Benazepril N=554	Amlodipine N=475	Placebo N=408
Cough	3.3	1.8	0.4	0.2
Headache	2.2	3.8	2.9	5.6
Dizziness	1.3	1.6	2.3	1.5
Edema*	2.1	0.9	5.1	2.2

*Edema refers to all edema, such as dependent edema, angioedema, facial edema.

The incidence of edema was statistically greater in patients treated with amlodipine monotherapy than in patients treated with the combination. Edema and certain other side effects are associated with amlodipine monotherapy in a dose-dependent manner, and appear to affect women more than men. The addition of benazepril resulted in lower incidences as shown in the following table; the protective effect of benazepril was independent of race and (within the range of doses tested) of dose.

[See table at left.]

PERCENT INCIDENCE BY SEX OF CERTAIN ADVERSE EVENTS

	Benazepril/ Amlodipine		Benazepril		Amlodipine		Placebo	
	Male N=329	Female N=431	Male N=269	Female N=285	Male N=277	Female N=198	Male N=217	Female N=191
Edema	0.6	3.2	0.0	1.8	2.2	9.1	1.4	3.1
Flushing	0.3	0.0	0.0	0.7	0.4	2.0	0.5	0.0
Palpitations	0.3	0.5	0.4	1.4	0.4	2.0	0.5	0.5
Somnolence	0.3	0.0	0.4	0.4	0.4	0.5	0.0	0.0

Other side effects considered possibly or probably related to study drug that occurred in U.S. placebo-controlled trials of patients treated with Lotrel were the following:
Angioedema: Includes edema of the lips or face without other manifestations of angioedema (see WARNINGS, Angioedema).
Body as a Whole: Asthenia and fatigue.
CNS: Insomnia, nervousness, anxiety, tremor, and decreased libido.
Dermatologic: Flushing, hot flashes, rash, skin nodule, and dermatitis. There have been rare reports of pemphigus in patients receiving ACE inhibitors.
Digestive: Dry mouth, nausea, abdominal pain, constipation, diarrhea, dyspepsia, and esophagitis. There have been rare reports of pancreatitis in patients receiving ACE inhibitors.
Hematologic: There have been rare reports of hemolytic anemia in patients receiving ACE inhibitors.
Metabolic and Nutritional: Hypokalemia.
Musculoskeletal: Back pain, musculoskeletal pain, cramps, and muscle cramps.
Respiratory: Pharyngitis.
Urogenital: Sexual problems such as impotence, and polyuria.
Other infrequently reported events were seen in clinical trials (causal relationship unlikely). These included chest pain, ventricular extrasystole, gout, neuritis, and tinnitus.
Fetal/Neonatal Morbidity and Mortality: See WARNINGS, Fetal/Neonatal Morbidity and Mortality.
Monotherapies of benazepril and amlodipine have been evaluated for safety in clinical trials in over 6000 and 11,000 patients, respectively. The observed adverse reactions to the monotherapies in these trials were similar to those seen in trials of Lotrel. In postmarketing experience with benazepril, there have been rare reports of Stevens-Johnson syndrome and thrombocytopenia. Jaundice and hepatic enzyme elevations (mostly consistent with cholestasis) severe enough to require hospitalization have been reported in association with use of amlodipine.

Clinical Laboratory Test Findings
Serum Electrolytes: See PRECAUTIONS.
Creatinine: Minor reversible increases in serum creatinine were observed in patients with essential hypertension treated with Lotrel. Increases in creatinine are more likely to occur in patients with renal insufficiency or those pretreated with a diuretic and, based on experience with other ACE inhibitors, would be expected to be especially likely in patients with renal artery stenosis (see PRECAUTIONS, General).
Other (causal relationships unknown): Clinically important changes in standard laboratory tests were rarely associated with Lotrel administration. Elevations of serum bilirubin and uric acid have been reported as have scattered incidents of elevations of liver enzymes.

OVERDOSAGE

Only a few cases of human overdose with amlodipine have been reported. One patient was asymptomatic after a 250-mg ingestion; another, who combined 70 mg of amlodipine with an unknown large quantity of a benzodiazepine, developed refractory shock and died.
Human overdoses with any combination of amlodipine and benazepril have not been reported. In scattered reports of human overdoses with benazepril and other ACE inhibitors, there are no reports of death.
When mice were given single oral doses of benazepril/amlodipine, mortality was 20% at 50:25 mg/kg, 10% at 100:50 mg/kg, and 100% at 500:250 mg/kg. In rats, mortality was 25% (pooling two studies) at 500:250 mg/kg and 100% at 900:450 mg/kg.
Treatment: To obtain up-to-date information about the treatment of overdose, a good resource is your certified Regional Poison-Control Center. Telephone numbers of certified poison-control centers are listed in the *Physicians' Desk Reference (PDR).* In managing overdose, consider the possibilities of multiple-drug overdoses, drug-drug interactions, and unusual drug kinetics in your patient.
The most likely effect of overdose with Lotrel is vasodilation, with consequent hypotension and tachycardia. Simple repletion of central fluid volume (Trendelenburg positioning, infusion of crystalloids) may be sufficient therapy, but pressor agents (norepinephrine or high-dose dopamine) may be required. Overdoses of other dihydropyridine calcium channel blockers are reported to have been treated with calcium chloride and glucagon, but evidence of a dose-response relation has not been seen, and these interventions must be regarded as unproven. With abrupt return of peripheral vascular tone, overdoses of other dihydropyridine calcium channel blockers have sometimes progressed to pulmonary edema, and patients must be monitored for this complication.
Analyses of bodily fluids for concentrations of amlodipine, benazepril, or their metabolites are not widely available. Such analyses are, in any event, not known to be of value in therapy or prognosis.
No data are available to suggest physiologic maneuvers (e.g., maneuvers to change the pH of the urine) that might accelerate elimination of amlodipine, benazepril, or their metabolites. Benazeprilat is only slightly dialyzable; attempted clearance of amlodipine by hemodialysis or hemoperfusion has not been reported, but amlodipine's high protein binding makes it unlikely that these interventions will be of value.
Angiotensin II could presumably serve as a specific antagonist-antidote to benazepril, but angiotensin II is essentially unavailable outside of scattered research laboratories.

DOSAGE AND ADMINISTRATION

Amlodipine is an effective treatment of hypertension in once-daily doses of 2.5–10 mg while benazepril is effective in doses of 10–80 mg. In clinical trials of amlodipine/benazepril combination therapy using amlodipine doses of 2.5–5 mg and benazepril doses of 10–20 mg, the antihypertensive effects increased with increasing dose of amlodipine in all patient groups, and the effects increased with increasing dose of benazepril in nonblack groups. All patient groups benefited from the reduction in amlodipine-induced edema (see below).
The hazards (see WARNINGS) of benazepril are generally independent of dose; those of amlodipine are a mixture of dose-dependent phenomena (primarily peripheral edema) and dose-independent phenomena, the former much more common than the latter. When benazepril is added to a regimen of amlodipine, the incidence of edema is substantially reduced. Therapy with any combination of amlodipine and benazepril will thus be associated with both sets of dose-independent hazards, but the incidence of edema will generally be less than that seen with similar (or higher) doses of amlodipine monotherapy.
Rarely, the dose-independent hazards of benazepril are serious. To minimize dose-independent hazards, it is usually appropriate to begin therapy with Lotrel only after a patient has either (a) failed to achieve the desired antihypertensive effect with one or the other monotherapy, or (b) demonstrated inability to achieve adequate antihypertensive effect with amlodipine therapy without developing edema.
Dose Titration Guided by Clinical Effect: A patient whose blood pressure is not adequately controlled with amlodipine (or another dihydropyridine) alone or with benazepril (or another ACE inhibitor) alone may be switched to combination therapy with Lotrel. The addition of benazepril to a regimen of amlodipine should not be expected to provide additional antihypertensive effect in African-Americans. However, all patient groups benefit from the reduction in amlodipine-induced edema. Dosage must be guided by clinical response; steady-state levels of benazepril and amlodipine will be reached after approximately 2 and 7 days of dosing, respectively.
In patients whose blood pressures are adequately controlled with amlodipine but who experience unacceptable edema, combination therapy may achieve similar (or better) blood-pressure control without edema. Especially in nonblacks, it may be prudent to minimize the risk of excessive response by reducing the dose of amlodipine as benazepril is added to the regimen.
Replacement Therapy: For convenience, patients receiving amlodipine and benazepril from separate tablets may instead wish to receive capsules of Lotrel containing the same component doses.
Use in Patients With Metabolic Impairments: Regimens of therapy with Lotrel need not take account of renal function as long as the patient's creatinine clearance is > 30 mL/min/1.73m^2 (serum creatinine roughly ≤ 3 mg/dL or 265 μmol/L). In patients with more severe renal impairment, the recommended initial dose of benazepril is 5 mg. Lotrel is not recommended in these patients.
In small, elderly, frail, or hepatically impaired patients, the recommended initial dose of amlodipine, as monotherapy or as a component of combination therapy, is 2.5 mg.

HOW SUPPLIED

Lotrel is available as capsules containing amlodipine/benazepril HCl 2.5/10 mg, 5/10 mg, and 5/20 mg. All three strengths are packaged with a desiccant in bottles of 100 capsules.
Capsules are imprinted with "Lotrel" and a portion of the NDC code. Samples, when available, are identified by the word *SAMPLE* appearing on each capsule.

Dose	Capsule Color	NDC Code Bottle of 100
2.5/10 mg	white capsule with 2 gold bands	NDC 0083-2255-30
5/10 mg	light brown capsule with 2 white bands	NDC 0083-2260-30
5/20 mg	pink capsule with 2 white bands	NDC 0083-2265-30

Storage: Do not store above 86°F (30°C). Protect from moisture and light.
Dispense in tight, light-resistant container (USP).
C96-34 (Rev. 3/96)

Dist. by:
Ciba-Geigy Corporation
Pharmaceuticals Division
Summit, New Jersey 07901
Shown in Product Identification Guide, page 309

LUDIOMIL® ℞
[loó-dee-oh-mill]
(maprotiline hydrochloride)
Tablets

DESCRIPTION

Ludiomil, maprotiline hydrochloride USP, is a tetracyclic antidepressant, available as 25-mg, 50-mg and 75-mg tablets for oral administration. Its chemical name is N-methyl-9,10-ethanoanthracene-9(10H)-propylamine hydrochloride.
Maprotiline hydrochloride USP is a fine, white to off-white, practically odorless crystalline powder. It is freely soluble in methanol and in chloroform, slightly soluble in water, and practically insoluble in isooctane. Its molecular weight is 313.87.
Inactive Ingredients. Calcium phosphate, cellulose compounds, colloidal silicon dioxide, FD&C Yellow No. 6 Aluminum Lake (25-mg and 50-mg tablets), lactose, magnesium stearate, povidone, shellac, starch, stearic acid, talc, and titanium dioxide.

CLINICAL PHARMACOLOGY

The mechanism of action of Ludiomil is not precisely known. It does not act primarily by stimulation of the central nervous system and is not a monoamine oxidase inhibitor. The postulated mechanism of Ludiomil is that it acts primarily by potentiation of central adrenergic synapses by blocking reuptake of norepinephrine at nerve endings. This pharmacologic action is thought to be responsible for the drug's antidepressant and anxiolytic effects.
The mean time to peak is 12 hours. The half-life of elimination averages 51 hours.
Steady-state levels measured prior to the morning dose on a one-dosage regimen are summarized as follows:

Regimen	Average Minimum Concentration ng/ml	95% Confidence Limits ng/ml
50 mg x 3 daily	238	181–295

INDICATIONS AND USAGE

Ludiomil is indicated for the treatment of depressive illness in patients with depressive neurosis (dysthymic disorder) and manic-depressive illness, depressed type (major depressive disorder). Ludiomil is also effective for the relief of anxiety associated with depression.

CONTRAINDICATIONS

Ludiomil is contraindicated in patients hypersensitive to Ludiomil and in patients with known or suspected seizure disorders. It should not be given concomitantly with monoamine oxidase (MAO) inhibitors. A minimum of 14 days should be allowed to elapse after discontinuation of MAO inhibitors before treatment with Ludiomil is initiated. Effects should be monitored with gradual increase in dosage until optimum response is achieved. The drug is not recommended for use during the acute phase of myocardial infarction.

WARNINGS

Seizures have been associated with the use of Ludiomil.
Most of the seizures have occurred in patients without a known history of seizures. However, in some of these cases, other confounding factors were present, including concomitant medications known to lower the seizure threshold, rapid escalation of the dosage of Ludiomil, and dosage that exceeded the recommended therapeutic range. The incidence of direct reports is less than $\frac{1}{10}$ of 1%. The risk of seizures may be increased when Ludiomil is taken concomitantly with phenothiazines, when the dosage of benzodiazepines is rapidly tapered in patients receiving Ludiomil or when the recommended dosage of Ludiomil is exceeded. While a cause-and-effect relationship has not been established, the risk of seizures in patients treated with Ludiomil may be reduced by (1) initiating therapy at a low dosage, (2) maintaining the initial dosage for 2 weeks before raising it gradually in small increments as necessitated by the long half-life of Ludiomil (average 51 hours), and (3) keeping the dosage at the minimally effective level during maintenance therapy. (See **DOSAGE AND ADMINISTRATION.)**
Extreme caution should be used when this drug is given to:
—patients with a history of myocardial infarction;
—patients with a history or presence of cardiovascular disease because of the possibility of conduction defects, arrhythmias, myocardial infarction, strokes and tachycardia.

PRECAUTIONS

General: The possibility of suicide in seriously depressed patients is inherent in their illness and may persist until

Continued on next page

CibaGeneva—Cont.

significant remission occurs. Therefore, patients must be carefully supervised during all phases of treatment with Ludiomil, and prescriptions should be written for the smallest number of tablets consistent with good patient management.

Hypomanic or manic episodes have been known to occur in some patients taking tricyclic antidepressant drugs, particularly in patients with cyclic disorders. Such occurrences have also been noted, rarely, with Ludiomil.

Prior to elective surgery, Ludiomil should be discontinued for as long as clinically feasible, since little is known about the interaction between Ludiomil and general anesthetics.

Ludiomil should be administered with caution in patients with increased intraocular pressure, history of urinary retention, or history of narrow-angle glaucoma because of the drug's anticholinergic properties.

Information for Patients: Patients should be warned of the association between seizures and the use of Ludiomil. Moreover, they should be informed that this association is enhanced in patients with a known history of seizures and in those patients who are taking certain other drugs. (See **WARNINGS.**)

Warn patients to exercise caution about potentially hazardous tasks, or operating automobiles or machinery since the drug may impair mental and/or physical abilities.

Ludiomil may enhance the response to alcohol, barbiturates, and other CNS depressants, requiring appropriate caution of administration.

Laboratory Tests: Ludiomil should be discontinued if there is evidence of pathological neutrophil depression. Leukocyte and differential counts should be performed in patients who develop fever and sore throat during therapy.

Drug Interactions: Close supervision and careful adjustment of dosage are required when administering Ludiomil concomitantly with anticholinergic or sympathomimetic drugs because of the possibility of additive atropine-like effects.

Concurrent administration of Ludiomil with electroshock therapy should be avoided because of the lack of experience in this area.

Caution should be exercised when administering Ludiomil to hyperthyroid patients or those on thyroid medication because of the possibility of enhanced potential for cardiovascular toxicity of Ludiomil.

Ludiomil should be used with caution in patients receiving guanethidine or similar agents since it may block the pharmacologic effects of these drugs.

The risk of seizures may be increased when Ludiomil is taken concomitantly with phenothiazines or when the dosage of benzodiazepines is rapidly tapered in patients receiving Ludiomil.

Because of the pharmacologic similarity of Ludiomil to the tricyclic antidepressants, the plasma concentration of Ludiomil may be increased when the drug is given concomitantly with hepatic enzyme inhibitors (e.g., cimetidine, fluoxetine) and decreased by concomitant administration with hepatic enzyme enducers (e.g., barbiturates, phenytoin), as has occurred with tricyclic antidepressants. Adjustment of the dosage of Ludiomil may therefore be necessary in such cases.

(See **Information for Patients.**)

Carcinogenesis, Mutagenesis, Impairment of Fertility: Carcinogenicity and chronic toxicity studies have been conducted in laboratory rats and dogs. No drug- or dose-related occurrence of carcinogenesis was evident in rats receiving daily oral doses up to 60 mg/kg of Ludiomil for eighteen months or in dogs receiving daily oral doses up to 30 mg/kg of Ludiomil for one year. In addition, no evidence of mutagenic activity was found in offspring of female mice mated with males treated with up to 60 times the maximum daily human dose.

Pregnancy Category B: Reproduction studies have been performed in female laboratory rabbits, mice, and rats at doses up to 1.3, 7, and 9 times the maximum daily human dose respectively and have revealed no evidence of impaired fertility or harm to the fetus due to Ludiomil. There are, however, no adequate and well-controlled studies in pregnant women. Because animal reproduction studies are not always predictive of human response, this drug should be used during pregnancy only if clearly needed.

Labor and Delivery: Although the effect of Ludiomil on labor and delivery is unknown, caution should be exercised as with any drug with CNS depressant action.

Nursing Mothers: Ludiomil is excreted in breast milk. At steady state, the concentrations in milk correspond closely to the concentrations in whole blood. Caution should be exercised when Ludiomil is administered to a nursing woman.

Pediatric Use: Safety and effectiveness in pediatric patients below the age of 18 have not been established.

ADVERSE REACTIONS

The following adverse reactions have been noted with Ludiomil and are generally similar to those observed with tricyclic antidepressants.

Cardiovascular: Rare occurrences of hypotension, hypertension, tachycardia, palpitation, arrhythmia, heart block, and syncope have been reported with Ludiomil.

Psychiatric: Nervousness (6%), anxiety (3%), insomnia (2%), and agitation (2%); rarely, confusional states (especially in the elderly), hallucinations, disorientation, delusions, restlessness, nightmares, hypomania, mania, exacerbation of psychosis, decrease in memory, and feelings of unreality.

Neurological: Drowsiness (16%), dizziness (8%), tremor (3%), and, rarely, numbness, tingling, motor hyperactivity, akathisia, seizures, EEG alterations, tinnitus, extrapyramidal symptoms, ataxia, and dysarthria.

Anticholinergic: Dry mouth (22%), constipation (6%), and blurred vision (4%); rarely, accommodation disturbances, mydriasis, urinary retention, and delayed micturition.

Allergic: Rare instances of skin rash, petechiae, itching, photosensitization, edema, and drug fever.

Gastrointestinal: Nausea (2%) and, rarely, vomiting, epigastric distress, diarrhea, bitter taste, abdominal cramps and dysphagia.

Endocrine: Rare instances of increased or decreased libido, impotence, and elevation or depression of blood sugar levels.

Other: Weakness and fatigue (4%) and headache (4%); rarely, altered liver function, jaundice, weight loss or gain, excessive perspiration, flushing, urinary frequency, increased salivation, nasal congestion and alopecia.

Note: Although there have been only isolated reports of the following adverse reactions with Ludiomil, its pharmacologic similarity to tricyclic antidepressants requires that each reaction be considered when administering Ludiomil.

—Bone marrow depression, including agranulocytosis, eosinophilia, purpura, and thrombocytopenia, myocardial infarction, stroke, peripheral neuropathy, sublingual adenitis, black tongue, stomatitis, paralytic ileus, gynecomastia in the male, breast enlargement and galactorrhea in the female, and testicular swelling.

Post-Introduction Reports: Several voluntary reports of interstitial pneumonitis, which were in some cases associated with eosinophilia and increased liver enzymes, have been received since market introduction. However, there is no clear causal relationship.

OVERDOSAGE

Deaths may occur from overdosage with this class of drugs. Multiple drug ingestion (including alcohol) is common in deliberate overdose. As the management is complex and changing, it is recommended that the physician contact a poison control center for current information on treatment. Signs and symptoms of toxicity develop rapidly after overdose. Therefore, hospital monitoring is required as soon as possible.

Animal Oral LD_{50}: The oral LD_{50} of Ludiomil is 600–750 mg/kg in mice, 760–900 mg/kg in rats, > 1000 mg/kg in rabbits, > 300 mg/kg in cats, and > 30 mg/kg in dogs.

Manifestations: Data dealing with overdosage in humans are limited with only a few cases on record. Signs and symptoms of Ludiomil overdose are similar to those seen with tricyclic overdose. Critical manifestations of overdose include cardiac dysrhythmias, severe hypotension, convulsions and CNS depression including coma. Changes in the electrocardiogram, particularly in QRS axis or width are clinically significant indicators of toxicity. Other clinical manifestations include drowsiness, tachycardia, ataxia, vomiting, cyanosis, shock, restlessness, agitation, hyperpyrexia, muscle rigidity, athetoid movements, and mydriasis. Since congestive heart failure has been seen with overdosages of tricyclic antidepressants, it should be considered with Ludiomil overdosage.

Management

Obtain an ECG and immediately initiate cardiac monitoring. Protect the patient's airway, establish an intravenous line and initiate gastric decontamination. A minimum of six hours of observation with cardiac monitoring and observation for signs of CNS or respiratory depression, hypotension, cardiac dysrhythmias and/or conduction blocks, and seizures is necessary. If signs of toxicity occur at any time during this period, extended monitoring is required. There are case reports of patients succumbing to fatal dysrhythmias late after tricyclic overdose; these patients had clinical evidence of significant poisoning prior to death and most received inadequate gastrointestinal decontamination. Monitoring of plasma drug levels should not guide management of the patient.

Gastrointestinal Decontamination: All patients suspected of overdose should receive gastrointestinal decontamination. This should include large volume gastric lavage followed by activated charcoal. If consciousness is impaired, the airway should be secured prior to lavage. Emesis is contraindicated.

Cardiovascular: A maximal limb-lead QRS duration of ≥ 0.10 seconds may be the best indication of the severity of the overdose. Serum alkalinization, to a pH of 7.45 to 7.55, using intravenous sodium bicarbonate and hyperventilation (as needed) should be instituted for patients with dysrhythmias and/or QRS widening. A pH > 7.60 or a Pco_2 < 20 mmHg is undesirable. Dysrhythmias unresponsive to sodium bicarbonate therapy/hyperventilation may respond to lidocaine, bretylium, or phenytoin. Type 1A and 1C antiarrhythmics are generally contraindicated (e.g., quinidine, disopyramide, and procainamide).

In rare instances, hemoperfusion may be beneficial in acute refractory cardiovascular instability in patients with acute toxicity. However, hemodialysis, peritoneal dialysis, exchange transfusions, and forced diuresis generally have been reported as ineffective.

CNS: In patients with CNS depression, early intubation is advised because of the potential for abrupt deterioration. Seizures should be controlled with benzodiazepines, or if these are ineffective, other anticonvulsants (e.g., phenobarbital, phenytoin). Physostigmine is not recommended except to treat life-threatening symptoms that have been unresponsive to other therapies, and then only in consultation with a poison control center.

Psychiatric Follow-up: Since overdosage is often deliberate, patients may attempt suicide by other means during the recovery phase. Psychiatric referral may be appropriate.

Pediatric Management: The principles of management of child and adult overdosages are similar. It is strongly recommended that the physician contact the local poison control center for specific pediatric treatment.

DOSAGE AND ADMINISTRATION

A single daily dose is an alternative to divided daily doses. Therapeutic effects are sometimes seen within 3 to 7 days, although as long as 2 to 3 weeks are usually necessary.

Initial Adult Dosage: An initial dosage of 75 mg daily is suggested for outpatients with mild-to-moderate depression. However, in some patients, particularly the elderly, an initial dosage of 25 mg daily may be used. Because of the long half-life of Ludiomil, the initial dosage should be maintained for two weeks. The dosage may then be increased gradually in 25-mg increments as required and tolerated. In most outpatients a maximum dose of 150 mg daily will result in therapeutic efficacy. It is recommended that this dose not be exceeded except in the most severely depressed patients. In such patients, dosage may be gradually increased to a maximum of 225 mg.

More severely depressed, hospitalized patients should be given an initial daily dose of 100 mg to 150 mg which may be gradually increased as required and tolerated. Most hospitalized patients with moderate-to-severe depression respond to a daily dosage of 150 mg although dosages as high as 225 mg may be required in some cases. Daily dosage of 225 mg should not be exceeded.

Elderly Patients: In general, lower dosages are recommended for patients over 60 years of age. Dosages of 50 mg to 75 mg daily are usually satisfactory as maintenance therapy for elderly patients who do not tolerate higher amounts.

Maintenance: Dosage during prolonged maintenance therapy should be kept at the lowest effective level. Dosage may be reduced to levels of 75 mg to 150 mg daily during such periods, with subsequent adjustment depending on therapeutic response.

HOW SUPPLIED

Tablets 25 mg—oval, dark orange, scored, coated (imprinted CIBA 110)

Bottles of 100 .... NDC 0083-0110-30

Tablets 50 mg—round, dark orange, scored, coated (imprinted CIBA 26)

Bottles of 100 .... NDC 0083-0026-30

Tablets 75 mg—oval, white, scored, coated (imprinted CIBA 135)

Bottles of 100 .... NDC 0083-0135-30

Do not store above 86°F (30°C).

Dispense in tight container (USP).

C96-2 (Rev. 1/96)

Shown in Product Identification Guide, page 309

PBZ-SR® ℞

tripelennamine hydrochloride USP
Extended-Release Tablets

DESCRIPTION

PBZ-SR, tripelennamine hydrochloride USP, is an antihistamine for oral administration available as 100-mg extended-release tablets that provide a gradual and prolonged release of drug from the wax matrix.

Tripelennamine hydrochloride is 2-[Benzyl[2-(dimethylamino)ethyl]amino] pyridine monohydrochloride.

Tripelennamine hydrochloride USP is a white, crystalline powder. Its solutions are practically neutral to litmus. It is freely soluble in water, in alcohol, and in chloroform; slightly soluble in acetone; and insoluble in benzene, in ether, and in ethyl acetate. Its molecular weight is 291.82.

Inactive Ingredients: Cellulose compounds, cetostearyl alcohol, D&C Red No. 30 lake, FD&C Blue No. 2 lake, magnesium stearate, mineral oil, titanium dioxide, and zein.

ACTIONS
Antihistamines are competitive antagonists of histamine, which also produce central nervous system effects (both stimulant and depressant) and peripheral anticholinergic, atropine-like effects (e.g., drying).

INDICATIONS
Perennial and seasonal allergic rhinitis; vasomotor rhinitis; allergic conjunctivitis due to inhalant allergens and foods; mild, uncomplicated allergic skin manifestations of urticaria and angioedema; amelioration of allergic reactions to blood or plasma; dermographism; anaphylactic reactions as adjunctive therapy to epinephrine and other standard measures after the acute manifestations have been controlled.

CONTRAINDICATIONS
PBZ-SR should not be used in premature infants, neonates, or nursing mothers; patients receiving MAO inhibitors; patients with narrow-angle glaucoma, stenosing peptic ulcer, symptomatic prostatic hypertrophy, bladder neck obstruction, pyloroduodenal obstruction, lower respiratory tract symptoms (including asthma), or hypersensitivity to tripelennamine or related compounds.

WARNINGS
Antihistamines often produce drowsiness and may reduce mental alertness in children and adults. Patients should be warned about engaging in activities requiring mental alertness (e.g., driving a car, operating machinery or hazardous appliances). In elderly patients, approximately 60 years or older, antihistamines are more likely to cause dizziness, sedation and hypotension. Patients should be warned that the central nervous system effects of PBZ-SR may be additive with those of alcohol and other CNS depressants (e.g., hypnotics, sedatives, tranquilizers, antianxiety agents).
Antihistamines may produce excitation, particularly in children.
Usage in Pregnancy: Although no tripelennamine-related teratogenic potential or other adverse effects on the fetus have been observed in limited animal reproduction studies, the safe use of this drug in pregnancy or during lactation has not been established. Therefore, the drug should not be used during pregnancy or lactation unless, in the judgment of the physician, the expected benefits outweigh the potential hazards.
Usage in Children: In infants and children particularly, antihistamines in overdosage may produce hallucinations, convulsions and/or death.

PRECAUTIONS
PBZ-SR, like other antihistamines, has atropine-like, anticholinergic activity and should be used with caution in patients with increased intraocular pressure, hyperthyroidism, cardiovascular disease, hypertension, or history of bronchial asthma.
Pediatric Use: Safety and effectiveness in pediatric patients have not been established.

ADVERSE REACTIONS
The most frequent adverse reactions to antihistamines are sedation or drowsiness; sleepiness; dryness of the mouth, nose, and throat; thickening of bronchial secretions; dizziness; disturbed coordination; epigastric distress.
Other adverse reactions which may occur are: fatigue; chills; confusion; restlessness; excitation; hysteria; nervousness; irritability; insomnia; euphoria; anorexia; nausea; vomiting; diarrhea; constipation; hypotension; tightness in the chest; wheezing; blurred vision; diplopia; vertigo; tinnitus; convulsions; headache; palpitations; tachycardia; extrasystoles; nasal stuffiness; urinary frequency; difficult urination; urinary retention; leukopenia; hemolytic anemia; thrombocytopenia; agranulocytosis; aplastic anemia; allergic or hypersensitivity reactions, including drug rash, urticaria, anaphylactic shock, and photosensitivity. Although the following may have been reported to occur in association with some antihistamines, they have not been known to result from the use of PBZ-SR: excessive perspiration, tremor, paresthesias, acute labyrinthitis, neuritis and early menses.

DOSAGE AND ADMINISTRATION
Dosage should be individualized according to the needs and response of the patient.
Adults: One 100-mg PBZ-SR tablet in the morning and one in the evening is generally adequate. In difficult cases, one 100-mg PBZ-SR tablet every 8 hours may be required.
Children: PBZ-SR tablets are not intended for use in children.
Note: PBZ-SR extended-release tablets must be swallowed whole and never crushed or chewed.

OVERDOSAGE
Signs and Symptoms: The greatest danger from acute overdosage with antihistamines is their central nervous system effects which produce depression and/or stimulation.
In children, stimulation predominates initially in a syndrome which may include excitement, hallucinations, ataxia, incoordination, athetosis, and convulsions followed by postictal depression. Dry mouth, fixed dilated pupils, flushing of the face, and fever are common and resemble the syndrome of atropine poisoning. In adults, CNS depression (i.e., drowsiness, coma) is more common. CNS stimulation is rare; fever and flushing are uncommon.
In both children and adults, there can be a terminal deepening of coma and cardiovascular collapse; death can occur, especially in infants and children.
Treatment: There is no specific therapy for acute overdosage with antihistamines. General symptomatic and supportive measures should be instituted promptly and maintained for as long as necessary.
In the conscious patient, vomiting should be induced even though it may have occurred spontaneously. If vomiting cannot be induced, gastric lavage is indicated. Adequate precautions must be taken to protect against aspiration, especially in infants and children. Charcoal slurry or other suitable agent should be instilled into the stomach after vomiting or lavage. Saline cathartics or milk of magnesia may be of additional benefit.
In the unconscious patient, the airway should be secured with a cuffed endotracheal tube before attempting to evacuate the gastric contents. Intensive supportive and nursing care is indicated, as for any comatose patient.
If breathing is significantly impaired, maintenance of an adequate airway and mechanical support of respiration is the safest and most effective means of providing for adequate oxygenation of tissues to prevent hypoxia (especially brain hypoxia during convulsions).
Hypotension is an early sign of impeding cardiovascular collapse and should be treated vigorously. Although general supportive measures are important, specific treatment with intravenous infusion of a vasopressor (e.g., levarterenol bitartrate) titrated to maintain adequate blood pressure may be necessary.
Do *not* use CNS stimulants.
Convulsions should be controlled by careful titration of a short-acting barbiturate, repeated as necessary.
Ice packs and cooling sponge baths can aid in reducing the fever commonly seen in children.

HOW SUPPLIED
Tablets (extended-release) 100 mg—round, lavender (imprinted Geigy 48)
Bottles of 100 ....NDC 0028-0048-01
Store at controlled room temperature (15°–30°C) (59°–86°F). Protect from moisture.
Dispense in tight container (USP).

C96-40 (Rev. 4/96)

Shown in Product Identification Guide, page 309

PBZ® ℞
tripelennamine hydrochloride
Tablets USP

Listed in USP, a Medicare designated compendium.

DESCRIPTION
PBZ, tripelennamine hydrochloride USP, is an antihistamine for oral administration. PBZ *tablets* contain 25 mg and 50 mg of the hydrochoride salt. Tripelennamine hydrochloride is 2-[Benzyl[2-(dimethylamino)ethyl]amino]pyridine monohydrochloride.
Tripelennamine hydrochloride USP is a white, crystalline powder. Its solutions are practically neutral to litmus. It is freely soluble in water, in alcohol, and in chloroform; slightly soluble in acetone; and insoluble in benzene, in ether, and in ethyl acetate. Its molecular weight is 291.82.
Inactive ingredients (PBZ Tablets 25 mg): Lactose, magnesium stearate, polyethylene glycol, starch, sucrose and talc. (PBZ Tablets 50 mg): Acacia, lactose, magnesium stearate, polyethylene glycol, talc and tragacanth.

ACTIONS
Antihistamines are competitive antagonists of histamine, which also produce central nervous system effects (both stimulant and depressant) and peripheral anticholinergic, atropine-like effects (e.g., drying).

INDICATIONS
Perennial and seasonal allergic rhinitis; vasomotor rhinitis; allergic conjunctivitis due to inhalant allergens and foods; mild, uncomplicated allergic skin manifestations of urticaria and angioedema; amelioration of allergic reactions to blood or plasma; dermographism; anaphylactic reactions as adjunctive therapy to epinephrine and other standard measures after the acute manifestations have been controlled.

CONTRAINDICATIONS
PBZ should not be used in premature infants, neonates, or nursing mothers; patients receiving MAO inhibitors; patients with narrow-angle glaucoma, stenosing peptic ulcer, symptomatic prostatic hypertrophy, bladder neck obstruction, pyloroduodenal obstruction, lower respiratory tract symptoms (including asthma), or hypersensitivity to tripelennamine or related compounds.

WARNINGS
Antihistamines often produce drowsiness and may reduce mental alertness in children and adults. Patients should be warned about engaging in activities requiring mental alertness (e.g., driving a car, operating machinery or hazardous appliances). In elderly patients, approximately 60 years or older, antihistamines are more likely to cause dizziness, sedation and hypotension.
Patients should be warned that the central nervous system effects of PBZ may be additive with those of alcohol and other CNS depressants (e.g., hypnotics, sedatives, tranquilizers, antianxiety agents).
Antihistamines may produce excitation, particularly in children.

Usage in Pregnancy
Although no tripelennamine-related teratogenic potential or other adverse effects on the fetus have been observed in limited animal reproduction studies, the safe use of this drug in pregnancy or during lactation has not been established. Therefore, the drug should not be used during pregnancy or lactation unless, in the judgment of the physician, the expected benefits outweigh the potential hazards.

Usage in Children
In infants and children particularly, antihistamines in overdosage may produce hallucinations, convulsions and/or death.

PRECAUTIONS
PBZ, like other antihistamines, has atropine-like, anticholinergic activity and should be used with caution in patients with increased intraocular pressure, hyperthyroidism, cardiovascular disease, hypertension, or history of bronchial asthma.

ADVERSE REACTIONS
The most frequent adverse reactions to antihistamines are sedation or drowsiness; sleepiness; dryness of the mouth, nose, and throat; thickening of bronchial secretions; dizziness; disturbed coordination; epigastric distress.
Other adverse reactions which may occur are: fatigue; chills; confusion; restlessness; excitation; hysteria; nervousness; irritability; insomnia; euphoria; anorexia; nausea; vomiting; diarrhea; constipation; hypotension; tightness in the chest; wheezing; blurred vision; diplopia; vertigo; tinnitus; convulsions; headache; palpitations; tachycardia; extrasystoles; nasal stuffiness; urinary frequency; difficult urination; urinary retention; leukopenia; hemolytic anemia; thrombocytopenia; agranulocytosis; aplastic anemia; allergic or hypersensitivity reactions, including drug rash, urticaria, anaphylactic shock, and photosensitivity. Although the following may have been reported to occur in association with some antihistamines, they have not been known to result from the use of PBZ: excessive perspiration, tremor, paresthesias, acute labyrinthitis, neuritis and early menses.

DOSAGE AND ADMINISTRATION
Dosage should be individualized.
Usual Adult Dose: 25 to 50 mg every four to six hours. As little as 25 mg may control symptoms, but as much as 600 mg daily may be given in divided doses, if necessary.
Children and Infants: 5 mg/kg/24 hours or 150 mg/m^2/24 hours divided into four to six doses. Do not exceed maximum total dose of 300 mg/24 hours.

OVERDOSAGE

Signs and Symptoms
The greatest danger from acute overdosage with antihistamines is their central nervous system effects which produce depression and/or stimulation.
In children, stimulation predominates initially in a syndrome which may include excitement, hallucinations, ataxia, incoordination, athetosis, and convulsions followed by postictal depression. Dry mouth, fixed dilated pupils, flushing of the face, and fever are common and resemble the syndrome of atropine poisoning.
In adults, CNS depression (i.e., drowsiness, coma) is more common. CNS stimulation is rare; fever and flushing are uncommon.
In both children and adults, there can be a terminal deepening of coma and cardiovascular collapse, death can occur, especially in infants and children.

Treatment
There is no specific therapy for acute overdosage with antihistamines. General symptomatic and supportive measures should be instituted promptly and maintained for as long as necessary.
In the conscious patient, vomiting should be induced even though it may have occurred spontaneously. If vomiting cannot be induced, gastric lavage is indicated. Adequate precautions must be taken to protect against aspiration, especially in infants and children. Charcoal slurry or other suitable agent should be instilled into the stomach after vomiting or lavage. Saline cathartics or milk of magnesia may be of additional benefit.

Continued on next page

CibaGeneva—Cont.

In the unconscious patient, the airway should be secured with a cuffed endotracheal tube before attempting to evacuate the gastric contents. Intensive supportive and nursing care is indicated, as for any comatose patient.

If breathing is significantly impaired, maintenance of an adequate airway and mechanical support of respiration is the safest and most effective means of providing for adequate oxygenation of tissues to prevent hypoxia (especially brain hypoxia during convulsions).

Hypotension is an early sign of impending cardiovascular collapse and should be treated vigorously. Although general supportive measures are important, specific treatment with intravenous infusion of a vasopressor (e.g., levarterenol bitartrate) titrated to maintain adequate blood pressure may be necessary.

Do *not* use CNS stimulants.

Convulsions should be controlled by careful titration of a short-acting barbiturate, repeated as necessary.

Ice packs and cooling sponge baths can aid in reducing the fever commonly seen in children.

HOW SUPPLIED

Tablets 25 mg—round, white to off-white, biconvex (scored on one side and imprinted Geigy 111 on the other side)

    Bottles of 100 ....NDC 0028-0111-01

Tablets 50 mg—round, white to off-white, biconvex (scored on one side and imprinted Geigy 117 on the other side)

    Bottles of 100 ....NDC 0028-0117-01

Do not store above 86°F (30°C). Protect from light.

Dispense in tight, light-resistant container.

                                  C92-21 (Rev. 4/96)

Shown in Product Identification Guide, page 309

PRISCOLINE® hydrochloride ℞

[*priss 'coe-leen*]

tolazoline hydrochloride USP

Ampuls

DESCRIPTION

Priscoline, tolazoline hydrochloride USP, is a peripheral vasodilator available in ampuls for intravenous administration. Each milliliter of sterile, aqueous solution contains tolazoline hydrochloride USP, 25 mg; tartaric acid ACS, 6.5 mg; and hydrous sodium citrate USP, 6.5 mg. Tolazoline hydrochloride is 4,5-dihydro-2-(phenylmethyl)-1H-imidazole monohydrochloride.

Tolazoline hydrochloride USP is a white to off-white crystalline powder. Its solutions are slightly acid to litmus. It is freely soluble in water and in alcohol. Its molecular weight is 196.68.

CLINICAL PHARMACOLOGY

Priscoline is a direct peripheral vasodilator with moderate competitive alpha-adrenergic blocking activity. It decreases peripheral resistance and increases venous capacitance. It has the following additional actions: (1) sympathomimetic, including cardiac stimulation; (2) parasympathomimetic, including gastrointestinal tract stimulation that is blocked by atropine; and (3) histamine-like, including stimulation of gastric secretion and peripheral vasodilatation. Priscoline given intravenously produces vasodilatation, primarily due to a direct effect on vascular smooth muscle, and cardiac stimulation; the blood pressure response depends on the relative contributions of the two effects. Priscoline usually reduces pulmonary arterial pressure and vascular resistance. In neonates the half-life of Priscoline ranges from 3 to 10 hours.

INDICATIONS AND USAGE

Priscoline is indicated for the treatment of persistent pulmonary hypertension of the newborn ("persistent fetal circulation") when systemic arterial oxygenation cannot be satisfactorily maintained by usual supportive care (supplemental oxygen and/or mechanical ventilation).

Priscoline should be used in a highly supervised setting, where vital signs, oxygenation, acid-base status, fluid, and electrolytes can be monitored and maintained.

CONTRAINDICATIONS

Priscoline is contraindicated in patients with hypersensitivity to tolazoline.

WARNINGS

Priscoline stimulates gastric secretion and may activate stress ulcers. Through this mechanism, it can produce significant hypochloremic alkalosis. Pretreatment of infants with antacids may prevent gastrointestinal bleeding.

Patients should be observed closely for signs of systemic hypotension, and supportive therapy should be instituted if needed.

In patients with mitral stenosis, parenterally administered Priscoline may produce a rise or fall in pulmonary artery pressure and total pulmonary resistance; therefore, it must be used with caution in patients with known or suspected mitral stenosis.

PRECAUTIONS

General: The effects of Priscoline on pulmonary vessels may be pH dependent. Acidosis may decrease the effect of Priscoline.

Carcinogenesis, Mutagenesis, Impairment of Fertility: Long-term carcinogenicity studies in animals have not been performed with Priscoline.

Pregnancy Category C: Animal reproduction studies have not been conducted with Priscoline. It is also not known whether Priscoline can cause fetal harm when administered to a pregnant woman or can affect reproduction capacity. Priscoline should be given to a pregnant woman only if clearly needed.

Nursing Mothers: It is not known whether this drug is excreted in human milk. Because many drugs are excreted in human milk, caution should be exercised when Priscoline is administered to a nursing woman.

ADVERSE REACTIONS

The following adverse reactions have been observed, but there are insufficient data to support an estimate of their frequency:

Cardiovascular: Hypotension, tachycardia, cardiac arrhythmias, hypertension, pulmonary hemorrhage.

Digestive and Hepatic: Gastrointestinal hemorrhage, nausea, vomiting, diarrhea, hepatitis.

Skin: Flushing, increased pilomotor activity with tingling or chilliness, rash.

Hematologic: Thrombocytopenia, leukopenia.

Renal: Edema, oliguria, hematuria.

OVERDOSAGE

Acute Toxicity

Oral LD$_{50}$'s (mg/kg): mice, 400; rats, 1200.

Signs and Symptoms

Signs and symptoms of overdosage may include increased pilomotor activity, peripheral vasodilatation, skin flushing, and, in rare instances, hypotension and shock.

Treatment

In treating hypotension, it is most important to place the patient's head low and administer intravenous fluids. Epinephrine should not be used, since large doses of Priscoline may cause "epinephrine reversal" (further reduction in blood pressure, followed by an exaggerated rebound).

DOSAGE AND ADMINISTRATION

An initial dose of 1 to 2 mg/kg, via scalp vein, followed by an infusion of 1 to 2 mg/kg per hour have usually resulted in significant increases in arterial oxygen. There is very little experience with infusions lasting beyond 36 to 48 hours. Response, if it occurs, can be expected within 30 minutes after the initial dose.

Note: Parenteral drug products should be inspected visually for particulate matter and discoloration prior to administration, whenever solution and container permit.

HOW SUPPLIED

Ampuls—4 ml—each milliliter contains 25 mg of tolazoline hydrochloride.

Carton of 4 ampuls .... NDC 0083-6733-04

Store between 15° and 30°C (59°–86°F). Protect from light.

                                  C89-33 (Rev. 8/89)

REGITINE® ℞

[*rej 'a-teen*]

phentolamine mesylate USP

Vials

DESCRIPTION

Regitine, phentolamine mesylate USP, is an antihypertensive, available in vials for intravenous and intramuscular administration. Each vial contains phentolamine mesylate USP, 5 mg, and mannitol USP, 25 mg, in sterile, lyophilized form.

Phentolamine mesylate is 4,5-dihydro-2-[N-(*m*-hydroxyphenyl)-N-(*p*-methylphenyl) aminomethyl]-1H-imidazole 1:1 methanesulfonate.

Phentolamine mesylate USP is a white or off-white, odorless crystalline powder with a molecular weight of 377.46. Its solutions are acid to litmus. It is freely soluble in water and in alcohol, and slightly soluble in chloroform. It melts at about 178°C.

CLINICAL PHARMACOLOGY

Regitine produces an alpha-adrenergic block of relatively short duration. It also has direct, but less marked, positive inotropic and chronotropic effects on cardiac muscle and vasodilator effects on vascular smooth muscle.

Regitine has a half-life in the blood of 19 minutes following intravenous administration. Approximately 13% of a single intravenous dose appears in the urine as unchanged drug.

INDICATIONS AND USAGE

Regitine is indicated for the prevention or control of hypertensive episodes that may occur in a patient with pheochromocytoma as a result of stress or manipulation during preoperative preparation and surgical excision.

Regitine is indicated for the prevention or treatment of dermal necrosis and sloughing following intravenous administration or extravasation of norepinephrine.

Regitine is also indicated for the diagnosis of pheochromocytoma by the Regitine blocking test.

CONTRAINDICATIONS

Myocardial infarction, history of myocardial infarction, coronary insufficiency, angina, or other evidence suggestive of coronary artery disease; hypersensitivity to phentolamine or related compounds.

WARNINGS

Myocardial infarction, cerebrovascular spasm, and cerebrovascular occlusion have been reported to occur following the administration of Regitine, usually in association with marked hypotensive episodes.

For screening tests in patients with hypertension, the generally available urinary assay of catecholamines or other biochemical assays have largely replaced the Regitine and other pharmacological tests for reasons of accuracy and safety. None of the chemical or pharmacological tests is infallible in the diagnosis of pheochromocytoma. The Regitine blocking test is not the procedure of choice and should be reserved for cases in which additional confirmatory evidence is necessary and the relative risks involved in conducting the test have been considered.

PRECAUTIONS

General

Tachycardia and cardiac arrhythmias may occur with the use of Regitine or other alpha-adrenergic blocking agents. When possible, administration of cardiac glycosides should be deferred until cardiac rhythm returns to normal.

Drug Interactions

See **DOSAGE AND ADMINISTRATION, Diagnosis of pheochromocytoma,** *Preparation.*

Carcinogenesis, Mutagenesis, Impairment of Fertility

Long-term carcinogenicity studies, mutagenicity studies, and fertility studies have not been conducted with Regitine.

Pregnancy Category C

Administration of Regitine to pregnant rats and mice at oral doses 24–30 times the usual daily human dose (based on a 60-kg human) resulted in slightly decreased growth and slight skeletal immaturity of the fetuses. Immaturity was manifested by increased incidence of incomplete or unossified calcanei and phalangeal nuclei of the hind limb and of incompletely ossified sternebrae. At oral doses 60 times the usual daily human dose (based on a 60-kg human), a slightly lower rate of implantation was found in the rat. Regitine did not affect embryonic or fetal development in the rabbit at oral doses 20 times the usual daily human dose (based on a 60-kg human). No teratogenic or embryotoxic effects were observed in the rat, mouse, or rabbit studies.

There are no adequate and well-controlled studies in pregnant women. Regitine should be used during pregnancy only if the potential benefit justifies the potential risk to the fetus.

Nursing Mothers

It is not known whether this drug is excreted in human milk. Because many drugs are excreted in human milk and because of the potential for serious adverse reactions in nursing infants from Regitine, a decision should be made whether to discontinue nursing or to discontinue the drug, taking into account the importance of the drug to the mother.

Pediatric Use

See **DOSAGE AND ADMINISTRATION.**

ADVERSE REACTIONS

Acute and prolonged hypotensive episodes, tachycardia, and cardiac arrhythmias have been reported. In addition, weakness, dizziness, flushing, orthostatic hypotension, nasal stuffiness, nausea, vomiting, and diarrhea may occur.

OVERDOSAGE

Acute Toxicity

No deaths due to acute poisoning with Regitine have been reported.

Oral LD$_{50}$'s (mg/kg): mice, 1000; rats, 1250.

Signs and Symptoms

Overdosage with Regitine is characterized chiefly by cardiovascular disturbances, such as arrhythmias, tachycardia, hypotension, and possibly shock. In addition, the following might occur: excitation, headache, sweating, pupillary contraction, visual disturbances; nausea, vomiting, diarrhea; hypoglycemia.

Treatment

There is no specific antidote.

A decrease in blood pressure to dangerous levels or other evidence of shocklike conditions should be treated vigorously and promptly. The patient's legs should be kept raised and a plasma expander should be administered. If necessary, intra-

venous infusion of norepinephrine, titrated to maintain blood pressure at the normotensive level, and all available supportive measures should be included. Epinephrine should not be used, since it may cause a paradoxical reduction in blood pressure.

DOSAGE AND ADMINISTRATION

The reconstituted solution should be used upon preparation and should not be stored.

Note: Parenteral drug products should be inspected visually for particulate matter and discoloration prior to administration, whenever solution and container permit.

1. Prevention or control of hypertensive episodes in the patient with pheochromocytoma.

For preoperative reduction of elevated blood pressure, 5 mg of Regitine (1 mg for children) is injected intravenously or intramuscularly 1 or 2 hours before surgery, and repeated if necessary.

During surgery, Regitine (5 mg for adults, 1 mg for children) is administered intravenously as indicated, to help prevent or control paroxysms of hypertension, tachycardia, respiratory depression, convulsions, or other effects of epinephrine intoxication. (Postoperatively, norepinephrine may be given to control the hypotension that commonly follows complete removal of a pheochromocytoma.)

2. Prevention or treatment of dermal necrosis and sloughing following intravenous administration or extravasation of norepinephrine.

For Prevention: 10 mg of Regitine is added to each liter of solution containing norepinephrine. The pressor effect of norepinephrine is not affected.

For Treatment: 5–10 mg of Regitine in 10 ml of saline is injected into the area of extravasation within 12 hours.

3. Diagnosis of pheochromocytoma—Regitine blocking test.

The test is most reliable in detecting pheochromocytoma in patients with sustained hypertension and least reliable in those with paroxysmal hypertension. False-positive tests may occur in patients with hypertension without pheochromocytoma.

a. Intravenous

Preparation

The CONTRAINDICATIONS, WARNINGS, and PRECAUTIONS sections should be reviewed. Sedatives, analgesics, and all other medications except those that might be deemed essential (such as digitalis and insulin) are withheld for at least 24 hours, and preferably 48–72 hours, prior to the test. Antihypertensive drugs are withheld until blood pressure returns to the untreated, hypertensive level. This test is not performed on a patient who is normotensive.

Procedure

The patient is kept at rest in the supine position throughout the test, preferably in a quiet, darkened room. Injection of Regitine is delayed until blood pressure is stabilized, as evidenced by blood pressure readings taken every 10 minutes for at least 30 minutes.

Five milligrams of Regitine is dissolved in 1 ml of Sterile Water for Injection. The dose for adults is 5 mg; for children, 1 mg.

The syringe needle is inserted into the vein, and injection is delayed until pressor response to venipuncture has subsided. Regitine is injected rapidly. Blood pressure is recorded immediately after injection, at 30-second intervals for the first 3 minutes, and at 60-second intervals for the next 7 minutes.

Interpretation

A positive response, suggestive of pheochromocytoma, is indicated when the blood pressure is reduced more than 35 mm Hg systolic and 25 mm Hg diastolic. A typical positive response is a reduction in pressure of 60 mm Hg systolic and 25 mm Hg diastolic. Usually, maximal effect is evident within 2 minutes after injection. A return to preinjection pressure commonly occurs within 15–30 minutes but may occur more rapidly.

If blood pressure decreases to a dangerous level, the patient should be treated as outlined under **OVERDOSAGE.**

A positive response should always be confirmed by other diagnostic procedures, preferably by measurement of urinary catecholamines or their metabolites.

A negative response is indicated when the blood pressure is elevated, unchanged, or reduced less than 35 mm Hg systolic and 25 mm Hg diastolic after injection of Regitine. A negative reponse to this test does not exclude the diagnosis of pheochromocytoma, especially in patients with paroxysmal hypertension in whom the incidence of false-negative responses is high.

b. Intramuscular

If the intramuscular test for pheochromocytoma is preferred, preparation is the same as for the intravenous test. Five milligrams of Regitine is then dissolved in 1 ml of Sterile Water for Injection. The dose for adults is 5 mg intramuscularly; for children, 3 mg. Blood pressure is recorded every 5 minutes for 30–45 minutes following injection. A positive response is indicated when the blood pressure is reduced 35 mm Hg systolic and 25 mm Hg diastolic, or more, within 20 minutes following injection.

HOW SUPPLIED

Vials —each containing 5 mg of phentolamine mesylate USP and 25 mg of mannitol USP, in lyophilized form

Cartons of 2 .... NDC 0083-6830-02
Cartons of 6 .... NDC 0083-6830-06

The reconstituted solution should be used upon preparation and should not be stored.

Store between 59° and 86°F.

Dist. by:
Ciba Pharmaceutical Company
Ciba-Geigy Corporation
Summit, NJ 07901

C85-2 (Rev. 8/85)

RIMACTANE® ℞
[re-mack 'tayne]
rifampin USP

DESCRIPTION

Rimactane, rifampin USP , is a semisynthetic antibiotic derivative of rifamycin B, available as 300-mg capsules for oral administration. It is also available in Dual Packs containing two 300-mg capsules of Rimactane and one 300-mg tablet of INH®, isoniazid USP. Rimactane is 3-[[(4-methyl-1-piperazinyl)imino]methyl] rifamycin.

Rifampin USP is a red-brown crystalline powder. It is very slightly soluble in water, freely soluble in chloroform, and soluble in ethyl acetate and in methanol. Its molecular weight is 822.95.

Inactive Ingredients: FD&C Blue No. 1, FD&C Red No. 40, FD&C Yellow No. 6, gelatin, lactose, magnesium stearate, methylparaben, propylparaben, silicon dioxide, sodium lauryl sulfate, starch, talc, and titanium dioxide.

ACTIONS

Rimactane inhibits DNA-dependent RNA polymerase activity in susceptible cells. Specifically, it interacts with bacterial RNA polymerase but does not inhibit the mammalian enzyme. This is the mechanism of action by which Rimactane exerts its therapeutic effect. Rimactane cross resistance has only been shown with other rifamycins.

Peak blood levels in normal adults vary widely from individual to individual. Peak levels occur between 2 and 4 hours following the oral administration of a 600-mg dose. The average peak value is 7 mcg/ml; however, the peak level may vary from 4 to 32 mcg/ml.

In normal subjects the $T\frac{1}{2}$ (biological half-life) of Rimactane in blood is approximately 3 hours. Elimination occurs mainly through the bile and, to a much lesser extent, the urine.

INDICATIONS

Pulmonary Tuberculosis

In the initial treatment and in the retreatment of pulmonary tuberculosis, Rimactane must be used in conjunction with at least one other antituberculous drug.

Frequently used regimens have been the following:

    isoniazid and Rimactane

    ethambutol and Rimactane

    isoniazid, ethambutol, and Rimactane

Neisseria Meningitidis Carriers

Rimactane is indicated for the treatment of asymptomatic carriers of *N. meningitidis* to eliminate meningococci from the nasopharynx.

Rimactane is not indicated for the treatment of meningococcal infection.

To avoid the indiscriminate use of Rimactane, diagnostic laboratory procedures, including serotyping and susceptibility testing, should be performed to establish the carrier state and the correct treatment. In order to preserve the usefulness of Rimactane in the treatment of asymptomatic meningococcal carriers, it is recommended that the drug be reserved for situations in which the risk of meningococcal meningitis is high.

Both in the treatment of tuberculosis and in the treatment of meningococcal carriers, small numbers of resistant cells, present within large populations of susceptible cells, can rapidly become the predominating type. Since rapid emergence of resistance can occur, culture and susceptibility tests should be performed in the event of persistent positive cultures.

CONTRAINDICATIONS

A history of previous hypersensitivity reaction to any of the rifamycins.

WARNINGS

Rifampin has been shown to produce liver dysfunction. There have been fatalities associated with jaundice in patients with liver disease or receiving rifampin concomitantly with other hepatotoxic agents. Since an increased risk may exist for individuals with liver disease, benefits must be weighed carefully against the risk of further liver damage. Periodic liver function monitoring is mandatory.

The possibility of rapid emergence of resistant meningococci restricts the use of Rimactane to short-term treatment of the asymptomatic carrier state. Rimactane is not to be used for the treatment of meningococcal disease.

Several studies of tumorigenicity potential have been done in rodents. In one strain of mice known to be particularly susceptible to the spontaneous development of hepatomas, rifampin given at a level 2–10 times the maximum dosage used clinically, resulted in a significant increase in the occurrence of hepatomas in female mice of this strain after one year of administration. There was no evidence of tumorigenicity in the males of this strain, in males or females of another mouse strain, or rats.

Usage in Pregnancy

Although rifampin has been reported to cross the placental barrier and appear in cord blood, the effect of Rimactane, alone or in combination with other antituberculous drugs, on the human fetus is not known. An increase in congenital malformations, primarily spina bifida and cleft palate, has been reported in the offspring of rodents given oral doses of 150-250 mg/kg/day of rifampin during pregnancy.

The possible teratogenic potential in women capable of bearing children should be carefully weighed against the benefits of therapy.

PRECAUTIONS

Rimactane is not recommended for intermittent therapy; the patient should be cautioned against intentional or accidental interruption of the daily dosage regimen since rare renal hypersensitivity reactions have been reported when therapy was resumed in such cases.

Rifampin has been observed to increase the requirements for anticoagulant drugs of the coumarin type. The cause of this phenomenon is unknown. In patients receiving anticoagulants and rifampin concurrently, it is recommended that the prothrombin time be performed daily or as frequently as necessary to establish and maintain the required dose of anticoagulant.

Urine, feces, saliva, sputum, sweat, and tears may be colored red-orange by rifampin and its metabolites. Soft contact lenses may be permanently stained. Individuals to be treated should be made aware of these possibilities.

It has been reported that the reliability of oral contraceptives may be affected in some patients being treated for tuberculosis with rifampin in combination with at least one other antituberculous drug. In such cases, alternative contraceptive measures may need to be considered.

Rifampin has been reported to diminish the effects of concurrently administered methadone, oral hypoglycemics, corticosteroids, dapsone, digitalis preparations and to reduce the bioavailability and efficacy of verapamil. Appropriate dosage adjustments may be necessary if indicated by the patient's clinical condition.

When rifampin is taken in combination with PAS, decreased rifampin serum levels may result. Therefore, the drugs should be given at least 4 hours apart.

Therapeutic levels of rifampin have been shown to inhibit standard assays for serum folate and vitamin B_{12}. Alternative methods must be considered when determining folate and vitamin B_{12} concentrations in the presence of rifampin. Since rifampin has been reported to cross the placental barrier and appear in cord blood, neonates of rifampin-treated mothers should be carefully observed for any evidence of adverse effects. Rifampin is excreted in breast milk.

ADVERSE REACTIONS

Gastrointestinal disturbances such as heartburn, epigastric distress, anorexia, nausea, vomiting, gas, cramps, and diarrhea have been noted in some patients. Rarely, pseudomembranous enterocolitis has been reported. Headache, drowsiness, fatigue, ataxia, dizziness, inability to concentrate, mental confusion, visual disturbances, muscular weakness, fever, pains in extremities, generalized numbness, and menstrual disturbances have also been noted.

Hypersensitivity reactions have been reported. Encountered occasionally have been pruritus, urticaria, rash, pemphigoid reaction, eosinophilia, sore mouth, sore tongue, and exudative conjunctivitis. Rarely, hepatitis or a shock-like syndrome with hepatic involvement and abnormal liver function tests have been reported. Transient abnormalities in liver function tests (eg, elevations in serum bilirubin, BSP, alkaline phosphatase, serum transaminases) have also been observed. The BSP test should be performed prior to the morning dose of rifampin to avoid false-positive results. Thrombocytopenia, transient leukopenia, hemolytic anemia, and decreased hemoglobin have been observed. Thrombocytopenia has occurred when rifampin and ethambutol were administered concomitantly according to an intermittent dose schedule twice weekly and in high doses.

Elevations in BUN and serum uric acid have occurred. Rarely, hemolysis, hemoglobinuria, hematuria, renal insufficiency or acute renal failure have been reported and are generally considered to be hypersensitivity reactions. These have usually occurred during intermittent therapy or when

Continued on next page

CibaGeneva—Cont.

treatment was resumed following intentional or accidental interruption of a daily dosage regimen and were reversible when rifampin was discontinued and appropriate therapy instituted.

Although rifampin has been reported to have an immunosuppressive effect in some animal experiments, available human data indicate that this has no clinical significance.

DOSAGE AND ADMINISTRATION

It is recommended that Rimactane be administered once daily, either one hour before or two hours after a meal. Data are not available for determination of dosage for children under 5.

Pulmonary Tuberculosis

Adults: 600 mg (two 300-mg Capsules) in a single daily administration.

Children: 10 to 20 mg/kg, not to exceed 600 mg/day.

In the treatment of pulmonary tuberculosis, Rimactane must be used in conjunction with at least one other antituberculous agent. In general, therapy should be continued until bacterial conversion and maximal improvement have occurred.

Meningococcal Carriers

It is recommended that Rimactane be administered once daily for four consecutive days in the following doses:

Adults: 600 mg (two 300-mg Capsules) in a single daily administration.

Children: 10 to 20 mg/kg, not to exceed 600 mg/day.

Susceptibility Testing

Pulmonary Tuberculosis: Rifampin susceptibility powders are available for both direct and indirect methods of determining the susceptibility of strains of mycobacteria. The MICs of susceptible clinical isolates when determined in 7H10 or other non-egg-containing media have ranged from 0.1 to 2 mcg/ml.

Meningococcal Carriers: Susceptibility discs containing 5 mcg rifampin are available for susceptibility testing of *N. meningitidis.*

Quantitative methods that require measurement of zone diameters give the most precise estimates of antibiotic susceptibility. One such procedure[1] has been recommended for use with discs for testing susceptibility to rifampin. Interpretations correlate zone diameters from the disc test with MIC (minimal inhibitory concentration) values for rifampin. A range of MIC's from 0.1 to 1 mcg/ml has been found *in vitro* for susceptible strains of *N. meningitidis.* With this procedure, a report from the laboratory of "resistant" indicates that the organism is not likely to be eradicated from the nasopharynx of asymptomatic carriers.

OVERDOSAGE

Signs and Symptoms

Nausea, vomiting, and increasing lethargy will probably occur within a short time after ingestion; actual unconsciousness may occur with severe hepatic involvement. Brownish-red or orange discoloration of the skin, urine, sweat, saliva, tears, and feces is proportional to amount ingested.

Liver enlargement, possibly with tenderness, can develop within a few hours after severe overdosage and jaundice may develop rapidly. Hepatic involvement may be more marked in patients with prior impairment of hepatic function. Other physical findings remain essentially normal.

Direct and total bilirubin levels may increase rapidly with severe overdosage; hepatic enzyme levels may be affected, especially with prior impairment of hepatic function. A direct effect upon hemopoietic system, electrolyte levels, or acid-base balance is unlikely.

Treatment

Since nausea and vomiting are likely to be present, gastric lavage is probably preferable to induction of emesis. Activated charcoal slurry instilled into the stomach following evacuation of gastric contents can help absorb any remaining drug in G.I. tract. Antiemetic medication may be required to control severe nausea/vomiting.

Active diuresis (with measured intake and output) will help promote excretion of the drug. Bile drainage may be indicated in presence of serious impairment of hepatic function lasting more than 24–48 hours; under these circumstances, extracorporeal hemodialysis may be required.

In patients with previously adequate hepatic function, reversal of liver enlargement and impaired hepatic excretory function probably will be noted within 72 hours, with rapid return toward normal thereafter.

HOW SUPPLIED

Capsules 300 mg—opaque, scarlet, caramel (imprinted CIBA 154)

Bottles of 30 ....NDC 0083-0154-26
Bottles of 60 ....NDC 0083-0154-29
Bottles of 100 ....NDC 0083-0154-30

Do not store above 86°F (30°C).

Keep tightly closed. Protect from heat and moisture.
Dispense in tight, light-resistant container (USP).
Also available—Rimactane®/INH® (isoniazid USP) Dual Pack. Each Dual Pack contains two Rimactane 300-mg capsules and one INH 300-mg tablet.

Cartons of 30 Dual Packs
(60 Rimactane capsules and
30 INH tablets)...NDC 0083-8912-23
Store between 59°–86°F (15°–30°C). Protect from light and moisture.

REFERENCE

1. Bauer AW, Kirby WMM, Sherris JC, et al: Antibiotic susceptibility testing by a standardized single disk method. *Am J Clin Path* 1966;45:493–496.

C92-7 (Rev. 3/92)

Shown in Product Identification Guide, page 309

RITALIN® hydrochloride   Ⓒ
[*rit'ah-lin*]
methylphenidate hydrochloride
tablets USP

RITALIN-SR®   Ⓒ
methylphenidate hydrochloride USP
sustained-release tablets

Prescribing Information

DESCRIPTION

Ritalin hydrochloride, methylphenidate hydrochloride USP, is a mild central nervous system (CNS) stimulant, available as tablets of 5, 10, and 20 mg for oral administration; Ritalin-SR is available as sustained-release tablets of 20 mg for oral administration. Methylphenidate hydrochloride is methyl α-phenyl-2-piperidineacetate hydrochloride.

Methylphenidate hydrochloride USP is a white, odorless, fine crystalline powder. Its solutions are acid to litmus. It is freely soluble in water and in methanol, soluble in alcohol, and slightly soluble in chloroform and in acetone. Its molecular weight is 269.77.

Inactive Ingredients. Ritalin tablets: D&C Yellow No. 10 (5-mg and 20-mg tablets), FD&C Green No. 3 (10-mg tablets), lactose, magnesium stearate, polyethylene glycol, starch (5-mg and 10-mg tablets), sucrose, talc, and tragacanth (20-mg tablets).

Ritalin-SR tablets: Cellulose compounds, cetostearyl alcohol, lactose, magnesium stearate, mineral oil, povidone, titanium dioxide, and zein.

CLINICAL PHARMACOLOGY

Ritalin is a mild central nervous system stimulant.

The mode of action in man is not completely understood, but Ritalin presumably activates the brain stem arousal system and cortex to produce its stimulant effect.

There is neither specific evidence which clearly establishes the mechanism whereby Ritalin produces its mental and behavioral effects in children, nor conclusive evidence regarding how these effects relate to the condition of the central nervous system.

Ritalin in the SR tablets is more slowly but as extensively absorbed as in the regular tablets. Relative bioavailability of the SR tablet compared to the Ritalin tablet, measured by the urinary excretion of Ritalin major metabolite (α-phenyl-2-piperidine acetic acid) was 105% (49%–168%) in children and 101% (85%–152%) in adults. The time to peak rate in children was 4.7 hours (1.3–8.2 hours) for the SR tablets and 1.9 hours (0.3–4.4 hours) for the tablets. An average of 67% of SR tablet dose was excreted in children as compared to 86% in adults. In a clinical study involving adult subjects who received SR tablets, plasma concentrations of Ritalin's major metabolite appeared to be greater in females than in males. No gender differences were observed for Ritalin plasma concentration in the same subjects.

INDICATIONS

Attention Deficit Disorders, Narcolepsy

Attention Deficit Disorders (previously known as Minimal Brain Dysfunction in Children). Other terms being used to describe the behavioral syndrome below include: Hyperkinetic Child Syndrome, Minimal Brain Damage, Minimal Cerebral Dysfunction, Minor Cerebral Dysfunction.

Ritalin is indicated as an integral part of a total treatment program which typically includes other remedial measures (psychological, educational, social) for a stabilizing effect in children with a behavioral syndrome characterized by the following group of developmentally inappropriate symptoms, moderate-to-severe distractibility, short attention span, hyperactivity, emotional lability, and impulsivity. The diagnosis of this syndrome should not be made with finality when these symptoms are only of comparatively recent origin. Nonlocalizing (soft) neurological signs, learning disability, and abnormal EEG may or may not be present, and a diagnosis of central nervous system dysfunction may or may not be warranted.

Special Diagnostic Considerations

Specific etiology of this syndrome is unknown, and there is no single diagnostic test. Adequate diagnosis requires the use not only of medical but of special psychological, educational, and social resources.

Characteristics commonly reported include: chronic history of short attention span, distractibility, emotional lability, impulsivity, and moderate-to-severe hyperactivity; minor neurological signs and abnormal EEG. Learning may or may not be impaired. The diagnosis must be based upon a complete history and evaluation of the child and not solely on the presence of one or more of these characteristics.

Drug treatment is not indicated for all children with this syndrome. Stimulants are not intended for use in the child who exhibits symptoms secondary to environmental factors and/or primary psychiatric disorders, including psychosis. Appropriate educational placement is essential and psychosocial intervention is generally necessary. When remedial measures alone are insufficient, the decision to prescribe stimulant medication will depend upon the physician's assessment of the chronicity and severity of the child's symptoms.

CONTRAINDICATIONS

Marked anxiety, tension, and agitation are contraindications to Ritalin, since the drug may aggravate these symptoms. Ritalin is contraindicated also in patients known to be hypersensitive to the drug, in patients with glaucoma, and in patients with motor tics or with a family history or diagnosis of Tourette's syndrome.

WARNINGS

Ritalin should not be used in children under six years, since safety and efficacy in this age group have not been established.

Sufficient data on safety and efficacy of long-term use of Ritalin in children are not yet available. Although a causal relationship has not been established, suppression of growth (ie, weight gain, and/or height) has been reported with the long-term use of stimulants in children. Therefore, patients requiring long-term therapy should be carefully monitored.

Ritalin should not be used for severe depression of either exogenous or endogenous origin. Clinical experience suggests that in phychotic childern, administration of Ritalin may exacerbate symptoms of behavior disturbance and thought disorder.

Ritalin should not be used for the prevention or treatment of normal fatigue states.

There is some clinical evidence that Ritalin may lower the convulsive threshold in patients with prior history of seizures, with prior EEG abnormalities in absence of seizures, and, very rarely, in absence of history of seizures and no prior EEG evidence of seizures. Safe concomitant use of anticonvulsants and Ritalin has not been established. In the presence of seizures, the drug should be discontinued.

Use cautiously in patients with hypertension. Blood pressure should be monitored at appropriate intervals in all patients taking Ritalin, especially those with hypertension.

Symptoms of visual disturbances have been encountered in rare cases. Difficulties with accommodation and blurring of vision have been reported.

Drug Interactions

Ritalin may decrease the hypotensive effect of guanethidine. Use cautiously with pressor agents and MAO inhibitors.

Human pharmacologic studies have shown that Ritalin may inhibit the metabolism of coumarin anticoagulants, anticonvulsants (phenobarbital, diphenylhydantoin, primidone), phenylbutazone, and tricyclic drugs (imipramine, clomipramine, desipramine). Downward dosage adjustments of these drugs may be required when given concomitantly with Ritalin.

Usage in Pregnancy

Adequate animal reproduction studies, to establish safe use of Ritalin during pregnancy have not been conducted. Therefore, until more information is available, Ritalin should not be prescribed for women of childbearing age unless, in the opinion of the physician, the potential benefits outweigh the possible risks.

Drug Dependence

Ritalin should be given cautiously to emotionally unstable patients, such as those with a history of drug dependence or alcoholism, because such patients may increase dosage on their own initiative.

Chronically abusive use can lead to marked tolerance and psychic dependence with varying degrees of abnormal behavior. Frank psychotic episodes can occur, especially with parenteral abuse. Careful supervision is required during drug withdrawal, since severe depression as well as the effects of chronic overactivity can be unmasked. Long-term follow-up may be required because of the patient's basic personality disturbances.

PRECAUTIONS

Patients with an element of agitation may react adversely; discontinue therapy if necessary.

Periodic CBC, differential, and platelet counts are advised during prolonged therapy.

Drug treatment is not indicated in all cases of this behavioral syndrome and should be considered only in light of the complete history and evaluation of the child. The decision to prescribe Ritalin should depend on the physician's assessment of the chronicity and severity of the child's symptoms and their appropriateness for his/her age. Prescription should not depend solely on the presence of one or more of the behavioral characteristics.

When these symptoms are associated with acute stress reactions, treatment with Ritalin is usually not indicated.

Long-term effects of Ritalin in children have not been well established.

Carcinogenesis/Mutagenesis

In a lifetime carcinogenicity study carried out in B6C3F1 mice, methylphenidate caused an increase in hepatocellular adenomas and, in males only, an increase in hepatoblastomas, at a daily dose of approximately 60 mg/kg/day. This dose is approximately 30 times and 2.5 times the maximum recommended human dose on a mg/kg and mg/m^2 basis, respectively. Hepatoblastoma is a relatively rare rodent malignant tumor type. There was no increase in total malignant hepatic tumors. The mouse strain used is sensitive to the development of hepatic tumors, and the significance of these results to humans is unknown.

Methylphenidate did not cause any increases in tumors in a lifetime carcinogenicity study carried out in F344 rats; the highest dose used was approximately 45 mg/kg/day, which is approximately 22 times and 4 times the maximum recommended human dose on a mg/kg and mg/m^2 basis, respectively.

Methylphenidate was not mutagenic in the in vitro Ames reverse mutation assay or in the in vitro mouse lymphoma cell forward mutation assay. Sister chromatid exchanges and chromosome aberrations were increased, indicative of a weak clastogenic response, in an in vitro assay in cultured Chinese Hamster Ovary (CHO) cells. The genotoxic potential of methylphenidate has not been evaluated in an in vivo assay.

ADVERSE REACTIONS

Nervousness and insomnia are the most common adverse reactions but are usually controlled by reducing dosage and omitting the drug in the afternoon or evening. Other reactions include hypersensitivity (including skin rash, urticaria, fever, arthralgia, exfoliative dermatitis, erythema multiforme with histopathological findings of necrotizing vasculitis, and thrombocytopenic purpura); anorexia; nausea; dizziness; palpitations; headache; dyskinesia; drowsiness; blood pressure and pulse changes, both up and down; tachycardia; angina; cardiac arrhythmia; abdominal pain; weight loss during prolonged therapy. There have been rare reports of Tourette's syndrome. Toxic psychosis has been reported. Although a definite causal relationship has not been established, the following have been reported in patients taking this drug: instances of abnormal liver function, ranging from transaminase elevation to hepatic coma; isolated cases of cerebral arteritis and/or occlusion; leukopenia and/or anemia; transient depressed mood; a few instances of scalp hair loss.

In children, loss of appetite, abdominal pain, weight loss during prolonged therapy, insomnia, and tachycardia may occur more frequently; however, any of the other adverse reactions listed above may also occur.

DOSAGE AND ADMINISTRATION

Dosage should be individualized according to the needs and responses of the patient.

Adults

Tablets: Administer in divided doses 2 or 3 times daily, preferably 30 to 45 minutes before meals. Average dosage is 20 to 30 mg daily. Some patients may require 40 to 60 mg daily. In others, 10 to 15 mg daily will be adequate. Patients who are unable to sleep if medication is taken late in the day should take the last dose before 6 p.m.

SR Tablets: Ritalin-SR tablets have a duration of action of approximately 8 hours. Therefore, Ritalin-SR tablets may be used in place of Ritalin tablets when the 8-hour dosage of Ritalin-SR corresponds to the titrated 8-hour dosage of Ritalin. Ritalin-SR tablets must be swallowed whole and never crushed or chewed.

Children (6 years and over)

Ritalin should be initiated in small doses, with gradual weekly increments. Daily dosage above 60 mg is not recommended.

If improvement is not observed after appropriate dosage adjustment over a one-month period, the drug should be discontinued.

Tablets: Start with 5 mg twice daily (before breakfast and lunch) with gradual increments of 5 to 10 mg weekly.

SR Tablets: Ritalin-SR tablets have a duration of action of approximately 8 hours. Therefore, Ritalin-SR tablets may be used in place of Ritalin tablets when the 8-hour dosage of Ritalin-SR corresponds to the titrated 8-hour dosage of Ritalin. Ritalin-SR tablets must be swallowed whole and never crushed or chewed.

If paradoxical aggravation of symptoms or other adverse effects occur, reduce dosage, or, if necessary, discontinue the drug.

Ritalin should be periodically discontinued to assess the child's condition. Improvement may be sustained when the drug is either temporarily or permanently discontinued.

Drug treatment should not and need not be indefinite and usually may be discontinued after puberty.

OVERDOSAGE

Signs and symptoms of acute overdosage, resulting principally from overstimulation of the central nervous system and from excessive sympathomimetic effects, may include the following, agitation, tremors, hyperreflexia, muscle twitching, convulsions (may be followed by coma), euphoria, confusion, hallucinations, delirium, sweating, flushing, headache, hyperpyrexia, tachycardia, palpitations, cardiac arrhythmias, hypertension, mydriasis, and dryness of mucous membranes.

Consult with a Certified Poison Control Center regarding treatment for up-to-date guidance and advice.

Treatment consists of appropriate supportive measures. The patient must be protected against self-injury and against external stimuli that would aggravate overstimulation already present. Gastic contents may be evacuated by gastric lavage. In the presence of severe intoxication, use a carefully titrated dosage of a *short-acting* barbiturate before performing gastric lavage. Other measures to detoxify the gut include administration of activated charcoal and a cathartic.

Intensive care must be provided to maintain adequate circulation and respiratory exchange; external cooling procedures may be required for hyperpyrexia.

Efficacy of peritoneal dialysis or extracorporeal hemodialysis for Ritalin overdosage has not been established.

HOW SUPPLIED

Tablets 5 mg—round, yellow (imprinted CIBA 7)

Bottles of 100 .... NDC 0083-0007-30

Tablets 10 mg—round, pale green, scored (imprinted CIBA 3)

Bottles of 100 .... NDC 0083-0003-30

Tablets 20 mg—round, pale yellow, scored (imprinted CIBA 34)

Bottles of 100 .... NDC 0083-0034-30

Protect from light.

Do not store above 86°F (30°C).

Dispense in tight, light-resistant container (USP).

SR Tablets 20 mg—round, white, coated (imprinted CIBA 16)

Bottles of 100 .... NDC 0083-0016-30

Note: SR Tablets are color-additive free.

Do not store above 86°F (30°C). Protect from moisture.

Dispense in tight, light-resistant container (USP).

C96-8 (Rev. 2/96)

Ciba-Geigy Corporation
Pharmaceuticals Division
Summit, New Jersey 07901

Shown in Product Identification Guide, page 309

SER-AP-ES® ℞

reserpine USP 0.1 mg
hydralazine hydrochloride USP 25 mg
hydrochlorothiazide USP 15 mg

Combination Tablets

PRESCRIBING INFORMATION

> **WARNING**
> This fixed-combination drug is not indicated for initial therapy of hypertension. Hypertension requires therapy titrated to the individual patient. If the fixed combination represents the dosage so determined, its use may be more convenient in patient management. The treatment of hypertension is not static but must be reevaluated as conditions in each patient warrant.

DESCRIPTION

Ser-Ap-Es is an antihypertensive-diuretic combination, available as tablets for oral administration. Each tablet contains Serpasil (reserpine USP), 0.1 mg; Apresoline (hydralazine hydrochloride USP), 25 mg; and Esidrix (hydrochlorothiazide USP), 15 mg.

Reserpine is methyl 18β-hydroxy-11, 17α-dimethoxy-3β, 20α-yohimban-16β-carboxylate 3,4,5-trimethoxybenzoate (ester).

Reserpine USP, a pure crystalline alkaloid of rauwolfia, is a white or pale buff to slightly yellowish, odorless crystalline powder. It darkens slowly on exposure to light, but more rapidly when in solution. It is insoluble in water, freely soluble in acetic acid and in chloroform, slightly soluble in benzene, and very slightly soluble in alcohol and in ether. Its molecular weight is 608.69.

Hydralazine hydrochloride is 1-hydrazinophthalazine monohydrochloride.

Hydralazine hydrochloride USP is a white to off-white, odorless crystalline powder. It is soluble in water, slightly soluble in alcohol, and very slightly soluble in ether. It melts at about 275°C, with decomposition, and has a molecular weight of 196.64.

Hydrochlorothiazide is 6-chloro-3,4-dihydro-2*H*-1,2,4-benzothiadiazine-7-sulfonamide 1, 1-dioxide.

Hydrochlorothiazide USP is a white, or practically white, practically odorless crystalline powder. It is slightly soluble in water; freely soluble in sodium hydroxide solution, in *n*-butylamine, and in dimethylformamide; sparingly soluble in methanol; and insoluble in ether, in chloroform, and in dilute mineral acids. Its molecular weight is 297.73.

Inactive Ingredients: Acacia, FD&C Blue No. 1, FD&C Green No. 3, FD&C Red No. 40, FD&C Yellow No. 6, lactose, polyethylene glycol, starch, stearic acid and sucrose.

CLINICAL PHARMACOLOGY

Reserpine: Reserpine depletes stores of catecholamines and 5-hydroxytryptamine in many organs, including the brain and adrenal medulla. Most of its pharmacological effects have been attributed to this action. Depletion is slower and less complete in the adrenal medulla than in other tissues.

The depression of sympathetic nerve function results in a decreased heart rate and a lowering of arterial blood pressure. The sedative and tranquilizing properties of reserpine are thought to be related to depletion of catecholamines and 5-hydroxytryptamine from the brain.

Reserpine, like other rauwolfia compounds, is characterized by slow onset of action and sustained effects. Both cardiovascular and central nervous system effects may persist for a period of time following withdrawal of the drug.

Mean maximum plasma levels of 1.54 ng/ml were attained after a median of 3.5 hours in six normal subjects receiving a single oral dose of four 0.25-mg Serpasil tablets. Bioavailability was approximately 50% of that of a corresponding intravenous dose. Plasma levels of reserpine after intravenous administration declined with a mean half-life of 33 hours. Reserpine is extensively bound (96%) to plasma proteins. No definitive studies on the human metabolism of reserpine have been made.

Hydralazine: Although the precise mechanism of action of hydralazine is not fully understood, the major effects are on the cardiovascular system. Hydralazine apparently lowers blood pressure by exerting a peripheral vasodilating effect through a direct relaxation of vascular smooth muscle. Hydralazine, by altering cellular calcium metabolism, interferes with the calcium movements within the vascular smooth muscle that are responsible for initiating or maintaining the contractile state.

The peripheral vasodilating effect of hydralazine results in decreased arterial blood pressure (diastolic more than systolic); decreased peripheral vascular resistance; and in increased heart rate, stroke volume, and cardiac output. The preferential dilatation of arterioles, as compared to veins, minimizes postural hypotension and promotes the increase in cardiac output. Hydralazine usually increases renin activity in plasma, presumably as a result of increased secretion of renin by the renal juxtaglomerular cells in response to reflex sympathetic discharge. This increase in renin activity leads to the production of angiotensin II, which then causes stimulation of aldosterone and consequent sodium reabsorption. Hydralazine also maintains or increases renal and cerebral blood flow.

Hydralazine is rapidly absorbed after oral administration, and peak plasma levels are reached at 1–2 hours. Plasma levels decline with a half-life of 3–7 hours. Binding to human plasma protein is 87%. Plasma levels of hydralazine vary widely among individuals. Hydralazine is subject to polymorphic acetylation; slow acetylators generally have higher plasma levels of hydralazine and require lower doses to maintain control of blood pressure. Hydralazine undergoes extensive hepatic metabolism; it is excreted mainly in the form of metabolites in the urine.

Administration of hydralazine with food results in higher levels of the drug in plasma.

Hydrochlorothiazide: Thiazides affect the renal tubular mechanism of electrolyte reabsorption. At maximal therapeutic dosage, all thiazides are approximately equal in their diuretic potency. Thiazides increase excretion of sodium and chloride in approximately equivalent amounts. Natriuresis causes a secondary loss of potassium.

The mechanism of the antihypertensive effect of thiazides is unknown. Thiazides do not affect normal blood pressure.

The onset of action of thiazides occurs in 2 hours, and the peak effect at about 4 hours. The action persists for approximately 6–12 hours. Hydrochlorothiazide is rapidly absorbed, as indicated by peak plasma concentrations 1–2.5 hours after

Continued on next page

CibaGeneva—Cont.

oral administration. Plasma levels of the drug are proportional to dose; the concentration in whole blood is 1.6–1.8 times higher than in plasma. Thiazides are eliminated rapidly by the kidney. After oral administration of 25- to 100-mg doses of hydrochlorothiazide, 72–97% of the dose is excreted in the urine, indicating dose-independent absorption. Hydrochlorothiazide is eliminated from plasma in a biphasic fashion with a terminal half-life of 10–17 hours. Plasma protein binding is 67.9%. Plasma clearance is 15.9–30.0 L/hr; volume of distribution is 3.6–7.8 L/kg.

Gastrointestinal absorption of hydrochlorothiazide is enhanced when administered with food. Absorption is decreased in patients with congestive heart failure, and the pharmacokinetics are considerably different in these patients.

INDICATIONS AND USAGE
Hypertension (see boxed WARNING).

CONTRAINDICATIONS
Reserpine: Hypersensitivity to reserpine; mental depression or history of mental depression (especially with suicidal tendencies); active peptic ulcer, ulcerative colitis; patients receiving electroconvulsive therapy.

Hydralazine: Hypersensitivity to hydralazine; coronary artery disease; mitral valvular rheumatic heart disease.

Hydrochlorothiazide: Anuria; hypersensitivity to this or other sulfonamide-derived drugs.

WARNINGS
Reserpine: Reserpine may cause mental depression. Recognition of depression may be difficult because this condition may often be disguised by somatic complaints. The drug should be discontinued at first signs of depression such as despondency, early morning insomnia, loss of appetite, impotence, or self-deprecation. Drug-induced depression may persist for several months after drug withdrawal and may be severe enough to result in suicide.

Hydralazine: In a few patients hydralazine may produce a clinical picture simulating systemic lupus erythematosus including glomerulonephritis. In such patients hydralazine should be discontinued unless the benefit-to-risk determination requires continued antihypertensive therapy with this drug. Signs and symptoms usually regress when the drug is discontinued, but residua have been detected many years later. Long-term treatment with steroids may be necessary. (See PRECAUTIONS, Laboratory Tests.)

Hydrochlorothiazide: Thiazides should be used with caution in patients with severe renal disease. In patients with renal disease, thiazides may precipitate azotemia. Cumulative effects of the drug may develop in patients with impaired renal function.

Thiazides should be used with caution in patients with impaired hepatic function or progressive liver disease, since minor alterations of fluid and electrolyte imbalance may precipitate hepatic coma.

Thiazides may add to or potentiate the action of other antihypertensive drugs. Potentiation occurs with ganglionic or peripheral adrenergic blocking drugs.

Sensitivity reactions are more likely to occur in patients with a history of allergy or bronchial asthma.

The possibility of exacerbation or activation of systemic lupus erythematosus has been reported.

PRECAUTIONS
General
Reserpine: Since reserpine increases gastrointestinal motility and secretion, it should be used cautiously in patients with a history of peptic ulcer, ulcerative colitis, or gallstones (billiary colic may be precipitated).

Caution should be exercised when treating hypertensive patients with renal insufficiency, since they adjust poorly to lowered blood pressure levels.

Preoperative withdrawal of reserpine does not assure that circulatory instability will not occur. It is important that the anesthesiologist be aware of the patient's drug intake and consider this in the overall management, since hypotension has occurred in patients receiving rauwolfia preparations. Anticholinergic and adrenergic drugs (e.g., metaraminol, norepinephrine) have been employed to treat adverse vagocirculatory effects.

Hydralazine: Myocardial stimulation produced by hydralazine can cause anginal attacks and ECG changes indicative of myocardial ischemia. The drug has been implicated in the production of myocardial infarction. It must, therefore, be used with caution in patients with suspected coronary artery disease.

The "hyperdynamic" circulation caused by hydralazine may accentuate specific cardiovascular inadequacies. For example, hydralazine may increase pulmonary artery pressure in patients with mitral valvular disease. The drug may reduce the pressor responses to epinephrine. Postural hypotension may result from hydralazine but is less common than with

ganglionic blocking agents. It should be used with caution in patients with cerebral vascular accidents.

In hypertensive patients with normal kidneys who are treated with hydralazine, there is evidence of increased renal blood flow and a maintenance of glomerular filtration rate. In some instances where control values were below normal, improved renal function has been noted after administration of hydralazine. However, as with any antihypertensive agent, hydralazine should be used with caution in patients with advanced renal damage.

Peripheral neuritis, evidenced by paresthesia, numbness, and tingling, has been observed. Published evidence suggests that hydralazine has an antipyridoxine effect and that pyridoxine should be added to the regimen if symptoms develop.

Hydrochlorothiazide: All patients receiving thiazide therapy should be observed for clinical signs of fluid or electrolyte imbalance, namely hyponatremia, hypochloremic alkalosis, and hypokalemia (see Laboratory Tests and Drug/Drug Interactions). Warning signs are dryness of mouth, thirst, weakness, lethargy, drowsiness, restlessness, muscle pains or cramps, muscular fatigue, hypotension, oliguria, tachycardia, and gastrointestinal disturbance, such as nausea or vomiting.

Hypokalemia may develop, especially in cases of brisk diuresis or severe cirrhosis.

Interference with adequate oral intake of electrolytes will also contribute to hypokalemia. Hypokalemia may be avoided or treated by use of potassium supplements or foods with a high potassium content.

Any chloride deficit is generally mild and usually does not require specific treatment, except under extraordinary circumstances (as in liver disease or renal disease). Dilutional hyponatremia may occur in edematous patients in hot weather; appropriate therapy is water restriction, rather than administration of salt, except in rare instances when the hyponatremia is life-threatening. In cases of actual salt depletion, appropriate replacement is the therapy of choice.

Hyperuricemia may occur or frank gout may be precipitated in certain patients receiving thiazide therapy.

Latant diabetes may become manifest during thiazide administration (see Drug/Drug Interactions).

The antihypertensive effects of the drug may be enhanced in the postsympathectomy patient.

If progressive renal impairment becomes evident, withholding or discontinuing diuretic therapy should be considered.

Calcium excretion is decreased by thiazides. Pathological changes in the parathyroid gland with hypercalcemia and hypophosphatemia have been observed in a few patients on prolonged thiazide therapy. The common complications of hyperparathyroidism, such as renal lithiasis, bone resorption, and peptic ulceration, have not been seen.

Thiazide diuretics have been shown to increase the urinary excretion of magnesium; this may result in hypomagnesemia.

Information for Patients: Patients should be informed of possible side effects and advised to take the medication regularly and continuously as directed.

Laboratory Tests
Hydralazine: Complete blood counts and antinuclear antibody titer determinations are indicated before and periodically during prolonged therapy with hydralazine even though the patient is asymptomatic. These studies are also indicated if the patient develops arthralgia, fever, chest pain, continued malaise, or other unexplained signs or symptoms. A positive antinuclear antibody titer requires that the physician carefully weigh the implications of the test results against the benefits to be derived from antihypertensive therapy with a combination drug containing hydralazine.

Blood dyscrasias, consisting of reduction in hemoglobin and red cell count, leukopenia, agranulocytosis, and purpura, have been reported. If such abnormalities develop, therapy should be discontinued.

Hydrochlorothiazide: Initial and periodic determinations of serum electrolytes to detect possible electrolyte imbalance should be performed at appropriate intervals.

Serum and urine electrolyte determinations are particularly important when the patient is vomiting excessively or receiving parenteral fluids.

Drug/Drug Interactions
Reserpine: MAO inhibitors should be avoided or used with extreme caution.

Reserpine should be used cautiously with digitalis and quinidine, since cardiac arrhythmias have occurred with rauwolfia preparations.

Concurrent use of tricyclic antidepressants may decrease the antihypertensive effect of reserpine (see CONTRAINDICATIONS).

Concurrent use of reserpine and direct or indirect-acting sympathomimetics should be closely monitored. The action of direct-acting amines (epinephrine, isoproterenol, phenylephrine, metaraminol) may be prolonged when given to patients taking reserpine. The action of indirect-acting amines (ephedrine, tyramine, amphetamines) is inhibited.

Hydralazine: MAO inhibitors should be used with caution in patients receiving hydralazine.

When other potent parenteral antihypertensive drugs, such as diazoxide, are used in combination with hydralazine, patients should be continuously observed for several hours for any excessive fall in blood pressure. Profound hypotensive episodes may occur when diazoxide injections and hydralazine are used concomitantly.

Hydrochlorothiazide: Hypokalemia can sensitize or exaggerate the response of the heart to the toxic effects of digitalis (e.g., increased ventricular irritability).

Hypokalemia may develop during concomitant use of steroids or ACTH.

Insulin requirements in diabetic patients may be increased, decreased, or unchanged.

Thiazides may decrease arterial responsiveness to norepinephrine, but not enough to preclude effectiveness of the pressor agent for therapeutic use.

Thiazides may increase the responsiveness to tubocurarine.

Lithium renal clearance is reduced by thiazides, increasing the risk of lithium toxicity.

There have been rare reports in the literature of hemolytic anemia occurring with the concomitant use of hydrochlorothiazide and methyldopa.

Concurrent administration of some nonsteroidal anti-inflammatory agents may reduce the diuretic, natriuretic and antihypertensive effects of thiazide diuretics.

Cholestyramine and colestipol resins: Absorption of hydrochlorothiazide is impaired in the presence of anionic exchange resins. Single doses of either cholestyramine or colestipol resins bind the hydrochlorothiazide and reduce its absorption from the gastrointestinal tract by up to 85% and 43%, respectively.

Drug/Laboratory Test Interactions: Thiazides may decrease serum levels of protein-bound iodine without signs of thyroid disturbance. Ser-Ap-Es should be discontinued before tests for parathyroid function are made (see General, Hydrochlorothiazide, Calcium excretion).

Carcinogenesis, Mutagenesis, Impairment of Fertility Carcinogenicity, mutagenicity, and fertility studies in animals have not been conducted with Ser-Ap-Es.

Reserpine: *Animal Tumorigenicity:* Rodent studies have shown that reserpine is an animal tumorigen, causing an increased incidence of mammary fibroadenomas in female mice, malignant tumors of the seminal vesicles in male mice, and malignant adrenal medullary tumors in male rats. These findings arose in 2-year studies in which the drug was administered in the feed at concentrations of 5 and 10 ppm—about 100 to 300 times the usual human dose. The breast neoplasms are thought to be related to reserpine's prolactin-elevating effect. Several other prolactin-elevating drugs have also been associated with an increased incidence of mammary neoplasia in rodents.

The extent to which these findings indicate a risk to humans is uncertain. Tissue culture experiments show that about one third of human breast tumors are prolactin-dependent in vitro, a factor of considerable importance if the use of the drug is contemplated in a patient with previously detected breast cancer. The possibility of an increased risk of breast cancer in reserpine users has been studied extensively; however, no firm conclusion has emerged. Although a few epidemiologic studies have suggested a slightly increased risk (less than twofold in all studies except one) in women who have used reserpine, other studies of generally similar design have not confirmed this. Epidemiologic studies conducted using other drugs (neuroleptic agents) that, like reserpine, increase prolactin levels and therefore would be considered rodent mammary carcinogens have not shown an association between chronic administration of the drug and human mammary tumorigenesis. While long-term clinical observation has not suggested such an association, the available evidence is considered too limited to be conclusive at this time. An association of reserpine intake with pheochromocytoma or tumors of the seminal vesicles has not been explored.

Hydralazine: In a lifetime study in Swiss albino mice, there was a statistically significant increase in the incidence of lung tumors (adenomas and adenocarcinomas) of both male and female mice given hydralazine continuously in their drinking water at a dosage of about 250 mg/kg/day (about 80 times the maximum recommended human dose). In a 2-year carcinogenicity study of rats given hydralazine by gavage at dose levels of 15, 30, and 60 mg/kg/day (approximately 5 to 20 times the recommended human daily dosage), microscopic examination of the liver revealed a small, but statistically significant, increase in benign neoplastic nodules in male and female rats from the high-dose group and in female rats from the intermediate-dose group. Benign interstitial cell tumors of the testes were also significantly increased in male rats from the high-dose group. The tumors observed are common in aged rats and a significantly increased incidence was not observed until 18 months of treatment. Hydralazine was shown to be mutagenic in bacterial systems (Gene Mutation and DNA Repair) and in one of two rat and one rabbit hepatocyte in vitro DNA repair studies. Additional in vivo and in vitro studies using lymphoma cells, germinal cells, and fibroblasts from mice, bone marrow cells from Chinese hamsters and fibroblasts from human cell lines did not demonstrate any mutagenic potential for hydralazine.

The extent to which these findings indicate a risk to man is uncertain. While long-term clinical observation has not suggested that human cancer is associated with hydralazine use, epidemiologic studies have so far been insufficient to arrive at any conclusions.

Fertility studies in animals have not been conducted with hydralazine.

Hydrochlorothiazide: Two-year feeding studies in mice and rats conducted under the auspices of the National Toxicology Program (NTP) uncovered no evidence of a carcinogenic potential of hydrochlorothiazide in female mice (at doses of up to approximately 600 mg/kg/day) or in male and female rats (at doses of up to approximately 100 mg/kg/day). The NTP, however, found equivocal evidence for hepatocarcinogenicity in male mice.

Hydrochlorothiazide was not genotoxic in in vitro assays using strains TA 98, TA 100, TA 1535, TA 1537, and TA 1538 of *Salmonella typhimurium* (Ames assay) and in the Chinese Hamster Ovary (CHO) test for chromosomal aberrations, or in in vivo assays using mouse germinal cell chromosomes, Chinese hamster bone marrow chromosomes, and the *Drosophila* sex-linked recessive lethal trait gene. Positive test results were obtained only in the in vitro CHO Sister Chromatid Exchange (clastogenicity) and in the Mouse Lymphoma Cell (mutagenicity) assays, using concentrations of hydrochlorothiazide from 43 to 1300 µg/mL, and in the *Aspergillus nidulans* nondisjunction assay at an unspecified concentration.

Hydrochlorothiazide had no adverse effects on the fertility of mice and rats of either sex in studies wherein these species were exposed, via their diet, to doses of up to 100 and 4 mg/kg/day, respectively, prior to mating, and throughout gestation.

Pregnancy: Teratogenic Effects. Pregnancy Category C: Animal reproduction studies have not been conducted with Ser-Ap-Es.

Reserpine. Reserpine administered parenterally has been shown to be teratogenic in rats at doses up to 2 mg/kg and to have an embryocidal effect in guinea pigs given dosages of 0.5 mg daily.

Hydralazine. Animal studies indicate that hydralazine is teratogenic in mice at 20-30 times the maximum daily human dose of 200-300 mg and possibly in rabbits at 10-15 times the maximum daily human dose, but that it is nonteratogenic in rats. Teratogenic effects observed were cleft palate and malformations of facial and cranial bones.

Hydrochlorothiazide. Studies in which hydrochlorothiazide was orally administered to pregnant mice and rats during their respective periods of major organogenesis at doses up to 3000 and 1000 mg/kg/day, respectively, provided no evidence of harm to the fetus. There are, however, no adequate and well-controlled studies of Ser-Ap-Es in pregnant women. Because animal reproduction studies are not always predictive of human response, this combination drug should be used during pregnancy only if clearly needed.

Nonteratogenic Effects. ***Reserpine.*** Reserpine crosses the placental barrier and increased respiratory tract secretions, nasal congestion, cyanosis, and anorexia may occur in neonates of mothers treated with reserpine.

Hydrochlorothiazide. Thiazides also cross the placental barrier and appear in cord blood, and there is a risk of fetal or neonatal jaundice, fibrocytopenia, and possibly other adverse reactions that have occurred in adults.

Nursing Mothers: Reserpine is excreted in maternal breast milk, and increased respiratory tract secretions, nasal congestion, cyanosis, and anorexia may occur in breast-fed infants. Thiazides are also excreted in breast milk. Because of the potential for serious adverse reactions in nursing infants and the potential for tumorigenicity shown for reserpine in animal studies, a decision should be made whether to discontinue nursing or to discontinue Ser-Ap-Es, taking into account the importance of the drug to the mother.

Pediatric Use: Safety and effectiveness of the combination drug in pediatric patients have not been established.

ADVERSE REACTIONS

Adverse reactions are usually reversible upon reduction of dosage or discontinuation of Ser-Ap-Es. Whenever adverse reactions are moderate or severe, it may be necessary to discontinue the drug.

The following adverse reactions have been observed, but there has not been enough systematic collection of data to support an estimate of their frequency. Consequently the reactions are categorized by organ system and are listed in decreasing order of severity and not frequency.

Reserpine: The following have been observed with rauwolfia preparations:

Digestive: Vomiting, diarrhea, nausea, anorexia, dryness of mouth, hypersecretion.

Cardiovascular: Arrhythmia (particularly when used concurrently with digitalis or quindine), syncope, angina-like symptoms, bradycardia, edema.

Respiratory: Dyspnea, epistaxis, nasal congestion.

Neurologic: Rare parkinsonian syndrome and other extrapyramidal tract symptoms; dizziness; headache; paradoxical anxiety; depression; nervousness; nightmares; dull sensorium; drowsiness.

Musculoskeletal: Muscular aches.

Genitourinary: Pseudolactation, impotence, dysuria, gynecomastia, decreased libido, breast engorgement.

Metabolic: Weight gain.

Special Senses: Deafness, optic atrophy, glaucoma, uveitis, conjunctival injection.

Hypersensitive Reactions: Purpura, rash, pruritus.

Hydralazine: *Digestive:* Hepatitis, paralytic ileus, vomiting, diarrhea, nausea, constipation, anorexia.

Cardiovascular: Angina pectoris, hypotension, paradoxical pressor response, tachycardia, palpitations, edema, flushing.

Respiratory: Dyspnea, nasal congestion.

Neurologic: Psychotic reactions characterized by depression, disorientation, or anxiety; peripheral neuritis, evidenced by paresthesia, numbness, and tingling; tremors; dizziness; headache.

Musculoskeletal: Muscle cramps, arthralgia.

Genitourinary: Difficulty in urination.

Hematologic: Blood dyscrasias, consisting of reduction in hemoglobin and red cell count, leukopenia, agranulocytosis; lymphadenopathy; splenomegaly; eosinophilia.

Special Senses: Conjunctivitis, lacrimation.

Hypersensitive Reactions: Purpura, fever, urticaria, rash, pruritus, chills.

Hydrochlorothiazide: *Digestive:* Pancreatitis, jaundice (intrahepatic cholestatic), sialadenitis, vomiting, diarrhea, cramping, nausea, gastric irritation, constipation, anorexia.

Cardiovascular: Orthostatic hypotension (may be potentiated by alcohol, barbiturates, or narcotics).

Neurologic: Vertigo, dizziness, transient blurred vision, headache, paresthesia, xanthopsia, weakness, restlessness.

Musculoskeletal: Muscle spasm.

Hematologic: Aplastic anemia, agranulocytosis, leukopenia, thrombocytopenia.

Metabolic: Hyperglycemia, glycosuria, hyperuricemia.

Hypersensitive Reactions: Necrotizing angiitis, Stevens-Johnson syndrome, respiratory distress including pneumonitis and pulmonary edema, purpura, urticaria, rash, photosensitivity.

OVERDOSAGE

Acute Toxicity: No deaths due to acute poisoning with Ser-Ap-Es have been reported.

Oral LD_{50}'s in animals (mg/kg): rats, 397; mice, 272.

Signs and Symptoms

Reserpine. The clinical picture of acute poisoning is characterized chiefly by signs and symptoms due to the reflex parasympathomimetic effect of reserpine.

Impairment of consciousness may occur and may range from drowsiness to coma, depending upon the severity of overdosage. Flushing of the skin, conjunctival injection, and pupillary constriction are to be expected. Hypotension, hypothermia, central respiratory depression, and bradycardia may develop in cases of severe overdosage. Increased salivary and gastric secretion and diarrhea may also occur.

Hydralazine. Signs and symptoms of overdosage include hypotension, tachycardia, headache, and generalized skin flushing.

Complications can include myocardial ischemia and subsequent myocardial infarction, cardiac arrhythmia, and profound shock.

Hydrochlorothiazide. The most prominent feature of poisoning is acute loss of fluid and electrolytes.

Cardiovascular: Trachycardia, hypotension, shock.

Neuromuscular: Weakness, confusion, dizziness, cramps of the calf muscles, paresthesia, fatigue, impairment of consciousness.

Digestive: Nausea, vomiting, thirst.

Renal: Polyuria, oliguria, or anuria (due to hemoconcentration).

Laboratory Findings: Hypokalemia, hyponatremia, hypochloremia, alkalosis; increased BUN (especially in patients with renal insufficiency).

Combined Poisoning: Signs and symptoms may be aggravated or modified by concomitant intake of antihypertensive medication, barbiturates, digitalis (hypokalemia), corticosteroids, narcotics, or alcohol.

Treatment: There is no specific antidote.

The gastric contents should be evacuated, taking adequate precautions against aspiration and for protection of the airway. An activated charcoal slurry may be instilled if conditions permit. Dialysis may not be effective for elimination of Ser-Ap-Es because of its plasma protein binding (see CLINICAL PHARMACOLOGY).

These manipulations may have to be omitted or carried out after cardiovascular status has been stabilized, since they might precipitate cardiac arrhythmias or increase the depth of shock.

If hypotension or shock occurs, the patient's legs should be kept raised and lost fluid and electrolytes (potassium, sodium) should be replaced.

Support of the cardiovascular system is of primary importance in suspected hydralazine overdosage. If possible, vasopressors should not be given, but if a vasopressor is required, care should be taken not to precipitate or aggravate cardiac arrhythmia. Tachycardia responds to beta blockers. Digitalization may be necessary.

If hypotension is severe enough to require treatment with a vasopressor, one having a direct action upon vascular smooth muscle (e.g., phenylephrine, levarterenol, metaraminol) should be used to treat the symptomatic effects of reserpine overdosage.

Fluid and electrolyte balance (especially serum potassium) and renal function should be monitored until conditions become normal. Since reserpine is long-acting, the patient should be observed carefully for at least 72 hours.

DOSAGE AND ADMINISTRATION

Dosage should be determined by individual titration (see boxed **WARNING**). Dosage regimens that exceed 0.25 mg of reserpine per day are not recommended.

HOW SUPPLIED

Tablets—round, salmon pink, dry-coated (imprinted CIBA 71) 0.1 mg of reserpine, 25 mg of hydralazine hydrochloride, 15 mg of hydrochlorothiazide.

Bottles of 100—NDC 0083-0071-30

Bottles of 1000—NDC 0083-0071-40

Do not store above 86°F (30°C).

Dispense in tight, light-resistant container (USP).

C96-29 (Rev. 3/96)

Shown in Product Identification Guide, page 309

SLOW-K® ℞

[sloe-kay]

potassium chloride

Extended-Release Tablets USP

DESCRIPTION

Slow-K, potassium chloride extended-release tablets USP, is a sugar-coated (not enteric-coated) tablet for oral administration, containing 600 mg of potassium chloride (equivalent to 8 mEq) in a wax matrix. This formulation is intended to provide an extended release of potassium from the matrix to minimize the likelihood of producing high, localized concentrations of potassium within the gastrointestinal tract.

Slow-K is an electrolyte replenisher. Its chemical name is potassium chloride, and its structural formula is KCl. Potassium chloride USP is a white, granular powder or colorless crystals. It is odorless and has a saline taste. Its solutions are neutral to litmus. It is freely soluble in water and insoluble in alcohol.

Inactive Ingredients. Acacia, cetostearyl alcohol, gelatin, iron oxide, magnesium stearate, polyvinylpyrrolidone, parabens, sodium benzoate, starch, sucrose, talc, and titanium dioxide.

CLINICAL PHARMACOLOGY

The potassium ion is the principal intracellular cation of most body tissues. Potassium ions participate in a number of essential physiological processes, including the maintenance of intracellular tonicity, the transmission of nerve impulses, the contraction of cardiac, skeletal, and smooth muscle, and the maintenance of normal renal function.

In adults normal plasma potassium concentration is 3.5–5.0 mEq/L.

Potassium depletion may occur whenever the rate of potassium loss through renal excretion and/or loss from the gastrointestinal tract exceeds the rate of potassium intake. Such depletion usually develops slowly as a consequence of prolonged therapy with oral diuretics, primary or secondary hyperaldosteronism, diabetic ketoacidosis, severe diarrhea, or inadequate replacement of potassium in patients on prolonged parenteral nutrition. Potassium depletion due to these causes is usually accompanied by a concomitant deficiency of chloride and is manifested by hypokalemia and metabolic alkalosis. Potassium depletion may produce weakness, fatigue, disturbances of cardiac rhythm (primarily ectopic beats), prominent U-waves in the electrocardiogram, and in advanced cases flaccid paralysis and/or impaired ability to concentrate urine.

Potassium depletion associated with metabolic alkalosis is managed by correcting the fundamental causes of the deficiency whenever possible and administering supplemental potassium chloride in the form of high potassium food or potassium chloride solution or tablets.

In rare circumstances (*e.g.,* patients with renal tubular acidosis) potassium depletion may be associated with metabolic acidosis and hyperchloremia. In such patients potassium replacement should be accomplished with potassium salts other than the chloride, such as potassium bicarbonate, potassium citrate, or potassium acetate.

The potassium chloride in Slow-K is completely absorbed before it leaves the small intestine. The wax matrix is not absorbed and is excreted in the feces; in some instances the empty matrices may be noticeable in the stool. When the

Continued on next page

CibaGeneva—Cont.

bioavailability of the potassium ion from Slow-K is compared to that of a true solution the extent of absorption is similar. The extended-release properties of Slow-K are demonstrated by the finding that a significant increase in time is required for renal excretion of the first 50% of the Slow-K dose as compared to the solution.

Increased urinary potassium excretion is first observed 1 hour after administration of Slow-K, reaches a peak at 4 hours, and extends up to 8 hours. Mean daily steady-state plasma levels of potassium following daily administration of Slow-K cannot be distinguished from those following administration of a potassium chloride solution or from control plasma levels of potassium ion.

INDICATIONS AND USAGE

BECAUSE OF REPORTS OF INTESTINAL AND GASTRIC ULCERATION AND BLEEDING WITH EXTENDED-RELEASE POTASSIUM CHLORIDE PREPARATIONS, THESE DRUGS SHOULD BE RESERVED FOR THOSE PATIENTS WHO CANNOT TOLERATE OR REFUSE TO TAKE LIQUID OR EFFERVESCENT POTASSIUM PREPARATIONS OR FOR PATIENTS IN WHOM THERE IS A PROBLEM OF COMPLIANCE WITH THESE PREPARATIONS.

1. For therapeutic use in patients with hypokalemia with or without metabolic alkalosis; in digitalis intoxication and in patients with hypokalemic familial periodic paralysis.

2. For prevention of potassium depletion when the dietary intake of potassium is inadequate in the following conditions: patients receiving digitalis and diuretics for congestive heart failure; hepatic cirrhosis with ascites; states of aldosterone excess with normal renal function; potassium-losing nephropathy, and certain diarrheal states.

3. The use of potassium salts in patients receiving diuretics for uncomplicated essential hypertension is often unnecessary when such patients have a normal dietary pattern. Serum potassium should be checked periodically, however, and, if hypokalemia occurs, dietary supplementation with potassium-containing foods may be adequate to control milder cases. In more severe cases supplementation with potassium salts may be indicated.

CONTRAINDICATIONS

Potassium supplements are contraindicated in patients with hyperkalemia, since a further increase in serum potassium concentration in such patients can produce cardiac arrest. Hyperkalemia may complicate any of the following conditions: chronic renal failure, systemic acidosis such as diabetic acidosis, acute dehydration, extensive tissue breakdown as in severe burns, adrenal insufficiency, or the administration of a potassium-sparing diuretic (e.g., spironolactone, triamterene) (see OVERDOSAGE).

All solid dosage forms of potassium supplements are contraindicated in any patient in whom there is cause for arrest or delay in tablet passage through the gastrointestinal tract. In these instances, potassium supplementation should be with a liquid preparation. Wax-matrix potassium chloride preparations have produced esophageal ulceration in certain cardiac patients with esophageal compression due to an enlarged left atrium.

WARNINGS

Hyperkalemia (See OVERDOSAGE.)

In patients with impaired mechanisms for excreting potassium, the administration of potassium salts can produce hyperkalemia and cardiac arrest. This occurs most commonly in patients given potassium by the intravenous route but may also occur in patients given potassium orally. Potentially fatal hyperkalemia can develop rapidly and be asymptomatic.

The use of potassium salts in patients with chronic renal disease, or any other condition which impairs potassium excretion, requires particularly careful monitoring of the serum potassium concentration and appropriate dosage adjustment.

Interaction with Potassium-Sparing Diuretics

Hypokalemia should not be treated by the concomitant administration of potassium salts and a potassium-sparing diuretic (e.g., spironolactone or triamterene), since the simultaneous administration of these agents can produce severe hyperkalemia.

Gastrointestinal lesions

Potassium chloride tablets have produced stenotic and/or ulcerative lesions of the small bowel and deaths. These lesions are caused by a high localized concentration of potassium ion in the region of a rapidly dissolving tablet, which injures the bowel wall and thereby produces obstruction, hemorrhage, or perforation. Slow-K is a wax-matrix tablet formulated to provide an extended rate of release of potassium chloride and thus to minimize the possibility of a high local concentration of potassium ion near the bowel wall. While the reported frequency of small-bowel lesions is much less with wax-matrix tablets (less than one per 100,000 patient-years) than with enteric-coated potassium chloride

tablets (40–50 per 100,000 patient-years) cases associated with wax-matrix tablets have been reported both in foreign countries and in the United States. In addition, perhaps because the wax-matrix preparations are not enteric-coated and release potassium in the stomach, there have been reports of upper gastrointestinal bleeding associated with these products. The total number of gastrointestinal lesions remains approximately one per 100,000 patient-years. Slow-K should be discontinued immediately and the possibility of bowel obstruction or perforation considered if severe vomiting, abdominal pain, distention, or gastrointestinal bleeding occurs.

Metabolic acidosis

Hypokalemia in patients with metabolic *acidosis* should be treated with an alkalinizing potassium salt such as potassium bicarbonate, potassium citrate, or potassium acetate.

PRECAUTIONS

General: The diagnosis of potassium depletion is ordinarily made by demonstrating hypokalemia in a patient with a clinical history suggesting some cause for potassium depletion. In interpreting the serum potassium level, the physician should bear in mind that acute alkalosis *per se* can produce hypokalemia in the absence of a deficit in total body potassium, while acute acidosis *per se* can increase the serum potassium concentration into the normal range even in the presence of a reduced total body potassium.

Information for Patients

Physicians should consider reminding the patient of the following:

To take each dose without crushing, chewing, or sucking the tablets.

To take this medicine only as directed. This is especially important if the patient is also taking both diuretics and digitalis preparations.

To check with the physician if there is trouble swallowing tablets or if the tablets seem to stick in the throat.

To check with the doctor at once if tarry stools or other evidence of gastrointestinal bleeding is noticed.

Laboratory Tests

Regular serum potassium determinations are recommended. In addition, during the treatment of potassium depletion, careful attention should be paid to acid-base balance, other serum electrolyte levels, the electrocardiogram, and the clinical status of the patient, particularly in the presence of cardiac disease, renal disease, or acidosis.

Drug Interactions

Potassium-sparing diuretics: see WARNINGS.

Carcinogenesis, Mutagenesis, Impairment of Fertility

Long-term carcinogenicity studies in animals have not been performed.

Pregnancy Category C

Animal reproduction studies have not been conducted with Slow-K. It is also not known whether Slow-K can cause fetal harm when administered to a pregnant woman or can affect reproduction capacity. Slow-K should be given to a pregnant woman only if clearly needed.

Nursing Mothers

The normal potassium ion content of human milk is about 13 mEq/L. It is not known if Slow-K has an effect on this content. Caution should be exercised when Slow-K is administered to a nursing woman.

Pediatric Use

Safety and effectiveness in pediatric patients have not been established.

ADVERSE REACTIONS

One of the most severe adverse effects is hyperkalemia (see CONTRAINDICATIONS, WARNINGS and OVERDOSAGE). There also have been reports of upper and lower gastrointestinal conditions including obstruction, bleeding, ulceration, and perforation (see CONTRAINDICATIONS and WARNINGS); other factors known to be associated with such conditions were present in many of these patients.

The most common adverse reactions to oral potassium salts are nausea, vomiting, abdominal discomfort, and diarrhea. These symptoms are due to irritation of the gastrointestinal tract and are best managed by taking the dose with meals or reducing the dose.

Skin rash has been reported rarely.

OVERDOSAGE

The administration of oral potassium salts to persons with normal excretory mechanisms for potassium rarely causes serious hyperkalemia. However, if excretory mechanisms are impaired or if potassium is administered too rapidly intravenously, potentially fatal hyperkalemia can result (see CONTRAINDICATIONS and WARNINGS). It is important to recognize that hyperkalemia is usually asymptomatic and may be manifested only by an increased serum potassium concentration (6.5–8.0 mEq/L) and characteristic electrocardiographic changes (peaking of T waves, loss of P wave, depression of S-T segment, and prolongation of the Q-T interval). Late manifestations include muscle paralysis and cardiovascular collapse from cardiac arrest (9–12 mEq/L).

Treatment measures for hyperkalemia include the following: (1) elimination of foods and medications containing po-

tassium and of potassium-sparing diuretics; (2) intravenous administration of 300–500 ml/hr of 10% dextrose solution containing 10–20 units of insulin per 1,000 ml; (3) correction of acidosis, if present, with intravenous sodium bicarbonate; (4) use of exchange resins, hemodialysis, or peritoneal dialysis.

In treating hyperkalemia in patients who have been stabilized on digitalis, too rapid a lowering of the serum potassium concentration can produce digitalis toxicity.

DOSAGE AND ADMINISTRATION

The usual dietary intake of potassium by the average adult is 40–80 mEq per day. Potassium depletion sufficient to cause hypokalemia usually requires the loss of 200 or more mEq of potassium from the total body store. Dosage must be adjusted to the individual needs of each patient but is typically in the range of 20 mEq per day for the prevention of hypokalemia to 40–100 mEq or more per day for the treatment of potassium depletion. Large numbers of tablets should be given in divided doses.

Note: Slow-K extended-release tablets must be swallowed whole and never crushed, chewed, or sucked.

HOW SUPPLIED

Tablets 600 mg potassium chloride (equivalent to 8 mEq) round, buff colored, sugar-coated (imprinted Slow-K)

Bottles of 100 .... NDC 57267-165-30
Bottles of 1000 .... NDC 57267-165-40
Consumer Pack—One Unit
   12 Bottles—100 tablets each .... NDC 57267-165-65
Samples, when available, are identified by the word *SAMPLE* appearing on each tablet.

Do not store above 86°F (30°C). Protect from moisture. Protect from light.

Dispense in tight, light-resistant container (USP).

Dist. by:
Summit Pharmaceuticals
Ciba-Geigy Corporation
Summit, NJ 07901

C96-30 (Rev. 3/96)

Shown in Product Identification Guide, page 309

TEGRETOL®   ℞
carbamazepine USP
Chewable Tablets of 100 mg—red-speckled, pink
Tablets of 200 mg—pink
Suspension of 100 mg/5 mL

TEGRETOL®-XR   ℞
(carbamazepine extended-release tablets)
100 mg, 200 mg, 400 mg

Prescribing Information

> #### WARNING
> APLASTIC ANEMIA AND AGRANULOCYTOSIS HAVE BEEN REPORTED IN ASSOCIATION WITH THE USE OF TEGRETOL. DATA FROM A POPULATION-BASED CASE CONTROL STUDY DEMONSTRATE THAT THE RISK OF DEVELOPING THESE REACTIONS IS 5–8 TIMES GREATER THAN IN THE GENERAL POPULATION. HOWEVER, THE OVERALL RISK OF THESE REACTIONS IN THE UNTREATED GENERAL POPULATION IS LOW, APPROXIMATELY SIX PATIENTS PER ONE MILLION POPULATION PER YEAR FOR AGRANULOCYTOSIS AND TWO PATIENTS PER ONE MILLION POPULATION PER YEAR FOR APLASTIC ANEMIA.
>
> ALTHOUGH REPORTS OF TRANSIENT OR PERSISTENT DECREASED PLATELET OR WHITE BLOOD CELL COUNTS ARE NOT UNCOMMON IN ASSOCIATION WITH THE USE OF TEGRETOL, DATA ARE NOT AVAILABLE TO ESTIMATE ACCURATELY THEIR INCIDENCE OR OUTCOME. HOWEVER, THE VAST MAJORITY OF THE CASES OF LEUKOPENIA HAVE NOT PROGRESSED TO THE MORE SERIOUS CONDITIONS OF APLASTIC ANEMIA OR AGRANULOCYTOSIS.
>
> BECAUSE OF THE VERY LOW INCIDENCE OF AGRANULOCYTOSIS AND APLASTIC ANEMIA, THE VAST MAJORITY OF MINOR HEMATOLOGIC CHANGES OBSERVED IN MONITORING OF PATIENTS ON TEGRETOL ARE UNLIKELY TO SIGNAL THE OCCURRENCE OF EITHER ABNORMALITY. NONETHELESS, COMPLETE PRETREATMENT HEMATOLOGICAL TESTING SHOULD BE OBTAINED AS A BASELINE. IF A PATIENT IN THE COURSE OF TREATMENT EXHIBITS LOW OR DECREASED WHITE BLOOD CELL OR PLATELET COUNTS, THE PATIENT SHOULD BE MONITORED CLOSELY. DISCONTINUATION OF THE DRUG SHOULD BE CONSIDERED IF ANY EVIDENCE OF SIGNIFICANT BONE MARROW DEPRESSION DEVELOPS.

Before prescribing Tegretol, the physician should be thoroughly familiar with the details of this prescribing information, particularly regarding use with other drugs, especially those which accentuate toxicity potential.

DESCRIPTION

Tegretol, carbamazepine USP, is an anticonvulsant and specific analgesic for trigeminal neuralgia, available for oral administration as chewable tablets of 100 mg, tablets of 200 mg, XR tablets of 100, 200, and 400 mg, and as a suspension of 100 mg/5 mL (teaspoon). Its chemical name is 5*H*-dibenz[b,f]azepine-5-carboxamide.

Carbamazepine USP is a white to off-white powder, practically insoluble in water and soluble in alcohol and in acetone. Its molecular weight is 236.27.

Inactive Ingredients. Tablets: Colloidal silicon dioxide, D&C Red No. 30 Aluminum Lake (chewable tablets only), FD&C Red No. 40 (200-mg tablets only), flavoring (chewable tablets only), gelatin, glycerin, magnesium stearate, sodium starch glycolate (chewable tablets only), starch, stearic acid, and sucrose (chewable tablets only). Suspension: Citric acid, FD&C Yellow No. 6, flavoring, polymer, potassium sorbate, propylene glycol, purified water, sorbitol, sucrose, and xanthan gum.

Tegretol-XR tablets: cellulose compounds, dextrates, iron oxides, magnesium stearate, mannitol, polyethylene glycol, sodium lauryl sulfate, titanium dioxide (200-mg tablets only).

CLINICAL PHARMACOLOGY

In controlled clinical trials, Tegretol has been shown to be effective in the treatment of psychomotor and grand mal seizures, as well as trigeminal neuralgia.

Mechanism of Action

Tegretol has demonstrated anticonvulsant properties in rats and mice with electrically and chemically induced seizures. It appears to act by reducing polysynaptic responses and blocking the post-tetanic potentiation. Tegretol greatly reduces or abolishes pain induced by stimulation of the infraorbital nerve in cats and rats. It depresses thalamic potential and bulbar and polysynaptic reflexes, including the linguomandibular reflex in cats. Tegretol is chemically unrelated to other anticonvulsants or other drugs used to control the pain of trigeminal neuralgia. The mechanism of action remains unknown.

The principal metabolite of Tegretol, carbamazepine-10, 11-epoxide, has anticonvulsant activity as demonstrated in several in vivo animal models of seizures. Though clinical activity for the epoxide has been postulated, the significance of its activity with respect to the safety and efficacy of Tegretol has not been established.

Pharmacokinetics

In clinical studies, Tegretol suspension, conventional tablets, and XR tablets delivered equivalent amounts of drug to the systemic circulation. However, the suspension was absorbed somewhat faster, and the XR tablet slightly slower, than the conventional tablet. The bioavailability of the XR tablet was 89% compared to suspension. Following a b.i.d. dosage regimen, the suspension provides higher peak levels and lower trough levels than those obtained from the conventional tablet for the same dosage regimen. On the other hand, following a t.i.d. dosage regimen, Tegretol suspension affords steady-state plasma levels comparable to Tegretol tablets given b.i.d. when administered at the same total mg daily dose. Following a b.i.d. dosage regimen, Tegretol-XR tablets afford steady-state plasma levels comparable to conventional Tegretol tablets given q.i.d., when administered at the same total mg daily dose. Tegretol in blood is 76% bound to plasma proteins. Plasma levels of Tegretol are variable and may range from 0.5–25 μg/mL, with no apparent relationship to the daily intake of the drug. Usual adult therapeutic levels are between 4 and 12 μg/mL. In polytherapy, the concentration of Tegretol and concomitant drugs may be increased or decreased during therapy, and drug effects may be altered (see PRECAUTIONS, Drug Interactions). Following chronic oral administration of suspension, plasma levels peak at approximately 1.5 hours compared to 4–5 hours after administration of conventional Tegretol tablets, and 3–12 hours after administration of Tegretol-XR tablets. The CSF/serum ratio is 0.22, similar to the 24% unbound Tegretol in serum. Because Tegretol induces its own metabolism, the half-life is also variable. Autoinduction is completed after 3–5 weeks of a fixed dosing regimen. Initial half-life values range from 25–65 hours, decreasing to 12–17 hours on repeated doses. Tegretol is metabolized in the liver. Cytochrome P450 3A4 was identified as the major isoform responsible for the formation of carbamazepine-10, 11-epoxide from Tegretol. After oral administration of ^{14}C-carbamazepine, 72% of the administered radioactivity was found in the urine and 28% in the feces. This urinary radioactivity was composed largely of hydroxylated and conjugated metabolites, with only 3% of unchanged Tegretol.

The pharmacokinetic parameters of Tegretol disposition are similar in children and in adults. However, there is a poor correlation between plasma concentrations of carbamazepine and Tegretol dose in children. Carbamazepine is more rapidly metabolized to carbamazepine-10, 11-epoxide (a metabolite shown to be equipotent to carbamazepine as an anticonvulsant in animal screens) in the younger age groups than in adults. In children below the age of 15, there is an inverse relationship between CBZ-E/CBZ ratio and increasing age (in one report from 0.44 in children below the age of 1 year to 0.18 in children between 10–15 years of age).

The effects of race and gender on carbamazepine pharmacokinetics have not been systematically evaluated.

INDICATIONS AND USAGE

Epilepsy

Tegretol is indicated for use as an anticonvulsant drug. Evidence supporting efficacy of Tegretol as an anticonvulsant was derived from active drug-controlled studies that enrolled patients with the following seizure types:

1. Partial seizures with complex symptomatology (psychomotor, temporal lobe). Patients with these seizures appear to show greater improvement than those with other types.
2. Generalized tonic-clonic seizures (grand mal).
3. Mixed seizure patterns which include the above, or other partial or generalized seizures.

   Absence seizures (petit mal) do not appear to be controlled by Tegretol (see PRECAUTIONS, General).

Trigeminal Neuralgia

Tegretol is indicated in the treatment of the pain associated with true trigeminal neuralgia.

Beneficial results have also been reported in glossopharyngeal neuralgia.

This drug is not a simple analgesic and should not be used for the relief of trivial aches or pains.

CONTRAINDICATIONS

Tegretol should not be used in patients with a history of previous bone marrow depression, hypersensitivity to the drug, or known sensitivity to any of the tricyclic compounds, such as amitriptyline, desipramine, imipramine, protriptyline, nortriptyline, etc. Likewise, on theoretical grounds its use with monoamine oxidase inhibitors is not recommended. Before administration of Tegretol, MAO inhibitors should be discontinued for a minimum of 14 days, or longer if the clinical situation permits.

WARNINGS

Patients with a history of adverse hematologic reaction to any drug may be particularly at risk.

Severe dermatologic reactions, including toxic epidermal necrolysis (Lyell's syndrome) and Stevens-Johnson syndrome, have been reported with Tegretol. These reactions have been extremely rare. However, a few fatalities have been reported.

Tegretol has shown mild anticholinergic activity; therefore, patients with increased intraocular pressure should be closely observed during therapy.

Because of the relationship of the drug to other tricyclic compounds, the possibility of activation of a latent psychosis and, in elderly patients, of confusion or agitation should be borne in mind.

PRECAUTIONS

General

Before initiating therapy, a detailed history and physical examination should be made.

Tegretol should be used with caution in patients with a mixed seizure disorder that includes atypical absence seizures, since in these patients Tegretol has been associated with increased frequency of generalized convulsions (see INDICATIONS AND USAGE).

Therapy should be prescribed only after critical benefit-to-risk appraisal in patients with a history of cardiac, hepatic, or renal damage; adverse hematologic reaction to other drugs; or interrupted courses of therapy with Tegretol.

Since a given dose of Tegretol suspension will produce higher peak levels than the same dose given as the tablet, it is recommended that patients given the suspension be started on lower doses and increased slowly to avoid unwanted side effects (see DOSAGE AND ADMINISTRATION).

Information for Patients

Patients should be made aware of the early toxic signs and symptoms of a potential hematologic problem, such as fever, sore throat, rash, ulcers in the mouth, easy bruising, petechial or purpuric hemorrhage, and should be advised to report to the physician immediately if any such signs or symptoms appear.

Since dizziness and drowsiness may occur, patients should be cautioned about the hazards of operating machinery or automobiles or engaging in other potentially dangerous tasks.

Laboratory Tests

Complete pretreatment blood counts, including platelets and possibly reticulocytes and serum iron, should be obtained as a baseline. If a patient in the course of treatment exhibits low or decreased white blood cell or platelet counts, the patient should be monitored closely. Discontinuation of the drug should be considered if any evidence of significant bone marrow depression develops.

Baseline and periodic evaluations of liver function, particularly in patients with a history of liver disease, must be performed during treatment with this drug since liver damage may occur. The drug should be discontinued immediately in cases of aggravated liver dysfunction or active liver disease.

Baseline and periodic eye examinations, including slit-lamp, funduscopy, and tonometry, are recommended since many phenothiazines and related drugs have been shown to cause eye changes.

Baseline and periodic complete urinalysis and BUN determinations are recommended for patients treated with this agent because of observed renal dysfunction.

Monitoring of blood levels (see CLINICAL PHARMACOLOGY) has increased the efficacy and safety of anticonvulsants. This monitoring may be particularly useful in cases of dramatic increase in seizure frequency and for verification of compliance. In addition, measurement of drug serum levels may aid in determining the cause of toxicity when more than one medication is being used.

Thyroid function tests have been reported to show decreased values with Tegretol administered alone.

Hyponatremia has been reported in association with Tegretol use, either alone or in combination with other drugs.

Interference with some pregnancy tests has been reported.

Drug Interactions

Clinically meaningful drug interactions have occurred with concomitant medications and include, but are not limited to, the following:

Agents That May Affect Tegretol Plasma Levels

CYP 3A4 inhibitors inhibit Tegretol metabolism and can thus increase plasma carbamazepine levels. Drugs that have been shown, or would be expected, to increase plasma carbamazepine levels include

cimetidine, danazol, diltiazem, macrolides, erythromycin, troleandomycin, clarithromycin, fluoxetine, loratadine, terfenadine, isoniazid, niacinamide, nicotinamide, propoxyphene, ketaconazole, itraconazole, verapamil, valproate.*

CYP 3A4 inducers can increase the rate of Tegretol metabolism. Drugs that have been shown, or that would be expected, to decrease plasma carbamazepine levels include

cisplatin, doxorubicin HCl, felbamate,† rifampin, phenobarbital, phenytoin, primidone, theophylline.

*increased levels of the active 10, 11-epoxide
†decreased levels of carbamazepine and increased levels of the 10, 11-epoxide

Effect of Tegretol on Plasma Levels of Concomitant Agents

Increased levels: clomipramine HCl, phenytoin, primidone

Tegretol induces hepatic CYP activity. Tegretol causes, or would be expected to cause, decreased levels of the following:

acetaminophen, alprazolam, clonazepam, clozapine, dicumarol, doxycycline, ethosuximide, haloperidol, methsuximide, oral contraceptives, phensuximide, phenytoin, theophylline, valproate, warfarin.

Concomitant administration of carbamazepine and lithium may increase the risk of neurotoxic side effects.

Alterations of thyroid function have been reported in combination therapy with other anticonvulsant medications.

Breakthrough bleeding has been reported among patients receiving concomitant oral contraceptives and their reliability may be adversely affected.

Carcinogenesis, Mutagenesis, Impairment of Fertility

Carbamazepine, when administered to Sprague-Dawley rats for two years in the diet at doses of 25, 75, and 250 mg/kg/day, resulted in a dose-related increase in the incidence of hepatocellular tumors in females and of benign interstitial cell adenomas in the testes of males.

Carbamazepine must, therefore, be considered to be carcinogenic in Sprague-Dawley rats. Bacterial and mammalian mutagenicity studies using carbamazepine produced negative results. The significance of these findings relative to the use of carbamazepine in humans is, at present, unknown.

Pregnancy Category C

Tegretol has been shown to have adverse effects in reproduction studies in rats when given orally in dosages 10–25 times the maximum human daily dosage of 1200 mg. In rat teratology studies, 2 of 135 offspring showed kinked ribs at 250 mg/kg and 4 of 119 offspring at 650 mg/kg showed other anomalies (cleft palate, 1; talipes, 1; anophthalmos, 2). In reproduction studies in rats, nursing offspring demonstrated a lack of weight gain and an unkempt appearance at a maternal dosage level of 200 mg/kg.

In humans, transplacental passage of Tegretol is rapid (30–60 minutes), and the drug is accumulated in fetal tissues, with higher levels found in liver and kidney than in brain and lung.

There are no adequate and well-controlled studies in pregnant women. Epidemiological data suggest that there may be an association between the use of carbamazepine during pregnancy and congenital malformations, including spina bifida. Tegretol should be used during pregnancy only if the potential benefit justifies the potential risk to the fetus.

Continued on next page

Ciba Geneva—Cont.

Retrospective case reviews suggest that, compared with monotherapy, there may be a higher prevalence of teratogenic effects associated with the use of anticonvulsants in combination therapy. Therefore, monotherapy is recommended for pregnant women.

It is important to note that anticonvulsant drugs should not be discontinued in patients in whom the drug is administered to prevent major seizures because of the strong possibility of precipitating status epilepticus with attendant hypoxia and threat to life. In individual cases where the severity and frequency of the seizure disorder are such that removal of medication does not pose a serious threat to the patient, discontinuation of the drug may be considered prior to and during pregnancy, although it cannot be said with any confidence that even minor seizures do not pose some hazard to the developing embryo or fetus.

Labor and Delivery

The effect of Tegretol on human labor and delivery is unknown.

Nursing Mothers

Tegretol and its epoxide metabolite are transferred to breast milk. The ratio of the concentration in breast milk to that in maternal plasma is about 0.4 for Tegretol and about 0.5 for the epoxide. The estimated doses given to the newborn during breast feeding are in the range of 2–5 mg daily for Tegretol and 1–2 mg daily for the epoxide.

Because of the potential for serious adverse reactions in nursing infants from carbamazepine, a decision should be made whether to discontinue nursing or to discontinue the drug, taking into account the importance of the drug to the mother.

Pediatric Use

Substantial evidence of Tegretol's effectiveness for use in the management of children with epilepsy (see Indications for specific seizure types) is derived from clinical investigations performed in adults and from studies in several in vitro systems which support the conclusion that (1) the pathogenetic mechanisms underlying seizure propagation are essentially identical in adults and children, and (2) the mechanism of action of carbamazepine in treating seizures is essentially identical in adults and children.

Taken as a whole, this information supports a conclusion that the generally accepted therapeutic range of total carbamazepine in plasma (i.e., 4–12 mcg/mL) is the same in children and adults.

The evidence assembled was primarily obtained from short-term use of carbamazepine. The safety of carbamazepine in children has been systematically studied up to 6 months. No longer-term data from clinical trials is available.

Geriatric Use

No systematic studies in geriatric patients have been conducted.

ADVERSE REACTIONS

If adverse reactions are of such severity that the drug must be discontinued, the physician must be aware that abrupt discontinuation of any anticonvulsant drug in a responsive epileptic patient may lead to seizures or even status epilepticus with its life-threatening hazards.

The most severe adverse reactions have been observed in the hemopoietic system (see boxed WARNING), the skin, and the cardiovascular system.

The most frequently observed adverse reactions, particularly during the initial phases of therapy, are dizziness, drowsiness, unsteadiness, nausea, and vomiting. To minimize the possibility of such reactions, therapy should be initiated at the low dosage recommended.

The following additional adverse reactions have been reported:

Hemopoietic System: Aplastic anemia, agranulocytosis, pancytopenia, bone marrow depression, thrombocytopenia, leukopenia, leukocytosis, eosinophilia, acute intermittent porphyria.

Skin: Pruritic and erythematous rashes, urticaria, toxic epidermal necrolysis (Lyell's syndrome) (see WARNINGS), Stevens-Johnson syndrome (see WARNINGS), photosensitivity reactions, alterations in skin pigmentation, exfoliative dermatitis, erythema multiforme and nodosum, purpura, aggravation of disseminated lupus erythematosus, alopecia, and diaphoresis. In certain cases, discontinuation of therapy may be necessary. Isolated cases of hirsutism have been reported, but a causal relationship is not clear.

Cardiovascular System: Congestive heart failure, edema, aggravation of hypertension, hypotension, syncope and collapse, aggravation of coronary artery disease, arrhythmias and AV block, thrombophlebitis, thromboembolism, and adenopathy or lymphadenopathy.

Some of these cardiovascular complications have resulted in fatalities. Myocardial infarction has been associated with other tricyclic compounds.

Liver: Abnormalities in liver function tests, cholestatic and hepatocellular jaundice, hepatitis.

Respiratory System: Pulmonary hypersensitivity characterized by fever, dyspnea, pneumonitis, or pneumonia.

Genitourinary System: Urinary frequency, acute urinary retention, oliguria with elevated blood pressure, azotemia, renal failure, and impotence. Albuminuria, glycosuria, elevated BUN, and microscopic deposits in the urine have also been reported.

Testicular atrophy occurred in rats receiving Tegretol orally from 4–52 weeks at dosage levels of 50–400 mg/kg/day. Additionally, rats receiving Tegretol in the diet for 2 years at dosage levels of 25, 75, and 250 mg/kg/day had a dose-related incidence of testicular atrophy and aspermatogenesis. In dogs, it produced a brownish discoloration, presumably a metabolite, in the urinary bladder at dosage levels of 50 mg/kg and higher. Relevance of these findings to humans is unknown.

Nervous System: Dizziness, drowsiness, disturbances of coordination, confusion, headache, fatigue, blurred vision, visual hallucinations, transient diplopia, oculomotor disturbances, nystagmus, speech disturbances, abnormal involuntary movements, peripheral neuritis and paresthesias, depression with agitation, talkativeness, tinnitus, and hyperacusis.

There have been reports of associated paralysis and other symptoms of cerebral arterial insufficiency, but the exact relationship of these reactions to the drug has not been established.

Isolated cases of neuroleptic malignant syndrome have been reported with concomitant use of psychotropic drugs.

Digestive System: Nausea, vomiting, gastric distress and abdominal pain, diarrhea, constipation, anorexia, and dryness of the mouth and pharynx, including glossitis and stomatitis.

Eyes: Scattered punctate cortical lens opacities, as well as conjunctivitis, have been reported. Although a direct causal relationship has not been established, many phenothiazines and related drugs have been shown to cause eye changes.

Musculoskeletal System: Aching joints and muscles, and leg cramps.

Metabolism: Fever and chills. Inappropriate antidiuretic hormone (ADH) secretion syndrome has been reported. Cases of frank water intoxication, with decreased serum sodium (hyponatremia) and confusion, have been reported in association with Tegretol use (see PRECAUTIONS, Laboratory Tests). Decreased levels of plasma calcium have been reported.

Other: Isolated cases of a lupus erythematosus-like syndrome have been reported. There have been occasional reports of elevated levels of cholesterol, HDL cholesterol, and triglycerides in patients taking anticonvulsants.

A case of aseptic meningitis, accompanied by myoclonus and peripheral eosinophilia, has been reported in a patient taking carbamazepine in combination with other medications. The patient was successfully dechallenged, and the meningitis reappeared upon rechallenge with carbamazepine.

DRUG ABUSE AND DEPENDENCE

No evidence of abuse potential has been associated with Tegretol, nor is there evidence of psychological or physical dependence in humans.

OVERDOSAGE

Acute Toxicity

Lowest known lethal dose: adults, > 60 g (39-year-old man). Highest known doses survived: adults, 30 g (31-year-old woman); children, 10 g (6-year-old boy); small children, 5 g (3-year-old girl).

Oral LD_{50} in animals (mg/kg): mice, 1100–3750; rats, 3850–4025; rabbits, 1500–2680; guinea pigs, 920.

Signs and Symptoms

The first signs and symptoms appear after 1-3 hours. Neuromuscular disturbances are the most prominent. Cardiovascular disorders are generally milder, and severe cardiac complications occur only when very high doses (> 60 g) have been ingested.

Respiration: Irregular breathing, respiratory depression.

Cardiovascular System: Tachycardia, hypotension or hypertension, shock, conduction disorders.

Nervous System and Muscles: Impairment of consciousness ranging in severity to deep coma. Convulsions, especially in small children. Motor restlessness, muscular twitching, tremor, athetoid movements, opisthotonos, ataxia, drowsiness, dizziness, mydriasis, nystagmus, adiadochokinesia,

---

Dosage Information

Indication	Initial Dose Tablet*	Initial Dose XR†	Initial Dose Suspension	Subsequent Dose Tablet*	Subsequent Dose XR†	Subsequent Dose Suspension	Maximum Daily Dose Tablet*	Maximum Daily Dose XR†	Maximum Daily Dose Suspension
Epilepsy Under 6 yr	10–20 mg/kg/day b.i.d. or t.i.d.		10–20 mg/kg/day q.i.d.	Increase weekly to achieve optimal clinical response, t.i.d. or q.i.d.		Increase weekly to achieve optimal clinical response, t.i.d. or q.i.d.	35 mg/kg/24 hr (see Dosage and Administration section above)		35 mg/kg/24 hr (see Dosage and Administration section above)
6–12 yr	100 mg b.i.d. (200 mg/day)	100 mg b.i.d. (200 mg/day)	½ tsp q.i.d. (200 mg/day)	Add up to 100 mg/day at weekly intervals, t.i.d. or q.i.d.	Add 100 mg/day at weekly intervals b.i.d.	Add up to 1 tsp (100 mg)/day at weekly intervals, t.i.d. or q.i.d.	1000 mg/24 hr		
Over 12 yr	200 mg b.i.d. (400 mg/day)	200 mg b.i.d. (400 mg/day)	1 tsp q.i.d. (400 mg/day)	Add up to 200 mg/day at weekly intervals, t.i.d. or q.i.d.	Add up to 200 mg/day at weekly intervals, b.i.d.	Add up to 2 tsp (200 mg)/day at weekly intervals, t.i.d. or q.i.d.	1000 mg/24 hr (12–15 yr) 1200 mg/24 hr (> 15 yr) 1600 mg/24 hr (adults, in rare instances)		
Trigeminal Neuralgia	100 mg b.i.d. (200 mg/day)	100 mg b.i.d. (200 mg/day)	½ tsp q.i.d. (200 mg/day)	Add up to 200 mg/day in increments of 100 mg every 12 hr	Add up to 200 mg/day in increments of 100 mg every 12 hr	Add up to 2 tsp (200 mg)/day in increments of 50 mg (½ tsp) q.i.d.	1200 mg/24 hr		

*Tablet = Chewable or conventional tablets
†XR = Tegretol®-XR extended-release tablets

ballism, psychomotor disturbances, dysmetria. Initial hyperreflexia, followed by hyporeflexia.
Gastrointestinal Tract: Nausea, vomiting.
Kidneys and Bladder: Anuria or oliguria, urinary retention.
Laboratory Findings: Isolated instances of overdosage have included leukocytosis, reduced leukocyte count, glycosuria, and acetonuria. EEG may show dysrhythmias.
Combined Poisoning: When alcohol, tricyclic antidepressants, barbiturates, or hydantoins are taken at the same time, the signs and symptoms of acute poisoning with Tegretol may be aggravated or modified.

Treatment
The prognosis in cases of severe poisoning is critically dependent upon prompt elimination of the drug, which may be achieved by inducing vomiting, irrigating the stomach, and by taking appropriate steps to diminish absorption. If these measures cannot be implemented without risk on the spot, the patient should be transferred at once to a hospital, while ensuring that vital functions are safeguarded. There is no specific antidote.
Elimination of the Drug: Induction of vomiting. Gastric lavage. Even when more than 4 hours have elapsed following ingestion of the drug, the stomach should be repeatedly irrigated, especially if the patient has also consumed alcohol.
Measures to Reduce Absorption: Activated charcoal, laxatives.
Measures to Accelerate Elimination: Forced diuresis. Dialysis is indicated only in severe poisoning associated with renal failure. Replacement transfusion is indicated in severe poisoning in small children.
Respiratory Depression: Keep the airways free; resort, if necessary, to endotracheal intubation, artificial respiration, and administration of oxygen.
Hypotension, Shock: Keep the patient's legs raised and administer a plasma expander. If blood pressure fails to rise despite measures taken to increase plasma volume, use of vasoactive substances should be considered.
Convulsions: Diazepam or barbiturates.
Warning: Diazepam or barbiturates may aggravate respiratory depression (especially in children), hypotension, and coma. However, barbiturates should *not* be used if drugs that inhibit monoamine oxidase have also been taken by the patient either in overdosage or in recent therapy (within 1 week).
Surveillance: Respiration, cardiac function (ECG monitoring), blood pressure, body temperature, pupillary reflexes, and kidney and bladder function should be monitored for several days.
Treatment of Blood Count Abnormalities: If evidence of significant bone marrow depression develops, the following recommendations are suggested: (1) stop the drug, (2) perform daily CBC, platelet, and reticulocyte counts, (3) do a bone marrow aspiration and trephine biopsy immediately and repeat with sufficient frequency to monitor recovery. Special periodic studies might be helpful as follows: (1) white cell and platelet antibodies, (2) ^{59}Fe—ferrokinetic studies, (3) peripheral blood cell typing, (4) cytogenetic studies on marrow and peripheral blood, (5) bone marrow culture studies for colony-forming units, (6) hemoglobin electrophoresis for A_2 and F hemoglobin, and (7) serum folic acid and B_{12} levels. A fully developed aplastic anemia will require appropriate, intensive monitoring and therapy, for which specialized consultation should be sought.

DOSAGE AND ADMINISTRATION
[See table on preceding page.]
Monitoring of blood levels has increased the efficacy and safety of anticonvulsants (see PRECAUTIONS, Laboratory Tests). Dosage should be adjusted to the needs of the individual patient. A low initial daily dosage with a gradual increase is advised. As soon as adequate control is achieved, the dosage may be reduced very gradually to the minimum effective level. Medication should be taken with meals.
Since a given dose of Tegretol suspension will produce higher peak levels than the same dose given as the tablet, it is recommended to start with low doses (children 6–12 years: $^1/_2$ teaspoon q.i.d.) and to increase slowly to avoid unwanted side effects.
Conversion of patients from oral Tegretol tablets to Tegretol suspension: Patients should be converted by administering the same number of mg per day in smaller, more frequent doses (i.e., b.i.d. tablets to t.i.d. suspension).
Tegretol-XR is an extended-release formulation for twice-a-day administration. When converting patients from Tegretol conventional tablets to Tegretol-XR, the same total daily mg dose of Tegretol-XR should be administered.
Tegretol-XR tablets must be swallowed whole and never crushed or chewed. Tegretol-XR tablets should be inspected for chips or cracks. Damaged tablets should not be consumed.
Epilepsy (See INDICATIONS AND USAGE)
Adults and children over 12 years of age—Initial: Either 200 mg b.i.d. for tablets and XR tablets, or 1 teaspoon q.i.d. for suspension (400 mg/day). Increase at weekly intervals by adding up to 200 mg/day using a b.i.d. regimen of

Tegretol-XR or a t.i.d. or q.i.d. regimen of the other formulations until the optimal response is obtained. Dosage generally should not exceed 1000 mg daily in children 12–15 years of age, and 1200 mg daily in patients above 15 years of age. Doses up to 1600 mg daily have been used in adults in rare instances. *Maintenance:* Adjust dosage to the minimum effective level, usually 800–1200 mg daily.
Children 6–12 years of age—Initial: Either 100 mg b.i.d. for tablets or XR tablets, or $^1/_2$ teaspoon q.i.d. for suspension (200 mg/day). Increase at weekly intervals by adding up to 100 mg/day using a b.i.d. regimen of Tegretol-XR or a t.i.d. or q.i.d. regimen of the other formulations until the optimal response is obtained. Dosage generally should not exceed 1000 mg daily. *Maintenance:* Adjust dosage to the minimum effective level, usually 400–800 mg daily.
Children under 6 years of age—Initial: 10–20 mg/kg/day b.i.d. or t.i.d. as tablets, or q.i.d. as suspension. Increase weekly to achieve optimal clinical response administered t.i.d. or q.i.d. *Maintenance:* Ordinarily, optimal clinical response is achieved at daily doses below 35 mg/kg. If satisfactory clinical response has not been achieved, plasma levels should be measured to determine whether or not they are in the therapeutic range. No recommendation regarding the safety of carbamazepine for use at doses above 35 mg/kg/24 hours can be made. Combination Therapy: Tegretol may be used alone or with other anticonvulsants. When added to existing anticonvulsant therapy, the drug should be added gradually while the other anticonvulsants are maintained or gradually decreased, except phenytoin, which may have to be increased (see PRECAUTIONS, Drug Interactions, and Pregnancy Category C).
Trigeminal Neuralgia (see INDICATIONS AND USAGE)
Initial: On the first day, either 100 mg b.i.d. for tablets or XR tablets, or $^1/_2$ teaspoon q.i.d. for suspension, for a total daily dose of 200 mg. This daily dose may be increased by up to 200 mg/day using increments of 100 mg every 12 hours for tablets or XR tablets, or 50 mg ($^1/_2$ teaspoon) q.i.d. for suspension, only as needed to achieve freedom from pain. Do not exceed 1200 mg daily. *Maintenance:* Control of pain can be maintained in most patients with 400–800 mg daily. However, some patients may be maintained on as little as 200 mg daily while others may require as much as 1200 mg daily. At least once every 3 months throughout the treatment period, attempts should be made to reduce the dose to the minimum effective level or even to discontinue the drug.

HOW SUPPLIED
Chewable Tablets 100 mg—round, red-speckled, pink, single-scored (imprinted Tegretol on one side and 52 twice on the scored side)
Bottles of 100 .... NDC 0083-0052-30
Unit Dose (blister pack)
Box of 100 (strips of 10) .... NDC 0083-0052-32
Do not store above 30°C (86°F). *Protect from light and moisture.*
Dispense in tight, light-resistant container (USP).
Tablets 200 mg—capsule-shaped, pink, single-scored (imprinted Tegretol on one side and 27 twice on the partially scored side)
Bottles of 100 .... NDC 0083-0027-30
Bottles of 1000 .... NDC 0083-0027-40
Unit Dose (blister pack)
Box of 100 (strips of 10) .... NDC 0083-0027-32
Do not store above 30°C (86°F). *Protect from moisture. Dispense in tight container (USP).*
XR Tablets 100 mg—round, yellow, coated (imprinted T on one side and 100 mg on the other), release portal on one side
Bottles of 100 .... NDC 0083-0061-30
Unit Dose (blister pack)
Box of 100 (strips of 10) .... NDC 0083-0061-32
XR Tablets 200 mg—round, pink, coated (imprinted T on one side and 200 mg on the other), release portal on one side
Bottles of 100 .... NDC 0083-0062-30
Unit Dose (blister pack)
Box of 100 (strips of 10) .... NDC 0083-0062-32
XR Tablets 400 mg—round, brown, coated (imprinted T on one side and 400 mg on the other), release portal on one side
Bottles of 100 .... NDC 0083-0060-30
Unit Dose (blister pack)
Box of 100 (strips of 10) .... NDC 0083-0060-32
Store at controlled room temperature 15°-30°C (59°-86°F). *Protect from moisture. Dispense in tight container (USP).*
Samples, when available, are identified by the word *SAMPLE* appearing on each tablet.
Suspension 100 mg/5 mL (teaspoon)—yellow-orange, citrus-vanilla flavored
Bottles of 450 mL .... NDC 0083-0019-76
Shake well before using.
Because of the possibility of component interaction, Tegretol suspension should not be administered simultaneously with other liquid medicinal agents or diluents.
Do not store above 30°C (86°F). *Dispense in tight, light-resistant container (USP).*
[See table on preceding page.]

C96-46 (Rev. 5/96)

Ciba-Geigy Corporation
Pharmaceuticals Division
Summit, NJ 07901
Tegretol Suspension Manufactured by
Ciba-Geigy Canada, Ltd.
Dorval, Quebec, Canada
Shown in Product Identification Guide, page 309

TOFRANIL®   ℞
[*toe-fray 'nill*]
imipramine hydrochloride USP
Ampuls
For intramuscular administration

Prescribing Information
DESCRIPTION
Tofranil, imipramine hydrochloride USP, the original tricyclic antidepressant, is available in ampuls for intramuscular administration. Each 2 mL ampul contains imipramine hydrochloride USP, 25 mg; ascorbic acid, 2 mg; sodium bisulfite, 1 mg; sodium sulfite, anhydrous, 1 mg. Tofranil is a member of the dibenzazepine group of compounds. It is designated 5-[3-(dimethylamino)propyl] -10,11-dihydro-5H-dibenz[b,f]azepine monohydrochloride.
Imipramine hydrochloride USP is a white to off-white, odorless, or practically odorless crystalline powder. It is freely soluble in water and in alcohol, soluble in acetone, and insoluble in ether and in benzene. Its molecular weight is 316.87.

CLINICAL PHARMACOLOGY
The mechanism of action of Tofranil is not definitely known. However, it does not act primarily by stimulation of the central nervous system. The clinical effect is hypothesized as being due to potentiation of adrenergic synapses by blocking uptake of norepinephrine at nerve endings. The mode of action of the drug in controlling childhood enuresis is thought to be apart from its antidepressant effect.

INDICATIONS AND USAGE
Depression: For the relief of symptoms of depression. Endogenous depression is more likely to be alleviated than other depressive states. One to three weeks of treatment may be needed before optimal therapeutic effects are evident.

CONTRAINDICATIONS
The concomitant use of monoamine oxidase inhibiting compounds is contraindicated. Hyperpyretic crises or severe convulsive seizures may occur in patients receiving such combinations. The potentiation of adverse effects can be serious, or even fatal. When it is desired to substitute Tofranil in patients receiving a monoamine oxidase inhibitor, as long an interval should elapse as the clinical situation will allow, with a minimum of 14 days. Initial dosage should be low and increases should be gradual and cautiously prescribed.
The drug is contraindicated during the acute recovery period after a myocardial infarction. Patients with a known hypersensitivity to this compound should not be given the drug. The possibility of cross-sensitivity to other dibenzazepine compounds should be kept in mind.

WARNINGS
Children: A dose of 2.5 mg/kg/day of imipramine hydrochloride should not be exceeded in childhood. ECG changes of unknown significance have been reported in pediatric patients with doses twice this amount.
Extreme caution should be used when this drug is given to: patients with cardiovascular disease because of the possibility of conduction defects, arrhythmias, congestive heart failure, myocardial infarction, strokes and tachycardia. These patients require cardiac surveillance at all dosage levels of the drug; patients with increased intraocular pressure, history of urinary retention, or history of narrow-angle glaucoma because of the drug's anticholinergic properties; hyperthyroid patients or those on thyroid medication because of the possibility of cardiovascular toxicity; patients with a history of seizure disorder because this drug has been shown to lower the seizure threshold; patients receiving guanethidine, clonidine, or similar agents, since imipramine hydrochloride may block the pharmacologic effects of these drugs; patients receiving methylphenidate hydrochloride. Since methylphenidate hydrochloride may inhibit the metabolism of imipramine hydrochloride, downward dosage adjustment of imipramine hydrochloride may be required when given concomitantly with methylphenidate hydrochloride.
Tofranil may enhance the CNS depressant effects of alcohol. Therefore, it should be borne in mind that the dangers inherent in a suicide attempt or accidental overdosage with the drug may be increased for the patient who uses excessive amounts of alcohol. (See PRECAUTIONS.)
Since imipramine hydrochloride may impair the mental and/or physical abilities required for the performance of potentially hazardous tasks, such as operating an automobile or machinery, the patient should be cautioned accordingly.

Continued on next page

CibaGeneva—Cont.

Contains sodium sulfite and sodium bisulfite, that may cause allergic-type reactions including anaphylactic symptoms and life-threatening or less severe asthmatic episodes in certain susceptible people. The overall prevalence of sulfite sensitivity in the general population is unknown and probably low. Sulfite sensitivity is seen more frequently in asthmatic than in nonasthmatic people.

PRECAUTIONS

General

An ECG recording should be taken prior to the initiation of larger-than-usual doses of imipramine hydrochloride and at appropriate intervals thereafter until steady state is achieved. (Patients with any evidence of cardiovascular disease require cardiac surveillance at all dosage levels of the drug. See WARNINGS.) Elderly patients and patients with cardiac disease or a prior history of cardiac disease are at special risk of developing the cardiac abnormalities associated with the use of imipramine hydrochloride.

It should be kept in mind that the possibility of suicide in seriously depressed patients is inherent in the illness and may persist until significant remission occurs. Such patients should be carefully supervised during the early phase of treatment with imipramine hydrochloride, and may require hospitalization. Prescriptions should be written for the smallest amount feasible.

Hypomanic or manic episodes may occur, particularly in patients with cyclic disorders.

Such reactions may necessitate discontinuation of the drug. If needed, imipramine hydrochloride may be resumed in lower dosage when these episodes are relieved.

Administration of a tranquilizer may be useful in controlling such episodes.

An activation of the psychosis may occasionally be observed in schizophrenic patients and may require reduction of dosage and the addition of a phenothiazine.

Concurrent administration of imipramine hydrochloride with electroshock therapy may increase the hazards; such treatment should be limited to those patients for whom it is essential, since there is limited clinical experience.

Patients taking imipramine hydrochloride should avoid excessive exposure to sunlight since there have been reports of photosensitization.

Both elevation and lowering of blood sugar levels have been reported with imipramine hydrocholoride use.

Imipramine hydrochloride should be used with caution in patients with significantly impaired renal or hepatic function.

Patients who develop a fever and a sore throat during therapy with imipramine hydrochloride should have leukocyte and differential blood counts performed. Imipramine hydrochloride should be discontinued if there is evidence of pathologic neutrophil depression.

Prior to elective surgery, imipramine hydrochloride should be discontinued for as long as the clinical situation will allow.

DRUG INTERACTIONS

Drugs Metabolized by P450 2D6: The biochemical activity of the drug metabolizing isozyme cytochrome P450 2D6 (debrisoquin hydroxylase) is reduced in a subset of the Caucasian population (about 7%–10% of Caucasians are so-called "poor metabolizers"); reliable estimates of the prevalence of reduced P450 2D6 isozyme activity among Asian, African, and other populations are not yet available. Poor metabolizers have higher than expected plasma concentrations of tricyclic antidepressants (TCAs) when given usual doses. Depending on the fraction of drug metabolized by P450 2D6, the increase in plasma concentration may be small, or quite large (8-fold increase in plasma AUC of the TCA).

In addition, certain drugs inhibit the activity of this isozyme and make normal metabolizers resemble poor metabolizers. An individual who is stable on a given dose of TCA may become abruptly toxic when given one of these inhibiting drugs as concomitant therapy. The drugs that inhibit cytochrome P450 2D6 include some that are not metabolized by the enzyme (quinidine; cimetidine) and many that are substrates for P450 2D6 (many other antidepressants, phenothiazines, and the Type 1C antiarrhythmics propafenone and flecainide). While all the selective serotonin reuptake inhibitors (SSRIs), e.g., fluoxetine, sertraline, and paroxetine, inhibit P450 2D6, they may vary in the extent of inhibition. The extent to which SSRI-TCA interactions may pose clinical problems will depend on the degree of inhibition and the pharmacokinetics of the SSRI involved. Nevertheless, caution is indicated in the co-administration of TCAs with any of the SSRIs and also in switching from one class to the other. Of particular importance, sufficient time must elapse before initiating TCA treatment in a patient being withdrawn from fluoxetine, given the long half-life of the parent and active metabolite (at least 5 weeks may be necessary).

Concomitant use of tricyclic antidepressants with drugs that can inhibit cytochrome P450 2D6 may require lower doses than usually prescribed for either the tricyclic antidepressant or the other drug. Furthermore, whenever one of these other drugs is withdrawn from co-therapy, an increased dose of tricyclic antidepressant may be required. It is desirable to monitor TCA plasma levels whenever a TCA is going to be co-administered with another drug known to be an inhibitor of P450 2D6.

The plasma concentration of imipramine may increase when the drug is given concomitantly with hepatic enzyme inhibitors (e.g., cimetidine, fluoxetine) and decrease by concomitant administration with hepatic enzyme inducers (e.g., barbiturates, phenytoin), and adjustment of the dosage of imipramine may therefore be necessary.

In occasional susceptible patients or in those receiving anticholinergic drugs (including antiparkinsonism agents) in addition, the atropine-like effects may become more pronounced (e.g., paralytic ileus). Close supervision and careful adjustment of dosage is required when imipramine hydrochloride is administered concomitantly with anticholinergic drugs.

Avoid the use of preparations, such as decongestants and local anesthetics, that contain any sympathomimetic amine (e.g., epinephrine, norepinephrine), since it has been reported that tricyclic antidepressants can potentiate the effects of catecholamines.

Caution should be exercised when impramine hydrochloride is used with agents that lower blood pressure. Imipramine hydrochloride may potentiate the effects of CNS depressant drugs.

Patients should be warned that imipramine hydrochloride may enhance the CNS depressant effects of alcohol (See WARNINGS.)

Usage During Pregnancy and Lactation: Animal reproduction studies have yielded inconclusive results. (See also ANIMAL PHARMACOLOGY & TOXICOLOGY.)

There have been no well-controlled studies conducted with pregnant women to determine the effect of imipramine hydrochloride on the fetus. However, there have been clinical reports of congenital malformations associated with the use of the drug. Although a causal relationship between these effects and the drug could not be established, the possibility of fetal risk from the maternal ingestion of imipramine hydrochloride cannot be excluded. Therefore, imipramine hydrochloride should be used in women who are or might become pregnant only if the clinical condition clearly justifies potential risk to the fetus.

Limited data suggest that imipramine hydrochloride is likely to be excreted in human breast milk. As a general rule, a woman taking a drug should not nurse since the possibility exists that the drug may be excreted in breast milk and be harmful to the child.

Usage in Children: The effectiveness of the drug in children for conditions other than nocturnal enuresis given orally has not been established.

ADVERSE REACTIONS

Note: Although the listing which follows includes a few adverse reactions which have not been reported with this specific drug, the pharmacological similarities among the tricyclic antidepressant drugs require that each of the reactions be considered when imipramine is administered.

Cardiovascular: Orthostatic hypotension, hypertension, tachycardia, palpitation, myocardial infarction, arrhythmias, heart block, ECG changes, precipitation of congestive heart failure, stroke.

Psychiatric: Confusional states (especially in the elderly) with hallucinations, disorientation, delusions; anxiety, restlessness, agitation; insomnia and nightmares; hypomania; exacerbation of psychosis.

Neurological: Numbness, tingling, paresthesias of extremities; incoordination, ataxia, tremors; peripheral neuropathy; extrapyramidal symptoms; seizures, alterations in EEG patterns; tinnitus.

Anticholinergic: Dry mouth, and, rarely, associated sublingual adenitis; blurred vision, disturbances of accommodation, mydriasis; constipation, paralytic ileus; urinary retention, delayed micturition, dilation of the urinary tract.

Allergic: Skin rash, petechiae, urticaria, itching, photosensitization; edema (general or of face and tongue); drug fever; cross-sensitivity with desipramine.

Hematologic: Bone marrow depression including agranulocytosis; eosinophilia; purpura; thrombocytopenia.

Gastrointestinal: Nausea and vomiting, anorexia, epigastric distress, diarrhea; peculiar taste, stomatitis, abdominal cramps, black tongue.

Endocrine: Gynecomastia in the male; breast enlargement and galactorrhea in the female; increased or decreased libido, impotence; testicular swelling; elevation or depression of blood sugar levels; inappropriate antidiuretic hormone (ADH) secretion syndrome.

Other: Jaundice (simulating obstructive); altered liver function; weight gain or loss; perspiration; flushing; urinary frequency; drowsiness, dizziness, weakness and fatigue; headache; parotid swelling; alopecia; proneness to falling.

Withdrawal Symptoms: Though not indicative of addiction, abrupt cessation of treatment after prolonged therapy may produce nausea, headache and malaise.

DOSAGE AND ADMINISTRATION

Initially, up to 100 mg/day intramuscularly in divided doses. Parenteral administration should be used only for starting therapy in patients unable or unwilling to use oral medication. The oral form should supplant the injectable as soon as possible.

Lower dosages are recommended for elderly patients and adolescents. Lower dosages are also recommended for outpatients as compared to hospitalized patients who will be under close supervision. Dosage should be initiated at a low level and increased gradually, noting carefully the clinical response and any evidence of intolerance. Following remission, oral maintenance medication may be required for a longer period of time, at the lowest dose that will maintain remission.

OVERDOSAGE

Children have been reported to be more sensitive than adults to an acute overdosage of imipramine hydrochloride. An acute overdose of any amount in infants or young children, especially, must be considered serious and potentially fatal.

Signs and Symptoms: These may vary in severity depending upon factors such as the amount of drug absorbed, the age of the patient, and the interval between drug ingestion and the start of treatment. Blood and urine levels of imipramine may not reflect the severity of poisoning; they have chiefly a qualitative rather than quantitative value, and are unreliable indicators in the clinical management of the patient.

CNS abnormalities may include drowsiness, stupor, coma, ataxia, restlessness, agitation, hyperactive reflexes, muscle rigidity, athetoid and choreiform movements, and convulsions.

Cardiac abnormalities may include arrhythmia, tachycardia, ECG evidence of impaired conduction, and signs of congestive failure. Respiratory depression, cyanosis, hypotension, shock, vomiting, hyperpyrexia, mydriasis, and diaphoresis may also be present.

Treatment: The recommended treatment for overdosage with tricyclic antidepressants may change periodically. Therefore, it is recommended that the physician contact a poison control center for current information on treatment.

Because CNS involvement, respiratory depression and cardiac arrhythmia can occur suddenly, hospitalization and close observation may be necessary, even when the amount ingested is thought to be small or the initial degree of intoxication appears slight or moderate. All patients with ECG abnormalities should have continuous cardiac monitoring and be closely observed until well after cardiac status has returned to normal; relapses may occur after apparent recovery.

In the alert patient, empty the stomach promptly by lavage. In the obtunded patient, secure the airway with a cuffed endotracheal tube before beginning lavage (do not induce emesis). Instillation of activated charcoal slurry may help reduce absorption of imipramine.

Minimize external stimulation to reduce the tendency to convulsions. If anticonvulsants are necessary, diazepam and phenytoin may be useful.

Maintain adequate respiratory exchange. Do not use respiratory stimulants.

Shock should be treated with supportive measures, such as appropriate position, intravenous fluids, and, if necessary, a vasopressor agent. The use of corticosteroids in shock is controversial and may be contraindicated in cases of overdosage with tricyclic antidepressants. Digitalis may increase conduction abnormalities and further irritate an already sensitized myocardium. If congestive heart failure necessitates rapid digitalization, particular care must be exercised.

Hyperpyrexia should be controlled by whatever external means are available, including ice packs and cooling sponge baths, if necessary.

Hemodialysis, peritoneal dialysis, exchange transfusions and forced diuresis have been generally reported as ineffective because of the rapid fixation of imipramine in tissues. Blood and urine levels of imipramine may not correlate with the degree of intoxication, and are unreliable indicators in the clinical management of the patient.

The slow intravenous administration of physostigmine salicylate has been used as a last resort to reverse severe CNS anticholinergic manifestations of overdosage with tricyclic antidepressants; however, it should not be used routinely, since it may induce seizures and cholinergic crises.

HOW SUPPLIED

Ampuls 2 ml—*For intramuscular administration only*

25 mg imipramine hydrochloride, 2 mg ascorbic acid, 1 mg sodium bisulfite, 1 mg sodium sulfite, anhydrous

Boxes of 10 .... NDC 0028-0065-23

Store between 59°–86°F (15°–30°C).

Note: Upon storage, minute crystals may form in some ampuls. This has no influence on the therapeutic efficacy of the

preparation, and the crystals redissolve when the affected ampuls are immersed in hot tap water for 1 minute.

ANIMAL PHARMACOLOGY & TOXICOLOGY

A. *Acute:* Oral LD$_{50}$ ranges are as follows:

Rat   355 to 682 mg/kg
Dog   100 to 215 mg/kg

Depending on the dosage in both species, toxic signs proceeded progressively from depression, irregular respiration and ataxia to convulsions and death.

B. *Reproduction/Teratogenic:* The overall evaluation may be summed up in the following manner:

Oral: Independent studies in three species (rat, mouse, and rabbit) revealed that when Tofranil is administered orally in doses up to approximately 2½ times the maximum human dose in the first 2 species and up to 25 times the maximum human dose in the third species, the drug is essentially free from teratogenic potential. In the three species studied, only one instance of fetal abnormality occurred (in the rabbit) and in that study there was likewise an abnormality in the control group. However, evidence does exist from the rat studies that some systemic and embryotoxic potential is demonstrable. This is manifested by reduced litter size, a slight increase in the stillborn rate and a reduction in the mean birth weight.

Parenteral: In contradistinction to the oral data, Tofranil does exhibit a slight but definite teratogenic potential when administered by the subcutaneous route. Drug effects on both the mother and fetus in the rabbit are manifested in higher resorption rates and decrease in mean fetal birth weights, while teratogenic findings occurred at a level of 5 times the maximum human dose. In the mouse, teratogenicity occurred at 1½ and 6½ times the maximum human dose, but no teratogenic effects were seen at levels 3 times the maximum human dose. Thus, in the mouse, the findings are equivocal.

C94-15 (Rev. 7/94)

Dist. by:
Geigy Pharmaceuticals
Ciba-Geigy Corporation
Ardsley, New York 10502

TOFRANIL®   ℞
imipramine hydrochloride tablets USP
Tablets of 10 mg
Tablets of 25 mg
Tablets of 50 mg
For oral administration

Prescribing Information

DESCRIPTION

Tofranil, imipramine hydrochloride USP, the original tricyclic antidepressant, is a member of the dibenzazepine group of compounds. It is designated 5-[3-(dimethylamino) propyl]-10,11-dihydro-5*H*-dibenz [b,f]azepine monohydrochloride. Imipramine hydrochloride USP is a white to off-white, odorless, or practically odorless crystalline powder. It is freely soluble in water and in alcohol, soluble in acetone, and insoluble in ether and in benzene. Its molecular weight is 316.87.
Inactive Ingredients: Calcium phosphate, cellulose compounds, docusate sodium, iron oxides, magnesium stearate, polyethylene glycol, povidone, sodium starch glycolate, sucrose, talc and titanium dioxide.

CLINICAL PHARMACOLOGY

The mechanism of action of Tofranil is not definitely known. However, it does not act primarily by stimulation of the central nervous system. The clinical effect is hypothesized as being due to potentiation of adrenergic synapses by blocking uptake of norepinephrine at nerve endings. The mode of action of the drug in controlling childhood enuresis is thought to be apart from its antidepressant effect.

INDICATIONS AND USAGE

Depression: For the relief of symptoms of depression. Endogenous depression is more likely to be alleviated than other depressive states. One to three weeks of treatment may be needed before optimal therapeutic effects are evident.
Childhood Enuresis: May be useful as temporary adjunctive therapy in reducing enuresis in children aged 6 years and older, after possible organic causes have been excluded by appropriate tests. In patients having daytime symptoms of frequency and urgency, examination should include voiding cystourethrography and cystoscopy, as necessary. The effectiveness of treatment may decrease with continued drug administration.

CONTRAINDICATIONS

The concomitant use of monoamine oxidase inhibiting compounds is contraindicated. Hyperpyretic crises or severe convulsive seizures may occur in patients receiving such combinations. The potentiation of adverse effects can be serious, or even fatal. When it is desired to substitute Tofranil in patients receiving a monoamine oxidase inhibitor, as long an interval should elapse as the clinical situation will allow,

---

with a minimum of 14 days. Initial dosage should be low and increases should be gradual and cautiously prescribed.
The drug is contraindicated during the acute recovery period after a myocardial infarction. Patients with a known hypersensitivity to this compound should not be given the drug. The possibility of cross-sensitivity to other dibenzazepine compounds should be kept in mind.

WARNINGS

Children: A dose of 2.5 mg/kg/day of Tofranil should not be exceeded in childhood. ECG changes of unknown significance have been reported in pediatric patients with doses twice this amount.

Extreme caution should be used when this drug is given to: patients with cardiovascular disease because of the possibility of conduction defects, arrhythmias, congestive heart failure, myocardial infarction, strokes and tachycardia. These patients require cardiac surveillance at all dosage levels of the drug; patients with increased intraocular pressure, history of urinary retention, or history of narrow-angle glaucoma because of the drug's anticholinergic properties; hyperthyroid patients or those on thyroid medication because of the possibility of cardiovascular toxicity; patients with a history of seizure disorder because this drug has been shown to lower the seizure threshold; patients receiving guanethidine, clonidine, or similar agents, since Tofranil may block the pharmacologic effects of these drugs; patients receiving methylphenidate hydrochloride. Since methylphenidate hydrochloride may inhibit the metabolism of Tofranil, downward dosage adjustment of imipramine hydrochloride may be required when given concomitantly with methylphenidate hydrochloride.
Tofranil may enhance the CNS depressant effects of alcohol. Therefore, it should be borne in mind that the dangers inherent in a suicide attempt or accidental overdosage with the drug may be increased for the patient who uses excessive amounts of alcohol. (See PRECAUTIONS.)
Since Tofranil may impair the mental and/or physical abilities required for the performance of potentially hazardous tasks, such as operating an automobile or machinery, the patient should be cautioned accordingly.

PRECAUTIONS
General
An ECG recording should be taken prior to the initiation of larger-than-usual doses of Tofranil and at appropriate intervals thereafter until steady state is achieved. (Patients with any evidence of cardiovascular disease require cardiac surveillance at all dosage levels of the drug. See WARNINGS.)
Elderly patients and patients with cardiac disease or a prior history of cardiac disease are at special risk of developing the cardiac abnormalities associated with the use of Tofranil.
It should be kept in mind that the possibility of suicide in seriously depressed patients is inherent in the illness and may persist until significant remission occurs. Such patients should be carefully supervised during the early phase of treatment with Tofranil, and may require hospitalization. Prescriptions should be written for the smallest amount feasible. Hypomanic or manic episodes may occur, particularly in patients with cyclic disorders. Such reactions may necessitate discontinuation of the drug. If needed, Tofranil may be resumed in lower dosage when these episodes are relieved.
Administration of a tranquilizer may be useful in controlling such episodes.
An activation of the psychosis may occasionally be observed in schizophrenic patients and may require reduction of dosage and the addition of a phenothiazine.
Concurrent administration of Tofranil with electroshock therapy may increase the hazards; such treatment should be limited to those patients for whom it is essential, since there is limited clinical experience.
Patients taking imipramine hydrochloride should avoid excessive exposure to sunlight since there have been reports of photosensitization.
Both elevation and lowering of blood sugar levels have been reported with imipramine hydrochloride use.
Imipramine hydrochloride should be used with caution in patients with significantly impaired renal or hepatic function.
Patients who develop a fever and a sore throat during therapy with imipramine hydrochloride should have leukocyte and differential blood counts performed. Imipramine hydrochloride should be discontinued if there is evidence of pathological neutrophil depression.
Prior to elective surgery, imipramine hydrochloride should be discontinued for as long as the clinical situation will allow.

Drug Interactions
Drugs Metabolized by P450 2D6: The biochemical activity of the drug metabolizing isozyme cytochrome P450 2D6 (debrisoquin hydroxylase) is reduced in a subset of the Caucasian population (about 7%–10% of Caucasians are so-called "poor metabolizers"); reliable estimates of the prevalence of reduced P450 2D6 isozyme activity among Asian, African, and other populations are not yet available. Poor metaboliz-

---

ers have higher than expected plasma concentrations of tricyclic antidepressants (TCAs) when given usual doses. Depending on the fraction of drug metabolized by P450 2D6, the increase in plasma concentration may be small, or quite large (8-fold increase in plasma AUC of the TCA).
In addition, certain drugs inhibit the activity of this isozyme and make normal metabolizers resemble poor metabolizers. An individual who is stable on a given dose of TCA may become abruptly toxic when given one of these inhibiting drugs as concomitant therapy. The drugs that inhibit cytochrome P450 2D6 include some that are not metabolized by the enzyme (quinidine; cimetidine) and many that are substrates for P450 2D6 (many other antidepressants, phenothiazines, and the Type 1C antiarrhythmics propafenone and flecainide). While all the selective serotonin reuptake inhibitors (SSRIs), e.g., fluoxetine, sertraline, and paroxetine, inhibit P450 2D6, they may vary in the extent of inhibition. The extent to which SSRI-TCA interactions may pose clinical problems will depend on the degree of inhibition and the pharmacokinetics of the SSRI involved. Nevertheless, caution is indicated in the co-administration of TCAs with any of the SSRIs and also in switching from one class to the other. Of particular importance, sufficient time must elapse before initiating TCA treatment in a patient being withdrawn from fluoxetine, given the long half-life of the parent and active metabolite (at least 5 weeks may be necessary).
Concomitant use of tricyclic antidepressants with drugs that can inhibit cytochrome P450 2D6 may require lower doses than usually prescribed for either the tricyclic antidepressant or the other drug. Furthermore, whenever one of these other drugs is withdrawn from co-therapy, an increased dose of tricyclic antidepressant may be required. It is desirable to monitor TCA plasma levels whenever a TCA is going to be co-administered with another drug known to be an inhibitor of P450 2D6.
The plasma concentration of imipramine may increase when the drug is given concomitantly with hepatic enzyme inhibitors (e.g., cimetidine, fluoxetine) and decrease by concomitant administration with hepatic enzyme inducers (e.g., barbiturates, phenytoin), and adjustment of the dosage of imipramine may therefore be necessary.
In occasional susceptible patients or in those receiving anticholinergic drugs (including antiparkinsonism agents) in addition, the atropine-like effects may become more pronounced (e.g., paralytic ileus). Close supervision and careful adjustment of dosage is required when imipramine hydrochloride is administered concomitantly with anticholinergic drugs.
Avoid the use of preparations, such as decongestants and local anesthetics, that contain any sympathomimetic amine (e.g., epinephrine, norepinephrine), since it has been reported that tricyclic antidepressants can potentiate the effects of catecholamines.
Caution should be exercised when imipramine hydrochloride is used with agents that lower blood pressure. Imipramine hydrochloride may potentiate the effects of CNS depressant drugs.
Patients should be warned that imipramine hydrochloride may enhance the CNS depressant effects of alcohol. (See WARNINGS.)
Pregnancy
Animal reproduction studies have yielded inconclusive results. (See also ANIMAL PHARMACOLOGY & TOXICOLOGY.)
There have been no well-controlled studies conducted with pregnant women to determine the effect of Tofranil on the fetus. However, there have been clinical reports of congenital malformations associated with the use of the drug. Although a causal relationship between these effects and the drug could not be established, the possibility of fetal risk from the maternal ingestion of Tofranil cannot be excluded. Therefore, Tofranil should be used in women who are or might become pregnant only if the clinical condition clearly justifies potential risk to the fetus.
Nursing Mothers
Limited data suggest that Tofranil is likely to be excreted in human breast milk. As a general rule, a woman taking a drug should not nurse since the possibility exists that the drug may be excreted in breast milk and be harmful to the child.
Pediatric Use
The effectiveness of the drug in children for conditions other than nocturnal enuresis has not been established.
The safety and effectiveness of the drug as temporary adjunctive therapy for nocturnal enuresis in children less than 6 years of age has not been established.
The safety of the drug for long-term, chronic use as adjunctive therapy for nocturnal enuresis in children 6 years of age or older has not been established; consideration should be given to instituting a drug-free period following an adequate therapeutic trial with a favorable response.

Continued on next page

CibaGeneva—Cont.

A dose of 2.5 mg/kg/day should not be exceeded in childhood. ECG changes of unknown significance have been reported in pediatric patients with doses twice this amount.

ADVERSE REACTIONS

Note: Although the listing which follows includes a few adverse reactions which have not been reported with this specific drug, the pharmacological similarities among the tricyclic antidepressant drugs require that each of the reactions be considered when Tofranil is administered.

Cardiovascular: Orthostatic hypotension, hypertension, tachycardia, palpitation, myocardial infarction, arrhythmias, heart block, ECG changes, precipitation of congestive heart failure, stroke.

Psychiatric: Confusional states (especially in the elderly) with hallucinations, disorientation, delusions; anxiety, restlessness, agitation; insomnia and nightmares; hypomania; exacerbation of psychosis.

Neurological: Numbness, tingling, paresthesias of extremities; incoordination, ataxia, tremors; peripheral neuropathy; extrapyramidal symptoms; seizures, alterations in EEG patterns; tinnitus.

Anticholinergic: Dry mouth, and, rarely, associated sublingual adenitis; blurred vision, disturbances of accommodation, mydriasis; constipation, paralytic ileus; urinary retention, delayed micturition, dilation of the urinary tract.

Allergic: Skin rash, petechiae, urticaria, itching, photosensitization; edema (general or of face and tongue); drug fever; cross-sensitivity with desipramine.

Hematologic: Bone marrow depression including agranulocytosis; eosinophilia; purpura; thrombocytopenia.

Gastrointestinal: Nausea and vomiting, anorexia, epigastric distress, diarrhea; peculiar taste, stomatitis, abdominal cramps, black tongue.

Endocrine: Gynecomastia in the male; breast enlargement and galactorrhea in the female; increased or decreased libido, impotence; testicular swelling; elevation or depression of blood sugar levels; inappropriate antidiuretic hormone (ADH) secretion syndrome.

Other: Jaundice (simulating obstructive); altered liver function; weight gain or loss; perspiration; flushing; urinary frequency; drowsiness, dizziness, weakness and fatigue; headache; parotid swelling; alopecia; proneness to falling.

Withdrawal Symptoms: Though not indicative of addiction, abrupt cessation of treatment after prolonged therapy may produce nausea, headache, and malaise.

Note: In enuretic children treated with Tofranil the most common adverse reactions have been nervousness, sleep disorders, tiredness, and mild gastrointestinal disturbances. These usually disappear during continued drug administration or when dosage is decreased. Other reactions which have been reported include constipation, convulsions, anxiety, emotional instability, syncope, and collapse. All of the adverse effects reported with adult use should be considered.

DOSAGE AND ADMINISTRATION

__Depression__

Lower dosages are recommended for elderly patients and adolescents. Lower dosages are also recommended for outpatients as compared to hospitalized patients who will be under close supervision. Dosage should be initiated at a low level and increased gradually, noting carefully the clinical response and any evidence of intolerance. Following remission, maintenance medication may be required for a longer period of time, at the lowest dose that will maintain remission.

Usual Adult Dose:

Hospitalized patients— Initially, 100 mg/day in divided doses gradually increased to 200 mg/day as required. If no response after two weeks, increase to 250–300 mg/day.

Outpatients—Initially, 75 mg/day increased to 150 mg/day. Dosages over 200 mg/day are not recommended. Maintenance, 50–150 mg/day.

Adolescent and geriatric patients—Initially, 30–40 mg/day; it is generally not necessary to exceed 100 mg/day.

__Childhood Enuresis__

Initially, an oral dose of 25 mg/day should be tried in children aged 6 and older. Medication should be given one hour before bedtime. If a satisfactory response does not occur within one week, increase the dose to 50 mg nightly in children under 12 years; children over 12 may receive up to 75 mg nightly. A daily dose greater than 75 mg does not enhance efficacy and tends to increase side effects. Evidence suggests that in early night bedwetters, the drug is more effective given earlier and in divided amounts, i.e., 25 mg in midafternoon, repeated at bedtime. Consideration should be given to instituting a drug-free period following an adequate therapeutic trial with a favorable response. Dosage should be tapered off gradually rather than abruptly discontinued; this may reduce the tendency to relapse. Children who relapse when the drug is discontinued do not always respond to a subsequent course of treatment.

A dose of 2.5 mg/kg/day should not be exceeded. ECG changes of unknown significance have been reported in pediatric patients with doses twice this amount.

The safety and effectiveness of Tofranil as temporary adjunctive therapy for nocturnal enuresis in children less than 6 years of age has not been established.

OVERDOSAGE

Deaths may occur from overdosage with this class of drug. Multiple drug ingestion (including alcohol) is common in deliberate tricyclic overdose. As the management is complex and changing, it is recommended that the physician contact a poison control center for current information on treatment. Signs and symptoms of toxicity develop rapidly after tricyclic overdose. Therefore, hospital monitoring is required as soon as possible.

Children have been reported to be more sensitive than adults to an acute overdosage of imipramine hydrochloride. An acute overdose of any amount in infants or young children, especially, must be considered serious and potentially fatal.

Manifestations

These may vary in severity depending upon factors such as the amount of drug absorbed, the age of the patient, and the interval between drug ingestion and the start of treatment. Critical manifestations of overdose include cardiac dysrhythmias, severe hypotension, convulsions, and CNS depression including coma. Changes in the electrocardiogram, particularly in QRS axis or width, are clinically significant indicators of tricyclic toxicity.

Other CNS manifestations may include drowsiness, stupor, ataxia, restlessness, agitation, hyperactive reflexes, muscle rigidity, athetoid and choreiform movements.

Cardiac abnormalities may include tachycardia and signs of congestive failure. Respiratory depression, cyanosis, shock, vomiting, hyperpyrexia, mydriasis, and diaphoresis may also be present.

Management

Obtain an ECG and immediately initiate cardiac monitoring. Protect the patient's airway, establish an intravenous line and initiate gastric decontamination. A minimum of 6 hours of observation with cardiac monitoring and observation for signs of CNS or respiratory depression, hypotension, cardiac dysrhythmias and/or conduction blocks, and seizures is necessary. If signs of toxicity occur at any time during this period, extended monitoring is required. There are case reports of patients succumbing to fatal dysrhythmias late after overdose; these patients had clinical evidence of significant poisoning prior to death and most received inadequate gastrointestinal decontamination. Monitoring of plasma drug levels should not guide management of the patient.

Gastrointestinal Decontamination: All patients suspected of tricyclic overdose should receive gastrointestinal decontamination. This should include large volume gastric lavage followed by activated charcoal. If consciousness is impaired, the airway should be secured prior to lavage. Emesis is contraindicated.

Cardiovascular: A maximal limb-lead QRS duration of ≥ 0.10 seconds may be the best indication of the severity of the overdose. Serum alkalinization, to a pH of 7.45 to 7.55, using intravenous sodium bicarbonate and hyperventilation (as needed) should be instituted for patients with dysrhythmias and/or QRS widening. A pH > 7.60 or a Pco_2 < 20 mmHg is undesirable. Dysrhythmias unresponsive to sodium bicarbonate therapy/hyperventilation may respond to lidocaine, bretylium, or phenytoin. Type 1A and 1C antiarrhythmics are generally contraindicated (e.g., quinidine, disopyramide, and procainamide).

In rare instances, hemoperfusion may be beneficial in acute refractory cardiovascular instability in patients with acute toxicity. However, hemodialysis, peritoneal dialysis, exchange transfusions, and forced diuresis generally have been reported as ineffective in tricyclic poisoning.

CNS: In patients with CNS depression, early intubation is advised because of the potential for abrupt deterioration. Seizures should be controlled with benzodiazepines, or if these are ineffective, other anticonvulsants (e.g., phenobarbital, phenytoin). Physostigmine is not recommended except to treat life-threatening symptoms that have been unresponsive to other therapies, and then only in consultation with a poison control center.

Psychiatric Follow-up: Since overdosage is often deliberate, patients may attempt suicide by other means during the recovery phase. Psychiatric referral may be appropriate.

Pediatric Management: The principles of management of child and adult overdosages are similar. It is strongly recommended that the physician contact the local poison control center for specific pediatric treatment.

HOW SUPPLIED

Tablets 10 mg—triangular, coral, sugar-coated (imprinted black Geigy 32)

Bottles of 100 .... NDC 0028-0032-01

Tablets 25 mg—round, biconvex, coral, sugar-coated (imprinted black Geigy 140)

Bottles of 100 .... NDC 0028-0140-01

Gy-Pak®—One Unit

12 bottles—100 tablets each

.... NDC 0028-0140-65

Tablets 50 mg—round, biconvex, coral, sugar-coated (imprinted black Geigy 136)

Bottles of 100 .... NDC 0028-0136-01

Store between 59°–86° F (15°–30° C)

Dispense in tight container (USP).

ANIMAL PHARMACOLOGY & TOXICOLOGY

A. *Acute:* Oral LD_{50} ranges are as follows:

Rat 355 to 682 mg/kg

Dog 100 to 215 mg/kg

Depending on the dosage in both species, toxic signs proceeded progressively from depression, irregular respiration and ataxia to convulsions and death.

B. *Reproduction/Teratogenic:* The overall evaluation may be summed up in the following manner:

Oral: Independent studies in three species (rat, mouse and rabbit) revealed that when Tofranil is administered orally in doses up to approximately 2½ times the maximum human dose in the first 2 species and up to 25 times the maximum human dose in the third species, the drug is essentially free from teratogenic potential. In the three species studied, only one instance of fetal abnormality occurred (in the rabbit) and in that study there was likewise an abnormality in the control group. However, evidence does exist from the rat studies that some systemic and embryotoxic potential is demonstrable. This is manifested by reduced litter size, a slight increase in the stillborn rate and a reduction in the mean birth weight.

C96-5 (Rev. 1/96)

Ciba-Geigy Corporation
Pharmaceuticals Division
Summit, NJ 07901

Shown in Product Identification Guide, page 309

TOFRANIL-PM® ℞

imipramine pamoate
Capsules of 75 mg
Capsules of 100 mg
Capsules of 125 mg
Capsules of 150 mg
For oral administration

Prescribing Information

DESCRIPTION

Tofranil-PM, imipramine pamoate, is a tricyclic antidepressant, available as capsules for oral administration. The 75-, 100-, 125-, and 150-mg capsules contain imipramine pamoate equivalent to 75, 100, 125, and 150 mg of imipramine hydrochloride. Imipramine pamoate is 5-[3-(dimethylamino)propyl]-10, 11-dihydro-5-*H*-dibenz[b,f]azepine 4,4′-methylenebis-(3-hydroxy-2-naphthoate) (2:1).

Imipramine pamoate is a fine, yellow, tasteless, odorless powder. It is soluble in ethanol, in acetone, in ether, in chloroform, and in carbon tetrachloride, and is insoluble in water. Its molecular weight is 949.21.

Inactive Ingredients. D&C Red No. 28, FD&C Blue No. 1, FD&C Yellow No. 6, D&C Yellow No. 10 (100 mg and 125 mg tablets only), gelatin, magnesium stearate, parabens, silicon dioxide, sodium lauryl sulfate, starch, talc, and titanium dioxide.

CLINICAL PHARMACOLOGY

The mechanism of action of imipramine is not definitely known. However, it does not act primarily by stimulation of the central nervous system. The clinical effect is hypothesized as being due to potentiation of adrenergic synapses by blocking uptake of norepinephrine at nerve endings.

INDICATIONS AND USAGE

For the relief of symptoms of depression. Endogenous depression is more likely to be alleviated than other depressive states. One to three weeks of treatment may be needed before optimal therapeutic effects are evident.

CONTRAINDICATIONS

The concomitant use of monoamine oxidase inhibiting compounds is contraindicated. Hyperpyretic crises or severe convulsive seizures may occur in patients receiving such combinations. The potentiation of adverse effects can be serious, or even fatal. When it is desired to substitute Tofranil-PM in patients receiving a monoamine oxidase inhibitor, as long an interval should elapse as the clinical situation will allow, with a minimum of 14 days. Initial dosage should be low and increases should be gradual and cautiously prescribed.

The drug is contraindicated during the acute recovery period after a myocardial infarction. Patients with a known hypersensitivity to this compound should not be given the drug. The possibility of cross-sensitivity to other dibenzazepine compounds should be kept in mind.

WARNINGS

Extreme caution should be used when this drug is given to: patients with cardiovascular disease because of the possibil-

ity of conduction defects, arrhythmias, congestive heart failure, myocardial infarction, strokes and tachycardia. These patients require cardiac surveillance at all dosage levels of the drug; patients with increased intraocular pressure, history of urinary retention, or history of narrow-angle glaucoma because of the drug's anticholinergic properties; hyperthyroid patients or those on thyroid medication because of the possibility of cardiovascular toxicity; patients with a history of seizure disorder because this drug has been shown to lower the seizure threshold; patients receiving guanethidine, clonidine, or similar agents, since imipramine pamoate may block the pharmacologic effects of these drugs; patients receiving methylphenidate hydrochloride. Since methylphenidate hydrochloride may inhibit the metabolism of imipramine pamoate, downward dosage adjustment of imipramine pamoate may be required when given concomitantly with methylphenidate hydrochloride.

Since imipramine pamoate may impair the mental and/or physical abilities required for the performance of potentially hazardous tasks, such as operating an automobile or machinery, the patient should be cautioned accordingly.

Tofranil-PM may enhance the CNS depressant effects of alcohol. Therefore, it should be borne in mind that the dangers inherent in a suicide attempt or accidental overdosage with the drug may be increased for the patient who uses excessive amounts of alcohol. (See PRECAUTIONS.)

Usage in Children: Tofranil-PM should not be used in children of any age because of the increased potential for acute overdosage due to the high unit potency (75 mg, 100 mg, 125 mg and 150 mg). Each capsule contains imipramine pamoate equivalent to 75 mg, 100 mg, 125 mg, or 150 mg imipramine hydrochloride.

PRECAUTIONS

General

An ECG recording should be taken prior to the initiation of larger-than-usual doses of imipramine pamoate and at appropriate intervals thereafter until steady state is achieved. (Patients with any evidence of cardiovascular disease require cardiac surveillance at all dosage levels of the drug. See WARNINGS.) Elderly patients and patients with cardiac disease or a prior history of cardiac disease are at special risk of developing the cardiac abnormalities associated with the use of imipramine pamoate. It should be kept in mind that the possibility of suicide in seriously depressed patients is inherent in the illness and may persist until significant remission occurs. Such patients should be carefully supervised during the early phase of treatment with imipramine pamoate and may require hospitalization. Prescriptions should be written for the smallest amount feasible.

Hypomanic or manic episodes may occur, particularly in patients with cyclic disorders. Such reactions may necessitate discontinuation of the drug. If needed, imipramine pamoate may be resumed in lower dosage when these episodes are relieved. Administration of a tranquilizer may be useful in controlling such episodes.

An activation of the psychosis may occasionally be observed in schizophrenic patients and may require reduction of dosage and the addition of a phenothiazine.

Concurrent administration of imipramine pamoate with electroshock therapy may increase the hazards: such treatment should be limited to those patients for whom it is essential, since there is limited clinical experience.

Patients taking imipramine pamoate should avoid excessive exposure to sunlight since there have been reports of photosensitization.

Both elevation and lowering of blood sugar levels have been reported with imipramine pamoate use.

Imipramine pamoate should be used with caution in patients with significantly impaired renal or hepatic function.

Patients who develop a fever and a sore throat during therapy with imipramine pamoate should have leukocyte and differential blood counts performed.

Imipramine pamoate should be discontinued if there is evidence of pathological neutrophil depression.

Prior to elective surgery, imipramine pamoate should be discontinued for as long as the clinical situation will allow.

Drug Interactions

Drugs Metabolized by P450 2D6: The biochemical activity of the drug metabolizing isozyme cytochrome P450 2D6 (debrisoquin hydroxylase) is reduced in a subset of the Caucasian population (about 7%-10% of Caucasians are so-called "poor metabolizers"); reliable estimates of the prevalence of reduced P450 2D6 isozyme activity among Asian, African, and other populations are not yet available. Poor metabolizers have higher than expected plasma concentrations of tricyclic antidepressants (TCAs) when given usual doses. Depending on the fraction of drug metabolized by P450 2D6, the increase in plasma concentration may be small, or quite large (8-fold increase in plasma AUC of the TCA).

In addition, certain drugs inhibit the activity of this isozyme and make normal metabolizers resemble poor metabolizers. An individual who is stable on a given dose of TCA may become abruptly toxic when given one of these inhibiting drugs as concomitant therapy. The drugs that inhibit cytochrome P450 2D6 include some that are not metabolized by the enzyme (quinidine; cimetidine) and many that are substrates for P450 2D6 (many other antidepressants, phenothiazines, and the Type 1C antiarrhythmics propafenone and flecainide). While all the selective serotonin reuptake inhibitors (SSRIs), e.g., fluoxetine, sertraline, and paroxetine, inhibit P450 2D6, they may vary in the extent of inhibition. The extent to which SSRI-TCA interactions may pose clinical problems will depend on the degree of inhibition and the pharmacokinetics of the SSRI involved. Nevertheless, caution is indicated in the co-administration of TCAs with any of the SSRIs and also in switching from one class to the other. Of particular importance, sufficient time must elapse before initiating TCA treatment in a patient being withdrawn from fluoxetine, given the long half-life of the parent and active metabolite (at least 5 weeks may be necessary).

Concomitant use of tricyclic antidepressants with drugs that can inhibit cytochrome P450 2D6 may require lower doses than usually prescribed for either the tricyclic antidepressant or the other drug. Furthermore, whenever one of these other drugs is withdrawn from co-therapy, an increased dose of tricyclic antidepressant may be required. It is desirable to monitor TCA plasma levels whenever a TCA is going to be coadministered with another drug known to be an inhibitor of P450 2D6.

The plasma concentration of imipramine may increase when the drug is given concomitantly with hepatic enzyme inhibitors (e.g., cimetidine, fluoxetine) and decrease by concomitant administration with hepatic enzyme inducers (e.g., barbiturates, phenytoin), and adjustment of the dosage of imipramine may therefore be necessary.

In occasional susceptible patients or in those receiving anticholinergic drugs (including antiparkinsonism agents) in addition, the atropine-like effects may become more pronounced (e.g., paralytic ileus). Close supervision and careful adjustment of dosage is required when imipramine pamoate is administered concomitantly with anticholinergic drugs.

Avoid the use of preparations, such as decongestants and local anesthetics, that contain any sympathomimetic amine (e.g., epinephrine, norepinephrine), since it has been reported that tricyclic antidepressants can potentiate the effects of catecholamines.

Caution should be exercised when imipramine pamoate is used with agents that lower blood pressure. Imipramine pamoate may potentiate the effects of CNS depressant drugs. Patients should be warned that imipramine pamoate may enhance the CNS depressant effects of alcohol. (See WARNINGS.)

Pregnancy

Animal reproduction studies have yielded inconclusive results. (See also ANIMAL PHARMACOLOGY & TOXICOLOGY.)

There have been no well-controlled studies conducted with pregnant women to determine the effect of imipramine on the fetus. However, there have been clinical reports of congenital malformations associated with the use of the drug. Although a causal relationship between these effects and the drug could not be established, the possibility of fetal risk from the maternal ingestion of imipramine cannot be excluded. Therefore, imipramine should be used in women who are or might become pregnant only if the clinical condition clearly justifies potential risk to the fetus.

Nursing Mothers

Limited data suggest that imipramine is likely to be excreted in human breast milk. As a general rule, a woman taking a drug should not nurse since the possibility exists that the drug may be excreted in breast milk and be harmful to the child.

Pediatric Use

See WARNINGS

ADVERSE REACTIONS

Note: Although the listing which follows includes a few adverse reactions which have not been reported with this specific drug, the pharmacological similarities among the tricyclic antidepressant drugs require that each of the reactions be considered when imipramine is administered.

Cardiovascular: Orthostatic hypotension, hypertension, tachycardia, palpitation, myocardial infarction, arrhythmias, heart block, ECG changes, precipitation of congestive heart failure, stroke.

Psychiatric: Confusional states (especially in the elderly) with hallucinations, disorientation, delusions; anxiety, restlessness, agitation; insomnia and nightmares; hypomania; exacerbation of psychosis.

Neurological: Numbness, tingling, paresthesias of extremities; incoordination, ataxia, tremors; peripheral neuropathy; extrapyramidal symptoms; seizures, alterations in EEG patterns; tinnitus.

Anticholinergic: Dry mouth, and, rarely, associated sublingual adenitis; blurred vision, disturbances of accommodation, mydriasis; constipation, paralytic ileus; urinary retention, delayed micturition, dilation of the urinary tract.

Allergic: Skin rash, petechiae, urticaria, itching, photosensitization; edema (general or of face and tongue); drug fever; cross-sensitivity with desipramine.

Hematologic: Bone marrow depression including agranulocytosis; eosinophilia; purpura; thrombocytopenia.

Gastrointestinal: Nausea and vomiting, anorexia, epigastric distress, diarrhea; peculiar taste, stomatitis, abdominal cramps, black tongue.

Endocrine: Gynecomastia in the male; breast enlargement and galactorrhea in the female; increased or decreased libido, impotence; testicular swelling; elevation or depression of blood sugar levels; inappropriate antidiuretic hormone (ADH) secretion syndrome.

Other: Jaundice (simulating obstructive); altered liver function; weight gain or loss; perspiration; flushing; urinary frequency; drowsiness, dizziness, weakness and fatigue; headache; parotid swelling; alopecia; proneness to falling.

Withdrawal Symptoms: Though not indicative of addiction, abrupt cessation of treatment after prolonged therapy may produce nausea, headache and malaise.

DOSAGE AND ADMINISTRATION

The following recommended dosages for Tofranil-PM should be modified as necessary by the clinical response and any evidence of intolerance.

Initial Adult Dosage:

Outpatients—Therapy should be initiated at 75 mg/day. Dosage may be increased to 150 mg/day which is the dose level at which optimum response is usually obtained. If necessary, dosage may be increased to 200 mg/day.

Dosage higher than 75 mg/day may also be administered on a once-a-day basis after the optimum dosage and tolerance have been determined. The daily dosage may be given at bedtime. In some patients it may be necessary to employ a divided-dose schedule.

As with all tricyclics, the antidepressant effect of imipramine may not be evident for one to three weeks in some patients.

Hospitalized Patients—Therapy should be initiated at 100–150 mg/day and may be increased to 200 mg/day. If there is no response after two weeks, dosage should be increased to 250–300 mg/day.

Dosage higher than 150 mg/day may also be administered on a once-a-day basis after the optimum dosage and tolerance have been determined. The daily dosage may be given at bedtime. In some patients it may be necessary to employ a divided-dose schedule.

As with all tricyclics, the antidepressant effect of imipramine may not be evident for one to three weeks in some patients.

Adult Maintenance Dosage: Following remission, maintenance medication may be required for a longer period of time at the lowest dose that will maintain remission after which the dosage should gradually be decreased.

The usual maintenance dosage is 75–150 mg/day. The total daily dosage can be administered on a once-a-day basis, preferably at bedtime. In some patients it may be necessary to employ a divided-dose schedule.

In cases of relapse due to premature withdrawal of the drug, the effective dosage of imipramine should be reinstituted.

Adolescent and Geriatric Patients: Therapy in these age groups should be initiated with Tofranil®, brand of imipramine hydrochloride, tablets at a total daily dosage of 25–50 mg, since Tofranil-PM capsules are not available in these strengths. Dosage may be increased according to response and tolerance, but it is generally unnecessary to exceed 100 mg/day in these patients. Tofranil-PM capsules may be used when total daily dosage is established at 75 mg or higher.

The total daily dosage can be administered on a once-a-day basis, preferably at bedtime. In some patients it may be necessary to employ a divided-dose schedule.

As with all tricyclics, the antidepressant effect of imipramine may not be evident for one to three weeks in some patients.

Adolescent and geriatric patients can usually be maintained at lower dosage. Following remission, maintenance medication may be required for a longer period of time at the lowest dose that will maintain remission after which the dosage should gradually be decreased.

The total daily maintenance dosage can be administered on a once-a-day basis, preferably at bedtime.

In some patients it may be necessary to employ a divided-dose schedule.

In cases of relapse due to premature withdrawal of the drug, the effective dosage of imipramine should be reinstituted.

OVERDOSAGE

Deaths may occur from overdosage with this class of drugs. Multiple drug ingestion (including alcohol) is common in deliberate tricyclic overdose. As the management is complex and changing, it is recommended that the physician contact a poison control center for current information on treatment. Signs and symptoms of toxicity develop rapidly after tricyclic overdose. Therefore, hospital monitoring is required as soon as possible.

Continued on next page

CibaGeneva—Cont.

Children have been reported to be more sensitive than adults to an acute overdosage of imipramine pamoate. An acute overdose of any amount in infants or young children, especially, must be considered serious and potentially fatal.

Manifestations
These may vary in severity depending upon factors such as the amount of drug absorbed, the age of the patient, and the interval between drug ingestion and the start of treatment. Critical manifestations of overdose include cardiac dysrhythmias, severe hypotension, convulsions, and CNS depression including coma. Changes in the electrocardiogram, particularly in QRS axis or width, are clinically significant indicators of tricyclic toxicity.
Other CNS manifestations may include drowsiness, stupor, ataxia, restlessness, agitation, hyperactive reflexes, muscle rigidity, athetoid and choreiform movements.
Cardiac abnormalities may include tachycardia, and signs of congestive failure. Respiratory depression, cyanosis, shock, vomiting, hyperpyrexia, mydriasis, and diaphoresis may also be present.

Management
Obtain an ECG and immediately initiate cardiac monitoring. Protect the patient's airway, establish an intravenous line, and initiate gastric decontamination. A minimum of 6 hours of observation with cardiac monitoring and observation for signs of CNS or respiratory depression, hypotension, cardiac dysrhythmias and/or conduction blocks, and seizures is necessary. If signs of toxicity occur at any time during this period, extended monitoring is required. There are case reports of patients succumbing to fatal dysrhythmias late after overdose; these patients had clinical evidence of significant poisoning prior to death and most received inadequate gastrointestinal decontamination. Monitoring of plasma drug levels should not guide management of the patient.

Gastrointestinal Decontamination: All patients suspected of tricyclic overdose should receive gastrointestinal decontamination. This should include large volume gastric lavage followed by activated charcoal. If consciousness is impaired, the airway should be secured prior to lavage. Emesis is contraindicated.

Cardiovascular: A maximal limb-lead QRS duration of ≥ 0.10 seconds may be the best indication of the severity of the overdose. Serum alkalinization, to a pH of 7.45 to 7.55, using intravenous sodium bicarbonate and the hyperventilation (as needed) should be instituted for patients with dysrhythmias and/or QRS widening. A pH > 7.60 or a $Pco_2 < 20$ mmHg is undesirable. Dysrhythmias unresponsive to sodium bicarbonate therapy/hyperventilation may respond to lidocaine, bretylium, or phenytoin. Type 1A and 1C antiarrhythmics are generally contraindicated (e.g., quinidine, disopyramide, and procainamide).
In rare instances, hemoperfusion may be beneficial in acute refractory cardiovascular instability in patients with acute toxicity. However, hemodialysis, peritoneal dialysis, exchange transfusions, and forced diuresis generally have been reported as ineffective in tricyclic poisoning.

CNS: In patients with CNS depression, early intubation is advised because of the potential for abrupt deterioration. Seizures should be controlled with benzodiazepines, or if these are ineffective, other anticonvulsants (e.g., phenobarbital, phenytoin). Physostigmine is not recommended except to treat life-threatening symptoms that have been unresponsive to other therapies, and then only in consultation with a poison control center.

Psychiatric Follow-up: Since overdosage is often deliberate, patients may attempt suicide by other means during the recovery phase.
Psychiatric referral may be appropriate.

Pediatric Management: The principles of management of child and adult overdosages are similar. It is strongly recommended that the physician contact the local poison control center for specific pediatric treatment.

HOW SUPPLIED

Capsules 75 mg—coral (imprinted black Geigy 20) equivalent to 75 mg imipramine hydrochloride
   Bottles of 30 .... NDC 0028-0020-26
   Bottles of 100 .... NDC 0028-0020-01
Capsules 100 mg—dark yellow/coral (imprinted black Geigy 40) equivalent to 100 mg imipramine hydrochloride
   Bottles of 30 .... NDC 0028-0040-26
   Bottles of 100 .... NDC 0028-0040-01
Capsules 125 mg—ivory/coral (imprinted black Geigy 45) equivalent to 125 mg imipramine hydrochloride
   Bottles of 30 .... NDC 0028-0045-26
   Bottles of 100 .... NDC 0028-0045-01
Capsules 150 mg—coral (imprinted black Geigy 22) equivalent to 150 mg imipramine hydrochloride
   Bottles of 30 .... NDC 0028-0022-26
   Bottles of 100 .... NDC 0028-0022-01
Do not store above 86°F (30°C).
Dispense in tight container (USP).

ANIMAL PHARMACOLOGY & TOXICOLOGY

A. *Acute:* Oral LD_{50}:
Mouse		2185 mg/kg
Rat	(F)	1142 mg/kg
	(M)	1807 mg/kg
Rabbit		1016 mg/kg
Dog		693 mg/kg (Emesis ED_{50})

B. *Subacute:*
Two three-month studies in dogs gave evidence of an adverse drug effect on the testes, but only at the highest dose level employed, i.e., 90 mg/kg (10 times the maximum human dose). Depending on the histological section of the testes examined, the findings consisted of a range of degenerative changes up to and including complete atrophy of the seminiferous tubules, with spermatogenesis usually arrested.
Human studies show no definitive effect on sperm count, sperm motility, sperm morphology or volume of ejaculate.
Rat
One three-month study was done in rats at dosage levels comparable to those of the dog studies. No adverse drug effect on the testes was noted in this study, as confirmed by histological examination.

C. *Reproduction/Teratogenic:*
Oral: Imipramine pamoate was fed to male and female albino rats for 28 weeks through two breeding cycles at dose levels of 15 mg/kg/day and 40 mg/kg/day (equivalent to $2^{1}/_{2}$ and 7 times the maximum human dose).
No abnormalities which could be related to drug administration were noted in gross inspection. Autopsies performed on pups from the second breeding likewise revealed no pathological changes in organs or tissues; however, a decrease in mean litter size from both matings was noted in the drug-treated groups and significant growth suppression occurred in the nursing pups of both sexes in the high group as well as in the females of the low-level group. Finally, the lactation index (pups weaned divided by number left to nurse) was significantly lower in the second litter of the high-level group.

C96-4 (Rev. 1/96)

Ciba-Geigy Corporation
Pharmaceuticals Division
Summit, NJ 07901
Shown in Product Identification Guide, page 309

TRANSDERM–NITRO® ℞
[trans'derm nye'trow]
nitroglycerin
Transdermal Therapeutic System

Prescribing Information
DESCRIPTION
Nitroglycerin is 1,2,3-propanetriol, trinitrate, an organic nitrate whose molecular weight is 227.09. The organic nitrates are vasodilators, active on both arteries and veins.
The Transderm-Nitro (nitroglycerin) transdermal system is a flat unit designed to provide continuous controlled release of nitroglycerin through intact skin.
The rate of release of nitroglycerin is linearly dependent upon the area of the applied system; each cm^2 of applied system delivers approximately 0.02 mg of nitroglycerin per hour. Thus, the 5-, 10-, 20-, and 30-cm^2 systems deliver approximately 0.1, 0.2, 0.4, and 0.6 mg of nitroglycerin per hour, respectively.
The remainder of the nitroglycerin in each system serves as a reservoir and is not delivered in normal use. After 12 hours, for example, each system has delivered 10% of its original content of nitroglycerin.
The Transderm-Nitro system comprises four layers as shown below. Proceeding from the visible surface towards the surface attached to the skin, these layers are: 1) a tan-colored backing layer (aluminized plastic) that is impermeable to nitroglycerin; 2) a drug reservoir containing nitroglycerin adsorbed on lactose, colloidal silicon dioxide, and silicone medical fluid; 3) an ethylene-vinyl acetate copolymer membrane that is permeable to nitroglycerin; and 4) a layer of hypoallergenic silicone adhesive. Prior to use, a protective peel strip is removed from the adhesive surface.
Cross section of the system:

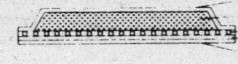

Backing
Drug Reservoir
Semipermeable Membrane
Adhesive
Protective Peel Strip

CLINICAL PHARMACOLOGY
The principal pharmacological action of nitroglycerin is relaxation of vascular smooth muscle, and consequent dilatation of peripheral arteries and veins, especially the latter. Dilatation of the veins promotes peripheral pooling of blood and decreases venous return to the heart, thereby reducing left ventricular end-diastolic pressure and pulmonary capillary wedge pressure (preload). Arteriolar relaxation reduces systemic vascular resistance, systolic arterial pressure, and mean arterial pressure (afterload). Dilatation of the coro-

nary arteries also occurs. The relative importance of preload reduction, afterload reduction, and coronary dilatation remains undefined.
Dosing regimens for most chronically used drugs are designed to provide plasma concentrations that are continuously greater than a minimally effective concentration. This strategy is inappropriate for organic nitrates. Several well-controlled clinical trials have used exercise testing to assess the antianginal efficacy of continuously-delivered nitrates. In the large majority of these trials, active agents were indistinguishable from placebo after 24 hours (or less) of continuous therapy. Attempts to overcome nitrate tolerance by dose escalation, even to doses far in excess of those used acutely, have consistently failed. Only after nitrates had been absent from the body for several hours was their antianginal efficacy restored.

Pharmacokinetics
The volume of distribution of nitroglycerin is about 3L/kg, and nitroglycerin is cleared from this volume at extremely rapid rates, with a resulting serum half-life of about 3 minutes. The observed clearance rates (close to 1L/kg/min) greatly exceed hepatic blood flow, known sites of extrahepatic metabolism include red blood cells and vascular walls. The first products in the metabolism of nitroglycerin are inorganic nitrate and the 1,2- and 1,3-dinitroglycerols. The dinitrates are less effective vasodilators than nitroglycerin, but they are longer-lived in the serum, and their net contribution to the overall effect of chronic nitroglycerin regimens is not known. The dinitrates are further metabolized to (nonvasoactive) mononitrates and, ultimately, to glycerol and carbon dioxide.
To avoid development of tolerance to nitroglycerin, drug-free intervals of 10–12 hours are known to be sufficient; shorter intervals have not been well studied. In one well-controlled clinical trial, subjects receiving nitroglycerin appeared to exhibit a rebound or withdrawal effect, so that their exercise tolerance at the end of the daily drug-free interval was *less* than that exhibited by the parallel group receiving placebo. In healthy volunteers, steady-state plasma concentrations of nitroglycerin are reached by about two hours after application of a patch and are maintained for the duration of wearing the system (observations have been limited to 24 hours). Upon removal of the patch, the plasma concentration declines with a half-life of about an hour.

Clinical Trials
Regimens in which nitroglycerin patches were worn for 12 hours daily have been studied in well-controlled trials up to 4 weeks in duration. Starting about 2 hours after application and continuing until 10–12 hours after application, patches that deliver at least 0.4 mg of nitroglycerin per hour have consistently demonstrated greater antianginal activity than placebo. Lower-dose patches have not been as well studied, but in one large, well-controlled trial in which higher-dose patches were also studied, patches delivering 0.2 mg/hr had significantly less antianginal activity than placebo.
It is reasonable to believe that the rate of nitroglycerin absorption from patches may vary with the site of application, but this relationship has not been adequately studied.
The onset of action of transdermal nitroglycerin is not sufficiently rapid for this product to be useful in aborting an acute anginal episode.

INDICATIONS AND USAGE
Transdermal nitroglycerin is indicated for the prevention of angina pectoris due to coronary artery disease. The onset of action of transdermal nitroglycerin is not sufficiently rapid for this product to be useful in aborting an acute attack.

CONTRAINDICATIONS
Allergic reactions to organic nitrates are extremely rare, but they do occur. Nitroglycerin is contraindicated in patients who are allergic to it. Allergy to the adhesives used in nitroglycerin patches has also been reported, and it similarly constitutes a contraindication to the use of this product.

WARNINGS
The benefits of transdermal nitroglycerin in patients with acute myocardial infarction or congestive heart failure have not been established. If one elects to use nitroglycerin in these conditions, careful clinical or hemodynamic monitoring must be used to avoid the hazards of hypotension and tachycardia.
A cardioverter/defibrillator should not be discharged through a paddle electrode that overlies a Transderm-Nitro patch. The arcing that may be seen in this situation is harmless in itself, but it may be associated with local current concentration that can cause damage to the paddles and burns to the patient.

PRECAUTIONS
General
Severe hypotension, particularly with upright posture, may occur with even small doses of nitroglycerin. This drug should therefore be used with caution in patients who may be volume depleted or who, for whatever reason, are already hypotensive. Hypotension induced by nitroglycerin may be

accompanied by paradoxical bradycardia and increased angina pectoris.

Nitrate therapy may aggravate the angina caused by hypertrophic cardiomyopathy.

As tolerance to other forms of nitroglycerin develops, the effect of sublingual nitroglycerin on exercise tolerance, although still observable, is somewhat blunted.

In industrial workers who have had long-term exposure to unknown (presumably high) doses of organic nitrates, tolerance clearly occurs. Chest pain, acute myocardial infarction, and even sudden death have occurred during temporary withdrawal of nitrates from these workers, demonstrating the existence of true physical dependence.

Several clinical trials in patients with angina pectoris have evaluated nitroglycerin regimens which incorporated a 10–12 hour nitrate-free interval. In some of these trials, an increase in the frequency of anginal attacks during the nitrate-free interval was observed in a small number of patients. In one trial, patients demonstrated decreased exercise tolerance at the end of the nitrate-free interval. Hemodynamic rebound has been observed only rarely; on the other hand, few studies were so designed that rebound, if it had occurred, would have been detected. The importance of these observations to the routine, clinical use of transdermal nitroglycerin is unknown.

Information for Patients

Daily headaches sometimes accompany treatment with nitroglycerin. In patients who get these headaches, the headaches may be a marker of the activity of the drug. Patients should resist the temptation to avoid headaches by altering the schedule of their treatment with nitroglycerin, since loss of headache may be associated with simultaneous loss of antianginal efficacy.

Treatment with nitroglycerin may be associated with lightheadedness on standing, especially just after rising from a recumbent or seated position. This effect may be more frequent in patients who have also consumed alcohol.

After normal use, there is enough residual nitroglycerin in discarded patches that they are a potential hazard to children and pets.

A patient leaflet is supplied with the systems.

Drug Interactions

The vasodilating effects of nitroglycerin may be additive with those of other vasodilators. Alcohol, in particular, has been found to exhibit additive effects of this variety.

Marked symptomatic orthostatic hypotension has been reported when calcium channel blockers and organic nitrates were used in combination. Dose adjustments of either class of agents may be necessary.

Carcinogenesis, Mutagenesis, Impairment of Fertility

Animal carcinogenesis studies with topically applied nitroglycerin have not been performed.

Rats receiving up to 434 mg/kg/day of dietary nitroglycerin for 2 years developed dose-related fibrotic and neoplastic changes in liver, including carcinomas, and interstitial cell tumors in testes. At high dose, the incidences of hepatocellular carcinomas in both sexes were 52% vs. 0% in controls, and incidences of testicular tumors were 52% vs. 8% in controls. Lifetime dietary administration of up to 1058 mg/kg/day of nitroglycerin was not tumorigenic in mice.

Nitroglycerin was weakly mutagenic in Ames tests performed in two different laboratories. Nevertheless, there was not evidence of mutagenicity in an in vivo dominant lethal assay with male rats treated with doses up to about 363 mg/kg/day, p.o., or in in vitro cytogenetic tests in rat and dog tissues.

In a three-generation reproduction study, rats received dietary nitroglycerin at doses up to about 434 mg/kg/day for six months prior to mating of the F_0 generation with treatment continuing through successive F_1 and F_2 generations. The high dose was associated with decreased feed intake and body weight gain in both sexes at all matings. No specific effect on the fertility of the F_0 generation was seen. Infertility noted in subsequent generations, however, was attributed to increased interstitial cell tissue and aspermatogenesis in the high-dose males. In this three-generation study there was no clear evidence of teratogenicity.

Pregnancy Category C

Animal teratology studies have not been conducted with nitroglycerin transdermal systems. Teratology studies in rats and rabbits, however, were conducted with topically applied nitroglycerin ointment at doses up to 80 mg/kg/day and 240 mg/kg/day, respectively. No toxic effects on dams or fetuses were seen at any dose tested. There are no adequate and well-controlled studies in pregnant women. Nitroglycerin should be given to a pregnant woman only if clearly needed.

Nursing Mothers

It is not known whether nitroglycerin is excreted in human milk. Because many drugs are excreted in human milk, caution should be exercised when nitroglycerin is administered to a nursing woman.

Pediatric Use

Safety and effectiveness in children have not been established.

ADVERSE REACTIONS

Adverse reactions to nitroglycerin are generally dose-related, and almost all of these reactions are the result of nitroglycerin's activity as a vasodilator. Headache, which may be severe, is the most commonly reported side effect. Headache may be recurrent with each daily dose, especially at higher doses. Transient episodes of lightheadedness, occasionally related to blood pressure changes, may also occur. Hypotension occurs infrequently, but in some patients it may be severe enough to warrant discontinuation of therapy. Syncope, crescendo angina, and rebound hypertension have been reported but are uncommon.

Allergic reactions to nitroglycerin are also uncommon, and the great majority of those reported have been cases of contact dematitis or fixed drug eruptions in patients receiving nitroglycerin in ointments or patches. There have been a few reports of genuine anaphylactoid reactions, and these reactions can probably occur in patients receiving nitroglycerin by any route.

Extremely rarely, ordinary doses of organic nitrates have caused methemoglobinemia in normal-seeming patients. Methemoglobinemia is so infrequent at these doses that further discussion of its diagnosis and treatment is deferred (see Overdosage).

Application-site irritation may occur but is rarely severe.

In two placebo-controlled trials of intermittent therapy with nitroglycerin patches at 0.2 to 0.8 mg/hr, the most frequent adverse reactions among 307 subjects were as follows:

	Placebo	Patch
Headache	18%	63%
Lightheadedness	4%	6%
Hypotension, and/or syncope	0%	4%
Increased angina	2%	2%

OVERDOSAGE

Hemodynamic Effects

The ill effects of nitroglycerin overdose are generally the result of nitroglycerin's capacity to induce vasodilatation, venous pooling, reduced cardiac output, and hypotension. These hemodynamic changes may have protean manifestations, including increased intracranial pressure, with any or all of persistent throbbing headache, confusion, and moderate fever; vertigo; palpitations; visual disturbances; nausea and vomiting (possibly with colic and even bloody diarrhea); syncope (especially in the upright posture); air hunger and dyspnea, later followed by reduced ventilatory effort; diaphoresis, with the skin either flushed or cold and clammy; heart block and bradycardia; paralysis; coma; seizures; and death.

Laboratory determinations of serum levels of nitroglycerin and its metabolites are not widely available, and such determinations have, in any event, no established role in the management of nitroglycerin overdose.

No data are available to suggest physiological maneuvers (e.g., maneuvers to change the pH of the urine) that might accelerate elimination of nitroglycerin and its active metabolites. Similarly, it is not known which, if any, of these substances can usefully be removed from the body by hemodialysis.

No specific antagonist to the vasodilator effects of nitroglycerin is known, and no intervention has been subject to controlled study as a therapy of nitroglycerin overdose. Because the hypotension associated with nitroglycerin overdose is the result of venodilatation and arterial hypovolemia, prudent therapy in this situation should be directed toward an increase in central fluid volume. Passive elevation of the patient's legs may be sufficient, but intravenous infusion of normal saline or similar fluid may also be necessary.

The use of epinephrine or other arterial vasoconstrictors in this setting is likely to do more harm than good.

In patients with renal disease or congestive heart failure, therapy resulting in central volume expansion is not without hazard. Treatment of nitroglycerin overdose in these patients may be subtle and difficult, and invasive monitoring may be required.

Methemoglobinemia

Nitrate ions liberated during metabolism of nitroglycerin can oxidize hemoglobin into methemoglobin. Even in patients totally without cytochrome b_5 reductase activity, however, and even assuming that the nitrate moieties of nitroglycerin are quantitatively applied to oxidation of hemoglobin, about 1 mg/kg of nitroglycerin should be required before any of these patients manifests clinically significant ($\geq 10\%$) methemoglobinemia. In patients with normal reductase function, significant production of methemoglobin should require even larger doses of nitroglycerin. In one study in which 36 patients received 2–4 weeks of continuous nitroglycerin therapy at 3.1 to 4.4 mg/hr, the average methemoglobin level measured was 0.2%; this was comparable to that observed in parallel patients who received placebo.

Notwithstanding these observations, there are case reports of significant methemoglobinemia in association with moderate overdoses of organic nitrates. None of the affected patients had been thought to be unusually susceptible.

Methemoglobin levels are available from most clinical laboratories. The diagnosis should be suspected in patients who exhibit signs of impaired oxygen delivery despite adequate cardiac output and adequate arterial pO_2. Classically, methemoglobinemic blood is described as chocolate brown, without color change on exposure to air.

When methemoglobinemia is diagnosed, the treatment of choice is methylene blue, 1–2 mg/kg intravenously.

DOSAGE AND ADMINISTRATION

The suggested starting dose is between 0.2 mg/hr*, and 0.4 mg/hr*. Doses between 0.4 mg/hr* and 0.8 mg/hr* have shown continued effectiveness for 10–12 hours daily for at least one month (the longest period studied) of intermittent administration. Although the minimum nitrate-free interval has not been defined, data show that a nitrate-free interval of 10–12 hours is sufficient (see CLINICAL PHARMACOLOGY). Thus, an appropriate dosing schedule for nitroglycerin patches would include a daily patch-on period of 12–14 hours and a daily patch-off period of 10–12 hours.

Although some well-controlled clinical trials using exercise tolerance testing have shown maintenance of effectiveness when patches are worn continuously, the large majority of such controlled trials have shown the development of tolerance (i.e., complete loss of effect) within the first 24 hours after therapy was initiated. Dose adjustment, even to levels much higher than generally used, did not restore efficacy.

PATIENT INSTRUCTIONS FOR APPLICATION OF SYSTEM

A patient leaflet is supplied with each carton.

HOW SUPPLIED

Nitroglycerin Transdermal System 0.1 mg/hr-tan, round (imprinted Transderm-Nitro 0.1 mg/hr), supplied in a foil-lined pouch

30 Systems	NDC 57267-902-26
**30 Systems	NDC 57267-902-42
**100 Systems	NDC 57267-902-30

Nitroglycerin Transdermal System 0.2 mg/hr-tan, oblong (imprinted Transderm-Nitro 0.2 mg/hr), supplied in a foil-lined pouch

30 Systems	NDC 57267-905-26
**30 Systems	NDC 57267-905-42
**100 Systems	NDC 57267-905-30

Nitroglycerin Transdermal System 0.4 mg/hr-tan, oblong (imprinted Transderm-Nitro 0.4 mg/hr), supplied in a foil-lined pouch

30 Systems	NDC 57267-910-26
**30 Systems	NDC 57267-910-42
**100 Systems	NDC 57267-910-30

Nitroglycerin Transdermal System 0.6 mg/hr-tan, oblong (imprinted Transderm-Nitro 0.6 mg/hr), supplied in a foil-lined pouch

30 Systems	NDC 57267-915-26
**30 Systems	NDC 57267-915-42
**100 Systems	NDC 57267-915-30

Nitroglycerin Transdermal System 0.8 mg/hr-tan, round (imprinted Transderm-Nitro 0.8 mg/hr), supplied in a foil-lined pouch

30 Systems	NDC 57267-920-26
**30 Systems	NDC 57267-920-42

*Rated release in vivo. Release rates were formerly described in terms of drug delivered per 24 hours. In these terms, the supplied Transderm-Nitro systems would be rated at 2.5 mg/24 hr (0.1 mg/hr), 5 mg/24 hr (0.2 mg/hr), 10 mg/24 hr (0.4 mg/hr), 15 mg/24 hr (0.6 mg/hr), and 20 mg/24 hr (0.8 mg/hr).

**Institutional Pack

Do not store above 86°F (30°C).

Do not store unpouched. Apply immediately upon removal from the pouch.

C95-25 (Rev. 6/95)

How to use

TRANSDERM-NITRO®

nitroglycerin

Transdermal Therapeutic System

for the prevention of angina

Transderm-Nitro is easy to use—it has a clear plastic backing, and a special adhesive that keeps the system firmly in place.

Where to place Transderm-Nitro.

Select any area of skin on the body, EXCEPT the extremities below the knee or elbow. The chest is the preferred site. The area should be clean, dry, and hairless. If hair is likely to interfere with system adhesion or removal, it can be clipped, but not shaved. Take care to avoid areas with cuts or irritations. Do NOT apply the system immediately after showering or bathing. It is best to wait until you are certain the skin is completely dry.

How to apply Transderm-Nitro® nitroglycerin

1. Each Transderm-Nitro system is individually sealed in a protective pouch. Tear open this pouch at the indicated indentations. Carefully pick up the system lengthwise with the tab up, and the clear plastic backing facing you. You should be able to see the white cream containing ni-

Continued on next page

CibaGeneva—Cont.

troglycerin. (On very rare occasions, you may find a system without any white medication in it. Do not use it. Simply apply another system.)

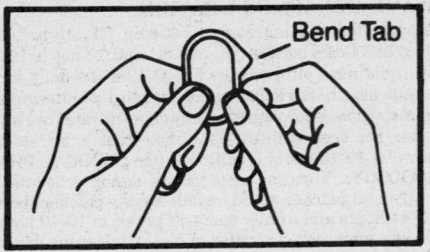

Figure A.

2. Firmly bend the tab <u>forward</u> with the thumb (Figure A). With both thumbs, begin to remove the <u>clear plastic</u> backing from the system at the tab (Figure B). Do not touch the inside of the exposed system, because the adhesive covers the entire surface.

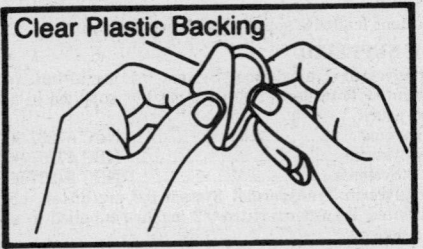

Figure B

3. Continue to remove the <u>clear plastic</u> backing <u>slowly</u> along the length of the system, allowing the system to rest on the outside of your fingers (Figure C).

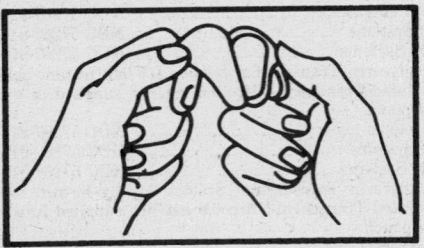

Figure C

4. Place the exposed, adhesive side of the system on the chosen skin site. <u>Press</u> firmly in place with the palm of your hand (Figure D). Once the system is in place, do not test the adhesion by pulling on it.

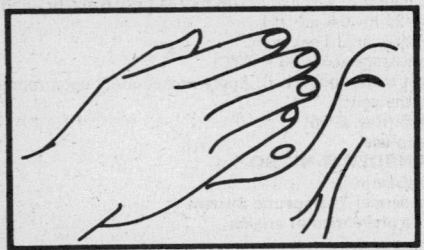

Figure D

When Transderm-Nitro is applied to your body, the nitroglycerin contained in the system begins to flow onto your skin through a unique rate-controlling membrane. This membrane allows the nitroglycerin to be released and available for absorption through your skin at a uniform rate.

5. At the time recommended by your doctor, remove and discard the system.

6. Place a new system on a different skin site, following Steps 1–4, according to your doctor's instructions.

Please note:
Contact with water, as in bathing, swimming, or showering will not affect the system. In the unlikely event that a system falls off, discard it and put a new one on a different skin site.

PRECAUTIONS

The most common side effect is headache, which often decreases as therapy is continued, but may require treatment with a mild analgesic. Although uncommon, faintness, flush-

ing, and dizziness may occur, especially when suddenly rising from the recumbent (lying horizontal) position. If these symptoms occur, remove the system and notify your physician.

Skin irritation may occur. If it persists, consult your physician.

Keep these systems and all drugs out of the reach of children.

Important: Your doctor may decide to increase or decrease the size of the system, or prescribe a combination of systems, to suit your particular needs. The dose may vary depending on your individual response to the system.

This system is to be used for <u>preventing</u> angina, not for treating an acute attack.

DO NOT STORE ABOVE 86°F (30°C).

Do not store unpouched. Apply immediately upon removal from the protective pouch.

Dist. by:
Summit Pharmaceuticals
Ciba-Geigy Corp.
Summit, NJ 07901

C93-19 (Rev. 7/93)

Shown in Product Identification Guide, page 309

VIVELLE™ ℞
estradiol transdermal system
Continuous delivery for twice-weekly application

Prescribing Information

> **1. ESTROGENS HAVE BEEN REPORTED TO INCREASE THE RISK OF ENDOMETRIAL CARCINOMA IN POSTMENOPAUSAL WOMEN.**
> Close clinical surveillance of all women taking estrogens is important. Adequate diagnostic measures, including endometrial sampling when indicated, should be undertaken to rule out malignancy in all cases of undiagnosed persistent or recurring abnormal vaginal bleeding. There is no evidence that "natural" estrogens are more or less hazardous than "synthetic" estrogens at equiestrogenic doses.
>
> **2. ESTROGENS SHOULD NOT BE USED DURING PREGNANCY.**
> Estrogen therapy during pregnancy is associated with an increased risk of congenital defects in the reproductive organs of the fetus, and possibly other birth defects. Studies of women who received diethylstilbestrol (DES) during pregnancy have shown that female offspring have an increased risk of vaginal adenosis, squamous cell dysplasia of the uterine cervix, and clear cell vaginal cancer later in life; male offspring have an increased risk of urogenital abnormalities and possibly testicular cancer later in life. The 1985 DES Task Force concluded that use of DES during pregnancy is associated with a subsequent increased risk of breast cancer in the mothers, although a causal relationship remains unproven and the observed level of excess risk is similar to that for a number of other breast cancer risk factors.
> There is no indication for estrogen therapy during pregnancy or during the immediate postpartum period. Estrogens are ineffective for the prevention or treatment of threatened or habitual abortion. Estrogens are not indicated for the prevention of postpartum breast engorgement.

DESCRIPTION

The Vivelle estradiol transdermal system contains estradiol in a multipolymeric adhesive. The system is designed to release 17β-estradiol continuously upon application to intact skin.

Four systems are available to provide nominal in vivo delivery of 0.0375, 0.05, 0.075, or 0.1 mg of estradiol per day via skin of average permeability. Each corresponding system having an active surface area of 11.0, 14.5, 22.0, or 29.0 cm² contains 3.28, 4.33, 6.57, or 8.66 mg of estradiol USP, respectively. The composition of the systems per unit area is identical.

Estradiol USP (17β-estradiol) is a white, crystalline powder, chemically described as estra-1,3,5(10)-triene-3,17β-diol.

The molecular formula of estradiol is $C_{18}H_{24}O_2$. The molecular weight is 272.39.

The Vivelle system comprises three layers. Proceeding from the visible surface toward the surface attached to the skin, these layers are (1) a translucent flexible film consisting of an ethylene vinyl alcohol copolymer film, a polyurethane film, urethane polymer and epoxy resin, (2) an adhesive formulation containing estradiol, acrylic adhesive, polyisobutylene, ethylene vinyl acetate copolymer, 1,3 butylene glycol, styrene-butadiene rubber, oleic acid, lecithin, propylene glycol, bentonite, mineral oil, and dipropylene glycol, and (3) a polyester release liner that is attached to the adhesive surface and must be removed before the system can be used.

[See Figure at top of next column.]

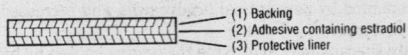

(1) Backing
(2) Adhesive containing estradiol
(3) Protective liner

The active component of the system is estradiol. The remaining components of the system are pharmacologically inactive.

CLINICAL PHARMACOLOGY

The Vivelle system releases estradiol, the major estrogenic hormone secreted by the human ovary. Although circulating estrogens exist in a dynamic equilibrium of metabolic interconversions, estradiol is the principal intracellular human estrogen and is substantially more potent than estrone or estriol at the receptor level.

Vivelle provides systemic estrogen replacement therapy. Estrogen receptors have been identified in tissues of the reproductive tract, breast, pituitary, hypothalamus, liver, and bone of women. Among numerous effects, estradiol is largely responsible for the development and maintenance of the female reproductive system and secondary sex characteristics. By a direct action, it causes growth and development of the vagina, uterus, and fallopian tubes. With other hormones, such as pituitary hormones and progesterone, it causes enlargement of the breasts through promotion of ductal growth, stromal development, and the accretion of fat. Estrogens contribute to the shaping of the skeleton, to the maintenance of tone and elasticity of urogenital structures, to changes in the epiphyses of the long bones that allow for the pubertal growth spurt and its termination, to the growth of axillary and pubic hair, and pigmentation of the nipples and genitals.

Estrogens are intricately involved with other hormones, especially progesterone, in the processes of the ovulatory menstrual cycle and pregnancy, and affect the release of pituitary gonadotropins.

Loss of ovarian estradiol secretion after menopause can result in instability of thermoregulation, causing hot flushes associated with sleep disturbance and excessive sweating, and urogenital atrophy, causing dyspareunia and urinary incontinence. Estradiol replacement therapy alleviates many of these symptoms of estradiol deficiency in the menopausal woman.

Pharmacokinetics

Transdermal administration produces therapeutic plasma levels of estradiol with lower circulating levels of estrone and estrone conjugates and requires smaller total doses than does oral therapy. Studies conducted with the Vivelle system show the drug has an apparent mean half-life of 4.4±2.3 hours.

In a multiple-dose study consisting of three consecutive patch applications of the Vivelle system, which was conducted in 17 healthy, postmenopausal women, blood levels of estradiol and estrone were compared following application of these units to sites on the abdomen and buttocks in a crossover fashion. Patches that deliver nominal estradiol doses of approximately 0.0375 mg/day and 0.1 mg/day were applied to abdominal application sites while the 0.1 mg/day doses were also applied to sites on the buttocks. These systems increased estradiol levels above baseline within 4 hours and maintained respective mean levels of 25 and 79 pg/mL above baseline following application to the abdomen; slightly higher mean levels of 88 pg/mL above baseline were observed following application to the buttocks. At the same time, increases in estrone plasma concentrations averaged about 12 and 50 pg/mL, respectively, following application to the abdomen and 61 pg/mL for the buttocks. While plasma concentrations of estradiol and estrone remained slightly above baseline at 12 hours following removal of the patches in this study, results from another study show these levels to return to baseline values within 24 hours following removal of the patches.

The graph illustrates the mean plasma concentrations of estradiol at steady-state during application of these patches at four different dosages.

Steady-State Estradiol Plasma Concentrations for Systems Applied to the Abdomen
Nonbaseline-corrected levels

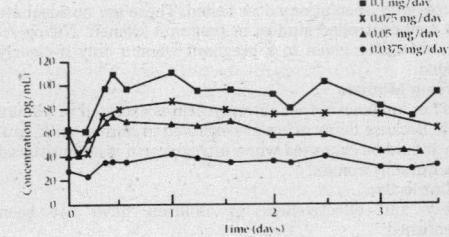

The corresponding pharmacokinetic parameters are summarized in the table below.

**Steady-State Estradiol Pharmacokinetic Parameters
for Systems Applied to the Abdomen
(mean ± standard deviation)
Nonbaseline-corrected data ***

Dosage (mg/day)	C_{max}† (pg/mL)	C_{avg}‡ (pg/mL)	C_{min}(84 hr)§ (pg/mL)
0.0375	46 ± 16	34 ± 10	30 ± 10
0.05	83 ± 41	57 ± 23#	41 ± 11#
0.075	99 ± 35	72 ± 24	60 ± 24
0.1	133 ± 51	89 ± 38	90 ± 44
0.1¶	145 ± 71	104 ± 52	85 ± 47

* Mean baseline estradiol concentration = 11.7 pg/mL
† Peak plasma concentration
‡ Average plasma concentration
§ Minimum plasma concentration at 84 hr
# Measured over 80 hr
¶ Applied to the buttocks

INDICATIONS AND USAGE

Vivelle™ (estradiol transdermal system) is indicated in the following:

1. Treatment of moderate-to-severe vasomotor symptoms associated with the menopause. There is no adequate evidence that estrogens are effective for nervous symptoms or depression that might occur during menopause and they should not be used to treat these conditions.
2. Treatment of vulval and vaginal atrophy.
3. Treatment of hypoestrogenism due to hypogonadism, castration, or primary ovarian failure.

CONTRAINDICATIONS

Patients with known hypersensitivity to any of the components of the therapeutic system should not use Vivelle.
Estrogens should not be used in individuals with any of the following conditions:

1. Known or suspected pregnancy (see Boxed Warning). Estrogen may cause fetal harm when administered to a pregnant woman.
2. Undiagnosed abnormal genital bleeding.
3. Known or suspected cancer of the breast.
4. Known or suspected estrogen-dependent neoplasia.
5. Active thrombophlebitis or thromboembolic disorders.

WARNINGS

1. Induction of Malignant Neoplasms. Some studies have suggested a possible increased incidence of breast cancer in those women taking estrogen therapy at higher doses or for prolonged periods of time. The majority of studies, however, have not shown an association with the usual doses used for estrogen replacement therapy. Women on this therapy should have regular breast examinations and should be instructed in breast self-examination. The reported endometrial cancer risk among unopposed estrogen users is about 2- to 12-fold greater than in nonusers and appears dependent on duration of treatment and on estrogen dose. Most studies show no significant increased risk associated with the use of estrogens for less than 1 year. The greatest risk appears associated with prolonged use with increased risks of 15- to 24-fold for 5 to 10 years or more. In three studies, persistence of risk was demonstrated for 8 to over 15 years after cessation of estrogen treatment. In one study, a significant decrease in the incidence of endometrial cancer occurred 6 months after estrogen withdrawal. Concurrent progestin therapy may offset this risk, but the overall health impact in postmenopausal women is not known (see PRECAUTIONS).
Estrogen therapy during pregnancy is associated with an increased risk of fetal congenital reproductive tract disorders. In female offspring, there is an increased risk of vaginal adenosis, squamous cell dysplasia of the cervix, and clear cell vaginal cancer later in life; in males, urogenital and possibly testicular abnormalities. Although some of these changes are benign, it is not known whether they are precursors of malignancy.
2. Gallbladder Disease. Two studies have reported a 2- to 4-fold increase in the risk of surgically confirmed gallbladder disease in postmenopausal women receiving oral estrogen replacement therapy, similar to the 2-fold increase previously noted in users of oral contraceptives.
3. Cardiovascular Disease. Large doses of estrogen (5 mg conjugated estrogens per day), comparable to those used to treat cancer of the prostate and breast, have been shown in a large prospective clinical trial in men to increase the risks of nonfatal myocardial infarction, pulmonary embolism, and thrombophlebitis. These risks cannot necessarily be extrapolated from men to women. However, to avoid the theoretical cardiovascular risk to women caused by high estrogen doses, the dose for estrogen replacement therapy should not exceed the lowest effective dose.
4. Elevated Blood Pressure. Occasional blood pressure increases during estrogen replacement therapy have been attributed to idiosyncratic reactions to estrogens. More of-

ten, blood pressure has remained the same or has dropped. Postmenopausal estrogen use does not increase the risk of stroke. Nonetheless, blood pressure should be monitored at regular intervals with estrogen use, especially if high doses are used. Ethinyl estradiol and conjugated estrogens have been shown to increase renin substrate. In contrast to these oral estrogens, transdermally administered estradiol does not affect renin substrate.
5. Hypercalcemia. Administration of estrogen may lead to severe hypercalcemia in patients with breast cancer and bone metastases. If this occurs, the drug should be stopped and appropriate measures taken to reduce the serum calcium level.

PRECAUTIONS

General

1. Addition of a Progestin. Studies of the addition of a progestin for 10 or more days of a cycle of estrogen administration have reported a lower incidence of endometrial hyperplasia than would be induced by estrogen treatment alone. Morphologic and biochemical studies of endometria suggest that 10 to 14 days of progestin are needed to provide maximal maturation of the endometrium and to reduce the likelihood of hyperplastic changes.
There are, however, possible risks that may be associated with the use of progestins in estrogen replacement regimens. These include
(1) adverse effects on lipoprotein metabolism (lowering HDL and raising LDL), which could diminish the purported cardioprotective effect of estrogen therapy (see PRECAUTIONS, below);
(2) impairment of glucose tolerance; and
(3) possible enhancement of mitotic activity in breast epithelial tissue, although few epidemiologic data are available to address this point (see PRECAUTIONS, below).
The choice of progestin, its dose, and its regimen may be important in minimizing these adverse effects, but these issues will require further study before they are clarified.
2. Cardiovascular Risk. A causal relationship between estrogen replacement therapy and reduction of cardiovascular disease in postmenopausal women has not been proven. Furthermore, the effect of added progestins on this putative benefit is not yet known.
In recent years, many published studies have suggested that there may be a cause-effect relationship between postmenopausal oral estrogen replacement therapy *without added progestins* and a decrease in cardiovascular disease in women. Although most of the observational studies which assessed this statistical association have reported a 20% to 50% reduction in coronary heart disease risk and associated mortality in estrogen takers, the following should be considered when interpreting these reports:
(1) Because only one of these studies was randomized and it was too small to yield statistically significant results, all relevant studies were subject to selection bias. Thus, the apparently reduced risk of coronary artery disease cannot be attributed with certainty to estrogen replacement therapy. It may instead have been caused by life-style and medical characteristics of the women studied with the result that healthier women were selected for estrogen therapy. In general, treated women were of higher socioeconomic and educational status, more slender, more physically active, more likely to have undergone surgical menopause, and less likely to have diabetes than the untreated women. Although some studies attempted to control for these selection factors, it is common for properly designed randomized trials to fail to confirm benefits suggested by less rigorous study designs. Thus, ongoing and future large-scale randomized trials may fail to confirm this apparent benefit.
(2) Current medical practice often includes the use of concomitant progestin therapy in women with intact uteri (see PRECAUTIONS and WARNINGS). While the effects of added progestins on the risk of ischemic heart disease are not known, all available progestins reverse at least some of the favorable effects of estrogens on HDL and LDL levels.
(3) While the effects of added progestins on the risk of breast cancer are also unknown, available epidemiologic evidence suggests that progestins do not reduce, and may enhance, the moderately increased breast cancer incidence that has been reported with prolonged estrogen replacement therapy (see WARNINGS, above).
Because relatively long-term use of estrogens by a woman with a uterus has been shown to induce endometrial cancer, physicians often recommend that women who are deemed candidates for hormone replacement should take progestins as well as estrogens. When considering prescribing concomitant estrogens and progestins for hormone replacement therapy, physicians and patients are advised to carefully weigh the potential benefits and risks of the added progestin. Large-scale randomized, placebo-controlled, prospective clinical trials are required to clarify these issues.
3. Physical Examination. A complete medical and family history should be taken prior to the initiation of any estrogen therapy. The pretreatment and periodic physical examinations should include special reference to blood pressure,

breasts, abdomen, and pelvic organs and should include a Papanicolaou smear. As a general rule, estrogen should not be prescribed for longer than 1 year without reexamining the patient.
4. Hypercoagulability. Some studies have shown that women taking estrogen replacement therapy have hypercoagulability, primarily related to decreased antithrombin activity. This effect appears dose- and duration-dependent and is less pronounced than that associated with oral contraceptive use. Also, postmenopausal women tend to have increased coagulation parameters at baseline compared to premenopausal women. There is some suggestion that low-dose postmenopausal mestranol may increase the risk of thromboembolism, although the majority of studies (primarily of users of conjugated estrogens) report no such increase. There is insufficient information on hypercoagulability in women who have had previous thromboembolic disease.
5. Familial Hyperlipoproteinemia. Estrogen therapy may be associated with massive elevations of plasma triglycerides leading to pancreatitis and other complications in patients with familial defects of lipoprotein metabolism.
6. Fluid Retention. Because estrogens may cause some degree of fluid retention, conditions that might be exacerbated by this factor, such as asthma, epilepsy, migraine, and cardiac or renal dysfunction, require careful observation.
7. Uterine Bleeding and Mastodynia. Certain patients may develop undesirable manifestations of estrogenic stimulation, such as abnormal uterine bleeding and mastodynia.
8. Impaired Liver Function. Estrogens may be poorly metabolized in patients with impaired liver function and should be administered with caution.

Information for the Patient

See text of Patient Package Insert, which appears after the HOW SUPPLIED section.

Laboratory Tests

Estrogen administration should generally be guided by clinical response at the smallest dose, rather than laboratory monitoring, for relief of symptoms for those indications in which symptoms are observable.

Drug/Laboratory Test Interactions

Some of these drug/laboratory test interactions have been observed only with estrogen-progestin combinations (oral contraceptives):
1. Accelerated prothrombin time, partial thromboplastin time, and platelet aggregation time; increased platelet count; increased factors II, VII antigen, VIII antigen, VIII coagulant activity, IX, X, XII, VII-X complex, II-VII-X complex; and beta-thromboglobulin; decreased levels of antifactor Xa and antithrombin III; decreased antithrombin III activity; increased levels of fibrinogen and fibrinogen activity; increased plasminogen antigen and activity.
2. Increased thyroid-binding globulin (TBG) leading to increased circulating total thyroid hormone, as measured by protein-bound iodine (PBI), T_4 levels (by column or by radioimmunoassay) or T_3 levels by radioimmunoassay. T_3 resin uptake is decreased, reflecting the elevated TBG. Free T_4 and free T_3 concentrations are unaltered.
3. Other binding proteins may be elevated in serum, i.e., corticosteroid binding globulin (CBG), sex hormone-binding globulin (SHBG), leading to increased circulating corticosteroids and sex steroids, respectively. Free or biologically active hormone concentrations are unchanged. Other plasma proteins may be increased (angiotensinogen/renin substrate, alpha-1-antitrypsin, ceruloplasmin).
4. Increased plasma HDL and HDL_2 subfraction concentrations, reduced LDL cholesterol concentration, increased triglycerides levels.
5. Impaired glucose tolerance.
6. Reduced response to metyrapone test.
7. Reduced serum folate concentration.

Carcinogenesis, Mutagenesis, Impairment of Fertility

Long-term, continuous administration of natural and synthetic estrogens in certain animal species increases the frequency of carcinomas of the breast, cervix, vagina, testis, and liver (see CONTRAINDICATIONS and WARNINGS).

Pregnancy Category X

Estrogens should not be used during pregnancy (see CONTRAINDICATIONS and Boxed Warning).

Nursing Mothers

As a general principle, the administration of any drug to nursing mothers should be done only when clearly necessary since many drugs are excreted in human milk. In addition, estrogen administration to nursing mothers has been shown to decrease the quantity and quality of the milk.

ADVERSE REACTIONS

See WARNINGS and Boxed Warning regarding the potential adverse effects on the fetus, the induction of malignant neoplasms, gallbladder disease, cardiovascular disease, elevated blood pressure, and hypercalcemia.
The most commonly reported systemic adverse event to the Vivelle system in controlled clinical trials was headache. This occurred in approximately 36% of patients treated with

Continued on next page

CibaGeneva—Cont.

active systems and in 30% of patients treated with placebo. The most common topical adverse events in these trials were erythema and pruritus at the application site. Most cases were considered mild. Fewer than 5% of patients on active drug at the final visit of the study had reactions of greater than mild intensity. Rash was reported rarely in these trials. Two patients out of 356 were discontinued from the trials due to skin irritation/erythema.

The following additional adverse reactions have been reported with estrogen therapy:

1. *Genitourinary System.* Changes in vaginal bleeding pattern and abnormal withdrawal bleeding or flow; breakthrough bleeding, spotting; increase in size of uterine leiomyomata; vaginal candidiasis; change in amount of cervical secretion.
2. *Breasts.* Tenderness, enlargement.
3. *Gastrointestinal.* Nausea, vomiting; abdominal cramps, bloating; cholestatic jaundice; gallbladder disease.
4. *Skin.* Chloasma or melasma that may persist when drug is discontinued; erythema multiforme; erythema nodosum; hemorrhagic eruption; loss of scalp hair; hirsutism.
5. *Eyes.* Steepening of corneal curvature; intolerance to contact lenses.
6. *Central Nervous System.* Headache, migraine, dizziness; mental depression; chorea.
7. *Miscellaneous.* Increase or decrease in weight; reduced carbohydrate tolerance; aggravation of porphyria; edema; changes in libido.

OVERDOSAGE

Serious ill effects have not been reported following acute ingestion of large doses of estrogen-containing oral contraceptives by young children. Overdosage of estrogen may cause nausea and vomiting, and withdrawal bleeding may occur in females.

DOSAGE AND ADMINISTRATION

The adhesive side of the Vivelle system should be placed on a clean, dry area of the skin on the trunk of the body (including the buttocks and abdomen). *Vivelle should not be applied to the breasts.* The Vivelle system should be replaced twice weekly. The sites of application must be rotated, with an interval of at least 1 week allowed between applications to a particular site. The area selected should not be oily, damaged, or irritated. The waistline should be avoided, since tight clothing may rub the system off. The system should be applied immediately after opening the pouch and removing the protective liner. The system should be pressed firmly in place with the palm of the hand for about 10 seconds, making sure there is good contact, especially around the edges. In the unlikely event that a system should fall off, the same system may be reapplied. If necessary, a new system may be applied. In either case, the original treatment schedule should be continued.

Initiation of Therapy

For treatment of moderate-to-severe vasomotor symptoms and vulval and vaginal atrophy associated with the menopause, start therapy with the Vivelle estradiol transdermal system 0.05 mg/day applied to the skin twice weekly. In order to use the lowest dosage necessary for the control of symptoms, decisions to increase dosage should not be made until after the first month of therapy. Some women taking the 0.0375 mg/day dosage may experience a delayed onset of efficacy. Attempts to discontinue or taper medication should be made at 3-month to 6-month intervals.

In women not currently taking oral estrogens or in women switching from another estradiol transdermal therapy, treatment with the Vivelle estradiol transdermal system may be initiated at once. In women who are currently taking oral estrogens, treatment with the Vivelle estradiol transdermal system should be initiated 1 week after withdrawal of oral hormone replacement therapy, or sooner if menopausal symptoms reappear in less than 1 week.

Therapeutic Regimen

Vivelle may be given continuously in patients who do not have an intact uterus. In those patients with an intact uterus, Vivelle may be given on a cyclic schedule (e.g., 3 weeks on drug followed by 1 week off drug).

HOW SUPPLIED

Vivelle estradiol transdermal system 0.0375 mg/day - each 11.0 cm² system contains 3.28 mg of estradiol USP for nominal* delivery of 0.0375 mg of estradiol per day.
Patient Calendar Pack of
8 systems .... NDC 0083-2325-08
Carton of 6 Patient Calendar Packs
of 8 systems .... NDC 0083-2325-62
Carton of 24 systems .... NDC 0083-2325-25
Vivelle estradiol transdermal system 0.05 mg/day - each 14.5 cm² system contains 4.33 mg of estradiol USP for nominal* delivery of 0.05 mg of estradiol per day.

Patient Calendar Pack of
8 systems .... NDC 0083-2326-08
Carton of 6 Patient Calendar Packs
of 8 systems .... NDC 0083-2326-62
Carton of 24 systems .... NDC 0083-2326-25
Vivelle estradiol transdermal system 0.075 mg/day - each 22.0 cm² system contains 6.57 mg of estradiol USP for nominal* delivery of 0.075 mg of estradiol per day.
Patient Calendar Pack of
8 systems .... NDC 0083-2327-08
Carton of 6 Patient Calendar Packs
of 8 systems .... NDC 0083-2327-62
Carton of 24 systems .... NDC 0083-2327-25
Vivelle estradiol transdermal system 0.1 mg/day - each 29.0 cm² system contains 8.66 mg of estradiol USP for nominal* delivery of 0.1 mg of estradiol per day.
Patient Calendar Pack of
8 systems .... NDC 0083-2328-08
Carton of 6 Patient Calendar Packs
of 8 systems .... NDC 0083-2328-62
Carton of 24 systems .... NDC 0083-2328-25

*See DESCRIPTION.
Do not store above 86°F (30°C). Do not store unpouched. Apply immediately upon removal from the protective pouch.
C95-40 (Rev. 9/95)

Information for the Patient

VIVELLE™
estradiol transdermal system

> **1. ESTROGENS INCREASE THE RISK OF CANCER OF THE UTERUS IN WOMEN WHO HAVE HAD THEIR MENOPAUSE ("CHANGE OF LIFE").**
> If you use any estrogen-containing drug, it is important to visit your doctor regularly and report any unusual vaginal bleeding right away. Vaginal bleeding after menopause may be a warning sign of uterine cancer. Your doctor should evaluate any unusual vaginal bleeding to find out the cause.
> **2. ESTROGENS SHOULD NOT BE USED DURING PREGNANCY.**
> Estrogens do not prevent miscarriage (spontaneous abortion) and are not needed in the days following childbirth. If you take estrogens during pregnancy, your unborn child has a greater than usual chance of having birth defects. The risk of developing these defects is small, but clearly larger than the risk in children whose mothers did not take estrogens during pregnancy. These birth defects may affect the baby's urinary system and sex organs. Daughters born to mothers who took DES (an estrogen drug) have a higher than usual chance of developing cancer of the vagina or cervix when they become teenagers or young adults. Sons may have a higher than usual chance of developing cancer of the testicles when they become teenagers or young adults.

INTRODUCTION

Your doctor has prescribed the Vivelle system for the treatment of your menopausal symptoms. During menopause, production of estrogen hormones by your body decreases well below the amounts normally produced during your fertile years. In many women, this decrease in estrogen production causes uncomfortable symptoms, most noticeably hot flushes and sleep disturbance. Estrogens can be given to reduce or eliminate these symptoms.

The Vivelle system that your doctor has prescribed for you releases small amounts of estradiol through the skin in a continuous way. Estradiol is the same hormone that your ovaries produce abundantly before menopause. The dose of estradiol you require will depend upon your individual response. The dose is adjusted by the size of the Vivelle system used; the systems are available in four sizes.

INFORMATION ABOUT VIVELLE

How Vivelle Works

Vivelle contains estradiol. When applied to the skin as directed below, the Vivelle system releases estradiol, which flows through the skin into the bloodstream.

How and Where to Apply Vivelle

Each system is individually sealed in a protective pouch. Tear open this pouch at the indentation (do not use scissors) and remove the system.

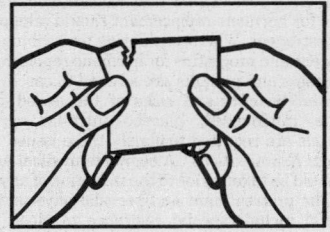

A stiff protective liner covers the adhesive side of the system—the side that will be placed against your skin. This liner must be removed before applying the system. Hold the unit with the protective liner facing you.

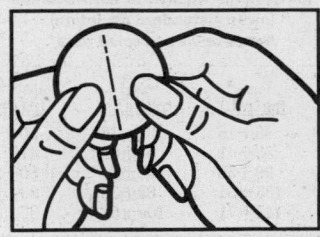

Peel off one side of the protective liner and discard it. Try to avoid touching the sticky side of the system with your fingers.

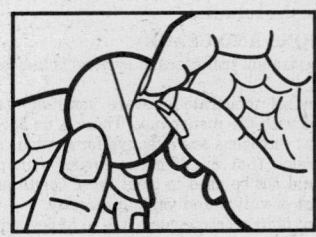

Using the other half of the liner as a handle, apply the sticky side of the system to a dry area of the skin on the trunk of the body (including the buttocks and abdomen). Press the sticky side on the skin and smooth down.

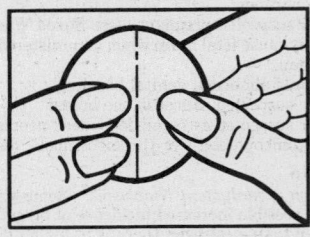

Fold back the remaining side of the system. Grasp the straight edge of the protective liner and pull it off the system.

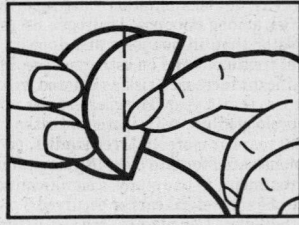

Press the system firmly in place.

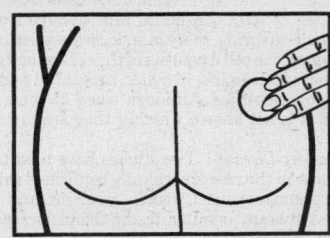

Some women may find that it is more comfortable to wear Vivelle on the buttocks. *Do not apply Vivelle to your breasts.* The sites of application must be rotated, with an interval of at least 1 week allowed between applications to a particular site. The area selected should not be oily, damaged, or irritated. Avoid the waistline, since tight clothing may rub the system off. Apply the system immediately after opening the pouch and removing the protective liner. Press the system firmly in place with the palm of your hand for about 10 seconds, making sure there is good contact, especially around the edges.

The Vivelle system should be worn continuously until it is time to replace it with a new system. You may wish to experiment with different locations when applying a new system, to find ones that are most comfortable for you and where clothing will not rub on the system.

When to Apply Vivelle

The Vivelle system should be replaced twice weekly. Your Vivelle package contains a calendar checklist on the back to help you remember a schedule. Mark the 2-day schedule you plan to follow. Always change the system on the 2 days of the week you have marked.

When changing the system, remove the used Vivelle system and discard it. Any adhesive that might remain on your skin can be easily rubbed off. Then place the new Vivelle system on a different skin site. (The same skin site should not be used again for at least 1 week after removal of the system.) Please note: Contact with water when you are bathing, swimming, or showering will not affect the system. In the unlikely event that a system should fall off, put this same system back on and continue to follow your original treatment schedule. If necessary, you may apply a new system but continue to follow your original schedule.

Benefits of Treatment With Vivelle

Regular use of Vivelle twice weekly offers relief of moderate-to-severe symptoms of menopause.

Small quantities of the naturally occurring hormone estradiol are absorbed through the skin from the Vivelle system, ensuring a continuous supply of circulating hormone in the body.

USES OF ESTROGEN

To reduce moderate-to-severe menopausal symptoms. Estrogens are hormones produced by the ovaries. The decrease in the amount of estrogen that occurs in all women, usually between ages 45 and 55, causes the menopause. Sometimes the ovaries are removed by an operation, causing "surgical menopause." When the amount of estrogen begins to decrease, some women develop very uncomfortable symptoms, such as feelings of warmth in the face, neck, and chest or sudden intense episodes of heat and sweating ("hot flashes"). The use of drugs containing estrogens can help the body adjust to lower estrogen levels.

Some women have only mild menopausal symptoms, or none at all, and do not need estrogen therapy for these particular symptoms. Other women may need estrogens for a few months while their bodies adjust to lower estrogen levels. For the treatment of menopausal symptoms only, most women need estrogen replacement therapy for no longer than 6 months.

To treat vulval and vaginal atrophy (itching, burning, dryness in or around the vagina, difficulty or burning on urination) *associated with menopause.*

To treat certain conditions in which a young woman's ovaries do not produce enough estrogen naturally.

WHEN ESTROGENS SHOULD NOT BE USED

During pregnancy (see Boxed Warning). If you think you may be pregnant, do not use any form of estrogen-containing drug. Using estrogens while you are pregnant may cause your unborn child to have birth defects. Estrogens do not prevent miscarriage.

If you have unusual vaginal bleeding that has not been evaluated by your doctor (see Boxed Warning). Unusual vaginal bleeding can be a warning sign of cancer of the uterus, especially if it happens after menopause. Your doctor must find out the cause of the bleeding so that he or she can recommend the proper treatment. Taking estrogens without visiting your doctor can cause you serious harm if your vaginal bleeding is caused by cancer of the uterus.

If you have had cancer. Since estrogens increase the risk of certain types of cancer, you should not use estrogens if you ever have had cancer of the breast or uterus.

If you have any circulation problems. Estrogen therapy should be used only after consultation with your doctor and only in recommended doses. Patients with a tendency for abnormal blood clotting should avoid estrogen use (see DANGERS OF ESTROGENS, below).

When they are ineffective. During menopause, some women develop nervous symptoms or depression. Estrogens do not relieve these symptoms. You may have heard that taking estrogens for years after menopause will keep your skin soft and supple and keep you feeling young. There is no evidence for these claims and such long-term estrogen use may have serious risks.

After childbirth or when breastfeeding a baby. Estrogens should not be used to try to stop the breasts from filling with milk after a baby is born. Such treatment may increase the risk of developing blood clots (see DANGERS OF ESTROGENS, below).

If you are breastfeeding, you should avoid using any drugs because many drugs pass through to the baby in the milk. While nursing a baby, you should take drugs only on the advice of your healthcare provider.

DANGERS OF ESTROGENS

Cancer of the uterus. The risk of developing cancer of the uterus gets higher the longer estrogens are used and when larger doses are taken. One study showed that when estrogens are discontinued, this increased risk of cancer seems to fall off quickly. Three other studies showed that the risk for uterine cancer stayed high for 8 to more than 15 years after stopping estrogen treatment. Because of this risk, *it is important to take the lowest dose that works and to take it only as long as you need it.* Using progestin therapy together with estrogen therapy may reduce the higher risk of uterine cancer related to estrogen use (but see OTHER INFORMATION, below).

If you have had your uterus removed (total hysterectomy), there is no danger of developing cancer of the uterus.

Cancer of the breast. The majority of studies have shown no association between the usual doses used for estrogen replacement therapy and breast cancer. Some studies have suggested a possible increased incidence of breast cancer in those women taking estrogens for prolonged periods of time and especially if higher doses are used.

Regular breast examinations by a health professional and monthly self-examination are recommended for women receiving estrogen therapy, as they are for all women.

Gallbladder disease. Women who use estrogens after menopause are more likely to develop gallbladder disease needing surgery than women who do not use estrogens.

Abnormal blood clotting. Taking estrogens may increase the risk of blood clots. These clots can cause a stroke, heart attack, or pulmonary embolus, any of which may be fatal. However, most studies of low-dose estrogen usage by women do not show an increased risk of these complications.

SIDE EFFECTS

In addition to the risks listed above, the following side effects have been reported with estrogen use:

- Headache.
- Nausea and vomiting.
- Breast tenderness or enlargement.
- Enlargement of benign tumors ("fibroids") of the uterus.
- Retention of excess fluid. This may make some conditions worsen, such as asthma, epilepsy, migraine, heart disease, or kidney disease.
- A spotty darkening of the skin, particularly on the face. Skin irritation, redness, or rash may occur at the site of application.

REDUCING RISK OF ESTROGEN USE

If you use estrogens, you can reduce your risks by doing these things: *See your doctor regularly.* While you are using estrogens, it is important to visit your doctor at least once a year for a check-up. If you develop vaginal bleeding while taking estrogens, you may need further evaluation. If members of your family have had breast cancer or if you have ever had breast lumps or an abnormal mammogram (breast x-ray), you may need to have more frequent breast examinations. *Reassess your need for estrogens.* You and your doctor should reevaluate whether or not you still need estrogens at least every 6 months.

Be alert for signs of trouble. Report these or any other unusual side effects to your doctor immediately:

- Abnormal bleeding from the vagina.
- Pains in the calves or chest, sudden shortness of breath, or coughing blood (indicating possible clots in the legs, heart, or lungs).
- Severe headache, dizziness, faintness, or changes in vision (indicating possible clots in the brain or eye).
- Breast lumps.
- Yellowing of the skin or eyes.
- Pain, swelling, or tenderness in the abdomen.
- Skin irritation, redness, or rash.

OTHER INFORMATION

If your uterus has not been removed, your doctor may choose to prescribe a progestin, a different hormonal drug to be used in association with estrogen treatment. Progestins lower the risk of developing endometrial hyperplasia, a possible precancerous condition of the uterine lining, which may occur while using estrogen. There are possible additional risks that may be associated with the inclusion of a progestin in estrogen treatment. The possible risks include unfavorable effects on blood fats and sugars, as well as a possible further increase in breast cancer risk that may be associated with long-term estrogen use.

Some research has suggested that estrogen taken *without progestins* may protect women against developing heart disease. However, this effect of estrogen is not certain.

You are cautioned to discuss very carefully with your doctor or healthcare provider all the possible risks and benefits of long-term estrogen and progestin treatment, as they affect you personally.

Your doctor has prescribed this drug for you and you alone. Do not give the drug to anyone else.

Keep this and all drugs out of the reach of children. In case of overdose, remove the system and call your doctor, hospital, or poison control center immediately.

This leaflet provides a summary of the most important information about estrogens. If you want more information, ask your doctor or pharmacist to show you the professional labeling.

C95-34 (Rev. 8/95)
C95-40/C95-34 (Rev. 9/95)

Dist. by:
Ciba-Geigy Corporation
Pharmaceuticals Division
Summit, NJ 07901
Shown in Product Identification Guide, page 310

Ciba Pharmaceutical Company
Ciba-Geigy Corporation
556 MORRIS AVENUE
SUMMIT, NJ 07901

For Information Contact:
Consumer Affairs Department:
(800) 742-2422
Medical Services Department:
556 Morris Avenue
Summit, NJ 07901

PLEASE NOTE:
Due to the alliance between Ciba Pharmaceuticals (which includes Basel Pharmaceuticals, Ciba Pharmaceutical Company, Geigy Pharmaceuticals, and Summit Pharmaceuticals) and Geneva Pharmaceuticals, Inc, please refer to **CibaGeneva** for product information.

See CibaGeneva Pharmaceuticals for information on the following products:
Anturane®
Apresazide®
Apresoline®
Aredia®
Cytadren®
Desferal®
Esidrix®
Esimil®
Estraderm®
Ismelin®
Lotensin®
Lotensin HCT®
Lotrel®
Ludiomil®
Priscoline®
Regitine®
Rimactane®
Ritalin®
Ritalin-SR®
Ser-Ap-Es®
Tegretol®
Tegretol®-XR
Vivelle™

Ciba Self-Medication, Inc.
Mack Woodbridge II
581 MAIN STREET
WOODBRIDGE, NJ 07095

Direct Inquiries to:
Consumer Affairs
1-800-452-0051

After Hours and Weekend Emergencies:
(908) 277-5000

DULCOLAX® OTC
[dul 'co-lax]
brand of bisacodyl USP

DESCRIPTION AND CLINICAL PHARMACOLOGY

Dulcolax is a contact stimulant laxative, administered either orally or rectally, which acts directly on the colonic mucosa to produce normal peristalsis throughout the large intestine. The active ingredient in Dulcolax, bisacodyl, is a colorless, tasteless compound that is practically insoluble in water or alkaline solution. Its chemical name is: bis(p-acetoxyphenyl)-2-pyridylmethane. Bisacodyl is very poorly absorbed, if at all, in the small intestine following oral administration, or in the large intestine following rectal administration. On contact

Continued on next page

Ciba Self-Medication, Inc.—Cont.

with the mucosa or submucosal plexi of the large intestine, bisacodyl stimulates sensory nerve endings to produce parasympathetic reflexes resulting in increased peristaltic contractions of the colon. It has also been shown to promote fluid and ion accumulation in the colon, which increases the laxative effect. A bowel movement is usually produced approximately 6 hours after oral administration (8–12 hours if taken at bedtime), and approximately 15 minutes to 1 hour after rectal administration, providing satisfactory cleansing of the bowel which may, under certain circumstances, obviate the need for colonic irrigation.
Dulcolax (brand of bisacodyl USP) is available as enteric coated tablets of 5 mg each or as suppositories of 10 mg each. Each tablet also contains: acacia, acetylated monoglyceride, carnauba wax, cellulose acetate phthalate, corn starch, D&C Red No. 30 aluminum lake, D&C Yellow No. 10 aluminum lake, dibutyl phthalate, docusate sodium, gelatin, glycerin, iron oxides, kaolin, lactose, magnesium stearate, methylparaben, pharmaceutical glaze, polyethylene glycol, povidone, propylparaben, sodium benzoate, sorbitan monooleate, sucrose, talc, titanium dioxide, and white wax. Each suppository also contains hydrogenated vegetable oil. Tablets and suppositories contain less than 0.2 mg sodium per dosage unit and are thus dietetically sodium-free.

INDICATIONS AND USAGE

For the relief of occasional constipation and irregularity. For use as part of a bowel cleansing regimen in preparing the patient for surgery or for preparing the colon for x-ray endoscopic examination. Dulcolax will not replace the colonic irrigations usually given patients before intracolonic surgery, but is useful in the preliminary emptying of the colon prior to those procedures. Dulcolax may also be used in postoperative care (i.e., restoration of normal bowel hygiene), antepartum care, postpartum care, and in preparation for delivery.

CONTRAINDICATIONS

Stimulant laxatives, such as Dulcolax, are contraindicated for patients with acute surgical abdomen, appendicitis, rectal bleeding, gastroenteritis, or intestinal obstruction.

WARNINGS AND PRECAUTIONS

Use of Dulcolax is not recommended when abdominal pain, nausea, or vomiting are present. Long term administration of Dulcolax is not recommended in the treatment of chronic constipation. This product should not be used beyond 7 days unless deemed necessary. Rectal bleeding or failure to have a bowel movement after Dulcolax use may indicate a serious condition. If this occurs, the patient should discontinue use of the product.
This and all medication should be kept out of the reach of children.
Pregnancy Category B
Teratology
Reproduction studies of oral doses of Dulcolax (bisacodyl) have been performed in rats administered up to 70 times the human dose, and have revealed no evidence of impaired fertility or damage to the fetus. At the dose which equated to 70 times the human dose, there was some evidence of lower litter survival at weaning. There are, however, no adequate and well-controlled studies in pregnant women, hence Dulcolax should be used during pregnancy only at the discretion of the physician.
Extent of Drug Absorption
In a pharmacokinetic (crossover) study involving 12 patients (Roth, 1988), plasma levels of bisacodyl were measured following oral administration of a 10 mg reference solution and two 5 mg Dulcolax tablets, and following rectal administration of one 10 mg Dulcolax suppository. With the solution dose, the average Cmax was 237 ng/ml; with the tablet dose, the average Cmax was 26 ng/ml (11% of the solution Cmax); with the suppository dose, in six patients the plasma level was below the limit of detection, and in the remaining six patients, the average Cmax was 31 ng/ml (13% of the solution Cmax in those particular patients). These data demonstrate the low level of systemic absorption of bisacodyl resulting from Dulcolax use.

ADVERSE DRUG REACTIONS

The process of restoring normal bowel function by use of a laxative may result in some abdominal discomfort.

OVERDOSAGE

There are no specific antidotes that are required to be administered in the event of overdosage; however, supportive care may be required in order to prevent dehydration and/or electrolyte imbalance.

DOSAGE AND ADMINISTRATION

Tablets
Adults and children 12 years of age and over: Take 2 or 3 tablets (usually 2) in a single dose once daily.
Children 6 to under 12 years of age: Take 1 tablet once daily. Expect results in 8–12 hours if taken at bedtime or within 6 hours if taken before breakfast. Do not chew or crush tablets. Do not administer tablets within 1 hour after taking an antacid or milk.
Children under 6 years of age: Oral administration is not recommended due to the requirement to swallow tablets whole.
Suppositories
Adults and children 12 years of age and over: Use 1 suppository once daily. Remove foil wrapper. Lie on your side and, with pointed end first, push suppository high into the rectum so it will not slip out. Retain it for 15 to 20 minutes. If you feel the suppository must come out immediately, it was not inserted high enough and should be pushed higher.
Children under 12 years of age: One half of one 10 mg suppository once daily.
If the suppository seems soft, hold in foil wrapper under cold water for one or two minutes. In the presence of anal fissures or hemorrhoids, suppository may be coated at the tip with petroleum jelly before insertion.
Preparation for x-ray endoscopy: For barium enemas, no food should be given following oral administration to prevent reaccumulation of material in the rectum, and a suppository should be administered one to two hours prior to examination.

HOW SUPPLIED

Dulcolax, brand of bisacodyl, is supplied as either light orange enteric coated tablets of 5 mg each in sample packages of 2 or boxes of 4, 10, 25, 50, 100 (OTC as well as hospital unit doses) and 1000, or as suppositories of 10 mg each in sample packages of 1 or boxes of 4, 8, 16, 50, and 500.
NDC 0067-6200 (tablets)
NDC 0067-6100 (suppositories)
Store Dulcolax tablets and suppositories at temperatures below 77°F (25°C). Avoid excessive humidity.
Dulcolax is also supplied in a Bowel Prep Kit. Each kit contains one Dulcolax suppository (10 mg), four Dulcolax tablets (5 mg each), and complete patient instructions.

BIBLIOGRAPHY

Roth, V.W. et al: "Pharmacokinetics and Laxative Effect of Bisacodyl after Administration of Various Dosage Forms"; Arzneim.-Forsch. *38* (I), No. 4, pp. 570–4 (1988).
Additional literature references available upon request.
Shown in Product Identification Guide, page 308

HABITROL® ℞
(nicotine transdermal system)
Systemic delivery of 21, 14, or 7 mg/day over 24 hours
Prescribing Information

DESCRIPTION

Habitrol is a transdermal system that provides systemic delivery of nicotine following its application to intact skin for 24 hours.
Nicotine is a tertiary amine composed of a pyridine and a pyrrolidine ring. It is a colorless-to-pale yellow, freely water-soluble, strongly alkaline, oily, volatile, hygroscopic liquid obtained from the tobacco plant. Nicotine has a characteristic pungent odor and turns brown on exposure to air or light. Of its two stereoisomers, S(-)-nicotine is the more active and is the more prevalent form in tobacco. The free alkaloid is absorbed rapidly through the skin and respiratory tract.
Structural Formula

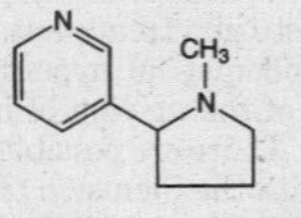

Chemical Name: S-3(1-methyl-2-pyrrolidinyl) pyridine
Molecular Formula: $C_{10}H_{14}N_2$
Molecular Weight: 162.23
Ionization Constants: $pK_{a1}=7.84$, $pK_{a2}=3.04$
Octanol-Water Partition Coefficient: 15:1 at pH 7

Habitrol systems are round, flat, 0.6-mm-thick multi-layer units containing nicotine as the active agent. Proceeding from the visible surface toward the surface attached to the skin are: (1) a tan-colored aluminized backing film; (2) a pressure-sensitive acrylate adhesive; (3) a layer containing a methacrylic acid copolymer solution of nicotine dispersed in a pad of nonwoven viscose and cotton; (4) an adhesive layer similar in composition to (2) above; (5) a protective aluminized release liner which overlays the adhesive layer and must be removed prior to use.
[See Figure at top of next column.]
Nicotine is the active ingredient; other components of the system are pharmacologically inactive.

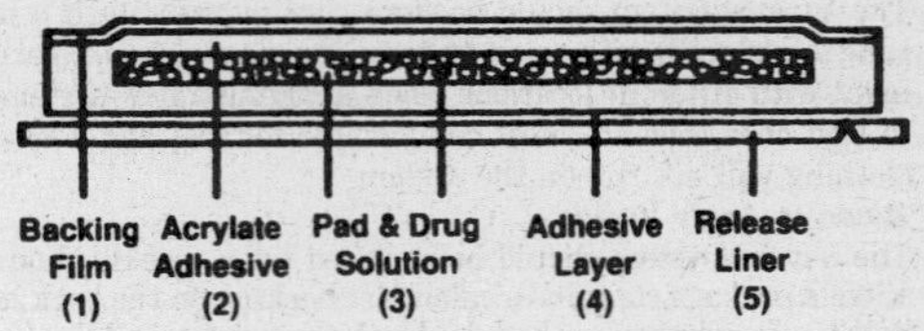

The amount of nicotine delivered to the patient from each system (29 mcg/cm^2-h) is nearly proportional to the surface area. About 60% of the total amount of nicotine remains in the system 24 hours after application. Habitrol systems are labeled as to the dose actually absorbed by the patient. The dose of nicotine absorbed from a Habitrol system represents 98% of the amount released from the system in 24 hours.

Dose Absorbed in 24 hours (mg/day)	System Surface Area (cm²)	Total Nicotine Content (mg)
21	30	52.5
14	20	35.0
7	10	17.5

CLINICAL PHARMACOLOGY

Pharmacologic Action
Nicotine, the chief alkaloid in tobacco products, binds stereoselectively to acetylcholine receptors at the autonomic ganglia, in the adrenal medulla, at neuromuscular junctions, and in the brain. Two types of central nervous system effects are believed to be the basis of nicotine's positively reinforcing properties. A stimulating effect, exerted mainly in the cortex via the locus ceruleus, produces increased alertness and cognitive performance. A "reward" effect via the "pleasure system" in the brain is exerted in the limbic system. At low doses the stimulant effects predominate while at high doses the reward effects predominate. Intermittent intravenous administration of nicotine activates neurohormonal pathways, releasing acetylcholine, norepinephrine, dopamine, serotonin, vasopressin, beta-endorphin, growth hormone, and ACTH.
Pharmacodynamics
The cardiovascular effects of nicotine include peripheral vasoconstriction, tachycardia, and elevated blood pressure. Acute and chronic tolerance to nicotine develops from smoking tobacco or ingesting nicotine preparations. Acute tolerance (a reduction in response for a given dose) develops rapidly (less than 1 hour), however, not at the same rate for different physiologic effects (skin temperature, heart rate, subjective effects). Withdrawal symptoms such as cigarette craving can be reduced in some individuals by plasma nicotine levels lower than those from smoking.
Withdrawal from nicotine in addicted individuals is characterized by craving, nervousness, restlessness, irritability, mood lability, anxiety, drowsiness, sleep disturbances, impaired concentration, increased appetite, minor somatic complaints (headache, myalgia, constipation, fatigue), and weight gain. Nicotine toxicity is characterized by nausea, abdominal pain, vomiting, diarrhea, diaphoresis, flushing, dizziness, disturbed hearing and vision, confusion, weakness, palpitations, altered respiration, and hypotension.
The cardiovascular effects of Habitrol 14 mg/day systems used continuously for 24 hours were compared with smoking every hour during waking hours, for 10 days. A small increase in blood pressure was detectable on the first day but not after 10 days. Heart rate was increased by 3%–7% and stroke volume decreased by 5%–12% on the 10th day of application. Habitrol treatment had no significant influence on cutaneous blood flow or skin temperature.
Both smoking and nicotine can increase circulating cortisol and catecholamines, and tolerance does not develop to the catecholamine-releasing effects of nicotine. Changes in the response to a concomitantly administered adrenergic agonist or antagonist should be watched for when nicotine intake is altered during Habitrol therapy and/or smoking cessation (see PRECAUTIONS, Drug Interactions).
Pharmacokinetics
The volume of distribution following IV administration of nicotine is approximately 2 to 3 L/kg and the half-life ranges from 1 to 2 hours. The major eliminating organ is the liver, and average plasma clearance is about 1.2 L/min; the kidney and lung also metabolize nicotine. There is no significant skin metabolism of nicotine. More than 20 metabolites of nicotine have been identified, all of which are believed to be less active than the parent compound. The primary metabolite of nicotine in plasma, cotinine, has a half-life of 15 to 20 hours and concentrations that exceed nicotine by 10-fold.
Plasma-protein binding of nicotine is <5%. Therefore, changes in nicotine binding from use of concomitant drugs or alterations of plasma proteins by disease states would not be expected to have significant consequences.
The primary urinary metabolites are cotinine (15% of the dose) and trans-3-hydroxycotinine (45% of the dose). About 10% of nicotine is excreted unchanged in the urine. As much as 30% may be excreted in the urine with high urine flow rates and urine acidification below pH 5.

The pharmacokinetic model which best fits the plasma nicotine concentrations from Habitrol systems is an open, two-compartment disposition model with a skin depot through which nicotine enters the central circulation compartment. The nicotine from the drug matrix is released slowly from the system. Therefore, the decline of plasma nicotine concentrations during the last 12 hours is determined primarily by release of nicotine from the system through the skin.

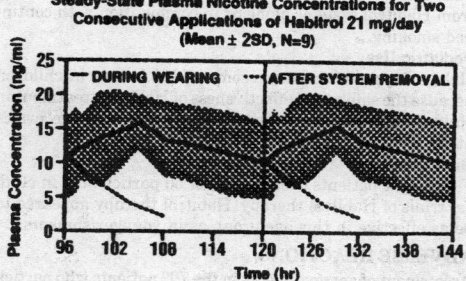

Steady-State Plasma Nicotine Concentrations for Two Consecutive Applications of Habitrol 21 mg/day (Mean ± 2SD, N=9)

Following an initial lag time of 1–2 hours, nicotine concentrations increase to a broad peak between 6 and 12 hours and then decrease gradually. Steady state for nicotine is attained within 2 days of initiating Habitrol treatment and average plasma nicotine concentrations are, on average, 25% higher compared to single dose applications. Upon application of a new system and removal of the old system there is, in some patients, a slight and transient (30–60 min.) increase in nicotine plasma concentration and its variability. Plasma nicotine concentrations are proportional to dose (ie, linear kinetics are observed) for the three dosages of Habitrol systems. Nicotine kinetics are similar for all sites of application on the back, abdomen, or side.

Following removal of Habitrol systems, plasma nicotine concentrations decline in an exponential fashion with an apparent mean half-life of 3–4 hours (see dotted line in graph) compared with 1–2 hours for IV administration, due to continued absorption from the skin depot. Most nonsmoking patients will have nondetectable nicotine concentrations in 10 to 12 hours.

Steady-State Nicotine Pharmacokinetic Parameters for Habitrol Systems
(mean, standard deviation, range)

Parameter (units)	14 mg/day (N=9) Mean	SD	Range	21 mg/day (N=9) Mean	SD	Range
C_{max} (ng/mL)	12	4	6–16	17	2	13–19
C_{avg} (ng/mL)	9	3	5–12	13	2	9–17
C_{min} (ng/mL)	6	2	3–10	9	2	7–14
T_{max} (hrs)	5	3	0–8	6	3	2–9

C_{max}: maximum observed plasma concentration
C_{avg}: average plasma concentration
C_{min}: minimum observed plasma concentration
T_{max}: time of maximum plasma concentration

Clinical Studies
The efficacy of Habitrol treatment as an aid to smoking cessation was demonstrated in three placebo-controlled, double-blind trials in otherwise healthy patients smoking at least one pack per day (N=792). In two of the trials Habitrol therapy was combined with concomitant support and in one trial Habitrol was used without concomitant support. In all three trials, patients were treated for 7 weeks (3 weeks of titration and 4 weeks of maintenance) followed by 3 weeks of weaning. Quitting was defined as total abstinence from smoking as measured by patient diary and verified by expired carbon monoxide. The "quit rates" are the proportions of all persons initially enrolled who abstained after week 3.

The two trials in otherwise healthy smokers with concomitant support showed that Habitrol therapy was more effective than placebo after 7 weeks. Quit rates were still significantly different after the additional 3-week weaning period. The quit rates varied approximately 3-fold among clinics for each treatment when Habitrol therapy was used with a concomitant support program. Data from these two studies (N=516) are combined in the Quit Rate table. Greater variability and decreased quit rates were demonstrated in both placebo and Habitrol treatment groups when concomitant support was not employed (N=276, see table).

[See table on top of page.]

Patients who used Habitrol treatment in clinical trials had a significant reduction in craving for cigarettes, a major nicotine withdrawal symptom, as compared to placebo-treated patients (see graph). Reduction in craving, as with quit rate, is quite variable. This variability is presumed to be due to inherent differences in patient populations, eg, patient motivation, concomitant illnesses, number of cigarettes smoked per day, number of years smoking, exposure to other smokers, socioeconomic status, etc, as well as differences among the clinics.

Quit Rates After Week 3 by Treatment

Concomitant Support	Treatment	Number of Patients	After 7 Weeks (range)	After Weaning (range)
Yes†	Habitrol	260	19–54%	8–43%
	Placebo*	256	9–30%	8–30%
No††	Habitrol	141	4–28%	4–20%
	Placebo*	135	0–24%	0–22%

*Sub Therapeutic (ST) Placebo systems contained 13% of the nicotine found in the respective-sized active system to allow blinding as to color and odor.
†Two trials with 9 clinics, number of patients per treatment ranged from 22 to 39.
††One trial with 5 clinics, number of patients per treatment ranged from 24 to 40.

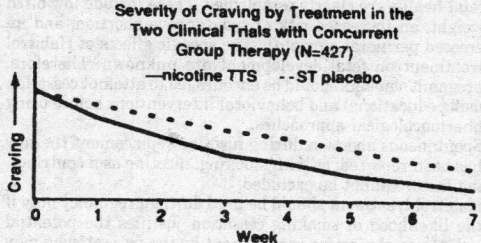

Severity of Craving by Treatment in the Two Clinical Trials with Concurrent Group Therapy (N=427)
—nicotine TTS   - -ST placebo

Patients using Habitrol systems dropped out of the trials less frequently than did patients receiving placebo. Quit rates for the 32 patients over age 60 were comparable to the quit rates for the 369 patients aged 60 and under.

Individualization of Dosage
It is important to make sure that patients read the instructions made available to them and have their questions answered. They should clearly understand the directions for applying and disposing of Habitrol systems. They should be instructed to stop smoking completely when the first system is applied.

The success or failure of smoking cessation depends heavily on the quality, intensity, and frequency of supportive care. Patients are more likely to quit smoking if they are seen frequently and participate in formal smoking cessation programs.

The goal of Habitrol therapy is complete abstinence. Significant health benefits have not been demonstrated for reduction of smoking. If a patient is unable to stop smoking by the fourth week of therapy, treatment should probably be discontinued. Patients who have not stopped smoking after 4 weeks of Habitrol therapy are unlikely to quit on that attempt.

Patients who fail to quit on any attempt may benefit from interventions to improve their chances for success on subsequent attempts. Patients who were unsuccessful should be counseled to determine why they failed. Patients should then probably be given a "therapy holiday" before the next attempt. A new quit attempt should be encouraged when the factors that contributed to failure can be eliminated or reduced, and conditions are more favorable.

Based on the clinical trials, a reasonable approach to assisting patients in their attempt to quit smoking is to assign their initial Habitrol dosage using the recommended dosing schedule (see Dosing Schedule). The need for dose adjustment should be assessed during the first 2 weeks. Patients should continue the dose selected with counseling and support over the following month. Those who have successfully stopped smoking during that time should be supported during 4 to 8 weeks of weaning, after which treatment should be terminated.

Therapy should generally begin with the Habitrol 21 mg/day dose (see Dosing Schedule below) except if the patient is small (less than 100 lbs), is a light smoker (less than 1/2 pack of cigarettes per day) or has cardiovascular disease.

Dosing Schedule

	Otherwise Healthy Patients	Other Patients*
Initial/Starting Dose	21 mg/day	14 mg/day
Duration of Treatment	4–8 weeks	4–8 weeks
First Weaning Dose	14 mg/day	7 mg/day
Duration of Treatment	2–4 weeks	2–4 weeks
Second Weaning Dose	7 mg/day	
Duration of Treatment	2–4 weeks	

* small patient (less than 100 lbs)
  or light smoker (less than 10 cigarettes/day)
  or patient with cardiovascular disease

The symptoms of nicotine withdrawal and excess overlap (see Pharmacodynamics and ADVERSE REACTIONS). Since patients using Habitrol treatment may also smoke intermittently, it may be difficult to determine if patients are experiencing nicotine withdrawal or nicotine excess. The controlled clinical trials using Habitrol therapy suggest that abnormal dreams are more often symptoms of nicotine excess while flatulence, anxiety, and depression are more often symptoms of nicotine withdrawal.

INDICATIONS AND USAGE
Habitrol treatment is indicated as an aid to smoking cessation for the relief of nicotine withdrawal symptoms. Habitrol treatment should be used as a part of a comprehensive behavioral smoking cessation program.
The use of Habitrol systems for longer than 3 months has not been studied.

CONTRAINDICATIONS
Use of Habitrol systems is contraindicated in patients with hypersensitivity or allergy to nicotine or to any of the components of the therapeutic system.

WARNINGS
Nicotine from any source can be toxic and addictive. Smoking causes lung cancer, heart disease, emphysema, and may adversely affect the fetus and the pregnant woman. For any smoker, with or without concomitant disease or pregnancy, the risk of nicotine replacement in a smoking cessation program should be weighed against the hazard of continued smoking while using Habitrol systems, and the likelihood of achieving cessation of smoking without nicotine replacement.

Pregnancy Warning
Tobacco smoke, which has been shown to be harmful to the fetus, contains nicotine, hydrogen cyanide, and carbon monoxide. Nicotine has been shown in animal studies to cause fetal harm. It is therefore presumed that Habitrol treatment can cause fetal harm when administered to a pregnant woman. The effect of nicotine delivery by Habitrol systems has not been examined in pregnancy (see PRECAUTIONS, Other Effects). Therefore, pregnant smokers should be encouraged to attempt cessation using educational and behavioral interventions before using pharmacological approaches. If Habitrol therapy is used during pregnancy, or if the patient becomes pregnant while using Habitrol treatment, the patient should be apprised of the potential hazard to the fetus.

Safety Note Concerning Children
The amounts of nicotine that are tolerated by adult smokers can produce symptoms of poisoning and could prove fatal if Habitrol systems are applied or ingested by children or pets. Used 21 mg/day systems contain about 60% (32 mg) of their initial drug content. Therefore, patients should be cautioned to keep both used and unused Habitrol systems out of the reach of children and pets.

PRECAUTIONS
General
The patient should be urged to stop smoking completely when initiating Habitrol therapy (see DOSAGE AND ADMINISTRATION). Patients should be informed that if they continue to smoke while using Habitrol systems, they may experience adverse effects due to peak nicotine levels higher than those experienced from smoking alone. If there is a clinically significant increase in cardiovascular or other effects attributable to nicotine, the Habitrol dose should be reduced or Habitrol treatment discontinued (see WARNINGS). Physicians should anticipate that concomitant medications may need dosage adjustment (see Drug Interactions). The use of Habitrol systems beyond 3 months by patients who stop smoking should be discouraged because the chronic consumption of nicotine by any route can be harmful and addicting.

Allergic Reactions: In a 12-week, open-label dermal irritation and sensitization study of Habitrol systems, 22 of 223 patients exhibited definite erythema at 24 hours after application. Upon rechallenge, 3 patients exhibited mild-to-moderate contact allergy. Patients with contact sensitization should be cautioned that a serious reaction could occur from exposure to other nicotine-containing products or smoking. In the efficacy trials, erythema following system removal was typically seen in about 17% of patients, some edema in 4%, and dropouts due to skin reactions occurred in 6% of patients.

Patients should be instructed to promptly discontinue the Habitrol treatment and contact their physicians if they experience severe or persistent local skin reactions at the site of

Continued on next page

Ciba Self-Medication, Inc.—Cont.

application (eg, severe erythema, pruritus, or edema) or a generalized skin reaction (eg, urticaria, hives, or generalized rash).

Skin Disease: Habitrol systems are usually well tolerated by patients with normal skin, but may be irritating for patients with some skin disorders (atopic or eczematous dermatitis).

Cardiovascular or Peripheral Vascular Diseases: The risks of nicotine replacement in patients with certain cardiovascular and peripheral vascular diseases should be weighed against the benefits of including nicotine replacement in a smoking cessation program for them. Specifically, patients with coronary heart disease (history of myocardial infarction and/or angina pectoris), serious cardiac arrhythmias, or vasospastic diseases (Buerger's disease, Prinzmetal's variant angina) should be carefully screened and evaluated before nicotine replacement is prescribed.

Tachycardia occurring in association with the use of Habitrol treatment was reported occasionally. If serious cardiovascular symptoms occur with Habitrol treatment, it should be discontinued.

Habitrol treatment should generally not be used in patients during the immediate post-myocardial infarction period, patients with serious arrhythmias, and patients with severe or worsening angina pectoris.

Renal or Hepatic Insufficiency: The pharmacokinetics of nicotine have not been studied in the elderly or in patients with renal or hepatic impairment. However, given that nicotine is extensively metabolized and that its total system clearance is dependent on liver blood flow, some influence of hepatic impairment on drug kinetics (reduced clearance) should be anticipated. Only severe renal impairment would be expected to affect the clearance of nicotine or its metabolites from the circulation (see CLINICAL PHARMACOLOGY, Pharmacokinetics).

Endocrine Diseases: Habitrol treatment should be used with caution in patients with hyperthyroidism, pheochromocytoma, or insulin-dependent diabetes since nicotine causes the release of catecholamines by the adrenal medulla.

Peptic Ulcer Disease: Nicotine delays healing in peptic ulcer disease; therefore, Habitrol treatment should be used with caution in patients with active peptic ulcers and only when the benefits of including nicotine replacement in a smoking cessation program outweigh the risks.

Accelerated Hypertension: Nicotine constitutes a risk factor for development of malignant hypertension in patients with accelerated hypertension; therefore, Habitrol treatment should be used with caution in these patients and only when the benefits of including nicotine replacement in a smoking cessation program outweigh the risks.

Information for Patients: A patient instruction sheet is included in the package of Habitrol systems dispensed to the patient. It contains important information and instructions on how to use and dispose of Habitrol systems properly. Patients should be encouraged to ask questions of the physician and pharmacist.

Patients must be advised to keep both used and unused systems out of the reach of children and pets.

Drug Interactions

Smoking cessation, with or without nicotine replacement, may alter the pharmacokinetics of certain concomitant medications.

[See table below.]

Carcinogenesis, Mutagenesis, Impairment of Fertility

Nicotine itself does not appear to be a carcinogen in laboratory animals. However, nicotine and its metabolites increased the incidence of tumors in the cheek pouches of hamsters and forestomach of F344 rats, respectively, when given in combination with tumor-initiators. One study, which could not be replicated, suggested that cotinine, the primary metabolite of nicotine, may cause lymphoreticular sarcoma in the large intestine in rats.

Nicotine and cotinine were not mutagenic in the Ames *Salmonella* test. Nicotine induced repairable DNA damage in an *E. coli* test system. Nicotine was shown to be genotoxic in a test system using Chinese hamster ovary cells. In rats and rabbits, implantation can be delayed or inhibited by a reduction in DNA synthesis that appears to be caused by nicotine. Studies have shown a decrease in litter size in rats treated with nicotine during gestation.

Pregnancy Category D (see WARNINGS)

The harmful effects of cigarette smoking on maternal and fetal health are clearly established. These include low birth weight, an increased risk of spontaneous abortion, and increased perinatal mortality. The specific effects of Habitrol treatment on fetal development are unknown. Therefore, pregnant smokers should be encouraged to attempt cessation using educational and behavioral interventions before using pharmacological approaches.

Spontaneous abortion during nicotine replacement therapy has been reported; as with smoking, nicotine as a contributing factor cannot be excluded.

Habitrol treatment should be used during pregnancy only if the likelihood of smoking cessation justifies the potential risk of use of nicotine replacement by the patient, who may continue to smoke.

Teratogenicity

Animal Studies: Nicotine was shown to produce skeletal abnormalities in the offspring of mice when given doses toxic to the dams (25 mg/kg/day IP or SC).

Human Studies: Nicotine teratogenicity has not been studied in humans except as a component of cigarette smoke (each cigarette smoked delivers about 1 mg of nicotine). It has not been possible to conclude whether cigarette smoking is teratogenic to humans.

Other Effects

Animal Studies: A nicotine bolus (up to 2 mg/kg) to pregnant rhesus monkeys caused acidosis, hypercarbia, and hypotension (fetal and maternal concentrations were about 20 times those achieved after smoking 1 cigarette in 5 minutes). Fetal breathing movements were reduced in the fetal lamb after intravenous injection of 0.25 mg/kg nicotine to the ewe (equivalent to smoking 1 cigarette every 20 seconds for 5 minutes). Uterine blood flow was reduced about 30% after infusion of 0.1 mg/kg/min nicotine for 20 minutes to pregnant rhesus monkeys (equivalent to smoking about six cigarettes every minute for 20 minutes).

Human Experience: Cigarette smoking during pregnancy is associated with an increased risk of spontaneous abortion, low-birth-weight infants and perinatal mortality. Nicotine and carbon monoxide are considered the most likely mediators of these outcomes. The effects of cigarette smoking on fetal cardiovascular parameters have been studied near term. Cigarettes increased fetal aortic blood flow and heart rate and decreased uterine blood flow and fetal breathing movements. Habitrol treatment has not been studied in pregnant humans.

Labor and Delivery

Habitrol systems are not recommended to be left on during labor and delivery. The effects of nicotine on the mother or the fetus during labor are unknown.

Nursing Mothers

Caution should be exercised when Habitrol therapy is administered to nursing women. The safety of Habitrol treatment in nursing infants has not been examined. Nicotine passes freely into breast milk; the milk-to-plasma ratio averages 2.9. Nicotine is absorbed orally. An infant has the ability to clear nicotine by hepatic first-pass clearance; however, the efficiency of removal is probably lowest at birth. The nicotine concentrations in milk can be expected to be lower with Habitrol treatment when used as directed than with cigarette smoking, as maternal plasma nicotine concentrations are generally reduced with nicotine replacement. The risk of exposure of the infant to nicotine from Habitrol systems should be weighed against the risks associated with the infant's exposure to nicotine from continued smoking by the mother (passive smoke exposure and contamination of breast milk with other components of tobacco smoke) and from Habitrol systems alone or in combination with continued smoking.

Pediatric Use

Habitrol systems are not recommended for use in children because the safety and effectiveness of Habitrol treatment in children and adolescents who smoke have not been evaluated.

Geriatric Use

Forty-eight patients over the age of 60 participated in clinical trials of Habitrol therapy. Habitrol therapy appeared to be as effective in this age group as in younger smokers.

ADVERSE REACTIONS

Assessment of adverse events in the 792 patients who participated in controlled clinical trials is complicated by the occurrence of GI and CNS effects of nicotine withdrawal as well as nicotine excess. The actual incidences of both are confounded by concurrent smoking by many of the patients. In the trials, when reporting adverse events, the investigators did not attempt to identify the cause of the symptom.

Topical Adverse Events

The most common adverse event associated with topical nicotine is a short-lived erythema, pruritus, or burning at the application site, which was seen at least once in 35% of patients on Habitrol treatment in the clinical trials. Local erythema after system removal was noted at least once in 17% of patients and local edema in 4%. Erythema generally resolved within 24 hours. Cutaneous hypersensitivity (contact sensitization) occurred in 2% of patients on Habitrol treatment (see PRECAUTIONS, Allergic Reactions).

Probably Causally Related

The following adverse events were reported more frequently in Habitrol-treated patients than in placebo-treated patients or exhibited a dose response in clinical trials.

Digestive system—Diarrhea*, dyspepsia*.
Mouth/Tooth disorders—Dry mouth.
Musculoskeletal system—Arthralgia*, myalgia*.
Nervous system—Abnormal dreams†, somnolence†.

Frequencies for 21 mg/day system
* Reported in 3% to 9% of patients.
† Reported in 1% to 3% of patients.
  Unmarked if reported in <1% of patients.

Causal Relationship Unknown

Adverse events reported in Habitrol- and placebo-treated patients at about the same frequency in clinical trials are listed below. The clinical significance of the association between Habitrol treatment and these events is unknown, but they are reported as alerting information for the clinician.

Body as a whole—Allergy†, back pain†.
Cardiovascular system—Hypertension*.
Digestive system—Abdominal pain†, constipation†, nausea*, vomiting.
Nervous system—Dizziness*, concentration impaired†, headache (17%), insomnia*.
Respiratory system—Cough increased†, pharyngitis†, sinusitis†.
Urogenital system—Dysmenorrhea*.

Frequencies for 21 mg/day system
* Reported in 3% to 9% of patients.
† Reported in 1% to 3% of patients.
  Unmarked if reported in <1% of patients.

DRUG ABUSE AND DEPENDENCE

Habitrol systems are likely to have a low abuse potential based on differences between it and cigarettes in four characteristics commonly considered important in contributing to abuse: much slower absorption, much smaller fluctuations in blood levels, lower blood levels of nicotine, and less frequent use (ie, once daily).

Dependence on nicotine polacrilex chewing gum replacement therapy has been reported. Such dependence might also occur from transference to Habitrol systems of tobacco-based nicotine dependence. The use of the system beyond 3 months has not been evaluated and should be discouraged. To minimize the risk of dependence, patients should be encouraged to withdraw gradually from Habitrol treatment after 4 to 8 weeks of usage. Recommended dose reduction is to progressively decrease the dose every 2 to 4 weeks (see DOSAGE AND ADMINISTRATION).

OVERDOSAGE

The effects of applying several Habitrol systems simultaneously or of swallowing Habitrol systems are unknown (see WARNINGS, Safety Note Concerning Children).

May Require a Decrease in Dose at Cessation of Smoking	Possible Mechanism
Acetaminophen, caffeine, imipramine, oxazepam, pentazocine, propranolol, theophylline	Deinduction of hepatic enzymes on smoking cessation
Insulin	Increase of subcutaneous insulin absorption with smoking cessation
Adrenergic antagonists (eg, prazosin, labetalol)	Decrease in circulating catecholamines with smoking cessation

May Require an Increase in Dose at Cessation of Smoking	Possible Mechanism
Adrenergic agonists (eg, isoproterenol, phenylephrine)	Decrease in circulating catecholamines with smoking cessation

The oral LD_{50} for nicotine in rodents varies with species but is in excess of 24 mg/kg; death is due to respiratory paralysis. The oral minimum lethal dose of nicotine in dogs is greater than 5 mg/kg. The oral minimum acute lethal dose for nicotine in human adults is reported to be 40 to 60 mg (<1 mg/kg).

Two or three Habitrol 30 cm^2 systems in capsules fed to dogs weighing 8–17 kg were emetic, but did not produce any other significant clinical signs. The administration of these patches corresponds to about 6–17 mg/kg of nicotine.

Signs and symptoms of an overdose of Habitrol systems would be expected to be the same as those of acute nicotine poisoning including: pallor, cold sweat, nausea, salivation, vomiting, abdominal pain, diarrhea, headache, dizziness, disturbed hearing and vision, tremor, mental confusion, and weakness. Prostration, hypotension, and respiratory failure may ensue with large overdoses. Lethal doses produce convulsions quickly and death follows as a result of peripheral or central respiratory paralysis or, less frequently, cardiac failure.

Overdose From Topical Exposure

The Habitrol system should be removed immediately if the patient shows signs of overdosage and the patient should seek immediate medical care. The skin surface may be flushed with water and dried. No soap should be used since it may increase nicotine absorption. Nicotine will continue to be delivered into the bloodstream for several hours (see CLINICAL PHARMACOLOGY, Pharmacokinetics) after removal of the system because of a depot of nicotine in the skin.

Overdose From Ingestion

Persons ingesting Habitrol systems should be referred to a health care facility for management. Due to the possibility of nicotine-induced seizures, activated charcoal should be administered. In unconscious patients with a secure airway, instill activated charcoal via nasogastric tube. A saline cathartic or sorbitol added to the first dose of activated charcoal may speed gastrointestinal passage of the system. Repeated doses of activated charcoal should be administered as long as the system remains in the gastrointestinal tract since it will continue to release nicotine for many hours.

Management of Nicotine Poisoning

Other supportive measures include diazepam or barbiturates for seizures, atropine for excessive bronchial secretions or diarrhea, respiratory support for respiratory failure, and vigorous fluid support for hypotension and cardiovascular collapse.

DOSAGE AND ADMINISTRATION

Patients must desire to stop smoking and should be instructed to *stop smoking immediately* as they begin using Habitrol therapy. The patient should read the patient instruction sheet on Habitrol treatment and be encouraged to ask any questions. Treatment should be initiated with Habitrol 21 mg/day or 14 mg/day systems (see CLINICAL PHARMACOLOGY, Individualization of Dosage). Dosage cannot be adjusted by cutting a Habitrol system.

Once the appropriate dosage is selected the patient should begin 4–6 weeks of therapy at that dosage. The patient should stop smoking cigarettes completely during this period. If the patient is unable to stop cigarette smoking within 4 weeks, Habitrol therapy should probably be stopped, since few additional patients in clinical trials were able to quit after this time.

Recommended Dosing Schedule for Healthy Patients[a]
(see Individualization of Dosage)

Dose	Duration
Habitrol 21 mg/day	First 6 Weeks
Habitrol 14 mg/day	Next 2 Weeks[b]
Habitrol 7 mg/day	Last 2 Weeks[c]

[a] Start with Habitrol 14 mg/day for 6 weeks for patients who:
—have cardiovascular disease
—weigh less than 100 pounds
—smoke less than $^1/_2$ a pack of cigarettes/day
Decrease dose to Habitrol 7 mg/day for the final 2–4 weeks.

[b] Patients who have successfully abstained from smoking should have their dose of Habitrol reduced after each 2–4 weeks of treatment until the 7 mg/day dose has been used for 2–4 weeks (see Individualization of Dosage).

[c] The entire course of nicotine substitution and gradual withdrawal should take 8–12 weeks, depending on the size of the initial dose. The use of Habitrol beyond 3 months has not been studied.

The Habitrol system should be applied promptly upon its removal from the protective pouch to prevent evaporative loss of nicotine from the system. Habitrol systems should be used only when the pouch is intact to assure that the product has not been tampered with.

Habitrol systems should be applied only once a day to a non-hairy, clean, and dry skin site on the trunk or upper, outer arm. After 24 hours, the used Habitrol system should be removed and a new system applied to an alternate skin site. Skin sites should not be reused for at least a week. Patients should be cautioned not to continue to use the same system for more than 24 hours.

Nicotine Delivery Rate *(in vivo)*	Nicotine in System	System Size	Package Size	NDC Number
21 mg/day	52.5 mg	30 cm^2	30 systems	0067-0810-21
14 mg/day	35.0 mg	20 cm^2	30 systems	0067-0820-14
7 mg/day	17.5 mg	10 cm^2	30 systems	0067-0830-07

Safety and Handling

Habitrol systems can be a dermal irritant and can cause contact sensitization. Although exposure of health care workers to nicotine from Habitrol systems should be minimal, care should be taken to avoid unnecessary contact with active systems. If active systems are handled, wash with water alone, since soap may increase nicotine absorption. Do not touch eyes. KEEP OUT OF THE REACH OF CHILDREN.

Disposal

When the used system is removed from the skin, it should be folded over and placed in the protective pouch which contained the new system. The used system should be immediately disposed of in such a way to prevent its access by children or pets. See patient information for further directions for handling and disposal.

HOW SUPPLIED

Habitrol systems are individually packaged in child-resistant pouches and should not be used if individual pouches are unsealed.

[See table above.]

How to Store

Do not store above 86°F (30°C) because Habitrol systems are sensitive to heat. A slight discoloration of the system is not significant.

Do not store unpouched. Once removed from the protective pouch, Habitrol systems should be applied promptly since nicotine is volatile and the system may lose strength.

The use of this product is covered by U.S. Patent No. 4,597,961.

CAUTION: Federal law prohibits dispensing without prescription.

(Rev. 2/96)

Ciba Self-Medication, Inc.
Dist. by:
Ciba Self-Medication, Inc.
Woodbridge, NJ 07095

HABITROL®

(nicotine transdermal system)
Patient Instructions

IMPORTANT

YOUR DOCTOR HAS PRESCRIBED THIS DRUG FOR YOUR USE ONLY. DO NOT LET ANYONE ELSE USE IT. KEEP THIS MEDICINE OUT OF THE REACH OF CHILDREN AND PETS. Nicotine can be very toxic and harmful. Small amounts of nicotine can cause serious illness in children. Even used Habitrol patches contain enough nicotine to poison children and pets. Be sure to throw Habitrol patches away out of the reach of children and pets. If a child puts on Habitrol patches or plays with a Habitrol patch that is out of the sealed pouch, take it away from the child and contact a poison control center, or contact a doctor immediately.

Women: Nicotine in any form may cause harm to your unborn baby if you use nicotine while you are pregnant. Do not use Habitrol patches if you are pregnant or nursing unless advised by your doctor. If you become pregnant while using Habitrol patches or if you think you might be pregnant, stop smoking and don't use Habitrol patches until you have talked to your doctor.

This leaflet will provide you with general information about nicotine and specific instructions about how to use Habitrol patches. It is important that you read it carefully and completely before you start using Habitrol patches. Be sure to read the PRECAUTIONS section before using Habitrol patches, because, as with all drugs, Habitrol treatment has side effects. Since this leaflet is only a summary of information, be sure to ask your doctor if you have any questions or want to know more.

INTRODUCTION

IT IS IMPORTANT THAT YOU ARE FIRMLY COMMITTED TO GIVING UP SMOKING.

Habitrol is a skin patch containing nicotine designed to help you quit smoking cigarettes. When you wear a Habitrol patch, it releases nicotine through the skin into your bloodstream while you're wearing it. The nicotine which is in your skin will still be entering your bloodstream for several hours after you take the patch off.

It is the nicotine in cigarettes that causes addiction to smoking. Habitrol therapy replaces some of the nicotine you crave when you are stopping smoking. Habitrol patches may also help relieve other symptoms of nicotine withdrawal that may occur when you stop smoking such as irritability, frustration, anger, anxiety, difficulty in concentration, and restlessness.

There are three doses of Habitrol. Your doctor has chosen the Habitrol patch with the correct dose for you and may adjust it during the first week or two. After about 6 weeks, your doctor will give you smaller Habitrol patches approximately every two weeks. The smaller patches give you less nicotine. In time, you will be completely off nicotine. You cannot adjust the nicotine dose by cutting a Habitrol patch.

INFORMATION ABOUT HABITROL PATCHES

How Habitrol Patches Work

Habitrol patches contain nicotine. When you put a Habitrol patch on your skin, nicotine passes from the patch through the skin and into your blood.

How to Apply a Habitrol Patch

Step 1. Choose a non-hairy, clean, dry area on your trunk or upper, outer part of your arm. Do not put a Habitrol patch on skin that is very oily, burned, broken out, cut, or irritated in any way.

Step 2. Do not remove the Habitrol patch from its sealed, child-resistant, protective pouch until you are ready to use it. Carefully cut open the child-resistant pouch. Discard the used patch you take off by folding it in half and putting it into the opened pouch. Throw it away in the trash out of the reach of children and pets (see Step 7).

Step 3. A shiny protective liner covers the sticky side of the Habitrol patch—the side that will be put on your skin. The liner has a precut slit to help you remove it from the patch. With the silver side facing you, pull the liner away from the Habitrol patch starting at the precut slit. Hold the Habitrol patch at the edge (touch the sticky side as little as possible) and pull off the other piece of the protective liner. Throw away this liner.

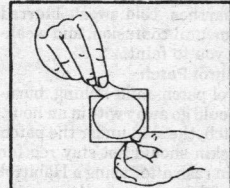

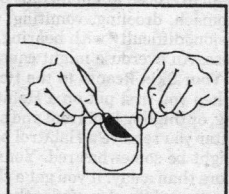

Step 4. Immediately apply the sticky side of the Habitrol patch to your skin. Press the Habitrol patch firmly on your skin with the palm of your hand for about 10 seconds. Make sure it sticks well to your skin, expecially around the edges.

Step 5. Wash your hands when you have finished applying the Habitrol patch. Nicotine on your hands could get into your eyes and nose and could cause stinging, redness, or more serious problems.

Step 6. After approximately 24 hours, remove the patch you have been wearing. Choose a *different* place on your skin to apply the next Habitrol patch and repeat Steps 1 to 5. Do not return to a previously used skin site for at least one week. Do not leave the Habitrol patch on for more than 24 hours because it may irritate your skin and because it loses strength after 24 hours.

Step 7. Fold the used Habitrol patch in half with the sticky side together. After you have put on a new Habitrol patch, take its pouch and place the used, folded Habitrol patch inside of it. Throw the pouch in the trash away from children and pets.

When to Apply a Habitrol Patch

If you apply the Habitrol patch at about the same time each day, it will help you to remember when to put on a new Habitrol patch. If you want to change the time when you put on your patch, you can do so. Just remove the Habitrol patch you are wearing and put on a new one. After that, apply the Habitrol patch at the new time each day.

If Your Habitrol Patch Gets Wet

Water will not harm the Habitrol patch you are wearing. You can bathe, swim, use a hot tub, or shower while you are wearing a Habitrol patch.

If Your Habitrol Patch Comes Off

If your Habitrol patch falls off, put on a new one. Remove the Habitrol patch at your regular time to keep your schedule the same, or 24 hours after applying the replacement patch if you wish to change the time each day that you apply a new patch. Before putting on a new patch, make sure you select a non-hairy area which is not irritated and is clean and dry.

Continued on next page

Ciba Self-Medication, Inc.—Cont.

Disposing of a Habitrol Patch
Fold the used Habitrol patch in half with the sticky side together. After you put on a new Habitrol patch, take its opened pouch or aluminum foil and place the used, folded Habitrol patch inside of it. THROW THE POUCH IN THE TRASH AWAY FROM CHILDREN AND PETS.

Storage Instructions
Keep the Habitrol patch in its protective pouch until you are ready to use it. Do not store your Habitrol patches above 86°F (30°C) because the patch is sensitive to heat. Remember, the inside of your car can reach temperatures much higher than this in the summer.

PRECAUTIONS
What to Ask Your Doctor
Ask your doctor about possible problems with Habitrol therapy. Be sure to tell your doctor if you have had any of the following:
- a recent heart attack (myocardial infarction)
- irregular heart beat (arrhythmia)
- severe or worsening heart pain (angina pectoris)
- allergies to drugs
- rashes from adhesive tape or bandages
- skin diseases
- very high blood pressure
- stomach ulcers
- overactive thyroid
- diabetes requiring insulin
- kidney or liver disease

If You Are Taking Medicines
Habitrol patch use, together with stopping smoking, may change the effect of other medicines. It is important to tell your doctor about all the medicines you are taking.

What to Watch For (Adverse Effects)
You should not smoke while using the Habitrol patch. It is possible to get too much nicotine (an overdose), especially if you use a Habitrol patch and smoke at the same time. Signs of an overdose would include bad headaches, dizziness, upset stomach, drooling, vomiting, diarrhea, cold sweat, blurred vision, difficulty with hearing, mental confusion, and weakness. An overdose might cause you to faint.

If Your Skin Reacts to the Habitrol Patch
When you first put on a Habitrol patch, mild itching, burning, or tingling is normal and should go away within an hour. After you remove a Habitrol patch, the skin under the patch might be somewhat red. Your skin should not stay red for more than a day. If you get a skin rash after using a Habitrol patch, or if the skin under the patch becomes swollen or very red, call your doctor. Do not put on a new patch. You may be allergic to one of the components of the Habitrol patch.
If you do become allergic to the nicotine in the Habitrol patch, you could get sick from using cigarettes or other nicotine-containing products.

What to Do When Problems Occur
IF YOU NOTICE ANY WORRISOME SYMPTOMS OR PROBLEMS, TAKE OFF THE HABITROL PATCH AND CALL YOUR DOCTOR AT ONCE.
CHILD-RESISTANT POUCH. DO NOT USE IF INDIVIDUAL POUCHES ARE UNSEALED.

(Rev. 2/96)

Dist. by:
Ciba Self-Medication, Inc.
Woodbridge, NJ 07095
Shown in Product Identification Guide, page 308

EXTRA STRENGTH
MAALOX® ANTACID/ANTI-GAS   OTC
Alumina, Magnesia and Simethicone Oral
Suspensions and Tablets, Antacid/Anti-Gas

Suspensions and Tablets
☐ Refreshing Lemon
  Smooth Cherry
  Cooling Mint
☐ Physician-proven Maalox® formula for antacid effectiveness.
☐ Simethicone, at a recognized clinical dose, for antiflatulent action.

DESCRIPTION
Extra Strength Maalox® Antacid/Anti-Gas, a balanced combination of magnesium and aluminum hydroxides plus simethicone, is a non-constipating antacid/anti-gas product to provide symptomatic relief of acid indigestion, heartburn, and gas and upset stomach associated with these symptoms. Available in suspensions in Refreshing Lemon, Smooth Cherry, and Cooling Mint flavors and in tablets in Cooling Mint and assorted (Refreshing Lemon/Smooth Cherry/Cooling Mint) flavors.

COMPOSITION
To provide symptomatic relief of hyperacidity plus alleviation of gas symptoms, each teaspoonful/tablet contains:

Active Ingredients	Extra Strength Maalox® Antacid/Anti-Gas	
	Per Tsp. (5 mL)	Per Tablet
Magnesium Hydroxide	450 mg	350 mg
Aluminum Hydroxide (equivalent to dried gel, USP)	500 mg	350 mg
Simethicone	40 mg	30 mg

INACTIVE INGREDIENTS
Suspensions: Calcium Saccharin, FD&C Red No. 40 (Smooth Cherry only), Flavors, Methylparaben, Propylparaben, Purified Water, Sorbitol and other ingredients.
Tablets: D&C Red No. 30, D&C Yellow No. 10, Dextrose, FD&C Blue No. 1, Flavors, Magnesium Stearate, Mannitol, Saccharin Sodium, Sorbitol, Starch, Sugar.

DIRECTIONS FOR USE
Suspensions; 2 to 4 teaspoonfuls, 4 times per day, or as directed by a physician. Tablets; chew 1 to 3 tablets, 4 times per day, or as directed by a physician.

PATIENT WARNINGS
Do not take more than 12 teaspoonfuls or 12 tablets in a 24-hour period or use the maximum dosage for more than 2 weeks or use if you have kidney disease except under the advice and supervision of a physician. Keep this and all drugs out of the reach of children.

DRUG INTERACTION PRECAUTION
Antacids may interact with certain prescription drugs. If you are presently taking a prescription drug, do not take this product without checking with your physician or other health professional.
To aid in establishing proper dosage schedules, the following information is provided:

	Minimum Recommended Dosage: Extra Strength Maalox® Antacid/Anti-Gas	
	Per 2 Tsp. (10 mL)	Per Tablet
Acid neutralizing capacity	52.2 mEq	NLT 16.7 mEq
Sodium content*	< 2 mg	< 1.4 mg

*Dietetically insignificant.

Professional Labeling
INDICATIONS
As an antacid for symptomatic relief of hyperacidity associated with the diagnosis of peptic ulcer, gastritis, peptic esophagitis, gastric hyperacidity, heartburn, or hiatal hernia. As an antiflatulent to alleviate the symptoms of gas, including postoperative gas pain.

ADVANTAGES
Among antacids, Extra Strength Maalox® Antacid/Anti-Gas Suspension and Extra Strength Maalox® Antacid/Anti-Gas Tablets are uniquely palatable—an important feature which encourages patients to follow your dosage directions. Extra Strength Maalox® Antacid/Anti-Gas Suspension and Extra Strength Maalox® Antacid/Anti-Gas Tablets have the time-proven, nonconstipating, sodium-free* Maalox® formula—useful for those patients suffering from the problems associated with hyperacidity. Additionally, Extra Strength Maalox® Antacid/Anti-Gas Suspension and Extra Strength Maalox® Antacid/Anti-Gas Tablets contain simethicone to alleviate discomfort associated with entrapped gas.
*Dietetically insignificant.

WARNINGS
Prolonged use of aluminum-containing antacids in patients with renal failure may result in or worsen dialysis osteomalacia. Elevated tissue aluminum levels contribute to the development of the dialysis encephalopathy and osteomalacia syndromes. Small amounts of aluminum are absorbed from the gastrointestinal tract and renal excretion of aluminum is impaired in renal failure. Aluminum is not well removed by dialysis because it is bound to albumin and transferrin, which do not cross dialysis membranes. As a result, aluminum is deposited in bone, and dialysis osteomalacia may develop when large amounts of aluminum are ingested orally by patients with impaired renal function. Aluminum forms insoluble complexes with phosphate in the gastrointestinal tract, thus decreasing phosphate absorption. Prolonged use of aluminum-containing antacids by normophosphatemic patients may result in hypophosphatemia if phosphate intake is not adequate. In its more severe forms, hypophosphatemia can lead to anorexia, malaise, muscle weakness, and osteomalacia.

HOW SUPPLIED
Extra Strength Maalox® Antacid/Anti-Gas Suspensions Available in Refreshing Lemon in the following sizes: 5 fl. oz. (148 mL) (0067-0333-62), 12 fl. oz. (355 mL) (0067-0333-71) and 26 fl. oz. (769 mL) (0067-0333-44).
Smooth Cherry is available in plastic bottles of 12 fl. oz. (355 mL) (0067-0336-71) and 26 fl. oz. (769 mL) (0067-0336-44).
Cooling Mint is available in plastic bottles of 12 fl. oz. (355 mL) (0067-0338-71) and 26 fl. oz. (769 mL) (0067-0338-44).
Extra Strength Maalox® Antacid/Anti-Gas Cooling Mint Tablets are available in bottles of 38 tablets (0067-0345-38) and 75 tablets (0067-0345-75).
Extra Strength Maalox® Antacid/Anti-Gas assorted flavors tablets are available in bottles of 38 tablets (0067-7214-38) and 75 tablets (0067-7214-75).

MAALOX®   OTC
Magnesia and Alumina
Oral Suspension
Antacid

Liquids
Mint Flavored
Cherry Creme

DESCRIPTION
Maalox® Antacid is used for the relief of acid indigestion, heartburn, sour stomach and upset stomach associated with these symptoms.

Active Ingredients	Maalox Suspension 5 mL teaspoon
Magnesium Hydroxide	200 mg
Aluminum Hydroxide (equivalent to dried gel, USP)	225 mg

INACTIVE INGREDIENTS
Calcium saccharin, flavors, methylparaben, propylparaben, sorbitol, purified water and other ingredients.

	Minimum Recommended Dosage: Maalox Suspension
	Per 2 Tsp. (10 mL)
Acid neutralizing capacity	NLT 26.6 mEq
Sodium content	NMT 3 mg

DIRECTIONS FOR USE
Two to four teaspoonfuls, four times a day or as directed by a physician.

PATIENT WARNINGS
Do not take more than 16 teaspoonfuls in a 24-hour period or use the maximum dosage for more than 2 weeks or use if you have kidney disease except under the advice and supervision of a physician. Keep this and all drugs out of the reach of children.

DRUG INTERACTION PRECAUTION
Antacids may interact with certain prescription drugs. If you are presently taking a prescription drug, do not take this product without checking with your physician or other health professional.

Professional Labeling
INDICATIONS
As an antacid for symptomatic relief of hyperacidity associated with the diagnosis of peptic ulcer, gastritis, peptic

esophagitis, gastric hyperacidity, heartburn, or hiatal hernia.

WARNINGS

Prolonged use of aluminum-containing antacids in patients with renal failure may result in or worsen dialysis osteomalacia. Elevated tissue aluminum levels contribute to the development of the dialysis encephalopathy and osteomalacia syndromes. Small amounts of aluminum are absorbed from the gastrointestinal tract and renal excretion of aluminum is impaired in renal failure. Aluminum is not well removed by dialysis because it is bound to albumin and transferrin, which do not cross dialysis membranes. As a result, aluminum is deposited in bone, and dialysis osteomalacia may develop when large amounts of aluminum are ingested orally by patients with impaired renal function.

Aluminum forms insoluble complexes with phosphate in the gastrointestinal tract, thus decreasing phosphate absorption. Prolonged use of aluminum-containing antacids by normophosphatemic patients may result in hypophosphatemia if phosphate intake is not adequate. In its more severe forms, hypophosphatemia can lead to anorexia, malaise, muscle weakness, and osteomalacia.

HOW SUPPLIED

Maalox® Mint Flavored Suspension is available in plastic bottles of 12 oz (0067-0330-71) and 26 oz (0067-0330-44).
Maalox® Cherry Creme Flavored Suspension is available in plastic bottles of 12 oz (0067-0331-71) and 26 oz (0067-0331-44).

MAALOX® ANTACID/ANTI-GAS   OTC
Alumina, Magnesia and Simethicone Tablets
Antacid/Anti-Gas

Tablets
Lemon, Cherry, and Mint Flavors

☐ **Physician-proven Maalox® formula for antacid effectiveness.**
☐ **Simethicone, at a recognized clinical dose, for antiflatulent action.**

DESCRIPTION

Maalox® Antacid/Anti-Gas, a balanced combination of magnesium and aluminum hydroxides plus simethicone, is a non-constipating antacid/anti-gas product which comes in pleasant tasting flavors.

COMPOSITION

To provide symptomatic relief of hyperacidity plus alleviation of gas symptoms, each tablet contains:

Active Ingredients	Maalox® Antacid/Anti-Gas Per Tablet
Magnesium Hydroxide	200 mg
Aluminum Hydroxide (equivalent to dried gel, USP)	200 mg
Simethicone	25 mg

INACTIVE INGREDIENTS

Maalox® Antacid/Anti-Gas Tablets: Confectioners' sugar, D&C Red No. 30, D&C Yellow No. 10, FD&C Blue No. 1, dextrose, flavors, glycerin, magnesium stearate, mannitol, saccharin sodium, sorbitol, starch, talc. May also contain citric acid.

To aid in establishing proper dosage schedules, the following information is provided:

Minimum Recommended Dosage:	Per Tablet
Acid neutralizing capacity	NLT 10.65 mEq
Sodium content*	NMT 1 mg
Sugar content	0.54 g
Lactose content	None

*Dietetically insignificant.

DIRECTIONS FOR USE

Chew 1 to 4 tablets 4 times a day or as directed by a physician.

PATIENT WARNINGS

Do not take more than 16 tablets in a 24-hour period or use the maximum dosage for more than 2 weeks or use if you have kidney disease except under the advice and supervision of a physician. Keep this and all drugs out of the reach of children.

DRUG INTERACTION PRECAUTION

Antacids may interact with certain prescription drugs. If you are presently taking a prescription drug, do not take this product without checking with your physician or other health professional.

Professional Labeling

INDICATIONS

As an antacid for symptomatic relief of hyperacidity associated with the diagnosis of peptic ulcer, gastritis, peptic esophagitis, gastric hyperacidity, heartburn, or hiatal hernia. As an antiflatulent to alleviate the symptoms of gas, including postoperative gas pain.

WARNINGS

Prolonged use of aluminum-containing antacids in patients with renal failure may result in or worsen dialysis osteomalacia. Elevated tissue aluminum levels contribute to the development of the dialysis encephalopathy and osteomalacia syndromes. Small amounts of aluminum are absorbed from the gastrointestinal tract and renal excretion of aluminum is impaired in renal failure. Aluminum is not well removed by dialysis because it is bound to albumin and transferrin, which do not cross dialysis membranes. As a result, aluminum is deposited in bone, and dialysis osteomalacia may develop when large amounts of aluminum are ingested orally by patients with impaired renal function.

Aluminum forms insoluble complexes with phosphate in the gastrointestinal tract, thus decreasing phosphate absorption. Prolonged use of aluminum-containing antacids by normophosphatemic patients may result in hypophosphatemia if phosphate intake is not adequate. In its more severe forms, hypophosphatemia can lead to anorexia, malaise, muscle weakness, and osteomalacia.

ADVANTAGES

Maalox® Antacid/Anti-Gas Tablets are uniquely palatable—an important feature which encourages patients to follow your dosage directions. Maalox® Antacid/Anti-Gas Tablets have the time-proven, nonconstipating, sodium-free* Maalox® formula—useful for those patients suffering from the problems associated with hyperacidity. Additionally, Maalox® Antacid/Anti-Gas Tablets contain simethicone to alleviate discomfort associated with entrapped gas.
*Dietetically insignificant.

HOW SUPPLIED

Maalox® Antacid/Anti-Gas Lemon Tablets are available in plastic bottles of 50 tablets (0067-0339-50) and 100 tablets (0067-0339-67), convenience packs of 12 tablets (0067-0339-19), tray of 12 rolls (0067-0339-23), and 3 roll packs of 36 tablets (0067-0339-33).

Maalox® Antacid/Anti-Gas Cherry Tablets are available in plastic bottles of 50 tablets (0067-0341-50) and 100 tablets (0067-0341-68).

Maalox® Antacid/Anti-Gas Tablets are also available in **assorted flavor** bottles of 50 tablets (0067-7346-50) and 100 tablets (0067-7346-68), tray of 12 rolls (0067-7346-23) and 3 roll packs of 36 tablets (0067-7346-33).

PERDIEM®   OTC
[pĕr'dē'ŭm]
Bulk Fiber Laxative Plus Natural, Vegetable Stimulant

ACTIONS

Perdiem®, with its 100% natural, gentle action provides comfortable, overnight relief from occasional constipation. Perdiem is a unique combination of natural bulk-forming fiber and natural stimulant. The vegetable mucilages of Perdiem soften the stool and provide overnight evacuation of the bowel with no chemical stimulants. Perdiem, which takes effect usually within 12 hrs., is also effective as an aid to elimination for the hemorrhoid or fissure patient prior to and following surgery.

ACTIVE INGREDIENTS

82% psyllium (Plantago hydrocolloid) and 18% senna (Cassia Pod concentrate). Each 6 gm rounded teaspoon contains 3.25 gm psyllium, 0.74 gm senna, and 1.8 mg sodium.

DIRECTIONS FOR USE

Perdiem requires no mixing in liquids for use.
Adults and Children 12 Years and Older: In the evening and/or before breakfast, 1 to 2 rounded teaspoonfuls placed in the mouth and swallowed with at least 8 oz. of cool liquid. Up to 2 tsp. every 6 hrs. not to exceed 5 tsp. per day may be taken for severe constipation.
Children 7–11 Years: One rounded teaspoonful one to two times daily with at least 8 oz. of cool liquid.

Perdiem is not intended for use in children under the age of 7 years. Perdiem should not be chewed. Taking this product without enough fluid may cause choking (see Warnings). This product should be used beyond 7 days only under professional medical supervision.

PRECAUTIONS

Pregnancy category B. Animal reproduction studies have been conducted and have not demonstrated a risk to the fetus. However, because there are no adequate and well-controlled studies in pregnant women, this product should be used during pregnancy only if clearly needed.

WARNINGS

Taking this product without adequate fluid may cause it to swell and block the throat or esophagus and may cause choking. This product should not be used if the patient has difficulty in swallowing. If the patient experiences chest pain, vomiting, or difficulty in swallowing or breathing after taking this product, use should be stopped and medical care provided.
Do not use if the patient has a history of psyllium allergy. Laxative products should not be used when abdominal pain, nausea or vomiting are present unless directed by a doctor.

HOW SUPPLIED

400 gm (14 oz.) canisters (NDC 0067-0690-39)
250 gm. (8.8 oz.) canisters (NDC 0067-0690-70)
6×6 gm. Individual packets (NDC 0067-0690-16)
24 gm sample

PERDIEM® FIBER   OTC
[pĕr'dē'ŭm]
Bulk Fiber Laxative

ACTIONS

Perdiem® Fiber is a 100% natural bulk-forming fiber laxative that gently helps restore regularity and treat occasional constipation. Its unique form is easy to swallow and requires no mixing with liquid. Perdiem Fiber's vegetable mucilage softens the stool and contains no chemical stimulants. Perdiem Fiber takes effect usually within 12 hrs. to 72 hrs.

ACTIVE INGREDIENTS

100% psyllium (Plantago hydrocolloid). Each 6 gm rounded teaspoon contains 4.03 gm psyllium and 1.8 mg sodium.

DIRECTIONS FOR USE

Perdiem requires no mixing in liquids for use.
Adults and Children 12 Years and Older: In the evening and/or before breakfast, 1 to 2 rounded teaspoonfuls placed in the mouth and swallowed with at least 8 oz. of cool liquid. Up to 2 tsp. every 6 hrs. not to exceed 5 tsp. per day may be taken for severe constipation.
Children 7–11 Years: One rounded teaspoonful one to two times daily with at least 8 oz. of cool liquid.
Perdiem is not intended for use in children under the age of 7 years. Perdiem should not be chewed. Taking this product without enough liquid may cause choking (see Warnings). This product should be used beyond 7 days only under professional medical supervision.

PRECAUTIONS

Pregnancy category B. Results from limited animal reproduction studies have not demonstrated a risk to the fetus. However, because there are no adequate and well-controlled studies in pregnant women, this product should be used during pregnancy only if clearly needed.

WARNINGS

Taking this product without adequate fluid may cause it to swell and block the throat or esophagus and may cause choking. This product should not be used if the patient has difficulty in swallowing. If the patient experiences chest pain, vomiting, or difficulty in swallowing or breathing after taking this product, use should be stopped and medical care provided.
Do not use if the patient has a history of psyllium allergy. Laxative products should not be used when abdominal pain, nausea or vomiting are present unless directed by a doctor.

HOW SUPPLIED

250 gm. (8.8 oz.) canisters (NDC 0067-0795-70)
24 gm Sample

SLOW FE®   OTC
Slow Release Iron Tablets

DESCRIPTION

SLOW FE supplies ferrous sulfate, for the treatment of iron deficiency and iron deficiency anemia with a significant reduction in the incidence of the common side effects associated with taking oral iron preparations. The wax matrix

Continued on next page

Ciba Self-Medication, Inc.—Cont.

delivery system of SLOW FE is designed to maximize the release of ferrous sulfate in the duodenum and the jejunum where it is best tolerated and absorbed. SLOW FE has been clinically shown to be associated with a lower incidence of constipation, diarrhea and abdominal discomfort when compared to an immediate release iron tablet[1] and a leading sustained release iron capsule.[2]

FORMULA
Each tablet contains: Active Ingredient: 160 mg dried ferrous sulfate USP, equivalent to 50 mg elemental iron. Inactive Ingredients: cetostearyl alcohol, hydroxypropyl methylcellulose, lactose, magnesium stearate, polysorbate 80, talc, titanium dioxide, yellow iron oxide, FD&C blue #2 aluminum lake.

DOSAGE
ADULTS—one or two tablets daily or as recommended by a physician. A maximum of four tablets daily may be taken. CHILDREN—one tablet daily. Tablets must be swallowed whole.

WARNING
The treatment of any anemic condition should be under the advice and supervision of a physician. As oral iron products interfere with absorption of oral tetracycline antibiotics, these products should not be taken within two hours of each other. As with any drug, if you are pregnant or nursing a baby, seek the advice of a health professional before using this product.
Keep this and all drugs out of the reach of children. Close bottles tightly. Contains iron, which can be harmful or fatal to children in large doses. In case of accidental overdose, seek professional assistance or contact a poison control center immediately.
Tamper-Evident Packaging.

HOW SUPPLIED
Blister Packages of 30 and 60, and bottles of 100 supplied in Child-Resistant packaging.
Do not store above 30°C (86°F). Protect from moisture.

REFERENCES
1. Brock C et al. Adverse effects of iron supplementation: A comparative trial of a wax-matrix iron preparation and conventional ferrous sulfate tablets. *Clin Ther.* 1985; 7:I-VI.
2. Brock C, Curry H. Comparative incidence of side effects of a wax-matrix and a sustained-release iron preparation. *Clin Ther.* 1985;7:492-496.
Shown in Product Identification Guide, page 308

SLOW FE® WITH FOLIC ACID   OTC
(Slow Release Iron – Folic Acid)

DESCRIPTION
Slow Fe + Folic Acid delivers 50 mg. elemental iron (160 mg. dried ferrous sulfate) using the unique wax matrix delivery system described above (for SLOW FE® Slow Release Iron Tablets) plus 400 mcg. folic acid.
Provides women of childbearing potential with the daily target level of folic acid to reduce the risk of neural tube birth defects. These birth defects are rare, but serious, and occur within 28 days of conception, often before a woman knows she's pregnant.

FORMULA
Each tablet contains: Active Ingredients: 160 mg. dried ferrous sulfate, USP (equivalent to 50 mg. elemental iron) and 400 mcg. folic acid. Inactive Ingredients: cetostearyl alcohol, hydroxypropyl methylcellulose, lactose, magnesium stearate, polysorbate 80, talc, titanium dioxide, yellow iron oxide.

DOSAGE
ADULTS—One or two tablets once a day or as recommended by a physician. A maximum of two tablets daily may be taken. CHILDREN UNDER 12—Consult a physician. Tablets must be swallowed whole.

WARNING
The treatment of any anemic condition should be under the advice and supervision of a physician. As oral iron products interfere with absorption of oral tetracycline antibiotics, these products should not be taken within two hours of each other. Intake of folic acid from all sources should be limited to 1000 mcg. per day to prevent the masking of Vitamin B_{12} deficiencies. Should you become pregnant while using this product, consult a physician as soon as possible about good prenatal care and the continued use of this product. If you are already pregnant or nursing a baby, seek the advice of a health care professional before using this product. KEEP THIS PRODUCT AND ALL MEDICATIONS OUT OF THE REACH OF CHILDREN:

Contains iron, which can be harmful or fatal to children in large doses. In case of accidental overdose, contact a physician or a poison control center immediately.

HOW SUPPLIED
Blister packages of 20 supplied in Child-Resistant packaging. Do not store above 30°C (86°F). Protect from moisture.

CHILD-RESISTANT
Blister packaged for your protection. Do not use if individual seals are broken.

Distributed by: Ciba Self-Medication, Inc.
Woodbridge, NJ 07095
Tablets made in Great Britain
© 1994 Ciba Self-Medication, Inc.
Shown in Product Identification Guide, page 308

TRANSDERM SCŌP®   Rx
[*trans-derm scōpe*]
scopolamine

Transdermal Therapeutic System

Programmed delivery in vivo of 0.5 mg of scopolamine over 3 days

Prescribing Information

DESCRIPTION
The Transderm Scōp patch is a circular flat disc designed for continuous release of scopolamine following application to an area of intact skin on the head, behind the ear. Clinical evaluation has demonstrated that the patch provides effective antiemetic and antinauseant actions when tested against motion-sickness stimuli in adults. The Transderm Scōp patch is a film 0.2 mm thick and 2.5 cm², with four layers. Proceeding from the visible surface towards the surface attached to the skin, these layers are: (1) a backing layer of tan-colored, aluminized, polyester film; (2) a drug reservoir of scopolamine, mineral oil, and polyisobutylene; (3) a microporous polypropylene membrane that controls the rate of delivery of scopolamine from the patch to the skin surface; and (4) an adhesive formulation of mineral oil, polyisobutylene, and scopolamine. A protective peel strip of siliconized polyester, which covers the adhesive layer, is removed before the patch is used. The inactive components, mineral oil (12.4 mg) and polyisobutylene (11.4 mg), are not released from the system.

Cross section of the patch:

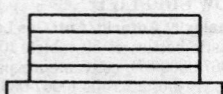

Backing Layer
Drug Reservoir
Rate-Controlling Membrane
Contact Adhesive
Protective Peel Strip

Release-Rate Concept: The Transderm Scōp patch contains 1.5 mg of scopolamine. The patch is programmed to deliver 0.5 mg of scopolamine at an approximately constant rate to the systemic circulation over the 3-day lifetime of the patch. An initial priming dose of scopolamine, released from the adhesive layer of the patch, saturates the skin binding sites and rapidly brings the plasma concentration of scopolamine to the required steady-state level. A continuous controlled release of scopolamine, which flows from the drug reservoir through the rate-controlling membrane, maintains the plasma level constant.

CLINICAL PHARMACOLOGY
The sole active agent of Transderm Scōp is scopolamine, a belladonna alkaloid with well-known pharmacological properties. The drug has a long history of oral and parenteral use for central anticholinergic activity, including prophylaxis of motion sickness. The mechanism of action of scopolamine in the central nervous system (CNS) is not definitely known but may include anticholinergic effects. The ability of scopolamine to prevent motion-induced nausea is believed to be associated with inhibition of vestibular input to the CNS, which results in inhibition of the vomiting reflex. In addition, scopolamine may have a direct action on the vomiting center within the reticular formation of the brain stem. Applied to the postauricular skin, Transderm Scōp provides for a gradual release of scopolamine from an adhesive matrix of mineral oil and polyisobutylene.

INDICATIONS AND USAGE
Transderm Scōp is indicated for prevention of nausea and vomiting associated with motion sickness in adults. The patch should be applied only to skin in the postauricular area.
Clinical Results: Transderm Scōp provides antiemetic protection within several hours following application of the patch behind the ear. In 195 adult subjects of different racial origins who participated in clinical efficacy studies at sea or in a controlled motion environment, there was a 75% reduc-

tion in the incidence of motion-induced nausea and vomiting. Transderm Scōp provided significantly greater protection than that obtained with oral dimenhydrinate.

CONTRAINDICATIONS
Transderm Scōp should not be used in patients with known hypersensitivity to scopolamine or any of the components of the adhesive matrix making up the therapeutic system, or in patients with glaucoma.

WARNINGS
Transderm Scōp should not be used in children and should be used with special caution in the elderly. See **PRECAUTIONS.**
Since drowsiness, disorientation, and confusion may occur with the use of scopolamine, patients should be warned of the possibility and cautioned against engaging in activities that require mental alertness, such as driving a motor vehicle or operating dangerous machinery.
Potentially alarming idiosyncratic reactions may occur with ordinary therapeutic doses of scopolamine.

PRECAUTIONS
General
Scopolamine should be used with caution in patients with pyloric obstruction, or urinary bladder neck obstruction. Caution should be exercised when administering an antiemetic or antimuscarinic drug to patients suspected of having intestinal obstruction.
Transderm Scōp should be used with special caution in the elderly or in individuals with impaired metabolic, liver, or kidney functions, because of the increased likelihood of CNS effects.
Information for Patients
Since scopolamine can cause temporary dilation of the pupils and blurred vision if it comes in contact with the eyes, patients should be strongly advised to wash their hands thoroughly with soap and water immediately after handling the patch.
Patients should be advised to remove the patch immediately and contact a physician in the unlikely event that they experience symptoms of acute narrow-angle glaucoma (pain in and reddening of the eyes accompanied by dilated pupils). Patients should be warned against driving a motor vehicle or operating dangerous machinery. A patient brochure is available.
Drug Interactions
Scopolamine should be used with care in patients taking drugs, including alcohol, capable of causing CNS effects. Special attention should be given to drugs having anticholinergic properties, e.g., belladonna alkaloids, antihistamines (including meclizine), and antidepressants.
Carcinogenesis, Mutagenesis, Impairment of Fertility
No long-term studies in animals have been performed to evaluate carcinogenic potential. Fertility studies were performed in female rats and revealed no evidence of impaired fertility or harm to the fetus due to scopolamine hydrobromide administered by daily subcutaneous injection. In the highest-dose group (plasma level approximately 500 times the level achieved in humans using a transdermal system), reduced maternal body weights were observed.
Pregnancy Category C
Teratogenic studies were performed in pregnant rats and rabbits with scopolamine hydrobromide administered by daily intravenous injection. No adverse effects were recorded in the rats. In the rabbits, the highest dose (plasma level approximately 100 times the level achieved in humans using a transdermal system) of drug administered had a marginal embryotoxic effect. Transderm Scōp should be used during pregnancy only if the anticipated benefit justifies the potential risk to the fetus.
Nursing Mothers
It is not known whether scopolamine is excreted in human milk. Because many drugs are excreted in human milk, caution should be exercised when Transderm Scōp is administered to a nursing woman.
Pediatric Use
Children are particularly susceptible to the side effects of belladonna alkaloids. Transderm Scōp should not be used in children because it is not known whether the patch will release an amount of scopolamine that could produce serious adverse effects in children.

ADVERSE REACTIONS
The most frequent adverse reaction to Transderm Scōp is dryness of the mouth. This occurs in about two thirds of patients on drug. A less frequent adverse reaction is drowsiness, which occurs in less than one sixth of patients on drug. Transient impairment of eye accommodation, including blurred vision and dilation of the pupils, is also observed. The following adverse reactions have also been reported on infrequent occasions during the use of Transderm Scōp: disorientation; memory disturbances; dizziness; restlessness; hallucinations; confusion; difficulty urinating; rashes and erythema; acute narrow-angle glaucoma; and dry, itchy, or red eyes.

Drug Withdrawal: Symptoms including dizziness, nausea, vomiting, headache and disturbances of equilibrium have been reported in a few patients following discontinuation of the use of the Transderm Scōp patch. These symptoms have occurred most often in patients who have used the patches for more than three days.

OVERDOSAGE

Overdosage with scopolamine may cause disorientation, memory disturbances, dizziness, restlessness, hallucinations, or confusion. Should these symptoms occur, the Transderm Scōp patch should be immediately removed. Appropriate parasympathomimetic therapy should be initiated if these symptoms are severe.

DOSAGE AND ADMINISTRATION

Initiation of Therapy: One Transderm Scōp patch (programmed to deliver 0.5 mg of scopolamine over 3 days) should be applied to the hairless area behind one ear at least 4 hours before the antiemetic effect is required. Only one patch should be worn at any time.

Handling: After the patch is applied on dry skin behind the ear, the hands should be washed thoroughly with soap and water and dried. Upon removal of the patch, it should be discarded, and the hands and application site washed thoroughly with soap and water and dried, to prevent any traces of scopolamine from coming into direct contact with the eyes. (A patient brochure is available.)

Continuation of Therapy: Should the patch become displaced, it should be discarded, and a fresh one placed on the hairless area behind the other ear. If therapy is required for longer than 3 days, the first patch should be discarded, and a fresh one placed on the hairless area behind the other ear.

Disposal: The patch will still contain some active ingredient after use. To avoid accidental contact or ingestion by children or pets, fold the used patch in half with the sticky side together and dispose in the trash out of the reach of children and pets.

HOW SUPPLIED

The Transderm Scōp patch is a tan-colored disc, 2.5 cm², on a clear, oversized, hexagonal peel strip, which is removed prior to use.

Each Transderm Scōp patch contains 1.5 mg of scopolamine and is programmed to deliver *in vivo* 0.5 mg of scopolamine over 3 days. Transderm Scōp is available in packages of four patches. Each patch is foil wrapped. Patient instructions are included.

1 Package (4 patches) .... NDC 0083-4345-04
The patch should be stored between 59° - 86°F (15° - 30°C).
CAUTION
Federal law prohibits dispensing without prescription.

C88-5 (Rev. 2/88)

Please read this instruction sheet carefully before opening the patch package.

Information for the Patient About—

TRANSDERM SCŌP®
Generic Name: scopolamine,
pronounced skoe-POL-a-meen

Transdermal Therapeutic System

The Transderm Scōp patch helps to prevent the nausea and vomiting of motion sickness for up to 3 days. It is an adhesive patch that you place behind your ear several hours before you travel. Wear only one patch at any time.

Be sure to wash your hands thoroughly with soap and water immediately after handling the patch, so that any drug that might get on your hands will not come into contact with your eyes.

Avoid drinking alcohol while using Transderm Scōp. Also, be careful about driving or operating any machinery while using the patch because the drug might make you drowsy.

DO NOT USE TRANSDERM SCŌP IF YOU ARE ALLERGIC TO SCOPOLAMINE OR HAVE GLAUCOMA. TRANSDERM SCŌP SHOULD NOT BE USED IN CHILDREN AND SHOULD BE USED WITH SPECIAL CAUTION IN THE ELDERLY.

How the Transderm Scōp Patch Works
A group of nerve fibers deep inside the ear helps people keep their balance. For some people, the motion of ships, airplanes, trains, automobiles, and buses increases the activity of these nerve fibers. This increased activity causes the *dizziness, nausea, and vomiting* of motion sickness. People may have one, some, or all of these symptoms.

Transderm Scōp contains the drug scopolamine, which helps reduce the activity of the nerve fibers in the inner ear. When a Transderm Scōp patch is placed on the skin behind one of the ears, scopolamine passes through the skin and into the bloodstream. One patch may be kept in place for 3 days if needed.

Precautions
Before using Transderm Scōp be sure to tell your doctor if you—

- Are pregnant or nursing (or planning to become pregnant)
- Have (or have had) glaucoma (increased pressure in the eyeball)
- Have (or have had) any metabolic, liver, or kidney disease
- Have any obstructions of the stomach or intestine
- Have trouble urinating or any bladder obstruction
- Have any skin allergy or have had a skin reaction such as a rash or redness to any drug, especially scopolamine, or chemical or food substance.

Any of these conditions could make Transderm Scōp unsuitable for you. Also tell your doctor if you are taking any other medicines.

In the unlikely event that you experience pain in the eye and reddened whites of the eye, which may be accompanied by widening of the pupil and blurred vision, remove the patch immediately and consult your physician. As indicated below under Side Effects, widening of the pupils and blurred vision without pain or reddened whites of the eye is usually temporary and not serious.

Transderm Scōp should not be used in children. The safety of its use in children has not been determined. Children and the elderly may be particularly sensitive to the effects of scopolamine.

Side Effects
The most common side effect experienced by people using Transderm Scōp is dryness of the mouth. This occurs in about two thirds of patch users. A less frequent side effect is drowsiness, which occurs in less than one sixth of patch users. Temporary blurring of vision and dilation (widening) of the pupils may occur, especially if the drug is on your hands and comes in contact with the eyes. On infrequent occasions, disorientation, memory disturbances, dizziness, restlessness, hallucinations, confusion, difficulty urinating, skin rashes or redness, dry, itchy, or red eyes and eye pain have been reported. If these effects do occur, remove the patch and call your doctor. Since drowsiness, disorientation, and confusion may occur with the use of scopolamine, be careful driving or operating any dangerous machinery, especially when you first start using the patch.

Drug Withdrawal: Symptoms including dizziness, nausea, vomiting, headache and disturbances of equilibrium have been reported in a few people following discontinuation of the Transderm Scōp patch. These symptoms have occurred most often in people who have used patches for more than three days. We recommend that you consult your doctor if these symptoms occur.

How to Use Transderm Scōp
Transderm Scōp should be stored between 59° - 86°F (15° - 30°C) until you are ready to use it.
1. Plan to apply one Transderm Scōp patch at least 4 hours before you need it. **Wear only one patch at a time.**
2. Select a hairless area of skin behind one ear, taking care to avoid any cuts or irritations. Wipe the area with a clean, dry tissue.
3. Peel the package open and remove the patch (Figure 1).

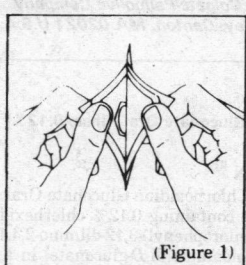

(Figure 1)

4. Remove the clear plastic six-sided backing from the patch. Try not to touch the adhesive surface on the patch with your hands (Figure 2).

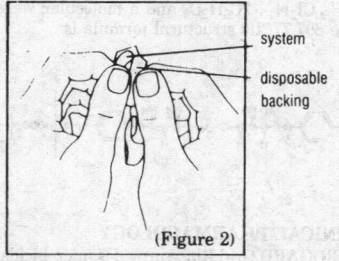

system

disposable backing

(Figure 2)

5. Firmly apply the adhesive surface (metallic side) to the dry area of skin behind the ear so that the tan-colored side is showing (Figure 3). Make good contact, especially around the edge. Once you have placed the patch behind your ear, do not move it for as long as you want to use it (up to 3 days).
[See Figure at top of next column.]

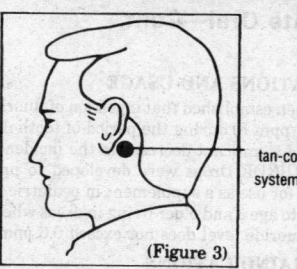

tan-colored system

(Figure 3)

6. *Important:* After the patch is in place, be sure to wash your hands thoroughly with soap and water to remove any scopolamine. If this drug were to contact your eyes, it could cause temporary blurring of vision and dilation (widening) of the pupils (the dark circles in the center of your eyes). This is not serious unless accompanied by eye pain and redness (see Precautions), and your pupils should return to normal.
7. Remove the patch after 3 days and throw it away. (You may remove it sooner if you are no longer concerned about motion sickness.) After removing the patch, be sure to wash your hands and the area behind your ear thoroughly with soap and water.
8. If you wish to control nausea for longer than 3 days, *remove* the first patch after 3 days and place a new one *behind the other ear*, repeating instructions 2 to 7.
9. Keep the patch dry, if possible, to prevent it from falling off. Limited contact with water, however, as in bathing or swimming, will not affect the system. In the unlikely event that the patch falls off, throw it away and put a new one behind the other ear.

Disposal
The patch will still contain some active ingredient after use. To avoid accidental contact or ingestion by children or pets, fold the used patch in half with the sticky side together and dispose in the trash out of the reach of children and pets.

This leaflet presents a summary of information about Transderm Scōp. If you would like more information or if you have any questions, ask your doctor or pharmacist. A more technical leaflet is available, written for your doctor. If you would like to read the leaflet, ask your pharmacist to show you a copy. You may need the help of your doctor or pharmacist to understand some of the information.

Dist. by:
Ciba Self-Medication, Inc.
Woodbridge, NJ 07095

C88-6 (Rev. 2/88)

Shown in Product Identification Guide, page 308

Colgate Oral Pharmaceuticals, Inc.
a subsidiary of Colgate-Palmolive Company
ONE COLGATE WAY
CANTON, MA 02021 U.S.A.

Direct Inquiries to:
Professional Services Department
(800) 226-5428

For Medical Information Contact:
In Emergencies:
Pittsburgh Poison Control
(412) 692-5596

LURIDE® DROPS
Brand of Sodium Fluoride

℞

DESCRIPTION

LURIDE® brand of sodium fluoride is available as liquid drops. Each ml contains 0.5 mg fluoride ion (F-) from 1.1 mg sodium fluoride (NaF). For use as a dental caries preventive in pediatric patients. Sugar-free. Saccharin-free.
ACTIVE INGREDIENT: Sodium fluoride 0.11% (w/v).
INACTIVE INGREDIENTS: Purified water, sorbitol solution 70%, propylene glycol, methyl paraben, propyl paraben, flavor, FD&C Yellow No. 6.

CLINICAL PHARMACOLOGY

Sodium fluoride acts systemically (before tooth eruption) and topically (post-eruption) by increasing tooth resistance to acid dissolution, by promoting remineralization and by inhibiting the cariogenic microbial process.

Continued on next page

Colgate Oral—Cont.

INDICATIONS AND USAGE
It has been established that ingestion of fluoridated drinking water (1 ppm F) during the period of tooth development results in a significant decrease in the incidence of dental caries.[1] LURIDE Drops were developed to provide systemic fluoride for use as a supplement in pediatric patients from 6 months to age 3 and older living in areas where the drinking water fluoride level does not exceed 0.6 ppm F.

CONTRAINDICATIONS
Do not use in areas where the drinking water exceeds 0.6 ppm F. Do not administer to pediatric patients under 6 months of age.

WARNINGS
See "Contraindications" above. As in the case of all medications, keep out of reach of infants and children. Contains FD&C Yellow No. 6.

PRECAUTIONS
See "Overdosage" section. Incompatibility of fluoride with dairy foods has been reported due to formation of calcium fluoride which is poorly absorbed. Not for use in the eyes.

ADVERSE REACTIONS
Allergic rash and other idiosyncrasies have been rarely reported.

OVERDOSAGE
Prolonged daily ingestion of excessive fluoride will result in varying degrees of dental fluorosis. (The total amount of sodium fluoride in a bottle of 50 ml LURIDE Drops (25 mg F) conforms with recommendations of the American Dental Association for the maximum to be dispensed at one time for safety purposes.)

DOSAGE[2] AND ADMINISTRATION
Daily oral dose (in areas where the drinking water contains less than 0.3 ppm F)—6 months to age 3: 0.5 ml (one half dropperful); age 3–6, 1 ml (one dropperful); age 6–16, 2 ml (two dropperful). When drinking water is partially fluoridated (0.3 to 0.6 ppm F inclusive) dose as follows: 6 months to age 3, fluoride supplementation not indicated; age 3–6, 0.5 ml (one half dropperful); age 6–16, 1 ml (one dropperful).

HOW SUPPLIED
50 ml bottles (peach flavor) — NDC #0126-0002-62.

CAUTION: Federal (U.S.A.) law prohibits dispensing without prescription.

REFERENCES: 1. Accepted Dental Therapeutics. Ed. 40. American Dental Association, Chicago, 1984. p. 399–402. 2. Jakush, J., New fluoride schedule adopted. ADA News. May 16, 1994. p.12, 14.

LURIDE LOZI-TABS ℞
brand of sodium fluoride

DESCRIPTION
LURIDE® brand of sodium fluoride Lozi-Tabs® brand of lozenge/chewable tablets for use as a dental caries preventive in pediatric patients. Sugar-free. Saccharin free. Erythrosine (FD&C Red dye #3)-free. Each LURIDE 1 mg tablet (full-strength) contains 1 mg fluoride ion (F) from 2.2 mg sodium fluoride (NaF).
Each LURIDE 0.5 mg F tablet (half-strength) contains 0.5 mg F from 1.1 mg NaF.
Each LURIDE 0.25 mg F tablet (quarter-strength) contains 0.25 mg F from 0.55 mg NaF.
Active Ingredient: Sodium Fluoride.
Other Ingredients: Sorbitol, Mannitol, Povidone, Citric Acid (0.5 mg and 1 mg strength tablets only), Magnesium Stearate, D&C Red Lake Blend (Cherry flavor only), Violet Lake Dye Blend (Grape flavor only), D&C Yellow #10 (Lemon and Lime flavors only), FD&C Blue #1 (Lime flavor only), FD&C Yellow No. 6 (Orange and Vanilla flavors only). Tablets (except Special Formula) also contain natural and artificial flavors in varying concentrations.

CLINICAL PHARMACOLOGY
Sodium fluoride acts systemically (before tooth eruption) and topically (post eruption) by increasing tooth resistance to acid dissolution, by promoting remineralization, and by inhibiting the cariogenic microbial process.

INDICATIONS AND USAGE
It has been established that ingestion of fluoridated drinking water (1 ppm F) during the period of tooth development results in significant decrease in the incidence of dental caries.[1] LURIDE tablets were developed to provide systemic fluoride for use as a supplement in pediatric patients from age 6 months to 16 years, living in areas where the drinking water fluoride level does not exceed 0.6 ppm F.

CONTRAINDICATIONS
LURIDE 1 mg F Tablets are contraindicated when the Fluoride content of drinking water is 0.3 ppm or more and should not be administered to pediatric patients under age 6. LURIDE 0.5 mg F Tablets are contraindicated when the F content of drinking water is 0.6 ppm or more and should not be administered to pediatric patients under age 3. LURIDE 0.25 mg F Tablets are contraindicated when the fluoride content of drinking water is 0.6 ppm or more and should not be administered to pediatric patients under age 6 months.

WARNINGS
See "Contraindications" above. As in the case of all medications, keep out of reach of infants and children.

PRECAUTIONS
See "Overdosage" section. Incompatibility of fluoride with dairy foods has been reported due to formation of calcium fluoride which is poorly absorbed.

ADVERSE REACTIONS
Allergic rash and other idiosyncrasies have been rarely reported.

OVERDOSAGE
Prolonged daily ingestion of excessive fluoride will result in varying degrees of dental fluorosis. (The total amount of sodium fluoride in a bottle of 120 LURIDE tablets [all strengths] conforms with the recommendations of the American Dental Association for the maximum to be dispensed at one time for safety purposes.)

DOSAGE[2] AND ADMINISTRATION
See schedule below to determine daily dosage. Dissolve in the mouth or chew before swallowing, preferably at bedtime after brushing teeth.

	Water F⁻ content		
AGE	**0–0.3 PPM**	**0.3–0.6 PPM**	**>0.6 PPM**
6 Mo–3 Yrs	0.25 mg	0	0
3–6 Yrs	0.5 mg	0.25 mg	0
6–16 Yrs	1 mg	0.5 mg	0

HOW SUPPLIED
LURIDE 1 mg F available in bottles of 120 and 1000*; Cherry and Assorted flavors.
LURIDE 0.5 mg F available in bottles of 120 and 1200*; Grape flavor.
LURIDE 0.25 mg F available in bottles of 120; Vanilla flavor and Special Formula (with no artificial color or flavor).
**FOR DISPENSING ONLY*

Caution: Federal (U.S.A.) law prohibits dispensing without prescription.

References: 1. Accepted Dental Therapeutics, Ed. 40. Americal Dental Association. Chicago, 1984, p. 399–402. 2. Jakush, J., New fluoride schedule adopted. ADA News. May 16, 1994, p. 12,14.

Manufactured for:
Colgate Oral Pharmaceuticals, Inc.
a subsidiary of Colgate-Palmolive Company
One Colgate Way, Canton, MA 02021 U.S.A.

PERIOGARD® ℞
(Chlorhexidine Gluconate Oral Rinse, 0.12%)

DESCRIPTION
PERIOGARD (Chlorhexidine Gluconate Oral Rinse, 0.12%) is an oral rinse containing 0.12% chlorhexidine gluconate [*N,N'*-bis (4-chlorophenyl)-3,12-diimino-2,4,11,13-tetraazatetradecanediimidamide di-*D*-gluconate] in a base containing water, 11.6% alcohol (%v/v), glycerin, PEG-40 sorbitan diisostearate, flavor, sodium saccharin, and FD&C Blue No. 1. PERIOGARD Oral Rinse is a near-neutral solution (pH ranges 5–7). Chlorhexidine gluconate is a salt of chlorhexidine and gluconic acid, with a molecular formula of $C_{22}H_{30}Cl_2N_{10} \cdot 2C_6H_{12}O_7$ and a molecular weight calculated to be 897.77. Its structural formula is:

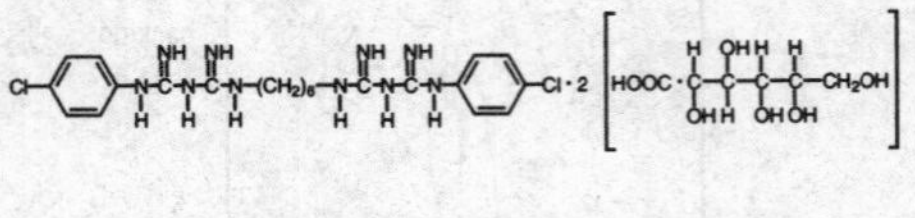

CLINICAL PHARMACOLOGY
PERIOGARD Oral Rinse provides microbicidal activity during oral rinsing. The clinical significance of 0.12% chlorhexidine gluconate oral rinse's anti-microbial activities is not clear. Microbiological sampling of plaque has shown a general reduction of counts of certain assayed bacteria, both aerobic and anaerobic, ranging from 54–97% through six months' use.
Use of a chlorhexidine gluconate oral rinse in a six-month clinical study did not result in any significant changes in bacterial resistance, overgrowth of potentially opportunistic organisms or other adverse changes in the oral microbial ecosystem. Three months after chlorhexidine gluconate use was discontinued, the number of bacteria in plaque had returned to baseline levels and resistance of plaque bacteria to chlorhexidine gluconate was equal to that at baseline.

PHARMACOKINETICS
Pharmacokinetic studies with a 0.12% chlorhexidine gluconate oral rinse indicate approximately 30% of the active ingredient is retained in the oral cavity following rinsing. This retained drug is slowly released into the oral fluids. Studies conducted on human subjects and animals demonstrate chlorehexidine gluconate is poorly absorbed from the gastrointestinal tract. The mean plasma level of chlorhexidine gluconate reached a peak of 0.206 μg/g in humans 30 minutes after they ingested a 300 mg dose of the drug. Detectable levels of chlorhexidine gluconate were not present in the plasma of these subjects 12 hours after the compound was administered. Excretion of chlorhexidine gluconate occurred primarily through the feces (~90%). Less than 1% of the chlorhexidine gluconate ingested by these subjects was excreted in the urine.

INDICATIONS AND USAGE
PERIOGARD Oral Rinse is indicated for use between dental visits as part of a professional program for the treatment of gingivitis as characterized by redness and swelling of the gingivae, including gingival bleeding upon probing. PERIOGARD Oral Rinse has not been tested among patients with acute necrotizing ulcerative gingivitis (ANUG). For patients having coexisting gingivitis and periodontitis, see PRECAUTIONS.

CONTRAINDICATIONS
PERIOGARD Oral Rinse should not be used by persons who are known to be hypersensitive to chlorhexidine gluconate.

WARNINGS
The effect of PERIOGARD Oral Rinse on periodontitis has not been determined. An increase in supragingival calculus was noted in clinical testing with users of chlorhexidine gluconate oral rinse compared with control users. It is not known if chlorhexidine gluconate use results in an increase in subgingival calculus. Calculus deposits should be removed by a dental prophylaxis at intervals not greater than six months.
Rare hypersensitivity and generalized allergic reactions have also been reported. PERIOGARD Oral Rinse should not be used by persons who have a sensitivity to it or its components.

PRECAUTIONS
GENERAL
1. For patients having coexisting gingivitis and periodontitis, the presence or absence of gingival inflammation following treatment with PERIOGARD Oral Rinse should not be used as a major indicator of underlying periodontitis.
2. PERIOGARD Oral Rinse can cause staining of oral surfaces, such tooth surfaces, restorations, and the dorsum of the tongue. Not all patients will experience a visually significant increase in toothstaining. In clinical testing, 56% of the chlorhexidine gluconate oral rinse users exhibited a measurable increase in facial anterior stain, compared to 35% of control users after six months; 15% of the chlorhexidine gluconate users developed what was judged to be heavy stain, compared to 1% of control users after six months. Stain will be more pronounced in patients who have heavier accumulations of unremoved plaque.
Stain resulting from the use of PERIOGARD Oral Rinse does not adversely affect health of the gingivae or other oral tissues. Stain can be removed from most tooth surfaces by conventional professional prophylactic techniques. Additional time may be required to complete the prophylaxis.
Discretion should be used when prescribing to patients with anterior facial restorations with rough surfaces or margins. If natural stain cannot be removed from these surfaces by a dental prophylaxis, patients should be excluded from PERIOGARD Oral Rinse treatment if permanent discoloration is unacceptable. Stain in these areas may be difficult to remove by dental prophylaxis and on rare occasions may necessitate replacement of these restorations.
3. Some patients may experience an alteration in taste perception while undergoing treatment with a chlorhexidine gluconate oral rinse. Most patients accommodate to this effect with continued use of PERIOGARD Oral Rinse. No instances of permanent taste alteration due to the use of a chlorhexidine gluconate oral rinse have been reported.
CARCINOGENESIS, MUTAGENESIS,
IMPAIRMENT OF FERTILITY:
In a drinking water study in rats, carcinogenesis was not observed. The highest dose of chlorhexidine gluconate used in this study, 38 mg/kg/day, is at least 500 times the amount that would be ingested from the recommended daily dose of PERIOGARD Oral Rinse.
In two mammalian *in vivo* mutagenic studies with chlorhexidine gluconate, mutagenesis was not observed. The highest dose of chlorhexidine gluconate used in a mouse dominant

lethal assay was 1000 mg/kg/day and in a hamster cytogenetics test was 250 m/kg/day, i.e. > 3200 times the amount that would be ingested from the recommended daily dose of PERIOGARD Oral Rinse.

PREGNANCY: Pregnancy Category B, Reproduction and fertility studies with chlorhexidine gluconate have been conducted. No evidence of impaired fertility was observed in rats at doses up to 100mg/kg/day, and no evidence of harm to the fetus was observed in rats and rabbits at doses up to 300 mg/kg/day and 40 mg/kg/day, respectively. These doses are approximately 100, 300, and 40 times that which would result from a person's ingesting 30 mL of PERIOGARD Oral Rinse per day. Since controlled studies in pregnant women have not been conducted, the benefits of the drug in pregnant women should be weighed against possible risk to the fetus.

NURSING MOTHERS: It is not known whether this drug is excreted in human milk. Because many drugs are excreted in human milk, caution should be exercised when PERIOGARD Oral Rinse is administered to a nursing woman. In parturition and lactation studies with rats, no evidence of impaired parturition or of toxic effects to suckling pups was observed when chlorhexidine gluconate was administered to dams at doses that were over 100 times greater than that which would result from a person's ingesting 30 mL (2 capfuls) of PERIOGARD Oral Rinse per day.

PEDIATRIC USE: Safety and effectiveness in pediatric patients have not been established.

ADVERSE REACTIONS

The most common side effects associated with chlorhexidine gluconate oral rinses are (1) an increase in staining of teeth and other oral surfaces, (2) an increase in calculus formation, and (3) an alteration in taste perception; see WARNINGS and PRECAUTIONS. No serious systemic adverse reactions associated with use of a 0.12% chlorhexidine gluconate oral rinse were observed in clinical testing.

Minor irritation and superficial desquamation of the oral mucosa have been noted in patients using chlorhexidine gluconate oral rinses, particularly among children.

Although there have been no reports of parotitis (inflammation or swelling of the salivary glands) among the users of chlorhexidine gluconate oral rinse in controlled clinical studies, transient parotitis has been reported in research studies with chlorhexidine-containing mouthrinses.

OVERDOSAGE

Ingestion of 1 or 2 ounces of PERIOGARD Oral Rinse by a small child (~10 kg body weight) might result in gastric distress, including nausea, or signs of alcohol intoxication. Medical attention should be sought if more than 4 ounces of PERIOGARD Oral Rinse is ingested by a small child or if signs of alcohol intoxication develop.

DOSAGE AND ADMINISTRATION

PERIOGARD Oral Rinse therapy should be initiated directly following a dental prophylaxis. Patients using PERIOGARD Oral Rinse should be reevaluated and given a thorough prophylaxis at intervals no longer than six months.

Recommended use is twice daily oral rinsing for 30 seconds, morning and evening after toothbrushing. Usual dosage is $^1/_2$ fl. oz. (marked on dosage cup) of undiluted PERIOGARD Oral Rinse. PERIOGARD Oral Rinse is not intended for ingestion and should be expectorated after rinsing.

HOW SUPPLIED

PERIOGARD Oral Rinse is supplied as a blue liquid in 16 fluid ounce amber plastic bottles with child-resistant closures and dosage cups. Store above freezing (32°F).
Revised 4/95
Manufactured for Colgate Oral Pharmaceuticals by PACO Pharm.,
Lakewood, NJ 08701
Colgate Oral Pharmaceuticals, Inc.
a subsidiary of
Colgate-Palmolive Company
One Colgate Way
Canton, MA 02021 U.S.A.

PREVIDENT® 5000 PLUS™   ℞
brand of 1.1% Sodium Fluoride
prescription dental cream

DESCRIPTION

Self-topical neutral 1.1% sodium fluoride for use as a dental caries preventive in adults and pediatric patients.

ACTIVE INGREDIENT

Sodium Fluoride, 1.1% (w/v)

INACTIVE INGREDIENTS

Purified water, sorbitol, hydrated silica, PEG-12, tetrapotassium pyrophosphate, xanthan gum, flavor, sodium benzoate, sodium lauryl sulfate, sodium saccharin, titanium dioxide, sodium hydroxide, FD&C blue #1.

CLINICAL PHARMACOLOGY

Frequent topical applications to the teeth with preparations having a relatively high fluoride content increase tooth resistance to acid dissolution and enhance penetration of the fluoride ion into tooth enamel.

INDICATIONS AND USAGE

It is well established that 1.1% sodium fluoride is safe and extraordinarily effective as a caries preventive when applied frequently with mouthpiece applicators.[1][4] PreviDent 5000 Plus brand of 1.1% sodium fluoride in a squeeze tube is easily applied on a toothbrush. This prescription dental cream should be used daily in place of your regular toothpaste unless otherwise instructed by your dental professional.

CONTRAINDICATIONS

None. (May be used in areas where drinking water is fluoridated or not, because topical fluoride cannot produce fluorosis.)

WARNINGS

DO NOT SWALLOW. As with all medications, keep out of reach of infants and children. Do not use in pediatric patients under age 6 because repeated swallowing of dental cream could cause dental fluorosis.

OVERDOSAGE

Accidental ingestion of a usual treatment dose is not harmful.

DOSAGE AND ADMINISTRATION

Follow these instructions unless otherwise instructed by your dental professional:
1. Adults and pediatric patients 6 years of age or older, apply daily a thin ribbon of PreviDent 5000 Plus to a toothbrush. Brush thoroughly for two minutes, preferably at bedtime.
2. After use, adults expectorate. For best results, do not eat, drink or rinse for 30 minutes. Pediatric patients, age 6-16, expectorate after use and rinse mouth thoroughly.

HOW SUPPLIED

2 oz. (56 g) net wt. tubes. NDC# 0126-0287-02.
STORAGE Store below 86° F (30° C).
CAUTION:
Federal (U.S.A.) law prohibits dispensing without prescription.

REFERENCES

1. Accepted Dental Therapeutics, Ed. 40, ADA, Chicago. P.405-407, 1984.
2. Englander HR, Keyes et al: JADA 75:638-644, 1967.
3. Englander HR, et al: JADA 78:783-787, 1969.
4. Englander HR, et al: JADA 83:354-358, 1971.
                                       Rev. 10/95 IN5037-02
Colgate Oral Pharmaceuticals, Inc.
A subsidiary of Colgate-Palmolive Company
One Colgate Way, Canton, MA 02021 U.S.A.

Connaught Laboratories, Inc.
A Pasteur Mérieux Company
SWIFTWATER, PA 18370

For Medical Information Contact:
Generally:
Medical Affairs
(800) VACCINE
(800) 822-2463
Adverse Drug Experiences:
Medical Director
(717) 839-7187
(800) 835-3592

Sales and Ordering:
Connaught Laboratories, Inc.
Customer Service
(800) VACCINE
(800) 822-2463
(717) 839-7187

HAEMOPHILUS b CONJUGATE VACCINE   ℞
(Tetanus Toxoid Conjugate)
ActHIB®

Caution: Federal (USA) law prohibits dispensing without prescription.
NOTE: Haemophilus b Conjugate Vaccine (Tetanus Toxoid Conjugate)—ActHIB® is identical to Haemophilus b Conjugate Vaccine (Tetanus Toxoid Conjugate)—OmniHIB™ (distributed by SmithKline Beecham Pharmaceuticals); both products are manufactured by Pasteur Mérieux Sérums & Vaccins S.A.

DESCRIPTION

ActHIB®, Haemophilus b Conjugate Vaccine (Tetanus Toxoid Conjugate), produced by Pasteur Mérieux Sérums & Vaccins S.A., is a sterile, lyophilized powder which is reconstituted at the time of use with either saline diluent (0.4% Sodium Chloride) or Connaught Laboratories, Inc. (CLI) Diphtheria and Tetanus Toxoids and Pertussis Vaccine Adsorbed (DTP) for intramuscular use only. The vaccine consists of the Haemophilus b polysaccharide, a high molecular weight polymer prepared from the *Haemophilus influenzae* type b strain 1482 grown in a semi-synthetic medium, covalently bound to tetanus toxoid.[1] The lyophilized ActHIB® powder and saline diluent contain no preservative. The tetanus toxoid is prepared by extraction, ammonium sulfate purification, and formalin inactivation of the toxin from cultures of *Clostridium tetani* (Harvard strain) grown in a modified Mueller and Miller medium.[2] The toxoid is filter sterilized prior to the conjugation process. Potency of ActHIB® is specified on each lot by limits on the content of PRP polysaccharide and protein in each dose and the proportion of polysaccharide and protein in the vaccine which is characterized as high molecular weight conjugate. Each single dose of 0.5 mL is formulated to contain 10 µg of purified capsular polysaccharide conjugated to 24 µg of inactivated tetanus toxoid, and 8.5% of sucrose when reconstituted with saline diluent. At the time ActHIB® is reconstituted with CLI DTP vaccine, each single dose of 0.5 mL is formulated to contain 10 µg of purified capsular polysaccharide conjugated to 24 µg of inactivated tetanus toxoid, 8.5% of sucrose, 6.7 Lf of diphtheria toxoid, 5 Lf of tetanus toxoid and an estimate of 4 protective units of pertussis vaccine. Thimerosal (mercury derivative) 1:10,000 is added as a preservative to CLI DTP vaccine.
(Refer to product insert for CLI whole-cell DTP.)
The reconstituted vaccine, using saline diluent, appears clear and colorless. The reconstituted vaccine, using CLI DTP vaccine, appears whitish in color.

CLINICAL PHARMACOLOGY

NOTE: Haemophilus b Conjugate Vaccine (Tetanus Toxoid Conjugate)—ActHIB® is identical to Haemophilus b Conjugate Vaccine (Tetanus Toxoid Conjugate)—OmniHIB™ (distributed by SmithKline Beecham Pharmaceuticals); both products are manufactured by Pasteur Mérieux Sérums & Vaccins S.A.

H influenzae type b was the leading cause of invasive bacterial disease among children in the United States prior to licensing of Haemophilus b conjugate vaccines. Based on its active surveillance areas, the Centers for Disease Control and Prevention (CDC) now estimate that *H influenzae* type b disease in children under the age of 5 years has been reduced by 95%.[3] Before effective vaccines were introduced, it was estimated that one in 200 children developed invasive *H influenzae* type b disease by the age of 5 years. In children less than 5 years of age, the mortality rate for invasive *H influenzae* type b disease ranged between 3% and 6%.[3] In more than 60% of these children, meningitis was the clinical syndrome and permanent sequelae ranging from mild hearing loss to mental retardation affecting 20% to 30% of all survivors.[3] Ninety-five percent of the cases of invasive *H influenzae* disease among children < 5 years of age were caused by organisms with the type b polysaccharide capsule. Approximately two-thirds of all cases of invasive *H influenzae* type b disease affected infants and children < 15 months of age, a group for which a vaccine was not available until late 1990.[4][5] Incidence rates of invasive *H influenzae* type b disease have been shown to be increased in certain high-risk groups, such as native Americans (both American Indians and Eskimos), blacks, individuals of lower socioeconomic status, and patients with asplenia, sickle cell disease, Hodgkin's disease, and antibody deficiency syndromes.[5][6] Studies also have suggested that the risk of acquiring primary invasive *H influenzae* type b disease for children under 5 years of age appears to be greater for those who attend day-care facilities.[7][8][9][10]
The potential for person to person transmission of the organism among susceptible individuals has been recognized. Studies of secondary spread of disease in household contacts of index patients have shown a substantially increased risk among exposed household contacts under 4 years of age.[11] Adults can be colonized with *H influenzae* type b from children infected with the organism.[12]
The response to ActHIB® is typical of a T-dependent immune response to antigen. The predominant isotype of anticapsular polysaccharide (polyribosyl-ribitol-phosphate or PRP) antibody induced by ActHIB® is IgG.[13] A substantial booster response has been demonstrated in children 12 months of age or older who previously received two or three doses. Bactericidal activity against *H influenzae* type b is demonstrated in serum after immunization and statistically correlates with the anti-PRP antibody response induced by ActHIB®.[14]
Antibody to *H influenzae* capsular polysaccharide (anti-PRP) titers of > 1.0 µg/mL following vaccination with unconjugated PRP vaccine correlated with long-term protection

Continued on next page

Connaught Laboratories—Cont.

against invasive *H influenzae* type b disease in children older than 24 months of age.[15] Although the relevance of this threshold to clinical protection after immunization with conjugate vaccines is not known, particularly in light of the induced, immunologic memory, this level continues to be considered as indicative of long-term protection.[4] The immunogenicity and safety of ActHIB® has been demonstrated in the United States and worldwide. ActHIB® induced, on average anti-PRP levels ≥ 1.0 µg/mL in 90% of infants after the primary series and in more than 98% of infants after a booster dose.[14]

Two clinical trials supported by the National Institutes of Health (NIH) have compared the anti-PRP antibody responses to three Haemophilus b conjugate vaccines in a racially mixed population of children. These studies were done in Tennessee[16] (Table 1) and in Minnesota, Missouri and Texas[17] (Table 2) in infants immunized with ActHIB® and other Haemophilus b conjugate vaccines at 2, 4 and 6 months of age. All Haemophilus b conjugate vaccines were administered concomitantly with Live Oral Poliovirus Vaccine and DTP vaccines at separate sites.

[See tables 1 and 2 below.]

Native American populations have high rates of *H influenzae* type b disease and have been observed to have low immune responses to Haemophilus b conjugate vaccines. Following three doses of ActHIB® at six weeks, four and six months of age, 75% of Native Americans in Alaska showed an anti-PRP antibody titer of ≥ 1.0 µg/mL.[18]

In three US trials in 12- to 15-month-old children and one trial in 17- to 24-month-old children who had not previously received Haemophilus b conjugate vaccination, a single dose of ActHIB® produced an anti-PRP antibody response comparable to those seen after three doses were administered in infants (Table 3).[18]

TABLE 3[18]
ANTI-PRP ANTIBODY RESPONSES IN 12- TO 24-MONTH-OLD CHILDREN IMMUNIZED WITH A SINGLE DOSE OF ActHIB®

AGE GROUP	N	GMT (µg/mL) Pre	GMT (µg/mL) Post	% SUBJECTS WITH ≥ 1.0 µg/mL Pre	% SUBJECTS WITH ≥ 1.0 µg/mL Post
12 to 15 months	256	0.06	5.12	1.6	90.2
17 to 24 months	81	0.10	4.4	3.7	81.5

TABLE 1[16]
ANTI-PRP ANTIBODY RESPONSES IN 2-MONTH-OLD INFANTS NIH TRIAL IN TENNESSEE

VACCINE	N*	GEOMETRIC MEAN TITER (GMT) (µg/mL) Pre-Immunization	Post Second Immunization	Post Third Immunization	Post Third§ Immunization % ≥ 1.0 µg/mL
PRP-T† (ActHIB®)	65	0.10	0.30	3.64	83%
PRP-OMP¶ (PedvaxHIB®)	64	0.11	0.84	N/A	50%**
HbOC‡ (HibTITER®)	61	0.07	0.13	3.08	75%

TABLE 2[17]
ANTI-PRP ANTIBODY RESPONSES IN 2-MONTH-OLD INFANTS NIH TRIAL IN MINNESOTA, MISSOURI AND TEXAS

VACCINE	N*	GEOMETRIC MEAN TITER (GMT) (µg/mL) Pre-Immunization	Post Second Immunization	Post Third Immunization	Post Third§ Immunization % ≥ 1.0 µg/mL
PRP-T† (ActHIB®)	142	0.25	1.25	6.37	97%
PRP-OMP¶ (PedvaxHIB®)	149	0.18	4.00	N/A	85%**
HbOC‡ (HibTITER®)	167	0.17	0.45	6.31	90%

* N = Number of Children
§ Sera were obtained after the third dose from 86 and 110 infants, in PRP-T and HbOC vaccine groups, respectively.
† Haemophilus b Conjugate Vaccine (Tetanus Toxoid Conjugate)
¶ Haemophilus b Conjugate Vaccine (Meningococcal Protein Conjugate)
** Seroconversion after the recommended 2-dose primary immunization series is shown.
‡ Haemophilus b Conjugate Vaccine (Diphtheria CRM197 Protein Conjugate)
N/A Not applicable in this comparison trial although third dose data have been published.[16,17]

TABLE 4[18]
ANTI-PRP ANTIBODY RESPONSES IN 2-MONTH-OLD INFANTS FOLLOWING IMMUNIZATION WITH ActHIB® RECONSTITUTED WITH CONNAUGHT LABORATORIES, INC. DTP

Study Site	N*	GEOMETRIC MEAN TITER (GMT) (µg/mL) Pre-Immunization	Post Second Immunization	Post Third Immunization	Post Third Immunization % ≥ 1.0 µg/mL
US	45	0.13	0.55	4.49	91
US	135	0.12	0.43	4.46	85
Chile	94	0.09	4.31	6.94	96

* N = Number of Children

These trials demonstrated that ActHIB® consistently conferred an anti-PRP antibody response previously shown to correlate with protection, when administered either as a regimen of three doses at least four to eight weeks apart in infants 2 to 6 months of age or as a single dose in children 12 months of age and older.[18]

ActHIB® has been found to be immunogenic in children with sickle cell anemia, a condition which may cause increased susceptibility to Haemophilus b disease. Two doses of ActHIB® given at two-month intervals induced anti-PRP antibody titers of ≥ 1.0 µg/mL in 89% of these children with a mean age of 11 months. This is comparable to anti-PRP antibody levels demonstrated in normal children of similar age following two doses of ActHIB®.[19]

Comparative clinical trials demonstrated that a similar anti-PRP response was achieved in infants as young as 2 months old when one dose of CLI whole-cell DTP vaccine was used to reconstitute one dose of lyophilized ActHIB® (Table 4).[14,18] [See table above.]

INDICATIONS AND USAGE

NOTE: Haemophilus b Conjugate Vaccine (Tetanus Toxoid Conjugate) — ActHIB® is identical to Haemophilus b Conjugate Vaccine (Tetanus Toxoid Conjugate) — OmniHIB™ (distributed by SmithKline Beecham Pharmaceuticals); both products are manufactured by Pasteur Mérieux Sérums & Vaccins S.A.

ActHIB® or ActHIB® reconstituted with CLI DTP vaccine is indicated for the active immunization of infants and children 2 months through 5 years of age for the prevention of invasive disease caused by *H influenzae* type b, and/or diphtheria, tetanus and pertussis.

Antibody levels associated with protection may not be achieved earlier than two weeks following the last recommended dose.

As with any vaccine, vaccination with ActHIB® reconstituted with CLI DTP vaccine or saline diluent (0.4% Sodium Chloride) may not protect 100% of susceptible individuals.

A single injection containing diphtheria, tetanus, pertussis and Haemophilus b conjugate antigens may be more acceptable to parents and may increase compliance with vaccination programs. Therefore, in those situations where, in the judgment of the physician, it is of benefit to administer a single injection of whole-cell DTP and Haemophilus b conjugate vaccines *only CLI whole-cell DTP vaccine may be used for reconstitution of lyophilized ActHIB®.*

CONTRAINDICATIONS

ActHIB® RECONSTITUTED WITH CLI DTP VACCINE OR SALINE DILUENT (0.4% SODIUM CHLORIDE) IS CONTRAINDICATED IN CHILDREN WITH A HISTORY OF HYPERSENSITIVITY TO ANY COMPONENT OF THE HAEMOPHILUS b CONJUGATE VACCINE AND DIPHTHERIA AND TETANUS TOXOIDS AND PERTUSSIS VACCINE ADSORBED (DTP). ANY CONTRAINDICATION FOR CLI DTP VACCINE IS A CONTRAINDICATION FOR ActHIB® RECONSTITUTED WITH CLI DTP VACCINE.

WARNINGS

If ActHIB® or ActHIB® reconstituted with CLI DTP is administered to immunosuppressed persons or persons receiving immunosuppressive therapy, the expected antibody responses may not be obtained. This includes patients with asymptomatic or symptomatic HIV-infection,[20] severe combined immunodeficiency, hypogammaglobulinemia, or agammaglobulinemia; altered immune states due to diseases such as leukemia, lymphoma, or generalized malignancy; or an immune system compromised by treatment with corticosteroids, alkylating drugs, antimetabolites or radiation.[21] *(Refer to product insert for CLI whole-cell DTP.)*

PRECAUTIONS

GENERAL

Care is to be taken by the health-care provider for the safe and effective use of this vaccine.

EPINEPHRINE INJECTION (1:1000) MUST BE IMMEDIATELY AVAILABLE SHOULD AN ANAPHYLACTIC OR OTHER ALLERGIC REACTIONS OCCUR DUE TO ANY COMPONENT OF THE VACCINE.

Prior to an injection of any vaccine, all known precautions should be taken to prevent adverse reactions. This includes a review of the patient's history with respect to possible sensitivity and any previous adverse reactions to the vaccine or similar vaccines, previous immunization history, current health status (see **CONTRAINDICATIONS; WARNINGS** sections), and a current knowledge of the literature concerning the use of the vaccine under consideration. *(Refer to product insert for CLI whole-cell DTP.)*

The health-care provider should ask the parent or guardian about the recent health status of the infant or child to be immunized including the infant's or child's previous immunization history prior to administration of ActHIB® and CLI DTP vaccines.

Minor illnesses such as upper respiratory infection with or without low-grade fever are not contraindications for use of ActHIB®.[22]

As reported with Haemophilus b polysaccharide vaccines,[23] cases of *H influenzae* type b disease may occur subsequent to vaccination and prior to the onset of protective effects of the vaccine.[18] (See **INDICATIONS AND USAGE** section.)

Antigenuria has been detected in some instances following receipt of ActHIB®; therefore, urine antigen detection may not have definitive diagnostic value in suspected *H influenzae* type b disease within one week of immunization.[24]

Special care should be taken to ensure that ActHIB® reconstituted with CLI DTP vaccine or saline diluent (0.4% Sodium Chloride) is not injected into a blood vessel.

Administration of ActHIB® reconstituted with CLI DTP vaccine or saline diluent (0.4% Sodium Chloride) is not contraindicated in individuals with HIV infection.[21]

A separate, sterile syringe and needle or a sterile disposable unit should be used for each patient to prevent transmission of hepatitis or other infectious agents from person to person. Needles should not be recapped and should be properly disposed.

INFORMATION FOR PATIENT

The health-care provider should inform the parent or guardian of the benefits and risks of the vaccine.

Prior to administration of ActHIB® reconstituted with CLI DTP vaccine or saline diluent (0.4% Sodium Chloride), the parent or guardian should be asked about the recent health status of the infant or child to be immunized.

The physician should inform the parent or guardian about the significant adverse reactions that have been temporally associated with ActHIB® reconstituted with CLI DTP vaccine administration. The parent or guardian should be instructed to report any serious adverse reactions to their health-care provider.

As part of the child's immunization record, the date, lot number and manufacturer of the vaccine administered should be recorded.[25,26,27]

The US Department of Health and Human Services has established a new Vaccine Adverse Event Reporting System (VAERS) to accept all reports of suspected adverse events after the administration of any vaccine, including but not limited to the reporting of events required by the National Childhood Vaccine Injury Act of 1986.[25] The toll-free number for VAERS forms and information is 1-800-822-7967.

The National Vaccine Injury Compensation Program, established by the National Childhood Vaccine Injury Act of 1986, requires physicians and other health-care providers who administer vaccines to maintain permanent vaccination records and to report occurrences of certain adverse events to the US Department of Health and Human Services. Reportable events include those listed in the Act for each vaccine and events specified in the package insert as contraindications to further doses of the vaccine.[26,27]

The health-care provider should inform the parent or guardian of the importance of completing the immunization series. The health-care provider should provide the Vaccine Information Materials (VIMs) which are required to be given with each immunization.

DRUG INTERACTIONS

When CLI DTP vaccine is used to reconstitute ActHIB® and administered to immunosuppressed persons or persons receiving immunosuppressive therapy, the expected antibody response may not be obtained.

Immunosuppressive therapies, including irradiation, antimetabolites, alkylating agents, cytotoxic drugs, and corticosteroids (used in greater than physiologic doses), may reduce the immune response to vaccines. Short-term (<2 weeks) corticosteroid therapy or intra-articular, bursal, or tendon injections with corticosteroids should not be immunosuppressive. Although no specific studies with pertussis vaccine are available, if immunosuppressive therapy will be discontinued shortly, it is reasonable to defer vaccination until the patient has been off therapy for one month; otherwise, the patient should be vaccinated while still on therapy.[22]

If ActHIB® reconstituted with DTP has been administered to persons receiving immunosuppressive therapy, a recent injection of immunoglobulin or having an immunodeficiency disorder, an adequate immunologic response may not be obtained.

As with other intramuscular injections, use with caution in patients on anticoagulant therapy.

In clinical trials, ActHIB® was routinely administered, at separate sites, concomitantly with one or more of the following vaccines: DTP vaccine, Oral Poliovirus Vaccine (OPV), Measles, Mumps and Rubella Vaccine (MMR), Hepatitis B Vaccine and occasionally Inactivated Poliovirus Vaccine (IPV). No significant impairment of the antibody response to any antigen of Connaught Laboratories, Inc. (CLI) DTP vaccine was observed in the three clinical trials when given either separately with ActHIB® or combined with ActHIB® in the same syringe.[18] Interference with the antibody response to the pertussis component has been suggested with a DTP vaccine unlicensed in the US.[28] No impairment of the antibody response to the individual antigens, diphtheria, tetanus and pertussis, was demonstrated when ActHIB® was given at the same time, at separate sites, with Inactivated Poliovirus Vaccine (IPV) or Measles, Mumps and Rubella Vaccine (MMR).[18] In addition, more than 47,000 infants in Finland have received a third dose of ActHIB® concomitantly with MMR vaccine with no increase in serious or unexpected adverse events.[18]

No data are available to the manufacturer concerning the effects on immune response of OPV or Hepatitis B vaccine when given concurrently with ActHIB® reconstituted with CLI DTP.

TABLE 6 [14]

PERCENTAGE OF INFANTS PRESENTING WITH LOCAL OR SYSTEMIC REACTIONS AT 6, 24, AND 48 HOURS OF IMMUNIZATION WITH ActHIB® ADMINISTERED SIMULTANEOUSLY, AT SEPARATE SITES, WITH CLI DTP VACCINE

REACTION	AGE AT IMMUNIZATION								
	2 Months (n=365)			4 Months (n=364)			6 Months (n=365)		
	6 Hrs.	24 Hrs.	48 Hrs.	6 Hrs.	24 Hrs.	48 Hrs.	6 Hrs.	24 Hrs.	48 Hrs.
Local§									
Tenderness	46.3%	11.5%	2.2%	23.4%	7.4%	1.1%	19.2%	6.0%	1.1%
Erythema	14.3%	4.1%	0.3%	8.8%	5.8%	0.6%	11.5%	6.9%	1.6%
Induration	22.5%	6.3%	1.9%	12.4%	4.7%	0.8%	9.6%	3.8%	1.1%
Systemic*									
Fever >100.8°F†	20.1%	1.3%	0.6%	14.6%	6.6%	1.4%	15.7%	8.8%	0.8%
Irritability	72.6%	21.9%	12.6%	48.4%	25.0%	13.2%	44.1%	25.2%	10.1%
Drowsiness	57.5%	29.9%	10.4%	44.2%	18.1%	7.4%	32.6%	13.4%	2.5%
Anorexia	15.3%	5.8%	4.9%	8.0%	5.05%	3.0%	5.5%	4.9%	2.2%
Diarrhea	4.4%	6.6%	5.2%	5.0%	4.7%	4.7%	4.7%	6.3%	3.6%
Vomiting	2.7%	4.1%	2.7%	2.5%	3.3%	2.8%	2.2%	2.7%	1.9%
Presistent Crying	Percentage of infants within 72 hours after immunization was 1.6% after dose one, 0.6% after dose two, and 0.3% after dose three.								

§ Local reactions were evaluated at the ActHIB® injection site.
* The adverse reaction profile is defined by the concomitant use of CLI DTP vaccine.
† The number of individuals observed at each time point for fever varied from 357 to 363.

CARCINOGENESIS, MUTAGENESIS, IMPAIRMENT OF FERTILITY

ActHIB® reconstituted with CLI DTP vaccine has not been evaluated for its carcinogenic, mutagenic potential or impairment of fertility.

PREGNANCY

REPRODUCTIVE STUDIES–PREGNANCY CATEGORY C

Animal reproduction studies have not been conducted with ActHIB® reconstituted with CLI DTP vaccine or saline diluent (0.4% Sodium Chloride). It is also not known whether ActHIB® reconstituted with CLI DTP vaccine or saline diluent (0.4% Sodium Chloride) can cause fetal harm when administered to a pregnant woman or can affect reproduction capacity. ActHIB® reconstituted with CLI DTP vaccine or saline diluent (0.4% Sodium Chloride) is NOT recommended for use in a pregnant woman and is not approved for use in children 5 years of age or older.

PEDIATRIC USE

SAFETY AND EFFECTIVENESS OF ActHIB® RECONSTITUTED WITH CLI DTP VACCINE OR SALINE DILUENT (0.4% SODIUM CHLORIDE) IN INFANTS BELOW THE AGE OF SIX WEEKS HAVE NOT BEEN ESTABLISHED. (See **DOSAGE AND ADMINISTRATION** section.)

ADVERSE REACTIONS

NOTE: Haemophilus b Conjugate Vaccine (Tetanus Toxoid Conjugate) – ActHIB® is identical to Haemophilus b Conjugate Vaccine (Tetanus Toxoid Conjugate) – OmniHIB™ (distributed by SmithKline Beecham Pharmaceuticals); both products are manufactured by Pasteur Mérieux Sérums & Vaccins S.A.

More than 7,000 infants and young children (≤2 years of age) have received at least one dose of ActHIB® during US clinical trials. Of these, 1,064 subjects 12 to 24 months of age who received ActHIB® alone reported no serious or life threatening adverse reactions.

Summarized in Table 5 are adverse reactions temporally associated with ActHIB® immunization in 188 subjects 12 to 15 months of age.[18]

TABLE 5 [18]

PERCENTAGE OF 12- TO 15-MONTH-OLD CHILDREN PRESENTING WITH LOCAL OR SYSTEMIC REACTIONS WITHIN THE FIRST 24 HOURS OF IMMUNIZATION WITH ActHIB® (n = 188)

REACTIONS	DOSE 1*	DOSE 2*
Local		
Pain	9.0%	6.4%
Erythema (1 to 5 cm)	24.0%	18.6%
Induration	9.6%	9.0%
Systemic		
Fever (>100.6°F)	7.4%	6.4%
Irritability	30.9%	28.2%
Lethargy	18.6%	17.0%
Anorexia	9.0%	8.5%
Rhinorrhea	24.5%	21.3%
Diarrhea	5.8%	8.5%
Vomiting	4.3%	3.7%
Cough	9.6%	4.3%

* DTP was not administered concomitantly with ActHIB®.

When ActHIB® was administered to infants at 2, 4, and 6 months of age concomitantly, at separate sites, with CLI DTP vaccine, the systemic adverse experience profile was not different from that seen when CLI DTP vaccine was administered alone.[18] *(Refer to product insert for CLI whole-cell DTP.)*

Adverse reactions from a US multicenter trial in 2-, 4- and 6-month-old infants are summarized in Table 6. Systemic adverse reactions listed in Table 6 are more prominent than those in Table 5 because infants also received concomitant immunization with DTP.[14,18]

[See table 6 above.]

In general, the rates of minor systemic reactions after ActHIB® and DTP immunization were comparable to those usually reported after DTP vaccine alone.[29,30,31,32]

When ActHIB® reconstituted with CLI whole-cell DTP was administered in infants at 2, 4, and 6 months of age, the systemic adverse experience profile (Table 7) was comparable to that observed when the two vaccines were given separately (Table 6). An increase in the rate of local reactions was observed in some instances within the 24-hour period after immunizations.[18]

[See table 7 at bottom of next page.]

In a third US trial where ActHIB® was reconstituted with DTP, approximately 1,450 doses were administered to infants starting at 2 months of age. Adverse reactions observed at 6 and 24 hours respectively after the first immunization (n=498) were tenderness 66.9% and 30.7%; erythema (>1″) 8.6% and 2.2%; induration 38.2% and 21.7%; irritability 77.9% and 35.7%; drowsiness 63.7% and 34.1%; anorexia 26.1% and 12.9%; diarrhea 6.8% and 9.0%; and vomiting 3.4% and 3.8%.[18] One hypotonic/hyporesponsive episode (HHE) was seen in an infant following the second dose in this trial. This is consistent with the HHE incidence rate observed with DTP vaccination alone.[4]

Adverse reactions associated with ActHIB® generally subsided after 24 hours and usually do not persist beyond 48 hours after immunization.

In a randomized, double-blind US clinical trial, ActHIB® was given concomitantly with DTP to more than 5,000 infants and hepatitis B vaccine was given with DTP to a similar number. In this large study, deaths due to sudden infant death syndrome (SIDS) and other causes were observed but were not different in the two groups. In the first 48 hours following immunization, two definite and three possible seizures were observed after ActHIB® and DTP in comparison with none after hepatitis B vaccine and DTP.[18] This rate of seizures following ActHIB® and DTP was not greater than previously reported in infants receiving DTP alone. Other adverse reactions reported with administration of other Haemophilus b conjugate vaccines include urticaria, seizures, hives, renal failure and Guillain-Barré syndrome (GBS).[18,33] A cause and effect relationship among any of these events and the vaccination has not been established.

When ActHIB® was given with DTP and inactivated poliovirus vaccine to more than 100,000 Finnish infants, the rate and extent of serious adverse reactions were not different from those seen when other Haemophilus b conjugate vaccines were evaluated in Finland (i.e. HibTITER®, ProHIBit®).[18]

Reporting of Adverse Events

Reporting by the parent or guardian of all adverse events occurring after vaccine administration should be encouraged. Adverse events following immunization with vaccine should be reported by the health-care provider to the US Department of Health and Human Services (DHHS) Vaccine Adverse Event Reporting System (VAERS). Reporting forms and information about reporting requirements on comple-

Continued on next page

Connaught Laboratories—Cont.

tion of the form can be obtained from VAERS through a toll-free number 1-800-822-7967.[24,25,26]

Health care providers also should report these events to the Director of Medical Affairs, Connaught Laboratories, Inc., Route 611, PO Box 187, Swiftwater, PA 18370 or call 1-800-822-2463.

DOSAGE AND ADMINISTRATION

NOTE: Haemophilus b Conjugate Vaccine (Tetanus Toxoid Conjugate)—ActHIB® is identical to Haemophilus b Conjugate Vaccine (Tetanus Toxoid Conjugate)—OmniHIB™ (distributed by SmithKline Beecham Pharmaceuticals); both products are manufactured by Pasteur Mérieux Sérums & Vaccins S.A.

Parenteral drug products should be inspected visually for particulate matter and/or discoloration prior to administration, whenever solution and container permit. If these conditions exist, the vaccine should not be administered.

RECONSTITUTION:

Using saline diluent (0.4% Sodium Chloride) cleanse the vaccine vial rubber barrier with a suitable germicide and inject the entire volume of diluent contained in the syringe into the vial of lyophilized vaccine. Thorough agitation is advised to ensure complete reconstitution. The entire volume of reconstituted vaccine is then drawn back into a new syringe before injection of one 0.5 mL dose. The vaccine will appear clear and colorless.

Reconstitution instructions for saline diluent (0.4% Sodium Chloride): see Figures 3, 4 and 5 below.

Administer ActHIB® reconstituted with saline diluent (0.4% Sodium Chloride) **intramuscularly. Vaccine should be used within 24 hours after reconstitution.**

Using Connaught Laboratories, Inc. DTP vaccine, cleanse both the DTP and ActHIB® vaccine vial rubber barriers with a suitable germicide prior to reconstitution. Thoroughly agitate the vial of CLI DTP vaccine, then withdraw a 0.6 mL dose and inject into the vial of lyophilized ActHIB® vaccine. After reconstitution and thorough agitation, ActHIB® will appear whitish in color. Withdraw and administer 0.5 mL dose of ActHIB® reconstituted with CLI DTP vaccine.

Administer ActHIB® reconstituted with CLI DTP vaccine **intramuscularly only. Vaccine should be used within 24 hours after reconstitution.**

INSTRUCTIONS FOR RECONSTITUTION OF ActHIB® WITH CLI DTP VACCINE OR SALINE DILUENT (0.4% SODIUM CHLORIDE):

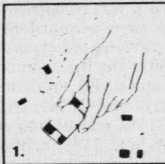

Figure 1. Using DTP for reconstitution, agitate CLI DTP vial thoroughly for resuspension.

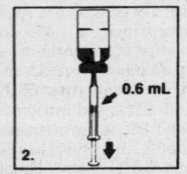

Figure 2. Withdraw 0.6 mL of DTP.

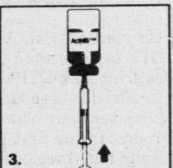

Figure 3. After cleansing the rubber barriers, insert syringe needle through the rubber barrier into the ActHIB® vial and inject 0.6 mL of DTP or saline diluent (0.4% Sodium Chloride).

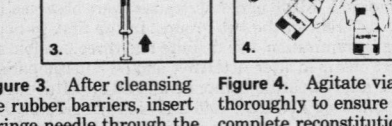

Figure 4. Agitate vial thoroughly to ensure complete reconstitution.

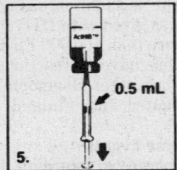

Figure 5. After reconstitution with DTP vaccine, withdraw 0.5 mL of reconstituted vaccine and administer **intramuscularly only.**

After reconstitution with saline diluent (0.4% Sodium Chloride), discard syringe and withdraw total volume of reconstituted vaccine in a new syringe and administer 0.5 mL intra-muscularly.

After reconstitution with CLI DTP, each 0.5 mL dose is formulated to contain 10 μg of purified capsular polysaccharide conjugated to 24 μg of inactivated tetanus toxoid, 8.5% of sucrose, 6.7 Lf of diphtheria toxoid, 5 Lf of tetanus toxoid and an estimate of 4 protective units of pertussis vaccine. *(Refer to product insert for CLI whole-cell DTP.)*

Before injection, the skin over the site to be injected should be cleansed with a suitable germicide. After insertion of the needle, aspirate to ensure that the needle has not entered a blood vessel.

DO NOT INJECT INTRAVENOUSLY.

Each dose of ActHIB® reconstituted with CLI DTP vaccine or saline diluent (0.4% Sodium Chloride) is administered intramuscularly in the outer aspect of the vastus lateralis (mid-thigh) or deltoid. The vaccine should not be injected into the gluteal area or areas where there may be a nerve trunk. During the course of primary immunizations, injections should not be made more than once at the same site. When ActHIB® or OmniHIB™ is reconstituted with CLI DTP vaccine, the combined vaccines are indicated for infants and children 2 months through 5 years of age for intramuscular administration in accordance with the schedule indicated in Table 8.[14]

[See table below.]

For Previously Unvaccinated Children

Immunization schedules should be considered on an individual basis for children not vaccinated according to the recommended schedule. Three doses of a product containing DTP, given at approximately 2-month intervals, are required followed by a fourth dose of a product containing DTP or DTaP approximately 12 months later and a fifth dose of a product containing DTP or DTaP at 4 to 6 years of age. If the fourth dose of a pertussis-containing vaccine is not given until after the fourth birthday, no further doses of a pertussis-containing vaccine are necessary.

The number of doses of Haemophilus b Conjugate Vaccine indicated depends on the age at which immunization is begun. A child 7 to 11 months of age should receive 2 doses of Haemophilus b Conjugate Vaccine at 8-week intervals and a booster dose at 15 to 18 months of age. A child 12 to 14 months of age should receive 1 dose of Haemophilus b Conjugate Vaccine followed by a booster dose at 15 to 18 months of age. A child 15 to 59 months of age should receive 1 dose of Haemophilus b Conjugate Vaccine.

Preterm infants should be vaccinated according to their chronological age from birth.[34]

Interruption of the recommended schedule with a delay between doses should not interfere with the final immunity achieved with ActHIB® reconstituted with CLI DIP vaccine or saline diluent (0.4% Sodium Chloride). There is no need to start the series over again, regardless of the time elapsed between doses.

It is recommended that the same conjugate vaccine be used throughout each immunization schedule, consistent with the data supporting approval and licensure of the vaccine. Since ActHIB® and OmniHIB™ are the same vaccine, these may be used interchangeably.

HOW SUPPLIED

Vial, 1 Dose, lyophilized vaccine (10 × 1 Dose vials per package), packaged with one 7.5 mL vial of Connaught Laboratories, Inc. Diphtheria and Tetanus Toxoids and Pertussis Vaccine as Diluent—Product No. 49281-549-10

Administer vaccine within 24 hours after reconstitution

STORAGE

Store lyophilized vaccine packaged with vial containing Diphtheria and Tetanus Toxoids and Pertussis and reconstituted vaccine, when not in use, between 2°–8°C (35°–46°F). DO NOT FREEZE. Discard vaccine within 24 hours after reconstitution.

REFERENCES

1. Chu CY, et al. Further studies on the immunogenicity of *Haemophilus influenzae* type b and pneumococcal type 6A polysaccharide-parotein conjugate. Infect immun 40: 245–246, 1983
2. Mueller JH, et al. Production of diphtheria toxin of high potency (100 Lf) on a reproducible medium. J Immunol 40: 21–32, 1941
3. Adams WG, et al. Decline of Childhood *Haemophilus influenzae* Type b (Hib) Disease in the Hib Vaccine Era. JAMA 269: 221–226, 1993
4. Recommendations of the Immunization Practices Advisory Committee (ACIP). Haemophilus b conjugate vaccines for prevention of *Haemophilus influenzae* type b disease among infants and children two months of age and older. MMWR 40: No. RR-1, 1991
5. Broome CV. Epidemiology of *Haemophilus influenzae* type b infections in the United States. Pediatr Infect Dis J 6: 779–782, 1987
6. ACIP. Polysaccharide vaccine for prevention of *Haemophilus influenzae* type b disease. MMWR 34: 201–205, 1985
7. Istre GR, et al. Risk factors for primary invasive *Haemophilus influenzae* disease: Increased risk from day care attendance and school-aged household members. J Pediatr 106: 190–195, 1985
8. Redmond SR, et al. *Hemophilus influenzae* type b disease. An epidemiologic study with special reference to day-care centers. JAMA 252: 2581–2584, 1984

TABLE 7[18] **PERCENTAGE OF INFANTS PRESENTING WITH LOCAL OR SYSTEMIC REACTIONS AT 6, 24, AND 48 HOURS OF IMMUNIZATION WITH ActHIB® RECONSTITUTED WITH CLI DTP VACCINE**

REACTION	2 Months (n=204) 6 Hrs.	24 Hrs.	48 Hrs.	4 Months (n=199) 6 Hrs.	24 Hrs.	48 Hrs.	6 Months (n=200) 6 Hrs.	24 Hrs.	48 Hrs.
Local									
Tenderness	47.1%	18.6%	3.4%	33.2%	17.6%	4.0%	25.0%	17.0%	3.5%
Erythema > 1″	11.8%	2.5%	0.0%	11.6%	9.1%	2.5%	10.5%	13.5%	3.5%
Induration	31.4%	17.2%	3.9%	26.1%	20.1%	7.5%	28.5%	22.5%	10.0%
Systemic									
Fever >100.4°F	24.6%	2.0%	0.5%	15.8%	6.1%	3.6%	13.0%	10.3%	3.1%
Irritability	70.6%	22.1%	12.8%	56.8%	31.2%	19.1%	40.5%	28.2%	15.9%
Drowsiness	60.3%	23.5%	11.3%	42.2%	20.6%	9.6%	30.3%	12.3%	5.6%
Anorexia	17.7%	6.4%	2.9%	10.1%	7.5%	5.5%	5.1%	4.6%	4.1%
Diarrhea	2.5%	5.4%	1.5%	3.5%	3.5%	2.5%	2.6%	4.1%	5.6%
Vomiting	2.9%	5.4%	2.9%	3.0%	5.0%	3.0%	3.6%	3.6%	1.5%
Presistent Crying	Percentage of infants within 72 hours after immunization was 0.0% after dose one, 0.0% after dose two, and 0.005% after dose three.								

TABLE 8[14] **RECOMMENDED IMMUNIZATION SCHEDULE FOR ActHIB® AND DTP** For Previously Unvaccinated Children

DOSE	AGE	IMMUNIZATION
First, Second and Third	At 2, 4 and 6 months	ActHIB® or OmniHIB™/reconstituted with DTP or with saline diluent (0.4% Sodium Chloride)
Fourth	At 15 to 18 months	ActHIB® or OmniHIB™/reconstituted with DTP or with saline diluent (0.4% Sodium Chloride)
Fifth	At 4 to 6 years	DTP or Acellular Pertussis (DTaP)*

*Acellular Pertussis (DTaP) should NOT be used to reconstitute ActHIB®/OmniHIB™. When administering DTaP for the fourth dose, *Haemophilus influenzae* type b vaccine also should be administered at this time in a separate syringe at a different site.

9. Murphy TV, et al. County-wide surveillance of invasive Haemophilus infections: Risk of associated cases in Child Care Programs (CCPs). Twenty-third Interscience Conference on Antimicrobial Agents and Chemotherapy (Abstract #788) 229, 1983
10. Fleming D, et al. *Haemophilus influenzae* b (Hib) disease—secondary spread in day care. Twenty-fourth Interscience Conference on Antimicrobial Agents and Chemotherapy (Abstract #967) 261, 1984
11. CDC. Prevention of secondary cases of *Haemophilus influenzae* type b disease. MMWR 31: 672–680, 1982
12. Michaels RH, et al. Pharyngeal colonization with *Haemophilus influenzae* type b: A longitudinal study of families with a child with meningitis or epiglottitis due to *H. influenzae* type b. J Infec Dis 136: 222–227, 1977
13. Holmes SJ, et al. Immunogenicity of four *Haemophilus influenzae* type b conjugate vaccines in 17- to 19-month-old children. J Pediatr 118: 364–371, 1991
14. Data on file, Pasteur Mérieux Sérums & Vaccins S.A.
15. Peltola H, et al. Prevention of *Haemophilus influenzae* type b bacteremic infections with the capsular polysaccharide vaccine. N Engl J Med 310: 1561–1566, 1984
16. Decker MD, et al. Comparative trial in infants of four conjugate *Haemophilus influenzae* type b vaccines. J Pediar 120: 184–189, 1992
17. Granoff DM, et al. Differences in the immunogenicity of three *Haemophilus influenzae* type b conjugate vaccines in infants. J Pediatr 121: 187–194, 1992
18. Data on file, Connaught Laboratories, Inc.
19. Kaplan SL, et al. Immunogenicity of *Haemophilus influenzae* type b polysaccharide-tetanus protein conjugate vaccine in children with sickle hemoglobinopathy or malignancies, and after systemic *Haemophilus influenzae* type b infection. J Pediatr 120: 367–370, 1992
20. Steinhoff MC, et al. Antibody responses to *Haemophilus influenzae* type b vaccines in men with human immunodeficiency virus infection. N Engl J Med 325(26): 1837–1842, 1991
21. ACIP. General recommendations on immunization. MMWR 38: 205–227, 1989
22. ACIP. Diphtheria, Tetanus, and Pertussis: Recommendations for Vaccine Use and Other Preventive Measures. MMWR 40: No. RR-10, 1991
23. FDA Workshop on Haemophilus b Polysaccharide Vaccine—A Preliminary Report. MMWR 36: 529–531, 1987
24. Rothstein EP, et al. Comparison of antigenuria after immunization with three *Haemophilus influenzae* type b conjugate vaccines. Pediatr Infect Dis J 10: 311–314, 1991
25. Vaccine Adverse Event Reporting System—United States. MMWR 39: 730–733, 1990
26. CDC. National Childhood Vaccine Injury Act: Requirements for permanent vaccination records and for reporting of selected events after vaccination. MMWR 37: 197–200, 1988
27. National Childhood Vaccine Injury Act of 1986 (Amended 1987)
28. Clemens JD, et al. Impact of *Haemophilus influenzae* Type b Polysaccharide-Tetanus Protein Conjugate Vaccine on responses to concurrently administered Diphtheria-Tetanus-Pertussis Vaccine. JAMA 267: 673–678, 1992
29. Cody CL, et al. Nature and rates of adverse reactions associated with DTP and DT immunizations in infants and children. Pediatr 68: 650–660, 1981
30. Barkin RM, et al. Diphtheria-tetanus-pertussis vaccine: reactogenicity of commercial products. Pediatr 63: 256–260, 1979
31. Baraff LJ, et al. DTP-associated reactions: an analysis by injection site, manufacturer, prior reactions and dose. Pediatr 73: 31–39, 1984
32. Long SS, et al. Longitudinal study of adverse reactions following diphtheria-tetanus-pertussis vaccine in infancy. Pediatr 85: 294–302, 1990
33. D'Cruz OF, et al. Acute inflammatory demyelinating polyradiculoneuropathy (Guillain-Barré Syndrome) after immunization with *Haemophilus influenzae* type b conjugate vaccine. J Pediatr 115: 743–746, 1989
34. American Academy of Pediatrics. Immunization in Special Clinical Circumstances. In: Peter G, ed. 1994 Red Book: Report of the Committee on Infectious Diseases. 23rd ed. Elk Grove Village, IL 51–52, 1994

Product information
as of November 1994

Manufactured by:
PASTEUR MERIEUX Sérums & Vaccins S.A.
Lyon, France US License No. 384

Distributed by:
CONNAUGHT LABORATORIES, INC
Swiftwater, Pennsylvania 18370, USA
1-800-VACCINE (1-800-822-2463)

DIPHTHERIA AND TETANUS TOXOIDS AND PERTUSSIS VACCINE ADSORBED USP (FOR PEDIATRIC USE) ℞

Caution: Federal (USA) law prohibits dispensing without prescription.

DESCRIPTION

Diphtheria and Tetanus Toxoids and Pertussis Vaccine Adsorbed USP (For Pediatric Use) combines diphtheria and tetanus toxoids adsorbed with pertussis vaccine, for intramuscular use, in a sterile isotonic sodium chloride solution containing sodium phosphate buffer to control pH. The vaccine, after shaking, is a turbid liquid, whitish-gray in color. When used to reconstitute Haemophilus b Conjugate Vaccine (Tetanus Toxoid Conjugate), ActHIB® or OmniHIB™, the combined vaccines appear whitish in color.

Corynebacterium diphtheriae cultures are grown in a modified Mueller and Miller medium.[1] *Clostridium tetani* cultures are grown in a peptone-based medium. Both toxins are detoxified with formaldehyde. The detoxified materials are separately purified by serial ammonium sulfate fractionation and diafiltration.

The pertussis vaccine component is derived from *Bordetella pertussis* cultures grown on blood-free Bordet Gengou media. The pertussis organisms are harvested and inactivated with thimerosal and resuspended in physiological saline and thimerosal.

The toxoids are adsorbed to aluminum potassium sulfate (alum). The adsorbed diphtheria and tetanus toxoids are combined with pertussis vaccine concentrate, and diluted to a final volume using sterile phosphate-buffered physiological saline. Each 0.5 mL dose contains, by assay, not more than 0.17 mg of aluminum and not more than 100 µg (0.02%) of residual formaldehyde. Thimerosal (mercury derivative) 1:10,000 is added as a preservative.

Each 0.5 mL dose is formulated to contain 6.7 Lf of diphtheria toxoid and 5 Lf of tetanus toxoid (both toxoids induce at least 2 units of antitoxin per mL in the guinea pig potency test).

The total human immunizing dose (the first three 0.5 mL doses administered) contains an estimate of 12 units of pertussis vaccine (4 protective units per single dose).[2] The potency of the pertussis component of each lot of DTP is tested in a mouse protection test.

At the time when Connaught Laboratories, Inc. (CLI) DTP vaccine is used to reconstitute ActHIB® or OmniHIB™, each single dose of the 0.5 mL mixture is formulated to contain 6.7 Lf of diphtheria toxoid, 5 Lf of tetanus toxoid, an estimate of 4 protective units of pertussis vaccine, 10 µg of purified capsular polysaccharide conjugated to 24 µg of inactivated tetanus toxoid, and 8.5% of sucrose.

NOTE: Haemophilus b Conjugate Vaccine (Tetanus Toxoid Conjugate)—ActHIB® is identical to Haemophilus b Conjugate Vaccine (Tetanus Toxoid Conjugate)—OmniHIB™ (distributed by SmithKline Beecham Pharmaceuticals); both products are manufactured by Pasteur Mérieux Sérums & Vaccins S.A.

HOW SUPPLIED

DTP Vial, 7.5 mL—Product No. 49281-280-84

One 7.5 mL vial of Connaught Laboratories, Inc. Diphtheria and Tetanus Toxoids and Pertussis Vaccine as Diluent packaged with Vial, 1 Dose lyophilized Haemophilus b Conjugate Vaccine (Tetanus Toxoid Conjugate) (10 × 1 Dose vials per package)—Product No. 49281-549-10

Administer vaccine immediately within 24 hours after reconstitution.

STORAGE

Store between 2°–8°C (35°–46°F). DO NOT FREEZE. Temperature extremes may adversely affect resuspendability of this vaccine.

Store lyophilized vaccine packaged with vial containing Diphtheria and Tetanus Toxoids and Pertussis vaccine and reconstituted vaccine, when not in use, between 2°–8°C (35°–46°F). DO NOT FREEZE. Discard vaccine within 24 hours after reconstitution.

INFLUENZA VIRUS VACCINE USP TRIVALENT Types A and B ℞
(Zonal Purified, Whole Subvirion)
1995–96 Formula—For 6 Months and Older
FLUZONE®

DESCRIPTION

Fluzone®, Influenza Virus Vaccine USP, (Zonal Purified, Subvirion) for intramuscular use, is a sterile suspension prepared from the aliantoic fluids of chicken embryos infected with a specific type of influenza virus. The virus-containing fluids are harvested and inactivated with formaldehyde. Influenza virus is concentrated and purified in a linear sucrose density gradient solution using a continuous flow centrifuge. The virus is then chemically disrupted using Glycol p-isooctylphenyl Ether (Triton® X-100—A registered trademark of Rohm and Haas, Co.) producing a "split-antigen." The split-antigen is then further purified by chemical means and suspended in sodium phosphate-buffered isotonic sodium chloride solution. Fluzone has been standardized according to USPHS requirements for the 1995-96 influenza season and contains 45 micrograms (µg) hemagglutinin (HA) per 0.5 mL dose, in the recommended ratio of 15 µg HA each, representative of the following three prototype strains: A/Texas/36/91 (H1N1), A/Wuhan/359/95 — Like (H3N2) and B/Beijing/184/93 — Like. Gelatin 0.05% is added as a stabilizer and thimerosal (mercury derivative) 1:10,000 is added as a preservative. Fluzone, after shaking syringe/vial well, is essentially clear and slightly opalescent in color.

ANTIBIOTICS ARE NOT USED IN THE MANUFACTURE OF FLUZONE.

HOW SUPPLIED

Syringe, 0.5 mL. (Shake syringe before administering.) (Do not use for administering 0.25 mL.)—Product No. 49281-352-11

Vial, 5 mL, for administration with needle and syringe (may be used with jet injector, although the desired number of doses may not be obtained). (Shake vial well before withdrawing each dose.)—Product No. 49281–352–15

Vial, 25 mL, recommended for JET INJECTOR USE (may be used in needle and syringe method of immunization; however, due to coring of the stopper do not insert needle into vial more than 20 times). (Available on special order only.) (Shake vial well before withdrawing each dose.)—Product No. 49281–350–50

RABIES IMMUNE GLOBULIN (HUMAN) U.S.P. IMOGAM® RABIES ℞
[Im 'o-gam]

DESCRIPTION

Rabies Immune Globulin (Human) IMOGAM® RABIES is a sterile solution of antirabies immunoglobulin (10–18% protein) for intramuscular administration. It is prepared by cold alcohol fractionation from pooled venous plasma of individuals immunized with Rabies Vaccine prepared from human diploid cells (HDCV). The product is stabilizied with 0.3 M glycine and contains 1:10,000 sodium ethylmercurithiosalicylate (thimerosal) as a preservative. The globulin solution has a pH of 6.860.4 adjusted with sodium hydroxide or hydrochloric acid.

The product is standardized against the U.S. Standard Rabies Immune Globulin. The U.S. unit of potency is equivalent to the International Unit (I.U.) for rabies antibody.

CLINICAL PHARMACOLOGY

Rabies antibody provides passive protection when given immediately to individuals exposed to rabies virus.[1,2] Rabies Immune Globulin (Human) [RIG(H)] of adequate potency[3] was used in conjunction with Rabies Vaccine of duck embryo origin.[3,4] When a globulin dose of 20 I.U./kg of rabies antibody was given simultaneously with the first dose of vaccine, adequate levels of passive rabies antibody were detected 24 hours after injection in all individuals. There was minimal or no interference with the immune response to the initial and subsequent doses of vaccine, including booster doses.

More recently studies of Rabies Immune Globulin (Human)[5] IMOGAM RABIES given with the first of five doses of Pasteur Mérieux Sérums et Vaccins S.A. HDCV[6] confirmed that passive immunization with 20 I.U./kg of Rabies Immune Globulin (Human) provides maximum circulating antibody with minimum interference of active immunization by HDCV.

INDICATIONS AND USAGE

Rabies Immune Globulin (Human) IMOGAM RABIES is indicated for individuals suspected of exposure to rabies, particularly severe exposure, with one exception: persons who have been previously immunized with Rabies Vaccine and have confirmed adequate rabies antibody titers should receive only vaccine.

Rabies Immune Globulin (Human) IMOGAM RABIES should be injected as promptly as possible after exposure. If initiation of treatment is delayed for any reason, Rabies Immune Globulin (Human) should still be given, regardless of the interval between exposure and treatment, up to the eighth day after the first dose of vaccine was given.

Rabies virus is usually transmitted by the bite of a rabid animal but can occasionally penetrate abraded skin contaminated with the saliva of infected animals. Progress of the virus after exposure is believed to follow a neural pathway and the time between exposure and clinical rabies is a function of the proximity of the bite (or abrasion) to the central nervous system and the dose of virus injected. The incubation is usually 2–6 weeks but can be longer. After severe bites about the face and neck and arms, it may be as short as 10

Continued on next page

Connaught Laboratories—Cont.

days. After initiation of the vaccine series (human diploid cell origin), it takes approximately one week for development of immunity to rabies; therefore, the value of immediate passive immunization with rabies antibodies in the form of Rabies Immune Globulin (Human) cannot be overemphasized.

Recommendations for passive and/or active immunization after exposure to an animal suspected of having rabies have been outlined by the W.H.O.[7] and by the United States Public Health Service Immunization Practices Advisory Committee (ACIP).[6]

I. Rationale of Treatment
In the United States and Canada the following factors should be considered before specific antirabies treatment is indicated:

1. Species of Biting Animal
Carnivorous animals (especially skunks, foxes, coyotes, raccoons, dogs, bobcats, and cats) and bats are more likely to be infected with rabies than other animals. Rats, mice, squirrels, hamsters, guinea pigs, gerbils, chipmunks and other rodents or rabbits and hares are rarely infected with rabies and have not been known to cause human rabies in the United States. Their bites almost never call for antirabies prophylaxis; therefore, before initiating antirabies prophylaxis, the local or state health department should be consulted.

2. Circumstances of Biting Incident
An UNPROVOKED attack is more likely than a provoked attack to indicate that the animal is rabid. Bites inflicted on a person attempting to feed or handle an apparently healthy animal should generally be regarded as PROVOKED.

3. Type of Exposure
Rabies is commonly transmitted by inoculation with infectious saliva. The likelihood that rabies infection will result from exposure to a rabid animal varies with the nature and extent of the exposure. Two categories of exposure should be considered:
Bite: Any penetration of the skin by teeth.
Nonbite: Scratches, abrasions, open wounds of mucous membranes contaminated with saliva or other potentially infectious material such as brain tissue from a rabid animal.
In addition, there have been two instances of airborne rabies acquired in the laboratory and probable airborne rabies acquired in one bat-infested cave (Frio Cave, Texas). Casual contact with a rabid animal, such as petting the animal (without a bite or nonbite exposure as described above) does not constitute an exposure and is not an indication for prophylaxis.
The only documented cases of rabies due to human-to-human transmission occurred in patients who received corneas transplanted from persons who died of rabies undiagnosed at the time of death.
Each exposure to possible rabies infection must be individually evaluated. Local or state public health officials should be consulted if questions arise about the need for rabies prophylaxis.

4. Vaccination Status of Biting Animal
A properly immunized animal has only a minimal chance of developing rabies and transmitting the virus.

II. Post-Exposure Treatment of Rabies
1. Local Treatment of Wounds
Immediate and thorough local treatment of all bite wounds and scratches is perhaps the most effective preventive measure. The wound should be thoroughly cleansed immediately with soap and water. Tetanus prophylaxis and measures to control bacterial infection should be given as indicated.

2. Specific Treatment
Post-exposure antirabies treatment should always include both passive (preferably Rabies Immune Globulin—Human) and active (preferably Rabies Vaccine prepared from human diploid cells) immunization with one exception: persons who have been previously immunized with Rabies Vaccine and have a documented adequate rabies antibody titer should receive only vaccine. The combination of globulin and vaccine is recommended for both bite exposures and nonbite exposures (as described under "Rationale for Treatment") and regardless of the interval between exposure and treatment. The sooner treatment is begun after exposure, the better.

3. Post-Exposure Treatment Guide
The following recommendations are only a guide. They should be applied in conjunction with knowledge of the animal species involved, circumstances of the bite or other exposure, vaccination status of the animal, and presence of rabies in the region. Local and state public health officials should be consulted if questions arise about the need for rabies prophylaxis.
[See table below.]

CONTRAINDICATIONS
Rabies Immune Globulin (Human) *should not* be administered in repeated doses once vaccine treatment has been initiated. Repeating the dose may interfere with maximum active immunity expected from the vaccine.

WARNINGS
Rabies Immune Globulin (Human) should be given with caution to patients with a history of prior systemic allergic reactions following the administration of human immune globulin preparations or those individuals allergic to thimerosal.
Persons with specific IgA deficiency have increased potential for developing antibodies to IgA and could have anaphylactic reactions to subsequent administration of blood products containing IgA.[8,9]

PRECAUTIONS
General—Rabies Immune Globulin (Human) should not be administered intravenously because of the potential for serious reactions. Injection should be made intramuscularly and care should be taken to draw back on the plunger of the syringe before injection in order to be certain that the needle is not in a blood vessel. Although systemic reactions to immunoglobulin preparations are rare, epinephrine should be available for treatment of acute anaphylactoid systems. As with all preparations given intramuscularly, bleeding complications may be encountered in patients with bleeding disorders.
Drug Interactions—Live virus vaccine such as measles vaccines should not be given close to the time of Rabies Immune Globulin (Human) administration because antibodies in the globulin preparation may interfere with the immune response to the vaccination. Immunization with live vaccines should not be given within three months after Rabies Immune Globulin (Human) administration.
Pregnancy Category C—Animal reproduction studies have not been conducted with Rabies Immune Globulin (Human). It is also not known whether RIG(H) can cause fetal harm when administered to a pregnant woman or can affect reproductive capacity. RIG(H) should be given to a pregnant woman only if clearly needed.

ADVERSE REACTIONS
Local or mild systemic adverse reactions to the globulin after intramuscular injection are uncommon [10,11] and may be treated symptomatically. Local tenderness, soreness or stiffness of the muscles may occur at the injection site and may persist for several hours after injection. Urticaria and angioedema may occur. Anaphylactic reactions, although rare, have been reported following injection of human immune globulin preparations.

DOSAGE AND ADMINISTRATION
IMOGAM RABIES should be used in conjunction with Rabies Vaccine such as Mérieux's IMOVAX® RABIES vaccine prepared from human diploid cell cultures. The recommended dose of IMOGAM RABIES is a single intramuscular administration of 20 I.U./kg (0.133 ml/kg) or 9 I.U./lb (0.06 ml/lb) of body weight at the time of administration of the first vaccine dose.[3,4] If possible up to half the dose should be used to infiltrate the wound, and the rest administered intramuscularly, in a different site from the rabies vaccine, preferably in the gluteal region.
Parenteral drug products should be inspected visually for particulate matter and discoloration prior to administration, when ever solution and container permit.

HOW SUPPLIED
Rabies Immune Globulin (Human) IMOGAM RABIES is supplied in 2 ml and 10 ml vials with average potency of 150 international Units per milliliter (I.U./ml). The 2 ml vial contains 300 I.U. which is sufficient for a child weighing 15 kg (33 lb). The 10 ml vial contains a total of 1,500 I.U. which is sufficient for an adult weighing 75 kg (165 lb).

STORAGE
IMOGAM® RABIES should be stored in the refrigerator between 2 and 8°C (35 to 47°F). Do not freeze.

REFERENCES
1. Baltazard M., Bahmanyar M., Ghodssi M., et al. Essai pratique du serum antirabique chez les mordus par loups enrages. *Bull WHO* 13:747–772 (1955).
2. Habel K., Koprowski H. Laboratory data supporting clinical trial of antirabies serum in persons bitten by rabid wolf. *Bull WHO* 13:773–779 (1955).
3. Cabasso V.J., Loofbourow J.C., Roby R.E., et al. Rabies immune globulin of human origin: preparation and dosage determination in non-exposed volunteer subjects. *Bull WHO* 45:303–315 (1971).
4. Loofbourow J.C., Cabasso VJ., Roby R.E., et al. Rabies immune globulin (human). Clinical trials and dose determination. *JAMA* 217:1825–1831 (1971).
5. Helmick C.G., et al. A clinical study of Merieux human rabies immune globulin. *J Biol Stand* 10:357–367 (1982).
6. Centers for Disease Control: ACIP recommendation: Rabies prevention. *Morbidity & Mortality Weekly Report* 29:265–272, 277–280 (1980).
7. WHO Expert Committee on Rabies. *WHO Tech Rep Ser* 523:50–51 (1973).
8. Fudenberg H.H. Sensitization to immunoglobulins and hazards of gamma globulin therapy, pp 211–220 in Merler E., Editor Immunoglobulins: biologic aspects and clinical uses. National Academy of Sciences, Wash., D.C. (1970).
9. Pineda A.A. and Taswell H.F. Transfusion reactions associated with anti-IgA antibodies: Report of four cases and review of the literature. *Transfusion* 15:10–15 (1975).
10. Janeway C.A., Rosen F.S. The gamma globulins. IV. Therapeutic uses of gamma globulins. *N Engl J Med* 275:826–831 (1966).
11. Kjellman H. Adverse reactions to human immune serum globulin in Sweden (1969–1978). pp 143–150. Immunoglobulins: Characteristics and uses of intravenous preparations. Alving B.M. and Finlayson J.S., Editors. U.S. Dept. Health & Human Services, DHHS Publ. No. (FDA) 80-9005, Wash., D.C. (1980).

Manufactured by:
PASTEUR MÉRIEUX Sérums & Vaccins S.A.
Lyon, France   U.S. License No. 384
Distributed by:
CONNAUGHT LABORATORIES, INC.
Swiftwater, Pennsylvania 18370, U.S.A.
800-VACCINE (800-822-2463)
CONNAUGHT
A PASTEUR MÉRIEUX COMPANY
Revised July 1991

Animal Species	Condition of Animal at Time of Attack	Treatment of Exposed Person (1). All bites and wounds should immediately be thoroughly cleansed with soap and water (see preceding text)
Domestic dog and cat	Healthy and available for 10 days of observation	None unless animal develops rabies (2)
	Rabid or suspected rabid	Rabies Immune Globulin (Human) [RIG(H)] and Rabies Vaccine (4)
	Unknown	Consultation with public health officials. If treatment is indicated, give [RIG(H)] (3) and Rabies Vaccine (4).
Wild Skunk, bat, fox, coyote, raccoon, bobcat and other carnivores	Regard as rabid unless proven negative by laboratory test (5)	[RIG(H)] (3) and Rabies Vaccine (4)
Other livestock, rodents, rabbits and hares.	Consider individually – provoked bites of squirrels, hamsters, guinea pigs, gerbils, chipmunks, rats, mice and other rodents or rabbits and hares almost never call for antirabies prophylaxis. Local or state public health officials should be consulted about questions that arise about the need for rabies prophylaxis.	

(1) If antirabies treatment is indicated, both RIG(H) and Rabies Vaccine should be given as soon as possible, *regardless* of the interval after exposure, excepts persons who have been previously immunized with rabies vaccine and have a confirmed adequate rabies antibody titer should receive only vaccine.
(2) Begin treatment with RIG(H) and Rabies Vaccine at first sign of rabies in biting domestic animals during the usual holding period of 10 days. The symptomatic animal should be killed immediately and tested.
(3) If RIG(H) is not available, use antirabies serum of equine origin. Do not use more than the recommended dosage.
(4) Discontinue vaccine if fluorescent antibody tests of animal are negative.
(5) The animal should be killed and tested as soon as possible. Holding for observation is not recommended.

RABIES VACCINE ℞
IMOVAX® RABIES
[Im 'o-vaks]
WISTAR RABIES VIRUS STRAIN PM-1503-3M GROWN IN HUMAN DIPLOID CELL STRUCTURES

DESCRIPTION

The Imovax® Rabies Vaccine produced by Pasteur Mérieux Sérums et Vaccins is a sterile, stable, freeze-dried suspension of rabies virus prepared from strain PM-1503-3M obtained from the Wistar Institute, Philadelphia, PA.
The virus is harvested from infected human diploid cells, MRC-5 strain, concentrated by ultrafiltration and is inactivated by beta propiolactone. One dose of reconstituted vaccine contains less than 100 mg albumin, less than 150 µg neomycin sulfate and 20 µg of phenol red indicator. This vaccine must only be used intramuscularly and as a single dose vial.
The vaccine contains no preservative or stabilizer. It should be used immediately after reconstitution, and if not administered promptly, discard contents.
The potency of one dose (1.0 ml) Merieux Imovax Rabies Vaccine is equal to or greater than 2.5 international units of rabies antigen.

CLINICAL PHARMACOLOGY

Pre-exposure immunization
High titer antibody responses of the Merieux Imovax Rabies Vaccine made in human diploid cells have been demonstrated in trials conducted in England (1), Germany (2, 3), France (4) and Belgium (5), Seroconversion was often obtained with only one dose. With two doses one month apart, 100% of the recipients developed specific antibody and the geometric mean titer of the group was approximately 10 international units. In the U.S., Merieux Imovax Rabies Vaccine resulted in geometric mean titers (GMT) of 12.9 I.U./ml at Day 49 and 5.1 I.U./ml at Day 90 when three doses were given intramuscularly during the course of one month. The range of antibody responses was 2.8 to 55.0 I.U./ml at Day 49 and 1.8 to 12.4 I.U. at Day 90. (6) The definition of a minimally accepted antibody titer varies among laboratories and is influenced by the type of test conducted. CDC currently specifies a 1:5 titer (complete inhibition) by the rapid fluorescent focus inhibition test (RFFIT) as acceptable. The World Health Organization (WHO) specifies a titer of 0.5 I.U.
Post-exposure immunization
Post-exposure efficacy of Merieux Imovax Rabies Vaccine was successfully proven during clinical experience in Iran (7) in conjunction with antirabies serum. Forty-five persons severely bitten by rabid dogs and wolves received Merieux vaccine within hours of and up to 14 days after the bites. All individuals were fully protected against rabies.
There have been reports of possible vaccine failure when the vaccine has been administered in the gluteal area. Presumably subcutaneous fat in the gluteal area may interfere with the immunogenicity of human diploid cell rabies vaccine (HDCV) (26, 29). For adults and children, Rabies Vaccine should be administered in the deltoid muscle. (See Dosage and Administration).

INDICATIONS AND USAGE

1. Rationale of treatment
Physicians must evaluate each possible rabies exposure. Local or state public health officials should be consulted if questions arise about the need for prophylaxis. (8)
In the United States and Canada, the following factors should be considered before antirabies treatment is initiated.
Species of biting animal
Carnivorous wild animals (especially skunks, raccoons, foxes, coyotes, and bobcats) and bats are the animals most commonly infected with rabies and have caused most of the indigenous cases of human rabies in the United States since 1960. Unless an animal is tested and shown not to be rabid, post-exposure prophylaxis should be initiated upon bite or nonbite exposure to the animals. (See definition in "Type of Exposure" below.) If treatment has been initiated and subsequent testing in a competent laboratory shows the exposing animal is not rabid, treatment can be discontinued. (8)
The likelihood that a domestic dog or cat is infected with rabies varies from region to region; hence the need for post-exposure prophylaxis also varies. (8)
Rodents (such as squirrels, hamsters, guinea pigs, gerbils, chipmunks, rats and mice) and lagomorphs (including rabbits and hares) are rarely found to be infected with rabies and have not been known to cause human rabies in the United States. In these cases, the state or local health department should be consulted before a decision is made to initiate post-exposure antirabies prophylaxis. (8)
Circumstances of biting incident
An UNPROVOKED attack is more likely than a provoked attack to indicate the animal is rabid. Bites inflicted on a person attempting to feed or handle an apparently healthy animal should generally be regarded as PROVOKED.
Type of exposure
Rabies is transmitted by introducing the virus into open cuts or wounds in skin or via mucous membranes. The likelihood of rabies infection varies with the nature and extent of exposure. Two categories of exposure should be considered.
Bite: Any penetration of the skin by teeth.
Nonbite: Scratches, abrasions, open wounds, or mucous membranes contaminated with saliva or other potentially infectious material, such as brain tissue, from a rabid animal. Casual contact, such as petting a rabid animal (without a bite or nonbite exposure as described above), does not constitute an exposure and is not an indication for prophylaxis. There have been two instances of airborne rabies acquired in laboratories and two probable airborne rabies cases acquired in a bat-infested cave in Texas. (8, 9)
The only documented cases for rabies from human-to-human transmission occured in four patients in the United States and overseas who received corneas transplanted from persons who died of rabies, undiagnosed at the time of death. (9,10) Stringent guidelines for acceptance of donor corneas should reduce this risk. Bite and nonbite exposure from humans with rabies theoretically could transmit rabies, although no cases of rabies acquired this way have been documented. Each potential exposure to human rabies should be carefully evaluated to minimize unnecessary rabies prophylaxis. (8, 11).

II. Pre- and post-exposure treatment of rabies
A. Pre-exposure—See Table 1
Pre-exposure immunization may be offered to persons in high risk groups, such as veterinarians, animal handlers, certain laboratory workers, and persons spending time (e.g. 1 month or more) in foreign countries where rabies is a constant threat. Persons whose vocational or avocational pursuits bring them into contact with potentially rabid dogs, cats, foxes, skunks, bats, or other species at risk of having rabies should also be considered for pre-exposure prophylaxis. (8)
Vaccination is recommended for children living in or visiting countries where exposure to rabid animals is a constant threat. Worldwide statistics indicate children are more at risk than adults.
Pre-exposure prophylaxis is given for several reasons. First, it may provide protection to persons with inapparent exposure to rabies. Secondly, it may protect persons whose post-exposure therapy might be expected to be delayed. Finally, although it does not eliminate the need for additional therapy after a rabies exposure, it simplifies therapy by eliminating the need for globulin and decreasing the number of doses of vaccine needed. This is of particular importance for persons at high risk of being exposed in countries where the available rabies immunizing products may carry a higher risk of adverse reactions.
Pre-exposure immunization does not eliminate the need for prompt prophylaxis following an exposure. It only reduces the post-exposure treatment regimen. (8)

TABLE 1 (8)

CRITERIA FOR PRE-EXPOSURE IMMUNIZATION

Risk category	Nature of risk	Typical populations	Pre-exposure regimen
Continuous	Virus present continuously often in high concentrations. Aerosol, mucus membrane, bite or nonbite exposure possible. Specific exposures may go unrecognized.	Rabies research lab workers*. Rabies biologics production workers.	Primary pre-exposure immunization course. Serology every 6 months. Booster immunization when antibody titer falls below acceptable level*.
Frequent	Exposure usually episodic, with source recognized, but exposure may also be unrecognized. Aerosol, mucous membrane, bite or nonbite exposure.	Rabies diagnostic lab workers*, spelunkers, veterinarians, and animal control and wildlife workers in rabies epizootic areas.	Primary pre-exposure immunization course. Booster immunization or serology every 2 years†
Infrequent (greater than population-at-large)	Exposure nearly always episodic with source recognized. Mucous membrane, bite or nonbite exposure.	Veterinarians and animal control and wildlife workers in areas of low rabies endemicity. Certain travelers to foreign rabies epizootic areas. Veterinary students.	Primary pre-exposure immunization course. No routine booster immunization or serology.
Rare (population-at-large)	Exposure always episodic, mucous membrane, or bite with source recognized.	U.S. population-at-large, including individuals in rabies epizootic areas.	No pre-exposure immunization.

* Judgement of relative risk and extra monitoring of immunization status of laboratory workers is the responsibility of the laboratory supervisor (see U.S. Department of Health and Human Service's Biosafety in Microbiological and Biomedical Laboratories, 1984).
† Pre-exposure booster immunization consists of one dose of HDCV, 1.0 ml/dose, IM (deltoid area). Acceptable antibody level is 1:5 titer (complete inhibition in RFFIT at 1:5 dilution). See Clinical Pharmacology. Boost if titer falls below 1:5.

PRE-EXPOSURE RABIES TREATMENT GUIDE

1. Pre-exposure immunization: Consists of the three doses of HDCV, 1.0 ml, intramuscularly (deltoid area), one each on Days 0,7 and 21 or 28. Administration of routine booster doses of vaccine depends on exposure risk category as noted in Table 1. Pre-exposure immunization of immunosuppressed persons is not recommended. (8)
[See Table 1 above.]
B. Post-exposure—See Table 2
The essential components of rabies post-exposure prophylaxis are local treatment of wounds and immunization, including administration, in most instances, of both globulin and vaccine (Table 2). (8, 13)
1. Local treatment of wounds: Immediate and thorough washing of all bite wounds and scratches with soap and water is perhaps the most effective measure for preventing rabies. In experimental animals, simple local wound cleansing has been shown to reduce markedly the likelihood of rabies. (8, 11)
Tetanus prophylaxis and measures to control bacterial infection should be given as indicated.
2. Specific treatment: Post-exposure antirabies immunization should always include administration of both antibody (preferably RIG) and vaccine, with one exception: persons who have been previously immunized with the recommended pre-exposure or post-exposure regimens with HDCV or who have been immunized with other types of vaccines and have a history of documented adequate rabies antibody titer should receive only vaccine. The combination of globulin and vaccine is recommended for both bite exposures and nonbite exposures regardless of the interval between exposure and treatment. (14,15) The sooner treatment is begun after exposure, the better. However, there have been instances in which the decision to begin treatment was made as late as 6 months or longer after the exposure due to delay in recognition that an exposure had occurred. (8, 13)
3. Treatment outside the United States: If post-exposure is begun outside the United States with locally produced biologics, it may be desirable to provide additional treatment when the patient reaches the U.S. State health departments should be contacted for specific advice in such cases. (8)

POST-EXPOSURE TREATMENT GUIDE

The following recommendations are only a guide. In applying them, take into account the animal species involved, the circumstances of the bite or other exposure, the vaccination status of the animal, and presence of rabies in the region. Local or state public health officials should be consulted if questions arise about the need for rabies prophylaxis. (8)
[See Table 2 at bottom of next page.]

Continued on next page

Connaught Laboratories—Cont.

CONTRAINDICATIONS

For post-exposure treatment, there are no known specific contraindications to the use of Merieux Imovax Rabies Vaccine. In cases of pre-exposure immunization, there are no known specific contraindications other than situations such as developing febrile illness, etc.

WARNINGS

Rabies Vaccine in this package is a unit dose to be delivered intramuscularly in the deltoid area. (8)

This vaccine must not be used intradermally or as a multiple dose dispensing unit. In both pre-exposure and post exposure immunization, the full 1.0 ml dose should be given intramuscularly.

In the case of pre-exposure immunization, recently a significant increase has been noted in "immune complex-like" reactions in persons receiving booster doses of HDCV. (16) The illness characterized by onset 2–21 days post-booster, presents with a generalized urticaria and may also include arthralgia, arthritis, angioedema, nausea, vomiting, fever, and malaise. In no cases were the illnesses life-threatening. Preliminary data suggest this "immune complex-like" illness may occur in up to 6% of persons receiving booster vaccines and much less frequently in persons receiving primary immunization. Additional experience with this vaccine is needed to define more clearly the risk of these adverse reactions. (8, 17)

Two cases of neurologic illness resembling Guillain-Barre syndrome (18, 19), a transient neuroparalytic illness, that resolved without sequelae in 12 weeks and a focal subacute central nervous system disorder temporally associated with HDCV, have been reported. (20)

All serious systemic neuroparalytic or anaphylactic reactions to a rabies vaccine should be immediately reported to the state health department or Connaught Laboratories, Inc., 800-VACCINE/800-822-2463. (8)

PRECAUTIONS

IN ADULTS AND CHILDREN THE VACCINE SHOULD BE INJECTED INTO THE DELTOID MUSCLE. IN INFANTS AND SMALL CHILDREN THE MID-LATERAL ASPECT OF THE THIGH MAY BE PREFERABLE.

General

When a person with a history of hypersensitivity must be given rabies vaccine, antihistamines may be given; epinephrine (1:1000) should be readily available to counteract anaphylactic reactions, and the person should be carefully observed after immunization.

While the concentration of antibiotics in each dose of vaccine is extremely small, persons with known hypersensitivity to any of these agents could manifest an allergic reaction. While the risk is small, it should be weighed in light of the potential risk of contracting rabies.

Drug interactions

Corticosteroids, other immunosuppressive agents, and immunosuppressive illnesses can interfere with the development of active immunity and predispose the patient to developing rabies. Immunosuppressive agents should not be administered during post-exposure therapy, unless essential for the treatment of other conditions. When rabies post-exposure prophylaxis is administered to persons receiving ste-roids or other immunosuppressive therapy, it is especially important that serum be tested for rabies antibody to ensure than an adequate response has developed. (8)

Usage in pregnancy

Pregnancy Category C. Animal reproduction studies have not been conducted with Imovax Rabies Vaccine. It is also not known whether the product can cause fetal harm when administered to a pregnant woman or can affect reproductive capacity. Rabies vaccine should be given to a pregnant woman only if clearly needed.

Because of the potential consequences of inadequately treated rabies exposure and limited data that indicate that fetal abnormalities have not been associated with rabies vaccination, pregnancy is not considered a contraindication to post-exposure prophylaxis. (8, 21) If there is substantial risk of exposure to rabies, pre-exposure prophylaxis may also be indicated during pregnancy. (8)

Pediatric use

Both safety and efficacy in children have been established.

ADVERSE REACTIONS

ALSO SEE WARNINGS AND CONTRAINDICATIONS SECTIONS FOR ADDITIONAL STATEMENTS

Once initiated, rabies prophylaxis should not be interrupted or discontinued because of local or mild systemic adverse reactions to rabies vaccine. Usually such reactions can be successfully managed with anti-inflammatory and antipyretic agents (e.g. aspirin).

Reactions after vaccination with HDCV are less common than with previously available vaccines. (12,16,17) In a study using five doses of HDCV, local reactions, such as pain, erythema, and swelling or itching at the injection site were reported in about 25% of recipients of HDCV, and mild systemic reactions such as headache, nausea, abdominal pain, muscle aches and dizziness were reported in about 20% of recipients. (8)

Serious systemic anaphylactic or neuroparalytic reactions occurring during the administration of rabies vaccines pose a dilemma for the attending physician. A patient's risk of developing rabies must be carefully considered before deciding to discontinue vaccination. Moreover, the use of corticosteroids to treat life-threatening neuroparalytic reactions carries the risk of inhibiting the development of active immunity to rabies. It is especially important in these cases that the serum of the patient be tested for rabies antibodies. Advice and assistance on the management of serious adverse reactions in persons receiving rabies vaccines may be sought from the state health department or Merieux Institute, Inc. (8)

DOSAGE AND ADMINISTRATION

Parenteral drug products should be inspected visually for particulate matter and discoloration prior to administration, whenever solution and container permit. Reconstitute the freeze-dried vaccine in its vial with the 1.0 ml of diluent supplied in the disposable syringe using the longer of the two needles. Gently swirl the contents until completely dissolved and withdraw the total amount of dissolved vaccine into the syringe by setting the vial in an upright position on the table. Remove the reconstitution needle and replace it with the smaller needle.

The reconstituted vaccine should be used immediately.

After preparation of the injection site, immediately inject the vaccine intramuscularly. For adults and children, the vaccine should be injected into the deltoid muscle (22 to 27, 29). In infants and small children, the mid lateral aspect of the thigh may be preferable. Care should be taken to avoid injection into or near blood vessels and nerves. After aspiration, if blood or any suspicious discoloration appears in the syringe, do not inject but discard contents and repeat procedure using a new dose of vaccine, at a different site.

NOTE: The freeze-dried vaccine is creamy white to orange. After reconstitution it is pink to red.

A. Pre-exposure dosage

1. Primary vaccination: In the United States, the Immunization Practices Avisory Committee (ACIP) recommends three injections of 1.0 ml each, one injection on Day 0 and one on Day 7 and one either on Day 21 or 28. (8)

2. Booster dose: Persons working with live rabies virus in research laboratories and in vaccine production facilities should have rabies antibody titers checked every six months and boosters given as needed to maintain an adequate titer. (For definition of adequate titer, see Clinical Pharmacology.) Only laboratory workers, such as those doing rabies diagnostic tests, spelunkers and veterinarians, animal control and wildlife officers in areas where rabies is epizootic should have boosters every 2 years or have their serum tested for rabies antibody every 2 years and, if the titer is inadequate, have a booster dose. Veterinarians and animal control and wildlife officers, if working in areas of low rabies endemicity, do not require routine booster doses of HDCV after completion of primary pre-exposure immunization (Table 1). (8)

Persons who have experienced "immune complex-like" hypersensitivity reactions should receive no further doses of HDCV unless they are exposed to rabies or they are truly likely to be inapparently and/or unavoidably exposed to rabies virus and have unsatisfactory antibody titers.

B. Post-exposure dosage

The World Health Organization established a recommendation for six intramuscular doses of human diploid cell vaccine (HDCV) based on studies in Germany and Iran. (3,7) Used in this way, a total of 6 injections of a 1.0 ml dose of vaccine are given according to the following schedule. On Day 0, 3, 7, 14, 30 and 90. The first dose should be accompanied by Rabies Immune Globulin (RIG) or Antirabies Serum (ARS). If possible, up to half the dose of RIG or ARS should be used to infiltrate the wound, and the rest administered intramuscularly, in a different site from the rabies vaccine, preferably in the gluteal region.

Studies conducted at the CDC in the United States have shown that a regimen of 1 dose of Rabies Immune Globulin (RIG) and 5 doses of HDCV induced an excellent antibody response in all recipients. Of 511 persons bitten by proven rabid animals and so treated, none developed rabies. (8)

Based on these data, the ACIP recommends a 5-dose regimen for post-exposure situations. Five 1.0 ml doses are given intramuscularly on Day 0, 3, 7, 14 and 28 in conjunction with RIG on Day 0. (8)

Because the antibody response following the recommended vaccination regimen with HDCV has been so satisfactory, routine post-vaccination serologic testing is not recommended. Serologic testing is indicated in unusual circumstances, as when the patient is known to be immunosuppressed. Contact state health department or CDC for recommendations. (8, 28)

C. Post-exposure therapy of previously immunized persons

When an immunized person who was vaccinated by the recommended regimen with HDCV or who had previously demonstrated rabies antibody is exposed to rabies, that person should receive two I.M. doses (1.0 ml each) of HDCV, one immediately and one 3 days later. RIG should not be given in these cases. If the immune status of a previously vaccinated person who did not receive the recommended HDCV regimen is not known, full primary post-exposure antirabies treatment (RIG plus 5 doses of HDCV) may be necessary. In such cases, if antibody can be demonstrated in a serum sample collected before vaccine is given, treatment can be discontinued after at least two doses of HDCV. (8)

HOW SUPPLIED

IMOVAX RABIES VACCINE is supplied in a tamperproof unit dose plastic box with:
—One vial of freeze-dried vaccine containing a single dose.
—One disposable needle and syringe containing diluent for reconstitution.
—One smaller disposable needle for administration.

STORAGE

The freeze-dried vaccine is stable if stored in the refrigerator between 2°C and 8°C (36°F to 46°F). Do not freeze.

TABLE 2 (8)

Animal species	Condition of animal at time of attack	Treatment of exposed person*
DOMESTIC: Dog and cat	Healthy and available for 10 days of observation	None unless animal develops rabies†
	Rabid or suspected rabid	RIG§ and HDCV
	Unknown (escaped)	Consult public health officials If treatment is indicated, give RIG§ and HDCV
WILD: Skunk, bat, fox, coyote, raccoon, bobcat and other carnivores	Regard as rabid unless proven negative by laboratory tests £	RIG§ and HDCV
OTHER: Livestock, rodents and lagomorphs (rabbits and hares)	Consider individually. Local and state public health officials should be consulted on questions about the need for rabies prophylaxis. Bites of squirrels, hamsters, guinea pigs, gerbils, chipmunks, rats, mice, other rodents, rabbits and hares, almost never call for antirabies prophylaxis.	

* All bites and wounds should immediately be thoroughly cleansed with soap and water. If antirabies treatment is indicated, both rabies immune globulin (RIG) and human diploid cell rabies vaccine (HDCV) should be given as soon as possible regardless of the interval from exposure. Local reactions to vaccines are common and do not contraindicate continuing treatment. Discontinue vaccine if fluorescent antibody tests of the animal are negative.

† During the usual holding period of 10 days, begin treatment with RIG and HDCV at first sign of rabies in a dog or cat that has bitten someone. The symptomatic animal should be killed immediately and tested.

§ If RIG is not available, use antirabies serum, equine (ARS). Do not use more than the recommended dosage.

£ The animal should be killed and tested as soon as possible. Holding for observation is not recommended.

REFERENCES

1. Aoki FY, Tyrell DAJ, Hill LE. Immunogenicity and acceptability of a human diploid cell culture rabies vaccine in volunteers. The Lancet, March 22, pp. 660–2 (1975).

2. Cox JH, Schneider LG. Prophylactic immunization of humans against rabies by intradermal inoculation of human diploid cell culture vaccine. J Clin Microbiol 3:96–101 (1976).

3. Kuwert EK, Marcus 1, Werner J, Iwand A, Thraenhart O. Some experiences with human diploid cell

strain—(HDCS) rabies vaccine in pre- and post-exposure vaccinated humans. Develop Biol Standard 40:79–88 (1978).

4. Ajjan N, Soulebot J-P, Stellmann C, Biron G, Charbonnier C, Triau R, Merieux C. Resultats de la vaccination antirabique preventive par le vaccin inactivé concentré souche PM/W138-1503-3M cultivés sur cellules diploïdes humaines. Develop Biol Standard 40:89–199 (1978).

5. Coty-Berger F. Vaccination antirabique préventive par du vaccin préparé sur cellules diploïdes humaines. Develop Biol Standard 40:101–4 (1978).

6. Bernard KW, Roberts MA, Sumner J, Winkler WG, Mallonee J, Baer GM, Chaney R. Human diploid cell rabies vaccine JAMA 247:1138–42 (1982).

7. Bahmanyar M, Fayaz A, Nour-Salehi S, Mohammadi M, Koprowski H. Successful protection of humans exposed to rabies infection. JAMA 236: 2751–4 (1976).

8. CDC. Recommendations of the Immunization Practices Advisory Committee (ACIP). Rabies Prevention—United States, 1984, MMWR 33: 393–402, 407–8 (1984).

9. Anderson U.,Nicholson KG, Tauxe RV, Winkler WG. Human rabies in the United States, 1960 to 1979, epidemiology, diagnosis and prevention. Ann Intern Med 100: 728–35 (1984).

10. WHO. Sixth report of the Expert Committee on Rabies. Geneva Switzerland: World Health Organization. (WHO technical report No. 523) (1973).

11. Baer GM, ed. The natural history of rabies. New York: Academic Press. (1975).

12. Greenberg M, Childress J. Vaccination against rabies with duck-embryo and Semple vaccines. JAMA 173:333–7 (1960).

13. Helmick CG. The epidemiology of human rabies post-exposure prophylaxis. JAMA 250: 1990–6 (1983).

14. Devriendt J, Staroukine M, Costy F, Vanderhaegen, J-J. Fatal encephalitis apparently due to rabies. JAMA 248: 2304–6 (1982).

15. CDC. Human Rabies—Rwanda. MMWR 31: 135 (1982).

16. CDC. Systemic allergic reactions following immunization with human diploid cell rabies vaccine. MMWR 33:185–7 (1984).

17. Rubin RH, Hattwick MAW, Jones S, Gregg MB, Schwartz VD. Adverse reactions to duck embryo rabies vaccine. Ann Intern Med 78: 643–9 (1973).

18. Boe E, Nyland H. Guillain-Barre syndrome after vaccination with human diploid cell rabies vaccine. Scand J Infect Dis 12:231–2 (1980).

19. CDC. Adverse reactions to human diploid cell rabies vaccine. MMWR 29: 609–10 (1980).

20. Bernard KW, Smith PW, Kader FJ, Moran MJ. Neuroparalytic illness and human diploid cell rabies vaccine. JAMA 248: 3136–8 (1982).

21. Varner MW, McGuinness GA, Galask RP. Rabies vaccination in pregnancy. Am J of Obst and Gyn 143:717–18 (1982).

22. Cockshott WP, Thompson GT, Howlett U, Seely ET. Intramuscular or intralipomatous injections? N Eng J Med 307: 356–58 (1982).

23. CDC. General Recommendations on Immunization, ACIP. MMWR 32: 1–8, 13–17 (1983).

24. Committee on Immunization Council of Medical Societies, American College of Physicians. Guide for Adult Immunizations. (1985).

25. CDC. Rabies post-exposure prophylaxis with HDCV: Lower neutralizing antibody titers with Wyeth vaccine. MMWR 34: 90–92 (1985).

26. Shill M, Baynes RD, Miller SD. Fatal rabies encephalitis despite appropriate post-exposure prophylaxis. N Engl J Med 316:1257–58 (1987).

27. Baer GM, Fishbein DB. Rabies post-exposure prophylaxis. N Engl J Med 316: 1270–72 (1987).

28. CDC. Recommendations of the Immunization Practices Advisory Committee (ACIP). Supplementary statement on rabies vaccine and serologic testing. MMWR 30: 535–6 (1981).

29. CDC. Human rabies despite treatment with Rabies Immune Globulin and Human Diploid Cell Rabies Vaccine—Thailand. MMWR 36: 759–765 (1987).

Manufactured by:
PASTEUR MERIEUX Sérums & Vaccins S.A.
Lyon, France   U.S. License No. 384
Distributed by:
CONNAUGHT LABORATORIES, INC.
Swiftwater, Pennsylvania 18370, U.S.A.
800-VACCINE (800-822-2463)
Revised: July 1991

RABIES VACCINE   ℞
IMOVAX® RABIES I.D.
[im'o-vaks I.D.]
Wistar Rabies Virus Strain PM–1503-3M
Grown in Human Diploid Cell Cultures

FOR PRE-EXPOSURE USE ONLY BY THE INTRADERMAL ROUTE (I.D.)

DESCRIPTION
The Imovax Rabies I.D., Rabies Vaccine, produced by Pasteur Mérieux Sérums et Vaccins is a sterile, stable, freeze-dried suspension of rabies virus prepared from strain PM-1503-3M obtained from the Wistar Institute, Philadelphia, PA.

The virus is harvested from infected human diploid cells, MRC-5 strain, concentrated by ultrafiltration and is inactivated by beta propiolactone. One dose of reconstituted vaccine contains less than 15 mg human albumin, less than 22 μg neomycin sulfate and 3 μg of phenol red indicator. *This vaccine dose is for intradermal use only.*

The vaccine contains no preservative or stabilizer. It should be used immediately after reconstitution.

The potency of Merieux Imovax Rabies I.D., Rabies Vaccine, is equal to or greater than 2.5 International Units/ml of rabies antigen. An intradermal dose contains at least 0.25 International Units (I.U.).

CLINICAL PHARMACOLOGY
Studies in Europe (1–6) and in the United States (7,8) to investigate the efficacy and safety of low dose intradermal vaccination schedules have shown that satisfactory levels of antibody were produced in all subjects with two or more inoculations.

Studies in the United States (7,8,9) using three doses of Merieux's Rabies Vaccine demonstrated adequate rabies antibody titers in 100% persons receiving intradermal injections. The geometric mean titer in these subjects 49 days after immunization was approximately 7.5 to 8.9 I.U. compared with 12.9 to 13.8 I.U. in controls receiving 1.0 ml of vaccine intramuscularly (7).

The definition of a minimally acceptable antibody titer varies both among laboratories and according to the purposes for which immunization is given. The Centers for Disease Control (CDC) currently specifies, complete virus neutralization at a 1:5 serum dilution in the rapid fluorescent focus inhibition test (RFFIT) as an acceptable response to pre-exposure immunization. After studies of post-exposure immunization, the World Health Organization (WHO) specifies a titer of 0.5 I.U. as an acceptable response.

INDICATIONS AND USAGE
For Pre-Exposure Use Only
Pre-exposure immunization should be considered for persons in high risk groups, such as veterinarians, animal handlers, certain laboratory workers, and those whose vocational or avocational pursuits bring them into contact with potentially rabid dogs, cats, foxes, skunks, bats, or other species at risk of having rabies. (See Table I).

For persons traveling abroad into endemic areas, Human Diploid Cell Vaccine (HDCV) may be administered by the I.D. dose and route if the 3 dose series is completed 30 days or more before departure. If pre-exposure vaccination is performed for travelers at other times, a vaccine intended for intramuscular use should be used.

Vaccination is recommended for children living in or visiting countries where exposure to rabid animals is a constant threat. Worldwide statistics indicate children are more at risk than adults.

Pre-exposure prophylaxis is given for several reasons. First, it may provide protection to persons with inapparent exposure to rabies. Secondly, it may protect persons, whose post-exposure therapy might be expected to be delayed. Finally, although it does not eliminate the need for additional therapy after a rabies exposure, it simplifies therapy by eliminating the need for globulin and decreasing the number of doses of vaccine needed. This is of particular importance for persons at high risk of being exposed in countries where the available rabies immunizing products may carry a higher risk of adverse reactions.

Pre-exposure immunization does not eliminate the need for prompt prophylaxis following an exposure. It only reduces the post-exposure treatment regimen.

Pre-Exposure Rabies Treatment Guide
Pre-exposure immunization consists of a total of three doses of HDCV given on Days 0, 7 and 21 or 28. Each dose is 0.1 given intradermally in the deltoid area of either arm. Administration of booster doses of vaccine following primary 3-dose immunization depends on exposure risk category as noted in Table I. Pre-exposure immunization of immunosuppressed persons is not recommended. (9)

[See Table 1 below.]

CONTRAINDICATIONS
There are no known specific contraindications other than situations such as developing febrile illness, etc.

WARNINGS
SYRINGES IN THIS PACKAGE TO DELIVER INTRADERMALLY ONE DOSE (0.1 ML) OF IMOVAX RABIES I.D., RABIES VACCINE MUST NOT BE USED FOR POST-EXPOSURE IMMUNIZATION
The full 0.1 ml dose should be given intradermally.

Recently a significant increase has been noted of "immune complex-like" reactions in persons receiving booster doses of HDCV by the intradermal (0.1 ml) or intramuscular (1.0 ml) route. (10.11). The illness characterized by onset 2-21 days post-booster, presents with a generalized urticaria and may

Table I (9)

Criteria for Pre-exposure Immunization

Risk category	Nature at risk	Typical populations	Pre-esposure regimen
Continuous	Virus present continuously, often in high concentrations. Aerosol, mucous membrane, bite, or nonbite exposure possible. Specific exposures may go unrecognized.	Rabies research lab worker.* Rabies biologics production workers.	Primary pre-exposure immunization course. Serology every 6 months. Booster immunization when antibody titer falls below acceptable level.†
Frequent	Exposure usually episodic. with source recognized, but exposure may also be unrecognized. Aerosol, mucous, membrane, bite, or nonbite exposure.	Rabies diagnostic lab workers, *spelunkers, veterinarians, and animal control and wildlife workers in rabies epizootic areas.	Primary pre-exposure immunization course. Booster immunization or serology every 2 years.†
Infrequent (greater than population-at-large)	Exposure nearly always episodic with source recognized Mucous membrane, bite, or nonbite exposure.	Veterinarians and animal control and wildlife workers in areas of low rabies endemnicity. Certain travelers to foreign rabies epizootic areas. Veterinary students.	Primary pre-exposure immunization course. No routine booster immunization or serology.
Rare (population-at-large).	Exposure always episodic, mucous membrane, or bite with source recognized.	U.S. population-at-large, including individuals in rabies epizootic areas.	No pre-exposure immunization.

* Judgment of relative risk and extra monitoring of immunization status of laboratory workers is the responsibility of the laboratory supervisor (see U.S. Department of Health and Human Service's Biosafety in Microbiological and Biomedical Laboratories, 1984).

† Pre-exposure booster immunization consists of one dose of HDCV, 0.1 ml I.D. or 1.0 ml I.M. (deltoid area). Acceptable antibody level is a titer of 1:5 (complete inhibition of infectious foci in RFFIT at 1:5 serum dilution). See Clinical Pharmacology. Boost if titer falls below 1:5.

Continued on next page

Connaught Laboratories—Cont.

also include arthralgia, arthritis, angioedema, nausea, vomiting, fever and malaise. In no cases were the illnesses life-threatening. Preliminary data suggest this "immune complex-like" illness may occur in up to 6% of persons receiving booster doses of Rabies Vaccines and much less frequently in persons receiving primary immunization. There is preliminary evidence that beta propiolactone altered human albumin induces most of the allergic reactions. (9, 12) Persons who travel from the U.S. to developing countries and receive their pre-exposure vaccination abroad or within 30 days before leaving should be immunized by the intramuscular (IM) route (3 × 1.0 ml).

Two cases of neurologic illness resembling Guillain-Barré syndrome (13, 14), a transient neuroparalytic illness, that resolved without sequelae in 12 weeks, and a focal subacute nervous system disorder temporarily associated with HDCV, have been reported. (15)

All serious systemic neuroparalytic or anaphylactic reactions to a Rabies Vaccine should be immediately reported to the state health department or the Division of Viral Diseases, Center for Infectious Diseases, CDC, 404-329-3095 during working hours, or 404-329-2888 at other times. (9)

Persons previously vaccinated successfully against rabies and who come in contact with a rabid or potentially rabid animal, should have the wounds cleansed and receive a post-exposure dose of 1.0 ml of Rabies Vaccine intramuscularly, followed by a second 1.0 ml dose on Day 3. Intradermal immunization must not be used. Rabies Immune Globulin should NOT be given.

PRECAUTIONS

General—When a person with a history of hypersensitivity must be given Rabies Vaccine, antihistamines may be given; epinephrine (1:1000) should be readily available to counteract anaphylactic reactions, and the person should be carefully observed after immunization.

While the concentration of antibiotics in each dose of vaccine is extremely small, persons with known hypersensitivity to any of these agents could manifest an allergic reaction. While the risk is small, it should be weighed in light of potential risk of contracting rabies.

Drug Interactions—Antimalarial drugs such as chloroquine have been associated with a reduction in the antibody response to Rabies Vaccine administered by the intradermal route. Although it is apparent that antimalarial agents are not the sole factor responsible for the reduced antibody response, it is recommended that persons on corticosteroids and other immunosuppressive drugs receive Rabies Vaccine (3 doses/1.0 ml each) by the intramuscular route until more definitive data is available. (16, 17, 18)

Pregnancy Category C—Animal reproduction studies have not been conducted with Imovax Rabies I.D., Rabies Vaccine. It is also not known whether the product can cause fetal harm when administered to a pregnant woman or can affect reproductive capacity. Rabies Vaccine should be given to a pregnant woman only if clearly needed. Pre-exposure immunization should be carefully considered and may be indicated if there is substantial risk of rabies exposure.

Pediatric Use—Although specific intradermal studies in children have not been conducted, vaccine given to children intramuscularly (1.0 ml) has been shown to be safe. There are no known specific hazards expected from intradermal use of the vaccine in children. (19)

ADVERSE REACTIONS

Also See Warnings and Contraindications Sections for Additional Statements

Reactions after vaccination with HDVC are less common than with previously available vaccines. (10, 12, 20). In a study using five doses of HDVC administered intramuscularly, local reactions such as pain, erythema and swelling or itching at the injection site were reported in about 25% of recipients; mild systemic reactions such as headache, nausea, abdominal pain, muscle aches and dizziness were reported in about 20% of recipients. (9)

Clinical experience with Merieux Imovax Rabies I.D., Rabies Vaccine, has resulted in a low incidence of adverse reactions comparable to those following intramuscular vaccination when administered by the intradermal route except that a slight increase in transient local reactions has been observed following intradermal vaccination, especially when the vaccine is given in the forearm rather than in the lateral aspect of the upper arm. Local reactions consist of redness, itching, mild pain and minimal swelling at the site of injection. Generalized reactions are uncommon.(7) Mild local or systemic reactions can be treated with anti-inflammatory, antipyretic agents, e.g., aspirin and antihistamines. Systemic allergic or anaphylactic reactions following primary immunization have been reported to be less than 1%.(14) If an anaphylactic reaction should occur, epinephrine is indicated.

For "immune complex-like" reactions in persons receiving booster doses of HDCV see WARNINGS.

Advice and assistance on the management of serious adverse reactions in persons receiving primary or booster rabies im-

munization may be sought from the state health department or CDC.(9)

DOSAGE AND ADMINISTRATION

PARENTERAL DRUG PRODUCTS SHOULD BE INSPECTED VISUALLY FOR PARTICULATE MATTER AND DISCOLORATION PRIOR TO ADMINISTRATION, WHENEVER SOLUTION AND CONTAINER PERMIT. THE FREEZE-DRIED VACCINE IS CREAMY WHITE TO ORANGE. AFTER RECONSTITUTION IT IS PINK TO RED.

Primary Vaccination—Based upon studies in Europe (3,4) and the United States (8,9) the Immunization Practices Advisory Committee (ACIP) recommends three injections of 0.1 ml each; one injection on Day 0, one on Day 7, and one either on Day 21 or 28. (9,21) The ACIP, in making this recommendation, cites studies conducted in the United States and Europe in which more than 1500 persons received 0.1 ml of vaccine intradermally as the 2 or 3-dose pre-exposure vaccination. All subjects developed antibody as shown by the rapid fluorescent focus inhibition test (RFFIT). The ACIP suggests that routine serologic testing to confirm a satisfactory antibody response is not necessary. (22)

Booster Dose—Persons working with live rabies virus in research laboratories and in vaccine production facilities should have rabies antibody titers checked every six months and boosters given as needed to maintain an adequate titer. (For definition of adequate titer, see Clinical Pharmacology.) Laboratory workers, such as those doing rabies diagnostic tests, spelunkers and veterinarians, animal control and wildlife officers in areas where rabies is epizootic should have boosters every 2 years or have their serum tested for rabies antibody every 2 years and, if the titer is inadequate, have a booster dose. Veterinarians and animal control and wildlife officers working in areas of low rabies endemicity do not require routine doses of HDCV after completion of primary pre-exposure immunization (Table 1).

Persons who have experienced "immune complex-like" hypersensitivity reactions should receive no further doses of HDCV unless they are exposed to rabies or they are truly likely to be inapparently and/or unavoidably exposed to rabies virus and have unsatisfactory antibody titers.

INSTRUCTIONS FOR USE—Please Read Carefully and Completely

This package contains:

A single dose syringe of freeze dried Imovax Rabies I.D., Rabies Vaccine, which after reconstitution must be completely given by the intradermal route.

If the intradermal inoculation was not performed satisfactorily (vaccine injected subcutaneously) another dose should be given intradermally at a different site.

One vial of diluent (Sterile Water for Injection USP). The quantity of diluent contained in the vial is in excess of the volume needed. The purpose of this excess is to permit withdrawal of diluent without introduction of air.

To Open Vial

1. Pull green metal flip top in direction of arrow. This will loosen outer seal enough to be removed. (Figure 1)
2. Remove gray stopper. (Figure 2)

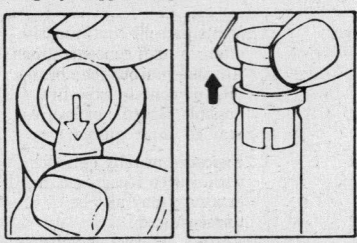

Figure 1   Figure 2

3. Carefully slide syringe out of glass vial.

To Prepare Diluent

1. Remove center of green protective cover at perforation on diluent vial. (Figure 3)

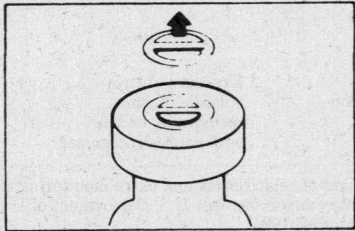

Figure 3

2. Disinfect pink stopper seal surface.

Reconstituting Vaccine

1. Remove protective rubber cap from needle. (Figure 4)

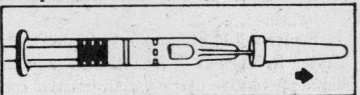

Figure 4

2. Push plunger so that the leading edge of the black stopper is even with the broken blue line (Figure 5)

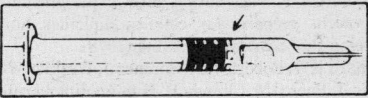

Figure 5

3. Insert needle into diluent bottle, keeping it upright. The needle must be in the liquid during withdrawal of the diluent to prevent air bubbles. (Fig. 6)
4. Withdraw diluent so that end of black stopper is at solid blue line. (Figure 7)

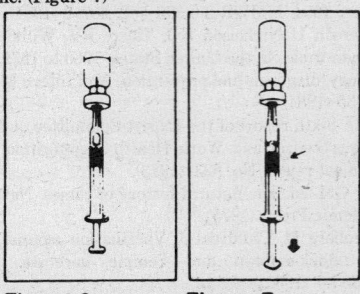

Figure 6   Figure 7

5. Replace protective rubber cap on needle and wait for freeze-dried vaccine to dissolve. Make sure that the freeze dried vaccine is completely dissolved. Shake if necessary. (Figure 8)

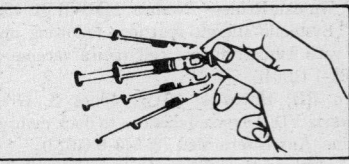

Figure 8

6. Remove protective cap and vaccine is ready to use.

After reconstitution, eliminate the air bubbles and bring together the droplets of vaccine either by flicking the syringe or, if necessary, grasp the covered needle end of the syringe and use a strong downward motion as indicated in Fig. 8 (as with a thermometer).

THE RECONSTITUTED VACCINE SHOULD BE USED IMMEDIATELY.

Remove the needle cover.

Push in the plunger to eliminate the air.

Disinfect the injection site.

Inject intradermally.

Destroy needle by clipping it off at the base of syringe.

HOW SUPPLIED

Imovax Rabies I.D., Rabies Vaccine—for pre-exposure use only by the intradermal route is supplied in a tamperproof unit with:

- One disposable syringe with integral needle containing a single dose of freeze-dried vaccine.
- One vial of Sterile Water for Injection USP for reconstitution.

STORAGE

The freeze-dried vaccine should be stored in the refrigerator between 2°C and 8°C (35°F to 47°F). Do not freeze.

REFERENCES

1. Aoki FY, Tyrell DA, Hill LE: Immunogenicity and acceptability of a human diploid cell rabies vaccine in volunteers. Lancet 1: 660-62(1975).
2. Turner GS, Aoki FY, Nicholson KG, Tyrrell DA, Hill LE: Human diploid cell strain rabies vaccine: Rapid prophylactic immunization of volunteers with small doses. Lancet 1: 1379-81 (1976).
3. Cox JH, Schneider LG: Prophylactic immunization of humans against rabies by intradermal inoculation of human diploid cell culture vaccine. J. Clin. Microbiol. 3: 96-101 (1976).
4. Nicholson KG, Turner GS, Aoki FY: Immunization with a human diploid cell strain of rabies virus vaccine: Two-year results, J. Infect. Dis. 137: 783-88 (1978).
5. Nicholson KG, Turner GS: Studies with human diploid cell strain rabies vaccine and human antirabies globulin in man. Dev. Biol. Stand. 40:115-20 (1978).

6. Ajjan N, Soulebot JP, Triau R, Biron G: Intradermal Immunization with rabies vaccine: Inactivated Wistar strain cultivated in human diploid cells. JAMA 244: 2528-31 (1980).

7. Bernard KW, Roberts MA, Sumner J, Winkler WG, Mallonee J, Baer GM, Chaney R: Human diploid cell rabies vaccine: Effectiveness of immunization with small intradermal or subcutaneous doses. JAMA 247: 1138-42 (1982).

8. Dreesen DW, Brown WJ, Kemp DT, Brown J, Reid FL, Baer GM: Pre-exposure rabies prophylaxis: efficacy of a new packaging and delivery system for intradermal administration of human diploid cell vaccine. Vaccine 2: 185-88 (1984).

9. CDC. Recommendations of the Immunization Practices Advisory Committee (ACIP). Rabies Prevention—United States, 1984. MMWR 33: 393-402, 407-8 (1984).

10. CDC. Systemic allergic reactions following immunization with human diploid cell rabies vaccine. MMWR 33: 185-87 (1984).

11. Dreesen DW, Bernard KW, Parker RA, Deutsch AJ, Brown J: Immune complex-like disease in 23 persons following a booster dose of rabies human diploid cell vaccine. Vaccine 4: 45-49 (1986).

12. Baer H, Anderson HC, Bernard K, Quinnan G: Beta propiolactone treated human serum albumin (BPL-HSA) an allergen for humans receiving rabies vaccine. (Abstract). J. Allergy and Clin. Immunol.75: (No. 1 Part 2 suppl) (1985).

13. Boe E, Nyland H: Guillain-Barré syndrome after vaccination with human diploid cell rabies vaccine. Scand. J. Infect. Dis. 12: 231-32 (1980).

14. CDC. Adverse reactions to human diploid cells rabies vaccine MMWR 29: 609-10 (1980).

15. Bernard KW, Smith PW, Kader FJ, Moran MJ: Neuroparalytic illness and human diploid cell rabies vaccine. JAMA 248: 3136-38 (1982).

16. Taylor DN, Wasi C, Bernard K: Chloroquine prophylaxis associated with a poor antibody reponse to human diploid cell rabies vaccine. Lancet 1: 1408 (1984).

17. Pappaioanou M, Fishbein DB, Dreesen DW, Schwartz IK, Campbell GH, Sumner JW, Patchen LC, Brown WJ: Antibody response to pre-exposure human diploid cell rabies vaccine given concurrently with chloroquine. N. Engl. J. Med. 314: 280-84 (1986).

18. Bernard KW, Fishbein DB, Miller KD, Parker RA, Watermon S, Sumner JW, Reid FL, Johnson BK, Rollins AJ, Oster CN, Schonberger LB, Baer GM, Winkler WG: Pre-exposure rabies immunization with human diploid cell vaccine. Decreased antibody reponses in persons immunized in developing countries. Am. J. Trop. Med. Hyg. 34: 633-47 (1985).

19. Fridell E, Grandien M, Johansson R: Pre-exposure prophylaxis against rabies in children by human diploid cell vaccine. Lancet 1: 623 (1984).

20. Greenberg M, Childress J: Vaccination against rabies with duck embryo and Semple vaccines. JAMA 173: 333-37 (1960).

21. CDC. ACIP Recommendations: Supplementary statement on pre-exposure rabies prophylaxis by the intradermal route. MMWR: 31: 279-85 (1982).

22. CDC. ACIP Recommendation: Supplementary statement on rabies vaccine and serologic testing. MMWR 30: 535-36 (1981).

A.H.F.S Category 80:12

Manufactured by:

PASTEUR MÉRIEUX Sérums & Vaccins S.A.

Lyon, France   U.S. License No. 384

Distributed by:

CONNAUGHT LABORATORIES, INC.

Swiftwater, Pennsylvania 18370, U.S.A.

800-VACCINE (800-822-2463)

CONNAUGHT

A PASTEUR MÉRIEUX COMPANY

Issued July 1991

IPOL®   ℞
POLIOVIRUS VACCINE INACTIVATED

DESCRIPTION

IPOL®, Poliovirus Vaccine Inactivated, produced by Pasteur Mérieux Sérums & Vaccins S.A., is a sterile suspension of three types of poliovirus: Type 1 (Mahoney), Type 2 (MEF-1), and Type 3 (Saukett). The viruses are grown in cultures of VERO cells, a continuous line of monkey kidney cells, by the microcarrier technique. The viruses are concentrated, purified, and made noninfectious by inactivation with formaldehyde. Each sterile immunizing dose (0.5 ml) of trivalent vaccine is formulated to contain 40 D antigen units of Type 1, 8 D antigen units of Type 2, and 32 D antigen units of Type 3 poliovirus, determined by comparison to a reference preparation. The poliovirus vaccine is dissolved in phosphate buffered saline. Also present are 0.5% of 2-phenoxyethanol and a maximum of 0.02% of formaldehyde per dose as preservatives. Neomycin, streptomycin and polymyxin B are used in vaccine production, and although purification procedures eliminate measurable amounts, less than 5 ng neomycin, 200 ng streptomycin and 25 ng polymyxin B per dose may

still be present. The vaccine is clear and colorless and should be administered subcutaneously.

CLINICAL PHARMACOLOGY

IPOL is a highly purified, inactivated poliovirus vaccine produced by microcarrier culture.[1,2] This culture technique and improvements in purification, concentration and standardization of poliovirus antigen have resulted in a more potent and more consistently immunogenic vaccine than the Poliovirus Vaccine Inactivated which was available in the U.S. prior to 1988. These new methods allow for the production of vaccine that induces antibody responses in most children after administering fewer doses[3] than with vaccine available prior to 1988.

Studies in developed[3] and developing[4,5] countries with a similar inactivated poliovirus vaccine produced by the same technology have shown that a direct relationship exists between the antigenic content of the vaccine, the frequency of seroconversion, and resulting antibody titer.

A study in the U.S. was carried out, which involved 219 two-month old infants who had received three doses of a Poliovirus Vaccine Inactivated manufactured by the same process as IPOL except the cell substrate was primary monkey kidney cells. Seroconversion to all three Types of poliovirus was demonstrated in 99% of these infants after two doses of vaccine. Following a third dose of vaccine at 18 months of age, high titers of neutralizing antibody were present in 99.1% of children to Type 1 and 100% of children to Types 2 and 3 polioviruses.[6]

Additional studies were carried out in the U.S. with IPOL. Results were reported for 120 infants who received two doses of IPOL at 2 and 4 months of age. Of these 120 children, detectable serum neutralizing antibody was induced after two doses of vaccine in 98.3% (Type 1), 100% (Type 2) and 97.5% (Type 3) of the children. In 83 children receiving three doses at 2, 4, and 12 months of age detectable serum neutralizing antibodies were detected in 97.6% (Type 1) and 100% (Types 2 and 3) of the children.[7,8]

Poliovirus Vaccine Inactivated reduces pharyngeal excretion of poliovirus.[9-12] Field studies in Europe have demonstrated immunity in populations thoroughly immunized with another IPV.[13-17] A survey of Swedish children and young adults given a Swedish IPV demonstrated persistence of circulating antibodies for at least 10 years to all three types of poliovirus.[13]

Paralytic polio has not been reported in association with administration of Poliovirus Vaccine Inactivated.

INDICATIONS AND USAGE

Poliovirus Vaccine Inactivated is indicated for active immunization of infants, children and adults for the prevention of poliomyelitis. Recommendations on the use of live and inactivated poliovirus vaccines are described in the ACIP Recommendations[18,19] and the 1988 American Academy of Pediatrics Red Book.[20]

INFANTS, CHILDREN AND ADOLESCENTS
General Recommendations

It is recommended that all infants, unimmunized children and adolescents not previously immunized be vaccinated routinely against paralytic poliomyelitis.[18] Poliovirus Vaccine Inactivated should be offered to individuals who have refused Poliovirus Vaccine Live Oral Trivalent (OPV) or in whom OPV is contraindicated. Parents should be adequately informed of the risks and benefits of both inactivated and oral polio vaccines so that they can make an informed choice (Report of An Evaluation of Poliomyelitis Vaccine Policy Options, Institute of Medicine, National Academy of Sciences, Washington, D.C., 1988).

OPV should not be used in households with immunodeficient individuals because OPV is excreted in the stool by healthy vaccinees and can infect an immunocompromised household member, which may result in paralytic disease. In a household with an immunocompromised member, only Poliovirus Vaccine Inactivated should be used for all those requiring poliovirus immunization.[20]

Children Incompletely Immunized

Children of all ages should have their immunization status reviewed and be considered for supplemental immunization as follows for adults. Time intervals between doses longer than those recommended for routine primary immunization do not necessitate additional doses as long as a final total of four doses is reached (see DOSAGE AND ADMINISTRATION).

Previous clinical poliomyelitis (usually due to only a single poliovirus type) or incomplete immunization with OPV are not contraindications to completing the primary series of immunization with Poliovirus Vaccine Inactivated.

ADULTS
General Recommendations

Routine primary poliovirus vaccination of adults (generally those 18 years of age or older) residing in the U.S. is not recommended. Adults who have increased risk of exposure to either vaccine or wild poliovirus and have not been adequately immunized should receive polio vaccination in accordance with the schedule given in the DOSAGE AND ADMINISTRATION section.[18]

The following categories of adults run an increased risk of exposure to wild polioviruses:[19]

- Travelers to regions or countries where poliomyelitis is endemic or epidemic.
- Health care workers in close contact with patients who may be excreting polioviruses.
- Laboratory workers handling specimens that may contain polioviruses.
- Members of communities or specific population groups with disease caused by wild polioviruses.
- Incompletely vaccinated or unvaccinated adults in a household (or other close contacts) with children given OPV provided that the immunization of the child can be assured and not unduly delayed. The adult should be informed of the small OPV related risk to the contact.

IMMUNODEFICIENCY AND ALTERED IMMUNE STATUS

Patients with recognized immunodeficiency are at greater risk of developing paralysis when exposed to live poliovirus than persons with a normal immune system. Under no circumstances should oral live poliovirus vaccine be used in such patients or introduced into a household where such a patient resides.[18]

Poliovirus Vaccine Inactivated should be used in all patients with immunodeficiency diseases and members of such patients' households when vaccination of such persons is indicated. This includes patients with asymptomatic HIV infection, AIDS or AIDS Related Complex, severe combined immunodeficiency, hypogammaglobulinemia, or aggammaglobulinemia; altered immune states due to diseases such as leukemia, lymphoma, or generalized malignancy; or an immune system compromised by treatment with corticosteroids, alkylating drugs, antimetabolites or radiation. Patients with an altered immune state may or may not develop a protective response against paralytic poliomyelitis after administration of Poliovirus Vaccine Inactivated.[21]

CONTRAINDICATIONS

Poliovirus Vaccine Inactivated is contraindicated in persons with a history of hypersensitivity to any component of the vaccine, including neomycin, streptomycin and polymyxin B.

If anaphylaxis or anaphylactic shock occurs within 24 hours of administration of a dose of vaccine, no further doses should be given.

Vaccination of persons with any acute, febrile illness should be deferred until after recovery; however, minor illnesses such as mild upper respiratory infections, are not in themselves reasons for postponing vaccine administration.

WARNINGS

Neomycin, streptomycin, and polymyxin B are used in the producton of this vaccine. Although purification procedures eliminate measurable amounts of these substances, traces may be present (see DESCRIPTION) and allergic reactions may occur in persons sensitive to these substances.

PRECAUTIONS

General

Before injection of the vaccine, the physician should carefully review the recommendations for product use and the patient's medical history including possible hypersensitivities and side effects that may have occurred following previous doses of the vaccine.

Epinephrine hydrochloride (1:1000) and other appropriate agents should be available to control immediate allergic reactions.

Concerns have been raised that stimulation of the immune system of a patient with HIV infection by immunization with inactivated vaccines might cause deterioration in immunologic function. However, such effects have not been noted thus far among children with AIDS or among immunosuppressed individuals after immunizations with inactivated vaccines. The potential benefits of immunization of these children outweigh the undocumented risk of such adverse events.[18]

Drug Interactions

There are no known interactions of Poliovirus Vaccine Inactivated with drugs or foods. Simultaneous administration of other parenteral vaccines is not contraindicated.

Carcinogenesis, Mutagenesis, Impairment of Fertility

Long term studies in animals to evaluate carcinogenic potential or impairment of fertility have not been conducted.

PREGNANCY

REPRODUCTIVE STUDIES—PREGNANCY CATEGORY C

Animal reproduction studies have not been conducted with Poliovirus Vaccine Inactivated. It is also not known whether Poliovirus Vaccine Inactivated can cause fetal harm when administered to a pregnant woman or can affect reproduction capacity. Poliovirus Vaccine Inactivated should be given to a pregnant woman only if clearly needed.

PEDIATRIC USE

Safety and efficacy of IPOL have been shown in children 6 weeks of age and older[6,8] (see DOSAGE AND ADMINISTRATION).

Continued on next page

Connaught Laboratories—Cont.

ADVERSE REACTIONS

In earlier studies with the vaccine grown in primary monkey kidney cells, transient local reactions at the site of injection were observed during a clinical trial.[6] Erythema, induration and pain occurred in 3.2%, 1% and 13%, respectively, of vaccinees within 48 hours post-vaccination. Temperatures ≥ 39°C (≥ 102°F) were reported in up to 38% of vaccinees. Other symptoms noted included sleepiness, fussiness, crying, decreased appetite, and spitting up of feedings. Because Poliovirus Vaccine Inactivated was given in a different site but concurrently with Diphtheria and Tetanus Toxoids and Pertussis Vaccine Adsorbed (DTP), systemic reactions could not be attributed to a specific vaccine. However, these systemic reactions were comparable in frequency and severity to that reported for DTP given without IPV.

In another study using IPOL in the United States, there were no significant local or systemic reactions following injection of the vaccine. There were 7% (6/86), 12% (8/65) and 4% (2/45) of children with temperatures over 100.6°F, following the first, second and third doses respectively. Most of the children received DTP at the same time as IPV and therefore it was not possible to attribute reactions to a particular vaccine; however, such reactions were not significantly different than when DTP is given alone.

Although no causal relationship between Poliovirus Vaccine Inactivated and Guillain-Barré Syndrome (GBS) has been established,[22] GBS has been temporally related to administration of another Poliovirus Vaccine Inactivated.

NOTE: The National Childhood Vaccine Injury Act of 1986 requires the keeping of certain records and the reporting of certain events occurring after the administration of vaccine, including the occurrence of any contraindicating reaction. Poliovirus Vaccines are listed vaccines covered by this Act and health care providers should ensure that they comply with the terms thereof.[23]

DOSAGE AND ADMINISTRATION

Parenteral drug products should be inspected visually for particulate matter and/or discoloration prior to administration. If these conditions exist, vaccine should not be administered.

After preparation of the injection site, immediately administer the vaccine subcutaneously. In infants and small children, the mid-lateral aspect of the thigh is the preferred site. In adults the vaccine should be administered in the deltoid area.

Care should be taken to avoid administering the injection into or near blood vessels and nerves. After aspiration, if blood or any suspicious discoloration appears in the syringe, do not inject but discard contents and repeat procedures using a new dose of vaccine administered at a different site.

DO NOT ADMINISTER VACCINE INTRAVENOUSLY.

CHILDREN

Primary Immunization

A primary series of IPOL consists of three 0.5 ml doses administered subcutaneously. The interval between the first two doses should be at least four weeks, but preferably eight weeks. The first two doses are usually administered with DTP immunization and are given at two and four months of age. The third dose should follow at least six months but preferably 12 months after the second dose. It may be desirable to administer this dose with MMR and other vaccines, but at a different site, in children 15–18 months of age. All children who received a primary series of Poliovirus Vaccine Inactivated, or a combination of IPV and OPV, should be given a booster dose of OPV or IPV before entering school, unless the final (third dose) of the primary series was administered on or after the fourth birthday.[18]

The need to routinely administer additional doses is unknown at this time.[18]

A final total of four doses is necessary to complete a series of primary and booster doses. Children and adolescents with a previously incomplete series of IPV should receive sufficient additional doses to reach this number.

ADULTS

Unvaccinated Adults

For unvaccinated adults at increased risk of exposure to poliovirus, a primary series of Poliovirus Vaccine Inactivated is recommended. While the responses of adults to primary series have not been studied, the recommended schedule for adults is two doses given at a 1 to 2 month interval and a third dose given 6 to 12 months later. If less than 3 months but more than 2 months are available before protection is needed, 3 doses of Poliovirus Vaccine Inactivated should be given at least 1 month apart. Likewise, if only 1 or 2 months are available, two doses of Poliovirus Vaccine Inactivated should be given at least 1 month apart. If less than 1 month is available, a single dose of either OPV or IPV is recommended.

Incompletely Vaccinated Adults

Adults who are at an increased risk of exposure to poliovirus and who have had at least one dose of OPV, fewer than 3 doses of conventional IPV or a combination of conventional IPV or OPV totalling fewer than 3 doses should receive at least 1 dose of OPV or Poliovirus Vaccine Inactivated. Additional doses needed to complete a primary series should be given if time permits.

Completely Vaccinated Adults

Adults who are at an increased risk of exposure to poliovirus and who have previously completed a primary series with one or a combination of polio vaccines can be given a dose of either OPV or IPV.[19]

HOW SUPPLIED

Syringe, 0.5 ml with integrated needle (1 × 1 Dose package—Product No. 49281-860-51 and 10 × 1 Dose package—Product No. 49281-860-52)

STORAGE

The vaccine is stable if stored in the refrigerator between 2°C and 8°C (35°F and 46°F). *The vaccine must not be frozen.*

REFERENCES

1. van Wezel, A.L., et al: Inactivated poliovirus vaccine: Current production methods and new developments. Rev Infect Dis 6 (Suppl 2): S335–S340, 1984
2. Montagnon, B.J., et al: Industrial scale production of inactivated poliovirus vaccine prepared by culture of Vero cells on microcarrier. Rev Infect Dis 6 (Suppl 2): S341–S344, 1984
3. Salk, J., et al: Antigen content of inactivated poliovirus vaccine for use in a one- or two-dose regimen. Ann Clin Res 14: 204–212, 1982
4. Salk, J., et al: Killed poliovirus antigen titration in humans. Develop Biol Standard 41: 110–132, 1978
5. Salk, J., et al: Theoretical and practical considerations in the application of killed poliovirus vaccine for the control of paralytic poliomyelitis. Develop Biol Standard 47: 181–198, 1981
6. McBean, A.M., et al: Serologic response to oral polio vaccine and enhanced-potency inactivated polio vaccines. Am J Epidemiol 128: 615–628, 1988
7. Unpublished data available from Pasteur Mérieux Sérums & Vaccins S.A.
8. Faden, H., et al: Comparative evaluation of immunization with live attenuated and enhanced potency inactivated trivalent poliovirus vaccines in childhood: Systemic and local immune responses. J Infect Dis 162: 1291–1297, 1990
9. Marine, W.M., et al: Limitation of fecal and pharyngeal poliovirus excretion in Salk-vaccinated children. A family study during a Type 1 poliomyelitis epidemic. Amer J Hyg 76: 173–175, 1962
10. Bottiger, M., et al: Vaccination with attenuated Type 1 poliovirus, the Chat strain. II. Transmission of virus in relation to age. Acta Paed Scand 55: 416–421, 1966
11. Dick, G.W.A., et al: Vaccination against poliomyelitis with live virus vaccines. Effect of previous Salk vaccination on virus excretion. Brit Med J 2: 266–269, 1961
12. Wehrle, P.F., et al: Transmission of poliovirus; III. Prevalence of polioviruses in pharyngeal secretions of infected household contacts of patients with clinical disease. Pediatrics 27: 762–764, 1961
13. Bottiger, M.: Long-term immunity following vaccination with killed poliovirus vaccine in Sweden, a country with no circulating poliovirus. Rev Infect Dis 6 (Suppl 2): S545–551, 1984
14. Chin, T.D.Y.: Immunity induced by inactivated poliovirus vaccine and excretion of virus. Rev Infect Dis 6 (Suppl 2): S369–S370, 1984
15. Salk, D.: Herd effect and virus eradication with use of killed poliovirus vaccine. Develop Biol Standard 47: 247–255, 1981
16. Bijerk, H.: Surveillance and control of poliomyelitis in the Netherlands. Rev Infect Dis 6 (Suppl 2): S451–S456, 1984
17. Lapinleimu, K.: Elimination of poliomyelitis in Finland. Rev Infect Dis 6 (Suppl 2): S457–S460, 1984
18. Immunization Practices Advisory Committee (ACIP), Poliomyelitis Prevention: Enhanced-Potency Inactivated Poliomyelitis Vaccine Supplementary Statement. MMWR 36: 795–798, 1987
19. ACIP: Poliomyelitis Prevention, MMWR 31: 22–26 and 31–34, 1982
20. Report of the Committee on Infectious Diseases, American Academy of Pediatrics, 21st ed: 334–342, 1988
21. ACIP: Immunization of children infected with human T-lymphotropic virus type III/lymphadenopathy-associated virus. MMWR 35: 595–606, 1986
22. WHO: Weekly Epidemiology Record 54: 82–83, 1979
23. National Childhood Vaccine Injury Act: Requirements for permanent vaccination records and for reporting of selected events after vaccination. MMWR 37: 197–200, 1988

Product information
as of December 1990

Manufactured by:
PASTEUR MÉRIEUX Sérums & Vaccins S.A.
Lyon, France
U.S. License No. 384

Distributed by:
Connaught Laboratories, Inc.
Swiftwater, Pennsylvania 18370, U.S.A.
800-VACCINE/800-822-2463

JE-VAX® ℞

JAPANESE ENCEPHALITIS VIRUS VACCINE INACTIVATED

CAUTION: Federal (U.S.A.) law prohibits dispensing without prescription.

DESCRIPTION

JE-VAX®, Japanese Encephalitis Virus Vaccine Inactivated, is a sterile, lyophilized vaccine for subcutaneous use, prepared by inoculating mice intracerebrally with Japanese encephalitis (JE) virus, "Nakayama-NIH" strain, manufactured by The Research Foundation for Microbial Diseases of Osaka University ("BIKEN®"). Infected brains are harvested and homogenized in phosphate buffered saline, pH 8.0. The homogenate is centrifuged and the supernatant inactivated with formaldehyde, then processed to yield a partially purified, inactivated virus suspension. This is further purified by ultra-centrifugation through 40 w/v% sucrose. The suspension is then lyophilized in final containers and sealed under dry nitrogen atmosphere. Thimerosal (mercury derivative) is added as a preservative to a final concentration of 0.007%. The diluent, Sterile Water for Injection, contains no preservative. Each 1.0 mL dose contains approximately 500 μg of gelatin, less than 100 μg of formaldehyde, and less than 50 ng of mouse serum protein. No myelin basic protein can be detected at the detection threshold of the assay (< 2 ng/mL). Prior to reconstitution, the vaccine is a white caked powder, and after reconstitution the vaccine is a colorless transparent liquid. The potency of JE vaccine is determined by immunizing mice with either the test vaccine or the JE reference vaccine. Neutralizing antibodies are measured in a plaque neutralization assay performed on sera from the immunized mice. The potency of the test vaccine must be no less than that of the reference vaccine.

CLINICAL PHARMACOLOGY

Japanese encephalitis (JE), a mosquito-borne arboviral Flavivirus infection, is the leading cause of viral encephalitis in Asia. Infection leads to overt encephalitis in 1 of 20 to 1000 cases. Encephalitis, usually is severe, resulting in a fatal outcome in 25% of cases and residual neuropsychiatric sequelae in 50% of cases. JE acquired during the first or second trimesters of pregnancy may cause intrauterine infection and miscarriage. Infections that occur during the third trimester of pregnancy have not been associated with adverse outcomes in newborns.[1]

The virus is transmitted in an enzootic cycle among mosquitoes and vertebrate amplifying hosts, chiefly domestic pigs and, in some areas, wild Ardeid (wading) birds. Viral infection rates in mosquitoes range from < 1% to 3%. These species are prolific in rural areas where their larvae breed in ground pools and flooded rice fields. Thus all elements of the transmission cycle are prevalent in rural areas of Asia and human infections occur principally in this setting. Because vertebrate amplifying hosts and agricultural activities may be situated within and at the periphery of cities, human cases occasionally are reported from urban locations.[1]

JE virus is transmitted seasonally in most areas of Asia. The seasonal patterns of viral transmission are correlated with the abundance of vector mosquitoes and of vertebrate amplifying hosts. Although the abundance of vector mosquitoes fluctuates with the amount of rainfall, and with the impact of the rainy season, in some tropical locations, irrigation associated with agricultural practices is a more important factor affecting vector abundance, and transmission may occur year-round. Thus the periods of greatest risk for JE viral transmission vary regionally and within countries, and from year to year.[1]

In areas where JE is endemic, annual incidence ranges from 1 to 10 per 10,000 people. Cases occur primarily in children under 10 years of age. Seroprevalence studies in these endemic areas indicate nearly universal exposure by adulthood (calculating from a ratio of asymptomatic to symptomatic infections of 200 to 1, approximately 10% of the susceptible population is infected per year). In addition to children < 10 years, an increase in JE incidence has been observed in the elderly.[1]

Challenge experiments in passively protected mice have defined the levels of neutralizing antibody that may be protective for humans.[2] Mice passively immunized to achieve a neutralizing antibody titer of ≥ 1:10 were protected from a JE virus challenge of $10^5 LD_{50}$, a viral dose thought to be transmitted by an infected mosquito.[2]

The efficacy of the BIKEN Nakayama-NIH strain Japanese Encephalitis Virus Vaccine Inactivated was demonstrated in a placebo-controlled, randomized clinical trial in Thai children, sponsored by the U.S. Army.[3] In this trial, children between 1 and 14 years of age received BIKEN monovalent

Nakayama-NIH strain (n=21,628) or a bivalent vaccine containing the Nakayama-NIH and Beijing JE virus strains (n=22,080) or tetanus toxoid as a placebo (n=21,516). Immunization consisted of two (2) subcutaneous 1.0 mL doses of vaccine, *except in children under 3 years of age who received two 0.5 mL doses.* One case (5 cases/100,000) of JE occurred in the monovalent vaccine group, one case (5 cases/100,000) in the bivalent vaccine group, and 11 cases (51 cases/100,000) in the placebo group. The observed efficacy of both monovalent and bivalent vaccines was 91% (95% confidence interval, 54% to 98%). Side effects of vaccination, including headache, sore arm, rash, and swelling were reported at rates similar to those in the placebo group, usually less than 1%. Symptoms did not increase after the second dose. It should be noted that a schedule of two doses, separated by seven days, as employed in this trial, may be appropriate for use in residents of endemic or epidemic areas, where pre-existing exposure to Flaviviruses may contribute to the immune response.[3]

A three-dose vaccination schedule is recommended for U.S. travelers and military personnel, based on the Centers for Disease Control and Prevention (CDC) experience and on a controlled immunogenicity trial performed in U.S. military personnel.[4,5] The CDC experience demonstrated that neutralizing antibody was produced in fewer than 80% of vaccinees following two doses of vaccine in U.S. travelers and antibody levels declined substantially in most vaccinees within six months. The U.S. Army studied the immunogenicity of JE-VAX in 538 volunteers. Two three-dose regimens were evaluated (Day 0, 7, and 14 or Day 0, 7, and 30). All vaccine recipients demonstrated neutralizing antibodies at 2 months and 6 months after initiation of vaccination. The schedule of Day 0, 7, and 30 produced higher antibody responses than the Day 0, 7, and 14 schedule. Two hundred and seventy-three of the original study participants were tested at 12 months post-vaccination and there was no longer a statistical difference in antibody titers between the two vaccination regimens.[5]

The full duration of protection is unknown. Of U.S. Army volunteers completing a three-dose regimen, 252 agreed to receive a booster dose of vaccine one year after the primary series. All boosted participants still had antibody 12 months after the booster. Protective levels of neutralizing antibody persisted for 24 months (2 years) in all 21 persons who had not received a booster.[5] Definitive recommendations cannot be given on the timing of booster doses at this time.

INDICATIONS AND USAGE

JE-VAX is indicated for active immunization against JE for persons one year of age and older. For recommended primary immunization series see DOSAGE AND ADMINISTRATION section.

JE-VAX should be considered for use in persons who plan to reside in or travel to areas where JE is endemic or epidemic during a transmission season. ***JE-VAX is NOT recommended for all persons traveling to or residing to Asia.*** The incidence of JE in the location of intended stay, the conditions of housing, nature of activities, duration of stay, and the possibility of unexpected travel to high-risk areas are factors that should be considered in the decision to administer vaccine. In general, vaccine should be considered for use in persons spending a month or longer in epidemic or endemic areas during the transmission season, especially if travel will include rural areas. Depending on the epidemic circumstances, vaccine should be considered for persons spending less than 30 days whose activities, such as extensive outdoor activities in rural areas, place them at particularly high risk for exposure.[1]

In all instances, travelers are advised to take personal precautions to reduce exposure to mosquito bites. (See INFORMATION FOR PATIENTS section)

Current CDC advisories should be consulted with regard to JE epidemicity in specific locales.[1]

The decision to use JE-VAX should balance the risks for exposure to the virus and for developing illness, the availability and acceptability of repellents and other alternative measures, and the side effects of vaccination. Assessments should be interpreted cautiously because risk can vary within areas and from year to year and available data are incomplete. Estimates suggest that risk of JE in highly endemic areas during the transmission season can reach 1 per 5000 per month of exposure; risk for most short-term travelers may be 1 per million or less. Although JE vaccine is reactogenic, rates of serious allergic reactions (generalized urticaria and/or angioedema) are low (approximately 1-104 per 10,000).[1]

Advanced age may be a risk factor for developing symptomatic illness after infection. JE acquired during pregnancy carries the potential for intrauterine infection and fetal death. These factors should be considered when advising elderly persons and pregnant women who plan visits to JE endemic areas.

There are no data on the safety and efficacy of JE vaccine in infants under one year of age. Whenever possible, immunization of infants should be deferred until they are one year of age or older.[1]

Research laboratory workers:

Laboratory acquired JE has been reported in 22 cases. JE virus may be transmitted in a laboratory setting through needle sticks and other accidental exposures. Vaccine-derived immunity presumably protects against exposure through these percutaneous routes. Exposure to aerosolized JE virus, and particularly to high concentrations of virus, such as may occur during viral purification, potentially could lead to infection through mucous membranes and possibly directly into the central nervous system through the olfactory mucosa. It is unknown whether vaccine-derived immunity protects against such exposures, but immunization is recommended for all laboratory workers with a potential for exposure to infectious JE virus.[1]

As with any vaccine, vaccination with JE-VAX may not result in protection in all individuals. Long-term protection, as demonstrated by persistence of neutralizing antibody for more than two years, has not yet been shown.

CONTRAINDICATIONS

Adverse reactions to a prior dose of JE vaccine manifesting as generalized urticaria and angioedema are considered to be contraindications to further vaccination.

Patients who develop allergic or unusual adverse events after vaccination should be reported through the Vaccine Adverse Event Reporting System (VAERS) 1-800-822-7967.[1]

JE vaccine is produced in mouse brains and should not be administered to persons with a proven or suspected hypersensitivity to proteins of rodent or neural origin. ***HYPERSENSITIVITY TO THIMEROSAL IS A CONTRAINDICATION TO VACCINATION.***[1]

WARNINGS

Adverse reactions to JE vaccine manifesting as generalized urticaria or angioedema may occur within minutes following vaccination. A possibly related reaction has occurred as late as 17 days after vaccination. Most reactions occur within 10 days with the majority occurring within 48 hours.[1] (See ADVERSE REACTIONS section)

Vaccinees should be observed for 30 minutes after vaccination and warned about the possibility of delayed generalized urticaria, often in a generalized distribution or angioedema of the extremities, face and oropharynx, especially of the lips.[1]

Vaccinees should be advised to remain in areas where they have ready access to medical care for 10 days after receiving a dose of JE vaccine. *Vaccinees should be instructed to seek medical attention immediately upon onset of any reaction.*[1]

***Persons should not embark on international travel within 10 days of JE-VAX immunization because of the possibility of delayed allergic reactions.*[1]**

Persons with a past history of urticaria after hymenoptera envenomation, drugs, physical or other provocations, or of idiopathic cause appear to have a greater risk of developing reactions to JE vaccine (relative risk 9.1, 95% confidence interval 1.8 to 50.9).[6] This history should be considered when weighing risks and benefits of the vaccine for an individual patient. When patients with such a history are offered JE vaccine, they should be alerted to their increased risk for reaction and monitored appropriately. There are no data supporting the efficacy of prophylactic antihistamines or steroids in preventing JE vaccine-ralated allergic reactions.[1]

Epinephrine and other medications and equipment to treat anaphylaxis should be available at vaccine administration centers.

PRECAUTIONS

GENERAL

Epinephrine Injection (1:1000) must be immediately available should an acute anaphylactic reaction occur due to any component of the vaccine.

Prior to injection of any vaccine, all known precautions should be taken to prevent adverse reactions. This includes a review of the patient's history with respect to possible sensitivity to this vaccine, a similar vaccine or allergic disorders in general (see CONTRAINDICATIONS section).

A separate, sterile syringe and needle or a disposable unit should be used for each patient to prevent transmission of infectious agents from person to person. Needles should not be recapped and should be disposed of properly.

Although substantial neutralizing antibody titers are elicited by JE-VAX in more than 90% of U.S. travelers without history of prior JE immunization or of prior exposure to JE, the precise relationship between antibody level and efficacy has not been established even though these titers persisted for at least two years after immunization.[7]

The decision to administer JE vaccine should balance the risks for exposure to the virus and for developing illness, the availability and acceptability of repellents and other alternative protective measures, and the side effects of vaccination.

INFORMATION FOR PATIENTS

Patients should be advised of the following:

- JE-VAX is given to provide immunization against Japanese encephalitis virus.
- A three-dose immunizing series should be completed, except in unusual circumstances. (See CONTRAINDICATIONS AND DOSAGE AND ADMINISTRATION sections)
- JE-VAX should be given to a pregnant women only if, in the opinion of a physician, withholding the vaccine entails even greater risk.
- Any adverse events following JE-VAX should be reported through the Vaccine Adverse Event Reporting System (VAERS) 1-800-822-7967 after contacting the physician immediately.
- If the patient has a past history of urticaria (hives) (following hymenoptera envenomation, drugs, physical or other provocation or of idiopathic origin), adverse effects are more likely.
- Adverse events consisting of arm soreness and local redness can occur shortly after vaccination.
- Adverse events consisting of headache, rash, edema and generalized urticaria or angioedema may occur shortly after vaccination or up to 17 days (usually within 10 days) following vaccination.
- International travel should not be initiated within 10 days of JE-VAX vaccination because of the possibility of delayed adverse reactions. Patients should be instructed to seek medical attention immediately upon onset of any adverse reaction.
- Personal precautions should be taken to avoid exposure to mosquito bites by the use of insect repellents, and protective clothing. Avoiding outdoor activity, especially during twilight periods and in the evening, will reduce risk even further.

DRUG INTERACTIONS

There are no data on the effect of concurrent administration of other vaccines, drugs (e.g. chloroquine, meflaquine) or biologicals on the safety and immunogenicity of JE vaccine.

CARCINOGENESIS, MUTAGENESIS, IMPAIRMENT OF FERTILITY

No studies have been performed to evaluate carcinogenicity, mutagenic potential, or impact on fertility.

PREGNANCY

REPRODUCTIVE STUDIES–PREGNANCY CATEGORY C

Animal reproduction studies have not been conducted with Japanese Encephalitis Virus Vaccine. It is not known whether Japanese Encephalitis Virus Vaccine can cause fetal harm when administered to a pregnant woman or can affect reproductive capacity. Pregnant women who must travel to an area where risk of JE is high should be immunized when the theoretical risks of immunization are outweighed by the risk of infection to the mother and developing fetus. Japanese Encephalitis Virus Vaccine should be given to a pregnant woman only if clearly needed.

NURSING MOTHERS

It is not known whether JE-VAX is excreted in human milk. Because many drugs are excreted in human milk, caution should be exercised when JE-VAX is administered to a nursing woman.

PEDIATRIC USE

Safety and efficacy of JE vaccine in infants under one year of age have not been established.

ADVERSE REACTIONS

JE vaccine is associated with a moderate frequency of local and mild systemic adverse effects.[3,4,5,8,9,10,11] Tenderness, redness, swelling and other local effects have been reported in about 20% of vaccinees (<1% to 31%). Systemic side effects, principally fever, headache, malaise, rash, and other reactions, such as chills, dizziness, myalgia, nausea, vomiting and abdominal pain have been reported in approximately 10% of vaccinees.

In a study conducted by the CDC less than 5% of the 1,756 U.S. travelers immunized with a three-dose regimen of the vaccine reported headache, flu-like symptoms, fever, and other systemic complaints. Hives and facial swelling were reported in 0.2% and 0.1% of vaccinees, respectively. Local soreness occurred in 5.9% and local redness in 2.9%. There was no increase in the number or severity of reactions with increasing numbers of doses.[7]

The U.S. Army studied 4,034 personnel from 1987 to 1989.[10] Using a two- or three-dose regimen of JE vaccine, arm soreness was described in 22.7%, local redness in 4.8%, headache in 15.2%, and a febrile episode in 5.5%. In another trial evaluating the safety and immunogenicity of a three-dose immunizing series (Day 0, 7, and 30 or Day 0, 7, and 14), performed in 538 adult volunteers in 1990, the Army determined that local soreness and redness occurred in 21% of vaccinees after the first dose, then decreased with subsequent injections ($p < 0.0001$, Chi-square for downward trend). Systemic symptoms including feverishness, headache and rash occurred in 5% of vaccinees after the first dose, then decreased with subsequent injections ($p < 0.001$, Chi-square for downward trend).[5] Participants who received the third dose on Day 14 reported more side effects than those who received the injection on Day 30. Among these volunteers, 252 received a booster injection of vaccine one year after receiving the first

Continued on next page

Connaught Laboratories—Cont.

dose of the primary series. Side effects reported after the booster injection included local symptoms of soreness (24.5%) and redness (6.1%) at the injection site and systemic complaints of headache (4.9%), fever (1.6%), and rash (0.8%). Less than 1% of all reported symptoms was graded as severe. No generalized urticaria or anaphylaxis was reported.
Since 1989, an apparently new pattern of adverse reactions has been reported among vaccinees in Europe, North America, and Australia.[11,12,13] The reactions have been characterized by urticaria, often in a generalized distribution, or angioedema of the extremities, face, especially of the lips and oropharynx. Three vaccine recipients developed respiratory distress. Distress or collapse due to hypotension or other causes led to hospitalization in several cases. Most reactions were treated successfully with antihistamines or oral steroids; however some patients were hospitalized for parenteral steroid therapy. Three patients developed an erythema multiforme or erythema nodosum and some patients have had joint swelling. Some vaccinees complained of generalized itching without objective evidence of a rash.
An important feature of the reactions has been the interval between vaccination and onset of symptoms. Reactions after a first vaccine dose occurred after a median of 12 hours after immunization (88% of reactions occurred within 3 days). The interval between administration of a second dose and onset of symptoms generally was longer, (median 3 days and possibly as long as 2 weeks). Reactions have occurred after a second or third dose, when preceding doses were received uneventfully.
Between November 1991 and May 1992, the U.S. Navy immunized 35,253 U.S. personnel (marines, other military and dependents) with JE-VAX on Okinawa. The overall reaction rate, 62.4 per 10,000 vaccinees (95% confidence interval 54.2 to 70.6) includes persons reporting urticaria, angioedema, generalized itching and wheezing. The reaction rate per 10,000 vaccinees was 26.7 (95% confidence interval 21.3 to 32.1), 30.8 (95% confidence interval 24.6 to 37.0) or 12.2 (95% confidence interval 7.9 to 16.5) after the first, second or third dose, respectively.[6] These reactions were generally mild to moderate in severity. Nine out of 35,253 persons immunized were hospitalized (2.6 per 10,000 vaccinees) primarily to allow administration of intravenous steroids for refractory urticaria. None of these reactions were considered life-threatening.
A case-control study conducted as part of the JE immunization campaign in Okinawa found that persons developing these reactions after JE vaccination were more likely to have had a past history of urticaria after hymenoptera envenomation, drugs, physical or other provocations or of idiopathic origins (relative risk 9.1, 95% confidence interval 1.8 to 50.9).[6] The vaccine constituents responsible for these adverse reactions have not been identified.
Other serious adverse events reported following vaccination include (1) one case of Guillain-Barré syndrome after JE vaccination has been reported in the United States since 1984, however, this patient was diagnosed as having mononucleosis three weeks before the onset of weakness; (2) one case of urticaria, hepatitis and respiratory failure one week after dose 2 (this person showed effusion and infiltrate on chest x-ray and eosinophilia); and (3) one case of respiratory and renal failure one week after a dose (this 26-month-old male had infiltrate on chest x-ray and acid fast bacilli in sputum); and (4) one case of newly diagnosed hypertension in a young adult male presenting with a headache several hours after receiving dose one. The etiology of these adverse events is unknown.
Sudden death occurred approximately 60 hours after receiving the first dose of JE vaccine in a 21-year-old U.S. military person with a history of recurrent hypersensitivity and an episode of possible anaphylaxis. This person also received the third dose of plague vaccine approximately 12–15 hours prior to the death. There was no evidence of urticaria or angioedema. Cause of death was not established at autopsy.
Surveillance of JE vaccine related complications in Japan from 1965 to 1973 disclosed neurologic events (primarily encephalitis, encephalopathy, seizures, and peripheral neuropathy) in 1 to 2.3 per million vaccinees.[14,15] Very rarely, deaths occurred with vaccine-associated encephalitis. Between 1987 and 1989, two cases of neurologic dysfunction were reported from Japan; one of these was a transverse myelitis, while the second included seizures, cranial nerve paresis, cerebellar ataxia, and behavior disorder.[15] In 1992, two cases of acute disseminated encephalomyelitis were reported from Japan; one occurred 14 days after the second dose and the second occurred 17 days after a booster dose of JE vaccine. Both cases recovered.[16] One case of Bell's Palsy was reported from Thailand.

Reporting of Adverse Events
Reporting by parents and patients of all adverse events occurring after antigen administration should be encouraged. Adverse events following immunization with vaccine should be reported by the health-care provider to the U.S. Department of Health and Human Services (DHHS) Vaccine Adverse Event Reporting System (VAERS). Reporting forms and information about reporting requirements or completion of the form can be obtained from VAERS through a toll-free number 1-800-822-7967.[17]
Health-care providers also should report these events to Director of Medical Affairs, Connaught Laboratories, Inc., Route 611, P.O. Box 187, Swiftwater, PA 18370 or call 1-800-822-2463.

DOSAGE AND ADMINISTRATION

Parenteral drug products should be inspected visually for extraneous particulate matter and/or discoloration prior to administration whenever solution and container permit. If either of these conditions exist, the vaccine should not be administered.
For persons 3 years of age and older, a single dose is 1.0 mL of vaccine. *For children 1 year to 3 years of age, a single dose is 0.5 mL of vaccine.* (See PRIMARY IMMUNIZATION SCHEDULE below.)
Single-Dose vial of lyophilized vaccine: Remove plastic tab of flip-off cap. DO NOT REMOVE RUBBER STOPPER. Cleanse stopper with a suitable disinfectant. Reconstitute only with the supplied 1.3 mL of diluent (Sterile Water for Injection). Shake vial thoroughly. After reconstitution the vaccine should be stored between 2°-8°C (35°-46°F) and used within 8 hours. DO NOT FREEZE RECONSTITUTED VACCINE.
10-Dose vial of lyophilized vaccine: Remove plastic tab of flip-off cap. DO NOT REMOVE RUBBER STOPPER. Cleanse stopper with a suitable disinfectant. Reconstitute only with the supplied 11 mL of diluent (Sterile Water for Injection). Shake vial thoroughly. After reconstitution the vaccine should be stored between 2°-8° C (35°-46° F) and used within 8 hours. DO NOT FREEZE RECONSTITUTED VACCINE.
A separate, sterile syringe and needle or a sterile disposable unit should be used for each patient to prevent transmission of infectious agents from person to person. Needles should not be recapped and should be disposed of properly.
SHAKE VIAL WELL
PRIMARY IMMUNIZATION SCHEDULE[1]
The recommended primary immunization series is three doses of 1.0 mL each for individuals > 3 years of age given subcutaneously on days 0, 7, and 30. *For children 1 to 3 years of age a series of three doses of 0.5 mL each should be given subcutaneously on days 0, 7, and 30.* An abbreviated schedule of days 0, 7, and 14 can be used when the longer schedule is impractical because of time constraints. (When it is impossible to follow one of the above recommended schedules, two doses given a week apart will induce antibodies in approximately 80% of vaccinees; however, this two-dose regimen should not be used except under unusual circumstances.)
The last dose should be given at least 10 days before the commencement of international travel to ensure an adequate immune response and access to medical care in the event of delayed adverse reactions.
A booster dose of 1.0 mL (*0.5 mL for children from 1 to 3 years of age*) may be given after two years. In the absence of firm data on the persistence of antibody after primary immunization, a definite recommendation cannot be made on the spacing of boosters beyond two years.
There are no data on the safety and efficacy of JE vaccine in infants under one year of age. Whenever possible, immunization of infants should be deferred until they are one year of age or older.[1]
The skin at the site of injection first should be cleansed and disinfected. Shake vial thoroughly before each use. Cleanse top of rubber stopper of the vial with a suitable antiseptic and wipe away all excess before withdrawing vaccine.
When JE-VAX and any other vaccines are given concurrently, separate syringes and separate sites should be used.

HOW SUPPLIED

Vial, Single Dose (3 per package) with vial of Diluent (3 per package) - Product No. 49281-680-30
Vial, Single Dose (5 per package) with vial of Diluent (5 per package) - Product No. 49281-680-50
Vial, 10 Dose with vial Diluent - Product No. 49281-680-20
For persons 3 years of age and older, a single dose is 1.0 mL of vaccine. *For children 1 year to 3 years of age, a single dose is 0.5 mL of vaccine.* (See PRIMARY IMMUNIZATION SCHEDULE above.)

STORAGE

The vaccine should be stored between 2°-8° C (35°-46° F). DO NOT FREEZE. After reconstitution the vaccine should be stored between 2°-8° C (35°-46° F) and used within 8 hours. DO NOT FREEZE RECONSTITUTED VACCINE.

REFERENCES

1. Recommendations of the Advisory Committee on Immunization Practices (ACIP). Inactivated Japanese Encephalitis Virus Vaccine. MMWR (In Press)
2. Oya A. Japanese Encephalitis Vaccine. Acta Paediatr Jpn 30: 175–184, 1988
3. Hoke CH, et al. Protection Against Japanese Encephalitis by Inactivated Vaccines. N Eng J Med 319: 608–614, 1988
4. Poland JD, et al. Evaluation of the Potency and Safety of Inactivated Japanese Encephalitis Vaccine in US Inhabitants. J Infect Dis 161: 878–882, 1990
5. DeFraites RF. Immunogenicity and Safety of Japanese Encephalitis Vaccine (Inactivated: Nakayama/BIKEN) in U.S. Army Soldiers: Evaluation of Three Consecutively Manufactured Lots of Vaccine Administered in Two Dosing Regimens. April 30, 1991, and November 12, 1992. Unpublished Data, on file with BIKEN and with Walter Reed Army Institute of Research, Washington, DC
6. Berg WS, Navy Environmental Health Center, Norfolk, VA June 16, 1992 (unpublished)
7. Unpublished data on file with "BIKEN" and CDC
8. Rojanasuphot S, et al. A field trial of Japanese encephalitis vaccine produced in Thailand. Southeast Asian J Trop Med Publ Health 20: 653–654, 1989
9. Rao Bhau LN, et al. Safety and efficacy of Japanese encephalitis vaccine produced in India. Indian J Med Res 88: 301–307, 1988
10. Sanchez JL, et al. Further Experience with Japanese Encephalitis Vaccine. Lancet 335: 972–973, 1990
11. Japanese Encephalitis Vaccine and Adverse Effects among Travelers. Canada Diseases Weekly Report. Vol. 17–32: 173–177, 1991
12. Anderson MM, et al. Side-Effects with Japanese Encephalitis Vaccine. Lancet 337: 1044, 1991
13. Ruff TA, et al. Adverse Reactions to Japanese Encephalitis Vaccine. Lancet 338: 881–882, 1991
14. Kitaoka M. Follow-up on use of vaccine in children in Japan, in McDHammon W, Kitaoka M, Downs WG eds. Immunization for Japanese encephalitis, Excerpta Medica, Amsterdam 275–277, 1972
15. Unpublished data on file with "BIKEN"
16. Ohtaki E, et al. Acute disseminated encephalomyelitis after Japanese B Encephalitis Vaccination. Pediatric Neurology Vol. 8 No. 2: 137–139, 1992
17. CDC. Vaccine Adverse Event Reporting System—United States. MMWR 39: 730–733, 1990

Manufactured by:
The Research Foundation for Microbial Diseases of Osaka University
Suita, Osaka, Japan
"BIKEN ®"
Distributed by:
CONNAUGHT LABORATORIES, INC.
Swiftwater, PA 18370, U.S.A.
1-800-VACCINE (1-800-822-2463)
Product Information as of December 1992
2533

MENOMUNE®—A/C/Y/W-135 ℞

[*mĕn-ō-mūne*]
MENINGOCOCCAL POLYSACCHARIDE VACCINE, GROUPS A, C, Y AND W-135 COMBINED

Caution: Federal (U.S.A.) law prohibits dispensing without prescription.

> For special instructions on use of Meningococcal Polysaccharide Vaccine Groups A, C, Y and W-135 Combined, for Jet Injector Use—see end of insert.

DESCRIPTION

Menomune®, Meningococcal Polysaccharide Vaccine, Groups A, C, Y and W-135 Combined, is a freeze-dried preparation of the group-specific polysaccharide antigens from *Neisseria meningitidis*, Group A, Group C, Group Y and Group W-135 for subcutaneous use. The diluent is sterile pyrogen-free distilled water to which thimerosal (mercury derivative) 1:10,000 is added as a preservative. After reconstitution with diluent as indicated on the label, each 0.5 ml dose contains 50 mcg of "isolated product" from each of Groups A, C, Y and W-135 in isotonic sodium chloride solution preserved with thimerosal (mercury derivative). Each dose of vaccine also contains 2.5 mg to 5 mg of lactose added as a stabilizer.[1] The vaccine when reconstituted is a clear colorless liquid.
THIS VACCINE CONFORMS TO WHO REQUIREMENTS.

CLINICAL PHARMACOLOGY

N. meningitidis causes both endemic and epidemic disease, principally meningitis and meningococcemia. It is the second most common cause of bacterial meningitis in the United States (approximately 20% of all cases), affecting an estimated 3,000–4,000 people each year. The case-fatality rate is approximately 10% for meningococcal meningitis and 20% for meningococcemia, despite therapy with antimicro-

bial agents, such as penicillin, to which all strains remain highly sensitive.[2]

Within the United States, serogroup B, for which a vaccine is not yet available, accounts for 50%–55% of all cases; serogroup C, for 20%–25%; and serogroup W-135, for 15%. Serogroups Y (10%) and A (1%–2%) account for nearly all remaining cases. Serogroup W-135 has emerged as a major cause of disease only since 1975. While serogroup A causes only a small proportion of endemic disease in the United States, it is the most common cause of epidemics elsewhere.[2]

A study performed using 4 lots of Meningococcal Polysaccharide Vaccine, Groups A, C, Y and W-135 Combined in 150 adults showed at least a 4-fold increase in bactericidal antibodies to all groups in greater than 90 percent of the subjects.[3,4]

A study was conducted in 73 children 2 to 12 years of age. Post-immunization sera were not obtained on four children. Therefore, the seroconversion rates were based on 69 paired samples. Seroconversion rates as measured by bactericidal antibody were: Group A—72 percent, Group C—58 percent, Group Y—90 percent and Group W-135—82 percent. Seroconversion rates as measured by a 2-fold rise in antibody titers based on Solid Phase Radioimmunoassay were: Group A—99 percent, Group C—99 percent, Group Y—97 percent and Group W-135—89 percent.[5]

As with any vaccine, vaccination with Meningococcal Polysaccharide Vaccine, Groups A, C, Y and W-135 Combined may not protect 100% of susceptible individuals.

Vaccine efficacy. Numerous studies have demonstrated the immunogenicity and clinical efficacy of the A and C vaccines. The serogroup A polysaccharide induces antibody in some children as young as 3 months of age, although a response comparable to that seen in adults is not achieved until 4 or 5 years of age; the serogroup C component does not induce a good antibody response before age 18–24 months. The serogroup A vaccine has been shown to have a clinical efficacy of 85%–95% and to be of use in controlling epidemics.[6] A similar level of clinical efficacy has been demonstrated for the serogroup C vaccine, both in American military recruits and in an epidemic. The group Y and W-135 polysaccharides have been shown to be safe and immunogenic in adults and in children over 2 years of age; clinical protection has not been demonstrated directly, but is assumed, based on the production of bactericidal antibody, which for group C has been correlated with clinical protection. The antibody responses to each of the four polysaccharides in the quadrivalent vaccine are serogroup-specific and independent.[2]

Duration of efficacy. Antibodies against the group A and C polysaccharides decline markedly over the first 3 years following a single dose of vaccine. This antibody decline is more rapid in infants and young children than in adults. Similarly, while vaccine-induced clinical protection probably persists in schoolchildren and adults for at least 3 years, a recent study in Africa has demonstrated a marked decline in the efficacy of the group A vaccine in young children over time. In this study, efficacy declined from greater than 90% to less than 10% over 3 years in those under 4 years of age at the time of vaccination; in older children, efficacy was still 67%, 3 years after vaccination.[2,7]

INDICATIONS AND USAGE

Meningococcal Polysaccharide Vaccine, Groups A, C, Y and W-135 Combined, is indicated for the following individuals:

1. Persons 2 years of age and above in epidemic or endemic areas as might be determined in a population delineated by neighborhood, school, dormitory, or other reasonable boundary. The prevalent serogroup in such a situation should match a serogroup in the vaccine.
2. Individuals at particular high-risk to include persons with terminal component complement deficiencies and those with anatomic or functional asplenia.
3. Travelers to countries recognized as having hyperendemic or epidemic disease such as the part of Sub-Saharan Africa known as the "meningitis belt", which extends from Mauritania in the west to Ethiopia in the east.

Vaccinations also should be considered for household or institutional contacts of persons with meningococcal disease as an adjunct to appropriate antibiotic chemoprophylaxis as well as medical and laboratory personnel at risk of exposure to meningococcal disease.

This vaccine will not stimulate protection against infections caused by organisms other than Groups A, C, Y and W-135 meningococci.

CONTRAINDICATIONS

Immunization should be deferred during the course of any acute illness. Pregnant women should not be immunized since effects of vaccine on the fetus are unknown.

IT IS A CONTRAINDICATION TO ADMINISTER MENOMUNE A/C/Y/W-135 TO INDIVIDUALS KNOWN TO BE SENSITIVE TO THIMEROSAL OR AN OTHER COMPONENT OF THE VACCINE.

WARNING

If the vaccine is used in persons receiving immunosuppressive therapy, the expected immune response may not be obtained.

PRECAUTIONS

GENERAL

Epinephrine Injection (1:1000) must be immediately available to combat unexpected anaphylactic or other allergic reactions.

Prior to an injection of any vaccine, all known precautions should be taken to prevent side reactions. This includes a review of the patient's history with respect to possible sensitivity to the vaccine or similar vaccines.

As with any vaccine, vaccination with Meningococcal Polysaccharide Vaccine, Groups A, C, Y and W-135 Combined may not protect 100% of susceptible individuals. Protective antibody levels may be achieved within 10–14 days after vaccination.[2]

Special care should be taken to avoid injecting the vaccine intradermally, intramuscularly, or intravenously since clinical studies have not been done to establish safety and efficacy of the vaccine using these routes of administration.

A separate, sterile syringe and needle or a sterile disposable unit should be used for each individual patient to prevent transmission of hepatitis and other infectious agents from one person to another.

During use it is possible that the nozzle of the Jet Injector Apparatus may become contaminated with blood or serum. In one instance, such contamination has been reported to be associated with transmission of hepatitis b disease. Therefore, if blood or serum contamination occurs, the nozzle should be disassembled, cleansed and sterilized before continued use to prevent the possibility of transmission of hepatitis or other infectious agents from one person to another.[8]

PREGNANCY [9]

REPRODUCTIVE STUDIES—PREGNANCY CATEGORY C

Animal reproduction studies have not been conducted with Meningococcal Polysaccharide Vaccine, Groups A, C, Y and W-135. It is also not known whether Meningococcal Polysaccharide Vaccine, Groups A, C, Y and W-135 can cause fetal harm when administered to a pregnant woman or can affect reproduction capacity.

EXPERIENCE IN HUMANS

There is no data on the safety of Menomune when administered to a pregnant woman. Therefore, Menomune should not be administered to a pregnant woman, particularly in the first trimester.

PEDIATRIC USE

THERE ARE NO DATA ON SAFETY AND EFFICACY OF MENOMUNE WHEN ADMINISTERED TO CHILDREN UNDER 2 YEARS OF AGE.

ADVERSE REACTIONS

Adverse reactions to meningococcal vaccine are mild and infrequent, consisting of localized erythema lasting 1–2 days. Up to 2% of young children develop fever transiently after vaccination.[2]

As with the administration of any vaccine, one should expect possible hypersensitivity reactions.

DOSAGE AND ADMINISTRATION

Parenteral drug products should be inspected visually for extraneous particulate matter and/or discoloration prior to administration whenever solution and container permit. If these conditions exist, vaccine should not be administered. Reconstitute the vaccine using only the diluent supplied for this purpose. Draw the volume of diluent shown on the diluent label into a suitable size syringe and inject into the vial containing the vaccine. Shake vial until the vaccine is dissolved. Administer the vaccine subcutaneously.

The immunizing dose is a single injection of 0.5 ml given subcutaneously.

Primary Immunization

For both adults and children, vaccine is administered subcutaneously as a single 0.5 ml dose. The vaccine can be given at the same time as other immunizations, if needed. Protective antibody levels may be achieved within 10–14 days after vaccination.[2]

REVACCINATION

Revaccination may be indicated for individuals at high risk of infection, particularly children who were first immunized under 4 years of age; such children should be considered for revaccination after 2 or 3 years if they remain at high risk. The need for revaccination in older children and adults remains unknown.[2]

HOW SUPPLIED

Vial, 1 Dose, with 0.78 ml vial of diluent—Product No. 49281-489-01

Vial, 10 Dose, with 6 ml vial of diluent, for administration with needle and syringe (may be used with jet injector although the desired number of doses may not be obtained). Product No. 49281-489-91

Vial, 50 Dose, with 27.5 ml of diluent, for JET INJECTOR USE ONLY. Product No. 49281-489-95

Additional package sizes available on special order.

STORAGE

Store freeze-dried vaccine and reconstituted vaccine, when not in use, between 2°–8°C (35°–46°F). Discard remainder of multidose vials of vaccine within 5 days after reconstitution. The single dose vial should be used within 24 hours of reconstitution.

Special instructions for 50 Dose Vial of Meningococcal Polysaccharide Vaccine, A, C, Y and W-135 Combined, for Jet Injector Use.

DOSAGE AND ADMINISTRATION

Parenteral drug products should be inspected visually for extraneous particular matter and/or discoloration prior to administration whenever solution and container permit. If these conditions exist, vaccine should not be administered.

Using a suitable size syringe and needle and aseptic precautions, transfer the volume of diluent shown on the diluent label into the vial containing the vaccine. Shake vial until the vaccine is dissolved.

Administer ONLY with automatic hypodermic jet apparatus. 50 DOSE VIAL NOT TO BE UTILIZED IN NEEDLE AND SYRINGE METHOD OF IMMUNIZATION. If absolutely necessary, syringes and needles may be used with such containers with caution. However, due to coring of the stopper do NOT insert needle into vial more than 20 times. Discard partially used vial of vaccine. Immunization consists of a single injection of 0.5 ml given subcutaneously. Special care should be taken to avoid injecting the vaccine intradermally, intramuscularly, or intravenously by using the deltoid area, since clinical studies have not been done to establish the safety and efficacy of the vaccine using these routes of administration.

Any partially used reconstituted vaccine which has been administered with a Jet Injector Apparatus should NOT be reused and should be discarded.

CAUTION

During use it is possible that the nozzle of the Jet Injector Apparatus may become contaminated with blood or serum. In one instance, such contamination has been reported to be associated with transmission of hepatitis b disease. Therefore, if blood or serum contamination occurs, the nozzle should be disassembled, cleansed and sterilized before continued use to prevent the possibility of transmission of hepatitis or other infectious agents from one person to another.[8]

REFERENCES

1. Tiesjema, R. H., et al: Enhanced stability of meningococcal polysaccharide vaccines by using lactose as a menstruum for lyophilization. Bull WHO 55: 43–48, 1977
2. Recommendation of the Immunization Practices Advisory Committee (ACIP). Meningococcal Vaccines. MMWR 34: 255–259, 1985
3. Hankins, W.A., et al: Clinical and serological evaluation of a meningococcal polysaccharide vaccine groups A, C, Y and W-135. Proc Soc Exper Biol Med 169: 54–57, 1982
4. Lepow, M. L., et al: Reactogenicity and immunogenicity of a quadrivalent combined meningococcal polysaccharide vaccine in children. J Infect Dis 154: 1033–1036, 1986
5. Unpublished data available from Connaught Laboratories, Inc., compiled 1982
6. Peltola, H., et al: Clinical efficacy of meningococcus Group A capsular polysaccharide vaccine in children three months to five years of age. N Engl J Med 297: 686–691, 1977
7. Reingold, A. L., et al: Age-specific differences in duration of clinical protection after vaccination with meningococcal polysaccharide A vaccine. Lancet. No. 8447: 114–118, 1985
8. CDC. Hepatitis B associated with jet gun injection—California. MMWR 35: 373–376, 1986
9. Code of Federal Regulations. 21CFR201.57 (f) (6) (c), 1989

CONNAUGHT © is a trademark owned by Connaught Laboratories Limited.

Manufactured by:

CONNAUGHT LABORATORIES, INC.
Swiftwater, Pennsylvania 18370, U.S.A.
Product Information as of July, 1990

1895

Continued on next page

Connaught Laboratories—Cont.

TETANUS AND DIPHTHERIA TOXOIDS ADSORBED FOR ADULT USE USP ℞

Caution: Federal (U.S.A.) law prohibits dispensing without prescription.

For special instructions on use of Tetanus and Diphtheria Toxoids Adsorbed For Adult Use USP for JET INJECTOR USE—see other side of insert.

DESCRIPTION

Tetanus and Diphtheria Toxoids Adsorbed For Adult Use USP, is a sterile suspension of alum precipitated tetanus toxoid and diphtheria toxoid in isotonic sodium chloride solution for intramuscular use. Thimerosal (mercury derivative) 1:10,000 is added as a preservative. The vaccine, in suspension, is a turbid liquid, whitish-gray in color. Each single dose of 0.5 ml is formulated to contain not more than 2 Lf units of diphtheria toxoid, 5 Lf units of tetanus toxoid and not more than 0.25 mg of aluminum added in the form of aluminum potassium sulfate.

HOW SUPPLIED

Vial, 5 ml for administration with needle and syringe—Product No. 49281-271-83

Vial, 30 ml for JET INJECTOR USE ONLY—Product No. 49281-271-92

DIPHTHERIA AND TETANUS TOXOIDS AND ACELLULAR PERTUSSIS VACCINE ADSORBED ℞

TRIPEDIA®

CAUTION: *Federal (U.S.A.) law prohibits dispensing without prescription.*

DESCRIPTION

Tripedia®, Diphtheria and Tetanus Toxoids and Acellular Pertussis Vaccine Adsorbed, for intramuscular use, is a sterile solution of diphtheria and tetanus toxoids adsorbed, with acellular pertussis vaccine in an isotonic sodium chloride solution containing thimerosal as a preservative and sodium phosphate to control pH. After shaking, the vaccine is a homogeneous white suspension.

The acellular pertussis vaccine components are isolated from culture fluids of Phase 1 *Bordetella pertussis* grown in a modified Stainer-Scholte medium.[1] After purification by salt precipitation, ultracentrifugation, and ultrafiltration, pertussis toxin (PT) and filamentous hemagglutinin (FHA) are combined to obtain a 1:1 ratio and treated with formaldehyde to inactivate PT. Thimerosal (mercury derivative) 1:10,000 is added as a preservative.

Corynebacterium diphtheriae cultures are grown in a modified Mueller and Miller medium. *Clostridium tetani* cultures are grown in a peptone-based medium. Both toxins are detoxified with formaldehyde. The detoxified materials are then separately purified by serial ammonium sulfate fractionation and diafiltration.

The toxoids are adsorbed using aluminum potassium sulfate (alum). The adsorbed diphtheria and tetanus toxoids are combined with acellular pertussis concentrate, and diluted to a final volume using sterile phosphate-buffered physiological saline. Thimerosal (mercury derivative) 1:10,000 is added as a preservative. Each 0.5 mL dose contains, by assay, not more than 0.170 mg of aluminum and not more than 100 μg (0.02%) of residual formaldehyde. The vaccine contains gelatin and polysorbate 80 (Tween-80) which are used in the production of the pertussis concentrate.

Each 0.5 mL dose is formulated to contain 6.7 Lf units of diphtheria toxoid and 5 Lf units of tetanus toxoid (both toxoids induce at least 2 units of antitoxin per mL in the guinea pig potency test), and 46.8 μg of pertussis antigens. This is represented in the final vaccine as 23.4 μg of inactivated pertussis toxin (PT—also referred to as lymphocytosis promoting factor of LPF) and 23.4 μg of filamentous hemagglutinin antigen (FHA).

The potency of the pertussis component is evaluated by measurement, using an ELISA system, of the antibody response to PT and FHA in immunized mice.

Acellular Pertussis Vaccine Concentrate (For Further Manufacturing Use) is produced by The Research Foundation for Microbial Diseases of Osaka University ("BIKEN®"), Osaka, Japan under U.S. license, and is combined with diphtheria and tetanus toxoids manufactured by Connaught Laboratories, Inc. The bulk vaccine is prepared by Connaught Laboratories, Inc. Tripedia is filled, labeled, packaged, and released by Connaught Laboratories, Inc. (CLI).

CLINICAL PHARMACOLOGY

Simultaneous immunization against diphtheria, tetanus, and pertussis, using a conventional "whole-cell" pertussis DTP vaccine (Diphtheria and Tetanus Toxoids and Pertussis Vaccine Adsorbed—For Pediatric Use), has been a routine practice during infancy and childhood in the United States since the late 1940s. This practice has played a major role in markedly reducing the incidence rates of cases and deaths from each of these diseases.[2]

Tripedia (Diphtheria and Tetanus Toxoids and Acellular Pertussis Vaccine Adsorbed) combines Connaught Laboratories, Inc. diphtheria and tetanus toxoids with purified pertussis antigens (inactivated PT and FHA). These pertussis antigens, produced by The Research Foundation for Microbial Diseases of Osaka University ("BIKEN®"), have been used routinely in Japan for approximately ten years[3,4,5,6] and have been under investigational use in Sweden,[1,7,8,9,10] as well as in the United States.[11,12,13,14]

DIPHTHERIA

Corynebacterium diphtheriae may cause both localized and generalized disease. The systemic intoxication is caused by diphtheria exotoxin, an extracellular protein metabolite of toxigenic strains of *C. diphtheriae.* Protection against disease is due to the development of antibody to diphtheria toxin.

At one time, diphtheria was common in the United States. More than 200,000 cases, primarily among children, were reported in 1921. Approximately 5% to 10% of cases were fatal; the highest case-fatality rates were in the very young and the elderly. Reported cases of diphtheria of all types declined from 306 in 1975 to 59 in 1979; most were cutaneous diphtheria reported from a single state. After 1979, cutaneous diphtheria was no longer reportable.[2] From 1980 to 1986, only 18 cases of respiratory diphtheria were reported in the United States; 14 occurred among persons 15 years of age or older.[15,16]

Diphtheria is currently a rare disease in the United States primarily because of the high level of appropriate vaccination among children (97% of children entering school have received ≥ three doses of diphtheria and tetanus toxoids and pertussis vaccine adsorbed [DTP]) and because of an apparent reduction in the circulation of toxigenic strains of *Corynebacterium diphtheriae.*[2] Most cases occur among unvaccinated or inadequately vaccinated persons.[2]

Both toxigenic and nontoxigenic strains of *C. diphtheriae* can cause disease, but only strains that produce diphtheria toxin cause severe manifestations, such as myocarditis and neuritis. Diphtheria remains a serious disease, with the highest case-fatality rates among infants and the elderly.[2]

Complete immunization significantly reduces the risk of developing diphtheria, and immunized persons who develop disease have milder illness. Protection is thought to last at least 10 years. Immunization does not, however, eliminate carriage of *C. diphtheriae* in the pharynx or nose or on the skin.[2]

The efficacy of the CLI's diphtheria toxoid used in Tripedia was determined on the basis of immunogenicity studies, with a comparison to a serological correlate of protection (0.01 antitoxin units/mL) established by the Panel on Review of Bacterial Vaccines & Toxoids.[17]

TETANUS

Tetanus is an intoxication manifested primarily by neuromuscular dysfunction caused by a potent exotoxin elaborated by *Clostridium tetani.*

The occurrence of tetanus in the United States has decreased dramatically from 560 reported cases in 1947 to a record low of 48 reported cases in 1987. Tetanus in the United States is primarily a disease of older adults. Of 99 tetanus patients with complete information reported to the Centers for Disease Control (CDC) during 1987 and 1988, 68% were ≥50 years of age, while only six were <20 years of age. Overall, the case-fatality rate was 21%. The disease continues to occur almost exclusively among persons who are unvaccinated or inadequately vaccinated or whose vaccination histories are unknown or uncertain.[2]

In 4% of tetanus cases reported during 1987 and 1988, no wound or other condition was implicated. Non-acute skin lesions, such as ulcers, or medical conditions, such as abscesses, were reported in 14% of cases.[2]

Spores of *C. tetani* are ubiquitous. Serological tests indicate that naturally acquired immunity to tetanus toxin does not occur in the United States. Thus, universal primary immunization, with subsequent maintenance of adequate antitoxin levels by means of appropriately timed boosters, is necessary to protect all age groups. Tetanus toxoid is a highly effective antigen, and a completed primary series generally induces protective levels of serum antitoxin that persist for 10 or more years.[2]

The efficacy of the CLI's tetanus toxoid used in Tripedia was determined on the basis of immunogenicity studies with a comparison to a serological correlate of protection (0.01 antitoxin units/mL) established by the Panel on Review of Bacterial Vaccines & Toxoids.[17]

PERTUSSIS

Pertussis (whooping cough) is a disease of the respiratory tract caused by *Bordetella pertussis.* This gram-negative coccobacillus produces a variety of biologically active components. One of these components, pertussis toxin (PT), has been associated with a number of effects such as lymphocytosis, leukocytosis, sensitivity to histamine, changes in glucose and/or insulin levels, neurological effects, and adjuvant activity.[18] The role of the different components produced by *B. pertussis* in either the pathogenesis of, or the immunity to, pertussis is not well understood. Immunization with vaccines containing inactivated PT and filamentous hemagglutinin (FHA), have been associated with protection in clinical studies. The pertussis component in Tripedia induces immunity against pertussis.[9] The acellular pertussis component, in Tripedia, contains not more than 50 endotoxin units/mL.

Pertussis is highly communicable (attack rates of >90% have been reported among unvaccinated household contacts)[19] and can cause severe disease, particularly among very young children. Of 10,749 patients <1 year of age reported nationally as having pertussis during the period 1980 to 1989, 69% were hospitalized, 22% had pneumonia, 3.0% had ≥one seizure, 0.9% had encephalopathy, and 0.6% died.[20] Because of the substantial risks of complications of the disease, completion of a primary series of DTP vaccine early in life is essential.[2]

In older children and adults, including in some instances those previously immunized, infection may result in nonspecific symptoms of bronchitis or an upper respiratory tract infection, and pertussis may not be diagnosed because classic signs, especially the inspiratory whoop, may be absent. Older preschool-aged children and school-aged siblings who are not fully immunized and develop pertussis can be important sources of infection for young infants, the group at highest risk of disease and disease severity.[2] The infected adult is important in the overall transmission of pertussis.[21,22]

General use of whole-cell pertussis DTP vaccines has resulted in a substantial reduction in cases and deaths from pertussis disease.[23,24] The use of Tripedia as the fourth or fifth dose evokes an antibody response at least as great as Connaught's whole-cell pertussis DTP vaccine following a primary series with commercially available U.S. whole-cell pertussis DTP with respect to PT and FHA antibodies.[1,11,12]

Acellular pertussis vaccines have been used in Japan since 1981, mostly in 2-year-old children. Evidence for the efficacy of these vaccines, as a group, is demonstrated by the decline in pertussis disease with their routine use in that country.[3,23] In addition, a review of epidemiological studies of the Japanese acellular pertussis vaccines estimated that these vaccines, as a group, were 88% efficacious in protecting against clinical pertussis on household exposure, with a 95% confidence interval of 79% to 93%.[25]

A large placebo-controlled efficacy trial of two BIKEN acellular pertussis vaccines was carried out in Sweden in 1986–1987. One of the vaccines contained a BIKEN two-component acellular pertussis vaccine comparable to that contained in Tripedia. In its first phase, the trial in Sweden was a randomized, blinded prospective trial using a standardized case definition and active case ascertainment. In this phase, 1,389 children, 5 to 11 months of age, received two doses of the BIKEN inactivated PT/FHA acellular pertussis vaccine 7 to 13 weeks apart and 954 received a placebo control. During the 15 months of follow-up from 30 days after the second dose, culture-confirmed whooping cough (cough and a positive culture of *Bordetella pertussis*) occurred in 40 placebo and 18 acellular pertussis vaccine recipients. The point estimate of protective efficacy for the vaccine was 69% (95% confidence interval; 47% to 82%) for all cases of culture-confirmed pertussis and 80% (95% confidence interval; 59% to 91%) for culture confirmed cases with cough of over 30 days duration.[9]

A three-year unblinded passive follow-up of vaccine and placebo recipients from the above Swedish study has shown a post-trial efficacy of 77% (95% confidence interval; 65% to 85%) for all culture-proven cases of pertussis, and an efficacy of 92% (95% confidence interval; 84% to 96%) for culture-proven cases with a cough of over 30 days duration.[26]

Anti-PT and anti-FHA antibody responses in children enrolled in the trial in Sweden were subsequently compared to responses observed in clinical trials of Tripedia conducted in the U.S. In the U.S. trials, children 15 to 20 months of age who had previously received three doses of licensed whole-cell pertussis DTP and children 4 to 6 years of age who had previously received four doses of licensed whole-cell pertussis DTP were immunized with a single dose of Tripedia. The anti-PT and anti-FHA antibody responses to Tripedia in the U.S. trials were found to be similar to the responses observed in children enrolled in the trial in Sweden.[1] Although the Swedish efficacy trial immunization with an inactivated PT/FHA vaccine was shown to protect against pertussis, no specific serological correlate or measure of protective immune response was found.[1,9] The role in clinical protection of specific serum antibodies is, therefore, not known at this time.

Additionally, the antibody responses in children immunized with Tripedia were compared to those in children immunized with CLI's licensed whole-cell pertussis DTP vaccine. Immunogenicity data from the clinical trials in the U.S. are summarized in Table 1. Anti-PT and anti-FHA responses to

Tripedia were significantly higher than those to CLI's whole-cell pertussis DTP vaccine. Serological responses to diphtheria and tetanus antigens, not shown in Table 1, were equal to or greater than those produced by CLI's whole-cell pertussis DTP vaccine.[1,11,12]
Clinical experience (immunogenicity) in the United States is summarized in Table 1.[1,11,12]
[See Table 1 at right.]
A total of 3,700 doses of Tripedia have been adminstered in U.S. clinical trials, in children 15–20 months of age and 4–6 years of age. When compared to CLI's whole-cell pertussis DTP vaccine, Tripedia produced fewer and milder local reactions such as erythema, swelling, and tenderness at the injection site; as well as fewer and milder systemic reactions such as fever, irritability, drowsiness, vomiting, anorexia and high-pitched unusual cry.[1] Rates of more serious and infrequent adverse experiences for Tripedia are not known at this time.

TABLE 1.[1,11,12] COMPARISON OF IgG ANTIBODY TO PT AND FHA IN ELISA UNITS (EU) AND CHO-CELL NEUTRALIZATION TITERS (CHO) INDUCED BY A SINGLE DOSE OF EITHER TRIPEDIA OR CLI'S WHOLE-CELL PERTUSSIS DTP VACCINE IN CHILDREN 15 TO 20 MONTHS OF AGE* AND 4 TO 6 YEARS OF AGE**

VACCINE	AGE GROUP (n=)	PT/GMT† (EU)		FHA/GMT† (EU)		CHO	
		Pre-Vaccination	Post-Vaccination‡	Pre-Vaccination	Post-Vaccination‡	Pre-Vaccination	Post-Vaccination†
Tripedia	15–20 Months (354)	14.5	443.0§	7.0	65.0§	25.3	300§
CLI's Whole-Cell DTP	15–20 Months (175)	14.5	67.0	6.0	19.0	24.8	119
Tripedia	4–6 Years (211)	14.5	408.0§	18.9	36.0§	23.6	210§
CLI's Whole-Cell DTP	4–6 Years (65)	15.2	81.0	19.2	104.0	27.9	107

* All children in the 15- to 20-month group received U.S. licensed whole-cell pertussis DTP vaccine for the first three doses of their primary series.
** All children in the 4- to 6-year group received U.S. licensed whole-cell pertussis DTP vaccine for the first four doses in their primary series.
† Geometric mean titer.
‡ Post-vaccination 4 to 6 weeks.
£ Post-vaccination GMT for the Tripedia group, (4 to 6 year olds), is significantly higher than that of the whole-cell pertussis DTP vaccine group ($P < 0.05$).
§ Post-vaccination GMT's for the Tripedia group, at 15 to 20 months and at 4 to 6 years, are significantly higher than those of the matching whole-cell DTP group, ($P < 0.001$ in each case).

INDICATIONS AND USAGE

Diphtheria and Tetanus Toxoids and Acellular Pertussis Vaccine Adsorbed, Tripedia, is indicated as a fourth and/or fifth dose for immunization of children 15 months to 7 years of age (prior to seventh birthday) who have previously been immunized against diphtheria, tetanus and pertussis with three or four doses of whole-cell pertussis DTP vaccine. However, in instances where the pertussis vaccine component is contraindicated, Diphtheria and Tetanus Toxoids Adsorbed (For Pediatric Use) (DT) should be used for each of the remaining doses.
If passive immunization is required, Tetanus Immune Globulin (Human) (TIG) and/or equine Diphtheria Antitoxin should be used.
Persons recovering from confirmed pertussis do not need additional doses of DTP but should receive additional doses of DT to complete the series.
Tripedia is not to be used for treatment of actual infection.
As with any vaccine, vaccination with Tripedia may not protect 100% of susceptible individuals.
THIS VACCINE IS NOT RECOMMENDED FOR USE IN CHILDREN BELOW THE AGE OF 15 MONTHS. THIS VACCINE IS NOT RECOMMENDED FOR USE AS A PRIMARY SERIES IN CHILDREN OF ANY AGE.

CONTRAINDICATIONS

Hypersensitivity to any component of the vaccine, including thimerosal, a mercury derivative, is a contraindication.
Immunization should be deferred during the course of any febrile illness or acute infection. A minor afebrile illness such as a mild upper respiratory infection is not usually reason to defer immunization.
Elective immunization procedures should be deferred during an outbreak of poliomyelitis.[27]
Data on the use of Tripedia in children for whom whole-cell pertussis DTP vaccine is contraindicated are not available. Until such data are available, it would be prudent to consider the Immunization Practices Advisory Committee (ACIP) and American Academy of Pediatrics (AAP) contraindications to whole-cell pertussis DTP vaccine to be contraindications to Tripedia.
Immunization with Tripedia is contraindicated if the child has experienced any event following previous immunization with pertussis vaccine (whole-cell DTP or acellular pertussis-containing DTP vaccine), which is considered by the ACIP or AAP to be a contraindication to further doses of pertussis vaccine. The ACIP states that if any of the following events listed in Table 2 occur in temporal relation to receipt of DTP, the decision to give subsequent doses of vaccine containing the pertussis component should be carefully considered.
It is a contraindication to use this or any other vaccine after a serious adverse reaction temporally associated with a previous dose, including an anaphylactic reaction.[2]
Encephalopathy not due to an identifiable cause, occurring within 7 days of a prior whole-cell pertussis DTP or acellular pertussis DTP immunization and consisting of major alterations of consciousness, unresponsiveness, generalized or focal seizures that persist for more than a few hours and failure to recover within 24 hours should be considered a contraindication to further use; this includes severe alterations in consciousness with generalized or focal neurologic signs. Even though causation cannot be established, no subsequent doses should be given.[2]

WARNINGS

This vaccine is not recommended for use in children below the age of 15 months. Efficacy data for Tripedia in infants is not available. Although antibody responses to diphtheria, tetanus, and pertussis toxin, and FHA in infants immunized with Tripedia were at least equivalent to those for CLI's whole-cell pertussis DTP vaccine, the role of serum antibodies in protection against pertussis is unknown.
Tripedia is not recommended for immunization on or after the seventh birthday.
If any of the following events occur in temporal relation to receipt of DTP, the decision to give subsequent doses of vaccine containing the pertussis component should be carefully considered. There may be circumstances, such as a high incidence of pertussis, when the potential benefits outweigh possible risks, particularly since these events are not associated with permanent sequelae.[2]
THE FOLLOWING EVENTS WERE PREVIOUSLY CONSIDERED CONTRAINDICATIONS AND ARE NOW CONSIDERED PRECAUTIONS BY THE ACIP:[2]
Temperature of ≥40.5°C (105°F) within 48 hours not due to another identifiable cause. Such a temperature is considered a precaution because of the likelihood that fever following a subsequent dose of DTP vaccine also will be high. Because such febrile reactions are usually attributed to the pertussis component, vaccination with DT should not be discontinued.[2]
Collapse or shock-like state (hypotonic-hyporesponsive episode) within 48 hours. Although these uncommon events have not been recognized to cause death nor to induce permanent neurological sequelae, it is prudent to continue vaccination with DT, omitting the pertussis component.[2]
Persistent, inconsolable crying lasting ≥3 hours, occurring within 48 hours of vaccination. Follow-up of infants who have cried inconsolably following DTP vaccination has indicated that this reaction, though unpleasant, is without long-term sequelae and not associated with other reactions of greater significance. Inconsolable crying occurs most frequently following the first dose and is less frequently reported following subsequent doses of DTP vaccine.[2]
Convulsions with or without fever occurring within three days. Short-lived convulsions, with or without fever, have not been shown to cause permanent sequelae. Furthermore, the occurrence of prolonged febrile seizures (i.e., status epilepticus—any seizure lasting >30 minutes or recurrent seizures lasting a total of 30 minutes without the child fully regaining consciousness), irrespective of their cause, involving an otherwise normal child does not substantially increase the risk for subsequent febrile (brief or prolonged) or afebrile seizures. The risk is significantly increased only among those children who are neurologically abnormal before their episode of status epilepticus.[2]
Tripedia should not be given to children with any coagulation disorder, including thrombocytopenia, that would contraindicate intramuscular injection unless the potential benefit clearly outweighs the risk of administration.
In the opinion of the manufacturer, use of this vaccine is also contraindicated if the child, siblings, or parents have a history of a seizure disorder. Recent studies suggest that infants and children with a history of convulsions in first-degree family members (i.e., siblings and parents) have a 3.2-fold increased risk for neurologic events compared with those without such histories.[25,29]
However, the ACIP has concluded that a family history of convulsions in parents and siblings is not a contraindication to pertussis vaccination and that children with such family histories should receive pertussis vaccine according to the recommended schedule.[2,23,28]
Acetaminophen should be given at the time of DTP vaccination and every four hours for 24 hours to reduce the possibility of post-vaccination fever.[2]
Studies have failed to provide evidence to support a causal relation between DTP vaccination and either serious acute neurologic illness or permanent neurologic injury.[2]
Infants and children with recognized possible or potential underlying neurologic conditions seem to be at enhanced risk for the appearance of manifestations of the underlying neurologic disorder within two or three days following vaccination. Whether to administer DTP (or Tripedia) to children with proven or suspected underlying neurologic disorders must be decided on an individual basis. Important considerations include the current local incidence of pertussis, the near absence of diphtheria in the United States and the low risk of infection with *C. tetani*.[2]
Only full doses (0.5 mL) of DTP (or Tripedia) vaccine should be given; if a specific contraindication to DTP exists, the vaccine should not be given.[2]
Controversy regarding the safety of pertussis vaccine during the 1970s led to several studies of the benefits and risks of this vaccination during the 1980s. These epidemiologic analyses clearly indicate that the benefits of the pertussis immunization program outweigh the risks.[2,30]

PRECAUTIONS

GENERAL

Care is to be taken by the health-care provider for the safe and effective use of this vaccine.
EPINEPHRINE INJECTION (1:1000) MUST BE IMMEDIATELY AVAILABLE SHOULD AN ACUTE ANAPHYLACTIC REACTION OCCUR DUE TO ANY COMPONENT OF THE VACCINE.
Previous immunization history should be ascertained to confirm that at least three doses of whole-cell pertussis DTP vaccine have been given.
Prior to an injection of any vaccine, all known precautions should be taken to prevent adverse reactions. This includes a review of the patient's history with respect to possible sensitivity and any previous adverse reactions to the vaccine or similar vaccines, previous immunization history, current health status (see **CONTRAINDICATIONS** section), and a current knowledge of the literature concerning the use of the vaccine under consideration. Immunosuppressed patients may not respond. Tripedia is not contraindicated based on the presence of HIV infection.[2]

TABLE 2.[2] Contraindications and Precautions to Further DTP (or acellular pertussis) Vaccination

Contraindications
An immediate anaphylactic reaction.
Encephalopathy occurring within 7 days following DTP (or acellular pertussis) vaccination.
Precautions
Temperature ≥40.5°C (105°F) within 48 hours not due to another identifiable cause.
Collapse or shock-like state (hypotonic-hyporesponsive episode) within 48 hours.
Persistent, inconsolable crying lasting ≥3 hours, occurring within 48 hours.
Convulsions with or without fever occurring within 3 days.

Special care should be taken to ensure that the injection does not enter a blood vessel.
A separate, sterile syringe and needle or a sterile disposable unit should be used for each patient to prevent transmission of hepatitis or other infectious agents from person to person. Needles should not be recapped and should be disposed of properly.

Continued on next page

Consult 1997 supplements and future editions for revisions

Connaught Laboratories—Cont.

INFORMATION FOR PATIENT
Parents should be fully informed of the benefits and risks of immunization with Tripedia. The health-care provider should provide the Vaccine Information Pamphlets (VIPs) which are required to be given with each immunization.
The physician should inform the parents or guardians about the potential for adverse reactions that have been temporally associated with whole-cell pertussis DTP vaccine and Tripedia administration and obtain informed consent. Parents or guardians should be instructed to report any serious adverse reactions to their health-care provider.
IT IS EXTREMELY IMPORTANT WHEN A CHILD IS RETURNED FOR THE NEXT DOSE IN THE SERIES, THAT THE PARENT SHOULD BE QUESTIONED CONCERNING OCCURRENCE OF ANY SYMPTOMS AND/OR SIGNS OF AN ADVERSE REACTION AFTER THE PREVIOUS DOSE (SEE CONTRAINDICATIONS; ADVERSE REACTIONS).
The health-care provider should inform the parent or guardian the importance of completing the immunization series, unless a contraindication to further immunization exists.
The U.S. Department of Health and Human Services has established a new Vaccine Adverse Event Reporting System (VAERS) to accept all reports of suspected adverse events after the administration of any vaccine, including but not limited to the reporting of events required by the National Childhood Vaccine Injury Act of 1986.[31] The toll-free number for VAERS forms and information is 1-800-822-7967.
The National Vaccine Injury Compensation Program, established by the National Childhood Vaccine Injury Act of 1986, requires physicians and other health-care providers who administer vaccines to maintain permanent vaccination records and to report occurrences of certain adverse events to the U.S. Department of Health and Human Services. Reportable events include those listed in the Act for each vaccine and events specified in the package insert as contraindications to further doses of the vaccine.[32,33]
DRUG INTERACTIONS
As with other IM injections use with caution in patients on anticoagulant therapy.
Influenza Virus Vaccine should not be given within three days of the administration of Tripedia.[30]
Immunosuppressive therapies, including irradiation, antimetabolites, alkylating agents, cytotoxic drugs, and corticosteroids (used in greater than physiologic doses), may reduce the immune response to vaccines. Although no specific studies with pertussis vaccine are available, if immunosuppressive therapy will be discontinued shortly, it would be reasonable to defer immunization until the patient has been off therapy for one month; otherwise, the patient should be vaccinated while still on therapy.[2]
If Tripedia has been administered to persons receiving immunosuppressive therapy, a recent injection of immune globulin or having an immunodeficiency disorder, an adequate immunologic response may not be obtained.
Tetanus Immune Globulin, or Diphtheria Antitoxin, if used, should be given in a separate site, with a separate needle and syringe.
CARCINOGENESIS, MUTAGENESIS, IMPAIRMENT OF FERTILITY
Tripedia has not been evaluated for its carcinogenic, mutagenic potentials or impairment of fertility.

THIS VACCINE IS NOT RECOMMENDED FOR PERSONS 7 YEARS OF AGE AND OLDER.
PEDIATRIC USE
Efficacy data for Tripedia in infants is not available. Although antibody responses to diphtheria, tetanus, and pertussis toxin and FHA in infants immunized with Tripedia were at least equivalent to those for CLI's whole-cell pertussis DTP vaccine, the role of serum antibodies in protection against pertussis is unknown at this time.
Tripedia is not recommended for use in children below 15 months of age. This vaccine is not recommended for use as a primary series in children of any age.
Tripedia is not recommended for individuals over 7 years of age. Tetanus and Diphtheria Toxoids Adsorbed For Adult Use (Td) is to be used in individuals 7 years of age or older. Diphtheria and Tetanus Toxoids and Acellular Pertussis Vaccine Adsorbed, should not be used to immunize children less than 15 months of age.

ADVERSE REACTIONS

Local adverse reactions which include pain, erythema, heat, edema, and induration, and systemic reactions such as fever, drowsiness, fretfulness, and anorexia may occur following vaccination. Table 3 lists the frequency of adverse reactions in 372 children who received Tripedia at 15 to 20 months and 239 children who received Tripedia at 4 to 6 years of age. These children had previously received three or four doses of whole-cell pertussis DTP vaccine at approximately 2, 4, 6 and 18 months of age.[1]
Rarely, an anaphylactic reaction (i.e., hives, swelling of the mouth, difficulty breathing, hypotension, or shock) has been reported after receiving preparations containing diphtheria, tetanus, and/or pertussis antigens.[2]
Arthus-type hypersensitivity reactions, characterized by severe local reactions (generally starting 2 to 8 hours after an injection), may follow receipt of tetanus toxoid. A few cases of peripheral neuropathy have been reported following tetanus toxoid administration, although a causal relationship has not been established.[2]
In the National Childhood Encephalopathy Study, (NCES), a large, case-control study in England, children 2 to 35 months of age with serious, acute neurologic disorders such as encephalopathy or complicated convulsion(s), were more likely to have received DTP in the 7 days preceding onset than their age-, sex-, and neighborhood-matched controls. Among children known to be neurologically normal before entering the study, the relative risk (estimated by odds ratio) of a neurologic illness occurring within the 7-day period following receipt of DTP dose, compared to children not receiving DTP vaccine in the 7-day period before onset of their illness, was 3.3 ($p < 0.001$).[2]
Within this 7-day period, the risk was significantly increased for immunized children only within 3 days of vaccination (relative risk 4.2, $p < 0.001$). The relative risk for illnesses occurring 4 to 7 days after vaccination was 2.1 ($.05 < p < 0.1$). Serious neurologic illnesses requiring hospitalization attributable to pertussis vaccine are rare. Final analysis of a comprehensive case-control study has estimated that the risk of such illnesses is 1 in 140,000 doses administered. An earlier analysis had estimated this risk at 1/110,000 doses. In contrast, final analysis of the case control study found that the risk of serious neurologic illness following pertussis disease was 1/11,000 pertussis cases.[34] Repeated evaluations have shown that the benefits of vaccination outweigh the risks; therefore, both the ACIP and the American Academy of Pediatrics continue to recommend the use of DTP vaccine.[2,30]

TABLE 3.[1] ADVERSE EVENTS OCCURRING 24, 48 AND 72 HOURS FOLLOWING DIPHTHERIA AND TETANUS TOXOIDS AND ACELLULAR PERTUSSIS VACCINE ADSORBED (TRIPEDIA) IMMUNIZATIONS GIVEN AT 15 TO 20 MONTHS AND 4 TO 6 YEARS OF AGE.

EVENT	FREQUENCY					
	15 to 20 Months Reaction % (n=372)			4 to 6 Years Reaction % (n=239)		
	24 hr.	48 hr.	72 hr.	24 hr.	48 hr.	72 hr.
Local						
Erythema*	13%	7%	3%	25%	23%	14%
Swelling**	6%	2%	1%	21%	20%	14%
Tenderness	6%	4%	2%	35%	20%	8%
Mild/Moderate Systemic						
Fever >101°F (rectal)	4%	1%	1%	3%	2%	1%
Gastrointestinal						
Diarrhea	3%	3%	2%	0%	0%	0%
Vomiting	2%	1%	0%	1%	1%	0%
Anorexia	6%	4%	3%	5%	3%	1%
Neurological						
Drowsiness	11%	4%	1%	13%	3%	2%
Irritability	15%	9%	5%	10%	7%	5%
High-pitched unusual cry	1%	1%	0%	0%	0%	0%

* Includes all occurrences of erythema.
** Includes all occurrences of swelling.

The methods and results of the NCES have been thoroughly scrutinized since publication of the study. This reassessment by multiple groups has determined that the number of patients was too small and their classification subject to enough uncertainty to preclude drawing valid conclusions about whether a causal relation exists between pertussis vaccine and permanent neurologic damage. Preliminary data from a 10-year follow-up study of some of the children studied in the original NCES study also suggested a relation between symptoms following DTP vaccination and permanent neurologic disability. However, details are not available to evaluate this study adequately, and the same concerns remain about DTP vaccine precipitating initial manifestations of pre-existing neurologic disorders.[2]
Sudden Infant Death Syndrome (SIDS) has occurred in infants following administration of DTP. Large case-control studies of SIDS in the United States have shown that receipt of DTP was not causally related to SIDS.[35,36,37] It should be recognized that the first three primary immunizing doses of DTP are usually administered to infants 2 to 6 months old and that approximately 85% of SIDS cases occur at ages 1 to 6 months, with the peak incidence occurring at 6 weeks to 4 months of age. By chance alone, some cases of SIDS can be expected to be related to recent receipt of DTP.[35] Recent evidence does not indicate a causal relation between DTP vaccine and SIDS.[38]
Onset of infantile spasms has occurred in infants who have recently received DTP or DT. Analysis of data from the NCES on children with infantile spasms showed that receipt of DT or DTP was not causally related to infantile spasms.[39] The incidence of onset of infantile spasms increases at 3 to 9 months of age, the time period in which the second and third doses of DTP are generally given. Therefore, some cases of infantile spasms can be expected to be related by chance alone to recent receipt of DTP.[2]
A bulging fontanelle associated with increased intracranial pressure which occurred within 24 hours following DTP immunization has been reported, although a causal relationship has not been established.[40,41,42]
[See Table 3 below.]
The following illnesses have been reported as temporally associated with vaccine containing tetanus toxoid: neurological complications[43,44] including cochlear lesion,[45] brachial plexus neuropathies,[45,46] paralysis of the radial nerve,[47] paralysis of the recurrent nerve,[45] accommodation paresis, and EEG disturbances with encephalopathy.[48] In the differential diagnosis of polyradiculoneuropathies following administration of a vaccine containing tetanus toxoid, tetanus toxoid should be considered as a possible etiology.[49,50]

Reporting of Adverse Events
Reporting by parents and patients of all adverse events occurring after vaccine administration should be encouraged. Adverse events following immunization with vaccine should be reported by the health-care provider to the U.S. Department of Health and Human Services (DHHS) Vaccine Adverse Event Reporting System (VAERS). Reporting forms and information about reporting requirements or completion of the form can be obtained from VAERS through a toll-free number 1-800-822-7967.[31,32,33]
The health-care provider also should report these events to Director of Medical Affairs, Connaught Laboratories, Inc., Route 611, P.O. Box 187, Swiftwater, PA 18370 or call 1-800-822-2463.

DOSAGE AND ADMINISTRATION

Parenteral drug products should be inspected visually for extraneous particulate matter and/or discoloration prior to administration whenever solution and container permit. If these conditions exist, the vaccine should not be administered.
SHAKE VIAL WELL *before withdrawing each dose.* Inject 0.5 mL of Tripedia intramuscularly only. The preferred injection sites are the anterolateral aspect of the thigh and the deltoid muscle of the upper arm. The vaccine should not be injected into the gluteal area or areas where there may be a major nerve trunk. During the course of immunizations, injections should not be made more than once at the same site.
The use of reduced volume (fractional doses) is not recommended. The effect of such practices on the frequency of serious adverse events and on protection against disease has not been determined.
Do NOT administer this product subcutaneously. Special care should be taken to ensure that the injection does not enter a blood vessel.
TRIPEDIA IS INDICATED FOR THE FOURTH DOSE OF THE DIPHTHERIA, TETANUS AND PERTUSSIS IMMUNIZATION SERIES. TRIPEDIA MAY BE GIVEN 6 TO 12 MONTHS AFTER THE THIRD DOSE OF WHOLE-CELL PERTUSSIS DTP TO MAINTAIN ADEQUATE IMMUNITY DURING THE PRESCHOOL YEARS. THIS DOSE IS AN INTEGRAL PART OF THE PRIMARY VACCINATING COURSE.
TRIPEDIA IS INDICATED FOR THE FIFTH DOSE OF THE DIPHTHERIA, TETANUS AND PERTUSSIS IMMUNIZATION SERIES. PRIOR IMMUNIZATIONS MAY CON-

SIST OF THREE DOSES OF WHOLE-CELL PERTUSSIS DTP AND ONE DOSE OF ACELLULAR PERTUSSIS DTP OR FOUR DOSES OF WHOLE-CELL PERTUSSIS DTP. TRIPEDIA MAY BE GIVEN TO CHILDREN 4 TO 6 YEARS OF AGE, BEFORE ENTERING KINDERGARTEN OR ELEMENTARY SCHOOL (NOT CONSIDERED NECESSARY IF FOURTH PRIMARY VACCINATING DOSE ADMINISTERED AFTER FOURTH BIRTHDAY).

The vial of vaccine should be shaken to ensure a proper suspension of the vaccine prior to use.

The simultaneous administration of DTaP, OPV, and MMR has not been evaluated. However, on the basis of studies using whole-cell DTP, the ACIP does not anticipate any differences in seroconversion rates and rates of side effects from those observed when the vaccines are administered separately. The ACIP recommends the simultaneous administration of all vaccines appropriate to the age and the previous vaccination status of the child, including the special circumstance of simultaneous administration of DTP or DTaP, OPV, HbCV, and MMR at age ≥ 15 months.[51]

HOW SUPPLIED

Vial 7.5 mL—Product No. 49281-282-15

STORAGE

Store between 2°–8°C (35°–46°F). DO NOT FREEZE. Temperature extremes may adversely affect resuspendability of this vaccine.

REFERENCES

1. Unpublished data available from Connaught Laboratories, Inc.
2. Recommendations of the Immunization Practices Advisory Committee (ACIP). Diphtheria, Tetanus, and Pertussis: Recommendations for vaccine use and other preventive measures. MMWR 40: No RR-10, 1991
3. Kimura M, et al. Developments in pertussis immunisation in Japan. The Lancet: 30–32, 1990
4. Kimura M, et al. Current epidemiology of pertussis in Japan. Pediatr Infect Dis J 9: 705–709, 1990
5. Aoyama T, et al. Efficacy and immunogenicity of acellular pertussis vaccine by manufacturer and patient age. AJDC 143: 655–659, 1989
6. Aoyama T, et al. Efficacy of an acellular pertussis vaccine in Japan. J Pediatr 107: 180–183, 1985
7. Blennow M, et al. Preliminary data from a clinical trial (phase 2) of an Acellular Pertussis Vaccine, J-NIH-6. Develop Biol Standard 65: 185–190, 1986
8. Blennow M, et al. Primary immunization of infants with an Acellular Pertussis Vaccine in a double-blind randomized clinical trial. Pediatr 82: 293–299, 1988
9. Kallings LO, et al. Placebo-controlled trial of two Acellular Pertussis Vaccines in Sweden—protective efficacy and adverse events. Lancet: 955–960, 1988
10. Storsaeter J, et al. Mortality and morbidity from invasive bacterial injections during a clinical trial of acellular pertussis vaccines in Sweden. Pediatr Infect Dis J 7: 637–645, 1988
11. Bernstein H, et al. Clinical reactions and immunogenicity of the BIKEN Acellular Diphtheria and Tetanus Toxoids and Pertussis Vaccine in 4- through 6-year-old US children. AJDC 146: 556–559, 1992
12. Feldman S, et al. Comparison of acellular (B-Type) and whole-cell pertussis-component diphtheria-tetanus-pertussis vaccines as the first booster immunization in 15- to 24-month-old children. J Pediatr, IN PRESS
13. Feldman S, et al. Comparison of two-component acellular and standard whole-cell pertussis vaccines, combined with diphtheria-tetanus toxoids, as the primary immunization series in infants. Southern Medical J, IN PRESS
14. Pichichero ME, et al. Acellular pertussis vaccination of 2-month-old infants in the United States. J Pediatr, Vol 89 No. 5, 882–887, 1992
15. Mortimer EA. Diphtheria Toxoid. Vaccines, W.B. Saunders Company: p 35, 1988
16. Karzon DT, et al. Diphtheria outbreaks in immunized populations. N Engl J Med 318: 41–43, 1988
17. Department of Health and Human Services, Food and Drug Administration. Biological Products; Bacterial Vaccines and Toxoids; Implementation of Efficacy Review; Proposed Rule. Federal Register Vol 50 No 240, pp 51002–51117, 1985
18. Manclark CR, et al. Pertussis. In: R. Germainier (ed), Bacterial Vaccines Academic Press Inc., NY 69–106, 1984
19. Report of the Committee on Infectious Diseases. Elk Grove Village, IL, American Academy of Pediatrics, 358–369, 1991
20. Farizo KM, et al. Epidemiologic features of pertussis in the United States, 1980–1989. Rev Infect Dis (IN PRESS)
21. Linnemann CC, et al. Use of pertussis vaccine in an epidemic involving hospital staff. The Lancet 2:540–544, 1975
22. Linnemann CC, et al. Pertussis in the adult. Ann Rev Med 28: 179–185, 1977
23. Pertussis. Report of the Committee on Infectious Diseases. American Academy of Pediatrics, Evanston, Illinois. Twenty-second Edition, 1991
24. CDC. Pertussis Surveillance—United States, 1986 and 1988. MMWR 39: 57–66, 1990
25. Noble GR, et al. Acellular and whole-cell pertussis vaccines in Japan. JAMA 257:1351–1356, 1987
26. Olin P, et al. Relative efficacy of two acellular pertussis vaccines during three years of passive surveillance. Vaccine 10:142–144, 1992
27. Wilson GS. The Hazards of Immunization. Provocation poliomyelitis. 270–274, 1967
28. ACIP. General recommendations on immunization. MMWR 38: 205–227, 1989
29. ACIP. Pertussis immunization: Family history of convulsions and use of antipyretics—Supplementary ACIP statement. MMWR 36: 281–282, 1987
30. Active Immunization Procedures. Report of the Committee on Infectious Diseases. American Academy of Pediatrics, Evanston, Illinois. Twenty-second Edition, 1991
31. CDC. Vaccine Adverse Event Reporting System—United States. MMWR 39: 730–733, 1990
32. CDC. National Childhood Vaccine Injury Act: requirements for permanent vaccination records and for reporting of selected events after vaccination. MMWR 37: 197–200, 1988
33. Food and Drug Administration. New reporting requirements for vaccine adverse events. FDA Drug Bull 18 (2), 16–18, 1988
34. Miller D, et al. Pertussis vaccine and whooping cough as risk factors for acute neurological illness and death in young children. Dev Biol Stand 61:389–394, 1985
35. Griffin MR, et al. Risk of sudden infant death syndrome after immunization with the Diphtheria-Tetanus-Pertussis Vaccine. N Engl J Med 618–623, 1988
36. Hoffman HJ, et al. Diphtheria-tetanus-pertussis immunization and sudden infant death: Results of the National Institute of Child Health and Human Development Cooperative Epidemiological Study of Sudden Infant Death Syndrome Risk Factors. Pediatr 79: 598–611, 1987
37. Walker AM, et al. Diphtheria-tetanus-pertussis immunization and sudden infant death syndrome. Am J Public Health 77: 945–951, 1987
38. Howson CP, et al. *Adverse Effects of Pertussis and Rubella Vaccines.* National Academy Press, Washington, DC, 1991
39. Bellman MH, et al. Infantile spasms and pertussis immunization. Lancet, i: 1031–1034, 1983
40. Jacob J, et al. Increased intracranial pressure after diphtheria, tetanus and pertussis immunization. Am J Dis Child Vol 133: 217–218, 1979
41. Mathur R, et al. Bulging fontanel following triple vaccine. Indian Pediatr 18 (6): 417–418, 1981
42. Shendurnikar, N, et al. Bulging fontanel following DTP vaccine. Indian Pediatr 23 (11): 960, 1986
43. Rutledge SL, et al. Neurological complications of immunizations. J Pediatr 109: 917–924, 1986
44. Walker AM, et al. Neurologic events following diphtheria-tetanus-pertussis immunization. Pediatr 81: 345–349, 1988
45. Wilson GS. The Hazards of Immunization. Allergic manifestations: Post-vaccinal neuritis. 153–156, 1967
46. Tsairis P, et al. Natural history of brachial plexus neuropathy. Arch Neurol 27: 109–117, 1972
47. Blumstein GI, et al. Peripheral neuropathy following tetanus toxoid administration. JAMA 198: 1030–1031, 1966
48. Cody CL, et al. Nature and rates of adverse reactions associated with DTP and DT immunizations in infants and children. Pediatr 68: 650–660, 1981
49. Schlenska GK. Unusual neurological complications following tetanus toxoid administration. J Neurol 215: 299–302, 1977
50. CDC. *Adverse events following immunization.* Surveillance Report No. 3, 1985–1986, Issued February 1989
51. ACIP. Pertussis Vaccination: Acellular Pertussis Vaccine for reinforcing and booster use—supplementary ACIP statement. MMWR 41: No. RR-1, 1992

Manufactured by:
CONNAUGHT LABORATORIES, INC.
Swiftwater, Pennsylvania 18370, U.S.A.
and
The Research Foundation for Microbial Diseases of Osaka University ("BIKEN®")
Suita, Osaka, Japan

Product information as of August 1992

1722

ProHIBiT®
HAEMOPHILUS b CONJUGATE VACCINE ℞
(Diphtheria Toxoid-Conjugate)

Caution: Federal (U.S.A.) law prohibits dispensing without prescription.

DESCRIPTION

ProHIBiT®, Haemophilus b Conjugate Vaccine (Diphtheria Toxoid-Conjugate), for intramuscular use, is a sterile solution, prepared from the purified capsular polysaccharide, a polymer of ribose, ribitol and phosphate (PRP) of the Eagen *Haemophilus influenzae* type b strain covalently bound to diphtheria toxoid (D) and dissolved in sodium phosphate buffered isotonic sodium chloride solution. The polysaccharide-protein conjugate molecule is referred to as PRP-D. Thimerosal (mercury derivative) 1:10,000 is added as a preservative. The vaccine is a clear, colorless solution. Each single dose of 0.5 mL is formulated to contain 25 μg of purified capsular polysaccharide and 18 μg of diphtheria toxoid protein.

HOW SUPPLIED

Syringe, 1 Dose (6 per package)—Product No. 49281-541-61
Vial, 1 Dose (5 per package)—Product No. 49281-541-01
Vial, 5 Dose—Product No. 49281-541-05
Vial, 10 Dose—Product No. 49281-541-10

BCG LIVE (INTRAVESICAL) THERACYS® ℞
For Treatment of Carcinoma In-situ of the Urinary Bladder

DESCRIPTION

BCG Live (Intravesical), TheraCys®, as prepared by Connaught Laboratories Limited, is a freeze-dried suspension of an attenuated strain of *Mycobacterium bovis* (Bacillus Calmette and Guérin), which has been grown on Sauton medium (potato and glycerin based medium), used in the non-specific active therapy of carcinoma in-situ of the urinary bladder.

CAUTION: TheraCys® is NOT intended to be used as an immunizing agent for the prevention of tuberculosis. TheraCys® is NOT a vaccine for the prevention of cancer.

TheraCys® is formulated to contain 81 mg (dry weight)/vial Bacillus of Calmette and Guérin (BCG) and 5% w/v monosodium glutamate. This product contains no preservative. A vial of TheraCys® is ready for use following reconstitution with the accompanying diluent (3.0 ml), which consists of approximately 0.85% sodium chloride, 0.025% Tween 80, 0.06% w/v sodium dihydrogen phosphate and 0.25% disodium hydrogen phosphate. The diluent contains no preservative. One dose consists of one vial of reconstituted material further diluted in sterile, preservative-free saline. The reconstituted product contains $10.5 \pm 8.7 \times 10^8$ colony-forming units (CFU) per vial when resuspended in the diluent provided.

To ensure viability of the product through to its labeled expiration date, it is very important that TheraCys® and diluent be stored continuously between 2° and 8°C (35° and 46°F) until use (see STORAGE). It should be used immediately after reconstitution.

CLINICAL PHARMACOLOGY

TheraCys® promotes a local inflammatory reaction with histiocytic and leukocytic infiltration in the urinary bladder.[1,2,3] The local inflammatory effects are associated with an apparent elimination or reduction of superficial cancerous lesions of the urinary bladder. The exact mechanism by which this is accomplished is unknown.

In a randomized, actively controlled multicenter study TheraCys® was compared to doxorubicin hydrochloride (Adriamycin®) in the treatment of carcinoma in-situ of the urinary bladder. The response of 114 eligible patients for evaluation is given in Table 1 below. Among the 54 patients receiving TheraCys®, 74% had a complete response (negative by cystoscopic examination and by urine cytology). The estimated median time to treatment failure (recurrence, progression or death) was 48.2 months (Table 2).[4]

TABLE 1: Response of Patients with Carcinoma In-Situ To Treatment with TheraCys® or Adriamycin®

	TheraCys® (n = 54)	Adriamycin® (n = 60)
Complete Response†	74%*	42%*
No Response††	11%	10%
Progressive Disease§	13%	42%
No Evaluation	2%	7%
Total	100%	100%

* Difference is statistically significant (P < 0.01).
† Confirmed by cytology and cystoscopic examination.
††Less than a CR or stable disease.
§ Increase of stage or grade.

Continued on next page

Connaught Laboratories—Cont.

TABLE 2: Time to Recurrence, Progression or Death: Time to Treatment Failure (TTF)

Treatment	Number Studied	Number Failures	Median TTF
TheraCys®	54	27	48.2 months*
Adriamycin®	60	46	5.9 months*

*Difference is statistically significant (P<0.01 by stratified logrank test).

TABLE 3: Prior Versus No Prior Treatment

Prior Treatment*	Study Arm	Response Rate	Median TTF (# Events/N)
Yes	TheraCys®	81%	Not reached (11/26)
Yes	Adriamycin®	53%	7.0 months (22/30)
No	TheraCys®	68%	32.8 months (16/28)
No	Adriamycin®	30%	3.7 months (24/30)

*Other than TheraCys® and Adriamycin®.

The effect of chemotherapy (other than TheraCys® or Adriamycin®) prior to entry into the controlled study was analysed. Patients in the TheraCys® treated arm who had received prior chemotherapy had a complete response rate of 81% (11/26) as compared to 68% (16/28) in the group who had not received prior chemotherapy (Table 3). This difference was not statistically significant.

No survival advantage for TheraCys® therapy[4] over that for Adriamycin®[4,5,6] was demonstrated after a 40–72 month follow-up. The median time to death for each group was 23 months and 21 months for TheraCys® and Adriamycin® respectively.

The clinical trials carried out with TheraCys® included percutaneous administration of 0.5 ml of BCG Live (Intravesical) solution, which was reconstituted in the diluent provided and further diluted in 50 ml sterile preservative-free saline, with each intravesical dose.[4] Some studies have suggested that this may not be necessary[15] and if severe reactions, such as ulceration, occurred the percutaneous treatment was discontinued.

INDICATIONS AND USAGE

TheraCys® is indicated for intravesical use in the treatment of primary and relapsed carcinoma in-situ of the urinary bladder to eliminate residual tumor cells and to reduce the frequency of tumor recurrence. It is indicated for the treatment of carcinoma in-situ with or without associated papillary tumors. TheraCys® is not indicated for the treatment of papillary tumors occurring alone. TheraCys® is also indicated as a therapy for patients with carcinoma in-situ of the bladder following failure to respond to other treatment regimens. CAUTION: TheraCys® is NOT indicated as an immunizing agent for the prevention of tuberculosis. TheraCys® is NOT a vaccine for the prevention of cancer.

CONTRAINDICATIONS

Patients on immunosuppressive therapy or with compromised immune systems should not receive TheraCys® due to the risk of overwhelming systemic mycobacterial sepsis.

TheraCys® should not be administered to patients with fever unless the cause of the fever is determined and evaluated. If the fever is due to an infection, TheraCys® should be withheld until the patient is afebrile and off all therapy.

Patients with urinary tract infection should not receive TheraCys® treatment because administration may result in the risk of disseminated BCG infection or in an increased severity of bladder irritation.

TheraCys® should NOT be administered as an immunizing agent for the prevention of tuberculosis. TheraCys® is NOT a vaccine for the prevention of cancer.

WARNINGS

TheraCys® should NOT be administered as an immunizing agent for the prevention of tuberculosis. TheraCys® is NOT a vaccine for the prevention of cancer.

Since administration of intravesical TheraCys® causes an inflammatory response in the bladder and has been associated with hematuria, urinary frequency, dysuria and bacterial urinary tract infection, careful monitoring of urinary status is required. If there is an increase in the patient's existing symptoms, or if their symptoms persist or if any of these symptoms develop, the patient should be evaluated and managed for urinary tract infection or BCG toxicity.

Since death has occurred due to systemic BCG infection, patients should be closely monitored for symptoms of such an infection (see PRECAUTIONS). BCG therapy should be withheld upon any suspicion of systemic infection, e.g. granulomatous hepatitis.

Drug combinations containing bone marrow depressants and/or immunosuppressants and/or radiation may either impair the response to TheraCys® or increase the risk of osteomyelitis or disseminated BCG infection (see DRUG INTERACTIONS).

Patients undergoing antimicrobial therapy for other infections should be evaluated to assess whether the therapy will obviate the effects of TheraCys® actions.

For patients with small bladder capacity, increased risk of severity of local irritation should be considered in decisions to treat with TheraCys®.

Intravesical treatment with TheraCys® may induce a sensitivity to tuberculin which could complicate future interpretations of skin test reactions to tuberculin in the diagnosis of suspected mycobacterial infections. Determination of a patient's reactivity to tuberculin prior to administration of TheraCys® may be desirable in this regard.

PRECAUTIONS

General

Contains viable attenuated mycobacteria. Handle as infectious. Use aseptic technique.

The possibility of allergic reactions in individuals sensitive to the components of the product should be borne in mind.

After usage all equipment and materials (e.g. syringes, catheters and containers that may have come into contact with TheraCys®) used for instillation of the product into the bladder, should be placed immediately into plastic bags which are labelled "Infectious Waste" and disposed of accordingly as biohazardous waste.

Aseptic technique must be used during administration of intravesical TheraCys® so as not to introduce contaminants into the urinary tract or to traumatize unduly the urinary mucosa.

Urine voided for 6 hours after instillation should be disinfected with an equal volume of 5% hypochlorite solution (undiluted household bleach) and allowed to stand for 15 minutes before flushing.

It is recommended that intravesical TheraCys® not be administered any sooner than one week following transurethral resection because fatalities due to disseminated BCG infection have been reported with use of TheraCys® after traumatic catheterization.

If the physician believes that the bladder catheterization has been traumatic (e.g., associated with bleeding or possible false passage), then TheraCys® should not be administered and there must be a treatment delay of at least one week. Subsequent treatment should be resumed as if no interruption in the schedule had occurred. That is, all doses of TheraCys® should be administered even after a temporary halt in administration.

If systemic BCG infection is suspected (i.e., if patients have fever over 39°C (103°F) or persistent fever above 38°C (101°F) over two days or severe malaise), an infectious disease specialist should be consulted and fast acting antituberculosis therapy should be initiated. It should be noted that BCG systemic infections are rarely evidenced by positive cultures.

INFORMATION FOR PATIENTS

Patients should be advised to check with their doctor as soon as possible if there is an increase in their existing symptoms, or if their symptoms persist even after receiving a number of treatments, or if any of the following symptoms develop:

More Common	Rare
Blood in Urine	Cough
Fever and Chills	Skin Rash
Frequent Urge to Urinate	
Increased Frequency of Urination	
Joint Pain	
Nausea and Vomiting	
Painful Urination	

A cough that develops after administration of TheraCys® could indicate a BCG systemic infection which is life-threatening. If systemic infection occurs it should be treated immediately with antituberculous antibiotics.

All patients should sit while voiding following instillation of solution.

Urine voided for 6 hours after instillation should be disinfected with an equal volume of 5% hypochlorite solution (undiluted household bleach) and allowed to stand for 15 minutes before flushing.

DRUG INTERACTIONS

Patients must also be advised that drug combinations containing bone marrow depressants and/or immunosuppressants and/or radiation may impair the response to TheraCys® or increase the risk of osteomyelitis or disseminated BCG infection.

TABLE 4: Local Reactions (% OF 112 Patients)

Reaction	Total	Severe*
Dysuria	51.8	3.6
Frequency	40.2	1.8
Hematuria	39.3	17.0
Cystitis	29.5	0.0
Urgency	17.9	0.0
Urinary Tract Infection	17.9	1.0
Urinary Incontinence	6.3	0.0
Cramps/Pain	6.3	0.0
Decreased Bladder Capacity	5.4	0.0
Tissue in Urine	0.9	0.0
Local Infection	0.9	0.0

*Severe is defined as grade 3 (severe) or grade 4 (life threatening).

PREGNANCY

Pregnancy Category C. TheraCys®. Animal reproduction studies have not been conducted with TheraCys®. It is also not known whether TheraCys® can cause fetal harm when administered to a pregnant woman or can affect reproduction capacity. TheraCys® should be given to a pregnant woman only if clearly needed. Women should be advised not be become pregnant while on therapy.

NURSING MOTHERS

It is not known whether TheraCys® is excreted in human milk. Because many drugs are excreted in human milk, caution should be exercised when TheraCys® is administered to a nursing mother.

TABLE 5: Systemic Reactions (% of 112 Patients)

Reaction	Total	Severe*
Malaise	40.2	2.0
Fever (>38°C)	38.4	2.6
Chills	33.9	2.6
Anemia	20.5	0.0
Nausea/Vomiting	16.1	0.0
Anorexia	10.7	0.0
Myalgia/Arthralgia/Arthritis	7.1	1.0
Diarrhea	6.3	0.0
Mild Liver Involvement	2.7	0.0
Mild Abdominal Pain	2.7	0.0
Systemic Infection**	2.7	2.0
Pulmonary Infection**	2.7	0.0
Cardiac	2.7	0.0
Headache	1.8	0.0
Hypersensitivity Skin Rash	1.8	0.0
Constipation	0.9	0.0
Dizziness	0.9	0.0
Fatigue	0.9	0.0
Leukopenia	5.4	0.0
Disseminated Intravascular Coagulation	2.7	0.0
Thrombocytopenia	0.9	0.0
Renal Toxicity	9.8	2.0
Genital Pain	9.8	0.0
Flank Pain	0.9	0.0

*Severe is defined as grade 3 (severe) or grade 4 (life threatening).

**Includes both BCG and other infections.

PEDIATRIC USE

Safety and effectiveness for carcinoma in-situ of the urinary bladder in children have not been established.

ADVERSE REACTIONS

TheraCys® therapy can affect several organs (or parts) of the body in addition to the cancer cells.

In a controlled multi-center clinical trial comparing BCG therapy and doxorubicin hydrochloride (Adriamycin®) for the intravesical treatment of superficial transitional cell carcinoma with and without carcinoma in-situ of the bladder, 112 patients received BCG.[4]

In another controlled study using TheraCys® for the treatment of superficial transitional cell carcinoma, with or without carcinoma in-situ, of the blader, similar adverse reactions were observed.[13] However, two deaths were noted in this study which may have been associated with traumatic catheterization.

The incidence of adverse reactions associated with intravesical TheraCys® therapy is given below. Most local adverse reactions occur following the third intravesical instillation. Symptoms usually begin two to four hours after instillation and persist for 24 to 72 hours. Systemic reactions usually last for 1–3 days after each intravesical instillation.[4,13,14]

No fatalities associated with the use of TheraCys® were reported in this study. Two fatalities have been reported with the use of TheraCys® in another study after traumatic catheterization or in the presence of urinary infection.[13]

An increased risk of additional primary malignancies has been reported following radiotherapy and chemotherapy for many types of malignancies. No increase in second primary malignancies after treatment with TheraCys® was reported in these studies.[4]

Irritative bladder symptoms associated with TheraCys® administration can be managed symptomatically with phenazopyridine hydrochloride (Pyridium), propantheline bromide (Pro-Banthine), and acetaminophen.[4]

Systemic side effects (such as malaise, fever and chills) may represent hypersensitivity reactions and can be treated with diphenhydramine hydrochloride.[4] Systemic infection as a result of the spread of BCG organisms has occasionally occurred with intravesical TheraCys® administration. The management of this condition is provided under PRECAUTIONS.

DOSAGE AND ADMINISTRATION

Intravesical treatment and prophylaxis for carcinoma in-situ of the urinary bladder should begin between 7 to 14 days after biopsy or transurethral resection if this procedure is done. A dose of TheraCys® is given intravesically under aseptic conditions once weekly for 6 weeks (induction therapy). Each dose (1 reconstituted vial) is further diluted in an additional 50 ml sterile, preservative-free saline for a total of 53 ml (see below). A urethral catheter is inserted into the bladder under aseptic conditions, the bladder drained and then 53 ml suspension of TheraCys® is instilled slowly by gravity following which the catheter is withdrawn. During the first hour following instillation, the patient should lie for 15 minutes each in the prone and supine positions and also on each side. The patient is then allowed to be up but retains the suspension for another 60 minutes for a total of 2 hours. All patients may not be able to retain the suspension for the 2 hours and should be instructed to void in less time if necessary. At the end of 2 hours all patients should void in a seated position for safety reasons. Patients should be instructed to maintain adequate hydration.

If the physician believes that the bladder catheterization has been traumatic (e.g., associated with bleeding or possible false passage), then TheraCys® should not be administered and there must be a treatment delay of at least one week. Subsequent treatment should be resumed as if no interruption in the schedule had occurred. That is, all doses of TheraCys® should be administered even after a temporary halt in administration.

The induction therapy should be followed by one treatment given 3, 6, 12, 18 and 24 months following the initial treatment.

After use, all equipment, materials and containers that may have come in contact with TheraCys® should be sterilized or disposed of properly as with any other biohazardous waste (see PRECAUTIONS).

Reconstitution of Freeze-Dried Product and Withdrawal from Rubber-Stoppered Vial.

TheraCys® SHOULD BE USED IMMEDIATELY AFTER RECONSTITUTION. KEEP REFRIGERATED UNTIL USE. DISCARD AFTER 2 HOURS.

DO NOT REMOVE THE RUBBER STOPPER FROM THE VIAL.

Reconstitute and dilute immediately prior to use.

Persons handling product should be masked and gloved.

TheraCys® should not be handled by persons with a known immunologic deficiency.

TheraCys® should be handled as infectious material.

Reconstitute and dilute using aseptic technique.

TheraCys® should be reconstituted only with the diluent provided to ensure proper dispersion of the organisms.

IMPORTANT RECONSTITUTION INSTRUCTIONS

Fig. (1) Apply a **sterile** pledget of cotton moistened with a suitable antiseptic to the surface of the rubber stoppers of vials of diluent and TheraCys®.

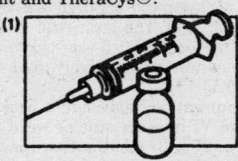

Fig. (1)

Fig. (2) Using a 5 ml **sterile** syringe and needle, draw into the syringe 3.0 ml of air. Pierce the center of the rubber stopper in the vial containing diluent with the **sterile** needle of the syringe, invert the vial and slowly inject some of the air in the syringe into the vial. Without removing the needle, alternately withdraw diluent and inject air into the vial until 3 ml of diluent has been withdrawn into the syringe. Then holding the syringe-plunger steady, withdraw the needle from the vial.

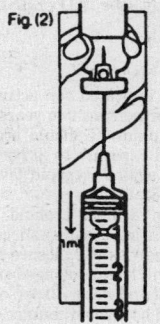

Fig. (2)

Fig. (3) Using the same syringe and needle, pierce the stopper in one vial of freeze-dried material with the needle.

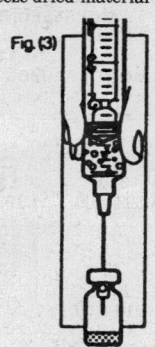

Fig. (3)

Fig. (4) Hold the vial of freeze-dried material upright and pull the plunger of the syringe back to the 5 ml marking on the barrel. This will create a mild vacuum in the vial.

Release the plunger and allow the vacuum to pull the diluent from the syringe into the vial of freeze-dried material. After all the diluent has passed into the vial of freeze-dried material, remove the needle and syringe.

Shake the vial gently until a fine, even suspension results.

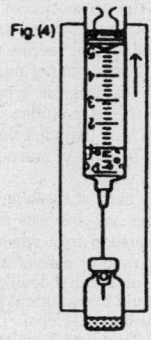

Fig. (4)

Fig. (5) Withdraw the entire contents of the reconstituted material from the vial again using the same 5 ml syringe.

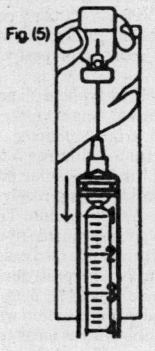

Fig. (5)

Fig. (6) Return the vial to an upright position before removing the syringe from the vial.

The reconstituted material from the vial (1 dose) is further diluted in an additional 50 ml **sterile**, preservative-free saline to a final volume of 53 ml for intravesical instillation (and percutaneous injection if it is given, see CLINICAL PHARMACOLOGY).

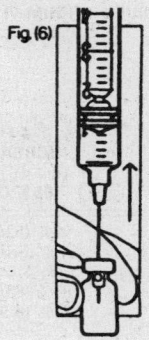

Fig. (6)

HOW SUPPLIED

TheraCys® is supplied in packages containing one vial of the freeze-dried product, containing 81 mg (dry weight) ($10.5 \pm 8.7 \times 10^8$ CFU), and one vial of diluent containing 3 ml. A 50 ml vial of Phosphate Buffered Saline is available for use as the final diluent.

STORAGE

TheraCys® and the accompanying diluent should be kept in a refrigerator at a temperature between 2°C and 8°C (35° and 46°F). It should not be used after the expiration date marked on the vial, otherwise it may be inactive. The product should be used **immediately** after reconstitution; however, it must not be used after 2 hours. Any reconstituted product which exhibits flocculation or clumping that cannot be dispersed with gentle shaking should not be used.

At no time should the freeze-dried or reconstituted TheraCys® be exposed to sunlight, direct or indirect. Exposure to artificial light should be kept to a minimum.[9]

REFERENCES

1. Old LJ, Clarke DA, Benacerraf B. Effect of bacillus Calmette-Guérin infection on transplanted tumors in the mouse. Nature 1959; 184: 291.

2. Lamm DL, Harris SC, Gittes RF. Bacillus Calmette-Guérin and dinitrochlorobenzene immunotherapy of chemically induced bladder tumors. Investigative Urology 1977; 14: 369.

3. Morales A. Ottenhof P, Emerson L. Treatment of residual non-infiltrating bladder cancer with bacillus Calmette-Guérin. J Urol 1981; 125: 649.

4. Unpublished clinical data available from Connaught Laboratories Limited.

5. Horn Y, Eidelman A, Walach N, Ilian M. Intravesical chemotherapy in controlled trial with thiotepa versus doxorubicin hydrochloride. J Urol 1981; 125: 652–654.

6. Zincke H, Utz DC, Taylor WF, Myers RP, Leary FJ. Influence of thiotepa and doxorubicin instillation at time of transurethral surgical treatment of bladder cancer on tumor recurrence: a prospective, randomized, double-blind, controlled trial. J Urol 1983; 129: 505–509.

7. Unpublished clinical data available from Connaught Laboratories Limited.

8. Lamm DL, et al. Complications of Bacillus Calmette-Guérin immunotherapy: review of 2602 patients and comparison of chemotherapy complications. EORTC GU Group Monograph 1989; 6: 335–355.

9. Landi S, Barbara C, Przykuta K, Held RH. Effect of light on freeze dried BCG Vaccines. J Biol Stand 1977; 5: 321-6.

10. Lamm DL, Blumenstein BA, Crawford ED, et al. South-West Oncology Group comparison of bacillus Calmette-Guérin and doxorubicin in the treatment and prophylaxis of superficial bladder cancer. J Urol 1987; 178A.

11. Mori K, Lamm DL, Crawford ED. A trial of Bacillus Calmette-Guérin versus Adriamycin in superficial bladder cancer: a South-West Oncology Group study. Urol Int 1986; 41: 254–259.

12. Soloway M. Evaluation and management of patients with superficial bladder cancer. Urol Clin North Am 1987; 14: 771.

13. Lamm DL, BCG in carcinoma in-situ and superficial bladder tumors. EORTC GU Group Monograph 1988; 5: 497.

14. Lamm DL. Complications of Bacillus Calmette-Guérin immunotherapy in 1,278 patients with bladder cancer. J Urol 1986; 135: 272.

15. Lamm DL, Sarodosy MS, DeHaven JI. Percutaneous, oral, or intravesical BCG administration: what is the optimal route? EORTC Genitourinary Group Monograph 6: BCG in Superficial Bladder Cancer. 1989; 301–310.

Manufactured by
CONNAUGHT LABORATORIES LIMITED
Willowdale, Ontario, Canada

Distributed by:
CONNAUGHT LABORATORIES, INC.
Swiftwater, Pennsylvania 18370, U.S.A.
©July 1993 Connaught Laboratories, Inc.
MKT 1916

Continued on next page

Connaught Laboratories—Cont.

TYPHOID Vi POLYSACCHARIDE VACCINE ℞
TYPHIM Vi®

Caution: Federal (U.S.A.) law prohibits dispensing without prescription.

DESCRIPTION

Typhim Vi®, Typhoid Vi Polysaccharide Vaccine, produced by Pasteur Mérieux Sérums & Vaccins S.A., for intramuscular use, is a sterile solution containing the cell surface Vi polysaccharide extracted from *Salmonella typhi* Ty2 strain. The organism is grown in a semi-synthetic medium without animal proteins. The capsular polysaccharide is precipitated from the concentrated culture supernatant by the addition of hexadecyltrimethylammonium bromide and the product is purified by differential centrifugation and precipitation. The potency of the purified polysaccharide is assessed by molecular size and O-acetyl content. Phenol, 0.25%, is added as a preservative. The vaccine contains residual polydimethylsiloxane-based antifoam. The vaccine is a clear, colorless solution. Each single-dose of 0.5 mL is formulated to contain 25 μg of purified Vi polysaccharide in a colorless isotonic phosphate buffered saline (pH 7 ± 0.3), 4.150 mg of Sodium Chloride, 0.065 mg of Disodium Phosphate ($2H_2O$), 0.023 mg of Monosodium Phosphate and 0.5 mL of Sterile Water for Injection.

CLINICAL PHARMACOLOGY

Typhoid fever is an infectious disease caused by *S. typhi.* Humans are the only natural host and reservoir for *S. typhi;* infections result from the consumption of food or water that has been contaminated by the excretions of an acute case or a carrier. *S. typhi* organisms efficiently invade the human intestinal mucosae ultimately leading to bacteremia; following a typical 10- to 14-day incubation period, a systemic illness occurs. The clinical presentation of typhoid fever exhibits a broad range of severity and can be debilitating. Classical cases have fever, myalgia, anorexia, abdominal discomfort and headaches; the fever increases step-wise over a period of days and then may remain at 102°F to 106°F over 10 to 14 days before decreasing in a step-wise manner. Skin lesions known as rose spots may be present. Constipation is common in older children and adults, while diarrhea may occur in younger children. Among the less common but most severe complications are intestinal perforation and hemorrhage, and death. The course is typically more severe without appropriate antimicrobial therapy. The case fatality rate was reported to be approximately 10% to 20% in the pre-antibiotic era.[1,2,3] During the period of 1983 to 1991 in the U.S., the case fatality rate reported to the Centers for Disease Control and Prevention (CDC) was 0.2% (9/4010).[4] Infection of the gallbladder can lead to the chronic carrier state.

Typhoid fever is still endemic in many countries of the world where it is predominantly a disease of school-age children and may be a major public health problem. Most cases of typhoid fever in the U.S. are thought to be acquired during foreign travel. During the periods of 1975 to 1984 and 1983 to 1984, respectively, 62% and 70% of the cases of typhoid fever reported to the CDC were acquired during foreign travel; this compares to 33% of cases during 1967-1972.[5]

In 1992, 414 cases of typhoid fever were reported to the CDC. Of these 414 cases, 1 (0.2%) case occurred in an infant under one year of age; 77 (18.6%) cases occurred in persons one to nine years of age; 81 (19.6%) cases occurred in persons 10 to 19 years of age; 251 (60.6%) cases occurred in individuals ≥ 20 years of age; the age was not available for 4 (1%) cases. One death was reported in 1991.[4] Domestic surveillance could underestimate the risk of typhoid fever in travelers since the disease is unlikely to be reported for persons who received diagnosis and treatment overseas.[6]

Approximately 2% to 4% of acute typhoid fever cases develop into a chronic carrier state. The chronic carrier state occurs more frequently with advanced age, and among females than males.[2,7] These non-symptomatic carriers are the natural reservoir for *S. typhi* and can serve to maintain the disease in its endemic state or to directly infect new individuals. Outbreaks of typhoid fever are often traced to food handlers who are asymptomatic carriers.[8]

Other vaccines used for the prevention of typhoid fever in selected populations include a parenteral vaccine containing killed *S. typhi* bacteria and an oral vaccine with live, attenuated *S. typhi.* Typhim Vi, consisting of purified *S. typhi* Vi capsular polysaccharide, is a different type of vaccine.

Two formulations were utilized in studies of the typhoid Vi polysaccharide vaccine. These included the liquid formulation which is identical to Typhim Vi and a lyophilized formulation.

The protective efficacy of each of these formulations of the typhoid Vi polysaccharide vaccine was assessed independently in two trials conducted in areas where typhoid fever is endemic. A single intramuscular dose of 25 μg was used in these efficacy studies. A randomized double-blind controlled trial with Typhim Vi (liquid formulation) was conducted in five villages west of Katmandu, Nepal. There were 6,908 vaccinated subjects: 3,454 received Typhim Vi and 3,454 in the control group received a 23-valent pneumococcal polysaccharide vaccine. Of the 6,908 subjects, 6,439 subjects were in the target population of 5 to 44 years of age. In addition, 165 children ages 2 to 4 years and 304 adults over 44 years of age were included in the study. The overall protective efficacy of Typhim Vi was 74% (95% confidence interval (CI): 49% to 87%) for blood culture confirmed cases of typhoid fever during 20 months of post-vaccination follow-up.[9,10,11]

The protective efficacy of the typhoid Vi polysaccharide vaccine, lyophilized formulation, was evaluated in a randomized double-blind controlled trial conducted in South Africa. There were 11,384 vaccinated children 5 to 15 years of age; 5,692 children received the Vi capsular polysaccharide vaccine and 5,692 in the control group received meningococcal polysaccharide (Groups A+C) vaccine. The protective efficacy for the Vi capsular polysaccharide (lyophilized formulation) group for blood culture confirmed cases of typhoid fever was 55% (95% CI: 30% to 70%) overall during 3 years of post-vaccination follow-up, and was 61%, 52% and 50%, respectively, for years 1, 2, and 3. Vaccination was associated with an increase in anti-Vi antibodies as measured by radioimmunoassay (RIA) and enzyme-linked immunosorbent assay. Antibody levels remained elevated at 6 and 12 months post-vaccination.[11,12]

Because of the very low incidence of typhoid fever in the U.S., efficacy studies are not currently feasible in this population.

Controlled comparative efficacy studies of Typhim Vi and other types of typhoid vaccines have not been performed.

An increase in serum anti-capsular antibodies is thought to be the basis of protection provided by Typhim Vi. However, a specific correlation of post-vaccination antibody levels with subsequent protection is not available and the level of Vi antibody that will provide protection has not been determined. Also, limitations exist for comparing immunogenicity results from subjects in endemic areas, where some subjects have baseline serological evidence of prior *S. typhi* exposure, to naive populations such as most American travelers.

In endemic regions (Nepal, South Africa, Indonesia) where trials were conducted, pre-vaccination geometric mean antibody levels suggest that infection with *S. typhi* has previously occurred in a large percentage of the vaccinees. In these populations, specific antibody levels increased four-fold or greater in 68% to 87.5% of older children and adult subjects following vaccination. For 43 persons 15 to 44 years of age in the Nepal pilot study, geometric mean specific antibody levels pre- and 3 weeks post-vaccination were, respectively, 0.38 and 3.68 μg antibody/mL by RIA; 79% had a four-fold or greater rise in Vi antibody levels.[9,12]

Immunogenicity and safety trials were conducted in a racially mixed U.S. population. A single dose of Typhim Vi vaccine induced a four-fold or greater increase in antibody levels in 88% and 96% of this adult population for 2 studies, respectively, following vaccination (see TABLE 1).[10,13]

[See table below.]

No studies of safety and immunogenicity have been conducted in U.S. children. A double-blind randomized controlled trial testing the safety and immunogenicity of Typhim Vi was performed in 175 Indonesian children. The percentage of 2- to 5-year-old children achieving a four-fold or greater increase in antibody levels at 4 weeks post-vaccination was 96.3% (52/54) (95% CI: 87.3% to 99.6%), and in the study subset of 2-year-old children was 94.4% (17/18) (95% CI:72.7% to 99.9%). The geometric mean levels (μg antibody/mL by RIA) for the 2-to 5-year-old children and the subset of 2-year-olds were, respectively, 5.81 (4.36 to 7.77) and 5.76 (3.48 to 9.53).[10,11]

In the U.S. Reimmunization Study, adults previously immunized with Typhim Vi in other studies were reimmunized with a 25 μg dose at 27 or 34 months after the primary dose. Data on antibody response to primary immunization, decline following primary immunization, and response to reimmunization are presented in TABLE 2. Antibody levels attained following reimmunization at 27 or 34 months after the primary dose were similar to levels attained following the primary immunization.[10,13] This response is typical for a T-cell independent polysaccharide vaccine in that reimmunization does not elicit higher antibody levels than primary immunization. The safety of reimmunization was also evaluated in this study (see **ADVERSE REACTIONS** section).

[See Table 2 above.]

TABLE 2.[10,13] U.S. STUDIES IN 18- TO 40-YEAR-OLD ADULTS: KINETICS AND PERSISTENCE OF Vi ANTIBODY* RESPONSE TO PRIMARY IMMUNIZATION WITH TYPHIM Vi, AND RESPONSE TO REIMMUNIZATION AT 27 OR 34 MONTHS

	PRE-DOSE 1	1 MONTH	11 MONTHS	18 MONTHS	27 MONTHS	34 MONTHS	1 MONTH POST-REIMMUNIZATION[e]
GROUP 1[a]							
N	43	43	39	ND[c]	43	ND	43
Level*	0.19	3.01	1.97		1.07[d]		3.04
95% CI	(0.14–0.26)	(2.22–4.06)	(1.31–3.00)		(0.71–1.62)		(2.17–4.26)
Group 2[b]							
N	12	12	ND	10	ND	12	12
Level	0.14	3.78		1.21		0.76[d]	3.31
95% CI	(0.11–0.18)	(2.18–6.56)		(0.63–2.35)		(0.37–1.55)	(1.61–6.77)

* μg antibody/mL by RIA
[a] Group 1: Reimmunized at 27 months following primary immunization.
[b] Group 2: Reimmunized at 34 months following primary immunization.
[c] Not Done
[d] Antibody levels pre-reimmunization.
[e] Includes available data from all reimmunized subjects (subjects initially randomized to Typhim Vi, and subjects initially randomized to placebo who received open label Typhim Vi two weeks later).

TABLE 1.[10,13] Vi ANTIBODY LEVELS IN U.S. ADULTS 18 TO 40 YEARS OF AGE GIVEN TYPHIM Vi

	N	GEOMETRIC MEAN ANTIBODY LEVELS (μg antibody/mL by RIA) Pre (95% CI)	Post (4 weeks) (95% CI)	% ≥ 4 FOLD INCREASE (95% CI)
Trial 1 (1 lot)	54	0.16 (0.13 to 0.21)	3.23 (2.59 to 4.03)	96% (52/54) (87% to 100%)
Trial 2 (2 lots combined)	97	0.17 (0.14 to 0.21)	2.86 (2.26 to 3.62)	88% (85/97) (81% to 94%)

INDICATIONS AND USAGE

Typhim Vi vaccine is indicated for active immunization against typhoid fever for persons two years of age or older.

Immunization with Typhim Vi should occur at least two weeks prior to expected exposure to *S. typhi.*

Routine immunization against typhoid fever is not recommended in the United States.[14]

Selective immunization against typhoid fever is recommended under the following circumstances: 1) travelers to areas where a recognized risk of exposure to typhoid exists, particularly ones who will have prolonged exposure to potentially contaminated food and water, 2) persons with intimate exposure (i.e., continued household contact) to a documented

typhoid carrier, and 3) workers in microbiology laboratories who frequently work with *S. typhi*.[14]

Typhoid vaccination is not required for international travel, but is recommended for travelers to areas where there is a recognized risk of exposure to *S. typhi*. *S. typhi* is prevalent in many countries of Africa, Asia, and Central and South America. Current CDC advisories should be consulted with regard to specific locales. Vaccination is particularly recommended for travelers who will have prolonged exposure to potentially contaminated food and water. However, even travelers who have been vaccinated should use caution in selecting food and water.[15]

Based on the available efficacy data, vaccination with Typhim Vi may not be expected to protect 100% of susceptible individuals.

There is no evidence to support the use of typhoid vaccine to control common source outbreaks, disease following natural disaster or in persons attending rural summer camps.[16]

An optimal reimmunization schedule has not been established. Reimmunization every two years under conditions of repeated or continued exposure to the *S. typhi* organism is recommended at this time.

Typhim Vi has efficacy against typhoid fever caused by *S. typhi* infection but will not afford protection against species of *Salmonella* other than *S. typhi* or other bacteria that cause enteric disease.

For recommended primary immunization and reimmunization see DOSAGE AND ADMINISTRATION section.

Typhim Vi should not be used to treat a patient with typhoid fever or a chronic typhoid carrier.

CONTRAINDICATIONS

TYPHIM Vi IS CONTRAINDICATED IN PATIENTS WITH A HISTORY OF HYPERSENSITIVITY TO ANY COMPONENT OF THIS VACCINE.

WARNINGS

Allergic reactions have been reported rarely in the French post-marketing experience (see ADVERSE REACTIONS section).

If Typhim Vi is administered to immunosuppressed persons or persons receiving immunosuppressive therapy, the expected immune response may not be obtained. This includes patients with asymptomatic or symptomatic HIV-infection, severe combined immunodeficiency, hypogammaglobulinemia, or agammaglobulinemia; altered immune states due to diseases such as leukemia, lymphoma, or generalized malignancy; or an immune system compromised by treatment with corticosteroids, alkylating drugs, antimetabolites or radiation.[11]

As with any intramuscular injection, Typhim Vi should be given with caution to individuals with thrombocytopenia or any coagulation disorder that would contraindicate intramuscular injection (see DRUG INTERACTIONS).

PRECAUTIONS

GENERAL

Care is to be taken by the health-care provider for the safe and effective use of Typhim Vi.

EPINEPHRINE INJECTION (1:1000) MUST BE IMMEDIATELY AVAILABLE FOLLOWING IMMUNIZATION SHOULD AN ANAPHYLACTIC OR OTHER ALLERGIC REACTIONS OCCUR DUE TO ANY COMPONENT OF THE VACCINE.

Prior to an injection of any vaccine, all known precautions should be taken to prevent adverse reactions. This includes a review of the patient's history with respect to possible hypersensitivity to the vaccine or similar vaccines.

Acute infection or febrile illness may be reason for delaying use of Typhim Vi except when in the opinion of the physician, withholding the vaccine entails a greater risk.

A separate, sterile syringe and needle or a sterile disposable unit must be used for each patient to prevent the transmission of infectious agents from person to person. Needles should not be recapped and should be properly disposed.

Special care should be taken to ensure that Typhim Vi is not injected into a blood vessel.

Safety and immunogenicity data from controlled trials are not available for Typhim Vi following previous immunization with whole-cell typhoid or live, oral typhoid vaccine (see ADVERSE REACTIONS section).

INFORMATION FOR PATIENTS

Patients, parents or guardians should be fully informed of the benefits and risks of immunization with Typhim Vi. Prior to administration of Typhim Vi, patients, parents and guardians should be asked about the recent health status of the patient to be immunized.

Typhim Vi is indicated in persons traveling to endemic or epidemic areas. Current CDC advisories should be consulted with regard to specific locales.

Travelers should take all necessary precautions to avoid contact with or ingestion of contaminated food and water.

One dose of vaccine should be given at least 2 weeks prior to expected exposure.

An optimal reimmunization schedule has not been established. Reimmunization consisting of a single dose for U.S. travelers every two years under conditions of repeated or continued exposure to the *S. typhi* organism is recommended at this time.

As part of the child's or adult's immunization record, the date, lot number and manufacturer of the vaccine administered should be recorded.[18]

The U.S. Department of Health and Human Services has established a new Vaccine Adverse Event Reporting System (VAERS) to accept reports of suspected adverse events after the administration of any vaccine, including but not limited to the reporting of events required by the National Childhood Vaccine Injury Act of 1986.[19,20] The toll-free number for VAERS forms and information is 1-800-822-7967.[18]

DRUG INTERACTIONS

There are no known interactions of Typhim Vi with drugs or foods.

No studies have been conducted in the U.S. to evaluate interactions or immunological interference between the concurrent use of Typhim Vi and drugs (including antibiotics and antimalarial drugs), immune globulins or common traveler's vaccines (e.g., vaccines for tetanus, poliomyelitis, yellow fever and meningococcus). (See ADVERSE REACTIONS section.)

As with other intramuscular injections, Typhim Vi should be given with caution to individuals on anticoagulant therapy.

CARCINOGENESIS, MUTAGENESIS, IMPAIRMENT OF FERTILITY

Typhim Vi has not been evaluated for its carcinogenic potential, mutagenic potential or impairment of fertility.

PREGNANCY

REPRODUCTIVE STUDIES–PREGNANCY CATEGORY C

Animal reproduction studies have not been conducted with Typhim Vi. It is not known whether Typhim Vi can cause fetal harm when administered to a pregnant woman or can affect reproduction capacity. Typhim Vi should be given to a pregnant woman only if clearly needed.[21]

When possible, delaying vaccination until the second or third trimester to minimize the possibility of teratogenicity is a reasonable precaution.[14]

NURSING MOTHERS

It is not known if Typhim Vi is excreted in human milk. There is no data to warrant the use of this product in nursing mothers for passive antibody transfer to an infant.

PEDIATRIC USE

Safety and effectiveness of Typhim Vi have been established in children 2 years of age and older.[10,11] (See DOSAGE AND ADMINISTRATION section.) FOR CHILDREN BELOW THE AGE OF 2 YEARS, SAFETY AND EFFECTIVENESS HAVE NOT BEEN ESTABLISHED.

ADVERSE REACTIONS

Safety of Typhim Vi, the U.S. licensed liquid formulation, has been assessed in clinical trials in more than 4,000 subjects both in countries of high and low endemicity. In addition, the safety of the lyophilized formulation has been assessed in more than 6,000 individuals. The adverse reactions were predominately minor and transient local reactions. Local reactions such as injection site pain, erythema and induration almost always resolved within 48 hours of vaccination. Elevated oral temperature, above 38°C (100.4°F), was observed in approximately 1% of vaccinees in all studies. No serious or life-threatening systemic events were reported in these clinical trials.[10,11]

Adverse reactions from two trials evaluating Typhim Vi lots in the U.S. (18- to 40-year-old adults) are summarized in TABLE 3. No severe or unusual side effects were observed. Most subjects reported pain and/or tenderness (pain upon direct pressure). Local adverse experiences were generally limited to the first 48 hours.[10,11]

TABLE 3.[10,11] PERCENTAGE OF 18- TO 40-YEAR-OLD U.S. ADULTS PRESENTING WITH LOCAL OR SYSTEMIC REACTIONS WITHIN 48 HOURS AFTER THE FIRST IMMUNIZATION WITH TYPHIM Vi

REACTION	Trial 1 Placebo N=54	Trial 1 Typhim Vi N=54 (1 Lot)	Trial 2 Typhim Vi N=98 (2 Lots combined)
Local			
Tenderness	7 (13.0%)	53 (98.0%)	95 (96.9%)
Pain	4 (7.4%)	22 (40.7%)	26 (26.5%)
Induration	0	8 (14.8%)	5 (5.1%)
Erythema	0	2 (3.7%)	5 (5.1%)
Systemic			
Malaise	8 (14.8%)	13 (24.0%)	4 (4.1%)
Headache	7 (13.0%)	11 (20.4%)	16 (16.3%)
Myalgia	0	4 (7.4%)	3 (3.1%)
Nausea	2 (3.7%)	1 (1.9%)	8 (8.2%)
Diarrhea	2 (3.7%)	0	3 (3.1%)
Feverish (subjective)	0	6 (11.1%)	3 (3.1%)
Fever ≥ 100°F	0	1 (1.9%)	0
Vomiting	0	1 (1.9%)	0

No studies were conducted in U.S. children. Adverse reactions from a trial in Indonesia in children one to twelve years of age are summarized in TABLE 4.[10,11] No severe or unusual side effects were observed.

TABLE 4.[10,11] PERCENTAGE OF INDONESIAN CHILDREN ONE TO TWELVE YEARS OF AGE PRESENTING WITH LOCAL OR SYSTEMIC REACTIONS WITHIN 48 HOURS AFTER THE FIRST IMMUNIZATION WITH TYPHIM Vi

REACTIONS	N = 175
Local	
Soreness	23 (13.0%)
Pain	25 (14.3%)
Erythema	12 (6.9%)
Induration	5 (2.9%)
Impaired Limb Use	0
Systemic	
Feverishness*	5 (2.9%)
Headache	
Decreased Activity	3 (1.7%)

*Subjective feeling of fever.

In the U.S. Reimmunization Study, subjects who had received Typhim Vi 27 or 34 months earlier, and subjects who had never previously received a typhoid vaccination, were randomized to placebo or Typhim Vi, in a double-blind study. Safety data from the U.S. Reimmunization Study are presented in TABLE 5.[10,11,13] In this study 5/30 (17%) primary immunization subjects and 10/45 (22%) reimmunization subjects had an objective local reaction. No severe or unusual side effects were observed. Most subjects reported pain and/or tenderness (pain upon direct pressure). Local adverse experiences were generally limited to the first 48 hours.[10,11,13]

TABLE 5.[10,11,13] U.S. REIMMUNIZATION STUDY. SUBJECTS PRESENTING WITH LOCAL AND SYSTEMIC REACTIONS WITHIN 48 HOURS AFTER IMMUNIZATION WITH TYPHIM Vi

REACTIONS	PLACEBO N=32	FIRST IMMUNIZATION (N=30)	REIMMUNIZATION (N=45*)
Local			
Tenderness	2 (6%)	28 (93%)	44 (98%)
Pain	1 (3%)	13 (43%)	25 (56%)
Induration	0	5 (17%)	8 (18%)
Erythema	0	1 (3%)	5 (11%)
Systemic			
Malaise	1 (3%)	11 (37%)	11 (24%)
Headache	5 (16%)	8 (27%)	5 (11%)
Myalgia	0	2 (7%)	1 (2%)
Nausea	0	1 (3%)	1 (2%)
Diarrhea	0	0	1 (2%)
Feverish (subjective)	0	3 (10%)	2 (4%)
Fever ≥ 100°F	1 (3%)	0	1 (2%)
Vomiting	0	0	0

*At 27 or 34 months following a previous dose given in different studies.

Post-marketing data from foreign countries are available. During the first 5.5 years following approval of Typhim Vi in France, approximately 3.89 million doses were distributed in France. An additional 10.8 million doses have been distributed to other countries worldwide. Reports of adverse events were received either by the French post-marketing surveillance system, which utilizes spontaneous reporting of adverse events, or directly by Pasteur Mérieux; 56 and 16 reports were received, respectively, from French and other foreign distribution. Local events reported included ery-

Continued on next page

Connaught Laboratories—Cont.

thema, induration and/or pain at the injection site and lymphadenopathy. Systemic events reported included fever, flu-like episode, headache, cervical pain, vomiting, diarrhea, abdominal pain, tremor, hypotension, loss of consciousness, allergic type reactions including urticaria, and other events described below.[10,11]

In the French post-marketing experience, there was one report of diffuse arthralgias and fever two weeks post-vaccination in a 44-year old female who had also received hepatitis B vaccine simultaneously; one report of glomerulonephritis seven days post-vaccination in a 23-year old male who had also received BCG vaccine; one report of neutropenia in a 29-year-old female two days post-vaccination who had also received yellow fever vaccine; one report of bilateral retinitis three weeks post-vaccination in a 26-year-old male who had also received hepatitis B vaccine; and one report of polyarthritis four days post-vaccination in an 18-year-old male who had also received Meningococcal Groups A + C vaccine and DT Polio (Diphtheria Tetanus Poliomyelitis) vaccine combination manufactured by Pasteur Mérieux Sérums & Vaccins.[10,11]

In the French post-marketing experience, the most severe allergic-type reaction occurred in a 24-year old female with known multiple allergies who had previously received two complete series with a whole-cell typhoid vaccine; she experienced sweats, myalgia and difficulty breathing starting two hours after an IM injection (deltoid) of Typhim Vi. She received 10 mg hydrocortisone and did not require hospitalization.[10,11]

Reporting of Adverse Events

Reporting by parents and patients of all adverse events occurring after vaccine administration should be encouraged. Adverse events following immunization with vaccine should be reported by the health-care provider to the U.S. Department of Health and Human Services (DHHS) Vaccine Adverse Event Reporting System (VAERS). Reporting forms and information about reporting requirements or completion of the form can be obtained from VAERS through a toll-free number 1-800-822-7967.[18]

Health-care providers also should report these events to the Director of Medical Affairs, Connaught Laboratories, Inc., Route 611, P.O. Box 187, Swiftwater, PA 18370, the U.S. distributor, or call 1 800-822-2463.

DOSAGE AND ADMINISTRATION

Parenteral drug products should be inspected visually for particulate matter and/or discoloration prior to administration. If either of these conditions exist, the vaccine should not be administered.

For intramuscular use only. Do NOT inject intravenously. Typhim Vi vaccine is indicated for persons two years of age and older.

The immunizing dose for adults and children is a single injection of 0.5 mL. The dose for adults is given intramuscularly in the deltoid, and the dose for children is given IM either in the deltoid or the vastus lateralis. The vaccine should not be injected into the gluteal area or areas where there may be a nerve trunk.

A reimmunization dose is 0.5 mL. An optimal reimmunization schedule has not been established. Reimmunization consisting of a single dose for U.S. travelers every two years under conditions of repeated or continued exposure to the *S. typhi* organism is recommended at this time.

The skin at the site of injection first should be cleansed and disinfected. Tear off upper aluminum seal of cap. Cleanse top of rubber stopper of the vial with a suitable antiseptic and wipe away all excess antiseptic before withdrawing vaccine. For single dose syringes, thread the plunger rod into stopper until the plunger rod bottoms out against the stopper and resistance is felt. Do not over tighten the plunger rod.

A separate, sterile syringe and needle or a sterile disposable unit should be used for each patient to prevent transmission of infectious agents from person to person. Needles should not be recapped and should be properly disposed.

There are no data on safety and efficacy of Typhim Vi administered with any jet injector apparatus and this method of delivery is not recommended.

HOW SUPPLIED

Syringe, 0.5 mL–Product No. 49281-790-01
Vial, 20 Dose (Available on speacial contract basis only.)–Product No. 49281-790-20
Vial, 50 Dose (Available on special contract basis only.)–Product No. 49281-790-50

STORAGE

Store between 2°–8°C (35°–46°F). DO NOT FREEZE.

REFERENCES

1. Levine MM, et al. New knowledge on pathogenesis of bacterial enteric infections as applied to vaccine development. Microbiol. Rev. 47: 510-550, 1983
2. Levine MM. Typhoid Fever Vaccines. p 333-361. In Vaccines, Plotkin SA, Mortimer EA, eds. W.B. Saunders, 1988
3. Levine MM. et al. Typhoid Fever Chapter 5, In: *Vaccines and Immunotherapy.* Stanley J. Cryz, Jr., Editor. pp 59-72 1991
4. CDC. Summary of Notifiable Diseases, United States 1992. MMWR 41: No. 55, 1993
5. Ryan CA, et al. *Salmonella typhi* infections in the United States, 1975-1984: Increasing Role of Foreign Travel. Rev Infect Dis 11:1-8, 1989
6. Woodruff BA, et al. A new look at typhoid vaccination. Information for the practicing physician. JAMA 265: 756-759, 1991
7. Ames WR, et al. Age and sex as factors in the development of the typhoid carrier state, and a method for estimating carrier prevalence. Am J Public Health 33: 221-230, 1943
8. CDC. Typhoid fever–Skagit County, Washington. MMWR 39: 749-751, 1990
9. Acharya, IL, et al. Prevention of typhoid fever in Nepal with the Vi capsular polysaccharide of *Salmonella typhi.* N Engl J Med 317: 1101-1104, 1987
10. Unpublished data available from Connaught Laboratories, Inc., compiled 1991
11. Unpublished data available from Pasteur Mérieux Sérums & Vaccins S.A.
12. Klugman KP, et al. Protective activity of Vi capsular polysaccharide vaccine against typhoid fever. The Lancet, 1165-1169, 1987
13. Keitel WA, et al. Clinical and serological responses following primary and booster immunization with *Salmonella typhi* Vi capsular polysaccharide vaccines. Vaccine 12: 195-199, 1994
14. Recommendations of the Advisory Committee on Immunization Practices (ACIP): Update on Adult Immunization. MMWR 40: No. RR-12, 1991
15. CDC. Health Information for International Travel 1992. U. S. Department of Health and Human Services, Public Health Service
16. Recommendations of the Immunization Practices Advisory Committee (ACIP). Typhoid Immunization. MMWR 39: No. RR-10, 1990
17. ACIP: Use of vaccines and immune globulins in persons with altered immunocompetence. MMWR 42: No. RR-4, 1993
18. CDC. Vaccine Adverse Event Reporting System–United States. MMWR 39: 730-733, 1990
19. National Childhood Vaccine Injury Act: Requirements for permanent vaccination records and for reporting of selected events after vaccination. MMWR 37: 197-200, 1988
20. National Childhood Vaccine Injury Act of 1986 (Amended 1987)
21. Recommendations of the ACIP. General recommendations on immunization. MMWR 43: No. RR-1, 1994

Manufactured by:
PASTEUR MÉRIEUX Sérums & Vaccins S.A.
Lyon, France   U.S. License No. 384

Distributed by:
CONNAUGHT LABORATORIES, INC.
Swiftwater, Pennsylvania 18370, U.S.A.
Product Information as of October 1994

YF-VAX®   ℞
[*Y-F-Văks'*]
YELLOW FEVER VACCINE

Caution: Federal (U.S.A.) law prohibits dispensing without prescription.

> For special instructions on use of Yellow Fever for JET INJECTOR USE—see other side of insert.

DESCRIPTION

YF-VAX®, Yellow Fever Vaccine, is prepared by culturing the 17D strain of yellow fever virus in living avian leukosis virus-free (ALV-free) chicken embryos for subcutaneous use. The vaccine, containing sorbitol and gelatin as a stabilizer, is lyophilized, and hermetically sealed under nitrogen. No preservative is added. The vaccine must be reconstitued immediately before use with the sterile diluent provided (Sodium Chloride Injection USP—contains no preservative). YF-VAX is formulated to contain not less than 5.04 Log$_{10}$ Plaque Forming Units (PFU) per 0.5 ml dose. The vaccine appears slightly opalescent and light orange in color after reconstitution.

YF-VAX complies with official potency tests and other requirements of the U.S. Food and Drug Administration, and the World Health Organization.

HOW SUPPLIED

Vial, 1 Dose (5 per package) with vial of diluent (5 per package) for administration with needle and syringe. Product No. 49281-915-01
Vial, 5 Dose, with vial of diluent, for administration with needle and syringe. Product No. 49281-915-05
Vial, 20 Dose, with vial of diluent, for administration with needle and syringe or jet injector use. Product No. 49281-915-20
Vial, 100 Dose, with vial of diluent, for JET INJECTOR USE ONLY; *this package size and others available on special contract basis only.*

> YF-VAX® (Yellow Fever Vaccine) in the United States is supplied only to designated Yellow Fever Vaccination Centers authorized to issue valid certificates of Yellow Fever Vaccination. Location of the nearest Yellow Fever Vaccination Centers may be obtained from the Centers for Disease Control, Atlanta, GA 30333, state or local health departments, or the USPHS booklet "Immunization Information for International Travel" (obtainable from the Superintendent of Documents, U.S. Government Printing Office, Washington, D.C. 20402).

CPH International
P.O. BOX 11439
OAKLAND, CA 94611

For Medical Information Contact:
FAX (510) 352-6009

Product Listing

The following products are available for export. Direct inquiries to CPH International, P.O. Box 11439, Oakland, CA 94611 FAX(510)352-6009

FOCAN (Liver Assistance) In boxes of 42	OTC
GERININ (Kidney Assistance) In boxes of 40	OTC
INTESNON-11 (Lactic Bacteria) In boxes of 30	OTC
MUCOS (Glucosamin & Calcium) In boxes of 30	OTC
ORTHOGEN (Bone Marrow & Collagen) In boxes of 30	OTC
SERIN-P (S.O.D. & Placenta) In boxes of 45	OTC
SHARKIN (Hydrolysate Shark Cartilage) In boxes of 50	OTC
TONSIN (Ginkgo & Blood Assistance) In boxes of 50	OTC
VEGE-ESSENSE (Vegetable Conc. & Minerals) In boxes of 60	OTC
VF-25 (Vegetable & Fruit Conc.) In boxes of 60	OTC
VITATONIN (Melatonin & Antioxidants) In boxes of 42	OTC

Curatek Pharmaceuticals
1965 PRATT BOULEVARD
ELK GROVE VILLAGE, IL 60007

Direct Inquiries to:
Professional Services Department
(800) 332-7680

For Medical Information Contact:
In Emergencies:
Robert J. Borgman, Ph.D.
(847) 806-7680

METROGEL-VAGINAL® ℞
(metronidazole vaginal gel)
0.75% Vaginal Gel
FOR INTRAVAGINAL USE ONLY
NOT FOR OPHTHALMIC, DERMAL, OR ORAL USE

DESCRIPTION
METROGEL-VAGINAL is the intravaginal dosage form of the synthetic antibacterial agent, metronidazole, USP at a concentration of 0.75%. Metronidazole is a member of the imidazole class of antibacterial agents and is classified therapeutically as an anti-protozoal and anti-bacterial agent. Chemically, metronidazole is 2-methyl-5-nitroimidazole-1-ethanol. It has a chemical formula of $C_6H_9N_3O_3$, a molecular weight of 171.16, and has the following structure:

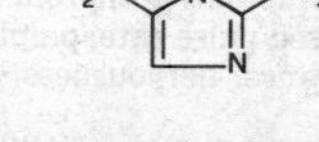

METROGEL-VAGINAL is a gelled, purified water solution, containing metronidazole at a concentration of 7.5 mg/g (0.75%). The gel is formulated at pH 4.0. The gel also contains carbomer 934P, edetate disodium, methyl paraben, propyl paraben, propylene glycol, and sodium hydroxide. Each applicator full of 5 grams of vaginal gel contains approximately 37.5 mg of metronidazole.

CLINICAL PHARMACOLOGY
Normal Subjects:
Following a single, intravaginal 5-gram dose of metronidazole vaginal gel (equivalent to 37.5 mg of metronidazole) to 12 normal subjects, a mean maximum serum metronidazole concentration of 237 ng/mL was reported (range: 152 to 368 ng/mL). This is approximately 2% of the mean maximum serum metronidazole concentration reported in the same subjects administered a single, oral 500-mg dose of metronidazole (mean C_{max}=12,785 ng/mL, range: 10,013 to 17,400 ng/mL). These peak concentrations were obtained in 6 to 12 hours after dosing with metronidazole vaginal gel and 1 to 3 hours after dosing with oral metronidazole.
The extent of exposure [area under the curve (A.U.C.)] of metronidazole, when administered as a single intravaginal 5-gram dose of metronidazole vaginal gel (equivalent to 37.5 mg of metronidazole), was approximately 4% of the A.U.C. of a single oral 500-mg metronidazole dose (4977 ng-hr/mL and approximately 125,000 ng-hr/mL, respectively). Dose adjusted comparisons of A.U.C.'s demonstrated that, on a mg to mg comparison basis, the absorption of metronidazole, when administered vaginally, was approximately half that of an equivalent oral dosage.
Patients with Bacterial Vaginosis:
Following single and multiple 5-gram doses of metronidazole vaginal gel to 4 patients with bacterial vaginosis, a mean maximum serum metronidazole concentration of 214 ng/mL on day 1 and 294 ng/mL (range: 228 to 349 ng/mL) on day five were reported. Steady state metronidazole serum concentrations following oral dosages of 400 to 500 mg B.I.D. have been reported to range from 6,000 to 20,000 ng/mL.
Microbiology:
The intracellular targets of action of metronidazole on anaerobes are largely unknown. The 5-nitro group of metronidazole is reduced by metabolically active anaerobes, and studies have demonstrated that the reduced form of the drug interacts with bacterial DNA. However, it is not clear whether interaction with DNA alone is an important component in the bactericidal action of metronidazole on anaerobic organisms.
Culture and sensitivity testing of bacteria are not routinely performed to establish the diagnosis of bacterial vaginosis. (See **INDICATIONS AND USAGE.**)
Standard methodology for the susceptibility testing of the potential bacterial vaginosis pathogens. *Gardnerella vaginalis, Mobiluncus* spp., and *Mycoplasma hominis,* has not been defined. Nonetheless, metronidazole is an antimicrobial agent active *in vitro* against most strains of the following organisms that have been reported to be associated with bacterial vaginosis:
Bacteroides spp.
Gardnerella vaginalis
Mobiluncus spp.
Peptostreptococcus spp.

INDICATIONS AND USAGE
METROGEL-VAGINAL is indicated in the treatment of bacterial vaginosis (formerly referred to as *Haemophilus* vaginitis, *Gardnerella* vaginitis, nonspecific vaginitis, *Corynebacterium* vaginitis, or anerobic vaginosis).
NOTE: For purposes of this indication, a clinical diagnosis of bacterial vaginosis is usually defined by the presence of a homogeneous vaginal discharge that (a) has a pH of greater than 4.5, (b) emits a "fishy" amine odor when mixed with a 10% KOH solution, and (c) contains clue cells on microscopic examination. Gram's stain results consistent with a diagnosis of bacterial vaginosis include (a) markedly reduced or absent *Lactobacillus* morphology, (b) predominace of *Gardnerella* morphotype, and (c) absent or few white blood cells. Other pathogens commonly associated with vulvovaginitis, e.g., *Trichomonas vaginalis, Chlamydia trachomatis, N. gonorrhoeae, Candida albicans,* and *Herpes simplex* virus should be ruled out.

CONTRAINDICATIONS
METROGEL-VAGINAL is contraindicated in patients with a prior history of hypersensitivity to metronidazole, parabens, other ingredients of the formulation, or other nitroimidazole derivatives.

WARNINGS
Convulsive Seizures and Peripheral Neuropathy:
Convulsive seizures and peripheral neuropathy, the latter characterized mainly by numbness or paresthesia of an extremity, have been reported in patients treated with oral metronidazole. The appearance of abnormal neurologic signs demands the prompt discontinuation of metronidazole vaginal gel therapy. Metronidazole vaginal gel should be administered with caution to patients with central nervous system diseases.
Psychotic Reactions:
Psychotic reactions have been reported in alcoholic patients who were using oral metronidazole and disulfiram concurrently. Metronidazole vaginal gel should not be administered to patients who have taken disulfiram within the last two weeks.

PRECAUTIONS
METROGEL-VAGINAL affords minimal peak serum levels and systemic exposure (A.U.C.'s) of metronidazole compared to 500 mg oral metronidazole dosing. Although these lower levels of exposure are less likely to produce the common reactions seen with oral metronidazole, the possibility of these and other reactions cannot be excluded presently. Data from well-controlled trials directly comparing metronidazole administered orally to metronidazole administered vaginally are not available.
General:
Patients with severe hepatic disease metabolize metronidazole slowly. This results in the accumulation of metronidazole and its metabolites in the plasma. Accordingly, for such patients, metronidazole vaginal gel should be administered cautiously.
Known or previously unrecognized vaginal candidiasis may present more prominent symptoms during therapy with metronidazole vaginal gel. Approximately 6% of patients treated with METROGEL-VAGINAL developed symptomatic *candida* vaginitis during or immediately after therapy.
Disulfiram-like reaction to alcohol has been reported with oral metronidazole, thus the possibility of such a reaction occurring while on metronidazole vaginal gel therapy cannot be excluded.
METROGEL-VAGINAL contains ingredients that may cause burning and irritation of the eye. In the event of accidental contact with the eye, rinse the eye with copious amounts of cool tap water.
Information for the Patient:
The patient should be informed not to drink alcohol while being treated with metronidazole vaginal gel. While blood levels are significantly lower with METROGEL-VAGINAL than with usual doses of oral metronidazole, a possible interaction with alcohol cannot be excluded.
The patient should also be instructed not to engage in vaginal intercourse during treatment with this product.
Drug Interactions:
Oral metronidazole has been reported to potentiate the anticoagulant effect of warfarin and other coumarin anticoagulants, resulting in a prolongation of prothrombin time. This possible drug interaction should be considered when metronidazole vaginal gel is prescribed for patients on this type of anticoagulant therapy.
Drug/Laboratory test interactions:
Metronidazole may interfere with certain types of determinations of serum chemistry values, such as aspartate aminotransferase (AST, SGOT), alanine aminotransferase (ALT, SGPT), lactate dehydrogenase (LDH), triglycerides, and glucose hexokinase. Values of zero may be observed. All of the assays in which interference has been reported involve enzymatic coupling of the assay to oxidation-reduction of nicotinamide-adenine dinucleotide (NAD+NADH). Interference is due to the similarity in absorbance peaks of NADH (340 nm) and metronidazole (322 nm) at pH 7.
Carcinogenesis, mutagenesis, impairment of fertility:
Metronidazole has shown evidence of carcinogenic activity in a number of studies involving chronic oral administration in mice and rats. Prominent among the effects in the mouse was the promotion of pulmonary tumorigenesis. This has been observed in all six reported studies in that species, including one study in which the animals were dosed on an intermittent schedule (administration during every fourth week only). At very high dose levels (approx. 500 mg/kg/day), there was a statistically significant increase in the incidence of malignant liver tumors in males. Also, the published results of one of the mouse studies indicate an increase in the incidence of malignant lymphomas as well as pulmonary neoplasms associated with lifetime feeding of the drug. All these effects are statistically significant. Several long-term oral dosing studies in the rat have been completed. There were statistically significant increases in the incidence of various neoplasms, particularly in mammary and hepatic tumors, among female rats administered metronidazole over those noted in the concurrent female control groups.
Two lifetime tumorigenicity studies in hamsters have been performed and reported to be negative. These studies have not been conducted with 0.75% metronidazole vaginal gel, which would result in significantly lower systemic blood levels than those obtained with oral formulations.
Although metronidazole has shown mutagenic activity in a number of *in vitro* assay systems, studies in mammals (*in vivo*) have failed to demonstrate a potential for genetic damage.
Fertility studies have been performed in mice up to six times the recommended human vaginal dose (based on mg/m^2) and have revealed no evidence of impaired fertility.
Pregnancy: Teratogenic Effects
Pregnancy Category B
There has been no experience to date with the use of METROGEL-VAGINAL in pregnant patients. Metronidazole crosses the placental barrier and enters the fetal circulation rapidly. No fetotoxicity or teratogenicity was observed when metronidazole was administered orally to pregnant mice at six times the recommended human vaginal dose (based on mg/m^2); however, in a single small study where the drug was administered intraperitoneally, some intrauterine deaths were observed. The relationship of these findings to the drug is unknown.
There are, however, no adequate and well-controlled studies in pregnant women. Because animal reproduction studies are not always predictive of human response, and because metronidazole is a carcinogen in rodents, this drug should be used during pregnancy only if clearly needed.
Nursing mothers:
Specific studies of metronidazole levels in human milk following intravaginally administered metronidazole have not been performed. However, metronidazole is secreted in human milk in concentrations similar to those found in plasma following oral administration of metronidazole.
Because of the potential for tumorigenicity shown for metronidazole in mouse and rat studies, a decision should be made whether to discontinue nursing or to discontinue the drug, taking into account the importance of the drug to the mother.
Pediatric use:
Safety and effectiveness in children have not been established.

ADVERSE REACTIONS
Clinical Trials:
There were no deaths or serious adverse events in clinical trials involving 295 patients; however, approximately 1% of non-pregnant patients treated with METROGEL-VAGINAL discontinued therapy early due to drug-related adverse events. One patient discontiued therapy due to abdominal pain after 2 days of therapy and one patient discontinued therapy due to a severe headache after 5 doses. Similar headaches of uncertain cause had been reported in the past by this patient.
Medical events judged to be related, probably related, or possibly related to administration of METROGEL-VAGINAL were reported for 50/295 (17%) non-pregnant patients. Unless percentages are otherwise stipulated, the incidence of individual adverse reactions listed below was less than 1%:

Continued on next page

Curatek—Cont.

Genital tract:
Symptomatic *Candida* cervicitis/vaginitis (6.1%),
Vaginal, perineal, or vulvar itching (1.4%),
Urinary frequency, vaginal or vulvar burning or irritation, vaginal discharge (not *candida*), and vulvar swelling.
Gastrointestinal:
Cramps/pain (abdominal/uterine) (3.4%),
Nausea (2.0%),
Metallic or bad taste (1.7%),
Constipation, decreased appetite, and diarrhea.
Central Nervous System:
Dizziness, headache, and lightheadedness.
Dermatologic:
Rash.
Laboratory:
Increased/decreased white blood cell counts (1.7%).
Other metronidazole formulations:
Other effects that have been reported in association with the use of **topical (dermal)** formulations of metronidazole include skin irritation, transient skin erythema, and mild skin dryness and burning. None of these adverse events exceeded an incidence of 2% of patients.
METROGEL-VAGINAL affords minimal peak serum levels and systemic exposure (A.U.C.'s) of metronidazole compared to 500 mg oral metronidazole dosing. Although these lower levels of exposure are less likely to produce the common reactions seen with oral metronidazole, the possibility of these and other reactions cannot be excluded presently. Data from well-controlled trials directly comparing metronidazole administered orally to metronidazole administered vaginally are not available.
The following adverse reactions and altered laboratory tests have been reported with the **oral or parenteral** use of metronidazole:
Cardiovascular: Flattening of the T-wave may be seen in electrocardiographic tracings.
Central Nervous System: (See **WARNINGS.**) Headache, dizziness, syncope, ataxia, confusion, convulsive seizures, peripheral neuropathy, vertigo, incoordination, irritability, depression, weakness, insomnia.
Gastrointestinal: Abdominal discomfort; nausea; vomiting; diarrhea; an unpleasant metallic taste; anorexia; epigastric distress; abdominal cramping; constipation; "furry" tongue; glossitis and stomatitis; pancreatitis; modification of taste of alcoholic beverages.
Genitourinary: Overgrowth of *Candida* in the vagina, dyspareunia, decreased libido, proctitis.
Hematopoietic: Reversible neutropenia, reversible thrombocytopenia.
Hypersensitivity Reactions: Urticaria; erythematous rash; flushing; nasal congestion; dryness of the mouth, vagina, or vulva; fever; pruritus; fleeting joint pains.
Renal: Dysuria, cystitis, polyuria, incontinence, a sense of pelvic pressure, darkened urine.

OVERDOSAGE
There is no human experience with overdosage of metronidazole vaginal gel. Vaginally applied metronidazole, 0.75% could be absorbed in sufficient amounts to produce systemic effect. (See **WARNINGS.**)

DOSAGE AND ADMINISTRATION
The recommended dose is one applicator full of METROGEL-VAGINAL (approximately 5 grams containing approximately 37.5 mg of metronidazole) intravaginally twice daily for 5 days. The medication should be applied once in the morning and once in the evening.

HOW SUPPLIED
METROGEL-VAGINAL (metronidazole vaginal gel) 0.75% Vaginal Gel is supplied in a 70 gram aluminum tube and packaged with a 5 gram vaginal applicator. NDC number is 55326-200-25.
Store at controlled room temperature 15° to 30°C (59° to 86°F). Protect from freezing.
Caution: Federal law prohibits dispensing without a prescription.
This package insert issued 5/94.
Curatek Pharmaceuticals
Limited Partnership
1965 Pratt Blvd.
Elk Grove Village, IL 60007
©1992 Curatek

Daniels Pharmaceuticals, Inc.
**2517 25TH AVENUE NORTH
ST. PETERSBURG, FL 33713-3918**

Direct Inquiries to:
(800) 237-7427

LEVOXYL™   ℞
**(LEVOTHYROXINE SODIUM TABLETS, USP)
FOR ORAL ADMINISTRATION**

DESCRIPTION
Each LEVOXYL (Levothyroxine Sodium, USP) tablet contains synthetic crystalline levothyroxine sodium (L-thyroxine). L-thyroxine is the principle hormone secreted by the normal thyroid gland. Chemically, L-thyroxine is designated as L-tyrosine, O- (4-hydroxy-3,5-diiodophenyl)-3,5-diiodo-, monosodium salt, hydrate. The molecular formula is $C_{15}H_{10}I_4N\,NaO_4$ and the structural formula is:

HO—⬡—O—⬡—$CH_2CHCOONa \cdot XH_2O$
                          |
                         NH_2

INACTIVE INGREDIENTS
lactose, microcrystalline cellulose, pregelatinized starch, magnesium stearate. The following are the color additives per tablet strength:

Strength (mcg)	Color Additive(s)
25	FD&C Yellow No. 6
50	none
75	FD&C Blue No. 1
	D&C Red No. 30
88	FD&C Yellow No. 6
	FD&C Blue No. 1
	D&C Yellow No. 10
100	FD&C Yellow No. 6
	D&C Yellow No. 10
112	FD&C Yellow No. 6
	FD&C Red No. 40
	D&C Red No. 30
125	FD&C Red No. 40
	D&C Yellow No. 10
137	FD&C Blue No. 1
150	FD&C Blue No. 1
	D&C Red No. 30
175	FD&C Blue No. 1
	D&C Yellow No. 10
200	D&C Red No. 30
	D&C Yellow No. 10
300	FD&C Yelllow No. 6
	FD&C Blue No. 1
	D&C Yellow No. 10

CLINICAL PHARMACOLOGY
The principal effect of thyroid hormones is to increase the metabolic rate of body tissues.
The thyroid hormones are also concerned with growth and development of tissues in the young.
The major thyroid hormones are L-thyroxine (T_4) and L-triiodothyronine (T_3). The amounts of T_4 and T_3 released from the normally functioning thyroid gland are regulated by the amount of thyrotropin (TSH) secreted from the anterior pituitary gland. T_4 is the major component of normal thyroid gland secretions and is therefore the primary determinant of normal thyroid functions. T_4 acts as a substrate for physiologic deiodination to T_3 in the peripheral tissues. The physiologic effects of thyroid hormones are mediated at the cellular level primarily by T_3.
LEVOXYL (L-thyroxine) tablets taken orally provide T_4 which upon absorption cannot be distinguished from T_4 that is secreted endogenously.

INDICATIONS AND USAGE
LEVOXYL (L-thyroxine) tablets are indicated:
1. As replacement or supplemental therapy for diminished or absent thyroid function (e.g., cretinism, myxedema, nontoxic goiter or hypothyroidism generally, including the hypothyroid state in children, in pregnancy and in the elderly) resulting from functional deficiency, primary atrophy, from partial or complete absence of the gland or from the effects of surgery, radiation or antithyroid agents. Therapy must be maintained continuously to control the symptoms of hypothyroidism.
2. As a pituitary TSH suppressant, in the treatment or prevention of various types of euthyroid goiters, including thyroid nodules, subacute or chronic lymphocytic thyroiditis (Hashimoto's), multinodular goiter, and in the management of thyroid cancer.

3. As a diagnostic agent in suppression tests to aid in the diagnosis of suspected mild hyperthyroidism or thyroid gland autonomy.

CONTRAINDICATIONS
L-thyroxine therapy is contraindicated in thyrotoxicosis, acute myocardial infarction and uncorrected adrenal insufficiency.

WARNINGS
Drugs with thyroid hormone activity, alone or together with other therapeutic agents, have been used for the treatment of obesity. In euthyroid patients, doses within the range of daily hormonal requirements are ineffective for weight reduction. Larger doses may produce serious or even life-threatening manifestations of toxicity, particularly when given in association with sympathomimetic amines such as those used for their anorectic effects.

PRECAUTIONS
General—Caution must be exercised in the administration of this drug to patients with cardiovascular disease. Development of chest pain or other aggravation of the cardiovascular disease requires a reduction of dosage.
Information For The Patient—Patients on thyroid preparations and parents of children on thyroid therapy should be informed that:
1. Replacement therapy is to be taken essentially for life, with the exception of cases of transient hypothyroidism, usually associated with thyroiditis, and in those patients receiving a therapeutic trial of the drug.
2. They should immediately report during the course of therapy any signs or symptoms of thyroid hormone toxicity, e.g., chest pain, increased pulse rate, palpitations, excessive sweating, heat intolerance, nervousness, or any other unusual event.
3. In case of concomitant diabetes mellitus, the daily dosage of antidiabetic medication may need readjustment as thyroid hormone replacement is achieved. If thyroid medication is stopped, a downward readjustment of the dosage of insulin or oral hypoglycemic agent may be necessary to avoid hypoglycemia. At all times, close monitoring of urinary or blood glucose levels is mandatory in such patients.
4. In case of concomitant oral anticoagulant therapy, the prothrombin time should be measured frequently to determine if the dosage of oral anticoagulants is to be readjusted.
5. Partial loss of hair may be experienced by children in the first few months of thyroid therapy, but this is usually a transient phenomenon and later recovery is usually the rule.
Laboratory Tests—The patient's response to thyroid replacement may be followed by laboratory tests such as serum thyroxine (T_4), serum triiodothyronine (T_3), free thyroxine index and thyroid stimulating hormone (TSH) blood levels.
Drug Interactions—In patients with diabetes mellitus, addition of thyroid hormone therapy may cause an increase in required dosage of insulin or oral hypoglycemic agents. Therefore, patients with diabetes mellitus should be observed closely for possible changes in antidiabetic drug dosage requirements.
Patients stabilized on oral anticoagulants who are found to require thyroid replacement therapy should be watched very closely when therapy is started. If a patient is truly hypothyroid, it is likely that a reduction in anticoagulant dosage will be required. No special precautions appear to be necessary when oral anticoagulant therapy is begun in a patient already stabilized on maintenance thyroid replacement therapy.
Cholestyramine binds both T_4 and T_3 in the intestine, thus impairing absorption of these thyroid hormones. In vitro studies indicate that the binding is not easily removed. Therefore, four to five hours should elapse between administration of cholestyramine and thyroid hormones.
Estrogens tend to increase serum thyroxine-binding globulin (TBG). In a patient with a non-functioning thyroid gland who is receiving thyroid replacement therapy, free thyroxine may be decreased when estrogens are started thus increasing thyroid requirements. However, if the patient's thyroid gland has sufficient function the decreased free thyroxine will result in a compensatory increase in thyroxine output by the thyroid. Therefore, patients without a functioning thyroid gland who are on thyroid replacement therapy may need to increase their thyroid dose if estrogens or estrogen containing oral contraceptives are given.
Drug/Laboratory Test Interactions—The following drugs or moieties are known to interfere with laboratory tests performed on patients taking thyroid hormone: androgens, corticosteroids, estrogens, oral contraceptives containing estrogens, iodine-containing preparations, and the numerous preparations containing salicylates.
1. Changes in TBG concentration should be taken into consideration in the interpretation of T_4 and T_3 values. In such cases, the unbound (free) hormone should be measured. Preg-

nancy, estrogens, and estrogen-containing oral contraceptives increase TBG concentrations. TBG may also be increased during infectious hepatitis. Decreases in TBG concentrations are observed in nephrosis, acromegaly, and after androgen or corticosteroid therapy. Familial hyper-or hypothyroxine-binding-globulinemias have been described. The incidence of TBG deficiency approximates 1 in 9000. The binding of thyroxine by thyroid-binding pre-albumin (TBPA) is inhibited by salicylates.

2. Medical or dietary iodine interferes with all in vivo tests of radio-iodine uptake, producing low uptakes which may not be reflective of a true decrease in hormone synthesis.

3. The persistence of clinical and laboratory evidence of hypothyroidism in spite of adequate dosage replacement indicates either poor patient compliance, poor absorption, excessive fecal loss, or inactivity of the preparation. Intracellular resistance to thyroid hormone is quite rare.

Carcinogenesis, Mutagenesis, And Impairment Of Fertility—A reportedly apparent association between prolonged thyroid therapy and breast cancer has not been confirmed and patients on thyroid for established indications should not discontinue therapy. No confirmatory long-term studies in animals have been performed to evaluate carcinogenic potential, mutagenicity, or impairment of fertility in either males or females.

Pregnancy—Category A—Thyroid hormones do not readily cross the placental barrier. The clinical experience to date does not indicate any adverse effect on fetuses when thyroid hormones are administered to pregnant women. On the basis of current knowledge, thyroid replacement therapy to hypothyroid women should not be discontinued during pregnancy.

Nursing Mothers—Minimal amounts of thyroid hormones are excreted in human milk. Thyroid is not associated with serious adverse reactions and does not have a known tumorigenic potential. However, caution should be exercised when thyroid is administered to a nursing woman.

Pediatric Use—Pregnant mothers provide little or no thyroid hormone to the fetus. The incidence of congenital hypothyroidism is relatively high (1:4,000) and the hypothyroid fetus would not derive any benefit from the small amounts of hormone crossing the placental barrier. Routine determinations of serum (T_4) and/or TSH is strongly advised in neonates in view of the deleterious effects of thyroid deficiency on growth and development.

Treatment should be initiated immediately upon diagnosis, and maintained for life, unless transient hypothyroidism is suspected; in which case, therapy may be interrupted for 2 to 8 weeks after the age of 3 years to reassess the condition. Cessation of therapy is justified in patients who have maintained a normal TSH during those 2 to 8 weeks.

ADVERSE REACTIONS

Adverse reactions are due to overdosage and are those of induced hyperthyroidism.

OVERDOSAGE

Excessive dosage of thyroid medication may result in symptoms of hyperthyroidism. Since, however, the effects do not appear at once, the symptoms may not appear for one to three weeks after the dosage regimen is begun. The most common signs and symptoms of overdosage are weight loss, palpitation, nervousness, diarrhea or abdominal cramps, sweating, tachycardia, cardiac arrhythmias, angina pectoris, tremors, headache, insomnia, intolerance to heat and fever. If symptoms of overdosage appear, discontinue medication for several days and reinstitute treatment at a lower dosage level.

Laboratory tests such as serum T_4, serum T_3 and the free thyroxine index will be elevated during the period of overdosage.

Complications as a result of the induced hypermetabolic state may include cardiac failure and death due to arrhythmia or failure.

TREATMENT OF OVERDOSAGE

Dosage should be reduced or therapy temporarily discontinued if signs and symptoms of overdosage appear. Treatment may be reinstituted at a lower dosage. In normal individuals, normal hypothalamic pituitary-thyroid axis function is restored in 6 to 8 weeks after thyroid suppression.

Treatment of acute massive thyroid hormone overdosage is aimed at reducing gastrointestinal absorption of the drugs and counteracting central and peripheral effects, mainly those of increased sympathetic activity. Vomiting may be induced initially if further gastrointestinal absorption can reasonably be prevented and barring contraindications such as coma, convulsions, or loss of the gagging reflex. Treatment is symptomatic and supportive. Oxygen may be administered and ventilation maintained. Cardiac glycosides may be indicated if congestive heart failure develops. Measures to control fever, hypoglycemia, or fluid loss should be instituted if needed. Antiadrenergic agents, particularly propranolol, have been used advantageously in the treatment of increased sympathetic activity. Propranolol may be administered intravenously at a dosage of 1 to 3 mg over a 10 minute

period or orally, 80 to 160 mg/day, especially when no contraindications exist for its use.

DOSAGE AND ADMINISTRATION

The goal of therapy should be the restoration of euthyroidism as judged by clinical response and confirmed by appropriate laboratory tests such as serum thyroxine (T_4), serum triiodothyronine (T_3), free thyroxine index and thyroid stimulating hormone (TSH) blood levels. The age and general condition of the patient and the severity and duration of hypothyroid symptoms determine the starting dosage and the rate of incremental dosage increase leading to a final maintenance dosage.

In otherwise healthy adults, the recommended initial dosage is 25 to 100 mcg (0.025 to 0.1 mg) daily, while the predicted full maintenance dose of 100 to 200 mcg (0.1 to 0.2 mg) daily may be achieved in two to three weeks.

In the elderly patient with long standing disease, evidence of myxedema, or evidence of cardiovascular dysfunction, the initial dose may be as little as 12.5 mcg (0.0125 mg) per day. Incremental increases of 25 mcg (0.025 mg) per day at 3 to 4 week intervals may be instituted depending on patient response. It is the physician's judgement of the severity of the disease and close observation of patient response which determine the rate and extent of dosage increase.

In infants and children there is a great urgency to achieve full thyroid replacement because of the critical importance of thyroid hormone in sustaining growth and maturation. Despite the smaller body size, the dosage needed to sustain a full rate of growth, development and general thriving is higher in the child than in the adult. The recommended daily replacement dosage of L-thyroxine in childhood is: 0–6 months: 8–10 mcg/kg; 6–12 months: 6–8 mcg/kg; 1–5 years: 5–6 mcg/kg; 6–12 years: 4–5 mcg/kg of body weight daily.

HOW SUPPLIED

LEVOXYL (L-thyroxine) tablets are supplied as oval, color coded, potency marked tablets in 12 strengths:

25 mcg (0.025 mg)—Orange:
Bottles of 100, 1000 and unit dose cartons of 100
50 mcg (0.05 mg)—White:
Bottles of 100, 1000 and unit dose cartons of 100
75 mcg (0.075 mg)—Purple:
Bottles of 100, 1000 and unit dose cartons of 100
88 mcg (0.088 mg)—Olive:
Bottles of 100 and 1000
100 mcg (0.1 mg)—Yellow:
Bottles of 100, 1000 and unit dose cartons of 100
112 mcg (0.112 mg)—Rose:
Bottles of 100 and 1000
125 mcg (0.125 mg)—Brown:
Bottles of 100, 1000 and unit dose cartons of 100
137 mcg (0.137 mg)—Dark Blue:
Bottles of 100 and 1000
150 mcg (0.15 mg)—Blue:
Bottles of 100, 1000 and unit dose cartons of 100
175 mcg (0.175 mg)—Turquoise:
Bottles of 100 and 1000
200 mcg (0.2 mg)—Pink:
Bottles of 100, 1000 and unit dose cartons of 100
300 mcg (0.3 mg)—Green:
Bottles of 100 and 1000
Daniels Pharmaceuticals, Inc.
2517 25th Avenue North
St. Petersburg, Florida 33713
Revised Sept. 1995

Shown in Product Identification Guide, page 310

TUSSIGON® Tablets Ⓒ ℞
(Hydrocodone bitartrate and Homatropine methylbromide)

DESCRIPTION

Each blue, scored tablet contains Hydrocodone bitartrate, USP, 5 mg, and Homatropine methylbromide, USP 1.5 mg.

HOW SUPPLIED

Tussigon tablets are supplied in bottles of 100 count NDC# 0689-0082-01 and bottles of 500 count NDC# 0689-0082-05.

WARNING

Hydrocodone bitartrate may be habit forming.

For EMERGENCY telephone numbers, consult the **Manufacturers Index.**

Dermik Laboratories, Inc.
500 ARCOLA ROAD, P.O. BOX 1200
COLLEGEVILLE, PA 19426-0107

Direct Inquiries to:
P.O. Box 1200
Collegeville, PA 19426-0107

5 BENZAGEL® ℞
[ben-za-jel]
(5% benzoyl peroxide) and
10 BENZAGEL® ℞
(10% benzoyl peroxide)
MICROGEL™ FORMULA
Acne Gels

DESCRIPTION

Each gram of **5 Benzagel®** and **10 Benzagel®** contains 50 mg and 100 mg respectively, of benzoyl peroxide in a gel vehicle of purified water, carbomer 940, 14% alcohol, sodium hydroxide, dioctyl sodium sulfosuccinate and fragrances. Benzoyl peroxide is an antibacterial and keratolytic agent.

HOW SUPPLIED

5 & 10 Benzagel® are available in 1.5 oz (42.5 g) and 3 oz (85 g) plastic tubes; 5 Benzagel® contains 50 mg benzoyl peroxide per gram and 10 Benzagel® contains 100 mg benzoyl peroxide per gram.
5-Benzagel 1.5 oz NDC 0066-0430-15
5-Benzagel 3.0 oz NDC 0066-0430-30
10-Benzagel 1.5 oz NDC 0066-0431-15
10 Benzagel 3.0 oz NDC 0066-0431-30
CR-5733M   Rev. 1/96

BENZAMYCIN® Topical Gel ℞
[ben 'za-mi "sin]
(erythromycin—benzoyl peroxide)

PRODUCT OVERVIEW

KEY FACTS

Benzamycin® is a topical gel containing 3% erythromycin and 5% benzoyl peroxide. Erythromycin is an antibiotic and benzoyl peroxide is an antibacterial and keratolytic agent.

MAJOR USES

Benzamycin® is indicated for the topical control of acne vulgaris.

SAFETY INFORMATION

Benzamycin® is contraindicated in patients with a history of hypersensitivity to erythromycin, benzoyl peroxide, or any of the other listed ingredients. Avoid contact with eyes and mucous membranes. Concomitant topical acne therapy should be used with caution. Adverse reactions may include dryness, erythema, and pruritus.

PRESCRIBING INFORMATION

BENZAMYCIN® Topical Gel ℞
[ben 'za-mi "sin]
(erythromycin-benzoyl peroxide topical gel)
Topical gel: erythromycin (3%), benzoyl peroxide (5%)
For Dermatological Use Only — Not for Ophthalmic Use
Reconstitute Before Dispensing

DESCRIPTION

BENZAMYCIN® Topical Gel contains erythromycin [(3R*, 4S*, 5S*, 6R*, 7R*, 9R*, 11R*, 12R*, 13S*, 14R*)-4-[(2,6-Dideoxy -3- C-methyl-3-O-methyl-a-L-ribo-hexopyranosyl)-oxy]-14 -ethyl-7,12,13-trihydroxy-3,5,7,9,11,13-hexa-methyl-6- [[3,4,6-trideoxy-3-(dimethylamino)-b-D-xylo-hexopyranosyl]oxy]oxacyclotetradecane-2,10-dione]. Erythromycin is a macrolide antibiotic produced from a strain of *Saccharopolyspora erythraea* (formerly *Streptomyces erythreus*). It is a base and readily forms salts with acids.
Chemically, erythromycin is ($C_{37}H_{67}NO_{13}$). It has the following structural formula: Erythromycin has the molecular weight of 733.94. It is a white crystalline powder and has a solubility of approximately 1 mg/mL in water and is soluble in alcohol at 25°C.
BENZAMYCIN Topical Gel also contains benzoyl peroxide for topical use. Benzoyl peroxide is an antibacterial and keratolytic agent.
Chemically, benzoyl peroxide is ($C_{14}H_{10}O_4$). It has the following structural formula: Benzoyl peroxide has the molecular weight of 242.23. It is a white granular powder and is sparingly soluble in water and alcohol and soluble in acetone, chloroform and ether.

Continued on next page

Dermik Laboratories—Cont.

Size (Net Weight)	NDC 0066-	Benzoyl Peroxide Gel	Active Erythromycin Powder (In Plastic Vial)	Ethyl Alcohol (70%) To Be Added
23.3 grams (as dispensed)	0510-23	20 grams	0.8 grams	3 mL
46.6 grams (as dispensed)	0510-46	40 grams	1.6 grams	6 mL

Each gram of BENZAMYCIN Topical Gel contains, as dispensed, 30 mg (3%) of erythromycin and 50 mg (5%) of benzoyl peroxide in a base of purified water USP, carbomer 940 NF, alcohol 20%, sodium hydroxide NF, docusate sodium and fragrance.

CLINICAL PHARMACOLOGY

The exact mechanism by which erythromycin reduces lesions of acne vulgaris is not fully known; however, the effect appears to be due in part to the antibacterial activity of the drug.

Benzoyl peroxide has a keratolytic and desquamative effect which may also contribute to its efficacy.

Benzoyl peroxide has been shown to be absorbed by the skin where it is converted to benzoic acid.

MICROBIOLOGY

Erythromycin acts by inhibition of protein synthesis in susceptible organisms by reversibly binding to 50 **S** ribosomal subunits, thereby inhibiting translocation of aminoacyl transfer-RNA and inhibiting polypeptide synthesis. Antagonism has been demonstrated *in vitro* between erythromycin, lincomycin, chloramphenicol and clindamycin.

Benzoyl peroxide is an antibacterial agent which has been shown to be effective against *Propionibacterium acnes*, an anaerobe found in sebaceous follicles and comedones. The antibacterial action of benzoyl peroxide is believed to be due to the release of active oxygen.

INDICATIONS AND USAGE

BENZAMYCIN Topical Gel is indicated for the topical treatment of acne vulgaris.

CONTRAINDICATIONS

BENZAMYCIN Topical Gel is contraindicated in those individuals who have shown hypersensitivity to any of its components.

WARNINGS

Pseudomembranous colitis has been reported with nearly all antibacterial agents, including erythromycin, and may range in severity from mild to life-threatening. Therefore, it is important to consider this diagnosis in patients who present with diarrhea subsequent to the administration of antibacterial agents.

Treatment with antibacterial agents alters the normal flora of the colon and may permit overgrowth of clostridia. Studies indicate that a toxin produced by *Clostridium difficile* is one primary cause of "antibiotic-associated colitis."

After the diagnosis of pseudomembranous colitis has been established, therapeutic measures should be initiated. Mild cases of pseudomembranous colitis usually respond to drug discontinuation alone. In moderate to severe cases, consideration should be given to management with fluids and electrolytes, protein supplementation and treatment with an antibacterial drug clinically effective against *C. difficile* colitis.

PRECAUTIONS

General: For topical use only; not for ophthalmic use. Concomitant topical acne therapy should be used with caution because a possible cumulative irritancy effect may occur, especially with the use of peeling, desquamating or abrasive agents. If severe irritation develops, discontinue use and institute appropriate therapy.

The use of antibiotic agents may be associated with the overgrowth of nonsusceptible organisms including fungi. If this occurs, discontinue use and take appropriate measures.

Avoid contact with eyes and all mucous membranes.

Information for Patients: Patients using BENZAMYCIN Topical Gel should receive the following information and instructions.

1. This medication is to be used as directed by the physician. It is for external use only. Avoid contact with the eyes, nose, mouth, and all mucous membranes.

2. This medication should not be used for any disorder other than that for which it was prescribed.

3. Patients should not use any other topical acne preparation unless otherwise directed by physician.

4. Patients should report to their physician any signs of local adverse reactions.

5. BENZAMYCIN® Topical Gel may bleach hair or colored fabric.

6. Keep product refrigerated and discard after 3 months.

Carcinogenesis, Mutagenesis and Impairment of Fertility

Data from a study using mice known to be highly susceptible to cancer suggests that benzoyl peroxide acts as a tumor promoter. The clinical significance of this is unknown.

No animal studies have been performed to evaluate the carcinogenic and mutagenic potential or effects on fertility of topical erythromycin. However, long-term (2-year) oral studies in rats with erythromycin ethylsuccinate and erythromycin base did not provide evidence of tumorigenicity. There was no apparent effect on male or female fertility in rats fed erythromycin (base) at levels up to 0.25% of diet.

Pregnancy: Teratogenic Effects: Pregnancy CATEGORY C: Animal reproduction studies have not been conducted with BENZAMYCIN Topical Gel or benzoyl peroxide.

There was no evidence of teratogenicity or any other adverse effect on reproduction in female rats fed erythromycin base (up to 0.25% diet) prior to and during mating, during gestation and through weaning of two successive litters.

There are no well-controlled trials in pregnant women with BENZAMYCIN Topical Gel. It also is not known whether BENZAMYCIN Topical Gel can cause fetal harm when administered to a pregnant woman or can affect reproductive capacity. BENZAMYCIN Topical Gel should be given to a pregnant woman only if clearly needed.

Nursing Women: It is not known whether BENZAMYCIN Topical Gel is excreted in human milk after topical application. However, erythromycin is excreted in human milk following oral and parenteral erythromycin administration. Therefore, caution should be exercised when erythromycin is administered to a nursing woman.

Pediatric Use: Safety and effectiveness of this product in pediatric patients below the age of 12 have not been established.

ADVERSE REACTIONS

In controlled clinical trials, the total incidence of adverse reactions associated with the use of BENZAMYCIN Topical Gel was approximately 3%. These were dryness and urticarial reaction.

The following additional local adverse reactions have been reported occasionally: irritation of the skin including peeling, itching, burning sensation, erythema, inflammation of the face, eyes and nose, and irritation of the eyes. Skin discoloration, oiliness and tenderness of the skin have also been reported.

DOSAGE AND ADMINISTRATION

BENZAMYCIN Topical Gel should be applied twice daily, morning and evening, or as directed by a physician, to affected areas after the skin is thoroughly washed, rinsed with warm water and gently patted dry.

How Supplied and Compounding Directions:

[See table above.]

Prior to dispensing, tap vial until powder flows freely. Add indicated amount of ethyl alcohol (70%) to vial (to the mark) and immediately shake to completely dissolve erythromycin. Add this solution to gel and stir until homogeneous in appearance (1 to 1¹/₂ minutes). BENZAMYCIN Topical Gel should then be stored under refrigeration. Do not freeze. Place a 3-month expiration date on the label.

NOTE: *Prior to reconstitution*, store at room temperature between 15° and 30°C (59°–86°F).

After reconstitution, store under refrigeration between 2° and 8°C (36°–46°F).

Do not freeze. Keep tightly closed. Keep out of the reach of children.

Caution: Federal (U.S.A.) law prohibits dispensing without prescription.

U.S. Patent Nos. 4,387,107 and 4,497,794.

Manufactured by Rhône-Poulenc Rorer Puerto Rico Inc. Manati, Puerto Rico

For **DERMIK LABORATORIES, INC.** A Rhône-Poulenc Rorer Company Collegeville, PA 19426 Rev. 12/95   IN-7121N

DRITHOCREME® ℞
(anthralin) 0.1%, 0.25%, 0.5%, 1.0% (HP)

DESCRIPTION

Drithocreme® is a pale yellow topical cream containing 0.1%, 0.25%, 0.5% or 1.0% (HP) anthralin USP in a base of white petrolatum, sodium lauryl sulfate, cetostearyl alcohol, ascorbic acid, salicylic acid, chlorocresol and purified water.

CLINICAL PHARMACOLOGY

Although the precise mechanism of anthralin's anti-psoriatic action is not fully understood, *in vitro* evidence suggests that its antimitotic effect results from inhibition of DNA synthesis. Additionally, the chemically reducing properties of anthralin may upset oxidative metabolic processes, providing a further slowing down of epidermal mitosis. Absorption in man has not been finally determined, but in a limited clinical study of Drithocreme, no traces of anthraquinone metabolites were detected in the urine of subjects treated; however, caution is advised in patients with renal disease.

INDICATIONS AND USAGE

An aid in the topical treatment of quiescent or chronic psoriasis. Treatment should be continued until the skin is entirely clear, *i.e.*, when there is nothing to feel with the fingers and the texture is normal.

CONTRAINDICATIONS

Do not use Drithocreme on the face, or for acute or actively inflamed psoriatic eruptions. Do not use if sensitive to any of the ingredients.

WARNINGS

Avoid contact with the eyes or mucous membranes. Drithocreme should not normally be applied to intertriginous skin areas and high strengths should not be used on these sites. Remove any unintended residue which may be deposited behind the ears. Avoid applying to the folds and creases of the skin. Discontinue use if a sensitivity reaction occurs or if excessive irritation develops on uninvolved skin areas. Keep out of the reach of children.

PRECAUTIONS

For external use only. To prevent the possibility of staining clothing or bed linen while gaining experience in using Drithocreme, it may be advisable to use protective dressings. To prevent the possibility of discoloration, particularly where Drithocreme HP (1.0%) has been used, always rinse the bath/shower with hot water immediately after washing/showering and then use a suitable cleanser to remove any deposit on the surface of the bath or shower. Contact with fabrics, plastics and other materials may cause staining and should be avoided. Always wash hands thoroughly after use. Long-term studies in animals have not been performed to evaluate the carcinogenic potential of the drug. Although anthralin has been found to have tumor-promoting properties on mouse skin, there have been no reports to suggest carcinogenic effects in humans after many years of clinical use.

As long-term use of topical corticosteroids may destabilize psoriasis, and withdrawal may also give rise to a 'rebound' phenomenon, an interval of at least one week should be allowed between the discontinuance of such steroids and the commencement of Drithocreme therapy. Petrolatum or a suitably bland emollient may usefully be applied during the intervening period.

PREGNANCY

Pregnancy Category C. Animal reproduction studies have not been conducted with Drithocreme. It is also not known whether Drithocreme can cause fetal harm when administered to a pregnant woman or can affect reproduction capacity. Drithocreme® should be given to a pregnant woman only if clearly needed.

Nursing Mothers

It is not known whether this drug is excreted in human milk. Because many drugs are excreted in milk and because of the potential for tumorigenicity shown for anthralin in animal studies, a decision should be made whether to discontinue nursing or to discontinue the drug, taking into account the importance of the drug to the mother.

Pediatric Use

Safety and effectiveness in children have not been specifically established.

ADVERSE REACTIONS

Very few instances of contact allergic reactions to anthralin have been reported. However, transient primary irritation of normal skin or uninvolved skin surrounding the treated lesions is more frequently seen and may occasionally be severe. Application of Drithocreme must be restricted to the psoriatic lesions. If the initial treatment produces excessive soreness or if the lesions spread, reduce frequency of application and, in extreme cases, discontinue use and consult physician. Some temporary discoloration of hair and fingernails may arise during the period of treatment but should be minimized by careful application.

DOSAGE AND ADMINISTRATION

Generally, it is recommended that Drithocreme be applied once a day or as directed by a physician. Anthralin is known to be a potential skin irritant. The irritant potential of anthralin is directly related to the strength being used and each patient's individual tolerance. Therefore, where the response to anthralin treatment has not previously been

established, always commence treatment for at least one week using 0.1% Drithocreme. Increase to the 0.25%, 0.5% and 1.0% (HP) strengths when directed by a physician.

To open the tube, unscrew the cap and invert to pierce membrane. Apply as directed and remove by washing or showering. The optimal period of contact will vary according to the strength used and the patient's response to treatment.

For the Skin

Apply sparingly only to the psoriatic lesions and rub gently and carefully into the skin until absorbed. It is most important to avoid applying an excessive quantity which may cause unnecessary soiling and staining of the clothing and/or bed linen. At the end of each period of treatment, a bath or shower should be taken to remove any surplus cream (which may have become red/brown in color). The margins of the lesions may gradually become stained purple/brown as treatment progresses, but this will disappear after cessation of treatment.

For the Scalp

Comb the hair to remove scalar debris and, after suitably parting, rub the cream well into the lesions. Keep Drithocreme away from the eyes. Care should be taken to avoid application of the cream to uninvolved scalp margins. Remove any unintended residue which may be deposited behind the ears. At the end of each period of contact, wash the hair and scalp to remove any surplus cream (which may have become red/brown in color). Keep tightly capped when not in use.

Store at controlled room temperature, 15°–30°C (59°–88°F).

HOW SUPPLIED

50g tubes
Drithocreme 0.1% NDC 0088-7200-50
Drithocreme 0.25% NDC 0066-7201-50
Drithocreme 0.5% NDC 0056-7202-50
Drithocreme HP 1% NDC 0086-7203-50

DRITHO-SCALP®   ℞
(anthralin) 0.25%, 0.5%

DESCRIPTION
Dritho-Scalp® is a pale yellow topical cream containing 0.25 or 0.5% anthralin USP in a base of white petrolatum, mineral oil, sodium lauryl sulfate, cetostearyl alcohol, ascorbic acid, salicylic acid, chlorocresol and purified water.

CLINICAL PHARMACOLOGY
Although the precise mechanism of anthralin's antipsoriatic action is not fully understood, *in vitro* evidence suggests that its antimitotic effect results from inhibition of DNA synthesis. Additionally, the chemically reducing properties of anthralin may upset oxidative metabolic processes, providing a further slowing down of epidermal mitosis.

Absorption in man has not been finally determined, but in a limited clinical study of anthralin cream, no traces of anthraquinone metabolites were detected in the urine of subjects treated; however, caution is advised in patients with renal disease.

INDICATIONS AND USAGE
An aid in the topical treatment of quiescent or chronic psoriasis of the scalp. Treatment should be continued until the skin is entirely clear, *i.e.*, when there is nothing to feel with the fingers and the texture is normal.

CONTRAINDICATIONS
In patients with acute psoriatic eruptions or a history of hypersensitivity to any of the ingredients.

WARNINGS
Avoid contact with the eyes or mucous membranes. Dritho-Scalp should not normally be applied to intertriginous skin area and high strengths should not be used on these sites. Remove any unintended residue which may be deposited behind the ears. Avoid applying to the folds and creases of the skin. Discontinue use if a sensitivity reaction occurs or if excessive irritation develops on uninvolved skin areas. Keep out of the reach of children.

PRECAUTIONS
For external use only. Dritho-Scalp may stain the hair and should be applied sparingly and carefully to psoriatic lesions only. Contact with fabrics, plastics and other materials may cause staining and should be avoided. To prevent the possibility of discoloration, always rinse the bath/shower with hot water immediately after washing/showering and then use a suitable cleanser to remove any deposit on the surface of the bath or shower. Always wash hands thoroughly after use. Long-term studies in animals have not been performed to evaluate the carcinogenic potential of the drug. Although anthralin has been found to have tumor-promoting properties on mouse skin, there have been no reports to suggest carcinogenic effects in humans after many years of clinical use.

As long-term use of topical corticosteroids may destabilize psoriasis, and withdrawal may also give rise to a 'rebound'

phenomenon, an interval of at least one week should be allowed between the discontinuance of such steroids and the commencement of Dritho-Scalp therapy. Petrolatum or a suitably bland emollient may usefully be applied during the intervening period.

Pregnancy
Pregnancy Category C. Animal reproduction studies have not been conducted with Dritho-Scalp. It is also not known whether Dritho-Scalp can cause fetal harm when administered to a pregnant women or can affect reproduction capacity. Dritho-Scalp should be given to a pregnant woman only if clearly needed.

Nursing Mothers
It is not known whether this drug is excreted in human milk. Because many drugs are excreted in milk and because of the potential for tumorigenicity shown for anthralin in animal studies, a decision should be made whether to discontinue nursing or to discontinue the drug, taking into account the importance of the drug to the mother.

Pediatric Use
Safety and effectiveness in children have not been specifically established.

ADVERSE REACTIONS
Very few instances of contact allergic reactions to anthralin have been reported. However, transient primary irritation of uninvolved skin surrounding the treated lesions is more frequently seen and may occasionally be severe. Application of Dritho-Scalp® must be restricted to the psoriatic lesions. If the initial treatment produces excessive soreness or if the lesions spread, reduce frequency of application and, in extreme cases, discontinue use and consult physician. Some temporary discoloration of hair and fingernails may arise during the period of treatment but should be minimized by careful application.

DOSAGE AND ADMINISTRATION
Generally, it is recommended that Dritho-Scalp be applied once a day or as directed by a physician. Anthralin is known to be a potential skin irritant. The irritant potential of anthralin is directly related to the strength being used and each patient's individual tolerance. Therefore, where the response to anthralin treatment has not previously been established, always commence treatment for at least one week using 0.25% Dritho-Scalp. Increase to the 0.5% strength only when directed by a physician.

Before initial use, the tube membrane should be pierced by inverting the white cap, which should then be discarded. The black applicator should then be screwed firmly onto the tube. This applicator includes a black cap which should always be replaced between treatments (see illustration).

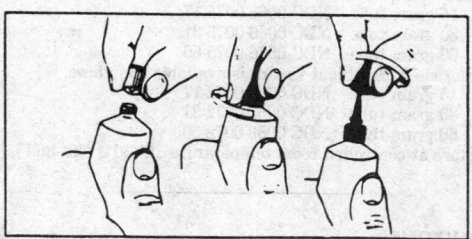

Apply as directed and remove by washing or showering. The optimal period of contact will vary according to the strength used and the patient's response to treatment.

Comb the hair to remove scalar debris and, after suitably parting, apply Dritho-Scalp only to the lesions and rub in well, taking care to prevent the cream spreading onto the forehead.

Keep Dritho-Scalp well away from the eyes.

Avoid application of the cream to uninvolved scalp margins. Remove any unintended residue which may be deposited behind the ears. At the end of each period of contact, wash the hair and scalp to remove any surplus cream (which may have become red/brown in color).

Always wash hands thoroughly after use.

Store at controlled room temperature, 15°–30°C (59°–85°F).

HOW SUPPLIED
50 g tube with special applicator
Dritho-Scalp 0.25% NDC 0066-7204-50
Dritho-Scalp 0.5% NDC 0055-7205-50

FLORONE®   ℞
[flŏr-ōhn]
(brand of diflorasone diacetate cream and
diflorasone diacetate ointment 0.05%)

FLORONE E®   ℞
(brand of diflorasone diacetate
emollient cream 0.05%)
Not For Ophthalmic Use

PRODUCT OVERVIEW

KEY FACTS
Florone is a topical corticosteroid containing 0.05% diflorasone diacetate in an emulsified, hydrophilic cream and in an ointment with an emollient, occlusive base. Florone Ointment contains no propylene glycol. Florone E Emollient Cream contains 0.5 mg diflorasone diacetate in a hydrophilic, vanishing cream base.

MAJOR USES
These products are indicated for the relief of the inflammatory and pruritic manifestations of corticosteroid-responsive dermatoses.

SAFETY INFORMATION
The Florone products are contraindicated in patients with a history of hypersensitivity to any of their components. Systemic absorption of topical corticosteroids has produced reversible HPA axis suppression. Therefore, patients receiving a large dose applied to a large area or under an occlusive dressing should be evaluated periodically. The most common adverse reactions are burning, itching, irritation, and dryness.

PRESCRIBING INFORMATION

FLORONE®   ℞
[flŏr-ōhn]
(brand of diflorasone diacetate cream and
diflorasone diacetate ointment 0.05%)

FLORONE E®   ℞
(brand of diflorasone diacetate
emollient cream 0.05%)
Not For Ophthalmic Use

DESCRIPTION
Each gram of FLORONE Cream and FLORONE Ointment contains 0.5 mg diflorasone diacetate in a cream or ointment base respectively. Each gram of Florone E Emollient Cream contains 0.5 mg diflorasone diacetate in an emollient cream base.

Chemically, diflorasone diacetate is: 6α, 9α-difluoro-11β, $17,21$-trihydroxy-16β-methylpregna-1,4-diene-3,20-dione 17,21 diacetate.

FLORONE Cream contains diflorasone diacetate in an emulsified and hydrophilic cream base consisting of propylene glycol, stearic acid, polysorbate 60, sorbitan monostearate and monooleate, sorbic acid, citric acid and water. The corticosteroid is formulated as a solution in the vehicle using 15 percent propylene glycol to optimize drug delivery.

FLORONE Ointment contains diflorasone diacetate in an emollient, occlusive base consisting of polyoxypropylene 15-stearyl ether, stearic acid, lanolin alcohol and white petrolatum.

Florone E Emollient Cream contains diflorasone diacetate in a hydrophilic, vanishing cream base of propylene glycol, stearyl alcohol, cetyl alcohol, sorbitan monostearate, polysorbate 60, mineral oil and water.

CLINICAL PHARMACOLOGY
Topical corticosteroids share anti-inflammatory, antipruritic and vasoconstrictive actions.

The mechanism of anti-inflammatory activity of the topical corticosteroids is unclear. Various laboratory methods, including vasoconstrictor assays, are used to compare and predict potencies and/or clinical efficacies of the topical corticosteroids. There is some evidence to suggest that a recognizable correlation exists between vasoconstrictor potency and therapeutic efficacy in man.

Pharmacokinetics: The extent of percutaneous absorption of topical corticosteroids is determined by many factors including the vehicle, the integrity of the epidermal barrier and the use of occlusive dressings.

Topical corticosteroids can be absorbed from normal intact skin. Inflammation and/or other disease processes in the skin increase percutaneous absorption. Occlusive dressings substantially increase the percutaneous absorption of topical corticosteroids. Thus, occlusive dressings may be a valuable therapeutic adjunct for treatment of resistant dermatoses. (See DOSAGE AND ADMINISTRATION.)

Once absorbed through the skin, topical corticosteroids are handled through pharmacokinetic pathways similar to systemically administered corticosteroids. Corticosteroids are bound to plasma proteins in varying degrees. They are metabolized primarily in the liver and are then excreted by the

Continued on next page

Dermik Laboratories—Cont.

kidneys. Some of the topical corticosteroids and their metabolites are also excreted into the bile.

INDICATIONS AND USAGE

Topical corticosteroids are indicated for relief of the inflammatory and pruritic manifestations of corticosteroid-responsive dermatoses.

CONTRAINDICATIONS

Topical steroids are contraindicated in those patients with a history of hypersensitivity to any of the components of the preparation.

PRECAUTIONS

General:
Systemic absorption of topical corticosteroids has produced reversible hypothalamic-pituitary-adrenal (HPA) axis suppression, manifestations of Cushing's syndrome, hyperglycemia, and glucosuria in some patients.
Conditions which augment systemic absorption include the application of the more potent steroids, use over large surface areas, prolonged use, and the addition of occlusive dressings.
Therefore, patients receiving a large dose of a potent topical steroid applied to a large surface area or under an occlusive dressing should be evaluated periodically for evidence of HPA axis suppression by using the urinary free-cortisol and ACTH stimulation tests. If HPA axis suppression is noted, an attempt should be made to withdraw the drug, to reduce the frequency of application, or to substitute a less potent steroid.
Recovery of HPA axis function is generally prompt and complete upon discontinuation of the drug. Infrequently, signs and symptoms of steroid withdrawal may occur, requiring supplemental systemic corticosteroids.
Children may absorb proportionally larger amounts of topical corticosteroids and thus be more susceptible to systemic toxicity. (See PRECAUTIONS—Pediatric Use.)
If irritation develops, topical corticosteroids should be discontinued and appropriate therapy instituted.
In the presence of dermatological infections, the use of an appropriate antifungal or antibacterial agent should be instituted. If a favorable response does not occur promptly, the corticosteroid should be discontinued until the infection has been adequately controlled.

Information for the Patient: Patients using topical corticosteroids should receive the following information and instructions:

1. This medication is to be used as directed by the physician. It is for external use only. Avoid contact with the eyes.
2. Patients should be advised not to use this medication for any disorder other than for which it was prescribed.
3. The treated skin area should not be bandaged or otherwise covered or wrapped as to be occlusive unless directed by the physician.
4. Patients should report any signs of local adverse reactions especially under occlusive dressing.
5. Parents of pediatric patients should be advised not to use tight-fitting diapers or plastic pants on a child being treated in the diaper area, as these garments may constitute occlusive dressings.

Laboratory Tests: The following tests may be helpful in evaluating the HPA axis suppression:
Urinary free cortisol test
ACTH stimulation test

Carcinogenesis, Mutagenesis, and Impairment of Fertility:
Long-term animal studies have not been performed to evaluate the carcinogenic potential or the effect on fertility of topical corticosteroids.
Studies to determine mutagenicity with prednisolone and hydrocortisone have revealed negative results.

Pregnancy Category C: Corticosteroids are generally teratogenic in laboratory animals when administered systemically at relatively low dosage levels. The more potent corticosteroids have been shown to be teratogenic after dermal application in laboratory animals. There are no adequate and well-controlled studies in pregnant women on teratogenic effects from topically applied corticosteroids. Therefore, topical corticosteroids should be used during pregnancy only if the potential benefit justifies the potential risk to the fetus. Drugs of this class should not be used extensively on pregnant patients, in large amounts, or for prolonged periods of time.

Nursing Mothers: It is not known whether topical administration of corticosteroids could result in sufficient systemic absorption to produce detectable quantities in breast milk. Systemically administered corticosteroids are secreted into breast milk in quantities **not** likely to have a deleterious effect on the infant. Nevertheless, caution should be exercised when topical corticosteroids are administered to a nursing woman.

Pediatric Use: *Pediatric patients may demonstrate greater susceptibility to topical corticosteroid-induced HPA axis suppression and Cushing's syndrome than mature patients because of a larger skin surface area to body weight ratio.*
Hypothalamic-pituitary-adrenal (HPA) axis suppression, Cushing's syndrome, and intracranial hypertension have been reported in children receiving topical corticosteroids. Manifestations of adrenal suppression in children include linear growth retardation, delayed weight gain, low plasma cortisol levels, and absence of response to ACTH stimulation. Manifestations of intracranial hypertension include bulging fontanelles, headaches, and bilateral papilledema.
Administration of topical corticosteroids to children should be limited to the least amount compatible with an effective therapeutic regimen. Chronic corticosteroid therapy may interfere with the growth and development of children.

ADVERSE REACTIONS

The following local adverse reactions have been reported with topical corticosteroids, but may occur more frequently with the use of occlusive dressings. These reactions are listed in an approximate decreasing order of occurrence:

1. Burning
2. Itching
3. Irritation
4. Dryness
5. Folliculitis
6. Hypertrichosis
7. Acneiform eruptions
8. Hypopigmentation
9. Perioral dermatitis
10. Allergic contact dermatitis
11. Maceration of the skin
12. Secondary infection
13. Skin atrophy
14. Striae
15. Miliaria

OVERDOSAGE

Topically applied corticosteroids can be absorbed in sufficient amounts to produce systemic effects (See PRECAUTIONS).

DOSAGE AND ADMINISTRATION

Florone Cream and Florone Ointment are generally applied to the affected areas as a thin film from one to four times daily depending on the severity of the condition.
Florone E Emollient Cream should be applied to the affected areas as a thin film from one to three times daily depending on the severity or resistant nature of the condition.
Occlusive dressings may be used for the management of psoriasis or recalcitrant conditions.
If an infection develops, the use of occlusive dressings should be discontinued and appropriate antimicrobial therapy instituted.

HOW SUPPLIED

FLORONE Cream 0.05% is available as follows:
15 gram tube NDC 0066-0074-17
30 gram tube NDC 0066-0074-31
60 gram tube NDC 0066-0074-60
FLORONE Ointment 0.05% is available as follows:
15 gram tube NDC 0066-0075-17
30 gram tube NDC 0066-0075-31
60 gram tube NDC 0066-0075-60
Florone E Emollient Cream is available as follows:
15 gram tube NDC 0066-0072-17
30 gram tube NDC 0066-0072-31
60 gram tube NDC 0066-0072-60
Store at controlled room temperature 15°–30°C (59°–86°F).

HYTONE® ℞
[*hī-tōne*]
(hydrocortisone)
Cream, Lotion

DESCRIPTION

Each gram of Hytone® (hydrocortisone) Cream 2½% contains 25 mg of hydrocortisone in a water-washable base of purified water, propylene glycol, glyceryl monostearate SE, cholesterol and related sterols, isopropyl myristate, polysorbate 60, cetyl alcohol, sorbitan monostearate, polyoxyl 40 stearate and sorbic acid.
Each mL of Hytone (hydrocortisone) Lotion 2½% contains 25 mg of hydrocortisone in a vehicle consisting of carbomer 940, propylene glycol, polysorbate 40, propylene glycol stearate, cholesterol and related sterols, isopropyl myristate, sorbitan palmitate, cetyl alcohol, triethanolamine, sorbic acid, simethicone, and purified water.
Chemically, hydrocortisone is [Pregn-4-ene-3,20-dione, 11, 17, 21- trihydroxy-, (11β)-] with the molecular formula ($C_{21}H_{30}O_5$).
Its molecular weight is 362.47 and its CAS Registry Number is 50-23-7. The topical corticosteroids, including hydrocortisone, constitute a class of primarily synthetic steroids used as anti-inflammatory and antipruritic agents.

CLINICAL PHARMACOLOGY

Topical corticosteroids share anti-inflammatory, antipruritic, and vasoconstrictive actions. The mechanism of anti-inflammatory activity of the topical corticosteroids is unclear. Various laboratory methods, including vasoconstrictor assays, are used to compare and predict potencies and/or clinical efficacies of the topical corticosteroids. There is some evidence to suggest that a recognizable correlation exists between vasoconstrictor potency and therapeutic efficacy in man.

Pharmacokinetics: The extent of percutaneous absorption of topical corticosteroids is determined by many factors including the vehicle, the integrity of the epidermal barrier, and the use of occlusive dressings.
Topical corticosteroids can be absorbed from normal intact skin. Inflammation and/or other disease processes in the skin increase percutaneous absorption. Occlusive dressings substantially increase the percutaneous absorption of topical corticosteroids. Thus, occlusive dressings may be a valuable therapeutic adjunct for treatment of resistant dermatoses. (See **DOSAGE AND ADMINISTRATION.**)
Once absorbed through the skin, topical corticosteroids are handled through pharmacokinetic pathways similar to systemically administered corticosteroids. Corticosteroids are bound to plasma proteins in varying degrees. Corticosteroids are metabolized primarily in the liver and are then excreted by the kidneys. Some of the topical corticosteroids and their metabolites are also excreted into the bile.

INDICATIONS AND USAGE

Topical corticosteroids are indicated for the relief of the inflammatory and pruritic manifestations of corticosteroid-responsive dermatoses.

CONTRAINDICATIONS

Topical corticosteroids are contraindicated in those patients with a history of hypersensitivity to any of the components of the preparation.

PRECAUTIONS

General: Systemic absorption of topical corticosteroids has produced reversible hypothalamic-pituitary-adrenal (HPA) axis suppression, manifestations of Cushing's syndrome, hyperglycemia, and glucosuria in some patients.
Conditions which augment systemic absorption include the application of the more potent steroids, use over large surface areas, prolonged use, and the addition of occlusive dressings.
Therefore, patients receiving a large dose of a potent topical steroid applied to a large surface area or under an occlusive dressing should be evaluated periodically for evidence of HPA axis suppression by using the urinary free cortisol and ACTH stimulation tests. If HPA axis suppression is noted, an attempt should be made to withdraw the drug, to reduce the frequency of application, or to substitute a less potent steroid.
Recovery of HPA axis function is generally prompt and complete upon discontinuation of the drug. Infrequently, signs and symptoms of steroid withdrawal may occur, requiring supplemental systemic corticosteroids.
Children may absorb proportionally larger amounts of topical corticosteroids and thus be more susceptible to systemic toxicity (see **PRECAUTIONS: Pediatric Use**).
If irritation develops, topical corticosteroids should be discontinued and appropriate therapy instituted.
In the presence of dermatological infections, the use of an appropriate antifungal or antibacterial agent should be instituted. If a favorable response does not occur promptly, the corticosteroid should be discontinued until the infection has been adequately controlled.

Information for the Patient: Patients using topical corticosteroids should receive the following information and instructions:

1. This medication is to be used as directed by the physician. It is for external use only. Avoid contact with the eyes.
2. Patients should be advised not to use this medication for any disorder other than for which it was prescribed.
3. The treated skin area should not be bandaged or otherwise covered or wrapped as to be occlusive unless directed by the physician.
4. Patients should report any signs of local adverse reactions, especially under occlusive dressing.
5. Parents of pediatric patients should be advised not to use tight-fitting diapers or plastic pants on a child being treated in the diaper area, as these garments may constitute occlusive dressings.

Laboratory Tests: The following tests may be helpful in evaluating the HPA axis suppression:
Urinary free cortisol test
ACTH stimulation test

Carcinogenesis, Mutagenesis and Impairment of Fertility:
Long-term animal studies have not been performed to evaluate the carcinogenic potential or the effect on fertility of topical corticosteroids.
Studies to determine mutagenicity with prednisolone and hydrocortisone have revealed negative results.

Pregnancy: *Teratogenic Effects:* Pregnancy Category C: Corticosteroids are generally teratogenic in laboratory animals when administered systemically at relatively low dosage levels. The more potent corticosteroids have been shown to be teratogenic after dermal application in laboratory animals. There are no adequate and well-controlled studies in pregnant women on teratogenic effects from topically applied corticosteroids. Therefore, topical corticosteroids should be used during pregnancy only if the potential benefit justifies the potential risk to the fetus. Drugs of this class should not be used extensively on pregnant patients, in large amounts, or for prolonged periods of time.

Nursing Mothers: It is not known whether topical administration of corticosteroids could result in sufficient systemic absorption to produce detectable quantities in breast milk. Systemically administered corticosteroids are secreted into breast milk in quantities *not* likely to have a deleterious effect on the infant. Nevertheless, caution should be exercised when topical corticosteroids are administered to a nursing woman.

Pediatric Use: *Pediatric patients may demonstrate greater susceptibility to topical corticosteroid-induced HPA axis suppression and Cushing's syndrome than mature patients because of a larger skin surface area to body weight ratio.*

Hypothalamic-pituitary-adrenal (HPA) axis suppression, Cushing's syndrome, and intracranial hypertension have been reported in children receiving topical corticosteroids. Manifestations of adrenal suppression in children include linear growth retardation, delayed weight gain, low plasma cortisol levels, and absence of response to ACTH stimulation. Manifestations of intracranial hypertension include bulging fontanelles, headaches, and bilateral papilledema.

Administration of topical corticosteroids to children should be limited to the least amount compatible with an effective therapeutic regimen. Chronic corticosteroid therapy may interfere with the growth and development of children.

ADVERSE REACTIONS

The following local adverse reactions are reported infrequently with topical corticosteroids, but may occur more frequently with the use of occlusive dressings. These reactions are listed in an approximate decreasing order of occurrence: burning, itching, irritation, dryness, folliculitis, hypertrichosis, acneiform eruptions, hypopigmentation, perioral dermatitis, allergic contact dermatitis, maceration of the skin, secondary infection, skin atrophy, striae, and miliaria.

OVERDOSAGE

Topically applied corticosteroids can be absorbed in sufficient amounts to produce systemic effects (see **PRECAUTIONS**).

DOSAGE AND ADMINISTRATION

Topical corticosteroids are generally applied to the affected area as a thin film from two to four times daily depending on the severity of the condition. Occlusive dressings may be used for the management of psoriasis or recalcitrant conditions.

If an infection develops, the use of occlusive dressings should be discontinued and appropriate antimicrobial therapy instituted.

HOW SUPPLIED

Cream—2½% Tube 1 OZ NDC 0066-0095-01; 2½% Tube 2 OZ NDC 0066-0095-02

Lotion—2½% bottle 2 FL OZ NDC 0066-0098-02

Caution: Federal law prohibits dispensing without prescription.

Marketed by

Dermik Laboratories, Inc.

A Rhône-Poulenc Rorer Company

Collegeville, PA 19426

Rev. 3/96   IN-7245C

HYTONE®   ℞

[*hī-tōne*]

(hydrocortisone)

Ointment

DESCRIPTION

The topical corticosteroids constitute a class of primarily synthetic steroids used as anti-inflammatory and antipruritic agents. Hytone® 2½% (hydrocortisone ointment, USP) contains Hydrocortisone [Pregn-4-ene-3,20-dione,11,17,21-trihydroxy-,(11β-], with the molecular formula $C_{21}H_{30}O_5$ and a molecular weight of 362.47. CAS 50-23-7. Each gram of the ointment contains 25 mg of hydrocortisone in a base of white petrolatum and mineral oil.

CLINICAL PHARMACOLOGY

Topical corticosteroids share anti-inflammatory, antipruritic, and vasoconstrictive actions.

The mechanism of anti-inflammatory activity of the topical corticosteroids is unclear. Various laboratory methods, including vasoconstrictor assays, are used to compare and predict potencies and/or clinical efficacies of the topical corticosteroids. There is some evidence to suggest that a recognizable correlation exists between vasoconstrictor potency and therapeutic efficacy in man.

Pharmacokinetics: The extent of percutaneous absorption of topical corticosteroids is determined by many factors including the vehicle, the integrity of the epidermal barrier, and the use of occlusive dressings.

Topical corticosteroids can be absorbed from normal intact skin. Inflammation and/or other disease processes in the skin increase percutaneous absorption. Occlusive dressings substantially increase the percutaneous absorption of topical corticosteroids. Thus, occlusive dressings may be a valuable therapeutic adjunct for treatment of resistant dermatoses. (See **DOSAGE AND ADMINISTRATION**.)

Once absorbed through the skin, topical corticosteroids are handled through pharmacokinetic pathways similar to systemically administered corticosteroids. Corticosteroids are bound to plasma proteins in varying degrees. Corticosteroids are metabolized primarily in the liver and are then excreted by the kidneys. Some of the topical corticosteroids and their metabolites are also excreted into the bile.

INDICATIONS AND USAGE

Hydrocortisone ointment is indicated for the relief of the inflammatory and pruritic manifestations of corticosteroid-responsive dermatoses.

CONTRAINDICATIONS

Hydrocortisone ointment is contraindicated in those patients with a history of hypersensitivity to any of the components of this preparation.

PRECAUTIONS

General: Systemic absorption of topical corticosteroids has produced reversible hypothalamic-pituitary-adrenal (HPA) axis suppression, manifestations of Cushing's syndrome, hyperglycemia, and glucosuria in some patients.

Conditions which augment systemic absorption include the application of the more potent steroids, use over large surface areas, prolonged use, and the addition of occlusive dressings.

Therefore, patients receiving a large dose of a potent topical steroid applied to a large surface area or under an occlusive dressing should be evaluated periodically for evidence of HPA axis suppression by using the urinary free cortisol and ACTH stimulation tests. If HPA axis suppression is noted, an attempt should be made to withdraw the drug, to reduce the frequency of application, or to substitute a less potent steroid.

Recovery of HPA axis function is generally prompt and complete upon discontinuation of the drug. Infrequently, signs and symptoms of steroid withdrawal may occur, requiring supplemental systemic corticosteroids.

Children may absorb proportionally larger amounts of topical corticosteroids and thus be more susceptible to systemic toxicity (see **PRECAUTIONS: Pediatric Use**).

If irritation develops, topical corticosteroids should be discontinued and appropriate therapy instituted.

In the presence of dermatological infections, the use of an appropriate antifungal or antibacterial agent should be instituted. If a favorable response does not occur promptly, the corticosteroid should be discontinued until the infection has been adequately controlled.

Information for the Patient: Patients using topical corticosteroids should receive the following information and instructions:

1. This medication is to be used as directed by the physician. It is for external use only. Avoid contact with the eyes.
2. Patients should be advised not to use this medication for any disorder other than for which it was prescribed.
3. The treated skin area should not be bandaged or otherwise covered or wrapped as to be occlusive unless directed by the physician.
4. Patients should report any signs of local adverse reactions, especially under occlusive dressing.
5. Parents of pediatric patients should be advised not to use tight-fitting diapers or plastic pants on a child being treated in the diaper area, as these garments may constitute occlusive dressings.

Laboratory Tests: The following tests may be helpful in evaluating the HPA axis suppression: Urinary free cortisol test; ACTH stimulation test.

Carcinogenesis, Mutagenesis and Impairment of Fertility: Long-term animal studies have not been performed to evaluate the carcinogenic potential or the effect on fertility of topical corticosteroids.

Studies to determine mutagenicity with prednisolone and hydrocortisone have revealed negative results.

Pregnancy: *Teratogenic Effects:* Pregnancy Category C: Corticosteroids are generally teratogenic in laboratory animals when administered systemically at relatively low dosage levels. The more potent corticosteroids have been shown to be teratogenic after dermal application in laboratory animals. There are no adequate and well-controlled studies in pregnant women on teratogenic effects from topically applied corticosteroids. Therefore, topical corticosteroids should be used during pregnancy only if the potential benefit justifies the potential risk to the fetus. Drugs of this class should not be used extensively on pregnant patients, in large amounts, or for prolonged periods of time.

Nursing Mothers: It is not known whether topical administration of corticosteroids could result in sufficient systemic absorption to produce detectable quantities in breast milk. Systemically administered corticosteroids are secreted into breast milk in quantities *not* likely to have a deleterious effect on the infant. Nevertheless, caution should be exercised when topical corticosteroids are administered to a nursing woman.

Pediatric Use: *Pediatric patients may demonstrate greater susceptibility to topical corticosteroid-induced hypothalamic-pituitary-adrenal (HPA) axis suppression and Cushing's syndrome than mature patients because of a larger skin surface area to body weight ratio.*

Hypothalamic-pituitary-adrenal (HPA) axis suppression, Cushing's syndrome, and intracranial hypertension have been reported in children receiving topical corticosteroids. Manifestations of adrenal suppression in children include linear growth retardation, delayed weight gain, low plasma cortisol levels, and absence of response to ACTH stimulation. Manifestations of intracranial hypertension include bulging fontanelles, headaches, and bilateral papilledema.

Administration of topical corticosteroids to children should be limited to the least amount compatible with an effective therapeutic regimen. Chronic corticosteroid therapy may interfere with the growth and development of children.

ADVERSE REACTIONS

The following local adverse reactions are reported infrequently with topical corticosteroids, but may occur more frequently with the use of occlusive dressings. These reactions are listed in an approximate decreasing order of occurrence: burning, itching, irritation, dryness, folliculitis, hypertrichosis, acneiform eruptions, hypopigmentation, perioral dermatitis, allergic contact dermatitis, maceration of the skin, secondary infection, skin atrophy, striae and miliaria.

OVERDOSAGE

Topically applied corticosteroids can be absorbed in sufficient amounts to produce systemic effects (see PRECAUTIONS).

DOSAGE AND ADMINISTRATION

Apply to the affected area as a thin film from 2 to 4 times daily depending on the severity of the condition.

Occlusive dressings may be used for the management of psoriasis or recalcitrant conditions. If an infection develops, the use of occlusive dressings should be discontinued and appropriate antimicrobial therapy instituted.

HOW SUPPLIED

Hytone® 2½% (hydrocortisone ointment, USP) in 1 oz (28.35 g) tubes, NDC 0066-9997-01.

Store at controlled room temperature 15°-30°C (59°-86°F).

Caution: Federal law prohibits dispensing without prescription.

Marketed by

Dermik Laboratories, Inc.

A Rhône-Poulenc Rorer Company

Collegeville, PA 19426

Rev. 3/96   IN-5609

PSORCON®   ℞

[*sŏr-kon*]

brand of diflorasone diacetate ointment

0.05%

Not For Ophthalmic Use

PRODUCT OVERVIEW

KEY FACTS

Psorcon® is a potent (Class I) topical corticosteroid containing 0.05% diflorasone diacetate in an optimized base.

MAJOR USES

Psorcon® is indicated for the relief of the inflammatory and pruritic manifestations of corticosteroid-responsive dermatoses.

SAFETY INFORMATION

Psorcon® is contraindicated in patients with a history of hypersensitivity to any of its components. Systemic absorption of topical corticosteroids has produced reversible HPA axis suppression. Therefore, patients receiving a large dose applied to a large area or under an occlusive dressing should be evaluated periodically. The most common adverse reactions are burning, itching, irritation, and dryness.

PRESCRIBING INFORMATION

PSORCON®   ℞

[*sŏr-kon*]

brand of diflorasone diacetate ointment

0.05%

Not For Ophthalmic Use

Continued on next page

Dermik Laboratories—Cont.

DESCRIPTION

Each gram of **psorcon** Ointment contains 0.5 mg diflorasone diacetate in an ointment base.

Chemically, diflorasone diacetate is 6α, 9α-difluoro-11β, 17, 21-trihydroxy-16β-methylpregna-1, 4-diene-3, 20-dione 17,21 diacetate.

Each gram of **psorcon** Ointment contains 0.5 mg diflorasone diacetate in an ointment base of propylene glycol, glyceryl monostearate and white petrolatum.

CLINICAL PHARMACOLOGY

Topical corticosteroids share anti-inflammatory, antipruritic and vasoconstrictive actions.

The mechanism of anti-inflammatory activity of the topical corticosteroids is unclear. Various laboratory methods, including vasoconstrictor assays, are used to compare and predict potencies and/or clinical efficacies of the topical corticosteroids. There is some evidence to suggest that a recognizable correlation exists between vasoconstrictor potency and therapeutic efficacy in man.

Pharmacokinetics

The extent of percutaneous absorption of topical corticosteroids is determined by many factors including the vehicle, the integrity of the epidermal barrier, and the use of occlusive dressings.

Topical corticosteroids can be absorbed from normal intact skin. Inflammation and/or other disease processes in the skin increase percutaneous absorption. Occlusive dressings substantially increase the percutaneous absorption of topical corticosteroids. Thus, occlusive dressings may be a valuable therapeutic adjunct for treatment of resistant dermatoses. (See DOSAGE AND ADMINISTRATION.)

Once absorbed through the skin, topical corticosteroids are handled through pharmacokinetic pathways similar to systemically administered corticosteroids. Corticosteroids are bound to plasma proteins in varying degrees. They are metabolized primarily in the liver and are then excreted by the kidneys. Some of the topical corticosteroids and their metabolites are also excreted into the bile.

INDICATIONS AND USAGE

Topical corticosteroids are indicated for relief of the inflammatory and pruritic manifestations of corticosteroid-responsive dermatoses.

CONTRAINDICATIONS

Topical steroids are contraindicated in those patients with a history of hypersensitivity to any of the components of the preparation.

PRECAUTIONS

General

Systemic absorption of topical corticosteroids has produced reversible hypothalamic-pituitary-adrenal (HPA) axis suppression, manifestations of Cushing's syndrome, hyperglycemia, and glucosuria in some patients.

Conditions which augment systemic absorption include the application of the more potent steroids, use over large surface areas, prolonged use, and the addition of occlusive dressings.

Therefore, patients receiving a large dose of a potent topical steroid applied to a large surface area or under an occlusive dressing should be evaluated periodically for evidence of HPA axis suppression by using the urinary free cortisol and ACTH stimulation tests. If HPA axis suppression is noted, an attempt should be made to withdraw the drug, to reduce the frequency of application, or to substitute a less potent steroid.

Recovery of HPA axis function is generally prompt and complete upon discontinuation of the drug. Infrequently, signs and symptoms of steroid withdrawal may occur, requiring supplemental systemic corticosteroids.

Children may absorb proportionally larger amounts of topical corticosteroids and thus be more susceptible to systemic toxicity. (See PRECAUTIONS—Pediatric Use.)

If irritation develops, topical corticosteroids should be discontinued and appropriate therapy instituted.

In the presence of dermatological infections, the use of an appropriate antifungal or antibacterial agent should be instituted. If a favorable response does not occur promptly, the corticosteroid should be discontinued until the infection has been adequately controlled.

Information for the Patient

Patients using topical corticosteroids should receive the following information and instructions:

1. This medication is to be used as directed by the physician. It is for external use only. Avoid contact with the eyes.
2. Patients should be advised not to use this medication for any disorder other than for which it was prescribed.
3. The treated skin area should not be bandaged or otherwise covered or wrapped as to be occlusive unless directed by the physician.
4. Patients should report any signs of local adverse reactions especially under occlusive dressing.
5. Parents of pediatric patients should be advised not to use tight-fitting diapers or plastic pants on a child being treated in the diaper area, as these garments may constitute occlusive dressings.

Laboratory Tests

The following tests may be helpful in evaluating the HPA axis suppression:

Urinary free cortisol test
ACTH stimulation test

Carcinogenesis, Mutagenesis, and Impairment of Fertility

Long-term animal studies have not been performed to evaluate the carcinogenic potential or the effect on fertility of topical corticosteroids.

Studies to determine mutagenicity with prednisolone and hydrocortisone have revealed negative results.

Pregnancy Category C

Corticosteroids are generally teratogenic in laboratory animals when administered systemically at relatively low dosage levels. The more potent corticosteroids have been shown to be teratogenic after dermal application in laboratory animals. There are no adequate and well-controlled studies in pregnant women on teratogenic effects from topically applied corticosteroids. Therefore, topical corticosteroids should be used during pregnancy only if the potential benefit justifies the potential risk to the fetus.

Nursing Mothers

It is not known whether topical administration of corticosteroids could result in sufficient systemic absorption to produce detectable quantities in breast milk. Systemically administered corticosteroids are secreted into breast milk in quantities **not** likely to have a deleterious effect on the infant. Nevertheless, caution should be exercised when topical corticosteroids are administered to a nursing woman.

Pediatric Use

Pediatric patients may demonstrate greater susceptibility to topical corticosteroid-induced HPA axis suppression and Cushing's syndrome than mature patients because of a large skin surface area to body weight ratio.

Hypothalamic-pituitary-adrenal (HPA) axis suppression, Cushing's syndrome, and intracranial hypertension have been reported in children receiving topical corticosteroids. Manifestations of adrenal suppression in children include linear growth retardation, delayed weight gain, low plasma cortisol levels, and absence of response to ACTH stimulation. Manifestations of intracranial hypertension include bulging fontanelles, headaches, and bilateral papilledema.

Administration of topical corticosteroids to children should be limited to the least amount compatible with an effective therapeutic regimen. Chronic corticosteroid therapy may interfere with the growth and development of children.

ADVERSE REACTIONS

The following local adverse reactions have been reported with topical corticosteroids, but may occur more frequently with the use of occlusive dressings. These reactions are listed in approximate decreasing order of occurrence.

1. Burning
2. Itching
3. Irritation
4. Dryness
5. Folliculitis
6. Hypertrichosis
7. Acneiform eruptions
8. Hypopigmentation
9. Perioral dermatitis
10. Allergic contact dermatitis
11. Maceration of the skin
12. Secondary infection
13. Skin atrophy
14. Striae
15. Miliaria

OVERDOSAGE

Topically applied corticosteroids can be absorbed in sufficient amounts to produce systemic effects. (See PRECAUTIONS.)

DOSAGE AND ADMINISTRATION

psorcon Ointment should be applied to the affected area as a thin film from one to three times daily depending on the severity or resistant nature of the condition.

Occlusive dressings may be used for the management of psoriasis or recalcitrant conditions.

If an infection develops, the use of occlusive dressings should be discontinued and appropriate antimicrobial therapy initiated.

HOW SUPPLIED

psorcon Ointment 0.05% is available in the following size tubes:

15 gram	NDC 0066-0071-17
30 gram	NDC 0066-0071-31
60 gram	NDC 0066-0071-60

Store at controlled room temperature 15°-30°C (59°-80°F).

DERMIK LABORATORIES, INC.
Dedicated to Dermatology™
A RHÔNE-POULENC RORER COMPANY
IN-7191G

PSORCON® (diflorasone diacetate) Cream 0.05% ℞

Caution: Federal law prohibits dispensing without prescription.

For Dermatological Use Only—Not for Ophthalmic Use.

DESCRIPTION

psorcon (diflorasone diacetate) Cream contains the active compound diflorasone diacetate, a synthetic corticosteroid for topical dermatological use.

Chemically, diflorasone diacetate is 6α, 9α-difluoro-11B, 17, 21-trihydroxy-16-methylpregna-1, 4-diene-3, 20-dione 17, 21 diacetate.

Each gram of **psorcon** Cream contains 0.5 mg diflorasone diacetate in a cream base consisting of purified water, propylene glycol, mineral oil (and) lanolin alcohol, glyceryl stearate SE (nonionic), isopropyl myristate, polysorbate 60, sorbitan monostearate, polyoxyl 40 stearate, cetyl alcohol, monobasic sodium phosphate, vegetable oil, monoglyceride citrate, BHT and citric acid.

CLINICAL PHARMACOLOGY

Like other topical corticosteroids, diflorasone diacetate has anti-inflammatory, anti-pruritic, and vasoconstrictive actions. The mechanism of the anti-inflammatory activity of the topical corticosteroids, in general, is unclear. However, corticosteroids are thought to act by the induction of phospholipase A_2 inhibitory proteins collectively called lipocortins. It is postulated that these proteins control the biosynthesis of potent mediators of inflammation such as prostaglandins and leukotrienes by inhibiting the release of their common precursor, arachidonic acid. Arachidonic acid is released from membrane phospholipids A_2

Pharmacokinetics: The extent of percutaneous absorption of topical corticosteroids is determined by many factors including the vehicle and the integrity of the epidermal barrier. Occlusive dressings with hydrocortisone for up to 24 hours have not been demonstrated to increase penetration; however, occlusion of hydrocortisone for 96 hours markedly enhances penetration. Topical corticosteroids can be absorbed from normal intact skin. Inflammation and/or other disease processes in the skin may increase percutaneous absorption. Studies performed with **psorcon** Cream indicate that it is in the high range of potency as compared with other topical corticosteroids.

INDICATION AND USAGE

psorcon (diflorasone diacetate) Cream, 0.05% is a high potency corticosteroid indicated for the relief of the inflammatory and pruritic manifestations of corticosteroid-responsive dermatoses.

CONTRAINDICATIONS

psorcon (diflorasone diacetate) Cream is contraindicated in those patients with a history of hypersensitivity to any of the components of the preparation.

PRECAUTIONS

General: Systemic absorption of topical corticosteroids can produce reversible hypothalamic-pituitary-adrenal (HPA) axis suppression with the potential for glucocorticosteroid insufficiency after withdrawal of treatment. Manifestations of Cushing's syndrome, hyperglycemia, and glucosuria can also be produced in some patients by systemic absorption of topical corticosteroids while on treatment.

Patients receiving a large dose of a higher potency topical steroid applied to a large surface area or under an occlusive dressing should be evaluated periodically for evidence of HPA axis suppression. This may be done by using the ACTH-stimulation, A.M. plasma cortisol, and urinary-free cortisol tests.

This product has a greater ability to produce adrenal suppression than does **psorcon** (diflorasone diacetate) Ointment, 0.05%. At 30 g per day (applied as 15 g twice daily) **psorcon** Cream, 0.05% was shown to cause inhibition of the HPA axis in one of two patients following application for one week to psoriatic skin. At 15 g per day (applied as 7.5 g twice daily) **psorcon** Cream was shown to cause mild inhibition of the HPA axis in one of five patients following application for one week to diseased skin (psoriasis or atopic dermatitis). These effects were reversible upon discontinuation of treatment. By comparison, **psorcon** (diflorasone diacetate) Ointment, 0.05% did not produce significant HPA axis suppression when used in divided doses at 30 g per day for one week in patients with psoriasis or atopic dermatitis.

If HPA axis suppression is noted, an attempt should be made to withdraw the drug, to reduce the frequency of application, or to substitute a less potent corticosteroid. Recovery of HPA axis function is generally prompt and complete upon discontinuation of topical corticosteroids. Infrequently, signs and

symptoms of glucocorticosteroid insufficiency may occur, requiring supplemental systemic corticosteroids. For information on systemic supplementation, see prescribing information for those products.

Children may be more susceptible to systemic toxicity from equivalent doses due to their larger skin surface to body mass ratios (See PRECAUTIONS: Pediatric Use).

If irritation develops, **psorcon** (diflorasone diacetate) Cream should be discontinued and appropriate therapy instituted. Allergic contact dermatitis with corticosteroids is usually diagnosed by observing failure to heal rather than noting a clinical exacerbation as with most topical products not containing corticosteroids. Such an observation should be corroborated with appropriate diagnostic patch testing.

If concomitant skin infections are present or develop, an appropriate antifungal or antibacterial agent should be used. If a favorable response does not occur promptly, use of **psorcon** (diflorasone diacetate) Cream should be discontinued until the infection has been adequately controlled.

psorcon (diflorasone diacetate) Cream should not be used in the treatment of rosacea or perioral dermatitis, and it should not be used on the face, groin, or axillae.

Information for Patients: Patients using topical corticosteroids should receive the following information and instructions:

1. The medication is to be used as directed by the physician. It is for external use only. Avoid contact with the eyes.
2. The medication should not be used for any disorder other than that for which it was prescribed.
3. The treated skin area should not be bandaged or otherwise covered or wrapped so as to be occlusive unless directed by the physician.
4. Patients should report to their physician any signs of local adverse reactions.

Laboratory Tests The following tests may be helpful in evaluating patients for HPA axis suppression: ACTH-stimulation test; A.M. plasma-cortisol test; Urinary-free cortisol test.

Carcinogenesis, Mutagenesis and Impairment of Fertility: Long-term animal studies have not been performed to evaluate the carcinogenic potential of diflorasone diacetate.

Diflorasone diacetate was not found to be mutagenic in a micronucleus test in rats at dosages of 2400 mg/kg.

Studies in the rat following topical administration at doses up to 0.5 mg/kg revealed no effects on fertility.

Pregnancy: Teratogenic effects. Pregnancy Category C. Corticosteroids have been shown to be teratogenic in laboratory animals when administered systemically at relatively low dosage levels. Some corticosteroids have been shown to be teratogenic after dermal application to laboratory animals.

Diflorasone diacetate has been shown to be teratogenic (cleft palate) in rats when applied topically at a dose of approximately 0.001 mg/kg/day to the shaven thorax of pregnant animals. This is approximately 0.3 times the human topical dose of **psorcon** (diflorasone diacetate) Cream. When pregnant rats were treated topically with approximately 0.5 mg/kg/day, uterine deaths were higher in the treated animals than in control animals.

In rabbits, cleft palate was seen when diflorasone diacetate was applied in topical doses as low as 20 mg/kg/day. In addition, fetal weight was depressed and litter sizes were smaller. There are no adequate and well-controlled studies of the teratogenic potential of diflorasone diacetate in pregnant women. **psorcon** Cream should be used during pregnancy only if the potential benefit justifies the potential risk to the fetus.

Nursing Mothers: Systemically administered corticosteroids appear in human milk and could suppress growth, interfere with endogenous corticosteroid production, or cause other untoward effects. It is not known whether topical administration of corticosteroids could result in sufficient systemic absorption to produce detectable quantities in human milk. Because many drugs are excreted in human milk, caution should be exercised when **psorcon** (diflorasone diacetate) Cream is administered to a nursing woman.

Pediatric Use: Safety and effectiveness of **psorcon** (diflorasone diacetate) Cream in children have not been established. Because of a higher ratio of skin surface area to body mass, children are at a greater risk than adults of HPA-axis suppression when they are treated with topical corticosteroids. They are, therefore, also at greater risk of glucocorticosteroid insufficiency after withdrawal of treatment and of Cushing's syndrome while on treatment. Adverse effects including striae have been reported with inappropriate use of topical corticosteroids in infants and children.

HPA axis suppression, Cushing's syndrome, and intracranial hypertension have been reported in children receiving topical corticosteroids. Manifestations of adrenal suppression in children include linear growth retardation, delayed weight gain, low plasma cortisol levels, and absence of response to ACTH stimulation. Manifestations of intracranial hypertension include bulging fontanelles, headaches, and bilateral papilledema.

ADVERSE REACTIONS

The following local adverse reactions have been reported infrequently with other topical corticosteroids, and they may occur more frequently with the use of occlusive dressings, especially with higher potency corticosteroids. These reactions are listed in an approximate decreasing order of occurrence: burning, itching, irritation, dryness, folliculitis, acneiform eruptions, hypopigmentation, perioral dermatitis, allergic contact dermatitis, secondary infections, skin atrophy, striae, and miliaria.

OVERDOSAGE

Topically applied **psorcon** (diflorasone diacetate) Cream can be absorbed in sufficient amounts to produce systemic effects (see PRECAUTIONS).

DOSAGE AND ADMINISTRATION

psorcon (diflorasone diacetate) Cream should be applied to the affected area twice daily.

HOW SUPPLIED

psorcon Cream 0.05% is available in the following size tubes:
15 gram NDC 0066-0069-17
30 gram NDC 0066-0069-31
60 gram NDC 0066-0069-60

Store at or below 25°C (77°F).

DERMIK LABORATORIES, INC.
Dedicated to Dermatology™
A RHÔNE-POULENC RORER COMPANY
IN-1193B

SULFACET-R® Lotion ℞

[*sul-fa-set*]
(sodium sulfacetamide 10% and sulfur 5%)

PRODUCT OVERVIEW

KEY FACTS

Sulfacet-R® contains sodium sulfacetamide 10% and sulfur 5% in a flesh-tinted lotion. Sodium sulfacetamide is an antibacterial, while sulfur acts as a keratolytic agent.

MAJOR USES

Sulfacet-R® is indicated in the topical control of acne rosacea, acne vulgaris, & seborrheic dermatitis.

SAFETY INFORMATION

Sulfacet-R® is contraindicated in patients with a known hypersensitivity to sulfonamides, sulfur, or any other of its ingredients. It should not be used in patients with kidney disease. Although rare, sensitivity to sodium sulfacetamide may occur. It contains sodium bisulfite which may cause allergic-type reactions. Sulfacet-R® may cause local irritation. If irritation develops, discontinue use of the product.

PRESCRIBING INFORMATION

SULFACET-R® Lotion
[*sul-fa-set*]
(sodium sulfacetamide 10% and sulfur 5%)

DESCRIPTION

Each mL of **Sulfacet-R® Lotion** (sodium sulfacetamide 10% and sulfur 5%) as dispensed contains 100 mg of sodium sulfacetamide and 50 mg of sulfur in a tinted lotion of 2–bromo-2-nitropropane-1, 3 diol, attapulgite, butylparaben, hydroxyethyl cellulose, iron oxides, lauramide DEA (and) diethanolamine, methylparaben, polyethylene glycol 400 monolaurate, propylene glycol, purified water, silicone emulsion, sodium chloride, sodium metabisulfite, sodium polynaphthalenesulfonate, talc, titanium dioxide, xanthan gum, and zinc oxide.

Sodium sulfacetamide is a sulfonamide with antibacterial activity while sulfur acts as a keratolytic agent. Chemically sodium sulfacetamide is N'-[(4-aminophenyl) sulfonyl]-acetamide, monosodium salt, monohydrate.

CLINICAL PHARMACOLOGY

The most widely accepted mechanism of action of sulfonamides is the Woods-Fildes theory which is based on the fact that sulfonamides act as competitive antagonists to para-aminobenzoic acid (PABA), an essential component for bacterial growth. While absorption through intact skin has not been determined, sodium sulfacetamide is readily absorbed from the gastrointestinal tract when taken orally and excreted in the urine, largely unchanged. The biological half-life has variously been reported as 7 to 12.8 hours.

The exact mode of action of sulfur in the treatment of acne is unknown, but it has been reported that it inhibits the growth of *p. acnes* and the formation of free fatty acids.

INDICATIONS

Sulfacet-R Lotion is indicated in the topical control of acne vulgaris, acne rosacea and seborrheic dermatitis.

CONTRAINDICATIONS

Sulfacet-R Lotion is contraindicated for use by patients having known hypersensitivity to sulfonamides, sulfur, or any other component of this preparation. **Sulfacet-R Lotion** is not to be used by patients with kidney disease.

WARNINGS

Although rare, sensitivity to sodium sulfacetamide may occur. Therefore, caution and careful supervision should be observed when prescribing this drug for patients who may be prone to hypersensitivity to topical sulfonamides. Systemic toxic reactions such as agranulocytosis, acute hemolytic anemia, purpura hemorrhagica, drug fever, jaundice, and contact dermatitis indicate hypersensitivity to sulfonamides. Particular caution should be employed if areas of denuded or abraded skin are involved.

Contains sodium metabisulfite, a sulfite that may cause allergic-type reactions including anaphylactic symptoms and life-threatening or less severe asthmatic episodes in certain susceptible people. The overall prevalence of sulfite sensitivity in the general population is unknown and probably low. Sulfite sensitivity is seen more frequently in asthmatic than in nonasthmatic people.

PRECAUTIONS

General — If irritation develops, use of the product should be discontinued and appropriate therapy instituted. For external use only. Keep away from eyes. Patients should be carefully observed for possible local irritation or sensitization during long-term therapy. The object of this therapy is to achieve desquamation without irritation, but sodium sulfacetamide and sulfur can cause reddening and scaling of epidermis. These side effects are not unusual in the treatment of acne vulgaris, but patients should be cautioned about the possibility.

Keep out of the reach of children.

Carcinogenesis, Mutagenesis and Impairment of Fertility — Long-term studies in animals have not been performed to evaluate carcinogenic potential.

Pregnancy — Category C. Animal reproduction studies have not been conducted with **Sulfacet-R Lotion**. It is also not known whether **Sulfacet-R Lotion** can cause fetal harm when administered to a pregnant woman or can affect reproduction capacity. **Sulfacet-R Lotion** should be given to a pregnant woman only if clearly needed.

Nursing Mothers — It is not known whether sodium sulfacetamide is excreted in the human milk following topical use of **Sulfacet-R Lotion**. However, small amounts of orally administered sulfonamides have been reported to be eliminated in human milk. In view of this and because many drugs are excreted in human milk, caution should be exercised when **Sulfacet-R Lotion** is administered to a nursing woman.

Pediatric Use — Safety and effectiveness in children under the age of 12 have not been established.

ADVERSE REACTIONS

Although rare, sodium sulfacetamide may cause local irritation.

DOSAGE AND ADMINISTRATION

Shake well before using. Apply a thin film to affected areas with light massaging to blend in each application 1 to 3 times daily. Each package contains a **Dermik Color Blender™** which enables the patient to alter the basic shade of the lotion so that it matches the skin color exactly.

(Important to the Pharmacist — At the time of dispensing, add contents of Sulfa-Pak™ vial* to the bottle. Shake well and/or stir with a glass rod to ensure uniform dispersion. Place expiration date of four (4) months on bottle label.)

*Sulfa-Pak™ vial contains 2.1 g of sodium sulfacetamide.

HOW SUPPLIED

25 g bottles (NDC 0066-0028-25).

CAUTION — Federal law prohibits dispensing without prescription.

Marketed by
Dermik Laboratories, Inc.,A Rhône-Poulenc Rorer Company, Collegeville, PA, U.S.A. 19426
Rev. 4/96 IN-5125L

SULFACET-R® TINT FREE LOTION ℞

[*sul-fă-set*]
(Sodium Sulfacetamide 10% and Sulfur 5%)

DESCRIPTION

Each mL of **Sulfacet-R® Tint Free Lotion** (sodium sulfacetamide 10% and sulfur 5%) as dispensed contains 100 mg of sodium sulfacetamide and 50 mg of sulfur in a lotion of 2-bromo-2-nitropropane-1, 3 diol, attapulgite, butylparaben, hydroxyethyl cellulose, iron oxides, lauramide DEA (and) diethanolamine, methylparaben, polyethylene glycol 400 monolaurate, propylene glycol, purified water, silicone emulsion, sodium chloride, sodium metabisulfite, sodium polynaphthalenesulfonate, talc, xanthan gum, and zinc oxide.

Continued on next page

Dermik Laboratories—Cont.

Sodium sulfacetamide is a sulfonamide with antibacterial activity while sulfur acts as a keratolytic agent.
Chemically sodium sulfacetamide is N' -[(4-aminophenyl)sulfonyl]-acetamide, monosodium salt, monohydrate.

CLINICAL PHARMACOLOGY

The most widely accepted mechanism of action of sulfonamides is the Woods-Fildes theory which is based on the fact that sulfonamides act as competitive antagonists to para-aminobenzoic acid (PABA), an essential component for bacterial growth. While absorption through intact skin has not been determined, sodium sulfacetamide is readily absorbed from the gastrointestinal tract when taken orally and excreted in the urine, largely unchanged. The biological half-life has variously been reported as 7 to 12.8 hours. The exact mode of action of sulfur in the treatment of acne is unknown, but it has been reported that it inhibits the growth of *p. acnes* and the formation of free fatty acids.

INDICATIONS

Sulfacet-R® Tint Free Lotion is indicated in the topical control of acne vulgaris, acne rosacea and seborrheic dermatitis.

CONTRAINDICATIONS

Sulfacet-R Tint Free Lotion is contraindicated for use by patients having known hypersensitivity to sulfonamides, sulfur, or any other component of this preparation. **Sulfacet-R Tint Free Lotion** is not to be used by patients with kidney disease.

WARNINGS

Although rare, sensitivity to sodium sulfacetamide may occur. Therefore, caution and careful supervision should be observed when prescribing this drug for patients who may be prone to hypersensitivity to topical sulfonamides. Systemic toxic reactions such as agranulocytosis, acute hemolytic anemia, purpura hemorrhagica, drug fever, jaundice, and contact dermatitis indicate hypersensitivity to sulfonamides. Particular caution should be employed if areas of denuded or abraded skin are involved.
Contains sodium bisulfite, a sulfite that may cause allergic-type reactions including anaphylactic symptoms and life-threatening or less severe asthmatic episodes in certain susceptible people. The overall prevalence of sulfite sensitivity in the general population is unknown and probably low. Sulfite sensitivity is seen more frequently in asthmatic than in nonasthmatic people.

PRECAUTIONS

General — If irritation develops, use of the product should be discontinued and appropriate therapy instituted. For external use only. Keep away from eyes. Patients should be carefully observed for possible local irritation or sensitization during long-term therapy. The object of this therapy is to achieve desquamation without irritation, but sodium sulfacetamide and sulfur can cause reddening and scaling of epidermis. These side effects are not unusual in the treatment of acne vulgaris, but patients should be cautioned about the possibility.
Keep out of the reach of children.
Carcinogenesis, Mutagenesis and Impairment of Fertility — Long-term studies in animals have not been performed to evaluate carcinogenic potential.
Pregnancy — Category C. Animal reproduction studies have not been conducted with **Sulfacet-R Tint Free Lotion**. It is also not known whether **Sulfacet-R Tint Free Lotion** can cause fetal harm when administered to a pregnant woman or can affect reproduction capacity. **Sulfacet-R Tint Free Lotion** should be given to a pregnant woman only if clearly needed.
Nursing Mothers — It is not known whether sodium sulfacetamide is excreted in the human milk following topical use of **Sulfacet-R Tint Free Lotion**. However, small amounts of orally administered sulfonamides have been reported to be eliminated in human milk. In view of this and because many drugs are excreted in human milk, caution should be exercised when **Sulfacet-R Tint Free Lotion** is administered to a nursing woman.
Pediatric Use — Safety and effectiveness in children under the age of 12 have not been established.

ADVERSE REACTIONS

Although rare, sodium sulfacetamide may cause local irritation.

DOSAGE AND ADMINISTRATION

Shake well before using. Apply a thin film to affected areas with light massaging, 1 to 3 times daily.
(**Important to the Pharmacist** — At the time of dispensing, add contents of vial* to the bottle. Shake well and/or stir with a glass rod to insure uniform dispersion. Place expiration date of four (4) months on bottle label.)
*Sulfa-Pak™ vial contains 2.1 g of sodium sulfacetamide.

HOW SUPPLIED

25 g bottles (NDC 0066-9028-25).
CAUTION — Federal law prohibits dispensing without prescription.
Dermik Laboratories, Inc.
A Rhône-Poulenc Rorer Company
Collegeville, PA, U.S.A. 19426
CR-5380   Rev. 5/95

VYTONE® CREAM   ℞
[vī-tone]
(hydrocortisone-iodoquinol)

DESCRIPTION

Each gram of Vytone® Cream 1% contains 10 mg of hydrocortisone, and 10 mg of iodoquinol in a greaseless base of purified water, propylene glycol, glyceryl monostearate SE, cholesterol and related sterols, isopropyl myristate, polysorbate 60, cetyl alcohol, sorbitan monostearate, polyoxyl 40 stearate, sorbic acid, and polysorbate 20.
Chemically, hydrocortisone is 11, 17, 21-trihydroxypregn-4-ene-3, 20-dione and iodoquinol, 5,7-diiodo-8-quinolinol. Hydrocortisone is an anti-inflammatory and antipruritic agent, while iodoquinol is an antifungal and antibacterial agent.

HOW SUPPLIED

1%-Tube 1 oz NDC 0066-0051-01

ZETAR® EMULSION (Coal Tar)   ℞
[zē-tar]

DESCRIPTION

Zetar® Emulsion, coal tar, is a liquid for topical application, following dilution in aqueous media. Each ml contains 300 mg whole coal tar in polysorbates. It is a topical anti-eczematic. The complete chemical composition of coal tar has not been ascertained; components are grouped into six categories: aromatic hydrocarbons, acidic phenolic compounds, cyclic nitrogen compounds, organic sulfur compounds, non-acidic phenolics and nonbasic nitrogen compounds.

HOW SUPPLIED

Zetar® Emulsion (coal tar) is available in 6 fl oz (177 ml) plastic bottles. The strength of the preparation is 300 mg coal tar/mL.

Dey Laboratories
2751 NAPA VALLEY CORPORATE DRIVE
NAPA, CA 94558

Direct Inquiries to:
Russ Johnston
(800) 755-5560
FAX: (707) 224-8918

For Medical Information Contact:
In Emergencies:
Allan Kaplan
(707) 224-3200
FAX: (707) 224-3235

Brand Name or Generic Name	Concentration Or Size	NDC or Product #
Mucosil™-10 (℞)	Acetylcysteine Solution 10%	
	Twelve 4 mL Vials	49502-181-04
	Three 10 mL Vials	49502-181-10
	Three 30 mL Vials	49502-181-30
Mucosil™-20 (℞)	Acetylcysteine Solution 20%	
	Twelve 4 mL Vials	49502-182-04
	Three 10 mL Vials	49502-182-10
	Three 30 mL Vials	49502-182-30
	One 100 mL Vial	49502-182-00
Albuterol Inhalation Aerosol ℞	One 17 g Inhaler 200 Metered Inhalations	49502-303-17
Albuterol Sulfate Inhalation Solution ℞	Twenty-Five 3 mL Vials 0.083% (expressed as Albuterol)	49502-697-03
	Sixty 3 mL Vials 0.083% (expressed as Albuterol)	49502-697-60

Shown in Product Identification Section, page 310

Albuterol Sulfate Inhalation Solution 0.5% ℞	One 20 mL Concentrate	49502-196-20
Albuterol Sulfate Syrup ℞	One 16 Fl Oz (1 pint) 2 mg/5mL	49502-795-16
Cromolyn Sodium Inhalation Solution USP (℞)	Sixty 2 mL Vials 20 mg/2mL	49502-689-02
	One Hundred Twenty 2 mL Vials 20 mg/2mL	49502-689-12

Shown in Product Identification Section, page 310

Isoetharine Inhalation Solution USP (℞)	Twenty-five 3 mL Vials 0.08%	49502-661-03
	Twenty-five 5 mL Vials 0.10%	49502-664-05
	Twenty-five 3 mL Vials 0.17%	49502-660-03
	Twenty-two 2 mL Vials 0.25%	49502-659-02
Metaproterenol Sulfate Inhalation Solution USP (℞)	Twenty-five 2.5 mL Vials 0.4%	49502-678-03
	Twenty-five 2.5 mL Vials 0.6%	49502-676-03

Shown in Product Identification Section, page 310

Dey Vial® (OTC)	Sodium Chloride Solutions	
	Two Hundred Fifty 3 mL Vials 0.9%	49502-030-03
	Two Hundred Fifty 5 mL Vials 0.9%	49502-030-05
	One Hundred Twenty-five 10 mL Vials 0.9%	49502-030-10
	One Hundred 20 mL Vials 0.9%	49502-030-20
Sodium Chloride Inhalation Solution, USP (OTC)	One Hundred 3 mL Vials 0.45%	49502-820-03
	One Hundred 5 mL Vials 0.45%	49502-820-05
	One Hundred 3 mL Vials 0.9%	49502-830-03
	One Hundred 5 mL Vials 0.9%	49502-830-05
	Twenty Four 15 mL Vials 0.9%	49502-830-15
(℞)	Fifty 15 mL Vials 3%	49502-640-15
	Fifty 15 mL Vials 10%	49502-641-15
Sterile Water For Inhalation USP (OTC)	One Hundred 3 mL Vials	49502-810-03
	One Hundred 5 mL Vials	49502-810-05

Dista Products and Eli Lilly and Company
LILLY CORPORATE CENTER
INDIANAPOLIS, IN 46285

Direct Inquiries to:
Dista Products and Eli Lilly and Company
Lilly Corporate Center
Indianapolis, IN 46285
(317) 276-4000

For Medical Information Contact:
Lilly Research Laboratories
Lilly Corporate Center
Indianapolis, IN 46285
(800) 545-5979

LEGEND

Identi-Code®—*Formula Identification Code, Dista*
Identi-Dose®—*Unit Dose Medication, Dista*
Pulvules®—*Filled Gelatin Capsules, Dista*
℞Pak—*Prescription Package, Dista*

IDENTI-CODE® Index
(formula identification code, Dista)
Provides Positive Product Identification

A letter-number symbol, a 4-digit number, the name of the product, the strength of the product, or a combination of these appears on each Dista capsule and tablet and on each

label of pediatric liquids and powders for oral suspension. The letter/number or 4-digit number identifies the product.

Identi-
Code® Product Name

Coated   **Tablets**

Pulvules®

3104 Prozac®
Composition (Each Pulvule®): fluoxetine hydrochloride, 10 mg (equiv. to fluoxetine)

3105 Prozac®
Composition (Each Pulvule®): fluoxetine hydrochloride, 20 mg (equiv. to fluoxetine)

3123 Co-Pyronil 2®
Composition (Each Pulvule®): chlorpheniramine maleate, 4 mg; pseudoephedrine hydrochloride, 60 mg

H09 Ilosone®
Composition (Each Pulvule®): Erythromycin Estolate, USP, 250 mg (equiv. to erythromycin)

H69 Keflex®
Composition (Each Pulvule®): Cephalexin, USP, 250 mg

H71 Keflex®
Composition (Each Pulvule®): Cephalexin, USP, 500 mg

H76 Nalfon® 200
Composition (Each Pulvule®): Fenoprofen Calcium, USP, 200 mg (equiv. to fenoprofen)

H77 Nalfon®
Composition (Each Pulvule®): Fenoprofen Calcium, USP, 300 mg (equiv. to fenoprofen)

Compressed Tablets

U26 Ilosone®
Composition (Each Compressed Tablet): Erythromycin Estolate, USP, 500 mg (equiv. to erythromycin)

4143 Keftab®
Composition (Each Compressed Tablet): Cephalexin Hydrochloride, USP, 500 mg (equiv. to cephalexin)

Miscellaneous

W15 Ilosone® Liquid, Oral Suspension
Composition: Each 5 mL contain erythromycin estolate equivalent to 125 mg erythromycin (USP).

W17 Ilosone® Liquid, Oral Suspension
Composition: Each 5 mL contain erythromycin estolate equivalent to 250 mg erythromycin (USP).

W21 Keflex®, for Oral Suspension
Composition (When Mixed as Directed): Each 5 mL contain 125 mg cephalexin (USP).

W68 Keflex®, for Oral Suspension
Composition (When Mixed as Directed): Each 5 mL contain 250 mg cephalexin (USP).

UNIT-DOSE PACKAGING

Identi-Dose® (unit dose medication, Dista) Closed-circuit control of medication from pharmacy to nurse to patient and return. Simplifies counting and dispensing whether in single-unit or prescription-size quantities. Fits into any dispensing system for ready identification and legibility, better inventory control, protection from contamination, easier handling and recording under Medicare, prevention of drug loss through pilferage or spilling, better control of Federal Controlled Substances, and less chance of medication errors. The following products are available through normal channels of supply:
Identi-Dose®
Pulvules®
No.
402 Keflex®, 250 mg
403 Keflex®, 500 mg
Ointments
No.
52 Ilotycin®, Ophthalmic
Miscellaneous
No.
M-202 Keflex®, for Oral Suspension, 250 mg/5 mL

ILOSONE®   ℞
[ī'lō-sōn]
(erythromycin estolate)
USP

WARNING

Hepatic dysfunction with or without jaundice has occurred, chiefly in adults, in association with erythromycin estolate administration. It may be accompanied by malaise, nausea, vomiting, abdominal colic, and fever. In some instances, severe abdominal pain may simulate an abdominal surgical emergency.
If the above findings occur, discontinue Ilosone® (Erythromycin Estolate, USP) promptly.
Ilosone is contraindicated for patients with a known history of sensitivity to this drug and for those with preexisting liver disease.

DESCRIPTION

Erythromycin is produced by a strain of *Streptomyces erythraeus* and belongs to the macrolide group of antibiotics. It is basic and readily forms salts with acids. The base, the stearate salt, and the esters are poorly soluble in water and are suitable for oral administration.
Ilosone is the lauryl sulfate salt of the propionyl ester of erythromycin.
The Pulvules® contain 250 mg (0.237 mmol) erythromycin estolate. They also contain FD&C Red No. 3, FD&C Yellow No. 6, gelatin, iron oxides, magnesium stearate, mineral oil, silica gel, talc, titanium dioxide, and other inactive ingredients.
The tablets contain 500 mg (0.473 mmol) erythromycin estolate. They also contain cornstarch, magnesium stearate, povidone, titanium dioxide, and other inactive ingredients. The suspensions contain 125 mg (0.118 mmol) or 250 mg (0.237 mmol) of erythromycin estolate per 5 mL. The suspensions also contain butylparaben, carboxymethylcellulose, cellulose, citric acid, edetate calcium disodium, flavors, methylparaben, propylparaben, silicone, sodium chloride, sodium citrate, sodium lauryl sulfate, sucrose, and water. The 125-mg suspension also contains FD&C Yellow No. 6. The 250-mg suspension also contains FD&C Red No. 40.

ACTIONS

Erythromycin inhibits protein synthesis without affecting nucleic acid synthesis. Some strains of *Haemophilus influenzae* and staphylococci have demonstrated resistance to erythromycin. Some strains of *H. influenzae* that are resistant in vitro to erythromycin alone are susceptible to erythromycin and sulfonamides used concomitantly. Culture and susceptibility testing should be done. If the Bauer-Kirby method of disk susceptibility testing is used, a 15-μg erythromycin disk should give a zone diameter of at least 18 mm when tested against an erythromycin-susceptible organism.
Orally administered erythromycin estolate is readily and reliably absorbed. Because of acid stability, serum levels are comparable whether the estolate is taken in the fasting state or after food. After a single 250-mg dose, blood concentrations average 0.29, 1.2, and 1.2 μg/mL respectively at 2, 4, and 6 hours. Following a 500-mg dose, blood concentrations average 3, 1.9, and 0.7 μg/mL respectively at 2, 6, and 12 hours.
After oral administration, serum antibiotic levels consist of erythromycin base and propionyl erythromycin ester. The propionyl ester continuously hydrolyzes to the base form of erythromycin to maintain an equilibrium ratio of approximately 20% base and 80% ester in the serum.
After absorption, erythromycin diffuses readily into most body fluids. In the absence of meningeal inflammation, low concentrations are normally achieved in the spinal fluid, but passage of the drug across the blood-brain barrier increases in meningitis. In the presence of normal hepatic function, erythromycin is concentrated in the liver and excreted in the bile; the effect of hepatic dysfunction on excretion of erythromycin by the liver into the bile is not known. After oral administration, less than 5% of the administered dose can be recovered as the active form in the urine.
Erythromycin crosses the placental barrier, but fetal plasma levels are low.

INDICATIONS

Streptococcus pyogenes (Group A β-hemolytic)—Upper and lower respiratory tract, skin, and soft-tissue infections of mild to moderate severity.
Injectable penicillin G benzathine is considered by the American Heart Association to be the drug of choice in the treatment and prevention of streptococcal pharyngitis and in long-term prophylaxis of rheumatic fever.

When oral medication is preferred for treating these conditions, penicillin G or V or erythromycin is the alternate drug of choice.
The importance of the patient's strict adherence to the prescribed dosage regimen must be stressed when oral medication is given. A therapeutic dose should be administered for at least 10 days.
α-Hemolytic Streptococci (viridans group) —Although no controlled clinical efficacy trials have been conducted, oral erythromycin has been suggested by the American Heart Association and American Dental Association for prophylactic use against bacterial endocarditis in patients hypersensitive to penicillin who have congenital heart disease or rheumatic or other acquired valvular heart disease when they undergo dental procedures and surgical procedures of the upper respiratory tract.[1] Erythromycin is not suitable for such prophylaxis prior to genitourinary or gastrointestinal tract surgery.
Note: When selecting antibiotics for the prevention of bacterial endocarditis, the physician or dentist should read the full joint statement of the American Heart Association and the American Dental Association.[1]
Staphylococcus aureus—Acute infections of skin and soft tissue that are mild to moderately severe. Resistance may develop during treatment.
Streptococcus pneumoniae —Infections of the upper respiratory tract (eg, otitis media, pharyngitis) and lower respiratory tract (eg, pneumonia) of mild to moderate severity.
Mycoplasma pneumoniae —In the treatment of respiratory tract infections due to this organism.
H. influenzae —May be used concomitantly with adequate doses of sulfonamides in treating upper respiratory tract infections of mild to moderate severity. Not all strains of this organism are susceptible at the erythromycin concentrations ordinarily achieved (see appropriate sulfonamide labeling for prescribing information).
Treponema pallidum —Erythromycin is an alternate choice of treatment for primary syphilis in penicillin-allergic patients. In primary syphilis, spinal-fluid examinations should be done before treatment and as part of follow-up after therapy.
Corynebacterium diphtheriae —As an adjunct to antitoxin, to prevent establishment of carriers, and to eradicate the organism in carriers.
Corynebacterium minutissimum —In the treatment of erythrasma.
Entamoeba histolytica —In the treatment of intestinal amebiasis only. Extraenteric amebiasis requires treatment with other agents.
Listeria monocytogenes —Infections due to this organism.
Bordetella pertussis —Erythromycin is effective in eliminating the organism from the nasopharynx of infected individuals, rendering them noninfectious. Some clinical studies suggest that erythromycin may be helpful in the prophylaxis of pertussis in exposed susceptible individuals.
Legionnaires' Disease —Although no controlled clinical efficacy studies have been conducted, in vitro and limited preliminary clinical data suggest that erythromycin may be effective in treating Legionnaires' disease.
Chlamydia trachomatis —Erythromycins are indicated for treatment of the following infections caused by *C. trachomatis*: conjunctivitis of the newborn, pneumonia of infancy, and urogenital infections during pregnancy (see Precautions). When tetracyclines are contraindicated or not tolerated, erythromycin is indicated for the treatment of adults with uncomplicated urethral, endocervical, or rectal infections due to *C. trachomatis*.[2]

CONTRAINDICATIONS

Erythromycin is contraindicated in patients with known hypersensitivity to this antibiotic.
Erythromycin is contraindicated in patients taking terfenadine or astemizole (see **Precautions—Drug Interactions**).

WARNINGS

(See boxed Warning.) The administration of erythromycin estolate has been associated with the infrequent occurrence of cholestatic hepatitis. Laboratory findings have been characterized by abnormal hepatic function test values, peripheral eosinophilia, and leukocytosis. Symptoms may include malaise, nausea, vomiting, abdominal cramps, and fever. Jaundice may or may not be present. In some instances, severe abdominal pain may simulate the pain of biliary colic, pancreatitis, perforated ulcer, or an acute abdominal surgical problem. In other instances, clinical symptoms and results of liver function tests have resembled findings in extrahepatic obstructive jaundice.

Continued on next page

This product information was prepared in June 1996. Current information on these and other products of Dista Products Products Company may be obtained by direct inquiry to Lilly Research Laboratories, Lilly Corporate Center, Indianapolis, Indiana 46285, (800) 545-5979.

Consult 1997 supplements and future editions for revisions

Dista—Cont.

Initial symptoms have developed in some cases after a few days of treatment but generally have followed 1 or 2 weeks of continuous therapy. Symptoms reappear promptly, usually within 48 hours after the drug is readministered to sensitive patients. The syndrome seems to result from a form of sensitization, occurs chiefly in adults, and has been reversible when medication is discontinued.
Pseudomembranous colitis has been reported with virtually all broad-spectrum antibiotics (including macrolides, semisynthetic penicillins, and cephalosporins); therefore, it is important to consider its diagnosis in patients who develop diarrhea in association with the use of antibiotics. Such colitis may range in severity from mild to life threatening.
Treatment with broad-spectrum antibiotics alters the normal flora of the colon and may permit overgrowth of clostridia. Studies indicate that a toxin produced by *Clostridium difficile* is a primary cause of antibiotic-associated colitis.
Mild cases of pseudomembranous colitis usually respond to drug discontinuance alone. In moderate to severe cases, management should include sigmoidoscopy, appropriate bacteriologic studies, and fluid, electrolyte, and protein supplementation. When the colitis does not improve after the drug has been discontinued, or when it is severe, oral vancomycin is the drug of choice for antibiotic-associated pseudomembranous colitis produced by *C. difficile*. Other causes of colitis should be ruled out.

PRECAUTIONS

General—Since erythromycin is excreted principally by the liver, caution should be exercised in administering the antibiotic to patients with impaired hepatic function.
Surgical procedures should be performed when indicated.
The antibacterial activity of erythromycin is markedly greater in alkaline than in neutral or acid media, and several investigators have recommended concomitant administration of urinary alkalinizing agents, such as sodium bicarbonate or acetazolamide (Diamox), when erythromycin is prescribed for treatment of urinary infections.
Laboratory Tests—There are reports that erythromycin interferes in some clinical laboratory tests and causes aberrant results. For example, evidence has been published indicating that high SGOT values recorded for some patients receiving erythromycin estolate may be artifacts and may not necessarily reflect changes in liver function.
Drug Interactions—Erythromycin has been reported to significantly alter the metabolism of the nonsedating antihistamines, terfenadine or astemizole, when taken concomitantly. Rare cases of serious cardiovascular adverse events, including electrocardiographic QT/QTc interval prolongation, cardiac arrest, torsades de pointes, and other ventricular arrhythmias, have been observed (*see* **Contraindications**). In addition, rare reports of death have also been reported with concomitant administration of terfenadine and erythromycin.
Since probenecid inhibits tubular reabsorption of erythromycin in animals, it prolongs maintenance of plasma levels.
Erythromycin and lincomycin or clindamycin may under some conditions be antagonistic. Lincomycin or clindamycin therapy should be avoided in treatment of infections due to erythromycin-resistant organisms.
Erythromycin use in patients who are receiving high doses of theophylline may be associated with an increase in serum theophylline levels and potential theophylline toxicity. In case of theophylline toxicity and/or elevated serum theophylline levels, the dose of theophylline should be reduced while the patient is receiving concomitant erythromycin therapy.
Concomitant administration of erythromycin and digoxin has been reported to result in elevated digoxin serum levels.
There have been reports of increased anticoagulant effects when erythromycin and oral anticoagulants were used concomitantly. Increased anticoagulation effects due to this drug interaction may be more pronounced in the elderly.
Concurrent use of erythromycin and ergotamine or dihydroergotamine has been associated in some patients with acute ergot toxicity characterized by severe peripheral vasospasm and dysesthesia.
Erythromycin has been reported to decrease the clearance of triazolam and midazolam and thus may increase the pharmacologic effect of these benzodiazepines.
The use of erythromycin in patients concurrently taking drugs metabolized by the cytochrome P-450 system may be associated with elevations in serum concentrations of these other drugs. Elevated serum concentrations of the following drugs have been reported when administered concurrently with erythromycin: carbamazepine, cyclosporine, hexobarbital, phenytoin, alfentanil, disopyramide, lovastatin, bromocriptine, and valproate. Serum concentrations of these and other drugs metabolized by the cytochrome P-450 system should be monitored closely in patients concurrently receiving erythromycin.
Usage in Pregnancy—Pregnancy Category B—Reproduction studies have been performed in rats, mice, and rabbits using erythromycin and its various salts and esters at doses several times the usual human dose. No evidence of impaired fertility or harm to the fetus that appeared to be related to erythromycin was reported in these studies. There are, however, no adequate and well-controlled studies in pregnant women. Because animal reproductive studies are not always predictive of human response, this drug should be used during pregnancy only if clearly needed.
Nursing Mothers—Erythromycin is excreted in breast milk. Caution should be exercised when erythromycin is administered to a nursing woman.
Pediatric Use—See Indications *and* Dosage and Administration.

ADVERSE REACTIONS

The most frequent side effects of erythromycin preparations are gastrointestinal (eg, abdominal cramping and discomfort) and are dose related. Nausea, vomiting, and diarrhea occur infrequently with usual oral doses.
During prolonged or repeated therapy, there is a possibility of overgrowth of nonsusceptible bacteria or fungi. If such infections arise, the drug should be discontinued and appropriate therapy instituted.
Mild allergic reactions, such as urticaria and other skin rashes, have occurred. Serious allergic reactions, including anaphylaxis, have been reported.
There have been isolated reports of hearing loss and/or tinnitus in patients receiving erythromycin. The ototoxic effect of the drug is usually reversible with drug discontinuance; however, in rare instances involving intravenous administration, the ototoxic effect has been irreversible. Ototoxic effects occur chiefly in patients with renal or hepatic insufficiency and in patients receiving high doses of erythromycin.
Rarely, erythromycin has been associated with the production of ventricular arrhythmias, including ventricular tachycardia and torsades de pointes, in individuals with prolonged QT intervals.

OVERDOSAGE

Signs and Symptoms—Symptoms of oral overdose of erythromycin estolate may include nausea, vomiting, epigastric distress, and diarrhea. The severity of the epigastric distress and the diarrhea are dose related. Reversible mild acute pancreatitis has been reported. Hearing loss, with or without tinnitus and vertigo, may occur, especially in patients with renal or hepatic insufficiency.
Treatment—To obtain up-to-date information about the treatment of overdose, a good resource is your certified Regional Poison Control Center. Telephone numbers of certified poison control centers are listed in the *Physicians' Desk Reference (PDR)*. In managing overdosage, consider the possibility of multiple drug overdoses, interaction among drugs, and unusual drug kinetics in your patient.
Unless 5 times the normal single dose of erythromycin estolate has been ingested, gastrointestinal decontamination should not be necessary. An accidental ingestion of erythromycin should not be predicted to have minimal toxicity unless there is a good approximation of how much was ingested and unless only a single medication was involved.
Protect the patient's airway and support ventilation and perfusion. Meticulously monitor and maintain, within acceptable limits, the patient's vital signs, blood gases, serum electrolytes, etc. Absorption of drugs from the gastrointestinal tract may be decreased by giving activated charcoal, which, in many cases, is more effective than emesis or lavage; consider charcoal instead of or in addition to gastric emptying. Repeated doses of charcoal over time may hasten elimination of some drugs that have been absorbed. Safeguard the patient's airway when employing gastric emptying or charcoal.
Forced diuresis, peritoneal dialysis, hemodialysis, or charcoal hemoperfusion have not been established as beneficial for an overdose of erythromycin estolate.

DOSAGE AND ADMINISTRATION

Adults —The usual dosage is 250 mg every 6 hours. This may be increased up to 4 g/day or more according to the severity of the infection.
Children —Age, weight, and severity of the infection are important factors in determining the proper dosage. The usual regimen is 30 to 50 mg/kg/day in divided doses. For more severe infections, this dosage may be doubled.
If administration is desired on a twice-a-day schedule in either adults or children, ½ of the total daily dose may be given every 12 hours.
Twice-a-day dosing is not recommended when doses larger than 1 g daily are administered.
Streptococcal Infections —For the treatment of streptococcal pharyngitis and tonsillitis, the usual dosage range is 20 to 50 mg/kg/day in divided doses.

Body Weight	Total Daily Dose
10 kg or less (less than 25 lb)	250 mg
11–18 kg (25–40 lb)	375 mg
18–25 kg (40–55 lb)	500 mg
25–36 kg (55–80 lb)	750 mg
36 kg or more (more than 80 lb)	1,000 mg (adult dose)

In the treatment of group A β-hemolytic streptococcal infections, a therapeutic dosage of erythromycin should be administered for at least 10 days. In continuous prophylaxis of streptococcal infections in persons with a history of rheumatic heart disease, the dosage is 250 mg twice a day.
For prophylaxis against bacterial endocarditis[1] in penicillin-allergic patients with congenital heart disease or rheumatic or other acquired valvular heart disease when undergoing dental procedures or surgical procedures of the upper respiratory tract, the dosage schedule for adults is 1 g (20 mg/kg for children) orally 1 hour before the procedure and then 500 mg (10 mg/kg for children) orally 6 hours later.
Primary Syphilis —A regimen of 20 g of erythromycin estolate in divided doses over a period of 10 days has been shown to be effective in the treatment of primary syphilis.
Dysenteric Amebiasis —Dosage for adults is 250 mg 4 times daily for 10 to 14 days; for children, 30 to 50 mg/kg/day in divided doses for 10 to 14 days.
Pertussis —Although optimum dosage and duration have not been established, the dosage of erythromycin utilized in reported clinical studies was 40 to 50 mg/kg/day, given in divided doses for 5 to 14 days.
Legionnaires' Disease —Although optimum doses have not been established, doses utilized in reported clinical data were those recommended above (1 to 4 g erythromycin estolate daily in divided doses).
Conjunctivitis of the Newborn Caused by C. trachomatis —Oral erythromycin suspension, 50 mg/kg/day in 4 divided doses for at least 2 weeks.[2]
Pneumonia of Infancy Caused by C. trachomatis —Although the optimum duration of therapy has not been established, the recommended therapy is oral erythromycin suspension, 50 mg/kg/day in 4 divided doses for at least 3 weeks.[2]
Urogenital Infections During Pregnancy Due to C. trachomatis—Although the optimum dose and duration of therapy have not been established, the suggested treatment is erythromycin, 500 mg orally 4 times a day for at least 7 days. For women who cannot tolerate this regimen, a decreased dose of 250 mg orally 4 times a day should be used for at least 14 days.[2]
For adults with uncomplicated urethral, endocervical, or rectal infections caused by *C. trachomatis* in whom tetracyclines are contraindicated or not tolerated: 500 mg orally 4 times a day for at least 7 days.[2]

REFERENCES

1. American Heart Association: Prevention of bacterial endocarditis. *Circulation*, 1984; 70:1123A.
2. Sexually Transmitted Diseases Treatment Guidelines 1982. Centers for Disease Control, Morbidity and Mortality Weekly Report, US Department of Health and Human Services, Atlanta, 1982; 31 (suppl): 355.

HOW SUPPLIED

℞ Pulvules, ivory and red
250 mg* (No. 375)—(100s) NDC 0777-0809-02
Tablets, specially coated, white (capsule-shaped, scored)
500 mg* (No. 1863)—(50s) NDC 0777-2126-50
Store at controlled room temperature, 59° to 86°F (15° to 30°C).
Liquid, Oral Suspension
125 mg*/5 mL, orange-flavored vehicle (M-148)†—(16 fl oz) NDC 0777-2315-05
250 mg*/5 mL, cherry-flavored vehicle (M-153)†—(100 mL) NDC 0777-2317-48; (16 fl oz) NDC 0777-2317-05

* Equivalent to erythromycin.
† Shake well before using. Refrigerate to maintain optimum taste.

[060993]

ILOTYCIN® ℞

[ī-lō-tī′-sĭn]
(erythromycin)
Ophthalmic Ointment, USP

DESCRIPTION

Ilotycin® (Erythromycin Ophthalmic Ointment, USP) belongs to the macrolide group of antibiotics. It is basic and readily forms a salt when combined with an acid. The base, as crystals or powder, is slightly soluble in water, moderately soluble in ether, and readily soluble in alcohol or chloroform. Erythromycin is an antibiotic produced from a strain of *Streptomyces erythraeus*. The special sterile ophthalmic ointment base flows freely over the conjunctiva.
Chemical Name: (3R*, 4S*, 5S*, 6R*, 7R*, 9R*, 11R*, 12R*, 13S*, 14R*)-4-[(2,6-Dideoxy-3-C-methyl-3-O-methyl-α-L-*ribo*-hexopyranosyl)oxy]-14-ethyl-7,12,13-trihydroxy-3, 5, 7, 9,

11, 13-hexamethyl-6-[[3,4,6-trideoxy-3-(dimethylamino)-β-D-*xylo*-hexopyranosyl]oxy]oxacyclotetradecane-2, 10-dione.
Each Gram Contains: ACTIVE: Erythromycin, USP, 5 mg (0.5%); INACTIVES: White Petrolatum, Mineral Oil.
It has the following structural formula:

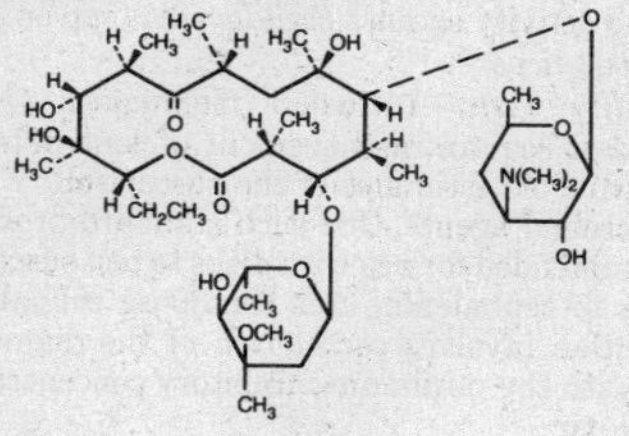

CLINICAL PHARMACOLOGY

Microbiology—Erythromycin inhibits protein synthesis without affecting nucleic acid synthesis. Erythromycin is usually active against the following organisms *in vitro* and in clinical infections:

Streptococcus pyogenes (group A β-hemolytic)
Alpha-hemolytic streptococci (viridans group)
Staphylococcus aureus, including penicillinase-producing strains (methicillin-resistant staphylococci are uniformly resistant to erythromycin)
Streptococcus pneumoniae
Mycoplasma pneumoniae (Eaton Agent, PPLO)
Haemophilus influenzae (not all strains of this organism are susceptible at the erythromycin concentrations ordinarily achieved)
Treponema pallidum
Corynebacterium diphtheriae
Neisseria gonorrhoeae
Chlamydia trachomatis

INDICATIONS AND USAGE

For the treatment of superficial ocular infections involving the conjunctiva and/or cornea caused by organisms susceptible to Ilotycin.
For prophylaxis of ophthalmia neonatorum due to *N. gonorrhoeae* or *C. trachomatis.*
The effectiveness of erythromycin in the prevention of ophthalmia caused by penicillinase-producing *N. gonorrhoeae* is not established.
For infants born to mothers with clinically apparent gonorrhea, intravenous or intramuscular injections of aqueous crystalline penicillin G should be given; a single dose of 50,000 units for term infants or 20,000 units for infants of low birth weight. Topical prophylaxis alone is inadequate for these infants.

CONTRAINDICATION

This drug is contraindicated in patients with a history of hypersensitivity to erythromycin.

PRECAUTIONS

General—The use of antimicrobial agents may be associated with the overgrowth of nonsusceptible organisms including fungi; in such a case, antibiotic administration should be stopped and appropriate measures taken.
Information for Patients—Avoid contaminating the tip of container with material from the eye, fingers, or other source.
Carcinogenesis Mutagenesis, Impairment of Fertility —Two year oral studies conducted in rats with erythromycin did not provide evidence of tumorigenicity. Mutagenicity studies have not been conducted. No evidence of impaired fertility or harm to the fetus that appeared related to erythromycin was reported in these studies.
Pregnancy—Pregnancy Category B—Reproduction studies have been performed in rats, mice, and rabbits using erythromycin and its various salts and esters, at doses that were several multiples of the usual human dose. There are, however, no adequate and well-controlled studies in pregnant women. Because animal reproductive studies are not always predictive of human response, the erythromycins should be used during pregnancy only if clearly needed.
Nursing Mothers—Caution should be exercised when erythromycin is administered to a nursing woman.
Pediatric Use—See INDICATIONS AND USAGE and DOSAGE AND ADMINISTRATION.

ADVERSE REACTIONS

The most frequently reported adverse reactions are minor ocular irritations, redness, and hypersensitivity reactions.

DOSAGE AND ADMINISTRATION

In the treatment of superficial ocular infections, Ophthalmic Ointment Ilotycin® (Erythromycin, USP) approximately 1 cm in length should be applied directly to the infected structure up to 6 times daily, depending on the severity of the infection.
For prophylaxis of neonatal gonococcal or chlamydial ophthalmia, a ribbon of ointment approximately 1 cm in length should be instilled into each lower conjunctival sac. The ointment should not be flushed from the eye following instillation. A new tube should be used for each infant.
Directions For Use for 1 Gram Plastic Tube: DO NOT PULL CAP OFF. Twist cap to verify that a click is heard and/or resistance is felt. Either indicates that the plastic tip under cap was intact. The twisting motion breaks the seal and the tip remains in the cap. Dispense product and discard after use.

HOW SUPPLIED

ILOTYCIN® (Erythromycin Ophthalmic Ointment, USP, 0.5%) No. 52 is available in the following sizes:
1/8 oz. (3.5 g) tamper-resistant tube—(NDC 0777-1863-17—Prod. No. FL09234

DO NOT USE IF BOTTOM RIDGE OF TUBE CAP IS EXPOSED.

1 g plastic container (in cartons of 50)—(NDC 0777-1863-52)—Prod. No. FL09232

DO NOT USE IF CLICK IS NOT HEARD AND/OR RESISTANCE IS NOT FELT.

Storage: Store between 15°–30°C (59°–86°F).
KEEP OUT OF REACH OF CHILDREN.
Caution: Federal law prohibits dispensing without prescription.

[050095]

ILOTYCIN® GLUCEPTATE ℞

[*ī-lō-tī 'sĭn gloo-sĕp 'tāt*]
(erythromycin gluceptate)
Sterile, USP
Intravenous

DESCRIPTION

Erythromycin is produced by a strain of*Streptomyces erythraeus* and belongs to the macrolide group of antibiotics. It is basic and readily forms a salt when combined with an acid.

ACTIONS

Erythromycin inhibits protein synthesis without affecting nucleic acid synthesis. Some strains of *Haemophilus influenzae* and staphylococci have demonstrated resistance to erythromycin. Culture and susceptibility testing should be done. If the Bauer-Kirby method of disk susceptibility testing is used, a 15-μg erythromycin disk should give a zone diameter of at least 18 mm when tested against an erythromycin-susceptible organism.
Intravenous injection of 200 mg of erythromycin produces peak serum levels of 3 to 4 μg/mL at 1 hour and 0.5 μg/mL at 6 hours.
Erythromycin diffuses readily into the body fluids. Only low concentrations are normally achieved in the spinal fluid, but passage of the drug across the blood-brain barrier increases in meningitis. In the presence of normal hepatic function, erythromycin is concentrated in the liver and excreted in the bile; the effect of hepatic dysfunction on excretion of erythromycin by the liver into the bile is not known. From 12% to 15% of intravenously administered erythromycin is excreted in active form in the urine.
Erythromycin crosses the placental barrier, but fetal plasma levels are low.

INDICATIONS AND USAGE

Streptococcus pyogenes (group A β-hemolytic)—Upper and lower respiratory tract, skin, and soft-tissue infections of mild to moderate severity.
Injectable penicillin G benzathine is considered by the American Heart Association to be the drug of choice in the treatment and prevention of streptococcal pharyngitis and in long-term prophylaxis of rheumatic fever.
Staphylococcus aureus —Acute infections of skin and soft tissue that are mild to moderately severe. Resistance may develop during treatment.
Streptococcus pneumoniae —Infections of the upper respiratory tract (eg, otitis media and pharyngitis) and lower respiratory tract (eg, pneumonia) of mild to moderate severity.
Mycoplasma pneumoniae —In the treatment of respiratory tract infections due to this organism.
H. influenzae —May be used concomitantly with adequate doses of sulfonamides in treating upper respiratory tract infections of mild to moderate severity. Not all strains of this organism are susceptible at the erythromycin concentrations ordinarily achieved (see appropriate sulfonamide labeling for prescribing information).
Corynebacterium diphtheriae —As an adjunct to antitoxin.
Listeria monocytogenes —Infections due to this organism.
Neisseria gonorrhoeae —In female patients with a history of sensitivity to penicillin, a parenteral erythromycin (such as the gluceptate) may be administered in conjunction with an oral erythromycin as alternate therapy in acute pelvic inflammatory disease caused by *N. gonorrhoeae.* In the treatment of gonorrhea, patients suspected of having concomitant syphilis should have microscopic examinations (by immunofluorescence or dark-field) before receiving erythromycin and monthly serologic tests for a minimum of 4 months.
Legionnaires' Disease —Although no controlled clinical efficacy studies have been conducted, in vitro and limited preliminary clinical data suggest that erythromycin may be effective in treating Legionnaires' disease.

CONTRAINDICATIONS

Intravenous erythromycin is contraindicated in patients with known hypersensitivity to this antibiotic.
Erythromycin is contraindicated in patients taking terfenadine or astemizole (*see* **Precautions—Drug Interactions**).

WARNINGS

Usage in Pregnancy —Safety of this drug for use during pregnancy has not been established.
Pseudomembranous colitis has been reported with virtually all broad-spectrum antibiotics (including macrolides, semisynthetic penicillins, and cephalosporins); therefore, it is important to consider its diagnosis in patients who develop diarrhea in association with the use of antibiotics. Such colitis may range in severity from mild to life threatening.
Treatment with broad-spectrum antibiotics alters the normal flora of the colon and may permit overgrowth of clostridia. Studies indicate that a toxin produced by *Clostridium difficile* is one primary cause of antibiotic-associated colitis.
Mild cases of pseudomembranous colitis usually respond to drug discontinuance alone. In moderate to severe cases, management should include sigmoidoscopy, appropriate bacteriologic studies, and fluid, electrolyte, and protein supplementation. When the colitis does not improve after the drug has been discontinued, or when it is severe, oral vancomycin is the drug of choice for antibiotic-associated pseudomembranous colitis produced by *C. difficile.* Other causes of colitis should be ruled out.

PRECAUTIONS

Surgical procedures should be performed when indicated.
Side effects following the use of intravenous erythromycin are rare. Occasional venous irritation has been encountered, but if the injection is given slowly, in dilute solution, preferably by continuous intravenous infusion over 20 to 60 minutes, pain and vessel trauma are minimized.
Since erythromycin is excreted principally by the liver, caution should be exercised in administering the antibiotic to patients with impaired hepatic function.
Drug Interactions —Erythromycin has been reported to significantly alter the metabolism of the nonsedating antihistamines, terfenadine or astemizole, when taken concomitantly. Rare cases of serious cardiovascular adverse events, including electrocardiographic QT/QTc interval prolongation, cardiac arrest, torsades de pointes, and other ventricular arrhythmias, have been observed (*see* **Contraindications**). In addition, rare reports of death have also been reported with concomitant administration of terfenadine and erythromycin.
Erythromycin use in patients who are receiving high doses of theophylline may be associated with an increase in serum theophylline levels and potential theophylline toxicity. In case of theophylline toxicity and/or elevated serum theophylline levels, the dose of theophylline should be reduced while the patient is receiving concomitant erythromycin therapy.
Concomitant administration of erythromycin and digoxin has been reported to result in elevated digoxin serum levels.
There have been reports of increased anticoagulant effects when erythromycin and oral anticoagulants were used concomitantly. Increased anticoagulation effects due to this drug interaction may be more pronounced in the elderly.
Concurrent use of erythromycin and ergotamine or dihydroergotamine has been associated in some patients with acute ergot toxicity characterized by severe peripheral vasospasm and dysesthesia.
Erythromycin has been reported to decrease the clearance of triazolam and midazolam and thus may increase the pharmacologic effect of these benzodiazepines.
The use of erythromycin in patients concurrently taking drugs metabolized by the cytochrome P-450 system may be associated with elevations in serum concentrations of these other drugs. Elevated serum concentrations of the following drugs have been reported when administered concurrently with erythromycin: carbamazepine, cyclosporine, hexobarbital, phenytoin, alfentanil, disopyramide, lovastatin, and bromocriptine. Serum concentrations of these and other drugs metabolized by the cytochrome P-450 system should

Continued on next page

This product information was prepared in June 1996. Current information on these and other products of Dista Products Products Company may be obtained by direct inquiry to Lilly Research Laboratories, Lilly Corporate Center, Indianapolis, Indiana 46285, (800) 545-5979.

Dista—Cont.

be monitored closely in patients concurrently receiving erythromycin.

ADVERSE REACTIONS

Allergic reactions, ranging from urticaria and mild skin eruptions to anaphylaxis, have occurred with intravenously administered erythromycin.

During prolonged or repeated therapy, there is a possibility of overgrowth of nonsusceptible bacteria or fungi. If such infections arise, the drug should be discontinued and appropriate therapy instituted.

Variations in liver function have been observed following daily doses at high levels or after prolonged therapy. Hepatic function tests should be performed when such therapy is given.

Reversible hearing loss associated with the intravenous infusion of 4 g/day or more of erythromycin has been reported rarely.

Rarely, erythromycin has been associated with the production of ventricular arrhythmias, including ventricular tachycardia and torsades de pointes, in individuals with prolonged QT intervals.

OVERDOSAGE

Signs and Symptoms—Experience with overdosage of Ilotycin Gluceptate is limited. Alterations in liver function tests and reversible hearing loss are possible, especially in patients with renal insufficiency.

Treatment—To obtain up-to-date information about the treatment of overdose, a good resource is your certified Regional Poison Control Center. Telephone numbers of certified poison control centers are listed in the *Physicians' Desk Reference (PDR)*. In managing overdosage, consider the possibility of multiple drug overdoses, interaction among drugs, and unusual drug kinetics in your patient.

Protect the patient's airway and support ventilation and perfusion. Meticulously monitor and maintain, within acceptable limits, the patient's vital signs, blood gases, serum electrolytes, etc.

Forced diuresis, peritoneal dialysis, hemodialysis, or charcoal hemoperfusion have not been established as beneficial for an overdose of erythromycin gluceptate.

DOSAGE AND ADMINISTRATION

Prepare the initial solution of Ilotycin Gluceptate by (1) adding at least 20 mL of Sterile Water for Injection to the 1-g vial of Ilotycin Gluceptate and (2) shaking the vial until all of the drug is dissolved.

It is important that the product be diluted only with Sterile Water for Injection without preservatives.

After reconstitution, the sterile solution should be stored in a refrigerator and used within 7 days.

When all of the drug is dissolved, the solution may then be added to 0.9% Sodium Chloride Injection or to 5% Dextrose in Water to give 1 g per liter for slow, continuous infusion. IV fluid admixtures with a pH below 5.5 tend to lose potency rapidly. Therefore, such solutions should be administered completely within 4 hours after dilution.

If the period of administration is prolonged, the pH of the infusion fluid should be buffered to neutrality with a sterile agent such as Neut® (Sodium Bicarbonate 4% Additive Solution, Abbott) or Buff™ (Phosphate-Carbonate Buffer, Travenol). For administration of the antibiotic in 500 or 1,000 mL of 5% Dextrose in Water, add 1 ampoule of full-strength Buff or 5 mL of Neut; for administration of the antibiotic in the same volumes of 0.9% Sodium Chloride Injection, add 1 ampoule of half-strength Buff or 5 mL of Neut. These solutions should be completely administered within 24 hours after dilution.

If the medication is to be given in 100 to 250 mL of fluid by a volume control set such as Metriset® (McGaw), Volu-Trole® "B" (Cutter), Soluset® (Abbott), or Buretrol® (Baxter-Travenol), the IV fluid should be buffered in its primary container before being added to the volumetric administration set.

If the medication is to be given by intermittent injection, one-fourth of the total daily dose can be given in 20 to 60 minutes by slow intravenous injection of 250 to 500 mg in 100 to 250 mL of 0.9% Sodium Chloride Injection or 5% Dextrose in Water. Injection should be sufficiently slow to avoid pain along the vein.

The recommended IV dosage for severe infections in adults and pediatric patients is 15 to 20 mg/kg of body weight/day. Higher doses (up to 4 g/day) may be given in very severe infections. Continuous infusion is preferable, but administration in divided doses at intervals of no more than every 6 hours is also effective.

For treatment of acute pelvic inflammatory disease caused by *N. gonorrhoeae*, administer 500 mg Ilotycin Gluceptate intravenously every 6 hours for at least 3 days, followed by 250 mg oral erythromycin every 6 hours for 7 days.

Patients receiving intravenous erythromycin should be transferred to the oral dosage form as soon as possible.

For Treatment of Legionnaires' Disease—Although optimum doses have not been established, doses utilized in reported clinical data were those recommended above (1 to 4 g daily in divided doses).

HOW SUPPLIED

Vials:

1 g,* 30-mL size (No. 646)—(1s) NDC 0777-1441-01

* Equivalent to erythromycin.

Prior to reconstitution, store at controlled room temperature, 59° to 86°F (15° to 30°C).

[040596]

KEFLEX® ℞

[*kĕf′lĕks*]

(cephalexin)

USP

DESCRIPTION

Keflex® (Cephalexin, USP) is a semisynthetic cephalosporin antibiotic intended for oral administration. It is 7-(D-α-amino-α-phenylacetamido)-3-methyl-3-cephem-4-carboxylic acid monohydrate. Cephalexin has the molecular formula $C_{16}H_{17}N_3O_4S \cdot H_2O$ and the molecular weight is 365.4.

Cephalexin has the following structural formula:

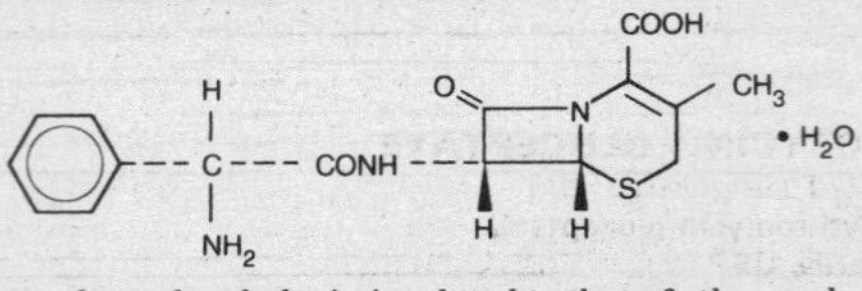

The nucleus of cephalexin is related to that of other cephalosporin antibiotics. The compound is a zwitterion; ie, the molecule contains both a basic and an acidic group. The isoelectric point of cephalexin in water is approximately 4.5 to 5.

The crystalline form of cephalexin which is available is a monohydrate. It is a white crystalline solid having a bitter taste. Solubility in water is low at room temperature; 1 or 2 mg/mL may be dissolved readily, but higher concentrations are obtained with increasing difficulty.

The cephalosporins differ from penicillins in the structure of the bicyclic ring system. Cephalexin has a *D*-phenylglycyl group as substituent at the 7-amino position and an unsubstituted methyl group at the 3-position.

Each Pulvule® contains cephalexin monohydrate equivalent to 250 mg (720 μmol) or 500 mg (1,439 μmol) of cephalexin. The Pulvules also contain cellulose, D & C Yellow No. 10, F D & C Blue No. 1, F D & C Yellow No. 6, gelatin, magnesium stearate, silicone, titanium dioxide, and other inactive ingredients.

After mixing, each 5 mL of Keflex, for Oral Suspension, will contain cephalexin monohydrate equivalent to 125 mg (360 μmol) or 250 mg (720 μmol) of cephalexin. The suspensions also contain flavors, methylcellulose, silicone, sodium lauryl sulfate, and sucrose. The 125-mg suspension contains F D & C Red No. 40, and the 250-mg suspension contains F D & C Yellow No. 6.

CLINICAL PHARMACOLOGY

Human Pharmacology—Keflex is acid stable and may be given without regard to meals. It is rapidly absorbed after oral administration. Following doses of 250 mg, 500 mg, and 1 g, average peak serum levels of approximately 9, 18, and 32 μg/mL respectively were obtained at 1 hour. Measurable levels were present 6 hours after administration. Cephalexin is excreted in the urine by glomerular filtration and tubular secretion. Studies showed that over 90% of the drug was excreted unchanged in the urine within 8 hours. During this period, peak urine concentrations following the 250-mg, 500-mg, and 1-g doses were approximately 1,000, 2,200, and 5,000 μg/mL respectively.

Microbiology—In vitro tests demonstrate that the cephalosporins are bactericidal because of their inhibition of cell-wall synthesis. Cephalexin has been shown to be active against most strains of the following microorganisms both *in vitro* and in clinical infections as described in the INDICATIONS AND USAGE section.

Aerobes, Gram-positive:

Staphylococcus aureus (including penicillinase-producing strains)

Staphylococcus epidermidis (penicillin-susceptible strains)

Streptococcus pneumoniae

Streptococcus pyogenes

Aerobes, Gram-negative:

Escherichia coli

Haemophilus influenzae

Klebsiella pneumoniae

Moraxella (Branhamella) catarrhalis

Proteus mirabilis

Note—Methicillin-resistant staphylococci and most strains of enterococci (*Enterococcus faecalis* [formerly *Streptococcus faecalis*]) are resistant to cephalosporins, including cephalexin. It is not active against most strains of *Enterobacter* spp, *Morganella morganii* and *Proteus vulgaris*. It has no activity against *Pseudomonas* spp or *Acinetobacter calcoaceticus*.

Susceptibility Tests—**Diffusion techniques:** Quantitative methods that require measurement of zone diameters provide reproducible estimates of the susceptibility of bacteria to antimicrobial agents. One such standard procedure[1] has been recommended for use with disks to test susceptibility of organisms to cephalexin, uses the 30-μg cephalothin disk. Interpretation involves correlation of the diameter in the disk test with the minimum inhibitory concentration (MIC) for cephalexin.

Reports from the laboratory giving results of the standard single-disk susceptibility test with a 30-μg cephalothin disk should be interpreted according to the following criteria:

Zone Diameter (mm)	Interpretation
≥18	(S) Susceptible
15–17	(I) Intermediate
≤14	(R) Resistant

A report of "Susceptible" indicates that the pathogen is likely to be inhibited by usually achievable concentrations of the antimicrobial compound in blood. A report of "Intermediate" indicates that the result should be considered equivocal, and, if the microorganism is not fully susceptible to alternative, clinically feasible drugs, the test should be repeated. This category implies possible clinical applicability in body sites where the drug is physiologically concentrated or in situations where high dosage of drug can be used. This category also provides a buffer zone that prevents small uncontrolled technical factors from causing major discrepancies in interpretation. A report of "Resistant" indicates that usually achievable concentrations of the antimicrobial compound in the blood are unlikely to be inhibitory and that other therapy should be selected.

Measurement of MIC or MBC and achieved antimicrobial compound concentrations may be appropriate to guide therapy in some infections. (See CLINICAL PHARMACOLOGY section for information on drug concentrations achieved in infected body sites and other pharmacokinetic properties of this antimicrobial drug product.)

Standardized susceptibility test procedures require the use of laboratory control microorganisms. The 30-μg cephalothin disk should provide the following zone diameters in these laboratory test quality control strains:

Microorganism	Zone Diameter (mm)
E. coli ATCC 25922	15–21
S. aureus ATCC 25923	29–37

Dilution techniques:

Quantitative methods that are used to determine MICs provide reproducible estimates of the susceptibility of bacteria to antimicrobial compounds. One such standardized procedure uses a standardized dilution method[2] (broth, agar, microdilution) or equivalent with cephalothin powder. The MIC values obtained should be interpreted according to the following criteria:

MIC (μg/mL)	Interpretation
≤8	(S) Susceptible
16	(I) Intermediate
≥32	(R) Resistant

As with standard diffusion techniques, dilution methods require the use of laboratory control organisms. Standard cephalothin powder should provide the following MIC values:

Organism	MIC (μg/mL)
E. coli ATCC 25922	4–16
E. faecalis ATCC 29212	8–32
S. aureus ATCC 29213	0.12–0.5

* Laboratory Standards: Performance standards for antimicrobial disk susceptibility tests—4th ed. Approved Standard NCCLS Document M2-A4, Vol 10, No 7, NCCLS, Villanova, PA, 1990.

† National Committee for Clinical Laboratory Standards: Methods for dilution antimicrobial susceptibility tests for bacteria that grow aerobically—2nd ed. Approved Standard NCCLS Document M7-A2, Vol 10, No 8, NCCLS, Villanova, PA, 1990.

INDICATIONS AND USAGE

Keflex is indicated for the treatment of the following infections when caused by susceptible strains of the designated microorganisms:

Respiratory tract infections caused by *S. pneumoniae* and *S. pyogenes* (Penicillin is the usual drug of choice in the treatment and prevention of streptococcal infections, including the prophylaxis of rheumatic fever. Keflex is generally effective in the eradication of streptococci from the nasopharynx; however, substantial data establishing the efficacy of Keflex in the subsequent prevention of rheumatic fever are not available at present.)

Otitis media due to *S. pneumoniae*, *H. influenzae*, staphylococci, streptococci, and *M. catarrhalis*
Skin and skin structure infections caused by staphylococci and/or streptococci
Bone infections caused by staphylococci and/or *P. mirabilis*
Genitourinary tract infections, including acute prostatitis, caused by *E. coli*, *P. mirabilis*, and *K. pneumoniae*
Note—Culture and susceptibility tests should be initiated prior to and during therapy. Renal function studies should be performed when indicated.

CONTRAINDICATIONS

Keflex is contraindicated in patients with known allergy to the cephalosporin group of antibiotics.

WARNINGS

BEFORE CEPHALEXIN THERAPY IS INSTITUTED, CAREFUL INQUIRY SHOULD BE MADE CONCERNING PREVIOUS HYPERSENSITIVITY REACTIONS TO CEPHALOSPORINS AND PENICILLIN. CEPHALOSPORIN C DERIVATIVES SHOULD BE GIVEN CAUTIOUSLY TO PENICILLIN-SENSITIVE PATIENTS.
SERIOUS ACUTE HYPERSENSITIVITY REACTIONS MAY REQUIRE EPINEPHRINE AND OTHER EMERGENCY MEASURES.
There is some clinical and laboratory evidence of partial cross-allergenicity of the penicillins and the cephalosporins. Patients have been reported to have had severe reactions (including anaphylaxis) to both drugs.
Any patient who has demonstrated some form of allergy, particularly to drugs, should receive antibiotics cautiously. No exception should be made with regard to Keflex.
Pseudomembranous colitis has been reported with nearly all antibacterial agents, including cephalexin, and may range from mild to life threatening. Therefore, it is important to consider this diagnosis in patients with diarrhea subsequent to the administration of antibacterial agents.
Treatment with antibacterial agents alter the normal flora of the colon and may permit overgrowth of clostridia. Studies indicate that a toxin produced by *Clostridium difficile* is one primary cause of antibiotic-associated colitis.
After the diagnosis of pseudomembranous colitis has been established, appropriate therapeutic measures should be initiated. Mild cases of pseudomembranous colitis usually respond to drug discontinuation alone. In moderate to severe cases, consideration should be given to management with fluids and electrolytes, protein supplementation, and treatment with an antibacterial drug clinically effective against *Clostridium difficile* colitis.
Usage in Pregnancy—Safety of this product for use during pregnancy has not been established.

PRECAUTIONS

General—Patients should be followed carefully so that any side effects or unusual manifestations of drug idiosyncrasy may be detected. If an allergic reaction to Keflex occurs, the drug should be discontinued and the patient treated with the usual agents (eg, epinephrine or other pressor amines, antihistamines, or corticosteroids).
Prolonged use of Keflex may result in the overgrowth of nonsusceptible organisms. Careful observation of the patient is essential. If superinfection occurs during therapy, appropriate measures should be taken.
Positive direct Coombs' tests have been reported during treatment with the cephalosporin antibiotics. In hematologic studies or in transfusion cross-matching procedures when antiglobulin tests are performed on the minor side or in Coombs' testing of newborns whose mothers have received cephalosporin antibiotics before parturition, it should be recognized that a positive Coombs' test may be due to the drug.
Keflex should be administered with caution in the presence of markedly impaired renal function. Under such conditions, careful clinical observation and laboratory studies should be made because safe dosage may be lower than that usually recommended.
Indicated surgical procedures should be performed in conjunction with antibiotic therapy.
As a result of administration of Keflex, a false-positive reaction for glucose in the urine may occur. This has been observed with Benedict's and Fehling's solutions and also with Clinitest® tablets but not with Tes-Tape® (Glucose Enzymatic Test Strip, USP).
Broad-spectrum antibiotics should be prescribed with caution in individuals with a history of gastrointestinal disease, particularly colitis.
Usage in Pregnancy—*Pregnancy Category B*—The daily oral administration of cephalexin to rats in doses of 250 or 500 mg/kg prior to and during pregnancy, or to rats and mice during the period of organogenesis only, had no adverse effect on fertility, fetal viability, fetal weight, or litter size. Note that the safety of cephalexin during pregnancy in humans has not been established.
Cephalexin showed no enhanced toxicity in weanling and newborn rats as compared with adult animals. Nevertheless, because the studies in humans cannot rule out the possibility of harm, Keflex should be used during pregnancy only if clearly needed.
Nursing Mothers—The excretion of cephalexin in the milk increased up to 4 hours after a 500-mg dose; the drug reached a maximum level of 4 μg/mL, then decreased gradually, and had disappeared 8 hours after administration. Caution should be exercised when Keflex is administered to a nursing woman.

ADVERSE REACTIONS

Gastrointestinal—Symptoms of pseudomembranous colitis may appear either during or after antibiotic treatment. Nausea and vomiting have been reported rarely. The most frequent side effect has been diarrhea. It was very rarely severe enough to warrant cessation of therapy. Dyspepsia, gastritis, and abdominal pain have also occurred. As with some penicillins and some other cephalosporins, transient hepatitis and cholestatic jaundice have been reported rarely.
Hypersensitivity—Allergic reactions in the form of rash, urticaria, angioedema, and, rarely, erythema multiforme, Stevens-Johnson syndrome, or toxic epidermal necrolysis have been observed. These reactions usually subsided upon discontinuation of the drug. In some of these reactions, supportive therapy may be necessary. Anaphylaxis has also been reported.
Other reactions have included genital and anal pruritus, genital moniliasis, vaginitis and vaginal discharge, dizziness, fatigue, headache, agitation, confusion, hallucinations, arthralgia, arthritis, and joint disorder. Reversible interstitial nephritis has been reported rarely. Eosinophilia, neutropenia, thrombocytopenia, and slight elevations in AST (SGOT) and ALT (SGPT) have been reported.

OVERDOSAGE

Signs and Symptoms—Symptoms of oral overdose may include nausea, vomiting, epigastric distress, diarrhea, and hematuria. If other symptoms are present, it is probably secondary to an underlying disease state, an allergic reaction, or toxicity due to ingestion of a second medication.
Treatment—To obtain up-to-date information about the treatment of overdose, a good resource is your certified Regional Poison Control Center. Telephone numbers of certified poison control centers are listed in the *Physicians' Desk Reference (PDR)*. In managing overdosage, consider the possibility of multiple drug overdoses, interaction among drugs, and unusual drug kinetics in your patient.
Unless 5 to 10 times the normal dose of cephalexin has been ingested, gastrointestinal decontamination should not be necessary.
Protect the patient's airway and support ventilation and perfusion. Meticulously monitor and maintain, within acceptable limits, the patient's vital signs, blood gases, serum electrolytes, etc. Absorption of drugs from the gastrointestinal tract may be decreased by giving activated charcoal, which, in many cases, is more effective than emesis or lavage; consider charcoal instead of or in addition to gastric emptying. Repeated doses of charcoal over time may hasten elimination of some drugs that have been absorbed. Safeguard the patient's airway when employing gastric emptying or charcoal.
Forced diuresis, peritoneal dialysis, hemodialysis, or charcoal hemoperfusion have not been established as beneficial for an overdose of cephalexin; however, it would be extremely unlikely that one of these procedures would be indicated.
The oral median lethal dose of cephalexin in rats is 5,000 mg/kg.

DOSAGE AND ADMINISTRATION

Keflex is administered orally.
Adults—The adult dosage ranges from 1 to 4 g daily in divided doses. The usual adult dose is 250 mg every 6 hours. For the following infections, a dosage of 500 mg may be administered every 12 hours: streptococcal pharyngitis, skin and skin structure infections, and uncomplicated cystitis in patients over 15 years of age. Cystitis therapy should be continued for 7 to 14 days. For more severe infections or those caused by less susceptible organisms, larger doses may be needed. If daily doses of Keflex greater than 4 g are required, parenteral cephalosporins, in appropriate doses, should be considered.
Children—The usual recommended daily dosage for children is 25 to 50 mg/kg in divided doses. For streptococcal pharyngitis in patients over 1 year of age and for skin and skin structure infections, the total daily dose may be divided and administered every 12 hours.

Keflex Suspension

Child's Weight	125 mg/5 mL	250 mg/5 mL
10 kg (22 lb)	1/2 to 1 tsp q.i.d.	1/4 to 1/2 tsp q.i.d.
20 kg (44 lb)	1 to 2 tsp q.i.d.	1/2 to 1 tsp q.i.d.
40 kg (88 lb)	2 to 4 tsp q.i.d.	1 to 2 tsp q.i.d.

or

Child's Weight	125 mg/5 mL	250 mg/5 mL
10 kg (22 lb)	1 to 2 tsp b.i.d.	1/2 to 1 tsp b.i.d.
20 kg (44 lb)	2 to 4 tsp b.i.d.	1 to 2 tsp b.i.d.
40 kg (88 lb)	4 to 8 tsp b.i.d.	2 to 4 tsp b.i.d.

In severe infections, the dosage may be doubled.
In the therapy of otitis media, clinical studies have shown that a dosage of 75 to 100 mg/kg/day in 4 divided doses is required.
In the treatment of β-hemolytic streptococcal infections, a therapeutic dosage of Keflex should be administered for at least 10 days.

HOW SUPPLIED

For Oral Suspension:
125 mg/5 mL (No. M-201)*—(100-mL size) NDC 0777-2321-48; (200-mL size) NDC 0777-2321-89
250 mg/5 mL (No. M-202)*—(100-mL size) NDC 0777-2368-48; (200-mL size) NDC 0777-2368-89; (5-mL size) (ID†100) NDC 0777-2368-33
Pulvules (white and dark green, size 2):
250 mg (No. 402)—(20s) NDC 0777-0869-20; (100s) NDC 0777-0869-02; (ID 100) NDC 0777-0869-33
Pulvules (light green and dark green, size 0):
500 mg (No. 403)—(20s) NDC 0777-0871-20; (100s) NDC 0777-0871-02; (ID 100) NDC 0777-0871-33

* After mixing, store in a refrigerator. May be kept for 14 days without significant loss of potency. Shake well before using. Keep tightly closed.
† Identi-Dose® (unit dose medication, Dista).

Store at controlled room temperature, 15° to 30°C (59° to 86°F).

REFERENCES

1. National Committee for Clinical Laboratory Standards: Performance standards for antimicrobial disk susceptibility tests—5th ed. Approved Standard NCCLS Document M2-A5, Vol 13, No 24, NCCLS, Villanova, PA, 1993.
2. National Committee for Clinical Laboratory Standards: Methods for dilution antimicrobial susceptibility tests for bacteria that grow aerobically—3rd ed. Approved Standard NCCLS Document M7-A3, Vol 13, No 25, NCCLS, Villanova, PA, 1993.

[091995]

KEFTAB® ℞
[*kĕf'tăb*]
(cephalexin hydrochloride)

DESCRIPTION

Keftab® (Cephalexin Hydrochloride) is a semisynthetic cephalosporin antibiotic intended for oral administration. Chemically, it is designated 7-(D-2-amino-2phenylacetamido)-3-methyl-3-cephem-4-carboxylic acid hydrochloride monohydrate, and the chemical formula is $C_{16}H_{17}N_3O_4S \cdot HCl \cdot H_2O$. The molecular weight is 401.86, and it has the following structural formula:

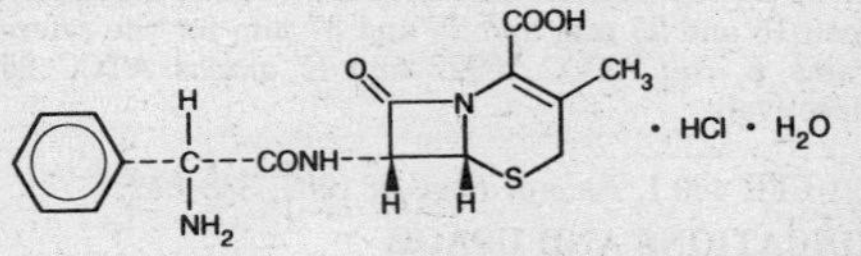

The nucleus of cephalexin hydrochloride is related to that of other cephalosporin antibiotics. The compound is the hydrochloride salt of cephalexin. The isoelectric point of cephalexin in water is approximately 4.5 to 5.
Cephalexin hydrochloride is in crystalline form and is a monohydrate. It is a white crystalline solid having a bitter taste. Solubility in water is high at room temperature; greater than 10 mg/mL may be dissolved readily.
The cephalosporins differ from penicillins in the structure of the bicyclic ring system. Cephalexin has a *D*-phenylglycyl group as substituent at the 7-amino position and an unsubstituted methyl group at the 3-position.
Each tablet contains cephalexin hydrochloride equivalent to 500 mg (1,439 μmol) cephalexin. The tablets also contain D & C Yellow No. 10, F D & C Blue No. 1, F D & C Red No. 40, magnesium stearate, silicon dioxide, stearic acid, sucrose, titanium dioxide, and other inactive ingredients.

CLINICAL PHARMACOLOGY

Human Pharmacology—Keftab is acid stable and may be given without regard to meals. It is rapidly absorbed after

Continued on next page

This product information was prepared in June 1996. Current information on these and other products of Dista Products Products Company may be obtained by direct inquiry to Lilly Research Laboratories, Lilly Corporate Center, Indianapolis, Indiana 46285, (800) 545-5979.

Dista—Cont.

oral administration. Following doses of 250 mg and 500 mg, average peak serum levels of approximately 9 and 18 μg/mL respectively were obtained at 1 hour and declined to 1.6 and 3.4 μg/mL respectively at 3 hours. Measurable levels were present 6 hours after administration. Cephalexin is excreted in the urine by glomerular filtration and tubular secretion. Studies showed that approximately 70% of the drug was excreted unchanged in the urine within 12 hours. During the first 6 hours, average urine concentrations following the 250-mg and 500-mg doses were approximately 200 μg/mL (range, 54 to 663) and 500 μg/mL (range, 137 to 1,306) respectively. The average serum half-life is 1.1 hours.

Microbiology—In vitro tests demonstrate that the cephalosporins are bactericidal because of their inhibition of cell-wall synthesis. Keftab is active against the following organisms in vitro:

β-hemolytic streptococci
Staphylococcus aureus, including penicillinase-producing strains
Streptococcus pneumoniae
Escherichia coli
Proteus mirabilis
Klebsiella sp
Haemophilus influenzae
Moraxella (Branhamella) catarrhalis

Note—Most strains of enterococci (*Enterococcus faecalis* [formerly *Streptococcus faecalis*]) and a few strains of staphylococci are resistant to Keftab. When tested by in vitro methods, staphylococci exhibit cross-resistance between Keftab and methicillin-type antibiotics. Keftab is not active against most strains of *Enterobacter* spp, *Morganella morganii* (formerly *Proteus morganii*), *Serratia* spp, and *Proteus vulgaris*. It has no activity against *Pseudomonas* or *Acinetobacter* spp.

Disk Susceptibility Tests—Quantitative methods that require measurement of zone diameters give the most precise estimates of antibiotic susceptibility. One such procedure[1] has been recommended for use with cephalosporin class (cephalothin) disks for testing susceptibility to cephalexin. The currently accepted zone diameter interpretation for the cephalothin disks[1] are appropriate for determining susceptibility to cephalexin. Interpretations correlate zone diameters of the disk test with MIC values for cephalexin. With this procedure, a report from the laboratory of "resistant" indicates a zone diameter of 14 mm or less and suggests that the infecting organism is not likely to respond to therapy. A report of "susceptibility" indicates a zone diameter of 18 mm or greater. A report of "intermediate susceptibility" indicates zone diameters between 15 and 17 mm and suggests that the organism would be susceptible if the infection is confined to the urine, in which high antibiotic levels can be obtained, or if high dosage is used in other types of infection. Standardized procedures require use of control organisms.[1] The 30-μg cephalothin disk should give zone diameters between 18 and 23 mm and 25 and 37 mm for the reference strains *E. coli* ATCC 25922 and *S. aureus* ATCC 25923 respectively.

[1] 21 CFR 460.1, *Federal Register* 1987; 838–842.

INDICATIONS AND USAGE

Keftab is indicated for the treatment of the following infections when caused by susceptible strains of the designated microorganisms:

Respiratory tract infections caused by *S. pneumoniae* and group A β-hemolytic streptococci (Penicillin is the usual drug of choice in the treatment and prevention of streptococcal infections, including the prophylaxis of rheumatic fever. Keftab is generally effective in the eradication of streptococci from the nasopharynx; however, substantial data establishing the efficacy of Keftab in the subsequent prevention of rheumatic fever are not available at present.)

Skin and skin structure infections caused by *S. aureus* and/or β-hemolytic streptococci.

Bone infections caused by *S. aureus* and/or *P. mirabilis.*

Genitourinary tract infections, including acute prostatitis, caused by *E. coli, P. mirabilis,* and *Klebsiella* spp.

Note—Culture and susceptibility tests should be initiated prior to and during therapy. Renal function studies should be performed when indicated.

CONTRAINDICATION

Keftab is contraindicated in patients with known allergy to the cephalosporin group of antibiotics.

WARNINGS

BEFORE CEPHALEXIN THERAPY IS INSTITUTED, CAREFUL INQUIRY SHOULD BE MADE CONCERNING PREVIOUS HYPERSENSITIVITY REACTIONS TO CEPHALOSPORINS AND PENICILLIN. CEPHALOSPORIN C DERIVATIVES SHOULD BE GIVEN CAUTIOUSLY TO PENICILLIN-SENSITIVE PATIENTS.

SERIOUS ACUTE HYPERSENSITIVITY REACTIONS MAY REQUIRE EPINEPHRINE AND OTHER EMERGENCY MEASURES.

There is some clinical and laboratory evidence of partial cross-allergenicity of the penicillins and the cephalosporins. Patients have been reported to have had severe reactions (including anaphylaxis) to both drugs.

Any patient who has demonstrated some form of allergy, particularly to drugs, should receive antibiotics cautiously. No exception should be made with regard to Keftab.

Pseudomembranous colitis has been reported with virtually all broad-spectrum antibiotics (including macrolides, semisynthetic penicillins, and cephalosporins); therefore, it is important to consider its diagnosis in patients who develop diarrhea in association with the use of antibiotics. Such colitis may range in severity from mild to life threatening.

Treatment with broad-spectrum antibiotics alters the normal flora of the colon and may permit overgrowth of clostridia. Studies indicate that a toxin produced by *Clostridium difficile* is a primary cause of antibiotic-associated colitis.

Mild cases of pseudomembranous colitis usually respond to drug discontinuance alone. In moderate to severe cases, management should include sigmoidoscopy, appropriate bacteriologic studies, and fluid, electrolyte, and protein supplementation. When the colitis does not improve after the drug has been discontinued or when it is severe, treatment with an oral antibacterial drug effective against *C. difficile* is recommended. Other causes of colitis should be ruled out.

PRECAUTIONS

General—Patients should be followed carefully so that any side effects or unusual manifestations of drug idiosyncrasy may be detected. If an allergic reaction to Keftab occurs, the drug should be discontinued and the patient treated with the usual agents (eg, epinephrine or other pressor amines, antihistamines, or corticosteroids).

Prolonged use of Keftab may result in the overgrowth of nonsusceptible organisms. Careful observation of the patient is essential. If superinfection occurs during therapy, appropriate measures should be taken.

Positive direct Coombs' tests have been reported during treatment with the cephalosporin antibiotics. In hematologic studies or in transfusion cross-matching procedures when antiglobulin tests are performed on the minor side or in Coombs' testing of newborns whose mothers have received cephalosporin antibiotics before parturition, it should be recognized that a positive Coombs' test may be due to the drug.

Keftab should be administered with caution in the presence of markedly impaired renal function. Under such conditions, careful clinical observation and laboratory studies should be made because safe dosage may be lower than that usually recommended.

As a result of administration of Keftab, a false-positive reaction for glucose in the urine may occur. This has been observed with Benedict's and Fehling's solutions and also with Clinitest® tablets but not with Tes-Tape® (Glucose Enzymatic Test Strip, USP).

Broad-spectrum antibiotics should be prescribed with caution in individuals with a history of gastrointestinal disease, particularly colitis.

Pregnancy—Pregnancy Category B—Reproduction studies have been performed on rats in doses of 250 or 500 mg/kg/day and have revealed no evidence of impaired fertility or harm to the fetus due to cephalexin. There are, however, no adequate and well-controlled studies in pregnant women. Because animal reproduction studies are not always predictive of human response, this drug should be used during pregnancy only if clearly needed.

Nursing Mothers—The excretion of cephalexin in the milk increased up to 4 hours after a 500-mg dose; the drug reached a maximum level of 4 μg/mL, then decreased gradually, and had disappeared 8 hours after administration. A decision should be considered to discontinue nursing temporarily during therapy with Keftab.

Pediatric Use—Safety and effectiveness in children have not been established.

ADVERSE REACTIONS

Gastrointestinal—Symptoms of pseudomembranous colitis may appear either during or after antibiotic treatment. Nausea and vomiting have been reported rarely. The most frequent side effect has been diarrhea. It was very rarely severe enough to warrant cessation of therapy. Abdominal pain, gastritis, and dyspepsia have also occurred. As with some penicillins and some other cephalosporins, transient hepatitis and cholestatic jaundice have been reported rarely.

Hypersensitivity—Allergic reactions in the form of rash, urticaria, angioedema, and, rarely, erythema multiforme, Stevens-Johnson syndrome, or toxic epidermal necrolysis have been observed. These reactions usually subsided upon discontinuation of the drug. In some of these reactions, supportive therapy may be necessary. Anaphylaxis has also been reported.

Other reactions have included genital and anal pruritus, genital moniliasis, vaginitis and vaginal discharge, dizziness, fatigue, headache, agitation, confusion, hallucinations, arthralgia, arthritis, and joint disorder. Reversible interstitial nephritis has been reported rarely. Eosinophilia, neutropenia, thrombocytopenia, slight elevations in aspartate aminotransferase (AST, SGOT) and alanine aminotransferase (ALT, SGPT), and elevated creatinine and BUN have been reported.

In addition to the adverse reactions listed above that have been observed in patients treated with Keftab, the following adverse reactions and altered laboratory tests have been reported for cephalosporin class antibiotics:

Adverse Reactions—Allergic reactions, including fever, colitis, renal dysfunction, toxic nephropathy, and hepatic dysfunction, including cholestasis.

Several cephalosporins have been implicated in triggering seizures, particularly in patients with renal impairment when the dosage was not reduced (*see* Indications and Usage *and* Precautions, General). If seizures associated with drug therapy should occur, the drug should be discontinued. Anticonvulsant therapy can be given if clinically indicated.

Altered Laboratory Tests—Increased prothrombin time, increased alkaline phosphatase, and leukopenia.

OVERDOSAGE

Signs and Symptoms—Symptoms of oral overdose may include nausea, vomiting, epigastric distress, diarrhea, and hematuria. If other symptoms are present, it is probably secondary to an underlying disease state, an allergic reaction, or toxicity due to ingestion of a second medication.

Treatment—To obtain up-to-date information about the treatment of overdose, a good resource is your certified Regional Poison Control Center. Telephone numbers of certified poison control centers are listed in the *Physicians' Desk Reference (PDR).* In managing overdosage, consider the possibility of multiple drug overdoses, interaction among drugs, and unusual drug kinetics in your patient.

Unless 5 to 10 times the normal dose of cephalexin has been ingested, gastrointestinal decontamination should not be necessary.

Protect the patient's airway and support ventilation and perfusion. Meticulously monitor and maintain, within acceptable limits, the patient's vital signs, blood gases, serum electrolytes, etc. Absorption of drugs from the gastrointestinal tract may be decreased by giving activated charcoal, which, in many cases, is more effective than emesis or lavage; consider charcoal instead of or in addition to gastric emptying. Repeated doses of charcoal over time may hasten elimination of some drugs that have been absorbed. Safeguard the patient's airway when employing gastric emptying or charcoal.

Forced diuresis, peritoneal dialysis, hemodialysis, or charcoal hemoperfusion have not been established as beneficial for an overdose of cephalexin; however, it would be extremely unlikely that one of these procedures would be indicated.

The oral median lethal dose of cephalexin in rats is 5,000 mg/kg.

DOSAGE AND ADMINISTRATION

Keftab is administered orally.

The adult dosage ranges from 1 to 4 g daily in divided doses. For the following infections, a dosage of 500 mg may be administered every 12 hours: streptococcal pharyngitis, skin and skin structure infections, and uncomplicated cystitis. Cystitis therapy should be continued for 7 to 14 days. For other infections, the usual dose is 250 mg every 6 hours. For more severe infections or those caused by less susceptible organisms, larger doses may be needed. If daily doses of Keftab greater than 4 g are required, parenteral cephalosporins, in appropriate doses, should be considered.

HOW SUPPLIED

Tablets (elliptical-shaped):

500 mg* (dark-green) (No. 4143)—(100s) NDC 0777-4143-02

Store at controlled room temperature, 59° to 86°F (15° to 30°C).

* Equivalent to cephalexin.

[050796]

METUBINE® IODIDE ℞

[*mĕ-tū 'bēn ī-ō-dīd*]

(Metocurine Iodide Injection, USP)

THIS DRUG SHOULD BE ADMINISTERED ONLY BY ADEQUATELY TRAINED INDIVIDUALS WHO ARE FAMILIAR WITH ITS ACTIONS, CHARACTERISTICS, AND HAZARDS.

DESCRIPTION

Metubine® Iodide (Metocurine Iodide Injection, USP) is a nondepolarizing muscle relaxant and is presented as a sterile isotonic solution for intravenous injection. It is (+)-*O, O'*-Dimethylchondrocurarine diiodide.

The empirical formula is $C_{40}H_{48}I_2N_2O_6$, and the molecular weight is 906.64.
The structural formula is as follows:

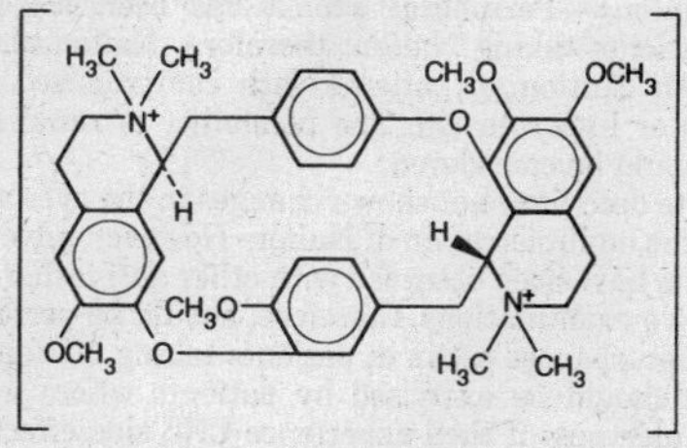

Each mL contains 2 mg (2.2 μmol) metocurine iodide and sodium chloride, 0.9%, with 0.5% phenol as a preservative. Sodium carbonate and/or hydrochloric acid may have been added during manufacture to adjust the pH in the range of 4 to 6.

CLINICAL PHARMACOLOGY

Metubine Iodide is a methyl analogue of tubocurarine which produces nondepolarizing (competitive) neuromuscular blockade at the myoneural junction. Recent animal studies suggest that Metubine Iodide does not produce the autonomic ganglionic blockade seen with other nondepolarizing muscle relaxants. Recent clinical findings suggest that Metubine Iodide reaches the neuromuscular junction more rapidly than does tubocurarine. After intravenous injection, there is rapid onset (1 to 4 minutes) of muscle relaxation with maximum twitch inhibition (96%) in 1.5 to 10 minutes. The maximum effect lasts 35 to 60 minutes. The time for recovery to 50% of control twitch response is in excess of 3 hours.
Following bolus injection of 0.05 mg/kg, the mean terminal half-life of Metubine Iodide was 3.6 hours (217 minutes). Approximately 50% of the dose was excreted as unchanged drug in the urine over 48 hours, and 2% was excreted unchanged in the bile. Approximately 35% is protein bound, mainly to the beta and gamma globulins.
The use of repeated doses may be accompanied by a cumulative effect. The duration of action and degree of muscle relaxation may be altered by dehydration, body temperature changes, hypocalcemia, excess magnesium, or acid-base imbalance. Concurrently administered general anesthetics, certain antibiotics, and neuromuscular disease may potentiate the neuromuscular blocking action of Metubine Iodide.
Histamine release with Metubine Iodide occurs less frequently than with *d*-tubocurarine and is related to dosage and rapidity of administration. Effects on the cardiovascular system (eg, changes in pulse rate, hypotension) are less than those reported with equipotent doses of *d*-tubocurarine and gallamine.
Because the main excretory pathway for Metubine Iodide is through the kidneys, severe renal disease or conditions associated with poor renal perfusion (shock states) may result in prolonged neuromuscular blockade.
Following intravenous injection in the mother, placental transfer of Metubine Iodide occurs rapidly, and, after 6 minutes, the fetal plasma concentration is approximately one-tenth the maternal level.

INDICATIONS AND USAGE

Metubine Iodide is indicated as an adjunct to anesthesia to induce skeletal-muscle relaxation. It may be employed to reduce the intensity of muscle contractions in pharmacologically or electrically induced convulsions. It may also be employed to facilitate the management of patients undergoing mechanical ventilation.

CONTRAINDICATIONS

Metubine Iodide is contraindicated in those persons with known hypersensitivity to the drug or to its iodide content.

WARNINGS

METUBINE IODIDE SHOULD BE ADMINISTERED IN CAREFULLY ADJUSTED DOSES BY OR UNDER THE SUPERVISION OF EXPERIENCED CLINICIANS WHO ARE FAMILIAR WITH THE COMPLICATIONS WHICH MAY OCCUR WITH THE USE OF THIS DRUG. Metubine Iodide should not be administered unless facilities for intubation, artificial ventilation, oxygen therapy, and reversal agents are immediately available. The clinician must be prepared to assist or control respiration.
Metubine Iodide should be used with extreme caution in patients with myasthenia gravis. In such patients, a peripheral nerve stimulator may be valuable in assessing the effects of administration.

PRECAUTIONS

General—Metubine Iodide should be used with caution in patients with poor renal perfusion or severe renal disease (*see* Clinical Pharmacology).
Rapid administration of large doses of Metubine Iodide may produce changes in blood pressure or heart rate or signs of histamine release.
Metubine Iodide has no effect on consciousness, pain threshold, or cerebration; therefore, it should be used with adequate anesthesia.
Drug Interactions—Synergistic or antagonistic effects may result when depolarizing and nondepolarizing muscle relaxants are administered simultaneously or sequentially.
Parenteral administration of high doses of certain antibiotics may intensify or resemble the neuroblocking action of muscle relaxants. These include neomycin, streptomycin, bacitracin, kanamycin, gentamicin, dihydrostreptomycin, polymyxin B, colistin, sodium colistimethate, and tetracyclines. If muscle relaxants and antibiotics must be administered simultaneously, the patient should be observed closely for any unexpected prolongation of respiratory depression.
Certain general anesthetics have a synergistic action with neuromuscular blocking agents. Diethyl ether, halothane, and isoflurane potentiate the neuromuscular blocking action of other nondepolarizing agents and may be presumed to do so with Metubine Iodide.
Administration of quinidine shortly after recovery may produce recurrent paralysis.
The effect of diazepam on neuromuscular blockade by Metubine Iodide is not clear. Until more information is available, patients should be carefully monitored for unexpected drug response and prolongation of action.
The use of magnesium sulfate in preeclamptic patients potentiates the effects of both depolarizing and nondepolarizing muscle relaxants.
Usage in Pregnancy—Pregnancy Category C—Intrauterine growth retardation and limb deformities resembling clubfoot were produced by *d*-tubocurarine chloride and succinylcholine chloride when administered to the rat fetus between the 16th and 19th days of gestation or when injected in chick embryos from the 5th to the 15th day of incubation. When *d*-tubocurarine was injected intramuscularly into the interscapular region of the fetuses on the 16th to the 19th day of gestation, the incidence of growth retardation and limb deformity ranged from 21 to 23% and 7 to 8% respectively.
There are no adequate and well-controlled studies of Metubine Iodide in pregnant women. Metubine Iodide should be used during pregnancy only if the potential benefit justifies the risk to the fetus.
Labor and Delivery—It is not known whether the use of muscle relaxants during labor or delivery has immediate or delayed adverse effects on the fetus, prolongs the duration of labor, or increases the likelihood that forceps delivery, obstetric intervention, or resuscitation of the newborn will be necessary.
Nursing Mothers—It is not known whether Metubine Iodide is excreted in human milk. Because many drugs are excreted in human milk, caution should be exercised when Metubine Iodide is administered to a nursing woman.
Usage in Children—A clinical study has shown that Metubine Iodide is twice as potent as *d*-tubocurarine in children, but the rate of recovery is the same. There may be a slight increase in heart rate, but no change occurs in blood pressure or ECG. Doses calculated on the basis of body weight or body surface area may be applicable when the advantages of nondepolarizing neuromuscular blockade are desired.

ADVERSE REACTIONS

The most frequently noted adverse reaction is prolongation of the drug's pharmacologic action. Neuromuscular effects may range from skeletal-muscle weakness to a profound relaxation that produces respiratory insufficiency or apnea.
Possible adverse reactions include allergic or hypersensitivity reactions to the drug or its iodide content and histamine release when large doses are administered rapidly. Signs of histamine release include erythema, edema, flushing, tachycardia, arterial hypotension, bronchospasm, and circulatory collapse.
Prolonged apnea and respiratory depression have occurred following the use of muscle relaxants. Many physiologic factors, drug interactions, and individual sensitivities may contribute to the development of respiratory paralysis (*see* Clinical Pharmacology *and* Precautions).

OVERDOSAGE

To obtain up-to-date information about the treatment of overdose, a good resource is your certified Regional Poison Control Center. Telephone numbers of certified poison control centers are listed in the *Physicians' Desk Reference (PDR).* In managing overdosage, consider the possibility of multiple drug overdoses, interaction among drugs, and unusual drug kinetics in your patient.
An overdose of Metubine Iodide may result in prolonged apnea, cardiovascular collapse, and sudden release of histamine.
Massive doses of metocurarine are not reversible by the antagonists edrophonium or neostigmine and atropine.
Overdosage may be avoided by the careful monitoring of response by means of a peripheral nerve stimulator.
The primary treatment for residual neuromuscular blockade with respiratory paralysis or inadequate ventilation is maintenance of the patient's airway and manual or mechanical ventilation.
Accompanying derangements of blood pressure, electrolyte imbalance, or circulating blood volume should be determined and corrected by appropriate fluid and electrolyte therapy.
Residual neuromuscular blockade following surgery may be reversed by the use of anticholinesterase inhibitors such as neostigmine or pyridostigmine bromide and atropine. Prescribing information should be consulted for the appropriate drug selection based on dosage and desired duration of action.

DOSAGE AND ADMINISTRATION

Metubine Iodide should be administered intravenously as a sustained injection over a period of 30 to 60 seconds. INTRAMUSCULAR ADMINISTRATION OF METUBINE IODIDE IS NOT RECOMMENDED. Care must be taken to avoid overdosage. The use of a peripheral nerve stimulator to monitor response will minimize the risk of overdosage. The type of anesthetic used and nature of the surgical procedure will influence the amount of Metubine Iodide required. Doses of 0.2 to 0.4 mg/ kg have been found satisfactory for endotracheal intubation. Relaxation following the initial dose may be expected to be effective for periods of 25 to 90 minutes, with an average of approximately 60 minutes. Supplemental administration may be made as indicated to provide needed surgical relaxation. Supplemental doses average 0.5 to 1 mg.
The use of strong anesthetics that potentiate the effect of neuromuscular blocking drugs such as halothane, diethyl ether, isoflurane, or enflurane reduces the requirement for Metubine Iodide. Incremental doses should be reduced by approximately one-third to one-half.
Recommended Doses for Use During Electroshock Therapy—Doses required for satisfactory relaxation range from 1.75 to 5.5 mg. When the patient is treated for the 1st time, the drug is administered slowly by the intravenous route as a sustained injection until a head-drop response ensues. After dosage has been established, subsequent injections are completed in 15 to 50 seconds. The average dose ranges from 2 to 3 mg.
Drug Incompatibilities—Metubine Iodide is unstable in alkaline solutions. When it is combined with barbiturate solutions, precipitation may occur. Solutions of barbiturates, meperidine, and morphine sulfate should not be administered from the same syringe.
Parenteral drug products should be inspected visually for particulate matter and discoloration prior to administration, whenever solution and container permit.

HOW SUPPLIED

Multiple-Dose Vials:
2 mg/mL, 20 mL (No. 586) (1s), NDC 0777-1421-01
Store at controlled room temperature, 59° to 86°F (15° to 30°C).
Metubine Iodide is a clear, colorless solution.

[060893]

NALFON® ℞
[*năl'fŏn*]
NALFON® 200
(fenoprofen calcium)
USP

DESCRIPTION

Nalfon® (Fenoprofen Calcium, USP) is a nonsteroidal, antiinflammatory, antiarthritic drug. Pulvules® Nalfon contain fenoprofen calcium as the dihydrate in an amount equivalent to 200 mg (0.826 mmol) or 300 mg (1.24 mmol) of fenoprofen. The Pulvules also contain cellulose, gelatin, iron oxides, silicone, titanium dioxide, and other inactive ingredients. The 300-mg Pulvules also contain D & C Yellow No. 10 and F D & C Yellow No. 6.
Tablets Nalfon contain fenoprofen calcium as the dihydrate in an amount equivalent to 600 mg (2.48 mmol) of fenoprofen. The tablets also contain amberlite, benzyl alcohol, calcium phosphate, cornstarch, D & C Yellow No. 10, F D & C Yellow No. 6, hydroxypropyl methylcellulose, magnesium stearate, polyethylene glycol, stearic acid, titanium dioxide, and other inactive ingredients.
Chemically, Nalfon is an arylacetic acid derivative.
The structural formula is as follows:
[See chemical structure at top of next column.]
Benzeneacetic acid, α-methyl-3-phenoxy-, calcium salt dihydrate, (±)-
Nalfon is a white crystalline powder that has the empirical formula $C_{30}H_{26}CaO_6 \cdot 2H_2O$ representing a molecular weight

Continued on next page

This product information was prepared in June 1996. Current information on these and other products of Dista Products Products Company may be obtained by direct inquiry to Lilly Research Laboratories, Lilly Corporate Center, Indianapolis, Indiana 46285, (800) 545-5979.

Dista—Cont.

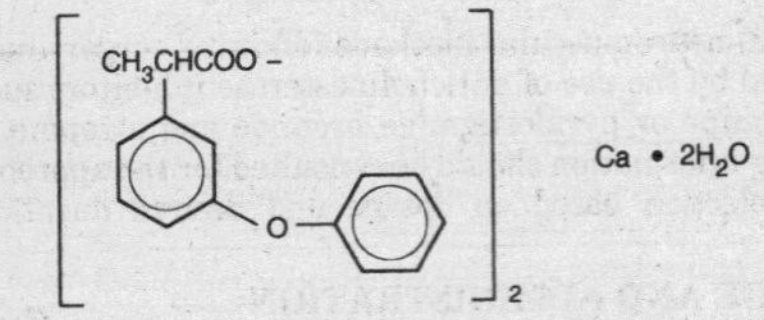

of 558.64. At 25°C, it dissolves to a 15 mg/mL solution in alcohol (95%). It is slightly soluble in water and insoluble in benzene.

The *p* Ka of Nalfon is 4.5 at 25°C.

CLINICAL PHARMACOLOGY

Nalfon is a nonsteroidal, anti-inflammatory, antiarthritic drug that also possesses analgesic and antipyretic activities. Its exact mode of action is unknown, but it is thought that prostaglandin synthetase inhibition is involved. Nalfon has been shown to inhibit prostaglandin synthetase isolated from bovine seminal vesicles. Reproduction studies in rats have shown Nalfon to be associated with prolonged labor and difficult parturition when given during late pregnancy. Evidence suggests that this may be due to decreased uterine contractility resulting from the inhibition of prostaglandin synthesis. Its action is not mediated through the adrenal gland.

Fenoprofen shows anti-inflammatory effects in rodents by inhibiting the development of redness and edema in acute inflammatory conditions and by reducing soft-tissue swelling and bone damage associated with chronic inflammation. It exhibits analgesic activity in rodents by inhibiting the writhing response caused by the introduction of an irritant into the peritoneal cavities of mice and by elevating pain thresholds that are related to pressure in edematous hindpaws of rats. In rats made febrile by the subcutaneous administration of brewer's yeast, fenoprofen produces antipyretic action. These effects are characteristic of nonsteroidal, anti-inflammatory, antipyretic, analgesic drugs.

The results in humans confirmed the anti-inflammatory and analgesic actions found in animals. The emergence and degree of erythemic response were measured in adult male volunteers exposed to ultraviolet irradiation. The effects of Nalfon, aspirin, and indomethacin were each compared with those of a placebo. All 3 drugs demonstrated antierythemic activity.

In patients with rheumatoid arthritis, the anti-inflammatory action of Nalfon has been evidenced by relief of pain, increase in grip strength, and reductions in joint swelling, duration of morning stiffness, and disease activity (as assessed by both the investigator and the patient). The anti-inflammatory action of Nalfon has also been evidenced by increased mobility (ie, a decrease in the number of joints having limited motion).

The use of Nalfon in combination with gold salts or corticosteroids has been studied in patients with rheumatoid arthritis. The studies, however, were inadequate in demonstrating whether further improvement is obtained by adding Nalfon to maintenance therapy with gold salts or steroids. Whether or not Nalfon used in conjunction with partially effective doses of a corticosteroid has a "steroid-sparing" effect is unknown.

In patients with osteoarthritis, the anti-inflammatory and analgesic effects of Nalfon have been demonstrated by reduction in tenderness as a response to pressure and reductions in night pain, stiffness, swelling, and overall disease activity (as assessed by both the patient and the investigator). These effects have also been demonstrated by relief of pain with motion and at rest and increased range of motion in involved joints.

In patients with rheumatoid arthritis and osteoarthritis, clinical studies have shown Nalfon to be comparable to aspirin in controlling the aforementioned measures of disease activity, but mild gastrointestinal reactions (nausea, dyspepsia) and tinnitus occurred less frequently in patients treated with Nalfon than in aspirin-treated patients. It is not known whether Nalfon causes less peptic ulceration than does aspirin.

In patients with pain, the analgesic action of Nalfon has produced a reduction in pain intensity, an increase in pain relief, improvement in total analgesia scores, and a sustained analgesic effect.

Under fasting conditions, Nalfon is rapidly absorbed, and peak plasma levels of 50 μg/mL are achieved within 2 hours after oral administration of 600-mg doses. Good dose proportionality was observed between 200-mg and 600-mg doses in fasting male volunteers. The plasma half-life is approximately 3 hours. About 90% of a single oral dose is eliminated within 24 hours as fenoprofen glucuronide and 4′-hydroxyfenoprofen glucuronide, the major urinary metabolites of fenoprofen. Fenoprofen is highly bound (99%) to albumin.

The concomitant administration of antacid (containing both aluminum and magnesium hydroxide) does not interfere with absorption of Nalfon.

There is less suppression of collagen-induced platelet aggregation with single doses of Nalfon than there is with aspirin.

INDICATIONS AND USAGE

Nalfon is indicated for relief of the signs and symptoms of rheumatoid arthritis and osteoarthritis. It is recommended for the treatment of acute flare-ups and exacerbations and for the long-term management of these diseases.

Nalfon is also indicated for the relief of mild to moderate pain.

CONTRAINDICATIONS

Nalfon® (Fenoprofen Calcium, USP) is contraindicated in patients who have shown hypersensitivity to it.

The drug should not be administered to patients with a history of significantly impaired renal function.

Nalfon should not be given to patients in whom aspirin and other nonsteroidal anti-inflammatory drugs induce the symptoms of asthma, rhinitis, or urticaria, because cross-sensitivity to these drugs occurs in a high proportion of such patients.

WARNINGS

Risk of GI Ulceration, Bleeding, and Perforation with NSAID Therapy—Serious gastrointestinal toxicity, such as bleeding, ulceration, and perforation, can occur at any time, with or without warning symptoms, in patients treated chronically with NSAID therapy. Although minor upper gastrointestinal problems, such as dyspepsia, are common, usually developing early in therapy, physicians should remain alert for ulceration and bleeding in patients treated chronically with NSAIDs, even in the absence of previous GI tract symptoms. In patients observed in clinical trials of several months to 2 years duration, symptomatic upper GI ulcers, gross bleeding, or perforation appear to occur in approximately 1% of patients treated for 3 to 6 months, and in about 2% to 4% of patients treated for 1 year. Physicians should inform patients about the signs and/or symptoms of serious GI toxicity and what steps to take if they occur.

Studies to date have not identified any subset of patients not at risk of developing peptic ulceration and bleeding. Except for a prior history of serious GI events and other risk factors known to be associated with peptic ulcer disease, such as alcoholism, smoking, etc, no risk factors (eg, age, sex) have been associated with increased risk. Elderly or debilitated patients seem to tolerate ulceration or bleeding less well than other individuals and most spontaneous reports of fatal GI events are in this population. Studies to date are inconclusive concerning the relative risk of various NSAIDs in causing such reactions. High doses of any NSAID probably carry a greater risk of these reactions, although controlled clinical trials showing this do not exist in most cases. In considering the use of relatively large doses (within the recommended dosage range), sufficient benefit should be anticipated to offset the potential increased risk of GI toxicity.

Since Nalfon has been marketed, there have been reports of genitourinary tract problems in patients taking it. The most frequently reported problems have been episodes of dysuria, cystitis, hematuria, interstitial nephritis, and nephrotic syndrome. This syndrome may be preceded by the appearance of fever, rash, arthralgia, oliguria, and azotemia and may progress to anuria. There may also be substantial proteinuria, and, on renal biopsy, electron microscopy has shown foot process fusion and T-lymphocyte infiltration in the renal interstitium. Early recognition of the syndrome and withdrawal of the drug have been followed by rapid recovery. Administration of steroids and the use of dialysis have also been included in the treatment. Because a syndrome with some of these characteristics has also been reported with other nonsteroidal anti-inflammatory drugs, it is recommended that patients who have had these reactions with other such drugs not be treated with Nalfon. In patients with possibly compromised renal function, periodic renal function examinations should be done.

PRECAUTIONS

General—Renal Effects—There have been reports of acute interstitial nephritis and nephrotic syndrome (*see* Contraindications *and* Warnings).

A second form of renal toxicity has been seen in patients with prerenal conditions leading to a reduction in renal blood flow or blood volume, in which renal prostaglandins play a supportive role in the maintenance of renal perfusion. In these patients, administration of an NSAID may cause a dose-dependent reduction in prostaglandin formation and may precipitate overt renal decompensation at any time. Patients at greatest risk for this reaction are those with impaired renal function, heart failure, liver dysfunction, those taking diuretics, and the elderly. Discontinuation of NSAID therapy is typically followed by recovery to the pretreatment state.

Since Nalfon is primarily eliminated by the kidneys, patients with possibly compromised renal function (such as the elderly) should be monitored periodically, especially during long-term therapy. For such patients, it may be anticipated that a lower daily dosage will avoid excessive drug accumulation.

Miscellaneous—Peripheral edema has been observed in some patients taking Nalfon; therefore, Nalfon should be used with caution in patients with compromised cardiac function or hypertension. The possibility of renal involvement should be considered.

Studies to date have not shown changes in the eyes attributable to the administration of Nalfon. However, adverse ocular effects have been observed with other anti-inflammatory drugs. Eye examinations, therefore, should be performed if visual disturbances occur in patients taking Nalfon.

Caution should be exercised by patients whose activities require alertness if they experience CNS side effects while taking Nalfon.

Since the safety of Nalfon has not been established in patients with impaired hearing, these patients should have periodic tests of auditory function during prolonged therapy with Nalfon.

Information for Patients—Nalfon, like other drugs of its class, is not free of side effects. The side effects of these drugs can cause discomfort and, rarely, there are more serious side effects, such as gastrointestinal bleeding, which may result in hospitalization and even fatal outcomes.

NSAIDs (Nonsteroidal Anti-Inflammatory Drugs) are often essential agents in the management of arthritis and have a major role in the treatment of pain, but they also may be commonly employed for conditions which are less serious. Physicians may wish to discuss with their patients the potential risks (*see* Warnings, Precautions, *and* Adverse Reactions sections) and likely benefits of NSAID treatment, particularly when the drugs are used for less serious conditions where treatment without NSAIDs may represent an acceptable alternative to both the patient and physician.

Laboratory Tests—In chronic studies in rats, high doses of Nalfon caused elevation of serum transaminase and hepatocellular hypertrophy. In clinical trials, some patients developed elevation of serum transaminase, LDH, and alkaline phosphatase that persisted for some months and usually, but not always, declined despite continuation of the drug. The significance of this is unknown. It is recommended, therefore, that Nalfon be discontinued if any significant liver abnormality occurs.

As with other nonsteroidal anti-inflammatory drugs, borderline elevations in 1 or more liver tests may occur in up to 15% of patients. These abnormalities may progress, may remain essentially unchanged, or may be transient with continued therapy. The SGPT (ALT) test is probably the most sensitive indicator of liver dysfunction. Meaningful (ie, 3 times the upper limit of normal) elevations of SGPT or SGOT (AST) occurred in controlled clinical trials in less than 1% of patients. A patient with symptoms and/or signs suggesting liver dysfunction, or in whom an abnormal liver test has occurred, should be evaluated for evidence of the development of more severe hepatic reactions while using Nalfon. Severe hepatic reactions, including jaundice and cases of fatal hepatitis, have been reported with Nalfon, as with other nonsteroidal anti-inflammatory drugs. As a result, during long-term therapy, liver function tests should be monitored periodically. Although such reactions are rare, if liver tests continue to be abnormal or worsen, if clinical signs and symptoms consistent with liver disease develop, or if systemic manifestations occur (eg, eosinophilia and rash), Nalfon should be discontinued. If this drug is to be used in the presence of impaired liver function, it must be done under strict observation.

Patients with initial low hemoglobin values who are receiving long-term therapy with Nalfon should have a hemoglobin determination made at reasonable intervals.

Nalfon decreases platelet aggregation and may prolong bleeding time. Patients who may be adversely affected by prolongation of the bleeding time should be carefully observed when Nalfon is administered.

Because serious GI tract ulceration and bleeding can occur without warning symptoms, physicians should follow chronically treated patients for the signs and symptoms of ulceration and bleeding and should inform them of the importance of this follow-up (*see* Risk of GI Ulceration, Bleeding, and Perforation with NSAID Therapy *under* Warnings).

Laboratory Test Interactions—Amerlex-M kit assay values of total and free triiodothyronine in patients receiving Nalfon have been reported as falsely elevated on the basis of a chemical cross-reaction that directly interferes with the assay. Thyroid-stimulating hormone, total thyroxine, and thyrotropin-releasing hormone response are not affected.

Drug Interactions—The coadministration of aspirin decreases the biologic half-life of fenoprofen because of an increase in metabolic clearance that results in a greater amount of hydroxylated fenoprofen in the urine. Although the mechanism of interaction between fenoprofen and aspirin is not totally known, enzyme induction and displacement of fenoprofen from plasma albumin binding sites are possibilities. Because Nalfon has not been shown to produce any additional effect beyond that obtained with aspirin alone and because aspirin increases the rate of excretion of Nalfon,

the concomitant use of Nalfon and salicylates is not recommended.

Chronic administration of phenobarbital, a known enzyme inducer, may be associated with a decrease in the plasma half-life of fenoprofen. When phenobarbital is added to or withdrawn from treatment, dosage adjustment of Nalfon may be required.

In vitro studies have shown that fenoprofen, because of its affinity for albumin, may displace from their binding sites other drugs that are also albumin bound, and this may lead to drug interaction. Theoretically, fenoprofen could likewise be displaced. Patients receiving hydantoin, sulfonamides, or sulfonylureas should be observed for increased activity of these drugs and, therefore, signs of toxicity from these drugs. In patients receiving coumarin-type anticoagulants, the addition of Nalfon to therapy could prolong the prothrombin time. Patients receiving both drugs should be under careful observation. Patients treated with Nalfon may be resistant to the effects of loop diuretics.

In patients receiving Nalfon and a steroid concomitantly, any reduction in steroid dosage should be gradual in order to avoid the possible complications of sudden steroid withdrawal.

Usage in Pregnancy—Safe use of Nalfon during pregnancy and lactation has not been established; therefore, administration to pregnant patients and nursing mothers is not recommended. Reproduction studies have been performed in rats and rabbits. When fenoprofen was given to rats during pregnancy and continued until the time of labor, parturition was prolonged. Similar results have been found with other nonsteroidal anti-inflammatory drugs that inhibit prostaglandin synthetase.

Usage in Children—Fenoprofen calcium is not recommended for use in children because documented clinical experience has been insufficient to establish safety and a suitable dosage regimen in the pediatric age group.

ADVERSE REACTIONS

During clinical studies for rheumatoid arthritis, osteoarthritis, or mild to moderate pain and studies of pharmacokinetics, complaints were compiled from a checklist of potential adverse reactions, and the following data emerged. These encompass observations in 6,786 patients, including 188 observed for at least 52 weeks. For comparison, data are also presented from complaints received from the 266 patients who received placebo in these same trials. During short-term studies for analgesia, the incidence of adverse reactions was markedly lower than that seen in longer-term studies.

INCIDENCE GREATER THAN 1%

Probable Causal Relationship

Digestive System—During clinical trials with Nalfon, the most common adverse reactions were gastrointestinal in nature and occurred in 20.8% of patients receiving Nalfon as compared to 16.9% of patients receiving placebo. In descending order of frequency, these reactions included dyspepsia (10.3%, Nalfon, vs 2.3%, placebo), nausea (7.7% vs 7.1%), constipation (7% vs 1.5%), vomiting (2.6% vs 1.9%), abdominal pain (2% vs 1.1%), and diarrhea (1.8% vs 4.1%).

The drug was discontinued because of adverse gastrointestinal reactions in less than 2% of patients during premarketing studies.

Nervous System—The most frequent adverse neurologic reactions were headache (8.7% treated vs 7.5% placebo) and somnolence (8.5% vs 6.4%). Dizziness (6.5% vs 5.6%), tremor (2.2% vs 0.4%), and confusion (1.4% vs none) were noted less frequently.

Nalfon was discontinued in less than 0.5% of patients because of these side effects during premarketing studies.

Skin and Appendages—Increased sweating (4.6% vs 0.4%), pruritus (4.2% vs 0.8%), and rash (3.7% vs 0.4%) were reported.

Nalfon was discontinued in about 1% of patients because of an adverse effect related to the skin during premarketing studies.

Special Senses—Tinnitus (4.5% vs 0.4%), blurred vision (2.2% vs none), and decreased hearing (1.6% vs none) were reported.

Nalfon was discontinued in less than 0.5% of patients because of adverse effects related to the special senses during premarketing studies.

Cardiovascular—Palpitations (2.5% vs 0.4%).

Nalfon was discontinued in about 0.5% of patients because of adverse cardiovascular reactions during premarketing studies.

Miscellaneous—Nervousness (5.7% vs 1.5%), asthenia (5.4% vs 0.4%), peripheral edema (5.0% vs 0.4%), dyspnea (2.8% vs none), fatigue (1.7% vs 1.5%), upper respiratory infection (1.5% vs 5.6%), and nasopharyngitis (1.2% vs none).

INCIDENCE LESS THAN 1%

Probable Causal Relationship

The following adverse reactions, occurring in less than 1% of patients, were reported in controlled clinical trials and voluntary reports made since Nalfon® (Fenoprofen Calcium, USP) was initially marketed. The probability of a causal relationship exists between Nalfon and these adverse reactions:

Digestive System—Gastritis, peptic ulcer with/without perforation, gastrointestinal hemorrhage, anorexia, flatulence, dry mouth, and blood in the stool. Increases in alkaline phosphatase, LDH, and SGOT, jaundice, and cholestatic hepatitis were observed (*see* Precautions).

Genitourinary Tract—Renal failure, dysuria, cystitis, hematuria, oliguria, azotemia, anuria, interstitial nephritis, nephrosis, and papillary necrosis (*see* Warnings).

Hypersensitivity—Angioedema (angioneurotic edema).

Hematologic—Purpura, bruising, hemorrhage, thrombocytopenia, hemolytic anemia, aplastic anemia, agranulocytosis, and pancytopenia.

Miscellaneous—Anaphylaxis, urticaria, malaise, insomnia, and tachycardia.

INCIDENCE LESS THAN 1%

Causal Relationship Unknown

Other reactions reported either in clinical trials or spontaneously, occurred in circumstances in which a causal relationship could not be established. However, with these rarely reported reactions, the possibility of such a relationship cannot be excluded. Therefore, these observations are listed to alert the physician.

Skin and Appendages—Exfoliative dermatitis, toxic epidermal necrolysis, Stevens-Johnson syndrome, and alopecia.

Digestive System—Aphthous ulcerations of the buccal mucosa, metallic taste, and pancreatitis.

Cardiovascular—Atrial fibrillation, pulmonary edema, electrocardiographic changes, and supraventricular tachycardia.

Nervous System—Depression, disorientation, seizures, and trigeminal neuralgia.

Special Senses—Burning tongue, diplopia, and optic neuritis.

Miscellaneous—Personality change, lymphadenopathy, mastodynia, and fever.

OVERDOSAGE

Signs and Symptoms—Symptoms of overdose appear within several hours and generally involve the gastrointestinal and central nervous systems. They include dyspepsia, nausea, vomiting, abdominal pain, dizziness, headache, ataxia, tinnitus, tremor, drowsiness, and confusion. Hyperpyrexia, tachycardia, hypotension, and acute renal failure may occur rarely following overdose. Respiratory depression and metabolic acidosis have also been reported following overdose with certain NSAIDs.

Treatment—To obtain up-to-date information about the treatment of overdose, a good resource is your certified Regional Poison Control Center. Telephone numbers of certified poison control centers are listed in the *Physicians' Desk Reference (PDR)*. In managing overdosage, consider the possibility of multiple drug overdoses, interaction among drugs, and unusual drug kinetics in your patient.

Protect the patient's airway and support ventilation and perfusion. Meticulously monitor and maintain, within acceptable limits, the patient's vital signs, blood gases, serum electrolytes, etc. Absorption of drugs from the gastrointestinal tract may be decreased by giving activated charcoal, which, in many cases, is more effective than emesis or lavage; consider charcoal instead of or in addition to gastric emptying. Repeated doses of charcoal over time may hasten elimination of some drugs that have been absorbed. Safeguard the patient's airway when employing gastric emptying or charcoal.

Alkalinization of the urine, forced diuresis, peritoneal dialysis, hemodialysis, and charcoal hemoperfusion do not enhance systemic drug elimination.

DOSAGE AND ADMINISTRATION

Analgesia—For the treatment of mild to moderate pain, the recommended dosage is 200 mg every 4 to 6 hours, as needed.

Rheumatoid Arthritis and Osteoarthritis—The suggested dosage is 300 to 600 mg, 3 or 4 times a day. The dose should be tailored to the needs of the patient and may be increased or decreased depending on the severity of the symptoms. Dosage adjustments may be made after initiation of drug therapy or during exacerbations of the disease. Total daily dosage should not exceed 3,200 mg.

If gastrointestinal complaints occur, Nalfon may be administered with meals or with milk. Although the total amount absorbed is not affected, peak blood levels are delayed and diminished.

Patients with rheumatoid arthritis generally seem to require larger doses of Nalfon than do those with osteoarthritis. The smallest dose that yields acceptable control should be employed.

Although improvement may be seen in a few days in many patients, an additional 2 to 3 weeks may be required to gauge the full benefits of therapy.

HOW SUPPLIED

Pulvules:

200 mg* (white and ocher) (No. 415)—(Identi-Code† H76) (RxPak‡ of 100) NDC 0777-0876-02

300 mg* (yellow and ocher) (No. 416)—(Identi-Code H77) (RxPak of 100) NDC 0777-0877-02; (500s) NDC 0777-0877-03

Tablets (DISTA imprinted on one side, NALFON on other side):

600 mg* (yellow, paracapsule-shaped, scored) (No. 1900)—(RxPak of 100) NDC 0777-2159-02; (500s) NDC 0777-2159-03

* Equivalent to fenoprofen.

† Identi-Code® (formula identification code, Dista).

‡ All RxPaks (prescription packages, Dista) have safey closures.

Store at controlled room temperature, 59° to 86°F (15° to 30°C).

[112095]

PROZAC® ℞

[prō′zăk]

(fluoxetine hydrochloride)

DESCRIPTION

Prozac® (Fluoxetine Hydrochloride) is an antidepressant for oral administration; it is chemically unrelated to tricyclic, tetracyclic, or other available antidepressant agents. It is designated (±)-N-methyl-3-phenyl-3-[(α,α,α-trifluoro-*p*-tolyl)oxy]propylamine hydrochloride and has the empirical formula of $C_{17}H_{18}F_3NO \cdot HCl$. Its molecular weight is 345.79. The structural formula is:

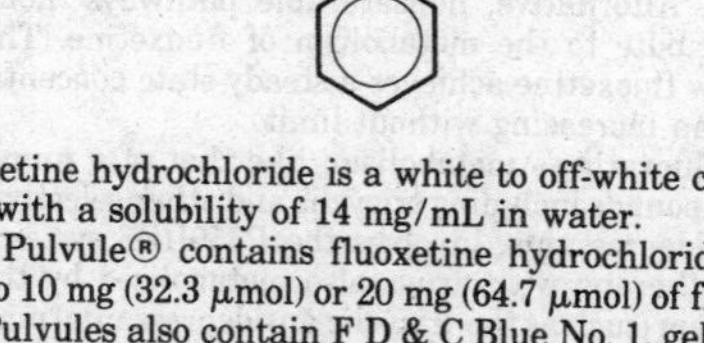

Fluoxetine hydrochloride is a white to off-white crystalline solid with a solubility of 14 mg/mL in water.

Each Pulvule® contains fluoxetine hydrochloride equivalent to 10 mg (32.3 μmol) or 20 mg (64.7 μmol) of fluoxetine. The Pulvules also contain F D & C Blue No. 1, gelatin, iron oxide, silicone, starch, titanium dioxide, and other inactive ingredients.

The oral solution contains fluoxetine hydrochloride equivalent to 20 mg/5 mL (64.7 μmol) of fluoxetine. It also contains alcohol 0.23%, benzoic acid, flavoring agent, glycerin, purified water, and sucrose.

CLINICAL PHARMACOLOGY

Pharmacodynamics: The antidepressant and antiobsessive-compulsive action of fluoxetine is presumed to be linked to its inhibition of CNS neuronal uptake of serotonin. Studies at clinically relevant doses in man have demonstrated that fluoxetine blocks the uptake of serotonin into human platelets. Studies in animals also suggest that fluoxetine is a much more potent uptake inhibitor of serotonin than of norepinephrine.

Antagonism of muscarinic, histaminergic, and α_1-adrenergic receptors has been hypothesized to be associated with various anticholinergic, sedative, and cardiovascular effects of classical tricyclic antidepressant drugs. Fluoxetine binds to these and other membrane receptors from brain tissue much less potently in vitro than do the tricyclic drugs.

Absorption, Distribution, Metabolism, and Excretion:

Systemic Bioavailability—In man, following a single oral 40 mg dose, peak plasma concentrations of fluoxetine from 15 to 55 ng/mL are observed after 6 to 8 hours.

The Pulvule and oral solution dosage forms of fluoxetine are bioequivalent. Food does not appear to affect the systemic bioavailability of fluoxetine, although it may delay its absorption inconsequentially. Thus, fluoxetine may be administered with or without food.

Protein Binding—Over the concentration range from 200 to 1,000 ng/mL, approximately 94.5% of fluoxetine is bound in vitro to human serum proteins, including albumin and α_1-glycoprotein. The interaction between fluoxetine and other highly protein-bound drugs has not been fully evaluated, but may be important (*see* Precautions).

Enantiomers—Fluoxetine is a racemic mixture (50/50) of *R*-fluoxetine and *S*-fluoxetine enantiomers. In animal models, both enantiomers are specific and potent serotonin uptake inhibitors with essentially equivalent pharmacologic activity. The *S*-fluoxetine enantiomer is eliminated more slowly and is the predominant enantiomer present in plasma at steady state.

Metabolism—Fluoxetine is extensively metabolized in the liver to norfluoxetine and a number of other, unidentified

Continued on next page

This product information was prepared in June 1996. Current information on these and other products of Dista Products Products Company may be obtained by direct inquiry to Lilly Research Laboratories, Lilly Corporate Center, Indianapolis, Indiana 46285, (800) 545-5979.

Dista—Cont.

metabolites. The only identified active metabolite, norfluoxetine, is formed by demethylation of fluoxetine. In animal models, *S*-norfluoxetine is a potent and selective inhibitor of serotonin uptake and has activity essentially equivalent to *R*- or *S*-fluoxetine. *R*-norfluoxetine is significantly less potent than the parent drug in the inhibition of serotonin uptake. The primary route of elimination appears to be hepatic metabolism to inactive metabolites excreted by the kidney.

Clinical Issues Related to Metabolism/Elimination—The complexity of the metabolism of fluoxetine has several consequences that may potentially affect fluoxetine's clinical use.

Variability in Metabolism—A subset (about 7%) of the population has reduced activity of the drug metabolizing enzyme cytochrome PA450IID6. Such individuals are referred to as "poor metabolizers" of drugs such as debrisoquin, dextromethorphan, and the tricyclic antidepressants. In a study involving labeled and unlabeled enantiomers administered as a racemate, these individuals metabolized *S*-fluoxetine at a slower rate and thus achieved higher concentrations of S-fluoxetine. Consequently, concentrations of *S*-norfluoxetine at steady state were lower. The metabolism of *R*-fluoxetine in these poor metabolizers appears normal. When compared with normal metabolizers, the total sum at steady state of the plasma concentrations of the 4 active enantiomers was not significantly greater among poor metabolizers. Thus, the net pharmacodynamic activities were essentially the same. Alternative, nonsaturable pathways (non-IID6) also contribute to the metabolism of fluoxetine. This explains how fluoxetine achieves a steady-state concentration rather than increasing without limit.

Because fluoxetine's metabolism, like that of a number of other compounds including tricyclic and other selective serotonin antidepressants, involves the P450IID6 system, concomitant therapy with drugs also metabolized by this enzyme system (such as the tricyclic antidepressants) may lead to drug interactions (*see* Drug Interactions *under* Precautions).

Accumulation and Slow Elimination—The relatively slow elimination of fluoxetine (elimination half-life of 1 to 3 days after acute administration and 4 to 6 days after chronic administration) and its active metabolite, norfluoxetine (elimination half-life of 4 to 16 days after acute and chronic administration), leads to significant accumulation of these active species in chronic use and delayed attainment of steady state, even when a fixed dose is used. After 30 days of dosing at 40 mg/ day, plasma concentrations of fluoxetine in the range of 91 to 302 ng/mL and norfluoxetine in the range of 72 to 258 ng/mL have been observed. Plasma concentrations of fluoxetine were higher than those predicted by single-dose studies, because fluoxetine's metabolism is not proportional to dose. Norfluoxetine, however, appears to have linear pharmacokinetics. Its mean terminal half-life after a single dose was 8.6 days and after multiple dosing was 9.3 days. Steady state levels after prolonged dosing are similar to levels seen at 4–5 weeks.

The long elimination half-lives of fluoxetine and norfluoxetine assure that, even when dosing is stopped, active drug substance will persist in the body for weeks (primarily depending on individual patient characteristics, previous dosing regimen, and length of previous therapy at discontinuation). This is of potential consequence when drug discontinuation is required or when drugs are prescribed that might interact with fluoxetine and norfluoxetine following the discontinuation of Prozac.

Liver Disease—As might be predicted from its primary site of metabolism, liver impairment can affect the elimination of fluoxetine. The elimination half-life of fluoxetine was prolonged in a study of cirrhotic patients, with a mean of 7.6 days compared to the range of 2 to 3 days seen in subjects without liver disease; norfluoxetine elimination was also delayed, with a mean duration of 12 days for cirrhotic patients compared to the range of 7 to 9 days in normal subjects. This suggests that the use of fluoxetine in patients with liver disease must be approached with caution. If fluoxetine is administered to patients with liver disease, a lower or less frequent dose should be used (*see* Precautions *and* Dosage and Administration).

Renal Disease—In single dose studies, the pharmacokinetics of fluoxetine and norfluoxetine were similar among subjects with all levels of impaired renal function including anephric patients on chronic hemodialysis. However, with chronic administration, additional accumulation of fluoxetine or its metabolites (possibly including some not yet identified) may occur in patients with severely impaired renal function and use of a lower or less frequent dose is advised (*see* Precautions).

Age—The disposition of single doses of fluoxetine in healthy elderly subjects (greater than 65 years of age) did not differ significantly from that in younger normal subjects. However, given the long half-life and nonlinear disposition of the drug, a single-dose study is not adequate to rule out the possibility of altered pharmacokinetics in the elderly, particularly if they have systemic illness or are receiving multiple drugs for concomitant diseases. The effects of age upon the metabolism of fluoxetine have been investigated in 260 elderly but otherwise healthy depressed patients ($\geq$ 60 years of age) who received 20 mg fluoxetine for 6 weeks. Combined fluoxetine plus norfluoxetine plasma concentrations were 209.3 ± 85.7 ng/mL at the end of 6 weeks. No unusual age-associated pattern of adverse events was observed in those elderly patients.

Clinical Trials:

Depression—The efficacy of Prozac for the treatment of patients with depression ($\geq$ 18 years of age) has been studied in 5- and 6-week placebo-controlled trials. Prozac was shown to be significantly more effective than placebo as measured by the Hamilton Depression Rating Scale (HAM-D). Prozac was also significantly more effective than placebo on the HAM-D subscores for depressed mood, sleep disturbance, and the anxiety subfactor.

Two 6-week controlled studies comparing Prozac, 20 mg, and placebo have shown Prozac, 20 mg daily, to be effective in the treatment of elderly patients ($\geq$ 60 years of age) with depression. In these studies, Prozac produced a significantly higher rate of response and remission as defined respectively by a 50% decrease in the HAM-D score and a total endpoint HAM-D score of $\leq$7. Prozac was well tolerated and the rate of treatment discontinuations due to adverse events did not differ between Prozac (12%) and placebo (9%).

Obsessive Compulsive Disorder.—The effectiveness of Prozac for the treatment for obsessive compulsive disorder (OCD) was demonstrated in two 13-week, multicenter, parallel group studies (Studies 1 and 2) of adult outpatients who received fixed Prozac doses of 20, 40, or 60 mg/day (on a once a day schedule, in the morning) or placebo. Patients in both studies had moderate to severe OCD (DSM-III-R), with mean baseline ratings on the Yale-Brown Obsessive Compulsive Scale (YBOCS, total score) ranging from 22 to 26. In Study 1, patients receiving Prozac experienced mean reductions of approximately 4 to 6 units on the YBOCS total score, compared to a 1-unit reduction for placebo patients. In Study 2, patients receiving Prozac experienced mean reductions of approximately 4 to 9 units on the YBOCS total score, compared to a 1-unit reduction for placebo patients. While there was no indication of a dose response relationship for effectiveness in Study 1, a dose response relationship was observed in Study 2, with numerically better responses in the 2 higher dose groups. The following table provides the outcome classification by treatment group on the Clinical Global Impression (CGI) improvement scale for studies 1 and 2 combined.

Outcome Classification (%) on CGI Improvement Scale for Completers in Pool of Two OCD Studies

Outcome Classification	Placebo	Prozac 20 mg	40 mg	60 mg
Worse	8%	0%	0%	0%
No Change	64%	41%	33%	29%
Minimally Improved	17%	23%	28%	24%
Much Improved	8%	28%	27%	28%
Very Much Improved	3%	8%	12%	19%

Exploratory analyses for age and gender effects on outcome did not suggest any differential responsiveness on the basis of age or sex.

INDICATIONS AND USAGE

Depression—Prozac is indicated for the treatment of depression. The efficacy of Prozac was established in 5- and 6-week trials with depressed outpatients ($\geq$ 18 years of age) whose diagnoses corresponded most closely to the DSM-III category of major depressive disorder (*see* Clinical Trials *under* Clinical Pharmacology).

A major depressive episode implies a prominent and relatively persistent depressed or dysphoric mood that usually interferes with daily functioning (nearly every day for at least 2 weeks); it should include at least 4 of the following 8 symptoms: change in appetite, change in sleep, psychomotor agitation or retardation, loss of interest in usual activities or decrease in sexual drive, increased fatigue, feelings of guilt or worthlessness, slowed thinking or impaired concentration, and a suicide attempt or suicidal ideation.

The antidepressant action of Prozac in hospitalized depressed patients has not been adequately studied.

The effectiveness of Prozac in long-term use, that is, for more than 5 to 6 weeks, has not been systematically evaluated in controlled trials. Therefore, the physician who elects to use Prozac for extended periods should periodically reevaluate the long-term usefulness of the drug for the individual patient.

Obsessive-Compulsive Disorder—Prozac is indicated for the treatment of obsessions and compulsions in patients with obsessive-compulsive disorder (OCD), as defined in the DSM-III-R; ie, the obsessions or compulsions cause marked distress, are time-consuming, or significantly interfere with social or occupational functioning.

The efficacy of Prozac was established in 13-week trials with obsessive-compulsive outpatients whose diagnoses corresponded most closely to the DSM-III-R category of obsessive-compulsive disorder (*see* Clinical Trials *under* Clinical Pharmacology).

Obsessive-compulsive disorder is characterized by recurrent and persistent ideas, thoughts, impulses, or images (obsessions) that are ego-dystonic and/or repetitive, purposeful, and intentional behaviors (compulsions) that are recognized by the person as excessive or unreasonable.

The effectiveness of Prozac in long-term use, ie, for more than 13 weeks, has not been systematically evaluated in placebo-controlled trials. Therefore, the physician who elects to use Prozac for extended periods should periodically reevaluate the long-term usefulness of the drug for the individual patient (*see* Dosage and Administration).

CONTRAINDICATIONS

Prozac is contraindicated in patients known to be hypersensitive to it.

Monoamine Oxidase Inhibitors—There have been reports of serious, sometimes fatal, reactions (including hyperthermia, rigidity, myoclonus, autonomic instability with possible rapid fluctuations of vital signs, and mental status changes that include extreme agitation progressing to delirium and coma) in patients receiving fluoxetine in combination with a monoamine oxidase inhibitor (MAOI), and in patients who have recently discontinued fluoxetine and are then started on an MAOI. Some cases presented with features resembling neuroleptic malignant syndrome. Therefore, Prozac should not be used in combination with an MAOI, or within 14 days of discontinuing therapy with an MAOI. Since fluoxetine and its major metabolite have very long elimination half-lives, at least 5 weeks (perhaps longer, especially if fluoxetine has been prescribed chronically and/or at higher doses [*see* Accumulation and Slow Elimination *under* Clinical Pharmacology]) should be allowed after stopping Prozac before starting an MAOI.

WARNINGS

Rash and Possibly Allergic Events—During premarketing testing of more than 5,600 US patients given fluoxetine, approximately 4% developed a rash and/or urticaria. Among these cases, almost a third were withdrawn from treatment because of the rash and/or systemic signs or symptoms associated with the rash. Clinical findings reported in association with rash include fever, leukocytosis, arthralgias, edema, carpal tunnel syndrome, respiratory distress, lymphadenopathy, proteinuria, and mild transaminase elevation. Most patients improved promptly with discontinuation of fluoxetine and/or adjunctive treatment with antihistamines or steroids, and all patients experiencing these events were reported to recover completely.

In premarketing clinical trials, 2 patients are known to have developed a serious cutaneous systemic illness. In neither patient was there an unequivocal diagnosis, but 1 was considered to have a leukocytoclastic vasculitis, and the other, a severe desquamating syndrome that was considered variously to be a vasculitis or erythema multiforme. Other patients have had systemic syndromes suggestive of serum sickness.

Since the introduction of Prozac, systemic events, possibly related to vasculitis, have developed in patients with rash. Although these events are rare, they may be serious, involving the lung, kidney, or liver. Death has been reported to occur in association with these systemic events.

Anaphylactoid events, including bronchospasm, angioedema, and urticaria alone and in combination, have been reported.

Pulmonary events, including inflammatory processes of varying histopathology and/or fibrosis, have been reported rarely. These events have occurred with dyspnea as the only preceding symptom.

Whether these systemic events and rash have a common underlying cause or are due to different etiologies or pathogenic processes is not known. Furthermore, a specific underlying immunologic basis for these events has not been identified. Upon the appearance of rash or of other possibly allergic phenomena for which an alternative etiology cannot be identified, Prozac should be discontinued.

PRECAUTIONS

General

Anxiety and Insomnia—Anxiety, nervousness, and insomnia were reported by 10% to 15% of patients treated with Prozac. These symptoms led to drug discontinuation in 5% of patients treated with Prozac.

In controlled clinical trials for obsessive-compulsive disorder, insomnia was reported in 30% of patients treated with Prozac and in 22% of patients treated with placebo. Anxiety was reported in 14% of patients treated with Prozac and in 7% of patients treated with placebo. These 2 symptoms led to drug discontinuation in 2% of patients treated with Prozac and no patients treated with placebo.

Altered Appetite and Weight—Significant weight loss, especially in underweight depressed patients, may be an undesirable result of treatment with Prozac.

In controlled clinical trials, approximately 9% of patients treated with Prozac experienced anorexia. This incidence is approximately sixfold that seen in placebo controls. A weight loss of greater than 5% of body weight occurred in 13% of patients treated with Prozac compared to 4% of placebo and 3% of patients treated with tricyclics. However, only rarely have patients discontinued treatment with Prozac because of weight loss.

In controlled clinical trials for OCD, 17% of patients treated with Prozac and 10% of patients treated with placebo reported anorexia. One patient discontinued treatment with Prozac because of anorexia.

Activation of Mania/Hypomania—During premarketing testing, hypomania or mania occurred in approximately 1% of fluoxetine treated patients. Activation of mania/hypomania has also been reported in a small proportion of patients with Major Affective Disorder treated with other marketed antidepressants. Mania/hypomania was reported in 1% of patients treated with fluoxetine in controlled clinical OCD trials.

Seizures—Twelve patients among more than 6,000 evaluated worldwide in the course of premarketing development of fluoxetine experienced convulsions (or events described as possibly having been seizures), a rate of 0.2% that appears to be similar to that associated with other marketed antidepressants. Prozac should be introduced with care in patients with a history of seizures.

In controlled clinical trials for OCD, 1 patient treated with fluoxetine experienced a seizure.

Suicide—The possibility of a suicide attempt is inherent in depression and may persist until significant remission occurs. Close supervision of high risk patients should accompany initial drug therapy. Prescriptions for Prozac should be written for the smallest quantity of capsules consistent with good patient management, in order to reduce the risk of overdose.

Because of well-established comorbidity between OCD and depression, the same precautions observed when treating patients with depression should be observed when treating patients with OCD.

The Long Elimination Half-Lives of Fluoxetine and Its Metabolites—Because of the long elimination half-lives of the parent drug and its major active metabolite, changes in dose will not be fully reflected in plasma for several weeks, affecting both strategies for titration to final dose and withdrawal from treatment (*see* Clinical Pharmacology *and* Dosage and Administration).

Use in Patients With Concomitant Illness—Clinical experience with Prozac in patients with concomitant systemic illness is limited. Caution is advisable in using Prozac in patients with diseases or conditions that could affect metabolism or hemodynamic responses.

Fluoxetine has **not** been evaluated or used to any appreciable extent in patients with a recent history of myocardial infarction or unstable heart disease. Patients with these diagnoses were systematically excluded from clinical studies during the product's premarket testing. However, the electrocardiograms of 312 patients who received Prozac in double-blind trials were retrospectively evaluated; no conduction abnormalities that resulted in heart block were observed. The mean heart rate was reduced by approximately 3 beats/min.

In subjects with cirrhosis of the liver, the clearances of fluoxetine and its active metabolite, norfluoxetine, were decreased, thus increasing the elimination half-lives of these substances. A lower or less frequent dose should be used in patients with cirrhosis.

Since fluoxetine is extensively metabolized, excretion of unchanged drug in urine is a minor route of elimination. However, until adequate numbers of patients with severe renal impairment have been evaluated during chronic treatment with fluoxetine, it should be used with caution in such patients.

In patients with diabetes, Prozac may alter glycemic control. Hypoglycemia has occurred during therapy with Prozac, and hyperglycemia has developed following discontinuation of the drug. As is true with many other types of medication when taken concurrently by patients with diabetes, insulin and/or oral hypoglycemic dosage may need to be adjusted when therapy with Prozac is instituted or discontinued.

Interference With Cognitive and Motor Performance—Any psychoactive drug may impair judgment, thinking, or motor skills, and patients should be cautioned about operating hazardous machinery, including automobiles, until they are reasonably certain that the drug treatment does not affect them adversely.

Information for Patients—Physicians are advised to discuss the following issues with patients for whom they prescribe Prozac:

Because Prozac may impair judgment, thinking, or motor skills, patients should be advised to avoid driving a car or operating hazardous machinery until they are reasonably certain that their performance is not affected.

Patients should be advised to inform their physician if they are taking or plan to take any prescription or over-the-counter drugs, or alcohol.

Patients should be advised to notify their physician if they become pregnant or intend to become pregnant during therapy.

Patients should be advised to notify their physician if they are breast feeding an infant.

Patients should be advised to notify their physician if they develop a rash or hives.

Laboratory Tests—There are no specific laboratory tests recommended.

Drug Interactions—As with all drugs, the potential for interaction by a variety of mechanisms (eg, pharmacodynamic, pharmacokinetic drug inhibition or enhancement, etc) is a possibility (*see* Accumulation and Slow Elimination *under* Clinical Pharmacology).

Drugs Metabolized by P450IID6—Approximately 7% of the normal population has a genetic defect that leads to reduced levels of activity of the cytochrome P450 isoenzyme P450IID6. Such individuals have been referred to as "poor metabolizers" of drugs such as debrisoquin, dextromethorphan, and tricyclic antidepressants. Many drugs, such as most antidepressants including fluoxetine and other selective uptake inhibitors of serotonin, are metabolized by this isoenzyme; thus, both the pharmacokinetic properties and relative proportion of metabolites are altered in poor metabolizers. However, for fluoxetine and its metabolite the sum of the plasma concentrations of the 4 active enantiomers is comparable between poor and extensive metabolizers (*see* Variability in Metabolism *under* Clinical Pharmacology).

Fluoxetine, like other agents that are metabolized by P450IID6, inhibits the activity of this isoenzyme, and thus may make normal metabolizers resemble "poor metabolizers." Therapy with medications that are predominantly metabolized by the P450IID6 system and that have a relatively narrow therapeutic index (*see* list below), should be initiated at the low end of the dose range if a patient is receiving fluoxetine concurrently or has taken it in the previous 5 weeks. Thus, his/her dosing requirements resemble those of "poor metabolizers." If fluoxetine is added to the treatment regimen of a patient already receiving a drug metabolized by P450IID6, the need for decreased dose of the original medication should be considered. Drugs with a narrow therapeutic index represent the greatest concern (eg, flecainide, vinblastine, carbamazepine, and tricyclic antidepressants).

Tryptophan—Five patients receiving Prozac in combination with tryptophan experienced adverse reactions, including agitation, restlessness, and gastrointestinal distress.

Monoamine Oxidase Inhibitors—*See* Contraindications.

Other Antidepressants—In two studies, previously stable plasma levels of imipramine and desipramine have increased greater than 2 to 10-fold when fluoxetine has been administered in combination. This influence may persist for three weeks or longer after fluoxetine is discontinued. Thus, the dose of tricyclic antidepressant (TCA) may need to be reduced and plasma TCA concentrations may need to be monitored temporarily when fluoxetine is coadministered or has been recently discontinued (*see* Accumulation and Slow Elimination *under* Clinical Pharmacology, and Drugs Metabolized by P450IID6 *under* Drug Interactions).

Lithium—There have been reports of both increased and decreased lithium levels when lithium was used concomitantly with fluoxetine. Cases of lithium toxicity have been reported. Lithium levels should be monitored when these drugs are administered concomitantly.

Diazepam Clearance—The half-life of concurrently administered diazepam may be prolonged in some patients (*see* Accumulation and Slow Elimination *under* Clinical Pharmacology).

Phenytoin—Patients on stable doses of phenytoin have developed elevated plasma phenytoin concentrations and clinical phenytoin toxicity following initiation of concomitant fluoxetine treatment.

Potential Effects of Coadministration of Drugs Tightly Bound to Plasma Proteins—Because fluoxetine is tightly bound to plasma protein, the administration of fluoxetine to a patient taking another drug that is tightly bound to protein (eg, Coumadin, digitoxin) may cause a shift in plasma concentrations potentially resulting in an adverse effect. Conversely, adverse effects may result from displacement of protein bound fluoxetine by other tightly bound drugs (*see* Accumulation and Slow Elimination *under* Clinical Pharmacology).

CNS Active Drugs—The risk of using Prozac in combination with other CNS active drugs has not been systematically evaluated. Consequently, caution is advised if the concomitant administration of Prozac and such drugs is required (*see* Accumulation and Slow Elimination *under* Clinical Pharmacology).

Electroconvulsive Therapy—There are no clinical studies establishing the benefit of the combined use of ECT and fluoxetine. There have been rare reports of prolonged seizures in patients on fluoxetine receiving ECT treatment.

Carcinogenesis, Mutagenesis, Impairment of Fertility—There is no evidence of carcinogenicity, mutagenicity, or impairment of fertility with Prozac.

The dietary administration of fluoxetine to rats and mice for 2 years at levels equivalent to approximately 7.5 and 9.0 times the maximum human dose (80 mg) respectively produced no evidence of carcinogenicity.

Fluoxetine and norfluoxetine have been shown to have no genotoxic effects based on the following assays: bacterial mutation assay, DNA repair assay in cultured rat hepatocytes, mouse lymphoma assay, and in vivo sister chromatid exchange assay in Chinese hamster bone marrow cells.

Two fertility studies conducted in rats at doses of approximately 5 and 9 times the maximum human dose (80 mg) indicated that fluoxetine had no adverse effects on fertility. A slight decrease in neonatal survival was noted, but this was probably associated with depressed maternal food consumption and suppressed weight gain.

Pregnancy—Teratogenic Effects—Pregnancy Category B: Reproduction studies have been performed in rats and rabbits at doses 9 and 11 times the maximum daily human dose (80 mg) respectively and have revealed no evidence of harm to the fetus due to Prozac® (Fluoxetine Hydrochloride). There are, however, no adequate and well-controlled studies in pregnant women. Because animal reproduction studies are not always predictive of human response, this drug should be used during pregnancy only if clearly needed.

Labor and Delivery—The effect of Prozac on labor and delivery in humans is unknown.

Nursing Mothers—Because Prozac is excreted in human milk, nursing while on Proazc is not recommended. In 1 breast milk sample, the concentration of fluoxetine plus norfluoxetine was 70.4 ng/mL. The concentration in the mother's plasma was 295.0 ng/mL. No adverse effects on the infant were reported. In another case, an infant nursed by a mother on Prozac developed crying, sleep disturbance, vomiting, and watery stools. The infant's plasma drug levels were 340 ng/mL of fluoxetine and 208 ng/mL of norfluoxetine on the second day of feeding.

Usage in Children—Safety and effectiveness in children have not been established.

Usage in the Elderly—Evaluation of patients over the age of 60 who received Prozac 20 mg daily revealed no unusual pattern of adverse events relative to the clinical experience in younger patients. However, these data are insufficient to rule out possible age-related differences during chronic use, particularly in elderly patients who have concomitant systemic illnesses or who are receiving concomitant drugs. (*see* Age *under* Clinical Pharmacology).

Hyponatremia—Several cases of hyponatremia (some with serum sodium lower than 110 mmol/L) have been reported. The hyponatremia appeared to be reversible when Prozac was discontinued. Although these cases were complex with varying possible etiologies, some were possibly due to the syndrome of inappropriate antidiuretic hormone secretion (SIADH). The majority of these occurrences have been in older patients and in patients taking diuretics or who were otherwise volume depleted. In a placebo-controlled, double-blind trial, 10 of 313 fluoxetine patients and 6 of 320 placebo recipients had a lowering of serum sodium below the reference range; this difference was not statistically significant. The lowest observed concentration was 129 mmol/L. The observed decreases were not clinically significant.

Platelet Function—There have been rare reports of altered platelet function and/or abnormal results from laboratory studies in patients taking fluoxetine. While there have been reports of abnormal bleeding in several patients taking fluoxetine, it is unclear whether fluoxetine had a causative role.

ADVERSE REACTIONS

Commonly Observed—The most commonly observed adverse events associated with the use of Prozac and not seen at an equivalent incidence among placebo-treated patients were: nervous system complaints, including anxiety, nervousness, and insomnia; drowsiness and fatigue or asthenia; tremor; sweating; gastrointestinal complaints, including anorexia, nausea, and diarrhea; and dizziness or lightheadedness.

In controlled clinical trials for OCD using fixed doses of 20, 40, or 60 mg daily, adverse events observed at an incidence of at least 5% for Prozac and for which the incidence was approximately twice or more the incidence among placebo-treated patients included: somnolence, anxiety, tremor, nausea, dyspepsia, gastrointestinal disorder, vasodilatation, dry mouth, sweating, rash, abnormal vision, yawn, decreased libido, and abnormal ejaculation.

Continued on next page

This product information was prepared in June 1996. Current information on these and other products of Dista Products Products Company may be obtained by direct inquiry to Lilly Research Laboratories, Lilly Corporate Center, Indianapolis, Indiana 46285, (800) 545-5979.

Dista—Cont.

Associated With Discontinuation of Treatment —Fifteen percent of approximately 4,000 patients who received Prozac in US premarketing clinical trials discontinued treatment due to an adverse event. The more common events causing discontinuation included: psychiatric (5.3%), primarily nervousness, anxiety, and insomnia; digestive (3.0%), primarily nausea; nervous system (1.6%), primarily dizziness; body as a whole (1.5%), primarily asthenia and headache; and skin (1.4%), primarily rash and pruritus.

In controlled clinical trials for OCD, 12% of patients treated with Prozac discontinued treatment due to adverse events. The most common events were anxiety (2%) and rash/urticaria (2%).

Incidence in Controlled Clinical Trials —

Depression—Table 1 enumerates adverse events that occurred at a frequency of 1% or more among patients treated with Prozac who participated in controlled trials comparing Prozac with placebo.

Obsessive-Compulsive Disorder—Table 2 enumerates adverse events that occurred at a frequency of 2% or more among patients on Prozac who participated in controlled trials comparing Prozac with placebo in the treatment of OCD.

The prescriber should be aware that the figures in Tables 1 and 2 cannot be used to predict the incidence of side effects in the course of usual medical practice where patient characteristics and other factors differ from those that prevailed in the clinical trials. Similarly, the cited frequencies cannot be compared with figures obtained from other clinical investigations involving different treatments, uses, and investigators. The cited figures, however, do provide the prescribing physician with some basis for estimating the relative contribution of drug and nondrug factors to the side effect incidence rate in the population studied.

[See table 1 below.]
[See table 2 at top of next page.]

Other Events Observed During Premarketing Evaluation of Prozac—During clinical testing in the US, multiple doses of Prozac were administered to approximately 5,600 subjects. Untoward events associated with this exposure were recorded by clinical investigators using descriptive terminology of their own choosing. Consequently, it is not possible to provide a meaningful estimate of the proportion of individuals experiencing adverse events without first grouping similar types of untoward events into a limited (ie, reduced) number of standardized event categories.

In the tabulations that follow, a standard COSTART Dictionary terminology has been used to classify reported adverse events. The frequencies presented, therefore, represent the proportion of the 5,600 individuals exposed to Prozac who experienced an event of the type cited on at least 1 occasion while receiving Prozac. All reported events are included except those already listed in Table 1, those COSTART terms so general as to be uninformative, and those events where a drug cause was remote. It is important to emphasize that, although the events reported did occur during treatment with Prozac, they were not necessarily caused by it.

Events are further classified within body system categories and enumerated in order of decreasing frequency using the following definitions: frequent adverse events are defined as those occurring on 1 or more occasions in at least 1/100 patients; infrequent adverse events are those occurring in 1/100 to 1/1,000 patients; rare events are those occurring in less than 1/1,000 patients.

Body as a Whole—*Frequent:* chills; *Infrequent:* chills and fever, cyst, face edema, hangover effect, jaw pain, malaise, neck pain, neck rigidity, and pelvic pain; *Rare:* abdomen enlarged, cellulitis, hydrocephalus, hypothermia, LE syndrome, moniliasis, and serum sickness.

Cardiovascular System—*Infrequent:* angina pectoris, arrhythmia, hemorrhage, hypertension, hypotension, migraine, postural hypotension, syncope, and tachycardia; *Rare:* AV block first degree, bradycardia, bundle branch block, cerebral ischemia, myocardial infarct, thrombophlebitis, vascular headache, and ventricular arrhythmia.

Digestive System—*Frequent:* increased appetite; *Infrequent:* aphthous stomatitis, dysphagia, eructation, esophagitis, gastritis, gingivitis, glossitis, liver function tests abnormal, melena, stomatitis, thirst; *Rare:* bloody diarrhea, cholecystitis, cholelithiasis, colitis, duodenal ulcer, enteritis, fecal incontinence, hematemesis, hepatitis, hepatomegaly, hyperchlorhydria, increased salivation, jaundice, liver tenderness, mouth ulceration, salivary gland enlargement, stomach ulcer, tongue discoloration, and tongue edema.

Endocrine System—*Infrequent:* hypothyroidism; *Rare:* goiter and hyperthyroidism.

Hemic and Lymphatic System—*Infrequent:* anemia and lymphadenopathy; *Rare:* bleeding time increased, blood dyscrasia, leukopenia, lymphocytosis, petechia, purpura, sedimentation rate increased, and thrombocythemia.

Metabolic and Nutritional—*Frequent:* weight loss; *Infrequent:* generalized edema, hypoglycemia, peripheral edema, and weight gain; *Rare:* dehydration, gout, hypercholesteremia, hyperglycemia, hyperlipemia, hypoglycemic reaction, hypokalemia, hyponatremia, and iron deficiency anemia.

Musculoskeletal System—*Infrequent:* arthritis, bone pain, bursitis, tenosynovitis, and twitching; *Rare:* bone necrosis, chondrodystrophy, muscle hemorrhage, myositis, osteoporosis, pathological fracture, and rheumatoid arthritis.

Nervous System—*Frequent:* abnormal dreams and agitation; *Infrequent:* abnormal gait, acute brain syndrome, akathisia, amnesia, apathy, ataxia, buccoglossal syndrome, CNS stimulation, convulsion, delusions, depersonalization, emotional lability, euphoria, hallucinations, hostility, hyperkinesia, hypesthesia, incoordination, libido increased, manic reaction, neuralgia, neuropathy, paranoid reaction, psychosis, and vertigo; *Rare:* abnormal electroencephalogram, antisocial reaction, chronic brain syndrome, circumoral paresthesia, CNS depression, coma, dysarthria, dystonia, extrapyramidal syndrome, hypertonia, hysteria, myoclonus, nystagmus, paralysis, reflexes decreased, stupor, and torticollis.

Respiratory System—*Frequent:* bronchitis, rhinitis, and yawn; *Infrequent:* asthma, epistaxis, hiccup, hyperventilation, and pneumonia; *Rare:* apnea, hemoptysis, hypoxia, larynx edema, lung edema, lung fibrosis/alveolitis, and pleural effusion.

Skin and Appendages—*Infrequent:* acne, alopecia, contact dermatitis, dry skin, herpes simplex, maculopapular rash, and urticaria; *Rare:* eczema, erythema multiforme, fungal dermatitis, herpes zoster, hirsutism, psoriasis, purpuric rash, pustular rash, seborrhea, skin discoloration, skin hypertrophy, subcutaneous nodule, and vesiculobullous rash.

Special Senses—*Infrequent:* amblyopia, conjunctivitis, ear pain, eye pain, mydriasis, photophobia, and tinnitus; *Rare:* blepharitis, cataract, corneal lesion, deafness, diplopia, eye hemorrhage, glaucoma, iritis, ptosis, strabismus, and taste loss.

Urogenital System—*Infrequent:* abnormal ejaculation, amenorrhea, breast pain, cystitis, dysuria, fibrocystic breast, leukorrhea, menopause, menorrhagia, ovarian disorder, urinary incontinence, urinary retention, urinary urgency, urination impaired, and vaginitis; *Rare:* abortion, albuminuria, breast enlargement, dyspareunia, epididymitis, female lactation, hematuria, hypomenorrhea, kidney calculus, metrorrhagia, orchitis, polyuria, pyelonephritis, pyuria, salpingitis, urethral pain, urethritis, urinary tract disorder, urolithiasis, uterine hemorrhage, uterine spasm, and vaginal hemorrhage.

Postintroduction Reports—Voluntary reports of adverse events temporally associated with Prozac that have been received since market introduction, that are not listed above, and that may have no causal relationship with the drug include the following: aplastic anemia, atrial fibrillation, cerebral vascular accident, cholestatic jaundice, confusion, dyskinesia (including, for example, a case of buccal-lingual-masticatory syndrome with involuntary tongue protrusion reported to develop in a 77-year-old female after 5 weeks of fluoxetine therapy and which completely resolved over the next few months following drug discontinuation), eosinophilic pneumonia, epidermal necrolysis, exfoliative dermatitis, gynecomastia, heart arrest, hepatic failure/necrosis, hyperprolactinemia, immune-related hemolytic anemia, kidney failure, misuse/abuse, movement disorders developing in patients with risk factors including drugs associated with such events and worsening of preexisting movement disorders, neuroleptic malignant syndrome-like events, pancreatitis, pancytopenia, priapism, pulmonary embolism, QT prolongation, sudden unexpected death, suicidal ideation, thrombocytopenia, thrombocytopenic purpura, vaginal bleeding after drug withdrawal, and violent behaviors.

DRUG ABUSE AND DEPENDENCE

Controlled Substance Class —Prozac is not a controlled substance.

Physical and Psychological Dependence —Prozac has not been systematically studied, in animals or humans, for its potential for abuse, tolerance, or physical dependence. While the premarketing clinical experience with Prozac did not reveal any tendency for a withdrawal syndrome or any drug seeking behavior, these observations were not systematic and it is not possible to predict on the basis of this limited

TABLE 1—TREATMENT-EMERGENT ADVERSE EXPERIENCE INCIDENCE IN PLACEBO-CONTROLLED CLINICAL TRIALS

Body System/ Preferred Term*	Percentage of Patients Reporting Event		Body System/ Preferred Term*	Percentage of Patients Reporting Event	
	Prozac (N=1,730)	Placebo (N=799)		Prozac (N=1,730)	Placebo (N=799)
Nervous			**Body as a Whole**		
Headache	20.3	15.5	Asthenia	4.4	1.9
Nervousness	14.9	8.5	Infection, viral	3.4	3.1
Insomnia	13.8	7.1	Pain, limb	1.6	1.1
Drowsiness	11.6	6.3	Fever	1.4	—
Anxiety	9.4	5.5	Pain, chest	1.3	1.1
Tremor	7.9	2.4	Allergy	1.2	1.1
Dizziness	5.7	3.3	Influenza	1.2	1.5
Fatigue	4.2	1.1	**Respiratory**		
Sedated	1.9	1.3	Upper respiratory infection	7.6	6.0
Sensation disturbance	1.7	2.0	Flu-like syndrome	2.8	1.9
Libido, decreased	1.6	—	Pharyngitis	2.7	1.3
Light-headedness	1.6	—	Nasal congestion	2.6	2.3
Concentration, decreased	1.5	—	Headache, sinus	2.3	1.8
Digestive			Sinusitis	2.1	2.0
Nausea	21.1	10.1	Cough	1.6	1.6
Diarrhea	12.3	7.0	Dyspnea	1.4	—
Mouth dryness	9.5	6.0	**Cardiovascular**		
Anorexia	8.7	1.5	Hot flushes	1.8	1.0
Dyspepsia	6.4	4.3	Palpitations	1.3	1.4
Constipation	4.5	3.3	**Musculoskeletal**		
Pain, abdominal	3.4	2.9	Pain, back	2.0	2.4
Vomiting	2.4	1.3	Pain, joint	1.2	1.1
Taste change	1.8	—	Pain, muscle	1.2	1.0
Flatulence	1.6	1.1	**Urogenital**		
Gastroenteritis	1.0	1.4	Menstruation, painful†	2.6	2.1
Skin and Appendages			Sexual dysfunction	1.9	—
Sweating, excessive	8.4	3.8	Impotence, sexual‡	1.7	0.4
Rash	2.7	1.8	Frequent micturition	1.6	—
Pruritus	2.4	1.4	Urinary tract infection	1.2	—
			Special Senses		
			Vision disturbance	2.8	1.8

* Events reported by at least 1% of patients treated with Prozac are included.
† Denominator used was females only (N = 1,210 Prozac; N = 523 placebo).
‡ Denominator used was males only (N = 520 Prozac; N = 276 placebo).
—Incidence less than 1%.

experience the extent to which a CNS active drug will be misused, diverted, and/or abused once marketed. Consequently, physicians should carefully evaluate patients for history of drug abuse and follow such patients closely, observing them for signs of misuse or abuse of Prozac (eg, development of tolerance, incrementation of dose, drug-seeking behavior).

OVERDOSAGE

Human Experience—As of December 1987, there were 2 deaths among approximately 38 reports of acute overdose with fluoxetine, either alone or in combination with other drugs and/or alcohol. One death involved a combined overdose with approximately 1,800 mg of fluoxetine and an undetermined amount of maprotiline. Plasma concentrations of fluoxetine and maprotiline were 4.57 mg/L and 4.18 mg/L, respectively. A second death involved 3 drugs yielding plasma concentrations as follows: fluoxetine, 1.93 mg/L; norfluoxetine, 1.10 mg/L; codeine, 1.80 mg/L; temazepam, 3.80 mg/L.

One other patient who reportedly took 3,000 mg of fluoxetine experienced 2 grand mal seizures that remitted spontaneously without specific anticonvulsant treatment (*see* Management of Overdose). The actual amount of drug absorbed may have been less due to vomiting.

Nausea and vomiting were prominent in overdoses involving higher fluoxetine doses. Other prominent symptoms of overdose included agitation, restlessness, hypomania, and other signs of CNS excitation. Except for the 2 deaths noted above, all other overdose cases recovered without residua.

Since introduction, reports of death attributed to overdosage of fluoxetine alone have been extremely rare.

Animal Experience—Studies in animals do not provide precise or necessarily valid information about the treatment of human overdose. However, animal experiments can provide useful insights into possible treatment strategies.

The oral median lethal dose in rats and mice was found to be 452 and 248 mg/kg respectively. Acute high oral doses produced hyperirritability and convulsions in several animal species.

Among 6 dogs purposely overdosed with oral fluoxetine, 5 experienced grand mal seizures. Seizures stopped immediately upon the bolus intravenous administration of a standard veterinary dose of diazepam. In this short term study, the lowest plasma concentration at which a seizure occurred was only twice the maximum plasma concentration seen in humans taking 80 mg/day, chronically.

In a separate single-dose study, the ECG in dogs given high doses did not reveal prolongation of the PR, QRS, or QT intervals. Tachycardia and an increase in blood pressure were observed. Consequently, the value of the ECG in predicting cardiac toxicity is unknown. Nonetheless, the ECG should ordinarily be monitored in cases of human overdose (*see* Management of Overdose).

Management of Overdose—Establish and maintain an airway; ensure adequate oxygenation and ventilation. Activated charcoal, which may be used with sorbitol, may be as or more effective than emesis or lavage, and should be considered in treating overdose.

Cardiac and vital signs monitoring is recommended, along with general symptomatic and supportive measures. Based on experience in animals, which may not be relevant to humans, fluoxetine-induced seizures that fail to remit spontaneously may respond to diazepam.

There are no specific antidotes for Prozac.

Due to the large volume of distribution of Prozac, forced diuresis, dialysis, hemoperfusion, and exchange transfusion are unlikely to be of benefit.

In managing overdosage, consider the possibility of multiple drug involvement. A specific caution involves patients taking or recently having taken fluoxetine who might ingest by accident or intent, excessive quantities of a tricyclic antidepressant. In such a case, accumulation of the parent tricyclic and an active metabolite may increase the possibility of clinically significant sequelae and extend the time needed for close medical observation (*see* Other Antidepressants *under* Precautions).

The physician should consider contacting a poison control center on the treatment of any overdose. Telephone numbers of certified poison control centers are listed in the *Physicians' Desk Reference (PDR)*.

DOSAGE AND ADMINISTRATION

Depression:

Initial Treatment—In controlled trials used to support the efficacy of fluoxetine, patients were administered morning doses ranging from 20 mg to 80 mg/day. Studies comparing fluoxetine 20, 40, and 60 mg/day to placebo indicate that 20 mg/day is sufficient to obtain a satisfactory antidepressant response in most cases. Consequently, a dose of 20 mg/day, administered in the morning, is recommended as the initial dose.

A dose increase may be considered after several weeks if no clinical improvement is observed. Doses above 20 mg/day may be administered on a once a day (morning) or b.i.d.

TABLE 2
TREATMENT EMERGENT ADVERSE EXPERIENCE INCIDENCE IN PLACEBO-CONTROLLED CLINICAL TRIALS FOR OBSESSIVE-COMPULSIVE DISORDER

Body System/ Preferred Team*	Percentage of Patients Reporting Event		Body System/ Preferred Team*	Percentage of Patients Reporting Event	
	Prozac (N=264)	Placebo (N=89)		Prozac (N=264)	Placebo (N=89)
Nervous			**Body as a Whole**		
Insomnia	30	22	Headache	33	24
Somnolence	17	7	Asthenia	15	11
Anxiety	14	7	Flu syndrome	10	7
Dizziness	14	11	Pain	6	4
Libido, decreased	11	2	Injury, accidental	4	2
Tremor	9	1	Surgical procedure	3	—
Abnormal dreams	5	2	Chest pain	3	1
Thinking, abnormal	4	2	Allergic reaction	3	—
Sleep disorder	3	1	Fever	2	1
Confusion	2	1	**Respiratory**		
Myoclonus	2	—	Pharyngitis	11	9
Agitation	2	1	Yawn	7	—
Amnesia	2	1	Sinusitis	5	2
Digestive			Cough, increased	3	2
Nausea	27	13	**Cardiovascular**		
Diarrhea	18	13	Vasodilatation	5	—
Anorexia	17	10	Palpitations	2	1
Dry mouth	12	3	**Musculoskeletal**		
Dyspepsia	10	4	Myalgia	5	4
Gastrointestinal disorder	6	1	Arthralgia	3	2
Melena	2	—	**Urogenital**		
Skin and Appendages			Urinary frequency	4	1
Sweating	7	—	Abnormal ejaculation†	7	—
Rash	6	3	**Hemic and Lymphatic**		
Pruritus	3	1	Lymphadenopathy	2	—
Acne	2	1	**Metabolic and Nutritional**		
			Weight loss	5	3
			Special Senses		
			Ambylopia	3	1
			Abnormal vision	2	—
			Taste perversion	2	1
			Tinnitus	2	—

* Events reported by at least 2% of patients treated with Prozac are included, except the following events which had an incidence on placebo ≥ Prozac: abdominal pain, back pain, constipation, depression, dysmenorrhea, flatulence, infection, menstrual disorder, nervousness, rhinitis, tooth disorder, and twitching.

† Denominator used was males only (N=116 Prozac; N=43 placebo).

— Adverse event not reported by placebo-treated patients.

schedule (ie, morning and noon) and should not exceed a maximum dose of 80 mg/day.

As with other antidepressants, the full antidepressant effect may be delayed until 4 weeks of treatment or longer.

As with many other medications, a lower or less frequent dosage should be used in patients with renal and/or hepatic impairment. A lower or less frequent dosage should also be considered for patients, such as the elderly (*see* Usage in the Elderly *under* Precautions), with concurrent disease or on multiple medications.

Maintenance/Continuation/Extended Treatment—There is no body of evidence available to answer the question of how long the patient treated with fluoxetine should remain on it. It is generally agreed among expert psychopharmacologists (circa 1987) that acute episodes of depression require several months or longer of sustained pharmacologic therapy. Whether the dose of antidepressant needed to induce remission is identical to the dose needed to maintain and/or sustain euthymia is unknown.

Obsessive-Compulsive Disorder:

Initial Treatment—In the controlled clinical trials of fluoxetine supporting its effectiveness in the treatment of obsessive-compulsive disorder, patients were administered fixed daily doses of 20, 40, or 60 mg of fluoxetine or placebo (*see* Clinical Trials *under* Clinical Pharmacology). In one of these studies, no dose response relationship for effectiveness was demonstrated. Consequently, a dose of 20 mg/day, administered in the morning, is recommended as the initial dose. Since there was a suggestion of a possible dose response relationship for effectiveness in the second study, a dose increase may be considered after several weeks if insufficient clinical improvement is observed. The full therapeutic effect may be delayed until 5 weeks of treatment or longer.

Doses above 20 mg/day may be administered on a once a day (ie, morning) or b.i.d. schedule (ie, morning and noon). A dose range of 20 to 60 mg/day is recommended, however, doses of up to 80 mg/day have been well tolerated in open studies of OCD. The maximum fluoxetine dose should not exceed 80 mg/day.

As with the use of Prozac in depression, a lower or less frequent dosage should be used in patients with renal and/or hepatic impairment. A lower or less frequent dosage should also be considered for patients, such as the elderly (*see* Usage in the Elderly *under* Precautions), with concurrent disease or on multiple medications.

Maintenance/Continuation Treatment—While there are no systematic studies that answer the question of how long to continue Prozac, OCD is a chronic condition and it is reasonable to consider continuation for a responding patient. Although the efficacy of Prozac after 13 weeks has not been documented in controlled trials, patients have been continued in therapy under double-blind conditions for up to an additional 6 months without loss of benefit. However, dosage adjustments should be made to maintain the patient on the lowest effective dosage, and patients should be periodically reassessed to determine the need for treatment.

Switching Patients to a Tricyclic Antidepressant (TCA)—Dosage of a TCA may need to be reduced, and plasma TCA concentrations may need to be monitored temporarily when fluoxetine is coadministered or has been recently discontinued (*see* Other Antidepressants *under* Drug Interactions).

Switching Patients to or from a Monoamine Oxidase Inhibitor—At least 14 days should elapse between discontinuation of an MAOI and initiation of therapy with Prozac. In addition, at least 5 weeks, perhaps longer, should be allowed after stopping Prozac before starting on MAOI (*see* Contraindications and Precautions).

HOW SUPPLIED

Pulvules:

10 mg*, green and green (No. 3104)—(100s) NDC 0777-3104-02; (2000s) NDC 0777-3104-07 (20 FlexPak§ blister cards of 31) NDC 0777-3104-82

20 mg*, green and off-white (No. 3105)—(30s) NDC 0777-3105-30;(100s) NDC 0777-3105-02; (2000s) NDC 0777-3105-07 (ID†100)NDC 0777-3105-33;(20 FlexPak§ blister cards of 31) NDC 0777-3105-82

Continued on next page

This product information was prepared in June 1996. Current information on these and other products of Dista Products Products Company may be obtained by direct inquiry to Lilly Research Laboratories, Lilly Corporate Center, Indianapolis, Indiana 46285, (800) 545-5979.

Dista—Cont.

Liquid, Oral Solution:
20 mg*/5 mL, mint flavor (M-5120‡)—(120 mL) NDC 0777-5120-58
* Fluoxetine base equivalent.
† Identi-Dose® (unit dose medication, Dista).
‡ Dispense in a tight, light-resistant container.
§FlexPak (flexible blister card, Lilly).
Store at controlled room temperature, 59° to 86°F (15° to 30°C).

ANIMAL TOXICOLOGY

Phospholipids are increased in some tissues of mice, rats, and dogs given fluoxetine chronically. This effect is reversible after cessation of fluoxetine treatment. Phospholipid accumulation in animals has been observed with many cationic amphiphilic drugs, including fenfluramine, imipramine, and ranitidine. The significance of this effect in humans is unknown.

[060396]

Shown in Product Identification Guide, page 310

Dow Hickam Pharmaceuticals Inc.
P.O. BOX 2006
SUGAR LAND, TX 77487-2006

Direct Inquiries to:
Professional Services Department
(713) 240-1000

GRANULEX ℞

COMPOSITION

Each 0.82 cc. of medication delivered to the wound site contains Trypsin crystallized 0.1 mg., Balsam Peru 72.5 mg., Castor Oil 650.0 mg., and an emulsifier.

ACTION

Trypsin is intended for debridement of eschar and other necrotic tissue. It appears that in many instances removal of wound debris strengthens humoral defense mechanisms sufficiently to retard proliferation of local pathogens. Balsam Peru is an effective capillary bed stimulant used to increase circulation in the wound site area. Also, Balsam Peru has a mildly bactericidal action. Castor Oil is used to improve epithelialization by reducing premature epithelial desiccation and cornification. Also, it can act as a protective covering and aids in the reduction of pain.

INDICATIONS

For the treatment of decubitus ulcers, varicose ulcers, debridement of eschar, dehiscent wounds and sunburn.

USES

Granulex is in aerosol form which can be important to healing. It must be remembered, healing starts with a thin sheath of epithelium no more than a cell or two thick. Any rough movement or trauma can quickly destroy the healing tissue. Aerosols have the advantage of eliminating all extraneous physical contact with the wound. Granulex is easy to apply and quickly reduces odor frequently accompanying a decubitus ulcer. The wound may be left open or a wet bandage may be applied. As a suggestion; keep in mind wounds heal poorly in the presence of hemoglobin or zinc deficiency.

WARNING

Do not spray on fresh arterial clots. Avoid spraying in eyes. Flammable, do not expose to fire or open flame. Contents under pressure. Do not puncture or incinerate. Do not store at temperature above 120°F. Keep out of reach of children. Use only as directed. Intentional misuse by deliberately concentrating and inhaling the contents can be harmful or fatal.

DOSAGE

Apply a minimum of twice daily or as often as necessary. Shake well, press the aerosol valve and coat the wound rapidly but not excessively.

HOW SUPPLIED

2 oz. Aerosol NDC 0514-0001-01
4 oz. Aerosol NDC 0514-0001-02

SULFAMYLON® CREAM ℞
Brand of MAFENIDE ACETATE CREAM, USP
Topical Antibacterial Agent for Adjunctive Therapy in Second- and Third-Degree Burns

DESCRIPTION

SULFAMYLON Cream is a soft, white, nonstaining, water-miscible, anti-infective cream for topical administration to burn wounds.

SULFAMYLON Cream spreads easily, and can be washed off readily with water. It has a slight acetic odor. Each gram of SULFAMYLON Cream contains mafenide acetate equivalent to 85 mg of the base. The cream vehicle consists of cetyl alcohol, stearyl alcohol, cetyl esters wax, polyoxyl 40 stearate, polyoxyl 8 stearate, glycerin, and water, with methylparaben, propylparaben, sodium metabisulfite, and edetate disodium as preservatives.

Chemically, mafenide acetate is α-Amino-ρ-toluenesulfonamide monoacetate and has the following structural formula:

$$H_2NO_2S \text{—} \bigcirc \text{—} CH_2NH_2 \cdot CH_3COOH$$

CLINICAL PHARMACOLOGY

SULFAMYLON Cream, applied topically, produces a marked reduction in the bacterial population present in the avascular tissues of second- and third-degree burns. Reduction in bacterial growth after application of SULFAMYLON Cream has also been reported to permit spontaneous healing of deep partial-thickness burns, and thus prevent conversion of burn wounds from partial thickness to full thickness. It should be noted, however, that delayed eschar separation has occurred in some cases.

Absorption and Metabolism. Applied topically, SULFAMYLON Cream diffuses through devascularized areas, is absorbed, and rapidly converted to a metabolite (ρ-carboxybenzenesulfonamide) which is cleared through the kidneys. SULFAMYLON is active in the presence of pus and serum, and its activity is not altered by changes in the acidity of the environment.

Antibacterial Activity. SULFAMYLON exerts bacteriostatic action against many gram-negative and gram-positive organisms, including *Pseudomonas aeruginosa* and certain strains of anaerobes.

INDICATIONS AND USAGE

SULFAMYLON Cream is a topical agent indicated for adjunctive therapy of patients with second- and third-degree burns.

CONTRAINDICATIONS

SULFAMYLON is contraindicated in patients who are hypersensitive to it. It is not known whether there is cross sensitivity to other sulfonamides.

WARNINGS

Fatal hemolytic anemia with disseminated intravascular coagulation, presumably related to a glucose-6-phosphate dehydrogenase deficiency, has been reported following therapy with SULFAMYLON Cream.

Contains sodium metabisulfite, a sulfite that may cause allergic-type reactions including anaphylactic symptoms and life-threatening or less severe asthmatic episodes in certain susceptible people. The overall prevalence of sulfite sensitivity in the general population is unknown and probably low. Sulfite sensitivity is seen more frequently in asthmatic than in nonasthmatic people.

PRECAUTIONS

SULFAMYLON and its metabolite, ρ-carboxybenzenesulfonamide, inhibit carbonic anhydrase, which may result in metabolic acidosis, usually compensated by hyperventilation. In the presence of impaired renal function, high blood levels of SULFAMYLON and its metabolite may exaggerate the carbonic anhydrase inhibition. Therefore, close monitoring of acid-base balance is necessary, particularly in patients with extensive second-degree or partial thickness burns and in those with pulmonary or renal dysfunction. Some burn patients treated with SULFAMYLON Cream have also been reported to manifest an unexplained syndrome of marked hyperventilation with resulting respiratory alkalosis (slightly aklaline blood pH, low arterial pCO_2, and decreased total CO_2); change in arterial pO_2 is variable. The etiology and significance of these findings are unknown.

Mafenide acetate cream should be used with caution in burn patients with acute renal failure.

SULFAMYLON Cream should be administered with caution to patients with history of hypersensitivity to mafenide. It is not known whether there is cross sensitivity to other sulfonamides.

Fungal colonization in and below the eschar may occur concomitantly with reduction of bacterial growth in the burn wound. However, fungal dissemination through the infected burn wound is rare.

Carcinogenesis, Mutagenesis, Impairment of Fertility. No long-term animal studies have been performed to evaluate the drug's potential in these areas.

Pregnancy Category C. Animal reproduction studies have not been conducted with SULFAMYLON. It is also not known whether SULFAMYLON can cause fetal harm when administered to a pregnant woman or can affect reproduction capacity. Therefore, the preparation is not recommended for the treatment of women of childbearing potential, unless the burned area covers more than 20% of the total body surface, or the need for the therapeutic benefit of SULFAMYLON Cream is, in the physician's judgment, greater than the possible risk to the fetus.

Nursing Mothers. It is not known whether mafenide acetate is excreted in human milk. Because many drugs are excreted in human milk and because of the potential for serious adverse reaction in nursing infants from SULFAMYLON, a decision should be made whether to discontinue nursing or to discontinue the drug, taking into account the importance of the drug to the mother.

Pediatric Use. Same as for adults. (See DOSAGE AND ADMINISTRATION.)

ADVERSE REACTIONS

It is frequently difficult to distinguish between an adverse reaction to SULFAMYLON Cream and the effect of a severe burn. A single case of bone marrow depression and a single case of an acute attack of porphyria have been reported following therapy with SULFAMYLON Cream. Fatal hemolytic anemia with disseminated intravascular coagulation, presumably related to a glucose-6-phosphate dehydrogenase deficiency, has been reported following therapy with SULFAMYLON Cream.

Dermatologic: The most frequently reported reaction was pain on application or a burning sensation. Rare occurrences are excoriation of new skin, and bleeding of skin.

Allergic: Rash, itching, facial edema, swelling, hives, blisters, erythema, and eosinophilia.

Respiratory: Tachypnea or hyperventilation, decrease in arterial pCO_2.

Metabolic: Acidosis, increase in serum chloride.

Accidental ingestion of SULFAMYLON Cream has been reported to cause diarrhea.

DOSAGE AND ADMINISTRATION

Prompt institution of appropriate measures for controlling shock and pain is of prime importance. The burn wounds are then cleansed and debrided, and SULFAMYLON Cream is applied with a sterile gloved hand. Satisfactory results can be achieved with application of the cream once or twice daily, to a thickness of approximately 1/16 inch; thicker application is not recommended. The burned areas should be covered with SULFAMYLON Cream at all times. Therefore, whenever necessary, the cream should be reapplied to any areas from which it has been removed (eg, by patient activity). The routine of administration can be accomplished in minimal time, since dressings usually are not required. If individual patient demands make them necessary, however, only a thin layer of dressing should be used.

When feasible, the patient should be bathed daily, to aid in debridement. A whirlpool bath is particularly helpful, but the patient may be bathed in bed or in a shower.

The duration of therapy with SULFAMYLON Cream depends on each patient's requirements. Treatment is usually continued until healing is progressing well or until the burn site is ready for grafting. *SULFAMYLON Cream should not be withdrawn from the therapeutic regimen while there is the possibility of infection.* However, if allergic manifestations occur during treatment with SULFAMYLON Cream, discontinuation of treatment should be considered.

If acidosis occurs and becomes difficult to control, particularly in patients with pulmonary dysfunction, discontinuing therapy with SULFAMYLON Cream for 24 to 48 hours while continuing fluid therapy may aid in restoring acid-base balance.

HOW SUPPLIED

16 ounce plastic jar (453.6 g)—NDC 0514-0101-54
Cans of 14.5 ounces (411 g)—NDC 0514-0101-53
Collapsible tubes of 4 ounces (113.4 g)—NDC 0514-0101-51
Collapsible tubes of 2 ounces (56.7 g)—NDC 0514-0101-50
Avoid exposure to excessive heat (temperatures above 104°F or 40°C).

Caution: U.S. Federal law prohibits dispensing without prescription.

DISTRIBUTED BY:
DOW HICKAM PHARMACEUTICALS INC.
P.O. Box 2006
Sugar Land, TX 77487
1-800-231-3052 or
713-240-1000 in Texas

Revised May 1995

DuPont Pharma
WILMINGTON, DE 19805

DUPONT PHARMA
DuPont Merck Plaza, Hickory Run
P.O. Box 80723
Wilmington, DE 19880-0723
(302) 992-5000

Address all product-related inquiries to:
Medical Affairs Department

*For Product Information/Adverse Drug
Experience Reporting, call*
Product Information
(302) 992-4240

COUMADIN® TABLETS ℞
(Warfarin Sodium Tablets, USP) Crystalline
Anticoagulant

COUMADIN® FOR INJECTION ℞
(Warfarin Sodium for Injection, USP)

DESCRIPTION
COUMADIN (crystalline warfarin sodium), is an anticoagulant which acts by inhibiting vitamin K-dependent coagulation factors. Chemically, it is 3-(α-acetonylbenzyl)-4-hydroxycoumarin and is a racemic mixture of the R and S enantiomers. Crystalline warfarin sodium is an isopropanol clathrate. The crystallization of warfarin sodium virtually eliminates trace impurities present in amorphous warfarin. Its empirical formula is $C_{19}H_{15}NaO_4$ and its structural formula may be represented by the following:

Crystalline warfarin sodium occurs as a white, odorless, crystalline powder, is discolored by light and is very soluble in water; freely soluble in alcohol; very slightly soluble in chloroform and in ether.
COUMADIN Tablets for oral use also contain:

All strengths:	Lactose, starch and magnesium stearate
1 mg:	D&C Red 6
2 mg:	FD&C Blue 2 and FD&C Red 40
2½ mg:	FD&C Blue 1 and D&C Yellow 10
4 mg:	FD&C Blue 1 Lake
5 mg:	FD&C Yellow 6
7½ mg:	D&C Yellow 10 and FD&C Yellow 6
10 mg:	Dye Free

COUMADIN for Injection is supplied as a sterile, lyophilized powder, which, after reconstitution with 2.7 mL sterile Water for Injection, contains:

Warfarin Sodium	2 mg/mL
Sodium Phosphate, Dibasic, Heptahydrate	4.98 mg/mL
Sodium Phosphate, Monobasic, Monohydrate	0.194 mg/mL
Sodium Chloride	0.1 mg/mL
Mannitol	38.0 mg/mL
Sodium Hydroxide, as needed for pH adjustment to	8.1 to 8.3

CLINICAL PHARMACOLOGY
COUMADIN and other coumarin anticoagulants act by inhibiting the synthesis of vitamin K dependent clotting factors, which include Factors II, VII, IX and X, and the anticoagulant proteins C and S. Half-lives of these clotting factors are as follows: Factor II—60 hours, VII—4-6 hours, IX—24 hours, and X—48-72 hours. The half-lives of proteins C and S are approximately 8 hours and 30 hours, respectively. The resultant *in vivo* effect is a sequential depression of Factors VII, IX, X and II activities. Vitamin K is an essential cofactor for the post ribosomal synthesis of the vitamin K dependent clotting factors. The vitamin promotes the biosynthesis of γ-carboxyglutamic acid residues in the proteins which are essential for biological activity. Warfarin is thought to interfere with clotting factor synthesis by inhibition of the regeneration of vitamin K_1 epoxide. The degree of depression is dependent upon the dosage administered. Therapeutic doses of warfarin decrease the total amount of the active form of each vitamin K dependent clotting factor made by the liver by approximately 30% to 50%.
An anticoagulation effect generally occurs within 24 hours after drug administration. However, peak anticoagulant effect may be delayed 72 to 96 hours. The duration of action of a single dose of racemic warfarin is 2 to 5 days. The effects of COUMADIN may become more pronounced as effects of daily maintenance doses overlap. Anticoagulants have no direct effect on an established thrombus, nor do they reverse ischemic tissue damage. However, once a thrombus has occurred, the goal of anticoagulant treatment is to prevent further extension of the formed clot and prevent secondary thromboembolic complications which may result in serious and possibly fatal sequelae.
Pharmacokinetics: COUMADIN is a racemic mixture of the R- and S-enantiomers. The S-enantiomer exhibits 2–5 times more anticoagulant activity than the R-enantiomer in humans, but generally has a more rapid clearance.
Absorption: COUMADIN is essentially completely absorbed after oral administration with peak concentration generally attained within the first 4 hours.
Distribution: There are no differences in the apparent volumes of distribution after intravenous and oral administration of single doses of warfarin solution. Warfarin distributes into a relatively small apparent volume of distribution of about 0.14 liter/kg. A distribution phase lasting 6 to 12 hours is distinguishable after rapid intravenous or oral administration of an aqueous solution. Using a one compartment model, and assuming complete bioavailability, estimates of the volumes of distribution of R- and S-warfarin are similar to each other and to that of the racemate. Concentrations in fetal plasma approach the maternal values, but warfarin has not been found in human milk (see WARNINGS—Lactation). Approximately 99% of the drug is bound to plasma proteins.
Metabolism: The elimination of warfarin is almost entirely by metabolism. COUMADIN is stereoselectively metabolized by hepatic microsomal enzymes (cytochrome P-450) to inactivate hydroxylated metabolites (predominant route) and by reductases to reduced metabolites (warfarin alcohols). The warfarin alcohols have minimal anticoagulant activity. The metabolites are principally excreted into the urine; and to a lesser extent into the bile. The metabolites of warfarin that have been identified include dehydrowarfarin, two diastereoisomer alcohols, 4'-, 6-, 7-, 8- and 10-hydroxywarfarin. The Cytochrome P-450 isozymes involved in the metabolism of warfarin include 2C9, 2C19, 2C8, 2C18, 1A2, and 3A4. 2C9 is likely to be the principal form of human liver P-450 which modulates the *in vivo* anticoagulant activity of warfarin.

Excretion: The terminal half-life of warfarin after a single dose is approximately one week; however, the effective half-life ranges from 20 to 60 hours, with a mean of about 40 hours. The clearance of R-warfarin is generally half that of S-warfarin, thus as the volumes of distribution are similar, the half-life of R-warfarin is longer than that of S-warfarin. The half-life of R-warfarin ranges from 37 to 89 hours, while that of S-warfarin ranges from 21 to 43 hours. Studies with radiolabeled drug have demonstrated that up to 92% of the orally administered dose is recovered in urine. Very little warfarin is excreted unchanged in urine. Urinary excretion is in the form of metabolites.
Elderly: There are no significant age-related differences in the pharmacokinetics of racemic warfarin. Limited information suggests that there is no difference in the clearance of S-warfarin in elderly versus young subjects. However, there may be a slight decrease in the clearance of R-warfarin in the elderly compared to the young. Older patients (60 years or older) appear to exhibit greater than expected PT/INR response to the anticoagulant effects of warfarin. As patient age increases, less warfarin is required to produce a therapeutic level of anticoagulation. The cause of this response to warfarin is not known.
Renal Dysfunction: Renal clearance is considered to be a minor determinant of anticoagulant response to warfarin. No dosage adjustment is necessary for patients with renal failure.
Hepatic Dysfunction: Hepatic dysfunction can potentiate the response to warfarin through impaired synthesis of clotting factors and decreased metabolism of warfarin.
The administration of COUMADIN via the intravenous (I.V.) route should provide the patient with the same concentration of an equal oral dose, but maximum plasma concentration will be reached earlier. However, the full anticoagulant effect of a dose of warfarin may not be achieved until 72–96 hours after dosing, indicating that the administration of I.V. COUMADIN should not provide any increased biological effect or earlier onset of action.
Clinical Trials
Atrial Fibrillation (AF): In five prospective randomized controlled clinical trials involving 3711 patients with nonrheumatic AF, warfarin significantly reduced the risk of systemic thromboembolism including stroke (See Table 1). The risk reduction ranged from 60% to 86% in all except one trial (CAFA: 45%) which stopped early due to published positive results from two of these trials. The incidence of major bleeding in these trials ranged from 0.6 to 2.7% (See Table 1). Meta-analysis findings of these studies revealed that the effects of warfarin in reducing thromboembolic events including stroke were similar at either moderately high INR (2.0–4.5) or low INR (1.4–3.0). There was a significant reduction in minor bleeds at the low INR. Similar data from clinical studies in valvular atrial fibrillation patients are not available.
[See Table 1 above.]
Myocardial Infarction: WARIS (The Warfarin Re-Infarction Study) was a double-blind, randomized study of 1214 patients 2 to 4 weeks post-infarction treated with warfarin to a target INR of 2.8 to 4.8. (But note that a lower INR was achieved and reduced bleeding was associated with INR's above 4.0; see Dosage and Administration.) The primary endpoint was a combination of total mortality and recurrent infarction. A secondary endpoint of cerebrovascular events was assessed. Mean follow-up of the patients was 37 months. The results for each endpoint separately, including an analysis of vascular death, are provided in the following table:
[See Table 2 at left.]
Mechanical and Bioprosthetic Heart Valves: In a prospective, randomized, open label, positive-controlled study (Mok et al, 1985) in 254 patients, the thromboembolic-free interval was found to be significantly greater in patients with mechanical prosthetic heart valves treated with warfarin alone compared with dipyridamole-aspirin (p < 0.005) and pentoxifylline-aspirin (p < 0.05) treated patients. Rates of thromboembolic events in these groups were 2.2, 8.6, and 7.9/100

TABLE 1
CLINICAL STUDIES OF WARFARIN IN NON-RHEUMATIC AF PATIENTS*

Study	N Warfarin-Treated Patients	N Control Patients	PT Ratio	INR	Thromboembolism %Risk Reduction	*p*-value	% Major Bleeding Warfarin-Treated Patients	Control Patients
AFASAK	335	336	1.5–2.0	2.8–4.2	60	0.027	0.6	0.0
SPAF	210	211	1.3–1.8	2.0–4.5	67	0.01	1.9	1.9
BAATAF	212	208	1.2–1.5	1.5–2.7	86	< 0.05	0.9	0.5
CAFA	187	191	1.3–1.6	2.0–3.0	45	0.25	2.7	0.5
SPINAF	260	265	1.2–1.5	1.4–2.8	79	0.001	2.3	1.5

*All study results of warfarin vs. control are based on intention-to-treat analysis and include ischemic stroke and systemic throboembolism, excluding hemorrhage and transient ischemic attacks.

TABLE 2

Event	Warfarin (N=607)	Placebo (N=607)	RR (95%CI)	% Risk Reduction (p-value)
Total Patient Years of Follow-up	2018	1944		
Total Mortality	94 (4.7/100 py)	123 (6.3/100 py)	0.76 (0.60, 0.97)	24 (p=0.030)
Vascular Death	82 (4.1/100 py)	105 (5.4/100 py)	0.78 (0.60, 1.02)	22 (p=0.068)
Recurrent MI	82 (4.1/100 py)	124 (6.4/100 py)	0.66 (0.51, 0.85)	34 (p=0.001)
Cerebrovascular Event	20 (1.0/100 py)	44 (2.3/100 py)	0.46 (0.28, 0.75)	54 (p=0.002)

RR=Relative risk; Risk reduction=(I–RR); CI=Confidence interval; MI=Myocardial infarction; py=patient years

Continued on next page

Consult 1997 supplements and future editions for revisions

DuPont Pharma—Cont.

patient years, respectively. Major bleeding rates were 2.5, 0.0, and 0.9/100 patient years, respectively.

In a prospective, open label, clinical trial (Saour et al, 1990) comparing moderate (INR 2.65) vs. high intensity (INR 9.0) warfarin therapies in 258 patients with mechanical prosthetic heart valves, thromboembolism occurred with similar frequency in the two groups (4.0 and 3.7 events/100 patient years, respectively). Major bleeding was more common in the high intensity group (2.1 events/100 patient years) vs 0.95 events/100 patient years in the moderate intensity group.

In a randomized trial (Turpie et al, 1988) in 210 patients comparing two intensities of warfarin therapy (INR 2.0–2.25 vs. INR 2.5–4.0) for a three month period following tissue heart value replacement, thromboembolism occurred with similar frequency in the two groups (major embolic events 2.0% vs. 1.9%, respectively and minor embolic events 10.8% vs. 10.2%, respectively). Major bleeding complications were more frequent with the higher intensity (major hemorrhages 4.6%) vs. none in the lower intensity.

INDICATIONS AND USAGE

COUMADIN (Warfarin Sodium) is indicated for the prophylaxis and/or treatment of venous thrombosis and its extension, and pulmonary embolism.

COUMADIN is indicated for the prophylaxis and/or treatment of the thromboembolic complications associated with atrial fibrillation and/or cardiac valve replacement.

COUMADIN is indicated to reduce the risk of death, recurrent myocardial infarction, and thromboembolic events such as stroke or systemic embolization after myocardial infarction.

CONTRAINDICATIONS

Anticoagulation is contraindicated in any localized or general physical condition or personal circumstance in which the hazard of hemorrhage might be greater than the potential clinical benefits of anticoagulation, such as:

Pregnancy: COUMADIN is contraindicated in women who are or may become pregnant because the drug passes through the placental barrier and may cause fatal hemorrhage to the fetus *in utero*. Furthermore, there have been reports of birth malformations in children born to mothers who have been treated with warfarin during pregnancy. Embryopathy characterized by nasal hypoplasia with or without stippled epiphyses (chondrodysplasia punctata) has been reported in pregnant women exposed to warfarin during the first trimester. Central nervous system abnormalities also have been reported, including dorsal midline dysplasia characterized by agenesis of the corpus callosum, Dandy-Walker malformation, and midline cerebellar atrophy. Ventral midline dysplasia, characterized by optic atrophy, and eye abnormalities have been observed. Mental retardation, blindness, and other central nervous system abnormalities have been reported in association with second and third trimester exposure. Although rare, teratogenic reports following *in utero* exposure to warfarin include urinary tract anomalies such as single kidney, asplenia, anencephaly, spina bifida, cranial nerve palsy, hydrocephalus, cardiac defects and congenital heart disease, polydactyly, deformities of toes, diaphragmatic hernia, corneal leukoma, cleft palate, cleft lip, schizencephaly, and microcephaly. Spontaneous abortion and still birth are known to occur and a higher risk of fetal mortality is associated with the use of warfarin. Low birth weight and growth retardation have also been reported.

Women of childbearing potential who are candidates for anticoagulant therapy should be carefully evaluated and the indications critically reviewed with the patient. If the patient becomes pregnant while taking this drug, she should be apprised of the potential risks to the fetus, and the possibility of termination of the pregnancy should be discussed in light of those risks.

Hemorrhagic tendencies or blood dyscrasias.

Recent or contemplated surgery of: (1) central nervous system; (2) eye; (3) traumatic surgery resulting in large open surfaces.

Bleeding tendencies associated with active ulceration or overt bleeding of: (1) gastrointestinal, genitourinary or respiratory tracts; (2) cerebrovascular hemorrhage; (3) aneurysms-cerebral, dissecting aorta; (4) pericarditis and pericardial effusions; (5) bacterial endocarditis.

Threatened abortion, eclampsia and preeclampsia.

Inadequate laboratory facilities.

Unsupervised patients with senility, alcoholism, or psychosis or other lack of patient cooperation.

Spinal puncture and other diagnostic or therapeutic procedures with potential for uncontrollable bleeding.

Miscellaneous: major regional, lumbar block anesthesia and malignant hypertension.

WARNINGS

The most serious risks associated with anticoagulant therapy with sodium warfarin are hemorrhage in any tissue or organ and, less frequently (< 0.1%), necrosis and/or gangrene of skin and other tissues. The risk of hemorrhage is related to the level of intensity and the duration of anticoagulant therapy. Hemorrhage and necrosis have in some cases been reported to result in death or permanent disability. Necrosis appears to be associated with local thrombosis and usually appears within a few days of the start of anticoagulant therapy. In severe cases of necrosis, treatment through debridement or amputation of the affected tissue, limb, breast or penis has been reported. Careful diagnosis is required to determine whether necrosis is caused by an underlying disease. Warfarin therapy should be discontinued when warfarin is suspected to be the cause of developing necrosis and heparin therapy may be considered for anticoagulation. Although various treatments have been attempted, no treatment for necrosis has been considered uniformly effective. See below for information on predisposing conditions. These and other risks associated with anticoagulant therapy must be weighed against the risk of thrombosis or embolization in untreated cases.

It cannot be emphasized too strongly that treatment of each patient is a highly individualized matter. COUMADIN, a narrow therapeutic range (index) drug, may be affected by factors such as other drugs and dietary Vitamin K. Dosage should be controlled by periodic determinations of prothrombin time (PT)/International Normalized Ratio (INR) or other suitable coagulation tests. Determinations of whole blood clotting and bleeding times are not effective measures for control of therapy. Heparin prolongs the one-stage PT. When heparin and COUMADIN are administered concomitantly, refer below to CONVERSION FROM HEPARIN THERAPY for recommendations.

Caution should be observed when COUMADIN is administered in any situation or in the presence of any predisposing condition where added risk of hemorrhage or necrosis is present.

Anticoagulation therapy with COUMADIN may enhance the release of atheromatous plaque emboli, thereby increasing the risk of complications from systemic cholesterol microembolization, including the "purple toes syndrome." Discontinuation of COUMADIN therapy is recommended when such phenomena are observed.

Systemic atheroemboli and cholesterol microemboli can present with a variety of signs and symptoms including purple toes syndrome, livedo reticularis, rash, gangrene, abrupt and intense pain in the leg, foot, or toes, foot ulcers, myalgia, penile gangrene, abdominal pain, flank or back pain, hematuria, renal insufficiency, hypertension, cerebral ischemia, spinal cord infarction, pancreatitis, symptoms simulating polyarteritis, or any other sequelae of vascular compromise due to embolic occlusion. The most commonly involved visceral organs are the kidneys followed by the pancreas, spleen, and liver. Some cases have progressed to necrosis or death.

Purple toes syndrome is a complication of oral anticoagulation characterized by a dark, purplish or mottled color of the toes, usually occurring between 3–10 weeks, or later, after the initiation of therapy with warfarin or related compounds. Major features of this syndrome include purple color of plantar surfaces and sides of the toes that blanches on moderate pressure and fades with elevation of the legs; pain and tenderness of the toes; waxing and waning of the color over time. While the purple toes syndrome is reported to be reversible, some cases progress to gangrene or necrosis which may require debridement of the affected area, or may lead to amputation.

A severe elevation (> 50 seconds) in activated partial thromboplastin time (aPTT) with a PT/INR in the desired range has been identified as an indication of increased risk of postoperative hemorrhage.

The decision to administer anticoagulants in the following conditions must be based upon clinical judgment in which the risks of anticoagulant therapy are weighed against the benefits:

Lactation: COUMADIN appears in the milk of nursing mothers in an inactive form. Infants nursed by COUMADIN treated mothers had no change in prothrombin times (PTs). Effects in premature infants have not been evaluated.

Severe to moderate hepatic or renal insufficiency.

Infectious diseases or disturbances of intestinal flora: sprue, antibiotic therapy.

Trauma which may result in internal bleeding.

Surgery or trauma resulting in large exposed raw surfaces.

Indwelling catheters.

Severe to moderate hypertension.

Known or suspected deficiency in protein C mediated anticoagulant response: Hereditary or acquired deficiencies of protein C or its cofactor, protein S, have been associated with tissue necrosis following warfarin administration. Not all patients with these conditions develop necrosis, and tissue necrosis occurs in patients without these deficiencies. Inherited resistance to activated protein C has been described in many patients with venous thromboembolic disorders but has not yet been evaluated as a risk factor for tissue necrosis. The risk associated with these conditions, both for recurrent thrombosis and for adverse reactions, is difficult to evaluate since it does not appear to be the same for everyone. Decisions about testing and therapy must be made on an individual basis. It has been reported that concurrent anticoagulation therapy with heparin for 5 to 7 days during initiation of therapy with COUMADIN may minimize the incidence of tissue necrosis. Warfarin therapy should be discontinued when warfarin is suspected to be the cause of developing necrosis and heparin therapy may be considered for anticoagulation.

Miscellaneous: polycythemia vera, vasculitis, and severe diabetes.

Minor and severe allergic/hypersensitivity reactions and anaphylactic reactions have been reported.

In patients with acquired or inherited warfarin resistance, decreased therapeutic responses to COUMADIN have been reported. Exaggerated therapeutic responses have been reported in other patients.

Patients with congestive heart failure may exhibit greater than expected PT/INR response to COUMADIN, thereby requiring more frequent laboratory monitoring, and reduced doses of COUMADIN.

Concurrent use of anticoagulants with streptokinase or urokinase is not recommended and may be hazardous. (Please note recommendations accompanying these preparations.)

PRECAUTIONS

Periodic determination of PT/INR or other suitable coagulation test is essential.

Numerous factors, alone or in combination, including travel, changes in diet, environment, physical state and medication may influence response of the patient to anticoagulants. It is generally good practice to monitor the patient's response with additional PT/INR determinations in the period immediately after discharge from the hospital, and whenever other medications are initiated, discontinued or taken irregularly. The following factors are listed for reference; however, other factors may also affect the anticoagulant response.

Drugs may interact with COUMADIN through pharmacodynamic or pharmacokinetic mechanisms. Pharmacodynamic mechanisms for drug interactions with COUMADIN are synergism (impaired hemostasis, reduced clotting factor synthesis), competitive antagonism (vitamin K), and altered physiologic control loop for vitamin K metabolism (hereditary resistance). Pharmacokinetic mechanisms for drug interactions with COUMADIN are mainly enzyme induction, enzyme inhibition, and reduced plasma protein binding. It is important to note that some drugs may interact by more than one mechanism.

The following factors, alone or in combination, may be responsible for INCREASED PT/INR response:

ENDOGENOUS FACTORS:
blood dyscrasias—see CONTRAINDICATIONS
cancer
collagen vascular disease
congestive heart failure
diarrhea
elevated temperature
hepatic disorders
    infectious hepatitis
    jaundice
hyperthyroidism
poor nutritional state
steatorrhea
vitamin K deficiency

EXOGENOUS FACTORS:
Potential drug interactions with COUMADIN are listed below by drug class and by specific drugs.
Classes of Drugs
Adrenergic Stimulants, Central
Alcohol Abuse Reduction Preparations
Analgesics
Anesthetics, Inhalation
Antiarrhythmics†
Antibiotics†
    Aminoglycosides (oral)
    Cephalosporins, parenteral
    Macrolides
    Miscellaneous
    Penicillins, intravenous, high dose
    Quinolones (fluoroquinolones)
    Sulfonamides, long acting
    Tetracyclines
Anticoagulants
Anticonvulsants†
Antidepressants†
Antimalarial Agents
Antineoplastics†
Antiparasitic/Antimicrobials
Antiplatelet Drugs/Effects

Antithyroid Drugs†
Beta-Adrenergic Blockers
Bromelains
Cholelitholytic Agents
Diabetes Agents, Oral
Diuretics†
Fungal Medications, Systemic†
Gastric Acidity and Peptic Ulcer Agents†
Gastrointestinal, Ulcerative Colitis Agents
Gout Treatment Agents
Hemorrheologic Agents
Hepatotoxic Drugs
Hyperglycemic Agents
Hypertensive Emergency Agents
Hypnotics†
Hypolipidemics†
Monoamine Oxidase Inhibitors
Narcotics, prolonged
Nonsteroidal Anti-Inflammatory Agents
Psychostimulants
Pyrazolones
Salicylates
Steroids, Adrenocortical†
Steroids, Anabolic (17-Alkyl Testosterone Derivatives)
Thrombolytics
Thyroid Drugs
Tuberculosis Agents†
Uricosuric Agents
Vaccines
Vitamins†

Specific Drugs Reported
acetaminophen
alcohol†
allopurinol
aminosalicylic acid
amiodarone HCl
aspirin
cefamandole
cefazolin
cefoperazone
cefotetan
cefoxitin
ceftriaxone
chenodiol
chloramphenicol
chloral hydrate†
chlorpropamide
cholestyramine†
cimetidine
ciprofloxacin
clarithromycin
clofibrate
COUMADIN overdose
cyclophosphamide†
danazol
dextran
dextrothyroxine
diazoxide
diclofenac
dicumarol
diflunisal
disulfiram
doxycycline
erythromycin
ethacrynic acid
fenoprofen
fluconazole
fluorouracil
glucagon
halothane
heparin
ibuprofen
ifosfamide
indomethacin
influenza virus vaccine
itraconazole
ketoprofen
ketorolac
levamisole
levothyroxine
liothyronine
lovastatin
mefenamic acid
methimazole†
methyldopa
methylphenidate
methylsalicylate ointment (topical)
metronidazole
miconazole
moricizine hydrochloride†
nalidixic acid
naproxen
neomycin
norfloxacin
ofloxacin

olsalazine
omeprazole
oxaprozin
oxymetholone
paroxetine
penicillin G, intravenous
pentoxifylline
phenylbutazone
phenytoin†
piperacillin
piroxicam
prednisone†
propafenone
propoxyphene
propranolol
propylthiouracil†
quinidine
quinine
ranitidine†
sertraline
simvastatin
stanozolol
streptokinase
sulfamethizole
sulfamethoxazole
sulfinpyrazone
sulfisoxazole
sulindac
tamoxifen
tetracycline
thyroid
ticarcillin
ticlopidine
tissue plasminogen activator (t-PA)
tolbutamide
trimethoprim/sulfamethoxazole
urokinase
valproate
vitamin E
also: other medications affecting blood elements which may
modify hemostasis
    dietary deficiencies
    prolonged hot weather
    unreliable PT/INR determinations
†Increased and decreased PT/INR responses have been reported.

The following factors, alone or in combination, may be responsible for DECREASED PT/INR response:

ENDOGENOUS FACTORS:
edema
hereditary coumarin resistance
hyperlipemia
hypothyroidism
nephrotic syndrome

EXOGENOUS FACTORS:
Potential drug interactions with COUMADIN are listed below by drug class and by specific drugs.
Classes of Drugs
Adrenal Cortical Steroid Inhibitors
Antacids
Antianxiety Agents
Antiarrhythmics†
Antibiotics†
Anticonvulsants†
Antidepressants†
Antihistamines
Antineoplastics†
Antipsychotic Medications
Antithyroid Drugs†
Barbiturates
Diuretics†
Enteral Nutritional Supplements
Fungal Medications, Systemic†
Gastric Acidity and Peptic Ulcer
  Agents†
Hypnotics†
Hypolipidemics†
Immunosuppressives
Oral Contraceptives, Estrogen Containing
Steroids, Adrenocortical†
Tuberculosis Agents†
Vitamins†

Specific Drugs Reported
alcohol†
aminoglutethimide
amobarbital
azathioprine
butabarbital
butalbital
carbamazepine
chloral hydrate†
chlordiazepoxide
chlorthalidone
cholestyramine†

corticotropin
cortisone
COUMADIN underdosage
cyclophosphamide†
dicloxacillin
ethchlorvynol
glutethimide
griseofulvin
haloperidol
meprobamate
methimazole†
moricizine hydrochloride†
nafcillin
paraldehyde
pentobarbital
phenobarbital
phenytoin†
prednisone†
primidone
propylthiouracil†
ranitidine†
rifampin
secobarbital
spironolactone
sucralfate
trazodone
vitamin C (high dose)
vitamin K
also: diet high in vitamin K
    unreliable PT/INR determinations
†Increased and decreased PT/INR responses have been reported.

Because a patient may be exposed to a combination of the above factors, the net effect of COUMADIN on PT/INR response may be unpredictable. More frequent PT/INR monitoring is therefore advisable. Medications of unknown interaction with coumarins are best regarded with caution. When these medications are started or stopped, more frequent PT/INR monitoring is advisable.

It has been reported that concomitant administration of warfarin and ticlopidine may be associated with cholestatic hepatitis.

Effect on Other Drugs: Coumarins may also affect the action of other drugs. Hypoglycemic agents (chlorpropamide and tolbutamide) and anticonvulsants (phenytoin and phenobarbital) may accumulate in the body as a result of interference with either their metabolism or excretion.

Special Risk Patients: COUMADIN is a narrow therapeutic range (index) drug, and caution should be observed when warfarin sodium is administered to certain patients such as the elderly or debilitated or when administered in any situation or physical condition where added risk of hemorrhage is present.

Intramuscular (I.M.) injections of concomitant medications should be confined to the upper extremities which permits easy access for manual compression, inspections for bleeding and use of pressure bandages.

Caution should be observed when COUMADIN (or warfarin) is administered concomitantly with nonsteroidal anti-inflammatory drugs (NSAIDs), including aspirin, to be certain that no change in anticoagulation dosage is required. In addition to specific drug interactions that might affect PT/INR, NSAIDs, including aspirin, can inhibit platelet aggregation, and can cause gastrointestinal bleeding, peptic ulceration and/or perforation.

Acquired or inherited warfarin resistance should be suspected if large daily doses of COUMADIN are required to maintain a patient's PT/INR within a normal therapeutic range.

Information for Patients: The objective of anticoagulant therapy is to decrease the clotting ability of the blood so that thrombosis is prevented, while avoiding spontaneous bleeding. Effective therapeutic levels with minimal complications are in part dependent upon cooperative and well-instructed patients who communicate effectively with their physician. Patients should be advised: Strict adherence to prescribed dosage schedule is necessary. Do not take or discontinue any other medication, including salicylates (e.g., aspirin and topical analgesics) and other over-the-counter medications except on advice of the physician. Avoid alcohol consumption. Do not take COUMADIN during pregnancy and do not become pregnant while taking it (see CONTRAINDICATIONS). Avoid any activity or sport that may result in traumatic injury. Prothrombin time tests and regular visits to physician or clinic are needed to monitor therapy. Carry identification stating that COUMADIN is being taken. If the prescribed dose of COUMADIN is forgotten, notify the physician immediately. Take the dose as soon as possible on the same day but do not take a double dose of COUMADIN the next day to make up for missed doses. The amount of vitamin K in food may affect therapy with COUMADIN. Eat a normal, balanced diet maintaining a consistent amount of vitamin K. Avoid drastic changes in dietary habits, such as eat-

Continued on next page

Consult 1997 supplements and future editions for revisions

DuPont Pharma—Cont.

ing large amounts of green leafy vegetables. Contact physician to report any illness, such as diarrhea, infection or fever. Notify physician immediately if any unusual bleeding or symptoms occur. Signs and symptoms of bleeding include: pain, swelling or discomfort, prolonged bleeding from cuts, increased menstrual flow or vaginal bleeding, nosebleeds, bleeding of gums from brushing, unusual bleeding or bruising, red or dark brown urine, red or tar black stools, headache, dizziness, or weakness. If therapy with COUMADIN is discontinued, patients should be cautioned that the anticoagulant effects of COUMADIN may persist for about 2 to 5 days.

Carcinogenesis, Mutagenesis, Impairment of Fertility: Carcinogenicity and mutagenicity studies have not been performed with COUMADIN. The reproductive effects of COUMADIN have not been evaluated.

Use in Pregnancy: Pregnancy Category X—See CONTRA-INDICATIONS.

Pediatric Use: Safety and effectiveness in pediatric patients below the age of 18 have not been established, in randomized, controlled clinical trials. However, the use of COUMADIN in pediatric patients is well-documented for the prevention and treatment of thromboembolic events. Difficulty achieving and maintaining therapeutic PT/INR ranges in the pediatric patient has been reported. More frequent PT/INR determinations are recommended because of possible changing warfarin requirements.

ADVERSE REACTIONS

Potential adverse reactions to COUMADIN may include:

- Fatal or nonfatal hemorrhage from any tissue or organ. This is a consequence of the anticoagulant effect. The signs, symptoms, and severity will vary according to the location and degree or extent of the bleeding. Hemorrhagic complications may present as paralysis; paresthesia; headache, chest, abdomen, joint, muscle or other pain; dizziness; shortness of breath, difficult breathing or swallowing; unexplained swelling; weakness; hypotension; or unexplained shock. Therefore, the possibility of hemorrhage should be considered in evaluating the condition of any anticoagulated patient with complaints which do not indicate an obvious diagnosis. Bleeding during anticoagulant therapy does not always correlate with PT/INR. (See OVERDOSAGE—Treatment.)
- Bleeding which occurs when the PT/INR is within the therapeutic range warrants diagnostic investigation since it may unmask a previously unsuspected lesion, e.g., tumor, ulcer, etc.
- Necrosis of skin and other tissues. (See WARNINGS.)
- Adverse reactions reported infrequently include: hypersensitivity reactions, systemic cholesterol microembolization, purple toes syndrome, vasculitis, hepatitis, cholestatic hepatic injury, jaundice, elevated liver enzymes, fever, dermatitis, including bullous eruptions, urticaria, abdominal pain including cramping, asthenia, nausea, vomiting, diarrhea, headache, pruritis, alopecia, and paresthesia.

Rare events of tracheal or tracheobronchial calcification have been reported in association with long-term warfarin therapy. The clinical significance of this event is unknown.

Priapism has been associated with anticoagulant administration, however, a causal relationship has not been established.

OVERDOSAGE

Signs and Symptoms: Suspected or overt abnormal bleeding (e.g., appearance of blood in stools or urine, hematuria, excessive menstrual bleeding, melena, petechiae, excessive bruising or persistent oozing from superficial injuries) are early manifestations of anticoagulation beyond a safe and satisfactory level.

Treatment: Excessive anticoagulation, with or without bleeding, may be controlled by discontinuing COUMADIN therapy and if necessary, by administration of oral or parenteral vitamin K_1. (Please see recommendations accompanying vitamin K_1 preparations prior to use.)

Such use of vitamin K_1 reduces response to subsequent COUMADIN therapy. Patients may return to a pretreatment thrombotic status following the rapid reversal of a prolonged PT/INR. Resumption of COUMADIN administration reverses the effect of vitamin K, and a therapeutic PT/INR can again be obtained by careful dosage adjustment. If rapid anticoagulation is indicated, heparin may be preferable for initial therapy.

If minor bleeding progresses to major bleeding, give 5 to 25 mg (rarely up to 50 mg) parenteral vitamin K_1. In emergency situations of severe hemorrhage, clotting factors can be returned to normal by administering 200 to 500 mL of fresh whole blood or fresh frozen plasma, or by giving commercial Factor IX complex.

A risk of hepatitis and other viral diseases is associated with the use of these blood products; Factor IX complex is also

associated with an increased risk of thrombosis. Therefore, these preparations should be used only in exceptional or life-threatening bleeding episodes secondary to COUMADIN overdosage.

Purified Factor IX preparations should not be used because they cannot increase the levels of prothrombin, Factor VII and Factor X which are also depressed along with the levels of Factor IX as a result of COUMADIN treatment. Packed red blood cells may also be given if significant blood loss has occurred. Infusions of blood or plasma should be monitored carefully to avoid precipitating pulmonary edema in elderly patients or patients with heart disease.

DOSAGE AND ADMINISTRATION

The dosage and administration of COUMADIN must be individualized for each patient according to the particular patient's PT/INR response to the drug. The dosage should be adjusted based upon the patient's PT/INR. (See LABORATORY CONTROL below for full discussion on INR.)

Venous Thromboembolism (including pulmonary embolism): Available clinical evidence indicates that an INR of 2.0–3.0 is sufficient for prophylaxis and treatment of venous thromboembolism and minimizes the risk of hemorrhage associated with higher INRs.

Atrial Fibrillation: Five recent clinical trials evaluated the effects of warfarin in patients with non-valvular atrial fibrillation (AF). Meta-analysis findings of these studies revealed that the effects of warfarin in reducing thromboembolic events including stroke were similar at either moderately high INR (2.0–4.5) or low INR (1.4–3.0). There was a significant reduction in minor bleeds at the low INR. Similar data from clinical studies in valvular atrial fibrillation patients are not available. The trials in non-valvular atrial fibrillation support the American College of Chest Physicians' (ACCP) recommendation that an INR of 2.0–3.0 be used for long term warfarin therapy in appropriate AF patients.

Post-Myocardial Infarction: In post myocardial infarction patients, COUMADIN therapy should be initiated early (2–4 weeks post-infarction) and dosage should be adjusted to maintain an INR of 2.5–3.5 long-term. The recommendation is based on the results of the WARIS study in which treatment was initiated 2 to 4 weeks after the infarction. In patients thought to be at an increased risk of bleeding complications or on aspirin therapy, maintenance of COUMADIN therapy at the lower end of this INR range is recommended.

Mechanical and Bioprosthetic Heart Valves: In patients with mechanical heart valve(s), long term prophylaxis with warfarin to an INR of 2.5–3.5 is recommended. In patients with bioprosthetic heart valve(s), based on limited data, the American College of Chest Physicians recommends warfarin therapy to an INR of 2.0–3.0 for 12 weeks after valve insertion. In patients with additional risk factors such as atrial fibrillation or prior thromboembolism, consideration should be given for longer term therapy.

Recurrent Systemic Embolism: In cases where the risk of thromboembolism is great, such as in patients with recurrent systemic embolism, a higher INR may be required.

An INR of greater than 4.0 appears to provide no additional therapeutic benefit in most patients and is associated with a higher risk of bleeding.

Initial Dosage: The dosing of COUMADIN must be individualized according to patient's sensitivity to the drug as indicated by the PT/INR. Use of a large loading dose may increase the incidence of hemorrhagic and other complications, does not offer more rapid protection against thrombi formation, and is not recommended. Low initiation doses are recommended for elderly and/or debilitated patients and patients with potential to exhibit greater than expected PT/INR response to COUMADIN (see PRECAUTIONS). It is recommended that COUMADIN therapy be initiated with a dose of 2 to 5 mg per day with dosage adjustments based on the results of PT/INR determinations.

Maintenance: Most patients are satisfactorily maintained at a dose of 2 to 10 mg daily. Flexibility of dosage is provided by breaking scored tablets in half. The individual dose and interval should be gauged by the patient's prothrombin response.

Duration of Therapy: The duration of therapy in each patient should be individualized. In general, anticoagulant therapy should be continued until the danger of thrombosis and embolism has passed.

Missed Dose: The anticoagulant effect of COUMADIN persists beyond 24 hours. If the patient forgets to take the prescribed dose of COUMADIN at the scheduled time, the dose should be taken as soon as possible on the same day. The patient should not take the missed dose by doubling the daily dose to make up for missed doses, but should refer back to his or her physician.

Intravenous Route of Administration: COUMADIN for Injection provides an alternate administration route for patients who cannot receive oral drugs. The I.V. dosages would be the same as those that would be used orally if the patient could take the drug by the oral route. COUMADIN for Injection should be administered as a slow bolus injection over 1 to 2 minutes into a peripheral vein. It

is not recommended for intramuscular administration. The vial should be reconstituted with 2.7 mL of sterile Water for Injection and inspected for particulate matter and discoloration immediately prior to use. Do not use if either particulate matter and/or discoloration is noted. After reconstitution, COUMADIN for Injection is chemically and physically stable for 4 hours at room temperature. It does not contain any antimicrobial preservative and, thus, care must be taken to assure the sterility of the prepared solution. The vial is not recommended for multiple use and unused solution should be discarded.

LABORATORY CONTROL The PT reflects the depression of vitamin K dependent Factors VII, X and II. There are several modifications of the one-stage PT and the physician should become familiar with the specific method used in his laboratory. The degree of anticoagulation indicated by any range of PTs may be altered by the type of thromboplastin used; the appropriate therapeutic range must be based on the experience of each laboratory. The PT should be determined daily after the administration of the initial dose until PT/INR results stabilize in the therapeutic range. Intervals between subsequent PT/INR determinations should be based upon the physician's judgment of the patient's reliability and response to COUMADIN in order to maintain the individual within the therapeutic range. Acceptable intervals for PT/INR determinations are normally within the range of one to four weeks after a stable dosage has been determined. To ensure adequate control, it is recommended that additional PT tests are done when other warfarin products are interchanged with COUMADIN and also if other medications are coadministered with COUMADIN (see PRECAUTIONS).

Different thromboplastin reagents vary substantially in their sensitivity to sodium warfarin-induced effects on PT. To define the appropriate therapeutic regimen it is important to be familiar with the sensitivity of the thromboplastin reagent used in the laboratory and its relationship to the International Reference Preparation (IRP), a sensitive thromboplastin reagent prepared from human brain.

A system of standardizing the PT in oral anticoagulant control was introduced by the World Health Organization in 1983. It is based upon the determination of an International Normalized Ratio (INR) which provides a common basis for communication of PT results and interpretations of therapeutic ranges. The INR system of reporting is based on a logarithmic relationship between the PT ratios of the test and reference preparation. The INR is the PT ratio that would be obtained if the International Reference Preparation (IRP), which has an ISI of 1.0, were used to perform the test. Early clinical studies of oral anticoagulants, which formed the basis for recommended therapeutic ranges of 1.5 to 2.5 times control mean normal PT, used sensitive human brain thromboplastin. When using the less sensitive rabbit brain thromboplastins commonly employed in PT assays today, adjustments must be made to the targeted PT range that reflect this decrease in sensitivity.

The INR can be calculated as:

$$INR = (\text{observed PT ratio})^{ISI}$$

where the ISI (International Sensitivity Index) is the correction factor in the equation that relates the PT ratio of the local reagent to the reference preparation and is a measure of the sensitivity of a given thromboplastin to reduction of vitamin K-dependent coagulation factors; the lower the ISI, the more "sensitive" the reagent and the closer the derived INR will be to the observed PT ratio.[1]

The proceedings and recommendations of the 1992 National Conference on Antithrombotic Therapy[2-4] review and evaluate issues related to oral anticoagulant therapy and the sensitivity of thromboplastin reagents and provide additional guidelines for defining the appropriate therapeutic regimen. The conversion of the INR to PT ratios for the less-intense (INR 2.0–3.0) and more intense (INR 2.5–3.5) therapeutic range recommended by the ACCP for thromboplastins over a range of ISI values is shown in Table 3.[5]

[See table at top of next page.]

TREATMENT DURING DENTISTRY AND SURGERY The management of patients who undergo dental and surgical procedures requires close liaison between attending physicians, surgeons and dentists. PT/INR determination is recommended just prior to any dental or surgical procedure. In patients undergoing minimal invasive procedures who must be anticoagulated prior to, during, or immediately following these procedures, adjusting the dosage of COUMADIN to maintain the PT/INR at the low end of the therapeutic range may safely allow for continued anticoagulation. The operative site should be sufficiently limited and accessible to permit the effective use of local procedures for hemostasis. Under these conditions, dental and minor surgical procedures may be performed without undue risk of hemorrhage. Some dental or surgical procedures may necessitate the interruption of COUMADIN therapy. When discontinuing COUMADIN even for a short period of time, the benefits and risks should be strongly considered.

CONVERSION FROM HEPARIN THERAPY Since the anticoagulant effect of COUMADIN is delayed, heparin is

TABLE 3
Relationship Between INR and PT Ratios
For Thromboplastins With Different ISI Values (Sensitivities)

		PT RATIOS			
	ISI 1.0	ISI 1.4	ISI 1.8	ISI 2.3	ISI 2.8
INR = 2.0–3.0	2.0–3.0	1.6–2.2	1.5–1.8	1.4–1.6	1.3–1.5
INR = 2.5–3.5	2.5–3.5	1.9–2.4	1.7–2.0	1.5–1.7	1.4–1.6

	30's	100's	1000's	Hospital Unit-Dose blister package of 100
1 mg pink		NDC 0056-0169-70	NDC 0056-0169-90	NDC 0056-0169-75
2 mg lavender	NDC 0056-0170-30	NDC 0056-0170-70	NDC 0056-0170-90	NDC 0056-0170-75
2½ mg green	NDC 0056-0176-30	NDC 0056-0176-70	NDC 0056-0176-90	NDC 0056-0176-75
4 mg blue		NDC 0056-0168-70	NDC 0056-0168-90	NDC 0056-0168-75
5 mg peach	NDC 0056-0172-30	NDC 0056-0172-70	NDC 0056-0172-90	NDC 0056-0172-75
7½ mg yellow		NDC 0056-0173-70		NDC 0056-0173-75
10 mg white		NDC 0056-0174-70		NDC 0056-0174-75

preferred initially for rapid anticoagulation. Conversion to COUMADIN may begin concomitantly with heparin therapy or may be delayed 3 to 6 days. To ensure continuous anticoagulation, it is advisable to continue full dose heparin therapy and that COUMADIN therapy be overlapped with heparin for 4 to 5 days, until COUMADIN has produced the desired therapeutic response as determined by PT/INR. When COUMADIN has produced the desired PT/INR or prothrombin activity, heparin may be discontinued.

COUMADIN may increase the aPTT test. During initial therapy with COUMADIN, the interference with heparin anticoagulation is of minimal clinical significance.

As heparin may affect the PT/INR, patients receiving both heparin and COUMADIN should have blood for PT/INR determination drawn at least:

* 5 hours after the last IV bolus dose of heparin, or
* 4 hours after cessation of a continuous IV infusion of heparin, or
* 24 hours after the last subcutaneous heparin injection.

HOW SUPPLIED

Tablets: For oral use, single scored, imprinted numerically and packaged in bottles with potencies and colors as follows: [See second table above.]

COUMADIN oral tablet is available in 1, 2, 2½, 4, 5, 7½ and 10 mg of warfarin sodium with one face inscribed with the word COUMADIN, single scored and imprinted numerically and with the 1, 2, 2½, 4, 5, 7½ or 10 superimposed, and on the other face inscribed with the word "DuPont."

Protect from light. Store in carton until contents have been used. Store at controlled room temperature (59°–86°F, 15°–30°C). Dispense in a tight, light-resistant container as defined in the USP.

Injection: Available for intravenous use only. Not recommended for intramuscular administration. Reconstitute with 2.7 mL of sterile Water for Injection to yield 2 mg/mL. Net contents 5.4 mg lyophilized powder. Maximum yield 2.5 mL.

5 mg vial (box of 6) NDC 0590-0324-35

Protect from light. Keep vial in box until used. Store at controlled room temperature (59°–86°F, 15°–30°C).

After reconstitution, store at controlled room temperature (59°–86°F, 15°–30°C) and use within 4 hours. Do not refrigerate. Discard any unused solution.

CAUTION: Federal law prohibits dispensing without a prescription.

REFERENCES

1. Poller, L.: Laboratory Control of Anticoagulant Therapy. Seminars in Thrombosis and Hemostasis, Vol. 12, No. 1, pp. 13-19, 1986.
2. Hirsh, J.: Is the Dose of Warfarin Prescribed by American Physicians Unnecessarily High? *Arch Int Med,* Vol. 147, pp. 769-771, 1987.
3. Cook, D.J., Guyatt, H.G., Laupacis, A., Sackett, D.L.: Rules of Evidence and Clinical Recommendations on the Use of Antithrombotic Agents. Chest ACCP Consensus Conference on Antithrombotic Therapy. *Chest,* Vol. 102(Suppl), pp. 305S-311S, 1992.
4. Hirsh, J., Dalen, J., Deykin, D., Poller, L: Oral Anticoagulants Mechanism of Action, Clinical Effectiveness, and Optimal Therapeutic Range. Chest ACCP Consensus Conference on Antithrombotic Therapy. *Chest,* Vol. 102(Suppl), pp. 312S-326S, 1992.
5. Hirsh, J., M.D., F.C.C.P.: Hamilton Civic Hospitals Research Center, Hamilton, Ontario, Personal Communication.

DuPont Pharma
Wilmington, Delaware 19880
COUMADIN® and the color and configuration of COUMADIN tablets are trademarks of The DuPont Merck Pharmaceutical Company. Any unlicensed use of these trademarks is expressly prohibited under the U.S. Trademark Act.
Copyright © DuPont Pharma 1995
6386-02/Rev. Sept., 1995   CU-31864-02
Shown in Product Identification Guide, page 310

HESPAN®   ℞

[*hes' pan*]
(6% hetastarch in
0.9% sodium chloride injection)

DESCRIPTION

HESPAN® (6% hetastarch in 0.9% sodium chloride injection) is a sterile, nonpyrogenic solution. The composition of each 100 mL is as follows:

Hetastarch .... 6.0 g
Sodium Chloride, USP .... 0.9 g
Water for Injection, USP .... qs
pH adjusted with Sodium Hydroxide NF
Concentration of Electrolytes (mEq/liter): Sodium 154, Chloride 154 pH: 3.5-7.0; Calc. Osmolarity: 310 mOsM/liter

Hetastarch is an artificial colloid derived from a waxy starch composed almost entirely of amylopectin. Hydroxyethyl ether groups are introduced into the glucose units of the starch and the resultant material is hydrolyzed to yield a product with a molecular weight suitable for use as a plasma volume expander and erythrocyte sedimenting agent. Hetastarch is characterized by its molar substitution, and also by its molecular weight. The molar substitution is 0.7 which means hetastarch has 7 hydroxyethyl groups for every 10 glucose units. The weight average molecular weight is approximately 480,000 with a range of 400,000 to 550,000 and with 80% of the polymers falling between the range of 30,000 and 2,400,000. Hydroxyethyl groups are attached by ether linkage primarily at C-2 of the glucose unit and to a lesser extent at C-3 and C-6. The polymer resembles glycogen, and the polymerized glucose units are joined primarily by 1-4 linkages with occasional 1-6 branching linkages. The degree of branching is approximately 1:20 which means that there is one 1-6 branch for every 20 glucose monomer units.
The chemical name for hetastarch is hydroxyethyl starch. The structural formula is as follows:

Amylopectin derivative in which R_2, R_3, and R_6 are H or CH_2CH_2OH, or R_6 is a branching point in the starch polymer connected through a 1-6 linkage to additional α-D-glucopyranosyl units.
HESPAN is a clear, pale yellow to amber solution. Exposure to prolonged adverse storage conditions may result in a change to a turbid deep brown or the formation of a crystalline precipitate. Do not use the solution if these conditions are evident.
The plastic container is made from a multi-layered film specifically developed for parenteral drugs. It contains no plasticizers and exhibits virtually no leachables. The solution contact layer is a rubberized copolymer of ethylene and propyl-ene. The container is nontoxic and biologically inert. The container-solution unit is a closed system and is not dependent upon entry of external air during administration. The container is overwrapped to provide protection from the physical environment and to provide an additional moisture barrier when necessary.
The closure system has two ports; the one for the administration set has a tamper evident plastic protector.

CLINICAL PHARMACOLOGY

The plasma volume expansion produced by HESPAN approximate those of 5% human albumin. Intravenous infusion of HESPAN results in expansion of plasma volume that decreases over the succeeding 24 to 36 hours. The degree of plasma volume expansion and improvement in hemodynamic state depend upon the patient's intravascular status. Hetastarch molecules below 50,000 molecular weight are rapidly eliminated by renal excretion. A single dose of approximately 500 mL of HESPAN (approximately 30 g) results in elimination in the urine of approximately 33% of the dose within 24 hours. This is a variable process but generally results in an intravascular hetastarch concentration of less than 10% of the total dose injected by two weeks. A study of the biliary excretion of HESPAN in 10 healthy males accounted for less than 1% of the dose over a 14-day period. The hydroxyethyl group is not cleaved by the body, but remains intact and attached to glucose units when excreted. Significant quantities of glucose are not produced as hydroxyethylation prevents complete metabolism of the smaller polymers.
The addition of HESPAN to whole blood increases the erythrocyte sedimentation rate. Therefore, HESPAN is used to improve the efficiency of granulocyte collection by centrifugal means.

INDICATIONS AND USAGE

HESPAN is indicated in the treatment of hypovolemia when plasma volume expansion is desired. It is not a substitute for blood or plasma.
The adjunctive use of HESPAN in leukapheresis has also been shown to be safe and efficacious in improving the harvesting and increasing the yield of granulocytes by centrifugal means.

CONTRAINDICATIONS

HESPAN is contraindicated in patients with known hypersensitivity to hydroxyethyl starch, or with bleeding disorders, or with congestive heart failure where volume overload is a potential problem. HESPAN should not be used in renal disease with oliguria or anuria not related to hypovolemia.

WARNINGS

Life threatening anaphylactic/anaphylactoid reactions have been rarely reported with HESPAN; death has occurred, but a causal relationship has not been established. Patients who develop severe anaphylactoid reactions may need continued supportive care until symptoms have resolved.
Hypersensitivity reactions can occur even after HESPAN has been discontinued.

Usage in Plasma Volume Expansion
Large volumes of HESPAN may transiently alter the coagulation mechanism due to hemodilution and a mild direct inhibitory action on Factor VIII. In addition, administration of HESPAN may result in transient prolongation of prothrombin time, activated partial thromboplastin, clotting, and bleeding times.
Hematocrit may be decreased and plasma proteins diluted excessively by administration of large volumes of HESPAN. Administration of packed red cells, platelets, and fresh frozen plasma should be considered if excessive dilution occurs. In randomized, controlled, comparative studies of HESPAN (n=92) and albumin (n=85) in surgical patients, no patient in either treatment group had a bleeding complication and no significant difference was found in the amount of blood loss between the treatment groups.[1-4]
Use over extended periods: HESPAN has not been adequately evaluated to establish its safety in situations other than leukapheresis that require frequent use of colloidal solutions over extended periods. In some cases, HESPAN has been associated with coagulation abnormalities in conjunction with an acquired, reversible von Willebrand's-like syndrome and/or Factor VIII deficiency when used over a period of days. Replacement therapy should be considered if a severe Factor VIII deficiency is identified. If a coagulopathy develops, it may take several days to resolve. Certain conditions may affect the safe use of HESPAN on a chronic basis. For example, in patients with subarachnoid hemorrhage where HESPAN is used repeatedly over a period of days for the prevention of cerebral vasospasm, significant clinical bleeding may occur. Intracranial bleeding resulting in death has been reported.[5]

Usage in Leukapheresis
Slight declines in platelet counts and hemoglobin levels have been observed in donors undergoing repeated leukapheresis procedures using HESPAN due to the volume expanding effects of HESPAN and to the collection of platelets and

Continued on next page

DuPont Pharma—Cont.

erythrocytes. Hemoglobin levels usually return to normal within 24 hours. Hemodilution by HESPAN and saline may also result in 24 hour declines of total protein, albumin, calcium and fibrinogen values. None of these decreases are to a degree recognized to be clinically significant risks to healthy donors.

PRECAUTIONS

General

Regular and frequent clinical evaluation and complete blood counts (CBC) are necessary for proper monitoring of HESPAN use during leukapheresis. If the frequency of leukapheresis is to exceed the guidelines for whole blood donation, you may wish to consider the following additional studies: total leukocyte and platelet counts, leukocyte differential count, hemoglobin and hematocrit, prothrombin time (PT), and partial thromboplastin time (PTT) tests.

The possibility of circulatory overload should be kept in mind. Caution should be used when the risk of pulmonary edema and/or congestive heart failure is increased. Special care should be exercised in patients who have impaired renal clearance since this is the principal way in which hetastarch is eliminated.

Indirect bilirubin levels of 8.3 mg/L (normal 0.0-7.0 mg/L) have been reported in 2 out of 20 normal subjects who received multiple HESPAN infusions. Total bilirubin was within normal limits at all times; indirect bilirubin returned to normal by 96 hours following the final infusion. The significance, if any, of these elevations is not known; however, caution should be observed before administering HESPAN to patients with a history of liver disease.

If a hypersensitivity effect occurs, administration of the drug should be discontinued and appropriate treatment and supportive measures should be undertaken (see **WARNINGS**). Caution should be used when administering HESPAN to patients allergic to corn because such patients can also be allergic to HESPAN.

The EXCEL® container has a natural gum rubber/latex-containing injection port. Unless medication addition occurs, a diaphragm prevents the latex from coming in contact with the HESPAN solution. In patients with latex hypersensitivity, caution should be exercised when adding medication through the port of the EXCEL® container.

Elevated serum amylase levels may be observed temporarily following administration of HESPAN, although no association with pancreatitis has been demonstrated. Serum amylase levels cannot be used to assess or to evaluate for pancreatitis for 3-5 days after administration of HESPAN. Elevated serum amylase levels persist for longer periods of time in patients with renal impairment. HESPAN has not been shown to increase serum lipase.

One report suggests that in the presence of renal glomerular damage, larger molecules of HESPAN can leak into the urine and elevate the specific gravity. The elevation of specific gravity can obscure the diagnosis of renal failure.

HESPAN is not eliminated by hemodialysis. The utility of other extracorporeal elimination techniques has not been evaluated.

If administration is by pressure infusion, all air should be withdrawn or expelled from the bag through the medication port prior to infusion.

Carcinogenesis, Mutagenesis, Impairment of Fertility

Long-term studies of animals have not been performed to evaluate the carcinogenic potential of hetastarch.

Teratogenic Effects

Pregnancy Category C. HESPAN has been shown to have an embryocidal effect on New Zealand rabbits when given intravenously over the entire organogenesis period in a daily dose ½ times the maximum recommended therapeutic human dose (1500 mL), and on BD rats when given intraperitoneally, from the 16th to the 21st day of pregnancy, in a daily dose 2.3 times the maximum recommended therapeutic human dose. When HESPAN was administered to New Zealand rabbits, BD rats, and swiss mice with intravenous daily doses of 2 times, ⅓ times and 1 time the maximum recommended therapeutic human dose respectively over several days during the period of gestation, no evidence of teratogenicity was evident. There are no adequate and well controlled studies in pregnant women. HESPAN should be used during pregnancy only if the potential benefit justifies the potential risk to the fetus.

Nursing Mothers

It is not known whether hetastarch is excreted in human milk. Because many drugs are excreted in human milk, caution should be exercised when HESPAN is administered to a nursing woman.

Pediatric Use

The safety and effectiveness of HESPAN in pediatric patients have not been established.

ADVERSE REACTIONS

Reported adverse reactions associated with HESPAN include:

General

Hypersensitivity (see **WARNINGS**).

Death, life-threatening anaphylactic/anaphylactoid reactions, cardiac arrest, ventricular fibrillation, severe hypotension, non-cardiac pulmonary edema, laryngeal edema, bronchospasm, angioedema, wheezing, restlessness, tachypnea, stridor, fever, chest pain, bradycardia, tachycardia, shortness of breath, chills, urticaria, pruritus, facial and periorbital edema, coughing, sneezing, flushing, erythema multiforme and rash.

Cardiovascular

Circulatory overload, congestive heart failure, and pulmonary edema (see **PRECAUTIONS**).

Hematologic

Intracranial bleeding, bleeding and/or anemia due to hemodilution (see **WARNINGS**) and/or Factor VIII deficiency, acquired von Willebrand's-like syndrome, and coagulopathy including rare cases of disseminated intravascular coagulopathy and hemolysis.

Metabolic

Metabolic acidosis.

Other

Vomiting, peripheral edema of the lower extremities, submaxillary and parotid glandular enlargement, mild influenza-like symptoms, headaches and muscle pains.

DOSAGE AND ADMINISTRATION

Dosage for Acute Use in Plasma Volume Expansion

HESPAN is administered by intravenous infusion only. Total dosage and rate of infusion depend upon the amount of blood or plasma lost and the resultant hemoconcentration. In adults, the amount usually administered is 500 to 1000 mL. Doses of more than 1500 mL per day for the typical 70 kg patient (approximately 20 mL per kg of body weight) are usually not required, although higher doses have been reported in postoperative and trauma patients where severe blood loss has occurred.

Dosage in Leukapheresis

250 to 700 mL of HESPAN to which citrate anticoagulant has been added is typically administered by aseptic addition to the input line of the centrifugation apparatus at a ratio of 1:8 to 1:13 to venous whole blood. The HESPAN and citrate should be thoroughly mixed to assure effective anticoagulation of blood as it flows through the leukapheresis machine. When stored at room temperature, HESPAN admixtures of 500-560 mL with citrate concentrations up to 2.5% were compatible for 24 hours. The safety and compatibility of additives other than citrate have not been established.

General Recommendations

Do not use plastic container in series connection.

If administration is controlled by a pumping device, care must be taken to discontinue pumping action before the container runs dry or air embolism may result.

This solution is intended for intravenous administration using sterile equipment. It is recommended that intravenous administration apparatus be replaced at least once every 24 hours.

Use only if solution is clear and container and seals are intact.

Parenteral drug products should be inspected visually for particulate matter and discoloration prior to administration whenever solution and container permit.

If administration is by pressure infusion, all air should be withdrawn or expelled from the bag through the medication port prior to infusion.

CAUTION: Before administering to the patient, review these directions:

To Open

Do not remove the plastic infusion container from its overwrap until immediately before use. To open, tear overwrap down at notch and remove solution container. Check for minute leaks by squeezing solution container firmly. If leaks are found, discard solution as sterility may be impaired.

Invert container and carefully inspect the solution in good light for cloudiness, haze, or particulate matter. Any container which is suspect should not be used.

Preparation for Administration (Use aseptic technique)

1. Close flow control clamp of administration set.
2. Twist off plug from port designated "Infusion Set Port".
3. Insert spike of infusion set into port with a twisting motion until the set is firmly seated.
4. Suspend container from hanger.
5. Follow manufacturer's recommended procedures for the administration set.
6. Discontinue administration and notify physician immediately if patient exhibits signs of adverse reactions.

HOW SUPPLIED

HESPAN® (6% hetastarch in 0.9% sodium chloride injection) is supplied sterile and nonpyrogenic in 500 mL and 250 mL EXCEL® Containers.

NDC	Size
HESPAN (6% hetastarch in 0.9% sodium chloride injection)	
0056-0037-46	500 mL (12 per case)
0056-0037-42	250 mL (24 per case)

Exposure of pharmaceutical products to heat should be minimized. Avoid excessive heat. Protect from freezing. It is recommended that the product be stored at room temperature (25°C); however, brief exposure up to 40°C does not adversely affect the product.

CAUTION: Federal (USA) law prohibits dispensing without prescription.

REFERENCES

1. Diehl J. et al, Clinical Comparison of Hetastarch and Albumin in Postoperative Cardiac Patients. *The Annals of Thoracic Surgery.* 1982;34(6):674-679.
2. Gold M. et al, Comparison of Hetastarch to Albumin for Perioperative Bleeding in Patients Undergoing Abdominal Aortic Aneurysm Surgery, *Annals of Surgery*, 1990;211(4):482-485.
3. Kirklin J. et al, Hydroxyethyl Starch versus Albumin for Colloid Infusion Following Cardiopulmonary Bypass in Patients Undergoing Myocardial Revascularization, *The Annals of Thoracic Surgery*, 1984;37(1):40-46.
4. Moggio RA. et al, Hemodynamic Comparison of Albumin and Hydroxyethyl Starch in Postoperative Cardiac Surgery Patients, *Critical Care Medicine*, 1983;11(12):943-945.
5. Damon L., Intracranial Bleeding During Treatment with Hydroxyethyl Starch, *New England Journal of Medicine*, 1987;317(15):964-965.

Marketed and Distributed by:
DuPont Pharma
Wilmington, Delaware 19880
Distributed and Manufactured by:
McGaw, Inc.
Irvine, CA USA 92714-5895
6253-3/Rev. January, 1996
U.S. Patent No. 4,803,102
EXCEL® is a registered trademark of McGaw, Inc.
HESPAN® is a registered trademark of The DuPont Merck Pharmaceutical Co.

HYCODAN®

[hī-kō-dan]

(hydrocodone bitartrate and homatropine methylbromide)
Tablets and Syrup
Antitussive

DESCRIPTION

HYCODAN contains hydrocodone (dihydrocodeinone) bitartrate, a semisynthetic centrally-acting narcotic antitussive. Homatropine methylbromide is included in a subtherapeutic amount to discourage deliberate overdosage.

Each HYCODAN tablet or teaspoonful (5 mL) contains:
Hydrocodone bitartrate, USP   5 mg
WARNING: May be habit forming.
Homatropine methylbromide, USP   1.5 mg
HYCODAN tablets also contain: calcium phosphate dibasic, colloidal silicon dioxide, lactose, magnesium stearate, starch and stearic acid.
HYCODAN syrup: caramel coloring, FD&C Red 40, liquid sugar, methylparaben, propylparaben, sorbitol solution and wild cherry imitation flavor.

The hydrocodone component is 4,5α-epoxy-3-methoxy-17-methylmorphinan-6-one tartrate (1:1) hydrate (2:5), a fine white crystal or crystalline powder, which is derived from the opium alkaloid, thebaine, has a molecular weight of (494.50) and may be represented by the following structural formula.

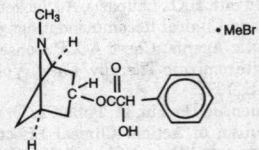

$$C_{18}H_{21}NO_3 \cdot C_4H_6O_6 \cdot 2\tfrac{1}{2}H_2O$$
HYDROCODONE BITARTRATE

$$C_{17}H_{24}BrNO_3$$
HOMATROPINE METHYLBROMIDE

Homatropine methylbromide is 8-Azoniabicyclo[3.2.1] octane, 3- [(hydroxyphenylacetyl) oxy] -8, 8-dimethyl-, bromide, endo-; a white crystal or fine white crystalline powder, with a molecular weight of (370.29).

CLINICAL PHARMACOLOGY

Hydrocodone is a semisynthetic narcotic antitussive and analgesic with multiple actions qualitatively similar to those of codeine. The precise mechanism of action of hydrocodone and other opiates is not known; however, hydrocodone is believed to act directly on the cough center. In excessive doses, hydrocodone, like other opium derivatives, will depress respiration. The effects of hydrocodone in therapeutic doses on the cardiovascular system are insignificant. Hydrocodone can produce miosis, euphoria, physical and physiological dependence.

Following a 10 mg oral dose of hydrocodone administered to five adult male subjects, the mean peak concentration was 23.6 $\pm$ 5.2 ng/mL. Maximum serum levels were achieved at 1.3 $\pm$ 0.3 hours and the half-life was determined to be 3.8 $\pm$ 0.3 hours. Hydrocodone exhibits a complex pattern of metabolism including O-demethylation, N-demethylation and 6-keto reduction to the corresponding 6-α- and 6-β- hydroxy-metabolites.

INDICATIONS AND USAGE

HYCODAN is indicated for the symptomatic relief of cough.

CONTRAINDICATIONS

HYCODAN should not be administered to patients who are hypersensitive to hydrocodone or homatropine methylbromide.

WARNINGS

May be habit forming. Hydrocodone can produce drug dependence of the morphine type and, therefore, has the potential for being abused. Psychic dependence, physical dependence and tolerance may develop upon repeated administration of HYCODAN and it should be prescribed and administered with the same degree of caution appropriate to the use of other narcotic drugs (see DRUG ABUSE AND DEPENDENCE).

Respiratory Depression: HYCODAN produces dose-related respiratory depression by directly acting on brain stem respiratory centers. If respiratory depression occurs, it may be antagonized by the use of naloxone hydrochloride and other supportive measures when indicated.

Head Injury And Increased Intracranial Pressure: The respiratory depression properties of narcotics and their capacity to elevate cerebrospinal fluid pressure may be markedly exaggerated in the presence of head injury, other intracranial lesions or a pre-existing increase in intracranial pressure. Furthermore, narcotics produce adverse reactions which may obscure the clinical course of patients with head injuries.

Acute Abdominal Conditions: The administration of HYCODAN or other narcotics may obscure the diagnosis or clinical course of patients with acute abdominal conditions.

Pediatric Use: In young children, as well as adults, the respiratory center is sensitive to the depressant action of narcotic cough suppressants in a dose-dependent manner. Benefit to risk ratio should be carefully considered especially in children with respiratory embarrassment (e.g., croup).

PRECAUTIONS

General: Before prescribing medication to suppress or modify cough, it is important to ascertain that the underlying cause of cough is identified, that modification of cough does not increase the risk of clinical or physiological complications, and that appropriate therapy for the primary disease is provided.

Special Risk Patients: HYCODAN should be given with caution to certain patients such as the elderly or debilitated, and those with severe impairment of hepatic or renal functions, hypothyroidism, Addison's disease, prostatic hypertrophy or urethral stricture, asthma, and narrow-angle glaucoma.

Information For Patients: Hydrocodone may impair the mental and/or physical abilities required for the performance of potentially hazardous tasks such as driving a car or operating machinery. The patient using HYCODAN should be cautioned accordingly.

Drug Interactions: Patients receiving narcotics, antihistamines, antipsychotics, antianxiety agents or other CNS depressants (including alcohol) concomitantly with HYCODAN may exhibit an additive CNS depression. When combined therapy is contemplated, the dose of one or both agents should be reduced. The use of MAO inhibitors or tricyclic antidepressants with hydrocodone preparations may increase the effect of either the antidepressant or hydrocodone.

Carcinogenesis, Mutagenesis, Impairment Of Fertility: Studies of HYCODAN in animals to evaluate the carcinogenic and mutagenic potential and the effect on fertility have not been conducted.

PREGNANCY

Teratogenic Effects: Pregnancy Category C; Animal reproduction studies have not been conducted with HYCODAN (hydrocodone bitartrate and homatropine methylbromide). It is also not known whether HYCODAN can cause fetal harm when administered to a pregnant woman or can affect reproduction capacity. HYCODAN should be given to a pregnant woman only if clearly needed.

Nonteratogenic Effects: Babies born to mothers who have been taking opioids regularly prior to delivery will be physically dependent. The withdrawal signs include irritability and excessive crying, tremors, hyperactive reflexes, increased respiratory rate, increased stools, sneezing, yawning, vomiting and fever. The intensity of the syndrome does not always correlate with the duration of maternal opioid use or dose.

Labor and Delivery: As with all narcotics, administration of HYCODAN to the mother shortly before delivery may result in some degree of respiratory depression in the newborn, especially if higher doses are used.

Nursing Mothers: It is not known whether this drug is excreted in human milk. Because many drugs are excreted in human milk and because of the potential for serious adverse reactions in nursing infants from HYCODAN, a decision should be made whether to discontinue nursing or to discontinue the drug, taking into account the importance of the drug to the mother.

Pediatric Use: Safety and effectiveness of HYCODAN in children under six have not been established.

ADVERSE REACTIONS

Central Nervous System: Sedation, drowsiness, mental clouding, lethargy, impairment of mental and physical performance, anxiety, fear, dysphoria, dizziness, psychic dependence, mood changes.

Gastrointestinal System: Nausea and vomiting may occur; they are more frequent in ambulatory than in recumbent patients. Prolonged administration of HYCODAN may produce constipation.

Genitourinary System: Ureteral spasm, spasm of vesicle sphincters and urinary retention have been reported with opiates.

Respiratory Depression: HYCODAN may produce dose-related respiratory depression by acting directly on brain stem respiratory centers (see OVERDOSAGE).

Dermatological: Skin rash, pruritus.

DRUG ABUSE AND DEPENDENCE

HYCODAN is a Schedule III narcotic. Psychic dependence, physical dependence and tolerance may develop upon repeated administration of narcotics; therefore, HYCODAN should be prescribed and administered with caution. However, psychic dependence is unlikely to develop when HYCODAN is used for a short time for the treatment of cough. Physical dependence, the condition in which continued administration of the drug is required to prevent the appearance of a withdrawal syndrome, assumes clinically significant proportions only after several weeks of continued oral narcotic use, although some mild degree of physical dependence may develop after a few days of narcotic therapy.

OVERDOSAGE

Signs and Symptoms: Serious overdosage with hydrocodone is characterized by respiratory depression (a decrease in respiratory rate and/or tidal volume, Cheyne-Stokes respiration, cyanosis), extreme somnolence progressing to stupor or coma, skeletal muscle flaccidity, cold and clammy skin, and sometimes bradycardia and hypotension. In severe overdosage, apnea, circulatory collapse, cardiac arrest and death may occur. The ingestion of very large amounts of HYCODAN may, in addition, result in acute homatropine intoxication.

Treatment: Primary attention should be given to the reestablishment of adequate respiratory exchange through provision of a patent airway and the institution of assisted or controlled ventilation. The narcotic antagonist naloxone hydrochloride is a specific antidote for respiratory depression which may result from overdosage or unusual sensitivity to narcotics including hydrocodone. Therefore, an appropriate dose of naloxone hydrochloride should be administered, preferably by the intravenous route, simultaneously with efforts at respiratory resuscitation. For further information, see full prescribing information for naloxone hydrochloride. An antagonist should not be administered in the absence of clinically significant respiratory depression. Oxygen, intravenous fluids, vasopressors and other supportive measures should be employed as indicated. Gastric emptying may be useful in removing unabsorbed drug.

DOSAGE AND ADMINISTRATION

Adults: One (1) tablet or one (1) teaspoonful (5 mL) of the syrup every 4 to 6 hours as needed; do not exceed six (6) tablets or six (6) teaspoonfuls in 24 hours.

Children 6 to 12 years of age: One-half (½) tablet or one-half (½) teaspoonful (2.5 mL) of the syrup every 4 to 6 hours as needed; do not exceed three (3) tablets or three (3) teaspoonfuls in 24 hours.

HOW SUPPLIED

As white tablets with one face scored and inscribed HYCODAN, and the other inscribed with DuPont name is available in:

Bottles of 100	NDC 0056-0042-70
Bottles of 500	NDC 0056-0042-85

As a clear red colored, wild cherry flavored syrup in:

Bottles of one pint	NDC 0056-0234-16

Store at controlled room temperature (59°–86° F, 15°–30° C).

Caution: Federal law prohibits dispensing without prescription.

Oral prescription where permitted by state law.

DuPont Pharma
Wilmington, Delaware 19880

HYCODAN® is a Registered Trademark of The DuPont Merck Pharmaceutical Co.
6132-9/Rev. Aug. 1994

HYCOMINE® Ⓒ III
(hydrocodone bitartrate and phenylpropanolamine hydrochloride)
Pediatric Syrup

HYCOMINE® Ⓒ III
(hydrocodone bitartrate and phenylpropanolamine hydrochloride)
Syrup

DESCRIPTION

HYCOMINE contains hydrocodone (dihydrocodeinone) bitartrate, a semi-synthetic centrally-acting narcotic antitussive and phenylpropanolamine hydrochloride, a sympathomimetic amine decongestant for oral administration.

The pH of HYCOMINE and HYCOMINE Pediatric Syrup is 3.2–4.2. The hydrocodone component is (5α)-4,5-epoxy-3-methoxy-17-methylmorphinan-6-one [R-(R*,R*)]-2,3-dihydroxybutanedioate (1:1) hydrate (2:5), a fine white crystal or crystalline powder, which is derived from the opium alkaloid, thebaine, and has a molecular weight of 494.50. The phenylpropanolamine component is ($\pm$)-(R*,S*)-α-(1-aminoethyl) benzenemethanol hydrochloride and has a molecular weight of 187.67. These may be represented by the following structural formulas:

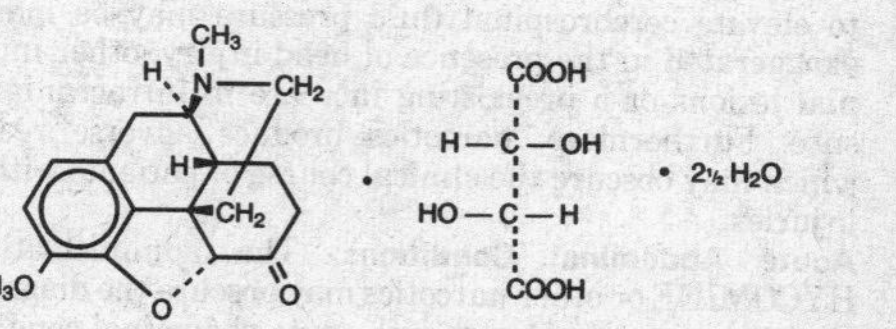

HYDROCODONE BITARTRATE

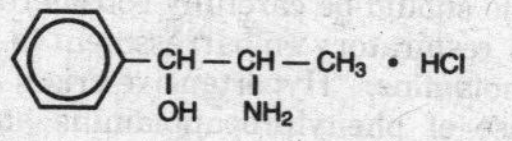

PHENYLPROPANOLAMINE HYDROCHLORIDE

	HYCOMINE Pediatric Syrup	HYCOMINE Syrup
Each teaspoonful (5 mL) contains:		
Hydrocodone bitartrate, USP WARNING: May be habit forming	2.5 mg	5 mg
Phenylpropanolamine hydrochloride, USP	12.5 mg	25 mg

Also, HYCOMINE, both strengths, contain: artificial cherry flavor, glycerin, methylparaben, propylparaben, saccharin sodium, and sorbitol solution. HYCOMINE Pediatric Syrup contains: D&C Yellow 10 and FD&C Green 3. HYCOMINE Syrup: FD&C Red 40 and FD&C Yellow 6.

CLINICAL PHARMACOLOGY

Hydrocodone is a semisynthetic narcotic antitussive and analgesic with multiple actions qualitatively similar to those of codeine. The precise mechanism of action of hydrocodone and other opiates is not known; however, hydrocodone is believed to act directly on the cough center. In excessive doses, hydrocodone, like other opium derivatives, will depress respiration. The effects of hydrocodone in therapeutic doses on the cardiovascular system are insignificant. Hydrocodone can produce miosis, euphoria, physical and physiological dependence.

Continued on next page

DuPont Pharma—Cont.

Following a 10 mg oral dose of hydrocodone administered to five adult male subjects, the mean peak concentration was 23.6 ± 5.2 ng/mL. Maximum serum levels were achieved at 1.3 ± 0.3 hours and the half-life was determined to be 3.8 ± 0.3 hours. Hydrocodone exhibits a complex pattern of metabolism including O-demethylation, N-demethylation and 6-keto reduction to the corresponding 6-α- and 6-β-hydroxymetabolites.

Phenylpropanolamine effects its vasoconstrictor activity by releasing noradrenaline from sympathetic nerve endings, and from direct stimulation of α-adrenoreceptors of blood vessels.

INDICATIONS AND USAGE

HYCOMINE is indicated for the symptomatic relief of cough and nasal congestion.

CONTRAINDICATIONS

HYCOMINE is contraindicated in patients hypersensitive to hydrocodone or phenylpropanolamine, and in patients on concurrent MAO inhibitor therapy. Patients known to be hypersensitive to other opioids or sympathomimetic amines may exhibit cross sensitivity to HYCOMINE. Phenylpropanolamine is contraindicated in patients with heart disease, hypertension, diabetes or hyperthyroidism. Hydrocodone is contraindicated in the presence of an intracranial lesion associated with increased intracranial pressure; and whenever ventilatory function is depressed.

WARNINGS

May be habit forming. Hydrocodone can produce drug dependence of the morphine type and, therefore, has the potential for being abused. Psychic dependence, physical dependence and tolerance may develop upon repeated administration of HYCOMINE and it should be prescribed and administered with the same degree of caution appropriate to the use of other narcotic drugs (see DRUG ABUSE AND DEPENDENCE).

Respiratory Depression: HYCOMINE produces dose-related respiratory depression by directly acting on brain stem respiratory centers. If respiratory depression occurs, it may be antagonized by the use of naloxone hydrochloride and other supportive measures when indicated.

Head Injury and Increased Intracranial Pressure: The respiratory depression properties of narcotics and their capacity to elevate cerebrospinal fluid pressure may be markedly exaggerated in the presence of head injury, other intracranial lesions or a preexisting increase in intracranial pressure. Furthermore, narcotics produce adverse reactions which may obscure the clinical course of patients with head injuries.

Acute Abdominal Conditions: The administration of HYCOMINE or other narcotics may obscure the diagnosis or clinical course of patients with acute abdominal conditions.

Pediatric Use: In young children, as well as adults, the respiratory center is sensitive to the depressant action of narcotic cough suppressants in a dose-dependent manner. Benefit to risk ratio should be carefully considered especially in children with respiratory embarrassment (e.g., croup).

Phenylpropanolamine: Hypertensive crises can occur with concurrent use of phenylpropanolamine and monoamine oxidase (MAO) inhibitors, indomethacin or with beta-blockers and methyldopa.

If a hypertensive crisis occurs, these drugs should be discontinued immediately and therapy to lower blood pressure should be instituted immediately. Fever should be managed by means of external cooling.

PRECAUTIONS

General: Before prescribing medication to suppress or modify cough, it is important to ascertain that the underlying cause of cough is identified, that modification of cough does not increase the risk of clinical or physiologic complications, and that appropriate therapy for the primary disease is provided.

Special Risk Patients: HYCOMINE should be given with caution to certain patients such as the elderly or debilitated, and those with severe impairment of hepatic or renal functions, hypothyroidism, Addison's disease, prostatic hypertrophy or urethral stricture, asthma, narrow-angle glaucoma, and uncontrolled hypertension.

Information for Patients: Hydrocodone may impair the mental and/or physical abilities required for the performance of potentially hazardous tasks such as driving a car or operating machinery; phenylpropanolamine may produce a rapid pulse, dizziness or palpitations. The patient using HYCOMINE should be cautioned accordingly.

Drug Interactions: Patients receiving other narcotic analgesics, general anesthetics, phenothiazines, other tranquilizers, sedative-hypnotics or other CNS depressants (including alcohol) concomitantly with hydrocodone may exhibit an additive CNS depression. When such combined therapy is contemplated, the dose of one or both agents should be reduced. The use of phenylpropanolamine with other sympathomimetic amines and MAO inhibitors may produce an additive elevation of blood pressure (see WARNINGS).

Carcinogenesis, Mutagenesis, Impairment of Fertility: Carcinogenicity, mutagenicity and reproduction studies have not been conducted with HYCOMINE.

Pregnancy: Teratogenic Effects: Pregnancy Category C: Animal reproduction studies have not been conducted with HYCOMINE. It is also not known whether HYCOMINE can cause fetal harm when administered to a pregnant woman or can affect reproductive capacity. HYCOMINE should be given to a pregnant woman only if clearly needed.

Nonteratogenic Effects: Babies born to mothers who have been taking opioids regularly prior to delivery will be physically dependent. The withdrawal signs include irritability and excessive crying, tremors, hyperactive reflexes, increased respiratory rate, increased stools, sneezing, yawning, vomiting and fever. The intensity of the syndrome does not always correlate with the duration of maternal opioid use or dose.

Labor and Delivery: As with all narcotics, administration of HYCOMINE to the mother shortly before delivery may result in some degree of respiratory depression in the newborn, especially if higher doses are used.

Nursing Mothers: It is not known whether this drug is excreted in human milk. Because many drugs are excreted in human milk and because of the potential for serious adverse reactions in nursing infants from HYCOMINE, a decision should be made whether to discontinue nursing or discontinue the drug, taking into account the importance of the drug to the mother.

Pediatric Use: Safety and effectiveness of HYCOMINE in children under six have not been established.

ADVERSE REACTIONS

Respiratory System: Hydrocodone produces dose-related respiratory depression by acting directly on brain stem respiratory centers. (See OVERDOSAGE).

Cardiovascular System: Hypertension, postural hypotension, tachycardia and palpitations.

Genitourinary System: Ureteral spasm, spasm of vesical sphincters and urinary retention have been reported with opiates.

Central Nervous System: Sedation, drowsiness, mental clouding, lethargy, impairment of mental and physical performance, anxiety, fear, dysphoria, dizziness, psychic dependence, mood changes and blurred vision.

Gastrointestinal System: Nausea and vomiting occur more frequently in ambulatory than in recumbent patients. Prolonged administration of HYCOMINE may produce constipation.

Dermatological: Skin rash, pruritus.

DRUG ABUSE AND DEPENDENCE

Hycomine is a Schedule III narcotic. Psychic dependence, physical dependence, and tolerance may develop upon repeated administration of narcotics; therefore, HYCOMINE should be prescribed and administered with caution. However, psychic dependence is unlikely to develop when HYCOMINE is used for a short time for the treatment of cough. Physical dependence, the condition in which continued administration of the drug is required to prevent the appearance of a withdrawal syndrome, assumes clinically significant proportions only after several weeks of continued oral narcotic use, although some mild degree of physical dependence may develop after a few days of narcotic therapy.

OVERDOSAGE

Signs and Symptoms: Serious overdosage with HYCOMINE is characterized by respiratory depression (a decrease in respiratory rate and/or tidal volume, Cheyne-Stokes respiration, cyanosis), extreme somnolence progressing to stupor or coma, skeletal muscle flaccidity, cold and clammy skin, and sometimes bradycardia and hypotension. In severe overdosage, apnea, circulatory collapse, cardiac arrest, and death may occur.

The signs and symptoms of overdosage of the individual components of HYCOMINE may be modified in varying degrees by the presence of other active ingredients. Overdosage with phenylpropanolamine alone may result in tremor, restlessness, increased motor activity, agitation and hallucinations.

Treatment: Primary attention should be given to the reestablishment of adequate respiratory exchange through provision of a patent airway and the institution of assisted or controlled ventilation. The narcotic antagonist naloxone hydrochloride is a specific antidote for respiratory depression which may result from overdosage or unusual sensitivity to narcotics including hydrocodone. Therefore, an appropriate dose of naloxone hydrochloride should be administered preferably by the intravenous route, simultaneously with efforts at respiratory resuscitation.

For further information, see full prescribing information for naloxone hydrochloride. An antagonist should not be administered in the absence of clinically significant respiratory depression. Oxygen, intravenous fluids, vasopressors, and other supportive measures should be employed as indicated. Gastric emptying may be useful in removing unabsorbed drug.

DOSAGE AND ADMINISTRATION

Adults: The usual dose for adults is one teaspoonful HYCOMINE Syrup (hydrocodone bitartrate 5 mg and phenylpropanolamine hydrochloride 25 mg/5 cc) every four hours as needed, not to exceed six teaspoonfuls in a 24 hour period. **Children 6 to 12 years of age:** The usual dose for children 6 to 12 years of age is one teaspoonful HYCOMINE Pediatric Syrup (hydrocodone bitartrate 2.5 mg and phenylpropanolamine hydrochloride 12.5 mg/5 cc) every four hours as needed, not to exceed six teaspoonfuls in a 24 hour period.

HOW SUPPLIED

HYCOMINE Syrup (5 mg hydrocodone bitartrate, USP and 25 mg phenylpropanolamine hydrochloride, USP—per 5 mL teaspoonful) is available as an orange-colored, cherry-flavored syrup in bottles as follows:

One Pint (473.2 mL): NDC 0056-0246-16

HYCOMINE Pediatric Syrup (2.5 mg hydrocodone bitartrate, USP and 12.5 mg phenylpropanolamine hydrochloride, USP—per 5 mL teaspoonful) is available as a green-colored, cherry-flavored syrup in bottles as follows:

One Pint (473.2 mL): NDC 0056-0247-16

Store at controlled room temperature (59°–86°F, 15°–30°C). Oral prescription where permitted by state law.

DuPont Pharma
Wilmington, Delaware 19880
HYCOMINE® is a Registered Trademark of The DuPont Merck Pharmaceutical Co.
6153-6/Rev. Aug., 1994

HYCOMINE® COMPOUND

[hĭ-ko-mēn kom'pound]

DESCRIPTION

HYCOMINE Compound tablets contain hydrocodone (dihydrocodeinone) bitartrate, a semi-synthetic centrally-acting narcotic antitussive; chlorpheniramine maleate, an antihistamine; phenylephrine hydrochloride, a sympathomimetic amine decongestant; acetaminophen, an analgesic/antipyretic; and caffeine, a centrally-acting stimulant; for oral administration.

HYDROCODONE BITARTRATE

CHLORPHENIRAMINE MALEATE

PHENYLEPHRINE HYDROCHLORIDE

ACETAMINOPHEN

CAFFEINE

Each HYCOMINE Compound tablet contains:

Hydrocodone bitartrate, USP	5 mg
WARNING: May be habit forming	
Chlorpheniramine maleate, USP	2 mg
Phenylephrine hydrochloride, USP	10 mg
Acetaminophen, USP	250 mg
Caffeine, anhydrous, USP	30 mg

HYCOMINE Compound tablets also contain: cherry flavor, colloidal silicon dioxide, FD&C Red 40, magnesium stearate, microcrystalline cellulose, povidone and starch.

CLINICAL PHARMACOLOGY

Clinical trials have proven hydrocodone bitartrate to be an effective antitussive agent which is pharmacologically 2 to 8 times as potent as codeine. At equi-effective doses, its sedative action is greater than codeine. The precise mechanism of action of hydrocodone and other opiates is not known, however, hydrocodone is believed to act by directly depressing the cough center. In excessive doses hydrocodone, like other opium derivatives, will depress respiration. The effects of hydrocodone in therapeutic doses on the cardiovascular system is insignificant. The constipation effects of hydrocodone are much weaker than that of morphine and no stronger than that of codeine. Hydrocodone can produce miosis, euphoria, physical and psychological dependence. At therapeutic antitussive doses, it does exert analgesic effects. Following a 10 mg oral dose of hydrocodone administered to five adult male human subjects, the mean peak concentration was 23.6 ± 5.2 ng/mL. Maximum serum levels were achieved at 1.3 ± 0.3 hours and the half-life was determined to be 3.8 ± 0.3 hours. Hydrocodone exhibits a complex pattern of metabolism including O-demethylation, N-demethylation and 6-keto reduction to the corresponding 6-α- and 6-β-hydroxymetabolites.

Chlorpheniramine maleate is a competitive H_1-receptor histamine blocking drug, thereby counteracting the effects of histamine release associated with allergic manifestations of upper respiratory tract inflammatory disorders. H_1-blocking drugs inhibit the actions of histamine on smooth muscle, capillary permeability, and can both stimulate and depress the central nervous system. Phenylephrine hydrochloride effects its vasoconstrictor activity by releasing noradrenaline from sympathetic nerve endings, and from direct stimulation of α-adrenoreceptors in blood vessels. Acetaminophen is an antipyretic and peripherally acting analgesic. Caffeine is a central nervous system stimulant.

INDICATIONS AND USAGE

HYCOMINE Compound is indicated for the symptomatic relief of cough, nasal congestion, and discomfort associated with upper respiratory tract infections.

CONTRAINDICATIONS

HYCOMINE Compound is contraindicated in patients hypersensitive to any component of the drug, and concurrent MAO inhibitor therapy. Patients known to be hypersensitive to other opioids, antihistamines, or sympathomimetic amines may exhibit cross sensitivity with HYCOMINE Compound. Phenylephrine is contraindicated in patients with heart disease, hypertension, diabetes or hyperthyroidism. Hydrocodone is contraindicated in the presence of an intracranial lesion associated with increased intracranial pressure, and whenever ventilatory function is depressed.

WARNINGS

May be habit forming. Hydrocodone can produce drug dependence of the morphine type and therefore has the potential for being abused. Psychic dependence, physical dependence and tolerance may develop upon repeated administration of HYCOMINE Compound and it should be prescribed and administered with the same degree of caution appropriate to the use of other narcotic drugs. (See DRUG ABUSE AND DEPENDENCE.)

Respiratory Depression: HYCOMINE Compound produces dose-related respiratory depression by directly acting on brain stem respiratory centers. If respiratory depression occurs, it may be antagonized by the use of NARCAN® (naloxone hydrochloride) and other supportive measures when indicated.

Head Injury and Increased Intracranial Pressure: The respiratory depressant properties of narcotics and their capacity to elevate cerebrospinal fluid pressure may be markedly exaggerated in the presence of head injury, other intracranial lesions or a pre-existing increase in intracranial pressure. Furthermore, narcotics produce adverse reactions which may obscure the clinical course of patients with head injuries.

Acute abdominal conditions: The administration of HYCOMINE Compound or other narcotics may obscure the diagnosis or clinical course of patients with acute abdominal conditions.

Phenylephrine: Hypertensive crises can occur with concurrent use of phenylephrine and monoamine oxidase (MAO) inhibitors, indomethacin or with beta-blockers and methyldopa.

If a hypertensive crisis occurs these drugs should be discontinued immediately and therapy to lower blood pressure should be instituted immediately. Fever should be managed by means of external cooling.

Chlorpheniramine: Antihistamines may produce drowsiness or excitation, particularly in children and elderly patients.

PRECAUTIONS

Before prescribing medication to suppress or modify cough, it is important to ascertain that the underlying cause of cough is identified, that modification of cough does not increase the risk of clinical or physiologic complications, and that appropriate therapy for the primary disease is provided.

Usage in Ambulatory Patients: Hydrocodone, like all narcotics, and antihistamines such as chlorpheniramine maleate, may impair the mental and/or physical abilities required for the performance of potentially hazardous tasks such as driving a car or operating machinery; phenylephrine may produce a rapid pulse, dizziness or palpitations; patients should be cautioned accordingly.

Drug Interactions: Patients receiving other narcotic analgesics, general anesthetics, phenothiazines, other tranquilizers, sedative-hypnotics or other CNS depressants (including alcohol) concomitantly with hydrocodone may exhibit an additive CNS depression. When such combined therapy is contemplated, the dose of one or both agents should be reduced. The use of phenylephrine with other sympathomimetic amines and MAO inhibitors may produce an additive elevation of blood pressure. MAO inhibitors may prolong the anticholinergic effects of antihistamines. (See WARNINGS.)

Carcinogenesis, mutagenesis, impairment of fertility: Carcinogenicity, mutagenicity, and reproduction studies have not been conducted with HYCOMINE Compound.

Usage in Pregnancy: Pregnancy Category C. Animal reproduction studies have not been conducted with HYCOMINE Compound. It is also not known whether HYCOMINE Compound can cause fetal harm when administered to a pregnant woman or can affect reproductive capacity. HYCOMINE Compound should be given to a pregnant woman only if clearly needed.

Nonteratogenic effects: Babies born to mothers who have been taking opioids regularly prior to delivery will be physically dependent. The withdrawal signs include irritability and excessive crying, tremors, hyperactive reflexes, increased respiratory rate, increased stools, sneezing, yawning, vomiting and fever. The intensity of the syndrome does not always correlate with the duration of maternal opioid use or dose. Chlorpromazine 0.7–1.0 mg/kg q 6 h, phenobarbital 2 mg/kg q 6 h, and paregoric 2–4 drops/kg q 4 h, have been used to treat withdrawal symptoms in infants. The duration of therapy is 4 to 28 days, with the dosages decreased as tolerated.

Nursing mothers: It is not known whether this drug is excreted in human milk. Because many drugs are excreted in human milk and because of the potential for serious adverse reactions in nursing infants from HYCOMINE Compound, a decision should be made whether to discontinue nursing or discontinue the drug, taking into account the importance of the drug to the mother.

Pediatric use: Safety and effectiveness in children below the age of 2 years have not been established.

ADVERSE REACTIONS

Respiratory System: Hydrocodone produces dose-related respiratory depression by acting directly on brain stem respiratory centers.

Cardiovascular System: Hypertension, postural hypotension, tachycardia and palpitations.

Genitourinary System: Ureteral spasm, spasm of vesical sphincters and urinary retention have been reported with opiates.

Central Nervous System: Sedation, drowsiness, mental clouding, lethargy, impairment of mental and physical performance, anxiety, fear, dysphoria, dizziness, psychic dependence, mood changes, and blurred vision.

Gastrointestinal System: Nausea and vomiting occur more frequently in ambulatory than in recumbent patients.

DRUG ABUSE AND DEPENDENCE

Special care should be exercised in prescribing hydrocodone for emotionally unstable patients and for those with a history of drug misuse. Such patients should be closely supervised when long-term therapy is contemplated.

HYCOMINE Compound is a Schedule III narcotic. Psychic dependence, physical dependence, and tolerance may develop upon repeated administration of narcotics; therefore, HYCOMINE Compound should always be prescribed and administered with caution. Physical dependence is the condition in which continued administration of the drug is required to prevent the appearance of a withdrawal syndrome.

Patients physically dependent on opioids will develop an abstinence syndrome upon abrupt discontinuation of the opioid or following the administration of a narcotic antagonist. The character and severity of the withdrawal symptoms are related to the degree of physical dependence. Manifestations of opioid withdrawal are similar to but milder than that of morphine and include lacrimation, rhinorrhea, yawning, sweating, restlessness, dilated pupils, anorexia, gooseflesh, irritability and tremor. In more severe forms, nausea, vomiting, intestinal spasm and diarrhea, increased heart rate and blood pressure, chills, and pains in bones and muscles of the back and extremities may occur. Peak effects will usually be apparent at 48 to 72 hours.

Treatment of withdrawal is usually managed by providing sufficient quantities of an opioid to suppress **severe** withdrawal symptoms and then gradually reducing the dose of opioid over a period of several days.

OVERDOSAGE

The signs and symptoms of overdosage of the individual components of HYCOMINE Compound may be modified in varying degrees by the presence of other active ingredients. Overdosage with phenylephrine alone may result in tremor, restlessness, increased motor activity, agitation and hallucinations.

Acetaminophen

Signs and Symptoms: In acute acetaminophen overdosage, dose-dependent, potentially fatal hepatic necrosis is the most serious adverse effect. Renal tubular necrosis, hypoglycemic coma and thrombocytopenia may also occur.

Acetaminophen in massive overdosage may cause hepatic toxicity in some patients. In cases of suspected overdose, you may wish to call your regional poison center for assistance in diagnosis and for directions in the use of N-acetylcysteine as an antidote.

In adults, hepatic toxicity has rarely been reported with acute overdoses of less than 10 grams and fatalities with less than 15 grams. Importantly, young children seem to be more resistant than adults to the hepatotoxic effect of an acetaminophen overdose. Despite this, the measures outlined below should be initiated in any adult or child suspected of having ingested an acetaminophen overdose.

Early symptoms following a potentially hepatotoxic overdose may include nausea, vomiting, diaphoresis and general malaise. Clinical and laboratory evidence of hepatic toxicity may not be apparent until 48 to 72 hours post-ingestion.

Treatment: The stomach should be emptied promptly by lavage or by induction of emesis with syrup of ipecac. Patient's estimates of the quantity of a drug ingested are notoriously unreliable. Therefore, if an acetaminophen overdose is suspected, a serum acetaminophen assay should be obtained as early as possible, but no sooner than four hours following ingestion. Liver function studies should be obtained initially and repeated at 24-hour intervals.

The antidote, N-acetylcysteine should be administered as early as possible, preferably within 16 hours of the overdose ingestions for optimal results, but in any case, within 24 hours. Following recovery, there are no residual structural or functional hepatic abnormalities.

Hydrocodone

Signs and Symptoms: Serious overdosage with hydrocodone is characterized by respiratory depression (a decrease in respiratory rate and/or tidal volume, Cheyne-Stokes respiration, cyanosis), extreme somnolence progressing to stupor or coma, skeletal muscle flaccidity, cold and clammy skin, and sometimes bradycardia and hypotension. In severe overdosage apnea, circulatory collapse, cardiac arrest and death may occur.

Treatment: Primary attention should be given to the reestablishment of adequate respiratory exchange through provision of a patent airway and the institution of assisted or controlled ventilation. The narcotic antagonist naloxone hydrochloride is a specific antidote for respiratory depression which may result from overdosage or unusual sensitivity to narcotics including hydrocodone. Therefore, an appropriate dose of naloxone hydrochloride should be administered, preferably by the intravenous route, simultaneously with efforts at respiratory resuscitation. For further information, see full prescribing information for naloxone hydrochloride. An antagonist should not be administered in the absence of clinically significant respiratory depression. Oxygen, intravenous fluids, vasopressors and other supportive measures should be employed as indicated. Gastric emptying may be useful in removing unabsorbed drug. Activated charcoal may be of benefit.

DOSAGE AND ADMINISTRATION

Usual dosage, not less than 4 hours apart:
Adults: 1 tablet 4 times a day
Children: 6 to 12 years: 1/2 tablet 4 times a day

HOW SUPPLIED

HYCOMINE® Compound is available as a coral pink, scored tablet in bottles as follows:

Bottles of 100	NDC 0056-0048-70
Bottles of 500	NDC 0056-0048-85

Store at controlled room temperature (59°–86° F, 15°–30° C)
Oral prescription where permitted by State Law.

DuPont Pharmaceuticals
Wilmington, Delaware 19880
HYCOMINE® is a Registered Trademark of The DuPont Merck Pharmaceutical Co.
NARCAN® is a Registered Trademark of The DuPont Merck Pharmaceutical Co.
6015-13/Rev. April, 1993

Continued on next page

DuPont Pharma—Cont.

HYCOTUSS® (CIII)

[*hī-kō-tus*]

Expectorant

DESCRIPTION

HYCOTUSS Expectorant Syrup contains hydrocodone (dihydrocodeinone) bitartrate, a semi-synthetic centrally-acting narcotic antitussive and guaifenesin, an expectorant for oral administration.

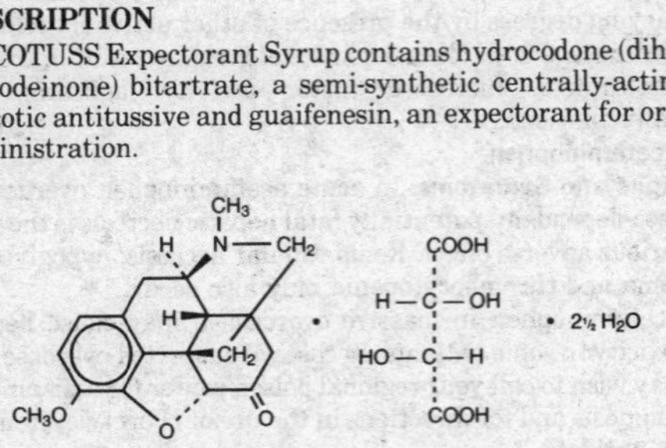

HYDROCODONE BITARTRATE

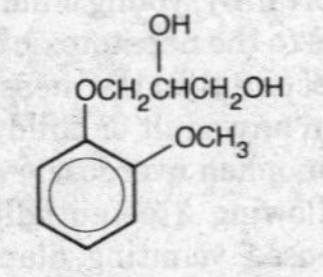

GUAIFENESIN

Each teaspoonful (5 mL) contains:

Hydrocodone bitartrate, USP	5 mg
WARNING: May be habit forming	
Guaifenesin, USP	100 mg
Alcohol, USP	10% v/v

HYCOTUSS Expectorant Syrup also contains: artificial butterscotch flavor, FD&C Red 40, FD&C Yellow 6, glycerin, liquid sugar, methylparaben, propylparaben, saccharin sodium, and sorbitol solution.

CLINICAL PHARMACOLOGY

Clinical trials have proven hydrocodone bitartrate to be an effective antitussive agent which is pharmacologically 2 to 8 times as potent as codeine. At equi-effective doses, its sedative action is greater than codeine. The precise mechanism of action of hydrocodone and other opiates is not known, however, hydrocodone is believed to act by directly depressing the cough center. In excessive doses hydrocodone, like other opium derivatives, can depress respiration. The effects of hydrocodone in therapeutic doses on the cardiovascular system is insignificant. The constipation effects of hydrocodone are much weaker than that of morphine and no stronger than that of codeine. Hydrocodone can produce miosis, euphoria, physical and psychological dependence. At therapeutic antitussive doses, it does exert analgesic effects. Following a 10 mg oral dose of hydrocodone administered to five male human subjects, the mean peak concentration was 23.6 ± 5.2 ng/mL. Maximum serum levels were achieved at 1.3 ± 0.3 hours and half-life was determined to be 3.8 ± 0.3 hours. Hydrocodone exhibits a complex pattern of metabolism including O-demethylation, N-demethylation and 6-keto reduction to the corresponding 6-α- and 6-β-hydroxy-metabolites.

The exact mechanism of action is not established but guaifenesin is believed to act by stimulating receptors in the gastric mucosa that initiates a reflex secretion of respiratory tract fluid, thereby increasing the volume and decreasing the viscosity of bronchial secretions. Studies with guaifenesin indicate that it is rapidly absorbed from the gastrointestinal tract and has a half-life of one hour.

INDICATIONS AND USAGE

HYCOTUSS Expectorant is indicated for the symptomatic relief of irritating non-productive cough associated with upper and lower respiratory tract congestion.

CONTRAINDICATIONS

HYCOTUSS Expectorant is contraindicated in patients hypersensitive to hydrocodone or guaifenesin. Patients known to be hypersensitive to other opioids may exhibit cross sensitivity to HYCOTUSS Expectorant. Hydrocodone is contraindicated in the presence of an intracranial lesion associated with increased intracranial pressure; and whenever ventilatory function is depressed.

WARNINGS

May be habit forming. Hydrocodone can produce drug dependence of the morphine type and therefore has the potential for being abused. Psychic dependence, physical dependence and tolerance may develop upon repeated administration of HYCOTUSS Expectorant and it should be prescribed and administered with the same degree of caution appropriate to the use of other narcotic drugs (see DRUG ABUSE AND DEPENDENCE).

Respiratory Depression: HYCOTUSS Expectorant produces dose-related respiratory depression by directly acting on the brain stem respiratory centers. If respiratory depression occurs, it may be antagonized by the use of NARCAN® (naloxone hydrochloride) and other supportive measures when indicated.

Head Injury and Increased Intracranial Pressure: The respiratory depressant properties of narcotics and their capacity to elevate cerebrospinal fluid pressure may be markedly exaggerated in the presence of head injury, other intracranial lesions or a pre-existing increase in intracranial pressure. Furthermore, narcotics produce adverse reactions which may obscure the clinical course of patients with head injuries.

Acute Abdominal Conditions: The administration of HYCOTUSS Expectorant or other opioids may obscure the diagnosis or clinical course of patients with acute abdominal conditions.

PRECAUTIONS

Before prescribing medication to suppress or modify cough, it is important to ascertain that the underlying cause of cough is identified, that modification of cough does not increase the risk of clinical or physiologic complications, and that appropriate therapy for the primary disease is provided.

Usage in Ambulatory Patients: Hydrocodone, like all narcotics, may impair the mental and/or physical abilities required for the performance of potentially hazardous tasks such as driving a car or operating machinery, and patients should be warned accordingly.

Drug Interactions: Patients receiving other narcotics, analgesics, general anesthetics, phenothiazines, other tranquilizers, sedative hypnotics or other CNS depressants (including alcohol) concomitantly with hydrocodone may exhibit an additive CNS depression. When such combined therapy is contemplated, the dose of one or both agents should be reduced (see WARNINGS).

Laboratory Interactions: The metabolite of guaifenesin has been found to produce an apparent increase in urinary 5-hydroxyindoleacetic acid, and guaifenesin therefore may interfere with the interpretation of this test for the diagnosis of carcinoid syndrome. Guaifenesin administration should be discontinued 24 hours prior to the collection of urine specimens for the determination of 5-hydroxyindoleacetic acid.

Carcinogenesis, Mutagenesis, Impairment of Fertility: Carcinogenicity, mutagenicity and reproduction studies have not been conducted with HYCOTUSS Expectorant.

Usage in Pregnancy: Pregnancy Category C. Animal reproduction studies have not been conducted with HYCOTUSS Expectorant. It is also not known whether HYCOTUSS Expectorant can cause fetal harm when administered to a pregnant woman or can affect reproductive capacity. HYCOTUSS Expectorant should be given to a pregnant woman only if clearly needed.

Nonteratogenic Effects: Babies born to mothers who have been taking opioids regularly prior to delivery will be physically dependent. The withdrawal signs include irritability and excessive crying, tremors, hyperactive reflexes, increased respiratory rate, increased stools, sneezing, yawning, vomiting and fever. The intensity of the syndrome does not always correlate with the duration of maternal opioid use or dose. There is no consensus on the best method of managing withdrawal. Chlorpromazine 0.7–1.0 mg/kg q 6 h, phenobarbital 2 mg/kg q 6 h, and paregoric 2–4 drops/kg q 4 h, have been used to treat withdrawal symptoms in infants. The duration of therapy is 4 to 28 days, with the dosages decreased as tolerated.

Nursing Mothers: It is not known whether this drug is excreted in human milk. Because many drugs are excreted in human milk and because of the potential for serious adverse reactions in nursing infants from HYCOTUSS Expectorant, a decision should be made whether to discontinue nursing or discontinue the drug, taking into account the importance of the drug to the mother.

ADVERSE REACTIONS

Respiratory System: Hydrocodone produces dose-related respiratory depression by acting directly on brain stem respiratory centers.

Cardiovascular System: Hypertension, postural hypotension and palpitations.

Genitourinary System: Ureteral spasm, spasm of vesical sphincters and urinary retention have been reported with opiates.

Central Nervous System: Sedation, drowsiness, mental clouding, lethargy, impairment of mental and physical performance, anxiety, fear, dysphoria, dizziness, psychic dependence, mood changes and blurred vision.

Gastrointestinal System: Nausea and vomiting occur more frequently in ambulatory than in recumbent patients.

DRUG ABUSE AND DEPENDENCE

Special care should be exercised in prescribing hydrocodone for emotionally unstable patients and for those with a history of drug misuse. Such patients should be closely supervised when long-term therapy is contemplated.

HYCOTUSS Expectorant is a Schedule III narcotic. Psychic dependence, physical dependence and tolerance may develop upon repeated administration of narcotics; therefore, HYCOTUSS Expectorant should always be prescribed and administered with caution. Physical dependence is the condition in which continued administration of the drug is required to prevent the appearance of a withdrawal syndrome. Patients physically dependent on opioids will develop an abstinence syndrome upon abrupt discontinuation of the opioid or following the administration of a narcotic antagonist. The character and severity of the withdrawal symptoms are related to the degree of physical dependence. Manifestations of opioid withdrawal are similar to but milder than that of morphine and include lacrimation, rhinorrhea, yawning, sweating, restlessness, dilated pupils, anorexia, gooseflesh, irritability and tremor. In more severe forms, nausea, vomiting, intestinal spasm and diarrhea, increased heart rate and blood pressure, chills, and pains in bones and muscles of the back and extremities may occur. Peak effects will usually be apparent at 48 to 72 hours.

Treatment of withdrawal is usually managed by providing sufficient quantities of an opioid to suppress **severe** withdrawal symptoms and then gradually reducing the dose of opioid over a period of several days.

OVERDOSAGE

Signs and Symptoms: Serious overdosage with HYCOTUSS Expectorant is characterized by respiratory depression (a decrease in respiratory rate and/or tidal volume, Cheyne-Stokes respiration, cyanosis), extreme somnolence progressing to stupor or coma, skeletal muscle flaccidity, cold and clammy skin, and sometimes bradycardia and hypotension. In severe overdosage, apnea, circulatory collapse, cardiac arrest, and death may occur.

Treatment: Primary attention should be given to the reestablishment of adequate respiratory exchange through provision of a patent airway and the institution of assisted or controlled ventilation. The narcotic antagonist naloxone hydrochloride is a specific antidote for respiratory depression which may result from overdosage or unusual sensitivity to narcotics including hydrocodone. Therefore, an appropriate dose of naloxone hydrochloride should be administered, preferably by the intravenous route, simultaneously with efforts at respiratory resuscitation. For further information, see full prescribing information for naloxone hydrochloride. An antagonist should not be administered in the absence of clinically significant respiratory depression. Oxygen, intravenous fluids, vasopressors and other supportive measures should be employed as indicated. Gastric emptying may be useful in removing unabsorbed drug. Activated charcoal may be of benefit.

DOSAGE AND ADMINISTRATION

Usual Adult Dose: One teaspoonful (5 mL) after meals and at bedtime, not less than 4 hours apart (not to exceed 6 teaspoonsful in a 24 hour period). Treatment should be initiated with one teaspoonful and subsequent doses, up to a maximum single dose of 3 teaspoonsful, adjusted if required.

Usual Children's Dose:

Over 12 years: Initial dose 1 teaspoonful; maximum single dose, 2 teaspoonsful.

6 to 12 years: Initial dose ½ teaspoonful; maximum single dose, 1 teaspoonful.

HOW SUPPLIED

HYCOTUSS Expectorant is available as an orange-colored, butterscotch flavored syrup in bottles as follows:

One pint: NDC 0056-0235-16

Store at controlled room temperature (59°–86° F, 15°–30° C).

Oral prescription where permitted by State Law.

DuPont Pharma
Wilmington, Delaware 19880

HYCOTUSS® is a Registered Trademark of The DuPont Merck Pharmaceutical Co.

NARCAN® is a Registered Trademark of The DuPont Merck Pharmaceutical Co.

6131-7/Rev. Aug., 1994

Copyright © DuPont Pharma 1994

NARCAN® ℞

[*nar'kan*]

(naloxone hydrochloride injection, USP)

Narcotic Antagonist

DESCRIPTION

NARCAN (naloxone hydrochloride injection, USP), a narcotic antagonist, is a synthetic congener of oxymorphone. In structure it differs from oxymorphone in that the methyl group on the nitrogen atom is replaced by an allyl group. [See chemical structure at top of next column.]

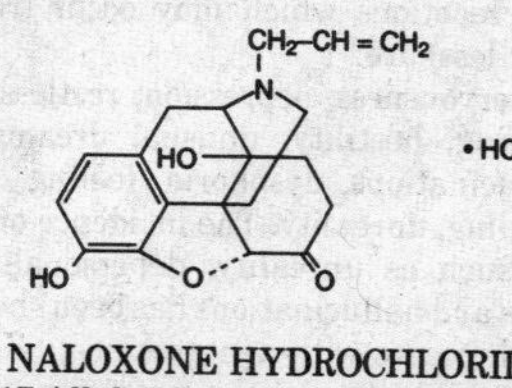

NALOXONE HYDROCHLORIDE
(-)-17-Allyl-4, 5α-epoxy-3, 14 - dihydroxy morphinan-6-one hydrochloride

Naloxone hydrochloride occurs as a white to slightly off-white powder, and is soluble in water, in dilute acids, and in strong alkali; slightly soluble in alcohol; practically insoluble in ether and in chloroform.

NARCAN injection is available as a sterile solution for intravenous, intramuscular and subcutaneous administration in three concentrations, 0.02 mg, 0.4 mg and 1.0 mg of naloxone hydrochloride per mL. One mL of the 0.02 mg and 0.4 mg strengths contains 8.6 mg of sodium chloride. One mL of the 1.0 mg strength contains 8.35 mg of sodium chloride. One mL of the 0.4 mg and 1.0 mg strengths also contains 2.0 mg of methylparaben and propylparaben as preservatives in a ratio of 9 to 1. pH is adjusted to 3.5 ± 0.5 with hydrochloric acid.

NARCAN injection is also available in a paraben-free formulation in three concentrations; 0.02 mg, 0.4 mg and 1.0 mg of naloxone hydrochloride per mL. One mL of each strength contains 9.0 mg of sodium chloride. pH is adjusted to 3.5 ± 0.5 with hydrochloric acid.

CLINICAL PHARMACOLOGY

Complete or Partial Reversal of Narcotic Depression NARCAN (naloxone hydrochloride injection, USP) prevents or reverses the effects of opioids including respiratory depression, sedation and hypotension. Also, it can reverse the psychotomimetic and dysphoric effects of agonist-antagonists such as pentazocine.

NARCAN (naloxone hydrochloride injection, USP) is an essentially pure narcotic antagonist, i.e., it does not possess the "agonistic" or morphine-like properties characteristic of other narcotic antagonists; NARCAN does not produce respiratory depression, psychotomimetic effects or pupillary constriction. In the absence of narcotics or agonistic effects of other narcotic antagonists it exhibits essentially no pharmacologic activity.

NARCAN has not been shown to produce tolerance nor to cause physical or psychological dependence.

In the presence of physical dependence on narcotics NARCAN will produce withdrawal symptoms.

While the mechanism of action of NARCAN is not fully understood, the preponderance of evidence suggests that NARCAN antagonizes the opioid effects by competing for the same receptor sites.

When NARCAN is administered intravenously the onset of action is generally apparent within two minutes; the onset of action is only slightly less rapid when it is administered subcutaneously or intramuscularly. The duration of action is dependent upon the dose and route of administration of NARCAN. Intramuscular administration produces a more prolonged effect than intravenous administration. The requirement for repeat doses of NARCAN, however, will also be dependent upon the amount, type and route of administration of the narcotic being antagonized.

Following parenteral administration NARCAN is rapidly distributed in the body. It is metabolized in the liver, primarily by glucuronide conjugation and excreted in urine. In one study the serum half-life in adults ranged from 30 to 81 minutes (mean 64 ± 12 minutes). In a neonatal study the mean plasma half-life was observed to be 3.1 ± 0.5 hours.

Adjunctive Use in Septic Shock Although the mechanism of action is not completely understood, NARCAN appears to block endorphine-mediated hypotension in septic shock patients.

NARCAN has been shown in some cases of septic shock to produce a rise in blood pressure that may last up to several hours; however, this pressor response has not been demonstrated to improve patient survival.

Patients who have responded to NARCAN received the drug early in the course of treatment of septic shock. Because of the limited number of patients who have been treated, optimal dosage and treatment regimens have not been established. Published reports demonstrating a pressor effect have evaluated single bolus injections of 0.4 mg over three (3) to five (5) minutes, which have been repeated for 3–5 doses depending on the response. Bolus infusion doses ranging from 0.03 mg/kg to 0.2 mg/kg over five (5) minutes have also been reported. If a response was elicited, treatment was continued by intravenous infusion of concentrations of 0.03 mg/kg/hour to 0.3 mg/kg/hour for 1–24 hours or more depending upon the clinical response.

INDICATIONS AND USAGE

NARCAN is indicated for the complete or partial reversal of narcotic depression, including respiratory depression, induced by opioids including natural and synthetic narcotics, propoxyphene, methadone and certain narcotic-antagonist analgesics: nalbuphine, pentazocine and butorphanol. NARCAN is also indicated for the diagnosis of suspected acute opioid overdosage.

NARCAN may be useful as an adjunctive agent to increase blood pressure in the management of septic shock.

CONTRAINDICATIONS

NARCAN is contraindicated in patients known to be hypersensitive to it.

WARNINGS

NARCAN should be administered cautiously to persons including newborns of mothers who are known or suspected to be physically dependent on opioids. In such cases an abrupt and complete reversal of narcotic effects may precipitate an acute abstinence syndrome.

The patient who has satisfactorily responded to NARCAN should be kept under continued surveillance and repeated doses of NARCAN should be administered, as necessary, since the duration of action of some narcotics may exceed that of NARCAN.

NARCAN is not effective against respiratory depression due to non-opioid drugs. Reversal of buprenorphine-induced respiratory depression may be incomplete. If an incomplete response occurs, respirations should be mechanically assisted.

PRECAUTIONS

In addition to NARCAN, other resuscitative measures such as maintenance of a free airway, artificial ventilation, cardiac massage, and vasopressor agents should be available and employed when necessary to counteract acute narcotic poisoning.

Several instances of hypotension, hypertension, ventricular tachycardia and fibrillation, and pulmonary edema have been reported. These have occurred in postoperative patients most of whom had pre-existing cardiovascular disorders or received other drugs which may have similar adverse cardiovascular effects. Although a direct cause and effect relationship has not been established, NARCAN should be used with caution in patients with pre-existing cardiac disease or patients who have received potentially cardiotoxic drugs.

Carcinogenesis, Mutagenesis, Impairment of Fertility Carcinogenicity and mutagenicity studies have not been performed with NARCAN. Reproductive studies in mice and rats demonstrated no impairment of fertility.

Use in Pregnancy Pregnancy Category B: Reproduction studies performed in mice and rats at doses up to 1,000 times the human dose, revealed no evidence of impaired fertility or harm to the fetus due to NARCAN. There are, however, no adequate and well controlled studies in pregnant women. Because animal reproduction studies are not always predictive of human response, NARCAN should be used during pregnancy only if clearly needed.

Nursing Mothers It is not known whether NARCAN (naloxone hydrochloride injection, USP) is excreted in human milk. Because many drugs are excreted in human milk, caution should be exercised when NARCAN is administered to a nursing woman.

Usage in Children and Neonates for Septic Shock The safety and effectiveness of NARCAN in the treatment of hypotension in children and neonates with septic shock have not been established.

ADVERSE REACTIONS

Abrupt reversal of narcotic depression may result in nausea, vomiting, sweating, tachycardia, increased blood pressure, tremulousness, seizures and cardiac arrest. In postoperative patients, larger than necessary dosage of NARCAN may result in significant reversal of analgesia, and in excitement. Hypotension, hypertension, ventricular tachycardia and fibrillation, and pulmonary edema have been associated with the use of NARCAN postoperatively (see PRECAUTIONS & USAGE IN ADULTS-POSTOPERATIVE NARCOTIC DEPRESSION).

OVERDOSAGE

There is no clinical experience with NARCAN overdosage in humans.

In the mouse and rat the intravenous LD_{50} is 150 ± 5 mg/kg and 109 ± 4 mg/kg respectively. In acute subcutaneous toxicity studies in newborn rats the LD_{50} (95% CL) is 260 (228–296) mg/kg. Subcutaneous injection of 100 mg/kg/day in rats for 3 weeks produced only transient salivation and partial ptosis following injection; no toxic effects were seen at 10 mg/kg/day for 3 weeks.

Some chemical impurities in naloxone, i.e., noroxymorphone and bisnaloxone, have been shown to produce emesis in dogs when administered alone i.v. at doses equivalent to impurity levels present in naloxone at 50x the recommended maximum naloxone dose or less.

DOSAGE AND ADMINISTRATION

NARCAN (naloxone hydrochloride injection, USP) may be administered intravenously, intramuscularly, or subcutaneously. The most rapid onset of action is achieved by intravenous administration and it is recommended in emergency situations.

Since the duration of action of some narcotics may exceed that of NARCAN the patient should be kept under continued surveillance and repeated doses of NARCAN should be administered, as necessary.

Intravenous Infusion NARCAN may be diluted for intravenous infusion in normal saline or 5% dextrose solutions. The addition of 2 mg of NARCAN in 500 mL of either solution provides a concentration of 0.004 mg/mL. Mixtures should be used within 24 hours. After 24 hours, the remaining unused solution must be discarded. The rate of administration should be titrated in accordance with the patient's response.

Parenteral drug products should be inspected visually for particulate matter and discoloration prior to administration whenever solution and container permit. NARCAN should not be mixed with preparations containing bisulfite, metabisulfite, long-chain or high molecular weight anions, or any solution having an alkaline pH. No drug or chemical agent should be added to NARCAN unless its effect on the chemical and physical stability of the solution has first been established.

USAGE IN ADULTS

Narcotic Overdose—Known or Suspected An initial dose of 0.4 mg to 2 mg of NARCAN may be administered intravenously. If the desired degree of counteraction and improvement in respiratory functions is not obtained, it may be repeated at 2 to 3 minute intervals. If no response is observed after 10 mg of NARCAN have been administered, the diagnosis of narcotic induced or partial narcotic induced toxicity should be questioned. Intramuscular or subcutaneous administration may be necessary if the intravenous route is not available.

Postoperative Narcotic Depression For the partial reversal of narcotic depression following the use of narcotics during surgery, smaller doses of NARCAN are usually sufficient. The dose of NARCAN should be titrated according to the patient's response. For the initial reversal of respiratory depression, NARCAN should be injected in increments of 0.1 to 0.2 mg intravenously at two to three minute intervals to the desired degree of reversal i.e., adequate ventilation and alertness without significant pain or discomfort. Larger than necessary dosage of NARCAN may result in significant reversal of analgesia and increase in blood pressure. Similarly, too rapid reversal may induce nausea, vomiting, sweating or circulatory stress.

Repeat doses of NARCAN may be required within one to two hour intervals depending upon the amount, type (i.e., short or long acting) and time interval since last administration of narcotic. Supplemental intramuscular doses have been shown to produce a longer lasting effect.

Septic Shock The optimal dosage of NARCAN or duration of therapy for the treatment of hypotension in septic shock patients has not been established (see CLINICAL PHARMACOLOGY).

USAGE IN CHILDREN

Narcotic Overdose—Known or Suspected The usual initial dose in children is 0.01 mg/kg body weight given I.V. If this dose does not result in the desired degree of clinical improvement, a subsequent dose of 0.1 mg/kg body weight may be administered. If an I.V. route of administration is not available, NARCAN may be administered I.M. or S.C. in divided doses. If necessary, NARCAN can be diluted with sterile water for injection.

Postoperative Narcotic Depression Follow the recommendations and cautions under **Adult Postoperative Depression.** For the initial reversal of respiratory depression NARCAN should be injected in increments of 0.005 mg to 0.01 mg intravenously at two to three minute intervals to the desired degree of reversal.

USAGE IN NEONATES

Narcotic-induced Depression The usual initial dose is 0.01 mg/kg body weight administered I.V., I.M., or S.C. This dose may be repeated in accordance with adult administration guidelines for postoperative narcotic depression.

HOW SUPPLIED

NARCAN (naloxone hydrochloride injection, USP) for intravenous, intramuscular and subcutaneous administration is available as:

0.4 mg/mL	10 mL multiple dose vial—box of 1	NDC 0590-0365-05
0.4 mg/mL (paraben-free)	1 mL ampul—box of 10	NDC 0590-0358-10
1.0 mg/mL	10 mL multiple dose vial—box of 1	NDC 0590-0368-05
1.0 mg/mL (paraben-free)	2 mL ampul—box of 10	NDC 0590-0377-10
0.02 mg/mL (paraben-free)	2 mL ampul—box of 10	NDC 0590-0359-10

Continued on next page

DuPont Pharma—Cont.

Store at controlled room temperature (59°–86°F, 15°–30°C)
NARCAN® is a Registered Trademark of The DuPont Merck Pharmaceutical Co.
Copyright © DuPont Pharma 1995
DuPont Pharma
DuPont Merck Pharma
Manati, Puerto Rico 00674
6108-12/Rev. Feb., 1995

NUBAIN® ℞
[*nū 'bān*]
(nalbuphine hydrochloride)

DESCRIPTION
NUBAIN (nalbuphine hydrochloride) is a synthetic narcotic agonist-antagonist analgesic of the phenanthrene series. It is chemically related to both the widely used narcotic antagonist, naloxone, and the potent narcotic analgesic, oxymorphone.

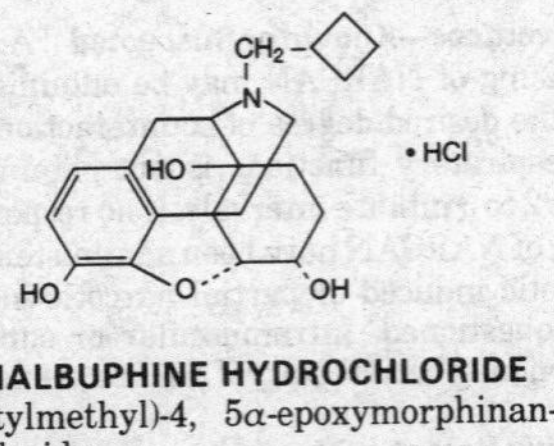

NALBUPHINE HYDROCHLORIDE
(-)-17-(cyclobutylmethyl)-4, 5α-epoxymorphinan-3, 6α, 14-triol, hydrochloride

NUBAIN is a sterile solution suitable for subcutaneous, intramuscular, or intravenous injection. NUBAIN is available in two concentrations, 10 mg and 20 mg of nalbuphine hydrochloride per mL. Both strengths in 10 mL vials contain 0.94% sodium citrate hydrous, 1.26% citric acid anhydrous, and 0.2% of a 9:1 mixture of methylparaben and propylparaben as preservatives; pH is adjusted, if necessary, to 3.5 to 3.7 with hydrochloric acid. The 10 mg/mL strength contains 0.2% sodium chloride.
NUBAIN is also available in ampuls in a sterile, paraben-free formulation in two concentrations, 10 mg and 20 mg of nalbuphine hydrochloride per mL. One mL of each strength contains 0.94% sodium citrate hydrous and 1.26% citric acid anhydrous; pH is adjusted, if necessary, to 3.5 to 3.7 with hydrochloric acid. The 10 mg/mL strength contains 0.2% sodium chloride.

ACTIONS
NUBAIN is a potent analgesic. Its analgesic potency is essentially equivalent to that of morphine on a milligram basis. Its onset of action occurs within 2 to 3 minutes after intravenous administration, and in less than 15 minutes following subcutaneous or intramuscular injection. The plasma half-life of nalbuphine is 5 hours and in clinical studies the duration of analgesic activity has been reported to range from 3 to 6 hours.
The narcotic antagonist activity of NUBAIN is one-fourth as potent as nalorphine and 10 times that of pentazocine.

INDICATIONS
NUBAIN is indicated for the relief of moderate to severe pain. NUBAIN can also be used as a supplement to balanced anesthesia, for preoperative and postoperative analgesia, and for obstetrical analgesia during labor and delivery.

CONTRAINDICATIONS
NUBAIN should not be administered to patients who are hypersensitive to it, or to any of the ingredients in NUBAIN.

WARNINGS
NUBAIN should be administered as a supplement to general anesthesia only by persons specifically trained in the use of intravenous anesthetics and management of the respiratory effects of potent opioids.
Naloxone, resuscitative and intubation equipment and oxygen should be readily available.
Drug Dependence NUBAIN has been shown to have a low abuse potential. When compared with drugs which are not mixed agonist-antagonists, it has been reported that nalbuphine's potential for abuse would be less than that of codeine and propoxyphene. Psychological and physical dependence and tolerance may follow the abuse or misuse of nalbuphine. Therefore, caution should be observed in prescribing it for emotionally unstable patients, or for individuals with a history of narcotic abuse. Such patients should be closely supervised when long-term therapy is contemplated.
Care should be taken to avoid increases in dosage or frequency of administration which in susceptible individuals might result in physical dependence.
Abrupt discontinuation of NUBAIN following prolonged use has been followed by symptoms of narcotic withdrawal, i.e., abdominal cramps, nausea and vomiting, rhinorrhea, lacrimation, restlessness, anxiety, elevated temperature and piloerection.
Use in Ambulatory Patients NUBAIN may impair the mental or physical abilities required for the performance of potentially dangerous tasks such as driving a car or operating machinery. Therefore, NUBAIN should be administered with caution to ambulatory patients who should be warned to avoid such hazards.
Use in Emergency Procedures Maintain patient under observation until recovered from NUBAIN effects that would affect driving or other potentially dangerous tasks.
Use in Children Clinical experience to support administration to patients under 18 years is not available at present.
Use in Pregnancy (other than labor) Safe use of NUBAIN in pregnancy has not been established. Although animal reproductive studies have not revealed teratogenic or embryotoxic effects, nalbuphine should only be administered to pregnant women when, in the judgement of the physician, the potential benefits outweigh the possible hazards.
Use During Labor and Delivery The placental transfer of nalbuphine is high, rapid, and variable with a maternal to fetal ratio ranging from 1:0.37 to 1:1.6. Fetal and neonatal adverse effects that have been reported following the administration of nalbuphine to the mother during labor include fetal bradycardia, respiratory depression at birth, apnea and cyanosis. Maternal administration of naloxone during labor has normalized these effects in some cases. Severe and prolonged fetal bradycardia has been reported. Permanent neurological damage attributed to fetal bradycardia has occurred. A sinusoidal fetal heart rate pattern associated with the use of nalbuphine has also been reported. NUBAIN should be used with caution in women during labor and delivery, and newborns should be monitored for respiratory depression, apnea, bradycardia, and arrhythmias if NUBAIN has been used.
Head Injury and Increased Intracranial Pressure The possible respiratory depressant effects and the potential of potent analgesics to elevate cerebrospinal fluid pressure (resulting from vasodilation following CO_2 retention) may be markedly exaggerated in the presence of head injury, intracranial lesions or a pre-existing increase in intracranial pressure. Furthermore, potent analgesics can produce effects which may obscure the clinical course of patients with head injuries. Therefore, NUBAIN should be used in these circumstances only when essential, and then should be administered with extreme caution.
Interaction With Other Central Nervous System Depressants Although NUBAIN possesses narcotic antagonist activity, there is evidence that in nondependent patients it will not antagonize a narcotic analgesic administered just before, concurrently, or just after an injection of NUBAIN. Therefore, patients receiving a narcotic analgesic, general anesthetics, phenothiazines, or other tranquilizers, sedatives, hypnotics, or other CNS depressants (including alcohol) concomitantly with NUBAIN may exhibit an additive effect. When such combined therapy is contemplated, the dose of one or both agents should be reduced.

PRECAUTIONS
Impaired Respiration At the usual adult dose of 10mg/70kg, NUBAIN (nalbuphine hydrochloride) causes some respiratory depression approximately equal to that produced by equal doses of morphine. However, in contrast to morphine, respiratory depression is not appreciably increased with higher doses of NUBAIN. Respiratory depression induced by NUBAIN can be reversed by NARCAN® (naloxone hydrochloride) when indicated. NUBAIN should be administered with caution at low doses to patients with impaired respiration (e.g., from other medication, uremia, bronchial asthma, severe infection, cyanosis, or respiratory obstructions).
Impaired Renal or Hepatic Function Because NUBAIN is metabolized in the liver and excreted by the kidneys, patients with renal or liver dysfunction may over-react to customary doses. Therefore, in these individuals, NUBAIN should be used with caution and administered in reduced amounts.
Myocardial Infarction As with all potent analgesics, NUBAIN should be used with caution in patients with myocardial infarction who have nausea or vomiting.
Biliary Tract Surgery As with all narcotic analgesics, NUBAIN should be used with caution in patients about to undergo surgery of the biliary tract since it may cause spasm of the sphincter of Oddi.
Cardiovascular System During evaluation of NUBAIN in anesthesia, a higher incidence of bradycardia has been reported in patients who did not receive atropine pre-operatively or in the pre-operative period.

ADVERSE REACTIONS
The most frequent adverse reaction in 1066 patients treated with NUBAIN is sedation 381 (36%).
Less frequent reactions are: sweaty/clammy 99 (9%), nausea/vomiting 68 (6%), dizziness/vertigo 58 (5%), dry mouth 44 (4%), and headache 27 (3%).
Other adverse reactions which may occur (reported incidence of 1% or less) are:
CNS Effects Nervousness, depression, restlessness, crying, euphoria, floating, hostility, unusual dreams, confusion, faintness, hallucinations, dysphoria, feeling of heaviness, numbness, tingling, unreality. The incidence of psychotomimetic effects, such as unreality, depersonalization, delusions, dysphoria and hallucinations has been shown to be less than that which occurs with pentazocine.
Cardiovascular Hypertension, hypotension, bradycardia, tachycardia, pulmonary edema.
Gastrointestinal Cramps, dyspepsia, bitter taste.
Respiration Depression, dyspnea, asthma.
Dermatological Itching, burning, urticaria.
Miscellaneous Speech difficulty, urinary urgency, blurred vision, flushing and warmth.
Allergic Reactions Anaphylactic/anaphylactoid and other serious hypersensitivity reactions have been reported following the use of nalbuphine and may require immediate, supportive medical treatment. These reactions may include shock, respiratory distress, respiratory arrest, bradycardia, cardiac arrest, hypotension, or laryngeal edema. Other allergic-type reactions reported include stridor, bronchospasm, wheezing, edema, rash, pruritus, nausea, vomiting, diaphoresis, weakness, and shakiness.

DOSAGE AND ADMINISTRATION
The usual recommended adult dose is 10 mg for a 70 kg individual, administered subcutaneously, intramuscularly or intravenously; this dose may be repeated every 3 to 6 hours as necessary. Dosage should be adjusted according to the severity of the pain, physical status of the patient, and other medications which the patient may be receiving. (See Interaction with Other Central Nervous System Depressants under WARNINGS). In non-tolerant individuals, the recommended single maximum dose is 20 mg, with a maximum total daily dose of 160 mg.
The use of NUBAIN as a supplement to balanced anesthesia requires larger doses than those recommended for analgesia. Induction doses of NUBAIN range from 0.3 mg/kg to 3.0 mg/kg intravenously to be administered over a 10 to 15 minute period with maintenance doses of 0.25 to 0.50 mg/kg in single intravenous administrations as required. The use of NUBAIN may be followed by respiratory depression which can be reversed with the narcotic antagonist NARCAN® (naloxone hydrochloride).
Patients Dependent on Narcotics Patients who have been taking narcotics chronically may experience withdrawal symptoms upon the administration of NUBAIN. If unduly troublesome, narcotic withdrawal symptoms can be controlled by the slow intravenous administration of small increments of morphine, until relief occurs. If the previous analgesic was morphine, meperidine, codeine, or other narcotic with similar duration of activity, one-fourth of the anticipated dose of NUBAIN can be administered initially and the patient observed for signs of withdrawal, i.e., abdominal cramps, nausea and vomiting, lacrimation, rhinorrhea, anxiety, restlessness, elevation of temperature or piloerection. If untoward symptoms do not occur, progressively larger doses may be tried at appropriate intervals until the desired level of analgesia is obtained with NUBAIN.
Management of Overdosage The immediate intravenous administration of NARCAN® (naloxone hydrochloride) is a specific antidote. Oxygen, intravenous fluids, vasopressors and other supportive measures should be used as indicated.
The administration of single doses of 72 mg of NUBAIN subcutaneously to eight normal subjects has been reported to have resulted primarily in symptoms of sleepiness and mild dysphoria.

HOW SUPPLIED
NUBAIN® (nalbuphine hydrochloride) injection for intramuscular, subcutaneous, or intravenous use is a sterile solution available in:

NDC 0590-0508-01	(sulfite-free) 10 mg/mL, 10 mL multiple dose vials (box of 1)
NDC 0590-0432-10	(sulfite/paraben-free) 10 mg/mL, 1 mL ampuls (box of 10)
NDC 0590-0509-01	(sulfite-free) 20 mg/mL, 10 mL multiple dose vials (box of 1)
NDC 0590-0433-10	(sulfite/paraben-free) 20 mg/mL, 1 mL ampuls (box of 10)

Store at controlled room temperature (59°–86°F, 15°–30°C). Protect from excessive light. Store in carton until contents have been used.
Parenteral drug products should be inspected visually for particulate matter and discoloration prior to administration whenever solution and container permit.
CAUTION: Federal law prohibits dispensing without prescription.
DuPont Pharma
DuPont Merck Pharma
P. O. Box 363
Manati, Puerto Rico 00674
NUBAIN® is a Registered Trademark of The DuPont Merck Pharmaceutical Co.

NARCAN® is a Registered Trademark of The DuPont Merck Pharmaceutical Co.
Copyright © DuPont Pharma 1996

6436/March, 1996

NUMORPHAN® (II)
[nū-mor'fan]
(oxymorphone hydrochloride)
injection
Narcotic Analgesic

DESCRIPTION
NUMORPHAN (oxymorphone hydrochloride), a semi-synthetic narcotic substitute for morphine, is a potent analgesic.

Oxymorphone hydrochloride is 4,5α-Epoxy-3,14- dihydroxy-17-methylmorphinan-6-one hydrochloride.
Oxymorphone hydrochloride occurs as a white or slightly off-white, odorless powder, sparingly soluble in alcohol and ether, but freely soluble in water.
NUMORPHAN injection is available in two concentrations, 1 mg and 1.5 mg of oxymorphone hydrochloride per mL. Both strengths contain sodium chloride 0.8%; with methylparaben 0.18%, propylparaben 0.02% and sodium dithionite 0.1%, as preservatives. pH is adjusted with sodium hydroxide.

ACTIONS
NUMORPHAN (oxymorphone hydrochloride) is a potent narcotic analgesic. Administered parenterally, 1 mg of NUMORPHAN is approximately equivalent in analgesic activity to 10 mg of morphine sulfate.
The onset of action is rapid; initial effects are usually perceived within 5 to 10 minutes. Its duration of action is approximately 3 to 6 hours.
NUMORPHAN produces mild sedation and causes little depression of the cough reflex. These properties make it particularly useful in postoperative patients.

INDICATIONS
NUMORPHAN (oxymorphone hydrochloride) is indicated for the relief of moderate to severe pain. This drug is also indicated parenterally for preoperative medication, for support of anesthesia, for obstetrical analgesia, and for relief of anxiety in patients with dyspnea associated with acute left ventricular failure and pulmonary edema.

CONTRAINDICATIONS
Safe use of NUMORPHAN (oxymorphone hydrochloride) in children under 12 years of age has not been established. This drug should not be used in patients known to be hypersensitive to morphine analogs.

WARNINGS
May be habit forming. As with other narcotic drugs, tolerance and addiction may develop. The addicting potential of the drug appears to be about the same as for morphine.
Like other narcotic-containing medications, NUMORPHAN is subject to the Federal Controlled Substances Act.
Interaction with other central nervous system depressants: Patients receiving other narcotic analgesics, general anesthetics, phenothiazines, other tranquilizers, sedatives, hypnotics or other CNS depressants (including alcohol) concomitantly with NUMORPHAN may exhibit an additive CNS depression. When such combined therapy is contemplated, the dose of one or both agents should be reduced.
Safe use in pregnancy has not been established (relative to possible adverse effects on fetal development). As with other analgesics, the use of NUMORPHAN (oxymorphone hydrochloride) in pregnancy, in nursing mothers, or in women of child-bearing potential requires that the possible benefits of the drug be weighed against the possible hazards to the mother and the child.
Sulfites Sensitivity: NUMORPHAN contains sodium dithionite, a sulfite that may cause allergic-type reactions including anaphylactic symptoms and life-threatening or less severe asthmatic episodes in certain susceptible people. The overall prevalence of sulfite sensitivity in the general population is unknown and probably low. Sulfite sensitivity is seen more frequently in asthmatic than in nonasthmatic people.

PRECAUTIONS
The same care and caution should be taken when administering NUMORPHAN (oxymorphone hydrochloride) as when other potent narcotic analgesics are used. It should be borne in mind that some respiratory depression may occur as with all potent narcotics especially when other analgesic and/or anesthetic drugs with depressant action have been given shortly before administration of NUMORPHAN.
The respiratory depressant effects of narcotics and their capacity to elevate cerebrospinal fluid pressure may be markedly exaggerated in the presence of head injury, other intracranial lesions or a pre-existing increase in intracranial pressure. Furthermore, narcotics produce adverse reactions which may obscure the clinical course of patients with head injuries.
As with other analgesics, caution must also be exercised in elderly and debilitated patients and in patients who are known to be sensitive to central nervous system depressants, such as those with cardiovascular, pulmonary, or hepatic disease, in hypothyroidism (myxedema), acute alcoholism, delirium tremens, convulsive disorders, bronchial asthma and kyphoscoliosis. Debilitated and elderly patients and those with severe liver diseases should receive smaller doses of NUMORPHAN (oxymorphone hydrochloride).

ADVERSE REACTIONS
As with all potent narcotic analgesics, possible side effects include drowsiness, nausea, vomiting, miosis, itching, dysphoria, light-headedness, and headache. Respiratory depression may occur with oxymorphone as with other narcotics.

DOSAGE AND ADMINISTRATION
Usual Adult Dosage of NUMORPHAN (oxymorphone hydrochloride) Injection: Subcutaneous or intramuscular administration: initially 1 mg to 1.5 mg, repeated every 4 to 6 hours as needed. Intravenous: 0.5 mg initially. In nondebilitated patients the dose can be cautiously increased until satisfactory pain relief is obtained. For analgesia during labor 0.5 mg to 1 mg intramuscularly is recommended.

MANAGEMENT OF OVERDOSAGE
Signs and Symptoms: Serious overdosage with NUMORPHAN is characterized by respiratory depression, (a decrease in respiratory rate and/or tidal volume, Cheyne-Stokes respiration, cyanosis), extreme somnolence progressing to stupor or coma, skeletal muscle flaccidity, cold and clammy skin, and sometimes bradycardia and hypotension. In severe overdosage, apnea, circulatory collapse, cardiac arrest and death may occur.
Treatment: Primary attention should be given to the reestablishment of adequate respiratory exchange through provision of a patent airway and the institution of assisted or controlled ventilation. The narcotic antagonist naloxone hydrochloride (NARCAN®) is a specific antidote against respiratory depression which may result from overdosage or unusual sensitivity to narcotics including oxymorphone. Therefore, an appropriate dose of naloxone hydrochloride should be administered (usual initial adult dose 0.4 mg–2 mg) preferably by the intravenous route and simultaneously with efforts at respiratory resuscitation. Since the duration of action of oxymorphone may exceed that of the antagonist, the patient should be kept under continued surveillance and repeated doses of the antagonist should be administered as needed to maintain adequate respiration.
Oxygen, intravenous fluids, vasopressors and other supportive measures should be employed as indicated.

HOW SUPPLIED
For Injection: DEA Order Form Required.
1 mg/mL   1 mL ampuls (box of 10)
NDC 0590-0370-10
1.5 mg/mL 1 mL ampuls (box of 10)
NDC 0590-0373-10
           10 mL multiple dose vial (box of 1)
NDC 0590-0374-01
Store at controlled room temperature (59°–86°F, 15°–30°C). Protect from light.
Caution: Federal law prohibits dispensing without prescription.
DuPont Pharma
DuPont Merck Pharma
Manati, Puerto Rico 00674
NUMORPHAN® is a Registered Trademark of The DuPont Merck Pharmaceutical Co.
NARCAN® is a Registered Trademark of The DuPont Merck Pharmaceutical Co.
6110-7/Rev. Oct., 1994
Copyright© DuPont Pharma 1994

NUMORPHAN® (II) ℞
(oxymorphone hydrochloride)
RECTAL SUPPOSITORIES
Narcotic
Analgesic

DESCRIPTION
NUMORPHAN (oxymorphone hydrochloride), a semi-synthetic narcotic substitute for morphine, is a potent analgesic.
[See structure at top of next column.]

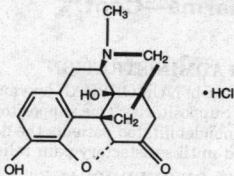

4,5α-Expoxy-3, 14-dihydroxy-17-methylmorphinan-6-one hydrochloride

Oxymorphone hydrochloride occurs as a white or slightly off-white, odorless powder, sparingly soluble in alcohol and ether, but freely soluble in water.
The NUMORPHAN rectal suppository is available in a concentration of 5 mg of oxymorphone hydrochloride in a base consisting of polyethylene glycol 1000 and polyethylene glycol 3350.

ACTIONS
NUMORPHAN (oxymorphone hydrochloride) is a potent narcotic analgesic. Administered parenterally, 1 mg of NUMORPHAN is approximately equivalent in analgesic activity to 10 mg of morphine sulfate.
The onset of action of parenterally administered NUMORPHAN is rapid; initial effects are usually perceived within 5 to 10 minutes. Its duration of action is approximately 3 to 6 hours.
NUMORPHAN produces mild sedation and causes little depression of the cough reflex. These properties make it particularly useful in postoperative patients.

INDICATIONS
For the relief of moderate to severe pain.

CONTRAINDICATIONS
Safe use of NUMORPHAN (oxymorphone hydrochloride) in children under 12 years of age has not been established. This drug should not be used in patients known to be hypersensitive to morphine analogs.

WARNINGS
May be habit forming. As with other narcotic drugs, tolerance and addiction may develop. The addicting potential of the drug appears to be about the same as for morphine.
Like other narcotic-containing medications, NUMORPHAN is subject to the Federal Controlled Substances Act.
Interaction with other central nervous system depressants: Patients receiving other narcotic analgesics, general anesthetics, phenothiazines, other tranquilizers, sedatives, hypnotics or other CNS depressants (including alcohol) concomitantly with NUMORPHAN may exhibit an additive CNS depression. When such combined therapy is contemplated, the dose of one or both agents should be reduced.
Safe use in pregnancy has not been established (relative to possible adverse effects on fetal development). As with other potent analgesics, the use of NUMORPHAN (oxymorphone hydrochloride) in pregnancy, in nursing mothers, or in women of child-bearing potential requires that the possible benefits of the drug be weighed against the possible hazards to the mother and child.

PRECAUTIONS
The same care and caution should be taken when administering NUMORPHAN (oxymorphone hydrochloride) as when other potent narcotic analgesics are used. It should be borne in mind that some respiratory depression may occur as with all potent narcotics especially when other analgesic and/or anesthetic drugs with depressant action have been given shortly before administration of NUMORPHAN.
The respiratory depressant effects of narcotics and their capacity to elevate cerebrospinal fluid pressure may be markedly exaggerated in the presence of head injury, other intracranial lesions or a pre-existing increase in intracranial pressure. Furthermore, narcotics produce adverse reactions which may obscure the clinical course of patients with head injuries.
As with other analgesics, caution must also be exercised in elderly and debilitated patients and in patients who are known to be sensitive to central nervous system depressants, such as those with cardiovascular, pulmonary, or hepatic disease, in hypothyroidism (myxedema), acute alcoholism, delirium tremens, convulsive disorders, bronchial asthma and kyphoscoliosis. Debilitated and elderly patients and those with severe liver diseases should receive smaller doses of NUMORPHAN.

ADVERSE REACTIONS
As with all potent narcotic analgesics, possible side effects include drowsiness, nausea, vomiting, miosis, itching, dysphoria, light-headedness, and headache. Respiratory depression may occur with oxymorphone as with other narcotics.

Continued on next page

DuPont Pharma—Cont.

DOSAGE AND ADMINISTRATION

Usual Adult Dosage of NUMORPHAN (oxymorphone hydrochloride) Rectal Suppositories: One suppository, 5 mg, every 4 to 6 hours. In nondebilitated patients the dose can be cautiously increased until satisfactory pain relief is obtained.

MANAGEMENT OF OVERDOSAGE

Signs and symptoms: Serious overdosage with NUMORPHAN is characterized by respiratory depression, (a decrease in respiratory rate and/or tidal volume, Cheyne-Stokes respiration, cyanosis), extreme somnolence progressing to stupor or coma, skeletal muscle flaccidity, cold and clammy skin, and sometimes bradycardia and hypotension. In severe overdosage, apnea, circulatory collapse, cardiac arrest and death may occur.

Treatment: Primary attention should be given to the reestablishment of adequate respiratory exchange through provision of a patent airway and the institution of assisted or controlled ventilation. The narcotic antagonist naloxone hydrochloride (NARCAN®) is a specific antidote against respiratory depression which may result from overdosage or unusual sensitivity to narcotics including oxymorphone. Therefore, an appropriate dose of naloxone hydrochloride should be administered (usual initial adult dose: 0.4 mg-2 mg) preferably by the intravenous route and simultaneously with efforts at respiratory resuscitation. Since the duration of action of oxymorphone may exceed that of the antagonist, the patient should be kept under continued surveillance and repeated doses of the antagonist should be administered as needed to maintain adequate respiration.

Oxygen, intravenous fluids, vasopressors and other supportive measures should be employed as indicated.

HOW SUPPLIED

Rectal Suppositories: DEA Order Form Required.
5 mg, wrapped in gold foil, box of 6 NDC 0590-0761-06
Store under refrigeration (36°–46°F, 2°–8°C).
Caution: Federal law prohibits dispensing without prescription.

DuPont Pharma
DuPont Merck Pharma
Manati, Puerto Rico 00674
NUMORPHAN® is a Registered Trademark of The DuPont Merck Pharmaceutical Co.
NARCAN® is a Registered Trademark of The DuPont Merck Pharmaceutical Co.

6111-6/Rev. Oct., 1994

Copyright© DuPont Pharma 1994

PENTASPAN®   ℞

(10% pentastarch in 0.9% sodium chloride injection)

DESCRIPTION

PENTASPAN (10% pentastarch in 0.9% sodium chloride injection) is a sterile, nonpyrogenic solution. The composition of each 100 mL is as follows:

Pentastarch... 10.0 g
Sodium Chloride USP... 0.9 g
Water for Injection USP.. qs
pH adjusted with Sodium Hydroxide, NF
Concentration of Electrolytes (mEq/Liter): Sodium 154, Chloride 154
pH: Approx. 4.8 (3.5-7.0); Calculated Osmolarity: Approx. 326 mOsM

Pentastarch is an artificial colloid derived from a waxy starch composed almost entirely of amylopectin. Hydroxyethyl ether groups are introduced into the glucose units of the starch and the resultant material is hydrolyzed to yield a product with a molecular weight suitable for use as an erythrocyte sedimenting agent. Pentastarch is characterized by its molar substitution, and also by its molecular weight. The degree of substitution is 0.45 which means pentastarch has 45 hydroxyethyl groups for every 100 glucose units. The weight average molecular weight of pentastarch is approximately 264,000 with a range of 150,000 to 350,000 and with 80% of the polymers falling between 10,000 and 2,000,000. Hydroxyethyl groups are attached by an ether linkage primarily at C-2 of the glucose unit and to a lesser extent at C-3 and C-6. The polymer resembles glycogen, and the polymerized glucose units are joined primarily by 1–4 linkages with occasional 1–6 branching linkages. The degree of branching is approximately 1:20 which means that there is one 1–6 branch for every 20 glucose monomer units.

The chemical name for pentastarch is hydroxyethyl starch. The structural formula is as follows:
[See chemical structure at top of next column.]
Amylopectin derivative in which R_2, R_3, and R_6 are H or CH_2CH_2OH, or R_6 is a branching point in the starch polymer connected through a 1–6 linkage to additional α-D-glucopyranosyl units.

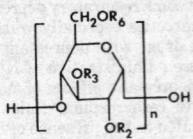

PENTASPAN is a clear, pale yellow to amber solution. Exposure to prolonged adverse storage conditions may result in a change to a turbid deep brown or the formation of a crystalline precipitate. Do not use the solution if these conditions are evident.

CLINICAL PHARMACOLOGY

The addition of PENTASPAN to whole blood increases the erythrocyte sedimentation rate. Therefore, 10% pentastarch in 0.9% sodium chloride injection is used to improve the efficiency of leukocyte collection by centrifugal means. Pentastarch molecules below 50,000 molecular weight are rapidly eliminated by renal excretion. A single dose of approximately 500 mL of PENTASPAN (approximately 50 g) results in elimination in the urine of approximately 70% of the dose within 24 hours, and approximately 80% of the dose within one week. An additional 5–6% of the pentastarch dose is recovered in the leukapheresis collection bag. The remaining 12–15% (approximately 6.8 g) of an administered dose is presumed to undergo slower elimination. This is a variable process but generally results in an intravascular pentastarch concentration below the level of detection by one week. The hydroxyethyl group is not cleaved by the body, but remains intact and attached to glucose units when excreted.

The colloidal properties of the related product HESPAN® (6% hetastarch in 0.9% sodium chloride injection) approximate those of 5% human albumin. Intravenous infusion of HESPAN results in expansion of plasma volume that decreases over the succeeding 24 to 36 hours. Similar, although reduced duration, volume expansion may be expected to occur following use of PENTASPAN® (10% pentastarch in 0.9% sodium chloride injection) in leukapheresis procedures.

INDICATIONS AND USAGE

PENTASPAN is indicated as an adjunct in leukapheresis, to improve the harvesting and increase the yield of leukocytes by centrifugal means.

CONTRAINDICATIONS

PENTASPAN is contraindicated in donors with known hypersensitivity to hydroxyethyl starch, or with bleeding disorders, or with congestive heart failure where volume overload is a potential problem. PENTASPAN should not be used in renal disease with oliguria or anuria.

WARNINGS

Slight declines in platelet counts and hemoglobin levels have been observed in donors undergoing repeated leukapheresis procedures using HESPAN due to the volume expanding effects of HESPAN and to the collection of platelets and erythrocytes. Hemoglobin levels usually return to normal within 24 hours. Similar effects may be expected with PENTASPAN. Hemodilution by PENTASPAN and saline may also result in 24 hour declines of total protein, albumin, calcium and fibrinogen values. None of these decreases are to a degree recognized to be clinically significant risks to healthy donors.

Large volumes of PENTASPAN may slightly alter the coagulation mechanism; *i.e.*, transient prolongation of prothrombin, partial thromboplastin and clotting times. The physician should also be alert to the possibility of transient prolongation of bleeding time.

PRECAUTIONS

General

Regular and frequent clinical evaluation and complete blood counts (CBC) are necessary for proper monitoring of PENTASPAN use during leukapheresis. If the frequency of leukapheresis is to exceed the guidelines for whole blood donation, you may wish to consider the following additional studies: total leukocyte and platelet counts, leukocyte differential count, hemoglobin and hematocrit, prothrombin time (PT), and partial thromboplastin time (PTT) tests.

The possibility of circulatory overload should be kept in mind. Caution should be used when the risk of pulmonary edema and/or congestive heart failure is increased. Special care should be exercised in patients who have impaired renal clearance since this is the principal way in which pentastarch is eliminated.

The serum chemistries of sixteen normal volunteers who were given 500 to 2000 mL infusions of PENTASPAN were essentially unchanged pre- and post-infusion, except for dilutional effects. However, indirect bilirubin levels of 8.3 mg/L (normal 0–7 mg/L) have been reported in 2 out of 20 normal subjects who received multiple HESPAN infusions. Total bilirubin was within normal limits at all times; indirect bilirubin returned to normal by 96 hours following the final infusion. The significance, if any, of these elevations is not

known; however, caution should be observed before administering PENTASPAN to patients with a history of liver disease.

PENTASPAN has been reported to produce hypersensitivity reactions such as wheezing, urticaria and hypotension. However, pentastarch has not been observed to stimulate antibody formation. If hypersensitivity effects occur, discontinue the drug and, if necessary, administer appropriate therapy.

Caution should be exercised when administering PENTASPAN to patients allergic to corn because such patients can also be allergic to PENTASPAN.

Elevated serum amylase levels may be observed temporarily following administration of PENTASPAN, although no association with pancreatitis has been demonstrated. HESPAN® (6% hetastarch in 0.9% sodium chloride injection) has not been shown to increase serum lipase. Similar effects may be expected with PENTASPAN.

Carcinogenesis, Mutagenesis, Impairment of Fertility
Long-term studies in animals have not been performed to evaluate the carcinogenic potential of pentastarch.

Teratogenic Effects
Pregnancy Category C. PENTASPAN has been shown to be embryocidal in New Zealand rabbits and in Swiss Mice when given in doses 5 times the human dose. PENTASPAN® was administered to mated New Zealand rabbits and Swiss Mice with intravenous doses of 10, 20, and 40 mL/kg/day during the period of gestation. The results demonstrated that at 10 and 20 mL/kg/day pentastarch produced no higher incidence of teratogenicity or embryotoxicity in either species than normal saline did in control animals. At 40 mL/kg/day, however, pentastarch increased the number of resorptions and minor visceral anomalies (diffuse edema of the trunk and extremities and diffuse whitish color of the heart, lungs, liver, and kidneys) in rabbits and reduced nidation in the mouse. There are no adequate and well-controlled clinical studies using pentastarch in pregnant women. PENTASPAN should be used during pregnancy only if the potential benefits justify the potential risk to the fetus.

Nursing mothers
It is not known whether pentastarch is excreted in human milk. Because many drugs are excreted in human milk, caution should be exercised when PENTASPAN is administered to a nursing woman.

Pediatric use
The safety and effectiveness of PENTASPAN in pediatric patients have not been established.

ADVERSE REACTIONS

PENTASPAN has been reported to produce hypersensitivity reactions such as wheezing, urticaria, and hypotension (see PRECAUTIONS).

The following have been reported in association with the use of PENTASPAN in leukapheresis: headache, diarrhea, nausea, weakness, temporary weight gain, insomnia, fatigue, fever, edema, paresthesia, acne, malaise, shakiness, dizziness, chest pain, chills, nasal congestion, anxiety, and increased heart rate. It is uncertain whether they are attributable to the drug, the procedure, additional adjunctive medication, or some combination of these factors.

DOSAGE AND ADMINISTRATION

250 to 700 mL of PENTASPAN to which citrate anticoagulant has been added is typically administered by aseptic addition to the input line of the centrifugation apparatus at a ratio of 1:8 to 1:13 to venous whole blood. The bottle containing PENTASPAN and citrate should be thoroughly mixed to assure effective anticoagulation of blood as it flows through the leukapheresis machine.

Parenteral drug products should be inspected visually for particulate matter and discoloration prior to administration whenever solution and container permit.

When stored at room temperature, PENTASPAN admixtures of 500–560 mL with citrate up to 2.5% were compatible for 24 hours. The safety and compatibility of other additives have not been established.

General Recommendations
This solution is intended for intravenous administration using sterile equipment. It is recommended that intravenous administration apparatus be replaced at least once every 24 hours.

Use only if solution is clear and container and seals are intact.

Directions for Use
Caution: Before administering to patient, perform the following checks:
1. Each container should be inspected before use. Read the label. Insure solution is the one ordered, is within the expiration date, and that label name agrees with the abbreviated name stamped on closure. Check the security of bail and band.
2. Invert container and carefully inspect the solution in good light for cloudiness, haze, or particulate matter; check the bottle for cracks or other damage. In checking for cracks, do not be confused by normal surface mold marks and seams on bottom and sides of bottle. These are not flaws. Look instead for bright reflections that have depth and

penetrate into the wall of the bottle. Reject any such bottle.

3. Check for vacuum, first by confirming the presence of depressions in the latex disk and then by audible hiss when the disk is removed. Reject any container that does not meet these criteria.
4. After admixtures and during administration, reinspect solution as frequently as possible. If any evidence of solution contamination or instability is found or if the patient exhibits any signs of fever or chills or other reaction not readily explainable, discontinue administration immediately and notify physician.

HOW SUPPLIED

NDC 0056-0081-95: PENTASPAN® (10% pentastarch in 0.9% sodium chloride injection) is supplied sterile and nonpyrogenic in 500 mL intravenous infusion bottles.

Exposure of pharmaceutical products to heat should be minimized. Avoid excessive heat. Protect from freezing. It is recommended that the product be stored at room temperature (25°C); however, brief exposure up to 40°C does not adversely affect the product.

Caution: Federal (U.S.A.) law prohibits dispensing without prescription.

Distributed by
DuPont Pharma
Wilmington, Delaware 19880
Manufactured by
McGaw, Inc.
Irvine, CA USA 92714-5895
6270-1/Rev. December, 1995
PENTASPAN® and HESPAN® are registered trademarks of
The DuPont Merck Pharmaceutical Co.

PERCOCET® Ⓒ II

[*perk 'o-set*]
(oxycodone and acetaminophen tablets, USP)

DESCRIPTION

Each tablet of PERCOCET contains:
Oxycodone hydrochloride .... 5 mg*
WARNING: May be habit forming
Acetaminophen, USP .... 325 mg
*5 mg oxycodone HCl is equivalent to 4.4815 mg of oxycodone.

PERCOCET Tablets also contain: microcrystalline cellulose, povidone, pregelatinized starch, stearic acid and other ingredients.

Acetaminophen occurs as a white, odorless, crystalline powder, possessing a slightly bitter taste.

The oxycodone component is 14-hydroxydihydrocodeinone, a white, odorless, crystalline powder having a saline, bitter taste. It is derived from the opium alkaloid thebaine, and may be represented by the following structural formula:

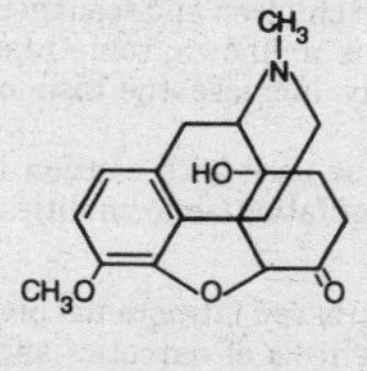

CLINICAL PHARMACOLOGY

The principal ingredient, oxycodone, is a semisynthetic narcotic analgesic with multiple actions qualitatively similar to those of morphine; the most prominent of these involve the central nervous system and organs composed of smooth muscle. The principal actions of therapeutic value of the oxycodone in PERCOCET are analgesia and sedation.

Oxycodone is similar to codeine and methadone in that it retains at least one-half of its analgesic activity when administered orally.

Acetaminophen is a non-opiate, non-salicylate analgesic and antipyretic.

INDICATIONS AND USAGE

PERCOCET is indicated for the relief of moderate to moderately severe pain.

CONTRAINDICATIONS

PERCOCET should not be administered to patients who are hypersensitive to oxycodone or acetaminophen.

WARNINGS

Drug Dependence: Oxycodone can produce drug dependence of the morphine type and, therefore, has the potential for being abused. Psychic dependence, physical dependence and tolerance may develop upon repeated administration of PERCOCET, and it should be prescribed and administered with the same degree of caution appropriate to the use of other oral narcotic-containing medications. Like other narcotic-containing medications, PERCOCET is subject to the Federal Controlled Substances Act (Schedule II).

PRECAUTIONS

General

Head Injury and Increased Intracranial Pressure: The respiratory depressant effects of narcotics and their capacity to elevate cerebrospinal fluid pressure may be markedly exaggerated in the presence of head injury, other intracranial lesions or a pre-existing increase in intracranial pressure. Furthermore, narcotics produce adverse reactions which may obscure the clinical course of patients with head injuries.

Acute Abdominal Conditions: The administration of PERCOCET or other narcotics may obscure the diagnosis or clinical course in patients with acute abdominal conditions.

Special Risk Patients: PERCOCET should be given with caution to certain patients such as the elderly or debilitated, and those with severe impairment of hepatic or renal function, hypothyroidism, Addison's disease, and prostatic hypertrophy or urethral stricture.

Information for Patients

Oxycodone may impair the mental and/or physical abilities required for the performance of potentially hazardous tasks such as driving a car or operating machinery. The patient using PERCOCET should be cautioned accordingly.

Drug Interactions

Patients receiving other narcotic analgesics, general anesthetics, phenothiazines, other tranquilizers, sedative-hypnotics or other CNS depressants (including alcohol) concomitantly with PERCOCET may exhibit an additive CNS depression. When such combined therapy is contemplated, the dose of one or both agents should be reduced.

The use of MAO inhibitors or tricyclic antidepressants with oxycodone preparations may increase the effect of either the antidepressant or oxycodone.

The concurrent use of anticholinergics with narcotics may produce paralytic ileus.

Usage In Pregnancy

Pregnancy Category C: Animal reproductive studies have not been conducted with PERCOCET. It is also not known whether PERCOCET can cause fetal harm when administered to a pregnant woman or can affect reproductive capacity. PERCOCET should not be given to a pregnant woman unless in the judgment of the physician, the potential benefits outweigh the possible hazards.

Nonteratogenic Effects: Use of narcotics during pregnancy may produce physical dependence in the neonate.

Labor and Delivery: As with all narcotics, administration of PERCOCET to the mother shortly before delivery may result in some degree of respiratory depression in the newborn and the mother, especially if higher doses are used.

Nursing Mothers

It is not known whether PERCOCET is excreted in human milk. Because many drugs are excreted in human milk, caution should be exercised when PERCOCET is administered to a nursing woman.

Pediatric Use

Safety and effectiveness in children have not been established.

ADVERSE REACTIONS

The most frequently observed adverse reactions include lightheadedness, dizziness, sedation, nausea and vomiting. These effects seem to be more prominent in ambulatory than in nonambulatory patients, and some of these adverse reactions may be alleviated if the patient lies down.

Other adverse reactions include euphoria, dysphoria, constipation, skin rash and pruritus. At higher doses, oxycodone has most of the disadvantages of morphine including respiratory depression.

DRUG ABUSE AND DEPENDENCE

PERCOCET Tablets are a Schedule II controlled substance. Oxycodone can produce drug dependence and has the potential for being abused. (See WARNINGS.)

OVERDOSAGE

Acetaminophen

Signs and Symptoms: In acute acetaminophen overdosage, dose-dependent, potentially fatal hepatic necrosis is the most serious adverse effect. Renal tubular necrosis, hypoglycemic coma and thrombocytopenia may also occur.

In adults, hepatic toxicity has rarely been reported with acute overdoses of less than 10 grams and fatalities with less than 15 grams. Importantly, young children seem to be more resistant than adults to the hepatotoxic effect of an acetaminophen overdose. Despite this, the measures outlined below should be initiated in any adult or child suspected of having ingested an acetaminophen overdose.

Early symptoms following a potentially hepatotoxic overdose may include: nausea, vomiting, diaphoresis and general malaise. Clinical and laboratory evidence of hepatic toxicity may not be apparent until 48 to 72 hours post-ingestion.

Treatment: The stomach should be emptied promptly by lavage or by induction of emesis with syrup of ipecac. Patient's estimates of the quantity of a drug ingested are notoriously unreliable. Therefore, if an acetaminophen overdose is suspected, a serum acetaminophen assay should be obtained as early as possible, but no sooner than four hours following ingestion. Liver function studies should be obtained initially and repeated at 24-hour intervals.

The antidote, N-acetylcysteine, should be administered as early as possible, preferably within 16 hours of the overdose ingestion for optimal results, but in any case, within 24 hours. Following recovery, there are no residual, structural, or functional hepatic abnormalities.

Oxycodone

Signs and Symptoms: Serious overdosage with oxycodone is characterized by respiratory depression (a decrease in respiratory rate and/or tidal volume, Cheyne-Stokes respiration, cyanosis), extreme somnolence progressing to stupor or coma, skeletal muscle flaccidity, cold and clammy skin, and sometimes bradycardia and hypotension. In severe overdosage, apnea, circulatory collapse, cardiac arrest and death may occur.

Treatment: Primary attention should be given to the reestablishment of adequate respiratory exchange through provision of a patent airway and the institution of assisted or controlled ventilation. The narcotic antagonist naloxone hydrochloride (Narcan®) is a specific antidote against respiratory depression which may result from overdosage or unusual sensitivity to narcotics, including oxycodone. Therefore, an appropriate dose of naloxone hydrochloride (usual initial adult dose 0.4 mg to 2 mg) should be administered preferably by the intravenous route, and simultaneously with efforts at respiratory resuscitation (see package insert). Since the duration of action of oxycodone may exceed that of the antagonist, the patient should be kept under continued surveillance and repeated doses of the antagonist should be administered as needed to maintain adequate respiration.

An antagonist should not be administered in the absence of clinically significant respiratory or cardiovascular depression. Oxygen, intravenous fluids, vasopressors and other supportive measures should be employed as indicated.

Gastric emptying may be useful in removing unabsorbed drug.

DOSAGE AND ADMINISTRATION

Dosage should be adjusted according to the severity of the pain and the response of the patient. It may occasionally be necessary to exceed the usual dosage recommended below in cases of more severe pain or in those patients who have become tolerant to the analgesic effect of narcotics. PERCOCET (oxycodone and acetaminophen tablets) is given orally. The usual adult dosage is one tablet every 6 hours as needed for pain.

HOW SUPPLIED

PERCOCET (5 mg oxycodone hydrochloride and 325 mg acetaminophen tablets), supplied as a white tablet, with one face scored and inscribed PERCOCET, and the other inscribed with DuPont name is available in:

Bottles of 100	NDC 0590-0127-70
Bottles of 500	NDC 0590-0127-85
Hospital Blister Pack of 25 (in units of 100)	NDC 0590-0127-75

Store at controlled room temperature (15°–30°C, 59°–86°F).
DEA Order Form Required
DuPont Pharma
DuPont Merck Pharma
Manati, Puerto Rico 00674
PERCOCET® is a Registered Trademark of The DuPont Merck Pharmaceutical Co.
NARCAN® is a Registered Trademark of The DuPont Merck Pharmaceutical Co.

6365/Aug., 1994

Shown in Product Identification Guide, page 310

---

†PERCODAN® Ⓒ II

[*perk 'o-dan*]
(oxycodone and aspirin tablets, USP)

DESCRIPTION

Each tablet of PERCODAN contains:
Oxycodone hydrochloride .... 4.50 mg*
WARNING: May be habit forming
Oxycodone terephthalate .... 0.38 mg**
WARNING May be habit forming
Aspirin, USP .... 325 mg
*4.50 mg oxycodone HCl is equivalent to 4.0338 mg of oxycodone.
**0.38 mg oxycodone terephthalate is equivalent to 0.3008 mg of oxycodone.

PERCODAN Tablets also contain: D&C Yellow 10, FD&C Yellow 6, microcrystalline cellulose and starch.

The oxycodone component is 14-hydroxydihydrocodeinone, a white odorless crystalline powder which is derived from the

Continued on next page

DuPont Pharma—Cont.

opium alkaloid, thebaine, and may be represented by the following structural formula:

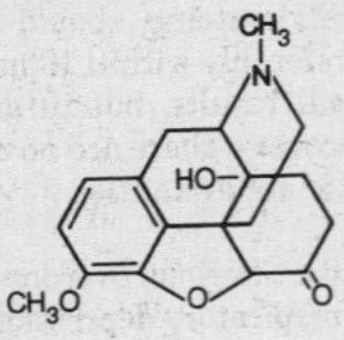

ACTIONS

The principal ingredient, oxycodone, is a semisynthetic narcotic analgesic with multiple actions qualitatively similar to those of morphine; the most prominent of these involve the central nervous system and organs composed of smooth muscle. The principal actions of therapeutic value of the oxycodone in PERCODAN are analgesia and sedation.
Oxycodone is similar to codeine and methadone in that it retains at least one-half of its analgesic activity when administered orally.
PERCODAN also contains the non-narcotic antipyretic-analgesic, aspirin.

INDICATIONS

For the relief of moderate to moderately severe pain.

CONTRAINDICATIONS

Hypersensitivity to oxycodone or aspirin.

WARNINGS

Drug Dependence: Oxycodone can produce drug dependence of the morphine type and, therefore, has the potential for being abused. Psychic dependence, physical dependence and tolerance may develop upon repeated administration of PERCODAN, and it should be prescribed and administered with the same degree of caution appropriate to the use of other oral narcotic-containing medications. Like other narcotic-containing medications, PERCODAN is subject to the Federal Controlled Substances Act.
Usage in ambulatory patients: Oxycodone may impair the mental and/or physical abilities required for the performance of potentially hazardous tasks such as driving a car or operating machinery. The patient using PERCODAN should be cautioned accordingly.
Interaction with other central nervous system depressants: Patients receiving other narcotic analgesics, general anesthetics, phenothiazines, other tranquilizers, sedative-hypnotics or other CNS depressants (including alcohol) concomitantly with PERCODAN may exhibit an additive CNS depression. When such combined therapy is contemplated, the dose of one or both agents should be reduced.
Usage in pregnancy: Safe use in pregnancy has not been established relative to possible adverse effects on fetal development. Therefore, PERCODAN should not be used in pregnant women unless, in the judgment of the physician, the potential benefits outweigh the possible hazards.
Usage in children: PERCODAN should not be administered to children. PERCODAN®-Demi, containing half the amount of oxycodone, can be considered. (See product prescribing information for PERCODAN-Demi).
Reye Syndrome is a rare but serious disease which can follow flu or chicken pox in children and teenagers. While the cause of Reye Syndrome is unknown, some reports claim aspirin (or salicylates) may increase the risk of developing this disease.
Salicylates should be used with caution in the presence of peptic ulcer or coagulation abnormalities.

PRECAUTIONS

Head injury and increased intracranial pressure: The respiratory depressant effects of narcotics and their capacity to elevate cerebrospinal fluid pressure may be markedly exaggerated in the presence of head injury, other intracranial lesions or a pre-existing increase in intracranial pressure. Furthermore, narcotics produce adverse reactions which may obscure the clinical course of patients with head injuries.
Acute abdominal conditions: The administration of PERCODAN (oxycodone and aspirin) or other narcotics may obscure the diagnosis or clinical course in patients with acute abdominal conditions.
Special risk patients: PERCODAN should be given with caution to certain patients such as the elderly or debilitated, and those with severe impairment of hepatic or renal function, hypothyroidism, Addison's disease, and prostatic hypertrophy or urethral stricture.

ADVERSE REACTIONS

The most frequently observed adverse reactions include lightheadedness, dizziness, sedation, nausea and vomiting. These effects seem to be more prominent in ambulatory than in nonambulatory patients, and some of these adverse reactions may be alleviated if the patient lies down.
Other adverse reactions include euphoria, dysphoria, constipation and pruritus.

DRUG ABUSE AND DEPENDENCE

PERCODAN tablets are a Schedule II controlled substance. Oxycodone can produce drug dependence and has the potential for being abused. (See WARNINGS.)

DOSAGE AND ADMINISTRATION

Dosage should be adjusted according to the severity of the pain and the response of the patient. It may occasionally be necessary to exceed the usual dosage recommended below in cases of more severe pain or in those patients who have become tolerant to the analgesic effect of narcotics. PERCODAN is given orally. The usual adult dose is one tablet every 6 hours as needed for pain.

DRUG INTERACTIONS

The CNS depressant effects of PERCODAN may be additive with that of other CNS depressants. (See WARNINGS.)
Aspirin may enhance the effect of anticoagulants and inhibit the uricosuric effects of uricosuric agents.

MANAGEMENT OF OVERDOSAGE

Signs and Symptoms: Serious overdose with PERCODAN is characterized by respiratory depression (a decrease in respiratory rate and/or tidal volume, Cheyne-Stokes respiration, cyanosis), extreme somnolence progressing to stupor or coma, skeletal muscle flaccidity, cold and clammy skin, and sometimes bradycardia and hypotension. In severe overdosage, apnea, circulatory collapse, cardiac arrest and death may occur. The ingestion of very large amounts of PERCODAN may, in addition, result in acute salicylate intoxication.
Treatment: Primary attention should be given to the reestablishment of adequate respiratory exchange through provision of a patent airway and the institution of assisted or controlled ventilation. The narcotic antagonist naloxone hydrochloride (NARCAN®) is a specific antidote against respiratory depression which may result from overdosage or unusual sensitivity to narcotics including oxycodone. Therefore, an appropriate dose of naloxone hydrochloride should be administered (usual initial adult dose: 0.4 mg–2 mg) preferably by the intravenous route, simultaneously with efforts at respiratory resuscitation. Since the duration of action of oxycodone may exceed that of the antagonist, the patient should be kept under continued surveillance and repeated doses of the antagonist should be administered as needed to maintain adequate respiration.
Oxygen, intravenous fluids, vasopressors and other supportive measures should be employed as indicated.
Gastric emptying may be useful in removing unabsorbed drug.

HOW SUPPLIED

PERCODAN (4.50 mg oxycodone hydrochloride, 0.38 mg oxycodone terephthalate, 325 mg Aspirin, USP), supplied as a yellow tablet, with one face scored and inscribed PERCODAN, and the other inscribed with DuPont name is available in:

Bottles of 100	NDC 0590-0135-70
Bottles of 500	NDC 0590-0135-85
Bottles of 1000	NDC 0590-0135-90
Hospital blister pack of 25 (in units of 250 tablets)	NDC 0590-0135-65

Store at controlled room temperature (15°–30°C, 59°–86°F).
DEA Order Form Required.

DuPont Pharma
DuPont Merck Pharma
Manati, Puerto Rico 00674

PERCODAN® is a Registered Trademark of The DuPont Merck Pharmaceutical Co.
NARCAN® is a Registered Trademark of The DuPont Merck Pharmaceutical Co.
6366/Aug., 1994

Shown in Product Identification Guide, page 310

PERCODAN®-DEMI Ⓒ

[perk 'o-dan]
(oxycodone and aspirin)

DESCRIPTION

Each tablet of PERCODAN-Demi contains:

Oxycodone hydrochloride	2.25 mg*
WARNING: May be habit forming	
Oxycodone terephthalate	0.19 mg**
WARNING: May be habit forming	
Aspirin, USP	325 mg

*2.25 mg oxycodone HCl is equivalent to 2.0169 mg of oxycodone.
**0.19 mg oxycodone terephthalate is equivalent to 0.1504 mg of oxycodone.

PERCODAN-Demi Tablets also contain: microcrystalline cellulose and starch.
The oxycodone component is 14-hydroxydihydrocodeinone, a white odorless crystalline powder which is derived from the opium alkaloid, thebaine, and may be represented by the following structural formula:

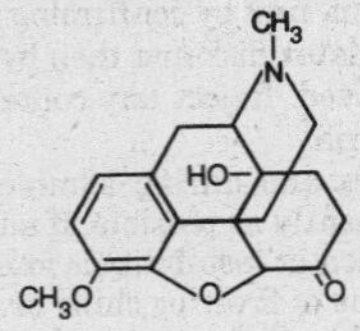

ACTIONS

The principal ingredient, oxycodone, is a semisynthetic narcotic analgesic with multiple actions qualitatively similar to those of morphine; the most prominent of these involve the central nervous system and organs composed of smooth muscle. The principal actions of therapeutic value of the oxycodone in PERCODAN-Demi are analgesia and sedation.
Oxycodone is similar to codeine and methadone in that it retains at least one half of its analgesic activity when administered orally.
PERCODAN-Demi also contains the non-narcotic antipyretic-analgesic, aspirin.

INDICATIONS

For the relief of moderate to moderately severe pain.

CONTRAINDICATIONS

Hypersensitivity to oxycodone or aspirin.

WARNINGS

Drug Dependence: Oxycodone can produce drug dependence of the morphine type and, therefore, has the potential for being abused. Psychic dependence, physical dependence and tolerance may develop upon repeated administration of PERCODAN-Demi, and it should be prescribed and administered with the same degree of caution appropriate to the use of other oral narcotic-containing medications. Like other narcotic-containing medications, PERCODAN-Demi is subject to the Federal Controlled Substances Act.
Usage in ambulatory patients: Oxycodone may impair the mental and/or physical abilities required for the performance of potentially hazardous tasks such as driving a car or operating machinery. The patient using PERCODAN-Demi should be cautioned accordingly.
Interaction with other central nervous system depressants: Patients receiving other narcotic analgesics, general anesthetics, phenothiazines, other tranquilizers, sedative-hypnotics or other CNS depressants (including alcohol) concomitantly with PERCODAN-Demi may exhibit an additive CNS depression. When such combined therapy is contemplated, the dose of one or both agents should be reduced.
Usage in pregnancy: Safe use in pregnancy has not been established relative to possible adverse effects on fetal development. Therefore, PERCODAN-Demi should not be used in pregnant women unless, in the judgement of the physician, the potential benefits outweigh the possible hazards.
Reye Syndrome is a rare but serious disease which can follow flu or chicken pox in children and teenagers. While the cause of Reye Syndrome is unknown, some reports claim aspirin (or salicylates) may increase the risk of developing this disease.
Salicylates should be used with caution in the presence of peptic ulcer or coagulation abnormalities.

PRECAUTIONS

Head Injury and Increased Intracranial pressure: The respiratory depressant effects of narcotics and their capacity to elevate cerebrospinal fluid pressure may be markedly exaggerated in the presence of head injury, other intracranial lesions or a pre-existing increase in intracranial pressure. Furthermore, narcotics produce adverse reactions which may obscure the clinical course of patients with head injuries.
Acute abdominal conditions: The administration of PERCODAN-Demi or other narcotics may obscure the diagnosis or clinical course in patients with acute abdominal conditions.
Special risk patients: PERCODAN-Demi (oxycodone and aspirin) should be given with caution to certain patients such as the elderly or debilitated, and those with severe impairment of hepatic or renal function, hypothyroidism, Addison's disease, and prostatic hypertrophy or urethral stricture.

ADVERSE REACTIONS

The most frequently observed adverse reactions include lightheadedness, dizziness, sedation, nausea and vomiting. These effects seem to be more prominent in ambulatory than in non-ambulatory patients, and some of these adverse reactions may be alleviated if the patient lies down.
Other adverse reactions include euphoria, dysphoria, constipation and pruritus.

DRUG ABUSE AND DEPENDENCE

PERCODAN-Demi tablets are a Schedule II controlled substance. Oxycodone can produce drug dependence and has the potential for being abused. (See WARNINGS)

DOSAGE AND ADMINISTRATION

Dosage should be adjusted according to the severity of the pain and the response of the patient. It may occasionally be necessary to exceed the usual dosage recommended below in cases of more severe pain or in those patients who have become tolerant to the analgesic effect of narcotics. PERCODAN-Demi is given orally.

Dosage: Adults—One or two tablets every six hours.
Children 12 years and older—One-half tablet every six hours.
Children 6 to 12 years—One-quarter tablet every six hours.
PERCODAN-Demi is not indicated for children under 6 years of age.

DRUG INTERACTIONS

The CNS depressant effects of PERCODAN-Demi may be additive with that of other CNS depressants. (See WARNINGS)
Aspirin may enhance the effect of anticoagulants and inhibit the uricosuric effect of uricosuric agents.

MANAGEMENT OF OVERDOSAGE

Signs and Symptoms: Serious overdose with PERCODAN-Demi is characterized by respiratory depression (a decrease in respiratory rate and/or tidal volume, Cheyne-Stokes respiration, cyanosis), extreme somnolence progressing to stupor or coma, skeletal muscle flaccidity, cold and clammy skin, and sometimes bradycardia and hypotension. In severe overdosage, apnea, circulatory collapse, cardiac arrest and death may occur. The ingestion of very large amounts of PERCODAN-Demi may, in addition, result in acute salicylate intoxication.

Treatment: Primary attention should be given to the reestablishment of adequate respiratory exchange through provision of a patent airway and the institution of assisted or controlled ventilation. The narcotic antagonist naloxone hydrochloride (NARCAN®) is a specific antidote against respiratory depression which may result from overdosage or unusual sensitivity to narcotics including oxycodone. Therefore, an appropriate dose of naloxone hydrochloride should be administered (usual initial adult dose 0.4 mg–2 mg) preferably by the intravenous route, simultaneously with efforts at respiratory resuscitation. Since the duration of action of oxycodone may exceed that of the antagonist, the patient should be kept under continued surveillance and repeated doses of the antagonist should be administered as needed to maintain adequate respiration.
Oxygen, intravenous fluids, vasopressors and other supportive measures should be employed as indicated.
Gastric emptying may be useful in removing unabsorbed drug.

HOW SUPPLIED

As white, scored tablets available in:
Bottles of 100 NDC 0590-0166-70
Store at controlled room temperature (15°–30°C, 59°–86°F).
DEA Order Form Required.

DuPont Pharmaceuticals
DuPont Merck Pharma
P.O. Box 363, Manati, Puerto Rico 00674

PERCODAN® is a Registered Trademark of The DuPont Merck Pharmaceutical Co.
NARCAN® is a Registered Trademark of The DuPont Merck Pharmaceutical Co.

6234-2/Rev. June, 1993

REVIA™ ℞

[*reh "vēē 'uh "*]
(naltrexone hydrochloride tablets)

DESCRIPTION

REVIA (naltrexone hydrochloride), an opioid antagonist, is a synthetic congener of oxymorphone with no opioid agonist properties. Naltrexone differs in structure from oxymorphone in that the methyl group on the nitrogen atom is replaced by a cyclopropylmethyl group. REVIA (naltrexone hydrochloride) is also related to the potent opioid antagonist, naloxone, or n-allylnoroxymorphone (NARCAN®).

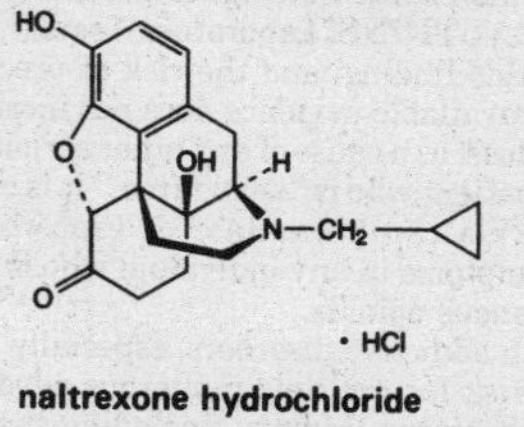

naltrexone hydrochloride

REVIA (naltrexone hydrochloride) is a white, crystalline compound. The hydrochloride salt is soluble in water to the extent of about 100 mg/cc. REVIA is available in scored tablets containing 50 mg of naltrexone hydrochloride.

REVIA Tablets also contain: lactose, microcrystalline cellulose, crospovidone, colloidal silicon dioxide, magnesium stearate, hydroxypropyl methylcellulose, titanium dioxide, polyethylene glycol, polysorbate 80, yellow iron oxide and red iron oxide.

CLINICAL PHARMACOLOGY

Pharmacodynamic actions: REVIA (naltrexone hydrochloride) is a pure opioid antagonist. It markedly attenuates or completely blocks, reversibly, the subjective effects of intravenously administered opioids.
When co-administered with morphine, on a chronic basis, REVIA blocks the physical dependence to morphine, heroin and other opioids.
REVIA has few, if any, intrinsic actions besides its opioid blocking properties. However, it does produce some pupillary constriction, by an unknown mechanism.
The administration of REVIA is not associated with the development of tolerance or dependence. In subjects physically dependent on opioids, REVIA will precipitate withdrawal symptomatology.
Clinical studies indicate that 50 mg of REVIA will block the pharmacologic effects of 25 mg of intravenously administered heroin for periods as long as 24 hours. Other data suggest that doubling the dose of REVIA provides blockade for 48 hours, and tripling the dose of REVIA provides blockade for about 72 hours.
REVIA blocks the effects of opioids by competitive binding (i.e., analogous to competitive inhibition of enzymes) at opioid receptors. This makes the blockade produced potentially surmountable, but overcoming full naltrexone blockade by administration of very high doses of opiates has resulted in excessive symptoms of histamine release in experimental subjects.
The mechanism of action of REVIA in alcoholism is not understood; however, involvement of the endogenous opioid system is suggested by preclinical data. REVIA, an opioid receptor antagonist, competitively binds to such receptors and may block the effects of endogenous opioids. Opioid antagonists have been shown to reduce alcohol consumption by animals, and REVIA has been shown to reduce alcohol consumption in clinical studies.
REVIA is not aversive therapy and does not cause a disulfiram-like reaction either as a result of opiate use or ethanol ingestion.

Pharmacokinetics
REVIA (naltrexone hydrochloride) is a pure opioid receptor antagonist. Although well absorbed orally, naltrexone is subject to significant first pass metabolism with oral bioavailability estimates ranging from 5 to 40%. The activity of naltrexone is believed to be due to both parent and the 6-β-naltrexol metabolite. Both parent drug and metabolites are excreted primarily by the kidney (53% to 79% of the dose), however, urinary excretion of unchanged naltrexone accounts for less than 2% of an oral dose and fecal excretion is a minor elimination pathway. The mean elimination half-life (T-1/2) values for naltrexone and 6-β-naltrexol are 4 hours and 13 hours, respectively. Naltrexone and 6-β-naltrexol are dose proportional in terms of AUC and C_{max} over the range of 50 to 200 mg and do not accumulate after 100 mg daily doses.

Absorption
Following oral administration, naltrexone undergoes rapid and nearly complete absorption with approximately 96% of the dose absorbed from the gastrointestinal tract. Peak plasma levels of both naltrexone and 6-β-naltrexol occur within one hour of dosing.

Distribution
The volume of distribution for naltrexone following intravenous administration is estimated to be 1350 liters. *In vitro* tests with human plasma show naltrexone to be 21% bound to plasma proteins over the therapeutic dose range.

Metabolism
The systemic clearance (after intravenous administration) of naltrexone is ~3.5 L/min, which exceeds liver blood flow (~1.2 L/min). This suggests both that naltrexone is a highly extracted drug (>98% metabolized) and that extra-hepatic sites of drug metabolism exist. The major metabolite of naltrexone is 6-β-naltrexol. Two other minor metabolites are 2-hydroxy-3-methoxy-6-β-naltrexol and 2-hydroxy-3-methyl-naltrexone. Naltrexone and its metabolites are also conjugated to form additional metabolic products.

Elimination
The renal clearance for naltrexone ranges from 30-127 mL/min and suggests that renal elimination is primarily by glomerular filtration. In comparison the renal clearance for 6-β-naltrexol ranges from 230-369 mL/min, suggesting an additional renal tubular secretory mechanism. The urinary excretion of unchanged naltrexone accounts for less than 2% of an oral dose; urinary excretion of unchanged and conjugated 6-β-naltrexol accounts for 43% of an oral dose. The pharmacokinetic profile of naltrexone suggests that naltrexone and its metabolites may undergo enterohepatic recycling.

Hepatic and Renal Impairment
Naltrexone appears to have extra-hepatic sites of drug metabolism and its major metabolite undergoes active tubular secretion (see **Metabolism** above). Adequate studies of naltrexone in patients with severe hepatic or renal impairment have not been conducted.

Clinical Trials:
Alcoholism:
The efficacy of REVIA as an aid to the treatment of alcoholism was tested in placebo-controlled, outpatient, double blind trials. These studies used a dose of REVIA 50 mg once daily for 12 weeks as an adjunct to social and psychotherapeutic methods when given under conditions that enhanced patient compliance. Patients with psychosis, dementia, and secondary psychiatric diagnoses were excluded from these studies. In one of these studies, 104 alcohol-dependent patients were randomized to receive either REVIA 50 mg once daily or placebo. In this study, REVIA proved superior to placebo in measures of drinking including abstention rates (51% vs. 23%), number of drinking days, and relapse (31% vs. 60%). In a second study with 82 alcohol-dependent patients, the group of patients receiving REVIA were shown to have lower relapse rates (21% vs. 41%), less alcohol craving, and fewer drinking days compared with patients who received placebo, but these results depended on the specific analysis used.
The clinical use of REVIA as adjunctive pharmacotherapy for the treatment of alcoholism was also evaluated in a multicenter safety study. This study of 865 individuals with alcoholism included patients with comorbid psychiatric conditions, concomitant medications, polysubstance abuse and HIV disease. Results of this study demonstrated that the side effect profile of REVIA appears to be similar in both alcoholic and opioid dependent populations, and that serious side effects are uncommon.
In the clinical studies, treatment with REVIA supported abstinence, prevented relapse and decreased alcohol consumption. In the uncontrolled study, the patterns of abstinence and relapse were similar to those observed in the controlled studies. REVIA was not uniformly helpful to all patients, and the expected effect of the drug is a modest improvement in the outcome of conventional treatment.

Treatment of Narcotic Addiction:
REVIA has been shown to produce complete blockade of the euphoric effects of opioids in both volunteer and addict populations. When administered by means that enforce compliance, it will produce an effective opioid blockade, but has not been shown to affect the use of cocaine or other non-opioid drugs of abuse.
There are no data that demonstrate an unequivocally beneficial effect of REVIA on rates of recidivism among detoxified,-formerly opioid-dependent individuals who self-administer the drug. The failure of the drug in this setting appears to be due to poor medication compliance.
The drug is reported to be of greatest use in good prognosis narcotic addicts who take the drug as part of a comprehensive occupational rehabilitative program, behavioral contract, or other compliance-enhancing protocol. REVIA, unlike methadone or LAAM (levo-alpha-acetylmethadol), does not reinforce medication compliance and is expected to have a therapeutic effect only when given under external conditions that support continued use of the medication.

Individualization of dosage:
DO NOT ATTEMPT TREATMENT WITH REVIA UNLESS, IN THE MEDICAL JUDGEMENT OF THE PRESCRIBING PHYSICIAN, THERE IS NO REASONABLE POSSIBILITY OF OPIOID USE WITHIN THE PAST 7-10 DAYS. IF THERE IS ANY QUESTION OF OCCULT OPIOID DEPENDENCE, PERFORM A NARCAN CHALLENGE TEST.

Treatment of Alcoholism:
The placebo-controlled studies that demonstrated the efficacy of REVIA as an adjunctive treatment of alcoholism used a dose regimen of REVIA 50 mg once daily for up to 12 weeks. Other dose regimens or durations of therapy were not studied in these trials.
Physicians are advised that 5-15% of patients taking REVIA for alcoholism will complain of non-specific side effects, chiefly gastrointestinal upset. Prescribing physicians have tried using an initial 25 mg dose, splitting the daily dose, and adjusting the time of dosing with limited success. No dose or pattern of dosing has been shown to be more effective than any other in reducing these complaints for all patients.

Treatment of Narcotic Dependence:
Once the patient has been started on REVIA, 50 mg once a day will produce adequate clinical blockade of the actions of parenterally administered opioids. As with many non-agonist treatments for addiction, REVIA is of proven value only when given as part of a comprehensive plan of management that includes some measure to ensure the patient takes the medication.
A flexible approach to a dosing regimen may be employed to enhance compliance. Thus, patients may receive 50 mg of REVIA every weekday with a 100 mg dose on Saturday or patients may receive 100 mg every other day, or 150 mg ev-

Continued on next page

DuPont Pharma—Cont.

ery third day. Several of the clinical studies reported in the literature have employed the following dosing regimen: 100 mg on Monday, 100 mg on Wednesday, and 150 mg on Friday. This dosing schedule appeared to be acceptable to many REVIA patients successfully maintaining their opioid-free state.

Experience with the supervised administration of a number of potentially hepatotoxic agents suggests that supervised administration and single doses of REVIA higher than 50 mg may have an associated increased risk of hepatocellular injury, even though three-times a week dosing has been well tolerated in the addict population and in initial clinical trials in alcoholism. Clinics using this approach should balance the possible risks against the probable benefits and may wish to maintain a higher index of suspicion for drug-associated hepatitis and ensure patients are advised of the need to report non-specific abdominal complaints (see **Information for Patients**).

INDICATIONS AND USAGE:

REVIA (naltrexone hydrochloride) is indicated :
In the treatment of alcohol dependence and for the blockade of the effects of exogenously administered opioids.

REVIA has not been shown to provide any therapeutic benefit except as part of an appropriate plan of management for the addictions.

CONTRAINDICATIONS

REVIA is contraindicated in:
1) Patients receiving opioid analgesics.
2) Patients currently dependent on opioids.
3) Patients in acute opioid withdrawal (see **WARNINGS**).
4) Any individual who has failed the NARCAN challenge test or who has a positive urine screen for opioids.
5) Any individual with a history of sensitivity to REVIA (naltrexone hydrochloride). It is not known if there is any cross-sensitivity with naloxone or the phenanthrene containing opioids.
6) Any individual with acute hepatitis or liver failure.

WARNINGS
Hepatotoxicity:

> REVIA has the capacity to cause hepatocellular injury when given in excessive doses.
>
> REVIA is contraindicated in acute hepatitis or liver failure, and its use in patients with active liver disease must be carefully considered in light of its hepatotoxic effects.
>
> The margin of separation between the apparently safe dose of REVIA and the dose causing hepatic injury appears to be only five-fold or less. REVIA does not appear to be a hepatotoxin at the recommended doses.
>
> Patients should be warned of the risk of hepatic injury and advised to stop the use of REVIA and seek medical attention if they experience symptoms of acute hepatitis.

Evidence of the hepatotoxic potential of REVIA is derived primarily from a placebo controlled study in which REVIA was administered to obese subjects at a dose approximately five-fold that recommended for the blockade of opiate receptors (300 mg per day). In that study, 5 of 26 REVIA recipients developed elevations of serum transaminases (i.e., peak ALT values ranging from a low of 121 to a high of 532; or 3 to 19 times their baseline values) after three to eight weeks of treatment. Although the patients involved were generally clinically asymptomatic and the transaminase levels of all patients on whom follow-up was obtained returned to (or toward) baseline values in a matter of weeks, the lack of any transaminase elevations of similar magnitude in any of the 24 placebo patients in the same study is persuasive evidence that REVIA is a direct (i.e., not idiosyncratic) hepatotoxin. This conclusion is also supported by evidence from other placebo controlled studies in which exposure to REVIA at doses above the amount recommended for the treatment of alcoholism or opiate blockade (50 mg/day) consistently produced more numerous and more significant elevations of serum transaminases than did placebo. Transaminase elevations in 3 of 9 patients with Alzheimer's Disease who received REVIA (at doses up to 300 mg/day) for 5 to 8 weeks in an open clinical trial have been reported.

Although no cases of hepatic failure due to REVIA administration have ever been reported, physicians are advised to consider this as a possible risk of treatment and to use the same care in prescribing REVIA as they would other drugs with the potential for causing hepatic injury.

Unintended Precipitation of Abstinence:
To prevent occurrence of an acute abstinence syndrome, or exacerbation of a pre-existing subclinical abstinence syndrome, patients must be opioid-free for a minimum of 7-10 days before starting REVIA. Since the absence of an opioid drug in the urine is often not sufficient proof that a patient is

opioid-free, a NARCAN challenge should be employed if the prescribing physician feels there is a risk of precipitating a withdrawal reaction following administration of REVIA .The NARCAN challenge test is described in the **DOSAGE AND ADMINISTRATION** section.

While REVIA is a potent antagonist with a prolonged pharmacologic effect (24 to 72 hours), the blockade produced by REVIA is surmountable. This is useful in patients who may require analgesia, but poses a potential risk to individuals who attempt, on their own, to overcome the blockade by administering large amounts of exogenous opioids. Indeed, any attempt by a patient to overcome the antagonism by taking opioids is very dangerous and may lead to a fatal overdose. Injury may arise because the plasma concentration of exogenous opioids attained immediately following their acute administration may be sufficient to overcome the competitive receptor blockade.

As a consequence, the patient may be in immediate danger of suffering life endangering opioid intoxication (e.g., respiratory arrest, circulatory collapse). Also, lesser amounts of exogenous opioids may prove dangerous if they are taken in a manner (i.e., relatively long after the last dose of naltrexone) and in an amount so that they persist in the body longer than effective concentrations of naltrexone and its metabolites. Patients should be told of the serious consequences of trying to overcome the opiate blockade. (See **Information for Patients** section.)

PRECAUTIONS: GENERAL

When Reversal of REVIA Blockade is Required: In an emergency situation in patients receiving fully blocking doses of REVIA, a suggested plan of management is regional analgesia, conscious sedation with a benzodiazepine, use of non-opioid analgesics or general anesthesia.

In a situation requiring opioid analgesia, the amount of opioid required may be greater than usual, and the resulting respiratory depression may be deeper and more prolonged. A rapidly acting opioid analgesic which minimizes the duration of respiratory depression is preferred. The amount of analgesic administered should be titrated to the needs of the patient. Non-receptor mediated actions may occur and should be expected (e.g., facial swelling, itching, generalized erythema, or bronchoconstriction) presumably due to histamine release.

Irrespective of the drug chosen to reverse REVIA (naltrexone hydrochloride) blockade, the patient should be monitored closely by appropriately trained personnel in a setting equipped and staffed for cardiopulmonary resuscitation.

When Withdrawal is Accidentally Precipitated With REVIA: Severe opioid withdrawal syndromes precipitated by the accidental ingestion of REVIA have been reported in opioid-dependent individuals. Symptoms of withdrawal have usually appeared within five minutes of ingestion of REVIA and have lasted for up to 48 hours. Mental status changes including confusion, somnolence and visual hallucinations have occurred. Significant fluid losses from vomiting and diarrhea have required intravenous fluid administration. In all cases patients were closely monitored and therapy with non-opioid medications was tailored to meet individual requirements.

Suicide: The risk of suicide is known to be increased in patients with substance abuse with or without concomitant depression. This risk is not abated by treatment with REVIA (see **ADVERSE REACTIONS**).

Information for Patients: It is recommended that the prescribing physician relate the following information to patients being treated with REVIA:

You have been prescribed REVIA (naltrexone hydrochloride) as part of the comprehensive treatment for your alcoholism or drug dependence. You should carry identification to alert medical personnel to the fact that you are taking REVIA. A REVIA medication card may be obtained from your physician and can be used for this purpose. Carrying the identification card should help to ensure that you can obtain adequate treatment in an emergency. If you require medical treatment, be sure to tell the treating physician that you are receiving REVIA therapy.

You should take REVIA as directed by your physician. If you attempt to self-administer heroin or any other opiate drug, in small doses, you will not perceive any effect. Most important, however, if you attempt to self-administer large doses of heroin or any other narcotic, you may die or sustain serious injury, including coma.

REVIA is well-tolerated in the recommended doses, but may cause liver injury when taken in excess or in people who develop liver disease from other causes. If you develop abdominal pain lasting more than a few days, white bowel movements, dark urine, or yellowing of your eyes, you should stop taking REVIA immediately and see your doctor as soon as possible.

Laboratory tests: A high index of suspicion for drug-related hepatic injury is critical if the occurrence of liver damage induced by REVIA is to be detected at the earliest possible time. Evaluations, using appropriate batteries of tests to detect liver injury are recommended at a frequency appropriate to the clinical situation and the dose of REVIA.

REVIA does not interfere with thin-layer, gas-liquid, and high pressure liquid chromatographic methods which may be used for the separation and detection of morphine, methadone or quinine in the urine. REVIA may or may not interfere with enzymatic methods for the detection of opioids depending on the specificity of the test. Please consult the test manufacturer for specific details.

Drug Interactions: Studies to evaluate possible interactions between REVIA and drugs other than opiates have not been performed. Consequently, caution is advised if the concomitant administration of REVIA and other drugs is required.

The safety and efficacy of concomitant use of REVIA and disulfiram is unknown, and the concomitant use of two potentially hepatotoxic medications is not ordinarily recommended unless the probable benefits outweigh the known risks.

Lethargy and somnolence have been reported following doses of REVIA (naltrexone hydrochloride) and thioridazine. Patients taking REVIA may not benefit from opioid containing medicines, such as cough and cold preparations, antidiarrheal preparations, and opioid analgesics. In an emergency situation when opioid analgesia must be administered to a patient receiving REVIA, the amount of opioid required may be greater than usual, and the resulting respiratory depression may be deeper and more prolonged (see **PRECAUTIONS**).

Carcinogenesis, Mutagenesis and Impairment of Fertility:
Carcinogenesis: In a two-year carcinogenicity study in rats, there were small increases in the numbers of mesotheliomas in males, and tumors of vascular origin in both sexes. The number of tumors were within the range seen in historical control groups, except for the vascular tumors in females, where the 4% incidence exceeded the historical maximum of 2%.

Mutagenesis: A total of twenty-two distinct tests were performed using bacterial, mammalian, and tissue culture systems. All tests were negative except for weakly positive findings in the Drosophila recessive lethal assay and non-specific DNA repair tests with E. coli. The significance of these findings is undetermined.

Impairment of Fertility: REVIA (100 mg/kg, approximately 140 times the human therapeutic dose) caused a significant increase in pseudo-pregnancy in the rat. A decrease in the pregnancy rate of mated female rats also occurred. The relevance of these observations to human fertility is not known.

Pregnancy: Category C. REVIA has been shown to have an embryocidal effect in the rat and rabbit when given in doses approximately 140 times the human therapeutic dose. This effect was demonstrated in rats dosed with REVIA (100 mg/kg) prior to and throughout gestation, and rabbits treated with 60 mg/kg of REVIA during the period of organogenesis. There are no adequate and well-controlled studies in pregnant women. REVIA should be used in pregnancy only when the potential benefit justifies the potential risk to the fetus.

Labor and Delivery: Whether or not REVIA affects the duration of labor and delivery is unknown.

Nursing Mothers: Whether or not REVIA is excreted in human milk is unknown. Because many drugs are excreted in human milk, caution should be exercised when REVIA is administered to a nursing woman.

Pediatric Use: The safe use of REVIA in subjects younger than 18 years old has not been established.

ADVERSE REACTIONS

During two randomized, double-blind placebo-controlled 12 week trials to evaluate the efficacy of REVIA as an adjunctive treatment of alcohol dependence, most patients tolerated REVIA well. In these studies, a total of 93 patients received REVIA at a dose of 50 mg once daily. Five of these patients discontinued REVIA because of nausea. No serious adverse events were reported during these two trials.

While extensive clinical studies evaluating the use of REVIA in detoxified, formerly opioid dependent individuals failed to identify any single, serious untoward risk of REVIA use, placebo controlled studies employing up to five-fold higher doses of REVIA (up to 300 mg per day) than that recommended for use in opiate receptor blockade have shown that REVIA causes hepatocellular injury in a substantial proportion of patients exposed at higher doses (see **WARNINGS AND PRECAUTIONS: Laboratory Tests**).

Aside from this finding, and the risk of precipitated opioid withdrawal, available evidence does not incriminate REVIA, used at any dose, as a cause of any other serious adverse reaction for the patient who is "opioid free." It is critical to recognize that REVIA can precipitate or exacerbate abstinence signs and symptoms in any individual who is not completely free of exogenous opioids.

Patients with addictive disorders, especially narcotic addiction, are at risk for multiple numerous adverse events and abnormal laboratory findings, including liver function abnormalities. Data from both controlled and observational studies suggest that these abnormalities, other than the dose-related hepatotoxicity described above, are not related to the use of REVIA.

Among opioid free individuals, REVIA administration at the recommended dose has not been associated with a predictable profile of serious adverse or untoward events. However, as mentioned above, among individuals using opioids, REVIA may cause serious withdrawal reactions (see **CONTRAINDICATIONS, WARNINGS, DOSAGE AND ADMINISTRATION).**

Reported Adverse Events

REVIA has not been shown to cause significant increases in complaints in placebo-controlled trials in patients known to be free of opioids for more than 7–10 days. Studies in alcoholic populations and in volunteers in clinical pharmacology studies have suggested that a small fraction of patients may experience an opioid withdrawal-like symptom complex consisting of tearfulness, mild nausea, abdominal cramps, restlessness, bone or joint pain, myalgia, and nasal symptoms. This may represent the unmasking of occult opioid use, or it may represent symptoms attributable to naltrexone. A number of alternative dosing patterns have been recommended to try to reduce the frequency of these complaints (see **Individualization of dosage**).

Alcoholism:

In an open label safety study with approximately 570 individuals with alcoholism receiving REVIA, the following new-onset adverse reactions occurred in 2% or more of the patients: nausea (10%), headache (7%), dizziness (4%), nervousness (4%), fatigue (4%), insomnia (3%), vomiting (3%), anxiety (2%) and somnolence (2%).

Depression (5-7%), suicidal ideation (2%), and attempted suicide (<1%) have been reported in individuals on REVIA, placebo and in concurrent control groups undergoing treatment for alcoholism. Although no causal relationship with REVIA is suspected, physicians should be aware that treatment with REVIA does not reduce the risk of suicide in these patients (see **PRECAUTIONS**).

Narcotic Addiction:

The following adverse reactions have been reported both at baseline and during the REVIA clinical trials in narcotic addiction at an incidence rate of more than 10%:

Difficulty sleeping, anxiety, nervousness, abdominal pain/cramps, nausea and/or vomiting, low energy, joint and muscle pain, and headache.

The incidence was less than 10% for:

Loss of appetite, diarrhea, constipation, increased thirst, increased energy, feeling down, irritability, dizziness, skin rash, delayed ejaculation, decreased potency, and chills.

The following events occurred in less than 1% of subjects:

Respiratory: nasal congestion, itching, rhinorrhea, sneezing, sore throat, excess mucus or phlegm, sinus trouble, heavy breathing, hoarseness, cough, shortness of breath.

Cardiovascular: nose bleeds, phlebitis, edema, increased blood pressure, non-specific ECG changes, palpitations, tachycardia.

Gastrointestinal: excessive gas, hemorrhoids, diarrhea, ulcer.

Musculoskeletal: painful shoulders, legs or knees; tremors, twitching.

Genitourinary: increased frequency of, or discomfort during, urination; increased or decreased sexual interest.

Dermatologic: oily skin, pruritus, acne, athlete's foot, cold sores, alopecia.

Psychiatric: depression, paranoia, fatigue, restlessness, confusion, disorientation, hallucinations, nightmares, bad dreams.

Special senses: eyes—blurred, burning, light sensitive, swollen, aching, strained; ears—"clogged", aching, tinnitus.

General: increased appetite, weight loss, weight gain, yawning, somnolence, fever, dry mouth, head "pounding", inguinal pain, swollen glands, "side" pains, cold feet, "hot spells."

Other: Depression, suicide, attempted suicide and suicidal ideation have been reported in the post-marketing experience with REVIA used in the treatment of narcotic dependence. No causal relationship has been demonstrated.

Laboratory tests: With the exception of liver test abnormalities (see **WARNINGS, PRECAUTIONS,** etc.), results of laboratory tests, like adverse reaction reports, have not shown consistent patterns of abnormalities that can be attributed to treatment with REVIA.

Idiopathic thrombocytopenic purpura was reported in one patient who may have been sensitized to REVIA in a previous course of treatment with REVIA. The condition cleared without sequelae after discontinuation of REVIA and corticosteroid treatment.

DRUG ABUSE AND DEPENDENCE

REVIA is a pure opioid antagonist. It does not lead to physical or psychological dependence. Tolerance to the opioid antagonist effect is not known to occur.

OVERDOSAGE

There is limited clinical experience with REVIA overdosage in humans. In one study, subjects who received 800 mg daily REVIA for up to one week showed no evidence of toxicity.

In the mouse, rat and guinea pig, the oral LD50s were 1,100 ± 96 mg/kg; 1,450 ± 265 mg/kg; and 1,490 ± 102 mg/kg, respectively.

In acute toxicity studies in the mouse, rat, and dog, cause of death was due to clonic-tonic convulsions and/or respiratory failure.

Treatment Of Overdosage: In view of the lack of actual experience in the treatment of REVIA overdose, patients should be treated symptomatically in a closely supervised environment. Physicians should contact a poison control center for the most up-to-date information.

DOSAGE AND ADMINISTRATION

IF THERE IS ANY QUESTION OF OCCULT OPIOID DEPENDENCE, PERFORM A NARCAN CHALLENGE TEST AND DO NOT INITIATE REVIA THERAPY UNTIL THE NARCAN CHALLENGE IS NEGATIVE.

Treatment of Alcoholism

A dose of 50 mg once daily is recommended for most patients (see **Individualization of dosage**).

REVIA should be considered as only one of many factors determining the success of treatment of alcoholism. Factors associated with a good outcome in the clinical trials with REVIA were the type, intensity, and duration of treatment; appropriate management of comorbid conditions; use of community-based support groups; and good medication compliance. To achieve the best possible treatment outcome, appropriate compliance-enhancing techniques should be implemented for all components of the treatment program, especially medication compliance.

Treatment of Narcotic Dependence

Initiate treatment with REVIA using the following guidelines:

1. Treatment should not be attempted unless the patient has remained opioid- free for at least 7–10 days. Self-reporting of abstinence from opioids in narcotic addicts should be verified by analysis of the patient's urine for absence of opioids. The patient should not be manifesting withdrawal signs or reporting withdrawal symptoms.
2. If there is any question of occult opioid dependence, perform a NARCAN challenge test. If signs of opioid withdrawal are still observed following NARCAN challenge, treatment with REVIA should not be attempted. The NARCAN challenge can be repeated in 24 hours.
3. Treatment should be initiated carefully, with an initial dose of 25 mg of REVIA. If no withdrawal signs occur, the patient may be started on 50 mg a day thereafter.

NARCAN Challenge Test: The NARCAN challenge test should not be performed in a patient showing clinical signs or symptoms of opioid withdrawal, or in a patient whose urine contains opioids. The NARCAN challenge test may be administered by either the intravenous or subcutaneous routes. Intravenous challenge: Following appropriate screening of the patient, 0.8 mg of NARCAN should be drawn into a sterile syringe. If the intravenous route of administration is selected, 0.2 mg of NARCAN should be injected, and while the needle is still in the patient's vein, the patient should be observed for 30 seconds for evidence of withdrawal signs or symptoms. If there is no evidence of withdrawal, the remaining 0.6 mg of NARCAN should be injected, and the patient observed for an additional period of 20 minutes for signs and symptoms of withdrawal.

Subcutaneous challenge: If the subcutaneous route is selected, 0.8 mg should be administered subcutaneously, and the patient observed for signs and symptoms of withdrawal for 20 minutes.

Conditions and technique for observation of patient: During the appropriate period of observation, the patient's vital signs should be monitored and the patient should be monitored for signs of withdrawal. It is also important to question the patient carefully. The signs and symptoms of opioid withdrawal include, but are not limited to, the following:

WITHDRAWAL SIGNS: stuffiness or running nose, tearing, yawning, sweating, tremor, vomiting or piloerection.

WITHDRAWAL SYMPTOMS: feeling of temperature change, joint or bone and muscle pain, abdominal cramps, skin crawling, etc.

Interpretation of the Challenge: Warning: the elicitation of the enumerated signs or symptoms indicates a potential risk for the subject, and REVIA should not be administered. If no signs or symptoms of withdrawal are observed, elicited, or reported, REVIA MAY BE ADMINISTERED. If there is any doubt in the observer's mind that the patient is not in an opioid-free state, or is in continuing withdrawal, REVIA should be withheld for 24 hours and the challenge repeated.

Alternative Dosing Schedules

Once the patient has been started on REVIA, 50 mg every 24 hours will produce adequate clinical blockade of the actions of parenterally administered opioids (i.e., this dose will block the effects of a 25 mg intravenous heroin challenge). A flexible approach to a dosing regimen may need to be employed in cases of supervised administration. Thus, patients may receive 50 mg of REVIA every weekday with a 100 mg dose on Saturday, 100 mg every other day, or 150 mg every third day. The degree of blockade produced by REVIA may be reduced by these extended dosing intervals.

There may be a higher risk of hepatocellular injury with single doses above 50 mg, and use of higher doses and extended dosing intervals should balance the possible risks against the probable benefits (see **WARNINGS** and **Individualization of dosage**).

Patient Compliance: REVIA should be considered as only one of many factors determining the success of treatment. To achieve the best possible treatment outcome, appropriate compliance-enhancing techniques should be implemented for all components of the treatment program, including medication compliance.

HOW SUPPLIED

REVIA (naltrexone hydrochloride) tablets are available in 50 mg capsule-shaped tablets, scored and imprinted with DuPont on one side and 11 on the other, as follows:

Bottles of 30 Tablets	NDC 0056-0011-30
Bottles of 100 Tablets	NDC 0056-0011-70
28 Daypak™ (blister package of 28 tablets)	NDC 0056-0011-22

DuPont Pharma
Wilmington, Delaware 19880

NARCAN® is a Registered U.S. Trademark of The DuPont Merck Pharmaceutical Co.

REVIA ™ is a Trademark of The DuPont Merck Pharmaceutical Co.

Daypak™ is a Trademark of The DuPont Merck Pharmaceutical Co.

Copyright© DuPont Pharma 1995. 6430/October, 1995

Shown in Product Identification Guide, page 310

SINEMET® ℞
(CARBIDOPA-LEVODOPA)
TABLETS

DESCRIPTION

When SINEMET* (Carbidopa-Levodopa) is to be given to patients who are being treated with levodopa, levodopa must be discontinued at least eight hours before therapy with SINEMET is started. In order to reduce adverse reactions, it is necessary to individualize therapy. See the WARNINGS and DOSAGE AND ADMINISTRATION sections before initiating therapy.

Carbidopa, an inhibitor of aromatic amino acid decarboxylation, is a white, crystalline compound, slightly soluble in water, with a molecular weight of 244.3. It is designated chemically as (—)-L-α-hydrazino -α- methyl -β- (3, 4- dihydroxybenzene) propanoic acid monohydrate, and has the following structural formula:

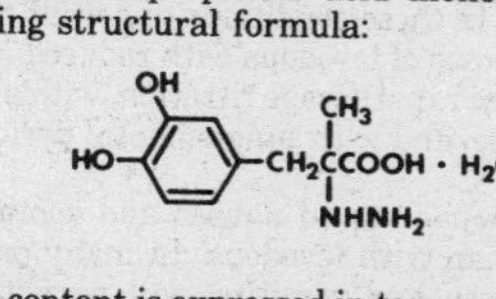

Tablet content is expressed in terms of anhydrous carbidopa which has a molecular weight of 226.3.

Levodopa, an aromatic amino acid, is a white, crystalline compound, slightly soluble in water, with a molecular weight of 197.2. It is designated chemically as (—)-L-α-amino-β-(3,4-dihydroxybenzene) propanoic acid, and has the following structural formula:

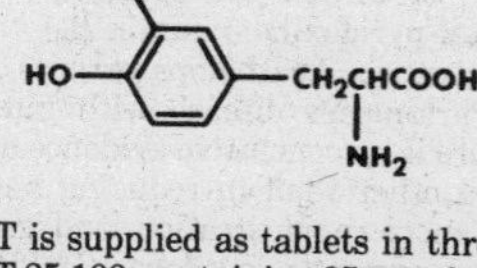

SINEMET is supplied as tablets in three strengths:

SINEMET 25-100, containing 25 mg of carbidopa and 100 mg of levodopa.

SINEMET 10-100, containing 10 mg of carbidopa and 100 mg of levodopa.

SINEMET 25-250, containing 25 mg of carbidopa and 250 mg of levodopa.

Inactive ingredients are cellulose, magnesium stearate, and starch. Tablets SINEMET 10-100 and 25-250 also contain FD&C Blue 2. Tablets SINEMET 25-100 also contain D&C Yellow 10 and FD&C Yellow 6.

---

*Registered trademark of MERCK & CO., INC. COPYRIGHT © MERCK & CO., INC. 1985.
All rights reserved

ACTIONS

Current evidence indicates that symptoms of Parkinson's disease are related to depletion of dopamine in the corpus striatum. Administration of dopamine is ineffective in the treatment of Parkinson's disease apparently because it does not cross the blood-brain barrier. However, levodopa, the metabolic precursor of dopamine, does cross the blood-brain

Continued on next page

DuPont Pharma—Cont.

barrier, and presumably is converted to dopamine in the basal ganglia. This is thought to be the mechanism whereby levodopa relieves symptoms of Parkinson's disease.

When levodopa is administered orally it is rapidly converted to dopamine in extracerebral tissues so that only a small portion of a given dose is transported unchanged to the central nervous system. For this reason, large doses of levodopa are required for adequate therapeutic effect and these may often be attended by nausea and other adverse reactions, some of which are attributable to dopamine formed in extracerebral tissues.

Since levodopa competes with certain amino acids, the absorption of levodopa may be impaired in some patients on a high protein diet.

Carbidopa inhibits decarboxylation of peripheral levodopa. It does not cross the blood-brain barrier and does not affect the metabolism of levodopa within the central nervous system.

Since its decarboxylase inhibiting activity is limited to extracerebral tissues, administration of carbidopa with levodopa makes more levodopa available for transport to the brain. In dogs, reduced formation of dopamine in extracerebral tissues, such as the heart, provides protection against the development of dopamine-induced cardiac arrhythmias. Clinical studies tend to support the hypothesis of a similar protective effect in humans although controlled data are too limited at the present time to draw firm conclusions.

Carbidopa reduces the amount of levodopa required by about 75 percent and, when administered with levodopa, increases both plasma levels and the plasma half-life of levodopa, and decreases plasma and urinary dopamine and homovanillic acid.

In clinical pharmacologic studies, simultaneous administration of carbidopa and levodopa produced greater urinary excretion of levodopa in proportion to the excretion of dopamine than administration of the two drugs at separate times.

Pyridoxine hydrochloride (vitamin B_6), in oral doses of 10 mg to 25 mg, may reverse the effects of levodopa by increasing the rate of aromatic amino acid decarboxylation. Carbidopa inhibits this action of pyridoxine.

INDICATIONS

SINEMET is indicated in the treatment of the symptoms of idiopathic Parkinson's disease (paralysis agitans), postencephalitic parkinsonism, and symptomatic parkinsonism which may follow injury to the nervous system by carbon monoxide intoxication and manganese intoxication. SINEMET is indicated in these conditions to permit the administration of lower doses of levodopa with reduced nausea and vomiting, with more rapid dosage titration, with a somewhat smoother response, and with supplemental pyridoxine (vitamin B_6).

The incidence of levodopa-induced nausea and vomiting is less with SINEMET than with levodopa. In many patients this reduction in nausea and vomiting will permit more rapid dosage titration.

In some patients a somewhat smoother antiparkinsonian effect results from therapy with SINEMET than with levodopa. However, patients with markedly irregular ("on-off") responses to levodopa have not been shown to benefit from SINEMET.

Since carbidopa prevents the reversal of levodopa effects caused by pyridoxine, SINEMET can be given to patients receiving supplemental pyridoxine (vitamin B_6).

Although the administration of carbidopa permits control of parkinsonism and Parkinson's disease with much lower doses of levodopa, there is no conclusive evidence at present that this is beneficial other than in reducing nausea and vomiting, permitting more rapid titration, and providing a somewhat smoother response to levodopa. *Carbidopa does not decrease adverse reactions due to central effects of levodopa. By permitting more levodopa to reach the brain, particularly when nausea and vomiting is not a dose-limiting factor, certain adverse CNS effects, e.g., dyskinesias, may occur at lower dosages and sooner during therapy with SINEMET than with levodopa.*

Certain patients who responded poorly to levodopa have improved when SINEMET was substituted. This is most likely due to decreased peripheral decarboxylation of levodopa which results from administration of carbidopa rather than to a primary effect of carbidopa on the nervous system. Carbidopa has not been shown to enhance the intrinsic efficacy of levodopa in parkinsonian syndromes.

In considering whether to give SINEMET to patients already on levodopa who have nausea and/or vomiting, the practitioner should be aware that, while many patients may be expected to improve, some do not. Since one cannot predict which patients are likely to improve, this can only be determined by a trial of therapy. It should be further noted that in controlled trials comparing SINEMET with levodopa, about half of the patients with nausea and/or vomiting on levodopa improved spontaneously despite being retained on the same dose of levodopa during the controlled portion of the trial.

CONTRAINDICATIONS

Monoamine oxidase inhibitors and SINEMET should not be given concomitantly. These inhibitors must be discontinued at least two weeks prior to initiating therapy with SINEMET.

SINEMET is contraindicated in patients with known hypersensitivity to this drug, and in narrow angle glaucoma.

Because levodopa may activate a malignant melanoma, it should not be used in patients with suspicious, undiagnosed skin lesions or a history of melanoma.

WARNINGS

When patients are receiving levodopa, it must be discontinued at least eight hours before SINEMET is started. SINEMET should be substituted at a dosage that will provide approximately 25 percent of the previous levodopa dosage (see DOSAGE AND ADMINISTRATION). Patients who are taking SINEMET should be instructed not to take additional levodopa unless it is prescribed by the physician.

As with levodopa, SINEMET may cause involuntary movements and mental disturbances. These reactions are thought to be due to increased brain dopamine following administration of levodopa. All patients should be observed carefully for the development of depression with concomitant suicidal tendencies. Patients with past or current psychoses should be treated with caution. *Because carbidopa permits more levodopa to reach the brain and, thus, more dopamine to be formed, dyskinesias may occur at lower dosages and sooner with SINEMET than with levodopa.* The occurrence of dyskinesias may require dosage reduction.

SINEMET should be administered cautiously to patients with severe cardiovascular or pulmonary disease, bronchial asthma, renal, hepatic or endocrine disease.

Care should be exercised in administering SINEMET, as with levodopa, to patients with a history of myocardial infarction who have residual atrial, nodal, or ventricular arrhythmias. In such patients, cardiac function should be monitored with particular care during the period of initial dosage adjustment, in a facility with provisions for intensive cardiac care.

As with levodopa there is a possibility of upper gastrointestinal hemorrhage in patients with a history of peptic ulcer.

A symptom complex resembling the neuroleptic malignant syndrome including muscular rigidity, elevated body temperature, mental changes, and increased serum creatine phosphokinase has been reported when antiparkinsonian agents were withdrawn abruptly. Therefore, patients should be observed carefully when the dosage of SINEMET is reduced abruptly or discontinued, especially if the patient is receiving neuroleptics.

Usage in Pregnancy and Lactation: Although the effects of SINEMET on human pregnancy and lactation are unknown, both levodopa and combinations of carbidopa and levodopa have caused visceral and skeletal malformations in rabbits. Use of SINEMET in women of childbearing potential requires that the anticipated benefits of the drug be weighed against possible hazards to mother and child. SINEMET should not be given to nursing mothers.

Usage in Children: The safety of SINEMET in patients under 18 years of age has not been established.

PRECAUTIONS

As with levodopa, periodic evaluations of hepatic, hematopoietic, cardiovascular, and renal function are recommended during extended therapy.

Patients with chronic wide angle glaucoma may be treated cautiously with SINEMET provided the intraocular pressure is well controlled and the patient is monitored carefully for changes in intraocular pressure during therapy.

Laboratory Tests

Abnormalities in laboratory tests may include elevations of liver function tests such as alkaline phosphatase, SGOT (AST), SGPT (ALT), lactic dehydrogenase, and bilirubin. Abnormalities in protein-bound iodine, blood urea nitrogen and positive Coombs test have also been reported. Commonly, levels of blood urea nitrogen, creatinine, and uric acid are lower during administration of SINEMET than with levodopa.

SINEMET may cause a false-positive reaction for urinary ketone bodies when a test tape is used for determination of ketonuria. This reaction will not be altered by boiling the urine specimen. False-negative tests may result with the use of glucose-oxidase methods of testing for glucosuria.

Drug Interactions

Caution should be exercised when the following drugs are administered concomitantly with SINEMET.

Symptomatic postural hypotension can occur when SINEMET is added to the treatment of a patient receiving antihypertensive drugs. Therefore, when therapy with SINEMET is started, dosage adjustment of the antihypertensive drug may be required. For patients receiving monoamine oxidase inhibitors, see CONTRAINDICATIONS. There have been rare reports of adverse reactions, including hypertension and dyskinesia, resulting from the concomitant use of tricyclic antidepressants and SINEMET.

Phenothiazines and butyrophenones may reduce the therapeutic effects of levodopa. In addition, the beneficial effects of levodopa in Parkinson's disease have been reported to be reversed by phenytoin and papaverine. Patients taking these drugs with SINEMET should be carefully observed for loss of therapeutic response.

ADVERSE REACTIONS

The most common serious adverse reactions occurring with SINEMET are choreiform, dystonic, and other involuntary movements. Other serious adverse reactions are mental changes including paranoid ideation and psychotic episodes, depression with or without development of suicidal tendencies, and dementia. Convulsions also have occurred; however, a causal relationship with SINEMET has not been established.

A common but less serious effect is nausea.

Less frequent adverse reactions are cardiac irregularities and/or palpitation, orthostatic hypotensive episodes, bradykinetic episodes (the "on-off" phenomenon), anorexia, vomiting, and dizziness.

Rarely, gastrointestinal bleeding, development of duodenal ulcer, hypertension, phlebitis, hemolytic and nonhemolytic anemia, thrombocytopenia, leukopenia, and agranulocytosis have occurred.

Laboratory tests which have been reported to be abnormal are alkaline phosphatase, SGOT (AST), SGPT (ALT), lactic dehydrogenase, bilirubin, blood urea nitrogen, protein-bound iodine, and Coombs test.

Other adverse reactions that have been reported with levodopa are:

Nervous System: ataxia, numbness, increased hand tremor, muscle twitching, muscle cramps, blepharospasm (which may be taken as an early sign of excess dosage, consideration of dosage reduction may be made at this time), trismus, activation of latent Horner's syndrome.

Psychiatric: confusion, sleepiness, insomnia, nightmares, hallucinations, delusions, agitation, anxiety, euphoria.

Gastrointestinal: dry mouth, bitter taste, sialorrhea, dysphagia, bruxism, hiccups, abdominal pain and distress, constipation, diarrhea, flatulence, burning sensation of tongue.

Metabolic: weight gain or loss, edema.

Integumentary: malignant melanoma (see also CONTRAINDICATIONS), flushing, increased sweating, dark sweat, skin rash, loss of hair.

Genitourinary: urinary retention, urinary incontinence, dark urine, priapism.

Special Senses: diplopia, blurred vision, dilated pupils, oculogyric crises.

Miscellaneous: weakness, faintness, fatigue, headache, hoarseness, malaise, hot flashes, sense of stimulation, bizarre breathing patterns, neuroleptic malignant syndrome.

DOSAGE AND ADMINISTRATION

The optimum daily dosage of SINEMET must be determined by careful titration in each patient. SINEMET tablets are available in a 1:4 ratio of carbidopa to levodopa (SINEMET 25-100) as well as 1:10 ratio (SINEMET 25-250 and SINEMET 10-100). Tablets of the two ratios may be given separately or combined as needed to provide the optimum dosage.

Studies show that peripheral dopa decarboxylase is saturated by carbidopa at approximately 70 to 100 mg a day. Patients receiving less than this amount of carbidopa are more likely to experience nausea and vomiting.

Usual Initial Dosage

Dosage is best initiated with one tablet of SINEMET 25-100 three times a day. This dosage schedule provides 75 mg of carbidopa per day. Dosage may be increased by one tablet every day or every other day, as necessary, until a dosage of eight tablets of SINEMET 25-100 a day is reached.

If SINEMET 10-100 is used, dosage may be initiated with one tablet three or four times a day. However, this will not provide an adequate amount of carbidopa for many patients. Dosage may be increased by one tablet every day or every other day until a total of eight tablets (2 tablets q.i.d.) is reached.

How to Transfer Patients from Levodopa

Levodopa must be discontinued at least eight hours before starting SINEMET (Carbidopa-Levodopa). A daily dosage of SINEMET should be chosen that will provide approximately 25 percent of the previous levodopa dosage. Patients who are taking less than 1500 mg of levodopa a day should be started on one tablet of SINEMET 25-100 three or four times a day. The suggested starting dosage for most patients taking more than 1500 mg of levodopa is one tablet of SINEMET 25-250 three or four times a day.

Maintenance

Therapy should be individualized and adjusted according to the desired therapeutic response. At least 70 to 100 mg of carbidopa per day should be provided. When a greater proportion of carbidopa is required, one tablet of SINEMET 25-100 may be substituted for each tablet of SINEMET 10-100. When more levodopa is required, SINEMET 25-250 should be substituted for SINEMET 25-100 or SINEMET 10-100. If necessary, the dosage of SINEMET 25-250 may be increased

by one-half or one tablet every day or every other day to a maximum of eight tablets a day. Experience with total daily dosages of carbidopa greater than 200 mg is limited.

Because both therapeutic and adverse responses occur more rapidly with SINEMET than with levodopa alone, patients should be monitored closely during the dose adjustment period. Specifically, involuntary movements will occur more rapidly with SINEMET than with levodopa. The occurrence of involuntary movements may require dosage reduction. Blepharospasm may be a useful early sign of excess dosage in some patients.

Current evidence indicates that other standard drugs for Parkinson's disease (except levodopa) may be continued while SINEMET is being administered, although their dosage may have to be adjusted.

If general anesthesia is required, SINEMET may be continued as long as the patient is permitted to take fluids and medication by mouth. If therapy is interrupted temporarily, the usual daily dosage may be administered as soon as the patient is able to take oral medication.

OVERDOSAGE

Management of acute overdosage with SINEMET is basically the same as management of acute overdosage with levodopa; however, pyridoxine is not effective in reversing the actions of SINEMET.

General supportive measures should be employed, along with immediate gastric lavage. Intravenous fluids should be administered judiciously and an adequate airway maintained. Electrocardiographic monitoring should be instituted and the patient carefully observed for the development of arrhythmias; if required, appropriate antiarrhythmic therapy should be given. The possibility that the patient may have taken other drugs as well as SINEMET should be taken into consideration. To date, no experience has been reported with dialysis; hence, its value in overdosage is not known.

HOW SUPPLIED

Tablets SINEMET 25-100 are yellow, oval, scored tablets, coded 650. They are supplied as follows:
NDC 0056-0650-68 bottles of 100
NDC 0056-0650-28 unit dose packages of 100.

Tablets SINEMET 10-100 are dark dapple-blue, oval, scored, uncoated tablets, coded 647. They are supplied as follows:
NDC 0056-0647-68 bottles of 100
NDC 0056-0647-28 unit dose packages of 100.

Tablets SINEMET 25-250 are light dapple-blue, oval, scored, uncoated tablets, coded 654. They are supplied as follows:
NDC 0056-0654-68 bottles of 100
NDC 0056-0654-28 unit dose packages of 100.

Storage

Tablets SINEMET 10-100 and Tablets SINEMET 25-250 must be protected from light.

Manufactured by:
MERCK & CO., INC.
WEST POINT, PA 19486, USA
For:
DuPont Pharma
Wilmington, Delaware 19880
AHFS Category: 92:00
6350-1/January 1995

Shown in Product Identification Guide, page 310

SINEMET® CR ℞
(Carbidopa-Levodopa)
Sustained-Release Tablets

DESCRIPTION

SINEMET* CR (Carbidopa-Levodopa) is a sustained-release combination of carbidopa and levodopa for the treatment of Parkinson's disease and syndrome.

Carbidopa, an inhibitor of aromatic amino acid decarboxylation, is a white, crystalline compound, slightly soluble in water, with a molecular weight of 244.3. It is designated chemically as (-)-*L*-α-hydrazino-α-methyl-β-(3,4-dihydroxybenzene) propanoic acid monohydrate. Its empirical formula is $C_{10}H_{14}N_2O_4 \cdot H_2O$ and its structural formula is:

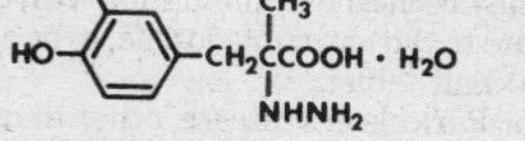

Tablet content is expressed in terms of anhydrous carbidopa, which has a molecular weight of 226.3.

Levodopa, an aromatic amino acid, is a white, crystalline compound, slightly soluble in water, with a molecular weight of 197.2. It is designated chemically as (-)-*L*-α-amino-β-(3,4-dihydroxybenzene) propanoic acid. Its empirical formula is $C_9H_{11}NO_4$ and its structural formula is:

[See chemical structure at top of next column.]

SINEMET CR is supplied as sustained-release tablets containing 50 mg of carbidopa and 200 mg of levodopa, or 25 mg of carbidopa and 100 mg of levodopa. Inactive ingredients in

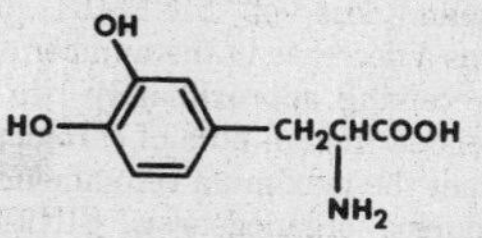

SINEMET CR 50–200 are: D&C Yellow 10, magnesium stearate, iron oxide, and other ingredients. Inactive ingredients in SINEMET CR 25–100 are: magnesium stearate, red ferric oxide, and other ingredients.

The 50–200 tablet is supplied as an oval, scored, biconvex, compressed tablet that is peach colored. The 25–100 tablet is supplied as an oval, biconvex, compressed tablet that is pink colored. The SINEMET CR tablet is a polymeric-based drug delivery system that controls the release of carbidopa and levodopa as it slowly erodes. SINEMET CR 25–100 is available to facilitate titration and as an alternative to the half-tablet of SINEMET CR 50–200.

CLINICAL PHARMACOLOGY

Pharmacodynamics

Current evidence indicates that symptoms of Parkinson's disease are related to depletion of dopamine in the corpus striatum. Administration of dopamine is ineffective in the treatment of Parkinson's disease apparently because it does not cross the blood-brain barrier. However, levodopa, the metabolic precursor of dopamine, does cross the blood-brain barrier, and presumably is converted to dopamine in the brain. This is thought to be the mechanism whereby levodopa relieves symptoms of Parkinson's disease.

When levodopa is administered orally it is rapidly decarboxylated to dopamine in extracerebral tissues so that only a small portion of a given dose is transported unchanged to the central nervous system. For this reason, large doses of levodopa are required for adequate therapeutic effect and these may often be attended by nausea and other adverse reactions, some of which are attributable to dopamine formed in extracerebral tissues.

Since levodopa competes with certain amino acids for transport across the gut wall, the absorption of levodopa may be impaired in some patients on a high protein diet.

Carbidopa inhibits decarboxylation of peripheral levodopa. It does not cross the blood-brain barrier and does not affect the metabolism of levodopa within the central nervous system.

Since its decarboxylase inhibiting activity is limited to extracerebral tissues, administration of carbidopa with levodopa makes more levodopa available for transport to the brain.

Patients treated with levodopa therapy for Parkinson's disease may develop motor fluctuations characterized by end-of-dose failure, peak dose dyskinesia, and akinesia. The advanced form of motor fluctuations ('on-off' phenomenon) is characterized by unpredictable swings from mobility to immobility. Although the causes of the motor fluctuations are not completely understood, *in some patients* they may be attenuated by treatment regimens that produce steady plasma levels of levodopa.

SINEMET CR contains either 50 mg of carbidopa and 200 mg of levodopa, or 25 mg of carbidopa and 100 mg of levodopa in a sustained-release dosage form designed to release these ingredients over a 4 to 6 hour period. With SINEMET CR there is less variation in plasma levodopa levels than with SINEMET* (Carbidopa-Levodopa), the conventional formulation. *However, SINEMET CR (Carbidopa-Levodopa, Sustained-Release) is less systemically bioavailable than SINEMET (Carbidopa-Levodopa) and may require increased daily doses to achieve the same level of symptomatic relief as provided by SINEMET (Carbidopa-Levodopa).*

In clinical trials, patients with moderate to severe motor fluctuations who received SINEMET CR *did not experience quantitatively significant reductions* in 'off' time when compared to SINEMET (Carbidopa-Levodopa). However, global ratings of improvement as assessed by both patient and physician were better during therapy with SINEMET CR than with SINEMET (Carbidopa-Levodopa). In patients without motor fluctuations, SINEMET CR, under controlled conditions, provided the same therapeutic benefit with less frequent dosing when compared to SINEMET (Carbidopa-Levodopa).

Pyridoxine hydrochloride (vitamin B_6), in oral doses of 10 mg to 25 mg, may reverse the effects of levodopa by increasing the rate of aromatic amino acid decarboxylation. Carbidopa inhibits this action of pyridoxine.

Pharmacokinetics

Carbidopa reduces the amount of levodopa required to produce a given response by about 75 percent and, when administered with levodopa, increases both plasma levels and the plasma half-life of levodopa, and decreases plasma and urinary dopamine and homovanillic acid.

Elimination half-life of levodopa in the presence of carbidopa is about 1.5 hours. Following SINEMET CR, the apparent half-life of levodopa may be prolonged because of continuous absorption.

In healthy elderly subjects (56–67 years old) the mean time to peak concentration of levodopa after a single dose of SINEMET CR 50–200 was about 2 hours as compared to 0.5 hours after standard SINEMET (Carbidopa-Levodopa). The maximum concentration of levodopa after a single dose of SINEMET CR was about 35% of the standard SINEMET (Carbidopa-Levodopa) (1151 vs 3256 ng/mL). The extent of availability of levodopa from SINEMET CR was about 70–75% relative to intravenous levodopa or standard SINEMET (Carbidopa-Levodopa) in the elderly. The absolute bioavailability of levodopa from SINEMET CR (relative to I.V.) in young subjects was shown to be only about 44%. The extent of availability and the peak concentrations of levodopa were comparable in the elderly after a single dose and at steady state after t.i.d. administration of SINEMET CR 50–200. In elderly subjects, the average trough levels of levodopa at steady state after the CR tablet were about 2 fold higher than after the standard SINEMET (Carbidopa-Levodopa) (163 vs 74 ng/mL).

In these studies, using similar total daily doses of levodopa, plasma levodopa concentrations with SINEMET CR fluctuated in a narrower range than with SINEMET (Carbidopa-Levodopa). Because the bioavailability of levodopa from SINEMET CR relative to SINEMET (Carbidopa-Levodopa) is approximately 70–75%, the daily dosage of levodopa necessary to produce a given clinical response with the sustained-release formulation will usually be higher.

The extent of availability and peak concentrations of levodopa after a single dose of SINEMET CR 50–200 increased by about 50% and 25%, respectively, when administered with food.

INDICATIONS AND USAGE

SINEMET CR is indicated in the treatment of the symptoms of idiopathic Parkinson's disease (paralysis agitans), postencephalitic parkinsonism, and symptomatic parkinsonism which may follow injury to the nervous system by carbon monoxide intoxication and manganese intoxication.

CONTRAINDICATIONS

Nonselective MAO inhibitors are contraindicated for use with SINEMET CR. These inhibitors must be discontinued at least two weeks prior to initiating therapy with SINEMET CR. SINEMET CR may be administered concomitantly with the manufacturer's recommended dose of an MAO inhibitor with selectivity for MAO type B (e.g., selegiline HCl).

SINEMET CR is contraindicated in patients with known hypersensitivity to any component of this drug and in patients with narrow-angle glaucoma.

Because levodopa may activate a malignant melanoma, SINEMET CR should not be used in patients with suspicious, undiagnosed skin lesions or a history of melanoma.

WARNINGS

When patients are receiving levodopa without a decarboxylase inhibitor, levodopa must be discontinued at least eight hours before SINEMET CR is started. In order to reduce adverse reactions, it is necessary to individualize therapy. SINEMET CR should be substituted at a dosage that will provide approximately 25 percent of the previous levodopa dosage (see DOSAGE AND ADMINISTRATION).

Carbidopa does not decrease adverse reactions due to central effects of levodopa. By permitting more levodopa to reach the brain, particularly when nausea and vomiting is not a dose-limiting factor, certain adverse CNS effects, e.g., dyskinesias, will occur at lower dosages and sooner during therapy with SINEMET CR (Carbidopa-Levodopa. Sustained-Release) than with levodopa alone.

As with levodopa, SINEMET CR may cause involuntary movements and mental disturbances. These reactions are thought to be due to increased brain dopamine following administration of levodopa. All patients should be observed carefully for the development of depression with concomitant suicidal tendencies. Patients with past or current psychoses should be treated with caution. The occurrence of dyskinesias may require dosage reduction.

Patients receiving SINEMET CR may develop increased dyskinesia compared to SINEMET (Carbidopa-Levodopa). SINEMET CR should be administered cautiously to patients with severe cardiovascular or pulmonary disease, bronchial asthma, renal, hepatic or endocrine disease.

As with levodopa, care should be exercised in administering SINEMET CR to patients with a history of myocardial infarction who have residual atrial, nodal, or ventricular arrhythmias. In such patients, cardiac function should be monitored with particular care during the period of initial dosage adjustment, in a facility with provisions for intensive cardiac care.

As with levodopa, treatment with SINEMET CR may increase the possibility of upper gastrointestinal hemorrhage in patients with a history of peptic ulcer.

A symptom complex resembling the neuroleptic malignant syndrome including muscular rigidity, elevated body tem-

Continued on next page

DuPont Pharma—Cont.

perature, mental changes, and increased serum creatine phosphokinase has been reported when antiparkinsonian agents were withdrawn abruptly. Therefore, patients should be observed carefully when the dosage of SINEMET CR is reduced abruptly or discontinued, especially if the patient is receiving neuroleptics.

PRECAUTIONS

General

As with levodopa, periodic evaluations of hepatic, hematopoietic, cardiovascular, and renal function are recommended during extended therapy.

Patients with chronic wide-angle glaucoma may be treated cautiously with SINEMET CR provided the intraocular pressure is well controlled and the patient is monitored carefully for changes in intraocular pressure during therapy.

Information for Patients

The patient should be informed that SINEMET CR is a sustained-release formulation of carbidopa-levodopa which releases these ingredients over a 4 to 6 hour period. It is important that SINEMET CR be taken at regular intervals according to the schedule outlined by the physician. The patient should be cautioned not to change the prescribed dosage regimen and not to add any additional antiparkinson medications, including other carbidopa-levodopa preparations, without first consulting the physician.

If abnormal involuntary movements appear or get worse during treatment with SINEMET CR, the physician should be notified, as dosage adjustment may be necessary.

Patients should be advised that sometimes the onset of effect of the first morning dose of SINEMET CR may be delayed for up to 1 hour compared with the response usually obtained from the first morning dose of SINEMET (Carbidopa-Levodopa). The physician should be notified if such delayed responses pose a problem in treatment.

Patients must be advised that the whole or half tablet should be swallowed without chewing or crushing.

NOTE: The suggested advice to patients being treated with SINEMET CR is intended to aid in the safe and effective use of this medication. It is not a disclosure of all possible adverse or intended effects.

Laboratory Tests

Abnormalities in laboratory tests may include elevations of liver function tests such as alkaline phosphatase, SGOT (AST), SGPT (ALT), lactic dehydrogenase, and bilirubin. Abnormalities in blood urea nitrogen and positive Coombs test have also been reported. Commonly, levels of blood urea nitrogen, creatinine, and uric acid are lower during administration of carbidopa-levodopa preparations than with levodopa.

Carbidopa-levodopa preparations may cause a false-positive reaction for urinary ketone bodies when a test tape is used for determination of ketonuria. This reaction will not be altered by boiling the urine specimen. False-negative tests may result with the use of glucose-oxidase methods of testing for glucosuria.

Drug Interactions

Caution should be exercised when the following drugs are administered concomitantly with SINEMET CR (Carbidopa-Levodopa, Sustained-Release).

Symptomatic postural hypotension has occurred when carbidopa-levodopa preparations were added to the treatment of patients receiving some antihypertensive drugs. Therefore, when therapy with SINEMET CR is started, dosage adjustment of the antihypertensive drug may be required. For patients receiving monoamine oxidase inhibitors, see CONTRAINDICATIONS.

There have been rare reports of adverse reactions, including hypertension and dyskinesia, resulting from the concomitant use of tricyclic antidepressants and carbidopa-levodopa preparations.

Phenothiazines and butyrophenones may reduce the therapeutic effects of levodopa. In addition, the beneficial effects of levodopa in Parkinson's disease have been reported to be reversed by phenytoin and papaverine. Patients taking these drugs with SINEMET CR should be carefully observed for loss of therapeutic response.

Carcinogenesis, Mutagenesis, Impairment of Fertility

In a two-year bioassay of SINEMET (Carbidopa-Levodopa), no evidence of carcinogenicity was found in rats receiving doses of approximately two times the maximum daily human dose of carbidopa and four times the maximum daily human dose of levodopa (equivalent to 8 SINEMET CR tablets).

In reproduction studies with SINEMET (Carbidopa-Levodopa), no effects on fertility were found in rats receiving doses of approximately two times the maximum daily human dose of carbidopa and four times the maximum daily human dose of levodopa (equivalent to 8 SINEMET CR tablets).

Pregnancy

Pregnancy Category C. No teratogenic effects were observed in a study in mice receiving up to 20 times the maximum recommended human dose of SINEMET (Carbidopa-Levodopa). There was a decrease in the number of live pups delivered by rats receiving approximately two times the maximum recommended human dose of carbidopa and approximately five times the maximum recommended human dose of levodopa during organogenesis. SINEMET (Carbidopa-Levodopa) caused both visceral and skeletal malformations in rabbits at all doses and ratios of carbidopa/levodopa tested, which ranged from 10 times/5 times the maximum recommended human dose of carbidopa/levodopa to 20 times/10 times the maximum recommended human dose of carbidopa/levodopa.

There are no adequate or well-controlled studies in pregnant women. Use of SINEMET CR in women of childbearing potential requires that the anticipated benefits of the drug be weighed against possible hazards to mother and child.

Nursing Mothers

It is not known whether this drug is excreted in human milk. Because many drugs are excreted in human milk, caution should be exercised when SINEMET CR is administered to a nursing mother.

Pediatric Use

Safety and effectiveness in infants and children have not been established, and use of the drug in patients below the age of 18 is not recommended.

ADVERSE REACTIONS

In controlled clinical trials, patients predominantly with moderate to severe motor fluctuations while on SINEMET (Carbidopa-Levodopa) were randomized to therapy with either SINEMET (Carbidopa-Levodopa) or SINEMET CR. The adverse experience frequency profile of SINEMET CR did not differ substantially from that of SINEMET (Carbidopa-Levodopa), as shown in Table I.

Table I.
Clinical Adverse Experiences Occurring in 1% or Greater of Patients

Adverse Experience	SINEMET CR n=491 %	SINEMET (Carbidopa-Levodopa) n=524 %
Dyskinesia	16.5	12.2
Nausea	5.5	5.7
Hallucinations	3.9	3.2
Confusion	3.7	2.3
Dizziness	2.9	2.3
Depression	2.2	1.3
Urinary tract infection	2.2	2.3
Headache	2.0	1.9
Dream abnormalities	1.8	0.8
Dystonia	1.8	0.8
Vomiting	1.8	1.9
Upper respiratory infection	1.8	1.0
Dyspnea	1.6	0.4
'On-Off' phenomena	1.6	1.1
Back pain	1.6	0.6
Dry mouth	1.4	1.1
Anorexia	1.2	1.1
Diarrhea	1.2	0.6
Insomnia	1.2	1.0
Orthostatic hypotension	1.0	1.1
Shoulder pain	1.0	0.6
Chest pain	1.0	0.8
Muscle cramps	0.8	1.0
Paresthesia	0.8	1.1
Urinary frequency	0.8	1.1
Dyspepsia	0.6	1.1
Constipation	0.2	1.5

Abnormal laboratory findings occurring at a frequency of 1% or greater in approximately 443 patients who received SINEMET CR and 475 who received SINEMET (Carbidopa-Levodopa) during controlled clinical trials included: decreased hemoglobin and hematocrit; elevated serum glucose; white blood cells, bacteria and blood in the urine.

The adverse experiences observed in patients in uncontrolled studies were similar to those seen in controlled clinical studies.

Other adverse experiences reported overall in clinical trials in 748 patients treated with SINEMET CR, listed by body system in order of decreasing frequency, include:

Nervous System/Psychiatric: Chorea, somnolence, falling, anxiety disorder, disorientation, decreased mental acuity, gait abnormalities, extrapyramidal disorder, agitation, nervousness, sleep disorders, memory impairment.

Body as a Whole: Asthenia, fatigue, abdominal pain, orthostatic effects.

Digestive: Gastrointestinal pain, dysphagia, heartburn.

Cardiovascular: Palpitation, essential hypertension, hypotension, myocardial infarction.

Special Senses: Blurred vision.

Metabolic: Weight loss.

Skin: Rash.

Respiratory: Cough, pharyngeal pain, common cold.

Urogenital: Urinary incontinence.

Musculoskeletal: Leg pain.

Laboratory Tests: Decreased white blood cell count and serum potassium; increased BUN, serum creatinine and serum LDH; protein and glucose in the urine.

Other adverse experiences have been reported with various carbidopa-levodopa formulations and may occur with SINEMET CR:

Nervous System/Psychiatric: Mental changes including paranoid ideation, psychotic episodes, depression with suicidal tendencies and dementia; convulsions (however, a causal relationship has not been established); bradykinetic episodes.

Gastrointestinal: Gastrointestinal bleeding, development of duodenal ulcer.

Cardiovascular: Cardiac irregularities, phlebitis.

Hematologic: Hemolytic and nonhemolytic anemia, thrombocytopenia, leukopenia, agranulocytosis.

Laboratory Tests: Abnormalities in alkaline phosphatase, SGOT (AST), SGPT (ALT), lactic dehydrogenase, bilirubin, protein-bound iodine, Coombs test.

Other adverse reactions that have been reported with levodopa are:

Nervous System: Numbness, increased hand tremor, muscle twitching, blepharospasm (which may be taken as an early sign of excess dosage, consideration of dosage reduction may be made at this time), trismus, activation of latent Horner's syndrome.

Psychiatric: Delusions, euphoria.

Gastrointestinal: Bitter taste, sialorrhea, bruxism, hiccups, flatulence, burning sensation of tongue.

Metabolic: Weight gain, edema.

Integumentary: Malignant melanoma (see also CONTRAINDICATIONS), flushing, increased sweating, dark sweat, loss of hair.

Genitourinary: Urinary retention, urinary incontinence, dark urine, priapism.

Miscellaneous: Faintness, hoarseness, malaise, hot flashes, sense of stimulation, bizarre breathing patterns, neuroleptic malignant syndrome.

OVERDOSAGE

Management of acute overdosage with SINEMET CR is the same as with levodopa. Pyridoxine is not effective in reversing the actions of SINEMET CR.

General supportive measures should be employed, along with immediate gastric lavage. Intravenous fluids should be administered judiciously and an adequate airway maintained. Electrocardiographic monitoring should be instituted and the patient carefully observed for the development of arrhythmias; if required, appropriate antiarrhythmic therapy should be given. The possibility that the patient may have taken other drugs as well as SINEMET CR should be taken into consideration. To date, no experience has been reported with dialysis; hence, its value in overdosage is not known.

Based on studies in which high doses of levodopa and/or carbidopa were administered, a significant proportion of rats and mice given single oral doses of levodopa of approximately 1500–2000 mg/kg are expected to die. A significant proportion of infant rats of both sexes are expected to die at a dose of 800 mg/kg. A significant proportion of rats are expected to die after treatment with similar doses of carbidopa. The addition of carbidopa in a 1:10 ratio with levodopa increases the dose at which a significant proportion of mice are expected to die to 3360 mg/kg.

DOSAGE AND ADMINISTRATION

SINEMET CR contains carbidopa and levodopa in a 1:4 ratio as either the 50–200 tablet or the 25–100 tablet. The daily dosage of SINEMET CR must be determined by careful titration. Patients should be monitored closely during the dose adjustment period, particularly with regard to appearance or worsening of involuntary movements, dyskinesias or nausea. SINEMET CR 50–200 may be administered as whole or as half-tablets which should not be chewed or crushed. SINEMET CR 25–100 may be used in combination with SINEMET CR 50–200 to titrate to the optimum dosage, or as an alternative to the 50–200 half tablet.

Standard drugs for Parkinson's disease, other than levodopa without a decarboxylase inhibitor, may be used concomitantly while SINEMET CR is being administered, although their dosage may have to be adjusted.

Since carbidopa prevents the reversal of levodopa effects caused by pyridoxine, SINEMET CR can be given to patients receiving supplemental pyridoxine (vitamin B_6).

Initial Dosage

Patients currently treated with conventional carbidopa-levodopa preparations: Dosage with SINEMET CR should be substituted at an amount that provides approximately 10% more levodopa per day, although this may need to be increased to a dosage that provides up to 30% more levodopa

per day depending on clinical response (see DOSAGE AND ADMINISTRATION, *Titration*). The interval between doses of SINEMET CR should be 4–8 hours during the waking day. (See CLINICAL PHARMACOLOGY, *Pharmacodynamics*.)
A guideline for initiation of SINEMET CR is shown in Table II.

Table II.
Guidelines for Initial Conversion from SINEMET (Carbidopa-Levodopa) to SINEMET CR

SINEMET (Carbidopa-Levodopa) Total Daily Dose* Levodopa (mg)	SINEMET CR Suggested Dosage Regimen
300–400	200 mg b.i.d.
500–600	300 mg b.i.d. or 200 mg t.i.d.
700–800	A total of 800 mg in 3 or more divided doses (e.g., 300 mg a.m., 300 mg early p.m. and 200 mg later p.m.)
900–1000	A total of 1000 mg in 3 or more divided doses (e.g., 400 mg a.m., 400 mg early p.m., and 200 mg later p.m.)

*For dosing ranges not shown in the table see DOSAGE AND ADMINISTRATION, *Initial Dosage—Patients currently treated with conventional carbidopa-levodopa preparations.*

Patients currently treated with levodopa without a decarboxylase inhibitor: Levodopa must be discontinued at least eight hours before therapy with SINEMET CR is started. SINEMET CR should be substituted at a dosage that will provide approximately 25% of the previous levodopa dosage. In patients with mild to moderate disease, the initial dose is usually 1 tablet of SINEMET CR b.i.d.

Patients not receiving levodopa: In patients with mild to moderate disease, the initial recommended dose is 1 tablet of SINEMET CR 50-200 b.i.d. Initial dosage should not be given at intervals of less than 6 hours.

Titration with SINEMET CR
Following initiation of therapy, doses and dosing intervals may be increased or decreased depending upon therapeutic response. Most patients have been adequately treated with doses of SINEMET CR that provide 400 to 1600 mg of levodopa per day, administered as divided doses at intervals ranging from 4 to 8 hours during the waking day. Higher doses of SINEMET CR (2400 mg or more of levodopa per day) and shorter intervals (less than 4 hours) have been used, but are not usually recommended.
When doses of SINEMET CR are given at intervals of less than 4 hours, and/or if the divided doses are not equal, it is recommended that the smaller doses be given at the end of the day.
An interval of at least 3 days between dosage adjustments is recommended.

Maintenance
Because Parkinson's disease is progressive, periodic clinical evaluations are recommended; adjustment of the dosage regimen of SINEMET CR may be required.

Addition of Other Antiparkinson Medications
Anticholinergic agents, dopamine agonists, and amantadine can be given with SINEMET CR. Dosage adjustment of SINEMET CR may be necessary when these agents are added.
A dose of SINEMET (Carbidopa-Levodopa) 25–100 or 10–100 (one half or a whole tablet) can be added to the dosage regimen of SINEMET CR in selected patients with advanced disease who need additional immediate-release levodopa for a brief time during daytime hours.

Interruption of Therapy
Patients should be observed carefully if abrupt reduction or discontinuation of SINEMET CR is required, especially if the patient is receiving neuroleptics. (See WARNINGS).
If general anesthesia is required, SINEMET CR may be continued as long as the patient is permitted to take oral medication. If therapy is interrupted temporarily, the usual dosage should be administered as soon as the patient is able to take oral medication.

HOW SUPPLIED

SINEMET CR 50–200 (Carbidopa-Levodopa) SUSTAINED-RELEASE TABLETS containing 50 mg of carbidopa and 200 mg of levodopa, are peach colored, oval, scored, biconvex, compressed tablets, coded 521. They are supplied as follows:
NDC 0056-0521-68 bottles of 100
(6505-01-343-3482, 100's)
NDC 0056-0521-28 unit dose package of 100.
(6505-01-343-3483, individually sealed 100's).
SINEMET CR 25–100 (Carbidopa-Levodopa) SUSTAINED-RELEASE TABLETS containing 25 mg carbidopa and 100 mg of levodopa, are pink colored, oval, biconvex, compressed tablets, coded 601. They are supplied as follows:
NDC 0056-0601-68 bottles of 100
NDC 0056-0601-28 unit dose packages of 100.

Storage
Avoid temperatures above 30°C (86°F). Store in a tightly closed container.

Manufactured by:
MERCK & CO., INC.
WEST POINT, PA 19486, USA
For:
DuPont Pharma
Wilmington, Delaware 19880
6351-1 Issued January 1995
Shown in Product Identification Guide, page 310

SYMMETREL® ℞
[sim 'e-trel"]
(amantadine hydrochloride)

DESCRIPTION

SYMMETREL is designated generically as amantadine hydrochloride and chemically as 1-adamantanamine hydrochloride.

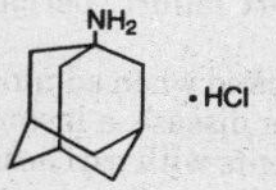

Amantadine hydrochloride is a stable white or nearly white crystalline powder, freely soluble in water and soluble in alcohol and in chloroform.
Amantadine hydrochloride has pharmacological actions as both an anti-Parkinson and an antiviral drug.
SYMMETREL syrup contains: artificial raspberry flavor, citric acid, methylparaben, propylparaben, and sorbitol solution.

CLINICAL PHARMACOLOGY

Mechanism of Action: Parkinson's Disease The mechanism of action of amantadine in the treatment of Parkinson's disease and drug-induced extrapyramidal reactions is not known. It has been shown to cause an increase in dopamine release in the animal brain. The drug does not possess anticholinergic activity in dogs at doses of 31.5 mg/kg, equivalent to an approximate human dose of 15.8 mg/kg (based on body surface area conversions).

Mechanism of Action: Antiviral The mechanism by which amantadine exerts its antiviral activity is not clearly understood. It appears to mainly prevent the release of infectious viral nucleic acid into the host cell by interfering with the function of the transmembrane domain of the viral M2 protein. In certain cases, amantadine is also known to prevent virus assembly during virus replication. It does not appear to interfere with the immunogenicity of inactivated influenza A virus vaccine.

Antiviral Activity: Amantadine inhibits the replication of influenza A virus isolates from each of the subtypes, i.e., H1N1, H2N2 and H3N2. It has very little or no activity against influenza B virus isolates. A quantitative relationship between the *in vitro* susceptibility of influenza A virus to amantadine and the clinical response to therapy has not been established in man. Sensitivity test results, expressed as the concentration of amantadine required to inhibit by 50% the growth of virus (ED_{50}) in tissue culture vary greatly (from 0.1 μg/mL to 25.0 μg/mL) depending upon the assay protocol used, size of virus inoculum, isolates of influenza A virus strains tested, and the cell type used. Host cells in tissue culture readily tolerated amantadine up to a concentration of 100 μg/mL.

Drug Resistance: Influenza A variants with reduced *in vitro* sensitivity to amantadine have been isolated from epidemic strains in areas where adamantane derivatives are being used. Influenza viruses with reduced *in vitro* sensitivity have been shown to be transmissible and to cause typical influenza illness. The quantitative relationship between the *in vitro* sensitivity of influenza A variants to amantadine and the clinical response to therapy has not been established.

Pharmacokinetics: SYMMETREL is well absorbed orally. Maximum plasma concentrations are directly related to dose for doses up to 200 mg/day. Doses above 200 mg/day may result in a greater than proportional increase in maximum plasma concentrations. It is primarily excreted unchanged in the urine by glomerular filtration and tubular secretion. Eight metabolites of amantadine have been identified in human urine. One metabolite, an N-acetylated compound, was quantified in human urine and accounted for 5–15% of the administered dose. Plasma acetylamantadine accounted for up to 80% of the concurrent amantadine plasma concentration in 5 of 12 healthy volunteers following the ingestion of a 200 mg dose of amantadine. Acetylamantadine was not detected in the plasma of the remaining seven volunteers. The contribution of this metabolite to efficacy or toxicity is not known.
There appears to be a relationship between plasma amantadine concentrations and toxicity. As concentration increases toxicity seems to be more prevalent, however absolute values of amantadine concentrations associated with adverse effects have not been fully defined.
Amantadine pharmacokinetics were determined in 24 normal adult male volunteers after the oral administration of a single SYMMETREL 100 mg capsule. The mean ± SD maximum plasma concentration was 0.22 ± 0.03 μg/mL (range: 0.18 to 0.32 μg/mL). The time to peak concentration was 3.3 ± 1.5 hours (range: 1.5 to 8.0 hours). The apparent oral clearance was 0.28 ± 0.11 L/hr/kg (range: 0.14 to 0.62 L/hr/kg). The half-life was 17 ± 4 hours (range: 10 to 25 hours). Across other studies, amantadine plasma half-life has averaged 16 ± 6 hours (range: 9 to 31 hours) in 19 healthy volunteers.
After oral administration of a single dose of 100 mg amantadine syrup to five healthy volunteers, the mean ± SD maximum plasma concentration C_{max} was 0.24 ± 0.04 μg/mL and ranged from 0.18 to 0.28 μg/mL. After 15 days of amantadine 100 mg b.i.d., the C_{max} was 0.47 ± 0.11 μg/mL in four of the five volunteers. The administration of amantadine tablets as a 200 mg single dose to 6 healthy subjects resulted in a C_{max} of 0.51 ± 0.14 μg/mL. Across studies, the time to C_{max} (T_{max}) averaged about 2 to 4 hours.
Plasma amantadine clearance ranged from 0.2 to 0.3 L/hr/kg after the administration of 5 mg to 25 mg intravenous doses of amantadine to 15 healthy volunteers.
In six healthy volunteers, the ratio of amantadine renal clearance to apparent oral plasma clearance was 0.79 ± 0.17 (mean ± SD).
The volume of distribution determined after the intravenous administration of amantadine to 15 healthy subjects was 3 to 8 L/kg, suggesting tissue binding. Amantadine, after single oral 200 mg doses to 6 healthy young subjects and to 6 healthy elderly subjects has been found in nasal mucus at mean ± SD concentrations of 0.15 ± 0.16, 0.28 ± 0.26, and 0.39 ± 0.34 μg/g at 1, 4, and 8 hours after dosing, respectively. These concentrations represented 31 ± 33%, 59 ± 61%, and 95 ± 86% of the corresponding plasma amantadine concentrations. Amantadine is approximately 67% bound to plasma proteins over a concentration range of 0.1 to 2.0 μg/mL. Following the administration of amantadine 100 mg as a single dose, the mean ± SD red blood cell to plasma ratio ranged from 2.7 ± 0.5 in 6 healthy subjects to 1.4 ± 0.2 in 8 patients with renal insufficiency.
The apparent oral plasma clearance of amantadine is reduced and the plasma half-life and plasma concentrations are increased in healthy elderly individuals age 60 and older. After single dose administration of 25 to 75 mg to 7 healthy, elderly male volunteers, the apparent plasma clearance of amantadine was 0.10 ± 0.04 L/hr/kg (range 0.06 to 0.17 L/hr/kg) and the half-life was 29 ± 7 hours (range 20 to 41 hours). Whether these changes are due to decline in renal function or other age related factors is not known.
Compared with otherwise healthy adult individuals, the clearance of amantadine is significantly reduced in adult patients with renal insufficiency. The elimination half-life increases two to three fold or greater when creatinine clearance is less than 40 mL/min/1.73 m^2 and averages eight days in patients on chronic maintenance hemodialysis. Amantadine is removed in negligible amounts by hemodialysis.
The pH of the urine has been reported to influence the excretion rate of SYMMETREL. Since the excretion rate of SYMMETREL increases rapidly when the urine is acidic, the administration of urine acidifying drugs may increase the elimination of the drug from the body.

INDICATIONS AND USAGE

SYMMETREL is indicated for the prophylaxis and treatment of signs and symptoms of infection caused by various strains of influenza A virus. SYMMETREL is also indicated in the treatment of parkinsonism and drug- induced extrapyramidal reactions.

Influenza A Prophylaxis: SYMMETREL is indicated for chemoprophylaxis against signs and symptoms of influenza A virus infection when early vaccination is not feasible or when the vaccine is contraindicated or not available. In the prophylaxis of influenza, early vaccination on an annual basis as recommended by the Centers for Disease Control's Immunization Practices Advisory Committee is the method of choice. Because SYMMETREL does not completely prevent the host immune response to influenza A infection, individuals who take this drug may still develop immune responses to natural disease or vaccination and may be protected when later exposed to antigenically related viruses. Following vaccination during an influenza A outbreak, SYMMETREL prophylaxis should be considered for the 2 to 4 week time period required to develop an antibody response.

Influenza A Treatment: SYMMETREL is also indicated in the treatment of uncomplicated respiratory tract illness caused by influenza A virus strains especially when administered early in the course of illness. There are no well-con-

Continued on next page

DuPont Pharma—Cont.

trolled clinical studies demonstrating that treatment with SYMMETREL will avoid the development of influenza A virus pneumonitis or other complications in high risk patients.

There is no clinical evidence indicating that SYMMETREL is effective in the prophylaxis or treatment of viral respiratory tract illnesses other than those caused by influenza A virus strains.

Parkinson's Disease/Syndrome: SYMMETREL is indicated in the treatment of idiopathic Parkinson's disease (Paralysis Agitans), postencephalitic parkinsonism, and symptomatic parkinsonism which may follow injury to the nervous system by carbon monoxide intoxication. It is indicated in those elderly patients believed to develop parkinsonism in association with cerebral arteriosclerosis. In the treatment of Parkinson's disease, SYMMETREL is less effective than levodopa, (-)-3-(3,4-dihydroxyphenyl)-L-alanine, and its efficacy in comparison with the anticholinergic antiparkinson drugs has not yet been established.

Drug-Induced Extrapyramidal Reactions: SYMMETREL is indicated in the treatment of drug-induced extrapyramidal reactions. Although anticholinergic-type side effects have been noted with SYMMETREL when used in patients with drug-induced extrapyramidal reactions, there is a lower incidence of these side effects than that observed with the anticholinergic antiparkinson drugs.

CONTRAINDICATIONS

SYMMETREL is contraindicated in patients with known hypersensitivity to the drug.

WARNINGS

Deaths: Deaths have been reported from overdose with SYMMETREL. The lowest reported acute lethal dose was 2 grams. Acute toxicity may be attributable to the anticholinergic effects of amantadine. Drug overdose has resulted in cardiac, respiratory, renal or central nervous system toxicity. Cardiac dysfunction includes arrhythmia, tachycardia and hypertension (see OVERDOSAGE).

Suicide Attempts: Suicide attempts, some of which have been fatal, have been reported in patients treated with SYMMETREL, many of whom received short courses for influenza treatment or prophylaxis. The incidence of suicide attempts is not known and the pathophysiologic mechanism is not understood. Suicide attempts and suicidal ideation have been reported in patients with and without prior history of psychiatric illness. SYMMETREL can exacerbate mental problems in patients with a history of psychiatric disorders or substance abuse. Patients who attempt suicide may exhibit abnormal mental states which include disorientation, confusion, depression, personality changes, agitation, aggressive behavior, hallucinations, paranoia, other psychotic reactions, and somnolence or insomnia. Because of the possibility of serious adverse effects, caution should be observed when prescribing SYMMETREL to patients being treated with drugs having CNS effects, or for whom the potential risks outweigh the benefit of treatment. Because some patients have attempted suicide by overdosing with amantadine, prescriptions should be written for the smallest quantity consistent with good patient management.

CNS Effects: Patients with a history of epilepsy or other "seizures" should be observed closely for possible increased seizure activity.

Patients receiving SYMMETREL who note central nervous system effects or blurring of vision should be cautioned against driving or working in situations where alertness and adequate motor coordination are important.

Other: Patients with a history of congestive heart failure or peripheral edema should be followed closely as there are patients who developed congestive heart failure while receiving SYMMETREL.

Patients with Parkinson's disease improving on SYMMETREL should resume normal activities gradually and cautiously, consistent with other medical considerations, such as the presence of osteoporosis or phlebothrombosis.

PRECAUTIONS

SYMMETREL should not be discontinued abruptly in patients with Parkinson's disease since a few patients have experienced a parkinsonian crisis, i.e., a sudden marked clinical deterioration, when this medication was suddenly stopped. The dose of anticholinergic drugs or of SYMMETREL should be reduced if atropine-like effects appear when these drugs are used concurrently.

Neuroleptic Malignant Syndrome (NMS): Sporadic cases of possible Neuroleptic Malignant Syndrome (NMS) have been reported in association with dose reduction or withdrawal of SYMMETREL therapy.

NMS is an uncommon but life-threatening syndrome characterized by fever or hyperthermia; neurologic findings including muscle rigidity, involuntary movements, altered consciousness; other disturbances such as autonomic dysfunction, tachycardia, tachypnea, hyper- or hypotension; labora-

tory findings such as creatine phosphokinase elevation, leukocytosis and increased serum myoglobin.

The early diagnosis of this condition is important for the appropriate management of these patients. Considering NMS as a possible diagnosis and ruling out other acute illnesses (e.g., pneumonia, systemic infection, etc.) is essential. This may be especially complex if the clinical presentation includes both serious medical illness and untreated or inadequately treated extrapyramidal signs and symptoms (EPS). Other important considerations in the differential diagnosis include central anticholinergic toxicity, heat stroke, drug fever and primary central nervous system (CNS) pathology. The management of NMS should include: 1) intensive symptomatic treatment and medical monitoring, and 2) treatment of any concomitant serious medical problems for which specific treatments are available. Dopamine agonists, such as bromocriptine, and muscle relaxants, such as dantrolene are often used in the treatment of NMS, however, their effectiveness has not been demonstrated in controlled studies.

Other: Because SYMMETREL is mainly excreted in the urine, it accumulates in the plasma and in the body when renal function declines. Thus, the dose of SYMMETREL should be reduced in patients with renal impairment and in individuals who are 65 years of age or older. The dose of SYMMETREL may need careful adjustment in patients with congestive heart failure, peripheral edema, or orthostatic hypotension.

Care should be exercised when administering SYMMETREL to patients with liver disease, a history of recurrent eczematoid rash, or to patients with psychosis or severe psychoneurosis not controlled by chemotherapeutic agents. Rare instances of reversible elevation of liver enzymes have been reported in patients receiving SYMMETREL, though a specific relationship between the drug and such changes has not been established.

Drug Interactions: Careful observation is required when SYMMETREL is administered concurrently with central nervous system stimulants.

Coadministration of thioridazine has been reported to worsen the tremor in elderly patients with Parkinson's disease, however, it is not known if other phenothiazines produce a similar response.

Coadministration of Dyazide (triamterene/hydrochlorothiazide) resulted in a higher plasma amantadine concentration in a 61 year old man receiving SYMMETREL 100 mg TID for Parkinson's disease.[1] It is not known which of the components of Dyazide contributed to the observation or if related drugs produce a similar response.

Carcinogenesis and Mutagenesis: Long-term *in vivo* animal studies designed to evaluate the carcinogenic potential of SYMMETREL have not been performed. In several *in vitro* assays for gene mutation, SYMMETREL did not increase the number of spontaneously observed mutations in four strains of *Salmonella typhimurium* (Ames Test) or in a mammalian cell line (Chinese Hamster Ovary cells) when incubations were performed either with or without a liver metabolic activation extract. Further, there was no evidence of chromosome damage observed in an *in vitro* test using freshly derived and stimulated human peripheral blood lymphocytes (with and without metabolic activation) or in an *in vivo* mouse bone marrow micronucleus test (140–550 mg/kg; estimated human equivalent doses of 11.7–45.8 mg/kg based on body surface area conversion).

Impairment of Fertility: In a three litter reproduction study in rats, SYMMETREL at a dose of 32 mg/kg/day (estimated human equivalent dose of 4.5 mg/kg/day, based on body surface area conversions) administered to both males and females slightly impaired fertility. There were no effects on fertility at a dose level of 10 mg/kg/day (estimated human equivalent dose of 1.4 mg/kg/day); intermediate doses were not tested.

Pregnancy Category C: SYMMETREL has been shown to be embryotoxic and teratogenic in rats at 50 mg/kg/day (estimated human equivalent dose of 7.1 mg/kg/day based on body surface area conversion), while a dose of 37 mg/kg/day (estimated human equivalent dose of 5.3 mg/kg/day) was without effect. Embryotoxic and teratogenic effects were not seen in rabbits that received 32 mg/kg/day (estimated human equivalent dose of 9.6 mg/kg/day, based on body surface area conversion). There are no adequate and well-controlled studies in pregnant women. SYMMETREL should be used during pregnancy only if the potential benefit justifies the potential risk to the embryo or fetus.

Nursing Mothers: SYMMETREL is excreted in human milk. Use is not recommended in nursing mothers.

Pediatric Use: The safety and efficacy of SYMMETREL in newborn infants and infants below the age of 1 year have not been established.

Usage in the Elderly: Because SYMMETREL is primarily excreted in the urine, it accumulates in the plasma and in the body when renal function declines. Thus, the dose of SYMMETREL should be reduced in patients with renal impairment and in individuals who are 65 years of age or older. The dose of SYMMETREL may need reduction in patients with congestive heart failure, peripheral edema, or ortho-

static hypotension (see DOSAGE AND ADMINISTRATION).

ADVERSE REACTIONS

The adverse reactions reported most frequently at the recommended dose of SYMMETREL (5–10%) are: nausea, dizziness (lightheadedness), and insomnia.

Less frequently (1–5%) reported adverse reactions are: depression, anxiety and irritability, hallucinations, confusion, anorexia, dry mouth, constipation, ataxia, livedo reticularis, peripheral edema, orthostatic hypotension, headache, somnolence, nervousness, dream abnormality, agitation, dry nose, diarrhea and fatigue.

Infrequently (0.1–1%) occurring adverse reactions are: congestive heart failure, psychosis, urinary retention, dyspnea, fatigue, skin rash, vomiting, weakness, slurred speech, euphoria, confusion, thinking abnormality, amnesia, hyperkinesia, hypertension, decreased libido, and visual disturbance, including punctuate subepithelial or other corneal opacity, corneal edema, decreased visual acuity, sensitivity to light, and optic nerve palsy.

Rare (less than 0.1%) occurring adverse reactions are: instances of convulsion, leukopenia, neutropenia, eczematoid dermatitis, oculogyric episodes, suicidal attempt, suicide, and suicidal ideation (see WARNINGS).

OVERDOSAGE

Deaths have been reported from overdose with SYMMETREL. The lowest reported acute lethal dose was 2 grams. Acute toxicity may be attributable to the anticholinergic effects of amantadine. Drug overdose has resulted in cardiac, respiratory, renal or central nervous system toxicity. Cardiac dysfunction includes arrhythmia, tachycardia and hypertension. Pulmonary edema and respiratory distress (including adult respiratory distress syndrome—ARDS) have been reported; renal dysfunction including increased BUN, decreased creatinine clearance and renal insufficiency can occur. Central nervous system effects that have been reported include insomnia, anxiety, aggressive behavior, hypertonia, hyperkinesia, tremor, confusion, disorientation, depersonalization, fear, delirium, hallucinations, psychotic reactions, lethargy, somnolence and coma. Seizures may be exacerbated in patients with prior history of seizure disorders. Hyperthermia has also been observed in cases where a drug overdose has occurred.

There is no specific antidote for an overdose of SYMMETREL. However, slowly administered intravenous physostigmine in 1 and 2 mg doses in an adult[2] at 1 to 2 hour intervals and 0.5 mg doses in a child[3] at 5 to 10 minute intervals up to a maximum of 2 mg/hour have been reported to be effective in the control of central nervous system toxicity caused by amantadine hydrochloride. For acute overdosing, general supportive measures should be employed along with immediate gastric lavage or induction of emesis. Fluids should be forced, and if necessary, given intravenously. Hemodialysis does not remove significant amounts of SYMMETREL; in patients with renal failure, a four hour hemodialysis removed 7 to 15 mg after a single 300 mg oral dose.[4] The pH of the urine has been reported to influence the excretion rate of SYMMETREL. Since the excretion rate of SYMMETREL increases rapidly when the urine is acidic, the administration of urine acidifying drugs may increase the elimination of the drug from the body. The blood pressure, pulse, respiration and temperature should be monitored. The patient should be observed for hyperactivity and convulsions; if required, sedation, and anticonvulsant therapy should be administered. The patient should be observed for the possible development of arrhythmias and hypotension; if required, appropriate antiarrhythmic and antihypotensive therapy should be given. The blood electrolytes, urine pH and urinary output should be monitored. If there is no record of recent voiding, catheterization should be done.

DOSAGE AND ADMINISTRATION

The dose of SYMMETREL may need reduction in patients with congestive heart failure, peripheral edema, orthostatic hypotension, or impaired renal function (see Dosage for Impaired Renal Function).

Dosage for Prophylaxis and Treatment of Uncomplicated Influenza A Virus Illness:

Adult: The adult daily dosage of SYMMETREL is 200 mg; four teaspoonfuls of syrup as a single daily dose. The daily dosage may be split into 100 mg (two teaspoonfuls of syrup) twice a day. If central nervous system effects develop in once-a-day dosage, a split dosage schedule may reduce such complaints. In persons 65 years of age or older, the daily dosage of SYMMETREL is 100 mg.

A 100 mg daily dose has also been shown in experimental challenge studies to be effective as prophylaxis in healthy adults who are not at high risk for influenza-related complications. However, it has not been demonstrated that a 100 mg daily dose is as effective as a 200 mg daily dose for prophylaxis, nor has the 100 mg daily dose been studied in the treatment of acute influenza illness. In recent clinical trials, the incidence of central nervous system (CNS) side effects associated with the 100 mg daily dose was at or near the level of placebo. The 100 mg dose is recommended for persons who

have demonstrated intolerance to 200 mg of SYMMETREL daily because of CNS or other toxicities.

Children: 1 yr.–9 yrs. of age: The total daily dose should be calculated on the basis of 2 to 4 mg/lb/day (4.4 to 8.8 mg/kg/day), but not to exceed 150 mg per day.

9 yrs.–12 yrs. of age: The total daily dose is 200 mg given as 100 mg (two teaspoonfuls of syrup) twice a day. The 100 mg daily dose has not been studied in children. Therefore, there are no data which demonstrate that this dose is as effective as or is safer than the 200 mg daily dose in this patient population.

Prophylactic dosing should be started in anticipation of an influenza A outbreak and before or after contact with individuals with influenza A virus respiratory tract illness.

SYMMETREL should be continued daily for at least 10 days following a known exposure. If SYMMETREL is used chemoprophylactically in conjunction with inactivated influenza A virus vaccine until protective antibody responses develop, then it should be administered for 2 to 4 weeks after the vaccine has been given. When inactivated influenza A virus vaccine is unavailable or contraindicated, SYMMETREL should be administered for the duration of known influenza A in the community because of repeated and unknown exposure.

Treatment of influenza A virus illness should be started as soon as possible, preferably within 24 to 48 hours after onset of signs and symptoms, and should be continued for 24 to 48 hours after the disappearance of signs and symptoms.

Dosage for Parkinsonism:

Adult: The usual dose of SYMMETREL is 100 mg twice a day when used alone. SYMMETREL has an onset of action usually within 48 hours.

The initial dose of SYMMETREL is 100 mg daily for patients with serious associated medical illnesses or who are receiving high doses of other antiparkinson drugs. After one to several weeks at 100 mg once daily, the dose may be increased to 100 mg twice daily, if necessary.

Occasionally, patients whose responses are not optimal with SYMMETREL at 200 mg daily may benefit from an increase up to 400 mg daily in divided doses. However, such patients should be supervised closely by their physicians.

Patients initially deriving benefit from SYMMETREL not uncommonly experience a fall-off of effectiveness after a few months. Benefit may be regained by increasing the dose to 300 mg daily. Alternatively, temporary discontinuation of SYMMETREL for several weeks, followed by reinitiation of the drug, may result in regaining benefit in some patients. A decision to use other antiparkinson drugs may be necessary.

Dosage for Concomitant Therapy: Some patients who do not respond to anticholinergic antiparkinson drugs may respond to SYMMETREL. When SYMMETREL or anticholinergic antiparkinson drugs are each used with marginal benefit, concomitant use may produce additional benefit.

When SYMMETREL and levodopa are initiated concurrently, the patient can exhibit rapid therapeutic benefits. SYMMETREL should be held constant at 100 mg daily or twice daily while the daily dose of levodopa is gradually increased to optimal benefit.

When SYMMETREL is added to optimal well-tolerated doses of levodopa, additional benefit may result, including smoothing out the fluctuations in improvement which sometimes occur in patients on levodopa alone. Patients who require a reduction in their usual dose of levodopa because of development of side effects may possibly regain lost benefit with the addition of SYMMETREL.

Dosage for Drug-Induced Extrapyramidal Reactions:

Adult: The usual dose of SYMMETREL is 100 mg twice a day. Occasionally, patients whose responses are not optimal with SYMMETREL at 200 mg daily may benefit from an increase up to 300 mg daily in divided doses.

Dosage for Impaired Renal Function:

Depending upon creatinine clearance, the following dosage adjustments are recommended:

CREATININE CLEARANCE (mL/min/1.73m^2)	SYMMETREL DOSAGE
30–50	200 mg 1st day and 100 mg each day thereafter
15–29	200 mg 1st day followed by 100 mg on alternate days
<15	200 mg every 7 days

The recommended dosage for patients on hemodialysis is 200 mg every 7 days.

HOW SUPPLIED

SYMMETREL is available as a syrup [each 5 mL (1 teaspoonful) contains 50 mg amantadine hydrochloride] in:

16 oz. (480 mL) bottles NDC 0056-0205-16

Store at controlled room temperature (59°–86°F, 15°–30°C).

REFERENCES

1. W.W. Wilson and A.H. Rajput, Amantadine-Dyazide Interaction, Can Med Assoc J. 129:974-975, 1983.
2. D.F. Casey, N. Engl. J. Med. 298:516, 1978.
3. C.D. Berkowitz, J. Pediatr. 95:144, 1979.
4. V.W. Horadam, et. al., Ann. Intern. Med. 94:454, 1981.

DuPont Pharma
Wilmington, Delaware 19880

SYMMETREL® is a Registered Trademark of DuPont Merck Pharmaceutical Co.

6448/March, 1996

SYMMETREL® ℞

[sim' e-trel ″]
(amantadine hydrochloride)
Capsules, USP

DESCRIPTION

SYMMETREL (amantadine hydrochloride) is designated chemically as 1-adamantanamine hydrochloride. Its molecular weight is 187.71 with a molecular formula $C_{10}H_{18}NCl$. It has the following structural formula:

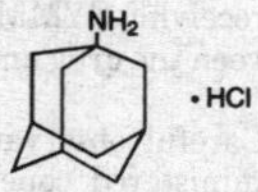

Amantadine hydrochloride is a stable white or nearly white crystalline powder, freely soluble in water and soluble in alcohol and in chloroform.

Amantadine has pharmacological actions as both an anti-Parkinson and an antiviral drug.

Each capsule intended for oral administration contains 100 mg amantadine hydrochloride and has the following inactive ingredients: Croscarmellose sodium, Ethylcellulose, FD&C Blue 1, FD&C Red 40, Gelatin, Magnesium stearate, Methylparaben, Microcrystalline cellulose, Pregelatinized starch, Propylparaben, Silicon dioxide, Sodium lauryl sulfate and Titanium dioxide.

CLINICAL PHARMACOLOGY

Mechanism of Action: Parkinson's Disease The mechanism of action of amantadine in the treatment of Parkinson's disease and drug-induced extrapyramidal reactions is not known. It has been shown to cause an increase in dopamine release in the animal brain. The drug does not possess anticholinergic activity in dogs at doses of 31.5 mg/kg, equivalent to an approximate human dose of 15.8 mg/kg (based on body surface area conversions).

Mechanism of Action: Antiviral The mechanism by which amantadine exerts its antiviral activity is not clearly understood. It appears to mainly prevent the release of infectious viral nucleic acid into the host cell by interfering with the function of the transmembrane domain of the viral M2 protein. In certain cases, amantadine is also known to prevent virus assembly during virus replication. It does not appear to interfere with the immunogenicity of inactivated influenza A virus vaccine.

Antiviral Activity: Amantadine inhibits the replication of influenza A virus isolates from each of the subtypes, i.e., H1N1, H2N2 and H3N2. It has very little or no activity against influenza B virus isolates. A quantitative relationship between the *in vitro* susceptibility of influenza A virus to amantadine and the clinical response to therapy has not been established in man. Sensitivity test results, expressed as the concentration of amantadine required to inhibit by 50% the growth of virus (ED_{50}) in tissue culture vary greatly (from 0.1 mcg/mL to 25.0 mcg/mL) depending upon the assay protocol used, size of virus inoculum, isolates of influenza A virus strains tested, and the cell type used. Host cells in tissue culture readily tolerated amantadine up to a concentration of 100 mcg/mL.

Drug Resistance: Influenza A variants with reduced *in vitro* sensitivity to amantadine have been isolated from epidemic strains in areas where adamantane derivatives are being used. Influenza viruses with reduced *in vitro* sensitivity have been shown to be transmissible and to cause typical influenza illness. The quantitative relationship between the *in vitro* sensitivity of influenza A variants to amantadine and the clinical response to therapy has not been established.

Pharmacokinetics: SYMMETREL is well absorbed orally. Maximum plasma concentrations are directly related to dose for doses up to 200 mg/day. Doses above 200 mg/day may result in a greater than proportional increase in maximum plasma concentrations. It is primarily excreted unchanged in the urine by glomerular filtration and tubular secretion. Eight metabolites of amantadine have been identified in human urine. One metabolite, an N-acetylated compound, was quantified in human urine and accounted for 5–15% of the administered dose. Plasma acetylamantadine accounted for up to 80% of the concurrent amantadine plasma concentration in 5 of 12 healthy volunteers following the ingestion of a 200 mg dose of amantadine. Acetylamantadine was not detected in the plasma of the remaining seven volunteers. The contribution of this metabolite to efficacy or toxicity is not known.

There appears to be a relationship between plasma amantadine concentrations and toxicity. As concentration increases toxicity seems to be more prevalent, however absolute values of amantadine concentrations associated with adverse effects have not been fully defined.

After the oral administration of a single 100 mg SYMMETREL capsule, several studies showed mean maximum plasma concentrations of 0.2 to 0.4 mcg/mL and mean times to peak concentration of 2.5 to 4 hours. Mean half-lives ranged from 10 to 14 hours. Across other studies, amantadine plasma half-life has averaged 16 $\pm$ 6 hours (range 9 to 31 hours) in 19 healthy volunteers.

Plasma amantadine clearance ranged from 0.2 to 0.3 L/hr/kg after the administration of 5 mg to 25 mg intravenous doses of amantadine to 15 healthy volunteers.

In six healthy volunteers, the ratio of amantadine renal clearance to apparent oral plasma clearance was 0.79 $\pm$ 0.17 (mean $\pm$ SD).

The volume of distribution determined after the intravenous administration of amantadine to 15 healthy subjects was 3 to 8 L/kg, suggesting tissue binding. Amantadine, after single oral 200 mg doses to 6 healthy young subjects and to 6 healthy elderly subjects has been found in nasal mucus at mean $\pm$ SD concentrations of 0.15 $\pm$ 0.16, 0.28 $\pm$ 0.26, and 0.39 $\pm$ 0.34 mcg/g at 1, 4, and 8 hours after dosing, respectively. These concentrations represented 31 $\pm$ 33%, 59 $\pm$ 61%, and 95 $\pm$ 86% of the corresponding plasma amantadine concentrations. Amantadine is approximately 67% bound to plasma proteins over a concentration range of 0.1 to 2.0 mcg/mL. Following the administration of amantadine 100 mg as a single dose, the mean $\pm$ SD red blood cell to plasma ratio ranged from 2.7 $\pm$ 0.5 in 6 healthy subjects to 1.4 $\pm$ 0.2 in 8 patients with renal insufficiency.

The apparent oral plasma clearance of amantadine is reduced and the plasma half-life and plasma concentrations are increased in healthy elderly individuals age 60 and older. After single dose administration of 25 to 75 mg to 7 healthy, elderly male volunteers, the apparent plasma clearance of amantadine was 0.10 $\pm$ 0.04 L/hr/kg (range 0.06 to 0.17 L/hr/kg) and the half-life was 29 $\pm$ 7 hours (range 20 to 41 hours). Whether these changes are due to decline in renal function or other age related factors is not known.

Compared with otherwise healthy adult individuals, the clearance of amantadine is significantly reduced in adult patients with renal insufficiency. The elimination half-life increases two to three fold or greater when creatinine clearance is less than 40 mL/min/1.73 m^2 and averages eight days in patients on chronic maintenance hemodialysis. Amantadine is removed in negligible amounts by hemodialysis.

The pH of the urine has been reported to influence the excretion rate of SYMMETREL. Since the excretion rate of SYMMETREL increases rapidly when the urine is acidic, the administration of urine acidifying drugs may increase the elimination of the drug from the body.

INDICATIONS AND USAGE

SYMMETREL is indicated for the prophylaxis and treatment of signs and symptoms of infection caused by various strains of influenza A virus. SYMMETREL capsules are also indicated in the treatment of parkinsonism and drug-induced extrapyramidal reactions.

Influenza A Prophylaxis: SYMMETREL capsules are indicated for chemoprophylaxis against signs and symptoms of influenza A virus infection when early vaccination is not feasible or when the vaccine is contraindicated or not available. In the prophylaxis of influenza, early vaccination on an annual basis as recommended by the Centers for Disease Control's Immunization Practices Advisory Committee is the method of choice. Because SYMMETREL does not completely prevent the host immune response to influenza A infection, individuals who take this drug may still develop immune responses to natural disease or vaccination and may be protected when later exposed to antigenically related viruses. Following vaccination during an influenza A outbreak, SYMMETREL prophylaxis should be considered for the 2 to 4 week time period required to develop an antibody response.

Influenza A Treatment: SYMMETREL capsules are also indicated in the treatment of uncomplicated respiratory tract illness caused by influenza A virus strains especially when administered early in the course of illness. There are no well-controlled clinical studies demonstrating that treatment with SYMMETREL will avoid the development of influenza A virus pneumonitis or other complications in high risk patients.

There is no clinical evidence indicating that SYMMETREL is effective in the prophylaxis or treatment of viral respiratory tract illnesses other than those caused by influenza A virus strains.

Parkinson's Disease/Syndrome: SYMMETREL is indicated in the treatment of idiopathic Parkinson's disease (Paralysis Agitans), postencephalitic parkinsonism, and symp-

Continued on next page

DuPont Pharma—Cont.

tomatic parkinsonism which may follow injury to the nervous system by carbon monoxide intoxication. It is indicated in those elderly patients believed to develop parkinsonism in association with cerebral arteriosclerosis. In the treatment of Parkinson's disease, SYMMETREL is less effective than levodopa, (-)-3-(3,4-dihydroxyphenyl)-L-alanine, and its efficacy in comparison with the anticholinergic antiparkinson drugs has not yet been established.

Drug-Induced Extrapyramidal Reactions: SYMMETREL is indicated in the treatment of drug-induced extrapyramidal reactions. Although anticholinergic-type side effects have been noted with SYMMETREL when used in patients with drug-induced extrapyramidal reactions, there is a lower incidence of these side effects than that observed with the anticholinergic antiparkinson drugs.

CONTRAINDICATIONS

SYMMETREL is contraindicated in patients with known hypersensitivity to the drug.

WARNINGS

Deaths: Deaths have been reported from overdose with SYMMETREL. The lowest reported acute lethal dose was 2 grams. Acute toxicity may be attributable to the anticholinergic effects of amantadine. Drug overdose has resulted in cardiac, respiratory, renal or central nervous system toxicity. Cardiac dysfunction includes arrhythmia, tachycardia and hypertension (see OVERDOSAGE).

Suicide Attempts: Suicide attempts, some of which have been fatal, have been reported in patients treated with SYMMETREL, many of whom received short courses for influenza treatment or prophylaxis. The incidence of suicide attempts is not known and the pathophysiologic mechanism is not understood. Suicide attempts and suicidal ideation have been reported in patients with and without prior history of psychiatric illness. SYMMETREL can exacerbate mental problems in patients with a history of psychiatric disorders or substance abuse. Patients who attempt suicide may exhibit abnormal mental states which include disorientation, confusion, depression, personality changes, agitation, aggressive behavior, hallucinations, paranoia, other psychotic reactions, and somnolence or insomnia. Because of the possibility of serious adverse effects, caution should be observed when prescribing SYMMETREL to patients being treated with drugs having CNS effects, or for whom the potential risks outweigh the benefit of treatment. Because some patients have attempted suicide by overdosing with amantadine, prescriptions should be written for the smallest quantity consistent with good patient management.

CNS Effects: Patients with a history of epilepsy or other "seizures" should be observed closely for possible increased seizure activity.

Patients receiving SYMMETREL who note central nervous system effects or blurring of vision should be cautioned against driving or working in situations where alertness and adequate motor coordination are important.

Other: Patients with a history of congestive heart failure or peripheral edema should be followed closely as there are patients who developed congestive heart failure while receiving SYMMETREL.

Patients with Parkinson's disease improving on SYMMETREL should resume normal activities gradually and cautiously, consistent with other medical considerations, such as the presence of osteoporosis or phlebothrombosis.

PRECAUTIONS

SYMMETREL should not be discontinued abruptly in patients with Parkinson's disease since a few patients have experienced a parkinsonian crisis, i.e., a sudden marked clinical deterioration, when this medication was suddenly stopped. The dose of anticholinergic drugs or of SYMMETREL should be reduced if atropine-like effects appear when these drugs are used concurrently.

Neuroleptic Malignant Syndrome (NMS): Sporadic cases of possible Neuroleptic Malignant Syndrome (NMS) have been reported in association with dose reduction or withdrawal of SYMMETREL therapy.

NMS is an uncommon but life-threatening syndrome characterized by fever or hyperthermia; neurologic findings including muscle rigidity, involuntary movements, altered consciousness; other disturbances such as autonomic dysfunction, tachycardia, tachypnea, hyper- or hypotension; laboratory findings such as creatine phosphokinase elevation, leukocytosis and increased serum myoglobin.

The early diagnosis of this condition is important for the appropriate management of these patients. Considering NMS as a possible diagnosis and ruling out other acute illnesses (e.g., pneumonia, systemic infection, etc.) is essential. This may be especially complex if the clinical presentation includes both serious medical illness and untreated or inadequately treated extrapyramidal signs and symptoms (EPS). Other important considerations in the differential diagnosis include central anticholinergic toxicity, heat stroke, drug fever and primary central nervous system (CNS) pathology.

The management of NMS should include: 1) intensive symptomatic treatment and medical monitoring, and 2) treatment of any concomitant serious medical problems for which specific treatments are available. Dopamine agonists, such as bromocriptine, and muscle relaxants, such as dantrolene are often used in the treatment of NMS, however, their effectiveness has not been demonstrated in controlled studies.

Other: Because SYMMETREL is mainly excreted in the urine, it accumulates in the plasma and in the body when renal function declines. Thus, the dose of SYMMETREL should be reduced in patients with renal impairment and in individuals who are 65 years of age or older. The dose of SYMMETREL may need careful adjustment in patients with congestive heart failure, peripheral edema, or orthostatic hypotension.

Care should be exercised when administering SYMMETREL to patients with liver disease, a history of recurrent eczematoid rash, or to patients with psychosis or severe psychoneurosis not controlled by chemotherapeutic agents. Rare instances of reversible elevation of liver enzymes have been reported in patients receiving SYMMETREL, though a specific relationship between the drug and such changes has not been established.

Drug Interactions: Careful observation is required when SYMMETREL is administered concurrently with central nervous system stimulants.

Coadministration of thioridazine has been reported to worsen the tremor in elderly patients with Parkinson's disease, however, it is not known if other phenothiazines produce a similar response.

Coadministration of triamterene and hydrochlorothiazide capsules resulted in a higher plasma amantadine concentration in a 61 year old man receiving SYMMETREL 100 mg TID for Parkinson's disease.[1] It is not known which of the components of triamterene and hydrochlorothiazide capsules contributed to the observation or if related drugs produce similar response.

Carcinogenesis, Mutagenesis, Impairment of Fertility: Long-term in vivo animal studies designed to evaluate the carcinogenic potential of SYMMETREL have not been performed. In several in vitro assays for gene mutation, SYMMETREL did not increase the number of spontaneously observed mutations in four strains of Salmonella typhimurium (Ames Test) or in a mammalian cell line (Chinese Hamster Ovary cells) when incubations were performed either with or without a liver metabolic activation extract. Further, there was no evidence of chromosome damage observed in an in vitro test using freshly derived and stimulated human peripheral blood lymphocytes (with and without metabolic activation) or in an in vivo mouse bone marrow micronucleus test (140–550 mg/kg; estimated human equivalent doses of 11.7–45.8 mg/kg based on body surface area conversion).

In a three litter reproduction study in rats, SYMMETREL at a dose of 32 mg/kg/day (estimated human equivalent dose of 4.5 mg/kg/day, based on body surface area conversions) administered to both males and females slightly impaired fertility. There were no effects on fertility at a dose level of 10 mg/kg/day (estimated human equivalent dose of 1.4 mg/kg/day); intermediate doses were not tested.

Pregnancy: Teratogenic Effects: Pregnancy Category C: SYMMETREL has been shown to be embryotoxic and teratogenic in rats at 50 mg/kg/day (estimated human equivalent dose of 7.1 mg/kg/day based on body surface area conversion), while a dose of 37 mg/kg/day (estimated human equivalent dose of 5.3 mg/kg/day) was without effect. Embryotoxic and teratogenic effects were not seen in rabbits that received 32 mg/kg/day (estimated human equivalent dose of 9.6 mg/kg/day, based on body surface area conversion). There are no adequate and well-controlled studies in pregnant women. SYMMETREL should be used during pregnancy only if the potential benefit justifies the potential risk to the embryo or fetus.

Nursing Mothers: SYMMETREL is excreted in human milk. Use is not recommended in nursing mothers.

Pediatric Use: The safety and efficacy of SYMMETREL in newborn infants and infants below the age of 1 year have not been established.

Usage in the Elderly: Because SYMMETREL is primarily excreted in the urine, it accumulates in the plasma and in the body when renal function declines. Thus, the dose of SYMMETREL should be reduced in patients with renal impairment and in individuals who are 65 years of age or older. The dose of SYMMETREL may need reduction in patients with congestive heart failure, peripheral edema, or orthostatic hypotension (see DOSAGE AND ADMINISTRATION).

ADVERSE REACTIONS

The adverse reactions reported most frequently at the recommended dose of SYMMETREL (5–10%) are: nausea, dizziness (lightheadedness), and insomnia.

Less frequently (1–5%) reported adverse reactions are: depression, anxiety, irritability, hallucinations, confusion, anorexia, dry mouth, constipation, ataxia, livedo reticularis, peripheral edema, orthostatic hypotension, headache, somnolence, nervousness, dream abnormality, agitation, dry nose, diarrhea and fatigue.

Infrequently (0.1–1%) occurring adverse reactions are: congestive heart failure, psychosis, urinary retention, dyspnea, fatigue, skin rash, vomiting, weakness, slurred speech, euphoria, confusion, thinking abnormality, amnesia, hyperkinesia, hypertension, decreased libido, and visual disturbance, including punctuate subepithelial or other corneal opacity, corneal edema, decreased visual acuity, sensitivity to light, and optic nerve palsy.

Rare (less than 0.1%) occurring adverse reactions are: instances of convulsion, leukopenia, neutropenia, eczematoid dermatitis, oculogyric episodes, suicidal attempt, suicide, and suicidal ideation (see WARNINGS).

OVERDOSAGE

Deaths have been reported from overdose with SYMMETREL. The lowest reported acute lethal dose was 2 grams. Acute toxicity may be attributable to the anticholinergic effects of amantadine. Drug overdose has resulted in cardiac, respiratory, renal or central nervous system toxicity. Cardiac dysfunction includes arrhythmia, tachycardia and hypertension. Pulmonary edema and respiratory distress (including adult respiratory distress syndrome —ARDS) have been reported; renal dysfunction including increased BUN, decreased creatinine clearance and renal insufficiency can occur. Central nervous system effects that have been reported include insomnia, anxiety, aggressive behavior, hypertonia, hyperkinesia, tremor, confusion, disorientation, depersonalization, fear, delirium, hallucinations, psychotic reactions, lethargy, somnolence and coma. Seizures may be exacerbated in patients with prior history of seizure disorders. Hyperthermia has also been observed in cases where a drug overdose has occurred.

There is no specific antidote for an overdose of SYMMETREL. However, slowly administered intravenous physostigmine in 1 and 2 mg doses in an adult[2] at 1 to 2 hour intervals and 0.5 mg doses in a child[3] at 5 to 10 minute intervals up to a maximum of 2 mg/hour have been reported to be effective in the control of central nervous system toxicity caused by amantadine hydrochloride. For acute overdosing, general supportive measures should be employed along with immediate gastric lavage or induction of emesis. Fluids should be forced, and if necessary, given intravenously. Hemodialysis does not remove significant amounts of SYMMETREL; in patients with renal failure, a four hour hemodialysis removed 7 to 15 mg after a single 300 mg oral dose.[4] The pH of the urine has been reported to influence the excretion rate of SYMMETREL. Since the excretion rate of SYMMETREL increases rapidly when the urine is acidic, the administration of urine acidifying drugs may increase the elimination of the drug from the body. The blood pressure, pulse, respiration and temperature should be monitored. The patient should be observed for hyperactivity and convulsions; if required, sedation, and anticonvulsant therapy should be administered. The patient should be observed for the possible development of arrhythmias and hypotension; if required, appropriate antiarrhythmic and antihypotensive therapy should be given. The blood electrolytes, urine pH and urinary output should be monitored. If there is no record of recent voiding, catheterization should be done.

DOSAGE AND ADMINISTRATION

The dose of SYMMETREL may need reduction in patients with congestive heart failure, peripheral edema, orthostatic hypotension, or impaired renal function (see Dosage for Impaired Renal Function).

Dosage for Prophylaxis and Treatment of Uncomplicated Influenza A Virus Illness: Adult: The adult daily dosage of SYMMETREL is 200 mg; two 100 mg capsules as a single daily dose. The daily dosage may be split into one capsule of 100 mg twice a day. If central nervous system effects develop in once-a-day dosage, a split dosage schedule may reduce such complaints. In persons 65 years of age or older, the daily dosage of SYMMETREL is 100 mg.

A 100 mg daily dose has also been shown in experimental challenge studies to be effective as prophylaxis in healthy adults who are not at high risk for influenza-related complications. However, it has not been demonstrated that a 100 mg daily dose is as effective as a 200 mg daily dose for prophylaxis, nor has the 100 mg daily dose been studied in the treatment of acute influenza illness. In recent clinical trials, the incidence of central nervous system (CNS) side effects associated with the 100 mg daily dose was at or near the level of placebo. The 100 mg dose is recommended for persons who have demonstrated intolerance to 200 mg of SYMMETREL daily because of CNS or other toxicities.

Children: 1 yr.–9 yrs. of age: The total daily dose should be calculated on the basis of 2 to 4 mg/lb/day (4.4 to 8.8 mg/kg/day), but not to exceed 150 mg per day.

Amantadine hydrochloride syrup should be used for ease and flexibility in administering doses not in 100 mg increments.

9 yrs.–12 yrs. of age: The total daily dose is 200 mg given as one capsule of 100 mg twice a day. The 100 mg daily dose has not been studied in children. Therefore, there are no data

which demonstrate that this dose is as effective as or is safer than the 200 mg daily dose in this patient population.

Prophylactic dosing should be started in anticipation of an influenza A outbreak and before or after contact with individuals with influenza A virus respiratory tract illness.

SYMMETREL should be continued daily for at least 10 days following a known exposure. If SYMMETREL is used chemoprophylactically in conjunction with inactivated influenza A virus vaccine until protective antibody responses develop, then it should be administered for 2 to 4 weeks after the vaccine has been given. When inactivated influenza A virus vaccine is unavailable or contraindicated, SYMMETREL should be administered for the duration of known influenza A in the community because of repeated and unknown exposure.

Treatment of influenza A virus illness should be started as soon as possible, preferably within 24 to 48 hours after onset of signs and symptoms, and should be continued for 24 to 48 hours after the disappearance of signs and symptoms.

Dosage for Parkinsonism:

Adult: The usual dose of SYMMETREL is 100 mg twice a day when used alone. SYMMETREL has an onset of action usually within 48 hours.

The initial dose of SYMMETREL is 100 mg daily for patients with serious associated medical illnesses or who are receiving high doses of other antiparkinson drugs. After one to several weeks at 100 mg once daily, the dose may be increased to 100 mg twice daily, if necessary.

Occasionally, patients whose responses are not optimal with SYMMETREL at 200 mg daily may benefit from an increase up to 400 mg daily in divided doses. However, such patients should be supervised closely by their physicians.

Patients initially deriving benefit from SYMMETREL not uncommonly experience a fall-off of effectiveness after a few months. Benefit may be regained by increasing the dose to 300 mg daily. Alternatively, temporary discontinuation of SYMMETREL for several weeks, followed by reinitiation of the drug, may result in regaining benefit in some patients. A decision to use other antiparkinson drugs may be necessary.

Dosage for Concomitant Therapy: Some patients who do not respond to anticholinergic antiparkinson drugs may respond to SYMMETREL. When SYMMETREL or anticholinergic antiparkinson drugs are each used with marginal benefit, concomitant use may produce additional benefit.

When SYMMETREL and levodopa are initiated concurrently, the patient can exhibit rapid therapeutic benefits. SYMMETREL should be held constant at 100 mg daily or twice daily while the daily dose of levodopa is gradually increased to optimal benefit.

When SYMMETREL is added to optimal well-tolerated doses of levodopa, additional benefit may result, including smoothing out the fluctuations in improvement which sometimes occur in patients on levodopa alone. Patients who require a reduction in their usual dose of levodopa because of development of side effects may possibly regain lost benefit with the addition of SYMMETREL.

Dosage for Drug-Induced Extrapyramidal Reactions:

Adult: The usual dose of SYMMETREL is 100 mg twice a day. Occasionally, patients whose responses are not optimal with SYMMETREL at 200 mg daily may benefit from an increase up to 300 mg daily in divided doses.

Dosage for Impaired Renal Function:

Depending upon creatinine clearance, the following dosage adjustments are recommended:

CREATININE CLEARANCE ($mL/min/1.73m^2$)	SYMMETREL DOSAGE
30–50	100 mg 1st day and 100 mg each day thereafter
15–29	200 mg 1st day followed by 100 mg on alternate days
<15	200 mg every 7 days

The recommended dosage for patients on hemodialysis is 200 mg every 7 days.

HOW SUPPLIED

SYMMETREL is available in bottles of 100 capsules. Each red, gelatin capsule contains 100 mg amantadine hydrochloride and is imprinted with DuPont PHARMA and SYMMETREL.

Bottles of 100   0056-0315-70

Store at controlled room temperature 15°–30°C (59°–86°F).

REFERENCES

[1] W.W. Wilson and A.H. Rajput, Amantadine-Dyazide Interaction, Can Med Assoc J. 129:974–975, 1983.

[2] D.F. Casey, N. Engl. J. Med. 298:516, 1978.

[3] C.D. Berkowitz, J. Pediatr. 95:144, 1979.

[4] V.W. Horadam, et. al., Ann. Intern. Med. 94:454, 1981.

CAUTION: Federal law prohibits dispensing without prescription.

Manufactured by: INVAMED, INC.
Dayton, New Jersey 08810 USA

Distributed by:
DuPont Pharma
Wilmington, Delaware 19880 USA
6437/February, 1996

SYMMETREL® is a registered trademark of the DuPont Merck Pharmaceutical Company

---

ZYDONE® Ⓒ III

[zī″dōn′]

(Hydrocodone Bitartrate and Acetaminophen) Capsules

DESCRIPTION

Each ZYDONE capsule contains:

Hydrocodone Bitartrate .... 5 mg
WARNING: May be habit forming
Acetaminophen .... 500 mg

Hydrocodone Bitartrate is an opioid analgesic and antitussive and occurs as fine, white crystals or as a crystalline powder. It is affected by light. The chemical name is: 4,5α-epoxy-3-methoxy-17-methylmorphinan-6-one tartrate (1:1) hydrate (2:5).

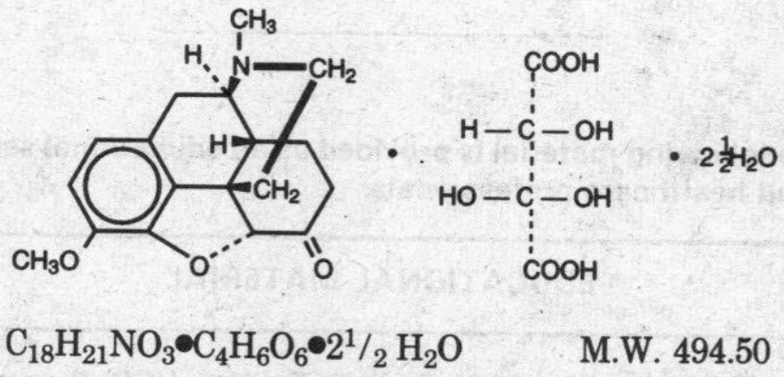

$C_{18}H_{21}NO_3 \bullet C_4H_6O_6 \bullet 2^1/_2 H_2O$ M.W. 494.50

Acetaminophen, 4′-hydroxyacetanilide, is a non-opiate, non-salicylate analgesic and antipyretic which occurs as a white, odorless crystalline powder possessing a slightly bitter taste.

ZYDONE capsules also contain: FD&C Red 7, FD&C Yellow 6, gelatin, pharmaceutical glaze, silicon dioxide, sodium lauryl sulfate and titanium dioxide.

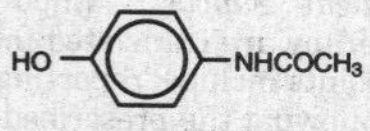

$C_8H_9NO_2$ M.W. 151.16

CLINICAL PHARMACOLOGY

Hydrocodone is a semisynthetic narcotic analgesic and antitussive with multiple actions qualitatively similar to those of codeine. Most of these involve the central nervous system and smooth muscle. The precise mechanism of action of hydrocodone and other opiates is not known, although it is believed to relate to the existence of opiate receptors in the central nervous system. In addition to analgesia, narcotics may produce drowsiness, changes in mood and mental clouding.

Radioimmunoassay techniques have recently been developed for the analysis of hydrocodone in human plasma. After a 10 mg oral dose of hydrocodone bitartrate, a mean peak serum drug level of 23.6 ng/mL and an elimination half-life of 3.8 hours were found.

The analgesic action of acetaminophen involves peripheral and central influences, but the specific mechanism is as yet undetermined. Antipyretic activity is mediated through hypothalamic heat regulating centers. Acetaminophen inhibits prostaglandin synthetase. Therapeutic doses of acetaminophen have negligible effects on the cardiovascular or respiratory systems; however, toxic doses may cause circulatory failure and rapid, shallow breathing. Acetaminophen is rapidly and almost completely absorbed from the gastrointestinal tract, producing maximum serum concentrations within 30 minutes to one hour. The plasma half-life in adults and children ranges from 0.90 hours to 3.25 hours with an average of approximately 2 hours. The drug distributes uniformly in most body fluids and is approximately 25% protein bound. Acetaminophen is conjugated in the liver, with less than 3% of the dose excreted unchanged in 24 hours. The primary metabolic pathway is conjugation to sulfate and glucuronide by-products. A minor oxidative pathway forms cysteine and mercapturic acid. These compounds are subsequently excreted by the kidneys into the urine.

INDICATIONS AND USAGE

For the relief of moderate to moderately severe pain.

CONTRAINDICATIONS

Hypersensitivity to acetaminophen or hydrocodone.

WARNINGS

Respiratory Depression: At high doses or in sensitive patients, hydrocodone may produce dose-related respiratory depression by acting directly on the brain stem respiratory center. Hydrocodone also affects the center that controls respiratory rhythm, and may produce irregular and periodic breathing.

Head Injury and Increased Intracranial Pressure: The respiratory depressant effects of narcotics and their capacity to elevate cerebrospinal fluid pressure may be markedly exaggerated in the presence of head injury, other intracranial lesions or a preexisting increase in intracranial pressure. Furthermore, narcotics produce adverse reactions which may obscure the clinical course of patients with head injuries.

Acute Abdominal Conditions: The administration of narcotics may obscure the diagnosis or clinical course of patients with acute abdominal conditions.

PRECAUTIONS

Special Risk Patients: As with any narcotic analgesic agent, Hydrocodone Bitartrate and Acetaminophen Capsules should be used with caution in elderly or debilitated patients and those with severe impairment of hepatic or renal function, hypothyroidism, Addison's disease, prostatic hypertrophy or urethral stricture. The usual precautions should be observed and the possibility of respiratory depression should be kept in mind.

Information for Patients: ZYDONE Capsules, like all narcotics, may impair the mental and/or physical abilities required for the performance of potentially hazardous tasks such as driving a car or operating machinery; patients should be cautioned accordingly.

Cough Reflex: Hydrocodone suppresses the cough reflex; as with all narcotics, caution should be exercised when ZYDONE Capsules are used postoperatively and in patients with pulmonary disease.

Drug Interactions: Patients receiving other narcotic analgesics, antipsychotics, antianxiety agents, or other CNS depressants (including alcohol) concomitantly with ZYDONE Capsules may exhibit an additive CNS depression. When combined therapy is contemplated, the dose of one or both agents should be reduced.

The use of MAO inhibitors or tricyclic antidepressants with hydrocodone preparations may increase the effect of either the antidepressant or hydrocodone.

The concurrent use of anticholinergics with hydrocodone may produce paralytic ileus.

Usage in Pregnancy: Teratogenic Effects: Pregnancy Category C. Hydrocodone has been shown to be teratogenic in hamsters when given in doses 700 times the human dose. There are no adequate and well-controlled studies in pregnant women. Hydrocodone Bitartrate and Acetaminophen Capsules should be used during pregnancy only if the potential benefit justifies the potential risk to the fetus.

Nonteratogenic Effects: Babies born to mothers who have been taking opioids regularly prior to delivery will be physically dependent. The withdrawal signs include irritability and excessive crying, tremors, hyperactive reflexes, increased respiratory rate, increased stools, sneezing, yawning, vomiting, and fever. The intensity of the syndrome does not always correlate with the duration of maternal opioid use or dose. There is no consensus on the best method of managing withdrawal. Chlorpromazine 0.7 to 1 mg/kg q6h, and paregoric 2 to 4 drops/kg q4h, have been used to treat withdrawal symptoms in infants. The duration of therapy is 4 to 28 days, with the dosage decreased as tolerated.

Labor and Delivery: As with all narcotics, administration of ZYDONE Capsules to the mother shortly before delivery may result in some degree of respiratory depression in the newborn, especially if higher doses are used.

Nursing Mothers: It is not known whether this drug is excreted in human milk. Because many drugs are excreted in human milk and because of the potential for serious adverse reactions in nursing infants from ZYDONE Capsules, a decision should be made whether to discontinue nursing or to discontinue the drug, taking into account the importance of the drug to the mother.

Pediatric Use: Safety and effectiveness in children have not been established.

ADVERSE REACTIONS

The most frequently observed adverse reactions include lightheadedness, dizziness, sedation, nausea and vomiting. These effects seem to be more prominent in ambulatory than in nonambulatory patients and some of these adverse reactions may be alleviated if the patient lies down.

Other adverse reactions include:

Central Nervous System: Drowsiness, mental clouding, lethargy, impairment of mental and physical performance, anxiety, fear, dysphoria, psychic dependence, mood changes.

Gastrointestinal System: The antiemetic phenothiazines are useful in suppressing the nausea and vomiting which may occur (see above); however, some phenothiazine derivatives seem to be antianalgesic and to increase the amount of narcotic required to produce pain relief, while other phenothiazines reduce the amount of narcotic required to produce a given level of analgesia. Prolonged administration of ZYDONE (Hydrocodone Bitartrate and Acetaminophen) Capsules may produce constipation.

Continued on next page

DuPont Pharma—Cont.

Genitourinary System: Ureteral spasm, spasm of vesical sphincters and urinary retention have been reported.

Respiratory Depression: Hydrocodone Bitartrate may produce dose-related respiratory depression by acting directly on the brain stem respiratory center. Hydrocodone also affects the center that controls respiratory rhythm, and may produce irregular and periodic breathing. If significant respiratory depression occurs, it may be antagonized by the use of naloxone hydrochloride. Apply other supportive measures when indicated.

DRUG ABUSE AND DEPENDENCE

ZYDONE Capsules are subject to the Federal Controlled Substances Act (Schedule III).

Psychic dependence, physical dependence, and tolerance may develop upon repeated administration of narcotics; therefore, ZYDONE Capsules should be prescribed and administered with caution. However, psychic dependence is unlikely to develop when ZYDONE Capsules are used for a short time for the treatment of pain.

Physical dependence, the condition in which continued administration of the drug is required to prevent the appearance of a withdrawal syndrome, assumes clinically significant proportions only after several weeks of continued narcotic use, although some mild degree of physical dependence may develop after a few days of narcotic therapy. Tolerance, in which increasingly large doses are required in order to produce the same degree of analgesia, is manifested initially by a shortened duration of analgesic effect, and subsequently by decreases in the intensity of analgesia. The rate of development of tolerance varies among patients.

OVERDOSAGE

Hydrocodone: Signs and Symptoms: Serious overdose with hydrocodone is characterized by respiratory depression (a decrease in respiratory rate and/or tidal volume, Cheyne-Stokes respiration, cyanosis), extreme somnolence progressing to stupor or coma, skeletal muscle flaccidity, cold and clammy skin, and sometimes bradycardia and hypotension. In severe overdosage, apnea, circulatory collapse, cardiac arrest and death may occur.

Treatment: Primary attention should be given to the reestablishment of adequate respiratory exchange through provision of a patent airway and the institution of assisted or controlled ventilation. The narcotic antagonist naloxone is a specific antidote against respiratory depression which may result from overdosage or unusual sensitivity to narcotics, including hydrocodone. Therefore, an appropriate dose of naloxone hydrochloride (see package insert) should be administered, preferably by the intravenous route, and simultaneously with efforts at respiratory resuscitation. Since the duration of action of hydrocodone may exceed that of the antagonist, the patient should be kept under continued surveillance and repeated doses of the antagonist should be administered as needed to maintain adequate respiration.

An antagonist should not be administered in the absence of clinically significant respiratory or cardiovascular depression. Oxygen, intravenous fluids, vasopressors and other supportive measures should be employed as indicated.

Gastric emptying may be useful in removing unabsorbed drug.

Acetaminophen: Signs and Symptoms: In acute acetaminophen overdosage, dose-dependent, potentially fatal hepatic necrosis is the most serious adverse effect. Renal tubular necrosis, hypoglycemic coma and thrombocytopenia may also occur.

In adults, hepatic toxicity has rarely been reported with acute overdoses of less than 10 grams and fatalities with less than 15 grams. Importantly, young children seem to be more resistant than adults to the hepatotoxic effect of an acetaminophen overdose. Despite this, the measures outlined below should be initiated in any adult or child suspected of having ingested an acetaminophen overdose.

Early symptoms following a potentially hepatotoxic overdose may include: nausea, vomiting, diaphoresis and general malaise. Clinical and laboratory evidence of hepatic toxicity may not be apparent until 48 to 72 hours post-ingestion.

Treatment: The stomach should be emptied promptly by lavage or by induction of emesis with syrup of ipecac. Patients' estimates of the quantity of a drug ingested are notoriously unreliable. Therefore, if an acetaminophen overdose is suspected, a serum acetaminophen assay should be obtained as early as possible, but no sooner than four hours following ingestion. Liver function studies should be obtained initially and repeated at 24-hour intervals.

The antidote, N-acetylcysteine, should be administered as early as possible, preferably within 16 hours of the overdose ingestion for optimal results, but in any case within 24 hours. Following recovery, there are no residual, structural or functional hepatic abnormalities.

DOSAGE AND ADMINISTRATION

Dosage should be adjusted according to the severity of the pain and the response of the patient. However, it should be

kept in mind that tolerance to hydrocodone can develop with continued use and that the incidence of untoward effects is dose related.

The usual adult dosage is one or two capsules every four to six hours as needed for pain. The total 24 hour dose should not exceed eight capsules.

HOW SUPPLIED

ZYDONE (Hydrocodone Bitratrate 5 mg and Acetaminophen 500 mg) is a white, hard gelatin capsule with red band. Each capsule is imprinted in red, DU PONT ZYDONE.
Bottles of 100: NDC 0056-0091-70
Storage: Store at controlled room temperature 15°–30°C (59°–86°F).
CAUTION: Federal law prohibits dispensing without prescription.

Manufactured by
D.M. Graham Laboratories, Inc., Hobart, New York 13788
for
Du Pont Pharmaceuticals
The DuPont Merck Pharmaceutical Co.
Wilmington, Delaware 19880
ZYDONE® is a Registered Trademark of The Du Pont Merck Pharmaceutical Co.

6173-7/Rev. Dec., 1990

The following material is provided as an educational service to all healthcare professionals:

EDUCATIONAL MATERIAL

COUMADIN® (Warfarin Sodium Tablets, USP) Crystalline

Books/Booklets/Brochures
"*COUMADIN® Patient Aid*". This booklet explains key points of anticoagulation therapy, how it affects the patient's lifestyle, warning signs, and Vitamin K information. It also includes a COUMADIN® ID card and a dosage calendar. Available in English and Spanish.
"*Multilingual Patient Support*". Important facts about COUMADIN® therapy are translated into 50 languages in this booklet. Key points include: reporting problems, having blood tested and following the prescribed weekly schedule.
"*Atrial Fibriwhat? Brochure*". This easy-to-read patient brochure outlines what atrial fibrillation is, the risks associated with the disorder, and treatment plans available in English and Spanish.

Video/Audio
"*COUMADIN® Therapy and You*". This 11 minute, ½-inch VHS video is designed to be shown by the physician to his/her patients on COUMADIN® in order to increase patient commitment and understanding of COUMADIN® therapy.
An audiocassette of the same program, "COUMADIN® Therapy and You," is available for patients to take home.

Both items are available in English and Spanish.

Charts
"*COUMADIN® Patient Anticoagulation Flow Sheet*". This laminated 8-½″ × 11″ chart provides a convenient way to record patient prothrombin times and COUMADIN® doses.
"*COUMADIN® Patient Education Easel Flip Chart*". An easel that allows the physician or nurse to educate the patient about COUMADIN® therapy in a practical question-and-answer format. Available in English and Spanish.

All of the above material is available at no charge to physicians, pharmacists, and other healthcare professionals involved with the management of patients on COUMADIN® therapy by calling 1-800-COUMADIN.

PERCOCET®
(oxycodone and acetaminophen tablets, USP)
PERCODAN®
(oxycodone and aspirin tablets, USP)
Brochures
"How to talk to Doctor About Pain" (PM-31871) Write DuPont Pharma and ask for material by PM # or call (302) 992-4240.

SINEMET®
(Carbidopa-Levodopa)
SINEMET® CR
(Carbidopa-Levodopa)
Sustained-Release Tablets
Booklets
"*A Patient's Guide to Parkinson's Disease and Sinemet® CR* (Carbidopa-Levopoda) Sustained Release" (CR-31412) "*Tips on taking Sinemet® CR*" (CR-31414)
Available at no charge. Write DuPont Pharma and ask for materials by CR # or call (302) 992-4240.

REVIA® (naltrexone HCl tablets)
Booklets/Brochures
"*REVIA® Patient Q & A*". This booklet answers the most commonly asked questions about REVIA®.

"*REVIA® Counselor Q & A*". Answers most commonly asked question in a more detailed level for counselors. Provides information needed on how to use REVIA®.
"*REVIA® Counselor Brochure*". A practical implementation piece on what a counselor should see when using REVIA®. Effectively and completely communicates the features and benefits of REVIA®.

Dura Pharmaceuticals, Inc.
SAN DIEGO, CA 92121-4204

Direct Inquiries to:
(619) 457-2553

For Medical Information Contact:
Generally:
(619) 457-2553
In Emergencies:
Medical Affairs Department
(619) 457-2553

CAPASTAT® SULFATE   ℞
STERILE CAPREOMYCIN SULFATE, USP

Not for Pediatric Use

WARNINGS
This preparation is for intramuscular use only.
The use of Capastat® Sulfate (Sterile Capreomycin Sulfate, USP) in patients with renal insufficiency or preexisting auditory impairment must be undertaken with great caution, and the risk of additional cranial nerve VIII impairment or renal injury should be weighed against the benefits to be derived from therapy. *Refer to ANIMAL PHARMACOLOGY for additional information.*
Since other parenteral antituberculosis agents (streptomycin, viomycin) also have similar and sometimes irreversible toxic effects, particularly on cranial nerve VIII and renal function, simultaneous administration of these agents with Capastat Sulfate is not recommended. Use with nonantituberculosis drugs (polymyxin A sulfate, colistin sulfate, amikacin, gentamicin, tobramycin, vancomycin, kanamycin, and neomycin) having ototoxic or nephrotoxic potential should be undertaken only with great caution.
Usage in Pregnancy: The safety of the use of Capastat Sulfate in pregnancy has not been determined.
Pediatric Usage: Safety and effectiveness in pediatric patients have not been established.

DESCRIPTION

Capastat Sulfate is a polypeptide antibiotic isolated from *Streptomyces capreolus*. It is a complex of 4 microbiologically active components which have been characterized in part; however, complete structural determination of all the components has not been established.

Capreomycin is supplied as the disulfate salt and is soluble in water. In complete solution, it is almost colorless.

Each vial contains the equivalent of 1 g capreomycin activity.

The structural formula is as follows:

	R	
Capreomycin IA	OH	$C_{25}H_{44}N_{14}O_8$
Capreomycin IB	H	$C_{25}H_{44}N_{14}O_7$

CLINICAL PHARMACOLOGY

Human Pharmacology: Capreomycin is not absorbed in significant quantities from the gastrointestinal tract and must be administered parenterally. In 2 studies of 10 patients each, peak serum concentrations following 1 g of capreomycin given intramuscularly were achieved in 1 to 2 hours after administration, and average peak levels reached were 28 and 32 µg/mL respectively (range, 20 to 47 µg/mL). Low

serum concentrations were present at 24 hours. However, 1 g of capreomycin daily for 30 days or more produced no significant accumulation in subjects with normal renal function. Two patients with marked reduction of renal function had high serum concentrations 24 hours after administration of the drug. When a 1-g dose of capreomycin was given intramuscularly to normal volunteers, 52% was excreted in the urine within 12 hours.

Paper chromatographic studies indicated that capreomycin is excreted essentially unaltered. Urine concentrations averaged 1.68 μg/mL (average urine volume, 228 mL) during the 6 hours following a 1-g dose.

Microbiology: Capreomycin is active against strains of *Mycobacterium tuberculosis* found in humans.

Susceptibility Tests: The in vitro susceptibility of strains of *M. tuberculosis* to capreomycin varies with the media and techniques employed. In general, the minimum inhibitory concentrations for *M. tuberculosis* are lowest in liquid media that are free of egg protein (7H10 or Dubos) and range from 1 to 5 μg/mL when the indirect method is used. Comparable inhibitory concentrations are obtained when 7H10 agar is used for direct susceptibility testing. When indirect susceptibility tests are performed on standard tube slants with 7H10 media, susceptible strains are inhibited by 10 to 25 μg/mL capreomycin. Egg-containing media, such as Löwenstein-Jensen or ATS, require concentrations of 25 to 50 μg/mL to inhibit susceptible strains.

Cross-Resistance: Frequent cross-resistance occurs between capreomycin and viomycin. Varying degrees of cross-resistance between capreomycin and kanamycin and neomycin have been reported. No cross-resistance has been observed between capreomycin and isoniazid, aminosalicylic acid, cycloserine, streptomycin, ethionamide, or ethambutol.

INDICATIONS AND USAGE

Capastat Sulfate, which is to be used concomitantly with other appropriate antituberculosis agents, is indicated in pulmonary infections caused by capreomycin-susceptible strains of *M. tuberculosis* when the primary agents (isoniazid, rifampin, ethambutol, aminosalicylic acid, and streptomycin) have been ineffective or cannot be used because of toxicity or the presence of resistant tubercle bacilli.

Susceptibility studies should be performed to determine the presence of a capreomycin-susceptible strain of *M. tuberculosis*.

CONTRAINDICATION

Capastat Sulfate is contraindicated in patients who are hypersensitive to capreomycin.

PRECAUTIONS

General: Audiometric measurements and assessment of vestibular function should be performed prior to initiation of therapy with Capastat Sulfate and at regular intervals during treatment.

Renal injury, with tubular necrosis, elevation of the blood urea nitrogen (BUN) or serum creatinine, and abnormal urinary sediment, has been noted. Slight elevation of the BUN and serum creatinine has been observed in a significant number of patients receiving prolonged therapy. The appearance of casts, red cells, and white cells in the urine has been noted in a high percentage of these cases. Elevation of the BUN above 30 mg/100 mL, or any other evidence of decreasing renal function with or without a rise in BUN levels calls for careful evaluation of the patient, and the dosage should be reduced or the drug completely withdrawn. The clinical significance of abnormal urine sediment and slight elevation in the BUN (or serum creatinine) observed during long-term therapy with Capastat Sulfate has not been established.

The peripheral neuromuscular blocking action that has been attributed to other polypeptide antibiotics (colistin sulfate, polymyxin A sulfate, paromomycin, and viomycin) and to aminoglycoside antibiotics (streptomycin, dihydrostreptomycin, neomycin, and kanamycin) has been studied with Capastat Sulfate. A partial neuromuscular blockade was demonstrated after large intravenous doses of Capastat Sulfate. This action was enhanced by ether anesthesia (as has been reported for neomycin) and was antagonized by neostigmine.

Caution should be exercised in the administration of antibiotics, including Capastat Sulfate, to any patient who has demonstrated some form of allergy, particularly to drugs.

Laboratory Tests: Regular tests of renal function should be made throughout the period of treatment, and reduced dosage should be employed in patients with known or suspected renal impairment.

Renal function studies should be made both before therapy with Capastat Sulfate is started and on a weekly basis during treatment.

Since hypokalemia may occur during therapy, serum potassium levels should be determined frequently.

Drug Interactions: For neuromuscular blocking action of this drug, *see* PRECAUTIONS, GENERAL.

Carcinogenesis, Mutagenesis, Impairment of Fertility: Studies have not been performed to determine potential for carcinogenicity, mutagenicity, or impairment of fertility.

Table 1. Estimated Dosages to Attain Steady-State Serum Capreomycin Concentration of 10 μg/mL (Based on Creatinine Clearance)

CrCl (mL/min)	Capreomycin Clearance L/kg/h × 10^{-2})	Half-Life (hours)	Dose[a](mg/kg) for the Following Dosing Intervals		
			24 h	48 h	72 h
0	0.54	55.5	1.29	2.58	3.87
10	1.01	29.4	2.43	4.87	7.30
20	1.49	20.0	3.58	7.16	10.7
30	1.97	15.1	4.72	9.45	14.2
40	2.45	12.2	5.87	11.7	
50	2.92	10.2	7.01	14.0	
60	3.40	8.8	8.16		
80	4.35	6.8	10.4[b]		
100	5.31	5.6	12.7[b]		
110	5.78	5.2	13.9[b]		

a. For patients with renal impairment, initial maintenance dose estimates are given for optional dosing intervals; longer dosing intervals are expected to provide greater peak and lower trough serum capreomycin levels than shorter dosing intervals.

b. The usual dosage for patients with *normal* renal function is 1,000 mg daily, not to exceed 20 mg/kg/day, for 60 to 120 days, then 1,000 mg 2 to 3 times weekly.

Parenteral drug products should be inspected visually for particulate matter and discoloration prior to administration, whenever solution and container permit.

Usage in Pregnancy—Pregnancy Category C: Capastat Sulfate has been shown to be teratogenic in rats when given in doses 3 1/2 times the human dose. There are no adequate and well-controlled studies in pregnant women. Capastat Sulfate should be used during pregnancy only if the potential benefit justifies the potential risk to the fetus (*see boxed* WARNINGS *and* ANIMAL PHARMACOLOGY).

Nursing Mothers: It is not known whether this drug is excreted in human milk. Because many drugs are excreted in human milk, caution should be exercised when Capastat Sulfate is administered to a nursing woman.

Pediatric Use: Safety and effectiveness in pediatric patients have not been established (*see boxed* WARNINGS).

ADVERSE REACTIONS

Nephrotoxicity: In 36% of 722 patients treated with Capastat Sulfate, elevation of the BUN above 20 mg/100 mL has been observed. In many instances, there was also depression of PSP excretion and abnormal urine sediment. In 10% of this series, the BUN elevation exceeded 30 mg/100 mL. Toxic nephritis was reported in 1 patient with tuberculosis and portal cirrhosis who was treated with Capastat Sulfate (1 g) and aminosalicylic acid daily for 1 month. This patient developed renal insufficiency and oliguria and died. Autopsy showed subsiding acute tubular necrosis.

Electrolyte disturbances resembling Bartter's syndrome have been reported in 1 patient.

Ototoxicity: Subclinical auditory loss was noted in approximately 11% of 722 patients undergoing treatment with Capastat Sulfate. This was a 5- to 10-decibel loss in the 4,000- to 8,000-CPS range. Clinically apparent hearing loss occurred in 3% of the 722 subjects. Some audiometric changes were reversible. Other cases with permanent loss were not progressive following withdrawal of Capastat Sulfate.

Tinnitus and vertigo have occurred.

Liver: Serial tests of liver function have demonstrated a decrease in BSP excretion without change in AST (SGOT) or ALT (SGPT) in the presence of preexisting liver disease. Abnormal results in liver function tests have occurred in many persons receiving Capstat Sulfate in combination with other antituberculosis agents that also are known to cause changes in hepatic function. The role of Capastat Sulfate in producing these abnormalities is not clear; however, periodic determinations of liver function are recommended.

Blood: Leukocytosis and leukopenia have been observed. The majority of patients treated have had eosinophilia exceeding 5% while receiving daily injections of Capastat Sulfate. This has subsided with reduction of the Capastat Sulfate dosage to 2 or 3 g weekly.

Pain and induration at the injection site have been observed. Excessive bleeding at the injection site has been reported. Sterile abscesses have been noted. Rare cases of thrombocytopenia have been reported.

Hypersensitivity: Urticaria and maculopapular skin rashes associated in some cases with febrile reactions have been reported when Capastat Sulfate and other antituberculosis drugs were given concomitantly.

OVERDOSAGE

Signs and Symptoms: Nephrotoxicity following the parenteral administration of Capastat Sulfate is most closely related to the area under the curve of the serum concentration versus time graph. The elderly patient, patients with abnormal renal function or dehydration, and patients receiving other nephrotoxic drugs are at much greater risk for developing acute tubular necrosis.

Damage to the auditory and vestibular divisions of cranial nerve VIII has been associated with Capastat Sulfate given to patients with abnormal renal function or dehydration and in those receiving medications with additive auditory toxicities. These patients often experience dizziness, tinnitus, vertigo, and a loss of high-tone acuity.

Neuromuscular blockage or respiratory paralysis may occur following rapid intravenous administration.

If capreomycin is ingested, toxicity would be unlikely because it is poorly absorbed (less than 1%) from an intact gastrointestinal system.

Hypokalemia, hypocalcemia, hypomagnesemia, and an electrolyte disturbance resembling Bartter's syndrome have been reported to occur in patients with capreomycin toxicity. The subcutaneous median lethal dose in mice was 514 mg/kg.

Treatment: To obtain up-to-date information about the treatment of overdose, a good resource is your certified Regional Poison Control Center. Telephone numbers of certified poison control centers are listed in the *Physicians' Desk Reference (PDR)*. In managing overdosage, consider the possibility of multiple drug overdoses, interaction among drugs, and unusual drug kinetics in your patient.

Protect the patient's airway and support ventilation and perfusion. Meticulously monitor and maintain, within acceptable limits, the patient's vital signs, blood gases, serum electrolyes, etc. Absorption of drugs from the gastrointestinal tract may be decreased by giving activated charcoal, which, in many cases, is more effective than emesis or lavage; consider charcoal instead of or in addition to gastric emptying. Repeated doses of charcoal over time may hasten elimination of some drugs that have been absorbed. Safeguard the patient's airway when employing gastric emptying or charcoal.

Patients who have received an overdose of capreomycin and have normal renal function should be carefully hydrated to maintain a urine output of 3 to 5 mL/kg/h. Fluid balance, electrolytes, and creatinine clearance should be carefully monitored.

Hemodialysis may be effectively used to remove capreomycin in patients with significant renal disease.

DOSAGE AND ADMINISTRATION

Capastat Sulfate is for intramuscular use only.

Capastat Sulfate should be given by deep intramuscular injection into a large muscle mass, since superficial injection may be associated with increased pain and the development of sterile abscesses.

Capastat Sulfate should be dissolved in 2 mL of 0.9% Sodium Chloride Injection or Sterile Water for Injection. Two to 3 minutes should be allowed for complete dissolution. For administration of a 1-g dose, the entire contents of the vial should be given. For doses lower than 1 g, the following dilution table may be used.

DILUTION TABLE

Diluent Added to 1-g, 10-mL Vial	Volume of Capastat Sulfate Solution	Concentration (Approx)
2.15 mL	2.85 mL	350 mg*/mL
2.63 mL	3.33 mL	300 mg*/mL
3.3 mL	4 mL	250 mg*/mL
4.3 mL	5 mL	200 mg*/mL

*Equivalent to capreomycin activity.

The solution may acquire a pale straw color and darken with time, but this is not associated with loss of potency or the development of toxicity. After reconstitution, solutions of Capastat Sulfate may be stored for 48 hours at room temperature and up to 14 days under refrigeration

Capreomycin is always administered in combination with at least 1 other antituberculosis agent to which the patient's strain of tubercle bacilli is susceptible. The usual dose is 1 g

Continued on next page

Dura—Cont.

daily (not to exceed 20 mg/kg/day) given intramuscularly for 60 to 120 days, followed by 1 g intramuscularly 2 or 3 times weekly. (*Note*—Therapy for tuberculosis should be maintained for 12 to 24 months. If facilities for administering injectable medication are not available, a change to appropriate oral therapy is indicated on the patient's release from the hospital.)

Patients with reduced renal function should have dosage reduction based on creatinine clearance using the guidelines included in Table 1. These dosages are designed to achieve a mean steady-state capreomycin level of 10 μg/mL.

[See table on top of preceding page.]

HOW SUPPLIED

Capastat® Sulfate, Sterile Capreomycin Sulfate, USP, is available in:

Vials: 1 g*/10 mL size (UC5001) (1s) NDC 51479-018-01

---

*Equivalent to capreomycin activity.

Store at controlled room temperature 59° to 86°F (15° to 30°C) prior to reconstitution.

ANIMAL PHARMACOLOGY

In addition to renal and cranial nerve VIII toxicity demonstrated in animal toxicology studies, cataracts developed in 2 dogs on doses of 62 mg/kg and 100 mg/kg for prolonged periods.

In teratology studies, a low incidence of "wavy ribs" was noted in litters of female rats treated with daily doses of 50 mg/kg or more of capreomycin.

CAUTION: Federal (USA) law prohibits dispensing without prescription.

Literature revised April 8, 1996

DURA PHARMACEUTICALS

Manufactured by: Eli Lilly and Company
Indianapolis, IN 46285
Distributed by: DURA Pharmaceuticals, Inc.
San Diego, CA 92121
PA 7951 UCP   CSV003B1095

D.A. CHEWABLE™ Tablets   ℞

DESCRIPTION

Each D.A. CHEWABLE TABLET for oral administration contains:

chlorpheniramine maleate............................... 2 mg
phenylephrine HCl....................................... 10 mg
methscopolamine nitrate .... 1.25 mg

in an orange-flavored and orange-colored chewable tablet.

Chlorpheniramine maleate is an antihistamine having the chemical name: 2-Pyridinepropanamine, γ-(4chlorophenyl)-N,N-dimethyl-,(Z)-2-butenedioate(1:1)

Phenylephrine HCl is a decongestant having the chemical name:

Benzenemethanol, 3-hydroxy-α[(methylamino) methyl]-, hydrochloride.

Methscopolamine nitrate is an anticholinergic having the chemical name: 3-Oxa-9-azoniatricyclo[3.3.1.0^{2,4}] nonane, 7-(3-hydroxy-1-oxo-2-phenylpropoxy)-9,9-dimethyl-, nitrate, [7(S)-(1 α, 2 β, 4 β, 5 α, 7 β)]-

Inactive ingredients: artificial orange flavor, aspartame, colloidal silicon dioxide, croscarmellose sodium, FD&C yellow #6 (aluminum lake), magnesium stearate, malic acid, mannitol, microcrystalline cellulose, vanillin.

CLINICAL PHARAMACOLOGY

Chlorpheniramine maleate is an alkylamine-type antihistamine with anticholinergic and sedative effects. Antihistamines competitively antagonize histamine at the H$_1$ receptor site. This prevents histamine mediated increased vascular permeability, increased mucus production, pruritis and sneezing.

Phenylephrine HCl is a sympathomimetic amine that causes vasoconstriction via the activation of post-junctional α-adrenergic receptors located on the precapillary and post-capillary blood vessels of the nasal mucosa. Activation of these receptors occurs directly by binding of phenylephrine or indirectly by binding of norepinephrine released from sympathomimetic nerve endings in response to phenylephrine. The resulting vasoconstriction decreases blood flow through the nasal mucosa and results in a shrinkage of this tissue. Methscopolamine nitrate is quaternary ammonium derivative of the anticholinergic scopolamine, which possesses the peripheral actions of the belladonna alkaloids, but does not exhibit the central actions because of its lack of ability to cross the blood-brain barrier. Its antimuscarinic effect causes dryining of mucous secretions.

INDICATIONS

D.A. CHEWABLE is indicated for the temporary relief of symptoms of allergic rhinitis, vasomotor rhinitis, sinusitis and the common cold.

CONTRAINDICATIONS

Patients with hypersensitivity or idiosyncrasy to any of its ingredients. Sympathomimetic amines are contraindicated in patients with severe hypertension, severe coronary artery disease and patients on monoamine oxidase (MAO) inhibitor therapy. Antihistamines and anticholinergics are contraindicated in patients with narrow-angle glaucoma, urinary retention, peptic ulcer disease and during an asthma attack.

WARNINGS

Sympathomimetic amines should be used cautiously with hypertension, diabetes mellitus, ischemic heart disease, hyperthyroidism, increased intraocular pressure and prostatic hypertrophy. **See Contraindications**. Sympathomimetic amines may produce CNS stimulation and convulsions or cardiovascular collapse with accompanying hypotension. The elderly (60 years and older) are more likely to exhibit adverse reactions. Antihistamines may cause excitability, especially in children. At dosages higher than the recommended dose, nervousness, dizziness or sleeplessness may occur. Do not exceed recommended dose.

PRECAUTIONS

General: Should be used with caution in patients with diabetes mellitus, hypertension, cardiovascular disease and hyperreactivity to sympathomimetic amines. The antihistamines may cause drowsiness, and ambulatory patients who operate machinery or motor vehicles should be cautioned accordingly.

Phenylketonurics: Contains phenylanine 7.5 mg per tablet.

Information for Patients: Antihistamines may impair mental and physicial abilities required for the performance of potentially hazardous tasks such as driving a vehicle or operating machinery. The antihistamine in this product may have additive effects with alcohol and other central nervous system depressants (hypnotics, sedatives, tranquilizers).

Drug Interactions: Monoamine oxidase (MAO) inhibitors and beta-adrenergic blockers increase the effects of sympathomimetic amines. Sympathomimetic amines may reduce the antihypertensive effects of methyldopa, mecamylamine, and reserpine. Concomitant use of antihistamines with alcohol, tricyclic antidepressants, barbiturates and other CNS depressants may have an additive effect.

Pregnancy Category C: Animal reproduction studies have not been conducted with D.A. CHEWABLE. It is also not known whether D.A. CHEWABLE can cause fetal harm when administered to a pregnant woman or can affect reproductive capacity. D.A. CHEWABLE should be given to a pregnant woman only if clearly needed.

Nursing Mothers: It is not known whether the drugs in D.A CHEWABLE are excreted in human milk. Because many drugs are excreted in human milk and because of the potential for serious adverse reactions in nursing infants, a decision should be made whether to discontinue nursing or discontinue the product, taking into account the importance of the drug to the mother.

Pediatric Use: Safety and effectiveness of D.A. CHEWABLE in pediatric patients younger than 6 years of age have not been established.

ADVERSE REACTIONS

Sympathomimetic amines may cause tachycardia, palpitations, nervousness, insomnia, restlessness, headache, gastric irritation, and irritability. Sympathomimetic amines have been associated with certain untoward reactions including fear, anxiety, tenseness, restlessness, tremor, weakness, pallor, respiratory difficulty, dysuria, insomnia, hallucinations, convulsions, CNS depression, arrhythmias and cardiovascular collapse with hypotension. Urinary retention may occur in patients with prostatic hypertrophy. Antihistamines and anticholinergics may cause drowsiness, dizziness, blurred vision, and excessive dryness of the nose, throat and mouth.

OVERDOSAGE

The treatment of overdosage should provide symptomatic and supportive care. Induction of emesis and gastric lavage may be performed if the patients is alert and seen within early hours after ingestion. Drug remaining in the stomach may be adsorbed by the administration of activated charcoal. Stimulants should not be used because they may precipitate convulsions. If convulsions or marked CNS excitement occurs, treatment with appropriate measures is indicated.

DOSAGE AND ADMINISTRATION

Adults and adolescents 12 years of age and older: 1–2 tablets every 4 hours. Children 6 to 12 years of age: 1 tablet every 4 hours. Tablets may be broken in half for ease of administration.

HOW SUPPLIED

D.A. CHEWABLE Tablets are available as orange flavored and orange colored scored tablets imprinted with *DURA* on one side and *CHEW* on the other.

Bottles of 100 (NDC 51479-013-01).

Store at room temperature, 15°–25°C (59°–77°F).

Dispense in a tight, light-resistant container (USP/NF) with a child-resistant closure.

CAUTION: Federal law prohibits dispensing without a prescription.

Manufactured for
Dura Pharmaceuticals, Inc.
San Diego, CA 92121
Manufactured by
Anabolic, Inc.
Irvine, CA 92614
© 1996 Dura Pharmaceuticals, Inc.
DACT005H0596

DURA–GEST®   ℞
DECONGESTANT/EXPECTORANT CAPSULE

DESCRIPTION

Each Dura-Gest gray and white capsule for oral administration contains:

phenylephrine hydrochloride..............................5 mg
phenylpropanolamine hydrochloride ....45 mg
guaifenesin ....200 mg

HOW SUPPLIED

DURA-GEST gray and white capsules are imprinted with "*DURA-GEST*" and "*51479005*".

Bottles of 100 (NDC 51479-005-01).

Bottles of 500 (NDC 51479-005-05).

Dispense in a tight, light-resistant container (USP/NF) with a child-resistant closure. Store at controlled temperature 15°–25°C (59°–77°F).

Caution: Federal law prohibits dispensing without prescription.

Manufactured for Dura Pharmaceuticals, Inc. San Diego, CA 92121

Manufactured by Anabolic, Inc. Irvine, CA 92614

© 1996 Dura Pharmaceuticals, Inc.   DG003E0396

DURA-TAP/PD®   ℞
Antihistamine/Decongestant

DESCRIPTION

Each Dura-Tap/PD opaque blue and clear capsule containing white beads for oral administration contains:

chlorpheniramine maleate .... 4 mg
pseudoephedrine hydrochloride .... 60 mg

In a specially-prepared base to provide a prolonged therapeutic effect. Chlorpheniramine maleate is an antihistamine having the chemical name:

2-Pyridinepropanamine, γ-(4-chlorophenyl)-N, N-dimethyl-, (Z)-2-butenedeioate(1:1)

Pseudoephedrine hydrochloride is a decongestant having the chemical name:

Benzenemethanol, α-[1-(methylamino)ethyl]-, [S-(R*,R*)]-, hydrochloride.

Inactive ingredients: corn starch, D&C Red #28, FD&C Blue #1, gelatin, pharmaceutical glaze, silicon dioxide, sodium lauryl sulfate, sucrose, titanium dioxide, and other proprietary ingredients.

CLINICAL PHARMACOLOGY

Chlorpheniramine maleate is an alkylamine-type antihistamine with anticholinergic and sedative effects. Antihistamines competitively antagonize histamine at the H$_1$ receptor site. This prevents histamine-mediated increased vascular permeability, increased mucus production, pruritis and sneezing. Pseudoephedrine HCl is an orally active sympathomimetic amine which predominantly effects alpha receptors. It provides relief of nasal congestion by causing constriction of blood vessels and a reduction of blood supply to nasal mucosa, thereby decreasing the volume of blood in the sinusoids and the amount of mucosal edema. Pseudoephedrine produces peripheral effects similar to those of epinephrine and central effects similar to, but less intense than, amphetamines. It has a potential for excitatory side effects.

INDICATIONS

For the temporary relief of symptoms associated with allergic rhinitis, vasomotor rhinitis, sinusitis and the common cold.

CONTRAINDICATIONS

Patients with hypersensitivity or idiosyncrasy to any of its ingredients. Sympathomimetic amines are contraindicated in patients with severe hypertension, severe coronary artery disease and patients on monoamine oxidase (MAO) inhibitor therapy.

Antihistamines are contraindicated in patients with narrow-angle glaucoma, urinary retention, peptic ulcer disease and during an asthma attack.

WARNINGS

Sympathomimetic amines should be used cautiously in patients with hypertension, diabetes mellitus, ischemic heart disease, hyperthyroidism, increased intraocular pressure or prostatic hypertrophy. **See Contraindications.** Sympathomimetic amines may produce CNS stimulation with convulsions or cardiovascular collapse with accompanying hypotension. The elderly (60 years and older) are more likely to exhibit adverse reactions. Antihistamines may cause excitability, especially in children. At doses higher than the recommended dose, nervousness, dizziness, or sleeplessness may occur. Do not exceed recommended dosage.

PRECAUTIONS

General: Should be used with caution in patients with diabetes mellitus, hypertension, cardiovascular disease and hyperreactivity to sympathomimetic amines. Antihistamines may cause drowsiness and ambulatory patients who operate machinery or motor vehicles should be cautioned accordingly.

Information for Patients: Antihistamines may impair mental and physical abilities required for the performance of potentially hazardous tasks, such as driving a vehicle or operating machinery. The antihistamine in this product may have additive effects with alcohol and other central nervous system depressants (hypnotics, sedatives, tranquilizers).

Drug Interactions: Monoamine oxidase (MAO) inhibitors and beta-adrenergic blockers increase the effect of sympathomimetic amines. Sympathomimetic amines may reduce the antihypertensive effects of methyldopa, mecamylamine and reserpine. Concomitant use of antihistamines with alcohol, tricyclic antidepressants, barbiturates and other CNS depressants may have an additive effect.

Pregnancy Category C: Animal reproduction studies have not been conducted with Dura-Tap/PD. It is also not known whether Dura-Tap/PD can cause fetal harm when administered to a pregnant woman or can affect reproductive capacity. Dura-Tap/PD should be given to a pregnant woman only if clearly needed.

Nursing Mothers: It is not known whether the drugs in Dura-Tap/PD are excreted in human milk. Because many drugs are excreted in human milk and because of the potential for serious adverse reactions in nursing infants, a decision should be made whether to discontinue nursing or discontinue the product, taking into account the importance of the drug to the mother.

Pediatric Use: Safety and effectiveness of Dura-Tap/PD in pediatric patients below the age of 6 years have not been established.

ADVERSE REACTIONS

Sympathomimetic amines may cause tachycardia, palpitations, nervousness, insomnia, restlessness, headache, gastric irritation, and irritability. Sympathomimetic amines have been associated with certain untoward reactions including fear, anxiety, tenseness, restlessness, tremor, weakness, pallor, respiratory difficulty, dysuria, insomnia, hallucinations, convulsions, CNS depression, arrhythmias and cardiovascular collapse with hypotension. Urinary retention may occur in patients with prostatic hypertrophy. Antihistamines may cause drowsiness, dizziness, blurred vision, and excessive dryness of the nose, throat and mouth.

OVERDOSAGE

The treatment of overdosage should provide symptomatic and supportive care. Induction of emesis and gastric lavage may be performed if the patient is alert and seen within early hours after ingestion. Drug remaining in the stomach may be absorbed by the administration of activated charcoal. Stimulants should not be used because they may precipitate convulsions. If convulsions or marked CNS excitement occur, treatment with appropriate measures is indicated. Since the effects of Dura-Tap/PD may last up to 12 hours, the patient should be monitored for at least that length of time and treated as necessary.

DOSAGE AND ADMINISTRATION

Adults and adolescents over 12 years of age: two capsules every 12 hours. Children 6 to 12 years of age: one capsule every 12 hours. Not recommended for pediatric patients under 6 years of age.

HOW SUPPLIED

Dura-Tap/PD is available as an opaque blue and clear capsule coded with the imprints 51479 and 007. Bottles of 100 (NDC 51479-007-01).
Store at room temperature, 15°–23°C (59°–73°F).
Dispense in a tight, light-resistant container (USP/NF) with a child-resistant closure.
CAUTION: Federal law prohibits dispensing without prescription.
Manufactured for
Dura Pharmaceuticals, Inc.
San Diego, CA 92121
Manufactured by
Central Pharmaceuticals, Inc.
Seymour, IN 47274

© 1996 Dura Pharmaceuticals, Inc.
DTPD002E0496

DURA-VENT® ℞
DECONGESTANT/EXPECTORANT TABLET

DESCRIPTION

Each DURA-VENT white, scored tablet for oral administration contains:
Phenylpropanolamine hydrochloride .... 75 mg
Guaifenesin .... 600 mg
in a special base to provide a prolonged therapeutic effect. Phenylpropanolamine hydrochloride is a decongestant having the chemical name:
Benzenemethanol, α-(1-aminoethyl)-, hydrochloride, (R^*, S^*)-,$(\pm)$.
Guaifenesin is an expectorant having the chemical name: 1,2-Propanediol, 3-(2-methoxyphenoxy)-.
Inactive ingredients: dicalcium phosphate, hydrogenated cottonseed oil, magnesium stearate, methylcellulose, microcrystalline cellulose, silicon dioxide, stearic acid, tricalcium phosphate.

CLINICAL PHARMACOLOGY

Phenylpropanolamine hydrochloride is a sympathomimetic amine that causes vasoconstriction via the activation of postjunctional α-adrenergic receptors located on the pre-capillary and post-capillary blood vessels of the nasal mucosa. Activation of these receptors occurs directly by binding of phenylpropanolamine or indirectly by binding of norepinephrine released from sympathomimetic nerve endings in response to phenylpropanolamine. The resulting vasoconstriction decreases blood flow through the nasal mucosa and results in a shrinkage of this tissue. Phenylpropanolamine also has beta adrenergic effects. This increases heart rate, force of contraction, cardiac output, and excitability. Phenylpropanolamine causes CNS stimulation and reportedly has an anorexigenic effect.
Guaifenesin promotes lower respiratory tract drainage by thinning bronchial secretions, and facilitates removal of viscous, inspissated mucus. By reducing the viscosity of secretions, guaifenesin increases the efficiency of the cough reflex and of the ciliary action in removing accumulated secretions from the trachea and bronchi.

INDICATIONS AND USAGE

DURA-VENT is indicated for the temporary symptomatic relief of sinusitis, bronchitis, pharyngitis, and the common cold when these conditions are associated with nasal congestion and viscous mucus in the lower respiratory tract.

CONTRAINDICATIONS

Patients with hypersensitivity or idiosyncrasy to any of its ingredients. Sympathomimetic amines are contraindicated in patients with severe hypertension, severe coronary artery disease and patients on monoamine oxidase (MAO) inhibitor therapy.

WARNINGS

Sympathomimetic amines should be used cautiously in patients with hypertension, diabetes mellitus, ischemic heart disease, hyperthyroidism, increased intraocular pressure and prostatic hypertrophy. **See Contraindications.** Sympathomimetic amines may produce CNS stimulation and convulsions or cardiovascular collapse with accompanying hypotension. The elderly (60 years and older) are more likely to exhibit adverse reactions. Do not exceed recommended dosage. Also, this produce should not be taken simultaneously with other products containing phenylpropanolamine, phenylephrine, pseudoephedrine, ephedrine, or amphetamines.

PRECAUTIONS

General: Should be used with caution in patients with diabetes mellitus, hypertension, cardiovascular disease and hyperreactivity to sympathomimetic amines.
Information for Patients: Do not crush or chew DURA-VENT tablets prior to swallowing.
Drug Interactions: Monoamine oxidase (MAO) inhibitors and beta-adrenergic blockers increase the effect of sympathomimetic amines. Sympathomimetic amines may reduce the antihypertensive effects of methyldopa, mecamylamine and reserpine.
Drug/Laboratory Test Interactions: Guaifenesin has been reported to interfere with clinical laboratory determinations of urinary 5-hydroxyindoleacetic acid (5-HIAA) and urinary vanillylmandelic acid (VMA).
Pregnancy Category C: Animal reproduction studies have not been conducted with DURA-VENT. It is also not known whether Dura-Vent can cause fetal harm when administered to a pregnant woman or can affect reproduction capacity. DURA-VENT should be given to a pregnant woman only if clearly needed.
Nursing Mothers: It is not known whether the drugs in DURA-VENT are excreted in human milk. Because many drugs are excreted in human milk and because of the potential for serious adverse reactions in nursing infants, a deci-

sion should be made whether to discontinue nursing or discontinue the product, taking into account the importance of the drug to the mother.
Pediatric Use: Safety and effectiveness of DURA-VENT in pediatric patients below the age of 6 years have not been established.

ADVERSE REACTIONS

Sympathomimetic amines may cause tachycardia, palpitations, nervousness, insomnia, restlessness, headache, gastric irritation, and irritability. Sympathomimetic amines have been associated with certain untoward reactions including fear, anxiety, tenseness, restlessness, tremor, weakness, pallor, respiratory difficulty, dysuria, insomnia, hallucinations, convulsions, CNS depression, arrhythmias and cardiovascular collapse with hypotension. Urinary retention may occur in patients with prostatic hypertrophy. Guaifenesin may cause nausea, vomiting, diarrhea, and gastric irritation.

OVERDOSAGE

The treatment of overdosage should provide symptomatic and supportive care. Induction of emesis and gastric lavage may be performed if the patient is alert and seen within early hours after ingestion. Drug remaining in the stomach may be absorbed by the administration of activated charcoal. Stimulants should not be used because they may precipitate convulsions. If convulsions or marked CNS excitement occur, treatment with appropriate measures is indicated. Since the effects of DURA-VENT may last up to 12 hours, the patient should be monitored for at least that length of time and treated as necessary.

DOSAGE AND ADMINISTRATION

Adults and adolescents 12 years of age and older: one tablet twice daily (every 12 hours). Children 6 to under 12 years: one-half ($^1/_2$) tablet twice daily (every 12 hours). DURA-VENT is not recommended for pediatric patients under 6 years of age. Tablets may be broken in half for ease of administration without affecting release of medication, but should not be crushed or chewed prior to swallowing.

HOW SUPPLIED

DURA-VENT is available as a white, scored tablet imprinted with 7.5/7.5 on one side and *DURA* on the other.
Bottles of 100 (NDC 51479-006-01).
Bottles of 600 (NDC 51479-006-06).
Store at room temperature, 15°–25°C (59°–77°F).
Dispense in a tight, light-resistant container (USP/NF) with a child-resistant closure.
Caution: Federal law prohibits dispensing without prescription.
Manufactured for
Dura Pharmaceuticals, Inc.
San Diego, CA 92121
Manufactured by
Anabolic, Inc.
Irvine, CA 92614
© 1996 Dura Pharmaceuticals, Inc.
DV001F0396

DURA-VENT®/A ℞
Decongestant/Antihistamine

DESCRIPTION

Each Dura-Vent/A clear capsule for oral administration contains:
phenylpropanolamine hydrochloride .... 75 mg
chlorpheniramine maleate .... 10 mg
Phenylpropanolamine hydrochloride is a decongestant having the chemical name:
Benzenemethanol, α-(1-amino-ethyl)-, hydrochloride, (R^*, S^*)-,$(\pm)$.
Chlorpheniramine maleate is an antihistamine having the chemical name:
2-Pyridinepropanamine, γ-(4-chlorophenyl)-N,N-dimethyl-, (Z)-2-butenedioate (1:1)
Inactive ingredients: benzyl alcohol, butylparaben, corn starch, edetate calcium disodium, gelatin, methylparaben, pharmaceutical glaze, propylparaben, sodium lauryl sulfate, sodium propionate, sucrose, and other proprietary ingredients.

HOW SUPPLIED

Dura-Vent/A clear capsules are imprinted with *DURA-VENT/A* and 51479002.
Bottles of 100 (NDC 51479-002-01).
Store at room temperature, 15°–23°C (59°–73°F).
Dispense in a tight, light-resistant container (USP/NF) with a child-resistant closure.

Continued on next page

Dura—Cont.

D.A. II™ Tablet
Dura-Vent®/DA Tablet ℞

DESCRIPTION

Antihistamine/decongestant/anticholinergic combination tablets for oral use.

D.A. II™ Tablet

Each white, capsule-shaped tablet contains:

chlorpheniramine maleate	4 mg
phenylephrine HCl	10 mg
methscopolamine nitrate	1.25 mg

In a specially prepared base to provide a prolonged therapeutic effect.

Inactive ingredients: dicalcium phosphate, hydrogenated cottonseed oil, magnesium stearate, methylcellulose, stearic acid, microcrystalline cellulose, and silicon dioxide.

Dura-Vent®/DA Tablet

Each light brown, scored tablet contains:

chlorpheniramine maleate	8 mg
phenylephrine HCl	20 mg
methscopolamine nitrate	2.5 mg

In a specially prepared base to provide a prolonged therapeutic effect.

Inactive ingredients: D&C yellow #10 (aluminum lake), dicalcium phosphate, FD&C blue #1 (aluminum lake), FD&C red #40 (aluminum lake), hydrogenated cottonseed oil, magnesium stearate, methylcellulose, silica gel, and stearic acid.

Chlorpheniramine maleate is an antihistamine having the chemical name: 2-Pyridinepropanamine, γ-(4-chlorophenyl)-N,N-dimethyl-, (Z)-2-butenedioate(1:1).

Phenylephrine HCl is a decongestant having the chemical name: Benzenemethanol, 3-hydroxy-α-[(methylamino) methyl]-, hydrochloride.

Methscopolamine nitrate is an anticholinergic having the chemical name: 3-Oxa-9-azonlatricyclo [3.3.1.0²⁴] nonane, 7-(3-hydroxy-1-oxo-2-phenylpropoxy)-9,9-dimethyl-,nitrate, [7(S)-(1α, 2β, 4β, 5α, 7β)]-.

CLINICAL PHARMACOLOGY

Chlorpheniramine maleate is an alkylamine-type antihistamine with anticholinergic and sedative effects. Antihistamines competitively antagonize histamine at the H_1 receptor site. This prevents histamine mediated increased vascular permeability, increased mucus production, pruritis and sneezing.

Phenylephrine HCl is a sympathomimetic amine that causes vasoconstriction via the activation of post-junctional α-adrenergic receptors located on the pre-capillary and post-capillary blood vessels of the nasal mucosa. Activation of these receptors occur directly by binding of phenylephrine or indirectly by binding of norepinephrine released from sympathomimetic nerve endings in response to phenylephrine. The resulting vasoconstriction decreases blood flow through the nasal mucosa and results in a shrinkage of this tissue.

Methscopolamine nitrate is a quaternary ammonium derivative of the anticholinergic scopolamine, which possesses the peripheral actions of the belladonna alkaloids, but does not exhibit the central actions because of its lack of ability to cross the blood-brain barrier. Its antimuscarinic effect causes drying of mucous secretions.

INDICATIONS AND USAGE

For the temporary relief of symptoms associated with allergic rhinitis, vasomotor rhinitis, sinusitis and the common cold.

CONTRAINDICATIONS

Patients with hypersensitivity or idiosyncrasy to any of its ingredients. Sympathomimetic amines are contraindicated in patients with severe hypertension, severe coronary artery disease and patients on monoamine oxidase (MAO) inhibitor therapy. Antihistamines and anticholinergics are contraindicated in patients with narrow-angle glaucoma, urinary retention, peptic ulcer disease and during an asthma attack.

WARNINGS

Sympathomimetic amines should be used cautiously in patients with hypertension, diabetes mellitus, ischemic heart disease, hyperthyroidism, increased intraocular pressure and prostatic hypertrophy. See Contraindications. Sympathomimetic amines may produce CNS stimulation and convulsions or cardiovascular collapse with accompanying hypotension. The elderly (60 years and older) are more likely to exhibit adverse reactions. Antihistamines may cause excitability, especially in children. At dosages higher than the recommended dose, nervousness, dizziness or sleeplessness may occur. Do not exceed recommended dose.

PRECAUTIONS

General: Should be used with caution in patients with diabetes mellitus, hypertension, cardiovascular disease and hyperreactivity to sympathomimetic amines. Antihistamines may cause drowsiness and ambulatory patients who operate machinery or motor vehicles should be cautioned accordingly.

Information for Patients: Antihistamines may impair mental and physical abilities required for the performance of potentially hazardous tasks, such as driving a vehicle or operating machinery. Do not crush or chew D.A. II or Dura-Vent/DA prior to swallowing. The antihistamine in this product may have additive effects with alcohol and other central nervous system depressants (hypnotics, sedatives, tranquilizers).

Drug Interactions: Monoamine oxidase (MAO) inhibitors and beta-adrenergic blockers increase the effect of sympathomimetic amines. Sympathomimetic amines may reduce the antihypertensive effects of methyldopa, mecamylamine and reserpine. Concomitant use of antihistamines with alcohol, tricyclic antidepressants, barbiturates and other CNS depressants may have an additive effect.

Pregnancy Category C: Animal reproduction studies have not been conducted with these products. It is also not known whether these products can cause fetal harm when administered to a pregnant woman or can affect reproductive capacity. Give to pregnant women only if clearly needed.

Nursing Mothers: It is not known whether the drugs in these products are excreted in human milk. Because many drugs are excreted in human milk and because of the potential for serious adverse reactions in nursing infants, a decision should be made whether to discontinue nursing or discontinue the product, taking into account the importance of the drug to the mother.

Pediatric Usage: Safety and effectiveness in pediatric patients below the age of 6 have not been established.

ADVERSE REACTIONS

Sympathomimetic amines may cause tachycardia, palpitations, nervousness, insomnia, restlessness, headache, gastric irritation, and irritability. Sympathomimetic amines have been associated with certain untoward reactions including fear, anxiety, tenseness, restlessness, tremor, weakness, pallor, respiratory difficulty, dysuria, insomnia, hallucinations, convulsions, CNS depression, arrhythmias, and cardiovascular collapse with hypotension. Urinary retention may occur in patients with prostatic hypertrophy. Antihistamines and anticholinergics may cause drowsiness, dizziness, blurred vision and excessive dryness of the nose, throat and mouth.

OVERDOSAGE

The treatment of overdosage should provide symptomatic and supportive care. Induction of emesis and gastric lavage may be performed if the patient is alert and seen within early hours after ingestion. Drug remaining in the stomach may be absorbed by the administration of activated charcoal. Stimulants should not be used because they may precipitate convulsions. If convulsions or marked CNS excitement occurs, treatment with appropriate measures is indicated. Since the effects of D.A. II and Dura-Vent/DA may last up to 12 hours, the patient should be monitored for at least that length of time and treated as necessary.

DOSAGE AND ADMINISTRATION

D.A. II Tablet

Adults and adolescents 12 years of age and older: two tablets twice daily (every 12 hours). Children 6 to 12 years of age: one tablet twice daily (every 12 hours). D.A. II is not recommended for pediatric patients under 6 years of age. Do not crush or chew tablets prior to swallowing.

Dura-Vent/DA Tablet

Adults and adolescents 12 years of age and older: one tablet twice daily (every 12 hours). Children 6 to 12 years of age: one-half ($^1/_2$) tablet twice daily (every 12 hours). Dura-Vent/DA is not recommended for pediatric patients under 6 years of age. Tablets may be broken in half for ease of administration without affecting release of medication, but should not be crushed or chewed prior to swallowing.

HOW SUPPLIED

D.A. II is available as a white, capsule-shaped tablet imprinted with *DURA* on one side and *DA II* on the other. Bottles of 100 (NDC 51479-028-01).

Dura-Vent/DA is available as a light brown, scored tablet imprinted with *DURA* on one side and *DA* on the other. Bottles of 100 (NDC 51479-008-01).

Store at room temperature 15°–25°C (59°–77°F). Dispense in a tight, light-resistant container (USP/NF) with a child-resistant closure.

CAUTION: Federal law prohibits dispensing without prescription.

Manufactured for
DURA Pharmaceuticals, Inc.
San Diego, CA 92121

Manufactured by
Anabolic, Inc.
Irvine, CA 92614
© 1996 Dura Pharmaceuticals, Inc.   DURA197A0496

ENTEX® capsules ℞

[n'tex]
(phenylephrine hydrochloride/
phenylpropanolamine
hydrochloride/guaifenesin)

DESCRIPTION

Each Entex orange and white capsule for oral administration contains

phenylephrine hydrochloride	5 mg
phenylpropanolamine hydrochloride	45 mg
guaifenesin	200 mg

This product contains ingredients of the following therapeutic classes: decongestant and expectorant.

HOW SUPPLIED

Entex orange and white capsules are imprinted "ENTEX" and "0149 0412".
NDC 51479-030-01 Bottles of 100
NDC 51479-030-05 Bottles of 500
Store below 86°F (30°C).

CAUTION

Federal law prohibits dispensing without prescription.

Manufactured by
Procter & Gamble Pharmaceuticals
Cincinnati, Ohio 45202
Manufactured for
DURA Pharmaceuticals, Inc.
San Diego, CA 92121
REVISED July 1996   EC003A0796

ENTEX® LIQUID ℞

[n'tex]
(phenylephrine hydrochloride/
phenylpropanolamine
hydrochloride/guaifenesin)

DESCRIPTION

Each 5 mL (one teaspoonful) for oral administration contains

phenylephrine hydrochloride	5 mg
phenylpropanolamine hydrochloride	20 mg
guaifenesin	100 mg
alcohol	5%

HOW SUPPLIED

Entex Liquid is available as an orange-colored, pleasant-tasting liquid.
NDC 51479-031-48 1 Pint (473 mL) bottle.
Store below 86°F (30°C). DO NOT REFRIGERATE.

CAUTION

Federal law prohibits dispensing without prescription.
Manufactured by
Procter & Gamble Pharmaceuticals
Cincinnati, Ohio 45202
Manufactured for
DURA Pharmaceuticals, Inc.
San Diego, CA 92121
Revised July 1996   EL002A0796

ENTEX® LA ℞

[n'tex]
(phenylpropanolamine
hydrochloride/guaifenesin)

DESCRIPTION

Each Entex LA orange, scored, long-acting tablet for oral administration contains

phenylpropanolamine hydrochloride	75 mg
guaifenesin	400 mg

in a special base to provide a prolonged therapeutic effect. This product contains ingredients of the following therapeutic classes: decongestant and expectorant.

Phenylpropanolamine hydrochloride is a decongestant having the chemical name, benzenemethanol, α-(1-aminoethyl)-, hydrochloride (R*, S*), (±), with the following structure:

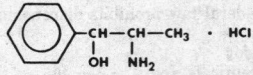

Guaifenesin is an expectorant having the chemical name, 1,2-propanediol, 3-(2-methoxyphenoxy)-, with the following structure:
[See chemical structure at top of next column.]

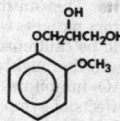

Inactive Ingredients: Each tablet contains carbomer 934 P, compressible sugar docusate sodium, FD&C Yellow No. 6 Aluminum Lake, hydroxypropyl cellulose, hydroxypropyl methylcellulose, polyethylene glycol, silicon dioxide, stearic acid, titanium dioxide, and zinc stearate.

CLINICAL PHARMACOLOGY

Phenylpropanolamine hydrochloride is an α-adrenergic receptor agonist (sympathomimetic) which produces vasoconstriction by stimulating α-receptors within the mucosa of the respiratory tract. Clinically, phenylpropanolamine shrinks swollen mucous membranes, reduces tissue hyperemia, edema, and nasal congestion, and increases nasal airway patency. Guaifenesin promotes lower respiratory tract drainage by thinning bronchial secretions, lubricates irritated respiratory tract membranes through increased mucous flow, and facilitates removal of viscous, inspissated mucus. As a result of these drugs, sinus and bronchial drainage is improved, and dry, nonproductive coughs become more productive and less frequent.

INDICATIONS AND USAGE

Entex LA is indicated for the symptomatic relief of sinusitis, bronchitis, pharyngitis, and coryza when these conditions are associated with nasal congestion and viscous mucus in the lower respiratory tract.

CONTRAINDICATIONS

Entex LA is contraindicated in individuals with known hypersensitivity to sympathomimetics, severe hypertension, or in patients receiving monoamine oxidase inhibitors.

WARNINGS

Sympathomimetic amines should be used with caution in patients with hypertension, diabetes mellitus, heart disease, peripheral vascular disease, increased intraocular pressure, hyperthyroidism, or prostatic hypertrophy.

PRECAUTIONS

Information for Patients: Do not crush or chew **Entex LA** tablets prior to swallowing.
Drug Interactions: **Entex LA** should not be used in patients taking monoamine oxidase inhibitors or other sympathomimetics.
Drug/Laboratory Test Interactions: Guaifenesin has been reported to interfere with clinical laboratory determinations of urinary 5-hydroxyindoleacetic acid (5-HIAA) and urinary vanillylmandelic acid (VMA).
Pregnancy: Pregnancy Category C. Animal reproduction studies have not been conducted with **Entex LA**. It is also not known whether **Entex LA** can cause fetal harm when administered to a pregnant woman or can affect reproduction capacity. **Entex LA** should be given to a pregnant woman only if clearly needed.
Nursing Mothers: It is not known whether the drugs in **Entex LA** are excreted in human milk. Because many drugs are excreted in human milk and because of the potential for serious adverse reactions in nursing infants, a decision should be made whether to discontinue nursing or to discontinue the product, taking into account the importance of the drug to the mother.
Pediatric Use: Safety and effectiveness of **Entex LA** tablets in pediatric patients below the age of 6 have not been established.

ADVERSE REACTIONS

Possible adverse reactions include nervousness, insomnia, restlessness, headache, nausea, or gastric irritation. These reactions seldom, if ever, require discontinuation of therapy. Urinary retention may occur in patients with prostatic hypertrophy.

OVERDOSAGE

The treatment of overdosage should provide symptomatic and supportive care. If the amount ingested is considered dangerous or excessive, induce vomiting with ipecac syrup unless the patient is convulsing, comatose, or has lost the gag reflex, in which case perform gastric lavage using a large-bore tube. If indicated, follow with activated charcoal and a saline cathartic. Since the effects of **Entex LA** may last up to 12 hours, treatment should be continued for at least that length of time.

DOSAGE AND ADMINISTRATION

Adults and adolescents 12 years of age and older: one tablet twice daily (every 12 hours).
Children 6 to under 12 years: one-half (1/2) tablet twice daily (every 12 hours). **Entex LA** is not recommended for pediatric patients under 6 years of age.
Tablets may be broken in half for ease of administration without affecting release of medication but should not be crushed or chewed prior to swallowing.

HOW SUPPLIED

Entex LA is available as an orange, scored tablet coded with "ENTEX LA" on one side and "0149 0436" on the scored side.
NDC 51479-033-01 bottles of 100
NDC 51479-033-05 bottles of 500
Dispense in tight, light-resistant containers as defined in USP.
Store below 86°F (30°C).
CAUTION: Federal law prohibits dispensing without prescription.
Manufactured by
Procter & Gamble Pharmaceuticals
Cincinnati, Ohio 45202
Manufactured for
DURA Pharmaceuticals, Inc.
San Diego, CA 92121
REVISED JULY 1996   ELA 004A796

ENTEX® PSE   ℞
[*n 'tex P-S-E*]
(pseudoephedrine hydrochloride/guaifenesin)

DESCRIPTION

Each Entex PSE yellow coated, scored, long-acting tablet for oral administration contains
pseudoephedrine hydrochloride..................... 120 mg
guaifenesin .... 600 mg
in a special base to provide a prolonged therapeutic effect. This product contains ingredients of the following therapeutic classes: decongestant and expectorant.
Pseudoephedrine hydrochloride is a decongestant having the chemical name, benzenemethanol,α-[1-(methylamino)ethyl]-[S-(R*, R*)]-, hydrochloride, with the following structure:

Guaifenesin is an expectorant having the chemical name, 1,2-propanediol, 3-(2-methoxyphenoxy)-, with the following structure:

Inactive Ingredients: Each tablet contains compressible sugar, D&C Yellow No. 10 Aluminum Lake, dioctyl sodium sulfosuccinate, FD&C Yellow No. 6 Aluminum Lake, hydroxypropyl cellulose, hydroxypropyl methylcellulose, magnesium stearate, polyethylene glycol, purified water, silicon dioxide, sodium citrate, stearic acid, and titanium dioxide.

CLINICAL PHARMACOLOGY

Pseudoephedrine hydrochloride is an α-adrenergic receptor agonist (sympathomimetic) which produces vasoconstriction by stimulating α-receptors within the mucosa of the respiratory tract. Clinically, pseudoephedrine shrinks swollen mucous membranes, reduces tissue hyperemia, edema, and nasal congestion, and increases nasal airway patency. Guaifenesin promotes lower respiratory tract drainage by thinning bronchial secretions, lubricates irritated respiratory tract membranes through increased mucous flow, and facilitates removal of viscous, inspissated mucus. As a result of these drugs, sinus and bronchial drainage is improved, and dry, nonproductive coughs become more productive and less frequent.

INDICATIONS AND USAGE

Entex PSE tablets are indicated for the relief of nasal congestion due to the common cold, hay fever or other upper respiratory allergies, and nasal congestion associated with sinusitis. To promote nasal or sinus drainage; for the symptomatic relief of respiratory conditions characterized by dry nonproductive cough and in the presence of tenacious mucus and/or mucous plugs in the respiratory tract.

CONTRAINDICATIONS

Entex PSE tablets are contraindicated in patients with a known hypersensitivity to any of its ingredients, in nursing mothers, or in patients with severe hypertension, severe coronary artery disease, prostatic hypertrophy, or in patients on MAO inhibitor therapy.

WARNINGS

Sympathomimetic amines should be used with caution in patients with hypertension, diabetes mellitus, heart disease, peripheral vascular disease, increased intraocular pressure, hyperthyroidism, or prostatic hypertrophy.

PRECAUTIONS

General: Hypertensive patients should use Entex PSE tablets only with medical advice, as they may experience a change in blood pressure due to added vasoconstriction.
Information for Patients: Persistent cough may indicate a serious condition. If cough persists for more than one week, tends to recur, or is accompanied by a high fever, rash, or persistent headache, consult a physician.
Drug Interactions: MAO inhibitors and beta adrenergic blockers increase effects of sympathomimetics. Sympathomimetics may reduce the antihypertensive effects if methyldopa, guanethidine, mecamylamine, reserpine and veratrum alkaloids.
Drug/Laboratory Test Interactions: Guaifenesin has been reported to interfere with clinical laboratory determinations of urinary 5-hydroxyindoleacetic acid (5-HIAA) and urinary vanillylmandelic acid (VMA).
Pregnancy: Pregnancy Category C. Animal reproduction studies have not been conducted with Entex PSE tablets. It is also not known whether Entex PSE tablets can cause fetal harm when administered to a pregnant woman or can affect reproduction capacity. Entex PSE tablets should be given to a pregnant woman only if clearly needed.
Nursing Mothers: Entex PSE tablets are contraindicated in the nursing mother because of the higher than usual risks to infants from sympathomimetic agents.
Usage in Elderly: Patients 60 years and older are more likely to experience adverse reactions to sympathomimetics. Overdose may cause hallucinations, convulsions, CNS depression and death. Demonstrate safe use of a short-acting sympathomimetic before use of a sustained action formulation in elderly patients.
Pediatric Use: Safety and effectiveness of Entex PSE tablets in pediatric patients below the age of 6 have not been established.

ADVERSE REACTIONS

Gastrointestinal: nausea and vomiting.
Central Nervous System: nervousness, dizziness, sleeplessness, lightheadedness, tremor, hallucinations, convulsions, CNS depression, fear, anxiety, headache, increased irritability or excitement.
Cardiovascular: palpitations, tachycardia, cardiovascular collapse and death.
General: weakness.
Respiratory: respiratory difficulties.

OVERDOSAGE

Symptoms: Overdose may cause hallucinations, convulsions, CNS depression, cardiovascular collapse and death.
Treatment: Treatment of overdosage should provide symptomatic care. If the amount ingested is considered dangerous or excessive, induce vomiting with ipecac syrup unless the patient is convulsing, comatose, or has lost the gag reflex, in which case, perform gastric lavage using a large-bore tube. If indicated, follow with activated charcoal and a saline cathartic. Since the effects of Entex PSE tablets may last up to 12 hours, treatment should be continued for at least that length of time.

DOSAGE AND ADMINISTRATION

Adults and adolescents 12 years of age and older: one tablet twice daily (every 12 hours).
Children 6 to under 12 years: one-half (1/2) tablet twice daily (every 12 hours). Entex PSE tablets are not recommended for pediatric patients under 6 years of age.
Tablets may be broken in half for ease of administration without affecting release of medication but should not be crushed or chewed prior to swallowing.

HOW SUPPLIED

Entex PSE tablets are coated yellow, scored and coded with "Entex PSE" on one side and "NE" on the scored side.
NDC 51479-032-01 Bottles of 100
Store at controlled room temperature (59°–86°F or 15°–30°C).
Dispense in tight, light-resistant containers as defined in USP.
CAUTION: Federal law prohibits dispensing without prescription.
Manufactured by
Procter & Gamble Pharmaceuticals
Cincinnati, Ohio 45202
Manufactured for
DURA Pharmaceuticals, Inc.
San Diego, CA 92121
REVISED July 1996
EPSE 003A0796

Continued on next page

Dura—Cont.

FENESIN™ ℞
ORAL EXPECTORANT TABLET

DESCRIPTION
Each light blue, scored, sustained-release tablet provides 600 mg guaifenesin in a specially-prepared base to provide a prolonged therapeutic effect. Guaifenesin is an expectorant having the chemical name: 1,2-Propanediol, 3-(2-methoxphenoxy)-.

Inactive Ingredients: colloidal silicon dioxide, FD&C Blue #1, partially hydrogenated cottonseed oil, dicalcium phosphate, hydroxypropyl methylcellulose, magnesium stearate, stearic acid.

HOW SUPPLIED
Fenesin is available as a light blue, scored tablet embossed with DURA on one side and 009 on the other.
Bottles of 100 (NDC 51479-009-01)
Bottles of 600 (NDC 51479-009-06)
Store at room temperature, 15°–25°C (59°–77°F).
Dispense in a tight, light-resistant container (USP/NF) with a child-resistant closure.

FENESIN™ DM ℞
ANTITUSSIVE/EXPECTORANT TABLET

DESCRIPTION
Each dark blue, scored tablet for oral administration contains:
dextromethorphan
hydrobromide .... 30 mg
guaifenesin .... 600 mg
in a special base to provide a prolonged therapeutic effect.

HOW SUPPLIED
Fenesin DM is available as a dark blue, scored tablet embossed with *Dura* on one side and *FDM 014* on the other.
Bottles of 100 (NDC 51479-014-01).
Store at controlled room temperature 15°–25°C (59°–77°F).
Dispense in a tight, light-resistant container (USP/NF) with a child-resistant closure.

FURADANTIN® ℞
(nitrofurantoin)
Oral Suspension

DESCRIPTION
Furadantin (nitrofurantoin), a synthetic chemical, is a stable, yellow, crystalline compound. Furadantin is an antibacterial agent for specific urinary tract infections. Furadantin is available in 25 mg/5 mL liquid suspension for oral administration.

$$O_2N-\text{furan}-CH=N-N\text{(imidazolidinedione)}$$

1-[[(5-nitro-2-furanyl)methylene]amino]-2,
4-imidazolidinedione

DOSAGE AND ADMINISTRATION
Furadantin should be given with food to improve drug absorption and, in some patients, tolerance.
Adults: 50–100 mg four times a day—the lower dosage level is recommended for uncomplicated urinary tract infections. Children: 5–7 mg/kg of body weight per 24 hours, given in four divided doses (contraindicated under one month of age). The following table is based on an average weight in each range receiving 5 to 6 mg/kg of body weight per 24 hours, given in four divided doses. It can be used to calculate an average dose of Furadantin Oral Suspension (25 mg/5 mL) for children (one 5–mL teaspoon of Furadantin Oral Suspension contains 25 mg of Furadantin):

| Body Weight | | No. Teaspoonfuls |
Pounds	Kilograms	4 Times Daily
15 to 26	7 to 11	1/2 (2.5 mL)
27 to 46	12 to 21	1 (5 mL)
47 to 68	22 to 30	1 1/2 (7.5 mL)
69 to 88	31 to 41	2 (10 mL)

Therapy should be continued for one week or for at least 3 days after sterility of the urine is obtained. Continued infection indicates the need for reevaluation.
For long-term suppressive therapy in adults, a reduction of dosage to 50–100 mg at bedtime may be adequate. For long-term suppressive therapy in children, doses as low as 1 mg/kg per 24 hours, given in a single dose or in two divided doses, may be adequate.
SEE WARNINGS SECTION REGARDING RISKS ASSOCIATED WITH LONG-TERM THERAPY.

HOW SUPPLIED
Furadantin Oral Suspension is available in:
NDC 51479-029-06   amber bottle of 60 mL
NDC 51479-029-47   amber bottle of 470 mL
Avoid exposure to strong light which may darken the drug. It is stable in storage. It should be dispensed in amber bottles.
CAUTION: Federal law prohibits dispensing without prescription.

GUAI-VENT™/PSE TABLETS ℞

DESCRIPTION
Each Guai-Vent/PSE white, scored tablet for oral administration contains:
pseudoephedrine HCl .... 120 mg
guaifenesin .... 600 mg
in a special base to provide a prolonged action.

HOW SUPPLIED
Guai-Vent/PSE is available as a white, scored tablet imprinted with Dura and 015.
NDC 51479-015-01   Bottle of 100
Dispense in tight containers as defined in USP/NF.
Store between 15°–25°C (59°–77°F).
Dispense in child-resistant containers.

RONDEC® Chewable Tablets ℞
with brompheniramine

DESCRIPTION
A scored, pink-colored, strawberry-tasting chewable tablet. Each tablet contains:
Brompheniramine maleate.............................. 4 mg
Pseudoephedrine hydrochloride .... 60 mg
Also contains as inactive ingredients artificial strawberry flavoring aspartame, colloidal silicon dioxide, crospovidone, D&C Red #7 (calcium lake), magnesium stearate, mannitol, microcrystalline cellulose, talc, ethylcellulose, povidone K-90, and paraffin wax.
A slight color change (i.e., from pink to peach) may occur over time, but has no effect on its quality or potency.
Rondec® Chewable Tablets with brompheniramine contain ingredients of the following therapeutic classes: antihistamine and nasal decongestant.

CLINICAL PHARMACOLOGY
Brompheniramine maleate is an alkylamine-type antihistamine. This group of antihistamines is among the most active histamine antagonists and is generally effective in relatively low doses. The drugs are not so prone to produce drowsiness and are among the most suitable agents for day time use; but again, a significant proportion of patients do experience this effect. Pseudoephedrine hydrochloride is a sympathomimetic which acts predominantly on alpha receptors and has some action on beta receptors.

INDICATIONS
For the temporary relief of symptoms of seasonal and perennial allergic rhinitis, and vasomotor rhinitis.

CONTRAINDICATIONS
Hypersensitivity to any of the ingredients. Also contraindicated in patients with severe hypertension, severe coronary artery disease, patients on MAO inhibitor therapy, patients with narrow-angle glaucoma, urinary retention, peptic ulcer and during an asthmatic attack.

WARNINGS
Considerable caution should be exercised in patients with hypertension, diabetes mellitus, ischemic heart disease, hyperthyroidism, increased intraocular pressure and prostatic hypertrophy. The elderly (60 years or older) are more likely to exhibit adverse reactions.
Antihistamines may cause excitability, especially in children. At dosages higher than the recommended dose, nervousness, dizziness or sleeplessness may occur.

PRECAUTIONS
General: Caution should be exercised in patients with high blood pressure, heart disease, diabetes or thyroid disease. The antihistamine in this product may exhibit additive effects with other CNS depressants, including alcohol.
Phenylketonurics: Contains phenylalanine 30.9 mg per tablet.

Information for Patients: This antihistamine may cause drowsiness and ambulatory patients who operate machinery or motor vehicles should be cautioned accordingly. Rondec Chewable must be chewed thoroughly before swallowing.
Drug Interactions: MAO inhibitors and beta adrenergic blockers increase the effects of sympathomimetics. Sympathomimetics may reduce the antihypertensive effects of methyldopa, mecamylamine, and reserpine. Concomitant use of antihistamines with alcohol and other CNS depressants may have an additive effect.
Pregnancy: The safety of use of this product in pregnancy has not been established.
Nursing Mothers: It is not known whether the drugs in Rondec Chewable are excreted in human milk. Because many drugs are excreted in human milk and because of the potential for serious adverse reactions in nursing infants, a decision should be made whether to discontinue nursing or discontinue the product, taking into account the importance of the drug to the mother.
Pediatric Use: Safety and effectiveness of Rondec Chewable tablets in pediatric patients below the age of 6 years have not been established.

ADVERSE REACTIONS
Adverse reactions include drowsiness, lassitude, nausea, giddiness, dryness of mouth, blurred vision, cardiac palpitations, flushing, increased irrritability or excitement (especially in children).

OVERDOSAGE
The treatment of overdosage should provide symptomatic and supportive care. Induction of emesis and gastric lavage may be performed if the patient is alert and seen within early hours after ingestion. Drug remaining in the stomach may be absorbed by the administration of activated charcoal. Stimulants should not be used because they may precipitate convulsions. If convulsions or marked CNS excitement occurs, treatment with appropriate measures is indicated.

DOSAGE AND ADMINISTRATION
Adults and adolescents 12 and over: One tablet every 4 hours not to exceed 6 doses in 24 hours. Children 6 to 12 years: One-half tablet every 4 hours not to exceed 6 doses in 24 hours.

HOW SUPPLIED
Bottles of 100 (NDC 51479-017-01). Each tablet is coded "DURA" on one side and "017" on the reverse side.
Dispense in a tight, light-resistant container as defined in USP/NF with a child-resistant closure. Store between 15°–23°C (59°–73°F).
CAUTION: FEDERAL LAW PROHIBITS DISPENSING WITHOUT A PRESCRIPTION.
Manufactured for Dura Pharmaceuticals, Inc.
San Diego, CA 92121
Manufactured by Central Pharmaceuticals, Inc.
Seymour, IN 47274
©1996 Dura Pharmaceuticals, Inc.
RC002B0296

RONDEC® Oral Drops ℞
RONDEC® Syrup ℞
RONDEC® Tablet ℞
RONDEC-TR® Tablet ℞

DESCRIPTION
Antihistamine/Decongestant
for oral use

for infants
RONDEC® Oral Drops ℞
each dropperful (1 mL) contains carbinoxamine maleate, 2 mg; pseudoephedrine hydrochloride, 25 mg.
Inactive Ingredients: Citric acid, DC Red No. 33, FDC Yellow No. 6, glycerin, methylparaben, propylparaben, purified water, sodium benzoate, sodium citrate, sorbitol and artificial flavoring.

for young children
RONDEC® Syrup ℞
each teaspoonful (5 mL) contains carbinoxamine maleate, 4 mg; pseudoephedrine hydrochloride, 60 mg.
Inactive Ingredients: Citric acid, DC Red No. 33, FDC Yellow No. 6, glycerin, methylparaben, propylparaben, purified water, sodium benzoate, sodium citrate, sorbitol and artificial flavoring.

for adults and children 6 years and over
RONDEC® Tablet ℞
each Filmtab® tablet contains carbinoxamine maleate, 4 mg; pseudoephedrine hydrochloride, 60 mg.
Inactive Ingredients: Cellulosic polymers, FDC Yellow No. 6, hydrogenated vegetable oil wax, lactose, magnesium stearate, microcrystalline cellulose, polyethylene glycol, povidine, propylene glycol, silicon dioxide, sodium starch glycolate, sorbitan monooleate, titanium dioxide and vanillin.

for adults and children 12 years and over
RONDEC-TR®Tablet   ℞

each timed-release Filmtab tablet contains carbinoxamine maleate, 8 mg; pseudoephedrine hydrochloride, 120 mg.
Inactive Ingredients: Castor oil, cellulosic polymers, confectioner's sugar, cornstarch, FDC Blue No. 1, lactose, magnesium stearate, methyl acrylate-methyl methacrylate copolymer, microcrystalline cellulose, povidone, propylene glycol, sorbitan monooleate and titanium dioxide.

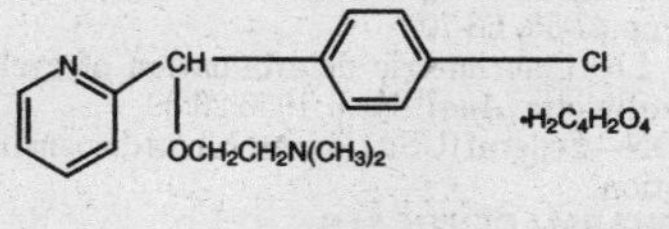

Carbinoxamine maleate (2-[p-Chloro-α-[2-(dimethylamino)ethoxy] benzyl] pyridine maleate) is one of the ethanolamine class of H_1 antihistamines.

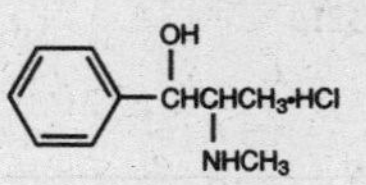

Pseudoephedrine hydrochloride (Benzene-methanol, α-[1-(methylamino)ethyl]-, [S-(R*,R*)]-, hydrochloride) is the hydrochloride of pseudoephedrine, a naturally occurring dextrorotatory stereoisomer of ephedrine.

CLINICAL PHARMACOLOGY
Antihistaminic and decongestant actions.
Carbinoxamine maleate possesses H_1 antihistaminic activity and mild anticholinergic and sedative effects. Serum half-life for carbinoxamine is estimated to be 10 to 20 hours. Virtually no intact drug is excreted in the urine.
Pseudoephedrine hydrochloride is an oral sympathomimetic amine that acts as a decongestant to respiratory tract mucous membranes. While its vasoconstrictor action is similar to that of ephedrine, pseudoephedrine has less pressor effect in normotensive adults. Serum half-life for pseudoephedrine is 6 to 8 hours. Acidic urine is associated with faster elimination of the drug. About one-half of the administered dose is excreted in the urine.

INDICATIONS AND USAGE
For symptomatic relief of seasonal and perennial allergic rhinitis and vasomotor rhinitis.
Rondec Oral Drops, Rondec Syrup and Rondec Tablet are immediate-release dosage forms allowing titration of dose up to four times a day.
Rondec-TR Tablet utilizes a gradual-release mechanism providing approximately a 12-hour therapeutic effect, thus allowing twice-daily dosage.

CONTRAINDICATIONS
Patients with hypersensitivity or idiosyncrasy to any ingredients, patients taking monoamine oxidase (MAO) inhibitors, patients with narrow-angle glaucoma, urinary retention, peptic ulcer, severe hypertension or coronary artery disease, or patients undergoing an asthmatic attack.

WARNINGS
Use in Pregnancy: Safety for use during pregnancy has not been established.
Nursing Mothers: Use with caution in nursing mothers.
Special Risk Patients: Use with caution in patients with hypertension or ischemic heart disease, and persons older than 60 years.

PRECAUTIONS
Use with caution in patients with hypertension, heart disease, asthma, hyperthyroidism, increased intraocular pressure, diabetes mellitus and prostatic hypertrophy.
Information for Patients: Avoid alcohol and other CNS depressants while taking these products. Patients sensitive to antihistamines may experience moderate to severe drowsiness. Patients sensitive to sympathomimetic amines may note mild CNS stimulation. While taking these products, exercise care in driving or operating appliances, machinery, etc.
Drug Interactions: Antihistamines may enhance the effects of tricyclic antidepressants, barbiturates, alcohol, and other CNS depressants. MAO inhibitors prolong and intensify the anticholinergic effects of antihistamines. Sympathomimetic amines may reduce the antihypertensive effects of reserpine, veratrum alkaloids, methyldopa and mecamylamine. Effects of sympathomimetics are increased with MAO inhibitors and beta-adrenergic blockers.
Pregnancy Category C.: Animal reproduction studies have not been conducted with these products. It is also not known whether these products can cause fetal harm when administered to a pregnant woman or affect reproduction capacity. Give to pregnant women only if clearly needed.

ADVERSE REACTIONS
Antihistamines: Sedation, dizziness, diplopia, vomiting, diarrhea, dry mouth, headache, nervousness, nausea, anorexia, heartburn, weakness, polyuria and dysuria and, rarely, excitability in children.
Sympathomimetic Amines: Convulsions, CNS stimulation, cardiac arrhythmias, respiratory difficulty, increased heart rate or blood pressure, hallucinations, tremors, nervousness, insomnia, weakness, pallor and dysuria.

OVERDOSAGE
No information is available as to specific results of an overdose of these products. The signs, symptoms and treatment described below are those of H_1 antihistamines and ephedrine overdose.
Symptoms: Should antihistamine effects predominate, central action constitutes the greatest danger. In the small child, symptoms include excitation, hallucination, ataxia, incoordination, tremors, flushed face and fever. Convulsions, fixed and dilated pupils, coma and death may occur in severe cases. In the adult, fever and flushing are uncommon; excitement leading to convulsions and postictal depression is often preceded by drowsiness and coma. Respiration is usually not seriously depressed; blood pressure is usually stable.
Should sympathomimetic symptoms predominate, central effects include restlessness, dizziness, tremor, hyperactive reflexes, talkativeness, irritability and insomnia. Cardiovascular and renal effects include difficulty in micturition, headache, flushing, palpitation, cardiac arrhythmias, hypertension with subsequent hypotension and circulatory collapse. Gastrointestinal effects include dry mouth, metallic taste, anorexia, nausea, vomiting, diarrhea and abdominal cramps.
Treatment: a) Evacuate stomach as condition warrants. Activated charcoal may be useful. b) Maintain a non-stimulating environment. c) Monitor cardiovascular status. d) Do not give stimulants. e) Reduce fever with cool sponging. f) Support respiration. g) Use sedatives or anticonvulsants to control CNS excitation and convulsions. h) Physostigmine may reverse anticholinergic symptoms. i) Ammonium chloride may acidify the urine to increase excretion of pseudoephedrine. j) Further care is symptomatic and supportive.

DOSAGE AND ADMINISTRATION

AGE	DOSE*	FREQUENCY*
Rondex Oral Drops		
for oral use only		
1–3 months	¼ dropperful (¼ mL)	q.i.d.
3–6 months	½ dropperful (½ mL)	q.i.d.
6–9 months	¾ dropperful (¾ mL)	q.i.d.
9–18 months	1 dropperful (1 mL)	q.i.d.
Rondex Syrup and		
Rondec Tablet		
18 months–6 years	½ teaspoonful (2.5 mL)	q.i.d.
adults and children 6 years and over	1 teaspoonful (5 mL) or 1 tablet	q.i.d.
Rondec-TR Tablet		
adults and children 12 years and over	1 tablet	b.i.d.

*In mild cases or in particularly sensitive patients, less frequent or reduced doses may be adequate.

HOW SUPPLIED
Rondec Oral Drops, berry-flavored, in 30-mL bottles for dropper dosage, **NDC** 0074-5783-30. Calibrated shatterproof dropper enclosed in each carton. Container meets safety closure requirements.
Rondec Syrup, berry-flavored, in 16-fl-oz (1-pint) bottles, **NDC** 0074-5782-16; and 4-fl-oz bottles, **NDC** 0074-5782-04. Dispense in USP tight glass container.
Rondec Tablet, Filmtab tablets, in bottles of 100, **NDC** 0074-5726-13; and bottles of 500, **NDC** 0074-5726-53. Each orange-colored tablet marked with Ross and the number 5726 for professional identification. Dispense in USP tight container.
Rondec-TR Tablet, Filmtab tablets, in bottles of 100, **NDC** 0074-6240-13. Each blue-colored tablet marked with Ross and the number 6240 for professional identification. Dispense in USP tight container.
Recommended storage: Store below 86°F (30°C).
Revised: October, 1991
Formerly distributed by
Ross Laboratories
(division of Abbott).
Now distributed by
Dura Pharmaceuticals.

RONDEC®-DM Syrup   ℞
RONDEC®-DM Oral Drops   ℞

DESCRIPTION
Antihistamine/Decongestant/Antitussive for oral use
for adults and children
RONDEC®-DM Syrup   ℞

each teaspoonful (5 mL) contains carbinoxamine maleate, 4 mg; pseudoephedrine hydrochloride, 60 mg; dextromethorphan hydrobromide, 15 mg.
Inactive Ingredients: Citric acid, DC Red No. 33, FDC Blue No. 1, glycerin, menthol, purified water, sodium benzoate, sodium citrate, sorbitol, natural and artificial flavoring and other ingredients.

for infants
RONDEC®-DM Oral Drops   ℞

each dropperful (1 mL) contains carbinoxamine maleate, 2 mg; pseudoephedrine hydrochloride, 25 mg; dextromethorphan hydrobromide, 4 mg.
Inactive Ingredients: Citric acid, DC Red No. 33, FDC Blue No. 1, glycerin, menthol, purified water, sodium benzoate, sodium citrate, sorbitol, natural and artificial flavoring and other ingredients.

DOSAGE AND ADMINISTRATION

AGE	DOSE*	FREQUENCY*
Rondec-DM Syrup		
18 months–6 years	½ teaspoonful (2.5 mL)	q.i.d.
adults and children 6 years and over	1 teaspoonful (5 mL)	q.i.d.
Rondec-DM Oral Drops		
for oral use only		
1–3 months	¼ dropperful (¼ mL)	q.i.d.
3–6 months	½ dropperful (½ mL)	q.i.d.
6–9 months	¾ dropperful (¾ mL)	q.i.d.
9–18 months	1 dropperful (1 mL)	q.i.d.

*In mild cases or in particularly sensitive patients, less frequent of reduced doses may be adequate.

HOW SUPPLIED
Rondec-DM Syrup, grape-flavored, in 16-fl-oz (1-pint) bottles, **NDC** 0074-5640-16; and 4-fl-oz bottles, **NDC** 0074-5640-04. Dispense in USP tight, light-resistant, glass container. Avoid exposure to excessive heat.
Rondec-DM Oral Drops, grape-flavored, in 30-mL bottles for dropper dosage. Calibrated, shatterproof dropper enclosed in each carton. Container meets safety closure requirements **NDC** 0074-5639-30. Avoid exposure to excessive heat.

SEROMYCIN®   ℞
CYCLOSERINE CAPSULES, USP

DESCRIPTION
Seromycin® (Cycloserine Capsules, USP), 3-isoxazolidinone, 4-amino-, (R)- is a broad spectrum antibiotic that is produced by a strain of *Streptomyces orchidaceus* and has also been synthesized. Cycloserine is a white to off-white powder that is soluble in water and stable in alkaline solution. It is rapidly destroyed at a neutral or acid pH.
Cycloserine has a pH between 5.5 and 6.5 in a solution containing 100 mg/mL. The molecular weight of cycloserine is 102.09, and it has an empirical formula of $C_3H_6N_2O_2$. The structural formula of cycloserine is as follows:

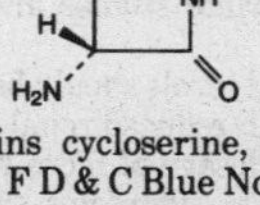

Each capsule contains cycloserine, 250 mg (2.45 mmol); D & C Yellow No. 10, F D & C Blue No. 1, F D & C Red No. 3, F D & C Yellow No. 6, gelatin, iron oxide, talc, titanium dioxide, and other inactive ingredients.

CLINICAL PHARMACOLOGY
After oral administration cycloserine is readily absorbed from the gastrointestinal tract, with peak blood levels occurring in 4 to 8 hours. Blood levels of 25 to 30 μg/mL can generally be maintained with the usual dosage of 250 mg twice a day, although the relationship of plasma levels to dosage is not always consistent. Concentrations in the cerebrospinal fluid, pleural fluid, fetal blood, and mother's milk approach those found in the serum. Detectable amounts are found in ascitic fluid, bile sputum, amniotic fluid, and lung and lymph tissues. Approximately 65% of a single dose of cycloserine can be recovered in the urine within 72 hours ofter oral administration. The remaining 35% is apparently metabolized to unknown substances. The maximum excretion rate occurs 2 to 6 hours after administration, with 50% of the drug eliminated in 12 hours.

Continued on next page

Dura—Cont.

Microbiology: Cycloserine inhibits cell-wall synthesis in susceptible strains of gram-positive and gram-negative bacteria and in *Mycobacterium tuberculosis*.

Susceptibility Tests: Cycloserine clinical laboratory standard powder is available for both direct and indirect methods[1] of determining the susceptibility of strains of mycobacteria. Cycloserine MICs for susceptible strains are 25 μg/mL or lower.

INDICATIONS AND USAGE

Seromycin is indicated in the treatment of active pulmonary and extrapulmonary tuberculosis (including renal disease) when the causative organisms are susceptible to this drug and when treatment with the primary medications (streptomycin, isoniazid, rifampin, and ethambutol) has proved inadequate. Like all antituberculosis drugs, Seromycin should be administered in conjuction with other effective chemotherapy and not as the sole therapeutic agent.

Seromycin may be effective in the treatment of acute urinary tract infections caused by susceptible strains of gram-positive and gram-negative bacteria, especially *Enterobacter* sp. and *Escherichia coli*. It is generally no more and is usually less effective than other antimicrobial agents in the treatment of urinary tract infections caused by bacteria other than mycobacteria. Use of Seromycin in these infections should be considered only when more conventional therapy has failed and when the organism has been demonstrated to be susceptible to the drug.

CONTRAINDICATIONS

Administration is contraindicated in patients with any of the following:

Hypersensitivity to cycloserine
Epilepsy
Depression, severe anxiety, or psychosis
Severe renal insufficiency
Excessive concurrent use of alcohol

WARNINGS

Administration of Seromycin should be discontinued or the dosage reduced if the patient develops allergic dermatitis or symptoms of CNS toxicity, such as convulsions, psychosis, somnolence, depression, confusion, hyperreflexia, headache, tremor, vertigo, paresis, or dysarthria.

The toxicity of Seromycin is closely related to excessive blood levels (above 30 μg/mL), as determined by high dosage or inadequate renal clearance. The ratio of toxic dose to effective dose in tuberculosis is small.

The risk of convulsions is increased in chronic alcoholics.

Patients should be monitored by hematologic, renal excretion, blood level, and liver function studies.

PRECAUTIONS

General: Before treatment with Seromycin is initiated, cultures should be taken and the organism's susceptibility to the drug should be established. In tuberculous infections, the organism's susceptibility to the other antituberculosis agents in the regimen should also be demonstrated.

Anticonvulsant drugs or sedatives may be effective in controlling symptoms of CNS toxicity, such as convulsions, anxiety, and tremor. Patients receiving more than 500 mg of Seromycin daily should be closely observed for such symptoms. The value of pyridoxine in preventing CNS toxicity from Seromycin has not been proved.

Administration of Seromycin and other antituberculosis drugs has been associated in a few instances with vitamin B_{12} and/or folic-acid deficiency, megaloblastic anemia, and sideroblastic anemia. If evidence of anemia develops during treatment, appropriate studies and therapy should be instituted.

Laboratory Tests: Blood levels should be determined at least weekly for patients with reduced renal function, for individuals receiving a daily dosage of more than 500 mg, and for those showing signs and symptoms suggestive of toxicity. The dosage should be adjusted to keep the blood level below 30 μg/mL.

Drug Interactions: Concurrent administration of ethionamide has been reported to potentiate neurotoxic side effects.

Alcohol and Seromycin are incompatible, especially during a regimen calling for large doses of the latter. Alcohol increases the possibility and risk of epileptic episodes.

Concurrent administration of isoniazid may result in increased incidence of CNS effects, such as dizziness or drowsiness. Dosage adjustments may be necessary and patients should be monitored closely for signs of CNS toxicity.

Carcinogenesis, Mutagenicity, and Impairment of Fertility: Studies have not been performed to determine potential for carcinogenicity. The Ames test and unscheduled DNA repair test were negative. A study in 2 generations of rats showed no impairment of fertility relative to controls for the first mating but somewhat lower fertility in the second mating.

Pregnancy Category C: A study in 2 generations of rats given doses up to 100 mg/kg/day demonstrated no teratogenic effect in offspring. It is not known whether Seromycin can cause fetal harm when administered to a pregnant woman or can affect reproduction capacity. Seromycin should be given to a pregnant woman only if clearly needed.

Nursing Mothers: Because of the potential for serious adverse reactions in nursing infants from Seromycin, a decision should be made to whether to discontinue nursing or discontinue the drug, taking into account the importance of the drug to the mother.

Usage in Pediatric Patients: Safety and effectiveness in pediatric patients have not been established.

ADVERSE REACTIONS

Most adverse reactions occurring during therapy with Seromycin involve the nervous system or are manifestations of drug hypersensitivity. The following side effects have been observed in patients receivng Seromycin:

Nervous system symptoms (which appear to be related to higher dosages of the drug, ie, more than 500 mg daily)

Convulsions
Drowsiness and somnolence
Headache
Tremor
Dysarthria
Vertigo
Confusion and disorientation with loss of memory
Psychoses, possibly with suicidal tendencies
Character changes
Hyperirritability
Aggression
Paresis
Hyperreflexia
Paresthesia
Major and minor (localized) clonic seizures
Coma

Cardiovascular

Sudden development of congestive heart failure in patients receiving 1 to 1.5 g of Seromycin daily has been reported

Allergy (apparently not related to dosage)

Skin Rash

Miscellaneous

Elevated serum transaminase, especially in patients with preexisting liver disease

OVERDOSAGE

Signs and Symptoms: Acute toxicity from cycloserine can occur if more than 1 g is ingested by an adult. Chronic toxicity from cycloserine is dose related and can occur if more than 500 mg is administered daily. Patients with renal impairment will accumulate cycloserine and may develop toxicity if the dosing regimen is not modified. Patients with severe renal impairment should not receive the drug. The central nervous system is the most common organ system involved with toxicity. Toxic effects may include headache, vertigo, confusion, drowsiness, hyperirritability, paresthesias, dysarthria, and psychosis. Following larger ingestions, paresis, convulsions, and coma often occur. Ethyl alcohol may increase the risk of seizures in patients receiving cycloserine.

The oral median lethal dose in mice is 5,290 mg/kg.

Treatment: To obtain up-to-date information about the treatment of overdose, a good resource is your certified Regional Poison Control Center. Telephone numbers of certified poison control centers are listed in the *Physicians' Desk Reference (PDR)*. In managing overdosage, consider the possibility of multiple drug overdoses, interaction among drugs, and unusual drug kinetics in your patient.

Overdoses of cycloserine have been reported rarely. The following is provided to serve as a guide should such an overdose be encountered.

Protect the patient's airway and support ventilation and perfusion. Meticulously monitor and maintain, within acceptable limits, the patient's vital signs, blood gases, serum electrolytes, etc. Absorption of drugs from the gastrointestinal tract may be decreased by giving activated charcoal, which, in many cases, is more effective than emesis or lavage; consider charcoal instead of or in addition to gastric emptying. Repeated doses of charcoal over time may hasten elimination of some drugs that have been absorbed. Safeguard the patient's airway when employing gastric emptying or charcoal.

In adults, many of the neurotoxic effects of cycloserine can be both treated and prevented with the administration of 200 to 300 mg of pyridoxine daily.

The use of hemodialysis has been shown to remove cycloserine from the bloodstream. This procedure should be reserved for patients with life-threatening toxicity that is unresponsive to less invasive therapy.

DOSAGE AND ADMINISTRATION

Seromycin is effective orally and is currently administered only by this route. The usual dosage is 500 mg to 1 g daily in divided doses monitored by blood levels.[2] The initial adult dosage most frequently given is 250 mg twice daily at 12-hour intervals for the first 2 weeks. A daily dosage of 1 g should not be exceeded.

HOW SUPPLIED

Seromycin® is available as a red and gray capsule coded with the imprints 51479-019 on each half.

Bottles of 40 (UC5000) (NDC 51479-019-01).

Store at controlled room temperature, 59° to 86°F (15° to 30°C).

REFERENCES

1. Kubica GP, Dye WE: Laboratory methods for clinical and public health—mycobacteriology. US Department of Health, Education and Welfare, Public Health Service, 1967, pp 47-55, 66-70.
2. Jones LR: Colorimetric determination of cycloserine, a new antibiotic. *Anal Chem* 1956;28:39.

CAUTION—Federal (USA) law prohibits dispensing without prescription.

DURA PHARMACEUTICALS

Literature revised May 7, 1996
Manufactured by: Eli Lilly and Company
Indianapolis, IN 46285
Distributed by: DURA Pharmaceuticals, Inc.
San Diego, CA 92121
PV 0681 UCP

SC002B0496

TORNALATE® ℞

(bitolterol mesylate)
Solution for Inhalation, 0.2%

DESCRIPTION

Tornalate (bitolterol mesylate) is the di-p-toluate ester of the β-adrenergic agonist bronchodilator *N*-t-butylarterenol (colterol). It has a molecular weight of 557.7 and the molecular formula is $C_{25}H_{31}NO \cdot CH_3SO_3H$. Bitolterol mesylate is known chemically as 4-[2-[(1,1-dimethylethyl) amino]-1-hydroxyethyl]-1,2-phenylene 4-methylbenzoate (ester) methanesulfonate (salt) and has the following structural formula:

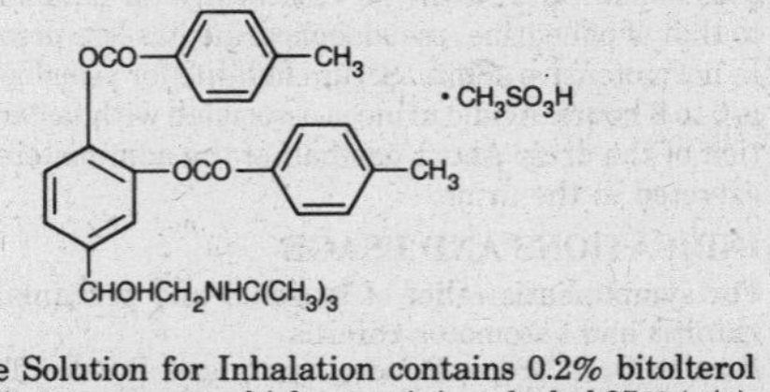

Tornalate Solution for Inhalation contains 0.2% bitolterol mesylate in an aqueous vehicle containing alcohol 25% (v/v), citric acid, propylene glycol, and sodium hydroxide. Tornalate's pH range is 3.0–3.4

Each mL of Tornalate Solution for Inhalation, 0.2% contains 2.0 mg of bitolterol mesylate.

CLINICAL PHARMACOLOGY

Tornalate is administered as a pro-drug which is hydrolyzed by esterases in tissue and blood to the active moiety colterol. Tornalate administered by nebulization has a rapid onset of activity (2 to 3 minutes) after administration in most patients based on interpolation between baseline and 5 minutes. The duration of action with Tornalate administered by nebulization is 6 hours or more in most patients and 8 hours in 40% of patients based on 15% or greater increase in forced expiratory volume in one second (FEV_1), as demonstrated in 3-month isoproterenol controlled multicenter trials in non-steroid dependent patients. Based on mid-maximal expiratory flow (MMEF) measurements, the duration of action is 7.5 to 8 hours in most patients. Median duration of effect in steroid-dependent asthmatic patients ranged from 4.3 to 7.1 hours based on 15% or greater increase in FEV_1. The mean maximum increase in FEV_1 over baseline in patients during the three-month studies was 49% to 55% and occurred by 30 to 60 minutes in most patients.

In vitro studies and in vivo pharmacologic studies have demonstrated that Tornalate has a preferential effect on beta-2 adrenergic receptors compared with isoproterenol. While it is recognized that beta-2 adrenergic receptors are the prominent receptors in bronchial smooth muscle, recent data indicate that there are between 10% to 50% beta-2 receptors in the human heart. The precise function of these, however, is not yet established. Tornalate has been shown in most controlled clinical trials to have more effect on the respiratory tract, in the form of bronchial smooth muscle relaxation than isoproterenol at comparable doses, while producing fewer cardiovascular effects. Controlled clinical studies and other clinical experience have shown the inhaled Tornalate, like other beta-adrenergic agonists, can produce a significant cardiovascular effect in some patients, as measured by pulse rate, blood pressure, symptoms and/or ECG changes.

The incidence of cardiovascular side effects such as tachycardia and palpitation was less in patients treated with bitolterol mesylate as compared with patients treated with isoproterenol hydrochloride. The incidence of tachycardia and

palpitation was 3.7% and 3.1%, respectively, in patients treated with bitolterol mesylate as compared with an incidence of 12.3% and 12.6% for tachycardia and palpitation for patients treated with isoproterenol.
Blood levels of colterol formed by gradual release from the pro-drug (bitolterol) in the lungs are too low to be measured by currently available assay methods and the bioavailability, pharmacokinetics and metabolism of bitolterol following administration as a solution for inhalation are not known. Data on disposition are available from oral studies in man. Following oral administration of 5.9 mg tritiated bitolterol to man, radioactivity measurements indicated mean maximum colterol concentration in blood of approximately 2.1 μg/mL one hour after medication. Urinary excretion data indicate that 83% of the radioactivity of this oral dose was excreted within the first 24 hours. By 72 hours, 85.6% of the tritium had been excreted in the urine and 8.1% in the feces. Most of the radioactivity was excreted as conjugated colterol; free colterol accounted for 2.1% to 3.7% of the total radioactivity excreted in the urine. No intact bitolterol was detected in urine.
The pharmacologic effects of β-adrenergic agonist drugs, including bitolterol mesylate, are at least in part attributable to stimulation through beta adrenergic receptors of intracellular adenyl cyclase, the enzyme which catalyzes the conversion of adenosine triphosphate (ATP) to cyclic-3′, 5′-adenosine monophosphate (c-AMP). Increased c-AMP levels are associated with relaxation of bronchial smooth muscle and inhibition of release of mediators of immediate hypersensitivity from cells, especially from mast cells.
In repetitive dosing studies, continued effectiveness was demonstrated throughout the three-month period of treatment in the majority of patients. In steroid-dependent asthmatics, the median duration of bronchodilator activity as measured by FEV_1 was greater on the first test day as compared with later test days, but patient response remained constant throughout the balance of the three-month period.
Recent studies in laboratory animals (minipigs, rodents, and dogs) recorded the occurrence of cardiac arrhythmias and sudden death (with histologic evidence of myocardial necrosis) when beta agonists and methylxanthines were administered concurrently. The significance of these findings when applied to humans is currently unknown.

INDICATIONS AND USAGE

Tornalate Solution for Inhalation, 0.2% is indicated for both prophylaxis and treatment of asthma or other conditions characterized by reversible bronchospasm. It may be used with or without concurrent theophylline and/or steroid therapy.

CONTRAINDICATIONS

Tornalate Solution for Inhalation, 0.2% is contraindicated in patients who are hypersensitive to bitolterol mesylate or any other ingredients of the formulation.

WARNINGS

As with other β-adrenergic agents, bitolterol mesylate should not be used in excess. Fatalities have been reported in association with excessive use of inhaled sympathomimetic drugs. The exact cause of death is unknown.Use of β-adrenergic drugs may have a deleterious cardiac effect. Paradoxical bronchoconstriction (which can be life-threatening) has been reported with administration of β-adrenergic agents. Immediate hypersensitivity reactions can occur after the administration of sympathomimetic agents. In such instances, the drug should be discontinued immediately and alternative therapy instituted.
In controlled clinical studies, clinically significant increases in pulse rate, increases and decreases in systolic and diastolic blood pressure have been demonstrated in individual patients after administration of Tornalate. Therefore, caution should be exercised when administering bitolterol mesylate to patients with underlying cardiovascular disease. Even though the changes may be significant in a small number of patients, these changes occur within a short period of time after administration and have not been shown to be persistent.
If an unusual smell or taste is noted with use of this product, the patient should discontinue use in consultation with his/her physician.

PRECAUTIONS

General As with all β-adrenergic stimulating agents, caution should be used when administering Tornalate to patients with cardiovascular disease such as ischemic heart disease or hypertension. Caution is also advised in patients with hyperthyroidism, diabetes mellitus, cardiac arrhythmias, convulsive disorders or unusual responsiveness to β-adrenergic agonists. Use of any β-adrenergic bronchodilator may produce significant changes in systolic and diastolic blood pressure in some patients.
Information for Patients The effects of Tornalate may last up to eight hours or longer. It should not be used more often than recommended and the patient should not increase the number of treatments or dose without first consulting with the physician. If symptoms of asthma get worse, adverse reactions occur, or the patient does not respond to the usual dose, the patient should be instructed to contact the physician immediately. Drug stability and safety of Tornalate when mixed with other drugs in a nebulizer have not been established. The patient should be advised as to the proper use of the equipment used for nebulization and to see the Illustrated Patient's Instructions for Use.
Drug Interactions Other sympathomimetic bronchodilators or epinephrine should not be used concomitantly with Tornalate because they may have additive effects.
Tornalate should be administered with caution to patients being treated with monoamine oxidase inhibitors or tricyclic antidepressants, since the action of bitolterol on the vascular system may be potentiated.
Carcinogenesis, Mutagenesis, and Impairment of Fertility No tumorigenicity (and specifically no increase in leiomyomas) was observed in a two-year oral study in Sprague-Dawley CD rats at doses of Tornalate corresponding to 12 or 62 times the maximal total daily human inhalational dose (8.0 mg bitolterol mesylate per day). Tornalate was not tumorigenic in an 18-month oral study in Swiss-Webster mice at doses up to 312 times the maximal daily human inhalational dose. Ames Salmonella and mouse lymphoma mutation assays in vitro revealed no mutagenesis due to Tornalate. Reproductive studies in male and female rats revealed no significant effects on fertility at doses of Tornalate up to 241 times the maximal daily human inhalational dose.
Teratogenic Effects—Pregnancy Category C No teratogenic effects were seen in rats and rabbits after oral doses of Tornalate up to 361 times the maximal daily human inhalational dose and in mice after oral doses up to 188 times the maximal daily human inhalational dose.
When Tornalate (as base) was injected subcutaneously into mice in doses of 2 mg/kg, 10 mg/kg, and 20 mg/kg (corresponding to 15, 75, and 151 times the maximal daily human inhalational dose) the incidence of cleft palate was 5.7%, 3.8%, and 3.3%, respectively. Occurrence of cleft palate with isoproterenol (as base) at 10 mg/kg subcutaneously was 10.7%. Since no well-controlled studies in pregnant women are available, Tornalate should be used during pregnancy only if the potential benefit justifies the potential risk to the fetus.
Nursing Mothers It is not known whether Tornalate is excreted in human milk. Because many drugs are excreted in human milk, caution should be exercised when Tornalate is administered to a nursing woman.
Pediatric Use Safety and effectiveness of Tornalate in children 12 years of age or younger has not been established.

ADVERSE REACTIONS

The adverse reactions observed with Tornalate are consistent with those seen with other beta-adrenergic agonists. The frequency of most cardiovascular effects was less after bitolterol mesylate than after isoproterenol in 3-month repetitive dose studies.
Like the findings noted after the administration of other beta-adrenergic agonist drugs, infrequent laboratory abnormalities with undetermined clinical significance were noted after administration of Tornalate. These include decreases in hemoglobin and hematocrit, decreases in WBC, elevation of liver enzymes, increases in blood sugar, decreases in serum potassium and abnormal urinalysis. In addition, one patient in a Tornalate controlled clinical trial had increased liver function tests and documented hepatomegaly.
The results of all clinical trials with Tornalate (323 patients) showed the following side effects:
Central/Peripheral Nervous System: Tremors (26.6%), nervousness (11.1%), headache (8.4%), lightheadedness (6.8%), dizziness (4.0%), paresthesia (1.5%), somnolence (1.2%). In three-month studies, the incidence of tremors decreased from 22% during the first month to 9% during the third month.
Cardiovascular: Tachycardia (3.7%), palpitation (3.1%), irregular pulse (1.2%).
Respiratory: Coughing (2.5%), bronchospasm (1.5%), chest discomfort (1.5%), rhinitis (1.5%).
Oro-Pharyngeal: Throat irritation (2.5%), mouth irritation (1.9%).
Gastrointestinal: Nausea (1.9%).
Other: Fatigue (1.5%).
The incidence of the following adverse reactions was less than one percent:
CNS: Vertigo, insomnia, euphoria, incoordination, hyperkinesia, hypoesthesia, anxiety.
Cardiovascular: Transient ECG changes (ventricular premature contractions, atrial arrhythmia, inverted T waves, junctional rhythm), chest discomfort, increase in blood pressure, chills, heart rate decrease, flushing.
Respiratory: Dyspnea, sputum increase.
Gastrointestinal: Vomiting, hepatomegalia.
Others: Pruritus, urticaria, asthenia, arthralgia, eye irritation, facial discomfort, taste loss.
Clinical relevance or relationship to administration of Tornalate and rarely reported elevations of SGOT, SGPT, LDH are not known.

OVERDOSAGE

Overdosage with Tornalate may be expected to result in exaggeration of those drug effects listed in the ADVERSE REACTIONS section. In such cases therapy with Tornalate and all β-adrenergic stimulating drugs should be stopped, supportive therapy provided, and judicious use of a cardioselective β-adrenergic blocking agent should be considered bearing in mind the possibility that such agents can produce profound bronchospasm. As with all sympathomimetic aerosol medications, cardiac arrest and even death may be associated with abuse.
The oral LD_{50} of Tornalate in rats was 5,650 mg/kg and in mice it was 6,575 mg/kg.

DOSAGE AND ADMINISTRATION

Tornalate Solution for Inhalation, 0.2% can be administered by nebulization to adults and children over 12 years of age. As with all medications, the physician should begin therapy with the lowest effective dose according to the individual patient's requirements following manufacturer's dosage recommendation. Tornalate should be administered during a ten to fifteen-minute period. The treatment period can be adjusted by varying the amount of diluent (normal saline solution) placed in the nebulizer with the medication. The total volume (medication plus diluent) is usually adjusted to 2.0 mL to 4.0 mL. Safety of the treatment should be monitored by measuring blood pressure and pulse.
Clinical studies were conducted with two types of nebulizer systems.
Intermittent Aerosol Flow (Patient-Activated Nebulizer) This nebulizer is operated by a patient-activated valve to permit the release of aerosol mist only during inspiration.
Continuous Aerosol Flow Nebulizer This nebulizer generates a continuous flow of mist while the patient inhales and exhales through the nebulizer resulting in the loss of some medication through an exhaust port.
When using these types of nebulizer systems the following dosing regimens are recommended:

Tornalate Solution for Inhalation, 0.2%

Doses	Continuous Flow Nebulization		Intermittent Flow Nebulization	
	Volume	Tornalate	Volume	Tornalate
Usual Dose	**1.25 mL**	**2.5 mg**	0.5 mL	1.0 mg
Decreased Dose	0.75 mL	1.5 mg	0.25 mL	0.5 mg
Increased Dose	1.75 mL	3.5 mg	0.75 mL	1.5 mg

Up to 1.0 mL of Tornalate Solution for Inhalation, 0.2% (2.0 mg Tornalate) can be administered with the intermittent flow system to severely-obstructed patients.
The usual frequency of treatments is three times a day. Treatments may be increased up to four times daily, however the interval between treatments should not be less than four hours. For some patients two treatments a day may be adequate. If a previously effective dosage regimen fails to provide the usual relief, the patient should be advised to seek medical advice immediately as this is often a sign of seriously-worsening asthma that would require reassessment of therapy.
The maximum daily dose should not exceed 8.0 mg Tornalate with an intermittent flow nebulization system or 14.0 mg Tornalate with a continuous flow nebulization system.
Tornalate Solution for Inhalation, 0.2% should be added to the nebulizer just prior to use and should not be left in the nebulizer.
Drug stability and safety of Tornalate (bitolterol mesylate) Solution for Inhalation, 0.2% when mixed with other drugs in a nebulizer have not been established. Tornalate Solution for Inhalation, 0.2% should not be mixed with other drugs such as cromolyn sodium or acetylcysteine at clinically-recommended doses due to chemical and/or physical incompatibilities.

HOW SUPPLIED

Amber Glass Bottle of 10 mL with .75 cc dropper (NDC 51479-011-01)
Amber Glass Bottle of 30 mL with 1.25 cc dropper (NDC 51479-011-03)
Amber Glass Bottle of 60 mL with 1.25 cc dropper (NDC 51479-011-06)
Included in each carton is an overwrapped graduated medicine dropper for use with Tornalate Solution for Inhalation, 0.2%.
Do not use the solution if it is discolored or contains a precipitate.
Store at controlled room temperature between 15°C–30°C (59°F–86°F).
CAUTION: Federal law prohibits dispensing without a prescription.
Distributed by DURA Pharmaceuticals, Inc., San Diego, CA 92121
Manufactured by Nycomed Puerto Rico Inc., Barceloneta, Puerto Rico 00617

Continued on next page

Dura—Cont.

DURA PHARMACEUTICALS
Revised December 1994
TS007D1294

TORNALATE® ℞
(bitolterol mesylate)
Metered Dose Inhaler
Bronchodilator for Oral Inhalation

DESCRIPTION

Tornalate (bitolterol mesylate) is the di-p-toluate ester of the β-adrenergic agonist bronchodilator *N-t*-butylarterenol (colterol). It has a molecular weight of 557.7. Bitolterol mesylate is known chemically as 4-[2-[(1,1-dimethylethyl) amino]-1-hydroxyethyl]-1,2-phenylene 4-methylbenzoate (ester) methanesulfonate (salt) and has the following structural formula:

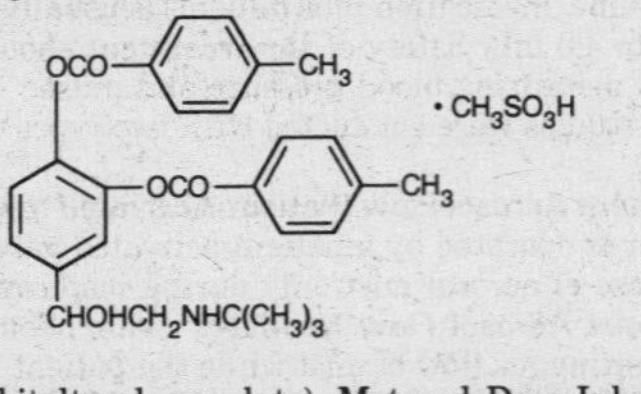

Tornalate (bitolterol mesylate), Metered Dose Inhaler is a complete aerosol unit for oral inhalation. It consists of a plastic-coated bottle of ready-to-use aerosol solution and a detachable plastic mouthpiece with built-in nebulizer. The bottle contains 16.4 g (15 mL) of 0.8% bitolterol mesylate in a vehicle containing 38% alcohol (w/w), inert propellants (dichlorodifluoromethane and dichlorotetrafluoroethane), ascorbic acid, saccharin, and menthol.

Each bottle provides at least 300 actuations. Each actuation delivers a measured dose of 0.37 mg of bitolterol mesylate as a fine, even mist.

CLINICAL PHARMACOLOGY

Tornalate (bitolterol mesylate) is administered as a pro-drug which is hydrolyzed by esterases in tissue and blood to the active moiety colterol. Tornalate administered as an inhaled aerosol has a rapid (3 to 4 minutes) onset of bronchodilator activity. The duration of action with Tornalate is at least 5 hours in most patients and 8 or more hours in 25% to 35% of patients, based on 15% or greater increase in forced expiratory volume in one second (FEV_1), as demonstrated in 3-month isoproterenol controlled multicenter trials. Based on mean maximal expiratory flow (MMEF) measurements, the duration of action is 6 to 7 hours. The duration of bronchodilator action with Tornalate in these trials is longer than that seen with isoproterenol, especially in steroid-dependent patients. Duration of effect was reduced over time in steroid-dependent asthmatic patients where the duration was 3.5 to 5 hours for FEV_1. The mean maximum increase in FEV_1 over baseline in the majority of patients was 39% to 42% and occurred by 30 to 60 minutes, similar to that seen in the isoproterenol group.

Tornalate is a beta-adrenergic agonist which has been shown by in vitro and in vivo pharmacological studies in animals to exert a preferential effect on $beta_2$ adrenergic receptors, such as those located in bronchial smooth muscle. However, controlled clinical trials in patients who were administered the drug have not revealed a preferential $beta_2$ adrenergic effect. At doses that produced long duration of bronchodilator activity (up to 8 hours in some patients) with a mean maximum bronchodilating effect of approximately 40% increase in FEV_1 (forced expiratory volume in one second), a less than 10 beat per minute mean maximum increase in heart rate was seen. The effect on the heart rate was transient and similar to the increases seen in the isoproterenol treated patients in these studies.

Although blood levels of colterol formed by gradual release from the pro-drug (bitolterol) in the lungs are too low to be measured by currently available assay methods, data on disposition are available from oral studies in man. Following oral administration of 5.9 mg tritiated bitolterol mesylate to man, radioactivity measurements indicated mean maximum colterol concentration in blood of approximately 2.1 μg/mL one hour after medication. Urinary excretion data indicate that 83 percent of the radioactivity of this oral dose was excreted within the first 24 hours. By 72 hours, 85.6 percent of the tritium had been excreted in the urine and 8.1 percent in the feces. Most of the radioactivity was excreted as conjugated colterol; free colterol accounted for 2.1 to 3.7 percent of the total radioactivity excreted in the urine. No intact bitolterol was detected in urine.

The pharmacologic effects of β-adrenergic drugs including Tornalate (bitolterol mesylate) are attributable to stimulation of adenyl cyclase, the enzyme which catalyzes the conversion of adenosine triphosphate (ATP) to cyclic-3′, 5′-adenosine monophosphate (c-AMP). Increased c-AMP levels are associated with relaxation of bronchial smooth muscle and with inhibition of release of mediators of immediate hypersensitivity from cells, especially from mast cells.

In a six-week clinical trial in which 24 asthmatic patients received Tornalate and theophylline concurrently, improvement in pulmonary function was enhanced over that seen with either drug alone. No potentiation of side effects was observed, and 24-hour ECG recordings (Holter monitoring) indicated no greater degree of cardiac toxicity with Tornalate alone or in combination with theophylline than that which occurred with theophylline alone.

Tornalate did not adversely affect arterial oxygen tension in a blood-gas study in 24 asthmatic patients. However, a decrease in arterial oxygen tension has been reported with other adrenergic bronchodilators and could be anticipated to occur with Tornalate as well.

In repetitive dosing studies, continued effectiveness was demonstrated throughout the 3-month period of treatment in the majority of patients. However, some overall decrease was observed in steroid-dependent asthmatics.

INDICATIONS AND USAGE

Tornalate (bitolterol mesylate) is indicated for both prophylactic and therapeutic use as a bronchodilator for bronchial asthma and for reversible bronchospasm. It may be used with or without concurrent theophylline and/or steroid therapy.

CONTRAINDICATIONS

Tornalate (bitolterol mesylate) is contraindicated in patients who are hypersensitive to any of its ingredients.

WARNINGS

As with other β-adrenergic aerosols, Tornalate (bitolterol mesylate) should not be used in excess. Fatalities have been reported in association with excessive use of inhaled sympathomimetic drugs. The exact cause of death is unknown. Use of aerosolized β-adrenergic drugs may have a deleterious cardiac effect. Paradoxical bronchoconstriction (which can be life-threatening) has been reported with administration of β-adrenergic agents. Immediate hypersensitivity (allergic) reactions can occur after the administration of Tornalate. In such instances, the drug should be discontinued immediately and alternative therapy instituted.

The contents of Tornalate Metered Dose Inhaler are under pressure. Do not puncture. Do not use or store near heat or open flame. Exposure to temperatures above 120°F may cause bursting. Never throw container into fire or incinerator. Keep out of reach of children.

If an unusual smell or taste is noted with the use of this product, the patient should discontinue use in consultation with his/her physician.

PRECAUTIONS

General As with all β-adrenergic stimulating agents, caution should be used when administering Tornalate (bitolterol mesylate) to patients with cardiovascular disease such as ischemic heart disease or hypertension. Caution is also advised in patients with hyperthyroidism, diabetes mellitus, cardiac arrhythmias, convulsive disorders or unusual responsiveness to β-adrenergic agonists. Significant changes in systolic and diastolic blood pressure have been seen in individual patients and could be expected to occur in some patients after use of any β-adrenergic aerosol bronchodilator.

Information for Patients The effects of Tornalate may last up to eight hours or longer. It should not be used more often than recommended and the patient should not increase the number of inhalations or frequency of use without first asking the physician. If symptoms of asthma get worse, adverse reactions occur, or the patient does not respond to the usual dose, the patient should be instructed to contact the physician immediately. The patient should be advised to see the illustrated Patients Instructions for Use.

Drug Interactions Other sympathomimetic aerosol bronchodilators should not be used concomitantly with Tornalate. If additional adrenergic drugs are to be administered by any route, they should be used with caution to avoid deleterious cardiovascular effects.

Carcinogenesis, Mutagenesis, and Impairment of Fertility No tumorigenicity (and specifically no increase in leiomyomas) was observed in a two-year oral study in Sprague-Dawley CD rats at doses of Tornalate corresponding to 23 or 114 times the maximal daily human inhalational dose. Tornalate was not tumorigenic in an 18-month oral study in Swiss-Webster mice at doses up to 568 times the maximal daily human inhalational dose.

Ames Salmonella and mouse lymphoma mutation assays in vitro revealed no mutagenesis due to Tornalate. Reproductive studies in male and female rats revealed no significant effects on fertility at doses of Tornalate up to 364 times the maximal daily human inhalational dose.

Teratogenic Effects—Pregnancy Category C No teratogenic effects were seen in rats and rabbits after oral doses of Tornalate up to 557 times the maximal daily human inhalational dose and in mice after oral doses up to 284 times the maximal daily human inhalational dose.

When Tornalate was injected subcutaneously into mice at doses of 2 mg/kg, 10 mg/kg, and 20 mg/kg (corresponding to 23, 114, and 227 times the maximal daily human inhalational dose) cleft palate incidences of 5.7 percent, 3.8 percent, and 3.3 percent (compared with 0.9 percent in controls) were found. Cleft palate induction with isoproterenol at 10 mg/kg SC as the positive control was 10.7 percent. Since no well-controlled studies in pregnant women are available, Tornalate should be used during pregnancy only if the potential benefit justifies the potential risk to the fetus.

Nursing Mothers It is not known whether Tornalate is excreted in human milk. Because many drugs are excreted in human milk, caution should be exercised when Tornalate is administered to a nursing woman.

Pediatric Use Safety and effectiveness of Tornalate in children 12 years of age or younger has not been established.

ADVERSE REACTIONS

The results of all clinical trials with Tornalate (bitolterol mesylate) in 492 patients showed the following side effects:

CNS: Tremors (14%), nervousness (5%), headache (4%), dizziness (3%), lightheadedness (3%), insomnia (<1%), hyperkinesia (<1%).

Gastrointestinal: Nausea (3%).

Oro-Pharyngeal: Throat irritation (5%).

Cardiovascular: The overall incidence of cardiovascular effects was approximately 5% of patients and these effects included palpitations (approximately 3%), and chest discomfort (approximately 1%). Tachycardia was seen in less than 1%. Premature ventricular contractions and flushing were rarely seen.

Respiratory: Coughing (4%), bronchospasm (<1%), dyspnea (<1%), chest tightness (<1%).

Clinical relevance or relationship to Tornalate administration of rarely reported elevations of SGOT, decrease in platelets, decrease in WBC levels or proteinuria are not known.

In comparing the adverse reactions for bitolterol mesylate treated patients to those of isoproterenol treated patients, during three-month clinical trials involving approximately 400 patients, the following moderate to severe reactions, as judged by the investigators, were reported for both steroid and non-steroid dependent patients. The table does not include mild reactions or those occurring only with the first dose.

PERCENT INCIDENCE OF MODERATE TO SEVERE ADVERSE REACTIONS

Reaction	Bitolterol N=197	Isoproterenol N=194
Central Nervous System		
Tremors	9.1%	1.5%
Nervousness	1.5%	1.0%
Headache	3.5%	6.1%
Dizziness	1.0%	1.5%
Insomnia	0.5%	0%
Cardiovascular		
Palpitations	1.5%	0%
PVC—Transient Increase	0.5%	0%
Chest Discomfort	0.5%	0%
Respiratory		
Cough	4.1%	1.0%
Bronchospasm	1.0%	0%
Dyspnea	1.0%	0%
Oro-Pharyngeal		
Throat Irritation	3.0%	3.1%
Gastrointestinal		
Nausea (Dyspepsia)	0.5%	0.5%

NOTE: In most patients, the total isoproterenol dosage was divided into three equally dosed inhalations, administered at three-minute intervals. This procedure may have reduced the incidence of adverse reactions observed with isoproterenol.

OVERDOSAGE

Overdosage with Tornalate (bitolterol mesylate) may be expected to result in exaggeration of those drug effects listed in the ADVERSE REACTIONS section. In such cases therapy with Tornalate and all β-adrenergic stimulating drugs should be stopped, supportive therapy provided, and judicious use of a cardioselective β-adrenergic blocking agent should be considered bearing in mind the possibility that such agents can produce profound bronchospasm. As with all sympathomimetic aerosol medications, cardiac arrest and even death may be associated with abuse.

The oral LD_{50} of Tornalate in rats was greater than 5,000 mg/kg and in mice greater than 6,000 mg/kg.

DOSAGE AND ADMINISTRATION

The usual dose to relieve bronchospasm for adults and children over 12 years of age is two inhalations at an interval of at least one to three minutes followed by a third inhalation if needed. For prevention of bronchospasm, the usual dose is two inhalations every 8 hours. The dose of Tornalate (bitolterol mesylate) should never exceed 3 inhalations every 6 hours or 2 inhalations every 4 hours. If a previously effective dosage regimen fails to provide the usual relief, the patient should be advised to seek medical advice immediately as this is often a sign of seriously worsening asthma that would require reassessment of therapy.

HOW SUPPLIED

Tornalate (bitolterol mesylate) Metered Dose Inhaler is supplied in 16.4 g (15mL) self-contained aerosol units (NDC 51479-012-01). Refill of 16.4 g (15mL) NDC 51479-012-02.

Note The indented statement below is required by the Federal government's Clean Air Act for all products containing or manufactured with chlorofluorocarbons (CFC's).

> **WARNING Contains dichlorodifluoromethane and dichlorotetrafluoroethane, substances which harm public health and environment by destroying ozone in the upper atmosphere.**

A notice similar to the above WARNING has been placed in the information for the patient of this product pursuant to EPA regulations.

Store at controlled room temperature between 15°C and 30°C (59°F and 86°F). Use of the product outside this temperature range may result in improper dosing.

Caution: Federal law prohibits dispensing without a prescription.

Copyright, Dura Pharmaceuticals, 1994

DURA PHARMACEUTICALS

Distributed by DURA Pharmaceuticals, Inc., San Diego, CA 92121

Manufactured by Nycomed Puerto Rico Inc., Barceloneta, Puerto Rico 00617

Revised Apr 1994   TM009EO494

Duramed Pharmaceuticals, Inc.
**5040 DURAMED DRIVE
CINCINNATI, OH 45213**

Direct Inquiries to:
Phillip J. Rose R.Ph.
V.P. Marketing and Managed Care
(513) 247-9500
1-800-543-8338

For Medical Information Contact:
In Emergenices:
Bill Stoltman
(800) 543-8338

PRODUCT LIST

NDC # 51285-	Strength	Color	Description	Brand Equivalent	Pkg Size
Acetaminophen and Codeine Phosphate Tablets #2 C-III (Rx)					
600-02	300/ 15 mg	White	Round	Tylenol w/codeine	100
Acetaminophen and Codeine Phosphate Tablets #3 C-III (Rx)					
601-02	300/	White	Round	Tylenol	100
601-05	30 mg			w/codeine	1000
Acetaminophen and Codeine Phosphate Tablets #4 C-III (Rx)					
602-02	300/	White	Round	Tylenol	100
602-05	60 mg			w/codeine	1000
Albuterol Sulfate Syrup (Rx)					
720-57	2 mg/ 5mL	Orange	Liquid	Proventil	16 oz
Amantadine Capsules (Rx)					
839-02	100 mg	Yellow	Capsule	Symmetrel	100
839-04					500
Atenolol Tablets (C.T.) (Rx)					
837-02	50 mg	White	Round, scored	Tenormin	100
837-05	50 mg	White	Round, scored	Tenormin	1000
838-02	100 mg	White	Round	Tenormin	100
Benztropine Mesylate Tablets (C.T.) (Rx)					
827-02	0.5 mg	White	Round	Cogentin	100
828-02	1 mg.	White	Oval	Cogentin	100
828-05					1000
829-02	2 mg.	White	Round	Cogentin	100
829-05					1000

Choline Magnesium Trisalicylate					
902-02	500 mg.	Pale Pink	Capsule	Trilisate	100
903-02	750 mg.	White	Capsule	Trilisate	100
904-02	1000 mg.	Pink	Capsule	Trilisate	100
Cyclobenzaprine HCl Tablets (F.C.) (Rx)					
913-02	10 mg.	White	Round	Flexeril	100
913-05					1000
Duradrin Capsules					
Acetaminophen 325 mg./Dichloralphenazone 100 mg./Isometheptene Mucate 65 mg					
Duradrin Capsules (Rx)					
364-02	—	Scarlet & White	Capsule	Midrin	100
Duratex Capsules					
Phenylephrine HCl 5 mg./Guaifenesin 200 mg./Phenylpropanolamine HCl 45 mg.					
Duratex Capsules (Rx)					
293-02	—	Orange & Beige	Capsule	Entex	100
Estropipate Tablets USP (C.T.) (Rx)					
875-02	0.75 mg	Light Orange	Diamond shaped	Ogen	100
876-02	1.5 mg	White	Diamond shaped	Ogen	100
Guaifenesin Tablets (Rx)					
417-02	600 mg	Light Green	Capsule shaped	Humibid L.A.	100
417-04					500
Isoniazid Tablets (Rx)					
277-30	300 mg.	White	Round, Scored	Isoniazid	30
277-02					100
277-05					1000
Levothyroxine Sodium Tablets (C.T.) (Rx)					
860-02	0.025 mg	Peach	Round, scored	Synthroid	100
860-05	0.025 mg	Peach	Round, scored	Synthroid	1000
861-02	0.05 mg	White	Round, scored	Synthroid	100
861-05	0.05 mg	White	Round, scored	Synthroid	1000
861-02	0.05 mg	White	round, scored	Synthroid	100
861-05					1000
862-02	0.075 mg	Purple	Round, scored	Synthroid	100
862-05					1000
863-02	0.1 mg	Yellow	Round, scored	Synthroid	100
863-05					1000
864-02	0.125 mg	Tan	Round, scored	Synthroid	100
864-05					1000
865-02	0.15 mg	Blue	Round, scored	Synthroid	100
865-05					1000
866-02	0.2 mg	Pink	Round, scored	Synthroid	100
866-05					1000
867-02	0.3 mg	Green	Round, scored	Synthroid	100
867-05					1000
Methylprednisolone Tablets (C.T.) (Rx)					
301-02	4 mg.	White	Oval, scored	Medrol	100
301-21					21 pk
Metoclopramide Tablets (C.T.) (Rx)					
805-02	10 mg.	White	Round Scored	Reglan	100
805-05					1000
834-02	5 mg.	White	Round	Reglan	100
834-04					500
Oxycodone and Acetaminophen Capsules USP C-II (Rx)					
644-02	5/500 mg	Red & White	Capsule	Tylox	100
Phenylpropanolamine HCl & Guaifenesin Long Acting Tablets (C.T.) (Rx)					
295-02	75/	Blue	Oval	Entex L.A.	100
295-04	400 mg.		shaped, scored		500
Pseudoephedrine HCl & Guaifenesin Extended Release Tablets (F.C.) (Rx)					
401-02	120/ 600 mg	Yellow	Capsule shaped, scored	Entex PSE	100
401-04					500
Salsalate Tablets (F.C.) (Rx)					
296-02	500 mg.	Blue	Round	Disalcid	100
296-04					500
297-02	750 mg.	Blue	Capsule shaped, scored	Disalcid	100
297-04					500
Tolmetin Sodium Capsules (Rx)					
846-02	200 mg	White	Round, scored	Tolectin	100
Tolmetin Sodium Capsules (Rx)					
847-02	400 mg	Orange	Capsule	Tolectin DS	100
847-04					500

Tolmetin Sodium Tablets (F.C.) (Rx)					
848-02	600 mg	Orange	Football shaped	Tolectin	100
Triotann Pediatric Suspension					
Phenylephrine Tannate 5 mg./Chlorpheniramine Tannate 2 mg./Pyrilamine Tannate 12.5 mg.					
Triotann Pediatric Suspension (Rx)					
717-57		Med. Pink		Rynatan	pint
Triotann-S Pediatric Suspension (Rx)					
717-55		Med. Pink		Rynatan-S	4×4 oz.
Triotann Tablets					
Phenylephrine Tannate 25 mg./Chlorpheniramine Tannate 8 mg./Pyrilamine Tannate 25 mg.					
Triotann Tablets (S.C.) (Rx)					
825-02	—	Buff	Capsule shaped	Rynatan	100

ECR Pharmaceuticals
**Distributor of ECR, &
Wm. P. Poythress Products
3981 DEEP ROCK ROAD
P. O. BOX 71600
RICHMOND, VA 23255**

Direct Inquiries to:
Professional Services Department
(804) 527-1950
FAX: (804) 527-1959

For Medical Information Contact:
In Emergencies:
Professional Services Department
(804) 527-1950
FAX: (804) 527-1959

NDC 0095	Product	
—0130	**Anaplex HD Cough Syrup** Each teaspoon (5 ml) contains: Hydrocodone Bitartrate, 1.7 mg; Phenylephrine HCl, 5 mg; Chlorpheniramine Maleate, 2 mg. Sugar Free. Alcohol Free.	Rx ⓒ
—0240	**Bupap Tablets** (Butalbital, 50 mg; Acetaminophen, 650 mg)	Rx
—0016	**Bensulfoid Cream** (Sulfur, 8%; Resorcinol 2%; Alcohol, 10%)	OTC
—6004	**Lodrane Liquid** Each teaspoon (5 ml) contains: Brompheniramine Maleate, 4 mg; Pseudoephedrine HCl, 60 mg. Sugar Free. Alcohol Free. Dye Free.	Rx
—6006	**Lodrane LD Capsules** (Brompheniramine Maleate, 6 mg; Pseudoephedrine HCl, 60 mg—Sustained Release, Dye Free)	Rx
—0050	**Mudrane Tablets** (Potassium Iodide, 195 mg; Aminophylline, 130 mg; Ephedrine HCl, 16 mg; Phenobarbital, 8 mg)	Rx
—0051	**Mudrane GG Tablets** (Aminophylline, 130 mg; Guaifenesin, 100 mg; Ephedrine HCl, 16 mg; Phenobarbital, 8 mg)	Rx
—0225	**Nasatab LA Tablets** (Guaifenesin, 500 mg; Pseudoephedrine HCl, 120 mg— Sustained Release, Dye Free)	Rx
—0131	**Panasal 5/500 Tablets** (Hydrocodone Bitartrate 5 mg; Aspirin 500 mg)	Rx ⓒ
—0021	**Panalgesic Gold Cream** (Methyl Salicylate, 35%; Menthol, 4%)	OTC
—0120	**Panalgesic Gold Liniment** (Methyl Salicylate, 55%; Camphor, 3%; Menthol, 1%)	OTC
—0600	**Pneumomist Tablets** (Guaifenesin, 600 mg—Sustained Release, Dye Free)	Rx
—0065	**Pneumotussin HC Cough Syrup** Each teaspoon (5 ml) contains: (Guaifenesin, 100 mg; Hydrocodone Bitartrate, 5 mg)	Rx ⓒ

Continued on next page

ECR—Cont.

—0023 **Solfoton Tablets** ℞ ©
(Phenobarbital, 16 mg)

—0031 **Uro-Phosphate Tablets** ℞
(Methenamine, 300 mg; Sodium Biphosphate, 500 mg)

Elkins-Sinn, Inc.
**2 ESTERBROOK LANE
CHERRY HILL, NJ 08003-4099**

Direct Inquiries to:
Professional Service
(610) 688-4400

For Emergency Medical Information Contact:
Day: (800) 934-5556 8:30 AM to 4:30 PM
(Eastern Standard Time), Weekdays only
Night: (610) 688-4400 (Emergencies only; non-emergencies should wait until the next day)
For Medical/Pharmacy Inquiries on Marketed Products Call:
(800) 934-5556 8:30 AM to 4:30 PM
(Eastern Standard Time), Weekdays only

Elkins-Sinn's DOSETTE® line offers a broad spectrum of injectable products in a variety of unit-of-use containers— DOSETTE® vials, DOSETTE® ampuls, DOSETTE® syringes, and DOSETTE® cartridge-needle units. Easily adaptable to any hospital pharmacy set-up, the DOSETTE® system combines easily identifiable, clearly printed product labeling with space-conserving packaging. Each DOSETTE® container is characterized by product name and strength in large, bold-faced type, important usage and storage data, lot identification number, and expiration date. Elkins-Sinn also produces a vast number of multiple dose vials. Listed below are the major ESI products. For prescribing information on products listed, write to Professional Service, Wyeth-Ayerst Laboratories, P.O. Box 8299, Philadelphia, PA 19101, or contact your local Wyeth-Ayerst representative.

AMIKACIN SULFATE INJECTION, USP
250 mg/mL	2 mL Dosette Vial
250 mg/mL	4 mL Vial

AMINOCAPROIC ACID INJECTION, USP
250 mg/mL	20 mL Multiple Dose Vial

ATROPINE SULFATE INJECTION, USP
400 mcg/mL (0.4 mg, 1/150 gr)	1 mL Dosette Vial
400 mcg/mL (0.4 mg, 1/150 gr)	1 mL Dosette Ampul
400 mcg/mL (0.4 mg, 1/150 gr)	20 mL Multiple Dose Vial
1 mg/mL (1/60 gr)	1 mL Dosette Vial

BRETYLIUM TOSYLATE INJECTION (Preservative-Free)
500 mg/10 mL	10 mL Single Use Vial

CHLORPROMAZINE HYDROCHLORIDE INJECTION, USP
25 mg/mL	1 mL Dosette Ampul
50 mg/2 mL	2 mL Dosette Ampul

CLINDAMYCIN PHOSPHATE INJECTION, USP
300 mg/2 mL	2 mL Dosette Vial
600 mg/4 mL	4 mL Single Use Vial
900 mg/6 mL	6 mL Single Use Vial
9 gram/60 mL (150 mg/mL)	Pharmacy Bulk Package

CODEINE PHOSPHATE INJECTION, USP©
30 mg/mL	1 mL Dosette Vial
60 mg/mL	1 mL Dosette Vial

CYANOCOBALAMIN INJECTION, USP
1 mg/mL (1000 mcg)	1 mL Dosette Vial
1 mg/mL (1000 mcg)	10 mL Multiple Dose Vial
1 mg/mL (1000 mcg)	30 mL Multiple Dose Vial

DEXAMETHASONE SODIUM PHOSPHATE INJECTION, USP
4 mg/mL	1 mL Dosette Vial
4 mg/mL	5 mL Multiple Dose Vial
10 mg/mL	1 mL Dosette Vial
10 mg/mL	10 mL Multiple Dose Vial

DIAZEPAM INJECTION, USP℞
5 mg/mL	1 mL Dosette Vial
5 mg/mL	10 mL Multiple Dose Vial
5 mg/mL	1 mL Dosette Syringe
10 mg/2 mL	2 mL Dosette Vial
10 mg/2 mL	2 mL Dosette Ampul
10 mg/2 mL	2 mL Dosette Syringe

DIAZEPAM INJECTION, USP℞
DOSETTE CARTRIDGE NEEDLE UNITS
5 mg/mL	1 mL Dosette Cartridge
10 mg/2 mL	2 mL Dosette Cartridge

DIGOXIN INJECTION, USP
500 mcg/2 mL (0.5 mg)	2 mL Dosette Ampul

DIPHENHYDRAMINE HYDROCHLORIDE INJECTION, USP
50 mg/mL	1 mL Dosette Vial

DOPAMINE HYDROCHLORIDE INJECTION, USP
200 mg/5 mL	5 mL Dosette Ampul
200 mg/5 mL	5 mL Single Use Vial
400 mg/5 mL	5 mL Dosette Ampul
400 mg/5 mL	5 mL Single Use Vial

DURAMORPH® (Morphine Sulfate Injection, USP)© (Preservative-Free for Epidural & Intrathecal Administration)
5 mg/10 mL (0.5 mg/mL)	10 mL Dosette Ampul
10 mg/10 mL (1 mg/mL)	10 mL Dosette Ampul

EPINEPHRINE INJECTION, USP
1 mg/mL (1:1000)	1 mL Dosette Ampul

FENTANYL CITRATE INJECTION, USP (Preservative-Free)©
100 mcg/2 mL (0.05 mg/mL)	2 mL Dosette Ampul
250 mcg/5 mL (0.05 mg/mL)	5 mL Dosette Ampul
500 mcg/10 mL (0.05 mg/mL)	10 mL Dosette Ampul
1000 mcg/20 mL (0.05 mg/mL)	20 mL Dosette Ampul
1500 mcg/30 mL	Single Dose Vial
2500 mcg/50 mL	Single Dose Vial

FUROSEMIDE INJECTION, USP (Preservative-Free)
20 mg/2 mL	2 mL Dosette Ampul
20 mg/2 mL	2 mL Single Use Vial
40 mg/4 mL	4 mL Dosette Ampul
40 mg/4 mL	4 mL Single Use Vial
100 mg/10 mL	10 mL Single Use Vial

GENTAMICIN SULFATE INJECTION, USP
20 mg/2 mL (10 mg/mL—Pediatric)	2 mL Dosette Vial
80 mg/2 mL (40 mg/mL)	2 mL Dosette Vial
800 mg/20 mL (40 mg/mL)	20 mL Multiple Dose Vial

GENTAMICIN SULFATE INJECTION, USP
DOSETTE CARTRIDGE NEEDLE UNITS
60 mg/1.5 mL	1.5 mL Dosette Cartridge
80 mg/2 mL	2 mL Dosette Cartridge

HEPARIN SODIUM INJECTION, USP (Porcine Derived)
1,000 Units/mL	1 mL Dosette Vial
1,000 Units/mL	30 mL Multiple Dose Vial
5,000 Units/mL	1 mL Dosette Vial
5,000 Units/mL	10 mL Multiple Dose Vial
10,000 Units/mL	1 mL Dosette Vial

HEPARIN SODIUM INJECTION, USP (Porcine Derived)
DOSETTE CARTRIDGE NEEDLE UNITS
5,000 Units/0.5 mL	0.5 mL Dosette Cartridge
5,000 Units/1 mL	1 mL Dosette Cartridge
10,000 Units/1 mL	1 mL Dosette Cartridge

HEP-LOCK® (Heparin Lock Flush Solution, USP)
10 Units/mL	1 mL Dosette Vial
10 Units/mL	2 mL Dosette Vial
10 Units/mL	10 mL Multiple Dose Vial
10 Units/mL	30 mL Multiple Dose Vial
100 Units/mL	1 mL Dosette Vial
100 Units/mL	2 mL Dosette Vial
100 Units/mL	10 mL Multiple Dose Vial
100 Units/mL	30 mL Multiple Dose Vial

HEP-LOCK® (Heparin Lock Flush Solution, USP)
DOSETTE CARTRIDGE NEEDLE UNITS
10 Units/1 mL	1 mL Dosette Cartridge
25 Units/2.5 mL	2.5 mL Dosette Cartridge
100 Units/1 mL	1 mL Dosette Cartridge
250 Units/2.5 mL	2.5 mL Dosette Cartridge

HEP-LOCK® (Preservative-Free Heparin Lock Flush Solution, USP)
10 Units/mL	1 mL Dosette Vial
100 Units/mL	1 mL Dosette Vial

HYDROMORPHONE HYDROCHLORIDE INJECTION, USP©
2 mg/mL	1 mL Dosette Vial
2 mg/mL	20 mL Multiple Dose Vial

HYDROXYZINE HYDROCHLORIDE I.M. INJECTION, USP
25 mg/mL	1 mL Dosette Vial
50 mg/mL	1 mL Dosette Vial
100 mg/2 mL	2 mL Dosette Vial
50 mg/mL	10 mL Multiple Dose Vial

INFUMORPH® 200
(Preservative-free Morphine Sulfate Sterile Solution)©
For Use in Continuous Microinfusion Devices
200 mg/20 mL (10 mg/mL)	20 mL Dosette Ampul

INFUMORPH® 500
(Preservative-free Morphine Sulfate Sterile Solution)©
For Use in Continuous Microinfusion Devices
500 mg/20 mL (25 mg/mL)	20 mL Dosette Ampul

ISOPROTERENOL HYDROCHLORIDE INJECTION, USP
(Refrigeration not required)
0.2 mg/mL (1:5000)	5 mL Dosette Ampul

LEUCOVORIN CALCIUM FOR INJECTION (Lyophilized)
50 mg	Single Use Vial
100 mg	Single Use Vial

LIDOCAINE HYDROCHLORIDE INJECTION, USP (Preserved)
1% (10 mg/mL)	30 mL Multiple Dose Vial
1% (10 mg/mL)	50 mL Multiple Dose Vial
2% (20 mg/mL)	30 mL Multiple Dose Vial
2% (20 mg/mL)	50 mL Multiple Dose Vial

LIDOCAINE HYDROCHLORIDE INJECTION, USP (Preservative-Free, Single Use)
1% (10 mg/mL)	5 mL Single Use Vial
2% (20 mg/mL)	5 mL Single Use Vial

LIDOCAINE HYDROCHLORIDE AND EPINEPHRINE INJECTION, USP (1:100,000) (Refrigeration not required)
1% (10 mg/mL)	30 mL Multiple Dose Vial
2% (20 mg/mL)	30 mL Multiple Dose Vial

MEPERIDINE HYDROCHLORIDE INJECTION, USP©
25 mg/mL	1 mL Dosette Vial
25 mg/mL	1 mL Dosette Ampul
50 mg/mL	1 mL Dosette Vial
50 mg/mL	1 mL Dosette Ampul
75 mg/mL	1 mL Dosette Vial
75 mg/mL	1 mL Dosette Ampul
100 mg/mL	1 mL Dosette Vial
100 mg/mL	1 mL Dosette Ampul

METRONIDAZOLE REDI-INFUSION™ (Preservative-Free, Single Use)
500 mg/100 mL	100 mL Single Use Vial

MORPHINE SULFATE INJECTION, USP©
1 mg/mL	60 mL Single Use Vial
5 mg/mL (1/12 gr)	1 mL Dosette Vial
8 mg/mL (1/8 gr)	1 mL Dosette Vial
8 mg/mL (1/8 gr)	1 mL Dosette Ampul
10 mg/mL (1/6 gr)	1 mL Dosette Vial
10 mg/mL (1/6 gr)	1 mL Dosette Ampul
10 mg/mL (1/6 gr)	10 mL Multiple Dose Vial
15 mg/mL (1/4 gr)	1 mL Dosette Vial
15 mg/mL (1/4 gr)	1 mL Dosette Ampul
15 mg/mL (1/4 gr)	20 mL Multiple Dose Vial

NALOXONE HYDROCHLORIDE INJECTION, USP
400 mcg/mL (0.4 mg/mL)	1 mL Dosette Vial
400 mcg/mL (0.4 mg/mL)	1 mL Dosette Ampul
400 mcg/mL (0.4 mg/mL)	10 mL Multiple Dose Vial

NEOSTIGMINE METHYLSULFATE INJECTION, USP
1:1000 (1 mg/mL)	10 mL Multiple Dose Vial
1:2000 (0.5 mg/mL)	10 mL Multiple Dose Vial

PANCURONIUM BROMIDE INJECTION
1 mg/mL	10 mL Multiple Dose Vial
2 mg/mL	2 mL Dosette Vial
2 mg/mL	2 mL Dosette Ampul
2 mg/mL	5 mL Dosette Ampul
2 mg/mL	5 mL Single Use Vial

PHENOBARBITAL SODIUM INJECTION, USP©
65 mg/mL (1 gr)	1 mL Dosette Vial
130 mg/mL (2 gr)	1 mL Dosette Vial

PHENYLEPHRINE HYDROCHLORIDE INJECTION, USP
10 mg/mL	1 mL Dosette Vial

PHENYTOIN SODIUM INJECTION, USP
100 mg/2 mL (50 mg/mL)	2 mL Dosette Vial
100 mg/2 mL (50 mg/mL)	2 mL Dosette Ampul
250 mg/5 mL (50 mg/mL)	5 mL Single Use Vial

PROCAINAMIDE HYDROCHLORIDE INJECTION, USP
100 mg/mL (1 gram/10 mL)	10 mL Multiple Dose Vial
500 mg/mL (1 gram/2 mL)	2 mL Multiple Dose Vial

PROCHLORPERAZINE EDISYLATE INJECTION, USP
10 mg/2 mL	2 mL Dosette Vial

PROMETHAZINE HYDROCHLORIDE INJECTION, USP
25 mg/mL	1 mL Dosette Ampul
50 mg/mL	1 mL Dosette Ampul

PROTAMINE SULFATE INJECTION, USP (Preservative-Free) (Refrigeration not required)
50 mg/5 mL	5 mL Dosette Ampul
250 mg/25 mL	25 mL Single Use Vial

SODIUM CHLORIDE INJECTION, USP (Preservative-Free, Single Use)
0.9%	2 mL Dosette Ampul
0.9%	5 mL Dosette Ampul
0.9%	10 mL Dosette Ampul

SODIUM CHLORIDE INJECTION, BACTERIOSTATIC, USP (Preserved with 0.9% Benzyl Alcohol)
0.9%	30 mL Multiple Dose Vial
0.9%	2 mL Dosette Cartridge

SODIUM NITROPRUSSIDE, STERILE, USP
50 mg	Single Use Vial

SOTRADECOL® (Sodium Tetradecyl Sulfate Injection)
1%	2 mL Dosette Ampul
3%	2 mL Dosette Ampul

SUFENTANIL CITRATE INJECTION, USP

500 mcg/mL	1 mL Dosette Ampul
100 mcg/2 mL	2 mL Dosette Ampul
250 mcg/5 mL	5 mL Dosette Ampul

SULFAMETHOXAZOLE & TRIMETHOPRIM CONCENTRATE FOR INJECTION, USP

80 mg/mL Sulfamethoxazole with 16 mg/mL Trimethoprim	5 mL Dosette Ampul
80 mg/mL Sulfamethoxazole with 16 mg/mL Trimethoprim	5 mL Single Use Vial
80 mg/mL Sulfamethoxazole with 16 mg/mL Trimethoprim	10 mL Single Use Vial
80 mg/mL Sulfamethoxazole with 16 mg/mL Trimethoprim	30 mL Multiple Dose Vial

THIAMINE HYDROCHLORIDE INJECTION, USP

100 mg/mL	1 mL Dosette Vial

WATER FOR INJECTION, BACTERIOSTATIC, USP
(Preserved with 0.9% Benzyl Alcohol)

	30 mL Multiple Dose Vial

AMIKACIN ℞
[ă'mĭ-că-sĭn]
SULFATE INJECTION, USP

WARNINGS

Patients treated with parenteral aminoglycosides should be under close clinical observation because of the potential ototoxicity and nephrotoxicity associated with their use. Safety for treatment periods which are longer than 14 days has not been established.

Neurotoxicity, manifested as vestibular and permanent bilateral auditory ototoxicity, can occur in patients with preexisting renal damage and in patients with normal renal function treated at higher doses and/or for periods longer than those recommended. The risk of aminoglycoside-induced ototoxicity is greater in patients with renal damage. High frequency deafness usually occurs first and can be detected only by audiometric testing. Vertigo may occur and may be evidence of vestibular injury. Other manifestations of neurotoxicity may include numbness, skin tingling, muscle twitching and convulsions. The risk of hearing loss due to aminoglycosides increases with the degree of exposure to either high peak or high trough serum concentrations. Patients developing cochlear damage may not have symptoms during therapy to warn them of developing eighth-nerve toxicity, and total or partial irreversible bilateral deafness may occur after the drug has been discontinued. Aminoglycoside-induced ototoxicity is usually irreversible.

Aminoglycosides are potentially nephrotoxic. The risk of nephrotoxicity is greater in patients with impaired renal function and in those who receive high doses or prolonged therapy.

Neuromuscular blockade and respiratory paralysis have been reported following parenteral injection, topical instillation (as in orthopedic and abdominal irrigation or in local treatment of empyema) and following oral use of aminoglycosides. The possibility of these phenomena should be considered if aminoglycosides are administered by any route, especially in patients receiving anesthetics; neuromuscular blocking agents such as tubocurarine, succinylcholine, decamethonium; or in patients receiving massive transfusions of citrate-anticoagulated blood. If blockage occurs, calcium salts may reverse these phenomena, but mechanical respiratory assistance may be necessary.

Renal and eighth-nerve function should be closely monitored especially in patients with known or suspected renal impairment at the onset of therapy and also in those whose renal function is initially normal but who develop signs of renal dysfunction during therapy. Serum concentrations of amikacin should be monitored when feasible to assure adequate levels and to avoid potentially toxic levels and prolonged peak concentrations above 35 micrograms per mL. Urine should be examined for decreased specific gravity, increased excretion of proteins and the presence of cells or casts. Blood urea nitrogen, serum creatinine or creatinine clearance should be measured periodically. Serial audiograms should be obtained where feasible in patients old enough to be tested, particularly high risk patients. Evidence of ototoxicity (dizziness, vertigo, tinnitus, roaring in the ears and hearing loss) or nephrotoxicity requires discontinuation of the drug or dosage adjustment.

Concurrent and/or sequential systemic, oral or topical use of other neurotoxic or nephrotoxic products, particularly bacitracin, cisplatin, amphotericin B, cephaloridine, paromomycin, viomycin, polymyxin B, colistin, vancomycin or other aminoglycosides should be avoided. Other factors that may increase risk of toxicity are advanced age and dehydration.

The concurrent use of amikacin with potent diuretics (ethacrynic acid or furosemide) should be avoided since diuretics by themselves may cause ototoxicity. In addition, when administered intravenously, diuretics may enhance aminoglycoside toxicity by altering antibiotic concentrations in serum and tissue.

DESCRIPTION

Amikacin sulfate, a semi-synthetic aminoglycoside antibiotic derived from kanamycin, has the following structural formula:

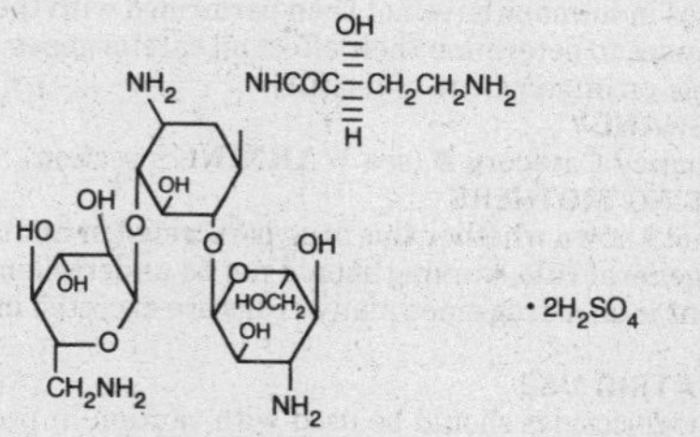

D-Streptamine, O-3-amino-3-deoxy-α-D-glucopyranosyl-(1→6)-O-[6-amino-6-deoxy-α-D-glucopyranosyl-(1→4)]-N^1-(4-amino-2-hydroxy-1-oxobutyl)-2-deoxy-, (S)-, sulfate (1:2) (salt)

$C_{22}H_{43}N_5O_{13} \cdot 2H_2SO_4$ Molecular weight 781.75

The dosage form is supplied as a sterile, colorless to light straw-colored solution for IM or IV use.

Each mL contains 250 mg amikacin as the sulfate, sodium citrate (dihydrate) 28.5 mg and sodium metabisulfite 6.6 mg in Water for Injection. pH 3.5–5.5; sodium hydroxide and/or sulfuric acid added, if needed, for pH adjustment. Sealed under nitrogen.

CLINICAL PHARMACOLOGY

INTRAMUSCULAR ADMINISTRATION

Amikacin is rapidly absorbed after intramuscular administration. In normal adult volunteers, average peak serum concentrations of about 12, 16 and 21 mcg/mL are obtained 1 hour after intramuscular administration of 250 mg (3.7 mg/kg), 375 mg (5 mg/kg), 500 mg (7.5 mg/kg), single doses, respectively. At 10 hours, serum levels are about 0.3 mcg/mL, 1.2 mcg/mL and 2.1 mcg/mL, respectively.

Tolerance studies in normal volunteers reveal that amikacin is well tolerated locally following repeated intramuscular dosing, and when given at maximally recommended doses, no ototoxicity or nephrotoxicity has been reported. There is no evidence of drug accumulation with repeated dosing for 10 days when administered according to recommended doses.

With normal renal function, about 91.9% of an intramuscular dose is excreted unchanged in the urine in the first 8 hours and 98.2% within 24 hours. Mean urine concentrations for 6 hours are 563 mcg/mL following a 250 mg dose, 697 mcg/mL following a 375 mg dose and 832 mcg/mL following a 500 mg dose.

Preliminary intramuscular studies in newborns of different weights (less than 1.5 kg, 1.5 to 2 kg, over 2 kg) at a dose of 7.5 mg/kg revealed that, like other aminoglycosides, serum half-life values were correlated inversely with post-natal age and renal clearances of amikacin. The volume of distribution indicates that amikacin, like other aminoglycosides, remains primarily in the extracellular fluid space of neonates. Repeated dosing every 12 hours in all the above groups did not demonstrate accumulation after 5 days.

INTRAVENOUS ADMINISTRATION

Single doses of 500 mg (7.5 mg/kg) administered to normal adults as an infusion over a period of 30 minutes produced a mean peak serum concentration of 38 mcg/mL at the end of the infusion and levels of 24 mcg/mL, 18 mcg/mL and 0.75 mcg/mL at 30 minutes, 1 hour and 10 hours post-infusion, respectively. Eighty-four percent of the administered dose was excreted in the urine in 9 hours and about 94% within 24 hours.

Repeat infusions of 7.5 mg/kg every 12 hours in normal adults were well tolerated and caused no drug accumulation.

GENERAL

Pharmacokinetic studies in normal adult subjects reveal the mean serum half-life to be slightly over 2 hours with a mean total apparent volume of distribution of 24 liters (28% of the body weight). By the ultrafiltration technique, reports of serum protein binding range from 0 to 11%. The mean serum clearance rate is about 100 mL/min and the renal clearance rate is 94 mL/min in subjects with normal renal function.

Amikacin is excreted primarily by glomerular filtration. Patients with impaired renal function or diminished glomerular filtration pressure excrete the drug much more slowly (effectively prolonging the serum half-life). Therefore, renal function should be monitored carefully and dosage adjusted accordingly (see suggested dosage schedule under **DOSAGE AND ADMINISTRATION**).

Following administration at the recommended dose, therapeutic levels are found in bone, heart, gallbladder and lung tissue in addition to significant concentrations in urine; bile; sputum; bronchial secretions; interstitial, pleural and synovial fluids.

Spinal fluid levels in normal infants are approximately 10 to 20% of the serum concentrations and may reach 50% when the meninges are inflamed. Amikacin has been demonstrated to cross the placental barrier and yield significant concentrations in amniotic fluid. The peak fetal serum concentration is about 16% of the peak maternal serum concentration and maternal and fetal serum half-life values are about 2 and 3.7 hours, respectively.

MICROBIOLOGY

Gram-negative—Amikacin is active *in vitro* against *Pseudomonas* species, *Escherichia coli, Proteus* species (indole-positive and indole-negative), *Providencia* species, *Klebsiella-Enterobacter-Serratia* species, *Acinetobacter* (formerly *Mima-Herellea*) species and *Citrobacter freundii.*

When strains of the above organisms are found to be resistant to other aminoglycosides, including gentamicin, tobramycin and kanamycin, many are susceptible to amikacin *in vitro.*

Gram-positive—Amikacin is active *in vitro* against penicillinase and non-penicillinase-producing *Staphylococcus* species, including methicillin-resistant strains. However, aminoglycosides in general have a low order of activity against other gram-positive organisms, viz., *Streptococcus pyogenes,* enterococci and *Streptococcus pneumoniae* (formerly *Diplococcus pneumoniae).*

Amikacin resists degradation by most aminoglycoside inactivating enzymes known to affect gentamicin, tobramycin and kanamycin.

In vitro studies have shown that amikacin sulfate combined with a beta-lactam antibiotic acts synergistically against many clinically significant gram-negative organisms.

Disc Susceptibility Tests—Quantitative methods that require measurement of zone diameters give the most precise estimates of antibiotic susceptibility. One such procedure* has been recommended for use with discs to test susceptibility to amikacin. Interpretation involves correlation of the diameters obtained in the disc test with MIC values for amikacin. When the causative organism is tested by the Kirby-Bauer method of disc susceptibility, a 30 mcg amikacin disc should give a zone of 17 mm or greater to indicate susceptibility. Zone sizes of 14 mm or less indicate resistance. Zone sizes of 15 to 16 mm indicate intermediate susceptibility. With this procedure, a report from the laboratory of "susceptible" indicates that the infecting organism is likely to respond to therapy. A report of "resistant" indicates that the infecting organism is not likely to respond to therapy. A report of "intermediate susceptibility" suggests that the organism would be susceptible if the infection is confined to tissues and fluids (e.g., urine) in which high antibiotic levels are attained.

INDICATIONS AND USAGE

Amikacin Sulfate Injection is indicated in the short-term treatment of serious infections due to susceptible strains of gram-negative bacteria, including *Pseudomonas* species, *Escherichia coli,* species of indole-positive and indole-negative *Proteus, Providencia* species, *Klebsiella-Enterobacter-Serratia* species and *Acinetobacter (Mima-Herellea)* species.

Clinical studies have shown Amikacin Sulfate Injection to be effective in bacterial septicemia (including neonatal sepsis); in serious infections of the respiratory tract, bones and joints, central nervous system (including meningitis) and skin and soft tissue; intra-abdominal infections (including peritonitis); and in burns and post-operative infections (including post-vascular surgery). Clinical studies have shown amikacin also to be effective in serious complicated and recurrent urinary tract infections due to these organisms. Aminoglycosides, including amikacin, are not indicated in uncomplicated initial episodes of urinary tract infections unless the causative organisms are not susceptible to antibiotics having less potential toxicity.

Bacteriologic studies should be performed to identify causative organisms and their susceptibilities to amikacin. Amikacin may be considered as initial therapy in suspected gram-negative infections, and therapy may be instituted before obtaining the results of susceptibility testing. Clinical trials demonstrated that amikacin was effective in infections caused by gentamicin- and/or tobramycin-resistant strains of gram-negative organisms, particularly *Proteus rettgeri, Providencia stuartii, Serratia marcescens* and *Pseudomonas aeruginosa.* The decision to continue therapy with the drug should be based on results of the susceptibility tests, the severity of the infection and the response of the patient, as well as important additional considerations (see **WARNINGS** box).

Amikacin has also been shown to be effective in staphylococcal infections and may be considered as initial therapy under certain conditions in the treatment of known or suspected

Continued on next page

Elkins-Sinn—Cont.

staphylococcal disease such as severe infections where the causative organism may be either a gram-negative bacterium or a staphylococcus, infections due to susceptible strains of staphylococci in patients allergic to other antibiotics and in mixed staphylococcal/gram-negative infections.
In certain severe infections such as neonatal sepsis, concomitant therapy with a penicillin-type drug may be indicated because of the possibility of infections due to gram-positive organisms such as streptococci or pneumococci.

CONTRAINDICATIONS

A history of hypersensitivity to amikacin is a contraindication for its use. A history of hypersensitivity or serious toxic reactions to aminoglycosides may contraindicate the use of any other aminoglycoside because of the known cross-sensitivities of patients to drugs in this class.

WARNINGS

See **WARNINGS** box above.
Aminoglycosides can cause fetal harm when administered to a pregnant woman. Aminoglycosides cross the placenta and there have been several reports of total irreversible, bilateral congenital deafness in children whose mothers received streptomycin during pregnancy. Although serious side effects to the fetus or newborns have not been reported in the treatment of pregnant women with other aminoglycosides, the potential for harm exists. Reproduction studies of amikacin have been performed in rats and mice and revealed no evidence of impaired fertility or harm to the fetus due to amikacin. There are no well-controlled studies in pregnant women, but investigational experience does not include any positive evidence of adverse effects to the fetus. If this drug is used during pregnancy, or if the patient becomes pregnant while taking this drug, the patient should be apprised of the potential hazard to the fetus.
Contains sodium metabisulfite, a sulfite that may cause allergic-type reactions including anaphylactic symptoms and life-threatening or less severe asthmatic episodes in certain susceptible people. The overall prevalence of sulfite sensitivity in the general population is unknown and probably low. Sulfite sensitivity is seen more frequently in asthmatic than nonasthmatic people.

PRECAUTIONS

Aminoglycosides are quickly and almost totally absorbed when they are applied topically, except to the urinary bladder, in association with surgical procedures. Irreversible deafness, renal failure and death due to neuromuscular blockade have been reported following irrigation of both small and large surgical fields with an aminoglycoside preparation.
Amikacin Sulfate Injection is potentially nephrotoxic, ototoxic and neurotoxic. The concurrent or serial use of other ototoxic or nephrotoxic agents should be avoided either systemically or topically because of the potential for additive effects. Increased nephrotoxicity has been reported following concomitant parenteral administration of aminoglycoside antibiotics and cephalosporins. Concomitant cephalosporins may spuriously elevate creatinine determinations.
Since amikacin is present in high concentrations in the renal excretory system, patients should be well-hydrated to minimize chemical irritation of the renal tubules. Kidney function should be assessed by the usual methods prior to starting therapy and daily during the course of treatment.
If signs of renal irritation appear (casts, white or red cells or albumin), hydration should be increased. A reduction in dosage (see **DOSAGE AND ADMINISTRATION**) may be desirable if other evidence of renal dysfunction occurs such as decreased creatinine clearance; decreased urine specific gravity; increased BUN, creatinine or oliguria. If azotemia increases or if a progressive decrease in urinary output occurs, treatment should be stopped.
Note: When patients are well hydrated and kidney function is normal, the risk of nephrotoxic reactions with amikacin is low if the dosage recommendations (see **DOSAGE AND ADMINISTRATION**) are not exceeded.
Elderly patients may have reduced renal function which may not be evident in routine screening tests such as BUN or serum creatinine. A creatinine clearance determination may be more useful. Monitoring of renal function during treatment with aminoglycosides is particularly important.
Aminoglycosides should be used with caution in patients with muscular disorders such as myasthenia gravis or parkinsonism since these drugs may aggravate muscle weakness because of their potential curare-like effect on the neuromuscular junction.
In vitro mixing of aminoglycosides with beta-lactam antibiotics (penicillin or cephalosporins) may result in a significant mutual inactivation. A reduction in serum half-life or serum level may occur when an aminoglycoside or penicillin-type drug is administered by separate routes. Inactivation of the aminoglycoside is clinically significant only in patients with severely impaired renal function. Inactivation may continue in specimens of body fluids collected for assay, resulting in inaccurate aminoglycoside readings. Such specimens should be properly handled (assayed promptly, frozen or treated with beta-lactamase).
Cross-allergenicity among aminoglycosides has been demonstrated.
As with other antibiotics, the use of amikacin may result in overgrowth of non-susceptible organisms. If this occurs, appropriate therapy should be instituted.
Aminoglycosides should not be given concurrently with potent diuretics (see **WARNINGS** box).

CARCINOGENESIS, MUTAGENESIS, IMPAIRMENT OF FERTILITY
Studies in humans have not been performed with the aminoglycosides to determine their effect on carcinogenesis, mutagenesis or impairment of fertility.

PREGNANCY
Pregnancy Category D (see **WARNINGS** section).

NURSING MOTHERS
It is not known whether this drug is excreted in human milk. As a general rule, nursing should not be undertaken while a patient is on a drug since many drugs are excreted in human milk.

PEDIATRIC USE
Aminoglycosides should be used with caution in premature and neonatal infants because of the renal immaturity of these patients and the resulting prolongation of serum half-life of these drugs.

ADVERSE REACTIONS

All aminoglycosides have the potential to induce auditory, vestibular and renal toxicity and neuromuscular blockade (see **WARNINGS** box). They occur more frequently in patients with present or past history of renal impairment, of treatment with other ototoxic or nephrotoxic drugs and in patients treated for longer periods and/or with higher doses than recommended.
Neurotoxicity-Ototoxicity—Toxic effects on the eighth cranial nerve can result in hearing loss, loss of balance or both. Amikacin primarily affects auditory function. Cochlear damage includes high frequency deafness and usually occurs before clinical hearing loss can be detected.
Neurotoxicity-Neuromuscular Blockage—Acute muscular paralysis and apnea can occur following treatment with aminoglycoside drugs.
Nephrotoxicity—Elevation of serum creatinine, albuminuria, presence of red and white cells, casts, azotemia and oliguria have been reported. Renal function changes are usually reversible when the drug is discontinued.
Other—In addition to those described above, other adverse reactions which have been reported on rare occasions are skin rash, drug fever, headache, paresthesia, tremor, nausea and vomiting, eosinophilia, arthralgia, anemia and hypotension.

OVERDOSAGE

In the event of overdosage or toxic reaction, peritoneal dialysis or hemodialysis will aid in the removal of amikacin from the blood. In the newborn infant, exchange transfusion may also be considered.

DOSAGE AND ADMINISTRATION

The patient's pretreatment body weight should be obtained for calculation of correct dosage. Amikacin Sulfate Injection may be given intramuscularly or intravenously.
The status of renal function should be estimated by measurement of the serum creatinine concentration or calculation of the endogenous creatinine clearance rate. The blood urea nitrogen (BUN) is much less reliable for this purpose. Reassessment of renal function should be made periodically during therapy.
Whenever possible, amikacin concentrations in serum should be measured to assure adequate but not excessive levels. It is desirable to measure both peak and trough serum concentrations intermittently during therapy. Peak concentrations (30–90 minutes after injection) above 35 micrograms per mL and trough concentrations (just prior to the next dose) above 10 micrograms per mL should be avoided. Dosage should be adjusted as indicated.

INTRAMUSCULAR ADMINISTRATION FOR PATIENTS WITH NORMAL RENAL FUNCTION
The recommended dosage for adults, children and older infants (see **WARNINGS** box) with normal renal function is 15 mg/kg/day divided into 2 or 3 equal doses administered at equally divided intervals, i.e., 7.5 mg/kg q12h or 5 mg/kg q8h. Treatment of patients in the heavier weight classes should not exceed 1.5 gram/day.
When amikacin is indicated in newborns (see **WARNINGS** box), it is recommended that a loading dose of 10 mg/kg be administered initially to be followed with 7.5 mg/kg every 12 hours.
The usual duration of treatment is 7 to 10 days. It is desirable to limit the duration of treatment to short-term whenever feasible. The total daily dose by all routes of administration should not exceed 15 mg/kg/day. In difficult and complicated infections where treatment beyond 10 days is considered, the use of amikacin should be reevaluated. If continued, amikacin serum levels and renal, auditory and vestibular functions should be monitored. At the recommended dosage level, uncomplicated infections due to amikacin-sensitive organisms should respond in 24 to 48 hours. If definite clinical response does not occur within 3 to 5 days, therapy should be stopped and the antibiotic susceptibility pattern of the invading organism should be rechecked. Failure of the infection to respond may be due to resistance of the organism or to the presence of septic foci requiring surgical drainage.
When amikacin is indicated in uncomplicated urinary tract infections, a dose of 250 mg twice daily may be used.

DOSAGE GUIDELINES
ADULTS AND CHILDREN WITH NORMAL RENAL FUNCTION

Patient Weight lbs	kg	Dosage 7.5 mg/kg q12h	OR	5 mg/kg q8h
99	45	337.5 mg		225 mg
110	50	375 mg		250 mg
121	55	412.5 mg		275 mg
132	60	450 mg		300 mg
143	65	487.5 mg		325 mg
154	70	525 mg		350 mg
165	75	562.5 mg		375 mg
176	80	600 mg		400 mg
187	85	637.5 mg		425 mg
198	90	675 mg		450 mg
209	95	712.5 mg		475 mg
220	100	750 mg		500 mg

INTRAMUSCULAR ADMINISTRATION FOR PATIENTS WITH IMPAIRED RENAL FUNCTION
Whenever possible, serum amikacin concentrations should be monitored by appropriate assay procedures. Doses may be adjusted in patients with impaired renal function either by administering normal doses at prolonged intervals or by administering reduced doses at a fixed interval.
Both methods are based on the patient's creatinine clearance or serum creatinine values since these have been found to correlate with aminoglycoside half-lives in patients with diminished renal function. These dosage schedules must be used in conjunction with careful clinical and laboratory observations of the patient and should be modified as necessary. Neither method should be used when dialysis is being performed.
Normal Dosage at Prolonged Intervals—If the creatinine clearance rate is not available and the patient's condition is stable, a dosage interval in hours for the normal dose can be calculated by multiplying the patient's serum creatinine by 9, e.g., if the serum creatinine concentration is 2 mg/100 mL, the recommended single dose (7.5 mg/kg) should be administered every 18 hours.
Reduced Dosage at Fixed Time Intervals—When renal function is impaired and it is desirable to administer amikacin at a fixed time interval, dosage must be reduced. In these patients, serum amikacin concentrations should be measured to assure accurate administration of amikacin and to avoid concentrations above 35 mcg/mL. If serum assay determinations are not available and the patient's condition is stable, serum creatinine and creatinine clearance values are the most readily available indicators of the degree of renal impairment to use as a guide for dosage.
First, initiate therapy by administering a normal dose, 7.5 mg/kg, as a loading dose. This loading dose is the same as the normally recommended dose which would be calculated for a patient with a normal renal function as described above.
To determine the size of maintenance doses administered every 12 hours, the loading dose should be reduced in proportion to the reduction in the patient's creatinine clearance rate:

$$\text{Maintenance Dose Every 12 hours} = \frac{\text{observed CC in mL/min}}{\text{normal CC in mL/min}} \times \text{calculated loading dose in mg}$$

(CC—creatinine clearance rate)
An alternate rough guide for determining reduced dosage at 12-hour intervals (for patients whose steady state serum creatinine values are known) is to divide the normally recommended dose by the patient's serum creatinine.
The above dosage schedules are not intended to be rigid recommendations but are provided as guides to dosage when the measurement of amikacin serum levels is not feasible.

INTRAVENOUS ADMINISTRATION

The individual dose, the total daily dose and the total cumulative dose of amikacin sulfate are identical to the dose recommended for intramuscular administration. The solution for intravenous use is prepared by adding the contents of a 500 mg vial to 100–200 mL of sterile diluent such as Normal Saline or 5% Dextrose in Water or any other compatible solution.
The solution is administered to adults over a 30 to 60 minute period. The total daily dose should not exceed 15 mg/kg/day and may be divided into either 2 or 3 equally divided doses at equally divided intervals.

In pediatric patients, the amount of fluid used will depend on the amount ordered for the patient. It should be a sufficient amount to infuse the amikacin over a 30 to 60 minute period. Infants should receive a 1 to 2 hour infusion.
Amikacin should not be physically premixed with other drugs but should be administered separately according to the recommended dose and route.
Stability in IV Fluids—Amikacin sulfate is stable for 24 hours at room temperature at concentrations of 0.25 and 5 mg/mL in the following solutions:

5% Dextrose Injection, USP
5% Dextrose and 0.2% Sodium Chloride Injection, USP
5% Dextrose and 0.45% Sodium Chloride Injection, USP
0.9% Sodium Chloride Injection, USP
Lactated Ringer's Injection, USP
Normosol® M in 5% Dextrose Injection (or Plasma-Lyte 56 Injection in 5% Dextrose in Water)
Normosol® R in 5% Dextrose Injection (or Plasma-Lyte 148 Injection in 5% Dextrose in Water)

Aminoglycosides administered by any of the above routes should not be physically premixed with other drugs but should be administered separately.
Because of the potential toxicity of aminoglycosides, "fixed dosage" recommendations which are not based upon body weight are not advised. Rather, it is essential to calculate the dosage to fit the needs of each patient.
Parenteral drug products should be inspected visually for particulate matter and discoloration prior to administration whenever the solution and container permit.

HOW SUPPLIED

Amikacin Sulfate Injection, USP is available in the following packages:
250 mg/mL
2 mL (500 mg) DOSETTE® vials packaged in 10s (*NDC* 0641-0123-23)
4 mL (1 gram) vials packaged in 10s (*NDC* 0641-2357-43)
STORAGE
Amikacin Sulfate Injection, USP is supplied as a colorless solution which requires no refrigeration. Store at controlled room temperature 15°–30°C (59°–86°F).
Store solutions for intravenous use as directed in **DOSAGE AND ADMINISTRATION.**
At times, the solution may become a very pale yellow; this does not indicate a decrease in potency.

* Bauer, AW; Kirby, WMM; Sherris, JC and Turck, M: Antibiotic Testing by a Standardized Single Disc Method, AM J CLIN PATHOL, 45:493, 1966; Standardized Disc Susceptibility Test, *FEDERAL REGISTER*, 37:20527-29, 1972.

DURAMORPH® Ⓒ II

[*dūr"a'mŏrf*]
(morphine sulfate injection, USP)
Preservative-Free

Warning: May be habit forming.

DESCRIPTION

Morphine is the most important alkaloid of opium and is a phenanthrene derivative. It is available as the sulfate salt, having the following structural formula:

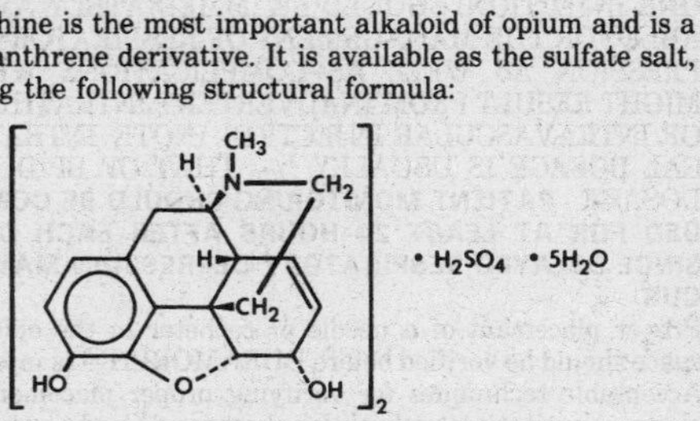

7,8 Didehydro-4,5-epoxy-17-methyl-(5α,6α)-morphinan-3,6-diol sulfate (2:1) (salt), pentahydrate

$(C_{17}H_{19}NO_3)_2 \cdot H_2SO_4 \cdot 5H_2O$ Molecular weight is 758.83.

Preservative-free DURAMORPH® (Morphine Sulfate Injection, USP) is a sterile, nonpyrogenic, isobaric solution of morphine sulfate, free of antioxidants, preservatives or other potentially neurotoxic additives and is intended for intravenous, epidural or intrathecal administration as a narcotic analgesic. Each milliliter contains morphine sulfate 0.5 mg or 1 mg and sodium chloride 9 mg in Water for Injection. pH range is 2.5–6.5. Ampuls are sealed under nitrogen. Each Dosette® ampul of DURAMORPH® is intended for **SINGLE USE ONLY.** *Discard any unused portion.* DO NOT HEAT-STERILIZE.

CLINICAL PHARMACOLOGY

Morphine produces a wide spectrum of pharmacologic effects including analgesia, dysphoria, euphoria, somnolence, respiratory depression, diminished gastrointestinal motility and physical dependence. Opiate analgesia involves at least three anatomical areas of the central nervous system: the periaqueductal-periventricular gray matter, the ventromedial medulla and the spinal cord. A systemically administered opiate may produce analgesia by acting at any, all or some combination of these distinct regions. Morphine interacts predominantly with the μ-receptor. The μ-binding sites of opioids are very discretely distributed in the human brain, with high densities of sites found in the posterior amygdala, hypothalamus, thalamus, nucleus caudatus, putamen and certain cortical areas. They are also found on the terminal axons of primary afferents within laminae I and II (substantia gelatinosa) of the spinal cord and in the spinal nucleus of the trigeminal nerve.
Morphine has an apparent volume of distribution ranging from 1.0 to 4.7 L/kg after *intravenous* dosage. Protein binding is low, about 36%, and muscle tissue binding is reported as 54%. A blood-brain barrier exists, and when morphine is introduced outside of the CNS (e.g. *intravenously*), plasma concentrations of morphine remain higher than the corresponding CSF morphine levels. Conversely, when morphine is injected into the *intrathecal space*, it diffuses out into the systemic circulation slowly, accounting for the long duration of action of morphine administered by this route. Morphine has a total plasma clearance which ranges from 0.9 to 1.2 L/kg/h (liters/kilogram/hour) in postoperative patients, but shows considerable interindividual variation. The major pathway of clearance is hepatic glucuronidation to morphine-3-glucuronide, which is pharmacologically inactive. The major excretion path of the conjugate is through the kidneys, with about 10% in the feces. Morphine is also eliminated by the kidneys, 2 to 12% being excreted unchanged in the urine. Terminal half-life is commonly reported to vary from 1.5 to 4.5 hours, although the longer half-lives were obtained when morphine levels were monitored over protracted periods with very sensitive radioimmunoassay methods. The accepted elimination half-life in normal subject is 1.5 to 2 hours.
"Selective" blockade of pain sensation is possible by neuraxial application of morphine. In addition, duration of analgesia may be much longer by this route compared to systemic administration. However, CNS effects, associated with systemic administration, are still seen. These include respiratory depression, sedation, nausea and vomiting, pruritus and urinary retention. In particular, both early and late respiratory depression (up to 24 hours post dosing) have been reported following neuraxial administration. Circulation of the spinal fluid may also result in high concentrations of morphine reaching the brain stem directly.
The incidence of unwanted CNS effects, including delayed respiratory depression, associated with neuraxial application of morphine, is related to the circulatory dynamics of the epidural venous plexus and the spinal fluid. The lipid solubility and degree of ionization of morphine plays an important part in both the onset and duration of analgesia and the CNS effects. Morphine has a pK_a 7.9, with an octanol/water partition coefficient of 1.42 at pH 7.4. At this pH, the tertiary amino group in each of the opioids is mostly ionized, making the molecule water soluble. Morphine, with additional hydroxyl groups on the molecule, is significantly more water soluble than any other opioid in clinical use.
Morphine, injected into the *epidural space*, is rapidly absorbed into the general circulation. Absorption is so rapid that the plasma concentration-time profiles closely resemble those obtained after intravenous or intramuscular administration. Peak plasma concentrations averaging 33–40 ng/mL (range 5–62 ng/mL) are achieved within 10 to 15 minutes after administration of 3 mg of morphine. Plasma concentrations decline in a multiexponential fashion. The terminal half-life is reported to range from 39 to 249 minutes (mean of 90±34.3 min) and, though somewhat shorter, is similar in magnitude as values reported after intravenous and intramuscular administration (1.5–4.5 h). CSF concentrations of morphine, after epidural doses of 2 to 6 mg in postoperative patients, have been reported to be 50 to 250 times higher than corresponding plasma concentrations. The CSF levels of morphine exceed those in plasma after only 15 minutes and are detectable for as long as 20 hours after the injection of 2 mg of epidural morphine. Approximately 4% of the dose injected epidurally reaches the CSF. This corresponds to the relative minimum effective epidural and intrathecal doses of 5 mg and 0.25 mg, respectively. The disposition of morphine in the CSF follows a biphasic pattern, with an early half-life of 1.5 h and a late phase half-life of about 6 h. Morphine crosses the dura slowly, with an absorption half-life across the dura averaging 22 minutes. Maximum CSF concentrations are seen 60–90 minutes after injection. Minimum effective CSF concentrations for postoperative analgesia average 150 ng/mL (range <1–380 ng/mL).
The *intrathecal route* of administration circumvents meningeal diffusion barriers and, therefore, lower doses of morphine produce comparable analgesia to that induced by the epidural route. After intrathecal bolus injection of morphine, there is a rapid initial distribution phase lasting 15–30 minutes and a half-life in the CSF of 42–136 min (mean 90±16 min). Derived from limited data, it appears that the disposition of morphine in the CSF, from 15 minutes postintrathecal administration to the end of a six-hour observation period, represents a combination of the distribution and elimination phases. Morphine concentrations in the CSF averaged 332±137 ng/mL at 6 hours, following a bolus dose of 0.3 mg of morphine. The apparent volume of distribution of morphine in the intrathecal space is about 22±8 mL.
Time-to-peak plasma concentrations, however, are similar (5–10 min) after either epidural or intrathecal bolus administration of morphine. Maximum plasma morphine concentrations after 0.3 mg intrathecal morphine have been reported from <1 to 7.8 ng/mL. The minimum analgesic morphine plasma concentration during Patient-Controlled Analgesia (PCA) has been reported as 20–40 ng/mL, suggesting that any analgesic contribution from systemic redistribution would be minimal after the first 30–60 minutes with epidural administration and virtually absent with intrathecal administration of morphine.

INDICATIONS AND USAGE

DURAMORPH® is a systemic narcotic analgesic for administration by the intravenous, epidural or intrathecal routes. It is used for the management of pain not responsive to non-narcotic analgesics. DURAMORPH®, administered epidurally or intrathecally, provides pain relief for extended periods without attendant loss of motor, sensory or sympathetic function.

CONTRAINDICATIONS

DURAMORPH® is contraindicated in those medical conditions which would preclude the administration of opioids by the intravenous route—allergy to morphine or other opiates, acute bronchial asthma, upper airway obstruction.

WARNINGS

Morphine sulfate may be habit forming. (See DRUG ABUSE AND DEPENDENCE.)
DURAMORPH® administration should be limited to use by those familiar with the management of respiratory depression. Rapid intravenous administration may result in chest wall rigidity.
Prior to any epidural or intrathecal drug administration, the physician should be familiar with patient conditions (such as infection at the injection site, bleeding diathesis, anticoagulant therapy, etc.) which call for special evaluation of the benefit versus risk potential.
In the case of epidural or intrathecal administration, DURAMORPH® should be administered by or under the direction of a physician experienced in the techniques and familiar with the patient management problems associated with epidural or intrathecal drug administration. Because epidural administration has been associated with less potential for immediate or late adverse effects than intrathecal administration, the epidural route should be used whenever possible.
SEVERE RESPIRATORY DEPRESSION UP TO 24 HOURS FOLLOWING EPIDURAL OR INTRATHECAL ADMINISTRATION HAS BEEN REPORTED.

BECAUSE OF THE RISK OF SEVERE ADVERSE EFFECTS WHEN THE EPIDURAL OR INTRATHECAL ROUTE OF ADMINISTRATION IS EMPLOYED, PATIENTS MUST BE OBSERVED IN A FULLY EQUIPPED AND STAFFED ENVIRONMENT FOR AT LEAST 24 HOURS AFTER THE INITIAL DOSE.

THE FACILITY MUST BE EQUIPPED TO RESUSCITATE PATIENTS WITH SEVERE OPIATE OVERDOSAGE, AND THE PERSONNEL MUST BE FAMILIAR WITH THE USE AND LIMITATIONS OF SPECIFIC NARCOTIC ANTAGONISTS (NALOXONE, NALTREXONE) IN SUCH CASES.

TOLERANCE AND MYOCLONIC ACTIVITY

PATIENTS SOMETIMES MANIFEST UNUSAL ACCELERATION OF NEURAXIAL MORPHINE REQUIREMENTS, WHICH MAY CAUSE CONCERN REGARDING SYSTEMIC ABSORPTION AND THE HAZARDS OF LARGE DOSES; THESE PATIENTS MAY BENEFIT FROM HOSPITALIZATION AND DETOXIFICATION. TWO CASES OF MYOCLONIC-LIKE SPASM OF THE LOWER EXTREMITIES HAVE BEEN REPORTED IN PATIENTS RECEIVING MORE THAN 20 MG/DAY OF INTRATHECAL MORPHINE. AFTER DETOXIFICATION, IT MIGHT BE POSSIBLE TO RESUME TREATMENT AT LOWER DOSES, AND SOME PATIENTS HAVE BEEN SUCCESSFULLY CHANGED FROM CONTINUOUS EPIDURAL MORPHINE TO CONTINUOUS INTRATHECAL MORPHINE. REPEAT DETOXIFICATION MAY BE INDICATED AT A LATER DATE. THE UPPER DAILY DOSAGE LIMIT FOR EACH PATIENT DURING CONTINUING TREATMENT MUST BE INDIVIDUALIZED.

PRECAUTIONS

GENERAL

Control of pain by neuraxial opiate delivery is always accompanied by considerable risk to the patients and requires a high level of skill to be successfully accomplished. The task of

Continued on next page

Elkins-Sinn—Cont.

treating these patients must be undertaken by experienced clinical teams, well-versed in patient selection, evolving technology and emerging standards of care. For safety reasons, it is recommended that administration of DURAMORPH® by the epidural or intrathecal routes be limited to the lumbar area. Intrathecal use has been associated with a higher incidence of respiratory depression than epidural use.

Seizures may result from high doses. Patients with known seizure disorders should be carefully observed for evidence of morphine-induced seizure activity.

USE IN PATIENTS WITH INCREASED INTRACRANIAL PRESSURE OR HEAD INJURY

DURAMORPH® should be used with extreme caution in patients with head injury or increased intracranial pressure. Pupillary changes (miosis) from morphine may obscure the existence, extent and course of intracranial pathology. High doses of neuraxial morphine may produce myoclonic events (see WARNINGS and ADVERSE REACTIONS). Clinicians should maintain a high index of suspicion for adverse drug reactions when evaluating altered mental status or movement abnormalities in patients receiving this modality of treatment.

USE IN CHRONIC PULMONARY DISEASE

Care is urged in using this drug in patients who have a decreased respiratory reserve (e.g., emphysema, severe obesity, kyphoscoliosis or paralysis of the phrenic nerve). DURAMORPH® should not be given in cases of chronic asthma, upper airway obstruction or in any other chronic pulmonary disorder without due consideration of the known risk of acute respiratory failure following morphine administration in such patients.

USE IN HEPATIC OR RENAL DISEASE

The elimination half-life of morphine may be prolonged in patients with reduced metabolic rates and with hepatic and/or renal dysfunction. Hence, care should be exercised in administering DURAMORPH® epidurally to patients with these conditions, since high blood morphine levels, due to reduced clearance, may take several days to develop.

USE IN BILIARY SURGERY OR DISORDERS OF THE BILIARY TRACT

As significant morphine is released into the systemic circulation from neuraxial administration, the ensuring smooth muscle hypertonicity may result in biliary colic.

USE WITH DISORDERS OF THE URINARY SYSTEM

Initiation of neuraxial opiate analgesia is frequently associated with disturbances of micturition, especially in males with prostatic enlargement. Early recognition of difficulty in urination and prompt intervention in cases of urinary retention is indicated.

USE IN AMBULATORY PATIENTS

Patients with reduced circulating blood volume, impaired myocardial function or on sympatholytic drugs should be monitored for the possible occurrence of orthostatic hypotension, a frequent complication in single-dose neuraxial morphine analgesia.

USE WITH OTHER CENTRAL NERVOUS SYSTEM DEPRESSANTS

The depressant effects of morphine are potentiated by the presence of other CNS depressants such as alcohol, sedatives, antihistaminics or psychotropic drugs. Use of neuroleptics in conjunction with neuraxial morphine may increase the risk of respiratory depression.

CARCINOGENESIS, MUTAGENESIS, IMPAIRMENT OF FERTILITY

Morphine is without known carcinogenic or mutagenic effects and is not known to impair fertility at non-narcotic doses in animals, but studies of the carcinogenic and mutagenic potential or the effect on fertility of DURAMORPH® have not been conducted.

PREGNANCY

Teratogenic Effects—Pregnancy Category C. Morphine sulfate is not teratogenic in rats at 35 mg/kg/day (thirty-five times the usual human dose) but does result in increased pup mortality and growth retardation at doses that narcotize the animal (> 10 mg/kg/day, ten times the usual human dose). DURAMORPH® should only be given to pregnant women when no other method of controlling pain is available and means are at hand to manage the delivery and perinatal care of the opiate-dependent infant.

Nonteratogenic Effects. Infants born to mothers who have been taking morphine chronically may exhibit withdrawal symptoms.

LABOR AND DELIVERY

Intravenous morphine readily passes into the fetal circulation and may result in respiratory depression in the neonate. Naloxone and resuscitative equipment should be available for reversal of narcotic-induced respiratory depression in the neonate. In addition, intravenous morphine may reduce the strength, duration and frequency of uterine contraction resulting in prolonged labor.

Epidurally and intrathecally administered morphine readily passes into the fetal circulation and may result in respiratory depression of the neonate. Controlled clinical studies have shown that *epidural* administration has little or no effect on the relief of labor pain.

NURSING MOTHERS

Morphine is excreted in maternal milk. Effects on the nursing infant are not known.

PEDIATRIC USE

Adequate studies, to establish the safty and effectiveness of spinal morphine in children, have not been performed, and usage in this population is not recommended.

USE IN THE AGED

The pharmacodynamic effects of neuraxial morphine in the aged are more variable than in the younger population. Patients will vary widely in the effective initial dose, rate of development of tolerance and the frequency and magnitude of associated adverse effects as the dose is increased. Initial doses should be based on careful clinical obsrvation following "test doses", after making due allowances for the effects of the patient's age and infirmity on his/her ability to clear the drug, particularly in patients receiving epidural morphine.

ADVERSE REACTIONS

The most serious adverse experience encountered during administration of DURAMORPH® is respiratory depression. This depression may be severe and could require intervention. (See WARNINGS AND OVERDOSAGE.) Because of delay in maximum CNS effect with intravenously administered drug (30 min), rapid administration may result in overdosing. Single-dose neuraxial administration may result in acute or delayed respiratory depression for periods at least as long as 24 hours.

Tolerance and myoclonus: See **WARNINGS** for discussion of these and related hazards.

While low doses of intravenously administered morphine have little effect on cardiovascular stability, high doses are excitatory, resulting from **sympathetic hyperactivity** and increase in circulating catecholamines. Excitation of the central nervous system, resulting in **convulsions**, may accompany high doses of morphine given intravenously. **Dysphoric reactions** may occur after any size dose and **toxic psychoses** have been reported.

Pruritus: Single-dose epidural or intrathecal administration is accompanied by a high incidence of *pruritus* that is dose-related but not confined to the site of administration. Pruritus, following continuous infusion of epidural or intrathecal morphine, is occasionally reported in the literature; these reactions are poorly understood as to their cause.

Urinary retention: Urinary retention, which may persist 10 to 20 hours following single epidural or intrathecal administration, is a frequent side effect and must be anticipated primarily in male patients, with a somewhat lower incidence in females. Also frequently reported in the literature is the occurrence of urinary retention during the first several days of hospitalization for the initiation of continuous intrathecal or epidural morphine therapy. Patients who develop urinary retention have responded to cholinomimetic treatment and/or judicious use of catheters (see PRECAUTIONS).

Constipation: Constipation is frequently encountered during continuous infusion of morphine; this can usually be managed by conventional therapy.

Headache: Lumbar puncture-type headache is encountered in a significant minority of cases for several days following intrathecal catheter implantation; this, generally, responds to bed rest and/or other conventional therapy.

Other: Other adverse experiences reported following morphine therapy include—**Dizziness, euphoria, anxiety, depression of cough reflex, interference with thermal regulation and oliguria.** Evidence of histamine release such as **urticaria, wheals** and/or **local tissue irritation** may occur. **Nausea** and **vomiting** are frequently seen in patients following morphine administration.

Pruritus, nausea/vomiting and urinary retention, if associated with continuous infusion therapy, may respond to intravenous administration of a low dose of naloxone (0.2 mg). The risks of using narcotic antagonists in patients chronicially receiving narcotic therapy should be considered.

In general, side effects are amenable to reversal by narcotic antagonists.

NALOXONE INJECTION AND RESUSCITATIVE EQUIPMENT SHOULD BE IMMEDIATELY AVAILABLE FOR ADMINISTRATION IN CASE OF LIFE-THREATENING OR INTOLERABLE SIDE EFFECTS AND WHENEVER DURAMORPH® THERAPY IS BEING INITIATED.

DRUG ABUSE AND DEPENDENCE

CONTROLLED SUBSTANCE

Morphine sulfate is a Schedule II narcotic under the United States Controlled Substance Act (21 U.S.C. 801–886).

Morphine is the most commonly cited prototype for narcotic substances that possess an addiction-forming or addiction-sustaining liability. A patient may be at risk for developing a dependence to morphine if used improperly or for overly long periods of time. As with all potent opioids which are μ-agonists, tolerance as well as psychological and physicial dependence to morphine may develop irrespective of the route of administration (intravenous, intramuscular, intrathecal, epidural or oral). Individuals with a prior history of opioid or other substance abuse or dependence, being more apt to respond to the euphorogenic and reinforcing properties of morphine, would be considered to be at greater risk.

Care must be taken to avert withdrawal in those patients who have been maintained on parenteral/oral narcotics when epidural or intrathecal administration is considered. Withdrawal symptoms may occur when morphine is discontinued abruptly or upon administration of a narcotic antagonist.

OVERDOSAGE

PARENTERAL ADMINISTRATION OF NARCOTICS IN PATIENTS RECEIVING EPIDURAL OR INTRATHECAL MORPHINE MAY RESULT IN OVERDOSAGE.

Overdosage of morphine is characterized by respiratory depression, with or without concomitant CNS depression. Since respiratory arrest may result either through direct depression of the respiratory center or as the result of hypoxia, primary attention should be given to the establishment of adequate respiratory exchange through provision of a patent airway and institution of assisted, or controlled, ventilation. The narcotic antagonist, naloxone, is a specific antidote. An initial dose of 0.4 to 2 mg of naloxone should be administered intravenously, simultaneously with respiratory resuscitation. If the desired degree of counteraction and improvement in respiratory function is not obtained, naloxone may be repeated at 2- to 3-minute intervals. If no response is observed after 10 mg of naloxone has been administered, the diagnosis of narcotic-induced, or partial narcotic-induced, toxicity should be questioned. Intramuscular or subcutaneous administration may be used if the intravenous route is not available.

As the duration of effect of naloxone is considerably shorter than that of epidural or intrathecal morphine, repeated administration may be necessary. Patients should be closely observed for evidence of renarcotization.

DOSAGE AND ADMINISTRATION

DURAMORPH® is intended for intravenous, epidural or intrathecal administration.

INTRAVENOUS ADMINISTRATION

Dosage: The initial dose of morphine should be 2 mg to 10 mg/70 kg of body weight. No information is available regarding the use of DURAMORPH® in patients under the age of 18.

EPIDURAL ADMINISTRATION

DURAMORPH® SHOULD BE ADMINISTERED EPIDURALLY BY OR UNDER THE DIRECTION OF A PHYSICIAN EXPERIENCED IN THE TECHNIQUE OF EPIDURAL ADMINISTRATION AND WHO IS THOROUGHLY FAMILIAR WITH THE LABELING. IT SHOULD BE ADMINISTERED ONLY IN SETTINGS WHERE ADEQUATE PATIENT MONITORING IS POSSIBLE. RESUSCITATIVE EQUIPMENT AND A SPECIFIC ANTAGONIST (NALOXONE INJECTION) SHOULD BE IMMEDIATELY AVAILABLE FOR THE MANAGEMENT OF RESPIRATORY DEPRESSION AS WELL AS COMPLICATIONS WHICH MIGHT RESULT FROM INADVERTENT INTRATHECAL OR INTRAVASCULAR INJECTION. (NOTE: INTRATHECAL DOSAGE IS USUALLY $^1/_{10}$ THAT OF EPIDURAL DOSAGE.) **PATIENT MONITORING SHOULD BE CONTINUED FOR AT LEAST 24 HOURS AFTER EACH DOSE, SINCE DELAYED RESPIRATORY DEPRESSION MAY OCCUR.**

Proper placement of a needle or catheter in the epidural space should be verified before DURAMORPH® is injected. Acceptable techniques for verifying proper placement include: a) aspiration to check for absence of blood or cerebrospinal fluid, or b) administration of 5 mL (3 mL in obstetric patients) of 1.5% PRESERVATIVE-FREE Lidocaine and Epinephrine (1:200,000) Injection and then observe the patient for lack of tachycardia (this indicates that vascular injection has *not* been made) and lack of sudden onset of segmental anesthesia (this indicates that intrathecal injection has *not* been made).

Epidural Adult Dosage: Initial injection of 5 mg in the lumbar region may provide satisfactory pain relief for up to 24 hours. If adequate pain relief is not achieved within one hour, careful administration of incremental doses of 1 to 2 mg at intervals sufficient to assess effectiveness may be given. No more than 10 mg/24 hr should be administered.

Thoracic administration has been shown to dramatically increase the incidence of early and late respiratory depression even at doses of 1 to 2 mg.

For continuous infusion, an initial dose of 2 to 4 mg/24 hours is recommended. Further doses of 1 to 2 mg may be given if pain relief is not achieved initially.

Aged patients—Administer with extreme caution. (See PRECAUTIONS.)

Epidural Pediatric Use: No information on use in pediatric patients is available. (See PRECAUTIONS.)

INTRATHECAL ADMINISTRATION

NOTE: INTRATHECAL DOSAGE IS USUALLY 1/10 THAT OF EPIDURAL DOSAGE.

DURAMORPH® SHOULD BE ADMINISTERED INTRATHECALLY BY OR UNDER THE DIRECTION OF A PHYSICIAN EXPERIENCED IN THE TECHNIQUE OF INTRATHECAL ADMINISTRATION AND WHO IS THOROUGHLY FAMILIAR WITH THE LABELING. IT SHOULD BE ADMINISTERED ONLY IN SETTINGS WHERE ADEQUATE PATIENT MONITORING IS POSSIBLE. RESUSCITATIVE EQUIPMENT AND A SPECIFIC ANTAGONIST (NALOXONE INJECTION) SHOULD BE IMMEDIATELY AVAILABLE FOR THE MANAGEMENT OF RESPIRATORY DEPRESSION AS WELL AS COMPLICATIONS WHICH MIGHT RESULT FROM INADVERTENT INTRAVASCULAR INJECTION. **PATIENT MONITORING SHOULD BE CONTINUED FOR AT LEAST 24 HOURS AFTER EACH DOSE, SINCE DELAYED RESPIRATORY DEPRESSION MAY OCCUR.** RESPIRATORY DEPRESSION (BOTH EARLY AND LATE ONSET) HAS OCCURRED MORE FREQUENTLY FOLLOWING INTRATHECAL ADMINISTRATION THAN EPIDURAL ADMINISTRATION.

Intrathecal Adult Dosage: A single injection of 0.2 to 1 mg may provide satisfactory pain relief for up to 24 hours. (CAUTION: THIS IS ONLY 0.4 TO 2 ML OF THE 5 MG/10 ML AMPUL OR 0.2 TO 1 ML OF THE 10 MG/10 ML AMPUL OF DURAMORPH®). DO NOT INJECT INTRATHECALLY MORE THAN 2 ML OF THE 5 MG/10 ML AMPUL OR 1 ML OF THE 10 MG/10 ML AMPUL. USE IN THE LUMBAR AREA ONLY IS RECOMMENDED. Repeated intrathecal injections of DURAMORPH® are not recommended. A constant intravenous infusion of naloxone, 0.6 mg/hr, for 24 hours after intrathecal injection may be used to reduce the incidence of potential side effects.

Aged patients—Administer with extreme caution. (See PRECAUTIONS.)

Repeat Dosage: If pain recurs, alternative routes of administration should be considered, since experience with repeated doses of morphine by the intrathecal route is limited.

Intrathecal Pediatric Use: No information on use in pediatric patients is available. (See PRECAUTIONS.)

SAFETY AND HANDLING INSTRUCTIONS

DURAMORPH® is supplied in sealed ampuls. Accidental dermal exposure should be treated by the removal of any contaminated clothing and rinsing the affected area with water.

Each ampul of DURAMORPH® contains a potent narcotic which has been associated with abuse and dependence among health care providers. **Due to the limited indications for this product, the risk of overdosage and the risk of its diversion and abuse, it is recommended that special measures be taken to control this product within the hospital or clinic. DURAMORPH® should be subject to rigid accounting, rigorous control of wastage and restricted access.**

Parenteral drug products should be inspected for particulate matter and discoloration prior to administration, whenever solution and container permit. DO NOT USE IF COLOR IS DARKER THAN PALE YELLOW, IF IT IS DISCOLORED IN ANY OTHER WAY OR IF IT CONTAINS A PRECIPITATE.

HOW SUPPLIED

Preservative-free DURAMORPH® (Morphine Sulfate Injection, USP) is available in amber DOSETTE® ampuls for intravenous, epidural or intrathecal administration:

5 mg/10 mL (0.5 mg/mL) packaged in 10s (NDC 0641-1112-33)

10 mg/10 mL (1 mg/1 mL) packaged in 10s (NDC 0641-1114-33)

Also available from Elkins-Sinn: INFUMORPH® (Preservative-free Morphine Sulfate Sterile Solution) 200 mg/20 mL (10 mg/mL) and 500 mg/20 mL (25 mg/mL) for epidural and intrathecal administration via a continuous microinfusion device. See insert J-1131.

STORAGE

Protect from light. Store in carton at controlled room temperature, 15° to 30°C (59° to 86°F) until ready to use. DO NOT FREEZE.

DURAMORPH® contains no preservative or antioxidant. DISCARD ANY UNUSED PORTION. DO NOT HEAT-STERILIZE.

* * * *

Manufactured by
ELKINS-SINN, INC., Cherry Hill, NJ 08003-4099

INFUMORPH® 200 Ⓒ
INFUMORPH® 500 Ⓒ

(Preservative-free Morphine Sulfate Sterile Solution)
WARNING: May be habit forming.
For Use in Continuous Microinfusion Devices

DESCRIPTION

Morphine is the most important alkaloid of opium and is a phenanthrene derivative. It is available as the sulfate salt, having the following structural formula:

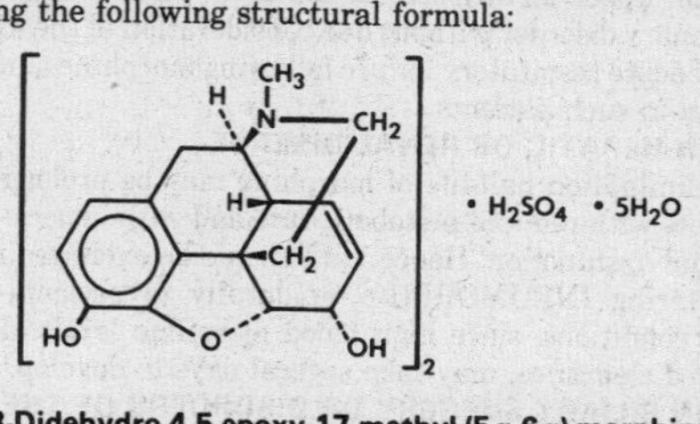

7,8-Didehydro-4,5-epoxy-17-methyl-(5α,6α)-morphinan-3,6-diol sulfate (2:1) (salt), pentahydrate

$(C_{17}H_{19}NO_3)_2 \cdot H_2SO_4 \cdot 5H_2O$ **MW 758.83.**

INFUMORPH® is a sterile, nonpyrogenic, isobaric, **high potency solution of morphine sulfate**, free of antioxidants, preservatives or other potentially neurotoxic additives. **INFUMORPH® is intended for use in continuous microinfusion devices for intraspinal administration in the management of pain.**

Each 20 mL ampul of **INFUMORPH® 200** contains morphine sulfate, USP 200 mg or 10 mg/mL and sodium chloride 8 mg/mL in Water for Injection, USP. Each 20 mL ampul of **INFUMORPH® 500** contains morphine sulfate, USP 500 mg or 25 mg/mL and sodium chloride 6.25 mg/mL in Water for Injection, USP. If needed, sodium hydroxide and/or sulfuric acid are added for pH adjustment to 4.5. Ampuls are sealed under nitrogen. Each 20 mL DOSETTE® ampul of **INFUMORPH®** is intended for **single use only.** *Discard any unused portion.* DO NO HEAT-STERILIZE.

CLINICAL PHARMACOLOGY

Morphine produces a wide spectrum of pharmacologic effects including analgesia, dysphoria, euphoria, somnolence, respiratory depression, diminished gastrointestinal motility and physical dependence. Opiate analgesia involves at least three anatomical areas of the central nervous system: the periaqueductal-periventricular gray matter, the ventromedial medulla and the spinal cord. A systemically administered opiate may produce analgesia by acting at any, all or some combination of these distinct regions. Morphine interacts predominantly with the μ-receptor. The μ-binding sites of opioids are very discretely distributed in the human brain, with high densities of sites found in the posterior amygdala, hypothalamus, thalamus, nucleus caudatus, putamen and certain cortical areas. They are also found on the terminal axons of primary afferents within laminae I and II (substantia gelatinosa) of the spinal cord and in the spinal nucleus of the trigeminal nerve.

Morphine has an apparent volume of distribution ranging from 1.0 to 4.7 L/kg after *intravenous* dosage. Protein binding is low, about 36%, and muscle tissue binding is reported as 54%. A blood-brain barrier exists, and when morphine is introduced outside of the CNS (e.g., *intravenously*), plasma concentrations of morphine remain higher than the corresponding CSF morphine levels. Conversely, when morphine is injected into the *intrathecal space*, it diffuses out into the systemic circulation slowly, accounting for the long duration of action of morphine administered by this route.

Morphine has a total plasma clearance which ranges from 0.9 to 1.2 L/kg/h (liters/kilogram/hour) in postoperative patients, but shows considerable interindividual variation. The major pathway of clearance is hepatic glucuronidation to morphine-3-glucuronide, which is pharmacologically inactive. The major excretion path of the conjugate is through the kidneys, with about 10% in the feces. Morphine is also eliminated by the kidneys, 2 to 12% being excreted unchanged in the urine. Terminal half-life is commonly reported to vary from 1.5 to 4.5 hours, although the longer half-lives were obtained when morphine levels were monitored over protracted periods with very sensitive radioimmunoassay methods. The accepted elimination half-life in normal subjects is 1.5 to 2 hours.

"Selective" blockade of pain sensation is possible by neuraxial application of morphine. In addition, duration of analgesia may be much longer by this route compared to systemic administration. However, CNS effects, associated with systemic administration, are still seen. These include respiratory depression, sedation, nausea and vomiting, pruritis and urinary retention. In particular, both early and late respiratory depression (up to 24 hours post dosing) have been reported following neuraxial administration. Circulation of the spinal fluid may also result in high concentrations of morphine reaching the brain stem directly.

The incidence of unwanted CNS effects, including delayed respiratory depression, associated with neuraxial application of morphine, is related to the circulatory dynamics of the epidural venous plexus and the spinal fluid. The lipid solubility and degree of ionization of morphine plays an important part in both the onset and duration of analgesia and the CNS effects. Morphine has a pK_a 7.9, with an octanol/water partition coefficient of 1.42 at pH 7.4. At this pH, the tertiary amino group in each of the opioids is mostly ionized, making the molecule water soluble. Morphine, with additional hydroxyl groups on the molecule, is significantly more water soluble than any other opioid in clinical use.

Morphine, injected into the *epidural space*, is rapidly absorbed into the general circulation. Absorption is so rapid that the plasma concentration-time profiles closely resembled those obtained after intravenous or intramuscular administration. Peak plasma concentrations averaging 33–40 ng/mL (range 5–62 ng/mL) are achieved within 10 to 15 minutes after administration of 3 mg of morphine. Plasma concentrations decline in a multiexponential fashion. The terminal half-life is reported to range from 39 to 249 minutes (mean of 90 ± 34.3 min) and, though somewhat shorter, is similar in magnitude as values reported after intravenous and intramuscular administration (1.5–4.5 h). CSF concentrations of morphine, after epidural doses of 2 to 6 mg in postoperative patients, have been reported to be 50 to 250 times higher than corresponding plasma concentrations. The CSF levels of morphine exceed those in plasma after only 15 minutes and are detectable for as long as 20 hours after the injection of 2 mg of epidural morphine. Approximately 4% of the dose injected epidurally reaches the CSF. This corresponds to the relative minimum effective epidural and intrathecal doses of 5 mg and 0.25 mg, respectively. The disposition of morphine in the CSF follows a biphasic pattern, with an early half-life of 1.5 h and a late phase half-life of about 6 h. Morphine crosses the dura slowly, with an absorption half-life across the dura averaging 22 minutes. Maximum CSF concentrations are seen 60–90 minutes after injection. Minimum effective CSF concentrations for postoperative analgesia average 150 ng/mL (range $<$1–380 ng/mL).

The *intrathecal route* of administration circumvents meningeal diffusion barriers and, therefore, lower doses of morphine produce comparable analgesia to that induced by the epidural route. After intrathecal bolus injection of morphine, there is a rapid initial distribution phase lasting 15–30 minutes and a half-life in the CSF of 42–136 min (mean 90 ± 16 min). Derived from limited data, it appears that the disposition of morphine in the CSF, from 15 minutes postintrathecal administration to the end of a six-hour observation period, represents a combination of the distribution and elimination phases. Morphine concentrations in the CSF averaged 332 ± 137 ng/mL at 6 hours, following a bolus dose of 0.3 mg of morphine. The apparent volume of distribution of morphine in the intrathecal space is about 22 ± 8 mL. Time-to-peak plasma concentrations, however, is similar (5–10 min) after either epidural or intrathecal bolus administration of morphine. Maximum plasma morphine concentrations after 0.3 mg intrathecal morphine have been reported from $<$1 to 7.8 ng/mL. The minimum analgesic morphine plasma concentration during Patient-Controlled Analgesia (PCA) has been reported as 20–40 ng/mL, suggesting that any analgesic contribution from systemic redistribution would be minimal after the first 30–60 minutes with epidural administration and virtually absent with intrathecal administration of morphine.

INDICATION AND USAGE

INFUMORPH® (Preservative-free Morphine Sulfate Sterile Solution) is indicated only for intrathecal or epidural infusion in the treatment of intractable chronic pain. It was developed for use in continuous microinfusion devices and may require dilution before use as dictated by the characteristics of the device and the dosage requirements of the individual patient.

INFUMORPH® IS NOT RECOMMENDED FOR SINGLE-DOSE INTRAVENOUS, INTRAMUSCULAR OR SUBCUTANEOUS ADMINISTRATION DUE TO THE VERY LARGE AMOUNT OF MORPHINE IN THE AMPUL AND THE ASSOCIATED RISK OF OVERDOSAGE.

CONTRAINDICATIONS

The only absolute contraindication to the use of INFUMORPH® is known allergy to morphine. Contraindications to the use of neuraxial analgesia include: the presence of infection at the injection microinfusion site, concomitant anticoagulant therapy, uncontrolled bleeding diathesis and the presence of any other concomitant therapy or medical condition which would render epidural or intrathecal administration of medication especially hazardous.

Continued on next page

Elkins-Sinn—Cont.

WARNINGS

THIS PRODUCT WAS DEVELOPED FOR USE (AFTER APPROPRIATE DILUTION, IF NECESSARY) IN CONTINUOUS MICROINFUSION DEVICES FOR INTRATHECAL OR EPIDURAL INFUSION OF NARCOTICS TO CONTROL SEVERE CANCER PAIN. CHRONIC NEURAXIAL OPIOID ANALGESIA IS APPROPRIATE ONLY WHEN LESS INVASIVE MEANS OF CONTROLLING PAIN HAVE FAILED AND SHOULD ONLY BE UNDERTAKEN BY THOSE WHO ARE EXPERIENCED IN APPLYING THE TREATMENT IN A SETTING WHERE ITS COMPLICATIONS CAN BE ADEQUATELY MANAGED.

> **BECAUSE OF THE RISK OF SEVERE ADVERSE EFFECTS, PATIENTS MUST BE OBSERVED IN A FULLY EQUIPPED AND STAFFED ENVIRONMENT FOR AT LEAST 24 HOURS AFTER THE INITIAL (SINGLE) TEST DOSE AND, AS APPROPRIATE, FOR THE FIRST SEVERAL DAYS AFTER CATHETER IMPLANTATION.**

THE FACILITY MUST BE EQUIPPED TO RESUSCITATE PATIENTS WITH SEVERE OPIATE OVERDOSAGE, AND THE PERSONNEL MUST BE FAMILIAR WITH THE USE AND LIMITATIONS OF SPECIFIC NARCOTIC ANTAGONISTS (NALOXONE, NALTREXONE) IN SUCH CASES. RESERVOIR FILLING MUST BE PERFORMED BY FULLY TRAINED AND QUALIFIED PERSONNEL, FOLLOWING THE DIRECTIONS PROVIDED BY THE DEVICE MANUFACTURER. CARE SHOULD BE TAKEN IN SELECTING THE PROPER REFILL FREQUENCY TO PREVENT DEPLETION OF THE RESERVOIR, WHICH WOULD RESULT IN EXACERBATION OF SEVERE PAIN AND/OR REFLUX OF CSF INTO SOME DEVICES. STRICT ASEPTIC TECHNIQUE IN FILLING IS REQUIRED TO AVOID BACTERIAL CONTAMINATION AND SERIOUS INFECTION. EXTREME CARE MUST BE TAKEN TO ENSURE THAT THE NEEDLE IS PROPERLY IN THE FILLING PORT OF THE DEVICE BEFORE ATTEMPTING TO REFILL THE RESERVOIR. INJECTING THE SOLUTION INTO THE TISSUE AROUND THE DEVICE OR (IN THE CASE OF DEVICES THAT HAVE MORE THAN ONE PORT) ATTEMPTING TO INJECT THE REFILL DOSE INTO THE DIRECT INJECTION PORT WILL RESULT IN A LARGE, CLINICALLY SIGNIFICANT, OVERDOSAGE TO THE PATIENT.

A PERIOD OF OBSERVATION APPROPRIATE TO THE CLINICAL SITUATION SHOULD FOLLOW EACH REFILL OR MANIPULATION OF THE DRUG RESERVOIR. BEFORE DISCHARGE, THE PATIENT AND ATTENDANT(S) SHOULD RECEIVE INSTRUCTION IN THE PROPER HOME CARE OF THE DEVICE AND INSERTION SITE AND IN THE RECOGNITION AND PRACTICAL TREATMENT OF AN OVERDOSE OF NEURAXIAL MORPHINE.

TOLERANCE AND MYOCLONIC ACTIVITY

PATIENTS SOMETIMES MANIFEST UNUSUAL ACCELERATION OF NEURAXIAL MORPHINE REQUIREMENTS, WHICH MAY CAUSE CONCERN REGARDING SYSTEMIC ABSORPTION AND THE HAZARDS OF LARGE DOSES; THESE PATIENTS MAY BENEFIT FROM HOSPITALIZATION AND DETOXIFICATION. TWO CASES OF MYOCLONIC-LIKE SPASM OF THE LOWER EXTREMITIES HAVE BEEN REPORTED IN PATIENTS RECEIVING MORE THAN 20 MG/DAY OF INTRATHECAL MORPHINE. AFTER DETOXIFICATION, IT MIGHT BE POSSIBLE TO RESUME TREATMENT AT LOWER DOSES, AND SOME PATIENTS HAVE BEEN SUCCESSFULLY CHANGED FROM CONTINUOUS EPIDURAL MORPHINE TO CONTINUOUS INTRATHECAL MORPHINE. REPEAT DETOXIFICATION MAY BE INDICATED AT A LATER DATE. THE UPPER DAILY DOSAGE LIMIT FOR EACH PATIENT DURING CONTINUING TREATMENT MUST BE INDIVIDUALIZED.

PRECAUTIONS

Control of pain by neuraxial opiate delivery, using a continuous microinfusion device, is always accompanied by considerable risk to the patients and requires a high level of skill to be successfully accomplished. The task of treating these patients must be undertaken by experienced clinical teams, well-versed in patient selection, evolving technology and emerging standards of care. For reasons of safety, it is recommended that administration of INFUMORPH® 200 and 500 (10 and 25 mg/mL, respectively) by the intrathecal route be limited to the lumber area.

USE IN PATIENTS WITH INCREASED INTRACRANIAL PRESSURE OR HEAD INJURY

INFUMORPH® (Preservative-free Morphine Sulfate Sterile Solution) should be used with extreme caution in patients with head injury or increased intracranial pressure. Pupillary changes (miosis) from morphine may obscure the existence, extent and course of intracranial pathology. High doses of neuraxial morphine may produce myoclonic events (see WARNINGS and ADVERSE REACTIONS). Clinicians

should maintain a high index of suspicion for adverse drug reactions when evaluating altered mental status or movement abnormalities in patients receiving this modality of treatment.

USE IN CHRONIC PULMONARY DISEASE

Care is urged in using this drug in patients who have a decreased respiratory reserve (e.g., emphysema, severe obesity, kyphoscoliosis or paralysis of the phrenic nerve). INFUMORPH® should not be given in cases of chronic asthma, upper airway obstruction or in any other chronic pulmonary disorder without due consideration of the known risk of acute respiratory failure following morphine administration in such patients.

USE IN HEPATIC OR RENAL DISEASE

The elimination half-life of morphine may be prolonged in patients with reduced metabolic rate and with hepatic and/or renal dysfunction. Hence, care should be exercised in administering INFUMORPH® epidurally to patients with these conditions, since high blood morphine levels, due to reduced clearance, may take several days to develop.

USE IN BILIARY SURGERY OR DISORDERS OF THE BILIARY TRACT

As significant morphine is released into the systemic circulation from neuraxial administration, the ensuing smooth muscle hypertonicity may result in biliary colic.

USE WITH DISORDERS OF THE URINARY SYSTEM

Initiation of neuraxial opiate analgesia is frequently associated with disturbances of micturition, especially in males with prostatic enlargement. Early recognition of difficulty in urination and prompt intervention in cases of urinary retention is indicated.

USE IN AMBULATORY PATIENTS

Patients with reduced circulating blood volume, impaired myocardial function or on sympatholytic drugs should be monitored for the possible occurrence of orthostatic hypotension, a frequent complication in single-dose neuraxial morphine analgesia.

USE WITH OTHER CENTRAL NERVOUS SYSTEM DEPRESSANTS

The depressant effects of morphine are potentiated by the presence of other CNS depressants such as alcohol, sedatives, antihistaminics or psychotropic drugs. Use of neuroleptics in conjunction with neuraxial morphine may increase the risk of respiratory depression.

CARCINOGENESIS, MUTAGENESIS, IMPAIRMENT OF FERTILITY

Morphine is without known carcinogenic or mutagenic effects and is not known to impair fertility at non-narcotic doses in animals, but studies of the carcinogenic and mutagenic potential or the effect on fertility of INFUMORPH® have not been conducted.

PREGNANCY CATEGORY C

Morphine sulfate is not teratogenic in rats at 35 mg/kg/day (thirty-five times the usual human dose) but does result in increased pup mortality and growth retardation at doses that narcotize the animal (>10 mg/kg/day, ten times the usual human dose). INFUMORPH® should only be given to pregnant women when no other method of controlling pain is available and means are at hand to manage the delivery and perinatal care of the opiate-dependent infant.

LABOR AND DELIVERY

INFUMORPH® 200 and 500 (10 and 25 mg/mL, respectively) are too highly concentrated for routine use in obstetric neuraxial analgesia.

NURSING MOTHERS

Morphine is excreted in maternal milk. Effects on the nursing infant are not known.

PEDIATRIC USE

Adequate studies, to establish the safety and effectiveness of spinal morphine in children, have not been performed, and usage in this population is not recommended.

USE IN THE AGED

The pharmacodynamic effects of neuraxial morphine in the aged are more variable than in the younger population. Patients will vary widely in the effective initial dose, rate of development of tolerance and the frequency and magnitude of associated adverse effects as the dose is increased. Initial doses should be based on careful clinical observation following "test doses", after making due allowances for the effects of the patient's age and infirmity on their ability to clear the drug, particularly in patients receiving epidural morphine.

ADVERSE REACTIONS

> **IMPROPER OR ERRONEOUS SUBSTITUTION OF INFUMORPH® 200 or 500 (10 or 25 mg/mL, respectively) FOR REGULAR DURAMORPH® (0.5 or 1 mg/mL) IS LIKELY TO RESULT IN SERIOUS OVERDOSAGE, LEADING TO SEIZURES, RESPIRATORY DEPRESSION AND, POSSIBLY, FATAL OUTCOME.**

The most serious adverse experiences encountered during continuous intrathecal or epidural infusion of INFUMORPH® are respiratory depression and myoclonus.

1. Single-dose neuraxial administration may result in acute or delayed respiratory depression for periods at least as long as 24 hours. **Severe respiratory depression, potentially life-threatening, can result from technical errors during refill, e.g., injection of INFUMORPH® outside the filling port, unintentional injection into the direct bypass-dosing port featured on some devices or local infiltration.**
2. **Tolerance and myoclonus:** See WARNINGS for discussion of these and related hazards.

While low doses of intravenously administered morphine have little effect on cardiovascular stability, high doses are excitatory, resulting from **sympathetic hyperactivity** and increase in circulatory catecholamines. Excitation of the central nervous system, resulting in **convulsions,** may accompany high doses of morphine given intravenously. **Dysphoric reactions** may occur after any size dose and **toxic psychoses** have been reported.

Pruritus: Single-dose epidural or intrathecal administration is accompanied by a high incidence of **pruritus** that is dose-related but not confined to the site of administration. Pruritus, following continuous infusion of epidural or intrathecal morphine, is occasionally reported in the literature; these reactions are poorly understood as to their cause.

Urinary retention: Urinary retention, which may persist 10 to 20 hours following single epidural or intrathecal administration, is a frequent side effect and must be anticipated primarily in male patients, with a somewhat lower incidence in females. Also frequently reported in the literature is the occurrence of urinary retention during the first several days of hospitalization for the initiation of continuous intrathecal or epidural morphine therapy. Patients who develop urinary retention have responded to cholinomimetic treatment and/or judicious use of catheters (see PRECAUTIONS).

Constipation: Constipation is frequently encountered during continuous infusion of morphine; this can usually be managed by conventional therapy.

Headache: Lumbar puncture-type headache is encountered in a significant minority of cases for several days following intrathecal catheter implantation; this, generally, responds to bed rest and/or other conventional therapy.

Peripheral edema: There are several reports of peripheral edema, including unexplained genital swelling in male patients, following infusion-device implant surgery.

Other: Other adverse experiences reported following morphine therapy include—**Dizziness, euphoria, anxiety, depression of cough reflex, interference with thermal regulation** and **oliguria.** Evidence of histamine release such as **urticaria, wheals** and/or **local tissue irritation** may occur.

Pruritus, nausea/vomiting and urinary retention, if associated with continuous infusion therapy, may respond to intravenous administration of a low dose of naloxone (0.2 mg). The risks of using narcotic antagonists in patients chronically receiving narcotic therapy should be considered.

> **NALOXONE INJECTION AND RESUSCITATIVE EQUIPMENT SHOULD BE IMMEDIATELY AVAILABLE FOR USE IN CASE OF LIFE-THREATENING OR INTOLERABLE SIDE EFFECTS AND WHENEVER INFUMORPH® THERAPY IS BEING INITIATED, THE RESERVOIR IS BEING REFILLED OR ANY MANIPULATION OF THE RESERVOIR SYSTEM IS TAKING PLACE.**

DRUG ABUSE AND DEPENDENCE

CONTROLLED SUBSTANCE

Morphine sulfate is a Schedule II narcotic under the United States Controlled Substance Act (21 U.S.C. 801–886).

Morphine is the most commonly cited prototype for narcotic substances that possess an addiction-forming or addiction-sustaining liability. A patient may be at risk for developing a dependence to morphine if used improperly or for overly long periods of time. As with all potent opioids which are μ-agonists, tolerance as well as psychological and physical dependence to morphine may develop irrespective of the route of administration (intravenous, intramuscular, intrathecal, epidural or oral). Individuals with a prior history of opioid or other substance abuse or dependence, being more apt to respond to the euphorogenic and reinforcing properties of morphine, would be considered to be a greater risk.

Care must be taken to avert withdrawal in patients who have been maintained on parenteral/oral narcotics when epidural or intrathecal administration is considered. Withdrawal symptoms may occur when morphine is discontinued abruptly or upon administration of a narcotic antagonist.

OVERDOSAGE

PARENTERAL ADMINISTRATION OF NARCOTICS IN PATIENTS RECEIVING EPIDURAL OR INTRATHECAL MORPHINE MAY RESULT IN OVERDOSAGE.

Overdosage of morphine is characterized by respiratory depression, with or without concomitant CNS depression. Since respiratory arrest may result either through direct depression of the respiratory center, or as the result of hypoxia, primary attention should be given to the establishment of adequate respiratory exchange through provision of a patent

airway and institution of assisted, or controlled, ventilation. The narcotic antagonist, naloxone, is a specific antidote. An initial dose of 0.4 to 2 mg of naloxone should be administered intravenously, simultaneously with respiratory resuscitation. If the desired degree of counteraction and improvement in respiratory function is not obtained, naloxone may be repeated at 2- to 3-minute intervals. If no response is observed after 10 mg of naloxone has been administered, the diagnosis of narcotic-induced, or partial narcotic-induced, toxicity should be questioned. Intramuscular or subcutaneous administration may be used if the intravenous route is not available.

As the duration of effect of naloxone is considerably shorter than that of epidural or intrathecal morphine, repeated administration may be necessary. Patients should be closely observed for evidence of renarcotization.

DOSAGE AND ADMINISTRATION

INFUMORPH® 200 AND 500 (10 AND 25 MG/ML, RESPECTIVELY) SHOULD NOT BE USED FOR SINGLE-DOSE NEURAXIAL INJECTION BECAUSE LOWER DOSES CAN BE MORE RELIABLY ADMINISTERED WITH THE STANDARD PREPARATION OF DURAMORPH® (0.5 AND 1 MG/ML).

CANDIDATES FOR NEURAXIAL ADMINISTRATION OF INFUMORPH® IN A CONTINUOUS MICROINFUSION DEVICE SHOULD BE HOSPITALIZED TO PROVIDE FOR ADEQUATE PATIENT MONITORING DURING ASSESSMENT OF RESPONSE TO SINGLE DOSES OF INTRATHECAL OR EPIDURAL MORPHINE. HOSPITALIZATION SHOULD BE MAINTAINED FOR SEVERAL DAYS AFTER SURGERY INVOLVING THE INFUSION DEVICE FOR ADDITIONAL MONITORING AND ADJUSTMENT OF DAILY DOSAGE. THE FACILITY MUST BE EQUIPPED WITH RESUSCITATIVE EQUIPMENT, OXYGEN, NALOXONE INJECTION AND OTHER RESUSCITATIVE DRUGS. BECAUSE OF THE RISK OF DELAYED RESPIRATORY DEPRESSION, PATIENTS SHOULD BE OBSERVED IN A FULLY EQUIPPED AND STAFFED ENVIRONMENT FOR AT LEAST 24 HOURS AFTER EACH TEST DOSE AND, AS INDICATED, FOR THE FIRST SEVERAL DAYS AFTER SURGERY.

Familiarization with the continuous microinfusion device is essential. The desired amount of morphine should be withdrawn from the ampul through a microfilter. **To minimize risk from glass or other particles, the product must be filtered through a 5 μ (or smaller) microfilter before injecting into the microinfusion device.** If dilution is required, 0.9% Sodium Chloride Injection is recommended.

Intrathecal Dosage: The starting dose must be individualized, based upon in-hospital evaluation of the response to serial single-dose intrathecal bolus injections of regular DURAMORPH® (Morphine Sulfate Injection, USP) 0.5 mg/mL or 1 mg/mL, with close observation of the analgesic efficacy and adverse effects *prior* to surgery involving the continuous microinfusion device.

The recommended initial lumbar intrathecal dose range in patients with no tolerance to opioids is 0.2 to 1 mg/day. The published range of doses for individuals who have some degree of opioid tolerance varies from 1 to 10 mg/day. The upper daily dosage limit for each patient must be individualized.

Limited experience with continuous intrathecal infusion of morphine has shown that the daily doses have to be increased over time. Although the rate of increase, over time, in the dose required to sustain analgesia is highly variable, an estimate of the expected rate of increase is shown in the following Figure.

Figure: Dose Trend in Continuous Infusions of Intrathecal Morphine (Mean and 95% Confidence Intervals)

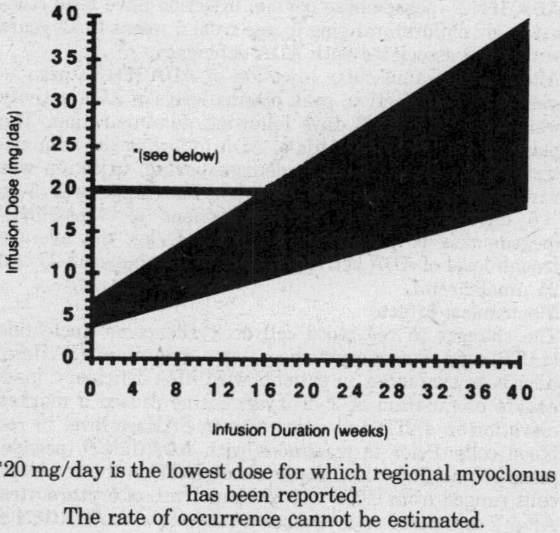

Infusion Dose (mg/day)
40
35
30
25
20
15
10
5
0
*(see below)
0 4 8 12 16 20 24 28 32 36 40
Infusion Duration (weeks)

*20 mg/day is the lowest dose for which regional myoclonus has been reported.
The rate of occurrence cannot be estimated.

Doses above 20 mg/day should be employed with caution since they may be associated with a higher likelihood of serious side effects (see WARNINGS concerning potential neurological hazards and ADVERSE REACTIONS).

Epidural Dosage: The starting dose must be individualized, based upon in-hospital evaluation of the response to serial single-dose epidural bolus injections of regular DURAMORPH® (Morphine Sulfate Injection, USP) 0.5 mg/mL or 1 mg/mL, with dose observation for analgesic efficacy and adverse effects *prior* to surgery involving the continuous microinfusion device.

The recommended initial epidural dose in patients who are not tolerant to opioids ranges from 3.5 to 7.5 mg/day. The usual starting dose for continuous epidural infusion, based upon limited data in patients who have some degree of opioid tolerance, is 4.5 to 10 mg/day. The dose requirements may increase significantly during treatment, frequently to 20–30 mg/day. The upper daily limit for each patient must be individualized.

SAFETY AND HANDLING INFORMATION

INFUMORPH® is supplied in sealed ampuls. Accidental dermal exposure should be treated by the removal of any contaminated clothing and rinsing the affected area with water.

Each ampul of INFUMORPH® contains a large amount of potent narcotic which has been associated with abuse and dependence among health care providers. **Due to the limited indications for this product, the risk of overdosage and the risk of its diversion and abuse, it is recommended that special measures be taken to control this product within the hospital or clinic. *INFUMORPH® should be subject to rigid accounting, rigorous control of wastage and restricted access.***

This parenteral drug product must be inspected for particulate matter before opening the amber ampul and again for color after removing contents from the ampul. Do not use if the solution in the unopened ampul contains a precipitate which does not disappear upon shaking. After removal, do not use unless the solution is colorless or pale yellow.

HOW SUPPLIED

Amber DOSETTE® ampuls for epidural or intrathecal via a continuous microinfusion device.

INFUMORPH® 200 (Preservative-free Morphine Sulfate Sterile Solution) 200 mg/20 mL (10 mg/mL) packaged individually (*NDC* 0641-1131-31)

INFUMORPH® 500 (Preservative-free Morphine Sulfate Sterile Solution) 500 mg/20 mL (25 mg/mL) packaged individually (*NDC* 0641-1132-31)

Also available from Elkins-Sinn, Inc. DURAMORPH® (Morphine Sulfate Injection, USP) 5 mg/10 mL (0.5 mg/mL) and 10 mg/10 mL (1 mg/mL). See insert J-1113.

STORAGE

Protect from light. Store in carton at controlled room temperature 15°–30°C (59°–86°F) until ready to use. DO NOT FREEZE. INFUMORPH® contains no preservative or antioxidant. DISCARD ANY UNUSED PORTION. DO NOT HEAT-STERILIZE.

• • • • •

Manufactured by
ELKINS-SINN, INC. Cherry Hill, NJ 08003-4099

SOTRADECOL® ℞
[*sō 'trah "de 'kol "*]
(Sodium Tetradecyl Sulfate Injection)
For Intravenous Use Only

DESCRIPTION

Sodium tetradecyl sulfate is an anionic surfactant which occurs as a white, waxy solid. The structural formula is as follows:

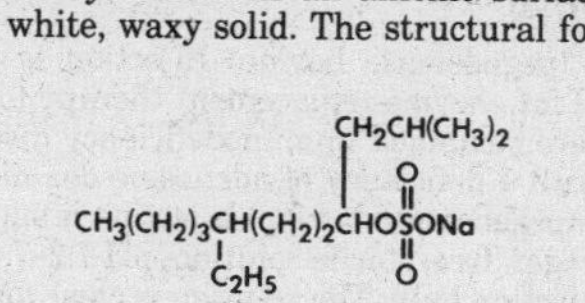

CH2CH(CH3)2
O
CH3(CH2)3CH(CH2)2CHOSONa
C2H5
O

$C_{14}H_{29}NaSO_4$
7-Ethyl-2-methyl-4-hendecanol sulfate sodium salt
M.W. 316.44

Sotradecol® (Sodium Tetradecyl Sulfate Injection) is a sterile nonpyrogenic solution for intravenous use as a sclerosing agent. Each mL contains sodium tetradecyl sulfate 10 mg or 30 mg, benzyl alcohol 0.02 mL and dibasic sodium phosphate, anhydrous 0.72 mg in Water for Injection. pH 7.9; monobasic sodium phosphate and/or sodium hydroxide added, if needed, for pH adjustment.

CLINICAL PHARMACOLOGY

Sotradecol® (Sodium Tetradecyl Sulfate Injection) is a mild sclerosing agent. Intravenous injection causes intima inflammation and thrombus formation. This usually occludes the injected vein. Subsequent formation of fibrous tissue results in partial or complete vein obliteration.

INDICATIONS AND USAGE

Indicated in the treatment of small uncomplicated varicose veins of the lower extremities that show simple dilation with competent valves. The benefit-to-risk ratio should be considered in selected patients who are great surgical risks due to conditions such as old age.

CONTRAINDICATIONS

Contraindicated in previous hypersensitivity reactions to the drug; in acute superficial thrombophlebitis; significant valvular or deep vein incompetence; huge superficial veins with wide open communications to deeper veins; phlebitis migrans; acute cellulitis; allergic conditions; acute infections; varicosities caused by abdominal and pelvic tumors unless the tumor has been removed; bedridden patients; such uncontrolled systemic diseases as diabetes, toxic hyperthyroidism, tuberculosis, asthma, neoplasm, sepsis, blood dyscrasias and acute respiratory or skin diseases.

WARNINGS

Since severe adverse local effects, including tissue necrosis, may occur following extravasation, Sotradecol® (Sodium Tetradecyl Sulfate Injection), should be administered only by a physician familiar with proper injection technique. Extreme care in needle placement and using the minimal effective volume at each injection site are, therefore, important. Allergic reactions have been reported. Therefore, as a precaution against anaphylactoid shock, it is recommended that 0.5 mL of Sotradecol® be injected into a varicosity, followed by observation of the patient for several hours before administration of a second or larger dose. The possibility of an anaphylactoid reaction should be kept in mind, and the physician should be prepared to treat it appropriately. In extreme emergencies, 0.25 mL of 1:1000 Epinephrine Injection (0.25 mg) intravenously should be used and side reactions controlled with antihistamines.

PRECAUTIONS

GENERAL

Venous sclerotherapy should not be undertaken if tests, such as the Trendelenberg and Perthes, and angiography show significant valvular or deep venous incompetence. The physician should bear in mind the fact that injection necrosis is likely to result from extravascular injection of sclerosing agents.

Extreme caution must be exercised in the presence of underlying arterial disease such as marked peripheral arteriosclerosis or thromboangiitis obliterans (Buerger's Disease).

The drug should only be administered by physicians who are familiar with an acceptable injection technique. Because of the danger of thrombosis extension into the deep venous system, thorough preinjection evaluation for valvular competency should be carried out and slow injections with a small amount (not over 2 mL) of the preparation should be injected into the varicosity. In particular, deep venous patency must be determined by angiography and/or the Perthes test before sclerotherapy is undertaken.

Embolism may occur as much as four weeks after injection of sodium tetradecyl sulfate.

The incidence of recurrence is low if the patient wears elastic stockings.

DRUG INTERACTIONS

No well-controlled studies have been performed on patients taking antiovulatory agents. The physician must use judgment and evaluate any patient taking antiovulatory drugs prior to initiating treatment with Sotradecol® (Sodium Tetradecyl Sulfate Injection). (See ADVERSE REACTIONS.) Heparin should not be included in the same syringe as Sotradecol® since the two are incompatible.

CARCINOGENESIS, MUTAGENESIS, IMPAIRMENT OF FERTILITY

When tested in the L5178YTK$^{+/-}$ mouse lymphoma assay, sodium tetradecyl sulfate did not induce a dose-related increase in the frequency of thymidine kinase-deficient mutants and, therefore, was judged to be nonmutagenic in this system. However, no long-term animal carcinogenicity studies with sodium tetradecyl sulfate have been performed.

PREGNANCY

Teratogenic Effects—Pregnancy Category C. Adequate reproduction studies have not been performed in animals to determine whether this drug affects fertility in males or females, has teratogenic potential, or has other adverse effects on the fetus. There are no well-controlled studies in pregnant women, but investigational and marketing experience does not include any positive evidence of adverse effects on the fetus. Although there is no clearly defined risk, such

Continued on next page

Elkins-Sinn—Cont.

experience cannot exclude the possibility of infrequent or subtle damage to the human fetus.

NURSING MOTHERS

It is not known whether this drug is excreted in human milk. Because many drugs are excreted in human milk, caution should be exercised when Sodium Tetradecyl Sulfate Injection is administered to a nursing woman.

ADVERSE REACTIONS

Local reactions consisting of pain, urticaria or ulceration may occur at the site of injection. A permanent discoloration, usually small and hardly noticeable but which may be objectionable from a cosmetic viewpoint, may remain along the path of the sclerosed vein segment. Sloughing and necrosis of tissue may occur following extravasation of the drug. Systemic reactions, except for allergic ones, have been slight. These include headache, nausea and vomiting. Allergic reactions such as hives, asthma, hayfever and anaphylactoid shock have been reported. (See WARNINGS.)

One death has been reported in a patient who received Sotradecol® (Sodium Tetradecyl Sulfate Injection) and who had been receiving an antiovulatory agent.

Another death (fatal pulmonary embolism) has been reported in a 36-year-old female treated with sodium tetradecyl *acetate* and who was **not** taking oral contraceptives.

DOSAGE AND ADMINISTRATION

For intravenous use only. Do not use if precipitated or discolored. The strength of solution required depends on the size and degree of varicosity. In general, the 1% solution will be found most useful with the 3% solution preferred for larger varicosities. The dosage should be kept small, using 0.5 to 2 mL (preferably 1 mL maximum) for each injection, and the maximum single treatment should not exceed 10 mL.

Parenteral drug products should be inspected visually for particulate matter and discoloration prior to administration, whenever solution and container permit.

HOW SUPPLIED

Sotradecol® (Sodium Tetradecyl Sulfate Injection)

1%—2 mL DOSETTE® ampuls packaged in 5s (NDC 0641-1514-34)

3%—2 mL DOSETTE® ampuls packaged in 5s (NDC 0641-1516-34)

STORAGE

Store at controlled room temperature 15°–30°C (59°–86°F).

ANIMAL TOXICOLOGY

The intravenous LD_{50} of sodium tetradecyl sulfate in mice was reported to be 90 ± 5 mg/kg.

In the rat, the acute intravenous LD_{50} of sodium tetradecyl sulfate was estimated to be between 72 mg/kg and 108 mg/kg.

Purified sodium tetradecyl sulfate was found to have an LD_{50} of 2 g/kg when administered orally by stomach tube as a 25% aqueous solution to rats. In rats given 0.15 g/kg in drinking water for 30 days, no appreciable toxicity was seen although some growth inhibition was discernible.

* * * *

Manufactured by
ELKINS-SINN, INC., Cherry Hill, NJ 08003-4099

Endo Laboratories, L.L.C.
DUPONT MERCK PLAZA
P.O. BOX 80390
WILMINGTON, DE 19880-0722

Direct Inquiries to:
During Business Hours (8:00 AM to 4:30 PM Eastern Time):
(302) 633-6887

For Medical Information Contact:
(302) 992-4240
Adverse Drug Experiences:
Business Hours Only:
(302) 992-4240

Products Available

Amantadine HCL Syrup, USP 50 mg 5 mL
Amiloride Hydrochloride and Hydrochlorothiazide Tablets, USP 5/50 mg
Captopril Tablets, USP 12.5 mg, 25 mg, 50 mg, 100 mg
Carbidopa and Levodopa Tablets, USP 10/100 mg, 25/100 mg, 25/250 mg
Chlorothiazide Tablets, USP 250 mg, 500 mg
Cimetidine Hydrochloride Injection, 300 mg/2mL
Cimetidine Hydrochloride Oral Solution, 300 mg/5mL
Cimetidine Tablets USP 200 mg, 300 mg, 400 mg, 800 mg
Cyclobenzaprine Hydrochloride Tablets, USP 10 mg

Dicyclomine HCl USP, 10 mg Capsules and 20 mg Tablets
Diflunisal Tablets, USP 250 mg, 500 mg
Endocet
  Oxycodone and Acetaminophen Tablets, USP CII
  Oxycodone HCl 5 mg, Acetaminophen 325 mg
Endodan
  Oxycodone and Aspirin Tablets, USP CII
  Oxycodone HCl 4.5 mg, Oxycodone Terephthalate 0.38 mg, Aspirin 325 mg
Glipizine Tablets 5 mg, 10 mg
Hydrochlorothiazide Tablets, USP 25 mg, 50 mg
Hydrocodone/APAP Tablets, USP CIII 5/500 mg, 7/5/650 mg, 7.5/750 mg
Indomethacin Capsules, USP 25 mg, 50 mg
Indomethacin Extended-Release Capsules, USP 75 mg
Methyldopa Tablets, USP 125 mg, 250 mg, 500 mg
Methyldopa/HCTZ Tablets, USP 250/15 mg, 250/25 mg
Oxycodone HCl USP, 5 mg Tablets
Sulindac Tablets, USP 150 mg, 200 mg
Timolol Maleate Tablets, USP 5 mg, 10 mg

Enzon, Inc.
20 KINGSBRIDGE RD.
PISCATAWAY, NJ 08854

Direct Inquiries to:
Toni L. Klich
(908) 980-4619
FAX: (908) 980-5911

For Medical Information Contact:
In Emergencies:
Anna T. Viau, Ph.D.
(908) 980-4677
(800) 836-4664
FAX: (908) 980-9642

ADAGEN® ℞
[ad-a-jen]
(pegademase bovine)
Injection

PRODUCT OVERVIEW

KEY FACTS

ADAGEN® (pegademase bovine) Injection is a modified enzyme used to provide direct and specific replacement of adenosine deaminase (ADA), an enzyme that is deficient in some patients with severe combined immunodeficiency disease (SCID). While regular administration of the compound can improve immune function and reduce the incidence of opportunistic infections in patients with ADA-deficient SCID, it is of no value in patients with immunodeficiency due to other causes. Further, it is not intended as a replacement for HLA-identical bone marrow transplant therapy.

MAJOR USES

ADAGEN® is to be used as enzyme replacement therapy in patients who have SCID associated with a deficiency of ADA, and who are not suitable candidates for-or who have failed-bone marrow transplantation. ADAGEN® should be used in infants from birth or in children of any age at the time of diagnosis.

SAFETY INFORMATION

ADAGEN® should be administered with caution to patients with thrombocytopenia and should not be given if thrombocytopenia is severe.

PRESCRIBING INFORMATION

ADAGEN® ℞
[ad-a-jen]
(pegademase bovine) Injection

DESCRIPTION

ADAGEN® (pegademase bovine) Injection is a modified enzyme used for enzyme replacement therapy for the treatment of severe combined immunodeficiency disease (SCID) associated with a deficiency of adenosine deaminase.

ADAGEN® (pegademase bovine) Injection is supplied in an isotonic, pyrogen free, sterile solution, pH 7.2–7.4, for intramuscular injection only. The solution is clear and colorless. It is supplied in 1.5 mL single-dose vials.

The chemical name for ADAGEN® (pegademase bovine) Injection is (monomethoxypolyethylene glycol succinimidyl)$_{11–17}$-adenosine deaminase. It is a conjugate of numerous strands of monomethoxypolyethylene glycol (PEG), molecular weight 5,000, covalently attached to the enzyme adenosine deaminase (ADA). ADA (adenosine deaminase EC 3.5.4.4) used in the manufacture of ADAGEN® (pegademase bovine) Injection is derived from bovine intestine.

The structural formula of ADAGEN® (pegademase bovine) Injection is:

$$[CH_3-(OCH_2CH_2)_x-O-\overset{O}{\underset{\|}{C}}-CH_2CH_2-\overset{O}{\underset{\|}{C}}-NH]_y-\text{adenosine deaminase}$$

x = 114 oxyethylene groups per PEG strand.
y = 11–17 primary amino groups of lysine onto which succinyl PEG is attached.

Each milliliter of ADAGEN® (pegademase bovine) Injection contains:
Pegademase bovine ....250 units*
Monobasic sodium phosphate, USP ....1.20 mg
Dibasic sodium phosphate, USP ....5.58 mg
Sodium Chloride, USP ....8.50 mg
Water for Injection, USP ....q.s. to 1.0 mL

*One unit of activity is defined as the amount of ADA that converts 1 μM of adenosine to inosine per minute at 25°C and pH 7.3.

CLINICAL PHARMACOLOGY

Severe Combined Immunodeficiency Disease Associated with ADA Deficiency

Severe combined immunodeficiency disease (SCID) associated with a deficiency of ADA is a rare, inherited, and often fatal disease. In the absence of the ADA enzyme, the purine substrates adenosine and 2'-deoxyadenosine accumulate, causing metabolic abnormalities that are directly toxic to lymphocytes.

The immune deficiency can be cured by bone marrow transplantation. When a suitable bone marrow donor is unavailable or when bone marrow transplantation fails, non-selective replacement of the ADA enzyme has been provided by periodic irradiated red blood cell transfusions. However, transmission of viral infections and iron overload are serious risks associated with irradiated red blood cell transfusions, and relatively few ADA deficient patients have benefitted from chronic transfusion therapy.

ADAGEN® (pegademase bovine) Injection provides specific and direct replacement of the deficient enzyme, but will not benefit patients with immunodeficiency due to other causes. In patients with ADA deficiency, rigorous adherence to a schedule of ADAGEN® (pegademase bovine) Injection administration can eliminate the toxic metabolites of ADA deficiency and result in improved immune function. It is imperative that treatment with ADAGEN® (pegademase bovine) Injection be carefully monitored by measurement of the level of ADA activity in plasma. Monitoring of the level of deoxyadenosine triphosphate (dATP) in erythrocytes is also helpful in determining that the dose of ADAGEN® (pegademase bovine) Injection is adequate.

Actions

ADAGEN® (pegademase bovine) Injection provides specific replacement of the deficient enzyme.

In the absence of the enzyme ADA, the purine substrates adenosine, 2'-deoxyadenosine and their metabolites are toxic to lymphocytes. The direct action of ADAGEN® (pegademase bovine) Injection is the correction of these metabolic abnormalities. Improvement in immune function and diminished frequency of opportunistic infections compared with the natural history of combined immunodeficiency due to ADA deficiency only occurs after metabolic abnormalities are corrected. There is a lag between the correction of the metabolic abnormalities and improved immune function. This period of time is variable, and has been reported to be from a few weeks to as long as 6 months. In contrast to the natural history of combined immunodeficiency disease due to ADA deficiency, a trend toward diminished frequency of opportunistic infections and fewer complications of infections has occurred in patients receiving ADAGEN® (pegademase bovine) Injection.

Pharmacokinetics

The pharmacokinetics and biochemical effects of ADAGEN® (pegademase bovine) Injection have been studied in six children ranging in age from 6 weeks to 12 years with SCID associated with ADA deficiency.

After the intramuscular injection of ADAGEN® (pegademase bovine) Injection, peak plasma levels of ADA activity were reached 2 to 3 days following administration. The plasma elimination half-life of ADA following the administration of ADAGEN® (pegademase bovine) Injection was variable, even for the same child. The range was 3 to >6 days. Following weekly injections of ADAGEN® (pegademase bovine) Injection at 15 U/kg, the average trough level of ADA activity in plasma was between 20 and 25 $\mu mol/hr/mL$.

Biochemical Effects

The changes in red blood cell deoxyadenosine nucleotide (dATP) and S-adenosylhomocysteine hydrolase (SAHase) have been evaluated. In patients with ADA deficiency, inadequate elimination of 2'-deoxyadenosine caused a marked elevation in dATP and a decrease in SAHase level in red blood cells. Prior to treatment with ADAGEN® (pegademase bovine) Injection, the levels of dATP in the red blood cells ranged from 0.056 to 0.899 $\mu mol/mL$ of erythrocytes. After 2 months of maintenance treatment with ADAGEN®

(pegademase bovine) Injection, the levels decreased to a range of 0.007 to 0.015 μmol/mL. The normal value of dATP is below 0.001 μmol/mL. In the same period of time, the levels of SAHase increased from the pretreatment range of 0.09 to 0.22 nmol/hr/mg protein to a range of 2.37 to 5.16 nmol/hr/mg protein. The normal value for SAHase is 4.18± 1.9 nmol/hr/mg protein.

The optimal dosage and schedule of administration of **ADAGEN®** (pegademase bovine) Injection should be established for each patient, based on monitoring of plasma ADA activity levels (trough levels before maintenance injection), biochemical markers of ADA deficiency (primarily red cell dATP content), and parameters of immune function. Since improvement in immune function follows correction of metabolic abnormalities, maintenance dosage in individual patients should be aimed at achieving the following biochemical goals: 1) maintain plasma ADA activity (trough levels) in the range of 15–35 μmol/hr/mL (assayed at 37°C); and 2) decline in erythrocyte dATP to ≤ 0.005–0.015 μmol/mL packed erythrocytes, or ≤ 1% of the total erythrocyte adenine nucleotide (ATP + dATP) content, with a normal ATP level, as measured in a pre-injection sample.

In vitro immunologic data (lymphocyte response to mitogens and lymphocyte surface antigens) were obtained, but their clinical significance is unknown. Prior to treatment with **ADAGEN®** (pegademase bovine) Injection, immune status was significantly below normal, as indicated by < 10% of normal mitogen responses and circulating mononuclear cells bearing T-cell surface antigens. These parameters improved, though not always to normal, within 2 to 6 months of therapy.

INDICATIONS AND USAGE

ADAGEN® (pegademase bovine) Injection is indicated for enzyme replacement therapy for adenosine deaminase (ADA) deficiency in patients with severe combined immunodeficiency disease (SCID) who are not suitable candidates for—or who have failed—bone marrow transplantation. **ADAGEN®** (pegademase bovine) Injection is recommended for use in infants from birth or in children of any age at the time of diagnosis. **ADAGEN®** (pegademase bovine) Injection is not intended as a replacement for HLA indentical bone marrow transplant therapy. **ADAGEN®** (pegademase bovine) Injection is also not intended to replace continued close medical supervision and the initiation of appropriate diagnostic tests and therapy (e.g., antibiotics, nutrition, oxygen, gammaglobulin) as indicated for intercurrent illnesses.

CONTRAINDICATIONS

There is no evidence to support the safety and efficacy of **ADAGEN®** (pegademase bovine) Injection as preparatory or support therapy for bone marrow transplantation. Since **ADAGEN®** (pegademase bovine) Injection is administered by intramuscular injection, it should be used with caution in patients with thrombocytopenia and should not be used if thrombocytopenia is severe.

PRECAUTIONS

Warnings

At present, testing prior to distribution may not assure the initial and continuing potency of each new lot of **ADAGEN®** (pegademase bovine) Injection. Any laboratory or clinical indication of a decrease in potency of **ADAGEN®** (pegademase bovine) Injection should be reported immediately by telephone to ENZON, Inc. Telephone 908-980-4500. Fax 908-980-5911.

General

There have been no reports of hypersensitivity reactions in patients who have been treated with **ADAGEN®** (pegademase bovine) Injection.

One of 12 patients showed an enhanced rate of clearance of plasma ADA activity after 5 months of therapy at 15 U/kg/week. Enhanced clearance was correlated with the appearance of an antibody that directly inhibited both unmodified ADA and **ADAGEN®** (pegademase bovine) Injection. Subsequently, the patient was treated with twice weekly intramuscular injections at an increased dose of 20 U/kg, or a total weekly dose of 40 U/kg. No adverse effects were observed at the higher dose and effective levels of plasma ADA were restored. After 4 months, the patient returned to a weekly dosage schedule of 20 U/kg and effective plasma levels have been maintained.

Appropriate care to protect immune deficient patients should be maintained until improvement in immune function has been documented. The degree of immune function improvement may vary from patient to patient and, therefore, each patient will require appropriate care consistent with immunologic status.

Laboratory Tests

The treatment of SCID associated with ADA deficiency with **ADAGEN®**](pegademase bovine) Injection should be monitored by measuring plasma ADA activity and red blood cell dATP levels.

Plasma ADA activity and red cell dATP should be determined prior to treatment. Once treatment with **ADAGEN®** (pegademase bovine) Injection has been initiated, a desirable range of plasma ADA activity (trough level before maintenance injection) should be 15–35 μmol/hr/mL. This minimum trough level will ensure that plasma ADA activity from injection to injection is maintained above the level of total erythrocyte ADA activity in the blood of normal individuals.

Plasma ADA activity (pre-injection) should be determined every 1–2 weeks during the first 8–12 weeks of treatment in order to establish an effective dose of **ADAGEN®** (pegademase bovine) Injection. After two months of maintenance treatment with **ADAGEN®** (pegademase bovine) Injection, red cell dATP levels should decrease to a range of ≤0.005 to 0.015 μmol/mL. The normal value of dATP is below 0.001 μmol/mL. Once the level of dATP has fallen adequately, it should be measured 2–4 times a year during the remainder of the first year and 2–3 times a year thereafter, assuming no interruption in therapy.

Between 3 and 9 months, plasma ADA should be determined twice a month, then monthly until after 18–24 months of treatment with **ADAGEN®** (pegademase bovine) Injection.

Patients who have successfully been maintained on therapy for two years should continue to have plasma ADA measured every 2–4 months and red cell dATP measured twice yearly. More frequent monitoring would be necessary if therapy were interrupted or if an enhanced rate of clearance of plasma ADA activity develops.

Once effective ADA plasma levels have been established, should a patient's plasma ADA activity level fall below 10 μmol/hr/mL (which cannot be attributed to improper dosing, sample handling or antibody development) then all patients receiving this lot of **ADAGEN®** (pegademase bovine) Injection will be required to have a blood sample for plasma ADA determination taken prior to their next injection of **ADAGEN®** (pegademase bovine) Injection. The index patient will require re-testing for determination of plasma ADA activity prior to his/her next injection of **ADAGEN®** (pegademase bovine) Injection. If this value, as well as the value from one of the other patients from a different site, is less than 10 μmol/hr/mL then the lot in use will be recalled and replaced with a new clinical lot by ENZON, Inc.

Immune function, including the ability to produce antibodies, generally improves after 2–6 months of therapy, and matures over a longer period. Compared with the natural history of combined immunodeficiency disease due to ADA deficiency, a trend toward diminished frequency of opportunistic infections and fewer complications of infections has occurred in patients receiving **ADAGEN®** (pegademase bovine) Injection. However, the lag between the correction of the metabolic abnormalities and improved immune function with a trend toward diminished frequency of infections and complications of infection is variable, and has ranged from a few weeks to approximately 6 months. Improvement in the general clinical status of the patient may be gradual (as evidenced by improvement in various clinical parameters) but should be apparent by the end of the first year of therapy.

Antibody to **ADAGEN®** (pegademase bovine) Injection may develop in patients and may result in more rapid clearance of **ADAGEN®** (pegademase bovine) Injection. Antibody to **ADAGEN®** (pegademase bovine) Injection should be suspected if a persistent fall in pre-injection levels of plasma ADA to ≤10 μmol/hr/mL occurs. If other causes for a decline in plasma ADA levels can be ruled out [such as improper storage of **ADAGEN®** (pegademase bovine) Injection vials (freezing or prolonged storage at temperatures above 8°C), or improper handling of plasma samples (e.g., repeated freezing and thawing during transport to laboratory)], then a specific assay for antibody to ADA and **ADAGEN®** (pegademase bovine) Injection (ELISA, enzyme inhibition) should be performed.

In patients undergoing treatment with **ADAGEN®** (pegademase bovine) Injection, a decline in immune function, with increased risk of opportunistic infections and complications of infection, will result from failure to maintain adequate levels of plasma ADA activity [whether due to the development of antibody to **ADAGEN®** (pegademase bovine) Injection, to improper calculation of **ADAGEN®** (pegademase bovine) Injection dosage, to interruption of treatment or to improper storage of **ADAGEN®** (pegademase bovine) Injection with subsequent loss of activity]. If a persistent decline in plasma ADA activity occurs, immune function and clinical status should be monitored closely and precautions should be taken to minimize the risk of infection. If antibody to ADA or **ADAGEN®** (pegademase bovine) Injection is found to be the cause of a persistent fall in plasma ADA activity, then adjustment in the dosage of **ADAGEN®** (pegademase bovine) Injection and other measures may be taken to induce tolerance and restore adequate ADA activity.

Drug Interactions

There are no known drug interactions with **ADAGEN®** (pegademase bovine) Injection. However, Vidarabine is a substrate for ADA and 2′-deoxycoformycin is a potent inhibitor of ADA. Thus, the activities of these drugs and **ADAGEN®** (pegademase bovine) Injection could be substantially altered if they are used in combination with one another.

Carcinogenesis, Mutagenesis, Impairment of Fertility

Long-term carcinogenic studies in animals have not been performed with **ADAGEN®** (pegademase bovine) Injection nor have studies been performed on impairment of fertility. **ADAGEN®** (pegademase bovine) Injection did not exhibit a mutagenic effect when tested against Salmonella typhimurium strains in the Ames assay.

Pregnancy

Pregnancy Category C. Animal reproduction studies have not been conducted with **ADAGEN®** (pegademase bovine) Injection. It is also not known whether **ADAGEN®** (pegademase bovine) Injection can cause fetal harm when administered to a pregnant woman or can affect reproduction capacity. **ADAGEN®** (pegademase bovine) Injection should be given to a pregnant woman only if clearly needed.

Nursing Mothers

It is not known whether **ADAGEN®** (pegademase bovine) Injection is excreted in human milk. Because many drugs are excreted in human milk, caution should be exercised when **ADAGEN®** (pegademase bovine) Injection is administered to a nursing woman.

ADVERSE REACTIONS

Clinical experience with **ADAGEN®** (pegademase bovine) Injection has been limited. The following adverse reactions have been reported: headache in one patient and pain at the injection site in two patients.

OVERDOSAGE

There is no documented experience with **ADAGEN®** (pegademase bovine) Injection overdosage. An intraperitoneal dose of 50,000 U/kg of **ADAGEN®** (pegademase bovine) Injection in mice resulted in weight loss up to 9%.

DOSAGE AND ADMINISTRATION

Before prescribing **ADAGEN®** (pegademase bovine) Injection the physician should be thoroughly familiar with the details of this prescribing information. For further information concerning the essential monitoring of **ADAGEN®** (pegademase bovine) Injection therapy, the prescribing physician should contact ENZON, Inc., 20 Kingsbridge Road, Piscataway, NJ 08854. Telephone 908-980-4500. Fax 908-980-5911.

ADAGEN® (pegademase bovine) Injection is recommended for use in infants from birth or in children of any age at the time of diagnosis.

Parenteral drug products should be inspected visually for particulate matter and discoloration prior to administration, whenever solution and container permits.

ADAGEN® (pegademase bovine) Injection should not be diluted nor mixed with any other drug prior to administration.

ADAGEN® (pegademase bovine) Injection should be administered every 7 days as an intramuscular injection. The dosage of **ADAGEN®** (pegademase bovine) Injection should be individualized. The recommended dosing schedule is 10 U/kg for the first dose, 15 U/kg for the second dose, and 20 U/kg for the third dose. The usual maintenance dose is 20 U/kg per week. Further increases of 5 U/kg/week may be necessary, but a maximum single dose of 30 U/kg should not be exceeded. Plasma levels of ADA more than twice the upper limit of 35 μmol/hr/mL have occurred on occasion in several patients, and have been maintained for several weeks in one patient who received twice weekly injections (20 U/kg per dose) of **ADAGEN®** (pegademase bovine) Injection. No adverse effects have been observed at these higher levels; there is no evidence that maintaining pre-injection plasma ADA above 35 μmol/hr/mL produces any additional clinical benefits.

Dose proportionality has not been established and patients should be closely monitored when the dosage is increased. **ADAGEN®** (pegademase bovine) Injection is not recommended for intravenous administration. The optimal dosage and schedule of administration should be established for each patient based on monitoring of plasma ADA activity levels (trough levels before maintenance injection) and biochemical markers of ADA deficiency (primarily red cell dATP content). Since improvement in immune function follows correction of metabolic abnormalities, maintenance dosage in individual patients should be aimed at achieving the following biochemical goals: 1) maintain plasma ADA activity (trough levels before maintenance injection) in the range of 15–35 μmol/hr/mL (assayed at 37°C); and 2) decline in erythrocyte dATP to ≤0.005–0.015 μmol/mL packed erythrocytes, or ≤1% of the total erythrocyte adenine nucleotide (ATP + dATP) content, with a normal ATP level, as measured in a pre-injection sample. In addition, continued monitoring of immune function and clinical status is essential in any patient with a primary immunodeficiency disease and should be continued in patients undergoing treatment with **ADAGEN®** (pegademase bovine) Injection.

HOW SUPPLIED

ADAGEN® (pegademase bovine) Injection is a clear, colorless solution for intramuscular injection. Each vial contains

Continued on next page

Enzon—Cont.

250 units/mL and is supplied as a 1.5 mL single-use vial, in boxes of 4 vials (NDC-57665-001-01).

Refrigerate. Store between +2°C and +8°C (36°F and 46°F). DO NOT FREEZE. **ADAGEN®** (pegademase bovine) Injection should not be stored at room temperature. This product should not be used if there are any indications that it may have been frozen.

REFERENCES

1. Hershfield MS, Buckley RH, Greenberg ML, et al. Treatment of adenosine deaminase deficiency with polyethylene glycol-modified adenosine deaminase. N Engl J Med 1987; 316:589–96.
2. Levy Y, Hershfield MS, Fernandez-Mejia C, Polmar ST, Scudiery D, Berger M, Sorensen RU. Adenosine deaminase deficiency with late onset of recurrent infections: response to treatment with polyethylene glycol-modified adenosine deaminase. J. Pediatr 1988; 113:312–17.
3. Kredich NM, Hershfield MS. Immunodeficiency diseases caused by adenosine deaminase deficiency and purine nucleoside phosphorylase deficiency. 6th ed. In: Scriver CR, Beaudet AL, Sly WS, Valle D, eds. The metabolic basis of inherited disease. New York: McGraw Hill, 1989; 1045–75.
4. Hirschhorn R. Inherited enzyme deficiencies and immunodeficiency: adenosine deaminase (ADA) and purine nucleoside phosphorylase (PNP) deficiencies. Clin Immunol Immunopathol 1986; 40:157–65.
5. Hirschhorn R, Roegner-Maniscalco V, Kuritsky L, Rosen FS. Bone marrow transplantation only partially restores purine metabolites to normal adenosine deaminase-deficient patients. J Clin Invest 1981; 68:1387–93.
6. Polmar AH, Stern RC, Schwartz AL, Wetzler EM, Chase PA, Hirschhorn R. Enzyme replacement therapy for adenosine deaminase deficiency and severe combined immunodeficiency. N Engl J Med 1976; 295:1337–43.
7. Rubinstein A, Hirschhorn R, Sicklick M, Murphy RA. In vivo and in vitro effects of thymosin and adenosine deaminase on adenosine-deaminase-deficient lymphocytes. N Engl J Med 1979; 300:387–92.
8. Hirschhorn R, Papageorgiou PS, Kesarwala HH, Taft LT. Amelioration of neurologic abnormalities after "enzyme replacement" in adenosine deaminase deficiency. N Engl J Med 1980; 303:377–80.
9. Hirshhorn R, Ratech H, Rubinstein A, et al. Increased excretion of modified adenine nucleosides by children with adenosine deaminase deficiency. Pediatr Res 1982; 16:362–9.
10. Polmar SH. Enzyme replacement and other biochemical approaches to the therapy of adenosine deaminase deficiency. In: Elliott K, Whelan J, eds. Enzyme defects and immune dysfunction. Amsterdam: Excerpta Medica, 1979; 213–30.

ESI Lederle Inc.
P.O. BOX 41502
PHILADELPHIA, PA 19101

Direct Inquiries to:
Professional Service
(610) 688-4400

For Emergency Medical Information Contact:
Day: (800) 934-5556 8:30 AM to 4:30 PM
      (Eastern Standard Time), Weekdays only
Night: (610) 688-4400 (Emergencies only; non-emergencies
      should wait until the next day)
For Medical/Pharmacy Inquiries on Marketed Products Call:
(800) 934-5556 8:30 AM to 4:30 PM
(Eastern Standard Time), Weekdays only

ESI Lederle Inc. was formerly known as ESI Pharma, Inc. Products previously listed under the ESI Pharma, Inc. heading are now products of ESI Lederle Inc. and are described below.

AYGESTIN®   ℞
[ā-jĕs'tin]
(norethindrone acetate tablets, USP)

Caution: Federal law prohibits dispensing without prescription.

WARNING:
THE USE OF Aygestin DURING THE FIRST FOUR MONTHS OF PREGNANCY IS NOT RECOMMENDED.

Progestational agents have been used beginning with the first trimester of pregnancy in an attempt to prevent habitual abortion. There is no adequate evidence that such use is effective when such drugs are given during the first four months of pregnancy. Furthermore, in the vast majority of women, the cause of abortion is a defective ovum which progestational agents could not be expected to influence. In addition, the use of progestational agents, with their uterine-relaxant properties, in patients with fertilized defective ova may cause a delay in spontaneous abortion. Therefore, the use of such drugs during the first four months of pregnancy is not recommended.

Several reports suggest an association between intrauterine exposure to progestational drugs in the first trimester of pregnancy and genital abnormalities in male and female fetuses. The risk of hypospadias, 5 to 8 per 1,000 male births in the general population, may be approximately doubled with exposure to these drugs. There are insufficient data to quantify the risk to exposed female fetuses, but insofar as some of these drugs induce mild virilization of the external genitalia of the female fetus, and because of the increased association of hypospadias in the male fetus, it is prudent to avoid the use of these drugs during the first trimester of pregnancy.

If the patient is exposed to Aygestin (norethindrone acetate tablets, USP) during the first four months of pregnancy or if she becomes pregnant while taking this drug, she should be apprised of the potential risks to the fetus.

DESCRIPTION
Aygestin (norethindrone acetate tablets, USP)—5 mg oral tablets.

Aygestin, (17-hydroxy-19-nor-17α-pregn-4-en-20-yn-3-one acetate), a synthetic, orally active progestin, is the acetic acid ester of norethindrone. It is a white, or creamy white, crystalline powder.

Aygestin Tablets contain the following inactive ingredients: lactose, magnesium stearate, and microcrystalline cellulose.

CLINICAL PHARMACOLOGY
Norethindrone acetate induces secretory changes in an estrogen-primed endometrium. It acts to inhibit the secretion of pituitary gonadotropins which, in turn, prevent follicular maturation and ovulation. On a weight basis, it is twice as potent as norethindrone.

INDICATIONS AND USAGE
Aygestin is indicated for the treatment of secondary amenorrhea, endometriosis, and abnormal uterine bleeding due to hormonal imbalance in the absence of organic pathology, such as submucous fibroids or uterine cancer.

CONTRAINDICATIONS
Thrombophlebitis, thromboembolic disorders, cerebral apoplexy, or a past history of these conditions.
Markedly impaired liver function or liver disease.
Known or suspected carcinoma of the breast.
Undiagnosed vaginal bleeding.
Missed abortion.
As a diagnostic test for pregnancy.

WARNINGS
1. Discontinue medication pending examination if there is a sudden partial or complete loss of vision or if there is sudden onset of proptosis, diplopia, or migraine. If examination reveals papilledema or retinal vascular lesions, medication should be withdrawn.
2. Because of the occasional occurrence of thrombophlebitis and pulmonary embolism in patients taking progestogens, the physician should be alert to the earliest manifestations of the disease.
3. Masculinization of the female fetus has occurred when progestogens have been used in pregnant women.

PRECAUTIONS
GENERAL PRECAUTIONS
1. The pretreatment physical examination should include special reference to breasts and pelvic organs, as well as a Papanicolaou smear.

2. Because this drug may cause some degree of fluid retention, conditions which might be influenced by this factor, such as epilepsy, migraine, asthma, cardiac or renal dysfunctions, require careful observation.
3. In cases of breakthrough bleeding, as in all cases of irregular bleeding per vaginam, nonfunctional causes should be borne in mind. In cases of undiagnosed vaginal bleeding, adequate diagnostic measures are indicated.
4. Patients who have a history of psychic depression should be carefully observed and the drug discontinued if the depression recurs to a serious degree.
5. Any possible influence of prolonged progestogen therapy on pituitary, ovarian, adrenal, hepatic, or uterine functions awaits further study.
6. Concomitant Use in Estrogen Replacement Therapy: In postmenopausal estrogen replacement therapy, studies of the addition of a progestin for 7 or more days of a cycle of estrogen administration have reported a lowered incidence of endometrial hyperplasia. Morphological and biochemical studies of the endometrium suggest that 10 to 13 days of progestin are needed to provide maximal maturation of the endometrium and to eliminate any hyperplastic changes. Whether this will provide protection from endometrial carcinoma has not been clearly established. There are possible additional risks which may be associated with the inclusion of progestin in estrogen replacement regimens. Progestin therapy may have an adverse effect on lipid metabolism.
7. A decrease in glucose tolerance has been observed in a small percentage of patients on estrogen-progestogen combination drugs. The mechanism of this decrease is obscure. For this reason, diabetic patients should be carefully observed while receiving progestogen therapy.
8. The age of the patient constitutes no absolute limiting factor, although treatment with progestogens may mask the onset of the climacteric.
9. The pathologist should be advised of progestogen therapy when relevant specimens are submitted.

INFORMATION FOR THE PATIENT.
See text which appears at the end of this insert.

CARCINOGENESIS, MUTAGENESIS, AND IMPAIRMENT OF FERTILITY.
Some beagle dogs treated with medroxyprogesterone acetate developed mammary nodules. Although nodules occasionally appeared in control animals, they were intermittent in nature, whereas nodules in treated animals were larger and more numerous, and persisted. There is no general agreement as to whether the nodules are benign or malignant. Their significance with respect to humans has not been established.

PREGNANCY CATEGORY X.
See Boxed Warning.

NURSING MOTHERS.
Detectable amounts of progestogens have been identified in the milk of mothers receiving them. The effect of this on the nursing infant has not been determined.

PEDIATRIC USE.
Safety and effectiveness in pediatric patients have not been established.

ADVERSE REACTIONS
The following adverse reactions have been observed in women taking progestins:
Breakthrough bleeding.
Spotting.
Change in menstrual flow.
Amenorrhea.
Edema.
Changes in weight (decreases, increases).
Changes in cervical erosion and cervical secretions.
Cholestatic jaundice.
Rash (allergic) with and without pruritus.
Melasma or chloasma.
Mental depression.
Progestins may alter the result of pregnanediol determinations. The following laboratory results may be altered by the concomitant use of estrogens with progestins:
Hepatic function.
Coagulation tests—increase in prothrombin, factors VII, VIII, IX, and X.
Increase in PBI, BEI, and a decrease in T^3 uptake.
Reduced response to metyrapone test.
A statistically significant association has been demonstrated between use of estrogen-progestogen combination drugs and the following serious adverse reactions: thrombophlebitis, pulmonary embolism, and cerebral thrombosis and embolism. For this reason, patients on progestogen therapy should be carefully observed. Although available evidence is suggestive of an association, such a relationship has been neither confirmed nor refuted for the following serious adverse reactions:
Neuro-ocular lesions, e.g., retinal thrombosis and optic neuritis.
The following adverse reactions have been observed in patients receiving estrogen-progestogen combination drugs:
1.   Rise in blood pressure in susceptible individuals.
2.   Premenstrual-like syndrome.

3. Changes in libido.
4. Changes in appetite.
5. Cystitis-like syndrome.
6. Headache.
7. Nervousness.
8. Dizziness.
9. Fatigue.
10. Backache.
11. Hirsutism.
12. Loss of scalp hair.
13. Erythema multiforme.
14. Erythema nodosum.
15. Hemorrhagic eruption.
16. Itching.

In view of these observations, patients on progestogen therapy should be carefully observed.

DOSAGE AND ADMINISTRATION

Therapy with Aygestin must be adapted to the specific indications and therapeutic response of the individual patient. This dosage schedule assumes the interval between menses to be 28 days.

Secondary amenorrhea, abnormal uterine bleeding due to hormonal imbalance in the absence of organic pathology: 2.5 to 10 mg Aygestin may be given daily for 5 to 10 days during the second half of the theoretical menstrual cycle to produce an optimum secretory transformation of an endometrium that has been adequately primed with either endogenous or exogenous estrogen.

Progestin withdrawal bleeding usually occurs within three to seven days after discontinuing Aygestin therapy. Patients with a past history of recurrent episodes of abnormal uterine bleeding may benefit from planned menstrual cycling with Aygestin.

Endometriosis: Initial daily dosage of 5 mg Aygestin for two weeks. Dosage should be increased by 2.5 mg per day every two weeks until 15 mg per day of Aygestin is reached. Therapy may be held at this level for six to nine months or until annoying breakthrough bleeding demands temporary termination.

HOW SUPPLIED

Each white, scored Aygestin® Tablet contains 5 mg norethindrone acetate, USP, in bottles of 50 (NDC 59911-5894-1).
Store at room temperature (approximately 25° C)
Dispense in a well-closed container as defined in the USP

INFORMATION FOR THE PATIENT

Your doctor has prescribed Aygestin (norethindrone acetate tablets, USP), a progestin, for you. Aygestin is similar to the progesterone hormones naturally produced by the body. Progestins are used to treat menstrual disorders and to test if the body is producing certain hormones.

Warning

Progesterone or progesterone-like drugs have been used to prevent miscarriage in the first few months of pregnancy. No adequate evidence is available to show that they are effective for this purpose. Furthermore, most cases of early miscarriage are due to causes which could not be helped by these drugs.

There is an increased risk of minor birth defects in children whose mothers take this drug during the first four months of pregnancy. Several reports suggest an association between mothers who take these drugs in the first trimester of pregnancy and genital abnormalities in male and female babies. The risk to the male baby is the possibility of being born with a condition in which the opening of the penis is on the underside rather than the tip of the penis (hypospadias). Hypospadias occurs in about 5 to 8 per 1,000 male births and is about doubled with exposure to these drugs. There is not enough information to quantify the risk to exposed female fetuses, but enlargement of the clitoris and fusion of the labia may occur, although rarely.

Therefore, since drugs of this type may induce mild masculinization of the external genitalia of the female fetus, as well as hypospadias in the male fetus, it is wise to avoid using the drug during the first trimester of pregnancy.

These drugs have been used as a test for pregnancy but such use is no longer considered safe because of possible damage to a developing baby. Also, more rapid methods for testing for pregnancy are now available.

If you take Aygestin (norethindrone acetate tablets, USP) and later find you were pregnant when you took it, be sure to discuss this with your doctor as soon as possible.

HOW SUPPLIED

Aygestin® (norethindrone acetate tablets, USP)—white, scored 5 mg tablets, in bottles of 50, for oral administration.

Shown in Product Identification Guide, page 310

CYCRIN®
℞
[sĭc′crĭn]
(medroxyprogesterone acetate tablets, USP)

WARNING

THE USE OF CYCRIN DURING THE FIRST FOUR MONTHS OF PREGNANCY IS NOT RECOMMENDED.

Progestational agents have been used, beginning with the first trimester of pregnancy, in an attempt to prevent habitual abortion. There is no adequate evidence that such use is effective when such drugs are given during the first 4 months of pregnancy. Furthermore, in the vast majority of women, the cause of abortion is a defective ovum, which progestational agents could not be expected to influence. In addition, the use of progestational agents with their uterine-relaxant properties, in patients with fertilized defective ova, may cause a delay in spontaneous abortion. Therefore, the use of such drugs during the first 4 months of pregnancy is not recommended.

Several reports suggest an association between intrauterine exposure to progestational drugs in the first trimester of pregnancy and genital abnormalities in male and female fetuses. The risk of hypospadias, 5 to 8 per 1,000 male births in the general population, may be approximately doubled with exposure to these drugs. There are insufficient data to quantify the risk to exposed female fetuses, but insofar as some of these drugs induce mild virilization of the external genitalia of the female fetus, and because of the increased association of hypospadias in the male fetus, it is prudent to avoid the use of these drugs during the first trimester of pregnancy.

If the patient is exposed to Cycrin (medroxyprogesterone acetate) during the first 4 months of pregnancy, or if she becomes pregnant while taking this drug, she should be apprised of the potential risks to the fetus.

DESCRIPTION

Cycrin tablets contain medroxyprogesterone acetate, which is a derivative of progesterone. It is a white to off-white, odorless, crystalline powder, stable in air, melting between 200°C and 210°C. It is freely soluble in chloroform, soluble in acetone and in dioxane, sparingly soluble in alcohol and in methanol, slightly soluble in ether, and insoluble in water. The chemical name for medroxyprogesterone acetate is pregn-4-ene-3,20-dione, 17-(acetyloxy)-6-methyl-, (6α)-. Its structural formula is:

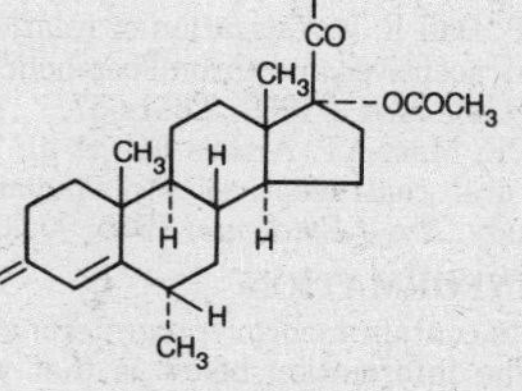

Cycrin is available in tablet form for oral administration. Each tablet contains 2.5 mg, 5 mg, or 10 mg of medroxyprogesterone acetate and the following inactive ingredients: lactose, magnesium stearate, methylcellulose, and microcrystalline cellulose. Each dosage strength also contains the following:

5 mg—D&C Red #30 and FD&C Blue #1;
10 mg—D&C Red #30 and D&C Yellow #10.

CLINICAL PHARMACOLOGY

Medroxyprogesterone acetate, administered orally or parenterally in the recommended doses to women with adequate endogenous estrogen, transforms proliferative into secretory endometrium. Androgenic and anabolic effects have been noted, but the drug is apparently devoid of significant estrogenic activity. While parenterally administered medroxyprogesterone acetate inhibits gonadotropin production, which in turn prevents follicular maturation and ovulation, available data indicate that this does not occur when the usually recommended oral dosage is given as single daily doses.

INDICATIONS AND USAGE

Secondary amenorrhea; abnormal uterine bleeding due to hormonal imbalance in the absence of organic pathology, such as fibroids or uterine cancer.

CONTRAINDICATIONS

1. Thrombophlebitis, thromboembolic disorders, cerebral apoplexy, or patients with a past history of these conditions.

---

2. Liver dysfunction or disease.
3. Known or suspected malignancy of breast or genital organs.
4. Undiagnosed vaginal bleeding.
5. Missed abortion.
6. As a diagnostic test for pregnancy.
7. Known sensitivity to medroxyprogesterone acetate.

WARNINGS

1. The physician should be alert to the earliest manifestations of thrombotic disorders (thrombophlebitis, cerebrovascular disorders, pulmonary embolism, and retinal thrombosis). Should any of these occur or be suspected, the drug should be discontinued immediately.
2. Beagle dogs treated with medroxyprogesterone acetate developed mammary nodules, some of which were malignant. Although nodules occasionally appeared in control animals, they were intermittent in nature, whereas the nodules in the drug-treated animals were larger, more numerous, persistent, and there were some breast malignancies with metastases. Their significance with respect to humans has not been established.
3. Discontinue medication pending examination if there is sudden partial or complete loss of vision, or if there is a sudden onset of proptosis, diplopia, or migraine. If examination reveals papilledema or retinal vascular lesions, medication should be withdrawn.
4. Detectable amounts of progestin have been identified in the milk of mothers receiving the drug. The effect of this on the nursing infant has not been determined.
5. Usage in pregnancy is not recommended (see Boxed Warning).
6. Retrospective studies of morbidity and mortality in Great Britain and studies of morbidity in the United States have shown a statistically significant association between thrombophlebitis, pulmonary embolism, and cerebral thrombosis and embolism and the use of oral contraceptives.[1-4] The estimate of the relative risk of thromboembolism in the study by Vessey and Doll[3] was about sevenfold, while Sartwell and associates[4] in the United States found a relative risk of 4.4, meaning that the users are several times as likely to undergo thromboembolic disease without evident cause as nonusers. The American study also indicated that the risk did not persist after discontinuation of administration, and that it was not enhanced by long, continued administration. The American study was not designed to evaluate a difference between products.

PRECAUTIONS

1. The pretreatment physical examination should include special reference to breasts and pelvic organs, as well as Papanicolaou smear.
2. Because progestogens may cause some degree of fluid retention, conditions which might be influenced by this factor, such as epilepsy, migraine, asthma, cardiac or renal dysfunction, require careful observation.
3. In cases of breakthrough bleeding, as in all cases of irregular bleeding per vaginum, nonfunctional causes should be borne in mind. In cases of undiagnosed vaginal bleeding, adequate diagnostic measures are indicated.
4. Patients who have a history of psychic depression should be carefully observed and the drug discontinued if the depression recurs to a serious degree.
5. Any possible influence of prolonged progestin therapy on pituitary, ovarian, adrenal, hepatic, or uterine functions awaits further study.
6. A decrease in glucose tolerance has been observed in a small percentage of patients on estrogen-progestin combination drugs. The mechanism of this decrease is obscure. For this reason, diabetic patients should be carefully observed while receiving progestin therapy.
7. The age of the patient constitutes no absolute limiting factor, although treatment with progestins may mask the onset of the climacteric.
8. The pathologist should be advised of progestin therapy when relevant specimens are submitted.
9. Because of the occasional occurrence of thrombotic disorders (thrombophlebitis, pulmonary embolism, retinal thrombosis, and cerebrovascular disorders) in patients taking estrogen-progestin combinations, and since the mechanism is obscure, the physician should be alert to the earliest manifestation of these disorders.
10. CONCOMITANT USE IN ESTROGEN REPLACEMENT THERAPY: Studies of the addition of a progestin product to an estrogen replacement regimen for 7 or more days of a cycle of estrogen administration have reported a lowered incidence of endometrial hyperplasia. Morphological and biochemical studies of the endometrium suggest that 10 to 13 days of progestin are needed to provide maximal maturation of the endometrium and to eliminate any hyperplastic changes. Whether this will provide protection from endometrial carcinoma has not been clearly established. There are possible additional risks which may be associated with

Continued on next page

Consult 1997 supplements and future editions for revisions

ESI Lederle—Cont.

the inclusion of progestin in estrogen replacement regimens. The potential risks include adverse effects on carbohydrate and lipid metabolism. The dosage used may be important in minimizing these adverse effects.

11. Aminoglutethimide administered concomitantly with Cycrin may significantly depress the bioavailability of Cycrin.

CARCINOGENESIS, MUTAGENESIS, IMPAIRMENT OF FERTILITY

Long-term intramuscular administration of medroxyprogesterone acetate has been shown to produce mammary tumors in beagle dogs (see **"Warnings"** above). There was no evidence of a carcinogenic effect associated with the oral administration of medroxyprogesterone acetate to rats and mice. Medroxyprogesterone acetate was not mutagenic in a battery of *in vitro* or *in vivo* genetic toxicity assays.

Medroxyprogesterone acetate at high doses is an antifertility drug and high doses would be expected to impair fertility until the cessation of treatment.

INFORMATION FOR THE PATIENT
See Patient Information at the end of insert.

ADVERSE REACTIONS

PREGNANCY: (See Boxed Warning for possible adverse effects on the fetus.)
BREAST: Breast tenderness or galactorrhea has been reported rarely.
SKIN: Sensitivity reactions consisting of urticaria, pruritus, edema, and generalized rash have occurred in an occasional patient. Acne, alopecia, and hirsutism have been reported in a few cases.
THROMBOEMBOLIC PHENOMENA: Thromboembolic phenomena, including thrombophlebitis and pulmonary embolism, have been reported.
The following adverse reactions have been observed in women taking progestins, including Cycrin (medroxyprogesterone acetate tablets):

   breakthrough bleeding
   spotting
   change in menstrual flow
   amenorrhea
   edema
   change in weight (increase or decrease)
   change in cervical erosion and cervical
      secretions
   cholestatic jaundice
   anaphylactoid reactions and anaphylaxis
   rash (allergic) with and without pruritus
   mental depression
   pyrexia
   insomnia
   nausea
   somnolence

A statistically significant association has been demonstrated between use of estrogen-progestin combination drugs and the following serious adverse reactions: thrombophlebitis; pulmonary embolism; and cerebral thrombosis and embolism. For this reason patients on progestin therapy should be carefully observed.
Although available evidence is suggestive of an association, such a relationship has been neither confirmed nor refuted for the following serious adverse reactions: neuro-ocular lesions, e.g., retinal thrombosis and optic neuritis.
The following adverse reactions have been observed in patients receiving estrogen-progestin combination drugs:

   rise in blood pressure in susceptible individuals
   premenstrual-like syndrome
   changes in libido
   changes in appetite
   cystitis-like syndrome
   headache
   nervousness
   dizziness
   fatigue
   backache
   hirsutism
   loss of scalp hair
   erythema multiforme
   erythema nodosum
   hemorrhagic eruption
   itching

In view of these observations, patients on progestin therapy should be carefully observed.
The following laboratory results may be altered by the use of estrogen-progestin combination drugs:
Increased sulfobromophthalein retention and other hepatic-function tests.
Coagulation tests: increase in prothrombin factors VII, VIII, IX, and X.

Metyrapone test.
Pregnanediol determination
Thyroid function: increase in PBI, and butanol extractable protein bound iodine and decrease in T_3 uptake values.

DOSAGE AND ADMINISTRATION

SECONDARY AMENORRHEA: Cycrin (medroxyprogesterone acetate tablets) may be given in dosages of 5 mg to 10 mg daily for from 5 to 10 days. A dose for inducing an optimum secretory transformation of an endometrium that has been adequately primed with either endogenous or exogenous estrogen is 10 mg of Cycrin daily for 10 days. In cases of secondary amenorrhea, therapy may be started at any time. Progestin withdrawal bleeding usually occurs within 3 to 7 days after discontinuing Cycrin therapy.
ABNORMAL UTERINE BLEEDING DUE TO HORMONAL IMBALANCE IN THE ABSENCE OF ORGANIC PATHOLOGY: Beginning on the calculated 16th or 21st day of the menstrual cycle, 5 to 10 mg of medroxyprogesterone acetate may be given daily for from 5 to 10 days. To produce an optimum secretory transformation of an endometrium that has been adequately primed with either endogenous or exogenous estrogen, 10 mg of medroxyprogesterone acetate daily for 10 days beginning on the 16th day of the cycle is suggested. Progestin withdrawal bleeding usually occurs within three to seven days after discontinuing therapy with Cycrin. Patients with a past history of recurrent episodes of abnormal uterine bleeding may benefit from planned menstrual cycling with Cycrin.

HOW SUPPLIED

Cycrin® (medroxyprogesterone acetate tablets, USP) is available for oral administration in the following dosage strengths:
2.5 mg, white, oval tablet with a score debossed on one side and opposing "C"s debossed on the reverse, in bottles of 100 tablets (NDC 59911-5898-1).
5 mg, light-purple, oval tablet with "CYCRIN" and a score debossed on one side and opposing "C"s debossed on the reverse, in bottles of 100 tablets (NDC 59911-5897-1).
10 mg, peach, oval tablet with "CYCRIN" and a score debossed on one side and opposing "C"s debossed on the reverse, in bottles of 100 tablets. (NDC 59911-5896-1).
The appearance of these tablets is a registered trademark.
Store at controlled room temperature, 20°–25° C (66°–77° F).
Dispense in a well-closed container as defined in the USP.
Caution: Federal law prohibits dispensing without prescription.

REFERENCES

1. Royal College of General Practitioners: Oral contraception and thromboembolic disease. *J Coll Gen Pract* 1967; 13:267-279.
2. Inman WHW, Vessey MP: Investigation of deaths from pulmonary, coronary, and cerebral thrombosis and embolism in women of childbearing age. *Br Med J* 1968; 2:193-199.
3. Vessey MP, Doll R: Investigation of relation between use of oral contraceptives and thromboembolic disease. A further report. *Br Med J* 1969; 2:651-657.
4. Sartwell PE, Masi AT, Arthes FG, et al: Thromboembolism and oral contraceptives: An epidemiological case-control study. *Am J Epidemiol* 1969; 90:365-380.

PATIENT INFORMATION

Cycrin tablets contain medroxyprogesterone acetate, a progesterone. The information below is that which the U.S. Food and Drug Administration requires be provided for all patients taking progesterones. The information below relates only to the risk to the unborn child associated with the use of progesterone during pregnancy. For further information on the use, side effects, and other risks associated with this product, ask your doctor.

Warning For Women

Progesterone or progesterone-like drugs have been used to prevent miscarriage in the first few months of pregnancy. No adequate evidence is available to show that they are effective for this purpose. Furthermore, most cases of early miscarriage are due to causes which could not be helped by these drugs.
There is an increased risk of minor birth defects in children whose mothers take this drug during the first four months of pregnancy. Several reports suggest an association between mothers who take these drugs in the first trimester of pregnancy and genital abnormalities in male and female babies. The risk to the male baby is the possibility of being born with a condition in which the opening of the penis is on the underside rather than the tip of the penis (hypospadias). Hypospadias occurs in about 5 to 8 per 1,000 male births and is about doubled with exposure to these drugs. There is not enough information to quantify the risk to exposed female fetuses, but enlargement of the clitoris and fusion of the labia may occur, although rarely.
Therefore, since drugs of this type may induce mild masculinization of the external genitalia of the female fetus, as well as hypospadias in the male fetus, it is wise to avoid using the drug during the first trimester of pregnancy.

These drugs have been used as a test for pregnancy, but such use is no longer considered safe because of possible damage to a developing baby. Also, more rapid methods for testing for pregnancy are now available.
If you take Cycrin (medroxyprogesterone acetate tablets, USP) and later find you were pregnant when you took it, be sure to discuss this with your doctor as soon as possible.
Shown in Product Identification Guide, page 310

GRISACTIN® Ultra   ℞
[grĭz-ăc'tĭn]
(griseofulvin ultramicrosize)

Caution: Federal law prohibits dispensing without prescription.

DESCRIPTION

Griseofulvin is an oral fungistatic antibiotic for the treatment of superficial mycoses. It is derived from a species of *Penicillium*.
Grisactin Ultra tablets contain griseofulvin ultramicrosize in 250 mg and 330 mg dosage strengths.
Grisactin Ultra tablets contain the following inactive ingredients: lactose, magnesium stearate, microcrystalline cellulose, sodium starch glycolate.

HOW SUPPLIED

Grisactin® Ultra tablets, 250 mg: white, square shaped, compressed tablets impressed with the trade name and dosage strength, in bottles of 100 (NDC 59911-5805-1).
Grisactin® Ultra tablets, 330 mg: white, wide-oval shaped, compressed tablets impressed with the trade name and dosage strength, in bottles of 100 (NDC 59911-5806-1).
Store at room temperature (approximately 25° C)
Dispense in a well-closed container as defined in the USP
For prescribing information write to Professional Service, Wyeth-Ayerst Laboratories, P.O. Box 8299, Philadelphia, PA 19101, or contact your local Wyeth-Ayerst representative.
Shown in Product Identification Guide, page 310

ESI Pharma, Inc.
P.O. BOX 41502
PHILADELPHIA, PA 19101

The name ESI Pharma, Inc. has been changed to ESI Lederle Inc. All products listed under the ESI Pharma company heading can now be found under ESI Lederle Inc. Please turn to page 990 of this 1997 PDR.

Everett Laboratories, Inc.
71 GLENWOOD PLACE
EAST ORANGE, NEW JERSEY 07017-3004

Direct Inquiries to:
Professional Service Department
(201) 674-8455
FAX: (201) 674-0933

CORTIC ear drops   ℞

Each 1 ml contains:
Chloroxylenol	1 mg
Pramoxine HCl	10 mg
Hydrocortisone	10 mg

SUPPLIED
Plastic dropper vials of 10 ml.

REPAN-CF Tablets   ℞

Each Tablet Contains:
Butalbital 50Mg.
(WARNING: May be habit forming),
Acetamenophen 650Mg.

HOW SUPPLIED
Bottles of 100 tablets, Imprinted EVERETT 166.

STROVITE FORTE CAPLETS   ℞
Sugar, Sodium and Yeast Free

Vitamin A (beta carotene & acetate)	4000 IU
Vitamin E (dl-alpha tocopheryl acetate)	60 IU
Vitamin C (ascorbic acid)	500 mg

Vitamin B1 (thiamine mononitrate)	20 mg
Vitamin B2 (riboflavin)	20 mg
Vitamin B6 (pyridoxine hydrochloride)	25 mg
Vitamin B12 (cyanocobalamin)	50 mcg
Niacinamide	100 mg
Biotin	0.15 mg
Pantothenic Acid (calcium pantothenate)	25 mg
Folic Acid	0.8 mg
Iron (ferrous fumarate)	10 mg
Chromium (chromium nitrate)	0.1 mg
Magnesium (magnesium oxide)	50 mg
Molybdenum (sodium molybdate)	25 mcg
Copper (cupric oxide)	3 mg
Selenium (L-selenomethionine)	50 mcg
Zinc (zinc gluconate)	15 mg

SUPPLIED
Bottle of 100—imprinted EV 0204

STROVITE FORTE SYRUP   ℞
Vitamin Mineral Supplement
Sugar, Sodium, and Yeast Free

SUPPLIED
Bottle 16 Oz.—Unit Dose 15 ml

STROVITE PLUS CAPLETS   ℞
Therapeutic Multivitamin Mineral Supplement
Sugar Free

SUPPLIED
Bottles of 100 imprinted EV 201.

TUSSAFED-HC   ⓒⅢ

Each 5 ml Contains:
Hydrocodone Bitarate	2.5 mg
Phenylephrine HCL	7.5 mg
Guaifenesin	50 mg

SUPPLIED
Bottle 16 Oz.

VITAFOL Caplets   ℞
Vitamins, Minerals, Iron, Folic Acid Supplement
Sugar Free

SUPPLIED
Bottles of 100 and 1000 tablets imprinted EV 0072.

VITAFOL-PN Caplets   ℞
(Prenatal)
Sugar, Sodium and Yeast Free

Vitamin A (acetate)	4000 IU
Vitamin D (cholecalciferol)	400 IU
Vitamin C (ascorbic acid)	60 mg
Vitamin E (dl-alpha-tocopheryl-acetate)	30 IU
Folic Acid	1 mg
Vitamin B1 (thiamine mononitrate)	1.6 mg
Vitamin B2 (riboflavin)	1.8 mg
Vitamin B6 (pyridoxine HCL)	2.5 mg
Vitamin B 12 (cyanocobalamin)	5 mcg
Niacinamide	15 mg
Calcium (calcium carbonate)	125 mg
Elemental Iron (ferrous fumarate)	65 mg
Magnesium (magnesium oxide)	25 mg
Selenium (L-selenomethionine)	65 mcg
Zinc (zinc gluconate)	15 mg

SUPPLIED
Bottle of 100-imprinted EV0078

VITAFOL Syrup   ℞
Vitamins, Minerals, Iron, Folic Acid Supplement
Sodium, Alcohol, and Yeast Free

SUPPLIED
Bottles of 16 oz.

Ferndale Laboratories, Inc.
780 W. EIGHT MILE ROAD
FERNDALE, MI 48220

Direct Inquiries to:
Mr. Thayer McMillan
(313) 548-0900
FAX: (313) 548-0708

For Medical Information Contact:
In Emergencies:
Mr. Pravin M. Patel
(313) 548-0900
FAX: (313) 548-0279

ANALPRAM–HC® CREAM   ℞
Rectal Cream

DESCRIPTION
Contains Hydrocortisone acetate 1% or 2.5% and Pramoxine HCl 1% in a washable, nongreasy base containing stearic acid, cetyl alcohol, aquaphor, isopropyl palmitate, polyoxyl 40 stearate, propylene glycol, potassium sorbate 0.1%, sorbic acid 0.1%, triethanolamine lauryl sulfate and water.
Topical corticosteroids are anti-inflammatory and antipruritic agents. The structural formula, the chemical name, molecular formula and molecular weight for active ingredients are presented below.

Hydrocortisone acetate
(Pregn-4-ene-3,20-dione,21 - (acetyloxy)-11, 17-dihydroxy-,(11 β)-.)
$C_{23}H_{32}O_6$; mol wt: 404.50

Pramoxine hydrochloride
(4-(3-(p-butoxyphenoxy)propyl)morpholine hydrochloride)
$C_{17}H_{27}NO_3 \cdot HCl$; mol wt: 329.87

CLINICAL PHARMACOLOGY
Topical corticosteroids share anti-inflammatory, anti-pruritic and vasoconstrictive actions.
The mechanism of anti-inflammatory activity of the topical corticosteroids is unclear. Various laboratory methods, including vasoconstrictor assays, are used to compare and predict potencies and/or clinical efficacies of the topical corticosteroids. There is some evidence to suggest that a recognizable correlation exists between vasoconstrictor potency and therapeutic efficacy in man.
Pramoxine hydrochloride is a topical anesthetic agent which provides temporary relief from itching and pain. It acts by stabilizing the neuronal membrane of nerve endings with which it comes into contact.
Pharmacokinetics: The extent of percutaneous absorption of topical corticosteroids is determined by many factors including the vehicle, the integrity of the epidermal barrier, and the use of occlusive dressings.
Topical corticosteroids can be absorbed from normal intact skin. Inflammation and/or other disease processes in the skin increase percutaneous absorption. Occlusive dressings substantially increase the percutaneous absorption of topical corticosteroids. Thus, occlusive dressings may be a valuable therapeutic adjunct for treatment of resistant dermatoses (See DOSAGE AND ADMINISTRATION).
Once absorbed through the skin, topical corticosteroids are handled through pharmacokinetic pathways similar to systemically administered corticosteroids. Corticosteroids are bound to plasma proteins in varying degrees. Corticosteroids are metabolized primarily in the liver and are then excreted by the kidneys. Some of the topical corticosteroids and their metabolites are also excreted into the bile.

INDICATIONS AND USAGE
Topical corticosteroids are indicated for the relief of the inflammatory and pruritic manifestations of corticosteroid-responsive dermatoses of the anal region.

CONTRAINDICATIONS
Topical corticosteroids are contraindicated in those patients with a history of hypersensitivity to any of the components of the preparation.

PRECAUTIONS
General: Systemic absorption of topical corticosteroids has produced reversible hypothalamic-pituitary-adrenal (HPA) axis suppression, manifestations of Cushing's syndrome, hyperglycemia, and glucosuria in some patients.
Conditions which augment systemic absorption include the application of the more potent steroids, use over large surface areas, prolonged use, and the addition of occlusive dressings.
Therefore, patients receiving a large dose of a potent topical steroid applied to a large surface area and under an occlusive dressing should be evaluated periodically for evidence of HPA axis suppression by using the urinary free cortisol and ACTH stimulation tests. If HPA axis suppression is noted, an attempt should be made to withdraw the drug, to reduce the frequency of application, or to substitute a less potent steroid.
Recovery of HPA axis function is generally prompt and complete upon discontinuation of the drug. Infrequently, signs and symptoms of steroid withdrawal may occur, requiring supplemental systemic corticosteroids.
Children may absorb proportionally larger amounts of topical corticosteroids and thus be more susceptible to systemic toxicity. (See PRECAUTIONS—Pediatric Use).
If irritation develops, topical corticosteroids should be discontinued and appropriate therapy instituted.
In the presence of dermatological infections, the use of an appropriate antifungal or antibacterial agent should be instituted. If a favorable response does not occur promptly, the corticosteroid should be discontinued until the infection has been adequately controlled.
Information for the Patient: Patients using topical corticosteroids should receive the following information and instructions:
1. This medication is to be used as directed by the physician. It is for external use only. Avoid contact with the eyes.
2. Patients should be advised not to use this medication for any disorder other than for which it was prescribed.
3. The treated skin area should not be bandaged or otherwise covered or wrapped as to be occlusive unless directed by the physician.
4. Patients should report any signs of local adverse reactions especially under occlusive dressing.
5. Parents of pediatric patients should be advised not to use tightfitting diapers or plastic pants on a child being treated in the diaper area, as these garments may constitute occlusive dressings.
Laboratory Tests: The following tests may be helpful in evaluating the HPA axis suppression:
   Urinary free cortisol test
   ACTH stimulation test
Carcinogenesis, Mutagenesis, and Impairment of Fertility: Long-term animal studies have not been performed to evaluate the carcinogenic potential or the effect on fertility of topical corticosteroids.
Studies to determine mutagenicity with prednisolone and hydrocortisone have revealed negative results.
Pregnancy Category C: Corticosteroids are generally teratogenic in laboratory animals when administered systemically at relatively low dosage levels. The more potent corticosteroids have been shown to be teratogenic after dermal application in laboratory animals. There are no adequate and well-controlled studies in pregnant women on teratogenic effects from topically applied corticosteroids. Therefore, topical corticosteroids should be used during pregnancy only if the potential benefit justifies the potential risk to the fetus. Drugs of this class should not be used extensively on pregnant patients, in large amounts, or for prolonged periods of time.
Nursing Mothers: It is not known whether topical administration of corticosteroids could result in sufficient systemic absorption to produce detectable amounts in breast milk. Systemically administered corticosteroids are secreted into breast milk in quantities NOT likely to have a deleterious effect on the infant. Nevertheless, caution should be exercised when topical corticosteroids are administered to a nursing woman.
Pediatric Use: PEDIATRIC PATIENTS MAY DEMONSTRATE GREATER SUSCEPTIBILITY TO TOPICAL CORTICOSTEROID-INDUCED HPA AXIS SUPPRESSION AND CUSHING'S SYNDROME THAN MATURE PATIENTS BECAUSE OF A LARGER SKIN SURFACE AREA TO BODY WEIGHT RATIO.
Hypothalamic-pituitary-adrenal (HPA) axis suppression, Cushing's syndrome, and intracranial hypertension have been reported in children receiving topical corticosteroids. Manifestations of adrenal suppression in children include linear growth retardation, delayed weight gain, low plasma cortisol levels, and absence of response to ACTH stimulation. Manifestations of intracranial hypertension include bulging fontanelles, headaches, and bilateral papilledema.
Administration of topical corticosteroids to children should be limited to the least amount compatible with an effective

Continued on next page

Ferndale Laboratories—Cont.

therapeutic regimen. Chronic corticosteroid therapy may interfere with the growth and development of children.

ADVERSE REACTIONS

The following local adverse reactions are reported infrequently with topical corticosteroids, but may occur more frequently with the use of occlusive dressings. These reactions are listed in an approximate decreasing order of occurrence:

Burning	Hypopigmentation
Itching	Perioral dermatitis
Irritation	Allergic contact dermatitis
Dryness	Maceration of the skin
Folliculitis	Secondary infection
Hypertrichosis	Skin Atrophy
Acneiform eruptions	Striae
	Miliaria

OVERDOSAGE

Topically applied corticosteroids can be absorbed in sufficient amounts to produce systemic effects (See PRECAUTIONS).

DOSAGE AND ADMINISTRATION

Topical corticosteroids are generally applied to the affected area as a thin film three or four times daily depending on the severity of the condition.

Occlusive dressings may be used for the management of psoriasis or recalcitrant conditions. If an infection develops, the use of occlusive dressings should be discontinued and appropriate antimicrobial therapy instituted.

HOW SUPPLIED

ANALPRAM-HC® Cream 1% or 2.5% in a 1 oz. tube with rectal applicator.

Dispense in a tight container as defined in the USP.

Store at controlled room temperature 15°–30°C (59°–86°F).

KRONOFED–A® Kronocaps ℞

Dye-Free

Decongestant plus Antihistamine

Each sustained release, white and clear capsule contains:

Pseudoephedrine HCl	120 mg
Chlorpheniramine Maleate	8 mg

KRONOFED–A–JR® Kronocaps ℞

Dye-Free

Decongestant plus Antihistamine

Each sustained release, white and clear capsule contains:

Pseudoephedrine HCl	60 mg
Chlorpheniramine Maleate	4 mg

INDICATIONS

For temporary relief of upper respiratory and nasal congestion associated with the common cold, hay fever and allergies, sinusitis and vasomotor and allergic rhinitis.

CONTRAINDICATIONS

Severe hypertension or severe cardiac disease. Sensitivity to antihistamines or sympathomimetic agents.

PRECAUTIONS

Use with caution in patients with hyperthyroidism. Patients susceptible to the soporific effects of chlorpheniramine should be warned against driving or operating of machinery which requires complete mental alertness.

PREGNANCY

Pregnancy Category C: Animal reproduction studies have not been conducted with **KRONOFED-A®** medications. It is also not known whether **KRONOFED-A®** medications can cause fetal harm when administered to a pregnant woman or can affect reproduction capacity. **KRONOFED-A®** medications should be given to a pregnant woman only if clearly needed.

Nursing Mothers: Due to the possible passage of pseudoephedrine and chlorpheniramine into breast milk, and, because of the higher than usual risk for infants from sympathomimetic amines and antihistamines, the benefit to the mother vs. the potential risk should be considered and a decision should be made whether to discontinue nursing or to discontinue the drug.

CAUTION

Federal law prohibits dispensing without prescription.

DOSAGE

Kronofed-A® Capsules: Adults and children over 12 years of age—1 capsule every 12 hours. **Kronofed-A-JR®** Capsules: Children 6–12 years of age—1 capsule every 12 hours. Adults 1 or 2 capsules every 12 hours.

HOW SUPPLIED

Bottles of 100 and 500 Capsules.

LOCOID® ℞

(hydrocortisone butyrate)
Cream 0.1%
Ointment 0.1%
Topical Solution 0.1%

CAUTION: Federal law prohibits dispensing without prescription.

DESCRIPTION

LOCOID® cream, ointment and topical solution contain the topical corticosteroid, hydrocortisone butyrate, a non-fluorinated hydrocortisone ester. It has the chemical name: pregn-4-ene-3.20-dione, 11.21-dihydroxy-17-[(1-oxobutyl)oxy]-, 11(β): the molecular formula: $C_{25}H_{36}O_6$; the molecular weight: 432.54; and the CAS registry number: 13609-67-1. Its structural formula is:

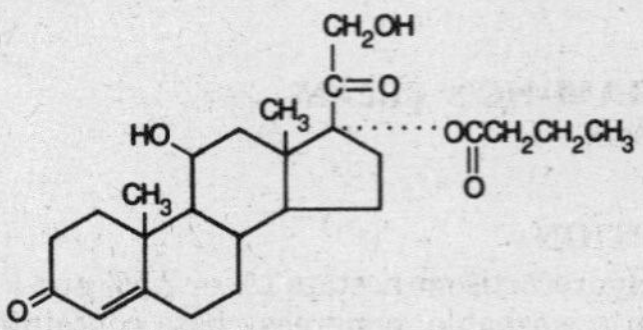

LOCOID® Cream 0.1%
Each gram of LOCOID® cream contains 1 mg of hydrocortisone butyrate in a hydrophilic base consisting of cetostearyl alcohol, ceteth-20, mineral oil, white petrolatum, citric acid, sodium citrate, methylparaben (preservative) and purified water.

LOCOID® Ointment 0.1%
Each gram of LOCOID® ointment contains 1 mg of hydrocortisone butyrate in a base consisting of mineral oil and polyethylene.

LOCOID® Solution 0.1%
Each mL of LOCOID® solution contains 1 mg of hydrocortisone butyrate in a vehicle consisting of isopropyl alcohol (50%), glycerin, povidone, citric acid, sodium citrate and purified water.

CLINICAL PHARMACOLOGY

Topical corticosteroids share anti-inflammatory, anti-pruritic and vasoconstrictive actions.

The mechanism of anti-inflammatory activity of the topical corticosteroids is unclear. Various laboratory methods, including vasoconstrictor assays, are used to compare and predict potencies and/or clinical efficacies of the topical corticosteroids. There is some evidence to suggest that a recognizable correlation exists between vasoconstrictor potency and therapeutic efficacy in man.

Pharmacokinetics
The extent of percutaneous absorption of topical corticosteroids is determined by many factors including the vehicle, the integrity of the epidermal barrier, and the use of occlusive dressings.

Topical corticosteroids can be absorbed from normal intact skin. Inflammation and/or other disease processes in the skin increase percutaneous absorption. Occlusive dressings substantially increase the percutaneous absorption of topical corticosteroids. Thus, occlusive dressings may be a valuable therapeutic adjunct for treatment of resistant dermatoses. (See DOSAGE AND ADMINISTRATION.)

Once absorbed through the skin, topical corticosteroids are handled through pharmacokinetic pathways similar to systemically administered corticosteroids. Corticosteroids are bound to plasma proteins in varying degrees. Corticosteroids are metabolized primarily in the liver and are then excreted by the kidneys. Some of the topical corticosteroids and their metabolites are also excreted into the bile.

INDICATIONS AND USAGE

LOCOID® cream 0.1% and ointment 0.1% (hydrocortisone butyrate) are indicated for the relief of the inflammatory and pruritic manifestations of corticosteroid-responsive dermatoses.

LOCOID® solution 0.1% (hydrocortisone butyrate) is indicated for the relief of the inflammatory and pruritic manifestations of seborrheic dermatitis.

CONTRAINDICATIONS

Topical corticosteroids are contraindicated in those patients with a history of hypersensitivity to any of the components of the preparation.

PRECAUTIONS

General: Systemic absorption of topical corticosteroids has produced reversible hypothalamic-pituitary-adrenal (HPA) axis suppression, manifestations of Cushing's syndrome, hyperglycemia, and glucosuria in some patients. Conditions which augment systemic absorption include the application of the more potent steroids, use over large surface areas, prolonged use, and the addition of occlusive dressings.

Therefore, patients receiving a large dose of a potent topical steroid applied to a large surface area or under an occlusive dressing should be evaluated periodically for evidence of HPA axis suppression by using the urinary free cortisol and ACTH stimulation tests. If HPA axis suppression is noted, an attempt should be made to withdraw the drug, to reduce the frequency of application, or to substitute a less potent steroid.

Recovery of HPA axis function is generally prompt and complete upon discontinuation of the drug. Infrequently, signs and symptoms of steroid withdrawal may occur, requiring supplemental systemic corticosteroids.

Children may absorb proportionally larger amounts of topical corticosteroids and thus be more susceptible to systemic toxicity (See PRECAUTIONS—PEDIATRIC USE.)

If irritation develops, topical corticosteroids should be discontinued and appropriate therapy instituted. In the presence of dermatological infections, the use of an appropriate antifungal or antibacterial agent should be instituted. If a favorable response does not occur promptly, the corticosteroid should be discontinued until the infection has been adequately controlled.

Information for the patient
Patients using topical corticosteroids should receive the following information and instructions:

1. This medication is to be used as directed by the physician. It is for external use only. Avoid contact with the eyes.
2. Patients should be advised not to use this medication for any disorder other than for which it was prescribed.
3. The treated skin area should not be bandaged or otherwise covered or wrapped as to be occlusive unless directed by the physician.
4. Patients should report any signs of local adverse reactions especially under occlusive dressing.
5. Parents of pediatric patients should be advised not to use tight-fitting diapers or plastic pants on a child being treated in the diaper area, as these garments may constitute occlusive dressings.

Laboratory tests
The following tests may be helpful in evaluating the HPA axis suppression:
Urinary free cortisol test
ACTH stimulation test

Carcinogenesis, Mutagenesis, and Impairment of Fertility
Long-term animal studies have not been performed to evaluate the carcinogenic potential or the effect on fertility of topical corticosteroids.

Studies to determine mutagenicity with prednisolone and hydrocortisone have revealed negative results.

Pregnancy Category C
Corticosteroids are generally teratogenic in laboratory animals when administered systemically at relatively low dosage levels. The more potent corticosteroids have been shown to be teratogenic after dermal application in laboratory animals. There are no adequate and well-controlled studies in pregnant women on teratogenic effects from topically applied corticosteroids. Therefore, topical corticosteroids should be used during pregnancy only if the potential benefit justifies the potential risk to the fetus. Drugs of this class should not be used extensively on pregnant patients, in large amounts, or for prolonged periods of time.

Nursing Mothers
It is not known whether topical administration of corticosteroids could result in sufficient systemic absorption to produce detectable quantities in breast milk. Systemically administered corticosteroids are secreted into breast milk, in quantities not likely to have a deleterious effect on the infant. Nevertheless, caution should be exercised when topical corticosteroids are administered to a nursing woman.

Pediatric Use
Pediatric patients may demonstrate greater susceptibility to topical corticosteroid-induced HPA axis suppression and Cushing's syndrome than mature patients because of a larger skin surface area to body weight ratio.

Hypothalamic-pituitary-adrenal (HPA) axis suppression, Cushing's syndrome, and intracranial hypertension have been reported in children receiving topical corticosteroids. Manifestations of adrenal suppression in children include linear growth retardation, delayed weight gain, low plasma cortisol levels, and absence of response to ACTH stimulation. Manifestations of intracranial hypertension include bulging fontanelles, headaches, and bilateral papilledema.

Administration of topical corticosteroids to children should be limited to the least amount compatible with an effective therapeutic regimen. Chronic corticosteroid therapy may interfere with the growth and development of children.

ADVERSE REACTIONS

The following local adverse reactions are reported infrequently with topical corticosteroids, but may occur more frequently with the use of occlusive dressings. These reactions are listed in an approximate decreasing order of occurrence: burning, itching, irritation, dryness, folliculitis, hypertrichosis, acneiform eruptions, hypopigmentation, perioral dermatitis, allergic contact dermatitis, maceration of the skin, secondary infection, skin atrophy, striae, miliaria.

OVERDOSAGE

Topically applied corticosteroids can be absorbed in sufficient amounts to produce systemic effects. (See PRECAUTIONS.)

DOSAGE AND ADMINISTRATION

LOCOID® cream 0.1% or LOCOID® ointment 0.1% (hydrocortisone butyrate) should be applied to the affected area as a thin film two to three times daily depending on the severity of the condition.

Occlusive dressings may be used for the management of psoriasis or recalcitrant conditions.

If an infection develops, the use of occlusive dressings should be discontinued and appropriate antimicrobial therapy instituted.

LOCOID® solution 0.1% (hydrocortisone butyrate) should be applied to the affected area as a thin film from two to three times daily depending on the severity of the condition.

HOW SUPPLIED

LOCOID® cream 0.1% (hydrocortisone butyrate) is supplied in tubes containing:
15 g NDC 0496-0802-15
45 g NDC 0496-0802-45
LOCOID® ointment 0.1% (hydrocortisone butyrate) is supplied in tubes containing:
15 g NDC 0496-0803-15
45 g NDC 0496-0803-45
LOCOID® solution 0.1% (hydrocortisone butyrate) is supplied in polyethylene bottles:
30 mL NDC 0496-0804-30
60 mL NDC 0496-0804-60

STORAGE

LOCOID® cream 0.1%: Store between 46° and 77°F (8° and 25°C).
LOCOID® ointment 0.1%: Store between 36°and 86°F (2°and 30°C).
LOCOID® solution 0.1%: Store between 41°and 77°F (5°and 25°C).

MARKETED BY:
FERNDALE LABORATORIES, INC.
FERNDALE, MICHIGAN 48220
MANUFACTURED BY:
Brocades Pharma bv
Leiderdorp/Netherlands
Revised: June 1991

PRAMOSONE® CREAM, LOTION AND OINTMENT   ℞

DESCRIPTION

Pramosone® Cream: Contains Hydrocortisone acetate 1% or 2.5% and Pramoxine HCl 1% in a hydrophilic base containing stearic acid, cetyl alcohol, aquaphor, isopropyl palmitate, polyoxyl 40 stearate, propylene glycol, potassium sorbate 0.1%, sorbic acid 0.1%, triethanolamine lauryl sulfate and water.

Pramosone® Lotion: Contains Hydrocortisone acetate 1% or 2.5% and Pramoxine HCl 1% in a base containing forlan-L, cetyl alcohol, stearic acid, di-isopropyl adipate, polyoxyl 40 stearate, silicon, triethanolamine, glycerine, polyvinylpyrolidone, potassium sorbate 0.1%, sorbic acid 0.1% and water.

Pramosone® Ointment: Contains Hydrocortisone acetate 1% or 2.5% and Pramoxine HCl 1% in an emollient ointment base containing Sorbitan sesquioleate, Water, Aquaphor and White petrolatum.

Topical corticosteroids are anti-inflammatory and antipruritic agents. The structural formula, the chemical name, molecular formula and molecular weight for active ingredients are presented below.

Hydrocortisone acetate
(Pregn-4-ene-3,20-dione,21 - (acetyloxy)-11, 17-dihydroxy-,(11 β)-).
$C_{23}H_{32}O_6$; mol wt: 404.50

Pramoxine hydrochloride
(4-(3-(p-butoxyphenoxy)propyl)morpholine hydrochloride)
$C_{17}H_{27}NO_3$·HCl; mol wt: 329.87

CLINICAL PHARMACOLOGY

Topical corticosteroids share anti-inflammatory, anti-pruritic and vasoconstrictive actions.

The mechanism of anti-inflammatory activity of the topical corticosteroids is unclear. Various laboratory methods, including vasoconstrictor assays, are used to compare and predict potencies and/or clinical efficacies of the topical corticosteroids. There is some evidence to suggest that a recognizable correlation exists between vasoconstrictor potency and therapeutic efficacy in man.

Pramoxine hydrochloride is a topical anesthetic agent which provides temporary relief from itching and pain. It acts by stabilizing the neuronal membrane of nerve endings with which it comes into contact.

Pharmacokinetics: The extent of percutaneous absorption of topical corticosteroids is determined by many factors including the vehicle, the integrity of the epidermal barrier, and the use of occlusive dressings.

Topical corticosteroids can be absorbed from normal intact skin. Inflammation and/or other disease processes in the skin increase percutaneous absorption. Occlusive dressings substantially increase the percutaneous absorption of topical corticosteroids. Thus, occlusive dressings may be a valuable therapeutic adjunct for treatment of resistant dermatoses (See DOSAGE AND ADMINISTRATION).

Once absorbed through the skin, topical corticosteroids are handled through pharmacokinetic pathways similar to systemically administered corticosteroids. Corticosteroids are bound to plasma proteins in varying degrees. Corticosteroids are metabolized primarily in the liver and are then excreted by the kidneys. Some of the topical corticosteroids and their metabolites are also excreted into the bile.

INDICATIONS AND USAGE

Topical corticosteroids are indicated for the relief of the inflammatory and pruritic manifestations of corticosteroid-responsive dermatoses.

CONTRAINDICATIONS

Topical corticosteroids are contraindicated in those patients with a history of hypersensitivity to any of the components of the preparation.

PRECAUTIONS

General: Systemic absorption of topical corticosteroids has produced reversible hypothalamic-pituitary-adrenal (HPA) axis suppression, manifestations of Cushing's syndrome, hyperglycemia, and glucosuria in some patients.

Conditions which augment systemic absorption include the application of the more potent steroids, use over large surface areas, prolonged use, and the addition of occlusive dressings.

Therefore, patients receiving a large dose of a potent topical steroid applied to a large surface area and under an occlusive dressing should be evaluated periodically for evidence of HPA axis suppression by using the urinary free cortisol and ACTH stimulation tests. If HPA axis suppression is noted, an attempt should be made to withdraw the drug, to reduce the frequency of application, or to substitute a less potent steroid.

Recovery of HPA axis function is generally prompt and complete upon discontinuation of the drug. Infrequently, signs and symptoms of steroid withdrawal may occur, requiring supplemental systemic corticosteroids.

Children may absorb proportionally larger amounts of topical corticosteroids and thus be more susceptible to systemic toxicity. (See PRECAUTIONS—Pediatric Use).

If irritation develops, topical corticosteroids should be discontinued and appropriate therapy instituted.

In the presence of dermatological infections, the use of an appropriate antifungal or antibacterial agent should be instituted. If a favorable response does not occur promptly, the corticosteroid should be discontinued until the infection has been adequately controlled.

Information for the Patient: Patients using topical corticosteroids should receive the following information and instructions:

1. This medication is to be used as directed by the physician. It is for external use only. Avoid contact with the eyes.
2. Patients should be advised not to use this medication for any disorder other than for which it was prescribed.
3. The treated skin area should not be bandaged or otherwise covered or wrapped as to be occlusive unless directed by the physician.
4. Patients should report any signs of local adverse reactions especially under occlusive dressing.
5. Parents of pediatric patients should be advised not to use tightfitting diapers or plastic pants on a child being treated in the diaper area, as these garments may constitute occlusive dressings.

Laboratory Tests: The following tests may be helpful in evaluating the HPA axis suppression:

Urinary free cortisol test
ACTH stimulation test

Carcinogenesis, Mutagenesis, and Impairment of Fertility: Long-term animal studies have not been performed to evaluate the carcinogenic potential or the effect on fertility of topical corticosteroids.

Studies to determine mutagenicity with prednisolone and hydrocortisone have revealed negative results.

Pregnancy Category C: Corticosteroids are generally teratogenic in laboratory animals when administered systemically at relatively low dosage levels. The more potent corticosteroids have been shown to be teratogenic after dermal application in laboratory animals. There are no adequate and well-controlled studies in pregnant women on teratogenic effects from topically applied corticosteroids. Therefore, topical corticosteroids should be used during pregnancy only if the potential benefit justifies the potential risk to the fetus. Drugs of this class should not be used extensively on pregnant patients, in large amounts, or for prolonged periods of time.

Nursing Mothers: It is not known whether topical administration of corticosteroids could result in sufficient systemic absorption to produce detectable amounts in breast milk. Systemically administered corticosteroids are secreted into breast milk in quantities NOT likely to have a deleterious effect on the infant. Nevertheless, caution should be exercised when topical corticosteroids are administered to a nursing woman.

Pediatric Use: PEDIATRIC PATIENTS MAY DEMONSTRATE GREATER SUSCEPTIBILITY TO TOPICAL CORTICOSTEROID-INDUCED HPA AXIS SUPPRESSION AND CUSHING'S SYNDROME THAN MATURE PATIENTS BECAUSE OF A LARGER SKIN SURFACE AREA TO BODY WEIGHT RATIO.

Hypothalamic-pituitary-adrenal (HPA) axis suppression, Cushing's syndrome, and intracranial hypertension have been reported in children receiving topical corticosteroids. Manifestations of adrenal suppression in children include linear growth retardation, delayed weight gain, low plasma cortisol levels, and absence of response to ACTH stimulation. Manifestations of intracranial hypertension include bulging fontanelles, headaches, and bilateral papilledema.

Administration of topical corticosteroids to children should be limited to the least amount compatible with an effective therapeutic regimen. Chronic corticosteroid therapy may interfere with the growth and development of children.

ADVERSE REACTIONS

The following local adverse reactions are reported infrequently with topical corticosteroids, but may occur more frequently with the use of occlusive dressings. These reactions are listed in an approximate decreasing order of occurrence:

Burning	Hypopigmentation
Itching	Perioral dermatitis
Irritation	Allergic contact dermatitis
Dryness	Maceration of the skin
Folliculitis	Secondary infection
Hypertrichosis	Skin Atrophy
Acneiform eruptions	Striae
	Miliaria

OVERDOSAGE

Topically applied corticosteroids can be absorbed in sufficient amounts to produce systemic effects (See PRECAUTIONS).

DOSAGE AND ADMINISTRATION

Topical corticosteroids are generally applied to the affected area as a thin film three or four times daily depending on the severity of the condition.

Occlusive dressings may be used for the management of psoriasis or recalcitrant conditions. If an infection develops, the use of occlusive dressings should be discontinued and appropriate antimicrobial therapy instituted.

HOW SUPPLIED

CREAM: 1% or 2½% in 1 oz. tubes, 2 oz. tubes.
LOTION: 1% in 2 fl. oz., 4 fl. oz. and 8 fl. oz. dispenser bottles. 2½% in 2 fl. oz. and 4 fl. oz. dispenser bottles.
OINTMENT: 1% or 2½% in 1 oz. tubes.
Dispense in a tight container as defined in the official compendium.

Store at controlled room temperature 15°- 30°C (59°- 86°F).

PRAX® LOTION*   OTC
(Pramoxine HCl 1% in an emollient hydrophilic base)

AVAILABLE

120 mL., and 240 mL. dispenser bottles.

---

*Additional information available upon request.

Ferring Laboratories, Inc.
400 RELLA BLVD, SUITE 201
SUFFERN, NY 10901-4249

Direct Inquiries to:
Ferring Laboratories, Inc.
Customer Service Department
400 Rella Blvd., Suite 201
Suffern, NY 10901-4249
(914) 368-7900
(800) 445-3690

For Medical Information Contact:
In Emergencies:
Ferring Laboratories, Inc.
Professional Services Department
400 Rella Blvd., Suite 201
Suffern, NY 10901-4249
(800) 822-8214

ACTHREL® ℞
(corticorelin ovine triflutate for injection)
For intravenous injection only
DIAGNOSTIC USE ONLY

HOW SUPPLIED
ACTHREL® is supplied as a sterile, nonpyrogenic, lyophilized, white cake containing 100 mcg corticorelin ovine (as the trifluoroacetate), 0.88 mg ascorbic acid, 10 mg lactose, and 20 mg human albumin. Trace amounts of chloride ion may be present from the manufacturing process. The package provides a single-dose, rubber-capped, 5-mL, brown-glass vial (NDC 55566-0301-1) containing 100 mcg corticorelin ovine (as the trifluoroacetate). ACTHREL® is stable in the lyophilized form when stored frozen at -20°C to -15°C (-4°F to +5°F) and protected from light. The reconstituted solution should be used immediately. Discard unused reconstituted solution.
Please see full prescribing information in the Diagnostic Product Information section.

DESMOPRESSIN ACETATE ℞
Injection

DESCRIPTION
DESMOPRESSIN ACETATE Injection is an antidiuretic hormone affecting renal water conservation and is a synthetic analogue of 8-arginine vasopressin. It is chemically defined as follows:
Mol. Wt. 1183.2
Empirical Formula: $C_{48}H_{74}N_{14}O_{17}S_2$

SCH₂CH₂CO-Tyr-Phe-Gln-Asn-Cys-Pro-D-Arg-Gly-NH₂ • C₂H₄O₂ • 3H₂O

1-(3-mercaptopropionic acid)-8-D-arginine vasopressin monoacetate (salt) trihydrate.
DESMOPRESSIN ACETATE Injection is provided as a sterile, aqueous solution for injection. Each mL provides:
Desmopressin acetate   4.0 mcg
Sodium chloride   9.0 mg
Hydrochloric acid to adjust pH to 4.0
The 10 mL vial contains chlorobutanol as a preservative (5.0 mg/mL).

CLINICAL PHARMACOLOGY
DESMOPRESSIN ACETATE Injection contains as active substance, 1-(3-mercaptopropionic acid)-8-D-arginine vasopressin, a synthetic analogue of the natural hormone arginine vasopressin. One mL (4 mcg) of desmopressin acetate solution has an antidiuretic activity of about 16 IU; 1 mcg of desmopressin acetate is equivalent to 4 IU.
Desmopressin acetate has been shown to be more potent than arginine vasopressin in increasing plasma levels of factor VIII activity in patients with hemophilia and von Willebrand's disease Type I.
Dose-response studies were performed in healthy persons, using doses of 0.1 to 0.4 mcg/kg body weight, infused over a 10-minute period. Maximal dose response occurred at 0.3 to 0.4 mcg/kg. The response to DESMOPRESSIN ACETATE Injection of factor VIII activity and plasminogen activator is dose-related, with maximal plasma levels of 300 to 400 per cent of initial concentrations obtained after infusion of 0.4 mcg/kg body weight. The increase is rapid and evident within 30 minutes, reaching a maximum at a point ranging from 90 minutes to two hours. The factor VIII related antigen and ristocetin cofactor activity were also increased to a smaller degree, but still are dose-dependent.

1. The biphasic half-lives of desmopressin acetate were 7.8 and 75.5 minutes for the fast and slow phases, respectively, compared with 2.5 and 14.5 minutes for lysine vasopressin, another form of the hormone. As a result, DESMOPRESSIN ACETATE Injection provides a prompt onset of antidiuretic action with a long duration after each administration.
2. The change in structure of arginine vasopressin to desmopressin acetate has resulted in a decreased vasopressor action and decreased actions on visceral smooth muscle relative to the enhanced antidiuretic activity, so that clinically effective antidiuretic doses are usually below threshold levels for effects on vascular or visceral smooth muscle.
3. When administered by injection, desmopressin acetate has an antidiuretic effect about ten times that of an equivalent dose administered intranasally.
4. The bioavailability of the subcutaneous route of administration was determined qualitatively using urine output data. The exact fraction of drug absorbed by that route of administration has not been quantitatively determined.
5. The percentage increase of factor VIII levels in patients with mild hemophilia A and von Willebrand's disease was not significantly different from that observed in normal healthy individuals when treated with 0.3 mcg/kg of desmopressin acetate infused over 10 minutes.
6. Plasminogen activator activity increases rapidly after desmopressin acetate infusion, but there has been no clinically significant fibrinolysis in patients treated with DESMOPRESSIN ACETATE Injection.
7. The effect of repeated DESMOPRESSIN ACETATE Injection administration when doses were given every 12 to 24 hours has generally shown a gradual diminution of the factor VIII activity increase noted with a single dose. The initial response is reproducible in any particular patient if there are 2 or 3 days between administrations.

INDICATION AND USAGE
Hemophilia A
DESMOPRESSIN ACETATE Injection is indicated for patients with hemophilia A with factor VIII coagulant activity levels greater than 5%.
DESMOPRESSIN ACETATE Injection will often maintain hemostasis in patients with hemophilia A during surgical procedures and postoperatively when administered 30 minutes prior to scheduled procedure.
DESMOPRESSIN ACETATE Injection will also stop bleeding in hemophilia A patients with episodes of spontaneous or trauma-induced injuries such as hemarthroses, intramuscular hematomas or mucosal bleeding.
DESMOPRESSIN ACETATE Injection is not indicated for the treatment of hemophilia A with factor VIII coagulant activity levels equal to or less than 5%, or for the treatment of hemophilia B, or in patients who have factor VIII antibodies. In certain clinical situations, it may be justified to try DESMOPRESSIN ACETATE Injection in patients with factor VIII levels between 2%–5%; however, these patients should be carefully monitored.
von Willebrand's Disease (Type I)
DESMOPRESSIN ACETATE Injection is indicated for patients with mild to moderate classic von Willebrand's disease (Type I) with factor VIII levels greater than 5%.
DESMOPRESSIN ACETATE Injection will often maintain hemostasis in patients with mild to moderate von Willebrand's disease during surgical procedures and postoperatively when administered 30 minutes prior to the scheduled procedure.
DESMOPRESSIN ACETATE Injection will usually stop bleeding in mild to moderate von Willebrand's patients with episodes of spontaneous or trauma-induced injuries such as hemarthroses, intramuscular hematomas or mucosal bleeding.
Those von Willebrand's disease patients who are least likely to respond are those with severe homozygous von Willebrand's disease with factor VIII coagulant activity and factor VIII von Willebrand factor antigen levels less than 1%. Other patients may respond in a variable fashion depending on the type of molecular defect they have. Bleeding time and factor VIII coagulant activity, ristocetin cofactor activity, and von Willebrand factor antigen should be checked during administration of DESMOPRESSIN ACETATE Injection to ensure that adequate levels are being achieved.
DESMOPRESSIN ACETATE Injection is not indicated for the treatment of severe classic von Willebrand's disease (Type I) and when there is evidence of an abnormal molecular form of factor VIII antigen. See Warning.
Diabetes Insipidus
DESMOPRESSIN ACETATE Injection is indicated as antidiuretic replacement therapy in the management of central (cranial) diabetes insipidus and for the management of the temporary polyuria and polydipsia following head trauma or surgery in the pituitary region. DESMOPRESSIN ACETATE Injection is ineffective for the treatment of nephrogenic diabetes insipidus.
Desmopressin acetate is also available as an intranasal preparation. However, this means of delivery can be compro-

mised by a variety of factors that can make nasal insufflation ineffective or inappropriate. These include poor intranasal absorption, nasal congestion and blockage, nasal discharge, atrophy of nasal mucosa, and severe atrophic rhinitis. Intranasal delivery may be inappropriate where there is an impaired level of consciousness. In addition, cranial surgical procedures, such as transphenoidal hypophysectomy, create situations where an alternative route of administration is needed as in cases of nasal packing or recovery from surgery.

CONTRAINDICATION
Known hypersensitivity to desmopressin acetate.

WARNINGS
Patients who do not have need of antidiuretic hormone for its antidiuretic effect, in particular those who are young or elderly, should be cautioned to ingest only enough fluid to satisfy thirst, in order to decrease the potential occurrence of water intoxication and hyponatremia.
Fluid intake should be adjusted, particularly in very young and elderly patients, in order to decrease the potential occurrence of water intoxication and hyponatremia. Particular attention should be paid to the possibility of the rare occurrence of an extreme decrease in plasma osmolality and resulting seizures which could lead to coma.
Desmopressin acetate should not be used to treat patients with Type IIB von Willebrand's disease since platelet aggregation may be induced.

PRECAUTIONS
General: For injection use only. DESMOPRESSIN ACETATE Injection has infrequently produced changes in blood pressure causing either a slight elevation in blood pressure or a transient fall in blood pressure and a compensatory increase in heart rate. The drug should be used with caution in patients with coronary artery insufficiency and/or hypertensive cardiovascular disease.
DESMOPRESSIN ACETATE Injection should be used with caution in patients with conditions associated with fluid and electrolyte imbalance, such as cystic fibrosis, because these patients are prone to hyponatremia.
There have been rare reports of thrombotic events following DESMOPRESSIN ACETATE Injection in patients predisposed to thrombus formation. No causality has been determined, however, the drug should be used with caution in these patients.
Severe allergic reactions have been reported rarely. Fatal anaphylaxis has been reported in one patient who received intravenous desmopressin acetate. It is not known whether antibodies to DESMOPRESSIN ACETATE Injection are produced after repeated injections.
Hemophilia A
Laboratory tests for assessing patient status include levels of factor VIII coagulant, factor VIII antigen and factor VIII ristocetin cofactor (von Willebrand factor) as well as activated partial thromboplastin time. Factor VIII coagulant activity should be determined before giving desmopressin acetate for hemostasis. If factor VIII coagulant activity is present at less than 5% of normal, desmopressin acetate should not be relied on.
von Willebrand's Disease
Laboratory tests for assessing patient status include levels of factor VIII coagulant activity, factor VIII ristocetin cofactor activity, and factor VIII von Willebrand factor antigen. The skin bleeding time may be helpful in following these patients.
Diabetes Insipidus
Laboratory tests for monitoring the patient include urine volume and osmolality. In some cases, plasma osmolality may be required.
Drug Interactions: Although the pressor activity of desmopressin acetate is very low compared with the antidiuretic activity, use of doses as large as 0.3 mcg/kg of desmopressin acetate with other pressor agents should be done only with careful patient monitoring.
Desmopressin acetate has been used with epsilon aminocaproic acid without adverse effects.
Carcinogenicity, Mutagenicity, Impairment of Fertility: Teratology studies in rats have shown no abnormalities. No further data are available.
Pregnancy (Pregnancy Category B): Reproduction studies performed in rats and rabbits with subcutaneous doses up to 12.5 times the human dose when used for factor VIII stimulation and 125 times the human dose when used in diabetes insipidus have revealed no evidence of harm to the fetus due to desmopressin acetate. There are several publications of management of diabetes insipidus in pregnant women with no harm to the fetus reported; however, there are no adequate and well-controlled studies in pregnant women. Published reports stress that, as opposed to preparations containing the natural hormones, desmopressin acetate in antidiuretic doses has no uterotonic action, but the physician will have to weigh possible therapeutic advantages against possible danger in each case.
Nursing Mothers: It is not known whether this drug is excreted in human milk. Because many drugs are excreted in

human milk, caution should be exercised when desmopressin acetate is administered to a nursing woman.

PEDIATRIC USE

Use in infants and children will require careful fluid intake restriction to prevent possible hyponatremia and water intoxication. *DESMOPRESSIN ACETATE Injection* should not be used in infants younger than three months in the treatment of hemophilia A or von Willebrand's disease; safety and effectiveness in children under 12 years of age with diabetes insipidus have not been established.

ADVERSE REACTIONS

Infrequently, desmopressin acetate has produced transient headache, nausea, mild abdominal cramps and vulval pain. These symptoms disappeared with reduction in dosage. Occasionally, injection of desmopressin acetate has produced local erythema, swelling or burning pain. Occasional facial flushing has been reported with the administration of desmopressin acetate.

DESMOPRESSIN ACETATE Injection has infrequently produced changes in blood pressure causing either a slight elevation or a transient fall and a compensatory increase in heart rate. Severe allergic reactions including anaphylaxis have been reported rarely with DESMOPRESSIN ACETATE Injection.

See **WARNINGS** for the possibility of water intoxication and hyponatremia.

There have been rare reports of thrombotic events (acute cerebrovascular thrombosis, acute myocardial infarction) following DESMOPRESSIN ACETATE Injection in patients predisposed to thrombus formation.

OVERDOSAGE

See **ADVERSE REACTIONS** above. In case of overdosage, the dosage should be reduced, frequency of administration decreased, or the drug withdrawn according to the severity of the condition.

There is no known specific antidote for desmopressin acetate.

An oral LD_{50} has not been established. An intravenous dose of 2 mg/kg in mice demonstrated no effect.

DOSAGE AND ADMINISTRATION

Hemophilia A and von Willebrand's Disease (Type I) DESMOPRESSIN ACETATE Injection is administered as an intravenous infusion at a dose of 0.3 mcg desmopressin acetate/kg body weight diluted in sterile physiological saline and infused slowly over 15 to 30 minutes. In adults and children weighing more than 10 kg, 50 mL of diluent is used; in children weighing 10 kg or less, 10 mL of diluent is used. Blood pressure and pulse should be monitored during infusion. If DESMOPRESSIN ACETATE Injection is used preoperatively, it should be administered 30 minutes prior to the scheduled procedure.

The necessity for repeat administration of desmopressin acetate or use of any blood products for hemostasis should be determined by laboratory response as well as the clinical condition of the patient. The tendency toward tachyphylaxis (lessening of response) with repeated administration given more frequently than every 48 hours should be considered in treating each patient.

Diabetes Insipidus This formulation is administered subcutaneously or by direct intravenous injection. DESMOPRESSIN ACETATE Injection dosage must be determined for each patient and adjusted according to the pattern of response. Response should be estimated by two parameters: adequate duration of sleep and adequate, not excessive, water turnover.

The usual dosage range in adults is 0.5 mL (2.0 mcg) to 1 mL (4.0 mcg) daily, administered intravenously or subcutaneously, usually in two divided doses. The morning and evening doses should be separately adjusted for an adequate diurnal rhythm of water turnover. For patients who have been controlled on intranasal desmopressin acetate and who must be switched to the injection form, either because of poor intranasal absorption or because of the need for surgery, the comparable antidiuretic dose of the injection is about one-tenth the intranasal dose.

Parenteral drug products should be inspected visually for particulate matter and discoloration prior to administration whenever solution and container permit.

HOW SUPPLIED

DESMOPRESSIN ACETATE Injection is available as a sterile solution in cartons of ten 1 mL single-dose ampules (NDC 55566-5030-1) and in 10 mL multiple-dose vials (NDC 55566-5040-1) each containing 4.0 mcg desmopressin acetate per mL. Keep refrigerated at about 4°C (39°F).

Caution: Federal (USA) law prohibits dispensing without prescription.

Manufactured for:
FERRING LABORATORIES, INC.
Suffern, NY 10901
By Ferring Pharmaceuticals, Malmö, Sweden
DC-140A Rev. 1/96

DESMOPRESSIN ACETATE RHINAL TUBE ℞

DESCRIPTION

Desmopressin Acetate Rhinal Tube is an antidiuretic hormone affecting renal water conservation and a synthetic analogue of 8-arginine vasopressin. It is chemically defined as follows:

Mol.wt. 1183.2
Empirical formula: $C_{48}H_{74}N_{14}O_{17}S_2$

SCH_2CH_2CO-Tyr-Phe-Gln-Asn-Cys-Pro-D-Arg-Gly-NH_2 • $C_2H_4O_2$ • $3H_2O$

1-(3-mercaptopropionic acid)-8-D-arginine vasopressin monoacetate (salt) trihydrate.

Desmopressin Acetate Rhinal Tube is provided as an aqueous solution for intranasal use. Each mL contains:

Desmopressin acetate	0.1 mg
Chlorobutanol	5.0 mg
Sodium Chloride	9.0 mg

Hydrochloric acid to adjust pH to approximately 4

CLINICAL PHARMACOLOGY

Desmopressin Acetate Rhinal Tube contains as active substance 1-(3-mercaptopropionic acid)-8-D-arginine vasopressin, which is a synthetic analogue of the natural hormone arginine vasopressin. One mL (0.1 mg) of Desmopressin Acetate Rhinal Tube has an antidiuretic activity of about 400 IU; 10 mcg of desmopressin acetate is equivalent to 40 IU.

1. The biphasic half-lives for Desmopressin Acetate Rhinal Tube were 7.8 and 75.5 minutes for the fast and slow phases, compared with 2.5 and 14.5 minutes for lysine vasopressin, another form of the hormone used in this condition. As a result, Desmopressin Acetate Rhinal Tube provides a prompt onset of antidiuretic action with a long duration after each administration.
2. The change in structure of arginine vasopressin to Desmopressin Acetate Rhinal Tube has resulted in a decreased vasopressor action and decreased actions on visceral smooth muscle relative to the enhanced antidiuretic activity, so that clinically effective antidiuretic doses are usually below threshold levels for effects on vascular or visceral smooth muscle.
3. Desmopressin Acetate Rhinal Tube administered intranasally has an antidiuretic effect about one-tenth that of an equivalent dose administered by injection.

INDICATIONS AND USAGE

Primary Noctural Enuresis: Desmopressin Acetate Rhinal Tube is indicated for the management of primary nocturnal enuresis. It may be used alone or adjunctive to behavioral conditioning or other non-pharmacological intervention. It has been shown to be effective in some cases that are refractory to conventional therapies.

Central Cranial Diabetes Insipidus: Desmopressin Acetate Rhinal Tube is indicated as antidiuretic replacement therapy in the management of central cranial diabetes insipidus and for management of the temporary polyuria and polydipsia following head trauma or surgery in the pituitary region. It is ineffective for the treatment of nephrogenic diabetes insipidus.

The use of Desmopressin Acetate Rhinal Tube in patients with an established diagnosis will result in a reduction in urinary ouput with increase in urine osmolality and a decrease in plasma osmolality. This will allow the resumption of a more normal life-style with a decrease in urinary frequency and nocturia.

There are reports of an occasional change in response with time, usually greater than 6 months. Some patients may show a decreased responsiveness, others a shortened duration of effect. There is no evidence this effect is due to the development of binding antibodies but may be due to a local inactivation of the peptide.

Patients are selected for therapy by establishing the diagnosis by means of the water deprivation test, the hypertonic saline infusion test, and/or the response to antidiuretic hormone. Continued response to Desmopressin Acetate Rhinal Tube can be monitored by urine volume and osmolality.

Desmopressin Acetate is also available as a solution for injection when the intranasal route may be compromised. These situations include nasal congestion and blockage, nasal discharge, atrophy of nasal mucosa, and severe atrophic rhinitis. Intranasal delivery may also be inappropriate where there is an impaired level of consciousness. In addition, cranial surgical procedures, such as transphenoidal hypophysectomy create situations where an alternative route of administration is needed as in cases of nasal packing or recovery from surgery.

CONTRAINDICATION

Known hypersensitivity to Desmopressin Acetate Rhinal Tube.

WARNINGS

1. For intranasal use only.
2. In very young and elderly patients in particular, fluid intake should be adjusted in order to decrease the potential occurrence of water intoxication and hyponatremia. Particular attention should be paid to the possibility of the rare occurrence of an extreme decrease in plasma osmolality and resulting seizures.

PRECAUTIONS

General: Desmopressin Acetate Rhinal Tube at high dosage has infrequently produced a slight elevation of blood pressure, which disappeared with a reduction in dosage. The drug should be used with caution in patients with coronary artery insufficiency and/or hypertensive cardiovascular disease because of possible rise in blood pressure.

Desmopressin Acetate Rhinal Tube should be used with caution in patients with conditions associated with fluid and electrolyte imbalance, such as cystic fibrosis, because these patients are prone to hyponatremia.

Central Cranial Diabetes Insipidus: Since Desmopressin Acetate Rhinal Tube is used intranasally, changes in the nasal mucosa such as scarring, edema, or other disease may cause erratic, unreliable absorption in which case Desmopressin Acetate Rhinal Tube should not be used. For such situations, Desmopressin Acetate Injection should be considered.

Primary Nocturnal Enuresis: If changes in the nasal mucosa have occurred, unreliable absorption may result. Desmopressin Acetate Rhinal Tube should be discontinued until the nasal problems resolve.

Laboratory Tests: Laboratory tests for following the patient with central cranial diabetes insipidus or post-surgical or head trauma-related polyuria and polydipsia include urine volume and osmolality. In some cases plasma osmolality may be required. For the healthy patient with primary nocturnal enuresis, serum electrolytes should be checked at least once if therapy is continued beyond 7 days.

Drug Interactions: Although the pressor activity of Desmopressin Acetate is very low compared to the antidiuretic activity, use of large doses of Desmopressin Acetate Rhinal Tube with other pressor agents should only be done with careful patient monitoring.

Carcinogenesis, Mutagenesis, Impairment of Fertility: Teratology studies in rats have shown no abnormalities. No further information is available.

Pregnancy-Category B: Reproduction studies performed in rats and rabbits with doses up to 12.5 times the human intranasal dose (i.e. about 125 times the total adult human dose given systemically) have revealed no evidence of harm to the fetus due to desmopressin acetate. There are several publications of management of diabetes insipidus in pregnant women with no harm to the fetus reported; however, no controlled studies in pregnant women have been carried out. Published reports stress that, as opposed to preparations containing the natural hormones, Desmopressin Acetate Rhinal Tube in antidiuretic doses has no uterotonic action, but the physician will have to weigh possible therapeutic advantages against possible dangers in each individual case.

Nursing Mothers: There have been no controlled studies in nursing mothers. A single study in a post-partum women demonstrated a marked change in plasma, but little if any change in assayable Desmopressin Acetate in breast milk following an intranasal dose of 10 mcg.

PEDIATRIC USE

Primary Nocturnal Enuresis: Desmopressin Acetate Rhinal Tube has been used in childhood nocturnal enuresis. Short-term (4–8 weeks) Desmopressin Acetate Rhinal Tube administration has been shown to be safe and modestly effective in children aged 6 years or older with severe childhood nocturnal enuresis. Adequately controlled studies with Desmopressin Acetate Rhinal Tube in primary nocturnal enuresis have not been conducted beyond 4–8 weeks. The dose should be individually adjusted to achieve the best results.

Central Cranial Diabetes Insipidus: Desmopressin Acetate Rhinal Tube has been used in children with diabetes insipidus. Use in infants and children will require careful fluid intake restriction to prevent possible hyponatremia and water intoxication. The dose must be individually adjusted to the patient with attention in the very young to the danger of an extreme decrease in plasma osmolality with resulting convulsions. Dose should start at 0.05 mL or less.

There are reports of an occasional change in response with time, usually greater than 6 months. Some patients may show a decreased responsiveness, others a shortened duration of effect. There is no evidence this effect is due to the development of binding antibodies but may be due to a local inactivation of the peptide.

Continued on next page

Ferring Laboratories—Cont.

ADVERSE REACTIONS

Infrequently, high dosages have produced transient headache and nausea. Nasal congestion, rhinitis and flushing have also been reported occasionally along with mild abdominal cramps. These symptoms disappeared with reduction in dosage. Nosebleed, sore throat, cough and upper respiratory infections have also been reported.

The following table lists the percent of patients having adverse experiences without regard to relationship to study drug from the pooled pivotal study data for nocturnal enuresis.

		DESMOPRESSIN	
	PLACEBO (N=59)	20 mcg (N=60)	40 mcg (N=61)
ADVERSE REACTION	%	%	%
BODY AS A WHOLE			
Abdominal Pain	0	2	2
Asthenia	0	0	2
Chills	0	0	2
Headache	0	2	5
Throat Pain	2	0	0
NERVOUS SYSTEM			
Depression	2	0	0
Dizziness	0	0	3
RESPIRATORY SYSTEM			
Epistaxis	2	3	0
Nostril Pain	0	2	0
Respiratory Infection	2	0	0
Rhinitis	2	8	3
CARDIOVASCULAR SYSTEM			
Vasodilation	2	0	0
DIGESTIVE SYSTEM			
Gastrointestinal Disorder	0	2	0
Nausea	0	0	2
SKIN & APPENDAGES			
Leg Rash	2	0	0
Rash	2	0	0
SPECIAL SENSES			
Conjunctivitis	0	2	0
Edema Eyes	0	2	0
Lachrymation Disorder	0	0	2

OVERDOSAGE

See adverse reactions above. In case of overdosage, the dose should be reduced, frequency of administration decreased, or the drug withdrawn according to the severity of the condition. There is no known specific antidote for Desmopressin Acetate Rhinal Tube.

An oral LD_{50} has not been established. An intravenous dose of 2 mg/kg in mice demonstrated no effect.

DOSAGE AND ADMINISTRATION

Primary Nocturnal Enuresis: Dosage should be adjusted according to the individual. The recommended initial dose for those 6 years of age and older is 20 mcg or 0.2 mL solution intranasally at bedtime. Adjustment up to 40 mcg is suggested if the patient does not respond. Some patients may respond to 10 mcg and adjustment to that lower dose may be done if the patient has shown a response to 20 mcg. It is recommended that one-half of the dose be administered per nostril. Adequately controlled studies with Desmopressin Acetate Rhinal Tube in primary nocturnal enuresis have not been conducted beyond 4–8 weeks.

Central Cranial Diabetes Insipidus: This drug is administered into the nose through a soft, flexible plastic rhinal tube which has four graduation marks on it that measure 0.2, 0.15, 0.1 and 0.05 mL. Desmopressin Acetate Rhinal Tube dosage must be determined for each individual patient and adjusted according to the diurnal pattern of response. Response should be estimated by two parameters: adequate duration of sleep and adequate, not excessive, water turnover. Patients with nasal congestion and blockage have often responded well to Desmopressin Acetate Rhinal Tube. The usual dosage range in adults is 0.1 to 0.4 mL daily, either as a single dose or divided into two or three doses. Most adults require 0.2 mL daily in two divided doses. The morning and evening doses should be separately adjusted for an adequate diurnal rhythm of water turnover. For children aged 3 months to 12 years, the usual dosage range is 0.05 to 0.3 mL daily, either as a single dose or divided into two doses.

About $^1/_4$ to $^1/_3$ of patients can be controlled by a single daily dose.

HOW SUPPLIED

2.5 mL per vial, packaged with two rhinal tube applicators per carton (NDC 55566-5020-1). Also available in shelf packs of 10 × 2.5 mL cartons (NDC 55566-5020-2).

KEEP REFRIGERATED AT ABOUT 4°C (39°F).

When traveling—controlled room temperature 22°C (72°F) closed sterile bottles will maintain stability for 3 weeks.

Caution: Federal (U.S.A.) law prohibits dispensing without prescription.

Manufactured for
FERRING LABORATORIES, INC.
Suffern, NY 10901
By Ferring Pharmaceuticals, Malmö, Sweden
DC 135A
Rev. 12/95

LUTREPULSE® for Injection ℞

(gonadorelin acetate)
Synthetic Gonadotropin-Releasing Hormone (GnRH)
For Pulsatile Intravenous Injection

DESCRIPTION

LUTREPULSE (gonadorelin acetate) for Injection is used for the induction of ovulation in women with primary hypothalamic amenorrhea. Gonadorelin acetate is a synthetic decapeptide that is identical in amino acid sequence to endogenous gonadotropin-releasing hormone (GnRH) synthesized in the human hypothalamus and in various neurons terminating in the hypothalamus. The molecular formula of gonadorelin acetate is:

$$C_{55}H_{75}N_{17}O_{13} \cdot xC_2H_4O_2 \cdot yH_2O$$

Its molecular weight is 1182.3 + x60 + y18, where x and y represent a non-stoichiometric ratio of acetate and water associated with the peptide, and x ranges from 1–2 and y ranges from 2–3. The amino acid sequence of GnRH is:

5-oxoPro-His-Trp-Ser-Tyr-Gly-Leu-Arg-Pro-Gly-NH_2

LUTREPULSE for Injection is a sterile, lyophilized powder intended for intravenous pulsatile injection after reconstitution. It is white and very soluble in water. Vials are available containing 0.8 mg or 3.2 mg gonadorelin acetate (expressed as the diacetate) and 10.0 mg mannitol as a carrier. After reconstituting with 8 mL of diluent (sterile 0.9% Sodium Chloride Solution and hydrochloric acid to adjust the pH) for LUTREPULSE for Injection, the concentration of gonadorelin acetate is 5 μg per 50 μL in each vial containing 0.8 mg lyophilized hormone, and 20 μg per 50 μL in each vial containing 3.2 mg lyophilized hormone. LUTREPULSE (gonadorelin acetate) for Injection is intended for use with the LUTREPULSE for Injection Kits and/or its individual components as listed below. The volumes and concentrations are specific for use with the LUTREPULSE PUMP for appropriate dosing.

CLINICAL PHARMACOLOGY

Under physiologic conditions, gonadotropin-releasing hormone (GnRH) is released by the hypothalamus in a pulsatile fashion. The primary effect of GnRH is the synthesis and release of luteinizing hormone (LH) in the anterior pituitary gland. GnRH also stimulates the synthesis and release of follicle stimulating hormone (FSH), but this effect is less pronounced. LH and FSH subsequently stimulate the gonads to produce steroids which are instrumental in regulating reproductive hormonal status. Unlike human menopausal gonadotropin (hMG) which supplies pituitary hormones, pulsatile administration of LUTREPULSE for Injection replaces defective hypothalamic secretion of GnRH. The pulsatile administration of LUTREPULSE for Injection approximates the natural hormonal secretory pattern, causing pulsatile release of pituitary gonadotropins. Accordingly, LUTREPULSE for Injection is useful in treating conditions of infertility caused by defective GnRH stimulation from the hypothalamus (See **INDICATIONS AND USAGE**). The following information summarizes clinical efficacy of gonadorelin acetate administered by pulsatile intravenous injection to patients with primary hypothalamic amenorrhea.

44 patients with primary hypothalamic amenorrhea (HA)
93% (41/44) patients ovulatory with gonadorelin acetate therapy
62% (24/39)* patients pregnant
100% (7/7) of those failing past attempts at ovulation induction by other methods were ovulatory on gonadorelin acetate.

*Five patients did not desire pregnancy.

Following intravenous injection of GnRH into normal subjects and/or hypogonadotropic patients, plasma GnRH concentrations rapidly decline with initial and terminal half-lives of 2–10 min. and 10–40 min., respectively. In these studies, high clearance values (500–1500 L/day) and low volumes of distribution (10–15 L) were calculated. The pharmacokinetics of GnRH in normal subjects and in hypogonadotropic patients were similar. GnRH was rapidly metabolized to various biologically inactive peptide fragments which are readily excreted in urine. Renal failure, but not hepatic disease, prolonged the half-life and reduced the clearance of GnRH.

INDICATIONS AND USAGE

LUTREPULSE (gonadorelin acetate) for Injection is indicated in the treatment of primary hypothalamic amenorrhea.

DIFFERENTIAL DIAGNOSIS: Proper diagnosis is critical for successful treatment with LUTREPULSE for Injection. It must be established that hypothalamic amenorrhea or hypogonadism is, in fact, due to a deficiency in quantity or pulsing of endogenous GnRH. The diagnosis of hypothalamic amenorrhea or hypogonadism is based on the exclusion of other causes of the dysfunction, since there is currently no practical technique to directly assess hypothalamic function. Prior to initiation of therapy with LUTREPULSE (gonadorelin acetate) for Injection, the physician should rule out disorders of general health, reproductive organs, anterior pituitary, and central nervous system, other than abnormalities of GnRH secretion.

CONTRAINDICATIONS

LUTREPULSE for Injection is contraindicated in women with any condition that could be exacerbated by pregnancy. For example, pituitary prolactinoma should be considered one such condition. Additionally, any history of sensitivity to gonadorelin acetate, gonadorelin hydrochloride or any component of LUTREPULSE for Injection is a contraindication.

Patients who have ovarian cysts or causes of anovulation other than those of hypothalamic origin should not receive LUTREPULSE for Injection.

LUTREPULSE for Injection is intended to initiate events including the production of reproductive hormones (e.g. estrogens and progestins). Therefore, any condition that may be worsened by reproductive hormones, such as hormonally-dependent tumor, is a contraindication to the use of LUTREPULSE for Injection.

WARNINGS

Therapy with LUTREPULSE (gonadorelin acetate) for Injection should be conducted by physicians familiar with pulsatile GnRH delivery and the clinical ramifications of ovulation induction. While there have been few cases of hyperstimulation(<1%) this possibility must be considered. If hyperstimulation should occur, therapy should be discontinued and spontaneous resolution can be expected. The preservation of the endogenous feedback mechanisms makes severe hyperstimulation (with ascites and pleural effusion) rare. However, the physician shoud be aware of the possibility and be alert for any evidence of ascites, pleural effusion, hemoconcentration, rupture of a cyst, fluid or electrolyte imbalance, or sepsis.

Multiple pregnancy is a possibility that can be minimized by careful attention to the recommended doses and ultrasonographic monitoring of the ovarian response to therapy. Following a baseline pelvic ultrasound, follow-up studies should be conducted at a minimum on day 7 and day 14 of therapy.

Serious hypersensitivity reactions (anaphylaxis) have been reported following gonadotropin-releasing hormone administration, including gonadorelin acetate. Clinical manifestations may include: cardiovascular collapse, hypotension, tachycardia, loss of consciousness, angioedema, bronchospasm, dyspnea, urticaria, flushing and pruritus. If any allergic reaction occurs, therapy with gonadorelin should be dicontinued. Serious acute hypersensitivity reactions may require emergency medical treatment.

As with any intravenous medication, scrupulous attention to asepsis is important. The infusion area must be monitored as with all indwelling parenteral approaches. The catheter and IV site should be monitored and changed at appropriate intervals for the type of intravenous catheter utilized for the delivery of therapy.

PRECAUTIONS

GENERAL: Ovarian hyperstimulation has been reported. This may be related to pulse dosage or concomitant use of other ovulation stimulators. Hyperstimulation may be a greater risk in patients where spontaneous variations in endogenous GnRH secretion occur. Multiple follicle development, multiple pregnancy, and spontaneous termination of pregnancy have been reported. Multiple pregnancy can be minimized by appropriate monitoring of follicle formation; nonetheless, the patient and her partner should be advised of the frequency (12%) and potential risks of multiple pregnancy before starting treatment.

Ovarian hyperstimulation, a syndrome of sudden ovarian enlargement, ascites with or without pain, and/or pleural effusion, is rare with pulsatile GnRH therapy. Among 268 patients participating in clinical trials, one case of moderate hyperstimulation has been reported, but this cycle included the concomitant use of clomiphene citrate.

Antibody formation (IgE and IgG) has been reported following administration of gonadorelin. The safety and efficacy implication of antibody development are uncertain (see: **WARNINGS**).

LUTREPULSE (gonadorelin acetate) for Injection should be administered only with the LUTREPULSE PUMP. The patient should be provided with detailed oral and written instructions regarding infusion pump usage and potential sepsis in order to minimize the frequency of infusion pump malfunction and inflammation, infection, mild phlebitis, or hematoma at the catheter site.

INFORMATION FOR PATIENTS: The patient should be advised to discontinue the drug and seek medical attention at the first sign of skin rash, urticaria, rapid heart beat, difficulty in swallowing and breathing, or any swelling which

may suggest angioedema (see: **WARNINGS** and **ADVERSE REACTIONS**).

LABORATORY TESTS: Following a diagnosis of primary hypothalamic amenorrhea, initiation of LUTREPULSE (gonadorelin acetate) for Injection therapy may be monitored by the following:

1) Ovarian ultrasound—baseline, therapy day 7, therapy day 14.
2) Mid-luteal phase serum progesterone.
3) Clinical observation of infusion site at each visit as needed.
4) Physical examination including pelvic at regularly scheduled visits.

DRUG INTERACTIONS: None are known. LUTREPULSE for Injection should not be used concomitantly with other ovulation stimulators.

DRUG/LABORATORY TEST INTERACTIONS: None are known.

CARCINOGENESIS, MUTAGENESIS, IMPAIRMENT OF FERTILITY: Since GnRH is a natural substance normally present in humans, long-term studies in animals have not been performed to evaluate carcinogenic potential. Mutagenicity testing was not done.

PREGNANCY: Pregnancy Category B
Reproduction studies (teratology and embryo-toxicity) performed in rats and rabbits have not revealed any evidence of harm to the fetus due to gonadorelin acetate. There was no evidence of teratogenicity when gonadorelin acetate was administered intravenously up to 120 μg/kg/day (> 70 times the recommended human dose of 5 μg per pulse) in rats and rabbits.

Studies in pregnant women have shown that gonadorelin acetate does not increase the risk of abnormalities when administered during the first trimester of pregnancy. It appears that the possibility of fetal harm is remote, if the drug is used during pregnancy. In clinical studies, 47 pregnant patients have used gonadorelin acetate during the first trimester of pregnancy (51 pregnancies) and the drug had no apparent adverse effect on the course of pregnancy. Available follow-up reports on infants born to these women reveal no adverse effects or complications that were attributable to gonadorelin acetate. Nevertheless, because the studies in humans cannot rule out the possibility of harm, gonadorelin acetate should be used during pregnancy only for maintenance of the corpus luteum in ovulation induction cycles.

NURSING MOTHERS: It is not known whether this drug is excreted in human milk. There is no indication for use of LUTREPULSE (gonadorelin acetate) for Injection in a nursing woman.

PEDIATRIC USE: Safety and effectiveness in children under the age of 18 have not been established.

ADVERSE REACTIONS

Adverse reactions have been reported in approximately 10% of treatment regimens. Ten of 268 patients interrupted therapy because of an adverse reaction but subsequently resumed treatment. One other subject did not resume treatment.

In clinical studies involving 268 women, one case of moderate ovarian hyperstimulation has been reported. This cycle included concomitant use of clomiphene citrate. This low incidence of hyperstimulation appears to be due to the preservation of normal feedback mechanisms of the pituitary-ovarian axis.

Despite the preservation of feedback mechanisms, some incidents of multiple follicle development, multiple pregnancy, and spontaneous termination of pregnancy have been reported. Multiple pregnancy can be minimized by appropriate monitoring of follicle formation; nonetheless, the patient and her partner should be advised of the frequency and potential hazards of multiple pregnancy before starting treatment. In clinical studies involving 142 pregnancies, delivery information was available on 89 pregnancies. Eleven of these LUTREPULSE (gonadorelin acetate) for Injection-induced pregnancies (12%) were multiple (10 sets of twins, 1 set of triplets).

The following adverse reactions have occurred at the injection site: urticaria, pruritus, inflammation, infection, mild phlebitis, or hematoma at the catheter site. Additionally, infusion set malfunction and interruption of infusion may occur; this has no known adverse effect other than interruption of therapy. Acute generalized (anaphylaxis, angio–edema, urticaria, etc.) hypersensitivity reactions have been reported (see: **WARNINGS** and **PRECAUTIONS**).

Anaphylaxis (bronchospasm, tachycardia, flushing, urticaria, induration at injection site) has also been reported with the related polypeptide hormone gonadorelin hydrochloride (FACTREL®).

® Registered trademark of Wyeth-Ayerst Laboratories.

OVERDOSAGE

Continuous, non-pulsatile exposure to gonadorelin acetate could temporarily reduce pituitary responsiveness. If the pump should malfunction and deliver the entire contents of the 3.2 mg system, no harmful effects would be expected. Bolus doses as high as 3000 μg of gonadorelin hydrochloride

have not been harmful. Pituitary hyperstimulation and multiple follicle development can be minimized by adhering to recommended doses, and appropriate monitoring of follicle formation (see **PRECAUTIONS**).

Administration of 640 μg/kg in monkeys as a single intravenous bolus resulted in no compound-related effects in clinical observations or gross morphologic evaluations.

DOSAGE AND ADMINISTRATION

DOSAGE: Dosages between 1 and 20 μg have been successfully used in clinical studies. The recommended dose in primary hypothalamic amenorrhea is 5 μg every 90 minutes. This is delivered by LUTREPULSE PUMP using the 0.8 mg solution at 50 μL per pulse (see physician pump manual). Sixty-eight percent of the 5 μg every 90 minute regimens induced ovulation in patients with primary hypothalamic amenorrhea.

The LUTREPULSE PUMP is capable of delivering 2.5, 5, 10, or 20 μg of gonadorelin acetate every 90 minutes. Some women may require a reduction in the recommended dose of 5 μg should laboratory testing and patient monitoring indicate an inappropriate response. While most primary hypothalamic amenorrhea patients will ovulate during the first cycle of 5 μg therapy, some may be refractory to this dose. The recommended treatment interval is 21 days. It may be necessary to raise the dose cautiously, and in stepwise fashion if there is no response after three treatment intervals. All dose changes should be carefully monitored for inappropriate response.

The following table can be used to calculate the dose per pulse when individualizing treatment:

Vial	Diluent	Volume/pulse	Dose/pulse
0.8 mg	8 mL	25 μL	2.5 μg
0.8 mg	8 mL	50 μL	5 μg
3.2 mg	8 mL	25 μL	10 μg
3.2 mg	8 mL	50 μL	20 μg

The response to LUTREPULSE (gonadorelin acetate) for Injection usually occurs within two to three weeks after therapy initiation. When ovulation occurs with the LUTREPULSE PUMP in place, therapy should be continued for another two weeks to maintain the corpus luteum. A comparison of LUTREPULSE for Injection to hCG or hCG + LUTREPULSE for Injection for corpus luteum maintenance revealed the following information:

hCG

Delivered $= \dfrac{43}{63} = 68\%$

Aborted $= \dfrac{20}{63} = 32\%$

LUTREPULSE for Injection

Delivered $= \dfrac{19}{26} = 73\%$

Aborted $= \dfrac{7}{26} = 27\%$

hCG + LUTREPULSE for Injection

Delivered $= \dfrac{19}{25} = 76\%$

Aborted $= \dfrac{6}{25} = 24\%$

LUTREPULSE (gonadorelin acetate) for Injection alone was able to maintain the corpus luteum during pregnancy.

ADMINISTRATION: LUTREPULSE for Injection is to be reconstituted aseptically with 8 mL of diluent for LUTREPULSE for Injection. *The drug product should be reconstituted immediately prior to use and transferred to the plastic reservoir.* First withdraw the required volume of the saline diluent and inject it gently onto the lyophile (drug product) cake. The product is gently rolled for a few seconds to produce a solution which should be clear, colorless, and free of particulate matter. Parenteral drug products should be inspected visually for particulate matter and discoloration prior to administration, whenever solution and container permit. If particulate matter or discoloration are present, the solution should not be used. A presterilized reservoir (bag) with the infusion catheter set supplied with the LUTREPULSE for Injection is filled with the reconstituted solution, and administered intravenously using the LUTREPULSE PUMP. The pump should be set to deliver 25 or 50 μL of solution, based upon the dose selected, over a pulse period of one minute and at a pulse frequency of 90 minutes. The solution will supply 90 minute pulsatile doses for approximately 7 or 14 consecutive days, depending upon the vial size and dose used.

HOW SUPPLIED

LUTREPULSE (gonadorelin acetate) for Injection is supplied in drug product alone, kits and LUTREPULSE Pump component packages. These packages are listed below:

Description	NDC Number
LUTREPULSE For Injection 0.8 mg Kit (1 each)	55566-7208-5
LUTREPULSE For Injection 3.2 mg Kit (1 each)	55566-7232-5
LUTREPULSE For Injection 0.8 mg Kit (12 each)	55566-7208-6
LUTREPULSE For Injection 3.2 mg Kit (12 each)	55566-7232-6
LUTREPULSE For Injection 0.8 mg (1 each)	55566-7208-0
LUTREPULSE For Injection 3.2 mg (1 each)	55566-7232-0
LUTREPULSE For Injection 0.8 mg (48 each)	55566-7208-1
LUTREPULSE For Injection 3.2 mg (48 each)	55566-7232-1
LUTREPULSE Pump (1 each)	55566-7210-0
LUTREPULSE Reservoir Catheter	55566-7215-0
LUTREPULSE Catheter Tubing	55566-7220-0
LUTREPULSE Pump Elastic Belt	55566-7225-0

Each LUTREPULSE for Injection drug product contains one 10 mL vial of 0.8 mg or 3.2 mg LUTREPULSE for Injection as a lyophilized, sterile powder and one 10 mL vial of LUTREPULSE for Injection Diluent. These should be stored at controlled room temperature (15–30°C, 59–86°F). The following components are included in each LUTREPULSE for Injection Kit:

Sterile catheter tubing
Sterile reservoir catheter with double-female luer adaptor
Sterile IV cannula units (four supplied)
Sterile 10 mL syringe
Sterile syringe needle
Alcohol swabs (four supplied)
Elastic belt
9-V battery
Physician package insert, physician pump manual, and patient instructions

The LUTREPULSE PUMP kit contains the following components:

LUTREPULSE Pump
9-V batteries (two supplied)
3-V lithium battery
Physician pump manual
Physician package insert
Warranty card
Manufactured for
FERRING LABORATORIES, INC.
Suffern, New York 10901
by FERRING ARZNEIMITTEL GmbH, Kiel, Germany
Revised March 1993 DC-110A

SECRETIN-FERRING   ℞
[si-krē′tin]

HOW SUPPLIED

Secretin-Ferring is supplied as a lyophilized sterile powder in 10 mL vials (NDC 55566-1075-1) containing 75 CU. The unreconstituted product should be stored at −20° C (freezer). However, the biological activity of Secretin-Ferring will not be significantly decreased by storage at temperatures up to 25° C for up to 3 weeks. Expiration date is marked on the label.
Please see full prescribing information in the Diagnostic Product Information section.

THYREL® TRH   ℞
(protirelin)
Injection
FOR INTRAVENOUS ADMINISTRATION

HOW SUPPLIED

As 1 mL ampuls—boxes of 5 (NDC 55566-0081-5). Each mL contains Thyrel TRH 0.50 mg (500 μg), sodium chloride 9.0 mg for isotonicity, hydrochloric acid and sodium hydroxide as needed to adjust pH.
Store at controlled room temperature (59° to 86°F).
Please see full prescribing information in the Diagnostic Product Information section.

For information on over-the-counter drugs, consult **PDR For Nonprescription Drugs**

The Fielding Company
112 WELDON PARKWAY
MARYLAND HEIGHTS, MO 63043

Direct Inquires to:
Professional Services Department
(314) 567-5462
For Medical Information Contact:
In Emergencies:
(314) 567-5462

GERIMED® Tablets   OTC

DESCRIPTION
A multivitamin-multimineral supplement useful as adjunctive therapy in osteoporosis. Provides a balanced ratio of calcium and phosphorus (2.8 to 1) with adequate Vitamin D for proper absorption.
Each tablet contains:

Dibasic Calcium Phosphate	600 mg.
Calcium Carbonate	200 mg.
Vitamin A	5000 I. U.
Vitamin D	400 I. U.
Vitamin E	30 I. U.
Vitamin C	120 mg.
Thiamine B_1	3 mg.
Riboflavin B_2	3 mg.
Niacinamide	25 mg.
Pyridoxine B_6	2 mg.
Vitamin B_{12}	6 mcg.
Zinc	15 mg.

*Total Calcium	370 mg.
*Total Phosphorus	130 mg.
Calcium/Phosphorus ratio 2.8 - 1	

DOSAGE
One tablet daily, or as prescribed by the physician.

HOW SUPPLIED
Bottle of 60 tablets.
NDC 0421-0080-60

IROSPAN® Tablets/Capsules   OTC

Each tablet or capsule contains:

Iron	65 mg.
(Ferrous Sulfate-Exsic. 200 mg.)	
Ascorbic Acid	150 mg.

DESCRIPTION
Irospan is a unique presentation of sustained release ferrous sulfate and ascorbic acid. Irospan is of particular value during pregnancy and lactation providing excellent tolerance and absorption.

DOSAGE
One tablet or capsule daily or as prescribed by the physician.

HOW SUPPLIED
Irospan Tablets—bottles of 100. NDC 0421-0360-01
Irospan Capsules—bottles of 60. NDC 0421-0361-60

LURLINE® PMS Tablets   OTC

Each tablet contains:

Acetaminophen	500 mg.
Pamabrom	25 mg.
Pyridoxine	50 mg.

DESCRIPTION
Lurline PMS is a safe and effective approach for relief of the multi-symptom complex of premenstrual syndrome. The medication combines an analgesic, a mild diuretic and pyridoxine, representing a safe first line treatment.
Lurline PMS contains no hormones, no sedatives and is aspirin free.

DOSAGE
Start Lurline PMS at the first sign of pain or discomfort, usually 7 to 10 days before menses. Usual dosage is one tablet 3 or 4 times daily. Do not exceed the maximum dose of 8 tablets a day.

HOW SUPPLIED
Lurline PMS—bottles of 24. NDC 0421-8787-24
Lurline PMS—bottles of 50. NDC 0421-8787-50
Physician samples and literature available.

NESTABS® FA Tablets   ℞
Prenatal Tablets

DESCRIPTION
East tablet contains:

Vitamin A	5000	Unit
Vitamin D	400	Units
Vitamin E	30	Units
Vitamin C	120	mg.
Folic Acid	1	mg.
Thiamine	3	mg.
Riboflavin	3	mg.
Niacinamide	20	mg.
Pyridoxine	3	mg.
Vitamin B12	8	mcg.
Calcium	200	mg.
(from calcium carbonate 500 mg.)		
Iodine	150	mcg.
Iron	36	mg.
(from ferrous fumarate 110 mg.)		
Zinc	15	mg.

A comprehensive vitamin-mineral supplement expressly formulated for use during pregnancy and lactation.

DOSAGE
One tablet daily, or as prescribed by the physician.

PRECAUTION
Folic acid may obscure pernicious anemia in that hematologic remission can occur while neurological manifestations remain progressive.

HOW SUPPLIED
Bottles of 100 tablets.
NDC 0421-1594-01

C. B. Fleet Co., Inc.
4615 MURRAY PL.
LYNCHBURG, VA 24502-2235

Direct Inquiries to:
David Vaughan
Director of Quality Assurance:
(804) 528-4000

FLEET® BABYLAX®, A LAXATIVE   OTC
FLEET GLYCERIN LAXATIVE RECTAL
APPLICATORS, A LAXATIVE   OTC

ACTIVE INGREDIENT
Glycerin (USP)

INDICATIONS
BABYLAX: For temporary relief of occasional constipation in young children. Children under 2 years old, consult physician.
GLYCERIN LAXATIVE RECTAL APPLICATORS: For temporary relief of occasional constipation in children 6 years of age and older and adults.

ACTIONS
This product generally produces a bowel movement within minutes. The exact mode of action of glycerin administered rectally as a laxative is not known. It has been suggested that glycerin causes dehydration of exposed tissues to produce an irritant effect which results in a laxative response.

WARNINGS
For rectal use only. Glycerin administered rectally may produce rectal discomfort or a burning sensation in some individuals. If use results in unusual pain or side effects, consult a physician.

GENERAL LAXATIVE WARNINGS
Do not use a laxative product when nausea, vomiting or abdominal pain are present unless directed by a physician. If you have noticed a sudden change in bowel habits that persists over two weeks, consult a physician before using a laxative. Laxative products should not be used longer than one week except under a physician's advice. Rectal bleeding or failure to have a bowel movement after use of a laxative may indicate a serious condition; discontinue use and consult a physician. Keep this and all drugs out of the reach of children. In case of accidental ingestion, seek professional assistance or contact a Poison Control Center immediately.

DOSAGE AND ADMINISTRATION
REMOVE PROTECTIVE SHIELD FROM TIP BEFORE ADMINISTERING.
Children under 2 years old: consult physician. Children 2-6 years of age: 1 BABYLAX rectal applicator containing 4 mL of glycerin in a single daily dose or as directed by physi-

cian. Children 6 years of age and older and adults: 1 GLYCERIN LAXATIVE RECTAL APPLICATOR containing 7.5 mL of glycerin in a single daily dose or as directed by a physician.
Hold unit upright. Gently insert stem with tip pointing toward navel. Squeeze unit until nearly all liquid is expelled. While continuing to squeeze the bulb, remove tip from rectum. Discontinue use if resistance is encountered. Forcing the tip can result in injury. Note: A small amount of liquid will remain in unit. Store and use at room temperature.

HOW SUPPLIED
BABYLAX: Six 4 mL rectal applicators per package.
GLYCERIN LAXATIVE RECTAL APPLICATORS: Four 7.5 mL rectal applicators per package.

IS THIS PRODUCT OTC?
Yes.

FLEET® BISACODYL ENEMA, A STIMULANT
LAXATIVE   OTC
(bisacodyl U.S.P.)

COMPOSITION
Each 30 mL (delivered dose) contains 10 mg. of bisacodyl, U.S.P. suspended in an aqueous medium. The FLEET® Bisacodyl Enema unit, with a 2-inch prelubricated Comfortip®, contains 1¼ fl. oz. (37 mL) of enema suspension in a ready-to-use plastic squeeze bottle. Designed for quick, convenient administration by nurse or patient according to instructions. Disposable after single use.

ACTION AND USES
FLEET® Bisacodyl Enema is a stimulant laxative acting directly on the colonic mucosa to produce peristalsis. FLEET® Bisacodyl Enema actually produces peristalsis and evacuation of the large intestine by stimulating sensory nerve endings in the colonic mucosa to produce parasympathetic reflexes. FLEET® Bisacodyl Enema is very effective usually producing an evacuation within 5 to 20 minutes. FLEET® Bisacodyl Enema may be used whenever a laxative or enema is indicated. It is useful as a laxative for occasional relief of constipation, in bowel cleansing in preparation for X-ray and endoscopic examination. May be used as a laxative in postoperative, antepartum, or postpartum care or in preparation for delivery.

WARNINGS
Do not use a laxative product when nausea, vomiting, or abdominal pain is present unless directed by a physician. If you have noticed a sudden change in bowel habits that persists over a period of 2 weeks, consult a physician before using a laxative. Rectal bleeding or failure to have a bowel movement after use of a laxative may indicate a serious condition. Discontinue use and consult a physician. Laxative products should not be used longer than 1 week unless directed by a physician. This product may cause abdominal discomfort, faintness, rectal burning, and mild cramps. Keep this and all drugs out of the reach of children. In case of accidental ingestion, seek professional assistance or contact a Poison Control Center immediately.

DOSAGE AND ADMINISTRATION
SHAKE BEFORE USING.
REMOVE PROTECTIVE SHIELD FROM TIP BEFORE ADMINISTERING.
Adults and children 12 years of age and older: 1 unit (30 mL) in a single daily dose.
Children 6 to under 12 years of age: one half unit (15 mL) in a single daily dose.
Children under 6 years of age: consult a physician.
Precaution: Do not administer to children under 2 years of age. **Administration:**   Preferred position—Lying on left side with left knee slightly bent and the right leg drawn up, or knee-chest position. Rubber diaphragm at base of tube prevents accidental leakage and assures controlled flow of the enema solution. May be used at room temperature.

PROFESSIONAL ADMINISTRATION
See FLEET® Ready-to-Use Enema.

HOW SUPPLIED
FLEET® Bisacodyl Enema is supplied in 1¼ fl. oz. (37 mL) ready-to-use squeeze bottle.

IS THIS PRODUCT OTC?
Yes.

LITERATURE AVAILABLE
Professional literature mailed on request.

FLEET® ENEMA, A SALINE LAXATIVE   OTC
FLEET® ENEMA FOR CHILDREN, A SALINE LAXATIVE

COMPOSITION
FLEET® ENEMA: Each 118 mL. (delivered dose) contains 19 g. monobasic sodium phosphate and 7 g. dibasic sodium phosphate. The FLEET® Enema unit, with a 2-inch, pre-lubricated Comfortip®, contains 4½ fl. oz. of enema solution in a hand-size plastic squeeze bottle. FLEET® ENEMA FOR CHILDREN: Each 59 mL (Delivered Dose) contains 9.5 g. monobasic sodium phosphate and 3.5 g. dibasic sodium phosphate. The FLEET® Enema for children unit, with a 2-inch, pre-lubricated Comfortip® contains 2¼ fl. oz. (66.5 mL) of enema solution in a hand-size plastic squeeze bottle. Designed for quick, convenient administration by nurse or patient according to instructions. Disposable after single use.

ACTION AND USES
FLEET® Enema is useful as a laxative in the relief of occasional constipation, and as part of a bowel cleansing regimen in preparing the patient for surgery or for preparing the colon for x-ray and endoscopic examination. Used as directed, FLEET® Enema provides thorough yet safe cleansing action and induces complete emptying of the left colon usually within 2 to 5 minutes without pain or spasm. Also used for general postoperative care and to help relieve fecal or barium impaction.

GENERAL LAXATIVE WARNINGS
Do not use laxative products when nausea, vomiting, or abdominal pain is present. If you notice a sudden change in bowel habits that persists over a period of 2 weeks, consult a physician. Rectal bleeding or failure to have a bowel movement after use of a laxative may indicate a serious condition. Discontinue use and consult a physician. Laxative products should not be used longer than 1 week unless directed by a physician. As with any drug, if you are pregnant or nursing a baby, seek the advice of a health professional before using this product. Keep this and all drugs out of the reach of children. In case of accidental ingestion or overdose, seek professional assistance or contact a Poison Control Center immediately.

PROFESSIONAL USE WARNINGS
Do not use in patients with congenital megacolon, imperforate anus or congestive heart failure as hypernatremic dehydration may occur. Use with caution in patients with impaired renal function, heart disease, or pre-existing electrolyte disturbances (such as dehydration or those secondary to the use of diuretics) or in patients on calcium channel blockers, diuretics or other medications which may affect electrolyte levels — or where colostomy exists, as hypocalcemia, hyperphosphatemia, hypernatremia and acidosis may occur. Calcium and phosphorus levels should be carefully monitored. Since FLEET® Ready-To-Use Enema contains dibasic sodium phosphate and monobasic sodium phosphate, there is a risk of acute elevation of sodium concentration in the serum and consequent dehydration, particularly in children with megacolon or any other condition where there is retention of enema solution. Additional fluids by mouth are recommended where appropriate (Fonkalsrud, E. and Keen, J.: "Hypernatremic Dehydration Hypertonic Enemas in Congenital Megacolon," *JAMA* 199:584–586, 1967. Zumoff, B. and Hellman, L.: "Rectal Absorption of Sodium from Hypertonic Sodium Phosphate Solutions," data on file, C. B. Fleet Company, Inc. Gilman, A., Goodman, L., Gilman, A., eds., *The Pharmacological Basis of Therapeutics*, Sixth Edition, 1980, p. 1005.) In addition, elevated levels of serum phosphates and decreased levels of serum calcium have been reported in patients with renal disease (and with prolonged use). (McConnell, T. H., "Fatal Hypocalcemia from Phosphate Absorption from Laxative Preparation," *JAMA*, 216:147–148, 1971.). SINCE FLEET® BRAND ENEMAS ARE AVAILABLE IN ADULT AND CHILDREN'S SIZES, PRESCRIBE CAREFULLY.

PRECAUTIONS
DO NOT ADMINISTER 4½ oz. ADULT SIZE TO CHILDREN UNDER 12 YEARS OF AGE. DO NOT ADMINISTER 2¼ OZ CHILDREN'S SIZE TO CHILDREN UNDER 2 YEARS OF AGE. IF AFTER THE ENEMA SOLUTION IS ADMINISTERED THERE IS NO RETURN OF LIQUID, CONTACT A PHYSICIAN IMMEDIATELY AS DEHYDRATION COULD OCCUR.

OVERDOSAGE
Overdosage with Fleet® Enema may cause hypocalcemia; hyperphosphatemia, hypernatremia, hypernatremic dehydration and acidosis.
1. Hypocalcemia, hyperphosphatemia, hypernatremia and acidosis
Calcium, Phosphate, Chloride and Sodium levels should be carefully monitored. Immediate corrective action should be taken to restore electrolyte balance with appropriate fluid replacements.

2. Hypernatremic Dehydration
Calcium, Phosphate, Chloride and Sodium levels should be carefully monitored. Prompt parenteral administration of fluids with lower concentrations of Sodium and Chloride than extracellular fluid (40–50 mEq/liter) and moderate concentration of Potassium (20–30 mEq/liter) administered at a rate of 3,000 to 4,000 cc/sq. m of body surface during the first 12 to 24 hours dependent on the severity of dehydration and the clinical response (Fonkalsrud, E. and Keen, J.: Hypernatremic Dehydration from Hypertonic Enemas in Congenital Megacolon, JAMA 199:584–586, 1967). See article for more details.

ADMINISTRATION AND DOSAGE
REMOVE PROTECTIVE SHIELD FROM TIP BEFORE ADMINISTERING.
Preferred position: Lying on left side with left knee slightly bent and the right leg drawn up, or knee-chest position. Dosage: Adults, 4 fl. oz. in a single daily dose. Child, 2 fl. oz. in a single daily dose. Rubber diaphragm at base of tube prevents accidental leakage and assures controlled flow of the enema solution. May be used at room temperature. Adult, each 118 mL (delivered dose) contains 4.4 g. (191 mEq) sodium. Child, each 59 mL (delivered dose) contains 2.2 g (95.5 mEq) sodium.

PROFESSIONAL DOSAGE AND ADMINISTRATION
Fleet® Ready-To-Use 4½ oz. Adult Size Enema should not be used in children under 12 years of age. In those cases where complications are reported, infants and young children are often involved. Fleet® Ready-To-Use Enema for Children should be used with caution in children of any age. Careful consideration of the use of enemas in general in children is recommended. The adult size enema should not be used in children under 12 years of age. For children 2 to 12 years of age, use Fleet® Ready-To-Use Enema for Children, which contains a dosage of one-half the adult size enema. For children less than 2 years of age, Fleet® Glycerin Suppositories for Children should be used.
Proper and safe use of Fleet® Ready-To-Use Enema also requires that the product be administered according to the Directions for Use. Health care professionals should remember, when administering the product, to *gently* insert the enema into the rectum with the tip pointing toward the navel. Insertion may be made easier by having the patient bear down as they would in having a bowel movement. Care during insertion is necessary due to lack of sensory innervation of the rectum and due to possibility of bowel perforation. Once inserted, squeeze the bottle until nearly all the liquid is expelled. If resistance is encountered on insertion of the nozzle or in administering the solution, the procedure should be discontinued. Forcing the enema can result in perforation and/or abrasion of the rectum.
If an enema containing phosphate or sodium is not advised, use FLEET Bisacodyl Enema. Please see complete prescribing instructions for Fleet Bisacodyl Enema.

HOW SUPPLIED
FLEET® Enema is supplied in a 4½ fl. oz. (133 mL) ready-to-use squeeze bottle. Children's size, 2¼ fl. oz. (66.5 mL) IMPORTANT: Fleet® Enema, Adult and Child size, ARE NOT INTENDED FOR ORAL CONSUMPTION, in any dosage size.

IS THIS PRODUCT OTC?
Yes.

LITERATURE AVAILABLE
Professional literature mailed on request.

FLEET® MINERAL OIL ENEMA   OTC
A LUBRICANT LAXATIVE

COMPOSITION
The FLEET® Mineral Oil Enema unit, with a 2-inch, pre-lubricated Comfortip®, delivers 118 mL of mineral oil USP in a hand-size plastic squeeze bottle.

ACTION AND INDICATIONS
Serves to soften and lubricate hard stools, easing their passage without irritating the mucosa. Results approximate a normal bowel movement in that only the rectum, sigmoid, and part or all of the descending colon are evacuated. Indicated for relief of fecal impaction; valuable in relief of occasional constipation when straining must be avoided (in hypertension, coronary occlusion, proctologic procedures, postoperative care); for removal of barium sulfate residues from the colon after barium administration for GI series or outlining the left atrium; to obtain the laxative benefits of mineral oil while avoiding possible untoward effects of oral administration such as (1) interference with intestinal absorption of fat-soluble vitamins A, D, E and K and other nutrients (2) danger of systemic absorption (3) possible risk of lipid pneumonia due to aspiration. Generally effective in 2 to 15 minutes.

WARNINGS
Do not use laxative products when nausea, vomiting, or abdominal pain is present unless directed by a physician. If you have noticed a sudden change in bowel habits that persists over a period of 2 weeks, consult a physician. Rectal bleeding or failure to have a bowel movement after use of a laxative may indicate a serious condition. Discontinue use and consult a physician. Laxative products should not be used longer than 1 week unless directed by a physician. As with any drug, if you are pregnant or nursing a baby, seek the advice of a health professional before using this product. Keep this and all drugs out of the reach of children. In case of accidental ingestion, seek professional assistance or contact a Poison Control Center immediately.

PRECAUTIONS
DO NOT ADMINISTER TO CHILDREN UNDER 2 YEARS OF AGE.

ADMINISTRATION AND DOSAGE
REMOVE PROTECTIVE SHIELD FROM TIP BEFORE ADMINISTERING.
Preferred position: Lying on left side with left knee slightly bent and the right leg drawn up, or knee-chest position. Dosage: Adults and children 12 and over: one bottle (118 ml delivered dose) in a single daily dose. Children 2 to under 12: ½ bottle (59 ml delivered dose) in a single daily dose. Rubber diaphragm at base of tube prevents accidental leakage and assures controlled flow of the enema solution. May be used at room temperature. Follow with regular Fleet® Enema according to dosage instructions contained in PDR for more thorough cleansing.

PROFESSIONAL DOSAGE AND ADMINISTRATION
Fleet® Ready-To-Use Mineral Oil Enema should not be used in children under 2 years of age. Fleet® Ready-To-Use Mineral Oil Enema should be used with caution in children of any age. Careful consideration of the use of enemas in general in children is recommended.
Proper and safe use of Fleet® Ready-To-Use Mineral Oil Enema also requires that the product be administered according to the Directions for Use. Health care professionals should remember, when administering the product, to gently insert the enema into the rectum with the tip pointing toward the naval. Insertion may be made easier by having the patient bear down as they would in having a bowel movement. Care during insertion is necessary due to lack of sensory innervation of the rectum and due to possibility of bowel perforation. Once inserted, squeeze the bottle until nearly all the liquid is expelled. If resistance is encountered on insertion of the nozzle or in administering the solution, the procedure should be discontinued. Forcing the enema can result in perforation and/or abrasion of the rectum.

HOW SUPPLIED
FLEET® Mineral Oil Enema is supplied in 4½ fl.oz. (133 mL) ready-to-use squeeze bottle.

IS THIS PRODUCT OTC?
Yes.

FLEET PAIN RELIEF   OTC
PREMOISTENED RECTAL PADS

ACTIVE INGREDIENTS
1% Pramoxine Hydrochloride (A Topical Anesthetic) and 12% Glycerin.

INDICATIONS
For fast temporary relief of **Pain, Soreness,** and **Burning** associated with hemorrhoids and other minor anorectal irritations. Temporarily protects inflamed perianal skin.

DIRECTIONS
For external use only.
Adults: When practical, cleanse the affected area with mild soap and warm water, and rinse thoroughly. Gently dry by patting or blotting with toilet tissue or soft cloth before each application of this product. Gently apply to affected area by patting and then discard. Apply to the affected area up to five times daily or after each bowel movement.
Children under 12 years of age: Consult a physician.
As a moist compress—For soothing pain relief, fold pad and place in contact with irritated tissue. Leave in place for 5 to 15 minutes. Repeat as needed up to five times daily.

WARNINGS
If condition worsens or does not improve within 7 days, consult a physician. Do not exceed recommended daily dosage unless directed by a physician. In case of bleeding, consult a physician promptly. Do not put this product into the rectum by using fingers or any mechanical device or applicator. Certain persons can develop allergic reactions to ingredients in this product. If the symptom being treated does not subside

Continued on next page

Fleet—Cont.

or if redness, irritation, swelling, pain, or other symptoms develop or increase, discontinue use and consult a physician. KEEP THIS AND ALL DRUGS OUT OF THE REACH OF CHILDREN. In case of accidental ingestion, seek professional assistance or contact a Poison Control Center immediately.

HOW SUPPLIED
100 ct. Jars.

FLEET® PHOSPHO®-SODA   OTC
A BUFFERED ORAL SALINE LAXATIVE

COMPOSITION
Each 5 mL of regular or flavored Phospho®-Soda contains 2.4 g. Monobasic Sodium Phosphate and 0.9 g. Dibasic Sodium Phosphate in a stable, buffered aqueous solution.

INDICATIONS
As a laxative, for the relief of occasional constipation. As a purgative, for use as part of a bowel cleansing regimen in preparing the patient for surgery or for preparing the colon for x-ray or endoscopic examination.

ACTION AND USES
Versatile in action as a gentle laxative or purgative, according to dosage. This product produces a bowel movement in ½ to 6 hours, depending on dosage. Especially useful as a preparation for colonoscopy. See DOSAGE AND ADMINISTRATION. Patient instruction pads available upon request.

CONTRAINDICATIONS
DO NOT USE THIS PRODUCT IF YOU HAVE KIDNEY DISEASE OR ARE ON A SODIUM RESTRICTED DIET UNLESS DIRECTED BY A PHYSICIAN.

PROFESSIONAL USE WARNINGS
DO NOT EXCEED RECOMMENDED DOSE UNLESS DIRECTED BY A PHYSICIAN. SERIOUS SIDE EFFECTS MAY OCCUR FROM EXCESS DOSAGE.
Do not use in patients with congenital megacolon or congestive heart failure, as hypernatremic dehydration may occur. Use with caution in patients with impaired renal function as hypocalcemia, hyperphosphatemia, hypernatremia and acidosis may occur. Since Fleet® Phospho®-soda contains dibasic sodium phosphate and monobasic sodium phosphate, there is a risk of acute elevation of sodium concentration in the serum and consequent dehydration, particularly in children with megacolon. Additional fluids by mouth are recommended where appropriate. (Fonkalsrud, E. and Keen, J.: "Hypernatremic Dehydration Hypertonic Enemas in Congenital Megacolon," *JAMA* 199:584–586, 1967. Zumoff, B. and Hellman, L.: "Rectal Absorption of Sodium from Hypertonic Sodium Phosphate Solutions," data on file, C. B. Fleet Company, Inc. Gilman, A., Goodman, L., Gilman, A., eds., *The Pharmacological Basis of Therapeutics*, Sixth Edition, 1980, p. 1005.) In addition, elevated levels of serum phosphates and decreased levels of serum calcium have been reported in patients with renal disease (and with prolonged use). (McConnell, T. H., "Fatal Hypocalcemia from Phosphate Absorption from Laxative Preparation," *JAMA*, 216:147–148, 1971.) SINCE FLEET® PHOSPHO®-SODA IS AVAILABLE IN TWO SIZES, PRESCRIBE BY VOLUMES. DO NOT PRESCRIBE "BY THE BOTTLE" AS SERIOUS SIDE EFFECTS FROM OVERDOSAGE MAY OCCUR.

GENERAL LAXATIVE WARNINGS
Do not use a laxative product when nausea, vomiting, or abdominal pain is present unless directed by a physician. If you have noticed a sudden change in bowel habits that persists over a period of 2 weeks, consult a physician before using a laxative. Rectal bleeding or failure to have a bowel movement may indicate a serious condition. Discontinue use and consult a physician. Laxative products should not be used longer than 1 week unless directed by a physician. Each teaspoonful (5 mL) contains 550 mg (24.1 milliequivalents) sodium. DO NOT USE THIS PRODUCT IF YOU ARE ON A SODIUM RESTRICTED DIET OR IF YOU HAVE KIDNEY DISEASE UNLESS DIRECTED BY A DOCTOR. SERIOUS SIDE EFFECTS FROM OVERDOSAGE MAY OCCUR. Keep this and all drugs out of the reach of children. In case of accidental overdose or ingestion, seek professional assistance or contact a Poison Control Center immediately. As with any drug, if you are pregnant or nursing a baby, seek the advice of a health professional before using this product.

OVERDOSAGE
Overdosage with Fleet® Phospho®-soda may cause hypocalcemia, hyperphosphatemia, hypernatremia, hypernatremic dehydration and acidosis.

1. Hypocalcemia, hyperphosphatemia, hypernatremia and acidosis
   Calcium, Phosphate, Chloride and Sodium levels should be carefully monitored. Immediate corrective action should be taken to restore electrolyte balance with appropriate fluid replacements.

2. Hypernatremic Dehydration
   Calcium, Phosphate, Chloride and Sodium levels should be carefully monitored. Prompt parenteral administration of fluids with lower concentrations of Sodium and Chloride than extracellular fluid (40–50 mEq./liter) and moderate concentration of Potassium (20–30 mEq./liter) administered at a rate of 3,000 to 4,000 cc/sq. m of body surface during the first 12 to 24 hours dependent on the severity of dehydration and the clinical response (Fonkalsrud, E. and Keen, J.: "Hypernatremic Dehydration from Hypertonic Enemas in Congenital Megacolon." JAMA 199:584-586, 1967). See article for more details.

DOSAGE AND ADMINISTRATION
For purgative or laxative, best taken on an empty stomach. Most effective when taken upon rising, at least 30 minutes before a meal, or at bedtime for overnight action. **Dilute recommended dosage with one-half glass (4 fl. oz.) cool water. Drink, then follow with one glass (8 fl. oz.) cool water.** DOSAGE: SINCE FLEET® PHOSPHO®-SODA IS AVAILABLE IN TWO SIZES, PRESCRIBE BY VOLUMES; DO NOT PRESCRIBE BY THE BOTTLE. DO NOT EXCEED RECOMMENDED DOSAGE AS SERIOUS SIDE EFFECTS MAY OCCUR.
SINGLE DAILY DOSAGE: DO NOT EXCEED.
LAXATIVE: Adults and children 12 years and over:
4 teaspoonfuls (20 mL).
Children 10 to under 12 years: 2 teaspoonfuls (10 mL).
Children 5 to under 10 years: 1 teaspoonful (5 mL).
PURGATIVE: Adults only: 3 tablespoonfuls (45 mL).
DO NOT GIVE TO CHILDREN UNDER 5 YEARS.
For colonoscopy, especially useful when taken as follows: 1½ fl. oz. (added to 4 fl. oz. water) 7 PM evening before exam (followed by three (3) 8 fl. oz. portions of clear liquids before retiring) and 1½ fl. oz. (added to 4 fl. oz. water) morning (6 AM) of exam. It is recommended that the prep be completed at least 3 hours in advance of appointment. Timing of dosage regimen can be adjusted by the physician.
Each teaspoonful (5 mL) contains: Active Ingredients: Monobasic Sodium Phosphate 2.4 g and Dibasic Sodium Phosphate 0.9 g. Each teaspoonful (5 mL) contains 550 mg (24.1 milliequivalents) sodium.

HOW SUPPLIED
Regular or Flavored, in bottles of 1½, and 3 fl. oz. Fleet® Phospho®-soda should not be confused with Fleet® Enema, a sodium phosphates disposable ready-to-use enema. Fleet® Enema, Adult and Child size, ARE NOT INTENDED FOR ORAL CONSUMPTION, in any dosage size.

IS THIS PRODUCT OTC?
Yes.

LITERATURE AVAILABLE
Professional literature mailed on request.

FLEET® PREP KITS   OTC
Bowel Evacuant

DESCRIPTION
FLEET® Prep Kit No. 1 contains:
1. FLEET® Phospho®-soda—1½ fl. oz. (45 mL). Ingredients: Each teaspoonful (5 mL) contains : Active Ingredients: monobasic sodium phosphate 2.4 g and dibasic sodium phosphate 0.9 g.
2. FLEET® Bisacodyl—4 laxative tablets. Ingredients: Each enteric-coated tablet contains Bisacodyl, USP, 5 mg.
3. FLEET® Bisacodyl—1 laxative suppository. Ingredients: Bisacodyl, USP, 10 mg.
4. 1 Patient Instruction Sheet.
FLEET® Prep Kit No. 2 contains:
1. FLEET® Phospho®-soda—1½ fl. oz. (45 mL).
2. FLEET® Bisacodyl—4 tablets.
3. FLEET® Bagenema—1.
4. 1 Patient Instruction Sheet.
FLEET® Prep Kit No. 3 contains:
1. FLEET® Phospho® —1 ½fl. oz. (45 mL)
2. FLEET® Bisacodyl—4 tablets.
3. FLEET® Bisacodyl Enema 1 ¼ fl. oz. (37 mL)—1 laxative enema. Ingredients: 1–30 mL. dose containing 10 mg. of Bisacodyl, USP.
4. 1 Patient Instruction Sheet.
FLEET® Prep Kit No. 4 contains:
1. FLEET® Magnesium Citrate Packet—Ingredients: When mixed with 8 oz water, delivers 18.7 g Magnesium Citrate.
2. FLEET® Bisacodyl—4 tablets.
3. FLEET® Bisacodyl—1 suppository.
4. 1 Patient Instruction Sheet.
FLEET® Prep Kit No. 5 contains:
1. FLEET® Magnesium Citrate Packet—Ingredients: When mixed with 8 oz. water, delivers 18.7 g Magnesium Citrate.

2. FLEET® Bisacodyl—4 tablets.
3. FLEET® Bagenema
4. 1 Patient Instruction Sheet.
FLEET® Prep Kit No. 6 contains:
1. FLEET® Magnesium Citrate Packet—Ingredients: When mixed with 8 oz. water, delivers 18.7 g Magnesium Citrate.
2. FLEET® Bisacodyl—4 tablets.
3. FLEET® Bisacodyl Enema—1 ¼ fl. oz. (37 mL)
4. 1 Patient Instruction Sheet.

ACTIONS
Bowel Cleansing System

INDICATIONS
For use as part of a bowel cleansing regimen in preparation of the colon for radiology (prior to barium enemas or I.V.P.'s), surgery, and many endoscopic and colonoscopic procedures.

WARNINGS
DO NOT EXCEED RECOMMENDED DOSE UNLESS DIRECTED BY A PHYSICIAN. SERIOUS SIDE EFFECTS MAY OCCUR FROM EXCESS DOSAGE.
Each recommended dose (1½ fl. oz.) (45 mL) of Phospho®-soda contains 216.9 milliequivalents (mEq) of sodium. **Persons on a sodium restricted diet or with kidney disease should consult a health professional before use.**
Bisacodyl products may cause abdominal discomfort, faintness, rectal burning, and mild cramps.

GENERAL LAXATIVE WARNINGS
Do not chew tablets or give to persons who cannot swallow without chewing unless directed by a physician. Do not take tablets within 1 hour after taking antacids and/or milk. Do not use a laxative product when nausea, vomiting, or abdominal pain is present unless directed by a physician. If you have noticed a sudden change in bowel habits that persists over a period of 2 weeks, consult a doctor before using a laxative. Rectal bleeding or failure to have a bowel movement may indicate a serious condition. Discontinue use and consult a physician. Laxative products should not be used longer than 1 week unless directed by a physician. Frequent or prolonged use of a laxative may result in dependence on laxatives. Keep this and all drugs out of the reach of children. In case of accidental overdose or ingestion, seek professional assistance or contact a Poison Control Center immediately.

PROFESSIONAL USE WARNINGS
Do not use in patients with congenital megacolon or congestive heart failure as hypernatremic dehydration may occur. Use with caution in patients with impaired renal function or where colostomy exists as hypocalcemia, hyperphosphatemia, hypermagnesium, hypernatremia and acidosis may occur. Since FLEET® Phospho®-soda contains monobasic sodium phosphate and dibasic sodium phosphate, there is a risk of acute elevation of sodium concentration in the serum and consequent dehydration, particularly in children with megacolon. Additional fluids by mouth are recommended where appropriate. (Fonkalsrud, E. and Keen, J.: "Hypernatremic Dehydration Hypertonic Enemas in Congenital Megacolon," *JAMA* 199:584–586, 1967. Zumoff, B. and Hellman, L.: "Rectal Absorption of Sodium from Hypertonic Sodium Phosphate Solutions," data on file, C. B. Fleet Company, Inc. Gilman, A., Goodman, L., Gilman, A., eds., *The Pharmacological Basis of Therapeutics*, Sixth Edition, 1980, p. 1005.) In addition, elevated levels of serum phosphates and decreased levels of serum calcium have been reported in patients with renal disease (and with prolonged use). (McConnell, T. H., "Fatal Hypocalcemia from Phosphate Absorption from Laxative Preparation," *JAMA*, 216:147–148, 1971.) If any of these complications occur following administration of FLEET® Phospho®-soda, immediate corrective action should be taken to restore electrolyte balance with appropriate fluid replacements. Calcium, magnesium, and phosphorous levels should be carefully monitored. **See individual listings (Fleet® Phospho®-soda, and Fleet® Bisacodyl Enema for additional warnings.**
THESE KITS SHOULD NOT BE USED BY PATIENTS UNDER 12 YEARS OF AGE.

DOSAGE AND ADMINISTRATION
SEE PATIENT INSTRUCTION SHEET FOR 18, 24, AND 48 HOUR PREPARATION SCHEDULE IN EACH KIT.

HOW SUPPLIED
See "Description" for contents of each kit.
Shipping Unit: 48 FLEET® Prep Kits per carton.
For full prescribing information on specific products, see individual listings (FLEET® Phospho®-soda, FLEET® Bisacodyl Enema).

IS THIS PRODUCT OTC?
Yes.

LITERATURE AVAILABLE
Yes.

FLEET SOF-LAX OVERNIGHT
LAXATIVE PLUS STOOL SOFTENER
OTC

ACTIVE INGREDIENTS
Docusate Sodium USP 100 mg, a stool softener and Casanthranol 30 mg, a stimulant laxative.

INDICATIONS
Fleet Sof-Lax Overnight is an effective combination of a gentle stool softener plus a mild laxative that provides overnight relief of occasional constipation. The stool softener facilitates absorption of water by the stool, making it softer and easier to pass. The laxative provides peristaltic stimulation to relieve constipation. Fleet Sof-Lax Overnight relieves straining associated with hemorrhoids, post-partum, or post-surgery. Fleet Sof-Lax Overnight works in 6 to 12 hours. To help prevent hard stools that may lead to constipation, take Fleet Sof-Lax Stool Softener gelcaps.

DIRECTIONS FOR USE
Adults and children 12 years and over: One or two gelcaps daily at bedtime. **Children 6 to under 12 years:** One gelcap daily.

WARNINGS
Do not use laxative products when abdominal pain, nausea, or vomiting are present unless directed by a physician. Do not take this product if you are presently taking mineral oil, unless directed by a physician. If you have noticed a sudden change in bowel habits that persists over a period of 2 weeks, consult a physician before using a laxative. Laxative products should not be used for a period longer than 1 week unless directed by a physician. Rectal bleeding or failure to have a bowel movement after use of a laxative may indicate a serious condition; discontinue use and consult a physician. Keep this and all drugs out of the reach of children. As with any drug, if you are pregnant or nursing a baby, seek the advice of a health professional before using this product. In case of accidental overdose or ingestion, seek professional assistance or contact a Poison Control Center immediately.

HOW SUPPLIED
Fleet Sof-Lax Overnight
Bottles of 30
Bottles of 60

SOF-LAX
A STOOL SOFTENER
OTC

ACTIVE INGREDIENT
Docusate Sodium USP 100 mg.

INDICATIONS
Fleet Sof-Lax is an effective aid to prevent the formation of hard stools that may lead to constipation. The stool softener facilitates absorption of water by the stool, making it softer and easier to pass. Fleet Sof-Lax relieves straining, minimizing painful bowel movements often associated with hemorrhoids, post-partum, or post-surgery. Fleet Sof-Lax works in 12 to 72 hours. For gentle overnight relief, Fleet Sof-Lax Overnight stool softner plus stimulant laxative works in 6 to 12 hours.

DIRECTIONS FOR USE
Adults and children 12 years and over: One or two gelcaps daily. **Children 6 to under 12 years:** One gelcap daily.

WARNINGS
Do not use when abdominal pain, nausea, or vomiting are present unless directed by a physician. Do not take this product if you are presently taking mineral oil, unless directed by a physician. If you have noticed a sudden change in bowel habits that persists over a period of 2 weeks, consult a physician before using this product. Rectal bleeding or failure to have a bowel movement after use may indicate a serious condition; discontinue use and consult a physician. Keep this and all drugs out of the reach of children. As with any drug, if you are pregnant or nursing a baby, seek the advice of a health professional before using this product. In case of accidental overdose or ingestion, seek professional assistance or contact a Poison Control Center immediately.

HOW SUPPLIED
Fleet Sof-Lax Gelcaps
Bottles of 60
Bottles of 100

Fleming & Company
1600 FENPARK DR.
FENTON, MO 63026

Direct Inquiries to:
H.C. Mansmann, Jr. MD
314-343-8200

AEROLATE SR & JR & III Capsules
(theophylline, anhydrous T.D.)
AEROLATE LIQUID
(theophylline, anhydrous)
℞

COMPOSITION
Contains theophylline 4 grs. (260 mg) as SR, 2 grs (130 mg) as JR, 1 gr. as III (65 mg), in red/clear capsules. Liquid has 150 mg theophylline/15cc in a non-sugar, non-alcoholic, non-saccharin tangerine flavored base.

ACTION AND USES
Timed action pellets by-pass stomach to prevent gastric upset. Bronchodilation is achieved through bowel absorption only. Liquid is for the acute attack primarily.

ADMINISTRATION AND DOSAGE
One capsule every 12 hours. Every 8 hours in severe attacks. Liquid—adults—40 ml (2.5 tablespoonfuls) for acute attack. Children—0.25 ml/lb. Maintainance therapy—adults—for the first 6 doses, 25 ml (1.5 tablespoonfuls) before breakfast, at 3 p.m., at bedtime. Then 15 ml doses at above times. Children—0.15 ml/lb at these times, then 0.1 ml/lb per dose.

SIDE EFFECTS
Nausea, vomiting, epigastric or substernal pain, palpitation, headache, dizziness may occur.

HOW SUPPLIED
Capsules in bottles of 100.
Liquid in pints and gallons.

CHLOR-3
OTC

DESCRIPTION
Medical condiment containing sodium chloride 50%; potassium chloride 30%; magnesium chloride 20%.

INDICATIONS AND USAGE
To reduce sodium intake for patients on diuretics; for potential hypertensives and cardiacs.
To encourage physicians to recommend a condiment to replace "table salt" for family use and gourmet cooking.

HOW SUPPLIED
Shaker 8 oz. plastic bottles.

CONGESS SR & JR Capsules
Expectorant/Decongestant T.D.
℞

COMPOSITION
Contains guaifenesin 250 mgs/pseudoephedrine 120 mgs as SR; guaifenesin 125 mgs/pseudoephedrine 60 mgs as JR in blue/pink capsules.

ACTION AND USES
To loosen mucus plugs in upper respiratory tract and congestion in acute pulmonary disorders, and in coughing. Nasal decongestion and alleviation of bronchospasm is also achieved up to 12 hrs. that accompany most coughs, especially during the nocturnal period.

INDICATIONS
Nasal congestion, sinusitis, acute aerotitis media, bronchial asthma, serous otitis media, and symptoms of the common cold.

DOSAGE
Adults and children over 12 yrs. one SR capsule every 12 hrs. Under 12 yrs. one JR capsule as prescribed by physician.

PRECAUTION AND SIDE EFFECTS
Use with care in severe hypertension, heart disease, hyperthyroidism, diabetes. Low grade sensitivity to drugs may be experienced.

CONTRAINDICATIONS
Prostatic hypertrophy, patients receiving MAO inhibitors.

HOW SUPPLIED
Plastic bottles of 100 and 1000 capsules.

EXTENDRYL
℞
T.D. Capsules SR & JR, Syrup and Tablets

Each timed action SR capsule contains phenylephrine HCl 20 mg; methscopolamine nitrate 2.5 mg; chlorpheniramine maleate 8 mg. The JR potency is exactly half-strength. Green/red color for both. Each 5 cc of root beer flavored syrup and tablet contains: phenylephrine HCl 10 mg; methscopolamine nitrate 1.25 mg; chlorpheniramine maleate 2 mg.

ACTION AND USES
Antihistaminic-decongestant for relief of respiratory congestion; allergic rhinitis; allergic skin reactions of urticaria and angioedema.

ADMINISTRATION AND DOSAGE
Capsules—one every 12 hrs of the SR for adults; one JR every 12 hrs for children 6–12 yrs. Syrup-two teaspoonfuls every 4 hrs for adults; children 1 teaspoonful every 4 hrs. Tablets—adults two and children one every 4 hrs. Do not exceed 4 doses in 24 hrs.
Children under 6 yrs. as recommended by a physician.

PRECAUTIONS
Withdraw therapy if drowsiness occurs. Patients are cautioned against driving or operating mechanical devices.

CONTRAINDICATIONS
Glaucoma, cardiac disease, hyperthyroidism and hypertension.

HOW SUPPLIED
Capsules and tablets in bottles of 100 and 1000. Syrup in pints and gallons.

IMPREGON Concentrate
OTC

ACTIVE INGREDIENT
Tetrachlorosalicylanilide 2%

INDICATIONS
Diaper Rash Relief, 'Staph' control, Mold inhibitor.

ACTIONS
This is a bacteriostatic/fungistatic agent for home usage and hospital usage.

WARNINGS
Impregon should not be exposed to direct sunlight for long periods after applications.

PRECAUTION
Addition of bleach prior to diaper treatment negates application effects.

DOSAGE AND ADMINISTRATION
One capful (5ml) per gallon of water to impregnate diapers in the diaper pail. Dilutions for many home areas accompany the full package.

NOTE
For disposable-type diapers, add one teaspoonful to 8 oz of water to a 'Windex-type' sprayer. Spray middle half area of diapers until damp, and allow to dry before using, to prevent rashes.

HOW SUPPLIED
Four ounce black plastic bottles.

MAGONATE TABLETS
MAGONATE LIQUID
OTC
Magnesium Gluconate (Dihydrate)

ACTIVE INGREDIENTS
Each tablet contains magnesium gluconate (dihydrate) 500mg (27mg of Mg^{++}). Each 5cc of Magonate Liquid contains magnesium gluconate (dihydrate) 1000mg (54mg of Mg^{++}).

INDICATIONS
For all patients in negative magnesium balance.

PRECAUTION
Excessive dosage may cause loose stools.

DOSAGE AND ADMINISTRATION
Magonate is recommended during and for three weeks after a course in chemotherapy, then monitored regularly.
Adults and children over 12 yrs.—one or two tablets or ½ to 1 teaspoon of liquid t.i.d. Under 12 yrs.—one tablet or ½ teaspoon of liquid t.i.d. Dosage may be increased in severe cases.

Continued on next page

Fleming—Cont.

HOW SUPPLIED

Magonate Tablets are supplied in bottles of 100 and 1000 tablets. Magonate Liquid is supplied in pints and gallons.

MARBLEN OTC
(calcium and magnesium carbonates)
ANTACID SUSPENSIONS AND TABLET

(See PDR For Nonprescription Drugs.)

NEPHROCAPS
Dialysis Vitamin Supplement

DESCRIPTION

Each black oval gelatin 'liquid' capsule provides:
Thiamin 1.5 mg; Riboflavin 1.7 mg; Niacin 20 mg; Pantothenic acid 5 mg; Biotin 150 mcg; Cyanocobalamin 6 mcg; Pyridoxin 10 mg; Ascorbic acid 100 mg and Folic acid 1.0 mg.

INDICATIONS

The wasting syndrome in chronic renal failure; uremia; impaired metabolic functions of the kidney.

DOSAGE

One capsule daily. On dialysis days, one Nephrocap must be taken after treatment.

SUPPLIED

Plastic bottles of 100 only.

NEPHROX SUSPENSION OTC
(aluminum hydroxide)
Antacid Suspension

(See PDR For Nonprescription Drugs.)

NICOTINEX Elixir OTC
nicotinic acid

(See PDR For Nonprescription Drugs.)

OCEAN MIST OTC
(buffered isotonic saline)

(See PDR For Nonprescription Drugs.)

PIMA Syrup ℞
(potassium iodide)

COMPOSITION

Contains KI 5 grs./tsp., in a black raspberry flavored base.

ACTION AND USES

An expectorant in the symptomatic treatment of chronic pulmonary diseases where tenacious mucus complicates the problem, including bronchial asthma, bronchitis and pulmonary emphysema.

ADMINISTRATION AND DOSAGE

Children—one half to one tsp. and adults one or two tsp. every 4-6 hours.

SIDE EFFECTS

May include gastrointestinal upset, metallic taste, minor skin eruptions, nausea, vomiting and epigastric pain. Therapy should be withdrawn.

PRECAUTIONS

In patients sensitive to iodides, in hyperthyroidism, and in rare cases iodine-induced goiter may occur.

HOW SUPPLIED

Plastic pints and gallons.

PURGE OTC
(flavored castor oil)

(See PDR For Nonprescription Drugs.)

RUM-K ℞
(potassium chloride 15% conc.)

DESCRIPTION

Each 10 ml. contains 1.5 Gm. potassium chloride (20 mEq) in a butter/rum synthetic flavored base that is alcohol and sugar free.

INDICATIONS

Hypokalemic-hypochloremic alkalosis; digitalis toxicity; hypokalemia prevention secondary to corticosteroid or diuretic administration.

CONTRAINDICATIONS

Impaired renal function, untreated Addison's Disease, acute dehydration, heat cramps, hyperkalemia.

PRECAUTIONS

Do not use in patients with low urinary output or renal decompensation. Potassium replacements vary and should be individualized. Patients should be checked frequently, ECG and plasma K^+ levels should be made. High serum concentrations of K^+ cause death thru cardiac depression, arrhythmias or arrest. Use with caution in cardiac disease.

ADVERSE REACTIONS

Vomiting, nausea, abdominal discomfort, diarrhea may occur. Symptoms and signs of potassium overdose include paresthesias of extremities, flaccid paralysis, listlessness, fall in blood pressure, weakness and heaviness of the legs, cardiac arrhythmias and heart block. Hyperkalemia may cause ECG changes as disappearance of the P wave, widening and slurring of QRS complex, changes of the S-T segment, tall peaked T waves.

DOSAGE AND ADMINISTRATION

Adults—two teaspoonsful (10ml) in 4–6 oz water 2 to 4 times daily after meals to supply 40–80 mEq of elemental potassium and chloride. Larger doses may be required and administered under close supervision due to possible potassium intoxication or saline laxative effect.

HOW SUPPLIED

Pints and gallons.

Forest Pharmaceuticals, Inc.
(Subsidiary of Forest Laboratories, Inc.)
13622 LAKEFRONT DRIVE
ST LOUIS, MO 63045

Direct Inquiries to:
Professional Services Department
13622 Lakefront Drive
St. Louis, MO 63045
(314) 344-8870

AEROBID® ℞
AEROBID®-M
(flunisolide)
Inhaler System
For oral inhalation only

DESCRIPTION

Flunisolide, the active component of **AEROBID** Inhaler System, is an anti-inflammatory steroid having the chemical name 6α-fluoro-11β, 16α, 17, 21-tetrahydroxypregna-1, 4-diene-3, 20-dione cyclic-16, 17-acetal with acetone.
It has the following structure:

Flunisolide is a white to creamy white crystalline powder with a molecular weight of 434.49. It is soluble in acetone, sparingly soluble in chloroform, slightly soluble in methanol, and practically insoluble in water. It has a melting point of about 245℃.
AEROBID Inhaler is delivered in a metered-dose aerosol system containing a microcrystalline suspension of flunisolide as the hemihydrate in propellants (trichloromonofluoromethane, dichlorodifluoromethane and dichlorotetrafluoroethane) with sorbitan trioleate as a dispersing agent.
AEROBID-M also contains menthol as a flavoring agent.
Each activation delivers approximately 250 mcg of fluniso-

lide to the patient. One **AEROBID** Inhaler System is designed to deliver at least 100 metered inhalations.

CLINICAL PHARMACOLOGY

Flunisolide has demonstrated marked anti-inflammatory and anti-allergic activity in classical test systems. It is a corticosteroid that is several hundred times more potent in animal anti-inflammatory assays than the cortisol standard. The molar dose of each activation of flunisolide in this preparation is approximately 2.5 to 7 times that of comparable inhaled corticosteroid products marketed for the same indication. The dose of flunisolide delivered per activation in this preparation is 10 times that per activation of Nasalide® (flunisolide) nasal solution. Clinical studies have shown therapeutic activity on bronchial mucosa with minimal evidence of systemic activity at recommended doses.
After oral inhalation of 1 mg flunisolide, total systemic availability was 40%. The flunisolide that is swallowed is rapidly and extensively converted to the 6β-OH metabolite and to water-soluble conjugates during the first pass through the liver. This offers a metabolic explanation for the low systemic activity of oral flunisolide itself since the metabolite has the low corticosteroid potency (on the order of the cortisol standard). The inhaled flunisolide absorbed through the bronchial tree is converted to the same metabolites. Repeated inhalation of 2.0 mg of flunisolide per day (the maximum recommended dose) for 14 days did not show accumulation of the drug in plasma. The plasma half-life of flunisolide is approximately 1.8 hours.
The following observations relevant to systemic absorption were made in clinical studies. In one uncontrolled study a statistically significant decrease in responsiveness to metyrapone was noted in 15 adult steroid-independent patients treated with 2.0 mg of flunisolide per day (the maximum recommended dose) for 3 months. A small but statistically significant drop in eosinophils from 11.5% to 7.4% of total circulating leucocytes was noted in another study in children who were not taking oral corticosteroids simultaneously. A 5% incidence of menstrual disturbances was reported during open studies, in which there were no control groups for comparison.
Aerosol administration of flunisolide 2.0 mg twice daily for one week to 6 healthy male subjects revealed neither suppression of adrenal function as measured by early morning cortisol levels nor impairment of HPA axis function as determined by insulin hypoglycemia tests.
Controlled clinical studies have included over 500 patients with asthma, among them 150 children age 6 and over. More than 120 patients have been treated in open trials for two years or more. No significant adrenal suppression attributed to flunisolide was seen in these studies.
Significant decreases of systemic steroid dosages have been possible in flunisolide-treated patients. Recommended doses of flunisolide appear to be the therapeutic equivalent of an average of 10 mg/day of oral prednisone. Asthma patients have had further symptomatic improvement with flunisolide treatment even while reducing concomitant medication.

INDICATIONS AND USAGE

AEROBID (flunisolide) Inhaler is indicated in the maintenance treatment of asthma as prophylactic therapy. **AEROBID** is also indicated for asthma patients who require corticosteroid administration, where adding **AEROBID** may reduce or eliminate the need for the systemic corticosteroids. **AEROBID** Inhaler is NOT indicated for the relief of acute bronchospasm.

CONTRAINDICATIONS

AEROBID (flunisolide) Inhaler is contraindicated in the primary treatment of status asthmaticus or other acute episodes of asthma where intensive measures are required. Hypersensitivity to any of the ingredients of this preparation contraindicates its use.

WARNINGS

Particular care is needed in patients who are transferred from systemically active corticosteroids to **AEROBID** Inhaler because deaths due to adrenal insufficiency have occurred in asthmatic patients during and after transfer from systemic corticosteroids to aerosol corticosteroids. After withdrawal from systemic corticosteroids, a number of months are required for recovery of hypothalamic-pituitary-adrenal (HPA) function. During this period of HPA suppression, patients may exhibit signs and symptoms of adrenal insufficiency when exposed to trauma, surgery or infections, particularly gastroenteritis. Although **AEROBID** Inhaler may provide control of asthmatic symptoms during these episodes, it does NOT provide the systemic steroid that is necessary for coping with these emergencies. During periods of stress or a severe asthmatic attack, patients who have been withdrawn from systemic corticosteroids should be instructed to resume systemic steroids (in large doses) immediately and to contact their physician for further instruction. These patients should also be instructed to carry a warning card indicating that they

may need supplementary systemic steroids during periods of stress or a severe asthma attack. To assess the risk of adrenal insufficiency in emergency situations, routine tests of adrenal cortical function, including measurement of early morning resting cortisol levels, should be performed periodically in all patients. An early morning resting cortisol level may be accepted as normal if it falls at or near the normal mean level.

Localized infections with *Candida albicans* or *Aspergillus niger* have occurred in the mouth and pharynx and occasionally in the larynx. Positive cultures for oral *Candida* may be present in up to 34% of patients. Although the frequency of clinically apparent infection is considerably lower, these infections may require treatment with appropriate antifungal therapy or discontinuance of treatment with **AEROBID** Inhaler.

AEROBID Inhaler is not to be regarded as a bronchodilator and is not indicated for rapid relief of bronchospasm.

Patients should be instructed to contact their physician immediately when episodes of asthma that are not responsive to bronchodilators occur during the course of treatment. During such episodes, patients may require therapy with systemic corticosteroids. Theoretically, the use of inhaled corticosteroids with alternate day prednisone systemic treatment should be accompanied by more HPA suppression than a therapeutically equivalent regimen of either alone.

Transfer of patients from systemic steroid therapy to **AEROBID** Inhaler may unmask allergic conditions previously suppressed by the systemic steroid therapy, e.g. rhinitis, conjunctivitis, and eczema.

Persons who are on drugs which suppress the immune system are more susceptible to infections than healthy individuals. Chicken pox and measles, for example, can have a more serious or even fatal course in non-immune children or adults on corticosteroids. In such children or adults who have not had these diseases, particular care should be taken to avoid exposure. How the dose, route and duration of corticosteriod administration affects the risk of developing a disseminated infection is not known. The contribution of the underlying disease and/or prior corticosteroid treatment to the risk is also not known. If exposed to chicken pox, prophylaxis with varicella zoster immune globulin (VZIG) may be indicated. If exposed to measles, prophylaxis with pooled intramuscular immunoglobulin (IG) may be indicated. (See the respective package inserts for complete VZIG and IG prescribing information). If chicken pox develops, treatment with antiviral agents may be considered.

PRECAUTIONS

General: Because of the relatively high molar dose of flunisolide per activation in this preparation, and because of the evidence suggesting higher levels of systemic absorption with flunisolide than with other comparable inhaled corticosteroids (see CLINICAL PHARMACOLOGY section), patients treated with **AEROBID** (flunisolide) should be observed carefully for any evidence of systemic corticosteroid effect, including suppression of bone growth in children.

Particular care should be taken in observing patients postoperatively or during periods of stress for evidence of a decrease in adrenal function. During withdrawal from oral steroids, some patients may experience symptoms of systemically active steroid withdrawal, e.g. joint and/or muscular pain, lassitude and depression, despite maintenance or even improvement of respiratory function. (See DOSAGE AND ADMINISTRATION for details.)

In responsive patients, flunisolide may permit control of asthmatic symptoms without suppression of HPA function.

Since flunisolide is absorbed into the circulation and can be systemically active, the beneficial effects of **AEROBID** Inhaler in minimizing or preventing HPA dysfunction may be expected only when recommended dosages are not exceeded.

The long-term local and systemic effects of **AEROBID** (flunisolide) in human subjects are still not fully known. In particular, the effects resulting from chronic use of **AEROBID** on developmental or immunologic processes in the mouth, pharynx, trachea, and lung are unknown.

Inhaled corticosteroids should be used with caution, if at all, in patients with active or quiescent tuberculosis infection of the respiratory tract; untreated systemic fungal, bacterial, parasitic or viral infections; or ocular herpes simplex.

Pulmonary infiltrates with eosinophilia may occur in patients on **AEROBID** Inhaler therapy. Although it is possible that in some patients this state may become manifest because of systemic steroid withdrawal when inhalational steroids are administered, a causative role for the drug and/or its vehicle cannot be ruled out.

Information for Patients:

Since the relief from **AEROBID** Inhaler depends on its regular use and on proper inhalation technique, patients must be instructed to take inhalations at regular intervals. They should also be instructed in the correct method of use (See Patient Instruction Leaflet.)

Patients whose systemic corticosteroids have been reduced or withdrawn should be instructed to carry a warning card indicating that they may need supplemental systemic steroids during periods of stress or a severe asthmatic attack that is not responsive to bronchodilators.

Persons who are on immunosuppressant doses of corticosteroids should be warned to avoid exposure to chicken pox or measles. Patients should also be advised that if they are exposed, medical advice should be sought without delay.

An illustrated leaflet of patient instructions for proper use accompanies each **AEROBID** Inhaler System.

CONTENTS UNDER PRESSURE

Do not puncture. Do not use or store near heat or open flame. Exposure to temperatures above 120°F (49°C) may cause container to explode. Never throw container into fire or incinerator. Keep out of reach of children.

Carcinogenesis: Long-term studies were conducted in mice and rats using oral administration to evaluate the carcinogenic potential of the drug. There was an increase in the incidence of pulmonary adenomas in mice, but not in rats.

Female rats receiving the highest oral dose had an increased incidence of mammary adenocarcinoma compared to control rats. An increased incidence of this tumor type has been reported for other corticosteroids.

Impairment of Fertility: Female rats receiving high doses of flunisolide (200 mcg/kg/day) showed some evidence of impaired fertility. Reproductive performance in the low- (8 mcg/kg/day) and mid-dose (40 mcg/kg/day) groups was comparable to controls.

Pregnancy: Pregnancy Category C. As with other corticosteroids, flunisolide has been shown to be teratogenic in rabbits and rats at doses of 40 and 200 mcg/kg/day respectively. It was also fetotoxic in these animal reproductive studies. There are no adequate and well-controlled studies in pregnant women. Flunisolide should be used during pregnancy only if the potential benefit justifies the potential risk to the fetus.

Nursing Mothers: It is not known whether this drug is excreted in human milk. Because other corticosteroids are excreted in human milk, caution should be exercised when flunisolide is administered to nursing women.

Pediatric Use: Safety and effectiveness have not been established in children below the age of 6. Oral corticoids have been shown to cause growth suppression in children and adolescents, particularly with higher doses over extended periods. If a child or adolescent on any corticoid appears to have growth suppression, the possibility that they are particularly sensitive to this effect of steroids should be considered.

ADVERSE REACTIONS

Adverse events reported in controlled clinical trials and long-term open studies in 514 patients treated with **AEROBID** (flunisolide) are described below. Of those patients, 463 were treated for 3 months or longer, 407 for 6 months or longer, 287 for 1 year or longer, and 122 for 2 years or longer.

Musculoskeletal reactions were reported in 35% of steroid-dependent patients in whom the dose of oral steroid was being tapered. This is a well-known effect of steroid withdrawal.

Incidence 10% or greater:

Gastrointestinal: diarrhea (10%), nausea and/or vomiting (25%), upset stomach (10%)
General: flu (10%)
Mouth and Throat: sore throat (20%)
Nervous System: headache (25%)
Respiratory: cold symptoms (15%), nasal congestion (15%), upper respiratory infection (25%)
Special Senses: unpleasant taste (10%)

Incidence 3–9%

Cardiovascular: palpitations
Gastrointestinal: abdominal pain, heartburn
General: chest pain, decreased appetite, edema, fever
Mouth and Throat: *Candida* infection
Nervous System: dizziness, irritability, nervousness, shakiness
Reproductive: menstrual disturbances
Respiratory: chest congestion, cough*, hoarseness, rhinitis, runny nose, sinus congestion, sinus drainage, sinus infection, sinusitis, sneezing, sputum, wheezing*
Skin: eczema, itching (pruritus), rash
Special Senses: ear infection, loss of smell or taste

Incidence 1–3%

General: chills, increased appetite and weight gain, malaise, peripheral edema, sweating, weakness
Cardiovascular: hypertension, tachycardia
Gastrointestinal: constipation, dyspepsia, gas
Hemic/Lymph: capillary fragility, enlarged lymph nodes
Mouth and Throat: dry throat, glossitis, mouth irritation, pharyngitis, phlegm, throat irritation
Nervous System: anxiety, depression, faintness, fatigue, hyperactivity, hypoactivity, insomnia, moodiness, numbness, vertigo
Respiratory: bronchitis, chest tightness*, dyspnea, epistaxis, head stuffiness, laryngitis, nasal irritation, pleurisy, pneumonia, sinus discomfort
Skin: acne, hives or urticaria
Special Senses: blurred vision, earache, eye discomfort, eye infection

Incidence less than 1%, judged by investigators as possibly or probably drug related: abdominal fullness, shortness of breath.

*The incidences as shown of cough, wheezing, and chest tightness were judged by investigators to be possibly or probably drug-related. In placebo-controlled trials, the *overall* incidences of these adverse events (regardless of investigators' judgment of drug relationship) were similar for drug and placebo-treated groups. They may be related to the vehicle or delivery system.

DOSAGE AND ADMINISTRATION

The **AEROBID** (flunisolide) Inhaler System is for oral inhalation only.

Adults: The recommended starting dose is 2 inhalations twice daily, morning and evening, for a total daily dose of 1 mg. The maximum daily dose should not exceed 4 inhalations twice a day for a total daily dose of 2 mg. When the drug is used chronically at 2 mg/day, patients should be monitored periodically for effects on the hypothalamic-pituitary-adrenal (HPA) axis.

Pediatric Patients: For children and adolescents 6–15 years of age, two inhalations may be administered twice daily for a total daily dose of 1 mg. Higher doses have not been studied. Insufficient information is available to warrant use in children under age 6. With chronic use, pediatric patients should be monitored for growth as well as for effects on the HPA axis.

Rinsing the mouth after inhalation is advised.

Different considerations must be given to the following groups of patients in order to obtain the full therapeutic benefit of **AEROBID** (flunisolide) Inhaler.

Patients Not Receiving Systemic Corticosteroids:

Patients who require maintenance therapy of their asthma may benefit from treatment with **AEROBID** at doses recommended above. In patients who respond to **AEROBID**, improvement in pulmonary function is usually apparent whithin one to four weeks after the start of therapy. Once the desired effect is achieved, consideration should be given to tapering to the lowest effective dose.

Patients Maintained on Systemic Corticosteroids:

Clinical studies have shown that **AEROBID** may be effective in the management of asthmatics dependent or maintained on systemic corticosteroids and may permit replacement or significant reduction in the dosage of systemic corticosteroids.

The patient's asthma should be reasonably stable before treatment with **AEROBID** is started. Initially, **AEROBID** should be used concurrently with the patient's usual maintenance dose of systemic corticosteroid. After approximately one week, gradual withdrawal of the systemic corticosteroid is started by reducing the daily or alternate daily dose. Reductions may be made after an interval of one or two weeks, depending on the response of the patient. A slow rate of withdrawal is strongly recommended. Generally, these decrements should not exceed 2.5 mg of prednisone or its equivalent. During withdrawal, some patients may experience symptoms of systemic corticosteroid withdrawal; e.g. joint and/or muscular pain, lassitude and depression, despite maintenance or even improvement of respiratory function. Such patients should be encouraged to continue with the inhaler but should be monitored for objective signs of adrenal insufficiency. If evidence of adrenal insufficiency occurs, the systemic corticosteroid doses should be increased temporarily and thereafter withdrawal should continue more slowly.

During periods of stress or a severe asthma attack, transfer patients may require supplementary treatment with systemic corticosteroids.

HOW SUPPLIED

AEROBID (flunisolide) Inhaler Systems are available in canisters of 100 metered inhalations.

NDC 0456-0672-99 **AEROBID**
NDC 0456-0670-99 **AEROBID-M**

"Note: The indented statement below is required by the Federal government's Clean Air Act for all products containing or manufactured with chlorofluorocarbons (CFC's)."

WARNING: Contains trichloromonofluoromethane, dichlorodifluoromethane and dichlorotetrafluoroethane, substances which harm public health and environment by destroying ozone in the upper atmosphere.

"A notice similar to the above WARNING has been placed in the information for the patient of this product pursuant to EPA regulations."

Caution: Federal Law prohibits dispensing without prescription.

Revised 4/96

mfd for
FOREST PHARMACEUTICALS, INC.
St. Louis, MO 63045

Continued on next page

Forest—Cont.

mfd by
3M Pharmaceuticals
St. Paul, MN

16053

Shown in Product Identification Guide, page 310

AeroChamber® ℞
AeroChamber® with *Mask—Small*
AeroChamber® with *Mask*
AeroChamber® with *Mask—Large*
Valved Aerosol Holding Chamber/Aerosol Holding Chamber
with *Mask* for Use With Metered Dose Inhalers.

Before using AeroChamber/AeroChamber with *Mask*, it is important to read these instructions very carefully, including the CAUTION sections that follow:

CAUTION

1. When cleaning, the only part of the AeroChamber/AeroChamber with Mask to be removed is the rubber like ring that holds the Metered Dose Inhaler and the protective mouthpiece cap from the AeroChamber. Do not remove the mouthpiece/face mask from the AeroChamber body.
2. Except as stated in 1 above, do not disassemble the AeroChamber/AeroChamber with Mask, as the overall reliability and safety of the product may be affected.
3. Replace AeroChamber/AeroChamber with Mask at once and do not use if the one-way valve becomes dislodged (partially or fully) or begins to harden or curl.
4. Running water through the AeroChamber/AeroChamber with Mask at high pressure may harm the valve. Examine AeroChamber/AeroChamber with Mask visually before and after cleaning to make sure the one-way valve and other parts are properly secured.
5. Disassembly may loosen or dislodge the one-way valve. Examine the AeroChamber/AeroChamber with Mask visually before and after use to make sure the one-way valve and other parts are properly secured.
6. Do not allow children to play with the AeroChamber/AeroChamber with Mask—allowing them to do so may alter its function and/or overall reliability. The mask membrane, the one-way valve, and the exhalation valve (Mask-Small) can be damaged as a result of pulling or poking.
7. As indicated, your AeroChamber/AeroChamber with Mask should be inspected visually before and after daily use and may need to be replaced after 6 to 12 months of use.

INTRODUCTION

The AeroChamber/AeroChamber with Mask line is a family of valved aerosol holding chambers available from Forest Pharmaceuticals, Inc., designed to be used with virtually all Metered Dose Inhalers [MDI's]. When you release a puff of aerosol into the AeroChamber/AeroChamber with Mask, the puff will be held there for a few seconds. The valved holding chamber selectively removes most large aerosol-drug particles that normally deposit in the mouth and throat, while allowing the smaller, therapeutic particles to pass through the patented one-way valve into the lungs. This provides effective treatment and helps to reduce unwanted side effects. In addition, the AeroChamber/AeroChamber with Mask is designed to make Metered Dose Inhalers easier to use.

CLEANING INSTRUCTIONS

The AeroChamber/AeroChamber with Mask is made of durable plastic materials and has one or two moving parts; the one-way valve and, in the AeroChamber with Mask-Small, an exhalation valve. With repeated use, residue may accumulate inside the AeroChamber/AeroChamber with Mask and around the one-way valve. This may eventually interfere with effective use. We suggest cleaning the Metered Dose Inhaler as instructed by the manufacturer and AeroChamber/AeroChamber with Mask about once a week or more often depending on your usage of the product.
To clean the AeroChamber/AeroChamber with Mask:

1. Remove the rubber-like ring from the end that holds the Metered Dose Inhaler and the protective mouthpiece cap from the AeroChamber. Do not remove the mouthpiece/face mask from the AeroChamber body.
2. Soak AeroChamber/AeroChamber with Mask, rubber-like ring, and the protective mouthpiece cap from the AeroChamber in basin filled with warm water, using mild detergent to dislodge or loosen any residue.
3. Rinse AeroChamber/AeroChamber with Mask, rubber-like ring, and the protective mouthpiece cap from the AeroChamber in basin filled with clean warm water, using a gentle motion.
4. Lightly shake away excess water droplets and leave on clean surface to air-dry.
5. Be sure the AeroChamber/AeroChamber with Mask is completely dry before use.

6. Replace the rubber-like ring on the AeroChamber/AeroChamber with Mask.

TECHNICAL INFORMATION

This apparently simple device is a product of considerable medical research and engineering. It was developed in a leading medical center.
The valved holding chamber selectively removes large aerosol particles that normally deposit in the mouth and throat, while allowing the smaller treatment particles to pass into the lungs. This provides effective treatment and helps reduce unwanted side effects.
AeroChamber

INSTRUCTIONS FOR USE

Please discuss the use of the AeroChamber with your physician, pharmacist, or other healthcare professional.

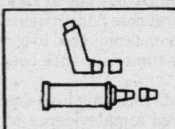 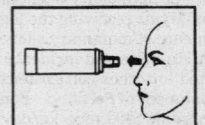

1. Remove the protective cap from Metered-Dose Inhaler [MDI]. Remove the protective cap from the mouthpiece of AeroChamber.
2. Visually check the AeroChamber for foreign objects. Ensure that all parts are secure, including the one-way valve.

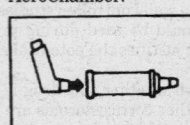 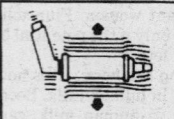

3. Insert inhaler mouthpiece into the round opening in the rubber-like ring at the end of the AeroChamber.
4. Holding the AeroChamber and Inhaler [MDI] firmly, shake vigorously 3 or 4 times.

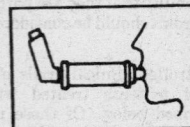 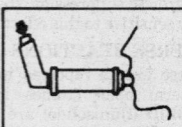

5. Exhale normally. Place the AeroChamber mouthpiece in mouth and close lips.
6. Spray only one puff from the inhaler [MDI] into the AeroChamber per inhalation maneuver. Spraying more than one puff into the AeroChamber before or during an inhalation maneuver will result in delivery of improper dose of medication.

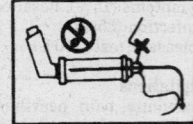

7. Breathe in slowly and deeply through mouth until you have taken a full breath. Do not breathe in so fast as to activate the flow signal whistle. A whistling sound from the flow signal indicates that you are breathing in too quickly.
8. Hold breath for 5 to 10 seconds.
9. Repeat steps 4 to 8 as prescribed by your physician.
10. Remove inhaler and examine the AeroChamber to make certain that the one-way valve is properly secured.
11. Replace protective cap on AeroChamber and MDI.

HELPFUL HINTS:

1. In order to obtain the maximum benefit from your Metered Dose Inhaler, it is extremely important to fill your lungs during inhalation by taking a *slow*, deep breath. If the flow signal makes a whistling sound, it is an indication that you are breathing in too quickly.
2. The one-way valve allows you to inhale at your own rate so that coordination of inhalation with the actuation of the inhaler is not a problem.
3. If you have trouble inhaling through your mouth, with the AeroChamber mouthpiece between your lips, it may be necessary to gently pinch your nose while inhaling the medication.
4. For the elderly and small children who may have difficulty using the AeroChamber, there is also an AeroCham-

ber available with Mask which allows another person to assist with coordination.
5. When using the AeroChamber with a corticosteroid Metered Dose Inhaler, it is recommended by the manufacturer of these drugs to rinse your mouth with water to remove any medication residue.

IMPORTANT INFORMATION

Package insert dosing instructions should be consulted for all Metered Dose Inhalers [MDIs] when used with AeroChamber®. Dosage and administration recommendations vary for different MDIs, and the limitations and conditions of use for each product should be considered before utilizing this device, particularly for younger and older patients.

This device helps deliver aerosol medication to the lungs more reliably. Should you have any problem using the AeroChamber please contact your doctor.
CAUTION: Federal law restricts this device to sale by, or on the order of, a physician.
Manufactured by Monaghan Medical Corporation, Plattsburgh, NY 12901
Assembled in USA of Canadian Components covered by one or more of the following patent numbers: 4,470,412; 5,042,467; 5,012,803; 4,809,692; 4,832,015; 5,012,804

AeroChamber with *Mask—Small*

INSTRUCTIONS FOR USE

Please discuss the use of the AeroChamber with Mask-Small with your physician, pharmacist, or other healthcare professional.

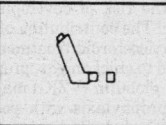 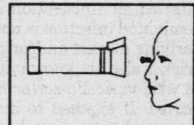

1. Remove the protective cap from Metered Dose Inhaler [MDI].
2. Visually check the AeroChamber with Mask-Small for foreign objects. Ensure that all parts are secure.

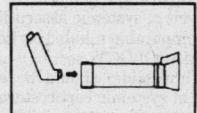 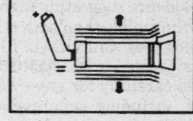

3. Insert inhaler mouthpiece into the round opening in the rubber-like end of the AeroChamber with Mask-Small.
4. Holding the AeroChamber with Mask-Small and inhaler firmly, shake vigorously 3 or 4 times.

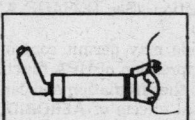 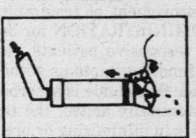

5. Place the soft mask gently to the face so that the mouth and nose are covered. Be certain to create a good seal; leaks will inhibit the delivery of the medication. The exhalation valve allows the patient to exhale comfortably while the mask is held firmly around their mouth and nose.
6. While the patient is exhaling, spray only one puff from the inhaler into the AeroChamber with Mask-Small. Spraying more than one puff into the AeroChamber with Mask-Small before or during an inhalation maneuver will result in delivery of improper dose of medication.

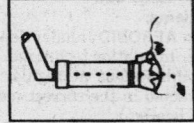

7. Hold the mask firmly to the patient's face for at least six (6) breaths.

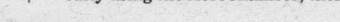

8. Repeat steps 4 to 7 as prescribed by your physician, waiting at least 30 seconds between puffs.
9. Remove inhaler and replace its protective cap.

AeroChamber with *Mask*

INSTRUCTIONS FOR USE

Please discuss the use of the AeroChamber with Mask with your physician, pharmacist, or other healthcare professional.

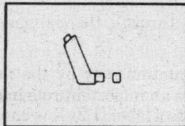

1. Remove the protective cap from Metered Dose Inhaler (MDI)

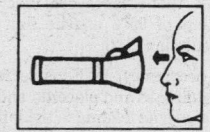

2. Visually check the AeroChamber® with Mask for foreign objects. Ensure that all parts are secure.

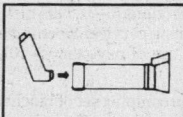

3. Insert inhaler mouthpiece into the opening in the soft rubber-like end of the AeroChamber® with Mask.

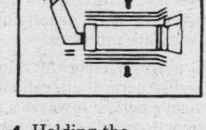

4. Holding the AeroChamber® with Mask and inhaler firmly. shake vigorously 3 or 4 times.

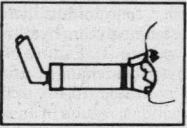

5. Place the soft mask gently to the face so that the mouth and nose are covered. Be certain to create a good seal: leaks will inhibit the delivery of the medication. The exhalation valve allows the patient to exhale comfortably while the mask is held firmly around their mouth and nose.

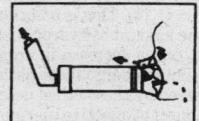

6. While the patient is exhaling, spray only one puff from the inhaler into the AeroChamber® with Mask. Spraying more that one puff into the AeroChamber® with Mask before or during an inhalation maneuver will result in delivery of improper dose of medication

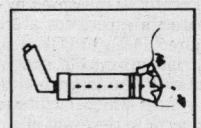

7. Hold the mask firmly to the patient's face for at least six (6) breaths.
8. Repeat steps 4 to 7 as prescribed by your physician, waiting at least 30 seconds between puffs.
9. Remove inhaler and replace its protective cap.

HELPFUL HINTS

1. Some children may resist their treatment by grabbing at the mask. Place the child on your lap and wrap one arm around the child to simplify placing the mask on the child's face.
2. In the case of a smaller child it may be more comfortable to lay the child on a bed while administering the medication.
3. If the child seems frightened by the AeroChamber with Mask-Small or AeroChamber with Mask, familiarize the child with the device by stroking his or her cheek with the soft mask. If the child cries during treatment with the AeroChamber with Mask-Small or AeroChamber with Mask, the medication will still be delivered as long as there is a good seal between the mask and the child's face. Remember, the child will inhale in after crying or screaming.
4. When using the AeroChamber with Mask-Small or AeroChamber with Mask with a corticosteroid Metered Dose Inhaler, it is recommended that the patient's face be cleaned with soap and water to remove any medication residue.

IMPORTANT INFORMATION:

Package insert dosing instructions should be consulted for all Metered Dose Inhalers [MDIs] when used with AeroChamber with Mask-Small or AeroChamber with Mask. Dosage and administration recommendations vary for different MDIs, and the limitations and conditions of use for each product should be considered before utilizing this device, particularly for younger and older patients.

This device helps deliver aerosol medication to the lungs more reliably. Should you have any problem using the Aero-Chamber with Mask-Small or AeroChamber with Mask, please contact your doctor.

CAUTION: Federal law restricts this device to sale by, or on the order of, a physician.
Manufactured by Monaghan Medical Corporation, Plattsburgh, NY 12901
Assembled in USA of Canadian Components covered by one or more of the following patent numbers: 4,470,412; 5,042,467; 5,012,803; 4,809,692; 4,832,015; 5,012,804

AeroChamber with *Mask—Large*

INSTRUCTIONS FOR USE:

Please discuss the use of the AeroChamber with Mask-Large with your physician, pharmacist, or other healthcare professional.

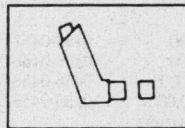

1. Remove the protective cap from Metered-Dose Inhaler [MDI].

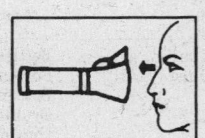

2. Visually check the AeroChamber with Mask-Large for foreign objects. Ensure that all parts are secure, including the one-way valve.

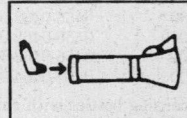

3. Insert inhaler mouth-piece into the round opening in the rubber-like ring at the end of the AeroChamber with Mask-Large.

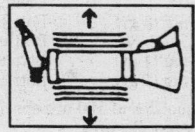

4. Holding the AeroChamber with Mask-Large and inhaler [MDI] firmly, shake vigorously 3 or 4 times.

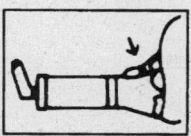

5. Place the soft mask gently to the face so that the mouth and nose are covered. Be certain to create a good seal. Leaks will inhibit the delivery of the medication. Seeing the diaphragm move is a helpful indication of a good seal.

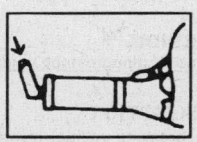

6. Spray only one puff from the inhaler [MDI] into the AeroChamber with Mask-Large per inhalation maneuver. Spraying more than one puff into the AeroChamber with Mask-Large before or during an inhalation maneuver will result in delivery of improper dose of medication.

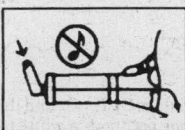

7. Breathe in slowly and deeply until you have taken a full breath. Do not breathe in so fast as to activate the flow signal whistle. A whistle sound from the flow signal indicates that you are breathing in too quickly.
8. Repeat steps 4 to 7 as prescribed by your physician.
9. Remove inhaler and examine the AeroChamber with Mask-Large to make certain that the one-way valve is properly secured.

HELPFUL HINTS

1. In order to obtain the maximum benefit from your Metered Dose Inhaler, it is extremely important to fill your lungs during inhalation by taking a *slow*, deep breath. If the flow signal makes a whistling sound, it is an indication that you are breathing in too quickly.
2. The one-way valve allows you to inhale at your own rate so that coordination of inhalation with the actuation of the inhaler is not a problem.
3. When using the AeroChamber with Mask-Large with a corticosteroid Metered Dose Inhaler, it is recommended that the patient's face be cleaned with soap and water to remove any medication residue.

IMPORTANT INFORMATION

Package insert dosing instructions should be consulted for all Metered Dose Inhalers [MDIs] when used with AeroChamber with Mask-Large. Dosage and administration recommendations vary for different MDIs and the limitations and conditions of use for each product should be considered before utilizing this device, particularly for younger and older patients.

This device helps deliver aerosol medication to the lungs more reliably. Should you have any problem using the AeroChamber with Mask-Large, please contact your doctor.
CAUTION: Federal law restricts this device to sale by, or on the order of, a physician.
Manufactured by Monaghan Medical Corporation, Plattsburgh, NY 12901
Assembled in USA of Canadian Components covered by one or more of the following patent numbers: 4,470,412; 5,042,467; 5,012,803; 4,809,692; 4,832,015; 5,012,804
Distributed by:
FOREST PHARMACEUTICALS, INC.
UAD LABORATORIES
St. Louis, Missouri 63045
REV 7/96 ACL
Shown in Product Identification Guide, page 310

ANTILIRIUM®   ℞
(Physostigmine Salicylate Injection)

DESCRIPTION

ANTILIRIUM (Physostigmine Salicylate) is a derivative of the Calabar bean, and its active moiety, physostigmine, is also known as eserine.
It is soluble in water and a 0.5% aqueous solution has a pH of 5.8.
ANTILIRIUM Injection is available in 2 ml ampuls, each ml containing 1 mg of Physostigmine Salicylate in a vehicle composed of sodium bisulfite 0.1%, benzyl alcohol 2.0% as a preservative in water for injection.

CLINICAL PHARMACOLOGY

ANTILIRIUM is a reversible anticholinesterase which effectively increases the concentration of acetylcholine at the sites of cholinergic transmission. The action of acetylcholine is normally very transient because of its hydrolysis by the enzyme, acetylcholinesterase. ANTILIRIUM inhibits the destructive action of acetylcholinesterase and thereby prolongs and exaggerates the effect of the acetylcholine.
ANTILIRIUM contains a tertiary amine and easily penetrates the blood brain barrier, while an anticholinesterase, such as neostigmine, which has a quaternary ammonium ion is not capable of crossing the barrier. ANTILIRIUM can reverse both central and peripheral anticholinergia. The anticholinergic syndrome has both central and peripheral signs and symptoms. Central toxic effects include anxiety, delirium, disorientation, hallucinations, hyper-activity and seizures. Severe poisoning may produce coma, medullary paralysis and death. Peripheral toxicity is characterized by tachycardia, hyperpyrexia, mydriasis, vasodilatation, urinary retention, diminution of gastrointestinal motility, decrease of secretion in salivary and sweat glands, and loss of secretions in the pharynx, bronchi, and nasal passages.
Dramatic reversal of the effects of anticholinergic symptoms can be expected in minutes after the intravenous administration of ANTILIRIUM, if the diagnosis is correct and the patient has not suffered anoxia or other insult. The duration of action of ANTILIRIUM is relatively short, approx. 45 to 60 minutes.
Numerous drugs and some plants produce the anticholinergic syndrome either directly or as a side effect; this undesirable or potentially dangerous phenomenon may be brought about by either therapeutic doses or overdoses of the drugs. Such drugs include among others, atropine, other derivatives of the belladonna alkaloids, tricyclic antidepressants, phenothiazines, and antihistamines.

Continued on next page

Forest—Cont.

INDICATIONS AND USAGES
To reverse the effect upon the central nervous system, caused by clinical or toxic dosages of drugs capable of producing the anticholinergic syndrome.

CONTRAINDICATIONS
ANTILIRIUM should not be used in the presence of asthma, gangrene, diabetes, cardiovascular disease, mechanical obstruction of the intestine or urogenital tract or any vagotonic state, and in patients receiving choline esters or depolarizing neuromuscular blocking agents (decamethonium succinylcholine).
For post-anesthesia, the concomitant use of atropine with the physostigmine salicylate is not recommended, since the atropine antagonizes the action of physostigmine.

WARNINGS
Contains sodium bisulfite, a sulfite that may cause allergic-type reactions including anaphylactic symptoms and life-threatening or less severe asthmatic episodes in certain susceptible people. The overall prevalence of sulfite sensitivity in the general population is unknown and probably low. Sulfite sensitivity is seen more frequently in asthmatic than in non-asthmatic people.
If excessive symptoms of salivation, emesis, urination and defecation occur, the use of ANTILIRIUM should be terminated. If excessive sweating or nausea occur, the dosage should be reduced.
Intravenous administration should be a slow, controlled rate, no more than 1 mg per minute (see dosage). Rapid administration can cause bradycardia, hypersalivation leading to respiratory difficulties and possible convulsions.
An overdosage of ANTILIRIUM can cause a cholinergic crisis.

PRECAUTIONS
Because of the possibility of hypersensitivity in an occasional patient, atropine sulfate injection should always be at hand since it is an antagonist and antidote for physostigmine.

USAGE IN PREGNANCY
Safe use in pregnancy and lactation has not been established; therefore, use in pregnant women, nursing mothers or women who may become pregnant requires that possible benefits be weighed against possible hazards to mother and child.

ADVERSE REACTIONS
Nausea, vomiting and salivation, can be offset by reducing dosage. Bradycardia and convulsions, if intravenous administration is too rapid. See DOSAGE AND ADMINISTRATION.

OVERDOSAGE
Can cause a cholinergic crisis. Appropriate antidote is atropine sulfate.

DOSAGE AND ADMINISTRATION
Post Anesthesia Care: 0.5 to 1.0 mg intramuscularly or intravenously. INTRAVENOUS ADMINISTRATION SHOULD BE AT A SLOW CONTROLLED RATE OF NO MORE THAN 1 MG PER MINUTE. Dosage may be repeated at intervals of 10 to 30 minutes if desired patient response is not obtained.
Overdosages of Drugs That Cause Anticholinergia: 2.0 mg intramuscularly or INTRAVENOUSLY AT SLOW CONTROLLED RATE (SEE ABOVE). Dosage may be repeated if life threatening signs, such as arrhythmia, convulsions or coma occurs.
Pediatric Dosage: Recommended dosage is 0.02 mg/kg, intramuscularly or by slow intravenous injection, no more than 0.5 mg per minute. If the toxic effects persist, and there is no sign of cholinergic effects, the dosage may be repeated at 5 to 10 minute intervals until a therapeutic effect is obtained or a maximum dose of 2 mg is attained.
IN ALL CASES OF POISONING, THE USUAL SUPPORTIVE MEASURES SHOULD BE UNDERTAKEN.

HOW SUPPLIED
Ampuls, 2 ml packed 12 per box, 1 mg per ml NDC-0456-1037-12.
Store at controlled room temperature 15°–30°C (59°–86°F).

CAUTION
Federal law prohibits dispensing without prescription.
SOME DRUGS WHICH PRODUCE THE ANTICHOLINERGIC SYNDROME
Amitriptyline, Amoxapine, Anisotropine, Atropine, Benztropine, Biperiden, Carbinoxamine, Clidinium, Cyclobenzaprine, Desipramine, Doxepin, Homatropine, Hyoscine, Hyoscyamine, Hyoscyamus, Imipramine, Lorazepam, Maprotiline, Mepenzolate, Nortriptyline, Propantheline, Protriptyline, Scopolamine, Trimipramine.
SOME PLANTS THAT PRODUCE THE ANTICHOLINERGIC SYNDROME
Black Henbane, Deadly Night Shade, Devil's Apple, Jimson Weed, Loco Seeds or Weeds, Matrimony Vine, Night Blooming Jessamine, Stinkweed.

ARMOUR® THYROID Tablets ℞
[thī'roid]
(THYROID TABLETS, U.S.P.)

DESCRIPTION
Armour® Thyroid Tablets (Thyroid Tablets, USP) for oral use are natural preparations derived from porcine thyroid glands. (T_3 liothyronine is approximately four times as potent as T_4 levothyroxine on a microgram for microgram basis.) They provide 38 mcg levothyroxine (T_4) and 9 mcg liothyronine (T_3) per grain of thyroid. The inactive ingredients are calcium stearate, dextrose and mineral oil.

HOW SUPPLIED
Armour Thyroid Tablets (thyroid tablets, USP) are supplied as follows:

Size	Available in	NDC No.
15 mg (1/4 gr)	Bottles of 100	0456-0457-01
30 mg (1/2 gr)	Bottles of 100	0456-0458-01
	Bottles of 1000	0456-0458-00
	Drums of 50,000	0456-0458-69
	Unit dose cartons of 100	0456-0458-63
60 mg (1 gr)	Bottles of 100	0456-0459-01
	Bottles of 1000	0456-0459-00
	Bottles of 5000	0456-0459-51
	Drums of 50,000	0456-0459-69
	Unit dose cartons of 100	0456-0459-63
90 mg (1 1/2 gr)	Bottles of 100	0456-0460-01
120 mg (2 gr)	Bottles of 100	0456-0461-01
	Bottles of 1000	0456-0461-00
	Drums of 50,000	0456-0461-69
180 mg (3 gr)	Bottles of 100	0456-0462-01
	Bottles of 1000	0456-0462-00
240 mg (4 gr)	Bottles of 100	0456-0463-01
300 mg (5 gr)	Bottles of 100	0456-0464-01

The bottles of 100 are special dispensing bottles with child-resistant closures.
Note: (T_3 liothyronine is approximately four times as potent as T_4 levothyroxine on a microgram for microgram basis.)
Tablets should be stored at controlled room temperature, 59°–86°F (15°–30°C), in capped bottles or unbroken plastic strip packing.
Shown in Product Identification Guide, page 310

CERVIDIL™ ℞
Brand of dinoprostone vaginal insert

DESCRIPTION
Dinoprostone vaginal insert is a thin, flat, polymeric slab which is rectangular in shape with rounded corners contained within the pouch of a knitted polyester retrieval system, an integral part of which is a long tape. Each slab is buff colored, semitransparent and contains 10 mg of dinoprostone. The hydrogel insert is contained within the pouch of an off-white knitted polyester retrieval system designed to aid retrieval at the end of the dosing interval. The finished product is a controlled release formulation which has been found to release dinoprostone *in vivo* at a rate of approximately 0.3 mg/hr.

The chemical name for dinoprostone (commonly known as prostaglandin E_2 or PGE_2) is 11α, 15S-dihydroxy-9-oxo-prosta-5Z, 13E-dien-1-oic acid and the structural formula is represented below:

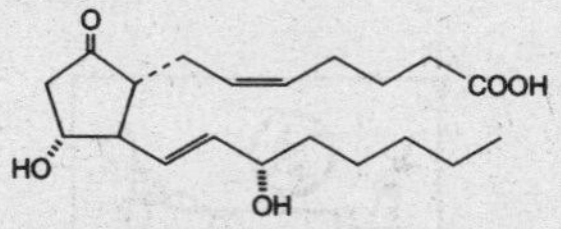

The molecular formula is $C_{20}H_{32}O_5$ and its molecular weight is 352.5. Dinoprostone occurs as a white to off-white crystalline powder. It has a melting point within the range of 65° to 69°C. Dinoprostone is soluble in ethanol and in 25% ethanol in water. Each insert contains 10 mg of dinoprostone in 236 mg of a cross-linked polyethylene oxide/urethane polymer which is a semi-opaque, beige colored, flat rectangular slab measuring 29 mm by 9.5 mm and 0.8 mm in thickness. The insert and its retrieval system, made of polyester yarn, are non-toxic and when placed in a moist environment, absorb water, swell, and release dinoprostone.

CLINICAL PHARMACOLOGY
Dinoprostone (PGE_2) is a naturally-occurring biomolecule. It is found in low concentrations in most tissues of the body and functions as a local hormone (1–3). As with any local hormone, it is very rapidly metabolized in the tissues of synthesis (the half-life estimated to be 2.5–5 minutes). The rate limiting step for inactivation is regulated by the enzyme 15-hydroxyprostaglandin dehydrogenase (PGDH) (1,4). Any PGE_2 that escapes local inactivation is rapidly cleared to the extent of 95% on the first pass through the pulmonary circulation (1,2).

In pregnancy, PGE_2 is secreted continuously by the fetal membranes and placenta and plays an important role in the final events leading to the initiation of labor (1,2). It is known that PGE_2 stimulates the production of $PGF_2\alpha$ which in turn sensitizes the myometrium to endogenous or exogenously administrated oxytocin. Although PGE_2 is capable of initiating uterine contractions and may interact with oxytocin to increase uterine contractility, the available evidence indicates that, in the concentrations found during the early part of labor, PGE_2 plays an important role in cervical ripening without affecting uterine contractions (5–7). This distinction serves as the basis for considering cervical ripening and induction of labor, usually by the use of oxytocin (8–10), as two separate processes.

PGE_2 plays an important role in the complex set of biochemical and structural alterations involved in cervical ripening. Cervical ripening involves a marked relaxation of the cervical smooth muscle fibers of the uterine cervix which must be transformed from a rigid structure to a softened, yielding and dilated configuration to allow passage of the fetus through the birth canal (11–13). This process involves activation of the enzyme collagenase, which is responsible for digestion of some of the structural collagen network of the cervix (1,14). This is associated with a concomitant increase in the amount of hydrophilic glycosaminoglycan, hyaluronic acid, and a decrease in dermatan sulfate (1). Failure of the cervix to undergo these natural physiologic changes, usually assessed by the method described by Bishop (15,16), prior to the onset of effective uterine contractions, results in an unfavorable outcome for successful vaginal delivery and may result in fetal compromise. It is estimated that in approximately 5% of pregnancies the cervix does not ripen normally (17). In an additional 10–11% of pregnancies, labor must be induced for medical or obstetric reasons prior to the time of cervical ripening (17).

The delivery rate of PGE_2 *in vivo* is about 0.3 mg/hour over a period of 12 hours. The controlled release of PGE_2 from the hydrogel insert is an attempt to provide sufficient quantities of PGE_2 to the local receptors to satisfy hormonal requirements. In the majority of patients, these local effects are manifested by changes in the consistency, dilatation and effacement of the cervix as measured by the Bishop score. Although some patients experience uterine hyperstimulation as a result of direct PGE_2- or $PGF_2\alpha$- mediated sensitization of the myometrium to oxytocin, systemic effects of PGE_2 are rarely encountered. The insert is fitted with a biocompatible retrieval system which facilitates removal at the conclusion of therapy or in the event of an adverse reaction.

No correlation could be established between PGE_2 release and plasma concentrations of PGE_m. The relative contributions of endogenously and exogenously released PGE_2 to the plasma levels of the metabolite PGE_m could not be determined. Moreover, it is uncertain as to whether the measured concentrations of PGE_m reflect the natural progression of PGE_m concentrations in blood as birth approaches or to what extent the measured concentrations following PGE_2 administration represent an increase over basal levels that might be measured in control patients.

INDICATIONS AND USAGE
Cervidil Vaginal Insert (dinoprostone, 10 mg) is indicated for the initiation and/or continuation of cervical ripening in patients at or near term in whom there is a medical or obstetrical indication for the induction of labor.

CONTRAINDICATIONS
Cervidil is contraindicated in:
- Patients with known hypersensitivity to prostaglandins.
- Patients in whom there is clinical suspicion or definite evidence of fetal distress where delivery is not imminent.
- Patients with unexplained vaginal bleeding during this pregnancy.
- Patients in whom there is evidence or strong suspicion of marked cephalopelvic disproportion.
- Patients in whom oxytocic drugs are contraindicated or when prolonged contraction of the uterus may be detrimental to fetal safety or uterine integrity (previous cesarean section or major uterine surgery).
- Patients already receiving intravenous oxytocic drugs.
- Multipara with 6 or more previous term pregnancies.

WARNINGS

For hospital use only

Cervidil should be administered only by trained obstetrical personnel in a hospital setting with appropriate obstetrical care facilities.

PRECAUTIONS

1. **General Precautions:** Since prostaglandins potentiate the effect of oxytocin, Cervidil must be removed before oxytocin administration is initiated and the patient's uterine activity carefully monitored for uterine hyperstimulation. If uterine hyperstimulation is encountered or if labor commences, the vaginal insert should be removed. Cervidil should also be removed prior to amniotomy.

   Caution should be exercised in the administration of Cervidil for cervical ripening in patients with ruptured membranes, in cases of non-vertex, or non-singleton presentation, and in patients with a history of previous uterine hypertony, glaucoma, or a history of childhood asthma, even though there have been no asthma attacks in adulthood.

   Uterine activity, fetal status and the progression of cervical dilatation and effacement should be carefully monitored whenever the dinoprostone vaginal insert is in place. Any evidence of uterine hyperstimulation, sustained uterine contractions, fetal distress, or other fetal or maternal adverse reactions, should be a cause for consideration of removal of the insert.

2. **Drug Interactions:** Cervidil may augment the activity of oxytocic agents and their concomitant use is not recommended. A dosing interval of at least 30 minutes is recommended for the sequential use of oxytocin following the removal of the dinoprostone vaginal insert. No other drug interactions have been identified.

3. **Carcinogenesis, Mutagenesis, Impairment of Fertility:** Long-term carcinogenicity and fertility studies have not been conducted with Cervidil (dinoprostone) Vaginal Insert. No evidence of mutagenicity has been observed with prostaglandin E_2 in the Unscheduled DNA Synthesis Assay, the Micronucleus Test, or Ames Assay.

4. **Pregnancy, Teratogenic Effects:**

   Pregnancy Category C:

   Prostaglandin E_2 has produced an increase in skeletal anomalies in rats and rabbits. No effect would be expected clinically, when used as indicated, since Cervidil (dinoprostone) Vaginal Insert is administered after the period of organogenesis. Prostaglandin E_2 has been shown to be embryotoxic in rats and rabbits, and any dose that produces sustained increased uterine tone could put the embryo or fetus at risk.

ADVERSE REACTIONS

Cervidil is well tolerated. In placebo-controlled trials in which 658 women were entered and 320 received active therapy (218 without retrieval system, 102 with retrieval system), the following events were reported.
[See Table 1 above.]

Drug related fever, nausea, vomiting, diarrhea, and abdominal pain were noted in less than 1% of patients who received Cervidil.

In study 101–801 (with the retrieval system) cases of hyperstimulation reversed within 2 to 13 minutes of removal of the product. Tocolytics were required in one of the five cases.

In cases of fetal distress, when product removal was thought advisable there was a return to normal rhythm and no neonatal sequelae.

Five minute Apgar scores were 7 or above in 98.2% (646/658) of studied neonates whose mothers received Cervidil. In a report of a 3 year pediatric follow-up study in 121 infants, 51 of whose mothers received Cervidil, there were no deleterious effects on physical examination or psychomotor evaluation (18).

DRUG ABUSE AND DEPENDENCE

No drug abuse or dependence has been seen with the use of the Cervidil.

OVERDOSAGE

Cervidil is used as a single dosage in a single application. Overdosage is usually manifested by uterine hyperstimulation which may be accompanied by fetal distress and is responsive to removal of the insert. Other treatment must be symptomatic since, to date, clinical experience with prostaglandin antagonists is insufficient.

The use of beta-adrenergic agents should be considered in the event of undesirable increased uterine activity.

DOSAGE AND ADMINISTRATION

The dosage of dinoprostone in the vaginal insert is 10 mg designed to be released at approximately 0.3 mg/hour over a 12 hour period. Cervidil should be removed upon onset of active labor or 12 hours after insertion.

One Cervidil is placed transversely in the posterior fornix of the vagina immediately after removal from its foil package. The insertion of the vaginal insert does not require sterile conditions. The vaginal insert must not be used without its retrieval system. There is no need for previous warming of the product. A minimal amount of K-Y® jelly (or other water-miscible lubricant) may be used to assist in insertion of Cervidil. Care should be taken not to permit excess contact or coating with the lubricant and thus prevent optimal swelling and release of dinoprostone from the vaginal insert. Patients should remain in the supine position for 2 hours following insertion, but thereafter may be ambulatory.

HOW SUPPLIED

Cervidil (NDC 0456-4123-63) contains 10 mg dinoprostone. The product is wound and enclosed in an aluminum sleeve which is contained in an aluminum/polyethylene pack.

Store in a freezer: between $-20°C$ and $-10°C$ ($-4°F$ and $14°F$). Cervidil is packed in foil and is stable when stored in a freezer for a period of three years. Vaginal inserts exposed to high humidity will absorb moisture from the air and thereby alter the release characteristics of dinoprostone. Once used, the vaginal insert should be discarded.

Caution: Federal law prohibits dispensing without prescription.

CLINICAL STUDIES

[See Table 2 below.]

REFERENCES

1. Physiology of Labor. In: Williams Obstetrics. Eds. Pritchard, J.A., MacDonald, P.C., and Gant, N.F. Appleton-Century-Crofts, Conn, Pp 295-321, (1985).
2. Rall, T.W. and Schliefer, L.S. Oxytocin, prostaglandin, ergot alkaloids, and other drugs; tocolytics agents, In: The Pharmacological Basis of Therapeutics. Eds. Gilman, A.G., Goodman, L.S., Rall, T.W., and Murad, F. MacMillan Publ. Co., New York, Pp. 926-945, (1985).
3. Casey, M.L. and MacDonald, P.C. The initiation of labor in women: Regulation of phospholipid and arachidonic acid metabolism and of prostaglandin production. Semin. Perinat. 10: 270-275, (1986).
4. Casey, M.L., MacDonald, P.C. and Mitchell, M.D. Stimulation of prostaglandin E_2 production in amnion cells in culture by a substance(s) in human fetal urine. Biochem. Biophys. Res. Comm. 114:1056, (1983).
5. Olson, C.M., Lye, S.J., Skinner, K., and Challis, J.R.G. Prostanoid concentrations in maternal/fetal plasma and amniotic fluid and intrauterine tissue prostanoid output in relation to myometrial contractility during the onset of Endocrinology. 116: 389-397, (1985).
6. Ledger, W.L., Ellwood, D.A., and Taylor, M.J. Cervical softening in late pregnant sheep by infusion of prostaglandin E-2 into cervical artery. J. Reprod. Fert. 69, 511-515, (1983).
7. Olson, D.M., Lye, S.J., Skinner, K., and Challis, J.R.G. Early changes in prostaglandin concentrations in ovine maternal and fetal plasma, amniotic fluid and from dispersed cells of intrauterine tissues before the onset of ACTH-induced pre-term labor. J. Reprod. Fert. 71: 45-55, (1984).
8. Caldero-Garcia, R. and Posiero, J. Oxytocin and the contractility of the human uterus, Ann, N.Y. Acad. Sci. 75:813, (1959).
9. Posiero, J. and Noriega-Guerra, L. Dose-response relationships in uterine effects of oxytocin infusion. Oxytocin. Eds., Caldero-Garcia, R. and Heller, J. Pergamon Press, New York, (1961).
10. Cibils, L. Enhancement of induction of labor. In: Risks in the Practice of Modern Obstetrics. Aldjem, S. Ed. Mosby Publishing, St. Louis, (1972).
11. Bryman, I., Lindblom, B., and Norstrom, A. Extreme sensitivity of cervical musculature to prostaglandin E_2 in early pregnancy. Lancet, 2:1471, (1982).
12. Thiery, M. Induction of labor with prostaglandins. In: Human Parturition. Eds. Keirse, M.J.N.C., Anderson, A.B.M.; and Gravenhorst, J.B. Martinus Nijhoff Publ., Boston, 155-164, (1979).
13. Thiery, M. and Amy, J.J. Induction of labor with prostaglandins. In:Advances in Prostaglandin Research. Prostaglandin and Reproduction. Karim, S.M.M., Ed., MTP, Lancaster, Pp. 149-228, (1975).
14. MacLennan, A.H., Katz, M., and Creasey, R. The morphologic characteristics of cervical ripening induced by the hormones relaxin and prostaglandin F_2 in a rabbit model. Am. J. Obstet. Gynecol, 152: 910696, (1985).
15. Bishop, E. Elective induction of labor. Obstet. & Gynecol. 5: 519-527, (1955).
16. Bishop, E. Pelvic scoring for elective induction. Obstet. & Gynecol.24: 266-268. (1969).
17. Thiery, M. Preinduction cervical ripening. In: Obstetrics and Gynecology Annual, Vol. 12 Ed. Wynn, R.M. Appleton-Century-Crofts, New York, Pp. 103-146, (1983).
18. MacKenzie, I.; Information on File: Controlled Therapeutics (Scotland).

Mfg by:
Controlled Therapeutics
East Kilbride, Scotland G74 5PB

Made in the U.K.

Distributed by:
FOREST PHARMACEUTICALS, INC.
Subsidiary of Forest Laboratories, Inc.
St. Louis, MO 63045 USA

RMS 311
Rev. 12/95
SAP 226

Shown in Product Identification Section, page 311

Table 1
Total Cervidil-Treated Drug Related Adverse Events

	Controlled Studies[1]		STUDY 101–801[2]	
	Active	Placebo	Active	Placebo
Uterine hyperstimulation with fetal distress	2.8%	0.3%	2.9%	0%
Uterine hyperstimulation without fetal distress	4.7%	0%	2.0%	0%
Fetal Distress without uterine hyperstimulation	3.8%	1.2%	2.9%	1.0%
N	320	338	102	104

[1] Controlled Studies (with and without retrieval system)
[2] Controlled Study (with retrieval system)

Table 2
Efficacy of Cervidil in Double Blind Studies

Parameter	Study #	Primip/Nullip		Multip		P-Value
		Cervidil	Placebo	Cervidil	Placebo	
Treatment	101–103 (N=81)	65%	28%	87%	29%	<0.001
Success*	101–003 (N=371)	68%	24%	77%	24%	<0.001
	101–801 (N=206)	72%	48%	55%	41%	0.003
Time to Delivery (hours)						
Average	101–103 (N=81)	33.7	48.6	14.0	28.6	
Median		25.7	34.5	12.3	24.6	0.001
Average	101–801 (N=206)	31.1	51.8	52.3	45.9	
Median		25.5	37.2	20.8	27.4	<0.001
Time to Onset of Labor (hours)						
Average	101–103 (N=81)	19.9	39.4	6.8	22.4	
Median		12.0	19.2	6.9	18.3	<0.001

*Treatment success was defined as Bishop score increase at 12 hours of ≥ 3, vaginal delivery within 12 hours or Bishop score at 12 hours ≥6. These studies were not designed with the power to show differences in cesarean section rates between Cervidil and placebo groups and none were noted.

DALALONE D.P.® ℞
(Sterile Dexamethasone Acetate Suspension, USP)
Equivalent to Dexamethasone 16 mg/mL

PRODUCT OVERVIEW

KEY FACTS

Dalalone D.P. injection is a synthetic, long-acting, repository adrenocorticosteroid agent that provides a prompt onset of

Continued on next page

Forest—Cont.

action. Each ml of suspension contains Dexamethasone Acetate equivalent to 16 mg of dexamethasone. It may be administered via intramuscular, intra-articular, or soft tissue injection, but must not be given intravenously or intralesionally.

MAJOR USES

Dexamethasone, a fluorinated derivative of prednisolone, is used primarily for its potent anti-inflammatory effects in disorders of many organ systems and other diseases responsive to glucocorticosteroids. At equipotent anti-inflammatory doses, dexamethasone almost lacks the sodium-retaining property of hydrocortisone.

SAFETY INFORMATION

Contraindicated in patients with systemic fungal infections. Corticosteroids can mask signs of existing or new infection. Repeated injections at the same site are to be avoided, as are subcutaneous injections, and injections into the deltoid muscle.

PRESCRIBING INFORMATION

DALALONE D.P.® ℞
(Sterile Dexamethasone Acetate Suspension, USP)
Equivalent to Dexamethasone 16 mg/mL

NOT FOR INTRAVENOUS OR INTRALESIONAL USE
FOR INTRAMUSCULAR, INTRA-ARTICULAR AND
SOFT TISSUE USE

DESCRIPTION

Dexamethasone acetate, a synthetic adrenocortical steroid, is a white to practically white, odorless powder. It is a practically insoluble ester of dexamethasone. The structural formula is

Dexamethasone acetate is present in sterile dexamethasone acetate suspension as the monohydrate, with the molecular formula, $C_{24}H_{31}FO_6 \cdot H_2O$, and molecular weight, 452.52. Dexamethasone acetate is designated chemically as 21-(acetyloxy)-9-fluoro-11β,17-dihydroxy-16α-methylpregna-1,4-diene-3,20-dione.

Sterile Dexamethasone Acetate suspension is a sterile white suspension (pH 5.0 to 7.5) that settles on standing, but is easily resuspended by mild shaking.

Each ml. contains: Dexamethasone Acetate equivalent to Dexamethasone 16 mg.
6.67 mg. Sodium Chloride
5 mg. Creatinine
0.5 mg Edetate Disodium
5 mg Carboxymethylcellulose Sodium
0.75 mg Polysorbate 80
1 mg Sodium Bisulfite
9 mg Benzyl Alcohol
as preservatives in Water for Injection q.s., Sodium Hydroxide may have been used to adjust pH.

CLINICAL PHARMACOLOGY

Sterile Dexamethasone Acetate suspension is a long-acting, repository adrenocorticosteroid preparation with a prompt onset of action. It is suitable for intramuscular or local injection, but not when an immediate effect of short duration is desired.

Naturally occurring glucocorticoids (hydrocortisone and cortisone), which also have salt-retaining properties, are used as replacement therapy in adrenocortical deficiency states. Their synthetic analogs, including dexamethasone, are primarily used for their potent anti-inflammatory effects in disorders of many organ systems.

Glucocorticoids cause profound and varied metabolic effects. In addition, they modify the body's immune responses to diverse stimuli.

At equipotent anti-inflammatory doses, dexamethasone almost completely lacks the sodium-retaining property of hydrocortisone.

INDICATIONS AND USAGE

A. By intramuscular injection when oral therapy is not feasible:

1. Endocrine disorders
Congenital adrenal hyperplasia
Nonsuppurative thyroiditis
Hypercalcemia associated with cancer

2. Rheumatic disorders
As adjunctive therapy for short-term administration (to tide the patient over an acute episode or exacerbation) in:
Post-traumatic osteoarthritis
Synovitis of osteoarthritis
Rheumatoid arthritis, including juvenile rheumatoid arthritis (selected cases may require low-dose maintenance therapy).
Acute and subacute bursitis
Epicondylitis
Acute nonspecific tenosynovitis
Acute gouty arthritis
Psoriatic arthritis
Ankylosing spondylitis

3. Collagen diseases
During an exacerbation or as maintenance therapy in selected cases of:
Systemic lupus erythematosus
Acute rheumatic carditis

4. Dermatologic diseases
Pemphigus
Severe erythema multiforme (Stevens-Johnson syndrome)
Exfoliative dermatitis
Bullous dermatitis herpetiformis
Severe seborrheic dermatitis
Severe psoriasis
Mycosis fungoides.

5. Allergic states
Control of severe or incapacitating allergic conditions intractable to adequate trials of conventional treatment in:
Bronchial asthma
Contact dermatitis
Atopic dermatitis
Serum sickness
Seasonal or perennial allergic rhinitis
Drug hypersensitivity reactions
Urticarial transfusion reactions

6. Ophthalmic diseases
Severe acute and chronic allergic and inflammatory processes involving the eye, such as:
Herpes zoster ophthalmicus
Iritis, Iridocyclitis
Chorioretinitis
Diffuse posterior uveitis and choroiditis
Optic neuritis
Sympathetic ophthalmia
Anterior segment inflammation
Allergic conjunctivitis
Keratitis
Allergic corneal marginal ulcers

7. Gastrointestinal diseases
To tide the patient over a critical period of disease in:
Ulcerative colitis—(Systemic therapy)
Regional enteritis—(Systemic therapy)

8. Respiratory diseases
Symptomatic sarcoidosis
Berylliosis
Loeffler's syndrome not manageable by other means.
Aspiration pneumonitis

9. Hematologic disorders
Acquired (autoimmune) hemolytic anemia
Secondary thrombocytopenia in adults
Erythroblastopenia (RBC anemia)
Congenital (erythroid) hypoplastic anemia.

10. Neoplastic diseases
For palliative management of leukemias and lymphomas in adults
Acute leukemia of childhood.

11. Edematous state
To induce diuresis or remission of proteinuria in the nephrotic syndrome without uremia, of the idiopathic type, or that due to lupus erythematosus.

12. Miscellaneous
Trichinosis with neurologic or myocardial involvement

B. By intra-articular or soft tissue injection as adjunctive therapy for short-term administration (to tide the patient over an acute episode of exacerbation) in:
Synovitis of osteoarthritis
Rheumatoid arthritis
Acute and subacute bursitis
Acute gouty arthritis
Epicondylitis
Acute nonspecific tenosynovitis
Post-traumatic osteoarthritis

CONTRAINDICATION

Systemic fungal infections.
Hypersensitivity to any component of this product, including sulfites (see WARNINGS)

WARNINGS

Do Not Inject Intravenously or Intralesionally.

Because rare instances of anaphylactoid reactions have occurred in patients receiving parenteral corticosteroid therapy, appropriate precautionary measures should be taken prior to administration, especially when the patient has a

history of allergy to any drug. Anaphylactoid and hypersensitivity reactions have been reported for sterile dexamethasone acetate suspension (See ADVERSE REACTIONS).

Sterile dexamethasone acetate suspension contains Sodium Bisulfite, a sulfite that may cause allergic-type reactions including anaphylactic symptoms and life-threatening or less severe asthmatic episodes in certain susceptible people. The overall prevalence of sulfite sensitivity in the general population is unknown and probably low. Sulfite sensitivity is seen more frequently in asthmatic than in nonasthmatic people.

In patients on corticosteroid therapy subjected to any unusual stress, increased dosage of rapidly acting corticosteroids before, during, and after the stressful situation is indicated.

Drug-induced secondary adrenocortical insufficiency may result from too rapid withdrawal of corticosteroids and may be minimized by gradual reduction of dosage. This type of relative insufficiency may persist for months after discontinuation of therapy; therefore, in any situation of stress occurring during that period, hormone therapy should be reinstituted. If the patient is receiving steroids already, dosage may have to be increased. Since mineralocorticoid secretion may be impaired, salt and/or a mineralocorticoid should be administered concurrently.

Corticosteroids may mask some signs of infection, and new infections may appear during their use. There may be decreased resistance and inability to localize infection when corticosteroids are used. Moreover, corticosteroids may affect the nitroblue-tetrazolium test for bacterial infectin and produce false negative results.

In cerebral malaria, a double-blind trial has shown that the use of corticosteroids is associated with prolongation of coma and a higher incidence of pneumonia and gastrointestinal bleeding.

Corticosteroids may activate latent amebiasis. Therefore, it is recommended that latent or active amebiasis be ruled out before initiating corticosteroid therapy in any patient who has spent time in the tropics or any patient with unexplained diarrhea.

Prolonged use of corticosteroids may produce posterior subcapsular cataracts, glaucoma with possible damage to the optic nerves, and may enhance the establishment of secondary ocular infections due to fungi or viruses.

Average and large doses of cortisone or hydrocortisone can cause elevation in blood pressure, salt and water retention, and increased excretion of potassium. These effects are less likely to occur with the synthetic derivatives except when used in large doses. Dietary salt restriction and potassium supplementation may be necessary. All corticosteroids increase calcium excretion.

Administration of live virus vaccines, including smallpox, is contraindicated in individuals receiving immunosuppressive doses of corticosteroids. If inactivated viral or bacterial vaccines are administered to individuals receiving immunosuppressive doses of corticosteroids, the expected serum antibody response may not be obtained.

Persons who are on drugs which suppress the immune system are more susceptible to infections than healthy individuals. Chickenpox and measles, for example, can have a more serious or even fatal course in non-immune children or adults on corticosteroids. In such children or adults who have not had these diseases, particular care should be taken to avoid exposure. How the dose, route and duration of corticosteroid administration affects the risk of developing a disseminated infection is not known. The contribution of the underlying disease and/or prior corticosteroid treatment to the risk is also not known. If exposed to chickenpox, prophylaxis with varicella zoster immune globulin (VZIG) may be indicated. If exposed to measles, prophylaxis with pooled intramuscular immunoglobulin (IG) may be indicated. (See the respective package inserts for complete VZIG and IG prescribing information). If chickenpox develops, treatment with antiviral agents may be considered.

If corticosteroids are indicated in patients with latent tuberculosis or tuberculin reactivity, close observation is necessary as reactivation of the disease may occur. During prolonged corticosteroid therapy, these patients should receive chemoprophylaxis.

Repository adrenocorticosteroid preparations may cause atrophy at the site of injection. To minimize the likelihood and/or severity of atrophy, do not inject subcutaneously, avoid injection into the deltoid muscle, and avoid repeated intramusuclar injections into the same site if possible.

Dosage in children under 12 has not been established.

Literature reports suggest an apparent association between use of corticosteroids and left ventricular free wall rupture after a recent myocardial infarction; therefore, therapy with corticosteroids should be used with great caution in these patients.

Usage in pregnancy: Since adequate human reproduction studies have not been done with corticosteroids, use of these drugs in pregnancy, or in women of childbearing potential requires that the anticipated benefits be weighed against the possible hazards to the mother and embryo or fetus. Infants born of mothers who have received substantial doses of corti-

costeroids during pregnancy should be carefully observed for signs of hypoadrenalism.

Corticosteroids appear in breast milk and could suppress growth interfere with endogenous corticosteroids production, or cause other unwanted effects. Mothers taking pharmacologic doses of corticosteroids should be advised not to nurse.

PRECAUTIONS

General: Sterile dexamethasone acetate suspension is not recommended as initial therapy in acute, life-threatening situations.

This product, like many other steroid formulations, is sensitive to heat. Therefore, it should not be autoclaved when it is desirable to sterilize the exterior of the vial.

Following prolonged therapy, withdrawal of corticosteroids may result in symptoms of the corticosteroid withdrawal syndrome including fever, myalgia, arthralgia, and malaise. This may occur in patients even without evidence of adrenal insufficiency.

There is an enhanced effect of corticosteroids in patients with hypothyroidism and in those with cirrhosis.

Corticosteroids should be used cautiously in patients with ocular herpes simplex for fear of corneal perforation.

Psychic derangements may appear when corticosteroids are used, ranging from euphoria, insomnia, mood swings, personality changes, and severe depression to frank psychotic manifestation. Also, existing emotional instability or psychotic tendencies may be aggravated by corticosteroids.

Aspirin should be used cautiously in conjunction with corticosteroids in hypoprothrombinemia.

Steroids should be used with caution in nonspecific ulcerative colitis, if there is a probability of impending perforation, abscess or other pyogenic infection, also in diverticulitis, fresh intestinal anastomoses, active or latent peptic ulcer, renal insufficiency, hypertension, osteoporosis, and myasthenia gravis. Signs of peritoneal irritation following gastrointestinal perforation in patients receiving large doses of corticosteroids may be minimal or absent. Fat embolism has been reported as a possible complication of hypercortisonism.

When large doses are given, some authorities advise that antacids be administered between meals to help prevent peptic ulcer.

Growth and development of infants and children on prolonged corticosteroid therapy should be carefully followed. Steroids may increase or decrease motility and number of spermatozoa in some patients.

Phenytoin, phenobarbital, ephedrine, and rifampin may enhance the metabolic clearance of corticosteroids, resulting in decreased blood levels and lessened physiologic activity, thus requiring adjustment in corticosteroid dosage.

The prothrombin time should be checked frequently in patients who are receiving corticosteroids and coumarin anticoagulants at the same time because of reports that corticosteroids have altered the response to these anticoagulants. Studies have shown that the usual effect produced by adding corticosteroids is inhibition of response to coumarins, although there have been some conflicting reports of potentiation not substantiated by studies.

When corticosteroids are administered concomitantly with potassium-depleting diuretics, patients should be observed closely for development of hypokalemia.

Intra-articular injection of a corticosteroid may produce systemic as well as local effects.

Appropriate examination of any joint fluid present necessary to exclude a septic process.

A marked increase in pain accompanied by local swelling, further restriction of joint motion, fever, and malaise are suggestive of septic arthritis. If this complication occurs and the diagnosis of sepsis is confirmed, appropriate antimicrobial therapy should be instituted.

Injection of a steroid into an infected site is to be avoided. Corticosteroids should not be injected into unstable joints. Patients should be impressed strongly with the importance of not over-using joints in which symptomatic benefit has been obtained as long as the inflammatory process remains active.

Frequent intra-articular injection may result in damage to joint tissues.

Information for Patients: Persons who are on immunosuppressant doses of corticosteroids should be warned to avoid exposure to chickenpox or measles. Patients should also be advised that if they are exposed, medical advice should be sought without delay.

ADVERSE REACTIONS

Fluid and electrolyte disturbances:
Sodium retention
Fluid retention
Congestive heart failure in susceptible patients
Potassium loss
Hypokalemic alkalosis
Hypertension
Musculoskeletal:
Muscle weakness

Steroid myopathy
Loss of muscle mass
Osteoporosis
Vertebral compression fractures
Aseptic necrosis of femoral and humeral heads
Pathologic fracture of long bones
Tendon Rupture
Gastrointestinal:
Peptic ulcer with possible subsequent perforation and hemorrhage
Perforation of the small and large bowel, particularly in patients with inflammatory bowel disease
Pancreatitis
Abdominal distention
Ulcerative esophagitis
Dermatologic:
Impaired wound healing
Thin fragile skin
Petechiae and ecchymoses
Erythema
Increased sweating
may suppress reactions to skin test
Other cutaneous reactions, such as allergic dermatitis, urticaria, angioneurotic edema
Neurologic:
Convulsions
Increased intracranial pressure with papilledema (pseudotumor cerebri) usually after treatment
Vertigo
Headache
Psychic disturbances
Endocrine:
Menstrual irregularities
Development of cushingoid state
Suppression of growth in children
Secondary adrenocortical and pituitary unresponsiveness, particularly in times of stress, as in trauma, surgery or illness
Decreased carbohydrate tolerance
Manifestations of latent diabetes mellitus
Increased requirements for insulin or oral hypoglycemic agents in diabetics
Hirsutism
Ophthalmic:
Posterior subcapsular cataracts
Increased intraocular pressure
Glaucoma
Exophthalmos
Metabolic:
Negative nitrogen balance due to protein catabolism
Cardiovascular:
Myocardial rupture following recent myocardial infarction (see WARNINGS)
Other:
Anaphylactoid or hypersensitivity reactions
Thromboembolism
Weight gain
Increased appetite
Nausea
Malaise
The following **additional** adverse reactions are related to parenteral corticosteroid therapy:
Rare instances of blindness associated with intralesional therapy around the face and head
Hyperpigmentation or hypopigmentation
Subcutaneous and cutaneous atrophy
Sterile abscess
Postinjection flare (following intra-articular use)
Charcot-like arthropathy
Scarring
Induration
Inflammation
Paresthesia
Delayed pain or soreness
Muscle twitching, ataxia, hiccups, and nystagmus have been reported in low incidence after injection of sterile Dexamethasone Acetate suspension

DRUG ABUSE AND DEPENDENCE

(See WARNINGS section).

OVERDOSAGE

Reports of acute toxicity and/or death following overdosage of glucocorticoids are rare. In the event of overdosage, no specific antidote is available; treatment is supportive and symptomatic.

The intraperitoneal LD_{50} of dexamethasone acetate in female mice was 424 mg/kg.

DOSAGE AND ADMINISTRATION

For intramuscular, intra-articular, and soft tissue injection.

Dosage Requirements Are Variable and Must Be Individualized on the Basis of the Disease Under Treatment and the Response of the Patient.

Dosage in children under 12 has not been established.

Intramuscular Injection
Dosage ranges from 0.5 to 1 mL, equivalent to 8 to 16 mg of dexamethasone. If further treatment is needed, dosage may be repeated at intervals of 1 to 3 weeks.
Intra-articular and Soft Tissue Injection
The dose varies, depending on the location and the severity of inflammation. The usual dose is 0.25 to 1 mL, equivalent to 4 to 16 mg of Dexamethasone. If further treatment is needed, dosage may be repeated at intervals of 1 to 3 weeks. Frequent intra-articular injection may result in damage to joint tissues.

Parenteral drug products should be inspected visually for particulate matter and discoloration prior to administration, whenever the solution and container permit.

HOW SUPPLIED

Sterile dexamethasone acetate suspension, equivalent to dexamethasone 16 mg/mL is available in:
1 mL vials, individually boxed;
5 mL multiple dose vials, individually boxed.
NDC 0456-1097-41
NDC 0456-1097-05
STORE AT CONTROLLED ROOM TEMPERATURE 15°–30° C (59°–86° F). DO NOT PERMIT TO FREEZE. SENSITIVE TO HEAT—DO NOT AUTOCLAVE. SHAKE WELL BEFORE USING.
PROTECT FROM LIGHT. Store in carton until contents are used.

CAUTION

Federal law prohibits dispensing without prescription.
Literature Revised: August 1994
Product No. 0669-01, 0669-05.
**Mfd. for
FOREST PHARMACEUTICALS, INC.
SUBSIDIARY OF FOREST LABORATORIES, INC.
ST. LOUIS, MISSOURI 63045**

ELIXOPHYLLIN® ℞
(theophylline anhydrous)
Elixir

DESCRIPTION

Elixophyllin® (theophylline anhydrous) Elixir
ELIXOPHYLLIN Elixir is available as a liquid intended for oral administration, containing 80 mg of theophylline anhydrous and 20% alcohol in each 15 mL (tablespoonful).
ELIXOPHYLLIN Elixir also contains the following inactive ingredients: citric acid, FD&C Red #40, flavoring agent, glycerin, saccharin sodium and purified water. Elixophyllin Elixir has a pH of 3.0–4.0.
Theophylline is a bronchodilator structurally classified as a xanthine derivative. It occurs as a white, odorless, crystalline powder having a bitter taste. Theophylline anhydrous has the chemical name, 1H- Purine-2, 6-dione, 3,7-dihydro-1,3-dimethyl-.

HOW SUPPLIED

ELIXOPHYLLIN® Elixir is a clear red solution with a mixed fruit flavor. Each tablespoonful (15 mL) contains 80 mg anhydrous theophylline.
ELIXOPHYLLIN® Elixir is available in bottles of
473 mL	NDC 0456-0644-16
946 mL	NDC 0456-0644-32
3785 mL	NDC 0456-0644-28

ELIXOPHYLLIN®–GG ℞
[ē "lix-off'fil-in gēē-gēē]
(theophylline-guaifenesin)
ORAL LIQUID

DESCRIPTION

Each 15 mL (tablespoonful) of ELIXOPHYLLIN®–GG (brand of theophylline-guaifenesin) Oral Liquid contains 100 mg anhydrous theophylline and 100 mg guaifenesin (glyceryl guaiacolate) in a cherry-berry flavored non-alcoholic liquid. ELIXOPHYLLIN®–GG Oral Liquid contains no sugar or dye.
Theophylline, a xanthine bronchodilator, is a white, odorless, crystalline powder having a bitter taste. Guaifenesin, a guaiacol compound is a white to slightly yellow crystalline powder with a bitter, aromatic taste.

HOW SUPPLIED

ELIXOPHYLLIN®–GG Oral Liquid is a clear, colorless, cherry-berry flavored non-alcoholic liquid. Each tablespoonful (15 mL) contains 100 mg anhydrous theophylline and 100 mg guaifenesin.
ELIXOPHYLLIN®–GG Oral Liquid is available in bottles of:
237 mL	NDC 0456-0648-08
473 mL	NDC 0456-0648-16

Continued on next page

Forest—Cont.

ELIXOPHYLLIN-KI® ℞
(brand of theophylline anhydrous
and potassium iodide)
Elixir

DESCRIPTION
Each 15 mL (tablespoonful) of ELIXOPHYLLIN-KI® (brand of theophylline anhydrous and potassium iodide) Elixir contains 80 mg anhydrous theophylline and 130 mg potassium iodide.

HOW SUPPLIED
ELIXOPHYLLIN-KI® Elixir is a clear yellowish amber solution with an anise aroma. Each tablespoonful (15 mL) contains 80 mg anhydrous theophylline and 130 mg potassium iodide.
ELIXOPHYLLIN-KI® Elixir is available in bottles of:
237 mL .... NDC 0456-0645-08

ENDAL™-HD Ⓒ ℞
[én dăl-HD]

DESCRIPTION
Each 5mL contains:
Hydrocodone Bitartrate .... 1.67 mg
  (WARNING: May Be Habit Forming)
Phenylephrine Hydrochloride .... 5 mg
Chlorpheniramine Maleate .... 2 mg

HOW SUPPLIED
Endal-HD is supplied in bottles of one pint (473 mL) NDC# 0785-6200-16.

ESGIC® Capsules ℞
[es'jik]
(Butalbital, Acetaminophen and Caffeine Capsules, USP)
50 mg/325 mg/40 mg

Shown in Product Identification Guide, page 311

ESGIC® Tablets ℞
(Butalbital, Acetaminophen and Caffeine Tablets, USP)
50 mg/325 mg/40 mg

ESGIC-PLUS™ ℞
CAPSULES AND TABLETS
Butalbital, Acetaminophen and Caffeine Capsules
and Tablets USP 50 mg/500 mg/40 mg

DESCRIPTION
Butalbial, acetaminophen and caffeine is supplied in capsule or tablet form for oral administration.
Butalbital (5-allyl-5-isobutylbarbituric acid), a slightly bitter, white, odorless, crystalline powder, is a short to intermediate-acting barbiturate. It has the following structural formula:

$C_{11}H_{16}N_2O_3$ MW=224.26

Acetaminophen (4'-hydroxyacetanilide), a slightly bitter, white, odorless, crystalline powder, is a non-opiate, non-salicylate analgesic and antipyretic. It has the following structural formula:

$C_8H_9NO_2$ MW=151.16

Caffeine (1,3,7-trimethylxanthine), a bitter, white powder or white-glistening needles, is a central nervous system stimulant. It has the following structural formula:
[See chemical structure at top of next column.]

$C_8H_{10}N_4O_2$ MW=194.19

Each capsule/tablet contains:
Butalbital .... 50 mg
WARNING: May be habit forming
Acetaminophen .... 500 mg
Caffeine .... 40 mg
In addition each capsule contains the following inactive ingredients: colloidal silicon dioxide, croscarmellose sodium, magnesium stearate and microcrystalline cellulose. Capsule shell composed of gelatin, titanium dioxide, D & C Red #33, D & C Yellow #10 and FD & C Red #3. Imprinting ink composed of ammonium hydroxide, dimethylpolysiloxane, isopropyl alcohol, n-butyl alcohol, pharmaceutical glaze, propylene glycol, and titanium dioxide.
In addition each tablet contains the following inactive ingredients: microcrystalline cellulose, croscarmellose sodium, colloidal silicon dioxide and stearic acid.

CLINICAL PHARMACOLOGY
This combination drug product is intended as a treatment for tension headache.
It consists of a fixed combination of butalbital, acetaminophen and caffeine. The role each component plays in the relief of the complex of symptoms known as tension headache is incompletely understood.
Pharmacokinetics: The behavior of the individual components is described below.
Butalbital: Butalbital is well absorbed from the gastrointestinal tract and is expected to distribute to most tissues in the body. Barbiturates in general may appear in breast milk and readily cross the placental barrier. They are bound to plasma and tissue proteins to a varying degree and binding increases directly as a function of lipid solubility.
Elimination of butalbital is primarily via the kidney (59% to 88% of the dose) as unchanged drug or metabolites. The plasma half-life is about 35 hours. Urinary excretion products include parent drug (about 3.6% of the dose), 5-isobutyl-5-(2,3-dihydroxypropyl) barbituric acid (about 24% of the dose), 5-allyl-5(3-hydroxy-2-methyl-1-propyl) barbituric acid (about 4.8% of the dose), products with the barbituric acid ring hydrolyzed with excretion of urea (about 14% of the dose), as well as unidentified materials. Of the materials excreted in the urine, 32% is conjugated.
See **OVERDOSAGE** for toxicity information.
Acetaminophen: Acetaminophen is rapidly absorbed from the gastrointestinal tract and is distributed throughout most body tissues. The plasma half-life is 1.25 to 3 hours, but may be increased by liver damage and following overdosage. Elimination of acetaminophen is principally by liver metabolism (conjugation) and subsequent renal excretion of metabolites. Approximately 85% of an oral dose appears in the urine within 24 hours of administration, most as the glucuronide conjugate, with small amounts of other conjugates and unchanged drug.
See **OVERDOSAGE** for toxicity information.
Caffeine: Like most xanthines, caffeine is rapidly absorbed and distributed in all body tissues and fluids, including the CNS, fetal tissues, and breast milk.
Caffeine is cleared through metabolism and excretion in the urine. The plasma half-life is about 3 hours. Hepatic biotransformation prior to excretion, results in about equal amounts of 1-methylxanthine and 1-methyluric acid. Of the 70% of the dose that is recovered in the urine, only 3% is unchanged drug.
See **OVERDOSAGE** for toxicity information.

INDICATIONS AND USAGE
Butalbital, acetaminophen and caffeine capsules/tablets are indicated for the relief of the symptom complex of tension (or muscle contraction) headache.
Evidence supporting the efficacy and safety of this combination product in the treatment of multiple recurrent headaches is unavailable. Caution in this regard is required because butalbital is habit-forming and potentially abusable.

CONTRAINDICATIONS
This product is contraindicated under the following conditions:
• Hypersensitivity or intolerance to any component of this product.
• Patients with porphyria.

WARNINGS
Butalbital is habit-forming and potentially abusable. Consequently, the extended use of this product is not recommended.

PRECAUTIONS
General: Butalbital, acetaminophen and caffeine capsules/tablets should be prescribed with caution in certain special-risk patients, such as the elderly or debilitated, and those with severe impairment of renal or hepatic function, or acute abdominal conditions.
Information for Patients: This product may impair mental and/or physical abilities required for the performance of potentially hazardous tasks such as driving a car or operating machinery. Such tasks should be avoided while taking this product.
Alcohol and other CNS depressants may produce an additive CNS depression, when taken with this combination product, and should be avoided.
Butalbital may be habit-forming. Patients should take the drug only for as long as it is prescribed, in the amounts prescribed, and no more frequently than prescribed.
Laboratory Tests: In patients with severe hepatic or renal disease, effects of therapy should be monitored with serial liver and/or renal function tests.
Drug Interactions: The CNS effects of butalbital may be enhanced by monoamine oxidase (MAO) inhibitors.
Butalbital, acetaminophen and caffeine may enhance the effects of: other narcotic analgesics, alcohol, general anesthetics, tranquilizers such as chlordiazepoxide, sedative-hypnotics, or other CNS depressants, causing increased CNS depression.
Drug/Laboratory Test Interactions: Acetaminophen may produce false-positive test results for urinary 5-hydroxyindoleacetic acid.
Carcinogenesis, Mutagenesis, Impairment of Fertility: No adequate studies have been conducted in animals to determine whether acetaminophen or butalbital have a potential for carcinogenesis, mutagenesis or impairment of fertility.
Pregnancy: *Teratogenic Effects:* Pregnancy Category C: Animal reproduction studies have not been conducted with this combination product. It is also not known whether butalbital, acetaminophen and caffeine can cause fetal harm when administered to a pregnant woman or can affect reproduction capacity. This product should be given to a pregnant woman only when clearly needed.
Nonteratogenic Effects: Withdrawal seizures were reported in a two-day-old male infant whose mother had taken a butalbital-containing drug during the last two months of pregnancy. Butalbital was found in the infant's serum. The infant was given phenobarbital 5 mg/kg, which was tapered without further seizure or other withdrawal symptoms.
Nursing Mothers: Caffeine, barbiturates and acetaminophen are excreted in breast milk in small amounts, but the significance of their effects on nursing infants is not known. Because of potential for serious adverse reactions in nursing infants from butalbital, acetaminophen and caffeine, a decision should be made whether to discontinue nursing or to discontinue drug, taking into account the importance of the drug to the mother.
Pediatric Use: Safety and effectiveness in pediatric patients below the age of 12 have not been established.

ADVERSE REACTIONS
Frequently Observed: The most frequently reported adverse reactions are drowsiness, lightheadedness, dizziness, sedation, shortness of breath, nausea, vomiting, abdominal pain, and intoxicated feeling.
Infrequently Observed: All adverse events tabulated below are classified as infrequent.
Central Nervous: headache, shaky feeling, tingling, agitation, fainting, fatigue, heavy eyelids, high energy, hot spells, numbness, sluggishness, seizure. Mental confusion, excitement or depression can also occur due to intolerance, particularly in elderly or debilitated patients, or due to overdosage of butalbital.
Autonomic Nervous: dry mouth, hyperhidrosis.
Gastrointestinal: difficulty swallowing, heartburn, flatulence, constipation.
Cardiovascular: tachycardia.
Musculoskeletal: leg pain, muscle fatigue.
Genitourinary: diuresis.
Miscellaneous: pruritus, fever, earache, nasal congestion, tinnitus, euphoria, allergic reactions.
Several cases of dermatological reactions, including toxic epidermal necrolysis and erythema multiforme, have been reported.
The following adverse drug events may be borne in mind as potential effects of the components of this product. Potential effects of high dosage are listed in the OVERDOSAGE section.
Acetaminophen: allergic reactions, rash, thrombocytopenia, agranulocytosis.
Caffeine: cardiac stimulation, irritability, tremor, dependence, nephrotoxicity, hyperglycemia.

DRUG ABUSE AND DEPENDENCE
Abuse and Dependence: Butalbital: *Barbiturates may be habit-forming:* Tolerance, psychological dependence, and physical dependence may occur especially following prolonged use of high doses of barbiturates. The average daily

dose for the barbiturate addict is usually about 1500 mg. As tolerance to barbiturates develops, the amount needed to maintain the same level of intoxication increases; tolerance to a fatal dosage, however, does not increase more than two-fold. As this occurs, the margin between an intoxication dosage and fatal dosage becomes smaller. The lethal dose of a barbiturate is far less if alcohol is also ingested. Major withdrawal symptoms (convulsions and delirium) may occur within 16 hours and last up to 5 days after abrupt cessation of these drugs. Intensity of withdrawal symptoms gradually declines over a period of approximately 15 days. Treatment of barbiturate dependence consists of cautious and gradual withdrawal of the drug. Barbiturate-dependent patients can be withdrawn by using a number of different withdrawal regimens. One method involves initiating treatment at the patient's regular dosage level and gradually decreasing the daily dosage as tolerated by the patient.

OVERDOSAGE

Following an acute overdosage of butalbital, acetaminophen and caffeine, toxicity may result from the barbiturate or the acetaminophen. Toxicity due to caffeine is less likely, due to the relatively small amounts in this formulation.

Signs and Symptoms: Toxicity from barbiturate poisoning include drowsiness, confusion, and coma; respiratory depression; hypotension; and hypovolemic shock.

In acetaminophen overdosage: dose-dependent, potentially fatal hepatic necrosis is the most serious adverse effect. Renal tubular necroses, hypoglycemic coma and thrombocytopenia may also occur. Early symptoms following a potentially hepatotoxic overdose may include: nausea, vomiting, diaphoresis and general malaise. Clinical and laboratory evidence of hepatic toxicity may not be apparent until 48 to 72 hours post-ingestion. In adults hepatic toxicity has rarely been reported with acute overdoses of less than 10 grams, or fatalities with less than 15 grams.

Acute caffeine poisoning may cause insomnia, restlessness, tremor, and delirium, tachycardia and extrasystoles.

Treatment: A single or multiple overdose with this combination product is a potentially lethal polydrug overdose, and consultation with a regional poison control center is recommended.

Immediate treatment includes support of cardiorespiratory function and measures to reduce drug absorption. Vomiting should be induced mechanically or with syrup of ipecac, if the patient is alert (adequate pharyngeal and laryngeal reflexes). Oral activated charcoal (1 g/kg) should follow gastric emptying. The first dose should be accompanied by an appropriate cathartic. If repeated doses are used, the cathartic might be included with alternate doses as required. Hypotension is usually hypovolemic and should respond to fluids. Pressors should be avoided. A cuffed endotracheal tube should be inserted before gastric lavage of the unconscious patient and, when necessary, to provide assisted respiration. If renal function is normal, forced diuresis may aid in the elimination of the barbiturate. Alkalinization of the urine increases renal excretion of some barbiturates, especially phenobarbital.

Meticulous attention should be given to maintaining adequate pulmonary ventilation. In severe cases of intoxication, peritoneal dialysis, or preferably hemodialysis may be considered. If hypoprothrombinemia occurs due to acetaminophen overdose, vitamin K should be administered intravenously.

If the dose of acetaminophen may have exceeded 140 mg/kg, acetylcysteine should be administered as early as possible. Serum acetaminophen levels should be obtained, since levels four or more hours following ingestion help predict acetaminophen toxicity. Do not await acetaminophen assay results before initiating treatment. Hepatic enzymes should be obtained initially, and repeated at 24-hour intervals.

Methemoglobinemia over 30% should be treated with methylene blue by slow intravenous administration.

Toxic Doses (for adults):

Butalbital:
    toxic dose 1 g (20 capsules/tablets)
Acetaminophen:
    toxic dose 10 g (20 capsules/tablets)
Caffeine:
    toxic dose 1 g (25 capsules/tablets)

DOSAGE AND ADMINISTRATION

50 mg/500 mg/40 mg:
    One capsule/tablet every four hours.
    Total daily dosage should not exceed 6 capsules/tablets.

Extended and repeated use of this product is not recommended because of the potential for physical dependence.

HOW SUPPLIED

Esgic-Plus™ (Butalbital [Warning—May be habit forming], Acetaminophen and Caffeine Capsules USP), 50 mg/500 mg/40 mg, are red, imprinted "Forest 0372" on the cap and "Esgic Plus" on the body in white. They are supplied in bottles of 20, NDC# 0456-0679-30, bottles of 100, NDC# 0456-0679-01, and bottles of 500, NDC# 0456-0679-02.

Esgic-plus™ (Butalbital 50 mg [Warning: May be habit forming], Acetaminophen 500 mg and Caffeine 40 mg) Tablets are white, capsule-shaped, single-scored, and are debossed "FOREST" on the upper side, "678" on one side of the score on the lower side. They are supplied as:
Bottles of 100-NDC 0456-0678-01
Bottles of 500-NDC 0456-0678-02

Storage: Store at controlled room temperature 15°–30°C (59°–86°F).

Dispense in a tight, light-resistant container with a child-resistant closure.

CAUTION: Federal law prohibits dispensing without prescription.

Manufactured by:
MIKART, INC.
Atlanta, GA 30318
Distributed by:
FOREST PHARMACEUTICALS, INC.
Subsidiary of Forest Laboratories, Inc.
St. Louis, MO 63045
Rev. 04/96 Code 646A00

Shown in Product Identification Section, page 311

FLUMADINE® TABLETS ℞
(rimantadine hydrochloride tablets)

FLUMADINE® SYRUP ℞
(rimantadine hydrochloride syrup)

DESCRIPTION

Flumadine® (rimantadine hydrochloride) is a synthetic antiviral drug available as a 100 mg film-coated tablet and as a syrup for oral administration. Each film-coated tablet contains 100 mg of rimantadine hydrochloride plus hydroxypropyl methylcellulose, magnesium stearate, microcrystalline cellulose, sodium starch glycolate, FD&C Yellow No. 6 Lake and FD&C Yellow No. 6. The film coat contains hydroxypropyl methylcellulose and polyethylene glycol. Each teaspoonful (5 mL) of the syrup contains 50 mg of rimantadine hydrochloride in an aqueous solution containing citric acid, parabens (methyl and propyl), saccharin sodium, sorbitol, D&C Red No. 33 and flavors.

Rimantadine hydrochloride is a white to off-white crystalline powder which is freely soluble in water (50 mg/mL at 20°C). Chemically, rimantadine hydrochloride is alpha-methyltricyclo-[3.3.1.1/3.7]decane-1-methanamine hydrochloride, with an empirical formula of $C_{12}H_{21}N \cdot HCl$, a molecular weight of 215.77 and the following structural formula:

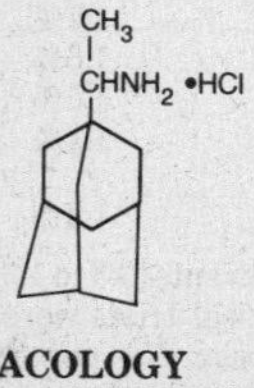

CLINICAL PHARMACOLOGY

Mechanism of Action: The mechanism of action of rimantadine is not fully understood. Rimantadine appears to exert its inhibitory effect early in the viral replicative cycle, possibly inhibiting the uncoating of the virus. Genetic studies suggest that a virus protein specified by the virion M_2 gene plays an important role in the susceptibility of influenza A virus to inhibition by rimantadine.

Microbiology: Rimantadine is inhibitory to the *in vitro* replication of influenza A virus isolates from each of the three antigenic subtypes, *i.e.*, H1N1, H2N2 and H3N2, that have been isolated from man. Rimantadine has little or no activity against influenza B virus (Ref. 1,2). Rimantadine does not appear to interfere with the immunogenicity of inactivated influenza A vaccine.

A quantitative relationship between the *in vitro* susceptibility of influenza A virus to rimantadine and clinical response to therapy has not been established.

Susceptibility test results, expressed as the concentration of the drug required to inhibit virus replication by 50% or more in a cell culture system, vary greatly (from 4 ng/mL to 20 μg/mL) depending upon the assay protocol used, size of the virus inoculum, isolates of the influenza A virus strains tested, and the cell type used (Ref. 2).

Rimantadine-resistant strains of influenza A virus have emerged among freshly isolated epidemic strains in closed settings where rimantadine has been used. Resistant viruses have been shown to be transmissible and to cause typical influenza illness (Ref. 3).

PHARMACOKINETICS

Although the pharmacokinetic profile of Flumadine has been described, no pharmacodynamic data establishing a correlation between plasma concentration and its antiviral effect are available.

The tablet and syrup formulations of Flumadine are equally absorbed after oral administration. The mean ± SD peak plasma concentration after a single 100 mg dose of Flumadine was 74 ± 22 ng/mL (range: 45 to 138 ng/mL). The time to peak concentration was 6 ± 1 hours in healthy adults (age 20 to 44 years). The single dose elimination half-life in this population was 25.4 ± 6.3 hours (range: 13 to 65 hours). The single dose elimination half-life in a group of healthy 71 to 79 year-old subjects was 32 ± 16 hours (range: 20 to 65 hours).

After the administration of rimantadine 100 mg twice daily to healthy volunteers (age 18 to 70 years) for 10 days, area under the curve (AUC) values were approximately 30% greater than predicted from a single dose. Plasma trough levels at steady state ranged between 118 and 468 ng/mL. In these patients no age-related differences in pharmacokinetics were detected. However, in a comparison of three groups of healthy older subjects (age 50-60, 61-70 and 71-79 years), the 71 to 79 year-old group had average AUC values, peak concentrations and elimination half-life values at steady state that were 20 to 30% higher than the other two groups. Steady-state concentrations in elderly nursing home patients (age 68 to 102 years) were 2- to 4-fold higher than those seen in healthy young and elderly adults.

The pharmacokinetic profile of rimantadine in children has not been established. In a group (n=10) of children 4 to 8 years old who were given a single dose (6.6 mg/kg) of Flumadine syrup, plasma concentrations of rimantadine ranged from 446 to 988 ng/mL at 5 to 6 hours and from 170 to 424 ng/mL at 24 hours. In some children drug was detected in plasma 72 hours after the last dose.

Following oral administration, rimantadine is extensively metabolized in the liver with less than 25% of the dose excreted in the urine as unchanged drug. Three hydroxylated metabolites have been found in plasma. These metabolites, an additional conjugated metabolite and parent drug account for 74 ± 10% (n=4) of a single 200 mg dose of rimantadine excreted in urine over 72 hours.

In a group (n=14) of patients with chronic liver disease, the majority of whom were stabilized cirrhotics, the pharmacokinetics of rimantadine were not appreciably altered following a single 200 mg oral dose compared to 6 healthy subjects who were sex, age and weight matched to 6 of the patients with liver disease. After administration of a single 200 mg dose to patients (n=10) with severe hepatic dysfunction, AUC was approximately 3-fold larger, elimination half-life was approximately 2-fold longer and apparent clearance was about 50% lower when compared to historic data from healthy subjects.

Studies of the effects of renal insufficiency on the pharmacokinetics of rimantadine have given inconsistent results. Following administration of a single 200 mg oral dose of rimantadine to 8 patients with a creatinine clearance (CrCl) of 31–50 mL/min and 6 patients with a CrCl of 11–30 mL/min, the apparent clearance was 37% and 16% lower, respectively, and plasma metabolite concentrations were higher when compared to weight-, age-, and sex-matched healthy subjects (n=9, CrCl > 50 mL/min). After a single 200 mg oral dose of rimantadine was given to 8 hemodialysis patients (CrCl 0–10 mL/min), there was a 1.6-fold increase in the elimination half-life and a 40% decrease in apparent clearance compared to age-matched healthy subjects. Hemodialysis did not contribute to the clearance of rimantadine.

The *in vitro* human plasma protein binding of rimantadine is about 40% over typical plasma concentrations. Albumin is the major binding protein.

INDICATIONS AND USAGE

Flumadine is indicated for the prophylaxis and treatment of illness caused by various strains of influenza A virus in adults.

Flumadine is indicated for prophylaxis against influenza A virus in children.

Prophylaxis: In controlled studies of children over the age of 1 year, healthy adults and elderly patients, Flumadine has been shown to be safe and effective in preventing signs and symptoms of infection caused by various strains of influenza A virus. Early vaccination on an annual basis as recommended by the Centers for Disease Control's Immunization Practices Advisory Committee is the method of choice in the prophylaxis of influenza unless vaccination is contraindicated, not available or not feasible. Since Flumadine does not completely prevent the host immune response to influenza A infection, individuals who take this drug may still develop immune responses to natural disease or vaccination and may be protected when later exposed to antigenically-related viruses. Following vaccination during an influenza outbreak, Flumadine prophylaxis should be considered for the 2 to 4 week time period required to develop an antibody response. However, the safety and effectiveness of Flumadine prophylaxis have not been demonstrated for longer than 6 weeks.

Treatment: Flumadine therapy should be considered for adults who develop an influenza-like illness during known or suspected influenza A infection in the community. When administered within 48 hours after onset of signs and symp-

Continued on next page

Forest—Cont.

toms of infection caused by influenza A virus strains, Flumadine has been shown to reduce the duration of fever and systemic symptoms.

CONTRAINDICATIONS

Flumadine is contraindicated in patients with known hypersensitivity to drugs of the adamantane class, including rimantadine and amantadine.

PRECAUTIONS

General: An increased incidence of seizures has been reported in patients with a history of epilepsy who received the related drug amantadine. In clinical trials of Flumadine, the occurrence of seizure-like activity was observed in a small number of patients with a history of seizures who were not receiving anticonvulsant medication while taking Flumadine. If seizures develop, Flumadine should be discontinued.

The safety and pharmacokinetics of rimantadine in renal and hepatic insufficiency have only been evaluated after single dose administration. In a single dose study of patients with anuric renal failure, the apparent clearance of rimantadine was approximately 40% lower and the elimination half-life was 1.6-fold greater than that in healthy age-matched controls. In a study of 14 persons with chronic liver disease (mostly stabilized cirrhotics), no alterations in the pharmacokinetics were observed after the administration of a single dose of rimantadine. However, the apparent clearance of rimantadine following a single dose to 10 patients with severe liver dysfunction was 50% lower than reported for healthy subjects. Because of the potential for accumulation of rimantadine and its metabolites in plasma, caution should be exercised when patients with renal or hepatic insufficiency are treated with rimantadine.

Transmission of rimantadine resistant virus should be considered when treating patients whose contacts are at high risk for influenza A illness. Influenza A virus strains resistant to rimantadine can emerge during treatment and such resistant strains have been shown to be transmissible and to cause typical influenza illness (Ref. 3). Although the frequency, rapidity, and clinical significance of the emergence of drug-resistant virus are not yet established, several small studies have demonstrated that 10% to 30% of patients with initially sensitive virus, upon treatment with rimantadine, shed rimantadine resistant virus (Ref. 3, 4, 5, 6).

Clinical response to rimantadine, although slower in those patients who subsequently shed resistant virus, was not significantly different from those who did not shed resistant virus (Ref. 3). No data are available in humans that address the activity or effectiveness of rimantadine therapy in subjects infected with resistant virus.

Drug Interactions: Cimetidine: The effects of chronic cimetidine use on the metabolism of rimantadine are not known. When a single 100 mg dose of Flumadine was administered one hour after the initiation of cimetidine (300 mg four times a day), the apparent total rimantadine clearance of this single dose in normal healthy adults was reduced by 18% (compared to the apparent total rimantadine clearance in the same subjects in the absence of cimetidine).

Acetaminophen: Flumadine, 100 mg, was given twice daily for 13 days to 12 healthy volunteers. On day 11, acetaminophen (650 mg four times daily) was started and continued for 8 days. The pharmacokinetics of rimantadine were assessed on days 11 and 13. Coadministration with acetaminophen reduced the peak concentration and AUC values for rimantadine by approximately 11%.

Aspirin: Flumadine, 100 mg, was given twice daily for 13 days to 12 healthy volunteers. On day 11, aspirin (650 mg, four times daily) was started and continued for 8 days. The pharmacokinetics of rimantadine were assessed on days 11 and 13. Peak plasma concentrations and AUC of rimantadine were reduced approximately 10% in the presence of aspirin.

Carcinogenesis, Mutagenesis, and Impairment of Fertility:

Carcinogenesis: Carcinogenicity studies in animals have not been performed.

Mutagenesis: No mutagenic effects were seen when rimantadine was evaluated in several standard assays for mutagenicity.

Impairment of Fertility: A reproduction study in male and female rats did not show detectable impairment of fertility at dosages up to 60 mg/kg/day (3 times the maximum human dose based on body surface area comparisons).

Pregnancy: Teratogenic Effects: Pregnancy Category C. There are no adequate and well-controlled studies in pregnant women. Rimantadine is reported to cross the placenta in mice. Rimantadine has been shown to be embryotoxic in rats when given at a dose of 200 mg/kg/day (11 times the recommended human dose based on body surface area comparisons). At this dose the embryotoxic effect consisted of increased fetal resorption in rats, this dose also produced a variety of maternal effects including ataxia, tremors, convulsions and significantly reduced weight gain. No embryotoxicity was observed when rabbits were given doses up to 50 mg/kg/day (5 times the recommended human dose based on body surface area comparisons). However, there was evidence of a developmental abnormality in the form of a change in the ratio of fetuses with 12 to 13 ribs. This ratio is normally about 50:50 in a litter but was 80:20 after rimantadine treatment.

Nonteratogenic Effects: Rimantadine was administered to pregnant rats in a peri- and postnatal reproduction toxicity study at doses of 30, 60 and 120 mg/kg/day (1.7, 3.4 and 6.8 times the recommended human dose based on body surface area comparisons). Maternal toxicity during gestation was noted at the two higher doses of rimantadine, and at the highest dose, 120 mg/kg/day, there was an increase in pup mortality during the first 2 to 4 days postpartum. Decreased fertility of the F1 generation was also noted for the two higher doses.

For these reasons, Flumadine should be used during pregnancy only if the potential benefit justifies the risk to the fetus.

Nursing Mothers: Flumadine should not be administered to nursing mothers because of the adverse effects noted in offspring of rats treated with rimantadine during the nursing period. Rimantadine is concentrated in rat milk in a dose-related manner: 2 to 3 hours following administration of rimantadine, rat breast milk levels were approximately twice those observed in the serum.

Pediatric Use: In children, Flumadine is recommended for the prophylaxis of influenza A. The safety and effectiveness of Flumadine in the treatment of symptomatic influenza infection in children have not been established. Prophylaxis studies with Flumadine have not been performed in children below the age of 1 year.

ADVERSE REACTIONS

In 1,027 patients treated with Flumadine in controlled clinical trials at the recommended dose of 200 mg daily, the most frequently reported adverse events involved the gastrointestinal and nervous systems.

Incidence > 1%: Adverse events reported most frequently (1-3%) at the recommended dose in controlled clinical trials are shown in the table below.

	Rimantadine (n=1027)	Control (n=986)
Nervous System		
Insomnia	2.1%	0.9%
Dizziness	1.9%	1.1%
Headache	1.4%	1.3%
Nervousness	1.3%	0.6%
Fatigue	1.0%	0.9%
Gastrointestinal System		
Nausea	2.8%	1.6%
Vomiting	1.7%	0.6%
Anorexia	1.6%	0.8%
Dry mouth	1.5%	0.6%
Abdominal Pain	1.4%	0.8%
Body as a Whole		
Asthenia	1.4%	0.5%

Less frequent adverse events (0.3 to 1%) at the recommended dose in controlled clinical trials were: *Gastrointestinal System:* diarrhea, dyspepsia; *Nervous System:* impairment of concentration, ataxia, somnolence, agitation, depression; *Skin and Appendages:* rash; *Hearing and Vestibular:* tinnitus; *Respiratory:* dyspena.

Additional adverse events (less than 0.3%) reported at recommended doses in controlled clinical trials were: Nervous System: gait abnormality, euphoria, hyperkinesia, tremor, hallucination, confusion, convulsions; *Respiratory:* bronchospasm, cough; *Cardiovascular:* pallor, palpitation, hypertension, cerebrovascular disorder, cardiac failure, pedal edema, heart block, tachycardia, syncope; *Reproduction:* non-puerperal lactation; *Special Senses;* taste loss/change, parosmia.

Rates of adverse events particularly those involving the gastrointestinal and nervous systems, increased significantly in controlled studies using higher than recommended doses of Flumadine. In most cases, symptoms resolved rapidly with discontinuation of treatment. In addition to the adverse events reported above, the following were also reported at higher than recommended doses: increased lacrimation, increased micturition frequency, fever, rigors, agitation, constipation, diaphoresis, dysphagia, stomatitis, hypesthesia and eye pain.

Adverse Reactions in Trials of Rimantadine and Amantadine: In a six-week prophylaxis study of 436 healthy adults comparing rimantadine with amantadine and placebo, the following adverse reactions were reported with an incidence > 1%.

	Rimantadine 200 mg/day (n=145)	Placebo (n=143)	Amantadine 200 mg/day (n=148)
Nervous System			
Insomnia	3.4%	0.7%	7.0%
Nervousness	2.1%	0.7%	2.8%
Impaired Concentration	2.1%	1.4%	2.1%
Dizziness	0.7%	0.0%	2.1%
Depression	0.7%	0.7%	3.5%
Total % of subjects with adverse reactions	6.9%	4.1%	14.7%
Total % of subjects withdrawn due to adverse reactions	6.9%	3.4%	14.0%

Usage in the Elderly: In general, the incidence of adverse events in controlled clinical trials in the elderly was higher in both the Flumadine and placebo-treated groups compared to younger adults and children. In a placebo-controlled study of 83 nursing home patients with influenza, 10.6% of those treated with Flumadine compared with 8.3% in the placebo group experienced events related to the central nervous system. The profile of these events was similar to that for the most frequent adverse events reported in other controlled trials (see list above).

Pooled data from controlled studies of prophylaxis and treatment of influenza with Flumadine in persons over 65 years of age showed an increase in adverse clinical events associated with the recommended dose of Flumadine (100 mg twice a day) compared to controls as follows: central and peripheral nervous systems, 12.5% for Flumadine versus 8.7% for control patients; gastrointestinal system, 17.0% for Flumadine versus 11.3% for controls.

OVERDOSAGE

As with any overdose, supportive therapy should be administered as indicated. Overdoses of a related drug, amantadine, have been reported with adverse reactions consisting of agitation, hallucinations, cardiac arrhythmia and death. The administration of intravenous physostigmine (a cholinergic agent) at doses of 1 to 2 mg in adults (Ref. 7) and 0.5 mg. in children (Ref. 8) repeated as needed as long as the dose did not exceed 2 mg/hour has been reported anecdotally to be beneficial in patients with central nervous system effects from overdoses of amantadine.

DOSAGE AND ADMINISTRATION

FOR PROPHYLAXIS IN ADULTS AND CHILDREN:

Adults: The recommended adult dose of Flumadine is 100 mg twice a day. In patients with severe hepatic dysfunction, renal failure (CrCl ≤ 10 mL/min.) and elderly nursing home patients, a dose reduction to 100 mg daily is recommended. There are currently no data available regarding the safety of rimantadine during multiple dosing in subjects with renal or hepatic impairment. Because of the potential for accumulation of rimantadine metabolites during multiple dosing, patients with any degree of renal insufficiency should be monitored for adverse effects, with dosage adjustments being made as necessary.

Children: In children less than 10 years of age, Flumadine should be administered once a day, at a dose of 5 mg/kg but not exceeding 150 mg. For children 10 years of age or older, use the adult dose.

FOR TREATMENT IN ADULTS: The recommended adult dose of Flumadine is 100 mg twice a day. In patients with severe hepatic dysfunction, renal failure (CrCl ≤ 10 mL/min) and elderly nursing home patients, a dose reduction to 100 mg daily is recommended. There are currently no data available regarding the safety of rimantadine during multiple dosing in subjects with renal or hepatic impairment. Because of the potential for accumulation of rimantadine metabolites during multiple dosing, patients with any degree of renal insufficiency should be monitored for adverse effects, with dosage adjustments being made as necessary. Flumadine therapy should be initiated as soon as possible, preferably within 48 hours after onset of signs and symptoms of influenza A infection. Therapy should be continued for approximately seven days from the initial onset of symptoms.

HOW SUPPLIED

Flumadine® tablets (rimantadine hydrochloride tablets) are supplied as 100 mg tablets (orange, oval-shaped, film-coated) in bottles of 20 (NDC 0456-0521-30), 100 (NDC 0456-0521-01), 500 (NDC 0456-0521-02) and 1000 (NDC 0456-0521-00). Imprint on tablets: (Front) FLUMADINE 100; (Back) FOREST.

Flumadine® syrup (rimantadine hydrochloride syrup) containing 50 mg of rimantadine hydrochloride per teaspoonful (5 mL) (purplish-red, raspberry-flavored) is supplied in bottles of 2 oz (NDC 0456-0527-21), 8 oz (NDC 0456-0527-08) and 16 oz (NDC 0456-0527-16).

Tablets and syrup should be stored at 15°– 30°C (59°– 86°F).

CAUTION: Federal (U.S.A.) law prohibits dispensing without prescription.

REFERENCES

1. Belshe, R.B., Burk, B., Newman, F., Cerruti, R.L. and Sim, I.S. (1989) J. Infect. Dis. 159, 430–435.
2. Sim, I.S., Cerruti, R.L. and Connell, E.V., (1989) J. Resp. Dis. (Suppl.), S46–S51.
3. Hayden, F.G., Belshe, R.B, Clover, R.D. et al (1989) N. Engl. J. Med. 321 (25), 1696–1702.
4. Hall, C.B., Dolin, R., Gala, C.L., et al (1987) Pediatrics 80, 275–282.

5. Thompson, J., Fleet, W., Lawrence, E. et al (1987) J. Med. Vir. 21, 249–255.
6. Belshe, R.B., Smith, M.H., Hall, C.B., et al (1988) J. Virol. 62, 1508–1512.
7. Casey, D.F.N. Engl. J. Med. 1978:298:516.
8. Berkowitz, C.D. J. Pediatrics. 1979:95:144
Rev. 11/95
MG#9040 (04)
FOREST PHARMACEUTICALS, INC.
Subsidiary of Forest Laboratories, Inc.
St. Louis, MO 63045
Shown in Product Identification Guide, page 311

LEVOTHROID® Tablets ℞
[lēv 'o-throid"]
(levothyroxine sodium tablets, USP)

Dist. by
FOREST PHARMACEUTICALS, INC.
A Subsidiary of Forest Laboratories, Inc.
St. Louis, MO 63045

DESCRIPTION
LEVOTHROID® TABLETS (levothyroxine sodium tablets, USP) provide crystalline sodium levothyroxine (T_4), a potent thyroid hormone, in twelve different strengths to permit easy, convenient dosage adjustment.
The structural formula for sodium levothyroxine as contained in Levothroid Tablets is:

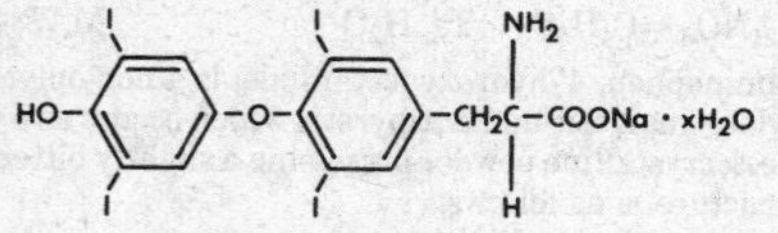
I
I
NH2
HO
O
CH2
C
COONa · xH2O
I
I
H

Sodium L-3, 3′, 5, 5′-tetraiodothyronine

CLINICAL PHARMACOLOGY
The major thyroid hormones are L-thyroxine (T_4) and L-triiodothyronine (T_3). The amounts of T_4 and T_3 released into the circulation from the normally functioning thyroid gland are regulated by the amount of thyrotropin (TSH) secreted from the anterior pituitary gland. TSH secretion is in turn regulated by the levels of circulating T_4 and T_3 and by secretion of thyrotropin releasing factor (TRH) from the hypothalamus. Recognition of this complex feedback system is important in the diagnosis and treatment of thyroid dysfunction.
The principal effect of exogenous thyroid hormone is to increase the metabolic rate of body tissues.
The thyroid hormones are also concerned with growth and differentiation of tissues. In deficiency states in the young there is retardation of growth and failure of maturation of the skeletal and other body systems, especially in failure of ossification in the epiphyses and in the growth and development of the brain.
The precise mechanism of action by which thyroid hormones affect thermogenesis and cellular growth and differentiation is not known. It is recognized that these physiologic effects are mediated at the cellular level primarily by T_3, a large part of which is derived from T_4 by deiodination in the peripheral tissues. Thyroxine (T_4) is the major component of normal secretions of the thyroid gland and is thus the primary determinant of normal thyroid function.
Depending on other factors, absorption has varied from 48 to 79 percent of the administered dose. Fasting increases absorption. Malabsorption syndromes, as well as dietary factors, (children's soybean formula, concomitant use of anionic exchange resins such as cholestyramine) cause excessive fecal loss.
More than 99 percent of circulating hormones are bound to serum proteins, including thyroid-binding globulin (TBg), thyroid-binding prealbumin (TBPA), and albumin (TBa), whose capacities and affinities vary for the hormones. L-thyroxine displays greater binding affinity than L-triiodothyronine, both in the circulation and at the cellular level, which explains its longer duration of action. The half-life of T_4 in normal plasma is 6–7 days while that of T_3 is about 1 day. The plasma half-lives of T_4 and T_3 are decreased in hyperthyroidism and increased in hypothyroidism.

INDICATIONS AND USAGE
Levothroid Tablets (levothyroxine sodium tablets, USP) are indicated as replacement or substitution therapy for diminished or absent thyroid function (e.g., cretinism, myxedema, non-toxic goiter or hypothyroidism generally, including the hypothyroid state in children, in pregnancy and in the elderly) resulting from functional deficiency, primary atrophy, from partial or complete absence of the gland or from the effects of surgery, radiation or antithyroid agents. Therapy must be maintained continuously to control the symptoms of hypothyroidism.
It may also be used to suppress the secretion of thyrotropin (TSH), action which may be beneficial in simple nonendemic goiter and in chronic lymphocytic thyroiditis. This may cause a reduction in the goiter size.
Thyroid hormone drugs are indicated as a diagnostic agent in suppression tests to differentiate suspected mild hyperthyroidism or thyroid gland autonomy.
Thyroid hormones may also be used with antithyroid drugs to treat thyrotoxicosis. This combination has been used to prevent goitrogenesis and hypothyroidism.

CONTRAINDICATIONS
Levothroid Tablets administration is contraindicated in untreated thyrotoxicosis and in acute myocardial infarction. Levothroid Tablets are contraindicated in the presence of uncorrected adrenal insufficiency because it increases the tissue demands for adrenocortical hormones and may cause an acute adrenal crisis in such patients. (See PRECAUTIONS).

WARNINGS

> Drugs with thyroid hormone activity, alone or together with other therapeutic agents, have been used for the treatment of obesity. In euthyroid patients, doses within the range of daily hormonal requirements are ineffective for weight reduction. Larger doses may produce serious or even life-threatening manifestations of toxicity, particularly when given in association with sympathomimetic amines such as those used for their anorectic effects.

The use of thyroid hormones in the therapy of obesity, alone or combined with other drugs, is unjustified and has been shown to be ineffective. Neither is their use justified for the treatment of male or female infertility unless this condition is accompanied by hypothyroidism.

PRECAUTIONS
GENERAL—Levothroid Tablets should be used with caution in patients with cardiovascular disease, including hypertension. The development of chest pain or other aggravation of cardiovascular disease will require a decrease in dosage.
Thyroid hormone therapy in patients with concomitant diabetes mellitus or diabetes insipidus or adrenal cortical insufficiency aggravates the intensity of their symptoms. Appropriate adjustments of the various therapeutic measures directed at these concomitant endocrine diseases are required. The therapy of myxedema coma requires simultaneous administration of glucocorticoids. (See DOSAGE AND ADMINISTRATION).
In infants, excessive doses of thyroid hormone preparations may produce craniosynostosis.
INFORMATION FOR THE PATIENT—Patients on thyroid preparations and parents of children on thyroid therapy should be informed that:
1. Replacement therapy is to be taken essentially for life, with the exception of cases of transient hypothyroidism, usually associated with thyroiditis, and in those patients receiving a therapeutic trial of the drug.
2. They should immediately report during the course of therapy any signs or symptoms of thyroid hormone toxicity, e.g., chest pain, increased pulse rate, palpitations, excessive sweating, heat intolerance, nervousness, or any other unusual event.
3. In case of concomitant diabetes mellitus, the daily dosage of antidiabetic medication may need readjustment as thyroid hormone replacement is achieved. If thyroid medication is stopped, a downward readjustment of the dosage of insulin or oral hypoglycemic agent may be necessary to avoid hypoglycemia. At all times, close monitoring of urinary glucose levels is mandatory in such patients.
4. In case of concomitant oral anticoagulant therapy, the prothrombin time should be measured frequently to determine if the dosage of oral anticoagulants is to be readjusted.
5. Partial loss of hair may be experienced by children in the first few months of thyroid therapy, but this is usually a transient phenomenon and later recovery is usually the rule.
LABORATORY TESTS—The patient's response to thyroid replacement may be followed by laboratory tests such as serum thyroxine (T_4), serum triiodothyronine (T_3), free thyroxine index and thyroid stimulating hormone (TSH) blood levels.
DRUG INTERACTIONS—In patients with diabetes mellitus, addition of thyroid hormone therapy may cause an increase in the required dosage of insulin or oral hypoglycemic agents. Conversely, decreasing the dose of thyroid hormone may possibly cause hypoglycemic reactions if the dosage of insulin or oral hypoglycemic agents is not adjusted.
Thyroid replacement may potentiate anticoagulant effects with agents such as warfarin or bishydroxycoumarin and reduction of one-third in anticoagulant dosage should be undertaken upon initiation of Levothroid Tablets therapy. Subsequent anticoagulant dosage adjustment should be made on the basis of frequent prothrombin determinations.
Injection of epinephrine in patients with coronary artery disease may precipitate an episode of coronary insufficiency. This may be enhanced in patients receiving thyroid preparations. Careful observation is required if catecholamines are administered to patients in this category.
Cholestyramine or colestipol binds both T_4 and T_3 in the intestine, thus impairing absorption of these thyroid hormones. *In vitro* studies indicate that the binding is not easily removed. Therefore, four to five hours should elapse between administration of cholestyramine or colestipol and thyroid hormones.
Estrogens tend to increase serum thyroxine-binding globulin (TBg). In a patient with a non-functioning thyroid gland who is receiving thyroid replacement therapy, free levothyroxine may be decreased when estrogens are started thus increasing thyroid requirements. However, if the patient's thyroid gland has sufficient function the decreased free thyroxine will result in a compensatory increase in thyroxine output by the thyroid. Therefore, patients without a functioning thyroid gland who are on thyroid replacement therapy may need to increase their thyroid dose if estrogens or estrogen-containing oral contraceptives are given.
DRUG/LABORATORY TEST INTERACTIONS—The following drugs or moieties are known to interfere with laboratory tests performed in patients on thyroid hormone therapy: androgens, corticosteroids, estrogens, oral contraceptives containing estrogens, iodine-containing preparations, and the numerous preparations containing salicylates.
1. Changes in TBg concentration should be taken into consideration in the interpretation of T_4 and T_3 values. In such cases, the unbound (free) hormone should be measured. Pregnancy, estrogens, and estrogen-containing oral contraceptives increase TBg concentrations. TBg may also be increased during infectious hepatitis. Decreases in TBg concentrations are observed in nephrosis, acromegaly, and after androgen or corticosteroid therapy. Familial hyper- or hypothyroxine-binding-globulinemias have been described. The incidence of TBg deficiency approximates 1 in 9000. The binding of thyroxine by thyroid-binding prealbumin (TBPA) is inhibited by salicylates.
2. Medical or dietary iodine interferes with all *in vivo* tests of radioiodine uptake, producing low uptakes which may not be reflective of a true decrease in hormone synthesis.
3. The persistence of clinical and laboratory evidence of hypothyroidism in spite of adequate dosage replacement indicates either poor patient compliance, poor absorption, excessive fecal loss, or inactivity of the preparation. Intracellular resistance to thyroid hormone is quite rare.
CARCINOGENESIS, MUTAGENESIS, AND IMPAIRMENT OF FERTILITY—A reportedly apparent association between prolonged thyroid therapy and breast cancer has not been confirmed and patients on thyroid for established indications should not discontinue therapy. No confirmatory long-term studies in animals have been performed to evaluate carcinogenic potential, mutagenicity, or impairment of fertility in either males or females.
PREGNANCY-CATEGORY A—Thyroid hormones do not readily cross the placental barrier. The clinical experience to date does not indicate any adverse effect on fetuses when thyroid hormones are administered to pregnant women. On the basis of current knowledge, thyroid replacement therapy to hypothyroid women should not be discontinued during pregnancy.
NURSING MOTHERS—Minimal amounts of thyroid hormones are excreted in human milk. Thyroid is not associated with serious adverse reactions and does not have a known tumorigenic potential. However, caution should be exercised when thyroid is administered to a nursing woman.
PEDIATRIC USE—The diagnosis and institution of therapy for cretinism should be done as soon after birth as feasible to prevent developmental deficiency. Screening tests for serum T_4 and TSH will identify this group of newborn patients.

ADVERSE REACTIONS
Patients who are sensitive to lactose may show intolerance to Levothroid Tablets since this substance is used in the manufacture of the product.
Adverse reactions other than those indicative of hyperthyroidism because of therapeutic overdosage, either initially or during the maintenance period, are rare. (See OVERDOSAGE).

OVERDOSAGE
Excessive dosage of thyroid medication may result in symptoms of hyperthyroidism. Since, however, the effects do not appear at once the symptoms may not appear for one to three weeks after the dosage regimen is begun. The most common signs and symptoms of overdosage are weight loss, palpitation, nervousness, diarrhea or abdominal cramps, sweating, tachycardia, cardiac arrhythmias, angina pectoris, tremors, headache, insomnia, intolerance to heat and fever. If symptoms of overdosage appear, discontinue medication for several days and reinstitute treatment at a lower dosage level. Laboratory tests such as serum T_4, and serum T_3 and the free thyroxine index will be elevated during the period of overdosage.

Continued on next page

Forest—Cont.

Complications as a result of the induced hypermetabolic state may include cardiac failure and death due to arrhythmia or failure.

TREATMENT OF OVERDOSAGE—Dosage should be reduced or therapy temporarily discontinued if signs and symptoms of overdosage appear. Treatment may be reinstituted at a lower dosage. In normal individuals, normal hypothalamic-pituitary-thyroid axis function is restored in 6 to 8 weeks after thyroid suppression.

Treatment of acute massive thyroid hormone overdosage is aimed at reducing gastrointestinal absorption of the drugs and counteracting central and peripheral effects, mainly those of increased sympathetic activity. Vomiting may be induced initially if further gastrointestinal absorption can reasonably be prevented and barring contraindications such as coma, convulsions, or loss of the gagging reflex. Treatment is symptomatic and supportive. Oxygen may be administered and ventilation maintained. Cardiac glycosides may be indicated if congestive heart failure develops. Measures to control fever, hypoglycemia, or fluid loss should be instituted if needed. Antiadrenergic agents, particularly propranolol, have been used advantageously in the treatment of increased sympathetic activity. Propranolol may be administered intravenously at a dosage of 1 to 3 mg over a 10-minute period or orally, 80 to 160 mg/day, initially, especially when no contraindications exist for its use. Other adjunctive measures may include administration of cholestyramine to interfere with thyroxine absorption, and glucocorticoids to inhibit conversion of T_4 to T_3.

DOSAGE AND ADMINISTRATION

The goal of therapy should be the restoration of euthyroidism as judged by clinical response and confirmed by appropriate laboratory values. In adults with no complicating endocrine or cardiovascular disease, the predicted full maintenance dose may be achieved immediately with adjustments made as indicated by clinical evaluation. The usual maintenance dose of Levothroid Tablets is 100 to 200 mcg.

In patients with known complications or in case of doubt, individual dose titration at 2- to 4-week intervals is recommended. The usual starting dose is 50 mcg with increases of 50 mcg at 2- to 4-week intervals until the patient is euthyroid or symptoms ensue which preclude further dose increase. In adult myxedema or hypothyroid patients with angina, the starting dose should be 25 mcg with increases at 2- to 4-week intervals of 25 to 50 mcg as determined by clinical response. Myxedema coma is usually precipitated in the hypothyroid patient of long-standing by intercurrent illness or drugs such as sedatives and anesthetics and should be considered a medical emergency. Therapy should be directed at the correction of electrolyte disturbances and possible infection besides the administration of thyroid hormones. Corticosteroids should be administered routinely. T_4 and T_3 may be administered via a nasogastric tube, but the preferred route of administration of both hormones is intravenous. Sodium levothyroxine (T_4) is given at a starting dose of 200–500 mcg (100 mcg/mL given rapidly), and is usually well tolerated, even in the elderly. This initial dose is followed by daily supplements of 100 to 200 mcg given IV. Normal T_4 levels are achieved in 24 hours followed in 3 days by threefold increase of T_3. Oral therapy with Levothroid Tablets should be resumed as soon as the clinical situation has been stabilized and the patient is able to take oral medication.

Pediatric dosage should follow the recommendations summarized in Table I. In infants with congenital hypothyroidism, therapy with full doses should be instituted as soon as the diagnosis has been made. Levothroid Tablets may be given to infants and children who cannot swallow intact tablets by crushing the proper dose tablet and suspending the **freshly crushed** tablet in a small amount of water or formula. The suspension can be given by spoon or dropper. DO NOT STORE THE SUSPENSION FOR ANY PERIOD OF TIME. The crushed tablet may also be sprinkled over a small amount of food, such as cooked cereal or apple sauce.

TABLE I
Recommended Pediatric Dosage
For Congenital Hypothyroidism*

LEVOTHROID TABLETS
(levothyroxine sodium tablets, USP)

Age	Dose per day	Daily dose per kg of body weight
0–6 mos	25–50 mcg	8–10 mcg
6–12 mos	50–75 mcg	6–8 mcg
1–5 yrs	75–100 mcg	5–6 mcg
6–12 yrs	100–150 mcg	4–5 mcg

* To be adjusted on the basis of clinical response and laboratory tests (See **Laboratory Tests**).

HOW SUPPLIED

Strength	Package Size	NDC Number
25 mcg	bottle of 100	0456-0320-01
50 mcg	bottle of 100	0456-0321-01
50 mcg	bottle of 5000	0456-0321-51
50 mcg	unit dose carton of 100	0456-0321-63
75 mcg	bottle of 100	0456-0322-01
88 mcg	bottle of 100	0456-0329-01
100 mcg	bottle of 100	0456-0323-01
100 mcg	bottle of 5000	0456-0323-51
100 mcg	unit dose carton of 100	0456-0323-63
112 mcg	bottle of 100	0456-0330-01
125 mcg	bottle of 100	0456-0324-01
125 mcg	unit dose carton of 100	0456-0324-63
137 mcg	bottle of 100	0456-0331-01
150 mcg	bottle of 100	0456-0325-01
150 mcg	bottle of 5000	0456-0325-51
150 mcg	unit dose carton of 100	0456-0325-63
175 mcg	bottle of 100	0456-0326-01
200 mcg	bottle of 100	0456-0327-01
200 mcg	bottle of 5000	0456-0327-51
200 mcg	unit dose carton of 100	0456-0327-63
300 mcg	bottle of 100	0456-0328-01
300 mcg	unit dose carton of 100	0456-0328-63

Strength	Tablet Color	Markings
25 mcg	Orange	25
50 mcg	White	50
75 mcg	Grey	75
88 mcg	Mint Green	88
100 mcg	Yellow	100
112 mcg	Rose	112
125 mcg	Purple	125
137 mcg	Blue	137
150 mcg	Light Blue	150
175 mcg	Turquoise	175
200 mcg	Pink	200
300 mcg	Lime Green	300

Tablets should be stored at controlled room temperature, 59°–86°F (15°–30°C) in capped bottles or unbroken plastic strip packing.

CAUTION: Federal law prohibits dispensing without prescription.

Rev. 1/96   03690196

Shown in Product Identification Section, page 311

LORCET®-HD
[lōr-sét h d]

DESCRIPTION

Each Lorcet-HD capsule contains 5 mg Hydrocodone* Bitartrate *(WARNING: May be habit forming) and 500 mg Acetaminophen.

HOW SUPPLIED

Lorcet-HD capsules are opaque maroon capsules imprinted with the UAD logo; 1120 and are supplied in bottles of 100 capsules. Each capsule contains Hydrocodone* Bitartrate, 5mg *(WARNING: May Be Habit Forming) and Acetaminophen (APAP), 500 mg. NDC# 0785-1120-01.

LORCET® PLUS
[lōr-sét plus]
Hydrocodone Bitartrate and Acetaminophen Tablets USP
7.5 mg/650 mg

DESCRIPTION

Each Lorcet Plus tablet contains:
Hydrocodone*Bitartrate .... 7.5 mg
        *(WARNING: May be habit forming)
Acetaminophen .... 650 mg

HOW SUPPLIED

Lorcet Plus, Hydrocodone Bitartrate and Acetaminophen Tablets USP, each tablet of which contains hydrocodone* bitartrate 7.5 mg *(WARNING: May be habit forming) and acetaminophen 650 mg, are white, capsule-shaped, scored tablets, debossed "U" on one side and "201" on the other side, and are supplied in containers of 100 tablets, NDC #0785-1122-01, containers of 500 tablets, NDC #0785-1122-50, and in unit-dose cartons of 100 tablets (4 cards of 25 tablets per card), NDC #0785-1122-63.

Shown in Product Identification Guide, page 311

LORCET® 10/650   CIII Rx
[lōr sēt]
Hydrocodone Bitartrate
and Acetaminophen Tablets USP
10 mg/650 mg

DESCRIPTION

Each Lorcet® 10/650 tablet contains:
Hydrocodone*
Bitartrate .... 10 mg
        *(WARNING: May be habit forming)
Acetaminophen .... 650 mg

Also contains colloidal silicon dioxide, croscarmellose sodium, crospovidone, microcrystalline cellulose, povidone, pregelatinized starch, stearic acid and FD &C Blue # 1 Lake. Hydrocodone bitartrate is an opioid analgesic and antitussive which occurs as fine, white crystals or as a crystalline powder. It is affected by light. The chemical name is: 4, 5α-epoxy-3-methoxy-17-methylmorphinan-6-one tartrate (1:1) hydrate (2:5).

Its structure is as follows:

$$C_{18}H_{21}NO_3 \cdot C_4H_6O_6 \cdot 2\frac{1}{2} H_2O \qquad \text{M.W. } 494.50$$

Acetaminophen, 4'-hydroxyacetanilide, is a non-opiate, non-salicylate analgesic and antipyretic which occurs as a white, odorless, crystalline powder possessing a slightly bitter taste. Its structure is as follows:

$$C_8H_9NO_2 \qquad \text{M.W. } 151.16$$

CLINICAL PHARMACOLOGY

Hydrocodone is a semisynthetic narcotic analgesic and antitussive with multiple actions qualitatively similar to those of codeine. Most of these involve the central nervous system and smooth muscle. The precise mechanism of action of hydrocodone and other opiates is not known, although it is believed to relate to the existence of opiate receptors in the central nervous system. In addition to analgesia, narcotics may produce drowsiness, changes in mood and mental clouding.

Radioimmunoassay techniques have recently been developed for the analysis of hydrocodone in human plasma. After a 10 mg oral dose of hydrocodone bitartrate, a mean peak serum drug level of 23.6 ng/mL and an elimination half-life of 3.8 hours were found.

The analgesic action of acetaminophen involves peripheral and central influences, but the specific mechanism is as yet undetermined. Antipyretic activity is mediated through hypothalamic heat regulating centers. Acetaminophen inhibits prostaglandin synthetase. Therapeutic doses of acetaminophen have negligible effects on the cardiovascular or respiratory systems; however, toxic doses may cause circulatory failure and rapid, shallow breathing. Acetaminophen is rapidly and almost completely absorbed from the gastrointestinal tract, producing maximum serum concentrations within 30 minutes to one hour. The plasma half-life in adults and children ranges from 0.90 hours to 3.25 hours with an average of approximately 2 hours. The drug distributes uniformly in most body fluids and is approximately 25% protein bound. Acetaminophen is conjugated in the liver, with less than 3% of the dose excreted unchanged in 24 hours. The primary metabolic pathway is conjugation to sulfate and glucuronide by-products. A minor oxidative pathway forms cysteine and mercapturic acid. These compounds are subsequently excreted by the kidneys into the urine.

INDICATIONS AND USAGE

For the relief of moderate to moderately severe pain.

CONTRAINDICATIONS

Hypersensitivity to acetaminophen or hydrocodone.

WARNINGS

Respiratory Depression:
At high doses or in sensitive patients, hydrocodone may produce dose-related respiratory depression by acting directly on the brain stem respiratory center. Hydrocodone also affects the center that controls respiratory rhythm, and may produce irregular and periodic breathing.

Head Injury and Increased Intracranial Pressure:
The respiratory depressant effects of narcotics and their capacity to elevate cerebrospinal fluid pressure may be markedly exaggerated in the presence of head injury, other intracranial lesions or a preexisting increase in intracranial

pressure. Furthermore, narcotics produce adverse reactions which may obscure the clinical course of patients with head injuries.

Acute Abdominal Conditions:
The administration of narcotics may obscure the diagnosis or clinical course of patients with acute abdominal conditions.

PRECAUTIONS

Special Risk Patients:
As with any narcotic analgesic agent, Lorcet® 10/650 should be used with caution in elderly or debilitated patients and those with severe impairment of hepatic or renal function, hypothyroidism, Addison's disease, prostatic hypertrophy or urethral stricture. The usual precautions should be observed and the possibility of respiratory depression should be kept in mind.

Information for Patients:
Lorcet® 10/650, like all narcotics, may impair the mental and/or physical abilities required for the performance of potentially hazardous tasks such as driving a car or operating machinery; patients should be cautioned accordingly.

Cough Reflex:
Hydrocodone suppresses the cough reflex; as with all narcotics, caution should be exercised when Lorcet® 10/650 is used postoperatively and in patients with pulmonary disease.

Drug Interactions:
Patients receiving other narcotic analgesics, antipsychotics, antianxiety agents, or other CNS depressants (including alcohol) concomitantly with Lorcet® 10/650 may exhibit an additive CNS depression. When combined therapy is contemplated, the dose of one or both agents should be reduced.

The use of MAO inhibitors or tricyclic antidepressants with hydrocodone preparations may increase the effect of either the antidepressant or hydrocodone.

The concurrent use of anticholinergics with hydrocodone may produce paralytic ileus.

Usage in Pregnancy:
Teratogenic Effects: Pregnancy Category C. Hydrocodone has been shown to be teratogenic in hamsters when given in doses 700 times the human dose. There are no adequate and well-controlled studies in pregnant women. Lorcet® 10/650 should be used during pregnancy only if the potential benefit justifies the potential risk to the fetus.
Nonteratogenic Effects: Babies born to mothers who have been taking opioids regularly prior to delivery will be physically dependent. The withdrawal signs include irritability and excessive crying, tremors, hyperactive reflexes, increased respiratory rate, increased stools, sneezing, yawning, vomiting, and fever. The intensity of the syndrome does not always correlate with the duration of maternal opioid use or dose. There is no consensus on the best method of managing withdrawal. Chlorpromazine 0.7 to 1 mg/kg q6h, and paregoric 2 to 4 drops/kg q4h, have been used to treat withdrawal symptoms in infants. The duration of therapy is 4 to 28 days, with the dosage decreased as tolerated.

Labor and Delivery:
As with all narcotics, administration of Lorcet® 10/650 to the mother shortly before delivery may result in some degree of respiratory depression in the newborn, especially if higher doses are used.

Nursing Mothers:
It is not known whether this drug is excreted in human milk. Because many drugs are excreted in human milk and because of the potential for serious adverse reactions in nursing infants from Lorcet® 10/650, a decision should be made whether to discontinue nursing or to discontinue the drug, taking into account the importance of the drug to the mother.

Pediatric Use:
Safety and effectiveness in children have not been established.

ADVERSE REACTIONS

The most frequently observed adverse reactions include lightheadedness, dizziness, sedation, nausea and vomiting. These effects seem to be more prominent in ambulatory than in nonambulatory patients and some of these adverse reactions may be alleviated if the patient lies down. Other adverse reactions include:

Central Nervous System:
Drowsiness, mental clouding, lethargy, impairment of mental and physical performance, anxiety, fear, dysphoria, psychic dependence, mood changes.

Gastrointestinal System:
The antiemetic phenothiazines are useful in suppressing the nausea and vomiting which may occur (see above); however, some phenothiazine derivatives seem to be antianalgesic and to increase the amount of narcotic required to produce pain relief, while other phenothiazines reduce the amount of narcotic required to produce a given level of analgesia. Prolonged administration of Lorcet® 10/650 may produce constipation.

Genitourinary System:
Ureteral spasm, spasm of vesical sphincters and urinary retention have been reported.

NITROGARD™

NDC 0456-0686-01	Bottles of 100	1 mg off white round standard convex, imprint: 1
NDC 0456-0687-01	Bottles of 100	2 mg off white round standard convex, imprint: 2
NDC 0456-0683-01	Bottles of 100	3 mg off white round standard convex, imprint: 3

Respiratory Depression:
Hydrocodone bitartrate may produce dose-related respiratory depression by acting directly on the brain stem respiratory center. Hydrocodone also affects the center that controls respiratory rhythm, and may produce irregular and periodic breathing. If significant respiratory depression occurs, it may be antagonized by the use of naloxone hydrochloride. Apply other supportive measures when indicated.

DRUG ABUSE AND DEPENDENCE

Lorcet® 10/650 is subject to the Federal Controlled Substances Act (Schedule III).
Psychic dependence, physical dependence, and tolerance may develop upon repeated administration of narcotics; therefore, Lorcet® 10/650 should be prescribed and administered with caution. However, psychic dependence is unlikely to develop when Lorcet® 10/650 is used for a short time for the treatment of pain.
Physical dependence, the condition in which continued administration of the drug is required to prevent the appearance of a withdrawal syndrome, assumes clinically significant proportions only after several weeks of continued narcotic use, although some mild degree of physical dependence may develop after a few days of narcotic therapy. Tolerance, in which increasingly large doses are required in order to produce the same degree of analgesia, is manifested initially by a shortened duration of analgesic effect, and subsequently by decreases in the intensity of analgesia. The rate of development of tolerance varies among patients.

OVERDOSAGE

Acetaminophen:
Signs and Symptoms: In acute acetaminophen overdosage, dose-dependent, potentially fatal hepatic necrosis is the most serious adverse effect. Renal tubular necrosis, hypoglycemic coma, and thrombocytopenia may also occur.
In adults, hepatic toxicity has rarely been reported with acute overdoses of less than 10 grams and fatalities with less than 15 grams. Importantly, young children seem to be more resistant than adults to the hepatotoxic effect of an acetaminophen overdose. Despite this, the measures outlined below should be initiated in any adult or child suspected of having ingested an acetaminophen overdose.
Early symptoms following a potentially hepatotoxic overdose may include: nausea, vomiting, diaphoresis and general malaise. Clinical and laboratory evidence of hepatic toxicity may not be apparent until 48 to 72 hours post-ingestion.
Treatment: The stomach should be emptied promptly by lavage or by induction of emesis with syrup of ipecac. Patients' estimates of the quantity of a drug ingested are notoriously unreliable. Therefore, if an acetaminophen overdose is suspected, a serum acetaminophen assay should be obtained as early as possible, but no sooner than four hours following ingestion. Liver function studies should be obtained initially and repeated at 24-hour intervals.
The antidote, N-acetylcysteine, should be administered as early as possible, preferably within 16 hours of the overdose ingestion for optimal results, but in any case, within 24 hours. Following recovery, there are no residual, structural or functional hepatic abnormalities.

Hydrocodone:
Signs and Symptoms: Serious overdose with hydrocodone is characterized by respiratory depression (a decrease in respiratory rate and/or tidal volume, Cheyne-Stokes respiration, cyanosis), extreme somnolence progressing to stupor or coma, skeletal muscle flaccidity, cold and clammy skin, and sometimes bradycardia and hypotension. In severe overdosage, apnea, circulatory collapse, cardiac arrest and death may occur.
Treatment: Primary attention should be given to the reestablishment of adequate respiratory exchange through provision of a patent airway and the institution of assisted or controlled ventilation. The narcotic antagonist naloxone is a specific antidote against respiratory depression which may result from overdosage or unusual sensitivity to narcotics, including hydrocodone. Therefore, an appropriate dose of naloxone hydrochloride (see package insert) should be administered, preferably by the intravenous route, and simultaneously with efforts at respiratory resuscitation. Since the duration of action of hydrocodone may exceed that of the antagonist, the patient should be kept under continued surveillance and repeated doses of the antagonist should be administered as needed to maintain adequate respiration.
An antagonist should not be administered in the absence of clinically significant respiratory or cardiovascular depression. Oxygen, intravenous fluids, vasopressors and other supportive measures should be employed as indicated.

Gastric emptying may be useful in removing unabsorbed drug.

DOSAGE AND ADMINISTRATION

Dosage should be adjusted according to the severity of the pain and the response of the patient. However, it should be kept in mind that tolerance to hydrocodone can develop with continued use and that the incidence of untoward effects is dose related.
The usual adult dosage is one tablet every four to six hours as needed for pain. The total 24 hour dose should not exceed 6 tablets.

HOW SUPPLIED

Lorcet® 10/650, Hydrocodone* Bitartrate and Acetaminophen Tablets USP 10 mg/650 mg, each tablet of which contains hydrocodone* bitartrate 10 mg *(**WARNING:** May be habit forming) and acetaminophen 650 mg, are light-blue, capsule-shaped, scored tablets, debossed "UAD" on one side and "63 50" on the other side, and are supplied in containers of 100 tablets, NDC 0785-6350-01, in containers of 500 tablets, NDC 0785-6350-50, and containers of unit dose (4 × 25's), NDC 0785-6350-63.
Storage: Store at controlled room temperature 15° – 30°C (59° – 86°F).
Dispense in a tight, light-resistant container, with a child-resistant closure.
CAUTION: Federal law prohibits dispensing without prescription.
A Schedule CIII Controlled Substance.
Manufactured by: MIKART, INC. ATLANTA, GA 30318

Manufactured for
UAD Laboratories
Division of Forest Pharmaceuticals, Inc.
St. Louis, MO 63045

Rev. 6/94   Code 558A00
Shown in Product Identification Guide, page 311

NITROGARD™   ℞
(Nitroglycerin
Extended-release)
Buccal Tablets

DESCRIPTION

Nitroglycerin is 1,2,3-propanetriol trinitrate, an organic nitrate whose molecular weight is 227.09. The organic nitrates are vasodilators, active on both arteries and veins.
NITROGARD (nitroglycerin) buccal tablets are an Extended-release preparation designed to deliver nitroglycerin through the oral mucosa over a sustained period of time. When a NITROGARD buccal tablet is placed under the lip or in the buccal pouch, it adheres to the mucosa. As the tablet gradually dissolves, it releases nitroglycerin to the systemic circulation.
Each extended-release tablet, for buccal administration contains 1 mg, 2 mg, or 3 mg of nitroglycerin.

HOW SUPPLIED

NITROGARD (Nitroglycerin Extended-release) Buccal tablets are supplied in three strengths as:
[See table above.]
CAUTION: Federal law prohibits dispensing without prescription.
Store at controlled room temperature 15°–30°C (59°–86°F).
Dispense in a tight container as defined in the USP.
FOREST PHARMACEUTICALS, INC.
Subsidiary of Forest Laboratories, Inc.
St. Louis, MO 63045
Rev. 3/91
MG #5832 (01)

SUS-PHRINE®   ℞
[sŭs 'frĭn '']
(epinephrine 5 mg/ml)
1:200
Injectable Suspension
For Subcutaneous Injection only

DESCRIPTION

Each mL of SUS-PHRINE® (epinephrine) contains 5 mg epinephrine in a sterile, non-pyrogenic aqueous vehicle containing ascorbic acid 10 mg and thioglycolic acid 6.6 mg (as sodium salts) phenol 5 mg and glycerin (USP) 325 mg. Sodium hydroxide is added to adjust the pH. Approximately

Continued on next page

Forest—Cont.

80% of the total epinephrine is in suspension. SUS-PHRINE® is sulfite-free.

$C_9H_{13}NO_3$ M.W. 183.21

Epinephrine is a white to off-white, odorless, microcrystalline powder or granules. It is affected by light. The chemical name is:
(R)-4-[1-hydroxy-2-(methylamino)ethyl]-1,2-benzenediol

CLINICAL PHARMACOLOGY

SUS-PHRINE® (epinephrine) acts at both the alpha and beta receptor sites. Beta stimulation provides bronchodilator action by relaxing bronchial muscle. Alpha stimulation increases vital capacity by relieving congestion of the bronchial mucosa and by constricting pulmonary vessels.

Recent studies in laboratory animals (minipigs, rodents, and dogs) recorded the occurrence of cardiac arrhythmias and sudden death (with histologic evidence of myocardial necrosis) when beta agonists and methylxanthines were administered concurrently. The significance of these findings when applied to humans is currently unknown.

SUS-PHRINE® (epinephrine) provides both rapid and sustained epinephrine activity. The rapid action is due to the epinephrine in solution, while the sustained activity is due to the crystalline epinephrine free base in suspension.

INDICATIONS AND USAGE

For the symptomatic treatment of bronchial asthma, and reversible bronchospasm associated with chronic bronchitis and emphysema.

CONTRAINDICATIONS

Hypersensitivity to any of the components.
Narrow angle glaucoma, shock, cerebral arteriosclerosis and organic heart disease. Epinephrine is also contraindicated during general anesthesia with halogenated hydrocarbons or cyclopropane, and in local anesthesia of certain areas, e.g., fingers, toes, because of the danger of vasoconstriction producing sloughing of tissue, and in labor because the drug may delay the second stage.

WARNINGS

SUS-PHRINE® (epinephrine) SHOULD NOT BE EMPLOYED TO CORRECT DRUG-INDUCED HYPOTENSION.
Administer with caution to elderly people; those with cardiovascular disease, diabetes, hypertension or hyperthyroidism; in psychoneurotic individuals and in pregnancy. Administer with extreme caution to patients with long-standing bronchial asthma and emphysema who have developed degenerative heart disease.
Cardiac arrhythmias may follow administration of epinephrine.
Anginal pain may be induced when coronary insufficiency is present.

PRECAUTIONS

Parenteral drug products should be inspected visually for foreign particulate matter and discoloration before administration whenever container permits.

DO NOT USE IF PRODUCT IS DISCOLORED. Discoloration indicates the oxidation of epinephrine and possible loss of potency.

Use of SUS-PHRINE® (eprinephrine) with digitalis, mercurial diuretics or other drugs that sensitize the heart to arrhythmias is not recommended.

Patients should be instructed to contact a physician immediately if severe pain at the site of injection develops.

SUS-PHRINE® (epinephrine) should not be administered concomitantly with other sympathomimetic agents, since their combined effects on the cardiovascular system may be deleterious to the patient.

The effects of epinephrine may be potentiated by tricyclic antidepressants; sodium L-thyroxine, and certain antihistamines (eg, diphenhydramine, tripelennamine or chlorpheniramine).

ADVERSE REACTIONS

In some individuals, restlessness, anxiety, headache, tremor, weakness, dizziness, pallor, respiratory difficulties, palpitation, nausea and vomiting may occur. These reactions may be exaggerated in hyperthyroidism. Occlusion of the central retinal artery, clostridial myonecrosis and shock have also been reported.

Also, urticaria, wheal and hemorrhage at the site of injection may occur. Repeated injections at the same site may result in necrosis from vascular constriction.

Tolerance to epinephrine may occur with prolonged use.

OVERDOSAGE

Overdose or inadvertent intravenous injection may cause cerebrovascular hemorrhage resulting from the sharp rise in blood pressure. Fatalities may also result from pulmonary edema because of peripheral constriction and cardiac stimulation produced. Rapidly acting vasodilators such as nitrites, or alpha blocking agents may counteract the marked pressor effects. Cardiac arrhythmias may be countered by administering rapidly acting antiarrhythmic or beta blocking agents.

DOSAGE AND ADMINISTRATION
NOTE: INJECT SUBCUTANEOUSLY.

As with all sterile products, failure to follow aseptic procedures may result in microbial contamination causing adverse consequences which could lead to life threatening illness.

It is suggested that SUS-PHRINE® (epinephrine) be administered with a tuberculin syringe and a 26 gauge, ½ inch needle.

A small initial test dose may be administered subcutaneously as a possible aid in determining patient sensitivity to epinephrine.

Site of injection should be varied to avoid necrosis at the site of injection.

Each time before withdrawing SUS-PHRINE® (epinephrine) into syringe, **SHAKE VIAL OR AMPUL THOROUGHLY** to disperse particles and obtain a uniform suspension. Inject promptly subcutaneously to avoid settling of suspension in the syringe.

ADULTS:
Adult dosage range is 0.1 to 0.3 mL depending on patient response.
Subsequent doses should be administered only when necessary and not more frequently than every six hours.
Infants 1 month to 2 years and Children 2 to 12 years:
Pediatric dose is 0.005 mL/kg (2.2 lb) body weight injected subcutaneously.
FOR CHILDREN 30 kg OR LESS MAXIMUM SINGLE DOSE IS 0.15 mL
Subsequent doses should be administered only when necessary and not more frequently than every six hours.

CLINICAL STUDIES

Controlled studies comparing the effectiveness of SUS-PHRINE® (epinephrine) 1:200 and an aqueous solution of epinephrine 1:1000 were conducted in both pediatric and adult asthmatics. The studies demonstrated rapid bronchodilator activity following administration of either SUS-PHRINE® (epinephrine) or epinephrine 1:1000; however during the 6 hour study period, a greater improvement in FEV_1 and $FEF_{25-75\%}$ was observed 4 to 6 hours subsequent to SUS-PHRINE® (epinephrine) administration. Improvement in Wright Peak Expiratory Flow Rate was greater for SUS-PHRINE® (epinephrine) than epinephrine 1:1000 3 to 8 hours following administration (10 hour study duration).

HOW SUPPLIED

In boxes of:
10 × 0.3 mL colorless glass ampuls ....NDC 0456-0664-39
25 × 0.3 mL colorless glass ampuls ....NDC 0456-0664-34
5.0 mL multiple dose colorless glass
vial ....NDC 0456-0664-05
Store under refrigeration between 2° and 8°C (36° and 46°F). Do not freeze.
Caution Statement:
Federal Law Prohibits Dispensing without a prescription
Revised 6/94
mfd by
Steris Laboratories, Inc.
Phoenix, AZ 85043
mfd for
Forest Pharmaceuticals, Inc.
Subsidiary of Forest Laboratories, Inc.
St. Louis, Missouri 63045

TESSALON®   ℞
(benzonatate USP)

DESCRIPTION

TESSALON®, a non-narcotic oral antitussive agent, is 2, 5, 8, 11, 14, 17, 20, 23, 26-nonaoxaoctacosan-28-yl p-(butylamino) benzoate; with a molecular weight of 603.7.

$C_{30}H_{53}NO_{11}$

Each TESSALON Perle contains:
Benzonatate, USP   100 mg
TESSALON Perles also contain: D&C Yellow 10, gelatin, glycerin, methylparaben and propylparaben.

CLINICAL PHARMACOLOGY

TESSALON acts peripherally by anesthetizing the stretch receptors located in the respiratory passages, lungs, and pleura by dampening their activity and thereby reducing the cough reflex at its source. It begins to act within 15 to 20 minutes and its effect lasts for 3 to 8 hours. TESSALON has no inhibitory effect on the respiratory center in recommended dosage.

INDICATIONS AND USAGE

TESSALON is indicated for the symptomatic relief of cough.

CONTRAINDICATIONS

Hypersensitivity to benzonatate or related compounds.

WARNINGS

Severe hypersensitivity reactions (including bronchospasm, laryngospasm and cardiovascular collapse) have been reported which are possibly related to local anesthesia from sucking or chewing the perle instead of swallowing it. Severe reactions have required intervention with vasopressor agents and supportive measures.

Isolated instances of bizarre behavior, including mental confusion and visual hallucinations, have also been reported in patients taking TESSALON in combination with other prescribed drugs.

PRECAUTIONS

Benzonatate is chemically related to anesthetic agents of the para-amino-benzoic acid class (e.g. procaine; tetracaine) and has been associated with adverse CNS effects possibly related to a prior sensitivity to related agents or interaction with concomitant medication.

Information for patients: Release of TESSALON from the perle in the mouth can produce a temporary local anesthesia of the oral mucosa and choking could occur. Therefore, the perles should be swallowed without chewing.

Usage in Pregnancy: Pregnancy Category C. Animal reproduction studies have not been conducted with TESSALON. It is also not known whether TESSALON can cause fetal harm when administered to a pregnant woman or can affect reproduction capacity. TESSALON should be given to a pregnant woman only if clearly needed.

Nursing mothers: It is not known whether this drug is excreted in human milk. Because many drugs are excreted in human milk caution should be exercised when TESSALON is administered to a nursing woman.

Carcinogenesis, mutagenesis, impairment of fertility: Carcinogenicity, mutagenicity, and reproduction studies have not been conducted with TESSALON.

Pediatric Use: Safety and effectiveness in children below the age of 10 has not been established.

ADVERSE REACTIONS

Potential Adverse Reactions to TESSALON may include: Hypersensitivity reactions including bronchospasm, laryngospasm, cardiovascular collapse possibly related to local anesthesia from chewing or sucking the perle.
CNS: sedation; headache; dizziness; mental confusion; visual hallucinations.
GI: constipation, nausea, GI upset.
Dermatologic: pruritus; skin eruptions.
Other: nasal congestion; sensation of burning in the eyes; vague "chilly" sensation; numbness of the chest; hypersensitivity.
Rare instances of deliberate or accidental overdose have resulted in death.

OVERDOSAGE

Overdose may result in death.
The drug is chemically related to tetracaine and other topical anesthetics and shares various aspects of their pharmacology and toxicology. Drugs of this type are generally well absorbed after ingestion.
Signs and Symptoms:
If perles are chewed or dissolved in the mouth, oropharyngeal anesthesia will develop rapidly. CNS stimulation may cause restlessness and tremors which may proceed to clonic convulsions followed by profound CNS depression.
Treatment:
Evacuate gastric contents and administer copious amounts of activated charcoal slurry. Even in the conscious patient, cough and gag reflexes may be so depressed as to necessitate special attention to protection against aspiration of gastric contents and orally administered materials. Convulsions should be treated with a short-acting barbiturate given intravenously and carefully titrated for the smallest effective dosage. Intensive support of respiration and cardiovascular-renal function is an essential feature of the treatment of severe intoxication from overdosage.
Do not use CNS stimulants.

DOSAGE AND ADMINISTRATION

Adults and Children over 10: Usual dose is one 100 mg perle t.i.d. as required. If necessary, up to 6 perles daily may be given.

HOW SUPPLIED

Perles, 100 mg (yellow); bottles of 100   NDC 0456-0688-01
Perles, 100 mg (yellow); bottles of 500   NDC 0456-0688-02
Store at controlled room temperature 15°–30°C (59°–86°F).

Rev. 9/95
MG #11385

Mfd by
R.P. Scherer-North America
St. Petersburg, Florida 33716
for
FOREST PHARMACEUTICALS, INC.
SUBSIDIARY OF FOREST LABORATORIES, INC.
ST. LOUIS, MISSOURI 63045
Shown in Product Identification Guide, page 311

THYROLAR® Tablets ℞
[*thī-rō-lär*]
(Liotrix Tablets, USP)

DESCRIPTION

Thyrolar® Tablets (Liotrix Tablets, USP) contain triiodothyronine (T_3 liothyronine) sodium and tetraiodothyronine (T_4 levothyroxine) sodium in the amounts listed in the "How Supplied" section. (T_3 liothyronine sodium is approximately four times as potent at T_4 thyroxine on a microgram for microgram basis.)

The inactive ingredients are calcium phosphate, microcrystalline cellulose, cornstarch, lactose, and magnesium stearate. The tablets also contain the following dyes: Thyrolar® ¼-FD&C Blue #1 and FD&C Red #40; Thyrolar® ½-FD&C Red #40 and D&C Yellow #10; Thyrolar® 1-FD&C Red #40; Thyrolar® 2-FD&C Blue #1, FD&C Red #40, and D&C Yellow #10; Thyrolar® 3-FD&C Red #40 and D&C Yellow #10.

STRUCTURAL FORMULAS

Liothyronine (T_3) Sodium

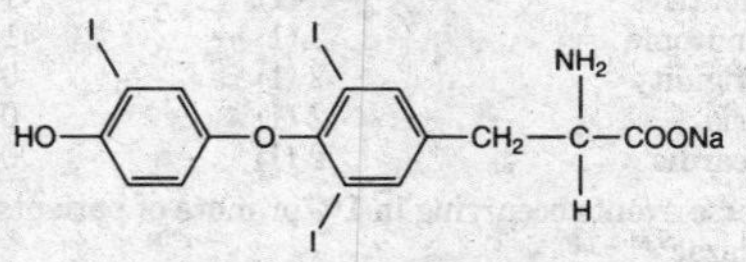

Levothyroxine (T_4) Sodium

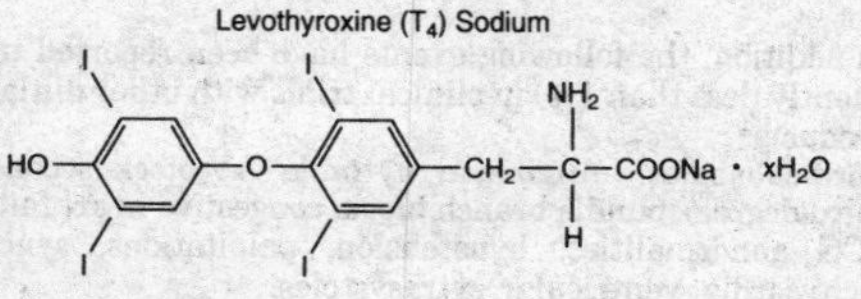

HOW SUPPLIED

Thyrolar® Tablets (Liotrix Tablets, USP) are available in five potencies, coded as follows: [See table above.]

Supplied in bottles of 100, two-layered compressed tablets.

Tablets should be stored at controlled room temperature, 59°–86°F (15°–30°C) in tight, light-resistant containers.

Note: (T_3) liothyronine sodium is approximately four times as potent as T_4 thyroxine on a microgram for microgram basis.)

Shown in Product Identification Guide, page 311

TIAZAC™ ℞
(diltiazem hydrochloride)
Extended Release Capsules

DESCRIPTION

Tiazac™ (diltiazem hydrochloride) is a calcium ion cellular influx inhibitor (slow channel blocker). Chemically, diltiazem hydrochloride is 1, 5-Benzothiazepin-4(5H)-one, 3-(acetyloxy)-5[2-(dimethylamino)ethyl]-2, -3-dihydro-2(4-methoxyphenyl)-, monohydrochloride, (+)-cis. The chemical structure is

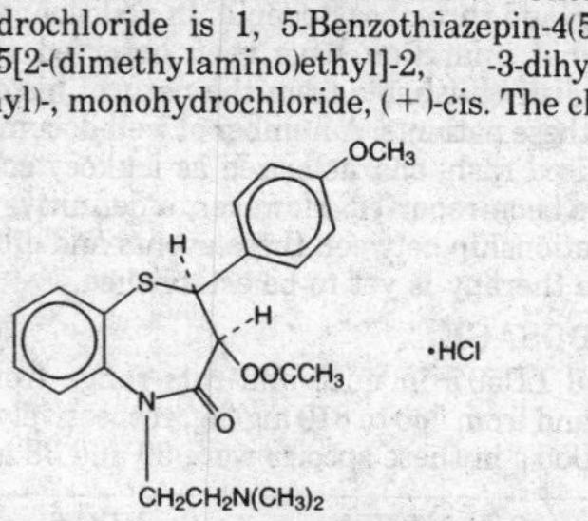

Diltiazem hydrochloride is a white to off-white crystalline powder with a bitter taste. It is soluble in water, methanol and chloroform and has a molecular weight of 450.98. Tiazac™ capsules contain diltiazem hydrochloride in extended release beads at doses of 120, 180, 240, 300 and 360 mg.

Tiazac™ also contains: Microcrystalline Cellulose NF, Sucrose Stearate, Eudragit, Povidone USP, Talc USP, Magnesium Stearate NF, Hydroxypropylmethylcellulose USP, Titanium Dioxide USP. Polysorbate NF, Simethicone USP, Gelatin NF, FD&C Blue #1, FD&C Red #40, D&C Red #28, FD&C Green #3, Black Iron Oxide USP, and other solids. For oral administration.

CLINICAL PHARMACOLOGY

The therapeutic effects of diltiazem hydrochloride are believed to be related to its ability to inhibit the cellular influx of calcium ions during membrane depolarization of cardiac and vascular smooth muscle.

THYROLAR® Tablets

Name	Composition (T_3/T_4 per tablet)	Color	Armacode®
Thyrolar®—¼(0456–0040–01)	3.1 mcg/12.5 mcg	Violet/White	YC
Thyrolar®—½(0456–0045–01)	6.25 mcg/25 mcg	Peach/White	YD
Thyrolar®—1 (0456–0050–01)	12.5 mcg/50 mcg	Pink/White	YE
Thyrolar®—2 (0456–0055–01)	25 mcg/100 mcg	Green/White	YF
Thyrolar®—3 (0456–0060–01)	37.5 mcg/150 mcg	Yellow/White	YH

Mechanisms of Action. Diltiazem produces its antihypertensive effect primarily by relaxation of vascular smooth muscle and the resultant decrease in peripheral vascular resistance. The magnitude of blood pressure reduction is related to the degree of hypertension: thus hypertensive individuals experience an antihypertensive effect, whereas there is only a modest fall in blood pressure in normotensives.

Hemodynamic and Electrophysiologic Effects. Like other calcium channel antagonists, diltiazem decreases sinoatrial and atrioventricular conduction in isolated tissues and has a negative inotropic effect in isolated preparations. In the intact animal, prolongation of the AH interval can be seen at higher doses.

In man, diltiazem prevents spontaneous and ergonovine-provoked coronary artery spasm. It causes a decrease in peripheral vascular resistance and a modest fall in blood pressure in normotensive individuals and, in exercise tolerance studies in patients with ischemic heart disease, reduces the heart rate-blood pressure product for any given work load. Studies to date, primarily in patients with good ventricular function, have not revealed evidence of a negative inotropic effect; cardiac output, ejection fraction, and left ventricular end diastolic pressure have not been affected. Such data has no predictive value with respect to effects in patients with poor ventricular function, and increased heart failure has been reported in patients with preexisting impairment of ventricular function. There are as yet few data on the interaction of diltiazem and beta-blockers in patients with poor ventricular function. Resting heart rate is usually slightly reduced by diltiazem.

Tiazac™ produces antihypertensive effects both in the supine and standing positions. Postural hypotension is infrequently noted upon suddenly assuming an upright position. No reflex tachycardia is associated with the chronic antihypertensive effects.

Diltiazem hydrochloride decreases vascular resistance, increases cardiac output (by increasing stroke volume), and produces a slight decrease or no change in heart rate. During dynamic exercise, increases in diastolic pressure are inhibited while maximum achievable systolic pressure is usually reduced. Chronic therapy with diltiazem hydrochloride produces no change or an increase in plasma catecholamines. No increased activity of the renin-angiotensin-aldosterone axis has been observed. Diltiazem hydrochloride reduces the renal and peripheral effects of angiotensin II. Hypertensive animal models respond to diltiazem with reductions in blood pressure and increased urinary output and natriuresis without a change in urinary sodium/potassium ratio. In man, transient natriuresis and kaliuresis have been reported, but only in high intravenous doses of 0.5 mg/kg of body weight.

Diltiazem-associated prolongation of the AH interval is not more pronounced in patients with first degree heart block. In patients with sick sinus syndrome, diltiazem significantly prolongs sinus cycle length (up to 50% in some cases). Intravenous diltiazem in doses of 20 mg prolongs AH conduction time and AV node functional and effective refractory periods by approximately 20%.

In two short term, double-blind, placebo-controlled studies in 256 hypertensive patients with doses up to 540 mg/day, Tiazac™ showed a clinically unimportant but statistically significant, dose-related increase in PR interval (0.008 seconds). There were no instances of greater than first-degree AV block in any of the clinical trials (See WARNINGS).

Pharmacodynamincs. In short term, double-blind, placebo-controlled clinical trials Tiazac™ demonstrated a dose-related antihypertensive response among patients with mild to moderate hypertension. In one parallel-group study of 198 patients Tiazac™ was given for four weeks. The changes in diastolic blood pressure measured at trough (24 hours after the dose) for placebo, 90mg, 180mg, 360mg and 540mg were −5.4, −6.3, −6.2, −8.2, and −11.8mm Hg, respectively. Supine diastolic blood pressure as well as standing diastolic and systolic blood pressures also showed statistically significant linear dose response effects.

In another clinical trial that followed a dose-escalation design, Tiazac™ also reduced blood pressure in a linear dose-related manner. Supine diastolic blood pressure measured following two week intervals of treatment was reduced by −3.7mm Hg with 120 mg/day versus −2.0mm Hg with placebo, by −7.6mm Hg after escalation to 240 mg/day versus −2.3mm Hg with placebo, by −8.1mm Hg after escalation to 360 mg/day versus −0.9mm Hg with placebo, and by −10.8mm Hg after escalation to 480/540 mg/day versus −2.2mm Hg with placebo.

Pharmacokinetics and Metabolism. Diltiazem is well absorbed from the gastrointestinal tract but undergoes substantial hepatic first-pass effect. The absolute bioavailability of an oral dose of an immediate release formulation (compared to intravenous administration) is approximately 40%. Only 2% to 4% of unchanged diltiazem appears in the urine. The plasma elimination half-life of diltiazem is approximately 3.0–4.5 h. Drugs which induce or inhibit hepatic microsomal enzymes may alter diltiazem disposition. Therapeutic blood levels of diltiazem appear to be in the range of 40–200 ng/mL. There is a departure from linearity when dose strengths are increased; the half-life is slightly increased with dose.

The two primary metabolites of diltiazem are desacetyldiltiazem and desmethyldiltiazem. The desacetyl metabolite is approximately 25% to 50% as potent a coronary vasodilator as diltiazem and is present in plasma at concentrations of 10% to 20% of parent diltiazem. However, recent studies employing sensitive and specific analytical methods have confirmed the existence of several sequential metabolic pathways of diltiazem. As many as nine diltiazem metabolites have been identified in the urine of humans. Total radioactivity measurements following single intravenous dose administration in healthy volunteers suggest the presence of other unidentified metabolites. These metabolites are more slowly excreted (with a half-life of total radioactivity of approximately 20 hours) and attain concentrations in excess of diltiazem.

In-vitro binding studies show diltiazem HCl is 70% to 80% bound to plasma proteins. Competitive *in-vitro* ligand binding studies have also shown diltiazem HCl binding is not altered by therapeutic concentrations of digoxin, hydrochlorothiazide, phenylbutazone, propranolol, salicylic acid, or warfarin. A study that compared patients with normal hepatic function to patients with cirrhosis who received immediate release diltiazem found an increase in diltiazem elimination half-life and a 69% increase in bioavailability in the hepatically impaired patients. Patients with severely impaired renal function (creatinine clearance <50 ml/min) who received immediate release diltiazem had modestly increased diltiazem concentrations compared to patients with normal renal function.

Tiazac™ Capsules. When compared to a regimen of immediate-release tablets at steady-state, approximately 93% of drug is absorbed from the Tiazac™ formulation. When Tiazac™ was coadministered with a high fat content breakfast, the extent of diltiazem absorption was not affected; T_{max}, however, occurred slightly earlier. The apparent elimination half-life after single or multiple dosing is 4 to 9.5 hours (mean 6.5 hours).

Tiazac™ demonstrates non-linear pharmacokinetics. As the daily dose of Tiazac™ capsules is increased from 120 to 540 mg, there was a more than proportional increase in diltiazem plasma concentrations as evidenced by an increase of AUC, C_{max} and C_{min} of 6.8, 6 and 8.6 times, respectively, for a 4.5 times increase in dose.

INDICATIONS AND USAGE

Tiazac™ is indicated for the treatment of hypertension. It may be used alone or in combination with other antihypertensive medications.

CONTRAINDICATIONS

Diltiazem is contraindicated in (1) patients with sick sinus syndrome except in the presence of a functioning ventricular pacemaker, (2) patients with second or third degree AV block except in the presence of a functioning ventricular pacemaker, (3) patients with severe hypotension (less than 90 mm Hg systolic), (4) patients who have demonstrated hypersensitivity to the drug, and (5) patients with acute myocardial infarction and pulmonary congestion documented by x-ray on admission.

WARNINGS

1. Cardiac Conduction. Diltiazem hydrochloride prolongs AV node refractory periods without significantly prolonging sinus node recovery time, except in patients with sick sinus syndrome. This effect may rarely result in abnormally slow heart rates (particularly in patients with sick sinus syndrome) or second- or third-degree AV block (13 of 3007 patients or 0.43%). Concomitant use of diltiazem with beta-blockers or digitalis may result in additive effects on cardiac conduction. A patient with Prinzmetal's angina developed

Continued on next page

Forest—Cont.

periods of asystole (2 to 5 seconds) after a single dose of 60 mg of diltiazem.

2. Congestive Heart Failure. Although diltiazem has a negative inotropic effect in isolated animal tissue preparations, hemodynamic studies in humans with normal ventricular function have not shown a reduction in cardiac index nor consistent negative effects on contractility (dp/dt). An acute study of oral diltiazem in patients with impaired ventricular function (ejection fraction 24%±6%) showed improvement in indices of ventricular function without significant decrease in contractile function (dp/dt). Worsening of congestive heart failure has been reported in patients with preexisting impairment of ventricular function. Experience with the use of diltiazem hydrochloride in combination with beta-blockers in patients with impaired ventricular function is limited. Caution should be exercised when using this combination.

3. Hypotension. Decreases in blood pressure associated with diltiazem hydrochloride therapy may occasionally result in symptomatic hypotension.

4. Acute Hepatic Injury. Mild elevations of transaminases with and without concomitant elevation in alkaline phosphatase and bilirubin have been observed in clinical studies. Such elevations were usually transient and frequently resolved even with continued diltiazem treatment. In rare instances, significant elevations in enzymes such as alkaline phosphatase, LDH, SGOT, and SGPT, and other phenomena consistent with acute hepatic injury have been noted. These reactions tended to occur early after therapy initiation (1 to 8 weeks) and have been reversible upon discontinuation of drug therapy. The relationship to diltiazem hydrochloride is uncertain in some cases, but probable in some (See PRECAUTIONS).

PRECAUTIONS

General. Diltiazem hydrochloride is extensively metabolized by the liver and excreted by the kidneys and in bile. As with any drug given over prolonged periods, laboratory parameters of renal and hepatic function should be monitored at regular intervals. The drug should be used with caution in patients with impaired renal or hepatic function. In subacute and chronic dog and rat studies designed to produce toxicity, high doses of diltiazem were associated with hepatic damage. In special subacute hepatic studies, oral doses of 125 mg/kg and higher in rats were associated with histological changes in the liver which were reversible when the drug was discontinued. In dogs, doses of 20 mg/kg were also associated with hepatic changes; however, these changes were reversible with continued dosing.

Dermatological events (see ADVERSE REACTIONS section) may be transient and may disappear despite continued use of diltiazem hydrochloride. However, skin eruptions progressing to erythema multiforme and/or exfoliative dermatitis have also been infrequently reported. Should a dermatologic reaction persist, the drug should be discontinued.

Drug Interactions. Due to the potential for additive effects, caution and careful titration are warranted in patients receiving diltiazem hydrochloride concomitantly with other agents known to affect cardiac contractility and/or conduction (See WARNINGS). Pharmacologic studies indicate that there may be additive effects in prolonging AV conduction when using beta-blockers or digitalis concomitantly with Tiazac™ (See WARNINGS). As with all drugs, care should be exercised when treating patients with multiple medications. Diltiazem hydrochloride undergoes biotransformation by cytochrome P-450 mixed function oxidase. Coadministration of diltiazem hydrochloride with other agents which follow the same route of biotransformation may result in the competitive inhibition of metabolism. Dosages of similarly metabolized drugs such as cyclosporine, particularly those of low therapeutic ratio or in patients with renal and/or hepatic impairment, may require adjustment when starting or stopping concomitantly administered diltiazem hydrochloride to maintain optimum therapeutic blood levels.

Beta Blockers. Controlled and uncontrolled domestic studies suggest that concomitant use of diltiazem hydrochloride and beta-blockers is usually well tolerated, but available data are not sufficient to predict the effects of concomitant treatment in patients with left ventricular dysfunction or cardiac conduction abnormalities. Administration of diltiazem hydrochloride concomitantly with propranolol in five normal volunteers resulted in increased propranolol levels in all subjects and bioavailability of propranolol was increased approximately 50%. *In vitro*, propranolol appears to be displaced from its binding sites by diltiazem. If combination therapy is initiated or withdrawn in conjunction with propranolol, an adjustment in the propranolol dose may be warranted (See WARNINGS).

Cimetidine. A study in six healthy volunteers has shown a significant increase in peak diltiazem plasma levels (58%) and area-under-the-curve (53%) after a 1-week course of cimetidine 1200 mg per day and a single dose of diltiazem 60 mg. Ranitidine produced smaller, nonsignificant increases. The effect may be mediated by cimetidine's known inhibition of hepatic cytochrome P-450, the enzyme system responsible for the first-pass metabolism of diltiazem. Patients currently receiving diltiazem therapy should be carefully monitored for a change in pharmacological effect when initiating and discontinuing therapy with cimetidine. An adjustment in the diltiazem dose may be warranted.

Digitalis. Administration of diltiazem hydrochloride with digoxin in 24 healthy male subjects increased plasma digoxin concentrations approximately 20%. Another investigator found no increase in digoxin levels in 12 patients with coronary artery disease. Since there have been conflicting results regarding the effect of digoxin levels, it is recommended that digoxin levels be monitored when initiating, adjusting, and discontinuing diltiazem hydrochloride therapy to avoid possible over- or under-digitalization (See WARNINGS).

Anesthetics. The depression of cardiac contractility, conductivity, and automaticity as well as the vascular dilation associated with anesthetics may be potentiated by calcium channel blockers. When used concomitantly, anesthetics and calcium blockers should be titrated carefully.

Cyclosporine. A pharmacokinetic interaction between diltiazem and cyclosporine has been observed during studies involving renal and cardiac transplant patients. In renal and cardiac transplant recipients, a reduction of cyclosporine dose ranging from 15% to 48% was necessary to maintain cyclosporine trough concentrations similar to those seen prior to the addition of diltiazem. If these agents are to be administered concurrently, cyclosporine concentrations should be monitored, especially when diltiazem therapy is initiated, adjusted, or discontinued.

The effect of cyclosporine on diltiazem plasma concentrations has not been evaluated.

Carbamazepine. Concomitant administration of diltiazem with carbamazepine has been reported to result in elevated serum levels of carbamazepine (40% to 72% increase), resulting in toxicity in some cases. Patients receiving these drugs concurrently should be monitored for a potential drug interaction.

Carcinogenesis, Mutagenesis, Impairment of Fertility. A 24 month study in rats at oral dosage levels of up to 100 mg/kg/day, and a 21 month study in mice at oral dosage levels of up to 30 mg/kg/day showed no evidence of carcinogenicity. There was also no mutagenic response *in vitro* or *in vivo* in mammalian cell assays or *in vitro* in bacteria. No evidence of impaired fertility was observed in a study performed in male and female rats at oral dosages of up to 100 mg/kg/day.

Pregnancy. Category C. Reproduction studies have been conducted in mice, rats, and rabbits. Administration of doses ranging from 4 to 6 times (depending on species) the upper limit of the optimum dosage range in clinical trials (480 mg q.d. or 8 mg/kg q.d. for a 60 kg patient) resulted in embryo and fetal lethality. These studies revealed, in one species or another, a propensity to cause abnormalities of the skeleton, heart, retina, and tongue. Also observed were reductions in early individual pup weights and pup survival, prolonged delivery and increased incidence of stillbirths. There are no well-controlled studies in pregnant women; therefore, use diltiazem hydrochloride in pregnant women only if the potential benefit justifies the potential risk to the fetus.

Nursing Mothers. Diltiazem is excreted in human milk. One report suggests that concentrations in breast milk may approximate serum levels. If use of Tiazac™ is deemed essential, an alternative method of infant feeding should be instituted.

Pediatric Use. Safety and effectiveness in children have not been established.

ADVERSE REACTIONS

Serious adverse reactions have been rare in studies with Tiazac™, as well as other diltiazem formulations. It should be recognized that patients with impaired ventricular function and cardiac conduction abnormalities have usually been excluded from these studies. The following table presents the most common adverse reactions reported in placebo-controlled trials in patients receiving Tiazac™ up to 540 mg with rates in placebo patients shown for comparison.

MOST COMMON ADVERSE EVENTS IN DOUBLE-BLIND PLACEBO-CONTROLLED HYPERTENSION TRIALS*

Adverse Events (COSTART Term)	Tiazac™ n=197 # pts (%)	Placebo n=57 # pts (%)
headache	35 (18)	11 (19)
edema, peripheral	15 (8)	1 (2)
pain	13 (7)	5 (9)
asthenia	10 (6)	6 (11)
dizziness	9 (5)	4 (7)
vasodilation	8 (4)	1 (2)
dyspepsia	7 (4)	0 (0)
pharyngitis	6 (3)	2 (4)
dyspnea	4 (2)	1 (2)
infection	4 (2)	2 (4)
nausea	4 (2)	2 (4)
rash	4 (2)	0 (0)
constipation	3 (2)	0 (0)
diarrhea	3 (2)	0 (0)
edema	3 (2)	1 (2)
nervousness	3 (2)	0 (0)
palpitations	3 (2)	0 (0)
parestehesia	3 (2)	2 (4)
rhinitis	3 (2)	2 (4)
somnolence	3 (2)	0 (0)
allergic reaction	2 (1)	0 (0)
anorexia	2 (1)	1 (2)
cough increase	2 (1)	0 (0)
dry mouth	2 (1)	1 (2)
flu syndrome	2 (1)	1 (2)
neck rigidity	2 (1)	0 (0)
polyuria	2 (1)	0 (0)
tachycardia	2 (1)	0 (0)

*Adverse events occurring in 1% or more of patients receiving Tiazac™

In addition, the following events have been reported infrequently (less than 1%) in clinical trials with other diltiazem products:

Cardiovascular. Angina, arrhythmia, AV block (second- or third-degree), bundle branch block, congestive heart failure, ECG abnormalities, hypotension, palpitations, syncope, tachycardia, ventricular extrasystoles.

Nervous System. Abnormal dreams, amnesia, depression, gait abnormality, hallucinations, insomnia, nervousness, paresthesia, personality change, somnolence, tinnitus, tremor.

Gastrointestinal. Anorexia, constipation, diarrhea, dry mouth, dysgeusia, mild elevations of SGOT, SGPT, LDH, and alkaline phosphatase (see hepatic warnings), thirst, vomiting, weight increase.

Dermatological. Petechiae, photosensitivity, pruritus.

Other. Amblyopia, CPK increase, dyspnea, epistaxis, eye irritation, hyperglycemia, hyperuricemia, impotence, muscle cramps, nasal congestion, nocturia, osteoarticular pain, polyuria, sexual difficulties.

In addition the following postmarketing events have been reported infrequently in patients receiving diltiazem hydrochloride: alopecia, erythema multiforme, exfoliative dermatitis, Stevens-Johnson syndrome, toxic epidermal necrolysis, extrapyramidal symptoms, gingival hyperplasia, hemolytic anemia, increased bleeding time, leukopenia, purpura, retinopathy, and thrombocytopenia. In addition, events such as myocardial infarction have been observed which are not readily distinguishable from the natural history of the disease in these patients. A number of well-documented cases of generalized rash, characterized as leukocytoclastic vasculitis, have been reported. However, a definitive cause and effect relationship between these events and diltiazem hydrochloride therapy is yet to be established.

OVERDOSAGE

The oral LD50's in mice and rats range from 415 to 740 mg/kg and from 560 to 810 mg/kg, respectively. The intravenous LD50's in these species were 60 and 38 mg/kg, respec-

STRENGTH	DESCRIPTION	QUANTITY	NDC#
120 mg	#3 lavender/lavender capsule imprinted "Tiazac" 120	30's	0456-2612-30
		90's	0456-2612-90
180 mg	#2 white/blue-green capsule imprinted "Tiazac" 180	30's	0456-2613-30
		90's	0456-2613-90
		1000's	0456-2613-00
			0456-2613-00
240 mg	#1 blue-green/lavender capsule imprinted "Tiazac" 240	30's	0456-2614-30
		90's	0456-2614-90
		1000's	0456-2614-00
300 mg	#0 white/lavender capsule imprinted "Tiazac" 300	30's	0456-2615-30
		90's	0456-2615-90
		1000's	0456-2615-00
360 mg	#0 blue-green/blue-green capsule imprinted "Tiazac" 360	30's	0456-2616-30
		90's	0456-2616-90

tively. The oral LD50 in dogs is considered to be in excess of 50 mg/kg, while lethality was seen in monkeys at 360 mg/kg. The toxic dose in man is not known. Due to extensive metabolism, blood levels after a standard dose of diltiazem can vary over tenfold, limiting the usefulness of blood levels in overdose cases. There have been 29 reports of diltiazem overdose in doses ranging from less than 1 gm to 10.8 gm. Sixteen of these reports involved multiple drug ingestions. Twenty-two reports indicated patients had recovered from diltiazem overdose ranging from less than 1 gm to 10.8 gm. There were seven reports with a fatal outcome; although the amount of diltiazem ingested was unknown, multiple drug ingestions were confirmed in six of the seven reports.

Events observed following diltiazem overdose included bradycardia, hypotension, heart block, and cardiac failure. Most reports of overdose described some supportive medical measure and/or drug treatment. Bradycardia frequently responded favorably to atropine as did heart block, although cardiac pacing was also frequently utilized to treat heart block. Fluids and vasopressors were used to maintain blood pressure, and in cases of cardiac failure, inotropic agents were administered. In addition, some patients received treatment with ventilatory support, activated charcoal, and/or intravenous calcium. Evidence of the effectiveness of intravenous calcium administration to reverse the pharmacological effects of diltiazem overdose was conflicting.

In the event of overdose or exaggerated response, appropriate supportive measures should be employed in addition to gastrointestinal decontamination. Diltiazem does not appear to be removed by peritoneal or hemodialysis. Based on the known pharmacological effects of diltiazem and/or reported clinical experiences, the following measures may be considered:

Bradycardia: Administer atropine (0.60 to 1.0 mg). If there is no response to vagal blockage, administer isoproterenol cautiously.

High-Degree AV Block: Treat as for bradycardia above. Fixed high-degree AV block should be treated with cardiac pacing.

Cardiac Failure: Administer inotropic agents (isoproterenol, dopamine, or dobutamine) and diuretics.

Hypotension: Vasopressors (e.g. dopamine or levarterenol bitartrate). Actual treatment and dosage should depend on the severity of the clinical situation and the judgment and experience of the treating physician.

Due to extensive metabolism, plasma concentrations after a standard dose of diltiazem can vary over tenfold, which significantly limits their value in evaluation cases of overdosage.

Charcoal hemoperfusion has been used successfully as an adjunct therapy to hasten drug elimination. Overdoses with as much as 10.8 gm of oral diltiazem have been successfully treated using appropriate supportive care.

DOSAGE AND ADMINISTRATION

Dosage needs to be adjusted by titration to individual patient needs. When used as monotherapy, usual starting doses are 120 to 240 mg once daily. Maximum antihypertensive effect is usually observed by 14 days of chronic therapy; therefore, dosage adjustments should be scheduled accordingly. The usual dosage range studied in clinical trials was 120 to 540 mg once daily. Current clinical experience with 540 mg dose is limited, however, the dose may be increased to 540 mg once daily.

Hypertensive patients controlled on diltiazem alone or in combination with other antihypertensive medications may be safely switched to Tiazac™ capsules at the nearest equivalent total daily dose. Subsequent titration to higher or lower doses may be necessary and should be initiated as clinically warranted.

Diltiazem hydrochloride has an additive antihypertensive effect when used with other antihypertensive agents. Therefore, the dosage of diltiazem hydrochloride or the concomitant antihypertensive may need to be adjusted when adding one to the other. See WARNINGS and PRECAUTIONS regarding use with beta-blockers.

HOW SUPPLIED

Tiazac™ (diltiazem hydrochloride) Extended-release Capsules

[See table on bottom of preceding page.]

Storage conditions: Store at controlled room temperature 20°–25°C (68°–77°F). Avoid excessive humidity.

CAUTION: Federal (U.S.A.) Law prohibits dispensing without prescription

Manufactured by:
BIOVAIL LABORATORIES INC., Carolina, Puerto Rico Encapsulated and Made in Canada

Manufactured for:
Forest Pharmaceuticals, Inc.
Subsidiary of Forest Laboratories, Inc.
St. Louis, Missouri 63045
Rev. 3/96   LB-0001-02
Shown in Product Identification Guide, page 311

ZONE–A CREAM 1%   ℞
[zōn 'ā]

DESCRIPTION

A topical preparation containing Hydrocortisone acetate 1% and Pramoxine HCl 1% in a hydrophilic cream base containing stearic acid, cetyl alcohol, aquaphor, isopropyl palmitate, polyoxyl 40 stearate, propylene glycol, potassium sorbate 0.1%, sorbic acid 0.1%, triethanolamine lauryl sulfate and water.

HOW SUPPLIED

1 oz. tube NDC 0785-5505-04

Fujisawa USA, Inc.
PARKWAY NORTH CENTER
3 PARKWAY NORTH
DEERFIELD, IL 60015-2548

For Medical Information Contact:
Generally:
Medical and Scientific Information
(800) 727-7003
In Emergencies:
Medical and Scientific Information
(800) 727-7003

ADENOCARD® IV   ℞
(adenosine)
For Rapid Bolus Intravenous Use

DESCRIPTION

Adenosine is an endogenous nucleoside occurring in all cells of the body. It is chemically 6-amino-9-β-D-ribofuranosyl-9-H-purine and has the following structural formula:

$C_{10}H_{13}N_5O_4$ 267.24

Adenosine is a white crystalline powder. It is soluble in water and practically insoluble in alcohol. Solubility increases by warming and lowering the pH. Adenosine is not chemically related to other antiarrhythmic drugs. Adenocard® (adenosine) is a sterile solution for rapid bolus intravenous injection. Each mL contains 3 mg adenosine and 9 mg sodium chloride in Water for Injection. The pH of the solution is between 5.5 and 7.5.

CLINICAL PHARMACOLOGY
Mechanism of Action
Adenocard (adenosine) slows conduction time through the A-V node, can interrupt the reentry pathways through the A-V node, and can restore normal sinus rhythm in patients with paroxysmal supraventricular tachycardia (PSVT), including PSVT associated with Wolff-Parkinson-White Syndrome.
Adenocard is antagonized competitively by methylxanthines such as caffeine and theophylline, and potentiated by blockers of nucleoside transport such as dipyridamole. Adenocard is not blocked by atropine.
Hemodynamics
The usual intravenous bolus dose of 6 or 12 mg Adenocard (adenosine) will have no systemic hemodynamic effects. When larger doses are given by infusion, adenosine decreases blood pressure by decreasing peripheral resistance.
Pharmacokinetics
Intravenously administered Adenocard (adenosine) is removed from the circulation very rapidly. Following an intravenous bolus, adenosine is taken up by erythrocytes and vascular endothelial cells. The half-life of intravenous adeno-

sine is estimated to be less than 10 seconds. Adenosine enters the body pool and is primarily metabolized to inosine and adenosine monophosphate (AMP).
Hepatic and Renal Failure
Hepatic and renal failure should have no effect on the activity of a bolus Adenocard (adenosine) injection. Since Adenocard (adenosine) has a direct action, hepatic and renal function are not required for the activity or the metabolism of a bolus adenosine injection.
Clinical Trial Results
In controlled studies in the United States, bolus doses of 3, 6, 9, and 12 mg were studied. A cumulative 60% of patients with paroxysmal supraventricular tachycardia had converted to normal sinus rhythm within one minute after an intravenous bolus dose of 6 mg Adenocard (some converted on 3 mg and failures were given 6 mg), and a cumulative 92% converted after a bolus dose of 12 mg. Seven to sixteen percent of patients converted after 1–4 placebo bolus injections. Similar responses were seen in a variety of patient subsets, including those using or not using digoxin, those with Wolff-Parkinson-White Syndrome, males, females, blacks, Caucasians, and Hispanics.
Adenosine is not effective in converting rhythms other than PSVT, such as atrial flutter, atrial fibrillation, or ventricular tachycardia, to normal sinus rhythm. To date, such patients have not had adverse consequences following administration of adenosine.

INDICATIONS AND USAGE

Intravenous Adenocard (adenosine) is indicated for the following.
Conversion to sinus rhythm of paroxysmal supraventricular tachycardia (PSVT), including that associated with accessory bypass tracts (Wolff-Parkinson-White Syndrome). When clinically advisable, appropriate vagal maneuvers (e.g., Valsalva maneuver), should be attempted prior to Adenocard administration.
It is important to be sure the Adenocard solution actually reaches the systemic circulation (see **Dosage and Administration**).
Adenocard does not convert atrial flutter, atrial fibrillation, or ventricular tachycardia to normal sinus rhythm. In the presence of atrial flutter or atrial fibrillation, a transient modest slowing of ventricular response may occur immediately following Adenocard administration.

CONTRAINDICATIONS

Intravenous Adenocard (adenosine) is contraindicated in:
1. Second- or third-degree A-V block (except in patients with a functioning artificial pacemaker).
2. Sick sinus syndrome (except in patients with a functioning artificial pacemaker).
3. Known hypersensitivity to adenosine.

WARNINGS
Heart Block
Adenocard (adenosine) exerts its effect by decreasing conduction through the A-V node and may produce a short lasting first-, second- or third-degree heart block. In extreme cases, transient asystole may result (one case has been reported in a patient with atrial flutter who was receiving carbamazepine). Appropriate therapy should be instituted as needed. Patients who develop high-level block on one dose of Adenocard should not be given additional doses. Because of the very short half-life of adenosine, these effects are generally self-limiting.
Rarely, ventricular fibrillation has been reported following Adenocard administration, including both resuscitated and fatal events. In most instances, these cases were associated with the concomitant use of digoxin. Although no causal relationship or drug-drug interaction has been established, Adenocard should be used with caution in patients receiving digoxin. Appropriate resuscitative measures should be available.
Arrhythmias at Time of Conversion
At the time of conversion to normal sinus rhythm, a variety of new rhythms may appear on the electrocardiogram. They generally last only a few seconds without intervention, and may take the form of premature ventricular contractions, atrial premature contractions, sinus bradycardia, sinus tachycardia, skipped beats, and varying degrees of A-V nodal block. Such findings were seen in 55% of patients.

PRECAUTIONS
Drug Interactions
Intravenous Adenocard (adenosine) has been effectively administered in the presence of other cardioactive drugs, such as quinidine, beta-adrenergic blocking agents, calcium channel blocking agents, and angiotensin converting enzyme inhibitors, without any change in the adverse reaction profile. The use of Adenocard in patients receiving digitalis may be rarely associated with ventricular fibrillation (see WARNINGS).
The effects of adenosine are antagonized by methylxanthines such as caffeine and theophylline. In the presence of

Continued on next page

Consult 1997 supplements and future editions for revisions

Fujisawa—Cont.

these methylxanthines, larger doses of adenosine may be required or adenosine may not be effective. Adenosine effects are potentiated by dipyridamole. Thus, smaller doses of adenosine may be effective in the presence of dipyridamole. Carbamazepine has been reported to increase the degree of heart block produced by other agents. As the primary effect of adenosine is to decrease conduction through the A-V node, higher degrees of heart block may be produced in the presence of carbamazepine.

Asthma

Most patients with asthma who have received intravenous Adenocard (adenosine) have not experienced exacerbation of their asthma. Cases of bronchospasm have been reported rarely in both asthmatic and non-asthmatic patients. Inhaled adenosine has been reported to induce bronchoconstriction in asthmatic patients, but not in normal individuals.

Carcinogenesis, Mutagenesis, Impairment of Fertility

Studies in animals have not been performed to evaluate the carcinogenic potential of Adenocard (adenosine). Adenosine was negative for genotoxic potential in the Salmonella (Ames Test) and Mammalian Microsome Assay.

Adenosine, however, like other nucleosides at millimolar concentrations present for several doubling times of cells in culture, is known to produce a variety of chromosomal alterations. In rats and mice, adenosine administered intraperitoneally once a day for five days at 50, 100, and 150 mg/kg [10–30 (rats) and 5–15 (mice) times human dosage on a mg/M^2 basis] caused decreased spermatogenesis and increased numbers of abnormal sperm, a reflection of the ability of adenosine to produce chromosomal damage.

Pregnancy Category C

Animal reproduction studies have not been conducted with adenosine; nor have studies been performed in pregnant women. As adenosine is a naturally occurring material, widely dispersed throughout the body, no fetal effects would be anticipated. However, since it is not known whether Adenocard can cause fetal harm when administered to pregnant women, Adenocard should be used during pregnancy only if clearly needed.

Pediatrics

No controlled studies have been conducted in pediatric patients.

ADVERSE REACTIONS

The following reactions were reported with intravenous Adenocard (adenosine) used in controlled U.S. clinical trials. The placebo group had a less than 1% rate of all of these reactions.

Cardiovascular	Facial flushing (18%), headache (2%), sweating, palpitations, chest pain, hypotension (less than 1%).
Respiratory	Shortness of breath/dyspnea (12%), chest pressure (7%), hyperventilation, head pressure (less than 1%).
Central Nervous System	Lightheadedness (2%), dizziness, tingling in arms, numbness (1%), apprehension, blurred vision, burning sensation, heaviness in arms, neck and back pain (less than 1%).
Gastrointestinal	Nausea (3%), metallic taste, tightness in throat, pressure in groin (less than 1%).

In post-market clinical experience with Adenocard, cases of prolonged asystole, ventricular tachycardia, ventricular fibrillation, transient increase in blood pressure, and bronchospasm, in association with Adenocard use, have been reported.

OVERDOSAGE

The half-life of Adenocard (adenosine) is less than 10 seconds. Thus, adverse effects are generally rapidly self-limiting. Treatment of any prolonged adverse effects should be individualized and be directed toward the specific effect. Methylxanthines, such as caffeine and theophylline, are competitive antagonists of adenosine.

DOSAGE AND ADMINISTRATION

For rapid bolus intravenous use only.

Adenocard (adenosine) Injection should be given as a rapid bolus by the peripheral intravenous route. To be certain the solution reaches the systemic circulation, it should be administered either directly into a vein or, if given into an IV line, it should be given as close to the patient as possible and followed by a rapid saline flush.

The dose recommendation is based on clinical studies with peripheral venous bolus dosing. Central venous (CVP or other) administration of Adenocard has not been systematically studied.

The recommended intravenous doses for adults are as follows:

Initial dose: 6 mg given as a rapid intravenous bolus (administered over a 1–2 second period).

Repeat administration: If the first dose does not result in elimination of the supraventricular tachycardia within 1–2 minutes, 12 mg should be given as a rapid intravenous bolus. This 12 mg dose may be repeated a second time if required.

Doses greater than 12 mg are not recommended.

NOTE: Parenteral drug products should be inspected visually for particulate matter and discoloration prior to administration.

HOW SUPPLIED

Adenocard® (adenosine) Injection is supplied as a sterile solution in normal saline.

NDC 0469-0871-02 Product Code 87102 6 mg/2 mL (3 mg/mL) in 2 mL flip-top vials, packaged in 10's.

NDC 0469-7234-12 Product Code 723412 6 mg/2 mL (3 mg/mL) in a 2 mL disposable syringe, in a package of five.

NDC 0469-7234-14 Product Code 723414 12 mg/4 mL (3 mg/mL) in a 5 mL disposable syringe, in a package of five.

Store at controlled room temperature 15°–30°C (59°–86°F).

DO NOT REFRIGERATE as crystallization may occur. If crystallization has occurred, dissolve crystals by warming to room temperature. The solution must be clear at the time of use.

Contains no preservatives. Discard unused portion.

CAUTION: Federal law prohibits dispensing without prescription.

Fujisawa USA, Inc., Deerfield, IL 60015
Under license from Medco Research, Inc.
Research Triangle Park, NC 27709
45514F
Revised: September 1995

ADENOSCAN® ℞

adenosine
For Intravenous Infusion Only

DESCRIPTION

Adenosine is an endogenous nucleoside occurring in all cells of the body. It is chemically 6-amino-9-beta-D-ribofuranosyl-9-H-purine and has the following structural formula:

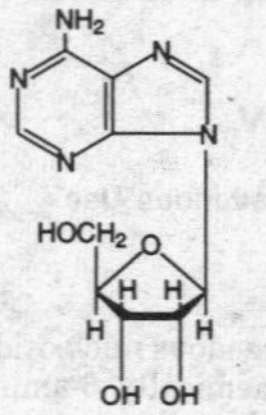

$C_{10}H_{13}N_5O_4$ 267.24

Adenosine is a white crystalline powder. It is soluble in water and practically insoluble in alcohol. Solubility increases by warming and lowering the pH of the solution.

Each Adenoscan vial contains a sterile, nonpyrogenic solution of adenosine 3 mg/mL and sodium chloride 9 mg/mL in Water for Injection, q.s. The pH of the solution is between 4.5 and 7.5.

CLINICAL PHARMACOLOGY

Mechanism of Action

Adenosine is a potent vasodilator in most vascular beds, except in renal afferent arterioles and hepatic veins where it produces vasoconstriction. Adenosine is thought to exert its pharmacological effects through activation of purine receptors (cell-surface A_1 and A_2 adenosine receptors). Although the exact mechanism by which adenosine receptor activation relaxes vascular smooth muscle is not known, there is evidence to support both inhibition of the slow inward calcium current reducing calcium uptake, and activation of adenylate cyclase through A_2 receptors in smooth muscle cells. Adenosine may also lessen vascular tone by modulating sympathetic neurotransmission. The intracellular uptake of adenosine is mediated by a specific transmembrane nucleoside transport system. Once inside the cell, adenosine is rapidly phosphorylated by adenosine kinase to adenosine monophosphate, or deaminated by adenosine deaminase to inosine. These intracellular metabolites of adenosine are not vasoactive.

Myocardial uptake of thallium-201 is directly proportional to coronary blood flow. Since Adenoscan significantly increases blood flow in normal coronary arteries with little or no increase in stenotic arteries, Adenoscan causes relatively less thallium-201 uptake in vascular territories supplied by stenotic coronary arteries i.e., a greater difference is seen after Adenoscan between areas served by normal and areas served by stenotic vessels than is seen prior to Adenoscan.

Hemodynamics

Adenosine produces a direct negative chronotropic, dromotropic and inotropic effect on the heart, presumably due to A_1-receptor agonism, and produces peripheral vasodilation, presumably due to A_2-receptor agonism. The net effect of Adenoscan in humans is typically a mild to moderate reduction in systolic, diastolic and mean arterial blood pressure associated with a reflex increase in heart rate. Rarely, significant hypotension and tachycardia have been observed.

Pharmacokinetics

Intravenously administered adenosine is rapidly cleared from the circulation via cellular uptake, primarily by erythrocytes and vascular endothelial cells. This process involves a specific transmembrane nucleoside carrier system that is reversible, nonconcentrative, and bidirectionally symmetrical. Intracellular adenosine is rapidly metabolized either via phosphorylation to adenosine monophosphate by adenosine kinase, or via deamination to inosine by adenosine deaminase in the cytosol. Since adenosine kinase has a lower K_m and V_{max} than adenosine deaminase, deamination plays a significant role only when cytosolic adenosine saturates the phosphorylation pathway. Inosine formed by deamination of adenosine can leave the cell intact or can be degraded to hypoxanthine, xanthine, and ultimately uric acid. Adenosine monophosphate formed by phosphorylation of adenosine is incorporated into the high-energy phosphate pool. While extracellular adenosine is primarily cleared by cellular uptake with a half-life of less than 10 seconds in whole blood, excessive amounts may be deaminated by an ecto-form of adenosine deaminase. As Adenoscan requires no hepatic or renal function for its activation or inactivation, hepatic and renal failure would not be expected to alter its effectiveness or tolerability.

Clinical Trials

In two crossover comparative studies involving 319 subjects who would exercise (including 106 healthy volunteers and 213 patients with known or suspected coronary disease), Adenoscan and exercise thallium images were compared by blinded observers. The images were concordant for the presence of perfusion defects in 85.5% of cases by global analysis (patient by patient) and up to 93% of cases based on vascular territories. In these two studies, 193 patients also had recent coronary arteriography for comparison (healthy volunteers were not catheterized). The sensitivity (true positive Adenoscan divided by the number of patients with positive (abnormal) angiography) for detecting angiographically significant disease (≥ 50% reduction in the luminal diameter of at least one major vessel) was 64% for Adenoscan and 64% for exercise testing, while the specificity (true negative divided by the number of patients with negative angiograms) was 54% for Andenoscan and 65% for exercise testing. The 95% confidence limits for Adenoscan sensitivity were 56% to 78% and for specificity were 37% to 71%.

Intracoronary Doppler flow catheter studies have demonstrated that a dose of intravenous Adenoscan of 140 mcg/kg/min produces maximum coronary hyperemia (relative to intracoronary papaverine) in approximately 95% of cases within two to three minutes of the onset of the infusion. Coronary blood flow velocity returns to basal levels within one to two minutes of discontinuing the Adenoscan infusion.

INDICATIONS AND USAGE

Intravenous Adenoscan is indicated as an adjunct to thallium-201 myocardial perfusion scintigraphy in patients unable to exercise adequately (See **WARNINGS**).

CONTRAINDICATIONS

Intravenous Adenoscan (adenosine) should not be administered to individuals with:

1. Second- or third-degree AV block (except in patients with a functioning artificial pacemaker).
2. Sinus node disease, such as sick sinus syndrome or symptomatic bradycardia (except in patients with a functioning artificial pacemaker).
3. Known or suspected bronchoconstrictive or bronchospastic lung disease (e.g., asthma).
4. Known hypersensitivity to adenosine.

WARNINGS

Fatal Cardiac Arrest, Life Threatening Ventricular Arrhythmias, and Myocardial Infarction.

Fatal cardiac arrest, sustained ventricular tachycardia (requiring resuscitation), and non-fatal myocardial infarction have been reported coincident with Adenoscan infusion. Patients with unstable angina may be at greater risk.

Sinoatrial and Atrioventricular Nodal Block

Adenoscan (adenosine) exerts a direct depressant effect on the SA and AV nodes and has the potential to cause first-, second- or third-degree AV block, or sinus bradycardia. Approximately 6.3% of patients develop AV block with Adenoscan, including first-degree (2.9%), second-degree (2.6%) and third-degree (0.8%) heart block. All episodes of AV block have been asymptomatic, transient, and did not require intervention. Adenoscan can cause sinus bradycardia. Adenoscan should be used with caution in patients with preexisting first-degree AV block or bundle branch block and should be avoided in patients with high-grade AV block or sinus node dysfunction (except in patients with a functioning artificial pacemaker). Adenoscan should be discontinued in any patient who develops persistent or symptomatic high-grade AV block. Sinus pause has been rarely observed with adenosine infusions.

Hypotension

Adenoscan (adenosine) is a potent peripheral vasodilator and can cause significant hypotension. Patients with an intact baroreceptor reflex mechanism are able to maintain blood pressure and tissue perfusion in response to Adenoscan by increasing heart rate and cardiac output. However, Adenoscan should be used with caution in patients with autonomic dysfunction, stenotic valvular heart disease, pericarditis or pericardial effusions, stenotic carotid artery disease with cerebrovascular insufficiency, or uncorrected hypovolemia, due to the risk of hypotensive complications in these patients. Adenoscan should be discontinued in any patient who develops persistent or symptomatic hypotension.

Hypertension

Increases in systolic and diastolic pressure have been observed (as great as 140 mm Hg systolic in one case) concomitant with Adenoscan infusion; most increases resolved spontaneously within several minutes, but in some cases, hypertension lasted for several hours.

Bronchoconstriction

Adenoscan (adenosine) is a respiratory stimulant (probably through activation of carotid body chemoreceptors) and intravenous administration in man has been shown to increase minute ventilation (Ve) and reduce arterial PCO_2 causing respiratory alkalosis. Approximately 28% of patients experience breathlessness (dyspnea) or an urge to breathe deeply with Adenoscan. These respiratory complaints are transient and only rarely require intervention.

Adenosine administered by inhalation has been reported to cause bronchoconstriction in asthmatic patients, presumably due to mast cell degranulation and histamine release. These effects have not been observed in normal subjects. Adenoscan has been administered to a limited number of patients with asthma and mild to moderate exacerbation of their symptoms has been reported. Respiratory compromise has occurred during adenosine infusion in patients with obstructive pulmonary disease. Adenoscan should be used with caution in patients with obstructive lung disease not associated with bronchoconstriction (e.g., emphysema, bronchitis, etc.) and should be avoided in patients with bronchoconstriction or bronchospasm (e.g., asthma). Adenoscan should be discontinued in any patient who develops severe respiratory difficulties.

PRECAUTIONS

Drug Interactions

Intravenous Adenoscan (adenosine) has been given with other cardioactive drugs (such as beta adrenergic blocking agents, cardiac glycosides, and calcium channel blockers) without apparent adverse interactions, but its effectiveness with these agents has not been systematically evaluated. Because of the potential for additive or synergistic depressant effects on the SA and AV nodes, however, Adenoscan should be used with caution in the presence of these agents. The vasoactive effects of Adenoscan are inhibited by adenosine receptor antagonists, such as alkylxanthines (e.g., caffeine and theophylline). The safety and efficacy of Adenoscan in the presence of these agents has not been systematically evaluated.

The vasoactive effects of Adenoscan are potentiated by nucleoside transport inhibitors, such as dipyridamole. The safety and efficacy of Adenoscan in the presence of dipyridamole has not been systematically evaluated.

Whenever possible, drugs that might inhibit or augment the effects of adenosine should be withheld for at least five half-lives prior to the use of Adenoscan.

Carcinogenesis, Mutagenesis, Impairment of Fertility

Studies in animals have not been performed to evaluate the carcinogenic potential of Adenoscan (adenosine). Adenosine was negative for genotoxic potential in the Salmonella (Ames Test) and Mammalian Microsome Assay.

Adenosine, however, like other nucleosides at millimolar concentrations present for several doubling times of cells in culture, is known to produce a variety of chromosomal alterations. In rats and mice, adenosine administered intraperitoneally once a day for five days at 50, 100, and 150 mg/kg [10–30 (rats) and 5–15 (mice) times human dosage on a mg/M^2 basis] caused decreased spermatogenesis and increased numbers of abnormal sperm, a reflection of the ability of adenosine to produce chromosomal damage.

Pregnancy Category C

Animal reproduction studies have not been conducted with adenosine; nor have studies been performed in pregnant women. Because it is not known whether Adenoscan can cause fetal harm when administered to pregnant women, Adenoscan should be used during pregnancy only if clearly needed.

Pediatric Use

The safety and effectiveness of Adenoscan in patients less than 18 years of age have not been established.

ADVERSE REACTIONS

The following reactions with an incidence of at least 1% were reported with intravenous Adenoscan among 1421 patients enrolled in controlled and uncontrolled U.S. clinical trials. Despite the short half-life of adenosine, 10.6% of the side effects occurred not with the infusion of Adenoscan but several hours after the infusion terminated. Also, 8.4% of the side effects that began coincident with the infusion persisted for up to 24 hours after the infusion was complete. In many cases, it is not possible to know whether these late adverse events are the result of Adenoscan infusion.

Flushing	44%
Chest discomfort	40%
Dyspnea or urge to breathe deeply	28%
Headache	18%
Throat, neck or jaw discomfort	15%
Gastrointestinal discomfort	13%
Lightheadedness/dizziness	12%
Upper extremity discomfort	4%
ST segment depression	3%
First-degree AV block	3%
Second-degree AV block	3%
Paresthesia	2%
Hypotension	2%
Nervousness	2%
Arrhythmias	1%

Adverse experiences of any severity reported in less than 1% of patients include:

Body as a Whole: back discomfort; lower extremity discomfort; weakness.

Cardiovascular System: nonfatal myocardial infarction; life-threatening ventricular arrhythmia; third-degree AV block; bradycardia; palpitation; sinus exit block; sinus pause; sweating; T-wave changes, hypertension (systolic blood pressure > 200 mm Hg).

Central Nervous System: drowsiness; emotional instability; tremors.

Genital/Urinary System: vaginal pressure; urgency.

Respiratory System: cough.

Special Senses: blurred vision; dry mouth; ear discomfort; metallic taste; nasal congestion; scotomas; tongue discomfort.

OVERDOSAGE

The half-life of adenosine is less than 10 seconds and side effects of Adenoscan (when they occur) usually resolve quickly when the infusion is discontinued, although delayed or persistent effects have been observed. Methylxanthines, such as caffeine and theophylline, are competitive adenosine receptor antagonists and theophylline has been used to effectively terminate persistent side effects. In controlled U.S. clinical trials, theophylline (50-125 mg slow intravenous injection) was needed to abort Adenoscan side effects in less than 2% of patients.

DOSAGE AND ADMINISTRATION

For intravenous infusion only.

Adenoscan should be given as a continuous peripheral intravenous infusion.

The recommended intravenous dose for adults is 140 mcg/kg/min infused for six minutes (total dose of 0.84 mg/kg). The required dose of thallium-201 should be injected at the midpoint of the Adenoscan infusion (i.e., after the first three minutes of Adenoscan). Thallium-201 is physically compatible with Adenoscan and may be injected directly into the Adenoscan infusion set.

The injection should be as close to the venous access as possible to prevent an inadvertent increase in the dose of Adenoscan (the contents of the IV tubing) being administered.

There are no data on the safety or efficacy of alternative Adenoscan infusion protocols.

The safety and efficacy of Adenoscan administered by the intracoronary route have not been established.

The following Adenoscan infusion nomogram may be used to determine the appropriate infusion rate corrected for total body weight:

Patient Weight		Infusion Rate
kg	lbs	mL/min
45	99	2.1
50	110	2.3
55	121	2.6
60	132	2.8
65	143	3.0
70	154	3.3
75	165	3.5
80	176	3.8
85	187	4.0
90	198	4.2

This nomogram was derived from the following general formula:

$$\frac{0.140 \ (mg/kg/min) \times total \ body \ weight \ (kg)}{Adenoscan \ concentration \ (3 \ mg/mL)} = infusion \ rate \ (mL/min)$$

Note: Parenteral drug products should be inspected visually for particulate matter and discoloration prior to administration.

HOW SUPPLIED

Adenoscan (adenosine) is supplied as a 30 mL vial of sterile nonpyrogenic solution in normal saline.

Product NDC

Code	NDC	
87130	0469–0871–30	90 mg/30 mL (3 mg/mL) in a 30 mL single-dose, flip-top glass vial, packaged individually and in packages of ten.

Store at controlled room temperature 15°–30°C (59°–86°F). Do not refrigerate as crystallization may occur. If crystallization has occurred, dissolve crystals by warming to room temperature. The solution must be clear at the time of use. Contains no preservative. Discard unused portion.

CAUTION: Federal law prohibits dispensing without prescription.

Fujisawa USA, Inc.
Deerfield, IL 60015
Under license from Medco Research, Inc.
Research Triangle Park, NC 27709
45558B/Issued: May 1995

ARISTOCORT® ℞

[a-ris-tō-cort]
**Sterile Triamcinolone Diacetate
Suspension
25 mg/mL
INTRALESIONAL
NOT FOR INTRAVENOUS USE**

DESCRIPTION

ARISTOCORT triamcinolone diacetate possesses glucocorticoid properties while being essentially devoid of mineralocorticoid activity thus causing little or no sodium retention. Supplied as a sterile suspension of 25 mg/mL micronized triamcinolone diacetate in the following vehicle:

Polysorbate 80	0.20%
Polyethylene Glycol 3350	3%
Sodium Chloride	0.85%
Benzyl Alcohol (preservative)	0.90%
Water for Injection q.s.	100%

Hydrochloric acid and/or sodium hydroxide may be used during manufacture to adjust pH of suspension to approximately 6.

Chemically triamcinolone diacetate is 9-Fluoro-11β,16α, 17,21-tetrahydroxypregna-1,4-diene-3,20-dione 16,21-diacetate.

Molecular weight is 478.51. Its structural formula is:

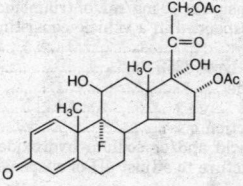

HOW SUPPLIED

ARISTOCORT® (sterile triamcinolone diacetate) suspension, 25 mg/mL, Intralesional, NOT FOR INTRAVENOUS USE.

NDC 0469-5117-05   Product Code 511705
5 mL Vial
Store at Controlled Room Temperature 15°–30°C (59°–86°F).
DO NOT FREEZE.
Manufactured for Fujisawa USA, Inc., Deerfield, IL 60015, by
Lederle Parenterals, Inc.,
Carolina, Puerto Rico 00987
41207-94/Issued April 1994
FP4

ARISTOCORT A® ℞

[a-ris-tō-cort]
**(triamcinolone acetonide)
0.025% CREAM
with AQUATAIN™ hydrophilic base**

DESCRIPTION

0.025% TOPICAL CREAM

Each gram of ARISTOCORT A Topical Cream contains 0.25 mg of the highly active steroid Triamcinolone Acetonide (a derivative of triamcinolone) in AQUATAIN, a specially formulated cream base composed of Emulsifying Wax, Isopro-

Continued on next page

Fujisawa—Cont.

pyl Palmitate, Glycerin, Sorbitol Solution, Lactic Acid, 2% Benzyl Alcohol and Purified Water. AQUATAIN is non-staining, water-washable, paraben-free, spermaceti-free and has a light texture and consistency.

Triamcinolone acetonide is $(11\beta, 16\alpha)$-9-Fluoro-11, 21-dihydroxy-16,17-[(1-methylethylidene)bis(oxy)]pregna-1, 4-diene-3,20-dione. Its structural formula is:

Molecular Weight 434.50 $C_{24}H_{31}FO_6$

The topical corticosteroids constitute a class of primarily synthetic steroids used as anti-inflammatory and antipruritic agents.

HOW SUPPLIED
ARISTOCORT A® (triamcinolone acetonide) Cream 0.025% (0.25 mg/g) with AQUATAIN™ hydrophilic base.
NDC 0469-5101-15   Product Code 510115
15 g tube
NDC 0469-5101-60   Product Code 510160
60 g tube
Store at Controlled Room Temperature 15°–30°C (59°–86°F).
DO NOT FREEZE.
Manufactured for Fujisawa USA, Inc., Deerfield, IL 60015,
by
Lederle Laboratories Division,
American Cyanamid Company,
Pearl River, NY 10965
CI 4546-1   Issued November 13, 1995

ARISTOCORT® Forte ℞
[a-ris-tō-cort]
(sterile triamcinolone diacetate)
Suspension 40 mg/mL
Parenteral
NOT FOR INTRAVENOUS USE

DESCRIPTION
A sterile suspension of 40 mg/mL of triamcinolone diacetate (micronized) suspended in a vehicle consisting of:
Polysorbate 80 .... 0.20%
Polyethylene Glycol 3350 .... 3%
Sodium Chloride 0.85%
Benzyl Alcohol 0.90%
Water for injection q.s. 100%
Hydrochloric acid and/or sodium hydroxide may be used during manufacture to adjust pH of suspension to approximately 6.
This preparation is a slightly soluble suspension suitable for parenteral administration through a 24-gauge needle (or larger), but NOT suitable for intravenous use. It may be administered by the intramuscular, intra-articular, or intra-synovial routes, depending upon the situation. The response to each glucocorticoid varies considerably with each type of disease indication and each corticosteroid prescribed. Irreversible clumping occurs when product is frozen.

Chemically triamcinolone diacetate is 9-Fluoro-11β, 16α, 17,21-tetrahydroxypregna-1,4-diene-3,20-dione   16,21-diacetate.

Molecular weight is 478.51. Its structural formula is:

HOW SUPPLIED
ARISTOCORT® FORTE (sterile triamcinolone diacetate) suspension, 40 mg/mL, Parenteral, NOT FOR INTRAVENOUS USE.
NDC 0469-5116-01   Product Code 511601
1 mL Vial
NDC 0469-5116-05   Product Code 511605
5 mL Vial
Store at Controlled Room Temperature 15°–30°C (59°–86°F).

DO NOT FREEZE.
Irreversible clumping occurs when product is frozen.
Manufactured for Fujisawa USA, Inc.,
Deerfield, IL 60015,
by
Lederle Parenterals, Inc.,
Carolina, Puerto Rico 00987
41233-94/Issued April 1994
FP5

ARISTOCORT A® ℞
[a-ris-tō-cort]
(triamcinolone acetonide)
0.1% OINTMENT
with PROPYLENE GLYCOL

DESCRIPTION
0.1% TOPICAL OINTMENT
Each gram of ARISTOCORT Topical Ointment contains 1 mg of the highly active steroid Triamcinolone Acetonide (a derivative of triamcinolone) in a specially formulated ointment base composed of White Petrolatum, Propylene Glycol, Emulsifying Wax, Tenox II (butylated hydroxanisole, propyl gallate, citric acid, propylene glycol) and Lactic Acid.
Triamcinolone acetonide is $(11\beta,16\alpha)$-9-Fluoro-11,21-dihydroxy -16,17- [(1-methylethylidene) bis (oxy)] pregna-1,4 - diene-3,20-dione.
Chemically triamcinolone acetonide is:

Molecular Weight 434.50 $C_{24}H_{31}FO_6$

The topical corticosteroids constitute a class of primarily synthetic steroids used as anti-inflammatory and anti-pruritic agents.

HOW SUPPLIED
ARISTOCORT A® (triamcinolone acetonide) Ointment 0.1% (1 mg/g) with Propylene Glycol
NDC 0469-5105-15   Product Code 510515
15 g tube
NDC 0469-5105-60   Product Code 510560
60 g tube
Store at Controlled Room Temperature 15°–30°C (59°–86°F).
Manufactured for Fujisawa USA, Inc., Deerfield, IL 60015,
by
Lederle Laboratories Division,
American Cyanamid Company,
Pearl River, NY 10965
CI 4564–1   Issued November 13, 1995

ARISTOCORT A® ℞
[a-ris-tō-cort]
(triamcinolone acetonide)
0.1% CREAM
with AQUATAIN™ hydrophilic base

DESCRIPTION
0.1% TOPICAL CREAM
Each gram of ARISTOCORT A Topical Cream contains 1 mg of the highly active steroid Triamcinolone Acetonide (a derivative of triamcinolone) in AQUATAIN, a specially formulated cream base composed of Emulsifying Wax, Isopropyl Palmitate, Glycerin, Sorbitol Solution, Lactic Acid, 2% Benzyl Alcohol and Purified Water. AQUATAIN is non-staining, water-washable, paraben-free, spermaceti-free and has a light texture and consistency.
Triamcinolone acetonide is $(11\beta,16\alpha)$-9-Fluoro-11,21-dihydroxy-16,17- [(1-methylethylidene)bis(oxy)]pregna-1,4-diene-3,20-dione. Its structural formula is:

Molecular Weight 434.50 $C_{24}H_{31}FO_6$

The topical corticosteroids constitute a class of primarily synthetic steroids used as anti-inflammatory and antipruritic agents.

HOW SUPPLIED
ARISTOCORT A® (triamcinolone acetonide) Cream 0.1% (1 mg/g) with AQUATAIN™ hydrophilic base
NDC 0469-5102-15   Product Code 510215
15 g tube
NDC 0469-5102-60   Product Code 510260
60 g tube
NDC 0469-5102-24   Product Code 510324
240 g jar
Store at Controlled Room Temperature 15°–30°C (59°–86°F).
DO NOT FREEZE.
Manufactured for Fujisawa USA, Inc., Deerfield, IL 60015,
by
Lederle Laboratories Division,
American Cyanamid Company,
Pearl River, NY 10965
CI 4428–1   Issued November 2, 1995

ARISTOCORT A® ℞
[a-ris-tō-cort]
(triamcinolone acetonide)
0.5% CREAM
with AQUATAIN™ hydrophilic base

DESCRIPTION
0.5% TOPICAL CREAM
Each gram of ARISTOCORT A Topical Cream contains 5 mg of the highly active steroid Triamcinolone Acetonide (a derivative of triamcinolone) in AQUATAIN, a specially formulated cream base composed of Emulsifying Wax, Isopropyl Palmitate, Glycerin, Sorbitol Solution, Lactic Acid, 2% Benzyl Alcohol and Purified Water. AQUATAIN is non-staining, water-washable, paraben-free, spermaceti-free and has a light texture and consistency.
Triamcinolone acetonide is $(11\beta, 16\alpha)$-9-Fluoro-11,21-dihydroxy-16, 17-[(1-methylethylidene)bis(oxy)]pregna-1,4-diene-3,20-dione. Its structural formula is:

Molecular Weight 434.50 $C_{24}H_{31}FO_6$

The topical corticosteroids constitute a class of primarily synthetic steroids used as anti-inflammatory and antipruritic agents.

HOW SUPPLIED
ARISTOCORT A® (triamcinolone acetonide) Cream 0.5% (5 mg/g) with AQUATAIN™ hydrophilic base
NDC 0469-5104-15   Product Code 510415
15 g tube
Store at Controlled Room Temperature 15°–30°C (59°–86°F).
DO NOT FREEZE.
Manufactured by Fujisawa USA, Inc., Deerfield, IL 60015,
by
Lederle Laboratories Division,
American Cyanamid Company,
Pearl River, NY 10965
CI 4425–1   Issued November 13, 1995

ARISTOSPAN® ℞
[a-ris-tō-span]
(sterile triamcinolone hexacetonide)
Suspension 5 mg/mL
Parenteral For Intralesional Use
NOT FOR INTRAVENOUS USE

DESCRIPTION
A sterile suspension containing 5 mg/mL of micronized triamcinolone hexacetonide in the following inactive ingredients:
Polysorbate 80 .... 0.20%
Sorbitol Solution 50%
Benzyl Alcohol (preservative) 0.90%
Water for Injection q.s. 100%
Hydrochloric Acid and Sodium Hydroxide, if required, to adjust pH to 4.5–6.5.
The hexacetonide ester of the potent glucocorticoid triamcinolone is relatively insoluble (0.0002% at 25°C in water).

When injected intralesionally or sublesionally, it can be expected to be absorbed slowly from the injection site.

Chemically triamcinolone hexacetonide is 9-Fluoro-11β, 16α, 17,21-tetrahydroxypregna-1,4-diene-3,20-dione cyclic 16,17-acetal with acetone 21-(3,3-dimethylbutyrate). Molecular weight is 532.65. The structural formula is:

HOW SUPPLIED

ARISTOSPAN® (sterile triamcinolone hexacetonide) suspension, 5 mg/mL, for Intralesional Use. NOT FOR INTRAVENOUS USE.

NDC 0469-5118-05   Product Code 511805
5 mL Vial

Store at Controlled Room Temperature 15–30°C (59–86°F). DO NOT FREEZE.

Manufactured for Fujisawa USA, Inc., Deerfield, IL 60015, by
Lederle Parenterals, Inc.,
Carolina, Puerto Rico 00987
41209-94/Issued April 1994
FP5

ARISTOSPAN®   ℞

[a-ris-tō-span]
(sterile triamcinolone hexacetonide)
Suspension 20 mg/mL
Parenteral For Intra-articular Use
NOT FOR INTRAVENOUS USE

DESCRIPTION

A sterile suspension containing 20 mg/mL of micronized triamcinolone hexacetonide in the following inactive ingredients:

Polysorbate 80	0.40%
Sorbitol Solution	50%
Benzyl Alcohol (preservative)	0.90%
Water for Injection qs	100%

Hydrochloric Acid and Sodium Hydroxide, if required, to adjust pH to 4.5–6.5.

The hexacetonide ester of the potent glucocorticoid triamcinolone is relatively insoluble (0.0002% at 25°C in water). When injected intra-articularly, it can be expected to be absorbed slowly from the injection site.

Chemically triamcinolone hexacetonide is 9-Fluoro-11β, 16α, 17,21-tetrahydroxypregna-1,4-diene-3,20-dione cyclic 16,17-acetal with acetone 21-(3,3-dimethylbutyrate). Molecular weight is 532.65. The structural formula is:

HOW SUPPLIED

ARISTOSPAN® (sterile triamcinolone hexacetonide) suspension 20 mg/mL, for Intra-articular Use. NOT FOR INTRAVENOUS USE.

NDC 0469-5119-01   Product Code 511901
1 mL Vial
NDC 0469-5119-05   Product Code 511905
5 mL vial

Store at Controlled Room Temperature 15–30°C (59–86°F). DO NOT FREEZE.

Manufactured for Fujisawa USA, Inc., Deerfield, IL 60015, by
Lederle Parenterals, Inc.,
Carolina, Puerto Rico 00987
41232-94/Issued April 1994
FP5

CEFIZOX®   ℞
(sterile ceftizoxime sodium)
For Intramuscular or Intravenous Use

DESCRIPTION

Cefizox® (sterile ceftizoxime sodium) is a sterile, semisynthetic, broad-spectrum, beta-lactamase resistant cephalosporin antibiotic for parenteral (I.V., I.M.) administration. It is the sodium salt of [6R-[6a, 7β(Z)]]-7-[[(2,3-dihydro-2-imino-4-thiazolyl) (methoxyimino) acetyl] amino]-8-oxo-5-thia-1-azabicyclo [4.2.0] oct-2-ene-2-carboxylic acid. Its sodium content is approximately 60 mg (2.6 mEq) per gram of ceftizoxime activity.

It has the following structural formula:

$C_{13}H_{12}N_5NaO_5S_2$ 405.38

Sterile ceftizoxime sodium is a white to pale yellow crystalline powder.

Cefizox is supplied in vials equivalent to 500 mg, 1 gram or 2 grams of ceftizoxime, and in "Piggyback" Vials for intravenous admixture equivalent to 1 gram or 2 grams of ceftizoxime.

CLINICAL PHARMACOLOGY

The table below demonstrates the serum levels and duration of Cefizox (sterile ceftizoxime sodium) following intramuscular administration of 500 mg and 1 gram doses, respectively, to normal volunteers.

Serum Concentrations After Intramuscular Administration
Serum Concentration (mcg/mL)

Dose	½ hr	1 hr	2 hr	4 hr	6 hr	8 hr
500 mg	13.3	13.7	9.2	4.8	1.9	0.7
1 gm	36.0	39.0	31.0	15.0	6.0	3.0

Following intravenous administration of 1, 2, and 3 gram doses of Cefizox to normal volunteers, the following serum levels were obtained.

Serum Concentrations After Intravenous Administration
Serum Concentration (mcg/mL)

Dose	5 min	10 min	30 min	1 hr	2 hr	4 hr	8 hr
1 gram	ND	ND	60.5	38.9	21.5	8.4	1.4
2 grams	131.8	110.9	77.5	53.6	33.1	12.1	2.0
3 grams	221.1	174.0	112.7	83.9	47.4	26.2	4.8

ND = Not Done

A serum half-life of approximately 1.7 hours was observed after intravenous or intramuscular administration.

Cefizox is 30% protein bound.

Cefizox is not metabolized, and is excreted virtually unchanged by the kidneys in 24 hours. This provides a high urinary concentration. Concentrations greater than 6000 mcg/mL have been achieved in the urine by 2 hours after a 1 gram dose of Cefizox intravenously. Probenecid slows tubular secretion and produces even higher serum levels, increasing the duration of measurable serum concentrations.

Cefizox achieves therapeutic levels in various body fluids, e.g., cerebrospinal fluid (in patients with inflamed meninges), bile, surgical wound fluid, pleural fluid, aqueous humor, ascitic fluid, peritoneal fluid, prostatic fluid and saliva, and in the following body tissues: heart, gallbladder, bone, biliary, peritoneal, prostatic, and uterine.

In clinical experience to date, no disulfiram-like reactions have been reported with Cefizox.

Microbiology

The bactericidal action of Cefizox (sterile ceftizoxime sodium) results from inhibition of cell-wall synthesis. Cefizox is highly resistant to a broad spectrum of beta-lactamases (penicillinase and cephalosporinase), including Richmond types I, II, III, TEM, and IV, produced by both aerobic and anaerobic gram-positive and gram-negative organisms. Cefizox is active against a wide range of gram-positive and gram-negative organisms, and is usually active against the following organisms in vitro and in clinical situations (see Indications and Usage.)

Gram-Positive Aerobes
Staphylococcus aureus (including penicillinase- and non-penicillinase-producing strains)
NOTE: Methicillin-resistant staphylococci are resistant to cephalosporins, including ceftizoxime.

Staphylococcus epidermidis (including penicillinase- and nonpenicillinase-producing strains)
Streptococcus agalactiae
Streptococcus pneumoniae
Streptococcus pyogenes
NOTE: Ceftizoxime is usually inactive against most strains of Enterococcus faecalis (formerly S. faecalis).

Gram-Negative Aerobes
Acinetobacter spp.
Enterobacter spp.
Escherichia coli
Haemophilus influenzae (including ampicillin-resistant strains)
Klebsiella pneumoniae
Morganella morganii (formerly Proteus morganii)
Neisseria gonorrhoeae
Proteus mirabilis
Proteus vulgaris
Providencia rettgeri (formerly Proteus rettgeri)
Pseudomonas aeruginosa
Serratia marcescens

Anaerobes
Bacteroides spp.
Peptococcus spp.
Peptostreptococcus spp.

Ceftizoxime is usually active against the following organisms in vitro, but the clinical significance of these data is unknown.

Gram-Positive Aerobes
Corynebacterium diphtheriae

Gram-Negative Aerobes
Aeromonas hydrophila
Citrobacter spp.
Moraxella spp.
Neisseria meningitidis
Pasteurella multocida
Providencia stuartii
Salmonella spp.
Shigella spp.
Yersinia enterocolitica

Anaerobes
Actinomyces spp.
Bifidobacterium spp.
Clostridium spp.
NOTE: Most strains of Clostridium difficile are resistant.
Eubacterium spp.
Fusobacterium spp.
Propionibacterium spp.
Veillonella spp.

Susceptibility Testing: Diffusion Techniques

Quantitative methods that require measurement of zone diameters give the most precise estimate of the susceptibility of bacteria to antimicrobial agents. One such standard procedure[1] has been recommended for use with disks to test susceptibility of organisms to ceftizoxime. Interpretation involves the correlation of the diameters obtained in the disk test with the minimum inhibitory concentration (MIC) for ceftizoxime.

Organisms should be tested with the ceftizoxime disk, since ceftizoxime has been shown by in vitro tests to be active against certain strains found resistant when other beta-lactam disks are used.

Reports from the laboratory giving results of the standard single-disk susceptibility test with a 30 mcg ceftizoxime disk should be interpreted according to the following criteria (with the exception of Pseudomonas aeruginosa).

Zone Diameter (mm)	Interpretation
≥ 20	(S) Susceptible
15–19	(MS) Moderately Susceptible
≤ 14	(R) Resistant

A report of "Susceptible" indicates that the pathogen is likely to be inhibited by generally achievable blood levels. A report of "Moderately Susceptible" suggests that the organism would be susceptible if high dosage is used or if the infection is confined to tissue and fluids (e.g., urine) in which high antibiotic levels are attained. A report of "Resistant" indicates that achievable concentrations of the antibiotic are unlikely to be inhibitory and other therapy should be selected.

Standardized procedures require the use of laboratory control organisms. The 30 mcg ceftizoxime disk should give the following zone diameters.

Organism	ATCC	Zone Diameter (mm)
Escherichia coli	25922	30–36
Pseudomonas aeruginosa	27853	12–17
Staphylococcus aureus	25923	27–35

Susceptibility Testing for Pseudomonas in Urinary Tract Infections

Most strains of Pseudomonas aeruginosa are moderately susceptible to ceftizoxime. Ceftizoxime achieves high levels in the urine (greater than 6000 mcg/mL at 2 hours with 1 gram I.V.) and, therefore, the following zone sizes should be used

Continued on next page

Fujisawa—Cont.

when testing ceftizoxime for treatment of urinary tract infections caused by *Pseudomonas aeruginosa*.

Susceptible organisms produce zones of 20 mm or greater, indicating that the test organism is likely to respond to therapy.

Organisms that produce zones of 11 to 19 mm are expected to be susceptible when the infection is confined to the urinary tract (in which high antibiotic levels are attained).

Resistant organisms produce zones of 10 mm or less, indicating that other therapy should be selected.

Susceptibility Testing: Dilution Techniques

When using the NCCLS agar dilution or broth dilution (including microdilution) method[2] or equivalent, the following MIC data should be used for interpretation.

MIC (mcg/mL)	Interpretation
≤8	(S) Susceptible
16–32	(MS) Moderately Susceptible
≥64	(R) Resistant

As with standard disk diffusion methods, dilution procedures require the use of laboratory control organisms. Standard ceftizoxime powder should give MIC values in the following ranges.

Organism	ATCC	MIC (mcg/mL)
Escherichia coli	25922	0.03–0.12
Pseudomonas aeruginosa	27853	16–64
Staphylococcus aureus	29213	2–8

INDICATIONS AND USAGE

Cefizox (sterile ceftizoxime sodium) is indicated in the treatment of infections due to susceptible strains of the microorganisms listed below.

Lower Respiratory Tract Infections caused by *Klebsiella* spp.; *Proteus mirabilis; Escherichia coli; Haemophilus influenzae* including ampicillin-resistant strains; *Staphylococcus aureus* (penicillinase- and nonpenicillinase-producing); *Serratia* spp.; *Enterobacter* spp.; *Bacteroides* spp.; and *Streptococcus* spp. including *S. pneumoniae*, but excluding enterococci.

Urinary Tract Infections caused by *Staphylococcus aureus* (penicillinase- and nonpenicillinase-producing); *Escherichia coli; Pseudomonas* spp. including *P. aeruginosa; Proteus mirabilis; P. vulgaris; Providencia rettgeri* (formerly *Proteus rettgeri*) and *Morganella morganii* (formerly *Proteus morganii*); *Klebsiella* spp.; *Serratia* spp. including *S. marcescens*; and *Enterobacter* spp.

Gonorrhea including uncomplicated cervical and urethral gonorrhea caused by *Neisseria gonorrhoeae*.

Pelvic Inflammatory Disease caused by *Neisseria gonorrhoeae, Escherichia coli* or *Streptococcus agalactiae*.

NOTE: Ceftizoxime, like other cephalosporins, has no activity against *Chlamydia trachomatis*. Therefore, when cephalosporins are used in the treatment of patients with pelvic inflammatory disease and *C. trachomatis* is one of the suspected pathogens, appropriate antichlamydial coverage should be added.

Intra-Abdominal Infections caused by *Escherichia coli; Staphylococcus epidermidis; Streptococcus* spp. (excluding enterococci); *Enterobacter* spp.; *Klebsiella* spp.; *Bacteroides* spp. including *B. fragilis*; and anaerobic cocci, including *Peptococcus* spp. and *Peptostreptococcus* spp.

Septicemia caused by *Streptococcus* spp. including *S. pneumoniae* (but excluding enterococci); *Staphylococcus aureus* (penicillinase- and nonpenicillinase-producing); *Escherichia coli; Bacteroides* spp. including *B. fragilis; Klebsiella* spp.; and *Serratia* spp.

Skin and Skin Structure Infections caused by *Staphylococcus aureus* (penicillinase- and nonpenicillinase-producing); *Staphylococcus epidermidis; Escherichia coli; Klebsiella* spp.; *Streptococcus* spp. including *Streptococcus pyogenes* (but excluding enterococci); *Proteus mirabilis; Serratia* spp.; *Enterobacter* spp.; *Bacteroides* spp. including *B. fragilis*; and anaerobic cocci, including *Peptococcus* spp. and *Peptostreptococcus* spp.

Bone and Joint Infections caused by *Staphylococcus aureus* (penicillinase- and nonpenicillinase-producing); *Streptococcus* spp. (excluding enterococci); *Proteus mirabilis; Bacteroides* spp.; and anaerobic cocci, including *Peptococcus* spp. and *Peptostreptococcus* spp.

Meningitis caused by *Haemophilus influenzae*. Cefizox has also been used successfully in the treatment of a limited number of pediatric and adult cases of meningitis caused by *Streptococcus pneumoniae*.

Cefizox has been effective in the treatment of seriously ill, compromised patients, including those who were debilitated, immunosuppressed, or neutropenic.

Infections caused by aerobic gram-negative and by mixtures of organisms resistant to other cephalosporins, aminoglycosides, or penicillins have responded to treatment with Cefizox.

Because of the serious nature of some urinary tract infections due to *P. aeruginosa* and because many strains of *Pseudomonas* species are only moderately susceptible to Cefizox,

higher dosage is recommended. Other therapy should be instituted if the response is not prompt.

Susceptibility studies on specimens obtained prior to therapy should be used to determine the response of causative organisms to Cefizox. Therapy with Cefizox may be initiated pending results of the studies; however, treatment should be adjusted according to study findings. In serious infections, Cefizox has been used concomitantly with aminoglycosides (see Precautions). Before using Cefizox concomitantly with other antibiotics, the prescribing information for those agents should be reviewed for contraindications, warnings, precautions, and adverse reactions. Renal function should be carefully monitored.

CONTRAINDICATIONS

Cefizox (sterile ceftizoxime sodium) is contraindicated in patients who have known allergy to the drug.

WARNINGS

BEFORE THERAPY WITH CEFIZOX IS INSTITUTED, CAREFUL INQUIRY SHOULD BE MADE TO DETERMINE WHETHER THE PATIENT HAS HAD PREVIOUS HYPERSENSITIVITY REACTIONS TO CEFIZOX, OTHER CEPHALOSPORINS, PENICILLINS, OR OTHER DRUGS. IF THIS PRODUCT IS TO BE GIVEN TO PENICILLIN-SENSITIVE PATIENTS, CAUTION SHOULD BE EXERCISED BECAUSE CROSS HYPERSENSITIVITY AMONG BETA-LACTAM ANTIBIOTICS HAS BEEN CLEARLY DOCUMENTED AND MAY OCCUR IN UP TO 10% OF PATIENTS WITH A HISTORY OF PENICILLIN ALLERGY. IF AN ALLERGIC REACTION TO CEFIZOX OCCURS, DISCONTINUE THE DRUG. SERIOUS ACUTE HYPERSENSITIVITY REACTIONS MAY REQUIRE TREATMENT WITH EPINEPHRINE AND OTHER EMERGENCY MEASURES, INCLUDING OXYGEN, INTRAVENOUS FLUIDS, INTRAVENOUS ANTIHISTAMINES, CORTICOSTEROIDS, PRESSOR AMINES, AND AIRWAY MANAGEMENT, AS CLINICALLY INDICATED.

Pseudomembranous colitis has been reported with nearly all antibacterial agents, including ceftizoxime, and may range in severity from mild to life threatening. Therefore, it is important to consider this diagnosis in patients who present with diarrhea subsequent to the administration of antibacterial agents.

Treatment with antibacterial agents alters the normal flora of the colon and may permit overgrowth of clostridia. Studies indicate that a toxin produced by *Clostridium difficile* is a primary cause of "antibiotic-associated" colitis.

After the diagnosis of pseudomembranous colitis has been established, appropriate therapeutic measures should be initiated. Mild cases of pseudomembranous colitis usually respond to drug discontinuation alone. In moderate to severe cases, consideration should be given to management with fluids and electrolytes, protein supplementation, and treatment with an antibacterial drug clinically effective against *Clostridium difficile* colitis.

PRECAUTIONS

General

As with all broad-spectrum antibiotics, Cefizox (sterile ceftizoxime sodium) should be prescribed with caution in individuals with a history of gastrointestinal disease, particularly colitis.

Although Cefizox has not been shown to produce an alteration in renal function, renal status should be evaluated, especially in seriously ill patients receiving maximum dose therapy. As with any antibiotic, prolonged use may result in overgrowth of nonsusceptible organisms. Careful observation is essential; appropriate measures should be taken if superinfection occurs.

Drug Interactions

Although the occurrence has not been reported with Cefizox, nephrotoxicity has been reported following concomitant administration of other cephalosporins and aminoglycosides.

Carcinogenesis, Mutagenesis, Impairment of Fertility

Long term studies in animals to evaluate the carcinogenic potential of ceftizoxime have not been conducted.

In an *in vitro* bacterial cell assay (i.e., Ames test), there was no evidence of mutagenicity at ceftizoxime concentrations of 0.001–0.5 mcg/plate. Ceftizoxime did not produce increases in micronuclei in the *in vivo* mouse micronucleus test when given to animals at doses up to 7500 mg/kg, approximately six times greater than the maximum human daily dose on a mg/M^2 basis.

Ceftizoxime had no effect on fertility when administered subcutaneously to rats at daily doses of up to 1000 mg/kg/day, approximately two times the maximum human daily dose on a mg/M^2 basis. Ceftizoxime produced no histological changes in the sexual organs of male and female dogs when given intravenously for thirteen weeks at a dose of 1000 mg/kg/day, approximately five times greater than the maximum human daily dose on a mg/M^2 basis.

Pregnancy: Teratogenic Effects: Pregnancy Category B.

Reproduction studies performed in rats and rabbits have revealed no evidence of impaired fertility or harm to the fetus due to Cefizox. There are, however, no adequate and well-controlled studies in pregnant women. Because animal reproduction studies are not always predictive of human

effects, this drug should be used during pregnancy only if clearly needed.

Labor and Delivery

Safety of Cefizox use during labor and delivery has not been established.

Nursing Mothers

Cefizox is excreted in human milk in low concentrations. Caution should be exercised when Cefizox is administered to a nursing woman.

Pediatric Use

Safety and efficacy in infants from birth to six months of age have not been established. In children six months of age and older, treatment with Cefizox has been associated with transient elevated levels of eosinophils, AST (SGOT), ALT (SGPT), and CPK (creatine phosphokinase). The CPK elevation may be related to I.M. administration.

The potential for the toxic effect in children from chemicals that may leach from the single-dose I.V. preparation in plastic has not been determined.

ADVERSE REACTIONS

Cefizox® (sterile ceftizoxime sodium) is generally well tolerated. The *most* frequent adverse reactions (*greater* than 1% but *less* than 5%) are:

Hypersensitivity—Rash, pruritus, fever.

Hepatic—Transient elevation in AST (SGOT), ALT (SGPT), and alkaline phosphatase.

Hematologic—Transient eosinophilia, thrombocytosis. Some individuals have developed a positive Coombs test.

Local—Injection site—Burning, cellulitis, phlebitis with I.V. administration, pain, induration, tenderness, paresthesia.

The *less* frequent adverse reactions (*less* than 1%) are:

Hypersensitivity—Numbness and anaphylaxis have been reported rarely.

Hepatic—Elevation of bilirubin has been reported rarely.

Renal—Transient elevations of BUN and creatinine have been occasionally observed with Cefizox.

Hematologic—Anemia, including hemolytic anemia with occasional fatal outcome, leukopenia, neutropenia, and thrombocytopenia have been reported rarely.

Urogenital—Vaginitis has occurred rarely.

Gastrointestinal—Diarrhea; nausea and vomiting have been reported occasionally.

Symptoms of pseudomembranous colitis can appear during or after antibiotic treatment (see Warnings).

In addition to the adverse reactions listed above which have been observed in patients treated with ceftizoxime, the following adverse reactions and altered laboratory tests have been reported for cephalosporin-class antibiotics:

Stevens-Johnson syndrome, erythema multiforme, toxic epidermal necrolysis, serum-sickness like reaction, toxic nephropathy, aplastic anemia, hemorrhage, prolonged prothrombin time, elevated LDH, pancytopenia, and agranulocytosis.

Several cephalosporins have been implicated in triggering seizures, particularly in patients with renal impairment, when the dosage was not reduced. (See DOSAGE AND ADMINISTRATION.) If seizures associated with drug therapy occur, the drug should be discontinued. Anticonvulsant therapy can be given if clinically indicated.

DOSAGE AND ADMINISTRATION

The usual adult dosage is 1 or 2 grams of Cefizox (sterile ceftizoxime sodium) every 8 to 12 hours. Proper dosage and route of administration should be determined by the condition of the patient, severity of the infection, and susceptibility of the causative organisms.

General Guidelines for Dosage of Cefizox

Type of Infection	Daily Dose (Grams)	Frequency and Route
Uncomplicated Urinary Tract	1	500 mg q12h I.M. or I.V.
Other Sites	2–3	1 gram q8–12h I.M. or I.V.
Severe or Refractory	3–6	1 gram q8h I.M. or I.V.
		2 grams q8–12h I.M.[a] or I.V.
PID[b]	6	2 grams q8h I.V.
Life-Threatening[c]	9–12	3–4 grams q8h I.V.

a) When administering 2 gram I.M. doses, the dose should be divided and given in different large muscle masses.

b) If *C. trachomatis* is a suspected pathogen, appropriate antichlamydial coverage should be added, because ceftizoxime has no activity against this organism.

c) In life-threatening infections, dosages up to 2 grams every 4 hours have been given.

Because of the serious nature of urinary tract infections due to *P. aeruginosa* and because many strains of *Pseudomonas* species are only moderately susceptible to Cefizox, higher dosage is recommended. Other therapy should be instituted if the response is not prompt.

A single, 1 gram I.M. dose is the usual dose for treatment of uncomplicated gonorrhea.

The intravenous route may be preferable for patients with bacterial septicemia, localized parenchymal abscesses (such as intra-abdominal abscess), peritonitis, or other severe or life-threatening infections.

In those with normal renal function, the intravenous dosage for such infections is 2 to 12 grams of Cefizox (sterile ceftizoxime sodium) daily. In conditions such as bacterial septicemia, 6 to 12 grams/day may be given initially by the intravenous route for several days, and the dosage may then be gradually reduced according to clinical response and laboratory findings.

Pediatric Dosage Schedule

	Unit Dose	Frequency
Children 6 months and older	50 mg/kg	q6-8h

Dosage may be increased to a total daily dose of 200 mg/kg (not to exceed the maximum adult dose for serious infection).

Impaired Renal Function

Modification of Cefizox dosage is necessary in patients with impaired renal function. Following an initial loading dose of 500 mg–1 gram I.M. or I.V., the maintenance dosing schedule shown below should be followed. Further dosing should be determined by therapeutic monitoring, severity of the infection, and susceptibility of the causative organisms.

When only the serum creatinine level is available, creatinine clearance may be calculated from the following formula. The serum creatinine level should represent current renal function at the steady state.

Males

$$\text{Clcr} = \frac{\text{Weight (kg)} \times (140 - \text{age})}{72 \times \text{serum creatinine (mg/100 mL)}}$$

Females are 0.85 of the calculated clearance values for males.

In patients undergoing hemodialysis, no additional supplemental dosing is required following hemodialysis; however, dosing should be timed so that the patient receives the dose (according to the table below) at the end of the dialysis.

Dosage in Adults with Reduced Renal Function

Creatinine Clearance mL/min	Renal Function	Less Severe Infections	Life-Threatening Infections
79–50	Mild impairment	500 mg q8h	0.75–1.5 grams q8h
49–5	Moderate to severe impairment	250–500 mg q12h	0.5–1 gram q12h
4–0	Dialysis patients	500 mg q48h or 250 mg q24h	0.5–1 gram q48h or 0.5 gram q24h

Preparation of Parenteral Solution

RECONSTITUTION

I.M. Administration: Reconstitute with Sterile Water for Injection. SHAKE WELL.

Vial Size	Diluent to Be Added	Approx. Avail. Vol.	Approx. Avg. Concentration
500 mg	1.5 mL	1.8 mL	280 mg/mL
1 gram	3.0 mL	3.7 mL	270 mg/mL
2 grams*	6.0 mL	7.4 mL	270 mg/mL

*When administering 2 gram I.M. doses, the dose should be divided and given in different large muscle masses.

I.V. Administration: Reconstitute with Sterile Water for Injection. SHAKE WELL.

Vial Size	Diluent to Be Added	Approx. Avail. Vol.	Approx. Avg. Concentration
500 mg	5 mL	5.3 mL	95 mg/mL
1 gram	10 mL	10.7 mL	95 mg/mL
2 grams	20 mL	21.4 mL	95 mg/mL

These solutions of Cefizox are stable 24 hours at room temperature or 96 hours if refrigerated (5°C).

Parenteral drug products should be inspected visually for particulate matter prior to administration. If particulate matter is evident in reconstituted fluids, then the drug solution should be discarded. Reconstituted solutions may range from yellow to amber without changes in potency.

"Piggyback" Vials: Reconstitute with 50 to 100 mL of Sodium Chloride Injection or any other I.V. solution listed below.

SHAKE WELL

Administer with primary I.V. fluids, as a single dose. These solutions of Cefizox are stable 24 hours at room temperature or 96 hours if refrigerated (5°C).

A solution of 1 gram Cefizox in 13 mL Sterile Water for Injection is isotonic.

I.M. Injection

Inject well within the body of a relatively large muscle. Aspiration is necessary to avoid inadvertent injection into a blood vessel. When administering 2 gram I.M. doses, the dose should be divided and given in different large muscle masses.

I.V. Administration

Direct (bolus) injection, slowly over 3 to 5 minutes, directly or through tubing for patients receiving parenteral fluids (see list below). Intermittent or continuous infusion, dilute reconstituted Cefizox in 50 to 100 mL of one of the following solutions:

- Sodium Chloride Injection
- 5% or 10% Dextrose Injection
- 5% Dextrose and 0.9%, 0.45%, or 0.2% Sodium Chloride Injection
- Ringer's Injection
- Lactated Ringer's Injection
- Invert Sugar 10% in Sterile Water for Injection
- 5% Sodium Bicarbonate in Sterile Water for Injection
- 5% Dextrose in Lactated Ringer's Injection (only when reconstituted with 4% Sodium Bicarbonate Injection)

In these fluids, Cefizox is stable 24 hours at room temperature or 96 hours if refrigerated (5°C).

HOW SUPPLIED

Cefizox® (sterile ceftizoxime sodium)

NDC 0469-7250-01   Product No. 725001
    Equivalent to 500 mg ceftizoxime in 10 mL, single-dose, flip-top vials, individually packaged

NDC 0469-7251-01   Product No. 725101
    Equivalent to 1 gram ceftizoxime in 20 mL, single-dose, flip-top vials, individually packaged

NDC 0469-7252-01   Product No. 725201
    Equivalent to 1 gram ceftizoxime in 100 mL, single-dose, Piggyback, flip-top vials, packaged in tens

NDC 0469-7253-02   Product No. 725302
    Equivalent to 2 grams ceftizoxime in 20 mL, single-dose, flip-top vials, individually packaged

NDC 0469-7254-02   Product No. 725402
    Equivalent to 2 grams ceftizoxime in 100 mL, single-dose, Piggyback, flip-top vials, packaged in tens

Unreconstituted Cefizox should be protected from excessive light, and stored at controlled room temperature (59°–86°F) in the original package until used.

Product of Japan

Manufactured for Fujisawa USA, Inc., Deerfield, IL 60015, by SmithKline Beecham, Philadelphia, PA 19101

REFERENCES

1. National Committee for Clinical Laboratory Standards, Approved Standard. *Performance Standards for Antimicrobial Disk Susceptibility Test*, 4th Edition, Vol 10 (7):M2-A4. Villanova, PA, April 1990.
2. National Committee for Clinical Laboratory Standards, Approved Standard. *Methods for Dilution Antimicrobial Susceptibility Tests for Bacteria that Grow Aerobically*, 2nd Edition, Vol 10 (8):M7-A2. Villanova, PA, April 1990.

CF:L2SV
675778
685563
         Revised May 1995

CEFIZOX®   ℞
(sterile ceftizoxime sodium)
For Intramuscular or Intravenous Use
PHARMACY BULK PACKAGE—NOT FOR DIRECT INFUSION

DESCRIPTION

Cefizox® (sterile ceftizoxime sodium) pharmacy bulk vial is a sterile dosage form which contains many single doses for use in a pharmacy admixture program in the preparation of parenteral fluids. Cefizox is a sterile, semi-synthetic, broad-spectrum, beta-lactamase resistant cephalosporin antibiotic for parenteral (I.V., I.M.) administration. It is the sodium salt of [6R-[6a, 7β(Z)]]7-[[(2,3-dihydro-2-imino-4-thiazolyl) (methoxyimino) acetyl] amino]-8-oxo-5-thia-1-azabicyclo [4.2.0] oct-2-ene-2-carboxylic acid. Its sodium content is approximately 60 mg (2.6 mEq) per gram of ceftizoxime activity.

It has the following structural formula:

$C_{13}H_{12}N_5NaO_5S_2$ 405.38

Sterile ceftizoxime sodium is a white to pale yellow crystalline powder. Cefizox is supplied in vials equivalent to 10 grams of ceftizoxime, in pharmacy bulk packaging.

HOW SUPPLIED

Cefizox® (sterile ceftizoxime sodium)

NDC 0469-7255-10   Product No. 725510
    Equivalent to 10 grams ceftizoxime in 100 mL, Pharmacy Bulk Package, packaged in tens

Unreconstituted Cefizox should be protected from excessive light, and stored at controlled room temperature (59°–86°F) in the original package until used.

Product of Japan

Manufactured for Fujisawa USA, Inc., Deerfield, IL 60015, by SmithKline Beecham, Philadelphia, PA 19101

CF L2PB
685620   Revised May 1995

CEFIZOX®   ℞
(sterile ceftizoxime sodium, USP)
For Intravenous Infusion

DESCRIPTION

Cefizox® (sterile ceftizoxime sodium, USP) is a sterile, semi-synthetic, broad-spectrum, beta-lactamase resistant cephalosporin antibiotic for parenteral (I.V., I.M.) administration. It is the sodium salt of [6R-[6a, 7β(Z)]]-7-[[(2.3-dihydro-2-imino-4-thiazolyl) (methoxyimino) acetyl] amino]-8-oxo-5-thia-1-azabicyclo [4.2.0] oct-2-ene-2-carboxylic acid. Its sodium content is approximately 60 mg (2.6 mEq) per gram of ceftizoxime activity.

It has the following structural formula:

$C_{13}H_{12}N_5NaO_5S_2$ 405.38

Sterile ceftizoxime sodium is a white to pale yellow crystalline powder.

Cefizox is supplied in ADD-Vantage® vials as ceftizoxime sodium equivalent to 1 gram and 2 grams of ceftizoxime.

HOW SUPPLIED

Cefizox® (sterile ceftizoxime sodium, USP) in ADD-Vantage® Vials

NDC 0469-7271-01   Product No. 727101
    equivalent to 1 gram ceftizoxime, packaged in tens

NDC 0469-7272-02   Product No. 727202
    equivalent to 2 grams ceftizoxime, packaged in tens

Unreconstituted Cefizox should be protected from excessive light, and stored at controlled room temperature 15°–30°C (59°–86°F) in the original package until used.

ADD-Vantage® is a registered trademark of Abbott Laboratories.

Product of Japan

U.S. Patent 4,427,674

Manufactured for Fujisawa USA, Inc., Deerfield, IL 60015, by SmithKline Beecham, Philadelphia, PA 19101.

CF:L2AV   Revised Dec. 1995

CEFIZOX®   ℞
(ceftizoxime sodium injection)
in Galaxy® Plastic Container (PL 2040)
For Intravenous Use

DESCRIPTION

Cefizox® (ceftizoxime sodium injection) in the Galaxy® plastic container (PL 2040) contains ceftizoxime as ceftizoxime sodium. It is a sterile, semisynthetic, broad spectrum, cephalosporin antibiotic for intravenous administration. Chemically, it is the sodium (6R, 7R-[2-(2-imino-4-thiazolin-4-yl), glyoxylamido]-8-oxo-5-thia-1-azabicyclo [4.2.0]oct-2-ene-2-carboxylate7²-(Z)-(O-methyloxime). The molecular formula is $C_{13}H_{12}N_5NaO_5S_2$ and the molecular weight is 405.38. The structural formula of ceftizoxime sodium is as follows:

Continued on next page

Fujisawa—Cont.

Cefizox (ceftizoxime sodium injection) in the Galaxy® plastic container is a frozen iso-osmotic, sterile, nonpyrogenic premixed 50 mL solution containing 1 g or 2 g of ceftizoxime as ceftizoxime sodium. Dextrose, USP has been added to these dosages to adjust osmolality (approximately 1.9 g and 950 mg to the 1 g and 2 g dosages as dextrose hydrous, respectively). Thawed solutions range from very pale yellow to yellow. The pH of thawed solutions range from 5.5 to 8.0. After thawing to room temperature, the solution is intended for intravenous use only.

The Galaxy® container is fabricated from a specially designed multilayer plastic (PL 2040). Solutions are in contact with the polyethylene layer of this container and can leach out certain chemical components of the plastic in very small amounts within the expiration dating period. The suitability of the plastic has been confirmed in tests in animals according to the USP biological tests for plastic containers, as well as by tissue culture toxicity studies.

HOW SUPPLIED

Cefizox® (ceftizoxime sodium injection) is supplied as a frozen, sio-osmotic, sterile, nonpyrogenic solution in 50 mL single dose Galaxy® plastic containers (PL2040) as follows:

NDC 0469-7220-01   Product No. 722001
   1 g ceftizoxime/50 mL container
NDC 0469-7221-02   Product No. 722102
   2 g ceftizoxime/50 mL container

Store at or below –20°C/–4°F.
See DIRECTIONS FOR USE OF CEFIZOX® (ceftizoxime sodium injection) IN GALAXY® PLASTIC CONTAINER (PL 2040).

Galaxy® is a registered trademark of Baxter International Inc.
Ceftizoxime sodium is a product of Japan.
Manufactured for Fujisawa USA, Inc.
Deerfield, IL 60015 by
Baxter Healthcare Corporation, Deerfield, IL 60015,
45621A/Issued April 1995

CYCLOCORT®   ℞
[amcinonide]

DESCRIPTION

The topical corticosteroids constitute a class of primarily synthetic steroids used as anti-inflammatory and antipruritic agents.
TOPICAL LOTION 0.1%
Each gram of CYCLOCORT (amcinonide) topical Lotion contains 1 mg of the active steroid amcinonide in AQUATAIN,* a white, smooth, homogeneous, opaque emulsion composed of Benzyl Alcohol 1% (wt/wt) as preservative, Emulsifying Wax, Glycerin, Isopropyl Palmitate, Lactic Acid, Purified Water, and Sorbitol Solution. In addition, contains Polyethylene Glycol 400.
Sodium hydroxide may be used to adjust pH to approximately 4.4 during manufacture.
TOPICAL CREAM 0.1%
Each gram of CYCLOCORT (amcinonide) topical Cream contains 1 mg of the active steroid amcinonide in AQUATAIN,* a white, smooth, homogeneous, opaque emulsion composed of Benzyl Alcohol 2% (wt/wt) as preservative, Emulsifying Wax, Glycerin, Isopropyl Palmitate, Lactic Acid, Purified Water, and Sorbitol Solution.
*AQUATAIN™ is non-staining, water-washable, paraben-free, spermaceti-free, and has a light texture and consistency.
TOPICAL OINTMENT 0.1%
Each gram of CYCLOCORT (amcinonide) topical Ointment contains 1 mg of the active steroid amcinonide in a specially formulated base composed of Benzyl Alcohol 2% (wt/wt) as preservative, White Petrolatum, Emulsifying Wax, and Tenox II (Butylated Hydroxyanisole, Propyl Gallate, Citric Acid, Propylene Glycol).
Chemically, amcinonide is:

Molecular Weight 502.58 $C_{28}H_{35}FO_7$

Pregna-1,4-diene-3,20-dione, 21-(acetyloxy)-16,17-[cyclopentylidenebis(oxy)]-9-fluoro-11-hydroxy-, (11β, 16α).

HOW SUPPLIED

CYCLOCORT® (amcinonide) Topical Lotion 0.1% (1 mg/g) with AQUATAIN™ hydrophilic base

NDC 0469-7404-20   Product Code 740420
20 mL (19.6 g) Bottle
NDC 0469-7404-60   Product Code 740460
60 mL (58.8 g) Bottle
CYCLOCORT® (amcinonide) Topical Cream 0.1% (1 mg/g) with AQUATAIN™ hydrophilic base
NDC 0469-7054-15   Product Code 705415
15 gram Tube
NDC 0469-7054-30   Product Code 705430
30 gram Tube
NDC 0469-7054-60   Product Code 705460
60 gram Tube
CYCLOCORT® (amcinonide) Topical Ointment 0.1% (1 mg/g)
NDC 0469-7115-15   Product Code 711515
15 gram Tube
NDC 0469-7115-30   Product Code 711530
30 gram Tube
NDC 0469-7115-60   Product Code 711560
60 gram Tube

Store at controlled room temperature 15°–30°C (59°–86°F).
DO NOT FREEZE.
Manufactured for Fujisawa USA, Inc., Deerfield, IL 60015 by
Lederle Laboratories Division,
American Cyanamid Company,
Pearl River, NY 10965
CI 4432–1   Issued November 20, 1995

ELASE® OINTMENT   ℞
[e'lāse]
(Fibrinolysin and Desoxyribonuclease, Combined, [Bovine] Ointment)

DESCRIPTION

Elase Ointment is a combination of two lytic enzymes, fibrinolysin and desoxyribonuclease, supplied in an ointment base of liquid petrolatum and polyethylene. The fibrinolysin component is derived from bovine plasma[1,2] and the desoxyribonuclease is isolated in a purified form from bovine pancreas. The fibrinolysin used in the combination is activated by chloroform.

HOW SUPPLIED

N0469-7004-30 Elase Ointment, 30-gram
The 30-gram tube contains 30 units of fibrinolysin and 20,000 units of desoxyribonuclease in a special ointment base of liquid petrolatum and polyethylene.
N0469-7004-10 Elase Ointment, 10-gram
The 10-gram tube contains 10 units of fibrinolysin and 6,666 units of desoxyribonuclease in a special ointment base of liquid petrolatum and polyethylene.
This product also contains sodium chloride and sucrose as incidental ingredients.
Storage: Store at no warmer than 30°C (86°F).
Caution—Federal law prohibits dispensing without prescription.
© 1994 Warner-Lambert Co.
December 1994
Manufactured by
PARKE-DAVIS
Div of Warner-Lambert Co/Morris Plains, NJ 07950 USA
Distributed by
Fujisawa USA, Inc.   9011G023
Deerfield, IL 60015   183

ELASE-CHLOROMYCETIN® OINTMENT   ℞
(Fibrinolysin and Desoxyribonuclease, Combined, [Bovine] with Chloramphenicol Ointment)

DESCRIPTION

Elase-Chloromycetin Ointment contains two lytic enzymes, fibrinolysin and desoxyribonuclease, combined with chloramphenicol in an ointment base.
The fibrinolysin component is derived from bovine plasma,[1,2] and the desoxyribonuclease is isolated in a purified form from bovine pancreas. The fibrinolysin used in the combination is activated by chloroform.
Chloramphenicol is a broad-spectrum antibiotic originally isolated from *Streptomyces venezuelae*. It is therapeutically active against a wide variety of susceptible organisms, both gram-positive and gram-negative. Chemically, chloramphenicol may be identified as D(-)-*threo*-1-*p*-nitrophenyl-2-dichloroacetamido-1,3-propanediol.

HOW SUPPLIED

Elase-Chloromycetin (fibrinolysin-desoxyribonuclease-chloramphenicol) is supplied in 30-g and 10-g ointment tubes. The 10-g tubes have an elongated nozzle to facilitate the application to surface lesions.

N0469-7006-30 Elase-Chloromycetin Ointment, 30-gram.
The 30-g tubes contain 30 units (Loomis) of fibrinolysin (bovine), 20,000 units* of desoxyribonuclease, and 0.3 g** chloramphenicol in a special ointment base of liquid petrolatum and polyethylene.
N0469-7006-10 Elase-Chloromycetin Ointment, 10-gram.
The 10-g tubes contain 10 units (Loomis) of fibrinolysin (bovine), 6,666 units* of desoxyribonuclease, and 0.1 g** chloramphenicol in a special ointment base of liquid petrolatum and polyethylene.
The ointment contains sodium chloride and sucrose used in its manufacture.
Storage: Store at no warmer than 30°C (86°F).
Caution—Federal law prohibits dispensing without prescription.
* Modified Christensen method.[4]
** 10 mg chloramphenicol per gram, or 1%.
© 1994, Warner-Lambert Co.
December 1994
Manufactured by
PARKE-DAVIS
Div of Warner-Lambert Co/
Morris Plains, NJ 07950 USA
Distributed by
Fujisawa USA, Inc.   9021G023
Deerfield, IL 60015   182

PROGRAF®   ℞
tacrolimus capsules
tacrolimus injection (for intravenous infusion only)

> **WARNING**
> Increased susceptibility to infection and the possible development of lymphoma may result from immunosuppression. Only physicians experienced in immunosuppressive therapy and management of organ transplant patients should prescribe Prograf. Patients receiving the drug should be managed in facilities equipped and staffed with adequate laboratory and supportive medical resources. The physician responsible for maintenance therapy should have complete information requisite for the follow-up of the patient.

DESCRIPTION

Prograf is available for oral administration as capsules (tacrolimus capsules) containing the equivalent of 1 mg or 5 mg of anhydrous tacrolimus. Inactive ingredients include lactose, hydroxypropyl methylcellulose, croscarmellose sodium, and magnesium stearate. The 1-mg capsule shell contains gelatin and titanium dioxide, and the 5-mg capsule shell contains gelatin, titanium dioxide and ferric oxide.
Prograf is also available as a sterile solution (tacrolimus injection) containing the equivalent of 5 mg anhydrous tacrolimus in 1 mL for administration by intravenous infusion only. Each mL contains polyoxyl 60 hydrogenated castor oil (HCO-60), 200 mg, and dehydrated alcohol, USP, 80.0% v/v. Prograf injection must be diluted with 0.9% Sodium Chloride Injection or 5% Dextrose Injection before use.
Tacrolimus, previously known as FK506, is the active ingredient in Prograf. Tacrolimus is a macrolide immunosuppressant produced by *Streptomyces tsukubaensis*. Chemically, tacrolimus is designated as [3S-[3R *[E (1S *,3S *,4S *)], 4S *,5R *,8S *,9E, 12R *, 14R *,15S *,16R *,18S *,19S *,26a-R *]]-5, 6, 8, 11, 12, 13, 14, 15, 16, 17, 18, 19, 24, 25, 26, 26a-hexadecahydro-5,19-dihydroxy-3-[2-(4- hydroxy-3-methoxycyclohexyl)-1-methylethenyl]-14, 16-dimethoxy 4,10,12,18-tetramethyl-8-(2-propenyl)-15,19-epoxy-3H-pyrido [2,1-c][1,4] oxaazacyclotricosine-1, 7, 20, 21 (4H,23H)-tetrone, monohydrate.
The chemical structure of tacrolimus is:

Tacrolimus has an empirical formula of $C_{44}H_{69}NO_{12} \cdot H_2O$ and a formula weight of 822.05. Tacrolimus appears as white crystals or crystalline powder. It is practically insoluble in

Population	No. of Subjs/Study	Dose mg/kg/12h	Cmax ng/mL	Tmax hours	AUC ng/ml.h	F%
Healthy Volunteers	27	0.07 (1x5mg)	28.6 (8.6)	1.4 (0.62)	271 (122)	14.4 (6.0)
		0.07 (5x1mg)	36.2 (13.8)	1.3 (0.43)	329 (174)	17.4 (7.0)
Liver Transplant Patients	17	0.15	68.5 (30.0)	2.3 (1.5)	519 (179)	21.8 (6.3)
	11 Effect of Food	0.15 (Food)	27.1 (14.7)	3.2 (1.3)	223 (125)	– –
		0.15 (Fasting)	52.4 (17.0)	1.5 (1.2)	290 (117)	– –

Mean (SD) Cmax maximum concentration; AUC area under the conc-time curve; Tmax time to maximum concentration; F absolute bioavailability

water, freely soluble in ethanol, and very soluble in methanol and chloroform.

CLINICAL PHARMACOLOGY

Mechanism of Action

Tacrolimus prolongs the survival of the host and transplanted graft in animal transplant models of liver, kidney, heart, bone marrow, small bowel and pancreas, lung and trachea, skin, cornea, and limb.

In animals, tacrolimus has been demonstrated to suppress some humoral immunity and, to a greater extent, cell-mediated reactions such as allograft rejection, delayed type hypersensitivity, collagen-induced arthritis, experimental allergic encephalomyelitis, and graft versus host disease.

Tacrolimus inhibits T-lymphocyte activation, although the exact mechanism of action is not known. Experimental evidence suggests that tacrolimus binds to an intracellular protein, FKBP-12. A complex of tacrolimus-FKBP-12, calcium, calmodulin, and calcineurin is then formed and the phosphatase activity of calcineurin inhibited. This effect may prevent the generation of nuclear factor of activated T-cells (NF-AT), a nuclear component thought to initiate gene transcription for the formation of lymphokines (interleukin-2, gamma interferon). The net result is the inhibition of T-lymphocyte activation (i.e., immunosuppression).

Pharmacokinetics

Absorption of tacrolimus from the gastrointestinal tract after oral administration is variable. The absorption half-life of tacrolimus in 16 liver transplant patients averaged 0.6 hour (standard deviation 1.0 hour). Peak concentrations (Cmax) in blood and plasma were achieved at approximately 1.5–3.5 hours. Mean (standard deviation) pharmacokinetic parameters of tacrolimus in whole blood after oral administration were:

[See table above.]

The disposition of tacrolimus from whole blood was biphasic with a terminal elimination half-life of 11.7 (±3.9) hours in liver transplant patients and 21.2 (±8.5) hours in healthy volunteers. The volume of distribution and total body clearance for tacrolimus following intravenous administration were:

Population	Number of Subjects	Dose (mg/kg/12h)	Vd (l/kg)	Cl (L/h/kg)
Health Volunteers	27	0.01	0.88 (0.31)	0.042 (0.016)
Liver Transplant Patients	17	0.05	0.85 (0.3)	0.053 (0.017)

Mean (SD) Vd Volume of distribution; Cl Total body clearance

Pharmacokinetic data indicate that whole blood rather than plasma may serve as the more appropriate medium to describe the pharmacokinetic characteristics of tacrolimus.

The results of a single-dose bioequivalence study conducted in 27 healthy volunteers indicated that the absolute bioavailability of the 5-mg capsule was 14.4% and that of five 1-mg capsules was 17.4%. This study failed to establish the bioequivalence of these two formulations.

The effect of food was studied in 11 liver transplant patients. Prograf was administered in the fasting state or 15 minutes after a breakfast of measured fat content (34% of 400 total calories). The results indicate that the presence of food reduces the absorption of tacrolimus (decrease in AUC and Cmax, and increase in Tmax). The relative oral bioavailability (whole blood) was reduced by 27.0 (±18.2%) when compared to administration in the fasting state.

The protein-binding of tacrolimus reported in two studies was 75% and 99% over a range of concentrations of 0.1–100 ng/mL. Tacrolimus is bound to proteins, mainly albumins and alpha-1-acid glycoprotein, and is highly bound to erythrocytes. The distribution of tacrolimus between whole blood and plasma depends on several factors such as hematocrit, temperature of separation of plasma, drug concentration, and plasma protein concentration. In a U.S. study, the ratio of whole blood concentration to plasma concentration ranged from 12 to 67 (mean 35).

Tacrolimus trough concentrations from 10 to 60 ng/mL measured at 10–12 hours post-dose (Cmin) correlated well with the area under the plasma or whole blood concentration-time curve (AUC). In 28 liver transplant patients, the correlation coefficient was 0.94.

Pharmacokinetic studies in pediatric patients have not been conducted. However, trough concentrations obtained from 30 children (less than 12 years old) showed that children need higher doses than adults to achieve similar tacrolimus trough concentrations, suggesting that the pharmacokinetic characteristics of tacrolimus are different in children as compared to adults. (See DOSAGE AND ADMINISTRATION).

Tacrolimus is extensively metabolized by the mixed-function oxidase system, primarily the cytochrome P-450 enzyme system (P-450 IIIA). In man, less than 1% of the dose administered is excreted unchanged in the urine. The major metabolic pathway has not been determined. Demethylation and hydroxylation were identified as the primary mechanisms of biotransformation *in vitro*. The major metabolite identified in incubations with human liver microsomes is 13-demethyl tacrolimus. Ten possible metabolites have been identified in human plasma. Two metabolites, a demethylated and a double-demethylated tacrolimus, were shown to retain 10% and 7%, respectively, of the inhibitory effect of tacrolimus on T-lymphocyte activation.

Clinical Studies

The safety and efficacy of Prograf-based immunosuppression following orthotopic liver transplantation were assessed in two prospective, randomized, non-blinded multicenter studies. The active control groups were treated with a cyclosporine-based immunosuppressive regimen. Both studies used concomitant adrenal corticosteroids as part of the immunosuppressive regimens. These studies were designed to evaluate whether the two regimens were therapeutically equivalent, with patient and graft survival at 12 months following transplantation as the primary endpoints. The Prograf-based immunosuppressive regimen was found to be equivalent to the cyclosporine-based immunosuppressive regimens.

In one trial, 529 patients were enrolled at 12 clinical sites in the United States; prior to surgery, 263 were randomized to the Prograf-based immunosuppressive regimen and 266 to a cyclosporine-based immunosuppressive regimen (CBIR). In 10 of the 12 sites, the same CBIR protocol was used, while 2 sites used different control protocols. This trial excluded patients with renal dysfunction, fulminant hepatic failure with Stage IV encephalopathy, and cancers; pediatric patients (≤ 12 years old) were allowed.

In the second trial, 545 patients were enrolled at 8 clinical sites in Europe; prior to surgery, 270 were randomized to the Prograf-based immunosuppressive regimen and 275 to a CBIR. In this study, each center used its local standard CBIR protocol in the active-control arm. This trial excluded pediatric patients, but did allow enrollment of subjects with renal dysfunction, fulminant hepatic failure in Stage IV encephalopathy, and cancers other than primary hepatic with metastases.

One-year patient survival and graft survival in the Prograf-based treatment groups were equivalent to those in the CBIR treatment groups in both studies. The overall one-year patient survival (CBIR and Prograf-based treatment groups combined) was 88% in the U.S. study and 78% in the European study. The overall one-year graft survival (CBIR and Prograf-based treatment groups combined) was 81% in the U.S. study and 73% in the European study. In both studies, the median time to convert from IV to oral Prograf dosing was 2 days.

Information on secondary outcomes (incidence of acute rejection, use of OKT3 for steroid-resistant rejection, and incidence of refractory rejection) was also collected. Because of the nature of the study designs, comparisons of differences between the study arms for these secondary endpoints could not be reliably assessed.

INDICATIONS AND USAGE

Prograf is indicated for the prophylaxis of organ rejection in patients receiving allogeneic liver transplants. It is recommended that Prograf be used concomitantly with adrenal corticosteroids. Because of the risk of anaphylaxis, Prograf injection should be reserved for patients unable to take Prograf capsules orally.

CONTRAINDICATIONS

Prograf is contraindicated in patients with a hypersensitivity to tacrolimus. Prograf injection is contraindicated in patients with a hypersensitivity to HCO-60 (polyoxyl 60 hydrogenated castor oil).

WARNINGS

(See boxed **WARNING**)

Prograf can cause neurotoxicity and nephrotoxicity, particularly when used in high doses. Nephrotoxicity has been noted in 40% and 33% of liver transplantation patients receiving Prograf in the U.S. and European randomized trials, respectively (see ADVERSE REACTIONS). More overt nephrotoxicity is seen early after transplantation, characterized by increasing serum creatinine and a decrease in urine output. Patients with impaired renal function should be monitored closely, and the dosage of Prograf may need to be reduced. In patients with persistent elevations of serum creatinine who are unresponsive to dosage adjustments, consideration should be given to changing to another immunosuppressive therapy. Care should be taken in using tacrolimus and other nephrotoxic drugs. **In particular, to avoid excess nephrotoxicity, Prograf should not be used simultaneously with cyclosporine. Prograf or cyclosporine should be discontinued at least 24 hours prior to initiating the other. In the presence of elevated Prograf of cyclosporine concentrations, dosing with the other drug usually should be further delayed.**

Mild to severe hyperkalemia has been noted in 44% and 10% of liver transplant recipients treated with Prograf in the U.S. and European randomized trials and may require treatment (see ADVERSE REACTIONS). **Serum potassium levels should be monitored and potassium-sparing diuretics should not be used during Prograf therapy (see PRECAUTIONS).**

Neurotoxicity, including tremor, headache, and other changes in motor function, mental status, and sensory function were reported in approximately 55% of liver transplant recipients in the two randomized studies (see ADVERSE REACTIONS). Tremor and headache have been associated with high whole-blood concentrations of tacrolimus and may respond to dosage adjustment. Seizures have occurred in adult and pediatric patients receiving Prograf (see ADVERSE REACTIONS). Coma and delirium also have been associated with high plasma concentrations of tacrolimus.

As in patients receiving other immunosuppressants, patients receiving Prograf are at increased risk of developing lymphomas and other malignancies, particularly of the skin. The risk appears to be related to the intensity and duration of immunosuppression rather than to the use of any specific agent. A lymphoproliferative disorder (LPD) related to Epstein-Barr Virus (EBV) infection has been reported in immunosuppressed organ transplant recipients. The risk of LPD appears greatest in young children who are at risk for primary EBV infection while immunosuppressed or who are switched to Prograf following long-term immunosuppression therapy. Because of the danger of oversuppression of the immune system, which can increase susceptibility to infection, Prograf should not be administered with other immunosuppressive agents except adrenal corticosteroids. The efficacy and safety of the use of Prograf in combination with other immunosuppressive agents has not been determined.

A few patients receiving Prograf injection have experienced anaphylactic reactions. Although the exact cause of these reactions is not known, other drugs with castor oil derivatives in the formulation have been associated with anaphylaxis in a small percentage of patients. Because of this potential risk of anaphylaxis, Prograf injection should be reserved for patients who are unable to take Prograf capsules.

Patients receiving Prograf injection should be under continuous observation for at least the first 30 minutes following the start of the infusion and at frequent intervals thereafter. If signs or symptoms of anaphylaxis occur, the infusion should be stopped. An aqueous solution of epinephrine 1:1000 should be available at the bedside as well as a source of oxygen.

Continued on next page

Fujisawa—Cont.

PRECAUTIONS
General
Hypertension is a common adverse effect of Prograf therapy (see ADVERSE REACTIONS). Mild or moderate hypertension is more frequently reported than severe hypertension. Antihypertensive therapy may be required; the control of blood pressure can be accomplished with any of the common antihypertensive agents. Since tacrolimus can cause hyperkalemia, potassium-sparing diuretics should be avoided. While calcium-channel blocking agents can be effective in treating Prograf-associated hypertension, care should be taken since interference with tacrolimus metabolism may require a dosage reduction (see *Drug Interactions*).

Hyperglycemia was associated with the use of Prograf in 47% and 29% of liver transplant recipients in the U.S. and European randomized studies, respectively, and may require treatment (see ADVERSE REACTIONS).

Renally and Hepatically Impaired Patients
For patients with renal insufficiency some evidence suggests that lower doses should be used (see **DOSAGE AND ADMINISTRATION**).

The use of Prograf in liver transplant recipients experiencing post-transplant hepatic impairment may be associated with increased risk of developing renal insufficiency related to high whole-blood levels of tacrolimus. These patients should be monitored closely and dosage adjustments should be considered. Some evidence suggests that lower doses should be used in these patients (see DOSAGE AND ADMINISTRATION).

Information for Patients
Patients should be informed of the need for repeated appropriate laboratory tests while they are receiving Prograf. They should be given complete dosage instructions, advised of the potential risks during pregnancy, and informed of the increased risk of neoplasia.

Laboratory Tests
Serum creatinine and potassium should be assessed regularly. Routine monitoring of metabolic and hematologic systems should be performed as clinically warranted.

Drug Interactions
Drug interaction studies with tacrolimus have not been conducted. Due to the potential for additive or synergistic impairment of renal function, care should be taken when administering Prograf with drugs that may be associated with renal dysfunction. These include, but are not limited to, aminoglycosides, amphotericin B, and cisplatin. Initial clinical experience with the co-administration of Prograf and cyclosporine resulted in additive/synergistic nephrotoxicity. Patients switched from cyclosporine to Prograf should receive the first Prograf dose no sooner than 24 hours after the last cyclosporine dose. Dosing may be further delayed in the presence of elevated cyclosporine levels.

Drugs that May Alter Tacrolimus Concentrations
Since tacrolimus is metabolized mainly by the cytochrome P-450 IIIA enzyme systems, substances known to inhibit these enzymes may decrease the metabolism of tacrolimus with resultant increases in whole blood or plasma levels. Drugs known to induce these enzyme systems may result in an increased metabolism of tacrolimus and decreased whole blood or plasma levels. Monitoring of blood levels and appropriate dosage adjustments are essential when such drugs are used concomitantly.

Drugs That May Increase Tacrolimus Blood Levels:

Calcium Channel Blockers	Antifungal Agents	Other Drugs
diltiazem	clotrimazole	bromocriptine
nicardipine	fluconazole	cimetidine
verapamil	itraconazole	clarithromycin
	ketoconazole	cyclosporine
		danazol
		erythromycin
		methylprednisolone
		metoclopramide

Drugs That May Decrease Tacrolimus Blood Levels:

Anticonvulsants	Antibiotics
carbamazepine	rifabutin
phenobarbital	rifampin
phenytoin	

Other Drug Interactions
Immunosuppressants may affect vaccination. Therefore, during treatment with Prograf, vaccination may be less effective. The use of live vaccines should be avoided; live vaccines may include, but are not limited to measles, mumps, rubella, oral polio, BCG, yellow fever, and TY 21a typhoid.[1]

Carcinogenesis, Mutagenesis and Impairment of Fertility
An increased incidence of malignancy is a recognized complication of immunosuppression in recipients of organ transplants. The most common forms of neoplasms are non-Hodgkin's lymphomas and carcinomas of the skin. As with other immunosuppressive therapies, the risk of malignan-

cies in Prograf recipients may be higher than in the normal, healthy population. Lymphoproliferative disorders associated with Epstein-Barr Virus infection have been seen. It has been reported that reduction or discontinuance of immunosuppression may cause the lesions to regress.

No evidence of genotoxicity was seen in bacterial (Salmonella and E. coli) or mammalian (Chinese hamster lung-derived cells) *in vitro* assays of mutagenicity, the *in vitro* CHO/HGPRT assay of mutagenicity, or *in vivo* clastogenicity assays performed in mice; tacrolimus did not cause unscheduled DNA synthesis in rodent hepatocytes.

Although studies are ongoing, no adequate studies to evaluate the carcinogenic potential of tacrolimus have been completed.

No impairment of fertility was demonstrated in studies of male and female rats. Tacrolimus, given orally in 1.0 mg/kg ($0.5\times$ the recommended clinical dose based on body surface area corrections) to male and female rats, prior to and during mating, as well as to dams during gestation and lactation, was associated with embryolethality and with adverse effects on female reproduction. Effects on female reproductive function (parturition) and embryolethal effects were indicated by a higher rate of pre-implantation loss and increased numbers of undelivered and nonviable pups. When given at 3.2 mg/kg ($1.5\times$ the recommended clinical dose based on body surface area correction), tacrolimus was associated with maternal and paternal toxicity as well as reproductive toxicity including marked adverse effects on estrus cycles, parturition, pup viability, and pup malformations.

Pregnancy: Category C
In reproduction studies in rats and rabbits, adverse effects on the fetus were observed mainly at dose levels that were toxic to dams. Tacrolimus at oral doses of 0.32 and 1.0 mg/kg during organogenesis in rabbits was associated with maternal toxicity as well as an increase in incidence of abortions; these doses are equivalent to 0.33X and 1.0X (based on body surface area corrections) the recommended clinical dose (0.3 mg/kg). At the higher dose only, an increased incidence of malformations and developmental variations was also seen. Tacrolimus, at oral doses of 3.2 mg/kg during organogenesis in rats, was associated with maternal toxicity and caused an increase in late resorptions, decreased numbers of live births, and decreased pup weight and viability. Tacrolimus, given orally at 1.0 and 3.2 mg/kg (equivalent to 0.5X and 1.5X the recommended clinical dose based on body surface area corrections) to pregnant rats after organogenesis and during lactation, was associated with reduced pup weights. No reduction in male or female fertility was evident.

There are no adequate and well-controlled studies in pregnant women. Tacrolimus is transferred across the placenta. The use of tacrolimus during pregnancy has been associated with neonatal hyperkalemia and renal dysfunction. Prograf should be used during pregnancy only if the potential benefit to the mother justifies potential risk to the fetus.

Nursing Mothers
Since tacrolimus is excreted in human milk, nursing should be avoided.

Pediatric Patients
Successful liver transplants have been performed in pediatric patients (age less than 12 years) using Prograf. One of the two randomized active-controlled trials of Prograf in primary liver transplantation included 51 pediatric patients. Thirty patients were randomized to Prograf-based and 21 to cyclosporine-based therapies. Additionally, 22 pediatric patients were studied in an uncontrolled trial of tacrolimus in living related donor liver transplantation. Pediatric patients generally required higher doses of Prograf to maintain blood trough levels of tacrolimus similar to adult patients (see **DOSAGE AND ADMINISTRATION**).

ADVERSE REACTIONS
The principal adverse reactions of Prograf are tremor, headache, diarrhea, hypertension, nausea, and renal dysfunction. These occur with oral and intravenous administration of Prograf and may respond to a reduction in dosing. Diarrhea was sometimes associated with other gastrointestinal complaints such as nausea and vomiting.

Hyperkalemia, hypomagnesemia and hyperuricemia have occurred in patients receiving Prograf therapy. Hyperglycemia has been noted in many patients; some may require insulin therapy.

The incidence of adverse events was determined in two randomized comparative liver transplant trials among 512 patients receiving tacrolimus and steroids and 511 patients receiving a cyclosporine-based regimen (CBIR). The proportion of patients reporting more than one adverse event was 99.8% in the tacrolimus group and 99.6% in the CBIR group. Precautions must be taken when comparing the incidence of adverse events in the U.S. study to that in the European study. Only adverse events occurring up to 12-months post-transplant in the U.S. study and up to 6-months in the European study are presented. The two studies also included different patient populations and patients were treated with immunosuppressive regimens of differing intensities. Adverse events reported in >15% in tacrolimus patients (com-

bined study results) are presented below for the two controlled trials in liver transplantation:
[See table at top of next page.]

The following adverse events, not mentioned above, were reported with greater than 3% incidence in tacrolimus-treated patients.

NERVOUS SYSTEM: (see WARNINGS) abnormal dreams, agitation, anxiety, confusion, convulsion, depression, dizziness, emotional lability, hallucinations, hypertonia, incoordination, myoclonus nervousness, neuropathy, psychosis, somnolence, thinking abnormal; SPECIAL SENSES: abnormal vision, amblyopia, tinnitus; GASTROINTESTINAL: cholangitis, cholestatic jaundice, dyspepsia, dysphasia, flatulence, gastrointestinal hemorrhage, GGT increase, GI perforation, hepatitis, ileus, increased appetite, jaundice, liver damage, oral moniliasis; CARDIOVASCULAR: chest pain, abnormal ECG, hemorrhage, hypotension, tachycardia; UROGENITAL: (see WARNINGS) hematuria, kidney failure; METABOLIC NUTRITIONAL: acidosis, alkaline phosphatase increased, alkalosis, bilirubinemia, healing abnormal, hyperlipemia, hyperphosphatemia, hyperuricemia, hypocalcemia, hypophosphatemia, hyponatremia, hypoproteinemia, AST (SGOT) increased, ALT (SGPT) increased; ENDOCRINE: (see PRECAUTIONS) diabetes mellitus; HEMIC/LYMPHATIC: coagulation disorder, ecchymosis, hypochromic anemia, leukopenia, prothrombin decreased; MISCELLANEOUS: abdomen enlarged, abscess, chills, hernia, peritonitis, photosensitivity reaction; MUSCULOSKELETAL: arthralgia, generalized spasm, leg cramps, myalgia, myasthenia, osteoporosis; RESPIRATORY: asthma, bronchitis, cough increased, lung disorder, pulmonary edema, pharyngitis, pneumonia, respiratory disorder, rhinitis, sinusitis, voice alteration; SKIN: alopecia, herpes simplex, hirsutism, skin disorder, sweating.

OVERDOSAGE
There is minimal experience with overdosage. In patients who have received inadvertent overdosage of Prograf, no adverse reactions different from those reported in patients receiving therapeutic doses have been described. General supportive measures and systemic treatment should be followed in all cases of overdosage. Based on the poor aqueous solubility and extensive erythrocyte and plasma protein binding, it is anticipated that tacrolimus is not dialyzable to any significant extent.

In acute oral and intravenous toxicity studies, mortalities were seen at and above the following doses: in adult rats, 52X the recommended human oral dose; in immature rats, 16X the recommended oral dose; and in adult rats, 16X the recommended human intravenous dose (all based on body surface area corrections).

DOSAGE AND ADMINISTRATION
Prograf injection (tacrolimus injection)
For Intravenous Infusion Only
NOTE: Anaphylactic reactions have occurred with injectables containing castor oil derivatives. See WARNINGS SECTION.

In patients unable to take oral Prograf capsules, therapy may be initiated with Prograf injection. The initial dose of Prograf should be administered no sooner than 6 hours after transplantation. The recommended starting dose of Prograf injection is 0.05–0.10 mg/kg/day as a continuous intravenous infusion. Adult patients receive doses at the lower end of the dosing range. Concomitant adrenal corticosteroid therapy is recommended early post-transplantation. Continuous intravenous infusion of Prograf injection should be continued only until the patient can tolerate oral administration of Prograf capsules.

Preparation for Administration/Stability
Prograf injection must be diluted with 0.9% Sodium Chloride Injection or 5% Dextrose Injection to a concentration between 0.004 mg/mL and 0.02 mg/mL prior to use. Diluted infusion solution should be stored in glass or polyethylene containers and should be discarded after 24 hours. The diluted infusion solution should not be stored in a PVC container due to decreased stability and the potential for extraction of phthalates. Parenteral drug products should be inspected visually for particulate matter and discoloration prior to administration, whenever solution and container permit.

Prograf capsules (tacrolimus capsules)
It is recommended that patients be converted from intravenous to oral Prograf capsules as soon as oral therapy can be tolerated. This usually occurs within 2–3 days. The first dose of oral therapy should be given 8–12 hours after discontinuing the IV infusion. The recommended starting oral dose of Prograf capsules is 0.15–0.30 mg/kg/day administered in two divided daily doses every 12 hours. The initial dose of Prograf should be administered no sooner than 6 hours after transplantation. Adult patients should receive doses at the lower end of the dosing range.

Dosing should be titrated based on clinical assessments of rejection and tolerability. Lower Prograf dosages may be sufficient as maintenance therapy. Adjunct therapy with adrenal corticosteroids is recommended early post transplant.

	U.S. STUDY(%)		EUROPEAN STUDY (%)	
	Prograf (N=250)	CBIR (N=250)	Prograf (N=262)	CBIR (N=261)
Nervous System				
Headache (See WARNINGS)	64	60	31	20
Tremor (See WARNINGS)	56	46	44	30
Insomnia	64	68	29	21
Paresthesia	40	30	15	13
Gastrointestinal				
Diarrhea	72	47	32	23
Nausea	46	37	30	22
Constipation	24	27	19	20
LFT Abnormal	36	30	5	2
Anorexia	34	24	6	4
Vomiting	27	15	12	9
Cardiovascular				
Hypertension (See PRECAUTIONS)	47	56	31	35
Urogenital				
Kidney Function Abnormal (See WARNINGS)	40	27	33	18
Creatinine Increased (See WARNINGS)	39	25	19	16
BUN Increased (See WARNINGS)	30	22	8	7
Urinary Tract Infection	16	18	19	18
Oliguria	18	15	16	8
Metabolic and Nutritional				
Hyperkalemia (See WARNINGS)	45	26	10	7
Hypokalemia	29	34	11	14
Hyperglycemia (See PRECAUTIONS)	47	38	29	16
Hypomagnesemia	48	45	15	8
Hemic and Lymphatic				
Anemia	47	38	4	1
Leukocytosis	32	26	8	7
Thrombocytopenia	24	20	10	14
Miscellaneous				
Abdominal Pain	59	54	26	20
Pain	63	57	19	14
Fever	48	56	15	18
Asthenia	52	48	7	4
Back Pain	30	29	13	14
Ascites	27	22	5	6
Peripheral Edema	26	26	10	11
Respiratory System				
Pleural Effusion	30	32	32	29
Atelectasis	28	30	5	4
Dyspnea	29	23	3	2
Skin and Appendages				
Pruritus	36	20	11	5
Rash	24	19	8	3

Pediatric Patients
Pediatric patients without pre-existing renal or hepatic dysfunction have required and tolerated higher doses than adults to achieve similar blood concentrations. Therefore, it is recommended that therapy be initiated in pediatric patients at the high end of the recommended adult intravenous and oral dosing ranges (0.1 mg/kg/day intravenous and 0.3 mg/kg/day oral). Dose adjustments may be required.

Patients with Hepatic or Renal Dysfunction
Due to the potential for nephrotoxicity, patients with renal or hepatic impairment should receive doses at the lowest value of the recommended intravenous and oral dosing ranges. Further reductions in dose below these ranges may be required. Prograf therapy usually should be delayed up to 48 hours or longer in patients with post-operative oliguria.

Conversion from one Immunosuppressive Regimen to Another
Prograf should not be used simultaneously with cyclosporine. Prograf or cyclosporine should be discontinued at least 24 hours before initiating the other. In the presence of elevated Prograf or cyclosporine concentrations, dosing with the other drug usually should be further delayed.

Blood Concentration Monitoring
Most study centers have found tacrolimus blood-concentration monitoring helpful in patient management. While no fixed relationship has been established, such blood monitoring may assist in the clinical evaluation of rejection and toxicity, dose adjustments, and the assessment of compliance. Various assays have been used to measure blood concentrations of tacrolimus. Comparison of the concentrations in published literature to patient concentrations using current assays must be made with detailed knowledge of the assay methods employed.
Data from the U.S. clinical trail show that tacrolimus whole blood concentrations, as measured by ELISA, were most variable during the first week post-transplantation. After this early period, the median trough blood concentrations, measured at intervals from the second week to one year post-transplantation, ranged from 9.8 ng/mL to 19.4 ng/mL.

HOW SUPPLIED

Prograf capsules (tacrolimus capsules) 1mg
Oblong, white, branded with red "1 mg" on the capsule cap and 617" on the capsule body, supplied in 100-count bottles (NDC 0469-0617-71), and ten blister cards of ten capsules (NDC 0469-0617-10,), containing the equivalent of 1 mg of anhydrous tacrolimus.

Prograf capsules (tacrolimus capsules) 5mg
Oblong, grayish/red, branded with white "5 mg" on the capsule cap and 657" on the capsule body, supplied in 100-count bottles (NDC 0469-0657-71) (NDC 0469-0657-10), containing the equivalent of 5 mg of anhydrous tacrolimus.
Store and Dispense
Store at controlled room temperature, 15°C-30°C (59°F-86°F).
Prograf injection (tacrolimus injection) 5mg (for intravenous infusion only)
Supplied as a sterile solution in 1-mL ampules containing the equivalent of 5 mg of anhydrous tacrolimus per mL, in boxes of 10 ampules (NDC 0469-3016-01).
Store and Dispense
Store between 5°C and 25°C (41°F and 77°F).

CAUTION: Federal law prohibits dispensing without prescription.

Made in Ireland
for Fujisawa USA, Inc.
Deerfield, IL 60015-2548
by Fujisawa Ireland, Ltd.
Killorglin, Co. Kerry Ireland

REFERENCE
1. CDC: Recommendations of the Advisory Committee on Immunization Practices: Use of vaccines and immune globulins in persons with altered immunocompetence. MMWR 1993;42(RR-4):1–18.
ZL40301
Shown in Product Identification Guide, page 311

IDENTIFICATION PROBLEM?
Turn to the **Product Identification** Guide, where you'll find more than 1600 products pictured in actual size and full color.

Galderma Laboratories, Inc.
P.O. BOX 331329
FT. WORTH, TX 76163

Direct Inquiries to:
(817) 263-2600

BENZAC® AC 2¹/₂, 5 & 10 ℞
(benzoyl peroxide gel)
BENZAC® AC Wash 2¹/₂, 5 & 10 ℞
(benzoyl peroxide)
BENZAC W® 2¹/₂, 5 & 10 Water Base Gel ℞
BENZAC W® WASH 5 & 10 ℞
(benzoyl peroxide)
BENZAC® 5 & 10 Gel ℞
(benzoyl peroxide)

DESCRIPTION
Benzac AC 2¹/₂, 5 and 10 (benzoyl peroxide gel), Benzac AC Wash 2¹/₂, 5 and 10 (benzoyl peroxide wash), Benzac W 2¹/₂, 5 and 10, (benzoyl peroxide) and Benzac W Wash 5 and 10, are topical, water-base, benzoyl peroxide containing preparations for use in the treatment of acne vulgaris. Benzac (benzoyl peroxide) 5 and 10 are topical alcohol-base preparations. Benzoyl peroxide is an oxidizing agent which possesses antibacterial properties and is classified as a keratolytic. Benzoyl peroxide ($C_{14}H_{10}O_4$) is represented by the following chemical structure:

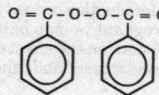

Benzac AC 2¹/₂, Benzac AC 5, and Benzac AC 10 contain, respectively, benzoyl peroxide 2¹/₂%, 5% and 10% as the active ingredient in a gel base containing docusate sodium, edetate disodium, poloxamer 182, carbomer 940, propylene glycol, acrylates copolymer, glycerin, colloidal silicon dioxide, sodium hydroxide and purified water. May contain citric acid to adjust pH.
Benzac AC Wash 2¹/₂, Benzac AC Wash 5 and Benzac AC Wash 10 contain, respectively, benzoyl peroxide 2¹/₂%, 5% and 10% as the active ingredient in a vehicle consisting of purified water, sodium C14–16 olefin sulfonate, acrylates copolymer, glycerin, sodium hydroxide, and carbomer 940. May contain citric acid to adjust pH.
Benzac 5 and Benzac 10 contain, respectively, benzoyl peroxide 5% and 10% as the active ingredient in a gel base containing alcohol 12% (w/w), laureth 4, dimethicone, carbomer 940, sodium hydroxide, fragrance and purified water. May contain citric acid to adjust pH.
Benzac W 2¹/₂, Benzac W 5 and Benzac W 10 contain, respectively, benzoyl peroxide 2¹/₂%, 5% and 10% as the active ingredient in a gel base containing docusate sodium, edetate disodium, poloxamer 182, carbomer 940, propylene glycol, colloidal silicon dioxide, sodium hydroxide and purified water. May contain citric acid to adjust pH.
Benzac W Wash 5 and Benzac W Wash 10 contain, respectively, benzoyl peroxide 5% and 10% as the active ingredient in a vehicle consisting of sodium C14–16 olefin sulfonate, carbomer 940, and purified water. May contain citric acid to adjust pH.

CLINICAL PHARMACOLOGY
The mechanism of action of benzoyl peroxide is not totally understood but its antibacterial activity against *Propionibacterium acnes* is thought to be a major mode of action. In addition, patients treated with benzoyl peroxide show a reduction in lipids and free fatty acids and mild desquamation (drying and peeling activity) with a simultaneous reduction in comedones and acne lesions.
Little is known about the percutaneous penetration, metabolism, and excretion of benzoyl peroxide, although it has been shown that benzoyl peroxide absorbed by the skin is metabolized to benzoic acid and then excreted as benzoate in the urine. There is no evidence of systemic toxicity caused by benzoyl peroxide in humans.

INDICATIONS AND USAGE
Benzac 5 and 10 and Benzac W 2¹/₂, 5 and 10 are indicated for the topical treatment of acne vulgaris. Benzac W Wash 5 and 10 are indicated for the topical treatment of mild to moderate acne vulgaris. In severe complicated acne. Benzac W

Continued on next page

Galderma Laboratories—Cont.

Wash 5 and 10 may be used as an adjunct to other therapeutic regimens.
Benzac AC $2^1/_2$, **5** and **10** and **Benzac AC Wash** $2^1/_2$, **5** and **10** are indicated for the topical treatment of acne vulgaris.

CONTRAINDICATIONS
These preparations are contraindicated in patients with a history of hypersensitivity to any of their components.

PRECAUTIONS
General: For external use only. If severe irritation develops, discontinue use and institute appropriate therapy. After the reaction clears, treatment may often be resumed with less frequent application. These preparations should not be used in or near the eyes or on mucous membranes.
Information for patients: Avoid contact with eyes, eyelids, lips and mucous membranes. If accidental contact occurs, rinse with water. Avoid contact with eyes, hair, fabric or carpet. Benzoyl peroxide will cause bleaching. If excessive irritation develops, discontinue use and consult your physician.
Carcinogenesis, Mutagenesis, Impairment of Fertility: Data from several studies employing a strain of mice that are highly susceptible to developing cancer suggest that benzoyl peroxide acts as a tumor promotor. The clinical significance of these findings to humans is unknown. Benzoyl peroxide has not been found to be mutagenic (Ames Test) and there are no published data indicating it impairs fertility.
Pregnancy: Teratogenic Effects: *Pregnancy Category C:* Animal reproduction studies have not been conducted with benzoyl peroxide. It is not known whether benzoyl peroxide can cause fetal harm when administered to a pregnant woman or can affect reproduction capacity. Benzoyl peroxide should be used by a pregnant woman only if clearly needed. There are no available data on the effect of benzoyl peroxide on the later growth, development and functional maturation of the unborn child.
Nursing Mothers: It is not known whether this drug is excreted in human milk. Because many drugs are excreted in human milk, caution should be exercised when benzoyl peroxide is administered to a nursing woman.
Pediatric Use: Safety and effectiveness in children have not been established.

ADVERSE REACTIONS
Allergic contact dermatitis and dryness have been reported with topical benzoyl peroxide therapy.

OVERDOSAGE
If excessive scaling, erythema or edema occur, the use of this preparation should be discontinued. To hasten resolution of the adverse effects, cool compresses may be used. After symptoms and signs subside, a reduced dosage schedule may be cautiously tried if the reaction is judged to be due to excessive use and not allergenicity.

DOSAGE AND ADMINISTRATION
Benzac AC $2^1/_2$, **5** or **10** should be applied once or twice daily to cover affected areas after washing with a mild cleanser and water.
Benzac AC Wash $2^1/_2$, **5** or **10.** Wash once or twice daily avoiding contact with the eyes and mucous membranes. Wet the area of application. Apply **Benzac AC Wash** $2^1/_2$, **5** or **10** to the hands and wash the affected areas. Rinse with water and pat dry.
Benzac 5 or **10** or **Benzac W** $2^1/_2$, **5** or **10** should be applied once or twice daily to cover affected areas after washing with a mild cleanser and water. Wash with **Benzac W Wash 5** or **10** once or twice daily, avoiding contact with eyes and mucous membranes. Wet the area of application. Apply **Benzac W Wash 5** or **10** to the hands and wash the affected areas. Rinse with water and dry. The degree of drying and peeling can be adjusted by modification of the dosage schedule.

HOW SUPPLIED
Benzac® AC $2^1/_2$ Water Base Gel
60 g tubes—**NDC** 0299-3620-60
90 g tubes—**NDC** 0299-3620-90
Benzac® AC 5 Water Base Gel
60 g tubes—**NDC** 0299-3625-60
90 g tubes—**NDC** 0299-3625-90
Benzac® AC 10 Water Base Gel
60 g tubes—**NDC** 0299-3630-60
90 g tubes—**NDC** 0299-3630-90
Benzac® AC Wash $2^1/_2$
8 oz. plastic bottles—**NDC** 0299-3635-08
Benzac® AC Wash 5
8 oz. plastic bottles—**NDC** 0299-3640-08
Benzac® AC Wash 10
8 oz. plastic bottles—**NDC** 0299-3645-08
Benzac® 5 Gel
60 g tubes—**NDC** 0299-3655-01
Benzac® 10 Gel
60 g tubes—**NDC** 0299-3665-01

Benzac W® $2^1/_2$ Water Base Gel
60 g tubes—**NDC** 0299-3590-60
90 g tubes—**NDC** 0299-3590-90
Benzac W® 5 Water Base Gel
60 g tubes—**NDC** 0299-3600-01
90 g tubes—**NDC** 0299-3600-09
Benzac W® 10 Water Base Gel
60 g tubes—**NDC** 0299-3610-01
90 g tubes—**NDC** 0299-3610-09
Benzac W® Wash 5
4 oz. plastic bottles—**NDC** 0299-3670-04
8 oz. plastic bottles—**NDC** 0299-3670-08
Benzac W® Wash 10
8 oz. plastic bottles—**NDC** 0299-3672-08

STORAGE
Store **Benzac AC** and **Benzac AC Wash** at controlled room temperature (59°–86°F).
Store Benzac W and Benzac W Wash at controlled room temperature (59°–86°F). Store Benzac® below 75°F.

CAUTION
Federal law prohibits dispensing without prescription.
Marketed by:
GALDERMA
LABORATORIES, INC. Fort Worth, Texas 76133
Mfd. by: DPT Laboratories, Inc.
San Antonio, Texas 78215
GALDERMA is a registered trademark.

CETAPHIL®   OTC
Gentle Skin Cleanser—Soap Substitute

COMPOSITION
Contains water, cetyl alcohol, propylene glycol, sodium lauryl sulfate, stearyl alcohol, methylparaben, propylparaben and butylparaben.

ACTION AND USES
CETAPHIL® Cleanser was formulated for dermatologists as a gentle, non-irritating cleanser for sensitive skin. **CETAPHIL** is completely non-alkaline, non-comedogenic fragrance free, and mild enough for all skin types. **CETAPHIL** soothes and softens as it cleanses, helping the skin retain needed moisture. **CETAPHIL** is also an excellent cleanser for the delicate skin of babies.

ADMINISTRATION AND DOSAGE
CETAPHIL can be used with or without water.
Without water: Apply a liberal amount to the skin and rub gently. The unique, low lathering formula allows gentle, yet thorough cleansing. Remove excess with a soft cloth, leaving a thin film of **CETAPHIL** on the skin. The emollient quality will leave the skin soft and moist.
With water: Apply to the skin and rub gently. Rinse.

HOW SUPPLIED
CETAPHIL® Cleanser 4 fl. oz. (UPC 0299-3921-40)
CETAPHIL® Cleanser 8 fl. oz. (UPC 0299-3921-08);
CETAPHIL® Cleanser 16 fl. oz. (UPC 0299-3921-16).

CETAPHIL®   OTC
Gentle Cleansing Bar

COMPOSITION
Contains sodium cocoyl isethionate, stearic acid, sodium tallowate, water, sodium stearate, sodium dodecylbenzene sulfonate, sodium cocoate, PEG-20, sodium chloride, masking fragrance, sodium isethionate, petrolatum, sodium isostearoyl lactylate, sucrose laurate, titanium dioxide, pentasodium pentetate, tetrasodium etidronate. May also contain sodium palm kernelate.

ACTION AND USES
Cetaphil® gentle cleansing bar's non-soap formulation is designed for cleansing dry, sensitive skin.

ADMINISTRATION AND DOSAGE
Cetaphil gentle cleansing bar is ideal for bath or shower.
Cetaphil gentle cleansing bar is non-comedogenic and contains no harsh detergents that might dry or irritate the skin.

HOW SUPPLIED
Cetaphil® gentle cleansing bar net wt. 4.5 oz. (UPC 0299-3923-04)

CETAPHIL®   OTC
[cē'-ta-phil]
Moisturizing Cream

COMPOSTION
Contains purified water, polyglycerylmethacrylate (and) propylene glycol, petrolatum, dicaprylyl ether, PEG-5 glyceryl stearate, glycerin, dimethicone (and) dimethiconol, cetyl alcohol, sweet almond oil, acrylates/C10–30 alkyl acrylate crosspolymer, tocopheryl acetate, phenoxyethanol, benzyl alcohol, disodium EDTA, sodium hydroxide, lactic acid.

ACTION AND USES
CETAPHIL® Moisturizing Cream was formulated specifically for chronic dry, sensitive skin. Contains a superior system of extra-strength emollients and humectants, clinically proven to bind water to skin and prevent moisture loss. Provides long-lasting relief to even severe dry skin. Free of lanolins, parabens and fragrances that can irritate sensitive skin. Non-comedogenic.

ADMINISTRATION AND DOSAGE
Apply liberally as often as needed, or as directed by physician.

HOW SUPPLIED
CETAPHIL® Moisturizing Cream 16 oz. (UPC 0299-3917-16)
CETAPHIL® Moisturizing Cream 3 oz. tube (UPC 0299-3917-02)

CETAPHIL®   OTC
[cē'-ta-phil]
Moisturizing Lotion

COMPOSITION
Contains purified water, glycerin, hydrogenated polyisobutene, cetearyl alcohol (and) ceteareth-20, macadamia nut oil, dimethicone, tocopheryl acetate, stearoxytrimethylsilane (and) stearyl alcohol. panthenol, farnesol, benzyl alcohol, phenoxyethanol, acrylates/C10–30 alkyl acrylate crosspolymer, sodium hydroxide, citric acid.

ACTION AND USES
CETAPHIL® Moisturizing Lotion was formulated specifically for chronic dry, sensitive skin.
Contains a superior system of extra-strength emollients and humectants, clinically proven to bind water to the skin and prevent moisture loss. Provides long-lasting relief to even severe dry skin. Free of lanolins, parabens and fragrances that can irritate sensitive skin. Non-comedogenic.

ADMINISTRATION AND DOSAGE
Apply daily to dry skin as needed or as directed by physician

HOW SUPPLIED
CETAPHIL® Moisturizing Lotion 16 fl oz (UPC 0299-3918-16)

DESOWEN®   ℞
(desonide cream, ointment
and lotion)
cream 0.05%
ointment 0.05%
and lotion 0.05%

For Dermatologic Use Only–
Not for Ophthalmic Use–

DESCRIPTION
DesOwen® Cream 0.05%, Ointment 0.05%, and Lotion 0.05% contain desonide (Pregna-1,4-diene-3,20-dione,11, 21-dihydroxy-16,17-[(1-methylethylidene)bis(oxy)]-,(11β, 16α-) a synthetic nonfluorinated corticosteroid for topical dermatologic use. The corticosteroids constitute a class of primarily synthetic steroids used topically as anti-inflammatory and anti-pruritic agents.
Chemically, desonide is $C_{24}H_{32}O_6$. It has the following structural formula:

Desonide has the molecular weight of 416.51. It is a white to off white odorless powder which is soluble in methanol and practically insoluble in water.
Each gram of **DesOwen** Cream contains 0.5 mg of desonide in a base of purified water, emulsifying wax, propylene glycol, stearic acid, isopropyl palmitate, synthetic beeswax, polysorbate 60, potassium sorbate, sorbic acid, propyl gallate, citric acid, and sodium hydroxide.
Each gram of **DesOwen** Ointment contains 0.5 mg of desonide in a base of mineral oil and polyethylene.
Each gram of **DesOwen** Lotion contains 0.5 mg of desonide in a base of sodium lauryl sulfate, light mineral oil, cetyl alcohol, stearyl alcohol, propylene glycol, methylparaben, propylparaben, sorbitan monostearate, glyceryl stearate SE,

edetate sodium and purified water. May contain citric acid and/or sodium hydroxide for pH adjustment.

CLINICAL PHARMACOLOGY

Like other topical corticosteroids, desonide has anti-inflammatory, antipruritic and vasoconstrictive properties. The mechanism of the anti-inflammatory activity of the topical steroids, in general, is unclear. However corticosteroids are thought to act by the induction of phospholipase A_2 inhibitory proteins, collectively called lipocortins. It is postulated that these proteins control the biosynthesis of potent mediators of inflammation such as prostaglandins and leukotrienes by inhibiting the release of their common precursor arachidonic acid. Arachidonic acid is released from membrane phospholipids by phospholipase A_2.

Pharmacokinetics: The extent of percutaneous absorption of topical corticosteroids is determined by many factors including the vehicle and the integrity of the epidermal barrier. Occulsive dressings with hydrocortisone for up to 24 hours have not been demonstrated to increase penetration; however, occlusion of hydrocortisone for 96 hours markedly enhances penetration. Topical corticosteroids can be absorbed from normal intact skin. Inflammation and/or other disease processes in the skin may increase percutaneous absorption.

Studies performed with **DesOwen** (desonide cream, ointment and lotion) Cream, Ointment, and Lotion indicate that they are in the low to medium range of potency as compared with other topical corticosteroids.

INDICATION AND USAGE

DesOwen Cream, Ointment and Lotion are low to medium potency corticosteroids indicated for the relief of the inflammatory and pruritic manifestations of corticosteroid responsive dermatoses.

CONTRAINDICATIONS

DesOwen Cream, Ointment and Lotion are contraindicated in those patients with a history of hypersensitivity to any of the components of the preparations.

PRECAUTIONS

General: Systemic absorption of topical corticosteroids can produce reversible hypothalamic-pituitary-adrenal (HPA) axis suppression with the potential for glucocorticosteroid insufficiency after withdrawal of treatment. Manifestations of Cushing's syndrome, hyperglycemia, and glucosuria can also be produced in some patients by systemic absorption of topical corticosteroids while on treatment.

Patients applying a topical steroid to a large surface area or to areas under occlusion should be evaluated periodically for evidence of HPA axis suppression. This may be done by using the ACTH stimulation, A.M. plasma cortisol, and urinary free cortisol tests. Patients receiving superpotent corticosteroids should not be treated for more than 2 weeks at a time and only small areas should be treated at any one time due to the increased risk of HPA axis suppression.

If HPA axis suppression is noted, an attempt should be made to withdraw the drug, to reduce the frequency of application, or to substitute a less potent corticosteroid. Recovery of HPA axis function is generally prompt and complete upon discontinuation of topical corticosteroids. Infrequently, signs and symptoms of glucocorticosteroid insufficiency may occur requiring supplemental systemic corticosteroids. For information on systemic supplementation, see prescribing information for those products.

Pediatric patients may be more susceptible to systemic toxicity from equivalent doses due to their larger skin surface to body mass ratios. (See PRECAUTIONS—Pediatric use).

If irritation develops, **DesOwen** Cream, Ointment or Lotion should be discontinued and appropriate therapy instituted. Allergic contact dermatitis with corticosteroids is usually diagnosed by observing *failure to heal* rather than noting a clinical exacerbation as with most topical products not containing corticosteroids. Such an observation should be corroborated with appropriate diagnostic patch testing.

If concomitant skin infections are present or develop, an appropriate antifungal or antibacterial agent should be used. If a favorable response does not occur promptly, use of **DesOwen** (desonide cream, ointment and lotion) Cream, Ointment or Lotion should be discontinued until the infection has been adequately controlled.

Information for patients: Patients using topical corticosteroids should receive the following information and instructions:

1. This medication is to be used as directed by the physician. It is for external use only. Avoid contact with the eyes.
2. This medication should not be used for any disorder other than that for which it was prescribed.
3. The treated skin area should not be bandaged or otherwise covered or wrapped so as to be occlusive unless directed by the physician.
4. Patients should report to their physician any signs of local adverse reactions.

Laboratory tests: The following tests may be helpful in evaluating patients for HPA axis suppression:

ACTH stimulation test
A.M. plasma cortisol test
Urinary free cortisol test

Carcinogenesis, mutagenesis, and impairment of fertility: Long-term animal studies have not been performed to evaluate the carcinogenic potential or the effect on reproduction with the use of **DesOwen** Cream, Ointment, and Lotion.

Pregnancy: *Teratogenic effects: Pregnancy category C:* Corticosteroids have been shown to be teratogenic in laboratory animals when administered systemically at relatively low dosage levels. Some corticosteroids have been shown to be teratogenic after dermal application in laboratory animals. Animal repoduction studies have not been conducted with **DesOwen** Cream, Ointment or Lotion. It is also not known whether **DesOwen** Cream, Ointment or Lotion can cause fetal harm when administered to a pregnant woman or can affect reproduction capacity. **DesOwen** Cream, Ointment and Lotion should be given to a pregnant woman only if clearly needed.

Nursing mothers: Systemically administered corticosteroids appear in human milk and could suppress growth, interfere with endogenous corticosteroid production, or cause other untoward effects. It is not known whether topical administration of corticosteroids could result in sufficient systemic absorption to produce detectable quantities in human milk. Because many drugs are excreted in human milk, caution should be exercised when **DesOwen** Cream, Ointment or Lotion is administered to a nursing woman.

Pediatric use: Safety and effectiveness in pediatric patients have not been established. Because of a higher ratio of skin surface area to body mass, pediatric patients are at a greater risk than adults of HPA axis suppression when they are treated with topical corticosteroids. They are therefore also at greater risk of glucocorticosteroid insufficiency after withdrawal of treatment and of Cushing's syndrome while on treatment. Adverse effects including striae have been reported with inappropriate use of topical corticosteroids in infants and children.

HPA axis suppression, Cushing's syndrome, linear growth retardation, delayed weight gain and intracranial hypertension have been reported in children receiving topical corticosteroids. Manifestations of adrenal suppression in children include low plasma cortisol levels, and absence of response to ACTH stimulation. Manifestations of intracranial hypertension include bulging fontanelles, headaches, and bilateral papilledema.

ADVERSE REACTIONS

In controlled clinical trials, the total incidence of adverse reactions associated with the use of desonide was approximately 8%. These were: stinging and burning approximately 3%, irritation, contact dermatitis, condition worsened, peeling of skin, itching, intense transient erythema, and dryness/scaliness, each less than 2%.

The following additional local adverse reactions have been reported infrequently with other topical corticosteroids, and they may occur more frequently with the use of occlusive dressings, especially with higher potency corticosteroids. These reactions are listed in an approximate decreasing order of occurrence: folliculitis, acneiform eruptions, hypopigmentation, perioral dermatitis, secondary infection, skin atrophy, striae, and miliaria.

OVERDOSAGE

Topically applied **DesOwen** (desonide cream, ointment, and lotion) Cream, Ointment and Lotion can be absorbed in sufficient amounts to produce systemic effects (See PRECAUTIONS).

DOSAGE AND ADMINISTRATION

DesOwen Cream, Ointment or Lotion should be applied to the affected areas as a thin film two or three times daily depending on the severity of the condition. SHAKE LOTION WELL BEFORE USING.

As with other corticosteroids, therapy should be discontinued when control is achieved. If no improvement is seen within 2 weeks, reassessment of diagnosis may be necessary. **DesOwen** Cream, Ointment and Lotion should not be used with occlusive dressings.

HOW SUPPLIED

DesOwen (desonide cream) Cream 0.05% is supplied in tubes containing:

15 g **NDC** 0299-5770-15
60 g **NDC** 0299-5770-60
90 g **NDC** 0299-5770-90

DesOwen (desonide ointment) Ointment 0.05% is supplied in tubes containing:

15 g **NDC** 0299-5775-15
60 g **NDC** 0299-5775-60

DesOwen (desonide lotion) Lotion 0.05% is supplied in bottles containing:

2 fl oz **NDC** 0299-5765-02
4 fl oz **NDC** 0299-5765-04

Storage Conditions: Store between 2° and 30°C (36° and 86°F).

CAUTION: Federal law prohibits dispensing without prescription.

Marketed by:
Galderma Laboratories, Inc.
Fort Worth, Texas 76133, USA
Mfd. by: DPT Laboratories, Inc.
San Antonio, Texas 78215, USA
GALDERMA is a registered trademark.
225025-0395 Revised: March 1995

DIFFERIN™ ℞

(adapalene gel)
Gel, 0.1%

DESCRIPTION

DIFFERIN™ Gel, containing adapalene, is used for the topical treatment of acne vulgaris. Each gram of DIFFERIN Gel contains adapalene 0.1% (1mg) in a vehicle consisting of propylene glycol, carbomer 940, poloxamer 182, edetate disodium, methylparaben, sodium hydroxide, and purified water. May contain hydrochloric acid to adjust pH.

The chemical name of adapalene is 6-[3-(1-adamantyl)-4-methoxyphenyl]-2-naphthoic acid. Adapalene is a white to off-white powder which is soluble in tetrahydrofuran, sparingly soluble in ethanol, and practically insoluble in water. The molecular formula is $C_{28}H_{28}O_3$ and molecular weight is 412.52. Adapalene is represented by the following structural formula:

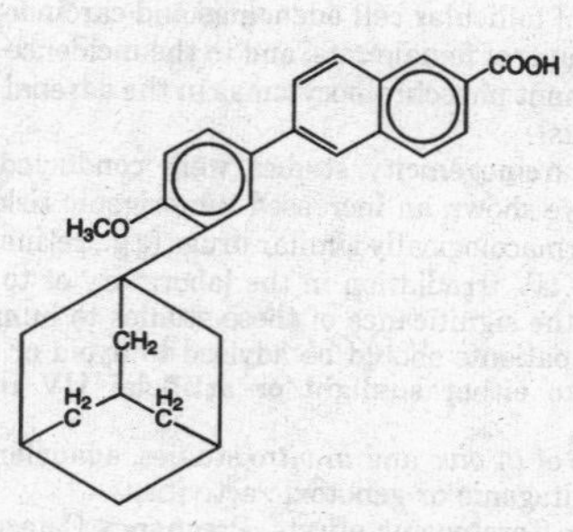

CLINICAL PHARMACOLOGY

Adapalene is a chemically stable, retinoid-like compound. Biochemical and pharmacological profile studies have demonstrated that adapalene is a modulator of cellular differentiation, keratinization, and inflammatory processes all of which represent important features in the pathology of acne vulgaris.

Mechanistically, adapalene binds to specific retinoic acid nuclear receptors but does not bind to the cytosolic receptor protein. Although the exact mode of action of adapalene is unknown, it is suggested that topical adapalene may normalize the differentiation of follicular epithelial cells resulting in decreased microcomedone formation.

Pharmacokinetics: Absorption of adapalene through human skin is low. Only trace amounts (<0.25 ng/mL) of parent substance have been found in the plasma of acne patients following chronic topical application of adapalene in controlled clinical trials. Excretion appears to be primarily by the biliary route.

INDICATIONS AND USAGE

DIFFERIN Gel is indicated for the topical treatment of acne vulgaris.

CONTRAINDICATIONS

DIFFERIN Gel should not be administered to individuals who are hypersensitive to adapalene or any of the components in the vehicle gel.

WARNINGS

Use of DIFFERIN Gel should be discontinued if hypersensitivity to any of the ingredients is noted. Patients with sunburn should be advised not to use the product until fully recovered.

PRECAUTIONS

General: If a reaction suggesting sensitivity or chemical irritation occurs, use of the medication should be discontinued. Exposure to sunlight, including sunlamps, should be minimized during the use of adapalene. Patients who normally experience high levels of sun exposure, and those with inherent sensitivity to sun, should be warned to exercise caution. Use of sunscreen products and protective clothing over treated areas is recommended when exposure cannot be avoided. Weather extremes, such as wind or cold, also may be irritating to patients under treatment with adapalene.

Continued on next page

Galderma Laboratories—Cont.

Avoid contact with the eyes, lips, angles of the nose, and mucous membranes. The product should not be applied to cuts, abrasions, eczematous skin, or sunburned skin.
Certain cutaneous signs and symptoms such as erythema, dryness, scaling, burning, or pruritus may be experienced during treatment. These are most likely to occur during the first two to four weeks and will usually lessen with continued use of the medication. Depending upon the severity of adverse events, patients should be instructed to reduce the frequency of application or discontinue use.
Drug Interactions: As DIFFERIN Gel has the potential to produce local irritation in some patients, concomitant use of other potentially irritating topical products (medicated or abrasive soaps and cleansers, soaps and cosmetics that have a strong drying effect, and products with high concentrations of alcohol, astringents, spices, or lime) should be approached with caution. Particular caution should be exercised in using preparations containing sulfur, resorcinol, or salicylic acid in combination with DIFFERIN Gel. If these preparations have been used, it is advisable not to start therapy with DIFFERIN Gel until the effects of such preparations in the skin have subsided.
Carcinogenesis, Mutagenesis, Impairment of Fertility: Carcinogenicity studies with adapalene have been conducted in mice at topical doses of 0.3, 0.9, and 2.6 mg/kg/day and in rats at oral doses of 0.15, 0.5, and 1.5 mg/kg/day, approximately 4–75 times the maximal daily human topical dose. In the oral study, positive linear trends were observed in the incidence of follicular cell adenomas and carcinomas in the thyroid glands of female rats, and in the incidence of benign and malignant pheochromocytomas in the adrenal medullas of male rats.
No photocarcinogenicity studies were conducted. Animal studies have shown an increased tumorigenic risk with the use of pharmacologically similar drugs (e.g., retinoids) when exposed to UV irradiation in the laboratory or to sunlight. Although the significance of these studies to human use is not clear, patients should be advised to avoid or minimize exposure to either sunlight or artificial UV irradiation sources.
In a series of *in vivo* and *in vitro* studies, adapalene did not exhibit mutagenic or genotoxic activities.
Pregnancy: Teratogenic effects. Pregnancy Category C. No teratogenic effects were seen in rats at oral doses of adapalene 0.15 to 5.0 mg/kg/day, up to 120 times the maximal daily human topical dose. Cutaneous route teratology studies conducted in rats and rabbits at doses of 0.6, 2.0, and 6.0 mg/kg/day, up to 150 times the maximal daily human topical dose exhibited no fetotoxicity and only minimal increases in supernumerary ribs in rats. There are no adequate and well-controlled studies in pregnant women. Adapalene should be used during pregnancy only if the potential benefit justifies the potential risk to the fetus.
Nursing Mothers: It is not known whether this drug is excreted in human milk. Because many drugs are excreted in human milk, caution should be exercised when DIFFERIN Gel is administered to a nursing woman.
Pediatric Use: Safety and effectiveness in pediatric patients below the age of 12 have not been established.

ADVERSE REACTIONS

Some adverse effects such as erythema, scaling, dryness, pruritus, and burning will occur in 10–40% of patients. Pruritus or burning immediately after application also occurs in approximately 20% of patients. The following additional adverse experiences were reported in approximately 1% or less of patients: skin irritation, burning/stinging, erythema, sunburn, and acne flares. These are most commonly seen during the first month of therapy and decrease in frequency and severity thereafter. All adverse effects with use of DIFFERIN Gel during clinical trials were reversible upon discontinuation of therapy.

OVERDOSAGE

DIFFERIN Gel is intended for cutaneous use only. If the medication is applied excessively, no more rapid or better results will be obtained and marked redness, peeling, or discomfort may occur. The acute oral toxicity of DIFFERIN Gel in mice and rats is greater than 10 mL/kg. Chronic ingestion of the drug may lead to the same side effects as those associated with excessive oral intake of Vitamin A.

DOSAGE AND ADMINISTRATION

DIFFERIN Gel should be applied once a day to affected areas after washing in the evening before retiring. A thin film of the gel should be applied, avoiding eyes, lips, and mucous membranes.
During the early weeks of therapy, an apparent exacerbation of acne may occur. This is due to the action of the medication on previously unseen lesions and should not be considered a reason to discontinue therapy. Therapeutic results should be noticed after eight to twelve weeks of treatment.

HOW SUPPLIED

DIFFERIN (adapalene gel) Gel, 0.1% is supplied in the following sizes:

15 g laminate tube-**NDC** 0299-5910-15
45 g laminate tube-**NDC** 0299-5910-45

Storage: Store at controlled room temperature 20°-25°C (68°-77°F).
CAUTION: Federal law prohibits dispensing without prescription.
Marketed by:
GALDERMA Laboratories, Inc.
Fort Worth, Texas 76133 USA
Mfd. by:
DPT Laboratories, Inc.
San Antonio, Texas 78215 USA
GALDERMA is a registered trademark.
225022-0596
Revised: May 1996

METROCREAM™ ℞

(metronidazole topical cream)
Topical Cream, 0.75%

FOR TOPICAL USE ONLY
(NOT FOR OPHTHALMIC USE)

DESCRIPTION

MetroCream™ Topical cream contains metronidazole, USP, at a concentration of 7.5 mg per gram (0.75%) in an emollient cream consisting of emulsifying wax, sorbitol solution, glycerin, isopropyl palmitate, benzyl alcohol, lactic acid and/or sodium hydroxide to adjust pH, and purified water. Metronidazol is a member of the imidazole class of antibacterial agents and is classified therapeutically as an antiprotozoal and antibacterial agent. Chemically, metronidazole is 2-methyl-5-nitro-1*H*-imidazole-1-ethanol. The molecular formula is $C_6H_9N_3O_3$ and molecular weight is 171.16. Metronidazole is represented by the following structural formula:

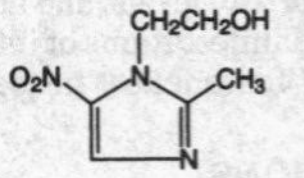
CH2CH2OH
O2N
N
CH3
N

CLINICAL PHARMACOLOGY

The mechanisms by which metronidazole acts in the treatment of rosacea are unknown, but appear to include an anti-inflammatory effect.

INDICATIONS AND USAGE

METROCREAM (metronidazole topical cream) Topical Cream is indicated for topical application in the treatment of inflammatory papules and pustules of rosacea.

CONTRAINDICATIONS

METROCREAM™ (metronidazole topical cream) Topical Cream is contraindicated in individuals with a history of hypersensitivity to metronidazole, or other ingredients of the formulation.

PRECAUTIONS

General: Topical metronidazole has been reported to cause tearing of the eyes. Therefore, contact with the eyes should be avoided. If a reaction suggesting local irritation occurs, patients should be directed to use the medication less frequently or discontinue use. Metronidazole is a nitroimidazole and should be used with care in patients with evidence of, or history of blood dyscrasia.
Information for patients: This medication is to be used as directed by the physician. It is for external use only. Avoid contact with the eyes.
Drug Interactions: Oral metronidazole has been reported to potentiate the anticoagulant effect of warfarin and coumarin anticoagulants, resulting in a prolongation of prothrombin time. The effect of topical metronidazole on prothrombin time is not known.
Carcinogenesis, mutagenesis, impairment of fertility: Metronidazole has shown evidence of carcinogenic activity in a number of studies involving chronic, oral administration in mice and rats but not in studies involving hamsters.
Metronidazole has shown evidence of mutagenic activity in several *in vitro* bacterial assay systems. In addition, a dose-response increase in the frequency of micronuclei was observed in mice after intraperitoneal injections and an increase in chromosome aberrations have been reported in patients with Crohn's disease who were treated with 200-1200 mg/day of metronidazole for 1 to 24 months. However, no excess chromosomal abberations in circulating human lymphocytes have been observed in patients treated for 8 months.
Pregnancy: *Teratogenic effects: Pregnancy category B:* There are no adequate and well-controlled studies with the *use of* METROCREAM™ (metronidazole topical cream) Topical Cream in pregnant women. Metronidazole crosses the placental barrier and enters the fetal circulation rapidly. No fetotoxicity was observed after oral metronidazole in rats or mice. However, because animal reproduction studies are not always predictive of human response and since oral metronidazole has been shown to be a carcinogen in some rodents, this drug should be used during pregnancy only if clearly needed.
Nursing Mothers: After oral administration, metronidazole is secreted in breast milk in concentrations similar to those found in the plasma. Even though blood levels are significantly lower with topically applied metronidazole than those achieved after oral administration of metronidazole, a decision should be made whether to discontinue nursing or to discontinue the drug, taking into account the importance of the drug to the mother.
Pediatric Use: Safety and effectiveness in pediatric patients have not been established.

ADVERSE REACTIONS

In controlled clinical trials, the total incidence of adverse reactions associated with the use of METROCREAM Topical Cream was approximately 10%. Skin discomfort (burning and stinging) was the most frequently reported event followed by erythema, skin irritation, pruritus and worsening of rosacea. All individual events occurred in less than 3% of patients.
The following additional adverse experiences have been reported with the topical use of metronidazole: dryness, transient redness, metallic taste, tingling or numbness of extremities and nausea.

DOSAGE AND ADMINISTRATION

Apply and rub in a thin layer of METROCREAM™ (metronidazole topical cream) Topical Cream twice daily, morning and evening, to entire affected areas after washing.
Areas to be treated should be washed with a mild cleanser before application. Patients may use cosmetics after application of METROCREAM Topical Cream.

HOW SUPPLIED

METROCREAM (metronidazole topical cream) Topical Cream, 0.75% is supplied in a 45 g aluminum tube–**NDC** 0299-3836-45.
Storage conditions: STORE AT CONTROLLED ROOM TEMPERATURE: 59° to 86°F (15° to 30°C).
Caution: Federal law prohibits dispensing without prescription.
Marketed by:
GALDERMA Laboratories, Inc.
Fort Worth, Texas 76133 USA
Manufactured by:
DPT Laboratories, Inc.
San Antonio, Texas 78215 USA
GALDERMA is a registered trademark.
225029-0695
Revised: June 1995

METROGEL® ℞

(metronidazole topical gel)
Topical Gel, 0.75%
FOR TOPICAL USE ONLY
(NOT FOR OPHTHALMIC USE)

DESCRIPTION

METROGEL® Topical Gel contains metronidazole, USP, at a concentration of 7.5 mg per gram (0.75%) in a gel consisting of purified water, methylparaben, propylparaben, propylene glycol, carbomer 940, sodium hydroxide, and edetate disodium. Metronidazole is classified therapeutically as an antiprotozoal and antibacterial agent. Chemically, metronidazole is named 2-methyl-5-nitro-1*H*-imidazole-1-ethanol and has the following structure:

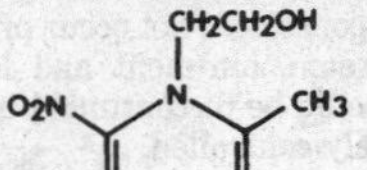
CH2CH2OH
O2N
N
CH3
N

CLINICAL PHARMACOLOGY

Bioavailability studies on the topical administration of 1 gram of METROGEL Topical Gel (7.5 mg of metronidazole) to the face of 10 rosacea patients showed a maximum serum concentration of 66 nanograms per milliliter in one patient. This concentration is approximately 100 times less than concentrations afforded by a single 250 mg oral tablet. The serum metronidazole concentrations were below the detectable limits of the assay at the majority of time points in all patients. Three of the patients had no detectable serum concentrations of metronidazole at any time point. The mean

dose of gel applied during clinical studies was 600 mg which represents 4.5 mg of metronidazole per application. Therefore, under normal usage levels, the formulation affords minimal serum concentrations of metronidazole. The mechanisms by which METROGEL (metronidazole topical gel) Topical Gel acts in the treatment of rosacea are unknown, but appear to include an anti-inflammatory effect.

INDICATIONS AND USAGE

METROGEL Topical Gel is indicated for topical application in the treatment of inflammatory papules and pustules of rosacea.

CONTRAINDICATIONS

METROGEL Topical Gel is contraindicated in individuals with a history of hypersensitivity to metronidazole, parabens, or other ingredients of the formulation.

PRECAUTIONS

General: METROGEL Topical Gel has been reported to cause tearing of the eyes. Therefore, contact with the eyes should be avoided. If a reaction suggesting local irritation occurs, patients should be directed to use the medication less frequently or discontinue use. Metronidazole is a nitroimidazole and should be used with care in patients with evidence of, or history of blood dyscrasia.

Information for patients: This medication is to be used as directed by the physician. It is for external use only. Avoid contact with the eyes.

Drug Interactions: Oral metronidazole has been reported to potentiate the anticoagulant effect of coumarin and warfarin resulting in a prolongation of prothrombin time. The effect of topical metronidazole on prothrombin time is not known.

Carcinogenesis, mutagenesis, impairment of fertility: Metronidazole has shown evidence of carcinogenic activity in a number of studies involving chronic, oral administration in mice and rats but not in studies involving hamsters.

Metronidazole has shown evidence of mutagenic activity in several *in vitro* bacterial assay systems. In addition, a dose-response increase in the frequency of micronuclei was observed in mice after intraperitoneal injections and an increase in chromosome aberrations have been reported in patients with Crohn's disease who were treated with 200–1200 mg/day of metronidazole for 1 to 24 months. However, no excess chromosomal aberrations in circulating human lymphocytes have been observed in patients treated for 8 months.

Pregnancy: *Teratogenic effects: Pregnancy category B:* There has been no experience to date with the use of METROGEL (metronidazole topical gel) Topical Gel in pregnant patients. Metronidazole crosses the placental barrier and enters the fetal circulation rapidly. No fetotoxicity was observed after oral metronidazole in rats or mice. However, because animal reproduction studies are not always predictive of human response and since oral metronidazole has been shown to be a carcinogen in some rodents, this drug should be used during pregnancy only if clearly needed.

Nursing mothers: After oral administration, metronidazole is secreted in breast milk in concentrations similar to those found in the plasma. Even though METROGEL Topical Gel blood levels are significantly lower than those achieved after oral metronidazole, a decision should be made whether to discontinue nursing or to discontinue the drug, taking into account the importance of the drug to the mother.

Pediatric use: Safety and effectiveness in pediatric patients have not been established.

ADVERSE REACTIONS

The following adverse experiences have been reported with the topical use of metronidazole: burning, skin irritation, dryness, transient redness, metallic taste, tingling or numbness of extremities and nausea.

DOSAGE AND ADMINISTRATION

Apply and rub in a thin film of METROGEL Topical Gel twice daily, morning and evening, to entire affected areas after washing.

Areas to be treated should be cleansed before application of METROGEL (metronidazole topical gel) Topical Gel. Patients may use cosmetics after application of METROGEL Topical Gel.

HOW SUPPLIED

METROGEL (metronidazole topical gel) Topical Gel is supplied in a 1 oz. (28.4 g) aluminum tube—**NDC** 0299-3835-28 and a 45 g aluminum tube—**NDC** 0299-3835-45.

Storage conditions: STORE AT CONTROLLED ROOM TEMPERATURE: 59° to 86°F (15° to 30°C).

Caution: Federal law prohibits dispensing without prescription.

GALDERMA

Marketed by:

GALDERMA Laboratories, Inc., Fort Worth, Texas 76133 USA

Manufactured by: DPT Laboratories, Inc.

San Antonio, Texas 78215 USA

GALDERMA is a registered trademark.

225032-0695

Revised: August 1995

GATE Pharmaceuticals

division of Teva Pharmaceuticals USA
650 CATHILL ROAD
SELLERSVILLE, PA 18960

Direct Inquiries to:
650 Cathill Road
Sellersville, PA 18960
(800) 292–4283

ADIPEX-P®   Ⓒ ℞

[ă 'dĭ-pĕx]

(Phentermine Hydrochloride USP, 37.5 mg)

DESCRIPTION

Phentermine hydrochloride USP has the chemical name of α, α-dimethylphenethylamine hydrochloride. The structural formula is as follows:

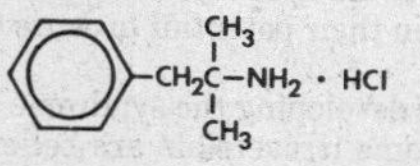

$C_{10}H_{15}N \cdot HCl$ M.W. 185.7

Phentermine hydrochloride is a white, odorless, hygroscopic, crystalline powder which is soluble in water and lower alcohols, slightly soluble in chloroform and insoluble in ether.

ADIPEX-P, an anorectic agent for oral administration, is available as a capsule or tablet containing 37.5 mg of phentermine hydrochloride (equivalent to 30 mg of phentermine base).

ADIPEX-P Capsules contain the inactive ingredients Corn Starch, Gelatin, Lactose, Magnesium Stearate, Titanium Dioxide, FD & C Blue #1 and FD & C Red #3.

ADIPEX-P Tablets contain the inactive ingredients Acacia, Confectioner's Sugar, Corn Starch, Lactose, Magnesium Stearate, Pregelatinized Starch, Stearic Acid, and FD & C Blue #1.

CLINICAL PHARMACOLOGY

Phentermine hydrochloride is a sympathomimetic amine with pharmacologic activity similar to the prototype drugs of this class used in obesity, the amphetamines. Actions include central nervous system stimulation and elevation of blood pressure. Tachyphylaxis and tolerance have been demonstrated with all drugs of this class in which these phenomena have been looked for.

Drugs of this class used in obesity are commonly known as "anorectics" or "anorexigenics". It has not been established, however, that the action of such drugs in treating obesity is primarily one of appetite suppression. Other central nervous system actions, or metabolic effects may be involved, for example.

Adult obese subjects instructed in dietary management and treated with "anorectic" drugs, lose more weight on the average than those treated with placebo and diet, as determined in relatively short-term clinical trials.

The magnitude of increased weight loss of drug-treated patients over placebo-treated patients is only a fraction of a pound a week. The rate of weight loss is greatest in the first weeks of therapy for both drug and placebo subjects and tends to decrease in succeeding weeks. The possible origins of the increased weight loss due to the various drug effects are not established. The amount of weight loss associated with the use of "anorectic" drugs varies from trial to trial, and the increased weight loss appears to be related in part to variables other than the drug prescribed, such as the physician-investigator, the population treated, and the diet prescribed. Studies do not permit conclusions as to the relative importance of the drug and non-drug factors on weight loss.

The natural history of obesity is measured in years, whereas the studies cited are restricted to a few weeks duration; thus, the total impact of drug-induced weight loss over that of diet alone must be considered clinically limited.

INDICATIONS AND USAGE

Adipex-P® (phentermine hydrochloride) is indicated in the management of exogenous obesity as a short term adjunct (a few weeks) in a regimen of weight reduction based on caloric restriction.

The limited usefulness of agents of this class (see CLINICAL PHARMACOLOGY) should be measured against possible risk factors inherent in their use such as those described below.

CONTRAINDICATIONS

Advanced arteriosclerosis, symptomatic cardiovascular disease, moderate to severe hypertension, hyperthyroidism, known hypersensitivity or idiosyncrasy to the sympathomimetic amines, glaucoma.

Agitated states.

Patients with a history of drug abuse.

During or within 14 days following the administration of monoamine oxidase inhibitors (hypertensive crises may result).

WARNINGS

Tolerance to the anorectic effect usually develops within a few weeks. When this occurs, the recommended dose should not be exceeded in an attempt to increase the effect; rather, the drug should be discontinued.

Phentermine hydrochloride may impair the ability of the patient to engage in potentially hazardous activities such as operating machinery or driving a motor vehicle; the patient should therefore be cautioned accordingly.

Usage in Pregnancy: Safe use in pregnancy has not been established. Use of phentermine hydrochloride by women who are or who may become pregnant, and those in the first trimester of pregnancy, requires that the potential benefit be weighed against the possible hazard to mother and infant.

Usage in Children: Phentermine hydrochloride is not recommended for use in children under 12 years of age.

Usage with Alcohol: Concomitant use of alcohol with phentermine hydrochloride may result in an adverse drug interaction.

PRECAUTIONS

Caution is to be exercised in prescribing phentermine hydrochloride for patients with even mild hypertension.

Insulin requirements in diabetes mellitus may be altered in association with the use of phentermine hydrochloride and the concomitant dietary regimen.

Phentermine hydrochloride may decrease the hypotensive effect of guanethidine.

The least amount feasible should be prescribed or dispensed at one time in order to minimize the possibility of overdosage.

ADVERSE REACTIONS

Cardiovascular: Palpitation, tachycardia, elevation of blood pressure.

Central Nervous System: Overstimulation, restlessness, dizziness, insomnia, euphoria, dysphoria, tremor, headache; rarely psychotic episodes at recommended doses.

Gastrointestinal: Dryness of the mouth, unpleasant taste, diarrhea, constipation, other gastrointestinal disturbances.

Allergic: Urticaria.

Endocrine: Impotence, changes in libido.

DRUG ABUSE AND DEPENDENCE

Phentermine hydrochloride is a Schedule IV controlled substance. Phentermine hydrochloride is related chemically and pharmacologically to the amphetamines. Amphetamines and related stimulant drugs have been extensively abused, and the possibility of abuse of phentermine hydrochloride should be kept in mind when evaluating the desirability of including a drug as part of a weight reduction program. Abuse of amphetamines and related drugs may be associated with intense psychological dependence and severe social dysfunction. There are reports of patients who have increased the dosage to many times that recommended. Abrupt cessation following prolonged high dosage administration results in extreme fatigue and mental depression; changes are also noted on the sleep EEG. Manifestations of chronic intoxication with anorectic drugs include severe dermatoses, marked insomnia, irritability, hyperactivity, and personality changes. The most severe manifestation of chronic intoxication is psychosis, often clinically indistinguishable from schizophrenia.

OVERDOSAGE

Manifestations of acute overdosage with phentermine hydrochloride include restlessness, tremor, hyperreflexia, rapid respiration, confusion, assaultiveness, hallucinations, panic states.

Fatigue and depression usually follow the central stimulation.

Cardiovascular effects include arrhythmias, hypertension or hypotension and circulatory collapse. Gastrointestinal symptoms include nausea, vomiting, diarrhea, and abdominal cramps. Fatal poisoning usually terminates in convulsions and coma.

Management of acute phentermine hydrochloride intoxication is largely symptomatic and includes lavage and sedation with a barbiturate. Experience with hemodialysis or peritoneal dialysis is inadequate to permit recommendation in this regard. Acidification of the urine increases phentermine excretion. Intravenous phentolamine has been suggested for possible acute, severe hypertension, if this complicates phentermine hydrochloride overdosage.

DOSAGE AND ADMINISTRATION

Dosage should be individualized to obtain an adequate response with the lowest effective dose.

Continued on next page

Gate—Cont.

The usual adult dose is one capsule or tablet (37.5 mg) daily, administered before breakfast or 1–2 hours after breakfast. For tablets, the dosage may be adjusted to the patient's need. For some patients ½ tablet (18.75 mg) daily may be adequate, while in some cases it may be desirable to give ½ tablet (18.75 mg) two times a day.
Late evening medication should be avoided because of the possibility of resulting insomnia.
Phentermine hydrochloride is NOT recommended for use in children under 12 years of age.

HOW SUPPLIED
Available in tablets and capsules containing 37.5 mg phentermine hydrochloride (equivalent to 30 mg phentermine base). Each blue and white, oblong, scored tablet is debossed with "LEMMON" and "9"-"9". The #3 capsule has an opaque white body and an opaque light blue cap. Each capsule is imprinted with "Adipex-P"-"37.5" on the cap and two blue stripes on the body.
Tablets are packaged in bottles of 100 (NDC 57844-009-01); 400 (NDC 57844-009-26); and 1000 (NDC 57844-009-10).
Capsules are packaged in bottles of 100 (NDC 57844-019-01).
Store at controlled room temperature 15°-30°C (59°-86°F).
CAUTION: Federal law prohibits dispensing without prescription.

Manufactured for:
GATE PHARMACEUTICALS
division of Lemmon Company
Sellersville, PA 18960
Manufactured by:
LEMMON COMPANY
Sellersville, Pa 18960

Rev. C 3/94

Shown in Product Identification Guide, page 311

MOBAN® ℞
[mō'ban]
(molindone hydrochloride)

DESCRIPTION
MOBAN (molindone hydrochloride) is a dihydroindolone compound which is not structurally related to the phenothiazines, the butyrophenones or the thioxanthenes.
MOBAN is 3-ethyl-6, 7-dihydro-2-methyl-5-(morpholinomethyl) indol-4 (5H)-one hydrochloride. It is a white to off-white crystalline powder, freely soluble in water and alcohol and has a molecular weight of 312.67.
MOBAN Tablets also contain:

All strengths: calcium sulfate, lactose, magnesium stearate, microcrystalline cellulose and povidone.
5 mg: alginic acid, colloidal silicon dioxide and FD&C Yellow 6.
10 mg: alginic acid, colloidal silicon dioxide, FD&C Blue 2 and FD&C Red 40.
25 mg: alginic acid, colloidal silicon dioxide, D&C Yellow 10, FD&C Blue 2, and FD&C Yellow 6.
50 mg: FD&C Blue 2 and sodium starch glycolate.
100 mg: FD&C Blue 2, FD&C Yellow 6 and sodium starch glycolate.

MOBAN Concentrate contains: alcohol, artificial cherry flavor, artificial cover flavor, edetate disodium, glycerin, liquid sugar, methylparaben, propylparaben, sodium metabisulfite, sorbitol solution, and hydrochloric acid reagent grade for pH adjustment.

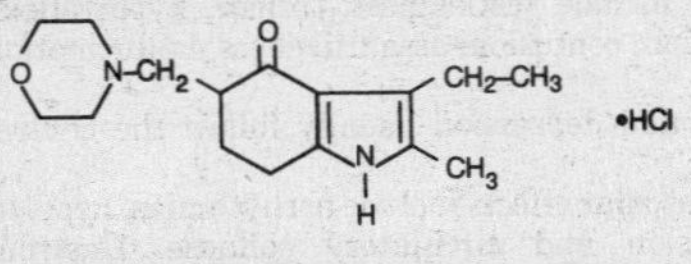

MOLINDONE HYDROCHLORIDE

ACTIONS
MOBAN (molindone hydrochloride) has a pharmacological profile in laboratory animals which predominantly resembles that of major tranquilizers causing reduction of spontaneous locomotion and aggressiveness, suppression of a conditioned response and antagonism of the bizarre stereotyped behavior and hyperactivity induced by amphetamines. In addition, MOBAN antagonizes the depression caused by the tranquilizing agent tetrabenazine.
In human clinical studies tranquilization is achieved in the absence of muscle relaxing or incoordinating effects. Based on EEG studies, MOBAN exerts its effect on the ascending reticular activating system.
Human metabolic studies show MOBAN (molindone hydrochloride) to be rapidly absorbed and metabolized when given orally. Unmetabolized drug reached a peak blood level at 1.5 hours. Pharmacological effect from a single oral dose persists for 24–36 hours. There are 36 recognized metabolites with less than 2–3% unmetabolized MOBAN being excreted in urine and feces.

INDICATIONS
MOBAN is indicated for the management of the manifestations of psychotic disorders. The antipsychotic efficacy of MOBAN was established in clinical studies which enrolled newly hospitalized and chronically hospitalized, acutely ill, schizophrenic patients as subjects.

CONTRAINDICATIONS
MOBAN (molindone hydrochloride) is contraindicated in severe central nervous system depression (alcohol, barbiturates, narcotics, etc.) or comatose states, and in patients with known hypersensitivity to the drug.

WARNINGS
Tardive Dyskinesia
Tardive dyskinesia, a syndrome consisting of potentially irreversible, involuntary, dyskinetic movements may develop in patients treated with neuroleptic (antipsychotic) drugs. Although the prevalence of the syndrome appears to be highest among the elderly, especially elderly women, it is impossible to rely upon prevalence estimates to predict, at the inception of neuroleptic treatment, which patients are likely to develop the syndrome. Whether neuroleptic drug products differ in their potential to cause tardive dyskinesia is unknown.
Both the risk of developing the syndrome and the likelihood that it will become irreversible are believed to increase as the duration of treatment and the total cumulative dose of neuroleptic drugs administered to the patient increase. However, the syndrome can develop, although much less commonly, after relatively brief treatment periods at low doses.
There is no known treatment for established cases of tardive dyskinesia, although the syndrome may remit, partially or completely, if neuroleptic treatment is withdrawn. Neuroleptic treatment, itself, however, may suppress (or partially suppress) the signs and symptoms of the syndrome and thereby may possibly mask the underlying disease process. The effect that symptomatic suppression has upon the long-term course of the syndrome is unknown.
Given these considerations, neuroleptics should be prescribed in a manner that is most likely to minimize the occurrence of tardive dyskinesia. Chronic neuroleptic treatment should generally be reserved for patients who suffer from a chronic illness that, 1) is known to respond to neuroleptic drugs, and 2) for whom alternative, equally effective, but potentially less harmful treatments are not available or appropriate. In patients who do require chronic treatment, the smallest dose and the shortest duration of treatment producing a satisfactory clinical response should be sought. The need for continued treatment should be reassessed periodically.
If signs and symptoms of tardive dyskinesia appear in a patient on neuroleptics, drug discontinuation should be considered. However, some patients may require treatment despite the presence of the syndrome.
(For further information about the description of tardive dyskinesia and its clinical detection, please refer to the section on Adverse Reactions.)
Neuroleptic Malignant Syndrome (NMS)
A potentially fatal symptom complex sometimes referred to as Neuroleptic Malignant Syndrome (NMS) has been reported in association with antipsychotic drugs. Clinical manifestations of NMS are hyperpyrexia, muscle rigidity, altered mental status and evidence of autonomic instability (irregular pulse or blood pressure, tachycardia, diaphoresis, and cardiac dysrhythmias).
The diagnostic evaluation of patients with this syndrome is complicated. In arriving at a diagnosis, it is important to identify cases where the clinical presentation includes both serious medical illness (e.g., pneumonia, systemic infection, etc.) and untreated or inadequately treated extrapyramidal signs and symptoms (EPS). Other important considerations in the differential diagnosis include central anticholinergic toxicity, heat stroke, drug fever and primary central nervous system (CNS) pathology.
The management of NMS should include, 1) immediate discontinuation of antipsychotic drugs and other drugs not essential to concurrent therapy, 2) intensive symptomatic treatment and medical monitoring, and 3) treatment of any concomitant serious medical problems for which specific treatments are available. There is no general agreement about specific pharmacological treatment regimens for uncomplicated NMS.
If a patient requires antipsychotic drug treatment after recovery from NMS, the potential reintroduction of drug therapy should be carefully considered. The patient should be carefully monitored, since recurrences of NMS have been reported.
Usage in Pregnancy: Studies in pregnant patients have not been carried out. Reproduction studies have been performed in the following animals:

Pregnant Rats oral dose—	
no adverse effect	20 mg/kg/day—10 days
no adverse effect	40 mg/kg/day—10 days
Pregnant Mice oral dose—	
slight increase resorptions	20 mg/kg/day—10 days
slight increase resorptions	40 mg/kg/day—10 days
Pregnant Rabbits oral dose—	
no adverse effect	5 mg/kg/day—12 days
no adverse effect	10 mg/kg/day—12 days
no adverse effect	20 mg/kg/day—12 days

Animal reproductive studies have not demonstrated a teratogenic potential. The anticipated benefits must be weighed against the unknown risks to the fetus if used in pregnant patients.
Nursing Mothers: Data are not available on the content of MOBAN (molindone hydrochloride) in the milk of nursing mothers.
Pediatric use: Use of MOBAN (molindone hydrochloride) in pediatric patients below the age of twelve years is not recommended because safe and effective conditions for its usage have not been established.
MOBAN has not been shown effective in the management of behavioral complications in patients with mental retardation.
Sulfites Sensitivity: MOBAN Concentrate contains sodium metabisulfite, a sulfite that may cause allergic-type reactions including anaphylactic symptoms and life-threatening or less severe asthmatic episodes in certain susceptible people. The overall prevalence of sulfite sensitivity in the general population is unknown and probably low. Sulfite sensitivity is seen more frequently in asthmatic than in nonasthmatic people.

PRECAUTIONS
Some patients receiving MOBAN (molindone hydrochloride) may note drowsiness initially and they should be advised against activities requiring mental alertness until their response to the drug has been established.
Increased activity has been noted in patients receiving MOBAN. Caution should be exercised where increased activity may be harmful.
MOBAN does not lower the seizure threshold in experimental animals to the degree noted with more sedating antipsychotic drugs. However, in humans convulsive seizures have been reported in a few instances.
The physician should be aware that this tablet preparation contains calcium sulfate as an excipient and that calcium ions may interfere with the absorption of preparations containing phenytoin sodium and tetracyclines.
MOBAN has an antiemetic effect in animals. A similar effect may occur in humans and may obscure signs of intestinal obstruction or brain tumor.
Neuroleptic drugs elevate prolactin levels; the elevation persists during chronic administration. Tissue culture experiments indicate that approximately one-third of human breast cancers are prolactin dependent in vitro, a factor of potential importance if the prescription of these drugs is contemplated in a patient with a previously detected breast cancer. Although disturbances such as galactorrhea, amenorrhea, gynecomastia, and impotence have been reported, the clinical significance of elevated serum prolactin levels is unknown for most patients. An increase in mammary neoplasms has been found in rodents after chronic administration of neuroleptic drugs. Neither clinical studies nor epidemiologic studies conducted to date, however, have shown an association between chronic administration of these drugs and mammary tumorigenesis; the available evidence is considered too limited to be conclusive at this time.

ADVERSE REACTIONS
CNS EFFECTS
The most frequently occurring effect is initial drowsiness that generally subsides with continued usage of the drug or lowering of the dose.
Noted less frequently were depression, hyperactivity and euphoria.
Neurological
Extrapyramidal Reactions
Extrapyramidal reactions noted below may occur in susceptible individuals and are usually reversible with appropriate management.
Akathisia
Motor restlessness may occur early.
Parkinson Syndrome
Akinesia, characterized by rigidity, immobility and reduction of voluntary movements and tremor, have been observed. Occurrence is less frequent than akathisia.
Dystonic Syndrome
Prolonged abnormal contractions of muscle groups occur infrequently. These symptoms may be managed by the addition of a synthetic antiparkinson agent (other than L-dopa), small doses of sedative drugs, and/or reduction in dosage.
Tardive Dyskinesia
Neuroleptic drugs are known to cause a syndrome of dyskinetic movements commonly referred to as tardive dyskinesia. The movements may appear during treatment or upon

withdrawal of treatment and may be either reversible or irreversible (i.e., persistent) upon cessation of further neuroleptic administration.

The syndrome is known to have a variable latency for development and the duration of the latency cannot be determined reliably. It is thus wise to assume that any neuroleptic agent has the capacity to induce the syndrome and act accordingly until sufficient data has been collected to settle the issue definitively for a specific drug product. In the case of neuroleptics known to produce the irreversible syndrome, the following has been observed:

Tardive dyskinesia has appeared in some patients on long-term therapy and has also appeared after drug therapy has been discontinued. The risk appears to be greater in elderly patients on high-dose therapy, especially females. The symptoms are persistent and in some patients appear to be irreversible. The syndrome is characterized by rhythmical involuntary movements of the tongue, face, mouth or jaw (e.g., protrusion of tongue, puffing of cheeks, puckering of mouth, chewing movements). There may be involuntary movements of extremities.

There is no known effective treatment of tardive dyskinesia; antiparkinsonism agents usually do not alleviate the symptoms of this syndrome. It is suggested that all antipsychotic agents be discontinued if these symptoms appear. Should it be necessary to reinstitute treatment, or increase the dosage of the agent, or switch to a different antipsychotic agent, the syndrome may be masked. It has been reported that fine vermicular movements of the tongue may be an early sign of the syndrome and if the mechanism is stopped at that time the syndrome may not develop (See WARNINGS).

Autonomic Nervous System

Occasionally blurring of vision, tachycardia, nausea, dry mouth and salivation have been reported. Urinary retention and constipation may occur particularly if anticholinergic drugs are used to treat extrapyramidal symptoms. One patient being treated with MOBAN experienced priapism which required surgical intervention, apparently resulting in residual impairment of erectile function.

Laboratory Tests

There have been rare reports of leucopenia and leucocytosis. If such reactions occur, treatment with MOBAN may continue if clinical symptoms are absent. Alterations of blood glucose, B.U.N., and red blood cells have not been considered clinically significant.

Metabolic and Endocrine Effects

Alteration of thyroid function has not been significant. Amenorrhea has been reported infrequently. Resumption of menses in previously amenorrheic women has been reported. Initially heavy menses may occur. Galactorrhea and gynecomastia have been reported infrequently. Increase in libido has been noted in some patients. Impotence has not been reported. Although both weight gain and weight loss have been in the direction of normal or ideal weight, excessive weight gain has not occurred with MOBAN.

Hepatic Effects

There have been rare reports of clinically significant alterations in liver function in association with MOBAN use.

Cardiovascular

Rare, transient, non-specific T wave changes have been reported on E.K.G. Association with a clinical syndrome has not been established. Rarely has significant hypotension been reported.

Ophthalmological

Lens opacities and pigmentary retinopathy have not been reported where patients have received MOBAN (molindone hydrochloride). In some patients, phenothiazine induced lenticular opacities have resolved following discontinuation of the phenothiazine while continuing therapy with MOBAN.

Skin

Early, non-specific skin rash, probably of allergic origin, has occasionally been reported. Skin pigmentation has not been seen with MOBAN usage alone.

MOBAN (molindone hydrochloride) has certain pharmacological similarities to other antipsychotic agents. Because adverse reactions are often extensions of the pharmacological activity of a drug, all of the known pharmacological effects associated with other antipsychotic drugs should be kept in mind when MOBAN is used. Upon abrupt withdrawal after prolonged high dosage an abstinence syndrome has not been noted.

DOSAGE AND ADMINISTRATION

Initial and maintenance doses of MOBAN (molindone hydrochloride) should be individualized.

Initial Dosage Schedule

The usual starting dosage is 50–75 mg/day.
—Increase to 100 mg/day in 3 or 4 days.
—Based on severity of symptomatology, dosage may be titrated up or down depending on individual patient response.
—An increase to 225 mg/day may be required in patients with severe symptomatology.

Elderly and debilitated patients should be started on lower dosage.

Maintenance Dosage Schedule

1. Mild-5 mg-15 mg three or four times a day.
2. Moderate-10 mg-25 mg three or four times a day.
3. Severe-225 mg/day may be required.

DRUG INTERACTIONS

Potentiation of drugs administered concurrently with MOBAN (molindone hydrochloride) has not been reported. Additionally, animal studies have not shown increased toxicity when MOBAN is given concurrently with representative members of three classes of drugs (i.e., barbiturates, chloral hydrate and antiparkinson drugs).

MANAGEMENT OF OVERDOSAGE

Symptomatic, supportive therapy should be the rule.

Gastric lavage is indicated for the reduction of absorption of MOBAN (molindone hydrochloride) which is freely soluble in water.

Since the adsorption of MOBAN (molindone hydrochloride) by activated charcoal has not been determined, the use of this antidote must be considered of theoretical value.

Emesis in a comatose patient is contraindicated. Additionally, while the emetic effect of apomorphine is blocked by MOBAN in animals, this blocking effect has not been determined in humans.

A significant increase in the rate of removal of unmetabolized MOBAN from the body by forced diuresis, peritoneal or renal dialysis would not be expected. (Only 2% of a single ingested dose of MOBAN is excreted unmetabolized in the urine). However, poor response of the patient may justify use of these procedures.

While the use of laxatives or enemas might be based on general principles, the amount of unmetabolized MOBAN in feces is less than 1%. Extrapyramidal symptoms have responded to the use of diphenhydramine (Benadryl*), Amantadine HCl (Symmetrel®*) and the synthetic anticholinergic antiparkinson agents, (i.e., Artane*, Cogentin*, Akineton*).

HOW SUPPLIED

As tablets in bottles of 100 with potencies and colors as follows:

5 mg orange	NDC 57844-914-01
10 mg lavender	NDC 57844-915-01
25 mg light green	NDC 57844-916-01
50 mg blue	NDC 57844-917-01
100 mg tan	NDC 57844-918-01

As a concentrate containing 20 mg molindone hydrochloride per mL in 4 oz. (120 mL) bottles, NDC 57844-920-12.

Store at controlled room temperature (59°–86°F, 15°–30°C). Protect from light.

*Benadryl-Trademark, Parke Davis and Co.
*Artane-Trademark, Lederle Laboratories
*Cogentin-Trademark, Merck Sharp & Dohme
*Akineton-Trademark, Knoll Pharmaceutical Co.
*Symmetrel-Trademark, The DuPont Merck Pharmaceutical Co.

Manufactured for:
GATE PHARMACEUTICALS
div. of Lemmon Company
Sellersville, PA 18960

Manufactured by:
DuPont Pharma
Wilmington, Delaware 19880

GATE PHARMACEUTICALS
division of Lemmon Company
Sellersville, PA 18960

MOBAN® is a Registered Trademark of The DuPont Merck Pharmaceutical Co.

6292-01/Rev. Feb., 1996

Shown in Product Identification Guide, page 311

ORAP® (Pimozide) ℞
Tablets

DESCRIPTION

ORAP (pimozide) is an orally active antipsychotic agent of the diphenylbutylpiperidine series. The structural formula of pimozide, 1-[1-[4,4-bis(4-fluorophenyl)butyl]-4-piperidinyl]-1,3-dihydro-2*H*-benzimidazol-2-one is:

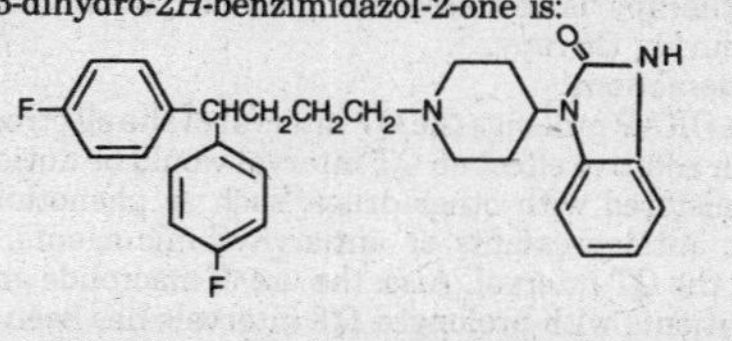

The solubility of pimozide in water is less than 0.01 mg/mL; it is slightly soluble in most organic solvents.

Each white ORAP tablet contains 2 mg of pimozide and the following inactive ingredients: calcium stearate, cellulose, lactose and corn starch.

CLINICAL PHARMACOLOGY

Pharmacodynamic Actions

ORAP (pimozide) is an orally active antipsychotic drug product which shares with other antipsychotics the ability to blockade dopaminergic receptors on neurons in the central nervous system. Although its exact mode of action has not been established, the ability of pimozide to suppress motor and phonic tics in Tourette's Disorder is thought to be a function of its dopaminergic blocking activity. However, receptor blockade is often accompanied by a series of secondary alterations in central dopamine metabolism and function which may contribute to both pimozide's therapeutic and untoward effects. In addition, pimozide, in common with other antipsychotic drugs, has various effects on other central nervous system receptor systems which are not fully characterized.

Metabolism and Pharmacokinetics

More than 50% of a dose of pimozide is absorbed after oral administration. Based on the pharmacokinetic and metabolic profile, pimozide appears to undergo significant first pass metabolism. Peak serum levels occur generally six to eight hours (range 4–12 hours) after dosing. Pimozide is extensively metabolized, primarily by N-dealkylation in the liver. Two major metabolites have been identified, 1-(4-piperidyl)-2-benzimidazolinone and 4,4-bis(4-fluorophenyl) butyric acid. The antipsychotic activity of these metabolites is undetermined. The major route of elimination of pimozide and its metabolites is through the kidney.

The mean serum elimination half-life of pimozide in schizophrenic patients was approximately 55 hours. There was a 13-fold inter individual difference in the area under the serum pimozide level-time curve and an equivalent degree of variation in peak serum levels among patients studied. The significance of this is unclear since there are few correlations between plasma levels and clinical findings.

Effects of food, disease or concomitant medication upon the absorption, distribution, metabolism and elimination of pimozide are not known.

INDICATIONS AND USAGE

ORAP (pimozide) is indicated for the suppression of motor and phonic tics in patients with Tourette's Disorder who have failed to respond satisfactorily to standard treatment. ORAP is not intended as a treatment of first choice nor is it intended for the treatment of tics that are merely annoying or cosmetically troublesome. ORAP should be reserved for use in Tourette's Disorder patients whose development and/or daily life function is severely compromised by the presence of motor and phonic tics.

Evidence supporting approval of pimozide for use in Tourette's Disorder was obtained in two controlled clinical investigations which enrolled patients between the ages of 8 and 53 years. Most subjects in the two trials were 12 or older.

CONTRAINDICATIONS

1. ORAP (pimozide) is contraindicated in the treatment of simple tics or tics other than those associated with Tourette's Disorder.
2. ORAP should not be used in patients taking drugs that may, themselves, cause motor and phonic tics (e.g., pemoline, methylphenidate and amphetamines) until such patients have been withdrawn from these drugs to determine whether or not the drugs, rather than Tourette's Disorder, are responsible for the tics.
3. Because ORAP prolongs the QT interval of the electrocardiogram it is contraindicated in patients with congenital long QT syndrome, patients with a history of cardiac arrhythmias, or patients taking other drugs which prolong the QT interval of the electrocardiogram (see DRUG INTERACTIONS).
4. ORAP is contraindicated in patients with severe toxic central nervous system depression or comatose states from any cause.
5. ORAP is contraindicated in patients with hypersensitivity to it. As it is not known whether cross-sensitivity exists among the antipsychotics, pimozide should be used with appropriate caution in patients who have demonstrated hypersensitivity to other antipsychotic drugs.
6. Ventricular arrhythmias have been rarely associated with the use of macrolide antibiotics in patients with prolonged QT intervals, as might be produced by ORAP. Specifically, two sudden deaths have been reported when clarithromycin was added to ongoing pimozide therapy. Therefore, ORAP is contraindicated in patients receiving the macrolide antibiotics clarithromycin, erythromycin, azithromycin, and dirithromycin.

WARNINGS

The use of ORAP (pimozide) in the treatment of Tourette's Disorder involves different risk/benefit considerations than when antipsychotic drugs are used to treat other conditions. Consequently, a decision to use ORAP should take into consideration the following (see also PRECAUTIONS—Information for Patients).

Continued on next page

Consult 1997 supplements and future editions for revisions

Gate—Cont.

Tardive Dyskinesia

A syndrome consisting of potentially irreversible, involuntary, dyskinetic movements may develop in patients treated with antipsychotic drugs. Although the prevalence of the syndrome appears to be highest among the elderly, especially elderly women, it is impossible to rely upon prevalence estimates to predict, at the inception of antipsychotic treatment, which patients are likely to develop the syndrome. Whether antipsychotic drug products differ in their potential to cause tardive dyskinesia is unknown.

Both the risk of developing tardive dyskinesia and the likelihood that it will become irreversible are believed to increase as the duration of treatment and the total cumulative dose of antipsychotic drugs administered to the patient increase. However, the syndrome can develop, although much less commonly, after relatively brief treatment periods at low doses.

There is no known treatment for established cases of tardive dyskinesia, although the syndrome may remit, partially or completely, if antipsychotic treatment is withdrawn. Antipsychotic treatment, itself, however, may suppress (or partially suppress) the signs and symptoms of the syndrome and thereby may possibly mask the underlying process. The effect that symptomatic suppression has upon the long-term course of the syndrome is unknown.

Given these considerations, antipsychotic drugs should be prescribed in a manner that is most likely to minimize the occurrence of tardive dyskinesia. Chronic antipsychotic treatment should generally be reserved for patients who suffer from a chronic illness that, 1) is known to respond to antipsychotic drugs, and 2) for whom alternative, equally effective, but potentially less harmful treatments are **not** available or appropriate. In patients who do require chronic treatment, the smallest dose and the shortest duration of treatment producing a satisfactory clinical response should be sought. The need for continued treatment should be reassessed periodically.

If signs and symptoms of tardive dyskinesia appear in a patient on antipsychotics, drug discontinuation should be considered. However, some patients may require treatment despite the presence of the syndrome.

(For further information about the description of tardive dyskinesia and its clinical detection, please refer to ADVERSE REACTIONS and PRECAUTIONS—Information for Patients.)

Neuroleptic Malignant Syndrome (NMS)

A potentially fatal symptom complex sometimes referred to as Neuroleptic Malignant Syndrome (NMS) has been reported in association with antipsychotic drugs. Clinical manifestations of NMS are hyperpyrexia, muscle rigidity, altered mental status (including catatonic signs) and evidence of autonomic instability (irregular pulse or blood pressure, tachycardia, diaphoresis, and cardiac dysrhythmias). Additional signs may include elevated creatine phosphokinase, myoglobinuria (rhabdomyolysis) and acute renal failure.

The diagnostic evaluation of patients with this syndrome is complicated. In arriving at a diagnosis, it is important to identify cases where the clinical presentation includes both serious medical illness (e.g., pneumonia, systemic infection, etc.) and untreated or inadequately treated extrapyramidal signs and symptoms (EPS). Other important considerations in the differential diagnosis include central anticholinergic toxicity, heat stroke, drug fever and primary central nervous system (CNS) pathology.

The management of NMS should include 1) immediate discontinuation of antipsychotic drugs and other drugs not essential to concurrent therapy, 2) intensive symptomatic treatment and medical monitoring, and 3) treatment of any concomitant serious medical problems for which specific treatments are available. There is no general agreement about specific pharmacological treatment regimens for uncomplicated NMS.

If a patient requires antipsychotic drug treatment after recovery from NMS, the potential reintroduction of drug therapy should be carefully considered. The patient should be carefully monitored, since recurrences of NMS have been reported.

Hyperpyrexia, not associated with the above symptom complex, has been reported with other antipsychotic drugs.

Other

Sudden, unexpected deaths have occurred in experimental studies of conditions other than Tourette's Disorder. These deaths occurred while patients were receiving dosages in the range of 1 mg per kg. One possible mechanism for such deaths is prolongation of the QT interval predisposing patients to ventricular arrhythmia. An electrocardiogram should be performed before ORAP treatment is initiated and periodically thereafter, especially during the period of dose adjustment.

ORAP may have a tumorigenic potential. Based on studies conducted in mice, it is known that pimozide can produce a dose related increase in pituitary tumors. The full significance of this finding is not known, but should be taken into consideration in the physician's and patient's decisions to use this drug product. This finding should be given special consideration when the patient is young and chronic use of pimozide is anticipated. (see PRECAUTIONS—Carcinogenesis, Mutagenesis, Impairment of Fertility)

PRECAUTIONS

General

ORAP (pimozide) may impair the mental and/or physical abilities required for the performance of potentially hazardous tasks, such as driving a car or operating machinery, especially during the first few days of therapy.

ORAP produces anticholinergic side effects and should be used with caution in individuals whose conditions may be aggravated by anticholinergic activity.

ORAP should be administered cautiously to patients with impairment of liver or kidney function, because it is metabolized by the liver and excreted by the kidneys.

Antipsychotics should be administered with caution to patients receiving anticonvulsant medication, with a history of seizures, or with EEG abnormalities, because they may lower the convulsive threshold. If indicated, adequate anticonvulsant therapy should be maintained concomitantly.

Information for Patients

Treatment with ORAP exposes the patient to serious risks. A decision to use ORAP chronically in Tourette's Disorder is one that deserves full consideration by the patient (or patient's family) as well as by the treating physician. Because the goal of treatment is symptomatic improvement, the patient's view of the need for treatment and assessment of response are critical in evaluating the impact of therapy and weighing its benefits against the risks. Since the physician is the primary source of information about the use of a drug in any disease, it is recommended that the following information be discussed with patients and/or their families.

ORAP is intended only for use in patients with Tourette's Disorder whose symptoms are severe and who cannot tolerate, or who do not respond to HALDOL® (haloperidol).

Given the likelihood that a proportion of patients exposed chronically to antipsychotics will develop tardive dyskinesia, it is advised that all patients in whom chronic use is contemplated be given, if possible, full information about this risk. The decision to inform patients and/or their guardians must obviously take into account the clinical circumstances and the competency of the patient to understand the information provided.

There is limited information available on the use of ORAP in children under 12 years of age.

The information available on ORAP from foreign marketing experience and from U.S. clinical trials indicates that ORAP has a side effect profile similar to that of other antipsychotic drugs. Patients should be informed that all types of side effects associated with the use of antipsychotics may be associated with the use of ORAP.

In addition, sudden, unexpected deaths have occurred in patients taking high doses of ORAP for conditions other than Tourette's Disorder. These deaths may have been the result of an effect of ORAP upon the heart. Therefore, patients should be instructed not to exceed the prescribed dose of ORAP and they should realize the need for the initial ECG and for follow-up ECG's during treatment.

Also, pimozide, at a dose about 15 times that given humans, caused an increase in the number of benign tumors of the pituitary gland in female mice. It is not possible to say how important this is. Similar tumors were not seen in rats given pimozide, nor at lower doses in mice, which is reassuring. However, any such finding must be considered to suggest a possible risk of long term use of the drug.

Laboratory Tests

An ECG should be done at baseline and periodically thereafter throughout the period of dose adjustment. Any indication of prolongation of QT_c interval beyond an absolute limit of 0.47 seconds (children) or 0.52 seconds (adults), or more than 25% above the patient's original baseline should be considered a basis for stopping further dose increase (see CONTRAINDICATIONS) and considering a lower dose.

Since hypokalemia has been associated with ventricular arrhythmias, potassium insufficiency, secondary to diuretics, diarrhea, or other cause, should be corrected before ORAP therapy is initiated and normal potassium maintained during therapy.

Drug Interactions

Because ORAP prolongs the QT interval of the electrocardiogram, an additive effect on QT interval would be anticipated if administered with other drugs, such as phenothiazines, tricyclic antidepressants or antiarrhythmic agents, which prolong the QT interval. Also, the use of macrolide antibiotics in patients with prolonged QT intervals has been rarely associated with ventricular arrhythmias. Such concomitant administration should not be undertaken (see CONTRAINDICATIONS).

ORAP may be capable of potentiating CNS depressants, including analgesics, sedatives, anxiolytics, and alcohol.

Carcinogenesis, Mutagenesis, Impairment of Fertility

Carcinogenicity studies were conducted in mice and rats. In mice, pimozide causes a dose-related increase in pituitary and mammary tumors.

When mice were treated for up to 18 months with pimozide, pituitary gland changes developed in females only. These changes were characterized as hyperplasia at doses approximating the human dose and adenoma at doses about fifteen times the maximum recommended human dose on a mg per kg basis. The mechanism for the induction of pituitary tumors in mice is not known.

Mammary gland tumors in female mice were also increased, but these tumors are expected in rodents treated with antipsychotic drugs which elevate prolactin levels. Chronic administration of an antipsychotic also causes elevated prolactin levels in humans. Tissue culture experiments indicate that approximately one-third of human breast cancers are prolactin-dependent *in vitro*, a factor of potential importance if the prescription of these drugs is contemplated in a patient with a previously detected breast cancer. Although disturbances such as galactorrhea, amenorrhea, gynecomastia, and impotence have been reported with antipsychotic drugs, the clinical significance of elevated serum prolactin levels is unknown for most patients. Neither clinical studies nor epidemiologic studies conducted to date have shown an association between chronic administration of these drugs and mammary tumorigenesis. The available evidence, however, is considered too limited to be conclusive at this time.

In a 24 month carcinogenicity study in rats, animals received up to 50 times the maximum recommended human dose. No increased incidence of overall tumors or tumors at any site was observed in either sex. Because of the limited number of animals surviving this study, the meaning of these results is unclear.

Pimozide did not have mutagenic activity in the Ames test with four bacterial test strains, in the mouse dominant lethal test or in the micronucleus test in rats.

Reproduction studies in animals were not adequate to assess all aspects of fertility. Nevertheless, female rats administered pimozide had prolonged estrus cycles, an effect also produced by other antipsychotic drugs.

Pregnancy

Category C. Reproduction studies performed in rats and rabbits at oral doses up to 8 times the maximum human dose did not reveal evidence of teratogenicity. In the rat, however, this multiple of the human dose resulted in decreased pregnancies and in the retarded development of fetuses. These effects are thought to be due to an inhibition or delay in implantation which is also observed in rodents administered other antipsychotic drugs. In the rabbit, maternal toxicity, mortality, decreased weight gain, and embryotoxicity including increased resorptions were dose related. Because animal reproduction studies are not always predictive of human response, pimozide should be given to a pregnant woman only if the potential benefits of treatment clearly outweigh the potential risks.

Labor and Delivery

This drug has no recognized use in labor or delivery.

Nursing Mothers

It is not known whether pimozide is excreted in human milk. Because many drugs are excreted in human milk and because of the potential for tumorigenicity and unknown cardiovascular effects in the infant, a decision should be made whether to discontinue nursing or to discontinue the drug, taking into account the importance of the drug to the mother.

Pediatric Use

Although Tourette's Disorder most often has its onset between the ages of 2 and 15 years, information on the use and efficacy of ORAP in patients less than 12 years of age is limited. A 24 week open label study in 36 children between the ages of 2 and 12 demonstrated that pimozide has a similar safety profile in this age group as in older patients and there were no safety findings that would preclude its use in this age group.

Because its use and safety have not been evaluated in other childhood disorders, ORAP is not recommended for use in any condition other than Tourette's Disorder.

ADVERSE REACTIONS

General

Extrapyramidal Reactions: Neuromuscular (extrapyramidal) reactions during the administration of ORAP (pimozide) have been reported frequently, often during the first few days of treatment. In most patients, these reactions involved Parkinson-like symptoms which, when first observed, were usually mild to moderately severe and usually reversible. Other types of neuromuscular reactions (motor restlessness, dystonia, akathisia, hyperreflexia, opisthotonos, oculogyric crises) have been reported far less frequently. Severe extrapyramidal reactions have been reported to occur at relatively low doses. Generally the occurrence and severity of most extrapyramidal symptoms are dose related since they occur at relatively high doses and have been shown to disappear or become less severe when the dose is reduced. Administration of antiparkinson drugs such as benztropine mesyl-

ate or trihexyphenidyl hydrochloride may be required for control of such reactions. It should be noted that persistent extrapyramidal reactions have been reported and that the drug may have to be discontinued in such cases.

Withdrawal Emergent Neurological Signs: Generally, patients receiving short term therapy experience no problems with abrupt discontinuation of antipsychotic drugs. However, some patients on maintenance treatment experience transient dyskinetic signs after abrupt withdrawal. In certain of these cases the dyskinetic movements are indistinguishable from the syndrome described below under "Tardive Dyskinesia" except for duration. It is not known whether gradual withdrawal of antipsychotic drugs will reduce the rate of occurrence of withdrawal emergent neurological signs but until further evidence becomes available, it seems reasonable to gradually withdraw use of ORAP.

Tardive Dyskinesia: ORAP may be associated with persistent dyskinesias. Tardive dyskinesia, a syndrome consisting of potentially irreversible, involuntary, dyskinetic movements, may appear in some patients on long-term therapy or may occur after drug therapy has been discontinued. The risk appears to be greater in elderly patients on high-dose therapy, especially females. The symptoms are persistent and in some patients appear irreversible. The syndrome is characterized by rhythmical involuntary movements of tongue, face, mouth or jaw (e.g., protrusion of tongue, puffing of cheeks, puckering of mouth, chewing movements). Sometimes these may be accompanied by involuntary movements of extremities and the trunk.

There is no known effective treatment for tardive dyskinesia; antiparkinson agents usually do not alleviate the symptoms of this syndrome. It is suggested that all antipsychotic agents be discontinued if these symptoms appear. Should it be necessary to reinstitute treatment, or increase the dosage of the agent, or switch to a different antipsychotic agent, this syndrome may be masked.

It has been reported that fine vermicular movement of the tongue may be an early sign of tardive dyskinesia and if the medication is stopped at that time the full syndrome may not develop.

Electrocardiographic Changes: Electrocardiographic changes have been observed in clinical trials of ORAP in Tourette's Disorder and schizophrenia. These have included prolongation of the QT interval, flattening, notching and inversion of the T wave and the appearance of U waves. Sudden, unexpected deaths and grand mal seizure have occurred at doses above 20 mg/day.

Neuroleptic Malignant Syndrome: Neuroleptic malignant syndrome (NMS) has been reported with ORAP. (See WARNINGS for further information concerning NMS.)

Hyperpyrexia: Hyperpyrexia has been reported with other antipsychotic drugs.

Clinical Trials

The following adverse reaction tabulation was derived from 20 patients in a 6 week long placebo controlled clinical trial of ORAP in Tourette's Disorder.

Body System/ Adverse Reactions	Pimozide (N = 20)	Placebo (N = 20)
Body as a Whole		
Headache	1	2
Gastrointestinal		
Dry mouth	5	1
Diarrhea	1	0
Nausea	0	2
Vomiting	0	1
Constipation	4	2
Eructations	0	1
Thirsty	1	0
Appetite increase	1	0
Endocrine		
Menstrual disorder	0	1
Breast secretions	0	1
Musculoskeletal		
Muscle cramps	0	1
Muscle tightness	3	0
Stooped posture	2	0
CNS		
Drowsiness	7	3
Sedation	14	5
Insomnia	2	2
Dizziness	0	1
Akathisia	8	0
Rigidity	2	0
Speech disorder	2	0
Handwriting change	1	0
Akinesia	8	0
Psychiatric		
Depression	2	3
Excitement	0	1
Nervous	1	0
Adverse behavior effect	5	0

Special Senses		
Visual disturbance	4	0
Taste change	1	0
Sensitivity of eyes to light	1	0
Decreased accommodation	4	1
Spots before eyes	0	1
Urogenital		
Impotence	3	0

The following adverse event tabulation was derived from 36 children (age 2 to 12) in a 24 week open trial of ORAP in Tourette's Disorder.

Body System Adverse Reaction	Number of Patients Experiencing Each Event(%)	
	All Events (N = 36)	Drug-Related Events (N = 36)
Body as a Whole		
Asthenia	9 (25.0)	5 (13.8)
Headache	8 (22.2)	1 (2.7)
Gastrointestinal		
Dysphagia	1 (2.7)	1 (2.7)
Increased Salivation	5 (13.8)	2 (5.5)
Musculoskeletal		
Myalgia	1 (2.7)	1 (2.7)
Central Nervous System		
Dreaming Abnormal	1 (2.7)	1 (2.7)
Hyperkinesia	2 (5.5)	1 (2.7)
Somnolence	10 (27.7)	9 (25.0)
Torticollis	1 (2.7)	1 (2.7)
Tremor Limbs	1 (2.7)	1 (2.7)
Psychiatric		
Adverse Behavior Effect	10 (27.7)	8 (22.2)
Nervous	3 (8.3)	2 (5.5)
Skin		
Rash	3 (8.3)	1 (2.7)
Special Senses		
Visual Disturbances	2 (5.5)	1 (2.7)
Cardiovascular		
ECG Abnormal	1 (2.7)	1 (2.7)

Because clinical investigational experience with ORAP in Tourette's Disorder is limited, uncommon adverse reactions may not have been detected. The physician should consider that other adverse reactions associated with antipsychotics may occur.

Other Adverse Reactions

In addition to the adverse reactions listed above, those listed below have been reported in U.S. clinical trials of ORAP in conditions other than Tourette's Disorder.

Body as a Whole: Asthenia, chest pain, periorbital edema
Cardiovascular/Respiratory: Postural hypotension, hypotension, hypertension, tachycardia, palpitations
Gastrointestinal: Increased salivation, nausea, vomiting, anorexia, GI distress
Endocrine: Loss of libido
Metabolic/Nutritional: Weight gain, weight loss
Central Nervous System: Dizziness, tremor, parkinsonism, fainting, dyskinesia
Psychiatric: Excitement
Skin: Rash, sweating, skin irritation
Special Senses: Blurred vision, cataracts
Urogenital: Nocturia, urinary frequency

Postmarketing Reports

The following experiences were described in spontaneous postmarketing reports. These reports do not provide sufficient information to establish a clear causal relationship with the use of ORAP.

Gastrointestinal: Gingival hyperplasia in one patient.
Hematologic: Hemolytic anemia.
Metabolic/Nutritional: Hyponatremia.
Other: Seizure.

OVERDOSAGE

In general, the signs and symptoms of overdosage with ORAP (pimozide) would be an exaggeration of known pharmacologic effects and adverse reactions, the most prominent of which would be: 1) electrocardiographic abnormalities, 2) severe extrapyramidal reactions, 3) hypotension, 4) a comatose state with respiratory depression.

In the event of overdosage, gastric lavage, establishment of a patent airway and, if necessary, mechanically-assisted respiration are advised. Electrocardiographic monitoring should commence immediately and continue until the ECG parameters are within the normal range. Hypotension and circulatory collapse may be counteracted by use of intravenous fluids, plasma, or concentrated albumin, and vasopressor agents such as metaraminol, phenylephrine and norepinephrine. Epinephrine should not be used. In case of severe extrapyramidal reactions, antiparkinson medication should be administered. Because of the long half-life of pimozide, patients who take an overdose should be observed for at least 4 days. As with all drugs, the physician should consider contacting a poison control center for additional information on the treatment of overdose.

DOSAGE AND ADMINISTRATION

General:
The suppression of tics by ORAP requires a slow and gradual introduction of the drug. The patient's dose should be carefully adjusted to a point where the suppression of tics and the relief afforded is balanced against the untoward side effects of the drug.

An ECG should be done at baseline and periodically thereafter, especially during the period of dose adjustment (see WARNINGS and PRECAUTIONS—Laboratory Tests).

Periodic attempts should be made to reduce the dosage of ORAP to see whether or not tics persist at the level and extent first identified. In attempts to reduce the dosage of ORAP, consideration should be given to the possibility that increases of tic intensity and frequency may represent a transient, withdrawal related phenomenon rather than a return of disease symptoms. Specifically, one to two weeks should be allowed to elapse before one concludes that an increase in tic manifestations is a function of the underlying disease syndrome rather than a response to drug withdrawal. A gradual withdrawal is recommended in any case.

Children:
Reliable dose response data for the effects of ORAP (pimozide) on tic manifestation in Tourette's Disorder patients below the age of twelve are not available.

Treatment should be initiated at a dose of 0.05 mg/kg preferably taken once at bedtime. The dose may be increased every third day to a maximum of 0.2 mg/kg not to exceed 10 mg/day.

Adults:
In general, treatment with ORAP should be initiated with a dose of 1 to 2 mg a day in divided doses. The dose may be increased thereafter every other day. Most patients are maintained at less than 0.2 mg/kg per day, or 10 mg/day, whichever is less. Doses greater than 0.2 mg/kg/day or 10 mg/day are not recommended.

ANIMAL PHARMACOLOGY

A chronic study in dogs indicated that pimozide caused gingival hyperplasia when administered for several months at about 5 times the maximum recommended human dose. This condition was reversible after withdrawal.

HOW SUPPLIED

ORAP® (pimozide) 2 mg tablets, white, scored, debossed "LEMMON" and "ORAP 2"—NDC 57844-187-01, bottles of 100.

Dispense in a tight, light-resistant container as defined in the official compendium.

Pharmacist: Dispense in a child-resistant container.

Manufactured for:
GATE PHARMACEUTICALS
Division of Lemmon Company
Sellersville, PA 18960
Manufactured by:
LEMMON COMPANY
Sellersville, PA 18960

Rev. E 2/96
Shown in Product Identification Guide, page 311

Gebauer Company
9410 ST. CATHERINE AVE.
CLEVELAND, OH 44104

Direct Inquiries to:
(800) 321-9348
(216) 271-5252

For Medical Information Contact:
In Emergencies:
(800) 321-9348
(216) 271-5252
After Hours and Weekend Emergencies:
Chemtrac:
(800) 424-9300

ETHYL CHLORIDE, U.S.P.   ℞
(Chloroethane)

INDICATIONS AND USAGE
Ethyl Chloride is a vapocoolant intended for topical application to control pain associated with minor surgical procedures (such as lancing boils, or incision and drainage of small abscesses), athletic injuries, injections, and for treatment of myofascial pain, restricted motion, and muscle spasm.

PRECAUTIONS
Inhalation of Ethyl Chloride should be avoided as it may produce narcotic and general anesthetic effects, and may produce deep anesthesia or fatal coma with respiratory or cardiac arrest. Ethyl Chloride is **FLAMMABLE** and should never be used in the presence of an open flame, or electrical cautery equipment. When used to produce local freezing of tissues, adjacent skin areas should be protected by application of petrolatum. The thawing process may be painful, and freezing may lower local resistance to infection and delay healing.

ADVERSE REACTIONS
Cutaneous sensitization may occur, but appears to be extremely rare. Freezing can occasionally alter pigmentation.

CONTRAINDICATIONS
Ethyl Chloride is contraindicated in individuals with a history of hypersensitivity to it. This product should not be used on patients having vascular impairment of the extremities.

WARNINGS
For external use only.
Skin absorption of Ethyl Chloride can occur; no cases of chronic poisoning have been reported. Ethyl Chloride is known as a liver and kidney toxin; long term exposure may cause liver or kidney damage.
Contents under pressure. Store in a cool place. Do not store above 120°F. Do not store on or near high frequency ultrasound equipment. Store upright only.

DOSAGE AND ADMINISTRATION
To apply Ethyl Chloride from amber bottle with dispenseal valve, invert over the treatment area approximately 12 inches (30 cm.) away from site of application. Open dispenseal spring valve completely allowing Ethyl Chloride to flow in a stream from the bottle.

1. TOPICAL ANESTHESIA IN MINOR SURGERY
The operative site should be cleansed with a suitable antiseptic. Apply petrolatum to protect the adjacent area. Spray Ethyl Chloride for a few seconds to the point of frost formation, when the tissue becomes white. Avoid prolonged spraying of skin beyond this state. The anesthetic action of Ethyl Chloride rarely lasts more than a few seconds to a minute. Quickly swab operative site with antiseptic and promptly make incision. Reapply as needed.

2. SPORTS INJURIES
The pain of bruises, contusions, abrasions, swelling, and minor sprains may be controlled with Ethyl Chloride.
Spray affected area for a few seconds until the tissue begins to frost and turn white. Avoid spraying of skin beyond this state. Use as you would ice. The amount of cooling depends on the dosage. The smallest dose needed to produce the desired effect should be used. Dosage varies with the nozzle size and duration of application.
Determine the extent of injury (fracture, sprain, etc.). The anesthetic effect of Ethyl Chloride rarely lasts more than a few seconds to a minute. This time interval is usually sufficient to help reduce or relieve the initial trauma of the injury.

3. FOR PRE-INJECTION ANESTHESIA
Prepare syringe and have it ready. Spray skin with Ethyl Chloride from a distance of about 12 inches (30 cm.) continuously for 3 to 5 seconds; do not frost skin. Swab skin with alcohol and quickly introduce needle with skin taut.

4. SPRAY and STRETCH TECHNIQUE for MYOFASCIAL PAIN
Ethyl Chloride may be used as a counterirritant in the management of myofascial pain, restricted motion, and muscle spasm. Clinical conditions that may respond to Ethyl Chloride include low back pain (due to muscle spasm), acute stiff neck, torticollis, acute bursitis of the shoulder, muscle spasm associated with osteoarthritis, tight hamstring, sprained ankle, masseter muscle spasm, certain types of headache, and referred pain due to irritated trigger point. Relief of pain facilitates early mobilization in restoration of muscle function. The Spray and Stretch technique is a therapeutic system which involves three stages: EVALUATION, SPRAYING, and STRETCHING.
The therapeutic value of Spray and Stretch becomes most effective when the practitioner has mastered all stages and applies them in the proper sequence.

I. EVALUATION
During the evaluation phase the cause of pain is determined as local spasm or an irritated trigger point. The method of applying the spray to a muscle spasm differs slightly from application to a trigger point. A trigger point is a deep hypersensitive localized spot in a muscle which causes a referred pain pattern. With trigger points the source of pain is seldom the site of the pain. A trigger point may be detected by a snapping palpation over the muscle, causing the muscle in which the irritated trigger point is situated to "jump".

II. SPRAYING
A. Patient should assume a comfortable position.
B. Take precautions to cover the patient's eyes, nose, mouth, if spraying near face.
C. Hold bottle in an upside down position 12 to 18 inches (30 to 45 cm.) away from the treatment surface allowing the jet stream of vapocoolant to meet the skin at an acute angle to lessen the shock of impact.
D. The spray is directed in parallel sweeps 1.5 to 2 cm. apart. The rate of spraying is approximately 10 cm/sec. and is continued until the entire muscle has been covered. The number of sweeps is determined by the size of the muscle. In the case of trigger point, the spray should be applied over the trigger point, through and over the reference zone. In case of muscle spasm, the spray should be applied from origin to insertion.

III. STRETCHING
During application of the spray, the muscle is passively stretched. Force is gradually increased with successive sweeps, and the slack is smoothly taken up as the muscle relaxes, establishing a new stretch length.
Reaching the full normal length of the muscle is necessary to completely inactivate trigger points and relieve pain.
After rewarming, the procedure may be repeated as necessary. Moist heat should be applied for 10 to 15 minutes following treatment. For lasting benefit, any factors that perpetuate the trigger mechanism must be eliminated.

HOW SUPPLIED
3.5 ounce amber glass bottle:
    Fine Spray...(NDC 0386-0001-04)
    Medium Spray.....................................(NDC 0386-0001-03)
3.0 ounce amber glass bottle:
    "Spra Pak"..(NDC 0386-0001-01)

CAUTION
Federal law restricts this device to sale by or on the order of a physician or other practitioner licensed by state law to use or order the use of the device.
©1994, Gebauer Company

FLUORI–METHANE®   ℞
(Dichlorodifluoromethane 15%
Trichloromonofluoromethane 85%)

INDICATIONS AND USAGE
Fluori-Methane Spray is a vapocoolant intended for topical application in the management of myofascial pain, restricted motion, and muscle spasm, and for the control of pain associated with injections.
Clinical conditions that may respond to Spray and Stretch include low back pain (due to muscle spasm), acute stiff neck, torticollis, muscle spasm associated with osteoarthritis, ankle sprain, tight hamstring, masseter muscle spasm, certain types of headache, and referred pain due to trigger points. Relief of pain facilitates early mobilization in restoration of muscle function.

PRECAUTIONS
Care should be taken to minimize inhalation of vapors, especially with application around head or neck. Avoid contact with eyes. Fluori-Methane should not be applied to the point of frost formation.

ADVERSE REACTIONS
Cutaneous sensitization may occur, but appears to be extremely rare. Freezing can occasionally alter pigmentation.

CONTRAINDICATIONS
Fluori-Methane is contraindicated in individuals with a history of hypersensitivity to dichlorodifluoromethane, and/or trichloromonofluoromethane. This product should not be used on patients having vascular impairment of the extremities.

WARNINGS
For external use only.
Dichlorodifluoromethane and trichloromonofluoromethane are not classified as carcinogens. Based on animal studies and human experience, these fluorocarbons pose no hazard to man relative to systemic toxicity, carcinogenicity, mutagenicity, or teratogenicity when occupational exposures are below 1000 p.p.m. over an 8 hour time weighted average. Contents under pressure. Store in a cool place. Do not store above 120°F. Do not store on or near high frequency ultrasound equipment.

DOSAGE AND ADMINISTRATION
To apply Fluori-Methane, invert the bottle over the treatment area approximately 12 inches (30 cm.) away from site of application. Open dispenseal spring valve completely, allowing the liquid to flow in a stream from the bottle.

1. SPRAY and STRETCH TECHNIQUE for MYOFASCIAL PAIN
Spray and Stretch technique is a therapeutic system which involves three stages: EVALUATION, SPRAYING, and STRETCHING.
The therapeutic value of Spray and Stretch becomes most effective when the practitioner has mastered all stages and applies them in proper sequence.

I. EVALUATION
During the evaluation phase the cause of pain is determined as local spasm or an irritated trigger point. The method of applying the spray to a muscle spasm differs slightly from application to a trigger point. A trigger point is a deep hypersensitive localized spot in a muscle which causes a referred pain pattern. With trigger points the source of pain is seldom the site of the pain. A trigger point may be detected by a snapping palpation over the muscle, causing the muscle in which the irritated trigger point is situated to "jump".

II. SPRAYING
A. Patient should assume a comfortable position.
B. Take precautions to cover the patient's eyes, nose, mouth, if spraying near face.
C. Hold bottle in an upside down position 12 to 18 inches (30 to 45 cm.) away from the treatment surface allowing the jet stream of vapocoolant to meet the skin at an acute angle to lessen the shock of impact.
D. The spray is directed in parallel sweeps 1.5 to 2 cm. apart. The rate of spraying is approximately 10 cm/sec. and is continued until the entire muscle has been covered. The number of sweeps is determined by the size of the muscle. In the case of a trigger point, the spray should be applied over the trigger point, through and over the reference zone. In the case of muscle spasm, the spray should be applied from origin to insertion.

III. STRETCHING
During application of the spray, the muscle is passively stretched. Force is gradually increased with successive sweeps, and the slack is smoothly taken up as the muscle relaxes, establishing a new stretch length.
Reaching the full normal length of the muscle is necessary to completely inactivate trigger points and relieve pain.
After rewarming, the procedure may be repeated as necessary. Moist heat should be applied for 10 to 15 minutes following treatment.
For lasting benefit, any factors that perpetuate the trigger mechanism must be eliminated.

2. PRE-INJECTION ANESTHESIA
Prepare syringe and have it ready. Spray skin with Fluori-Methane, from a distance of about 12 inches (30 cm.) continuously for 3 to 5 seconds; do not frost the skin. Swab skin with alcohol and quickly introduce needle with skin taut.

HOW SUPPLIED
3.5 ounce amber glass bottle.
Calibrated Fine Spray.............................(NDC 0386-0003-04)
Calibrated Medium Spray.......................(NDC 0386-0003-05)

CAUTION
Federal law restricts this device to sale by or on the order of a physician or other practitioner licensed by state law to use or order the use of the device.
©1994, Gebauer Company

EDUCATIONAL MATERIAL

For supporting educational materials contact Gebauer Company.

Geigy Pharmaceuticals
Ciba-Geigy Corporation
556 MORRIS AVENUE
SUMMIT, NJ 07901

For Information Contact:
Consumer Affairs Department:
(800) 742-2422
Medical Services Department:
556 Morris Avenue
Summit, NJ 07901

PLEASE NOTE:
Due to the alliance between Ciba Pharmaceuticals (which includes Basel Pharmaceuticals, Ciba Pharmaceutical Company, Geigy Pharmaceuticals, and Summit Pharmaceuticals) and Geneva Pharmaceuticals, Inc, please refer to **CibaGeneva** for product information.

See CibaGeneva Pharmaceuticals for information on the following products:
Brethaire®
Brethine®
Cataflam®
Lamprene®
Lioresal®
Lopressor®
Lopressor HCT®
PBZ®
PBZ-SR®
Tofranil®
Tofranil-PM®
Voltaren®
Voltaren®-XR

GenDerm Corporation
600 KNIGHTSBRIDGE PARKWAY
LINCOLNSHIRE, IL 60069

Direct Inquiries to:
Medical Information Department
(847) 634-7373

DOLORAC™   OTC
(capsaicin) cream, 0.25%
TOPICAL ANALGESIC CREAM

PRODUCT OVERVIEW

KEY FACTS
Dolorac is a highly concentrated cream formulation of capsaicin shown to have greater analgesic efficacy and a more rapid onset of action than conventional strengths of capsaicin cream.

MAJOR USES
Dolorac applied twice daily has been shown to be clinically effective in controlling pain from arthritis.

SAFETY INFORMATION
Patients are likely to experience a burning sensation at the site of Dolorac application, but the severity and duration of this effect are similar to those of lower strength capsaicin creams. Inhalation of airborne material from dried cream residue can cause coughing, sneezing or respiratory irritation and should be avoided. Patients should be instructed to wash hands after applying Dolorac. If applying to hands wait at least 30 minutes, then wash hands to avoid spreading cream to contact lenses, eyes, mouth or other sensitive mucous membranes.

PRESCRIBING INFORMATION

DOLORAC™   OTC
(capsaicin) cream, 0.25%
TOPICAL ANALGESIC CREAM

DESCRIPTION
Dolorac contains capsaicin, in an emollient base containing benzyl alcohol, cetyl alcohol, glyceryl monostearate, isopropyl myristate, PEG-100 stearate, purified water, sorbitol solution, and white petrolatum.

ACTION
Although the precise mechanism of action of capsaicin is not fully understood, current evidence suggests that capsaicin renders skin and joints insensitive to pain by depleting and preventing reaccumulation of substance P in peripheral sensory neurons. Substance P is thought to be the principal chemomediator of pain impulses from the periphery to the central nervous system. In addition, substance P has been shown to be released into joint tissues and activate inflammatory mediators involved in the pathogenesis of rheumatoid arthritis.

INDICATIONS
For the temporary relief of pain from arthritis. For use in painful neuralgias, consult a physician.

WARNINGS
FOR EXTERNAL USE ONLY. Avoid contact with eyes and broken (open) or irritated skin. Avoid inhaling airborne material from dried residue. Contact a physician immediately if difficulty breathing or swallowing occurs. Do not bandage tightly. If condition worsens, or does not improve after 7 days, discontinue use of this product and consult your physician. **Keep this and all drugs out of the reach of children.** In case of accidental ingestion, seek professional assistance or contact a Poison Control Center immediately.

DIRECTIONS
For adults and children 12 years of age and older: apply a thin film of Dolorac to affected area 2 times daily. For children under 12 years of age: consult with a physician. Substantial burning initially occurs at the site of application, but generally subsides after several days of use as directed. Application schedules of less than 2 times a day may cause this burning sensation to persist longer and may not provide optimum pain relief. **Wash hands after applying Dolorac. If applying to hands wait at least 30 minutes, then wash hands.**

HOW SUPPLIED
Dolorac™
1.0 oz (28 g) tube (NDC 52761-571-30)
Store at room temperature 15°–30°C (59°–86°F)
U.S. Patent Nos. 4486450 and 4536404

NOVACET® LOTION   ℞
[nov'a set]
(Sodium Sulfacetamide 10% and Sulfur 5%)
ACNE MEDICATION

DESCRIPTION
Each gram of Novacet Lotion (sodium sulfacetamide 10% and sulfur 5%) contains 100 mg of sodium sulfacetamide and 50 mg of sulfur in a lotion containing propylene glycol, isopropyl myristate, propylene glycol stearate, cetyl alcohol, PEG-8 stearate, benzyl alcohol, sodium thiosulfate, EDTA disodium, buffering agent, emulsifying wax, and purified water.
Sodium sulfacetamide is a sulfonamide with antibacterial activity while sulfur acts as a keratolytic agent. Chemically sodium sulfacetamide is N′-[(4-aminophenyl) sulfonyl]-acetamide, monosodium salt, monohydrate. The structural formula is:

$$NH_2 - \langle\!\langle \ \rangle\!\rangle - SO_2NCOCH_3 \cdot H_2O$$

with Na on the nitrogen.

CLINICAL PHARMACOLOGY
The most widely accepted mechanism of action of sulfonamides is the Woods-Fildes theory which is based on the fact that sulfonamides act as competitive antagonists to para-aminobenzoic acid (PABA), an essential component for bacterial growth. While absorption through intact skin has not been determined, sodium sulfacetamide is readily absorbed from the gastrointestinal tract when taken orally and excreted in the urine, largely unchanged. The biological half-life has variously been reported as 7 to 12.8 hours.
The exact mode of action of sulfur in the treatment of acne is unknown, but it has been reported that it inhibits the growth of **P. acnes** and the formation of free fatty acids.

INDICATIONS
Novacet Lotion is indicated in the topical control of acne vulgaris, acne rosacea and seborrheic dermatitis.

CONTRAINDICATIONS
Novacet Lotion is contraindicated for use by patients having known hypersensitivity to sulfonamides, sulfur or any other component of this preparation. Novacet Lotion is not to be used by patients with kidney disease.

WARNINGS
Although rare, sensitivity to sodium sulfacetamide may occur. Therefore, caution and careful supervision should be observed when prescribing this drug for patients who may be prone to hypersensitivity to topical sulfonamides. Systemic toxic reactions such as agranulocytosis, acute hemolytic anemia, purpura hemorrhagica, drug fever, jaundice, and contact dermatitis indicate hypersensitivity to sulfonamides. Particular caution should be employed if areas of denuded or abraded skin are involved.

PRECAUTIONS
General—If irritation develops, use of the product should be discontinued and appropriate therapy instituted. For external use only. Keep away from eyes. Patients should be carefully observed for possible local irritation or sensitization during long-term therapy. The object of this therapy is to achieve desquamation without irritation, but sodium sulfacetamide and sulfur can cause reddening and scaling of epidermis. These side effects are not unusual in the treatment of acne vulgaris, but patients should be cautioned about the possibility. Keep out of the reach of children.
Carcinogenesis, Mutagenesis and Impairment of Fertility—Long-term studies in animals have not been performed to evaluate carcinogenic potential.
Pregnancy—Category C. Animal reproduction studies have not been conducted with Novacet Lotion. It is also not known whether Novacet Lotion can cause fetal harm when administered to a pregnant woman or can affect reproduction capacity.
Novacet Lotion should be given to a pregnant woman only if clearly needed.
Nursing Mothers—It is not known whether sodium sulfacetamide is excreted in the human milk following topical use of Novacet Lotion. However, small amounts of orally administered sulfonamides have been reported to be eliminated in human milk. In view of this and because many drugs are excreted in human milk, caution should be exercised when Novacet Lotion is administered to a nursing woman.
Pediatric Use—Safety and effectiveness in children under the age of 12 have not been established.

ADVERSE REACTIONS
Although rare, sodium sulfacetamide may cause local irritation.

DOSAGE AND ADMINISTRATION
Apply a thin film of Novacet Lotion to affected areas 1 to 3 times daily.

HOW SUPPLIED
30 g tubes (NDC 52761-530-30) and 60 g tubes (NDC 52761-530-60)
Store at controlled room temperature 15°–30°C (59°–86°F).

CAUTION
Federal law prohibits dispensing without prescription.

OCCLUSAL®-HP   OTC
[ŏ-kloo'sal]
Salicylic Acid, USP, 17%
Wart Remover
FOR EXTERNAL USE ONLY

DESCRIPTION
Occlusal-HP is a topical wart remover preparation containing 17% salicylic acid, in a polyacrylic vehicle containing ethyl acetate, isopropyl alcohol, butyl acetate, polyvinyl butyral, dibutyl phthalate, acrylates copolymer and nitrocellulose. The pharmacologic activity of Occlusal-HP is generally attributed to the keratolytic action of salicylic acid. The structural formula of salicylic acid is:

COOH
OH (on benzene ring)

CLINICAL PHARMACOLOGY
Although the exact mode of action of salicylic acid in the treatment of warts is not known, its activity appears to be associated with its keratolytic action which results in mechanical removal of epidermal cells infected with wart viruses.

INDICATIONS AND USAGE
Occlusal-HP is indicated for the treatment and removal of common and plantar warts. The common wart is easily recognized by the rough 'cauliflower-like' appearance of the surface. The plantar wart is recognized by its location only on the bottom of the foot, its tenderness, and the interruption of the footprint pattern.

WARNINGS
Occlusal-HP is for external use only. Occlusal-HP is flammable and should be kept away from fire or flame. Keep bottle

Continued on next page

GenDerm—Cont.

tightly capped and store at room temperature away from heat when not in use.

Occlusal-HP should not be used on irritated skin, on any area that is infected or reddened, if you are a diabetic or if you have poor blood circulation. Occlusal-HP should not be used on moles, birthmarks, warts with hair growing from them, genital warts, or warts on the face or mucous membranes. Do not permit Occlusal-HP to contact eyes or mucous membranes. If contact with eyes or mucous membranes occurs, immediately flush with water for 15 minutes. Occlusal-HP should not be allowed to contact normal skin surrounding warts. Treatment should be discontinued if excessive irritation occurs. If discomfort persists, see your doctor. Avoid inhaling vapors.

Keep this and all drugs out of the reach of children. In case of accidental ingestion, seek professional assistance or contact a Poison Control Center immediately.

ADVERSE REACTIONS

A localized irritant reaction may occur if Occlusal-HP is applied to the normal skin surrounding the wart. Any irritation may normally be controlled by temporarily discontinuing use of Occlusal-HP, and by applying the medication only to the wart site when treatment is resumed.

DIRECTIONS

Prior to application of Occlusal-HP, may soak wart in warm water for five minutes. Remove any loosened tissue by rubbing with a brush, wash cloth, or emery board. Dry area thoroughly. Using the brush applicator supplied, apply small amount at a time with brush to sufficiently cover each wart. Let dry and repeat application. Be careful not to apply to surrounding skin.

Repeat this procedure once or twice daily as needed (until wart is removed) for up to 12 weeks.

You should see improvement in 1 to 2 weeks. Maximum resolution may be expected after 4 to 6 weeks of daily Occlusal-HP use. If skin irritation develops or there is no improvement after several weeks, contact your physician.

HOW SUPPLIED

Occlusal-HP is supplied in a 10 mL bottle with brush applicator (NDC 52761-185-10)

Store at controlled room temperature 15°–30°C (59°–86°F).

PENTRAX®   OTC
[pen'trax]
Anti-dandruff Tar Shampoo

DESCRIPTION

Pentrax Tar Shampoo contains 7.71% w/w Fractar® an extract of coal tar, equivalent to Coal Tar 4.3%, a blend of highly concentrated detergents, and conditioning agents. Spectrophotometric standardization, based on hydrocarbon analysis, assures uniform therapeutic activity from batch to batch. Pentrax Tar Shampoo does not contain parabens or other preservatives. Pentrax Tar Shampoo contains the highest concentration of coal tar currently available. Fractar consists of the desirable crude coal tar fractions without undesirable residues. It has excellent lathering qualities and leaves hair clean and manageable.

ACTION AND INDICATIONS

Coal tar helps correct abnormalities of keratinization by decreasing epidermal proliferation and dermal infiltration. Pentrax Tar Shampoo is indicated for relief of itching, redness, and/or scaling associated with dandruff, seborrheic dermatitis and psoriasis of the scalp.

WARNINGS

FOR EXTERNAL USE ONLY. Avoid contact with the eyes. If contact occurs, rinse eyes thoroughly with water. Do not use for prolonged periods without consulting a physician. If condition worsens or does not improve after regular use of this product as directed, consult a physician. Use caution in exposing skin to sunlight after applying this product. It may increase your tendency to sunburn for up to 24 hours after application. Do not use this product with other forms of psoriasis therapy such as ultraviolet radiation or prescription drugs unless directed to do so by a doctor. If condition covers a large area of the body, consult your doctor before using this product. Keep this and all drugs out of the reach of children. In case of accidental ingestion, seek professional assistance or contact a Poison Control Center immediately.

DIRECTIONS

Massage into wet hair and scalp. Rinse. Reapply, leaving lather on hair and scalp for up to 10 minutes. Rinse thoroughly. For best results, use at least twice a week or as directed by a physician.

ACTIVE INGREDIENTS

Contains 7.71% w/w Fractar®, an extract of coal tar, equivalent to Coal Tar 4.3%.

INACTIVE INGREDIENTS

Sodium lauryl sulfate, laureth-23, cocamide DEA, lauramine oxide, PEG-8, dioctyl sodium sulfosuccinate.

HOW SUPPLIED

4 fl oz plastic bottle (NDC 52761-665-04)
8 fl oz plastic bottle (NDC 52761-665-08)

PRAMEGEL®   OTC
[pram'eh-gel]
Antipruritic

DESCRIPTION

PrameGel is an antipruritic containing pramoxine hydrochloride USP 1% and menthol USP 0.5% in a water soluble emollient base with a naturally derived humectant. PrameGel is paraben, propylene glycol and fragrance free.

INDICATIONS

For the prompt temporary relief of itching associated with mild eczemas (including poison ivy and poison oak), insect bites, heat rash, sunburn, and other pruritic skin conditions, as well as for external anal itching.

WARNINGS

FOR EXTERNAL USE ONLY

Avoid contact with eyes. If itching worsens or if symptoms persist for more than 7 days, discontinue use of this product and consult a physician. Stinging or burning may occur if applied to broken skin. Keep this and all drugs out of the reach of children. In case of accidental ingestion, seek professional assistance or contact a Poison Control Center immediately.

DIRECTIONS

Adults and children 2 years of age and older: Apply liberally to affected area no more than 3 to 4 times daily. Children under 2 years of age: Consult a physician.

ACTIVE INGREDIENTS

Pramoxine Hydrochloride 1% and Menthol 0.5%.

INACTIVE INGREDIENTS

Benzyl alcohol, carbomer 940, methyl gluceth-20, SD alcohol 40, sodium hydroxide and water.

HOW SUPPLIED

4 fl oz plastic bottle (NDC 52761-395-04).

SALAC®   OTC
[sal'ak]
Acne Medication Cleanser

DESCRIPTION

SalAc is an acne medication cleanser containing 2% salicylic acid USP in a surfactant blend especially formulated to remove excess sebum.

INDICATIONS

For the management of acne. Helps prevent new blackheads and whiteheads (comedones) and acne pimples (papules and pustules).

WARNINGS

For external use only.

Keep cleanser out of eyes. Using other topical acne medications at the same time or immediately following use of this product may increase dryness or irritation of the skin. If this occurs, only one medication should be used unless directed by a physician. Keep this and all drugs out of the reach of children. In case of accidental ingestion, seek professional assistance or contact a Poison Control Center immediately.

DIRECTIONS

Wash affected area 2 to 3 times daily. Lather with warm water and massage into skin. Rinse and dry.

ACTIVE INGREDIENT

Salicylic Acid, 2%

INACTIVE INGREDIENTS

Benzyl alcohol, lauramide DEA, PEG-7 glyceryl cocoate, polystyrene dispersion, purified water, sodium C_{14-16} olefin sulfonate and sodium chloride.

HOW SUPPLIED

6 fl oz plastic bottle (NDC 52761-077-06).

ZONALON® CREAM   ℞
[zŏn a lon]
(doxepin hydrochloride cream), 5%
FOR TOPICAL DERMATOLOGIC USE ONLY—
NOT FOR OPHTHALMIC, ORAL, OR INTRAVAGINAL USE.

DESCRIPTION

ZONALON CREAM (doxepin hydrochloride cream) is a topical antipruritic cream. Each gram contains: 50 mg of doxepin hydrochloride (equivalent to 44.3 mg of doxepin).

Doxepin hydrochloride is one of a class of agents known as dibenzoxepin tricyclic compounds. It is an isomeric mixture of

N,N-Dimethyldibenz[b,e]oxepin-$\Delta^{11(6H),\gamma}$-propylamine hydrochloride

Doxepin hydrochloride has an empirical formula of $C_{19}H_{21}NO \cdot HCl$ and a molecular weight of 316.

The base is a cream of pH 3.5 to 5.5 that includes the inactive ingredients: sorbitol, cetyl alcohol, isopropyl myristate, glyceryl stearate, PEG-100 stearate, petrolatum, benzyl alcohol, titanium dioxide, and purified water.

CLINICAL PHARMACOLOGY

The exact mechanism by which doxepin exerts its antipruritic effect is unknown. Doxepin HCl does have potent H1 and potent H2 receptor blocking actions. Histamine-blocking drugs appear to compete at histamine receptor sites and inhibit the biological activation of histamine receptors. In addition, doxepin produces drowsiness in significant numbers of patients. Sedation may have an effect on certain pruritic symptoms. In 19 pruritic eczema patients treated with ZONALON CREAM, PLASMA doxepin concentrations ranged from nondetectable to 47 ng/mL from percutaneous absorption. Target therapeutic plasma levels of ORAL doxepin HCl for the treatment of depression range from 30 to 150 ng/mL.

Once absorbed into the systemic circulation, doxepin undergoes hepatic metabolism that results in conversion to pharmacologically-active desmethyldoxepin. Further glucuronidation results in urinary excretion of the parent drug and its metabolites. Desmethyldoxepin has a half life reportedly that ranges from 28 to 52 hours and is not affected by multiple dosing. Plasma levels of both doxepin and desmethyldoxepin are highly variable and are poorly correlated with dosage. Wide distribution occurs in body tissues including lungs, heart, brain, and liver. Renal disease, genetic factors, age, and other medications affect the metabolism and subsequent elimination of doxepin. (See Precautions—Drug Interactions.)

INDICATIONS AND USAGE

ZONALON CREAM is indicated for the short-term (up to 8 days) management of moderate pruritus in adult patients with the following forms of eczematous dermatitis: atopic dermatitis and lichen simplex chronicus. (See Dosage and Administration.)

CONTRAINDICATIONS

Because doxepin HCl has an anticholinergic effect and because significant plasma levels of doxepin are detectable after topical ZONALON CREAM application, the use of ZONALON CREAM is contraindicated in patients with untreated narrow angle glaucoma or a tendency to urinary retention.

ZONALON CREAM is contraindicated in individuals who have shown previous sensitivity to any of its components.

WARNINGS

Drowsiness occurs in over 20% of patients treated with ZONALON CREAM, especially in patients receiving treatment to greater than 10% of their body surface area. Patients should be warned of this possibility and cautioned against driving a motor vehicle or operating hazardous machinery while being treated with ZONALON CREAM. Patients should also be warned that the effects of alcoholic beverages can be potentiated when using ZONALON CREAM.

If excessive drowsiness occurs it may be necessary to reduce the number of applications, the amount of cream applied, and/or the percentage of body surface area treated, or discontinue the drug.

Keep this product away from the eyes.

PRECAUTIONS

Drug Interactions

Studies have not been performed examining drug interactions with ZONALON CREAM. However, data are available regarding potentially significant drug interactions regarding doxepin. As plasma levels of doxepin similar to therapeutic ranges for antidepressant therapy can be obtained following topical application of ZONALON CREAM, it would not be unexpected for the following drug interactions to be possible following topical ZONALON CREAM application.

MAO Inhibitors

Serious side effects and even death have been reported following the concomitant use of certain orally administered

drugs chemically related to doxepin and MAO inhibitors. Therefore, MAO inhibitors should be discontinued at least two weeks prior to the initiation of treatment with ZONALON CREAM.

Cimetidine
Cimetidine has been reported to produce clinically significant fluctuations in steady-state serum concentrations of various tricyclic antidepressants. Serious anticholinergic symptoms have been associated with elevations in the serum levels of tricyclic antidepressants when cimetidine therapy is initiated. Additionally, higher than expected tricyclic antidepressant levels have been observed in patients already taking cimetidine. In patients who have been reported to be well-controlled on tricyclic antidepressants receiving concurrent cimetidine therapy, discontinuation of cimetidine has been reported to decrease established steady-state serum tricyclic antidepressant levels and compromise their therapeutic effects.

Alcohol
Alcohol ingestion may exacerbate the potential sedative effects of ZONALON CREAM.

Drugs Metabolized by P$_{450}$IID6
A subset (3% to 10%) of the population has reduced activity of certain drug metabolizing enzymes such as the cytochrome P$_{450}$ isozyme P$_{450}$IID6. Such individuals are referred to as "poor metabolizers" of drug such as debrisoquin, dextromethorphan, and the tricyclic antidepressants. These individuals may have higher than expected plasma concentrations of tricyclic antidepressant when given usual doses. In addition, certain drugs that are metabolized by this isozyme, including many antidepressants (tricyclic antidepressants, selective serotonin reuptake inhibitors, and others), may inhibit the activity of this isozyme, and thus may make normal metabolizers resemble poor metabolizers with regard to concomitant therapy with other drugs metabolized by this enzyme system, leading to drug interactions.
Concomitant use of tricyclic antidepressants with other drugs metabolized by cytochrome P$_{450}$IID6 may require lower doses than usually prescribed for either the tricyclic antidepressant or the other drug. Therefore, co-administration of tricyclic antidepressants with other drugs that are metabolized by this isoenzyme, including other antidepressants, phenothiazines, carbamazepine, and Type 1C antiarrhythmics (e.g., propafenone, flecainide and encainide), or that inhibit this enzyme (e.g., quinidine), should be approached with caution. Concomitant use of ZONALON CREAM with drugs metabolized by cytochrome P$_{450}$IID6 has not been formally studied.

Carcinogenesis, Mutagenesis, Impairment of Fertility
Carcinogenesis, mutagenesis, and impairment of fertility studies have not been conducted with doxepin hydrochloride.

Pregnancy Pregnancy Category B:
Teratology studies have been performed in rats and rabbits at oral doses up to 8 times the topical human dose (based on a mg/kg basis) and have revealed no evidence of impaired fertility or harm to the fetus due to doxepin. There are, however, no adequate and well-controlled studies in pregnant women. Because animal reproduction studies are not always predictive of human response, this drug should be used during pregnancy only if clearly needed.

Nursing Mothers
Doxepin is excreted in human milk after oral administration. There have been no studies conducted to date to determine if doxepin is excreted in human milk after topical administration; however, it is known that significant systemic levels of doxepin are obtained after topical administration. It is therefore possible that doxepin could be secreted in human milk following topical administration.
One case has been reported of apnea and drowsiness in a nursing infant whose mother was taking an oral dosage form of doxepin HCl.
Because of the potential for serious adverse reactions in nursing infants from doxepin, a decision should be made whether to discontinue nursing or to discontinue the drug, taking into account the importance of the drug to the mother.

Pediatric Use
Safety and effectiveness of ZONALON CREAM in children have not been established.

ADVERSE REACTIONS
CONTROLLED CLINICAL TRIALS:
Systemic Adverse Effects:
In controlled clinical trials of patients treated with ZONALON CREAM, the most common systemic adverse effect reported was drowsiness. Drowsiness occurred in 22% of patients treated with ZONALON CREAM (and 2% of patients treated with placebo cream) and resulted in the premature discontinuation of the drug in approximately 5% of patients treated.
Other systemic adverse effects reported in approximately 1 to 10% of these patients included:
Dry mouth, dry lips, thirst, headache, fatigue, dizziness, emotional changes, and taste changes.
Other systemic adverse effects reported in less than 1% of these patients included:

Nausea, anxiety, and fever.
Local Site Adverse Effects:
In controlled clinical trials of patients treated with ZONALON CREAM, the most common local site adverse effect reported was burning and/or stinging at the site of application. These occurred in approximately 21% of these patients. Most of these reactions were categorized as "mild"; however, approximately 25% of patients who reported burning and/or stinging reported the reaction as "severe". Four patients treated with ZONALON CREAM withdrew from the study because of the burning and/or stinging.
Other local site adverse effects reported in approximately 1 to 10% of these patients included:
Pruritus exacerbation, eczema exacerbation, dryness and tightness to skin, paresthesias, and edema.
Other local site adverse effects reported in less than 1% of these patients included:
Irritation, tingling, scaling, and cracking.

OVERDOSAGE
Overdosage with a topical product is unlikely, should it occur, the signs and symptoms include:
Mild: Drowsiness, stupor, blurred vision, excessive dryness of mouth.
Severe: Respiratory depression, hypotension, coma, convulsions, cardiac arrhythmias and tachycardias. Also, urinary retention (bladder atony), decreased gastrointestinal motility (paralytic ileus), hyperthermia (or hypothermia), hypertension, dilated pupils, hyperactive reflexes.
Management and Treatment
Mild: Observation and supportive therapy is all that is usually necessary. It may be necessary to reduce the percent of body surface area treated or the frequency of application or apply a thinner layer of cream.
Severe: Medical management of severe doxepin overdosage consists of aggressive supportive therapy. The area covered with doxepin HCl cream should be thoroughly washed. An adequate airway should be established in comatose patients and assisted ventilation used if necessary. EKG monitoring may be required for several days, because relapse after apparent recovery has been reported with oral doxepin HCl. Arrhythmias should be treated with the appropriate antiarrhythmic agent. It has been reported that many of the cardiovascular and CNS symptoms of tricyclic antidepressant poisoning in adults may be reversed by the slow intravenous administration of 1 mg to 3 mg of physostigmine salicylate. Because physostigmine is rapidly metabolized, the dosage should be repeated as required. Convulsions may respond to standard anticonvulsant therapy; however, **barbiturates may potentiate any respiratory depression.**
Dialysis and forced diuresis generally are not of value in the management of overdosage due to high tissue and protein binding of doxepin HCl.

DOSAGE AND ADMINISTRATION
A thin film of ZONALON CREAM should be applied four times each day with at least a 3 to 4 hour interval between applications. There are no data to establish the safety and effectivness of ZONALON CREAM when used for greater than 8 days. Chronic use beyond eight days may result in higher systemic levels.
Clinical experience has shown that **drowsiness is significantly more common in patients applying ZONALON CREAM to over 10% of body surface area;** therefore, patients with greater than 10% of body surface area affected should be particularly cautioned concerning possible drowsiness and other systemic adverse effects of doxepin. If excessive drowsiness occurs it may be necessary to do one or more of the following: reduce the body surface area treated, reduce the number of applications per day, reduce the amount of cream applied, or discontinue the drug.
Occlusive dressings may increase absorption of most topical drugs; therefore, occlusive dressings with ZONALON CREAM should not be utilized.

HOW SUPPLIED
ZONALON CREAM is available in 30g (NDC 52761-523-30) and 45g (NDC 52761-523-45) aluminum tubes. Store at or below 27°C (80°F).

CAUTION
Federal law prohibits dispensing without prescription.

ZOSTRIX®   OTC
Purified capsaicin 0.025%
ZOSTRIX-HP
High Potency
Purified capsaicin 0.075%
TOPICAL ANALGESIC CREAM

PRODUCT OVERVIEW

KEY FACTS
Zostrix and Zostrix-HP contain purified capsaicin. Although the precise mechanism of action of capsaicin is not fully understood, current evidence suggests that capsaicin renders skin and joints insensitive to pain by depleting and preventing reaccumulation of substance P in peripheral sensory neurons.

MAJOR USES
Zostrix and Zostrix-HP have proven to be clinically effective in the relief of pain from arthritis and neuralgias such as painful diabetic neuropathy and postherpetic neuralgia.

SAFETY INFORMATION
Patients may experience a warm, stinging, or burning sensation at the site of application, especially during the initial few days of use. This effect is related to the pharmacologic action of capsaicin. Avoid contact with eyes, contact lenses or broken (open) or irritated skin. Thick applications of Zostrix/Zostrix-HP should be avoided. The cream should be massaged into the skin until no residue remains. Inhalation of dried cream residue can cause coughing, sneezing or respiratory irritation.

PRESCRIBING INFORMATION

ZOSTRIX®
(Capsaicin 0.025%)
ZOSTRIX®-HP
High Potency
(Capsaicin 0.075%)
TOPICAL ANALGESIC CREAM

DESCRIPTION
Zostrix/Zostrix-HP contain capsaicin in an emollient base containing benzyl alcohol, cetyl alcohol, glyceryl monostearate, isopropyl myristate, PEG-100 stearate, purified water, sorbitol solution and white petrolatum.

INDICATION
Zostrix/Zostrix-HP are indicated for the temporary relief of pain from arthritis. For use in painful neuralgias, consult a physician.

WARNINGS
FOR EXTERNAL USE ONLY. Avoid contact with eyes and broken or irritated skin. Do not bandage tightly. If condition worsens, or does not improve after 7 days, discontinue use of this product and consult your physician. **Keep this and all drugs out of the reach of children. In case of accidental ingestion, seek professional assistance or contact a Poison Control Center immediately.**

DIRECTIONS
Adults and children 2 years of age and older: Apply a thin film of Zostrix/Zostrix-HP to affected area 3 to 4 times daily. For children under 2 years of age, consult a physician. A passing burning sensation may occur upon application, but generally disappears in several days. Application schedules of less than 3 to 4 times a day may not provide optimum pain relief and the burning sensation may persist. Unless treating hands, wash hands after application.

HOW SUPPLIED
Zostrix 2.0-oz tube
(NDC 52761-552-02)
Zostrix-HP 2.0-oz tube
(NDC 52761-501-02)
Store at room temperature. 15°–30°C (59°–86°F).
U.S. Patents No. 4486450, 4536404

Genentech, Inc.
460 POINT SAN BRUNO BLVD.
SOUTH SAN FRANCISCO, CA 94080-4990

For Medical Information Contact:
Medical Information or Drug Experience Departments (24 hours):
(800) 821-8590
(415) 225-1000

Or write:
Medical Information or Drug Experience Departments
Genetech, Inc.
460 Point San Bruno Blvd.
South San Francisco, CA 94080

ACTIMMUNE®   ℞
(Interferon gamma-1b)
Injection

DESCRIPTION
ACTIMMUNE® (Interferon gamma-1b), a biologic response modifier, is a single-chain polypeptide containing 140 amino acids. Production of ACTIMMUNE is achieved by fermentation of a genetically engineered *Escherichia coli* bacterium containing the DNA which encodes for the human protein.

Continued on next page

Genentech—Cont.

Purification of the product is achieved by conventional column chromatography. ACTIMMUNE is a highly purified sterile solution consisting of non-covalent dimers of two identical 16,465 dalton monomers; with a specific activity of 30 million U/mg.

ACTIMMUNE (Interferon gamma-1b) is a sterile, clear, colorless solution filled in a single-dose vial for subcutaneous injection. Each 0.5 mL of ACTIMMUNE contains: **100 mcg (3 million U)** of Interferon gamma-1b formulated in 20 mg mannitol, 0.36 mg sodium succinate, 0.05 mg polysorbate 20 and Sterile Water for Injection.

CLINICAL PHARMACOLOGY

General

Interferons are a family of functionally related, species-specific proteins synthesized by eukaryotic cells in response to viruses and a variety of natural and synthetic stimuli. The most striking differences between interferon-gamma and other classes of interferon concern the immunomodulatory properties of this molecule. While gamma, alpha and beta interferons share certain properties, interferon-gamma has potent phagocyte-activating effects not seen with other interferon preparations. These effects include the generation of toxic oxygen metabolites within phagocytes, which are capable of mediating the killing of microorganisms such as *Staphylococcus aureus, Toxoplasma gondii, Leishmania donovani, Listeria monocytogenes,* and *Mycobacterium avium intracellulare.*

Clinical studies in patients using interferon-gamma have revealed a broad range of biological activities including the enhancement of the oxidative metabolism of tissue macrophages, enhancement of antibody-dependent cellular cytotoxicity (ADCC) and natural killer (NK) cell activity. Additionally, effects on Fc receptor expression on monocytes and major histocompatibility antigen expression have been noted.[1,2]

To the extent that interferon-gamma is produced by antigen-stimulated T lymphocytes and regulates the activity of immune cells, it is appropriate to characterize interferon-gamma as a lymphokine of the interleukin type. There is growing evidence that interferon-gamma interacts functionally with other interleukin molecules such as interleukin-2 and that all of the interleukins form part of a complex, lymphokine regulatory network.[3] For example, interferon-gamma and interleukin-4 appear to reciprocally interact to regulate murine IgE levels; interferon-gamma can suppress IgE levels in humans.[4,5] Interferon-gamma also inhibits the production of collagen at the transcription level in human systems.[6]

More specifically, with respect to Chronic Granulomatous Disease (an inherited disorder characterized by deficient phagocyte oxidative metabolism), pilot clinical trials of the systemic administration of ACTIMMUNE in patients with Chronic Granulomatous Disease were initiated which provided evidence for a treatment-related enhancement of phagocyte function including elevation of superoxide levels and improved killing of *Staphylococcus aureus.*[7,8] Based on this evidence, a randomized, double-blind, placebo-controlled clinical study was initiated to further delineate the effects of ACTIMMUNE in Chronic Granulomatous Disease.

Pharmacokinetics

The intravenous, intramuscular, and subcutaneous pharmacokinetics of ACTIMMUNE have been investigated in 24 healthy male subjects following single-dose administration of 100 mcg/m^2. ACTIMMUNE is rapidly cleared after intravenous administration (1.4 liters/minute) and slowly absorbed after intramuscular or subcutaneous injection. After intramuscular or subcutaneous injection, the apparent fraction of dose absorbed was greater than 89%. The mean elimination half-life after intravenous administration of 100 mcg/m^2 in healthy male subjects was 38 minutes. The mean elimination half-lives for intramuscular and subcutaneous dosing with 100 mcg/m^2 were 2.9 and 5.9 hours, respectively. Peak plasma concentrations, determined by ELISA, occurred approximately 4 hours (1.5 ng/mL) after intramuscular dosing and 7 hours (0.6 ng/mL) after subcutaneous dosing. Multiple dose subcutaneous pharmacokinetic studies were conducted in 38 healthy male subjects. There was no accumulation of ACTIMMUNE after 12 consecutive daily injections of 100 mcg/m^2. Pharmacokinetic studies in patients with Chronic Granulomatous Disease have not been performed.

Excretion studies of ACTIMMUNE have been performed. Trace amounts of interferon-gamma were detected in the urine of squirrel monkeys following intravenous administration of 500 mcg/kg. Interferon-gamma was not detected in the urine of healthy human volunteers following administration of 100 mcg/m^2 of ACTIMMUNE by the intravenous, intramuscular and subcutaneous routes. *In vitro* perfusion studies utilizing rabbit livers and kidneys demonstrate that these organs are capable of clearing interferon-gamma from perfusate. Studies of the administration of interferon-gamma to nephrectomized mice and squirrel monkeys demonstrate a reduction in clearance of interferon-gamma from blood; however, prior nephrectomy did not prevent elimination.

Effects of Chronic Granulomatous Disease

A randomized, double-blind, placebo-controlled study of ACTIMMUNE in patients with Chronic Granulomatous Disease, was performed to determine whether ACTIMMUNE administered subcutaneously on a three times weekly schedule could decrease the incidence of serious infectious episodes and improve existing infectious and inflammatory conditions in patients with Chronic Granulomatous Disease. One hundred twenty-eight eligible patients were enrolled on this study including patients with different patterns of inheritance. Most patients received prophylactic antibiotics. Patients ranged in age from 1 to 44 years with the mean age being 14.6 years. The study was terminated early following demonstration of a highly statistically significant benefit of ACTIMMUNE® (Interferon gamma-1b) therapy compared to placebo with respect to time to serious infection ($p=0.0036$), the primary endpoint of the investigation. Serious infection was defined as a clinical event requiring hospitalization and the use of parenteral antibiotics. The final analysis provided further support for the primary endpoint ($p=0.0006$). There was a 67 percent reduction in relative risk of serious infection in patients receiving ACTIMMUNE ($n=63$) compared to placebo ($n=65$). Additional supportive evidence of treatment benefit included a twofold reduction in the number of primary serious infections in the ACTIMMUNE group (30 on placebo versus 14 on ACTIMMUNE, $p=0.002$) and the total number and rate of serious infections including recurrent events (56 on placebo versus 20 on ACTIMMUNE, $p= <0.0001$). Moreover, the length of hospitalization for the treatment of all clinical events provided evidence highly supportive of an ACTIMMUNE treatment benefit. Placebo patients required three times as many inpatient hospitalization days for treatment of clinical events compared to patients receiving ACTIMMUNE (1493 versus 497 total days, $p=0.02$). An ACTIMMUNE treatment benefit with respect to time to serious infection was consistently demonstrated in all subgroup analyses according to stratification factors, including pattern of inheritance, use of prophylactic antibiotics, as well as age. There was a 67 percent reduction in relative risk of serious infection in patients receiving ACTIMMUNE compared to placebo across all groups. The beneficial effect of ACTIMMUNE therapy was observed throughout the entire study, in which the mean duration of ACTIMMUNE administration was 8.9 months/patient.

INDICATIONS AND USAGE

ACTIMMUNE is indicated for reducing the frequency and severity of serious infections associated with Chronic Granulomatous Disease. The safety and effectiveness in children under the age of 1 year has not been established.

CONTRAINDICATIONS

ACTIMMUNE is contraindicated in patients who develop or have known hypersensitivity to interferon-gamma, *E. coli* derived products, or any component of the product.

WARNINGS

ACTIMMUNE should be used with caution in patients with pre-existing cardiac disease, including symptoms of ischemia, congestive heart failure or arrhythmia. No direct cardiotoxic effect has been demonstrated but it is possible that acute and transient "flu-like" or constitutional symptoms such as fever and chills frequently associated with ACTIMMUNE administration at doses of 250 mcg/m^2/day or higher may exacerbate pre-existing cardiac conditions.

Caution should be exercised when treating patients with known seizure disorders and or compromised central nervous system function. Central nervous system adverse reactions including decreased mental status, gait disturbance and dizziness have been observed, particularly in patients receiving doses greater than 250 mcg/m^2/day. Most of these abnormalities were mild and reversible within a few days upon dose reduction or discontinuation of therapy.

Caution should be exercised when administering ACTIMMUNE to patients with myelosuppression. Reversible neutropenia and elevation of hepatic enzymes can be dose limiting above 250mcg/m^2/day. Thrombocytopenia and proteinuria have also been seen rarely.

PRECAUTIONS

General

Acute serious hypersensitivity reactions have not been observed in patients receiving ACTIMMUNE; however, if such an acute reaction develops the drug should be discontinued immediately and appropriate medical therapy instituted. Transient cutaneous rashes have occurred in some patients following injection but have rarely necessitated treatment interruption.

Information for Patients

Patients being treated with ACTIMMUNE and/or their parents should be informed regarding the potential benefits and risks associated with treatment. If home use is determined to be desirable by the physician, instructions on appropriate use should be given, including review of the contents of the Patient Information Insert. This information is intended to aid in the safe and effective use of the medication. It is not a disclosure of all possible adverse or intended effects.

If home use is prescribed, a puncture resistant container for the disposal of used syringes and needles should be supplied to the patient. Patients should be thoroughly instructed in the importance of proper disposal and cautioned against any reuse of needles and syringes. The full container should be disposed of according to the directions provided by the physician (see Patient Information Insert).

The most common adverse experiences occurring with ACTIMMUNE therapy are "flu-like" or constitutional symptoms such as fever, headache, chills, myalgia or fatigue (see ADVERSE REACTIONS Section) which may decrease in severity as treatment continues. Some of the "flu-like" symptoms may be minimized by bedtime administration. Acetaminophen may be used to prevent or partially alleviate the fever and headache.

The long-term effects of ACTIMMUNE therapy on growth, development or other parameters, are not known.

Laboratory Tests

In addition to those tests normally required for monitoring patients with Chronic Granulomatous Disease, the following laboratory tests are recommended for all patients on ACTIMMUNE therapy prior to the beginning of and at three month intervals during treatment.

- Hematologic tests—including complete blood counts, differential and platelet counts.
- Blood chemistries—including renal and liver function tests.
- Urinalysis.

Drug Interactions

Interactions between ACTIMMUNE® (Interferon gamma-1b) and other drugs have not been fully evaluated. Caution should be exercised when administering ACTIMMUNE in combination with other potentially myelosuppressive agents (see WARNINGS).

Preclinical studies in rodents using species-specific interferon-gamma have demonstrated a decrease in hepatic microsomal cytochrome P-450 concentrations. This could potentially lead to a depression of the hepatic metabolism of certain drugs that utilize this degradative pathway.

Carcinogenesis, Mutagenesis, and Impairment of Fertility

Carcinogenesis: ACTIMMUNE has not been tested for its carcinogenic potential.

Mutagenesis: Ames tests using five different tester strains of bacteria with and without metabolic activation revealed no evidence of mutagenic potential. ACTIMMUNE was tested in a micronucleus assay for its ability to induce chromosomal damage in bone marrow cells of mice following two intravenous doses of 20 mg/kg. No evidence of chromosomal damage was noted.

Impairment of Fertility: Female cynomolgus monkeys treated with daily subcutaneous doses of 150 mcg/kg ACTIMMUNE (approximately 100 times the human dose) exhibited irregular menstrual cycles or absence of cyclicity during treatment. Similar findings were not observed in animals treated with 3 or 30 mcg/kg ACTIMMUNE. No studies have been performed assessing any potential effects of ACTIMMUNE on male fertility.

Pregnancy

Teratogenic Effects: Pregnancy Category C. ACTIMMUNE has shown an increased incidence of abortions in primates when given in doses approximately 100 × the human dose. A study in pregnant primates treated with intravenous doses 2-100 × the human dose failed to demonstrate teratogenic activity for ACTIMMUNE. There are no adequate and well-controlled studies in pregnant women. ACTIMMUNE should be used during pregnancy only if the potential benefit justifies the potential risk to the fetus. In addition, studies evaluating recombinant murine interferon-gamma in pregnant mice, revealed increased incidences of uterine bleeding and abortifacient activity and decreased neonatal viability at maternally toxic doses. The clinical significance of this latter observation with recombinant murine interferon-gamma tested in a homologus system is uncertain.

Nursing Mothers

It is not known whether ACTIMMUNE is excreted in human milk. Because many drugs are excreted in human milk and because of the potential for serious adverse reactions in nursing infants from ACTIMMUNE, a decision should be made whether to discontinue nursing or to discontinue the drug, dependent upon the importance of the drug to the mother.

Pediatric Use

Safety and effectiveness in children under the age of 1 year has not been established.

ADVERSE REACTIONS

The following data on adverse reactions are based on the subcutaneous administration of ACTIMMUNE at a dose of 50 mcg/m^2, three times weekly, in 63 patients with Chronic Granulomatous Disease during an investigational trial in the United States and Europe. Sixty-five additional patients with Chronic Granulomatous Disease received placebo on this study. The following table represents the percentage of

patients experiencing common adverse reactions observed on this study.

| Clinical Toxicity | Percent of Patients | |
	ACTIMMUNE	Placebo
Fever	52	28
Headache	33	9
Rash	17	6
Chills	14	0
Injection site erythema or tenderness	14	2
Fatigue	14	11
Diarrhea	14	12
Vomiting	13	5
Nausea	10	2
Weight loss	6	6
Myalgia	6	0
Anorexia	3	5
Arthralgia	2	0
Injection site pain	0	2

Miscellaneous adverse events which occurred infrequently and may have been related to underlying disease included back pain (2 percent versus 0 percent), abdominal pain (8 percent versus 3 percent) and depression (3 percent versus 0 percent) for ACTIMMUNE and placebo treated patients, respectively.

ACTIMMUNE has also been evaluated in additional disease states in studies in which patients have generally received higher doses ($>100 \text{ mcg/m}^2$/day) administered by intramuscular injection or intravenous infusion. All of the previously described adverse reactions which occurred in patients with Chronic Granulomatous Disease have also been observed in patients receiving higher doses. Adverse reactions not observed in patients with Chronic Granulomatous Disease receiving doses less than 100 mcg/m^2/day but seen rarely in patients receiving ACTIMMUNE in other studies include: *Cardiovascular*—hypotension, syncope, tachyarrhythmia, heart block, heart failure, and myocardial infarction. *Central Nervous System*—confusion, disorientation, gait disturbance, Parkinsonian symptoms, seizure, hallucinations, and transient ischemic attacks. *Gastrointestinal*—hepatic insufficiency, gastrointestinal bleeding, and pancreatitis. *Renal*—reversible renal insufficiency. *Hematologic*—deep venous thrombosis and pulmonary embolism. *Pulmonary*—tachypnea, bronchospasm, and interstitial pneumonitis. *Metabolic*—hyponatremia and hyperglycemia. *Other*—exacerbation of dermatomyositis.

Abnormal Laboratory Test Values: No statistically significant differences between the ACTIMMUNE® (Interferon gamma-1b) and placebo treatment groups were observed with regard to effect of treatment on hematologic, coagulation, hepatic and renal laboratory studies.

No neutralizing antibodies to ACTIMMUNE have been detected in any Chronic Granulomatous Disease patient receiving ACTIMMUNE.

DOSAGE AND ADMINISTRATION

The recommended dosage of ACTIMMUNE (Interferon gamma-1b) for the treatment of patients with Chronic Granulomatous Disease is 50 mcg/m^2 (1.5 million U/m²) for patients whose body surface area is greater than 0.5m² and 1.5 mcg/kg/dose for patients whose body surface area is equal to or less than 0.5 m². Injections should be administered subcutaneously three times weekly (for example, Monday, Wednesday, Friday). The optimum sites of injection are the right and left deltoid and anterior thigh. ACTIMMUNE can be administered by a physician, nurse, family member or patient when trained in the administration of subcutaneous injections. Parenteral drug products should be inspected visually for particulate matter and discoloration prior to administration, whenever solution and container permit.

The formulation does not contain a preservative. A vial of ACTIMMUNE is suitable for a single dose only. The unused portion of any vial should be discarded.

Higher doses are not recommended. Safety and efficacy has not been established for ACTIMMUNE given in doses greater or less than the recommended dose of 50 mcg/m^2. The minimum effective dose of ACTIMMUNE has not been established.

If severe reactions occur, the dosage should be modified (50 percent reduction) or therapy should be discontinued until the adverse reaction abates.

ACTIMMUNE (Interferon gamma-1b) may be administered using either sterilized glass or plastic disposable syringes.

HOW SUPPLIED

ACTIMMUNE® (Interferon gamma-1b) is a sterile, clear, colorless solution filled in a single-dose vial for subcutaneous injection. Each 0.5 mL of ACTIMMUNE contains: **100 mcg (3 million U)** of Interferon gamma-1b, formulated in 20 mg mannitol, 0.36 mg sodium succinate, 0.05 mg polysorbate 20 and Sterile Water for Injection.

Single vial (NDC 50242-052-14)
Cartons of 12 (NDC 50242-052-23)

Stability and Storage

Vials of ACTIMMUNE (Interferon gamma-1b) must be placed in a 2–8°C (36–46°F) refrigerator immediately upon receipt to insure optimal retention of physical and biochemical integrity. DO NOT FREEZE. Avoid excessive or vigorous agitation. DO NOT SHAKE. An unentered vial of ACTIMMUNE should not be left at room temperature for a total time exceeding 12 hours prior to use. Vials exceeding this time period should not be returned to the refrigerator; such vials should be discarded.

Do not use beyond the expiration date stamped on the vial.

REFERENCES

1. Maluish AE, Urba WJ, Longo DL, *et al:* The determination of an immunologically active dose of interferon gamma in patients with melanoma. J Clin Onc 6: 434–445, 1988.
2. Nathan CF, Kaplan G, Levis W, *et al:* Local and systemic effects of intradermal recombinant interferon gamma in patients with lepromatous leprosy. NEJM 315: 6–11, 1986.
3. Fauci AS, Rosenberg SA, Sherwin SA, *et al:* Immunomodulators in clinical medicine. Ann Internal Med. 106: 421–433, 1987.
4. Snapper CM, Paul WE: Interferon-gamma and B cell stimulatory factor-1 reciprocally regulate Ig isotype production. Science 236: 944–947, 1987.
5. King CL, Gallin JI, Malech HL, *et al:* Regulation of immunoglobulin production in hyperimmunoglobulin E recurrent-infection syndrome by interferon gamma. PNAS USA 86: 10085–10089, 1989.
6. Rosenbloom J, Feldman G, Freundlich B, Jimenez SA: Inhibition of excessive scleroderma fibroblast collagen production by recombinant gamma-interferon. Arth Rheum 29: 851–856, 1986.
7. Ezekowitz RAB, Dinauer MC, Jaffe HS, *et al:* Partial correction of the phagocyte defect in patients with X-linked chronic granulomatous disease by subcutaneous interferon gamma. NEJM 319: 146–151, 1988.
8. Sechler JMG, Malech HL, White CJ, Gallin JI: Recombinant human interferon-gamma reconstitutes defective phagocyte function in patients with chronic granulomatous disease of childhood. PNAS USA 85: 4874–4878, 1988.

ACTIMMUNE®
(Interferon gamma-1b)
Injection
Manufactured by
GENENTECH, INC.   G48026-R1
460 Point San Bruno Blvd.   Revised December, 1995
South San Francisco, CA 94080   ©1995 Genentech, Inc.
Shown in Product Identification Guide, page 311

ACTIVASE®   ℞
Alteplase
recombinant

DESCRIPTION

Activase®, Alteplase, is a tissue plasminogen activator produced by recombinant DNA technology. It is a sterile, purified glycoprotein of 527 amino acids. It is synthesized using the complementary DNA (cDNA) for natural human tissue-type plasminogen activator obtained from a human melanoma cell line. The manufacturing process involves the secretion of the enzyme alteplase into the culture medium by an established mammalian cell line (Chinese Hamster Ovary cells) into which the cDNA for alteplase has been genetically inserted. Fermentation is carried out in a nutrient medium containing the antibiotic gentamycin, 100 mg/L. However, the presence of the antibiotic is not detectable in the final product.

Phosphoric acid and/or sodium hydroxide may be used prior to lyophilization for pH adjustment.

Activase is a sterile, white to off-white, lyophilized powder for intravenous administration after reconstitution with Sterile Water for Injection, USP.

[See table below.]

Biological potency is determined by an in vitro clot lysis assay and is expressed in International Units as tested against the WHO standard. The specific activity of Activase is 580,000 IU/mg.

CLINICAL PHARMACOLOGY

Activase is an enzyme (serine protease) which has the property of fibrin-enhanced conversion of plasminogen to plasmin. It produces limited conversion of plasminogen in the absence of fibrin. When introduced into the systemic circulation at pharmacologic concentration, Activase binds to fibrin in a thrombus and converts the entrapped plasminogen to plasmin. This initiates local fibrinolysis with limited systemic proteolysis. Following administration of 100 mg Activase, there is a decrease (16%–36%) in circulating fibrinogen.[1,2] In a controlled trial, 8 of 73 patients (11%) receiving Activase (1.25 mg/kg body weight over 3 hours) experienced a decrease in fibrinogen to below 100 mg/dL.[2]

The clearance of Alteplase in AMI patients has shown that it is rapidly cleared from the plasma with an initial half-life of less than 5 minutes. There is no difference in the dominant initial plasma half-life between the 3-Hour and accelerated regimens for AMI. The plasma clearance of Alteplase is 380–570 mL/min.[3,4] The clearance is mediated primarily by the liver. The initial volume of distribution approximates plasma volume.

Acute Myocardial Infarction (AMI) Patients

Coronary occlusion due to a thrombus is present in the infarct-related coronary artery in approximately 80% of patients experiencing a transmural myocardial infarction evaluated within 4 hours of onset of symptoms.[5,6]

Two Activase dose regimens have been studied in patients experiencing acute myocardial infarction. (Please see DOSAGE AND ADMINISTRATION.) The comparative efficacy of these two regimens has not been evaluated.

Accelerated Infusion in AMI Patients

Accelerated infusion of Activase was studied in an international, multi-center trial (GUSTO) that randomized 41,021 patients with acute myocardial infarction to four thrombolytic regimens. Entry criteria included onset of chest pain within 6 hours of treatment and ST segment elevation of ECG. The regimens included accelerated infusion of Activase (≤100 mg over 90 minutes, see DOSAGE AND ADMINISTRATION) plus intravenous (IV) heparin (accelerated infusion of Alteplase, n=10,396), or the Kabikinase brand of Streptokinase (1.5 million units over 60 minutes) plus IV heparin (SK [IV], n=10,410), or Streptokinase (as above) plus subcutaneous (SQ) heparin (SK [SQ], n=9841). A fourth regimen combined Alteplase and Streptokinase. Aspirin and heparin use was directed by the GUSTO study protocol as follows: All patients were to receive 160 mg chewable aspirin administered as soon as possible, followed by 160–325 mg daily. IV heparin was directed to be a 5000 U IV bolus initiated as soon as possible, followed by a 1000 U/hour continuous IV infusion for at least 48 hours; subsequent heparin therapy was at the discretion of the attending physician. SQ heparin was directed to be 12,500 U administered 4 hours after initiation of SK therapy, followed by 12,500 U twice daily for 7 days or until discharge, whichever came first. Many of the patients randomized to receive SQ heparin received some IV heparin, usually in response to recurrent chest pain and/or the need for a medical procedure. Some received IV heparin on arrival to the emergency room prior to enrollment and randomization.

Results for the primary endpoint of the study, 30-day mortality, are shown in Table 1. The incidence of 30-day mortality for accelerated infusion of Alteplase was 1.0% lower than for SK (IV) and 1.0% lower than for SK (SQ). The secondary endpoints of combined 30-day mortality or nonfatal stroke, and 24-hour mortality, as well as the safety endpoints of total stroke and intracerebral hemorrhage are also shown in Table 1. The incidence of combined 30-day mortality or nonfatal stroke for the Alteplase accelerated infusion was 1.0% lower than for SK (IV) and 0.8% lower than for SK (SQ).

[See Table 1 at bottom of next page.]

Subgroup analysis of patients by age, infarct location, time from symptom onset to thrombolytic treatment, and treatment in the U.S. or elsewhere showed consistently lower 30-day mortality for the Alteplase accelerated infusion group. For patients who were over 75 years of age, a predefined subgroup consisting of 12% of patients enrolled, the incidence of stroke was 4.0% for the Alteplase accelerated infusion group, 2.8% for SK (IV), and 3.2% for SK (SQ); the incidence of combined 30-day mortality or nonfatal stroke was 20.6%

Quantitative Composition of the Lyophilized Product

	100 mg Vial	50 mg Vial
Alteplase	100 mg (58 million IU)	50 mg (29 million IU)
L-Arginine	3.5 g	1.7 g
Phosphoric Acid	1 g	0.5 g
Polysorbate 80	less than or equal to 11 mg	less than or equal to 4 mg
Vacuum	No	Yes

Continued on next page

Genentech—Cont.

for accelerated infusion of Alteplase, 21.5% for SK (IV), and 22.0% for SK (SQ).

An angiographic substudy of the GUSTO trial provided data on infarct-related artery patency. Table 2 presents 90-minute, 180-minute, 24 hour, and 5–7 day patency values by TIMI flow grade for the three treatment regimens. Reocclusion rates were similar for all three treatment regimens. [See Table 2 at right.]

The safety and efficacy of the accelerated infusion of Alteplase have not been evaluated using antithrombotic or antiplatelet regimens other than those used in the GUSTO trial.

3-Hour Infusion in AMI Patients

In patients studied in a controlled trial with coronary angiography at 90 and 120 minutes following infusion of Activase, infarct artery patency was observed in 71% and 85% of patients (n=85), respectively.[2] In a second study, where patients received coronary angiography prior to and following infusion of Activase within 6 hours of the onset of symptoms, reperfusion of the obstructed vessel occurred within 90 minutes after the commencement of therapy in 71% of 83 patients.[1]

In a double-blind, randomized trial (138 patients) comparing Activase to placebo, patients infused with Activase within 4 hours of onset of symptoms experienced improved left ventricular function at day 10 compared to the placebo group, when ejection fraction was measured by gated blood pool scan (53.2% vs 46.4%, p=0.018). Relative to baseline (day 1) values, the net changes in ejection fraction were +3.6% and −4.7% for the treated and placebo groups, respectively (p=0.0001). Also documented was a reduced incidence of clinical congestive heart failure in the treated group (14%) compared to the placebo group (33%) (p=0.009).[7]

In a double-blind, randomized trial (145 patients) comparing Activase to placebo, patients infused with Activase within 2.5 hours of onset of symptoms experienced improved left ventricular function at a mean of 21 days compared to the placebo group, when ejection fraction was measured by gated blood pool scan (52% vs 48%, p=0.08) and by contrast ventriculogram (61% vs 54%, p=0.006).

Although the contribution of Activase alone is unclear, the incidence of nonischemic cardiac complications when taken as a group (i.e., congestive heart failure, pericarditis, atrial fibrillation, and conduction disturbance) was reduced when compared to those patients treated with placebo (p <0.01).[8]

In a double-blind, randomized trial (5013 patients) comparing Activase to placebo (ASSET study), patients infused with Activase within 5 hours of the onset of symptoms of acute myocardial infarction experienced improved 30-day survival compared to those treated with placebo. At 1 month, the overall mortality rates were 7.2% for the Activase-treated group and 9.8% for the placebo-treated group (p=0.001).[9,10] This benefit was maintained at 6 months for Activase-treated patients (10.4%) compared to those treated with placebo (13.1%, p=0.008).[10]

In a double-blind, randomized trial (721 patients) comparing Activase to placebo, patients infused with Activase within 5 hours of the onset of symptoms experienced improved ventricular function 10–22 days after treatment compared to the placebo group, when global ejection fraction was measured by contrast ventriculography (50.7% vs 48.5%, p=0.01). Patients treated with Activase had a 19% reduction in infarct size, as measured by cumulative release of HBDH (α-hydroxybutyrate dehydrogenase) activity compared to placebo-treated patients (p=0.001). Patients treated with Activase had significantly fewer episodes of cardiogenic shock (p=0.02), ventricular fibrillation (p<0.04) and pericarditis (p=0.01) compared to patients treated with placebo. Mortality at 21 days in Activase-treated patients was reduced to 3.7% compared to 6.3% in placebo-treated patients (1-sided p=0.05).[11] Although these data do not demonstrate unequivocally a significant reduction in mortality for this study, they do indicate a trend that is supported by the results of the ASSET study.

Acute Ischemic Stroke Patients

Two placebo-controlled, double-blind trials (The NINDS t-PA Stroke Trial, Part 1 and Part 2) have been conducted in patients with acute ischemic stroke.[12] Both studies enrolled patients with measurable neurological deficit who could complete screening and begin study treatment within 3 hours from symptom onset. A cranial computerized tomography (CT) scan was performed prior to treatment to rule out the presence of intracranial hemorrhage (ICH). Patients were also excluded for the presence of conditions related to risks of bleeding (see CONTRAINDICATIONS), for minor neurological deficit, for rapidly improving symptoms prior to initiating study treatment, or for blood glucose of <50 or >400 mg/dL.

Patients were randomized to receive either 0.9 mg/kg Activase (maximum of 90 mg), or placebo. Activase was administered as a 10% initial bolus over 1 minute followed by continuous intravenous infusion of the remainder over 60 minutes (see DOSAGE AND ADMINISTRATION). In patients without recent use of oral anticoagulants or heparin, study treatment was initiated prior to the availability of coagulation study results. However, the infusion was discontinued if either a pre-treatment prothrombin time (PT) >15 seconds or an elevated activated partial thromboplastin time (aPTT) was identified. Although patients with or without prior aspirin use were enrolled, administration of anticoagulants and antiplatelet agents was prohibited for the first 24 hours following symptom onset.

The initial study (NINDS-Part 1, n=291) evaluated neurological improvement at 24 hours after stroke onset. The primary endpoint, the proportion of patients with a 4 or more point improvement in the National Institutes of Health Stroke Scale (NIHSS) score or complete recovery (NIHSS score=0), was not significantly different between treatment groups. A secondary analysis suggested improved 3-month outcome associated with Activase treatment using the following stroke assessment scales: Barthel Index, Modified Rankin Scale, Glasgow Outcome Scale, and the NIHSS.

A second study (NINDS-Part 2, n=333) assessed clinical outcome at 3 months as the primary outcome. A favorable outcome was defined as minimal or no disability using the four stroke assessment scales: Barthel Index (score ≥95), Modified Rankin Scale (score ≤1), Glasgow Outcome Scale (score=1), and NIHSS (score ≤1). The results comparing Activase- and placebo-treated patients for the four outcome scales together (Generalized Estimating Equations) and individually are presented in Table 3. In this study, depending upon the scale, the favorable outcome of minimal or no disability occurred in at least 11 per 100 more patients treated with Activase than those receiving placebo. Secondary analyses demonstrated consistent functional and neurological improvement within all four stroke scales as indicated by median scores. These results were highly consistent with the 3-month outcome treatment effects observed in the Part 1 study.

[See Table 3 at top of next page.]

The incidences of all-cause 90-day mortality, ICH, and new ischemic stroke following Activase treatment compared to placebo are presented in Table 4 as a combined safety analysis (n=624) for Parts 1 and 2. These data indicated a significant increase in ICH following Activase treatment, particularly symptomatic ICH within 36 hours. In Activase-treated patients, there were no increases compared to placebo in the incidences of 90-day mortality or severe disability.

[See Table 4 at bottom of next page.]

In a prespecified subgroup analysis in patients receiving aspirin prior to onset of stroke symptoms, there was preserved favorable outcome for Activase-treated patients.

Exploratory, multivariate analyses of both studies combined (n=624) to investigate potential predictors of ICH and treatment effect modifiers were performed. In Activase-treated patients presenting with severe neurological deficit (e.g., NIHSS >22) or of advanced age (e.g., >77 years of age), the trends toward increased risk for symptomatic ICH within the first 36 hours were more prominent. Similar trends were also seen for total ICH and for all-cause 90-day mortality in these patients. When risk was assessed by the combination of death and severe disability in these patients, there was no difference between placebo and Activase groups. Analyses for efficacy suggested a reduced but still favorable clinical outcome for Activase-treated patients with severe neurological deficit or advanced age at presentation.

Pulmonary Embolism Patients

In a comparative randomized trial (n=45),[13] 59% of patients (n=22) treated with Activase (100 mg over 2 hours) experienced moderate or marked lysis of pulmonary emboli when assessed by pulmonary angiography 2 hours after treatment initiation. Activase-treated patients also experienced a significant reduction in pulmonary embolism-induced pulmonary hypertension within 2 hours of treatment (p=0.003). Pulmonary perfusion at 24 hours, as assessed by radionuclide scan, was significantly improved (p=0.002).

Table 2

Patency (TIMI 2 or 3)	Accelerated Activase	SK (IV)	p-Value	SK (SQ)	p-Value
90-Minute	n=272 81.3%	n=261 59.0%	<0.0001	n=260 53.5%	<0.0001
180-Minute	n=80 76.3%	n=76 72.4%	0.58	n=95 71.6%	0.48
24 Hour	n=81 88.9%	n=72 87.5%	0.24	n=67 82.1%	0.79
5–7 Day	n=72 83.3%	n=77 90.9%	0.47	n=75 78.7%	0.17

Table 1

Event	Accelerated Activase	SK (IV)	p-Value[1]	SK (SQ)	p-Value[1]
30-Day Mortality	6.3%	7.3%	0.003	7.3%	0.007
30-Day Mortality or Nonfatal Stroke	7.2%	8.2%	0.006	8.0%	0.036
24-Hour Mortality	2.4%	2.9%	0.009	2.8%	0.029
Any Stroke	1.6%	1.4%	0.32	1.2%	0.03
Intracerebral Hemorrhage	0.7%	0.6%	0.22	0.5%	0.02

[1] Two-tailed p-value is for comparison of Accelerated Activase®, Alteplase, recombinant to the respective SK control arm.

INDICATIONS AND USAGE

Acute Myocardial Infarction

Activase is indicated for use in the management of acute myocardial infarction in adults for the improvement of ventricular function following AMI, the reduction of the incidence of congestive heart failure, and the reduction of mortality associated with AMI. Treatment should be initiated as soon as possible after the onset of AMI symptoms (see CLINICAL PHARMACOLOGY).

Acute Ischemic Stroke

Activase is indicated for the management of acute ischemic stroke in adults for improving neurological recovery and reducing the incidence of disability. **Treatment should only be initiated within 3 hours after the onset of stroke symptoms, and after exclusion of intracranial hemorrhage by a cranial computerized tomography (CT) scan or other diagnostic imaging method sensitive for the presence of hemorrhage (see CONTRAINDICATIONS).**

Pulmonary Embolism

Activase is indicated in the management of acute massive pulmonary embolism (PE) in adults for:

- the lysis of acute pulmonary emboli, defined as obstruction of blood flow to a lobe or multiple segments of the lungs, and
- the lysis of pulmonary emboli accompanied by unstable hemodynamics, e.g., failure to maintain blood pressure without supportive measures.

The diagnosis should be confirmed by objective means, such as pulmonary angiography or noninvasive procedures such as lung scanning.

CONTRAINDICATIONS

Acute Myocardial Infarction or Pulmonary Embolism

Activase therapy in patients with acute myocardial infarction or pulmonary embolism is contraindicated in the following situations because of an increased risk of bleeding:

- **Active internal bleeding**
- **History of cerebrovascular accident**
- **Recent intracranial or intraspinal surgery or trauma (see WARNINGS)**
- **Intracranial neoplasm, arteriovenous malformation, or aneurysm**
- **Known bleeding diathesis**
- **Severe uncontrolled hypertension**

Acute Ischemic Stroke

Activase therapy in patients with acute ischemic stroke is contraindicated in the following situations because of an increased risk of bleeding, which could result in significant disability or death:

- **Evidence of intracranial hemorrhage on pretreatment evaluation**
- **Suspicion of subarachnoid hemorrhage**
- **Recent intracranial surgery or serious head trauma or recent previous stroke**
- **History of intracranial hemorrhage**
- **Uncontrolled hypertension at time of treatment (e.g., >185 mm Hg systolic or >110 mm Hg diastolic)**
- **Seizure at the onset of stroke**
- **Active internal bleeding**

- Intracranial neoplasm, arteriovenous malformation, or aneurysm
- Known bleeding diathesis including but not limited to:
  —Current use of oral anticoagulants (e.g., warfarin sodium) with prothrombin time (PT) > 15 seconds
  —Administration of heparin within 48 hours preceding the onset of stroke and have an elevated activated partial thromboplastin time (aPTT) at presentation
  —Platelet count < 100,000/mm^3

WARNINGS

Bleeding

The most common complication encountered during Activase®, Alteplase, recombinant therapy is bleeding. The type of bleeding associated with thrombolytic therapy can be divided into two broad categories:

- Internal bleeding, involving intracranial and retroperitoneal sites, or the gastrointestinal, genitourinary, or respiratory tracts.
- Superficial or surface bleeding, observed mainly at invaded or disturbed sites (e.g., venous cutdowns, arterial punctures, sites of recent surgical intervention).

The concomitant use of heparin anticoagulation may contribute to bleeding. Some of the hemorrhage episodes occurred 1 or more days after the effects of Activase had dissipated, but while heparin therapy was continuing.

As fibrin is lysed during Activase therapy, bleeding from recent puncture sites may occur. Therefore, thrombolytic therapy requires careful attention to all potential bleeding sites (including catheter insertion sites, arterial and venous puncture sites, cutdown sites, and needle puncture sites). Intramuscular injections and nonessential handling of the patient should be avoided during treatment with Activase. Venipunctures should be performed carefully and only as required.

Should an arterial puncture be necessary during an infusion of Activase, it is preferable to use an upper extremity vessel that is accessible to manual compression. Pressure should be applied for at least 30 minutes, a pressure dressing applied, and the puncture site checked frequently for evidence of bleeding.

Should serious bleeding (not controllable by local pressure) occur, the infusion of Activase and any concomitant heparin should be terminated immediately.

Each patient being considered for therapy with Activase should be carefully evaluated and anticipated benefits weighed against potential risks associated with therapy. In the following conditions, the risks of Activase therapy for all approved indications may be increased and should be weighed against the anticipated benefits:

- Recent major surgery, e.g., coronary artery bypass graft, obstetrical delivery, organ biopsy, previous puncture of noncompressible vessels
- Cerebrovascular disease
- Recent gastrointestinal or genitourinary bleeding
- Recent trauma
- Hypertension: systolic BP ≥ 180 mm Hg and/or diastolic BP ≥ 110 mm Hg
- High likelihood of left heart thrombus, e.g., mitral stenosis with atrial fibrillation
- Acute pericarditis
- Subacute bacterial endocarditis
- Hemostatic defects including those secondary to severe hepatic or renal disease
- Significant hepatic dysfunction
- Pregnancy
- Diabetic hemorrhagic retinopathy, or other hemorrhagic ophthalmic conditions
- Septic thrombophlebitis or occluded AV cannula at seriously infected site
- Advanced age, (e.g., over 75 years old)
- Patients currently receiving oral anticoagulants, e.g., warfarin sodium

- Any other condition in which bleeding constitutes a significant hazard or would be particularly difficult to manage because of its location

Cholesterol Embolization

Cholesterol embolism has been reported rarely in patients treated with all types of thrombolytic agents; the true incidence is unknown. This serious condition, which can be lethal, is also associated with invasive vascular procedures (e.g., cardiac catheterization, angiography, vascular surgery) and/or anticoagulant therapy. Clinical features of cholesterol embolism may include livedo reticularis, "purple toe" syndrome, acute renal failure, gangrenous digits, hypertension, pancreatitis, myocardial infarction, cerebral infarction, spinal cord infarction, retinal artery occlusion, bowel infarction, and rhabdomyolysis.

Arrhythmias

Coronary thrombolysis may result in arrhythmias associated with reperfusion. These arrhythmias (such as sinus bradycardia, accelerated idioventricular rhythm, ventricular premature depolarizations, ventricular tachycardia) are not different from those often seen in the ordinary course of acute myocardial infarction and may be managed with standard antiarrhythmic measures. It is recommended that antiarrhythmic therapy for bradycardia and/or ventricular irritability be available when infusions of Activase®, Alteplase, recombinant are administered.

Use in Acute Ischemic Stroke

In addition to the previously listed conditions, the risks of Activase therapy to treat acute ischemic stroke may be increased in the following conditions and should be weighed against the anticipated benefits:

- Patients with severe neurological deficit (e.g., NIHSS > 22) at presentation. There is an increased risk of intracranial hemorrhage in these patients.
- Patients with major early infarct signs on a computerized cranial tomography (CT) scan (e.g., substantial edema, mass effect, or midline shift).

In patients without recent use of oral anticoagulants or heparin, Activase treatment can be initiated prior to the availability of coagulation study results. However, infusion should be discontinued if either a pre-treatment prothrombin time (PT) > 15 seconds or an elevated activate partial thromboplastin time (aPTT) is identified.

Treatment should be limited to facilities that can provide appropriate evaluation and management of ICH.

In acute ischemic stroke, neither the incidence of intracranial hemorrhage nor the benefits of therapy are known in patients treated with Activase more than 3 hours after the onset of symptoms. Therefore, treatment of patients with acute ischemic stroke more than 3 hours after symptom onset is not recommended.

The safety and efficacy of treatment with Activase in patients with minor neurological deficit or with rapidly improving symptoms prior to the start of Activase administration has not been evaluated.

Use in Pulmonary Embolism

It should be recognized that the treatment of pulmonary embolism with Activase has not been shown to constitute adequate clinical treatment of underlying deep vein thrombosis. Furthermore, the possible risk of reembolization due to the lysis of underlying deep venous thrombi should be considered.

PRECAUTIONS

General

Standard management of myocardial infarction or pulmonary embolism should be implemented concomitantly with Activase treatment. Noncompressible arterial puncture must be avoided and internal jugular and subclavian venous punctures should be avoided to minimize bleeding from noncompressible sites. Arterial and venous punctures should be minimized. In the event of serious bleeding, Activase and heparin should be discontinued immediately. Heparin effects can be reversed by protamine.

Readministration

There is no experience with readministration of Activase. If an anaphylactoid reaction occurs, the infusion should be discontinued immediately and appropriate therapy initiated.

Although sustained antibody formation in patients receiving one dose of Activase has not been documented, readministration should be undertaken with caution. Detectable levels of antibody (a single point measurement) were reported in one patient, but subsequent antibody test results were negative.

Drug-Laboratory Test Interactions

During Activase therapy, if coagulation tests and/or measures of fibrinolytic activity are performed, the results may be unreliable unless specific precautions are taken to prevent in vitro artifacts. Activase is an enzyme that when present in blood in pharmacologic concentrations remains active under in vitro conditions. This can lead to degradation of fibrinogen in blood samples removed for analysis. Collection of blood samples in the presence of aprotinin (150–200 units/mL) can to some extent mitigate this phenomenon.

Drug Interactions

The interaction of Activase with other cardioactive or cerebroactive drugs has not been studied. In addition to bleeding associated with heparin and vitamin K antagonists, drugs that alter platelet function (such as acetylsalicylic acid, dipyridamole and Abciximab) may increase the risk of bleeding if administered prior to, during, or after Activase therapy.

Use of Antithrombotics

Aspirin and heparin have been administered concomitantly with and following infusions of Activase in the management of acute myocardial infarction or pulmonary embolism. Because heparin, aspirin, or Activase may cause bleeding complications, careful monitoring for bleeding is advised, especially at arterial puncture sites.

The concomitant use of heparin or aspirin during the first 24 hours following symptom onset were prohibited in The NINDS t-PA Stroke Trial. The safety of such concomitant use with Activase for the management of acute ischemic stroke is unknown.

Blood Pressure Control

Blood pressure should be monitored frequently and controlled during and following Activase administration in the

---

Table 3
The NINDS t-PA Stroke Trial, Part 2
3-Month Efficacy Outcomes

Analysis	Frequency of Favorable Outcome[1]				
	Placebo (n=165)	Activase (n=168)	Absolute Difference (95% CI)	Relative Frequency[2] (95% CI)	p-Value[3]
Generalized Estimating Equations (Multivariate)	—	—	—	1.34 (1.05, 1.72)	0.02
Barthel Index	37.6%	50.0%	12.4% (3.0, 21.9)	1.33 (1.04, 1.71)	0.02
Modified Rankin Scale	26.1%	38.7%	12.6% (3.7, 21.6)	1.48 (1.08, 2.04)	0.02
Glasgow Outcome Scale	31.5%	44.0%	12.5% (3.3, 21.8)	1.40 (1.05, 1.85)	0.02
NIHSS	20.0%	31.0%	11.0% (2.6, 19.3)	1.55 (1.06, 2.26)	0.02

[1] Favorable Outcome is defined as recovery with minimal or no disability.
[2] Value >1 indicates frequency of recovery in favor of Activase treatment.
[3] p-Value for Relative Frequency is from Generalized Estimating Equations with log link.

Table 4
The NINDS t-PA Stroke Trial
Safety Outcome

	Part 1 and Part 2 Combined		
	Placebo (n=312)	Activase (n=312)	p-Value[2]
All-Cause 90-day Mortality	64 (20.5%)	54 (17.3%)	0.36
Total ICH[1]	20 (6.4%)	48 (15.4%)	<0.01
Symptomatic	4 (1.3%)	25 (8.0%)	<0.01
Asymptomatic	16 (5.1%)	23 (7.4%)	0.32
Symptomatic ICH within 36 hours	2 (0.6%)	20 (6.4%)	<0.01
New Ischemic Stroke (3-months)	17 (5.4%)	18 (5.8%)	1.00

[1] Within trial follow-up period. Symptomatic ICH was defined as the occurrence of sudden clinical worsening followed by subsequent verification of ICH on CT scan. Asymptomatic ICH was defined as ICH detected on a routine repeat CT scan without preceding clinical worsening.
[2] Fisher's Exact Test

Continued on next page

Genentech—Cont.

management of acute ischemic stroke. In The NINDS t-PA Stroke Trial, blood pressure was monitored for 24 hours and was actively controlled (≤185/110 mm Hg) during this period with appropriate medication.

Carcinogenesis, Mutagenesis, Impairment of Fertility
Long-term studies in animals have not been performed to evaluate the carcinogenic potential or the effect on fertility. Short-term studies, which evaluated tumorigenicity of Activase and effect on tumor metastases in rodents, were negative.

Studies to determine mutagenicity (Ames test) and chromosomal aberration assays in human lymphocytes were negative at all concentrations tested. Cytotoxicity, as reflected by a decrease in mitotic index, was evidenced only after prolonged exposure and only at the highest concentrations tested.

Pregnancy (Category C)
Animal reproduction studies have not been conducted with Activase. It is also not known whether Activase can cause fetal harm when administered to a pregnant woman or can affect reproduction capacity. Activase should be given to a pregnant woman only if clearly needed.

Nursing Mothers
It is not known whether Activase is excreted in human milk. Because many drugs are excreted in human milk, caution should be exercised when Activase is administered to a nursing woman.

Pediatric Use
Safety and effectiveness of Activase in pediatric patients have not been established.

ADVERSE REACTIONS
Bleeding
The most frequent adverse reaction associated with Activase in all approved indications is bleeding (see WARNINGS)[14,15].

Should serious bleeding in a critical location (intracranial, gastrointestinal, retroperitoneal, pericardial) occur, Activase therapy should be discontinued immediately, along with any concomitant therapy with heparin. Death and permanent disability are not uncommonly reported in patients that have experienced stroke (including intracranial bleeding) and other serious bleeding episodes.

In the GUSTO trial for the treatment of acute myocardial infarction, using the accelerated infusion regimen the incidence of all strokes for the Activase-treated patients was 1.6%, while the incidence of nonfatal stroke was 0.9%. The incidence of hemorrhagic stroke was 0.7%, not all of which were fatal. The incidence of all strokes, as well as that for hemorrhagic stroke, increased with increasing age (see CLINICAL PHARMACOLOGY: Accelerated Infusion in AMI Patients). Data from previous trials utilizing a 3-hour infusion of ≤100 mg indicated that the incidence of total stroke in six randomized double-blind placebo controlled trials[2,7–11,16] was 1.2% (37/3161) in Alteplase-treated patients compared with 0.9% (27/3092) in placebo-treated patients.

For the 3-hour infusion regimen, the incidence of significant internal bleeding (estimated as >250 cc blood loss) has been reported in studies in over 800 patients. These data do not include patients treated with the Alteplase accelerated infusion:

	Total Dose ≤100 mg
gastrointestinal	5%
genitourinary	4%
ecchymosis	1%
retroperitoneal	<1%
epistaxis	<1%
gingival	<1%

The incidence of intracranial hemorrhage (ICH) in acute myocardial infarction patients treated with Activase is as follows:

Dose	Number of Patients	ICH (%)
100 mg, 3-hours	3272	0.4
≤100 mg, accelerated	10,396	0.7
150 mg	1779	1.3
1–1.4 mg/kg	237	0.4

These data indicate that a dose of 150 mg of Activase should not be used in the treatment of AMI because it has been associated with an increase in intracranial bleeding[17].

For acute massive pulmonary embolism, bleeding events were consistent with the general safety profile observed with Activase in acute myocardial infarction patients receiving the 3-hour infusion regimen.

The incidence of ICH, especially symptomatic ICH, in patients with acute ischemic stroke was higher in Activase-treated patients than placebo patients (see CLINICAL PHARMACOLOGY).

A study of another alteplase product, Actilyse, in acute ischemic stroke, suggested that doses greater than 0.9 mg/kg may be associated with an increased incidence of ICH[18]. **Doses greater than 0.9 mg/kg (maximum 90 mg) should not be used in the management of acute schemic stroke.**

Bleeding events other than ICH were noted in the studies of acute ischemic stroke and were consistent with the general safety profile of Activase. In The NINDS t-PA Stroke Trial (Parts 1 and 2), the frequency of bleeding requiring red blood cell transfusions was 6.4% for Activase-treated patients compared to 3.8% for placebo (p=0.19, using Mantel-Haenszel Chi-Square).

Fibrin which is part of the hemostatic plug formed at needle puncture sites will be lysed during Activase therapy. Therefore, Activase therapy requires careful attention to potential bleeding sites, e.g., catheter insertion sites, and arterial puncture sites.

Allergic Reactions
Allergic-type reactions, e.g., anaphylactoid reaction, laryngeal edema, rash, and urticaria have been reported very rarely (<0.02%). A cause and effect relationship to Activase therapy has not been established. When such reactions occur, they usually respond to conventional therapy.

Other Adverse Reactions
Patients with myocardial infarction or pulmonary embolism can experience disease-related events such as cardiogenic shock, arrhythmias, pulmonary edema, heart failure, cardiac arrest, recurrent ischemia, reinfarction, myocardial rupture, mitral regurgitation, pericardial effusion, pericarditis, cardiac tamponade, venous thrombosis and embolism, and electromechanical dissociation. These events can be life-threatening and may lead to death. Other adverse reactions have been reported, principally nausea and/or vomiting, hypotension, and fever. These reactions are frequent sequelae of myocardial infarction and may or may not be attributable to Activase therapy.

DOSAGE AND ADMINISTRATION
Activase®, Alteplase, recombinant is for intravenous administration only. Extravasation of Activase infusion can cause ecchymosis and/or inflammation. Management consists of terminating the infusion at that IV site and application of local therapy.

Acute Myocardial Infarction
Administer Activase as soon as possible after the onset of symptoms.

There are two Activase dose regimens for use in the management of acute myocardial infarction; controlled studies to compare clinical outcomes with these regimens have not been conducted.

A DOSE OF 150 mg OF ACTIVASE SHOULD NOT BE USED FOR THE TREATMENT OF ACUTE MYOCARDIAL INFARCTION BECAUSE IT HAS BEEN ASSOCIATED WITH AN INCREASE IN INTRACRANIAL BLEEDING.

Accelerated Infusion
The recommended total dose is based upon patient weight, not to exceed 100 mg. For patients weighing >67 kg, the recommended dose administered is 100 mg as a 15 mg intravenous bolus, followed by 50 mg infused over the next 30 minutes, and then 35 mg infused over the next 60 minutes. For patients weighing ≤67 kg, the recommended dose is administered as a 15 mg intravenous bolus, followed by 0.75 mg/kg infused over the next 30 minutes not to exceed 50 mg, and then 0.50 mg/kg over the next 60 minutes not to exceed 35 mg.

The safety and efficacy of this accelerated infusion of Alteplase regimen has only been investigated with concomitant administration of heparin and aspirin as described in CLINICAL PHARMACOLOGY.
a. The bolus dose may be prepared in one of the following ways:
1. By removing 15 mL from the vial of reconstituted (1 mg/mL) Activase using a syringe and needle. If this method is used with the 50 mg vials, the syringe should not be primed with air and the needle should be inserted into the Activase vial stopper. If the 100 mg vial is used, the syringe should not be primed with air and the needle should be inserted away from the puncture mark made by the transfer device.
2. By removing 15 mL from a port (second injection site) on the infusion line after the infusion set is primed.
3. By programming an infusion pump to deliver a 15 mL (1 mg/mL) bolus at the initiation of the infusion.
b. The remainder of the Activase®, Alteplase, recombinant dose may be administered as follows:
50 mg vials—administer using either a polyvinyl chloride bag or glass vial and infusion set
100 mg vial—insert the spike end of an infusion set through the same puncture site created by the transfer device in the stopper of the vial of reconstituted Activase. Hang the Activase vial from the plastic molded capping attached to the bottom of the vial.

3-Hour Infusion
The recommended dose is 100 mg administered as 60 mg (34.8 million IU) in the first hour (of which 6 to 10 mg is administered as a bolus), 20 mg (11.6 million IU) over the sec-

ond hour, and 20 mg (11.6 million IU) over the third hour. For smaller patients (<65 kg), a dose of 1.25 mg/kg administered over 3 hours, as described above, may be used[14].

Although the value of the use of anticoagulants during and following administration of Activase has not been fully studied, heparin has been administered concomitantly for 24 hours or longer in more than 90% of patients.

Aspirin and/or dipyridamole have been given to patients receiving Alteplase during and/or following heparin treatment.
a. The bolus dose may be prepared in one of the following ways:
1. By removing 6 to 10 mL from the vial of reconstituted (1 mg/mL) Activase using a syringe and needle. If this method is used with the 50 mg vials, the syringe should not be primed with air and the needle should be inserted into the Activase vial stopper. If the 100 mg vial is used, the syringe should not be primed with air and the needle should be inserted away from the puncture mark made by the transfer device.
2. By removing 6 to 10 mL from a port (second injection site) on the infusion line after the infusion set is primed.
3. By programming an infusion pump to deliver a 6 to 10 mL (1 mg/mL) bolus at the initiation of the infusion.
b. The remainder of the Activase dose may be administered as follows:
50 mg vials—administer using either a polyvinyl chloride bag or glass vial and infusion set
100 mg vial—insert the spike end of an infusion set through the same puncture site created by the transfer device in the stopper of the vial of reconstituted Activase. Hang the Activase vial from the plastic molded capping attached to the bottom of the vial.

Acute Ischemic Stroke
The recommended dose is 0.9 mg/kg (maximum of 90 mg) infused over 60 minutes with 10% of the total dose administered as an initial intravenous bolus over 1 minute.

The safety and efficacy of this regimen with concomitant administration of heparin and aspirin during the first 24 hours after symptom onset has not been investigated.

THE DOSE FOR TREATMENT OF ACUTE ISCHEMIC STROKE SHOULD NOT EXCEED 90 mg.
a. The bolus dose may be prepared in one of the following ways:
1. By removing the appropriate volume from the vial of reconstituted (1 mg/mL) Activase using a syringe and needle. If this method is used with the 50 mg vials, the syringe should not be primed with air and the needle should be inserted into the Activase vial stopper. If the 100 mg vial is used, the syringe should not be primed with air and the needle should be inserted away from the puncture mark made by the transfer device.
2. By removing the appropriate volume from a port (second injection site) on the infusion line after the infusion set is primed.
3. By programming an infusion pump to deliver the appropriate volume as a bolus at the initiation of the infusion.
b. The remainder of the Activase dose may be administered as follows:
50 mg vials—administer using either a polyvinyl chloride bag or glass vial and infusion set
100 mg vial—remove from the vial any quantity of drug in excess of that specified for patient treatment. Insert the spike end of an infusion set through the same puncture site created by the transfer device in the stopper of the vial of reconstituted Activase. Hang the Activase vial from the plastic molded capping attached to the bottom of the vial.

Pulmonary Embolism
The recommended dose is 100 mg administered by intravenous infusion over 2 hours. Heparin therapy should be instituted or reinstituted near the end of or immediately following the Activase infusion when the partial thromboplastin time or thrombin time returns to twice normal or less. The Activase dose may be administered as follows:
50 mg vials—administer using either a polyvinyl chloride bag or glass vial and infusion set
100 mg vial—insert the spike end of an infusion set through the same puncture site created by the transfer device in the stopper of the vial of reconstituted Activase. Hang the Activase vial from the plastic molded capping attached to the bottom of the vial.

Reconstitution and Dilution
Activase should be reconstituted by aseptically adding the appropriate volume of the accompanying Sterile Water for Injection, USP to the vial. It is important that Activase be reconstituted only with Sterile Water for Injection, USP, without preservatives. Do not use Bacteriostatic Water for Injection, USP. The reconstituted preparation results in a colorless to pale yellow transparent solution containing Activase 1 mg/mL at approximately pH 7.3. The osmolality of this solution is approximately 215 mOsm/kg. Because Activase contains no antibacterial preservatives, it should be reconstituted immediately before use. The solution may be used for intravenous administration within 8 hours following reconstitution when stored between 2–30°C (36–86°F). Before further dilution or administration, the

product should be visually inspected for particulate matter and discoloration prior to administration whenever solution and container permit.

Activase may be administered as reconstituted at 1 mg/mL. As an alternative, the reconstituted solution may be diluted further immediately before administration in an equal volume of 0.9% Sodium Chloride Injection, USP or 5% Dextrose Injection, USP to yield a concentration of 0.5 mg/mL. Either polyvinyl chloride bags or glass vials are acceptable. Activase is stable for up to 8 hours in these solutions at room temperature. Exposure to light has no effect on the stability of these solutions. Excessive agitation during dilution should be avoided; mixing should be accomplished with gentle swirling and/or slow inversion. Do not use other infusion solutions, e.g., Sterile Water for Injection, USP or preservative-containing solutions for further dilution.

50 mg Vials

Reconstitution should be carried out using a large bore needle (e.g.,18 gauge) and a syringe, directing the stream of Sterile Water for Injection, USP into the lyophilized cake. DO NOT USE IF VACUUM IS NOT PRESENT. Slight foaming upon reconstitution is not unusual; standing undisturbed for several minutes is usually sufficient to allow dissipation of any large bubbles.

No other medication should be added to infusion solutions containing Activase®, Alteplase. Any unused infusion solution should be discarded.

100 mg Vial

Reconstitution should be carried out using the transfer device provided, adding the contents of the accompanying 100 mL vial of Sterile Water for Injection, USP to the contents of the 100 mg vial of Activase powder. Slight foaming upon reconstitution is not unusual; standing undisturbed for several minutes is usually sufficient to allow dissipation of any large bubbles. Please refer to the accompanying Instructions for Reconstitution and Administration. **100 mg VIALS DO NOT CONTAIN VACUUM.**

100 mg VIAL RECONSTITUTION

1. Use aseptic technique throughout.
2. Remove the protective flip-caps from one vial of Activase and one vial of Sterile Water for Injection, USP (SWFI).
3. Open the package containing the transfer device by peeling the paper label off the package.
4. Remove the protective cap from one end of the transfer device and keeping the vial of SWFI upright, insert the piercing pin vertically into the center of the stopper of the vial of SWFI.
5. Remove the protective cap from the other end of the transfer device. **DO NOT INVERT THE VIAL OF SWFI.**
6. Holding the vial of Activase®, Alteplase, recombinant upside-down, position it so that the center of the stopper is directly over the exposed piercing pin of the transfer device.
7. Push the vial of Activase down so that the piercing pin is inserted through the center of the Activase vial stopper.
8. Invert the two vials so that the vial of Activase is on the bottom (upright) and the vial of SWFI is upside-down, allowing the SWFI to flow down through the transfer device. Allow the entire contents of the vial of SWFI to flow into the Activase vial (approximately 0.5 cc of SWFI will remain in the diluent vial). Approximately 2 minutes are required for this procedure.
9. Remove the transfer device and the empty SWFI vial from the Activase vial. Safely discard both the transfer device and the empty diluent vial according to institutional procedures.
10. Swirl gently to dissolve the Activase powder. **DO NOT SHAKE.**

No other medication should be added to infusion solutions containing Activase®, Alteplase. Any unused infusion solution should be discarded.

HOW SUPPLIED

Activase is supplied as a sterile, lyophilized powder in 50 mg vials containing vacuum and in 100 mg vials without vacuum.

Each 50 mg Activase vial (29 million IU) is packaged with diluent for reconstitution (50 mL Sterile Water for Injection, USP): NDC 50242-044-13..

Each 100 mg Activase vial (58 million IU) is packaged with diluent for reconstitution (100 mL Sterile Water for Injection, USP), and one transfer device: NDC 50242-085-27.

Storage

Store lyophilized Activase at controlled room temperature not to exceed 30°C (86°F), or under refrigeration (2–8°C/36–46°F). Protect the lyophilized material during extended storage from excessive exposure to light.

Do not use beyond the expiration date stamped on the vial.

REFERENCES

1. Mueller H, Rao AK, Forman SA, et al. Thrombolysis in myocardial infarction (TIMI): comparative studies of coronary reperfusion and systemic fibrinogenolysis with two forms of recombinant tissue-type plasminogen activator. J Am Coll Cardiol. 1987;10:479–90.
2. Topol EJ, Morriss DC, Smalling RW, et al. A multicenter, randomized, placebo-controlled trial of a new form of intravenous recombinant tissue-type plasminogen activator (Activase®) in acute myocardial infarction. J Am Coll Cardiol. 1987;9:1205–13.
3. Seifried E, Tanswell P, Ellbrück D, et al. Pharmacokinetics and haemostatic status during consecutive infusions of recombinant tissue-type plasminogen activator in patients with acute myocardial infarction. Thromb Haemostas. 1989;61:497–501.
4. Tanswell P, Tebbe U, Neuhaus K-L, et al. Pharmacokinetics and fibrin specificity of Alteplase during accelerated infusions in acute myocardial infarction. J Am Coll Cardiol. 1992;19:1071–5.
5. De Wood MA, Spores J, Notske R, et al. Prevalence of total coronary occlusion during the early hours of transmural myocardial infarction. New Engl J Med. 1980;303:897–902.
6. Chesebro JH, Knatterud G, Roberts R, et al. Thrombolysis in myocardial infarction (TIMI) trial, Phase I: a comparison between intravenous tissue plasminogen activator and intravenous streptokinase. Circulation. 1987;76(1):142–54.
7. Guerci AD, Gerstenblith G, Brinker JA, et al. A randomized trial of intravenous tissue plasminogen activator for acute myocardial infarction with subsequent randomization to elective coronary angioplasty. New Engl J Med. 1987;317:1613–18.
8. O'Rourke M, Baron D, Keogh A, et al. Limitation of myocardial infarction by early infusion of recombinant tissue-plasminogen activator. Circulation. 1988;77:1311–15.
9. Wilcox RG, von der Lippe G, Olsson CG, et al. Trial of tissue plasminogen activator for mortality reduction in acute myocardial infarction: ASSET. Lancet. 1988;2:525–30.
10. Hampton JR, The University of Nottingham. Personal communication.
11. Van de Werf F, Arnold AER, et al. Effect of intravenous tissue-plasminogen activator on infarct size, left ventricular function and survival in patients with acute myocardial infarction. Br Med J. 1988;297:1374–9.
12. The National Institute of Neurological Disorders and Stroke t-PA Stroke Study Group. Tissue plasminogen activator for acute ischemic stroke. New Engl J Med. 1995;333:1581–7.
13. Goldhaber SZ, Kessler CM, Heit J, et al. A randomized controlled trial of recombinant tissue plasminogen activator versus urokinase in the treatment of acute pulmonary embolism. Lancet. 1988;2:293–8.
14. Califf RM, Topol EJ, George BS, et al. Hemorrhagic complications associated with the use of intravenous tissue plasminogen activator in treatment of acute myocardial infarction. Am J Med. 1988;85:353–9.
15. Bovill EG, Terrin ML, Stump DC, et al. Hemorrhagic events during therapy with recombinant tissue-type plasminogen activator, heparin, and aspirin for acute myocardial infarction: results from the thrombolysis in myocardial infarction (TIMI), Phase II trial. Ann Int Med. 1991;115(4):256–65.
16. National Heart Foundation of Australia Coronary Thrombolysis Group. Coronary thrombolysis and myocardial infarction salvage by tissue plasminogen activator given up to 4 hours after onset of myocardial infarction. Lancet. 1988;1:203–7.
17. Gore JM, Sloan M, Price TR, et al. and the TIMI Investigators. Intracerebral hemorrhage, cerebral infarction, and subdural hematoma after acute myocardial infarction and thrombolytic therapy in the thrombolysis in myocardial infarction study. Circulation. 1991;83:448–59.
18. Hacke W, Kaste M, Fieschi C, Toni D, Lesaffre E, von Kummer R, et al. for the ECASS Study Group. Intravenous thrombolysis with recombinant tissue plasminogen activator for acute hemispheric stroke. The European Cooperative Acute Stroke Study (ECASS). JAMA. 1995;274:1017–25.

Activase®, Alteplase, recombinant   G48005-R9

Manufactured by
GENENTECH, INC.
460 Point San Bruno Boulevard   Revised June 1996
South San Francisco, CA 94080-4990

© 1996 Genentech, Inc.

Shown in Product Identification Guide, page 311

NUTROPIN®   ℞

[somatropin (rDNA origin) for injection]

DESCRIPTION

Nutropin® [somatropin (rDNA origin) for injection], is a human growth hormone (hGH) produced by recombinant DNA technology. Nutropin has 191 amino acid residues and a molecular weight of 22,125 daltons. The amino acid sequence of the product is identical to that of pituitary-derived human growth hormone. The protein is synthesized by a specific laboratory strain of *E. coli* as a precursor consisting of the rhGH molecule preceded by the secretion signal from an *E. coli* protein. This precursor is directed to the plasma membrane of the cell. The signal sequence is removed and the native protein is secreted into the periplasm so that the protein is folded appropriately as it is synthesized.

Nutropin is a highly purified preparation. Biological potency is determined by measuring the increase in body weight induced in hypophysectomized rats.

Nutropin is a sterile, white, lyophilized powder intended for subcutaneous administration after reconstitution with Bacteriostatic Water for Injection, USP (benzyl alcohol preserved). The reconstituted product is nearly isotonic at a concentration of 5 mg/mL growth hormone and has a pH of approximately 7.4.

Each 5 mg Nutropin vial contains 5 mg (approximately 15 IU) somatropin, lyophilized with 45 mg mannitol, 1.7 mg sodium phosphates (0.4 mg sodium phosphate monobasic and 1.3 mg sodium phosphate dibasic), and 1.7 mg glycine.

Each 10 mg Nutropin vial contains 10 mg (approximately 30 IU) somatropin, lyophilized with 90 mg mannitol, 3.4 mg sodium phosphates (0.8 mg sodium phosphate monobasic and 2.6 mg sodium phosphate dibasic), and 3.4 mg glycine.

The specific activity of somatropin is defined as International Units (IU) per mg of protein. Nutropin was previously labeled based on a specific activity of 2.6 IU/mg and is now labeled based on a specific activity of 3 IU/mg. The change in units is a result of harmonizing the defined specific activity of the current reference standard with the international World Health Organization (WHO) reference standard. Therefore, the units per vial of Nutropin have changed from approximately 13 IU to 15 IU and 26 IU to 30 IU. This does not represent a change in product purity or the quantity (mg) of somatropin per vial nor does it affect the recommended weekly dosage of somatropin per kg of body weight.

Bacteriostatic Water for Injection, USP is sterile water containing 0.9 percent benzyl alcohol per mL as an antimicrobial preservative packaged in a multidose vial. The diluent pH is 4.5–7.0.

CLINICAL PHARMACOLOGY

General

In vitro and in vivo preclinical, and clinical testing have demonstrated that Nutropin is therapeutically equivalent to pituitary-derived human growth hormone. Treatment of children who lack adequate endogenous growth hormone secretion with Nutropin resulted in an increase in growth rate and an increase in insulin-like growth factor-I levels similar to that seen with pituitary-derived human growth hormone.

Actions that have been demonstrated for Nutropin, somatrem and/or pituitary-derived human growth hormone include:

A. **Tissue Growth**—1) Skeletal Growth: Nutropin stimulates skeletal growth in children with growth failure due to a lack of adequate secretion of endogenous growth hormone or secondary to chronic renal insufficiency. Skeletal growth is accomplished at the epiphyseal plates at the ends of a growing bone. Growth and metabolism of epiphyseal plate cells are directly stimulated by growth hormone and one of its mediators, insulin-like growth factor-I. Serum levels of insulin-like growth factor-I are low in children and adolescents who are growth hormone deficient, but increase during treatment with Nutropin. New bone is formed at the epiphyses in response to growth hormone. This results in linear growth until these growth plates fuse at the end of puberty. 2) Cell Growth: Treatment with pituitary-derived human growth hormone results in an increase in both the number and the size of skeletal muscle cells. 3) Organ Growth: Growth hormone of human pituitary origin influences the size of internal organs, including kidneys, and increases red cell mass. Treatment of hypophysectomized or genetic dwarf rats with Nutropin results in organ growth that is proportional to the overall body growth. In normal rats subjected to nephrectomy-induced uremia, Nutropin promoted skeletal and body growth.

B. **Protein Metabolism**—Linear growth is facilitated in part by growth hormone-stimulated protein synthesis. This is reflected by nitrogen retention as demonstrated by a decline in urinary nitrogen excretion and blood urea nitrogen during growth hormone therapy.

C. **Carbohydrate Metabolism**—Growth hormone is a modulator of carbohydrate metabolism. For example, children with inadequate secretion of growth hormone sometimes experience fasting hypoglycemia that is improved by treatment with growth hormone. Nutropin therapy may decrease glucose tolerance. Administration of Nutropin to normal adults, patients with chronic renal insufficiency, and patients who lacked adequate secretion of endogenous growth hormone resulted in increases in mean serum fasting and postprandial insulin levels. However, mean glu-

Continued on next page

Genentech—Cont.

cose and hemoglobin A_{1C} levels remained in the normal range.

D. Lipid Metabolism—Acute administration of pituitary-derived human growth hormone to humans resulted in lipid mobilization. Nonesterified fatty acids increased in plasma within two hours of pituitary-derived human growth hormone administration. In growth hormone deficient patients, long-term growth hormone administration often decreases body fat. Mean cholesterol levels decreased in patients treated with Nutropin.

E. Mineral Metabolism—The retention of total body potassium in response to growth hormone administration apparently results from cellular growth. Serum levels of inorganic phosphorus may increase slightly in patients with inadequate secretion of endogenous growth hormone or chronic renal insufficiency after growth hormone therapy due to metabolic activity associated with bone growth as well as increased tubular reabsorption of phosphate by the kidney. Serum calcium is not significantly altered in these patients. Sodium retention also occurs. (See PRECAUTIONS: Laboratory Tests.)

F. Connective Tissue Metabolism—Growth hormone stimulates the synthesis of chondroitin sulfate and collagen as well as the urinary excretion of hydroxyproline.

Pharmacokinetics: The pharmacokinetics of Nutropin have been investigated in healthy men after the subcutaneous administration of 0.1 mg/kg of body weight. A mean peak concentration (C_{max}) of 56.1 ng/mL occurred at a mean time of 7.5 hrs. The extent of absorption of Nutropin® [somatropin (rDNA origin) for injection], assessed by area under the concentration versus time curve (AUC), was 626 ng·hr/mL and closely compares with that of somatrem (590 ng·hr/mL). The AUC of Nutropin is similar regardless of injection site.

Growth hormone localizes to highly perfused organs, most notably liver and kidney. In the kidney, growth hormone is filtered by the glomerulus, reabsorbed in the proximal tubule, and is broken down within renal cells into amino acids which return to the circulation.

In both normal and growth hormone deficient adults and children, the intramuscular and subcutaneous pharmacokinetic profiles of somatropin are similar regardless of type of growth hormone or dosing regimen used. The subcutaneous pharmacokinetic profile of Nutropin is comparable to estimates in the published literature. A small number of dose-ranging studies suggest that clearance and AUC of somatropin is proportional to dose in the therapeutic dose range. Consistent with the role of the liver and kidney as major elimination organs for exogenously administered human growth hormone, there is a reduction in growth hormone clearance in patients with severe liver or kidney dysfunction.

Effects of Nutropin on Growth Failure Due to Chronic Renal Insufficiency (CRI)

Two multicenter, randomized, controlled clinical trials were conducted to determine whether treatment with Nutropin prior to renal transplantation in children with chronic renal insufficiency could improve their growth rates and height deficits. One study was a double-blinded, placebo-controlled trial and the other was an open-label, randomized trial. The dose of Nutropin in both controlled studies was 0.05 mg/kg/day (0.35 mg/kg/wk) administered daily by subcutaneous injection. Combining the data from those patients completing two years in the two controlled studies results in 62 children treated with Nutropin and 28 children in the control groups (either placebo-treated or untreated). The mean first year growth rate was 10.8 cm/yr for Nutropin-treated patients, compared with a mean growth rate of 6.5 cm/yr for placebo/untreated controls (p < 0.00005). The mean second year growth rate was 7.8 cm/yr for the Nutropin-treated group, compared with 5.5 cm/yr for controls (p < 0.00005). There was a significant increase in mean height standard deviation score in the Nutropin group (−2.9 at baseline to −1.5 at Month 24, n = 62) but no significant change in the controls (−2.8 at baseline to −2.9 at Month 24, n = 28). The mean third year growth rate of 7.6 cm/yr in the Nutropin-treated patients (n = 27) suggests that Nutropin stimulates growth beyond two years. However, there are no control data for the third year because control patients crossed over to growth hormone treatment after two years of participation. The gains in height were accompanied by appropriate advancement of skeletal age. These data demonstrate that Nutropin therapy improves growth rate and corrects the acquired height deficit associated with chronic renal insufficiency. Currently there are insufficient data regarding the benefit of treatment beyond three years. Although predicted final height was improved during Nutropin therapy, the effect of Nutropin on final adult height remains to be determined.

Post-Transplant Growth

The North American Pediatric Renal Transplant Cooperative Study (NAPRTCS) has reported data for growth post-transplant in children who did not receive growth hormone. The average change in height SD score during the initial two years post-transplant was 0.18 (n = 300, J Ped 1993; 122:397–402).

Controlled studies of growth hormone treatment for the short stature associated with CRI were not designed to compare the growth of treated or untreated patients after they received renal transplants. However, growth data are available from a small number of patients who have been followed for at least 11 months. Of the 7 control patients, 4 increased their height SD score and 3 had either no significant change or a decrease in height SD score. The 13 patients treated with Nutropin prior to transplant had either no significant change or an increase in height SD score after transplantation, indicating that the individual gains achieved with growth hormone therapy prior to transplant were maintained after transplantation. The differences in the height deficit narrowed between the treated and untreated groups in the post-transplant period.

INDICATIONS AND USAGE

Nutropin® [somatropin (rDNA origin) for injection] is indicated for the long-term treatment of children who have growth failure due to a lack of adequate endogenous growth hormone secretion.

Nutropin® [somatropin (rDNA origin) for injection] is also indicated for the treatment of children who have growth failure associated with chronic renal insufficiency up to the time of renal transplantation. Nutropin therapy should be used in conjunction with optimal management of chronic renal insufficiency.

CONTRAINDICATIONS

Nutropin should not be used in subjects with closed epiphyses.

Nutropin should not be used in patients with active neoplasia. Growth hormone therapy should be discontinued if evidence of neoplasia develops.

Nutropin, when reconstituted with Bacteriostatic Water for Injection, USP (benzyl alcohol preserved) should not be used in patients with a known sensitivity to benzyl alcohol.

WARNINGS

Benzyl alcohol as a preservative in Bacteriostatic Water for Injection, USP has been associated with toxicity in newborns. When administering Nutropin to newborns, reconstitute with Sterile Water for Injection, USP. USE ONLY ONE DOSE PER NUTROPIN VIAL AND DISCARD THE UNUSED PORTION.

PRECAUTIONS

General: Nutropin should be prescribed by physicians experienced in the diagnosis and management of patients with chronic renal insufficiency or growth failure. No studies have been performed of Nutropin therapy in children who have received renal transplants. Currently, treatment of patients with functioning renal allografts is not indicated. Because Nutropin may induce a state of insulin resistance, patients should be monitored for evidence of glucose intolerance.

Patients with a history of an intracranial lesion taking Nutropin should be examined frequently for progression or recurrence of the lesion.

Patients with growth failure secondary to chronic renal insufficiency should be examined periodically for evidence of progression of renal osteodystrophy. Slipped capital femoral epiphysis or avascular necrosis of the femoral head may be seen in children with advanced renal osteodystrophy, and it is uncertain whether these problems are affected by growth hormone therapy. X-rays of the hip should be obtained prior to initiating therapy. Physicians and parents should be alert to the development of a limp or complaints of hip or knee pain in patients treated with Nutropin® [somatropin (rDNA origin) for injection].

Slipped capital femoral epiphysis may occur more frequently in patients with endocrine disorders or in patients undergoing rapid growth.

Progression of scoliosis can occur in children who experience rapid growth. Because growth hormone increases growth rate, patients with a history of scoliosis who are treated with growth hormone should be monitored for progression of scoliosis. Growth hormone has not been shown to increase the incidence of scoliosis.

Intracranial hypertension (IH) with papilledema, visual changes, headache, nausea and/or vomiting has been reported in a small number of patients treated with growth hormone products. Symptoms usually occurred within the first eight (8) weeks of the initiation of growth hormone therapy. In all reported cases, IH-associated signs and symptoms resolved after termination of therapy or a reduction of the

growth hormone dose. Funduscopic examination of patients is recommended at the initiation and periodically during the course of growth hormone therapy.

See WARNINGS for use of Bacteriostatic Water for Injection, USP (benzyl alcohol preserved) in newborns.

As with any protein, local or systemic allergic reactions may occur. Parents/Patient should be informed that such reactions are possible and that prompt medical attention should be sought if allergic reactions occur.

Laboratory Tests: Serum levels of inorganic phosphorus, alkaline phosphatase, and parathyroid hormone (PTH) may increase with Nutropin therapy. Changes in thyroid hormone laboratory measurements may develop during Nutropin treatment in children who lack adequate endogenous growth hormone secretion. Untreated hypothyroidism prevents optimal response to Nutropin. Therefore, patients should have periodic thyroid function tests and should be treated with thyroid hormone when indicated.

Drug Interaction: The use of Nutropin in patients with chronic renal insufficiency receiving glucocorticoid therapy has not been evaluated. Concomitant glucocorticoid therapy may inhibit the growth promoting effect of Nutropin. If glucocorticoid replacement is required, the dose should be carefully adjusted.

There was no evidence in the controlled studies of Nutropin's interaction with drugs commonly used in chronic renal insufficiency patients. However, formal drug interaction studies have not been conducted.

Carcinogenesis, Mutagenesis, Impairment of Fertility: Carcinogenicity, mutagenicity and reproduction studies have not been conducted with Nutropin.

Pregnancy: Pregnancy (Category C). Animal reproduction studies have not been conducted with Nutropin. It is also not known whether Nutropin can cause fetal harm when administered to a pregnant woman or can affect reproduction capacity. Nutropin should be given to a pregnant woman only if clearly needed.

Nursing Mothers: It is not known whether Nutropin is excreted in human milk. Because many drugs are excreted in human milk, caution should be exercised when Nutropin is administered to a nursing mother.

Information for Patients: Patients being treated with growth hormone and/or their parents should be informed of the potential benefits and risks associated with treatment. If home use is determined to be desirable by the physician, instructions on appropriate use should be given, including a review of the contents of the Patient Information Insert. This information is intended to aid in the safe and effective administration of the medication. It is not a disclosure of all possible adverse or intended effects.

If home use is prescribed, a puncture resistant container for the disposal of used syringes and needles should be recommended to the patient. Patients and/or parents should be thoroughly instructed in the importance of proper disposal and cautioned against any reuse of needles and syringes (see Patient Information Insert).

ADVERSE REACTIONS

As with all protein pharmaceuticals, a small percentage of patients may develop antibodies to the protein. Growth hormone antibody binding capacities below 2 mg/L have not been associated with growth attenuation. In some cases when binding capacity exceeds 2 mg/L, growth attenuation has been observed. In clinical studies of patients that were treated with Nutropin for the first time, 0/107 growth hormone inadequate (GHI) patients and 0/125 CRI patients screened for antibody production developed antibodies with binding capacities ≥ 2 mg/L at six months.

Additional short-term immunologic and renal function studies were carried out in a group of patients with chronic renal insufficiency after approximately one year of treatment to detect other potential adverse effects of antibodies to growth hormone. Testing included measurements of C1q, C3, C4, rheumatoid factor, creatinine, creatinine clearance and BUN. No adverse effects of growth hormone antibodies were noted.

In addition to an evaluation of compliance with the prescribed treatment program and thyroid status, testing for antibodies to human growth hormone should be carried out in any patient who fails to respond to therapy.

In studies in children treated with Nutropin, injection site pain was reported infrequently.

Leukemia has been reported in a small number of growth hormone deficient patients treated with growth hormone. It is uncertain whether this increased risk is related to the pathology of growth hormone deficiency itself, growth hormone therapy, or other associated treatments such as radiation therapy for intracranial tumors. On the basis of current evidence, experts cannot conclude that growth hormone therapy is responsible for these occurrences. There have been no reports of leukemia in growth hormone-treated CRI

patients. The risk to GHI and CRI patients, if any, remains to be established.

Other adverse drug reactions that have been reported in growth hormone-treated patients included the following: 1) Metabolic: Infrequent, mild and transient peripheral edema. 2) Musculoskeletal: Rare carpal tunnel syndrome. 3) Skin: Rare increased growth of pre-existing nevi. Malignant nevi transformation has not been reported. 4) Endocrine: Rare gynecomastia. Rare pancreatitis.

OVERDOSAGE

The recommended dosage for GHI is 0.30 mg/kg (approximately 0.90 IU/kg) of body weight weekly. The recommended dosage for CRI is 0.35 mg/kg (approximately 1.05 IU/kg) of body weight weekly. Long-term overdosage could result in signs and symptoms of gigantism and/or acromegaly consistent with the known effects of excess human growth hormone.

DOSAGE AND ADMINISTRATION

Growth Hormone Inadequacy (GHI)

A weekly dosage of 0.30 mg/kg (approximately 0.90 IU/kg) of body weight administered by daily subcutaneous injection is recommended.

The Nutropin® [somatropin (rDNA origin) for injection] dosage and administration schedule for GHI should be individualized for each patient. Therapy should not be continued if final height is achieved or epiphyseal fusion occurs. Patients who fail to respond adequately while on Nutropin therapy should be evaluated to determine the cause of unresponsiveness.

Chronic Renal Insufficiency (CRI)

A weekly dosage of 0.35 mg/kg (approximately 1.05 IU/kg) of body weight administered by daily subcutaneous injection is recommended.

The duration of Nutropin therapy for CRI should be individualized for each patient.

Nutropin therapy may be continued up to the time of renal transplantation. Therapy should not be continued if final height is achieved or epiphyseal fusion occurs. Patients who fail to respond adequately while on Nutropin therapy should be evaluated to determine the cause of unresponsiveness. In order to optimize therapy for patients who require dialysis, the following guidelines for injection schedule are recommended:

1. Hemodialysis patients should receive their injection at night just prior to going to sleep or at least 3-4 hours after their hemodialysis to prevent hematoma formation due to the heparin.
2. Chronic Cycling Peritoneal Dialysis (CCPD) patients should receive their injection in the morning after they have completed dialysis.
3. Chronic Ambulatory Peritoneal Dialysis (CAPD) patients should receive their injection in the evening at the time of the overnight exchange.

After the dose has been determined, reconstitute as follows: each 5 mg vial should be reconstituted with 1–5 mL of Bacteriostatic Water for Injection, USP (benzyl alcohol preserved); or each 10 mg vial should be reconstituted with 1–10 mL of Bacteriostatic Water for Injection, USP (benzyl alcohol preserved) only. For use in newborns see WARNINGS. The pH of Nutropin after reconstitution with Bacteriostatic Water for Injection, USP (benzyl alcohol preserved) is approximately 7.4.

To prepare the Nutropin solution, inject the Bacteriostatic Water for Injection, USP (benzyl alcohol preserved) into the Nutropin vial, aiming the stream of liquid against the glass wall. Then swirl the product vial with a GENTLE rotary motion until the contents are completely dissolved. DO NOT SHAKE. Because Nutropin is a protein, shaking can result in a cloudy solution. The Nutropin solution should be clear immediately after reconstitution. Occasionally, after refrigeration, you may notice that small colorless particles of protein are present in the Nutropin solution. This is not unusual for solutions containing proteins. If the solution is cloudy immediately after reconstitution or refrigeration, the contents MUST NOT be injected.

Before needle insertion, wipe the septum of both the Nutropin and diluent vials with rubbing alcohol or an antiseptic solution to prevent contamination of the contents by microorganisms that may be introduced by repeated needle insertions. It is recommended that Nutropin be administered using sterile, disposable syringes and needles. The syringes should be of small enough volume that the prescribed dose can be drawn from the vial with reasonable accuracy.

STABILITY AND STORAGE

Before Reconstitution—Nutropin® [somatropin (rDNA origin) for injection], and Bacteriostatic Water for Injection, USP (benzyl alcohol preserved), must be stored at 2–8°C/36–46°F (under refrigeration). Avoid freezing the vials of Nutropin and Bacteriostatic Water for Injection, USP (benzyl

alcohol preserved). Expiration dates are stated on the labels. After Reconstitution—Vial contents are stable for 14 days when reconstituted with Bacteriostatic Water for Injection, USP (benzyl alcohol preserved) and stored at 2–8°C/36–46°F (under refrigeration). Store the unused portion of Bacteriostatic Water for Injection, USP (benzyl alcohol preserved) at 2–8°C/36–46°F (under refrigeration). Avoid freezing the reconstituted vial of Nutropin and the Bacteriostatic Water for Injection, USP (benzyl alcohol preserved).

HOW SUPPLIED

Nutropin is supplied as 5 mg (approximately 15 IU) or 10 mg (approximately 30 IU) of lyophilized, sterile somatropin per vial.

Each 5 mg carton contains two vials of Nutropin® [somatropin (rDNA origin) for injection] (5 mg per vial) and one 10 mL multiple dose vial of Bacteriostatic Water for Injection, USP (benzyl alcohol preserved). NDC 50242-072-02

Each 10 mg carton contains two vials of Nutropin [somatropin (rDNA origin) for injection] (10 mg per vial) and two 10 mL multiple dose vials of Bacteriostatic Water for Injection, USP (benzyl alcohol preserved). NDC 50242-018-20

Nutropin® [somatropin (rDNA origin) for injection] manufactured by:
Genentech, Inc.
460 Point San Bruno Boulevard
South San Francisco, CA 94080-4990
Bacteriostatic Water for Injection, USP (benzyl alcohol preserved) Manufactured for:
Genentech, Inc.
Nutropin®
[somatropin (rDNA origin) for injection]
From Genentech, Inc.   G48086-R2
© 1995 Genentech, Inc.   Revised July, 1995
Shown in Product Identification Guide, page 311

NUTROPIN AQ™   ℞
[somatropin (rDNA origin) injection]

DESCRIPTION

Nutropin AQ™ [somatropin (rDNA origin) injection], is a human growth hormone (hGH) produced by recombinant DNA technology. Nutropin AQ has 191 amino acid residues and a molecular weight of 22,125 daltons. The amino acid sequence of the product is identical to that of pituitary-derived human growth hormone. The protein is synthesized by a specific laboratory strain of *E. coli* as a precursor consisting of the rhGH molecule preceded by the secretion signal from an *E. coli* protein. This precursor is directed to the plasma membrane of the cell. The signal sequence is removed and the native protein is secreted into the periplasm so that the protein is folded appropriately as it is synthesized.

Nutropin AQ is a highly purified preparation. Biological potency is determined by measuring the increase in body weight induced in hypophysectomized rats. Nutropin AQ may contain not more than fifteen percent deamidated growth hormone at expiration. The deamidated form of growth hormone has been extensively characterized and has been shown to be safe and fully active.

Nutropin AQ is a sterile liquid intended for subcutaneous administration. The product is nearly isotonic at a concentration of 5 mg of growth hormone per mL and has a pH of approximately 6.0.

Each 2 mL vial contains 10 mg (approximately 30 IU) somatropin, formulated in 17.4 mg sodium chloride, 5 mg phenol, 4 mg polysorbate 20, and 10 mM sodium citrate.

CLINICAL PHARMACOLOGY
General

In vitro, preclinical, and clinical testing have demonstrated that Nutropin AQ is therapeutically equivalent to pituitary-derived human growth hormone. Treatment of children who lack adequate endogenous growth hormone secretion with Nutropin AQ resulted in an increase in growth rate and an increase in insulin-like growth factor-I levels similar to that seen with pituitary-derived human growth hormone.

Actions that have been demonstrated for Nutropin AQ, somatropin, somatrem and/or pituitary-derived human growth hormone include:

A. Tissue Growth—1) Skeletal Growth: Nutropin AQ stimulates skeletal growth in children with growth failure due to a lack of adequate secretion of endogenous growth hormone. Skeletal growth is accomplished at the epiphyseal plates at the ends of a growing bone. Growth and metabolism of epiphyseal plate cells are directly stimulated by growth hormone and one of its mediators, insulin-like growth factor-I. Serum levels of insulin-like growth factor-I are low in children and adolescents who are growth

hormone inadequate, but increase during treatment with Nutropin AQ. New bone is formed at the epiphyses in response to growth hormone. This results in linear growth until these growth plates fuse at the end of puberty. 2) Cell Growth: Treatment with pituitary-derived human growth hormone results in an increase in both the number and the size of skeletal muscle cells. 3) Organ Growth: Growth hormone of human pituitary origin influences the size of internal organs, including kidneys, and increases red cell mass. Treatment of hypophysectomized or genetic dwarf rats with somatropin results in organ growth that is proportional to the overall body growth. In normal rats subjected to nephrectomy-induced uremia, somatropin promoted skeletal and body growth.

B. Protein Metabolism—Linear growth is facilitated in part by growth hormone-stimulated protein synthesis. This is reflected by nitrogen retention as demonstrated by a decline in urinary nitrogen excretion and blood urea nitrogen concentration during growth hormone therapy.

C. Carbohydrate Metabolism—Growth hormone is a modulator of carbohydrate metabolism. For example, children with inadequate secretion of growth hormone sometimes experience fasting hypoglycemia that is improved by treatment with growth hormone. Administration of somatropin to normal adults, patients with chronic renal insufficiency, and patients who lack adequate secretion of endogenous growth hormone resulted in increases in mean serum fasting and postprandial insulin levels. There were no clinically significant persistent abnormalities in any of these measurements of glucose regulation that were related to growth hormone treatment. Mean values remained well within the normal range.

D. Lipid Metabolism—Acute administration of pituitary-derived human growth hormone to humans results in lipid mobilization. Nonesterified fatty acids increased in plasma within two hours of pituitary-derived human growth hormone administration. In growth hormone inadequate patients, long-term growth hormone administration often decreases body fat. Mean cholesterol levels decreased in patients treated with Nutropin AQ™ [somatropin (rDNA origin) injection].

E. Mineral Metabolism—The retention of total body potassium in response to growth hormone administration apparently results from cellular growth. Serum levels of inorganic phosphorus may increase slightly in patients with inadequate secretion of endogenous growth hormone or chronic renal insufficiency after growth hormone therapy due to metabolic activity associated with bone growth as well as increased tubular reabsorption of phosphate by the kidney. Serum calcium is not significantly altered in these patients. Sodium retention also occurs. (See PRECAUTIONS: Laboratory Tests.)

F. Connective Tissue Metabolism—Growth hormone stimulates the synthesis of chondroitin sulfate and collagen as well as the urinary excretion of hydroxyproline.

Pharmacokinetics

Subcutaneous absorption—The absolute bioavailability of rhGH after subcutaneous administration in healthy adult males has been determined to be 81 ± 20 %. The mean terminal $t^1/_2$ after subcutaneous administration is significantly longer than that seen after intravenous administration (2.3 ± 0.42 hrs vs. 19.5 ± 3.1 min) indicating that the subcutaneous absorption of the compound is slow and rate-limiting.

Distribution—Animal studies with rhGH showed that growth hormone localizes to highly perfused organs, particularly the liver and kidney. The volume of distribution at steady state for rhGH in healthy adult males is about 50 mL/kg body weight, approximating the serum volume.

Metabolism—Both the liver and kidney have been shown to be important metabolizing organs for pituitary-derived human growth hormone. Animal studies suggest that the kidney is the dominant organ of clearance. Growth hormone is filtered at the glomerulus and reabsorbed in the proximal tubules. It is then cleaved within renal cells into its constituent amino acids, which return to the systemic circulation.

Elimination—The mean terminal $t^1/_2$ after intravenous administration of rhGH in healthy adult males is estimated to be 19.5 ± 3.1 minutes. Clearance of rhGH after intravenous administration in healthy adults and children is reported to be in the range of 116–174 mL/hr/kg.

Bioequivalence of Formulations—Nutropin AQ™ [somatropin (rDNA origin) injection] has been determined to be bioequivalent to Nutropin based on the statistical evaluation of AUC and C_{max}.

Special Populations

Pediatric—Available literature data suggest that rhGH clearances are similar in adults and children.

Continued on next page

Genentech—Cont.

Gender—No data are available for rhGH. Available data for methionyl recombinant growth hormone and pituitary-derived human growth hormone suggest no consistent gender-based differences in rhGH clearance.

Race—No data are available.

Growth Hormone Insufficiency (GHI)—Reported values for clearance of rhGH in adults and children with GHI range from 138–245 mL/hr/kg and are similar to those observed in healthy adults and children. Mean terminal $t^1/_2$ values following intravenous and subcutaneous administration in adult and pediatric GHI patients are also similar to those observed in healthy adult males.

Renal Insufficiency—Children and adults with chronic renal failure (CRF) tend to have decreased clearance as compared to normals. However, no rhGH accumulation has been reported in children with CRF or end-stage renal disease (ESRD) dosed with current regimens.

Hepatic Insufficiency—A reduction in rhGH clearance has been noted in patients with severe liver dysfunction. The clinical significance of this decrease is unknown.

Effects of Nutropin® [somatropin (rDNA origin) for injection] on Growth Failure Due to Chronic Renal Insufficiency (CRI)

Two multicenter, randomized, controlled clinical trials were conducted to determine whether treatment with Nutropin prior to renal transplantation in children with chronic renal insufficiency could improve their growth rates and height deficits. One study was a double-blinded, placebo-controlled trial and the other was an open-label, randomized trial. The dose of Nutropin in both controlled studies was 0.05 mg/kg/day (0.35 mg/kg/wk) administered daily by subcutaneous injection. Combining the data from those patients completing two years in the two controlled studies results in 62 children treated with Nutropin and 28 children in the control groups (either placebo-treated or untreated). The mean first year growth rate was 10.8 cm/yr for Nutropin-treated patients, compared with a mean growth rate of 6.5 cm/yr for placebo/untreated controls (p < 0.00005). The mean second year growth rate was 7.8 cm/yr for the Nutropin-treated group, compared with 5.5 cm/yr for controls (p < 0.00005). There was a significant increase in mean height standard deviation score in the Nutropin group (–2.9 at baseline to –1.5 at Month 24, n=62) but no significant change in the controls (–2.8 at baseline to –2.9 at Month 24, n=28). The mean third year growth rate of 7.6 cm/yr in the Nutropin-treated patients (n=27) suggests that Nutropin stimulates growth beyond two years. However, there are no control data for the third year because control patients crossed over to growth hormone treatment after two years of participation. The gains in height were accompanied by appropriate advancement of skeletal age. These data demonstrate that Nutropin therapy improves growth rate and corrects the acquired height deficit associated with chronic renal insufficiency. Currently there are insufficient data regarding the benefit of treatment beyond three years. Although predicted final height was improved during Nutropin therapy, the effect of Nutropin on final adult height remains to be determined.

Post-Transplant Growth

The North American Pediatric Renal Transplant Cooperative Study (NAPRTCS) has reported data for growth post-transplant in children who did not receive growth hormone. The average change in height SD score during the initial two years post-transplant was 0.18 (n=300, J Ped 1993; 122:397–402).

Controlled studies of growth hormone treatment for the short stature associated with CRI were not designed to compare the growth of treated or untreated patients after they received renal transplants. However, growth data are available from a small number of patients who have been followed for at least 11 months. Of the 7 control patients, 4 increased their height SD score and 3 had either no significant change or a decrease in height SD score. The 13 patients treated with Nutropin [somatropin (rDNA origin) for injection] prior to transplant had either no significant change or an increase in height SD score after transplantation, indicating that the individual gains achieved with growth hormone therapy prior to transplant were maintained after transplantation. The differences in the height deficit narrowed between the treated and untreated groups in the post-transplant period.

INDICATIONS AND USAGE

Nutropin AQ™ [somatropin (rDNA origin) injection] is indicated for the long-term treatment of children who have growth failure due to a lack of adequate endogenous growth hormone secretion.

Nutropin AQ™ [somatropin (rDNA origin) injection] is also indicated for the treatment of children who have growth failure associated with chronic renal insufficiency up to the time of renal transplantation. Nutropin AQ therapy should be used in conjunction with optimal management of chronic renal insufficiency.

CONTRAINDICATIONS

Nutropin AQ™ [somatropin (rDNA origin) injection] should not be used in subjects with closed epiphyses.

Nutropin AQ™ [somatropin (rDNA origin) injection] should not be used in patients with active neoplasia. Growth hormone therapy should be discontinued if evidence of neoplasia develops.

WARNINGS

None.

PRECAUTIONS

General: Nutropin AQ should be prescribed by physicians experienced in the diagnosis and management of patients with CRI or growth failure. No studies have been performed of Nutropin AQ in children who have received renal transplants. Currently, treatment of patients with functioning renal allografts is not indicated.

Because Nutropin AQ may induce a state of insulin resistance, patients should be monitored for evidence of glucose intolerance.

Patients with a history of an intracranial lesion taking somatropin and/or somatropin liquid should be examined frequently for progression or recurrence of the lesion.

Patients with growth failure secondary to CRI should be examined periodically for evidence of progression of renal osteodystrophy. Slipped capital femoral epiphysis or avascular necrosis of the femoral head may be seen in children with advanced renal osteodystrophy, and it is uncertain whether these problems are affected by growth hormone therapy. X-rays of the hips should be obtained prior to initiating therapy for CRI patients.

Slipped capital femoral epiphysis may also occur more frequently in patients with endocrine disorders or in patients undergoing rapid growth. Therefore, physicians and parents should be alert to the development of a limp or complaints of hip or knee pain in GHI or CRI patients treated with Nutropin AQ.

Progression of scoliosis can occur in children who experience rapid growth. Because growth hormone increases growth rate, patients with a history of scoliosis who are treated with growth hormone should be monitored for progression of scoliosis. Growth hormone has not been shown to increase the incidence of scoliosis.

Intracranial hypertension (IH) with papilledema, visual changes, headache, nausea and/or vomiting has been reported in a small number of patients treated with growth hormone products. Symptoms usually occurred within the first eight (8) weeks of the initiation of growth hormone therapy. In all reported cases, IH-associated signs and symptoms resolved after termination of therapy or a reduction of the growth hormone dose. Funduscopic examination of patients is recommended at the initiation and periodically during the course of growth hormone therapy.

As for any protein, local or systemic allergic reactions may occur. Parents/Patient should be informed that such reactions are possible and that prompt medical attention should be sought if allergic reactions occur.

Laboratory Tests: Serum levels of inorganic phosphorus, alkaline phosphatase, and parathyroid hormone (PTH) may increase with Nutropin AQ therapy. Changes in thyroid hormone laboratory measurements may develop during Nutropin AQ treatment in children who lack adequate endogenous growth hormone secretion. Untreated hypothyroidism prevents optimal response to Nutropin AQ. Therefore, patients should have periodic thyroid function tests and should be treated with thyroid hormone when indicated.

Drug Interaction: The use of Nutropin AQ™ [somatropin (rDNA origin) injection] in patients with CRI receiving glucocorticoid therapy has not been evaluated. Concomitant glucocorticoid therapy may inhibit the growth promoting effect of Nutropin AQ. If glucocorticoid replacement is required, the dose should be carefully adjusted.

There was no evidence in the controlled studies of somatropin's interaction with drugs commonly used in chronic renal insufficiency patients. However, formal drug interaction studies have not been conducted.

Carcinogenesis, Mutagenesis, Impairment of Fertility: Carcinogenicity, mutagenicity and reproduction studies have not been conducted with Nutropin AQ.

Pregnancy: Pregnancy (Category C). Animal reproduction studies have not been conducted with Nutropin AQ. It is also not known whether Nutropin AQ can cause fetal harm when administered to a pregnant woman or can affect reproduction capacity. Nutropin AQ should be given to a pregnant woman only if clearly needed.

Nursing Mothers: It is not known whether Nutropin AQ is excreted in human milk. Because many drugs are excreted in human milk, caution should be exercised when Nutropin AQ is administered to a nursing mother.

Information for Patients: Patients being treated with growth hormone and/or their parents should be informed of the potential benefits and risks associated with treatment. If home use is determined to be desirable by the physician, instructions on appropriate use should be given, including a review of the contents of the Patient Information Insert.

This information is intended to aid in the safe and effective administration of the medication. It is not a disclosure of all possible adverse or intended effects.

If home use is prescribed, a puncture resistant container for the disposal of used syringes and needles should be recommended to the patient. Patients and/or parents should be thoroughly instructed in the importance of proper disposal and cautioned against any reuse of needles and syringes (see Patient Information Insert).

ADVERSE REACTIONS

As with all protein pharmaceuticals, a small percentage of patients may develop antibodies to the protein. Growth hormone antibody binding capacities below 2 mg/L have not been associated with growth attenuation. In some cases when binding capacity exceeds 2 mg/L, growth attenuation has been observed. In clinical studies of patients that were treated with Nutropin® [somatropin (rDNA origin) for injection] for the first time, 0/107 growth hormone inadequate (GHI) patients and 0/125 CRI patients screened for antibody production developed antibodies with binding capacities ≥ 2 mg/L at six months. In a clinical study of patients that were treated with Nutropin AQ™ [somatropin (rDNA origin) injection] for the first time, 0/38 GHI patients screened for antibody production, for up to 15 months, developed antibodies with binding capacities ≥ 2 mg/L.

Additional short-term immunologic and renal function studies were carried out in a group of patients with chronic renal insufficiency after approximately one year of treatment to detect other potential adverse effects of antibodies to growth hormone. Testing included measurements of C1q, C3, C4, rheumatoid factor, creatinine, creatinine clearance and BUN. No adverse effects of growth hormone antibodies were noted.

In addition to an evaluation of compliance with the prescribed treatment program and thyroid status, testing for antibodies to human growth hormone should be carried out in any patient who fails to respond to therapy.

In studies in children treated with somatropin, injection site pain was reported infrequently.

Leukemia has been reported in a small number of growth hormone deficient patients treated with growth hormone. It is uncertain whether this increased risk is related to the pathology of growth hormone deficiency itself, growth hormone therapy, or other associated treatments such as radiation therapy for intracranial tumors. On the basis of current evidence, experts cannot conclude that growth hormone therapy is responsible for these occurrences. There have been no reports of leukemia in CRI patients treated with growth hormone. The risk to GHI and CRI patients, if any, remains to be established.

Other adverse drug reactions that have been reported in growth hormone-treated patients include the following: 1) Metabolic: Infrequent, mild and transient peripheral edema. 2) Musculoskeletal: Rare carpal tunnel syndrome. 3) Skin: Rare increased growth of pre-existing nevi. Malignant nevi transformation has not been reported. 4) Endocrine: Rare gynecomastia. Rare pancreatitis.

OVERDOSAGE

The recommended dosage for GHI is 0.30 mg/kg (approximately 0.90 IU/kg) of body weight weekly. The recommended dosage for CRI is 0.35 mg/kg (approximately 1.05 IU/kg) of body weight weekly. Long-term overdosage could result in signs and symptoms of gigantism and/or acromegaly consistent with the known effects of excess human growth hormone.

DOSAGE AND ADMINISTRATION

Growth Hormone Inadequacy (GHI)

A weekly dosage of 0.30 mg/kg (approximately 0.90 IU/kg) of body weight administered by daily subcutaneous injection is recommended.

The Nutropin AQ™ [somatropin (rDNA origin) injection] dosage and administration schedule for GHI should be individualized for each patient. Therapy should not be continued if final height is achieved or epiphyseal fusion occurs. Patients who fail to respond adequately while on Nutropin AQ should be evaluated to determine the cause of unresponsiveness.

Chronic Renal Insufficiency (CRI)

A weekly dosage of 0.35 mg/kg (approximately 1.05 IU/kg) of body weight administered by daily subcutaneous injection is recommended.

The duration of Nutropin AQ therapy for CRI should be individualized for each patient.

Nutropin AQ therapy may be continued up to the time of renal transplantation. Therapy should not be continued if final height is achieved or epiphyseal fusion occurs. Patients who fail to respond adequately while on Nutropin AQ therapy should be evaluated to determine the cause of unresponsiveness.

In order to optimize therapy for patients who require dialysis, the following guidelines for injection schedule are recommended:

1. Hemodialysis patients should receive their injection at night just prior to going to sleep or at least 3–4 hours after

their hemodialysis to prevent hematoma formation due to the heparin.
2. Chronic Cycling Peritoneal Dialysis (CCPD) patients should receive their injection in the morning after they have completed dialysis.
3. Chronic Ambulatory Peritoneal Dialysis (CAPD) patients should receive their injection in the evening at the time of the overnight exchange.

The solution should be clear immediately after removal from the refrigerator. Occasionally, after refrigeration, you may notice that small colorless particles of protein are present in the solution. This is not unusual for solutions containing proteins. Allow the vial to come to room temperature and gently swirl. If the solution is cloudy the contents **MUST NOT** be injected.
Before needle insertion, wipe the septum of the Nutropin AQ™ [somatropin (rDNA origin) injection] vial with rubbing alcohol or an antiseptic solution to prevent contamination of the contents by microorganisms that may be introduced by repeated needle insertions. It is recommended that Nutropin AQ be administered using sterile, disposable syringes and needles. The syringes should be of small enough volume that the prescribed dose can be drawn from the vial with reasonable accuracy.

STABILITY AND STORAGE

Vial contents are stable for 28 days after initial use when stored at 2–8°C/36–46°F (under refrigeration). **Avoid freezing the vial of Nutropin AQ.**

HOW SUPPLIED

Nutropin AQ is supplied as 10 mg (approximately 30 IU) of sterile liquid somatropin per vial.
Each carton contains six single vial cartons containing one 2 mL vial of Nutropin AQ™ [somatropin (rDNA origin) injection] (5 mg/mL).
NDC 50242-114-11

Nutropin AQ™ [somatropin (rDNA origin) injection]
Manufactured by:
Genentech, Inc. G48109-R0
460 Pt San Bruno Blvd January, 1996
So San Francisco, CA 94080-4990 ©1996 Genentech, Inc.
Shown in Product Identification Guide, page 311

PROTROPIN® ℞
(somatrem for injection)

DESCRIPTION

Protropin® (somatrem for injection), is a polypeptide hormone produced by recombinant DNA technology. Protropin has 192 amino acid residues and a molecular weight of about 22,000 daltons. The product contains the identical sequence of 191 amino acids constituting pituitary-derived human growth hormone plus an additional amino acid, methionine, on the N-terminus of the molecule. Protropin is synthesized in a special laboratory strain of *E. coli* bacteria which has been modified by the addition of the gene for human growth hormone production.
Protropin is a highly purified preparation. Biological potency is determined by measuring the increase in body weight induced in hypophysectomized rats.
Protropin is a sterile, white, lyophilized powder intended for intramuscular or subcutaneous administration after reconstitution with Bacteriostatic Water for Injection, USP (benzyl alcohol preserved).
Each 5 mg Protropin vial 5 mg (approximately 15 IU) somatrem, lyophilized with 40 mg mannitol, and 1.7 mg sodium phosphates (0.1 mg sodium phosphate monobasic and 1.6 mg sodium phosphate dibasic).
Each 10 mg Protropin vial contains 10 mg (approximately 30 IU) somatrem, lyophilized with 80 mg mannitol, and 3.4 mg sodium phosphates (0.2 mg sodium phosphate monobasic and 3.2 mg sodium phosphate dibasic).
Phosphoric acid may be used for pH adjustment.
Bacteriostatic Water for Injection, USP is a sterile water containing 0.9 percent benzyl alcohol per mL as an antimicrobial preservative packaged in a multi-dose vial. The diluent pH is 4.5–7.0.

CLINICAL PHARMACOLOGY

General

In vitro and in vivo preclinical, and clinical testing have demonstrated that Protropin is therapeutically equivalent to pituitary-derived human growth hormone. Treatment of children who lack adequate endogenous growth hormone secretion with Protropin resulted in an increase in growth rate and an increase in insulin-like growth factor-l levels similar to that seen with pituitary-derived human growth hormone.
Actions that have been demonstrated for Protropin, somatropin and/or pituitary-derived human growth hormone include:

A. Tissue Growth—1) Skeletal Growth: Protropin stimulates skeletal growth in children with growth failure due to a lack of adequate secretion of endogenous growth hormone. Skeletal growth is accomplished at the epiphyseal plates at the ends of a growing bone. Growth and metabolism of epiphyseal plate cells are directly stimulated by growth hormone and one of its mediators, insulin-like growth factor-l. Serum levels of insulin-like growth factor-l are low in children and adolescents who are growth hormone deficient, but increase during treatment with Protropin. New bone is formed at the epiphyses in response to growth hormone. This results in linear growth until these growth plates fuse at the end of puberty. 2) Cell Growth: Treatment with pituitary-derived human growth hormone results in an increase in both the number and the size of skeletal muscle cells. 3) Organ Growth: Growth hormone of human pituitary origin influences the size of internal organs, including kidneys, and increases red cell mass. Treatment of hypophysectomized or genetic dwarf rats with somatropin results in organ growth that is proportional to the overall body growth.

B. Protein Metabolism—Linear growth is facilitated in part by growth hormone-stimulated protein synthesis. This is reflected by nitrogen retention as demonstrated by a decline in urinary nitrogen excretion and blood urea nitrogen during growth hormone therapy.

C. Carbohydrate Metabolism—Growth hormone is a modulator of carbohydrate metabolism. For example, children with inadequate secretion of growth hormone sometimes experience fasting hypoglycemia that is improved by treatment with growth hormone. Protropin therapy may decrease glucose tolerance. Administration of Protropin to normal adults and patients who lacked adequate secretion of endogenous growth hormone resulted in increases in mean serum fasting and postprandial insulin levels. However, mean glucose and hemoglobin A_{1C} levels remained in the normal range.

D. Lipid Metabolism—Acute administration of pituitary-derived human growth hormone to humans resulted in lipid mobilization. Nonesterified fatty acids increased in plasma within two hours of pituitary-derived human growth hormone administration. In growth hormone deficient patients, long-term growth hormone administration often decreases body fat. Mean cholesterol levels decreased in patients treated with growth hormone.

E. Mineral Metabolism—The retention of total body potassium in response to growth hormone administration apparently results from cellular growth. Serum levels of inorganic phosphorus may increase slightly in patients with inadequate secretion of endogenous growth hormone after growth hormone therapy due to metabolic activity associated with bone growth as well as increased tubular reabsorption of phosphate by the kidney. Serum calcium is not significantly altered in these patients. Sodium retention also occurs. (See PRECAUTIONS: Laboratory Tests.)

F. Connective Tissue Metabolism—Growth hormone stimulates the synthesis of chondroitin sulfate and collagen as well as the urinary excretion of hydroxyproline.

INDICATIONS AND USAGE

Protropin® (somatrem for injection) is indicated only for the long- term treatment of children who have growth failure due to a lack of adequate endogenous growth hormone secretion. Other etiologies of short stature should be excluded.

CONTRAINDICATIONS

Protropin should not be used in subjects with closed epiphyses.
Protropin should not be used in patients with active neoplasia. Growth hormone therapy should be discontinued if evidence of neoplasia develops.
Protropin, when reconstituted with Bacteriostatic Water for Injection, USP (benzyl alcohol preserved) should not be used in patients with a known sensitivity to benzyl alcohol.

WARNINGS

Benzyl alcohol as a preservative in Bacteriostatic Water for Injection, USP has been associated with toxicity in newborns. When administering Protropin to newborns, reconstitute with Sterile Water for Injection, USP. USE ONLY ONE DOSE PER PROTROPIN VIAL AND DISCARD THE UNUSED PORTION.

PRECAUTIONS

General: Protropin should be prescribed by physicians experienced in the diagnosis and management of patients with growth failure.
Because Protropin may induce a state of insulin resistance, patients should be observed for evidence of glucose intolerance.
Patients with a history of an intracranial lesion should be examined frequently for progression or recurrence of the lesion.
Slipped capital femoral epiphysis may occur more frequently in patients with endocrine disorders or in patients undergoing rapid growth. Physicians and parents should be alert to the development of a limp or complaints of hip or knee pain in Protropin-treated patients.
Progression of scoliosis can occur in children who experience rapid growth. Because growth hormone increases growth rate, patients with a history of scoliosis who are treated with growth hormone should be monitored for progression of scoliosis. Growth hormone has not been shown to increase the incidence of scoliosis.
Intracranial hypertension (IH) with papilledema, visual changes, headache, nausea and/or vomiting has been reported in a small number of patients treated with growth hormone products. Symptoms usually occurred within the first eight (8) weeks of the initiation of growth hormone therapy. In all reported cases, IH-associated signs and symptoms resolved after termination of therapy or a reduction of the growth hormone dose. Funduscopic examination of patients is recommended at the initiation and periodically during the course of growth hormone therapy.
See WARNINGS for use of Bacteriostatic Water for Injection, USP (benzyl alcohol preserved) in newborns.
As with any protein, local or systemic allergic reactions may occur. Parents/Patient should be informed that such reactions are possible and that prompt medical attention should be sought if allergic reactions occur.
Laboratory Tests: Serum levels of inorganic phosphorus, alkaline phosphatase, and parathyroid hormone (PTH) may increase with Protropin therapy. Changes in thyroid hormone laboratory measurements may develop during Protropin treatment of children who lack adequate endogenous growth hormone secretion. Untreated hypothyroidism prevents optimal response to Protropin. Therefore, patients should have periodic thyroid function tests and should be treated with thyroid hormone when indicated.
Drug Interactions: Concomitant glucocorticoid therapy may inhibit the growth promoting effect of Protropin. If glucocorticoid replacement is required, the dose should be carefully adjusted.
Carcinogenesis, Mutagenesis, Impairment of Fertility: Carcinogenicity, mutagenicity and reproduction studies have not been conducted with Protropin.
Pregnancy: Pregnancy (Category C). Animal reproduction studies have not been conducted with Protropin. It is also not known whether Protropin can cause fetal harm when administered to a pregnant woman or can affect reproduction capacity. Protropin should be given to a pregnant woman only if clearly needed.
Nursing Mothers: It is not known whether this drug is excreted in human milk. Because many drugs are excreted in human milk, caution should be exercised when Proptropin is administered to a nursing mother.
Information for Patients: Patients being treated with growth hormone and/or their parents should be informed of the potential benefits and risks associated with treatment. If home use is determined to be desirable by the physician, instructions on appropriate use should be given, including a review of the contents of the Patient Information Insert. This information is intended to aid in the safe and effective administration of the medication. It is not a disclosure of all possible adverse or intended effects.
If home use is prescribed, a puncture resistant container for the disposal of used syringes and needles should be recommended to the patient. Patients and/or parents should be thoroughly instructed in the importance of proper disposal and cautioned against any reuse of needles and syringes (see Patient Information Insert).

ADVERSE REACTIONS

As with all protein pharmaceuticals, a small percentage of patients may develop antibodies to the protein. Growth hormone antibody binding capacities below 2 mg/L have not been associated with growth attenuation. In some cases when binding capacity exceeds 2 mg/L, growth attenuation has been observed. In clinical studies and postmarketing experience of patients treated with Protropin, approximately 0.4 percent of patients screened for antibody production developed antibodies with binding capacities > 2 mg/L at six months. Out of approximately 26,000 patients who have been treated with Protropin, 5 patients have had growth deceleration associated with binding capacities > 2 mg/L. If growth deceleration is observed that is not attributable to another cause, the patient should be tested for antibodies to growth hormone. Although no evidence exists to indicate that the methionine on the N-terminus of somatrem causes antibodies to growth hormone, the physician should consider transferring the patient to somatropin (rDNA origin) for injection, if a patient has antibody binding capacity > 2 mg/L, and has exhibited growth attenuation.
In addition to an evaluation of compliance with the prescribed treatment program and thyroid status, testing for antibodies to human growth hormone should be carried out in any patient who fails to respond to therapy.
Additional short-term immunologic and renal function studies were carried out in a group of patients after approximately two years of treatment to detect other potential ad-

Continued on next page

Genentech—Cont.

verse effects of antibodies to growth hormone. The antibody was determined to be of the IgG class; no antibodies to growth hormone of the IgE class were detected. Testing included immune complex determination, measurement of total hemolytic complement and specific complement components, and immunochemical analyses. No adverse effects of growth hormone antibody formation were observed.

These findings are supported by a toxicity study conducted in a primate model in which a similar antibody response to growth was observed. Protropin, administered to monkeys by intramuscular injection at doses of 125 and 625 ug/kg TIW, was compared to pituitary-human growth hormone at the same doses and with placebo over a period of 90 days. Most monkeys treated with high-dose Protropin developed persistent antibodies at week four. There were no biologically significant drug related changes in standard laboratory variables. Histopathologic examination of the kidney and other selected organs (pituitary, lungs, liver and pancreas) showed no treatment related toxicity. There was no evidence of immune complexes or immune complex toxicity when the kidney was also examined for the presence of immune complexes and possible toxic effects of immune complexes by immunohistochemistry and electron microscopy.

In studies in children treated with Protropin, injection site pain was reported infrequently.

Leukemia has been reported in a small number of growth hormone deficient patients treated with growth hormone. It is uncertain whether this increased risk is related to the pathology of growth hormone deficiency itself, growth hormone therapy, or other associated treatments such as radiation therapy for intracranial tumors. On the basis of current evidence, experts cannot conclude that growth hormone therapy is responsible for these occurrences. The risk to an individual patient, if any, remains to be established.

Other adverse drug reactions that have been reported in growth hormone-treated patients include the following: 1) Metabolic: Infrequent, mild and transient peripheral edema. 2) Musculoskeletal: Rare carpal tunnel syndrome. 3) Skin: Rare increased growth of pre-existing nevi. Malignant nevi transformation has not been reported. 4) Endocrine: Rare gynecomastia. Rare pancreatitis.

OVERDOSAGE
The recommended dosage of up to 0.30 mg/kg (approximately 0.90 IU/kg) of body weight weekly should not be exceeded due to the potential risk of known effects of excess human growth hormone.

DOSAGE AND ADMINISTRATION
A weekly dosage of 0.30 mg/kg (approximately 0.90 IU/kg) of body weight administered by daily intramuscular or subcutaneous injection is recommended.

The Protropin dosage and administration schedule should be individualized for each patient. Therapy should not be continued if final height is achieved or epiphyseal fusion occurs. Patients who fail to respond adequately while on Protropin therapy should be evaluated to determine the cause of unresponsiveness.

After the dose has been determined, reconstitute as follows: each 5 mg vial should be reconstituted with 1–5 mL of Bacteriostatic Water for Injection, USP (benzyl alcohol preserved); or each 10 mg vial should be reconstituted with 1–10 mL Bacteriostatic Water for Injection, USP (benzyl alcohol preserved) only. For use in newborns see WARNINGS. The pH of Protropin after reconstitution with Bacteriostatic Water for Injection, USP (benzyl alcohol preserved) is approximately 7.8.

To prepare the Protropin solution, inject the Bacteriostatic Water for Injection, USP (benzyl alcohol preserved) into the Protropin vial, aiming the stream of liquid against the glass wall. Then swirl the product vial with a **GENTLE** rotary motion until the contents are completely dissolved. **DO NOT SHAKE.** Because Protropin is a protein, shaking can result in a cloudy solution. The Protropin solution should be clear immediately after reconstitution. Occasionally, after refrigeration, you may notice that small colorless particles of protein are present in the Protropin solution. This is not unusual for solutions containing proteins. If the solution is cloudy immediately after reconstitution or refrigeration, the contents **MUST NOT** be injected.

Before needle insertion, wipe the septum of both the Protropin and diluent vials with rubbing alcohol or an antiseptic solution to prevent contamination of the contents by microorganisms that may be introduced by repeated needle insertions. It is recommended that Protropin be administered using sterile, disposable syringes and needles. The syringes should be of small enough volume that the prescribed dose can be drawn from the vial with reasonable accuracy.

STABILITY AND STORAGE
Before Reconstitution—Protropin® (somatrem for injection), and Bacteriostatic Water for Injection, USP (benzyl alcohol preserved), must be stored at 2–8°C/36–46°F (under refrigeration). **Avoid freezing the vials of Protropin and**

Bacteriostatic Water for Injection, USP (benzyl alcohol preserved). Expiration dates are stated on the labels.

After Reconstitution—Vial contents are stable for 14 days when reconstituted with Bacteriostatic Water for Injection, USP (benzyl alcohol preserved) at 2–8°C/36–46°F (under refrigeration. Store the unused portion of Bacteriostatic Water for Injection, USP (benzyl alcohol preserved) at 2–8°C/36–46°F (under refrigeration). **Avoid freezing the vials of Protropin and Bacteriostatic Water for Injection, USP (benzyl alcohol preserved).**

HOW SUPPLIED
Protropin® (somatrem for injection) is supplied as 5 mg (approximately 15 IU) or 10 mg (approximately 30 IU) of lyophilized, sterile, somatrem per vial.

Each 5 mg carton contains two vials of Protropin (somatrem for injection) (5 mg per vial) and one 10 mL multiple dose vial of Bacteriostatic Water for Injection, USP (benzyl alcohol preserved). NDC 50242-015-02

Each 10 mg carton contains two vials of Protropin (somatrem for injection) (10 mg per vial) and two 10 mL multiple dose vials of Bacteriostatic Water for Injection, USP (benzyl alcohol preserved). NDC 50242-016-20

Protropin® (somatrem for injection) Manufactured by:
Genetech, Inc.
460 Point San Bruno Boulevard
South San Francisco, CA 94080-4990
Bacteriostatic Water for Injection, USP (benzyl alcohol preserved)
Manufactured for:
Genentech, Inc.
Protropin®
(somatrem for injection)
From Genentech, Inc. G40053-R9
©1995 Genentech, Inc. Revised July, 1995
Shown in Product Identification Guide, page 311

PULMOZYME® ℞
(dornase alfa)
recombinant
INHALATION SOLUTION

DESCRIPTION
PULMOZYME (dornase alfa) INHALATION SOLUTION is a sterile, clear, colorless, highly purified solution of recombinant human deoxyribonuclease I (rhDNase), an enzyme which selectively cleaves DNA. The protein is produced by genetically engineered Chinese Hamster Ovary (CHO) cells containing DNA encoding for the native human protein, deoxyribonuclease I (DNase). The product is purified by tangential flow filtration and column chromatography. The purified glycoprotein contains 260 amino acids with an approximate molecular weight of 37,000 daltons (1). The primary amino acid sequence is identical to that of the native human enzyme.

PULMOZYME is administered by inhalation of an aerosol mist produced by a compressed air driven nebulizer system (see Clinical Experience; DOSAGE AND ADMINISTRATION). Each PULMOZYME single-use ampule will deliver 2.5 mL of the solution to the nebulizer bowl. The aqueous solution contains 1.0 mg/mL dornase alfa, 0.15 mg/mL calcium chloride dihydrate and 8.77 mg/mL sodium chloride. The solution contains no preservative. The nominal pH of the solution is 6.3.

CLINICAL PHARMACOLOGY
General
In cystic fibrosis (CF) patients, retention of viscous purulent secretions in the airways contributes both to reduced pulmonary function and to exacerbations of infection (2,3).

Purulent pulmonary secretions contain very high concentrations of extracellular DNA released by degenerating leukocytes that accumulate in response to infection (4). In vitro, PULMOZYME hydrolyzes the DNA in sputum of CF patients and reduces sputum viscoelasticity (1).

Pharmacokinetics
When 2.5 mg PULMOZYME was administered by inhalation to eighteen CF patients, mean sputum concentrations of 3 μg/mL DNase were measurable within 15 minutes. Mean sputum concentrations declined to an average of 0.6 μg/mL two hours following inhalation. Inhalation of up to 10 mg TID of PULMOZYME by 4 CF patients for six consecutive days, did not result in a significant elevation of serum concentrations of DNase above normal endogenous levels (5,6). After administration of up to 2.5 mg of PULMOZYME twice daily for six months to 321 CF patients, no accumulation of serum DNase was noted.

Clinical Experience
PULMOZYME has been evaluated in a large, randomized, placebo-controlled trial of clinically stable cystic fibrosis patients, 5 years of age and older, with baseline forced vital capacity (FVC) greater than or equal to 40% of predicted and receiving standard therapies for cystic fibrosis (7). Patients were treated with placebo (325 patients), 2.5 mg of

---

PULMOZYME once a day (322 patients), or 2.5 mg of PULMOZYME twice a day (321 patients) for six months administered via a Hudson T Up-draft II nebulizer with a Pulmo-Aide compressor.

Both doses of PULMOZYME resulted in significant reductions compared with the placebo group in the number of patients experiencing respiratory tract infections requiring use of parenteral antibiotics. Administration of PULMOZYME reduced the relative risk of developing a respiratory tract infection by 27% and 29% for the 2.5 mg daily dose and the 2.5 mg twice daily dose, respectively (see Table 1). The data suggest that the effects of PULMOZYME on respiratory tract infections in older patients (> 21 years) may be smaller than in younger patients, and that twice daily dosing may be required in the older patients. Patients with baseline FVC>85% may also benefit from twice a day dosing (see Table 1). The reduced risk of respiratory infection observed in PULMOZYME treated patients did not directly correlate with improvement in FEV₁ during the initial two weeks of therapy.

Within 8 days of the start of treatment with PULMOZYME, mean FEV_1 increased 7.9% in those treated once a day and 9.0% in those treated twice a day compared to the baseline values. The mean FEV_1 observed during long-term therapy increased 5.8% from baseline at the 2.5 mg daily dose level and 5.6% from baseline at the 2.5 mg twice daily dose level. Placebo recipients did not show significant mean changes in pulmonary function testing (see Figure 1).

For patients 5 years of age or older, with baseline FVC greater than or equal to 40%, administration of PULMOZYME decreased the incidence of occurrence of first respiratory tract infection requiring parenteral antibiotics, and improved mean FEV_1, regardless of age or baseline FVC.

Table 1
Incidence of First Respiratory Tract Infection
Requiring Parenteral Antibiotics in a Controlled Trial

	Placebo N=325	2.5 mg QD N=322	2.5 mg BID N=321
Percent of Patients Infected	43%	34%	33%
Relative Risk (vs placebo)		0.73	0.71
p-value (vs placebo)		0.015	0.007

Subgroup by Age and Baseline FVC	Placebo (N)	2.5 mg QD (N)	2.5 mg BID (N)
Age			
5–20 years	42% (201)	25% (199)	28% (184)
21 years and older	44% (124)	48% (123)	39% (137)
Baseline FVC			
40–85% Predicted	54% (194)	41% (201)	44% (203)
>85% Predicted	27% (131)	21% (121)	14% (118)

Figure 1: Mean Percent Change from Baseline FEV₁ in a Controlled Trial

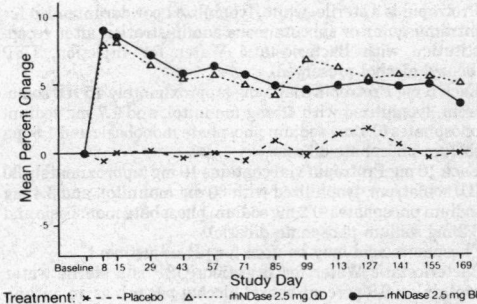

Treatment: ✻ - - Placebo   △ ········ rhDNase 2.5 mg QD   ● —— rhNDase 2.5 mg BID

Other Studies
PULMOZYME (dornase alfa) did not produce a pulmonary function benefit in short-term usage in patients with FVC less than 40% of predicted. Studies are in progress to assess the impact of chronic use on pulmonary function and infection risk in this population.

Clinical trials have indicated that PULMOZYME therapy can be continued or initiated during an acute respiratory exacerbation.

Short-term dose ranging studies demonstrated that doses in excess of 2.5 mg BID did not provide further improvement in FEV_1. Patients who have received drug on a cyclical regimen (ie, administration of PULMOZYME 10 mg BID for 14 days, followed by a 14 day wash out period) showed rapid improvement in FEV_1 with the initiation of each cycle and a return to baseline with each PULMOZYME withdrawal.

INDICATIONS AND USAGE

Daily administration of PULMOZYME in conjunction with standard therapies is indicated in the management of cystic fibrosis patients to reduce the frequency of respiratory infections requiring parenteral antibiotics and to improve pulmonary function. Safety and efficacy of daily administration have not been demonstrated in patients under the age of 5 years, or with FVC < 40% of predicted, or for longer than twelve months.

CONTRAINDICATIONS

PULMOZYME is contraindicated in patients with known hypersensitivity to dornase alfa, Chinese Hamster Ovary cell products, or any component of the product.

WARNINGS

None.

PRECAUTIONS

General

PULMOZYME should be used in conjunction with standard therapies for CF.

Information for Patients

PULMOZYME must be stored in the refrigerator at 2–8°C (36–46°F) and protected from strong light. It should be kept refrigerated during transport and should not be exposed to room temperatures for a total time of 24 hours. The solution should be discarded if it is cloudy or discolored. PULMOZYME contains no preservative and, once opened, the entire ampule must be used or discarded. Patients should be instructed in the proper use and maintenance of the nebulizer and compressor system used in its delivery.

PULMOZYME should not be diluted or mixed with other drugs in the nebulizer. Mixing of PULMOZYME with other drugs could lead to adverse physicochemical and/or functional changes in PULMOZYME or the admixed compound.

Drug Interactions

Clinical trials have indicated that PULMOZYME® (dornase alfa) can be effectively and safely used in conjunction with standard cystic fibrosis therapies including oral, inhaled and parenteral antibiotics, bronchodilators, enzyme supplements, vitamins, oral and inhaled corticosteroids, and analgesics. No formal drug interaction studies have been performed.

Carcinogenesis, Mutagenesis, Impairment of Fertility

Carcinogenesis: A two year inhalation (head-only) toxicity study of PULMOZYME in rats to assess oncogenic potential is in progress.

Mutagenesis: Ames tests using six different tester strains of bacteria (4 of S. typhimurium and 2 of E. coli) at concentrations up to 5000 μg/plate, a cytogenetic assay using human peripheral blood lymphocytes at concentrations up to 2000 μg/plate, and a mouse lymphoma assay at concentrations up to 1000 μg/plate, with and without metabolic activation, revealed no evidence of mutagenesis potential. PULMOZYME was tested in a micronucleus (in vivo) assay for its potential to produce chromosome damage in bone marrow cells of mice following a bolus intravenous dose of 10 mg/kg on two consecutive days. No evidence of chromosomal damage was noted.

Impairment of Fertility: In studies with rats receiving up to 10 mg/kg/day, a dose representing systemic exposures greater than 600 times that expected following the recommended human dose, fertility and reproductive performance of both males and females was not affected.

Pregnancy (Category B)

Reproduction studies have been performed in rats and rabbits with intravenous doses up to 10 mg/kg/day, representing systemic exposures greater than 600 times that expected following the recommended human dose. These studies have revealed no evidence of impaired fertility, harm to the fetus, or effects on development due to PULMOZYME. There are, however, no adequate and well-controlled studies in pregnant women. Because animal reproductive studies are not always predictive of the human response, this drug should be used during pregnancy only if clearly needed.

Nursing Mothers

It is not known whether the drug is excreted in human milk. Because many drugs are excreted in human milk, caution should be exercised when PULMOZYME is administered to a nursing woman.

Pediatric Use

Safety and effectiveness of PULMOZYME in children under the age of 5 years has not been studied.

ADVERSE REACTIONS

Patients have been exposed to PULMOZYME for up to 12 months in clinical trials. In a large, randomized, placebo-controlled clinical trial, over 600 patients received PULMOZYME once or twice daily for six months; most adverse events were not more common on PULMOZYME than on placebo and probably reflected the sequelae of the underlying lung disease. In most cases events that were increased were mild, transient in nature, and did not require alterations in dosing. Few patients experienced adverse events resulting in permanent discontinuation from PULMOZYME, and the discontinuation rate was similar for placebo (2%) and PULMOZYME (3%).

Events that were more frequent in PULMOZYME treated patients than in placebo treated patients are listed in Table 2.

Table 2
Adverse Events Reported in a Controlled Trial

Adverse Event	Placebo n=325	PULMOZYME QD n=322	PULMOZYME BID n=321
Voice alteration	7%	12%	16%
Pharyngitis	33%	36%	40%
Laryngitis	1%	3%	4%
Rash	7%	10%	12%
Chest pain	16%	18%	21%
Conjunctivitis	2%	4%	5%

EVENTS OBSERVED AT SIMILAR RATES IN PULMOZYME® (DORNASE ALFA) AND PLACEBO TREATED PATIENTS

Body as a Whole	Abdominal pain, Asthenia, Fever, Flu syndrome, Malaise, Sepsis
Digestive System	Intestinal Obstruction, Gall Bladder disease, Liver disease, Pancreatic disease
Metabolic Nutritional System	Diabetes Mellitus, Hypoxia, Weight Loss
Respiratory System	Apnea, Bronchiectasis, Bronchitis, Change in Sputum, Cough Increase, Dyspnea, Hemoptysis, Lung Function Decrease, Nasal Polyps, Pneumonia, Pneumothorax, Rhinitis, Sinusitis, Sputum Increase, Wheeze

Mortality rates observed in a controlled trial were similar for the placebo (1%) and PULMOZYME® (dornase alfa) (1%). Causes of death were consistent with progression of cystic fibrosis and included apnea, cardiac arrest, cardiopulmonary arrest, cor pulmonale, heart failure, massive hemoptysis, pneumonia, pneumothorax, and respiratory failure.

Allergic Reactions

There have been no reports of anaphylaxis attributed to the administration of PULMOZYME to date. Skin rash and urticaria have been observed, and were mild and transient in nature. Within all of the studies, a small percentage (average of 2–4%) of patients treated with PULMOZYME developed serum antibodies to PULMOZYME. None of these patients developed anaphylaxis, and the clinical significance of serum antibodies to PULMOZYME is unknown.

OVERDOSAGE

Single-dose inhalation studies in rats and monkeys at doses up to 180-times higher than doses routinely used in clinical studies are well tolerated. Single dose oral administration of PULMOZYME in doses up to 200 mg/kg are also well tolerated by rats.

Cystic fibrosis patients have received up to 20 mg BID for up to 6 days and 10 mg BID intermittently (2 weeks on/2 weeks off drug) for 168 days. These doses were well tolerated.

DOSAGE AND ADMINISTRATION

The recommended dose for use in most cystic fibrosis patients is one 2.5 mg single-use ampule inhaled once daily using a recommended nebulizer. Some patients may benefit from twice daily administration (see Clinical Experience, Table 1). Clinical trials have been performed with the following nebulizers and compressors: the disposable jet nebulizer Hudson T Up-draft II and disposable jet nebulizer Marquest Acorn II in conjunction with a Pulmo-Aide compressor, and the reusable PARI LC Jet^{+} nebulizer, in conjunction with the PARI PRONEB compressor. Safety and efficacy have been demonstrated only with these recommended nebulizer systems. No clinical data are currently available that support the safety and efficacy of administration of PULMOZYME with other nebulizer systems. The patient should follow the manufacturer's instructions on the use and maintenance of the equipment.

PULMOZYME should not be diluted or mixed with other drugs in the nebulizer. Mixing of PULMOZYME with other drugs could lead to adverse physicochemical and/or functional changes in PULMOZYME or the admixed compound.

HOW SUPPLIED

PULMOZYME Inhalation Solution is supplied in single-use ampules. Each ampule delivers 2.5 mL of a sterile, clear, colorless, aqueous solution containing 1.0 mg/mL dornase alfa, 0.15 mg/mL calcium chloride dihydrate and 8.77 mg/mL sodium chloride with no preservative. The nominal pH of the solution is 6.3.

PULMOZYME is supplied in:

- 14 unit cartons, containing 14 single-use ampules in single-unit foil pouches: NDC 50242-100-38
- 30 unit cartons containing 5 foil pouches of 6 single-use ampules: NDC 50242-100-40.

Storage

PULMOZYME should be stored under refrigeration (2-8°C/36-46°F). Ampules should be protected from light. Do not use beyond the expiration date stamped on the ampule. Unused ampules should be stored in their protective foil pouch under refrigeration.

REFERENCES

1. Shak S, Capon DJ, Hellmiss R, Marsters SA, Baker CL. Recombinant human DNase I reduces the viscosity of cystic fibrosis sputum. Proc Natl Acad Sci USA 1990; 87:9188-92.
2. Boat TF. Cystic Fibrosis. In: Murray JF, Nadel JA, editors. Textbook of respiratory medicine. Philadelphia: Saunders WB, 1988;1:1126-52.
3. Collins FS. Cystic Fibrosis: molecular biology and therapeutic implications. Science 1992;256:774-9.
4. Potter JL, Spector S, Matthews LW, Lemm J. Studies of pulmonary secretions. Amer Rev of Respiratory Disease 1969;99:909-15.
5. Hubbard RC, McElvaney NG, Birrer P, Shak S, Robinson WW, Jolley C, et al. A preliminary study of aerosolized recombinant human deoxyribonuclease I in the treatment of cystic fibrosis. New Eng J Med 1992;326:812-5.
6. Aitken ML, Burke W, McDonald G, Shak S, Montgomery AB, Smith A. Recombinant human DNase inhalation in normal subjects and patients with cystic fibrosis. JAMA 1992;267(14):1947-51.
7. Fuchs HJ, Borowitz D, Christianson D, Morris E, Nash M, Ramsey B, et al. Aerosolized recombinant human DNase reduces pulmonary exacerbations and improves pulmonary function in patients with cystic fibrosis. Presented by Mary Ellen Wohl, M.D. at the 36th Annual Conference on Chest Disease, Intermountain Thoracic Society, January 26, 1993.

PULMOZYME® (dornase alfa) recombinant — G48124-R1, Revised October, 1995

Manufactured by
GENENTECH, Inc.
460 Point San Bruno Boulevard
South San Francisco, CA 94080-4990

Shown in Product Identification Guide, page 311

Genzyme Corporation
ONE KENDALL SQUARE
CAMBRIDGE, MA 02139

Direct Inquiries to:
Clinical Services
(800) 745-4447
FAX: (617) 252-7700

For Medical Information Contact:
In Emergencies:
(800) 745-4447

CEREDASE® ℞
[sĕr 'ĕ-dāse]
(alglucerase injection)

DESCRIPTION

Ceredase® (alglucerase injection) is a modified form of the enzyme, β-glucocerebrosidase (β-D-glucosyl-N-acylsphingosine glucohydrolase, EC 3.2.1.45). Alglucerase is a monomeric glycoprotein of 497 amino acids with carbohydrates making up approximately 6% of the molecule (M_r = 59,300 as determined by SDS-PAGE). The unmodified enzyme (β-glucocerebrosidase) also contains 497 amino acids and contains approximately 12% carbohydrate (M_r = 67,000). The carbohydrates on the unmodified enzyme consist of N-linked carbohydrate chains of the complex and high mannose type. Glucocerebrosidase and alglucerase catalyze the hydrolysis of the glycolipid, glucocerebroside, within the lysosomes of the reticuloendothelial system.

Alglucerase is prepared by modification of the oligosaccharide chains of human β-glucocerebrosidase. The modification alters the sugar residues at the non-reducing ends of the oligosaccharide chains of the glycoprotein so that they are predominantly terminated with mannose residues which are specifically recognized by carbohydrate receptors on macrophage cells. **Ceredase®** is supplied as a clear sterile non-pyrogenic solution of alglucerase in a citrate buffered solution (53 mM citrate, 143 mM sodium) containing 1% albumin human USP. The enzyme is supplied in two concentrations, 400 units per bottle (80 units/mL) and 50 units per bottle (10 units/mL) with a fill volume of 5 mL per bottle. An enzyme unit (U) is defined as the amount of enzyme required

Continued on next page

Genzyme—Cont.

to hydrolyze in one minute one micromole of the synthetic substrate, 4 methylumbelliferyl-β-glucoside.

Ceredase® is purified from a large pool of human placental tissue collected from selected donors. Steps have been introduced into the manufacturing process to reduce further the risk of viral contamination. However, no procedure has been shown to be totally effective in removing viral infectivity. (See PRECAUTIONS). Each lot of product has been tested and found negative for hepatitis B surface antigen (HBsAg) and for human immunodeficiency virus antigen (HIV-1) and antibody (HIV-1/2).

Human chorionic gonadotropin (hCG), a naturally occurring hormone in human placenta, has been detected in **Ceredase®**. Although it is likely the hCG is partially deglycosylated, *in vitro* studies demonstrate biological activity of approximately 3 units of hCG activity per unit of **Ceredase®**. Preliminary studies suggest that the deglycosylated hCG in **Ceredase®** is rapidly cleared at a rate which is approximately forty times greater than that of native hCG. Therefore, *in vivo* biological activity and clearance of the material may be different to the naturally occurring hormone and is currently under investigation.

CLINICAL PHARMACOLOGY

Ceredase® (alglucerase injection) catalyzes the hydrolysis of the glycolipid, glucocerebroside, to glucose and ceramide as part of the normal degradation pathway for membrane lipids. Glucocerebroside is primarily derived from hematologic cell turnover. Gaucher disease is characterized by a functional deficiency in β-glucocerebrosidase enzymatic activity and the resultant accumulation of lipid glucocerebroside in tissue macrophages which become engorged and are termed Gaucher cells. Gaucher cells are typically found in liver, spleen and bone marrow and occasionally, as well, in lung, kidney and intestine. Secondary hematologic sequelae include severe anemia and thrombocytopenia in addition to the characteristic progressive hepatosplenomegaly. Skeletal complications, including osteonecrosis and osteopenia with secondary pathological fractures, are a common feature of Gaucher disease.

Pharmacokinetics

Following an intravenous infusion of different doses (between 0.6 and 234 units/kg) of **Ceredase®** (alglucerase injection) over a 4-hour period, steady-state enzymatic activity was achieved by 60 minutes. Individual steady-state enzymatic activity and area under the curve of the activity increased linearly with the infused dose (0.6 to 121 units/kg). Following infusion termination, plasma enzymatic activity declined rapidly with elimination half-life ranging between 3.6 and 10.4 minutes. Plasma clearance of **Ceredase®**, calculated from its plasma enzymatic activity, was variable and ranged between 6.34 and 25.39 mL/min/kg, whereas the volume of distribution ranged from 49.4 to 282.1 mL/kg. Within the dosage range of 0.6 and 121 units/kg, elimination half-life, plasma clearance, and volume of distribution values appear to be independent of the infused dose.

Pharmacologic Actions

Chronic administration of **Ceredase®** (alglucerase injection) in 13 patients with Type 1 Gaucher disease from initial studies induced the following effects:

1. **Splenomegaly and hepatomegaly** were significantly reduced, presumably by disruption of the lysosomal storage sites and metabolism of glucocerebroside in Gaucher cells. This effect was demonstrated within 6 months of initiation of therapy.
2. **Hematologic deficiencies** in hemoglobin, hematocrit, erythrocyte and platelet counts were significantly improved. In most patients a change in hemoglobin was the first observable effect. In some patients hemoglobin levels were normalized after six months of therapy.
3. **Improved mineralization** of bone, as revealed by plain radiographs of long bones, occurred in three patients after prolonged treatment as a result of a reduction in the osteolytic actions of lipid-laden Gaucher cells in the marrow.
4. **Cachexia and wasting** in children were reduced.

INDICATIONS AND USAGE

Ceredase® (alglucerase injection) is indicated for use as long-term enzyme replacement therapy for patients with a confirmed diagnosis of Type 1 Gaucher disease who exhibit signs and symptoms that are severe enough to result in one or more of the following conditions:

a) moderate-to-severe anemia;
b) thrombocytopenia with bleeding tendency;
c) bone disease;
d) significant hepatomegaly or splenomegaly.

CONTRAINDICATIONS

There are no known contraindications to the use of **Ceredase®** (alglucerase injection).

WARNINGS

Approximately 14% of 538 patients treated clinically and tested to date have developed IgG antibody to **Ceredase®** during the first year of therapy. It appears that patients who will develop IgG antibody are most likely to do so within 6 months of treatment and will rarely develop antibodies to **Ceredase®** after 12 months of therapy. **Approximately 25% of patients with detectable IgG antibodies experienced symptoms of hypersensitivity.**

Thus, patients with antibody to **Ceredase®** have a higher risk of hypersensitivity reaction. Conversely, not all patients with symptoms of hypersensitivity have detectable antibody and further evaluation of their antibody isotypes and mechanisms is continuing. It is suggested that patients be monitored periodically for IgG antibody formation.

At present, should a patient experience a reaction with symptoms suggestive of hypersensitivity, it is recommended that a serum sample for tryptase levels and complement activation be drawn within two hours of the event after appropriate treatment of the symptoms. Subsequent serum for testing antibody to **Ceredase®** would be helpful. Decreased efficacy has been noted in less than 0.5% of treated patients due to antibodies to Ceredase®.

PRECAUTIONS

General

Therapy with **Ceredase®** (alglucerase injection) should be directed by physicians knowledgeable in the management of patients with Gaucher disease.

Treatment with **Ceredase®** should be approached with caution in patients who have exhibited symptoms of hypersensitivity to the product. Pre-treatment with antihistamines has allowed continued use of **Ceredase®** in some patients (See **ADVERSE REACTIONS**). As hCG has been detected in **Ceredase®** physicians should be alert for signs of early virilization in males under the age of ten, although no cases of precocious puberty have been reported to date. **Ceredase®** should also be used with caution in patients with androgen sensitive malignancies e.g. prostate cancer and patients with known prior allergies to hCG.

Ceredase® is prepared from pooled human placental tissue that may contain the causative agents of some viral diseases. Manufacturing steps have been designed to reduce the risk of transmitting viral infectious agents. These steps have demonstrated *in vitro* inactivation of a panel of model viruses, including human immunodeficiency virus (HIV-1). The risk of contamination from slowly acting or latent viruses, including the Creutzfeldt-Jacob disease agent, is believed to be remote but has not been tested. Accordingly, the benefits and the risks of treatment with this product should be assessed prior to use.

Carcinogenesis, Mutagenesis, Impairment of Fertility

Studies have not been conducted to assess the potential effects of **Ceredase®** on carcinogenesis, mutagenesis, or impairment of fertility in animals or man.

Pregnancy Category C

Animal reproductive studies have not been conducted with **Ceredase®**. It is also not known whether **Ceredase®** can cause fetal harm when administered to a pregnant woman, or can affect reproductive capacity. **Ceredase®** should only be given to a pregnant woman if clearly needed.

Nursing Mothers

Since Ceredase® may be excreted in human milk, caution should be exercised when Ceredase® is administered to a nursing woman.

ANIMAL TOXICOLOGY

A three month toxicity study in rats revealed testicular changes of focal atrophy and necrosis of seminiferous tubules consistent with currently known effects of hCG, which is present in Ceredase®. Current experience suggests these testicular effects are specific to rats and unlikely to occur in humans.

ADVERSE REACTIONS

Experience in over 1000 patients treated with Ceredase® has revealed a small number of adverse events. Some of these events were related to the route of administration including discomfort, pruritus, burning and swelling or sterile abscess at the site of venipuncture. The remaining experiences consisted of slight fever, chills, abdominal discomfort, nausea or vomiting. None of these events were judged to require medical intervention.

Symptoms suggestive of hypersensitivity have been noted in a limited number of patients. Onset of such symptoms has occurred during or shortly after infusions; these symptoms have included pruritus, flushing, urticaria/angioedema (a small number of patients have had upper airway involvement), chest discomfort, respiratory symptoms, nausea and abdominal cramping. Hypotension has been reported to occur during a few of these events (see WARNINGS).

Pre-treatment with antihistamines and reduced rate of infusion has allowed continued use of **Ceredase®** in most patients. Additional adverse symptoms which have been reported include: fatigue, vasomotor irritability or hot flash, weakness, headache, light headedness, dysosmia, oral ulcerations, backache and transient peripheral edema, menstrual abnormalities and diarrhea.

Because it contains human chorionic gonadotropin. **Ceredase®** may cause a false positive pregnancy test.

OVERDOSE

No obvious toxicity was detected after single doses up to 234 U/kg. There is no experience with larger doses.

DOSAGE AND ADMINISTRATION

Ceredase® (alglucerase injection) is administered by intravenous infusion over 1–2 hours. Dosage should be individualized for each patient. Initial dosage may be as little as 2.5 units/kg of body weight 3 times a week up to as much as 60 units/kg administered as frequently as once a week or as infrequently as every 4 weeks. 60 units/kg every 2 weeks is the dose for which the most data is available. Disease severity may dictate that the drug be initiated with relatively high doses or relatively frequent administration. After patient response is well-established, a reduction in dosage may be attempted for maintenance therapy. Progressive reductions can be made at intervals of 3–6 months while carefully monitoring response parameters.

Ceredase® should not be shaken. Each bottle should be inspected visually for particulate matter and discoloration before use. Any bottles exhibiting particulate matter or discoloration should not be used. DO NOT USE **Ceredase®** after the expiration date on the bottle.

On the day of use, the appropriate amount of Ceredase® for each patient is diluted with 0.9% sodium chloride IV solution to a final volume not to exceed 200 mL. Aseptic techniques should be used when diluting the dose. Ceredase®, when diluted to 100 to 200 mL, has been shown to be stable for up to 18 hours when stored at 2–8°C. The use of an in-line particulate filter is recommended for the infusion apparatus. Since **Ceredase®** does not contain any preservative, after opening, bottles should not be stored for subsequent use.

Relatively low toxicity, combined with the extended time course of response, allows small dosage adjustments to be made occasionally to avoid discarding partially used bottles. Thus, the dosage administered in individual infusions may be slightly increased or decreased to utilize fully each bottle as long as the monthly administered dosage remains substantially unaltered.

HOW SUPPLIED

Ceredase® (alglucerase injection) is supplied as a clear sterile citrate buffered solution (53 mM citrate, 143 mM sodium) containing 1% albumin human USP. The following packages are available:

—The 400 unit bottle contains 5 mL in a 10 mL glass bottle. NDC 58468-1060-1.

—The 50 unit bottle contains 5 mL in a 6 mL glass bottle. NDC 58468-1781-1. Store at 2–8°C.

CAUTION! FEDERAL (U.S.A.) LAW PROHIBITS DISPENSING WITHOUT A PRESCRIPTION.

Ceredase® (alglucerase injection) is manufactured by:
Genzyme Corporation
One Kendall Square
Cambridge, MA 02139

Certain manufacturing operations have been performed by other firms.

1811/REV 6 (1/95)

CEREZYME™ ℞

[*sĕr'ĕ-zīm*]
imiglucerase for injection

DESCRIPTION

Cerezyme™ (imiglucerase for injection) is an analogue of the human enzyme, β-glucocerebrosidase produced by recombinant DNA technology. β-Glucocerebrosidase (β-D-glucosyl-N-acylsphingosine glucohydrolase, E.C. 3.2.1.45) is a lysosomal glycoprotein enzyme which catalyzes the hydrolysis of the glycolipid glucocerebroside to glucose and ceramide.

Cerezyme™ is produced by recombinant DNA technology using mammalian cell culture (Chinese hamster ovary). Purified imiglucerase is a monomeric glycoprotein of 497 amino acids, containing 4 N-linked glycosylation sites (Mr = 60,430). Imiglucerase differs from placental glucocerebrosidase by one amino acid at position 495 where histidine is substituted for arginine. The oligosaccharide chains at the glycosylation sites have been modified to terminate in mannose sugars. The modified carbohydrate structures on imiglucerase are somewhat different from those on placental glucocerebrosidase. These mannose-terminated oligosaccharide chains of imiglucerase are specifically recognized by endocytic carbohydrate receptors on macrophages, the cells that accumulate lipid in Gaucher disease.

Cerezyme™ is supplied as a sterile, non-pyrogenic, white to off-white lyophilized product. The quantitative composition of the lyophilized drug per vial is:

Imiglucerase 212 units (total amount)*
Mannitol 155 mg
Sodium Citrates 70 mg
(Trisodium Citrate 52 mg and Disodium Hydrogen Citrate 18 mg)
Polysorbate 80, NF 0.53 mg

Citric Acid and/or Sodium Hydroxide may have been added at the time of manufacture to adjust pH.

*This provides a withdrawal dose of 200 units of imiglucerase.

An enzyme unit (U) is defined as the amount of enzyme that catalyzes the hydrolysis of one micromole of the synthetic substrate para-nitrophenyl β-D-glucopyranoside (pNP-Glc) per minute at 37°C. The product is stored at 2–8°C (36–46°F.) After reconstitution with 5.1 mL of Sterile Water for Injection, USP, the imiglucerase concentration is 40 U/mL in a final volume of 5.3 mL which provides a withdrawal volume of 5.0 mL (200 enzyme units). Reconstituted solutions have a pH of approximately 6.1.

In addition, Haemaccel™ (cross-linked gelatin polypeptides), which is used as a stabilizing agent during the manufacturing process, may also be present in very small amounts in the final product.

CLINICAL PHARMACOLOGY
Mechanism of Action/Pharmacodynamics
Gaucher disease is characterized by a deficiency of β-glucocerebrosidase activity, resulting in accumulation of glucocerebroside in tissue macrophages which become engorged and are typically found in the liver, spleen, and bone marrow and occasionally in lung, kidney, and intestine. Secondary hematologic sequelae include severe anemia and thrombocytopenia in addition to the characteristic progressive hepatosplenomegaly, skeletal complications, including osteonecrosis and osteopenia with secondary pathological fractures. Cerezyme™ (imiglucerase for injection) catalyzes the hydrolysis of glucocerebroside to glucose and ceramide. In clinical trials, Cerezyme™ improved anemia and thrombocytopenia, reduced spleen and liver size, and decreased cachexia to a degree similar to that observed with Ceredase™.

Pharmacokinetics
During one hour intravenous infusions of four doses (7.5, 15, 30, 60 U/Kg) of Cerezyme™ (imiglucerase for injection) steady-state enzymatic activity was achieved by 30 minutes. Following infusion, plasma enzymatic activity declined rapidly with a half-life ranging from 3.6 to 10.4 minutes. Plasma clearance ranged from 9.8 to 20.3 mL/min/Kg, (mean $\pm$ S.D. 14.5 $\pm$ 4.0 mL/min/Kg). The volume of distribution corrected for weight ranged from 0.09 to 0.15 L/Kg (0.12 $\pm$ 0.02 L/Kg). These variables do not appear to be influenced by dose or duration of infusion. However, only one or two patients were studied at each dose level and infusion rate. The pharmacokinetics of Cerezyme™ do not appear to be different from placental-derived alglucerase (Ceredase™).

In patients who developed IgG antibody to Cerezyme™, an apparent effect on serum enzyme levels resulted in diminished volume of distribution and clearance and increased elimination half-life compared to patients without antibody (see WARNINGS).

INDICATIONS AND USAGE
Cerezyme™ (imiglucerase for injection) is indicated for long-term enzyme replacement therapy for patients with a confirmed diagnosis of Type 1 Gaucher disease that results in one or more of the following conditions:
a. anemia
b. thrombocytopenia
c. bone disease
d. hepatomegaly or splenomegaly

CONTRAINDICATIONS
There are no known contraindications to the use of Cerezyme™ (imiglucerase for injection). Treatment with Cerezyme™ should be carefully re-evaluated if there is significant clinical evidence of hypersensitivity to the product.

WARNINGS
During the clinical trials (duration 9 months), 4 of 25 patients (16%) treated with Cerezyme™ (imiglucerase for injection) developed IgG antibodies reactive with Cerezyme™. During the same clinical trial, 6 of 15 patients (40%) treated with placental-derived alglucerase (Ceredase™ developed IgG antibodies to Ceredase™, and one of these patients had clinical allergic signs and symptoms resulting in withdrawal from the study.

Of those patients treated with Cerezyme™, only one patient developed a transient rash. No patients treated with Cerezyme™, either initially or after changing over from Ceredase™, have exhibited serious symptoms of immediate hypersensitivity, although a risk for such reactions may be present.

Treatment with Cerezyme™ should be approached with caution in patients who have exhibited symptoms of hypersensitivity to the product.

PRECAUTIONS
General
Therapy with Cerezyme™ (imiglucerase for injection) should be directed by physicians knowledgeable in the management of patients with Gaucher disease.

Caution may be advisable in administration of Cerezyme™ to patients previously treated with Ceredase™ and who

---

have developed antibody to Ceredase™ or who have exhibited symptoms of hypersensitivity to Ceredase™.

Carcinogenesis, Mutagenesis, Impairment of Fertility
Studies have not been conducted in either animals or humans to assess the potential effects of Cerezyme™ (imiglucerase for injection) on carcinogenesis, mutagenesis, or impairment of fertility.

Teratogenic Effects: Pregnancy Category C
Animal reproduction studies have not been conducted with Cerezyme™ (imiglucerase for injection). It is also not known whether Cerezyme™ can cause fetal harm when administered to a pregnant woman, or can affect reproductive capacity. Cerezyme™ should not be administered during pregnancy except when the indication and need are clear and the potential benefit is judged by the physician to substantially justify the risk.

Nursing Mothers
It is not known whether this drug is excreted in human milk. Because many drugs are excreted in human milk, caution should be exercised when Cerezyme™ (imiglucerase for injection) is administered to a nursing woman.

ADVERSE REACTIONS
During clinical trials with Cerezyme™ (imiglucerase for injection) involving 25 patients with Gaucher disease, the following adverse events were noted that were possibly related to Cerezyme™.

Headache was noted in three patients. Nausea, abdominal discomfort, dizziness, pruritus, and rash occurred in one patient each. One patient was noted to have a mild decrease in blood pressure and another a decrease in urinary frequency. None of these events was judged to be serious or to warrant medical intervention or interruption of therapy. All proved transient and did not recur frequently.

Symptoms suggestive of allergic hypersensitivity have been noted in a number of patients treated with Ceredase™ (see WARNINGS).

OVERDOSE
Effects of dosages exceeding 120 U/kg per four weeks have not been studied and therefore dosages above 120 U/kg are not recommended.

DOSAGE AND ADMINISTRATION
Cerezyme™ (imiglucerase for injection) is administered by intravenous infusion over 1–2 hours. Dosage should be individualized to each patient. Initial dosage may be as little as 2.5 units/kg of body weight 3 times a week up to as much as 60 U/kg administered as frequently as once a week or as infrequently as every 4 weeks. 60 units/kg every 2 weeks is the dosage for which the most data are available. Disease severity may dictate that treatment be initiated at a relatively high dose or relatively frequent administration. After patient response is well established, a reduction in dosage may be attempted for maintenance therapy. Progressive reductions can be made at intervals of 3–6 months while carefully monitoring response parameters.

Cerezyme™ should be stored at 2–8°C (36–46°F). Each vial, after reconstitution with 5.1 mL Sterile Water for Injection, USP, should be inspected visually for particulate matter and discoloration before use. Any vials exhibiting particulate matter or discoloration should not be used. DO NOT USE Cerezyme™ after the expiration date on the vial.

On the day of use, after the correct amount of Cerezyme™ to be administered to the patient has been determined, the appropriate number of vials are each reconstituted with 5.1 mL of Sterile Water for Injection, USP, to give a reconstituted volume of 5.3 mL. A nominal 5.0 mL volume is then withdrawn from each vial and pooled with 0.9% Sodium Chloride Injection, USP, to a final volume of 100 to 200 mL. Cerezyme™ is administered by intravenous infusion over 1 to 2 hours. Alternatively, the appropriate dose of Cerezyme™ may be administered such that a rate of no greater than 1 unit per kg body weight per minute is infused. Aseptic techniques should be used when diluting the dose. Since Cerezyme™ does not contain any preservative, after reconstitution, vials should be promptly diluted and not stored for subsequent use. Cerezyme™, when diluted to 50 mL has been shown to be stable for up to 24 hours when stored at 2–8°C (36–46°F).

Relatively low toxicity, combined with the extended time course of response, allows small dosage adjustments to be made occasionally to avoid discarding partially used bottles. Thus, the dosage administered in individual infusions may be slightly increased or decreased to utilize fully each vial as long as the monthly administered dosage remains substantially unaltered.

HOW SUPPLIED
Cerezyme™ (imiglucerase for injection) is supplied as a sterile, non-pyrogenic, lyophilized product. It is available as follows:

---

200 Units per Vial
NDC 58468–1983–1
Store at 2–8°C (36–46°F).
CAUTION: FEDERAL (U.S.A.) LAW PROHIBITS DISPENSING WITHOUT A PRESCRIPTION.
Cerezyme™ (imiglucerase for injection) is manufactured by:
Genzyme Corporation
One Kendall Square
Cambridge, MA 02139
Certain manufacturing operations have been performed by other firms.

4156 (5/94)

Gilead Sciences
**333 LAKESIDE DRIVE
FOSTER CITY, CA 94404**

Direct Inquiries To:
Customer Service
(800) GILEAD5

Medical Emergency Contact:
Director, Medical Information
(800) GILEAD5
FAX: (800) 693–9009

VISTIDE® (cidofovir injection)   ℞
**FOR INTRAVENOUS INFUSION ONLY.
NOT FOR INTRAOCULAR INJECTION.**

RENAL IMPAIRMENT IS THE MAJOR TOXICITY OF VISTIDE. TO MINIMIZE POSSIBLE NEPHROTOXICITY, INTRAVENOUS PREHYDRATION WITH NORMAL SALINE AND ADMINISTRATION OF PROBENECID MUST BE USED WITH EACH VISTIDE INFUSION. RENAL FUNCTION (SERUM CREATININE AND URINE PROTEIN) SHOULD BE MONITORED PRIOR TO EACH DOSE OF VISTIDE AND THE DOSE OF VISTIDE MODIFIED FOR CHANGES IN RENAL FUNCTION AS APPROPRIATE (SEE DOSAGE AND ADMINISTRATION). GRANULOCYTOPENIA HAS BEEN OBSERVED IN ASSOCIATION WITH VISTIDE TREATMENT AND NEUTROPHIL COUNTS SHOULD BE MONITORED DURING VISTIDE THERAPY.
VISTIDE IS INDICATED ONLY FOR THE TREATMENT OF CMV RETINITIS IN PATIENTS WITH THE ACQUIRED IMMUNODEFICIENCY SYNDROME.
IN ANIMAL STUDIES CIDOFOVIR WAS CARCINOGENIC, TERATOGENIC AND CAUSED HYPOSPERMIA (SEE CARCINOGENESIS, MUTAGENESIS, & IMPAIRMENT OF FERTILITY).

DESCRIPTION
VISTIDE® is the brand name for cidofovir injection. The chemical name of cidofovir is 1-[(S)-3-hydroxy-2-(phosphonomethoxy)propyl]cytosine dihydrate (HPMPC), with the molecular formula of $C_8H_{14}N_3O_6P \bullet 2H_2O$ and a molecular weight of 315.22 (279.19 for anhydrous). The chemical structure is:

Cidofovir is a white crystalline powder with an aqueous solubility of $\geq$ 170 mg/mL at pH 6–8 and a log P (octanol/aqueous buffer, pH 7.1) value of -3.3.

VISTIDE is a sterile, hypertonic aqueous solution for intravenous infusion only. The solution is clear and colorless. It is supplied in clear glass vials, each containing 375 mg of anhydrous cidofovir in 5 mL aqueous solution at a concentration of 75 mg/mL. The formulation is pH-adjusted to 7.4 with sodium hydroxide and/or hydrochloric acid and contains no preservatives. The appropriate volume of VISTIDE must be removed from the single-use vial and diluted prior to administration (see DOSAGE AND ADMINISTRATION).

Continued on next page

Gilead—Cont.

MICROBIOLOGY

Mechanism of Action: Cidofovir suppresses cytomegalovirus (CMV) replication by selective inhibition of viral DNA synthesis. Biochemical data support selective inhibition of CMV DNA polymerase by cidofovir diphosphate, the active intracellular metabolite of cidofovir. Cidofovir diphosphate inhibits herpesvirus polymerases at concentrations that are 8- to 600-fold lower than those needed to inhibit human cellular DNA polymerases alpha, beta, and gamma[1, 2, 3].
Incorporation of cidofovir into the growing viral DNA chain results in reductions in the rate of viral DNA synthesis.
In Vitro Susceptibility: Cidofovir is active *in vitro* against a variety of laboratory and clinical isolates of CMV and other herpesviruses (Table 1). Controlled clinical studies of efficacy have been limited to patients with AIDS and CMV retinitis.

Table 1. Cidofovir Inhibition of Virus Multiplication in Cell Culture

Virus	IC_{50} (μM)
Wild-type CMV Isolates	0.5–2.8
HSV-1, HSV-2	12.7–31.7
VZV*	0.79
EBV	0.03
HHV-6	<6.3

*mean result for 4 human VZV strains

Resistance: CMV isolates with reduced susceptibility to cidofovir have been selected *in vitro* in the presence of high concentrations of cidofovir[4]. IC_{50} values for selected resistant isolates ranged from 7–15 μM.
There are insufficient data at this time to assess the frequency or the clinical significance of the development of resistant isolates following VISTIDE administration to patients.
Cross Resistance: Cidofovir-resistant isolates selected *in vitro* following exposure to increasing concentrations of cidofovir were assessed for susceptibility to ganciclovir and foscarnet[4]. All were cross resistant to ganciclovir, but remained susceptible to foscarnet. Ganciclovir- or ganciclovir/foscarnet-resistant isolates that are cross resistant to cidofovir have been obtained from drug naive patients and from patients following ganciclovir or ganciclovir/foscarnet therapy. To date, the majority of ganciclovir-resistant isolates are UL97 gene product (phosphokinase) mutants and remain susceptible to cidofovir[5]. Reduced susceptibility to cidofovir, however, has been reported for DNA polymerase mutants of CMV which are resistant to ganciclovir[6–8]. To date, all clinical isolates which exhibit high level resistance to ganciclovir, due to mutations in the DNA polymerase gene, have been shown to be cross resistant to cidofovir. Cidofovir is active against some, but not all, CMV isolates which are resistant to foscarnet[9–11]. The incidence of foscarnet-resistant isolates that are resistant to cidofovir is not known.
A few triple-drug resistant isolates have been described. Genotypic analysis of two of these triple-resistant isolates revealed several point mutations in the CMV DNA polymerase gene. The clinical significance of the development of these cross-resistant isolates is not known.

CLINICAL PHARMACOLOGY

PHARMACOKINETICS

VISTIDE must be administered with probenecid. The pharmacokinetics of cidofovir, administered both without and with probenecid, are described below.
The pharmacokinetics of cidofovir without probenecid were evaluated in 27 HIV-infected patients with or without asymptomatic CMV infection. Dose-independent pharmacokinetics were demonstrated after one hr infusions of 1.0 (n = 5), 3.0 (n = 10), 5.0 (n = 2) and 10.0 (n = 8) mg/kg (See Table 2 for pharmacokinetic parameters). There was no evidence of cidofovir accumulation after 4 weeks of repeated administration of 3 mg/kg/week (n = 5) without probenecid. In patients with normal renal function, approximately 80 to 100% of the VISTIDE dose was recovered unchanged in urine within 24 hr (n = 27). The renal clearance of cidofovir was greater than creatinine clearance, indicating renal tubular secretion contributes to the elimination of cidofovir.
The pharmacokinetics of cidofovir administered with probenecid were evaluated in 12 HIV-infected patients with or without asymptomatic CMV infection and 10 patients with relapsing CMV retinitis. Dose-independent pharmacokinetics were observed for cidofovir, administered with probenecid, after one hr infusions of 3.0 (n = 12), 5.0 (n = 6), and 7.5 (n = 4) mg/kg (See Table 2). Approximately 70 to 85% of the VISTIDE dose administered with concomitant probenecid was excreted as unchanged drug within 24 hr. When VISTIDE was administered with probenecid, the renal clearance of cidofovir was reduced to a level consistent with creatinine clearance, suggesting that probenecid blocks active renal tubular secretion of cidofovir.
[See Table 2 below.]

In vitro, cidofovir was less than 6% bound to plasma or serum proteins over the cidofovir concentration range 0.25 to 25 μg/mL. CSF concentrations of cidofovir following intravenous infusion of VISTIDE 5 mg/kg with concomitant probenecid and intravenous hydration were undetectable (< 0.1 μg/mL, assay detection threshold) at 15 minutes after the end of a 1 hr infusion in one patient whose corresponding serum concentration was 8.7 μg/mL.

DRUG-DRUG INTERACTIONS

Zidovudine
The pharmacokinetics of zidovudine were evaluated in 10 patients receiving zidovudine alone or with intravenous cidofovir (without probenecid). There was no evidence of an effect of cidofovir on the pharmacokinetics of zidovudine.

SPECIAL POPULATIONS

Renal Insufficiency
Cidofovir pharmacokinetics have not been investigated in patients with renal insufficiency. No data are currently available on the pharmacokinetics of cidofovir in patients with creatinine clearance values below 55 mL/min. The effect of dialysis on cidofovir pharmacokinetics is not known.
Geriatric/Gender/Race
The effects of age, gender, and race on cidofovir pharmacokinetics have not been investigated.

INDICATION AND USAGE

VISTIDE is indicated for the treatment of CMV retinitis in patients with acquired immunodeficiency syndrome (AIDS). THE SAFETY AND EFFICACY OF VISTIDE HAVE NOT BEEN ESTABLISHED FOR TREATMENT OF OTHER CMV INFECTIONS (SUCH AS PNEUMONITIS OR GASTROENTERITIS), CONGENITAL OR NEONATAL CMV DISEASE, OR CMV DISEASE IN NON-HIV-INFECTED INDIVIDUALS.

DESCRIPTION OF CLINICAL TRIALS

Two phase 2/3 controlled trials of VISTIDE have been conducted in HIV-infected patients with CMV retinitis.
Delayed Versus Immediate Therapy (Study 106): In an open-label trial, forty-eight previously untreated patients with peripheral CMV retinitis were randomized to either immediate treatment with VISTIDE (5 mg/kg once a week for 2 weeks, then 5 mg/kg every other week), or to have VISTIDE delayed until progression of CMV retinitis. Patient baseline characteristics and disposition are shown in Table 3. Of 25 and 23 patients in the immediate and delayed groups respectively, 23 and 21 were evaluable for retinitis progression as determined by retinal photography. Based on masked readings of retinal photographs, the median [95% confidence interval (CI)] times to retinitis progression were 120 days (40, 134) and 22 days (10, 27) for the immediate and delayed therapy groups, respectively. This difference was statistically significant. However, because of the limited number of patients remaining on treatment over time (3 of 25 patients received VISTIDE for 120 days or longer), the median time to progression for the immediate therapy group was difficult to precisely estimate. Median (95% CI) times to the alternative endpoint of retinitis progression or study drug discontinuation (including adverse events, withdrawn consent, and systemic CMV disease) were 52 days (37, 85) and 22 days (13, 27) for the immediate and delayed therapy groups, respectively. This difference was statistically significant. Time to progression estimates from this study may not be directly comparable to estimates reported for other therapies.

Table 3. Patient Characteristics and Disposition (Study 106)

	Immediate Therapy (n=25)	Delayed Therapy (n=23)
Baseline Characteristics		
Age (years)	38	38
Sex (M/F)	24/1	22/1
Median CD4 Cell Count	6	9
Endpoints		
CMV Retinitis Progression	10	18
Discontinued Due to Adverse Event	6	0
Withdrew Consent	3[a]	1
Discontinued Due to Intercurrent Illness	2[b]	1[b]
Discontinued Based on Ophthalmological Examination	1[c]	1[c]
No progression at Study Completion	1	0
Not Evaluable at Baseline	2	2

[a] One patient died 2 weeks after withdrawing consent.
[b] Two patients on immediate therapy were diagnosed with CMV disease and discontinued from study. One patient on delayed therapy was diagnosed with CMV gastrointestinal disease.
[c] CMV retinitis progression not confirmed by retinal photography.

Dose-response study of VISTIDE (Study 107): In an open-label trial, one-hundred patients with relapsing CMV retinitis were randomized to receive 5 mg/kg once a week for 2 weeks and then either 5 mg/kg (n = 49) or 3 mg/kg (n = 51) every other week. Enrolled patients had been diagnosed with CMV retinitis approximately 1 year prior to randomization and had received a median of 4 prior courses of systemic CMV therapy. Eighty-four of the 100 patients were considered evaluable for progression by serial retinal photographs (43 randomized to 5 mg/kg and 41 randomized to 3 mg/kg). Twenty-three and 20 patients discontinued therapy due to either an adverse event, intercurrent illness, excluded medication, or withdrawn consent in the 5 mg/kg and 3 mg/kg groups, respectively. Based on masked readings of retinal photographs, the median (95% CI) times to retinitis progression for the 5 mg/kg and 3 mg/kg groups were 115 days (70, not reached) and 49 days (35, 52), respectively. This difference was statistically significant. Similar to Study 106, the median time to retinitis progression for the 5 mg/kg group was difficult to precisely estimate due to the limited number of patients remaining on treatment over time (4 of the 49 patients in the 5 mg/kg group were treated for 115 days or longer). Median (95% CI) times to the alternative endpoint of retinitis progression or study drug discontinuation were 49 days (38, 63) and 35 days (27, 39) for the 5 mg/kg and 3 mg/kg groups, respectively. This difference was statistically significant.

CONTRAINDICATIONS

VISTIDE is contraindicated in patients with hypersensitivity to cidofovir.
VISTIDE is contraindicated in patients with a history of clinically severe hypersensitivity to probenecid or other sulfa-containing medications.
Direct intraocular injection of VISTIDE is contraindicated; direct injection may be associated with significant decreases in intraocular pressure and impairment of vision.

WARNINGS

Nephrotoxicity: Dose-dependent nephrotoxicity is the major dose-limiting toxicity related to VISTIDE administration. Dose adjustment or discontinuation is required for changes in renal function while on therapy. Proteinuria, as measured by urinalysis in a clinical laboratory, may be an early indicator of VISTIDE-related nephrotoxicity. Continued administration of VISTIDE may lead to additional proximal tubular cell injury, which may result in glycosuria, and decreases in serum phosphate, uric acid, and bicarbonate, and elevations in serum creatinine. Patients with these adverse events occurring concurrently and meeting a criteria of Fanconi's syndrome have been reported. Renal function that did not return to baseline after drug discontinuation has been observed in clinical studies of VISTIDE.
Intravenous normal saline hydration and oral probenecid must accompany each VISTIDE infusion. Probenecid is known to interact with the metabolism or renal tubular excretion of many drugs (see PRECAUTIONS). The safety of VISTIDE has not been evaluated in patients receiving other

Table 2. Cidofovir Pharmacokinetic Parameters Following 3.0 and 5.0 mg/kg Infusions, Without and With Probenecid*

PARAMETERS	VISTIDE ADMINISTERED WITHOUT PROBENECID		VISTIDE ADMINISTERED WITH PROBENECID	
	3 mg/kg (n=10)	5 mg/kg (n=2)	3 mg/kg (n=12)	5 mg/kg (n=6)
AUC (μg.hr/mL)	20.0 ± 2.3	28.3	25.7 ± 8.5	40.8 ± 9.0
Cmax (end of infusion) (μg/mL)	7.3 ± 1.4	11.5	9.8 ± 3.7	19.6 ± 7.2
Vdss (mL/kg)	537 ± 126 (n = 12)		410 ± 102 (n = 18)	
Clearance (mL/min/1.73 m²)	179 ± 23.1 (n = 12)		148 ± 38.8 (n = 18)	
Renal Clearance (mL/min/1.73 m²)	150 ± 26.9 (n = 12)		98.6 ± 27.9 (n = 11)	

*See DOSAGE AND ADMINISTRATION

known potentially nephrotoxic agents, such as aminoglycosides, amphotericin B, foscarnet, and intravenous pentamidine (see DOSAGE AND ADMINISTRATION).

Preexisting Renal Impairment: VISTIDE has not been studied in patients with baseline serum creatinine concentrations > 1.5 mg/dL or calculated creatinine clearances ≤ 55 mL/min. The most appropriate initial and maintenance doses of VISTIDE for patients with moderate to severe renal impairment are not known.

It is recommended that VISTIDE not be initiated in patients with baseline serum creatinine > 1.5 mg/dL or creatinine clearances ≤ 55 mL/min. In these patients, VISTIDE therapy should only be used when the potential benefits exceed the potential risks.

Hematological Toxicity: Neutropenia may occur during VISTIDE therapy. Neutrophil count should be monitored while receiving VISTIDE therapy.

Metabolic Acidosis: Fanconi's syndrome and decreases in serum bicarbonate associated with evidence of renal tubular damage have been reported in patients receiving VISTIDE (see ADVERSE EVENTS). Serious metabolic acidosis, in association with liver failure, pancreatitis, mucormycosis, aspergillus, disseminated mycobacterial infection, and progression to death occurred in 1 patient (< 1%) receiving VISTIDE.

PRECAUTIONS

General

Due to the potential for increased nephrotoxicity, doses greater than the recommended dose should not be administered and the frequency or rate of administration should not be exceeded (see DOSAGE AND ADMINISTRATION).

VISTIDE is formulated for intravenous infusion only and must not be administered by intraocular injection. Administration of VISTIDE by infusion must be accompanied by oral probenecid and intravenous saline prehydration (see DOSAGE AND ADMINISTRATION).

Information for Patients

Patients should be advised that VISTIDE is not a cure for CMV retinitis, and that they may continue to experience progression of retinitis during and following treatment. Patients receiving VISTIDE should be advised to have regular follow-up ophthalmologic examinations. Patients may also experience other manifestations of CMV disease despite VISTIDE therapy.

HIV-infected patients may continue taking antiretroviral therapy, but those taking zidovudine should be advised to temporarily discontinue zidovudine administration or decrease their zidovudine dose by 50%, on days of VISTIDE administration only, because probenecid reduces metabolic clearance of zidovudine.

Patients should be informed of the major toxicity of VISTIDE, namely renal impairment, and that dose modification, including reduction, interruption, and possibly discontinuation, may be required. Close monitoring of renal function (routine urinalysis and serum creatinine) while on therapy should be emphasized.

The importance of completing a full course of probenecid with each VISTIDE dose should be emphasized. Patients should be warned of potential adverse events caused by probenecid (e.g., headache, nausea, vomiting, and hypersensitivity reactions). Hypersensitivity/allergic reactions may include rash, fever, chills and anaphylaxis. Administration of probenecid after a meal or use of antiemetics may decrease the nausea. Prophylactic or therapeutic antihistamines and/or acetaminophen can be used to ameliorate hypersensitivity reactions.

Patients should be advised that cidofovir causes tumors, primarily mammary adenocarcinomas, in rats. VISTIDE should be considered a potential carcinogen in humans (See Carcinogenesis, Mutagenesis, & Impairment of Fertility). Women should be advised of the limited enrollment of women in clinical trials of VISTIDE.

Patients should be advised that VISTIDE caused reduced testes weight and hypospermia in animals. Such changes may occur in humans and cause infertility. Women of childbearing potential should be advised that cidofovir is embryotoxic in animals and should not be used during pregnancy. Women of childbearing potential should be advised to use effective contraception during and for 1 month following treatment with VISTIDE. Men should be advised to practice barrier contraceptive methods during and for 3 months after treatment with VISTIDE.

Drug Interactions

Probenecid: Probenecid is known to interact with the metabolism or renal tubular excretion of many drugs (e.g., acetaminophen, acyclovir, angiotensin-converting enzyme inhibitors, aminosalicylic acid, barbiturates, benzodiazepines, bumetanide, clofibrate, methotrexate, famotidine, furosemide, nonsteroidal anti-inflammatory agents, theophylline, and zidovudine). Concomitant medications should be carefully assessed.

Nephrotoxic agents: Concomitant administration of VISTIDE and agents with nephrotoxic potential (e.g., amphotericin B, aminoglycosides, foscarnet, and intravenous pentamidine) should be avoided.

Carcinogenesis, Mutagenesis, & Impairment of Fertility

Chronic, two-year carcinogenicity studies in rats and mice have not been carried out to evaluate the carcinogenic potential of cidofovir. However, a 26-week toxicology study evaluating once weekly subscapular subcutaneous injections of cidofovir in rats was terminated at 19 weeks because of the induction, in females, of palpable masses, the first of which was detected after six doses. The masses were diagnosed as mammary adenocarcinomas which developed at doses as low as 0.6 mg/kg/week, equivalent to 0.04 times the human systemic exposure at the recommended intravenous VISTIDE dose based on AUC comparisons.

In a 26-week intravenous toxicology study in which rats received 0.6, 3, or 15 mg/kg cidofovir once weekly, a significant increase in mammary adenocarcinomas in female rats as well as a significant incidence of Zymbal's gland carcinomas in male and female rats were seen at the high dose but not at the lower two doses. The high dose was equivalent to 1.1 times the human systemic exposure at the recommended dose of VISTIDE, based on comparisons of AUC measurements. In light of the results of these studies, cidofovir should be considered to be a carcinogen in rats as well as a potential carcinogen in humans.

Cynomolgus monkeys received intravenous cidofovir, alone and in conjunction with concomitant oral probenecid, intravenously once weekly for 52 weeks at doses resulting in exposures of approximately 0.7 times the human systemic exposure at the recommended dose of VISTIDE. No tumors were detected. However, the study was not designed as a carcinogenicity study due to the small number of animals at each dose and the short duration of treatment.

No mutagenic response was observed in microbial mutagenicity assays involving *Salmonella typhimurium* (Ames) and *Escherichia coli* in the presence and absence of metabolic activation. An increase in micronucleated polychromatic erythrocytes *in vivo* was seen in mice receiving ≥ 2000 mg/kg, a dosage approximately 65-fold higher than the maximum recommended clinical intravenous VISTIDE dose based on body surface area estimations. Cidofovir induced chromosomal aberrations in human peripheral blood lymphocytes *in vitro* without metabolic activation. At the 4 cidofovir levels tested, the percentage of damaged metaphases and number of aberrations per cell increased in a concentration-dependent manner.

Studies showed that cidofovir caused inhibition of spermatogenesis in rats and monkeys. However, no adverse effects on fertility or reproduction were seen following once weekly intravenous injections of cidofovir in male rats for 13 consecutive weeks at doses up to 15 mg/kg/week (equivalent to 1.1 times the recommended human dose based on AUC comparisons). Female rats dosed intravenously once weekly at 1.2 mg/kg/week (equivalent to 0.09 times the recommended human dose based on AUC) or higher, for up to 6 weeks prior to mating and for 2 weeks post mating had decreased litter sizes and live births per litter and increased early resorptions per litter. Peri- and post-natal development studies in which female rats received subcutaneous injections of cidofovir once daily at doses up to 1.0 mg/kg/day from day 7 of gestation through day 21 postpartum (approximately 5 weeks) resulted in no adverse effects on viability, growth, behavior, sexual maturation or reproductive capacity in the offspring.

Pregnancy: Category C

Cidofovir was embryotoxic (reduced fetal body weights) in rats at 1.5 mg/kg/day and in rabbits at 1.0 mg/kg/day, doses which were also maternally toxic, following daily intravenous dosing during the period of organogenesis. The no-observable-effect levels for embryotoxicity in rats (0.5 mg/kg/day) and in rabbits (0.25 mg/kg/day) were approximately 0.04 and 0.05 times the clinical dose (5 mg/kg every other week) based on AUC, respectively. An increased incidence of fetal external, soft tissue and skeletal anomalies (meningocele, short snout, and short maxillary bones) occurred in rabbits at the high dose (1.0 mg/kg/day) which was also maternally toxic. There are no adequate and well-controlled studies in pregnant women. VISTIDE should be used during pregnancy only if the potential benefit justifies the potential risk to the fetus.

Nursing Mothers

It is not known whether cidofovir is excreted in human milk. Since many drugs are excreted in human milk and because of the potential for adverse reactions as well as the potential for tumorigenicity shown for cidofovir in animal studies, VISTIDE should not be administered to nursing mothers. The U.S. Public Health Service Centers for Disease Control and Prevention advises HIV-infected women not to breastfeed to avoid postnatal transmission of HIV to a child who may not yet be infected.

Pediatric Use

Safety and effectiveness in children have not been studied. The use of VISTIDE in children with AIDS warrants extreme caution due to the risk of long-term carcinogenicity and reproductive toxicity. Administration of VISTIDE to children should be undertaken only after careful evaluation and only if the potential benefits of treatment outweigh the risks.

Use in Elderly Patients

No studies of the safety or efficacy of VISTIDE in patients over the age of 60 have been conducted. Since elderly individuals frequently have reduced glomerular filtration, particular attention should be paid to assessing renal function before and during VISTIDE administration (see DOSAGE AND ADMINISTRATION).

ADVERSE REACTIONS

1. *Nephrotoxicity:* Renal toxicity, as manifested by >1+ proteinuria, serum creatinine elevations of ≥ 0.4 mg/dL, or decreased creatinine clearance ≤ 55 mL/min, occurred in 47 of 89 (53%) patients receiving VISTIDE at a maintenance dose of 5 mg/kg every other week. Maintenance dose reductions from 5 mg/kg to 3 mg/kg due to proteinuria or serum creatinine elevations were made for 12 of 41 (29%) patients who had not received prior therapy for CMV retinitis (Study 106) and 11 of 48 (23%) patients who had received prior therapy for CMV retinitis (Study 107). Prior foscarnet use has been associated with an increased risk of nephrotoxicity, therefore such patients should be monitored closely.

2. *Neutropenia:* In clinical trials, at the 5 mg/kg maintenance dose, neutropenia to ≤ 500 cells/mm³ occurred in 20% of patients. Granulocyte colony stimulating factor (GCSF) was used in 34% of patients.

3. *Ocular hypotony:* Among the subset of patients monitored for intraocular pressure changes, ocular hypotony (≥ 50% change from baseline) was reported in 5 patients. Hypotony was reported in 1 patient with concomitant diabetes mellitus. Risk of ocular hypotony may be increased in patients with preexisting diabetes.

4. *Metabolic Acidosis:* A diagnosis of Fanconi's syndrome, as manifested by multiple abnormalities of proximal tubule function, was reported in 2% of patients. Decreases in serum bicarbonate to ≤ 16 meq/L associated with evidence of renal tubular damage occurred in approximately 9% of patients. Serious metabolic acidosis, in association with liver failure, pancreatitis, mucormycosis, aspergillus, disseminated mycobacterial infection, and progression to death occurred in 1 patient (< 1%) receiving VISTIDE.

In clinical trials, VISTIDE was withdrawn due to adverse events in approximately 25% of patients treated with 5 mg/kg every other week as maintenance therapy.

The incidence of adverse reactions reported as serious in two controlled clinical studies in patients with CMV retinitis, regardless of presumed relationship to drug, is listed in Table 4.

Table 4. Serious Clinical Adverse Events or Laboratory Abnormalities Occurring in > 5% of Patients

	N = 89[a]	%
Proteinuria (≥ 100 mg/dL)	42	48
Neutropenia (≤ 500 cells/mm³)	18	20
Creatinine Elevation	13	15
Fever	13	15
Infection	11	12
Dyspnea	9	10
Pneumonia	8	9
Decreased Serum Bicarbonate (≤ 16 meq/L)	8	9
Creatinine Elevation (to ≥ 2.0 mg/dL)	7	8
Nausea with Vomiting	7	8
Diarrhea	6	7
Asthenia	6	7
Ocular Hypotony[b]	5	12

[a] Patients receiving 5 mg/kg maintenance regimen in Studies 106 and 107.

[b] Incidence based on 42 patients receiving 5 mg/kg maintenance regimen in Studies 106 and 107 with pretreatment baseline intraocular pressure reading and follow-up evaluation ≤50% of baseline.

The most frequently reported adverse events regardless of relationship to study drugs (cidofovir or probenecid) or severity are shown in Table 5.

Table 5. All clinical Adverse Events, Laboratory Abnormalities or Intercurrent Illnesses Regardless of Severity Occurring in > 15% of Patients

	N = 89[a]	%
Any Adverse Event	89	100
Proteinuria	71	80
Nausea +/− Vomiting	58	65
Fever	51	57
Asthenia	41	46
Neutropenia (< 750/mm³)	28	31
Rash	27	30
Headache	24	27
Diarrhea	24	27

Continued on next page

Gilead—Cont.

Alopecia	22	25
Infections	22	25
Chills	21	24
Anorexia	20	22
Dyspnea	20	22
Anemia	18	20
Creatinine Elevation (to > 1.5 mg/dL)	16	18
Abdominal Pain	15	17

[a] Patients receiving 5 mg/kg maintenance regimen in Studies 106 and 107.

The following additional list of adverse events/intercurrent illnesses have been observed in clinical studies of VISTIDE and are listed below regardless of causal relationship to VISTIDE.

Body as a Whole: allergic reaction, face edema, malaise, back pain, chest pain, neck pain, sarcoma, sepsis

Cardiovascular System: hypotension, postural hypotension, pallor, syncope, tachycardia

Digestive System: colitis, constipation, tongue discoloration, dyspepsia, dysphagia, flatulence, gastritis, hepatomegaly, abnormal liver function tests, melena, oral candidiasis, rectal disorder, stomatitis, aphthous stomatitis, mouth ulceration

Hemic & Lymphatic System: thrombocytopenia

Metabolic & Nutritional System: edema, dehydration, hyperglycemia, hyperlipemia, hypocalcemia, hypokalemia, increased alkaline phosphatase, increased SGOT, increased SGPT, weight loss

Musculoskeletal System: arthralgia, myasthenia, myalgia

Nervous System: amnesia, anxiety, confusion, convulsion, depression, dizziness, dry mouth, abnormal gait, hallucinations, insomnia, neuropathy, paresthesia, somnolence, vasodilatation

Respiratory System: asthma, bronchitis, coughing, dyspnea, hiccup, increased sputum, lung disorder, pharyngitis, pneumonia, rhinitis, sinusitis

Skin & Appendages: alopecia, acne, skin discoloration, dry skin, herpes simplex, pruritus, rash, sweating, urticaria

Special Senses: amblyopia, conjunctivitis, eye disorder, hypotony, iritis, retinal detachment, taste perversion, uveitis, abnormal vision

Urogenital System: decreased creatinine clearance, glycosuria, hematuria, urinary incontinence, urinary tract infection

Reporting of Adverse Reactions

Malignancies or serious adverse reactions that occur in patients who have received VISTIDE should be reported to Gilead in writing to the Director of Clinical Research, Gilead Sciences, Inc., 333 Lakeside Drive, Foster City, CA 94404 or by calling 1-800-GILEAD-5 (445-3235), or to FDA MedWatch 1-800-FDA-1088/fax 1-800-FDA-0178.

OVERDOSAGE

Overdosage with VISTIDE has not been reported; however, hemodialysis and hydration may reduce drug plasma concentrations in patients who receive an overdosage of VISTIDE. Probenecid may reduce the potential for nephrotoxicity in patients who receive an overdose of VISTIDE through reduction of active tubular secretion.

DOSAGE AND ADMINISTRATION

VISTIDE MUST NOT BE ADMINISTERED BY INTRAOCULAR INJECTION.

Dosage

THE RECOMMENDED DOSAGE, FREQUENCY, OR INFUSION RATE MUST NOT BE EXCEEDED. VISTIDE MUST BE DILUTED IN 100 MILLILITERS 0.9% (NORMAL) SALINE PRIOR TO ADMINISTRATION. TO MINIMIZE POTENTIAL NEPHROTOXICITY, PROBENECID AND INTRAVENOUS SALINE PREHYDRATION MUST BE ADMINISTERED WITH EACH VISTIDE INFUSION.

Induction Treatment. The recommended dose of VISTIDE is 5 mg/kg body weight (given as an intravenous infusion at a constant rate over 1 hr) administered once weekly for two consecutive weeks.

Maintenance Treatment. The recommended maintenance dose of VISTIDE is 5 mg/kg body weight (given as an intravenous infusion at a constant rate over 1 hr) administered once every two weeks.

Probenecid. Probenecid must be administered orally with each VISTIDE dose. Two grams must be administered 3 hr prior to the VISTIDE dose and one gram administered at 2 and again at 8 hr after completion of the 1 hr VISTIDE infusion (for a total of 4 grams).

Ingestion of food prior to each dose of probenecid may reduce drug-related nausea and vomiting. Administration of an antiemetic may reduce the potential for nausea associated with probenecid ingestion. In patients who develop allergic or hypersensitivity symptoms to probenecid, the use of an appropriate prophylactic or therapeutic antihistamine and/or acetaminophen should be considered (see CONTRAINDICATIONS).

Hydration. Patients should receive a total of one liter of 0.9% (normal) saline solution intravenously with each infusion of VISTIDE. The saline solution should be infused over a 1–2 hr period immediately before the VISTIDE infusion. Patients who can tolerate the additional fluid load should receive a second liter. If administered, the second liter of saline should be initiated either at the start of the VISTIDE infusion or immediately afterwards, and infused over a 1 to 3 hr period.

Dose Adjustment

Changes in Renal Function During VISTIDE Therapy: For clinically significant increases in serum creatinine (0.3–0.4 mg/dL), the VISTIDE dose should be reduced from 5 mg/kg to 3 mg/kg. VISTIDE therapy should be discontinued for an increase in serum creatinine of ≥ 0.5 mg/dL or development of ≥ 3+ proteinuria.

Preexisting Renal Impairment: VISTIDE has not been studied in patients with preexisting renal impairment. The most appropriate initial and maintenance doses of VISTIDE for patients with serum creatinine concentrations > 1.5 mg/dL or creatinine clearances ≤ 55 mL/min are not known. When the potential benefits of therapy exceed the potential risks, dose adjustments should be made based on the following table:

VISTIDE DOSE*

Creatinine Clearance (mL/min)	Induction (once weekly for 2 weeks)	Maintenance (once every 2 weeks)
41–55	2.0 mg/kg	2.0 mg/kg
30–40	1.5 mg/kg	1.5 mg/kg
20–29	1.0 mg/kg	1.0 mg/kg
≤ 19	0.5 mg/kg	0.5 mg/kg

* These recommended dose adjustments are based on pharmacokinetic estimates, not on actual clinical data.

Intravenous normal saline and oral probenecid must accompany each VISTIDE infusion. VISTIDE has not been studied in patients receiving dialysis.

Because no clinical efficacy, safety or pharmacokinetic data are available from patients with moderate to severe renal impairment (creatinine clearance ≤ 55 mL/min), careful monitoring of disease progression and patient safety is required.

Method of Preparation and Administration

Inspect vials visually for particulate matter and discoloration prior to administration. If particulate matter or discoloration are observed, the vial should not be used.

With a syringe, extract the appropriate volume of VISTIDE from the vial and transfer the dose to an infusion bag containing 100 mL 0.9% (normal) saline solution. Infuse the entire volume intravenously into the patient at a constant rate over a 1 hr period. Use of a standard infusion pump for administration is recommended.

It is recommended that VISTIDE infusion admixtures be administered within 24 hr of preparation and that refrigerator or freezer storage not be used to extend this 24 hr limit.

If admixtures are not intended for immediate use, they may be stored under refrigeration (2–8°C) for no more than 24 hr. Refrigerated admixtures should be allowed to equilibrate to room temperature prior to use.

The chemical stability of VISTIDE admixtures was demonstrated in polyvinyl chloride composition and ethylene/propylene copolymer composition commercial infusion bags, and in glass bottles. **No data are available to support the addition of other drugs or supplements to the cidofovir admixture for concurrent administration.**

VISTIDE is supplied in single-use vials. Partially used vials should be discarded (see Handling and Disposal).

Compatibility with Ringer's solution, Lactated Ringer's solution or bacteriostatic infusion fluids has not been evaluated.

Handling and Disposal

Due to the mutagenic properties of cidofovir, adequate precautions including the use of appropriate safety equipment are recommended for the preparation, administration, and disposal of VISTIDE. The National Institutes of Health presently recommends that the preparation of such agents be prepared in a Class II laminar flow biological safety cabinet and that personnel preparing drugs of this class wear surgical gloves and a closed front surgical-type gown with knit cuffs. If VISTIDE contacts the skin, wash membranes and flush thoroughly with water. Excess VISTIDE and all other materials used in the admixture preparation and administration should be placed in a leak-proof, puncture-proof container. The recommended method of disposal is high temperature incineration.

Patient Monitoring

Serum creatinine, urine protein, and white blood cell counts with differential should be monitored prior to each dose. In patients with proteinuria, intravenous hydration should be administered and the test repeated. Intraocular pressure, visual acuity and ocular symptoms should be monitored periodically.

HOW SUPPLIED

VISTIDE (cidofovir injection) 75 mg/mL for intravenous infusion, is supplied as a non-preserved solution in single-use clear glass vials as follows:

NDC 61958-0101-1 375 mg in a 5 mL vial in a single unit carton.

VISTIDE should be stored at controlled room temperature 20°–25°C (68°–77°F).

CAUTION: Federal law prohibits dispensing without prescription.

Manufactured by:
Ben Venue Laboratories, Inc.
Bedford, OH 44146-0568

Manufactured for and distributed by:
Gilead Sciences, Inc.
333 Lakeside Drive
Foster City, CA 94404

VISTIDE® (cidofovir injection) is covered by U.S. Patent No. 5,142,051 and its foreign counterparts. Other patents pending.

REFERENCES

1. Ho HT, Woods KL, Bronson JJ, De Boeck H, Martin JC and Hitchcock MJM. Intracellular Metabolism of the Antiherpesvirus Agent (S)-1-[3-hydroxy-2-(phosphonylmethoxy)propyl]cytosine. *Mol Pharmacol*, **41**:197-202, 1992.
2. Cherrington JM, Allen SJW, McKee BH, and Chen MS. Kinetic Analysis of the Interaction Between the Diphosphate of (S)-1-(3-hydroxy-2-phosphonylmethoxypropyl)-cytosine, zalcitabineTP, zidovudineTP, and FIAUTP with Human DNA Polymerases β and γ. *Biochem Pharmacol*, **48**:1986-1988, 1994.
3. Xiong X, Kim C, Huang E, Smith JL, and Chen MS. Kinetic Analysis of the Interaction of Cidofovir Diphosphate with Human Cytomegalovirus DNA Polymerase. *Biochem Pharmacol*, 1996 (in press).
4. Cherrington JM, Mulato AS, Fuller MD, Chen MS. *In Vitro* Selection of a Human Cytomegalovirus (HCMV) that is Resistant to Cidofovir. 35th International Conference on Antimicrobial Agents and Chemotherapy (ICAAC), San Francisco, CA. Abstract H117, 1995.
5. Stanat SC, Reardon JE, Erice A, Jordan MC, Drew WL, and Biron KK. Ganciclovir-Resistant Cytomegalovirus Clinical Isolates: Mode of Resistance to Ganciclovir. *Antimicrob Agents Chemother*, **35**:2191-2197, 1991.
6. Sullivan V, Biron KK, Talarico C, Stanat SC, Davis M, Pozzi M, and Coen DM. A Point Mutation in the Human Cytomegalovirus DNA Polymerase Gene Confers Resistance to Ganciclovir and phosphonylmethoxyalkyl Derivatives. *Antimicrob Agents Chemother*, **37**:19-25, 1993.
7. Tatarowicz WA, Lurain NS, and Thompson KD. A Ganciclovir-Resistant Clinical Isolate of Human Cytomegalovirus Exhibiting Cross-Resistance to other DNA Polymerase Inhibitors. *J Infect Dis*, **166**:904-907, 1992.
8. Lurain NS, Thompson KD, Holmes EW, and Read GS. Point Mutations in the DNA Polymerase Gene of Human Cytomegalovirus that Result in Resistance to Antiviral Agents. *J Virol*, **66**:7146-7152, 1992.
9. Sullivan V and Coen DM. Isolation of Foscarnet-Resistant Human Cytomegalovirus Patterns of Resistance and Sensitivity to Other Antiviral Drugs. *J Infect Dis*, **164**:781-784, 1991.
10. Snoeck R, Andrei G, and De Clercq E. Human Cytomegalovirus (HCMV) Strains Selected Under Selective Pressure of Phosphonoformate (PFA) are Resistant for Both PFA and phosphonylmethoxyethyl (PME) Derivatives *In Vitro. Antiviral Res*, **26**, Abstract 177, 1995.
11. Baldanti F, Underwood MR, Stanat SC, Biron KK, Chou S, Sarasini A, Silini E, and Gerna G. Single Amino Acid Changes in the DNA Polymerase Confer Foscarnet Resistance and Slow-Growth Phenotype, While Mutations in the UL97-Encoded Phosphotransferase Confer Ganciclovir Resistance in Three Double-Resistant Human Cytomegalovirus Strains Recovered from Patients with AIDS. *J Virol*, **70**:1390-1395, 1996.

Part Number: RM-1078 June 1996

For information on over-the-counter drugs, consult **PDR For Nonprescription Drugs**

Glaxo Wellcome Inc.
FIVE MOORE DRIVE
RESEARCH TRIANGLE PARK, NC 27709

For Medical Information Contact:
Generally:
Medical Services Department
1-800-334-0089
In Emergencies:
Medical Services Department
1-800-334-0089
For Consumer Inquiries Contact:
1-800-722-9292

ACLOVATE® ℞
[a'klō-vāt"]
(alclometasone dipropionate cream)
Cream, 0.05%

ACLOVATE® ℞
(alclometasone dipropionate ointment)
Ointment, 0.05%
For Dermatologic Use Only—
Not for Ophthalmic Use.

DESCRIPTION

ACLOVATE Cream and Ointment contain alclometasone dipropionate (7α-chloro- 11β,17,21-trihydroxy -16α- methylpregna-1,4-diene-3,20-dione 17,21-dipropionate), a synthetic corticosteroid for topical dermatologic use. The corticosteroids constitute a class of primarily synthetic steroids used topically as anti-inflammatory and antipruritic agents. Chemically, alclometasone dipropionate is $C_{28}H_{37}ClO_7$.
Alclometasone dipropionate has the molecular weight of 521. It is a white powder, insoluble in water, slightly soluble in propylene glycol, and moderately soluble in hexylene glycol.
Each gram of ACLOVATE Cream contains 0.5 mg of alclometasone dipropionate in a hydrophilic, emollient cream base of propylene glycol, white petrolatum, cetearyl alcohol, glyceryl stearate, PEG 100 stearate, Ceteth-20, monobasic sodium phosphate, chlorocresol, phosphoric acid, and purified water.
Each gram of ACLOVATE Ointment contains 0.5 mg of alclometasone dipropionate in an ointment base of hexylene glycol, white wax, propylene glycol stearate, and white petrolatum.

CLINICAL PHARMACOLOGY

Like other topical corticosteroids, alclometasone dipropionate has anti-inflammatory, antipruritic, and vasoconstrictive properties. The mechanism of the anti-inflammatory activity of the topical steroids, in general, is unclear. However, corticosteroids are thought to act by the induction of phospholipase A_2 inhibitory proteins, collectively called lipocortins. It is postulated that these proteins control the biosynthesis of potent mediators of inflammation such as prostaglandins and leukotrienes by inhibiting the release of their common precursor, arachidonic acid. Arachidonic acid is released from membrane phospholipids by phospholipase A_2.
Pharmacokinetics: The extent of percutaneous absorption of topical corticosteroids is determined by many factors, including the vehicle and the integrity of the epidermal barrier. Occlusive dressings with hydrocortisone for up to 24 hours have not been demonstrated to increase penetration; however, occlusion of hydrocortisone for 96 hours markedly enhances penetration.
Topical corticosteroids can be absorbed from normal intact skin. Inflammation and/or other disease processes in the skin may increase percutaneous absorption. A study utilizing a radiolabeled alclometasone dipropionate ointment formulation was performed to measure systemic absorption and excretion. Results indicated that approximately 3% of the steroid was absorbed during 8 hours of contact with intact skin of normal volunteers.
Studies performed with ACLOVATE Cream and Ointment indicate that these products are in the low to medium range of potency as compared with other topical corticosteroids.

INDICATIONS AND USAGE

ACLOVATE Cream and Ointment are low to medium potency corticosteroids indicated for the relief of the inflammatory and pruritic manifestations of corticosteroid-responsive dermatoses. ACLOVATE Cream and Ointment may be used in pediatric patients 1 year of age or older, although the safety and efficacy of drug use for longer than 3 weeks have not been established (see PRECAUTIONS: Pediatric Use). Since the safety and efficacy of ACLOVATE Cream and Ointment have not been established in pediatric patients below 1 year of age, their use in this age-group is not recommended.

CONTRAINDICATIONS

ACLOVATE Cream and Ointment are contraindicated in those patients with a history of hypersensitivity to any of the components in these preparations.

PRECAUTIONS

General: Systemic absorption of topical corticosteroids can produce reversible hypothalamic-pituitary-adrenal (HPA) axis suppression with the potential for glucocorticosteroid insufficiency after withdrawal of treatment. Manifestations of Cushing's syndrome, hyperglycemia, and glucosuria can also be produced in some patients by systemic absorption of topical corticosteroids while on treatment.
Patients applying a topical steroid to a large surface area or to areas under occlusion should be evaluated periodically for evidence of HPA axis suppression. This may be done by using the ACTH stimulation, A.M. plasma cortisol, and urinary free cortisol tests.
The effects of ACLOVATE Cream and Ointment on the HPA axis have been evaluated. In one study, ACLOVATE Cream and Ointment were applied to 30% of the body twice daily for 7 days, and occlusive dressings were used in selected patients either 12 hours or 24 hours daily. In another study, ACLOVATE Cream was applied to 80% of the body surface of normal subjects twice daily for 21 days with daily 12-hour periods of whole body occlusion. Average plasma and urinary free cortisol levels and urinary levels of 17-hydroxysteroids were decreased (about 10%), suggesting suppression of the HPA axis under these conditions. Plasma cortisol levels have also been demonstrated to decrease in pediatric patients treated twice daily for 3 weeks without occlusion.
If HPA axis suppression is noted, an attempt should be made to withdraw the drug, to reduce the frequency of application, or to substitute a less potent corticosteroid. Recovery of HPA axis function is generally prompt upon discontinuation of topical corticosteroids. Infrequently, signs and symptoms of glucocorticosteroid insufficiency may occur, requiring supplemental systemic corticosteroids. For information on systemic supplementation, see prescribing information for those products.
Pediatric patients may be more susceptible to systemic toxicity from equivalent doses due to their larger skin surface area to body mass ratios (see PRECAUTIONS: Pediatric Use).
If irritation develops, ACLOVATE Cream or Ointment should be discontinued and appropriate therapy instituted. Allergic contact dermatitis with corticosteroids is usually diagnosed by observing *a failure to heal* rather than noting a clinical exacerbation, as with most topical products not containing corticosteroids. Such an observation should be corroborated with appropriate diagnostic patch testing.
If concomitant skin infections are present or develop, an appropriate antifungal or antibacterial agent should be used. If a favorable response does not occur promptly, use of ACLOVATE Cream or Ointment should be discontinued until the infection has been adequately controlled.
Information for Patients: Patients using topical corticosteroids should receive the following information and instructions:

1. This medication is to be used as directed by the physician. It is for external use only. Avoid contact with the eyes.
2. This medication should not be used for any disorder other than that for which it was prescribed.
3. The treated skin area should not be bandaged, otherwise covered or wrapped so as to be occlusive, unless directed by the physician.
4. Patients should report to their physician any signs of local adverse reactions.
5. Parents of pediatric patients should be advised not to use ACLOVATE Cream or Ointment in the treatment of diaper dematitis. ACLOVATE Cream or Ointment should not be applied in the diaper area as diapers or plastic pants may constitute occlusive dressing (see DOSAGE AND ADMINISTRATION).
6. This medication should not be used on the face, underarms, or groin areas unless directed by the physician.
7. As with other corticosteroids, therapy should be discontinued when control is achieved. If no improvement is seen within 2 weeks, contact the physician.

Laboratory Tests: The following tests may be helpful in evaluating patients for HPA axis suppression:
ACTH stimulation test
A.M. plasma cortisol test
Urinary free cortisol test
Carcinogenesis, Mutagenesis, Impairment of Fertility: Long-term animal studies have not been performed to evaluate the carcinogenic potential or the effect on fertility of topical corticosteroids.
Pregnancy: ***Teratogenic Effects: Pregnancy Category C:*** Corticosteroids have been shown to be teratogenic in laboratory animals when administered systemically at relatively low dosage levels. Some corticosteroids have been shown to be teratogenic after dermal application in laboratory animals. There are no adequate and well-controlled studies in pregnant women. ACLOVATE Cream or Ointment should be used during pregnancy only if the potential benefit justifies the potential risk to the fetus.
Nursing Mothers: Systemically administered corticosteroids appear in human milk and could suppress growth, interfere with endogenous corticosteroid production, or cause other untoward effects. It is not known whether topical administration of topical corticosteroids could result in sufficient systemic absorption to produce detectable quantities in human milk. Because many drugs are excreted in human milk, caution should be exercised when ACLOVATE Cream or Ointment is administered to a nursing woman.
Pediatric Use: ACLOVATE Cream and Ointment may be used with caution in pediatric patients 1 year of age or older, although the safety and efficacy of drug use for longer than 3 weeks have not been established. Use of ACLOVATE Cream and Ointment is supported by results from adequate and well-controlled studies in pediatric patients with corticosteroid-responsive dermatoses. Since the safety and efficacy of ACLOVATE Cream and Ointment have not been established in pediatric patients below 1 year of age, its use in this age-group is not recommended. Because of a higher ratio of skin surface area to body mass, pediatric patients are at a greater risk than adults of HPA axis suppression and Cushing's syndrome when they are treated with topical corticosteroids. They are therefore also at greater risk of adrenal insufficiency during and/or after withdrawal of treatment. Adverse effects, including striae, have been reported with use of topical corticosteroids in infants and children. Pediatric patients applying ACLOVATE Cream or Ointment to > 20% of the body surface area are at higher risk for HPA axis suppression.
HPA axis suppression, Cushing's syndrome, linear growth retardation, delayed weight gain, and intracranial hypertension have been reported in pediatric patients receiving topical corticosteroids. Manifestations of adrenal suppression in pediatric patients include low plasma cortisol levels and absence of response to ACTH stimulation. Manifestations of intracranial hypertension include bulging fontanelles, headaches, and bilateral papilledema.
ACLOVATE Cream or Ointment should not be used in the treatment of diaper dermatitis.

ADVERSE REACTIONS

The following local adverse reactions have been reported with ACLOVATE Cream in approximately 2% of patients: itching and burning, erythema, dryness, irritation, and papular rashes.
The following local adverse reactions have been reported with ACLOVATE Ointment in approximately 1% of patients: itching, burning, and erythema.
The following additional local adverse reactions have been reported infrequently with topical corticosteroids, but may occur more frequently with the use of occlusive dressings. These reactions are listed in approximate decreasing order of occurrence: folliculitis, acneiform eruptions, hypopigmentation, perioral dermatitis, allergic contact dermatitis, secondary infection, skin atrophy, striae, and miliaria.

OVERDOSAGE

Topically applied ACLOVATE Cream and Ointment can be absorbed in sufficient amounts to produce systemic effects (see PRECAUTIONS).

DOSAGE AND ADMINISTRATION

Apply a thin film of ACLOVATE Cream or Ointment to the affected skin areas two or three times daily; massage gently until the medication disappears.
ACLOVATE Cream and Ointment may be used in pediatric patients 1 year of age or older. Safety and effectiveness of ACLOVATE Cream or Ointment in pediatric patients for more than 3 weeks of use have not been established. Use in pediatric patients under 1 year of age is not recommended
As with other corticosteroids, therapy should be discontinued when control is achieved. If no improvement is seen within 2 weeks, reassessment of diagnosis may be necessary.
ACLOVATE Cream or Ointment should not be used with occlusive dressings unless directed by a physician. ACLOVATE Cream or Ointment should not be applied in the diaper area if the child still requires diapers or plastic pants as these garments may constitute occlusive dressing.

HOW SUPPLIED

ACLOVATE Cream, 0.05% is supplied in 15-g (NDC 0173-0401-00), 45-g (NDC 0173-0401-01), and 60-g (NDC 0173-0401-06) tubes.
ACLOVATE Ointment, 0.05% is supplied in 15-g (NDC 0173-0402-00), 45-g (NDC 0173-0402-01), and 60-g (NDC 0173-0402-06) tubes.
Store between 2° and 30° C (36° and 86° F)
April 1996/RL-217

Shown in Product Identification Guide, page 312

Continued on next page

Glaxo Wellcome—Cont.

ANECTINE® ℞
[ă-nĕk'tēn]
(succinylcholine chloride)
Injection, USP

ANECTINE® ℞
(succinylcholine chloride)
Sterile Powder Flo-Pack®

WARNING

RISK OF CARDIAC ARREST FROM HYPERKALEMIC RHABDOMYOLYSIS

There have been rare reports of acute rhabdomyolysis with hyperkalemia followed by ventricular dysrhythmias, cardiac arrest, and death after the administration of succinylcholine to apparently healthy children who were subsequently found to have undiagnosed skeletal muscle myopathy, most frequently Duchenne's muscular dystrophy.

This syndrome often presents as peaked T-waves and sudden cardiac arrest within minutes after the administration of the drug in healthy appearing children (usually, but not exclusively, males, and most frequently 8 years of age or younger). There have also been reports in adolescents.

Therefore, when a healthy appearing infant or child develops cardiac arrest soon after administration of succinylcholine, not felt to be due to inadequate ventilation, oxygenation or anesthetic overdose, immediate treatment for hyperkalemia should be instituted. This should include administration of intravenous calcium, bicarbonate, and glucose with insulin, with hyperventilation. Due to the abrupt onset of this syndrome, routine resuscitative measures are likely to be unsuccessful. However, extraordinary and prolonged resuscitative efforts have resulted in successful resuscitation in some reported cases. In addition, in the presence of signs of malignant hyperthermia, appropriate treatment should be instituted concurrently.

Since there may be no signs or symptoms to alert the practitioner to which patients are at risk, it is recommended that the use of succinylcholine in children should be reserved for emergency intubation or instances where immediate securing of the airway is necessary, e.g., laryngospasm, difficult airway, full stomach, or for intramuscular use when a suitable vein is inaccessible (see PRECAUTIONS: Pediatric Use and DOSAGE AND ADMINISTRATION).

This drug should be used only by individuals familiar with its actions, characteristics, and hazards.

DESCRIPTION

ANECTINE (succinylcholine chloride) is an ultra short-acting depolarizing-type, skeletal muscle relaxant for intravenous administration.

Succinylcholine chloride is a white, odorless, slightly bitter powder and very soluble in water. The drug is unstable in alkaline solutions but relatively stable in acid solutions, depending upon the concentration of the solution and the storage temperature. Solutions of succinylcholine chloride should be stored under refrigeration to preserve potency.

ANECTINE Injection is a sterile non-pyrogenic solution for intravenous injection, containing 20 mg succinylcholine chloride in each mL and made isotonic with sodium chloride. The pH is adjusted to 3.5 with hydrochloric acid. Methylparaben (0.1%) is added as a preservative. ANECTINE Flo-Pack is a sterile powder, containing either 500 mg or 1000 mg of succinylcholine chloride in each vial.

The chemical name for succinylcholine chloride is 2,2′-[(1,4-dioxo-1,4-butanediyl)bis(oxy)]bis[*N,N,N*-trimethylethanaminium] dichloride.

CLINICAL PHARMACOLOGY

Succinylcholine is a depolarizing skeletal muscle relaxant. As does acetylcholine, it combines with the cholinergic receptors of the motor end plate to produce depolarization. This depolarization may be observed as fasciculations. Subsequent neuromuscular transmission is inhibited so long as adequate concentration of succinylcholine remains at the receptor site. Onset of flaccid paralysis is rapid (less than one minute after intravenous administration), and with single administration lasts approximately 4 to 6 minutes.

Succinylcholine is rapidly hydrolyzed by plasma cholinesterase to succinylmonocholine (which possesses clinically insignificant depolarizing muscle relaxant properties) and then more slowly to succinic acid and choline (see PRECAUTIONS). About 10% of the drug is excreted unchanged in the urine. The paralysis following administration of succinylcholine is progressive, with differing sensitivities of different muscles. This initially involves consecutively the levator muscles of the face, muscles of the glottis and finally the intercostals and the diaphragm and all other skeletal muscles.

Succinylcholine has no direct action on the uterus or other smooth muscle structures. Because it is highly ionized and has low fat solubility, it does not readily cross the placenta.

Tachyphylaxis occurs with repeated administration (see PRECAUTIONS).

Depending on the dose and duration of succinylcholine administration, the characteristic depolarizing neuromuscular block (Phase I block) may change to a block with characteristics superficially resembling a non-depolarizing block (Phase II block). This may be associated with prolonged respiratory muscle paralysis or weakness in patients who manifest the transition to Phase II block. When this diagnosis is confirmed by peripheral nerve stimulation, it may sometimes be reversed with anticholinesterase drugs such as neostigmine (See PRECAUTIONS). Anticholinesterase drugs may not always be effective. If given before succinylcholine is metabolized by cholinesterase, anticholinesterase drugs may prolong rather than shorten paralysis.

Succinylcholine has no direct effect on the myocardium. Succinylcholine stimulates both autonomic ganglia and muscarinic receptors which may cause changes in cardiac rhythm, including cardiac arrest. Changes in rhythm, including cardiac arrest, may also result from vagal stimulation, which may occur during surgical procedures, or from hyperkalemia, particularly in children (see PRECAUTIONS: Pediatric Use). These effects are enhanced by halogenated anesthetics.

Succinylcholine causes an increase in intraocular pressure immediately after its injection and during the fasciculation phase, and slight increases which may persist after onset of complete paralysis (see WARNINGS). Succinylcholine may cause slight increases in intracranial pressure immediately after its injection and during the fasciculation phase (see PRECAUTIONS).

As with other neuromuscular blocking agents, the potential for releasing histamine is present following succinylcholine administration. Signs and symptoms of histamine mediated release such as flushing, hypotension and bronchoconstriction are, however, uncommon in normal clinical usage.

Succinylcholine has no effect on consciousness, pain threshold or cerebration. It should be used only with adequate anesthesia (see WARNINGS).

INDICATIONS AND USAGE

Succinylcholine chloride is indicated as an adjunct to general anesthesia, to facilitate tracheal intubation, and to provide skeletal muscle relaxation during surgery or mechanical ventilation.

CONTRAINDICATIONS

Succinylcholine is contraindicated in persons with personal or familial history of malignant hyperthermia, skeletal muscle myopathies, and known hypersensitivity to the drug. It is also contraindicated in patients after the acute phase of injury following major burns, multiple trauma, extensive denervation of skeletal muscle, or upper motor neuron injury, because succinylcholine administered to such individuals may result in severe hyperkalemia which may result in cardiac arrest (see WARNINGS). The risk of hyperkalemia in these patients increases over time and usually peaks at 7 to 10 days after the injury. The risk is dependent on the extent and location of the injury. The precise time of onset and the duration of the risk period are not known.

WARNINGS

SUCCINYLCHOLINE SHOULD BE USED ONLY BY THOSE SKILLED IN THE MANAGEMENT OF ARTIFICIAL RESPIRATION AND ONLY WHEN FACILITIES ARE INSTANTLY AVAILABLE FOR TRACHEAL INTUBATION AND FOR PROVIDING ADEQUATE VENTILATION OF THE PATIENT, INCLUDING THE ADMINISTRATION OF OXYGEN UNDER POSITIVE PRESSURE AND THE ELIMINATION OF CARBON DIOXIDE. THE CLINICIAN MUST BE PREPARED TO ASSIST OR CONTROL RESPIRATION.

TO AVOID DISTRESS TO THE PATIENT, SUCCINYLCHOLINE SHOULD NOT BE ADMINISTERED BEFORE UNCONSCIOUSNESS HAS BEEN INDUCED. IN EMERGENCY SITUATIONS, HOWEVER, IT MAY BE NECESSARY TO ADMINISTER SUCCINYLCHOLINE BEFORE UNCONSCIOUSNESS IS INDUCED.

SUCCINYLCHOLINE IS METABOLIZED BY PLASMA CHOLINESTERASE AND SHOULD BE USED WITH CAUTION, IF AT ALL, IN PATIENTS KNOWN TO BE OR SUSPECTED OF BEING HOMOZYGOUS FOR THE ATYPICAL PLASMA CHOLINESTERASE GENE.

Hyperkalemia: (SEE BOX WARNING) Succinylcholine should be administered with **GREAT CAUTION** to patients suffering from electrolyte abnormalities and those who may have massive digitalis toxicity, because in these circumstances succinylcholine may induce serious cardiac arrhythmias or cardiac arrest due to hyperkalemia.

GREAT CAUTION should be observed if succinylcholine is administered to patients during the acute phase of injury following major burns, multiple trauma, extensive denervation of skeletal muscle, or upper motor neuron injury (see CONTRAINDICATIONS). The risk of hyperkalemia in these patients increases over time and usually peaks at 7 to 10 days after the injury. The risk is dependent on the extent and location of the injury. The precise time of onset and the duration of the risk period are undetermined. Patients with chronic abdominal infection, subarachnoid hemorrhage, or conditions causing degeneration of central and peripheral nervous systems should receive succinylcholine with **GREAT CAUTION** because of the potential for developing severe hyperkalemia.

Malignant Hyperthermia: Succinylcholine administration has been associated with acute onset of malignant hyperthermia, a potentially fatal hypermetabolic state of skeletal muscle. The risk of developing malignant hyperthermia following succinylcholine administration increases with the concomitant administration of volatile anesthetics. Malignant hyperthermia frequently presents as intractable spasm of the jaw muscles (masseter spasm) which may progress to generalized rigidity, increased oxygen demand, tachycardia, tachypnea and profound hyperpyrexia. Successful outcome depends on recognition of early signs, such as jaw muscle spasm, acidosis, or generalized rigidity to initial administration of succinylcholine for tracheal intubation, or failure of tachycardia to respond to deepening anesthesia. Skin mottling, rising temperature and coagulopathies may occur later in the course of the hypermetabolic process. Recognition of the syndrome is a signal for discontinuance of anesthesia, attention to increased oxygen consumption, correction of acidosis, support of circulation, assurance of adequate urinary output and institution of measures to control rising temperature. Intravenous dantrolene sodium is recommended as an adjunct to supportive measures in the management of this problem. Consult literature references and the dantrolene prescribing information for additional information about the management of malignant hyperthermic crisis. Continuous monitoring of temperature and expired CO_2 is recommended as an aid to early recognition of malignant hyperthermia.

Other: In both adults and children the incidence of bradycardia, which may progress to asystole, is higher following a second dose of succinylcholine. The incidence and severity of bradycardia is higher in children than adults. Pretreatment with anticholinergic agents (e.g., atropine) may reduce the occurrence of bradyarrhythmias.

Succinylcholine causes an increase in intraocular pressure. It should not be used in instances in which an increase in intraocular pressure is undesirable (e.g., narrow angle glaucoma, penetrating eye injury) unless the potential benefit of its use outweighs the potential risk.

Succinylcholine is acidic (pH = 3.5) and should not be mixed with alkaline solutions having a pH greater than 8.5 (e.g., barbiturate solutions).

PRECAUTIONS: (SEE BOX WARNING)

General: When succinylcholine is given over a prolonged period of time, the characteristic depolarization block of the myoneural junction (Phase I block) may change to a block with characteristics superficially resembling a non-depolarizing block (Phase II block). Prolonged respiratory muscle paralysis or weakness may be observed in patients manifesting this transition to Phase II block. The transition from Phase I to Phase II block has been reported in 7 of 7 patients studied under halothane anesthesia after an accumulated dose of 2 to 4 mg/kg succinylcholine (administered in repeated, divided doses). The onset of Phase II block coincided with the onset of tachyphylaxis and prolongation of spontaneous recovery. In another study, using balanced anesthesia (N_2O/O_2/narcotic-thiopental) and succinylcholine infusion, the transition was less abrupt, with great individual variability in the dose of succinylcholine required to produce Phase II block. Of 32 patients studied, 24 developed Phase II block. Tachyphylaxis was not associated with the transition to Phase II block, and 50% of the patients who developed Phase II block experienced prolonged recovery.

When Phase II block is suspected in cases of prolonged neuromuscular blockade, positive diagnosis should be made by peripheral nerve stimulation, prior to administration of any anticholinesterase drug. Reversal of Phase II block is a medical decision which must be made upon the basis of the individual, clinical pharmacology and the experience and judgment of the physician. The presence of Phase II block is indicated by fade of responses to successive stimuli (preferably "train of four"). The use of an anticholinesterase drug to reverse Phase II block should be accompanied by appropriate doses of an anticholinergic drug to prevent disturbances of cardiac rhythm. After adequate reversal of Phase II block with an anticholinesterase agent, the patient should be continually observed for at least 1 hour for signs of return of muscle relaxation. Reversal should not be attempted unless: (1) a peripheral nerve stimulator is used to determine the presence of Phase II block (since anticholinesterase agents will potentiate succinylcholine-induced Phase I block), and (2) spontaneous recovery of muscle twitch has been observed for at least 20 minutes and has reached a plateau with further recovery proceeding slowly; this delay is to ensure complete hydrolysis of succinylcholine by plasma cholinesterase

prior to administration of the anticholinesterase agent. Should the type of block be misdiagnosed, depolarization of the type initially induced by succinylcholine (i.e., Phase I block) will be prolonged by an anticholinesterase agent.

Succinylcholine should be employed with caution in patients with fractures or muscle spasm because the initial muscle fasciculations may cause additional trauma.

Succinylcholine may cause a transient increase in intracranial pressure; however, adequate anesthetic induction prior to administration of succinylcholine will minimize this effect.

Succinylcholine may increase intragastric pressure, which could result in regurgitation and possible aspiration of stomach contents.

Neuromuscular blockade may be prolonged in patients with hypokalemia or hypocalcemia.

Reduced Plasma Cholinesterase Activity: Succinylcholine should be used carefully in patients with reduced plasma cholinesterase (pseudocholinesterase) activity. The likelihood of prolonged neuromuscular block following administration of succinylcholine must be considered in such patients (see DOSAGE AND ADMINISTRATION).

Plasma cholinesterase activity may be diminished in the presence of genetic abnormalities of plasma cholinesterase (e.g., patients heterozygous or homozygous for atypical plasma cholinesterase gene), pregnancy, severe liver or kidney disease, malignant tumors, infections, burns, anemia, decompensated heart disease, peptic ulcer, or myxedema. Plasma cholinesterase activity may also be diminished by chronic administration of oral contraceptives, glucocorticoids, or certain monoamine oxidase inhibitors and by irreversible inhibitors of plasma cholinesterase (e.g., organophosphate insecticides, echothiophate, and certain antineoplastic drugs).

Patients homozygous for atypical plasma cholinesterase gene (1 in 2500 patients) are extremely sensitive to the neuromuscular blocking effect of succinylcholine. In these patients, a 5 to 10 mg test dose of succinylcholine may be administered to evaluate sensitivity to succinylcholine, or neuromuscular blockade may be produced by the cautious administration of a 1 mg/mL solution of succinylcholine by slow intravenous infusion. Apnea or prolonged muscle paralysis should be treated with controlled respiration.

Drug Interactions: Drugs which may enhance the neuromuscular blocking action of succinylcholine include: promazine, oxytocin, aprotinin, certain non-penicillin antibiotics, quinidine, β-adrenergic blockers, procainamide, lidocaine, trimethaphan, lithium carbonate, magnesium salts, quinine, chloroquine, diethylether, isoflurane, desflurane, metoclopramide and terbutaline. The neuromuscular blocking effect of succinylcholine may be enhanced by drugs that reduce plasma cholinesterase activity (e.g., chronically administered oral contraceptives, glucocorticoids, or certain monoamine oxidase inhibitors) or by drugs that irreversibly inhibit plasma cholinesterase (see PRECAUTIONS).

If other neuromuscular blocking agents are to be used during the same procedure, the possibility of a synergistic or antagonistic effect should be considered.

Carcinogenesis, Mutagenesis, Impairment of Fertility: There have been no long-term studies performed in animals to evaluate carcinogenic potential.

Pregnancy: ***Teratogenic Effects:*** Pregnancy Category C. Animal reproduction studies have not been conducted with succinylcholine chloride. It is also not known whether succinylcholine can cause fetal harm when administered to a pregnant woman or can affect reproduction capacity. Succinylcholine should be given to a pregnant woman only if clearly needed.

Nonteratogenic Effects: Plasma cholinesterase levels are decreased by approximately 24% during pregnancy and for several days postpartum. Therefore, a higher proportion of patients may be expected to show increased sensitivity (prolonged apnea) to succinylcholine when pregnant than when nonpregnant.

Labor and Delivery: Succinylcholine is commonly used to provide muscle relaxation during delivery by cesarean section. While small amounts of succinylcholine are known to cross the placental barrier, under normal conditions the quantity of drug that enters fetal circulation after a single dose of 1 mg/kg to the mother should not endanger the fetus. However, since the amount of drug that crosses the placental barrier is dependent on the concentration gradient between the maternal and fetal circulations, residual neuromuscular blockade (apnea and flaccidity) may occur in the newborn after repeated high doses to, or in the presence of atypical plasma cholinesterase in, the mother.

Nursing Mothers: It is not known whether succinylcholine is excreted in human milk. Because many drugs are excreted in human milk, caution should be exercised following succinylcholine administration to a nursing woman.

Pediatric Use: There are rare reports of ventricular dysrhythmias and cardiac arrest secondary to acute rhabdomyolysis with hyperkalemia in apparently healthy children who receive succinylcholine (see BOX WARNING). Many of these children were subsequently found to have a skeletal muscle myopathy such as Duchenne's muscular dystrophy whose clinical signs were not obvious. The syndrome often presents as sudden cardiac arrest within minutes after the administration of succinylcholine. These children are usually, but not exclusively, males, and most frequently 8 years of age or younger. There have also been reports in adolescents. There may be no signs or symptoms to alert the practitioner to which patients are at risk. A careful history and physical may identify developmental delays suggestive of a myopathy. A preoperative creatine kinase could identify some but not all patients at risk. Due to the abrupt onset of this syndrome, routine resuscitative measures are likely to be unsuccessful. Careful monitoring of the electrocardiogram may alert the practitioner to peaked T-waves (an early sign). Administration of intravenous calcium, bicarbonate, and glucose with insulin, with hyperventilation have resulted in successful resuscitation in some of the reported cases. Extraordinary and prolonged resuscitative efforts have been effective in some cases. In addition, in the presence of signs of malignant hyperthermia, appropriate treatment should be initiated concurrently (see WARNINGS). Since it is difficult to identify which patients are at risk, it is recommended that the use of succinylcholine in children should be reserved for emergency intubation or instances where immediate securing of the airway is necessary, e.g., laryngospasm, difficult airway, full stomach, or for intramuscular use when a suitable vein is inaccessible.

As in adults, the incidence of bradycardia in children is higher following the second dose of succinylcholine. The incidence and severity of bradycardia is higher in children than adults. Pretreatment with anticholinergic agents, e.g., atropine, may reduce the occurrence of bradyarrhythmias.

ADVERSE REACTIONS

Adverse reactions to succinylcholine consist primarily of an extension of its pharmacological actions. Succinylcholine causes profound muscle relaxation resulting in respiratory depression to the point of apnea; this effect may be prolonged. Hypersensitivity reactions, including anaphylaxis, may occur in rare instances. The following additional adverse reactions have been reported: cardiac arrest, malignant hyperthermia, arrhythmias, bradycardia, tachycardia, hypertension, hypotension, hyperkalemia, prolonged respiratory depression or apnea, increased intraocular pressure, muscle fasciculation, jaw rigidity, postoperative muscle pain, rhabdomyolysis with possible myoglobinuric acute renal failure, excessive salivation, and rash.

OVERDOSAGE

Overdosage with succinylcholine may result in neuromuscular block beyond the time needed for surgery and anesthesia. This may be manifested by skeletal muscle weakness, decreased respiratory reserve, low tidal volume, or apnea. The primary treatment is maintenance of a patent airway and respiratory support until recovery of normal respiration is assured. Depending on the dose and duration of succinylcholine administration, the characteristic depolarizing neuromuscular block (Phase I) may change to a block with characteristics superficially resembling a non-depolarizing block (Phase II) (see PRECAUTIONS).

DOSAGE AND ADMINISTRATION

The dosage of succinylcholine should be individualized and should always be determined by the clinician after careful assessment of the patient (see WARNINGS).

Parenteral drug products should be inspected visually for particulate matter and discoloration prior to administration whenever solution and container permit. Solutions which are not clear and colorless should not be used.

Adults:

For Short Surgical Procedures: The average dose required to produce neuromuscular blockade and to facilitate tracheal intubation is 0.6 mg/kg ANECTINE (succinylcholine chloride) Injection given intravenously. The optimum dose will vary among individuals and may be from 0.3 to 1.1 mg/kg for adults. Following administration of doses in this range, neuromuscular blockade develops in about 1 minute; maximum blockade may persist for about 2 minutes, after which recovery takes place within 4 to 6 minutes. However, very large doses may result in more prolonged blockade. A 5 to 10 mg test dose may be used to determine the sensitivity of the patient and the individual recovery time (see PRECAUTIONS).

For Long Surgical Procedures: The dose of succinylcholine administered by infusion depends upon the duration of the surgical procedure and the need for muscle relaxation. The average rate for an adult ranges between 2.5 and 4.3 mg per minute.

Solutions containing from 1 to 2 mg per mL succinylcholine have commonly been used for continuous infusion. The more dilute solution (1 mg per mL) is probably preferable from the standpoint of ease of control of the rate of administration of the drug and, hence, of relaxation. This intravenous solution containing 1 mg per mL may be administered at a rate of 0.5 mg (0.5 mL) to 10 mg (10 mL) per minute to obtain the required amount of relaxation. The amount required per minute will depend upon the individual response as well as the degree of relaxation required. Avoid overburdening the circulation with a large volume of fluid. It is recommended that neuromuscular function be carefully monitored with a peripheral nerve stimulator when using succinylcholine by infusion in order to avoid overdose, detect development of Phase II block, follow its rate of recovery, and assess the effects of reversing agents (see PRECAUTIONS).

Intermittent intravenous injections of succinylcholine may also be used to provide muscle relaxation for long procedures. An intravenous injection of 0.3 to 1.1 mg/kg may be given initially, followed, at appropriate intervals, by further injections of 0.04 to 0.07 mg/kg to maintain the degree of relaxation required.

Pediatrics: For emergency tracheal intubation or in instances where immediate securing of the airway is necessary, the intravenous dose of succinylcholine is 2 mg/kg for infants and small children; for older children and adolescents the dose is 1 mg/kg (see BOX WARNING and PRECAUTIONS: Pediatric Use.)

Rarely, IV bolus administration of succinylcholine in infants and children may result in malignant ventricular arrythmias and cardiac arrest secondary to acute rhabdomyolysis with hyperkalemia. In such situations, an underlying myopathy should be suspected.

Intravenous bolus administration of succinylcholine in infants or children may result in profound bradycardia or, rarely, asystole. As in adults, the incidence of bradycardia in children is higher following a second dose of succinylcholine. The occurrence of bradyarrhythmias may be reduced by pretreatment with atropine (see PRECAUTIONS: Pediatric Use).

Intramuscular Use: If necessary, succinylcholine may be given intramuscularly to infants, older children or adults when a suitable vein is inaccessible. A dose of up to 3 to 4 mg/kg may be given, but not more than 150 mg total dose should be administered by this route. The onset of effect of succinylcholine given intramuscularly is usually observed in about 2 to 3 minutes.

Compatibility and Admixtures: Succinylcholine is acidic (pH 3.5) and should not be mixed with alkaline solutions having a pH greater than 8.5 (e.g., barbiturate solutions). Admixtures containing 1 to 2 mg/mL may be prepared by adding 1 g succinylcholine (the contents of one ANECTINE Sterile Powder Flo-Pack unit containing 1 g succinylcholine chloride) to 1000 or 500 mL sterile solution, such as 5% Dextrose Injection USP or 0.9% Sodium Chloride Injection USP. Admixtures of ANECTINE must be used within 24 hours after preparation. Aseptic techniques should be used to prepare the diluted product. Admixtures of ANECTINE should be prepared for single patient use only. The unused portion of diluted Anectine should be discarded.

HOW SUPPLIED

For immediate injection of single doses for short procedures:
ANECTINE (succinylcholine chloride) Injection, 20 mg in each mL.
Multiple-dose vials of 10 mL.
Box of 12 vials (NDC-0173-0071-95).
Store in refrigerator at 2° to 8°C (36° to 46°F). The multi-dose vials are stable for up to 14 days at room temperature without significant loss of potency.
For preparation of intravenous solutions only:
ANECTINE Flo-Pack, 500 mg sterile succinylcholine chloride powder.
Box of 12 vials (NDC-0173-0085-15).
ANECTINE Flo-Pack, 1000 mg sterile succinylcholine chloride powder.
Box of 12 vials (NDC-0173-0086-15).
ANECTINE Flo-Pack does not require refrigeration. Store at 15° to 25°C (59° to 77°F). Solutions of succinylcholine must be used within 24 hours after preparation. Discard unused solutions.

January 1996/RL-238

Shown in Product Identification Guide, page 312

BECLOVENT® ℞
[*be 'klō-vent "*]
(beclomethasone dipropionate, USP)
Inhalation Aerosol
For Oral Inhalation Only

DESCRIPTION

Beclomethasone dipropionate, USP, the active component of Beclovent® Inhalation Aerosol, is an anti-inflammatory steroid having the chemical name 9-chloro-11β, 17, 21-trihydroxy-16β-methylpregna-1, 4-diene-3, 20-dione 17, 21-dipropionate.

Beclovent Inhalation Aerosol is a metered-dose aerosol unit containing a microcrystalline suspension of beclomethasone dipropionate-trichloromonofluoromethane clathrate in a mixture of propellants (trichloromonofluoromethane and dichlorodifluoromethane) with oleic acid. Each canister contains beclomethasone dipropionate-trichloromono-

Continued on next page

Glaxo Wellcome—Cont.

fluoromethane clathrate having a molecular proportion of beclomethasone dipropionate to trichloromonofluoromethane between 3:1 and 3:2. Each actuation delivers from the mouthpiece a quantity of clathrate equivalent to 42 mcg of beclomethasone dipropionate, USP. The contents of one 6.7-g canister provide at least 80 oral inhalations, and the contents of one 16.8-g canister provide at least 200 oral inhalations.

CLINICAL PHARMACOLOGY

Beclomethasone 17, 21-dipropionate is a diester of beclomethasone, a synthetic halogenated corticosteroid. Animal studies show that beclomethasone dipropionate has potent anti-inflammatory activity. When beclomethasone dipropionate was administered systemically to mice, the anti-inflammatory activity was accompanied by other features typical of glucocorticoid action, including thymic involution, liver glycogen deposition, and pituitary-adrenal suppression. However, after systemic administration of beclomethasone dipropionate to rats, the anti-inflammatory action was associated with little or no effect on other tests of glucocorticoid activity.

Beclomethasone dipropionate is sparingly soluble and is poorly mobilized from subcutaneous or intramuscular injection sites. However, systemic absorption occurs after all routes of administration. When given to animals in the form of an aerosolized suspension of the trichloromonofluoromethane clathrate, the drug is deposited in the mouth and nasal passages, the trachea and principal bronchi, and the lung; a considerable portion of the drug is also swallowed. Absorption occurs rapidly from all respiratory and gastrointestinal tissues, as indicated by the rapid clearance of radioactively labeled drug from local tissues and appearance of tracer in the circulation. There is no evidence of tissue storage of beclomethasone dipropionate or its metabolites. Lung slices can metabolize beclomethasone dipropionate rapidly to beclomethasone 17-monopropionate and more slowly to free beclomethasone (which has very weak anti-inflammatory activity). However, irrespective of the route of administration (injection, oral, or aerosol), the principal route of excretion of the drug and its metabolites is the feces. Less than 10% of the drug and its metabolites is excreted in the urine. In humans, 12% to 15% of an orally administered dose of beclomethasone dipropionate was excreted in the urine as both conjugated and free metabolites of the drug.

The mechanisms responsible for the anti-inflammatory action of beclomethasone dipropionate are unknown. The precise mechanism of the aerosolized drug's action in the lung is also unknown.

INDICATIONS AND USAGE

Beclovent® (beclomethasone dipropionate) Inhalation Aerosol is indicated only for patients who require chronic treatment with corticosteroids for control of the symptoms of bronchial asthma. Such patients would include those already receiving systemic corticosteroids, and selected patients who are inadequately controlled on a nonsteroid regimen and in whom steroid therapy has been withheld because of concern over potential adverse effects.

Beclovent Inhalation Aerosol is NOT indicated:
1. For relief of asthma that can be controlled by bronchodilators and other nonsteroid medications.
2. In patients who require systemic corticosteroid treatment infrequently.
3. In the treatment of nonasthmatic bronchitis.

CONTRAINDICATIONS

Beclovent® (beclomethasone dipropionate) Inhalation Aerosol is contraindicated in the primary treatment of status asthmaticus or other acute episodes of asthma where intensive measures are required.

Hypersensitivity to any of the ingredients of this preparation contraindicates its use.

WARNINGS

Particular care is needed in patients who are transferred from systemically active corticosteroids to Beclovent® (beclomethasone dipropionate) Inhalation Aerosol because deaths due to adrenal insufficiency have occurred in asthmatic patients during and after transfer from systemic corticosteroids to aerosol beclomethasone dipropionate. After withdrawal from systemic corticosteroids, a number of months are required for recovery of hypothalamic-pituitary-adrenal (HPA) function. During this period of HPA suppression, patients may exhibit signs and symptoms of adrenal insufficiency when exposed to trauma, surgery, or infections, particularly gastroenteritis. Although Beclovent Inhalation Aerosol may provide control of asthmatic symptoms during these episodes, it does NOT provide the systemic steroid that is necessary for coping with these emergencies.

During periods of stress or a severe asthmatic attack, patients who have been withdrawn from systemic corticosteroids should be instructed to resume systemic steroids (in large doses) immediately and to contact their physician for further instruction. These patients should also be instructed to carry a warning card indicating that they may need supplementary systemic steroids during periods of stress or a severe asthma attack. To assess the risk of adrenal insufficiency in emergency situations, routine tests of adrenal cortical function, including measurement of early morning resting cortisol levels, should be performed periodically in all patients. An early morning resting cortisol level may be accepted as normal only if it falls at or near the normal mean level.

Studies have shown that the combined administration of alternate-day prednisone systemic treatment and orally inhaled beclomethasone increases the likelihood of HPA suppression compared to a therapeutic dose of either one alone.

Because of the possibility of systemic absorption of orally inhaled corticosteroids, including beclomethasone, patients should be monitored for symptoms of systemic effects such as mental disturbances, increased bruising, weight gain, cushingoid features, acneiform lesions, and cataracts. Therefore, if such changes occur, Beclovent Inhalation Aerosol should be discontinued slowly, consistent with accepted procedures for discontinuing oral steroids.

Persons who are on drugs that suppress the immune system are more susceptible to infections than healthy individuals. Chickenpox and measles, for example, can have a more serious or even fatal course in nonimmune children or adults on corticosteroids. In such children or adults who have not had these diseases, particular care should be taken to avoid exposure. How the dose, route, and duration of corticosteroid administration affects the risk of developing a disseminated infection is not known. The contribution of the underlying disease and/or prior corticosteroid treatment to the risk is also not known. If exposed to chickenpox, prophylaxis with varicella zoster immune globulin (VZIG) may be indicated. If exposed to measles, prophylaxis with pooled intramuscular immunoglobulin (IG) may be indicated. (See the respective package inserts for complete VZIG and IG prescribing information.) If chickenpox develops, treatment with antiviral agents may be considered.

Localized infections with *Candida albicans* or *Aspergillus niger* have occurred frequently in the mouth and pharynx and occasionally in the larynx. Positive cultures for oral *Candida* may be present in up to 75% of patients. Although the frequency of clinically apparent infection is considerably lower, these infections may require treatment with appropriate antifungal therapy or discontinuation of treatment with Beclovent Inhalation Aerosol.

Beclovent Inhalation Aerosol is not to be regarded as a bronchodilator and is not indicated for rapid relief of bronchospasm.

Patients should be instructed to contact their physician immediately when episodes of asthma that are not responsive to bronchodilators occur during the course of treatment with Beclovent Inhalation Aerosol. During such episodes, patients may require therapy with systemic corticosteroids. There is no evidence that control of asthma can be achieved by the administration of Beclovent Inhalation Aerosol in amounts greater than the recommended doses.

The management of asthma should follow a stepwise program, and patient response should be monitored clinically and by lung function tests. Increasing use of short-acting inhaled beta₂-agonists to control symptoms indicates deterioration of asthma control. Under these conditions, the patient's therapy plan should be reassessed. In patients considered at risk, daily flow monitoring may be instituted.

If patients find that short-acting relief bronchodilator treatment becomes less effective or they need more inhalations than usual, medical attention must be sought.

Transfer of patients from systemic steroid therapy to Beclovent Inhalation Aerosol may unmask allergic conditions previously suppressed by the systemic steroid therapy, e.g., rhinitis, conjunctivitis, and eczema.

PRECAUTIONS

During withdrawal from oral steroids, some patients may experience symptoms of systemically active steroid withdrawal, e.g., joint and/or muscular pain, lassitude, and depression, despite maintenance or even improvement of respiratory function (see DOSAGE AND ADMINISTRATION).

In responsive patients, beclomethasone dipropionate may permit control of asthmatic symptoms without suppression of HPA function, as discussed below (see CLINICAL STUDIES). Since beclomethasone dipropionate is absorbed into the circulation and can be systemically active, the beneficial effects of Beclovent® (beclomethasone dipropionate) Inhalation Aerosol in minimizing or preventing HPA dysfunction may be expected only when recommended dosages are not exceeded.

Children should be monitored for a reduction in growth velocity, although the relationship between growth velocity and final adult height is not known.

The long-term effects of beclomethasone dipropionate in human subjects are still unknown. In particular, the local effects of the agent on developmental or immunologic processes in the mouth, pharynx, trachea, and lung are unknown. There is also no information about the possible long-term systemic effects of the agent.

The potential effects of Beclovent Inhalation Aerosol on acute, recurrent, or chronic pulmonary infections, including active or quiescent tuberculosis, are not known. Similarly, the potential effects of long-term administration of the drug on lung or other tissues are unknown.

Rare instances of wheezing, cataracts, glaucoma, and increased intraocular pressure have been reported following the oral inhalation of beclomethasone dipropionate.

Pulmonary infiltrates with eosinophilia may occur in patients on Beclovent Inhalation Aerosol therapy. Although it is possible that in some patients this state may become manifest because of systemic steroid withdrawal when inhalational steroids are administered, a causative role for beclomethasone dipropionate and/or its vehicle cannot be ruled out.

Information for Patients: Persons who are on immunosuppressant doses of corticosteroids should be warned to avoid exposure to chickenpox or measles. Patients should also be advised that if they are exposed, medical advice should be sought without delay.

Patients should be made aware of the prophylactic nature of therapy with inhaled beclomethasone dipropionate and that it should be taken regularly even when they are asymptomatic.

Pregnancy: *Teratogenic Effects:* Glucocorticoids are known teratogens in rodent species and beclomethasone dipropionate is no exception.

Teratology studies were done in rats, mice, and rabbits treated with subcutaneous beclomethasone dipropionate. Beclomethasone dipropionate was found to produce fetal resorption, cleft palate, agnathia, microstomia, absence of tongue, delayed ossification, and partial agenesis of the thymus. Well-controlled trials relating to fetal risk in humans are not available. Glucocorticoids are secreted in human milk. It is not known whether beclomethasone dipropionate would be secreted in human milk, but it is safe to assume that it is likely. The use of beclomethasone dipropionate in pregnant women, nursing mothers, or women of childbearing potential requires that the possible benefits of the drug be weighed against the potential hazards to the mother, embryo, or fetus. Infants born of mothers who have received substantial doses of corticosteroids during pregnancy should be carefully observed for hypoadrenalism.

ADVERSE REACTIONS

Deaths due to adrenal insufficiency have occurred in asthmatic patients during and after transfer from systemic corticosteroids to aerosol beclomethasone dipropionate (see WARNINGS).

Suppression of HPA function (reduction of early morning plasma cortisol levels) has been reported in adult patients who received 1,600-mcg daily doses of Beclovent® (beclomethasone dipropionate) Inhalation Aerosol for 1 month. A few patients on Beclovent Inhalation Aerosol have complained of hoarseness or dry mouth.

Rare cases of immediate and delayed hypersensitivity reactions, including urticaria, angioedema, rash, and bronchospasm, have been reported after the use of beclomethasone oral or intranasal inhalers.

Rare instances of wheezing, cataracts, glaucoma, and increased intraocular pressure have been reported following the oral inhalation of beclomethasone dipropionate.

Reports of headache, light-headedness, dryness and irritation of the nose and throat, and unpleasant taste and smell have been received. There are rare reports of loss of taste and smell.

DOSAGE AND ADMINISTRATION

Adults and Children 12 Years of Age and Older: The usual recommended dosage is two inhalations (84 mcg) given three or four times a day. Alternatively, four inhalations (168 mcg) given twice daily have been shown to be effective in some patients. In patients with severe asthma, it is advisable to start with 12 to 16 inhalations a day and adjust the dosage downward according to the response of the patient. The maximal daily intake should not exceed 20 inhalations, 840 mcg (0.84 mg), in adults.

Children 6 to 12 Years of Age: The usual recommended dosage is one or two inhalations (42 to 84 mcg) given three or four times a day according to the response of the patient. Alternatively, four inhalations (168 mcg) given twice daily have been shown to be effective in some patients. The maximal daily intake should not exceed 10 inhalations, 420 mcg (0.42 mg), in children 6 to 12 years of age. Insufficient clinical data exist with respect to the administration of Beclovent® (beclomethasone dipropionate) Inhalation Aerosol in children below the age of 6.

Rinsing the mouth after inhalation is advised.

Treatment with Beclovent Inhalation Aerosol should not be stopped abruptly.

Patients receiving bronchodilators by inhalation should be advised to use the bronchodilator before Beclovent Inhalation Aerosol in order to enhance penetration of beclomethasone dipropionate into the bronchial tree. After use of an aerosol bronchodilator, several minutes should elapse before use of the Beclovent Inhalation Aerosol to reduce the potential toxicity from the inhaled fluorocarbon propellants in the two aerosols.

Different considerations must be given to the following groups of patients in order to obtain the full therapeutic benefit of Beclovent Inhalation Aerosol.

Patients Not Receiving Systemic Steroids: The use of Beclovent Inhalation Aerosol is straightforward in patients who are inadequately controlled with nonsteroid medications but in whom systemic steroid therapy has been withheld because of concern over potential adverse reactions. In patients who respond to Beclovent Inhalation Aerosol, an improvement in pulmonary function is usually apparent within 1 to 4 weeks after the start of Beclovent Inhalation Aerosol.

Patients Receiving Systemic Steroids: In those patients dependent on systemic steroids, transfer to Beclovent Inhalation Aerosol and subsequent management may be more difficult because recovery from impaired adrenal function is usually slow. Such suppression has been known to last for up to 12 months. Clinical studies, however, have demonstrated that Beclovent Inhalation Aerosol may be effective in the management of these asthmatic patients and may permit replacement or significant reduction in the dosage of systemic corticosteroids.

The patient's asthma should be reasonably stable before treatment with Beclovent Inhalation Aerosol is started. Initially, the aerosol should be used concurrently with the patient's usual maintenance dose of systemic steroid. After approximately 1 week, gradual withdrawal of the systemic steroid is started by reducing the daily or alternate-daily dose. The next reduction is made after an interval of 1 or 2 weeks, depending on the response of the patient. Generally, these decrements should not exceed 2.5 mg of prednisone or its equivalent. A slow rate of withdrawal cannot be overemphasized. During withdrawal some patients may experience symptoms of systemically active steroid withdrawal, e.g., joint and/or muscular pain, lassitude, and depression, despite maintenance or even improvement of respiratory function. Such patients should be encouraged to continue with the inhaler but should be watched carefully for objective signs of adrenal insufficiency such as hypotension and weight loss. If evidence of adrenal insufficiency occurs, the systemic steroid dose should be boosted temporarily and thereafter further withdrawal should continue more slowly. During periods of stress or a severe asthma attack, transfer patients will require supplementary treatment with systemic steroids. Exacerbations of asthma that occur during the course of treatment with Beclovent Inhalation Aerosol should be treated with a short course of systemic steroid that is gradually tapered as these symptoms subside. There is no evidence that control of asthma can be achieved by administration of Beclovent Inhalation Aerosol in amounts greater than the recommended doses.

Directions for Use: Illustrated Patient's Instructions for Use accompany each package of Beclovent Inhalation Aerosol.

CONTENTS UNDER PRESSURE: Do not puncture. Do not use or store near heat or open flame. Exposure to temperatures above 120°F may cause bursting. Never throw container into fire or incinerator. Keep out of reach of children.

HOW SUPPLIED

Beclovent® Inhalation Aerosol is supplied in a 6.7-g canister containing 80 metered inhalations with oral adapter and patient's instructions (NDC 0173-0469-00) and in a 16.8-g canister containing 200 metered inhalations with oral adapter and patient's instructions (NDC 0173-0312-88). Also available, Beclovent® Inhalation Aerosol Refill 16.8-g canister only with patient's instructions (NDC 0173-0312-98).

Store between 2° and 30°C (36° and 86°F). As with most inhaled medications in aerosol canisters, the therapeutic effect of this medication may decrease when the canister is cold. Shake well before using.

ANIMAL PHARMACOLOGY AND TOXICOLOGY

Studies in a number of animal species, including rats, rabbits, and dogs, have shown no unusual toxicity during acute experiments. However, the effects of beclomethasone dipropionate in producing signs of glucocorticoid excess during chronic administration by various routes were dose related.

CLINICAL STUDIES

The effects of beclomethasone dipropionate on HPA function have been evaluated in adult volunteers. There was no suppression of early morning plasma cortisol concentrations when beclomethasone dipropionate was administered in a dose of 1,000 mcg per day for 1 month as an aerosol or for 3 days by intramuscular injection. However, partial suppression of plasma cortisol concentration was observed when beclomethasone dipropionate was administered in doses of 2,000 mcg per day either intramuscularly or by aerosol. Immediate suppression of plasma cortisol concentrations was observed after single doses of 4,000 mcg of beclomethasone dipropionate.

In one study the effects of beclomethasone dipropionate on HPA function were examined in patients with asthma. There was no change in basal early morning plasma cortisol concentrations or in the cortisol responses to tetracosactrin (ACTH 1:24) stimulation after daily administration of 400, 800, or 1,200 mcg of beclomethasone dipropionate for 28 days. After daily administration of 1,600 mcg each day for 28 days, there was slight reduction in basal cortisol concentrations and a statistically significant ($p<.01$) reduction in plasma cortisol responses to tetracosactrin stimulation. The effects of a more prolonged period of beclomethasone dipropionate administration on HPA function have not been evaluated. However, a number of investigators have noted that when systemic corticosteroid therapy in asthmatic subjects can be replaced with recommended doses of beclomethasone dipropionate, there is gradual recovery of endogenous cortisol concentrations to the normal range. There is still no documented evidence of recovery from other adverse systemic corticosteroid-induced reactions during prolonged therapy of patients with beclomethasone dipropionate.

Clinical experience has shown that some patients with bronchial asthma who require corticosteroid therapy for control of symptoms can be partially or completely withdrawn from systemic corticosteroids if therapy with beclomethasone dipropionate aerosol is substituted. Beclomethasone dipropionate aerosol is not effective for all patients with bronchial asthma or at all stages of the disease in a given patient.

The early clinical experience has revealed several new problems that may be associated with the use of beclomethasone dipropionate by inhalation for treatment of patients with bronchial asthma.

1. There is a risk of adrenal insufficiency when patients are transferred from systemic corticosteroids to aerosol beclomethasone dipropionate. Although the aerosol may provide adequate control of asthma during the transfer period, it does not provide the systemic steroid that is needed during acute stress situations. Deaths due to adrenal insufficiency have occurred in asthmatic patients during and after transfer from systemic corticosteroids to aerosol beclomethasone dipropionate (see WARNINGS).
2. Transfer of patients from systemic steroid therapy to beclomethasone dipropionate aerosol may unmask allergic conditions that were previously controlled by the systemic steroid therapy, e.g., rhinitis, conjunctivitis, and eczema.
3. Localized infections with *Candida albicans* or *Aspergillus niger* have occurred frequently in the mouth and pharynx and occasionally in the larynx. It has been reported that up to 75% of the patients who receive prolonged treatment with beclomethasone dipropionate have positive oral cultures for *Candida albicans.* The incidence of clinically apparent infection is considerably lower but may require therapy with appropriate antifungal agents or discontinuation of treatment with beclomethasone dipropionate aerosol.

The long-term effects of beclomethasone dipropionate in human subjects are still unknown. In particular, the local effects of the agent on developmental or immunologic processes in the mouth, pharynx, trachea, and lung are unknown. There is also no information about the possible long-term systemic effects of the agent. The possible relevance of the data in animal studies to results in human subjects cannot be evaluated.

September 1995/RL-214

Shown in Product Identification Guide, page 312

BECONASE® ℞
[be'kō-nāz"]
(beclomethasone dipropionate, USP)
Inhalation Aerosol
For Nasal Inhalation Only

BECONASE AQ®
[be'kō-nāz"AQ]
(beclomethasone dipropionate, monohydrate)
Nasal Spray, 0.042%*
***Calculated on the dried basis.** **SHAKE WELL**
For Intranasal Use Only **BEFORE USE.**

DESCRIPTION

Beconase® Inhalation Aerosol:

Beclomethasone dipropionate, USP, the active component of Beconase Inhalation Aerosol, is an anti-inflammatory steroid having the chemical name 9-chloro-11β,17,21-trihydroxy-16β-methylpregna-1, 4-diene-3, 20-dione 17,21-dipropionate.

Beclomethasone dipropionate is a white to creamy-white, odorless powder with a molecular weight of 521.25. It is very slightly soluble in water, very soluble in chloroform, and freely soluble in acetone and in alcohol.

Beconase Inhalation Aerosol is a metered-dose aerosol unit containing a microcrystalline suspension of beclomethasone dipropionate-trichloromonofluoromethane clathrate in a mixture of propellants (trichloromonofluoromethane and dichlorodifluoromethane) with oleic acid. Each canister contains beclomethasone dipropionate-trichloromonofluoromethane clathrate having a molecular proportion of beclomethasone dipropionate to trichloromonofluoromethane between 3:1 and 3:2. Each actuation delivers from the compact actuator a quantity of clathrate equivalent to 42 mcg of beclomethasone dipropionate, USP. The contents of one 6.7-g canister provide at least 80 metered doses, and the contents of one 16.8-g canister provide at least 200 metered doses.

Beconase AQ Nasal Spray:

Beclomethasone dipropionate, monohydrate, the active component of Beconase AQ Nasal Spray, is an anti-inflammatory steroid having the chemical name 9-chloro-11β, 17,21-trihydroxy- 16β-methylpregna-1,4-diene-3,20-dione 17,21-dipropionate, monohydrate.

Beclomethasone dipropionate, monohydrate is a white to creamy-white, odorless powder with a molecular weight of 539.06. It is very slightly soluble in water, very soluble in chloroform, and freely soluble in acetone and in alcohol.

Beconase AQ Nasal Spray is a metered-dose, manual pump spray unit containing a microcrystalline suspension of beclomethasone dipropionate, monohydrate equivalent to 0.042% w/w beclomethasone dipropionate, calculated on the dried basis, in an aqueous medium containing microcrystalline cellulose, carboxymethylcellulose sodium, dextrose, benzalkonium chloride, polysorbate 80, and 0.25% v/w phenylethyl alcohol. Hydrochloric acid may be added to adjust pH. The pH is between 4.5 and 7.0.

After initial priming (three to four actuations), each actuation of the pump delivers from the nasal adapter 100 mg of suspension containing beclomethasone dipropionate, monohydrate equivalent to 42 mcg of beclomethasone dipropionate. Each bottle of Beconase AQ Nasal Spray will provide at least 200 metered doses.

CLINICAL PHARMACOLOGY

Beclomethasone 17,21-dipropionate is a diester of beclomethasone, a synthetic halogenated corticosteroid. Animal studies show that beclomethasone dipropionate has potent glucocorticoid and weak mineralocorticoid activity.

The mechanisms responsible for the anti-inflammatory action of beclomethasone dipropionate are unknown. The precise mechanism of the aerosolized drug's action in the nose is also unknown. Biopsies of nasal mucosa obtained during clinical studies showed no histopathologic changes when beclomethasone dipropionate was administered intranasally.

The effects of beclomethasone dipropionate on hypothalamic-pituitary-adrenal (HPA) function have been evaluated in adult volunteers by other routes of administration. Studies with beclomethasone dipropionate by the intranasal route may demonstrate that there is more or that there is less absorption by this route of administration. There was no suppression of early morning plasma cortisol concentrations when beclomethasone dipropionate was administered in a dose of 1,000 mcg per day for 1 month as an oral aerosol or for 3 days by intramuscular injection. However, partial suppression of plasma cortisol concentrations was observed when beclomethasone dipropionate was administered in doses of 2,000 mcg per day either by oral aerosol or intramuscular injection. Immediate suppression of plasma cortisol concentrations was observed after single doses of 4,000 mcg of beclomethasone dipropionate. Suppression of HPA function (reduction of early morning plasma cortisol levels) has been reported in adult patients who received 1,600-mcg daily doses of oral beclomethasone dipropionate for 1 month. In clinical studies using beclomethasone dipropionate intranasally, there was no evidence of adrenal insufficiency. The effect of Beconase AQ® (beclomethasone dipropionate, monohydrate) Nasal Spray on HPA function was not evaluated but would not be expected to differ from intranasal beclomethasone dipropionate aerosol.

In one study in asthmatic children, the administration of inhaled beclomethasone at recommended daily doses for at least 1 year was associated with a reduction in nocturnal cortisol secretion. The clinical significance of this finding is not clear. It reinforces other evidence, however, that topical beclomethasone may be absorbed in amounts that can have systemic effects and that physicians should be alert for evidence of systemic effects, especially in chronically treated patients (see PRECAUTIONS).

Beclomethasone dipropionate is sparingly soluble. When given by nasal inhalation in the form of an aqueous or aerosolized suspension, the drug is deposited primarily in the nasal passages. A portion of the drug is swallowed. Absorption occurs rapidly from all respiratory and gastrointestinal tissues. There is no evidence of tissue storage of beclomethasone dipropionate or its metabolites. *In vitro* studies have shown that tissue other than the liver (lung slices) can rapidly metabolize beclomethasone dipropionate to beclometha-

Continued on next page

Glaxo Wellcome—Cont.

sone 17-monopropionate and more slowly to free beclomethasone (which has very weak anti-inflammatory activity). However, irrespective of the route of entry, the principal route of excretion of the drug and its metabolites is the feces. In humans, 12% to 15% of an orally administered dose of beclomethasone dipropionate is excreted in the urine as both conjugated and free metabolites of the drug.

Studies have shown that the degree of binding to plasma proteins is 87%.

INDICATIONS AND USAGE

Beconase® (beclomethasone dipropionate) Inhalation Aerosol is indicated for the relief of the symptoms of seasonal or perennial rhinitis in those cases poorly responsive to conventional treatment. Beconase AQ® (beclomethasone dipropionate, monohydrate) Nasal Spray is indicated for the relief of the symptoms of seasonal or perennial allergic and nonallergic (vasomotor) rhinitis.

Both preparations are also indicated for the prevention of recurrence of nasal polyps following surgical removal.

Clinical studies with Beconase Inhalation Aerosol in patients with seasonal or perennial rhinitis have shown that improvement is usually apparent within a few days. Results from two clinical trials have shown that significant symptomatic relief was obtained with Beconase AQ Nasal Spray within 3 days. With either preparation, however, symptomatic relief may not occur in some patients for as long as 2 weeks. Although systemic effects are minimal at recommended doses, Beconase Inhalation Aerosol and Beconase AQ Nasal Spray should not be continued beyond 3 weeks in the absence of significant symptomatic improvement. Both preparations should not be used in the presence of untreated localized infection involving the nasal mucosa.

Clinical studies have shown that treatment of the symptoms associated with nasal polyps may have to be continued for several weeks or more before a therapeutic result can be fully assessed. Recurrence of symptoms due to polyps can occur after stopping treatment, depending on the severity of the disease.

CONTRAINDICATIONS

Hypersensitivity to any of the ingredients of either preparation contraindicates its use.

WARNINGS

The replacement of a systemic corticosteroid with Beconase® (beclomethasone dipropionate) Inhalation Aerosol or Beconase AQ® (beclomethasone dipropionate, monohydrate) Nasal Spray can be accompanied by signs of adrenal insufficiency.

Careful attention must be given when patients previously treated for prolonged periods with systemic corticosteroids are transferred to Beconase Inhalation Aerosol or Beconase AQ Nasal Spray. This is particularly important in those patients who have associated asthma or other clinical conditions where too rapid a decrease in systemic corticosteroids may cause a severe exacerbation of their symptoms. Studies have shown that the combined administration of alternate-day prednisone systemic treatment and orally inhaled beclomethasone increases the likelihood of HPA suppression compared to a therapeutic dose of either one alone. Therefore, Beconase Inhalation Aerosol and Beconase AQ Nasal Spray treatment should be used with caution in patients already on alternate-day prednisone regimens for any disease.

If recommended doses of intranasal beclomethasone are exceeded or if individuals are particularly sensitive or predisposed by virtue of recent systemic steroid therapy, symptoms of hypercorticism may occur, including very rare cases of menstrual irregularities, acneiform lesions, cataracts, and cushingoid features. If such changes occur, Beconase Inhalation Aerosol and Beconase AQ Nasal Spray should be discontinued slowly consistent with accepted procedures for discontinuing oral steroid therapy.

Persons who are on drugs that suppress the immune system are more susceptible to infections than healthy individuals. Chickenpox and measles, for example, can have a more serious or even fatal course in nonimmune children or adults on corticosteroids. In such children or adults who have not had these diseases, particular care should be taken to avoid exposure. How the dose, route, and duration of corticosteroid administration affects the risk of developing a disseminated infection is not known. The contribution of the underlying disease and/or prior corticosteroid treatment to the risk is also not known. If exposed to chickenpox, prophylaxis with varicella zoster immune globulin (VZIG) may be indicated. If exposed to measles, prophylaxis with pooled intramuscular immunoglobulin (IG) may be indicated. (See the respective package inserts for complete VZIG and IG prescribing information.) If chickenpox develops, treatment with antiviral agents may be considered.

PRECAUTIONS

General: During withdrawal from oral steroids, some patients may experience symptoms of withdrawal, e.g., joint and/or muscular pain, lassitude, and depression.

Rare instances of nasal septum perforation have been spontaneously reported.

Rare instances of wheezing, cataracts, glaucoma, and increased intraocular pressure have been reported following the intranasal use of beclomethasone dipropionate.

In clinical studies with beclomethasone dipropionate administered intranasally, the development of localized infections of the nose and pharynx with *Candida albicans* has occurred only rarely. When such an infection develops, it may require treatment with appropriate local therapy or discontinuation of treatment with Beconase® (beclomethasone dipropionate) Inhalation Aerosol or Beconase AQ® (beclomethasone dipropionate, monohydrate) Nasal Spray.

Beclomethasone dipropionate is absorbed into the circulation. Use of excessive doses of Beconase Inhalation Aerosol or Beconase AQ Nasal Spray may suppress HPA function. Beconase Inhalation Aerosol and Beconase AQ Nasal Spray should be used with caution, if at all, in patients with active or quiescent tuberculous infections of the respiratory tract; untreated fungal, bacterial, or systemic viral infections; or ocular herpes simplex.

For either preparation to be effective in the treatment of nasal polyps, the aerosol or spray must be able to enter the nose. Therefore, treatment of nasal polyps with these preparations should be considered adjunctive therapy to surgical removal and/or the use of other medications that will permit effective penetration of Beconase Inhalation Aerosol or Beconase AQ Nasal Spray into the nose. Nasal polyps may recur after any form of treatment.

As with any long-term treatment, patients using Beconase Inhalation Aerosol or Beconase AQ Nasal Spray over several months or longer should be examined periodically for possible changes in the nasal mucosa.

Because of the inhibitory effect of corticosteroids on wound healing, patients who have experienced recent nasal septum ulcers, nasal surgery, or trauma should not use a nasal corticosteroid until healing has occurred.

Although systemic effects have been minimal with recommended doses, this potential increases with excessive doses. Therefore, larger than recommended doses of Beconase Inhalation Aerosol and Beconase AQ Nasal Spray should be avoided.

Beconase AQ Nasal Spray: Rarely, immediate hyersensitivity reactions may occur after the intranasal administration of beclomethasone (see ADVERSE REACTIONS).

If persistent nasopharyngeal irritation occurs, it may be an indication for stopping Beconase AQ Nasal Spray.

Information for Patients: Patients being treated with Beconase Inhalation Aerosol or Beconase AQ Nasal Spray should receive the following information and instructions. This information is intended to aid in the safe and effective use of these medications. It is not a disclosure of all possible adverse or intended effects. Patients should use these preparations at regular intervals since their effectiveness depends on their regular use. The patient should take the medication as directed. It is not acutely effective, and the prescribed dosage should not be increased. Instead, nasal vasoconstrictors or oral antihistamines may be needed until the effects of Beconase Inhalation Aerosol or Beconase AQ Nasal Spray are fully manifested. One to 2 weeks may pass before full relief is obtained. The patient should contact the physician if symptoms do not improve, if the condition worsens, or if sneezing or nasal irritation occurs. For the proper use of either unit and to attain maximum improvement, the patient should read and follow carefully the patient's instructions section of the package insert.

Persons who are on immunosuppressant doses of corticosteroids should be warned to avoid exposure to chickenpox or measles. Patients should also be advised that if they are exposed, medical advice should be sought without delay.

Carcinogenesis, Mutagenesis, Impairment of Fertility: Treatment of rats for a total of 95 weeks, 13 weeks by inhalation and 82 weeks by the oral route, resulted in no evidence of carcinogenic activity. Mutagenic studies have not been performed.

Impairment of fertility, as evidenced by inhibition of the estrous cycle in dogs, was observed following treatment by the oral route. No inhibition of the estrous cycle in dogs was seen following treatment with beclomethasone dipropionate by the inhalation route.

Pregnancy: *Teratogenic Effects: Pregnancy Category C:* Like other corticoids, parenteral (subcutaneous) beclomethasone dipropionate has been shown to be teratogenic and embryocidal in the mouse and rabbit when given in doses approximately 10 times the human dose. In these studies, beclomethasone was found to produce fetal resorption, cleft palate, agnathia, microstomia, absence of tongue, delayed ossification, and agenesis of the thymus. No teratogenic or embryocidal effects have been seen in the rat when beclomethasone dipropionate was administered by inhalation at 10 times the human dose or orally at 1,000 times the human

dose. There are no adequate and well-controlled studies in pregnant women. Beclomethasone dipropionate should be used during pregnancy only if the potential benefit justifies the potential risk to the fetus.

Nonteratogenic Effects: Hypoadrenalism may occur in infants born of mothers receiving corticosteroids during pregnancy. Such infants should be carefully observed.

Nursing Mothers: It is not known whether beclomethasone dipropionate is excreted in human milk. Because other corticosteroids are excreted in human milk, caution should be exercised when Beconase Inhalation Aerosol or Beconase AQ Nasal Spray is administered to a nursing woman.

Pediatric Use: Safety and effectiveness in children below 6 years of age have not been established.

ADVERSE REACTIONS

In general, side effects in clinical studies with both preparations have been primarily associated with irritation of the nasal mucous membranes.

Beconase® (beclomethasone dipropionate) Inhalation Aerosol: Adverse reactions reported in controlled clinical trials and long-term open studies in patients treated with Beconase Inhalation Aerosol are described below.

Sensations of irritation and burning in the nose (11 per 100 patients) following the use of Beconase Inhalation Aerosol have been reported. Also, occasional sneezing attacks (10 per 100 adult patients) have occurred immediately following the use of the intranasal inhaler. This symptom may be more common in children. Rhinorrhea may occur occasionally (1 per 100 patients).

Localized infections of the nose and pharynx with *Candida albicans* have occurred rarely (see PRECAUTIONS).

Transient episodes of epistaxis have been reported in 2 per 100 patients.

Rare cases of ulceration of the nasal mucosa and instances of nasal septum perforation have been spontaneously reported (see PRECAUTIONS).

Reports of headache, light-headedness, dryness and irritation of the nose and throat, and unpleasant taste and smell have been received. There are rare reports of loss of taste and smell.

Rare instances of wheezing, cataracts, glaucoma, and increased intraocular pressure have been reported following the use of intranasal beclomethasone dipropionate (see PRECAUTIONS).

Rare cases of immediate and delayed hypersensitivity reactions, including urticaria, angioedema, rash, and bronchospasm, have been reported following the oral and intranasal inhalation and administration of beclomethasone.

Systemic corticosteroid side effects were not reported during the controlled clinical trials. If recommended doses are exceeded, however, or if individuals are particularly sensitive, symptoms of hypercorticism, i.e., Cushing's syndrome, could occur.

Beconase AQ® (beclomethasone dipropionate, monohydrate) Nasal Spray: Rare cases of immediate and delayed hypersensitivity reactions, including urticaria, angioedema, rash, and bronchospasm, have been reported following the oral and intranasal inhalation of beclomethasone dipropionate.

Adverse reactions reported in controlled clinical trials and open studies in patients treated with Beconase AQ Nasal Spray are described below.

Mild nasopharyngeal irritation following the use of beclomethasone aqueous nasal spray has been reported in up to 24% of patients treated, including occasional sneezing attacks (about 4%) occurring immediately following use of the spray. In patients experiencing these symptoms, none had to discontinue treatment. The incidence of transient irritation and sneezing was approximately the same in the group of patients who received placebo in these studies, implying that these complaints may be related to vehicle components of the formulation.

Fewer than 5 per 100 patients reported headache, nausea, or light-headedness following the use of Beconase AQ Nasal Spray. Fewer than 3 per 100 patients reported nasal stuffiness, nosebleeds, rhinorrhea, or tearing eyes.

Rare cases of ulceration of the nasal mucosa and instances of nasal septum perforation have been spontaneously reported (see PRECAUTIONS).

Rare instances of wheezing, cataracts, glaucoma, and increased intraocular pressure have been reported following the use of intranasal beclomethasone dipropionate (see PRECAUTIONS).

OVERDOSAGE

When used at excessive doses, systemic corticosteroid effects such as hypercorticism and adrenal suppression may appear. If such changes occur, Beconase® (beclomethasone dipropionate) Inhalation Aerosol and Beconase AQ® (beclomethasone dipropionate, monohydrate) Nasal Spray should be discontinued slowly consistent with accepted procedures for discontinuing oral steroid therapy. The oral LD_{50} of beclomethasone dipropionate is greater than 1 g/kg in rodents. One canister of Beconase Inhalation Aerosol contains 8.4 mg of beclomethasone dipropionate, and one bottle of Beconase AQ

Nasal Spray contains beclomethasone dipropionate, monohydrate equivalent to 10.5 mg of beclomethasone dipropionate; therefore, acute overdosage is unlikely.

DOSAGE AND ADMINISTRATION

Beconase® (beclomethasone dipropionate) Inhalation Aerosol: *Adults and Children 12 Years of Age and Older:* The usual dosage is one inhalation (42 mcg) in each nostril two to four times a day (total dose, 168 to 336 mcg per day). Patients can often be maintained on a maximum dose of one inhalation in each nostril three times a day (252 mcg per day). *Children 6 to 12 Years of Age:* The usual dosage is one inhalation in each nostril three times a day (252 mcg per day). Beconase Inhalation Aerosol is *not* recommended for children below 6 years of age since safety and efficacy studies have not been conducted in this age-group.

CONTENTS UNDER PRESSURE: Do not puncture. Do not use or store near heat or open flame. Exposure to temperatures above 120°F may cause bursting. Never throw container into fire or incinerator. Keep out of reach of children.

Beconase AQ® (beclomethasone dipropionate, monohydrate) Nasal Spray: *Adults and Children 6 Years of Age and Older:* The usual dosage is one or two inhalations (42 to 84 mcg) in each nostril twice a day (total dose, 168 to 336 mcg per day).

Beconase AQ Nasal Spray is *not* recommended for children below 6 years of age.

In patients who respond to Beconase Inhalation Aerosol and to Beconase AQ Nasal Spray, an improvement of the symptoms of seasonal or perennial rhinitis usually becomes apparent within a few days after the start of therapy. However, symptomatic relief may not occur in some patients for as long as 2 weeks. Beconase Inhalation Aerosol and Beconase AQ Nasal Spray should not be continued beyond 3 weeks in the absence of significant symptomatic improvement.

The therapeutic effects of corticosteroids, unlike those of decongestants, are not immediate. This should be explained to the patient in advance in order to ensure cooperation and continuation of treatment with the prescribed dosage regimen.

In the presence of excessive nasal mucous secretion or edema of the nasal mucosa, the drug may fail to reach the site of intended action. In such cases it is advisable to use a nasal vasoconstrictor during the first 2 to 3 days of Beconase Inhalation Aerosol or Beconase AQ Nasal Spray therapy.

Directions for Use: Illustrated Patient's Instructions for Use accompany each package of Beconase Inhalation Aerosol and Beconase AQ Nasal Spray.

HOW SUPPLIED

Beconase® (beclomethasone dipropionate) Inhalation Aerosol is supplied in a 6.7-g canister containing 80 metered doses (NDC 0173-0468-00) and in a 16.8-g canister containing 200 metered doses (NDC 0173-0336-02), each with beige compact actuator and patient's instructions. **Store between 2° and 30°C (36° and 86°F). As with most inhaled medications in aerosol canisters, the therapeutic effect of this medication may decrease when the canister is cold. Shake well before using.**

Beconase AQ® (beclomethasone dipropionate, monohydrate) Nasal Spray, 0.042%* is supplied in an amber glass bottle fitted with a metering atomizing pump and nasal adapter in a box of one (NDC 0173-0388-79) with patient's instructions for use. Each bottle contains 25 g of suspension. **Store between 15° and 30°C (59° and 86°F).**

*Calculated on the dried basis.

October 1995   RL-215/216
Shown in Product Identification Guide, page 312

CEFTIN® Tablets   ℞
[sef'tin]
(cefuroxime axetil tablets)

CEFTIN® for Oral Suspension   ℞
(cefuroxime axetil powder for oral suspension)

DESCRIPTION

CEFTIN Tablets and CEFTIN for Oral Suspension contain cefuroxime as cefuroxime axetil. CEFTIN is a semisynthetic, broad-spectrum cephalosporin antibiotic for oral administration.

Chemically, cefuroxime axetil, the 1-(acetyloxy) ethyl ester of cefuroxime, is (RS)-1-hydroxyethyl $(6R,7R)$-7-[2-(2-furyl)glyoxylamido]-3-(hydroxymethyl)-8-oxo-5-thia-1-azabicyclo[4.2.0]oct-2-ene-2-carboxylate, 7^2-(Z)-(O-methyl-oxime), 1-acetate 3-carbamate. Its molecular formula is $C_{20}H_{22}N_4O_{10}S$, and it has a molecular weight of 510.48. Cefuroxime axetil is in the amorphous form.

CEFTIN Tablets are film-coated and contain the equivalent of 125, 250, or 500 mg of cefuroxime as cefuroxime axetil. CEFTIN Tablets contain the inactive ingredients colloidal silicon dioxide, croscarmellose sodium, FD&C Blue No. 1 (250- and 500-mg tablets only), hydrogenated vegetable oil,

---

Postprandial Pharmacokinetics of Cefuroxime Administered as CEFTIN Tablets to Adults*

Dose† (Cefuroxime Equivalent)	Peak Plasma Concentration (mcg/mL)	Time of Peak Plasma Concentration (h)	Mean Elimination Half-Life (h)	A.U.C. (mcg-h mL)
125 mg	2.1	2.2	1.2	6.7
250 mg	4.1	2.5	1.2	12.9
500 mg	7.0	3.0	1.2	27.4
1,000 mg	13.6	2.5	1.3	50.0

* Mean values of 12 healthy adult volunteers.
† Drug administered immediately after a meal.

Postprandial Pharmacokinetics of Cefuroxime Administered as CEFTIN for Oral Suspension to Pediatric Patients*

Dose† (Cefuroxime Equivalent)	n	Peak Plasma Concentration (mcg/mL)	Time of Peak Plasma Concentration (h)	Mean Elimination Half-Life (h)	A.U.C. (mcg-h mL)
10 mg/kg	8	3.3	3.6	1.4	12.4
15 mg/kg	12	5.1	2.7	1.9	22.5
20 mg/kg	8	7.0	3.1	1.9	32.8

* Mean age = 23 months.
† Drug administered with milk or milk products.

hydroxypropyl methylcellulose, methylparaben, microcrystalline cellulose, propylene glycol, propylparaben, sodium benzoate (125-mg tablets only), sodium lauryl sulfate, and titanium dioxide.

CEFTIN for Oral Suspension, when reconstituted with water, provides the equivalent of 125 mg of cefuroxime (as cefuroxime axetil) per 5 mL of suspension. CEFTIN for Oral Suspension contains the inactive ingredients povidone K30, stearic acid, sucrose, and tutti-fruitti flavoring.

CLINICAL PHARMACOLOGY

Absorption and Metabolism: After oral administration, cefuroxime axetil is absorbed from the gastrointestinal tract and rapidly hydrolyzed by nonspecific esterases in the intestinal mucosa and blood to cefuroxime. Cefuroxime is subsequently distributed throughout the extracellular fluids. The axetil moiety is metabolized to acetaldehyde and acetic acid.

Serum Pharmacokinetics: Serum cefuroxime pharmacokinetic parameters for CEFTIN Tablets and CEFTIN for Oral Suspension are shown in the tables below.
[See tables above.]

Approximately 50% of serum cefuroxime is bound to protein.

Comparative Pharmacokinetic Properties: CEFTIN for Oral Suspension was not bioequivalent to CEFTIN Tablets when tested in healthy adults. The tablet and powder for oral suspension formulations are NOT substitutable on a mg/mg basis. The area under the curve for the suspension averaged 91% of that for the tablet, and the peak plasma concentration for the suspension averaged 71% of the peak plasma concentration of the tablets. Therefore, the safety and effectiveness of both the tablet and oral suspension formulations had to be established in separate clinical trials.

Food Effect on Pharmacokinetics: Absorption of the tablet is greater when taken after food (absolute bioavailability of CEFTIN Tablets increases from 37% to 52%). Despite this difference in absorption, the clinical and bacteriologic responses of patients were independent of food intake at the time of tablet administration in two studies where this was assessed.

All pharmacokinetic and clinical effectiveness and safety studies in pediatric patients using the suspension formulation were conducted in the fed state. No data are available on the absorption kinetics of the suspension formulation when administered to fasted pediatric patients.

Renal Excretion: Cefuroxime is excreted unchanged in the urine; in adults, approximately 50% of the administered dose is recovered in the urine within 12 hours. The pharmacokinetics of cefuroxime in the urine of pediatric patients have not been studied at this time. Until further data are available, the renal pharmacokinetic properties of cefuroxime axetil established in adults should not be extrapolated to pediatric patients.

Because cefuroxime is renally excreted, the serum half-life is prolonged in patients with reduced renal function. In a study of 20 elderly patients (mean age = 83.9 years) having a mean creatinine clearance of 34.9 mL/min, the mean serum elimination half-life was 3.5 hours. Despite the lower elimination of cefuroxime in geriatric patients, dosage adjustment based on age is not necessary (see PRECAUTIONS: Geriatric Use).

Microbiology: The *in vivo* bactericidal activity of cefuroxime axetil is due to cefuroxime's binding to essential target proteins and the resultant inhibition of cell-wall synthesis.

Cefuroxime has bactericidal activity against a wide range of common pathogens, including many beta-lactamase–producing strains. Cefuroxime is stable to many bacterial beta-lactamases, especially plasmid-mediated enzymes that are commonly found in enterobacteriaceae.

Cefuroxime has been demonstrated to be active against most strains of the following microorganisms both *in vitro* and in clinical infections as described in the INDICATIONS AND USAGE section (see INDICATIONS AND USAGE section).

Aerobic Gram-positive Microorganisms:
Staphylococcus aureus (including beta-lactamase–producing strains)
Streptococcus pneumoniae
Streptococcus pyogenes
Aerobic Gram-negative Microorganisms:
Escherichia coli
Haemophilus influenzae (including beta-lactamase–producing strains)
Haemophilus parainfluenzae
Klebsiella pneumoniae
Moraxella catarrhalis (including beta-lactamase–producing strains)
Neisseria gonorrhoeae (beta-lactamase negative strains only)
Cefuroxime has been shown to be active *in vitro* against most strains of the following microorganisms; however, the clinical significance of these findings is unknown.

Cefuroxime exhibits *in vitro* minimum inhibitory concentrations (MICs) of 4.0 mcg/mL or less (systemic susceptible breakpoint) against most ($\geq 90\%$) strains of the following microorganisms; however, the safety and effectiveness of cefuroxime in treating clinical infections due to these microorganisms have not been established in adequate and well-controlled trials.

Aerobic Gram-positive Microorganisms:
Staphylococcus epidermidis
Staphylococcus saprophyticus
Streptococcus agalactiae
NOTE: Certain strains of enterococci, e.g., *Enterococcus faecalis* (formerly *Streptococcus faecalis*), are resistant to cefuroxime. Methicillin-resistant staphylococci are resistant to cefuroxime.

Aerobic Gram-negative Microorganisms:
Morganella morganii
Neisseria gonorrhoeae (beta-lactamase–producing strains only)
Proteus inconstans
Proteus mirabilis
Providencia rettgeri
NOTE: *Pseudomonas* spp., *Campylobacter* spp., *Acinetobacter calcoaceticus*, and most strains of *Serratia* spp. and *Proteus vulgaris* are resistant to most first- and second-generation cephalosporins. Some strains of *Morganella morganii*, *Enterobacter cloacae*, and *Citrobacter* spp. have been shown by *in vitro* tests to be resistant to cefuroxime and other cephalosporins.

Anaerobic Microorganisms:
Peptococcus niger
NOTE: Most strains of *Clostridium difficile* and *Bacteroides fragilis* are resistant to cefuroxime.

Susceptibility Tests: *Dilution Techniques:* Quantitative methods that are used to determine MICs provide reproducible estimates of the susceptibility of bacteria to antimicro-

Continued on next page

Glaxo Wellcome—Cont.

bial compounds. One such standardized procedure uses a standardized dilution method[1] (broth, agar, or microdilution) or equivalent with cefuroxime powder. The MIC values obtained should be interpreted according to the following criteria:

MIC (mcg/mL)	Interpretation
≤4	(S) Susceptible
8–16	(I) Intermediate
≥32	(R) Resistant

A report of "Susceptible" indicates that the pathogen, if in the blood, is likely to be inhibited by usually achievable concentrations of the antimicrobial compound in blood. A report of "Intermediate" indicates that inhibitory concentrations of the antibiotic may be achieved if high dosage is used or if the infection is confined to tissues or fluids in which high antibiotic concentrations are attained. This category also provides a buffer zone that prevents small, uncontrolled technical factors from causing major discrepancies in interpretation. A report of "Resistant" indicates that usually achievable concentrations of the antimicrobial compound in the blood are unlikely to be inhibitory and that other therapy should be selected.

Standardized susceptibility test procedures require the use of laboratory control microorganisms. Standard cefuroxime powder should give the following MIC values:

Microorganism	MIC (mcg/mL)
Escherichia coli ATCC 25922	2–8
Staphylococcus aureus ATCC 29213	0.5–2

Diffusion Techniques: Quantitative methods that require measurement of zone diameters provide estimates of the susceptibility of bacteria to antimicrobial compounds. One such standardized procedure[2] that has been recommended (for use with disks) to test the susceptibility of microorganisms to cefuroxime uses the 30-mcg cefuroxime disk. Interpretation involves correlation of the diameter obtained in the disk test with the MIC for cefuroxime.

Reports from the laboratory providing results of the standard single-disk susceptibility test with a 30-mcg cefuroxime disk should be interpreted according to the following criteria:

Zone Diameter (mm)	Interpretation
≥23	(S) Susceptible
15–22	(I) Intermediate
≤14	(R) Resistant

Interpretation should be as stated above for results using dilution techniques.

As with standard dilution techniques, diffusion methods require the use of laboratory control microorganisms. The 30-mcg cefuroxime disk provides the following zone diameters in these laboratory test quality control strains:

Microorganism	Zone Diameter (mm)
Escherichia coli ATCC 25922	20–26
Staphylococcus aureus ATCC 25923	27–35

INDICATIONS AND USAGE

NOTE: CEFTIN TABLETS AND CEFTIN FOR ORAL SUSPENSION ARE NOT BIOEQUIVALENT AND ARE NOT SUBSTITUTABLE ON A MG/MG BASIS (SEE CLINICAL PHARMACOLOGY).

CEFTIN Tablets: CEFTIN Tablets are indicated for the treatment of patients with mild to moderate infections caused by susceptible strains of the designated microorganisms in the conditions listed below:

1. **Pharyngitis/Tonsillitis** caused by *Streptococcus pyogenes*.
   NOTE: The usual drug of choice in the treatment and prevention of streptococcal infections, including the prophylaxis of rheumatic fever, is penicillin given by the intramuscular route. CEFTIN Tablets are generally effective in the eradication of streptococci from the nasopharynx; however, substantial data establishing the efficacy of cefuroxime in the subsequent prevention of rheumatic fever are not available. Please also note that in all clinical trials, all isolates had to be sensitive to both penicillin and cefuroxime. There are no data from adequate and well-controlled trials to demonstrate the effectiveness of cefuroxime in the treatment of penicillin-resistant strains of *Streptococcus pyogenes*.

2. **Acute Bacterial Otitis Media** caused by *Streptococcus pneumoniae*, *Haemophilus influenzae* (including beta-lactamase–producing strains), *Moraxella catarrhalis* (including beta-lactamase–producing strains), or *Streptococcus pyogenes*.

3. **Acute Bacterial Maxillary Sinusitis** caused by *Streptococcus pneumoniae* or *Haemophilus influenzae* (non-beta-lactamase–producing strains only). (See CLINICAL STUDIES section.)
   NOTE: In view of the insufficient numbers of isolates of beta-lactamase–producing strains of *Haemophilus influenzae* and *Moraxella catarrhalis* that were obtained from clinical trials with CEFTIN Tablets for patients with acute bacterial maxillary sinusitis, it was not possible to adequately evaluate the effectiveness of CEFTIN Tablets for sinus infections known, suspected, or considered potentially to be caused by beta-lactamase–producing *Haemophilus influenzae* or *Moraxella catarrhalis*.

4. **Acute Bacterial Exacerbations of Chronic Bronchitis and Secondary Bacterial Infections of Acute Bronchitis** caused by *Streptococcus pneumoniae*, *Haemophilus influenzae* (beta-lactamase negative strains), or *Haemophilus parainfluenzae* (beta-lactamase negative strains).

5. **Uncomplicated Skin and Skin-Structure Infections** caused by *Staphylococcus aureus* (including beta-lactamase–producing strains) or *Streptococcus pyogenes*.

6. **Uncomplicated Urinary Tract Infections** caused by *Escherichia coli* or *Klebsiella pneumoniae*.

7. **Uncomplicated Gonorrhea** (urethral and endocervical) caused by non-penicillinase–producing strains of *Neisseria gonorrhoeae*.

CEFTIN for Oral Suspension: CEFTIN for Oral Suspension is indicated for the treatment of pediatric patients 3 months to 12 years of age with mild to moderate infections caused by susceptible strains of the designated microorganisms in the conditions listed below. The safety and effectiveness of CEFTIN for Oral Suspension in the treatment of infections other than those specifically listed below have not been established either by adequate and well-controlled trials or by pharmacokinetic data with which to determine an effective and safe dosing regimen.

1. **Pharyngitis/Tonsillitis** caused by *Streptococcus pyogenes*.
   NOTE: The usual drug of choice in the treatment and prevention of streptococcal infections, including the prophylaxis of rheumatic fever, is penicillin given by the intramuscular route. CEFTIN for Oral Suspension is generally effective in the eradication of streptococci from the nasopharynx; however, substantial data establishing the efficacy of cefuroxime in the subsequent prevention of rheumatic fever are not available. Please also note that in all clinical trials, all isolates had to be sensitive to both penicillin and cefuroxime. There are no data from adequate and well-controlled trials to demonstrate the effectiveness of cefuroxime in the treatment of penicillin-resistant strains of *Streptococcus pyogenes*.

2. **Acute Bacterial Otitis Media** caused by *Streptococcus pneumoniae*, *Haemophilus influenzae* (including beta-lactamase–producing strains), *Moraxella catarrhalis* (including beta-lactamase–producing strains), or *Streptococcus pyogenes*.

3. **Impetigo** caused by *Staphylococcus aureus* (including beta-lactamase–producing strains) or *Streptococcus pyogenes*.

Culture and susceptibility testing should be performed when appropriate to determine susceptibility of the causative microorganism(s) to cefuroxime. Therapy may be started while awaiting the results of this testing. Antimicrobial therapy should be appropriately adjusted according to the results of such testing.

CONTRAINDICATIONS

CEFTIN products are contraindicated in patients with known allergy to the cephalosporin group of antibiotics.

WARNINGS

CEFTIN TABLETS AND CEFTIN FOR ORAL SUSPENSION ARE NOT BIOEQUIVALENT AND ARE THEREFORE NOT SUBSTITUTABLE ON A MG/MG BASIS (SEE CLINICAL PHARMACOLOGY).

BEFORE THERAPY WITH CEFTIN PRODUCTS IS INSTITUTED, CAREFUL INQUIRY SHOULD BE MADE TO DETERMINE WHETHER THE PATIENT HAS HAD PREVIOUS HYPERSENSITIVITY REACTIONS TO CEFTIN PRODUCTS, OTHER CEPHALOSPORINS, PENICILLINS, OR OTHER DRUGS. IF THIS PRODUCT IS TO BE GIVEN TO PENICILLIN-SENSITIVE PATIENTS, CAUTION SHOULD BE EXERCISED BECAUSE CROSS-HYPERSENSITIVITY AMONG BETA-LACTAM ANTIBIOTICS HAS BEEN CLEARLY DOCUMENTED AND MAY OCCUR IN UP TO 10% OF PATIENTS WITH A HISTORY OF PENICILLIN ALLERGY. IF A CLINICALLY SIGNIFICANT ALLERGIC REACTION TO CEFTIN PRODUCTS OCCURS, DISCONTINUE THE DRUG AND INSTITUTE APPROPRIATE THERAPY. SERIOUS ACUTE HYPERSENSITIVITY REACTIONS MAY REQUIRE TREATMENT WITH EPINEPHRINE AND OTHER EMERGENCY MEASURES, INCLUDING OXYGEN, INTRAVENOUS FLUIDS, INTRAVENOUS ANTIHISTAMINES, CORTICOSTEROIDS, PRESSOR AMINES, AND AIRWAY MANAGEMENT, AS CLINICALLY INDICATED.

Pseudomembranous colitis has been reported with nearly all antibacterial agents, including cefuroxime, and may range from mild to life threatening. Therefore, it is important to consider this diagnosis in patients who present with diarrhea subsequent to the administration of antibacterial agents.

Treatment with antibacterial agents alters normal flora of the colon and may permit overgrowth of clostridia. Studies indicate that a toxin produced by *Clostridium difficile* is one primary cause of antibiotic-associated colitis.

After the diagnosis of pseudomembranous colitis has been established, appropriate therapeutic measures should be initiated. Mild cases of pseudomembranous colitis usually respond to drug discontinuation alone. In moderate to severe cases, consideration should be given to management with fluids and electrolytes, protein supplementation, and treatment with an antibacterial drug effective against *Clostridium difficile*.

PRECAUTIONS

General: As with other broad-spectrum antibiotics, prolonged administration of cefuroxime axetil may result in overgrowth of nonsusceptible microorganisms. If superinfection occurs during therapy, appropriate measures should be taken.

Cephalosporins, including cefuroxime axetil, should be given with caution to patients receiving concurrent treatment with potent diuretics because these diuretics are suspected of adversely affecting renal function.

Cefuroxime axetil, as with other broad-spectrum antibiotics, should be prescribed with caution in individuals with a history of colitis. The safety and effectiveness of cefuroxime axetil have not been established in patients with gastrointestinal malabsorption. Patients with gastrointestinal malabsorption were excluded from participating in clinial trials of cefuroxime axetil.

Information for Patients/Caregivers (Pediatric): 1. During clinical trials, the tablet was tolerated by pediatric patients old enough to swallow the cefuroxime axetil tablet whole. The crushed tablet has a strong, persistent, bitter taste and should not be administered to pediatric patients in this manner. Pediatric patients who cannot swallow the tablet whole should receive the oral suspension.

2. Discontinuation of therapy due to taste and/or problems of administering this drug occurred in 1.4% of pediatric patients given the oral suspension. Complaints about taste (which may impair compliance) occurred in 5% of pediatric patients.

Drug/Laboratory Test Interactions: A false-positive reaction for glucose in the urine may occur with copper reduction tests (Benedict's or Fehling's solution or with CLINITEST® tablets), but not with enzyme-based tests for glycosuria (e.g., CLINISTIX®, TES-TAPE®). As a false-negative result may occur in the ferricyanide test, it is recommended that either the glucose oxidase or hexokinase method be used to determine blood/plasma glucose levels in patients receiving cefuroxime axetil. The presence of cefuroxime does not interfere with the assay of serum and urine creatinine by the alkaline picrate method.

Drug/Drug Interactions: Concomitant administration of probenecid with cefuroxime axetil tablets increases the area under the serum concentration versus time curve by 50%. The peak serum cefuroxime concentration after a 1.5-g single dose is greater when taken with 1 g of probenecid (mean = 14.8 mcg/mL) than without probenecid (mean = 12.2 mcg/mL).

Drugs that reduce gastric acidity may result in a lower bioavailability of CEFTIN compared with that of fasting state and tend to cancel the effect of postprandial absorption.

Carcinogenesis, Mutagenesis, Impairment of Fertility: Although lifetime studies in animals have not been performed to evaluate carcinogenic potential, no mutagenic potential was found for cefuroxime axetil in the micronucleus test and a battery of bacterial mutation tests. Reproduction studies in rats at doses up to 1,000 mg/kg per day (nine times the recommended maximum human dose based on mg/m^2) have revealed no evidence of impaired fertility.

Pregnancy: *Teratogenic Effects: Pregnancy Category B:* Reproduction studies have been performed in rats and mice at doses up to 3,200 mg/kg per day (23 times the recommended maximum human dose based on mg/m^2) and have revealed no evidence of harm to the fetus due to cefuroxime axetil. There are, however, no adequate and well-controlled studies in pregnant women. Because animal reproduction studies are not always predictive of human response, this drug should be used during pregnancy only if clearly needed.

Labor and Delivery: Cefuroxime axetil has not been studied for use during labor and delivery.

Nursing Mothers: Because cefuroxime is excreted in human milk, consideration should be given to discontinuing nursing temporarily during treatment with cefuroxime axetil.

Pediatric Use: In controlled clinical trials, cefuroxime axetil has been administered to pediatric patients ranging in age from 3 months to 12 years (see INDICATIONS AND USAGE and DOSAGE AND ADMINISTRATION sections).

Geriatric Use: In clinical trials when 12- to 64-year-old patients and geriatric patients (65 years of age or older) were treated with usual recommended dosages (i.e., 125 to 500 mg b.i.d., depending on type of infections), no overall differences

CEFTIN Tablets
(May be administered without regard to meals.)

Population/Infection	Dosage	Duration (days)
Adolescents and Adults (13 years and older)		
Pharyngitis/tonsillitis	250 mg b.i.d.	10
Acute bacterial maxillary sinusitis	250 mg b.i.d.	10
Acute bacterial exacerbations of chronic bronchitis and secondary bacterial infections of acute bronchitis	250 or 500 mg b.i.d.	10
Uncomplicated skin and skin-structure infections	250 or 500 mg b.i.d.	10
Uncomplicated urinary tract infections	125 or 250 mg b.i.d.	7–10
Uncomplicated gonorrhea	1,000 mg once	single dose
Children (who can swallow tablets whole)		
Pharyngitis/tonsillitis	125 mg b.i.d.	10
Acute otitis media	250 mg b.i.d.	10

in effectiveness were observed between the two age-groups. The geriatric patients reported somewhat fewer gastrointestinal events and less frequent vaginal candidiasis compared with patients aged 12 to 64 years old; however, no clinically significant differences were reported between the two age-groups. Therefore, no adjustment of the usual adult dose is necessary based on age alone.

ADVERSE REACTIONS

CEFTIN TABLETS (MULTIPLE-DOSE DOSING REGIMENS): *In Clinical Trials:* In clinical trials using multiple doses of cefuroxime axetil tablets, 912 patients were treated with the recommended dosages of cefuroxime axetil (125 to 500 mg twice a day). There were no deaths or permanent disabilities thought related to drug toxicity. Twenty (2.2%) patients discontinued medication due to adverse events thought by the investigators to be possibly, probably, or almost certainly related to drug toxicity. Seventeen (85%) of the 20 patients who discontinued therapy did so because of gastrointestinal disturbances, including diarrhea, nausea, vomiting, and abdominal pain. The percentage of cefuroxime axetil tablet-treated patients who discontinued study drug because of adverse events was very similar at daily doses of 1,000, 500, and 250 mg (2.3%, 2.1%, and 2.2%, respectively). However, the incidence of gastrointestinal adverse events increased with the higher recommended doses.

The following adverse events were thought by the investigators to be possibly, probably, or almost certainly related to cefuroxime axetil tablets in multiple-dose clinical trials (n = 912 cefuroxime axetil-treated patients).

Adverse Reactions
CEFTIN Tablets
Multiple-Dose Dosing Regimens—
Clinical Trials

Incidence ≥1%	Diarrhea/loose stools	3.7%
	Nausea/vomiting	3.0%
	Transient elevation in AST	2.0%
	Transient elevation in ALT	1.6%
	Eosinophilia	1.1%
	Transient elevation in LDH	1.0%
Incidence <1% but >0.1%	Abdominal pain	
	Abdominal cramps	
	Flatulence	
	Indigestion	
	Headache	
	Vaginitis	
	Vulvar itch	
	Rash	
	Hives	
	Itch	
	Dysuria	
	Chills	
	Chest Pain	
	Shortness of breath	
	Mouth ulcers	
	Swollen tongue	
	Sleepiness	
	Thirst	
	Anorexia	
	Positive Coombs' test	

In Postmarketing Experience: In addition to the events reported during clinical trials with CEFTIN Tablets, the following adverse experiences have been reported from domestic and foreign sources during worldwide postmarketing surveillance: hypersensitivity reactions, including Stevens-Johnson syndrome, erythema multiforme, toxic epidermal necrolysis, serum sickness–like reactions, anaphylaxis, and angioedema. Jaundice has been reported very rarely. Onset of pseudomembranous colitis symptoms may occur during or after treatment (see WARNINGS).

CEFTIN TABLETS (SINGLE-DOSE REGIMEN FOR UNCOMPLICATED GONORRHEA: *In Clinical Trials:* In clinical trials using a single dose of cefuroxime axetil tablets, 644 patients were treated with the recommended dosage of cefuroxime axetil (1,000 mg) for the treatment of uncomplicated gonorrhea. There were no deaths or permanent disabilities thought related to drug toxicity in these studies.

The following adverse events were thought by the investigators to be possibly, probably, or almost certainly related to cefuroxime axetil in 1,000-mg single-dose clinical trials of cefuroxime axetil tablets in the treatment of uncomplicated gonorrhea conducted in the US.

Adverse Reactions
CEFTIN Tablets
1-g Single-Dose Regimen for Uncomplicated
Gonorrhea—Clinical Trials

Incidence ≥1%	Nausea/vomiting	6.7%
	Diarrhea	4.7%
Incidence <1% but >0.1%	Abdominal pain	
	Dyspepsia	
	Erythema	
	Rash	
	Pruritus	
	Vaginal candidiasis	
	Vaginal itch	
	Vaginal discharge	
	Headache	
	Dizziness	
	Somnolence	
	Muscle cramps	
	Muscle stiffness	
	Muscle spasm of neck	
	Tightness/pain in chest	
	Bleeding/pain in urethra	
	Kidney pain	
	Tachycardia	
	Lockjaw-type reaction	

CEFTIN FOR ORAL SUSPENSION (MULTIPLE-DOSE DOSING REGIMENS): *In Clinical Trials:* In clinical trials using multiple doses of cefuroxime axetil powder for oral suspension, pediatric patients (96.7% of whom were younger than 12 years of age) were treated with the recommended dosages of cefuroxime axetil (20 to 30 mg/kg per day divided twice a day up to a maximum dose of 500 or 1,000 mg/day, respectively). There were no deaths or permanent disabilities in any of the patients in these studies. Eleven US patients (1.2%) discontinued medication due to adverse events thought by the investigators to be possibly, probably, or almost certainly related to drug toxicity. The discontinuations were primarily for gastrointestinal disturbances, usually diarrhea or vomiting. During clinical trials, discontinuation of therapy due to the taste and/or problems with administering this drug occurred in 13 (1.4%) pediatric patients enrolled at centers in the US.

The following adverse events were thought by the investigators to be possibly, probably, or almost certainly related to cefuroxime axetil for oral suspension in multiple-dose clinical trials (n = 931 cefuroxime axetil-treated US patients).

Adverse Reactions
CEFTIN for Oral Suspension
Multiple-Dose Dosing Regimens—
Clinical Trials

Incidence ≥1%	Diarrhea/loose stools	8.6%
	Dislike of taste	5.0%
	Diaper rash	3.4%
	Nausea/vomiting	2.6%
Incidence <1% but >0.1%	Abdominal pain	
	Flatulence	
	Gastrointestinal infection	
	Candidiasis	
	Vaginal irritation	
	Rash	
	Hyperactivity	
	Irritable behavior	
	Eosinophilia	
	Positive direct Coombs' test	
	Elevated liver enzymes	
	Viral illness	
	Upper respiratory infection	
	Sinusitis	
	Cough	
	Urinary tract infection	
	Joint swelling	
	Arthralgia	
	Fever	
	Ptyalism	

In Postmarketing Experience: In addition to the events reported during clinical trials with CEFTIN for Oral Suspension, the following adverse experiences have been reported in postmarketing surveillance: hypersensitivity reactions (including rash, pruritus, urticaria, and anaphylaxis).

CEPHALOSPORIN-CLASS ADVERSE REACTIONS: In addition to the adverse reactions listed above that have been observed in patients treated with cefuroxime axetil, the following adverse reactions and altered laboratory tests have been reported for cephalosporin-class antibiotics: renal dysfunction, toxic nephropathy, hepatic cholestasis, aplastic anemia, hemolytic anemia, hemorrhage, increased prothrombin time, increased BUN, increased creatinine, false-positive test for urinary glucose, increased alkaline phosphatase, neutropenia, thrombocytopenia, leukopenia, elevated bilirubin, pancytopenia, and agranulocytosis.

Several cephalosporins have been implicated in triggering seizures, particularly in patients with renal impairment when the dosage was not reduced (see DOSAGE AND ADMINISTRATION and OVERDOSAGE). If seizures associated with drug therapy occur, the drug should be discontinued. Anticonvulsant therapy can be given if clinically indicated.

OVERDOSAGE

Overdosage of cephalosporins can cause cerebral irritation leading to convulsions. Serum levels of cefuroxime can be reduced by hemodialysis and peritoneal dialysis.

DOSAGE AND ADMINISTRATION

NOTE: CEFTIN TABLETS AND CEFTIN FOR ORAL SUSPENSION ARE NOT BIOEQUIVALENT AND ARE NOT SUBSTITUTABLE ON A MG/MG BASIS (SEE CLINICAL PHARMACOLOGY).

[See table above at top left.]

CEFTIN for Oral Suspension: CEFTIN for Oral Suspension may be administered to infants and children ranging in age from 3 months to 12 years, according to dosages in the following table:

[See table at top of next page.]

Patients With Renal Failure: The safety and efficacy of cefuroxime axetil in patients with renal failure have not been established. Since cefuroxime is renally eliminated, its half-life will be prolonged in patients with renal failure.

Directions for Mixing CEFTIN for Oral Suspension: Prepare a suspension at the time of dispensing as follows:
1. Shake the bottle to loosen the powder.
2. Remove the cap.
3. Add the total amount of water for reconstitution (see table below) and replace the cap.
4. Invert the bottle and vigorously rock the bottle from side to side so that water rises through the powder.
5. Once the sound of the powder against the bottle disappears, turn the bottle upright and vigorously shake it in a diagonal direction.

Bottle Size	Amount of Water Required for Reconstitution
50 mL	20 mL
100 mL	37 mL
200 mL	74 mL

Continued on next page

Glaxo Wellcome—Cont.

CEFTIN for Oral Suspension
(Must be administered with food. Shake well each time before using.)

Population/Infection	Dosage	Daily Maximum Dose	Duration (days)
Infants and children (3 months to 12 years)			
Pharyngitis/tonsillitis	20 mg/kg/day divided b.i.d.	500 mg	10
Acute otitis media	30 mg/kg/day divided b.i.d.	1,000 mg	10
Impetigo	30 mg/kg/day divided b.i.d.	1,000 mg	10

Each teaspoonful (5 mL) will contain the equivalent of 125 mg of cefuroxime as cefuroxime axetil.

NOTE: SHAKE THE ORAL SUSPENSION WELL BEFORE EACH USE. Replace cap securely after each opening. Reconstituted suspension should be stored between 2° and 25°C (36° and 77°F) (either in the refrigerator or at room temperature). DISCARD AFTER 10 DAYS.

HOW SUPPLIED

CEFTIN Tablets: CEFTIN Tablets, 125 mg of cefuroxime (as cefuroxime axetil), are white, capsule-shaped, film-coated tablets engraved with "395" on one side and "Glaxo" on the other side as follows:

20 Tablets/Bottle	NDC 0173-0395-00
60 Tablets/Bottle	NDC 0173-0395-01
Unit Dose Packs of 100	NDC 0173-0395-02

CEFTIN Tablets, 250 mg of cefuroxime (as cefuroxime axetil), are light blue, capsule-shaped, film-coated tablets engraved with "387" on one side and "Glaxo" on the other side as follows:

20 Tablets/Bottle	NDC 0173-0387-00
60 Tablets/Bottle	NDC 0173-0387-42
Unit Dose Packs of 100	NDC 0173-0387-01

CEFTIN Tablets, 500 mg of cefuroxime (as cefuroxime axetil), are dark blue, capsule-shaped, film-coated tablets engraved with "394" on one side and "Glaxo" on the other side as follows:

20 Tablets/Bottle	NDC 0173-0394-00
60 Tablets/Bottle	NDC 0173-0394-42
Unit Dose Packs of 50	NDC 0173-0394-01

Store the tablets between 15° and 30°C (59° and 86°F). Replace cap securely after each opening. Protect unit dose packs from excessive moisture.

CEFTIN for Oral Suspension: CEFTIN for Oral Suspension is provided as dry, white to pale yellow, tutti-frutti–flavored powder. When reconstituted as directed, CEFTIN for Oral Suspension provides the equivalent of 125 mg of cefuroxime (as cefuroxime axetil) per 5 mL of suspension. It is supplied in amber glass bottles as follows:

50-mL Suspension	NDC 0173-0406-01
100-mL Suspension	NDC 0173-0406-00
200-mL Suspension	NDC 0173-0406-04

Before reconstitution, store dry powder between 2° and 30°C (36° and 86°F).

After reconstitution, store suspension between 2° and 25°C (36° and 77°F), in a refrigerator or at room temperature. DISCARD AFTER 10 DAYS.

CLINICAL STUDIES

CEFTIN Tablets: ***Acute Bacterial Maxillary Sinusitis:*** One adequate and well-controlled study was performed in patients with acute bacterial maxillary sinusitis. In this study each patient had a maxillary sinus aspirate collected by sinus puncture before treatment was initiated for presumptive acute bacterial sinusitis. All patients had to have radiographic and clinical evidence of acute maxillary sinusitis. As shown in the following summary of the study, the general clinical effectiveness of CEFTIN Tablets was comparable to an oral antimicrobial agent that contained a specific beta-lactamase inhibitor in treating acute maxillary sinusitis. However, sufficient microbiology data were obtained to demonstrate the effectiveness of CEFTIN Tablets in treating acute maxillary sinusitis due only to *Streptococcus pneumoniae* or non-beta-lactamase–producing *Haemophilus influenzae.* An insufficient number of beta-lactamase–producing *Haemophilus influenzae* and *Moraxella catarrhalis* isolates were obtained in this trial to adequately evaluate the effectiveness of CEFTIN Tablets in the treatment of acute bacterial maxillary sinusitis due to these two organisms.

This study enrolled 317 adult patients, 132 patients in the United States and 185 patients in South America. Patients were randomized in a 1:1 ratio to cefuroxime axetil 250 mg b.i.d. or an oral microbial agent that contained a specific beta-lactamase inhibitor. An intent-to-treat analysis of the submitted clinical data yielded the following results:

Clinical Effectiveness of CEFTIN Tablets Compared to Beta-Lactamase Inhibitor-Containing Control Drug in the Treatment of Acute Bacterial Maxillary Sinusitis

	U.S. Patients*		South American Patients†	
	CEFTIN n=49	Control n=43	CEFTIN n=87	Control n=89
Clinical success (cure + improvement)	65%	53%	77%	74%
Clinical cure	53%	44%	72%	64%
Clinical improvement	12%	9%	5%	10%

* 95% Confidence interval around the success difference [−0.08, +0.32].

† 95% Confidence interval around the success difference [−0.10, +0.16].

In this trial and in a supporting maxillary puncture trial, 15 evaluable patients had non-beta-lactamase–producing *Haemophilus influenzae* as the identified pathogen. Ten (10) of these 15 patients (67%) had their pathogen (non-beta-lactamase–producing *Haemophilus influenzae*) eradicated. Eighteen (18) evaluable patients had *Streptococcus pneumoniae* as the identified pathogen. Fifteen (15) of these 18 patients (83%) had their pathogen (*Streptococcus pneumoniae*) eradicated.

Safety: The incidence of drug-related gastrointestinal adverse effects was statistically significantly higher in the control arm (an oral antimicrobial agent that contained a specific beta-lactamase inhibitor) versus the cefuroxime axetil arm (12% versus 1%, respectively; $p < 0.001$), particularly drug-related diarrhea (8% versus 1%, respectively; $p = 0.001$).

REFERENCES

1. National Committee for Clinical Laboratory Standards. *Methods for Dilution Antimicrobial Susceptibility Tests for Bacteria that Grow Aerobically.* 3rd ed. Approved Standard NCCLS Document M7-A3, Vol. 13, No. 25. Villanova, Pa: NCCLS; 1993.

2. National Committee for Clinical Laboratory Standards. *Performance Standards for Antimicrobial Disk Susceptibility Tests.* 4th ed. Approved Standard NCCLS Document M2-A4, Vol. 10, No. 7. Villanova, Pa: NCCLS; 1990.

U.S. Patents 4,267,320; 4,562,181; 4,865,851; and 4,897,270.

March 1996/RL-294

Shown in Product Identification Guide, page 312

CEPTAZ® ℞
[*sĕp' tăz*]
(ceftazidime for injection)
L-arginine formulation
For Intravenous or Intramuscular Use

DESCRIPTION

Ceftazidime is a semisynthetic, broad-spectrum, beta-lactam antibiotic for parenteral administration. It is the pentahydrate of pyridinium, 1-[[7-[[(2-amino-4-thiazolyl)[(1-carboxy-1-methylethoxy) imino]acetyl] amino]-2-carboxy-8-oxo-5-thia -1- azabicyclo[4.2.0]oct-2-en-3-yl]methyl]-, hydroxide, inner salt, [6R-[6α,7β(Z)]].

The empirical formula is $C_{22}H_{32}N_6O_{12}S_2$, representing a molecular weight of 636.6.

CEPTAZ is a sterile, dry mixture of ceftazidime pentahydrate and L-arginine. The L-arginine is at a concentration of 349 mg/g of ceftazidime activity. CEPTAZ dissolves without the evolution of gas. The product contains no sodium ion. Solutions of CEPTAZ range in color from light yellow to amber, depending on the diluent and volume used. The pH of freshly constituted solutions usually ranges from 5 to 7.5.

CLINICAL PHARMACOLOGY

After intravenous (IV) administration of 500-mg and 1-g doses of ceftazidime over 5 minutes to normal adult male volunteers, mean peak serum concentrations of 45 and 90 mcg/mL, respectively, were achieved. After IV infusion of 500-mg, 1-g, and 2-g doses of ceftazidime over 20 to 30 minutes to normal adult male volunteers, mean peak serum concentrations of 42, 69, and 170 mcg/mL, respectively, were achieved. The average serum concentrations following IV infusion of 500-mg, 1-g, and 2-g doses to these volunteers over an 8-hour interval are given in Table 1.

Table 1

Ceftazidime IV Dose	Serum Concentrations (mcg/mL) 0.5 h	1 h	2 h	4 h	8 h
500 mg	42	25	12	6	2
1 g	60	39	23	11	3
2 g	129	75	42	13	5

The absorption and elimination of ceftazidime were directly proportional to the size of the dose. The half-life following IV administration was approximately 1.9 hours. Less than 10% of ceftazidime was protein bound. The degree of protein binding was independent of concentration. There was no evidence of accumulation of ceftazidime in the serum in individuals with normal renal function following multiple IV doses of 1 and 2 g every 8 hours for 10 days.

Following intramuscular (IM) administration of 500-mg and 1-g doses of ceftazidime to normal adult volunteers, the mean peak serum concentrations were 17 and 39 mcg/mL, respectively, at approximately 1 hour. Serum concentrations remained above 4 mcg/mL for 6 and 8 hours after the IM administration of 500-mg and 1-g doses, respectively. The half-life of ceftazidime in these volunteers was approximately 2 hours.

The presence of hepatic dysfunction had no effect on the pharmacokinetics of ceftazidime in individuals administered 2 g intravenously every 8 hours for 5 days. Therefore, a dosage adjustment from the normal recommended dosage is not required for patients with hepatic dysfunction, provided renal function is not impaired.

Approximately 80% to 90% of an IM or IV dose of ceftazidime is excreted unchanged by the kidneys over a 24-hour period. After the IV administration of single 500-mg or 1-g doses, approximately 50% of the dose appeared in the urine in the first 2 hours. An additional 20% was excreted between 2 and 4 hours after dosing, and approximately another 12% of the dose appeared in the urine between 4 and 8 hours later. The elimination of ceftazidime by the kidneys resulted in high therapeutic concentrations in the urine.

The mean renal clearance of ceftazidime was approximately 100 mL/min. The calculated plasma clearance of approximately 115 mL/min indicated nearly complete elimination of ceftazidime by the renal route. Administration of probenecid before dosing had no effect on the elimination kinetics of ceftazidime. This suggested that ceftazidime is eliminated by glomerular filtration and is not actively secreted by renal tubular mechanisms.

Since ceftazidime is eliminated almost solely by the kidneys, its serum half-life is significantly prolonged in patients with impaired renal function. Consequently, dosage adjustments in such patients as described in the DOSAGE AND ADMINISTRATION section are suggested.

Ceftazidime concentrations achieved in specific body tissues and fluids are depicted in Table 2.

[See table at top of next page.]

Microbiology: Ceftazidime is bactericidal in action, exerting its effect by inhibition of enzymes responsible for cell-wall synthesis. A wide range of gram-negative organisms is susceptible to ceftazidime *in vitro,* including strains resistant to gentamicin and other aminoglycosides. In addition, ceftazidime has been shown to be active against gram-positive organisms. It is highly stable to most clinically important beta-lactamases, plasmid or chromosomal, which are produced by both gram-negative and gram-positive organisms and, consequently, is active against many strains resistant to ampicillin and other cephalosporins.

Ceftazidime has been shown to be active against the following organisms both *in vitro* and in clinical infections (see INDICATIONS AND USAGE).

Aerobes, Gram-negative: *Citrobacter* spp., including *Citrobacter freundii* and *Citrobacter diversus; Enterobacter* spp., including *Enterobacter cloacae* and *Enterobacter aerogenes; Escherichia coli; Haemophilus influenzae,* including ampicillin-resistant strains; *Klebsiella* spp. (including *Klebsiella pneumoniae); Neisseria meningitidis; Proteus mirabilis; Proteus vulgaris; Pseudomonas* spp. (including *Pseudomonas aeruginosa*); and *Serratia* spp.

Aerobes, Gram-positive: *Staphylococcus aureus,* including penicillinase- and non–penicillinase-producing strains; *Streptococcus agalactiae* (group B streptococci); *Streptococcus*

pneumoniae; and *Streptococcus pyogenes* (group A beta-hemolytic streptococci).

Anaerobes: *Bacteroides* spp. (NOTE: many strains of *Bacteroides fragilis* are resistant).

Ceftazidime has been shown to be active *in vitro* against most strains of the following organisms; however, the clinical significance of this activity is unknown: *Acinetobacter* spp., *Clostridium* spp. (not including *Clostridium difficile), Haemophilus parainfluenzae, Morganella morganii* (formerly *Proteus morganii), Neisseria gonorrhoeae, Peptococcus* spp., *Peptostreptococcus* spp., *Providencia* spp. (including *Providencia rettgeri,* formerly *Proteus rettgeri*), *Salmonella* spp., *Shigella* spp., *Staphylococcus epidermidis,* and *Yersinia enterocolitica.*

Ceftazidime and the aminoglycosides have been shown to be synergistic *in vitro* against *Pseudomonas aeruginosa* and the enterobacteriaceae. Ceftazidime and carbenicillin have also been shown to be synergistic *in vitro* against *Pseudomonas aeruginosa.*

Ceftazidime is not active *in vitro* against methicillin-resistant staphylococci, *Streptococcus faecalis* and many other enterococci, *Listeria monocytogenes, Campylobacter* spp., or *Clostridium difficile.*

Susceptibility Tests: ***Diffusion Techniques:*** Quantitative methods that require measurement of zone diameters give an estimate of antibiotic susceptibility. One such procedure[1–3] has been recommended for use with disks to test susceptibility to ceftazidime.

Reports from the laboratory giving results of the standard single-disk susceptibility test with a 30-mcg ceftazidime disk should be interpreted according to the following criteria:

Susceptible organisms produce zones of 18 mm or greater, indicating that the test organism is likely to respond to therapy.

Organisms that produce zones of 15 to 17 mm are expected to be susceptible if high dosage is used or if the infection is confined to tissues and fluids (e.g., urine) in which high antibiotic levels are attained.

Resistant organisms produce zones of 14 mm or less, indicating that other therapy should be selected.

Organisms should be tested with the ceftazidime disk since ceftazidime has been shown by *in vitro* tests to be active against certain strains found resistant when other beta-lactam disks are used.

Standardized procedures require the use of laboratory control organisms. The 30-mcg ceftazidime disk should give zone diameters between 25 and 32 mm for *Escherichia coli* ATCC 25922. For *Pseudomonas aeruginosa* ATCC 27853, the zone diameters should be between 22 and 29 mm. For *Staphylococcus aureus* ATCC 25923, the zone diameters should be between 16 and 20 mm.

Dilution Techniques: In other susceptibility testing procedures, e.g., ICS agar dilution or the equivalent, a bacterial isolate may be considered susceptible if the minimum inhibitory concentration (MIC) value for ceftazidime is not more than 16 mcg/mL. Organisms are considered resistant to ceftazidime if the MIC ≥ 64 mcg/mL. Organisms having an MIC value of < 64 mcg/mL but > 16 mcg/mL are expected to be susceptible if high dosage is used or if the infection is confined to tissues and fluids (e.g., urine) in which high antibiotic levels are attained.

As with standard diffusion methods, dilution procedures require the use of laboratory control organisms. Standard ceftazidime powder should give MIC values in the range of 4 to 16 mcg/mL for *Staphylococcus aureus* ATCC 25923. For *Escherichia coli* ATCC 25922, the MIC range should be between 0.125 and 0.5 mcg/mL. For *Pseudomonas aeruginosa* ATCC 27853, the MIC range should be between 0.5 and 2 mcg/mL.

INDICATIONS AND USAGE

CEPTAZ is indicated for the treatment of patients with infections caused by susceptible strains of the designated organisms in the following diseases:

1. **Lower Respiratory Tract Infections,** including pneumonia, caused by *Pseudomonas aeruginosa* and other *Pseudomonas* spp.; *Haemophilus influenzae,* including ampicillin-resistant strains; *Klebsiella* spp.; *Enterobacter* spp.; *Proteus mirabilis; Escherichia coli; Serratia* spp.; *Citrobacter* spp.; *Streptococcus pneumoniae;* and *Staphylococcus aureus* (methicillin-susceptible strains).
2. **Skin and Skin-Structure Infections** caused by *Pseudomonas aeruginosa; Klebsiella* spp.; *Escherichia coli; Proteus* spp., including *Proteus mirabilis* and indole-positive *Proteus; Enterobacter* spp.; *Serratia* spp.; *Staphylococcus aureus* (methicillin-susceptible strains); and *Streptococcus pyogenes* (group A beta-hemolytic streptococci).
3. **Urinary Tract Infections,** both complicated and uncomplicated, caused by *Pseudomonas aeruginosa; Enterobacter* spp.; *Proteus* spp., including *Proteus mirabilis* and indole-positive *Proteus; Klebsiella* spp.; and *Escherichia coli.*
4. **Bacterial Septicemia** caused by *Pseudomonas aeruginosa, Klebsiella* spp., *Haemophilus influenzae, Escherichia coli, Serratia* spp., *Streptococcus pneumoniae,* and *Staphylococcus aureus* (methicillin-susceptible strains).

Table 2: Ceftazidime Concentrations in Body Tissues and Fluids

Tissue or Fluid	Dose/ Route	No. of Patients	Time of Sample Postdose	Average Tissue or Fluid Level (mcg/mL or mcg/g)
Urine	500 mg IM	6	0–2 h	2,100.0
	2 g IV	6	0–2 h	12,000.0
Bile	2 g IV	3	90 min	36.4
Synovial fluid	2 g IV	13	2 h	25.6
Peritoneal fluid	2 g IV	8	2 h	48.6
Sputum	1 g IV	8	1 h	9.0
Cerebrospinal fluid	2 g q8h IV	5	120 min	9.8
(inflamed meninges)	2 g q8h IV	6	180 min	9.4
Aqueous humor	2 g IV	13	1–3 h	11.0
Blister fluid	1 g IV	7	2–3 h	19.7
Lymphatic fluid	1 g IV	7	2–3 h	23.4
Bone	2 g IV	8	0.67 h	31.1
Heart muscle	2 g IV	35	30–280 min	12.7
Skin	2 g IV	22	30–180 min	6.6
Skeletal muscle	2 g IV	35	30–280 min	9.4
Myometrium	2 g IV	31	1–2 h	18.7

5. **Bone and Joint Infections** caused by *Pseudomonas aeruginosa, Klebsiella* spp., *Enterobacter* spp., and *Staphylococcus aureus* (methicillin-susceptible strains).
6. **Gynecologic Infections,** including endometritis, pelvic cellulitis, and other infections of the female genital tract caused by *Escherichia coli.*
7. **Intra-abdominal Infections,** including peritonitis caused by *Escherichia coli, Klebsiella* spp., and *Staphylococcus aureus* (methicillin-susceptible strains) and polymicrobial infections caused by aerobic and anaerobic organisms and *Bacteroides* spp. (many strains of *Bacteroides fragilis* are resistant).
8. **Central Nervous System Infections,** including meningitis, caused by *Haemophilus influenzae* and *Neisseria meningitidis.* Ceftazidime has also been used successfully in a limited number of cases of meningitis due to *Pseudomonas aeruginosa* and *Streptococcus pneumoniae.*

Specimens for bacterial cultures should be obtained before therapy in order to isolate and identify causative organisms and to determine their susceptibility to ceftazidime. Therapy may be instituted before results of susceptibility studies are known; however, once these results become available, the antibiotic treatment should be adjusted accordingly.

As with other extended-spectrum cephalosporins and penicillins, some strains of *Enterobacter* spp. can develop resistance during ceftazidime therapy due to induced type-1 beta-lactamase production. When clinically appropriate during therapy of *Enterobacter* spp. infections, periodic susceptibility testing should be considered.

CEPTAZ may be used alone in cases of confirmed or suspected sepsis. Ceftazidime has been used successfully in clinical trials as empiric therapy in cases where various concomitant therapies with other antibiotics have been used.

CEPTAZ may also be used concomitantly with other antibiotics, such as aminoglycosides, vancomycin, and clindamycin; in severe and life-threatening infections; and in the immunocompromised patient (see COMPATIBILITY AND STABILITY). When such concomitant treatment is appropriate, prescribing information in the labeling for the other antibiotics should be followed. The dosage depends on the severity of the infection and the patient's condition.

CONTRAINDICATIONS

CEPTAZ is contraindicated in patients who have shown hypersensitivity to ceftazidime or the cephalosporin group of antibiotics.

WARNINGS

BEFORE THERAPY WITH CEPTAZ IS INSTITUTED, CAREFUL INQUIRY SHOULD BE MADE TO DETERMINE WHETHER THE PATIENT HAS HAD PREVIOUS HYPERSENSITIVITY REACTIONS TO CEFTAZIDIME, CEPHALOSPORINS, PENICILLINS, OR OTHER DRUGS. IF THIS PRODUCT IS GIVEN TO PENICILLIN-SENSITIVE PATIENTS, CAUTION SHOULD BE EXERCISED BECAUSE CROSS-HYPERSENSITIVITY AMONG BETA-LACTAM ANTIBIOTICS HAS BEEN CLEARLY DOCUMENTED AND MAY OCCUR IN UP TO 10% OF PATIENTS WITH A HISTORY OF PENICILLIN ALLERGY. IF AN ALLERGIC REACTION TO CEPTAZ OCCURS, DISCONTINUE THE DRUG. SERIOUS ACUTE HYPERSENSITIVITY REACTIONS MAY REQUIRE TREATMENT WITH EPINEPHRINE AND OTHER EMERGENCY MEASURES, INCLUDING OXYGEN, IV FLUIDS, IV ANTIHISTAMINES, CORTICOSTEROIDS, PRESSOR AMINES, AND AIRWAY MANAGEMENT, AS CLINICALLY INDICATED.

Pseudomembranous colitis has been reported with nearly all antibacterial agents, including ceftazidime, and may range from mild to life threatening. Therefore, it is important to consider this diagnosis in patients who present with diarrhea subsequent to the administration of antibacterial agents.

Treatment with antibacterial agents alters the normal flora of the colon and may permit overgrowth of clostridia. Studies indicate that a toxin produced by *Clostridium difficile* is one primary cause of "antibiotic-associated colitis."

After the diagnosis of pseudomembranous colitis has been established, appropriate therapeutic measures should be initiated. Mild cases of pseudomembranous colitis usually respond to drug discontinuation alone. In moderate to severe cases, consideration should be given to management with fluids and electrolytes, protein supplementation, and treatment with an antibacterial drug clinically effective against *Clostridium difficile colitis.*

Elevated levels of ceftazidime in patients with renal insufficiency can lead to seizures, encephalopathy, asterixis, and neuromuscular excitability (see PRECAUTIONS).

PRECAUTIONS

General: Ceftazidime has not been shown to be nephrotoxic; however, high and prolonged serum antibiotic concentrations can occur from usual dosages in patients with transient or persistent reduction of urinary output because of renal insufficiency. The total daily dosage should be reduced when ceftazidime is administered to patients with renal insufficiency (see DOSAGE AND ADMINISTRATION). Elevated levels of ceftazidime in these patients can lead to seizures, encephalopathy, asterixis, and neuromuscular excitability. Continued dosage should be determined by degree of renal impairment, severity of infection, and susceptibility of the causative organisms.

As with other antibiotics, prolonged use of CEPTAZ may result in overgrowth of nonsusceptible organisms. Repeated evaluation of the patient's condition is essential. If superinfection occurs during therapy, appropriate measures should be taken.

Cephalosporins may be associated with a fall in prothrombin activity. Those at risk include patients with renal or hepatic impairment, or poor nutritional state, as well as patients receiving a protracted course of antimicrobial therapy. Prothrombin time should be monitored in patients at risk and exogenous vitamin K administered as indicated.

CEPTAZ should be prescribed with caution in individuals with a history of gastrointestinal disease, particularly colitis.

Arginine has been shown to alter glucose metabolism and elevate serum potassium transiently when administered at 50 times the recommended dose. The effect of lower dosing is not known.

Distal necrosis can occur after inadvertent intra-arterial administration of ceftazidime.

Drug Interactions: Nephrotoxicity has been reported following concomitant administration of cephalosporins with aminoglycoside antibiotics or potent diuretics such as furosemide. Renal function should be carefully monitored, especially if higher dosages of the aminoglycosides are to be administered or if therapy is prolonged, because of the potential nephrotoxicity and ototoxicity of aminoglycosidic antibiotics. Nephrotoxicity and ototoxicity were not noted when ceftazidime was given alone in clinical trials.

Chloramphenicol has been shown to be antagonistic to beta-lactam antibiotics, including ceftazidime, based on *in vitro* studies and time kill curves with enteric gram-negative bacilli. Due to the possibility of antagonism *in vivo,* particularly when bactericidal activity is desired, this drug combination should be avoided.

Drug/Laboratory Test Interactions: The administration of ceftazidime may result in a false-positive reaction for glucose

Continued on next page

Glaxo Wellcome—Cont.

in the urine when using CLINITEST® tablets. Benedict's solution, or Fehling's solution. It is recommended that glucose tests based on enzymatic glucose oxidase reactions (such as CLINISTIX® or TES-TAPE®) be used.

Carcinogenesis, Mutagenesis, Impairment of Fertility: Long-term studies in animals have not been performed to evaluate carcinogenic potential. However, a mouse Micronucleus test and an Ames test were both negative for mutagenic effects.

Pregnancy: *Teratogenic Effects: Pregnancy Category B:* Reproduction studies have been performed in mice and rats at doses up to 40 times the human dose and have revealed no evidence of impaired fertility or harm to the fetus due to ceftazidime. CEPTAZ at 23 times the human dose was not teratogenic or embryotoxic in a rat reproduction study. There are, however, no adequate and well-controlled studies in pregnant women. Because animal reproduction studies are not always predictive of human response, this drug should be used during pregnancy only if clearly needed.

Nursing Mothers: Ceftazidime is excreted in human milk in low concentrations. It is not known whether the arginine component of this product is excreted in human milk. Because many drugs are excreted in human milk and because safety of the arginine component of CEPTAZ in nursing infants has not been established, a decision should be made whether to discontinue nursing or to discontinue the drug, taking into account the importance of the drug to the mother.

Pediatric Use: Safety of the arginine component of CEPTAZ in neonates, infants, and children has not been established. This product is for use in patients 12 years and older. If treatment with ceftazidime is indicated for neonates, infants, or children, a sodium carbonate formulation should be used.

ADVERSE REACTIONS

The following adverse effects from clinical trials were considered to be either related to ceftazidime therapy or were of uncertain etiology. The most common were local reactions following IV injection and allergic and gastrointestinal reactions. No disulfiramlike reactions were reported.

Local Effects, reported in fewer than 2% of patients, were phlebitis and inflammation at the site of injection (1 in 69 patients).

Hypersensitivity Reactions, reported in 2% of patients, were pruritus, rash, and fever. Immediate reactions, generally manifested by rash and/or pruritus, occurred in 1 in 285 patients. Toxic epidermal necrolysis, Stevens-Johnson syndrome, and erythema multiforme have also been reported with cephalosporin antibiotics, including ceftazidime. Angioedema and anaphylaxis (bronchospasm and/or hypotension) have been reported very rarely.

Gastrointestinal Symptoms, reported in fewer than 2% of patients, were diarrhea (1 in 78), nausea (1 in 156), vomiting (1 in 500), and abdominal pain (1 in 416). The onset of pseudomembranous colitis symptoms may occur during or after treatment (see WARNINGS).

Central Nervous System Reactions (fewer than 1%) included headache, dizziness, and paresthesia. Seizures have been reported with several cephalosporins, including ceftazidime. In addition, encephalopathy, asterixis, and neuromuscular excitability have been reported in renally impaired patients treated with unadjusted dosing regimens of ceftazidime (see PRECAUTIONS: General).

Less Frequent Adverse Events (fewer than 1%) were candidiasis (including oral thrush) and vaginitis.

Hematologic: Rare cases of hemolytic anemia have been reported.

Laboratory Test Changes noted during ceftazidime clinical trials were transient and included: eosinophilia (1 in 13), positive Coombs' test without hemolysis (1 in 23), thrombocytosis (1 in 45), and slight elevations in one or more of the hepatic enzymes, aspartate aminotransferase (AST, SGOT) (1 in 16), alanine aminotransferase (ALT, SGPT) (1 in 15), LDH (1 in 18), GGT (1 in 19), and alkaline phosphatase (1 in 23). As with some other cephalosporins, transient elevations of blood urea, blood urea nitrogen, and/or serum creatinine were observed occasionally. Transient leukopenia, neutropenia, agranulocytosis, thrombocytopenia, and lymphocytosis were seen very rarely. Elevations in hepatic enzymes (SGOT, SGPT, LDH, GGT, alkaline phosphatase) have been reported postmarketing.

In addition to the adverse reactions listed above that have been observed in patients treated with ceftazidime, the following adverse reactions and altered laboratory tests have been reported for cephalosporin-class antibiotics:

Adverse Reactions: Urticaria, colitis, renal dysfunction, toxic nephropathy, hepatic dysfunction including cholestasis, aplastic anemia, hemorrhage.

Altered Laboratory Tests: Prolonged prothrombin time, false-positive test for urinary glucose, elevated bilirubin, pancytopenia.

OVERDOSAGE

Ceftazidime overdosage has occurred in patients with renal failure. Reactions have included seizure activity, encephalopathy, asterixis, and neuromuscular excitability. Patients who receive an acute overdosage should be carefully observed and given supportive treatment. In the presence of renal insufficiency, hemodialysis or peritoneal dialysis may aid in the removal of ceftazidime from the body.

DOSAGE AND ADMINISTRATION

Dosage: The usual adult dosage is 1 gram administered intravenously or intramuscularly every 8 to 12 hours. The dosage and route should be determined by the susceptibility of the causative organisms, the severity of infection, and the condition and renal function of the patient.

The guidelines for dosage of CEPTAZ are listed in Table 3. The following dosage schedule is recommended.

[See table 3 below.]

Impaired Hepatic Function: No adjustment in dosage is required for patients with hepatic dysfunction.

Impaired Renal Function: Ceftazidime is excreted by the kidneys, almost exclusively by glomerular filtration. Therefore, in patients with impaired renal function (glomerular filtration rate [GFR] <50 mL/min), it is recommended that the dosage of ceftazidime be reduced to compensate for its slower excretion. In patients with suspected renal insufficiency, an initial loading dose of 1 gram of CEPTAZ may be given. An estimate of GFR should be made to determine the appropriate maintenance dosage. The recommended dosage is presented in Table 4.

Table 4: Recommended Maintenance Dosages of CEPTAZ in Renal Insufficiency

NOTE: IF THE DOSE RECOMMENDED IN TABLE 3 ABOVE IS LOWER THAN THAT RECOMMENDED FOR PATIENTS WITH RENAL INSUFFICIENCY AS OUTLINED IN TABLE 4, THE LOWER DOSE SHOULD BE USED.

Creatinine Clearance (mL/min)	Recommended Unit Dose of CEPTAZ	Frequency of Dosing
50–31	1 gram	q12h
30–16	1 gram	q24h
15–6	500 mg	q24h
<5	500 mg	q48h

When only serum creatinine is available, the following formula (Cockcroft's equation)[4] may be used to estimate creatinine clearance. The serum creatinine should represent a steady state of renal function:

Males:
$$\text{Creatinine clearance (mL/min)} = \frac{\text{Weight (kg)} \times (140 - \text{age})}{72 \times \text{serum creatinine (mg/dL)}}$$

Females: $0.85 \times$ male value

In patients with severe infections who would normally receive 6 grams of CEPTAZ daily were it not for renal insufficiency, the unit dose given in the table above may be increased by 50% or the dosing frequency may be increased appropriately. Further dosing should be determined by therapeutic monitoring, severity of the infection, and susceptibility of the causative organism.

In patients undergoing hemodialysis, a loading dose of 1 gram is recommended, followed by 1 gram after each hemodialysis period.

CEPTAZ can also be used in patients undergoing intraperitoneal dialysis and continuous ambulatory peritoneal dialysis. In such patients, a loading dose of 1 gram of CEPTAZ may be given, followed by 500 mg every 24 hours. It is not known whether or not CEPTAZ can be safely incorporated into dialysis fluid.

Note: Generally CEPTAZ should be continued for 2 days after the signs and symptoms of infection have disappeared, but in complicated infections longer therapy may be required.

Administration: CEPTAZ may be given intravenously or by deep IM injection into a large muscle mass such as the upper outer quadrant of the gluteus maximus or lateral part of the thigh. Intra-arterial administration should be avoided (see PRECAUTIONS).

Intramuscular Administration: For IM administration, CEPTAZ should be constituted with one of the following diluents: sterile water for injection, bacteriostatic water for injection, or 0.5% or 1% lidocaine hydrochloride injection. Refer to Table 5.

Intravenous Administration: The IV route is preferable for patients with bacterial septicemia, bacterial meningitis, peritonitis, or other severe or life-threatening infections, or for patients who may be poor risks because of lowered resistance resulting from such debilitating conditions as malnutrition, trauma, surgery, diabetes, heart failure, or malignancy, particularly if shock is present or pending.

For direct intermittent IV administration, constitute CEPTAZ as directed in Table 5 with sterile water for injection, 5% dextrose injection, or 0.9% sodium chloride injection. Slowly inject directly into the vein over a period of 3 to 5 minutes or give through the tubing of an administration set while the patient is also receiving one of the compatible IV fluids (see COMPATIBILITY AND STABILITY).

For IV infusion, constitute the 1- or 2-gram infusion pack with 100 mL of sterile water for injection or one of the compatible IV fluids listed under the COMPATIBILITY AND STABILITY section. Alternatively, constitute the 1- or 2-gram vial and add an appropriate quantity of the resulting solution to an IV container with one of the compatible IV fluids.

Intermittent IV infusion with a Y-type administration set can be accomplished with compatible solutions. However, during infusion of a solution containing ceftazidime, it is desirable to discontinue the other solution.

[See table 5 at top of next page.]

Solutions of CEPTAZ, like those of most beta-lactam antibiotics, should not be added to solutions of aminoglycoside antibiotics because of potential interaction.

However, if concurrent therapy with CEPTAZ and an aminoglycoside is indicated, each of these antibiotics can be administered separately to the same patient.

Instructions for Constitution: Vials of CEPTAZ as supplied are under a slightly reduced pressure. This may assist entry of the diluent. No gas-relief needle is required when adding the diluent, except for the infusion pack where it is required during the latter stages of addition (in order to preserve product sterility, a gas-relief needle should not be inserted until an overpressure is produced in the vial). No evolution of gas occurs on constitution. When the vial contents are dissolved, vials other than infusion packs may still be under a reduced pressure. This reduced pressure is particularly noticeable for the 10-g pharmacy bulk package.

COMPATIBILITY AND STABILITY

Intramuscular: CEPTAZ , when constituted as directed with sterile water for injection, bacteriostatic water for injection, or 0.5% or 1% lidocaine hydrochloride injection, maintains satisfactory potency for 18 hours at room temperature or for 7 days under refrigeration. Solutions in sterile water for injection that are frozen immediately after constitution in the original container are stable for 6 months when

Table 3: Recommended Dosage Schedule

	Dose	Frequency
Adults 12 years and older*		
Usual recommended dosage	**1 gram IV or IM**	**q8–12h**
Uncomplicated urinary tract infections	250 mg IV or IM	q12h
Bone and joint infections	2 grams IV	q12h
Complicated urinary tract infections	500 mg IV or IM	q8–12h
Uncomplicated pneumonia; mild skin and skin-structure infections	500 mg–1 gram IV or IM	q8h
Serious gynecologic and intra-abdominal infections	2 grams IV	q8h
Meningitis	2 grams IV	q8h
Very severe life-threatening infections, especially in immunocompromised patients	2 grams IV	q8h
Lung infections caused by *Pseudomonas* spp. in patients with cystic fibrosis with normal renal function†	30–50 mg/kg IV to a maximum of 6 grams per day	q8h

*This product is for use in patients 12 years and older. If treatment with ceftazidime is indicated for pediatric patients, a sodium carbonate formulation should be used.

†Although clinical improvement has been shown, bacteriologic cures cannot be expected in patients with chronic respiratory disease and cystic fibrosis.

Table 5: Preparation of CEPTAZ Solutions

Size	Amount of Diluent to Be Added (mL)	Volume to Be Withdrawn (mL)	Approximate Ceftazidime Concentration (mg/mL)
Intramuscular			
1-gram vial	3.0	Total	250
Intravenous			
1-gram vial	10.0	Total	90
2-gram vial	10.0	Total	170
Infusion pack			
1-gram vial	100	—	10
2-gram vial	100	—	20
Pharmacy bulk package			
10-gram vial	40	Amount needed	200

stored at −20°C. Components of the solution may precipitate in the frozen state and will dissolve on reaching room temperature with little or no agitation. Potency is not affected. Frozen solutions should only be thawed at room temperature. Do not force thaw by immersion in water baths or by microwave irradiation. Once thawed, solutions should not be refrozen. Thawed solutions may be stored for up to 12 hours at room temperature or for 7 days in a refrigerator.

Intravenous: *Ceftazidime concentration greater than 100 mg/mL (2-g vial or 10-g pharmacy bulk package):* CEPTAZ, when constituted as directed with sterile water for injection. 0.9% sodium chloride injection, or 5% dextrose injection, maintains satisfactory potency for 18 hours at room temperature or for 7 days under refrigeration. Solutions of a similar concentration in sterile water for injection that are frozen immediately after constitution in the original container are stable for 6 months when stored at −20°C. Components of the solution may precipitate in the frozen state and will dissolve on reaching room temperature with little or no agitation. Potency is not affected. Frozen solutions should only be thawed at room temperature. Do not force thaw by immersion in water baths or by microwave irradiation. Once thawed, solutions should not be refrozen. Thawed solutions may be stored for up to 12 hours at room temperature or for 7 days in a refrigerator.

Ceftazidime concentration of 100 mg/mL or less (1-g vial or infusion packs): CEPTAZ, when constituted as directed with sterile water for injection, 0.9% sodium chloride injection, or 5% dextrose injection, maintains satisfactory potency for 24 hours at room temperature or for 7 days under refrigeration. Solutions, prepared by a pharmacist, of the approved arginine formulation of ceftazidime of a similar concentration in sterile water for injection, 0.9% sodium chloride injection, or 5% dextrose injection in the original container or in 0.9% sodium chloride injection in VIAFLEX® (PL 146® Plastic) small-volume containers that are frozen immediately after constitution by the pharmacist are stable for 6 months when stored at −20°C. Solutions in the PL 146 Plastic small-volume containers are in contact with the polyvinyl chloride layer of this container and can leach out certain chemical components of the plastic in very small amounts within the expiration period. The suitability of the plastic has been confirmed in tests in animals according to USP biological tests for plastic containers as well as by tissue culture toxicity studies. Stability of the frozen solution in other containers has not been confirmed. Frozen solutions should only be thawed at room temperature. Do not force thaw by immersion in water baths or by microwave irradiation. For the larger volumes of IV infusion solutions where it may be necessary to warm the frozen product, care should be taken to avoid heating after thawing is complete. Once thawed, solutions should not be refrozen. Thawed solutions may be stored for up to 18 hours at room temperature or for 7 days in a refrigerator.

Components of the solution may precipitate in the frozen state and will dissolve upon reaching room temperature with little or no agitation. Potency is not affected. Check for minute leaks in plastic containers by squeezing bag firmly. Discard bag if leaks are found as sterility may be impaired. Do not add supplementary medication to bags. Do not use unless solution is clear and seal is intact.
Use sterile equipment.

Caution: Do not use plastic containers in series connections. Such use could result in air embolism due to residual air being drawn from the primary container before administration of the fluid from the secondary container is complete.

Preparation for Administration:
1. Suspend container from eyelet support.
2. Remove protector from outlet port at bottom of container.
3. Attach administration set. Refer to complete directions accompanying set.

CEPTAZ is compatible with the more commonly used IV infusion fluids. Solutions at concentrations between 1 and 40 mg/mL in 0.9% sodium chloride injection; 1/6 M sodium lactate injection; 5% dextrose injection; 5% dextrose and 0.225% sodium chloride injection; 5% dextrose and 0.45% sodium chloride injection; 5% dextrose and 0.9% sodium chloride injection; 10% dextrose injection; ringer's injec-

tion, USP; lactated ringer's injection, USP; 10% invert sugar in sterile water for injection; and NORMOSOL®-M in 5% dextrose injection may be stored for up to 24 hours at room temperature or for 7 days if refrigerated.

CEPTAZ is less stable in sodium bicarbonate injection than in other IV fluids. It is not recommended as a diluent. Solutions of CEPTAZ in 5% dextrose injection and 0.9% sodium chloride injection are stable for at least 6 hours at room temperature in plastic tubing, drip chambers, and volume control devices of common IV infusion sets.

Ceftazidime at a concentration of 4 mg/mL has been found compatible for 24 hours at room temperature or for 7 days under refrigeration in 0.9% sodium chloride injection or 5% dextrose injection when admixed with: cefuroxime sodium (ZINACEF®) 3 mg/mL; heparin sodium in concentrations up to 50 U/mL; or potassium chloride in concentrations up to 40 mEq/L. Ceftazidime may be constituted at a concentration of 20 mg/mL with metronidazole injection 5 mg/mL, and the resultant solution may be stored for 24 hours at room temperature or for 7 days under refrigeration. Ceftazidime at a concentration of 20 mg/mL has been found compatible for 24 hours at room temperature or for 7 days under refrigeration in 0.9% sodium chloride injection or 5% dextrose injection when admixed with 6 mg/mL clindamycin (as clindamycin phosphate).

Vancomycin solution exhibits a physical incompatibility when mixed with a number of drugs, including ceftazidime. The likelihood of precipitation with ceftazidime is dependent on the concentrations of vancomycin and ceftazidime present. It is therefore recommended, when both drugs are to be administered by intermittent IV infusion, that they be given separately, flushing the IV lines (with one of the compatible IV fluids) between the administration of these two agents.

Note: Parenteral drug products should be inspected visually for particulate matter before administration whenever solution and container permit.

As with other cephalosporins, CEPTAZ powder as well as solutions tend to darken, depending on storage conditions; within the stated recommendations, however, product potency is not adversely affected.

Directions for Dispensing: *Pharmacy Bulk Package—Not for Direct Infusion:* The pharmacy bulk package is for use in a pharmacy admixture service only under a laminar flow hood. Entry into the vial must be made with a sterile transfer set or other sterile dispensing device, and the contents dispensed in aliquots using aseptic technique. The use of syringe and needle is not recommended as it may cause leakage (see DOSAGE AND ADMINISTRATION). GOOD PHARMACY PRACTICE DICTATES THAT THE CLOSURE BE PENETRATED ONLY ONE TIME AFTER CONSTITUTION. AFTER INITIAL PENETRATION OF THE CLOSURE, USE ENTIRE CONTENTS OF VIAL PROMPTLY. ANY UNUSED PORTION MUST BE DISCARDED WITHIN 18 HOURS OF CONSTITUTION.

HOW SUPPLIED
CEPTAZ in the dry state should be stored between 15° and 30°C (59° and 86°F) and protected from light. CEPTAZ is a dry, white to off-white powder supplied in vials and infusion packs as follows:
NDC 0173-0414-00 1-g* Vial (Tray of 25)
NDC 0173-0415-00 2-g* Vial (Tray of 25)
NDC 0173-0416-00 1-g* Infusion Pack (Tray of 10)
NDC 0173-0417-00 2-g* Infusion Pack (Tray of 10)
NDC 0173-0418-00 10-g* Pharmacy Bulk Package (Tray of 6)
* Equivalent to anhydrous ceftazidime.

REFERENCES
1. Bauer AW, Kirby WMM, Sherris JC, Turck M. Antibiotic susceptibility testing by a standardized single disk method. *Am J Clin Pathol.* 1966;45:493–496.
2. National Committee for Clinical Laboratory Standards. *Approved Standard: Performance Standards for Antimicrobial Disc Susceptibility Tests.* (M2-A3). December 1984.

3. Certification procedure for antibiotic sensitivity discs (21 CFR 460.1). *Federal Register.* May 30, 1974;39:19182–19184.
4. Cockcroft DW, Gault MH. Prediction of creatinine clearance from serum creatinine. *Nephron.* 1976;16:31–41.

CEPTAZ and ZINACEF are registered trademarks of Glaxo Wellcome.
CLINITEST and CLINISTIX are registered trademarks of Ames Division, Miles Laboratories, Inc.
TES-TAPE is a registered trademark of Eli Lilly and Company.
VIAFLEX and PL 146 Plastic are registered trademarks of Baxter International Inc.
U.S. Patents 4,258,041; 4,329,453; and 4,582,830
February 1996/RL-230
Shown in Product Identification Guide, page 312

CORTISPORIN® Cream ℞

[kor'tĭ-spor"ĭn krēm]
(neomycin and polymyxin B sulfates and hydrocortisone acetate cream, USP)

DESCRIPTION
CORTISPORIN Cream (neomycin and polymyxin B sulfates and hydrocortisone acetate, USP) is a topical antibacterial cream. Each gram contains: neomycin sulfate equivalent to 3.5 mg neomycin base, and polymyxin B sulfate equivalent to 10,000 polymixin B units, hydrocortisone acetate 5 mg (0.5%). The inactive ingredients are liquid petrolatum, white petrolatum, propylene glycol, polyoxyethylene polyoxypropylene compound, emulsifying wax, purified water, and 0.25% methylparaben added as a preservative. Sodium hydroxide or sulfuric acid may be added to adjust pH.

Neomycin sulfate is the sulfate salt of neomycin B and C, which are produced by the growth of *Streptomyces fradiae* Waksman (Fam. Streptomycetaceae). It has a potency equivalent of not less than 600 μg of neomycin standard per mg, calculated on an anhydrous basis.

Polymyxin B sulfate is the sulfate salt of polymyxin B_1 and B_2, which are produced by the growth of *Bacillus polymyxa* (Prazmowski) Migula (Fam. Bacillaceae). It has a potency of not less than 6,000 polymyxin B units per mg, calculated on an anhydrous basis.

Hydrocortisone acetate is the acetate ester of hydrocortisone, an anti-inflammatory hormone. Its chemical name is 21-(acetyloxy)-11β,17-dihydroxypregn-4-ene-3,20-dione.

The base is a smooth vanishing cream with a pH of approximately 5.0.

CLINICAL PHARMACOLOGY
Corticoids suppress the inflammatory response to a variety of agents and they may delay healing. Since corticoids may inhibit the body's defense mechanism against infection, a concomitant antimicrobial drug may be used when this inhibition is considered to be clinically significant in a particular case.

The anti-infective components in the combination are included to provide action against specific organisms susceptible to them. Polymyxin B sulfate and neomycin sulfate together are considered active against the following microorganisms: *Staphylococcus aureus, Escherichia coli, Haemophilus influenzae, Klebsiella-Enterobacter* species, *Neisseria* species, and *Pseudomonas aeruginosa.* The product does not provide adequate coverage against *Serratia marcescens* and streptococci, including *Streptococcus pneumoniae.*

The relative potency of corticosteroids depends on the molecular structure, concentration, and release from the vehicle. The acid pH helps restore normal cutaneous acidity. Owing to its excellent spreading and penetrating properties, the cream facilitates treatment of hairy and intertriginous areas. It may also be of value in selective cases where the lesions are moist.

INDICATIONS AND USAGE
For the treatment of corticosteroid-responsive dermatoses with secondary infection. It has not been demonstrated that this steroid-antibiotic combination provides greater benefit than the steroid component alone after 7 days of treatment (see WARNINGS).

CONTRAINDICATIONS
Not for use in the eyes or in the external ear canal if the eardrum is perforated. This product is contraindicated in tuberculous, fungal, or viral lesions of the skin (herpes simplex, vaccinia, and varicella). This product is contraindicated in those individuals who have shown hypersensitivity to any of its components.

WARNINGS
Because of the concern of nephrotoxicity and ototoxicity associated with neomycin, this combination should not be used over a wide area or for extended periods of time.

Continued on next page

Glaxo Wellcome—Cont.

PRECAUTIONS

General: As with any antibacterial preparation, prolonged use may result in overgrowth of nonsusceptible organisms, including fungi. Appropriate measures should be taken if this occurs. Use of steroids on infected areas should be supervised with care as anti-inflammatory steroids may encourage spread of infection. If this occurs, steroid therapy should be stopped and appropriate antibacterial drugs used. Generalized dermatological conditions may require systemic corticosteroid therapy.

Signs and symptoms of exogenous hyperadrenocorticism can occur with the use of topical corticosteroids, including adrenal suppression. Systemic absorption of topically applied steroids will be increased if extensive body surface areas are treated or if occlusive dressings are used. Under these circumstances, suitable precautions should be taken when long-term use is anticipated.

Information for Patients: If redness, irritation, swelling or pain persists or increases, discontinue use and notify physician. Do not use in the eyes.

Laboratory Tests: Systemic effects of excessive levels of hydrocortisone may include a reduction in the number of circulating eosinophils and a decrease in urinary excretion of 17-hydroxycorticosteroids.

Carcinogenesis, Mutagenesis, Impairment of Fertility: Long-term studies in animals (rats, rabbits, mice) showed no evidence of carcinogenicity attributable to oral administration of corticosteroids.

Pregnancy: *Teratogenic Effects:* Pregnancy Category C. Corticosteroids have been shown to be teratogenic in rabbits when applied topically at concentrations of 0.5% on days 6 to 18 of gestation and in mice when applied topically at a concentration of 15% on days 10 to 13 of gestation. There are no adequate and well-controlled studies in pregnant women. Corticosteroids should be used during pregnancy only if the potential benefit justifies the potential risk to the fetus.

Nursing Mothers: Hydrocortisone acetate appears in human milk following oral administration of the drug. Since systemic absorption of hydrocortisone may occur when applied topically, caution should be exercised when CORTISPORIN Cream is used by a nursing woman.

Pediatric Use: Sufficient percutaneous absorption of hydrocortisone can occur in infants and children during prolonged use to cause cessation of growth, as well as other systemic signs and symptoms of hyperadrenocorticism.

ADVERSE REACTIONS

Neomycin occasionally causes skin sensitization. Ototoxicity and nephrotoxicity have also been reported (see WARNINGS). Adverse reactions have occurred with topical use of antibiotic combinations including neomycin and polymyxin B. Exact incidence figures are not available since no denominator of treated patients is available. The reaction occurring most often is allergic sensitization. In one clinical study using a 20% neomycin patch, neomycin-induced allergic skin reactions occurred in two of 2,175 (0.09%) individuals in the general population.[1] In another study, the incidence was found to be approximately 1%.[2]

The following local adverse reactions have been reported with topical corticosteroids, especially under occlusive dressings: burning, itching, irritation, dryness, folliculitis, hypertrichosis, acneiform eruptions, hypopigmentation, perioral dermatitis, allergic contact dermatitis, maceration of the skin, secondary infection, skin atrophy, striae, and miliaria.

When steroid preparations are used for long periods of time in intertriginous areas or over extensive body areas, with or without occlusive non-permeable dressings, striae may occur; also there exists the possibility of systemic side effects when steroid preparations are used over large areas or for a long period of time.

DOSAGE AND ADMINISTRATION

A small quantity of the cream should be applied 2 to 4 times daily, as required. The cream should, if conditions permit, be gently rubbed into the affected areas.

HOW SUPPLIED

Tube of 7.5 g (NDC 0173-0185-98).
Store at 15° to 25°C (59° to 77°F).

REFERENCES

1. Leyden JJ, Kligman AM. Contact dermatitis to neomycin sulfate. *JAMA* 1979;242:1276–1278.
2. Prystowsky SD, Allen AM, Smith RW, et al: Allergic contact hypersensitivity to nickel, neomycin, ethylenediamine, and benzocaine. *Arch Dermatol.* 1979;115: 959–962.

February 1996/RL-266

Shown in Product Identification Guide, page 312

CORTISPORIN® Ointment ℞

[*kor'tĭ-spor"ĭn*]

(neomycin and polymyxin B sulfates, bacitracin zinc, and hydrocortisone ointment, USP)

DESCRIPTION

CORTISPORIN Ointment (neomycin and polymyxin B sulfates, bacitracin zinc, and hydrocortisone ointment, USP) is a topical antibacterial ointment. Each gram contains: neomycin sulfate equivalent to 3.5 mg neomycin base, polymyxin B sulfate equivalent to 5,000 polymyxin B units, bacitracin zinc equivalent to 400 bacitracin units, hydrocortisone 10 mg (1%), and white petrolatum, qs.

Neomycin sulfate is the sulfate salt of neomycin B and C, which are produced by the growth of *Streptomyces fradiae* Waksman (Fam. Streptomycetaceae). It has a potency equivalent of not less than 600 μg of neomycin standard per mg, calculated on an anhydrous basis.

Polymyxin B sulfate is the sulfate salt of polymyxin B_1 and B_2, which are produced by the growth of *Bacillus polymyxa* (Prazmowski) Migula (Fam. Bacillaceae). It has a potency of not less than 6,000 polymyxin B units per mg, calculated on an anhydrous basis.

Bacitracin zinc is the zinc salt of bacitracin, a mixture of related cyclic polypeptides (mainly bacitracin A) produced by the growth of an organism of the *licheniformis* group of *Bacillus subtilis* (Fam. Bacillaceae). It has a potency of not less than 40 bacitracin units per mg.

Hydrocortisone, 11β, 17, 21-trihydroxypregn-4-ene-3, 20-dione, is an anti-inflammatory hormone.

CLINICAL PHARMACOLOGY

Corticoids suppress the inflammatory response to a variety of agents and they may delay healing. Since corticoids may inhibit the body's defense mechanism against infection, a concomitant antimicrobial drug may be used when this inhibition is considered to be clinically significant in a particular case.

The anti-infective components in the combination are included to provide action against specific organisms susceptible to them. Polymyxin B sulfate, bacitracin zinc, and neomycin sulfate together are considered active against the following microorganisms: *Staphylococcus aureus,* streptococci, including *Streptococcus pneumoniae, Escherichia coli, Haemophilus influenzae, Klebsiella-Enterobacter* species, *Neisseria* species, and *Pseudomonas aeruginosa.*

The product does not provide adequate coverage against *Serratia marcescens.*

The relative potency of corticosteroids depends on the molecular structure, concentration, and release from the vehicle.

INDICATIONS AND USAGE

For the treatment of corticosteroid-responsive dermatoses with secondary infection. It has not been demonstrated that this steroid-antibiotic combination provides greater benefit than the steroid component alone after 7 days of treatment (see WARNINGS).

CONTRAINDICATIONS

Not for use in the eyes or in the external ear canal if the eardrum is perforated. This product is contraindicated in tuberculous, fungal, or viral lesions of the skin (herpes simplex, vaccinia, and varicella). This product is contraindicated in those individuals who have shown hypersensitivity to any of its components.

WARNINGS

Because of the concern of nephrotoxicity and ototoxicity associated with neomycin, this combination should not be used over a wide area or for extended periods of time.

PRECAUTIONS

General: As with any antibiotic preparation, prolonged use may result in the overgrowth of nonsusceptible organisms, including fungi. Appropriate measures should be taken if this occurs. Use of steroids on infected areas should be supervised with care as anti-inflammatory steroids may encourage spread of infection. If this occurs, steroid therapy should be stopped and appropriate antibacterial drugs used. Generalized dermatological conditions may require systemic corticosteroid therapy.

Signs and symptoms of exogenous hyperadrenocorticism can occur with the use of topical corticosteroids, including adrenal suppression. Systemic absorption of topically applied steroids will be increased if extensive body surface areas are treated or if occlusive dressings are used. Under these circumstances, suitable precautions should be taken when long-term use is anticipated.

Information for Patients: If redness, irritation, swelling, or pain persists or increases, discontinue use and notify physician. Do not use in the eyes.

Laboratory Tests: Systemic effects of excessive levels of hydrocortisone may include a reduction in the number of circulating eosinophils and a decrease in urinary excretion of 17-hydroxycorticosteroids.

Carcinogenesis, Mutagenesis, Impairment of Fertility: Long-term studies in animals (rats, rabbits, mice) showed no evidence of carcinogenicity attributable to oral administration of corticosteroids.

Pregnancy: *Teratogenic Effects:* Pregnancy Category C. Corticosteroids have been shown to be teratogenic in rabbits when applied topically at concentrations of 0.5% on days 6 to 18 of gestation and in mice when applied topically at a concentration of 15% on days 10 to 13 of gestation. There are no adequate and well-controlled studies in pregnant women. Corticosteroids should be used during pregnancy only if the potential benefit justifies the potential risk to the fetus.

Nursing Mothers: Hydrocortisone appears in human milk following oral administration of the drug. Since systemic absorption of hydrocortisone may occur when applied topically, caution should be exercised when CORTISPORIN Ointment is used by a nursing woman.

Pediatric Use: Sufficient percutaneous absorption of hydrocortisone can occur in infants and children during prolonged use to cause cessation of growth, as well as other systemic signs and symptoms of hyperadrenocorticism.

ADVERSE REACTIONS

Neomycin occasionally causes skin sensitization. Ototoxicity and nephrotoxicity have also been reported (see WARNINGS). Adverse reactions have occurred with topical use of antibiotic combinations including neomycin, bacitracin, and polymyxin B. Exact incidence figures are not available since no denominator of treated patients is available. The reaction occurring most often is allergic sensitization. In one clinical study, using a 20% neomycin patch, neomycin-induced allergic skin reactions occurred in two of 2,175 (0.09%) individuals in the general population.[1] In another study, the incidence was found to be approximately 1%.[2]

The following local adverse reactions have been reported with topical corticosteroids, especially under occlusive dressings: burning, itching, irritation, dryness, folliculitis, hypertrichosis, acneiform eruptions, hypopigmentation, perioral dermatitis, allergic contact dermatitis, maceration of the skin, secondary infection, skin atrophy, striae, and miliaria.

When steroid preparations are used for long periods of time in intertriginous areas or over extensive body areas, with or without occlusive non-permeable dressings, striae may occur; also there exists the possibility of systemic side effects when steroid preparations are used over large areas or for a long period of time.

DOSAGE AND ADMINISTRATION

A thin film is applied 2 to 4 times daily to the affected area.

HOW SUPPLIED

Tube of 1/2 oz with applicator tip (NDC 0173-0196-88).
Store at 15° to 25°C (59° to 77°F).

REFERENCES

1. Leyden JJ, Kligman AM. Contact dermatitis to neomycin sulfate. *JAMA.* 1979;242:1276–1278.
2. Prystowsky SD, Allen AM, Smith RW, et al: Allergic contact hypersensitivity to nickel, neomycin, ethylenediamine, and benzocaine. *Arch Dermatol.* 1979;115: 959–962.

February 1996/RL-267

Shown in Product Identification Guide, page 312

CORTISPORIN® ℞

[*kor'tĭ-spor"ĭn*]

Ophthalmic Ointment Sterile

(neomycin and polymyxin B sulfates, bacitracin zinc, and hydrocortisone ophthalmic ointment, USP)

DESCRIPTION

CORTISPORIN® Ophthalmic Ointment (neomycin and polymyxin B sulfates, bacitracin zinc, and hydrocortisone ophthalmic ointment) is a sterile antimicrobial and anti-inflammatory ointment for ophthalmic use. Each gram contains: neomycin sulfate equivalent to 3.5 mg neomycin base, polymyxin B sulfate equivalent to 10,000 polymyxin B units, bacitracin zinc equivalent to 400 bacitracin units, hydrocortisone 10 mg (1%), and white petrolatum, q.s.

Neomycin sulfate is the sulfate salt of neomycin B and C, which are produced by the growth of *Streptomyces fradiae* Waksman (Fam. Streptomycetaceae). It has a potency equivalent of not less than 600 μg of neomycin standard per mg, calculated on an anhydrous basis.

Polymyxin B sulfate is the sulfate salt of polymyxin B_1 and B_2, which are produced by the growth of *Bacillus polymyxa* (Prazmowski) Migula (Fam. Bacillaceae). It has a potency of not less than 6,000 polymyxin B units per mg, calculated on an anhydrous basis.

Bacitracin zinc is the zinc salt of bacitracin, a mixture of related cyclic polypeptides (mainly bacitracin A) produced by the growth of an organism of the *licheniformis* group of *Bacillus subtilis* var Tracy. It has a potency of not less than 40 bacitracin units per mg.

Hydrocortisone, 11β, 17, 21-trihydroxypregn-4-ene-3, 20-dione, is an anti-inflammatory hormone.

CLINICAL PHARMACOLOGY

Corticosteroids suppress the inflammatory response to a variety of agents and they probably delay or slow healing. Since corticosteroids may inhibit the body's defense mechanism against infection, concomitant antimicrobial drugs may be used when this inhibition is considered to be clinically significant in a particular case.

When a decision to administer both a corticosteroid and antimicrobials is made, the administration of such drugs in combination has the advantage of greater patient compliance and convenience, with the added assurance that the appropriate dosage of all drugs is administered. When each type of drug is in the same formulation, compatibility of ingredients is assured and the correct volume of drug is delivered and retained.

The relative potency of corticosteroids depends on the molecular structure, concentration, and release from the vehicle.

Microbiology: The anti-infective components in CORTISPORIN Ophthalmic Ointment are included to provide action against specific organisms susceptible to it. Neomycin sulfate and polymyxin B sulfate are active in vitro against susceptible strains of the following microorganisms: *Staphylococcus aureus*, streptococci including *Streptococcus pneumoniae, Escherichia coli, Haemophilus influenzae, Klebsiella/Enterobacter* species, *Neisseria* species, and *Pseudomonas aeruginosa*. The product does not provide adequate coverage against *Serratia marcescens* (see INDICATIONS AND USAGE).

INDICATIONS AND USAGE

CORTISPORIN Ophthalmic Ointment is indicated for steroid-responsive inflammatory ocular conditions for which a corticosteroid is indicated and where bacterial infection or a risk of bacterial infection exists.

Ocular corticosteroids are indicated in inflammatory conditions of the palpebral and bulbar conjunctiva, cornea, and anterior segment of the globe where the inherent risk of corticosteroid use in certain infective conjunctivitides is accepted to obtain a diminution in edema and inflammation. They are also indicated in chronic anterior uveitis and corneal injury from chemical, radiation, or thermal burns, or penetration of foreign bodies.

The use of a combination drug with an anti-infective component is indicated where the risk of infection is high or where there is an expectation that potentially dangerous numbers of bacteria will be present in the eye (see CLINICAL PHARMACOLOGY: Microbiology).

The particular anti-infective drugs in this product are active against the following common bacterial eye pathogens: *Staphylococcus aureus*, streptococci, including *Streptococcus pneumoniae, Escherichia coli, Haemophilus influenzae, Klebsiella/Enterobacter* species, *Neisseria* species, and *Pseudomonas aeruginosa*.

The product does not provide adequate coverage against *Serratia marcescens*.

CONTRAINDICATIONS

CORTISPORIN Ophthalmic Ointment is contraindicated in most viral diseases of the cornea and conjunctiva including: epithelial herpes simplex keratitis (dendritic keratitis), vaccinia, varicella, and also in mycobacterial infection of the eye and fungal diseases of ocular structures.

CORTISPORIN Ophthalmic Ointment is also contraindicated in individuals who have shown hypersensitivity to any of its components. Hypersensitivity to the antibiotic component occurs at a higher rate than for other components.

WARNINGS

NOT FOR INJECTION INTO THE EYE. CORTISPORIN Ophthalmic Ointment should never be directly introduced into the anterior chamber of the eye. Ophthalmic ointments may retard corneal wound healing.

Prolonged use of corticosteroids may result in ocular hypertension and/or glaucoma, with damage to the optic nerve, defects in visual acuity and fields of vision, and in posterior subcapsular cataract formation.

Prolonged use may suppress the host response and thus increase the hazard of secondary ocular infections. In those diseases causing thinning of the cornea or sclera, perforations have been known to occur with the use of topical corticosteroids. In acute purulent conditions of the eye, corticosteroids may mask infection or enhance existing infection. If these products are used for 10 days or longer, intraocular pressure should be routinely monitored even though it may be difficult in uncooperative patients. Corticosteroids should be used with caution in the presence of glaucoma.

The use of corticosteroids afer cataract surgery may delay healing and increase the incidence of filtering blebs.

Use of ocular corticosteroids may prolong the course and may exacerbate the severity of many viral infections of the eye (including herpes simplex). Employment of corticosteroid medication in the treatment of herpes simplex requires great caution.

Topical antibiotics, particularly neomycin sulfate, may cause cutaneous sensitization. A precise incidence of hypersensitivity reactions (primarily skin rash) due to topical antibiotics is not known.

The manifestations of sensitization to topical antibiotics are usually itching, reddening, and edema of the conjunctiva and eyelid. A sensitization reaction may manifest simply as a failure to heal. During long-term use of topical antibiotic products, periodic examination for such signs is advisable, and the patient should be told to discontinue the product if they are observed. Symptoms usually subside quickly on withdrawing the medication. Applications of products containing these ingredients should be avoided for the patient thereafter (see PRECAUTIONS: General).

PRECAUTIONS

General: The initial prescription and renewal of the medication order beyond 8 grams should be made by a physician only after examination of the patient with the aid of magnification, such as slit lamp biomicroscopy and, where appropriate, fluorescein staining. If signs and symptoms fail to improve after two days, the patient should be re-evaluated.

The possibility of fungal infections of the cornea should be considered after prolonged corticosteroid dosing. Fungal cultures should be taken when appropriate.

If this product is used for 10 days or longer, intraocular pressure should be monitored (see WARNINGS).

There have been reports of bacterial keratitis associated with the use of topical ophthalmic products in multiple-dose containers which have been inadvertently contaminated by patients, most of whom had a concurrent corneal disease or a disruption of the ocular epithelial surface (see PRECAUTIONS: Information for Patients).

Allergic cross-reactions may occur which could prevent the use of any or all of the following antibiotics for the treatment of future infections: kanamycin, paromomycin, streptomycin, and possibly gentamicin.

Information for Patients: Patients should be instructed to avoid allowing the tip of the dispensing container to contact the eye, eyelid, fingers, or any other surface. The use of this product by more than one person may spread infection.

Patients should also be instructed that ocular products, if handled improperly, can become contaminated by common bacteria known to cause ocular infections. Serious damage to the eye and subsequent loss of vision may result from using contaminated products (see PRECAUTIONS: General).

If the condition persists or gets worse, or if a rash or allergic reaction develops, the patient should be advised to stop use and consult a physician. Do not use this product if you are allergic to any of the listed ingredients.

Keep tightly closed when not in use. Keep out of the reach of children.

Carcinogenesis, Mutagenesis, Impairment of Fertility: Long-term studies in animals to evaluate carcinogenic or mutagenic potential have not been conducted with polymyxin B sulfate or bacitracin. Treatment of cultured human lymphocytes in vitro with neomycin increased the frequency of chromosome aberrations at the highest concentrations (80 μg/mL) tested; however, the effects of neomycin on carcinogenesis and mutagenesis in humans are unknown.

Long-term studies in animals (rats, rabbits, mice) showed no evidence of carcinogenicity or mutagenicity attributable to oral administration of corticosteroids. Long-term animal studies have not been performed to evaluate the carcinogenic potential of topical corticosteroids. Studies to determine mutagenicity with hydrocortisone have revealed negative results.

Polymyxin B has been reported to impair the motility of equine sperm, but its effects on male or female fertility are unknown. No adverse effects on male or female fertility, litter size, or survival were observed in rabbits given bacitracin zinc 100 gm/ton of diet. Long-term animal studies have not been performed to evaluate the effect on fertility of topical corticosteroids.

Pregnancy: *Teratogenic Effects:* Pregnancy Category C. Corticosteroids have been found to be teratogenic in rabbits when applied topically at concentrations of 0.5% on days 6 to 18 of gestation and in mice when applied topically at a concentration of 15% on days 10 to 13 of gestation. There are no adequate and well-controlled studies in pregnant women. CORTISPORIN Ophthalmic Ointment should be used during pregnancy only if the potential benefit justifies the potential risk to the fetus.

Nursing Mothers: It is not known whether topical administration of corticosteroids could result in sufficient systemic absorption to produce detectable quantities in human milk. Systemically administered corticosteroids appear in human milk and could suppress growth, interfere with endogenous corticosteroid production, or cause other untoward effects. Because of the potential for serious adverse reactions in nursing infants from CORTISPORIN Ophthalmic Ointment, a decision should be made whether to discontinue nursing or to discontinue the drug, taking into account the importance of the drug to the mother.

Pediatric Use: Safety and effectiveness in pediatric patients have not been established.

ADVERSE REACTIONS

Adverse reactions have occurred with corticosteroid/anti-infective combination drugs which can be attributed to the corticosteroid component, the anti-infective component, or the combination. The exact incidence is not known.

Reactions occurring most often from the presence of the anti-infective ingredient are allergic sensitization reactions including itching, swelling, and conjunctival erythema (see WARNINGS). More serious hypersensitivity reactions, including anaphylaxis, have been reported rarely.

The reactions due to the corticosteroid component in decreasing order of frequency are: elevation of intraocular pressure (IOP) with possible development of glaucoma, and infrequent optic nerve damage; posterior subcapsular cataract formation; and delayed wound healing.

Secondary Infection: The development of secondary infection has occurred after use of combinations containing corticosteroids and antimicrobials. Fungal and viral infections of the cornea are particularly prone to develop coincidentally with long-term applications of a corticosteroid. The possibility of fungal invasion must be considered in any persistent corneal ulceration where corticosteroid treatment has been used.

Local irritation on instillation has been reported.

DOSAGE AND ADMINISTRATION

Apply the ointment in the affected eye every 3 or 4 hours, depending on the severity of the condition.

Not more than 8 grams should be prescribed initially and the prescription should not be refilled without further evaluation as outlined in PRECAUTIONS above.

HOW SUPPLIED

Tube of 1/8 oz (3.5 g) with ophthalmic tip (NDC 0081-0197-86).

Caution: Federal law prohibits dispensing without a prescription.

Store at 15° to 25°C (59° to 77°F).

June 1995

Shown in Product Identification Guide, page 312

CORTISPORIN® ℞

[kor'ti-spor"in]

Ophthalmic Suspension Sterile

(neomycin and polymyxin B sulfates and hydrocortisone ophthalmic suspension, USP)

DESCRIPTION

CORTISPORIN Ophthalmic Suspension (neomycin and polymyxin B sulfates and hydrocortisone ophthalmic suspension) is a sterile antimicrobial and anti-inflammatory suspension for ophthalmic use. Each mL contains: neomycin sulfate equivalent to 3.5 mg neomycin base, polymyxin B sulfate equivalent to 10,000 polymyxin B units, and hydrocortisone 10 mg (1%). The vehicle contains thimerosal 0.001% (added as a preservative) and the inactive ingredients cetyl alcohol, glyceryl monostearate, mineral oil, polyoxyl 40 stearate, propylene gylcol, and Water for Injection. Sulfuric acid may be added to adjust pH.

Neomycin sulfate is the sulfate salt of neomycin B and C, which are produced by the growth of *Streptomyces fradiae* Waksman (Fam. Streptomycetaceae). It has a potency equivalent of not less than 600 μg of neomycin standard per mg, calculated on an anhydrous basis.

Polymyxin B sulfate is the sulfate salt of polymyxin B_1 and B_2, which are produced by the growth of *Bacillus polymyxa* (Prazmowski) Migula (Fam. Bacillaceae). It has a potency of not less than 6,000 polymyxin B units per mg, calculated on an anhydrous basis.

Hydrocortisone, 11β, 17, 21-trihydroxypregn-4-ene-3,20-dione, is an anti-inflammatory hormone.

CLINICAL PHARMACOLOGY

Corticosteroids suppress the inflammatory response to a variety of agents, and they probably delay or slow healing. Since corticosteroids may inhibit the body's defense mechanism against infection, concomitant antimicrobial drugs may be used when this inhibition is considered to be clinically significant in a particular case.

When a decision to administer both a corticosteroid and antimicrobials is made, the administration of such drugs in combination has the advantage of greater patient compliance and convenience, with the added assurance that the appropriate dosage of all drugs is administered. When each type of drug is in the same formulation, compatibility of ingredients is assured, and the correct volume of drug is delivered and retained.

The relative potency of corticosteroids depends on the molecular structure, concentration, and release from the vehicle.

Microbiology: The anti-infective components in CORTISPORIN Ophthalmic Suspension are included to provide action against specific organisms susceptible to it. Neo-

Continued on next page

Glaxo Wellcome—Cont.

mycin sulfate and polymyxin B sulfate are active in vitro against susceptible strains of the following microorganisms: *Staphylococcus aureus, Escherichia coli, Haemophilus influenzae, Klebsiella/Enterobacter* species, *Neisseria* species, and *Pseudomonas aeruginosa.* The product does not provide adequate coverage against *Serratia marscescens* and streptococci, including *Streptococcus pneumoniae* (see INDICATIONS AND USAGE).

INDICATIONS AND USAGE

CORTISPORIN Ophthalmic Suspension is indicated for steroid-responsive inflammatory ocular conditions for which a corticosteroid is indicated and where bacterial infection or a risk of bacterial infection exists.

Ocular corticosteroids are indicated in inflammatory conditions of the palpebral and bulbar conjunctiva, cornea, and anterior segment of the globe where the inherent risk of corticosteroid use in certain infective conjunctivitides is accepted to obtain a diminution in edema and inflammation. They are also indicated in chronic anterior uveitis and corneal injury from chemical, radiation, or thermal burns, or penetration of foreign bodies.

The use of a combination drug with an anti-infective component is indicated where the risk of infection is high or where there is an expectation that potentially dangerous numbers of bacteria will be present in the eye (see CLINICAL PHARMACOLOGY: Microbiology).

The particular anti-infective drugs in this product are active against the following common bacterial eye pathogens: *Staphylococcus aureus, Escherichia coli, Haemophilus influenzae, Klebsiella/Enterobacter* species, *Neisseria* species, and *Pseudomonas aeruginosa.*

The product does not provide adequate coverage against *Serratia marcescens* and streptococci, including *Streptococcus pneumoniae.*

CONTRAINDICATIONS

CORTISPORIN Ophthalmic Suspension is contraindicated in most viral diseases of the cornea and conjunctiva including: epithelial herpes simplex keratitis (dendritic keratitis), vaccinia and varicella, and also in mycobacterial infection of the eye and fungal diseases of ocular structures. CORTISPORIN Ophthalmic Suspension is also contraindicated in individuals who have shown hypersensitivity to any of its components. Hypersensitivity to the antibiotic component occurs at a higher rate than for other components.

WARNINGS

NOT FOR INJECTION INTO THE EYE. CORTISPORIN Ophthalmic Suspension should never be directly introduced into the anterior chamber of the eye.

Prolonged use of corticosteroids may result in ocular hypertension and/or glaucoma, with damage to the optic nerve, defects in visual acuity and fields of vision, and in posterior subcapsular cataract formation. Prolonged use may suppress the host response and thus increase the hazard of secondary ocular infections. In those diseases causing thinning of the cornea or sclera, perforations have been known to occur with the use of topical corticosteroids. In acute purulent conditions of the eye, corticosteroids may mask infection or enhance existing infection.

If these products are used for 10 days or longer, intraocular pressure should be routinely monitored even though it may be difficult in uncooperative patients. Corticosteroids should be used with caution in the presence of glaucoma.

The use of corticosteroids after cataract surgery may delay healing and increase the incidence of filtering blebs.

Use of ocular corticosteroids may prolong the course and may exacerbate the severity of many viral infections of the eye (including herpes simplex). Employment of corticosteroid medication in the treatment of herpes simplex requires great caution.

Topical antibiotics, particularly neomycin sulfate, may cause cutaneous sensitization. A precise incidence of hypersensitivity reactions (primarily skin rash) due to topical antibiotics is not known. The manifestations of sensitization to topical antibiotics are usually itching, reddening, and edema of the conjunctiva and eyelid. A sensitization reaction may manifest simply as a failure to heal. During long-term use of topical antibiotic products, periodic examination for such signs is advisable, and the patient should be told to discontinue the product if they are observed. Symptoms usually subside quickly on withdrawing the medication. Application of products containing these ingredients should be avoided for the patient thereafter (see PRECAUTIONS: General).

PRECAUTIONS

General: The initial prescription and renewal of the medication order beyond 20 milliliters should be made by a physician only after examination of the patient with the aid of magnification, such as slit lamp biomicroscopy and, where appropriate, fluorescein staining. If signs and symptoms fail to improve after 2 days, the patient should be re-evaluated.

The possibility of fungal infections of the cornea should be considered after prolonged corticosteroid dosing. Fungal cultures should be taken when appropriate.

If this product is used for 10 days or longer, intraocular pressure should be monitored (see WARNINGS).

There have been reports of bacterial keratitis associated with the use of topical ophthalmic products in multiple-dose containers which have been inadvertently contaminated by patients, most of whom had a concurrent corneal disease or a disruption of the ocular epithelial surface (see PRECAUTIONS: Information for Patients).

Allergic cross-reactions may occur which could prevent the use of any or all of the following antibiotics for the treatment of future infections: kanamycin, paromomycin, streptomycin, and possible gentamicin.

Information for Patients: Patients should be instructed to avoid allowing the tip of the dispensing container to contact the eye, eyelid, fingers, or any other surface. The use of this product by more than one person may spread infection.

Patients should also be instructed that ocular products, if handled improperly, can become contaminated by common bacteria known to cause ocular infections. Serious damage to the eye and subsequent loss of vision may result from using contaminated products (see PRECAUTIONS: General).

If the condition persists or gets worse, or if a rash or allergic reaction develops, the patient should be advised to stop use and consult a physician. Do not use this product if you are allergic to any of the listed ingredients.

Keep tightly closed when not in use. Keep out of reach of children.

Carcinogenesis, Mutagenesis, Impairment of Fertility: Long-term studies in animals to evaluate carcinogenic or mutagenic potential have not been conducted with polymyxin B sulfate. Treatment of cultured human lymphocytes in vitro with neomycin increased the frequency of chromosome aberrations at the highest concentrations (80 μg/mL) tested: however, the effects of neomycin on carcinogenesis and mutagenesis in humans are unknown.

Long-term studies in animals (rats, rabbits, mice) showed no evidence of carcinogenicity or mutagenicity attributable to oral administration of corticosteroids. Long-term animal studies have not been performed to evaluate the carcinogenic potential of topical corticosteroids. Studies to determine mutagenicity with hydrocortisone have revealed negative results.

Polymyxin B has been reported to impair the motility of equine sperm, but its effects on male or female fertility are unknown. Long-term animal studies have not been performed to evaluate the effect on fertility of topical corticosteroids.

Pregnancy: ***Teratogenic Effects:*** Pregnancy Category C. Corticosteroids have been found to be teratogenic in rabbits when applied topically at concentrations of 0.5% on days 6 to 18 of gestation and in mice when applied topically at a concentration of 15% on days 10 to 13 of gestation. There are no adequate and well-controlled studies in pregnant women. CORTISPORIN Ophthalmic Suspension should be used during pregnancy only if the potential benefit justifies the potential risk to the fetus.

Nursing Mothers: It is not known whether topical administration of corticosteroids could result in sufficient systemic absorption to produce detectable quantities in human milk. Systemically administered corticosteroids appear in human milk and could suppress growth, interfere with endogenous corticosteroid production, or cause other untoward effects. Because of the potential for serious adverse reactions in nursing infants from CORTISPORIN Ophthalmic Suspension, a decision should be made whether to discontinue nursing or to discontinue the drug, taking into account the importance of the drug to the mother.

Pediatric Use: Safety and effectiveness in pediatric patients have not been established.

ADVERSE REACTIONS

Adverse reactions have occurred with corticosteroid/anti-infective combination drugs which can be attributed to the corticosteroid component, the anti-infective component, or the combination. The exact incidence is not known.

Reactions occurring most often from the presence of the anti-infective ingredient are allergic sensitization reactions, including itching, swelling, and conjunctival erythema (see WARNINGS). More serious hypersensitivity reactions, including anaphylaxis, have been reported rarely.

The reactions due to the corticosteroid component in decreasing order of frequency are: elevation of intraocular pressure (IOP) with possible development of glaucoma, and infrequent optic nerve damage; posterior subcapsular cataract formation; and delayed wound healing.

Secondary Infection: The development of secondary infection has occurred after use of combinations containing corticosteroids and antimicrobials. Fungal and viral infections of the cornea are particularly prone to develop coincidentally with long-term applications of a corticosteroid. The possibility of fungal invasion must be considered in any persistent corneal ulceration where corticosteroid treatment has been used.

Local irritation on instillation has also been reported.

DOSAGE AND ADMINISTRATION

One or two drops in the affected eye every 3 or 4 hours, depending on the severity of the condition. The suspension may be used more frequently if necessary.

Not more than 20 milliliters should be prescribed initially and the prescription should not be refilled without further evaluation as outlined in PRECAUTIONS above.

SHAKE WELL BEFORE USING.

HOW SUPPLIED

Plastic DROP DOSE® dispenser bottle of 7.5 mL (NDC 0173-0193-02).

Caution: Federal law prohibits dispensing without a prescription.

Store at 15° to 25°C (59° to 77°F).

May 1996/RL-292

Shown in Product Identification Guide, page 312

CORTISPORIN® ℞

[*kor 'tĭ-spor "ĭn ō 'tĭk*]

Otic Solution Sterile

(neomycin and polymyxin B sulfates and hydrocortisone otic solution, USP)

DESCRIPTION

CORTISPORIN Otic Solution (neomycin and polymyxin B sulfates and hydrocortisone otic solution, USP) is a sterile antibacterial and anti-inflammatory solution for otic use. Each mL contains: neomycin sulfate equivalent to 3.5 mg neomycin base, polymyxin B sulfate equivalent to 10,000 polymyxin B units, and hydrocortisone 10 mg (1%). The vehicle contains potassium metabisulfite 0.1% (added as a preservative) and the inactive ingredients cupric sulfate, glycerin, hydrochloric acid, propylene glycol, and Water for Injection.

Neomycin sulfate is the sulfate salt of neomycin B and C, which are produced by the growth of *Streptomyces fradiae* Waksman (Fam. Streptomycetaceae). It has a potency equivalent of not less than 600 μg of neomycin standard per mg, calculated on an anhydrous basis.

Polymyxin B sulfate is the sulfate salt of polymyxin B_1 and B_2, which are produced by the growth of *Bacillus polymyxa* (Prazmowski) Migula (Fam. Bacillaceae). It has a potency of not less than 6,000 polymyxin B units per mg, calculated on an anhydrous basis.

Hydrocortisone, 11β, 17, 21-trihydroxypregn-4-ene-3, 20-dione, is an anti-inflammatory hormone.

CLINICAL PHARMACOLOGY

Corticoids suppress the inflammatory response to a variety of agents and they may delay healing. Since corticoids may inhibit the body's defense mechanism against infection, a concomitant antimicrobial drug may be used when this inhibition is considered to be clinically significant in a particular case.

The anti-infective components in the combination are included to provide action against specific organisms susceptible to them. Neomycin sulfate and polymyxin B sulfate together are considered active against the following microorganisms: *Staphylococcus aureus, Escherichia coli, Haemophilus influenzae, Klebsiella, Enterobacter* species, *Neisseria* species, and *Pseudomonas aeruginosa.* This product does not provide adequate coverage against *Serratia marcescens* and streptococci, including *Streptococcus pneumonia.*

The relative potency of corticosteroids depends on the molecular structure, concentration, and release from the vehicle.

INDICATIONS AND USAGE

For the treatment of superficial bacterial infections of the external auditory canal caused by organisms susceptible to the action of the antibiotics.

CONTRAINDICATIONS

This product is contraindicated in those individuals who have shown hypersensitivity to any of its components, and in herpes simplex, vaccinia, and varicella infections.

WARNINGS

This product should be used with care when the integrity of the tympanic membrane is in question because of the possibility of ototoxicity, and because stinging and burning may occur when this product gains access to the middle ear.

Neomycin sulfate may cause cutaneous sensitization. A precise incidence of hypersensitivity reactions (primarily skin rash) due to topical neomycin is not known.

When using neomycin-containing products to control secondary infection in the chronic dermatoses, such as chronic otitis externa or stasis dermatitis, it should be borne in mind that the skin in these conditions is more liable than is normal skin to become sensitized to many substances, including neomycin. The manifestation of sensitization to neomycin is usually a low-grade reddening with swelling, dry scaling, and itching; it may be manifest simply as a failure to heal. Periodic examination for such signs is advisable, and the

patient should be told to discontinue the product if they are observed. These symptoms regress quickly on withdrawing the medication. Neomycin-containing applications should be avoided for the patient thereafter.

Contains potassium metabisulfite, a sulfite that may cause allergic-type reactions including anaphylactic symptoms and life-threatening or less severe asthmatic episodes in certain susceptible people. The overall prevalence of sulfite sensitivity in the general population is unknown and probably low. Sulfite sensitivity is seen more frequently in asthmatic than in nonasthmatic people.

PRECAUTIONS

General: As with other antibiotic preparations, prolonged use may result in overgrowth of nonsusceptible organisms, including fungi.

If the infection is not improved after 1 week, cultures and susceptibility tests should be repeated to verify the identity of the organism and to determine whether therapy should be changed.

Treatment should not be continued for longer than 10 days.

Allergic cross-reactions may occur which could prevent the use of any or all of the following antibiotics for the treatment of future infections: kanamycin, paromomycin, streptomycin, and possibly gentamicin.

Information for Patients: Avoid contaminating the dropper with material from the ear, fingers, or other source. This caution is necessary if the sterility of the drops is to be preserved.

If sensitization or irritation occurs, discontinue use immediately and contact your physician.

Do not use in the eyes.

Laboratory Tests: Systemic effects of excessive levels of hydrocortisone may include a reduction in the number of circulating eosinophils and a decrease in urinary excretion of 17-hydroxycorticosteroids.

Carcinogenesis, Mutagenesis, Impairment of Fertility: Long-term studies in animals (rats, rabbits, mice) showed no evidence of carcinogenicity attributable to oral administration of corticosteroids.

Pregnancy: Teratogenic Effects: Pregnancy Category C. Corticosteroids have been shown to be teratogenic in rabbits when applied topically at concentrations of 0.5% on days 6 to 18 of gestation and in mice when applied topically at a concentration of 15% on days 10 to 13 of gestation. There are no adequate and well-controlled studies in pregnant women. Corticosteroids should be used during pregnancy only if the potential benefit justifies the potential risk to the fetus.

Nursing Mothers: Hydrocortisone appears in human milk following oral administration of the drug. Since systemic absorption of hydrocortisone may occur when applied topically, caution should be exercised when CORTISPORIN Otic Solution is used by a nursing woman.

Pediatric Use: See DOSAGE AND ADMINISTRATION.

ADVERSE REACTIONS

Neomycin occasionally causes skin sensitization. Ototoxicity and nephrotoxicity have also been reported (see WARNINGS). Adverse reactions have occurred with topical use of antibiotic combinations including neomycin and polymyxin B. Exact incidence figures are not available since no denominator of treated patients is available. The reaction occurring most often is allergic sensitization. In one clinical study, using a 20% neomycin patch, neomycin-induced allergic skin reactions occurred in two of 2,175 (0.09%) individuals in the general population.[1] In another study, the incidence was found to be approximately 1%.[2]

The following local adverse reactions have been reported with topical corticosteroids, especially under occlusive dressings: burning, itching, irritation, dryness, folliculitis, hypertrichosis, acneiform eruptions, hypopigmentation, perioral dermatitis, allergic contact dermatitis, maceration of the skin, secondary infection, skin atrophy, striae, and miliaria. Stinging and burning have been reported when this product has gained access to the middle ear.

DOSAGE AND ADMINISTRATION

The external auditory canal should be thoroughly cleansed and dried with a sterile cotton applicator.

For adults, four drops of the solution should be instilled into the affected ear 3 or 4 times daily. For infants and children, three drops are suggested because of the smaller capacity of the ear canal.

The patient should lie with the affected ear upward and then the drops should be instilled. This position should be maintained for 5 minutes to facilitate penetration of the drops into the ear canal. Repeat, if necessary, for the opposite ear.

If preferred, a cotton wick may be inserted into the canal and then the cotton may be saturated with the solution. This wick should be kept moist by adding further solution every 4 hours. The wick should be replaced at least once every 24 hours.

HOW SUPPLIED

Bottle of 10 mL with sterilized dropper (NDC 0173-0199-92). Store at 15° to 25°C (59° to 77°F).

Also Available: CORTISPORIN Otic Suspension bottle of 10 mL with sterilized dropper.

PEDIOTIC® Suspension bottle of 7.5 mL with sterilized dropper.

REFERENCES

1. Leyden JJ, Kligman AM. Contact dermatitis to neomycin sulfate. *JAMA.* 1979;242: 1276–1278.
2. Prystowsky SD, Allen AM, Smith RW, Nonomura JH, Odom RB, Akers WA. Allergic contact hypersensitivity to nickel, neomycin, ethylenediamine, and benzocaine: relationships between age, sex, history of exposure, and reactivity to standard patch tests and use tests in a general population. *Arch Dermatol.* 1979; 115: 959–962.

May 1996/RL-291

Shown in Product Identification Guide, page 312

CORTISPORIN® ℞

[*kor'tĭ-spor"ĭn ō'tĭk*]

Otic Suspension Sterile

(neomycin and polymyxin B sulfates and hydrocortisone otic suspension, USP)

DESCRIPTION

CORTISPORIN Otic Suspension (neomycin and polymyxin B sulfates and hydrocortisone otic suspension, USP) is a sterile antibacterial and anti-inflammatory suspension for otic use. Each mL contains: neomycin sulfate equivalent to 3.5 mg neomycin base, polymyxin B sulfate equivalent to 10,000 polymyxin B units, and hydrocortisone 10 mg (1%). The vehicle contains thimerosal 0.01% (added as a preservative) and the inactive ingredients cetyl alcohol, propylene glycol, polysorbate 80, and Water for Injection. Sulfuric acid may be added to adjust pH.

Neomycin sulfate is the sulfate salt of neomycin B and C, which are produced by the growth of *Streptomyces fradiae* Waksman (Fam. Streptomycetaceae). It has a potency equivalent of not less than 600 µg of neomycin standard per mg, calculated on an anhydrous basis.

Polymyxin B sulfate is the sulfate salt of polymyxin B_1 and B_2, which are produced by the growth of *Bacillus polymyxa* (Prazmowski) Migula (Fam. Bacillaceae). It has a potency of not less than 6,000 polymyxin B units per mg, calculated on an anhydrous basis.

Hydrocortisone, 11β,17,21-trihydroxypregn-4-ene-3,20-dione, is an anti-inflammatory hormone.

CLINICAL PHARMACOLOGY

Corticoids suppress the inflammatory response to a variety of agents and they may delay healing. Since corticoids may inhibit the body's defense mechanism against infection, a concomitant antimicrobial drug may be used when this inhibition is considered to be clinically significant in a particular case.

The anti-infective components in the combination are included to provide action against specific organisms susceptible to them. Neomycin sulfate and polymyxin B sulfate together are considered active against the following microorganisms: *Staphylococcus aureus, Escherichia coli, Haemophilus influenzae, Klebsiella-Enterobacter* species, *Neisseria* species, and *Pseudomonas aeruginosa*. This product does not provide adequate coverage against *Serratia marcescens* and streptococci, including *Streptococcus pneumonia*.

The relative potency of corticosteroids depends on the molecular structure, concentration, and release from the vehicle.

INDICATIONS AND USAGE

For the treatment of superficial bacterial infections of the external auditory canal caused by organisms susceptible to the action of the antibiotics, and for the treatment of infections of mastoidectomy and fenestration cavities caused by organisms susceptible to the antibiotics.

CONTRAINDICATIONS

This product is contraindicated in those individuals who have shown hypersensitivity to any of its components, and in herpes simplex, vaccinia, and varicella infections.

WARNINGS

This product should be used with care in cases of perforated eardrum and in long-standing cases of chronic otitis media because of the possibility of ototoxicity.

Neomycin sulfate may cause cutaneous sensitization. A precise incidence of hypersensitivity reactions (primarily skin rash) due to topical neomycin is not known.

When using neomycin-containing products to control secondary infection in the chronic dermatoses, such as chronic otitis externa or stasis dermatitis, it should be borne in mind that the skin in these conditions is more liable than is normal skin to become sensitized to many substances, including neomycin. The manifestation of sensitization to neomycin is usually a low-grade reddening with swelling, dry scaling, and itching; it may be manifest simply as a failure to heal. Periodic examination for such signs is advisable, and the patient should be told to discontinue the product if they are observed. These symptoms regress quickly on withdrawing the medication. Neomycin-containing applications should be avoided for the patient thereafter.

PRECAUTIONS

General: As with other antibiotic preparations, prolonged use may result in overgrowth of nonsusceptible organisms, including fungi.

If the infection is not improved after 1 week, cultures and susceptibility tests should be repeated to verify the identity of the organism and to determine whether therapy should be changed.

Treatment should not be continued for longer than 10 days.

Allergic cross-reactions may occur which could prevent the use of any or all of the following antibiotics for the treatment of future infections: kanamycin, paromomycin, streptomycin, and possibly gentamicin.

Information for Patients: Avoid contaminating the dropper with material from the ear, fingers, or other source. This caution is necessary if the sterility of the drops is to be preserved.

If sensitization or irritation occurs, discontinue use immediately and contact your physician.

Do not use in the eyes.

SHAKE WELL BEFORE USING.

Laboratory Tests: Systemic effects of excessive levels of hydrocortisone may include a reduction in the number of circulating eosinophils and a decrease in urinary excretion of 17-hydroxycorticosteroids.

Carcinogenesis, Mutagenesis, Impairment of Fertility: Long-term studies in animals (rats, rabbits, mice) showed no evidence of carcinogenicity attributable to oral administration of corticosteroids.

Pregnancy: Teratogenic Effects: Pregnancy Category C. Corticosteroids have been shown to be teratogenic in rabbits when applied topically at concentrations of 0.5% on days 6 to 18 of gestation and in mice when applied topically at a concentration of 15% on days 10 to 13 of gestation. There are no adequate and well-controlled studies in pregnant women. Corticosteroids should be used during pregnancy only if the potential benefit justifies the potential risk to the fetus.

Nursing Mothers: Hydrocortisone appears in human milk following oral administration of the drug. Since systemic absorption of hydrocortisone may occur when applied topically, caution should be exercised when CORTISPORIN Otic Suspension is used by a nursing woman.

Pediatric Use: See DOSAGE AND ADMINISTRATION.

ADVERSE REACTIONS

Neomycin occasionally causes skin sensitization. Ototoxicity and nephrotoxicity have also been reported (see WARNINGS section). Adverse reactions have occurred with topical use of antibiotic combinations including neomycin and polymyxin B. Exact incidence figures are not available since no denominator of treated patients is available. The reaction occurring most often is allergic sensitization. In one clinical study, using a 20% neomycin patch, neomycin-induced allergic skin reactions occurred in two of 2,175 (0.09%) individuals in the general population.[1] In another study, the incidence was found to be approximately 1%.[2]

The following local adverse reactions have been reported with topical corticosteroids, especially under occlusive dressings: burning, itching, irritation, dryness, folliculitis, hypertrichosis, acneiform eruptions, hypopigmentation, perioral dermatitis, allergic contact dermatitis, maceration of the skin, secondary infection, skin atrophy, striae, and miliaria. Stinging and burning have been reported rarely when this drug has gained access to the middle ear.

DOSAGE AND ADMINISTRATION

The external auditory canal should be thoroughly cleansed and dried with a sterile cotton applicator.

For adults, 4 drops of the suspension should be instilled into the affected ear 3 or 4 times daily.

For infants and children, 3 drops are suggested because of the smaller capacity of the ear canal.

The patient should lie with the affected ear upward and then the drops should be instilled. This position should be maintained for 5 minutes to facilitate penetration of the drops into the ear canal. Repeat, if necessary, for the opposite ear.

If preferred, a cotton wick may be inserted into the canal and then the cotton may be saturated with the suspension. This wick should be kept moist by adding further suspension every 4 hours. The wick should be replaced at least once every 24 hours.

SHAKE WELL BEFORE USING.

HOW SUPPLIED

Bottle of 10 mL with sterilized dropper. (NDC 0173-0198-92). Store at 15° to 25°C (59° to 77°F).

Also Available: CORTISPORIN Otic Solution bottle of 10 mL with sterilized dropper.

Continued on next page

Glaxo Wellcome—Cont.

PEDIOTIC® Suspension bottle of 7.5 mL with sterilized dropper.

REFERENCES

1. Leyden JJ, Kligman AM. Contact dermatitis to neomycin sulfate. *JAMA.* 1979;242:1276–1278.
2. Prystowsky SD, Allen AM, Smith RW, Nonomura JH, Odom RB, Akers WA. Allergic contact hypersensitivity to nickel, neomycin, ethylenediamine, and benzocaine: relationship between age, sex, history of exposure, and reactivity to standard patch tests and use tests in a general population. *Arch Dermatol.* 1979;115:959–962.

February 1996/RL-268

Shown in Product Identification Guide, page 312

CUTIVATE® ℞

[kyōōt 'ə-vāt ″]
(fluticasone propionate cream)
Cream, 0.05%
For Dermatologic Use Only—
Not for Ophthalmic Use.

DESCRIPTION

Cutivate® Cream, 0.05% contains fluticasone propionate [(6α,11β,16α,17α)-6,9,-difluoro-11-hydroxy-16-methyl-3-oxo-17-(1-oxopropoxy) androsta-1,4-diene-17-carbothioic acid, S-fluoromethyl ester], a synthetic fluorinated corticosteroid, for topical dermatologic use. The topical corticosteroids constitute a class of primarily synthetic steroids used as anti-inflammatory and antipruritic agents.
Chemically, fluticasone propionate is $C_{25}H_{31}F_3O_5S$.
Fluticasone propionate has a molecular weight of 500.6. It is a white to off-white powder and is insoluble in water.
Each gram of Cutivate Cream, 0.05% contains fluticasone propionate 0.5 mg in a base of propylene glycol, mineral oil, cetostearyl alcohol, Ceteth-20, isopropyl myristate, dibasic sodium phosphate, citric acid, purified water, and imidurea as preservative.

CLINICAL PHARMACOLOGY

Like other topical corticosteroids, fluticasone propionate has anti-inflammatory, antipruritic, and vasoconstrictive properties. The mechanism of the anti-inflammatory activity of the topical steroids, in general, is unclear. However, corticosteroids are thought to act by the induction of phospholipase A_2 inhibitory proteins, collectively called lipocortins. It is postulated that these proteins control the biosynthesis of potent mediators of inflammation such as prostaglandins and leukotrienes by inhibiting the release of their common precursor, arachidonic acid, which is released from membrane phospholipids by phospholipase A_2.
Pharmacokinetics: The extent of percutaneous absorption of topical corticosteroids is determined by many factors, including the vehicle and the integrity of the epidermal barrier. Occlusive dressing with hydrocortisone for up to 24 hours has not been demonstrated to increase penetration; however, occlusion of hydrocortisone for 96 hours markedly enhances penetration. Topical corticosteroids can be absorbed from normal intact skin, while inflammation and/or other disease processes in the skin increase percutaneous absorption.
Studies performed with Cutivate® (fluticasone propionate cream) Cream, 0.05% indicate that it is in the medium range of potency as compared with other topical corticosteroids.

INDICATIONS AND USAGE

Cutivate® (fluticasone propionate cream) Cream, 0.05% is a medium potency corticosteroid indicated for the relief of the inflammatory and pruritic manifestations of corticosteroid-responsive dermatoses.

CONTRAINDICATIONS

Fluticasone propionate cream, 0.05% is contraindicated in those patients with a history of hypersensitivity to any of the components of the preparation.

PRECAUTIONS

General: Systemic absorption of topical corticosteroids can produce reversible hypothalamic-pituitary-adrenal (HPA) axis suppression with the potential for glucocorticosteroid insufficiency after withdrawal from treatment. Manifestations of Cushing's syndrome, hyperglycemia, and glucosuria can also be produced in some patients by systemic absorption of topical corticosteroids while on therapy.
Patients receiving a large dose of a potent topical steroid applied to a large surface area or under an occlusive dressing should be evaluated periodically for evidence of HPA axis suppression. This may be done by using the ACTH stimulation, A.M. plasma cortisol, and urinary free cortisol tests.
Fluticasone propionate cream, 0.05% produced HPA axis suppression within 7 days when used at a dose of 30 g per day in diseased patients. In a study of the effects of fluticasone propionate cream, 0.05% on the HPA axis, a total of 30 g per day was used in two applications daily for 7 days to six patients with psoriasis or atopic dermatitis involving at least 30% of the body surface. One patient developed evidence of adrenal suppression after 6 days of treatment with a below normal plasma cortisol level that returned to low normal levels the following day. Another patient developed a 60% decrease (although never below normal) in the plasma cortisol level from pretreatment values after 2 days of treatment. This suppression persisted at this level for 48 hours before recovering by day 6 of treatment. The results of this study indicate that fluticasone propionate cream, 0.05% may be able to suppress the HPA axis within a few days with a dose of 30 g per day.
If HPA axis suppression is noted, an attempt should be made to withdraw the drug, to reduce the frequency of application, or to substitute a less potent steroid. Recovery of HPA axis function is generally prompt and complete upon discontinuation of topical corticosteroids. Infrequently, signs and symptoms of glucocorticosteroid insufficiency may occur that require supplemental systemic corticosteroids. For information on systemic supplementation, see prescribing information for those products.
Children may be more susceptible to systemic toxicity from equivalent doses due to their larger skin surface to body mass ratios (see PRECAUTIONS: Pediatric Use).
If irritation develops, fluticasone propionate cream, 0.05% should be discontinued and appropriate therapy instituted. Allergic contact dermatitis with corticosteroids is usually diagnosed by observing *failure to heal* rather than noting a clinical exacerbation as with most topical products not containing corticosteroids. Such an observation should be corroborated with appropriate diagnostic patch testing.
If concomitant skin infections are present or develop, an appropriate antifungal or antibacterial agent should be used. If a favorable response does not occur promptly, use of fluticasone propionate cream, 0.05% should be discontinued until the infection has been adequately controlled.
Fluticasone propionate cream, 0.05% should not be used in the treatment of rosacea and perioral dermatitis.
Information for Patients: Patients using topical corticosteroids should receive the following information and instructions:
1. This medication is to be used as directed by the physician. It is for external use only. Avoid contact with the eyes.
2. This medication should not be used for any disorder other than that for which it was prescribed.
3. The treated skin area should not be bandaged or otherwise covered or wrapped so as to be occlusive unless directed by the physician.
4. Patients should report to their physician any signs of local adverse reactions.

Laboratory Tests: The following tests may be helpful in evaluating patients for HPA axis suppression:
ACTH stimulation test
A.M. plasma cortisol test
Urinary free cortisol test
Carcinogenesis, Mutagenesis, Impairment of Fertility: Long-term animal studies have not been performed to evaluate the carcinogenic potential of fluticasone propionate.
Fluticasone propionate was not mutagenic in the standard Ames test, *E. coli* fluctuation test, *S. cerevisiae* gene conversion test, or Chinese Hamster ovarian cell assay. It was not clastogenic in mouse micronucleus or cultured human lymphocyte tests.
In a fertility and general reproductive performance study in rats, fluticasone propionate administered subcutaneously to females at up to 50 μg/kg per day and to males at up to 100 μg/kg per day (later reduced to 50 μg/kg per day) had no effect upon mating performance or fertility. These doses are approximately 15 and 30 times, respectively, the human systemic exposure following use of the recommended human topical dose of fluticasone propionate cream, 0.05%, assuming human percutaneous absorption of approximately 3% and the use in a 70-kg person of 15 g per day.
Pregnancy: ***Teratogenic Effects: Pregnancy Category C:*** Corticosteroids have been shown to be teratogenic in laboratory animals when administered systemically at relatively low dosage levels. The more potent corticosteroids have been shown to be teratogenic after dermal application in laboratory animals. Teratology studies in the mouse demonstrated fluticasone propionate to be teratogenic (cleft palate) when administered subcutaneously in doses of 45 μg/kg per day and 150 μg/kg per day. This dose is approximately 14 and 45 times, respectively, the human topical dose of fluticasone propionate cream, 0.05%. There are no adequate and well-controlled studies in pregnant women. Fluticasone propionate cream, 0.05% should be used during pregnancy only if the potential benefit justifies the potential risk to the fetus.
Nursing Mothers: Systemically administered corticosteroids appear in human milk and could suppress growth, interfere with endogenous corticosteroid production, or cause other untoward effects. It is not known whether topical administration of corticosteroids could result in sufficient systemic absorption to produce detectable quantities in human milk. Because many drugs are excreted in human milk, caution should be exercised when fluticasone propionate cream, 0.05% is administered to a nursing woman.
Pediatric Use: Safety and effectiveness in children and infants have not been established. Because of a higher ratio of skin surface area to body mass, children are at a greater risk than adults of HPA axis suppression when they are treated with topical corticosteroids. They are therefore also at greater risk of glucocorticosteroid insufficiency after withdrawal of treatment and of Cushing's syndrome while on treatment. Adverse effects including striae have been reported with inappropriate use of topical corticosteroids in infants and children (see PRECAUTIONS).
HPA axis suppression, Cushing's syndrome, and intracranial hypertension have been reported in children receiving topical corticosteroids. Manifestations of adrenal suppression in children include linear growth retardation, delayed weight gain, low plasma cortisol levels, and absence of response to ACTH stimulation. Manifestations of intracranial hypertension include bulging fontanelles, headaches, and bilateral papilledema.

ADVERSE REACTIONS

In controlled clinical trials, the total incidence of adverse reactions associated with the use of fluticasone propionate cream, 0.05% was approximately 4%. These adverse reactions were mild, usually self-limiting, and consisted primarily of pruritus, dryness, numbness of fingers, and burning. These events occurred in 2.9%, 1.2%, 1.0%, and 0.6% of patients, respectively.
The following additional local adverse reactions have been reported infrequently with other topical corticosteroids, and they may occur more frequently with the use of occlusive dressings, especially with higher potency corticosteroids. These reactions are listed in an approximately decreasing order of occurrence: irritation, folliculitis, acneiform eruptions, hypopigmentation, perioral dermatitis, allergic contact dermatitis, secondary infection, skin atrophy, striae, and miliaria. Also, there are reports of the development of pustular psoriasis from chronic plaque psoriasis following reduction or discontinuation of potent topical corticosteroid products.

OVERDOSAGE

Topically applied fluticasone propionate cream, 0.05% can be absorbed in sufficient amounts to produce systemic effects (see PRECAUTIONS).

DOSAGE AND ADMINISTRATION

Apply a thin film of Cutivate® (fluticasone propionate cream) Cream, 0.05% to the affected skin areas twice daily. Rub in gently.

HOW SUPPLIED

Cutivate® (fluticasone propionate cream) Cream, 0.05% is supplied in 15-g (NDC 0173-0430-00), 30-g (NDC 0173-0430-01), and 60-g (NDC 0173-0430-02) tubes.
Store between 2° and 30°C (36° and 86°F).
February 1995/RL-181

Shown in Product Identification Guide, page 312

CUTIVATE® ℞

[kyoot 'ə-vāt ″]
(fluticasone propionate ointment)
Ointment, 0.005%
For Dermatologic Use Only—
Not for Ophthalmic Use.

DESCRIPTION

Cutivate® Ointment, 0.005% contains fluticasone propionate [(6α,11β,16α,17α)-6,9,-difluoro-11-hydroxy-16-methyl-3-oxo-17-(1-oxopropoxy) androsta-1,4-diene-17-carbothioic acid, S-fluoromethyl ester], a synthetic fluorinated corticosteroid, for topical dermatologic use. The topical corticosteroids constitute a class of primarily synthetic steroids used as anti-inflammatory and antipruritic agents.
Chemically, fluticasone propionate is $C_{25}H_{31}F_3O_5S$.
Fluticasone propionate has a molecular weight of 500.6. It is a white to off-white powder and is insoluble in water.
Each gram of Cutivate Ointment contains fluticasone propionate 0.05 mg in a base of propylene glycol, sorbitan sesquioleate, microcrystalline wax, and liquid paraffin.

CLINICAL PHARMACOLOGY

Like other topical corticosteroids, fluticasone propionate has anti-inflammatory, antipruritic, and vasoconstrictive properties. The mechanism of the anti-inflammatory activity of the topical steroids, in general, is unclear. However, corticosteroids are thought to act by the induction of phospholipase A_2 inhibitory proteins, collectively called lipocortins. It is postulated that these proteins control the biosynthesis of potent mediators of inflammation such as prostaglandins and leukotrienes by inhibiting the release of their common precursor, arachidonic acid. Archidonic acid is released from membrane phospholipids by phospholipase A_2.
Pharmacokinetics: The extent of percutaneous absorption of topical corticosteroids is determined by many factors, in-

cluding the vehicle and the integrity of the epidermal barrier. Occlusive dressing with hydrocortisone for up to 24 hours has not been demonstrated to increase penetration; however, occlusion of hydrocortisone for 96 hours markedly enhances penetration. Topical corticosteroids can be absorbed from normal intact skin. Inflammation and/or other disease processes in the skin increase percutaneous absorption.
Studies performed with Cutivate® (fluticasone propionate ointment) Ointment indicate that it is in the medium range of potency as compared with other topical corticosteroids.

INDICATIONS AND USAGE

Cutivate® (fluticasone propionate ointment) Ointment is a medium potency corticosteroid indicated for the relief of the inflammatory and pruritic manifestations of corticosteroid-responsive dermatoses.

CONTRAINDICATIONS

Cutivate® (fluticasone propionate ointment) Ointment is contraindicated in those patients with a history of hypersensitivity to any of the components of the preparation.

PRECAUTIONS

General: Systemic absorption of topical corticosteroids can produce reversible hypothalamic-pituitary-adrenal (HPA) axis suppression with the potential for glucocorticosteroid insufficiency after withdrawal from treatment. Manifestations of Cushing's syndrome, hyperglycemia, and glucosuria can also be produced in some patients by systemic absorption of topical corticosteroids while on treatment.
Patients applying a topical steroid to a large surface area or to areas under occlusion should be evaluated periodically for evidence of HPA axis suppression. This may be done by using the ACTH stimulation, A.M. plasma cortisol, and urinary free cortisol tests.
Fluticasone propionate ointment, 0.05% (a concentration 10 times that of fluticasone propionate ointment, 0.005%) suppressed 24-hour urinary free cortical levels in two of six patients when used at a dose of 30 g per day for a week in patients with psoriasis or atopic eczema. In a second study, fluticasone propionate ointment, 0.05% caused depression of A.M. plasma cortisol levels in 3 of 12 normal volunteers when applied at doses of 50 g per day for 21 days. Morning plasma levels returned to normal levels within the first week upon discontinuation of fluticasone propionate. In this study there was no corresponding decrease in 24-hour urinary free cortisol levels.
If HPA axis suppression is noted, an attempt should be made to withdraw the drug, to reduce the frequency of application, or to substitute a less potent corticosteroid. Recovery of HPA axis function is generally prompt upon discontinuation of topical corticosteroids. Infrequently, signs and symptoms of glucocorticosteroid insufficiency may occur, requiring supplemental systemic corticosteroids. For information on systemic supplementation, see prescribing information for those products.
Children may be more susceptible to systemic toxicity from equivalent doses due to their larger skin surface to body mass ratios (see PRECAUTIONS: Pediatric Use).
If irritation develops, Cutivate® (fluticasone propionate ointment) Ointment should be discontinued and appropriate therapy instituted. Allergic contact dermatitis with corticosteroids is usually diagnosed by observing failure to heal rather than noting a clinical exacerbation as with most topical products not containing corticosteroids. Such an observation should be corroborated with appropriate diagnostic patch testing.
If concomitant skin infections are present or develop, an appropriate antifungal or antibacterial agent should be used. If a favorable response does not occur promptly, use of Cutivate Ointment should be discontinued until the infection has been adequately controlled.
Cutivate Ointment should not be used in the treatment of preexisting skin atrophy and should not be used where infection is present at the treatment site. Cutivate Ointment should not be used in the treatment of rosacea and perioral dermatitis.
Information for Patients: Patients using topical corticosteroids should receive the following information and instructions:

1. This medication is to be used as directed by the physician. It is for external use only. Avoid contact with the eyes.
2. This medication should not be used for any disorder other than that for which it was prescribed.
3. The treated skin area should not be bandaged or otherwise covered or wrapped so as to be occlusive unless directed by the physician.
4. Patients should report to their physician any signs of local adverse reactions.

Laboratory Tests: The following tests may be helpful in evaluating patients for HPA axis suppression:
ACTH stimulation test
A.M. plasma cortisol test
Urinary free cortisol test
Carcinogenesis, Mutagenesis, and Impairment of Fertility: Two 18-month studies were performed in mice to evaluate the carcinogenic potential of fluticasone propionate when given topically (as an 0.05% ointment) and orally, No evidence of carcinogenicity was found in either study.
Fluticasone propionate was not mutagenic in the standard Ames test, *E. coli* fluctuation test, *S. cerevisiae* gene conversion test, or Chinese Hamster ovarian cell assay. It was not clastogenic in mouse micronucleus or cultured human lymphocyte tests.
In a fertility and general reproductive performance study in rats, fluticasone propionate administered subcutaneously to females at up to 50 μg/kg per day and to males at up to 100 μg/kg per day (later reduced to 50 μg/kg per day) had no effect upon mating performance or fertility. These doses are approximately 150 and 300 times, respectively, the human systemic exposure following use of the recommended human topical dose of fluticasone propionate ointment, 0.005%, assuming human percutaneous absorption of approximately 3% and the use in a 70-kg person of 15 g per day.
Pregnancy: ***Teratogenic Effects: Pregnancy Category C:*** Corticosteroids have been shown to be teratogenic in laboratory animals when administered systemically at relatively low dosage levels. Some corticosteroids have been shown to be teratogenic after dermal application in laboratory animals. Teratology studies in the mouse demonstrated fluticasone propionate to be teratogenic (cleft palate) when administered subcutaneously in doses of 45 μg/kg per day and 150 μg/kg per day. This dose is approximately 140 and 450 times, respectively, the human topical dose of fluticasone propionate ointment, 0.005%. There are no adequate and well-controlled studies in pregnant women. Cutivate Ointment should be used during pregnancy only if the potential benefit justifies the potential risk to the fetus.
Nursing Mothers: Systemically administered corticosteroids appear in human milk and could suppress growth, interfere with endogenous corticosteroid production, or cause other untoward effects. It is not known whether topical administration of corticosteroids could result in sufficient systemic absorption to produce detectable quantities in human milk. Because many drugs are excreted in human milk, caution should be exercised when Cutivate Ointment is administered to a nursing woman.
Pediatric Use: Safety and effectiveness in pediatric patients have not been established. Because of a higher ratio of skin surface area to body mass, pediatric patients are at a greater risk than adults of HPA axis suppression and Cushing's syndrome when they are treated with topical corticosteroids. They are therefore also at greater risk of adrenal insufficiency during or after withdrawal of treatment. Adverse effects including striae have been reported with inappropriate use of topical corticosteroids in pediatric patients.
HPA axis suppression, Cushing's syndrome, linear growth retardation, delayed weight gain, and intracranial hypertension have been reported in pediatric patients receiving topical corticosteroids. Manifestations of adrenal suppression in pediatric patients include low plasma cortisol levels and an absence of response to ACTH stimulation. Manifestations of intracranial hypertension include bulging fontanelles, headaches, and bilateral papilledema.

ADVERSE REACTIONS

In controlled clinical trials, the total incidence of adverse reactions associated with the use of Cutivate® (fluticasone propionate ointment) Ointment was approximately 4%. These adverse reactions were usually mild, self-limiting, and consisted primarily of pruritus, burning, hypertrichosis, increased erythema, hives, irritation, and lightheadedness. Each of these events occurred individually in less than 1% of patients.
The following additional local adverse reactions have been reported infrequently with topical corticosteroids, including fluticasone propionate, and they may occur more frequently with the use of occlusive dressings and higher potency corticosteroids. These reactions are listed in an approximately decreasing order of occurrence: dryness, folliculitis, acneiform eruptions, hypopigmentation, perioral dermatitis, allergic contact dermatitis, secondary infection, skin atrophy, striae, and miliaria. Also, there are reports of the development of pustular psoriasis from chronic plaque psoriasis following reduction or discontinuation of potent topical corticosteroid products.

OVERDOSAGE

Topically applied Cutivate® (fluticasone propionate ointment) Ointment can be absorbed in sufficient amounts to produce systemic effects (see PRECAUTIONS).

DOSAGE AND ADMINISTRATION

Apply a thin film of Cutivate® (fluticasone propionate ointment) Ointment to the affected skin areas twice daily. Rub in gently.

HOW SUPPLIED

Cutivate® (fluticasone propionate ointment) Ointment, 0.005% is supplied in 15-g (NDC 0173-0431-00), 30-g (NDC 0173-0431-01), and 60-g (NDC 0173-0431-02) tubes.
Store between 2° and 30°C (36° and 86°F).
August 1995/ RL-220
Shown in Product Identification Guide, page 312

DIGIBIND® ℞
[*dī'gi-bīnd*]
DIGOXIN IMMUNE FAB (OVINE)

DESCRIPTION

DIGIBIND, Digoxin Immune Fab (Ovine), is a sterile lyophilized powder of antigen binding fragments (Fab) derived from specific antidigoxin antibodies raised in sheep. Production of antibodies specific for digoxin involves conjugation of digoxin as a hapten to human albumin. Sheep are immunized with this material to produce antibodies specific for the antigenic determinants of the digoxin molecule. The antibody is then papain digested and digoxin-specific Fab fragments of the antibody are isolated and purified by affinity chromatography. These antibody fragments have a molecular weight of approximately 46,200.
Each vial, which will bind approximately 0.5 mg of digoxin (or digitoxin), contains 38 mg of digoxin-specific Fab fragments derived from sheep plus 75 mg of sorbitol as a stabilizer and 28 mg of sodium chloride. The vial contains no preservatives.
DIGIBIND is administered by intravenous injection after reconstitution with Sterile Water for Injection (4 mL per vial).

CLINICAL PHARMACOLOGY

After intravenous injection of Digoxin Immune Fab (Ovine) in the baboon, digoxin-specific Fab fragments are excreted in the urine with a biological half-life of about 9 to 13 hours.[1] In humans with normal renal function the half-life appears to be 15 to 20 hours.[2] Experimental studies in animals indicate that these antibody fragments have a large volume of distribution in the extracellular space, unlike whole antibody which distributes in a space only about twice the plasma volume.[1] Ordinarily, following administration of DIGIBIND, improvement in signs and symptoms of digitalis intoxication begins within one-half hour or less.[2,3,4,5]
The affinity of DIGIBIND for digoxin is in the range of 10^9 to 10^{11} M^{-1}, which is greater than the affinity of digoxin for (sodium, potassium) ATPase, the presumed receptor for its toxic effects. The affinity of DIGIBIND for digitoxin is about 10^8 to 10^9 M^{-1}.
DIGIBIND binds molecules of digoxin, making them unavailable for binding at their site of action on cells in the body. The Fab fragment-digoxin complex accumulates in the blood, from which it is excreted by the kidney. The net effect is to shift the equilibrium away from binding of digoxin to its receptors in the body, thereby reversing its effects.

INDICATIONS AND USAGE

DIGIBIND, Digoxin Immune Fab (Ovine), is indicated for treatment of potentially life-threatening digoxin intoxication.[3] Although designed specifically to treat life-threatening digoxin overdose, it has also been used successfully to treat life-threatening digitoxin overdose.[3] Since human experience is limited and the consequences of repeated exposures are unknown, DIGIBIND is not indicated for milder cases of digitalis toxicity.
Manifestations of life-threatening toxicity include severe ventricular arrhythmias such as ventricular tachycardia or ventricular fibrillation, or progressive bradyarrhythmias such as severe sinus bradycardia or second or third degree heart block not responsive to atropine.
Ingestion of more than 10 mg of digoxin in previously healthy adults or 4 mg of digoxin in previously healthy children, or ingestion causing steady-state serum concentrations greater than 10 ng/mL, often results in cardiac arrest. Digitalis-induced progressive elevation of the serum potassium concentration also suggests imminent cardiac arrest. If the potassium concentration exceeds 5 mEq/L in the setting of severe digitalis intoxication, DIGIBIND therapy is indicated.

CONTRAINDICATIONS

There are no known contraindications to the use of DIGIBIND.

WARNINGS

Suicidal ingestion often involves more than one drug; thus, toxicity from other drugs should not be overlooked.
One should consider the possibility of anaphylactic, hypersensitivity, or febrile reactions. If an anaphylactoid reaction occurs, the drug infusion should be discontinued and appropriate therapy initiated using aminophylline, oxygen, volume expansion, diphenhydramine, corticosteroids, and airway management as indicated. The need for epinephrine should be balanced against its potential risk in the setting of digitalis toxicity.
Since the Fab fragment of the antibody lacks the antigenic determinants of the Fc fragment, it should pose less of an

Continued on next page

Glaxo Wellcome—Cont.

immunogenic threat to patients than does an intact immunoglobulin molecule. Patients with known allergies would be particularly at risk, as would individuals who have previously received antibodies or Fab fragments raised in sheep. Papain is used to cleave the whole antibody into Fab and Fc fragments, and traces of papain or inactivated papain residues may be present in DIGIBIND. Patients with allergies to papain, chymopapain, or other papaya extracts also may be particularly at risk.

Skin testing for allergy was performed during the clinical investigation of DIGIBIND. Only one patient developed erythema at the site of skin testing, with no accompanying wheal reaction; this individual had no adverse reaction to systemic treatment with DIGIBIND. Since allergy testing can delay urgently needed therapy, it is not routinely required before treatment of life-threatening digitalis toxicity with DIGIBIND.

Skin testing may be appropriate for high risk individuals, especially patients with known allergies or those previously treated with Digoxin Immune Fab (Ovine). The intradermal skin test can be performed by: 1. Diluting 0.1 mL of reconstituted DIGIBIND (9.5 mg/mL) in 9.9 mL sterile isotonic saline (1:100 dilution, 95 μg/mL). 2. Injecting 0.1 mL of the 1:100 dilution (95 μg) intradermally and observing for an urticarial wheal surrounded by a zone of erythema. The test should be read at 20 minutes.

The scratch test procedure is performed by placing one drop of a 1:100 dilution of DIGIBIND on the skin and then making a $^1/_4$-inch scratch through the drop with a sterile needle. The scratch site is inspected at 20 minutes for an urticarial wheal surrounded by erythema.

If skin testing causes a systemic reaction, a tourniquet should be applied above the site of testing and measures to treat anaphylaxis should be instituted. Further administration of DIGIBIND should be avoided unless its use is absolutely essential, in which case the patient should be pretreated with corticosteroids and diphenhydramine. The physician should be prepared to treat anaphylaxis.

PRECAUTIONS

General: Standard therapy for digitalis intoxication includes withdrawal of the drug and correction of factors that may contribute to toxicity, such as electrolyte disturbances, hypoxia, acid-base disturbances and agents such as catecholamines. Also, treatment of arrhythmias may include judicious potassium supplements, lidocaine, phenytoin, procainamide and/or propranolol; treatment of sinus bradycardia or atrioventricular block may involve atropine or pacemaker insertion. Massive digitalis intoxication can cause hyperkalemia; administration of potassium supplements in the setting of massive intoxication may be hazardous (see Laboratory Tests). After treatment with DIGIBIND, the serum potassium concentration may drop rapidly[2] and must be monitored frequently, especially over the first several hours after DIGIBIND is given (see Laboratory Tests).

The elimination half-life in the setting of renal failure has not been clearly defined. Patients with renal dysfunction have been successfully treated with DIGIBIND.[4] There is no evidence to suggest the time-course of therapeutic effect is any different in these patients than in patients with normal renal function, but excretion of the Fab fragment-digoxin complex from the body is probably delayed. In patients who are functionally anephric, one would anticipate failure to clear the Fab fragment-digoxin complex from the blood by glomerular filtration and renal excretion. Whether failure to eliminate the Fab fragment-digoxin complex in severe renal failure can lead to reintoxication following release of newly unbound digoxin into the blood is uncertain. Such patients should be monitored for a prolonged period for possible recurrence of digitalis toxicity.

Patients with intrinsically poor cardiac function may deteriorate from withdrawal of the inotropic action of digoxin. Studies in animals have shown that the reversal of inotropic effect is relatively gradual, occurring over hours. When needed, additional support can be provided by use of intravenous inotropes, such as dopamine or dobutamine, or vasodilators. One must be careful in using catecholamines not to aggravate digitalis toxic rhythm disturbances. Clearly, other types of digitalis glycosides should not be used in this setting. Redigitalization should be postponed, if possible, until the Fab fragments have been eliminated from the body, which may require several days. Patients with impaired renal function may require a week or longer.

Laboratory Tests: DIGIBIND will interfere with digitalis immunoassay measurements.[6] Thus, the standard serum digoxin concentration measurement can be clinically misleading until the Fab fragment is eliminated from the body. Serum digoxin or digitoxin concentration should be obtained before DIGIBIND administration if at all possible. These measurements may be difficult to interpret if drawn soon after the last digitalis dose, since at least 6 to 8 hours are required for equilibration of digoxin between serum and tissue. Patients should be closely monitored, including temperature, blood pressure, electrocardiogram and potassium concentration, during and after administration of DIGIBIND. The total serum digoxin concentration may rise precipitously following administration of DIGIBIND but this will be almost entirely bound to the Fab fragment and therefore not able to react with receptors in the body.

Potassium concentrations should be followed carefully. Severe digitalis intoxication can cause life-threatening elevation in serum potassium concentration by shifting potassium from inside to outside the cell. The elevation in serum potassium concentration can lead to increased renal excretion of potassium. Thus, these patients may have hyperkalemia with a total body deficit of potassium. When the effect of digitalis is reversed by DIGIBIND, potassium shifts back inside the cell, with a resulting decline in serum potassium concentration.[4] Hypokalemia may thus develop rapidly. For these reasons, serum potassium concentration should be monitored repeatedly, especially over the first several hours after DIGIBIND is given, and cautiously treated when necessary.

Carcinogenesis, Mutagenesis, Impairment of Fertility: There have been no long-term studies performed in animals to evaluate carcinogenic potential.

Pregnancy: Pregnancy Category C. Animal reproduction studies have not been conducted with DIGIBIND. It is also not known whether DIGIBIND can cause fetal harm when administered to a pregnant woman or can affect reproduction capacity. DIGIBIND should be given to a pregnant woman only if clearly needed.

Nursing Mothers: It is not known whether this drug is excreted in human milk. Because many drugs are excreted in human milk, caution should be exercised when DIGIBIND is administered to a nursing woman.

Pediatric Use: DIGIBIND has been successfully used in infants with no apparent adverse sequelae. As in all other circumstances, use of this drug in infants should be based on careful consideration of the benefits of the drug balanced against the potential risk involved.

ADVERSE REACTIONS

Allergic reactions to DIGIBIND have been reported rarely. Patients with a history of allergy, especially to antibiotics, appear to be at particular risk (see WARNINGS). In a few instances, low cardiac output states and congestive heart failure could have been exacerbated by withdrawal of the inotropic effects of digitalis. Hypokalemia may occur from reactivation of (sodium, potassium) ATPase (see Laboratory Tests). Patients with atrial fibrillation may develop a rapid ventricular response from withdrawal of the effects of digitalis on the atrioventricular node.[4]

DOSAGE AND ADMINISTRATION

GENERAL GUIDELINES:

The dosage of DIGIBIND varies according to the amount of digoxin (or digitoxin) to be neutralized. The average dose used during clinical testing was 10 vials.

Dosage for Acute Ingestion of Unknown Amount: Twenty (20) vials (760 mg) of DIGIBIND is adequate to treat most life-threatening ingestions in both **adults and children.** However, in children it is important to monitor for volume overload. In general, a large DIGIBIND dose has a faster onset of effect but may enhance the possibility of a febrile reaction. The physician may consider administering 10 vials, observing the patient's response, and following with an additional 10 vials if clinically indicated.

Dosage for Toxicity During Chronic Therapy: For adults, 6 vials (228 mg) usually is adequate to reverse most cases of toxicity. This dose can be used in patients who are in acute distress or for whom a serum digoxin or digitoxin concentration is not available. In infants and small children (≤ 20 kg) a single vial usually should suffice.

Methods for calculating the dose of DIGIBIND required to neutralize the known or estimated amount of digoxin or digitoxin in the body are given below (see DOSAGE CALCULATION section).

When determining the dose for DIGIBIND, the following guidelines should be considered:

—Erroneous calculations may result from inaccurate estimates of the amount of digitalis ingested or absorbed or from nonsteady-state serum digitalis concentrations. Inaccurate serum digitalis concentration measurements are a possible source of error. Most serum digoxin assay kits are designed to measure values less than 5 ng/mL. Dilution of samples is required to obtain accurate measures above 5 ng/mL.

—Dosage calculations are based on a steady-state volume of distribution of approximately 5 L/kg for digoxin (0.5 L/kg for digitoxin) to convert serum digitalis concentration to the amount of digitalis in the body. The conversion is based on the principle that body load equals drug steady-state serum concentration multiplied by volume of distribution. These volumes are population averages and vary widely among individuals. Many patients may require higher doses for complete neutralization. Doses should ordinarily be rounded up to the next whole vial.

—If toxicity has not adequately reversed after several hours or appears to recur, readministration of DIGIBIND at a dose guided by clinical judgment may be required.

—Failure to respond to DIGIBIND raises the possibility that the clinical problem is not caused by digitalis intoxication. If there is no response to an adequate dose of DIGIBIND, the diagnosis of digitalis toxicity should be questioned.

DOSAGE CALCULATION:

Acute Ingestion of Known Amount: Each vial of DIGIBIND contains 38 mg of purified digoxin-specific Fab fragments which will bind approximately 0.5 mg of digoxin (or digitoxin). Thus one can calculate the total number of vials required by dividing the total digitalis body load in mg by 0.5 mg/vial (see Formula 1).

For toxicity from an acute ingestion, total body load in milligrams will be approximately equal to the amount ingested in milligrams for digoxin capsules and digitoxin, or the amount ingested in milligrams multiplied by 0.80 (to account for incomplete absorption) for digoxin tablets.

Table 1 gives dosage estimates in number of vials for **adults and children** who have ingested a single large dose of digoxin and for whom the approximate number of tablets or capsules is known. The DIGIBIND dose (in number of vials) represented in Table 1 can be approximated using the following formula:

Formula 1

$$\text{Dose (in \# of vials)} = \frac{\text{Total digitalis body load in mg}}{\text{0.5 mg of digitalis bound/vial}}$$

TABLE 1: Approximate DIGIBIND Dose for Reversal of a Single Large Digoxin Overdose

NUMBER of DIGOXIN Tablets or Capsules Ingested*	DIGIBIND Dose # of Vials
25	10
50	20
75	30
100	40
150	60
200	80

*0.25 mg tablets with 80% bioavailability or 0.2 mg LANOXICAPS® Capsules with 100% bioavailability.

Calculations Based on Steady-State Serum Digoxin Concentrations: Table 2 gives dosage estimates in number of vials for **adult patients** for whom a steady-state serum digoxin concentration is known. The DIGIBIND dose (in number of vials) represented in Table 2 can be approximated using the following formula:

Formula 2

$$\text{Dose (in \# of vials)} = \frac{\text{(Serum digoxin concentration in ng/mL) (weight in kg)}}{100}$$

[See Table 2 at left.]

TABLE 2: Adult Dose Estimate of DIGIBIND (in # of vials) from Steady-State Serum Digoxin Concentration

Patient Weight (kg)	Serum Digoxin Concentration (ng/mL) 1	2	4	8	12	16	20
40	0.5 V	1 V	2 V	3 V	5 V	7 V	8 V
60	0.5 V	1 V	3 V	5 V	7 V	10 V	12 V
70	1 V	2 V	3 V	6 V	9 V	11 V	14 V
80	1 V	2 V	3 V	7 V	10 V	13 V	16 V
100	1 V	2 V	4 V	8 V	12 V	16 V	20 V

V = vials

Table 3 gives dosage estimates in milligrams **for infants and small children** based on the steady-state serum digoxin concentration. The DIGIBIND dose represented in Table 3 can be estimated by multiplying the dose (in number of vials) calculated from Formula 2 by the amount of DIGIBIND contained in a vial (38 mg/vial) (see Formula 3). Since infants and small children can have much smaller dosage requirements, it is recommended that the 38 mg vial be reconstituted as directed and administered with a tuberculin syringe. For very small doses, a reconstituted vial can be di-

TABLE 3: Infants and Small Children Dose Estimates of DIGIBIND (in mg) from Steady-State Serum Digoxin Concentration

Patient Weight (kg)	Serum Digoxin Concentration (ng/mL)						
	1	2	4	8	12	16	20
1	0.4* mg	1* mg	1.5* mg	3* mg	5 mg	6 mg	8 mg
3	1* mg	2* mg	5 mg	9 mg	14 mg	18 mg	23 mg
5	2* mg	4 mg	8 mg	15 mg	23 mg	30 mg	38 mg
10	4 mg	8 mg	15 mg	30 mg	46 mg	61 mg	76 mg
20	8 mg	15 mg	30 mg	61 mg	91 mg	122 mg	152 mg

*Dilution of reconstituted vial of 1 mg/mL may be desirable.

luted with 34 mL of sterile isotonic saline to achieve a concentration of 1 mg/mL.

Formula 3

Dose (in mg) = (Dose [in # of vials]) (38 mg/vial)
[See table 3 above.]

Calculation Based on Steady-State Digitoxin Concentration: The DIGIBIND dose for digitoxin toxicity can be approximated using the following formula:

Formula 4

$$\text{Dose (in \# of vials)} = \frac{\text{(Serum digitoxin concentration in ng/mL) (weight in kg)}}{1000}$$

If the dose based on ingested amount differs substantially from that calculated from the serum digoxin or digitoxin concentration, it may be preferable to use the higher dose.

ADMINISTRATION: The contents in each vial to be used should be dissolved with 4 mL of Sterile Water for Injection, by gentle mixing, to give a clear, colorless, approximately isosmotic solution with a protein concentration of 9.5 mg/mL. Reconstituted product should be used promptly. If it is not used immediately, it may be stored under refrigeration at 2 to 8°C (36 to 46°F) for up to 4 hours. The reconstituted product may be diluted with sterile isotonic saline to a convenient volume. Parenteral drug products should be inspected visually for particulate matter and discoloration prior to administration, whenever solution and container permit.

DIGIBIND, Digoxin Immune Fab (Ovine), is administered by the intravenous route over 30 minutes. It is recommended that it be infused through a 0.22 micron membrane filter to ensure no undissolved particulate matter is administered. If cardiac arrest is imminent, it can be given as a bolus injection.

HOW SUPPLIED

Vials containing 38 mg of purified lyophilized digoxin-specific Fab fragments. Box of 1. (NDC 0081-0230-44).

STORAGE

Refrigerate at 2 to 8°C (36 to 46°F). Unreconstituted vials can be stored at up to 30°C (86°F) for a total of 30 days.

REFERENCES

1. Smith TW, Lloyd BL, Spicer N, Haber E. Immunogenicity and kinetics of distribution and elimination of sheep digoxin-specific IgG and Fab fragments in the rabbit and baboon. *Clin Exp Immunol* 1979; 36:384–396.
2. Smith TW, Haber E, Yeatman L, Butler VP Jr. Reversal of advanced digoxin intoxication with Fab fragments of digoxin-specific antibodies. *N Engl J Med* 1976; 294:797–800.
3. Smith TW, Butler VP Jr, Haber E, Fozzard H, Marcus Fl, Bremner WF, Schulman IC, Phillips A. Treatment of life-threatening digitalis intoxication with digoxin-specific Fab antibody fragments: Experience in 26 cases. *N Engl J Med* 1982; 307:1357–1362.
4. Wenger TL, Butler VP Jr, Haber E, Smith TW. Treatment of 63 severely digitalis-toxic patients with digoxin-specific antibody fragments. *J Am Coll Cardiol* 1985; 5:118A–123A.
5. Spiegel A, Marchlinski FE. Time course for reversal of digoxin toxicity with digoxin-specific antibody fragments. *Am Heart J* 1985;109:1397–1399.
6. Gibb I, Adams PC, Parnham AJ, Jennings K. Plasma digoxin: Assay anomalies in Fab-treated patients. *Br J Clin Pharmacol* 1983; 16:445–447.

May 1994

Shown in Product Identification Guide, page 312

EMGEL®   ℞
(erythromycin) 2%
Topical Gel
For Dermatologic Use Only—
Not for Ophthalmic Use.

DESCRIPTION

Emgel® Topical Gel contains erythromycin. Erythromycin is a macrolide antibiotic obtained from cultures of *Streptomyces erythreus*.
Erythromycin has the empirical formula $C_{37}H_{67}NO_{13}$ and a molecular weight of 733.94.

Emgel Topical Gel contains erythromycin, USP 2% (20 mg/g) with SD 40-2 alcohol 77%, propylene glycol, and hydroxypropyl cellulose.

CLINICAL PHARMACOLOGY

The exact mechanism by which erythromycin reduces lesions of acne vulgaris is not fully known; however, the effect appears to be due in part to the antibacterial activity of the drug.

Microbiology: Erythromycin appears to inhibit protein synthesis in susceptible organisms by reversibly binding to ribosomal subunits, thereby inhibiting translocation of aminoacyl transfer-RNA and inhibiting polypeptide synthesis. Antagonism has been demonstrated between erythromycin, lincomycin, chloramphenicol, and clindamycin.

INDICATIONS AND USAGE

Emgel® (erythromycin) Topical Gel is indicated for the topical treatment of acne vulgaris.

CONTRAINDICATIONS

Emgel® (erythromycin) Topical Gel is contraindicated in those individuals who have shown hypersensitivity to any of its components.

PRECAUTIONS

General: For topical use only; not for ophthalmic use. Concomitant topical acne therapy should be used with caution since a possible cumulative irritancy effect may occur, especially with the use of peeling, desquamating, or abrasive agents.
Avoid contact with eyes and all mucous membranes. The use of antibiotic agents may be associated with the overgrowth of antibiotic-resistant organisms. If this occurs, discontinue use and take appropriate measures.

Carcinogenesis, Mutagenesis, Impairment of Fertility: Animal studies to evaluate carcinogenic and mutagenic potential or effects on fertility have not been performed with erythromycin.

Pregnancy Category B: There was no evidence of teratogenicity or any other adverse effect on reproduction in female rats fed erythromycin base (up to 0.25% of diet) before and during mating, during gestation, and through weaning of two successive litters. There are, however, no adequate and well-controlled studies in pregnant women. Because animal reproduction studies are not always predictive of human response, this drug should be used in pregnancy only if clearly needed. Erythromycin has been reported to cross the placental barrier in humans, but fetal plasma levels are generally low.

Nursing Mothers: It is not known whether topically applied erythromycin is excreted in human milk. A decision should be made whether to discontinue nursing or to discontinue the drug, taking into account the importance of the drug to the mother.

Pediatric Use: Safety and effectiveness in children have not been established.

ADVERSE REACTIONS

The most common adverse reaction reported with Emgel® (erythromycin) Topical Gel was burning. The following have been reported occasionally: peeling, dryness, itching, erythema, and oiliness. Irritation of the eyes and tenderness of the skin have also been reported with the topical use of erythromycin. A generalized urticarial reaction, which was possibly related to the use of erythromycin and required systemic steroid therapy, has been reported.

DOSAGE AND ADMINISTRATION

Apply sparingly as a thin layer to affected area(s) twice a day, in the morning and the evening, after the skin has been thoroughly washed with soap and water and patted dry. The hands should be washed after application. If there has been no improvement after 6 to 8 weeks, or if the condition becomes worse, treatment should be discontinued, and the physician should be reconsulted. Spread the medication lightly rather than rubbing it in.

HOW SUPPLIED

Emgel® (erythromycin) 2% Topical Gel is supplied in plastic bottles containing 27 g (NDC 0173-0440-01) and 50 g (NDC 0173-0440-02).

Note: FLAMMABLE: Keep away from heat and flame.

Keep bottle tightly closed. Store at room temperature.
August 1994/RL-136
Shown in Product Identification Guide, page 312

EXOSURF NEONATAL®   ℞
[ĕx ′ō-sŭrf nē-ō ′nātal]
(colfosceril palmitate, cetyl alcohol, tyloxapol)
For Intratracheal Suspension

DESCRIPTION

EXOSURF NEONATAL (colfosceril palmitate, cetyl alcohol, tyloxapol) for Intratracheal Suspension is a protein-free synthetic lung surfactant stored under vacuum as a sterile lyophilized powder. EXOSURF NEONATAL is reconstituted with preservative-free Sterile Water for Injection prior to administration by intratracheal instillation. Each 10 mL vial contains 108 mg colfosceril palmitate, commonly known as dipalmitoylphosphatidylcholine (DPPC), 12 mg cetyl alcohol, 8 mg tyloxapol, and 47 mg sodium chloride. Sodium hydroxide or hydrochloric acid may have been added to adjust pH. When reconstituted with 8 mL Sterile Water for Injection, the EXOSURF NEONATAL suspension contains 13.5 mg/mL colfosceril palmitate, 1.5 mg/mL cetyl alcohol, and 1 mg/mL tyloxapol in 0.1 N NaCl. The suspension appears milky white with a pH of 5 to 7 and an osmolality of 185 mOsm/kg.

The chemical names of EXOSURF NEONATAL are colfosceril palmitate R)-4-hydroxy-N, N, N-trimethyl-10-oxo-7-[(1-oxohexadecyl) oxy]-3,5,9-trioxa-4-phosphapentacosan-1-aminium hydroxide inner salt, 4-oxide; cetyl alcohol (1-hexadecanol); and tyloxapol 4-(1,1,3,3-tetramethylbutyl)phenol polymer with formaldehyde and oxirane.

CLINICAL PHARMACOLOGY

Surfactant deficiency is an important factor in the development of the neonatal respiratory distress syndrome (RDS). Thus, surfactant replacement therapy early in the course of RDS should ameliorate the disease and improve symptoms. Natural surfactant, a combination of lipids and apoproteins, exhibits not only surface tension reducing properties (conferred by the lipids), but also rapid spreading and adsorption (conferred by the apoproteins). The major fraction of the lipid component of natural surfactant is DPPC, which comprises up to 70% of natural surfactant by weight.

Although DPPC reduces surface tension, DPPC alone is ineffective in RDS because DPPC spreads and adsorbs poorly. In EXOSURF NEONATAL, which is protein free, cetyl alcohol acts as the spreading agent for the DPPC on the air-fluid interface. Tyloxapol, a polymeric long-chain repeating alcohol, is a nonionic surfactant which acts to disperse both DPPC and cetyl alcohol. Sodium chloride is added to adjust osmolality.

Pharmacokinetics: EXOSURF NEONATAL is administered directly into the trachea. Human pharmacokinetic studies of the absorption, biotransformation, and excretion of the components of EXOSURF NEONATAL have not been performed. Nonclinical studies, however, have shown that DPPC can be absorbed from the alveolus into lung tissue where it can be catabolized extensively and reutilized for further phospholipid synthesis and secretion. In the developing rabbit, 90% of alveolar phospholipids are recycled. In premature rabbits, the alveolar half-life of intratracheally administered H^3-labeled phosphatidylcholine is approximately 12 hours.

Animal Studies: In animal models of RDS, treatment with EXOSURF NEONATAL significantly improved lung volume, compliance, and gas exchange in premature rabbits and lambs. The amount and distribution of lung water were not affected by treatment with EXOSURF NEONATAL of premature rabbit pups. The extent of lung injury in premature rabbit pups undergoing mechanical ventilation was reduced significantly by treatment with EXOSURF NEONATAL. In premature lambs, neither systemic blood flow nor flow through the ductus arteriosus were affected by treatment with EXOSURF NEONATAL. Survival was significantly better in both premature rabbits and premature lambs treated with EXOSURF NEONATAL.

Clinical Studies: EXOSURF NEONATAL has been studied in the U.S. and Canada in controlled clinical trials involving more than 4400 infants. Over 10,000 infants have received EXOSURF NEONATAL through an open, uncontrolled, North American study designed to provide the drug to premature infants who might benefit and to obtain additional safety information (EXOSURF NEONATAL Treatent IND).

Prophylactic Treatment: The efficacy of a single dose of EXOSURF NEONATAL in prophylactic treatment of infants at risk of developing respiratory distress syndrome (RDS) was examined in three double-blind, placebo-controlled studies, one involving 215 infants weighing 500 to 700 grams, one involving 385 infants weighing 700 to 1350 grams, and one involving 446 infants weighing 700 to 1100 grams. The infants were intubated and placed on mechanical

Continued on next page

Glaxo Wellcome—Cont.

ventilation and received 5 mL/kg EXOSURF NEONATAL or placebo (air) within 30 minutes of birth.

The efficacy of one versus three doses of EXOSURF NEONATAL in prophylactic treatment of infants at risk of developing RDS was examined in a double-blind, placebo-controlled study of 823 infants weighing 700 to 1100 grams. The infants were intubated and placed on mechanical ventilation and received a first 5 mL/kg dose of EXOSURF NEONATAL within 30 minutes. Repeat 5 mL/kg doses of EXOSURF NEONATAL or placebo (air) were given to all infants who remained on mechanical ventilation at approximately 12 and 24 hours of age. An initial analysis of 716 infants is available.

The major efficacy parameters from these studies are presented in Table 1.

[See table below.]

Rescue Treatment: The efficacy of EXOSURF NEONATAL in the rescue treatment of infants with RDS was examined in two double-blind, placebo-controlled studies. One study enrolled 419 infants weighing 700 to 1350 grams; the second enrolled 1237 infants weighing 1250 grams and above. In the rescue treatment studies, infants received an initial dose (5 mL/kg) of EXOSURF NEONATAL or placebo (air) between 2 and 24 hours of life followed by a second dose (5 mL/kg) approximately 12 hours later to infants who remained on mechanical ventilation. The major efficacy parameters from these studies are presented in Table 2.

[See table above.]

Clinical Results: In these six controlled clinical studies, infants in the group receiving EXOSURF NEONATAL showed significant improvements in FiO_2 and ventilator settings which persisted for at least 7 days. Pulmonary air leaks were significantly reduced in each study. Five of the studies also showed a significant reduction in death from RDS. Further, overall mortality was reduced for all infants weighing >700 grams. The one- versus three-dose prophylactic treatment study in 700 to 1100 gram infants showed a further reduction in overall mortality with two additional doses.

Safety information is presented in Tables 3 and 4 (see ADVERSE REACTIONS). Beneficial effects in the group receiving EXOSURF NEONATAL were observed for some safety assessments. Various forms of pulmonary air leak and use of pancuronium were reduced in infants receiving EXOSURF NEONATAL in all six studies.

Follow-up data at one year adjusted age are available on 1094 of 2470 surviving infants. Growth and development of infants who received EXOSURF NEONATAL in this sample were comparable to infants who received placebo.

INDICATIONS AND USAGE

EXOSURF NEONATAL is indicated for:
1. Prophylactic treatment of infants with birth weights of less than 1350 grams who are at risk of developing RDS (see PRECAUTIONS),
2. Prophylactic treatment of infants with birth weights greater than 1350 grams who have evidence of pulmonary immaturity, and
3. **Rescue** treatment of infants who have developed RDS.

For **prophylactic** treatment, the first dose of EXOSURF NEONATAL should be administered as soon as possible after birth (see DOSAGE AND ADMINISTRATION: General Guidelines for Administration).

Infants considered as candidates for **rescue** treatment with EXOSURF NEONATAL should be on mechanical ventilation and have a diagnosis of RDS by both of the following criteria:
1. Respiratory distress not attributable to causes other than RDS, based on clinical and laboratory assessments.
2. Chest radiographic findings consistent with the diagnosis of RDS.

During the clinical development of EXOSURF NEONATAL, all infants who received the drug were intubated and on mechanical ventilation. For three-dose prophylactic treatment with EXOSURF NEONATAL, the first dose of drug was administered as soon as possible after birth and repeat doses were given at approximately 12 and 24 hours after birth if infants remained on mechanical ventilation at those times. For rescue treatment, two doses were given; one between 2 and 24 hours of life, and a second approximately 12 hours later if infants remained on mechanical ventilation. Infants who received rescue treatment with EXOSURF NEONATAL had a documented arterial to alveolar oxygen tension ratio (a/A) <0.22.

CONTRAINDICATIONS

There are no known contraindications to treatment with EXOSURF NEONATAL.

WARNINGS

Intratracheal Administration Only: EXOSURF NEONATAL should be administered only by instillation into the trachea (see DOSAGE AND ADMINISTRATION).

General:
The use of EXOSURF NEONATAL requires expert clinical care by experienced neonatologists and other clinicians who are accomplished at neonatal intubation and ventilatory management. Adequate personnel, facilities, equipment, and medications are required to optimize perinatal outcome in premature infants.

Installation of EXOSURF NEONATAL should be performed **only** by trained medical personnel experienced in airway and clinical management of unstable premature infants. Vigilant clinical attention should be given to all infants prior to, during, and after administration of EXOSURF NEONATAL.

Acute Effects: EXOSURF NEONATAL can rapidly affect oxygenation and lung compliance.

Lung Compliance: If chest expansion improves substantially after dosing, peak ventilator inspiratory pressures should be reduced immediately, without waiting for confirmation of respiratory improvement by blood gas assessment. Failure to reduce inspiratory ventilator pressures rapidly in such instances can result in lung overdistention and fatal pulmonary air leak.

Hyperoxia: If the infant becomes pink and transcutaneous oxygen saturation is in excess of 95%, FiO_2 should be reduced in small but repeated steps (until saturation is 90% to 95%) without waiting for confirmation of elevated arterial pO_2 by blood gas assessment. Failure to reduce FiO_2 in such instances can result in hyperoxia.

Hypocarbia: If arterial or transcutaneous CO_2 measurements are <30 torr, the ventilator rate should be reduced at once. Failure to reduce ventilator rates in such instances can result in marked hypocarbia, which is known to reduce brain blood flow.

Pulmonary Hemorrhage: In the single study conducted in infants weighing <700 grams at birth, the incidence of pulmonary hemorrhage (10% vs 2% in the placebo group) was significantly increased in the group receiving EXOSURF NEONATAL. None of the five studies involving infants with birth weights >700 grams showed a significant increase in pulmonary hemorrhage in the group receiving EXOSURF NEONATAL. In a cross-study analysis of these five studies, pulmonary hemorrhage was reported for 1% (14/1420) of infants in the placebo group and 2% (27/1411) of infants in the group receiving EXOSURF NEONATAL. Fatal pulmonary hemorrhage occurred in three infants; two in the group receiving EXOSURF NEONATAL and one in the placebo group. Mortality from all causes among infants who developed pulmonary hemorrhage was 43% in the placebo group and 37% in the group receiving EXOSURF NEONATAL.

Pulmonary hemorrhage in infants treated with either EXOSURF NEONATAL or placebo was more frequent in infants who were younger, smaller, male, or who had a patent ductus arteriosus. Pulmonary hemorrhage typically occurred in the first 2 days of life in both treatment groups. In more than 7700 infants in the open, uncontrolled study, pulmonary hemorrhage was reported in 4%, but fatal pulmonary hemorrhage was reported rarely (0.4%).

In the controlled clinical studies, infants treated with EXOSURF NEONATAL who received steroids more than 24 hours prior to delivery or indomethacin postnatally had a lower rate of pulmonary hemorrhage than other infants treated with EXOSURF NEONATAL. Attention should be paid to early and aggressive diagnosis and treatment (unless contraindicated) of patent ductus arteriosus during the first 2 days of life (while the ductus arteriosus is often clinically silent). Other potentially protective measures include attempting to decrease FiO_2 preferentially over ventilator pressures during the first 24 to 48 hours after dosing, and attempting to decrease PEEP minimally for at least 48 hours after dosing.

Table 2. Efficacy Assessments—Rescue Treatment

Number of Doses: Birth Weight Range:	2 Doses 700 to 1350 grams		2 Doses 1250 grams and above	
Treatment Group Number of Infants:	Placebo (Air) n=213	EXOSURF® n=206	Placebo (Air) n=623	EXOSURF n=614
	% of Infants		% of Infants	
Death ≤ Day 28[a]	23	11*	7	4†
Death through 1 Year[a]	27	15*	9	6‡
Death from RDS[b]	10	3§	3	1†
Intact Cardiopulmonary Survival[a,c]	62	75§	88	93§
Bronchopulmonary Dysplasia (BPD)[a,d]	18	15	6	3†

[a] "Intent-to-treat" analyses (as randomized)
[b] "As-treated" analyses
[c] Defined by survival through 28 days of life without bronchopulmonary dysplasia
[d] Defined by a combination of clinical and radiographic criteria

* $P<0.001$
† $P<0.05$
‡ $P<0.067$
§ $P<0.01$

Table 1. Efficacy Assessments—Prophylactic Treatment

Number of Doses: Birth Weight Range:	Single Dose 500 to 700 grams		Single Dose 700 to 1350 grams		Single Dose 700 to 1100 grams		1 vs 3 Doses 700 to 1100 grams	
Treatment Group: Number of Infants:	Placebo (Air) n=106	EXOSURF® n=109	Placebo (Air) n=185	EXOSURF n=176	Placebo (Air) n=222	EXOSURF n=224	EXOSURF 1 Dose n=356	EXOSURF 3 Doses n=360
	% of Infants		% of Infants		% of Infants		% of Infants	
Death ≤ Day 28[a]	53	50	11	6	21	15	16	9*
Death through 1 Year[a]	59	60	14	11	30	20†	17	12*
Death from RDS[b]	25	13*	4	3	10	5‡	3	2
Intact Cardiopulmonary Survival[a,c]	29	25	69	78*	65	68	74	78
Bronchopulmonary Dysplasia (BPD)[a,d]	43	44	23	18	19	21	8	12
RDS Incidence[b]	73	81	46	42	55	55	63	68

[a] "Intent-to-treat" analyses (as randomized) except for the 700 to 1350 gram, single-dose study in which infants with congenital infections and anomalies were excluded
[b] "As-treated" analyses
[c] Defined by survival through 28 days of life without bronchopulmonary dysplasia
[d] Defined by a combination of clinical and radiographic criteria

* $P<0.05$
† $P<0.01$
‡ $P=0.051$

Table 3. Safety Assessments^a—Prophylactic Treatment

Number of Doses: Birth Weight Range:	Single Dose 500 to 700 grams		Single Dose 700 to 1350 grams		Single Dose 700 to 1100 grams		1 vs 3 Doses 700 to 1100 grams	
Treatment Group: Number of Infants:	Placebo (Air) n=108	EXOSURF® n=107	Placebo (Air) n=193	EXOSURF n=192	Placebo (Air) n=222	EXOSURF n=224	EXOSURF 1 Dose n=356	EXOSURF 3 Doses n=360
	% of Infants		% of Infants		% of Infants		% of Infants	
Intraventricular Hemorrhage (IVH)								
Overall	51	57	31	27	36	36	38	35
Severe IVH	26	25	10	8	13	14	9	9
Pulmonary Air Leak (PAL)								
Overall	52	48	16	11	32	25	29	27
Pneumothorax	23	10*	5	6	19	11*	14	12
Pneumopericardium	1	4	2	0	<1	1	1	1
Pneumomediastinum	2	1	2	3	7	1†	3	2
Pulmonary Interstitial Emphysema	43	44	13	7*	26	20	23	22
Death from PAL	4	6	<1	<1	2	1	2	1
Patent Ductus Arteriosus	49	53	66	70	50	55	59	57
Necrotizing Enterocolitis	2	4	11	13	3	4	6	2*
Pulmonary Hemorrhage	2	10†	2	4	1	4	4	6
Congenital Pneumonia	4	4	2	4	2	2	2	1
Nosocomial Pneumonia	10	10	2	4	4		14	15
Non-Pulmonary Infections	33	35	34	39	28	29	35	34
Sepsis	30	34	30	34	23	24	30	27
Death From Sepsis	4	4	3	3	1	2	3	2
Meningitis	4	6	3	1	2	3	1	2
Other Infections	7	4	5	3	6	10	10	11
Major Anomalies	3	1	2	4	7	4	4	4
Hypotension	70	77	52	47	59	62	54	50
Hyperbilirubinemia	22	21	63	61	27	31	20	21
Exchange Transfusion	4	3	1	2	2	2	3	1
Thrombocytopenia^b	21	25	not available		9	8	12	10
Persistent Fetal Circulation	0	1	1	1	0	2*	1	<1
Seizures	11	8	2	2	11	9	6	5
Apnea	34	33	76	73	55	65*	62	68
Drug Therapy								
Antibiotics	96	99	98	96	98	99	>99	99
Diuretics	55	60	39	37	59	63	64	65
Anticonvulsants	14	18	23	24	20	16	9	8
Inotropes	46	40	20	20	26	20	28	27
Sedatives	62	71	65	64	63	57	52	52
Pancuronium	19	11	22	14*	19	13*	15	11
Methylxanthines	38	43	77	77	61	72*	75	82*

^a All parameters were examined with "as-treated" analyses.
^b Thrombocytopenia requiring platelet transfusion.

* $P < 0.05$
† $P < 0.01$

Mucous Plugs: Infants whose ventilation becomes markedly impaired during or shortly after dosing may have mucous plugging of the endotracheal tube, particularly if pulmonary secretions were prominent prior to drug administration. Suctioning of all infants prior to dosing may lessen the chance of mucous plugs obstructing the endotracheal tube. If endotracheal tube obstruction from such plugs is suspected, and suctioning is unsuccessful in removing the obstruction, the blocked endotracheal tube should be replaced immediately.

PRECAUTIONS

General: In the controlled clinical studies, infants known prenatally or postnatally to have major congenital anomalies, or who were suspected of having congenital infection were excluded from entry. However, these disorders cannot be recognized early in life in all cases, and a few infants with these conditions were entered. The benefits of EXOSURF NEONATAL in the affected infants who received drug appeared to be similar to the benefits observed in infants without anomalies or occult infection.

Prophylactic Treatment—Infants <700 Grams: In infants weighing 500 to 700 grams, a single prophylactic dose of EXOSURF NEONATAL significantly: improved FiO2 and ventilator settings, reduced pneumothorax, and reduced death from RDS, but increased pulmonary hemorrhage (see WARNINGS). Overall mortality did not differ significantly between the group receiving placebo and the group receiving EXOSURF NEONATAL (see Table 1). Data on multiple doses in infants in this weight class are not yet available. Accordingly, clinicians should carefully evaluate the potential risks and benefits of administration of EXOSURF NEONATAL in these infants.

Rescue Treatment—Number of Doses: A small number of infants with RDS have received more than two doses of EXOSURF NEONATAL as rescue treatment. Definitive data on the safety and efficacy of these additional doses are not available.

Carcinogenesis, Mutagenesis, Impairment of Fertility: EXOSURF NEONATAL at concentrations up to 10,000 μg/plate was not mutagenic in the Ames Salmonella assay.

Long-term studies have not been performed in animals to evaluate the carcinogenic potential of EXOSURF NEONATAL.

The effects of EXOSURF NEONATAL on fertility have not been studied.

ADVERSE REACTIONS

General: Premature birth is associated with a high incidence of morbidity and mortality. Despite significant reductions in overall mortality associated with EXOSURF NEONATAL, some infants who received EXOSURF NEONATAL developed severe complications and either survived with permanent handicaps or died.

In controlled clinical studies evaluating the safety and efficacy of EXOSURF NEONATAL, numerous safety assessments were made. In infants receiving EXOSURF NEONATAL, pulmonary hemorrhage, apnea, and use of methylxanthines were increased. A number of other adverse events were significantly reduced in the group receiving EXOSURF NEONATAL, particularly various forms of pulmonary air leak and use of pancuronium (see CLINICAL PHARMACOLOGY: Clinical Results). Tables 3 and 4 summarize the results of the major safety evaluations from the controlled clinical studies.

[See table 3 above.]

[See table 4 at top of next page.]

Pulmonary Hemorrhage: See WARNINGS.

Abnormal Laboratory Values: Abnormal laboratory values are common in critically ill, mechanically ventilated, premature infants. A higher incidence of abnormal laboratory values in the group receiving EXOSURF NEONATAL was not reported.

Events During Dosing: Data on events during dosing are available from more than 8800 infants in the open, uncontrolled clinical study (Table 5).

[See table 5 on next page.]

Reflux: Reflux of EXOSURF NEONATAL into the endotracheal tube during dosing has been observed and may be associated with rapid drug administration. If reflux occurs, drug administration should be halted and, if necessary, peak in-spiratory pressure on the ventilator should be increased by 4 to 5 cm H2O until the endotracheal tube clears.

>20% Drop in Transcutaneous Oxygen Saturation: If transcutaneous oxygen saturation declines during dosing, drug administration should be halted and, if necessary, peak inspiratory pressure on the ventilator should be increased by 4 to 5 cm H2O for 1 to 2 minutes. In addition, increases of FiO2 may be required for 1 to 2 minutes.

Mucous Plugs: See WARNINGS.

OVERDOSAGE

There have been no reports of massive overdosage with EXOSURF NEONATAL.

DOSAGE AND ADMINISTRATION

Preparation of Suspension: EXOSURF NEONATAL is best reconstituted immediately before use because it does not contain antibacterial preservatives. However, the reconstituted suspension is chemically and physically stable and remains sterile (when reconstituted using aseptic techniques) when stored at 2° to 30°C (36° to 86°F) for up to 12 hours following reconstitution.

Solutions containing buffers or preservatives should not be used for reconstitution. **Do Not Use Bacteriostatic Water for Injection, USP.** Each vial of EXOSURF NEONATAL should be reconstituted with **8 mL** of the accompanying diluent (preservative-free Sterile Water for Injection) as follows:

1. Fill a 10 mL or 12 mL syringe with 8 mL preservative-free Sterile Water for Injection using an 18 or 19 gauge needle;
2. Allow the vacuum in the vial to draw the sterile water into the vial;
3. Aspirate as much as possible of the 8 mL out of the vial into the syringe (while maintaining the vacuum), then SUDDENLY release the syringe plunger.

Step 3 should be repeated three or four times to assure adequate mixing of the vial contents. If vacuum is not present, the vial of EXOSURF NEONATAL should not be used.

The appropriate dosage volume for the entire dose (5 mL/kg) should then be drawn into the syringe from **below** the froth in the vial (again maintaining the vacuum). If the infant weighs less than 1600 grams, unused EXOSURF NEONA-

Continued on next page

Glaxo Wellcome—Cont.

TAL suspension will remain in the vial after the entire dose is drawn into the syringe. If the infant weighs more than 1600 grams, at least two vials will be required for each dose. Reconstituted EXOSURF NEONATAL is a milky white suspension with a total volume of 8 mL per vial. Each mL of reconstituted EXOSURF NEONATAL contains 13.5 mg colfosceril palmitate, 1.5 mg cetyl alcohol, 1 mg tyloxapol, and sodium chloride to provide a 0.1 N concentration. If the suspension appears to separate, gently shake or swirl the vial to resuspend the preparation. The reconstituted product should be inspected visually for homogeneity immediately before administration; if persistent large flakes or particulates are present, the vial should not be used.

Dosage: Accurate determination of weight at birth is the key to accurate dosing.

Prophylactic Treatment: The first dose of EXOSURF NEONATAL should be administered as a single 5 mL/kg dose as soon as possible after birth. Second and third doses should be administered approximately 12 and 24 hours later to all infants who remain on mechanical ventilation at those times.

Rescue Treatment: EXOSURF NEONATAL should be administered in two 5 mL/kg doses. The initial dose should be administered as soon as possible after the diagnosis of RDS is confirmed. The second dose should be administered approximately 12 hours following the first dose, provided the infant remains on mechanical ventilation. A small number of infants with RDS have received more than two doses of EXOSURF NEONATAL as rescue treatment. Definitive data on the safety and efficacy of these additional doses are not available (see PRECAUTIONS).

Use of Special Endotracheal Tube Adapter: With each vial of EXOSURF NEONATAL for Intratracheal Suspension, five different sized endotracheal tube adapters each with a special right angle Luer®-lock sideport are supplied. The adapters are clean but not sterile. The adapters should be used as follows:

1. Select an adapter size which correponds to the inside diameter of the endotracheal tube.
2. Insert the adapter into the endotracheal tube with a firm push-twist motion.
3. Connect the breathing circuit wye to the adapter.
4. Remove the cap from the sideport on the adapter. Attach the syringe containing drug to the sideport.
5. After completion of dosing, remove the syringe and RE-CAP THE SIDEPORT.

Administration: The infant should be suctioned prior to administration of EXOSURF NEONATAL.

EXOSURF NEONATAL suspension is administered via the sideport on the special endotracheal tube adapter **WITHOUT INTERRUPTING MECHANICAL VENTILATION.**

Each dose of EXOSURF NEONATAL is administered in two 2.5 mL/kg half-doses. Each half-dose is instilled slowly over 1 to 2 minutes (30 to 50 mechanical breaths) in small bursts timed with inspiration. After the first 2.5 mL/kg half-dose is administered in the midline position, the infant's head and torso are turned 45° to the **right** for 30 seconds while mechanical ventilation is continued. After the infant is returned to the midline position, the second 2.5 mL/kg half-dose is given in an identical fashion over another 1 to 2 minutes. The infant's head and torso are then turned 45° to the **left** for 30 seconds while mechanical ventilation is continued, and the infant is then turned back to the midline position. These maneuvers allow gravity to assist in the distribution of EXOSURF NEONATAL in the lungs.

During dosing, heart rate, color, chest expansion, facial expressions, the oximeter, and the endotracheal tube patency and position should be monitored. If heart rate slows, the infant becomes dusky or agitated, transcutaneous oxygen saturation falls more than 15%, or EXOSURF NEONATAL backs up in the endotracheal tube, dosing should be slowed or halted and, if necessary, the peak inspiratory pressure, ventilator rate, and/or FiO₂ turned up. On the other hand, rapid improvements in lung function may require immediate reductions in peak inspiratory pressure, ventilator rate, and/or FiO₂. (See WARNINGS and see below for additional information concerning administration.)

Suctioning should not be performed for two hours after EXOSURF NEONATAL is administered, except when dictated by clinical necessity.

General Guidelines for Administration: Administration of EXOSURF NEONATAL should not take precedence over clinical assessment and stabilization of critically ill infants.

Intubation: Prior to dosing with EXOSURF NEONATAL, it is important to ensure that the endotracheal tube tip is in the trachea and not in the esophagus or right or left mainstem bronchus. Brisk and symmetrical chest movement with each mechanical inspiration should be confirmed prior to dosing, as should equal breath sounds in the two axillae. In prophylactic treatment, dosing with EXOSURF

NEONATAL need not be delayed for radiographic confirmation of the endotracheal tube tip position. In rescue treatment, bedside confirmation of endotracheal tube tip position is usually sufficient, if at least one chest radiograph subsequent to the last intubation confirmed proper position of the endotracheal tube tip. Some lung areas will remain undosed if the endotracheal tube tip is too low.

Monitoring: Continuous ECG and transcutaneous oxygen saturation monitoring during dosing are essential. In most infants treated prophylactically, it should be possible to initiate such monitoring prior to administration of the first dose of EXOSURF NEONATAL. For subsequent prophylactic and all rescue doses, arterial blood pressure monitoring during dosing is also highly desirable. After both prophylactic and rescue dosing, frequent arterial blood gas sampling is required to prevent post-dosing hyperoxia and hypocarbia (see WARNINGS).

Ventilatory Support During Dosing: The 5 mL/kg dosage volume may cause transient impairment of gas exchange by physical blockage of the airway, particularly in infants on low ventilator settings. As a result, infants may exhibit a drop in oxygen saturation during dosing, especially if they are on low ventilator settings prior to dosing. These transient effects are easily overcome by increasing peak inspiratory pressure on the ventilator by 4 to 5 cm H₂O for 1 to 2 minutes during dosing. FiO₂ can also be increased if necessary. In infants who are particularly fragile or reactive to external stimuli, increasing peak inspiratory pressure by 4 to 5 cm H₂O and/or FiO₂ 20% just prior to dosing may minimize any transient deterioration in oxygenation. However, in virtually all cases it should be possible to return the infant to pre-dose settings within a very short time of dose completion.

Post-Dosing: At the end of dosing, position of the endotracheal tube should be confirmed by listening for equal breath sounds in the two axillae. Attention should be paid to chest expansion, color, transcutaneous saturation, and arterial blood gases. Some infants who receive EXOSURF NEONATAL and other surfactants respond with rapid improvements in pulmonary compliance, minute ventilation, and gas exchange (see WARNINGS). Constant bedside attention of an experienced clinician for at least 30 minutes after dosing is essential. Frequent blood gas sampling also is absolutely essential. Rapid changes in lung function require im-

Table 4. Safety Assessments[a]—Rescue Treatment

Number of Doses:	2 Doses		2 Doses	
Birth Weight Range:	700 to 1350 grams		1250 grams and above	
Treatment Group:	Placebo (Air)	EXOSURF®	Placebo (Air)	EXOSURF
Number of Infants:	n=213	n=206	n=622	n=615
	% of Infants		% of Infants	
Intraventricular Hemorrhage (IVH)				
Overall	48	52	23	18*
Severe IVH	13	9	5	4
Pulmonary Air Leak (PAL)				
Overall	54	34†	30	18†
Pneumothorax	29	20*	20	10†
Pneumopericardium	4	1	1	2
Pneumomediastinum	8	4	5	2‡
Pulmonary Interstitial Emphysema	48	25†	24	13†
Death from PAL	7	3	<1	1
Patent Ductus Arteriosus	66	57	54	45*
Necrotizing Enterocolitis	3	3	1	2
Pulmonary Hemorrhage	3	1	<1	1
Congenital Pneumonia	2	3	2	2
Nosocomial Pneumonia	5	7	2	2
Non-Pulmonary Infections	19	22	13	13
Sepsis	15	17	8	8
Death From Sepsis	<1	<1	1	<1
Meningitis	1	<1	1	<1*
Other Infections	5	8	5	6
Major Anomalies	3	3	4	4
Hypotension	62	57	50	39‡
Hyperbilirubinemia	17	19	12	10
Exchange Transfusion	3	4	1	2
Thrombocytopenia[b]	10	11	4	<1‡
Persistent Fetal Circulation	1	1	6	2‡
Seizures	10	10	6	3*
Apnea	48	65‡	37	44*
Drug Therapy				
Antibiotics	100	99	98	98
Diuretics	60	65	45	32.34†
Anticonvulsants	17	17	10	5‡
Inotropes	36	31	27	16†
Sedatives	72	68	76	64†
Pancuronium	34	17‡	33	15†
Methylxanthines	62	74‡	49	53

[a] All parameters were examined with "as-treated" analyses.
[b] Thrombocytopenia requiring platelet transfusion.

* P<0.05
† P<0.001
‡ P<0.01

Table 5. Events During Dosing in the Open, Uncontrolled Study[a]

Treatment Type:	Prophylactic Treatment	Rescue Treatment
Number of Infants:	n=1127	n=7711
	% of Infants	% of Infants
Reflux of EXOSURF NEONATAL	20	31
Drop in O₂ saturation (≥20%)	6	22
Rise in O₂ saturation (≥10%)	5	6
Drop in transcutaneous pO₂ (≥20 mm Hg)	1	8
Rise in transcutaneous pO₂ (≥20 mm Hg)	2	5
Drop in transcutaneous pCO₂ (≥20 mm Hg)	<1	1
Rise in transcutaneous pCO₂ (≥20 mm Hg)	1	3
Bradycardia (<60 beats/min)	1	3
Tachycardia (>200 beats/min)	<1	<1
Gagging	1	5
Mucous Plugs	<1	<1

[a] Infants may have experienced more than one event.
Investigators were prohibited from adjusting FiO₂ and/or ventilator settings during dosing unless significant clinical deterioration occurred.

mediate changes in peak inspiratory pressure, ventilator rate, and/or FiO_2.

HOW SUPPLIED

EXOSURF NEONATAL for Intratracheal Suspension is supplied in a carton containing one 10 mL vial of EXOSURF NEONATAL for Intratracheal Suspension, one 10 mL vial of Sterile Water for Injection, and five endotracheal tube adapters (2.5, 3.0, 3.5, 4.0, and 4.5 mm I.D.) (NDC 0173-0207-01)

Store EXOSURF NEONATAL for Intratracheal Suspension at 15° to 30°C (59° to 86°F) in a dry place.

EDUCATIONAL MATERIAL

A videotape on dosing is available from your Glaxo Wellcome Inc. representative. This videotape demonstrates techniques for safe administration of EXOSURF NEONATAL and should be viewed by healthcare professionals who will administer the drug.

Licensed under U.S. Patent Nos. 4312860, 4826821, and 5110806

U.S. Patents No. 5207220 (Method) and 5309903 (Method)

May 1996/RL-311

Shown in Product Identification Guide, page 312

FLOLAN® ℞

[flō 'lan]

(epoprostenol sodium)

for Injection

DESCRIPTION

FLOLAN (epoprostenol sodium) for Injection is a sterile sodium salt formulated for intravenous administration. Each vial of FLOLAN contains epoprostenol sodium equivalent to either 0.5 mg (500,000 ng) or 1.5 mg (1,500,000 ng) epoprostenol, 3.76 mg glycine, 2.93 mg sodium chloride, and 50 mg mannitol. Sodium hydroxide may have been added to adjust pH.

Epoprostenol (PGI_2, PGX, prostacyclin), a metabolite of arachidonic acid, is a naturally occurring prostaglandin with potent vasodilatory activity and inhibitory activity of platelet aggregation.

Epoprostenol is (5Z,9α,11α,13*E*,15*S*)-6,9-epoxy-11,15-dihydroxyprosta-5,13-dien-1-oic acid.

Epoprostenol sodium has a molecular weight of 374.45 and a molecular formula of $C_{20}H_{31}NaO_5$. The structural formula is:

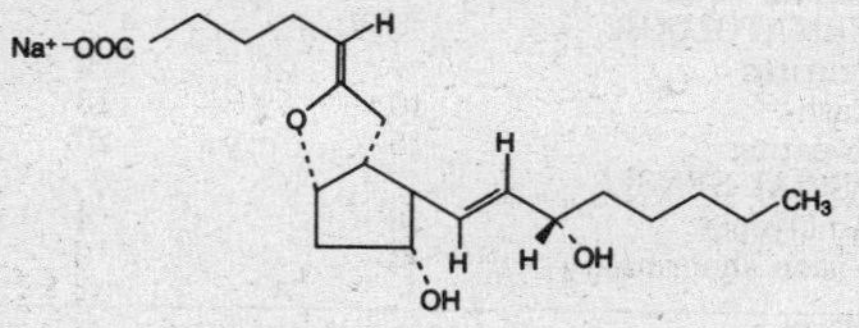

FLOLAN is a white to off-white powder that must be reconstituted with STERILE DILUENT for FLOLAN. STERILE DILUENT for FLOLAN is supplied in 50 mL glass vials containing 94 mg glycine, 73.5 mg sodium chloride, sodium hydroxide (added to adjust pH), and Water for Injection, USP. The reconstituted solution of FLOLAN has a pH of 10.2 to 10.8 and is increasingly unstable at a lower pH.

CLINICAL PHARMACOLOGY

General: Epoprostenol has two major pharmacological actions: (1) direct vasodilation of pulmonary and systemic arterial vascular beds, and (2) inhibition of platelet aggregation. In animals, the vasodilatory effects reduce right and left ventricular afterload and increase cardiac output and stroke volume. The effect of epoprostenol on heart rate in animals varies with dose. At low doses, there is vagally mediated bradycardia, but at higher doses, epoprostenol causes reflex tachycardia in response to direct vasodilation and hypotension. No major effects on cardiac conduction have been observed. Additional pharmacologic effects of epoprostenol in animals include bronchodilation, inhibition of gastric acid secretion, and decreased gastric emptying.

Pharmacokinetics: Epoprostenol is rapidly hydrolyzed at neutral pH in blood and is also subject to enzymatic degradation. Animal studies using tritium-labelled epoprostenol have indicated a high clearance (93 mL/min/kg), small volume of distribution (357 mL/kg), and a short half-life (2.7 minutes). During infusions in animals, steady-state plasma concentrations of tritium-labelled epoprostenol were reached within 15 minutes and were proportional to infusion rates.

No available chemical assay is sufficiently sensitive and specific to assess the in vivo human pharmacokinetics of epoprostenol. The in vitro half-life of epoprostenol in human blood at 37°C and pH 7.4 is approximately 6 minutes; the in vivo half-life of epoprostenol in man is therefore expected to be no greater than 6 minutes. The in vitro pharmacologic half-life of epoprostenol in human plasma, based on inhibition of platelet aggregation, was similar for males (n=954) and females (n=1024).

Tritium-labelled epoprostenol has been administered to humans in order to identify the metabolic products of epoprostenol. Epoprostenol is metabolized to two primary metabolites: 6-keto-$PGF_{1\alpha}$ (formed by spontaneous degradation) and 6,15-diketo-13,14-dihydro-$PGF_{1\alpha}$ (enzymatically formed), both of which have pharmacological activity orders of magnitude less than epoprostenol in animal test systems. The recovery of radioactivity in urine and feces over a one-week period was 82% and 4% of the administered dose, respectively. Fourteen additional minor metabolites have been isolated from urine, indicating that epoprostenol is extensively metabolized in man.

Clinical Trials in Primary Pulmonary Hypertension (PPH):

Hemodynamic Effects: Acute intravenous infusions of FLOLAN for up to 15 minutes in patients with secondary and primary pulmonary hypertension produce dose-related increases in cardiac index (CI) and stroke volume (SV), and dose-related decreases in pulmonary vascular resistance (PVR), total pulmonary resistance (TPR), and mean systemic arterial pressure (SAPm). The effects of FLOLAN on mean pulmonary artery pressure (PAPm) in patients with PPH were variable and minor.

Chronic continuous infusions of FLOLAN in patients with PPH were studied in two prospective, open, randomized trials of 8 and 12 weeks duration comparing FLOLAN plus standard therapy to standard therapy alone. Dosage of FLOLAN was determined as described in DOSAGE AND ADMINISTRATION and averaged 9.2 ng/kg/min at study end. Standard therapy varied among patients and included some or all of the following: anticoagulants in essentially all patients; oral vasodilators, diuretics, and digoxin in one-half to two-thirds of patients; and supplemental oxygen in about half the patients. Except for two New York Heart Association (NYHA) functional Class II patients, all patients were either functional Class III or Class IV. As results were similar in the two studies, the pooled results are described. Chronic hemodynamic effects were generally similar to acute effects. CI, SV, and arterial oxygen saturation were increased, and PAPm, right atrial pressure (RAP), TPR, and systemic vascular resistance (SVR) were decreased in patients who received FLOLAN chronically compared to those who did not. Table 1 illustrates the treatment-related hemodynamic changes in these patients after 8 or 12 weeks of treatment.

[See table above.]

Table 1
Hemodynamics During Chronic Administration of FLOLAN

Hemodynamic Parameter	Baseline		Mean change from baseline at end of treatment period*	
	FLOLAN® (n = 52)	Standard Therapy (n = 54)	FLOLAN (n = 48)	Standard Therapy (n = 41)
CI (L/min/m^2)	2.0	2.0	0.3**	−0.1
PAPm (mm Hg)	60	60	−5**	1
PVR (Wood U)	16	17	−4**	1
SAPm (mm Hg)	89	91	−4	−3
SV (mL/beat)	44	43	6**	−1
TPR (Wood U)	20	21	−5**	1

* At 8 weeks: FLOLAN n = 10; Standard Therapy n = 11.
At 12 weeks: FLOLAN n = 38; Standard Therapy n = 30.

** Denotes statistically significant change between FLOLAN and Standard Therapy groups.

CI = cardiac index; PAPm = mean pulmonary arterial pressure; PVR = pulmonary vascular resistance; SAPm = mean systemic arterial pressure; SV = stroke volume; TPR = total pulmonary resistance.

These hemodynamic improvements appeared to persist when FLOLAN was administered for at least 36 months in an open, non-randomized study.

Clinical Effects: Exercise capacity, as measured by the 6-minute walk test, improved significantly in patients receiving continuous intravenous FLOLAN plus standard therapy for 8 or 12 weeks compared to those receiving standard therapy alone. Improvements were apparent as early as the first week of therapy. Increases in exercise capacity were accompanied by significant improvement in dyspnea and fatigue, as measured by the Congestive Heart Failure Questionnaire and the Dyspnea Fatigue Index.

Survival was improved in NYHA functional Class III and Class IV PPH patients treated with FLOLAN for 12 weeks in a multicenter, open, randomized, parallel study. At the end of the treatment period, 8 of 40 patients receiving standard therapy alone died, whereas none of the 41 patients receiving FLOLAN died ($P = 0.003$).

INDICATIONS AND USAGE

FLOLAN is indicated for the long-term intravenous treatment of primary pulmonary hypertension in NYHA Class III and Class IV patients (see CLINICAL PHARMACOLOGY: Clinical Trials).

CONTRAINDICATIONS

A large study evaluating the effect of FLOLAN on survival in NYHA Class III and IV patients with CHF due to severe left ventricular systolic dysfunction was terminated after an interim analysis of 471 patients revealed a higher mortality in patients receiving FLOLAN plus standard therapy than in those receiving standard therapy alone. The chronic use of FLOLAN in patients with CHF due to severe left ventricular systolic dysfunction is therefore contraindicated.

FLOLAN is also contraindicated in patients with known hypersensitivity to the drug or to structurally-related compounds.

WARNINGS

FLOLAN must be reconstituted only as directed using STERILE DILUENT for FLOLAN. FLOLAN must not be reconstituted or mixed with any other parenteral medications or solutions prior to or during adminstration.

Abrupt Withdrawal: Abrupt withdrawal (including interruptions in drug delivery) or sudden large reductions in dosage of FLOLAN may result in symptoms associated with rebound pulmonary hypertension, including dyspnea, dizziness, and asthenia. In clinical trials, one Class III PPH patient's death was judged attributable to the interruption of FLOLAN. Abrupt withdrawal should be avoided.

Pulmonary Edema: Some patients with primary pulmonary hypertension have developed pulmonary edema during dose ranging, which may be associated with pulmonary veno-occlusive disease. FLOLAN should not be used chronically in patients who develop pulmonary edema during dose ranging.

Sepsis: See ADVERSE REACTIONS: Adverse Events Attributable to the Drug Delivery System.

PRECAUTIONS

General: FLOLAN should be used only by clinicians experienced in the diagnosis and treatment of PPH. The diagnosis of PPH should be carefully established by standard clinical tests to exclude secondary causes of pulmonary hypertension.

FLOLAN is a potent pulmonary and systemic vasodilator. Dose ranging with FLOLAN must be performed in a setting with adequate personnel and equipment for physiologic monitoring and emergency care. Although dose ranging in clinical trials was performed during right heart catheterization employing a pulmonary artery catheter, in uncontrolled studies utilizing FLOLAN, acute dose ranging was performed without cardiac catheterization. The risk of cardiac catheterization in patients with PPH should be carefully weighed against the potential benefits. During acute dose ranging, asymptomatic increases in pulmonary artery pressure coincident with increases in cardiac output occurred rarely. In such cases, dose reduction should be considered, but such an increase does not imply that chronic treatment is contraindicated.

During chronic use, FLOLAN is delivered continuously on an ambulatory basis through a permanent indwelling central venous catheter. Unless contraindicated, anticoagulant therapy should be administered to PPH patients receiving FLOLAN to reduce the risk of pulmonary thromboembolism or systemic embolism through a patent foramen ovale. In order to reduce the risk of infection, aseptic technique must be used in the reconstitution and administration of FLOLAN as well as in routine catheter care. Because FLOLAN is metabolized rapidly, even brief interruptions in the delivery of FLOLAN may result in symptoms associated with rebound pulmonary hypertension including dyspnea, dizziness, and asthenia. The decision to initiate therapy with FLOLAN should be based upon the understanding that there is a high likelihood that intravenous therapy with FLOLAN will be needed for prolonged periods, possibly years, and the patient's ability to accept and care for a permanent intrave-

Continued on next page

Glaxo Wellcome—Cont.

nous catheter and infusion pump should be carefully considered.

Based on clinical trials, the acute hemodynamic response to FLOLAN did not correlate well with improvement in exercise tolerance or survival during chronic use of FLOLAN. Dosage of FLOLAN during chronic use should be adjusted at the first sign of recurrence or worsening of symptoms attributable to PPH or the occurrence of adverse events associated with FLOLAN (see DOSAGE AND ADMINISTRATION). Following dosage adjustments, standing and supine blood pressure and heart rate should be monitored closely for several hours.

Information for Patients: Patients receiving FLOLAN should receive the following information: **FLOLAN must be reconstituted only with STERILE DILUENT for FLOLAN.** FLOLAN is infused continuously through a permanent indwelling central venous catheter via a small, portable infusion pump. Thus, therapy with FLOLAN requires commitment by the patient to drug reconstitution, drug administration, and care of the permanent central venous catheter. Sterile technique must be adhered to in preparing the drug and in the care of the catheter, and even brief interruptions in the delivery of FLOLAN may result in rapid symptomatic deterioration. The decision to receive FLOLAN for PPH should be based upon the understanding that there is a high likelihood that therapy with FLOLAN will be needed for prolonged periods, possibly years, and the patient's ability to accept and care for a permanent intravenous catheter and infusion pump should be carefully considered.

Drug Interactions: Additional reductions in blood pressure may occur when FLOLAN is administered with diuretics, antihypertensive agents, or other vasodilators. When other anti-platelet agents or anticoagulants are used concomitantly, there is a potential for FLOLAN to increase the risk of bleeding. However, patients receiving infusions of FLOLAN in clinical trials were maintained on anticoagulants without evidence of increased bleeding. In clinical trials, FLOLAN was used with digoxin, diuretics, anticoagulants, oral vasodilators, and supplemental oxygen.

Carcinogenesis, Mutagenesis, Impairment of Fertility: Long-term studies in animals have not been performed to evaluate carcinogenic potential. A micronucleus test in rats revealed no evidence of mutagenicity. The Ames test and DNA elution tests were also negative, although the instability of epoprostenol makes the significance of these tests uncertain. Fertility was not impaired in rats given FLOLAN by subcutaneous injection at doses up to 100 μg/kg/day [600 μg/m^2/day, 2.5 times the recommended human dose (4.6 ng/kg/min or 245.1 μg/m^2/day, i.v.) based on body surface area].

Pregnancy: Pregnancy Category B. Reproductive studies have been performed in pregnant rats and rabbits at doses up to 100 μg/kg/day (600 μg/m^2/day in rats, 2.5 times the recommended human dose, and 1180 μg/m^2/day in rabbits, 4.8 times the recommended human dose based on body surface area) and have revealed no evidence of impaired fertility or harm to the fetus due to FLOLAN. There are, however, no adequate and well-controlled studies in pregnant women. Because animal reproduction studies are not always predictive of human response, this drug should be used during pregnancy only if clearly needed.

Labor and Delivery: The use of FLOLAN during labor, vaginal delivery, or caesarean section has not been adequately studied in humans.

Nursing Mothers: It is not known whether this drug is excreted in human milk. Because many drugs are excreted in human milk, caution should be exercised when FLOLAN is administered to a nursing woman.

Pediatric Use: Safety and effectiveness in pediatric patients have not been established.

Geriatric Use: Clinical studies of FLOLAN did not include sufficient numbers of patients aged 65 and over to determine whether they respond differently from younger patients. In general, dose selection for an elderly patient should be cautious, reflecting the greater frequency of decreased hepatic, renal, or cardiac function and of concomitant disease or other drug therapy.

ADVERSE REACTIONS

During clinical trials, adverse events were classified as follows: (1) adverse events during acute dose ranging, (2) adverse events during chronic dosing, and (3) adverse events associated with the drug delivery system.

Adverse Events During Acute Dose Ranging: During acute dose ranging, FLOLAN was administered in 2 ng/kg/min increments until the patients developed symptomatic intolerance. The most common adverse events and the adverse events that limited further increases in dose were generally related to the major pharmacologic effect of FLOLAN, vasodilation. The most common dose-limiting adverse events (occurring in ≥ 1% of patients) were nausea, vomiting, headache, hypotension, and flushing, but also include chest pain, anxiety, dizziness, bradycardia, dyspnea, abdominal pain, musculoskeletal pain, and tachycardia. Table 2 lists the ad-

verse events reported during acute dose ranging in decreasing order of frequency.

Table 2
Adverse Events During Acute Dose Ranging

Adverse Events Occurring in ≥1% of Patients	FLOLAN® (% of patients) (n=391)
Flushing	58
Headache	49
Nausea/Vomiting	32
Hypotension	16
Anxiety, nervousness, agitation	11
Chest pain	11
Dizziness	8
Bradycardia	5
Abdominal pain	5
Musculoskeletal pain	3
Dyspnea	2
Back pain	2
Sweating	1
Dyspepsia	1
Hypesthesia/Paresthesia	1
Tachycardia	1

Adverse Events During Chronic Administration: Interpretation of adverse events is complicated by the clinical features of PPH, which are similar to some of the pharmacologic effects of FLOLAN (e.g., dizziness, syncope). Adverse events probably related to the underlying disease include dyspnea, fatigue, chest pain, right ventricular failure, and pallor. Several adverse events, on the other hand, can clearly be attributed to FLOLAN. These include headache, jaw pain, flushing, diarrhea, nausea and vomiting, flu-like symptoms, and anxiety/nervousness. In an effort to separate the adverse effects of the drug from the adverse effects of the underlying disease, table 3 lists adverse events that occurred at a rate at least 10% different in the two groups in controlled trials.

Table 3
Adverse Events Regardless of Attribution Occurring with ≥ 10% Difference Between FLOLAN and Standard Therapy Alone

Adverse Event	FLOLAN® (% of patients) (n=52)	Standard Therapy (% of patients) (n=54)
Occurrence More Common with FLOLAN		
GENERAL		
Chills/Fever/Sepsis/ Flu-like symptoms	25	11
CARDIOVASCULAR		
Tachycardia	35	24
Flushing	42	2
GASTROINTESTINAL		
Diarrhea	37	6
Nausea/Vomiting	67	48
MUSCULOSKELETAL		
Jaw Pain	54	0
Myalgia	44	31
Non-specific musculoskeletal pain	35	15
NEUROLOGICAL		
Anxiety/nervousness/ tremor	21	9
Dizziness	83	70
Headache	83	33
Hypesthesia, Hyperesthesia, Paresthesia	12	2
Occurrence More Common With Standard Therapy		
CARDIOVASCULAR		
Heart Failure	31	52
Syncope	13	24
Shock	0	13
RESPIRATORY		
Hypoxia	25	37

Thrombocytopenia has been reported during uncontrolled clinical trials in patients receiving FLOLAN.
Table 4 lists additional adverse events reported in PPH patients receiving FLOLAN plus standard therapy or standard therapy alone during controlled clinical trials.
[See table on top of next column.]

Adverse Events Attributable to the Drug Delivery System: Chronic infusions of FLOLAN are delivered using a small, portable infusion pump through an indwelling central venous catheter. During controlled trials of up to 12 weeks duration, 21% of patients reported a local infection and 13% of

Table 4
Adverse Events Regardless of Attribution Occurring with < 10% Difference Between FLOLAN and Standard Therapy Alone

Adverse Event	FLOLAN® (% of patients) (n = 52)	Standard Therapy (% of patients) (n = 54)
GENERAL		
Asthenia	87	81
CARDIOVASCULAR		
Angina pectoris	19	20
Arrhythmia	27	20
Bradycardia	15	9
Supraventricular tachycardia	8	0
Pallor	21	30
Cyanosis	31	39
Palpitation	63	61
Cerebrovascular accident	4	0
Hemorrhage	19	11
Hypotension	27	31
Myocardial ischemia	2	6
GASTROINTESTINAL		
Abdominal pain	27	31
Anorexia	25	30
Ascites	12	17
Constipation	6	2
METABOLIC		
Edema	60	63
Hypokalemia	6	4
Weight reduction	27	24
Weight gain	6	4
MUSCULOSKELETAL		
Arthralgia	6	0
Bone pain	0	4
Chest pain	67	65
NEUROLOGICAL		
Confusion	6	11
Convulsion	4	0
Depression	37	44
Insomnia	4	4
RESPIRATORY		
Cough increase	38	46
Dyspnea	90	85
Epistaxis	4	2
Pleural effusion	4	2
DERMATOLOGIC		
Pruritus	4	0
Rash	10	13
Sweating	15	20
SPECIAL SENSES		
Amblyopia	8	4
Vision abnormality	4	0

patients reported pain at the injection site. During long-term follow-up, sepsis was reported at least once in 14% of patients and occurred at a rate of 0.32 infections per patient per year in patients treated with FLOLAN. This rate was higher than reported in patients using chronic indwelling central venous catheters to administer parenteral nutrition, but lower than reported in oncology patients using these catheters. Malfunctions in the delivery system resulting in an inadvertent bolus of or a reduction in FLOLAN were associated with symptoms related to excess or insufficient FLOLAN, respectively (see ADVERSE REACTIONS: Adverse Events During Chronic Administration).

OVERDOSAGE

Signs and symptoms of excessive doses of FLOLAN during clinical trials are the expected dose-limiting pharmacologic effects of FLOLAN, including flushing, headache, hypotension, tachycardia, nausea, vomiting, and diarrhea. Treatment will ordinarily require dose reduction of FLOLAN.

One patient with secondary pulmonary hypertension accidentally received 50 mL of an unspecified concentration of FLOLAN. The patient vomited and became unconscious with an initially unrecordable blood pressure. FLOLAN was discontinued and the patient regained consciousness within seconds. No fatal events have been reported following overdosage of FLOLAN.

Single intravenous doses of FLOLAN at 10 and 50 mg/kg (2,703 and 27,027 times the recommended acute phase human dose based on body surface area) were lethal to mice and rats, respectively. Symptoms of acute toxicity were hypoactivity, ataxia, loss of righting reflex, deep slow breathing, and hypothermia.

DOSAGE AND ADMINISTRATION

Important Note: FLOLAN must be reconstituted only with **STERILE DILUENT for FLOLAN.** Reconstituted solutions of FLOLAN must not be diluted or administered with other parenteral solutions or medications (see WARNINGS).

Table 5

To make 100 mL of solution with final Concentration (ng/mL) of:	Directions:
3,000 ng/mL	Dissolve contents of one 0.5 mg vial with 5 mL of STERILE DILUENT for FLOLAN®. Withdraw 3 mL and add to sufficient STERILE DILUENT for FLOLAN to make a total of 100 mL.
5,000 ng/mL	Dissolve contents of one 0.5 mg vial with 5 mL of STERILE DILUENT for FLOLAN. Withdraw entire vial contents and add sufficient STERILE DILUENT for FLOLAN to make a total of 100 mL.
10,000 ng/mL	Dissolve contents of two 0.5 mg vials each with 5 mL of STERILE DILUENT for FLOLAN. Withdraw entire vial contents and add sufficient STERILE DILUENT for FLOLAN to make a total of 100 mL.
15,000 ng/mL*	Dissolve contents of one 1.5 mg vial with 5 mL of STERILE DILUENT for FLOLAN. Withdraw entire vial contents and add sufficient STERILE DILUENT for FLOLAN to make a total of 100 mL.

* Higher concentrations may be required for patients who receive FLOLAN long-term.

Dosage:

Acute Dose Ranging:

The initial chronic infusion rate of FLOLAN is determined by an acute dose-ranging procedure. During controlled clinical trials, this procedure was performed during cardiac catheterization (see PRECAUTIONS), but in subsequent uncontrolled clinical trials, acute dose ranging was performed without cardiac catheterization. In either case, the infusion rate is initiated at 2 ng/kg/min and increased in increments of 2 ng/kg/min every 15 minutes or longer until dose-limiting pharmacologic effects are elicited. The most common dose-limiting pharmacologic effects (occurring in ≥1% of patients) during dose ranging are nausea, vomiting, headache, hypotension, and flushing, but also include chest pain, anxiety, dizziness, bradycardia, dyspnea, abdominal pain, musculoskeletal pain, and tachycardia. During acute dose ranging in clinical trials, the mean maximum dose which did not elicit dose-limiting pharmacologic effects was 8.6 ± 0.3 ng/kg/min.

Continuous Chronic Infusion:

Chronic continuous infusion of FLOLAN should be administered through a central venous catheter. Temporary peripheral intravenous infusion may be used until central access is established. Chronic infusions of FLOLAN should be initiated at 4 ng/kg/min less than the maximum-tolerated infusion rate determined during acute dose ranging. If the maximum-tolerated infusion rate is less than 5 ng/kg/min, the chronic infusion should be started at one-half the maximum-tolerated infusion rate. During clinical trials, the mean initial chronic infusion rate was 5 ng/kg/min.

Dosage Adjustments:

Changes in the chronic infusion rate should be based on persistence, recurrence, or worsening of the patient's symptoms of PPH and the occurrence of adverse events due to excessive doses of FLOLAN. In general, increases in dose from the initial chronic dose should be expected. In the controlled 12-week trial, for example, the dose increased from a mean starting dose of 5.2 ng/kg/min (4 ng/kg/min less than the new tolerated dose) to 9.2 ng/kg/min by the end of week 12, just 1.6 ng/kg/min less than the mean non-tolerated dose.

Increments in dose should be considered if symptoms of PPH persist or recur after improving. The infusion should be increased by 1 to 2 ng/kg/min increments at intervals sufficient to allow assessment of clinical response; these intervals should be at least 15 minutes. Following establishment of a new chronic infusion rate, the patient should be observed, and standing and supine blood pressure and heart rate monitored for several hours to ensure that the new dose is tolerated.

During chronic infusion, the occurrence of dose-related pharmacological events similar to those observed during acute dose ranging may necessitate a decrease in infusion rate, but the adverse event may occasionally resolve without dosage adjustment. Dosage decreases should be made gradually in 2 ng/kg/min decrements every 15 minutes or longer until the dose-limiting effects resolve. Abrupt withdrawal of FLOLAN or sudden large reductions in infusion rates should be avoided. Except in life-threatening situations (e.g., unconsciousness, collapse, etc.), infusion rates of FLOLAN should be adjusted only under the direction of a physician.

In patients receiving lung transplants, doses of FLOLAN were tapered after the initiation of cardiopulmonary bypass.

Administration: FLOLAN is administered by continuous intravenous infusion via a central venous catheter using an ambulatory infusion pump. During dose ranging, FLOLAN may be administered peripherally.

The ambulatory infusion pump used to administer FLOLAN should: (1) be small and lightweight, (2) be able to adjust infusion rates in 2 ng/kg/min increments, (3) have occlusion, end of infusion, and low battery alarms, (4) be accurate to ±6% of the programmed rate, and (5) be positive pressure driven (continuous or pulsatile) with intervals between pulses not exceeding 3 minutes at infuson rates used to deliver FLOLAN. The reservoir should be made of polyvinyl chloride, polypropylene, or glass. Infusion pumps used in clinical trials were the CADD-1 HFX 5100 (Pharmacia Deltec), Walk-

Med 410 C (Medfusion, Inc.), and the Auto Syringe AS2F (Baxter Health Care).

To avoid potential interruptions in drug delivery, the patient should have access to a backup infusion pump and intravenous infusion sets. A multi-lumen catheter should be considered if other intravenous therapies are routinely administered.

To facilitate extended use at ambient temperatures exceeding 25°C (77°F), a cold pouch with frozen gel packs was used in clinical trials (see DOSAGE AND ADMINISTRATION: Storage and Stability). The cold pouches and gel packs used in clinical trials were obtained from Palco Labs, Palo Alto, California. Any cold pouch used must be capable of maintaining the temperature of reconstituted FLOLAN between 2° and 8°C for 12 hours.

Reconstitution: FLOLAN is stable only when reconstituted with STERILE DILUENT for FLOLAN. FLOLAN must not be reconstituted or mixed with any other parenteral medications or solutions prior to or during administration.

A concentration for the solution of FLOLAN for acute dose ranging or chronic therapy should be selected which is compatible with the infusion pump being used with respect to minimum and maximum flow rates, reservoir capacity, and the infusion pump criteria listed above. FLOLAN, when administered chronically, should be prepared in a drug delivery reservoir appropriate for the infusion pump with a total reservoir volume of at least 100 mL. FLOLAN should be prepared using 2 vials of STERILE DILUENT for FLOLAN for use during a 24-hour period. Table 5 gives directions for preparing several different concentrations of FLOLAN:

[See table 5 above.]

More than one solution strength may be required to accommodate the range of infusions anticipated during acute dose ranging. Generally, 3,000 ng/mL and 10,000 ng/mL are satisfactory concentrations to deliver between 2 to 16 ng/kg/min in adults. Infusion rates may be calculated using the following formula:

Infusion Rate (mL/hr) =

$$\frac{\text{Dose (ng/kg/min)} \times \text{Weight (kg)} \times 60 \text{ min/hr}}{\text{Final Concentration (ng/mL)}}$$

Tables 6 through 9 provide infusion delivery rates for doses up to 16 ng/kg/min based upon patient weight, drug delivery rate, and concentration of the solution of FLOLAN to be used. These tables may be used to select the most appropriate concentration of FLOLAN that will result in an infusion rate between the minimum and maximum flow rates of the infusion pump and which will allow the desired duration of infusion from a given reservoir volume. Higher infusion rates, and therefore, more concentrated solutions may be necessary with long-term administration of FLOLAN.

Table 6

Infusion Rates for FLOLAN® at a Concentration of 3,000 ng/mL

Patient Weight (kg)	Dose or Drug Delivery Rate (ng/kg/min)							
	2	4	6	8	10	12	14	16
	Infusion Delivery Rate (mL/hr)							
10	—	—	1.2	1.6	2.0	2.4	2.8	3.2
20	—	1.6	2.4	3.2	4.0	4.8	5.6	6.4
30	1.2	2.4	3.6	4.8	6.0	7.2	8.4	9.6
40	1.6	3.2	4.8	6.4	8.0	9.6	11.2	12.8
50	2.0	4.0	6.0	8.0	10.0	12.0	14.0	16.0
60	2.4	4.8	7.2	9.6	12.0	14.4	16.8	19.2
70	2.8	5.6	8.4	11.2	14.0	16.8	19.6	22.4
80	3.2	6.4	9.6	12.8	16.0	19.2	22.4	25.6
90	3.6	7.2	10.8	14.4	18.0	21.6	25.2	28.8
100	4.0	8.0	12.0	16.0	20.0	24.0	28.0	32.0

Table 7

Infusion Rates for FLOLAN® at a Concentration of 5,000 ng/mL

Patient Weight (kg)	Dose or Drug Delivery Rate (ng/kg/min)							
	2	4	6	8	10	12	14	16
	Infusion Delivery Rate (mL/hr)							
10	—	—	—	1.0	1.2	1.4	1.7	1.9
20	—	1.0	1.4	1.9	2.4	2.9	3.4	3.8
30	—	1.4	2.2	2.9	3.6	4.3	5.0	5.8
40	1.0	1.9	2.9	3.8	4.8	5.8	6.7	7.7
50	1.2	2.4	3.6	4.8	6.0	7.2	8.4	9.6
60	1.4	2.9	4.3	5.8	7.2	8.6	10.1	11.5
70	1.7	3.4	5.0	6.7	8.4	10.1	11.8	13.4
80	1.9	3.8	5.8	7.7	9.6	11.5	13.4	15.4
90	2.2	4.3	6.5	8.6	10.8	13.0	15.1	17.3
100	2.4	4.8	7.2	9.6	12.0	14.4	16.8	19.2

Table 8

Infusion Rates for FLOLAN® at a Concentration of 10,000 ng/mL

Patient Weight (kg)	Dose or Drug Delivery Rate (ng/kg/min)					
	4	6	8	10	12	14 16
	Infusion Delivery Rate (mL/hr)					
20	—	—	1.0	1.2	1.4	1.7 1.9
30	—	1.1	1.4	1.8	2.2	2.5 2.9
40	1.0	1.4	1.9	2.4	2.9	3.4 3.8
50	1.2	1.8	2.4	3.0	3.6	4.2 4.8
60	1.4	2.2	2.9	3.6	4.3	5.0 5.8
70	1.7	2.5	3.4	4.2	5.0	5.9 6.7
80	1.9	2.9	3.8	4.8	5.8	6.7 7.7
90	2.2	3.2	4.3	5.4	6.5	7.6 8.6
100	2.4	3.6	4.8	6.0	7.2	8.4 9.6

Table 9

Infusion Rates for FLOLAN® at a Concentration of 15,000 ng/mL

Patient Weight (kg)	Dose or Drug Delivery Rate (ng/kg/min)					
	4	6	8	10	12	14 16
	Infusion Delivery Rate (mL/hr)					
30	—	—	1.0	1.2	1.4	1.7 1.9
40	—	1.0	1.3	1.6	1.9	2.2 2.6
50	—	1.2	1.6	2.0	2.4	2.8 3.2
60	1.0	1.4	1.9	2.4	2.9	3.4 3.8
70	1.1	1.7	2.2	2.8	3.4	3.9 4.5
80	1.3	1.9	2.6	3.2	3.8	4.5 5.1
90	1.4	2.2	2.9	3.6	4.3	5.0 5.8
100	1.6	2.4	3.2	4.0	4.8	5.6 6.4

Storage and Stability: Unopened vials of FLOLAN are stable until the date indicated on the package when stored at 15° to 25°C (59° to 77°F) and protected from light in the carton. Unopened vials of STERILE DILUENT for FLOLAN are stable until the date indicated on the package when stored at 15° to 25°C (59° to 77°F).

Prior to use, reconstituted solutions of FLOLAN must be protected from light and must be refrigerated at 2° to 8°C (36° to 46°F) if not used immediately. **Do not freeze reconstituted solutions of FLOLAN. Discard any reconstituted solution that has been frozen. Discard any reconstituted solution if it has been refrigerated for more than 48 hours.**

During use, a single reservoir of reconstituted solution of FLOLAN can be administered at room temperature for a total duration of 8 hours, or it can be used with a cold pouch and administered up to 24 hours with the use of two frozen 6-oz gel packs in a cold pouch. When stored or in use, reconstituted FLOLAN must be insulated from temperatures greater than 25°C (77°F) and less than 0°C (32°F), and must not be exposed to direct sunlight.

Continued on next page

Glaxo Wellcome—Cont.

Use at Room Temperature: Prior to use at room temperature, 15° to 25°C (59° to 77°F), reconstituted solutions of FLOLAN may be stored refrigerated at 2° to 8°C (36° to 46°F) for no longer than 40 hours. When administered at room temperature, reconstituted solutions may be used for no longer than 8 hours. This 48-hour period allows the patient to reconstitute a 2-day supply (200 mL) of FLOLAN. Each 100 mL daily supply may be divided into three equal portions. Two portions are stored refrigerated at 2° to 8°C (36° to 46°F) until they are used.

Use with a Cold Pouch: Prior to infusion with the use of a cold pouch, solutions may be stored refrigerated at 2° to 8°C (36° to 46°F) for up to 24 hours. When a cold pouch is employed during the infusion, reconstituted solutions of FLOLAN may be used no longer than 24 hours. The gel packs should be changed every 12 hours. Reconstituted solutions may be kept at 2° to 8°C (36° to 46°F), either in refrigerated storage or in a cold pouch or a combination of the two, for no more than 48 hours.

Parenteral drug products should be inspected visually for particulate matter and discoloration prior to administration whenever solution and container permit. If either occurs, FLOLAN should not be administered.

HOW SUPPLIED

FLOLAN for Injection is supplied as a sterile freeze-dried powder in 17 mL flint glass vials with gray butyl rubber closures, individually packaged in a carton.

17 mL vial containing epoprostenol sodium equivalent to 0.5 mg (500,000 ng), carton of 1, (NDC 0173-0517-00).

17 mL vial containing epoprostenol sodium equivalent to 1.5 mg (1,500,000 ng), carton of 1, (NDC 0173-0519-00).

Store the vials of FLOLAN at 15° to 25°C (59° to 77°F). Protect from light.

The STERILE DILUENT for FLOLAN is supplied in 50 mL flint glass vials with fluororesin faced butyl rubber closures.

50 mL vial of STERILE DILUENT for FLOLAN, tray of 4 (NDC 0173-0518-00).

Store the vials of STERILE DILUENT for FLOLAN at 15° to 25°C (59° to 77°F). DO NOT FREEZE.

Caution: Federal law prohibits dispensing without prescription.

U.S. Patent Nos. 4335139, 4539333, and 4883812 (Use Patent)

Licensed Under U.S. Patent No. 4338325

January 1996/RL-263

Shown in Product Identification Guide, page 313

FLONASE® ℞

[flō-nāz]

(fluticasone propionate)

Nasal Spray, 0.05% w/w

For Intranasal Use Only.

SHAKE GENTLY BEFORE USE.

DESCRIPTION

Fluticasone propionate, the active ingredient of Flonase® Nasal Spray, is a glucocorticoid with the chemical name of S-fluoromethyl 6α,9α-difluoro-11β-hydroxy-16α-methyl-3-oxo-17α-propionyloxyandrosta-1,4-diene-17β-carbothioate and the following chemical structure:

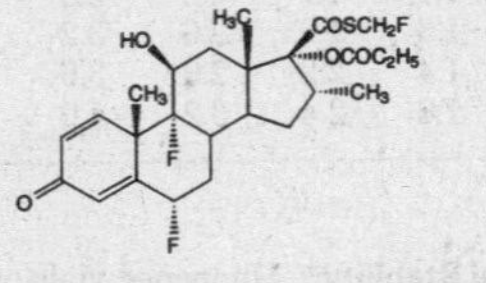

Fluticasone propionate is a white to off-white powder with a molecular weight of 500.6. It is practically insoluble in water, freely soluble in dimethyl sulfoxide and dimethylformamide, and slightly soluble in methanol and 95% ethanol.

Flonase Nasal Spray (0.05% w/w) is an aqueous suspension of microfine fluticasone propionate for topical administration to the nasal mucosa by means of a metering, atomizing spray pump. Flonase Nasal Spray also contains microcrystalline cellulose and carboxymethylcellulose sodium, dextrose, 0.02% w/w benzalkonium chloride, polysorbate 80, and 0.25% w/w phenylethyl alcohol.

After initial priming (three to four actuations), each 100-mg spray delivered by the nasal adapter contains 50 mcg of fluticasone propionate. Each 16-g bottle of Flonase Nasal Spray will provide at least 120 metered sprays. Each 9-g bottle will provide at least 60 metered sprays.

CLINICAL PHARMACOLOGY

Fluticasone propionate is a synthetic, trifluorinated glucocorticoid with anti-inflammatory activity. *In vitro* dose response studies on a cloned human glucocorticoid receptor system involving binding and gene expression afforded 50% responses at 1.25 and 0.17 nM concentrations, respectively. Fluticasone propionate was three- to five-fold more potent than dexamethasone in these assays. Data from the McKenzie vasoconstrictor assay in man also support its potent glucocorticoid activity.

In preclinical studies, fluticasone propionate revealed progesteronelike activity similar to the natural hormone. However, the clinical significance of these findings in relation to the low plasma levels (see Pharmacokinetics) is not known.

The precise mechanism through which glucocorticoids affect allergic rhinitis symptoms is not known. Glucocorticoids have been shown to have a wide range of effects on multiple cell types (e.g., mast cells, eosinophils, neutrophils, macrophages, and lymphocytes) and mediators (e.g., histamine, eicosanoids, leukotrienes, and cytokines) involved in inflammation. In seven trials, Flonase® (fluticasone propionate) Nasal Spray has decreased nasal mucosal eosinophils in 66% (35% for placebo) of patients and basophils in 39% (28% for placebo) of patients. The direct relationship of these findings to long-term symptom relief is not known.

Flonase Nasal Spray, like other glucocorticoids, is an agent that does not have an immediate effect on allergic symptoms. A decrease in nasal symptoms has been noted in some patients 12 hours after initial treatment with Flonase Nasal Spray. Maximum benefit may not be reached for several days. Similarly, when glucocorticoids are discontinued, symptoms may not return for several days.

Pharmacokinetics: ***Absorption:*** The activity of Flonase Nasal Spray is due to the parent drug, fluticasone propionate. Indirect calculations indicate that fluticasone propionate delivered by the intranasal route has an absolute bioavailability averaging less than 2%. After intranasal treatment of patients with allergic rhinitis for 3 weeks, fluticasone propionate plasma concentrations were above the level of detection (50 pg/mL) only when recommended doses were exceeded and then only in occasional samples at low plasma levels. Due to the low bioavailability by the intranasal route, the majority of the pharmacokinetic data was obtained via other routes of administration. Studies using oral dosing of radiolabeled drug have demonstrated that fluticasone propionate is highly extracted from plasma and absorption is low. Oral bioavailability is negligible, and the majority of the circulating radioactivity is due to an inactive metabolite.

Distribution: Following intravenous administration, the distribution of fluticasone propionate follows a three-compartment open model with an apparent volume of distribution of approximately 3.7 L/kg. The percentage of fluticasone propionate bound to human plasma proteins averaged 91% with no obvious concentration relationship. Fluticasone propionate is weakly and reversibly bound to erythrocytes and freely equilibrates between erythrocytes and plasma. Fluticasone propionate is not significantly bound to human transcortin.

Metabolism: The total blood clearance of fluticasone propionate approximates that of liver blood flow, with renal clearance accounting for less than 1% of total. The only circulating metabolite detected in man is the 17β-carboxylic acid derivative of fluticasone propionate. This metabolite has been shown to have negligible pharmacological activity in animal studies. Other metabolites detected *in vitro* using cultured human hepatoma cells have not been detected in man.

Excretion: Following intravenous dosing, fluticasone propionate had an elimination half-life of approximately 3 hours. Less than 5% of a radiolabeled oral dose was excreted in the urine as metabolites, with the remainder excreted in the feces as parent drug and metabolites.

Special Populations: Fluticasone propionate was not studied in any special populations, and no gender-specific pharmacokinetic data have been obtained.

Pharmacodynamics: In a trial to evaluate the potential systemic and topical effects of Flonase Nasal Spray on allergic rhinitis symptoms, the benefits of comparable drug blood levels produced by Flonase Nasal Spray and oral fluticasone propionate were compared. The doses used were 200 mcg of Flonase Nasal Spray, the nasal spray vehicle (plus oral placebo), and 5 and 10 mg of oral fluticasone propionate (plus nasal spray vehicle) per day for 14 days. Plasma levels were undetectable in the majority of patients after intranasal dosing, but present at low levels in the majority after oral dosing. Flonase Nasal Spray was significantly more effective in reducing symptoms of allergic rhinitis than either the oral fluticasone propionate or the nasal vehicle. This trial demonstrated that the therapeutic effect of Flonase Nasal Spray can be attributed to the topical effects of fluticasone propionate.

In another trial, the potential systemic effects of Flonase Nasal Spray on the hypothalamic-pituitary-adrenal (HPA) axis were also studied in allergic patients. Flonase Nasal Spray given as 200 mcg once daily or 400 mcg twice daily was compared with placebo or oral prednisone 7.5 or 15 mg given in the morning. Flonase Nasal Spray at either dose for 4 weeks did not affect the adrenal response to 6-hour cosyntropin stimulation, while both doses of oral prednisone significantly reduced the response to cosyntropin.

Clinical Trials: A total of 11 pivotal, randomized, double-blind, parallel, multicenter, vehicle-controlled clinical trials were conducted in adults and adolescents (children over 12 years of age) with seasonal or perennial allergic rhinitis. The trials included 2,633 adults (1,439 men and 1,194 women) with mean age of 37 years (range, 18 to 79). A total of 440 adolescents (405 boys and 35 girls), mean age of 14 (range, 12 to 17), were also studied. The overall racial distribution was 88% white, 4% black, and 8% other. These trials evaluated the total nasal symptoms scores (TNSS) that included rhinorrhea, nasal obstruction, sneezing, and nasal itching in known allergic patients who were treated for 2 to 24 weeks. Subjects treated with Flonase Nasal Spray noted relief of these symptoms and exhibited significant decrease in TNSS. Nasal mucosal basophils and eosinophils were also reduced at the end of treatment; however, the clinical significance of this decrease is not known.

There were no significant differences between fluticasone propionate regimens whether administered as a single daily dose of 200 mcg (two 50-mcg sprays in each nostril) or as 100 mcg (one 50-mcg spray in each nostril) twice daily in six clinical trials. A clear dose response could not be identified in clinical trials. In one trial, 200 mcg per day was slightly more effective than 50 mcg per day during the first few days of treatment; thereafter, no difference was seen. Doses higher than 200 mcg per day were not more effective.

Individualization of Dosage: Patients may be started on a 200-mcg once-a-day regimen (two 50-mcg sprays in each nostril once a day). An alternative 200-mcg per day dosage regimen can be given as 100 mcg twice daily (one 50-mcg spray in each nostril twice a day). Individual patients will experience a variable time to onset and different degree of symptom relief. A decrease in nasal symptoms may occur as soon as 12 hours after treatment onset. Maximum effect may take several days. Patients who have responded may be able to be maintained (after 4 to 7 days) on 100 mcg per day (one spray in each nostril once daily). Most adolescents (12 years of age and older) should be started with 100 mcg (one spray in each nostril). Treatment with 200 mcg (two sprays in each nostril once daily or one spray in each nostril twice daily) should be reserved for adolescents not adequately responding to 100 mcg daily or as a starting dosage for adolescents with more severe symptoms. In the latter case, depending upon the patient's response, dosage may be decreased to 100 mcg (one spray in each nostril) daily. Maximum total daily doses should not exceed two sprays in each nostril (total dose, 200 mcg per day). There is no evidence that exceeding the recommended dose is more effective.

INDICATIONS AND USAGE

Flonase® (fluticasone propionate) Nasal Spray is indicated for the management of seasonal and perennial allergic rhinitis in adults and adolescents 12 years of age and older.

It is not indicated for the treatment of nonallergic rhinitis since efficacy has not been adequately demonstrated in patients with this condition.

Children: It is not recommended for treatment of children below the age of 12 years with either seasonal rhinitis or allergic or nonallergic perennial rhinitis. Safety and effectiveness of Flonase Nasal Spray in children below 12 years of age have not been adequately established.

CONTRAINDICATIONS

Flonase® (fluticasone propionate) Nasal Spray is contraindicated in patients with a hypersensitivity to any of its ingredients.

WARNINGS

The replacement of a systemic glucocorticoid with a topical glucocorticoid can be accompanied by signs of adrenal insufficiency, and in addition some patients may experience symptoms of withdrawal, e.g., joint and/or muscular pain, lassitude, and depression. Patients previously treated for prolonged periods with systemic glucocorticoids and transferred to topical glucocorticoids should be carefully monitored for acute adrenal insufficiency in response to stress. In those patients who have asthma or other clinical conditions requiring long-term systemic glucocorticoid treatment, too rapid a decrease in systemic glucocorticoids may cause a severe exacerbation of their symptoms.

The use of Flonase® (fluticasone propionate) Nasal Spray with alternate-day systemic prednisone could increase the likelihood of HPA suppression compared with a therapeutic dose of either one alone. Therefore, Flonase Nasal Spray should be used with caution in patients already receiving alternate-day prednisone treatment for any disease. In addition, the concomitant use of Flonase Nasal Spray with other inhaled glucocorticoids could increase the risk of signs or symptoms of hypercorticism and/or suppression of the HPA axis.

Patients who are on immunosuppressant drugs are more susceptible to infections than healthy individuals. Chickenpox and measles, for example, can have a more serious or even fatal course in patients on immunosuppressant doses of corticosteroids. In such patients who have not had these dis-

eases, particular care should be taken to avoid exposure. How the dose, route, and duration of corticosteroid administration affects the risk of developing a disseminated infection is not known. The contribution of the underlying disease and/or prior corticosteroid treatment to the risk is also not known. If exposed to chickenpox, prophylaxis with varicella zoster immune globulin (VZIG) may be indicated. If exposed to measles, prophylaxis with pooled intramuscular immunoglobulin (IG) may be indicated. (See the respective package inserts for complete VZIG and IG prescribing information.) If chickenpox develops, treatment with antiviral agents may be considered.

PRECAUTIONS

General: Rarely, immediate hypersensitivity reactions or contact dermatitis may occur after the intranasal administration of fluticasone propionate. Rare instances of wheezing, nasal septum perforation, cataracts, glaucoma, and increased intraocular pressure have been reported following the intranasal application of glucocorticoids.

Use of excessive doses of glucocorticoids may lead to signs or symptoms of hypercorticism, suppression of HPA function, and/or suppression of growth in children or teenagers. Knemometry studies in asthmatic children on orally inhaled glucocorticoids showed inhibitory effects on short-term growth rate. The relationship between short-term changes in lower leg growth and long-term effects on growth is unclear at this time. Physicians should closely follow the growth of adolescents taking glucocorticoids, by any route, and weigh the benefits of glucocorticoid therapy against the possibility of growth suppression if an adolescent's growth appears slowed.

Although systemic effects have been minimal with recommended doses of Flonase® (fluticasone propionate) Nasal Spray, potential risk increases with larger doses. Therefore, larger than recommended doses of Flonase Nasal Spray should be avoided.

When used at larger doses, systemic glucocorticoid effects such as hypercorticism and adrenal suppression may appear. If such changes occur, the dosage of Flonase Nasal Spray should be discontinued slowly consistent with accepted procedures for discontinuing oral glucocorticoid therapy.

In clinical studies with fluticasone propionate administered intranasally, the development of localized infections of the nose and pharynx with *Candida albicans* has occurred only rarely. When such an infection develops, it may require treatment with appropriate local therapy and discontinuation of treatment with Flonase Nasal Spray. Patients using Flonase Nasal Spray over several months or longer should be examined periodically for evidence of *Candida* infection or other signs of adverse effects on the nasal mucosa.

Flonase Nasal Spray should be used with caution, if at all, in patients with active or quiescent tuberculous infections; untreated fungal, bacterial, or systemic viral infections; or ocular herpes simplex.

Because of the inhibitory effect of glucocorticoids on wound healing, patients who have experienced recent nasal septal ulcers, nasal surgery, or nasal trauma should not use a nasal glucocorticoid until healing has occurred.

Information for Patients: Patients being treated with Flonase Nasal Spray should receive the following information and instructions. This information is intended to aid them in the safe and effective use of this medication. It is not a disclosure of all possible adverse or intended effects.

Patients should be warned to avoid exposure to chickenpox or measles and, if exposed, to consult their physician without delay.

Patients should use Flonase Nasal Spray at regular intervals as directed since its effectiveness depends on its regular use. A decrease in nasal symptoms may occur as soon as 12 hours after starting therapy with Flonase Nasal Spray. Results in several clinical trials indicate statistically significant improvement within the first day or two of treatment; however, the full benefit of Flonase Nasal Spray may not be achieved until treatment has been administered for several days. The patient should not increase the prescribed dosage but should contact the physician if symptoms do not improve or if the condition worsens. For the proper use of the nasal spray and to attain maximum improvement, the patient should read and follow carefully the patient's instructions accompanying the product.

Carcinogenesis, Mutagenesis, Impairment of Fertility: Fluticasone propionate demonstrated no tumorigenic potential in studies of oral doses up to 1.0 mg/kg (3 mg/m² as calculated on a surface area basis) for 78 weeks in the mouse or inhalation of up to 57 mcg/kg (336 mcg/m²) for 104 weeks in the rat.

Fluticasone propionate did not induce gene mutation in prokaryotic or eukaryotic cells *in vitro*. No significant clastogenic effect was seen in cultured human peripheral lymphocytes *in vitro* or in the mouse micronucleus test when administered at high doses by the oral or subcutaneous routes. Furthermore, the compound did not delay erythroblast division in bone marrow.

No evidence of impairment of fertility was observed in reproductive studies conducted in rats dosed subcutaneously with doses up to 50 mcg/kg (295 mcg/m²) in males and females. However, prostate weight was significantly reduced in rats.

Pregnancy: *Teratogenic Effects: Pregnancy Category C:* Subcutaneous studies in the mouse and rat at 45 and 100 mcg/kg, respectively (135 and 590 mcg/m², respectively, as calculated on a surface area basis), revealed fetal toxicity characteristic of potent glucocorticoid compounds, including embryonic growth retardation, omphalocele, cleft palate, and retarded cranial ossification.

In the rabbit, fetal weight reduction and cleft palate were observed following subcutaneous doses of 4 mcg/kg (48 mcg/m²).

However, following oral administration of up to 300 mcg/kg (3.6 mg/m²) of fluticasone propionate to the rabbit, there were no maternal effects nor increased incidence of external, visceral, or skeletal fetal defects. No fluticasone propionate was detected in the plasma in this study, consistent with the established low bioavailability following oral administration (see CLINICAL PHARMACOLOGY).

Less than 0.008% of the dose crosses the placenta following oral administration to rats (100 mcg/kg, 590 mcg/m²) or rabbits (300 mcg/kg, 3.6 mg/m²).

There are no adequate and well-controlled studies in pregnant women. Fluticasone propionate should be used during pregnancy only if the potential benefit justifies the potential risk to the fetus. Experience with oral glucocorticoids since their introduction in pharmacologic, as opposed to physiologic, doses suggests that rodents are more prone to teratogenic effects from glucocorticoids than humans. In addition, because there is a natural increase in glucocorticoid production during pregnancy, most women will require a lower exogenous glucocorticoid dose and many will not need glucocorticoid treatment during pregnancy.

Nursing Mothers: It is not known whether fluticasone propionate is excreted in human breast milk. Subcutaneous administration of tritiated drug to lactating rats (10 mcg/kg, 59 mcg/m²) resulted in measurable radioactivity in both plasma and milk. Because other glucocorticoids are excreted in human milk, caution should be exercised when Flonase Nasal Spray is administered to a nursing woman.

Pediatric Use: The safety and effectiveness of Flonase Nasal Spray in children below 12 years of age have not been established. Oral glucocorticoids have been shown to cause growth suppression in children and teenagers with extended use. If a child or teenager on any glucocorticoid appears to have growth suppression, the possibility that they are particularly sensitive to this effect of glucocorticoids should be considered (see PRECAUTIONS).

Geriatric Use: A limited number of patients above 60 years of age (n=132) have been treated with Flonase Nasal Spray in US and non-US clinical trials. While the number of patients is too small to permit separate analysis of efficacy and safety, the adverse reactions reported in this population were similar to those reported by younger patients.

ADVERSE REACTIONS

In controlled US studies, 2,427 patients received treatment with intranasal fluticasone propionate. In general, adverse reactions in clinical studies have been primarily associated with irritation of the nasal mucous membranes, and the adverse reactions were reported with approximately the same frequency by patients treated with the vehicle itself. The complaints did not usually interfere with treatment. Less than 2% of patients in clinical trials discontinued because of adverse events; this rate was similar for vehicle and active comparators.

Systemic glucocorticoid side effects were not reported during controlled clinical studies up to 6 months' duration with Flonase® (fluticasone propionate) Nasal Spray. If recommended doses are exceeded, however, or if individuals are particularly sensitive or if in conjunction with systemically administered glucocorticoids, symptoms of hypercorticism, e.g., Cushing's syndrome, could occur.

The following incidence of common adverse reactions is based upon seven controlled clinical trials in which 536 patients (57 girls and 108 boys aged 4 to 11 years, 137 female and 234 male adolescents and adults) were treated with Flonase Nasal Spray 200 mcg once daily over 2 to 4 weeks and two controlled clinical trials in which 246 patients (119 female and 127 male adolescents and adults) were treated with Flonase Nasal Spray 200 mcg once daily over 6 months.

Incidence Greater than 1% (Causal Relationship Possible):
Respiratory: Epistaxis, nasal burning (incidence 3% to 6%); blood in nasal mucus, pharyngitis, nasal irritation (incidence 1% to 3%).
Neurological: Headache (incidence 1% to 3%).

Incidence Less than 1% (Causal Relationship Possible):
Respiratory: Sneezing, runny nose, nasal dryness, sinusitis, nasal congestion, bronchitis, nasal ulcer, nasal septum excoriation.
Neurological: Dizziness.
Special Senses: Eye disorder, unpleasant taste.

Digestive: Nausea and vomiting, xerostomia.
Skin and Appendages: Urticaria.

Postmarketing Experience: In addition to the events from clinical trials, the following have been reported during postmarketing experience.

Hypersensitivity reactions, including skin rash, edema of the face and tongue, and rarely bronchospasm, have been reported.

OVERDOSAGE

There are no data available on the effects of acute or chronic overdosage with Flonase® (fluticasone propionate) Nasal Spray. Intranasal administration of 2 mg (10 times the recommended dose) of fluticasone propionate twice daily for 7 days to healthy human volunteers was well tolerated. Single oral doses up to 16 mg have been studied in human volunteers with no acute toxic effects reported. Repeat oral doses up to 80 mg daily for 10 days in volunteers and repeat oral doses up to 10 mg daily for 14 days in patients were well tolerated. Adverse reactions were of mild or moderate severity, and incidences were similar in active and placebo treatment groups. Acute overdosage with this dosage form is unlikely since one bottle of Flonase Nasal Spray contains approximately 8 mg of fluticasone propionate. Chronic overdosage may result in signs/symptoms of hypercorticism (see PRECAUTIONS).

DOSAGE AND ADMINISTRATION

Patients should use Flonase® (fluticasone propionate) Nasal Spray at regular intervals as directed since its effectiveness depends on its regular use.

Adults and Adolescents 12 Years of Age and Older: The recommended starting dosage in **adults** is two sprays (50 mcg of fluticasone propionate each) in each nostril once a day (total daily dose, 200 mcg). The same dosage divided into 100 mcg given twice a day (e.g., 8 a.m. and 8 p.m.) is also effective. After the first few days, patients may be able to reduce their dosage to 100 mcg (one spray in each nostril) once daily for maintenance therapy.

Most **adolescents** should be started with 100 mcg (one spray in each nostril). Adolescents not adequately responding to 100 mcg or adolescents with more severe symptoms may use 200 mcg (two sprays in each nostril). Depending upon the patient's response, dosage may be decreased to 100 mcg (one spray in each nostril) daily.

The maximum total daily dosage should not exceed two sprays in each nostril (200 mcg per day). (See Individualization of Dosage and Clinical Trials Sections.)

Flonase Nasal Spray is not recommended for children under 12 years of age or for patients with nonallergic rhinitis.

Directions for Use: Illustrated patient's instructions for proper use accompany each package of Flonase Nasal Spray.

HOW SUPPLIED

Flonase® (fluticasone propionate) Nasal Spray, 0.05% w/w is supplied in a 16-g amber glass bottle providing 120 actuations (NDC 0173-0453-01) and in a 9-g amber glass bottle providing 60 actuations (NDC 0173-0472-00). Each actuation delivers 100 mg of the suspension, which contains 50 mcg of fluticasone propionate. Each bottle is fitted with a metering atomizing pump, nasal adapter, and dust cover in a box of one with patient's instructions for use.

Store between 4° and 30°C (39° and 86°F).

October 1995/RL-221

Shown in Product Identification Guide, page 313

FLOVENT® 44 mcg ℞
(fluticasone propionate, 44 mcg)
Inhalation Aerosol

FLOVENT® 110 mcg
(fluticasone propionate, 110 mcg)
Inhalation Aerosol

FLOVENT® 220 mcg
(fluticasone propionate, 220 mcg)
Inhalation Aerosol
For Oral Inhalation Only

DESCRIPTION

The active component of FLOVENT 44 mcg Inhalation Aerosol, FLOVENT 110 mcg Inhalation Aerosol, and FLOVENT 220 mcg Inhalation Aerosol is fluticasone propionate, a glucocorticoid having the chemical name S-(fluoromethyl)6α,-9-difluoro-11β, 17-dihydroxy-16α-methyl-3-oxoandrosta-1,4-diene-17β-carbothioate, 17-propionate.

Fluticasone propionate is a white to off-white powder with a molecular weight of 500.6. It is practically insoluble in water, freely soluble in dimethyl sulfoxide and dimethylformamide, and slightly soluble in methanol and 95% ethanol.

FLOVENT 44 mcg Inhalation Aerosol, FLOVENT 110 mcg Inhalation Aerosol, and FLOVENT 220 mcg Inhalation Aerosol are pressurized, metered-dose aerosol units intended for oral inhalation only. Each unit contains a microcrystalline

Continued on next page

Glaxo Wellcome—Cont.

suspension of fluticasone propionate (micronized) in a mixture of two chlorofluorocarbon propellants (trichlorofluoromethane and dichlorodifluoromethane) with lecithin. Each actuation of the inhaler delivers 50, 125, or 250 mcg of fluticasone propionate from the valve, and 44, 110, or 220 mcg, respectively, of fluticasone propionate from the actuator.

CLINICAL PHARMACOLOGY

Fluticasone propionate is a synthetic, trifluorinated glucocorticoid with potent anti-inflammatory activity. *In vitro* assays using human lung cytosol preparations have established fluticasone propionate as a human glucocorticoid receptor agonist with an affinity 18 times greater than dexamethasone, almost twice that of beclomethasone-17-monopropionate (BMP), the active metabolite of beclomethasone dipropionate, and over three times that of budesonide. Data from the McKenzie vasoconstrictor assay in man are consistent with these results.

The precise mechanisms of glucocorticoid action in asthma are unknown. Inflammation is recognized as an important component in the pathogenesis of asthma. Glucocorticoids have been shown to inhibit multiple cell types (e.g., mast cells, eosinophils, basophils, lymphocytes, macrophages, and neutrophils) and mediator production or secretion (e.g., histamine, eicosanoids, leukotrienes, and cytokines) involved in the asthmatic response. These anti-inflammatory actions of glucocorticoids may contribute to their efficacy in asthma.

Though highly effective for the treatment of asthma, glucocorticoids do not affect asthma symptoms immediately. However, improvement following inhaled administration of fluticasone propionate can occur within 24 hours of beginning treatment, although maximum benefit may not be achieved for 1 to 2 weeks or longer after starting treatment. When glucocorticoids are discontinued, asthma stability may persist for several days or longer.

Pharmacokinetics: ***Absorption:*** The activity of FLOVENT Inhalation Aerosol is due to the parent drug, fluticasone propionate. Studies using oral dosing of labeled and unlabeled drug have demonstrated that the oral systemic bioavailability of fluticasone propionate is negligible (<1%), primarily due to incomplete absorption and pre-systemic metabolism in the gut and liver. In contrast, the majority of the fluticasone propionate delivered to the lung is systemically absorbed. The systemic bioavailability of fluticasone propionate inhalation aerosol averaged about 30% of the dose delivered from the actuator.

Peak plasma concentrations after an 800-mcg inhaled dose ranged from 0.1 to 1.0 ng/mL.

Distribution: Following intravenous administration, the initial disposition phase for fluticasone propionate was rapid and consistent with its high lipid solubility and tissue binding. The volume of distribution averaged 4.2 L/kg. The percentage of fluticasone propionate bound to human plasma proteins averaged 91%. Fluticasone propionate is weakly and reversibly bound to erythrocytes. Fluticasone propionate is not significantly bound to human transcortin.

Metabolism: The total clearance of fluticasone propionate is high (average, 1,093 mL/min), with renal clearance accounting for less than 0.02% of the total. The only circulating metabolite detected in man is the 17β-carboxylic acid derivative of fluticasone propionate, which is formed through the cytochrome P450 3A4 pathway. This metabolite had approximately 2,000 times less affinity than the parent drug for the glucocorticoid receptor of human lung cytosol *in vitro* and negligible pharmacological activity in animal studies. Other metabolites detected *in vitro* using cultured human hepatoma cells have not been detected in man.

Excretion: Following intravenous dosing, fluticasone propionate showed polyexponential kinetics and had a terminal elimination half-life of approximately 7.8 hours. Less than 5% of a radiolabeled oral dose was excreted in the urine as metabolites, with the remainder excreted in the feces as parent drug and metabolites.

Special Populations: Formal pharmacokinetic studies using fluticasone propionate were not carried out in any special populations. In a clinical study using fluticasone propionate inhalation powder, trough fluticasone propionate plasma concentrations were collected in 76 males and 74 females after inhaled administration of 100 and 500 mcg twice daily. Full pharmacokinetic profiles were obtained from 7 female patients and 13 male patients at these doses, and no overall differences in pharmacokinetic behavior were found.

Pharmacodynamics: To confirm that systemic absorption does not play a role in the clinical response to inhaled fluticasone propionate, a double-blind clinical study comparing inhaled and oral fluticasone propionate was conducted. Doses of 100 and 500 mcg twice daily of fluticasone propionate inhalation powder were compared to oral fluticasone propionate, 20,000 mcg given once daily, and placebo for 6 weeks. Plasma levels of fluticasone propionate were detectable in all three active groups, but the mean values were highest in the oral group. Both doses of inhaled fluticasone propionate were effective in maintaining asthma stability and improving lung function while oral fluticasone propionate and placebo were ineffective. This demonstrates that the clinical effectiveness of inhaled fluticasone propionate is due to its direct local effect and not to an indirect effect through systemic absorption.

The potential systemic effects of inhaled fluticasone propionate on the hypothalamic-pituitary-adrenal (HPA) axis were also studied in asthma patients. Fluticasone propionate given by inhalation aerosol at doses of 220, 440, 660, or 880 mcg twice daily was compared with placebo or oral prednisone 10 mg given once daily for 4 weeks. For most patients, the ability to increase cortisol production in response to stress, as assessed by 6-hour cosyntropin stimulation, remained intact with inhaled fluticasone propionate treatment. No patient had a abnormal response (peak less than 18 mcg/dL) after dosing with placebo or 220 mcg twice daily. Ten percent (10%) to 16% of patients treated with fluticasone propionate at doses of 440 mcg or more twice daily had an abnormal response as compared to 29% of patients treated with prednisone.

Clinical Trials: Double-blind, parallel, placebo-controlled, US clinical trials were conducted in 1,818 adolescent and adult asthma patients to assess the efficacy and/or safety of FLOVENT Inhalation Aerosol in the treatment of asthma. Fixed doses ranging from 44 to 880 mcg twice daily were compared to placebo to provide information about appropriate dosing to cover a range of asthma severity. Asthmatic patients included in these studies were those not adequately controlled with beta-agonists alone, those already maintained on daily inhaled corticosteroids, and those requiring oral corticosteroid therapy. In all efficacy trials, at all doses, measures of pulmonary function (forced expiratory volume in 1 second [FEV_1] and morning peak expiratory flow rate [AM PEFR]) were statistically significantly improved as compared with placebo.

In two clinical trials of 660 asthmatic patients inadequately controlled on bronchodilators alone, fluticasone propionate administered by inhalation aerosol was evaluated at doses of 44 and 88 mcg twice daily. Both doses of fluticasone propionate improved asthma control significantly as compared with placebo.

Displayed in the figure below are results of pulmonary function tests for the recommended starting dosage of fluticasone propionate inhalation aerosol (88 mcg twice daily) and placebo from a 12-week trial in asthma patients inadequately controlled on bronchodilators alone. Because this trial used predetermined criteria for lack of efficacy, which caused more patients in the placebo group to be withdrawn, pulmonary function results at Endpoint, which is the last evaluable FEV_1 result and includes most patients' lung function data, are also provided. Pulmonary function improved significantly with fluticasone propionate compared with placebo by the second week of treatment, and this improvement was maintained over the duration of the trial.

A 12-Week Clinical Trial In Patients Inadequately Controlled on Bronchodilators Alone: Mean Percent Change From Baseline in FEV_1 Prior to AM Dose

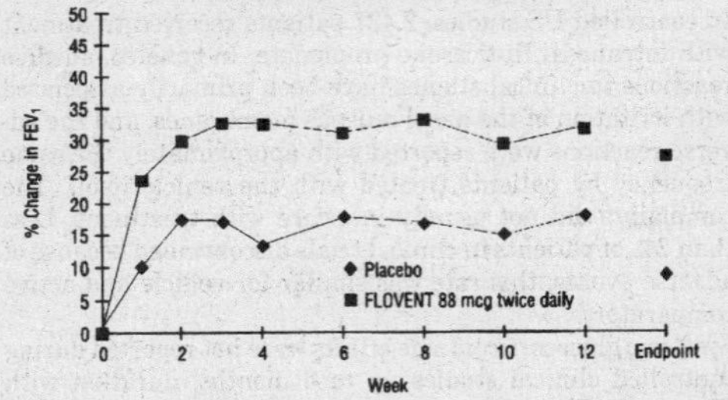

In clinical trials of 924 asthmatic patients already receiving daily inhaled corticosteriod therapy (doses of at least 336 mcg/day of beclomethasone dipropionate) in addition to as-needed albuterol and theophylline (46% of all patients), fluticasone propionate inhalation aerosol doses of 22 to 440 mcg twice daily were also evaluated. All doses of fluticasone propionate were efficacious when compared to placebo on major endpoints including lung function and symptom scores. Patients treated with fluticasone propionate were also less likely to discontinue study participation due to asthma deterioration (as defined by predetermined criteria for lack of efficacy including lung function and patient-recorded variables such as AM PEFR, albuterol use, and nighttime awakenings due to asthma).

Displayed in the figure below are results of pulmonary function from a 12-week clinical trial in asthma patients already receiving daily inhaled corticosteroid therapy (beclomethasone dipropionate 336 to 672 mcg/day). The mean percent change from baseline in lung function results for fluticasone propionate inhalation aerosol dosages of 88, 220, and 440 mcg twice daily and placebo are shown over the 12-week trial. Because this trial also used predetermined criteria for lack of efficacy, which caused more patients in the placebo group to be withdrawn, pulmonary function results at Endpoint are included. Pulmonary function improved significantly with fluticasone propionate compared with placebo by the first week of treatment, and the improvement was maintained over the duration of the trial. Analysis of the Endpoint results that adjusted for differential withdrawal rates indicated that pulmonary function significantly improved with fluticasone propionate compared with placebo treatment. Similar improvements in lung function were seen in the other two trials in patients treated with inhaled corticosteroids at baseline.

A 12-Week Clinical Trial With Patients Already Receiving Inhaled Corticosteroids: Mean Percent Change From Baseline in FEV_1 Prior to AM Dose

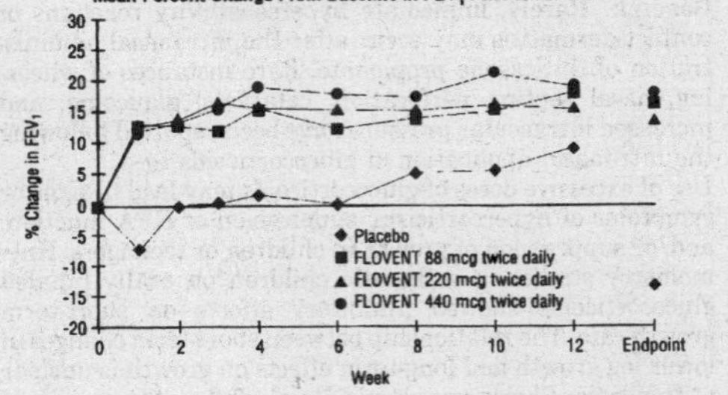

In a clinical trial of 96 severe asthmatic patients requiring chronic oral prednisone therapy (average baseline daily prednisone dose was 10 mg), FLOVENT Inhalation Aerosol doses of 660 and 880 mcg twice daily were evaluated. Both doses enabled a statistically significantly larger percentage of patients to wean successfully from oral prednisone as compared with placebo (69% of the patients on 660 mcg twice daily and 88% of the patients on 880 mcg twice daily as compared with 3% of patients on placebo). Accompanying the reduction in oral corticosteroid use, patients treated with FLOVENT Inhalation Aerosol had significantly improved lung function and fewer asthma symptoms as compared with the placebo group.

A 16-Week Clinical Trial in Patients Requiring Chronic Oral Prednisone Therapy: Change in Maintenance Prednisone Dose

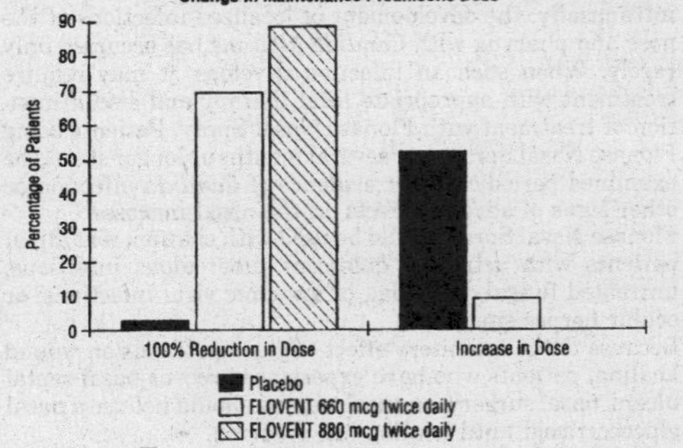

INDICATIONS AND USAGE

FLOVENT Inhalation Aerosol is indicated for the maintenance treatment of asthma as prophylactic therapy. It is also indicated for patients requiring oral corticosteroid therapy for asthma. Many of these patients may be able to reduce or eliminate their requirement for oral corticosteroids over time.

FLOVENT Inhalation Aerosol is NOT indicated for the relief of acute bronchospasm.

CONTRAINDICATIONS

FLOVENT Inhalation Aerosol is contraindicated in the primary treatment of status asthmaticus or other acute episodes of asthma where intensive measures are required. Hypersensitivity to any of the ingredients of these preparations contraindicates their use.

WARNINGS

Particular care is needed for patients who are transferred from systemically active corticosteroids to FLOVENT Inhalation Aerosol because deaths due to adrenal insufficiency have occurred in asthmatic patients during and after transfer from systemic corticosteroids to less systemically available inhaled corticosteroids. After withdrawal from systemic corticosteroids, a number of months are required for recovery of HPA function.

Patients who have been previously maintained on 20 mg or more per day of prednisone (or its equivalent) may be most susceptible, particularly when their systemic corticosteroids have been almost completely withdrawn. During this period of HPA suppression, patients may exhibit signs and symptoms of adrenal insufficiency when exposed to trauma, surgery, or infection (particularly gastroenteritis) or other conditions associ-

ated with severe electrolyte loss. Although fluticasone propionate inhalation aerosol may provide control of asthma symptoms during these episodes, in recommended doses it supplies less than normal physiological amounts of glucocorticoid systemically and does NOT provide the mineralocorticoid activity that is necessary for coping with these emergencies.

During periods of stress or a severe asthma attack, patients who have been withdrawn from systemic corticosteroids should be instructed to resume oral corticosteroids (in large doses) immediately and to contact their physicians for further instruction. These patients should also be instructed to carry a warning card indicating that they may need supplementary systemic corticosteroids during periods of stress or a severe asthma attack.

Patients requiring oral corticosteroids should be weaned slowly from systemic corticosteroids use after transferring to fluticasone propionate inhalation aerosol. In a trial of 96 patients, prednisone reduction was successfully accomplished by reducing the daily prednisone dose by 2.5 mg on a weekly basis during transfer to inhaled fluticasone propionate. Successive reduction of prednisone dose was allowed only when lung function, symptoms, and as-needed beta-agonist use were better than or comparable to that seen before initiation of prednisone dose reduction. Lung function (FEV_1 or AM PEFR), beta-agonist use, and asthma symptoms should be carefully monitored during withdrawal of oral corticosteroids. In addition to monitoring asthma signs and symptoms, patients should be observed for signs and symptoms of adrenal insufficiency such as fatigue, lassitude, weakness, nausea and vomiting, and hypotension.

Transfer of patients from systemic corticosteroid therapy to fluticasone propionate inhalation aerosol may unmask conditions previously suppressed by the systemic corticosteroid therapy, e.g., rhinitis, conjunctivitis, eczema, and arthritis.

Persons who are on drugs that suppress the immune system are more susceptible to infections than healthy individuals. Chickenpox and measles, for example, can have a more serious or even fatal course in susceptible children or adults on corticosteroids. In such children or adults who have not had these diseases, particular care should be taken to avoid exposure. How the dose, route, and duration of corticosteroid administration affects the risk of developing a disseminated infection is not known. The contribution of the underlying disease and/or prior corticosteroid treatment to the risk is also not known. If exposed to chickenpox, prophylaxis with varicella zoster immune globulin (VZIG) may be indicated. If exposed to measles, prophylaxis with pooled intramuscular immunoglobulin (IG) may be indicated. (See the respective package inserts for complete VZIG and IG prescribing information.) If chickenpox develops, treatment with antiviral agents may be considered.

Fluticasone propionate inhalation aerosol is not to be regarded as a bronchodilator and is not indicated for rapid relief of bronchospasm.

As with other inhaled asthma medications, bronchospasm may occur with an immediate increase in wheezing after dosing. If bronchospasm occurs following dosing with FLOVENT Inhalation Aerosol, it should be treated immediately with a fast-acting inhaled bronchodilator. Treatment with FLOVENT Inhalation Aerosol should be discontinued and alternative therapy instituted.

Patients should be instructed to contact their physicians immediately when episodes of asthma that are not responsive to bronchodilators occur during the course of treatment with fluticasone propionate inhalation aerosol. During such episodes, patients may require therapy with oral corticosteroids.

PRECAUTIONS

General: During withdrawal from oral corticosteroids, some patients may experience symptoms of systemically active corticosteroid withdrawal, e.g., joint and/or muscular pain, lassitude, and depression, despite maintenance or even improvement of respiratory function.

Fluticasone propionate will often permit control of asthma symptoms with less suppression of HPA function than therapeutically equivalent oral doses of prednisone. Since fluticasone propionate is absorbed into the circulation and can be systemically active at higher doses, the beneficial effects of fluticasone propionate inhalation aerosol in minimizing HPA dysfunction may be expected only when recommended dosages are not exceeded and individual patients are titrated to the lowest effective dose. A relationship between plasma levels of fluticasone propionate and inhibitory effects on stimulated cortisol production has been shown after 4 weeks of treatment with fluticasone propionate inhalation aerosol. Since individual sensitivity to effects on cortisol production exists, physicians should consider this information when prescribing fluticasone propionate inhalation aerosol.

Because of the possibility of systemic absorption of inhaled corticosteroids, patients treated with these drugs should be observed carefully for any evidence of systemic corticosteroid effects. Particular care should be taken in observing patients postoperatively or during periods of stress for evidence of inadequate adrenal response.

It is possible that systemic corticosteroid effects such as hypercorticism and adrenal suppression may appear in a small number of patients, particularly at higher doses. If such changes occur, fluticasone propionate inhalation aerosol should be reduced slowly, consistent with accepted procedures for reducing systemic corticosteroids and for management of asthma symptoms.

A reduction of growth velocity in children or teenagers may occur as a result of inadequate control of chronic diseases such as asthma or from use of corticosteroids for treatment. Physicians should closely follow the growth of adolescents taking corticosteroids by any route and weigh the benefits of corticosteroid therapy and asthma control against the possibility of growth suppression if an adolescent's growth appears slowed.

The long-term effects of fluticasone propionate in human subjects are not fully known. In particular, the effects resulting from chronic use of fluticasone propionate on developmental or immunologic processes in the mouth, pharynx, trachea, and lung are unknown. Some patients have received fluticasone propionate inhalation aerosol on a continuous basis for periods of 3 years or longer. In clinical studies with patients treated for nearly 2 years with inhaled fluticasone propionate, no apparent differences in the type or severity of adverse reactions were observed after long- versus short-term treatment.

Rare instances of glaucoma, increased intraocular pressure, and cataracts have been reported following the inhaled administration of corticosteroids.

In clinical studies with inhaled fluticasone propionate, the development of localized infections of the pharynx with *Candida albicans* has occurred. When such an infection develops, it should be treated with appropriate local or systemic (i.e., oral antifungal) therapy while remaining on treatment with fluticasone propionate inhalation aerosol, but at times therapy with fluticasone propionate may need to be interrupted.

Inhaled corticosteroids should be used with caution, if at all, in patients with active or quiescent tuberculosis infection of the respiratory tract; untreated systemic fungal, bacterial, viral or parasitic infections; or ocular herpes simplex.

Information for Patients: Patients being treated with FLOVENT Inhalation Aerosol should receive the following information and instructions. This information is intended to aid them in the safe and effective use of this medication. It is not a disclosure of all possible adverse or intended effects.

Patients should use FLOVENT Inhalation Aerosol at regular intervals as directed. Results of clinical trials indicated significant improvement may occur within the first day or two of treatment; however, the full benefit may not be achieved until treatment has been administered for 1 to 2 weeks or longer. The patient should not increase the prescribed dosage but should contact the physician if symptoms do not improve or if the condition worsens.

Patients should be warned to avoid exposure to chickenpox or measles and, if they are exposed, to consult their physicians without delay.

For the proper use of FLOVENT Inhalation Aerosol and to attain maximum improvement, the patient should read and follow carefully the accompanying Patient's Instructions for Use.

Carcinogenesis, Mutagenesis, Impairment of Fertility: Fluticasone propionate demonstrated no tumorigenic potential in studies of oral doses up to 1,000 mcg/kg (approximately two times the maximum human daily inhalation dose base on mcg/m^2) for 78 weeks in the mouse or inhalation of up to 57 mcg/kg (approximately ¼ the maximum human daily inhalation dose based on mcg/m^2) for 104 weeks in the rat.

Fluticasone propionate did not induce gene mutation in prokaryotic or eukaryotic cells *in vitro*. No significant clastogenic effect was seen in cultured human peripheral lymphocytes *in vitro* or in the mouse micronucleus test when administered at high doses by the oral or subcutaneous routes. Furthermore, the compound did not delay erythroblast division in bone marrow.

No evidence of impairment of fertilty was observed in reproductive studies conducted in rats dosed subcutaneously with doses up to 50 mcg/kg (approximately ¼ the maximum human daily inhalation dose based on mcg/m^2) in males and females. However, prostate weight was significantly reduced in rats.

Pregnancy: ***Teratogenic Effects: Pregnancy Category C:*** Subcutaneous studies in the mouse and rat at 45 and 100 mcg/kg, respectively (approximately $\frac{1}{10}$ and ½ the maximum human daily inhalation dose based on mcg/m^2, respectively), revealed fetal toxicity characteristic of potent glucocorticoid compounds, including embryonic growth retardation, omphalocele, cleft palate, and retarded cranial ossification.

In the rabbit, fetal weight reduction and cleft palate were observed following subcutaneous doses of 4 mcg/kg (approximately $\frac{1}{25}$ the maximum human daily inhalation dose based on mcg/m^2). However, following oral administration of up to 300 mcg/kg (approximately 3 times the maximum human daily inhalation dose based on mcg/m^2) of fluticasone propionate to the rabbit, there were no maternal effects nor increased incidence of external, visceral, or skeletal fetal defects. No fluticasone propionate was detected in the plasma in this study, consistent with the established low bioavailability following oral administration (see CLINICAL PHARMACOLOGY).

Less than 0.008% of the administered dose crossed the placenta following oral administration of 100 mcg/kg to rats or 300 mcg/kg to rabbits (approximately ½ and 3 times the maximum human daily inhalation dose based on mcg/m^2, respectively).

There are no adequate and well-controlled studies in pregnant women. Fluticasone propionate should be used during pregnancy only if the potential benefit justifies the potential risk to the fetus.

Experience with oral glucocorticoids since their introduction in pharmacologic, as opposed to physiologic, doses suggests that rodents are more prone to teratogenic effects from glucocorticoids than humans. In addition, because there is a natural increase in glucocorticoid production during pregnancy, most women will require a lower exogenous glucocorticoid dose and many will not need glucocorticoid treatment during pregnancy.

Nursing Mothers: It is not known whether fluticasone propionate is excreted in human breast milk. Subcutaneous administration of 10 mcg/kg tritiated drug to lactating rats (approximately $\frac{1}{20}$ the maximum human daily inhalation dose based on mcg/m^2) resulted in measurable radioactivity in both plasma and milk. Because glucocorticoids are excreted in human milk, caution should be exercised when fluticasone propionate inhalation aerosol is administered to a nursing woman.

Pediatric Use: One hundred thirty-seven (137) patients between the ages of 12 and 16 years were treated with fluticasone propionate inhalation aerosol in the US pivotal clinical trials. The safety and effectiveness of FLOVENT Inhalation Aerosol in children below 12 years of age have not been established. Oral corticosteroids have been shown to cause a reduction in growth velocity in children and teenagers with extended use. If a child or teenager on any corticosteroid appears to have growth suppression, the possibility that they are particularly sensitive to this effect of corticosteroids should be considered (see PRECAUTIONS).

Geriatric Use: Five hundred seventy-four (574) patients 65 years of age or older have been treated with fluticasone propionate inhalation aerosol in US and non-US clinical trials. There were no differences in adverse reactions compared to those reported by younger patients.

ADVERSE REACTIONS

The following incidence of common adverse experiences is based upon seven placebo-controlled US clinical trials in which 1,243 patients (509 female and 734 male adolescents and adults previously treated with as-needed bronchodilators and/or inhaled corticosteroids) were treated with fluticasone propionate inhalation aerosol (doses of 88 to 440 mcg twice daily for up to 12 weeks) or placebo.

[See table at bottom of next page.]

The table above includes all events (whether considered drug-related or nondrug-related by the investigator) that occurred at a rate of over 3% in the combined fluticasone propionate inhalation aerosol groups and were more common than in the placebo group. In considering these data, differences in average duration of exposure should be taken into account.

These adverse reactions were mostly mild to moderate in severity, with ≤2% of patients discontinuing the studies because of adverse events. Rare cases of immediate and delayed hypersensitivity reactions, including urticaria and rash and other rare events of angioedema and bronchospasm, have been reported.

Systemic glucocorticoid side effects were not reported during controlled clinical trials with fluticasone propionate inhalation aerosol. If recommended doses are exceeded, however, or if individuals are particularly sensitive, symptoms of hypercorticism, e.g., Cushing's syndrome, could occur.

Other adverse events that occurred in these clinical trials using fluticasone propionate inhalation aerosol with an incidence of 1% to 3% and which occurred at a greater incidence than with placebo were:

Ear, Nose, and Throat: Pain in nasal sinus(es), rhinitis.

Eye: Irritation of the eye(s).

Gastrointestinal: Nausea and vomiting, diarrhea, dyspepsia and stomach disorder.

Miscellaneous: Fever.

Mouth and Teeth: Dental problem.

Musculoskeletal: Pain in joint, sprain/strain, aches and pains, pain in limb.

Continued on next page

Glaxo Wellcome—Cont.

Previous Therapy	Recommended Starting Dose	Highest Recommended Dose
Bronchodilators alone	88 mcg twice daily	440 mcg twice daily
Inhaled corticosteroids	88-220 mcg twice daily*	440 mcg twice daily
Oral corticosteroids†	880 mcg twice daily	880 mcg twice daily

*Starting doses above 88 mcg twice daily may be considered for patients with poorer asthma control or those who have previously required doses of inhaled corticosteroids that are in the higher range for that specific agent.
NOTE: In all patients, it is desirable to titrate to the lowest effective dose once asthma stability is achieved.
†**For Patients Currently Receiving Chronic Oral Corticosteroid Therapy:** Prednisone should be reduced no faster than 2.5 mg/day on a weekly basis, beginning after at least 1 week of therapy with FLOVENT Inhalation Aerosol. Patients should be carefully monitored for signs of asthma instability, including serial objective measures of airflow, and for signs of adrenal insufficiency (see WARNINGS). Once prednisone reduction is complete, the dosage of fluticasone propionate should be reduced to the lowest effective dosage.

Neurological: Dizziness/giddiness.
Respiratory: Bronchitis, chest congestion.
Skin: Dermatitis, rash/skin eruption.
Urogenital: Dysmenorrhea.
In a 16-week study in asthmatics requiring oral corticosteroids, the effects of fluticasone propionate inhalation aerosol, 660 mcg twice daily (n = 32) and 880 mcg twice daily (n = 32), were compared with placebo. Adverse events (whether considered drug-related or nondrug-related by the investigator) reported by more than three patients in either fluticasone propionate group and which were more common with fluticasone propionate than placebo are shown below:
Ear, Nose, and Throat: Pharyngitis (9% and 25%); nasal congestion (19% and 22%); sinusitis (19% and 22%); nasal discharge (16% and 16%); dysphonia (16% and 9%); pain in nasal sinus(es) (13% and 0%); Candida-like oral lesions (16% and 9%); oropharyngeal candidiasis (25% and 19%).
Respiratory: Upper respiratory infection (31% and 19%); influenza (0% and 13%).
Other: Headache (28% and 34%); pain in joint (19% and 13%); nausea and vomiting (22% and 16%); muscular soreness (22% and 13%); malaise/fatigue (22% and 28%): insomnia (3% and 13%).

OVERDOSAGE
There are no data available on the effects of acute or chronic overdosage with FLOVENT Inhalation Aerosol. Inhalation by healthy volunteers of a single dose of 1,760 or 3,520 mcg of fluticasone propionate inhalation aerosol was well tolerated. Fluticasone propionate given by inhalation aerosol at doses of 1,320 mcg twice daily for 7 to 15 days to healthy human volunteers was also well tolerated. Repeat oral doses up to 80 mg daily for 10 days in healthy volunteers and repeat oral doses up to 20 mg daily for 42 days in patients were well tolerated. Adverse reactions were of mild or moderate severity, and incidences were similar in active and placebo treatment groups. Chronic overdosage may result in signs/symptoms of hypercorticism (see PRECAUTIONS). The oral and subcutaneous median lethal doses in rats and mice were > 1,000 mg/kg (> 2,000 times the maximum human daily inhalation dose based on mg/m²).

DOSAGE AND ADMINISTRATION
FLOVENT Inhalation Aerosol should be administered by the orally inhaled route in patients 12 years of age and older. Individual patients will experience a variable time to onset and degree of symptom relief. Generally, fluticasone propionate inhalation aerosol has a relatively rapid onset of action for an inhaled glucocorticoid. Improvement in asthma control following inhaled administration of fluticasone propio-

nate can occur within 24 hours of beginning treatment, although maximum benefit may not be achieved for 1 to 2 weeks or longer after starting treatment.
After asthma stability has been achieved at the starting dose (see below), it is always desirable to titrate to the lowest effective dose to reduce the possibility of side effects. For patients who do not respond adequately to the starting dose after 2 weeks of therapy, higher doses may provide additional asthma control. The safety and efficacy of FLOVENT Inhalation Aerosol when administered in excess of recommended doses has not been established.
Rinsing the mouth after inhalation is advised.
The recommended starting dose and the highest recommended dose of fluticasone propionate inhalation aerosol, based on prior antiasthma therapy, are listed in the following table.
[See table above.]

Geriatric Use: In studies where geriatric patients (65 years of age or older, see PRECAUTIONS) have been treated with fluticasone propionate inhalation aerosol, efficacy and safety did not differ from that in younger patients. Consequently, no dosage adjustment is recommended.

Directions for Use: Illustrated Patient's Instructions for Use accompany each package of FLOVENT Inhalation Aerosol.

HOW SUPPLIED
FLOVENT 44 mcg Inhalation Aerosol is supplied in 7.9-g canisters containing 60 metered inhalations in boxes of one (NDC 0173-0497-00) and in 13-g canisters containing 120 metered inhalations in boxes of one (NDC 0173-0491-00). Each canister is supplied with a dark orange-colored oral actuator with a peach-colored strapcap and patient's instructions. Each actuation of the inhaler delivers 44 mcg of fluticasone propionate from the actuator.
FLOVENT 110 mcg Inhalation Aerosol is supplied in 13-g canisters containing 120 metered inhalations in boxes of one (NDC 0173-0494-00). Each canister is supplied with a dark orange-colored oral actuator with a peach-colored strapcap and patient's instructions. Each actuation of the inhaler delivers 110 mcg of fluticasone propionate from the actuator.
FLOVENT 220 mcg Inhalation Aerosol is supplied in 13-g canisters containing 120 metered inhalations in boxes of one (NDC 0173-0495-00). Each canister is supplied with a dark orange-colored oral actuator with a peach-colored strapcap and patient's instructions. Each actuation of the inhaler delivers 220 mcg of fluticasone propionate from the actuator.

FLOVENT canisters are for use with FLOVENT Inhalation Aerosol actuators only. The actuators should not be used with other aerosol medications.
Store between 2° and 30°C (36° and 86°F). Store canister with nozzle end down. Protect from freezing temperatures and direct sunlight.
Avoid spraying in eyes. Contents under pressure. Do not puncture or incinerate. Do not store at temperatures above 120°F. Keep out of reach of children. For best results, the canister should be at room temperature before use. Shake well before using.
March 1996/RL-300
Shown in Product Identification Guide, page 313

FORTAZ® ℞
[for′ taz]
(ceftazidime for injection)

FORTAZ® ℞
(ceftazidime sodium injection)
For Intravenous or Intramuscular Use

DESCRIPTION
Ceftazidime is a semisynthetic, broad-spectrum, beta-lactam antibiotic for parenteral administration. It is the pentahydrate of pyridinium, 1-[[7-[[(2-amino-4-thiazolyl)][(1-carboxy-1-methylethoxy) imino]acetyl] amino]-2-carboxy-8-oxo-5-thia -1- azabicyclo[4.2.0]oct-2-en-3-yl]methyl]-, hydroxide, inner salt, [6R-[6α,7β(Z)]].
The empirical formula is $C_{22}H_{32}N_6O_{12}S_2$, representing a molecular weight of 636.6.
FORTAZ is a sterile, dry powdered mixture of ceftazidime pentahydrate and sodium carbonate. The sodium carbonate at a concentration of 118 mg/g of ceftazidime activity has been admixed to facilitate dissolution. The total sodium content of the mixture is approximately 54 mg (2.3 mEq)/g of ceftazidime activity.
FORTAZ in sterile crystalline form is supplied in vials equivalent to 500 mg, 1 g, 2 g, or 6 g of anhydrous ceftazidime and in ADD-Vantage® vials equivalent to 1 or 2 g of anhydrous ceftazidime. Solutions of FORTAZ range in color from light yellow to amber, depending on the diluent and volume used. The pH of freshly constituted solutions usually ranges from 5 to 8.
FORTAZ is available as a frozen, iso-osmotic, sterile, non-pyrogenic solution with 1 or 2 g of ceftazidime as ceftazidime sodium premixed with approximately 2.2 or 1.6 g, respectively, of dextrose hydrous, USP. Dextrose has been added to adjust the osmolality. Sodium hydroxide is used to adjust pH and neutralize ceftazidime pentahydrate free acid to the sodium salt. The pH may have been adjusted with hydrochloric acid. Solutions of premixed FORTAZ range in color from light yellow to amber. The solution is intended for intravenous (IV) use after thawing to room temperature. The osmolality of the solution is approximately 300 mOsml/kg, and the pH of thawed solutions ranges from 5 to 7.5.
The plastic container for the frozen solution is fabricated from a specially designed multilayer plastic, PL 2040. Solutions are in contact with the polyethylene layer of this container and can leach out certain chemical components of the plastic in very small amounts within the expiration period. The suitability of the plastic has been confirmed in tests in animals according to USP biological tests for plastic containers as well as by tissue culture toxicity studies.

CLINICAL PHARMACOLOGY
After IV administration of 500-mg and 1-g doses of ceftazidime over 5 minutes to normal adult male volunteers, mean peak serum concentrations of 45 and 90 mcg/mL, respectively, were achieved. After IV infusion of 500-mg, 1-g, and 2-g doses of ceftazidime over 20 to 30 minutes to normal adult male volunteers, mean peak serum concentrations of 42, 69, and 170 mcg/mL, respectively, were achieved. The average serum concentrations following IV infusion of 500-mg, 1-g, and 2-g doses to these volunteers over an 8-hour interval are given in Table 1.

Table 1

Ceftazidime IV Dose	Serum Concentrations (mcg/mL)				
	0.5 h	1 h	2 h	4 h	8 h
500 mg	42	25	12	6	2
1 g	60	39	23	11	3
2 g	129	75	42	13	5

The absorption and elimination of ceftazidime were directly proportional to the size of the dose. The half-life following IV

Overall Adverse Experiences With > 3% Incidence on Fluticasone Propionate in US Contolled Clinical Trials With MDI in Patients Previously Receiving Bronchodilators and/or Inhaled Corticosteroids

Adverse Event	Placebo (n = 475) %	FLOVENT 88 mcg twice daily (n = 488) %	FLOVENT 220 mcg twice daily (n = 95) %	FLOVENT 440 mcg twice daily (n = 185) %
Ear, nose, and throat				
Pharyngitis	7	10	14	14
Nasal congestion	8	8	16	10
Sinusitis	4	3	6	5
Nasal discharge	3	5	4	4
Dysphonia	1	4	3	8
Allergic rhinitis	4	5	3	3
Oral candidiasis	1	2	3	5
Respiratory				
Upper respiratory infection	12	15	22	16
Influenza	2	3	8	5
Neurological				
Headache	14	17	22	17
Average duration of exposure (days)	44	66	64	59

administration was approximately 1.9 hours. Less than 10% of ceftazidime was protein bound. The degree of protein binding was independent of concentration. There was no evidence of accumulation of ceftazidime in the serum in individuals with normal renal function following multiple IV doses of 1 and 2 g every 8 hours for 10 days.

Following intramuscular (IM) administration of 500-mg and 1-g doses of ceftazidime to normal adult volunteers, the mean peak serum concentrations were 17 and 39 mcg/mL, respectively, at approximately 1 hour. Serum concentrations remained above 4 mcg/mL for 6 and 8 hours after the IM administration of 500-mg and 1-g doses, respectively. The half-life of ceftazidime in these volunteers was approximately 2 hours.

The presence of hepatic dysfunction had no effect on the pharmacokinetics of ceftazidime in individuals administered 2 g intravenously every 8 hours for 5 days. Therefore, a dosage adjustment from the normal recommended dosage is not required for patients with hepatic dysfunction, provided renal function is not impaired.

Approximately 80% to 90% of an IM or IV dose of ceftazidime is excreted unchanged by the kidneys over a 24-hour period. After the IV administration of single 500-mg or 1-g doses, approximately 50% of the dose appeared in the urine in the first 2 hours. An additional 20% was excreted between 2 and 4 hours after dosing, and approximately another 12% of the dose appeared in the urine between 4 and 8 hours later. The elimination of ceftazidime by the kidneys resulted in high therapeutic concentrations in the urine.

The mean renal clearance of ceftazidime was approximately 100 mL/min. The calculated plasma clearance of approximately 115 mL/min indicated nearly complete elimination of ceftazidime by the renal route. Administration of probenecid before dosing had no effect on the elimination kinetics of ceftazidime. This suggested that ceftazidime is eliminated by glomerular filtration and is not actively secreted by renal tubular mechanisms.

Since ceftazidime is eliminated almost solely by the kidneys, its serum half-life is significantly prolonged in patients with impaired renal function. Consequently, dosage adjustments in such patients as described in the DOSAGE AND ADMINISTRATION section are suggested.

Therapeutic concentrations of ceftazidime are achieved in the following body tissues and fluids.

[See table 2 above.]

Table 2: Ceftazidime Concentrations in Body Tissues and Fluids

Tissue or Fluid	Dose/ Route	No. of Patients	Time of Sample Postdose	Average Tissue or Fluid Level (mcg/mL or mcg/g)
Urine	500 mg IM	6	0–2 h	2,100.0
	2 g IV	6	0–2 h	12,000.0
Bile	2 g IV	3	90 min	36.4
Synovial fluid	2 g IV	13	2 h	25.6
Peritoneal fluid	2 g IV	8	2 h	48.6
Sputum	1 g IV	8	1 h	9.0
Cerebrospinal fluid	2 g q8h IV	5	120 min	9.8
(inflamed meninges)	2 g q8h IV	6	180 min	9.4
Aqueous humor	2 g IV	13	1–3 h	11.0
Blister fluid	1 g IV	7	2–3 h	19.7
Lymphatic fluid	1 g IV	7	2–3 h	23.4
Bone	2 g IV	8	0.67 h	31.1
Heart muscle	2 g IV	35	30–280 min	12.7
Skin	2 g IV	22	30–180 min	6.6
Skeletal muscle	2 g IV	35	30–280 min	9.4
Myometrium	2 g IV	31	1–2 h	18.7

Microbiology: Ceftazidime is bactericidal in action, exerting its effect by inhibition of enzymes responsible for cell-wall synthesis. A wide range of gram-negative organisms is susceptible to ceftazidime *in vitro*, including strains resistant to gentamicin and other aminoglycosides. In addition, ceftazidime has been shown to be active against gram-positive organisms. It is highly stable to most clinically important beta-lactamases, plasmid or chromosomal, which are produced by both gram-negative and gram-positive organisms and, consequently, is active against many strains resistant to ampicillin and other cephalosporins.

Ceftazidime has been shown to be active against the following organisms both *in vitro* and in clinical infections (see INDICATIONS AND USAGE).

Aerobes, Gram-negative: *Citrobacter* spp., including *Citrobacter freundii* and *Citrobacter diversus; Enterobacter* spp., including *Enterobacter cloacae* and *Enterobacter aerogenes; Escherichia coli; Haemophilus influenzae*, including ampicillin-resistant strains; *Klebsiella* spp. (including *Klebsiella pneumoniae*); *Neisseria meningitidis; Proteus mirabilis; Proteus vulgaris; Pseudomonas* spp. (including *Pseudomonas aeruginosa*); and *Serratia* spp.

Aerobes, Gram-positive: *Staphylococcus aureus*, including penicillinase- and non–penicillinase-producing strains; *Streptococcus agalactiae* (group B streptococci); *Streptococcus pneumoniae;* and *Streptococcus pyogenes* (group A beta-hemolytic streptococci).

Anaerobes: *Bacteroides* spp. (NOTE: many strains of *Bacteroides fragilis* are resistant).

Ceftazidime has been shown to be active *in vitro* against most strains of the following organisms; however, the clinical significance of these data is unknown: *Acinetobacter* spp., *Clostridium* spp. (not including *Clostridium difficile*), *Haemophilus parainfluenzae, Morganella morganii* (formerly *Proteus morganii*), *Neisseria gonorrhoeae, Peptococcus* spp., *Peptostreptococcus* spp., *Providencia* spp. (including *Providencia rettgeri*, formerly *Proteus rettgeri*), *Salmonella* spp., *Shigella* spp., *Staphylococcus epidermidis*, and *Yersinia enterocolitica*.

Ceftazidime and the aminoglycosides have been shown to be synergistic *in vitro* against *Pseudomonas aeruginosa* and the enterobacteriaceae. Ceftazidime and carbenicillin have also been shown to be synergistic *in vitro* against *Pseudomonas aeruginosa*.

Ceftazidime is not active *in vitro* against methicillin-resistant staphylococci, *Streptococcus faecalis* and many other enterococci, *Listeria monocytogenes, Campylobacter* spp., or *Clostridium difficile*.

Susceptibility Tests: ***Diffusion Techniques:*** Quantitative methods that require measurement of zone diameters give an estimate of antibiotic susceptibility. One such procedure[1–3] has been recommended for use with disks to test susceptibility to ceftazidime.

Reports from the laboratory giving results of the standard single-disk susceptibility test with a 30-mcg ceftazidime disk should be interpreted according to the following criteria:

Susceptible organisms produce zones of 18 mm or greater, indicating that the test organism is likely to respond to therapy.

Organisms that produce zones of 15 to 17 mm are expected to be susceptible if high dosage is used or if the infection is confined to tissues and fluids (e.g., urine) in which high antibiotic levels are attained.

Resistant organisms produce zones of 14 mm or less, indicating that other therapy should be selected.

Organisms should be tested with the ceftazidime disk since ceftazidime has been shown by *in vitro* tests to be active against certain strains found resistant when other beta-lactam disks are used.

Standardized procedures require the use of laboratory control organisms. The 30-mcg ceftazidime disk should give zone diameters between 25 and 32 mm for *Escherichia coli* ATCC 25922. For *Pseudomonas aeruginosa* ATCC 27853, the zone diameters should be between 22 and 29 mm. For *Staphylococcus aureus* ATCC 25923, the zone diameters should be between 16 and 20 mm.

Dilution Techniques: In other susceptibility testing procedures, e.g., ICS agar dilution or the equivalent, a bacterial isolate may be considered susceptible if the minimum inhibitory concentration (MIC) value for ceftazidime is not more than 16 mcg/mL. Organisms are considered resistant to ceftazidime if the MIC is ≥ 64 mcg/mL. Organisms having an MIC value of < 64 mcg/mL but > 16 mcg/mL are expected to be susceptible if high dosage is used or if the infection is confined to tissues and fluids (e.g., urine) in which high antibiotic levels are attained.

As with standard diffusion methods, dilution procedures require the use of laboratory control organisms. Standard ceftazidime powder should give MIC values in the range of 4 to 16 mcg/mL for *Staphylococcus aureus* ATCC 25923. For *Escherichia coli* ATCC 25922, the MIC range should be between 0.125 and 0.5 mcg/mL. For *Pseudomonas aeruginosa* ATCC 27853, the MIC range should be between 0.5 and 2 mcg/mL.

INDICATIONS AND USAGE

FORTAZ is indicated for the treatment of patients with infections caused by susceptible strains of the designated organisms in the following diseases:

1. **Lower Respiratory Tract Infections,** including pneumonia, caused by *Pseudomonas aeruginosa* and other *Pseudomonas* spp.; *Haemophilus influenzae*, including ampicillin-resistant strains; *Klebsiella* spp.; *Enterobacter* spp.; *Proteus mirabilis; Escherichia coli; Serratia* spp.; *Citrobacter* spp.; *Streptococcus pneumoniae*; and *Staphylococcus aureus* (methicillin-susceptible strains).
2. **Skin and Skin-Structure Infections** caused by *Pseudomonas aeruginosa; Klebsiella* spp.; *Escherichia coli; Proteus* spp., including *Proteus mirabilis* and indole-positive *Proteus; Enterobacter* spp.; *Serratia* spp.; *Staphylococcus aureus* (methicillin-susceptible strains); and *Streptococcus pyogenes* (group A beta-hemolytic streptococci).
3. **Urinary Tract Infections,** both complicated and uncomplicated, caused by *Pseudomonas aeruginosa; Enterobacter* spp.; *Proteus* spp., including *Proteus mirabilis* and indole-positive *Proteus; Klebsiella* spp.; and *Escherichia coli.*
4. **Bacterial Septicemia** caused by *Pseudomonas aeruginosa, Klebsiella* spp., *Haemophilus influenzae, Escherichia coli, Serratia* spp., *Streptococcus pneumoniae*, and *Staphylococcus aureus* (methicillin-susceptible strains).
5. **Bone and Joint Infections** caused by *Pseudomonas aeruginosa, Klebsiella* spp., *Enterobacter* spp., and *Staphylococcus aureus* (methicillin-susceptible strains).
6. **Gynecologic Infections,** including endometritis, pelvic cellulitis, and other infections of the female genital tract caused by *Escherichia coli.*
7. **Intra-abdominal Infections,** including peritonitis caused by *Escherichia coli, Klebsiella* spp., and *Staphylococcus aureus* (methicillin-susceptible strains) and polymicrobial infections caused by aerobic and anaerobic organisms and *Bacteroides* spp. (many strains of *Bacteroides fragilis* are resistant).
8. **Central Nervous System Infections,** including meningitis, caused by *Haemophilus influenzae* and *Neisseria meningitidis*. Ceftazidime has also been used successfully in a limited number of cases of meningitis due to *Pseudomonas aeruginosa* and *Streptococcus pneumoniae.*

Specimens for bacterial cultures should be obtained before therapy in order to isolate and identify causative organisms and to determine their susceptibility to ceftazidime. Therapy may be instituted before results of susceptibility studies are known; however, once these results become available, the antibiotic treatment should be adjusted accordingly.

As with other extended-spectrum cephalosporins and penicillins, some strains of *Enterobacter* spp. can develop resistance during ceftazidime therapy due to induced type-1 beta-lactamase production. When clinically appropriate during therapy of *Enterobacter* spp. infections, periodic susceptibility testing should be considered.

FORTAZ may be used alone in cases of confirmed or suspected sepsis. Ceftazidime has been used successfully in clinical trials as empiric therapy in cases where various concomitant therapies with other antibiotics have been used.

FORTAZ may also be used concomitantly with other antibiotics, such as aminoglycosides, vancomycin, and clindamycin; in severe and life-threatening infections; and in the immunocompromised patient. When such concomitant treatment is appropriate, prescribing information in the labeling for the other antibiotics should be followed. The dose depends on the severity of the infection and the patient's condition.

CONTRAINDICATIONS

FORTAZ is contraindicated in patients who have shown hypersensitivity to ceftazidime or the cephalosporin group of antibiotics.

WARNINGS

BEFORE THERAPY WITH FORTAZ IS INSTITUTED, CAREFUL INQUIRY SHOULD BE MADE TO DETERMINE WHETHER THE PATIENT HAS HAD PREVIOUS HYPERSENSITIVITY REACTIONS TO CEFTAZIDIME, CEPHALOSPORINS, PENICILLINS, OR OTHER DRUGS. IF THIS PRODUCT IS TO BE GIVEN TO PENICILLIN-SENSITIVE PATIENTS, CAUTION SHOULD BE EXERCISED BECAUSE CROSS-HYPERSENSITIVITY AMONG BETA-LACTAM ANTIBIOTICS HAS BEEN CLEARLY DOCUMENTED AND MAY OCCUR IN UP TO 10% OF PATIENTS WITH A HISTORY OF PENICILLIN ALLERGY. IF AN ALLERGIC REACTION TO FORTAZ OCCURS, DISCONTINUE THE DRUG. SERIOUS ACUTE HYPERSENSITIVITY REACTIONS MAY REQUIRE TREATMENT WITH EPINEPHRINE AND OTHER EMERGENCY MEASURES, INCLUDING OXYGEN, IV FLUIDS, IV ANTIHISTAMINES, CORTICOSTEROIDS, PRESSOR AMINES, AND AIRWAY MANAGEMENT, AS CLINICALLY INDICATED.

Pseudomembranous colitis has been reported with nearly all antibacterial agents, including ceftazidime, and may range in severity from mild to life threatening. Therefore, it is im-

Continued on next page

Glaxo Wellcome—Cont.

portant to consider this diagnosis in patients who present with diarrhea subsequent to the administration of antibacterial agents.

Treatment with antibacterial agents alters the normal flora of the colon and may permit overgrowth of clostridia. Studies indicate that a toxin produced by *Clostridium difficile* is one primary cause of "antibiotic-associated colitis."

After the diagnosis of pseudomembranous colitis has been established, therapeutic measures should be initiated. Mild cases of pseudomembranous colitis usually respond to drug discontinuation alone. In moderate to severe cases, consideration should be given to management with fluids and electrolytes, protein supplementation, and treatment with an antibacterial drug clinically effective against *Clostridium difficile colitis*.

Elevated levels of ceftazidime in patients with renal insufficiency can lead to seizures, encephalopathy, asterixis, and neuromuscular excitability (see PRECAUTIONS).

PRECAUTIONS

General: Ceftazidime has not been shown to be nephrotoxic; however, high and prolonged serum antibiotic concentrations can occur from usual dosages in patients with transient or persistent reduction of urinary output because of renal insufficiency. The total daily dosage should be reduced when ceftazidime is administered to patients with renal insufficiency (see DOSAGE AND ADMINISTRATION). Elevated levels of ceftazidime in these patients can lead to seizures, encephalopathy, asterixis, and neuromuscular excitability. Continued dosage should be determined by degree of renal impairment, severity of infection, and susceptibility of the causative organisms.

As with other antibiotics, prolonged use of FORTAZ may result in overgrowth of nonsusceptible organisms. Repeated evaluation of the patient's condition is essential. If superinfection occurs during therapy, appropriate measures should be taken.

Cephalosporins may be associated with a fall in prothrombin activity. Those at risk include patients with renal and hepatic impairment, or poor nutritional state, as well as patients receiving a protracted course of antimicrobial therapy. Prothrombin time should be monitored in patients at risk and exogenous vitamin K administered as indicated.

FORTAZ should be prescribed with caution in individuals with a history of gastrointestinal disease, particularly colitis. Distal necrosis can occur after inadvertent intra-arterial administration of ceftazidime.

Drug Interactions: Nephrotoxicity has been reported following concomitant administration of cephalosporins with aminoglycoside antibiotics or potent diuretics such as furosemide. Renal function should be carefully monitored, especially if higher dosages of the aminoglycosides are to be administered or if therapy is prolonged, because of the potential nephrotoxicity and ototoxicity of aminoglycosidic antibiotics. Nephrotoxicity and ototoxicity were not noted when ceftazidime was given alone in clinical trials.

Chloramphenicol has been shown to be antagonistic to beta-lactam antibiotics, including ceftazidime, based on *in vitro* studies and time kill curves with enteric gram-negative bacilli. Due to the possibility of antagonism *in vivo*, particularly when bactericidal activity is desired, this drug combination should be avoided.

Drug/Laboratory Test Interactions: The administration of ceftazidime may result in a false-positive reaction for glucose in the urine using CLINITEST ® tablets, Benedict's solution, or Fehling's solution. It is recommended that glucose tests based on enzymatic glucose oxidase reactions (such as CLINISTIX® or TES-TAPE®) be used.

Carcinogenesis, Mutagenesis, Impairment of Fertility: Long-term studies in animals have not been performed to evaluate carcinogenic potential. However, a mouse Micronucleus test and an Ames test were both negative for mutagenic effects.

Pregnancy: *Teratogenic Effects: Pregnancy Category B:* Reproduction studies have been performed in mice and rats at doses up to 40 times the human dose and have revealed no evidence of impaired fertility or harm to the fetus due to FORTAZ. There are, however, no adequate and well-controlled studies in pregnant women. Because animal reproduction studies are not always predictive of human response, this drug should be used during pregnancy only if clearly needed.

Nursing Mothers: Ceftazidime is excreted in human milk in low concentrations. Caution should be exercised when FORTAZ is administered to a nursing woman.

Pediatric Use: (see DOSAGE AND ADMINISTRATION).

ADVERSE REACTIONS

Ceftazidime is generally well tolerated. The incidence of adverse reactions associated with the administration of ceftazidime was low in clinical trials. The most common were local reactions following IV injection and allergic and gastrointestinal reactions. Other adverse reactions were encountered infrequently. No disulfiramlike reactions were reported.

The following adverse effects from clinical trials were considered to be either related to ceftazidime therapy or were of uncertain etiology:

Local Effects, reported in fewer than 2% of patients, were phlebitis and inflammation at the site of injection (1 in 69 patients).

Hypersensitivity Reactions, reported in 2% of patients, were pruritus, rash, and fever. Immediate reactions, generally manifested by rash and/or pruritus, occurred in 1 in 285 patients. Toxic epidermal necrolysis, Stevens-Johnson syndrome, and erythema multiforme have also been reported with cephalosporin antibiotics, including ceftazidime. Angioedema and anaphylaxis (bronchospasm and/or hypotension) have been reported very rarely.

Gastrointestinal Symptoms, reported in fewer than 2% of patients, were diarrhea (1 in 78), nausea (1 in 156), vomiting (1 in 500), and abdominal pain (1 in 416). The onset of pseudomembranous colitis symptoms may occur during or after treatment (see WARNINGS).

Central Nervous System Reactions (fewer than 1%) included headache, dizziness, and paresthesia. Seizures have been reported with several cephalosporins, including ceftazidime. In addition, encephalopathy, asterixis, and neuromuscular excitability have been reported in renally impaired patients treated with unadjusted dosing regimens of ceftazidime (see PRECAUTIONS: General).

Less Frequent Adverse Events (fewer than 1%) were candidiasis (including oral thrush) and vaginitis.

Hematologic: Rare cases of hemolytic anemia have been reported.

Laboratory Test Changes noted during FORTAZ clinical trials were transient and included: eosinophilia (1 in 13), positive Coombs' test without hemolysis (1 in 23), thrombocytosis (1 in 45), and slight elevations in one or more of the hepatic enzymes, aspartate aminotransferase (AST, SGOT) (1 in 16), alanine aminotransferase (ALT, SGPT) (1 in 15), LDH (1 in 18), GGT (1 in 19), and alkaline phosphatase (1 in 23). As with some other cephalosporins, transient elevations of blood urea, blood urea nitrogen, and/or serum creatinine were observed occasionally. Transient leukopenia, neutropenia, agranulocytosis, thrombocytopenia, and lymphocytosis were seen very rarely. Elevations in hepatic enzymes (SGOT, SGPT, LDH, GGT, alkaline phosphatase) have been reported postmarketing.

In addition to the adverse reactions listed above that have been observed in patients treated with ceftazidime, the following adverse reactions and altered laboratory tests have been reported for cephalosporin-class antibiotics:

Adverse Reactions: Urticaria, colitis, renal dysfunction, toxic nephropathy, hepatic dysfunction including cholestasis, aplastic anemia, hemorrhage.

Altered Laboratory Tests: Prolonged prothrombin time, false-positive test for urinary glucose, elevated bilirubin, pancytopenia.

OVERDOSAGE

Ceftazidime overdosage has occurred in patients with renal failure. Reactions have included seizure activity, encephalopathy, asterixis, and neuromuscular excitability. Patients who receive an acute overdosage should be carefully observed and given supportive treatment. In the presence of renal insufficiency, hemodialysis or peritoneal dialysis may aid in the removal of ceftazidime from the body.

DOSAGE AND ADMINISTRATION

Dosage: The usual adult dosage is 1 gram administered intravenously or intramuscularly every 8 to 12 hours. The dosage and route should be determined by the susceptibility of the causative organisms, the severity of infection, and the condition and renal function of the patient.

The guidelines for dosage of FORTAZ are listed in Table 3. The following dosage schedule is recommended.

[See table 3 below.]

Impaired Hepatic Function: No adjustment in dosage is required for patients with hepatic dysfunction.

Impaired Renal Function: Ceftazidime is excreted by the kidneys, almost exclusively by glomerular filtration. Therefore, in patients with impaired renal function (glomerular filtration rate [GFR] <50 mL/min), it is recommended that the dosage of ceftazidime be reduced to compensate for its slower excretion. In patients with suspected renal insufficiency, an initial loading dose of 1 gram of FORTAZ may be given. An estimate of GFR should be made to determine the appropriate maintenance dose. The recommended dosage is presented in Table 4.

Table 4: Recommended Maintenance Dosages of FORTAZ in Renal Insufficiency
NOTE: IF THE DOSE RECOMMENDED IN TABLE 3 ABOVE IS LOWER THAN THAT RECOMMENDED FOR PATIENTS WITH RENAL INSUFFICIENCY AS OUTLINED IN TABLE 4, THE LOWER DOSE SHOULD BE USED.

Creatinine Clearance (mL/min)	Recommended Unit Dose of FORTAZ	Frequency of Dosing
50–31	1 gram	q12h
30–16	1 gram	q24h
15–6	500 mg	q24h
<5	500 mg	q48h

When only serum creatinine is available, the following formula (Cockcroft's equation)[4] may be used to estimate creatinine clearance. The serum creatinine should represent a steady state of renal function:

Males:
$$\text{Creatinine clearance (mL/min)} = \frac{\text{Weight (kg)} \times (140 - \text{age})}{72 \times \text{serum creatinine (mg/dL)}}$$

Females: 0.85 × male value

In patients with severe infections who would normally receive 6 grams of FORTAZ daily were it not for renal insufficiency, the unit dose given in the table above may be increased by 50% or the dosing frequency may be increased appropriately. Further dosing should be determined by therapeutic monitoring, severity of the infection, and susceptibility of the causative organism.

In pediatric patients as for adults, the creatinine clearance should be adjusted for body surface area or lean body mass, and the dosing frequency should be reduced in cases of renal insufficiency.

Table 3: Recommended Dosage Schedule

	Dose	Frequency
Adults		
Usual recommended dosage	1 gram IV or IM	q8–12h
Uncomplicated urinary tract infections	250 mg IV or IM	q12h
Bone and joint infections	2 grams IV	q12h
Complicated urinary tract infections	500 mg IV or IM	q8–12h
Uncomplicated pneumonia; mild skin and skin-structure infections	500 mg–1 gram IV or IM	q8h
Serious gynecologic and intra-abdominal infections	2 grams IV	q8h
Meningitis	2 grams IV	q8h
Very severe life-threatening infections, especially in immunocompromised patients	2 grams IV	q8h
Lung infections caused by *Pseudomonas* spp. in patients with cystic fibrosis with normal renal function*	30–50 mg/kg IV to a maximum of 6 grams per day	q8h
Neonates (0–4 weeks)	30 mg/kg IV	q12h
Infants and Children (1 month–12 years)	30–50 mg/kg IV to a maximum of 6 grams per day†	q8h

*Although clinical improvement has been shown, bacteriologic cures cannot be expected in patients with chronic respiratory disease and cystic fibrosis.
†The higher dose should be reserved for immunocompromised pediatric patients or pediatric patients with cystic fibrosis or meningitis.

In patients undergoing hemodialysis, a loading dose of 1 gram is recommended, followed by 1 gram after each hemodialysis period.

FORTAZ can also be used in patients undergoing intraperitoneal dialysis and continuous ambulatory peritoneal dialysis. In such patients, a loading dose of 1 gram of FORTAZ may be given, followed by 500 mg every 24 hours. In addition to IV use, FORTAZ can be incorporated in the dialysis fluid at a concentration of 250 mg for 2 L of dialysis fluid.

Note: Generally FORTAZ should be continued for 2 days after the signs and symptoms of infection have disappeared, but in complicated infections longer therapy may be required.

Administration: FORTAZ may be given intravenously or by deep IM injection into a large muscle mass such as the upper outer quadrant of the gluteus maximus or lateral part of the thigh. Intra-arterial administration should be avoided (see PRECAUTIONS).

Intramuscular Administration: For IM administration, FORTAZ should be constituted with one of the following diluents: sterile water for injection, bacteriostatic water for injection, or 0.5% or 1% lidocaine hydrochloride injection. Refer to Table 5.

Intravenous Administration: The IV route is preferable for patients with bacterial septicemia, bacterial meningitis, peritonitis, or other severe or life-threatening infections, or for patients who may be poor risks because of lowered resistance resulting from such debilitating conditions as malnutrition, trauma, surgery, diabetes, heart failure, or malignancy, particularly if shock is present or pending.

For direct intermittent IV administration, constitute FORTAZ as directed in Table 5 with sterile water for injection. Slowly inject directly into the vein over a period of 3 to 5 minutes or give through the tubing of an administration set while the patient is also receiving one of the compatible IV fluids (see COMPATIBILITY AND STABILITY).

For IV infusion, constitute the 1- or 2-gram infusion pack with 100 mL of sterile water for injection or one of the compatible IV fluids listed under the COMPATIBILITY AND STABILITY section. Alternatively, constitute the 500-mg, 1-gram, or 2-gram vial and add an appropriate quantity of the resulting solution to an IV container with one of the compatible IV fluids.

Intermittent IV infusion with a Y-type administration set can be accomplished with compatible solutions. However, during infusion of a solution containing ceftazidime, it is desirable to discontinue the other solution.

ADD-Vantage vials are to be constituted only with 50 or 100 mL of 5% dextrose injection, 0.9% sodium chloride injection, or 0.45% sodium chloride injection in Abbott ADD-Vantage flexible diluent containers (see Instructions for Constitution section of the product package insert). ADD-Vantage vials that have been joined to Abbott ADD-Vantage diluent containers and activated to dissolve the drug are stable for 24 hours at room temperature or for 7 days under refrigeration. Joined vials that have not been activated may be used within a 14-day period; this period corresponds to that for use of Abbott ADD-Vantage containers following removal of the outer packaging (overwrap). Freezing solutions of FORTAZ in the ADD-Vantage system is not recommended.

[See table 5 above.]

All vials of FORTAZ as supplied are under reduced pressure. When FORTAZ is dissolved, carbon dioxide is released and a positive pressure develops. For ease of use please follow the recommended techniques of constitution described on the detachable Instructions for Constitution section of the product package insert.

Solutions of FORTAZ, like those of most beta-lactam antibiotics, should not be added to solutions of aminoglycoside antibiotics because of potential interaction.

However, if concurrent therapy with FORTAZ and an aminoglycoside is indicated, each of these antibiotics can be administered separately to the same patient.

Directions for Use of FORTAZ Frozen in GALAXY® Plastic Containers: FORTAZ supplied as a frozen, sterile, iso-osmotic, nonpyrogenic solution in plastic containers is to be administered after thawing either as a continuous or intermittent IV infusion. The thawed solution is stable for 24 hours at room temperature or for 7 days if stored under refrigeration. **Do not Refreeze.**

Thaw container at room temperature (25°C) or under refrigeration (5°C). Do not force thaw by immersion in water baths or by microwave irradiation. Components of the solution may precipitate in the frozen state and will dissolve upon reaching room temperature with little or no agitation. Potency is not affected. Mix after solution has reached room temperature. Check for minute leaks by squeezing bag firmly. Discard bag if leaks are found as sterility may be impaired. Do not add supplementary medication. Do not use unless solution is clear and seal is intact. Use sterile equipment.

Caution: Do not use plastic containers in series connections. Such use could result in air embolism due to residual air being drawn from the primary container before administration of the fluid from the secondary container is complete.

Table 5: Preparation of FORTAZ Solutions

Size	Amount of Diluent to Be Added (mL)	Approximate Available Volume (mL)	Approximate Ceftazidime Concentration (mg/mL)
Intramuscular			
500-mg vial	1.5	1.8	280
1-gram vial	3.0	3.6	280
Intravenous			
500-mg vial	5.0	5.3	100
1-gram vial	10.0	10.6	100
2-gram vial	10.0	11.5	170
Infusion pack			
1-gram vial	100*	100	10
2-gram vial	100*	100	20
Pharmacy bulk package			
6-gram vial	26	30	200

* Note: Addition should be in two stages (see Instructions for Constitution accompanying the product package insert).

Preparation for Administration:
1. Suspend container from eyelet support.
2. Remove protector from outlet port at bottom of container.
3. Attach administration set. Refer to complete directions accompanying set.

COMPATIBILITY AND STABILITY

Intramuscular: FORTAZ, when constituted as directed with sterile water for injection, bacteriostatic water for injection, or 0.5% or 1% lidocaine hydrochloride injection, maintains satisfactory potency for 24 hours at room temperature or for 7 days under refrigeration. Solutions in sterile water for injection that are frozen immediately after constitution in the original container are stable for 3 months when stored at −20°C. Once thawed, solutions should not be refrozen. Thawed solutions may be stored for up to 8 hours at room temperature or for 4 days in a refrigerator.

Intravenous: FORTAZ, when constituted as directed with sterile water for injection, maintains satisfactory potency for 24 hours at room temperature or for 7 days under refrigeration. Solutions in sterile water for injection in the infusion vial or in 0.9% sodium chloride injection in VIAFLEX® small-volume containers that are frozen immediately after constitution are stable for 6 months when stored at −20°C. Do not force thaw by immersion in water baths or by microwave irradiation. Once thawed, solutions should not be refrozen. Thawed solutions may be stored for up to 24 hours at room temperature or for 7 days in a refrigerator. More concentrated solutions in sterile water for injection in the original container that are frozen immediately after constitution are stable for 3 months when stored at −20°C. Once thawed, solutions should not be refrozen. Thawed solutions may be stored for up to 8 hours at room temperature or for 4 days in a refrigerator.

FORTAZ is compatible with the more commonly used IV infusion fluids. Solutions at concentrations between 1 and 40 mg/mL in 0.9% sodium chloride injection; 1/6 M sodium lactate injection; 5% dextrose injection; 5% dextrose and 0.225% sodium chloride injection; 5% dextrose and 0.45% sodium chloride injection; 5% dextrose and 0.9% sodium chloride injection; 10% dextrose injection; ringer's injection, USP; lactated ringer's injection, USP; 10% invert sugar in water for injection; and NORMOSOL®-M in 5% dextrose injection may be stored for up to 24 hours at room temperature or for 7 days if refrigerated.

The 1- and 2-g FORTAZ ADD-Vantage vials, when diluted in 50 or 100 mL of 5% dextrose injection, 0.9% sodium chloride injection, or 0.45% sodium chloride injection, may be stored for up to 24 hours at room temperature or for 7 days under refrigeration.

FORTAZ is less stable in sodium bicarbonate injection than in other IV fluids. It is not recommended as a diluent. Solutions of FORTAZ in 5% dextrose injection and 0.9% sodium chloride injection are stable for at least 6 hours at room temperature in plastic tubing, drip chambers, and volume control devices of common IV infusion sets.

Ceftazidime at a concentration of 4 mg/mL has been found compatible for 24 hours at room temperature or for 7 days under refrigeration in 0.9% sodium chloride injection or 5% dextrose injection when admixed with: cefuroxime sodium (ZINACEF®) 3 mg/mL; heparin 10 or 50 U/mL; or potassium chloride 10 or 40 mEq/L.

Vancomycin solution exhibits a physical incompatibility when mixed with a number of drugs, including ceftazidime. The likelihood of precipitation with ceftazidime is dependent on the concentrations of vancomycin and ceftazidime present. It is therefore recommended, when both drugs are to be administered by intermittent IV infusion, that they be given separately, flushing the IV lines (with one of the compatible IV fluids) between the administration of these two agents.

Note: Parenteral drug products should be inspected visually for particulate matter before administration whenever solution and container permit.

As with other cephalosporins, FORTAZ powder as well as solutions tend to darken, depending on storage conditions; within the stated recommendations, however, product potency is not adversely affected.

HOW SUPPLIED

FORTAZ in the dry state should be stored between 15° and 30°C (59° and 86°F) and protected from light. FORTAZ is a dry, white to off-white powder supplied in vials and infusion packs as follows:

NDC 0173-0377-31 500-mg* Vial (Tray of 25)
NDC 0173-0378-35 1-g* Vial (Tray of 25)
NDC 0173-0379-34 2-g* Vial (Tray of 10)
NDC 0173-0380-32 1-g* Infusion Pack (Tray of 10)
NDC 0173-0381-32 2-g* Infusion Pack (Tray of 10)
NDC 0173-0382-37 6-g* Pharmacy Bulk Package (Tray of 6)
NDC 0173-0434-00 1-g ADD-Vantage® Vial (Tray of 25)
NDC 0173-0435-00 2-g ADD-Vantage® Vial (Tray of 10)
(The above ADD-Vantage vials are to be used only with Abbott ADD-Vantage diluent containers.)

FORTAZ frozen as a premixed solution of ceftazidime sodium should not be stored above −20° C. FORTAZ is supplied frozen in 50-mL, single-dose, plastic containers as follows:

NDC 0173-0412-00 1-g* Plastic Container (Carton of 24)
NDC 0713-0413-00 2-g* Plastic Container (Carton of 24)
*Equivalent to anhydrous ceftazidime.

REFERENCES

1. Bauer AW, Kirby WMM, Sherris JC, Turck M. Antibiotic susceptibility testing by a standardized single disk method. *Am J Clin Pathol.* 1966;45:493–496.
2. National Committee for Clinical Laboratory Standards. *Approved Standard: Performance Standards for Antimicrobial Disc Susceptibility Tests.* (M2-A3). December 1984.
3. Certification procedure for antibiotic sensitivity discs (21 CFR 460.1). *Federal Register.* May 30, 1974;39:19182-19184.
4. Cockcroft DW, Gault MH. Prediction of creatinine clearance from serum creatinine. *Nephron.* 1976;16:31-41.

FORTAZ and ZINACEF are registered trademarks of Glaxo Wellcome.
ADD-Vantage is a registered trademark of Abbott Laboratories.
CLINITEST and CLINISTIX are registered trademarks of Ames Division, Miles Laboratories, Inc.
TES-TAPE is a registered trademark of Eli Lilly and Company.
GALAXY and VIAFLEX are registered trademarks of Baxter International Inc.
U.S. Patents, 4,258,041; 4,329,453; and 4,582,830
February 1996/RL-231

Shown in Product Identification Guide, page 313

IMITREX® ℞

[ĭm´-ĭ-trĕx″]
(sumatriptan succinate)
Injection
For Subcutaneous Use Only.

DESCRIPTION

IMITREX Injection is a selective 5-hydroxytryptamine₁ receptor subtype agonist. Sumatriptan succinate is chemically designated as 3-[2-(dimethylamino)ethyl]-N-methyl-1H-indole-5-methanesulfonamide butane-1,4-dioate(1:1).
The empirical formula is $C_{14}H_{21}N_3O_2S \cdot C_4H_6O_4$, representing a molecular weight of 413.5.
Sumatriptan succinate is a white to off-white powder that is readily soluble in water and in saline.
IMITREX Injection is a clear, colorless to pale yellow, sterile, nonpyrogenic solution for subcutaneous injection. Each

Continued on next page

Glaxo Wellcome—Cont.

0.5 mL of solution contains 6 mg of sumatriptan (base) as the succinate salt and 3.5 mg of sodium chloride, USP in water for injection, USP. The pH range of the solution is approximately 4.2 to 5.3. The osmolality of the injection is 291 mOsmol.

CLINICAL PHARMACOLOGY

Mechanism of Action: Sumatriptan has been demonstrated to be a selective agonist for a vascular 5-hydroxytryptamine$_1$ receptor subtype (probably a member of the 5-HT$_{1D}$ family) with no significant affinity (as measured using standard radioligand binding assays) or pharmacological activity at 5-HT$_2$, 5-HT$_3$ receptor subtypes or at alpha$_1$-, or alpha$_2$-, or beta-adrenergic; dopamine$_1$; dopamine$_2$; muscarinic; or benzodiazepine receptors.

The vascular 5-HT$_1$ receptor subtype to which sumatriptan binds selectively, and through which it presumably exerts its antimigrainous effect, has been shown to be present on cranial arteries in both dog and primate, on the human basilar artery, and in the vasculature of the isolated dura mater of humans. In these tissues, sumatriptan activates this receptor to cause vasoconstriction, an action in humans correlating with the relief of migraine and cluster headache. In the anesthetized dog, sumatriptan selectively reduces the carotid arterial blood flow with little or no effect on arterial blood pressure or total peripheral resistance. In the cat, sumatriptan selectively constricts the carotid anastomoses while having little effect on blood flow or resistance in cerebral or extracerebral tissues.

Corneal Opacities: Dogs receiving oral sumatriptan developed corneal opacities and defects in the corneal epithelium. Corneal opacities were seen at the lowest dosage tested, 2 mg/kg per day, and were present after 1 month of treatment. Defects in the corneal epithelium were noted in a 60-week study. Earlier examinations for these toxicities were not conducted and no-effect doses were not established; however, the relative exposure at the lowest dose tested was approximately five times the human exposure after a 100-mg oral dose or three times the human exposure after a 6-mg subcutaneous dose.

Melanin Binding: In rats with a single subcutaneous dose (0.5 mg/kg) of radiolabeled sumatriptan, the elimination half-life of radioactivity from the eye was 15 days, suggesting that sumatriptan and its metabolites bind to the melanin of the eye. The clinical significance of this binding is unknown.

Pharmacokinetics: Pharmacokinetic parameters following a 6-mg subcutaneous injection into the deltoid area of the arm in nine males (mean age, 33 years; mean weight, 77 kg) were systemic clearance: 1,194 ± 149 mL/min (mean ±S.D.), distribution half-life: 15 ± 2 minutes, terminal half-life: 115 ± 19 minutes, and volume of distribution central compartment: 50 ± 8 liters. Of this dose, 22% ± 4% was excreted in the urine as unchanged sumatriptan and 38% ± 7% as the indole acetic acid metabolite.

After a single 6-mg subcutaneous manual injection into the deltoid area of the arm in 18 healthy males (age, 24 ±6 years; weight, 70 mg), the maximum serum concentration (C_{max}) was (mean ±standard deviation) 74 ± 15 ng/mL and the time to peak concentration (T_{max}) was 12 minutes after injection (range, 5 to 20 minutes). In this study, the same dose injected subcutaneously in the thigh gave a C_{max} of 61 ± 15 ng/mL by manual injection versus 52 ± 15 ng/mL by autoinjector techniques. The T_{max} or amount absorbed were not significantly altered by either the site or technique of injection.

The bioavailability of sumatriptan via subcutaneous site injection to 18 healthy male subjects was 97% ± 16% of that obtained following intravenous injection. Protein binding, determined by equilibrium dialysis over the concentration range of 10 to 1,000 ng/mL, is low, approximately 14% to 21%. The effect of sumatriptan on the protein binding of other drugs has not been evaluated.

Special Populations: *Renal Impairment:* The effect of renal impairment on the pharmacokinetics of sumatriptan has not been examined, but little clinical effect would be expected as sumatriptan is largely metabolized to an inactive substance.

Hepatic Impairment: The effect of hepatic disease on the pharmacokinetics of subcutaneously and orally administered sumatriptan has been evaluated. There were no statistically significant differences in the pharmacokinetics of subcutaneously administered sumatriptan in hepatically impaired patients compared to healthy controls. However, the liver plays an important role in the presystemic clearance of orally administered sumatriptan. Accordingly, the bioavailability of sumatriptan following oral administration may be markedly increased in patients with liver disease. In one small study of hepatically impaired patients (n = 8) matched for sex, age, and weight with healthy subjects, the hepatically impaired patients had an approximately 70% increase in AUC and C_{max} and a T_{max} minutes earlier compared to the healthy subjects.

Age: The pharmacokinetics of sumatriptan in the elderly (mean age, 72 years; two males and four females) and in patients with migraine (mean age, 38 years; 25 males and 155 females) were similar to that in healthy male subjects (mean age, 30 years).

Race: The systemic clearance and C_{max} of sumatriptan were similar in black (n = 34) and Caucasian (n = 38) healthy male subjects.

Drug Interactions: *MAO Inhibitors:* In vitro studies with human microsomes suggest that sumatriptan is metabolized by monoamine oxidase (MAO), predominantly the A isoenzyme. In a study of 14 healthy females, pretreatment with MAO-A inhibitor decreased the clearance of sumatriptan. Under the conditions of this experiment, the result was a twofold increase in the area under the sumatriptan plasma concentration × time curve (AUC), corresponding to a 40% increase in elimination half-life. No significant effect was seen with an MAO-B inhibitor.

Pharmacodynamics
Typical Physiologic Responses:
Blood Pressure: (see WARNINGS)

Peripheral (small) Arteries: In healthy volunteers (n = 18), a study evaluating the effects of sumatriptan on peripheral (small vessel) arterial reactivity failed to detect a clinically significant increase in peripheral resistance.

Heart Rate: Transient increases in blood pressure observed in some patients in clinical studies carried out during sumatriptan's development as a treatment for migraine were not accompanied by any clinically significant changes in heart rate.

Respiratory Rate: Experience gained during the clinical development of sumatriptan as a treatment for migraine failed to detect an effect of the drug on respiratory rate.

Clinical Studies: *Migraine:* In US controlled clinical trials enrolling more than 1,000 patients during migraine attacks who were experiencing moderate or severe pain and one or more of the symptoms enumerated in Table 2 below, onset of relief began as early as 10 minutes following a 6-mg IMITREX Injection. Smaller doses of sumatriptan may also prove effective, although the proportion of patients obtaining adequate relief is decreased and the latency to that relief is greater.

In one well-controlled study where placebo (n = 62) was compared to six different doses of IMITREX Injection (n = 30 each group) in a single-attack, parallel-group design, the dose response relationship was found to be as shown in the following Table 1.
[See table below.]

In two US well-controlled clinical trials in 1,104 migraine patients with moderate and severe migraine pain, the onset of relief was rapid (less than 10 minutes). Headache relief, as evidenced by a reduction in pain from severe or moderately severe to mild or no headache, was achieved in 70% of the patients within 1 hour of a single 6-mg subcutaneous dose of IMITREX Injection. Headache relief was achieved in approximately 82% of patients within 2 hours, and 65% of all patients were pain free within 2 hours.
The following table shows the 1- and 2-hour efficacy results.
[See table 2 above.]

IMITREX Injection also relieved photophobia, phonophobia (sound sensitivity), nausea, and vomiting associated with migraine attacks. Similar efficacy was seen when patients self-administered IMITREX Injection using an autoinjector. The efficacy of IMITREX Injection is unaffected by whether or not migraine is associated with aura, duration of attack, gender or age of the patient, or concomitant use of common migraine prophylactic drugs (e.g., beta-blockers).

Cluster Headache: The efficacy of IMITREX Injection in the acute treatment of cluster headache was demonstrated in two randomized, double-blind, placebo-controlled, two-period crossover trials. Patients age 21 to 65 were enrolled and were instructed to treat a moderate to very severe headache within 10 minutes of onset. Headache relief was defined as a reduction in headache severity to mild or no pain. In both trials, the proportion of individuals gaining relief at 10 or 15 minutes was significantly greater among patients receiving 6 mg of IMITREX Injection compared to those who received placebo (see Table 3, below). One study evaluated a

Table 2: Efficacy Data From US Phase III Trials

One-Hour Data	Study 1		Study 2	
	Placebo (n = 190)	IMITREX 6 mg (n = 384)	Placebo (n = 180)	IMITREX 6 mg (n = 350)
Patients with pain relief (grade 0/1)	18%	70%*	26%	70%*
Patients with no pain	5%	48%*	13%	49%*
Patients without nausea	48%	73%*	50%	73%*
Patients without photophobia	23%	56%*	25%	58%*
Patients with little or no clinical disability§	34%	76%*	34%	76%*

Two-Hour Data	Study 1		Study 2	
	Placebo†	IMITREX 6 mg‡	Placebo†	IMITREX 6 mg‡
Patients with pain relief (grade 0/1)	31%	81%*	39%	82%*
Patients with no pain	11%	63%*	19%	65%*
Patients without nausea	56%	82%*	63%	81%*
Patients without photophobia	31%	72%*	35%	71%*
Patients with little or no clinical disability§	42%	85%*	49%	84%*

* $p < 0.05$ versus placebo.
† Includes patients that may have received an additional placebo injection 1 hour after the initial injection.
‡ Includes patients that may have received an additional 6 mg of IMITREX Injection 1 hour after the initial injection.
§ A successful outcome in terms of clinical disability was defined prospectively as ability to work mildly impaired or ability to work and function normally.

Table 1: Dose Response Relationship For Efficacy

IMITREX Dose (mg)	% Patients With Relief* at 10 Minutes	% Patients With Relief* at 30 Minutes	% Patients With Relief* at 1 Hour	% Patients With Relief* at 2 Hours	Adverse Events Incidence (%)
placebo	5	15	24	21	55
1	10	40	43	40	63
2	7	23	57	43	63
3	17	47	57	60	77
4	13	37	50	57	80
6	10	63	73	70	83
8	23	57	80	83	93

* Relief is defined as the reduction of moderate or severe pain to no or mild pain after dosing without use of rescue medication.

12-mg dose; there was no statistically significant difference in outcome between patients randomized to the 6- and 12-mg doses.

[See table 3 at right.]

The Kaplan Meier (product limit) Survivorship Plot below (Figure 1) provides an estimate of the cumulative probability of a patient with cluster headache obtaining relief after being treated with either sumatriptan or placebo.

Figure 1: Time to Relief From Time of Injection*

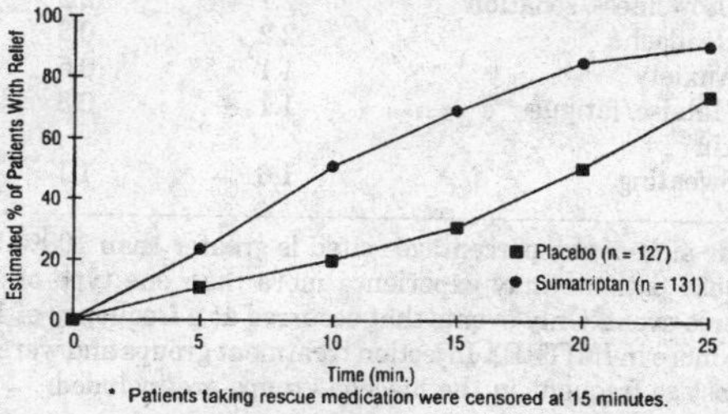

* Patients taking rescue medication were censored at 15 minutes.

The plot was constructed with data from patients who either experienced relief or did not require (request) rescue medication within a period of 2 hours following treatment. As a consequence, the data in the plot are derived from only a subset of the 258 headaches treated (rescue medication was required in 52 of the 127 placebo-treated headaches and 18 of the 131 sumatriptan-treated headaches).

Other data suggest that sumatriptan treatment is not associated with an increase in early recurrence of headache, and that treatment with sumatriptan has little effect on the incidence of latter occurring headaches (i.e., those occurring after 2, but before 18 or 24 hours).

INDICATIONS AND USAGE

IMITREX Injection is indicated for 1) the acute treatment of migraine attacks with or without aura and 2) the acute treatment of cluster headache episodes.

IMITREX Injection is not for use in the management of hemiplegic or basilar migraine (see CONTRAINDICATIONS).

CONTRAINDICATIONS

IMITREX Injection should not be given intravenously because of its potential to cause coronary vasospasm.

IMITREX Injection should not be given subcutaneously to patients with ischemic heart disease (angina pectoris, history of myocardial infarction, or documented silent ischemia) or to patients with Prinzmetal's variant angina.

IMITREX Injection should not be given subcutaneously to patients who are determined to have symptoms or findings consistent with coronary artery vasospasm, ischemic myocardial disease, or other significant underlying cardiovascular disease (see WARNINGS).

Because IMITREX Injection may increase blood pressure, it should not be given to patients with uncontrolled hypertension.

IMITREX Injection should not be used within 24 hours of treatment with an ergotamine-containing or ergot-type medication like dihydroergotamine or methysergide.

IMITREX Injection should not be administered to patients with hemiplegic or basilar migraine.

IMITREX Injection is contraindicated in patients with hypersensitivity to sumatriptan or any of its components.

WARNINGS

IMITREX Injection should only be used where a clear diagnosis of migraine or cluster headache has been established.

Risk of Myocardial Ischemia and/or Infarction and Other Adverse Cardiac Events: It is strongly recommended that sumatriptan not be given to patients in whom unrecognized coronary artery disease (CAD) is predicted by the presence of risk factors (e.g., hypertension, hypercholesterolemia, smoker, obesity, diabetes, strong family history of CAD, female who is surgically or physiologically postmenopausal, or male who is over 40 years of age) unless a cardiovascular evaluation provides satisfactory clinical evidence that the patient is reasonably free of coronary artery and ischemic myocardial disease or other significant underlying cardiovascular disease. The sensitivity of cardiac diagnostic procedures to detect cardiovascular disease or predisposition to coronary artery vasospasm is unknown. In considering this recommendation, it is noted that patients with cluster headache often possess one or more predictive risk factors for CAD. If, during the cardiovascular evaluation, the patient's medical history or electrocardiographic investigations reveal findings indicative of or consistent with coronary artery vasospasm or myocardial ischemia, sumatriptan should not be administered (see CONTRAINDICATIONS).

For patients with risk factors predictive of CAD who are determined to have a satisfactory cardiovascular evaluation, it is strongly recommended that administration of the first dose of sumatriptan injection take place in the setting of a physician's office or similar medically staffed and equipped facility. Because cardiac ischemia can occur in the absence of clinical symptoms, consideration should be given

Table 3: Efficacy Data From the Pivotal Cluster Headache Studies

	Study 1		Study 2	
	Placebo (n=39)	IMITREX 6 mg (n=39)	Placebo (n=88)	IMITREX 6 mg (n=92)
Patients with pain relief (no/mild)				
5 minutes postinjection	8%	21%*	7%	23%*
10 minutes postinjection	10%	49%*	25%	49%*
15 minutes postinjection	26%	74%*	35%	75%*

* $p < 0.05$.

(n=Number of headaches treated.)

to obtaining on the first occasion of use an electrocardiogram (ECG) during the interval immediately following IMITREX Injection, in these patients with risk factors.

It is recommended that patients who are intermittent long-term users of IMITREX Injection and who have or acquire risk factors predictive of CAD, as described above, undergo periodic interval cardiovascular evaluation as they continue to use IMITREX Injection. In considering this recommendation for periodic cardiovascular evaluation, it is noted that patients with cluster headache are predominantly male and over 40 years of age, which are risk factors for CAD.

The systematic approach described above is intended to reduce the likelihood that patients with unrecognized cardiovascular disease will be inadvertently exposed to sumatriptan.

Drug-Associated Cardiac Events and Fatalities: Serious adverse cardiac events, including acute myocardial infarction, life-threatening disturbances of cardiac rhythm, and death have been reported to have occurred within 1 hour following the administration of IMITREX Injection. Considering the extent of use of sumatriptan in patients with migraine, the incidence of these events is extremely low. The fact that sumatriptan can cause coronary vasospasm gives credence to the possibility that at least some of the cases reported in close temporal association with the use of IMITREX may have been caused by the drug.

Premarketing Experience: Among the more than 1,900 patients with migraine who participated in premarketing controlled clinical trials of sumatriptan, there were eight patients who sustained clinical events during or shortly after receiving subcutaneous sumatriptan that may have reflected coronary artery vasospasm. Six of these eight patients had ECG changes consistent with transient ischemia, but without accompanying clinical symptoms or signs. Of these eight patients, four had either findings suggestive of CAD or risk factors predictive of CAD prior to study enrollment.

Postmarketing Experience: Serious cardiovascular events, some resulting in death, have been reported in association with the use of IMITREX Injection. The uncontrolled nature of postmarketing surveillance, however, makes it impossible to determine definitively the proportion of the reported cases that were actually caused by sumatriptan or to reliably assess causation in individual cases. On clinical grounds, the longer the latency between the administration of IMITREX and the onset of the clinical event, the less likely the association is to be causative. Accordingly, interest has focused on events occurring within 1 hour of the administration of IMITREX.

Cardiac events that have been observed to have onset within 1 hour of sumatriptan administration include: coronary artery vasospasm, transient ischemia, myocardial infarction, ventricular tachycardia and ventricular fibrillation, cardiac arrest, and death.

Some of these events occurred in patients who had no findings of CAD and may represent sequellae of coronary artery vasospasm. However, among domestic cases reported prior to January 1996 involving patients with serious cardiac events within 1 hour of sumatriptan administration, the majority had risk factors predictive of CAD, and use of sumatriptan may have been contraindicated. The presence of significant underlying CAD was established in most of these cases.

Drug-Associated Cerebrovascular Events and Fatalities: Cerebral hemorrhage, subarachnoid hemorrhage, stroke, and other cerebrovascular events have been reported in patients treated with oral and subcutaneous sumatriptan, and some have resulted in fatalities. In a number of cases, it appears possible that the cerebrovascular events were primary, sumatriptan having been administered in the incorrect belief the symptoms experienced were a consequence of migraine when they were not. Accordingly, sumatriptan should not be administered if the headache being experienced is atypical. In this regard, it should be noted that patients with migraine may be at increased risk of certain cerebrovascular events (e.g. cerebrovascular accident, transient ischemic attack).

Increase in Blood Pressure: Significant elevation in blood pressure, including hypertensive crisis, has been reported on rare occasions in patients with and without a history of hypertension. Sumatriptan in contraindicated in patients with uncontrolled hypertension (see CONTRAINDICATIONS).

Concomitant Drug Use: In patients taking MAO-A inhibitors, sumatriptan plasma levels attained after treatment with recommended doses are nearly double those obtained under other conditions. Accordingly, the co-administration of sumatriptan and an MAO-A inhibitor is not generally recommended. If such therapy is clinically warranted, however, suitable dose adjustment and appropriate observation of the patient is advised (see CLINICAL PHARMACOLOGY).

Use in Women of Childbearing Potential: (see PRECAUTIONS)

Hypersensitivity: Hypersensitivity (anaphylaxis/anaphylactoid) reactions have occurred on rare occasions in patients receiving sumatriptan. Such reactions can be life threatening or fatal. In general, hypersensitivity reactions to drugs are more likely to occur in individuals with a history of sensitivity to multiple allergens (see CONTRAINDICATIONS).

PRECAUTIONS

General: Chest, jaw, or neck tightness is relatively common after administration of IMITREX Injection, but has only rarely been associated with ischemic ECG changes. However, because sumatriptan may cause coronary artery vasospasm, patients who experience signs or symptoms suggestive of angina following sumatriptan should be evaluated for the presence of CAD or a predisposition to variant angina before receiving additional doses of sumatriptan (see WARNINGS).

IMITREX Injection should also be administered with caution to patients with diseases that may alter the absorption, metabolism, or excretion of drugs, such as impaired hepatic or renal function.

There have been rare reports of seizure following administration of sumatriptan.

Care should be taken to exclude other potentially serious neurologic conditions before treating headache in patients not previously diagnosed with migraine or cluster headache or who experience a headache that is atypical for them. There have been rare reports where patients received sumatriptan for severe headaches that were subsequently shown to have been secondary to an evolving neurologic lesion (see WARNINGS). For a given attack, if a patient does not respond to the first dose of sumatriptan, the diagnosis of migraine or cluster headache should be reconsidered before administration of a second dose.

Binding to Melanin-Containing Tissues: Because sumatriptan binds to melanin, it could accumulate in melanin-rich tissues (such as the eye) over time. This raises the possibility that sumatriptan could cause toxicity in these tissues after extended use. However, no effects on the retina related to treatment with sumatriptan were noted in any of the toxicity studies. Although no systematic monitoring of ophthalmologic function was undertaken in clinical trials, and no specific recommendations for ophthalmologic function was undertaken in clinical trials, and no specific recommendations for ophthalmologic monitoring are offered, prescribers should be aware of the possibility of long-term ophthalmologic effects (see CLINICAL PHARMACOLOGY).

Corneal Opacities: Sumatriptan causes corneal opacities and defects in the corneal epithelium in dogs; this raises the possibility that these changes may occur in humans. While patients were not systematically evaluated for these changes in clinical trials, and no specific recommendations for monitoring are being offered, prescribers should be aware of the possibility of these changes (see CLINICAL PHARMACOLOGY).

Continued on next page

Glaxo Wellcome—Cont.

Although written instructions are supplied with the autoinjector, patients who are advised to self-administer IMITREX Injection in medically unsupervised situations should receive instruction on the proper use of the product from the physician or other suitably qualified health care professional prior to doing so for the first time.

Information for Patients: See PATIENT INFORMATION at the end of this labeling for the text of the separate leaflet provided for patients.

Laboratory Tests: No specific laboratory tests are recommended for monitoring patients prior to and/or after treatment with IMITREX Injection.

Drug Interactions: There is no evidence that concomitant use of migraine prophylactic medications has any effect on the efficacy or unwanted effects of sumatriptan. In two Phase III trials in the US, a retrospective analysis of 282 patients who had been using prophylactic drugs (verapamil n = 63, amitriptyline n = 57, propranolol n = 94, for 45 other drugs n = 123) were compared to those who had not used prophylaxis (n = 452). There were no differences in relief rates at 60 minutes postdose for IMITREX Injection, whether or not prophylactic medications were used. There were also no differences in overall adverse event rates between the two groups.

Ergot-containing drugs have been reported to cause prolonged vasospastic reactions. Because there is a theoretical basis that these effects may be additive, use of ergotamine-containing or ergot-type medications (like dihydroergotamine or methysergide) and sumatriptan within 24 hours of each other should be avoided (see CONTRAINDICATIONS).

MAO-A inhibitors reduce sumatriptan clearance, significantly increasing systemic exposure. Therefore, the use of sumatriptan in patients receiving MAO-A inhibitors is not ordinarily recommended. If the clinical situation warrants the combined use of sumatriptan and an MAOI, the dose of sumatriptan employed should be reduced (see CLINICAL PHARMACOLOGY and WARNINGS).

There have been rare postmarketing reports describing patients with weakness, hyperreflexia, and incoordination following the use of a selective serotonin reuptake inhibitor (SSRI) and sumatriptan. If concomitant treatment with sumatriptan and an SSRI (e.g., fluoxetine, fluvoxamine, paroxetine, sertraline) is clinically warranted, appropriate observation of the patient is advised.

Drug/Laboratory Test Interactions: IMITREX Injection is not known to interfere with commonly employed clinical laboratory tests.

Carcinogenesis, Mutagenesis, Impairment of Fertility: In carcinogenicity studies, rats and mice were given sumatriptan by oral gavage (rats, 104 weeks) or drinking water (mice, 78 weeks). Average exposures achieved in mice receiving the highest dose were approximately 110 times the exposure attained in humans after the maximum recommended single dose of 6 mg. The highest dose to rats was approximately 260 times the maximum single dose of 6 mg on a mg/m^2 basis. There was no evidence of an increase in tumors in either species related to sumatriptan administration.

Sumatriptan was not mutagenic in the presence or absence of metabolic activation when tested in two gene mutation assays (the Ames test and the *in vitro* mammalian Chinese hamster V79/HGPRT assay). In two cytogenetics assays (the *in vitro* human lymphocyte assay and the *in vivo* rat micronucleus assay) sumatriptan was not associated with clastogenic activity.

A fertility study (Segment I) by the subcutaneous route, during which male and female rats were dosed daily with sumatriptan prior to and throughout the mating period, has shown no evidence of impaired fertility at doses equivalent to approximately 100 times the maximum recommended single human dose of 6 mg on a mg/m^2 basis. However, following oral administration, a treatment-related decrease in fertility, secondary to a decrease in mating, was seen for rats treated with 50 and 500 mg/kg per day. The no-effect dose for this finding was approximately eight times the maximum recommended single human dose of 6 mg on a mg/m^2 basis. It is not clear whether the problem is associated with the treatment of males or females or both.

Pregnancy: ***Pregnancy Category C:*** Sumatriptan has been shown to be embryolethal in rabbits when given daily at a dose approximately equivalent to the maximum recommended single human subcutaneous dose of 6 mg on a mg/m^2 basis. There is no evidence that establishes that sumatriptan is a human teratogen; however, there are no adequate and well-controlled studies in pregnant women. IMITREX Injection should be used during pregnancy only if the potential benefit justifies the potential risk to the fetus. In assessing this information, the following additional findings should be considered.

Embryolethality: When given intravenously to pregnant rabbits daily throughout the period of organogenesis, sumatriptan caused embyolethality at doses at or close to those producing maternal toxicity. The mechanism of the embryolethality is not known. These doses were approximately equivalent to the maximum single human dose of 6 mg on a mg/m^2 basis.

The intravenous administration of sumatriptan to pregnant rats throughout organogenesis at doses that are approximately 20 times a human dose of 6 mg on a mg/m^2 basis, did not cause embryolethality. Additionally, in a study of pregnant rats given subcutaneous sumatriptan daily prior to and throughout pregnancy, there was no evidence of increased embryo/fetal lethality.

Teratogenicity: Term fetuses from Dutch Stride rabbits treated during organogenesis with oral sumatriptan exhibited an increased incidence of cervicothoracic vascular and skeletal abnormalities. The functional significance of these abnormalities is not known. The highest no-effect dose for these effects was 15 mg/kg per day, approximately 50 times the maximum single dose of 6 mg on a mg/m^2 basis.

In a study in rats dosed daily with subcutaneous sumatriptan prior to and throughout pregnancy, there was no evidence of teratogenicity.

To monitor fetal outcomes of pregnant women exposed to IMITREX, Glaxo Wellcome Inc. maintains a Sumatriptan Pregnancy Registry. Physicians are encouraged to register patients by calling (800) 722-9292, ext. 58465.

Nursing Mothers: Sumatriptan is excreted in human breast milk. Therefore, caution should be exercised when considering the administration of IMITREX Injection to a nursing woman.

Pediatric Use: Safety and effectiveness of IMITREX Injection in pediatric patients have not been established.

Use in the Elderly: Although the pharmacokinetic disposition of the drug in elderly is similar to that seen in younger adults, there is no information about the safety and effectiveness of sumatriptan in this population because patients over age 65 were excluded from the controlled clinical trials.

ADVERSE REACTIONS

Serious cardiac events, including some that have been fatal, have occurred following use of IMITREX Injection, but are extremely rare. Events reported have included coronary artery vasospasm, transient myocardial ischemia, myocardial infarction, ventricular tachycardia, and ventricular fibrillation (see CONTRAINDICATIONS, WARNINGS, and PRECAUTIONS).

Significant hypertensive episodes, including hypertensive crises, have been reported on rare occasions in patients with or without a history of hypertension (see WARNINGS).

Among patients in clinical trials of subcutaneous IMITREX Injection (n = 6,218), up to 3.5% of patients withdrew for reasons related to adverse events.

Incidence in Controlled Clinical Trials of Migraine Headache: The following Table 4 lists adverse events that occurred in two large US, Phase III, placebo-controlled clinical trials in migraine patients following either a single dose of IMITREX Injection or placebo. Only events that occurred at a frequency of 1% or more in IMITREX Injection treatment groups and were at least as frequent as in the placebo group are included in Table 4.

Table 4: Treatment-Emergent Adverse Experience Incidence in Two Large Placebo-Controlled Migraine Clinical Trials: Events Reported by at Least 1% of IMITREX Injection Patients

	Percent of Patients Reporting	
Adverse Event Type	IMITREX Injection 6 mg SC n = 547	Placebo n = 370
Atypical sensations	42.0	9.2
Tingling	13.5	3.0
Warm/hot sensation	10.8	3.5
Burning sensation	7.5	0.3
Feeling of heaviness	7.3	1.1
Pressure sensation	7.1	1.6
Feeling of tightness	5.1	0.3
Numbness	4.6	2.2
Feeling strange	2.2	0.3
Tight feeling in head	2.2	0.3
Cold sensation	1.1	0.5
Cardiovascular		
Flushing	6.6	2.4
Chest discomfort	4.5	1.4
Tightness in chest	2.7	0.5
Pressure in chest	1.8	0.3
Ear, nose, and throat		
Throat discomfort	3.3	0.5
Discomfort: nasal cavity/sinuses	2.2	0.3
Eye		
Vision alterations	1.1	0.0
Gastrointestinal		
Abdominal discomfort	1.3	0.8
Dysphagia	1.1	0.0
Injection site reaction	58.7	23.8
Miscellaneous		
Jaw discomfort	1.8	0.0
Mouth and teeth		
Discomfort of mouth/tongue	4.9	4.6
Musculoskeletal		
Weakness	4.9	0.3
Neck pain/stiffness	4.8	0.5
Myalgia	1.8	0.5
Muscle cramp(s)	1.1	0.0
Neurological		
Dizziness/vertigo	11.9	4.3
Drowsiness/sedation	2.7	2.2
Headache	2.2	0.3
Anxiety	1.1	0.5
Malaise/fatigue	1.1	0.8
Skin		
Sweating	1.6	1.1

The sum of the percentages cited is greater than 100% because patients may experience more than one type of adverse event. Only events that occurred at a frequency of 1% or more in IMITREX Injection treatment groups and were at least as frequent in the placebo groups are included.

The incidence of adverse events in controlled clinical trials was not affected by gender or age of the patients. There was insufficient data to assess the impact of race on the incidence of adverse events.

Incidence in Controlled Trials of Cluster Headache: In the controlled trials assessing sumatriptan's efficacy as a treatment for cluster headache, no new significant adverse events associated with the use of sumatriptan were detected that had not already been identified in association of the drug's use in migraine.

Overall, the frequency of adverse events reported in the studies of cluster headache were generally lower. Exceptions include reports of paresthesia (5% IMITREX, 0% placebo), nausea and vomiting (4% IMITREX, 0% placebo) and bronchospasm (1% IMITREX, 0% placebo).

Other Events Observed in Association With the Administration of IMITREX Injection: In the paragraphs that follow, the frequencies of less commonly reported adverse clinical events are presented. Because the reports cite events observed in open and uncontrolled studies, the role of IMITREX Injection in their causation cannot be reliably determined. Furthermore, variability associated with reporting requirements, the terminology used to describe adverse events, etc., limit the value of the quantitative frequency estimates provided.

Event frequencies are calculated as the number of patients reporting an event divided by the total number of patients (n = 6,218) exposed to subcutaneous IMITREX Injection. Given their imprecision, frequencies for specific adverse event occurrences are defined as follows: "infrequent" indicates a frequency estimated as falling between 1/1,000 and 1/100; "rare," a frequency of less than 1/1,000.

Cardiovascular: Infrequent were hypertension, hypotension, bradycardia, tachycardia, palpitations, pulsating sensations, various transient ECG changes (nonspecific ST or T wave changes, prolongation of PR or QTc intervals, sinus arrhythmia, nonsustained ventricular premature beats, isolated junctional ectopic beats, atrial ectopic beats, delayed activation of the right ventricle), and syncope. Rare were pallor, arrhythmia, abnormal pulse, vasodilatation, and Raynaud's syndrome.

Endocrine and Metabolic: Infrequent was thirst. Rare was polydipsia and dehydration.

Eye: Infrequent was irritation of the eye.

Gastrointestinal: Infrequent were gastroesophageal reflux, diarrhea, and disturbances of liver function tests. Rare were peptic ulcer, retching, flatulence/eructation, and gallstones.

Musculoskeletal: Infrequent were various joint disturbances (pain, stiffness, swelling, ache). Rare were muscle stiffness, need to flex calf muscles, backache, muscle tiredness, and swelling of the extremities.

Neurological: Infrequent were mental confusion, euphoria, agitation, relaxation, chills, sensation of lightness, tremor, shivering, disturbances of taste, prickling sensations, paresthesia, stinging sensations, headaches, facial pain, photophobia, and lacrimation. Rare were transient hemiplegia, hysteria, globus hystericus, intoxication, depression, myoclonia, monoplegia/diplegia, sleep disturbance, difficulties in concentration, disturbances of smell, hyperesthesia, dysesthesia, simultaneous hot and cold sensations, tickling sensations, dysarthria, yawning, reduced appetite, hunger, and dystonia.

Respiratory: Infrequent was dyspnea. Rare were influenza, diseases of the lower respiratory tract, and hiccoughs.

Dermatological: Infrequent were erythema, pruritus, and skin rashes and eruptions. Rare was skin tenderness.

Urogenital: Rare were dysuria, frequency, dysmenorrhea, and renal calculus.

Miscellaneous: Infrequent were miscellaneous laboratory abnormalities, including minor disturbances in liver function tests, "serotonin agonist effect", and hypersensitivity to various agents. Rare was fever.

Postmarketing Experience: The following are spontaneously reported adverse events from postmarketing experience except those events already listed previously in the ADVERSE REACTIONS section or those too general to be informative. Because the reports cite events reported spontaneously from worldwide postmarketing experience, frequency of events and the role of IMITREX Injection in their causation cannot be reliably determined.

Episodes of Prinzmetal's variant angina, acute renal failure, seizure, cerebrovascular accident, dysphasia, subarachnoid hemorrhage, photosensitivity, exacerbation of sunburn, and death (see WARNINGS); bronchospasm has been reported in patients with and without a history of asthma.

The following hypersensitivity reactions have been reported: urticaria and shortness of breath. In addition, severe anaphylaxis/anaphylactoid reactions have been reported (see WARNINGS).

Rarely, lipoatrophy (depression in the skin) or lipohypertrophy (enlargement of thickening of tissue) has been reported following subcutaneous administration of sumatriptan.

DRUG ABUSE AND DEPENDENCE

The abuse potential of IMITREX Injection cannot be fully delineated in advance of extensive marketing experience. One clinical study enrolling 12 patients with a history of substance abuse failed to induce subjective behavior and/or physiologic response ordinarily associated with drugs that have an established potential for abuse.

OVERDOSAGE

Patients ($n = 269$) have received single injections of 8 to 12 mg without significant adverse effects. Volunteers ($n = 47$) have received single subcutaneous doses of up to 16 mg without serious adverse events.

No gross overdoses in clinical practice have been reported. Coronary vasospasm was observed after intravenous administration of IMITREX Injection (see CONTRAINDICATIONS). Overdoses would be expected from animal data (dogs at 0.1 g/kg, rats at 2 g/kg) to possibly cause convulsions, tremor, inactivity, erythema of the extremities, reduced respiratory rate, cyanosis, ataxia, mydriasis, injection site reactions (desquamation, hair loss, and scab formation), and paralysis. The half-life of elimination of sumatriptan is about 2 hours (see CLINICAL PHARMACOLOGY), and therefore monitoring of patients after overdose with IMITREX Injection should continue while symptoms or signs persist, and for at least 10 hours.

It is unknown what effect hemodialysis or peritoneal dialysis has on the serum concentrations of sumatriptan.

DOSAGE AND ADMINISTRATION

The maximum single recommended adult dose of IMITREX Injection is 6 mg injected subcutaneously. Controlled clinical trials have failed to show that clear benefit is associated with the administration of a second 6-mg dose in patients who have failed to respond to a first injection.

The maximum recommended dose that may be given in 24 hours is two 6-mg injections separated by at least 1 hour. Although the recommended dose is 6 mg, if side effects are dose limiting, then lower doses may be used (see CLINICAL PHARMACOLOGY). In patients receiving MAO inhibitors, decreased doses of sumatriptan should be considered (see WARNINGS and CLINICAL PHARMACOLOGY). In patients receiving doses lower than 6 mg, only the single-dose vial dosage form should be used. An autoinjection device is available for use with 6-mg prefilled syringes to facilitate self-administration in patients in whom this dose is deemed necessary.

Parenteral drug products should be inspected visually for particulate matter and discoloration before administration whenever solution and container permit.

HOW SUPPLIED

IMITREX Injection 6 mg (12 mg/mL) containing sumatriptan (base) as the succinate salt is supplied as a clear, colorless to pale yellow, sterile, nonpyrogenic solution as follows.

(NDC 0173-0449-01) unit-of-use syringes (0.5 mL in 1 mL) in cartons of two syringes

(NDC 0173-0449-03) IMITREX® SELFdose System kit containing two unit-of-use syringes, one IMITREX® SELFdose Unit, and instructions for use

(NDC 0173-0449-02) 6-mg single-dose vials (0.5 mL in 2 mL) in cartons of five vials

Store between 2° and 30°C (36° and 86°F). Protect from light.

Caution: Federal law prohibits dispensing without a prescription.

PATIENT INFORMATION

The following wording is contained in a separate leaflet provided for patients.

Information for the Consumer

IMITREX (sumatriptan succinate) Injection

Please read this leaflet carefully before you take IMITREX Injection. This provides a summary of the information available on your medicine. Please do not throw away this leaflet until you have finished your medicine. You may need to read this leaflet again. This leaflet does not contain all the information on IMITREX Injection. For further information or advice, ask your doctor or pharmacist.

Information About Your Medicine:

The name of your medicine is IMITREX Injection. It can be obtained only by prescription from your doctor. The decision to use IMITREX Injection is one that you and your doctor should make jointly, taking into account your individual preferences and medical circumstances. If you have risk factors for heart disease (such as high blood pressure, high cholesterol, obesity, diabetes, smoking, strong family history of heart disease, or you are postmenopausal or a male over 40), you should tell your doctor, who should evaluate you for heart disease in order to determine if IMITREX is appropriate for you. Although the vast majority of those who have taken IMITREX have not experienced any significant side effects, some individuals have experienced problems and, rarely, deaths have been reported. In all but a few instances, however, IMITREX does not appear to have been a contributory factor in these deaths.

1. The Purpose of Your Medicine:

IMITREX Injection is intended to relieve your migraine or cluster headache, but not to prevent or reduce the number of attacks you experience. Use IMITREX Injection only to treat an actual migraine or cluster headache attack.

2. Important Questions to Consider Before Taking IMITREX Injection:

If the answer to any of the following questions is **YES** or if you do not know the answer, then please discuss with your doctor before you use IMITREX Injection.

- Are you pregnant? Do you think you might be pregnant? Are you trying to become pregnant? Are you using inadequate contraception? Are you breast-feeding?
- Do you have any chest pain, heart disease, shortness of breath, or irregular heartbeats? Have you had a heart attack?
- Do you have risk factors for heart disease (such as high blood pressure, high cholesterol, obesity, diabetes, smoking, strong family history of heart disease, or you are postmenopausal or a male over 40)?
- Do you have high blood pressure?
- Have you ever had to stop taking this or any other medication because of an allergy or other problems?
- Are you taking any medications, including migraine medications containing ergotamine, dihydroergotamine, or methysergide?
- Are you taking any medication for depression (monoamine oxidase inhibitors or selective serotonin reuptake inhibitors [SSRIs])?
- Have you had, or do you have, any disease of the liver or kidney?
- Have you had, or do you have, epilepsy or seizures?
- Is this headache different from your usual migraine attacks?

Remember, if you answered **YES** to any of the above questions, then discuss it with your doctor.

3. The Use of IMITREX Injection During Pregnancy:

Do not use IMITREX Injection if you are pregnant, think you might be pregnant, are trying to become pregnant, or are not using adequate contraception, unless you have discussed this with your doctor.

4. How to Use IMITREX Injection:

Before using the autoinjector, see the enclosed instruction pamphlet on loading your autoinjector and discarding the empty syringes.

For adults, the usual dose is a single injection given just below the skin. It should be given as soon as the symptoms of your migraine appear, but it may be given at any time during an attack. A second injection may be given if your symptoms of migraine come back. If your symptoms do not improve following the first injection, do not give a second injection for the same attack without first consulting with your doctor. Do not have more than two injections in any 24 hours and allow at least 1 hour between each dose.

5. Side Effects to Watch for:

- Some patients experience pain or tightness in the chest or throat when using IMITREX Injection. If this happens to you, then discuss it with your doctor before using any more IMITREX Injection. If the chest pain is severe or does not go away, call your doctor immediately.
- Shortness of breath; wheeziness; heart throbbing; swelling of eyelids, face, or lips; or a skin rash, skin lumps, or hives happens rarely. If it happens to you, then tell your doctor immediately. Do not take any more IMITREX Injection unless your doctor tells you to do so.
- Some people may have feelings of tingling, heat, flushing (redness of face lasting a short time), heaviness or pressure after treatment with IMITREX Injection. A few people may feel drowsy, dizzy, tired, or sick. Tell your doctor of these symptoms at your next visit.
- You may experience pain or redness at the site of injection, but this usually lasts less than an hour.
- If you feel unwell in any other way or have any symptoms that you do not understand, you should contact your doctor immediately.

6. What to Do If an Overdose Is Taken:

If you have taken more medication than you have been told, contact either your doctor, hospital emergency department, or nearest poison control center immediately.

7. Storing Your Medicine:

Keep your medicine in a safe place where children cannot reach it. It may be harmful to children.

Store your medication away from heat and light. Keep your medication in the case provided and do not store at temperatures above 86°F (30°C).

If your medication has expired (the expiration date is printed on the treatment pack), throw it away as instructed. Do not throw away your autoinjector.

If your doctor decides to stop your treatment, do not keep any leftover medicine unless your doctor tells you to. Throw away your medicine as instructed.

©Copyright 1996 Glaxo Wellcome Inc. All rights reserved.

May 1996/RL-309

Shown in Product Identification Guide, page 313

IMITREX® ℞

[*ĭm ′-ĭ-trĕx″*]

(sumatriptan succinate)

Tablets

DESCRIPTION

Imitrex® (sumatriptan succinate) Tablets contain sumatriptan (as the succinate), which is a selective 5-hydroxytryptamine$_1$ receptor subtype agonist, as the active ingredient. Sumatriptan succinate is chemically designated as 3-[2-(dimethylamino)ethyl] -N- methyl-1H-indole-5-methanesulfonamide butane-1,4-dioate(1:1).

The empirical formula is $C_{14}H_{21}N_3O_2S \cdot C_4H_6O_4$, representing a molecular weight of 413.5.

Sumatriptan succinate is a white to off-white powder that is readily soluble in water and in saline.

Each Imitrex Tablet for oral administration contains 35 or 70 mg of sumatriptan succinate equivalent to 25 or 50 mg of sumatriptan, respectively. Each tablet also contains the inactive ingredients croscarmellose sodium, lactose, magnesium stearate, microcrystalline cellulose, and titanium dioxide dye.

CLINICAL PHARMACOLOGY

Mechanism of Action: Sumatriptan has been demonstrated to be a selective agonist for a vascular 5-hydroxytryptamine$_1$ receptor subtype (probably a member of the 5-HT$_{1D}$ family) with no significant affinity (as measured using standard radioligand binding assays) or pharmacological activity at 5-HT$_2$, 5-HT$_3$ receptor subtypes or at alpha$_1$-, alpha$_2$-, or beta-adrenergic; dopamine$_1$; dopamine$_2$; muscarinic; or benzodiazepine receptors.

The vascular 5-HT$_1$ receptor subtype to which sumatriptan binds selectively, and through which it presumably exerts its antimigrainous effect, has been shown to be present on cranial arteries in both dog and primate, on the human basilar artery, and in the vasculature of the isolated dura mater of humans. In these tissues, sumatriptan activates this receptor to cause vasoconstriction, an action in humans correlating with the relief of migraine. In the anesthetized dog, sumatriptan selectively reduces the carotid arterial blood flow with little or no effect on arterial blood pressure or total peripheral resistance. In the cat, sumatriptan selectively constricts the carotid arteriovenous anastomoses while having little effect on blood flow or resistance in cerebral or extracerebral tissues.

Corneal Opacities: Dogs receiving oral sumatriptan developed corneal opacities and defects in the corneal epithelium. Corneal opacities were seen at the lowest dosage tested, 2 mg/kg per day, and were present after 1 month of treatment. Defects in the corneal epithelium were noted in a 60-week study. Earlier examinations for these toxicities were not conducted and no-effect doses were not established; however, the relative exposure at the lowest dose tested was approximately five times the human exposure after a 100-mg oral dose.

Melanin Binding: In rats treated with a single oral dose (2 mg/kg) of radiolabeled sumatriptan, the elimination half-life of radioactivity from the eye was 23 days, suggesting that sumatriptan and its metabolites bind to the melanin of the eye. The clinical significance of this binding is unknown.

Pharmacokinetics: ***Absorption and Elimination:*** Sumatriptan is rapidly absorbed after oral administration, with low absolute bioavailability, approximately 15%, primarily due to presystemic metabolism and partly due to incomplete absorption. The mean maximum concentration (C_{max}) following a 100-mg oral dose is 51 ng/mL. This compares with a C_{max} of about 75 ng/mL after a 6-mg subcutaneous dose. C_{max} is similar during a migraine attack and during a migraine-free period, but the T_{max} is slightly later during the attack, approximately 2.5 hours compared to 2.0 hours. When given as a single dose, sumatriptan displays dose pro-

Continued on next page

Glaxo Wellcome—Cont.

portionality in its extent of absorption (area under the curve [AUC]) over the dose range of 25 to 200 mg, but the C_{max} after 100 mg is approximately 25% less than expected (based on the 25-mg dose).

Food has no significant effect on the bioavailability of sumatriptan, but delays the T_{max} slightly (by about 0.5 hours). Plasma protein binding is low (14% to 21%).

The apparent volume of distribution is 2.4 L/kg.

The elimination half-life of sumatriptan is approximately 2.5 hours. Radiolabeled ^{14}C-sumatriptan administered orally is largely renally excreted (about 60%) with about 40% found in the feces. Most of the radiolabeled compound excreted in the urine is the major metabolite, indole acetic acid (IAA), which is inactive, or the IAA glucuronide. Only 3% of the dose can be recovered as unchanged sumatriptan.

In vitro studies with human microsomes suggest that sumatriptan is metabolized by monoamine oxidase (MAO), predominantly the A isoenzyme, and inhibitors of that enzyme may alter sumatriptan pharmacokinetics to increase systemic exposure. No significant effect was seen with a MAO-B inhibitor (see CONTRAINDICATIONS, WARNINGS, and PRECAUTIONS: Drug Interactions).

Special Populations: *Renal Impairment:* The effect of renal impairment on the pharmacokinetics of sumatriptan has not been examined, but little clinical effect would be expected as sumatriptan is largely metabolized to an inactive substance.

Hepatic Impairment: The liver plays an important role in the presystemic clearance of orally administered sumatriptan. Accordingly, the bioavailability of sumatriptan following oral administration may be markedly increased in patients with liver disease. In one small study of hepatically impaired patients (n=8) matched for sex, age, and weight with healthy subjects, the hepatically impaired patients had an approximately 70% increase in AUC and C_{max} and a T_{max} 40 minutes earlier compared to the healthy subjects (see DOSAGE AND ADMINISTRATION).

Age: Elderly: Sumatriptan pharmacokinetics in healthy elderly subjects were similar to those in healthy young volunteers.

Gender: In a study comparing females to males, no pharmacokinetic differences were observed between genders for AUC, C_{max}, T_{max}, and half-life.

Race: The effect of race on the pharmacokinetics of sumatriptan has not been examined.

Drug Interactions: *MAO Inhibitors:* Because of the important role played by MAO in the presystemic clearance of sumatriptan, MAO inhibitors can markedly increase sumatriptan systemic exposure after oral dosing. MAO inhibitors also affect its elimination. For example, in a study of women given subcutaneous sumatriptan, pretreatment with an MAO-A inhibitor resulted in a *marked* increase in sumatriptan AUC, *marked* increase in half-life, and a *marked* decrease in CI_p/F. No significant effect was seen with an MAO-B inhibitor. Although studies of this interaction have not been performed with oral sumatriptan, as noted above, the effects of an MAO inhibitor on oral sumatriptan bioavailability would be expected to be at least as great, if not greater, than those on subcutaneous sumatriptan (see CONTRAINDICATIONS, WARNINGS).

Pharmacodynamics: *Typical Physiological Responses: Cardiovascular:*

Blood Pressure: Transient increases in systolic and diastolic blood pressure may be observed after treatment with oral sumatriptan. Elderly (67 to 79 years of age) subjects given 100 or 200 mg of sumatriptan as a single oral dose had statistically significant increases in mean peak systolic blood pressure of up to 14 mmHg over the first 3 hours after dosing, with some evidence of increasing effect with dose. In the same study, however, a younger group of patients (19 to 37 years) had no change in systolic blood pressure after doses of up to 200 mg. In this study, there were small, but statistically significant, increases in diastolic blood pressure of between 2 and 6 mmHg compared to placebo in young and elderly subjects after administration of sumatriptan (50, 100, and 200 mg), but other studies did not confirm this finding. In controlled US studies in migraine patients, no consistent effects on blood pressure or heart rate were observed.

Heart and Respiratory: There have been no clinically significant effects of oral sumatriptan on heart or respiratory rates.

CLINICAL STUDIES

Two US controlled trials evaluated 25-, 50-, and 100-mg single doses of oral sumatriptan in a total of 446 patients with migraine attacks who were experiencing moderate or severe pain and one or more of the symptoms enumerated in Table 1 below. Onset of relief (defined as no or mild pain) was seen as early as 1 to 1.5 hours after all three doses. Statistically significant differences from placebo were seen in the proportion of patients achieving relief at all time points starting at 1 to 2 hours and persisting out to 4 hours postdosing. There was no evidence of a dose response for pain and other measures of effectiveness. At 2 hours, approximately 54% (range, 50% to 57%) of patients on any dose of oral sumatriptan had achieved relief, compared to 17% and 26% placebo response rates. By 4 hours postdosing, response rates in drug-treated patients were approximately 71% (range, 65% to 78%), compared to placebo rates of 19% and 38%. Imitrex® (sumatriptan succinate) Tablets also relieved nausea and photophobia associated with migraine attacks. The following table shows the 2- and 4-hour efficacy results:

[See table 1 below.]

The efficacy of Imitrex Tablets is unaffected by whether or not migraine is associated with aura, duration of attack, gender or age of the patient, relationship to menses, or concomitant use of common migraine prophylactic drugs (e.g., beta-blockers, calcium channel blockers, or tricyclic antidepressants). There was insufficient data to assess the impact of race on the efficacy of Imitrex Tablets.

INDICATIONS AND USAGE

Imitrex® (sumatriptan succinate) Tablets are indicated for the acute treatment of migraine attacks with or without aura.

Imitrex Tablets are not for use in the management of hemiplegic or basilar migraine (see WARNINGS). Safety and effectiveness also have not been established for cluster headache, which is present in an older, predominantly male population.

CONTRAINDICATIONS

Because of rare reports of coronary vasospasm, Imitrex® (sumatriptan succinate) Tablets should not be given to patients with ischemic heart disease (angina pectoris, history of myocardial infarction, or documented silent ischemia) or to patients with Prinzmetal's angina. Also, patients with symptoms or signs consistent with ischemic heart disease should not receive Imitrex Tablets. Because Imitrex Tablets can give rise to increases in blood pressure (usually small), they should not be given to patients with uncontrolled hypertension.

Concurrent administration of MAO inhibitors or use within 2 weeks of discontinuation of MAO inhibitor therapy is contraindicated (see CLINICAL PHARMACOLOGY: Drug Interactions and PRECAUTIONS: Drug Interactions).

Imitrex Tablets should not be used within 24 hours of an ergotamine-containing or ergot-type medication like dihydro-ergotamine or methysergide.

Imitrex Tablets are contraindicated in patients with hypersensitivity to sumatriptan or any of the ingredients.

WARNINGS

Imitrex® (sumatriptan succinate) Tablets should only be used where a clear diagnosis of migraine has been established.

Imitrex Tablets should not be administered to patients with basilar or hemiplegic migraine.

Hypersensitivity (anaphylaxis/anaphylactoid) reactions have occurred on rare occasions in patients receiving sumatriptan. Such reactions can be life threatening or fatal. In general, hypersensitivity reactions to drugs are more likely to occur in individuals with a history of sensitivity to multiple allergens.

Cardiac Events/Coronary Constriction: Serious coronary events, including some that have been fatal, following Imitrex Tablets have occurred but are extremely rare. Although it is not clear how many of these can be attributed to Imitrex® (sumatriptan succinate), because of their potential to cause coronary vasospasm, Imitrex Tablets should not be given to patients in whom unrecognized coronary artery disease (CAD) is likely without a prior evaluation for underlying cardiovascular disease. Such patients include postmenopausal women, males over 40, and patients with other risk factors for CAD such as hypertension, hypercholesterolemia, obesity, diabetes, smokers, and strong family history. Following a satisfactory cardiovascular assessment, it is recommended that the first dose of Imitrex Tablets be given in the physician's office for patients with underlying risk factors for CAD unless these patients have previously received sumatriptan. If symptoms consistent with angina occur, electrocardiographic (ECG) evaluation should be carried out to look for ischemic changes.

Sumatriptan may cause coronary vasospasm in patients with a history of CAD, who are known to be more susceptible than others to coronary artery vasospasm, and, rarely, in patients without prior history suggestive of CAD. Of 6,348 patients in clinical trials of oral sumatriptan, two experienced clinical adverse events shortly after receiving oral sumatriptan that may have reflected coronary vasospasm. Neither of these adverse events was associated with a serious clinical outcome.

There have been rare reports from countries where Imitrex Tablets are already on the market of serious adverse events, including myocardial infarction, ECG changes suggestive of myocardial ischemia, and symptoms consistent with angina pectoris.

Drug-Associated Fatalities: In extensive worldwide postmarketing experience, deaths have been reported following the use of Imitrex Tablets. In most cases, the deaths occurring after treatment with Imitrex Tablets occurred well after sumatriptan use (i.e., 3 or more hours postdose) and probably reflect underlying disease and spontaneous events. There have, however, been several fatalities that occurred within a few hours after the use of sumatriptan. The specific contribution of sumatriptan to most of these deaths cannot be determined, but in one case with Imitrex® (sumatriptan succinate) Injection, a 41-year-old woman with a 6-day history of unilateral headache, uncertain history of cardiovascular disease with known risk factors (positive family history, postmenopausal woman, and smoking) and a history of asthma and codeine allergy, experienced nausea, vomiting, a sense of warmth, chest pressure, and sweating within 7 minutes of dosing. This was followed by hypotension at about one-half hour, and ventricular tachycardia/ventricular fi-

Table 1: Imitrex Tablets Dose Response Relationship for Efficacy

	Study 1				Study 2			
	Placebo (n=65)	Imitrex 25 mg (n=66)	Imitrex 50 mg (n=62)	Imitrex 100 mg (n=66)	Placebo (n=47)	Imitrex 25 mg (n=48)	Imitrex 50 mg (n=46)	Imitrex 100 mg (n=46)
Results at 2 Hours								
Patients with pain relief (grade 0/1)	26%	52%*	50%*	56%*	17%	52%*	54%*	57%*
Patients with no pain	8%	21%*	16%	23%*	6%	21%	17%	24%*
Patients with meaningful relief†	34%	59%*	55%*	56%*	21%	54%*	54%*	57%*
Patients without nausea	57%	67%	68%	65%	40%	56%	61%	72%*
Patients without photophobia	22%	41%*	37%*	44%*	13%	29%	26%	39%*
Patients with little or no clinical disability‡	35%	58%*	60%*	59%*	28%	58%*	52%*	67%*
Results at 4 Hours								
Patients with pain relief (grade 0/1)	38%	70%*	68%*	71%*	19%	65%*	72%*	78%*
Patients with no pain	15%	45%*	32%*	52%*	11%	35%*	41%*	41%*
Patients with meaningful relief†	45%	71%*	71%*	79%*	26%	69%*	72%*	83%*
Patients without nausea	60%	76%	79%*	83%*	45%	73%*	70%*	91%*
Patients without photophobia	40%	62%*	66%*	71%*	28%	69%*	65%*	65%*
Patients with little or no clinical disability‡	40%	68%*	71%*	71%*	23%	73%*	70%*	83%*

*$p < 0.05$ vs. placebo. Once patients received rescue medication, they were considered treatment failures from that point onward.

†Meaningful relief is a patient assessment of when he/she felt onset of relief of headache pain.

‡A successful outcome in terms of clinical disability was defined prospectively as ability to work mildly impaired or ability to work and function normally.

brillation leading to death. In most other cases, death was attributed to myocardial infarctions occurring hours after drug administration.

Deaths attributed to strokes, cerebral hemorrhage, and other cerebrovascular events have also been reported in patients treated with oral and subcutaneous sumatriptan. In many cases, it appears possible that the cerebrovascular events were primary, sumatriptan having been administered in the incorrect belief that the symptoms experienced were migrainous in origin when they were not. Accordingly, it is important to advise patients not to administer sumatriptan if a headache being experienced is atypical.

Use in Women of Childbearing Potential: (see PRECAUTIONS).

PRECAUTIONS

General: Atypical sensations over the precordium (tightness, pressure, heaviness) have been reported after Imitrex® (sumatriptan succinate) Tablets, but have only rarely been associated with ischemic ECG changes.

Sumatriptan may cause mild, transient elevation of blood pressure (see CLINICAL PHARMACOLOGY).

Imitrex Tablets should also be administered with caution to patients with impaired hepatic function (see CLINICAL PHARMACOLOGY and DOSAGE AND ADMINISTRATION).

There have been rare reports of seizure following administration of sumatriptan.

As with other acute migraine therapies, before treating headaches in patients not previously diagnosed as migraineurs and in migraineurs who present with atypical symptoms, care should be taken to exclude other potentially serious neurological conditions. There have been rare reports where patients received sumatriptan for severe headaches that were subsequently shown to have been secondary to an evolving neurological lesion (cerebrovascular accident, subarachnoid hemorrhage). For a given attack, if a patient has no response to the first dose, the diagnosis of migraine should be reconsidered before administration of a second dose. In this regard, it should be noted that migraineurs may be at increased risk of certain cerebrovascular events (e.g., cerebrovascular accident, transient ischemic attack).

Binding to Melanin-Containing Tissues: Because sumatriptan binds to melanin, it could acumulate in melanin-rich tissues (such as the eye) over time. This raises the possibility that sumatriptan could cause toxicity in these tissues after extended use. However, no effects on the retina related to treatment with sumatriptan were noted in any of the toxicity studies. Although no systematic monitoring of ophthalmologic function was undertaken in clinical trials, and no specific recommendations for ophthalmologic monitoring are offered, prescribers should be aware of the possibility of long-term ophthalmologic effects (see CLINICAL PHARMACOLOGY).

Corneal Opacities: Sumatriptan causes corneal opacities and defects in the corneal epithelium in dogs; this raises the possibility that these changes may occur in humans. While patients were not systematically evaluated for these changes in clinical trials, and no specific recommendations for monitoring are being offered, prescribers should be aware of the possibility of these changes (see CLINICAL PHARMACOLOGY).

Information for Patients: See PATIENT INFORMATION at the end of this labeling for the text of the separate leaflet provided for patients.

Laboratory Tests: No specific laboratory tests are recommended for monitoring patients prior to and/or after treatment with Imitrex Tablets.

Drug Interactions:

Note: The combined use of oral sumatriptan and MAO inhibitors is contraindicated (see CONTRAINDICATIONS). There is no evidence that concomitant use of migraine prophylactic medications has any effect on the efficacy or unwanted effects of sumatriptan. In controlled trials, a retrospective analysis compared 199 patients who had been using Imitrex Tablets and prophylactic drgus (calcium channel blockers, n=76; tricyclic antidepressants, n=43; beta blockers, n=70) to those who had not used prophylaxis (n=1,220). There were no differences in overall adverse event rates between the two groups.

Ergot-containing drugs have been reported to cause prolonged vasospastic reactions. Because there is a theoretical basis that these effects may be additive, use of ergot-containing or ergot-type medications (like dihydroergotamine or methysergide) and sumatriptan within 24 hours of each other should be avoided (see CONTRAINDICATIONS).

Propranolol: Pretreatment with propranolol 80 mg twice daily for 7 days had no effect on the pharmacokinetic, blood pressure, or pulse rate of oral sumatriptan administered as a single 300-mg dose.

Alcohol: Alcohol consumed 30 minutes prior to sumatriptan ingestion had no effect on the pharmacokinetics of sumatriptan.

Drug/Laboratory Test Interactions: Imitrex Tablets are not known to interfere with commonly employed clinical laboratory tests.

Table 2: Treatment-Emergent Adverse Events in Controlled US Clinical Trials Reported by at Least 1% of Patients With Migraine*

	Percent of Patients Reporting			
Adverse Event Type	Placebo (n=112)	Imitrex 25 mg (n=114)	Imitrex 50 mg (n=108)	Imitrex 100 mg (n=112)
Atypical sensations				
Feeling of heaviness	<1	<1	<1	2
Feeling of tightness	0	<1	2	2
Pressure sensation	0	<1	2	2
Tingling	4	8	4	5
Warm/hot sensation	<1	2	3	3
Cardiovascular				
Flushing	<1	0	4	2
Palpitations	<1	0	<1	2
Ear, nose and throat				
Discomfort: nasal	4	5	5	7
Eye				
Irritation of eye(s)	0	0	0	2
Visual disturbance	<1	0	<1	3
Musculoskeletal				
Weakness	0	2	<1	2
Neurological				
Agitation	0	0	0	2
Urogenital				
Dysuria	<1	0	0	2

* Events that occurred at a frequency of 1% or more in the Imitrex Tablets 100-mg group and that occurred more frequently in that group than the placebo group.

Carcinogenesis, Mutagenesis, Impairment of Fertility: In carcinogenicity studies, rats and mice were given sumatriptan by oral gavage (rats, 104 weeks) or in drinking water (mice, 78 weeks). Average exposures achieved in mice receiving the highest dose were approximately 40 times the exposure attained in humans after the maximum recommended single dose of 100 mg. The highest dose to rats was approximately 15 times the maximum single human dose of 100 mg on a mg/m^2 basis. There was no evidence of an increase in tumors in either species related to sumatriptan administration.

Sumatriptan was not mutagenic in the presence or absence of metabolic activation when tested in two gene mutation assays (the Ames test and the in vitro mammalian Chinese hamster V79/HGPRT assay). In two cytogenetics assays (the in vitro human lymphocyte assay and the in vivo rat micronucleus assay) sumatriptan was not associated with clastogenic activity.

In a study in which male and female rats were dosed daily with oral sumatriptan prior to and throughout the mating period, there was a treatment-related decrease in fertility secondary to a decrease in mating in animals treated with 50 and 500 mg/kg per day. The no-effect dose for this finding was approximately one-half of the maximum recommended single human dose of 100 mg on a mg/m^2 basis. It is not clear whether the problem is associated with treatment of the males or females or both combined.

Pregnancy: Pregnancy Category C: In reproductive toxicity studies in rats and rabbits, oral treatment with sumatriptan was associated with embryolethality, fetal abnormalities, and pup mortality. There is no evidence that establishes that sumatriptan is a human teratogen; however, there are no adequate and well-controlled studies in pregnant women. Imitrex Tablets should be used during pregnancy only if the potential benefit justifies the potential risk to the fetus. In assessing this information, the following findings should be considered.

Embryolethality: When given orally to pregnant rabbits daily throughout the period of organogenesis, sumatriptan caused embryolethality only at a dose that clearly resulted in maternal toxicity, 100 mg/kg per day. The no-effect dose for embryolethality was 50 mg/kg per day, which is approximately nine times the maximum single human dose of 100 mg on a mg/m^2 basis.

Teratogenicity: A study in which rats were dosed daily with oral sumatriptan prior to and throughout gestation demonstrated fetal toxicity and a small increased incidence of a syndrome of malformations (short tail/short body and vertebral disorganization) after long-term treatment with 500 mg/kg per day. The no-effect dose for this effect was 50 mg/kg per day, approximately five times the maximum single human dose of 100 mg on a mg/m^2 basis.

Oral treatment of pregnant rats with sumatriptan during the period of organogenesis resulted in an increased incidence of blood vessel abnormalities (cervicothoracic and umbilical) at doses of approximately 250 mg/kg per day or higher. The no-effect dose for this was approximately 60 mg/kg per day, approximately six times the maximum single human dose of 100 mg on a mg/m^2 basis.

Oral treatment of pregnant rabbits with sumatriptan during the period of organogenesis resulted in an increased incidence of cervicothoracic vascular and skeletal abnormalities. The highest no-effect dose established for these effects was 15 mg/kg per day, approximately three times the human dose of 100 mg on a mg/m^2 basis.

Pup Deaths: Oral treatment of pregnant rats with sumatriptan during the period of organogenesis resulted in a decrease in pup survival between birth and postnatal day 4 at doses of approximately 250 mg/kg per day or higher. The no-effect dose for this effect was approximately 60 mg/kg per day, or six times the human dose of 100 mg on a mg/m^2 basis. Oral treatment of pregnant rats with sumatriptan from gestational day 17 through postnatal day 21 demonstrated a decrease in pup survival measured at postnatal days 2, 4, and 20 at the dose of 1,000 mg/kg per day. The no-effect dose for this finding was 100 mg/kg per day, approximately 10 times the human dose of 100 mg on a mg/m^2 basis.

Nursing Mothers: Sumatriptan is excreted in human breast milk. Therefore, caution should be exercised when considering the administration of Imitrex Tablets to nursing women.

Pediatric Use: Safety and effectiveness of Imitrex Tablets in pediatric patients have not been established.

Use in the Elderly: The safety and effectiveness of Imitrex Tablets in individuals over age 65 have not been systematically evaluated, but the pharmacokinetic disposition of Imitrex Tablets in the elderly is similar to that seen in younger adults.

ADVERSE REACTIONS (see also PRECAUTIONS)

Sumatriptan may cause coronary vasospasm in patients with a history of CAD, known to be susceptible to coronary artery vasospasm, and, very rarely, without prior history suggestive of CAD.

There have been rare reports from countries in which Imitrex® (sumatriptan succinate) Tablets have been marketed of serious and/or life-threatening arrhythmias including atrial fibrillation, ventricular fibrillation, ventricular tachycardia; myocardial infarction; ECG changes suggestive of myocardial ischemia; and symptoms consistent with angina pectoris after oral sumatriptan. Chest discomfort, when it occurs, is usually noncardiac in origin.

Other untoward clinical events associated with the use of Imitrex Tablets are: warm/hot sensations, tingling/paresthesia, pressure sensations, flushing, sensations of heaviness, chest symptoms (tightness and sensations of heaviness), dizziness/vertigo, bad taste in mouth, weakness, myalgias, neck stiffness; all these untoward effects are transient, although they may be severe in occasional patients.

Incidence in Controlled Clinical Trials: The following Table 2 lists adverse events that occurred in two large US placebo-controlled clinical trials. Only events that occurred at a frequency of 1% or more in the Imitrex Tablets 100-mg group and that occurred more frequently in that group than the placebo group are included in Table 2.

[See table above.]

Other events that occurred at least as often on placebo as in the 100-mg dose group included abdominal discomfort, mouth or tongue discomfort, neck stiffness, anxiety, taste disturbance, nausea and/or vomiting, migraine, headache,

Continued on next page

Glaxo Wellcome—Cont.

drowsiness/sedation, dizziness/vertigo, and malaise/fatigue. Imitrex Tablets are generally well tolerated. Across all doses, most adverse reactions are mild and transient and do not lead to long-lasting effects. The incidence of adverse events in controlled clinical trials was not affected by gender or age of the patients. There was insufficient data to assess the impact of race on the incidence of adverse events.

Other Events Observed in Association With Oral Sumatriptan: In the paragraphs that follow, the frequencies of less commonly reported adverse clinical events are presented. Because the reports cite events observed in open and uncontrolled studies, the role of Imitrex Tablets in their causation cannot be reliably determined. Furthermore, variability associated with reporting requirements, the terminology used to describe adverse events, etc., limit the value of quantitative frequency estimates provided.

Event frequencies are calculated as the number of patients reporting an event divided by the total number of patients (n=6,348) exposed to oral sumatriptan. All reported events are included except those already listed in the previous table, those too general to be informative, and those not reasonably associated with the use of the drug. Events are further classified within body system categories and enumerated in order of decreasing frequency using the following definitions: frequent adverse events are defined as those occurring in at least 1/100 patients; infrequent adverse events are those occurring in 1/100 to 1/1,000 patients; rare adverse events are those occurring in fewer than 1/1,000 patients.

Atypical Sensations: Frequent were burning sensation, numbness, paresthesia. Infrequent was tight feeling in head. Rare were dysesthesia, hot and cold sensation.

Cardiovascular: Frequent were chest discomfort, chest pressure/heaviness, chest tightness. Infrequent were arrhythmia, changes in ECG, hypertension, hypotension, pallor, pulsating sensations, tachycardia. Rare were angina, atherosclerosis, bradycardia, cerebral ischemia, cerebrovascular lesion, heart block, peripheral cyanosis, thrombosis, transient myocardial ischemia, vasodilation.

Ear, Nose, and Throat: Frequent were throat symptoms. Infrequent were hearing disturbances, otalgia. Rare was feeling of fullness in the ear(s).

Endocrine and Metabolic: Infrequent was thirst. Rare were elevated thyrotropin stimulating hormone (TSH) levels, galactorrhea, hyperglycemia, hypoglycemia, hypothyroidism, polydipsia, weight gain, weight loss.

Eye: Rare were disorders of sclera, mydriasis.

Gastrointestinal: Frequent were diarrhea, gastric symptoms. Infrequent were constipation, dysphagia, gastroesophageal reflux. Rare were gastrointestinal bleeding, hematemesis, melena, peptic ulcer.

Hematological Disorders: Rare was anemia.

Musculoskeletal: Frequent was myalgia. Infrequent was muscle cramps. Rare was tetany.

Neurological: Frequent were phonophobia, photophobia. Infrequent were confusion, depression, difficulty concentrating, disturbance of smell, dysarthria, euphoria, facial pain, heat sensitivity, incoordination, lacrimation, monoplegia, sleep disturbance, shivering, syncope, tremor. Rare were aggressiveness, apathy, bradylogia, cluster headache, convulsions, decreased appetite, drug abuse, dystonic reaction, facial paralysis, hallucinations, hunger, hyperesthesia, hysteria, increased alertness, memory disturbance, neuralgia, paralysis, personality change, phobia, radiculopathy, rigidity, suicide, twitching.

Respiratory: Frequent was dyspnea. Infrequent was asthma. Rare was hiccoughs.

Skin: Frequent was sweating. Infrequent were erythema, pruritus, rash, skin tenderness. Rare were dry/scaly skin, tightness of skin, wrinkling of skin.

Breasts: Infrequent was tenderness. Rare was nipple discharge.

Urogenital: Infrequent were dysmenorrhea, increased urination, intermenstrual bleeding. Rare were abortion, hematuria.

Miscellaneous: Frequent was hypersensitivity. Infrequent were cough, fever, fluid retention, overdose. Rare were edema, hematoma, lymphadenopathy, speech disturbance, voice disturbances.

Postmarketing Experience: The following are spontaneously reported adverse events from postmarketing experience except those events already listed previously in the ADVERSE REACTIONS section or those too general to be informative. Because the reports cite events reported spontaneously from worldwide postmarketing experience, frequency of events and the role of Imitrex Tablets in their causation cannot be reliably determined.

Episodes of acute renal failure, angioneurotic edema, cardiomyopathy, cerebrovascular accident, cyanosis, deafness, death, disturbances of liver function tests, exacerbation of sunburn, hepatic impairment, intraocular disorders, ischemic optic neuropathy, pancytopenia, panic disorder, peri-orbital edema, photosensitivity, pulmonary embolism, retinal artery occlusion, shock, subarachnoid hemorrhage, temporal arteritis, thrombocytopenia, and xerostomia. The following hypersensitivity reactions have been reported: rash, urticaria, pruritus, erythema, and shortness of breath. In addition, severe anaphylaxis/anaphylactoid reactions have been reported (see WARNINGS).

DRUG ABUSE AND DEPENDENCE

The abuse potential of Imitrex® (sumatriptan succinate) Tablets cannot be fully delineated in advance of extensive marketing experience. One clinical study with Imitrex® (sumatriptan succinate) Injection enrolling 12 patients with a history of substance abuse failed to induce subjective behavior and/or physiologic response ordinarily associated with drugs that have an established potential for abuse.

OVERDOSAGE

Patients (n=670) have received single oral doses of 140 to 300 mg without significant adverse effects. Volunteers (n=174) have received single oral doses of 140 to 400 mg without serious adverse events.

No gross overdoses in clinical practice have been reported. Coronary vasospasm was observed after intravenous administration of sumatriptan (see CONTRAINDICATIONS). Overdoses would be expected from animal data to possibly cause tremor, lethargy, erythema of the extremities, abnormal respiration, cyanosis, ataxia, mydriasis, and paralysis. The elimination half-life of sumatriptan is about 2.5 hours (see CLINICAL PHARMACOLOGY), and therefore monitoring of patients after overdose with Imitrex® (sumatriptan succinate) Tablets should continue for at least 10 hours or while symptoms or signs persist.

It is unknown what effect hemodialysis or peritoneal dialysis has on the serum concentrations of sumatriptan.

DOSAGE AND ADMINISTRATION

The recommended adult dose of Imitrex® (sumatriptan succinate) Tablets is a single 25-mg tablet taken with fluids; the maximum single dose recommended is 100 mg. There is no evidence that an initial dose of 100 mg provides substantially greater relief than 25 mg.

If a satisfactory response has not been obtained at 2 hours, a second dose of up to 100 mg may be given. Controlled trials have not examined the effectiveness of a second dose if an initial dose of 25 mg is ineffective. If headache returns, additional doses may be taken at intervals of at least 2 hours up to a daily maximum dose of 300 mg. If headache returns following an initial treatment with Imitrex® (sumatriptan succinate) Injection, additional doses of single Imitrex Tablets (up to 200 mg per day) may be given with an interval of at least 2 hours between tablet doses.

The maximum dose given in a 24-hour period to patients with migraine headaches has been 300 mg. This dose has been delivered either as a single 300-mg dose, or as three 100-mg single doses given at intervals no less than every 2 hours. While these doses have been generally well tolerated, there is no evidence that these higher doses afford greater relief than the recommended dose.

Imitrex Tablets are equally effective at whatever stage of the attack they are administered, though it is advisable that Imitrex Tablets be given as early as possible after the onset of an attack of migraine.

Because of the potential of MAO inhibitors to cause unpredictable elevations in the bioavailability of oral sumatriptan, their combined use is contraindicated (see CONTRAINDICATIONS).

Hepatic disease/functional impairment may also cause unpredictable elevations in the bioavailability of orally administered sumatriptan. Consequently, if treatment is deemed advisable in the presence of liver disease, the maximum single dose should in general not exceed 50 mg (see CLINICAL PHARMACOLOGY for the basis of this recommendation).

HOW SUPPLIED

Imitrex® (sumatriptan succinate) Tablets, 25 and 50 mg of sumatriptan (base) as the succinate. Imitrex Tablets, 25 mg are white, round, film-coated tablets embossed with "I" on one side and "25" on the other in blister packs of 9 tablets (NDC 0173-0460-02). Imitrex Tablets, 50 mg are white, capsule-shaped, film-coated tablets embossed with "Imitrex" on one side and "50" on the other in blister packs of 9 tablets (NDC 0173-0459-00).

Store between 2° and 30°C (36° and 86°F).

PATIENT INFORMATION: The following wording is contained in a separate leaflet provided for patients.

Information for the Consumer
Imitrex® (sumatriptan succinate) Tablets

Please read this leaflet carefully before you take Imitrex Tablets. This provides a summary of the information available on your medicine. Please do not throw away this leaflet until you have finished your medicine. You may need to read this leaflet again. This leaflet does not contain all the information on Imitrex Tablets. For further information or advice, ask you doctor or pharmacist.

Information About Your Medicine:
The name of your medicine is Imitrex® (sumatriptan succinate) Tablets. It can be obtained only by prescription from your doctor. The decision to use Imitrex Tablets is one that you and your doctor should make jointly, taking into account your individual preferences and medical circumstances. If you have risk factors for heart disease (such as high blood pressure, high cholesterol, obesity, diabetes, smoking, strong family history of heart disease, or you are postmenopausal or a male over 40), you should tell your doctor, who should evaluate you for heart disease in order to determine if Imitrex® (sumatriptan succinate) is appropriate for you. Although the vast majority of those who have taken Imitrex have not experienced any significant side effects, some individuals have experienced problems and, rarely, considering the extensiveness of Imitrex use worldwide, deaths have been reported. In all but a few instances, however, Imitrex does not appear to have been a contributory factor in these deaths.

1. The Purpose of Your Medicine:
Imitrex Tablets are intended to relieve your migraine, but not to prevent or reduce the number of attacks you experience. Use Imitrex Tablets only to treat an actual migraine attack.

2. Important Questions to Consider Before Taking Imitrex Tablets:
If the answer to any of the following questions is **YES** or if you do not know the answer, then please discuss with your doctor before you use Imitrex Tablets.
- Are you pregnant? Do you think you might be pregnant? Are you trying to become pregnant? Are you using inadequate contraception? Are you breastfeeding?
- Do you have any chest pain, heart disease, shortness of breath, or irregular heartbeats? Have you had a heart attack?
- Do you have risk factors for heart disease (such as high blood pressure, high cholesterol, obesity, diabetes, smoking, strong family history of heart disease, or you are postmenopausal or a male over 40)?
- Do you have high blood pressure?
- Have you ever had to stop taking this or any other medication because of an allergy or other problems?
- Are you taking any other migraine medications, including migraine medications containing ergotamine or dihydroergotamine, or any medications containing monoamine oxidase inhibitors?
- Have you had, or do you have, any disease of the liver or kidney?
- Have you had, or do you have, epilepsy or seizures?
- Is this headache different from your usual migraine attacks?

Remember, if you answered **YES** to any of the above questions, then discuss it with your doctor.

3. The Use of Imitrex Tablets During Pregnancy:
Do not use Imitrex Tablets if you are pregnant, think you might be pregnant, are trying to become pregnant, or are not using adequate contraception, unless you have discussed this with your doctor.

4. How to Use Imitrex Tablets:
For adults, the usual dose is a single tablet taken whole with fluids. It should be given as soon as the symptoms of your migraine appear, but it may be given at any time during an attack. A second tablet may be taken if your symptoms of migraine come back, but not sooner than 2 hours following the first tablet. For a given attack, if you have no response to the first tablet, do not take a second tablet without first consulting with your doctor. Do not take more than a total of 300 mg of Imitrex Tablets in any 24-hour period.

5. Side Effects to Watch for:
- Some patients experience pain or tightness in the chest or throat when using Imitrex Tablets. If this happens to you, then discuss it with your doctor before using any more Imitrex Tablets. If the chest pain is severe or does not go away, call your doctor immediately.
- Shortness of breath; wheeziness; heart throbbing; swelling of eyelids, face, or lips; or a skin rash, skin lumps, or hives happens rarely. If it happens to you, then tell your doctor immediately. Do not take any more Imitrex Tablets unless your doctor tells you to do so.
- Some people may have feelings of tingling, heat, flushing (redness of face lasting a short time), heaviness or pressure after treatment with Imitrex Tablets. A few people may feel drowsy, dizzy, tired, or sick. Tell your doctor these symptoms at your next visit.
- If you feel unwell in any other way or have any symptoms that you do not understand, you should contact your doctor immediately.

6. What to Do if an Overdose is Taken:
If you have taken more medication than you have been told, contact either your doctor, hospital emergency department, or nearest poison control center immediately.

7. Storing Your Medicine:
Keep your medicine in a safe place where children cannot reach it. It may be harmful to children.
Store your medication away from heat and light. Do not store at temperatures above 86°F (30°C).

If your medication has expired (the expiration date is printed on the treatment pack), throw it away as instructed.
If your doctor decides to stop your treatment, do not keep any leftover medicine unless your doctor tells you to. Throw away your medicine as instructed.
June 1995/RL-197
Shown in Product Identification Guide, page 313

IMURAN® ℞
[*ĭm 'ū-ran"*]
(azathioprine)
50 mg Scored Tablets
100 mg (as the sodium salt) for I.V. injection, equivalent to 100 mg azathioprine sterile lyophilized material.

WARNING
Chronic immunosuppression with this purine antimetabolite increases *risk of neoplasia* in humans. Physicians using this drug should be very familiar with this risk as well as with the mutagenic potential to both men and women and with possible hematologic toxicities. See WARNINGS.

DESCRIPTION
IMURAN (azathioprine), an immunosuppressive antimetabolite, is available in tablet form for oral administration and 100 mg vials for intravenous injection. Each scored tablet contains 50 mg azathioprine and the inactive ingredients lactose, magnesium stearate, potato starch, povidone, and stearic acid. Each 100 mg vial contains azathioprine, as the sodium salt, equivalent to 100 mg azathioprine sterile lyophilized material and sodium hydroxide to adjust pH.
Azathioprine is chemically 6-[(1-methyl-4-nitro-1*H*-imidazol-5-yl)thio]-1*H*-purine. It is an imidazolyl derivative of 6-mercaptopurine (PURINETHOL®) and many of its biological effects are similar to those of the parent compound.
Azathioprine is insoluble in water, but may be dissolved with addition of one molar equivalent of alkali. The sodium salt of azathioprine is sufficiently soluble to make a 10 mg/mL water solution which is stable for 24 hours at 59° to 77°F (15° to 25°C). Azathioprine is stable in solution at neutral or acid pH but hydrolysis to mercaptopurine occurs in excess sodium hydroxide (0.1N), especially on warming. Conversion to mercaptopurine also occurs in the presence of sulfhydryl compounds such as cysteine, glutathione, and hydrogen sulfide.

CLINICAL PHARMACOLOGY
Metabolism[1]: Azathioprine is well absorbed following oral administration. Maximum serum radioactivity occurs at 1 to 2 hours after oral ^{35}S-azathioprine and decays with a half-life of 5 hours. This is not an estimate of the half-life of azathioprine itself but is the decay rate for all ^{35}S-containing metabolites of the drug. Because of extensive metabolism, only a fraction of the radioactivity is present as azathioprine. Usual doses produce blood levels of azathioprine, and of mercaptopurine derived from it, which are low (<1 μg/mL). Blood levels are of little predictive value for therapy since the magnitude and duration of clinical effects correlate with thiopurine nucleotide levels in tissues rather than with plasma drug levels. Azathioprine and mercaptopurine are moderately bound to serum proteins (30%) and are partially dialyzable.
Azathioprine is cleaved in vivo to mercaptopurine. Both compounds are rapidly eliminated from blood and are oxidized or methylated in erythrocytes and liver; no azathioprine or mercaptopurine is detectable in urine after 8 hours. Conversion to inactive 6-thiouric acid by xanthine oxidase is an important degradative pathway, and the inhibition of this pathway in patients receiving allopurinol (ZYLOPRIM®) is the basis for the azathioprine dosage reduction required in these patients (see PRECAUTIONS: Drug Interactions). Proportions of metabolites are different in individual patients, and this presumably accounts for variable magnitude and duration of drug effects. Renal clearance is probably not important in predicting biological effectiveness or toxicities, although dose reduction is practiced in patients with poor renal function.
Homograft Survival[1,2]: Summary information from transplant centers and registries indicates relatively universal use of IMURAN with or without other immunosuppressive agents.[3,4,5] Although the use of azathioprine for inhibition of renal homograft rejection is well established, the mechanism(s) for this action are somewhat obscure. The drug suppresses hypersensitivities of the cell-mediated type and causes variable alterations in antibody production. Suppression of T-cell effects, including ablation of T-cell suppression, is dependent on the temporal relationship to antigenic stimulus or engraftment. This agent has little effect on established graft rejections or secondary responses.
Alterations in specific immune responses or immunologic functions in transplant recipients are difficult to relate specifically to immunosuppression by azathioprine. These patients have subnormal responses to vaccines, low numbers of T-cells, and abnormal phagocytosis by peripheral blood cells, but their mitogenic responses, serum immunoglobulins, and secondary antibody responses are usually normal.
Immunoinflammatory Response: Azathioprine suppresses disease manifestations as well as underlying pathology in animal models of autoimmune disease. For example, the severity of adjuvant arthritis is reduced by azathioprine.
The mechanisms whereby azathioprine affects autoimmune diseases are not known. Azathioprine is immunosuppressive, delayed hypersensitivity and cellular cytotoxicity tests being suppressed to a greater degree than are antibody responses. In the rat model of adjuvant arthritis, azathioprine has been shown to inhibit the lymph node hyperplasia which precedes the onset of the signs of the disease. Both the immunosuppressive and therapeutic effects in animal models are dose-related. Azathioprine is considered a slow-acting drug and effects may persist after the drug has been discontinued.

INDICATIONS AND USAGE
IMURAN is indicated as an adjunct for the prevention of rejection in renal homotransplantation. It is also indicated for the management of severe, active rheumatoid arthritis unresponsive to rest, aspirin, or other nonsteroidal anti-inflammatory drugs, or to agents in the class of which gold is an example.
Renal Homotransplantation: IMURAN is indicated as an adjunct for the prevention of rejection in renal homotransplantation. Experience with over 16,000 transplants shows a 5-year patient survival of 35% to 55%, but this is dependent on donor, match for HLA antigens, anti-donor or anti B-cell alloantigen antibody, and other variables. The effect of IMURAN on these variables has not been tested in controlled trials.
Rheumatoid Arthritis[6,7]: IMURAN is indicated only in adult patients meeting criteria for classic or definite rheumatoid arthritis as specified by the American Rheumatism Association.[8] IMURAN should be restricted to patients with severe, active and erosive disease not responsive to conventional management including rest, aspirin, or other nonsteroidal drugs or to agents in the class of which gold is an example. Rest, physiotherapy, and salicylates should be continued while IMURAN is given, but it may be possible to reduce the dose of corticosteroids in patients on IMURAN. The combined use of IMURAN with gold, antimalarials, or penicillamine has not been studied for either added benefit or unexpected adverse effects. The use of IMURAN with these agents cannot be recommended.

CONTRAINDICATIONS
IMURAN should not be given to patients who have shown hypersensitivity to the drug.
IMURAN should not be used for treating rheumatoid arthritis in pregnant women.
Patients with rheumatoid arthritis previously treated with alkylating agents (cyclophosphamide, chlorambucil, melphalan, or others) may have a prohibitive risk of neoplasia if treated with IMURAN.[9]

WARNINGS
Severe *leukopenia and/or thrombocytopenia* may occur in patients on IMURAN. Macrocytic anemia and severe bone marrow depression may also occur. Hematologic toxicities are dose related and may be more severe in renal transplant patients whose homograft is undergoing rejection. It is suggested that patients on IMURAN have complete blood counts, including platelet counts, weekly during the first month, twice monthly for the second and third months of treatment, then monthly or more frequently if dosage alterations or other therapy changes are necessary. Delayed hematologic suppression may occur. Prompt reduction in dosage or temporary withdrawal of the drug may be necessary if there is a rapid fall in, or persistently low leukocyte count or other evidence of bone marrow depression. Leukopenia does not correlate with therapeutic effect; therefore the dose should not be increased intentionally to lower the white blood cell count.
Serious infections are a constant hazard for patients receiving chronic immunosuppression, especially for homograft recipients. Fungal, viral, bacterial and protozoal infections may be fatal and should be treated vigorously. Reduction of azathioprine dosage and/or use of other drugs should be considered.
IMURAN is mutagenic in animals and humans, carcinogenic in animals, and may increase the patient's *risk of neoplasia.* Renal transplant patients are known to have an increased risk of malignancy, predominantly skin cancer and reticulum cell or lymphomatous tumors.[10] The risk of post-transplant lymphomas may be increased in patients who receive aggressive treatment with immunosuppressive drugs.[11] The degree of immunosuppression is determined not only by the immunosuppressive regimen but also by a number of other patient factors. The number of immunosuppressive agents may not necessarily increase the risk of post-transplant lymphomas. However, transplant patients who receive multiple immunosuppressive agents may be at risk for over-immunosuppression; therefore, immunosuppressive drug therapy should be maintained at the lowest effective levels. Information is available on the spontaneous neoplasia risk in rheumatoid arthritis,[12,13] and on neoplasia following immunosuppressive therapy of other autoimmune diseases.[14,15] It has not been possible to define the precise risk of neoplasia due to IMURAN.[16] The data suggest the risk may be elevated in patients with rheumatoid arthritis, though lower than for renal transplant patients.[11,13] However, acute myelogenous leukemia as well as solid tumors have been reported in patients with rheumatoid arthritis who have received azathioprine. Data on neoplasia in patients receiving IMURAN can be found under ADVERSE REACTIONS.
IMURAN has been reported to cause temporary depression in spermatogenesis and reduction in sperm viability and sperm count in mice at doses 10 times the human therapeutic dose[17]; a reduced percentage of fertile matings occurred when animals received 5 mg/kg.[18]
Pregnancy: Pregnancy Category D. IMURAN can cause fetal harm when administered to a pregnant woman. IMURAN should not be given during pregnancy without careful weighing of risk versus benefit. Whenever possible, use of IMURAN in pregnant patients should be avoided. This drug should not be used for treating rheumatoid arthritis in pregnant women.[19]
IMURAN is teratogenic in rabbits and mice when given in doses equivalent to the human dose (5 mg/kg daily). Abnormalities included skeletal malformations and visceral anomalies.[18]
Limited immunologic and other abnormalities have occurred in a few infants born of renal allograft recipients on IMURAN. In a detailed case report,[20] documented lymphopenia, diminished IgG and IgM levels, CMV infection, and a decreased thymic shadow were noted in an infant born to a mother receiving 150 mg azathioprine and 30 mg prednisone daily throughout pregnancy. At 10 weeks most features were normalized. DeWitte et al[21] reported pancytopenia and severe immune deficiency in a preterm infant whose mother received 125 mg azathioprine and 12.5 mg prednisone daily. There have been two published reports of abnormal physical findings. Williamson and Karp[22] described an infant born with preaxial polydactyly whose mother received azathioprine 200 mg daily and prednisone 20 mg every other day during pregnancy. Tallent et al[23] described an infant with a large myelomeningocele in the upper lumbar region, bilateral dislocated hips, and bilateral talipes equinovarus. The father was on long-term azathioprine therapy.
Benefit versus risk must be weighed carefully before use of IMURAN in patients of reproductive potential. There are no adequate and well-controlled studies in pregnant women. If this drug is used during pregnancy or if the patient becomes pregnant while taking this drug, the patient should be apprised of the potential hazard to the fetus. Women of childbearing age should be advised to avoid becoming pregnant.

PRECAUTIONS
General: A gastrointestinal hypersensitivity reaction characterized by severe nausea and vomiting has been reported.[24,25,26] These symptoms may also be accompanied by diarrhea, rash, fever, malaise, myalgias, elevations in liver enzymes, and occasionally, hypotension. Symptoms of gastrointestinal toxicity most often develop within the first several weeks of IMURAN therapy and are reversible upon discontinuation of the drug. The reaction can recur within hours after rechallenge with a single dose of IMURAN.
Information for Patients:
Patients being started on IMURAN should be informed of the necessity of periodic blood counts while they are receiving the drug and should be encouraged to report any unusual bleeding or bruising to their physician. They should be informed of the danger of infection while receiving IMURAN and encouraged to report signs and symptoms of infection to their physician. Careful dosage instructions should be given to the patient, especially when IMURAN is being administered in the presence of impaired renal function or concomitantly with allopurinol (see Drug Interactions subsection and DOSAGE AND ADMINISTRATION). Patients should be advised of the potential risks of the use of IMURAN during pregnancy and during the nursing period. The increased risk of neoplasia following IMURAN therapy should be explained to the patient.
Laboratory Tests: See WARNINGS and ADVERSE REACTIONS sections.
Drug Interactions:
Use with Allopurinol: The principal pathway for detoxification of IMURAN is inhibited by allopurinol. Patients receiving IMURAN and allopurinol concomitantly should have a dose reduction of IMURAN, to approximately ⅓ to ¼ the usual dose.
Use with Other Agents Affecting Myelopoesis: Drugs which may affect leukocyte production, including co-trimoxazole, may lead to exaggerated leukopenia, especially in renal transplant recipients.[27]

Continued on next page

Glaxo Wellcome—Cont.

Use with Angiotensin Converting Enzyme Inhibitors: The use of angiotensin converting enzyme inhibitors to control hypertension in patients on azathioprine has been reported to induce anemia and severe leukopenia.

Use with Warfarin: IMURAN may inhibit the anticoagulant effect of warfarin.

Carcinogenesis, Mutagenesis, Impairment of Fertility: See WARNINGS section.

Pregnancy: *Teratogenic Effects:* Pregnancy Category D. See WARNINGS section.

Nursing Mothers: The use of IMURAN in nursing mothers is not recommended. Azathioprine or its metabolites are transferred at low levels, both transplacentally and in breast milk.[29,30,31] Because of the potential for tumorigenicity shown for azathioprine, a decision should be made whether to discontinue nursing or discontinue the drug, taking into account the importance of the drug to the mother.

Pediatric Use: Safety and efficacy of azathioprine in pediatric patients have not been established.

ADVERSE REACTIONS

The principal and potentially serious toxic effects of IMURAN are hematologic and gastrointestinal. The risks of secondary infection and neoplasia are also significant (see WARNINGS). The frequency and severity of adverse reactions depend on the dose and duration of IMURAN as well as on the patient's underlying disease or concomitant therapies. The incidence of hematologic toxicities and neoplasia encountered in groups of renal homograft recipients is significantly higher than that in studies employing IMURAN for rheumatoid arthritis. The relative incidences in clinical studies are summarized below:

Toxicity	Renal Homograft	Rheumatoid Arthritis
Leukopenia		
Any Degree	>50%	28%
<2500/mm^3	16%	5.3%
Infections	20%	<1%
Neoplasia		*
Lymphoma	0.5%	
Others	2.8%	

*Data on the rate and risk of neoplasia among persons with rheumatoid arthritis treated with azathioprine are limited. The incidence of lymphoproliferative disease in patients with RA appears to be significantly higher than that in the general population.[12] In one completed study, the rate of lymphoproliferative disease in RA patients receiving higher than recommended doses of azathioprine (5 mg/kg/day) was 1.8 cases per 1000 patient years of follow-up, compared with 0.8 cases per 1000 patient years of follow-up in those not receiving azathioprine.[13] However, the proportion of the increased risk attributable to the azathioprine dosage or to other therapies (i.e., alkylating agents) received by patients treated with azathioprine cannot be determined.

Hematologic: Leukopenia and/or thrombocytopenia are dose dependent and may occur late in the course of therapy with IMURAN. Dose reduction or temporary withdrawal allows reversal of these toxicities. Infection may occur as a secondary manifestation of bone marrow suppression or leukopenia, but the incidence of infection in renal homotransplantation is 30 to 60 times that in rheumatoid arthritis. Macrocytic anemia and/or bleeding have been reported. There are rare individuals with an inherited deficiency of the enzyme thiopurine methyltransferase (TPMT) who may be unusually sensitive to the myelosuppressive effect of azathioprine and prone to developing rapid bone marrow suppression following the initiation of treatment with IMURAN.

Gastrointestinal: Nausea and vomiting may occur within the first few months of therapy with IMURAN, and occurred in approximately 12% of 676 rheumatoid arthritis patients. The frequency of gastric disturbance often can be reduced by administration of the drug in divided doses and/or after meals. However, in some patients, nausea and vomiting may be severe and may be accompanied by symptoms such as diarrhea, fever, malaise, and myalgias (see PRECAUTIONS). Vomiting with abdominal pain may occur rarely with a hypersensitivity pancreatitis. Hepatotoxicity manifest by elevation of serum alkaline phosphatase, bilirubin, and/or serum transaminases is known to occur following azathioprine use, primarily in allograft recipients. Hepatotoxicity has been uncommon (less than 1%) in rheumatoid arthritis patients. Hepatotoxicity following transplantation most often occurs within 6 months of transplantation and is generally reversible after interruption of IMURAN. A rare, but life-threatening hepatic veno-occlusive disease associated with chronic administration of azathioprine has been

described in transplant patients and in one patient receiving IMURAN for panuveitis.[32,33,34] Periodic measurement of serum transaminases, alkaline phosphatase, and bilirubin is indicated for early detection of hepatotoxicity. If hepatic veno-occlusive disease is clinically suspected, IMURAN should be permanently withdrawn.

Others: Additional side effects of low frequency have been reported. These include skin rashes, alopecia, fever, arthralgias, diarrhea, steatorrhea, negative nitrogen balance, and reversible interstitial pneumonitis.

OVERDOSAGE

The oral LD$_{50}$s for single doses of IMURAN in mice and rats are 2500 mg/kg and 400 mg/kg, respectively. Very large doses of this antimetabolite may lead to marrow hypoplasia, bleeding, infection, and death. About 30% of IMURAN is bound to serum proteins, but approximately 45% is removed during an 8-hour hemodialysis.[35] A single case has been reported of a renal transplant patient who ingested a single dose of 7500 mg IMURAN. The immediate toxic reactions were nausea, vomiting, and diarrhea, followed by mild leukopenia and mild abnormalities in liver function. The white blood cell count, SGOT, and bilirubin returned to normal 6 days after the overdose.

DOSAGE AND ADMINISTRATION

Renal Homotransplantation: The dose of IMURAN required to prevent rejection and minimize toxicity will vary with individual patients; this necessitates careful management. The initial dose is usually 3 to 5 mg/kg daily, beginning at the time of transplant. IMURAN is usually given as a single daily dose on the day of, and in a minority of cases 1 to 3 days before, transplantation. IMURAN is often initiated with the intravenous administration of the sodium salt, with subsequent use of tablets (at the same dose level) after the postoperative period. Intravenous administration of the sodium salt is indicated only in patients unable to tolerate oral medications. Dose reduction to maintenance levels of 1 to 3 mg/kg daily is usually possible. The dose of IMURAN should not be increased to toxic levels because of threatened rejection. Discontinuation may be necessary for severe hematologic or other toxicity, even if rejection of the homograft may be a consequence of drug withdrawal.

Rheumatoid Arthritis: IMURAN is usually given on a daily basis. The initial dose should be approximately 1.0 mg/kg (50 to 100 mg) given as a single dose or on a twice daily schedule. The dose may be increased, beginning at 6 to 8 weeks and thereafter by steps at 4-week intervals, if there are no serious toxicities and if initial response is unsatisfactory. Dose increments should be 0.5 mg/kg daily, up to a maximum dose of 2.5 mg/kg/day. Therapeutic response occurs after several weeks of treatment, usually 6 to 8; an adequate trial should be a minimum of 12 weeks. Patients not improved after 12 weeks can be considered refractory. IMURAN may be continued long-term in patients with clinical response, but patients should be monitored carefully, and gradual dosage reduction should be attempted to reduce risk of toxicities. Maintenance therapy should be at the lowest effective dose, and the dose given can be lowered decrementally with changes of 0.5 mg/kg or approximately 25 mg daily every 4 weeks while other therapy is kept constant. The optimum duration of maintenance IMURAN has not been determined. IMURAN can be discontinued abruptly, but delayed effects are possible.

Use in Renal Dysfunction: Relatively oliguric patients, especially those with tubular necrosis in the immediate postcadaveric transplant period, may have delayed clearance of IMURAN or its metabolites, may be particularly sensitive to this drug, and are usually given lower doses.

Parenteral Administration: Add 10 mL of Sterile Water for Injection, and swirl until a clear solution results. This solution, equivalent to 100 mg azathioprine, is for intravenous use only; it has a pH of approximately 9.6, and it should be used within 24 hours. Further dilution into sterile saline or dextrose is usually made for infusion; the final volume depends on time for the infusion, usually 30 to 60 minutes, but as short as 5 minutes and as long as 8 hours for the daily dose.

Parenteral drug products should be inspected visually for particulate matter and discoloration prior to administration, whenever solution and container permit.

Procedures for proper handling and disposal of this immunosuppressive antimetabolite drug should be considered. Several guidelines on this subject have been published.[36-42] There is no general agreement that all of the procedures recommended in the guidelines are necessary or appropriate.

HOW SUPPLIED

50 mg overlapping circle-shaped, yellow to off-white, scored tablets imprinted with "IMURAN" and "50" on each tablet; bottle of 100 (NDC 0173-0597-55).

Store at 15° to 25°C (59° to 77°F) in a dry place and protect from light.

20 mL vial, each containing the equivalent of 100 mg azathioprine (as the sodium salt), (NDC 0173-0598-71).

Store at 15° to 25°C (59° to 77°F) and protect from light. The sterile, lyophilized sodium salt is yellow, and should be dissolved in Sterile Water for Injection (see DOSAGE AND ADMINISTRATION: Parenteral Administration).

REFERENCES

1. Elion GB, Hitchings GH. Azathioprine. In: Sartorelli AC, Johns DG, eds. *Antineoplastic and Immunosuppressive Agents Pt II.* New York, NY: Springer Verlag; 1975: chap 48.
2. McIntosh J, Hansen P, Ziegler J, et al. Defective immune and phagocytic functions in uraemia and renal transplantation. *Int Arch Allergy Appl Immunol.* 1976;15:544–549.
3. Renal Transplant Registry Advisory Committee. The 12th report of the Human Renal Transplant Registry. *JAMA.* 1975;233:787–796.
4. McGeown M. Immunosuppression for kidney transplantation. *Lancet.* 1973;2:310–312.
5. Simmons RL, Thompson EJ, Yunis EJ, et al. 115 patients with first cadaver kidney transplants followed two to seven and a half years: a multifactorial analysis. *Am J Med.* 1977;62:234–242.
6. Fye K, Talal N. Cytotoxic drugs in the treatment of rheumatoid arthritis. *Ration Drug Ther.* 1975;9:1–5.
7. Davis JD, Muss HB, Turner RA. Cytotoxic agents in the treatment of rheumatoid arthritis. *South Med J.* 1978;71:58–64.
8. McEwen C. The diagnosis and differential diagnosis of rheumatoid arthritis. In: Hollander JL, ed. *Arthritis and Allied Conditions: A Textbook of Rheumatology.* 8th ed. Philadelphia, PA: Lea and Febiger; 1972:403–418.
9. Hoover R, Fraumeni, JF. Drug-induced cancer. *Cancer.* 1981;47:1071–1080.
10. Hoover R, Fraumeni JF Jr. Risk of cancer in renal transplant recipients. *Lancet.* 1973;2:55–57.
11. Wilkinson AH, Smith JL, Hunsicker LG, et al. Increased frequency of post-transplant lymphomas in patients treated with cyclosporine, azathioprine, and prednisone. *Transplantation.* 1989;47:293–296.
12. Prior P, Symmons DPM, Hawkins CF, et al. Cancer morbidity in rheumatoid arthritis. *Ann Rheum Dis* 1984; 43:128–131.
13. Silman, AJ, Petrie J, Hazelman B, et al. Lymphoproliferative cancer and other malignancy in patients with rheumatoid arthritis treated with azathioprine: a 20 year follow up study. *Ann Rheum Dis.* 1988; 47:988–992.
14. Louie S, Schwartz RS. Immunodeficiency and pathogenesis of lymphoma and leukemia. *Semin Hematol.* 1978;15:117-138.
15. Wang KK, Czaja AJ, Beaver SJ, et al. Extra hepatic malignancy following long-term immunosuppressive therapy of severe hepatitis B surface antigen-negative chronic active hepatitis. *Hepatology.* 1989; 10:39–43.
16. Sieber SM, Adamson RH. Toxicity of antineoplastic agents in man: chromosomal aberrations, antifertility effects, congenital malformations, and carcinogenic potential. In: Klein G, Weinhouse S, eds. *Advances in Cancer Research.* New York, NY: Academic Press; 1975;22:57-155.
17. Clark JM. The mutagenicity of azathioprine in mice, *Drosophila Melanogaster* and *Neurospora Crassa. Mut Res.* 1975; 28:87–99.
18. Data on file, Glaxo Wellcome Inc.
19. Tagatz GE, Simmons RL. Pregnancy after renal transplantation. *Ann Intern Med.* 1975:82:113-114. Editorial Notes.
20. Coté CJ, Meuwissen HJ, Pickering RJ. Effects on the neonate of prednisone and azathioprine administered to the mother during pregnancy. *J Pediatr.* 1974; 85:324–328.
21. DeWitte DB, Buick MK, Stephen EC, et al. Neonatal pancytopenia and severe combined immunodeficiency associated with antenatal administration of azathioprine and prednisone. *J Pediatr.* 1984;105:625–628.
22. Williamson RA, Karp LE. Azathioprine teratogenicity: review of the literature and case report. *Obstet Gynecol.* 1981;58:247–250.
23. Tallent MB, Simmons RL, Najarian JS. Birth defects in child of male recipient of kidney transplant. *JAMA.* 1970;211:1854–1855.
24. Assini JF, Hamilton R, Strosberg JM. Adverse reactions to azathioprine mimicking gastroenteritis. *J Rheumatol.* 1986;13:1117–1118.
25. Cochrane D, Adamson AR, Halsey JP. Adverse reactions to azathioprine mimicking gastroenteritis. *J Rheumatol.* 1987;14:1075.
26. Cox J, Daneshmend JK, Hawkey CJ, et al. Devastating diarrhoea caused by azathioprine: management difficulty in inflammatory bowel disease. *Gut.* 1988;29:686–688.
27. Bradley PP, Warden GD, Maxwell JG, et al. Neutropenia and thrombocytopenia in renal allograft recipients treated with trimethoprim-sulfamethoxazole. *Ann Int Med.* 1980;93:560–562.

28. Kirchertz EJ, Grone HJ, Rieger J, et al. Successful low dose captopril rechallenge following drug-induced leucopenia. *Lancet.* 1981;1362–1363.
29. Nelson D, Bugge C. Data on file, Glaxo Wellcome Inc..
30. Saarikoski S, Seppälä M. Immunosuppression during pregnancy: transmission of azathioprine and its metabolites from the mother to the fetus. *Am J Obstet Gynecol.* 1973:115:1100-1106.
31. Coulam CB, Moyer TP, Jiang NS, et al. Breast-feeding after renal transplantation. *Transplant Proc.* 1982;14:605–609.
32. Read AE, Wiesner RH, LaBrecque DR, et al. Hepatic veno-occlusive disease associated with renal transplantation and azathioprine therapy. *Ann Intern Med.* 1986;104:651-655.
33. Katzka DA, Saul SH, Jorkasky D, et al. Azathioprine and hepatic venocclusive disease in renal transplant patients. *Gastroenterology.* 1986:90:446–454.
34. Weitz H. Gokel JM, Loeschke K, et al. Veno-occlusive disease of the liver in patients receiving immunosuppressive therapy. *Virchows Arch A.* 1982:395:245-256.
35. Schusziarra V, Ziekursch V, Schlamp R, et al. Pharmacokinetics of azathioprine under haemodialysis. *Int J Clin Pharmacol Biopharm.* 1976;14:298–302.
36. Recommendations for the safe handling of parenteral antineoplastic drugs. Washington, DC: Division of Safety, National Institutes of Health; 1983. US Dept of Health and Human Services, Public Health Service publication NIH 83-2621.
37. AMA Council on Scientific Affairs. Guidelines for handling parenteral antineoplastics. *JAMA.* 1985;253:1590-1591.
38. National Study Commission on Cytotoxic Exposure. Recommendations for handling cytotoxic agents. 1987. Available from Louis P. Jeffrey, Chairman, National Study Commission on Cytotoxic Exposure. Massachusetts College of Pharmacy and Allied Health Sciences, 179 Longwood Avenue, Boston, Massachusetts, 02115.
39. Clinical Oncological Society of Australia. Guidelines and recommendations for safe handling of antineoplastic agents. *Med J Australia.* 1983;1:426-428.
40. Jones RB, Frank R, Mass T. Safe handling of chemotherapeutic agents: a report from the Mount Sinai Medical Center. *CA-A Cancer J for Clin.* 1983;33:258-263.
41. American Society of Hospital Pharmacists. ASHP technical assistance bulletin on handling cytotoxic and hazardous drugs. *Am J Hosp Pharm.* 1990;47:1033–1049.
42. Yodaiken RE, Bennett D. OSHA work-practice guidelines for personnel dealing with cytotoxic (antineoplastic) drugs. *Am J Hosp Pharm.* 1986;43:1193–1204.

January 1996/RL-261

Shown in Product Identification Guide, page 313

KEMADRIN® ℞

[*kĕm 'ah-drĭn*]
(procyclidine hydrochloride)
5 mg Scored Tablets

DESCRIPTION

KEMADRIN (procyclidine hydrochloride) is a synthetic antispasmodic compound of relatively low toxicity. It has been shown to be useful for the symptomatic treatment of parkinsonism (paralysis agitans) and extrapyramidal dysfunction caused by tranquilizer therapy. Procyclidine hydrochloride was developed at The Wellcome Research Laboratories as the most promising of a series of antiparkinsonism compounds produced by chemical modification of antihistamines. Procyclidine hydrochloride is a white crystalline substance which is soluble in water and almost tasteless. It is known chemically as α-cyclohexyl-α-phenyl-1-pyrrolidinepropanol hydrochloride.

KEMADRIN is available in tablet form for oral administration. Each scored tablet contains 5 mg procyclidine hydrochloride and the inactive ingredients corn and potato starch, lactose, and magnesium stearate.

CLINICAL PHARMACOLOGY

Pharmacologic tests have shown that procyclidine hydrochloride has an atropine-like action and exerts an antispasmodic effect on smooth muscle. It is a potent mydriatic and inhibits salivation. It has no sympathetic ganglion-blocking activity in doses as high as 4 mg/kg, as measured by the lack of inhibition of the response of the nictitating membrane to preganglionic electrical stimulation.

The intravenous LD_{50} in mice was about 60 mg/kg. Subcutaneously, doses of 300 mg/kg were not toxic. In dogs the intraperitoneal administration of procyclidine hydrochloride in doses of 5 mg/kg caused maximal dilation of the pupil and inhibition of salivation, but had no toxic action. When the dose was increased to 20 mg/kg the same symptoms occurred, and in addition there were tremors and ataxia lasting 4 to 5 hours. In one animal, convulsions occurred which were controlled by pentobarbital. In all animals behavior returned to normal within 24 hours.

Chronic toxicity tests in rats showed that the compound caused only a very slight retardation in growth, and no change in the erythrocyte count or the histological appearance of the lungs, liver, spleen, and kidney when as much as 10 mg/kg body weight was given subcutaneously daily for 9 weeks.

INDICATIONS

KEMADRIN (procyclidine hydrochloride) is indicated in the treatment of parkinsonism including the postencephalitic, arteriosclerotic, and idiopathic types. Partial control of the parkinsonism symptoms is the usual therapeutic accomplishment. Procyclidine hydrochloride is usually more efficacious in the relief of rigidity than tremor; but tremor, fatigue, weakness, and sluggishness are frequently beneficially influenced. It can be substituted for all the previous medications in mild and moderate cases. For the control of more severe cases, other drugs may be added to procyclidine therapy as indications warrant.

Clinical reports indicate that procyclidine often successfully relieves the symptoms of extrapyramidal dysfunction (dystonia, dyskinesia, akathisia, and parkinsonism) which accompany the therapy of mental disorders with phenothiazine and rauwolfia compounds. In addition to minimizing the symptoms induced by tranquilizing drugs, the drug effectively controls sialorrhea resulting from neuroleptic medication. At the same time, freedom from the side effects induced by tranquilizer drugs, as provided by the administration of procyclidine, permits a more sustained treatment of the patient's mental disorder.

Clinical results in the treatment of parkinsonism indicate that most patients experience subjective improvement characterized by a feeling of well-being and increased alertness, together with diminished salivation and a marked improvement in muscular coordination as demonstrated by objective tests of manual dexterity and by increased ability to carry out ordinary self-care activities. While the drug exerts a mild atropine-like action and therefore causes mydriasis, this may be kept minimal by careful adjustment of the daily dosage.

CONTRAINDICATIONS

Procyclidine hydrochloride should not be used in angle-closure glaucoma although simple type glaucomas do not appear to be adversely affected.

WARNINGS

Use in Children:
Safety and efficacy have not been established in the pediatric age group; therefore, the use of procyclidine hydrochloride in this age group requires that the potential benefits be weighed against the possible hazards to the child.

Pregnancy Warning: The safe use of this drug in pregnancy has not been established; therefore, the use of procyclidine hydrochloride in pregnancy, lactation, or in women of childbearing age requires that the potential benefits be weighed against the possible hazards to the mother and child.

PRECAUTIONS

Conditions in which inhibition of the parasympathetic nervous system is undesirable, such as tachycardia and urinary retention (such as may occur with marked prostatic hypertrophy), require special care in the administration of the drug. Hypotensive patients who receive the drug should be observed closely. Occasionally, particularly in older patients, mental confusion and disorientation may occur with the development of agitation, hallucinations, and psychotic-like symptoms.

Patients with mental disorders occasionally experience a precipitation of a psychotic episode when the dosage of antiparkinsonism drugs is increased to treat the extrapyramidal side effects of phenothiazine and rauwolfia derivatives.

ADVERSE REACTIONS

Anticholinergic effects can be produced by therapeutic doses although these can frequently be minimized or eliminated by careful dosage. They include: dryness of the mouth, mydriasis, blurring of vision, giddiness, lightheadedness, and gastrointestinal disturbances such as nausea, vomiting, epigastric distress, and constipation. Occasionally an allergic reaction such as a skin rash may be encountered. Feelings of muscular weakness may occur. Acute suppurative parotitis as a complication of dry mouth has been reported.

DOSAGE AND ADMINISTRATION

For Parkinsonism: The dosage of the drug for the treatment of parkinsonism depends upon the age of the patient, the etiology of the disease, and individual responsiveness. Therefore, the dosage must remain flexible to permit adjustment to the individual tolerance and requirements of each patient. In general, younger and postencephalitic patients require and tolerate a somewhat higher dosage than older patients and those with arteriosclerosis.

For Patients Who Have Received No Other Therapy: The usual dose of procyclidine hydrochloride for initial treatment is 2.5 mg administered three times daily after meals. If well tolerated, this dose may be gradually increased to 5 mg three times a day and occasionally 5 mg given before retiring. In some cases smaller doses may be employed with good therapeutic results.

Occasionally a patient is encountered who cannot tolerate a bedtime dose of the drug. In such cases it may be desirable to adjust dosage so that the bedtime dose is omitted and the total daily requirement is administered in three equal daytime doses. It is best administered during or after meals to minimize the development of side reactions.

To Transfer Patients to KEMADRIN from Other Therapy: Patients who have been receiving other drugs may be transferred to procyclidine hydrochloride. This is accomplished gradually by substituting 2.5 mg three times a day for all or part of the original drug. The dose of procyclidine is then increased as required while that of the other drug is correspondingly omitted or decreased until complete replacement is achieved. The total daily dosage may then be adjusted to the level which produces maximum benefit.

For Drug-Induced Extrapyramidal Symptoms: For treatment of symptoms of extrapyramidal dysfunction induced by tranquilizer drugs during the therapy of mental disorders, the dosage of procyclidine hydrochloride will depend on the severity of side effects associated with tranquilizer administration. In general the larger the dosage of the tranquilizer the more severe will be the associated symptoms, including rigidity and tremors. Accordingly, the drug dosage should be adjusted to suit the needs of the individual patient and to provide maximum relief of the induced symptoms. A convenient method to establish the daily dosage of procyclidine is to begin with the administration of 2.5 mg three times daily. This may be increased by 2.5 mg daily increments until the patient obtains relief of symptoms. In most cases excellent results will be obtained with 10 to 20 mg daily.

HOW SUPPLIED

White, scored tablets containing 5 mg procyclidine hydrochloride, imprinted with "KEMADRIN" and "S3A" in bottles of 100 (NDC 0081-0604-55).
Store at 15° to 25°C (59° to 77°F) in a dry place.
April 1994

Shown in Product Identification Guide, page 313

LAMICTAL® ℞

[*la-mik 'tal*]
(lamotrigine)
Tablets

DESCRIPTION

LAMICTAL (lamotrigine), an antiepileptic drug of the phenyltriazine class, is chemically unrelated to existing antiepileptic drugs. Its chemical name is 6-(2,3-dichlorophenyl)-1,2,4-triazine-3,5-diamine, its molecular formula is $C_9H_7Cl_2N_5$ and its molecular weight is 256.09. Lamotrigine is a white to pale cream-colored powder and has a Pka of 5.7. Lamotrigine is very slightly soluble in water (0.17 mg/mL at 25°C) and slightly soluble in 0.1 M HCl (4.1 mg/mL at 25°C).

LAMICTAL is supplied for oral administration as 25 mg (white), 100 mg (peach), 150 mg (cream), and 200 mg (blue) tablets. Each tablet contains the labeled amount of lamotrigine and the following inactive ingredients: lactose; magnesium stearate; microcrystalline cellulose; povidone; sodium starch glycolate; FD&C Yellow No. 6 Lake (100 mg tablet only); ferric oxide, yellow (150 mg tablet only); FD&C Blue No. 2 Lake (200 mg tablet only).

CLINICAL PHARMACOLOGY

Mechanism of Action: The precise mechanism(s) by which lamotrigine exerts its anticonvulsant action are unknown. In animal models designed to detect anticonvulsant activity, lamotrigine was effective in preventing seizure spread in the maximum electroshock (MES) and pentylenetetrazol (scMet) tests, and prevented seizures in the visually and electrically evoked after-discharge (EEAD) tests for antiepileptic activity. The relevance of these models to human epilepsy, however, is not known.

One proposed mechanism of action of LAMICTAL, the relevance of which remains to be established in humans, involves an effect on sodium channels. In vitro pharmacological studies suggest that lamotrigine inhibits voltage-sensitive sodium channels thereby stabilizing neuronal membranes and consequently modulating presynaptic transmitter release of excitatory amino acids (e.g., glutamate and aspartate).

Pharmacological Properties: Although the relevance for human use is unknown, the following data characterize the performance of LAMICTAL in receptor binding assays. Lamotrigine had a weak inhibitory effect on the serotonin 5-HT_3 receptor (IC_{50}=18 μM). It does not exhibit high affinity binding (IC_{50}>100 μM) to the following neurotransmitter receptors: adenosine A_1 and A_2, adrenergic α_1, α_2, and β; dopamine D_1 and D_2; γ-aminobutyric acid (GABA) A and B; histamine H_1; kappa opioid; muscarinic acetylcholine; and

Continued on next page

Glaxo Wellcome—Cont.

serotonin 5-HT$_2$. Studies have failed to detect an effect of lamotrigine on dihydropyridine-sensitive calcium channels. It had weak effects at sigma opioid receptors (IC$_{50}$=145 μM). Lamotrigine did not inhibit the uptake of norepinephrine, dopamine, serotonin, or aspartic acid (IC$_{50}$ > 100 μM).

Effect of lamotrigine on NMDA-mediated activity: Lamotrigine did not inhibit NMDA-induced depolarizations in rat cortical slices or NMDA-induced cyclic GMP formation in immature rat cerebellum nor did lamotrigine displace compounds that are either competitive or non-competitive ligands at this glutamate receptor complex (CNQX, CGS, TCHP). The IC$_{50}$ for lamotrigine effects on NMDA-induced currents (in the presence of 3 μM glycine) in cultured hippocampal neurons exceeded 100 μM.

Folate Metabolism: In vitro, lamotrigine was shown to be an inhibitor of dihydrofolate reductase, the enzyme that catalyzes the reduction of dihydrofolate to tetrahydrofolate. Inhibition of this enzyme may interfere with the biosynthesis of nucleic acids and proteins. When oral daily doses of lamotrigine were given to pregnant rats during organogenesis, fetal, placental, and maternal folate concentrations were reduced. Significantly reduced concentrations of folate are associated with teratogenesis (see PRECAUTIONS: Pregnancy). Folate concentrations were also reduced in male rats given repeated oral doses of lamotrigine. Reduced concentrations were partially returned to normal when supplemented with folinic acid.

Accumulation in Kidneys: Lamotrigine was found to accumulate in the kidney of the male rat causing chronic progressive nephrosis, necrosis, and mineralization. These findings are attributed to α-2 microglobulin, a species and sex specific protein that has not been detected in humans or other animal species.

Melanin Binding: Lamotrigine binds to melanin-containing tissues, e.g., in the eye and pigmented skin. It has been found in the uveal tract up to 52 weeks after a single dose in rodents.

Cardiovascular: In dogs, lamotrigine is extensively metabolized to a 2-N-methyl metabolite. This metabolite causes dose-dependent prolongations of the PR interval, widening of the QRS complex, and, at higher doses, complete AV conduction block. Similar cardiovascular effects are not anticipated in humans because only trace amounts of the 2-N-methyl metabolite (< 0.6% of lamotrigine dose) have been found in human urine (see Drug Disposition below). However, it is conceivable that plasma concentrations of this metabolite could be increased in patients with a reduced capacity to glucuronidate lamotrigine (e.g., in patients with liver disease).

Pharmacokinetics and Drug Metabolism: The pharmacokinetics of lamotrigine have been studied in patients with epilepsy, healthy young and elderly volunteers, and volunteers with chronic renal failure. Lamotrigine pharmacokinetic parameters for adult patients and healthy normal volunteers are summarized in Table 1.
[See table below.]

The clearance of lamotrigine is affected by the co-administration of antiepileptic drugs. Lamotrigine is eliminated more rapidly in patients who have been taking hepatic enzyme inducing antiepileptic drugs (EIAEDs), including carbamazepine, phenytoin, phenobarbital, and primidone. Most clinical experience is derived from this population.

Valproic acid (VPA), however, actually decreases the clearance of lamotrigine (i.e., more than doubles the elimination t$_{1/2}$ of lamotrigine), whether given with or without EIAEDs. Accordingly, if lamotrigine is to be administered to a patient receiving VPA, lamotrigine must be given at a reduced dosage, less than half the dose used in patients not receiving VPA (see DOSAGE AND ADMINISTRATION and PRECAUTIONS: Drug Interactions).

Absorption: Lamotrigine is rapidly and completely absorbed after oral administration with negligible first-pass metabolism (absolute bioavailability is 98%). The bioavailability is not affected by food. Peak plasma concentrations occur anywhere from 1.4 to 4.8 hours following drug administration.

Distribution: Estimates of the mean apparent volume of distribution (Vd/F) of lamotrigine following oral administration ranged from 0.9 to 1.3 L/kg. Vd/F is independent of dose and is similar following single and multiple doses in both patients with epilepsy and in healthy volunteers.

Protein Binding: Data from in vitro studies indicate that lamotrigine is approximately 55% bound to human plasma proteins at plasma lamotrigine concentrations from 1 to 10 μg/mL (10 μg/mL is 4 to 6 times the trough plasma concentration observed in the controlled efficacy trials). Because lamotrigine is not highly bound to plasma proteins, clinically significant interactions with other drugs through competition for protein binding sites are unlikely. The binding of lamotrigine to plasma proteins did not change in the presence of therapeutic concentrations of phenytoin, phenobarbital, or valproic acid. Lamotrigine did not displace other antiepileptic drugs (carbamazepine, phenytoin, phenobarbital) from protein binding sites.

Drug Disposition: Lamotrigine is metabolized predominantly by glucuronic acid conjugation; the major metabolite is an inactive 2-N-glucuronide conjugate. After oral administration of 240 mg ^{14}C-lamotrigine (15 μCi) to six healthy volunteers, 94% was recovered in the urine and 2% was recovered in the feces. The radioactivity in the urine consisted of unchanged lamotrigine (10%), a 2-N-glucuronide (76%), a 5-N-glucuronide (10%), a 2-N-methyl metabolite (0.14%), and other unidentified minor metabolites (4%).

Enzyme Induction: The effects of lamotrigine on specific families of mixed-function oxidase isozymes have not been systematically evaluated.

Following multiple administrations (150 mg b.i.d.) to normal volunteers taking no other medications, lamotrigine induced its own metabolism resulting in a 25% decrease in t$_{1/2}$ and a 37% increase in CL/F at steady state compared to values obtained in the same volunteers following a single dose. Evidence gathered from other sources suggests that self induction by LAMICTAL may not occur when LAMICTAL is given as add-on therapy in patients receiving enzyme-inducing AEDs.

Dose Proportionality: In healthy volunteers not receiving any other medications and given single doses, the plasma concentrations of lamotrigine increased in direct proportion to the dose administered over the range of 50 to 400 mg. In two small studies (n=7 and 8) of patients with epilepsy who were maintained on other antiepileptic drugs there also was a linear relationship between dose and lamotrigine plasma concentrations at steady state following doses of 50 mg to 350 mg b.i.d.

Elimination: (See Table 1)

Special Populations:
Patients with renal insufficiency: Twelve volunteers with chronic renal failure (mean creatinine clearance=13 mL/min; range 6 to 23) and another six individuals undergoing hemodialysis were each given a single 100 mg dose of LAMICTAL. The mean plasma half-lives determined in the study were 42.9 hours (chronic renal failure), 13.0 hours (during hemodialysis), and 57.4 hours (between hemodialysis) compared to 26.2 hours in healthy volunteers. On average, approximately 20% (range = 5.6 to 35.1) of the amount of lamotrigine present in the body was eliminated during a 4-hour hemodialysis session.

Hepatic disease: The pharmacokinetic parameters of lamotrigine in patients with impaired liver function have not been studied.

Age:
Elderly: In a single-dose study (150 mg LAMICTAL), the pharmacokinetics of lamotrigine in twelve elderly volunteers between the ages of 65 and 76 years (mean creatinine clearance=61 mL/min; range=33 to 108) were similar to those of young healthy volunteers in other studies.

Gender: The clearance of lamotrigine is not affected by gender.

Race: The apparent oral clearance of lamotrigine was 25% lower in noncaucasians than caucasians.

Clinical Studies: The effectiveness of LAMICTAL as adjunctive therapy (added to other antiepileptic drugs) was established in three multi-center placebo-controlled double-blind clinical trials in 355 adults with refractory partial seizures. The patients had a history of at least 4 partial seizures per month in spite of receiving one or more antiepileptic drugs at therapeutic concentrations and, in 2 of the studies, were observed on their established antiepileptic drug regimen during baselines that varied between 8 to 12 weeks. In the third, patients were not observed in a prospective baseline. In patients continuing to have at least 4 seizures per month during the baseline, LAMICTAL or placebo was then added to the existing therapy. In all three studies, change from baseline in seizure frequency was the primary measure of effectiveness. The results given below are for all partial seizures in the intent to treat (all patients who received at least one dose of treatment) population in each study, unless otherwise indicated. The median seizure frequency at baseline was 3 per week while the mean at baseline was 6.6 per week for all patients enrolled in efficacy studies.

One study (n=216) was a double-bind placebo-controlled parallel trial consisting of a 24-week treatment period. Patients could not be on more than two other anticonvulsants and valproic acid was not allowed. Patients were random-

TABLE 1:
MEAN[1] PHARMACOKINETIC PARAMETERS IN ADULT PATIENTS WITH EPILEPSY OR HEALTHY VOLUNTEERS

Adult Study Population	Number of Subjects	T$_{max}$: Time of Maximum Plasma Concentration (hours)	t$_{1/2}$ Elimination Half-life (hours)	CL/F: Plasma Clearance (mL/min/kg)
Patients Taking Enzyme-inducing Antiepileptic Drugs[2]:				
Single-Dose LAMICTAL®	24	2.3 (0.5–5.0)	14.4 (6.4–30.4)	1.10 (0.51–2.22)
Multiple-Dose LAMICTAL	17	2.0 (0.75–5.93)	12.6 (7.5–23.1)	1.21 (0.66–1.82)
Patients Taking Enzyme-Inducing Antiepileptic Drugs +Valproic Acid:				
Single-Dose LAMICTAL	25	3.8 (1.0–10.0)	27.2 (11.2–51.6)	0.53 (0.27–1.04)
Patients Taking Valproic Acid Only:				
Single-Dose LAMICTAL	4	4.8 (1.8–8.4)	58.8 (30.5–88.8)	0.28 (0.16–0.40)
Healthy Volunteers Taking Valproic Acid:				
Single-Dose LAMICTAL	6	1.8 (1.0–4.0)	48.3 (31.5–88.6)	0.30 (0.14–0.42)
Multiple Dose LAMICTAL	18	1.9 (0.5–3.5)	70.3 (41.9–113.5)	0.18 (0.12–0.33)
Healthy Volunteers Taking No Other Medications:				
Single-Dose LAMICTAL	179	2.2 (0.25–12.0)	32.8 (14.0–103.0)	0.44 (0.12–1.10)
Multiple-Dose LAMICTAL	36	1.7 (0.5–4.0)	25.4 (11.6–61.6)	0.58 (0.24–1.15)

[1] The majority of parameter means determined in each study had coefficients of variation between 20% and 40% for t$_{1/2}$ and plasma clearance, and between 30% and 70% for T$_{max}$. The overall mean values were calculated from individual study means that were weighted based on the number of volunteers/patients in each study. The numbers in parentheses below each parameter mean represent the range of individual volunteer/patient values across studies.

[2] Examples of enzyme-inducing antiepileptic drugs are carbamazepine, phenobarbital, phenytoin, and primidone.

ized to receive placebo, a target dose of 300 mg/day of LAMICTAL, or a target dose of 500 mg/day of LAMICTAL. The median reductions in the frequency of all partial seizures relative to baseline were 8% in patients receiving placebo, 20% in patients receiving 300 mg/day of LAMICTAL, and 36% in patients receiving 500 mg/day of LAMICTAL. The seizure frequency reduction was statistically significant in the 500 mg/day group compared to the placebo group, but not in the 300 mg/day group.

A second study (n=98) was a double-blind, placebo-controlled, randomized crossover trial consisting of two 14-week treatment periods (the last 2 weeks of which consisted of dose tapering), separated by a 4-week washout period. Patients could not be on more than two other anticonvulsants and valproic acid was not allowed. The target dose of LAMICTAL was 400 mg/day. When the first twelve weeks of the treatment periods were analyzed, the median change in seizure frequency was a 25% reduction on LAMICTAL compared to placebo ($P < 0.001$).

The third study (n=41) was a double-blind placebo-controlled crossover trial consisting of two 12-week treatment periods, separated by a 4-week washout period. Patients could not be on more than two other anticonvulsants. Thirteen patients were on concomitant valproic acid; these patients received 150 mg/day of LAMICTAL. The 28 other patients had a target dose of 300 mg/day of LAMICTAL. The median change in seizure frequency was a 26% reduction on LAMICTAL compared to a placebo ($P < 0.01$).

No differences in efficacy based on age, sex, or race, as measured by change in seizure frequency, were detected.

INDICATIONS AND USAGE

LAMICTAL (lamotrigine) is indicated as adjunctive therapy in the treatment of partial seizures in adults with epilepsy.

CONTRAINDICATIONS

LAMICTAL is contraindicated in patients who have demonstrated hypersensitivity to the drug or its ingredients.

WARNINGS

Dermatologic Events: Approximately 10% of all LAMICTAL exposed individuals develop a rash. However, not all cases of rash can be attributed to LAMICTAL; five percent (5%) of patients exposed to placebo developed a rash. Typically, rash occurs in the first 4 to 6 weeks of treatment initiation. The incidence of rash appears to be increased among patients being treated with a multi-drug regimen that includes both valproate and EIAEDs. When valproate and LAMICTAL have been used as a two-drug combination, the incidence of rash is even higher; note, dosing recommendations for the use of LAMICTAL and valproate alone cannot be provided because of insufficient experience with that combination (see DOSAGE AND ADMINISTRATION). The incidence of rash also appears to increase with the magnitude of the initial dose and the subsequent rate of dose escalation (see DOSAGE AND ADMINISTRATION).

LAMICTAL associated rashes do not appear to have unique identifying features. Maculopapular and/or erythematous eruptions are common. Rarely, more serious rashes with systemic involvement occur (see below). A benign initial appearance of a rash cannot predict an entirely benign outcome; however, a substantial number of patients developing a rash on LAMICTAL have continued treatment without ill effect.

Prior to initiation of treatment, patients should be instructed (1) that rash may occur, (2) that it may herald a serious medical event, and (3) that should it occur, it must be reported promptly to their physician.

Reports of rash should be promptly evaluated to determine whether treatment withdrawal is necessary. If a decision is made to continue treatment in the face of rash, close monitoring is essential.

Serious rash leading to hospitalization: Rash resulting in hospitalization occurred in 0.3% of the approximately 3400 subjects who participated in premarketing clinical trials. No fatalities occurred among these individuals, but rash has been associated with a fatal outcome in reports from non-domestic post-marketing experience.

Among the rashes leading to hospitalization were Stevens-Johnson syndrome, toxic epidermal necrolysis, angioedema, and a rash associated with a variable number of the following systemic manifestations: fever, lymphadenopathy, facial swelling, hematologic, and hepatologic abnormalities.

There is evidence that the inclusion of valproate in a multi-drug regimen increases the risk of serious, potentially life-threatening rash. Specifically, of 584 patients administered LAMICTAL with VPA in clinical trials, 6 (1%) were hospitalized in association with rash; in contrast, 4 (0.16%) of 2398 clinical trial patients and volunteers administered LAMICTAL in the absence of VPA were hospitalized.

Other examples of serious and potentially life-threatening rash that did not lead to hospitalization also occurred in premarketing development. Among these, one case was reported to be Stevens-Johnson like.

Rash leading to LAMICTAL withdrawal: Although not a certain indicator of severity, the clinician's decision to with-

draw a patient from LAMICTAL in the face of rash provides some insight into the clinical importance attributed to the finding. Rash leading to withdrawal was more common in patients on drug regimens including valproate as a component and has been reported to be even more common when LAMICTAL is co-administered with valproate alone (see DOSAGE AND ADMINISTRATION).

Because rash occurs frequently in association with a number of other signs and symptoms, it is impossible to discern reliably in what proportion of patients withdrawn with rash, the rash was the primary reason for withdrawal. The overall rate of discontinuation due to rash in patients participating in clinical trials (n=3501) was 3.8%.

In assessing the importance of a rash, consideration should be given to the fact that a substantial number of patients with rash were continued on treatment and had an uneventful course.

Acute Hepatic Failure/Multiorgan Failure: A case of fulminant hepatic failure has been reported in non-domestic post-marketing use. A 23-year-old woman receiving concomitant valproic acid and carbamazepine developed headache, fever, and a maculopapular rash 3 weeks after starting LAMICTAL. Hepatic coma followed within 3 days; despite apparent subsequent clinical improvement, the patient died unexpectedly from pulmonary embolus 2 months later.

Fatalities associated with multiorgan failure and various degrees of hepatic failure have been reported in five patients from among 7000 exposed during pre-marketing development of LAMICTAL. These cases occurred in association with other serious medical events (e.g., status epilepticus, overwhelming sepsis) making it impossible to identify the initiating cause.

Additionally, in the absence of any obvious precipitating event, a 45-year-old woman treated with carbamazepine and clonazepam developed DIC, rhabdomyolysis, renal failure, rash, ataxia, and elevated AST 14 days after LAMICTAL was added to her antiepileptic drug regimen. She subsequently recovered with supportive care after LAMICTAL treatment was discontinued.

Pure Red Cell Aplasia (PRCA): A case of PRCA was reported in a 32-year-old male with a history of β-thalassemia. The patient had a microcytic anemia (hemoglobin 11 g/dL) which was stable while receiving carbamazepine but which had become more severe in the three months after LAMICTAL was added. A bone marrow aspirate revealed markedly decreased erythropoiesis but normal granulopoiesis and thrombopoiesis. Erythropoiesis resumed after discontinuation of LAMICTAL and transfusions of packed red cells. Although PRCA is known to occur in patients with hemoglobinopathies, it is not known if β-thalassemia is a specific risk factor for the development of PRCA.

Sudden Unexplained Death in Epilepsy (SUDEP): During the premarketing development of LAMICTAL, 20 sudden and unexplained deaths were recorded among a cohort of 4700 patients with epilepsy (5747 patient-years of exposure). Some of these could represent seizure-related deaths in which the seizure was not observed, e.g., at night. This represents an incidence of .0035 deaths per patient-year. Although this rate exceeds that expected in a healthy population matched for age and sex, it is within the range of estimates for the incidence of sudden unexplained deaths in patients with epilepsy not receiving LAMICTAL (ranging from 0.0005 for the general population of patients with epilepsy, to 0.004 for a recently studied clinical trial population similar to that in the clinical development program for LAMICTAL, to 0.005 for patients with refractory epilepsy). Consequently, whether these figures are reassuring or suggest concern depends on the comparability of the populations reported upon to the cohort receiving LAMICTAL and the accuracy of the estimates provided. Probably most reassuring is the similarity of estimated SUDEP rates in patients receiving LAMICTAL and those receiving another antiepileptic drug that underwent clinical testing in a similar population at about the same time. Importantly, that drug is chemically unrelated to LAMICTAL. This evidence suggests, although it certainly does not prove, that the high SUDEP rates reflect population rates, not a drug effect.

Withdrawal Seizures: As a rule, antiepileptic drugs should not be abruptly discontinued because of the possibility of increasing seizure frequency. Unless safety concerns require a more rapid withdrawal, the dose of LAMICTAL should be tapered over a period of at least 2 weeks (see DOSAGE AND ADMINISTRATION).

Status Epilepticus: Valid estimates of the incidence of treatment emergent status epilepticus among LAMICTAL treated patients are difficult to obtain because reporters participating in clinical trials did not all employ identical rules for identifying cases. At a minimum, 7 of 2343 adult patients had episodes that could unequivocally be described as status. In addition, a number of reports of variably defined episodes of seizure exacerbation (e.g., seizure clusters, seizure flurries, etc.) were made.

PRECAUTIONS

Addition of LAMICTAL to a multi-drug regimen that includes valproate: dosage reduction.

Because valproic acid (VPA) reduces the clearance of lamotrigine, the dosage of lamotrigine in the presence of VPA is less than half of that required in its absence (see DOSAGE AND ADMINISTRATION).

Use in Patients with Concomitant Illness: Clinical experience with LAMICTAL in patients with concomitant illness is limited. Caution is advised when using LAMICTAL in patients with diseases or conditions that could affect metabolism or elimination of the drug, such as renal, hepatic, or cardiac functional impairment.

Hepatic metabolism to the glucuronide followed by renal excretion is the principal route of elimination of lamotrigine (see CLINICAL PHARMACOLOGY).

A study in individuals with severe chronic renal failure (mean creatinine clearance=13 mL/min) not receiving other AEDs indicated that the elimination half-life of unchanged lamotrigine is prolonged relative to individuals with normal renal function. Until adequate numbers of patients with severe renal impairment have been evaluated during chronic treatment with LAMICTAL, it should be used with caution in these patients, generally using a reduced maintenance dose for patients with significant impairment.

Because there is no experience with the use of LAMICTAL in patients with impaired liver function, the use in such patients may be associated with as yet unrecognized risks.

Dermatological Events (see WARNINGS): In controlled add-on studies the incidence of rash in patients receiving LAMICTAL was 10% compared to 5% in placebo patients. Usually, rashes were maculopapular and/or erythematous, occurred within the first 6 weeks of therapy, and resolved during continued administration of LAMICTAL. Approximately 4% of patients in all studies were discontinued because of rash. Serious, potentially life-threatening, dermatological events have occurred in patients taking LAMICTAL; rash, including serious rash, is more likely to occur in patients taking concomitant valproic acid (see WARNINGS). In patients receiving concomitant valproic acid, available data suggest that exceeding the recommended dose at the initiation of therapy with LAMICTAL may be associated with an increased incidence of rash requiring withdrawal of therapy.

Binding in the Eye and Other Melanin-containing Tissues: Because lamotrigine binds to melanin, it could accumulate in melanin rich tissues over time. This raises the possibility that lamotrigine may cause toxicity in these tissues after extended use. Although ophthalmological testing was performed in one controlled clinical trial, the testing was inadequate to exclude subtle effects or injury occurring after long-term exposure. Moreover, the capacity of available tests to detect potentially adverse consequences, if any, of lamotrigine's binding to melanin is unknown.

Accordingly, although there are no specific recommendations for periodic ophthalmological monitoring, prescribers should be aware of the possibility of long-term ophthalmologic effects.

Information for Patients: Patients should be advised to notify their physician immediately if they develop a skin rash while taking LAMICTAL, or if they acutely develop any worsening of seizure control.

Patients should be advised that LAMICTAL may cause dizziness, somnolence, and other symptoms and signs of CNS depression. Accordingly, they should be advised neither to drive a car nor to operate other complex machinery until they have gained sufficient experience on LAMICTAL to gauge whether or not it affects their mental and/or motor performance adversely.

Patients should be advised to notify their physician if they become pregnant or intend to become pregnant during therapy. Patients should be advised to notify their physician if they intend to breast-feed or are breast-feeding an infant.

Laboratory Tests: The value of monitoring plasma concentrations of LAMICTAL has not been established. Because of the possible pharmacokinetic interactions between LAMICTAL and other AEDs being taken concomitantly (see Table 2), monitoring of the plasma levels of LAMICTAL and concomitant AEDs may be indicated, particularly during dosage adjustments. In general, clinical judgment should be exercised regarding monitoring of plasma levels of LAMICTAL and other anti-seizure drugs and whether or not dosage adjustments are necessary.

Drug Interactions:

Antiepileptic Drugs (AEDs):

The use of antiepileptic drugs in combination is complicated by the potential for pharmacokinetic interactions.

The interaction of lamotrigine with phenytoin, carbamazepine, and valproic acid has been characterized. With the exception of valproic acid, the addition of lamotrigine to these AEDs does not affect their steady-state plasma concentrations. The net effects of these various AED combinations on individual AED plasma concentrations are summarized in Table 2.

Continued on next page

Glaxo Wellcome—Cont.

TABLE 2:
SUMMARY OF AED INTERACTIONS WITH LAMICTAL (lamotrigine)

Antiepileptic Drug (AED)	AED Plasma Concentration with Add-on LAMICTAL®[a]	Lamotrigine Plasma Concentration with Add-on AEDs[b]
Phenytoin (PHT)	↔	↓
Carbamazepine (CBZ)	↔	↓
CBZ epoxide[c]	?[d]	
Valproic Acid (VPA)	↓	↑
VPA+PHT and/or CBZ	NE[e]	↔

↔ No significant effect.

a From add-on clinical trials and volunteer studies.
b Net effects were estimated by comparing the mean clearance values obtained in add-on clinical trials and volunteers studies.
c Not administered, but an active metabolite of carbamazepine.
d Conflicting data.
e NE=not evaluated.

Specific effects of lamotrigine on the pharmacokinetics of other antiepileptic drug products:

LAMICTAL added to phenytoin: LAMICTAL has no appreciable effect on steady-state phenytoin plasma concentration.

LAMICTAL added to carbamazepine: LAMICTAL has no appreciable effect on steady-state carbamazepine plasma concentration. Limited clinical data suggest there is a higher incidence of dizziness, diplopia, ataxia, and blurred vision in patients receiving carbamazepine with LAMICTAL than in patients receiving other enzyme-inducing AEDs with LAMICTAL (see ADVERSE REACTIONS). The mechanism of this interaction is unclear. The effect of lamotrigine on plasma concentrations of carbamazepine-epoxide is unclear. In a small subset of patients (n=7) studied in a placebo-controlled trial, lamotrigine had no effect on carbamazepine-epoxide plasma concentrations, but in a small uncontrolled study (n=9), carbamazepine-epoxide levels were seen to increase.

LAMICTAL added to valproic acid: When LAMICTAL was administered to healthy volunteers already receiving valproic acid (VPA), the trough steady-state VPA concentrations in plasma decreased by an average of 25% over a 3-week period, and then stabilized.

LAMICTAL added to valproic acid + phenytoin and/or carbamazepine: Although the effects of LAMICTAL on plasma levels of these AEDs given in combination has not been systematically evaluated, it is expected that the effects would be similar to those when LAMICTAL is added to each independently (e.g., valproic levels decrease, phenytoin and carbamazepine do not change).

Specific effects of other antiepileptic drug products on the pharmacokinetics of lamotrigine:

Phenytoin added to LAMICTAL: The addition of phenytoin decreases lamotrigine steady-state concentrations by approximately 45% to 54% depending upon the total daily dose of phenytoin (i.e., from 100 to 400 mg).

Carbamazepine added to LAMICTAL: The addition of carbamazepine decreases lamotrigine steady-state concentrations by approximately 40%.

Phenobarbital or primidone added to LAMICTAL: The addition of phenobarbital or primidone decreases lamotrigine steady-state concentrations by approximately 40%.

Valproic acid added to LAMICTAL: The addition of valproic acid (VPA) increases lamotrigine steady-state concentrations in normal volunteers by slightly more than two-fold.

Interactions with drug products other than antiepileptics:

Folate Inhibitors: Lamotrigine is an inhibitor of dihydrofolate reductase. Prescribers should be aware of this action when prescribing other medications which inhibit folate metabolism.

Drug/Laboratory Test Interactions: None known.

Carcinogenesis, Mutagenesis, Impairment of Fertility: No evidence of carcinogenicity was seen in one mouse study or two rat studies following oral administration of lamotrigine for up to 2 years at maximum tolerated doses (30 mg/kg/day for mice and 10 to 15 mg/kg/day for rats, doses which are equivalent to 90 mg/m^2, and 60 to 90 mg/m^2, respectively). Steady-state plasma concentrations ranged from 1 to 4 µg/mL in the mouse study and 1 to 10 µg/mL in the rat study. Plasma concentrations associated with the recommended human doses of 300 to 500 mg/day are generally in the range of 2 to 5 µg/mL, but concentrations as high as 19 µg/mL have been recorded.

Lamotrigine was not mutagenic in the presence or absence of metabolic activation when tested in two gene mutation assays (the Ames test and the in vitro mammalian mouse lymphoma assay). In two cytogenetic assays (the in vitro human lymphocyte assay and the in vivo rat bone marrow assay), lamotrigine did not increase the incidence of structural or numerical chromosomal abnormalities.

No evidence of impairment of fertility was detected in rats given oral doses of lamotrigine up to 2.4 times the highest usual human maintenance dose of 8.33 mg/kg/day or 0.4 times the human dose on a mg/m^2 basis. The effect of lamotrigine on human fertility is unknown.

Pregnancy: ***Pregnancy Category C.*** No evidence of teratogenicity was found in mice, rats, or rabbits when lamotrigine was orally administered to pregnant animals during the period of organogenesis at doses up to 1.2, 0.5, and 1.1 times, respectively, on a mg/m^2 basis, the highest usual human maintenance dose (i.e., 500 mg/day). However, maternal toxicity and secondary fetal toxicity producing reduced fetal weight and/or delayed ossification were seen in mice and rats, but not in rabbits at these doses. Teratology studies were also conducted using bolus intravenous (I.V.) administration of the isethionate salt of lamotrigine in rats and rabbits. In rat dams administered an I.V. dose at 0.6 times the highest usual human maintenance dose, the incidence of intrauterine death without signs of teratogenicity was increased.

A behavioral teratology study was conducted in rats dosed during the period of organogenesis. At day 21 postpartum offspring of dams receiving 5 mg/kg/day or higher displayed a significantly longer latent period for open field exploration and a lower frequency of rearing. In a swimming maze test performed on days 39 to 44 postpartum, time to completion was increased in offspring of dams receiving 25 mg/kg/day. These doses represent 0.1 and 0.5 times the clinical dose on a mg/m^2 basis, respectively.

Lamotrigine did not affect fertility, teratogenesis, or postnatal development when rats were dosed prior to and during mating, and throughout gestation and lactation at doses equivalent to 0.4 times the highest usual human maintenance dose on a mg/m^2 basis.

When pregnant rats were orally dosed at 0.1, 0.14, or 0.3 times the highest human maintenance dose (on a mg/m^2 basis) during the latter part of gestation (days 15 to 20), maternal toxicity and fetal death were seen. In dams, food consumption and weight gain were reduced, and the gestation period was slightly prolonged (22.6 vs. 22.0 days in the control group). Stillborn pups were found in all three drug-treated groups with the highest number in the high dose group. Post-natal death was also seen but only in the two highest doses and occurred between day 1 and 20. Some of these deaths appear to be drug-related and not secondary to the maternal toxicity. A no observed effect level (NOEL) could not be determined for this study.

Although LAMICTAL was not found to be teratogenic in the above studies, lamotrigine decreases fetal folate concentrations in rats, an effect known to be associated with teratogenesis in animals and humans. There are no adequate and well-controlled studies in pregnant women. Because animal reproduction studies are not always predictive of human response, this drug should be used during pregnancy only if the potential benefit justifies the potential risk to the fetus.

Pregnancy Exposure Registry: To monitor fetal outcomes of pregnant women exposed to lamotrigine, Glaxo Wellcome Inc. maintains a Lamotrigine Pregnancy Registry. Physicians are encouraged to register patients by calling (800) 722-9292. ext. 39441.

Labor and Delivery: The effect of LAMICTAL on labor and delivery in humans is unknown.

Use in Nursing Mothers: Preliminary data indicate that lamotrigine passes into human milk. Because the effects on the infant exposed to LAMICTAL by this route are unknown, breast-feeding while taking LAMICTAL is not recommended.

Pediatric Use: Safety and effectiveness in pediatric patients below the age of 16 have not been established.

Geriatric Use: Because few patients over the age of 65 (approximately 20) were exposed to LAMICTAL during its premarket evaluation, no specific statements about the safety or effectiveness of LAMICTAL in this age group can be made.

ADVERSE REACTIONS

The most commonly observed adverse experiences associated with the use of LAMICTAL in combination with other antiepileptic drugs, not seen at an equivalent frequency among placebo-treated patients, were: dizziness, ataxia, somnolence, headache, diplopia, blurred vision, nausea, vomiting, and rash. Dizziness, diplopia, ataxia, blurred vision, nausea, and vomiting were dose-related. Dizziness, diplopia, ataxia, and blurred vision occurred more commonly in patients receiving carbamazepine with LAMICTAL than in patients receiving other enzyme-inducing AEDs with LAMICTAL. Clinical data suggest a higher incidence of rash, including serious rash, in patients receiving concomitant valproic acid than in patients not receiving valproic acid (see WARNINGS).

Approximately 10% of the 3501 individuals who received LAMICTAL in premarketing clinical trials discontinued treatment because of an adverse experience. The adverse events most commonly associated with discontinuation were: rash (3.8%), dizziness (1.3%), and headache (1.3%).

In a dose response study, the rate of discontinuation of LAMICTAL for dizziness, ataxia, diplopia, blurred vision, nausea, and vomiting was dose-related.

Incidence in Controlled Clinical Studies: Table 3 lists treatment-emergent signs and symptoms that occurred in at least 1% of patients with epilepsy treated with LAMICTAL participating in placebo-controlled trials and were numerically more common in the patients treated with LAMICTAL. In these studies, either LAMICTAL or placebo was added to the patient's current antiepileptic drug therapy. Adverse events were usually mild to moderate in intensity.

The prescriber should be aware that these figures, obtained when LAMICTAL was added to concurrent antiepileptic drug therapy, cannot be used to predict the frequency of adverse experiences in the course of usual medical practice where patient characteristics and other factors may differ from those prevailing during clinical studies. Similarly, the cited frequencies cannot be directly compared with figures obtained from other clinical investigations involving different treatments, uses, or investigators. An inspection of these frequencies, however, does provide the prescriber with one basis to estimate the relative contribution of drug and non-drug factors to the adverse event incidences in the population studied.

TABLE 3
TREATMENT-EMERGENT ADVERSE EVENT INCIDENCE IN PLACEBO-CONTROLLED ADD-ON TRIALS[1]
(Events in at least 1% of patients treated with LAMICTAL and numerically more frequent than in the placebo group.)

Body System/ Adverse Experience[2]	Percent of Patients Receiving LAMICTAL® (n=711)	Percent of Patients Receiving Placebo (n=419)
BODY AS A WHOLE		
Headache	29.1	19.1
Accidental Injury	9.1	8.6
Flu Syndrome	7.0	5.5
Fever	5.5	3.6
Abdominal Pain	5.2	3.6
Infection	4.4	4.1
Neck Pain	2.4	1.2
Malaise	2.3	1.9
Reaction Aggravated (Seizure Exacerbation)	2.3	0.5
Chills	1.3	0.5
CARDIOVASCULAR		
Hot Flashes	1.3	0.0
Palpitations	1.0	0.5
DIGESTIVE		
Nausea	18.6	9.5
Vomiting	9.4	4.3
Diarrhea	6.3	4.1
Dyspepsia	5.3	2.1
Constipation	4.1	3.1
Tooth Disorder	3.2	1.7
Anorexia	1.8	1.4
Dry Mouth	1.0	0.2
MUSCULOSKELETAL		
Arthralgia	2.0	0.2
Joint Disorder	1.3	1.0
Myasthenia	1.3	0.0
NERVOUS		
Dizziness	38.4	13.4
Ataxia	21.7	5.5
Somnolence	14.2	6.9
Incoordination	6.0	2.1
Insomnia	5.6	1.9
Tremor	4.4	1.4
Depression	4.2	2.6
Anxiety	3.8	2.6
Convulsion	3.2	1.2
Irritability	3.0	1.9
Speech Disorder	2.5	0.2
Memory Decreased	2.4	1.9
Confusion	1.8	1.7
Concentration Disturbance	1.7	0.7
Sleep Disorder	1.4	0.5
Emotional Lability	1.3	0.2
Vertigo	1.1	0.2
Mind Racing	1.0	0.5
Nystagmus	1.0	0.5
Dysarthria	1.0	0.2
Muscle Spasm	1.0	0.2
RESPIRATORY		
Rhinitis	13.6	9.3
Pharyngitis	9.8	8.8
Cough Increased	7.5	5.7
Dyspnea	1.1	0.2

SKIN AND APPENDAGES		
Rash	10.0	5.0
Pruritus	3.1	1.7
Alopecia	1.3	1.2
Acne	1.3	0.5
SPECIAL SENSES		
Diplopia	27.6	6.7
Blurred Vision	15.5	4.5
Vision Abnormality	3.4	1.0
Ear Pain	1.8	1.7
Tinnitus	1.1	1.0
UROGENITAL		
Female Patients Only	(n=365)	(n=207)
Dysmenorrhea	6.6	6.3
Vaginitis	4.1	0.5
Amenorrhea	1.9	0.5

[1] Patients in these add-on studies were receiving 1 to 3 concomitant enzyme-inducing antiepileptic drugs in addition to LAMICTAL or placebo. Patients may have reported multiple adverse experiences during the study or at discontinuation; thus, patients may be included in more than one category.
[2] Adverse Experiences reported by at least 1% of patients treated with LAMICTAL are included.

In a randomized parallel study comparing placebo, 300 mg, and 500 mg per day of LAMICTAL, some of the more common drug-related adverse events were dose-related (see Table 4).

TABLE 4
Dose-related Adverse Events from a Randomized Placebo-controlled Trial

	Percent of Patients Experiencing AE		
Adverse Experience (AE)	**Placebo (n=73)**	**LAMICTAL® 300 mg (n=71)**	**LAMICTAL 500 mg (n=72)**
Ataxia	10	10	28[1,2]
Blurred Vision	10	11	25[1,2]
Diplopia	8	24[1]	49[1,2]
Dizziness	27	31	54[1,2]
Nausea	11	18	25[1]
Vomiting	4	11	18[1]

[1] Significantly greater than placebo group ($P < 0.05$)
[2] Significantly greater than group receiving LAMICTAL 300 mg ($P < 0.05$)

Other events which occurred in more than 1% of patients but equally or more frequently in the placebo group included: asthenia, back pain, chest pain, flatulence, menstrual disorder, myalgia, paresthesia, respiratory disorder, and urinary tract infection.

The overall adverse experience profile for LAMICTAL was similar between females and males, and was independent of age. Because the largest non-white racial subgroup was only 6% of patients exposed to LAMICTAL (46/711) in placebo-controlled trials, there are insufficient data to support a statement regarding the distribution of adverse experience reports by race. Generally, females receiving either add-on LAMICTAL or placebo were more likely to report adverse experiences than males. The only adverse experience for which the reports on LAMICTAL were greater than 10% more frequent in females than males (without a corresponding difference by gender on placebo) was dizziness (difference=16.5%). There was little difference between females and males in the rates of discontinuation of LAMICTAL for individual adverse experiences.

Other Adverse Events Observed During All Clinical Trials:
Other Adverse Events: LAMICTAL has been administered to 3501 individuals during all clinical trials, only some of which were placebo-controlled. During these trials, all adverse events were recorded by the clinical investigators using terminology of their own choosing. To provide a meaningful estimate of the proportion of individuals having adverse events, similar types of events were grouped into a smaller number of standardized categories using modified COSTART dictionary terminology. The frequencies presented represent the proportion of the 3501 individuals exposed to LAMICTAL who experienced an event of the type cited on at least one occasion while receiving LAMICTAL. All reported events are included except those already listed in the previous table, those too general to be informative, and those not reasonably associated with the use of the drug.

TABLE 5
LAMICTAL® Dose Recommendations (mg/day) for Adults (over 16 Years)

	WEEKS 1 and 2	**WEEKS 3 and 4**	**USUAL MAINTENANCE DOSE**
With EIAEDs & No valproic acid	50 mg (once a day)	100 mg (two divided doses)	300 mg to 500 mg/day (two divided doses) Escalate dose by 100 mg/day every week.
With EIAEDs & valproic acid	25 mg every other day	25 mg (once a day)	100 mg to 150 mg/day (in two divided doses) Escalate dose by 25 to 50 mg/day every 1 or 2 weeks.

Events are further classified within body system categories and enumerated in order of decreasing frequency using the following definitions: *frequent* adverse events are defined as those occurring in at least $^1/_{100}$ patients; *infrequent* adverse events are those occurring in $^1/_{100}$ to $^1/_{1000}$ patients; *rare* adverse events are those occurring in fewer than $^1/_{1000}$ patients.

Body as a Whole: *Infrequent:* allergic reaction, face edema, and halitosis. *Rare:* abdomen enlarged, abscess, photosensitivity, and suicide attempt.

Cardiovascular System: *Infrequent:* flushing, migraine, postural hypotension, syncope, tachycardia, and vasodilation. *Rare:* angina pectoris, atrial fibrillation, deep thrombophlebitis, hemorrhage, hypertension, and myocardial infarction.

Dermatological: *Infrequent:* dry skin, eczema, erythema, hirsutism, maculopapular rash, sweating, vesiculobullous rash, and urticaria. *Rare:* angioedema, fungal dermatitis, herpes zoster, leukoderma, petechial rash, pustular rash, seborrhea, skin discoloration, and Stevens-Johnson syndrome.

Digestive System: *Infrequent:* dysphagia, gingivitis, glossitis, gum hyperplasia, increased appetite, increased salivation, liver function tests abnormal, mouth ulceration, stomatitis, and thirst. *Rare:* eructation, gastritis, gastrointestinal hemorrhage, gum hemorrhage, hemorrhagic colitis, hepatitis, melena, stomach ulcer, and tongue edema.

Endocrine System: *Rare:* goiter and hypothyroidism.

Hematologic and Lymphatic System: *Infrequent:* anemia, ecchymosis, eosinophilia, leukocytosis, leukopenia, lymphadenopathy, and petechia. *Rare:* fibrin decrease, fibrinogen decrease, iron deficiency anemia, macrocytic anemia, and thrombocytopenia.

Metabolic and Nutritional Disorders: *Frequent:* weight gain. *Infrequent:* alkaline phosphatase increase, peripheral edema, and weight loss. *Rare:* alcohol intolerance, bilirubinemia, general edema, and hyperglycemia.

Musculoskeletal System: *Infrequent:* twitching. *Rare:* arthritis, bursitis, leg cramps, tendinous contracture, and pathological fracture.

Nervous System: *Frequent:* amnesia, hostility, nervousness, thinking abnormality. *Infrequent:* abnormal dreams, abnormal gait, agitation, akathisia, apathy, aphasia, CNS depression, depersonalization, dyskinesia, dysphoria, euphoria, faintness, hallucinations, hyperkinesia, hypesthesia, myoclonus, panic attack, paranoid reaction, personality disorder, psychosis, and stupor. *Rare:* cerebrovascular accident, cerebellar syndrome, cerebral sinus thrombosis, choreoathetosis, CNS stimulation, delirium, delusions, dystonia, grand mal convulsions, hemiplegia, hyperalgesia, hyperesthesia, hypertonia, hypokinesia, hypomania, hypotonia, libido decreased, libido increased, manic depression reaction, movement disorder, neuralgia, neurosis, paralysis, and suicidal ideation.

Respiratory System: *Infrequent:* epistaxis and hyperventilation. *Rare:* bronchospasm, hiccup, and pneumonia.

Special Senses: *Infrequent:* abnormality of accommodation, conjunctivitis, oscillopsia, photophobia, and taste perversion. *Rare:* deafness, dry eyes, lacrimation disorder, parosmia, ptosis, strabismus, taste loss, and uveitis.

Urogenital System: *Infrequent:* breast pain, female lactation, hematuria, impotence, polyuria, urinary frequency, urinary incontinence, urinary retention, and vaginal moniliasis. *Rare:* abnormal ejaculation, acute kidney failure, breast abscess, cystitis, dysuria, breast neoplasm, creatinine increase, epididymitis, kidney failure, kidney pain, menorrhagia, and urine abnormality.

Postmarketing and Other Experience: In addition to the adverse experiences reported during clinical testing of LAMICTAL, the following adverse experiences have been reported in patients receiving marketed LAMICTAL in other countries and from worldwide non-controlled investigational use. These adverse experiences have not been listed above and data are insufficient to support an estimate of their incidence or to establish causation. The listing is alphabetized: Aplastic anemia, apnea, erythema multiforme, esophagitis, hematemesis, hemolytic anemia, neutropenia, pancreatitis, pancytopenia and progressive immunosuppression.

DRUG ABUSE AND DEPENDENCE

The abuse and dependence potential of LAMICTAL have not been evaluated in human studies.

OVERDOSAGE

Human Overdose Experience: Experience with single or daily doses greater than 700 mg is limited. During the clinical development of LAMICTAL, the highest known overdoses were in two women who each ingested doses greater than 4000 mg. The plasma concentration of lamotrigine in one woman was 52 μg/mL four hours after the ingestion (a value more than 10 times greater than that seen in clinical trials). She became comatose and remained comatose for 8 to 12 hours; no electrocardiographic abnormalities were detected. The other patient had dizziness, headache, and somnolence. Both women recovered without sequelae.

Management of Overdose: There are no specific antidotes for LAMICTAL. Following a suspected overdose, hospitalization of the patient is advised. General supportive care is indicated, including frequent monitoring of vital signs and close observation of the patient. If indicated, emesis should be induced or gastric lavage should be performed; usual precautions should be taken to protect the airway. It should be kept in mind that lamotrigine is rapidly absorbed (see CLINICAL PHARMACOLOGY). It is uncertain whether hemodialysis is an effective means of removing lamotrigine from the blood. In six renal failure patients, about 20% of the amount of lamotrigine in the body was removed during 4 hours of hemodialysis. A Poison Control Center should be contacted for information on the management of overdosage of LAMICTAL.

DOSAGE AND ADMINISTRATION

LAMICTAL (lamotrigine) is recommended as add-on therapy in patients over 16 years of age. Evidence bearing on its safety and effectiveness in children is not available.

General Dosing Considerations:

Patients receiving enzyme inducing antiepileptic drugs, but not valproate:
The initial dose of LAMICTAL in patients not taking valproic acid is 50 mg once a day for 2 weeks, followed by 100 mg/day given in two divided doses for 2 weeks. Thereafter, the usual maintenance dose is 300 to 500 mg/day given in two divided doses (see Table 5).

Patients receiving valproic acid as one component of a combination regimen also including enzyme inducing antiepileptic drugs:
In patients taking valproic acid as one component of a combination regimen also including enzyme inducing antiepileptic drugs, the initial dose of LAMICTAL is 25 mg every other day for 2 weeks, followed by 25 mg once a day for 2 weeks. Because the clearance of lamotrigine is decreased about 50% in the presence of valproate, the daily dose of LAMICTAL should ordinarily be no more than 150 mg a day, and should be administered on a b.i.d. schedule (see Table 5).
[See table above.]
Due to the increased risk of rash, the initial dose of LAMICTAL in patients receiving VPA should not exceed 25 mg every other day.
The Usual Maintenance Doses identified in the table above are derived from dosing regimens employed in the placebo controlled add-on studies in which the efficacy of LAMICTAL was established. In patients receiving multi-drug regimens employing EIAEDs **without VPA**, maintenance doses of LAMICTAL as high as 700 mg/day have been used. In patients receiving multi-drug regimens employed EIAEDs **with VPA**, maintenance doses of LAMICTAL as high as 200 mg/day have been used. The advantage of using doses above those recommended in the table above has not been established in controlled trials.

Note: The efficacy of add-on LAMICTAL in patients taking VPA alone has not been evaluated in controlled trials although it has been used in some patients. Consequently, an effective and safe dosing recommendation for the use of

Continued on next page

Glaxo Wellcome—Cont.

LAMICTAL and VPA as a two-drug regimen cannot be offered. If this regimen is nonetheless used, it should be noted that blood concentrations of LAMICTAL appear to be twice those associated with the use of LAMICTAL in a regimen containing both EIAEDs and VPA.

Patients with Renal Functional Impairment: Initial doses of LAMICTAL should be based on patients' antiepileptic drug regimen (see above); reduced maintenance doses may be effective for patients with significant renal functional impairment (see CLINICAL PHARMACOLOGY). Few patients with severe renal impairment have been evaluated during chronic treatment with LAMICTAL. Because there is inadequate experience in this population, LAMICTAL should be used with caution in these patients.

Discontinuation Strategy: For patients receiving LAMICTAL in combination with other AEDs, a re-evaluation for all AEDs in the regimen should be considered if a change in seizure control or an appearance or worsening of adverse experiences is observed.

If a decision is made to discontinue therapy with LAMICTAL, a step-wise reduction of dose over at least 2 weeks (approximately 50% per week) is recommended unless safety concerns require a more rapid withdrawal (see PRECAUTIONS).

Discontinuing an EIAED should prolong the half-life of lamotrigine; discontinuing valproic acid should shorten the half-life of lamotrigine.

Target plasma levels: A therapeutic plasma concentration range has not been established for lamotrigine. Dosing of LAMICTAL should be based on therapeutic response.

HOW SUPPLIED

25 mg (white) scored, shield-shaped tablets engraved with "LAMICTAL" and "25": Bottle of 25 (NDC 0173-0633-25). Store at 15° to 25°C (59° to 77°F) in a dry place.

100 mg (peach) scored, shield-shaped tablets engraved with "LAMICTAL" and "100": Bottle of 100 (NDC 0173-0642-55).

150 mg (cream) scored, shield-shaped tablets engraved with "LAMICTAL" and "150": Bottle of 60 (NDC 0173-0643-60).

200 mg (blue) scored, shield-shaped tablets engraved with "LAMICTAL" and "200": Bottle of 60 (NDC 0173-0644-60).

Store at 15° to 25°C (59° to 77°F) in a dry place and protect from light.

Caution: Federal law prohibits dispensing without prescription.

U.S. Patent No. 4602017

February 1996/RL-272

Shown in Product Identification Guide, page 313

LANOXICAPS® ℞

[*lă-nŏx 'ĭ-kăps"*]

(digoxin solution in capsules)

50 μg (0.05 mg) I.D. Imprint A2C (red)

100 μg (0.1 mg) I.D. Imprint B2C (yellow)

200 μg (0.2 mg) I.D. Imprint C2C (green)

DESCRIPTION

Digoxin is one of the cardiac (or digitalis) glycosides, a closely related group of drugs having in common specific effects on the myocardium. These drugs are found in a number of plants. Digoxin is extracted from the leaves of *Digitalis lanata*. The term "digitalis" is used to designate the whole group. The glycosides are composed of two portions: a sugar and a cardenolide (hence "glycosides").

Digoxin has the molecular formula $C_{41}H_{64}O_{14}$, a molecular weight of 780.95 and melting and decomposition points above 235°C. The drug is practically insoluble in water and in ether; slightly soluble in diluted (50%) alcohol and in chloroform; and freely soluble in pyridine. Digoxin powder is composed of odorless white crystals.

Digoxin has the chemical name: (3β, 5β, 12β)-3-[(*O*-2, 6-dideoxy-*β-D-ribo*-hexopyranosyl-(1→4)-*O*-2, 6-dideoxy-*β-D-ribo*-hexopyranosyl-(1→4)-2,6-dideoxy-*β-D-ribo*-hexopyranosyl) oxy]-12, 14-dihydroxycard-20(22)-enolide.

LANOXICAPS is a stable solution of digoxin enclosed within a soft gelatin capsule for oral use. Each capsule contains the labeled amount of digoxin USP dissolved in a solvent comprised of polyethylene glycol 400 USP, 8 percent ethyl alcohol, propylene glycol USP, and purified water USP. Inactive ingredients in the capsule shell include FD&C Red No. 40 (0.05 mg Capsule), D&C Yellow No. 10 (0.1 mg and 0.2 mg Capsules), FD&C Blue No. 1 (0.2 mg Capsule), gelatin, glycerin, methylparaben and propylparaben (added as preservatives), purified water and sorbitol. Capsules printed with edible ink.

CLINICAL PHARMACOLOGY

Mechanism of Action: The influence of digitalis glycosides on the myocardium is dose-related, and involves both a direct action on cardiac muscle and the specialized conduction system, and indirect actions on the cardiovascular system mediated by the autonomic nervous system. The indirect actions mediated by the autonomic nervous system involve a vagomimetic action, which is responsible for the effects of digitalis on the sino-atrial (SA) and atrioventricular (AV) nodes; and also a baroreceptor sensitization which results in increased carotid sinus nerve activity and enhanced sympathetic withdrawal for any given increment in mean arterial pressure. The pharmacologic consequences of these direct and indirect effects are: 1) an increase in the force and velocity of myocardial systolic contraction (positive inotropic action); 2) a slowing of heart rate (negative chronotropic effect); and 3) decreased conduction velocity through the AV node. In higher doses, digitalis increases sympathetic outflow from the central nervous system (CNS) to both cardiac and peripheral sympathetic nerves. This increase in sympathetic activity may be an important factor in digitalis cardiac toxicity. Most of the extracardiac manifestations of digitalis toxicity are also mediated by the CNS.

Pharmacokinetics:

Absorption: Gastrointestinal absorption of digoxin is a passive process. Absorption of digoxin from LANOXICAPS capsules has been demonstrated to be 90% to 100% complete compared to an identical intravenous dose of digoxin. Conventional digoxin tablets are absorbed 60% to 80%. The enhanced absorption from LANOXICAPS compared to digoxin tablets and elixir is associated with reduced between-patient and within-patient variability in steady-state serum concentrations. The peak serum concentrations are higher than those observed after tablets. When digoxin tablets or capsules are taken after meals, the rate of absorption is slowed, but the total amount of digoxin absorbed is usually unchanged. When taken with meals high in bran fiber, however, the amount absorbed from an oral dose may be reduced. Comparisons of the systemic availability and equivalent doses for digoxin preparations are shown in the following table:

[See table below.]

PRODUCT	BIOAVAILABILITY	EQUIVALENT DOSES (IN MG)*		
LANOXIN® Tablets	60% to 80%	0.125	0.25	0.5
LANOXIN Elixir	70% to 85%	0.125	0.25	0.5
LANOXIN Injection/I.M.	70% to 85%	0.125	0.25	0.5
LANOXIN Injection/I.V.	100%	0.1	0.2	0.4
LANOXICAPS® Capsules	90% to 100%	0.1	0.2	0.4

*1 mg = 1000 μg

In some patients, orally administered digoxin is converted to cardioinactive reduction products (e.g., dihydrodigoxin) by colonic bacteria in the gut. Data suggest that one in ten patients treated with digoxin tablets will degrade 40% or more of the ingested dose. This phenomenon is minimized with LANOXICAPS because they are rapidly absorbed in the upper gastrointestinal tract.

Distribution: Following drug administration, a 6 to 8 hour distribution phase is observed. This is followed by a much more gradual serum concentration decline, which is dependent on digoxin elimination from the body. The peak height and slope of the early portion (absorption/distribution phases) of the serum concentration-time curve are dependent upon the route of administration and the absorption characteristics of the formulation. Clinical evidence indicates that the early high serum concentrations (particularly high for digoxin capsules) do not reflect the concentration of digoxin at its site of action, but that with chronic use, the steady-state post-distribution serum levels are in equilibrium with tissue levels and correlate with pharmacologic effects. In individual patients, these post-distribution serum concentrations are linearly related to maintenance dosage and may be useful in evaluating therapeutic and toxic effects (see DOSAGE AND ADMINISTRATION: Serum Digoxin Concentrations).

Digoxin is concentrated in tissues and therefore has a large apparent volume of distribution. Digoxin crosses both the blood-brain barrier and the placenta. At delivery, serum digoxin concentration in the newborn is similar to the serum level in the mother. Approximately 20% to 25% of plasma digoxin is bound to protein. Serum digoxin concentrations are not significantly altered by large changes in fat tissue weight, so that its distribution space correlates best with lean (ideal) body weight, not total body weight.

Pharmacologic Response: The approximate times to onset of effect and to peak effect of all the LANOXIN and LANOXICAPS preparations are given in the following table:

[See table above.]

PRODUCT	TIME TO ONSET OF EFFECT*	TIME TO PEAK EFFECT*
LANOXIN® Tablets	0.5 to 2 hours	2 to 6 hours
LANOXIN Elixir	0.5 to 2 hours	2 to 6 hours
LANOXIN Injection/I.M.	0.5 to 2 hours	2 to 6 hours
LANOXIN Injection/I.V.	5 to 30 minutes†	1 to 4 hours
LANOXICAPS® Capsules	0.5 to 2 hours	2 to 6 hours

*Documented for ventricular response rate in atrial fibrillation, inotropic effect and electrocardiographic changes.

†Depending upon rate of infusion.

Excretion: Elimination of digoxin follows first-order kinetics (that is, the quantity of digoxin eliminated at any time is proportional to the total body content). Following intravenous administration to normal subjects, 50% to 70% of a digoxin dose is excreted unchanged in the urine. Renal excretion of digoxin is proportional to glomerular filtration rate and is largely independent of urine flow. In subjects with normal renal function, digoxin has a half-life of 1.5 to 2.0 days. The half-life in anuric patients is prolonged to 4 to 6 days. Digoxin is not effectively removed from the body by dialysis, exchange transfusion or during cardiopulmonary by-pass because most of the drug is in tissue rather than circulating in the blood.

INDICATIONS AND USAGE

Heart Failure: The increased cardiac output resulting from the inotropic action of digoxin ameliorates the disturbances characteristic of heart failure (venous congestion, edema, dyspnea, orthopnea, and cardiac asthma).

Digoxin is more effective in "low output" (pump) failure than in "high output" heart failure secondary to arteriovenous fistula, anemia, infection or hyperthyroidism.

Digoxin is usually continued after failure is controlled, unless some known precipitating factor is corrected. Studies have shown, however, that even though hemodynamic effects can be demonstrated in almost all patients, corresponding improvement in the signs and symptoms of heart failure is not necessarily apparent. Therefore, in patients in whom digoxin may be difficult to regulate, or in whom the risk of toxicity may be great (e.g., patients with unstable renal function or whose potassium levels tend to fluctuate) a cautious withdrawal of digoxin may be considered. If digoxin is discontinued, the patient should be regularly monitored for clinical evidence of recurrent heart failure.

Atrial Fibrillation: Digoxin reduces ventricular rate and thereby improves hemodynamics. Palpitation, precordial distress or weakness are relieved and concomitant congestive failure ameliorated. Digoxin should be continued in doses necessary to maintain the desired ventricular rate.

Atrial Flutter: Digoxin slows the heart and regular sinus rhythm may appear. Frequently the flutter is converted to atrial fibrillation with a controlled ventricular response. Digoxin treatment should be maintained if atrial fibrillation persists. (Electrical cardioversion is often the treatment of choice for atrial flutter. See discussion of cardioversion in PRECAUTIONS.)

Paroxysmal Atrial Tachycardia (PAT): Digoxin may convert PAT to sinus rhythm by slowing conduction through the AV node. If heart failure has ensued or paroxysms recur frequently, digoxin should be continued. In infants, digoxin is usually continued for 3 to 6 months after a single episode of PAT to prevent recurrence.

CONTRAINDICATIONS

Digitalis glycosides are contraindicated in ventricular fibrillation.

In a given patient, an untoward effect requiring permanent discontinuation of other digitalis preparations usually constitutes a contraindication to digoxin. Hypersensitivity to digoxin itself is a contraindication to its use. Allergy to digoxin, though rare, does occur. It may not extend to all such preparations, and another digitalis glycoside may be tried with caution.

WARNINGS

Digitalis alone or with other drugs has been used in the treatment of obesity. This use of digoxin or other digitalis glycosides is unwarranted. Moreover, since they may cause potentially fatal arrhythmias or other adverse effects, the

use of these drugs solely for the treatment of obesity is dangerous.

It is recommended that digoxin in soft capsules be administered in divided daily doses to minimize any potential adverse reactions, since peak serum digoxin concentrations resulting from the capsules are approximately twice those after bioequivalent tablet doses (400 μg of LANOXICAPS are bioequivalent to 500 μg of tablets). Studies are underway to determine if there are any increased risks associated with the higher peaks that occur with single daily dosing of soft gelatin capsules.

Anorexia, nausea, vomiting and arrhythmias may accompany heart failure or may be indications of digitalis intoxication. Clinical evaluation of the cause of these symptoms should be attempted before further digitalis administration. In such circumstances determination of the serum digoxin concentration may be an aid in deciding whether or not digitalis toxicity is likely to be present. If the possibility of digitalis intoxication cannot be excluded, cardiac glycosides should be temporarily withheld, if permitted by the clinical situation.

Patients with renal insufficiency require smaller than usual maintenance doses of digoxin (see DOSAGE AND ADMINISTRATION).

Heart failure accompanying acute glomerulonephritis requires extreme care in digitalization. Relatively low loading and maintenance doses and concomitant use of antihypertensive drugs may be necessary and careful monitoring is essential. Digoxin should be discontinued as soon as possible. Patients with severe carditis, such as carditis associated with rheumatic fever or viral myocarditis, are especially sensitive to digoxin-induced disturbances of rhythm.

Newborn infants display considerable variability in their tolerance to digoxin. Premature and immature infants are particularly sensitive, and dosage must not only be reduced but must be individualized according to their degree of maturity.

Note: Digitalis glycosides are an important cause of accidental poisoning in children.

PRECAUTIONS

General: Digoxin toxicity develops more frequently and lasts longer in patients with renal impairment because of the decreased excretion of digoxin. Therefore, it should be anticipated that dosage requirements will be decreased in patients with moderate to severe renal disease (see DOSAGE AND ADMINISTRATION section). Because of the prolonged half-life, a longer period of time is required to achieve an initial or new steady-state concentration in patients with renal impairment than in patients with normal renal function.

In patients with hypokalemia, toxicity may occur despite serum digoxin concentrations within the "normal range," because potassium depletion sensitizes the myocardium to digoxin. Therefore, it is desirable to maintain normal serum potassium levels in patients being treated with digoxin. Hypokalemia may result from diuretic, amphotericin B or corticosteroid therapy, and from dialysis or mechanical suction of gastrointestinal secretions. It may also accompany malnutrition, diarrhea, prolonged vomiting, old age and long-standing heart failure. In general, rapid changes in serum potassium or other electrolytes should be avoided, and intravenous treatment with potassium should be reserved for special circumstances as described below (see OVERDOSAGE: Treatment Of Arrhythmias Produced By Overdosage).

Calcium, particularly when administered rapidly by the intravenous route, may produce serious arrhythmias in digitalized patients. Hypercalcemia from any cause predisposes the patient to digitalis toxicity. On the other hand, hypocalcemia can nullify the effects of digoxin in man; thus, digoxin may be ineffective until serum calcium is restored to normal. These interactions are related to the fact that calcium affects contractility and excitability of the heart in a manner similar to digoxin.

Hypomagnesemia may predispose to digitalis toxicity. If low magnesium levels are detected in a patient on digoxin, replacement therapy should be instituted.

Quinidine, verapamil, amiodarone, propafenone, indomethacin, itraconazole, and alprazolam may cause a rise in serum digoxin concentration, with the implication that digitalis intoxication may result. This rise appears to be proportional to the dose. The effect is mediated by a reduction in the digoxin clearance and, in the case of quinidine, decreased volume of distribution as well.

Erythromycin and clarithromycin (and possibly other macrolide antibiotics) and tetracycline may increase digoxin absorption (see CLINICAL PHARMACOLOGY: Pharmacokinetics). Recent studies have shown that specific colonic bacteria in the lower gastrointestinal tract convert digoxin to cardioinactive reduction products, thereby reducing its bioavailability. Although inactivation of these bacteria by antibiotics is rapid, the serum digoxin concentration will rise at a rate consistent with the elimination half-life of digoxin. The magnitude of rise in serum digoxin concentration relates to the extent of bacterial inactivation, and may be as much as two-fold in some cases. This interaction is significantly reduced if digoxin is given as LANOXICAPS.

Patients with acute myocardial infarction or severe pulmonary disease may be unusually sensitive to digoxin-induced disturbances of rhythm.

Atrial arrhythmias associated with hypermetabolic states (e.g., hyperthyroidism) are particularly resistant to digoxin treatment. Large doses of digoxin are not recommended as the only treatment of these arrhythmias and care must be taken to avoid toxicity if large doses of digoxin are required. In hypothyroidism, the digoxin requirements are reduced. Digoxin responses in patients with compensated thyroid disease are normal.

Reduction of digoxin dosage may be desirable prior to electrical cardioversion to avoid induction of ventricular arrhythmias, but the physician must consider the consequences of rapid increase in ventricular response to atrial fibrillation if digoxin is withheld 1 to 2 days prior to cardioversion. If there is a suspicion that digitalis toxicity exists, elective cardioversion should be delayed. If it is not prudent to delay cardioversion, the energy level selected should be minimal at first and carefully increased in an attempt to avoid precipitating ventricular arrhythmias.

Incomplete AV block, especially in patients with Stokes-Adams attacks, may progress to advanced or complete heart block if digoxin is given.

In some patients with sinus node disease (i.e., Sick Sinus Syndrome), digoxin may worsen sinus bradycardia or sinoatrial block.

In patients with Wolff-Parkinson-White Syndrome and atrial fibrillation, digoxin can enhance transmission of impulses through the accessory pathway. This effect may result in extremely rapid ventricular rates and even ventricular fibrillation.

Digoxin may worsen the outflow obstruction in patients with idiopathic hypertrophic subaortic stenosis (IHSS). Unless cardiac failure is severe, it is doubtful whether digoxin should be employed.

Patients with chronic constrictive pericarditis may fail to respond to digoxin. In addition, slowing of the heart rate by digoxin in some patients may further decrease cardiac output.

Patients with heart failure from amyloid heart disease or constrictive cardiomyopathies respond poorly to treatment with digoxin.

Digoxin is not indicated for the treatment of sinus tachycardia unless it is associated with heart failure.

Digoxin may produce false positive ST-T changes in the electrocardiogram during exercise testing.

Intramuscular injection of digoxin is extremely painful and offers no advantages unless other routes of administration are contraindicated.

Laboratory Tests: Patients receiving digoxin should have their serum electrolytes and renal function (BUN and/or serum creatinine) assessed periodically; the frequency of assessments will depend on the clinical setting. For discussion of serum digoxin concentrations, see DOSAGE AND ADMINISTRATION.

Drug Interactions: Potassium-depleting *corticosteroids* and *diuretics* may be major contributing factors to digitalis toxicity. *Calcium*, particularly if administered rapidly by the intravenous route, may produce serious arrhythmias in digitalized patients. *Quinidine, verapamil, amiodarone, propafenone, indomethacin, itraconazole,* and *alprazolam* may cause a rise in serum digoxin concentration, with the implication that digitalis intoxication may result. Serum levels of digoxin may be increased by concomitant administration of *erythromycin* and *clarithromycin* (and possibly other *macrolide antibiotics*) and *tetracycline*. *Propantheline* and *diphenoxylate*, by decreasing gut motility, may increase digoxin absorption. *Antacids, kaolin-pectin, sulfasalazine, neomycin, cholestyramine*, and certain *anticancer drugs* may interfere with intestinal digoxin absorption, resulting in unexpectedly low serum concentrations. There have been inconsistent reports regarding the effects of other drugs on the serum digoxin concentration. *Thyroid* administration to a digitalized, hypothyroid patient may increase the dose requirement of digoxin. Concomitant use of digoxin and *sympathomimetics* increases the risk of cardiac arrhythmias, because both enhance ectopic pacemaker activity. *Succinylcholine* may cause a sudden extrusion of potassium from muscle cells, and may thereby cause arrhythmias in digitalized patients. Although β adrenergic blockers or calcium channel blockers and digoxin may be useful in combination to control atrial fibrillation, their additive effects on AV node conduction can result in complete heart block.

Due to the considerable variability of these interactions, digoxin dosage should be carefully individualized when patients receive coadministered medications. Furthermore, caution should be exercised when combining digoxin with any drug that may cause a significant deterioration in renal function, since this may impair the excretion of digoxin.

Carcinogenesis, Mutagenesis, Impairment of Fertility: There have been no long-term studies performed in animals to evaluate carcinogenic potential.

Pregnancy: *Teratogenic Effects:* Pregnancy Category C. Animal reproduction studies have not been conducted with digoxin. It is also not known whether digoxin can cause fetal

harm when administered to a pregnant woman or can affect reproduction capacity. Digoxin should be given to a pregnant woman only if clearly needed.

Nursing Mothers: Studies have shown that digoxin concentrations in the mother's serum and milk are similar. However, the estimated daily dose to a nursing infant will be far below the usual infant maintenance dose. Therefore, this amount should have no pharmacologic effect upon the infant. Nevertheless, caution should be exercised when digoxin is administered to a nursing woman.

ADVERSE REACTIONS

The frequency and severity of adverse reactions to digoxin depend on the dose and route of administration, as well as on the patient's underlying disease or concomitant therapies (see PRECAUTIONS and DOSAGE AND ADMINISTRATION: Serum Digoxin Concentrations). The overall incidence of adverse reactions has been reported as 5% to 20%, with 15% to 20% of them being considered serious (one to four percent of patients receiving digoxin). Evidence suggests that the incidence of toxicity has decreased since the introduction of the serum digoxin assay and improved standardization of digoxin tablets. Cardiac toxicity accounts for about one-half, gastrointestinal disturbances for about one-fourth, and CNS and other toxicity for about one-fourth of these adverse reactions.

Adults:

Cardiac: Unifocal or multiform ventricular premature contractions, especially in bigeminal or trigeminal patterns, are the most common arrhythmias associated with digoxin toxicity in adults with heart disease. Ventricular tachycardia may result from digitalis toxicity. Atrioventricular (AV) dissociation, accelerated junctional (nodal) rhythm and atrial tachycardia with block are also common arrhythmias caused by digoxin overdosage.

Excessive slowing of the pulse is a clinical sign of digoxin overdosage. AV block (Wenckebach) of increasing degree may proceed to complete heart block.

Note: The electrocardiogram is fundamental in determining the presence and nature of these cardiac disturbances. Digoxin may also induce other changes in the ECG (e.g., PR prolongation, ST depression), which represent digoxin effect and may or may not be associated with digitalis toxicity.

Gastrointestinal: Anorexia, nausea, vomiting and less commonly diarrhea are common early symptoms of overdosage. However, uncontrolled heart failure may also produce such symptoms. Digitalis toxicity very rarely may cause abdominal pain and hemorrhagic necrosis of the intestines.

CNS: Visual disturbances (blurred or yellow vision), headache, weakness, dizziness, apathy and psychosis can occur.

Other: Gynecomastia is occasionally observed. Maculopapular rash or other skin reactions are rarely observed.

Infants and Children: Toxicity differs from the adult in a number of respects. Anorexia, nausea, vomiting, diarrhea and CNS disturbances may be present but are rare as initial symptoms in infants. Cardiac arrhythmias are more reliable signs of toxicity. Digoxin in children may produce any arrhythmia. The most commonly encountered are conduction disturbances or supraventricular tachyarrhythmias, such as atrial tachycardia with or without block, and junctional (nodal) tachycardia. Ventricular arrhythmias are less common. Sinus bradycardia may also be a sign of impending digoxin intoxication, especially in infants, even in the absence of first degree heart block. Any arrhythmia or alteration in cardiac conduction that develops in a child taking digoxin should initially be assumed to be a consequence of digoxin intoxication.

OVERDOSAGE

Treatment of Arrhythmias Produced by Overdosage:

Adults: Digoxin should be discontinued until all signs of toxicity are gone. Discontinuation may be all that is necessary if toxic manifestations are not severe and appear only near the expected time for maximum effect of the drug.

Correction of factors that may contribute to toxicity such as electrolyte disturbances, hypoxia, acid-base disturbances and removal of aggravating agents such as catecholamines, should also be considered. Potassium salts may be indicated, particularly if hypokalemia is present. Potassium administration may be dangerous in the setting of massive digitalis overdosage (see Massive Digitalis Overdosage subsection below). Potassium chloride in divided oral doses totaling 3 to 6 grams of the salt (40 to 80 mEq K +) for adults may be given provided renal function is adequate (see below for potassium recommendations in Infants and Children).

When correction of the arrhythmia is urgent and the serum potassium concentration is low or normal, potassium should be administered intravenously in 5% dextrose injection. For adults, a total of 40 to 80 mEq (diluted to a concentration of 40 mEq per 500 mL) may be given at a rate not exceeding 20 mEq per hour or slower if limited by pain due to local irritation. Additional amounts may be given if the arrhythmia is uncontrolled and potassium well-tolerated. ECG monitoring

Continued on next page

Glaxo Wellcome—Cont.

should be performed to watch for any evidence of potassium toxicity (e.g., peaking of T waves) and to observe the effect on the arrhythmia. The infusion may be stopped when the desired effect is achieved.

Note: Potassium should not be used and may be dangerous in heart block due to digoxin, unless primarily related to supraventricular tachycardia.

Other agents that have been used for the treatment of digoxin intoxication include lidocaine, procainamide, propranolol; and phenytoin, although use of the latter must be considered experimental. In advanced heart block, atropine and/or temporary ventricular pacing may be beneficial. DIGIBIND®, Digoxin Immune Fab (Ovine), can be used to reverse potentially life-threatening digoxin (or digitoxin) intoxication. Improvement in signs and symptoms of digitalis toxicity usually begins within $^1/_2$ hour of DIGIBIND administration. Each 38 mg vial of DIGIBIND will neutralize 0.5 mg of digoxin (which is a usual body store of an adequately digitalized 70 kg patient).

Infants and Children: See Adult section for general recommendations for the treatment of arrhythmias produced by overdosage and for cautions regarding the use of potassium. If a potassium preparation is used to treat toxicity, it may be given orally in divided doses totaling 1 to 1.5 mEq K^+ per kilogram (kg) body weight (1 gram of potassium chloride contains 13.4 mEq K^+).

When correction of the arrhythmia with potassium is urgent, approximately 0.5 mEq/kg of potassium per hour may be given intravenously, with careful ECG monitoring. The intravenous solution of potassium should be dilute enough to avoid local irritation; however, especially in infants, care must be taken to avoid intravenous fluid overload.

Massive Digitalis Overdosage: Manifestations of life-threatening toxicity include severe ventricular arrhythmias such as ventricular tachycardia or ventricular fibrillation, or progessive bradyarrhythmias such as severe sinus bradycardia or second or third degree heart block not responsive to atropine. An overdosage of more than 10 mg of digoxin in previously healthy adults or 4 mg in previously healthy children or overdosage resulting in steady-state serum concentrations greater than 10 ng/mL, often results in cardiac arrest.

Severe digitalis intoxication can cause life-threatening elevation in serum potassium concentration by shifting potassium from inside to outside the cell resulting in hyperkalemia. Administration of potassium supplements in the setting of massive intoxication may be hazardous.

DIGIBIND, Digoxin Immune Fab (Ovine), may be used at a dose equimolar to digoxin in the body to reverse the effects of ingestion of a massive overdose. The decision to administer DIGIBIND before the onset of toxic manifestations will depend on the likelihood that life-threatening toxicity will occur (see above).

Patients with massive digitalis ingestion should receive large doses of activated charcoal to prevent absorption and bind digoxin in the gut during enteroenteric recirculation. Emesis or gastric lavage may be indicated especially if ingestion has occurred within 30 minutes of the patient's presentation at the hospital. Emesis should not be induced in patients who are obtunded. If a patient presents more than 2 hours after ingestion or already has toxic manifestations, it may be unsafe to induce vomiting or attempt passage of a gastric tube, because such maneuvers may induce an acute vagal episode that can worsen digitalis-toxic arrhythmias.

DOSAGE AND ADMINISTRATION

Recommended dosages are average values that may require considerable modification because of individual sensitivity or associated conditions. Diminished renal function is the most important factor requiring modification of recommended doses.

Due to the more complete absorption of digoxin from soft capsules, recommended oral doses are only 80 percent of those for Tablets, Elixir, and I.M. Injection.

Because the significance of the higher peak serum concentrations associated with once daily capsules is not established, divided daily dosing is presently recommended for:

1. Infants and children under 10 years of age;
2. Patients requiring a daily dose of 300 μg (0.3 mg) or greater;
3. Patients with a previous history of digitalis toxicity;
4. Patients considered likely to become toxic;
5. Patients in whom compliance is not a problem.

Where compliance is considered a problem, single daily dosing may be appropriate.

In deciding the dose of digoxin, several factors must be considered:

1. The disease being treated. Atrial arrhythmias may require larger doses than heart failure.
2. The body weight of the patient. Doses should be calculated based upon lean or ideal body weight.
3. The patient's renal function, preferably evaluated on the basis of creatinine clearance.
4. Age is an important factor in infants and children.
5. Concomitant disease states, drugs or other factors likely to alter the expected clinical response to digoxin (see PRECAUTIONS and Drug Interactions subsection).

Digitalization may be accomplished by either of two general approaches that vary in dosage and frequency of administration, but reach the same endpoint in terms of total amount of digoxin accumulated in the body.

1. Rapid digitalization may be achieved by administering a loading dose based upon projected peak body digoxin stores, then calculating the maintenance dose as a percentage of the loading dose.
2. More gradual digitalization may be obtained by beginning an appropriate maintenance dose, thus allowing digoxin body stores to accumulate slowly. Steady-state serum digoxin concentrations will be achieved in approximately 5 half-lives of the drug for the individual patient. Depending upon the patient's renal function, this will take between one and three weeks.

Adults:

Adults: Rapid Digitalization with a Loading Dose: Peak body digoxin stores of 8 to 12 μg/kg should provide therapeutic effect with minimum risk of toxicity in most patients with heart failure and normal sinus rhythm. Larger stores (10 to 15 μg/kg) are often required for adequate control of ventricular rate in patients with atrial flutter or fibrillation. Because of altered digoxin distribution and elimination, projected peak body stores for patients with renal insufficiency should be conservative (i.e., 6 to 10 μg/kg) (see PRECAUTIONS).

The loading dose should be based on the projected peak body stores and administered in several portions, with roughly half the total given as the first dose. Additional fractions of this planned total dose may be given at 6 to 8 hour intervals, **with careful assessment of clinical response before each additional dose.**

If the patient's clinical response necessitates a change from the calculated dose of digoxin, then calculation of the maintenance dose should be based upon the amount actually given.

In previously undigitalized patients, a single initial LANOXICAPS dose of 400 to 600 μg (0.4 to 0.6 mg) usually produces a detectable effect in 0.5 to 2 hours that becomes maximal in 2 to 6 hours. Additional doses of 100 to 300 μg (0.1 to 0.3 mg) may be given cautiously at 6 to 8 hour intervals until clinical evidence of an adequate effect is noted. The usual amount of LANOXICAPS that a 70 kg patient requires to achieve 8 to 15 μg/kg peak body stores is 600 to 1000 μg (0.6 to 1.0 mg).

Although peak body stores are mathematically related to loading doses and are utilized to calculate maintenance doses, they do not correlate with measured serum concentrations. This discrepancy is caused by digoxin distribution within the body during the first 6 to 8 hours following a dose. Serum concentrations drawn during this time are usually not interpretable.

Usual LANOXICAPS® Daily Maintenance Dose Requirements (μg) for Estimated Peak Body Stores of 10 μg/kg

		Lean Body Weight (kg/lbs)							
		50/110	60/132	70/154	80/176	90/198	100/220		
Corrected Ccr (mL/min per 70 kg)	0	50	100	100	100	150	150	22	Number of Days Before Steady-State Achieved
	10	100	100	100	150	150	150	19	
	20	100	100	150	150	150	200	16	
	30	100	150	150	150	200	200	14	
	40	100	150	150	200	200	250	13	
	50	150	150	200	200	250	250	12	
	60	150	150	200	200	250	300	11	
	70	150	200	200	250	250	300	10	
	80	150	200	200	250	300	300	9	
	90	150	200	250	250	300	350	8	
	100	200	200	250	300	300	350	7	

The maintenance dose should be based upon the percentage of the peak body stores lost each day through elimination. The following formula has had wide clinical use:

$$\text{Maintenance Dose} = \text{Peak Body Stores (i.e., Loading Dose)} \times \frac{\%\text{Daily Loss}}{100}$$

$$\text{Where: } \%\text{ Daily Loss} = 14 + \text{Ccr}/5$$

Ccr is creatinine clearance, corrected to 70 kg body weight or 1.73 m^2 body surface area. **For adults,** if only serum creatinine concentrations (Scr) are available, a Ccr (corrected to 70 kg body weight) may be estimated in men as (140 − Age)/Scr. For women, this result should be multiplied by 0.85.

Note: This equation cannot be used for estimating creatinine clearance in infants or children.

A common practice involves the use of LANOXIN Injection to achieve rapid digitalization, with conversion to LANOXICAPS or LANOXIN Tablets for maintenance therapy. If patients are switched from intravenous to oral digoxin formulations, allowances must be made for differences in bioavailability when calculating maintenance dosages (see Table, CLINICAL PHARMACOLOGY).

Adults: Gradual Digitalization with a Maintenance Dose: The following table provides average LANOXICAPS daily maintenance dose requirements for patients with heart failure based upon lean body weight and renal function:

[See table below.]

Example: Based on the above table, a patient in heart failure with an estimated lean body weight of 70 kg and a Ccr of 60 mL/min, should be given 200 μg (0.2 mg) of LANOXICAPS per day, usually taken as a 100 μg (0.1 mg) capsule after the morning and evening meals. Steady-state serum concentrations should not be anticipated before 11 days.

Infants and Children: Digitalization must be individualized. Divided daily dosing is recommended for infants and young children. In these patients, where dosage adjustment is frequent and outside the fixed dosages available, LANOXICAPS may not be the formulation of choice. Children over 10 years of age require adult dosages in proportion to their body weight.

In the newborn period, renal clearance of digoxin is diminished and suitable dosage adjustments must be observed. This is especially pronounced in the premature infant. Beyond the immediate newborn period, children generally require proportionally larger doses than adults on the basis of body weight or body surface area.

LANOXIN Injection Pediatric can be used to achieve rapid digitalization, with conversion to an oral LANOXIN formulation for maintenance therapy. If patients are switched from intravenous to oral digoxin tablets or elixir, allowances must be made for differences in bioavailability when calculating maintenance dosages (see bioavailability table in CLINICAL PHARMACOLOGY and dosing table below).

Intramuscular injection of digoxin is extremely painful and offers no advantages unless other routes of administration are contraindicated.

Digitalizing and daily maintenance doses for each age group are given below and should provide therapeutic effect with minimum risk of toxicity in most patients with heart failure and normal sinus rhythm. Larger doses are often required for adequate control of ventricular rate in patients with atrial flutter or fibrillation.

The loading dose should be administered in several portions, with roughly half the total given as the first dose. Additional fractions of this planned total dose may be given at 6 to 8 hour intervals, **with careful assessment of clinical response before each additional dose.** If the patient's clinical response necessitates a change from the calculated dose of digoxin, then calculation of the maintenance dose should be based upon the amount actually given.

[See table at top of next page.]

More gradual digitalization can also be accomplished by beginning an appropriate maintenance dose. The range of percentages provided above can be used in calculating this dose for patients with normal renal function. In children with renal disease, digoxin dosing must be carefully titrated based upon desired clinical response.

Long-term use of digoxin is indicated in many children who have been digitalized for acute heart failure, unless the cause is transient. Children with severe congenital heart disease, even after surgery, may require digoxin for prolonged periods.

It cannot be overemphasized that both the adult and pediatric dosage guidelines provided are based upon average patient response and substantial individual variation can be expected. Accordingly, ultimate dosage selection must be based upon clinical assessment of the patient.

Serum Digoxin Concentrations: Measurement of serum digoxin concentrations can be helpful to the clinician in determining the state of digitalization and in assigning certain probabilities to the likelihood of digoxin intoxication. Studies in adults considered adequately digitalized (without evidence of toxicity) show that about two-thirds of such patients have serum digoxin levels ranging from 0.8 to 2.0 ng/mL. Patients with atrial fibrillation or atrial flutter require and

Usual Digitalizing and Maintenance Dosages for LANOXICAPS® in Children with Normal Renal Function Based on Lean Body Weight

Age	Digitalizing* Dose (µg/kg)	Daily † Maintenance Dose (µg/kg)
2 to 5 Years	25 to 35	25% to 35% of the oral or I.V.
5 to 10 Years	15 to 30	loading dose ‡
Over 10 years	8 to 12	

*I.V. digitalizing doses are the same as LANOXICAPS digitalizing doses.
†Divided daily dosing is recommended for children under 10 years of age.
‡Projected or actual digitalizing dose providing desired clinical response.

appear to tolerate higher levels than do patients with other indications. On the other hand, in adult patients with clinical evidence of digoxin toxicity, about two-thirds will have serum digoxin levels greater than 2.0 ng/mL. Thus, whereas levels less than 0.8 ng/mL are infrequently associated with toxicity, levels greater than 2.0 ng/mL are often associated with toxicity. Values in between are not very helpful in deciding whether a certain sign or symptom is more likely caused by digoxin toxicity or by something else. There are rare patients who are unable to tolerate digoxin even at serum concentrations below 0.8 ng/mL. Some researchers suggest that infants and young children tolerate slightly higher serum concentrations than do adults.

To allow adequate time for equilibration of digoxin between serum and tissue, **sampling of serum concentrations for clinical use should be at least 6 to 8 hours after the last dose,** regardless of the route of administration or formulation used. On a twice daily dosing schedule, there will be only minor differences in serum digoxin concentrations whether sampling is done at 8 or 12 hours after a dose. After a single daily dose, the concentration will be 10% to 25% lower when sampled at 24 versus 8 hours, depending upon the patient's renal function. Ideally, sampling for assessment of steady-state concentrations should be done just before the next dose.

If a discrepancy exists between the reported serum concentration and the observed clinical response, the clinician should consider the following possibilities:

1. Analytical problems in the assay procedure.
2. Inappropriate serum sampling time.
3. Administration of a digitalis glycoside other than digoxin.
4. Conditions (described in WARNINGS and PRECAUTIONS) causing an alteration in the sensitivity of the patient to digoxin.
5. The patient falls outside the norm in his response to or handling of digoxin. This decision should only be reached after exclusion of the other possibilities and generally should be confirmed by additional correlations of clinical observations with serum digoxin concentrations.

The serum concentration data should always be interpreted in the overall clinical context and an isolated serum concentration value should not be used alone as a basis for increasing or decreasing digoxin dosage.

Adjustment of Maintenance Dose in Previously Digitalized Patients: LANOXICAPS maintenance doses in individual patients on steady-state digoxin can be adjusted upward or downward in proportion to the ratio of the desired versus the measured serum concentration. For example, a patient at steady-state on 100 µg (0.1 mg) of LANOXICAPS per day with a measured serum concentration of 0.7 ng/mL, should have the dose increased to 200 µg (0.2 mg) per day to achieve a steady-state serum concentration of 1.4 ng/mL, **assuming the serum digoxin concentration measurement is correct, renal function remains stable during this time and the needed adjustment is not the result of a problem with compliance.**

Dosage Adjustment When Changing Preparations: The absolute bioavailability of the capsule formulation is greater than that of the standard tablets and very near that of the intravenous dosage form. As a result the doses recommended for LANOXICAPS capsules are the same as those for LANOXIN Injection (see CLINICAL PHARMACOLOGY).

Adjustments in dosage will seldom be necessary when converting a patient from intravenous to LANOXICAPS formulation. The differences in bioavailability between injectable LANOXIN or LANOXICAPS, and LANOXIN Elixir Pediatric or LANOXIN Tablets must be considered when changing patients from one dosage form to another.

LANOXIN Injection and LANOXICAPS doses of 100 µg (0.1 mg) and 200 µg (0.2 mg) are approximately equivalent to 125 µg (0.125 mg) and 250 µg (0.25 mg) doses of LANOXIN Tablets and Elixir Pediatric (see Table in CLINICAL PHARMACOLOGY). Intramuscular injection of digoxin is extremely painful and offers no advantages unless other routes of administration are contraindicated.

HOW SUPPLIED

LANOXICAPS® (digoxin solution in capsules), 50 µg (0.05 mg): Bottle of 100 (NDC 0173-0270-55). Imprint A2C (red).
LANOXICAPS (digoxin solution in capsules), 100 µg (0.1 mg): Bottle of 100 (NDC 0173-0272-55). Imprint B2C (yellow).
LANOXICAPS (digoxin solution in capsules), 200 µg (0.2 mg): Bottle 100 (NDC 0173-0274-55). Imprint C2C (green).
Store at 15° to 25°C (59° to 77°F) in a dry place and protect from light.
Also Available:
LANOXIN® (digoxin) Tablets, Scored 125 µg (0.125 mg): bottles of 100 and 1000; unit dose pack of 100.
LANOXIN (digoxin) Tablets, Scored 250 µg (0.25 mg): bottles of 100, package of 12 bottles × 100 (with child-resistant cap), 1000 and 5000; unit dose pack of 100.
LANOXIN (digoxin) Elixir Pediatric, 50 µg (0.05 mg) per mL: bottle of 60 mL with calibrated dropper.
LANOXIN (digoxin) Injection, 500 µg (0.5 mg) in 2 mL (250 µg [0.25 mg] per mL): boxes of 10 and 20 ampuls.
LANOXIN (digoxin) Injection Pediatric, 100 µg (0.1 mg) in 1 mL: box of 10 ampuls.
February 1996/RL-274

Shown in Product Identification Guide, page 313

LANOXIN® Elixir Pediatric ℞

[lă-nŏx 'ĭn ″]
(digoxin)
50 µg (0.05 mg) per mL

DESCRIPTION

Digoxin is one of the cardiac (or digitalis) glycosides, a closely related group of drugs having in common specific effects on the myocardium. These drugs are found in a number of plants. Digoxin is extracted from the leaves of *Digitalis lanata*. The term "digitalis" is used to designate the whole group. The glycosides are composed of two portions: a sugar and a cardenolide (hence "glycosides").

Digoxin has the molecular formula $C_{41}H_{64}O_{14}$, a molecular weight of 780.95 and melting and decomposition points above 235°C. The drug is practically insoluble in water and in ether; slightly soluble in diluted (50%) alcohol and in chloroform; and freely soluble in pyridine. Digoxin powder is composed of odorless white crystals.

Digoxin has the chemical name: (3β,5β,12β)-3-[O-2,6-dideoxy-β-D-ribo-hexopyranosyl-(1→4)-O-2,6-dideoxy-β-D-ribo-hexopyranosyl-(1→4)-2,6-dideoxy-β-D-ribo-hexopyranosyl)oxy]-12,14-dihydroxycard-20(22)-enolide.

LANOXIN Elixir Pediatric is a stable solution of digoxin specially formulated for oral use in infants and children. Each mL contains 50 µg (0.05 mg) digoxin USP. The lime-flavored elixir contains the inactive ingredients alcohol 10%, methylparaben 0.1% (added as a preservative), citric acid, D&C Green No. 5 and Yellow No. 10, flavor, propylene glycol, sodium phosphate, and sucrose. Each package is supplied with a specially calibrated dropper to facilitate the administration of accurate dosage even in premature infants. Starting at 0.2 mL, this 1 mL dropper is marked in divisions of 0.1 mL, each corresponding to 5 µg (0.005 mg) digoxin.

CLINICAL PHARMACOLOGY

Mechanism of Action: The influence of digitalis glycosides on the myocardium is dose-related, and involves both a direct action on cardiac muscle and the specialized conduction system, and indirect actions on the cardiovascular system mediated by the autonomic nervous system. The indirect actions mediated by the autonomic nervous system involve a vago-mimetic action, which is responsible for the effects of digitalis on the sino-atrial (SA) and atrioventricular (AV) nodes; and also a baroreceptor sensitization which results in increased carotid sinus nerve activity and enhanced sympathetic withdrawal for any given increment in mean arterial pressure. The pharmacologic consequences of these direct and indirect effects are: 1) an increase in the force and velocity of myocardial systolic contraction (positive inotropic action); 2) a slowing of heart rate (negative chronotropic effect); and 3) decreased conduction velocity through the AV node. In higher doses, digitalis increases sympathetic outflow from the central nervous system (CNS) to both cardiac and peripheral sympathetic nerves. This increase in sympathetic activity may be an important factor in digitalis cardiac toxicity. Most of the extracardiac manifestations of digitalis toxicity are also mediated by the CNS.

Pharmacokinetics: Note: The following data are from studies performed in adults, unless otherwise stated.

Absorption: Gastrointestinal absorption of digoxin is a passive process. Absorption of digoxin from LANOXIN Elixir Pediatric formulation has been demonstrated to be 70% to 85% complete compared to an identical intravenous dose of digoxin. When the Elixir is taken after meals, the rate of absorption is slowed, but the total amount of digoxin absorbed is usually unchanged. When taken with meals high in bran fiber, however, the amount absorbed from an oral dose may be reduced. Comparisons of the systemic availability and equivalent doses for digoxin preparations are shown in the following table:
[See table below.]
In some patients, orally administered digoxin is converted to cardioinactive reduction products (e.g., dihydrodigoxin) by colonic bacteria in the gut. Data suggest that one in ten patients treated with digoxin tablets will degrade 40% or more of the ingested dose.

Distribution: Following drug administration, a 6 to 8 hour distribution phase is observed. This is followed by a much more gradual serum concentration decline, which is dependent on digoxin elimination from the body. The peak height and slope of the early portion (absorption/distribution phases) of the serum concentration-time curve are dependent upon the route of administration and the absorption characteristics of the formulation. Clinical evidence indicates that the early high serum concentrations do not reflect the concentration of digoxin at its site of action, but that with chronic use, the steady-state post-distribution serum levels are in equilibrium with tissue levels and correlate with pharmacologic effects. In individual patients, these post-distribution serum concentrations are linearly related to maintenance dosage and may be useful in evaluating therapeutic and toxic effects (see DOSAGE AND ADMINISTRATION: Serum Digoxin Concentrations).

Digoxin is concentrated in tissues and therefore has a large apparent volume of distribution. Digoxin crosses both the blood-brain barrier and the placenta. At delivery, serum digoxin concentration in the newborn is similar to the serum level in the mother. Approximately 20% to 25% of plasma digoxin is bound to protein. Serum digoxin concentrations are not significantly altered by large changes in fat tissue weight, so that its distribution space correlates best with lean (ideal) body weight, not total body weight.

Pharmacologic Response: The approximate times to onset of effect and to peak effect of all the LANOXIN preparations are given in the following table:
[See table at bottom of next page.]

Excretion: Elimination of digoxin follows first-order kinetics (that is, the quantity of digoxin eliminated at any time is proportional to the total body content). Following intravenous administration to normal subjects, 50% to 70% of a digoxin dose is excreted unchanged in the urine. Renal excretion of digoxin is proportional to glomerular filtration rate and is largely independent of urine flow. In subjects with normal renal function, digoxin has a half-life of 1.5 to 2.0 days. The half-life in anuric patients is prolonged to 4 to 6 days. Digoxin is not effectively removed from the body by dialysis, exchange transfusion or during cardiopulmonary by-pass because most of the drug is in tissue rather than circulating in the blood.

INDICATIONS AND USAGE

Heart Failure: The increased cardiac output resulting from the inotropic action of digoxin ameliorates the disturbances characteristic of heart failure (venous congestion, edema, dyspnea, orthopnea and cardiac asthma).

PRODUCT	ABSOLUTE BIOAVAILABILITY	EQUIVALENT DOSES (IN MG)*		
LANOXIN® Tablets	60% to 80%	0.125	0.25	0.5
LANOXIN Elixir	70% to 85%	0.125	0.25	0.5
LANOXIN Injection/I.M.	70% to 85%	0.125	0.25	0.5
LANOXIN Injection/I.V.	100%	0.1	0.2	0.4
LANOXICAPS® Capsules	90% to 100%	0.1	0.2	0.4

*1 mg = 1000 µg

Continued on next page

Glaxo Wellcome—Cont.

Digoxin is more effective in "low output" (pump) failure than in "high output" heart failure secondary to arteriovenous fistula, anemia, infection or hyperthyroidism.
Digoxin is usually continued after failure is controlled, unless some known precipitating factor is corrected. Studies have shown, however, that even though hemodynamic effects can be demonstrated in almost all patients, corresponding improvement in the signs and symptoms of heart failure is not necessarily apparent. Therefore, in patients in whom digoxin may be difficult to regulate, or in whom the risk of toxicity may be great (e.g., patients with unstable renal function or whose potassium levels tend to fluctuate), a cautious withdrawal of digoxin may be considered. If digoxin is discontinued, the patient should be regularly monitored for clinical evidence of recurrent heart failure.

Atrial Fibrillation: Digoxin reduces ventricular rate and thereby improves hemodynamics. Palpitation, precordial distress or weakness are relieved and concomitant congestive failure ameliorated. Digoxin should be continued in doses necessary to maintain the desired ventricular rate.

Atrial Flutter: Digoxin slows the heart and regular sinus rhythm may appear. Frequently the flutter is converted to atrial fibrillation with a controlled ventricular response. Digoxin treatment should be maintained if atrial fibrillation persists. (Electrical cardioversion is often the treatment of choice for atrial flutter. See discussion of cardioversion in PRECAUTIONS.)

Paroxysmal Atrial Tachycardia (PAT): Digoxin may convert PAT to sinus rhythm by slowing conduction through the AV node. If heart failure has ensued or paroxysms recur frequently, digoxin should be continued. In infants, digoxin is usually continued for 3 to 6 months after a single episode of PAT to prevent recurrence.

CONTRAINDICATIONS

Digitalis glycosides are contraindicated in ventricular fibrillation.
In a given patient, an untoward effect requiring permanent discontinuation of other digitalis preparations usually constitutes a contraindication to digoxin. Hypersensitivity to digoxin itself is a contraindication to its use. Allergy to digoxin, though rare, does occur. It may not extend to all such preparations, and another digitalis glycoside may be tried with caution.

WARNINGS

Anorexia, nausea, vomiting and arrhythmias may accompany heart failure or may be indications of digitalis intoxication. Clinical evaluation of the cause of these symptoms should be attempted before further digitalis administration. In such circumstances determination of the serum digoxin concentration may be an aid in deciding whether or not digitalis toxicity is likely to be present. If the possibility of digitalis intoxication cannot be excluded, cardiac glycosides should be temporarily withheld, if permitted by the clinical situation.
Patients with renal insufficiency require smaller than usual maintenance doses of digoxin (see DOSAGE AND ADMINISTRATION).
Heart failure accompanying acute glomerulonephritis requires extreme care in digitalization. Relatively low loading and maintenance doses and concomitant use of antihypertensive drugs may be necessary and careful monitoring is essential. Digoxin should be discontinued as soon as possible.
Patients with severe carditis, such as carditis associated with rheumatic fever or viral myocarditis, are especially sensitive to digoxin-induced disturbances of rhythm.
Newborn infants display considerable variability in their tolerance to digoxin. Premature and immature infants are particularly sensitive, and dosage must not only be reduced but must be individualized according to their degree of maturity.
Note: Digitalis glycosides are an important cause of accidental poisoning in children.

PRECAUTIONS

General: Digoxin toxicity develops more frequently and lasts longer in patients with renal impairment because of the decreased excretion of digoxin. Therefore, it should be anticipated that dosage requirements will be decreased in patients with moderate to severe renal disease (see DOSAGE AND ADMINISTRATION). Because of the prolonged half-life, a longer period of time is required to achieve an initial or new steady-state concentration in patients with renal impairment than in patients with normal renal function.
In patients with hypokalemia, toxicity may occur despite serum digoxin concentrations within the "normal range," because potassium depletion sensitizes the myocardium to digoxin. Therefore, it is desirable to maintain normal serum potassium levels in patients being treated with digoxin. Hypokalemia may result from diuretic, amphotericin B or corticosteroid therapy, and from dialysis or mechanical suction of gastrointestinal secretions. It may also accompany malnutrition, diarrhea, prolonged vomiting, old age, and long-standing heart failure. In general, rapid changes in serum potassium or other electrolytes should be avoided, and intravenous treatment with potassium should be reserved for special circumstances as described below (see OVERDOSAGE: Treatment of Arrhythmias Produced by Overdosage).
Calcium, particularly when administered rapidly by the intravenous route, may produce serious arrhythmias in digitalized patients. Hypercalcemia from any cause predisposes the patient to digitalis toxicity. On the other hand, hypocalcemia can nullify the effects of digoxin in humans; thus, digoxin may be ineffective until serum calcium is restored to normal. These interactions are related to the fact that calcium affects contractility and excitability of the heart in a manner similar to digoxin.
Hypomagnesemia may predispose to digitalis toxicity. If low magnesium levels are detected in a patient on digoxin, replacement therapy should be instituted.
Quinidine, verapamil, amiodarone, propafenone, indomethacin, itraconazole, and alprazolam may cause a rise in serum digoxin concentration, with the implication that digitalis intoxication may result. This rise appears to be proportional to the dose. The effect is mediated by a reduction in the digoxin clearance and, in the case of quinidine, decreased volume of distribution as well.
Erythromycin and clarithromycin (and possibly other macrolide antibiotics) and tetracycline may increase digoxin absorption (see CLINICAL PHARMACOLOGY: Pharmacokinetics). Recent studies have shown that specific colonic bacteria in the lower gastrointestinal tract convert digoxin to cardioinactive reduction products, thereby reducing its bioavailability. Although inactivation of these bacteria by antibiotics is rapid, the serum digoxin concentration will rise at a rate consistent with the elimination half-life of digoxin. The magnitude of rise in serum digoxin concentration relates to the extent of bacterial inactivation, and may be as much as two-fold in some cases.
Patients with acute myocardial infarction or severe pulmonary disease may be unusually sensitive to digoxin-induced disturbances of rhythm.
Atrial arrhythmias associated with hypermetabolic states (e.g., hyperthyroidism) are particularly resistant to digoxin treatment. Large doses of digoxin are not recommended as the only treatment of these arrhythmias and care must be taken to avoid toxicity if large doses of digoxin are required.
In hypothyroidism, the digoxin requirements are reduced. Digoxin responses in patients with compensated thyroid disease are normal.
Reduction of digoxin dosage may be desirable prior to electrical cardioversion to avoid induction of ventricular arrhythmias, but the physician must consider the consequences of rapid increase in ventricular response to atrial fibrillation if digoxin is withheld 1 to 2 days prior to cardioversion. If there is a suspicion that digitalis toxicity exists, elective cardioversion should be delayed. If it is not prudent to delay cardioversion, the energy level selected should be minimal at first and carefully increased in an attempt to avoid precipitating ventricular arrhythmias.
Incomplete AV block, especially in patients with Stokes-Adams attacks, may progress to advanced or complete heart block if digoxin is given.
In some patients with sinus node disease (i.e., Sick Sinus Syndrome), digoxin may worsen sinus bradycardia or sinoatrial block.
In patients with Wolff-Parkinson-White Syndrome and atrial fibrillation, digoxin can enhance transmission of impulses through the accessory pathway. This effect may result in extremely rapid ventricular rates and even ventricular fibrillation.
Digoxin may worsen the outflow obstruction in patients with idiopathic hypertrophic subaortic stenosis (IHSS). Unless cardiac failure is severe, it is doubtful whether digoxin should be employed.
Patients with chronic constrictive pericarditis may fail to respond to digoxin. In addition, slowing of the heart rate by digoxin in some patients may further decrease cardiac output.
Patients with heart failure from amyloid heart disease or constrictive cardiomyopathies respond poorly to treatment with digoxin.
Digoxin is not indicated for the treatment of sinus tachycardia unless it is associated with heart failure.
Digoxin may produce false positive ST-T changes in the electrocardiogram during exercise testing.
Intramuscular injection of digoxin is extremely painful and offers no advantages unless other routes of administration are contraindicated.

Laboratory Tests: Patients receiving digoxin should have their serum electrolytes and renal function (BUN and/or serum creatinine) assessed periodically; the frequency of assessments will depend on the clinical setting. For discussion of serum digoxin concentrations, see DOSAGE AND ADMINISTRATION section.

Drug Interactions: Potassium-depleting *corticosteroids* and *diuretics* may be major contributing factors to digitalis toxicity. *Calcium*, particularly if administered rapidly by the intravenous route, may produce serious arrhythmias in digitalized patients. *Quinidine, verapamil, amiodarone, propafenone, indomethacin, itraconazole,* and *alprazolam* may cause a rise in serum digoxin concentration, with the implication that digitalis intoxication may result. Serum levels of digoxin may be increased by concomitant administration of *erythromycin* and *clarithromycin* (and possibly other *macrolide antibiotics*) and *tetracycline. Propantheline* and *diphenoxylate*, by decreasing gut motility, may increase digoxin absorption. *Antacids, kaolin-pectin, sulfasalazine, neomycin, cholestyramine,* and *certain anticancer drugs* may interfere with intestinal digoxin absorption, resulting in unexpectedly low serum concentrations. There have been inconsistent reports regarding the effects of other drugs on the serum digoxin concentration. *Thyroid* administration to a digitalized, hypothyroid patient may increase the dose requirement of digoxin. Concomitant use of digoxin and *sympathomimetics* increases the risk of cardiac arrhythmias, because both enhance ectopic pacemaker activity. *Succinylcholine* may cause a sudden extrusion of potassium from muscle cells, and may thereby cause arrhythmias in digitalized patients. Although β adrenergic blockers or calcium channel blockers and digoxin may be useful in combination to control atrial fibrillation, their additive effects on AV node conduction can result in complete heart block.
Due to the considerable variability of these interactions, digoxin dosage should be carefully individualized when patients receive coadministered medications. Furthermore, caution should be exercised when combining digoxin with any drug that may cause a significant deterioration in renal function, since this may impair the excretion of digoxin.

Carcinogenesis, Mutagenesis, Impairment of Fertility: There have been no long-term studies performed in animals to evaluate carcinogenic potential.

ADVERSE REACTIONS

The frequency and severity of adverse reactions to digoxin depend on the dose and route of administration, as well as on the patient's underlying disease or concomitant therapies (see PRECAUTIONS and DOSAGE AND ADMINISTRATION: Serum Digoxin Concentrations). The overall incidence of adverse reactions has been reported as 5% to 20%, with 15% to 20% of them being considered serious (one to four percent of patients receiving digoxin). Evidence suggests that the incidence of toxicity has decreased since the introduction of the serum digoxin assay and improved standardization of digoxin tablets. Cardiac toxicity accounts for about one-half, gastrointestinal disturbances for about one-fourth, and CNS and other toxicity for about one-fourth of these adverse reactions.

Cardiac: Conduction disturbances or supraventricular tachyarrhythmias, such as atrioventricular (AV) block (Wenckebach), atrial tachycardia with or without block and junctional (nodal) tachycardia are the most common arrhythmias associated with digoxin toxicity in children. Ventricular arrhythmias, such as unifocal or multiform ventricular premature contractions, especially in bigeminal or trigeminal patterns, are less common. Ventricular tachycardia may result from digitalis toxicity. Sinus bradycardia may also be a sign of impending digoxin intoxication, especially in infants, even in the absence of first degree heart block. Any arrhythmias or alteration in cardiac conduction that develops in a child taking digoxin should initially be assumed to be a consequence of digoxin intoxication.
Note: The electrocardiogram is fundamental in determining the presence and nature of these cardiac disturbances. Digoxin may also induce other changes in the ECG (e.g., PR prolongation, ST depression), which represent digoxin effect and may or may not be associated with digitalis toxicity.

Gastrointestinal: Anorexia, nausea, vomiting, and diarrhea may be early symptoms of overdosage. However, uncon-

PRODUCT	TIME TO ONSET OF EFFECT*	TIME TO PEAK EFFECT*
LANOXIN® Tablets	0.5 to 2 hours	2 to 6 hours
LANOXIN Elixir	0.5 to 2 hours	2 to 6 hours
LANOXIN Injection/I.M.	0.5 to 2 hours	2 to 6 hours
LANOXIN Injection/I.V.	5 to 30 minutes†	1 to 4 hours
LANOXICAPS® Capsules	0.5 to 2 hours	2 to 6 hours

*Documented for ventricular response rate in atrial fibrillation, inotropic effect, and electrocardiographic changes.
†Depending upon rate of infusion.

trolled heart failure may also produce such symptoms. Digitalis toxicity very rarely may cause abdominal pain and hemorrhagic necrosis of the intestines.
CNS: Visual disturbances (blurred or yellow vision), headache, weakness, dizziness, apathy, and psychosis can occur. These may be difficult to recognize in infants and children.
Other: Gynecomastia is occasionally observed. Maculopapular rash or other skin reactions are rarely observed.

OVERDOSAGE

Treatment of Arrhythmias Produced by Overdosage: Digoxin should be discontinued until all signs of toxicity are gone. Discontinuation may be all that is necessary if toxic manifestations are not severe and appear only near the expected time for maximum effect of the drug.
Correction of factors that may contribute to toxicity such as electrolyte disturbances, hypoxia, acid-base disturbances and removal of aggravating agents such as catecholamines, should also be considered. Potassium salts may be indicated, particularly if hypokalemia is present. Potassium administration may be dangerous in the setting of massive digitalis overdosage (see Massive Digitalis Overdosage subsection below). Potassium chloride in divided oral doses totaling 1 to 1.5 mEq K+ per kilogram (kg) body weight may be given provided renal function is adequate (1 gram of potassium chloride contains 13.4 mEq K+).
When correction of the arrhythmia with potassium is urgent and the serum potassium concentration is low or normal, approximately 0.5 mEq/kg of potassium per hour may be given intravenously in 5% dextrose injection. The intravenous solution of potassium should be dilute enough to avoid local irritation; however, especially in infants, care must be taken to avoid intravenous fluid overload. ECG monitoring should be performed to watch for any evidence of potassium toxicity (e.g., peaking of T waves) and to observe the effect on the arrhythmia. The infusion may be stopped when the desired effect is achieved.
Note: Potassium should not be used and may be dangerous in heart block due to digoxin, unless primarily related to supraventricular tachycardia.
Other agents that have been used for the treatment of digoxin intoxication include lidocaine, procainamide, propranolol, and phenytoin, although use of the latter must be considered experimental. In advanced heart block, atropine and/or temporary ventricular pacing may be beneficial.
DIGIBIND®, Digoxin Immune Fab (Ovine), can be used to reverse potentially life-threatening digoxin (or digitoxin) intoxication. Improvement in signs and symptoms of digitalis toxicity usually begins within 1/2 hour of administration of DIGIBIND. Each 38 mg vial of DIGIBIND will neutralize 0.5 mg of digoxin (which is a usual body store of an adequately digitalized 70 kg patient).
Massive Digitalis Overdosage: Manifestations of life-threatening toxicity include severe ventricular arrhythmias such as ventricular tachycardia or ventricular fibrillation, or progressive bradyarrhythmias such as severe sinus bradycardia or second or third degree heart block not responsive to atropine. An overdosage of more than 10 mg of digoxin in previously healthy adults or 4 mg in previously healthy children or overdosage resulting in steady-state serum concentrations greater than 10 ng/mL, often results in cardiac arrest.
Severe digitalis intoxication can cause life-threatening elevation in serum potassium concentration by shifting potassium from inside to outside the cell resulting in hyperkalemia. Administration of potassium supplements in the setting of massive intoxication may be hazardous.
DIGIBIND, Digoxin Immune Fab (Ovine), may be used at a dose equimolar to digoxin in the body to reverse the effects of ingestion of a massive overdose. The decision to administer DIGIBIND before the onset of toxic manifestations will depend on the likelihood that life-threatening toxicity will occur (see above).
Patients with massive digitalis ingestion should receive large doses of activated charcoal to prevent absorption and bind digoxin in the gut during enteroenteric recirculation. Emesis or gastric lavage may be indicated especially if ingestion has occurred within 30 minutes of the patient's presentation at the hospital. Emesis should not be induced in patients who are obtunded. If a patient presents more than 2 hours after ingestion or already has toxic manifestations, it may be unsafe to induce vomiting or attempt passage of a gastric tube, because such maneuvers may induce an acute vagal episode that can worsen digitalis-toxic arrhythmias.

DOSAGE AND ADMINISTRATION

Recommended dosages are average values that may require considerable modification because of individual sensitivity or associated conditions. Diminished renal function is the most important factor requiring modification of recommended doses.
Adults: See the LANOXIN Tablets package insert for specific recommendations.
Infants and Children: Digitalization must be individualized. Divided daily dosing is recommended for infants and young children. Children over 10 years of age require adult dosages in proportion to their body weight.
In the newborn period, renal clearance of digoxin is diminished and suitable dosage adjustments must be observed. This is especially pronounced in the premature infant. Beyond the immediate newborn period, children generally require proportionally larger doses than adults on the basis of body weight or body surface area.
In deciding the dose of digoxin, several factors must be considered:

1. The disease being treated. Atrial arrhythmias may require larger doses than heart failure.
2. The body weight of the patient. Doses should be calculated based upon lean or ideal body weight.
3. The patient's renal function, preferably evaluated on the basis of creatinine clearance.
4. Age is an important factor in infants and children.
5. Concomitant disease states, drugs or other factors likely to alter the expected clinical response to digoxin (see PRECAUTIONS and Drug Interactions subsection).

Digitalization may be accomplished by either of two general approaches that vary in dosage and frequency of administration, but reach the same endpoint in terms of total amount of digoxin accumulated in the body.

1. Rapid digitalization may be achieved by administering a loading dose based upon projected peak body digoxin stores, then calculating the maintenance dose as a percentage of the loading dose.
2. More gradual digitalization may be obtained by beginning an appropriate maintenance dose, thus allowing digoxin body stores to accumulate slowly. Steady-state serum digoxin concentrations will be achieved in approximately 5 half-lives of the drug for the individual patient. Depending upon the patient's renal function, this will take between 1 and 3 weeks.

Infants and Children: Rapid Digitalization With a Loading Dose: LANOXIN Injection Pediatric can be used to achieve rapid digitalization, with conversion to an oral formulation of LANOXIN for maintenance therapy. If patients are switched from intravenous to oral digoxin tablets or elixir, allowances must be made for differences in bioavailability when calculating maintenance dosages (see bioavailability table in CLINICAL PHARMACOLOGY and dosing table below).
Intramuscular injection of digoxin is extremely painful and offers no advantages unless other routes of administration are contraindicated.
Digitalizing and daily maintenance doses for each age group are given below and should provide therapeutic effect with minimum risk of toxicity in most patients with heart failure and normal sinus rhythm. Larger doses are often required for adequate control of ventricular rate in patients with atrial flutter or fibrillation.
The loading dose should be administered in several portions, with roughly half the total given as the first dose. Additional fractions of this planned total dose may be given at 6 to 8 hour intervals, **with careful assessment of clinical response before each additional dose.** If the patient's clinical response necessitates a change from the calculated dose of digoxin, then calculation of the maintenance dose should be based upon the amount actually given.
[See table above.]

Usual Digitalizing and Maintenance Dosages for LANOXIN® Elixir Pediatric in Children with **Normal Renal Function Based on Lean Body Weight**

Age	Digitalizing* Dose (μg/kg)	Daily† Maintenance Dose (μg/kg)
Premature	20 to 30	20% to 30% of *oral* loading dose‡
Full Term	25 to 35	25% to 35% of *oral* loading dose‡
1 to 24 Months	35 to 60	
2 to 5 Years	30 to 40	
5 to 10 Years	20 to 35	
Over 10 Years	10 to 15	

*I.V. digitalizing doses are 80% of oral digitalizing doses.
†Divided daily dosing is recommended for children under 10 years of age.
‡Projected or actual digitalizing dose providing clinical response.

Infants and Children: Gradual Digitalization With A Maintenance Dose: More gradual digitalization can also be accomplished by beginning an appropriate maintenance dose. The range of percentages provided above can be used in calculating this dose for patients with normal renal function. In children with renal disease, digoxin dosing must be carefully titrated based upon desired clinical reponse.
Long-term use of digoxin is indicated in many children who have been digitalized for acute heart failure, unless the cause is transient. Children with severe congenital heart disease, even after surgery, may require digoxin for prolonged periods.
It cannot be overemphasized that these pediatric dosage guidelines are based upon average patient response and substantial individual variation can be expected. Accordingly, ultimate dosage selection must be based upon clinical assessment of the patient.
Serum Digoxin Concentrations: Measurement of serum digoxin concentrations can be helpful to the clinician in determining the state of digitalization and in assigning certain probabilities to the likelihood of digoxin intoxication. Studies in adults considered adequately digitalized (without evidence of toxicity) show that about two-thirds of such patients have serum digoxin levels ranging from 0.8 to 2.0 ng/mL. Patients with atrial fibrillation or atrial flutter require and appear to tolerate higher levels than do patients with other indications. On the other hand, in adult patients with clinical evidence of digoxin toxicity, about two-thirds will have serum digoxin levels greater than 2.0 ng/mL. Thus, whereas levels less than 0.8 ng/mL are infrequently associated with toxicity, levels greater than 2.0 ng/mL are often associated with toxicity. Values in between are not very helpful in deciding whether a certain sign or symptom is more likely caused by digoxin toxicity or by something else. There are rare patients who are unable to tolerate digoxin even at serum concentrations below 0.8 ng/mL. Some researchers suggest that infants and young children tolerate slightly higher serum concentrations than do adults.
To allow adequate time for equilibration of digoxin between serum and tissue, **sampling of serum concentrations for clinical use should be at least 6 to 8 hours after the last dose,** regardless of the route of administration or formulation used. On a twice daily dosing schedule, there will be only minor differences in serum digoxin concentrations whether sampling is done at 8 or 12 hours after a dose. After a single daily dose, the concentration will be 10% to 25% lower when sampled at 24 versus 8 hours, depending upon the patient's renal function. Ideally, sampling for assessment of steady-state concentrations should be done just before the next dose.
If a discrepancy exists between the reported serum concentration and the observed clinical response, the clinician should consider the following possibilities:

1. Analytical problems in the assay procedure.
2. Inappropriate serum sampling time.
3. Administration of a digitalis glycoside other than digoxin.
4. Conditions (described in WARNINGS and PRECAUTIONS) causing an alteration in the sensitivity of the patient to digoxin.
5. The patient falls outside the norm in his response to or handling of digoxin. This decision should only be reached after exclusion of the other possibilities and generally should be confirmed by additional correlations of clinical observations with serum digoxin concentrations.

The serum concentration data should always be interpreted in the overall clinical context and an isolated serum concentration value should not be used alone as a basis for increasing or decreasing digoxin dosage.
Adjustment of Maintenance Dose in Previously Digitalized Patients: LANOXIN Elixir Pediatric maintenance doses in individual patients on steady-state digoxin can be adjusted upward or downward in proportion to the ratio of the desired versus the measured serum concentration. For example, a patient at steady-state on 125 μg (0.125 mg) of LANOXIN Elixir per day with a measured serum concentration of 0.7 ng/mL, should have the dose increased to 250 μg (0.250 mg) per day to achieve a steady-state serum concentration of 1.4 ng/mL, **assuming the serum digoxin concentration measurement is correct, renal function remains stable during this time and the needed adjustment is not the result of a problem with compliance.**
Dosage Adjustment When Changing Preparations: The differences in bioavailability between injectable LANOXIN or LANOXICAPS® and LANOXIN Elixir Pediatric or LANOXIN Tablets must be considered when changing patients from one dosage form to another.
LANOXIN Injection and LANOXICAPS doses of 100 μg (0.1 mg) and 200 μg (0.2 mg) are approximately equivalent to 125

Continued on next page

Glaxo Wellcome—Cont.

μg (0.125 mg) and 250 μg (0.25 mg) doses of LANOXIN Elixir Pediatric and LANOXIN Tablets (see table in CLINICAL PHARMACOLOGY section). Intramuscular injection of digoxin is extremely painful and offers no advantages unless other routes of administration are contraindicated.

HOW SUPPLIED
LANOXIN (digoxin) Elixir Pediatric, 50 μg (0.05 mg) per mL; Bottle of 60 mL with calibrated dropper. (NDC 0173-0264-27). Store at 15° to 25°C (59° to 77°F) and protect from light.
Also Available:
LANOXIN (digoxin) Tablets, Scored 125 μg (0.125 mg): bottles of 100 and 1000; unit dose pack of 100.
LANOXIN (digoxin) Tablets, Scored 250 μg (0.25 mg): bottles of 100, package of 12 bottles × 100 (with child-resistant cap), 1000 and 5000; unit dose pack of 100.
LANOXIN (digoxin) Injection, 500 μg (0.5 mg) in 2 mL (250 μg [0.25 mg] per mL): boxes of 10 and 50 ampuls.
LANOXIN (digoxin) Injection Pediatric, 100 μg (0.1 mg) in 1 mL: box of 10 ampuls.
LANOXICAPS (digoxin solution in capsules), 50 μg (0.05 mg) bottle of 100; 100 μg (0.1 mg) bottles of 100; 200 μg (0.2 mg) bottle of 100.
February 1996/RL-254

Shown in Product Identification Guide, page 313

LANOXIN®
[lă-nŏx'ĭn"]
(digoxin)
Injection
500 μg (0.5 mg) in 2 mL (250 μg [0.25 mg] per mL)

DESCRIPTION
Digoxin is one of the cardiac (or digitalis) glycosides, a closely related group of drugs having in common specific effects on the myocardium. These drugs are found in a number of plants. Digoxin is extracted from the leaves of *Digitalis lanata*. The term "digitalis" is used to designate the whole group. The glycosides are composed of two portions: a sugar and a cardenolide (hence "glycosides").
Digoxin has the molecular formula $C_{41}H_{64}O_{14}$, a molecular weight of 780.95 and melting and decomposition points above 235°C. The drug is practically insoluble in water and in ether; slightly soluble in diluted (50%) alcohol and in chloroform; and freely soluble in pyridine. Digoxin powder is composed of odorless white crystals.
Digoxin has the chemical name: (3β,5β,12β)-3-[(O-2,6-dideoxy-β-D-ribo -hexopyranosyl-(1→4)-O-2,6-dideoxy-β-D-ribo-hexopyranosyl-(1→4)-2,6-dideoxy-β-D-ribo--hexopyranosyl) oxy]-12,14-dihydroxycard-20(22)-enolide.
LANOXIN (digoxin) Injection is a sterile solution of digoxin for intravenous or intramuscular injection. The vehicle contains 40% propylene glycol and 10% alcohol. The injection is buffered to a pH of 6.8 to 7.2 with 0.17% sodium phosphate and 0.08% anhydrous citric acid. Each 2 mL ampul contains 500 μg (0.5 mg) digoxin (250 μg [0.25 mg] per mL). Dilution is not required.

CLINICAL PHARMACOLOGY
Mechanism of Action: The influence of digitalis glycosides on the myocardium is dose-related, and involves both a direct action on cardiac muscle and the specialized conduction system, and indirect actions on the cardiovascular system mediated by the autonomic nervous system. The indirect actions mediated by the autonomic nervous system involve a vagomimetic action, which is responsible for the effects of digitalis on the sino-atrial (SA) and atrioventricular (AV) nodes; and also a baroreceptor sensitization which results in increased carotid sinus nerve activity and enhanced sympathetic withdrawal for any given increment in mean arterial pressure. The pharmacologic consequences of these direct and indirect effects are: 1) an increase in the force and velocity of myocardial systolic contraction (positive inotropic action); 2) a slowing of heart rate (negative chronotropic effect); and 3) decreased conduction velocity through the AV node. In higher doses, digitalis increases sympathetic outflow from the central nervous system (CNS) to both sympathetic and peripheral sympathetic nerves. This increase in sympathetic activity may be an important factor in digitalis cardiac toxicity. Most of the extracardiac manifestations of digitalis toxicity are also mediated by the CNS.
Pharmacokinetics:
Absorption: A comparison of the systemic availability and equivalent doses for digoxin preparations are shown in the following table:
[See table above.]
Distribution: Following drug administration, a 6 to 8 hour distribution phase is observed. This is followed by a much more gradual serum concentration decline, which is dependent on digoxin elimination from the body. The peak height

PRODUCT	TIME TO ONSET OF EFFECT*	TIME TO PEAK EFFECT*
LANOXIN® Tablets	0.5 to 2 hours	2 to 6 hours
LANOXIN Elixir	0.5 to 2 hours	2 to 6 hours
LANOXIN Injection/I.M.	0.5 to 2 hours	2 to 6 hours
LANOXIN Injection/I.V.	5 to 30 minutes†	1 to 4 hours
LANOXICAPS Capsules	0.5 to 2 hours	2 to 6 hours

*Documented for ventricular response rate in atrial fibrillation, inotropic effect and electrocardiographic changes.
†Depending upon rate of infusion.

and slope of the early portion (absorption/distribution phases) of the serum concentration-time curve are dependent upon the route of administration and the absorption characteristics of the formulation. Clinical evidence indicates that the early high serum concentrations do not reflect the concentration of digoxin at its site of action, but that with chronic use, the steady-state post-distribution serum levels are in equilibrium with tissue levels and correlate with pharmacologic effects. In individual patients, these post-distribution serum concentrations are linearly related to maintenance dosage and may be useful in evaluating therapeutic and toxic effects (see: DOSAGE AND ADMINISTRATION: Serum Digoxin Concentrations).
Digoxin is concentrated in tissues and therefore has a large apparent volume of distribution. Digoxin crosses both the blood-brain barrier and the placenta. At delivery, serum digoxin concentration in the newborn is similar to the serum level in the mother. Approximately 20% to 25% of plasma digoxin is bound to protein. Serum digoxin concentrations are not significantly altered by large changes in fat tissue weight, so that its distribution space correlates best with lean (ideal) body weight, not total body weight.
Pharmacologic Response: The approximate times to onset of effect and to peak effect of all the preparations of LANOXIN are given in the following table:
[See table below.]
Excretion: Elimination of digoxin follows first-order kinetics (that is, the quantity of digoxin eliminated at any time is proportional to the total body content). Following intravenous administration to normal subjects, 50% to 70% of a digoxin dose is excreted unchanged in the urine. Renal excretion of digoxin is proportional to glomerular filtration rate and is largely independent of urine flow. In subjects with normal renal function, digoxin has a half-life of 1.5 to 2.0 days. The half-life in anuric patients is prolonged to 4 to 6 days. Digoxin is not effectively removed from the body by dialysis, exchange transfusion, or during cardiopulmonary by-pass because most of the drug is in tissue rather than circulating in the blood.

INDICATIONS AND USAGE
Heart Failure: The increased cardiac output resulting from the inotropic action of digoxin ameliorates the disturbances characteristic of heart failure (venous congestion, edema, dyspnea, orthopnea, and cardiac asthma).
Digoxin is more effective in "low output" (pump) failure than in "high output" heart failure secondary to arteriovenous fistula, anemia, infection or hyperthyroidism.
Digoxin is usually continued after failure is controlled, unless some known precipitating factor is corrected. Studies have shown, however, that even though hemodynamic effects can be demonstrated in almost all patients, corresponding improvement in the signs and symptoms of heart failure is not necessarily apparent. Therefore, in patients in whom digoxin may be difficult to regulate, or in whom the risk of toxicity may be great (e.g., patients with unstable renal function or whose potassium levels tend to fluctuate) a cautious withdrawal of digoxin may be considered. If digoxin is discontinued, the patient should be regularly monitored for clinical evidence of recurrent heart failure.
Atrial Fibrillation: Digoxin reduces ventricular rate and thereby improves hemodynamics. Palpitation, precordial distress or weakness are relieved and concomitant congestive failure ameliorated. Digoxin should be continued in doses necessary to maintain the desired ventricular rate.
Atrial Flutter: Digoxin slows the heart and regular sinus rhythm may appear. Frequently the flutter is converted to atrial fibrillation with a controlled ventricular response. Digoxin treatment should be maintained if atrial fibrillation persists. (Electrical cardioversion is often the treatment of choice for atrial flutter. See discussion of cardioversion in PRECAUTIONS.)

Paroxysmal Atrial Tachycardia (PAT): Digoxin may convert PAT to sinus rhythm by slowing conduction through the AV node. If heart failure has ensued or paroxysms recur frequently, digoxin should be continued. In infants, digoxin is usually continued for 3 to 6 months after a single episode of PAT to prevent recurrence.

CONTRAINDICATIONS
Digitalis glycosides are contraindicated in ventricular fibrillation.
In a given patient, an untoward effect requiring permanent discontinuation of other digitalis preparations usually constitutes a contraindication to digoxin. Hypersensitivity to digoxin itself is a contraindication to its use. Allergy to digoxin, though rare, does occur. It may not extend to all such preparations, and another digitalis glycoside may be tried with caution.

WARNINGS
Digitalis alone or with other drugs has been used in the treatment of obesity. This use of digoxin or other digitalis glycosides is unwarranted. Moreover, since they may cause potentially fatal arrhythmias or other adverse effects, the use of these drugs solely for the treatment of obesity is dangerous. Anorexia, nausea, vomiting and arrhythmias may accompany heart failure or may be indications of digitalis intoxication. Clinical evaluation of the cause of these symptoms should be attempted before further digitalis administration. In such circumstances determination of the serum digoxin concentration may be an aid in deciding whether or not digitalis toxicity is likely to be present. If the possibility of digitalis intoxication cannot be excluded, cardiac glycosides should be temporarily withheld, if permitted by the clinical situation.
Patients with renal insufficiency require smaller than usual maintenance doses of digoxin (see DOSAGE AND ADMINISTRATION).
Heart failure accompanying acute glomerulonephritis requires extreme care in digitalization. Relatively low loading and maintenance doses and concomitant use of antihypertensive drugs may be necessary and careful monitoring is essential. Digoxin should be discontinued as soon as possible. Patients with severe carditis, such as carditis associated with rheumatic fever or viral myocarditis, are especially sensitive to digoxin-induced disturbances of rhythm.
Newborn infants display considerable variability in their tolerance to digoxin. Premature and immature infants are particularly sensitive, and dosage must not only be reduced but must be individualized according to their degree of maturity.
Note: Digitalis glycosides are an important cause of accidental poisoning in children.

PRECAUTIONS
General: Digoxin toxicity develops more frequently and lasts longer in patients with renal impairment because of the decreased excretion of digoxin. Therefore, it should be anticipated that dosage requirements will be decreased in patients with moderate to severe renal disease (see DOSAGE AND ADMINISTRATION). Because of the prolonged half-life, a longer period of time is required to achieve an initial or new steady-state concentration in patients with renal impairment than in patients with normal renal function.
In patients with hypokalemia, toxicity may occur despite serum digoxin concentrations within the "normal range," because potassium depletion sensitizes the myocardium to digoxin. Therefore, it is desirable to maintain normal serum potassium levels in patients being treated with digoxin. Hypokalemia may result from diuretic, amphotericin B or corticosteroid therapy, and from dialysis or mechanical suction of gastrointestinal secretions. It may also accompany malnutrition, diarrhea, prolonged vomiting, old age

PRODUCT	ABSOLUTE BIOAVAILABILITY	EQUIVALENT DOSES (IN MG)*		
LANOXIN® Tablets	60% to 80%	0.125	0.25	0.5
LANOXIN Elixir	70% to 85%	0.125	0.25	0.5
LANOXIN Injection/I.M.	70% to 85%	0.125	0.25	0.5
LANOXIN Injection/I.V.	100%	0.1	0.2	0.4
LANOXICAPS® Capsules	90% to 100%	0.1	0.2	0.4

*1 mg = 1000 μg

and long-standing heart failure. In general, rapid changes in serum potassium or other electrolytes should be avoided, and intravenous treatment with potassium should be reserved for special circumstances as described below (see OVERDOSAGE: Treatment of Arrhythmias Produced by Overdosage). Calcium, particularly when administered rapidly by the intravenous route, may produce serious arrhythmias in digitalized patients. Hypercalcemia from any cause predisposes the patient to digitalis toxicity. On the other hand, hypocalcemia can nullify the effects of digoxin in man; thus, digoxin may be ineffective until serum calcium is restored to normal. These interactions are related to the fact that calcium affects contractility and excitability of the heart in a manner similar to digoxin.

Hypomagnesemia may predispose to digitalis toxicity. If low magnesium levels are detected in a patient on digoxin, replacement therapy should be instituted.

Quinidine, verapamil, amiodarone, propafenone, indomethacin, itraconazole, and alprazolam may cause a rise in serum digoxin concentration, with the implication that digitalis intoxication may result. This rise appears to be proportional to the dose. The effect is mediated by a reduction in the digoxin clearance and, in the case of quinidine, decreased volume of distribution as well.

Patients with acute myocardial infarction or severe pulmonary disease may be unusually sensitive to digoxin-induced disturbances of rhythm.

Atrial arrhythmias associated with hypermetabolic states (e.g., hyperthyroidism) are particularly resistant to digoxin treatment. Large doses of digoxin are not recommended as the only treatment of these arrhythmias and care must be taken to avoid toxicity if large doses of digoxin are required.

In hypothyroidism, the digoxin requirements are reduced. Digoxin responses in patients with compensated thyroid disease are normal.

Reduction of digoxin dosage may be desirable prior to electrical cardioversion to avoid induction of ventricular arrhythmias, but the physician must consider the consequences of rapid increase in ventricular response to atrial fibrillation if digoxin is withheld 1 to 2 days prior to cardioversion. If there is a suspicion that digitalis toxicity exists, elective cardioversion should be delayed. If it is not prudent to delay cardioversion, the energy level selected should be minimal at first and carefully increased in an attempt to avoid precipitating ventricular arrhythmias.

Incomplete AV block, especially in patients with Stokes-Adams attacks, may progress to advanced or complete heart block if digoxin is given.

In some patients with sinus node disease (i.e., Sick Sinus Syndrome), digoxin may worsen sinus bradycardia or sino-atrial block.

In patients with Wolff-Parkinson-White Syndrome and atrial fibrillation, digoxin can enhance transmission of impulses through the accessory pathway. This effect may result in extremely rapid ventricular rates and even ventricular fibrillation.

Digoxin may worsen the outflow obstruction in patients with idiopathic hypertrophic subaortic stenosis (IHSS). Unless cardiac failure is severe, it is doubtful whether digoxin should be employed.

Patients with chronic constrictive pericarditis may fail to respond to digoxin. In addition, slowing of the heart rate by digoxin in some patients may further decrease cardiac output.

Patients with heart failure from amyloid heart disease or constrictive cardiomyopathies respond poorly to treatment with digoxin.

Digoxin is not indicated for the treatment of sinus tachycardia unless it is associated with heart failure.

Digoxin may produce false positive ST-T changes in the electrocardiogram during exercise testing.

Intramuscular injection of digoxin is extremely painful and offers no advantages unless other routes of administration are contraindicated.

Laboratory Tests: Patients receiving digoxin should have their serum electrolytes and renal function (BUN and/or serum creatinine) assessed periodically; the frequency of assessments will depend on the clinical setting. For discussion of serum digoxin concentrations, see DOSAGE AND ADMINISTRATION section.

Drug Interactions: Potassium-depleting *corticosteroids* and *diuretics* may be major contributing factors to digitalis toxicity. *Calcium*, particularly if administered rapidly by the intravenous route, may produce serious arrhythmias in digitalized patients. *Quinidine, verapamil, amiodarone, propafenone, indomethacin, itraconazole,* and *alprazolam* may cause a rise in serum digoxin concentration, with the implication that digitalis intoxication may result. Serum levels of digoxin may be increased by concomitant administration of *erythromycin* and *clarithromycin* (and possible other *macrolide antibiotics*) and *tetracycline*. *Propantheline* and *diphenoxylate*, by decreasing gut motility, may increase digoxin absorption. *Antacids, kaolin-pectin, sulfasalazine, neomycin, cholestyramine* and certain *anticancer drugs* may interfere with intestinal digoxin absorption, resulting in unexpectedly low serum concentrations. There have been inconsistent reports regarding the effects of other drugs on the serum digoxin concentration. *Thyroid* administration to a digitalized, hypothyroid patient may increase the dose requirement of digoxin. Concomitant use of digoxin and *sympathomimetics* increases the risk of cardiac arrhythmias because both enhance ectopic pacemaker activity. *Succinylcholine* may cause a sudden extrusion of potassium from muscle cells, and may thereby cause arrhythmias in digitalized patients. Although β adrenergic blockers or calcium channel blockers and digoxin may be useful in combination to control atrial fibrillation, their additive effects on AV node conduction can result in complete heart block.

Due to the considerable variability of these interactions, digoxin dosage should be carefully individualized when patients receive coadministered medications. Furthermore, caution should be exercised when combining digoxin with any drug that may cause a significant deterioration in renal function, since this may impair the excretion of digoxin.

Carcinogenesis, Mutagenesis, Impairment of Fertility: There have been no long-term studies performed in animals to evaluate carcinogenic potential.

Pregnancy: ***Teratogenic Effects:*** Pregnancy Category C. Animal reproduction studies have not been conducted with digoxin. It is also not known whether digoxin can cause fetal harm when administered to a pregnant woman or can affect reproduction capacity. Digoxin should be given to a pregnant woman only if clearly needed.

Nursing Mothers: Studies have shown that digoxin concentrations in the mother's serum and milk are similar. However, the estimated daily dose to a nursing infant will be far below the usual infant maintenance dose. Therefore, this amount should have no pharmacologic effect upon the infant. Nevertheless, caution should be exercised when digoxin is administered to a nursing woman.

ADVERSE REACTIONS

The frequency and severity of adverse reactions to digoxin depend on the dose and route of administration, as well as on the patient's underlying disease or concomitant therapies (see PRECAUTIONS and ADMINISTRATION: Serum Digoxin Concentrations). The overall incidence of adverse reactions has been reported as 5% to 20%, with 15% to 20% of them being considered serious (one to four percent of patients receiving digoxin). Evidence suggests that the incidence of toxicity has decreased since the introduction of the serum digoxin assay and improved standardization of digoxin tablets. Cardiac toxicity accounts for about one-half, gastrointestinal disturbances for about one-fourth, and CNS and other toxicity for about one-fourth of these adverse reactions.

Adults:

Cardiac: Unifocal or multiform ventricular premature contractions, especially in bigeminal or trigeminal patterns, are the most common arrhythmias associated with digoxin toxicity in adults with heart disease. Ventricular tachycardia may result from digitalis toxicity. Atrioventricular (AV) dissociation, accelerated junctional (nodal) rhythm and atrial tachycardia with block are also common arrhythmias caused by digoxin overdosage.

Excessive slowing of the pulse is a clinical sign of digoxin overdosage. AV block (Wenckebach) of increasing degree may proceed to complete heart block.

Note: The electrocardiogram is fundamental in determining the presence and nature of these cardiac disturbances. Digoxin may also induce other changes in the ECG (e.g., PR prolongation, ST depression), which represent digoxin effect and may or may not be associated with digitalis toxicity.

Gastrointestinal: Anorexia, nausea, vomiting and less commonly diarrhea are common early symptoms of overdosage. However, uncontrolled heart failure may also produce such symptoms. Digitalis toxicity very rarely may cause abdominal pain and hemorrhagic necrosis of the intestines.

CNS: Visual disturbances (blurred or yellow vision), headache, weakness, dizziness, apathy and psychosis can occur.

Other: Gynecomastia is occasionally observed. Maculopapular rash or other skin reactions are rarely observed.

Infants and Children: Toxicity differs from the adult in a number of respects. Anorexia, nausea, vomiting, diarrhea and CNS disturbances may be present but are rare as initial symptoms in infants. Cardiac arrhythmias are more reliable signs of toxicity. Digoxin in children may produce any arrhythmia. The most commonly encountered are conduction disturbances or supraventricular tachyarrhythmias, such as atrial tachycardia with or without block, and junctional (nodal) tachycardia. Ventricular arrhythmias are less common. Sinus bradycardia may also be a sign of impending digoxin intoxication, expecially in infants, even in the absence of first degree heart block. Any arrhythmia or alteration in cardiac conduction that develops in a child taking digoxin should initially be assumed to be a consequence of digoxin intoxication.

OVERDOSAGE

Treatment of Arrhythmias Produced by Overdosage:

Adults: Digoxin should be discontinued until all signs of toxicity are gone. Discontinuation may be all that is necessary if toxic manifestations are not severe and appear only near the expected time for maximum effect of the drug.

Correction of factors that may contribute to toxicity such as electrolyte disturbances hypoxia, acid-base disturbances and removal of aggravating agents such as catecholamines, should also be considered. Potassium salts may be indicated, particularly if hypokalemia is present. Potassium administration may be dangerous in the setting of massive digitalis overdosage (see Massive Digitalis Overdosage subsection below). Potassium chloride in divided oral doses totaling 3 to 6 grams of the salt (40 to 80 mEq K+) for adults may be given provided renal function is adequate (see Infants and Children below for potassium recommendations).

When correction of the arrhythmia is urgent and the serum potassium concentration is low or normal, potassium should be administered intravenously in 5% dextrose injection. For adults, a total of 40 to 80 mEq (diluted to a concentration of 40 mEq per 500 mL) may be given at a rate not exceeding 20 mEq per hour, or slower if limited by pain due to local irritation. Additional amounts may be given if the arrhythmia is uncontrolled and potassium well-tolerated. ECG monitoring should be performed to watch for any evidence of potassium toxicity (e.g., peaking of T waves) and to observe the effect on the arrhythmia. The infusion may be stopped when the desired effect is achieved.

Note: Potassium should not be used and may be dangerous in heart block due to digoxin, unless primarily related to supraventricular tachycardia.

Other agents that have been used for the treatment of digoxin intoxication include lidocaine, procainamide, propranolol, and phenytoin, although use of the latter must be considered experimental. In advanced heart block, atropine and/or temporary ventricular pacing may be beneficial. DIGIBIND®, Digoxin Immune Fab (Ovine), can be used to reverse potentially life-threatening digoxin (or digitoxin) intoxication. Improvement in signs and symptoms of digitalis toxicity usually begins within ½ hour of administration of DIGIBIND. Each 38 mg vial of DIGIBIND will neutralize 0.5 mg of digoxin (which is a usual body store of an adequately digitalized 70 kg patient).

Infants and Children: See Adults section for general recommendations for the treatment of arrhythmias produced by overdosage and for cautions regarding the use of potassium. If a potassium preparation is used to treat toxicity, it may be given orally in divided doses totaling 1 to 1.5 mEq K+ per kilogram (kg) body weight (1 gram of potassium chloride contains 13.4 mEq K+).

When correction of the arrhythmia with potassium is urgent, approximately 0.5 mEq/kg of potassium per hour may be given intravenously, with careful ECG monitoring. The intravenous solution of potassium should be dilute enough to avoid local irritation; however, especially in infants, care must be taken to avoid intravenous fluid overload.

Massive Digitalis Overdosage: Manifestations of life-threatening toxicity include severe ventricular arrhythmias such as ventricular tachycardia or ventricular fibrillation, or progressive bradyarrhythmias such as severe sinus bradycardia or second or third degree heart block not responsive to atropine. An overdosage of more than 10 mg of digoxin in previously healthy adults or 4 mg in previously healthy children or overdosage resulting in steady-state serum concentrations greater than 10 ng/mL, often results in cardiac arrest.

Severe digitalis intoxication can cause life-threatening elevation in serum potassium concentration by shifting potassium from inside to outside the cell resulting in hyperkalemia. Administration of potassium supplements in the setting of massive intoxication may be hazardous.

DIGBIND, Digoxin Immune Fab (Ovine), may be used at a dose equimolar to digoxin in the body to reverse the effects of ingestion of a massive overdose. The decision to administer DIGBIND before the onset of toxic manifestations will depend on the likelihood that life-threatening toxicity will occur (see above).

Patients with massive digitalis ingestion should receive large doses of activated charcoal to prevent absorption and bind digoxin in the gut during enteroenteric recirculation. Emesis or gastric lavage may be indicated especially if ingestion has occurred within 30 minutes of the patient's presentation at the hospital. Emesis should not be induced in patients who are obtunded. If a patient presents more than 2 hours after ingestion or already has toxic manifestations, it may be unsafe to induce vomiting or attempt passage of a gastric tube, because such maneuvers may induce an acute vagal episode that can worsen digitalis-toxic arrhythmias.

DOSAGE AND ADMINISTRATION

Recommended dosages are average values that may require considerable modification because of individual sensitivity

Continued on next page

Glaxo Wellcome—Cont.

or associated conditions. Diminished renal function is the most important factor requiring modification of recommended doses.

Parenteral administration of digoxin should be used only when the need for rapid digitalization is urgent or when the drug cannot be taken orally. Intramuscular injection can lead to severe pain at the injection site, thus intravenous administration is preferred. If the drug must be administered by the intramuscular route, it should be injected deep into the muscle followed by massage. No more than 500 µg (2 mL) should be injected into a single site.

LANOXIN Injection can be administered undiluted or diluted with a 4-fold or greater volume of Sterile Water for Injection, 0.9% Sodium Chloride Injection or 5% Dextrose Injection. The use of less than a 4-fold volume of diluent could lead to precipitation of the digoxin. Immediate use of the diluted product is recommended.

If tuberculin syringes are used to measure very small doses, one must be aware of the problem of inadvertent overadministration of digoxin. The syringe should *not* be flushed with the parenteral solution after its contents are expelled into an indwelling vascular catheter.

Slow infusion of LANOXIN Injection is preferable to bolus administration. Rapid infusion of digitalis glycosides has been shown to cause systemic and coronary arteriolar constriction, which may be clinically undesirable. Caution is thus advised and LANOXIN Injection should probably be administered over a period of 5 minutes or longer. Mixing of LANOXIN Injection with other drugs in the same container or simultaneous administration in the same intravenous line is not recommended.

In deciding the dose of digoxin, several factors must be considered:
1. The disease being treated. Atrial arrhythmias may require larger doses than heart failure.
2. The body weight of the patient. Doses should be calculated based upon lean or ideal body weight.
3. The patient's renal function, preferably evaluated on the basis of creatinine clearance.
4. Age is an important factor in infants and children.
5. Concomitant disease states, drugs or other factors likely to alter the expected clinical response to digoxin (see PRECAUTIONS and Drug Interactions subsection).

Digitalization may be accomplished by either of two general approaches that vary in dosage and frequency of administration, but reach the same endpoint in terms of total amount of digoxin accumulated in the body.
1. Rapid digitalization may be achieved by administering a loading dose based upon projected peak body digoxin stores, then calculating the maintenance dose as a percentage of the loading dose.
2. More gradual digitalization may be obtained by beginning an appropriate maintenance dose, thus allowing digoxin body stores to accumulate slowly. Steady-state serum digoxin concentrations will be achieved in approximately 5 half-lives of the drug for the individual patient. Depending upon the patient's renal function, this will take between one and three weeks.

Adults:

Rapid Digitalization with a Loading Dose: Peak body digoxin stores of 8 to 12 µg/kg should provide therapeutic effect with minimum risk of toxicity in most patients with heart failure and normal sinus rhythm. Larger stores (10 to 15 µg/kg) are often required for adequate control of ventricular rate in patients with atrial flutter or fibrillation. Because of altered digoxin distribution and elimination, projected peak body stores for patients with renal insufficiency should be conservative (i.e., 6 to 10 µg/kg) (see PRECAUTIONS).
The loading dose should be based on the projected peak body stores and administered in several portions, with roughly half the total given as the first dose. Additional fractions of this planned total dose may be given at 4 to 8 hour intervals, **with careful assessment of clinical response before each additional dose.** If the patient's clinical response necessitates a change from the calculated dose of digoxin, then calculation of the main-

tenance dose should be based upon the amount actually given.

In previously undigitalized patients, a single initial intravenous LANOXIN Injection dose of 400 to 600 µg (0.4 to 0.6 mg) usually produces a detectable effect in 5 to 30 minutes that becomes maximal in 1 to 4 hours. Additional doses of 100 to 300 µg (0.1 to 0.3 mg) may be given cautiously at 4 to 8 hour intervals until clinical evidence of an adequate effect is noted. The usual amount of LANOXIN Injection that a 70 kg patient requires to achieve 8 to 15 µg/kg peak body stores is 600 to 1000 µg (0.6 to 1.0 mg).

Although peak body stores are mathematically related to loading doses and are utilized to calculate maintenance doses, they do not correlate with measured serum concentrations. This discrepancy is caused by digoxin distribution within the body during the first 6 to 8 hours following a dose. Serum concentrations drawn during this time are usually not interpretable.

The maintenance dose should be based upon the percentage of the peak body stores lost each day through elimination. The following formula has had wide clinical use:

$$\text{Maintenance Dose} = \text{Peak Body Stores (i.e., Loading Dose)} \times \frac{\% \text{ Daily Loss}}{100}$$

Where % Daily Loss = 14 + Ccr/5

Ccr is creatinine clearance, corrected to 70 kg body weight or 1.73 m² body surface area. *For adults,* if only serum creatinine concentrations (Scr) are available, a Ccr (corrected to 70 kg body weight) may be estimated in men as (140 −Age)/Scr. For women, this result should be multiplied by 0.85.
Note: This equation cannot be used for estimating creatinine clearance in infants or children.

A common practice involves the use of LANOXIN Injection to achieve rapid digitalization, with conversion to LANOXIN Tablets or LANOXICAPS for maintenance therapy. If patients are switched from intravenous to oral digoxin formulations, allowances must be made for differences in bioavailability when calculating maintenance dosages (see table in CLINICAL PHARMACOLOGY).

Infants and Children: Digitalization must be individualized. Divided daily dosing is recommended for infants and young children. Children over 10 years of age require adult dosages in proportion to their body weight.
In the newborn period, renal clearance of digoxin is diminished and suitable dosage adjustments must be observed. This is especially pronounced in the premature infant. Beyond the immediate newborn period, children generally require proportionally larger doses than adults on the basis of body weight or body surface area.

Infants and Children: Rapid Digitalization with a Loading Dose: LANOXIN Injection Pediatric can be used to achieve rapid digitalization, with conversion to an oral LANOXIN formulation for maintenance therapy. If patients are switched from intravenous to oral digoxin tablets or elixir, allowances must be made for differences in bioavailability when calculating maintenance dosages (see bioavailability table in CLINICAL PHARMACOLOGY and dosing table next page). Intramuscular injection of digoxin is extremely painful and offers no advantages unless other routes of administration are contraindicated.

Digitalizing and daily maintenance doses for each age group are given below and should provide therapeutic effect with minimum risk of toxicity in most patients with heart failure and normal sinus rhythm. Larger doses are often required for adequate control of ventricular rate in patients with atrial flutter or fibrillation.
The loading dose should be administered in several portions, with roughly half the total given as the first dose. Additional fractions of this planned total dose may be given at 4 to 8 hour intervals, **with careful assessment of clinical response before each additional dose.** If the patient's clinical response necessitates a change from the calculated dose of digoxin, then calculation of the maintenance dose should be based upon the amount actually given.
[See table below.]

Infants and Children: Gradual Digitalization With A Maintenance Dose: More gradual digitalization can also be accomplished by beginning an appropriate maintenance dose. The range of percentages provided above can be used in calculating this dose for patients with normal renal function. In chil-

dren with renal disease, digoxin dosing must be carefully titrated based upon clinical response.

Long-term use of digoxin is indicated in many children who have been digitalized for acute heart failure, unless the cause is transient. Children with severe congenital heart disease, even after surgery, may require digoxin for prolonged periods.
It cannot be overemphasized that both the adult and pediatric dosage guidelines provided are based upon average patient response and substantial individual variation can be expected. Accordingly, ultimate dosage selection must be based upon clinical assessment of the patient.

Serum Digoxin Concentrations: Measurement of serum digoxin concentrations can be helpful to the clinician in determining the state of digitalization and in assigning certain probabilities to the likelihood of digoxin intoxication. Studies in adults considered adequately digitalized (without evidence of toxicity) show that about two-thirds of such patients have serum digoxin levels ranging from 0.8 to 2.0 ng/mL. Patients with atrial fibrillation or atrial flutter require and appear to tolerate higher levels than do patients with other indications. On the other hand, in adult patients with clinical evidence of digoxin toxicity, about two-thirds will have serum digoxin levels greater than 2.0 ng/mL. Thus, whereas levels less than 0.8 ng/mL are infrequently associated with toxicity, levels greater than 2.0 ng/mL are often associated with toxicity. Values in between are not very helpful in deciding whether a certain sign or symptom is more likely caused by digoxin toxicity or by something else. There are rare patients who are unable to tolerate digoxin even at serum concentrations below 0.8 ng/mL. Some researchers suggest that infants and young children tolerate slightly higher serum concentrations than do adults.

To allow adequate time for equilibration of digoxin between serum and tissue, **sampling of serum concentrations for clinical use should be at least 6 to 8 hours after the last dose,** regardless of the route of administration or formulation used. On a twice daily dosing schedule, there will be only minor differences in serum digoxin concentrations whether sampling is done at 8 or 12 hours after a dose. After a single daily dose, the concentration will be 10% to 25% lower when sampled at 24 versus 8 hours, depending upon the patient's renal function. Ideally, sampling for assessment of steady-state concentrations should be done just before the next dose.

If a discrepancy exists between the reported serum concentration and the observed clinical response, the clinician should consider the following possibilities:
1. Analytical problems in the assay procedure.
2. Inappropriate serum sampling time.
3. Administration of a digitalis glycoside other than digoxin.
4. Conditions (described in WARNINGS and PRECAUTIONS) causing an alteration in the sensitivity of the patient to digoxin.
5. The patient falls outside the norm in his response to or handling of digoxin. This decision should only be reached after exclusion of the other possibilities and generally should be confirmed by additional correlations of clinical observations with serum digoxin concentrations.

The serum concentration data should always be interpreted in the overall clinical context and an isolated serum concentration value should not be used alone as a basis for increasing or decreasing digoxin dosage.

Adjustment of Maintenance Dose in Previously Digitalized Patients: LANOXIN Injection maintenance doses in individual patients on steady-state digoxin can be adjusted upward or downward in proportion to the ratio of the desired versus the measured serum concentration. For example, a patient at steady-state on 100 µg (0.1 mg) of LANOXIN Injection per day with a measured serum concentration of 0.7 ng/mL, should have the dose increased to 200 µg (0.2 mg) per day to achieve a steady-state serum concentration of 1.4 ng/mL, **assuming the serum digoxin concentration measurement is correct, renal function remains stable during this time, and the needed adjustment is not the result of a problem with compliance.**

Dosage Adjustment When Changing Preparations: The difference in bioavailability between injectable LANOXIN or LANOXICAPS and LANOXIN Elixir Pediatric or LANOXIN Tablets must be considered when changing patients from one dosage form to another.
Doses of LANOXIN Injection and LANOXICAPS of 100 µg (0.1 mg) and 200 µg (0.2 mg) are approximately equivalent to 125 µg (0.125 mg) and 250 µg (0.25 mg) doses of LANOXIN Tablets and Elixir Pediatric (see table of CLINICAL PHARMACOLOGY). Intramuscular injection of digoxin is extremely painful and offers no advantages unless other routes of administration are contraindicated.

HOW SUPPLIED

LANOXIN (digoxin) Injection, 500 µg (0.5 mg) in 2 mL (250 µg [0.25 mg] per mL); Boxes of 10 (NDC 0173-0260-10) and 50 ampuls (NDC 0173-0260-35).

Usual Digitalizing and Maintenance Dosages for LANOXIN® Injection in Children with **Normal Renal Function Based on Lean Body Weight**

Age	Digitalizing* Dose (µg/kg)	Daily† I.V. Maintenance Dose (µg/kg)
2 to 5 Years	25 to 35	
5 to 10 Years	15 to 30	25% to 35% of the I.V. loading dose‡
Over 10 years	8 to 12	

* I.V. digitalizing doses are 80% of oral digitalizing doses.
† Divided daily dosing is recommended for children under 10 years of age.
‡ Projected or actual digitalizing dose providing clinical response.

Store at 15° to 25°C (59° to 77°F) and protect from light.
Also available:
LANOXIN (digoxin) Tablets, Scored 125 µg (0.125 mg): bottles of 100 package of 12 bottles × 100 with child-resistant cap and 1000; unit dose pack of 100.
LANOXIN (digoxin) Tablets, Scored 250 µg (0.25 mg): bottles of 100, 1000 and 5000; unit dose pack of 100.
LANOXIN (digoxin) Elixir Pediatric, 50 µg (0.05 mg) per mL: bottle of 60 mL with calibrated dropper.
LANOXIN (digoxin) Injection Pediatric, 100 µg (0.1 mg) in 1 mL: box of 10 ampuls.
LANOXICAPS (digoxin solution in Capsules), 50 µg (0.05 mg) bottle of 100; 100 µg (0.1 mg) bottle of 100; 200 µg (0.2 mg) bottle of 100.
February 1996/RL-253
Shown in Product Identification Guide, page 313

LANOXIN® ℞
[*lă-nŏx 'ĭn"*]
(digoxin)
Injection Pediatric
100 µg (0.1 mg) in 1 mL

DESCRIPTION

Digoxin is one of the cardiac (or digitalis) glycosides, a closely related group of drugs having in common specific effects on the myocardium. These drugs are found in a number of plants. Digoxin is extracted from the leaves of *Digitalis lanata.* The term "digitalis" is used to designate the whole group. The glycosides are composed of two portions: a sugar and a cardenolide (hence "glycosides").
Digoxin has the molecular formula $C_{41}H_{64}O_{14}$, a molecular weight of 780.95 and melting and decomposition points above 235°C. The drug is practically insoluble in water and in ether; slightly soluble in diluted (50%) alcohol and in chloroform; and freely soluble in pyridine. Digoxin powder is composed of odorless white crystals.
Digoxin has the chemical name: (3β, 5β, 12β)-3-[(*O*-2,6-dideoxy-*β-D-ribo*-hexopyranosyl-(1→4)- *O*-2,6-dideoxy -*β-D-ribo*-hexopyranosyl-(1→4) -2,6-dideoxy-*β -D-ribo*-hexopyranosyl)- oxy]-12, 14-dihydroxycard-20(22)-enolide.
LANOXIN (digoxin) Injection Pediatric is a sterile solution of digoxin for intravenous or intramuscular injection. The vehicle contains 40% propylene glycol and 10% alcohol. The injection is buffered to a pH of 6.8 to 7.2 with 0.17% sodium phosphate and 0.08% anhydrous citric acid. Each 1 mL ampul contains 100 µg (0.1 mg) digoxin. Dilution is not required.

CLINICAL PHARMACOLOGY

Mechanism of Action: The influence of digitalis glycosides on the myocardium is dose-related, and involves both a direct action on cardiac muscle and the specialized conduction system, and indirect actions on the cardiovascular system mediated by the autonomic nervous system. The indirect actions mediated by the autonomic nervous system involve a vagomimetic action, which is responsible for the effects of digitalis on the sino-atrial (SA) and atrioventricular (AV) nodes; and also a baroreceptor sensitization which results in increased carotid sinus nerve activity and enhanced sympathetic withdrawal for any given increment in mean arterial pressure. The pharmacologic consequences of these direct and indirect effects are: 1) an increase in the force and velocity of myocardial systolic contraction (positive inotropic action); 2) a slowing of heart rate (negative chronotropic effect); and 3) decreased conduction velocity through the AV node. In higher doses, digitalis increases sympathetic outflow from the central nervous system (CNS) to both cardiac and peripheral sympathetic nerves. This increase in sympathetic activity may be an important factor in digitalis cardiac toxicity. Most of the extracardiac manifestations of digitalis toxicity are also mediated by the CNS.
Pharmacokinetics: Note: The following data are from studies performed in adults, unless otherwise stated.
Absorption: A comparison of the systemic availability and equivalent doses for digoxin preparations are shown in the following table: [See table above.]

PRODUCT	ABSOLUTE BIOAVAILABILITY	EQUIVALENT DOSES (IN MG*)		
LANOXIN® Tablets	60% to 80%	0.125	0.25	0.5
LANOXIN Elixir	70% to 85%	0.125	0.25	0.5
LANOXIN Injection/I.M.	70% to 85%	0.125	0.25	0.5
LANOXIN Injection/I.V.	100%	0.1	0.2	0.4
LANOXICAPS® Capsules	90% to 100%	0.1	0.2	0.4

*1 mg = 1000 µg

Distribution: Following drug administration, a 6 to 8 hour distribution phase is observed. This is followed by a much more gradual serum concentration decline, which is dependent on digoxin elimination from the body. The peak height and slope of the early portion (absorption/distribution phases) of the serum concentration-time curve are dependent upon the route of administration and the absorption characteristics of the formulation. Clinical evidence indicates that the early high serum concentrations do not reflect the concentration of digoxin at its site of action, but that with chronic use, the steady-state post-distribution serum levels are in equilibrium with tissue levels and correlate with pharmacologic effects. In individual patients, these post-distribution serum concentrations are linearly related to maintenance dosage and may be useful in evaluating therapeutic and toxic effects (see DOSAGE AND ADMINISTRATION: Serum Digoxin Concentrations).
Digoxin is concentrated in tissues and therefore has a large apparent volume of distribution. Digoxin crosses both the blood-brain barrier and the placenta. At delivery, serum digoxin concentration in the newborn is similar to the serum level in the mother. Approximately 20% to 25% of plasma digoxin is bound to protein. Serum digoxin concentrations are not significantly altered by large changes in fat tissue weight, so that its distribution space correlates best with lean (ideal) body weight, not total body weight.
Pharmacologic Response: The approximate times to onset of effect and to peak effect of all the LANOXIN preparations are given in the following table:
[See table below.]
Excretion: Elimination of digoxin follows first-order kinetics (that is, the quantity of digoxin eliminated at any time is proportional to the total body content). Following intravenous administration to normal subjects, 50% to 70% of a digoxin dose is excreted unchanged in the urine. Renal excretion of digoxin is proportional to glomerular filtration rate and is largely independent of urine flow. In subjects with normal renal function, digoxin has a half-life of 1.5 to 2.0 days. The half-life in anuric patients is prolonged to 4 to 6 days. Digoxin is not effectively removed from the body by dialysis, exchange transfusion or during cardiopulmonary by-pass because most of the drug is in tissue rather than circulating in the blood.

INDICATIONS AND USAGE

Heart Failure: The increased cardiac output resulting from the inotropic action of digoxin ameliorates the disturbances characteristic of heart failure (venous congestion, edema, dyspnea, orthopnea, and cardiac asthma).
Digoxin is more effective in "low output" (pump) failure than in "high output" heart failure secondary to arteriovenous fistula, anemia, infection or hyperthyroidism.
Digoxin is usually continued after failure is controlled, unless some known precipitating factor is corrected. Studies have shown, however, that even though hemodynamic effects can be demonstrated in almost all patients, corresponding improvement in the signs and symptoms of heart failure is not necessarily apparent. Therefore, in patients in whom digoxin may be difficult to regulate, or in whom the risk of toxicity may be great (e.g., patients with unstable renal function or whose potassium levels tend to fluctuate), a cautious withdrawal of digoxin may be considered. If digoxin is discontinued, the patient should be regularly monitored for clinical evidence of recurrent heart failure.
Atrial Fibrillation: Digoxin reduces ventricular rate and thereby improves hemodynamics. Palpitation, precordial distress or weakness are relieved and concomitant congestive failure ameliorated. Digoxin should be continued in doses necessary to maintain the desired ventricular rate.
Atrial Flutter: Digoxin slows the heart and regular sinus rhythm may appear. Frequently the flutter is converted to atrial fibrillation with a controlled ventricular response. Digoxin treatment should be maintained if atrial fibrillation persists. (Electrical cardioversion is often the treatment of choice for atrial flutter. See discussion of cardioversion in PRECAUTIONS)
Paroxysmal Atrial Tachycardia (PAT): Digoxin may convert PAT to sinus rhythm by slowing conduction through the AV node. If heart failure has ensued or paroxysms recur frequently, digoxin should be continued. In infants, digoxin is usually continued for 3 to 6 months after a single episode of PAT to prevent recurrence.

CONTRAINDICATIONS

Digitalis glycosides are contraindicated in ventricular fibrillation.
In a given patient, an untoward effect requiring permanent discontinuation of other digitalis preparations usually constitutes a contraindication to digoxin. Hypersensitivity to digoxin itself is a contraindication to its use. Allergy to digoxin, though rare, does occur. It may not extend to all such preparations, and another digitalis glycoside may be tried with caution.

WARNINGS

Anorexia, nausea, vomiting, and arrhythmias may accompany heart failure or may be indications of digitalis intoxication. Clinical evaluation of the cause of these symptoms should be attempted before further digitalis administration. In such circumstances determination of the serum digoxin concentration may be an aid in deciding whether or not digitalis toxicity is likely to be present. If the possibility of digitalis intoxication cannot be excluded, cardiac glycosides should be temporarily withheld, if permitted by the clinical situation.
Patients with renal insufficiency require smaller than usual maintenance doses of digoxin (see DOSAGE AND ADMINISTRATION).
Heart failure accompanying acute glomerulonephritis requires extreme care in digitalization. Relatively low loading and maintenance doses and concomitant use of antihypertensive drugs may be necessary and careful monitoring is essential. Digoxin should be discontinued as soon as possible.
Patients with severe carditis, such as carditis associated with rheumatic fever or viral myocarditis, are especially sensitive to digoxin-induced disturbances of rhythm.
Newborn infants display considerable variability in their tolerance to digoxin. Premature and immature infants are particularly sensitive, and dosage must not only be reduced but must be individualized according to their degree of maturity.
Note: Digitalis glycosides are an important cause of accidental poisoning in children.

PRECAUTIONS

General: Digoxin toxicity develops more frequently and lasts longer in patients with renal impairment because of the decreased excretion of digoxin. Therefore, it should be anticipated that dosage requirements will be decreased in patients with moderate to severe renal disease (see DOSAGE AND ADMINISTRATION). Because of the prolonged half-life, a longer period of time is required to achieve an initial or new steady-state concentration in patients with renal impairment than in patients with normal renal function.
In patients with hypokalemia, toxicity may occur despite serum digoxin concentrations within the "normal range," because potassium depletion sensitizes the myocardium to digoxin. Therefore, it is desirable to maintain normal serum potassium levels in patients being treated with digoxin. Hypokalemia may result from diuretic, amphotericin B or corticosteroid therapy, and from dialysis or mechanical suction of gastrointestinal secretions. It may also accompany malnutrition, diarrhea, prolonged vomiting, old age and long-standing heart failure. In general, rapid changes in serum potassium or other electrolytes should be avoided, and intravenous treatment with potassium should be reserved for special circumstances as described below (see OVERDOSAGE: Treatment Of Arrhythmias Produced By Overdosage).
Calcium, particularly when administered rapidly by the intravenous route, may produce serious arrythmias in digitalized patients. Hypercalcemia from any cause predisposes the patient to digitalis toxicity. On the other hand, hypocalcemia can nullify the effects of digoxin in humans; thus, digoxin may be ineffective until serum calcium is restored to normal. These interactions are related to the fact that calcium affects contractility and excitability of the heart in a manner similar to digoxin.

PRODUCT	TIME TO ONSET OF EFFECT*	TIME TO PEAK EFFECT*
LANOXIN® Tablets	0.5 to 2 hours	2 to 6 hours
LANOXIN Elixir	0.5 to 2 hours	2 to 6 hours
LANOXIN Injection/I.M.	0.5 to 2 hours	2 to 6 hours
LANOXIN Injection/I.V.	5 to 30 minutes†	1 to 4 hours
LANOXICAPS® Capsules	0.5 to 2 hours	2 to 6 hours

*Documented for ventricular response rate in atrial fibrillation, inotropic effect and electrocardiographic changes.
†Depending upon rate of infusion.

Continued on next page

Consult 1997 supplements and future editions for revisions

Glaxo Wellcome—Cont.

Hypomagnesemia may predispose to digitalis toxicity. If low magnesium levels are detected in a patient on digoxin, replacement therapy should be instituted.
Quinidine, verapamil, amiodarone, propafenone, indomethacin, itraconazole, and alprazolam may cause a rise in serum digoxin concentration, with the implication that digitalis intoxication may result. This rise appears to be proportional to the dose. The effect is mediated by a reduction in the digoxin clearance and, in the case of quinidine, decreased volume of distribution as well.
Patients with acute myocardial infarction or severe pulmonary disease may be unusually sensitive to digoxin-induced disturbances of rhythm.
Atrial arrhythmias associated with hypermetabolic states (e.g., hyperthyroidism) are particularly resistant to digoxin treatment. Large doses of digoxin are not recommended as the only treatment of these arrhythmias and care must be taken to avoid toxicity if large doses of digoxin are required.
In hypothyroidism, the digoxin requirements are reduced. Digoxin responses in patients with compensated thyroid disease are normal.
Reduction of digoxin dosage may be desirable prior to electrical cardioversion to avoid induction of ventricular arrhythmias, but the physician must consider the consequences of rapid increase in ventricular response to atrial fibrillation if digoxin is withheld 1 to 2 days prior to cardioversion. If there is a suspicion that digitalis toxicity exists, elective cardioversion should be delayed. If it is not prudent to delay cardioversion, the energy level selected should be minimal at first and carefully increased in an attempt to avoid precipitating ventricular arrhythmias.
Incomplete AV block, especially in patients with Stokes-Adams attacks, may progress to advanced or complete heart block if digoxin is given.
In some patients with sinus node disease (i.e., Sick Sinus Syndrome), digoxin may worsen sinus bradycardia or sinoatrial block.
In patients with Wolff-Parkinson-White Syndrome and atrial fibrillation, digoxin can enhance transmission of impulses through the accessory pathway. This effect may result in extremely rapid ventricular rates and even ventricular fibrillation.
Digoxin may worsen the outflow obstruction in patients with idiopathic hypertrophic subaortic stenosis (IHSS). Unless cardiac failure is severe, it is doubtful whether digoxin should be employed.
Patients with chronic constrictive pericarditis may fail to respond to digoxin. In addition, slowing of the heart rate by digoxin in some patients may further decrease cardiac output.
Patients with heart failure from amyloid heart disease or constrictive cardiomyopathies respond poorly to treatment with digoxin.
Digoxin is not indicated for the treatment of sinus tachycardia unless it is associated with heart failure.
Digoxin may produce false positive ST-T changes in the electrocardiogram during exercise testing.
Intramuscular injection of digoxin is extremely painful and offers no advantages unless other routes of administration are contraindicated.
Laboratory Tests: Patients receiving digoxin should have their serum electrolytes and renal function (BUN and/or serum creatinine) assessed periodically; the frequency of assessments will depend on the clinical setting. For discussion of serum digoxin concentrations, see DOSAGE AND ADMINISTRATION.
Drug Interactions: Potassium-depleting *corticosteroids* and *diuretics* may be major contributing factors to digitalis toxicity. *Calcium*, particularly if administered rapidly by the intravenous route, may produce serious arrhythmias in digitalized patients. *Quinidine, verapamil, amiodarone, propafenone, indomethacin, itraconazole, and alprazolam* may cause a rise in serum digoxin concentration, with the implication that digitalis intoxication may result. Serum levels of digoxin may be increased by concomitant administration of *erythromycin* and *clarithromycin* (and possibly other *macrolide antibiotics* and *tetracycline*. *Propantheline* and *diphenoxylate*, by decreasing gut motility, may increase digoxin absorption. *Antacids, kaolin-pectin, sulfasalazine, neomycin, cholestyramine* and certain *anticancer drugs* may interfere with intestinal digoxin absorption, resulting in unexpectedly low serum concentrations. There have been inconsistent reports regarding the effects of other drugs on the serum digoxin concentration. *Thyroid* administration to a digitalized, hypothyroid patient may increase the dose requirement of digoxin. Concomitant use of digoxin and *sympathomimetics* increases the risk of cardiac arrhythmias because both enhance ectopic pacemaker activity. *Succinylcholine* may cause a sudden extrusion of potassium from muscle cells and may thereby cause arrhythmias in digitalized patients. Although β adrenergic blockers or calcium channel blockers and digoxin may be useful in combination to control atrial fibrillation, their additive effects on AV node conduction can result in complete heart block.
Due to the considerable variability of these interactions, digoxin dosage should be carefully individualized when patients receive coadministered medications. Furthermore, caution should be exercised when combining digoxin with any drug that may cause a significant deterioration in renal function, since this may impair the excretion of digoxin.
Carcinogenesis, Mutagenesis, Impairment of Fertility: There have been no long-term studies performed in animals to evaluate carcinogenic potential.

ADVERSE REACTIONS

The frequency and severity of adverse reactions to digoxin depend on the dose and route of administration, as well as on the patient's underlying disease or concomitant therapies (see PRECAUTIONS and DOSAGE AND ADMINISTRATION: Serum Digoxin Concentrations). The overall incidence of adverse reactions in adults has been reported as 5% to 20%, with 15% to 20% of them being considered serious (one to four percent of patients receiving digoxin). Evidence suggests that the incidence of toxicity has decreased since the introduction of the serum digoxin assay and improved standardization of digoxin tablets. Cardiac toxicity accounts for about one-half, gastrointestinal disturbances for about one-fourth, and CNS and other toxicity for about one-fourth of these adverse reactions.
Cardiac: Conduction disturbances or supraventricular tachyarrhythmias, such as atrioventricular (AV) block (Wenckebach), atrial tachycardia with or without block and junctional (nodal) tachycardia are the most common arrhythmias associated with digoxin toxicity in children. Ventricular arrhythmias, such as unifocal or multiform ventricular premature contractions, especially in bigeminal or trigeminal patterns, are less common. Ventricular tachycardia may result from digitalis toxicity. Sinus bradycardia may also be a sign of impending digoxin intoxication, especially in infants, even in the absence of first degree heart block. Any arrhythmias or alteration in cardiac conduction that develops in a child taking digoxin should initially be assumed to be a consequence of digoxin intoxication.
Note: The electrocardiogram is fundamental in determining the presence and nature of these cardiac disturbances. Digoxin may also induce other changes in the ECG (e.g., PR prolongation, ST depression), which represent digoxin effect and may or may not be associated with digitalis toxicity.
Gastrointestinal: Anorexia, nausea, vomiting and diarrhea may be early symptoms of overdosage. However, uncontrolled heart failure may also produce such symptoms. Digitalis toxicity very rarely may cause abdominal pain and hemorrhagic necrosis of the intestines.
CNS: Visual disturbances (blurred or yellow vision), headache, weakness, dizziness, apathy and psychosis can occur. These may be difficult to recognize in infants and children.
Other: Gynecomastia is occasionally observed. Maculopapular rash or other skin reactions are rarely observed.

OVERDOSAGE

Treatment of Arrhythmias Produced by Overdosage: Digoxin should be discontinued until all signs of toxicity are gone. Discontinuation may be all that is necessary if toxic manifestations are not severe and appear only near the expected time for maximum effect of the drug.
Correction of factors that may contribute to toxicity such as electrolyte disturbances, hypoxia, acid-base disturbances and removal of aggravating agents such as catecholamines, should also be considered. Potassium salts may be indicated, particularly if hypokalemia is present. Potassium administration may be dangerous in the setting of massive digitalis overdosage (see Massive Digitalis Overdosage subsection below). Potassium chloride in divided oral doses totaling 1 to 1.5 mEq K+ per kilogram (kg) body weight may be given provided renal function is adequate (1 gram of potassium chloride contains 13.4 mEq K+).
When correction of the arrhythmia with potassium is urgent and the serum potassium concentration is low or normal, approximately 0.5 mEq/kg of potassium per hour may be given intravenously in 5% dextrose injection. The intravenous solution of potassium should be dilute enough to avoid local irritation; however, especially in infants, care must be taken to avoid intravenous fluid overload. ECG monitoring should be performed to watch for any evidence of potassium toxicity (e.g., peaking of T waves) and to observe the effect on the arrhythmia. The infusion may be stopped when the desired effect is achieved.
Note: Potassium should not be used and may be dangerous in heart block due to digoxin, unless primarily related to supraventricular tachycardia.
Other agents that have been used for the treatment of digoxin intoxication include lidocaine, procainamide, propranolol, and phenytoin, although use of the latter must be considered experimental. In advanced heart block, atropine and/or temporary ventricular pacing may be beneficial. DIGIBIND®, Digoxin Immune Fab (Ovine), can be used to reverse potentially life-threatening digoxin (or digitoxin) intoxication. Improvement in signs and symptoms of digitalis toxicity usually begins within $^1/_2$ hour of administration of DIGIBIND. Each 38 mg vial of DIGIBIND will neutralize 0.5 mg of digoxin (which is a usual body store of an adequately digitalized 70 kg patient).
Massive Digitalis Overdosage: Manifestations of life-threatening toxicity include severe ventricular arrhythmias such as ventricular tachycardia or ventricular fibrillation, or progressive bradyarrhythmias such as severe sinus bradycardia or second or third degree heart block not responsive to atropine. An overdosage of more than 10 mg of digoxin in previously healthy adults or 4 mg in previously healthy children or overdosage resulting in steady-state serum concentrations greater than 10 ng/mL, often results in cardiac arrest.
Severe digitalis intoxication can cause life-threatening elevation in serum potassium concentration by shifting potassium from inside to outside the cell resulting in hyperkalemia. Administration of potassium supplements in the setting of massive intoxication may be hazardous.
DIGIBIND, Digoxin Immune Fab (Ovine), may be used at a dose equimolar to digoxin in the body to reverse the effects of ingestion of a massive overdose. The decision to administer DIGIBIND before the onset of toxic manifestations will depend on the likelihood that life-threatening toxicity will occur (see above).
Patients with massive digitalis ingestion should receive large doses of activated charcoal to prevent absorption and bind digoxin in the gut during enteroenteric recirculation. Emesis or gastric lavage may be indicated especially if ingestion has occurred within 30 minutes of the patient's presentation at the hospital. Emesis should not be induced in patients who are obtunded. If a patient presents more than 2 hours after ingestion or already has toxic manifestations, it may be unsafe to induce vomiting or attempt passage of a gastric tube, because such maneuvers may induce an acute vagal episode that can worsen digitalis-toxic arrhythmias.

DOSAGE AND ADMINISTRATION

Recommended dosages are average values that may require considerable modification because of individual sensitivity or associated conditions. Diminished renal function is the most important factor requiring modification of recommended doses.
Parenteral administration of digoxin should be used only when the need for rapid digitalization is urgent or when the drug cannot be taken orally. Intramuscular injection can lead to severe pain at the injection site, thus intravenous administration is preferred. If the drug must be administered by the intramuscular route, it should be injected deep into the muscle followed by massage. No more than 200 µg (2 mL) should be injected into a single site.
LANOXIN Injection Pediatric can be administered undiluted or diluted with a 4-fold or greater volume of Sterile Water for Injection, 0.9% Sodium Chloride Injection or 5% Dextrose Injection. The use of less than a 4-fold volume of diluent could lead to precipitation of the digoxin. Immediate use of the diluted product is recommended.
If tuberculin syringes are used to measure very small doses, one must be aware of the problem of inadvertent overadministration of digoxin. The syringe should *not* be flushed with the parenteral solution after its contents are expelled into an indwelling vascular catheter.
Slow infusion of LANOXIN Injection Pediatric is preferable to bolus administration. Rapid infusion of digitalis glycosides has been shown to cause systemic and coronary arteriolar constriction, which may be clinically undesirable. Caution is thus advised and LANOXIN Injection Pediatric should probably be administered over a period of 5 minutes or longer.
Mixing of LANOXIN Injection Pediatric with other drugs in the same container or simultaneous administration in the same intravenous line is not recommended.
Adults: See the LANOXIN Injection package insert for specific recomendations.
Infants and Children: Digitalization must be individualized. Divided daily dosing is recommended for infants and young children. Children over 10 years of age require adult dosages in proportion to their body weight.
In the newborn period, renal clearance of digoxin is diminished and suitable dosage adjustments must be observed. This is especially pronounced in the premature infant. Beyond the immediate newborn period, children generally require proportionally larger doses than adults on the basis of body weight or body surface area.
In deciding the dose of digoxin, several factors must be considered:

1. The disease being treated. Atrial arrhythmias may require larger doses than heart failure.
2. The body weight of the patient. Doses should be calculated based upon lean or ideal body weight.
3. The patient's renal function, preferably evaluated on the basis of creatinine clearance.
4. Age is an important factor in infants and children.
5. Concomitant disease states, drugs or other factors likely to alter the expected clinical response to digoxin (see PRECAUTIONS and Drug Interactions subsection).

Usual Digitalizing and Maintenance Dosages for LANOXIN® Injection Pediatric in Children with **Normal Renal Function Based on Lean Body Weight**

Age	Digitalizing* Dose (μg/kg)	Daily† I.V. Maintenance Dose (μg/kg)
Premature	15 to 25	20% to 30% of the I.V. loading dose‡
Full-Term	20 to 30	
1 to 24 Months	30 to 50	
2 to 5 Years	25 to 35	
5 to 10 Years	15 to 30	25% to 35% of the I.V. loading dose‡
Over 10 Years	8 to 12	

* I.V. digitalizing doses are 80% of oral digitalizing doses.
† Divided daily dosing is recommended for children under 10 years of age.
‡ Projected or actual digitalizing dose providing clinical response.

Digitalization may be accomplished by either of two general approaches that vary in dosage and frequency of administration, but reach the same endpoint in terms of total amount of digoxin accumulated in the body.

1. Rapid digitalization may be achieved by administering a loading dose based upon projected peak body digoxin stores, then calculating the maintenance dose as a percentage of the loading dose.

2. More gradual digitalization may be obtained by beginning an appropriate maintenance dose, thus allowing digoxin body stores to accumulate slowly. Steady-state serum digoxin concentrations will be achieved in approximately 5 half-lives of the drug for the individual patient. Depending upon the patient's renal function, this will take between one and three weeks.

Infants and Children: Rapid Digitalization with a Loading Dose: LANOXIN Injection Pediatric can be used to achieve rapid digitalization, with conversion to an oral formulation of LANOXIN for maintenance therapy. If patients are switched from intravenous to oral digoxin tablets or elixir, allowances must be made for differences in bioavailability when calculating maintenance dosages (see bioavailability table in CLINICAL PHARMACOLOGY and dosing table below).

Intramuscular injection of digoxin is extremely painful and offers no advantages unless other routes of administration are contraindicated.

Digitalizing and daily maintenance doses for each age group are given below and should provide therapeutic effect with minimum risk of toxicity in most patients with heart failure and normal sinus rhythm. Larger doses are often required for adequate control of ventricular rate in patients with atrial flutter or fibrillation.

The loading dose should be administered in several portions, with roughly half the total given as the first dose. Additional fractions of this planned total dose may be given at 4 to 8 hour intervals, **with careful assessment of clinical response before each additional dose.** If the patient's clinical response necessitates a change from the calculated dose of digoxin, then calculation of the maintenance dose should be based upon the amount actually given.

[See table above.]

Infants and Children: Gradual Digitalization With A Maintenance Dose: More gradual digitalization can also be accomplished by beginning an appropriate maintenance dose. The range of percentages provided above can be used in calculating this dose for patients with normal renal function. In children with renal disease, digoxin dosing must be carefully titrated based upon clinical response.

Long-term use of digoxin is indicated in many children who have been digitalized for acute heart failure, unless the cause is transient. Children with severe congenital heart disease, even after surgery, may require digoxin for prolonged periods.

It cannot be overemphasized that these pediatric dosage guidelines are based upon average patient response and substantial individual variation can be expected. Accordingly, ultimate dosage selection must be based upon clinical assessment of the patient.

Serum Digoxin Concentrations: Measurement of serum digoxin concentrations can be helpful to the clinician in determining the state of digitalization and in assigning certain probabilities to the likelihood of digoxin intoxication. Studies in adults considered adequately digitalized (without evidence of toxicity) show that about two-thirds of such patients have serum digoxin levels ranging from 0.8 to 2.0 ng/mL. Patients with atrial fibrillation or atrial flutter require and appear to tolerate higher levels than do patients with other indications. On the other hand, in adult patients with clinical evidence of digoxin toxicity, about two-thirds will have serum digoxin levels greater than 2.0 ng/mL. Thus, whereas levels less than 0.8 ng/mL are infrequently associated with toxicity, levels greater than 2.0 ng/mL are often associated with toxicity. Values in between are not very helpful in deciding whether a certain sign or symptom is more likely caused by digoxin toxicity or by something else. There are rare patients who are unable to tolerate digoxin even at

serum concentrations below 0.8 ng/mL. Some researchers suggest that infants and young children tolerate slightly higher serum concentrations than do adults.

To allow adequate time for equilibration of digoxin between serum and tissue, **sampling of serum concentrations for clinical use should be at least 6 to 8 hours after the last dose,** regardless of the route of administration or formulation used. On a twice-daily dosing schedule, there will be only minor differences in serum digoxin concentrations whether sampling is done at 8 or 12 hours after a dose. After a single daily dose, the concentration will be 10% to 25% lower when sampled at 24 versus 8 hours, depending upon the patient's renal function. Ideally, sampling for assessment of steady-state concentrations should be done just before the next dose.

If a discrepancy exists between the reported serum concentration and the observed clinical response, the clinician should consider the following possibilities:

1. Analytical problems in the assay procedure.
2. Inappropriate serum sampling time.
3. Administration of a digitalis glycoside other than digoxin.
4. Conditions (described in WARNINGS and PRECAUTIONS) causing an alteration in the sensitivity of the patient to digoxin.
5. The patient falls outside the norm in his response to or handling of digoxin. This decision should only be reached after exclusion of the other possibilities and generally should be confirmed by additional correlations of clinical observations with serum digoxin concentrations.

The serum concentration data should always be interpreted in the overall clinical context and an isolated serum concentration value should not be used alone as a basis for increasing or decreasing digoxin dosage.

Adjustment of Maintenance Dose in Previously Digitalized Patients: LANOXIN Injection Pediatric maintenance doses in individual patients on steady-state digoxin can be adjusted upward or downward in proportion to the ratio of the desired versus the measured serum concentrations. For example, a patient at steady-state on 100 μg (0.1 mg) of LANOXIN Injection Pediatric per day with a measured serum concentration of 0.7 ng/mL, should have the dose increased to 200 μg (0.2 mg) per day to achieve a steady-state serum concentration of 1.4 ng/mL, **assuming the serum digoxin concentration measurement is correct, renal function remains stable during this time and the needed adjustment is not the result of a problem with compliance.**

Dosage Adjustment When Changing Preparations: The differences in bioavailability between injectable LANOXIN or LANOXICAPS and LANOXIN Elixir Pediatric or LANOXIN Tablets must be considered when changing patients from one dosage form to another.

LANOXIN Injection and LANOXICAPS doses of 100 μg (0.1 mg) and 200 μg (0.2 mg) are approximately equivalent to 125 μg (0.125 mg) and 250 μg (0.25 mg) doses of LANOXIN Tablets and LANOXIN Elixir Pediatric (see table in CLINICAL PHARMACOLOGY). Intramuscular injection of digoxin is extremely painful and offers no advantages unless other routes of administration are contraindicated.

HOW SUPPLIED

LANOXIN (digoxin) Injection Pediatric, 100 μg (0.1 mg) in 1 mL; box of ampuls (NDC 0173-0262-10).
Store at 15° to 25°C (59° to 77°F) and protect from light.
Also available:
LANOXIN (digoxin) Tablets, Scored 125 μg (0.125 mg): bottles of 100 and 1000; unit dose pack of 100.
LANOXIN (digoxin) Tablets, Scored 250 μg (0.25 mg): bottles of 100, package of 12 bottles × 100 (with child-resistant cap), 1000 and 5000; unit dose pack of 100.
LANOXIN (digoxin) Elixir Pediatric, 50 μg (0.05 mg) per mL; bottle of 60 mL with calibrated dropper.
LANOXIN (digoxin) Injection, 500 μg (0.5 mg) in 2 mL (250 μg [0.25 mg] per mL): boxes of 10 and 50 ampuls.
LANOXICAPS (digoxin solution in capsules), 50 μg (0.05 mg) bottle of 100; 100 μg (0.1 mg) bottle of 100; 200 μg (0.2 mg) bottle of 100.
February 1996/RL-252

Shown in Product Identification Guide, page 313

LANOXIN® ℞
[lă-nŏx′ĭn″]
(digoxin)
Tablets
125 μg (0.125 mg) Scored I.D. Imprint Y3B (yellow)
250 μg (0.25 mg) Scored I.D. Imprint X3A (white)
500 μg (0.5 mg) Scored I.D. Imprint T9A (green)

DESCRIPTION

Digoxin is one of the cardiac (or digitalis) glycosides, a closely related group of drugs having in common specific effects on the myocardium. These drugs are found in a number of plants. Digoxin is extracted from the leaves of *Digitalis lanata.* The term "digitalis" is used to designate the whole group. The glycosides are composed of two portions: a sugar and a cardenolide (hence "glycosides").

Digoxin has the molecular formula $C_{41}H_{64}O_{14}$, a molecular weight of 780.95 and melting and decomposition points above 235°C. The drug is practically insoluble in water and in ether; slightly soluble in diluted (50%) alcohol and in chloroform; and freely soluble in pyridine. Digoxin powder is composed of odorless white crystals.

Digoxin has the chemical name: $(3\beta,5\beta,12\beta)$-3-[(O-2,6-dideoxyβ-D-ribo -hexopyranosyl-(1→4)-O-2, 6-dideoxy-β-D-ribo-hexopyranosyl-(1→4)-2,6-dideoxy-β-D-ribo -hexopyranosyl)oxy]-12, 14-dihydroxycard-20(22)-enolide.

LANOXIN Tablets with 125 μg (0.125 mg), 250 μg (0.25 mg) or 500 μg (0.5 mg) digoxin USP are intended for oral use. Each tablet contains the labeled amount of digoxin USP and the inactive ingredients: 0.125 mg tablet—corn and potato starch, D&C Yellow No. 10, FD&C Yellow No. 6, lactose, and magnesium stearate; 0.25 mg tablet—corn and potato starch, lactose, magnesium stearate, and stearic acid; 0.5 mg tablet—corn and potato starch, D&C Green No. 5 and Yellow No. 10, FD&C Red No. 40, lactose, magnesium stearate, and stearic acid.

CLINICAL PHARMACOLOGY

Mechanism of Action: The influence of digitalis glycosides on the myocardium is dose-related, and involves both a direct action on cardiac muscle and the specialized conduction system, and indirect actions on the cardiovascular system mediated by the autonomic nervous system. The indirect actions mediated by the autonomic nervous system involve a vagomimetic action, which is responsible for the effects of digitalis on the sino-atrial (SA) and atrioventricular (AV) nodes; and also a baroreceptor sensitization which results in increased carotid sinus nerve activity and enhanced sympathetic withdrawal for any given increment in mean arterial pressure. The pharmacologic consequences of these direct and indirect effects are: 1) an increase in the force and velocity of myocardial systolic contraction (positive inotropic action); 2) a slowing of heart rate (negative chronotropic effect); and 3) decreased conduction velocity through the AV node. In higher doses, digitalis increases sympathetic outflow from the central nervous system (CNS) to both cardiac and peripheral sympathetic nerves. This increase in sympathetic activity may be an important factor in digitalis cardiac toxicity. Most of the extracardiac manifestations of digitalis toxicity are also mediated by the CNS.

Pharmacokinetics:

Absorption: Gastrointestinal absorption of digoxin is a passive process. Absorption of digoxin from the LANOXIN tablet formulation has been demonstrated to be 60% to 80% complete compared to an identical intravenous dose of digoxin (absolute bioavailability). When digoxin tablets are taken after meals, the rate of absorption is slowed, but the total amount of digoxin absorbed is usually unchanged. When taken with meals high in bran fiber, however, the amount absorbed from an oral dose may be reduced. Comparison of the systemic availability and equivalent doses for digoxin preparations are shown in the following table:
[See table at bottom of next page.]

In some patients, orally administered digoxin is converted to cardioinactive reduction products (e.g., dihydrodigoxin) by colonic bacteria in the gut. Data suggest that one in ten patients treated with digoxin tablets will degrade 40% or more of the ingested dose.

Distribution: Following drug administration, a 6 to 8 hour distribution phase is observed. This is followed by a much more gradual serum concentration decline, which is dependent on digoxin elimination from the body. The peak height and slope of the early portion (absorption/distribution phases) of the serum concentration-time curve are dependent upon the route of administration and the absorption characteristics of the formulation. Clinical evidence indicates that the early high serum concentrations do not reflect the concentration of digoxin at its site of action, but that with chronic use, the steady-state post-distribution serum levels

Continued on next page

Glaxo Wellcome—Cont.

PRODUCT	TIME TO ONSET OF EFFECT*	TIME TO PEAK EFFECT*
LANOXIN® Tablets	0.5 to 2 hours	2 to 6 hours
LANOXIN Elixir	0.5 to 2 hours	2 to 6 hours
LANOXIN Injection/I.M.	0.5 to 2 hours	2 to 6 hours
LANOXIN Injection/I.V.	5 to 30 minutes†	1 to 4 hours
LANOXICAPS® Capsules	0.5 to 2 hours	2 to 6 hours

*Documented for ventricular response rate in atrial fibrillation, inotropic effect and electrocardiographic changes.
†Depending upon rate of infusion.

are in equilibrium with tissue levels and correlate with pharmacologic effects. In individual patients, these post-distribution serum concentrations are linearly related to maintenance dosage and may be useful in evaluating therapeutic and toxic effects (see DOSAGE AND ADMINISTRATION: Serum Digoxin Concentrations).

Digoxin is concentrated in tissues and therefore has a large apparent volume of distribution. Digoxin crosses both the blood-brain barrier and the placenta. At delivery, serum digoxin concentration in the newborn is similar to the serum level in the mother. Approximately 20% to 25% of plasma digoxin is bound to protein. Serum digoxin concentrations are not significantly altered by large changes in fat tissue weight, so that its distribution space correlates best with lean (ideal) body weight, not total body weight.

Pharmacologic Response: The approximate times to onset of effect and to peak effect of all the LANOXIN preparations are given in the following table:

[See table above.]

Excretion: Elimination of digoxin follows first-order kinetics (that is, the quantity of digoxin eliminated at any time is proportional to the total body content). Following intravenous administration to normal subjects, 50% to 70% of a digoxin dose is excreted unchanged in the urine. Renal excretion of digoxin is proportional to glomerular filtration rate and is largely independent of urine flow. In subjects with normal renal function, digoxin has a half-life of 1.5 to 2.0 days. The half-life in anuric patients is prolonged to 4 to 6 days. Digoxin is not effectively removed from the body by dialysis, exchange transfusion or during cardiopulmonary by-pass because most of the drug is in tissue rather than circulating in the blood.

INDICATIONS AND USAGE

Heart Failure: The increased cardiac output resulting from the inotropic action of digoxin ameliorates the disturbances characteristic of heart failure (venous congestion, edema, dyspnea, orthopnea and cardiac asthma).

Digoxin is more effective in "low output" (pump) failure than in "high output" heart failure secondary to arteriovenous fistula, anemia, infection, or hyperthyroidism.

Digoxin is usually continued after failure is controlled, unless some known precipitating factor is corrected. Studies have shown, however, that even though hemodynamic effects can be demonstrated in almost all patients, corresponding improvement in the signs and symptoms of heart failure is not necessarily apparent. Therefore, in patients in whom digoxin may be difficult to regulate, or in whom the risk of toxicity may be great (e.g., patients with unstable renal function or whose potassium levels tend to fluctuate), cautious withdrawal of digoxin may be considered. If digoxin is discontinued, the patient should be regularly monitored for clinical evidence of recurrent heart failure.

Atrial Fibrillation: Digoxin reduces ventricular rate and thereby improves hemodynamics. Palpitation, precordial distress or weakness are relieved and concomitant congestive failure ameliorated. Digoxin should be continued in doses necessary to maintain the desired ventricular rate.

Atrial Flutter: Digoxin slows the heart and regular sinus rhythm may appear. Frequently the flutter is converted to atrial fibrillation with a controlled ventricular response. Digoxin treatment should be maintained if atrial fibrillation persists. (Electrical cardioversion is often the treatment of choice for atrial flutter. See discussion of cardioversion in PRECAUTIONS.)

Paroxysmal Atrial Tachycardia (PAT): Digoxin may convert PAT to sinus rhythm by slowing conduction through the AV node. If heart failure has ensued or paroxysms recur frequently, digoxin should be continued. In infants, digoxin is usually continued for 3 to 6 months after a single episode of PAT to prevent recurrence.

CONTRAINDICATIONS

Digitalis glycosides are contraindicated in ventricular fibrillation.

In a given patient, an untoward effect requiring permanent discontinuation of other digitalis preparations usually constitutes a contraindication to digoxin. Hypersensitivity to digoxin itself is a contraindication to its use. Allergy to digoxin, though rare, does occur. It may not extend to all such preparations, and another digitalis glycoside may be tried with caution.

WARNINGS

Digitalis alone or with other drugs has been used in the treatment of obesity. This use of digoxin or other digitalis glycosides is unwarranted. Moreover, since they may cause potentially fatal arrhythmias or other adverse effects, the use of these drugs solely for the treatment of obesity is dangerous.

Anorexia, nausea, vomiting and arrhythmias may accompany heart failure or may be indications of digitalis intoxication. Clinical evaluation of the cause of these symptoms should be attempted before further digitalis administration. In such circumstances determination of the serum digoxin concentration may be an aid in deciding whether or not digitalis toxicity is likely to be present. If the possibility of digitalis intoxication cannot be excluded, cardiac glycosides should be temporarily withheld, if permitted by the clinical situation.

Patients with renal insufficiency require smaller than usual maintenance doses of digoxin (see DOSAGE AND ADMINISTRATION).

Heart failure accompanying acute glomerulonephritis requires extreme care in digitalization. Relatively low loading and maintenance doses and concomitant use of antihypertensive drugs may be necessary and careful monitoring is essential. Digoxin should be discontinued as soon as possible. Patients with severe carditis, such as carditis associated with rheumatic fever or viral myocarditis, are especially sensitive to digoxin-induced disturbances of rhythm.

Newborn infants display considerable variability in their tolerance to digoxin. Premature and immature infants are particularly sensitive, and dosage must not only be reduced but must be individualized according to their degree of maturity.

Note: Digitalis glycosides are an important cause of accidental poisoning in children.

PRECAUTIONS

General: Digoxin toxicity develops more frequently and lasts longer in patients with renal impairment because of the decreased excretion of digoxin. Therefore, it should be anticipated that dosage requirements will be decreased in patients with moderate to severe renal disease (see DOSAGE AND ADMINISTRATION). Because of the prolonged half-life, a longer period of time is required to achieve an initial or new steady-state concentration in patients with renal impairment than in patients with normal renal function.

In patients with hypokalemia, toxicity may occur despite serum digoxin concentrations within the "normal range," because potassium depletion sensitizes the myocardium to digoxin. Therefore, it is desirable to maintain normal serum potassium levels in patients being treated with digoxin. Hypokalemia may result from diuretic, amphotericin B or corticosteroid therapy, and from dialysis or mechanical suction of gastrointestinal secretions. It may also accompany malnutrition, diarrhea, prolonged vomiting, old age and long-standing heart failure. In general, rapid changes in serum potassium or other electrolytes should be avoided, and intravenous treatment with potassium should be reserved for special circumstances as described below (see OVERDOSAGE: Treatment of Arrhythmias Produced by Overdosage). Calcium, particularly when administered rapidly by the intravenous route, may produce serious arrhythmias in digitalized patients. Hypercalcemia from any cause predisposes the patient to digitalis toxicity. On the other hand, hypocalcemia can nullify the effects of digoxin in man; thus, digoxin may be ineffective until serum calcium is restored to normal. These interactions are related to the fact that calcium affects contractility and excitability of the heart in a manner similar to digoxin.

Hypomagnesemia may predispose to digitalis toxicity. If low magnesium levels are detected in a patient on digoxin, replacement therapy should be instituted.

Quinidine, verapamil, amiodarone, propafenone, indomethacin, itraconazole, and alprazolam may cause a rise in serum digoxin concentration, with the implication that digitalis intoxication may result. This rise appears to be proportional to the dose. The effect is mediated by a reduction in the digoxin clearance and, in the case of quinidine, decreased volume of distribution as well.

Erythromycin and clarithromycin (and possibly other macrolide antibiotics) and tetracycline may increase digoxin absorption (see CLINICAL PHARMACOLOGY: Pharmacokinetics). Recent studies have shown that specific colonic bacteria in the lower gastrointestinal tract convert digoxin to cardioinactive reduction products, thereby reducing its bioavailability. Although inactivation of these bacteria by antibiotics is rapid, the serum digoxin concentration will rise at a rate consistent with the elimination half-life of digoxin. The magnitude of rise in serum digoxin concentration relates to the extent of bacterial inactivation, and may be as much as two-fold in some cases.

Patients with acute myocardial infarction or severe pulmonary disease may be unusually sensitive to digoxin-induced disturbances of rhythm.

Atrial arrhythmias associated with hypermetabolic states (e.g., hyperthyroidism) are particularly resistant to digoxin treatment. Large doses of digoxin are not recommended as the only treatment of these arrhythmias and care must be taken to avoid toxicity if large doses of digoxin are required. In hypothyroidism, the digoxin requirements are reduced. Digoxin responses in patients with compensated thyroid disease are normal.

Reduction of digoxin dosage may be desirable prior to electrical cardioversion to avoid induction of ventricular arrhythmias, but the physician must consider the consequences of rapid increase in ventricular response to atrial fibrillation if digoxin is withheld 1 to 2 days prior to cardioversion. If there is a suspicion that digitalis toxicity exists, elective cardioversion should be delayed. If it is not prudent to delay cardioversion, the energy level selected should be minimal at first and carefully increased in an attempt to avoid precipitating ventricular arrhythmias.

Incomplete AV block, especially in patients with Stokes-Adams attacks, may progress to advanced or complete heart block if digoxin is given.

In some patients with sinus node disease (i.e., Sick Sinus Syndrome), digoxin may worsen sinus bradycardia or sinoatrial block.

In patients with Wolff-Parkinson-White Syndrome and atrial fibrillation, digoxin can enhance transmission of impulses through the accessory pathway. This effect may result in extremely rapid ventricular rates and even ventricular fibrillation.

Digoxin may worsen the outflow obstruction in patients with idiopathic hypertrophic subaortic stenosis (IHSS). Unless cardiac failure is severe, it is doubtful whether digoxin should be employed.

Patients with chronic constrictive pericarditis may fail to respond to digoxin. In addition, slowing of the heart rate by digoxin in some patients may further decrease cardiac output.

Patients with heart failure from amyloid heart disease or constrictive cardiomyopathies respond poorly to treatment with digoxin.

Digoxin is not indicated for the treatment of sinus tachycardia unless it is associated with heart failure.

Digoxin may produce false positive ST-T changes in the electrocardiogram during exercise testing.

Intramuscular injection of digoxin is extremely painful and offers no advantages unless other routes of administration are contraindicated.

Laboratory Tests: Patients receiving digoxin should have their serum electrolytes and renal function (BUN and/or serum creatinine) assessed periodically; the frequency of assessments will depend on the clinical setting. For discussion of serum digoxin concentrations, see DOSAGE AND ADMINISTRATION.

Drug Interactions: Potassium-depleting *corticosteroids* and *diuretics* may be major contributing factors to digitalis toxicity. *Calcium*, particularly if administered rapidly by the intravenous route, may produce serious arrhythmias in digitalized patients. *Quinidine, verapamil, amiodarone, propafenone, indomethacin, itraconazole,* and *alprazolam* may cause a rise in serum digoxin concentration, with the implication that digitalis intoxication may result. Serum levels of di-

PRODUCT	ABSOLUTE BIOAVAILABILITY	EQUIVALENT DOSES (IN MG*)		
LANOXIN® Tablets	60% to 80%	0.125	0.25	0.5
LANOXIN Elixir	70% to 85%	0.125	0.25	0.5
LANOXIN Injection/I.M.	70% to 85%	0.125	0.25	0.5
LANOXIN Injection/I.V.	100%	0.1	0.2	0.4
LANOXICAPS® Capsules	90% to 100%	0.1	0.2	0.4

*1 mg = 1000 μg

goxin may be increased by concomitant administration of *erythromycin* and *clarithromycin* (and possibly other *macrolide antibiotics*) and *tetracycline*. *Propantheline* and *diphenoxylate*, by decreasing gut motility, may increase digoxin absorption. *Antacids, kaolin-pectin, sulfasalazine, neomycin, cholestyramine*, certain *anticancer drugs*, and *metoclopramide* may reduce intestinal digoxin absorption, resulting in unexpectedly low serum concentrations. There have been inconsistent reports regarding the effects of other drugs on the serum digoxin concentration. *Thyroid* administration to a digitalized, hypothyroid patient may increase the dose requirement of digoxin. Concomitant use of digoxin and *sympathomimetics* increases the risk of cardiac arrhythmias because both enhance ectopic pacemaker activity. *Succinylcholine* may cause a sudden extrusion of potassium from muscle cells, and may thereby cause arrhythmias in digitalized patients. Although β adrenergic blockers or calcium channel blockers and digoxin may be useful in combination to control atrial fibrillation, their additive effects on AV node conduction can result in complete heart block.

Due to the considerable variability of these interactions, digoxin dosage should be carefully individualized when patients receive coadministered medications. Furthermore, caution should be exercised when combining digoxin with any drug that may cause a significant deterioration in renal function, since this may impair the excretion of digoxin.

Carcinogenesis, Mutagenesis, Impairment of Fertility: There have been no long-term studies performed in animals to evaluate carcinogenic potential.

Pregnancy: ***Teratogenic Effects:*** Pregnancy Category C. Animal reproduction studies have not been conducted with digoxin. It is also not known whether digoxin can cause fetal harm when administered to a pregnant woman or can affect reproduction capacity. Digoxin should be given to a pregnant woman only if clearly needed.

Nursing Mothers: Studies have shown that digoxin concentrations in the mother's serum and milk are similar. However, the estimated daily dose to a nursing infant will be far below the usual infant maintenance dose. Therefore, this amount should have no pharmacologic effect upon the infant. Nevertheless, caution should be exercised when digoxin is administered to a nursing woman.

ADVERSE REACTIONS

The frequency and severity of adverse reactions to digoxin depend on the dose and route of administration, as well as on the patient's underlying disease or concomitant therapies (see PRECAUTIONS and DOSAGE AND ADMINISTRATION: Serum Digoxin Concentrations). The overall incidence of adverse reactions has been reported as 5% to 20%, with 15% to 20% of them being considered serious (one to four percent of patients receiving digoxin). Evidence suggests that the incidence of toxicity has decreased since the introduction of the serum digoxin assay and improved standardization of digoxin tablets. Cardiac toxicity accounts for about one-half, gastrointestinal disturbances for about one-fourth, and CNS and other toxicity for about one-fourth of these adverse reactions.

Adults:

Cardiac: Unifocal or multiform ventricular premature contractions, especially in bigeminal or trigeminal patterns, are the most common arrhythmias associated with digoxin toxicity in adults with heart disease.

Ventricular tachycardia may result from digitalis toxicity. Atrioventricular (AV) dissociation, accelerated junctional (nodal) rhythm and atrial tachycardia with block are also common arrhythmias caused by digoxin overdosage.

Excessive slowing of the pulse is a clinical sign of digoxin overdosage. AV block (Wenckebach) of increasing degree may proceed to complete heart block.

Note: The electrocardiogram is fundamental in determining the presence and nature of these cardiac disturbances. Digoxin may also induce other changes in the ECG (e.g., PR prolongation, ST depression), which represent digoxin effect and may or may not be associated with digitalis toxicity.

Gastrointestinal: Anorexia, nausea, vomiting, and less commonly diarrhea are common early symptoms of overdosage. However, uncontrolled heart failure may also produce such symptoms. Digitalis toxicity very rarely may cause abdominal pain and hemorrhagic necrosis of the intestines.

CNS: Visual disturbances (blurred or yellow vision), headache, weakness, dizziness, apathy and psychosis can occur.

Other: Gynecomastia is occasionally observed. Maculopapular rash or other skin reactions are rarely observed.

Infants and Children: Toxicity differs from the adult in a number of respects. Anorexia, nausea, vomiting, diarrhea and CNS disturbances may be present but are rare as initial symptoms in infants. Cardiac arrhythmias are more reliable signs of toxicity. Digoxin in children may produce any arrhythmia. The most commonly encountered are conduction disturbances or supraventricular tachyarrythmias, such as atrial tachycardia with or without block and junctional (nodal) tachycardia. Ventricular arrhythmias are less common. Sinus bradycardia may also be a sign of impending digoxin intoxication, especially in infants, even in the absence of first-degree heart block. Any arrhythmia or alteration in cardiac conduction that develops in a child taking digoxin should initially be assumed to be a consequence of digoxin intoxication.

OVERDOSAGE

Treatment of Arrhythmias Produced by Overdosage:

Adults: Digoxin should be discontinued until all signs of toxicity are gone. Discontinuation may be all that is necessary if toxic manifestations are not severe and appear only near the expected time for maximum effect of the drug.

Correction of factors that may contribute to toxicity such as electrolyte disturbances, hypoxia, acid-base disturbances and removal of aggravating agents such as catecholamines, should also be considered. Potassium salts may be indicated, particularly if hypokalemia is present. Potassium administration may be dangerous in the setting of massive digitalis overdosage (see Massive Digitalis Overdosage subsection below). Potassium chloride in divided oral doses totaling 3 to 6 grams of the salt (40 to 80 mEq K+) for adults may be given provided renal function is adequate (see Infants and Children subsection below for potassium recommendations).

When correction of the arrhythmia is urgent and the serum potassium concentration is low or normal, potassium should be administered intravenously in 5% dextrose injection. For adults, a total of 40 to 80 mEq (diluted to a concentration of 40 mEq per 500 mL) may be given at a rate not exceeding 20 mEq per hour, or slower if limited by pain due to local irritation. Additional amounts may be given if the arrhythmia is uncontrolled and potassium well-tolerated. ECG monitoring should be performed to watch for any evidence of potassium toxicity (e.g., peaking of T waves) and to observe the effect on the arrhythmia. The infusion may be stopped when the desired effect is achieved.

Note: Potassium should not be used and may be dangerous in heart block due to digoxin, unless primarily related to supraventricular tachycardia.

Other agents that have been used for the treatment of digoxin intoxication include lidocaine, procainamide, propranolol, and phenytoin, although use of the latter must be considered experimental. In advanced heart block, atropine and/or temporary ventricular pacing may be beneficial. DIGIBIND®, Digoxin Immune Fab (Ovine), can be used to reverse potentially life-threatening digoxin (or digitoxin) intoxication. Improvement in signs and symptoms of digitalis toxicity usually begins within ½ hour of DIGIBIND administration. Each 38 mg vial of DIGIBIND will neutralize 0.5 mg of digoxin (which is a usual body store of an adequately digitalized 70 kg patient).

Infants and Children: See Adult section for general recommendations for the treatment of arrhythmias produced by overdosage and for cautions regarding the use of potassium. If a potassium preparation is used to treat toxicity, it may be given orally in divided doses totaling 1 to 1.5 mEq K+ per kilogram (kg) body weight (1 gram of potassium chloride contains 13.4 mEq K+).

When correction of the arrhythmia with potassium is urgent, approximately 0.5 mEq/kg of potassium per hour may be given intravenously, with careful ECG monitoring. The intravenous solution of potassium should be dilute enough to avoid local irritation; however, especially in infants, care must be taken to avoid intravenous fluid overload.

Massive Digitalis Overdosage: Manifestations of life-threatening toxicity include severe ventricular arrhythmias such as ventricular tachycardia or ventricular fibrillation, or progressive bradyarrhythmias such as severe sinus bradycardia or second or third degree heart block not responsive to atropine. An overdosage of more than 10 mg of digoxin in previously healthy adults or 4 mg in previously healthy children or overdosage resulting in steady-state serum concentrations greater than 10 ng/mL, often results in cardiac arrest.

Severe digitalis intoxication can cause life-threatening elevation in serum potassium concentration by shifting potassium from inside to outside the cell resulting in hyperkalemia. Administration of potassium supplements in the setting of massive intoxication may be hazardous.

DIGIBIND, Digoxin Immune Fab (Ovine), may be used at a dose equimolar to digoxin in the body to reverse the effects of ingestion of a massive overdose. The decision to administer DIGIBIND before the onset of toxic manifestations will depend on the likelihood that life threatening toxicity will occur (see above).

Patients with massive digitalis ingestion should receive large doses of activated charcoal to prevent absorption and bind digoxin in the gut during enteroenteric recirculation. Emesis or gastric lavage may be indicated especially if ingestion has occurred within 30 minutes of the patient's presentation at the hospital. Emesis should not be induced in patients who are obtunded. If a patient presents more than 2 hours after ingestion or already has toxic manifestations, it may be unsafe to induce vomiting or attempt passage of a gastric tube, because such maneuvers may induce an acute vagal episode that can worsen digitalis-toxic arrhythmias.

DOSAGE AND ADMINISTRATION

Recommended dosages are average values that may require considerable modification because of individual sensitivity or associated conditions. Diminished renal function is the most important factor requiring modification of recommended doses.

In deciding the dose of digoxin, several factors must be considered:

1. The disease being treated. Atrial arrhythmias may require larger doses than heart failure.
2. The body weight of the patient. Doses should be calculated based upon lean or ideal body weight.
3. The patient's renal function, preferably evaluated on the basis of creatinine clearance.
4. Age is an important factor in infants and children.
5. Concomitant disease states, drugs or other factors likely to alter the expected clinical response to digoxin (see PRECAUTIONS and Drug Interactions subsection).

Digitalization may be accomplished by either of two general approaches that vary in dosage and frequency of administration, but reach the same endpoint in terms of total amount of digoxin accumulated in the body.

1. Rapid digitalization may be achieved by administering a loading dose based upon projected peak body digoxin stores, then calculating the maintenance dose as a percentage of the loading dose.
2. More gradual digitalization may be obtained by beginning an appropriate maintenance dose, thus allowing digoxin body stores to accumulate slowly. Steady-state serum digoxin concentrations will be achieved in approximately 5 half-lives of the drug for the individual patient. Depending upon the patient's renal function, this will take between one and three weeks.

Adults:

Rapid Digitalization with a Loading Dose. Peak body digoxin stores of 8 to 12 μg/kg should provide therapeutic effect with minimum risk of toxicity in most patients with heart failure and normal sinus rhythm. Larger stores (10 to 15 μg/kg) are often required for adequate control of ventricular rate in patients with atrial flutter or fibrillation. Because of altered digoxin distribution and elimination, projected peak body stores for patients with renal insufficiency should be conservative (i.e., 6 to 10 μg/kg) (see PRECAUTIONS section).

The loading dose should be based on the projected peak body stores and administered in several portions, with roughly half the total given as the first dose. Additional fractions of this planned total dose may be given at 6 to 8 hour intervals, **with careful assessment of clinical response before each additional dose.**

If the patient's clinical response necessitates a change from the calculated dose of digoxin, then calculation of the maintenance dose should be based upon the amount actually given.

In previously undigitalized patients, a single initial LANOXIN Tablet dose of 500 to 750 μg (0.5 to 0.75 mg) usually produces a detectable effect in 0.5 to 2 hours that becomes maximal in 2 to 6 hours. Additional doses of 125 to 375 μg (0.125 to 0.375 mg) may be given cautiously at 6 to 8 hour intervals until clinical evidence of an adequate effect is noted. The usual amount of LANOXIN Tablets that a 70 kg patient requires to achieve 8 to 15 μg/kg peak body stores is 750 to 1250 μg (0.75 to 1.25 mg).

Although peak body stores are mathematically related to loading doses and are utilized to calculate maintenance doses, they do not correlate with measured serum concentrations. This discrepancy is caused by digoxin distribution within the body during the first 6 to 8 hours following a dose. Serum concentrations drawn during this time are usually not interpretable.

The maintenance dose should be based upon the percentage of the peak body stores lost each day through elimination. The following formula has had wide clinical use:

$$\text{Maintenance Dose} = \text{Peak Body Stores (i.e., Loading Dose)} \times \frac{\%\ \text{Daily Loss}}{100}$$

$$\text{Where: } \%\ \text{Daily Loss} = 14 + \text{Ccr}/5$$

Ccr is creatinine clearance, corrected to 70 kg body weight or 1.73 m^2 body surface area. *For adults*, if only serum creatinine concentrations (Scr) are available, a Ccr (corrected to 70 kg body weight) may be estimated in men as (140 − Age)/Scr. For women, this result should be multiplied by 0.85.

Note: This equation cannot be used for estimating creatinine clearance in infants or children.

A common practice involves the use of LANOXIN Injection to achieve rapid digitalization, with conversion to LANOXIN Tablets or LANOXICAPS for maintenance therapy. If patients are switched from intravenous to oral digoxin formulations, allowances must be made for differences in bioavailability when calculating maintenance dosages (see table in CLINICAL PHARMACOLOGY).

Adults: Gradual Digitalization with a Maintenance Dose: The following table provides average LANOXIN Tablet daily

Continued on next page

Glaxo Wellcome—Cont.

maintenance dose requirements for patients with heart failure based upon lean body weight and renal function:
[See table below.]

Example: Based on the above table, a patient in heart failure with an estimated lean body weight of 70 kg and a Ccr of 60 mL/min, should be given a 250 μg (0.25 mg) LANOXIN Tablet each day, usually taken after the morning meal. Steady-state serum concentrations should not be anticipated before 11 days.

Infants and Children: Digitalization must be individualized. Divided daily dosing is recommended for infants and young children. Children over 10 years of age require adult dosages in proportion to their body weight.

In the newborn period, renal clearance of digoxin is diminished and suitable dosage adjustments must be observed. This is especially pronounced in the premature infant. Beyond the immediate newborn period, children generally require proportionally larger doses than adults on the basis of body weight or body surface area.

LANOXIN Injection Pediatric can be used to achieve rapid digitalization, with conversion to an oral LANOXIN formulation for maintenance therapy. If patients are switched from intravenous to oral digoxin tablets or elixir, allowances must be made for differences in bioavailability when calculating maintenance dosages (see bioavailability table in CLINICAL PHARMACOLOGY and dosing table below).

Intramuscular injection of digoxin is extremely painful and offers no advantages unless other routes of administration are contraindicated.

Digitalizing and daily maintenance doses for each age group are given below and should provide therapeutic effect with minimum risk of toxicity in most patients with heart failure and normal sinus rhythm. Larger doses are often required for adequate control of ventricular rate in patients with atrial flutter or fibrillation.

The loading dose should be administered in several portions, with roughly half the total given as the first dose. Additional fractions of this planned total dose may be given at 6 to 8 hour intervals, **with careful assessment of clinical response before each additional dose.** If the patient's clinical response necessitates a change from the calculated dose of digoxin, then calculation of the maintenance dose should be based upon the amount actually given.

[See table above.]

More gradual digitalization can also be accomplished by beginning an appropriate maintenance dose. The range of percentages provided above can be used in calculating this dose for patients with normal renal function. In children with renal disease, digoxin dosing must be carefully titrated based upon clinical response.

Long-term use of digoxin is indicated in many children who have been digitalized for acute heart failure, unless the cause is transient. Children with severe congenital heart disease, even after surgery, may require digoxin for prolonged periods.

It cannot be overemphasized that both the adult and pediatric dosage guidelines provided are based upon average patient response and substantial individual variation can be expected. Accordingly, ultimate dosage selection must be based upon clinical assessment of the patient.

Serum Digoxin Concentrations: Measurement of serum digoxin concentrations can be helpful to the clinician in determining the state of digitalization and in assigning certain probabilities to the likelihood of digoxin intoxication. Studies in adults considered adequately digitalized (without evidence of toxicity) show that about two-thirds of such patients have serum digoxin levels ranging from 0.8 to 2.0 ng/mL. Patients with atrial fibrillation or atrial flutter require and appear to tolerate higher levels than do patients with other indications. On the other hand, in adult patients with clinical evidence of digoxin toxicity, about two-thirds will have serum digoxin levels greater than 2.0 ng/mL. Thus, whereas levels less than 0.8 ng/mL are infrequently associated with toxicity, levels greater than 2.0 ng/mL are often associated with toxicity. Values in between are not very helpful in deciding whether a certain sign or symptom is more likely caused by digoxin toxicity or by something else. There are rare patients who are unable to tolerate digoxin even at serum concentrations below 0.8 ng/mL. Some researchers suggest that infants and young children tolerate slightly higher serum concentrations than do adults.

Usual Digitalizing and Maintenance Dosages for LANOXIN® Tablets in Children with **Normal Renal Function Based on Lean Body Weight**

Age	Digitalizing* Dose (μg/kg)	Daily† Maintenance Dose (μg/kg)
2 to 5 Years	30 to 40	25% to 35% of *oral* loading dose‡
5 to 10 Years	20 to 35	
Over 10 years	10 to 15	

* I.V. digitalizing doses are 80% of oral digitalizing doses.
† Divided daily dosing is recommended for children under 10 years of age.
‡ Projected or actual digitalizing dose providing clinical response.

To allow adequate time for equilibration of digoxin between serum and tissue, **sampling of serum concentrations for clinical use should be at least 6 to 8 hours after the last dose,** regardless of the route of administration or formulation used. On a twice daily dosing schedule, there will be only minor differences in serum digoxin concentrations whether sampling is done at 8 or 12 hours after a dose. After a single daily dose, the concentration will be 10% to 25% lower when sampled at 24 versus 8 hours, depending upon the patient's renal function. Ideally, sampling for assessment of steady-state concentrations should be done just before the next dose.

If a discrepancy exists between the reported serum concentration and the observed clinical response, the clinician should consider the following possibilities:

1. Analytical problems in the assay procedure.
2. Inappropriate serum sampling time.
3. Administration of a digitalis glycoside other than digoxin.
4. Conditions (described in WARNINGS and PRECAUTIONS) causing an alteration in the sensitivity of the patient to digoxin.
5. The patient falls outside the norm in his response to or handling of digoxin. This decision should only be reached after exclusion of the other possibilities and generally should be confirmed by additional correlations of clinical observations with serum digoxin concentrations.

The serum concentration data should always be interpreted in the overall clinical context and an isolated serum concentration value should not be used alone as a basis for increasing or decreasing digoxin dosage.

Adjustment of Maintenance Dose in Previously Digitalized Patients: LANOXIN Tablet maintenance doses in individual patients on steady-state digoxin can be adjusted upward or downward in proportion to the ratio of the desired versus the measured serum concentration. For example, a patient at steady-state on 125 μg (0.125 mg) of LANOXIN Tablets per day with a measured serum concentration of 0.7 ng/mL, should have the dose increased to 250 μg (0.25 mg) per day to achieve a steady-state serum concentration of 1.4 ng/mL, **assuming the serum digoxin concentration measurement is correct, renal function remains stable during this time, and the needed adjustment is not the result of a problem with compliance.**

Dosage Adjustment When Changing Preparations: The difference in bioavailability between injectable LANOXIN or LANOXICAPS and LANOXIN Elixir Pediatric or LANOXIN Tablets must be considered when changing patients from one dosage form to another.

LANOXIN Injection and LANOXICAPS doses of 100 μg (0.1 mg) and 200 μg (0.2 mg) are approximately equivalent to 125 μg (0.125 mg) and 250 μg (0.25 mg) doses of LANOXIN Tablets and Elixir Pediatric (see Table CLINICAL PHARMACOLOGY). Intramuscular injection of digoxin is extremely painful and offers no advantages unless other routes of administration are contraindicated.

HOW SUPPLIED

LANOXIN (digoxin) Tablets, Scored 125 μg (0.125 mg): Bottles of 100 (NDC 0173-0242-55) and 1000 (NDC 0173-0242-75); unit dose pack of 100 (NDC 0173-0242-56). Imprinted with LANOXIN and Y3B (yellow). Store at 15° to 25°C (59° to 77°F) in a dry place and protect from light.

LANOXIN (digoxin) Tablets, Scored 250 μg (0.25 mg): Bottles of 100 (NDC 0173-0249-55), package of 12 bottles × 100 with child-resistant cap (NDC 0173-0249-01), 1000 (NDC 0173-0249-75) and 5000 (NDC 0173-0249-80); unit dose pack of 100 (NDC 0173-0249-56). Imprinted with LANOXIN and X3A (white). Store at 15° to 25°C (59° to 77°F) in a dry place.

Also Available:
LANOXIN (digoxin) Elixir Pediatric, 50 μg (0.05 mg) per mL; bottle of 60 mL with calibrated dropper.
LANOXIN (digoxin) Injection, 500 μg (0.5 mg) in 2 mL (250 μg [0.25 mg] per mL); boxes of 10 and 50 ampuls.
LANOXIN (digoxin) Injection Pediatric, 100 μg (0.1 mg) in 1 mL; box of 10 ampuls.
LANOXICAPS (digoxin solution in capsules) 50 μg (0.05 mg) bottle of 100; 100 μg (0.1 mg) bottle of 100; 200 μg (0.2 mg) bottle of 100.

February 1996/RL-240

Shown in Product Identification Guide, page 313

MANTADIL® ℞

[*măn 'ta-dĭl"*]
Cream

DESCRIPTION

MANTADIL® Cream contains the antihistamine, chlorcyclizine hydrochloride 2%, and the corticosteroid, hydrocortisone acetate 0.5%, with methylparaben 0.25% (added as a preservative) in a vanishing cream base. The inactive ingredients are liquid and white petrolatum, emulsifying wax, and purified water.

MANTADIL Cream is an ANTIPRURITIC-ANTI-INFLAMMATORY-ANESTHETIC for topical administration.

Chlorcyclizine hydrochloride is known chemically as 1-[(4-chlorophenyl)phenylmethyl]- 4-methylpiperazine monohydrochloride.

Hydrocortisone acetate is the acetate ester of cortisol, known chemically as 21- (acetyloxy) -11β,17-dihydroxypregn- 4 -ene-3, 20-dione.

The pH of this product is approximately 4.5.

CLINICAL PHARMACOLOGY

Chlorcyclizine hydrochloride is an H_1 histamine-receptor antagonist that will occupy receptor sites in effector cells to the exclusion of histamine. It blocks most of the effects of histamine mediated by H_1 receptors, including contraction of smooth muscle and increased capillary permeability. Absorption of chlorcyclizine hydrochloride into the skin is rapid following topical application, whereas systemic absorption from the skin is minimal. Chlorcyclizine hydrochloride prevents local edema and provides local anesthetic and antipruritic action in the skin.

Hydrocortisone acetate administered topically suppresses most inflammatory and allergic responses in the skin. Following topical application, it is absorbed rapidly into the skin, where it reduces local heat, redness, swelling, and tenderness. A small part of the dose applied to broken skin is absorbed systemically and metabolized by the liver.

INDICATIONS AND USAGE

MANTADIL Cream is indicated for the treatment of pruritic skin eruptions and other dermatoses including: eczema (allergic, nuchal, and nummular); dermatitis (atopic, lichenoid, and seborrheic); contact dermatitis including poison ivy, poison oak, and poison sumac; localized neurodermatitis; insect bites; sunburn; intertrigo; and anogenital pruritus.

Usual LANOXIN® Daily Maintenance Dose Requirements (μg)
For Estimated Peak Body Stores of 10 μg/kg

Corrected Ccr (mL/min per 70 kg)	Lean Body Weight (kg/lbs) 50/110	60/132	70/154	80/176	90/198	100/220	Number of Days Before Steady-State Achieved
0	63*†	125	125	125	188‡	188	22
10	125	125	125	188	188	188	19
20	125	125	188	188	188	250	16
30	125	188	188	188	250	250	14
40	125	188	188	250	250	250	13
50	188	188	250	250	250	250	12
60	188	188	250	250	250	375	11
70	188	250	250	250	250	375	10
80	188	250	250	250	375	375	9
90	188	250	250	250	375	500	8
100	250	250	250	375	375	500	7

* 63 μg = 0.063 mg.
† ½ of 125 μg tablet or 125 μg every other day.
‡ 1½ of 125 μg tablet.

CONTRAINDICATIONS

This preparation is contraindicated in patients who are hypersensitive to any of its components; in tuberculosis of the skin, vaccinia, varicella, and herpes simplex. As with other topical products containing hydrocortisone, the cream should not be used in bacterial infections of the skin unless antibacterial therapy is concomitant.

Not for ophthalmic use.

WARNINGS

Oral chlorcyclizine is teratogenic in animals. Long-term reproduction studies of topical chlorcyclizine have not been conducted in humans.

PRECAUTIONS

General: If signs of irritation develop with use of this cream, treatment should be discontinued and appropriate therapy instituted.

Any of the side effects reported following systemic use of corticosteroids, including adrenal suppression, may also occur following their topical use, especially in infants and children. Systemic absorption of topically applied steroids will be increased if extensive body surface areas are treated or if the occlusive technique is used. Under these circumstances, suitable precautions should be taken when long-term use is anticipated, particularly in infants and children.

Carcinogenesis, Mutagenesis, Impairment of Fertility: Oral chlorcyclizine is teratogenic in animals. Long-term reproduction studies of topical chlorcyclizine have not been conducted. It is poorly absorbed percutaneously.

Pregnancy: *Teratogenic Effects:* Pregnancy Category C. Animal reproduction studies have not been conducted with MANTADIL Cream. It is also not known whether MANTADIL Cream can cause fetal harm when administered to a pregnant woman or can affect reproduction capacity. MANTADIL Cream should be given to a pregnant woman only if clearly needed.

Nursing Mothers: Hydrocortisone acetate appears in human milk following oral administration of the drug.

Caution should be exercised when hydrocortisone acetate is administered to a nursing woman.

It is not known whether chlorcyclizine hydrochloride is excreted in human milk. Because many drugs are excreted in human milk, caution should be exercised when chlorcyclizine hydrochloride is administered to a nursing woman.

ADVERSE REACTIONS

Allergic contact dermatitis may occur with topical application of chlorcyclizine hydrochloride. Systemic side effects have been reported after topical application of antihistamines to large areas of skin.

The following local adverse reactions have been reported with topical corticosteroids, especially under occlusive dressings: irritation, folliculitis, hypertrichosis, acneiform eruptions, hypopigmentation, allergic contact dermatitis, secondary infection, skin atrophy, striae, and miliaria.

OVERDOSAGE

With continued application of topical corticosteroid on large areas of damaged skin and under occlusion, there is a remote possibility that sufficient absorption could occur to produce Cushing's syndrome. This is more likely in children.

Systemic toxicity following topical application of chlorcyclizine has never been reported.

The oral LD_{50} of chlorcyclizine hydrochloride in the mouse is 300 mg/kg.

The intraperitoneal LD_{50} of hydrocortisone acetate in the mouse is 2300 mg/kg.

DOSAGE AND ADMINISTRATION

Apply to the skin two to five times daily. If the condition of the skin will permit, the cream should be well rubbed in.

HOW SUPPLIED

MANTADIL Cream (chlorcyclizine hydrochloride 2% and hydrocortisone acetate 0.5%) is available in 15 gram tubes (NDC 0173-0650-94).

Store at 15° to 25°C (59° to 77°F).

February 1996/RL-288

Shown in Product Identification Guide, page 313

MIVACRON® INJECTION
MIVACRON® PREMIXED INFUSION ℞

[mĭv'ah-krŏn]

(mivacurium chloride)

This drug should be administered only by adequately trained individuals familiar with its actions, characteristics, and hazards.

DESCRIPTION

MIVACRON (mivacurium chloride) is a short-acting, nondepolarizing skeletal muscle relaxant for intravenous administration. Mivacurium chloride is [R-[R*,R*-(E)]]-2,2'-[(1,8-dioxo-4-octene-1,8-diyl)bis(oxy-3,1-propanediyl)]bis[1,2,3,4-tetrahydro-6,7-dimethoxy-2-methyl-1-[(3,4,5-trimethoxyphenyl)methyl]isoquinolinium]dichloride. The molecular

formula is $C_{58}H_{80}Cl_2N_2O_{14}$ and the molecular weight is 1100.18.

The partition coefficient of the compound is 0.015 in a 1-octanol/distilled water system at 25°C.

Mivacurium chloride is a mixture of three stereoisomers: (1R, 1'R, 2S, 2'S), the *trans-trans* diester; (1R, 1'R, 2R, 2'S), the *cis-trans* diester; and (1R, 1'R, 2R, 2'R), the *cis-cis* diester. The *trans-trans* and *cis-trans* stereoisomers comprise 92% to 96% of mivacurium chloride and their neuromuscular blocking potencies are not significantly different from each other or from mivacurium chloride. The *cis-cis* diester has been estimated from studies in cats to have one-tenth the neuromuscular blocking potency of the other two stereoisomers.

MIVACRON Injection is a sterile, non-pyrogenic solution (pH 3.5 to 5.0) containing mivacurium chloride equivalent to 2 mg/mL mivacurium in Water for Injection. Hydrochloric acid may have been added to adjust pH. Multiple dose vials contain 0.9% w/v benzyl alcohol. MIVACRON Premixed Infusion is a sterile, non-pyrogenic solution (pH 3.5 to 5.0; 260 mOsmol/L-measured) containing mivacurium chloride equivalent to 0.5 mg/mL mivacurium in 5% Dextrose Injection USP. Hydrochloric acid may have been added to adjust pH.

CLINICAL PHARMACOLOGY

MIVACRON (a mixture of three stereoisomers) binds competitively to cholinergic receptors on the motor end-plate to antagonize the action of acetylcholine, resulting in a block of neuromuscular transmission. This action is antagonized by acetylcholinesterase inhibitors, such as neostigmine.

Pharmacodynamics: The time to maximum neuromuscular block is similar for recommended doses of MIVACRON and intermediate-acting agents (e.g., atracurium), but longer than for the ultra-short-acting agent, succinylcholine. The clinically effective duration of action of the stereoisomers in MIVACRON (a mixture of three stereoisomers) is one-third to one-half that of intermediate-acting agents and 2 to 2.5 times that of succinylcholine.

The average ED_{95} (dose required to produce 95% suppression of the adductor pollicis muscle twitch response to ulnar nerve stimulation) of MIVACRON is 0.07 mg/kg (range: 0.06 to 0.09) in adults receiving opioid/nitrous oxide/oxygen anesthesia. The pharmacodynamics of doses of MIVACRON $\geq ED_{95}$ administered over 5 to 15 seconds during opioid/nitrous oxide/oxygen anesthesia are summarized in Table 1. The mean time for spontaneous recovery of the twitch response from 25% to 75% of control amplitude is about 6 minutes (range: 3 to 9, n=32) following an initial dose of 0.15 mg/kg MIVACRON and 7 to 8 minutes (range: 4 to 24, n=85) following initial doses of 0.20 or 0.25 mg/kg MIVACRON.

Volatile anesthetics may decrease the dosing requirement for MIVACRON and prolong the duration of action; the magnitude of these effects may be increased as the concentration of the volatile agent is increased. Isoflurane and enflurane (administered with nitrous oxide/oxygen to achieve 1.25 MAC [Minimum Alveolar Concentration]) may decrease the

effective dose of MIVACRON by as much as 25%, and may prolong the clinically effective duration of action and decrease the average infusion requirement by as much as 35% to 40%. At equivalent MAC values, halothane has little or no effect on the ED_{50} of MIVACRON, but may prolong the duration of action and decrease the average infusion requirement by as much as 20% (see CLINICAL PHARMACOLOGY: **Individualization of Dosages** subsection and PRECAUTIONS: **Drug Interactions**).

[See Table 1 above.]

Administration of MIVACRON over 30 to 60 seconds does not alter the time to maximum neuromuscular block or the duration of action. The duration of action of the stereoisomers in MIVACRON may be prolonged in patients with reduced plasma cholinesterase (pseudocholinesterase) activity (see PRECAUTIONS: **Reduced Plasma Cholinesterase Activity** and CLINICAL PHARMACOLOGY **Individualization of Dosages** subsection).

Interpatient variability in duration of action occurs with MIVACRON as with other neuromuscular blocking agents. However, analysis of data from 224 patients in clinical studies receiving various doses of MIVACRON during opioid/nitrous oxide/oxygen anesthesia with a variety of premedicants and varying lengths of surgery indicated that approximately 90% of the patients had clinically effective durations of block within 8 minutes of the median duration predicted from the dose-response data shown in Table 1. Variations in plasma cholinesterase activity, including values within the normal range and values as low as 20% below the lower limit of the normal range, were not associated with clinically significant effects on duration. The variability in duration, however, was greater in patients with plasma cholinesterase activity at or slightly below the lower limit of the normal range.

When administered during the induction of adequate anesthesia using thiopental or propofol, nitrous oxide/oxygen, and co-induction agents such as fentanyl and/or midazolam, doses of 0.15 mg/kg ($2 \times ED_{95}$) MIVACRON administered over 5 to 15 seconds or 0.20 mg/kg MIVACRON administered over 30 seconds produced generally good-to-excellent tracheal intubation conditions in 2.5 to 3 and 2 to 2.5 minutes, respectively. A dose of 0.25 mg/kg MIVACRON administered as a divided dose (0.15 mg/kg followed 30 sec later by 0.10 mg/kg) produced generally good-to-excellent intubation conditions in 1.5 to 2 minutes after initiating the dosing regimen.

Repeated administration of maintenance doses or continuous infusion of MIVACRON for up to 2.5 hours is not associated with development of tachyphylaxis or cumulative neuromuscular blocking effects in ASA Physical Status I–II patients. Limited data are available from patients receiving infusions for longer than 2.5 hours. Spontaneous recovery of neuromuscular function after infusion is independent of the

Table 1
Pharmacodynamic Dose Response During Opioid/Nitrous Oxide/Oxygen Anesthesia

Initial MIVACRON® Dose* (mg/kg)		Time to Maximum Block† (min)	Time to Spontaneous Recovery†			
			5% Recovery (min)	25% Recovery‡ (min)	95% Recovery§ (min)	T_4/T_1 Ratio ≥ 75%§ (min)
Adults						
0.07 to 0.10	[n=47]	4.9 (2.0-7.6)	11 (7-19)	13 (8-24)	21 (10-36)	21 (10-36)
0.15	[n=50]	3.3 (1.5-8.8)	13 (6-31)	16 (9-38)	26 (16-41)	26 (15-45)
0.20 "	[n=50]	2.5 (1.2-6.0)	16 (10-29)	20 (10-36)	31 (15-51)	34 (19-56)
0.25 "	[n=48]	2.3 (1.0-4.8)	19 (11-29)	23 (14-38)	34 (22-64)	43 (26-75)
Children 2 to 12 Years						
0.11 to 0.12	[n=17]	2.8 (1.2-4.6)	5 (3-9)	7 (4-10)	–	–
0.20	[n=18]	1.9 (1.3-3.3)	7 (3-12)	10 (6-15)	19 (14-26)	16 (12-23)
0.25	[n=9]	1.6 (1.0-2.2)	7 (4-9)	9 (5-12)	–	–

* Doses administered over 5 to 15 seconds.

† Values shown are medians of means from individual studies (range of individual patient values).

‡ Clinically effective duration of neuromuscular block.

§ Data available for as few as 40% of adults in specific dose groups and for 22% of children in the 0.20 mg/kg dose group due to administration of reversal agents or additional doses of MIVACRON prior to 95% recovery or T_4/T_1 ratio recovery to ≥ 75%.

" Rapid administration not recommended due to possibility of decreased blood pressure. Administer 0.20 mg/kg over 30 sec; administer 0.25 mg/kg as divided dose (0.15 mg/kg followed 30 sec later by 0.10 mg/kg). See DOSAGE AND ADMINISTRATION.

Continued on next page

Glaxo Wellcome—Cont.

duration of infusion and comparable to recovery reported for single doses (Table 1).

The neuromuscular block produced by the stereoisomers in MIVACRON is readily antagonized by anticholinesterase agents. As seen with other nondepolarizing neuromuscular blocking agents, the more profound the neuromuscular block at the time of reversal, the longer the time and the greater the dose of anticholinesterase agent required for recovery of neuromuscular function.

In children (2 to 12 years), MIVACRON has a higher ED_{95} (0.10 mg/kg), faster onset, and shorter duration of action than in adults. The mean time for spontaneous recovery of the twitch response from 25% to 75% of control amplitude is about 5 minutes (n=4) following an initial dose of 0.20 mg/kg MIVACRON. Recovery following reversal is faster in children than in adults (Table 1).

Hemodynamics: Administration of MIVACRON in doses up to and including 0.15 mg/kg ($2 \times ED_{95}$) over 5 to 15 seconds to ASA Physical Status I–II patients during opioid/nitrous oxide/oxygen anesthesia is associated with minimal changes in mean arterial blood pressure (MAP) or heart rate (HR) (Table 2).

Table 2
Cardiovascular Dose Response During Opioid/Nitrous Oxide/Oxygen Anesthesia

Initial MIVACRON® Dose* (mg/kg)		% of Patients With ≥30% Change: MAP Dec	MAP Inc	HR Dec	HR Inc
Adults					
0.07 to 0.10	[n=49]	0%	2%	0%	0%
0.15	[n=53]	4%	4%	4%	2%
0.20†	[n=53]	30%	0%	0%	8%
0.25†	[n=44]	39%	2%	0%	14%
Children 2 to 12 years					
0.11 to 0.12	[n=17]	0%	6%	0%	0%
0.20	[n=17]	0%	0%	0%	0%
0.25	[n=8]	13%	0%	0%	0%

* Doses administered over 5 to 15 seconds.
† Rapid administration not recommended due to possibility of decreased blood pressure. Administer 0.20 mg/kg over 30 sec; administer 0.25 mg/kg as divided dose (0.15 mg/kg followed 30 sec later by 0.10 mg/kg). See DOSAGE AND ADMINISTRATION.

Higher doses of ≥0.20 mg/kg ($\geq 3 \times ED_{95}$) may be associated with transient decreases in MAP and increases in HR in some patients. These decreases in MAP are usually maximal within 1 to 3 minutes following the dose, typically resolve without treatment in an additional 1 to 3 minutes, and are usually associated with increases in plasma histamine concentration. Decreases in MAP can be minimized by administering MIVACRON over 30 to 60 seconds (see CLINICAL PHARMACOLOGY: **Individualization of Dosages** subsection and PRECAUTIONS: **General**).

Analysis of 426 patients in clinical studies receiving initial doses of MIVACRON up to and including 0.30 mg/kg during opioid/nitrous oxide/oxygen anesthesia showed that high initial doses and a rapid rate of injection contributed to a greater probability of experiencing a decrease of ≥30% in MAP after MIVACRON administration. Obese patients also had a greater probability of experiencing a decrease of ≥30% in MAP when dosed on the basis of actual body weight, thereby receiving a larger dose than if dosed on the basis of ideal body weight (see CLINICAL PHARMACOLOGY: **Individualization of Dosages** subsection and PRECAUTIONS: **General**).

Children experience minimal changes in MAP or HR after administration of MIVACRON doses up to and including 0.20 mg/kg over 5 to 15 seconds, but higher doses (≥0.25 mg/kg) may be associated with transient decreases in MAP (Table 2).

Following a dose of 0.15 mg/kg MIVACRON administered over 60 seconds, adult patients with significant cardiovascular disease undergoing coronary artery bypass grafting or valve replacement procedures showed no clinically important changes in MAP or HR. Transient decreases in MAP were observed in some patients after doses of 0.20 to 0.25 mg/kg MIVACRON administered over 60 seconds. The number of patients in whom these decreases in MAP required treatment was small.

Pharmacokinetics: Table 3 describes the results from a study of 9 ASA Physical Status I–II adult patients (31 to 48 years) receiving an infusion of MIVACRON at 5 μg/kg/min for 60 minutes followed by 10 μg/kg/min for 60 minutes. MIVACRON is a mixture of isomers which do not interconvert in vivo. The mivacurium pharmacokinetic parameters presented in Table 3 were determined using a stereospecific assay. The two more potent isomers, *cis-trans* (36% of the mixture) and *trans-trans* (57% of the mixture), have very high clearances that exceed cardiac output, reflecting the extensive metabolism by plasma cholinesterase. The volume of distribution is relatively small, reflecting limited tissue distribution secondary to the polarity and large molecular weight of mivacurium. The combination of high metabolic clearance and low distribution volume results in the short elimination half-life of approximately 2 minutes for the two active isomers. The short elimination half-lives and high metabolic clearances of the active isomers are consistent with the short duration of action of MIVACRON. The steady-state concentrations of the *cis-trans* and *trans-trans* isomers doubled after the infusion rate was increased from 5 to 10 μg/kg/min, indicating that their pharmacokinetics is dose-proportional.

Table 3
Stereoisomer Pharmacokinetic Parameters* of MIVACRON® in ASA Physical Status I–II Adult Patients† [n=9] During Opioid/Nitrous Oxide/Oxygen Anesthesia

Parameter	*trans-trans* isomer	*cis-trans* isomer
Elimination Half-life ($t_{1/2}$, min)	2.3 (1.4–3.6)	2.1 (0.8–4.8)
Volume of Distribution (L/kg)	0.15 (0.06–0.24)	0.27 (0.08–0.56)
Plasma Clearance (mL/min/kg)	53 (32–105)	99 (52–230)

* Values shown are mean (range).
† Ages 31 to 48 years.

The *cis-cis* isomer (6% of the mixture) has approximately one-tenth the neuromuscular blocking potency of the *trans-trans* and *cis-trans* isomers in cats. In the nine patients shown in Table 3, the volume of distribution of the *cis-cis* isomer averaged 0.31 L/kg (range: 0.18 to 0.46), the clearance averaged 4.2 mL/min/kg (range: 2.4 to 5.4), and the half-life averaged 55 minutes (range: 32 to 102). The neuromuscular blocking potency of the *cis-cis* isomer in humans has not been established; however, modeling of clinical pharmacokinetic-pharmacodynamic data suggests that the *cis-cis* isomer produces minimal (<5%) neuromuscular block during a 2-hour infusion. In studies in which infusions of up to 2.5 hours were administered to ASA Physical Status I–II patients, the 25% to 75% recovery times were independent of the duration of infusion, suggesting that the *cis-cis* isomer does not contribute significant neuromuscular block during use for up to 2.5 hours. Limited data are available from infusions of longer duration or from patients with compromised elimination capacities (hepatic or renal failure).

Metabolism and Excretion: Enzymatic hydrolysis by plasma cholinesterase is the primary mechanism for inactivation of mivacurium and yields a quaternary alcohol and a quaternary monoester metabolite. Renal and biliary excretion of unchanged mivacurium are minor elimination pathways; urine and bile are important elimination pathways for the two metabolites. Tests in which these two metabolites were administered to cats and dogs suggest that each metabolite is unlikely to produce clinically significant neuromuscular, autonomic, or cardiovascular effects following administration of MIVACRON.

Special Populations: The pharmacokinetics of mivacurium isomers has not been studied in the elderly or in patients with renal or hepatic disease using a stereospecific assay. The non-stereospecific, total mivacurium assay used in pharmacokinetic-pharmacodynamic studies in these populations provided preliminary evidence that reduced clearance of one or more isomers is responsible for the longer duration of action of MIVACRON seen in patients with end-stage kidney or liver disease. The data did not provide a pharmacokinetic explanation for the 15% to 20% longer duration of block seen in the elderly. Tables 4 and 5 summarize the pharmacodynamic results in these special populations as compared with young adults (ages 18 to 49 years). No data are available from patients with kidney or liver disease not requiring transplantation.

[See Table 4 below.]

Renal: The clinically effective duration of action of 0.15 mg/kg MIVACRON was about 1.5 times longer in patients with end-stage kidney disease than in healthy patients, presumably due to reduced clearance of one or more isomers.

Hepatic: The clinically effective duration of action of 0.15 mg/kg MIVACRON was three times longer in patients with end-stage liver disease than in healthy patients and is likely related to the markedly decreased plasma cholinesterase activity (30% of healthy patient values) which could decrease the clearance of one or more isomers (see PRECAUTIONS: **Reduced Plasma Cholinesterase Activity**).

[See Table 5 at top of next page.]

Individualization of Dosages: DOSES OF MIVACRON SHOULD BE INDIVIDUALIZED AND A PERIPHERAL NERVE STIMULATOR SHOULD BE USED TO MEASURE NEUROMUSCULAR FUNCTION DURING MIVACRON ADMINISTRATION IN ORDER TO MONITOR DRUG EFFECT, DETERMINE THE NEED FOR ADDITIONAL DOSES, AND CONFIRM RECOVERY FROM NEUROMUSCULAR BLOCK.

Based on the known actions of MIVACRON (a mixture of three stereoisomers) and other neuromuscular blocking agents, the following factors should be considered when administering MIVACRON:

Renal or Hepatic Impairment: A dose of 0.15 mg/kg MIVACRON is recommended for facilitation of tracheal intubation in patients with renal or hepatic impairment. However, the clinically effective duration of block produced by this dose is about 1.5 times longer in patients with end-stage kidney disease and about 3 times longer in patients with end-stage liver disease than in patients with normal renal and hepatic function. Infusion rates should be decreased by as much as 50% in these patients depending on the degree of renal or hepatic impairment (see PRECAUTIONS: **Renal and Hepatic Disease**).

Reduced Plasma Cholinesterase Activity: The possibility of prolonged neuromuscular block following administration of MIVACRON must be considered in patients with reduced plasma cholinesterase (pseudocholinesterase) activity. MIVACRON should be used with great caution, if at all, in patients known or suspected of being homozygous for the atypical plasma cholinesterase gene (see WARNINGS). Doses of 0.03 mg/kg produced complete neuromuscular block for 26 to 128 minutes in three such patients; thus initial doses greater than 0.03 mg/kg are not recommended in homozygous patients. Infusions of MIVACRON are not recommended in homozygous patients.

MIVACRON has been used safely in patients heterozygous for the atypical plasma cholinesterase gene and in genotypically normal patients with reduced plasma cholinesterase activity. After an initial dose of 0.15 mg/kg MIVACRON, the clinically effective duration of block in heterozygous patients may be approximately 10 minutes longer than in patients with normal genotype and normal plasma cholinesterase

Table 4
Pharmacodynamic Parameters* of MIVACRON® in ASA Physical Status I–II Young Adult Patients and Elderly Patients During Isoflurane/Nitrous Oxide/Oxygen Anesthesia

Parameter	Young Adult Patients (18–49 years)		Elderly Patients (68–77 years)
Initial Dose†	0.10 mg/kg [n=9]	0.25 mg/kg‡ [n=9]	0.10 mg/kg [n=8]
Maximum Block (%)	98 (83–100)	100 (100–100)	99 (95–100)
Time to Maximum Block (min)	3.2 (2.0–6.0)	1.7 (1.3–2.5)	4.8 (3.0–7.0)
Clinically Effective Duration of Block§ (min)	17 (9–29)	27 (18–34)	20 (14–28)

* Values shown are mean (range).
† Doses administered over 5 to 15 seconds.
‡ Rapid administration not recommended due to possibility of decreased blood pressure. Administer 0.25 mg/kg as divided dose (0.15 mg/kg followed 30 sec later by 0.10 mg/kg). See DOSAGE AND ADMINISTRATION.
§ Time from injection to 25% recovery of the control twitch height.

activity. Lower MIVACRON infusion rates are recommended in these patients (see PRECAUTIONS: **Reduced Plasma Cholinesterase Activity**).

Drugs or Conditions Causing Potentiation of or Resistance to Neuromuscular Block: As with other neuromuscular blocking agents, MIVACRON may have profound neuromuscular blocking effects in cachectic or debilitated patients, patients with neuromuscular diseases, and patients with carcinomatosis. In these or other patients in whom potentiation of neuromuscular block or difficulty with reversal may be anticipated, the initial dose should be decreased. A test dose of not more than 0.015 to 0.020 mg/kg, which represents the lower end of the dose-response curve for MIVACRON, is recommended in such patients (see PRECAUTIONS: **General**).

The neuromuscular blocking action of the stereoisomers in MIVACRON is potentiated by isoflurane or enflurane anesthesia. Recommended initial MIVACRON doses (see DOSAGE AND ADMINISTRATION) may be used for intubation prior to the administration of these agents. If MIVACRON is first administered after establishment of stable-state isoflurane or enflurane anesthesia (administered with nitrous oxide/oxygen to achieve 1.25 MAC), the initial MIVACRON dose should be reduced by as much as 25%, and the infusion rate reduced by as much as 35% to 40%. A greater potentiation of the neuromuscular blocking action of the stereoisomers in MIVACRON may be expected with higher concentrations of enflurane or isoflurane. The use of halothane requires no adjustment of the initial dose of MIVACRON, but may prolong the duration of action and decrease the average infusion rate by as much as 20% (see PRECAUTIONS: **Drug Interactions**).

When MIVACRON is administered to patients receiving certain antibiotics, magnesium salts, lithium, local anesthetics, procainamide and quinidine, longer durations of neuromuscular block may be expected and infusion requirements may be lower (see PRECAUTIONS: **Drug Interactions**).

When MIVACRON is administered to patients chronically receiving phenytoin or carbamazepine, slightly shorter durations of neuromuscular block may be anticipated and infusion rate requirements may be higher (see PRECAUTIONS: **Drug Interactions**).

Severe acid-base and/or electrolyte abnormalities may potentiate or cause resistance to the neuromuscular blocking action of the stereoisomers in MIVACRON. No data are available in such patients and no dosing recommendations can be made (see PRECAUTIONS: **General**).

Burns: While patients with burns are known to develop resistance to nondepolarizing neuromuscular blocking agents, they may also have reduced plasma cholinesterase activity. Consequently, in these patients, a test dose of not more than 0.015 to 0.020 mg/kg MIVACRON is recommended, followed by additional appropriate dosing guided by the use of a neuromuscular block monitor (see PRECAUTIONS: **General**).

Cardiovascular Disease: In patients with clinically significant cardiovascular disease, the initial dose of MIVACRON should be 0.15 mg/kg or less, administered over 60 seconds (see CLINICAL PHARMACOLOGY: **Hemodynamics** subsection and PRECAUTIONS: **General**).

Obesity: Obese patients (patients weighing ≥ 30% more than their ideal body weight) dosed on the basis of actual body weight, thereby receiving a larger dose than if dosed on the basis of ideal body weight, had a greater probability of experiencing a decrease of ≥ 30% in MAP (see CLINICAL PHARMACOLOGY: **Hemodynamics** subsection and PRECAUTIONS: **General**). Therefore, in obese patients, the initial dose should be determined using the patient's ideal body weight (IBW), according to the following formulae:
Men: IBW in kg = (106 + [6 × inches in height above 5 feet])/2.2
Women: IBW in kg = (100 + [5 × inches in height above 5 feet])/2.2

Allergy and Sensitivity: In patients with any history suggestive of a greater sensitivity to the release of histamine or related mediators (e.g., asthma), the initial dose of MIVACRON should be 0.15 mg/kg or less, administered over 60 seconds (see PRECAUTIONS: **General**).

INDICATIONS AND USAGE
MIVACRON is a short-acting neuromuscular blocking agent indicated for inpatients and outpatients, as an adjunct to general anesthesia, to facilitate tracheal intubation and to provide skeletal muscle relaxation during surgery or mechanical ventilation.

CONTRAINDICATIONS
MIVACRON is contraindicated in patients known to have an allergic hypersensitivity to mivacurium chloride or other benzylisoquinolinium agents, as manifested by reactions such as urticaria or severe respiratory distress or hypotension. Use of MIVACRON from multiple dose vials containing benzyl alcohol as a preservative is contraindicated in patients with a known hypersensitivity to benzyl alcohol.

Table 5
Pharmacodynamic Parameters* of MIVACRON® in ASA Physical Status I–II Patients and in Patients Undergoing Kidney or Liver Transplantation During Isoflurane/Nitrous Oxide/Oxygen Anesthesia

Parameter	Young Adult Patients	Kidney Transplant Patients	Liver Transplant Patients‡
Initial Dose	0.15 mg/kg [n=8]	0.15 mg/kg [n=9]	0.15 mg/kg [n=8]
Maximum Block (%)	99.8 (98–100)	100 (100–100)	100 (100–100)
Time to Maximum Block (min)	1.9 (0.8–3.5)	2.6 (1.0–4.5)	2.1 (1.0–4.0)
Clinically Effective Duration of Block† (min)	19 (12–30)	30 (19–58)	57 (29–80)

* Values shown are mean (range).
† Time from injection to 25% recovery of the control twitch height.
‡ Liver transplant patients received isoflurane without nitrous oxide.

WARNINGS
MIVACRON SHOULD BE ADMINISTERED IN CAREFULLY ADJUSTED DOSAGE BY OR UNDER THE SUPERVISION OF EXPERIENCED CLINICIANS WHO ARE FAMILIAR WITH THE DRUG'S ACTIONS AND THE POSSIBLE COMPLICATIONS OF ITS USE. THE DRUG SHOULD NOT BE ADMINISTERED UNLESS PERSONNEL AND FACILITIES FOR RESUSCITATION AND LIFE SUPPORT (TRACHEAL INTUBATION, ARTIFICIAL VENTILATION, OXYGEN THERAPY), AND AN ANTAGONIST OF MIVACRON ARE IMMEDIATELY AVAILABLE. IT IS RECOMMENDED THAT A PERIPHERAL NERVE STIMULATOR BE USED TO MEASURE NEUROMUSCULAR FUNCTION DURING THE ADMINISTRATION OF MIVACRON IN ORDER TO MONITOR DRUG EFFECT, DETERMINE THE NEED FOR ADDITIONAL DRUG, AND CONFIRM RECOVERY FROM NEUROMUSCULAR BLOCK.
MIVACRON HAS NO KNOWN EFFECT ON CONSCIOUSNESS, PAIN THRESHOLD, OR CEREBRATION. TO AVOID DISTRESS TO THE PATIENT, NEUROMUSCULAR BLOCK SHOULD NOT BE INDUCED BEFORE UNCONSCIOUSNESS.
MIVACRON IS METABOLIZED BY PLASMA CHOLINESTERASE AND SHOULD BE USED WITH GREAT CAUTION, IF AT ALL, IN PATIENTS KNOWN TO BE OR SUSPECTED OF BEING HOMOZYGOUS FOR THE ATYPICAL PLASMA CHOLINESTERASE GENE.
MIVACRON Injection and MIVACRON Premixed Infusion are acidic (pH 3.5 to 5.0) and may not be compatible with alkaline solutions having a pH greater than 8.5 (e.g., barbiturate solutions).
Multiple dose vials of MIVACRON contain benzyl alcohol. In newborn infants, benzyl alcohol has been associated with an increased incidence of neurological and other complications which are sometimes fatal. Single-use vials and MIVACRON Premixed Infusion do not contain benzyl alcohol (see PRECAUTIONS: **Pediatric Use**).

PRECAUTIONS
General: Although MIVACRON (a mixture of three stereoisomers) is not a potent histamine releaser, the possibility of substantial histamine release must be considered. Release of histamine is related to the dose and speed of injection.
Caution should be exercised in administering MIVACRON to patients with clinically significant cardiovascular disease and patients with any history suggesting a greater sensitivity to the release of histamine or related mediators (e.g., asthma). In such patients, the initial dose of MIVACRON should be 0.15 mg/kg or less, administered over 60 seconds; assurance of adequate hydration and careful monitoring of hemodynamic status are important (see CLINICAL PHARMACOLOGY: **Hemodynamics** and **Individualization of Dosages**).
Obese patients may be more likely to experience clinically significant transient decreases in MAP than non-obese patients when the dose of MIVACRON is based on actual rather than ideal body weight. Therefore, in obese patients, the initial dose should be determined using the patient's ideal body weight (see CLINICAL PHARMACOLOGY: **Hemodynamics** and **Individualization of Dosages**).
Recommended doses of MIVACRON have no clinically significant effects on heart rate; therefore, MIVACRON will not counteract the bradycardia produced by many anesthetic agents or by vagal stimulation.
Neuromuscular blocking agents may have a profound effect in patients with neuromuscular diseases (e.g., myasthenia gravis and the myasthenic syndrome). In these and other conditions in which prolonged neuromuscular block is a possibility (e.g., carcinomatosis), the use of a peripheral nerve stimulator and a dose of not more than 0.015 to 0.020 mg/kg MIVACRON is recommended to assess the level of neuromuscular block and to monitor dosage requirements (see CLINICAL PHARMACOLOGY: **Individualization of Dosages**).
MIVACRON has not been studied in patients with burns. Resistance to nondepolarizing neuromuscular blocking agents may develop in patients with burns, depending upon the time elapsed since the injury and the size of the burn. Patients with burns may have reduced plasma cholinesterase activity which may offset this resistance (see CLINICAL PHARMACOLOGY: **Individualization of Dosages**).
Acid-base and/or serum electrolyte abnormalities may potentiate or antagonize the action of neuromuscular blocking agents. The action of neuromuscular blocking agents may be enhanced by magnesium salts administered for the management of toxemia of pregnancy (see CLINICAL PHARMACOLOGY: **Individualization of Dosages**).
No data are available to support the use of MIVACRON by intramuscular injection.
Renal and Hepatic Disease: The possibility of prolonged neuromuscular block must be considered when MIVACRON is used in patients with renal or hepatic disease (see CLINICAL PHARMACOLOGY: **Pharmacokinetics**). Most patients with chronic hepatic disease such as hepatitis, liver abscess, and cirrhosis of the liver exhibit a marked reduction in plasma cholinesterase activity. Patients with acute or chronic renal disease may also show a reduction in plasma cholinesterase activity (see CLINICAL PHARMACOLOGY: **Individualization of Dosages**).
Reduced Plasma Cholinesterase Activity: The possibility of prolonged neuromuscular block following administration of MIVACRON must be considered in patients with reduced plasma cholinesterase (pseudocholinesterase) activity.
Plasma cholinesterase activity may be diminished in the presence of genetic abnormalities of plasma cholinesterase (e.g., patients heterozygous or homozygous for the atypical plasma cholinesterase gene), pregnancy, liver or kidney disease, malignant tumors, infections, burns, anemia, decompensated heart disease, peptic ulcer, or myxedema. Plasma cholinesterase activity may also be diminished by chronic administration of oral contraceptives, glucocorticoids, or certain monoamine oxidase inhibitors and by irreversible inhibitors of plasma cholinesterase (e.g., organophosphate insecticides, echothiophate, and certain antineoplastic drugs).
MIVACRON has been used safely in patients heterozygous for the atypical plasma cholinesterase gene. At doses of 0.10 to 0.20 mg/kg MIVACRON, the clinically effective duration of action was 8 to 11 minutes longer in patients heterozygous for the atypical gene than in genotypically normal patients. As with succinylcholine, patients homozygous for the atypical plasma cholinesterase gene (1 in 2500 patients) are extremely sensitive to the neuromuscular blocking effect of MIVACRON. In three such adult patients, a small dose of 0.03 mg/kg (approximately the ED_{10-20} in genotypically normal patients) produced complete neuromuscular block for 26 to 128 minutes. Once spontaneous recovery had begun, neuromuscular block in these patients was antagonized with conventional doses of neostigmine. One adult patient, who was homozygous for the atypical plasma cholinesterase gene, received a dose of 0.18 mg/kg MIVACRON and exhibited complete neuromuscular block for about 4 hours. Response to post-tetanic stimulation was present after 4 hours, all four responses to train-of-four stimulation were present after 6 hours, and the patient was extubated after 8 hours. Reversal was not attempted in this patient.
Malignant Hyperthermia (MH): In a study of MH-susceptible pigs, MIVACRON did not trigger MH. MIVACRON has not been studied in MH-susceptible patients. Because MH can develop in the absence of established triggering agents, the

Continued on next page

Glaxo Wellcome—Cont.

clinician should be prepared to recognize and treat MH in any patient undergoing general anethesia.

Long-Term Use in the Intensive Care Unit (ICU): No data are available on the long-term use of MIVACRON in patients undergoing mechanical ventilation in the ICU.

Drug Interactions: Although MIVACRON (a mixture of three stereoisomers) has been administered safely following succinylcholine-facilitated tracheal intubation, the interaction between the stereoisomers in MIVACRON and succinylcholine has not been systematically studied. Prior administration of succinylcholine can potentiate the neuromuscular blocking effects of nondepolarizing agents. Evidence of spontaneous recovery from succinylcholine should be observed before the administration of MIVACRON.

The use of MIVACRON before succinylcholine to attenuate some of the side effects of succinylcholine has not been studied.

There are no clinical data on the use of MIVACRON with other nondepolarizing neuromuscular blocking agents.

Isoflurane and enflurane (administered with nitrous oxide/oxygen to achieve 1.25 MAC) decrease the ED_{50} of MIVACRON by as much as 25% (see CLINICAL PHARMACOLOGY: **Pharmacodynamics** and **Individualization of Dosages**). These agents may also prolong the clinically effective duration of action and decrease the average infusion requirement of MIVACRON by as much as 35% to 40%. A greater potentiation of the neuromuscular blocking effects of the stereoisomers in MIVACRON may be expected with higher concentrations of enflurane or isoflurane. Halothane has little or no effect on the ED_{50}, but may prolong the duration of action and decrease the average infusion requirement by as much as 20%.

Other drugs which may enhance the neuromuscular blocking action of nondepolarizing agents such as the stereoisomers in MIVACRON include certain antibiotics (e.g., aminoglycosides, tetracyclines, bacitracin, polymyxins, lincomycin, clindamycin, colistin, and sodium colistimethate), magnesium salts, lithium, local anesthetics, procainamide, and quinidine. The neuromuscular blocking effect of MIVACRON may be enhanced by drugs that reduce plasma cholinesterase activity (e.g., chronically administered oral contraceptives, glucocorticoids, or certain monoamine oxidase inhibitors) or by drugs that irreversibly inhibit plasma cholinesterase (see PRECAUTIONS: **Reduced Plasma Cholinesterase Activity** subsection).

Resistance to the neuromuscular blocking action of nondepolarizing neuromuscular blocking agents has been demonstrated in patients chronically administered phenytoin or carbamazepine. While the effects of chronic phenytoin or carbamazepine therapy on the action of the stereoisomers in MIVACRON are unknown, slightly shorter durations of neuromuscular block may be anticipated and infusion rate requirements may be higher.

Carcinogenesis, Mutagenesis, Impairment of Fertility: Carcinogenesis and fertility studies have not been performed. MIVACRON was evaluated in a battery of four short-term mutagenicity tests. It was non-mutagenic in the Ames Salmonella assay, the mouse lymphoma assay, the human lymphocyte assay, and the in vivo rat bone marrow cytogenetic assay.

Pregnancy: ***Teratogenic Effects:*** Pregnancy Category C. Teratology testing in nonventilated pregnant rats and mice treated subcutaneously with maximum subparalyzing doses of MIVACRON revealed no maternal or fetal toxicity or teratogenic effects. There are no adequate and well-controlled studies of MIVACRON in pregnant women. Because animal studies are not always predictive of human response, and the doses used were subparalyzing, MIVACRON should be used during pregnancy only if the potential benefit justifies the potential risk to the fetus.

Labor and Delivery: The use of MIVACRON during labor, vaginal delivery, or cesarean section has not been studied in humans and it is not known whether MIVACRON administered to the mother has effects on the fetus. Doses of 0.08 and 0.20 mg/kg MIVACRON given to female beagles undergoing cesarean section resulted in negligible levels of the stereoisomers in MIVACRON in umbilical vessel blood of neonates and no deleterious effects on the puppies.

Nursing Mothers: It is not known whether any of the stereoisomers of mivacurium are excreted in human milk. Because many drugs are excreted in human milk, caution should be exercised following administration of MIVACRON to a nursing woman.

Pediatric Use: MIVACRON has not been studied in pediatric patients below the age of 2 years (see CLINICAL PHARMACOLOGY and DOSAGE AND ADMINISTRATION for clinical experience and recommendations for use in children 2 to 12 years of age).

Geriatric Use: MIVACRON was safely administered during clinical trials to 64 elderly (≥ 65 years) patients, including 31 patients with significant cardiovascular disease (see PRECAUTIONS: **General** subsection). The duration of neuromuscular block may be slightly longer in elderly patients than in young adult patients (see CLINICAL PHARMACOLOGY).

ADVERSE REACTIONS

Observed in Clinical Trials: MIVACRON (a mixture of three stereoisomers) was well tolerated during extensive clinical trials in inpatients and outpatients. Prolonged neuromuscular block, which is an important adverse experience associated with neuromuscular blocking agents as a class, was reported as an adverse experience in 3 of 2074 patients administered MIVACRON. The most commonly reported adverse experience following the administration of MIVACRON was transient, dose-dependent cutaneous flushing about the face, neck, and/or chest. Flushing was most frequently noted after the initial dose of MIVACRON and was reported in about 25% of adult patients who received 0.15 mg/kg MIVACRON over 5 to 15 seconds. When present, flushing typically began within 1 to 2 minutes after the dose of MIVACRON and lasted for 3 to 5 minutes. Of 105 patients who experienced flushing after 0.15 mg/kg MIVACRON, two patients also experienced mild hypotension that was not treated, and one patient experienced moderate wheezing that was successfully treated.

Overall, hypotension was infrequently reported as an adverse experience in the clinical trials of MIVACRON. One of 332 (0.3%) healthy adults who received 0.15 mg/kg MIVACRON over 5 to 15 seconds and none of 37 cardiac surgery patients who received 0.15 mg/kg MIVACRON over 60 seconds was treated for a decrease in blood pressure in association with the administration of MIVACRON. One to two percent of healthy adults given ≥0.20 mg/kg MIVACRON over 5 to 15 seconds, 2% to 3% of healthy adults given 0.20 mg/kg over 30 seconds, none of 100 healthy adults given 0.25 mg/kg as a divided dose (0.15 mg/kg followed in 30 sec by 0.10 mg/kg), and 2% to 4% of cardiac surgery patients given ≥0.20 mg/kg over 60 seconds were treated for a decrease in blood pressure. None of the 63 children who received the recommended dose of 0.20 mg/kg MIVACRON was treated for a decrease in blood pressure in association with the administration of MIVACRON.

The following adverse experiences were reported in patients administered MIVACRON (all events judged by investigators during the clinical trials to have a possible causal relationship):

Incidence Greater Than 1%—

Cardiovascular: Flushing (16%)

Incidence Less Than 1%—

Cardiovascular: Hypotension, Tachycardia, Bradycardia, Cardiac Arrhythmia, Phlebitis

Respiratory: Bronchospasm, Wheezing, Hypoxemia

Dermatological: Rash, Urticaria, Erythema, Injection Site Reaction

Nonspecific: Prolonged Drug Effect

Neurologic: Dizziness

Musculoskeletal: Muscle Spasms

Observed in Clinical Practice: Based on initial clinical practice experience in patients who received MIVACRON, spontaneously reported adverse events are uncommon. Some of these events occurred at recommended doses and required treatment. There are insufficient data to establish a causal relationship or to support an estimate of their incidence. Adverse events reported during clinical practice include:

General: Allergic Reactions which, in rare instances, were severe

Musculoskeletal: Diminished Drug Effect, Prolonged Drug Effect

Cardiovascular: Hypotension (rarely severe), Flushing

Respiratory: Bronchospasm

Integumentary: Rash

OVERDOSAGE

Overdosage with neuromuscular blocking agents may result in neuromuscular block beyond the time needed for surgery and anesthesia. The primary treatment is maintenance of a patent airway and controlled ventilation until recovery of normal neuromuscular function is assured. Once evidence of recovery from neuromuscular block is observed, further recovery may be facilitated by administration of an anticholinesterase agent (e.g., neostigmine, edrophonium) in conjunction with an appropriate anticholinergic agent (see **Antagonism of Neuromuscular Block** subsection below).

Overdosage may increase the risk of hemodynamic side effects, especially decreases in blood pressure. If needed, cardiovascular support may be provided by proper positioning of the patient, fluid administration, and/or vasopressor agent administration.

Antagonism of Neuromuscular Block: ANTAGONISTS (SUCH AS NEOSTIGMINE) SHOULD NOT BE ADMINISTERED WHEN COMPLETE NEUROMUSCULAR BLOCK IS EVIDENT OR SUSPECTED. THE USE OF A PERIPHERAL NERVE STIMULATOR TO EVALUATE RECOVERY AND ANTAGONISM OF NEUROMUSCULAR BLOCK IS RECOMMENDED.

Administration of 0.030 to 0.064 mg/kg neostigmine or 0.5 mg/kg edrophonium at approximately 10% recovery from neuromuscular block (range: 1 to 15) produced 95% recovery of the muscle twitch response and a T_4/T_1 ratio ≥75% in about 10 minutes. The times from 25% recovery of the muscle twitch response to T_4/T_1 ratio ≥75% following these doses of antagonists averaged about 7 to 9 minutes. In comparison, average times for spontaneous recovery from 25% to T_4/T_1 ≥75% were 12 to 13 minutes.

Patients administered antagonists should be evaluated for adequate clinical evidence of antagonism, e.g., 5-second head lift and grip strength. Ventilation must be supported until no longer required.

Antagonism may be delayed in the presence of debilitation, carcinomatosis, and the concomitant use of certain broad spectrum antibiotics, or anesthetic agents and other drugs which enhance neuromuscular block or separately cause respiratory depression (see PRECAUTIONS: **Drug Interactions**). Under such circumstances the management is the same as that of prolonged neuromuscular block (see OVERDOSAGE).

DOSAGE AND ADMINISTRATION

MIVACRON SHOULD ONLY BE ADMINISTERED INTRAVENOUSLY.

The dosage information provided below is intended as a guide only. Doses of MIVACRON should be individualized (see CLINICAL PHARMACOLOGY: **Individualization of Dosages**). Factors that may warrant dosage adjustment include but may not be limited to: the presence of significant kidney, liver, or cardiovascular disease, obesity (patients weighing ≥30% more than ideal body weight for height), asthma, reduction in plasma cholinesterase activity, and the presence of inhalational anesthetic agents.

When using MIVACRON or other neuromuscular blocking agents to facilitate tracheal intubation, it is important to recognize that the most important factors affecting intubation are the depth of general anesthesia and the level of neuromuscular block. Satisfactory intubating conditions can usually be achieved before complete neuromuscular block is attained if there is adequate anesthesia.

The use of a peripheral nerve stimulator will permit the most advantageous use of MIVACRON, minimize the possibility of overdosage or underdosage, and assist in the evaluation of recovery. When using a stimulator to monitor onset of neuromuscular block, clinical studies have shown that all four twitches of the train-of-four response may be present, with little or no fade, at the times recommended for intubation. Therefore, as with other neuromuscular blocking agents, it is important to use other criteria, such as clinical evaluation of the status of relaxation of jaw muscles and vocal cords, in conjunction with peripheral muscle twitch monitoring, to guide the appropriate time of intubation.

The onset of conditions suitable for tracheal intubation occurs earlier after a conventional intubating dose of succinylcholine than after recommended doses of MIVACRON.

Adults:

Initial Doses: Doses of 0.15 mg/kg administered over 5 to 15 seconds, 0.20 mg/kg administered over 30 seconds, or 0.25 mg/kg administered in divided doses (0.15 mg/kg followed in 30 sec by 0.10 mg/kg) are recommended for facilitation of tracheal intubation for most patients (see Table 6).

[See table at top of next page.]

The purpose of slowed or divided dosing of MIVACRON at doses above 0.15 mg/kg is to minimize the transient decreases in blood pressure observed in some patients given these doses over 5 to 15 seconds (see CLINICAL PHARMACOLOGY, PRECAUTIONS, and ADVERSE REACTIONS).

The quality of intubation conditions does not significantly differ for the times and doses of MIVACRON recommended in Table 6, but the onset of suitable intubation conditions may be reached earlier with higher doses. The choice of a particular dose and regimen should be based on individual circumstances and patient requirements (see CLINICAL PHARMACOLOGY: **Individualization of Dosages**).

In patients with clinically significant cardiovascular disease and in patients with any history suggesting a greater sensitivity to the release of histamine or other mediators (e.g., asthma), the dose of MIVACRON should be 0.15 mg/kg or less, administered over 60 seconds (see PRECAUTIONS). No data are available on the use of doses of MIVACRON above 0.15 mg/kg in patients with clinically significant kidney or liver disease.

Clinically effective neuromuscular block may be expected to last for 15 to 20 minutes (range: 9 to 38) and spontaneous recovery may be expected to be 95% complete in 25 to 30 minutes (range: 16 to 41) following 0.15 mg/kg MIVACRON administered to patients receiving opioid/nitrous oxide/oxygen anesthesia. The expected duration of clinically effective block and time to 95% spontaneous recovery following 0.20 mg/kg MIVACRON are approximately 20 and 30 minutes, respectively, and following 0.25 mg/kg MIVACRON are approximately 25 and 35 minutes. Initiation of maintenance dosing during opioid/nitrous oxide/oxygen anesthesia is generally required approximately 15, 20, and 25 minutes following initial doses of 0.15, 0.20, and 0.25 mg/kg MIVACRON, respectively (see Table 1). Maintenance doses of 0.10 mg/kg each provide approximately 15 minutes of additional clinically effective block. For shorter or longer

Table 6
Recommended Initial Dosing Regimens for Adults

Dosing Paradigm*	Anesthetic Induction Technique Studied	Time to Generally Good-to-Excellent Intubating Conditions
0.15 mg/kg, i.v. (over 5 to 15 sec)	Thiopental/opioid/ N$_2$O/O$_2$ or propofol/opioid	2.5 to 3 min after completion of dose
0.20 mg/kg, i.v. (over 30 sec)	Thiopental/opioid/ N$_2$O/O$_2$ or propofol/opioid	2 to 2.5 min after completion of dose
0.25 mg/kg, i.v. (0.15 mg/kg followed in 30 sec by 0.10 mg/kg)	Propofol/opioid	1.5 to 2 min after completion of 0.15 mg/kg dose

* Dosing instituted after induction of adequate general anesthesia.

durations of action, smaller or larger maintenance doses may be administered.

The neuromuscular blocking action of MIVACRON is potentiated by isoflurane or enflurane anesthesia. Recommended initial doses of MIVACRON may be used to facilitate tracheal intubation prior to the administration of these agents; however, if MIVACRON is first administered after establishment of stable-state isoflurane or enflurane anesthesia (administered with nitrous oxide/oxygen to achieve 1.25 MAC), the initial MIVACRON dose may be reduced by as much as 25%. Greater reductions in the MIVACRON dose may be required with higher concentrations of enflurane or isoflurane. With halothane, which has only a minimal potentiating effect on MIVACRON, a smaller dosage reduction may be considered.

Continuous Infusion: Continuous infusion of MIVACRON may be used to maintain neuromuscular block. Upon early evidence of spontaneous recovery from an initial dose, an initial infusion rate of 9 to 10 µg/kg/min is recommended. If continuous infusion is initiated simultaneously with the administration of an initial dose, a lower initial infusion rate should be used (e.g., 4 µg/kg/min). In either case, the initial infusion rate should be adjusted according to the response to peripheral nerve stimulation and to clinical criteria. On average, an infusion rate of 6 to 7 µg/kg/min (range: 1 to 15) may be expected to maintain neuromuscular block within the range of 89% to 99% for extended periods in adults receiving opioid/nitrous oxide/oxygen anesthesia. Reduction of the infusion rate by up to 35% to 40% should be considered when MIVACRON is administered during stable-state conditions of isoflurane or enflurane anesthesia (administered with nitrous oxide/oxygen to achieve 1.25 MAC). Greater reductions in the MIVACRON infusion rate may be required with greater concentrations of enflurane or isoflurane. With halothane, smaller reductions in infusion rate may be required.

Children:

Initial Doses: Dosage requirements for MIVACRON on a mg/kg basis are higher in children than adults. Onset and recovery of neuromuscular block occur more rapidly in children than adults (see CLINICAL PHARMACOLOGY).

The recommended dose of MIVACRON for facilitating tracheal intubation in children 2 to 12 years of age is 0.20 mg/kg administered over 5 to 15 seconds. When administered during stable opioid/nitrous oxide/oxygen anesthesia, 0.20 mg/kg of MIVACRON produces maximum neuromuscular block in an average of 1.9 minutes (range: 1.3 to 3.3) and clinically effective block for 10 minutes (range: 6 to 15). Maintenance doses are generally required more frequently in children than in adults. Administration of MIVACRON doses above the recommended range (>0.20 mg/kg) is associated with transient decreases in MAP in some children (see CLINICAL PHARMACOLOGY: Hemodynamics). MIVACRON has not been studied in pediatric patients below the age of 2 years.

Continuous Infusion: Children require higher MIVACRON infusion rates than adults. During opioid/nitrous oxide/oxygen anesthesia the infusion rate required to maintain 89% to 99% neuromuscular block averages 14 µg/kg/min (range: 5 to 31). The principles for infusion of MIVACRON in adults are also applicable to children (see above).

Infusion Rate Tables:
For adults and children the amount of infusion solution required per hour depends upon the clinical requirements of the patient, the concentration of MIVACRON in the infusion solution, and the patient's weight. The contribution of the infusion solution to the fluid requirements of the patient must be considered. Tables 7 and 8 provide guidelines for delivery in mL/hr (equivalent to microdrops/min when 60 microdrops = 1 mL) of MIVACRON Premixed Infusion (0.5 mg/mL) and of MIVACRON Injection (2 mg/mL).

Table 7
Infusion Rates for Maintenance of Neuromuscular Block During Opioid/Nitrous Oxide/Oxygen Anesthesia Using MIVACRON® Premixed Infusion (0.5 mg/mL)

Patient Weight (kg)	Drug Delivery Rate (µg/kg/min)									
	4	5	6	7	8	10	14	16	18	20
	Infusion Delivery Rate (mL/hr)									
10	5	6	7	8	10	12	17	19	22	24
15	7	9	11	13	14	18	25	29	32	36
20	10	12	15	17	19	24	34	38	43	48
25	12	15	18	21	24	30	42	48	54	60
35	17	21	26	29	34	42	59	67	76	84
50	24	30	36	42	48	60	84	96	108	120
60	29	36	43	50	58	72	101	115	130	144
70	34	42	50	59	67	84	118	134	151	168
80	39	48	58	67	77	96	134	154	173	192
90	44	54	65	76	86	108	151	173	194	216
100	48	60	72	84	96	120	168	192	216	240

[See table 8 below.]

MIVACRON Premixed Infusion in Flexible Plastic Containers:

The flexible plastic container is fabricated from a specially formulated, nonplasticized, thermoplastic co-polyester (CR3). Water can permeate from inside the container into the overwrap but not in amounts sufficient to affect the solution significantly. Solutions inside the plastic container also can leach out certain of the chemical components in very small amounts before the expiration period is attained. However, the safety of the plastic has been confirmed by tests in animals according to USP biological standards for plastic containers.

Instructions for Use:
1. Tear outer wrap at notch and remove solution container. Check for minute leaks by squeezing container firmly. If leaks are found, discard solution as sterility may be impaired.
2. Close flow control clamp of administration set.
3. Remove cover from outlet port at bottom of container.
4. Insert piercing pin of administration set into port with a twisting motion until the pin is firmly seated. NOTE: See full directions on administration set carton.
5. Suspend container from hanger.
6. Squeeze and release drip chamber to establish proper fluid level in chamber during infusion.

7. Open flow control clamp to expel air from set. Close clamp.
8. Attach set to intravenous tubing.
9. Regulate rate of administration with flow control clamp.

Caution: Additives should not be introduced into this solution. Do not administer unless solution is clear and container is undamaged. MIVACRON Premixed Infusion is intended for single patient use only. The unused portion of the solution should be discarded.

Warning: Do not use flexible plastic container in series connections.

MIVACRON Injection Compatibility and Admixtures:

Y-site Administration: MIVACRON Injection may not be compatible with alkaline solutions having a pH greater than 8.5 (e.g., barbiturate solutions).

Studies have shown that MIVACRON Injection is compatible with:
- 5% Dextrose Injection USP
- 0.9% Sodium Chloride Injection USP
- 5% Dextrose and 0.9% Sodium Chloride Injection USP
- Lactated Ringer's Injection USP
- 5% Dextrose in Lactated Ringer's Injection
- Sufenta® (sufentanil citrate) Injection, diluted as directed
- Alfenta® (alfentanil hydrochloride) Injection, diluted as directed
- Sublimaze® (fentanyl citrate) Injection, diluted as directed
- Versed® (midazolam hydrochloride) Injection, diluted as directed
- Inapsine® (droperidol) Injection, diluted as directed

Compatibility studies with other parenteral products have not been conducted.

Dilution Stability: MIVACRON Injection diluted to 0.5 mg mivacurium per mL in 5% Dextrose Injection USP, 5% Dextrose and 0.9% Sodium Chloride Injection USP, 0.9% Sodium Chloride Injection USP, Lactated Ringer's Injection USP, or 5% Dextrose in Lactated Ringer's Injection is physically and chemically stable when stored in PVC (polyvinyl chloride) bags at 5° to 25°C (41° to 77°F) for up to 24 hours. Aseptic techniques should be used to prepare the diluted product. Admixtures of MIVACRON should be prepared for single patient use only and used within 24 hours of preparation. The unused portion of diluted MIVACRON should be discarded after each case.

NOTE: Parenteral drug products should be inspected visually for particulate matter and discoloration prior to administration whenever solution and container permit. Solutions which are not clear and colorless should not be used.

HOW SUPPLIED

MIVACRON Injection, 2 mg mivacurium in each mL.
5 mL Single Use Vials. Tray of 10 (NDC 0173-0705-44).
10 mL Single Use Vials. Tray of 10 (NDC 0173-0705-95).
20 mL Multiple Dose Vials containing 0.9% w/v benzyl alcohol as a preservative (see WARNINGS concerning newborn infants). Tray of 10 (NDC 0173-0542-00).
50 mL Multiple Dose Vials containing 0.9% w/v benzyl alcohol as a preservative (see WARNINGS concerning newborn infants). Tray of 3 (NDC 0173-0538-00).
MIVACRON Premixed Infusion in 5% Dextrose Injection USP, 0.5 mg mivacurium in each mL.
50 mL (in a 100 mL unit) Flexible Plastic Containers. (NDC 0173-0709-01).
100 mL (in a 100 mL unit) Flexible Plastic Containers (NDC 0173-0709-02).

STORAGE

Store MIVACRON Injection at room temperature of 15° to 25°C (59° to 77°F). Avoid exposure to direct ultraviolet light. DO NOT FREEZE.

Recommended storage for MIVACRON Premixed Infusion is room temperature (15° to 25°C/59° to 77°F). Avoid excessive

Table 8
Infusion Rates for Maintenance of Neuromuscular Block During Opioid/Nitrous Oxide/Oxygen Anesthesia Using MIVACRON® Injection (2 mg/mL)

Patient Weight (kg)	Drug Delivery Rate (µg/kg/min)									
	4	5	6	7	8	10	14	16	18	20
	Infusion Delivery Rate (mL/hr)									
10	1.2	1.5	1.8	2.1	2.4	3.0	4.2	4.8	5.4	6.0
15	1.8	2.3	2.7	3.2	3.6	4.5	6.3	7.2	8.1	9.0
20	2.4	3.0	3.6	4.2	4.8	6.0	8.4	9.6	10.8	12.0
25	3.0	3.8	4.5	5.3	6.0	7.5	10.5	12.0	13.5	15.0
35	4.2	5.3	6.3	7.4	8.4	10.5	14.7	16.8	18.9	21.0
50	6.0	7.5	9.0	10.5	12.0	15.0	21.0	24.0	27.0	30.0
60	7.2	9.0	10.8	12.6	14.4	18.0	25.2	28.8	32.4	36.0
70	8.4	10.5	12.6	14.7	16.8	21.0	29.4	33.6	37.8	42.0
80	9.6	12.0	14.4	16.8	19.2	24.0	33.6	38.4	43.2	48.0
90	10.8	13.5	16.2	18.9	21.6	27.0	37.8	43.2	48.6	54.0
100	12.0	15.0	18.0	21.0	24.0	30.0	42.0	48.0	54.0	60.0

Continued on next page

Glaxo Wellcome—Cont.

heat. Avoid exposure to direct ultraviolet light. Protect from freezing.
U.S. Patent No. 4761418
July 1996/RL-327
Shown in Product Identification Guide, page 313

NEOSPORIN® ℞
[nē″ō-spor′in]
G.U. Irrigant
Sterile
(neomycin sulfate-polymyxin B sulfate
solution for irrigation)
NOT FOR INJECTION

DESCRIPTION
NEOSPORIN G.U. Irrigant is a concentrated sterile antibiotic solution to be diluted for urinary bladder irrigation. Each mL contains neomycin sulfate equivalent to 40 mg neomycin base, 200,000 units polymyxin B sulfate, and Water for Injection. The 20-mL multiple-dose vial contains, in addition to the above, 1 mg methylparaben (0.1%) added as a preservative.
Neomycin sulfate, an antibiotic of the aminoglycoside group, is the sulfate salt of neomycin B and C produced by *Streptomyces fradiae*. It has a potency equivalent to not less than 600 μg of neomycin per mg.
Polymyxin B sulfate, a polypeptide antibiotic, is the sulfate salt of polymyxin B_1 and B_2 produced by the growth of *Bacillus polymyxa*. It has a potency of not less than 6,000 polymyxin B units per mg.

CLINICAL PHARMACOLOGY
After prophylactic irrigation of the intact urinary bladder, neomycin and polymyxin B are absorbed in clinically insignificant quantities. A neomycin serum level of 0.1 μg/mL was observed in three of 33 patients receiving the rinse solution. This level is well below that which has been associated with neomycin-induced toxicity.
When used topically, polymyxin B sulfate and neomycin are rarely irritating.
Microbiology: The prepared NEOSPORIN G.U. Irrigant Sterile solution is bactericidal. The aminoglycosides act by inhibiting normal protein synthesis in susceptible microorganisms. Polymyxins increase the permeability of bacterial cell wall membranes. The solution is active in vitro against
Escherichia coli
Staphylococcus aureus
Haemophilus influenzae
Klebsiella and *Enterobacter* species
Neisseria species, and
Pseudomonas aeruginosa
It is not active in vitro against *Serratia marcescens* and streptococci.
Bacterial resistance may develop following the use of the antibiotics in the catheter-rinse solution.

INDICATIONS AND USAGE
NEOSPORIN G.U. Irrigant is indicated for short-term use (up to 10 days) as a continuous irrigant or rinse in the urinary bladder of abacteriuric patients to help prevent bacteriuria and gram-negative rod septicemia associated with the use of indwelling catheters.
Since organisms gain entrance to the bladder by way of, through, and around the catheter, significant bacteriuria is induced by bacterial multiplication in the bladder urine, in the mucoid film often present between catheter and urethra, and in other sites. Urinary tract infection may result from the repeated presence in the urine of large numbers of pathogenic bacteria. The use of closed systems with indwelling catheters has been shown to reduce the risk of infection. A three-way closed catheter system with constant neomycin-polymyxin B bladder rinse is indicated to prevent the development of infection while using indwelling catheters.
If uropathogens are isolated, they should be identified and tested for susceptibility so that appropriate antimicrobial therapy for systemic use can be initiated.

CONTRAINDICATIONS
Hypersensitivity to neomycin, the polymyxins, or any ingredient in the solution is a contraindication to its use. A history of hypersensitivity or serious toxic reaction to an aminoglycoside may also contraindicate the use of any other aminoglycoside because of the known cross-sensitivity of patients to drugs of this class.

WARNINGS
PROPHYLACTIC BLADDER CARE WITH NEOSPORIN G.U. IRRIGANT STERILE SHOULD NOT BE GIVEN WHERE THERE IS A POSSIBILITY OF SYSTEMIC ABSORPTION. NEOSPORIN G.U. IRRIGANT STERILE SHOULD NOT BE USED FOR IRRIGATION OTHER THAN FOR THE URINARY BLADDER. Systemic absorp-

tion after topical application of neomycin to open wounds, burns, and granulating surfaces is significant and serum concentrations comparable to and often higher than those attained following oral and parenteral therapy have been reported. Absorption of neomycin from the denuded bladder surface has been reported.
However, the likelihood of toxicity following topical irrigation of the intact urinary bladder with NEOSPORIN G.U. Irrigant Sterile is low since no appreciable amounts of these antibiotics enter the systemic circulation by this route if irrigation does not exceed 10 days.
NEOSPORIN G.U. Irrigant is intended for continuous prophylactic irrigation of the lumen of the intact urinary bladder of patients with indwelling catheters. Patients should be under constant supervision by a physician. Irrigation should be avoided in patients with defects in the bladder mucosa or bladder wall, such as vesical rupture, or in association with operative procedures on the bladder wall, because of the risk of toxicity due to systemic absorption following diffusion into absorptive tissues and spaces. When absorbed, neomycin and polymyxin B are nephrotoxic antibiotics, and the nephrotoxic potentials are additive. In addition, both antibiotics, when absorbed, are neurotoxins; neomycin can destroy fibers of the acoustic nerve causing permanent bilateral deafness; neomycin and polymyxin B are additive in their neuromuscular blocking effects, not only in terms of potency and duration but also in terms of characteristics of the blocks produced.
Aminoglycosides, when absorbed, can cause fetal harm when administered to a pregnant woman. Aminoglycoside antibiotics cross the placenta, and there have been several reports of total, irreversible, bilateral, congenital deafness in children whose mothers received streptomycin during pregnancy. Although serious side effects have not been reported in the treatment of pregnant women with other aminoglycosides, the potential for harm exists. If NEOSPORIN G.U. Irrigant Sterile is used during pregnancy, the patient should be apprised of the potential hazard to the fetus (see PRECAUTIONS).

PRECAUTIONS
General: Ototoxicity, nephrotoxicity, and neuromuscular blockade may occur if NEOSPORIN G.U. Irrigant ingredients are systemically absorbed (see WARNINGS). Absorption of neomycin from the denuded bladder surface has been reported. Patients with impaired renal function, infants, dehydrated patients, elderly patients, and patients receiving high doses of prolonged treatment are especially at risk for the development of toxicity.
Irrigation of the bladder with NEOSPORIN G.U. Irrigant may result in overgrowth of nonsusceptible organisms, including fungi. Appropriate measures should be taken if this occurs. The safety and effectiveness of the preparation for use in the care of patients with recent lower urinary tract surgery have not been established.
Urine specimens should be collected during prophylactic bladder care for urinalysis, culture, and susceptibility testing. Positive cultures suggest the presence of organisms which are resistant to the bladder rinse antibiotics.
Pregnancy: *Teratogenic Effects:* Pregnancy Category D. See WARNINGS section.

ADVERSE REACTIONS
Neomycin occasionally causes skin sensitization when applied topically; however, topical application to mucus membranes rarely results in local or systemic hypersensitivity reactions.
Irritation of the urinary bladder mucosa has been reported. Signs of ototoxicity and nephrotoxicity have been reported following parenteral use of these drugs and following the oral and topical use of neomycin (see WARNINGS).

DOSAGE AND ADMINISTRATION
This preparation is specifically designed for use with "three-way" catheters or with other catheter systems permitting **continuous** irrigation of the urinary bladder. The usual irrigation dose is one 1-mL ampul a day for up to 10 days.
Using strict aseptic techniques, the contents of one 1-mL ampul of NEOSPORIN G.U. Irrigant Sterile (neomycin sulfate-polymyxin B sulfate solution for irrigation) should be added to a 1,000-mL container of isotonic saline solution. This container should then be connected to the inflow lumen of the "three-way" catheter which has been inserted with full aseptic precautions; use of a sterile lubricant is recommended during insertion of the catheter. The outflow lumen should be connected, via a sterile disposable plastic tube, to a disposable plastic collection bag. Stringent procedures, such as taping the inflow and outflow junction at the catheter, should be observed when necessary to ensure the junctional integrity of the system.
For most patients, the inflow rate of the 1,000-mL saline solution of neomycin and polymyxin B should be adjusted to a slow drip to deliver about 1,000 mL every 24 hours. If the patient's urine output exceeds 2 liters per day, it is recommended that the inflow rate be adjusted to deliver 2,000 mL of the solution in a 24-hour period.

It is important that the rinse of the bladder be **continuous**; the inflow or rinse solution should not be interrupted for more than a few minutes.
Preparation of the irrigation solution should be performed with strict aseptic techniques. The prepared solution should be stored at 4℃ and should be used within 48 hours following preparation to reduce the risk of contamination with resistant microorganisms.

HOW SUPPLIED
1-mL ampuls, boxes of 10 (NDC 0173-0748-10) and 50 ampuls (NDC 0173-0748-35); 20-mL multi-dose vial (NDC 0173-0544-00).
Store at 2° to 8℃ (36° to 46°F).
May 1996/RL-293
Shown in Product Identification Guide, page 313

NEOSPORIN® ℞
[nē″ō-spor′in]
Ophthalmic Ointment Sterile
(neomycin and polymyxin B sulfates and
bacitracin zinc ophthalmic ointment, USP).

DESCRIPTION
NEOSPORIN Ophthalmic Ointment (neomycin and polymyxin B sulfates and bacitracin zinc ophthalmic ointment) is a sterile antimicrobial ointment for ophthalmic use. Each gram contains: neomycin sulfate equivalent to 3.5 mg neomycin base, polymyxin B sulfate equivalent to 10,000 polymyxin B units, bacitracin zinc equivalent to 400 bacitracin units, and white petrolatum, q.s.
Neomycin sulfate is the sulfate salt of neomycin B and C, which are produced by the growth of *Streptomyces fradiae* Waksman (Fam, Streptomycetaceae). It has a potency equivalent of not less than 600 μg of neomycin standard per mg, calculated on an anhydrous basis.
Polymyxin B sulfate is the sulfate salt of polymyxin B_1 and B_2 which are produced by the growth of *Bacillus polymyxa* (Prazmowski) Miguia (Fam. Bacillaceae). It has a potency of not less than 6,000 polymyxin B units per mg, calculated on an anhydrous basis.
Bacitracin zinc is the zinc salt of bacitracin, a mixture of related cyclic polypeptides (mainly bacitracin A) produced by the growth of an organism of the *licheniformis* group of *Bacillus subtilis* var Tracy. It has a potency of not less than 40 bacitracin units per mg.

CLINICAL PHARMACOLOGY
A wide range of antibacterial action is provided by the overlapping spectra of neomycin, polymyxin B sulfate, and bacitracin.
Neomycin is bactericidal for many gram-positive and gram-negative organisms. It is an aminoglycoside antibiotic which inhibits protein synthesis by binding with ribosomal RNA and causing misreading of the bacterial genetic code.
Polymyxin B is bactericidal for a variety of gram-negative organisms. It increases the permeability of the bacterial cell membrane by interacting with the phospholipid components of the membrane.
Bacitracin is bactericidal for a variety of gram-positive and gram-negative organisms. It interferes with bacterial cell wall synthesis by inhibition of the regeneration of phospholipid receptors involved in peptidoglycan synthesis.

MICROBIOLOGY
Neomycin sulfate, polymyxin B sulfate, and bacitracin zinc together are considered active against the following microorganisms. *Staphylococcus aureus*, streptococci including *Streptococcus pneumoniae*, *Escherichia coli*, *Haemophilus influenzae*, *Klebsiella/Enterobacter* species, *Neisseria* species, and *Pseudomonas aeruginosa*. The product does not provide adequate coverage against *Serratia marcescens*.

INDICATIONS AND USAGE
NEOSPORIN Ophthalmic Ointment is indicated for the topical treatment of superficial infections of the external eye and its adnexa caused by susceptible bacteria. Such infections encompass conjunctivitis, keratitis and keratoconjunctivitis, blepharitis and blepharoconjunctivitis.

CONTRAINDICATIONS
NEOSPORIN Ophthalmic Ointment is contraindicated in individuals who have shown hypersensitivity to any of its components.

WARNINGS
NOT FOR INJECTION INTO THE EYE. NEOSPORIN Ophthalmic Ointment should never be directly introduced into the anterior chamber of the eye. Ophthalmic ointments may retard corneal wound healing.
Topical antibiotics particularly neomycin sulfate, may cause cutaneous sensitization. A precise incidence of hypersensitivity reactions (primarily skin rash) due to topical antibiotics is not known. The manifestations of sensitization to topical antibiotics are usually itching, reddening, and edema of the conjunctiva and eyelid. A sensitization reaction may

manifest simply as a failure to heal. During long-term use of topical antibiotic products, periodic examination for such signs is advisable, and the patient should be told to discontinue the product if they are observed. Symptoms usually subside quickly on withdrawing the medication. Application of products containing these ingredients should be avoided for the patient thereafter (see PRECAUTIONS: General).

PRECAUTIONS

General: As with other antibiotic preparations, prolonged use of NEOSPORIN Ophthalmic Ointment may result in overgrowth of nonsusceptible organisms including fungi. If superinfection occurs, appropriate measures should be initiated.

Bacterial resistance to NEOSPORIN Ophthalmic Ointment may also develop. If purulent discharge, inflammation, or pain becomes aggravated, the patient should discontinue use of the medication and consult a physician.

There have been reports of bacterial keratitis associated with the use of topical ophthalmic products in multiple-dose containers which have been inadvertently contaminated by patients, most of whom had a concurrent corneal disease or a disruption of the ocular epithelial surface (see PRECAUTIONS: Information for Patients).

Allergic cross-reactions may occur which could prevent the use of any or all of the following antibiotics for the treatment of future infections: kanamycin, paromomycin, streptomycin, and possibly gentamicin.

Information for Patients: Patients should be instructed to avoid allowing the tip of the dispensing container to contact the eye, eyelid, fingers, or any other surface. The use of this product by more than one person may spread infection.

Patients should also be instructed that ocular products, if handled improperly, can become contaminated by common bacteria known to cause ocular infections. Serious damage to the eye and subsequent loss of vision may result from using contaminated products (see PRECAUTIONS: General).

If the condition persists or gets worse, or if a rash or allergic reaction develops, the patient should be advised to stop use and consult a physician. Do not use this product if you are allergic to any of the listed ingredients.

Keep tightly closed when not in use. Keep out of reach of children.

Carcinogenesis, Mutagenesis, Impairment of Fertility: Long-term studies in animals to evaluate carcinogenic or mutagenic potential have not been conducted with polymyxin B sulfate or bacitracin. Treatment of cultured human lymphocytes in vitro with neomycin increased the frequency of chromosome abberrations at the highest concentration (80 μg/mL) tested; however, the effect of neomycin on carcinogenesis and mutagenesis in humans are unknown.

Polymyxin B has been reported to impair the motility of equine sperm, but its effects on male or female fertility are unknown. No adverse effects on male or female fertility, litter size, or survival were observed in rabbits given bacitracin zinc 100 gm/ton of diet.

Pregnancy: *Teratogenic Effects:* Pregnancy Category C. Animal reproduction studies have not been conducted with neomycin sulfate, polymyxin B sulfate, or bacitracin. It is also not known whether NEOSPORIN Ophthalmic Ointment can cause fetal harm when administered to a pregnant woman, or can affect reproduction capacity. NEOSPORIN Ophthalmic Ointment should be given to a pregnant woman only if clearly needed.

Nursing Mothers: It is not known whether this drug is excreted in human milk. Because many drugs are excreted in human milk, caution should be exercised when NEOSPORIN Ophthalmic Ointment is administered to a nursing woman.

Pediatric Use: Safety and effectiveness in pediatric patients have not been established.

ADVERSE REACTIONS

Adverse reactions have occurred with the anti-infective components of NEOSPORIN Ophthalmic Ointment. The exact incidence is not known. Reactions occurring most often are allergic sensitization reactions including itching, swelling, and conjunctival erythema (see WARNINGS). More serious hypersensitivity reactions, including anaphylaxis, have been reported rarely.

Local irritation on instillation has also been reported.

DOSAGE AND ADMINISTRATION

Apply the ointment every 3 or 4 hours for 7 to 10 days, depending on the severity of the infection.

HOW SUPPLIED

Tube of $^1/_8$ oz (3.5 g) with ophthalmic tip (NDC 0081-0732-86).

Caution Federal law prohibits dispensing without a prescription.

Store at 15° to 25°C (59° to 77°F).

June 1995

Shown in Product Identification Guide, page 314

NEOSPORIN® ℞

[*nē″ō-spor′ĭn*]

Ophthalmic Solution Sterile

(neomycin and polymyxin B sulfates and gramicidin ophthalmic solution, USP)

DESCRIPTION

NEOSPORIN Ophthalmic Solution (neomycin and polymyxin B sulfates and gramicidin ophthalmic solution) is a sterile antimicrobial solution for ophthalmic use. Each mL contains: neomycin sulfate equivalent to 1.75 mg neomycin base, polymyxin B sulfate equivalent to 10,000 polymyxin B units, and gramicidin 0.025 mg. The vehicle contains alcohol 0.5%, thimerosal 0.001% (added as a preservative) and the inactive ingredients propylene glycol, polyoxyethylene polyoxypropylene compound, sodium chloride, and Water for Injection.

Neomycin sulfate is the sulfate salt of neomycin B and C, which are produced by the growth of *Streptomyces fradiae* Waksman (Fam. Streptomycetaceae). It has a potency equivalent of not less than 600 μg of neomycin standard per mg, calculated on an anhydrous basis.

Polymyxin B sulfate is the sulfate salt of polymyxin B_1 and B_2 which are produced by the growth of *Bacillus polymyxa* (Prazmowski) Migula (Fam. Bacillaceae). It has a potency of not less than 6,000 polymyxin B units per mg, calculated on an anhydrous basis.

Gramicidin (also called Gramicidin D) is a mixture of three pairs of antibacterial substances (Gramicidin A, B, and C) produced by the growth of *Bacillus brevis* Dubos (Fam. Bacillaceae). It has a potency of not less than 900 μg of standard gramicidin per mg.

CLINICAL PHARMACOLOGY

A wide range of antibacterial action is provided by the overlapping spectra of neomycin, polymyxin B sulfate, and gramicidin.

Neomycin is bactericidal for many gram-positive and gram-negative organisms. It is an aminoglycoside antibiotic which inhibits protein synthesis by binding with ribosomal RNA and causing misreading of the bacterial genetic code.

Polymyxin B is bactericidal for a variety of gram-negative organisms. It increases the permeability of the bacterial cell membrane by interacting with the phospholipid components of the membrane.

Gramicidin is bactericidal for a variety of gram-positive organisms. It increases the permeability of the bacterial cell membrane to inorganic cations by forming a network of channels through the normal lipid bilayer of the membrane.

Microbiology: Neomycin sulfate, polymyxin B sulfate, and gramicidin together are considered active against the following microorganisms: *Staphylococcus aureus,* streptococci, including *Streptococcus pneumoniae, Escherichia coli, Haemophilus influenzae, Klebsiella/Enterobacter* species, *Neisseria* species and *Pseudomonas aeruginosa.* The product does not provide adequate coverage against *Serratia marcescens.*

INDICATIONS AND USAGE

NEOSPORIN Ophthalmic Solution is indicated for the topical treatment of superficial infections of the external eye and its adnexa caused by susceptible bacteria. Such infections encompass conjunctivitis, keratitis and keratoconjunctivitis, blepharitis and blepharoconjunctivitis.

CONTRAINDICATIONS

NEOSPORIN Ophthalmic Solution is contraindicated in individuals who have shown hypersensitivity to any of its components.

WARNINGS

NOT FOR INJECTION INTO THE EYE. NEOSPORIN Ophthalmic Solution should never be directly introduced into the anterior chamber of the eye or injected subconjunctivally.

Topical antibiotics, particularly neomycin sulfate, may cause cutaneous sensitization. A precise incidence of hypersensitivity reactions (primarily skin rash) due to topical antibiotics is not known. The manifestations of sensitization to topical antibiotics are usually itching, reddening, and edema of the conjunctiva and eyelid. A sensitization reaction may manifest simply as a failure to heal. During long-term use of topical antibiotic products, periodic examination for such signs is advisable, and the patient should be told to discontinue the product if they are observed. Symptoms usually subside quickly on withdrawing the medication. Application of products containing these ingredients should be avoided for the patient thereafter (see PRECAUTIONS: General).

PRECAUTIONS

General: As with other antibiotic preparations, prolonged use of NEOSPORIN Ophthalmic Solution may result in overgrowth of nonsusceptible organisms including fungi. If superinfection occurs, appropriate measures should be initiated.

Bacterial resistance to NEOSPORIN Ophthalmic Solution may also develop. If purulent discharge, inflammation, or pain becomes aggravated, the patient should discontinue use of the medication and consult a physician.

There have been reports of bacterial keratitis associated with the use of topical ophthalmic products in multiple-dose containers which have been inadvertently contaminated by patients, most of whom had a concurrent corneal disease or a disruption of the ocular epithelial surface (see PRECAUTIONS: Information for Patients).

Allergic cross-reactions may occur which could prevent the use of any or all of the following antibiotics for the treatment of future infections: kanamycin, paromomycin, streptomycin, and possibly gentamicin.

Information for Patients: Patients should be instructed to avoid allowing the tip of the dispensing container to contact the eye, eyelid, fingers, or any other surface. The use of this product by more than one person may spread infection.

Patients should also be instructed that ocular products, if handled improperly, can become contaminated by common bacteria known to cause ocular infections. Serious damage to the eye and subsequent loss of vision may result from using contaminated products (see PRECAUTIONS: General).

If the condition persists or gets worse, or if a rash or other allergic reaction develops, the patient should be advised to stop use and consult a physician. Do not use this product if you are allergic to any of the listed ingredients.

Keep tightly closed when not in use. Keep out of reach of children.

Carcinogenesis, Mutagenesis, Impairment of Fertility: Long-term studies in animals to evaluate carcinogenic or mutagenic potential have not been conducted with polymyxin B sulfate or gramicidin. Treatment of cultured human lymphocytes in vitro with neomycin increased the frequency of chromosome aberrations at the highest concentration (80 μg/mL) tested. However, the effects of neomycin on carcinogenesis and mutagenesis in humans are unknown.

Polymyxin B has been reported to impair the motility of equine sperm, but its effects on male or female fertility are unknown.

Pregnancy: *Teratogenic Effects:* Pregnancy Category C. Animal reproduction studies have not been conducted with neomycin sulfate, polymyxin B sulfate, or gramicidin. It is also not known whether NEOSPORIN Ophthalmic Solution can cause fetal harm when administered to a pregnant woman or can affect reproduction capacity. NEOSPORIN Ophthalmic Solution should be given to a pregnant woman only if clearly needed.

Nursing Mothers: It is not known whether this drug is excreted in human milk. Because many drugs are excreted in human milk, caution should be exercised when NEOSPORIN Ophthalmic Solution is administered to a nursing woman.

Pediatric Use: Safety and effectiveness in pediatric patients have not been established.

ADVERSE REACTIONS

Adverse reactions have occurred with the anti-infective components of NEOSPORIN Ophthalmic Solution. The exact incidence is not known. Reactions occurring most often are allergic sensitization reactions including itching, swelling, and conjunctival erythema (see WARNINGS). More serious hypersensitivity reactions, including anaphylaxis, have been reported rarely.

Local irritation on instillation has also been reported.

DOSAGE AND ADMINISTRATION

Instill one or two drops into the affected eye every 4 hours for 7 to 10 days. In severe infections, dosage may be increased to as much as two drops every hour.

HOW SUPPLIED

Drop Dose® of 10 mL (plastic dispenser bottle) (NDC 0173-0728-69).

Caution: Federal law prohibits dispensing without prescription.

Store at 15° to 25°C (59° to 77°F) and protect from light.

February 1996/RL-273

Shown in Product Identification Guide, page 314

NIMBEX™ ℞

[*nim′bex*]

(cisatracurium besylate)

Injection

This drug should be administered only by adequately trained individuals familiar with its actions, characteristics, and hazards.

DESCRIPTION

NIMBEX (cisatracurium besylate) is a nondepolarizing skeletal muscle relaxant for intravenous administration. Compared to other neuromuscular blocking agents, it is intermediate in its onset and duration of action. Cisatracurium besylate is one of 10 isomers of atracurium besylate and constitutes approximately 15% of that mixture. Cisatracur-

Continued on next page

Glaxo Wellcome—Cont.

ium besylate is [1R-[1α,2α(1'R*,2'R*)]]-2,2'-[1,5-pentanediyl-bis[oxy(3-oxo-3,1-propanediyl)]]bis[1-[(3,4-dimethoxyphenyl)-methyl]-1,2,3,4-tetrahydro-6,7-dimethoxy-2-methylisoquino-linium] dibenzenesulfonate. The molecular formula of the cisatracurium parent bis-cation is $C_{53}H_{72}N_2O_{12}$ and the molecular weight is 929.2. The molecular formula of cisatracurium as the besylate salt is $C_{65}H_{82}N_2O_{18}S_2$ and the molecular weight is 1243.50.

The log of the partition coefficient of cisatracurium besylate is -2.12 in a 1-octanol/distilled water system at 25°C.

NIMBEX Injection is a sterile, non-pyrogenic aqueous solution provided in 5 mL, 10 mL, and 20 mL vials. The pH is adjusted to 3.25 to 3.65 with benzenesulfonic acid. The 5 mL and 10 mL vials each contain cisatracurium besylate, equivalent to 2 mg/mL cisatracurium. The 20 mL vial, **intended for ICU use only**, contains cisatracurium besylate, equivalent to 10 mg/mL cisatracurium. The 10 mL vial, intended for multiple-dose use, contains 0.9% benzyl alcohol as a preservative. The 5 mL and 20 mL vials are single use vials and do not contain benzyl alcohol.

Cisatracurium besylate slowly loses potency with time at a rate of approximately 5% per *year* under refrigeration (5°C). NIMBEX should be refrigerated at 2° to 8°C (36° to 46°F) in the carton to preserve potency. The rate of loss in potency increases to approximately 5% per *month* at 25°C (77°F). Upon removal from refrigeration to room temperature storage conditions (25°C/77°F), use NIMBEX within 21 days, even if rerefrigerated.

CLINICAL PHARMACOLOGY

NIMBEX binds competitively to cholinergic receptors on the motor end-plate to antagonize the action of acetylcholine, resulting in block of neuromuscular transmission. This action is antagonized by acetylcholinesterase inhibitors such as neostigmine.

Pharmacodynamics: The neuromuscular blocking potency of NIMBEX is approximately threefold that of atracurium besylate. The time to maximum block is up to 2 minutes longer for equipotent doses of NIMBEX compared to atracurium besylate. The clinically effective duration of action and rate of spontaneous recovery from equipotent doses of NIMBEX and atracurium besylate are similar.

The average ED_{95} (dose required to produce 95% suppression of the adductor pollicis muscle twitch response to ulnar nerve stimulation) of cisatracurium is 0.05 mg/kg (range: 0.048 to 0.053) in adults receiving opioid/nitrous oxide/oxygen anesthesia. For comparison, the average ED_{95} for

atracurium when also expressed as the parent bis-cation is 0.17 mg/kg under similar anesthetic conditions.

The pharmacodynamics of $2 \times ED_{95}$ to $8 \times ED_{95}$ doses of cisatracurium administered over 5 to 10 seconds during opioid/nitrous oxide/oxygen anesthesia are summarized in Table 1. When the dose is doubled, the clinically effective duration of block increases by approximately 25 minutes. Once recovery begins, the rate of recovery is independent of dose.

Isoflurane or enflurane administered with nitrous oxide/oxygen to achieve 1.25 MAC [Minimum Alveolar Concentration] may prolong the clinically effective duration of action of initial and maintenance doses, and decrease the average infusion rate requirement of NIMBEX. The magnitude of these effects may depend on the duration of administration of the volatile agents. Fifteen to 30 minutes of exposure to 1.25 MAC isoflurane or enflurane had minimal effects on the duration of action of initial doses of NIMBEX and therefore, no adjustment to the initial dose should be necessary when NIMBEX is administered shortly after initiation of volatile agents. In long surgical procedures during enflurane or isoflurane anesthesia, less frequent maintenance dosing, lower maintenance doses, or reduced infusion rates of NIMBEX may be necessary. The average infusion rate requirement may be decreased by as much as 30% to 40%.

The onset, duration of action, and recovery profiles of NIMBEX during propofol/oxygen or propofol/nitrous oxide/oxygen anesthesia are similar to those during opioid/nitrous oxide/oxygen anesthesia.

[See table 1 below.]

When administered during the induction of adequate anesthesia using propofol, nitrous oxide/oxygen, and co-induction agents (e.g., fentanyl and midazolam), good or excellent conditions for tracheal intubation occurred in 67/71 (94%) patients in 1.5 to 2.0 minutes following 0.15 mg/kg cisatracurium and in 69/80 (87%) patients in 1.5 minutes following 0.2 mg/kg cisatracurium.

Repeated administration of maintenance doses or a continuous infusion of NIMBEX for up to 3 hours is not associated with development of tachyphylaxis or cumulative neuromuscular blocking effects. The time needed to recover from successive maintenance doses does not change with the number of doses administered as long as partial recovery is allowed to occur between doses. Maintenance doses can therefore be administered at relatively regular intervals with predictable results. The rate of spontaneous recovery from neuromuscular function after infusion is independent of the duration of infusion and comparable to the rate of recovery following initial doses (Table 1).

Long-term infusion (up to 6 days) of NIMBEX during mechanical ventilation in the ICU has been evaluated in two

studies. In a randomized, double-blind study using presence of a single twitch during train-of-four (TOF) monitoring to regulate dosage, patients treated with NIMBEX (n=19) recovered neuromuscular function ($T_4:T_1$ ratio ≥70%) following termination of infusion in approximately 55 minutes (range: 20 to 270) whereas those treated with vecuronium (n=12) recovered in 178 minutes (range: 40 minutes to 33 hours). In another study comparing NIMBEX and atracurium, patients recovered neuromuscular function in approximately 50 minutes for both NIMBEX (range: 20 to 175; n=34) and atracurium (range: 35 to 85; n=15).

The neuromuscular block produced by NIMBEX is readily antagonized by anticholinesterase agents once recovery has started. As with other nondepolarizing neuromuscular blocking agents, the more profound the neuromuscular block at the time of reversal, the longer the time required for recovery of neuromuscular function.

In children (2 to 12 years) cisatracurium has a lower ED_{95} than in adults (0.04 mg/kg, halothane/nitrous oxide/oxygen anesthesia). At 0.1 mg/kg during opioid anesthesia, cisatracurium had a faster onset and shorter duration of action in children than in adults (Table 1). Recovery following reversal is faster in children than in adults.

Hemodynamics Profile: Cisatracurium has no dose-related effects on mean arterial blood pressure (MAP) or heart rate (HR) following doses ranging from 2 to $8 \times ED_{95}$ (0.1 to 0.4 mg/kg), administered over 5 to 10 seconds, in healthy adult patients (Figure 1).

In patients with serious cardiovascular disease, NIMBEX has no clinically significant effects on MAP or HR following doses up to and including $6 \times ED_{95}$ (0.3 mg/kg), administered over 5 to 10 seconds (Figure 2). In two comparative studies involving patients undergoing coronary artery bypass grafting (CABG), there were no clinically significant differences in the hemodynamic effects following equipotent doses ranging from 0.1 to 0.3 mg/kg cisatracurium or vecuronium. Doses higher than $6 \times ED_{95}$ have not been studied in patients with serious cardiovascular disease.

Unlike atracurium, cisatracurium, at therapeutic doses of 2 $\times ED_{95}$ to $8 \times ED_{95}$ (0.1 to 0.4 mg/kg), administered over 5 to 10 seconds, does not cause dose-related elevations in mean plasma histamine concentration. The cardiovascular profile of NIMBEX allows it to be administered by rapid bolus at higher multiples of the ED_{95} than atracurium.

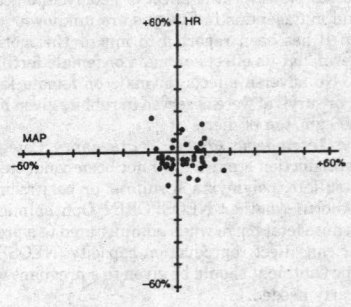

Figure 1

Maximum Percent Change from Preinjection in Heart Rate (HR) and Mean Arterial Pressure (MAP) During First 5 Minutes after Initial 4 x ED95 to 8 x ED95 Doses of NIMBEX™ in Healthy Adult Patients Receiving Opioid/Nitrous Oxide/Oxygen Anesthesia (n=44)

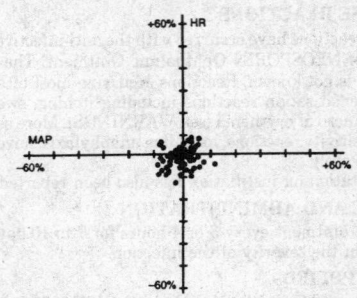

Figure 2

Percent Change from Preinjection in Heart Rate (HR) and Mean Arterial Pressure (MAP) 2 Minutes Following Administration of NIMBEX (2 to 6 x ED95) to Patients Undergoing CABG Surgery Receiving Etomidate/Fentanyl/Midazolam/Oxygen Anesthesia (n=90)

No clinically significant changes in MAP or HR were observed following administration of doses up to 0.1 mg/kg cisatracurium over 5 to 10 seconds in 2- to 12-year-old children receiving either halothane/nitrous oxide/oxygen or opioid/nitrous oxide/oxygen anesthesia.

Table 1
Pharmacodynamic Dose Response* of NIMBEX™
During Opioid/Nitrous Oxide/Oxygen Anesthesia

Initial Dose of NIMBEX (mg/kg)	Time to 90% Block (min)	Time to Maximum Block (min)	Time to Spontaneous Recovery				
			5% Recovery (min)	25% Recovery[†] (min)	95% Recovery (min)	$T_4:T_1$ Ratio[‡] ≥70% (min)	25%–75% Recovery Index (min)
Adults							
0.1 (2 × ED95) (n[§]=98)	3.3 (1.0–8.7)	5.0 (1.2–17.2)	33 (15–51)	42 (22–63)	64 (25–93)	64 (32–91)	13 (5–30)
0.15[ǁ] (3 × ED95) (n=39)	2.6 (1.0–4.4)	3.5 (1.6–6.8)	46 (28–65)	55 (44–74)	76 (60–103)	75 (63–98)	13 (11–16)
0.2 (4 × ED95) (n=30)	2.4 (1.5–4.5)	2.9 (1.9–5.2)	59 (31–103)	65 (43–103)	81 (53–114)	85 (55–114)	12 (2–30)
0.25 (5 × ED95) (n=15)	1.6 (0.8–3.3)	2.0 (1.2–3.7)	70 (58–85)	78 (66–86)	91 (76–109)	97 (82–113)	8 (5–12)
0.4 (8 × ED95) (n=15)	1.5 (1.3–1.8)	1.9 (1.4–2.3)	83 (37–103)	91 (59–107)	121 (110–134)	126 (115–137)	14 (10–18)
Children (2–12 yr)							
0.08[¶] (2 × ED95) (n=60)	2.2 (1.2–6.8)	3.3 (1.7–9.7)	22 (11–38)	29 (20–46)	52 (37–64)	50 (37–62)	11 (7–15)
0.1 (n=16)	1.7 (1.3–2.7)	2.8 (1.8–6.7)	21 (13–31)	28 (21–38)	46 (37–58)	44 (36–58)	10 (7–12)

* Values shown are medians of means from individual studies. Values in parentheses are ranges of individual patient values.
† Clinically effective duration of block
‡ Train-of-four ratio
§ n = the number of patients with Time to Maximum block data.
ǁ Propofol anesthesia
¶ Halothane anesthesia

Pharmacokinetics:

General: The neuromuscular blocking activity of NIMBEX is due to parent drug. Cisatracurium plasma concentration-time data following IV bolus administration are best described by a two-compartment open model (with elimination from both compartments) with an elimination half-life ($t_{1/2}\beta$) of 22 minutes, a plasma clearance (CL) of 4.57 mL/min/kg, and a volume of distribution at steady state (V_{ss}) of 145 mL/kg. Cisatracurium undergoes organ-independent Hofmann elimination (a chemical process dependent on pH and temperature) to form the monoquaternary acrylate metabolite and laudanosine, neither of which has any neuromuscular blocking activity (see **Pharmacokinetics: *Metabolism*** section). Following administration of radiolabeled cisatracurium, 95% of the dose was recovered in the urine; less than 10% of the dose was excreted as unchanged parent drug. Laudanosine, a metabolite of cisatracurium (and atracurium) has been noted to cause transient hypotension and, in higher doses, cerebral excitatory effects when administered to several animal species. The relationship between CNS excitation and laudanosine concentrations in humans has not been established (see **PRECAUTONS: Long-term use in the Intensive Care Unit**). Because cisatracurium is three times more potent than atracurium and lower doses are required, the corresponding laudanosine concentrations following cisatracurium are one-third those that would be expected following an equipotent dose of atracurium (see **Pharmacokinetics:** ***Special Populations:*** *Intensive Care Unit Patients*).

Results from population pharmacokinetic/pharmacodynamic (PK/PD) analyses from 241 healthy surgical patients are summarized in Table 2.

Table 2
Key Population PK/PD Parameter Estimates for Cisatracurium in Healthy Surgical Patients* Following 0.1 (2 × ED_{95}) to 0.4 mg/kg (8 × ED_{95}) NIMBEX™

Parameter	Estimate†	Magnitude of Interpatient Variability (CV)‡
CL (mL/min/kg)	4.57	16%
V_{ss}(mL/kg)§	145	27%
k_{eo}(min^{-1})II	0.0575	61%
EC_{50} (ng/mL)¶	141	52%

* Healthy male nonobese patients 19–64 years of age with creatinine clearance values greater than 70 mL/min who received cisatracurium during opioid anesthesia and had venous samples collected.

† The percent standard error of the mean (%SEM) ranged from 3 to 12% indicating good precision for the PK/PD estimates.

‡ Expressed as a coefficient of variation; the %SEM ranged from 20 to 35% indicating adequate precision for the estimates of interpatient variability.

§ V_{ss} is the volume of distribution at steady state estimated using a two-compartment model with elimination from both compartments. V_{ss} is equal to the sum of the volume in the central compartment (V_c) and the volume in the peripheral compartment (V_p); interpatient variability could only be estimated for V_c.

II Rate constant describing the equilibration between plasma concentrations and neuromuscular block

¶ Concentration required to produce 50% T_1 suppression; an index of patient sensitivity.

The magnitude of interpatient variability in CL was low (16%), as expected based on the importance of Hofmann elimination (see **Pharmacokinetics: *Elimination***). The magnitudes of interpatient variability in CL and volume of distribution were low in comparison to those for k_{eo} and EC_{50}. This suggests that any alterations in the time course of cisatracurium-induced block are more likely to be due to variability in the pharmacodynamic parameters than in the pharmacokinetic parameters. Parameter estimates from the population pharmacokinetic analyses were supported by noncompartmental pharmacokinetic analyses on data from healthy patients and from special patient populations.

Conventional pharmacokinetic analyses have shown that the pharmacokinetics of cisatracurium are proportional to dose between 0.1 (2 × ED_{95}) and 0.2 (4 × ED_{95}) mg/kg cisatracurium. In addition, population pharmacokinetic analyses revealed no statistically significant effect of initial dose on CL for doses between 0.1 (2 × ED_{95}) and 0.4 (8 × ED_{95}) mg/kg cisatracurium.

Distribution: The volume of distribution of cisatracurium is limited by its large molecular weight and high polarity. The V_{ss} was equal to 145 mL/kg (Table 2) in healthy 19- to 64-year-old surgical patients receiving opioid anesthesia. The V_{ss} was 21% larger in similar patients receiving inhalation anesthesia (see **Pharmacokinetics:** ***Special Populations:*** *Other Patient Factors*).

Protein Binding: The binding of cisatracurium to plasma proteins has not been successfully studied due to its rapid degradation at physiologic pH. Inhibition of degradation requires nonphysiological conditions of temperature and pH which are associated with changes in protein binding.

Metabolism: The degradation of cisatracurium is largely independent of liver metabolism. Results from in vitro experiments suggest that cisatracurium undergoes Hofmann elimination (a pH and temperature-dependent chemical process) to form laudanosine (see **PRECAUTIONS: Long-term Use in the Intensive Care Unit**) and the monoquaternary acrylate metabolite. The monoquaternary acrylate undergoes hydrolysis by non-specific plasma esterases to form the monoquaternary alcohol (MQA) metabolite. The MQA metabolite can also undergo Hofmann elimination but at a much slower rate than cisatracurium. Laudanosine is further metabolized to desmethyl metabolites which are conjugated with glucuronic acid and excreted in the urine.

Organ-independent Hofmann elimination is the predominant pathway for the elimination of cisatracurium. The liver and kidney play a minor role in the elimination of cisatracurium but are primary pathways for the elimination of metabolites. Therefore, the $t_{1/2}\beta$ values of metabolites (including laudanosine) are longer in patients with kidney or liver dysfunction and metabolite concentrations may be higher after long-term administration (see **PRECAUTIONS: Long-term Use in the Intensive Care Unit**). Most importantly, C_{max} values of laudanosine are significantly lower in healthy surgical patients receiving infusions of NIMBEX than in patients receiving infusions of atracurium (mean ± S.D. C_{max}: 60 ± 52 and 342 ± 93 ng/mL, respectively)

Elimination:

Clearance and Half-life: Mean CL values for cisatracurium ranged from 4.5 to 5.7 mL/min/kg in studies of healthy surgical patients. Compartmental pharmacokinetic modeling suggests that approximately 80% of the CL is accounted for by Hofmann elimination and the remaining 20% by renal and hepatic elimination. These findings are consistent with the low magnitude of interpatient variability in CL (16%) estimated as part of the population PK/PD analyses and with the recovery of parent and metabolites in urine. Following ^{14}C-cisatracurium administration to 6 healthy male patients, 95% of the dose was recovered in the urine (mostly as conjugated metabolites) and 4% in the feces; less than 10% of the dose was excreted as unchanged parent drug in the urine. In 12 healthy surgical patients receiving non-radiolabeled cisatracurium who had Foley catheters placed for surgical management, approximately 15% of the dose was excreted unchanged in the urine.

In studies of healthy surgical patients, mean $t_{1/2}\beta$ values of cisatracurium ranged from 22 to 29 minutes and were consistent with the $t_{1/2}\beta$ of cisatracurium in vitro (29 min). The mean ± SD $t_{1/2}\beta$ values of laudanosine were 3.1 ± 0.4 and 3.3 ± 2.1 hours in healthy surgical patients receiving NIMBEX (n=10) or atracurium (n=10), respectively. During IV infusions of NIMBEX, peak plasma concentrations (C_{max}) of laudanosine and the MQA metabolite are approximately 6% and 11% of the parent compound, respectively.

Special Populations:

Elderly Patients (≥65 years): The results of conventional pharmacokinetic analysis from a study of 12 healthy elderly patients and 12 healthy young adult patients receiving a single IV dose of 0.1 mg/kg NIMBEX are summarized in Table 3. Plasma clearances of cisatracurium were not affected by age; however, the volumes of distribution were slightly larger in elderly patients than in young patients resulting in slightly longer $t_{1/2}\beta$ values for cisatracurium. The rate of equilibration between plasma cisatracurium concentrations and neuromuscular block was slower in elderly patients than in young patients (mean ± SD k_{eo}: 0.071 ± 0.036 and 0.105 ± 0.021 min^{-1}, respectively); there was no difference in the patient sensitivity to cisatracurium-induced block, as indicated by EC_{50} values (mean ± SD EC_{50}: 91 ± 22 and 89 ± 23 ng/mL, respectively). These changes were consistent with the one-minute slower times to maximum block in elderly patients receiving 0.1 mg/kg NIMBEX, when compared to young patients receiving the same dose. The minor differences in PK/PD parameters of cisatracurium between elderly patients and young patients were not associated with clinically significant differences in the recovery profile of NIMBEX.

Table 3
Pharmacokinetic Parameters* of Cisatracurium in Healthy Elderly and Young Adult Patients Following 0.1 mg/kg (2 × ED_{95}) NIMBEX™ (Isoflurane/Nitrous Oxide/Oxygen Anesthesia)

Parameter	Healthy Elderly Patients	Healthy Young Adult Patients
Elimination Half-Life ($t_{1/2}\beta$, min)	25.8 ± 3.6†	22.1 ± 2.5
Volume of Distribution at Steady State‡(mL/kg)	156 ± 17†	133 ± 15
Plasma Clearance (mL/min/kg)	5.7 ± 1.0	5.3 ± 0.9

* Values presented are mean ± S.D.

† $P < 0.05$ for comparisons between healthy elderly and healthy young adult patients.

‡ Volume of distribution is underestimated because elimination from the peripheral compartment is ignored.

Patients with Hepatic Disease: Table 4 summarizes the conventional pharmacokinetic analysis from a study of NIMBEX in 13 patients with end-stage liver disease undergoing liver transplantation and 11 healthy adult patients undergoing elective surgery. The slightly larger volumes of distribution in liver transplant patients were associated with slightly higher plasma clearances of cisatracurium. The parallel changes in these parameters resulted in no difference in $t_{1/2}\beta$ values. There were no differences in k_{eo} or EC_{50} between patient groups. The times to maximum block were approximately one minute faster in liver transplant patients than in healthy adult patients receiving 0.1 mg/kg NIMBEX. These minor differences in pharmacokinetics were not associated with clinically significant differences in the recovery profile of NIMBEX.

The $t_{1/2}\beta$ values of metabolites are longer in patients with hepatic disease and concentrations may be higher after long-term administration (see **Pharmacokinetics: *Special Populations:*** *Intensive Care Unit Patients*).

Table 4
Pharmacokinetic Parameters* of Cisatracurium in Healthy Adult Patients and in Patients Undergoing Liver Transplantation Following 0.1 mg/kg (2 × ED_{95}) NIMBEX™ (Isoflurane/Nitrous Oxide/Oxygen Anesthesia)

Parameter	Liver Transplant Patients	Healthy Adult Patients
Elimination Half-Life ($t_{1/2}\beta$, min)	24.4 ± 2.9	23.5 ± 3.5
Volume of Distribution at Steady State‡(L/kg)	195 ± 38†	161 ± 23
Plasma Clearance (mL/min/kg)	6.6 ± 1.1†	5.7 ± 0.8

* Values presented are mean ± S.D.

† $P < 0.05$ for comparisons between liver transplant patients and healthy adult patients

‡ Volume of distribution is underestimated because elimination from the peripheral compartment is ignored.

Patients with Renal Dysfunction: Results from a conventional pharmacokinetic study of NIMBEX in 13 healthy adult patients and 15 patients with end-stage renal disease (ESRD) undergoing elective surgery are summarized in Table 5. The PK/PD parameters of cisatracurium were similar in healthy adult patients and ESRD patients. The times to 90% block were approximately one minute slower in ESRD patients following 0.1 mg/kg NIMBEX. There were no differences in the durations or rates of recovery of NIMBEX between ESRD and healthy adult patients.

The $t_{1/2}\beta$ values of metabolites are longer in patients with renal failure and concentrations may be higher after long-term administration (see **Pharmacokinetics: *Special Populations:*** *Intensive Care Unit Patients*).

Table 5
Pharmacokinetic Parameters* for Cisatracurium in Healthy Adult Patients and Patients with End-Stage Renal Disease (ESRD) Receiving 0.1 mg/kg (2 × ED_{95}) NIMBEX™ (Opioid/Nitrous Oxide/Oxygen Anesthesia)

Parameter	Healthy Adult Patients	ESRD Patients
Elimination Half-Life ($t_{1/2}\beta$, min)	29.4 ± 4.1	32.3 ± 6.3
Volume of Distribution at Steady State†(mL/kg)	149 ± 35	160 ± 32
Plasma Clearance (mL/min/kg)	4.66 ± 0.86	4.26 ± 0.62

* Values presented as mean ± S.D.

† Volume of distribution is underestimated because elimination from the peripheral compartment is ignored.

Population pharmacokinetic analyses revealed that patients with creatinine clearances ≤70 mL/min had a slower rate of equilibration between plasma concentrations and neuromuscular block than patients with normal renal function; this change was associated with a slightly slower (∼40 sec) predicted time to 90% T_1 suppression in patients with renal dysfunction following 0.1 mg/kg NIMBEX. There was no clinically significant alteration in the recovery profile of

Continued on next page

Glaxo Wellcome—Cont.

NIMBEX in patients with renal dysfunction. The recovery profile of NIMBEX is unchanged in the presence of renal or hepatic failure, which is consistent with predominantly organ-independent elimination.

Intensive Care Unit (ICU) Patients: The pharmacokinetics of cisatracurium, atracurium, and their metabolites were determined in 6 ICU patients receiving NIMBEX and in 6 ICU patients receiving atracurium and are presented in Table 6. The plasma clearances of cisatracurium and atracurium are similar. The volume of distribution was larger and the $t_{1/2}\beta$ was longer for cisatracurium than for atracurium. The relationships between plasma cisatracurium or atracurium concentrations and neuromuscular block have not been evaluated in ICU patients. The minor differences in pharmacokinetics were not associated with any differences in the recovery profiles of NIMBEX and atracurium in ICU patients.

[See table 6 below.]

Plasma metabolite pharmacokinetics are listed in Table 6. Limited pharmacokinetic data are available for patients with liver/kidney dysfunction receiving NIMBEX. Data from studies of atracurium demonstrate that renal/hepatic failure in ICU patients produces little to no effect on its pharmacokinetics, but decreases the biotransformation and elimination of the metabolites. Following atracurium, $t_{1/2}\beta$ values for laudanosine were longer in ICU patients with renal failure than in ICU patients with normal renal function (15 and 6 hrs, respectively). The $t_{1/2}\beta$ values of laudanosine were 39 ± 14 hrs in ICU patients with liver failure receiving atracurium after an unsuccessful liver transplantation and 5 ± 2 hrs in similar ICU patients after successful liver transplantation. Therefore, relative to ICU patients with normal renal and hepatic function receiving NIMBEX, metabolite concentrations (plasma and tissues) may be higher in ICU patients with renal or hepatic failure (see **Precautions: Long-term Use in the Intensive Care Unit**). Consistent with the decreased infusion rate requirements for NIMBEX, metabolite concentrations were lower in patients receiving NIMBEX than in patients receiving atracurium besylate.

Pediatric Patients: The population PK/PD of cisatracurium were described in 20 healthy pediatric patients during halothane anesthesia, using the same model developed for healthy adult patients. The CL was higher in healthy pediatric patients (5.89 mL/min/kg) than in healthy adult patients (4.57 mL/min/kg) during opioid anesthesia. The rate of equilibration between plasma concentrations and neuromuscular block, as indicated by K_{eo}, was faster in healthy pediatric patients receiving halothane anesthesia (0.1330 min^{-1}) than in healthy adult patients receiving opioid anesthesia (0.0575 min^{-1}). The EC_{50} in healthy pediatric patients (125 ng/mL) was similar to the value in healthy adult patients (141 ng/mL) during opioid anesthesia. The minor differences in the PK/PD parameters of cisatracurium were associated with a faster time to onset and a shorter duration of cisatracurium-induced neuromuscular block in pediatric patients.

Other Patient Factors: Population PK/PD analyses revealed that gender and obesity were associated with statistically significant effects on the pharmacokinetics and/or pharmacodynamics of cisatracurium; these factors were not associated with clinically significant alterations in the predicted onset or recovery profile of NIMBEX. The use of inhalation agents was associated was 21% larger V_{ss}, a 78% larger k_{eo}, and 15% lower EC_{50} for cisatracurium. These changes resulted in a slightly faster (~45 sec) predicted time to 90% T_1 suppression in patients receiving 0.1 mg/kg cisatracurium during inhalation anesthesia than in patients receiving the same dose of cisatracurium during opioid anesthesia; however, there were no clinically significant differences in the predicted recovery profile of NIMBEX between patients groups.

Individualization of Dosages: DOSES OF **NIMBEX** SHOULD BE INDIVIDUALIZED AND A PERIPHERAL NERVE STIMULATOR SHOULD BE USED TO MEASURE NEUROMUSCULAR FUNCTION DURING ADMINISTRATION OF **NIMBEX** IN ORDER TO MONITOR DRUG EFFECT, TO DETERMINE THE NEED FOR ADDITIONAL DOSES, AND TO CONFIRM RECOVERY FROM NEUROMUSCULAR BLOCK.

Based on the known action of NIMBEX and other neuromuscular blocking agents, the following factors should be considered when administering NIMBEX:

Renal and Hepatic Disease: See PRECAUTIONS section.

Long-Term Use in the Intensive Care Unit (ICU): The long-term infusion (up to 6 days) of NIMBEX during mechanical ventilation in the ICU has been evaluated in two studies. Average infusion rates of approximately 3 μg/kg/min (range: 0.5 to 10.2) were required to achieve adequate neuromuscular block. As with other neuromuscular blocking agents, these data indicate the presence of wide interpatient variability in dosage requirements. In addition, dosage requirements may increase or decrease with time (see PRECAUTIONS). Use of NIMBEX in the ICU for longer than 6 days has not been studied.

Drugs or Conditions Causing Potentiation of or Resistance to Neuromuscular Block: Persons with certain pre-existing conditions or receiving certain drugs may require individualization of dosing (see PRECAUTIONS).

Burns: Patients with burns have been shown to develop resistance to nondepolarizing neuromuscular blocking agents, and may require individualization of dosing (see PRECAUTIONS).

INDICATIONS AND USAGE

NIMBEX is an intermediate-onset/intermediate-duration neuromuscular blocking agent indicated for inpatients and outpatients as an adjunct to general anesthesia, to facilitate tracheal intubation, and to provide skeletal muscle relaxation during surgery or mechanical ventilation in the ICU.

CONTRAINDICATIONS

NIMBEX is contraindicated in patients known to have an allergic hypersensitivity to NIMBEX or other bis-benzylisoquinolinium agents. Use of NIMBEX from vials containing benzyl alcohol as a preservative is contraindicated in patients with a known hypersensitivity to benzyl alcohol.

WARNINGS

NIMBEX SHOULD BE ADMINISTERED IN CAREFULLY ADJUSTED DOSAGE BY OR UNDER THE SUPERVISION OR EXPERIENCED CLINICIANS WHO ARE FAMILIAR WITH THE DRUG'S ACTIONS AND THE POSSIBLE COMPLICATIONS OF ITS USE. THE DRUG SHOULD NOT BE ADMINISTERED UNLESS PERSONNEL AND FACILITIES FOR RESUSCITATION AND LIFE SUPPORT (TRACHEAL INTUBATION, ARTIFICIAL VENTILATION, OXYGEN THERAPY), AND AN ANTAGONIST OF **NIMBEX** ARE IMMEDIATELY AVAILABLE. IT IS RECOMMENDED THAT A PERIPHERAL NERVE STIMULATOR BE USED TO MEASURE NEUROMUSCULAR FUNCTION DURING THE ADMINISTRATION OF **NIMBEX** IN ORDER TO MONITOR DRUG EFFECT, DETERMINE THE NEED FOR ADDITIONAL DOSES, AND CONFIRM RECOVERY FROM NEUROMUSCULAR BLOCK.

NIMBEX HAS NO KNOWN EFFECT ON CONSCIOUSNESS, PAIN THRESHOLD, OR CEREBRATION. TO AVOID DISTRESS TO THE PATIENT, NEUROMUSCULAR BLOCK SHOULD NOT BE INDUCED BEFORE UNCONSCIOUSNESS.

NIMBEX Injection is acidic (pH 3.25 to 3.65) and may not be compatible with alkaline solutions having a pH greater than 8.5 (e.g., barbiturate solutions).

The 10 mL multiple dose vials of NIMBEX contain benzyl alcohol. In newborn infants, benzyl alcohol has been associated with an increased incidence of neurological and other complications which are sometimes fatal. Single use vials (5 mL and 20 mL) of NIMBEX do not contain benzyl alcohol (see PRECAUTIONS: **Pediatric Use**).

PRECAUTIONS

Because of its intermediate onset of action, NIMBEX is not recommended for rapid sequence endotracheal intubation.

Recommended doses of NIMBEX have no clinically significant effects on heart rate; therefore, NIMBEX will not counteract the bradycardia produced by many anesthetic agents or by vagal stimulation.

Neuromuscular blocking agents may have a profound effect in patients with neuromuscular diseases (e.g., myasthenia gravis and the myasthenic syndrome). In these and other conditions in which prolonged neuromuscular block is a possibility (e.g., carcinomatosis), the use of a peripheral nerve stimulator and a dose of not more than 0.02 mg/kg NIMBEX is recommended to assess the level of neuromuscular block and to monitor dosage requirements.

Patients with burns have been shown to develop resistance to nondepolarizing neuromuscular blocking agents, including atracurium. The extent of altered response depends upon the size of the burn and the time elapsed since the burn injury. NIMBEX has not been studied in patients with burns; however, based on its structural similarity to atracurium, the possibility of increased dosing requirements and shortened duration of action must be considered if NIMBEX is administered to burn patients.

Patients with hemiparesis or paraparesis also may demonstrate resistance to nondepolarizing muscle relaxants in the affected limbs. To avoid inaccurate dosing, neuromuscular monitoring should be performed on a non-paretic limb.

Acid-base and/or serum electrolye abnormalities may potentiate or antagonize the action of neuromuscular blocking agents.

No data are available to support the use of NIMBEX by intramuscular injection.

Renal and Hepatic Disease: No clinically significant alterations in the recovery profile were observed in patients with renal dysfunction or in patients with end-stage liver disease following a 0.1 mg/kg dose of cisatracurium. The onset time was approximately 1 minute faster in patients with end-stage liver disease and approximately 1 minute slower in patients with renal dysfunction than in healthy adult control patients.

Malignant Hyperthermia (MH): In a study of MH-susceptible pigs, cisatracurium besylate (highest dose 2000 μg/kg equivalent to 3 × ED_{95} in pigs and 40 × ED_{95} in humans) did not trigger MH. Cisatracurium besylate has not been studied in MH-susceptible patients. Because MH can develop in the absence of established triggering agents, the clinican should be prepared to recognize and treat MH in any patient undergoing general anesthesia.

Long-Term Use in the Intensive Care Unit (ICU): Long-term infusion (up to 6 days) of NIMBEX during mechanical ventilation in the ICU has been safely used to two studies. Dosage requirements may increase or decrease with time (see CLINICAL PHARMACOLOGY: **Individualization of Doses**).

Little information is available on the plasma levels and clinical consequences of cisatracurium metabolites that may accumulate during days to weeks of cisatracurium administration in ICU patients. Laudanosine, a major, biologically active metabolite of atracurium and cisatracurium without neuromuscular blocking activity, produces transient hypotension and, in higher doses, cerebral excitatory effects (generalized muscle twitching and seizures) when administered to several species of animals. There have been rare spontaneous reports of seizures in ICU patients who have received atracurium or other agents. These patients usually had predisposing causes (such as cranial trauma, cerebral edema, hypoxic encephalopathy, viral encephalitis, uremia). There are insufficient data to determine whether or not laudanosine contributes to seizures in ICU patients. Consistent with the decreased infusion rate requirements for NIMBEX, laudanosine concentrations were lower in patients receiving NIMBEX than in patients receiving atracurium for up to 48 hours (see **Pharmacokinetics: *Special Populations: Intensive Care Unit Patients***).

In a randomized, double-blind study using train-of-four nerve stimulator monitoring to maintain at least one visible twitch, evaluable patients treated with NIMBEX (n=19) recovered neuromuscular function (T_4: T_1 ratio ≥70%) following termination of infusion in approximately 55 minutes (range: 20 to 270) whereas evaluable vercuronium-treated patients (n=12) recovered in 178 minutes (range: 40 minutes to 33 hours). In another study comparing NIMBEX and atracurium, patients recovered neuromuscular function in approximately 50 minutes for both NIMBEX (range: 20 to 175; n=34) and atracurium (range: 35 to 85; n=15).

WHENEVER THE USE OF **NIMBEX** OR ANY OTHER NEUROMUSCULAR BLOCKING AGENT IN THE ICU IS CONTEMPLATED, IT IS RECOMMENDED THAT NEUROMUSCULAR FUNCTION BE MONITORED DURING ADMINISTRATION WITH A NERVE STIMULATOR. ADDITIONAL DOSES OF **NIMBEX** OR ANY OTHER NEUROMUSCULAR BLOCKING AGENT SHOULD NOT BE GIVEN BEFORE THERE IS A DEFINITE RESPONSE TO

Table 6

Parameter Estimates* for Cisatracurium, Atracurium and Metabolites in ICU Patients After Long-Term (24–48 hr) Administration of NIMBEX™ or Atracurium Besylate

	Parameter	Cisatracurium (n=6)	Atracurium (n=6)
Parent Compound	CL (mL/min/kg)	7.45 ± 1.02	7.49 ± 0.66†
	$t_{1/2}\beta$(min)	26.8 ± 11.1	16.5 ± 6.0†
	Vβ (mL/kg)‡	280 ± 103	178 ± 71†
Laudanosine	C_{max} (ng/mL)	707 ± 360	2318 ± 1498
	$t_{1/2}\beta$ (hrs)	6.6 ± 4.1	8.4 ± 7.3
MQA metabolite	C_{max} (ng/mL)	152 – 181§	943 ± 333‖
	$t_{1/2}\beta$ (min)	26 – 31§	21 – 58§

* presented as mean ± standard deviation

† n=5

‡ Volume of distribution during the terminal elimination phase, and underestimate because elimination from the peripheral compartment is ignored.

§ n=2, range presented

‖ n=3

NERVE STIMULATION. IF NO RESPONSE IS ELICITED, INFUSION ADMINISTRATION SHOULD BE DISCONTINUED UNTIL A RESPONSE RETURNS.

The effects of hemofiltration, hemodialysis, and hemoperfusion on plasma levels of NIMBEX and its metabolites are unknown.

Drug Interactions: NIMBEX has been used safely following varying degrees of recovery from succinylcholine-induced neuromuscular block. Administration of 0.1 mg/kg (2 × ED_{95}) NIMBEX at 10% or 95% recovery following an intubating dose of succinylcholine (1 mg/kg) produced ≥95% neuromuscular block. The time to onset of maxmium block following NIMBEX is approximately 2 minutes faster with prior administration of succinylcholine. Prior administration of succinylcholine had no effect on the duration of neuromuscular block following initial or maintenance bolus doses of NIMBEX. Infusion requirements of NIMBEX in patients administered succinylcholine prior to infusions of NIMBEX were comparable to or slightly greater than when succinylcholine was not administered.

The use of NIMBEX before succinylcholine to attenuate some of the side effects of succinylcholine has not been studied.

Although not studied systematically in clinical trials, no drug interactions were observed when vecuronium, pancuronium, or atracurium were administered following varying degrees of recovery from single doses or infusions of NIMBEX.

Isoflurane or enflurane administered with nitrous oxide/oxygen to achieve 1.25 MAC [Minimum Alveolar Concentration] may prolong the clinically effective duration of action of initial and maintenance doses of NIMBEX and decrease the required infusion rate of NIMBEX. The magnitude of these effects may depend on the duration of administration of the volatile agents. Fifteen to 30 minutes of exposure to 1.25 MAC isoflurane or enflurane had minimal effects on the duration of action of initial doses of NIMBEX and therefore, no adjustment to the initial dose should be necessary when NIMBEX is administered shortly after initiation of volatile agents. In long surgical procedures during enflurane or isoflurane anesthesia, less frequent maintenance dosing, lower maintenance doses, or reduced infusion rates of NIMBEX may be necessary. The average infusion rate requirement may be decreased by as much as 30% to 40%.

In clinical studies propofol had no effect on the duration of action or dosing requirements for NIMBEX.

Other drugs which may enhance the neuromuscular blocking action of nondepolarizing agents such as NIMBEX include certain antibiotics (e.g., aminoglycosides, tetracyclines, bacitracin, polymyxins, lincomycin, clindamycin, colistin, and sodium colistemethate), magnesium salts, lithium, local anesthetics, procainamide, and quinidine.

Resistance to the neuromuscular blocking action of nondepolarizing neuromuscular blocking agents has been demonstrated in patients chronically administered phenytoin or carbamazepine. While the effects of chronic phenytoin or carbamazepine therapy on the action of NIMBEX are unknown, slightly shorter durations of neuromuscular block may be anticipated and infusion rate requirements may be higher.

Drug/Laboratory Test Interactions: None known

Carcinogenesis, Mutagenesis, Impairment of Fertility: Carcinogenesis and fertility studies have not been performed. Cisatracurium besylate was evaluated in a battery of four short-term mutagenicity tests. It was non-mutagenic in the Ames Salmonella assay, a rat bone marrow cytogenetic assay, and an in vitro human lymphocyte cytogenetics assay. As was the case with atracurium, the mouse lymphoma assay was positive both in the presence and absence of exogenous metabolic activation (rat liver S-9). In the absence of S-9, cisatracurium besylate was positive at in vitro cisatracurium concentrations of 40 μg/mL and higher. The highest non-mutagenic concentration (30 μg/mL) and incubation time (4 hours) resulted in an AUC approximately 120 times that noted in clinical studies and approximately 8.5 times the mean peak clinical concentration noted. In the presence of S-9, cisatracurium besylate was positive at a cisatracurium concentration of 300 μg/mL but not at lower or higher concentrations.

Pregnancy: ***Teratogenic Effects:*** Pregnancy Category B. Teratology testing in nonventilated pregnant rats treated subcutaneously with maximum subparalyzing doses (4 mg/kg daily; equivalent to 8 × the human ED_{95} following a bolus dose of 0.2 mg/kg IV) and in ventilated rats treated intravenously with paralyzing doses of NIMBEX at 0.5 and 1.0 mg/kg; equivalent to 10 × and 20 × the human ED_{95} dose, respectively, revealed no maternal or fetal toxicity or teratogenic effects. There are no adequate and well-controlled studies of NIMBEX in pregnant women. Because animal studies are not always predictive of human response, NIMBEX should be used during pregnancy only if clearly needed.

Labor and Delivery: The use of NIMBEX during labor, vaginal delivery, or cesarean section has not been studied in humans and it is not known whether NIMBEX administered to the mother has effects on the fetus. Doses of 0.2 or 0.4 mg/kg cisatracurium given to female beagles undergoing cesarean section resulted in negligible levels of cisatracurium in umbilical vessel blood of neonates and no deleterious effects on the puppies. The action of neuromuscular blocking agents may be enhanced by magnesium salts administered for the management of toxemia of pregnancy.

Nursing Mothers: It is not known whether cisatracurium besylate is excreted in human milk. Because many drugs are excreted in human milk, caution should be exercised following administration of NIMBEX to a nursing woman.

Pediatric Use: NIMBEX has not been studied in pediatric patients below the age of 2 years (see CLINICAL PHARMACOLOGY and DOSAGE AND ADMINISTRATION for clinical experience and recommendations for use in children 2 to 12 years of age).

Geriatric Use: NIMBEX was safely administered during clinical trials to 145 elderly (≥65 years) patients, including a subset of patients with significant cardiovascular disease (see CLINICAL PHARMACOLOGY, **Elderly Patients and Hemodynamics Profile** sections).

Minor differences in the pharmacokinetics of cisatracurium between elderly and young adult patients are not associated with clinically significant differences in the recovery profile of NIMBEX following a single 0.1 mg/kg dose; the time to maximum block is approximately 1 minute slower in elderly patients (see CLINICAL PHARMACOLOGY: **Pharmacokinetics**).

ADVERSE REACTIONS

Observed in Clinical Trials of Surgical Patients: Adverse experiences were uncommon among the 945 surgical patients who received NIMBEX in conjunction with other drugs in U.S. and European clinical studies in the course of a wide variety of procedures in patients receiving opioid, propofol, or inhalation anesthesia. The following adverse experiences were judged by investigators during the clinical trials to have a possible causal relationship to administration of NIMBEX:

Incidence Greater than 1%: None

Incidence Less than 1%:

Cardiovascular: bradycardia (0.4%), hypotension (0.2%), flushing (0.2%)

Respiratory: bronchospasm (0.2%)

Dermatological: rash (0.1%)

Observed in Clinical Trials of Intensive Care Unit Patients: Adverse experiences were uncommon among the 68 ICU patients who received NIMBEX in conjunction with other drugs in U.S. and European clinical studies. One patient experienced bronchospasm. In one of the two ICU studies, a randomized and double-blind study of ICU patients using TOF neuromuscular monitoring, there were 2 reports of prolonged recovery (167 and 270 mins) among 28 patients administered NIMBEX and 13 reports of prolonged recovery (range: 90 mins to 33 hrs) among 30 patients administered vecuronium.

OVERDOSAGE

Overdosage with neuromuscular blocking agents may result in neuromuscular block beyond the time needed for surgery and anesthesia. The primary treatment is maintenance of a patent airway and controlled ventilation until recovery of normal neuromuscular function is assured. Once recovery from neuromuscular block begins, further recovery may be facilitated by administration of an anticholinesterase agent (e.g., neostigmine, edrophonium) in conjunction with an appropriate anticholinergic agent (see **Antagonism of Neuromuscular Block** below).

Antagonism of Neuromuscular Block:

ANTAGONISTS (SUCH AS NEOSTIGMINE AND EDROPHONIUM) SHOULD NOT BE ADMINISTERED WHEN COMPLETE NEUROMUSCULAR BLOCK IS EVIDENT OR SUSPECTED. THE USE OF A PERIPHERAL NERVE STIMULATOR TO EVALUATE RECOVERY AND ANTAGONISM OF NEUROMUSCULAR BLOCK IS RECOMMENDED.

Administration of 0.04 to 0.07 mg/kg neostigmine at approximately 10% recovery from neuromuscular block (range: 0 to 15%) produced 95% recovery of the muscle twitch response and a T_4:T_1 ratio ≥70% in an average of 9 to 10 minutes. The times from 25% recovery of the muscle twitch response to a T_4:T_1 ratio ≥70% following these doses of neostigmine averaged 7 minutes. The mean 25% to 75% recovery index following reversal was 3 to 4 minutes.

Administration of 1.0 mg/kg edrophonium at approximately 25% recovery from neuromuscular block (range: 16% to 30%) produced 95% recovery and a T_4:T_1 ratio ≥70% in an average of 3 to 5 minutes.

Patients administered antagonists should be evaluated for evidence of adequate clinical recovery (e.g., 5-second head lift and grip strength). Ventilation must be supported until no longer required.

The onset of antagonism may be delayed in the presence of debilitation, cachexia, carcinomatosis, and the concomitant use of certain broad spectrum antibiotics, or anesthetic agents and other drugs which enhance neuromuscular block or separately cause respiratory depression (see PRECAUTIONS: **Drug Interactions**). Under such circumstances the management is the same as that of prolonged neuromuscular block (see OVERDOSAGE).

DOSAGE AND ADMINISTRATION

NIMBEX SHOULD ONLY BE ADMINISTERED INTRAVENOUSLY. The dosage information provided below is intended as a guide only. Doses of NIMBEX should be individualized (see CLINICAL PHARMACOLOGY: Individualization of Dosages). The use of a peripheral nerve stimulator will permit the most advantageous use of NIMBEX, minimize the possibility of overdosage or underdosage, and assist in the evaluation of recovery.

Adults:

Initial Doses: One of two intubating doses of NIMBEX may be chosen, based on the desired time to intubation and the anticipated length of surgery. Doses of 0.15 (3 × ED_{95}) and 0.20 (4 × ED_{95}) mg/kg NIMBEX, as components of a propofol/nitrous oxide/oxygen induction-intubation technique, may produce generally good or excellent conditions for tracheal intubation in 2.0 and 1.5 minutes, respectively. The clinically effective durations of action for 0.15 and 0.20 mg/kg NIMBEX during propofol anesthesia are 55 minutes (range: 44 to 74 min) and 61 minutes (range: 41 to 81 min), respectively. Lower doses may result in a longer time for the development of satisfactory intubation conditions. In addition to the dose of the neuromuscular blocking agent, the presence or co-induction agents (e.g., fentanyl and midazolam) and the depth of anesthesia are factors that can influence intubation conditions. Doses up to 8 × ED_{95} NIMBEX have been safely administered to healthy adult patients and the larger doses are associated with longer clinically effective durations of action (see CLINICAL PHARMACOLOGY).

Because slower times to onset of complete neuromuscular block were observed in elderly patients and patients with renal dysfunction, extending the interval between administration of NIMBEX and the intubation attempt for these patients may be required to achieve adequate intubation conditions.

A dose of 0.03 mg/kg NIMBEX is recommended for maintenance of neuromuscular block during prolonged surgical procedures. Maintenance doses of 0.03 mg/kg each sustain neuromuscular block for approximately 20 minutes. Maintenance dosing is generally required 40 to 50 minutes following an initial dose of 0.15 mg/kg NIMBEX and 50 to 60 minutes following an initial dose of 0.20 mg/kg NIMBEX, but the need for maintenance doses should be determined by clinical criteria. For shorter or longer durations of action, smaller or larger maintenance doses may be administered.

Isoflurane or enflurane administered with nitrous oxide/oxygen to achieve 1.25 MAC (Minimum Alveolar Concentration) may prolong the clinically effective duration of action of initial and maintenance doses. The magnitude of these effects may depend on the duration of administration of the volatile agents. Fifteen to 30 minutes of exposure to 1.25 MAC isoflurane or enflurane had minimal effects on the duration of action of initial doses of NIMBEX and therefore, no adjustment to the initial dose should be necessary when NIMBEX is administered shortly after initiation of volatile agents. In long surgical procedures during enflurane or isoflurane anesthesia, less frequent maintenance dosing or lower maintenance doses of NIMBEX may be necessary. No adjustments to the initial dose of NIMBEX are required when used in patients receiving propofol anesthesia.

Children:

Initial Doses: The recommended dose of NIMBEX for children 2 to 12 years of age is 0.10 mg/kg administered over 5 to 10 seconds during either halothane or opioid anesthesia. When administered during stable opioid/nitrous oxide/oxygen anesthesia, 0.10 mg/kg NIMBEX produces maximum neuromuscular block in an average of 2.8 minutes (range: 1.8 to 6.7 min) and clinically effective block for 28 minutes (range: 21 to 38 min). NIMBEX has not been studied in children below the age of 2 years.

Use by Continuous Infusion:

Infusion in the Operating Room (OR): After administration of an initial bolus dose of NIMBEX, a diluted solution of NIMBEX can be administered by continuous infusion to adults and children aged 2 or more years for maintenance of neuromuscular block during extended surgical procedures. Infusion of NIMBEX should be individualized for each patient. The rate of administration should be adjusted according to the patient's response as determined by peripheral nerve stimulation. Accurate dosing is best achieved using a precision infusion device.

Infusion of NIMBEX should be initiated only after early evidence of spontaneous recovery from the initial bolus dose. An initial infusion rate of 3 μg/kg/min may be required to rapidly counteract the spontaneous recovery of neuromuscular function. Thereafter, a rate of 1 to 2 μg/kg/min should be adequate to maintain continuous neuromuscular block in the range of 89% to 99% in most pediatric and adult patients under opioid/nitrous oxide/oxygen anesthesia.

Continued on next page

Glaxo Wellcome—Cont.

Reduction of the infusion rate by up to 30% to 40% should be considered when NIMBEX is administered during stable isoflurane or enflurane anesthesia (administered with nitrous oxide/oxygen at the 1.25 MAC level). Greater reductions in the infusion rate of NIMBEX may be required with longer durations of administration of isoflurane or enflurane.
The rate of infusion of atracurium required to maintain adequate surgical relaxation in patients undergoing coronary artery bypass surgery with induced hypothermia (25° to 28°C) is approximately half the rate required during normothermia. Based on the structural similarity between NIMBEX and atracurium, a similar effect on the infusion rate of NIMBEX may be expected.
Spontaneous recovery from neuromuscular block following discontinuation of infusion of NIMBEX may be expected to proceed at a rate comparable to that following administration of a single bolus dose.
Infusion in the Intensive Care Unit (ICU): The principles for infusion of NIMBEX in the OR are also applicable to use in the ICU. An infusion rate of approximately 3 μg/kg/min (range: 0.5 to 10.2 μg/kg/min) should provide adequate neuromuscular block in adult patients in the ICU. There may be wide interpatient variability in dosage requirements and these may increase or decrease with time (see **PRECAUTIONS: Long-term Use in the Intensive Care Unit [ICU]**). Following recovery from neuromuscular block, readministration of a bolus dose may be necessary to quickly re-establish neuromuscular block prior to reinstitution of the infusion.
Infusion Rate Tables: The amount of infusion solution required per minute will depend upon the concentration of NIMBEX in the infusion solution, the desired dose of NIMBEX, and the patient's weight. The contribution of the infusion solution to the fluid requirements of the patient also must be considered. Tables 7 and 8 provide guidelines for delivery, in mL/hr (equivalent to microdrops/min when 60 microdrops = 1 mL), of NIMBEX solutions in concentrations of 0.1 mg/mL (10 mg/100 mL) or 0.4 mg/mL (40 mg/100 mL).

Table 7
Infusion Rates of NIMBEX™ for Maintenance of Neuromuscular Block During Opioid/Nitrous Oxide/Oxygen Anesthesia for a Concentration of 0.1 mg/mL

Patient Weight (kg)	DRUG DELIVERY RATE (μg/kg/min) 1.0	1.5	2.0	3.0	5.0
	Infusion Delivery Rate (mL/hr)				
10	6	9	12	18	30
45	27	41	54	81	135
70	42	63	84	126	210
100	60	90	120	180	300

Table 8
Infusion Rates of NIMBEX™ for Maintenance of Neuromuscular Block During Opioid/Nitrous Oxide/Oxygen Anesthesia for a Concentration of 0.4 mg/mL

Patient Weight (kg)	DRUG DELIVERY RATE (μg/kg/min) 1.0	1.5	2.0	3.0	5.0
	Infusion Delivery Rate (mL/hr)				
10	1.5	2.3	3.0	4.5	7.5
45	6.8	10.1	13.5	20.3	33.8
70	10.5	15.8	21.0	31.5	52.5
100	15.0	22.5	30.0	45.0	75.0

NIMBEX Injection Compatibility and Admixtures:
Y-site Administration: NIMBEX Injection is acidic (pH = 3.25 to 3.65) and may not be compatible with alkaline solution having a pH greater than 8.5 (e.g., barbiturate solutions).
Studies have shown than NIMBEX Injection is compatible with:

- 5% Dextrose Injection USP
- 0.9% Sodium Chloride Injection USP
- 5% Dextrose and 0.9% Sodium Chloride Injection USP
- Sufenta® (sufentanil citrate) Injection, diluted as directed
- Alfenta® (alfentanil hydrochloride) Injection, diluted as directed
- Sublimaze® (fentanyl citrate) Injection, diluted as directed
- Versed® (midazolam hydrochloride) Injection, diluted as directed
- Droperidol Injecion, diluted as directed

NIMBEX Injection is not compatible with Diprivan® (propofol) Injection or Toradol® (ketorolac) Injection for Y-site administration. Studies of other parenteral products have not been conducted.
Dilution Stability:
NIMBEX Injection diluted in 5% Dextrose Injection USP, 0.9% Sodium Chloride Injection USP, or 5% Dextrose and 0.9% Sodium Chloride Injection USP to 0.1 mg/mL may be stored either under refrigeration or at room temperature for 24 hours without significant loss of potency. Dilutions to 0.1 mg/mL or 0.2 mg/mL in 5% Dextrose and Lactated Ringer's Injection may be stored under refrigeration for 24 hours. NIMBEX Injection should not be diluted in Lactated Ringer's Injection USP due to chemical instability.
NOTE: Parenteral drug products should be inspected visually for particulate matter and discoloration prior to administration whenever solution and container permit. Solutions which are not clear, or contain visible particulates, should not be used. NIMBEX Injection is a colorless to slightly yellow or greenish-yellow solution.

HOW SUPPLIED

NIMBEX Injection, 2 mg cisatracurium in each mL.
5 mL Single Use Vials. Package of 10 (NDC 0173-0540-50).
10 mL Multiple Dose Vials containing 0.9% w/v benzyl alcohol as a preservative (see **WARNINGS** concerning newborn infants). Package of 10 (NDC 0173-0546-00).
NIMBEX Injection, 10 mg cisatracurium in each mL.
20 mL Single Use vials **intended only for use in the ICU.** Carton of 1 (NDC 0173-0543-01).
Storage
NIMBEX Injection should be refrigerated at 2° to 8°C (36° to 46°F) in the carton to preserve potency. Protect from light. DO NOT FREEZE. Upon removal from refrigeration to room temperature storage conditions (25°C/77°F), use NIMBEX Injection within 21 days even if rerefrigerated.
U.S. Patent No. 5,453,510
June 1995/RL-326
Shown in Product Identification Guide, page 314

NUROMAX® ℞

[*nōō 'rō-măks*]
(doxacurium chloride)
Injection

This drug should be administered only by adequately trained individuals familiar with its actions, characteristics, and hazards.

DESCRIPTION

NUROMAX (doxacurium chloride) is a long-acting, nondepolarizing skeletal muscle relaxant for intravenous administration. Doxacurium chloride is [1α,2β(1'*S**,2'*R**)]-2,2'-[(1,4-dioxo-1,4-butanediyl)bis(oxy-3,1-propanediyl)]bis[1,2,3,4-tetrahydro-6,7,8-trimethoxy-2-methyl-1-[(3,4,5-trimethoxypyhenyl)methyl]isoquinolinium]dichloride(meso form). The molecular formula is $C_{56}H_{78}Cl_2N_2O_{16}$ and the molecular weight is 1106.14. The compound does not partition into the 1-octanol phase of a distilled water/1-octanol system, *i.e.,* the n-octanol:water partition coefficient is 0.
Doxacurium chloride is a mixture of the three *trans, trans* stereoisomers, a *dl* pair [(1*R*, 1' *R*, 2*S*, 2' *S*) and (1*S*, 1' *S*, 2*R*, 2' *R*)] and a meso form (1*R*, 1' *S*, 2*S*, 2' *R*).
NUROMAX Injection is a sterile, non-pyrogenic aqueous solution (pH 3.9 to 5.0) containing doxacurium chloride equivalent to 1 mg/mL doxacurium in Water for Injection. Hydrochloric acid may have been added to adjust pH. NUROMAX Injection contains 0.9% w/v benzyl alcohol.

CLINICAL PHARMACOLOGY

NUROMAX binds competitively to cholinergic receptors on the motor end-plate to antagonize the action of acetylcholine, resulting in a block of neuromuscular transmission. This action is antagonized by acetylcholinesterase inhibitors, such as neostigmine.
Pharmacodynamics: NUROMAX is approximately 2.5 to 3 times more potent than pancuronium and 10 to 12 times more potent than metocurine. NUROMAX in doses of 1.5 to 2 x ED_{95} has a clinical duration of action (range and variability) similar to that of equipotent doses of pancuronium and metocurine (historic data and limited comparison). The average ED_{95} (dose required to produce 95% suppression of the adductor pollicis muscle twitch response to ulnar nerve stimulation) of NUROMAX is 0.025 mg/kg (range: 0.020 to 0.033) in adults receiving balanced anesthesia.
The onset and clinically effective duration (time from injection to 25% recovery) of NUROMAX administered alone or after succinylcholine during stable balanced anesthesia are shown in Table 1.

TABLE 1
Pharmacodynamic Dose Response*
Balanced Anesthesia

	Initial NUROMAX® Dose (mg/kg) 0.025† (n=34)	0.05 (n=27)	0.08 (n=9)
Time to Maximum Block (min)	9.3 (5.4–16)	5.2 (2.5–13)	3.5 (2.4–5)
Clinical Duration (min) (Time to 25% Recovery)	55 (9–145)	100 (39–232)	160 (110–338)

* Values shown are means (range).
† NUROMAX administered after 10% to 100% recovery from an intubating dose of succinylcholine.

Initial doses of 0.05 mg/kg (2 x ED_{95}) and 0.08 mg/kg (3 x ED_{95}) NUROMAX administered during the induction of thiopental-narcotic anesthesia produced good-to-excellent conditions for tracheal intubation in 5 minutes (13 of 15 cases studied) and 4 minutes (8 of 9 cases studied) (which are before maximum block), respectively.
As with other long-acting agents, the clinical duration of neuromuscular block associated with NUROMAX shows considerable interpatient variability. An analysis of 390 cases in U.S. clinical trials utilizing a variety of premedications, varying lengths of surgery, and various anesthetic agents, indicates that approximately two-thirds of the patients had clinical durations within 30 minutes of the duration predicted by dose (based on mg/kg actual body weight). Patients ≥ 60 years old are approximately twice as likely to experience prolonged clinical duration (30 minutes longer than predicted) than patients < 60 years old; thus, care should be used in older patients when prolonged recovery is undesirable (see PRECAUTIONS: **Geriatric Use** and CLINICAL PHARMACOLOGY: **Individualization of Dosages** subsection). In addition, obese patients (patients weighing ≥ 30% more than ideal body weight for height) were almost twice as likely to experience prolonged clinical duration than non-obese patients; therefore, dosing should be based on ideal body weight (IBW) for obese patients (see CLINICAL PHARMACOLOGY: **Individualization of Dosages** subsection).
The mean time for spontaneous T_1 recovery from 25% to 50% of control following initial doses of NUROMAX is approximately 26 minutes (range: 7 to 104, n = 253) during balanced anesthesia. The mean time for spontaneous T_1 recovery from 25% to 75% is 54 minutes (range: 14 to 184, n = 184).
Most patients receiving NUROMAX in clinical trials required pharmacologic reversal prior to full spontaneous recovery from neuromuscular block (see OVERDOSAGE: **Antagonism of Neuromuscular Block**); therefore, relatively few data are available on the time from injection to 95% spontaneous recovery of the twitch response. As with other long-acting neuromuscular blocking agents, NUROMAX may be associated with prolonged times to full spontaneous recovery. Following an initial dose of 0.025 mg/kg NUROMAX, some patients may require as long as 4 hours to exhibit full spontaneous recovery.
Cumulative neuromuscular blocking effects are not associated with repeated administration of maintenance doses of NUROMAX at 25% T_1 recovery. As with initial doses, however, the duration of action following maintenance doses of NUROMAX may vary considerably among patients.
The NUROMAX ED_{95} for children 2 to 12 years of age receiving halothane anesthesia is approximately 0.03 mg/kg. Children require higher doses of NUROMAX on a mg/kg basis than adults to achieve comparable levels of block. The onset time and duration of block are shorter in children than adults. During halothane anesthesia, doses of 0.03 mg/kg and 0.05 mg/kg NUROMAX produce maximum block in approximately 7 and 4 minutes, respectively. The duration of clinically effective block is approximately 30 minutes after an initial dose of 0.03 mg/kg and approximately 45 minutes after 0.05 mg/kg. NUROMAX has not been studied in pediatric patients below the age of 2 years.
The neuromuscular block produced by NUROMAX may be antagonized by anticholinesterase agents. As with other nondepolarizing neuromuscular blocking agents, the more profound the neuromuscular block at reversal, the longer the time and the greater the dose of anticholinesterase required for recovery of neuromuscular function.
Hemodynamics: Administration of NUROMAX doses up to and including 0.08 mg/kg (∼3 x ED_{95}) over 5 to 15 seconds to healthy adult patients during stable state balanced anesthesia and to patients with serious cardiovascular disease undergoing coronary artery bypass grafting, cardiac valvular repair, or vascular repair produced no dose-related effects on mean arterial blood pressure (MAP) or heart rate (HR).

No dose-related changes in MAP and HR were observed following administration of up to 0.05 mg/kg NUROMAX over 5 to 15 seconds in 2- to 12-year-old children receiving halothane anesthesia.

Doses of 0.03 to 0.08 mg/kg (1.2 to 3 x ED$_{95}$) were not associated with dose-dependent changes in mean plasma histamine concentration. Clinical experience with more than 1,000 patients indicates that adverse experiences typically associated with histamine release (*e.g.*, bronchospasm, hypotension, tachycardia, cutaneous flushing, urticaria, *etc.*) are very rare following the administration of NUROMAX (see ADVERSE REACTIONS).

Pharmacokinetics: Pharmacokinetic and pharmacodynamic results from a study of 24 healthy young adult patients and 8 healthy elderly patients are summarized in Table 2. The pharmacokinetics are linear over the dosage range tested (i.e., plasma concentrations are approximately proportional to dose). The pharmacokinetics of NUROMAX are similar in healthy young adult and elderly patients. Some healthy elderly patients tend to be more sensitive to the neuromuscular blocking effects of NUROMAX than healthy young adult patients receiving the same dose. The time to maximum block is longer in elderly patients than in young adult patients (11.2 minutes versus 7.7 minutes at 0.025 mg/kg NUROMAX). In addition, the clinically effective durations of block are more variable and tend to be longer in healthy elderly patients than in healthy young adult patients receiving the same dose.
[See table 2 above.]

Table 3 summarizes the pharmacokinetic and pharmacodynamic results from a study of 9 healthy young adult patients, 8 patients with end-stage kidney disease undergoing kidney transplantation, and 7 patients with end-stage liver disease undergoing liver transplantation. The results suggest that a longer t$_{1/2}$ can be expected in patients with end-stage kidney disease; in addition, these patients may be more sensitive to the neuromuscular blocking effects of NUROMAX. The time to maximum block was slightly longer and the clinically effective duration of block was prolonged in patients with end-stage kidney disease.
[See table 3 at right.]

No data are available from patients with liver disease not requiring transplantation. There are no significant alterations in the pharmacokinetics of NUROMAX in liver transplant patients. Sensitivity to the neuromuscular blocking effects of NUROMAX was highly variable in patients undergoing liver transplantation. Three of 7 patients developed ≤50% block, indicating that a reduced sensitivity to NUROMAX may occur in such patients. In those patients who developed >50% neuromuscular block, the time to maximum block and the clinically effective duration tended to be longer than in healthy young adult patients (see CLINICAL PHARMACOLOGY: **Individualization of Dosages** subsection).

Consecutively administered maintenance doses of 0.005 mg/kg NUROMAX, each given at 25% T$_1$ recovery following the preceding dose, do not result in a progressive increase in the plasma concentration of doxacurium or a progressive increase in the depth or duration of block produced by each dose.

NUROMAX is not metabolized *in vitro* in fresh human plasma. Plasma protein binding of NUROMAX is approximately 30% in human plasma.

In vivo data from humans suggest that NUROMAX is not metabolized and that the major elimination pathway is excretion of unchanged drug in urine and bile. In studies of healthy adult patients, 24% to 38% of an administered dose was recovered as parent drug in urine over 6 to 12 hours after dosing. High bile concentrations of NUROMAX (relative to plasma) have been found 35 to 90 minutes after administration. The overall extent of biliary excretion is unknown. The data derived from analysis of human urine and bile are consistent with data from in vivo studies in the rat, cat, and dog, which indicate that all of an administered dose of NUROMAX is recovered as parent drug in the urine and bile of these species.

Individualization of Dosages: In elderly patients or patients who have impaired renal function, the potential for a prolongation of block may be reduced by decreasing the initial dose of NUROMAX and by titrating the dose to achieve the desired depth of block. In obese patients (patients weighing ≥30% more than ideal body weight for height), the dose of NUROMAX should be determined using the patient's ideal body weight (IBW), according to the following formulae:

Men: IBW in kg=[106 +(6 x inches in height above 5 feet)]/2.2

Women: IBW in kg=[100 +(5 x inches in height above 5 feet)]/2.2

Dosage requirements for patients with severe liver disease are variable; some patients may require a higher than normal initial dose of NUROMAX to achieve clinically effective block. Once adequate block is established, the clinical duration of block may be prolonged in such patients relative to patients with normal liver function.

TABLE 2
Pharmacokinetic and Pharmacodynamic Parameters* of NUROMAX® in Young Adult and Elderly Patients
(Isoflurane Anesthesia)

Parameter	Healthy Young Adult Patients (22 to 49 yrs)			Healthy Elderly Patients (67 to 72 yrs)
	0.025 mg/kg (n=8)	0.05 mg/kg (n=8)	0.08 mg/kg (n=8)	0.025 mg/kg (n=8)
t$_{1/2}$ elimination (min)	86 (25–171)	123 (61–163)	98 (47–163)	96 (50–114)
Volume of Distribution at Steady State (L/kg)	0.15 (0.10–0.21)	0.24 (0.13–0.30)	0.22 (0.16–0.33)	0.22 (0.14–0.40)
Plasma Clearance (mL/min/kg)	2.22 (1.02–3.95)	2.62 (1.21–5.70)	2.53 (1.88–3.38)	2.47 (1.58–3.60)
Maximum Block (1%)	97 (88–100)	100 (100–100)	100 (100–100)	96 (90–100)
Clinically Effective Duration of Block† (min)	68 (35–90)	91 (47–132)	177 (74–268)	97 (36–179)

* Values shown are means (range).
† Time from injection to 25% recovery of the control twitch height.

TABLE 3
Pharmacokinetic and Pharmacodynamic Parameters* of NUROMAX® in Healthy Patients and in Patients Undergoing Kidney or Liver Transplantation
(Isoflurane Anesthesia)

Parameter	Healthy Young Adult Patients	Kidney Transplant Patients	Liver Transplant Patients
	0.015 mg/kg (n=9)	0.015 mg/kg (n=8)	0.015 mg/kg (n=7)
t$_{1/2}$ elimination (min)	99 (48–193)	221 (84–592)	115 (69–148)
Volume of Distribution at Steady State (L/kg)	0.22 (0.11–0.43)	0.27 (0.17–0.55)	0.29 (0.17–0.35)
Plasma Clearance (mL/min/kg)	2.66 (1.35–6.66)	1.23 (0.48–2.40)	2.30 (1.96–3.05)
Maximum Block (%)	86 (59–100)	98 (95–100)	70 (0–100)
Clinically Effective Duration of Block (min)	36 (19–80)	80 (29–133)	52 (20–91)

* Values shown are means (range).

As with pancuronium, metocurine, and vecuronium, resistance to NUROMAX, manifested by a reduced intensity and/or shortened duration of block, must be considered when NUROMAX is selected for use in patients receiving phenytoin or carbamazepine (see PRECAUTIONS: **Drug Interactions**).

As with other nondepolarizing neuromuscular blocking agents, a reduction in dosage of NUROMAX must be considered in cachectic or debilitated patients, in patients with neuromuscular diseases, severe electrolyte abnormalities, or carcinomatosis, and in other patients in whom potentiation of neuromuscular block or difficulty with reversal is anticipated. Increased doses of NUROMAX may be required in burn patients (see PRECAUTIONS).

INDICATIONS AND USAGE
NUROMAX is a long-acting neuromuscular blocking agent, indicated to provide skeletal muscle relaxation as an adjunct to general anesthesia, for endotracheal intubation or to facilitate mechanical ventilation.

CONTRAINDICATIONS
NUROMAX is contraindicated in patients known to have hypersensitivity to it. Use of NUROMAX from multiple dose vials containing benzyl alcohol as a preservative is contraindicated in patients with a known hypersensitivity to benzyl alcohol.

WARNINGS
NUROMAX SHOULD BE ADMINISTERED IN CAREFULLY ADJUSTED DOSAGE BY OR UNDER THE SUPERVISION OF EXPERIENCED CLINICIANS WHO ARE FAMILIAR WITH THE DRUG'S ACTIONS AND THE POSSIBLE COMPLICATIONS OF ITS USE. THE DRUG SHOULD NOT BE ADMINISTERED UNLESS FACILITIES FOR INTUBATION, ARTIFICIAL RESPIRATION, OXYGEN THERAPY, AND AN ANTAGONIST ARE WITHIN IMMEDIATE REACH. IT IS RECOMMENDED THAT CLINICIANS ADMINISTERING LONG-ACTING NEUROMUSCULAR BLOCKING AGENTS SUCH AS NUROMAX EMPLOY A PERIPHERAL NERVE STIMULATOR TO MONITOR DRUG RESPONSE, NEED FOR ADDITIONAL RELAXANTS, AND ADEQUACY OF SPONTANEOUS RECOVERY OR ANTAGONISM.

NUROMAX HAS NO KNOWN EFFECT ON CONSCIOUSNESS, PAIN THRESHOLD, OR CEREBRATION. TO AVOID DISTRESS TO THE PATIENT, NEUROMUSCULAR BLOCK SHOULD NOT BE INDUCED BEFORE UNCONSCIOUSNESS.

NUROMAX Injection is acidic (pH 3.9 to 5.0) and may not be compatible with alkaline solutions having a pH greater than 8.5 (e.g., barbiturate solutions).

NUROMAX Injection contains benzyl alcohol. In newborn infants, benzyl alcohol has been associated with an increased incidence of neurological and other complications which are sometimes fatal (see PRECAUTIONS: **Pediatric Use**).

PRECAUTIONS
General: NUROMAX has no clinically significant effects on heart rate; therefore, NUROMAX will not counteract the bradycardia produced by many anesthetic agents or by vagal stimulation.

Neuromuscular blocking agents may have a profound effect in patients with neuromuscular diseases (e.g., myasthenia gravis and the myasthenic syndrome). In these and other conditions in which prolonged neuromuscular block is a possibility (e.g., carcinomatosis), the use of a peripheral nerve stimulator and a small test dose of NUROMAX is recommended to assess the level of neuromuscular block and to monitor dosage requirements. Shorter acting muscle relax-

Continued on next page

Glaxo Wellcome—Cont.

ants than NUROMAX may be more suitable for these patients.

Resistance to nondepolarizing neuromuscular blocking agents may develop in patients with burns depending upon the time elapsed since the injury and the size of the burn. NUROMAX has not been studied in patients with burns.

Acid-base and/or serum electrolyte abnormalities may potentiate or antagonize the action of neuromuscular blocking agents. The action of neuromuscular blocking agents may be enhanced by magnesium salts administered for the management of toxemia of pregnancy.

NUROMAX has not been studied in patients with asthma.

No data are available to support the use of NUROMAX by intramuscular injection.

Renal and Hepatic Disease: NUROMAX has been studied in patients with end-stage kidney (n=8) or liver (n=7) disease undergoing transplantation procedures (see CLINICAL PHARMACOLOGY). The possibility of prolonged neuromuscular block in patients undergoing renal transplantation and the possibility of a variable onset and duration of neuromuscular block in patients undergoing liver transplantation must be considered when NUROMAX is used in such patients.

Obesity: Administration of NUROMAX on the basis of actual body weight is associated with a prolonged duration of action in obese patients (patients weighing ≥30% more than ideal body weight for height) (see CLINICAL PHARMACOLOGY). Therefore, the dose of NUROMAX should be based upon ideal body weight in obese patients (see CLINICAL PHARMACOLOGY: **Individualization of Dosages**).

Malignant Hyperthermia (MH): In a study of MH-susceptible pigs, NUROMAX did not trigger MH. NUROMAX has not been studied in MH-susceptible patients. Since MH can develop in the absence of established triggering agents, the clinician should be prepared to recognize and treat MH in any patient scheduled for general anesthesia.

Long-term Use in the Intensive Care Unit (ICU): Information on the use of NUROMAX in the ICU is limited. In a double-blind, randomized study, 17 patients received NUROMAX by intermittent bolus injection for a mean of 2.7 ± 0.5 days (range: 0.8 to 6.8 days) to facilitate mechanical ventilation. No evidence of tachyphylaxis, accumulation, or prolonged recovery was observed. The adverse experiences in patients receiving NUROMAX were consistent in type, severity, and frequency to those expected in a critically ill patient population. Since many ICU patients have hepatic and/or renal failure, a prolonged duration of block should be anticipated in these patients after administration of NUROMAX.

WHENEVER THE USE OF NUROMAX OR ANY OTHER NEUROMUSCULAR BLOCKING AGENT IS CONTEMPLATED IN THE ICU, IT IS RECOMMENDED THAT NEUROMUSCULAR TRANSMISSION BE MONITORED CONTINUOUSLY DURING ADMINISTRATION WITH THE HELP OF A NERVE STIMULATOR. ADDITIONAL DOSES OF NUROMAX OR ANY OTHER NEUROMUSCULAR BLOCKING AGENT SHOULD NOT BE GIVEN BEFORE THERE IS A DEFINITE RESPONSE TO T_1, OR TO THE FIRST TWITCH. IF NO RESPONSE IS ELICITED, BOLUS ADMINISTRATION SHOULD BE DELAYED UNTIL A RESPONSE RETURNS.

Drug Interactions: Prior administration of succinylcholine has no clinically important effect on the neuromuscular blocking action of NUROMAX.

The use of NUROMAX before succinylcholine to attenuate some of the side effects of succinylcholine has not been studied.

There are no clinical data on concomitant use of NUROMAX and other nondepolarizing neuromuscular blocking agents.

Isoflurane, enflurane, and halothane decrease the ED_{50} of NUROMAX by 30% to 45%. These agents may also prolong the clinically effective duration of action by up to 25%.

Other drugs which may enhance the neuromuscular blocking action of nondepolarizing agents such as NUROMAX include certain antibiotics (e.g., aminoglycosides, tetracyclines, bacitracin, polymyxins, lincomycin, clindamycin, colistin, and sodium colistimethate), magnesium salts, lithium, local anesthetics, procainamide, and quinidine.

As with some other nondepolarizing neuromuscular blocking agents, the time of onset of neuromuscular block induced by NUROMAX is lengthened and the duration of block is shortened in patients receiving phenytoin or carbamazepine.

Carcinogenesis, Mutagenesis, Impairment of Fertility: Carcinogenesis and fertility studies have not been performed. NUROMAX was evaluated in a battery of four short-term mutagenicity tests. It was non-mutagenic in the Ames Salmonella assay, in the mouse lymphoma assay, and in the human lymphocyte assay. In the in vivo rat bone marrow cytogenetic assay, statistically significant increases in the incidence of structural abnormalities, relative to vehicle controls, were observed in male rats dosed with 0.1 mg/kg (0.625 mg/m²) NUROMAX and sacrificed at 6 hours, but not at 24 or 48 hours, and in female rats dosed with 0.2 mg/kg (1.25 mg/m²) NUROMAX and sacrificed at 24 hours, but not at 6 or 48 hours. There was no increase in structural abnormalities in either male or female rats given 0.3 mg/kg (1.875 mg/m²) NUROMAX and sacrificed at 6, 24, or 48 hours. Thus, the incidence of abnormalities in the in vivo rat bone marrow cytogenetic assay was not dose-dependent and, therefore, the likelihood that the observed abnormalities were treatment-related or clinically significant is low.

Pregnancy: Teratogenic Effects: Pregnancy Category C. Teratology testing in nonventilated pregnant rats and mice treated subcutaneously with maximum subparalyzing doses of NUROMAX revealed no maternal or fetal toxicity or teratogenic effects. There are no adequate and well-controlled studies of NUROMAX in pregnant women. Because animal studies are not always predictive of human response and the doses used were subparalyzing, NUROMAX should be used during pregnancy only if the potential benefit justifies the potential risk to the fetus.

Labor and Delivery: The use of NUROMAX during labor, vaginal delivery, or cesarean section has not been studied. It is not known whether NUROMAX administered to the mother has immediate or delayed effects on the fetus. The duration of action of NUROMAX exceeds the usual duration of operative obstetrics (cesarean section). Therefore, NUROMAX is not recommended for use in patients undergoing C-section.

Nursing Mothers: It is not known whether NUROMAX is excreted in human milk. Because many drugs are excreted in human milk, caution should be exercised following NUROMAX administration to a nursing woman.

Pediatric Use: NUROMAX has not been studied in pediatric patients below the age of 2 years. See CLINICAL PHARMACOLOGY and DOSAGE AND ADMINISTRATION for clinical experience and recommendations for use in children 2 to 12 years of age.

Geriatric Use: NUROMAX has been used in elderly patients, including patients with significant cardiovascular disease. In elderly patients the onset of maximum block is slower and the duration of neuromuscular block produced by NUROMAX is more variable and, in some cases, longer than in young adult patients (see CLINICAL PHARMACOLOGY: **Pharmacodynamics** and **Individualization of Dosages**).

ADVERSE REACTIONS

The most frequent adverse effect of nondepolarizing blocking agents as a class consists of an extension of the pharmacological action beyond the time needed for surgery and anesthesia. This effect may vary from skeletal muscle weakness to profound and prolonged skeletal muscle paralysis resulting in respiratory insufficiency and apnea which require manual or mechanical ventilation until recovery is judged to be clinically adequate (see OVERDOSAGE). Inadequate reversal of neuromuscular block from NUROMAX is possible, as with all nondepolarizing agents. Prolonged neuromuscular block and inadequate reversal may lead to postoperative complications.

Observed in Clinical Trials: Adverse experiences were uncommon among the 1034 surgical patients and volunteers who received NUROMAX and other drugs in U.S. clinical studies in the course of a wide variety of procedures conducted during balanced or inhalational anesthesia. The following adverse experiences were reported in patients administered NUROMAX (all events judged by investigators during the clinical trials to have a possible causal relationship):

Incidence Greater than 1%—None

Incidence Less than 1%—

Cardiovascular*: hypotension,† flushing,† ventricular fibrillation, myocardial infarction

Respiratory: bronchospasm, wheezing

Dermatological: urticaria, injection site reaction

Special Senses: diplopia

Nonspecific: difficult neuromuscular block reversal, prolonged drug effect, fever

* Reports of ventricular fibrillation (n=1) and myocardial infarction (n=1) were limited to ASA Class 3–4 patients undergoing cardiac surgery (n=142).

† 0.3% incidence. All other reactions unmarked were ≤0.1%.

OVERDOSAGE

Overdosage with neuromuscular blocking agents may result in neuromuscular block beyond the time needed for surgery and anesthesia. The primary treatment is maintenance of a patent airway and controlled ventilation until recovery of normal neuromuscular function is assured. Once evidence of recovery from neuromuscular block is observed, further recovery may be facilitated by administration of an anticholinesterase agent (e.g., neostigmine, edrophonium) in conjunction with an appropriate anticholinergic agent (see **Antagonism of Neuromuscular Block** below).

Antagonism of Neuromuscular Block:

ANTAGONISTS (SUCH AS NEOSTIGMINE) SHOULD NOT BE ADMINISTERED PRIOR TO THE DEMONSTRATION OF SOME SPONTANEOUS RECOVERY FROM NEUROMUSCULAR BLOCK. THE USE OF A NERVE STIMULATOR TO DOCUMENT RECOVERY AND ANTAGONISM OF NEUROMUSCULAR BLOCK IS RECOMMENDED. T_4/T_1 SHOULD BE > ZERO BEFORE ANTAGONISM IS ATTEMPTED.

In an analysis of patients in whom antagonism of neuromuscular block was evaluated following administration of single doses of neostigmine averaging 0.06 mg/kg (range: 0.05 to 0.075) administered at approximately 25% T_1 spontaneous recovery during balanced anesthesia, 71% of patients exhibited $T_4/T_1 \geq 0.7$ before monitoring was discontinued. For these patients, the mean time to $T_4/T_1 \geq 0.7$ was 19 minutes (range: 7 to 55). As with other long-acting nondepolarizing neuromuscular blocking agents, the time for recovery of neuromuscular function following administration of neostigmine is dependent upon the level of residual neuromuscular block at the time of attempted reversal; longer recovery times than those cited above may be anticipated when neostigmine is administered at more profound levels of block (i.e., at <25% T_1 recovery).

Patients should be evaluated for adequate clinical evidence of antagonism, *e.g.,* 5-second head lift, and grip strength. Ventilation must be supported until no longer required. As with other neuromuscular blocking agents, physicians should be alert to the possibility that the action of the drugs used to antagonize neuromuscular block may wear off before the effects of NUROMAX on the neuromuscular junction have declined sufficiently.

Antagonism may be delayed in the presence of debilitation, carcinomatosis, and the concomitant use of certain broad spectrum antibiotics, or anesthetic agents and other drugs which enhance neuromuscular block or separately cause respiratory depression (see PRECAUTIONS: **Drug Interactions**). Under such circumstances the management is the same as that of prolonged neuromuscular block.

In clinical trials, a dose of 1 mg/kg edrophonium was not as effective as a dose of 0.06 mg/kg neostigmine in antagonizing moderate to deep levels of neuromuscular block (i.e., <60% T_1 recovery). Therefore, the use of 1 mg/kg edrophonium is not recommended for reversal from moderate to deep levels of block. The use of pyridostigmine has not been studied.

DOSAGE AND ADMINISTRATION

NUROMAX SHOULD ONLY BE ADMINISTERED INTRAVENOUSLY.

NUROMAX, like other long-acting neuromuscular blocking agents, displays variability in the duration of its effect. The potential for a prolonged clinical duration of neuromuscular block must be considered when NUROMAX is selected for administration. The dosage information provided below is intended as a guide only. Doses should be individualized (see CLINICAL PHARMACOLOGY: **Individualization of Dosages**). Factors that may warrant dosage adjustment include: advancing age, the presence of kidney or liver disease, or obesity (patients weighing ≥30% more than ideal body weight for height). The use of a peripheral nerve stimulator will permit the most advantageous use of NUROMAX, minimize the possibility of overdosage or underdosage, and assist in the evaluation of recovery.

Parenteral drug products should be inspected visually for particulate matter and discoloration prior to administration whenever solution and container permit.

Adults:

Initial Doses: When administered as a component of a thiopental/narcotic induction-intubation paradigm as well as for production of long-duration neuromuscular block during surgery, 0.05 mg/kg (2 x ED_{95}) NUROMAX produces good-to-excellent conditions for tracheal intubation in 5 minutes in approximately 90% of patients. Lower doses of NUROMAX may result in a longer time for development of satisfactory intubation conditions. Clinically effective neuromuscular block may be expected to last approximately 100 minutes on average (range: 39 to 232) following 0.05 mg/kg NUROMAX administered to patients receiving balanced anesthesia.

An initial NUROMAX dose of 0.08 mg/kg (3 x ED_{95}) should be reserved for instances in which a need for very prolonged neuromuscular block is anticipated. In approximately 90% of patients, good-to-excellent intubation conditions may be expected in 4 minutes after this dose; however, clinically effective block may be expected to persist for as long as 160 minutes or more (range: 110 to 338) (see CLINICAL PHARMACOLOGY).

If NUROMAX is administered during steady-state isoflurane, enflurane, or halothane anesthesia, reduction of the dose of NUROMAX by one-third should be considered.

When succinylcholine is administered to facilitate tracheal intubation in patients receiving balanced anesthesia, an initial dose of 0.025 mg/kg (ED_{95}) NUROMAX provides about 60 minutes (range: 9 to 145) of clinically effective neuromuscular block for surgery. For a longer duration of action, a larger initial dose may be administered.

Maintenance Doses: Maintenance dosing will generally be required about 60 minutes after an initial dose of 0.025 mg/kg NUROMAX or 100 minutes after an initial dose of 0.05 mg/kg NUROMAX during balanced anesthesia. Repeated maintenance doses administered at 25% T_1 recovery may be expected to be required at relatively regular intervals in

each patient. The interval may vary considerably between patients. Maintenance doses of 0.005 and 0.01 mg/kg NUROMAX each provide an average 30 minutes (range: 9 to 57) and 45 minutes (range: 14 to 108), respectively, of additional clinically effective neuromuscular block. For shorter or longer desired durations, smaller or larger maintenance doses may be administered.

Children:

When administered during halothane anesthesia, an initial dose of 0.03 mg/kg (ED_{95}) produces maximum neuromuscular block in about 7 minutes (range: 5 to 11) and clinically effective block for an average of 30 minutes (range: 12 to 54). Under halothane anesthesia, 0.05 mg/kg produces maximum block in about 4 minutes (range: 2 to 10) and clinically effective block for 45 minutes (range: 30 to 80). Maintenance doses are generally required more frequently in children than in adults. Because of the potentiating effect of halothane seen in adults, a higher dose of NUROMAX may be required in children receiving balanced anesthesia than in children receiving halothane anesthesia to achieve a comparable onset and duration of neuromuscular block.

NUROMAX has not been studied in pediatric patients below the age of 2 years.

Compatibility:

Y-site Administration: NUROMAX Injection may not be compatible with alkaline solutions with a pH greater than 8.5 (*e.g.*, barbiturate solutions).

NUROMAX is compatible with:

- 5% Dextrose Injection USP
- 0.9% Sodium Chloride Injection USP
- 5% Dextrose and 0.9% Sodium Chloride Injection USP
- Lactated Ringer's Injection USP
- 5% Dextrose and Lactated Ringer's Injection
- Sufenta® (sufentanil citrate) Injection, diluted as directed
- Alfenta® (alfentanil hydrochloride) Injection, diluted as directed
- Sublimaze® (fentanyl citrate) Injection, diluted as directed

Dilution Stability: NUROMAX diluted up to 1:10 in 5% Dextrose Injection USP or 0.9% Sodium Chloride Injection USP has been shown to be physically and chemically stable when stored in polypropylene syringes at 5° to 25°C (41° to 77°F), for up to 24 hours. Since dilution diminishes the preservative effectiveness of benzyl alcohol, aseptic techniques should be used to prepare the diluted product. Immediate use of the diluted product is preferred, and any unused portion of diluted NUROMAX should be discarded after 8 hours.

HOW SUPPLIED

NUROMAX Injection, 1 mg doxacurium in each mL.
5 mL Multiple Dose vials containing 0.9% w/v benzyl alcohol as a preservative (see WARNINGS). Tray of 10 (NDC 0173-0763-44).

STORAGE

Store NUROMAX Injection at room temperature of 15° to 25°C (59° to 77°F). DO NOT FREEZE.
U.S. Patent No. 4701460
February 1996/RL-255

Shown in Product Identification Guide, page 314

OXISTAT® ℞

[*äx′-e-stat″*]

(oxiconazole nitrate cream)
Cream, 1%*

OXISTAT®

(oxiconazole nitrate lotion)
Lotion, 1%*

*** Potency expressed as oxiconazole**

FOR TOPICAL DERMATOLOGIC USE ONLY—
NOT FOR OPHTHALMIC OR INTRAVAGINAL USE

DESCRIPTION

Oxistat® (oxiconazole nitrate cream) Cream and Oxistat® (oxiconazole nitrate lotion) Lotion formulations contain the antifungal active compound oxiconazole nitrate. Both formulations are for topical dermatologic use only.

Chemically, oxiconazole nitrate is 2′,4′-dichloro-2-imidazol-1-ylacetophenone (Z)-[*O*-(2,4-dichlorobenzyl)oxime], mononitrate. The compound has the empirical formula $C_{18}H_{13}Cl_4N_3 \cdot HNO_3$, a molecular weight of 492.15.

Oxiconazole nitrate is a nearly white crystalline powder, soluble in methanol; sparingly soluble in ethanol, chloroform, and acetone; and very slightly soluble in water.

Oxistat Cream contains 10 mg of oxiconazole per gram of cream in a white to off-white, opaque cream base of purified water USP, white petrolatum USP, stearyl alcohol NF, propylene glycol USP, polysorbate 60 NF, cetyl alcohol NF, and benzoic acid USP 0.2% as a preservative.

Oxistat Lotion contains 10 mg of oxiconazole per gram of lotion in a white to off-white, opaque lotion base of purified water USP, white petrolatum USP, stearyl alcohol NF, propylene glycol USP, polysorbate 60 NF, cetyl alcohol NF, and benzoic acid USP 0.2% as a preservative.

CLINICAL PHARMACOLOGY

Five hours after application of 2.5 mg/cm^2 of oxiconazole nitrate cream onto human skin, the concentration of oxiconazole nitrate was demonstrated to be 16.2 μmol in the epidermis, 3.64 μmol in the upper corium, and 1.29 μmol in the deeper corium. Systemic absorption of oxiconazole nitrate appears to be low. Less than 0.3% of the applied dose of oxiconazole nitrate was recovered in the urine of volunteer subjects up to 5 days after application of the cream formulation.

Neither *in vitro* nor *in vivo* studies have been conducted to establish relative activity between the lotion and cream formulations.

Microbiology: Oxiconazole nitrate is an imidazole derivative whose antifungal activity is derived primarily from the inhibition of ergosterol biosynthesis, which is critical for cellular membrane integrity. It has *in vitro* activity against a wide range of pathogenic fungi.

Oxiconazole has been shown to be active against most strains of the following organisms both *in vitro* and in clinical infections at indicated body sites: (See **INDICATIONS AND USAGE.**)

Epidermophyton floccosum
Trichophyton mentagrophytes
Trichophyton rubrum

The following *in vitro* data are available: *however, their clinical significance is unknown.* Oxiconazole exhibits satisfactory *in vitro* minimum inhibitory concentrations (MIC's) against most strains of the following organisms; however, the safety and efficacy of oxiconazole in treating clinical infections due to these organisms have not been established in adequate and well-controlled clinical trials:

Candida albicans
Malassezia furfur
Microsporum audouini
Microsporum canis
Microsporum gypseum
Trichophyton tonsurans
Trichophyton violaceum

INDICATIONS AND USAGE

Oxistat® (oxiconazole nitrate cream) Cream and Oxistat® (oxiconazole nitrate lotion) Lotion are indicated for the topical treatment of the following dermal infections: tinea pedis, tinea cruris, and tinea corporis due to *Trichophyton rubrum, Trichophyton mentagrophytes,* or *Epidermophyton floccosum.* (see **DOSAGE AND ADMINISTRATION** and **CLINICAL STUDIES).**

CONTRAINDICATIONS

Oxistat® (oxiconazole nitrate cream) Cream and Oxistat® (oxiconazole nitrate lotion) Lotion are contraindicated in individuals who have shown hypersensitivity to any of their components.

WARNINGS

Oxistat® (oxiconazole nitrate cream) Cream and Oxistat® (oxiconazole nitrate lotion) Lotion are not for ophthalmic or intravaginal use.

PRECAUTIONS

General: If a reaction suggesting sensitivity or chemical irritation should occur with the use of Oxistat® (oxiconazole nitrate cream) Cream or Oxistat® (oxiconazole nitrate lotion) Lotion, treatment should be discontinued and appropriate therapy instituted. Oxistat Cream and Lotion are for external dermal use only. Avoid introduction of Oxistat Cream or Lotion into the eyes or vagina.

Carcinogenesis, Mutagenesis, Impairment of Fertility: Although no long-term studies in animals have been performed to evaluate carcinogenic potential, no evidence of mutagenic effect was found in two mutation assays (Ames test and Chinese hamster V79 *in vitro* cell mutation assay) or in two cytogenetic assays (human peripheral blood lymphocyte *in vitro* chromosome aberration assay and *in vivo* micronucleus assay in mice).

Reproductive studies revealed no impairment of fertility in rats at oral doses of 3 mg/kg per day in females (one time the human dose based on mg/m^2) and 15 mg/kg per day in males (four times the human dose based on mg/m^2). However, at doses above this level, the following effects were observed: a reduction in the fertility parameters of males and females, a reduction in the number of sperm in vaginal smears, extended estrous cycle, and a decrease in mating frequency.

Pregnancy: Teratogenic Effects: *Pregnancy Category B:* Reproduction studies have been performed in rabbits, rats, and mice at oral doses up to 100, 150, and 200 mg/kg per day (57, 40, and 27 times the human dose based on mg/m^2), respectively, and revealed no evidence of harm to the fetus due to oxiconazole nitrate. There are, however, no adequate and well-controlled studies in pregnant women. Because animal reproduction studies are not always predictive of human response, this drug should be used during pregnancy only if clearly needed.

Nursing Mothers: Because oxiconazole is excreted in human milk, caution should be exercised when the drug is administered to a nursing woman.

ADVERSE REACTIONS

(Numbers in this section include patients treated both once daily and twice daily combined.)

During clinical trials, 41 (4.3%) of 955 patients treated with oxiconazole nitrate cream, 1% reported adverse reactions thought to be related to drug therapy. These reactions included pruritus (1.6%); burning (1.4%); irritation and allergic contact dermatitis (0.4% each); folliculitis (0.3%); erythema (0.2%); and papules, fissure, maceration, rash, stinging, and nodules (0.1% each).

In a controlled, multicenter clinical trial, 7 (2.6%) of 269 patients treated with oxiconazole nitrate lotion, 1% reported adverse reactions thought to be related to drug therapy. These reactions included burning and stinging (0.7% each) and pruritus, scaling, tingling, pain, and dyshidrotic eczema (0.4% each).

OVERDOSAGE

When a 5% oxiconazole cream was applied at a rate of 1 g/kg to approximately 10% of body surface area of a group of 40 male and female rats for 35 days, three deaths and severe dermal inflammation were reported.

DOSAGE AND ADMINISTRATION

Oxistat® (oxiconazole nitrate cream) Cream or Oxistat® (oxiconazole nitrate lotion) Lotion should be applied to cover affected and immediately surrounding areas once to twice daily in patients with tinea pedis, tinea corporis, or tinea cruris. Tinea corporis and tinea cruris should be treated for 2 weeks and tinea pedis for 1 month to reduce the possibility of recurrence. If a patient shows no clinical improvement after the treatment period, the diagnosis should be reviewed.

HOW SUPPLIED

Oxistat® (oxiconazole nitrate cream) Cream, 1% is supplied in 15-g tubes (NDC 0173-0423-00), 30-g tubes (NDC 0173-0423-01), and 60-g tubes (NDC 0173-0423-04). Oxistat® (oxiconazole nitrate lotion) Lotion, 1% is supplied in a 30-mL bottle (NDC 0173-0448-01).

Store between 15° and 30°C (59° and 86°F). Shake well before using.

CLINICAL STUDIES

Tinea Pedis Studies: The following definitions were applied to the clinical and microbiological outcomes in patients enrolled in the clinical trials that form the basis for the approvals of Oxistat® (oxiconazole nitrate lotion) Lotion and Oxistat® (oxiconazole nitrate cream) Cream.

THERE ARE NO HEAD-TO-HEAD COMPARISON TRIALS OF THE OXISTAT CREAM AND LOTION FORMULATIONS IN THE TREATMENT OF TINEA PEDIS.

Definitions: 1. Clinical Improvement: Greater than 50% improvement in the clinical signs and symptoms above the baseline assessment.

2. Clinical Cure: Greater than 90% improvement in the clinical signs and symptoms above the baseline assessment.

3. Mycological Cure: No evidence (culture and KOH preparation) of the baseline (original) pathogen in a specimen from the affected area taken at the 2-week post-treatment visit.

4. Overall Cure: Both a clinical cure (see above) and a microbiologic eradication (see above) at the 2-week post-treatment visit.

Lotion Formulation: The clinical trial for the lotion formulation line extension involved 332 evaluable patients with clinically and microbiologically established tinea pedis. Of these evaluable patients, 64% were diagnosed with hyperkeratotic plantar tinea pedis and 28% with interdigital tinea pedis. Seventy-seven percent had disease secondary to infection with *Trichophyton rubrum,* 18% had disease secondary to infection with *Trichophyton mentagrophytes,* and 4% had disease secondary to infection with *Epidermophyton floccosum.*

The results of this clinical trial at the 2-week post-treatment follow-up visit are shown in the following table:

Patient Outcome	Oxistat Lotion		
Category	b.i.d.	q.d.	Vehicle
Clinical improvement	82%	80%	50%
Clinical cure	52%	43%	18%
Mycological cure	67%	64%	28%
Overall cure	41%	34%	10%

In this study, the improvement and cure rates of the b.i.d.- and q.d.-treated groups did not differ significantly (95% confidence interval) from each other but were statistically (95% confidence interval) superior to the vehicle-treated group.

Continued on next page

Glaxo Wellcome—Cont.

Cream Formulation: The two pivotal trials for the cream formulation involved 281 evaluable patients (total from both trials) with clinically and microbiologically established tinea pedis.

The combined results of these two clinical trials at the 2-week post-treatment follow-up visit are shown in the following table:

Patient Outcome	Oxistat Cream		
Category	b.i.d	q.d.	Vehicle
Clinical improvement	84%	83%	49%
Mycological cure	77%	79%	33%
Overall cure	52%	43%	14%

All the improvement and cure rates of the b.i.d.- and q.d.-treated groups did not differ significantly (95% confidence interval) from each other but were statistically (95% confidence interval) superior to the vehicle-treated group.
May 1995/RL-190

Shown in Product Identification Guide, page 314

PEDIOTIC® ℞
[pĕd-ē-ō'tik]
Suspension Sterile
(neomycin and polymyxin B sulfates and hydrocortisone otic suspension, USP)

DESCRIPTION

PEDIOTIC Suspension (neomycin and polymyxin B sulfates and hydrocortisone otic suspension) is a sterile antibacterial and anti-inflammatory suspension for otic use. Each mL contains: neomycin sulfate equivalent to 3.5 mg neomycin base, polymyxin B sulfate equivalent to 10,000 polymyxin B units, and hydrocortisone 10 mg (1%). The vehicle contains thimerosal 0.001% (added as a preservative) and the inactive ingredients cetyl alcohol, glyceryl monostearate, mineral oil, polyoxyl 40 stearate, propylene glycol, and Water for Injection. Sulfuric acid may be added to adjust pH. PEDIOTIC Suspension has a minimum pH of 4.1, which is less acidic than the minimum pH of 3.0 for CORTISPORIN® Otic Suspension.

Neomycin sulfate is the sulfate salt of neomycin B and C, which are produced by the growth of *Streptomyces fradiae* Waksman (Fam. Streptomycetaceae). It has a potency equivalent of not less than 600 μg of neomycin standard per mg, calculated on an anhydrous basis.

Polymyxin B sulfate is the sulfate salt of polymyxin B_1 and B_2, which are produced by the growth of *Bacillus polymyxa* (Prazmowski) Migula (Fam. Bacillaceae). It has a potency of not less than 6,000 polymyxin B units per mg, calculated on an anhydrous basis.

Hydrocortisone, 11β,17,21-trihydroxypregn-4-ene-3,20-dione, is an anti-inflammatory hormone.

CLINICAL PHARMACOLOGY

Corticoids suppress the inflammatory response to a variety of agents and they may delay healing. Since corticoids may inhibit the body's defense mechanism against infection, a concomitant antimicrobial drug may be used when this inhibition is considered to be clinically significant in a particular case.

The anti-infective components in the combination are included to provide action against specific organisms susceptible to them. Neomycin sulfate and polymyxin B sulfate together are considered active against the following microorganisms: *Staphylococcus aureus, Escherichia coli, Haemophilus influenzae, Klebsiella-Enterobacter* species, *Neisseria* species, and *Pseudomonas aeruginosa*. This product does not provide adequate coverage against *Serratia marcescens* and streptococci, including *Streptococcus pneumonia*.

The relative potency of corticosteroids depends on the molecular structure, concentration, and release from the vehicle.

INDICATIONS AND USAGE

For the treatment of superficial bacterial infections of the external auditory canal caused by organisms susceptible to the action of the antibiotics, and for the treatment of infections of mastoidectomy and fenestration cavities caused by organisms susceptible to the antibiotics.

CONTRAINDICATIONS

This product is contraindicated in those individuals who have shown hypersensitivity to any of its components, and in herpes simplex, vaccinia, and varicella infections.

WARNINGS

This product should be used with care in cases of perforated eardrum and in long-standing cases of chronic otitis media because of the possibility of ototoxicity.

Neomycin sulfate may cause cutaneous sensitization. A precise incidence of hypersensitivity reactions (primarily skin rash) due to topical neomycin is not known.

When using neomycin-containing products to control secondary infection in the chronic dermatoses, such as chronic otitis externa or stasis dermatitis, it should be borne in mind that the skin in these conditions is more liable than is normal skin to become sensitized to many substances, including neomycin. The manifestation of sensitization to neomycin is usually a low-grade reddening with swelling, dry scaling, and itching; it may be manifest simply as a failure to heal. Periodic examination for such signs is advisable, and the patient should be told to discontinue the product if they are observed. These symptoms regress quickly on withdrawing the medication. Neomycin-containing applications should be avoided for the patient thereafter.

PRECAUTIONS

General: As with other antibacterial preparations, prolonged use may result in overgrowth of non-susceptible organisms, including fungi.

If the infection is not improved after 1 week, cultures and susceptibility tests should be repeated to verify the identity of the organism and to determine whether therapy should be changed.

Treatment should not be continued for longer than 10 days.

Allergic cross-reactions may occur which could prevent the use of any or all of the following antibiotics for the treatment of future infections: kanamycin, paromomycin, streptomycin, and possibly gentamicin.

Information for Patients: Avoid contaminating the dropper with material from the ear, fingers, or other source. This caution is necessary if the sterility of the drops is to be preserved.

If sensitization or irritation occurs, discontinue use immediately and contact your physician.

Do not use in the eyes.

SHAKE WELL BEFORE USING.

Laboratory Tests: Systemic effects of excessive levels of hydrocortisone may include a reduction in the number of circulating eosinophils and a decrease in urinary excretion of 17-hydroxycorticosteroids.

Carcinogenesis, Mutagenesis, Impairment of Fertility: Long-term studies in animals (rats, rabbits, mice) showed no evidence of carcinogenicity attributable to oral administration of corticosteroids.

Pregnancy:*Teratogenic Effects:* Pregnancy Category C. Corticosteroids have been shown to be teratogenic in rabbits when applied topically at concentrations of 0.5% on days 6–18 of gestation and in mice when applied topically at a concentration of 15% on days 10 to 13 of gestation. There are no adequate and well-controlled studies in pregnant women. Corticosteroids should be used during pregnancy only if the potential benefit justifies the potential risk to the fetus.

Nursing Mothers: Hydrocortisone appears in human milk following oral administration of the drug. Since systemic absorption of hydrocortisone may occur when applied topically, caution should be exercised when PEDIOTIC is used by a nursing woman.

Pediatric Use: See DOSAGE AND ADMINISTRATION.

ADVERSE REACTIONS

Neomycin occasionally causes skin sensitization. Ototoxicity and nephrotoxicity have also been reported (see WARNINGS). Adverse reactions have occurred with topical use of antibiotic combinations including neomycin and polymyxin B. Exact incidence figures are not available since no denominator of treated patients is available. The reaction occurring most often is allergic sensitization. In one clinical study, using a 20% neomycin patch, neomycin-induced allergic skin reactions occurred in two of 2,175 (0.09%) individuals in the general population.[1] In another study, the incidence was found to be approximately 1%.[2]

The following local adverse reactions have been reported with topical corticosteroids, especially under occlusive dressings: burning, itching, irritation, dryness, folliculitis, hypertrichosis, acneiform eruptions, hypopigmentation, perioral dermatitis, allergic contact dermatitis, maceration of the skin, secondary infection, skin atrophy, striae, and miliaria. Stinging and burning have been reported rarely when this drug has gained access to the middle ear.

DOSAGE AND ADMINISTRATION

The external auditory canal should be thoroughly cleansed and dried with a sterile cotton applicator.

For adults, 4 drops of the suspension should be instilled into the affected ear 3 or 4 times daily. For infants and children, 3 drops are suggested because of the smaller capacity of the ear canal.

The patient should lie with the affected ear upward and then the drops should be instilled. This position should be maintained for 5 minutes to facilitate penetration of the drops into the ear canal. Repeat, if necessary, for the opposite ear. If preferred, a cotton wick may be inserted into the canal and then the cotton may be saturated with the suspension. This wick should be kept moist by adding further suspension every 4 hours. The wick should be replaced at least once every 24 hours.

SHAKE WELL BEFORE USING.

HOW SUPPLIED

Bottle of 7.5 ml with sterilized dropper (NDC 0173-0910-02). Store at 15° to 25°C (59° to 77°F).

REFERENCES

1. Leyden JJ, Kligman AM. Contact dermatitis to neomycin sulfate. *JAMA.* 1979;242:1276–1278.
2. Prystowsky SD, Allen AM, Smith RW, Nonomura JH, Odom RB, Akers WA. Allergic contact hypersensitivity to nickel, neomycin, ethylenediamine, and benzocaine: relationships between age, sex, history of exposure, and reactivity to standard patch tests and use tests in a general population. *Arch Dermatol.* 1979;115:959–962.
January 1996/RL-257

Shown in Product Identification Guide, page 314

POLYSPORIN® ℞
[pah "l ē-spor'ĭn]
Ophthalmic Ointment Sterile
(bacitracin zinc and polymyxin B sulfate ophthalmic ointment, USP)

DESCRIPTION

POLYSPORIN Ophthalmic Ointment (bacitracin zinc and polymyxin B sulfate ophthalmic ointment) is a sterile antimicrobial ointment for ophthalmic use. Each gram contains: bacitracin zinc equivalent to 500 bacitracin units, polymyxin B sulfate equivalent to 10,000 polymyxin B units, and white petrolatum, q.s.

Bacitracin zinc is the zinc salt of bacitracin, a mixture of related cyclic polypeptides (mainly bacitracin A) produced by the growth of an organism of the *licheniformis* group of *Bacillus subtilis* var Tracy. It has a potency of not less than 40 bacitracin units per mg.

Polymyxin B sulfate is the sulfate salt of polymyxin B_1 and B_2 which are produced by the growth of *Bacillus polymyxa* (Prazmowski) Migula (Fam. Bacillaceae). It has a potency of not less than 6,000 polymyxin B units per mg, calculated on an anhydrous basis.

CLINICAL PHARMACOLOGY

A wide range of antibacterial action is provided by the overlapping spectra of bacitracin and polymyxin B sulfate.

Bacitracin is bactericidal for a variety of gram-positive and gram-negative organisms. It interferes with bacterial cell wall synthesis by inhibition of the regeneration of phospholipid receptors involved in peptidoglycan synthesis.

Polymyxin B is bactericidal for a variety of gram-negative organisms. It increases the permeability of the bacterial cell membrane by interacting with the phospholipid components of the membrane.

Microbiology: Bacitracin zinc and polymyxin B sulfate together are considered active against the following microorganisms: *Staphylococcus aureus*, streptococci including *Streptococcus pneumoniae, Escherichia coli, Haemophilus influenzae, Klebsiella/Enterobacter* species. *Neisseria* species, and *Pseudomonas aeruginosa*. The product does not provide adequate coverage against *Serratia marcescens*.

INDICATIONS AND USAGE

POLYSPORIN Ophthalmic Ointment is indicated for the topical treatment of superficial infections of the external eye and its adnexa caused by susceptible bacteria. Such infections encompass conjunctivitis, keratitis and keratoconjunctivitis, blepharitis and blepharoconjunctivitis.

CONTRAINDICATIONS

POLYSPORIN Ophthalmic Ointment is contraindicated in individuals who have shown hypersensitivity to any of its components.

WARNINGS

NOT FOR INJECTION INTO THE EYE. POLYSPORIN Ophthalmic Ointment should never be directly introduced into the anterior chamber of the eye. Ophthalmic ointments may retard corneal wound healing.

Topical antibiotics may cause cutaneous sensitization. A precise incidence of hypersensitivity reactions (primarily skin rash) due to topical antibiotics is not known. The manifestations of sensitization to topical antibiotics are usually itching, reddening, and edema of the conjunctiva and eyelid. A sensitization reaction may manifest simply as a failure to heal. During long-term use of topical antibiotic products, periodic examination for such signs is advisable, and the patient should be told to discontinue the product if they are observed. Symptoms usually subside quickly on withdrawing the medication. Application of products containing these

ingredients should be avoided for the patient thereafter (see PRECAUTIONS: General).

PRECAUTIONS

General: As with other antibiotic preparations, prolonged use of POLYSPORIN Ophthalmic Ointment may result in overgrowth of nonsusceptible organisms including fungi. If superinfection occurs, appropriate measures should be initiated.

Bacterial resistance to POLYSPORIN Ophthalmic Ointment may also develop. If purulent discharge, inflammation, or pain become aggravated, the patient should discontinue use of the medication and consult a physician.

There have been reports of bacterial keratitis associated with the use of topical ophthalmic products in multiple-dose containers which have been inadvertently contaminated by patients, most of whom had a concurrent corneal disease or a disruption of the ocular epithelial surface (see PRECAUTIONS: Information for Patients).

Allergic cross-reactions may occur which could prevent the use of any or all of the following antibiotics for the treatment of future infections: kanamycin, paromomycin, streptomycin, and possibly gentamicin.

Information for Patients: Patients should be instructed to avoid allowing the tip of the dispensing container to contact the eye, eyelid, fingers, or any other surface. the use of this product by more than one person may spread infection.

Patients should also be instructed that ocular products, if handled improperly, can become contaminated by common bacteria known to cause ocular infections. Serious damage to the eye and subsequent loss of vision may result from using contaminated products (see PRECAUTIONS: General).

If the condition persists or gets worse, or if a rash or other allergic reaction develops, the patient should be advised to stop use and consult a physician. Do not use this product if you are allergic to any of the listed ingredients.

Keep tightly closed when not in use. Keep out of reach of children.

Carcinogenesis, Mutagenesis, Impairment of Fertility: Long-term studies in animals to evaluate carcinogenic or mutagenic potential have not been conducted with polymyxin B sulfate or bacitracin. Polymyxin B has been reported to impair the motility of equine sperm, but its effects on male or female fertility are unknown. No adverse effects on male or female fertility, litter size, or survival were observed in rabbits given bacitracin zinc 100 gm/ton of diet.

Pregnancy: ***Teratogenic Effects:*** Pregnancy Category C. Animal reproduction studies have not been conducted with polymyxin B sulfate or bacitracin. It is also not known whether POLYSPORIN Ophthalmic Ointment can cause fetal harm when administered to a pregnant woman or can affect reproduction capacity. POLYSPORIN Ophthalmic Ointment should be given to a pregnant woman only if clearly needed.

Nursing Mothers: It is not known whether this drug is excreted in human milk. Because many drugs are excreted in human milk, caution should be exercise when POLYSPORIN Ophthalmic Ointment is administered to a nursing woman.

Pediatric Use: Safety and effectiveness in pediatric patients have not been established.

ADVERSE REACTIONS

Adverse reactions have occurred with the anti-infective components of POLYSPORIN Ophthalmic Ointment. The exact incidence is not known. Reactions occurring most often are allergic sensitization reactions including itching, swelling, and conjunctival erythema (see WARNINGS). More serious hypersensitivity reactions, including anaphylaxis, have been reported rarely.

Local irritation on instillation has also been reported.

DOSAGE AND ADMINISTRATION

Apply the ointment every 3 or 4 hours for 7 to 10 days, depending on the severity of the infection.

HOW SUPPLIED

POLYSPORIN Ophthalmic Ointment (bacitracin zinc and polymyxin B sulfate ophthalmic ointment, USP) is available as a tube of 1/8 oz (3.5 g) with ophthalmic tip (NDC 0173-0797-86).

Caution: Federal law prohibits dispensing without prescription.

Store at 15° to 25°C (59° to 77°F).

February 1996/RL-275

Shown in Product Identification Guide, page 314

PROLOPRIM® ℞

[prō'lah-prīm"]

(trimethoprim)

100 mg and 200 mg Scored Tablets

DESCRIPTION

PROLOPRIM (trimethoprim) is a synthetic antibacterial available in tablet form for oral administration. Each scored white tablet contains 100 mg trimethoprim and the inactive ingredients corn starch, lactose, magnesium stearate, and sodium starch glycolate. Each scored yellow tablet contains 200 mg trimethoprim and the inactive ingredients corn starch, D & C Yellow No. 10, magnesium stearate, and sodium starch glycolate.

Trimethoprim is 5-[(3,4,5,-trimethoxyphenyl)methyl]-2,4-pyrimidinediamine. It is a white to light yellow, odorless, bitter compound with a molecular weight of 290.32 and the molecular formula $C_{14}H_{18}N_4O_3$.

CLINICAL PHARMACOLOGY

Trimethoprim is rapidly absorbed following oral administration. It exists in the blood as unbound, protein-bound, and metabolized forms. Ten to twenty percent of trimethoprim is metabolized, primarily in the liver; the remainder is excreted unchanged in the urine. The principal metabolites of trimethoprim are the 1- and 3-oxides and the 3'- and 4'-hydroxy derivatives. The free form is considered to be the therapeutically active form. Approximately 44% of trimethoprim is bound to plasma proteins.

Mean peak plasma concentrations of approximately 1.0 μg/mL occur 1 to 4 hours after oral administration of a single 100 mg dose. A single 200 mg dose will result in serum levels approximately twice as high. The half-life of trimethoprim ranges from 8 to 10 hours. However, patients with severely impaired renal function exhibit an increase in the half-life of trimethoprim, which requires either dosage regimen adjustment or not using the drug in such patients (see DOSAGE AND ADMINISTRATION). During a 13-week study of trimethoprim administered at a daily dosage of 200 mg (50 mg qid), the mean minimum steady-state concentration of the drug was 1.1 μg/mL. Steady-state concentrations were achieved within 2 to 3 days of chronic administration and were maintained throughout the experimental period.

Excretion of trimethoprim is primarily by the kidneys through glomerular filtration and tubular secretion. Urine concentrations of trimethoprim are considerably higher than are the concentrations in the blood. After a single oral dose of 100 mg, urine concentrations of trimethoprim ranged from 30 to 160 μg/mL during the 0- to 4-hour period and declined to approximately 18 to 91 μg/mL during the 8- to 24-hour period. A 200 mg single oral dose will result in trimethoprim urine levels approximately twice as high. After oral administration, 50% to 60% of trimethoprim is excreted in the urine within 24 hours, approximately 80% of this being unmetabolized trimethoprim.

Since normal vaginal and fecal flora are the source of most pathogens causing urinary tract infections, it is relevant to consider the distribution of trimethoprim into these sites. Concentrations of trimethoprim in vaginal secretions are consistently greater than those found simultaneously in the serum, being typically 1.6 times the concentrations of simultaneously obtained serum samples. Sufficient trimethoprim is excreted in the feces to markedly reduce or eliminate trimethoprim-susceptible organisms from the fecal flora.

Trimethoprim also passes the placental barrier and is excreted in human milk.

Microbiology: PROLOPRIM blocks the production of tetrahydrofolic acid from dihydrofolic acid by binding to and reversibly inhibiting the required enzyme, dihydrofolate reductase. This binding is very much stronger for the bacterial enzyme than for the corresponding mammalian enzyme. Thus, PROLOPRIM selectively interferes with bacterial biosynthesis of nucleic acids and proteins.

In vitro serial dilution tests have shown that the spectrum of antibacterial activity of PROLOPRIM includes the common urinary tract pathogens with the exception of *Pseudomonas aeruginosa*.

The dominant non-*Enterobacteriaceae* fecal organisms, *Bacteroides* spp. and *Lactobacillus* spp., are not susceptible to trimethoprim concentrations obtained with the recommended dosage.

REPRESENTATIVE MINIMUM INHIBITORY CONCENTRATIONS FOR TRIMETHOPRIM-SUSCEPTIBLE ORGANISMS

Bacteria	Trimethoprim MIC—μg/mL (Range)
Escherichia coli	0.05–1.5
Proteus mirabilis	0.5 –1.5
Klebsiella pneumoniae	0.5 –5.0
Enterobacter species	0.5 –5.0
Staphylococcus species, coagulase-negative	0.15–5.0

Susceptibility Testing: The recommended quantitative disc susceptibility method[1,2] may be used for estimating the susceptibility of bacteria to PROLOPRIM. With this procedure, reports from the laboratory giving results using the 5 μg trimethoprim disc should be interpreted according to the following criteria: Organisms producing zones of 16 mm or greater are classified as susceptible, whereas those producing zones of 11 to 15 mm are classified as having intermediate susceptibility. A report from the laboratory of "Susceptible to trimethoprim" or "Intermediate susceptibility to trimethoprim" indicates that the infection is likely to respond when, as in uncomplicated urinary tract infections, effective therapy is dependent upon the urine concentration of trimethoprim. Organisms producing zones of 10 mm or less are reported as resistant, indicating that other therapy should be selected.

Dilution methods for determining susceptibility are also used, and results are reported as the minimum drug concentration inhibiting microbial growth (MIC).[3] If the MIC is 8 μg/mL or less, the microorganism is considered "susceptible." If the MIC is 16 μg/mL or greater, the microorganism is considered "resistant."

INDICATIONS AND USAGE

For the treatment of initial episodes of uncomplicated urinary tract infections due to susceptible strains of the following organisms: *Escherichia coli, Proteus mirabilis, Klebsiella pneumoniae, Enterobacter* species, and coagulase-negative *Staphylococcus* species, including *S. saprophyticus*.

Cultures and susceptibility tests should be performed to determine the susceptibility of the bacteria to trimethoprim. Therapy may be initiated prior to obtaining the results of these tests.

CONTRAINDICATIONS

PROLOPRIM is contraindicated in individuals hypersensitive to trimethoprim and in those with documented megaloblastic anemia due to folate deficiency.

WARNINGS

Serious hypersensitivity reactions have been reported rarely in patients on trimethoprim therapy. Trimethoprim has been reported rarely to interfere with hematopoiesis, especially when administered in large doses and/or for prolonged periods.

The presence of clinical signs such as sore throat, fever, pallor, or purpura may be early indications of serious blood disorders (see OVERDOSAGE: Chronic).

Complete blood counts should be obtained if any of these signs are noted in a patient receiving trimethoprim and the drug discontinued if a significant reduction in the count of any formed blood element is found.

PRECAUTIONS

General: Trimethoprim should be given with caution to patients with possible folate deficiency. Folates may be administered concomitantly without interfering with the antibacterial action of trimethoprim. Trimethoprim should also be given with caution to patients with impaired renal or hepatic function (see CLINICAL PHARMACOLOGY and DOSAGE AND ADMINISTRATION).

Drug Interactions: PROLOPRIM may inhibit the hepatic metabolism of phenytoin. Trimethoprim, given at a common clinical dosage, increased the phenytoin half-life by 51% and decreased the phenytoin metabolic clearance rate by 30%. When administering these drugs concurrently, one should be alert for possible excessive phenytoin effect.

Drug/Laboratory Test Interactions: Trimethoprim can interfere with a serum methotrexate assay as determined by the Competitive Binding Protein Technique (CBPA) when a bacterial dihydrofolate reductase is used as the binding protein. No interference occurs, however, if methotrexate is measured by a radioimmunoassay (RIA).

The presence of trimethoprim may also interfere with the Jaffé alkaline picrate reaction assay for creatinine, resulting in overestimations of about 10% in the range of normal values.

Carcinogenesis, Mutagenesis, Impairment of Fertility:

Carcinogenesis: Long-term studies in animals to evaluate carcinogenic potential have not been conducted with trimethoprim.

Mutagenesis: Trimethoprim was demonstrated to be non-mutagenic in the Ames assay. In studies at two laboratories no chromosomal damage was detected in cultured Chinese hamster ovary cells at concentrations approximately 500 times human plasma levels; at concentrations approximately 1000 times human plasma levels in these same cells, a low level of chromosomal damage was induced at one of the laboratories. No chromosomal abnormalities were observed in cultured human leukocytes at concentrations of trimethoprim up to 20 times human steady-state plasma levels. No chromosomal effects were detected in peripheral lymphocytes of human subjects receiving 320 mg of trimethoprim in combination with up to 1600 mg of sulfamethoxazole per day for as long as 112 weeks.

Impairment of Fertility: No adverse effects on fertility or general reproductive performance were observed in rats given trimethoprim in oral dosages as high as 70 mg/kg/day for males and 14 mg/kg/day for females.

Pregnancy: ***Teratogenic Effects:*** Pregnancy Category C. Trimethoprim has been shown to be teratogenic in the rat when given in doses 40 times the human dose. In some rabbit

Continued on next page

Glaxo Wellcome—Cont.

studies, the overall increase in fetal loss (dead and resorbed and malformed conceptuses) was associated with doses six times the human therapeutic dose.

While there are no large, well-controlled studies on the use of trimethoprim in pregnant women, Brumfitt and Pursell,[4] in a retrospective study, reported the outcome of 186 pregnancies during which the mother received either placebo or trimethoprim in combination with sulfamethoxazole. The incidence of congenital abnormalities was 4.5% (3 of 66) in those who received placebo and 3.3% (4 of 120) in those receiving trimethoprim and sulfamethoxazole. There were no abnormalities in the 10 children whose mothers received the drug during the first trimester. In a separate survey, Brumfitt and Pursell also found no congenital abnormalities in 35 children whose mothers had received trimethoprim and sulfamethoxazole at the time of conception or shortly thereafter.

Because trimethoprim may interfere with folic acid metabolism, PROLOPRIM should be used during pregnancy only if the potential benefit justifies the potential risk to the fetus.
Nonteratogenic Effects: The oral administration of trimethoprim to rats at a dose of 70 mg/kg/day commencing with the last third of gestation and continuing through parturition and lactation caused no deleterious effects on gestation or pup growth and survival.
Nursing Mothers: Trimethoprim is excreted in human milk. Because trimethoprim may interfere with folic acid metabolism, caution should be exercised when PROLOPRIM is administered to a nursing woman.
Pediatric Use: The safety of trimethoprim in pediatric patients under 2 months has not been demonstrated. The effectiveness of trimethoprim as a single agent has not been established in pediatric patients under 12 years of age.

ADVERSE REACTIONS

The adverse effects encountered most often with trimethoprim were rash and pruritus.
Dermatologic: Rash, pruritus, and phototoxic skin eruptions. At the recommended dosage regimens of 100 mg bid or 200 mg qd, each for 10 days, the incidence of rash is 2.9% to 6.7%. In clinical studies which employed high doses of PROLOPRIM, an elevated incidence of rash was noted. These rashes were maculopapular, morbilliform, pruritic, and generally mild to moderate, appearing 7 to 14 days after the initiation of therapy.
Hypersensitivity: Rare reports of exfoliative dermatitis, erythema multiforme, Stevens-Johnson syndrome, toxic epidermal necrolysis (Lyell Syndrome), and anaphylaxis have been received.
Gastrointestinal: Epigastric distress, nausea, vomiting, and glossitis. Elevation of serum transaminase and bilirubin has been noted, but the significance of this finding is unknown. Cholestatic jaundice has been rarely reported.
Hematologic: Thrombocytopenia, leukopenia, neutropenia, megaloblastic anemia, and methemoglobinemia.
Metabolic: Hyperkalemia, hyponatremia.
Neurologic: Aseptic meningitis has been rarely reported.
Miscellaneous: Fever, and increases in BUN and serum creatinine levels.

OVERDOSAGE

Acute: Signs of acute overdosage with trimethoprim may appear following ingestion of 1 gram or more of the drug and include nausea, vomiting, dizziness, headaches, mental depression, confusion, and bone marrow depression (see Chronic subsection).
Treatment consists of gastric lavage and general supportive measures. Acidification of the urine will increase renal elimination of trimethoprim. Peritoneal dialysis is not effective and hemodialysis only moderately effective in eliminating the drug.
Chronic: Use of trimethoprim at high doses and/or for extended periods of time may cause bone marrow depression manifested as thrombocytopenia, leukopenia, and/or megaloblastic anemia. If signs of bone marrow depression occur, trimethoprim should be discontinued and the patient should be given leucovorin; 5 to 15 mg leucovorin daily has been recommended by some investigators.

DOSAGE AND ADMINISTRATION

The usual oral adult dosage is 100 mg of PROLOPRIM every 12 hours or 200 mg PROLOPRIM every 24 hours, each for 10 days. The use of trimethoprim in patients with a creatinine clearance of less than 15 mL/min is not recommended. For patients with a creatinine clearance of 15 to 30 mL/min, the dose should be 50 mg every 12 hours.
The effectiveness of trimethoprim has not been established in pediatric patients under 12 years of age.

HOW SUPPLIED

100 mg Tablets (white, scored, round-shaped), containing 100 mg trimethoprim—bottle of 100 (NDC 0173-0820-55). Imprint on tablets "PROLOPRIM 09A." Store at 15° to 25°C (59° to 77°F) in a dry place.
200 mg Tablets (yellow, scored, round-shaped), containing 200 mg trimethoprim—bottle of 100 (NDC 0173-0825-55).

Imprint on tablets "PROLOPRIM 200." Store at 15° to 25°C (59° to 77°F) in a dry place and protect from light.

REFERENCES
1. Bauer AW, Kirby WMM, Sherris JC, Turck M. Antibiotic susceptibility testing by a standardized single disk method. *Am J Clin Pathol.* 1966;45:493–496.
2. National Committee for Clinical Laboratory Standards. Performance standards for antimicrobial disk susceptibility tests, 2nd ed. Villanova, PA. 1979.
3. Ericsson HM, Sherris JC. Antibiotic sensitivity testing: report of an international collaborative study. *Acta Pathol Microbiol Scand* [B]. 1971;217(suppl):1–90.
4. Brumfitt W, Pursell R. Trimethoprim-sulfamethoxazole in the treatment of bacteriuria in women. *J Infect Dis.* 1973;128(suppl):S657–S663.

April 1996/RL-305

Shown in Product Identification Guide, page 314

SEPTRA® ℞
[sĕp'tra]
I.V. Infusion
(trimethoprim and sulfamethoxazole)

DESCRIPTION

SEPTRA I.V. Infusion (trimethoprim and sulfamethoxazole), a sterile solution for intravenous infusion only, is a synthetic antibacterial combination product. Each mL contains 16 mg trimethoprim and 80 mg sulfamethoxazole compounded with 40% propylene glycol, 10% ethyl alcohol, and 0.3% diethanolamine; 1% benzyl alcohol and 0.1% sodium metabisulfite added as preservatives, Water for Injection, and pH adjusted to approximately 10 with sodium hydroxide.
Trimethoprim is 5-[(3,4,5-trimethoxyphenyl)methyl]-2,4-pyrimidinediamine. It is a white to light yellow, odorless, bitter compound with a molecular weight of 290.32 and the molecular formula $C_{14}H_{18}N_4O_3$.
Sulfamethoxazole is 4-amino-N-(5-methyl-3-isoxazolyl)benzenesulfonamide. It is an almost white, odorless, tasteless compound with a molecular weight of 253.28 and the molecular formula $C_{10}H_{11}N_3O_3S$.

CLINICAL PHARMACOLOGY

Following a 1-hour intravenous infusion of a single dose of 160 mg trimethoprim and 800 mg sulfamethoxazole to 11 patients whose weight ranged from 105 lb to 165 lb (mean, 143 lb), the mean peak plasma concentrations of trimethoprim and sulfamethoxazole were 3.4 ± 0.3 μg/mL and 46.3 ± 2.7 μg/mL, respectively. Following repeated intravenous administration of the same dose at 8-hour intervals, the mean plasma concentrations just prior to and immediately after each infusion at steady-state were 5.6 ± 0.6 μg/mL and 8.8 ± 0.9 μg/mL for trimethoprim and 70.6 ± 7.3 μg/mL and 105.6 ± 10.9 μg/mL for sulfamethoxazole. The mean plasma half-life was 11.3 ± 0.7 hours for trimethoprim and 12.8 ± 1.8 hours for sulfamethoxazole. All of these 11 patients had normal renal function and their ages ranged from 17 to 78 years (median, 60 years)[1].
Pharmacokinetic studies in children and adults suggest an age-dependent half-life of trimethoprim as indicated in the following table.[2]

Age (years)	No. of Patients	Mean TMP Half-life (hours)
<1	2	7.67
1–10	9	5.49
10–20	5	8.19
20–63	6	12.82

Patients with severely impaired renal function exhibit an increase in the half-lives of both components, requiring dosage regimen adjustment (see DOSAGE AND ADMINISTRATION).
Both trimethoprim and sulfamethoxazole exist in the blood as unbound, protein-bound, and metabolized forms; sulfamethoxazole also exists as the conjugated form. The metabolism of sulfamethoxazole occurs predominately by N_4-acetylation, although the glucuronide conjugate has been identified. The principal metabolites of trimethoprim are the 1- and 3- oxides and the 3'- and 4'-hydroxy derivatives. The free forms of trimethoprim and sulfamethoxazole are considered to be the therapeutically active forms. Approximately 44% of trimethoprim and 70% of sulfamethoxazole are bound to plasma proteins. The presence of 10 mg percent sulfamethoxazole in plasma decreases the protein binding of trimethoprim by an insignificant degree; trimethoprim does not influence the protein binding of sulfamethoxazole.
Excretion of trimethoprim and sulfamethoxazole is primarily by the kidneys through both glomerular filtration and tubular secretion. Urine concentrations of both trimethoprim and sulfamethoxazole are considerably higher than are the concentrations in the blood. The percent of dose excreted in urine over a 12-hour period following the intravenous administration of the first dose of 240 mg of trimethoprim and 1200 mg of sulfamethoxazole on day 1 ranged from 17% to 42.4% as free trimethoprim; 7% to 12.7% as free sulfamethoxazole; and 36.7% to 56% as total (free plus the N_4-acetylated metabolite) sulfamethoxazole. When administered together as SEPTRA, neither trimethoprim nor sulfamethoxazole affects the urinary excretion pattern of the other.
Both trimethoprim and sulfamethoxazole distribute to sputum and vaginal fluid; trimethoprim also distributes to bronchial secretions and both pass the placental barrier and are excreted in human milk.

Microbiology: Sulfamethoxazole inhibits bacterial synthesis of dihydrofolic acid by competing with *para*- aminobenzoic acid (PABA). Trimethoprim blocks the production of tetrahydrofolic acid from dihydrofolic acid by binding to and reversibly inhibiting the required enzyme, dihydrofolate reductase. Thus, SEPTRA blocks two consecutive steps in the biosynthesis of nucleic acids and proteins essential to many bacteria.
In vitro studies have shown that bacterial resistance develops more slowly with SEPTRA than with trimethoprim or sulfamethoxazole alone.
In vitro serial dilution tests have shown that the spectrum of antibacterial activity of SEPTRA includes common bacterial pathogens with the exception of *Pseudomonas aeruginosa.* The following organisms are usually susceptible: *Escherichia coli, Klebsiella* species, *Enterobacter* species, *Morganella morganii, Proteus mirabilis,* indole-positive *Proteus* species, including *Proteus vulgaris, Haemophilus influenzae* (including ampicillin-resistant strains), *Streptococcus pneumoniae, Shigella flexneri,* and *Shigella sonnei.* It should be noted, however, that there are little clinical data on the use of SEPTRA I.V. Infusion in serious systemic infections due to *Haemophilus influenzae* and *Streptococcus pneumoniae.*

[See table below.]

Susceptibility Testing: The recommended quantitative disc susceptibility method may be used for estimating the susceptibility of bacteria to SEPTRA.[3,4] With this procedure, a report from the laboratory of "Susceptible to trimethoprim and sulfamethoxazole" indicates that the infection is likely to respond to therapy with SEPTRA. If the infection is confined to the urine, a report of "Intermediate susceptibility to

REPRESENTATIVE MINIMUM INHIBITORY CONCENTRATION VALUES FOR ORGANISMS SUSCEPTIBLE TO SEPTRA
(MIC-μg/mL)

Bacteria	TMP Alone	SMX Alone	TMP/SMX (1:19) TMP	TMP/SMX (1:19) SMX
Escherichia coli	0.05–1.5	1.0–245	0.05–0.5	0.95–9.5
Proteus species (indole positive)	0.5–5.0	7.35–300	0.05–1.5	0.95–28.5
Morganella morganii	0.5–5.0	7.35–300	0.05–1.5	0.95–28.5
Proteus mirabilis	0.5–1.5	7.35–30	0.05–0.15	0.95–2.85
Klebsiella species	0.15–5.0	2.45–245	0.05–1.5	0.95–28.5
Enterobacter species	0.15–5.0	2.45–245	0.05–1.5	0.95–28.5
Haemophilus influenzae	0.15–1.5	2.85–95	0.015–0.15	0.285–2.85
Streptococcus pneumoniae	0.15–1.5	7.35–24.5	0.05–0.15	0.95–2.85
Shigella flexneri *	<0.01–0.04	<0.16–>320	<0.002–0.03	0.04–0.625
Shigella sonnei *	0.02–0.08	0.625–>320	0.004–0.06	0.08–1.25

TMP = trimethoprim
SMX = sulfamethoxazole
* Rudoy RC, Nelson JD, Haltalin KC. *Antimicrobial Agents and Chemotherapy.* 1974;5:439-443.

trimethoprim and sulfamethoxazole" also indicates that the infection is likely to respond. A report of "Resistant to trimethoprim and sulfamethoxazole" indicates that the infection is unlikely to respond to therapy with SEPTRA.

INDICATIONS AND USAGE

PNEUMOCYSTIS CARINII PNEUMONIA: SEPTRA I.V. Infusion is indicated in the treatment of *Pneumocystis carinii* pneumonia in children and adults.

SHIGELLOSIS: SEPTRA I.V. Infusion is indicated in the treatment of enteritis caused by susceptible strains of *Shigella flexneri* and *Shigella sonnei* in children and adults.

URINARY TRACT INFECTIONS: SEPTRA I.V. Infusion is indicated in the treatment of severe or complicated urinary tract infections due to susceptible strains of *Escherichia coli, Klebsiella* species, *Enterobacter* species, *Morganella morganii,* and *Proteus* species when oral administration of SEPTRA is not feasible and when the organism is not susceptible to single agent antibacterials effective in the urinary tract.

Although appropriate culture and susceptibility studies should be performed, therapy may be started while awaiting the results of these studies.

CONTRAINDICATIONS

SEPTRA is contraindicated in patients with a known hypersensitivity to trimethoprim or sulfonamides and in patients with documented megaloblastic anemia due to folate deficiency. SEPTRA is also contraindicated in pregnant patients at term and in nursing mothers, because sulfonamides pass the placenta and are excreted in the milk and may cause kernicterus. SEPTRA is contraindicated in infants less than two months of age.

WARNINGS

FATALITIES ASSOCIATED WITH THE ADMINISTRATION OF SULFONAMIDES, ALTHOUGH RARE, HAVE OCCURRED DUE TO SEVERE REACTIONS, INCLUDING STEVENS-JOHNSON SYNDROME, TOXIC EPIDERMAL NECROLYSIS, FULMINANT HEPATIC NECROSIS, AGRANULOCYTOSIS, APLASTIC ANEMIA, OTHER BLOOD DYSCRASIAS, AND HYPERSENSITIVITY OF THE RESPIRATORY TRACT.

SEPTRA SHOULD BE DISCONTINUED AT THE FIRST APPEARANCE OF SKIN RASH OR ANY SIGN OF ADVERSE REACTION. Clinical signs, such as rash, sore throat, fever, arthralgia, cough, shortness of breath, pallor, purpura, or jaundice may be early indications of serious reactions. Cough, shortness of breath, and/or pulmonary infiltrates may be indicators of pulmonary hypersensitivity to sulfonamides. In rare instances, a skin rash may be followed by more severe reactions, such as Stevens-Johnson syndrome, toxic epidermal necrolysis, hepatic necrosis, or serious blood disorder. Complete blood counts should be done frequently in patients receiving sulfonamides.

SEPTRA SHOULD NOT BE USED IN THE TREATMENT OF STREPTOCOCCAL PHARYNGITIS. Clinical studies have documented that patients with group A β-hemolytic streptococcal tonsillopharyngitis have a greater incidence of bacteriologic failure when treated with SEPTRA than do those patients treated with penicillin, as evidenced by failure to eradicate this organism from the tonsillopharyngeal area.

Contains sodium metabisulfite, a sulfite that may cause allergic-type reactions including anaphylactic symptoms and life-threatening or less severe asthmatic episodes in certain susceptible people. The overall prevalence of sulfite sensitivity in the general population is unknown and probably low. Sulfite sensitivity is seen more frequently in asthmatic than in nonasthmatic people.

Contains benzyl alcohol. In newborn infants, benzyl alcohol has been associated with an increased incidence of neurological and other complications which are sometimes fatal.

PRECAUTIONS

General: SEPTRA should be given with caution to patients with impaired renal or hepatic function, to those with possible folate deficiency (e.g., the elderly, chronic alcoholics, patients receiving anticonvulsant therapy, patients with malabsorption syndrome, and patients in malnutrition states), and to those with severe allergy or bronchial asthma. In glucose-6-phosphate dehydrogenase-deficient individuals, hemolysis may occur. This reaction is frequently dose-related. Adequate fluid intake must be maintained in order to prevent crystalluria and stone formation (see CLINICAL PHARMACOLOGY and DOSAGE AND ADMINISTRATION).

Local irritation and inflammation due to extravascular infiltration of the infusion has been observed with SEPTRA I.V. Infusion. If these occur, the infusion should be discontinued and restarted at another site.

Use in the Elderly: There may be an increased risk of severe adverse reactions in elderly patients, particularly when complicating conditions exist, e.g., impaired kidney and/or liver function, or concomitant use of other drugs. Severe skin reactions, or generalized bone marrow suppression (see WARNINGS and ADVERSE REACTIONS), or a specific decrease in platelets (with or without purpura) are the most frequently reported severe adverse reactions in elderly patients. In those concurrently receiving certain diuretics, primarily thiazides, an increased incidence of thrombocytopenia with purpura has been reported. Appropriate dosage adjustments should be made for patients with impaired kidney function (see DOSAGE AND ADMINISTRATION).

Use in the Treatment of *Pneumocystis carinii* Pneumonia in Patients with Acquired Immunodeficiency Syndrome (AIDS): The incidence of side effects, particularly rash, fever, leukopenia, elevated aminotransferase (transaminase) values in AIDS patients who are being treated with SEPTRA for *Pneumocystis carinii* pneumonia has been reported to be greatly increased compared with the incidence normally associated with the use of SEPTRA in non-AIDS patients. The incidence of hyperkalemia and hyponatremia appears to be increased in AIDS patients receiving SEPTRA.

The concomitant use of leucovorin with trimethoprim-sulfamethoxazole for the acute treatment of *Pneumocystis carinii* pneumonia in patients with HIV infection was associated with increased rates of treatment failure and morbidity in a placebo-controlled study.

Laboratory Tests: Appropriate culture and susceptibility studies should be performed before and throughout treatment. Complete blood counts should be done frequently in patients receiving SEPTRA; if a significant reduction in the count of any formed blood element is noted, SEPTRA should be discontinued. Urinalyses with careful microscopic examination and renal function tests should be performed during therapy, particularly for those patients with impaired renal function.

Drug Interactions: In elderly patients concurrently receiving certain diuretics, primarily thiazides, an increased incidence of thrombocytopenia with purpura has been reported.

It has been reported that SEPTRA may prolong the prothrombin time in patients who are receiving the anticoagulant warfarin. This interaction should be kept in mind when SEPTRA is given to patients already on anticoagulant therapy, and the coagulation time should be reassessed.

SEPTRA may inhibit the hepatic metabolism of phenytoin. SEPTRA, given at a common clinical dosage, increased the phenytoin half-life by 39% and decreased the phenytoin metabolic clearance rate by 27%. When administering these drugs concurrently, one should be alert for possible excessive phenytoin effect.

Sulfonamides can also displace methotrexate from plasma protein binding sites, thus increasing free methotrexate concentrations.

Drug/Laboratory Test Interactions: SEPTRA, specifically the trimethoprim component, can interfere with a serum methotrexate assay as determined by the competitive binding protein technique (CBPA) when a bacterial dihydrofolate reductase is used as the binding protein. No interference occurs, however, if methotrexate is measured by a radioimmunoassay (RIA).

The presence of trimethoprim and sulfamethoxazole may also interfere with the Jaffé alkaline picrate reaction assay for creatinine, resulting in over-estimations of about 10% in the range of normal values.

Carcinogenesis, Mutagenesis, Impairment of Fertility:

Carcinogenesis: Long-term studies in animals to evaluate carcinogenic potential have not been conducted with SEPTRA I.V. Infusion.

Mutagenesis: Bacterial mutagenic studies have not been performed with sulfamethoxazole and trimethoprim in combination. Trimethoprim was demonstrated to be non-mutagenic in the Ames assay. In studies at two laboratories, no chromosomal damage was detected in cultured Chinese hamster ovary cells at concentrations approximately 500 times human plasma levels; at concentrations approximately 1000 times human plasma levels in these same cells, a low level of chromosomal damage was induced at one of the laboratories. No chromosomal abnormalities were observed in cultured human leukocytes at concentrations of trimethoprim up to 20 times human steady-state plasma levels. No chromosomal effects were detected in peripheral lymphocytes of human subjects receiving 320 mg of trimethoprim in combination with up to 1600 mg of sulfamethoxazole per day for as long as 112 weeks.

Impairment of Fertility: SEPTRA I.V. Infusion has not been studied in animals for evidence of impairment of fertility. However, studies in rats at oral dosages as high as 70 mg/kg trimethoprim plus 350 mg/kg sulfamethoxazole daily showed no adverse effects on fertility or general reproductive performance.

Pregnancy: *Teratogenic Effects:* Pregnancy Category C. In rats, oral doses of 533 mg/kg sulfamethoxazole or 200 mg/kg trimethoprim produced teratological effects manifested mainly as cleft palates. The highest dose which did not cause cleft palates in rats was 512 mg/kg sulfamethoxazole or 192 mg/kg trimethoprim when administered separately. In two studies in rats, no teratology was observed when 512 mg/kg of sulfamethoxazole was used in combination with 128 mg/kg of trimethoprim. In one study, however, cleft palates were observed in one litter out of nine when 355 mg/kg of sulfamethoxazole was used in combination with 88 mg/kg of trimethoprim.

In some rabbit studies, an overall increase in fetal loss (dead and resorbed and malformed conceptuses) was associated with doses of trimethoprim six times the human therapeutic dose.

While there are no large, well-controlled studies on the use of trimethoprim and sulfamethoxazole in pregnant women, Brumfitt and Pursell[5], in a retrospective study, reported the outcome of 186 pregnancies during which the mother received either placebo or oral trimethoprim and sulfamethoxazole. The incidence of congenital abnormalities was 4.5% (3 of 66) in those who received placebo and 3.3% (4 of 120) in those receiving trimethoprim and sulfamethoxazole. There were no abnormalities in the 10 children whose mothers received the drug during the first trimester. In a separate survey, Brumfitt and Pursell also found no congenital abnormalities in 35 children whose mothers had received oral trimethoprim and sulfamethoxazole at the time of conception or shortly thereafter.

Because trimethoprim and sulfamethoxazole may interfere with folic acid metabolism, SEPTRA I.V. Infusion should be used during pregnancy only if the potential benefit justifies the potential risk to the fetus.

Nonteratogenic Effects: See CONTRAINDICATIONS section.

Nursing Mothers: See CONTRAINDICATIONS section.

Pediatric Use: SEPTRA I.V. Infusion is not recommended for infants younger than two months of age (see CONTRAINDICATIONS).

ADVERSE REACTIONS

The most common adverse effects are gastrointestinal disturbances (nausea, vomiting, anorexia) and allergic skin reactions (such as rash and urticaria). **FATALITIES ASSOCIATED WITH THE ADMINISTRATION OF SULFONAMIDES, ALTHOUGH RARE, HAVE OCCURRED DUE TO SEVERE REACTIONS, INCLUDING STEVENS-JOHNSON SYNDROME, TOXIC EPIDERMAL NECROLYSIS, FULMINANT HEPATIC NECROSIS, AGRANULOCYTOSIS, APLASTIC ANEMIA, OTHER BLOOD DYSCRASIAS, AND HYPERSENSITIVITY OF THE RESPIRATORY TRACT (SEE WARNINGS).** Local reaction, pain, and slight irritation on I.V. administration are infrequent. Thrombophlebitis has rarely been observed.

Hematologic: Agranulocytosis, aplastic anemia, thrombocytopenia, leukopenia, neutropenia, hemolytic anemia, megaloblastic anemia, hypoprothrombinemia, methemoglobinemia, eosinophilia.

Allergic: Stevens-Johnson syndrome, toxic epidermal necrolysis, anaphylaxis, allergic myocarditis, erythema multiforme, exfoliative dermatitis, angioedema, drug fever, chills, Henoch-Schönlein purpura, serum sickness-like syndrome, generalized allergic reactions, generalized skin eruptions, conjunctival and scleral injection, photosensitivity, pruritus, urticaria, and rash. In addition, periarteritis nodosa and systemic lupus erythematosus have been reported.

Gastrointestinal: Hepatitis, including cholestatic jaundice and hepatic necrosis, elevation of serum transaminase and bilirubin, pseudomembranous enterocolitis, pancreatitis, stomatitis, glossitis, nausea, emesis, abdominal pain, diarrhea, anorexia.

Genitourinary: Renal failure, interstitial nephritis, BUN and serum creatinine elevation, toxic nephrosis with oliguria and anuria, and crystalluria.

Metabolic: Hyperkalemia, hyponatremia.

Neurologic: Aseptic meningitis, convulsions, peripheral neuritis, ataxia, vertigo, tinnitus, headache.

Psychiatric: Hallucinations, depression, apathy, nervousness.

Endocrine: The sulfonamides bear certain chemical similarities to some goitrogens, diuretics (acetazolamide and the thiazides), and oral hypoglycemic agents. Cross-sensitivity may exist with these agents. Diuresis and hypoglycemia have occurred rarely in patients receiving sulfonamides.

Musculoskeletal: Arthralgia and myalgia.

Respiratory System: Pulmonary infiltrates, cough, shortness of breath.

Miscellaneous: Weakness, fatigue, insomnia.

OVERDOSAGE

Acute: Since there has been no extensive experience in humans with single doses of SEPTRA I.V. Infusion in excess of 25 mL (400 mg trimethoprim and 2000 mg sulfamethoxazole), the maximum tolerated dose in humans is unknown. Signs and symptoms of overdosage reported with sulfonamides include anorexia, colic, nausea, vomiting, dizziness, headache, drowsiness, and unconsciousness. Pyrexia, hematuria, and crystalluria may be noted. Blood dyscrasias and jaundice are potential late manifestations of overdosage. Signs of acute overdosage with trimethoprim include nausea, vomiting, dizziness, headache, mental depression, confusion, and bone marrow depression.

General principles of treatment include the administration of intravenous fluids if urine output is low and renal func-

Continued on next page

Glaxo Wellcome—Cont.

tion is normal. Acidification of the urine will increase renal elimination of trimethoprim.

The patient should be monitored with blood counts and appropriate blood chemistries, including electrolytes. If a significant blood dyscrasia or jaundice occurs, specific therapy should be instituted for these complications. Peritoneal dialysis is not effective and hemodialysis is only moderately effective in eliminating trimethoprim and sulfamethoxazole.

Chronic: Use of SEPTRA I.V. Infusion at high doses and/or for extended periods of time may cause bone marrow depression manifested as thrombocytopenia, leukopenia, and/or megaloblastic anemia. If signs of bone marrow depression occur, the patient should be given leucovorin; 5 to 15 mg leucovorin daily has been recommended by some investigators.

Animal Toxicity: The LD_{50} of SEPTRA I.V. Infusion in mice is 700 mg/kg or 7.3 mL/kg; in rats and rabbits the LD_{50} is >500 mg/kg or >5.2 mL/kg. The vehicle produced the same LD_{50} in each of these species as the active drug.

The signs and symptoms noted in mice, rats, and rabbits with SEPTRA I.V. Infusion or its vehicle at the high I.V. doses used in acute toxicity studies included ataxia, decreased motor activity, loss of righting reflex, tremors or convulsions, and/or respiratory depression.

DOSAGE AND ADMINISTRATION

CONTRAINDICATED IN INFANTS LESS THAN TWO MONTHS OF AGE. CAUTION—SEPTRA I.V. INFUSION MUST BE DILUTED IN 5% DEXTROSE IN WATER SOLUTION PRIOR TO ADMINISTRATION. DO NOT MIX SEPTRA I.V. INFUSION WITH OTHER DRUGS OR SOLUTIONS. RAPID INFUSION OR BOLUS INJECTION MUST BE AVOIDED.

DOSAGE

Children and Adults:

PNEUMOCYSTIS CARINII PNEUMONIA: Total daily dose is 15 to 20 mg/kg (based on the trimethoprim component) given in three to four equally divided doses every 6 or 8 hours for up to 14 days. One investigator noted that a total daily dose of 10 to 15 mg/kg was sufficient in 10 adult patients with normal renal function.[6]

SEVERE URINARY TRACT INFECTIONS AND SHIGELLOSIS: Total daily dose is 8 to 10 mg/kg (based on the trimethoprim component) given in two to four equally divided doses every 6, 8, or 12 hours for up to 14 days for severe urinary tract infections and 5 days for shigellosis. The maximum recommended daily dose is 60 mL per day.

For Patients with Impaired Renal Function: When renal function is impaired, a reduced dosage should be employed using the following table:

Creatinine Clearance (mL/min)	Recommended Dosage Regimen
Above 30	Use Standard Regimen
15–30	$^1/_2$ the Usual Regimen
Below 15	Use Not Recommended

Method of Preparation: SEPTRA I.V. Infusion must be diluted. EACH 5 mL SHOULD BE ADDED TO 125 mL OF 5% DEXTROSE IN WATER. After diluting with 5% dextrose in water, the solution should not be refrigerated and should be used within 6 hours. If a dilution of 5 mL per 100 mL of 5% dextrose in water is desired, it should be used within 4 hours. If upon visual inspection there is cloudiness or evidence of crystallization after mixing, the solution should be discarded and a fresh solution prepared.

Multiple Dose Vial: After initial entry into the vial, the remaining contents must be used within 48 hours.

The following infusion systems have been tested and found satisfactory: unit-dose glass containers; unit-dose polyvinyl chloride and polyolefin containers. No other systems have been tested and, therefore, no others can be recommended.

Dilution: EACH 5 mL OF SEPTRA I.V. INFUSION SHOULD BE ADDED TO 125 mL OF 5% DEXTROSE IN WATER.

NOTE: In those instances where fluid restriction is desirable, each 5 mL may be added to 75 mL of 5% dextrose in water. Under these circumstances the solution should be mixed just prior to use and should be administered within two (2) hours. If upon visual inspection there is cloudiness or evidence of crystallization after mixing, the solution should be discarded and a fresh solution prepared.

DO NOT MIX SEPTRA I.V. INFUSION-5% DEXTROSE IN WATER WITH DRUGS OR SOLUTIONS IN THE SAME CONTAINER.

ADMINISTRATION

The solution should be given by intravenous infusion over a period of 60 to 90 minutes. Rapid infusion or bolus injections

must be avoided. SEPTRA I.V. Infusion should not be given intramuscularly.

HOW SUPPLIED

5 mL vials, containing 80 mg trimethoprim (16 mg/mL) and 400 mg sulfamethoxazole (80 mg/mL) for infusion with 5% dextrose in water. Contains benzyl alcohol (see WARNINGS). Tray of 10 (NDC 0173-0856-44).

10 mL multiple dose vials, containing 160 mg trimethoprim (16 mg/mL) and 800 mg sulfamethoxazole (80 mg/mL) for infusion with 5% dextrose in water. Contains benzyl alcohol (see WARNINGS). Tray of 10 (NDC 0173-0856-95).

20 mL multiple dose vials, containing 320 mg trimethoprim (16 mg/mL) and 1600 mg sulfamethoxazole (80 mg/mL) for infusion with 5% dextrose in water. Contains benzyl alcohol (see WARNINGS). Tray of 10 (NDC 0173-0856-01).

STORE AT 15° to 25°C (59° to 77°F). DO NOT REFRIGERATE.

Also available in tablets containing 80 mg trimethoprim and 400 mg sulfamethoxazole (bottle of 100); DS (double strength) tablets containing 160 mg trimethoprim and 800 mg sulfamethoxazole (bottles of 100 and 250); and oral suspension containing 40 mg trimethoprim and 200 mg sulfamethoxazole in each 5 mL (pink, cherry-flavored: bottle of 1 pint [473 mL], 100 mL—package of 6; and purple, grape-flavored: bottle of 1 pint [473 mL]).

REFERENCES

1. Grose WE, Bodey GP, Loo TL. Clinical pharmacology of intravenously administered trimethoprim-sulfamethoxazole. *Antimicrob Agents Chemother.* 1979;15:447–451.
2. Siber GR, Gorham C, Durbin W, Lesko L, Levin MJ. Pharmacology of intravenous trimethoprim-sulfamethoxazole in children and adults. In: Nelson JD, Grassi C, eds. *Current Chemotherapy of Infectious Disease.* Washington, DC: American Society for Microbiology; 1980;1:691–692.
3. Bauer AW, Kirby WMM, Sherris JC, Turck M. Antibiotic susceptibility testing by standardized single disk method. *Am J Clin Pathol.* 1966;45:493–496.
4. National Committee for Clinical Laboratory Standards. Performance standards for antimicrobial disk susceptibility tests, 2nd ed. Villanova, PA. 1979.
5. Brumfitt W, Pursell R. Trimethoprim-sulfamethoxazole in the treatment of bacteriuria in women. *J Infect Dis.* 1973;128 (suppl):S657–S663.
6. Winston DJ, Lau WK, Gale RP, Young LS. Trimethoprim-sulfamethoxazole for the treatment of *Pneumocystis carinii* pneumonia. *Ann Intern Med.* 1980;92:762–769.

March 1996/RL-295

Shown in Product Identification Guide, page 314

SEPTRA® I.V. Infusion   ℞

[sĕp'tra]

ADD-Vantage® Vials

(trimethoprim and sulfamethoxazole)

DESCRIPTION

SEPTRA I.V. Infusion (trimethoprim and sulfamethoxazole), a sterile solution for intravenous infusion only, is a synthetic antibacterial combination product. Each mL contains 16 mg trimethoprim and 80 mg sulfamethoxazole compounded with 40% propylene glycol, 10% ethyl alcohol, and 0.3% diethanolamine; 1% benzyl alcohol and 0.1% sodium metabisulfite added as preservatives, Water for Injection, and pH adjusted to approximately 10 with sodium hydroxide.

Trimethoprim is 5-[(3,4,5-trimethoxyphenyl)methyl]-2,4-pyrimidinediamine. It is a white to light yellow, odorless, bitter compound with a molecular weight of 290.32 and the molecular formula $C_{14}H_{18}N_4O_3$.

Sulfamethoxazole is 4-amino-*N*-(5-methyl-3-isoxazolyl) benzenesulfonamide. It is an almost white, odorless, tasteless compound with a molecular weight of 253.28 and the molecular formula $C_{10}H_{11}N_3O_3S$.

CLINICAL PHARMACOLOGY

Following a 1-hour intravenous infusion of a single dose of 160 mg trimethoprim and 800 mg sulfamethoxazole to 11 patients whose weight ranged from 105 lb to 165 lb (mean, 143 lb), the mean peak plasma concentrations of trimethoprim and sulfamethoxazole were 3.4 ± 0.3 µg/mL and 46.3 ± 2.7 µg/mL, respectively. Following repeated intravenous administration of the same dose at 8-hour intervals, the mean plasma concentrations just prior to and immediately after each infusion at steady state were 5.6 ± 0.6 µg/mL and 8.8 ± 0.9 µg/mL for trimethoprim and 70.6 ± 7.3 µg/mL and 105.6 ± 10.9 µg/mL for sulfamethoxazole. The mean plasma half-life was 11.3 ± 0.7 hours for trimethoprim and 12.8 ± 1.8 hours for sulfamethoxazole. All of these 11 patients had normal renal function and their ages ranged from 17 to 78 years (median, 60 years)[1].

Pharmacokinetic studies in children and adults suggest an age-dependent half-life of trimethoprim as indicated in the following table.[2]

Age (yrs.)	No. of Patients	Mean Trimethoprim Half-life (hours)
<1	2	7.67
1–10	9	5.49
10–20	5	8.19
20–63	6	12.82

Patients with severely impaired renal function exhibit an increase in the half-lives of both components, requiring dosage regimen adjustment (see DOSAGE AND ADMINISTRATION).

Both trimethoprim and sulfamethoxazole exist in the blood as unbound, protein-bound, and metabolized forms; sulfamethoxazole also exists as the conjugated form. The metabolism of sulfamethoxazole occurs predominately by N_4-acetylation, although the glucuronide conjugate has been identified. The principal metabolites of trimethoprim are the 1- and 3- oxides and the 3'- and 4'-hydroxy derivatives. The free forms of trimethoprim and sulfamethoxazole are considered to be the therapeutically active forms. Approximately 44% of trimethoprim and 70% of sulfamethoxazole are bound to plasma proteins. The presence of 10 mg percent sulfamethoxazole in plasma decreases the protein binding of trimethoprim by an insignificant degree; trimethoprim does not influence the protein binding of sulfamethoxazole.

Excretion of trimethoprim and sulfamethoxazole is primarily by the kidneys through both glomerular filtration and tubular secretion. Urine concentrations of both trimethoprim and sulfamethoxazole are considerably higher than are the concentrations in the blood. The percent of dose excreted in urine over a 12-hour period following the intravenous administration of the first dose of 240 mg of trimethoprim and 1200 mg of sulfamethoxazole on day 1 ranged from 17% to 42.4% as free trimethoprim; 7% to 12.7% as free sulfamethoxazole; and 36.7% to 56% as total (free plus the N_4-acetylated metabolite) sulfamethoxazole. When administered together as SEPTRA, neither trimethoprim nor sulfamethoxazole affects the urinary excretion pattern of the other.

Both trimethoprim and sulfamethoxazole distribute to sputum and vaginal fluid; trimethoprim also distributes to bronchial secretions and both pass the placental barrier and are excreted in breast milk.

Microbiology: Sulfamethoxazole inhibits bacterial synthesis of dihydrofolic acid by competing with *para*-aminobenzoic acid (PABA). Trimethoprim blocks the production of tetrahydrofolic acid from dihydrofolic acid by binding to and reversibly inhibiting the required enzyme, dihydrofolate reductase. Thus, SEPTRA blocks two consecutive steps in the biosynthesis of nucleic acids and proteins essential to many bacteria.

In vitro studies have shown that bacterial resistance develops more slowly with SEPTRA than with trimethoprim or sulfamethoxazole alone.

In vitro serial dilution tests have shown that the spectrum of antibacterial activity of SEPTRA includes common bacterial pathogens with the exception of *Pseudomonas aeruginosa.* The following organisms are usually susceptible: *Escherichia coli, Klebsiella* species, *Enterobacter* species, *Morganella morganii, Proteus mirabilis,* indole-positive *Proteus* species, including *Proteus vulgaris, Haemophilus influenzae* (including ampicillin-resistant strains), *Streptococcus pneumoniae, Shigella flexneri,* and *Shigella sonnei.* It should be noted, however, that there are little clinical data on the use of SEPTRA I.V. Infusion in serious systemic infections due to *Haemophilus influenzae* and *Streptococcus pneumoniae.*

[See table at top of next page.]

Susceptibility Testing: The recommended quantitative disc susceptibility method may be used for estimating the susceptibility of bacteria to SEPTRA.[3,4] With this procedure, a report from the laboratory of "Susceptible to trimethoprim and sulfamethoxazole" indicates that the infection is likely to respond to therapy with SEPTRA. If the infection is confined to the urine, a report of "Intermediate susceptibility to trimethoprim and sulfamethoxazole" also indicates that the infection is likely to respond. A report of "Resistant to trimethoprim and sulfamethoxazole" indicates that the infection is unlikely to respond to therapy with SEPTRA.

INDICATIONS AND USAGE

PNEUMOCYSTIS CARINII PNEUMONIA: SEPTRA I.V. Infusion is indicated in the treatment of *Pneumocystis carinii* pneumonia in children and adults.

SHIGELLOSIS: SEPTRA I.V. Infusion is indicated in the treatment of enteritis caused by susceptible strains of *Shigella flexneri* and *Shigella sonnei* in children and adults.

URINARY TRACT INFECTIONS: SEPTRA I.V. Infusion is indicated in the treatment of severe or complicated urinary tract infections due to susceptible strains of *Escherichia coli, Klebsiella* species, *Enterobacter* species, *Morganella morganii,* and *Proteus* species when oral administration of SEPTRA is not feasible and when the organism is not susceptible to single agent antibacterials effective in the urinary tract.

Although appropriate culture and susceptibility studies should be performed, therapy may be started while awaiting the results of these studies.

REPRESENTATIVE MINIMUM INHIBITORY CONCENTRATION VALUES FOR ORGANISMS SUSCEPTIBLE TO SEPTRA (MIC-μg/mL)

Bacteria	Trimethoprim Alone	Sulfamethoxazole Alone	Trimethoprim/Sulfamethoxazole (1:19) Trimethoprim	Sulfamethoxazole
Escherichia coli	0.05–1.5	1.0–245	0.05–0.5	0.95–9.5
Proteus species (indole positive)	0.5–5.0	7.35–300	0.05–1.5	0.95–28.5
Morganella morganii	0.5–5.0	7.35–300	0.05–1.5	0.95–28.5
Proteus mirabilis	0.5–1.5	7.35–30	0.05–0.15	0.95–2.85
Klebsiella species	0.15–5.0	2.45–245	0.05–1.5	0.95–28.5
Enterobacter species	0.15–5.0	2.45–245	0.05–1.5	0.95–28.5
Haemophilus influenzae	0.15–1.5	2.85–95	0.015–0.15	0.285–2.85
Streptococcus pneumoniae	0.15–1.5	7.35–24.5	0.05–0.15	0.95–2.85
Shigella flexneri *	< 0.01–0.04	< 0.16–> 320	< 0.002–0.03	0.04–0.625
Shigella sonnei *	0.02–0.08	0.625–> 320	0.004–0.06	0.08–1.25

* Rudoy RC, Nelson JD, Haltalin KC. *Antimicrobial Agents and Chemotherapy.* 1974; 5:439-443.

CONTRAINDICATIONS

SEPTRA is contraindicated in patients with a known hypersensitivity to trimethoprim or sulfonamides and in patients with documented megaloblastic anemia due to folate deficiency. SEPTRA is also contraindicated in pregnant patients at term and in nursing mothers, because sulfonamides pass the placenta and are excreted in the milk and may cause kernicterus. SEPTRA is contraindicated in infants less than two months of age.

WARNINGS

FATALITIES ASSOCIATED WITH THE ADMINISTRATION OF SULFONAMIDES, ALTHOUGH RARE, HAVE OCCURRED DUE TO SEVERE REACTIONS, INCLUDING STEVENS-JOHNSON SYNDROME, TOXIC EPIDERMAL NECROLYSIS, FULMINANT HEPATIC NECROSIS, AGRANULOCYTOSIS, APLASTIC ANEMIA, OTHER BLOOD DYSCRASIAS, AND HYPERSENSITIVITY OF THE RESPIRATORY TRACT.

SEPTRA SHOULD BE DISCONTINUED AT THE FIRST APPEARANCE OF SKIN RASH OR ANY SIGN OF ADVERSE REACTION. Clinical signs, such as rash, sore throat, fever, arthralgia, cough, shortness of breath, pallor, purpura, or jaundice may be early indications of serious reactions. Cough, shortness of breath, and/or pulmonary infiltrates may be indicators of pulmonary hypersensitivity to sulfonamides. In rare instances, a skin rash may be followed by more severe reactions, such as Stevens-Johnson syndrome, toxic epidermal necrolysis, hepatic necrosis, or serious blood disorder. Complete blood counts should be done frequently in patients receiving sulfonamides.

SEPTRA SHOULD NOT BE USED IN THE TREATMENT OF STREPTOCOCCAL PHARYNGITIS. Clinical studies have documented that patients with group A β-hemolytic streptococcal tonsillopharyngitis have a greater incidence of bacteriologic failure when treated with SEPTRA than do those patients treated with penicillin, as evidenced by failure to eradicate this organism from the tonsillopharyngeal area.

Contains sodium metabisulfite, a sulfite that may cause allergic-type reactions including anaphylactic symptoms and life-threatening or less severe asthmatic episodes in certain susceptible people. The overall prevalence of sulfite sensitivity in the general population is unknown and probably low. Sulfite sensitivity is seen more frequently in asthmatic than in nonasthmatic people.

Contains benzyl alcohol. In newborn infants, benzyl alcohol has been associated with an increased incidence of neurological and other complications which are sometimes fatal.

PRECAUTIONS

General: SEPTRA should be given with caution to patients with impaired renal or hepatic function, to those with possible folate deficiency (e.g., the elderly, chronic alcoholics, patients receiving anticonvulsant therapy, patients with malabsorption syndrome, and patients in malnutrition states), and to those with severe allergy or bronchial asthma. In glucose-6-phosphate dehydrogenase-deficient individuals, hemolysis may occur. This reaction is frequently dose-related.

Adequate fluid intake must be maintained in order to prevent crystalluria and stone formation (see CLINICAL PHARMACOLOGY and DOSAGE AND ADMINISTRATION).

Local irritation and inflammation due to extravascular infiltration of the infusion has been observed with SEPTRA I.V. Infusion. If these occur, the infusion should be discontinued and restarted at another site.

Use in the Elderly: There may be an increased risk of severe adverse reactions in elderly patients, particularly when complicating conditions exist, e.g., impaired kidney and/or liver function, or concomitant use of other drugs. Severe skin reactions, or generalized bone marrow suppression (see WARNINGS and ADVERSE REACTIONS), or a specific decrease in platelets (with or without purpura) are the most frequently reported severe adverse reactions in elderly patients. In those concurrently receiving certain diuretics, primarily thiazides, an increased incidence of thrombocytopenia with purpura has been reported. Appropriate dosage adjustments should be made for patients with impaired kidney function (see DOSAGE AND ADMINISTRATION).

Use in the Treatment of *Pneumocystis carinii* Pneumonia in Patients with Acquired Immunodeficiency Syndrome (AIDS): The incidence of side effects, particularly rash, fever, leukopenia, elevated aminotransferase (transaminase) values in AIDS patients who are being treated with SEPTRA for *Pneumocystis carinii* pneumonia has been reported to be greatly increased compared with the incidence normally associated with the use of SEPTRA in non-AIDS patients. The incidence of hyperkalemia and hyponatremia appears to be increased in AIDS patients receiving SEPTRA. The concomitant use of leucovorin with trimethoprim-sulfamethoxazole for the acute treatment of *Pneumocystis carinii* pneumonia in patients with HIV infection was associated with increased rates of treatment failure and morbidity in a placebo-controlled study.

Laboratory Tests: Appropriate culture and susceptibility studies should be performed before and throughout treatment. Complete blood counts should be done frequently in patients receiving SEPTRA; if a significant reduction in the count of any formed blood element is noted, SEPTRA should be discontinued. Urinalyses with careful microscopic examination and renal function tests should be performed during therapy, particularly for those patients with impaired renal function.

Drug Interactions: In elderly patients concurrently receiving certain diuretics, primarily thiazides, an increased incidence of thrombocytopenia with purpura has been reported. It has been reported that SEPTRA may prolong the prothrombin time in patients who are receiving the anticoagulant warfarin. This interaction should be kept in mind when SEPTRA is given to patients already on anticoagulant therapy, and the coagulation time should be reassessed.

SEPTRA may inhibit the hepatic metabolism of phenytoin. SEPTRA, given at a common clinical dosage, increased the phenytoin half-life by 39% and decreased the phenytoin metabolic clearance rate by 27%. When administering these drugs concurrently, one should be alert for possible excessive phenytoin effect.

Sulfonamides can also displace methotrexate from plasma protein binding sites, thus increasing free methotrexate concentrations.

Drug/Laboratory Test Interactions: SEPTRA, specifically the trimethoprim component, can interfere with a serum methotrexate assay as determined by the competitive binding protein technique (CBPA) when a bacterial dihydrofolate reductase is used as the binding protein. No interference occurs, however, if methotrexate is measured by a radioimmunoassay (RIA).

The presence of trimethoprim and sulfamethoxazole may also interfere with the Jaffé alkaline picrate reaction assay for creatinine, resulting in over-estimations of about 10% in the range of normal values.

Carcinogenesis, Mutagenesis, Impairment of Fertility:

Carcinogenesis: Long-term studies in animals to evaluate carcinogenic potential have not been conducted with SEPTRA I.V. Infusion.

Mutagenesis: Bacterial mutagenic studies have not been performed with sulfamethoxazole and trimethoprim in combination. Trimethoprim was demonstrated to be non-mutagenic in the Ames assay. In studies at two laboratories, no chromosomal damage was detected in cultured Chinese hamster ovary cells at concentrations approximately 500 times human plasma levels; at concentrations approximately 1000 times human plasma levels in these same cells, a low level of chromosomal damage was induced at one of the laboratories. No chromosomal abnormalities were observed in cultured human leukocytes at concentrations of trimethoprim up to 20 times human steady-state plasma levels. No chromosomal effects were detected in peripheral lymphocytes of human subjects receiving 320 mg of trimethoprim in combination with up to 1600 mg of sulfamethoxazole per day for as long as 112 weeks.

Impairment of Fertility: SEPTRA I.V. Infusion has not been studied in animals for evidence of impairment of fertility. However, studies in rats at oral dosages as high as 70 mg/kg trimethoprim plus 350 mg/kg sulfamethoxazole daily showed no adverse effects on fertility or general reproductive performance.

Pregnancy: ***Teratogenic Effects:*** Pregnancy Category C. In rats, oral doses of 533 mg/kg sulfamethoxazole or 200 mg/kg trimethoprim produced teratological effects manifested mainly as cleft palates. The highest dose which did not cause cleft palates in rats was 512 mg/kg sulfamethoxazole or 192 mg/kg trimethoprim when administered separately. In two studies in rats, no teratology was observed when 512 mg/kg of sulfamethoxazole was used in combination with 128 mg/kg of trimethoprim. In one study, however, cleft palates were observed in one litter out of nine when 355 mg/kg of sulfamethoxazole was used in combination with 88 mg/kg of trimethoprim.

In some rabbit studies, an overall increase in fetal loss (dead and resorbed and malformed conceptuses) was associated with doses of trimethoprim six times the human therapeutic dose.

While there are no large, well-controlled studies on the use of trimethoprim and sulfamethoxazole in pregnant women, Brumfitt and Pursell,[5] in a retrospective study, reported the outcome of 186 pregnancies during which the mother received either placebo or oral trimethoprim and sulfamethoxazole. The incidence of congenital abnormalities was 4.5% (3 of 66) in those who received placebo and 3.3% (4 of 120) in those receiving trimethoprim and sulfamethoxazole. There were no abnormalities in the 10 children whose mothers received the drug during the first trimester. In a separate survey, Brumfitt and Pursell also found no congenital abnormalities in 35 children whose mothers had received oral trimethoprim and sulfamethoxazole at the time of conception or shortly thereafter.

Because trimethoprim and sulfamethoxazole may interfere with folic acid metabolism, SEPTRA I.V. Infusion should be used during pregnancy only if the potential benefit justifies the potential risk to the fetus.

Nonteratogenic Effects: See CONTRAINDICATIONS section.

Nursing Mothers: See CONTRAINDICATIONS section.

Pediatric Use: SEPTRA I.V. Infusion is not recommended for infants younger than two months of age (see CONTRAINDICATIONS).

ADVERSE REACTIONS

The most common adverse effects are gastrointestinal disturbances (nausea, vomiting, anorexia) and allergic skin reactions (such as rash and urticaria). **FATALITIES ASSOCIATED WITH THE ADMINISTRATION OF SULFONAMIDES, ALTHOUGH RARE, HAVE OCCURRED DUE TO SEVERE REACTIONS, INCLUDING STEVENS-JOHNSON SYNDROME, TOXIC EPIDERMAL NECROLYSIS, FULMINANT HEPATIC NECROSIS, AGRANULOCYTOSIS, APLASTIC ANEMIA, OTHER BLOOD DYSCRASIAS, AND HYPERSENSITIVITY OF THE RESPIRATORY TRACT (SEE WARNINGS).** Local reaction, pain, and slight irritation on I.V. administration are infrequent. Thrombophlebitis has rarely been observed.

Hematologic: Agranulocytosis, aplastic anemia, thrombocytopenia, leukopenia, neutropenia, hemolytic anemia, megaloblastic anemia, hypoprothrombinemia, methemoglobinemia, eosinophilia.

Allergic: Stevens-Johnson syndrome, toxic epidermal necrolysis, anaphylaxis, allergic myocarditis, erythema multiforme, exfoliative dermatitis, angioedema, drug fever, chills, Henoch-Schönlein purpura, serum sickness-like syndrome, generalized allergic reactions, generalized skin eruptions, conjunctival and scleral injection, photosensitivity, pruritus, urticaria, and rash. In addition, periarteritis nodosa and systemic lupus erythematosus have been reported.

Gastrointestinal: Hepatitis, including cholestatic jaundice and hepatic necrosis, elevation of serum transaminase and bilirubin, pseudomembranous enterocolitis, pancreatitis, stomatitis, glossitis, nausea, emesis, abdominal pain, diarrhea, anorexia.

Genitourinary: Renal failure, interstitial nephritis, BUN and serum creatinine elevation, toxic nephrosis with oliguria and anuria, and crystalluria.

Metabolic: Hyperkalemia, hyponatremia.

Neurologic: Aseptic meningitis, convulsions, peripheral neuritis, ataxia, vertigo, tinnitus, headache.

Psychiatric: Hallucinations, depression, apathy, nervousness.

Endocrine: The sulfonamides bear certain chemical similarities to some goitrogens, diuretics (acetazolamide and the thiazides), and oral hypoglycemic agents. Cross-sensitivity may exist with these agents. Diuresis and hypoglycemia have occurred rarely in patients receiving sulfonamides.

Continued on next page

Glaxo Wellcome—Cont.

Musculoskeletal: Arthralgia and myalgia.
Respiratory System: Pulmonary infiltrates, cough, shortness of breath.
Miscellaneous: Weakness, fatigue, insomnia.

OVERDOSAGE

Acute: Since there has been no extensive experience in humans with single doses of SEPTRA I.V. Infusion in excess of 25 mL (400 mg trimethoprim and 2000 mg sulfamethoxazole), the maximum tolerated dose in humans is unknown. Signs and symptoms of overdosage reported with sulfonamides include anorexia, colic, nausea, vomiting, dizziness, headache, drowsiness, and unconsciousness. Pyrexia, hematuria, and crystalluria may be noted. Blood dyscrasias and jaundice are potential late manifestations of overdosage. Signs of acute overdosage with trimethoprim include nausea, vomiting, dizziness, headache, mental depression, confusion, and bone marrow depression.
General principles of treatment include the administration of intravenous fluids if urine output is low and renal function is normal. Acidification of the urine will increase renal elimination of trimethoprim. The patient should be monitored with blood counts and appropriate blood chemistries, including electrolytes. If a significant blood dyscrasia or jaundice occurs, specific therapy should be instituted for these complications. Peritoneal dialysis is not effective and hemodialysis is only moderately effective in eliminating trimethoprim and sulfamethoxazole.
Chronic: Use of SEPTRA I.V. Infusion at high doses and/or for extended periods of time may cause bone marrow depression manifested as thrombocytopenia, leukopenia, and/or megaloblastic anemia. If signs of bone marrow depression occur, the patient should be given leucovorin; 5 to 15 mg leucovorin daily has been recommended by some investigators.
Animal Toxicity: The LD_{50} of SEPTRA I.V. Infusion in mice is 700 mg/kg or 7.3 mL/kg; in rats and rabbits the LD_{50} is >500 mg/kg or >5.2 mL/kg. The vehicle produced the same LD_{50} in each of these species as the active drug.
The signs and symptoms noted in mice, rats, and rabbits with SEPTRA I.V. Infusion or its vehicle at the high I.V. doses used in acute toxicity studies included ataxia, decreased motor activity, loss of righting reflex, tremors or convulsions, and/ or respiratory depression.

DOSAGE AND ADMINISTRATION

CONTRAINDICATED IN INFANTS LESS THAN TWO MONTHS OF AGE. CAUTION—SEPTRA I.V. INFUSION MUST BE DILUTED IN 5% DEXTROSE IN WATER SOLUTION PRIOR TO ADMINISTRATION. DO NOT MIX SEPTRA I.V. INFUSION WITH OTHER DRUGS OR SOLUTIONS. RAPID INFUSION OR BOLUS INJECTION MUST BE AVOIDED.

DOSAGE

Children and Adults:
PNEUMOCYSTIS CARINII PNEUMONIA: Total daily dose is 15 to 20 mg/kg (based on the trimethoprim component) given in three to four equally divided doses every 6 or 8 hours for up to 14 days. One investigator noted that a total daily dose of 10 to 15 mg/kg was sufficient in 10 adult patients with normal renal function.[6]
SEVERE URINARY TRACT INFECTIONS AND SHIGELLOSIS: Total daily dose is 8 to 10 mg/kg (based on the trimethoprim component) given in two to four equally divided doses every 6, 8, or 12 hours for up to 14 days for severe urinary tract infections and 5 days for shigellosis. The maximum recommended daily dose is 60 mL per day.
For Patients with Impaired Renal Function: When renal function is impaired, a reduced dosage should be employed using the following table:

Creatinine Clearance (mL/min)	Recommended Dosage Regimen
Above 30	Use Standard Regimen
15–30	$1/2$ the Usual Regimen
Below 15	Use Not Recommended

Method of Preparation: SEPTRA I.V. Infusion must be diluted. EACH 10 ML ADD-Vantage VIAL SHOULD BE ADDED TO 250 ML OF 5% DEXTROSE IN WATER AND USED WITHIN 6 HOURS. If upon visual inspection there is cloudiness or evidence of crystallization after mixing, the solution should be discarded and a fresh solution prepared. DO NOT MIX SEPTRA I.V. INFUSION-5% DEXTROSE IN WATER WITH DRUGS OR SOLUTIONS IN THE SAME CONTAINER.
After diluting with 5% dextrose in water, the solution should not be refrigerated and should be administered within the specified time.

ADMINISTRATION

The solution should be given by intravenous infusion over a period of 60 to 90 minutes. Rapid infusion or bolus injections must be avoided. SEPTRA I.V. Infusion should not be given intramuscularly.

INSTRUCTIONS FOR USE

To Open Diluent Container:
Peel overwrap from the corner and remove container. Some opacity of the plastic due to moisture absorption during the sterilization process may be observed. This is normal and does not affect the solution quality or safety. The opacity will diminish gradually.
To Assemble ADD-Vantage® Vial and Flexible Diluent Container:
(Use Aseptic Technique)
1. Remove the protective covers from the top of the vial and the vial port on the diluent container as follows:
   a. To remove the breakaway vial cap, swing the pull ring over the top of the vial and pull down far enough to start the opening (see Figure 1), then pull straight up to remove the cap. (see Figure 2.) **NOTE:** Once the breakaway cap has been removed, do not access vial with syringe.

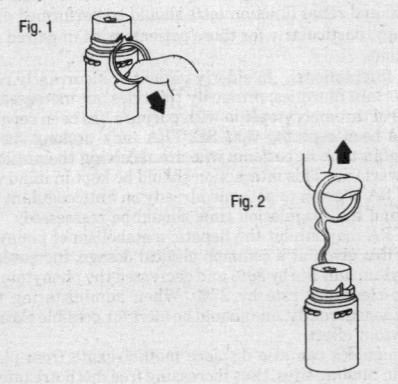

Fig. 1

Fig. 2

   b. To remove the vial port cover, grasp the tab on the pull ring, pull up to break the three tie strings, then pull back to remove the cover (see Figure 3).
2. Screw the vial into the vial port until it will go no further. THE VIAL MUST BE SCREWED IN TIGHTLY TO ASSURE A SEAL. This occurs approximately $1/2$ turn (180°) after the first audible click (see Figure 4). The clicking sound does not assure a seal; the vial must be turned as far as it will go. **NOTE:** Once vial is seated, do not attempt to remove (see Figure 4).
3. Recheck the vial to assure that it is tight by trying to turn it further in the direction of assembly.
4. Label appropriately.

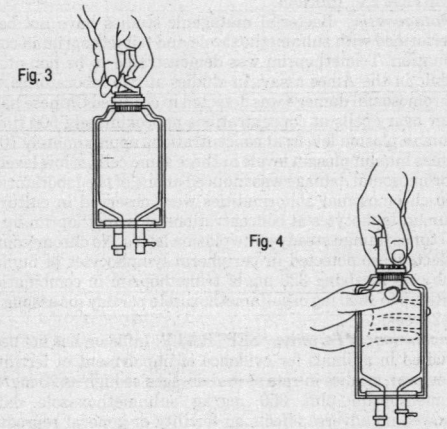

Fig. 3

Fig. 4

To Prepare Admixture:
1. Squeeze the bottom of the diluent container gently to inflate the portion of the container surrounding the end of the drug vial.
2. With the other hand, push the drug vial down into the container telescoping the walls of the container. Grasp the inner cap of the vial through the walls of the container (see Figure 5).
3. Pull the inner cap from the drug vial (see Figure 6.) Verify that the rubber stopper has been pulled out, allowing the drug and diluent to mix.
4. Mix container contents thoroughly and use within the specified time.
[See Figure at top of next column.]

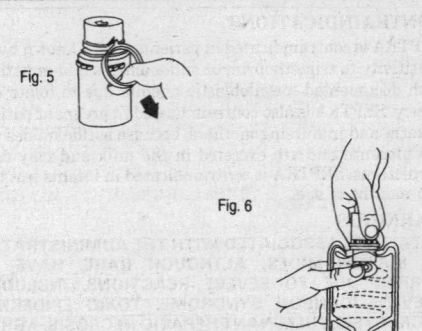

Fig. 5

Fig. 6

Preparation for Administration:
(Use Aseptic Technique)
1. Confirm the activation and admixture of vial contents.
2. Check for leaks by squeezing container firmly. If leaks are found, discard unit as sterility may be impaired.
3. Close flow control clamp of administration set.
4. Remove cover from outlet port at bottom of container.
5. Insert piercing pin of administration set into port with a twisting motion until the pin is firmly seated. **NOTE:** See full directions on administration set carton.
6. Lift the free end of the hanger loop on the bottom of the vial, breaking the two tie strings. Bend the loop outward to lock it in the upright position, then suspend container from hanger.
7. Squeeze and release drip chamber to establish proper fluid level in chamber.
8. Open flow control clamp and clear air from set. Close clamp.
9. Attach set to venipuncture device. If device is not indwelling, prime and make venipuncture.
10. Regulate rate of administration with flow control clamp.

WARNING

Do not use flexible container in series connections.

HOW SUPPLIED

10 mL ADD-Vantage® Vial containing 160 mg trimethoprim (16 mg/mL) and 800 mg sulfamethoxazole (80 mg/mL) for infusion with 5% dextrose in water. Contains benzyl alcohol (see WARNINGS). Box of 10 (NDC 0173-0856-47).
Store at 15° to 25°C (59° to 77°F).
DO NOT REFRIGERATE.
Also Available:
SEPTRA I.V. infusion: 5 mL vials, containing 80 mg trimethoprim (16 mg/mL) and 400 mg sulfamethoxazole (80 mg/mL), tray of 10; 10 mL multiple dose vials containing 160 mg trimethoprim (16 mg/mL) and 800 mg sulfamethoxazole (80 mg/mL), tray of 10; 20 mL multiple dose vials containing 320 mg trimethoprim (16 mg/mL) and 1600 mg sulfamethoxazole (80 mg/mL), tray of 10.

REFERENCES

1. Grose WE, Bodey GP, Loo TL. Clinical pharmacology of intravenously administered trimethoprim-sulfamethoxazole. *Antimicrob Agents Chemother.* 1979;15:447–451.
2. Siber GR, Gorham C, Durbin W, Lesko L, Levin MJ. Pharmacology of intravenous trimethoprim-sulfamethoxazole in children and adults. In: Nelson JD, Grassi C, eds. *Current Chemotherapy of Infectious Disease.* Washington, DC: American Society for Microbiology; 1980;1:691–692.
3. Bauer AW, Kirby WMM, Sherris JC, Turck M. Antibiotic susceptibility testing by a standardized single disk method. *Am J Clin Pathol.* 1966;45:493–496.
4. National Committee for Clinical Laboratory Standards, Performance standards for antimicrobial disk susceptibility tests, 2nd ed. Villanova, Pa. 1979.
5. Brumfitt W, Pursell R. Trimethoprim/sulfamethoxazole in the treatment of bacteriuria in women. *J Infect Dis.* 1973;128(suppl):S657–S663.
6. Winston DJ, Lau WK, Gale RP, Young LS. Trimethoprim-sulfamethoxazole for the treatment of *Pneumocystis carinii* pneumonia. *Ann Intern Med.* 1980;92:762–769.

March 1996/RL-296
Shown in Product Identification Guide, page 314

SEPTRA® Tablets   ℞
[sĕp 'tra]
SEPTRA® DS (Double Strength) Tablets   ℞
SEPTRA® Suspension   ℞
SEPTRA® Grape Suspension   ℞
(trimethoprim and sulfamethoxazole)

DESCRIPTION

SEPTRA (trimethoprim and sulfamethoxazole) is a synthetic antibacterial combination product. Each SEPTRA Tablet

contains 80 mg trimethoprim and 400 mg sulfamethoxazole and the inactive ingredients docusate sodium, FD&C Red No. 40, magnesium stearate, povidone, and sodium starch glycolate.

Each SEPTRA DS (double strength) Tablet contains 160 mg trimethoprim and 800 mg sulfamethoxazole and the inactive ingredients docusate sodium, FD&C Red No. 40, magnesium stearate, povidone, and sodium starch glycolate.

Each teaspoonful (5 mL) of SEPTRA Suspension contains 40 mg trimethoprim and 200 mg sulfamethoxazole and the inactive ingredients alcohol 0.26%, methylparaben 0.1%, and sodium benzoate 0.1% (added as preservatives), carboxymethylcellulose sodium, citric acid, FD&C Red No. 40 and Yellow No. 6, flavor, glycerin, microcrystalline cellulose, polysorbate 80, saccharin sodium, and sorbitol. Each teaspoonful (5 mL) of SEPTRA Grape Suspension contains 40 mg trimethoprim and 200 mg sulfamethoxazole and the inactive ingredients alcohol 0.26%, methylparaben 0.1%, and sodium benzoate 0.1% (added as preservatives), carboxymethylcellulose sodium, citric acid, FD&C Red No. 40 and Blue No. 1, flavor, glycerin, microcrystalline cellulose, polysorbate 80, saccharin sodium, and sorbitol. Both tablet and suspension forms are for oral administration.

Trimethoprim is 5-[(3,4,5-trimethoxyphenyl)methyl]-2,4-pyrimidinediamine. It is a white to light yellow, odorless, bitter compound with a molecular weight of 290.32, and the molecular formula $C_{14}H_{18}N_4O_3$.

Sulfamethoxazole is 4-amino-*N*-(5-methyl-3-isoxazolyl) benzenesulfonamide. It is an almost white, odorless, tasteless compound with a molecular weight of 253.28, and the molecular formula $C_{10}H_{11}N_3O_3S$.

CLINICAL PHARMACOLOGY

SEPTRA is rapidly absorbed following oral administration. Both sulfamethoxazole and trimethoprim exist in the blood as unbound, protein-bound, and metabolized forms: sulfamethoxazole also exists as the conjugated form. The metabolism of sulfamethoxazole occurs predominately by N_4-acetylation, although the glucuronide conjugate has been identified. The principal metabolites of trimethoprim are the 1- and 3-oxides and the 3′- and 4′- hydroxy derivatives. The free forms of sulfamethoxazole and trimethoprim are considered to be the therapeutically active forms. Approximately 44% of trimethoprim and 70% of sulfamethoxazole are bound to plasma proteins. The presence of 10 mg percent sulfamethoxazole in plasma decreases the protein binding of trimethoprim by an insignificant degree; trimethoprim does not influence the protein binding of sulfamethoxazole.

Peak blood levels for the individual components occur 1 to 4 hours after oral administration. The mean serum half-lives of sulfamethoxazole and trimethoprim are 10 and 8 to 10 hours, respectively. However, patients with severely impaired renal function exhibit an increase in the half-lives of both components, requiring dosage regimen adjustment (see DOSAGE AND ADMINISTRATION section). Detectable amounts of trimethoprim and sulfamethoxazole are present in the blood 24 hours after drug administration. During administration of 160 mg trimethoprim and 800 mg sulfamethoxazole bid, the mean steady-state plasma concentration of trimethoprim was 1.72 μg/mL. The steady state minimal plasma levels of free and total sulfamethoxazole were 57.4 μg/mL and 68.0 μg/mL, respectively. These steady-state levels were achieved after three days of drug administration.[1]

Excretion of sulfamethoxazole and trimethoprim is primarily by the kidneys through both glomerular filtration and tubular secretion. Urine concentrations of both sulfamethoxazole and trimethoprim are considerably higher than are the concentrations in the blood. The average percentage of the dose recovered in urine from 0 to 72 hours after a single oral dose is 84.5% for total sulfonamide and 66.8% for free trimethoprim. Thirty percent of the total sulfonamide is excreted as free sulfamethoxazole, with the remaining as N_4-acetylated metabolite.[2] When administered together as SEPTRA, neither sulfamethoxazole nor trimethoprim affects the urinary excretion pattern of the other.

Both trimethoprim and sulfamethoxazole distribute to sputum, vaginal fluid, and middle ear fluid; trimethoprim also distributes to bronchial secretions, and both pass the placental barrier and are excreted in human milk.

Microbiology: Sulfamethoxazole inhibits bacterial synthesis of dihydrofolic acid by competing with *para*-aminobenzoic acid (PABA). Trimethoprim blocks the production of tetrahydrofolic acid from dihydrofolic acid by binding to and reversibly inhibiting the required enzyme, dihydrofolate reductase. Thus, SEPTRA blocks two consecutive steps in the biosynthesis of nucleic acids and proteins essential to many bacteria.

In vitro studies have shown that bacterial resistance develops more slowly with SEPTRA than with either trimethoprim or sulfamethoxazole alone.

In vitro serial dilution tests have shown that the spectrum of antibacterial activity of SEPTRA includes the common urinary tract pathogens with the exception of *Pseudomonas aeruginosa*. The following organisms are usually susceptible: *Escherichia coli*, *Klebsiella* species, *Enterobacter* species,

REPRESENTATIVE MINIMUM INHIBITORY CONCENTRATION VALUES FOR ORGANISMS SUSCEPTIBLE TO SEPTRA (MIC·μg/mL)

Bacteria	TMP Alone	SMX Alone	TMP/SMX (1:19)	
			TMP	SMX
Escherichia coli	0.05-1.5	1.0-245	0.05-0.5	0.95-9.5
Escherichia coli (enterotoxigenic strains)	0.015-0.15	0.285->950	0.005-0.15	0.095-2.85
Proteus species (indole positive)	0.5-5.0	7.35-300	0.05-1.5	0.95-28.5
Morganella morganii	0.5-5.0	7.35-300	0.05-1.5	0.95-28.5
Proteus mirabilis	0.5-1.5	7.35-30	0.05-0.15	0.95-2.85
Klebsiella species	0.15-5.0	2.45-245	0.05-1.5	0.95-28.5
Enterobacter species	0.15-5.0	2.45-245	0.05-1.5	0.95-28.5
Haemophilus influenzae	0.15-1.5	2.85-95	0.015-0.15	0.285-2.85
Streptococcus pneumoniae	0.15-1.5	7.35-24.5	0.05-0.15	0.95-2.85
Shigella flexneri *	<0.01-0.04	<0.16->320	<0.002-0.03	0.04-0.625
Shigella sonnei *	0.02-0.08	0.625->320	0.004-0.06	0.08-1.25

TMP = trimethoprim   SMX = sulfamethoxazole

*Rudoy RC, Nelson JD, Haltalin KC, *Antimicrobial Agents and Chemotherapy*. 1974; 5:439–443.

Morganella morganii, *Proteus mirabilis*, and indole-positive *Proteus* species including *Proteus vulgaris*.

The usual spectrum of antimicrobial activity of SEPTRA includes bacterial pathogens isolated from middle ear exudate and from bronchial secretions (*Haemophilus influenzae*, including ampicillin-resistant strains, and *Streptococcus pneumoniae*), and enterotoxigenic strains of *Escherichia coli* (ETEC) causing bacterial gastroenteritis. *Shigella flexneri* and *Shigella sonnei* are also usually susceptible.

[See table above.]

Susceptibility Testing: The recommended quantitative disc susceptibility method may be used for estimating the susceptibility of bacteria to SEPTRA.[3,4] With this procedure, a report from the laboratory of "Susceptible to trimethoprim and sulfamethoxazole" indicates that the infection is likely to respond to therapy with SEPTRA. If the infection is confined to the urine, a report of "Intermediate susceptibility to trimethoprim and sulfamethoxazole" also indicates that the infection is likely to respond. A report of "Resistant to trimethoprim and sulfamethoxazole" indicates that the infection is unlikely to respond to therapy with SEPTRA.

INDICATIONS AND USAGE

URINARY TRACT INFECTIONS: For the treatment of urinary tract infections due to susceptible strains of the following organisms: *Escherichia coli*, *Klebsiella* species, *Enterobacter* species, *Morganella morganii*, *Proteus mirabilis*, and *Proteus vulgaris*. It is recommended that initial episodes of uncomplicated urinary tract infections be treated with a single effective antibacterial agent rather than the combination.

ACUTE OTITIS MEDIA: For the treatment of acute otitis media in children due to susceptible strains of *Streptococcus pneumoniae* or *Haemophilus influenzae* when, in the judgment of the physician, SEPTRA offers some advantage over the use of other antimicrobial agents. To date, there are limited data on the safety of repeated use of SEPTRA in children under two years of age. SEPTRA is not indicated for prophylactic or prolonged administration in otitis media at any age.

ACUTE EXACERBATIONS OF CHRONIC BRONCHITIS IN ADULTS: For the treatment of acute exacerbations of chronic bronchitis due to susceptible strains of *Streptococcus pneumoniae* or *Haemophilus influenzae* when, in the judgment of the physician, SEPTRA offers some advantage over the use of a single antimicrobial agent.

TRAVELERS' DIARRHEA IN ADULTS: For the treatment of travelers' diarrhea due to susceptible strains of enterotoxigenic *E. coli*.

SHIGELLOSIS: For the treatment of enteritis caused by susceptible strains of *Shigella flexneri* and *Shigella sonnei* when antibacterial therapy is indicated.

PNEUMOCYSTIS CARINII PNEUMONIA: For the treatment of documented *pneumocystis carinii* pneumonia.

For prophylaxis against *Pneumocystis carinii* pneumonia in individuals who are immunosuppressed and considered to be at an increased risk of developing *Pneumocystis carinii* pneumonia.

CONTRAINDICATIONS

SEPTRA is contraindicated in patients with a known hypersensitivity to trimethoprim or sulfonamides and in patients with documented megaloblastic anemia due to folate deficiency. SEPTRA is also contraindicated in pregnant patients at term and in nursing mothers, because sulfonamides pass the placenta and are excreted in the milk and may cause kernicterus. SEPTRA is contraindicated in infants less than two months of age.

WARNINGS

FATALITIES ASSOCIATED WITH THE ADMINISTRATION OF SULFONAMIDES, ALTHOUGH RARE, HAVE OCCURRED DUE TO SEVERE REACTIONS, INCLUDING STEVENS-JOHNSON SYNDROME, TOXIC EPIDERMAL NECROLYSIS, FULMINANT HEPATIC NECROSIS, AGRANULOCYTOSIS, APLASTIC ANEMIA, OTHER BLOOD DYSCRASIAS, AND HYPERSENSITIVITY OF THE RESPIRATORY TRACT.

SEPTRA SHOULD BE DISCONTINUED AT THE FIRST APPEARANCE OF SKIN RASH OR ANY SIGN OF ADVERSE REACTION. Clinical signs, such as rash, sore throat, fever, arthralgia, cough, shortness of breath, pallor, purpura, or jaundice may be early indications of serious reactions. Cough, shortness of breath, and/or pulmonary infiltrates may be indicators of pulmonary hypersensitivity to sulfonamides. In rare instances a skin rash may be followed by more severe reactions, such as Stevens-Johnson syndrome, toxic epidermal necrolysis, hepatic necrosis, or serious blood disorder. Complete blood counts should be done frequently in patients receiving sulfonamides.

SEPTRA SHOULD NOT BE USED IN THE TREATMENT OF STREPTOCOCCAL PHARYNGITIS. Clinical studies have documented that patients with group A β-hemolytic streptococcal tonsillopharyngitis have a greater incidence of bacteriologic failure when treated with SEPTRA than do those patients treated with penicillin, as evidenced by failure to eradicate this organism from the tonsillopharyngeal area.

PRECAUTIONS

General: SEPTRA should be given with caution to patients with impaired renal or hepatic function, to those with possible folate deficiency (e.g., the elderly, chronic alcoholics, patients receiving anticonvulsant therapy, patients with malabsorption syndrome, and patients in malnutrition states), and to those with severe allergy or bronchial asthma. In glucose-6-phosphate dehydrogenase-deficient individuals, hemolysis may occur. This reaction is frequently dose-related. (see CLINICAL PHARMACOLOGY and DOSAGE AND ADMINISTRATION).

Use in the Elderly: There may be an increased risk of severe adverse reactions in elderly patients, particularly when complicating conditions exist, e.g., impaired kidney and/or liver function, or concomitant use of other drugs. Severe skin reactions, or generalized bone marrow suppression (see WARNINGS and ADVERSE REACTIONS), or a specific decrease in platelets (with or without purpura) are the most frequently reported severe adverse reactions in elderly patients. In those concurrently receiving certain diuretics, primarily thiazides, an increased incidence of thrombocytopenia with purpura has been reported. Appropriate dosage adjustments should be made for patients with impaired kidney function (see DOSAGE AND ADMINISTRATION).

Use in the Treatment of and Prophylaxis for *Pneumocystis carinii* Pneumonia in Patients with Acquired Immunodeficiency Syndrome (AIDS): The incidence of side effects, particularly rash, fever, leukopenia, and elevated aminotransferase (transaminase) values in AIDS patients who are being treated with SEPTRA for *Pneumocystis carinii* pneumonia has been reported to be greatly increased compared with the incidence normally associated with the use of SEPTRA in non-AIDS patients. The incidence of hyperkalemia and hyponatremia appears to be increased in AIDS patients receiving SEPTRA. Adverse effects are generally less severe in patients receiving SEPTRA for prophylaxis. A history of mild intolerance to SEPTRA in AIDS patients does not appear to predict intolerance of subsequent secondary prophylaxis. However, if a patient develops skin rash or any sign of adverse reaction, therapy with SEPTRA should be re-evaluated (see WARNINGS).

The concomitant use of leucovorin with trimethoprim-sulfamethoxazole for the acute treatment of *Pneumocystis carinii* pneumonia in patients with HIV infection was associated with increased rates of treatment failure and morbidity in a placebo-controlled study.

Continued on next page

Glaxo Wellcome—Cont.

Information for Patients: Patients should be instructed to maintain an adequate fluid intake in order to prevent crystalluria and stone formation.

Laboratory Tests: Complete blood counts should be done frequently in patients receiving SEPTRA; if a significant reduction in the count of any formed blood element is noted, SEPTRA should be discontinued. Urinalyses with careful microscopic examination and renal function tests should be performed during therapy, particularly for those patients with impaired renal function.

Drug Interactions: In elderly patients concurrently receiving certain diuretics, primarily thiazides, an increased incidence of thrombocytopenia with purpura has been reported. It has been reported that SEPTRA may prolong the prothrombin time in patients who are receiving the anticoagulant warfarin. This interaction should be kept in mind when SEPTRA is given to patients already on anticoagulant therapy, and the coagulation time should be reassessed.

SEPTRA may inhibit the hepatic metabolism of phenytoin. SEPTRA, given at a common clinical dosage, increased the phenytoin half-life by 39% and decreased the phenytoin metabolic clearance rate by 27%. When administering these drugs concurrently, one should be alert for possible excessive phenytoin effect.

Sulfonamides can also displace methotrexate from plasma protein binding sites, thus increasing free methotrexate concentrations.

Drug/Laboratory Test Interactions: SEPTRA, specifically the trimethoprim component, can interfere with a serum methotrexate assay as determined by the competitive binding protein technique (CBPA) when a bacterial dihydrofolate reductase is used as the binding protein. No interference occurs, however, if methotrexate is measured by a radioimmunoassay (RIA).

The presence of trimethoprim and sulfamethoxazole may also interfere with the Jaffé alkaline picrate reaction assay for creatinine, resulting in overestimations of about 10% in the range of normal values.

Carcinogenesis, Mutagenesis, Impairment of Fertility:

Carcinogenesis: Long-term studies in animals to evaluate carcinogenic potential have not been conducted with SEPTRA.

Mutagenesis Bacterial mutagenic studies have not been performed with sulfamethoxazole and trimethoprim in combination. Trimethoprim was demonstrated to be non-mutagenic in the Ames assay. In studies at two laboratories, no chromosomal damage was detected in cultured Chinese hamster ovary cells at concentrations approximately 500 times human plasma levels; at concentrations approximately 1000 times human plasma levels in these same cells, a low level of chromosomal damage was induced at one of the laboratories. No chromosomal abnormalities were observed in cultured human leukocytes at concentrations of trimethoprim up to 20 times human steady-state plasma levels. No chromosomal effects were detected in peripheral lymphocytes of human subjects receiving 320 mg of trimethoprim in combination with up to 1600 mg of sulfamethoxazole per day for as long as 112 weeks.

Impairment of Fertility: No adverse effects on fertility or general reproductive performance were observed in rats given oral dosages as high as 70 mg/kg/day trimethoprim plus 350 mg/kg/day sulfamethoxazole.

Pregnancy: Teratogenic Effects: Pregnancy Category C. In rats, oral doses of 533 mg/kg sulfamethoxazole or 200 mg/kg trimethoprim produced teratological effects manifested mainly as cleft palates. The highest dose which did not cause cleft palates in rats was 512 mg/kg sulfamethoxazole or 192 mg/kg trimethoprim when administered separately. In two studies in rats, no teratology was observed when 512 mg/kg of sulfamethoxazole was used in combination with 128 mg/kg of trimethoprim. In one study, however, cleft palates were observed in one litter out of 9 when 355 mg/kg of sulfamethoxazole was used in combination with 88 mg/kg of trimethoprim.

In some rabbit studies, an overall increase in fetal loss (dead and resorbed and malformed conceptuses) was associated with doses of trimethoprim 6 times the human therapeutic dose.

While there are no large, well-controlled studies on the use of trimethoprim and sulfamethoxazole in pregnant women, Brumfitt and Pursell,[5] in a retrospective study, reported the outcome of 186 pregnancies during which the mother received either placebo or trimethoprim and sulfamethoxazole. The incidence of congenital abnormalities was 4.5% (3 of 66) in those who received placebo and 3.3% (4 of 120) in those receiving trimethoprim and sulfamethoxazole. There were no abnormalities in the 10 children whose mothers received the drug during the first trimester. In a separate survey, Brumfitt and Pursell also found no congenital abnormalities in 35 children whose mothers had received oral trimethoprim and sulfamethoxazole at the time of conception or shortly thereafter.

Because trimethoprim and sulfamethoxazole may interfere with folic acid metabolism, SEPTRA should be used during pregnancy only if the potential benefit justifies the potential risk to the fetus.

Nonteratogenic Effects: See CONTRAINDICATIONS section.

Nursing Mothers: See CONTRAINDICATIONS section.

Pediatric Use: SEPTRA is not recommended for infants younger than two months of age (see INDICATIONS AND USAGE and CONTRAINDICATIONS).

ADVERSE REACTIONS

The most common adverse effects are gastrointestinal disturbances (nausea, vomiting, anorexia) and allergic skin reactions (such as rash and urticaria). **FATALITIES ASSOCIATED WITH THE ADMINISTRATION OF SULFONAMIDES, ALTHOUGH RARE, HAVE OCCURRED DUE TO SEVERE REACTIONS, INCLUDING STEVENS-JOHNSON SYNDROME, TOXIC EPIDERMAL NECROLYSIS, FULMINANT HEPATIC NECROSIS, AGRANULOCYTOSIS, APLASTIC ANEMIA, OTHER BLOOD DYSCRASIAS, AND HYPERSENSITIVITY OF THE RESPIRATORY TRACT (SEE WARNINGS).**

Hematologic: Agranulocytosis, aplastic anemia, thrombocytopenia, leukopenia, neutropenia, hemolytic anemia, megaloblastic anemia, hypoprothrombinemia, methemoglobinemia, eosinophilia.

Allergic: Stevens-Johnson syndrome, toxic epidermal necrolysis, anaphylaxis, allergic myocarditis, erythema multiforme, exfoliative dermatitis, angioedema, drug fever, chills, Henoch-Schönlein purpura, serum sickness-like syndrome, generalized allergic reactions, generalized skin eruptions, photosensitivity, conjunctival and scleral injection, pruritus, urticaria, and rash. In addition, periarteritis nodosa and systemic lupus erythematosus have been reported.

Gastrointestinal: Hepatitis, including cholestatic jaundice and hepatic necrosis, elevation of serum transaminase and bilirubin, pseudomembranous enterocolitis, pancreatitis, stomatitis, glossitis, nausea, emesis, abdominal pain, diarrhea, anorexia.

Genitourinary: Renal failure, interstitial nephritis, BUN and serum creatinine elevation, toxic nephrosis with oliguria and anuria, and crystalluria.

Metabolic: Hyperkalemia, hyponatremia.

Neurologic: Aseptic meningitis, convulsions, peripheral neuritis, ataxia, vertigo, tinnitus, headache.

Psychiatric: Hallucinations, depression, apathy, nervousness.

Endocrine: The sulfonamides bear certain chemical similarities to some goitrogens, diuretics (acetazolamide and the thiazides), and oral hypoglycemic agents. Cross-sensitivity may exist with these agents. Diuresis and hypoglycemia have occurred rarely in patients receiving sulfonamides.

Musculoskeletal: Arthralgia and myalgia.

Respiratory System: Pulmonary infiltrates, cough, shortness of breath.

Miscellaneous: Weakness, fatigue, insomnia.

OVERDOSAGE

Acute: The amount of a single dose of SEPTRA that is either associated with symptoms of overdosage or is likely to be life-threatening has not been reported. Signs and symptoms of overdosage reported with sulfonamides include anorexia, colic, nausea, vomiting, dizziness, headache, drowsiness, and unconsciousness. Pyrexia, hematuria, and crystalluria may be noted. Blood dyscrasias and jaundice are potential late manifestations of overdosage. Signs of acute overdosage with trimethoprim include nausea, vomiting, dizziness, headache, mental depression, confusion, and bone marrow depression.

General principles of treatment include the institution of gastric lavage or emesis: forcing oral fluids: and the administration of intravenous fluids if urine output is low and renal function is normal. Acidification of the urine will increase renal elimination of trimethoprim. The patient should be monitored with blood counts and appropriate blood chemistries, including electrolytes. If a significant blood dyscrasia or jaundice occurs, specific therapy should be instituted for these complications. Peritoneal dialysis is not effective and hemodialysis is only moderately effective in eliminating trimethoprim and sulfamethoxazole.

Chronic: Use of SEPTRA at high doses and/or for extended periods of time may cause bone marrow depression manifested as thrombocytopenia, leukopenia, and/or megaloblastic anemia. If signs of bone marrow depression occur, the patient should be given leucovorin; 5 to 15 mg leucovorin daily has been recommended by some investigators.

DOSAGE AND ADMINISTRATION

Not recommended for use in infants less than two months of age.

URINARY TRACT INFECTIONS AND SHIGELLOSIS IN ADULTS AND CHILDREN AND ACUTE OTITIS MEDIA IN CHILDREN:

Adults: The usual adult dosage in the treatment of urinary tract infections is one SEPTRA DS (double strength) tablet, two SEPTRA tablets, or four teaspoonfuls (20 mL) SEPTRA Suspension every 12 hours for 10 to 14 days. An identical daily dosage is used for 5 days in the treatment of shigellosis.

Children: The recommended dose for children with urinary tract infections or acute otitis media is 8 mg/kg trimethoprim and 40 mg/kg sulfamethoxazole per 24 hours, given in two divided doses every 12 hours for 10 days. An identical daily dosage is used for 5 days in the treatment of shigellosis. The following table is a guideline for the attainment of this dosage:

Children: *Two months of age or older*

Weight		Dose—every 12 hours	
lb	kg	Teaspoonfuls	Tablets
22	10	1 (5 mL)	
44	20	2 (10 mL)	1
66	30	3 (15 mL)	1$\frac{1}{2}$
88	40	4 (20 mL)	2 (or 1 DS Tablet)

For patients with impaired renal function: When renal function is impaired, a reduced dosage should be employed using the following table:

Creatinine Clearance (mL/min)	Recommended Dosage Regimen
Above 30	Use Standard Regimen
15–30	$\frac{1}{2}$ the Usual Regimen
Below 15	Use Not Recommended

ACUTE EXACERBATIONS OF CHRONIC BRONCHITIS IN ADULTS: The usual adult dosage in the treatment of acute exacerbations of chronic bronchitis is one SEPTRA DS (double strength) tablet, two SEPTRA tablets or four teaspoonfuls (20 mL) SEPTRA Suspension every 12 hours for 14 days.

TRAVELERS' DIARRHEA IN ADULTS: For the treatment of travelers' diarrhea, the usual adult dosage is one SEPTRA DS (double strength) tablet, two SEPTRA tablets, or four teaspoonfuls (20 mL) of SEPTRA Suspension every 12 hours for 5 days.

PNEUMOCYSTIS CARINII PNEUMONIA:

Treatment:

Adults and Children:

The recommended dosage for treatment of patients with documented *Pneumocystis carinii* pneumonia is 15 to 20 mg/kg trimethoprim and 75 to 100 mg/kg sulfamethoxazole per 24 hours given in equally divided doses every 6 hours for 14 to 21 days. The following table is a guideline for the upper limit of this dosage:

Weight		Dose—every 6 hours	
lb	kg	Teaspoonfuls	Tablets
18	8	1 (5 mL)	
35	16	2 (10 mL)	1
53	24	3 (15 mL)	1$\frac{1}{2}$
70	32	4 (20 mL)	2 (or 1 DS Tablet)
88	40	5 (25 mL)	2$\frac{1}{2}$
106	48	6 (30 mL)	3 (or 1$\frac{1}{2}$ DS Tablets)
141	64	8 (40 mL)	4 (or 2 DS Tablets)
176	80	10 (50 mL)	5 (or 2$\frac{1}{2}$ DS Tablets)

For the lower limit dose (15 mg/kg trimethoprim and 75 mg/kg sulfamethoxazole per 24 hours) administer 75% of the dose in the above table.

Prophylaxis:

Adults:

The recommended dosage for prophylaxis in adults is one SEPTRA DS (double strength) tablet daily.

Children:

For children, the recommended dose is 150 mg/m²/day trimethoprim with 750 mg/m²/day sulfamethoxazole given orally in equally divided doses twice a day, on 3 consecutive days per week. The total daily dose should not exceed 320 mg trimethoprim and 1600 mg sulfamethoxazole. The following table is a guideline for the attainment of this dosage in children:

Body Surface Area (m²)		Dose—every 12 hours	
	Teaspoonfuls		Tablets
0.26	1/2 (2.5 mL)		
0.53	1 (5 mL)		1/2
1.06	2 (10 mL)		1

HOW SUPPLIED

TABLETS (pink, scored, round-shaped) containing 80 mg trimethoprim and 400 mg sulfamethoxazole: Bottles of 100 (NDC 0173-0852-55). Imprint on tablets "SEPTRA" and "Y2B."

DS (DOUBLE STRENGTH) TABLETS (pink, scored, oval-shaped) containing 160 mg trimethoprim and 800 mg sulfamethoxazole: Bottles of 100 (NDC 0173-0853-55) and 250 (NDC 0173-0853-65). Imprint on tablets "SEPTRA DS" and "O2C."

ORAL SUSPENSIONS (pink, cherry-flavored) containing 40 mg trimethoprim and 200 mg sulfamethoxazole in each teaspoonful (5 mL): Bottle of 1 pint (473 mL) (NDC 0173-0855-96) and 100 mL—package of 6 (NDC 0173-0855-03) and (purple, grape-flavored) containing 40 mg trimethoprim and 200 mg sulfamethoxazole in each teaspoonful (5 mL): Bottle of 1 pint (473 mL) (NDC 0173-0854-96).

Tablets should be stored at 15° to 25°C (59° to 77°F) in a dry place and protected from light.

Suspensions should be stored at 15° to 25°C (59° to 77°F) and protected from light.

Also available:

SEPTRA I.V. Infusion: 5 mL vials, containing 80 mg trimethoprim (16 mg/mL) and 400 mg sulfamethoxazole (80 mg/mL), tray of 10; 10 mL multiple dose vials containing 160 mg trimethoprim (16 mg/mL) and 800 mg sulfamethoxazole (80 mg/mL), tray of 10; 20 mL multiple dose vials containing 320 mg trimethoprim (16 mg/mL) and 1600 mg sulfamethoxazole (80 mg/mL), tray of 10.

REFERENCES

1. Kremers P, Duvivier J, Heusghem C. Pharmacokinetic studies of co-trimoxazole in man after single and repeated doses. *J Clin Pharmacol*. 1974; 14:112–117.
2. Kaplan SA, Weinfeld RE, Abruzzo CW, McFaden K, Jack ML, Weissman L. Pharmacokinetic profile of trimethoprim-sulfamethoxazole in man. *J Infect Dis*. 1973; 128(suppl):S547–S555.
3. Antibiotic susceptibility discs: certification procedure. *Federal Register*. 1972;37:20527–20529.
4. Bauer AW, Kirby WMM, Sherris JC, Turck M. Antibiotic susceptibility testing by standardized single disk method. *Am J Clin Pathol*. 1966; 45:493–496.
5. Brumfitt W, Pursell R. Trimethoprim-sulfamethoxazole in the treatment of bacteriuria in women. *J Infect Dis*. 1973; 128(suppl):S657–S663.

U.S. Patent No. 4,209,513 (Tablet)

March 1996/RL-297

Shown in Product Identification Guide, page 314

SEREVENT®

[ser 'ə-vent "]

(salmeterol xinafoate)
Inhalation Aerosol
Bronchodilator Aerosol
For Oral Inhalation Only

℞

DESCRIPTION

Serevent® (salmeterol xinafoate) Inhalation Aerosol contains salmeterol xinafoate as the racemic form of the 1-hydroxy-2-naphthoic acid salt of salmeterol. The active component of the formulation is salmeterol base, a highly selective beta$_2$-adrenergic bronchodilator. The chemical name of salmeterol xinafoate is 4-hydroxy-α^1-[[[6-(4-phenyl-butoxy)hexyl]amino]methyl]-1,3-benzenedimethanol, 1-hydroxy-2-naphthalenecarboxylate.

The molecular weight of salmeterol xinafoate is 603.8, and the empirical formula is $C_{25}H_{37}NO_4 \cdot C_{11}H_8O_3$. Salmeterol xinafoate is a white to off-white powder. It is freely soluble in methanol; slightly soluble in ethanol, chloroform, and isopropanol; and sparingly soluble in water.

Serevent Inhalation Aerosol is a pressurized, metered-dose aerosol unit for oral inhalation. It contains a microcrystalline suspension of salmeterol xinafoate in a mixture of two chlorofluorocarbon propellants (trichlorofluoromethane and dichlorodifluoromethane) with lecithin. 36.25 mcg of salmeterol xinafoate is equivalent to 25 mcg of salmeterol base. Each actuation delivers 25 mcg of salmeterol base (as salmeterol xinafoate) from the valve and 21 mcg of salmeterol base (as salmeterol xinafoate) from the actuator.

CLINICAL PHARMACOLOGY

Mechanism of Action: Salmeterol is a long-acting beta-adrenergic agonist. *In vitro* studies and *in vivo* pharmacologic studies demonstrate that salmeterol is selective for beta$_2$-adrenoceptors compared with isoproterenol, which has approximately equal agonist activity on beta$_1$- and beta$_2$-adrenoceptors. *In vitro* studies show salmeterol to be at least 50 times more selective for beta$_2$-adrenoceptors than albuterol. Although beta$_2$-adrenoceptors are the predominant adrenergic receptors in bronchial smooth muscle and beta$_1$-adrenoceptors are the predominant receptors in the heart, there are also beta$_2$-adrenoceptors in the human heart com-

prising 10% to 50% of the total beta-adrenoceptors. The precise function of these is not yet established, but they raise the possibility that even highly selective beta$_2$-agonists may have cardiac effects.

The pharmacologic effects of beta$_2$-adrenoceptor agonist drugs, including salmeterol, are at least in part attributable to stimulation of intracellular adenyl cyclase, the enzyme that catalyzes the conversion of adenosine triphosphate (ATP) to cyclic-3',5'-adenosine monophosphate (cyclic AMP). Increased cyclic AMP levels cause relaxation of bronchial smooth muscle and inhibition of release of mediators of immediate hypersensitivity from cells, especially from mast cells.

In vitro tests show that salmeterol is a potent and long-lasting inhibitor of the release of mast cell mediators, such as histamine, leukotrienes, and prostaglandin D$_2$, from human lung. Salmeterol inhibits histamine-induced plasma protein extravasation and inhibits platelet activating factor-induced eosinophil accumulation in the lungs of guinea pigs when administered by the inhaled route. In humans, salmeterol inhibits both the early- and late-phase responses to inhaled allergens, the latter persisting for over 30 hours after a single dose when the bronchodilator effect is no longer evident. Single doses of salmeterol also attenuate allergen-induced bronchial hyper-responsiveness.

Pharmacokinetics: Salmeterol acts locally in the lung; plasma levels therefore do not predict therapeutic effect. Because of the low therapeutic dose, systemic levels of salmeterol are low or undetectable after inhalation of recommended doses (42 mcg twice daily). Following chronic administration of an inhaled dose of 42 mcg twice daily, salmeterol was detected in plasma within 5 to 10 minutes in six asthmatic patients; plasma concentrations were very low, with peak concentrations of 150 pg/mL and no accumulation with repeated doses. Larger inhaled doses gave approximately proportionally increased blood levels. In these patients, a second peak concentration of 115 pg/mL occurred at about 45 minutes, probably due to absorption of the swallowed portion of the dose (most of the dose delivered by a metered-dose inhaler is swallowed). Oral administration of 1 mg of radiolabeled salmeterol (as salmeterol xinafoate) to two healthy subjects gave peak plasma salmeterol concentrations of about 650 pg/mL at about 45 minutes; the terminal elimination half-life was about 5.5 hours (one volunteer only).

Salmeterol xinafoate, as ionic salt, dissociates in solution so that the salmeterol and 1-hydroxy-2-naphthoic acid (xinafoate) moieties are absorbed, distributed, metabolized, and excreted independently. Salmeterol base is extensively metabolized by hydroxylation, with subsequent elimination predominantly in the feces. In the two subjects discussed above, approximately 25% and 60% of orally administered radioactivity was eliminated in urine and feces, respectively, over a period of 7 days. No significant amount of unchanged salmeterol base was detected in either urine or feces.

Salmeterol is 94% to 98% bound to human plasma proteins *in vitro* over the concentration range of 8 to 7,722 ng of base per milliliter, much higher concentrations than those achieved following therapeutic doses of salmeterol.

The xinafoate moiety has no apparent pharmacologic activity, is highly protein bound (>99%), and has a long elimination half-life of 11 days.

The pharmacokinetics of salmeterol base have not been studied in elderly patients nor in patients with hepatic or renal impairment. Since salmeterol is predominantly cleared by hepatic metabolism, liver function impairment may lead to accumulation of salmeterol in plasma. Therefore, patients with hepatic disease should be closely monitored.

Pharmacodynamics and Clinical Trials: Inhaled salmeterol, like other beta-adrenergic agonist drugs, can in some patients produce cardiovascular effects (see PRECAUTIONS). The cardiovascular effects (heart rate, blood pressure) associated with salmeterol administration occur with similar frequency, and are of similar type and severity, as those noted following albuterol administration.

The effects of rising inhaled doses of salmeterol and standard inhaled doses of albuterol were studied in volunteers and in patients with asthma. Salmeterol doses up to 84 mcg resulted in heart rate increases of 3 to 16 beats/minute, about the same as albuterol (4 to 10 beats/minute). In two double-blind studies, patients receiving either salmeterol (n=81) or albuterol (n=80) underwent continuous electrocardiographic monitoring during four 24-hour periods; no clinically significant dysrhythmias were noted.

Beta-agonists and methylxanthines administered concurrently in laboratory animals (minipigs, rodents, and dogs) cause cardiac arrhythmias and sudden death (with histologic evidence of myocardial necrosis). Whether these findings are relevant to humans is not known.

In placebo- and albuterol-controlled, single-dose clinical trials with Serevent® (salmeterol xinafoate) Inhalation Aerosol, the time to onset of effective bronchodilatation (>15% improvement in forced expiratory volume in 1 second [FEV$_1$]) was 10 to 20 minutes after a 42-mcg dose. Maximum improvement in FEV$_1$ generally occurred within 180 minutes, and clinically significant improvement continued for 12 hours in most patients.

In two large, randomized, double-blind studies, Serevent Inhalation Aerosol was compared with albuterol and placebo in patients with mild-to-moderate asthma, including both patients who did and who did not receive concomitant inhaled corticosteroids. The efficacy of Serevent Inhalation Aerosol was demonstrated over the 12-week period with no change in effectiveness over this period of time. There were no gender-related differences in safety or efficacy. No development of tachyphylaxis to the bronchodilator effect has been noted in these studies. FEV$_1$ measurements (percent of predicted) from these two 12-week trials are shown below for both the first and last treatment days.

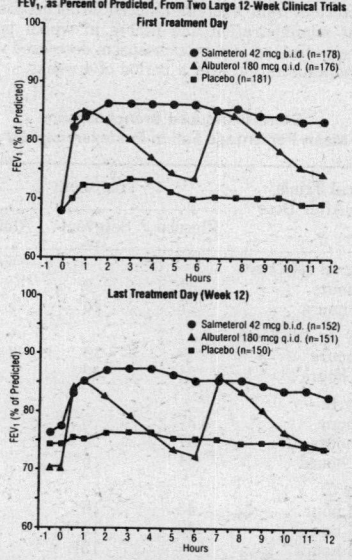

FEV$_1$, as Percent of Predicted, From Two Large 12-Week Clinical Trials

During daily treatment with Serevent Inhalation Aerosol for 12 weeks in patients with asthma, the following treatment effects were seen:

Two Large 12-Week Clinical Trials: Efficacy Parameters

Multicenter Study 1

Parameter	Time	Placebo	Serevent	Albuterol
Mean AM PEFR (L/min)	baseline	410	420	404
	12 weeks	409	443*	395
Mean % days with no symptoms	baseline	12	15	15
	12 weeks	17	35*	27
Mean % nights with no awakenings	baseline	71	77	70
	12 weeks	79	89†	75
Rescue medications (mean no. of inhalations per day)	baseline	3.9	3.8	4.0
	12 weeks	2.9	1.2‡	1.9
Asthma exacerbations		53%	16%	31%

* Statistically superior to placebo ($p=0.002$).
† Statistically superior to placebo ($p=0.008$).
‡ Statistically superior to placebo ($p<0.001$).

Multicenter Study 2

Parameter	Time	Placebo	Serevent	Albuterol
Mean AM PEFR (L/min)	baseline	409	406	390
	12 weeks	412	451*	388
Mean % days with no symptoms	baseline	11	8	14
	12 weeks	17	36*	21
Mean % nights with no awakenings	baseline	64	59	62
	12 weeks	70	85*	74
Rescue medications (mean no. of inhalations per day)	baseline	4.7	4.3	4.0
	12 weeks	3.6	1.4*	1.8
Asthma exacerbations		57%	17%	26%

* Statistically superior to placebo ($p<0.001$).

Continued on next page

Consult 1997 supplements and future editions for revisions

Glaxo Wellcome—Cont.

Safe usage with maintenance of efficacy for periods up to 1 year has been documented.
Protection against exercise-induced bronchospasm was examined in three controlled studies. Based on median values, patients who received Serevent Inhalation Aerosol had consistently less exercise-induced fall in FEV_1 than patients who received placebo, and they were protected for a longer period of time than patients who received albuterol (see table below). There were, however, some patients who were not protected from exercise-induced bronchospasm after Serevent administration and others in whom protection against exercise-induced bronchospasm decreased with continued administration over a period of 4 weeks.

Exercise-Induced Bronchospasm
Mean Percentage Fall in Postexercise FEV_1

Clinical Trials/ Time After Dose	Treatment		
	Placebo	Serevent	Albuterol
Study A: 1st Dose			
6 hours	37	9*	
12 hours	27	16*	
Study A: 4th Week			
6 hours	30	19	
12 hours	24	12	
Study B:			
1 hour	37	0*	2*
6 hours	37	5*†	27
12 hours	34	6*†	33
Study C:			
0.5 hour	43	16*	8*
2.5 hours	33	12*†	30
4.5 hours	—	12†	36
6.0 hours	—	19†	41

* Statistically superior to placebo ($p \leq 0.05$).
† Statistically superior to albuterol ($p \leq 0.05$).

INDICATIONS AND USAGE

Serevent® (salmeterol xinafoate) Inhalation Aerosol is indicated for long-term, twice-daily (morning and evening) administration in the maintenance treatment of asthma and in the prevention of bronchospasm in patients 12 years of age and older with reversible obstructive airway disease, including patients with symptoms of nocturnal asthma, who require regular treatment with inhaled, short-acting $beta_2$-agonists. It should not be used in patients whose asthma can be managed by occasional use of short-acting, inhaled $beta_2$-agonists.
Serevent Inhalation Aerosol may be used with or without concurrent inhaled or systemic corticosteroid therapy.
Serevent Inhalation Aerosol is also indicated for prevention of exercise-induced bronchospasm in patients 12 years of age and older.

CONTRAINDICATIONS

Serevent® (salmeterol xinafoate) Inhalation Aerosol is contraindicated in patients with a history of hypersensitivity to any of the components.

WARNINGS

IMPORTANT INFORMATION: SEREVENT® (SALMETEROL XINAFOATE) INHALATION AEROSOL SHOULD NOT BE INITIATED IN PATIENTS WITH SIGNIFICANTLY WORSENING OR ACUTELY DETERIORATING ASTHMA, WHICH MAY BE A LIFE-THREATENING CONDITION. Serious acute respiratory events, including fatalities, have been reported, both in the US and worldwide, when Serevent Inhalation Aerosol has been initiated in this situation.
Although it is not possible from these reports to determine whether Serevent Inhalation Aerosol contributed to these adverse events or simply failed to relieve the deteriorating asthma, the use of Serevent Inhalation Aerosol in this setting is inappropriate.
SEREVENT INHALATION AEROSOL SHOULD NOT BE USED TO TREAT ACUTE SYMPTOMS. It is crucial to inform patients of this and prescribe a short-acting, inhaled $beta_2$-agonist for this purpose as well as warn them that increasing inhaled $beta_2$-agonist use is a signal of deteriorating asthma.
SEREVENT INHALATION AEROSOL IS NOT A SUBSTITUTE FOR INHALED OR ORAL CORTICOSTEROIDS. Corticosteroids should not be stopped or reduced when Serevent Inhalation Aerosol is initiated.
(See PRECAUTIONS: Information for Patients and PATIENT'S INSTRUCTIONS FOR USE.)

1. Do Not Introduce Serevent Inhalation Aerosol as a Treatment for Acutely Deteriorating Asthma: Serevent Inhalation Aerosol is intended for the maintenance treatment of asthma (see INDICATIONS AND USAGE) and should not be introduced in acutely deteriorating asthma, which is a potentially life-threatening condition. There are no data demonstrating that Serevent Inhalation Aerosol provides greater efficacy than or additional efficacy to short-acting, inhaled $beta_2$-agonists in patients with worsening asthma. Serious acute respiratory events, including fatalities, have been reported, both in the US and worldwide, in patients receiving Serevent Inhalation Aerosol. In most cases, these have occurred in patients with severe asthma (e.g., patients with a history of corticosteroid dependence, low pulmonary function, intubation, mechanical ventilation, frequent hospitalizations, or previous life-threatening acute asthma exacerbations) and/or in some patients in whom asthma has been acutely deteriorating (e.g., unresponsive to usual medications, increasing need for inhaled short-acting $beta_2$-agonists, increasing need for systemic corticosteroids, significant increase in symptoms, recent emergency room visits, sudden or progressive deterioration in pulmonary function). However, they have occurred in a few patients with less severe asthma as well. It was not possible from these reports to determine whether Serevent Inhalation Aerosol contributed to these events or simply failed to relieve the deteriorating asthma.
2. Do Not Use Serevent Inhalation Aerosol to Treat Acute Symptoms: A short-acting, inhaled $beta_2$-agonist, not Serevent Inhalation Aerosol, should be used to relieve acute asthma symptoms. When prescribing Serevent Inhalation Aerosol, the physician must also provide the patient with a short-acting, inhaled $beta_2$-agonist (e.g., albuterol) for treatment of symptoms that occur acutely, despite regular twice daily (morning and evening) use of Serevent Inhalation Aerosol.
When beginning treatment with Serevent Inhalation Aerosol, patients who have been taking short-acting, inhaled $beta_2$-agonists on a regular basis (e.g., q.i.d.) should be instructed to discontinue the regular use of these drugs and use them only for symptomatic relief if they develop acute asthma symptoms while taking Serevent Inhalation Aerosol (see PRECAUTIONS: Information for Patients).
3. Watch for Increasing Use of Short-Acting, Inhaled $Beta_2$-Agonists, Which Is a Marker of Deteriorating Asthma: Asthma may deteriorate acutely over a period of hours or chronically over several days or longer. If the patient's short-acting, inhaled $beta_2$-agonist becomes less effective or the patient needs more inhalations than usual, this may be a marker of destabilization of asthma. In this setting, the patient requires immediate re-evaluation with reassessment of the treatment regimen, giving special consideration to the possible need for corticosteroids. If the patient uses four or more inhalations per day of a short-acting, inhaled $beta_2$-agonist for 2 or more consecutive days, or if more than one canister (200 inhalations per canister) of short-acting, inhaled $beta_2$-agonist is used in an 8-week period in conjunction with Serevent Inhalation Aerosol, then the patient should consult the physician for re-evaluation. **Increasing the daily dosage of Serevent Inhalation Aerosol in this situation is not appropriate. Serevent Inhalation Aerosol should not be used more frequently than twice daily (morning and evening) at the recommended dose of two inhalations.**
4. Do Not Use Serevent Inhalation Aerosol as a Substitute for Oral or Inhaled Corticosteroids: There are no data demonstrating that Serevent Inhalation Aerosol has a clinical anti-inflammatory effect and could be expected to take the place of, or reduce the dose of, corticosteroids. Patients who already require oral or inhaled corticosteroids for treatment of asthma should be continued on this type of treatment even if they feel better as a result of initiating Serevent Inhalation Aerosol. Any change in corticosteroid dosage should be made ONLY after clinical evaluation (see PRECAUTIONS: Information for Patients).
5. Do Not Exceed Recommended Dosage: As with other inhaled $beta_2$-adrenergic drugs, Serevent Inhalation Aerosol should not be used more often or at higher doses than recommended. Fatalities have been reported in association with excessive use of inhaled sympathomimetic drugs. Large doses of inhaled or oral salmeterol (12 to 20 times the recommended dose) have been associated with clinically significant prolongation of the QTc interval, which has the potential for producing ventricular arrhythmias.
6. Paradoxical Bronchospasm: As with other inhaled asthma medications, paradoxical bronchospasm (which can be life threatening) has been reported following the use of Serevent Inhalation Aerosol. If it occurs, treatment with Serevent Inhalation Aerosol should be discontinued immediately and alternative therapy instituted.
7. Immediate Hypersensitivity Reactions: Immediate hypersensitivity reactions may occur after administration of Serevent Inhalation Aerosol, as demonstrated by rare cases of urticaria, angioedema, rash, and bronchospasm.
8. Upper Airway Symptoms: Symptoms of laryngeal spasm, irritation, or swelling, such as stridor and choking, have been reported rarely in patients receiving Serevent Inhalation Aerosol.

PRECAUTIONS

General: 1. Use With Spacer or Other Devices: The safety and effectiveness of Serevent® (salmeterol xinafoate) Inhalation Aerosol when used with a spacer or other devices have not been adequately studied.
2. Cardiovascular and Other Effects: No effect on the cardiovascular system is usually seen after the administration of inhaled salmeterol in recommended doses, but the cardiovascular and central nervous system effects seen with all sympathomimetic drugs (e.g., increased blood pressure, heart rate, excitement) can occur after use of Serevent Inhalation Aerosol and may require discontinuation of the drug. Salmeterol, like all sympathomimetic amines, should be used with caution in patients with cardiovascular disorders, especially coronary insufficiency, cardiac arrhythmias, and hypertension; in patients with convulsive disorders or thyrotoxicosis; and in patients who are unusually responsive to sympathomimetic amines.
As has been described with other beta-adrenergic agonist bronchodilators, clinically significant changes in systolic and/or diastolic blood pressure, pulse rate, and electrocardiograms have been seen infrequently in individual patients in controlled clinical studies with salmeterol.
3. Metabolic Effects: Doses of the related $beta_2$-adrenoceptor agonist albuterol, when administered intravenously, have been reported to aggravate preexisting diabetes mellitus and ketoacidosis. No effects on glucose have been seen with Serevent Inhalation Aerosol at recommended doses.
Administration of $beta_2$-adrenoceptor agonists may cause a decrease in serum potassium, possibly through intracellular shunting, which has the potential to increase the likelihood of arrhythmias. The decrease is usually transient, not requiring supplementation.
Clinically significant changes in blood glucose and/or serum potassium were seen rarely during clinical studies with long-term administration of Serevent Inhalation Aerosol at recommended doses.
Information for Patients: See illustrated Patient's Instructions for Use. **SHAKE WELL BEFORE USING.**
It is important that patients understand how to use Serevent Inhalation Aerosol appropriately and how it should be used in relation to other asthma medications they are taking. Patients should be given the following information:
1. Shake well before using.
2. The recommended dosage (two inhalations twice daily, morning and evening) should not be exceeded.
3. Serevent Inhalation Aerosol is not meant to relieve acute asthma symptoms and extra doses should not be used for that purpose. Acute symptoms should be treated with a short-acting, inhaled $beta_2$-agonist such as albuterol (the physician should provide the patient with such medication and instruct the patient in how it should be used).
4. The physician should be notified immediately if any of the following situations occur, which may be a sign of seriously worsening asthma.
- Decreasing effectiveness of short-acting, inhaled $beta_2$-agonists
- Need for more inhalations than usual of short-acting, inhaled $beta_2$-agonists
- Use of four or more inhalations per day of a short-acting $beta_2$-agonist for 2 or more days consecutively
- Use of more than one canister of a short-acting, inhaled $beta_2$-agonist in an 8-week period (i.e., canister with 200 inhalations)

5. Serevent Inhalation Aerosol should not be used as a substitute for oral or inhaled corticosteroids. The dosage of these medications should not be changed and they should not be stopped without consulting the physician, even if the patient feels better after initiating treatment with Serevent Inhalation Aerosol.
6. Patients should be cautioned regarding potential adverse cardiovascular effects, such as palpitations or chest pain, related to the use of additional $beta_2$-agonist.
7. In patients receiving Serevent Inhalation Aerosol, other inhaled medications should be used only as directed by the physician.
8. When using Serevent Inhalation Aerosol to prevent exercise-induced bronchospasm, patients should take the dose at least 30 to 60 minutes before exercise.

Drug Interactions: ***Short-Acting Beta-Agonists:*** In the two 3-month, repetitive-dose clinical trials (n=184), the mean daily need for additional $beta_2$-agonist use was 1 to 1½ inhalations per day, but some patients used more. Eight percent of patients used at least eight inhalations per day at least on one occasion. Six percent used 9 to 12 inhalations at least once. There were 15 patients (8%) who averaged over four inhalations per day. Four of these used an average of 8 to 11 inhalations per day. In these 15 patients there was no observed increase in frequency of cardiovascular adverse events. The safety of concomitant use of more than eight inhalations per day of short-acting $beta_2$-agonists with Serevent Inhalation Aerosol has not been established. In 15 patients who experienced worsening of asthma while receiv-

ing Serevent Inhalation Aerosol, nebulized albuterol (one dose in most) led to improvement in FEV_1 and no increase in occurrence of cardiovascular adverse events.

Monoamine Oxidase Inhibitors and Tricyclic Antidepressants: Salmeterol should be administered with extreme caution to patients being treated with monoamine oxidase inhibitors or tricyclic antidepressants because the action of salmeterol on the vascular system may be potentiated by these agents.

Corticosteroids and Cromoglycate: In clinical trials, inhaled corticosteroids and/or inhaled cromolyn sodium did not alter the safety profile of Serevent Inhalation Aerosol when administered concurrently.

Methylxanthines: The concurrent use of intravenously or orally administered methylxanthines (e.g., aminophylline, theophylline) by patients receiving Serevent Inhalation Aerosol has not been completely evaluated. In one clinical trial, 87 patients receiving Serevent Inhalation Aerosol 42 mcg twice daily concurrently with a theophylline product had adverse event rates similar to those in 71 patients receiving Serevent Inhalation Aerosol without theophylline. Resting heart rates were slightly higher in the patients on theophylline but were little affected by Serevent Inhalation Aerosol therapy.

Carcinogenesis, Mutagenesis, Impairment of Fertility: In an 18-month oral carcinogenicity study in CD-mice, salmeterol xinafoate caused a dose-related increase in the incidence of smooth muscle hyperplasia, cystic glandular hyperplasia, and leiomyomas of the uterus and a dose-related increase in the incidence of cysts in the ovaries. A higher incidence of leiomyosarcomas was not statistically significant; tumor findings were observed at oral doses of 1.4 and 10 mg/kg, which gave 9 and 63 times, respectively, the human exposure based on rodent:human AUC comparisons. Salmeterol caused a dose-related increase in the incidence of mesovarian leiomyomas and ovarian cysts in Sprague Dawley rats in a 24-month inhalation/oral carcinogenicity study. Tumors were observed in rats receiving doses of 0.68 and 2.58 mg/kg per day (about 55 and 215 times the recommended clinical dose $[mg/m^2]$). These findings in rodents are similar to those reported previously for other beta-adrenergic agonist drugs. The relevance of these findings to human use is unknown.

No significant effects occurred in mice at 0.2 mg/kg (1.3 times the recommended clinical dose based on comparisons of the AUCs) and in rats at 0.21 mg/kg (15 times the recommended clinical dose on a mg/m^2 basis).

Salmeterol xinafoate produced no detectable or reproducible increases in microbial and mammalian gene mutation *in vitro*. No blastogenic activity occurred *in vitro* in human lymphocytes or *in vivo* in a rat micronucleus test. No effects on fertility were identified in male and female rats treated orally with salmeterol xinafoate at doses up to 2 mg/kg orally (about 160 times the recommended clinical dose on a mg/m^2 basis).

Pregnancy: *Teratogenic Effects: Pregnancy Category C:* No significant effects of maternal exposure to oral salmeterol xinafoate occurred in the rat at doses up to the equivalent of about 160 times the recommended clinical dose on a mg/m^2 basis. Dutch rabbit fetuses exposed to salmeterol xinafoate *in utero* exhibited effects characteristically resulting from beta-adrenoceptor stimulation; these included precocious eyelid openings, cleft palate, sternebral fusion, limb and paw flexures, and delayed ossification of the frontal cranial bones. No significant effects occurred at 0.6 mg/kg given orally (12 times the recommended clinical dose based on comparison of the AUCs).

New Zealand White rabbits were less sensitive since only delayed ossification of the frontal bones was seen at 10 mg/kg given orally (approximately 1,600 times the recommended clinical dose on a mg/m^2 basis). Extensive use of other beta-agonists has provided no evidence that these class effects in animals are relevant to use in humans. There are no adequate and well-controlled studies with Serevent Inhalation Aerosol in pregnant women. Serevent Inhalation Aerosol should be used during pregnancy only if the potential benefit justifies the potential risk to the fetus.

Use in Labor and Delivery: There are no well-controlled human studies that have investigated effects of salmeterol on preterm labor or labor at term. Because of the potential for beta-agonist interference with uterine contractility, use of Serevent Inhalation Aerosol during labor should be restricted to those patients in whom the benefits clearly outweigh the risks.

Nursing Mothers: Plasma levels of salmeterol after inhaled therapeutic doses are very low (85 to 200 pg/mL) in humans. In lactating rats dosed with radiolabeled salmeterol, levels of radioactivity were similar in plasma and milk. In rats, concentrations of salmeterol in plasma and milk were similar. The xinafoate moiety is also transferred to milk in rats at concentrations of about half the corresponding level in plasma. However, since there is no experience with use of Serevent Inhalation Aerosol by nursing mothers, a decision should be made whether to discontinue nursing or to discontinue the drug, taking into account the importance of the

drug to the mother. Caution should be exercised when salmeterol xinafoate is administered to a nursing woman.

Pediatric Use: The safety and effectiveness of Serevent Inhalation Aerosol in children younger than 12 years of age have not been established.

Geriatric Use: Of the total number of patients who received Serevent Inhalation Aerosol in all clinical studies, 241 were 65 years and older. Geriatric patients (65 years and older) with reversible obstructive airway disease were evaluated in four well-controlled studies of 3 weeks' to 3 months' duration. Two placebo-controlled, crossover studies evaluated twice-daily dosing with salmeterol for 21 to 28 days in 45 patients. An additional 75 geriatric patients were treated with salmeterol for 3 months in two large parallel-group, multicenter studies. These 120 patients experienced increases in AM and PM peak expiratory flow rate and decreases in diurnal variation in peak expiratory flow rate similar to responses seen in the total populations of the two latter studies. The adverse event type and frequency in geriatric patients were not different from those of the total populations studied.

No apparent differences in the efficacy and safety of Serevent Inhalation Aerosol were observed when geriatric patients were compared with younger patients in clinical trials. As with other beta$_2$-agonists, however, special caution should be observed when using Serevent Inhalation Aerosol in elderly patients who have concomitant cardiovascular disease that could be adversely affected by this class of drug. Based on available data, no adjustment of salmeterol dosage in geriatric patients is warranted.

ADVERSE REACTIONS

Adverse reactions to salmeterol are similar in nature to reactions to other selective beta$_2$-adrenoceptor agonists, i.e., tachycardia; palpitations; immediate hypersensitivity reactions, including urticaria, angioedema, rash, bronchospasm (see WARNINGS); headache; tremor; nervousness; and paradoxical bronchospasm (see WARNINGS).

Two multicenter, 12-week, controlled studies have evaluated twice-daily doses of Serevent® (salmeterol xinafoate) Inhalation Aerosol in patients 12 years of age and older with asthma. The following table reports the incidence of adverse events in these two studies.

Adverse Experience Incidence in Two Large 12-Week Clinical Trials*

Adverse Event Type	Percent of Patients		
	Placebo n=187	Serevent 42 mcg b.i.d. n=184	Albuterol 180 mcg q.i.d. n=185
Ear, nose, and throat			
Upper respiratory tract infection	13	14	16*
Nasopharyngitis	12	14	11
Disease of nasal cavity/sinus	4	6	1
Sinus headache	2	4	<1
Gastrointestinal			
Stomachache	0	4	0
Neurological			
Headache	23	28	27
Tremor	2	4	3
Respiratory			
Cough	6	7	3
Lower respiratory infection	2	4	2

* The only adverse experience classified as serious was one case of upper respiratory tract infection in a patient treated with albuterol.

The table above includes all events (whether considered drug related or nondrug related by the investigator) that occurred at a rate of over 3% in the Serevent Inhalation Aerosol treatment group and were more common in the Serevent Inhalation Aerosol group than in the placebo group.

Pharyngitis, allergic rhinitis, dizziness/giddiness, and influenza occurred at 3% or more but were equally common on placebo. Other events occurring in the Serevent Inhalation Aerosol treatment group at a frequency of 1% to 3% were as follows:

Cardiovascular: Tachycardia, palpitations.
Ear, Nose, and Throat: Rhinitis, laryngitis.
Gastrointestinal: Nausea, viral gastroenteritis, nausea and vomiting, diarrhea, abdominal pain.
Hypersensitivity: Urticaria.
Mouth and Teeth: Dental pain.
Musculoskeletal: Pain in joint, back pain, muscle cramp/contraction, myalgia/myositis, muscular soreness.

Neurological: Nervousness, malaise/fatigue.
Respiratory: Tracheitis/bronchitis.
Skin: Rash/skin eruption.
Urogenital: Dysmenorrhea.
In small dose-response studies, tremor, nervousness, and palpitations appeared to be dose related.

Postmarketing Experience: In extensive US and worldwide postmarketing experience, serious exacerbations of asthma, including some that have been fatal, have been reported. In most cases, these have occurred in patients with severe asthma and/or in some patients in whom asthma has been acutely deteriorating (see WARNINGS no. 1), but they have occurred in a few patients with less severe asthma as well. It was not possible from these reports to determine whether Serevent Inhalation Aerosol contributed to these events or simply failed to relieve the deteriorating asthma.

Postmarketing experience includes rare reports of upper airway symptoms of laryngeal spasm, irritation, or swelling, such as stridor and choking. Hypertension and arrhythmias have been reported.

OVERDOSAGE

Overdosage with salmeterol may be expected to result in exaggeration of the pharmacologic adverse effects associated with beta-adrenoceptor agonists, including tachycardia and/or arrhythmia, tremor, headache, and muscle cramps. Overdosage with salmeterol can lead to clinically significant prolongation of the QT_c interval, which can produce ventricular arrhythmias. Other signs of overdosage may include hypokalemia and hyperglycemia.

In these cases, therapy with Serevent® (salmeterol xinafoate) Inhalation Aerosol and all beta-adrenergic-stimulant drugs should be stopped, supportive therapy provided, and judicious use of a beta-adrenergic blocking agent should be considered, bearing in mind the possibility that such agents can produce bronchospasm. Cardiac monitoring is recommended in cases of overdosage.

As with all sympathomimetic pressurized aerosol medications, cardiac arrest and even death may be associated with abuse of Serevent Inhalation Aerosol.

Rats and dogs survived the maximum practicable inhalation doses of salmeterol of 2.9 and 0.7 mg/kg, respectively. The maximum nonlethal oral doses in mice and rats were approximately 150 mg/kg and >1,000 mg/kg, respectively. Dialysis is not appropriate treatment for overdosage of Serevent Inhalation Aerosol.

DOSAGE AND ADMINISTRATION

Serevent® (salmeterol xinafoate) Inhalation Aerosol should be administered by the orally inhaled route only (see Patient's Instructions for Use). For maintenance of bronchodilatation and prevention of symptoms of asthma, including the symptoms of nocturnal asthma, the usual dosage for adults and children 12 years of age and older is two inhalations (42 mcg) twice daily (morning and evening, approximately 12 hours apart). Adverse effects are more likely to occur with higher doses of salmeterol, and more frequent administration or administration of a larger number of inhalations is not recommended.

To gain full therapeutic benefit, Serevent Inhalation Aerosol should be administered twice daily (morning and evening) in the treatment of reversible airway obstruction.

If a previously effective dosage regimen fails to provide the usual response, medical advice should be sought immediately as this is often a sign of destabilization of asthma. Under these circumstances, the therapeutic regimen should be re-evaluated and additional therapeutic options, such as inhaled or systemic corticosteroids, should be considered. If symptoms arise in the period between doses, a short-acting, inhaled beta$_2$-agonist should be taken for immediate relief.

Prevention of Exercise-Induced Bronchospasm: Two inhalations at least 30 to 60 minutes before exercise have been shown to protect against exercise-induced bronchospasm in many patients for up to 12 hours. Additional doses of Serevent Inhalation Aerosol should not be used for 12 hours after the administration of this drug. Patients who are receiving Serevent Inhalation Aerosol twice daily (morning and evening) should not use additional Serevent Inhalation Aerosol for prevention of exercise-induced bronchospasm. If this dose is not effective, other appropriate therapy for exercise-induced bronchospasm should be considered.

Geriatric Use: In studies where geriatric patients (65 years of age or older, see PRECAUTIONS) have been treated with Serevent Inhalation Aerosol, efficacy and safety of 42 mcg given twice daily (morning and evening) did not differ from that in younger patients. Consequently, no dosage adjustment is recommended.

HOW SUPPLIED

Serevent® (salmeterol xinafoate) Inhalation Aerosol is supplied in 13-g canisters containing 120 metered actuations in boxes of one. Each actuation delivers 25 mcg of salmeterol base (as salmeterol xinafoate) from the valve and 21 mcg of salmeterol base (as salmeterol xinafoate) from the actuator. Each canister is supplied with a green plastic actuator with a

Continued on next page

Glaxo Wellcome—Cont.

teal-colored strapcap and patient's instructions (NDC 0173-0464-00). Also available, Serevent Inhalation Aerosol Refill (NDC 0173-0465-00), a 13-g canister only with patient's instructions.
Serevent Inhalation Aerosol is also supplied in a pack that consists of a 6.5-g canister containing 60 metered actuations in boxes of one. Each actuation delivers 25 mcg of salmeterol base (as salmeterol xinafoate) from the valve and 21 mcg of salmeterol base from the actuator (as salmeterol xinafoate). Each canister is supplied with a green plastic actuator with a teal-colored strapcap and patient's instructions (NDC 0173-0467-00).
For use with Serevent Inhalation Aerosol actuator only. The actuator should not be used with other aerosol medications.
Store between 2° and 30°C (36° and 86°F). Store canister with nozzle end down. Protect from freezing temperatures and direct sunlight.
Avoid spraying in eyes. Contents under pressure. Do not puncture or incinerate. Do not store at temperatures above 120°F. Keep out of reach of children. As with most inhaled medications in aerosol canisters, the therapeutic effect of this medication may decrease when the canister is cold; for best results, the canister should be at room temperature before use. Shake well before using.
December 1995/RL-227

Shown in Product Identification Guide, page 315

TEMOVATE® ℞
[tim 'ō-vāt"]
(clobetasol propionate cream)
Cream, 0.05%

TEMOVATE® ℞
(clobetasol propionate ointment)
Ointment, 0.05%
For Dermatologic Use Only—
Not for Ophthalmic Use.

DESCRIPTION
Temovate® (clobetasol propionate cream and ointment) Cream and Ointment contain the active compound clobetasol propionate, a synthetic corticosteroid, for topical dermatologic use. Clobetasol, an analog of prednisolone, has a high degree of glucocorticoid activity and a slight degree of mineralocorticoid activity.
Chemically, clobetasol propionate is (11β,16β)-21-chloro-9-fluoro-11-hydroxy-16-methyl -17- (1-oxopropoxy)-pregna-1,4-diene-3,20-dione.
Clobetasol propionate has the empirical formula $C_{25}H_{32}ClFO_5$ and a molecular weight of 467. It is a white to cream-colored crystalline powder insoluble in water.
Temovate Cream contains clobetasol propionate 0.5 mg/g in a cream base of propylene glycol, glyceryl monostearate, cetostearyl alcohol, glyceryl stearate, PEG 100 stearate, white wax, chlorocresol, sodium citrate, citric acid monohydrate, and purified water.
Temovate Ointment contains clobetasol propionate 0.5 mg/g in a base of propylene glycol, sorbitan sesquioleate, and white petrolatum.

CLINICAL PHARMACOLOGY
Like other topical corticosteroids, clobetasol propionate has anti-inflammatory, antipruritic, and vasoconstrictive properties. The mechanism of the anti-inflammatory activity of the topical steroids, in general, is unclear. However, corticosteroids are thought to act by the induction of phospholipase A_2 inhibitory proteins, collectively called lipocortins. It is postulated that these proteins control the biosynthesis of potent mediators of inflammation such as prostaglandins and leukotrienes by inhibiting the release of their common precursor, arachidonic acid. Arachidonic acid is released from membrane phospholipids by phospholipase A_2.
Pharmacokinetics: The extent of percutaneous absorption of topical corticosteroids is determined by many factors, including the vehicle and the integrity of the epidermal barrier. Occlusive dressing with hydrocortisone for up to 24 hours has not been demonstrated to increase penetration; however, occlusion of hydrocortisone for 96 hours markedly enhances penetration. Topical corticosteroids can be absorbed from normal intact skin. Inflammation and/or other disease processes in the skin may increase percutaneous absorption.
Studies performed with Temovate® Cream and Ointment indicate that they are in the super-high range of potency as compared with other topical corticosteroids.

INDICATIONS AND USAGE
Temovate® Cream and Ointment are super-high potency corticosteroid formulations indicated for the relief of the inflammatory and pruritic manifestations of corticosteroid-responsive dermatoses. Treatment beyond 2 consecutive weeks is not recommended, and the total dosage should not exceed 50 g per week because of the potential for the drug to suppress the hypothalamic-pituitary-adrenal (HPA) axis. Use in children under 12 years of age is not recommended.
As with other highly active corticosteroids, therapy should be discontinued when control has been achieved. If no improvement is seen within 2 weeks, reassessment of the diagnosis may be necessary.

CONTRAINDICATIONS
Temovate® Cream and Ointment are contraindicated in those patients with a history of hypersensitivity to any of the components of the preparations.

PRECAUTIONS
General: Temovate® Cream and Ointment should not be used in the treatment of rosacea or perioral dermatitis, and should not be used on the face, groin, or axillae.
Systemic absorption of topical corticosteroids can produce reversible HPA axis suppression with the potential for glucocorticosteroid insufficiency after withdrawal from treatment. Manifestations of Cushing's syndrome, hyperglycemia, and glucosuria can also be produced in some patients by systemic absorption of topical corticosteroids while on therapy.
Patients applying a topical steroid to a large surface area or to areas under occlusion should be evaluated periodically for evidence of HPA axis suppression. This may be done by using the ACTH stimulation, A.M. plasma cortisol, and urinary free cortisol tests. Patients receiving super-potent corticosteroids should not be treated for more than 2 weeks at a time, and only small areas should be treated at any one time due to the increased risk of HPA suppression.
Temovate Cream and Ointment produced HPA axis suppression when used at doses as low as 2 g per day for 1 week in patients with eczema.
If HPA axis suppression is noted, an attempt should be made to withdraw the drug, to reduce the frequency of application, or to substitute a less potent corticosteroid. Recovery of HPA axis function is generally prompt upon discontinuation of topical corticosteroids. Infrequently, signs and symptoms of glucocorticosteroid insufficiency may occur, requiring supplemental systemic corticosteroids. For information on systemic supplementation, see prescribing information for those products.
Pediatric patients may be more susceptible to systemic toxicity from equivalent doses due to their larger skin surface to body mass ratios (see PRECAUTIONS: Pediatric Use).
If irritation develops, Temovate Cream and Ointment should be discontinued and appropriate therapy instituted. Allergic contact dermatitis with corticosteroids is usually diagnosed by observing *failure to heal* rather than noting a clinical exacerbation as with most topical products not containing corticosteroids. Such an observation should be corroborated with appropriate diagnostic patch testing.
If concomitant skin infections are present or develop, an appropriate antifungal or antibacterial agent should be used. If a favorable response does not occur promptly, use of Temovate Cream and Ointment should be discontinued until the infection has been adequately controlled.
Information for Patients: Patients using topical corticosteroids should receive the following information and instructions:
1. This medication is to be used as directed by the physician. It is for external use only. Avoid contact with the eyes.
2. This medication should not be used for any disorder other than that for which it was prescribed.
3. The treated skin area should not be bandaged, otherwise covered, or wrapped so as to be occlusive unless directed by the physician.
4. Patients should report any signs of local adverse reactions to the physician.

Laboratory Tests: The following tests may be helpful in evaluating patients for HPA axis suppression:
ACTH stimulation test
A.M. plasma cortisol test
Urinary free cortisol test
Carcinogenesis, Mutagenesis, Impairment of Fertility: Long-term animal studies have not been performed to evaluate the carcinogenic potential of clobetasol propionate.
Studies in the rat following oral administration at dosage levels up to 50 mg/kg per day revealed that the females exhibited an increase in the number of resorbed embryos and a decrease in the number of living fetuses at the highest dose.
Clobetasol propionate was nonmutagenic in three different test systems: the Ames test, the *Saccharomyces cerevisiae* gene conversion assay, and the *E. coli* B WP2 fluctuation test.
Pregnancy: ***Teratogenic Effects: Pregnancy Category C:*** Corticosteroids have been shown to be teratogenic in laboratory animals when administered systemically at relatively low dosage levels. Some corticosteroids have been shown to be teratogenic after dermal application to laboratory animals.
Clobetasol propionate has not been tested for teratogenicity when applied topically; however, it is absorbed percutaneously, and when administered subcutaneously it was a significant teratogen in both the rabbit and mouse. Clobetasol propionate has greater teratogenic potential than steroids that are less potent.
Teratogenicity studies in mice using the subcutaneous route resulted in fetotoxicity at the highest dose tested (1 mg/kg) and teratogenicity at all dose levels tested down to 0.03 mg/kg. These doses are approximately 0.33 and 0.01 times, respectively, the human topical dose of Temovate Cream and Ointment. Abnormalities seen included cleft palate and skeletal abnormalities.
In rabbits, clobetasol propionate was teratogenic at doses of 3 and 10 mcg/kg. These doses are approximately 0.001 and 0.003 times, respectively, the human topical dose of Temovate Cream and Ointment. Abnormalities seen included cleft palate, cranioschisis, and other skeletal abnormalities.
There are no adequate and well-controlled studies of the teratogenic potential of clobetasol propionate in pregnant women. Temovate Cream and Ointment should be used during pregnancy only if the potential benefit justifies the potential risk to the fetus.
Nursing Mothers: Systemically administered corticosteroids appear in human milk and could suppress growth, interfere with endogenous corticosteroid production, or cause other untoward effects. It is not known whether topical administration of corticosteroids could result in sufficient systemic absorption to produce detectable quantities in human milk. Because many drugs are excreted in human milk, caution should be exercised when Temovate Cream or Ointment is administered to a nursing woman.
Pediatric Use: Safety and effectiveness of Temovate in pediatric patients have not been established. Use in children under 12 years of age is not recommended. Because of a higher ratio of skin surface area to body mass, pediatric patients are at a greater risk than adults of HPA axis suppression and Cushing's syndrome when they are treated with topical corticosteroids. They are therefore also at greater risk of adrenal insufficiency during or after withdrawal of treatment. Adverse effects including striae have been reported with inappropriate use of topical corticosteroids in infants and children.
HPA axis suppression, Cushing's syndrome, linear growth retardation, delayed weight gain, and intracranial hypertension have been reported in children receiving topical corticosteroids. Manifestations of adrenal suppression in children include low plasma cortisol levels and an absence of response to ACTH stimulation. Manifestations of intracranial hypertension include bulging fontanelles, headaches, and bilateral papilledema.

ADVERSE REACTIONS
In controlled clinical trials, the most frequent adverse reactions reported for Temovate® Cream were burning and stinging sensation in 1% of treated patients. Less frequent adverse reactions were itching, skin atrophy, and cracking and fissuring of the skin.
In controlled clinical trials, the most frequent adverse events reported for Temovate® Ointment were burning sensation, irritation, and itching in 0.5% of treated patients. Less frequent adverse reactions were stinging, cracking, erythema, folliculitis, numbness of fingers, skin atrophy, and telangiectasia.
Cushing's syndrome has been reported in infants and adults as a result of prolonged use of topical clobetasol propionate formulations.
The following additional local adverse reactions have been reported with topical corticosteroids, and they may occur more frequently with the use of occlusive dressings and higher potency corticosteroids. These reactions are listed in an approximately decreasing order of occurrence: dryness, acneiform eruptions, hypopigmentation, perioral dermatitis, allergic contact dermatitis, secondary infection, irritation, striae, and miliaria.

OVERDOSAGE
Topically applied Temovate® Cream and Ointment can be absorbed in sufficient amounts to produce systemic effects (see PRECAUTIONS).

DOSAGE AND ADMINISTRATION
Apply a thin layer of Temovate® Cream or Ointment to the affected skin areas twice daily and rub in gently and completely.
Temovate Cream and Ointment are super-high potency topical corticosteroids; therefore, **treatment should be limited to 2 consecutive weeks, and amounts greater than 50 g per week should not be used.**
As with other highly active corticosteroids, therapy should be discontinued when control has been achieved. If no improvement is seen within 2 weeks, reassessment of diagnosis may be necessary.
Temovate Cream and Ointment should not be used with occlusive dressings.

HOW SUPPLIED

Temovate® Cream, 0.05% is supplied in 15-g (NDC 0173-0375-73), 30-g (NDC 0173-0375-72), 45-g (NDC 0173-0375-01), and 60-g (NDC 0173-0375-02) tubes.

Temovate® Ointment, 0.05% is supplied in 15-g (NDC 0173-0376-73), 30-g (NDC 0173-0376-72), 45-g (NDC 0173-0376-01), and 60-g (NDC 0173-0376-02) tubes.

Store between 15° and 30°C (59° and 86°F). Temovate Cream should not be refrigerated.
August 1995/RL-219
Shown in Product Identification Guide, page 314

TEMOVATE® ℞

[tim 'ō-vāt"]
(clobetasol propionate gel)
Gel, 0.05%*
*potency expressed as clobetasol propionate

**FOR TOPICAL DERMATOLOGIC USE ONLY—
NOT FOR OPHTHALMIC, ORAL, OR INTRAVAGINAL USE**

DESCRIPTION

Temovate® Gel (clobetasol propionate gel) contains the active compound clobetasol propionate, a synthetic corticosteroid, for topical dermatologic use. Clobetasol, an analog of prednisolone, has a high degree of glucocorticoid activity and a slight degree of mineralocorticoid activity.

Chemically, clobetasol propionate is (11β,16β)-21-chloro-9-fluoro-11-hydroxy-16-methyl-17- (1-oxopropoxy)-pregna-1,4-diene-3,20-dione.

Clobetasol propionate has the empirical formula $C_{25}H_{32}ClFO_5$ and a molecular weight of 467. It is a white to cream-colored crystalline powder insoluble in water.

Temovate Gel contains clobetasol propionate 0.5 mg/g in a base of propylene glycol, carbomer 934P, sodium hydroxide, and purified water.

CLINICAL PHARMACOLOGY

Like other topical corticosteroids, clobetasol propionate has anti-inflammatory, antipruritic, and vasoconstrictive properties. The mechanism of the anti-inflammatory activity of the topical steroids, in general, is unclear. However, corticosteroids are thought to act by the induction of phospholipase A_2 inhibitory proteins, collectively called lipocortins. It is postulated that these proteins control the biosynthesis of potent mediators of inflammation such as prostaglandins and leukotrienes by inhibiting the release of their common precursor, arachidonic acid. Arachidonic acid is released from membrane phospholipids by phospholipase A_2.

Pharmacokinetics: The extent of percutaneous absorption of topical corticosteroids is determined by many factors, including the vehicle and the integrity of the epidermal barrier. Occlusive dressing with hydrocortisone for up to 24 hours has not been demonstrated to increase penetration; however, occlusion of hydrocortisone for 96 hours markedly enhances penetration. Topical corticosteroids can be absorbed from normal intact skin, while inflammation and/or other disease processes in the skin may increase percutaneous absorption. Greater absorption was observed for the Temovate® gel formulation as compared to the cream formulation in in vitro human skin penetration studies.

Studies performed with Temovate® Gel indicate that it is in the super-high range of potency as compared with other topical corticosteroids.

INDICATIONS AND USAGE

Temovate® Gel is a super-high potency corticosteroid formulation indicated for the relief of the inflammatory and pruritic manifestations of corticosteroid-responsive dermatoses. Treatment beyond 2 consecutive weeks is not recommended, and the total dosage should not exceed 50 g per week because of the potential for the drug to suppress the hypothalamic-pituitary- adrenal (HPA) axis. Use in children under 12 years of age is not recommended.

CONTRAINDICATIONS

Temovate® Gel is contraindicated in those patients with a history of hypersensitivity to any of the components of the preparation.

PRECAUTIONS

General: Clobetasol propionate is a highly potent topical corticosteroid that has been shown to suppress the HPA axis at doses as low as 2 g per day.
Systemic absorption of topical corticosteroids can produce reversible HPA axis suppression with the potential for glucocorticosteroid insufficiency after withdrawal from treatment. Manifestations of Cushing's syndrome, hyperglycemia, and glucosuria can also be produced in some patients by systemic absorption of topical corticosteroids while on therapy.

Patients receiving a large dose applied to a large surface area should be evaluated periodically for evidence of HPA axis suppression. This may be done by using the ACTH stimula-

tion, a.m. plasma cortisol, and urinary free cortisol tests. Patients receiving super-potent corticosteroids should not be treated for more than 2 weeks at a time, and only small areas should be treated at any one time due to the increased risk of HPA suppression.

If HPA axis suppression is noted, an attempt should be made to withdraw the drug, to reduce the frequency of application, or to substitute a less potent corticosteroid. Recovery of HPA axis function is generally prompt and complete upon discontinuation of topical corticosteroids. Infrequently, signs and symptoms of glucocorticosteroid insufficiency may occur that require supplemental systemic corticosteroids. For information on systemic supplementation, see prescribing information for those products.

Children may be more susceptible to systemic toxicity from equivalent doses due to their larger skin surface to body mass ratios (see PRECAUTIONS: Pediatric Use).

If irritation develops, Temovate® Gel should be discontinued and appropriate therapy instituted. Allergic contact dermatitis with corticosteroids is usually diagnosed by observing *failure to heal* rather than noting a clinical exacerbation as with most topical products not containing corticosteroids. Such an observation should be corroborated with appropriate diagnostic patch testing.

If concomitant skin infections are present or develop, an appropriate antifungal or antibacterial agent should be used. If a favorable response does not occur promptly, use of Temovate Gel should be discontinued until the infection has been adequately controlled.

Temovate Gel should not be used in the treatment of rosacea or perioral dermatitis, and should not be used on the face, groin, or axillae.

Information for Patients: Patients using topical corticosteroids should receive the following information and instructions:
1. This medication is to be used as directed by the physician. It is for external use only. Avoid contact with the eyes.
2. This medication should not be used for any disorder other than that for which it was prescribed.
3. The treated skin area should not be bandaged or otherwise covered or wrapped so as to be occlusive unless directed by the physician.
4. Patients should report any signs of local adverse reactions to the physician.
5. Patients should inform their physicians that they are using Temovate if surgery is contemplated.

Laboratory Tests: The following tests may be helpful in evaluating patients for HPA axis suppression:
ACTH stimulation test
A.M. plasma cortisol test
Urinary free cortisol test

Carcinogenesis, Mutagenesis, Impairment of Fertility: Long-term animal studies have not been performed to evaluate the carcinogenic potential of clobetasol propionate.

Studies in the rat following oral administration at dosage levels up to 50 mg/kg per day revealed no significant effect on the males. The females exhibited an increase in the number of resorbed embryos and a decrease in the number of living fetuses at the highest dose.

Clobetasol propionate was nonmutagenic in three different test systems: the Ames test, the *Saccharomyces cerevisiae* gene conversion assay, and the *E. coli* B WP2 fluctuation test.

Pregnancy: *Teratogenic Effects: Pregnancy Category C:* Corticosteroids have been shown to be teratogenic in laboratory animals when administered systemically at relatively low dosage levels. Some corticosteroids have been shown to be teratogenic after dermal application to laboratory animals.

Clobetasol propionate has not been tested for teratogenicity by this route; however, it is absorbed percutaneously, and when administered subcutaneously it was a significant teratogen in both the rabbit and mouse. Clobetasol propionate has greater teratogenic potential than steroids that are less potent.

Teratogenicity studies in mice using the subcutaneous route resulted in fetotoxicity at the highest dose tested (1 mg/kg) and teratogenicity at all dose levels tested down to 0.03 mg/kg. These doses are approximately 0.33 and 0.01 times, respectively, the human topical dose of Temovate Gel. Abnormalities seen included cleft palate and skeletal abnormalities.

In rabbits, clobetasol propionate given by the same route was teratogenic at doses of 3 and 10 mcg/kg. These doses are approximately 0.001 and 0.003 times, respectively, the human topical dose of Temovate Gel. Abnormalities seen included cleft palate, cranioschisis, and other skeletal abnormalities. There are no adequate and well-controlled studies of the teratogenic potential of clobetasol propionate in pregnant women. Temovate Gel should be used during pregnancy only if the potential benefit justifies the potential risk to the fetus.

Nursing Mothers: Systemically administered corticosteroids appear in human milk and could suppress growth, interfere with endogenous corticosteroid production, or cause other untoward effects. It is not known whether topical ad-

ministration of corticosteroids could result in sufficient systemic absorption to produce detectable quantities in human milk. Because many drugs are excreted in human milk, caution should be exercised when Temovate Gel is administered to a nursing woman.

Pediatric Use: Safety and effectiveness of Temovate Gel in children and infants have not been established; therefore, use in children under 12 years of age is not recommended. Because of a higher ratio of skin surface area to body mass, children are at a greater risk than adults of HPA axis suppression when they are treated with topical corticosteroids. They are therefore also at greater risk of glucocorticosteroid insufficiency after withdrawal of treatment and of Cushing's syndrome while on treatment. Adverse effects including striae have been reported with inappropriate use of topical corticosteroids in infants and children (see PRECAUTIONS).

HPA axis suppression, Cushing's syndrome, and intracranial hypertension have been reported in children receiving topical corticosteroids. Manifestations of adrenal suppression in children include linear growth retardation, delayed weight gain, low plasma cortisol levels, and absence of response to ACTH stimulation. Manifestations of intracranial hypertension include bulging fontanelles, headaches, and bilateral papilledema.

ADVERSE REACTIONS

In a controlled trial with Temovate® Gel, the only reported adverse reaction that was considered to be drug related was a report of burning sensation (1.8% of treated patients).

In larger controlled clinical trials with other clobetasol propionate formulations, the most frequently reported adverse reactions have included burning, stinging, irritation, pruritus, erythema, folliculitis, cracking and fissuring of the skin, numbness of fingers, skin atrophy, and telangiectasia (all less than 2%).

Cushing's syndrome has been reported in infants and adults as a result of prolonged use of topical clobetasol propionate formulations.

The following additional local adverse reactions are reported infrequently with topical corticosteroids, but may occur more frequently with super-high potency corticosteroids such as Temovate Gel. These reactions are listed in approximate decreasing order of occurrence: dryness, hypertrichosis, acneiform eruptions, hypopigmentation, perioral dermatitis, allergic contact dermatitis, secondary infection, irritation, striae, and miliaria.

OVERDOSAGE

Topically applied Temovate® Gel can be absorbed in sufficient amounts to produce systemic effects (see PRECAUTIONS).

DOSAGE AND ADMINISTRATION

Apply a thin layer of Temovate® Gel to the affected skin areas twice daily and rub in gently and completely (see INDICATIONS AND USAGE).

Temovate Gel is a super-high potency topical corticosteroid; therefore, **treatment should be limited to 2 consecutive weeks, and amounts greater than 50 g per week should not be used.**

As with other highly active corticosteroids, therapy should be discontinued when control has been achieved. If no improvement is seen within 2 weeks, reassessment of diagnosis may be necessary.

Temovate Gel should not be used with occlusive dressings.

HOW SUPPLIED

Temovate® Gel, 0.05% is supplied in 15-g (NDC 0173-0455-01), 30-g (NDC 0173-0455-02), and 60-g (NDC 0173-0455-03) tubes.

Store between 15° and 30°C (59° and 86°F). Temovate Gel should not be refrigerated.
June 1994/RL-165
Shown in Product Identification Guide, page 314

TEMOVATE® ℞

[tim 'ō-vāt"]
(clobetasol propionate scalp application)
Scalp Application, 0.05%
(Potency expressed as clobetasol propionate.)

**For Dermatologic Use Only—
Not for Ophthalmic Use.**

DESCRIPTION

Temovate® Scalp Application contains the active compound clobetasol propionate, a synthetic corticosteroid, for topical dermatologic use. Clobetasol, an analog of prednisolone, has a high degree of glucocorticoid activity and a slight degree of mineralocorticoid activity.

Continued on next page

Glaxo Wellcome—Cont.

Chemically, clobetasol propionate is (11β,16β)-21-chloro-9-fluoro-11-hydroxy-16-methyl-17-(1-oxopropoxy)pregna-1,4-diene-3,20-dione.
Clobetasol propionate has the empirical formula $C_{25}H_{32}ClFO_5$ and a molecular weight of 467. It is a white to cream-colored crystalline powder insoluble in water.
Temovate Scalp Application contains clobetasol propionate 0.5 mg/g in a base composed of purified water, isopropyl alcohol (39.3%), carbomer 934P, and sodium hydroxide.

CLINICAL PHARMACOLOGY

The corticosteroids are a class of compounds comprising steroid hormones secreted by the adrenal cortex and their synthetic analogs. In pharmacologic doses, corticosteroids are used primarily for their anti-inflammatory and/or immunosuppressive effects. Topical corticosteroids such as clobetasol propionate are effective in the treatment of corticosteroid-responsive dermatoses primarily because of their anti-inflammatory, antipruritic, and vasoconstrictive actions. However, while the physiologic, pharmacologic, and clinical effects of the corticosteroids are well known, the exact mechanisms of their actions in each disease are uncertain.
Clobetasol propionate, a corticosteroid, has been shown to have topical (dermatologic) and systemic pharmacologic and metabolic effects characteristic of this class of drugs.
Pharmacokinetics: The extent of percutaneous absorption of topical corticosteroids, including clobetasol propionate, is determined by many factors, including the vehicle, the integrity of the epidermal barrier, and the use of occlusive dressings (see DOSAGE AND ADMINISTRATION).
As with all topical corticosteroids, clobetasol propionate can be absorbed from normal intact skin. Inflammation and/or other disease processes in the skin may increase percutaneous absorption. Occlusive dressings substantially increase the percutaneous absorption of topical corticosteroids (see DOSAGE AND ADMINISTRATION).
Once absorbed through the skin, topical corticosteroids enter pharmacokinetic pathways similarly to systemically administered corticosteroids. Corticosteroids are bound to plasma proteins in varying degrees. Corticosteroids are metabolized primarily in the liver and are then excreted by the kidneys. Some of the topical corticosteroids, including clobetasol propionate and its metabolites, are also excreted into the bile.
Following repeated nonocclusive application in the treatment of scalp psoriasis, there is some evidence that Temovate® Scalp Application has the potential to depress plasma cortisol levels in some patients. However, hypothalamic-pituitary-adrenal (HPA) axis effects produced by systemically absorbed clobetasol propionate have been shown to be transient and reversible upon completion of a 2-week course of treatment.

INDICATIONS AND USAGE

Temovate® Scalp Application is indicated for short-term topical treatment of inflammatory and pruritic manifestations of moderate to severe corticosteroid-responsive dermatoses of the scalp. Treatment beyond 2 consecutive weeks is not recommended, and the total dosage should not exceed 50 mL per week because of the potential for the drug to suppress the HPA axis.
This product is not recommended for use in children under 12 years of age.

CONTRAINDICATIONS

Temovate® Scalp Application is contraindicated in patients with primary infections of the scalp, or in patients who are hypersensitive to clobetasol propionate, other corticosteroids, or any ingredient in this preparation.

PRECAUTIONS

General: Clobetasol propionate is a highly potent topical corticosteroid that has been shown to suppress the HPA axis at doses as low as 2 g (of ointment) per day.
Systemic absorption of topical corticosteroids has resulted in reversible HPA axis suppression, manifestations of Cushing's syndrome, hyperglycemia, and glucosuria in some patients.
Conditions that augment systemic absorption include the application of the more potent corticosteroids, use over large surface areas, prolonged use, and the addition of occlusive dressings. Therefore, patients receiving a large dose of a potent topical steroid applied to a large surface area should be evaluated periodically for evidence of HPA axis suppression by using the urinary free cortisol and ACTH stimulation tests. If HPA axis suppression is noted, an attempt should be made to withdraw the drug, to reduce the frequency of application, or to substitute a less potent steroid.
Recovery of HPA axis function is generally prompt and complete upon discontinuation of the drug. Infrequently, signs and symptoms of steroid withdrawal may occur, requiring supplemental systemic corticosteroids.
Children may absorb proportionally larger amounts of topical corticosteroids and thus be more susceptible to systemic toxicity (see PRECAUTIONS: Pediatric Use).
If irritation develops, topical corticosteroids should be discontinued and appropriate therapy instituted. Irritation is possible if Temovate® Scalp Application contacts the eye. If that should occur, immediate flushing of the eye with a large volume of water is recommended.
If the inflammatory lesion becomes infected, the use of an appropriate antifungal or antibacterial agent should be instituted. If a favorable response does not occur promptly, the corticosteroid should be discontinued until the infection has been adequately controlled.
Although Temovate Scalp Application is intended for the treatment of inflammatory conditions of the scalp, it should be noted that certain areas of the body, such as the face, groin, and axillae, are more prone to atrophic changes than other areas of the body following treatment with corticosteroids. Frequent observation of the patient is important if these areas are to be treated.
As with other potent topical corticosteroids, Temovate Scalp Application should not be used in the treatment of rosacea and perioral dermatitis. Topical corticosteroids in general should not be used in the treatment of acne or as sole therapy in widespread plaque psoriasis.
Information For Patients: Patients using Temovate Scalp Application should receive the following information and instructions:
1. This medication is to be used as directed by the physician and should not be used longer than the prescribed time period. It is for external use only. Avoid contact with the eyes.
2. This medication should not be used for any disorder other than that for which it was prescribed.
3. The treated skin area should not be bandaged or otherwise covered or wrapped so as to be occlusive.
4. Patients should report any signs of local adverse reactions to the physician.

Laboratory Tests: The following tests may be helpful in evaluating HPA axis suppression:
Urinary free cortisol test
ACTH stimulation test
Carcinogenesis, Mutagenesis, Impairment of Fertility: Long-term animal studies have not been performed to evaluate the carcinogenic potential or the effect on fertility of topical corticosteroids.
Studies to determine mutagenicity with prednisolone have revealed negative results.
Pregnancy: ***Teratogenic Effects: Pregnancy Category C:*** The more potent corticosteroids have been shown to be teratogenic in animals after dermal application. Clobetasol propionate has not been tested for teratogenicity by this route; however, it is absorbed percutaneously, and when administered subcutaneously it was a significant teratogen in both the rabbit and the mouse. Clobetasol propionate has greater teratogenic potential than steroids that are less potent.
There are no adequate and well-controlled studies of the teratogenic effects of topically applied corticosteroids, including clobetasol, in pregnant women. Therefore, clobetasol and other topical corticosteroids should be used during pregnancy only if the potential benefit justifies the potential risk to the fetus, and they should not be used extensively on pregnant patients, in large amounts, or for prolonged periods of time.
Nursing Mothers: It is not known whether topical administration of corticosteroids could result in sufficient systemic absorption to produce detectable quantities in breast milk. Systemically administered corticosteroids are secreted into breast milk in quantities not likely to have a deleterious effect on the infant. Nevertheless, caution should be exercised when topical corticosteroids are prescribed for a nursing woman.
Pediatric Use: Use of Temovate Scalp Application in children under 12 years of age is not recommended.
Pediatric patients may demonstrate greater susceptibility to topical corticosteroid-induced HPA axis suppression and Cushing's syndrome than mature patients because of a larger skin surface area to body weight ratio.
HPA axis suppression, Cushing's syndrome, and intracranial hypertension have been reported in children receiving topical corticosteroids. Manifestations of adrenal suppression in children include linear growth retardation, delayed weight gain, low plasma cortisol levels, and absence of response to ACTH stimulation. Manifestations of intracranial hypertension include bulging fontanelles, headaches, and bilateral papilledema.

ADVERSE REACTIONS

Temovate® Scalp Application is generally well tolerated when used for 2-week treatment periods.
The most frequent adverse events reported for Temovate Scalp Application have been local and have included burning and/or stinging sensation, which occurred in 29 of 294 patients; scalp pustules, which occurred in 3 of 294 patients; and tingling and folliculitis, each of which occurred in 2 of 294 patients. Less frequent adverse events were itching and tightness of the scalp, dermatitis, tenderness, headache, hair loss, and eye irritation, each of which occurred in 1 of 294 patients.
The following local adverse reactions are reported infrequently when topical corticosteroids are used as recommended. These reactions are listed in an approximately decreasing order of occurrence: burning, itching, irritation, dryness, folliculitis, hypertrichosis, acneiform eruptions, hypopigmentation, perioral dermatitis, allergic contact dermatitis, maceration of the skin, secondary infection, skin atrophy, striae, and miliaria. Systemic absorption of topical corticosteroids has produced reversible HPA axis suppression, manifestations of Cushing's syndrome, hyperglycemia, and glucosuria in some patients. In rare instances, treatment (or withdrawal of treatment) of psoriasis with corticosteroids is thought to have exacerbated the disease or provoked the pustular form of the disease, so careful patient supervision is recommended.

OVERDOSAGE

Topically applied Temovate® Scalp Application can be absorbed in sufficient amounts to produce systemic effects (see PRECAUTIONS).

DOSAGE AND ADMINISTRATION

Temovate® Scalp Application should be applied to the affected scalp areas twice daily, once in the morning and once at night.
Temovate Scalp Application is potent; therefore, **treatment must be limited to 2 consecutive weeks, and amounts greater than 50 mL per week should not be used. Temovate Scalp Application is not to be used with occlusive dressings.**

HOW SUPPLIED

Temovate® Scalp Application, 0.05% is supplied in plastic squeeze bottles, 25 mL (NDC 0173-0432-00) and 50 mL (NDC 0173-0432-01).
Store between 4° and 25°C (39° and 77°F). Do not use near an open flame.
July 1995/RL-208
Shown in Product Identification Guide, page 314

TEMOVATE® E ℞

[tim 'ō-vāt"]
(clobetasol propionate emollient cream)
Emollient, 0.05%*
*** potency expressed as clobetasol propionate**
FOR TOPICAL DERMATOLOGIC USE ONLY—NOT FOR OPHTHALMIC, ORAL, OR INTRAVAGINAL USE

DESCRIPTION

TEMOVATE E Emollient contains the active compound clobetasol propionate, a synthetic corticosteroid, for topical dermatologic use. Clobetasol, an analog of prednisolone, has a high degree of glucocorticoid activity and a slight degree of mineralocorticoid activity.
Chemically, clobetasol propionate is (11β,16β)-21-chloro-9-fluoro-11-hydroxy-16-methyl-17-(1-oxopropoxy)-pregna-1,4-diene-3,20-dione.
Clobetasol propionate has the empirical formula $C_{25}H_{32}ClFO_5$ and a molecular weight of 467. It is a white to cream-colored crystalline powder insoluble in water.
TEMOVATE E Emollient contains clobetasol propionate 0.5 mg/g in an emollient base of cetostearyl alcohol, isopropyl myristate, propylene glycol, cetomacrogol 1000, dimethicone 360, citric acid, sodium citrate, purified water, and imidurea as a preservative.

CLINICAL PHARMACOLOGY

Like other topical corticosteroids, clobetasol propionate has anti-inflammatory, antipruritic, and vasoconstrictive properties. The mechanism of the anti-inflammatory activity of the topical steroids, in general, is unclear. However, corticosteroids are thought to act by the induction of phospholipase A_2 inhibitory proteins, collectively called lipocortins. It is postulated that these proteins control the biosynthesis of potent mediators of inflammation such as prostaglandins and leukotrienes by inhibiting the release of their common precursor, arachidonic acid. Arachidonic acid is released from membrane phospholipids by phospholipase A_2.
Pharmacokinetics: The extent of percutaneous absorption of topical corticosteroids is determined by many factors, including the vehicle and the integrity of the epidermal barrier. Occlusive dressing with hydrocortisone for up to 24 hours has not been demonstrated to increase penetration; however, occlusion of hydrocortisone for 96 hours markedly enhances penetration. Topical corticosteroids can be absorbed from normal intact skin. Inflammation and/or other disease processes in the skin may increase percutaneous absorption.
Studies performed with TEMOVATE E Emollient indicate that it is in the super-high range of potency as compared with other topical corticosteroids.

INDICATIONS AND USAGE

TEMOVATE E Emollient is a super-high potency corticosteroid formulation indicated for the relief of the inflammatory and pruritic manifestions of corticosteroid-responsive dermatoses. Treatment beyond 2 consecutive weeks is not

recommended, and the total dosage should not exceed 50 g/week because of the potential for the drug to suppress the hypothalamic-pituitary-adrenal (HPA) axis. Use in children under 12 years of age is not recommended.

In the treatment of moderate to severe plaque-type psoriasis, TEMOVATE E Emollient applied to 5% to 10% of body surface area can be used up to 4 consecutive weeks. The total dosage should not exceed 50 g/week. When dosing for more than 2 weeks, any additional benefits of extending treatment should be weighed against the risk of HPA suppression. Treatment beyond 4 consecutive weeks is not recommended. Patients should be instructed to use TEMOVATE E Emollient for the minimum amount of time necessary to achieve the desired results (see PRECAUTIONS and INDICATIONS AND USAGE). Use in pediatric patients under 16 years of age has not been studied.

CONTRAINDICATIONS

TEMOVATE E Emollient is contraindicated in those patients with a history of hypersensitivity to any of the components of the preparation.

PRECAUTIONS

General: Clobetasol propionate is a highly potent topical corticosteroid that has been shown to suppress the HPA axis at doses as low as 2 g/day.

Systemic absorption of topical corticosteroids can produce reversible HPA axis suppression with the potential for glucocorticosteroid insufficiency after withdrawal from treatment. Manifestations of Cushing's syndrome, hyperglycemia, and glucosuria can also be produced in some patients by systemic absorption of topical corticosteroids while on therapy.

Patients applying a dose to a large surface area or to areas under occlusion should be evaluated periodically for evidence of HPA axis suppression. This may be done by using the ACTH stimulation, A.M. plasma cortisol, and urinary free cortisol tests. Patients receiving super-potent corticosteroids should not be treated for more than 2 weeks at a time, and only small areas should be treated at any one time due to the increased risk of HPA suppression.

In a controlled clinical trial involving patients with moderate to severe plaque-type psoriasis, TEMOVATE E Emollient applied to 5% to 10% of body surface area resulted in additional benefits in the treatment of patients for 4 consecutive weeks. In this trial, there were no clobetasol-treated patients with clinically significant decreases in morning cortisol levels after 4 weeks of treatment; however, morning cortisol levels may not identify patients with adrenal dysfunction. Therefore, the additional benefits of extending treatment beyound 2 weeks should be weighed against the potential for HPA suppression. Therapy should be discontinued when control has been achieved. Treatment beyound 4 consecutive weeks is not recommended.

If HPA axis suppression in noted, an attempt should be made to withdraw the drug, to reduce the frequency of application, or to substitute a less potent corticosteroid. Recovery of HPA axis function is generally prompt upon discontinuation of topical corticosteroids. Infrequently, signs and symptoms of glucocorticosteroid insufficiency may occur that require supplemental systemic corticosteroids. For information on systemic supplementation, see prescribing information for those products.

Pediatric patients may be more susceptible to systemic toxicity from equivalent doses due to their larger skin surface to body mass ratios (see PRECAUTIONS: Pediatric Use). The use of TEMOVATE E Emollient for 4 consecutive weeks has not been studied in pediatric patients under 16 years of age. If irritation develops, TEMOVATE E Emollient should be discontinued and appropriate therapy instituted. Allergic contact dermatitis with corticosteroids is usually diagnosed by observing *failure to heal* rather than noting a clinical exacerbation as with most topical products not containing corticosteroids. Such an observation should be corroborated with appropriate diagnostic patch testing.

If concomitant skin infections are present or develop, an appropriate antifungal or antibacterial agent should be used. If a favorable response does not occur promptly, use of TEMOVATE E Emollient should be discontinued until the infection has been adequately controlled.

TEMOVATE E Emollient should not be used in the treatment of rosacea or perioral dermatitis, and should not be used on the face, groin, or axillae.

Information for Patients: Patients using topical corticosteroids should receive the following information and instructions:

1. This medication is to be used as directed by the physician. It is for external use only. Avoid contact with the eyes.
2. This medication should not be used for any disorder other than that for which it was prescribed.
3. The treated skin area should not be bandaged, otherwise covered, or wrapped so as to be occlusive unless directed by the physician.
4. Patients should report any signs of local adverse reactions to the physician.

5. Patients should inform their physicians that they are using TEMOVATE if surgery is contemplated.
6. This medication should not be used on the face, underarms, or groin areas.
7. As with other corticosteroids, therapy should be discontinued when control has been achieved. If no improvement is seen within 2 weeks, contact the physician.

Laboratory Tests: The following tests may be helpful in evaluating patients for HPA axis suppression:
ACTH stimulation test
A.M. plasma cortisol test
Urinary free cortisol test

Carcinogenesis, Mutagenesis, Impairment of Fertility: Long-term animal studies have not been performed to evaluate the carcinogenic potential of clobetasol propionate.

Studies in the rat following oral administration at dosage levels up to 50 mg/kg per day revealed no significant effect on the males. The females exhibited an increase in the number of resorbed embryos and a decrease in the number of living fetuses at the highest dose.

Clobetasol propionate was nonmutagenic in three different test systems: the Ames test, the *Saccharomyces cerevisiae* gene conversion assay, and the *E. coli* B WP2 fluctuation test.

Pregnancy: *Teratogenic Effects: Pregnancy Category C:* Corticosteroids have been shown to be teratogenic in laboratory animals when administered systemically at relatively low dosage levels. Some corticosteroids have been shown to be teratogenic after dermal application to laboratory animals.

Clobetasol propionate has not been tested for teratogenicity by this route; however, it is absorbed percutaneously, and when administered subcutaneously it was a significant teratogen in both the rabbit and mouse. Clobetasol propionate has greater teratogenic potential than steroids that are less potent.

Teratogenicity studies in mice using the subcutaneous route resulted in fetotoxicity at the highest dose tested (1 mg/kg) and teratogenicity at all dose levels tested down to 0.03 mg/kg. These doses are approximately 0.33 and 0.01 times, respectively, the human topical dose of TEMOVATE E Emollient. Abnormalities seen included cleft palate and skeletal abnormalities.

In rabbits, clobetasol propionate was teratogenic at doses of 3 and 10 mcg/kg. These doses are approximately 0.001 and 0.003 times, respectively, the human topical dose of TEMOVATE E Emollient. Abnormalities seen included cleft palate, cranioschisis, and other skeletal abnormalities.

There are no adequate and well-controlled studies of the teratogenic potential of clobetasol propionate in pregnant women. TEMOVATE E Emollient should be used during pregnancy only if the potential benefit justifies the potential risk to the fetus.

Nursing Mothers: Systemically administered corticosteroids appear in human milk and could suppress growth, interfere with endogenous corticosteroid production, or cause other untoward effects. It is not known whether topical administration of corticosteroids could result in sufficient systemic absorption to produce detectable quantities in human milk. Because many drugs are excreted in human milk, caution should be exercised when TEMOVATE E Emollient is administered to a nursing woman.

Pediatric Use: Safety and effectiveness of TEMOVATE E Emollient in pediatric patients have not been established, and its use in pediatric patients under 12 years of age is not recommended. For continued use beyond 2 consecutive weeks, the safety of TEMOVATE E Emollient has not been studied. Because of a higher ratio of skin surface area to body mass, pediatric patients are at a greater risk than adults of HPA axis suppression and Cushing's syndrome when they are treated with topical corticosteroids. They are therefore also at greater risk of glucocorticosteroid insufficiency during or after withdrawal of treatment. Adverse effects including striae have been reported with inappropriate use of topical corticosteroids in infants and children.

HPA axis suppression, Cushing's syndrome, linear growth retardation, delayed weight gain, and intracranial hypertension have been reported in children receiving topical corticosteroids. Manifestations of adrenal suppression in children include low plasma cortisol levels and absence of response to ACTH stimulation. Manifestations of intracranial hypertension include bulging fontanelles, headaches, and bilateral papilledema.

ADVERSE REACTIONS

In controlled trials with all clobetasol propionate formulations, the following adverse reactions have been reported: burning/stinging, pruritus, irritation, erythema, folliculitis, cracking and fissuring of the skin, numbness of the fingers, tenderness in the elbow, skin atrophy, and telangiectasia. The incidence of local adverse reactions reported in the trials with TEMOVATE E Emollient was < 2% of patients treated with the exception of burning/stinging, which occured in 5% of treated patients.

Cushing's syndrome has been reported in infants and adults as a result of prolonged use of topical clobetasol propionate formulations.

The following additional local adverse reactions are reported infrequently with topical corticosteroids, but may occur more frequently with super-high potency corticosteroids such as TEMOVATE E Emollient. These reactions are listed in an approximately decreasing order of occurrence: dryness, hypertrichosis, acneiform eruptions, hypopigmentation, perioral dermatitis, allergic contact dermatitis, secondary infection, striae, and miliaria.

OVERDOSAGE

Topically applied TEMOVATE E Emollient can be absorbed in sufficient amounts to produce systemic effects.

DOSAGE AND ADMINISTRATION

Apply a thin layer of TEMOVATE E Emollient to the affected skin areas twice daily and rub in gently and completely (see INDICATIONS AND USAGE).

TEMOVATE E Emollient is a super-high potency topical corticosteroid; therefore, **treatment should be limited to 2 consecutive weeks and amounts greater than 50 g/week should not be used.** Use in children under 12 years of age is not recommended.

In moderate to severe plaque-type psoriasis, TEMOVATE E Emollient applied to 5% to 10% of body surface area can be used up to 4 weeks. The total dosage should not exceed 50 g/week. When dosing for more than 2 weeks, any additional benefits of extending treatment should be weighed against the risk of HPA suppression. Therapy should be discontinued when control has been achieved. If no improvement is seen within 2 weeks, reassessment of diagnosis may be necessary. Treatment beyond 4 consecutive weeks is not recommended. Use in pediatric patients under 16 years of age has not been studied.

TEMOVATE E Emollient should not be used with occlusive dressings.

HOW SUPPLIED

TEMOVATE E Emollient, 0.05% is supplied in 15-g (NDC 0173-0454-01), 30-g (NDC 0173-0454-02), and 60-g (NDC 0173-0454-03) tubes.

Store between 15° and 30°C (59° and 86°F). **TEMOVATE E Emollient should not be refrigerated.**
May 1996/RL-318

Shown in Product Identification Guide, page 314

TRACRIUM® Injection   ℞
[trā'krē"um]
(atracurium besylate)

This drug should be used only by adequately trained individuals familiar with its actions, characteristics, and hazards.

DESCRIPTION

TRACRIUM (atracurium besylate) is an intermediate-duration, nondepolarizing, skeletal muscle relaxant for intravenous administration. Atracurium besylate is designated as 2,2'-[1,5 - pentanediylbis[oxy(3 - oxo-3,1- propanediyl)]]bis[1-[(3,4 - dimethoxyphenyl)methyl] - 1,2,3,4 -tetrahydro - 6,7-dimethoxy-2-methylisoquinolinium] dibenzenesulfonate. It has a molecular weight of 1243.51, and its molecular formula is $C_{65}H_{82}N_2O_{18}S_2$.

Atracurium besylate is a complex molecule containing four sites at which different stereochemical configurations can occur. The symmetry of the molecule, however, results in only ten, instead of sixteen, possible different isomers. The manufacture of atracurium besylate results in these isomers being produced in unequal amounts but with a consistent ratio. Those molecules in which the methyl group attached to the quaternary nitrogen projects on the opposite side to the adjacent substituted-benzyl moiety predominate by approximately 3:1.

TRACRIUM Injection is a sterile, non-pyrogenic aqueous solution. Each mL contains 10 mg atracurium besylate. The pH is adjusted to 3.25 to 3.65 with benzenesulfonic acid. The multiple dose vial contains 0.9% benzyl alcohol added as a preservative.

TRACRIUM slowly loses potency with time at the rate of approximately 6% per *year* under refrigeration (5°C). TRACRIUM Injection should be refrigerated at 2° to 8°C (36° to 46°F) to preserve potency. Rate of loss in potency increases to approximately 5% per *month* at 25°C (77°F). Upon removal from refrigeration to room temperature storage conditions (25°C/77°F), use TRACRIUM Injection within 14 days even if rerefrigerated.

CLINICAL PHARMACOLOGY

TRACRIUM is a nondepolarizing skeletal muscle relaxant. Nondepolarizing agents antagonize the neurotransmitter action of acetylcholine by binding competitively with cholinergic receptor sites on the motor end-plate. This antagonism is inhibited, and neuromuscular block reversed, by acetyl-

Continued on next page

Glaxo Wellcome—Cont.

cholinesterase inhibitors such as neostigmine, edrophonium, and pyridostigmine.

TRACRIUM can be used most advantageously if muscle twitch response to peripheral nerve stimulation is monitored to assess degree of muscle relaxation.

The duration of neuromuscular block produced by TRACRIUM is approximately one-third to one-half the duration of block by d-tubocurarine, metocurine, and pancuronium at initially equipotent doses. As with other nondepolarizing neuromuscular blockers, the time to onset of paralysis decreases and the duration of maximum effect increases with increasing doses of TRACRIUM.

The ED_{95} (dose required to produce 95% suppression of the muscle twitch response with balanced anesthesia) has averaged 0.23 mg/kg (0.11 to 0.26 mg/kg in various studies). An initial dose of TRACRIUM 0.4 to 0.5 mg/kg generally produces maximum neuromuscular block within 3 to 5 minutes of injection, with good or excellent intubation conditions within 2 to 2.5 minutes in most patients. Recovery from neuromuscular block (under balanced anesthesia) can be expected to begin approximately 20 to 35 minutes after injection. Under balanced anesthesia, recovery to 25% of control is achieved approximately 35 to 45 minutes after injection, and recovery is usually 95% complete approximately 60 to 70 minutes after injection. The neuromuscular blocking action of TRACRIUM is enhanced in the presence of potent inhalation anesthetics. Isoflurane and enflurane increase the potency of TRACRIUM and prolong neuromuscular block by approximately 35%; however, halothane's potentiating effect (approximately 20%) is marginal (see DOSAGE AND ADMINISTRATION).

Repeated administration of maintenance doses of TRACRIUM has no cumulative effect on the duration of neuromuscular block if recovery is allowed to begin prior to repeat dosing. Moreover, the time needed to recover from repeat doses does not change with additional doses. Repeat doses can therefore be administered at relatively regular intervals with predictable results. After an initial dose of 0.4 to 0.5 mg/kg under balanced anesthesia, the first maintenance dose (suggested maintenance dose is 0.08 to 0.10 mg/kg) is generally required within 20 to 45 minutes, and subsequent maintenance doses are usually required at approximately 15 to 25 minute intervals.

Once recovery from the neuromuscular blocking effects of TRACRIUM begins, it proceeds more rapidly than recovery from d-tubocurarine, metocurine, and pancuronium. Regardless of the dose of TRACRIUM, the time from start of recovery (from complete block) to complete (95%) recovery is approximately 30 minutes under balanced anesthesia, and approximately 40 minutes under halothane, enflurane, or isoflurane. Repeated doses have no cumulative effect on recovery rate.

Reversal of neuromuscular block produced by TRACRIUM can be achieved with an anticholinesterase agent such as neostigmine, edrophonium, or pyridostigmine, in conjunction with an anticholinergic agent such as atropine or glycopyrrolate. Under balanced anesthesia, reversal can usually be attempted approximately 20 to 35 minutes after an initial TRACRIUM dose of 0.4 to 0.5 mg/kg, or approximately 10 to 30 minutes after a 0.08 to 0.10 mg/kg maintenance dose, when recovery of muscle twitch has started. Complete reversal is usually attained within 8 to 10 minutes of the administration of reversing agents. Rare instances of breathing difficulties, possibly related to incomplete reversal, have been reported following attempted pharmacologic antagonism of TRACRIUM-induced neuromuscular block. As with other agents in this class, the tendency for residual neuromuscular block is increased if reversal is attempted at deep levels of block or if inadequate doses of reversal agents are employed.

The pharmacokinetics of TRACRIUM in man are essentially linear within the 0.3 to 0.6 mg/kg dose range. The elimination half-life is approximately 20 minutes. THE DURATION OF NEUROMUSCULAR BLOCK PRODUCED BY TRACRIUM DOES NOT CORRELATE WITH PLASMA PSEUDOCHOLINESTERASE LEVELS AND IS NOT ALTERED BY THE ABSENCE OF RENAL FUNCTION. This is consistent with the results of in vitro studies which have shown that TRACRIUM is inactivated in plasma via two nonoxidative pathways: ester hydrolysis, catalyzed by nonspecific esterases; and Hofmann elimination, a nonenzymatic chemical process which occurs at physiological pH. Some placental transfer occurs in humans.

Radiolabel studies demonstrated that TRACRIUM undergoes extensive degradation in cats, and that neither kidney nor liver plays a major role in its elimination. Biliary and urinary excretion were the major routes of excretion of radioactivity (totaling >90% of the labeled dose within 7 hours of dosing), of which TRACRIUM represented only a minor fraction. The metabolites in bile and urine were similar, including products of Hofmann elimination and ester hydrolysis.

Elderly patients may have slightly altered pharmacokinetic parameters compared to younger patients, with a slightly decreased total plasma clearance which is offset by a corresponding increase in volume of distribution. The net effect is that there has been no significant difference in clinical duration and recovery from neuromuscular block observed between elderly and younger patients receiving TRACRIUM. TRACRIUM is a less potent histamine releaser than d-tubocurarine or metocurine. Histamine release is minimal with initial TRACRIUM doses up to 0.5 mg/kg, and hemodynamic changes are minimal within the recommended dose range. A moderate histamine release and significant falls in blood pressure have been seen following 0.6 mg/kg of TRACRIUM. The histamine and hemodynamic responses were poorly correlated. The effects were generally short-lived and manageable, but the possibility of substantial histamine release in sensitive individuals or in patients in whom substantial histamine release would be especially hazardous (e.g., patients with significant cardiovascular disease) must be considered.

It is not known whether the prior use of other nondepolarizing neuromuscular blocking agents has any effect on the activity of TRACRIUM. The prior use of succinylcholine decreases by approximately 2 to 3 minutes the time to maximum block induced by TRACRIUM, and may increase the depth of block. TRACRIUM should be administered only after a patient recovers from succinylcholine-induced neuromuscular block.

INDICATIONS AND USAGE

TRACRIUM is indicated, as an adjunct to general anesthesia, to facilitate endotracheal intubation and to provide skeletal muscle relaxation during surgery or mechanical ventilation.

CONTRAINDICATIONS

TRACRIUM is contraindicated in patients known to have a hypersensitivity to it. Use of TRACRIUM from multiple dose vials containing benzyl alcohol as a preservative is contraindicated in patients with a known hypersensitivity to benzyl alcohol.

WARNINGS

TRACRIUM SHOULD BE USED ONLY BY THOSE SKILLED IN AIRWAY MANAGEMENT AND RESPIRATORY SUPPORT. EQUIPMENT AND PERSONNEL MUST BE IMMEDIATELY AVAILABLE FOR ENDOTRACHEAL INTUBATION AND SUPPORT OF VENTILATION, INCLUDING ADMINISTRATION OF POSITIVE PRESSURE OXYGEN. ADEQUACY OF RESPIRATION MUST BE ASSURED THROUGH ASSISTED OR CONTROLLED VENTILATION. ANTICHOLINESTERASE REVERSAL AGENTS SHOULD BE IMMEDIATELY AVAILABLE.
DO NOT GIVE TRACRIUM BY INTRAMUSCULAR ADMINISTRATION.
TRACRIUM has no known effect on consciousness, pain threshold, or cerebration. It should be used only with adequate anesthesia.
TRACRIUM Injection, which has an acid pH, should not be mixed with alkaline solutions (e.g., barbiturate solutions) in the same syringe or administered simultaneously during intravenous infusion through the same needle. Depending on the resultant pH of such mixtures, TRACRIUM may be inactivated and a free acid may be precipitated.
TRACRIUM Injection 10 mL multiple dose vials contain benzyl alcohol. In newborn infants, benzyl alcohol has been associated with an increased incidence of neurological and other complications which are sometimes fatal. TRACRIUM Injection 5 mL single use vials do not contain benzyl alcohol (see PRECAUTIONS: **Pediatric Use**).

PRECAUTIONS

General: Although TRACRIUM is a less potent histamine releaser than d-tubocurarine or metocurine, the possibility of substantial histamine release in sensitive individuals must be considered. Special caution should be exercised in administering TRACRIUM to patients in whom substantial histamine release would be especially hazardous (e.g., patients with clinically significant cardiovascular disease) and in patients with any history (e.g., severe anaphylactoid reactions or asthma) suggesting a greater risk of histamine release. In these patients, the recommended initial TRACRIUM dose is lower (0.3 to 0.4 mg/kg) than for other patients and should be administered slowly or in divided doses over one minute.
Since TRACRIUM has no clinically significant effects on heart rate in the recommended dosage range, it will not counteract the bradycardia produced by many anesthetic agents or vagal stimulation. As a result, bradycardia during anesthesia may be more common with TRACRIUM than with other muscle relaxants.
TRACRIUM may have profound effects in patients with myasthenia gravis, Eaton-Lambert syndrome, or other neuromuscular diseases in which potentiation of nondepolarizing agents has been noted. The use of a peripheral nerve stimulator is especially important for assessing neuromuscular block in these patients. Similar precautions should be

taken in patients with severe electrolyte disorders or carcinomatosis.
Multiple factors in anesthesia practice are suspected of triggering malignant hyperthermia (MH), a potentially fatal hypermetabolic state of skeletal muscle. Halogenated anesthetic agents and succinylcholine are recognized as the principal pharmacologic triggering agents in MH-susceptible patients; however, since MH can develop in the absence of established triggering agents, the clinician should be prepared to recognize and treat MH in any patient scheduled for general anesthesia. Reports of MH have been rare in cases in which TRACRIUM has been used. In studies of MH-susceptible animals (swine) and in a clinical study of MH-susceptible patients, TRACRIUM did not trigger this syndrome.
Resistance to nondepolarizing neuromuscular blocking agents may develop in burn patients. Increased doses of nondepolarizing muscle relaxants may be required in burn patients and are dependent on the time elapsed since the burn injury and the size of the burn.
The safety of TRACRIUM has not been established in patients with bronchial asthma.

Long-Term Use in Intensive Care Unit (ICU): When there is a need for long-term mechanical ventilation, the benefits-to-risk ratio of neuromuscular block must be considered. The long-term (1 to 10 days) infusion of TRACRIUM during mechanical ventilation in the ICU has been evaluated in several studies. Average infusion rates of 11 to 13 µg/kg/min (range: 4.5 to 29.5) were required to achieve adequate neuromuscular block. These data suggest that there is wide interpatient variability in dosage requirements. In addition, these studies have shown that dosage requirements may decrease or increase with time. Following discontinuation of infusion of TRACRIUM in these ICU studies, spontaneous recovery of four twitches in a train-of-four occurred in an average of approximately 30 minutes (range: 15 to 75 min) and spontaneous recovery to a train-of-four ratio > 75% (the ratio of the height of the fourth to the first twitch in a train-of-four) occurred in an average of approximately 60 minutes (range: 32 to 108 min).
Little information is available on the plasma levels and clinical consequences of atracurium metabolites that may accumulate during days to weeks of atracurium administration in ICU patients. Laudanosine, a major biologically active metabolite of atracurium without neuromuscular blocking activity, produces transient hypotension and, in higher doses, cerebral excitatory effects (generalized muscle twitching and seizures) when administered to several species of animals. There have been rare spontaneous reports of seizures in ICU patients who have received atracurium or other agents. These patients usually had predisposing causes (such as head trauma, cerebral edema, hypoxic encephalopathy, viral encephalitis, uremia). There are insufficient data to determine whether or not laudanosine contributes to seizures in ICU patients.
WHENEVER THE USE OF TRACRIUM OR ANY NEUROMUSCULAR BLOCKING AGENT IS CONTEMPLATED IN THE ICU, IT IS RECOMMENDED THAT NEUROMUSCULAR TRANSMISSION BE MONITORED CONTINUOUSLY DURING ADMINISTRATION WITH THE HELP OF A NERVE STIMULATOR. ADDITIONAL DOSES OF TRACRIUM OR ANY OTHER NEUROMUSCULAR BLOCKING AGENT SHOULD NOT BE GIVEN BEFORE THERE IS A DEFINITE RESPONSE TO T_1 OR TO THE FIRST TWITCH. IF NO RESPONSE IS ELICITED, INFUSION ADMINISTRATION SHOULD BE DISCONTINUED UNTIL A RESPONSE RETURNS.
Hemofiltration has a minimal effect on plasma levels of atracurium and its metabolites, including laudanosine. The effects of hemodialysis and hemoperfusion on plasma levels of atracurium and its metabolites are unknown.

Drug Interactions: Drugs which may enhance the neuromuscular blocking action of TRACRIUM include: enflurane; isoflurane; halothane; certain antibiotics, especially the aminoglycosides and polymyxins; lithium; magnesium salts; procainamide; and quinidine.
If other muscle relaxants are used during the same procedure, the possibility of a synergistic or antagonist effect should be considered.
The prior administration of succinylcholine does not enhance the duration, but quickens the onset and may increase the depth, of neuromuscular block induced by TRACRIUM. TRACRIUM should not be administered until a patient has recovered from succinylcholine-induced neuromuscular block.

Carcinogenesis, Mutagenesis, Impairment of Fertility: Carcinogenesis and fertility studies have not been performed. Atracurium was evaluated in a battery of three short-term mutagenicity tests. It was non-mutagenic in both the Ames Salmonella assay at concentrations up to 1000 µg/plate, and in a rat bone marrow cytogenicity assay at up to paralyzing doses. A positive response was observed in the mouse lymphoma assay under conditions (80 and 100 µg/mL, in the absence of metabolic activation) which killed over 80% of the treated cells; there was no mutagenicity at 60 µg/mL and lower, concentrations which killed up to half of the treated cells. A far weaker response was observed in the presence of

metabolic activation at concentrations (1200 μg/mL and higher) which also killed over 80% of the treated cells.
Mutagenicity testing is intended to simulate chronic (years to lifetime) exposure in an effort to determine potential carcinogenicity. Thus, a single positive mutagenicity response for a drug used infrequently and/or briefly is of questionable clinical relevance.

Pregnancy: *Teratogenic Effects:* Pregnancy Category C. TRACRIUM has been shown to be potentially teratogenic in rabbits when given in doses up to approximately one-half the human dose. There are no adequate and well-controlled studies in pregnant women. TRACRIUM should be used during pregnancy only if the potential benefit justifies the potential risk to the fetus.
TRACRIUM was administered subcutaneously on days 6 through 18 of gestation to non-ventilated Dutch rabbits. Treatment groups were given either 0.15 mg/kg once daily or 0.10 mg/kg twice daily. Lethal respiratory distress occurred in two 0.15 mg/kg animals and in one 0.10 mg/kg animal, with transient respiratory distress or other evidence of neuromuscular block occurring in 10 of 19 and in 4 of 20 of the 0.15 mg/kg and 0.10 mg/kg animals, respectively. There was an increased incidence of certain spontaneously occurring visceral and skeletal anomalies or variations in one or both treated groups when compared to non-treated controls. The percentage of male fetuses was lower (41% vs. 51%) and the post-implantation losses were increased (15% vs. 8%) in the group given 0.15 mg/kg once daily when compared to the controls; the mean numbers of implants (6.5 vs. 4.4) and normal live fetuses (5.4 vs. 3.8) were greater in this group when compared to the control group.

Labor and Delivery: It is not known whether muscle relaxants administered during vaginal delivery have immediate or delayed adverse effects on the fetus or increase the likelihood that resuscitation of the newborn will be necessary. The possibility that forceps delivery will be necessary may increase.
TRACRIUM (0.3 mg/kg) has been administered to 26 pregnant women during delivery by cesarean section. No harmful effects were attributable to TRACRIUM in any of the newborn infants, although small amounts of TRACRIUM were shown to cross the placental barrier. The possibility of respiratory depression in the newborn infant should always be considered following cesarean section during which a neuromuscular blocking agent has been administered. In patients receiving magnesium sulfate, the reversal of neuromuscular block may be unsatisfactory and the dose of TRACRIUM should be lowered as indicated.

Nursing Mothers: It is not known whether this drug is excreted in human milk. Because many drugs are excreted in human milk, caution should be exercised when TRACRIUM is administered to a nursing woman.

Pediatric Use: Safety and effectiveness in pediatric patients below the age of 1 month have not been established.

Use in the Elderly: Since marketing in 1983, uncontrolled clinical experience and limited data from controlled trials have not identified differences in effectiveness, safety, or dosage requirements between healthy elderly and younger patients (see CLINICAL PHARMACOLOGY); however, as with other neuromuscular blocking agents, the use of a peripheral nerve stimulator to monitor neuromuscular function is suggested (see DOSAGE AND ADMINISTRATION).

ADVERSE REACTIONS

Observed in Controlled Clinical Studies: TRACRIUM was well tolerated and produced few adverse reactions during extensive clinical trials. Most adverse reactions were suggestive of histamine release. In studies including 875 patients, TRACRIUM was discontinued in only one patient (who required treatment for bronchial secretions), and six other patients required treatment for adverse reactions attributable to TRACRIUM (wheezing in one, hypotension in five). Of the five patients who required treatment for hypotension, three had a history of significant cardiovascular disease. The overall incidence rate for clinically important adverse reactions, therefore, was 7/875 or 0.8%. The table below includes all adverse reactions reported attributable to TRACRIUM during clinical trials with 875 patients.
[See table above.]

PERCENT OF PATIENTS REPORTING ADVERSE REACTIONS

Adverse Reaction	Initial TRACRIUM Dose (mg/kg)			
	0.00-0.30 (n=485)	0.31-0.50* (n=366)	≥0.60 (n=24)	Total (n=875)
Skin Flush	1.0%	8.7%	29.2%	5.0%
Erythema	0.6%	0.5%	0%	0.6%
Itching	0.4%	0%	0%	0.2%
Wheezing/Bronchial Secretions	0.2%	0.3%	0%	0.2%
Hives	0.2%	0%	0%	0.1%

*Includes the recommended initial dosage range for most patients.

Most adverse reactions were of little clinical significance unless they were associated with significant hemodynamic changes. The table below summarizes the incidences of substantial vital sign changes noted during TRACRIUM clinical trials with 530 patients, without cardiovascular disease, in whom these parameters were assessed.
[See table at right.]

PERCENT OF PATIENTS SHOWING ≥30% VITAL SIGN CHANGES FOLLOWING ADMINISTRATION OF TRACRIUM

Vital Sign Change	Initial TRACRIUM Dose (mg/kg)			
	0.00-0.30 (n=365)	0.31-0.50* (n=144)	≥0.60 (n=21)	Total (n=530)
Mean Arterial Pressure				
Increase	1.9%	2.8%	0%	2.1%
Decrease	1.1%	2.1%	14.3%	1.9%
Heart Rate				
Increase	1.6%	2.8%	4.8%	2.1%
Decrease	0.8%	0%	0%	0.6%

*Includes the recommended initial dosage range for most patients.

Observed in Clinical Practice: Based on initial clinical practice experience in approximately 3 million patients who received TRACRIUM in the U.S. and in the United Kingdom, spontaneously reported adverse reactions were uncommon (approximately 0.01% to 0.02%). The following adverse reactions are among the most frequently reported, but there are insufficient data to support an estimate of their incidence:
General: Allergic reactions (anaphylactic or anaphylactoid responses) which, in rare instances, were severe (e.g., cardiac arrest)
Musculoskeletal: Inadequate block, prolonged block
Cardiovascular: Hypotension, vasodilatation (flushing), tachycardia, bradycardia
Respiratory: Dyspnea, bronchospasm, laryngospasm
Integumentary: Rash, urticaria, reaction at injection site
There have been rare spontaneous reports of seizures in ICU patients following long-term infusion of atracurium to support mechanical ventilation. There are insufficient data to define the contribution, if any, of atracurium and/or its metabolite laudanosine. (See PRECAUTIONS: Long-Term Use in Intensive Care Unit [ICU]).

OVERDOSAGE

There has been limited experience with overdosage of TRACRIUM. The possibility of iatrogenic overdosage can be minimized by carefully monitoring muscle twitch response to peripheral nerve stimulation. Excessive doses of TRACRIUM can be expected to produce enhanced pharmacological effects. Overdosage may increase the risk of histamine release and cardiovascular effects, especially hypotension. If cardiovascular support is necessary, this should include proper positioning, fluid administration, and the use of vasopressor agents if necessary. The patient's airway should be assured, with manual or mechanical ventilation maintained as necessary. A longer duration of neuromuscular block may result from overdosage and a peripheral nerve stimulator should be used to monitor recovery. Recovery may be facilitated by administration of an anticholinesterase reversing agent such as neostigmine, edrophonium, or pyridostigmine, in conjunction with an anticholinergic agent such as atropine or glycopyrrolate. The appropriate package inserts should be consulted for prescribing information.
Three pediatric patients (3 weeks, 4 and 5 months of age) unintentionally received doses of 0.8 mg/kg to 1.0 mg/kg of TRACRIUM. The time to 25% recovery (50 to 55 minutes) following these doses, which were 5 to 6 times the ED_{95} dose, was moderately longer than the corresponding time observed following doses 2.0 to 2.5 times the TRACRIUM ED_{95} dose in infants (22 to 36 minutes). Cardiovascular changes were minimal. Nonetheless the possibility of cardiovascular changes must be considered in the case of overdose.
An adult patient (17 years of age) unintentionally received an initial dose of 1.3 mg/kg of TRACRIUM. The time from injection to 25% recovery (83 minutes) was approximately twice that observed following maximum recommended doses in adults (35 to 45 minutes). The patient experienced moderate hemodynamic changes (13% increase in mean arterial pressure and 27% increase in heart rate) which persisted for 40 minutes and did not require treatment.
The intravenous LD_{50}s determined in non-ventilated male and female albino mice and male Wistar rats were 1.9, 2.01, and 1.31 mg/kg, respectively. Deaths occurred within 2 minutes and were caused by respiratory paralysis. The subcutaneous LD_{50} determined in non-ventilated male Wistar rats was 282.8 mg/kg. Tremors, ptosis, loss of reflexes, and respiratory failure preceded death which occurred 45 to 120 minutes after injection.

DOSAGE AND ADMINISTRATION

To avoid distress to the patient, TRACRIUM should not be administered before unconsciousness has been induced. TRACRIUM should not be mixed in the same syringe, or administered simultaneously through the same needle, with alkaline solutions (e.g., barbiturate solutions).
TRACRIUM should be administered intravenously. DO NOT GIVE TRACRIUM BY INTRAMUSCULAR ADMINISTRATION. Intramuscular administration of TRACRIUM may result in tissue irritation and there are no clinical data to support this route of administration.
As with other neuromuscular blocking agents, the use of a peripheral nerve stimulator will permit the most advantageous use of TRACRIUM, minimizing the possibility of overdosage or underdosage, and assist in the evaluation of recovery.
Parenteral drug products should be inspected visually for particulate matter and discoloration prior to administration, whenever solution and container permit.

Bolus Doses for Intubation and Maintenance of Neuromuscular Block:
Adults: A dose of TRACRIUM of 0.4 to 0.5 mg/kg (1.7 to 2.2 times the ED_{95}), given as an intravenous bolus injection, is the recommended initial dose for most patients. With this dose, good or excellent conditions for nonemergency intubation can be expected in 2 to 2.5 minutes in most patients, with maximum neuromuscular block achieved approximately 3 to 5 minutes after injection. Clinically required neuromuscular block generally lasts 20 to 35 minutes under balanced anesthesia. Under balanced anesthesia, recovery to 25% of control is achieved approximately 35 to 45 minutes after injection, and recovery is usually 95% complete approximately 60 minutes after injection.
TRACRIUM is potentiated by isoflurane or enflurane anesthesia. The same initial dose of TRACRIUM of 0.4 to 0.5 mg/kg may be used for intubation prior to administration of these inhalation agents; however, if TRACRIUM is first administered under steady state of isoflurane or enflurane, the initial dose of TRACRIUM should be reduced by approximately one-third, i.e., to 0.25 to 0.35 mg/kg, to adjust for the potentiating effects of these anesthetic agents. With halothane, which has only a marginal (approximately 20%) potentiating effect on TRACRIUM, smaller dosage reductions may be considered.
Doses of TRACRIUM of 0.08 to 0.10 mg/kg are recommended for maintenance of neuromuscular block during prolonged surgical procedures. The first maintenance dose will generally be required 20 to 45 minutes after the initial TRACRIUM Injection, but the need for maintenance doses should be determined by clinical criteria. Because TRACRIUM lacks cumulative effects, maintenance doses may be administered at relatively regular intervals for each patient, ranging approximately from 15 to 25 minutes under balanced anesthesia, slightly longer under isoflurane or enflurane. Higher doses of TRACRIUM (up to 0.2 mg/kg) permit maintenance dosing at longer intervals.
Children and Infants: No TRACRIUM dosage adjustments are required for pediatric patients two years of age or older. A dose of TRACRIUM 0.3 to 0.4 mg/kg is recommended as the initial dose for infants (1 month to 2 years of age) under halothane anesthesia. Maintenance doses may be required with slightly greater frequency in infants and children than in adults.
Special Considerations: An initial dose of TRACRIUM 0.3 to 0.4 mg/kg, given slowly or in divided doses over one minute, is recommended for adults, children, or infants with significant cardiovascular disease and for adults, children, or

Continued on next page

Glaxo Wellcome—Cont.

infants with any history (e.g., severe anaphylactoid reactions or asthma) suggesting a greater risk of histamine release.

Dosage reductions must be considered also in patients with neuromuscular disease, severe electrolyte disorders, or carcinomatosis in which potentiation of neuromuscular block or difficulties with reversal have been demonstrated. There has been no clinical experience with TRACRIUM in these patients, and no specific dosage adjustments can be recommended. No TRACRIUM dosage adjustments are required for patients with renal disease.

An initial dose of TRACRIUM of 0.3 to 0.4 mg/kg is recommended for adults following the use of succinylcholine for intubation under balanced anesthesia. Further reductions may be desirable with the use of potent inhalation anesthetics. The patient should be permitted to recover from the effects of succinylcholine prior to administration of TRACRIUM. Insufficient data are available for recommendation of a specific initial dose of TRACRIUM for administration following the use of succinylcholine in children and infants.

Use by Continuous Infusion:

Infusion in the Operating Room (OR): After administration of a recommended initial bolus dose of TRACRIUM (0.3 to 0.5 mg/kg), a diluted solution of TRACRIUM can be administered by continuous infusion to adults and children aged 2 or more years for maintenance of neuromuscular block during extended surgical procedures.

Infusion of TRACRIUM should be individualized for each patient. The rate of administration should be adjusted according to the patient's response as determined by peripheral nerve stimulation. Accurate dosing is best achieved using a precision infusion device.

Infusion of TRACRIUM should be initiated only after early evidence of spontaneous recovery from the bolus dose. An initial infusion rate of 9 to 10 μg/kg/min may be required to rapidly counteract the spontaneous recovery of neuromuscular function. Thereafter, a rate of 5 to 9 μg/kg/min should be adequate to maintain continuous neuromuscular block in the range of 89% to 99% in most pediatric and adult patients under balanced anesthesia. Occasional patients may require infusion rates as low as 2 μg/kg/min or as high as 15 μg/kg/min.

The neuromuscular blocking effect of TRACRIUM administered by infusion is potentiated by enflurane or isoflurane and, to a lesser extent, by halothane. Reduction in the infusion rate of TRACRIUM should, therefore, be considered for patients receiving inhalation anesthesia. The rate of TRACRIUM infusion should be reduced by approximately one-third in the presence of steady-state enflurane or isoflurane anesthesia; smaller reductions should be considered in the presence of halothane.

In patients undergoing cardiopulmonary bypass with induced hypothermia, the rate of infusion of TRACRIUM required to maintain adequate surgical relaxation during hypothermia (25° to 28°C) has been shown to be approximately half the rate required during normothermia.

Spontaneous recovery from neuromuscular block following discontinuation of TRACRIUM infusion may be expected to proceed at a rate comparable to that following administration of a single bolus dose.

Infusion in the Intensive Care Unit (ICU): The principles for infusion of TRACRIUM in the OR are also applicable to use in the ICU.

An infusion rate of 11 to 13 μg/kg/min (range: 4.5 to 29.5) should provide adequate neuromuscular block in adult patients in an ICU. Limited information suggests that infusion rates required for pediatric patients in the ICU may be higher than in adult patients. There may be wide interpatient variability in dosage requirements and these requirements may increase or decrease with time (see PRECAUTIONS: Long-Term Use in Intensive Care Unit [ICU]). Following recovery from neuromuscular block, readministration of a bolus dose may be necessary to quickly re-establish neuromuscular block prior to reinstitution of the infusion.

Infusion Rate Tables: The amount of infusion solution required per minute will depend upon the concentration of TRACRIUM in the infusion solution, the desired dose of TRACRIUM, and the patient's weight. The following tables provide guidelines for delivery, in mL/hr (equivalent to microdrops/min when 60 microdrops = 1 mL), of TRACRIUM solutions in concentrations of 0.2 mg/mL (20 mg in 100 mL) or 0.5 mg/mL (50 mg in100 mL) with an infusion pump or a gravity flow device.

[See tables on top of next column.]

Compatibility and Admixtures: TRACRIUM Infusion solutions may be prepared by admixing TRACRIUM Injection with an appropriate diluent such as 5% Dextrose Injection USP, 0.9% Sodium Chloride Injection USP, or 5% Dextrose and 0.9% Sodium Chloride Injection USP. Infusion solutions should be used within 24 hours of preparation. Unused solutions should be discarded. Solutions containing 0.2 mg/mL or 0.5 mg/mL TRACRIUM in the above diluents may be stored either under refrigeration or at room temperature for 24 hours without significant loss of potency. Care should be taken during admixture to prevent inadvertent contamination. Visually inspect prior to administration.

TRACRIUM (atracurium besylate) Infusion Rates for a Concentration of 0.2 mg/mL

Patient Weight (Kg)	Drug Delivery Rate (μg/kg/min) 5	6	7	8	9	10	11	12	13
	Infusion Delivery Rate (mL/hr)								
30	45	54	63	72	81	90	99	108	117
35	53	63	74	84	95	105	116	126	137
40	60	72	84	96	108	120	132	144	156
45	68	81	95	108	122	135	149	162	176
50	75	90	105	120	135	150	165	180	195
55	83	99	116	132	149	165	182	198	215
60	90	108	126	144	162	180	198	216	234
65	98	117	137	156	176	195	215	234	254
70	105	126	147	168	189	210	231	252	273
75	113	135	158	180	203	225	248	270	293
80	120	144	168	192	216	240	264	288	312
90	135	162	189	216	243	270	297	324	351
100	150	180	210	240	270	300	330	360	390

TRACRIUM (atracurium besylate) Infusion Rates for a Concentration of 0.5 mg/mL

Patient Weight (Kg)	Drug Delivery Rate (μg/kg/min) 5	6	7	8	9	10	11	12	13
	Infusion Delivery Rate (mL/hr)								
30	18	22	25	29	32	36	40	43	47
35	21	25	29	34	38	42	46	50	55
40	24	29	34	38	43	48	53	58	62
45	27	32	38	43	49	54	59	65	70
50	30	36	42	48	54	60	66	72	78
55	33	40	46	53	59	66	73	79	86
60	36	43	50	58	65	72	79	86	94
65	39	47	55	62	70	78	86	94	101
70	42	50	59	67	76	84	92	101	109
75	45	54	63	72	81	90	99	108	117
80	48	58	67	77	86	96	106	115	125
90	54	65	76	86	97	108	119	130	140
100	60	72	84	96	108	120	132	144	156

Spontaneous degradation of TRACRIUM has been demonstrated to occur more rapidly in lactated Ringer's solution than in 0.9% sodium chloride solution. Therefore, it is recommended that Lactated Ringer's Injection USP not be used as a diluent in preparing solutions of TRACRIUM for infusion.

HOW SUPPLIED

TRACRIUM Injection, 10 mg atracurium besylate in each mL.

5 mL Single Use Vial (50 mg atracurium besylate per vial). Tray of 10 (NDC 0173-0940-44).

10 mL Multiple Dose Vial (100 mg atracurium besylate per vial). Contains benzyl alcohol (see WARNINGS). Tray of 10 (NDC 0173-0545-00).

STORAGE:

TRACRIUM Injection should be refrigerated at 2° to 8°C (36° to 46°F) to preserve potency. DO NOT FREEZE. Upon removal from refrigeration to room temperature storage conditions (25°C/77°F), use TRACRIUM Injection within 14 days even if rerefrigerated.

U.S. Patent No. 4179507

June 1996/RL-328

Shown in Product Identification Guide, page 314

TRANDATE® Tablets ℞

[tran 'dāt]

(labetalol hydrochloride)

TRANDATE® Injection

[tran 'dāt]

(labetalol hydrochloride)

DESCRIPTION

Trandate® (labetalol hydrochloride) Tablets and Trandate® (labetalol hydrochloride) Injection are adrenergic receptor blocking agents that have both selective $alpha_1$-adrenergic and nonselective beta-adrenergic receptor blocking actions in a single substance.

Labetalol hydrochloride (HCl) is a racemate chemically designated as 2-hydroxy-5-[1-hydroxy-2-[(1-methyl-3-phenylpropyl)amino]ethyl]benzamide monohydrochloride.

Labetalol HCl has the empirical formula $C_{19}H_{24}N_2O_3 \cdot HCl$ and a molecular weight of 364.9. It has two asymmetric centers and therefore exists as a molecular complex of two diastereoisomeric pairs. Dilevalol, the R,R' stereoisomer, makes up 25% of racemic labetalol.

Labetalol HCl is a white or off-white crystalline powder, soluble in water.

Trandate Tablets contain 100, 200, or 300 mg of labetalol HCl and are taken orally. The tablets also contain the inactive ingredients corn starch, FD&C Yellow No. 6 (100- and 300-mg tablets only), hydroxypropyl methylcellulose, lactose, magnesium stearate, methylparaben, pregelatinized corn starch, propylparaben, sodium benzoate (200-mg tablet only), talc (100-mg tablet only), and titanium dioxide.

Trandate Injection is a clear, colorless to light yellow, aqueous, sterile, isotonic solution for intravenous (IV) injection. It has a pH range of 3 to 4. Each milliliter contains 5 mg of labetalol HCl, 45 mg of anhydrous dextrose, 0.1 mg of edetate disodium; 0.8 mg of methylparaben and 0.1 mg of propylparaben as preservatives; and citric acid monohydrate and sodium hydroxide, as necessary, to bring the solution into the pH range.

CLINICAL PHARMACOLOGY

Labetalol HCl combines both selective, competitive, $alpha_1$-adrenergic blocking and nonselective, competitive, beta-adrenergic blocking activity in a single substance. In man, the ratios of alpha- to beta-blockade have been estimated to be approximately 1:3 and 1:7 following oral and IV administration, respectively. $Beta_2$-agonist activity has been demonstrated in animals with minimal $beta_1$-agonist (ISA) activity detected. In animals, at doses greater than those required for alpha- or beta-adrenergic blockade, a membrane stabilizing effect has been demonstrated.

Pharmacodynamics: The capacity of labetalol HCl to block alpha receptors in man has been demonstrated by attenuation of the pressor effect of phenylephrine and by a significant reduction of the pressor response caused by immersing the hand in ice-cold water ("cold-pressor test"). Labetalol HCl's $beta_1$-receptor blockade in man was demonstrated by a small decrease in the resting heart rate, attenuation of tachycardia produced by isoproterenol or exercise, and by attenuation of the reflex tachycardia to the hypotension produced by amyl nitrite. $Beta_2$-receptor blockade was demonstrated by inhibition of the isoproterenol-induced fall in diastolic blood pressure. Both the alpha- and beta-blocking actions of orally administered labetalol HCl contribute to a decrease in blood pressure in hypertensive patients. Labetalol HCl consistently, in dose-related fashion, blunted increases in exercise-induced blood pressure and heart rate, and in their double product. The pulmonary circulation during exercise was not affected by labetalol HCl dosing.

Single oral doses of labetalol HCl administered to patients with coronary artery disease had no significant effect on sinus rate, intraventricular conduction, or QRS duration. The atrioventricular (A-V) conduction time was modestly prolonged in two of seven patients. In another study, IV labetalol HCl slightly prolonged A-V nodal conduction time and atrial effective refractory period with only small changes in heart rate. The effects on A-V nodal refractoriness were inconsistent.

Labetalol HCl produces dose-related falls in blood pressure without reflex tachycardia and without significant reduction in heart rate, presumably through a mixture of its alpha- and beta-blocking effects. Hemodynamic effects are variable, with small, nonsignificant changes in cardiac output seen in some studies but not others, and small decreases in total peripheral resistance. Elevated plasma renins are reduced.

Doses of labetalol HCl that controlled hypertension did not affect renal function in mildly to severely hypertensive patients with normal renal function.

Due to the $alpha_1$-receptor blocking activity of labetalol HCl, blood pressure is lowered more in the standing than in the supine position, and symptoms of postural hypotension (2%), including rare instances of syncope, can occur. Following oral administration, when postural hypotension has occurred, it has been transient and is uncommon when the recommended starting dose and titration increments are closely followed (see DOSAGE AND ADMINISTRATION). Symptomatic postural hypotension is most likely to occur 2 to 4 hours after a dose, especially following the use of large initial doses or upon large changes in dose. During dosing with IV labetalol HCl, the contribution of the postural component should be considered when positioning the patient for treatment, and the patient should not be allowed to move to an erect position unmonitored until his ability to do so is established.

The peak effects of single oral doses of labetalol HCl occur within 2 to 4 hours. The duration of effect depends upon dose, lasting at least 8 hours following single oral doses of 100 mg and more than 12 hours following single oral doses of 300 mg. The maximum, steady-state blood pressure response upon oral, twice-a-day dosing occurs within 24 to 72 hours.

The antihypertensive effect of labetalol has a linear correlation with the logarithm of labetalol plasma concentration, and there is also a linear correlation between the reduction

in exercise-induced tachycardia occurring at 2 hours after oral administration of labetalol HCl and the logarithm of the plasma concentration.

About 70% of the maximum beta-blocking effect is present for 5 hours after the administration of a single oral dose of 400 mg with suggestion that about 40% remains at 8 hours.

The antianginal efficacy of labetalol HCl has not been studied. In 37 patients with hypertension and coronary artery disease, labetalol HCl did not increase the incidence or severity of angina attacks.

In a clinical pharmacologic study in severe hypertensives, an initial 0.25-mg/kg injection of labetalol HCl administered to patients in the supine position decreased blood pressure by an average of 11/7 mmHg. Additional injections of 0.5 mg/kg at 15-minute intervals up to a total cumulative dose of 1.75 mg/kg of labetalol HCl caused further dose-related decreases in blood pressure. Some patients required cumulative doses of up to 3.25 mg/kg. The maximal effect of each dose level occurred within 5 minutes. Following discontinuation of IV treatment with labetalol HCl, the blood pressure rose gradually and progressively, approaching pretreatment baseline values within an average of 16 to 18 hours in the majority of patients.

Similar results were obtained in the treatment of patients with severe hypertension who required urgent blood pressure reduction with an initial dose of 20 mg (which corresponds to 0.25 mg/kg for an 80-kg patient) followed by additional doses of either 40 or 80 mg at 10-minute intervals to achieve the desired effect, or up to a cumulative dose of 300 mg.

Labetalol HCl administered as a continuous IV infusion, with a mean dose of 136 mg (27 to 300 mg) over a period of 2 to 3 hours (mean of 2 hours and 39 minutes), lowered the blood pressure by an average of 60/35 mmHg.

Exacerbation of angina and, in some cases, myocardial infarction and ventricular dysrhythmias have been reported after abrupt discontinuation of therapy with beta-adrenergic blocking agents in patients with coronary artery disease. Abrupt withdrawal of these agents in patients without coronary artery disease has resulted in transient symptoms, including tremulousness, sweating, palpitation, headache, and malaise. Several mechanisms have been proposed to explain these phenomena, among them increased sensitivity to catecholamines because of increased numbers of beta receptors.

Although beta-adrenergic receptor blockade is useful in the treatment of angina and hypertension, there are also situations in which sympathetic stimulation is vital. For example, in patients with severely damaged hearts, adequate ventricular function may depend on sympathetic drive. Beta-adrenergic blockade may worsen A-V block by preventing the necessary facilitating effects of sympathetic activity on conduction. $Beta_2$-adrenergic blockade results in passive bronchial constriction by interfering with endogenous adrenergic bronchodilator activity in patients subject to bronchospasm, and it may also interfere with exogenous bronchodilators in such patients.

Pharmacokinetics and Metabolism: Labetalol HCl is completely absorbed from the gastrointestinal tract with peak plasma levels occurring 1 to 2 hours after oral administration. The relative bioavailability of labetalol HCl tablets compared to an oral solution is 100%. The absolute bioavailability (fraction of drug reaching systemic circulation) of labetalol when compared to an IV infusion is 25%; this is due to extensive "first-pass" metabolism. Despite "first-pass" metabolism, there is a linear relationship between oral doses of 100 to 3,000 mg and peak plasma levels. The absolute bioavailability of labetalol is increased when administered with food.

Following IV infusion of labetalol, the elimination half-life is about 5.5 hours and the total body clearance is approximately 33 mL/min/kg. The plasma half-life of labetalol following oral administration is about 6 to 8 hours. Steady-state plasma levels of labetalol during repetitive dosing are reached by about the third day of dosing. In patients with decreased hepatic or renal function, the elimination half-life of labetalol is not altered; however, the relative bioavailability in hepatically impaired patients is increased due to decreased "first-pass" metabolism.

The metabolism of labetalol is mainly through conjugation to glucuronide metabolites. These metabolites are present in plasma and are excreted in the urine and, via the bile, into the feces. Approximately 55% to 60% of a dose appears in the urine as conjugates or unchanged labetalol within the first 24 hours of dosing.

Labetalol has been shown to cross the placental barrier in humans. Only negligible amounts of the drug crossed the blood-brain barrier in animal studies. Labetalol is approximately 50% protein bound. Neither hemodialysis nor peritoneal dialysis removes a significant amount of labetalol HCl from the general circulation (<1%).

Elderly Patients: Some pharmacokinetic studies indicate that the elimination of labetalol is reduced in elderly patients. Therefore, although elderly patients may initiate therapy with Trandate Tablets at the currently recommended dosage of 100 mg b.i.d., elderly patients will generally require lower maintenance dosages than nonelderly patients.

INDICATIONS AND USAGE

Trandate® (labetalol HCl) Tablets are indicated in the management of hypertension. Trandate Tablets may be used alone or in combination with other antihypertensive agents, especially thiazide and loop diuretics.

Trandate® (labetalol HCl) Injection is indicated for control of blood pressure in severe hypertension.

CONTRAINDICATIONS

Trandate® (labetalol HCl) Tablets and Trandate® (labetalol HCl) Injection are contraindicated in bronchial asthma, overt cardiac failure, greater-than-first-degree heart block, cardiogenic shock, severe bradycardia, other conditions associated with severe and prolonged hypotension, and in patients with a history of hypersensitivity to any component of the product (see WARNINGS).

WARNINGS

Hepatic Injury: Severe hepatocellular injury, confirmed by rechallenge in at least one case, occurs rarely with labetalol therapy. The hepatic injury is usually reversible, but hepatic necrosis and death have been reported. Injury has occurred after both short- and long-term treatment and may be slowly progressive despite minimal symptomatology. Similar hepatic events have been reported with a related research compound, dilevalol HCl, including two deaths. Dilevalol HCl is one of the four isomers of labetalol HCl. Thus, for patients taking labetalol, periodic determination of suitable hepatic laboratory tests would be appropriate. Appropriate laboratory testing should be done at the first symptom/sign of liver dysfunction (e.g., pruritus, dark urine, persistent anorexia, jaundice, right upper quadrant tenderness, or unexplained "flu-like" symptoms). If the patient has laboratory evidence of liver injury or jaundice, labetalol should be stopped and not restarted.

Cardiac Failure: Sympathetic stimulation is a vital component supporting circulatory function in congestive heart failure. Beta-blockade carries a potential hazard of further depressing myocardial contractility and precipitating more severe failure. Although beta-blockers should be avoided in overt congestive heart failure, if necessary, labetalol HCl can be used with caution in patients with a history of heart failure who are well compensated. Congestive heart failure has been observed in patients receiving labetalol HCl. Labetalol HCl does not abolish the inotropic action of digitalis on heart muscle.

In Patients Without a History of Cardiac Failure: In patients with latent cardiac insufficiency, continued depression of the myocardium with beta-blocking agents over a period of time can, in some cases, lead to cardiac failure. At the first sign or symptom of impending cardiac failure, patients should be fully digitalized and/or be given a diuretic, and the response should be observed closely. If cardiac failure continues despite adequate digitalization and diuretic, Trandate® (labetalol HCl) Tablets and Trandate® (labetalol HCl) Injection therapy should be withdrawn (gradually, if possible).

Exacerbation of Ischemic Heart Disease Following Abrupt Withdrawal: Trandate Tablets: Angina pectoris has not been reported upon labetalol HCl discontinuation. However, hypersensitivity to catecholamines has been observed in patients withdrawn from beta-blocker therapy; exacerbation of angina and, in some cases, myocardial infarction have occurred after *abrupt* discontinuation of such therapy. When discontinuing chronically administered Trandate Tablets, particularly in patients with ischemic heart disease, the dosage should be gradually reduced over a period of 1 to 2 weeks and the patient should be carefully monitored. If angina markedly worsens or acute coronary insufficiency develops, Trandate Tablets therapy should be reinstituted promptly, at least temporarily, and other measures appropriate for the management of unstable angina should be taken. Patients should be warned against interruption or discontinuation of therapy without the physician's advice. Because coronary artery disease is common and may be unrecognized, it may be prudent not to discontinue Trandate Tablets therapy abruptly in patients being treated for hypertension.

Ischemic Heart Disease: Trandate Injection: Angina pectoris has not been reported upon labetalol HCl discontinuation. However, following abrupt cessation of therapy with some beta-blocking agents in patients with coronary artery disease, exacerbations of angina pectoris and, in some cases, myocardial infarction have been reported. Therefore, such patients should be cautioned against interruption of therapy without the physician's advice. Even in the absence of overt angina pectoris, when discontinuation of Trandate Injection is planned, the patient should be carefully observed and should be advised to limit physical activity. If angina markedly worsens or acute coronary insufficiency develops, Trandate Injection administration should be reinstituted promptly, at least temporarily, and other measures appropriate for the management of unstable angina should be taken.

Nonallergic Bronchospasm (e.g., Chronic Bronchitis and Emphysema): Patients with bronchospastic disease should, in general, not receive beta-blockers. Trandate Tablets may be used with caution, however, in patients who do not respond to, or cannot tolerate, other antihypertensive agents. It is prudent, if Trandate Tablets are used, to use the smallest effective dose, so that inhibition of endogenous or exogenous beta-agonists is minimized. Since Trandate Injection at the usual IV therapeutic doses has not been studied in patients with nonallergic bronchospastic disease, it should not be used in such patients.

Pheochromocytoma: Labetalol HCl has been shown to be effective in lowering blood pressure and relieving symptoms in patients with pheochromocytoma; higher than usual IV doses may be required. However, paradoxical hypertensive responses have been reported in a few patients with this tumor; therefore, use caution when administering labetalol HCl to patients with pheochromocytoma.

Diabetes Mellitus and Hypoglycemia: Beta-adrenergic blockade may prevent the appearance of premonitory signs and symptoms (e.g., tachycardia) of acute hypoglycemia. This is especially important with labile diabetics. Beta-blockade also reduces the release of insulin in response to hyperglycemia; it may therefore be necessary to adjust the dose of antidiabetic drugs.

Major Surgery: The necessity or desirability of withdrawing beta-blocking therapy before major surgery is controversial. Protracted severe hypotension and difficulty in restarting or maintaining a heartbeat have been reported with beta-blockers. The effect of labetalol HCl's alpha-adrenergic activity has not been evaluated in this setting.

A synergism between labetalol HCl and halothane anesthesia has been shown (see PRECAUTIONS: Drug Interactions).

Rapid Decreases of Blood Presure: Caution must be observed when reducing severely elevated blood pressure. Although such findings have not been reported with IV labetalol HCl, a number of adverse reactions, including cerebral infarction, optic nerve infarction, angina, and ischemic changes in the electrocardiogram, have been reported with other agents when severely elevated blood pressure was reduced over time courses of several hours to as long as 1 or 2 days. The desired blood pressure lowering should therefore be achieved over as long a period of time as is compatible with the patient's status.

PRECAUTIONS

General: Trandate® (labetalol HCl) Tablets: ***Impaired Hepatic Function:*** Trandate Tablets should be used with caution in patients with impaired hepatic function since metabolism of the drug may be diminished.

Jaundice or Hepatic Dysfunction: (see WARNINGS).

Trandate® (labetalol HCl) Injection: ***Impaired Hepatic Function:*** Trandate Injection should be used with caution in patients with impaired hepatic function since metabolism of the drug may be diminished.

Hypotension: Symptomatic postural hypotension (incidence, 58%) is likely to occur if patients are tilted or allowed to assume the upright position within 3 hours of receiving Trandate Injection. Therefore, the patient's ability to tolerate an upright position should be established before permitting any ambulation.

Following Coronary Artery Bypass Surgery: In one uncontrolled study, patients with low cardiac indices and elevated systemic vascular resistance following IV labetalol HCl experienced significant declines in cardiac output with little change in systemic vascular resistance. One of these patients developed hypotension following labetalol treatment. Therefore, use of labetalol HCl should be avoided in such patients.

High Dose Labetalol: Administration of up to 3 g per day as an infusion for up to 2 to 3 days has been anecdotally reported; several patients have experienced hypotension or bradycardia.

Jaundice or Hepatic Dysfunction: (see WARNINGS).

Information for Patients: As with all drugs with beta-blocking activity, certain advice to patients being treated with labetalol HCl is warranted. This information is intended to aid in the safe and effective use of this medication. It is not a disclosure of all possible adverse or intended effects. While no incident of the abrupt withdrawal phenomenon (exacerbation of angina pectoris) has been reported with labetalol HCl, dosing with Trandate Tablets should not be interrupted or discontinued without a physician's advice. Patients being treated with Trandate Tablets should consult a physician at any signs or symptoms of impending cardiac failure or hepatic dysfunction (see WARNINGS). Also, transient scalp tingling may occur, usually when treatment with Trandate Tablets is initiated (see ADVERSE REACTIONS).

During and immediately following (for up to 3 hours) Trandate Injection, the patient should remain supine. Subsequently, the patient should be advised on how to proceed gradually to become ambulatory and should be observed at the time of first ambulation.

When the patient is started on Trandate Tablets following adequate control of blood pressure with Trandate Injection,

Continued on next page

Glaxo Wellcome—Cont.

appropriate directions for titration of dosage should be provided (see DOSAGE AND ADMINISTRATION).

Laboratory Tests: As with any new drug given over prolonged periods, laboratory parameters should be observed over regular intervals. In patients with concomitant illnesses, such as impaired renal function, appropriate tests should be done to monitor these conditions.

Routine laboratory tests are ordinarily not required before or after IV labetalol HCl.

Drug Interactions: Since Trandate Injection may be administered to patients already being treated with other medications, including other antihypertensive agents, careful monitoring of these patients is necessary to detect and treat promptly any undesired effect from concomitant administration.

In one survey, 2.3% of patients taking labetalol HCl orally in combination with tricyclic antidepressants experienced tremor, as compared to 0.7% reported to occur with labetalol HCl alone. The contribution of each of the treatments to this adverse reaction is unknown, but the possibility of a drug interaction cannot be excluded.

Drugs possessing beta-blocking properties can blunt the bronchodilator effect of beta-receptor agonist drugs in patients with bronchospasm; therefore, doses greater than the normal antiasthmatic dose of beta-agonist bronchodilator drugs may be required.

Cimetidine has been shown to increase the bioavailability of labetalol HCl administered orally. Since this could be explained either by enhanced absorption or by an alteration of hepatic metabolism of labetalol HCl, special care should be used in establishing the dose required for blood pressure control in such patients.

Synergism has been shown between halothane anesthesia and intravenously administered labetalol HCl. During controlled hypotensive anesthesia using labetalol HCl in association with halothane, high concentrations (3% or above) of halothane should not be used because the degree of hypotension will be increased and because of the possibility of a large reduction in cardiac output and an increase in central venous pressure. The anesthesiologist should be informed when a patient is receiving labetalol HCl.

Labetalol HCl blunts the reflex tachycardia produced by nitroglycerin without preventing its hypotensive effect. If labetalol HCl is used with nitroglycerin in patients with angina pectoris, additional antihypertensive effects may occur. Care should be taken if labetalol is used concomitantly with calcium antagonists of the verapamil type.

Risk of Anaphylactic Reaction: While taking beta-blockers, patients with a history of severe anaphylactic reaction to a variety of allergens may be more reactive to repeated challenge, either accidental, diagnostic, or therapeutic. Such patients may be unresponsive to the usual doses of epinephrine used to treat allergic reaction.

Drug/Laboratory Test Interactions: The presence of labetalol metabolites in the urine may result in falsely elevated levels of urinary catecholamines, metanephrine, normetanephrine, and vanillylmandelic acid when measured by fluorimetric or photometric methods. In screening patients suspected of having a pheochromocytoma and being treated with labetalol HCl, a specific method, such as a high performance liquid chromatographic assay with solid phase extraction (e.g., *J Chromatogr* 385:241,1987) should be employed in determining levels of catecholamines.

Labetalol HCl has also been reported to produce a false-positive test for amphetamine when screening urine for the presence of drugs using the commercially available assay methods Toxi-Lab A® (thin-layer chromatographic assay) and Emit-d.a.u.® (radioenzymatic assay). When patients being treated with labetalol have a positive urine test for amphetamine using these techniques, confirmation should be made by using more specific methods, such as a gas chromatographic-mass spectrometer technique.

Carcinogenesis, Mutagenesis, Impairment of Fertility: Long-term oral dosing studies with labetalol HCl for 18 months in mice and for 2 years in rats showed no evidence of carcinogenesis. Studies with labetalol HCl using dominant lethal assays in rats and mice and exposing microorganisms according to modified Ames tests showed no evidence of mutagenesis.

Pregnancy: *Teratogenic Effects: Pregnancy Category C:* Teratogenic studies were performed with labetalol in rats and rabbits at oral doses up to approximately six and four times the maximum recommended human dose (MRHD), respectively. No reproducible evidence of fetal malformations was observed. Increased fetal resorptions were seen in both species at doses approximating the MRHD. A teratology study performed with labetalol in rabbits at IV doses up to 1.7 times the MRHD revealed no evidence of drug-related harm to the fetus. There are no adequate and well-controlled studies in pregnant women. Labetalol should be used during pregnancy only if the potential benefit justifies the potential risk to the fetus.

Nonteratogenic Effects: Hypotension, bradycardia, hypoglycemia, and respiratory depression have been reported in infants of mothers who were treated with labetalol HCl for hypertension during pregnancy. Oral administration of labetalol to rats during late gestation through weaning at doses of two to four times the MRHD caused a decrease in neonatal survival.

Labor and Delivery: Labetalol HCl given to pregnant women with hypertension did not appear to affect the usual course of labor and delivery.

Nursing Mothers: Small amounts of labetalol (approximately 0.004% of the maternal dose) are excreted in human milk. Caution should be exercised when Trandate is administered to a nursing woman.

Pediatric Use: Safety and effectiveness in pediatric patients have not been established.

Elderly Patients: As in the general population, some elderly patients (60 years of age and older) have experienced orthostatic hypotension, dizziness, or lightheadedness during treatment with labetalol. Because elderly patients are generally more likely than younger patients to experience orthostatic symptoms, they should be cautioned about the possibility of such side effects during treatment with Trandate Tablets.

ADVERSE REACTIONS

Trandate® (labetalol HCl) Tablets: Most adverse effects are mild and transient and occur early in the course of treatment. In controlled clinical trials of 3 to 4 months' duration, discontinuation of Trandate Tablets due to one or more adverse effects was required in 7% of all patients. In these same trials, other agents with solely beta-blocking activity used in the control groups led to discontinuation in 8% to 10% of patients, and a centrally acting alpha-agonist led to discontinuation in 30% of patients.

The incidence rates of adverse reactions listed in the following table were derived from multicenter, controlled clinical trials comparing labetalol HCl, placebo, metoprolol, and propranolol over treatment periods of 3 and 4 months. Where the frequency of adverse effects for labetalol HCl and placebo is similar, causal relationship is uncertain. The rates

	Labetalol HCl (n=227) %	Placebo (n=98) %	Propranolol (n=84) %	Metoprolol (n=49) %
Body as a whole				
Fatigue	5	0	12	12
Asthenia	1	1	1	0
Headache	2	1	1	2
Gastrointestinal				
Nausea	6	1	1	2
Vomiting	<1	0	0	0
Dyspepsia	3	1	1	0
Abdominal pain	0	0	1	2
Diarrhea	<1	0	2	0
Taste distortion	1	0	0	0
Central and peripheral nervous systems				
Dizziness	11	3	4	4
Paresthesia	<1	0	0	0
Drowsiness	<1	2	2	2
Autonomic nervous system				
Nasal stuffiness	3	0	0	0
Ejaculation failure	2	0	0	0
Impotence	1	0	1	3
Increased sweating	<1	0	0	0
Cardiovascular				
Edema	1	0	0	0
Postural hypotension	1	0	0	0
Bradycardia	0	0	5	12
Respiratory				
Dyspnea	2	0	1	2
Skin				
Rash	1	0	0	0
Special senses				
Vision abnormality	1	0	0	0
Vertigo	2	1	0	0

are based on adverse reactions considered probably drug related by the investigator. If all reports are considered, the rates are somewhat higher (e.g., dizziness, 20%; nausea, 14%; fatigue, 11%), but the overall conclusions are unchanged.

[See table above.]

The adverse effects were reported spontaneously and are representative of the incidence of adverse effects that may be observed in a properly selected hypertensive patient population, i.e., a group excluding patients with bronchospastic disease, overt congestive heart failure, or other contraindications to beta-blocker therapy.

Clinical trials also included studies utilizing daily doses up to 2,400 mg in more severely hypertensive patients. Certain of the side effects increased with increasing dose, as shown in the following table that depicts the entire US therapeutic trials data base for adverse reactions that are clearly or possibly dose related.

[See table below.]

In addition, a number of other less common adverse events have been reported:

Body as a Whole: Fever.

Cardiovascular: Hypotension, and rarely, syncope, bradycardia, heart block.

Central and Peripheral Nervous Systems: Paresthesia, most frequently described as scalp tingling. In most cases, it was mild and transient and usually occurred at the beginning of treatment.

Collagen Disorders: Systemic lupus erythematosus, positive antinuclear factor.

Eyes: Dry eyes.

Immunological System: Antimitochondrial antibodies.

Liver and Biliary System: Hepatic necrosis, hepatitis, cholestatic jaundice, elevated liver function tests.

Musculoskeletal System: Muscle cramps, toxic myopathy.

Respiratory System: Bronchospasm.

Skin and Appendages: Rashes of various types, such as generalized maculopapular, lichenoid, urticarial, bullous lichen planus, psoriaform, and facial erythema; Peyronie's disease; reversible alopecia.

Urinary System: Difficulty in micturition, including acute urinary bladder retention.

Labetalol HCl Daily Dose (mg)	200	300	400	600	800	900	1,200	1,600	2,400
Number of patients	522	181	606	608	503	117	411	242	175
Dizziness (%)	2	3	3	3	5	1	9	13	16
Fatigue	2	1	4	4	5	3	7	6	10
Nausea	<1	0	1	2	4	0	7	11	19
Vomiting	0	0	<1	<1	<1	0	1	2	3
Dyspepsia	1	1	2	2	1	1	2	2	4
Paresthesia	2	0	2	2	1	1	2	5	5
Nasal stuffiness	1	1	2	2	2	2	4	5	6
Ejaculation failure	0	2	1	1	2	1	3	4	5
Impotence	1	1	1	1	2	4	3	4	3
Edema	1	0	1	1	1	0	1	2	2

Hypersensitivity: Rare reports of hypersensitivity (e.g., rash, urticaria, pruritus, angioedema, dyspnea) and anaphylactoid reactions.

Following approval for marketing in the United Kingdom, a monitored release survey involving approximately 6,800 patients was conducted for further safety and efficacy evaluation of this product. Results of this survey indicate that the type, severity, and incidence of adverse effects were comparable to those cited above.

Potential Adverse Effects: In addition, other adverse effects not listed above have been reported with other beta-adrenergic blocking agents.

Central Nervous System: Reversible mental depression progressing to catatonia, an acute reversible syndrome characterized by disorientation for time and place, short-term memory loss, emotional lability, slightly clouded sensorium, and decreased performance on psychometrics.

Cardiovascular: Intensification of A-V block (see CONTRAINDICATIONS).

Allergic: Fever combined with aching and sore throat, laryngospasm, respiratory distress.

Hematologic: Agranulocytosis, thrombocytopenic or nonthrombocytopenic purpura.

Gastrointestinal: Mesenteric artery thrombosis, ischemic colitis.

Trandate® (labetalol HCl) Injection: Trandate Injection is usually well tolerated. Most adverse effects have been mild and transient and, in controlled trials involving 92 patients, did not require labetalol HCl withdrawal. Symptomatic postural hypotension (incidence, 58%) is likely to occur if patients are tilted or allowed to assume the upright position within 3 hours of receiving Trandate Injection. Moderate hypotension occurred in 1 of 100 patients while supine. Increased sweating was noted in 4 of 100 patients, and flushing occurred in 1 of 100 patients.

The following also were reported with Trandate Injection with the incidence per 100 patients as noted:

Cardiovascular System: Ventricular arrhythmia in 1.
Central and Peripheral Nervous Systems: Dizziness in 9, tingling of the scalp/skin in 7, hypoesthesia (numbness) and vertigo in 1 each.
Gastrointestinal System: Nausea in 13, vomiting in 4, dyspepsia and taste distortion in 1 each.
Metabolic Disorders: Transient increases in blood urea nitrogen and serum creatinine levels occurred in 8 of 100 patients; these were associated with drops in blood pressure, generally in patients with prior renal insufficiency.
Psychiatric Disorders: Somnolence/yawning in 3.
Respiratory System: Wheezing in 1.
Skin: Pruritus in 1.

The incidence of adverse reactions depends upon the dose of labetalol HCl. The largest experience is with oral labetalol HCl (see above for details). Certain of the side effects increased with increasing oral dose, as shown in the above table that depicts the entire US therapeutic trials data base for adverse reactions that are clearly or possibly dose related. In addition, a number of other less common adverse events have been reported:

Cardiovascular: Hypotension, and rarely, syncope, bradycardia, heart block.
Liver and Biliary System: Hepatic necrosis, hepatitis, cholestatic jaundice, elevated liver function tests.
Hypersensitivity: Rare reports of hypersensitivity (e.g., rash, urticaria, pruritus, angioedema, dyspnea) and anaphylactoid reactions.

The oculomucocutaneous syndrome associated with the beta-blocker practolol has not been reported with labetalol HCl.

Clinical Laboratory Tests: Among patients dosed with Trandate Tablets, there have been reversible increases of serum transaminases in 4% of patients tested and, more rarely, reversible increases in blood urea.

OVERDOSAGE

Overdosage with labetalol HCl causes excessive hypotension that is posture sensitive and, sometimes, excessive bradycardia. Patients should be placed supine and their legs raised if necessary to improve the blood supply to the brain. If overdosage with labetalol HCl follows oral ingestion, gastric lavage or pharmacologically induced emesis (using syrup of ipecac) may be useful for removal of the drug shortly after ingestion. The following additional measures should be employed if necessary: *Excessive bradycardia*—administer atropine or epinephrine. *Cardiac failure*—administer a digitalis glycoside and a diuretic. Dopamine or dobutamine may also be useful. *Hypotension*—administer vasopressors, e.g., norepinephrine. There is pharmacologic evidence that norepinephrine may be the drug of choice. *Bronchospasm*—administer epinephrine and/or an aerosolized beta2-agonist. *Seizures*—administer diazepam.

In severe beta-blocker overdose resulting in hypotension and/or bradycardia, glucagon has been shown to be effective when administered in large doses (5 to 10 mg rapidly over 30 seconds, followed by continuous infusion of 5 mg per hour that can be reduced as the patient improves).

Neither hemodialysis nor peritoneal dialysis removes a significant amount of labetalol HCl from the general circulation (<1%).

The oral LD$_{50}$ value of labetalol HCl in the mouse is approximately 600 mg/kg and in the rat is greater than 2 g/kg. The IV LD$_{50}$ in these species is 50 to 60 mg/kg.

DOSAGE AND ADMINISTRATION

Trandate® (labetalol HCl) Tablets: DOSAGE MUST BE INDIVIDUALIZED. The recommended *initial* dosage is 100 mg *twice* daily whether used alone or added to a diuretic regimen. After 2 or 3 days, using standing blood pressure as an indicator, dosage may be titrated in increments of 100 mg b.i.d. every 2 or 3 days. The usual *maintenance* dosage of labetalol HCl is between 200 and 400 mg *twice* daily.

Since the full antihypertensive effect of labetalol HCl is usually seen within the first 1 to 3 hours of the initial dose or dose increment, the assurance of a lack of an exaggerated hypotensive response can be clinically established in the office setting. The antihypertensive effects of continued dosing can be measured at subsequent visits, approximately 12 hours after a dose, to determine whether further titration is necessary.

Patients with severe hypertension may require from 1,200 to 2,400 mg per day, with or without thiazide diuretics. Should side effects (principally nausea or dizziness) occur with these doses administered twice daily, the same total daily dose administered three times daily may improve tolerability and facilitate further titration. Titration increments should not exceed 200 mg twice daily.

When a diuretic is added, an additive antihypertensive effect can be expected. In some cases this may necessitate a labetalol HCl dosage adjustment. As with most antihypertensive drugs, optimal dosages of Trandate Tablets are usually lower in patients also receiving a diuretic.

When transferring patients from other antihypertensive drugs, Trandate Tablets should be introduced as recommended and the dosage of the existing therapy progressively decreased.

Elderly Patients: As in the general patient population, labetalol therapy may be initiated at 100 mg twice daily and titrated upwards in increments of 100 mg b.i.d. as required for control of blood pressure. Since some elderly patients eliminate labetalol more slowly, however, adequate control of blood pressure may be achieved at a lower maintenance dosage compared to the general population. The majority of elderly patients will require between 100 and 200 mg b.i.d.

Trandate® (labetalol HCl) Injection: Trandate Injection is intended for IV use in hospitalized patients. DOSAGE MUST BE INDIVIDUALIZED depending upon the severity of hypertension and the response of the patient during dosing. **Patients should always be kept in a supine position during the period of IV drug administration. A substantial fall in blood pressure on standing should be expected in these patients. The patient's ability to tolerate an upright position should be established before permitting any ambulation, such as using toilet facilities.**

Either of two methods of administration of Trandate Injection may be used: a) repeated IV injection, or b) slow continuous infusion.

Repeated Intravenous Injection: Initially, Trandate Injection should be given in a 20-mg dose (which corresponds to 0.25 mg/kg for an 80-kg patient) by slow IV injection over a 2-minute period.

Immediately before the injection and at 5 and 10 minutes after injection, supine blood pressure should be measured to evaluate response. Additional injections of 40 or 80 mg can be given at 10-minute intervals until a desired supine blood pressure is achieved or a total of 300 mg of labetalol HCl has been injected. The maximum effect usually occurs within 5 minutes of each injection.

Slow Continuous Infusion: Trandate Injection is prepared for continuous IV infusion by diluting the vial contents with commonly used IV fluids (see below). Examples of two methods of preparing the infusion solution are:

Add 40 mL of Trandate Injection to 160 mL of a commonly used IV fluid such that the resultant 200 mL of solution contains 200 mg of labetalol HCl, 1 mg/mL. The diluted solution should be administered at a rate of 2 mL per minute to deliver 2 mg per minute.

Alternatively, add 40 mL of Trandate Injection to 250 mL of a commonly used IV fluid. The resultant solution will contain 200 mg of labetalol HCl, approximately 2 mg/3 mL. The diluted solution should be administered at a rate of 3 mL per minute to deliver approximately 2 mg per minute.

The rate of infusion of the diluted solution may be adjusted according to the blood pressure response, at the discretion of the physician. To facilitate a desired rate of infusion, the diluted solution can be infused using a controlled administration mechanism, e.g., graduated burette or mechanically driven infusion pump.

Since the half-life of labetalol is 5 to 8 hours, steady-state blood levels (in the face of a constant rate of infusion) would not be reached during the usual infusion time period. The infusion should be continued until a satisfactory response is obtained and should then be stopped and oral labetalol HCl started (see below). The effective IV dose is usually in the range of 50 to 200 mg. A total dose of up to 300 mg may be required in some patients.

Blood Pressure Monitoring: The blood pressure should be monitored during and after completion of the infusion or IV injection. Rapid or excessive falls in either systolic or diastolic blood pressure during IV treatment should be avoided. In patients with excessive systolic hypertension, the decrease in systolic pressure should be used as an indicator of effectiveness in addition to the response of the diastolic pressure.

Initiation of Dosing With Trandate Tablets: Subsequent oral dosing with Trandate Tablets should begin when it has been established that the supine diastolic blood pressure has begun to rise. The recommended initial dose is 200 mg, followed in 6 to 12 hours by an additional dose of 200 or 400 mg, depending on the blood pressure response. Thereafter, **inpatient titration with Trandate Tablets** may proceed as follows:

Inpatient Titration Instructions

Regimen	Daily Dose*
200 mg b.i.d.	400 mg
400 mg b.i.d.	800 mg
800 mg b.i.d.	1,600 mg
1,200 mg b.i.d.	2,400 mg

*If needed, the total daily dose may be given in three divided doses.

The dosage of Trandate Tablets used in the hospital may be increased at 1-day intervals to achieve the desired blood pressure reduction.

For subsequent outpatient titration or maintenance dosing, see Trandate Tablets dosage and administration information above for recommendations.

Compatibility With Commonly Used Intravenous Fluids: Parenteral drug products should be inspected visually for particulate matter and discoloration before administration whenever solution and container permit.

Trandate Injection was tested for compatibility with commonly used IV fluids at final concentrations of 1.25 to 3.75 mg of labetalol HCl per milliliter of the mixture. Trandate Injection was found to be compatible with and stable (for 24 hours refrigerated or at room temperature) in mixtures with the following solutions: ringer's injection, USP; lactated ringer's injection, USP; 5% dextrose and ringer's injection; 5% lactated ringer's and 5% dextrose injection; 5% dextrose injection, USP; 0.9% sodium chloride injection, USP; 5% dextrose and 0.2% sodium chloride injection, USP; 2.5% dextrose and 0.45% sodium chloride injection, USP; 5% dextrose and 0.9% sodium chloride injection, USP; and 5% dextrose and 0.33% sodium chloride injection, USP.

Trandate Injection was NOT compatible with 5% sodium bicarbonate injection, USP. Care should be taken when administering alkaline drugs, including furosemide, in combination with labetalol. Compatibility should be assured prior to administering these drugs together.

HOW SUPPLIED

Trandate® (labetalol HCl) Tablets, 100 mg, light orange, round, scored, film-coated tablets engraved on one side with "TRANDATE 100," bottles of 100 (NDC 0173-0346-43) and 500 (NDC 0173-0346-44) and unit dose packs of 100 tablets (NDC 0173-0346-47).

Trandate Tablets, 200 mg, white, round, scored, film-coated tablets engraved on one side with "TRANDATE 200," bottles of 100 (NDC 0173-0347-43) and 500 (NDC 0173-0347-44) and unit dose packs of 100 tablets (NDC 0173-0347-47).

Trandate Tablets, 300 mg, peach, round, scored, film-coated tablets engraved on one side with "TRANDATE 300," bottles of 100 (NDC 0173-0348-43) and 500 (NDC 0173-0348-44) and unit dose packs of 100 tablets (NDC 0173-0348-47).

Trandate Tablets should be stored between 2° and 30°C (36° and 86°F). Trandate Tablets in the unit dose boxes should be protected from excessive moisture.

Trandate® (labetalol HCl) Injection, 5 mg/mL, is supplied in 20-mL (100-mg) vials, box of one (NDC 0173-0350-58) and 40-mL (200-mg) vials, box of one (NDC 0173-0350-57).

Store between 2° and 30°C (36° and 86°F). Do not freeze. Protect from light.

July 1995/RL-099,207

Shown in Product Identification Guide, page 314

Continued on next page

Glaxo Wellcome—Cont.

Allergen Patch Test
T.R.U.E. TEST®
*Thin-layer Rapid Use Epicutaneous Test
FOR TOPICAL USE ONLY

℞

DESCRIPTION
T.R.U.E. Test® (Thin-layer Rapid Use Epicutaneous Test) is a ready-to-use patch test system containing 24 of the most common allergens suspected of causing allergic contact dermatitis.[1]

The source materials for the T.R.U.E. Test allergens are obtained from outside suppliers who certify that the materials meet specific standards of purity. The manufacturer then determines the purity and identity of the source materials using validated in-house chemical analyses.

Each test consists of two pieces of surgical tape (5.2 cm x 13.0 cm), each with 12 polyester patches of approximately 0.81 cm² each. Twelve patches are coated with a film containing a uniformly dispersed specific allergen or allergen mix. The test is covered by a protective sheet and sealed in a pouch of laminated foil.

The allergens are homogenized in one or more of the following materials to produce the allergen films that coat the patches: hydroxypropyl cellulose, methylcellulose, polyvidone, β-cyclodextrin. No other excipients are used to produce the patches.

T.R.U.E. Test is subjected to microbial load testing to assure that no more than 10² microorganisms per test are present. In addition, T.R.U.E. Test is further analyzed to assure the absence of *Staphylococcus aureus* and *Pseudomonas aeruginosa.*

Each patch is analytically tested and contains ±20% of its labeled value at the time of batch release. These values are maintained through expiry except for colophony, which maintains ±30% of label value under the recommended storage conditions.

The components of the patches containing mixtures, e.g., thiuram mix, have the potential to chemically interact, resulting in the formation of new substances.

Components: The individual components of T.R.U.E. Test, Panels 1 and 2 are listed below along with a quantitative description of the patch formulation.

Panel 1 Allergens

1. *Nickel Sulfate:* Nickel sulfate hexahydrate (purity 98.5% to 101.5%) is used to formulate this patch. The active allergenic component is nickel. The gel vehicle is hydroxypropyl cellulose. The product is formulated to contain 0.20 mg of nickel sulfate hexahydrate per square centimeter, which calculates to 0.036 mg of nickel per patch. Nickel is one of the most common metals in the environment and is found in most metal and metal-plated objects.

2. *Wool Alcohols:* Wool alcohols (lanolin) is a natural product obtained from the fleece of sheep. This allergen is a highly complex mixture of alcohols containing cholesterol, lanosterol, agnosterol, and their dihydro derivatives plus straight- and branched-chain aliphatic alcohols. The active allergenic component has not been identified. The gel vehicle is polyvidone. The product is formulated to contain 1.00 mg of wool alcohols per square centimeter, which calculates to 0.81 mg of wool alcohols per patch. Wool alcohols (lanolin) is a common constituent of many ointments, creams, lotions, and soaps.

3. *Neomycin Sulfate:* Neomycin sulfate, USP, an antibiotic drug substance, is used to formulate this patch. The gel vehicle is methylcellulose. The product is formulated to contain 0.23 mg of neomycin sulfate per square centimeter, which calculates to 0.19 mg of neomycin sulfate per patch. Neomycin is a common antibiotic and is found in topical antibiotic creams, lotions, ointments, eye drops, and ear drops.

4. *Potassium Dichromate:* Potassium dichromate (purity 98.5% to 101.5%) is used to formulate this patch. The active allergenic component is chromium. The gel vehicle is hydroxypropyl cellulose. The product is formulated to contain 0.023 mg of potassium dichromate per square centimeter, which calculates to 0.0067 mg of chromium per patch. Chromium is found in cement, as well as in many industrial chemicals.

5. *Caine Mix:* Caine mix is composed of three drug substances: benzocaine, USP; tetracaine hydrochloride, USP; and dibucaine hydrochloride, USP. The gel vehicle is polyvidone. The product is formulated to contain 0.63 mg of caine mix per square centimeter, which calculates to 0.364 mg of benzocaine, 0.063 mg of tetracaine, and 0.064 mg of dibucaine per patch. Benzocaine, tetracaine, and dibucaine are found in many topical anesthetic medications.

6. *Fragrance Mix:* Fragrance mix is composed of eight substances: geraniol (purity ≥ 95%, identity of impurities unknown), cinnamaldehyde (purity ≥ 95%, contains trace amounts of cinnamyl alcohol), hydroxycitronellal (purity ≥ 95%, identity of impurities unknown), cinnamyl alcohol (purity ≥ 95%, identity of impurities unknown), eugenol (purity ≥ 95%, identity of impurities unknown), isoeugenol

(purity ≥ 88%, identity of impurities unknown), α-amyl-cinnamaldehyde (purity ≥ 90%, identity of impurities unknown), and oak moss. Oak moss, a dark green sticky paste, is a solvent extract of the lichen *Evernia prunastri.* The chemical composition is very complex. The acid fraction (95% of the extracted material) is made up of depsides including atranorin, evernic acid, usnic acid, chloratranorin, and degradation products of these depsides. Atranorin is suspected as a prime allergenic component, and its peak (measured with gas chromatography) is used to determine the amount of oak moss in the fragrance mix patch.[2]

The gel vehicles used in this patch are hydroxypropyl cellulose and β-cyclodextrin. The product is formulated to contain 0.43 mg of fragrance mix per square centimeter, which calculates to 0.070 mg of geraniol, 0.034 mg of cinnamaldehyde, 0.054 mg of hydroxycitronellal, 0.054 mg of cinnamyl alcohol, 0.034 mg of eugenol, 0.015 mg of isoeugenol, 0.015 mg of α-amyl-cinnamaldehyde, and 0.070 mg of oak moss per patch. The components of fragrance mix are commonly used in toiletries, fragrances, and flavorings.

7. *Colophony:* Colophony is produced from the resin of the pine trees *Pinus massoniana* and *Pinus tabuliformis.* It is translucent, pale yellow or brownish yellow, brittle, and glassy in appearance. Colophony consists of 75% to 85% resin acids, 10% neutral fractions (i.e., terpenes), with the remaining part oxidation products. Oxidation products of abietic acid and other resin acids have been identified as the active allergenic components. The UV-absorbance measurement of one of the primary components, abietic acid, is used to quantify colophony. The gel vehicle is hydroxypropyl cellulose. The product is formulated to contain 0.85 mg of colophony per square centimeter, which calculates to 0.69 mg of colophony per patch. Colophony is found in adhesives, sealants, and pine oil cleaners.

8. *Epoxy Resin:* Epoxy resin, a clear viscous liquid, is used to formulate this patch. It consists of 75% to 85% diglycidylether of bisphenol A (the active allergenic component), which is a monomer used for the preparation of polymer epoxy resins. The remaining part consists of the dimer and the trimer. The gel vehicle is hydroxypropyl cellulose. This patch is formulated to contain 0.050 mg of epoxy resin per square centimeter, which calculates to 0.032 mg of diglycidylether of bisphenol A per patch. This resin is found in adhesives, surface coatings, and paints.

9. *Quinoline Mix:* Quinoline mix is a germicide and consists of equal parts of clioquinol (3-hydroxy-5-chloro-7-iodine-quinoline, purity ≥ 90%) and chlorquinaldol (2-methyl-5,7-dichlor-8-hydroxy-quinoline, purity ≥ 95%). The gel vehicle is hydroxypropyl cellulose. This patch is formulated to contain 0.19 mg of quinoline mix per square centimeter, which calculates to 0.154 mg of quinoline mix per patch. The components of quinoline mix are found mostly in veterinary products, in certain types of paste bandages, and in some medicated creams and ointments.

10. *Balsam of Peru:* Balsam of Peru is a resin from a South American tree, *Myroxylon balsamum pereirae.* The resin consists of a mixture of fragrances and other substances that have not all been identified. Balsam of Peru patch content is quantitated by gas chromatography of its two major constituents, benzyl cinnamate and benzyl benzoate. Several components of Balsam of Peru have been identified as allergens, including cinnamic acid, benzyl alcohol, and vanillin. The gel vehicle is polyvidone. This patch is formulated to contain 0.80 mg of Balsam of Peru resin per square centimeter, which calculates to 0.65 mg of Balsam of Peru resin per patch. This resin is found in many cosmetics and perfumes and is also used as a flavoring agent in cough syrups, lozenges, chewing gum, and candies.

11. *Ethylenediamine Dihydrochloride:* Ethylenediamine dihydrochloride (purity 98.5% to 101.5%) is used to formulate this patch. The active allergenic component is ethylenediamine. The gel vehicle is methylcellulose. The product is formulated to contain 0.050 mg of ethylenediamine dihydrochloride per square centimeter, which calculates to 0.018 mg of ethylenediamine per patch. Ethylenediamine is used as a stabilizer, emulsifier, and preservative in topical fungicides, antibiotic creams, eye drops, and nose drops.

12. *Cobalt Dichloride:* Cobalt dichloride hexahydrate (purity 98.5% to 101.5%) is used to formulate this patch. The active allergenic component is cobalt. The gel vehicle is hydroxypropyl cellulose. The product is formulated to contain 0.020 mg of cobalt dichloride hexahydrate per square centimeter, which calculates to 0.0040 mg of cobalt per patch. Cobalt is found in metal-plated objects and costume jewelry.

Panel 2 Allergens

13. *p-tert Butylphenol Formaldehyde Resin:* *p*-tert Butylphenol formaldehyde resin (purity 95% to 105%) is used to formulate this patch. The active allergenic components have been identified as *p*-tert butylphenol formaldehyde and numerous other compounds. The gel vehicle is hydroxypropyl cellulose. The product is formulated to contain 0.040 mg of *p*-tert butylphenol formaldehyde resin per square centimeter, which calculates to 0.032 mg of *p*-tert butylphenol formaldehyde resin per patch. This resin is found in many waterproof glues used in the leather goods, furniture, and shoe industries.

14. *Paraben Mix:* Paraben mix contains the five ester derivatives of parahydroxybenzoic acid, methyl, ethyl, propyl, butyl, and benzyl parahydroxybenzoate, in equal parts (purity of each derivative 98.5% to 101.5%). The gel vehicle is polyvidone. The product is formulated to contain 1.00 mg of paraben mix per square centimeter, which calculates to 0.81 mg of paraben mix per patch. The components of paraben mix can be found in cosmetics, dermatological creams, and paste bandages.

15. *Carba Mix:* Carba mix contains three chemicals used to stabilize rubber products: diphenylguanidine (purity 96% to 102%), zincdibutyldithiocarbamate (purity 96% to 102%), and zincdiethyldithiocarbamate (purity 96% to 102%) in equal parts. The gel vehicle is hydroxypropyl cellulose. The product is formulated to contain 0.25 mg of carba mix per square centimeter, which calculates to 0.20 mg of carba mix per patch. These chemical stabilizers are found in almost all rubber products, many pesticides, and some glues.

16. *Black Rubber Mix:* Black rubber mix contains the antioxidant and antiozonate chemicals N-isopropyl-N'-phenyl paraphenylenediamine (purity 95% to 102%), N-cyclohexyl-N'-phenyl paraphenylenediamine (purity ≥ 90%), and N, N'-diphenyl paraphenylenediamine (purity ≥ 90%) in the ratio 2:5:5. The gel vehicle is polyvidone. The product is formulated to contain 0.075 mg of black rubber mix per square centimeter, which calculates to 0.061 mg of black rubber mix per patch. The components of black rubber mix are found in almost all black rubber products, e.g., tires, handles, hoses.

17. *Cl+ Me- Isothiazolinone:* Cl+ Me- Isothiazolinone is an antibacterial preservative that consists of two active ingredients, 5-chloro-2-methyl-4-isothiazolin-3-one (1.05% to 1.25% w/w) and 2-methyl-4-isothiazolin-3-one (0.25% to 0.40% w/w) in a 3:1 ratio at a concentration of 1.5% in aqueous magnesium salts. The gel vehicle is polyvidone. The product is formulated to contain 0.0040 mg of Cl+ Me- isothiazolinone per square centimeter, which calculates to 0.0032 mg of Cl+ Me- isothiazolinone per patch. This preservative is found in many shampoos, creams, lotions, and other skin care products.

18. *Quaternium-15:* Quaternium-15, 1-(3-chloroallyl)-3,5,7,-triaza-1-azonium-adamantane chloride (purity 94% to 102%), is a preservative. The gel vehicle is hydroxypropyl cellulose. The product is formulated to contain 0.100 mg of Quaternium-15 per square centimeter, which calculates to 0.081 mg of Quaternium-15 per patch. This preservative is found in creams, lotions, shampoos, soaps, and other cosmetics and skin care products.

19. *Mercaptobenzothiazole:* Mercaptobenzothiazole (purity 98.5% to 101.5%) is a vulcanization accelerator used in rubber products. The gel vehicle is polyvidone. The product is formulated to contain 0.075 mg of mercaptobenzothiazole per square centimeter, which calculates to 0.061 mg of mercaptobenzothiazole per patch. This chemical is found in most rubber products, some adhesives, and is used as an industrial anticorrosive agent.

20. *p-Phenylenediamine:* *p*-Phenylenediamine (purity 97.5% to 101.5%), a blue-black aniline dye, is used to formulate this patch. The gel vehicle is polyvidone. The product is formulated to contain 0.090 mg of *p*-phenylenediamine per square centimeter, which calculates to 0.073 mg of *p*-phenylenediamine per patch. This dye is found most often in permanent and semipermanent hair dyes.

21. *Formaldehyde:* Formaldehyde is released from the proallergen N-hydroxymethyl succinimide, which is cleaved into succinimide and formaldehyde when it comes in contact with the transepidermal water on the surface of the skin. Formaldehyde is the active allergenic compound. The content of formaldehyde in the proallergen is 22.1% to 24.1%. The gel vehicle is polyvidone. The product is formulated to contain 0.18 mg of formaldehyde per square centimeter, which calculates to 0.15 mg of formaldehyde per patch. Formaldehyde is found in many building materials and plastic industries.

22. *Mercapto Mix:* Mercapto mix is composed of three chemical accelerators that are benzothiazole sulfenamide derivatives. N-cyclohexylbenzothiazyl-sulfenamide (purity ≥ 85%), dibenzothiazyl disulfide (purity 97% to 102%), and morpholinylmercaptobenzothiazole (purity ≥ 85%) and are present in equal parts. The gel vehicle is polyvidone. The product is formulated to contain 0.075 mg of mercapto mix per square centimeter, which calculates to 0.061 mg of mercapto mix per patch. This group of chemicals is found in many rubber products, e.g., shoes, gloves, elastic.

23. *Thimerosal:* Thimerosal (purity 97% to 101%) is a preservative that contains mercury. The gel vehicle is hydroxypropyl cellulose. The product is formulated to contain 0.0080 mg of thimerosal per square centimeter, which calculates to 0.0065 mg of thimerosal per patch. Thimerosal is found in some cosmetics, nose drops, and ear drops.

24. *Thiuram Mix:* Thiuram mix is composed of four substances in equal parts; tetramethylthiuram monosulfide (purity ≥ 95%, contains small amounts of tetramethylthiuram disulfide), tetramethylthiuram disulfide (purity ≥ 95%, contains small amounts of tetramethylthiuram monosulfide); disulfiram, USP (tetraethylthiuram disulfide, purity ≥ 95%), and dipentamethylenethiuram disulfide (pu-

rity ≥95%, impurities unknown). The components of thiuram mix can chemically interact, resulting in the formation of mixed disulfides. Thiuram monosulfides and disulfides are the active allergens. The gel vehicle is polyvidone. The product is formulated to contain 0.025 mg of thiuram mix per square centimeter, which calculates to 0.0051 mg of tetramethylthiuram monosulfide, 0.0051 mg of tetramethylthiuram disulfide, 0.0051 mg of disulfiram, and 0.0051 mg of dipentamethylenethiuram disulfide per patch. These antimicrobial and antioxidant substances are found in almost all rubber products.

CLINICAL PHARMACOLOGY

A positive response to the patch test is a classical delayed cell-mediated hypersensitivity reaction (type IV), which normally appears within 9 to 96 hours after exposure.[3]

Following primary contact, an allergen penetrates the skin and binds covalently or noncovalently to epidermal Langerhans cells. The processed allergen is presented to helper T-lymphocytes, resulting in the release of lymphokines, including interleukin 2. Interleukin 2 stimulates the production of other lymphocytes, chemotactic factors that recruit macrophages, basophils, eosinophils, and migration inhibitory factor, all which induce macrophages to remain at the reaction site. The resulting inflammation produces a papular, vesicular, or bullous response with erythema and itching at the site of application.[3,4]

Signs and symptoms of allergic contact dermatitis vary in intensity. Some patients may present with mild redness while others may present with severe swelling and bullae formation. Itching and vesiculation are common. The exposed areas of the skin, e.g., hands, forearm, face, neck, and dorsal surface of the feet, are primary initial sites of contact dermatitis. However, any area of the skin that comes into contact with a sensitizing allergen may also be affected.

The allergens in T.R.U.E. Test® were selected from those substances that have been widely reported to induce allergic contact dermatitis. They represent approximately 80% of the most common allergens. Nickel sulfate normally induces the greatest number of positive patch test responses when screening prospective patients. The frequency of positive responses to the various allergens can change depending upon the specific patient population as well as occupational and environmental influences. The epidemiology of allergic contact dermatitis and the frequency of positive patch test reactions to various causative allergens have been the subject of several extensive studies.[1,3,5,6,7]

Clinical Studies: A basic description of the interpretation method used to evaluate the patch reactions obtained during the clinical studies is as follows. Please refer to the DOSAGE AND ADMINISTRATION: Interpretation section for a complete description of this evaluation method.

? Doubtful reaction
\+ Weak (nonvesicular) positive reaction
++ Strong (vesicular) positive reaction
+++ Extreme positive reaction
- Negative reaction
IR Irritant reaction of different types

Four studies were done in North America to evaluate the clinical relevance of T.R.U.E. Test. Patients with suspected allergic contact dermatitis, based on history or clinical signs, were tested in all studies. Results of each study are described below. Note that the doubtful (?) and irritant (IR) reaction scores were combined in most studies because of the difficulty in interpretation between these two types of reactions. If there is allergen variation from the current patch, it is noted in the tables. Where there was a change in allergen vehicle, clinical studies were done to demonstrate equivalence. In the case of *p*-phenylenediamine, the patch was reformulated to utilize the base rather than the dihydrochloride form of the chemical. Dose response and irritation studies were used to support this reformulation. The results from the equivalency study done to compare the two formulations showed that *p*-phenylenediamine base gives higher bioavailability than the dihydrochloride form. Table 5 summarizes the data of reaction frequencies in the four studies and compares those frequencies to the results seen in the North American Contact Dermatitis Group (NACDG) studies.[8–14] Data on adverse reactions and itching and burning at the patch test site from the four clinical studies are shown in Tables 10 and 11 in the ADVERSE REACTIONS section.

Study No. 1: This study was conducted by six independent investigators to demonstrate the performance of T.R.U.E. Test Panel 1. A total of 128 patients with suspected contact dermatitis were recruited. Patients ranged in age from 17 to 79 years (mean age, 40.6 years). Females accounted for 86 (67%) of the 128 patients; 110 were Caucasian, 12 were Afro-American, and 6 were of other racial origin. The study period was approximately 8 months.

T.R.U.E. Test Panel 1, containing 12 allergens, was applied to the patient's back and remained there for 48 hours. The results were evaluated after 48, 72, or 96 hours.

Forty-five patients showed a total of 64 reactions to 11 of the 12 allergens in Panel 1. There were 18 weak (+), 37 strong (++), and 9 extreme (+++) positive reactions. There were

Table 1: Allergen Reaction Frequencies Observed in Study No. 1

Allergen	+ (% Frequency)	++ (% Frequency)	+++ (% Frequency)	+, ++, +++ Reaction Frequency (%)	IR/?	Missing
Nickel sulfate	8 (6.3)	9 (7.0)	4 (3.1)	16.4	1	
Neomycin sulfate	3 (2.3)	0	0	2.3	1	
Potassium dichromate	0	0	0	0	1	1
Caine mix	2 (1.6)	0	0	1.6	0	
Fragrance mix	1 (0.8)	7 (5.5)	1 (0.8)	7.1	1	
Colophony	0	3 (2.3)	1 (0.8)	3.1	0	
Epoxy resin	1 (0.8)	1 (0.8)	1 (0.8)	2.4	0	
Balsam of Peru*	1 (0.8)	4 (3.1)	0	3.9	1	
Ethylenediamine dihydrochloride	0	2 (1.6)	0	1.6	0	
Cobalt dichloride	2 (1.6)	6 (4.7)	1 (0.8)	7.1	1	
p-Phenylenediamine †	†	†	†	†	†	†
Thiuram mix ‡	0	5 (3.9)	1 (0.8)	4.7	0	

* Balsam of Peru vehicle is hydroxypropyl cellulose; vehicle in current patch is polyvidone.
† *p*-Phenylenediamine patch is dihydrochloride salt, 0.050 mg/cm^2; vehicle is hydroxypropyl cellulose. One patient experienced a 2+ reaction for a reaction frequency of 0.8%. Current patch contains 0.073 mg/cm^2 of *p*-phenylenediamine base; vehicle is polyvidone.
‡ Thiuram mix vehicle is hydroxypropyl cellulose; vehicle in current patch is polyvidone.

Table 2: Allergen Reaction Frequencies Observed in Study No. 2

Allergen	+ (% Frequency)	++ (% Frequency)	+++ (% Frequency)	+, ++, +++ Reaction Frequency (%)	IR/?
Wool alcohols	1 (0.8)	1 (0.8)	0	1.6	0
Quinoline mix	0	0	0	0	3
p-tert Butylphenol formaldehyde resin	1 (0.8)	3 (2.5)	1 (0.8)	4.1	0
Paraben mix	0	0	0	0	2
Carba mix	2 (1.6)	0	0	1.6	2
Black rubber mix*	1 (0.8)	2 (1.6)	0	2.4	5
CI+ Me- Isothiazolinone	3 (2.5)	1 (0.8)	0	3.3	1
Quaternium-15	2 (1.6)	5 (4.1)	0	5.7	1
Mercaptobenzothiazole†	2 (1.6)	4 (3.3)	0	4.9	0
Mercapto mix	0	5 (4.1)	0	4.1	0
Thimerosal	7 (5.7)	4 (3.3)	2 (1.6)	10.6	3

* Black rubber mix vehicle is hydroxypropyl cellulose; vehicle in current patch is polyvidone.
† Mercaptobenzothiazole vehicle is hydroxypropyl cellulose; vehicle in current patch is polyvidone.

positive test reactions to all allergens except chromium (see Table 1 below). In a follow-up of positive test reactors, 35% reported mild transient hyperpigmentation. No scarring was reported. Three patients required treatment for their reactions.

In all 128 patients there was good adhesion of the test tape to the skin. Some itching and burning sensations were reported (see Table 11). Such reactions are not unexpected and are considered a normal part of patch testing. Four patients (3%) experienced tape irritation.

[See Table 1 above.]

Study No. 2: This study was done to evaluate the performance of T.R.U.E. Test Panel 2. A total of 122 patients with suspected contact dermatitis were recruited. Patients ranged in age from 10 to 77 years (mean age, 41.2 years). Females accounted for 83 (68%) of the 122 patients; 107 were Caucasian, 14 were Afro-American, and 1 was of other racial origin. Five investigators participated in this study that was completed in approximately 8 months.

T.R.U.E. Test Panel 2, containing 11 allergens and a negative control, was applied to the patient's back and remained there for 48 hours. The results were evaluated after 72 or 96 hours. Thirty-three patients showed a total of 47 positive test reactions: 19 weak (+), 25 strong (++), and 3 extreme (+++). There were positive responses to all of the allergens except quinoline mix and paraben mix (see Table 2 below). Healing times for positive reactions ranged from 2 to 21 days; five patients required treatment.

In 108 patients (89%) there was satisfactory adhesion of the test tape to the skin. In 14 patients (11%), however, tape adhesion was not satisfactory. This was subsequently attributed to the particular lot of adhesive used to manufacture the clinical test tape. One patient (0.8%) experienced a tape irritation.

[See Table 2 above.]

Study No. 3: This study was conducted to demonstrate the performance of T.R.U.E. Test Panels 1 and 2 in a North American patient population referred for patch testing. One hundred twenty-two patients were enrolled. Patients ranged in age from 13 to 76 years (mean age, 42.6 years). Females accounted for 89 (73%) of the 122 patients; 100 were Caucasian, 13 were Afro-American, and 9 were of other racial origin. Five investigators participated in this study that was completed in approximately 8 months.

T.R.U.E. Test Panels 1 and 2, containing 24 allergens, were applied to the patient's back and remained there for 48 hours. The results were evaluated at either 72 or 96 hours after application.

Results show that 71 patients had a total of 122 positive test reactions: 50 weak (+), 58 strong (++), and 14 extreme (+++). Eleven patients demonstrated a total of 14 doubtful (?) reactions. Three patients experienced an irritant (IR) reaction. There were positive test responses to all of the allergens. See Table 3 below for distribution of allergen reactivities.

No unexpected adverse effects were reported. Healing times reported ranged from 1 to 34 days. Nineteen patients (16%) were prescribed medication to either promote healing or to relieve itching and/or burning sensations.

Two patients in this study reported reactions that are interpreted as possible sensitizations. One patient displayed a 1+ reaction to *p*-tert butylphenol formaldehyde resin at a follow-up visit on day 25. A potential positive reaction to wool alcohols on day 23 was observed for the second patient, although no description of the reaction was recorded. Neither patient was retested to verify whether these delayed reactions were indeed sensitizations.

In 120 patients (98%) there was good adhesion of the test tape to the skin. Seven patients (6%) reported an irritation related to the tape adhesive. Few itching and burning events were reported.

[See Table 3 on top of next page.]

Study No. 4: An open, multicenter, within-patient study was done to evaluate the clinical relevance of T.R.U.E. Test and to obtain information on late reactions and persistent local responses at a day 21 safety visit. A total number of 50 prospective patients with suspected contact dermatitis were recruited. The most common dermatitis site was hand, and the most common dermatitis type was allergic. Patients ranged in age from 19 to 82 years (mean age, 44.3 years). Females accounted for 36 (72%) of the 50 patients; 46 were Caucasian, 2 were Afro-American, and 2 were of other racial origin.

T.R.U.E. Test Panels 1 and 2 were applied to the patient's back and remained there for 48 hours. The results were evaluated after 72, 96, 120, or 168 hours. The patch sites were reexamined after 21 days for persistent local responses and late reactions. No additional safety data were collected after 21 days.

The tape adhered perfectly in 45 patients. The incidence of itching and burning sensation was absent for 34 patients, mild for 14, and moderate for 2. One of 50 patients had a weak irritation from the test tape.

Continued on next page

Glaxo Wellcome—Cont.

Table 3: Allergen Reaction Frequencies Observed in Study No. 3

Allergen	+ (% Frequency)	++ (% Frequency)	+++ (% Frequency)	+, ++, +++ Reaction Frequency (%)	?	IR
1. Nickel sulfate	11 (9.2)	10 (8.3)	8 (6.7)	24.2	1	0
2. Wool alcohols	0	1 (0.8)	0	0.8	0	0
3. Neomycin sulfate	3 (2.5)	5 (4.2)	0	6.7	0	0
4. Potassium dichromate	1 (0.8)	1 (0.8)	1 (0.8)	2.4	1	0
5. Caine mix	1 (0.8)	3 (2.5)	0	3.3	0	0
6. Fragrance mix	6 (5.0)	3 (2.5)	1 (0.8)	8.3	1	0
7. Colophony	1 (0.8)	0	1 (0.8)	1.6	0	0
8. Epoxy resin	1 (0.8)	0	0	0.8	0	0
9. Quinoline mix	0	2 (1.7)	0	1.7	2	0
10. Balsam of Peru	3 (2.5)	0	1 (0.8)	3.3	1	0
11. Ethylenediamine dihydrochloride	2 (1.7)	0	1 (0.8)	2.5	0	0
12. Cobalt chloride	4 (3.3)	3 (2.5)	1 (0.8)	6.6	0	2
13. p-tert Butylphenol formaldehyde resin	1 (0.8)	1 (0.8)	0	1.6	3	0
14. Paraben mix	3 (2.5)	1 (0.8)	0	3.3	0	0
15. Carba mix	1 (0.8)	2 (1.7)	0	2.5	3	0
16. Black rubber mix	2 (1.7)	0	0	1.7	0	0
17. Cl+ Me- Isothiazolinone	1 (0.8)	2 (1.7)	0	2.5	0	0
18. Quaternium-15	0	6 (5.0)	0	5.0	0	0
19. Mercapto- benzothiazole*	1 (0.8)	0	0	0.8	0	0
20. p-Phenylenediamine†	†	†	†	†	†	†
21. Formaldehyde	2 (1.7)	3 (2.5)	0	4.2	0	1
22. Mercapto mix	1 (0.8)	1 (0.8)	0	1.6	0	0
23. Thimerosal	3 (2.5)	10 (8.3)	0	10.8	1	0
24. Thiuram mix‡	2 (1.7)	4 (3.3)	0	5.0	1	0

* Mercaptobenzothiazole vehicle is hydroxypropyl cellulose; vehicle in current patch is polyvidone.

† p-Phenylenediamine patch tested in this study is dihydrochloride salt, 0.05 mg/cm^2; vehicle is hydroxypropyl cellulose. Two patients experienced a 1+ reaction and three patients experienced a 2+ reaction for an overall reaction frequency of 4.2%. The current patch contains 0.073 mg/cm^2 of p-phenylenediamine base; vehicle is polyvidone.

‡ Thiuram mix vehicle is hydroxypropyl cellulose; vehicle in current patch is polyvidone.

Table 4: Allergen Reaction Frequencies Observed in Study No. 4

Allergen	+ (% Frequency)	++ (% Frequency)	+++ (% Frequency)	+, ++, +++ Reaction Frequency (%)	?	ME*
1. Nickel sulfate	4 (8.0)	5 (10.0)	0	18.0	0	0
2. Wool alcohols	1 (2.0)	0	0	2.0	0	0
3. Neomycin sulfate	2 (4.0)	0	0	4.0	0	0
4. Potassium dichromate	1 (2.0)	1 (2.0)	0	4.0	0	0
5. Caine mix	0	0	0	0	0	0
6. Fragrance mix	1 (2.0)	1 (2.0)	0	4.0	0	3
7. Colophony	1 (2.0)	0	1 (2.0)	4.0	0	0
8. Epoxy resin	0	0	0	0	0	0
9. Quinoline mix	0	0	0	0	0	0
10. Balsam of Peru	3 (6.0)	2 (4.0)	0	10.0	0	0
11. Ethylenediamine dihydrochloride	1 (2.0)	1 (2.0)	0	4.0	0	0
12. Cobalt chloride	5 (10.0)	0	0	10.0	0	0
13. p-tert Butylphenol formaldehyde resin	1 (2.0)	1 (2.0)	0	4.0	0	0
14. Paraben mix	1 (2.0)	0	0	2.0	0	0
15. Carba mix	0	1 (2.0)	0	2.0	0	0
16. Black rubber mix	0	0	0	0	0	1
17. Cl+ Me- Isothiazolinone	0	1 (2.0)	0	2.0	0	0
18. Quaternium-15	5 (10.0)	2 (4.0)	0	14.0	0	0
19. Mercapto- benzothiazole	1 (2.0)	0	0	2.0	0	0
20. p-Phenylenediamine	2 (4.0)	0	0	4.0	0	0
21. Formaldehyde	3 (6.0)	2 (4.0)	0	10.0	0	0
22. Mercapto mix	2 (4.0)	0	0	4.0	0	1
23. Thimerosal	2 (4.0)	2 (4.0)	1 (2.0)	10.0	0	0
24. Thiuram mix	4 (8.0)	0	0	8.0	0	0

* Macular erythema only.

Thirty-two patients showed a total of 66 reactions to 21 of the 24 allergens included in T.R.U.E. Test (see Table 4 below). The following allergens gave no reactions: caine mix, epoxy resin, and quinoline mix. The allergen that gave most reactions was nickel sulfate, 9/66 (13.6%) reactions. Quaternium-15 showed 7/66 (10.6%) reactions, and fragrance mix, Balsam of Peru, cobalt dichloride, formaldehyde, and thimerosal showed 5/66 (7.6%) reactions each.

Eight patients had a total of 10 persistent local responses at the day 21 examination. One of these patients had a late reaction, a 2+ reaction to Cl+ Me- isothiazolinone, moderate erythema, and a persistent local response. There were no other adverse events reported in this study.

[See Table 4 above.]

These studies demonstrate that T.R.U.E. Test is a clinically relevant method for diagnosing allergic contact dermatitis. The persistent local responses, as well as the occurrence of late reactions, are within the normal range expected for patch testing. Although there is no specific data, in general, more severe positive reactions can be expected to require longer healing times. Of course, healing time can be influenced by many factors, especially the general health of the patient.

To further demonstrate the clinical relevance of the T.R.U.E. Test method for diagnosing allergic contact dermatitis, a comparison was made to data in a screening tray recommended by the NACDG.[8-14] The frequency of reactivities observed in the four North American clinical studies have been summarized in Table 5.[15]

Also listed in Table 5 are the frequency of reactivities for allergens in a screening tray recommended by the NACDG.[8-14] These data were collected over 4 years by 14 independent investigators in North America after testing 4,055 patients with suspected contact dermatitis. Forty-three percent of the patients tested were male. Eighty-seven percent of the patients assessed were Caucasian, 7% were Afro-American, 3% were Asian, and 2% were Hispanic; the average age of the patients was 43.8 years.[11]

These data in Table 5 demonstrate that most allergens have very similar reactivities in the two methods. Differences noted are most likely due to patient selection in the clinical trials and to the fact that there is approximately a 10-fold difference in size between the sample populations. Nickel sulfate, thimerosal, Quaternium-15, formaldehyde, thiuram mix, and Balsam of Peru are the most commonly reported reactive allergens in both series. Average concordance in clinical studies that tested both the T.R.U.E. Test method and allergens in petrolatum ranged from 60% to 77%.[15]

[See Table 5 at top of next page.]

Formaldehyde reflects data from studies 3 and 4 and p-phenylenediamine from study 4.

Nickel Use Test: Results from another clinical trial, a nickel use test, are described below.

A study was performed to investigate the relationship between reactions caused by a natural sensitizer, such as nickel-containing costume jewelry, and T.R.U.E. Test. Nickel is often implicated as a major cause of cutaneous reactions to jewelry.[16]

Fifty-one patients with history of cutaneous reactions to jewelry were tested with T.R.U.E. Test Panel 1 (identical to that used in study no. 1). A medallion containing approximately 20% nickel served as a positive control and a stainless steel earring post was intended to serve as a negative control. It was subsequently discovered that the earring post contained up to 14% nickel on the outer surface.

Patients ranged in age from 16 to 68 years (mean age, 39.3 years). Females accounted for 50 (98%) of the 51 patients and, except for one Mexican-American, all were Caucasian. One patient was excluded from the evaluation because of a dislocation of the test. In addition, 12 patients (24%) reported minor problems with the test adhering properly to the skin. This was subsequently attributed to a particular lot of adhesive used to manufacture the clinical test lot. Seven patients (14%) experienced a tape irritation. Thirty-six of the remaining 50 patients (72%) experienced a total of 51 reactions to various T.R.U.E. Test patches as shown below.

Table 6: Allergen Reactions Observed in the Nickel Use Test

Allergen	Reactions	Frequency (%)
Nickel sulfate	31	60.8
Cobalt dichloride	7	13.7
Fragrance mix	2	3.9
p-Phenylenediamine	1	2.0
Neomycin sulfate	3	5.9
Colophony	3	5.9
Epoxy resin	1	2.0
Thiuram mix	2	3.9
Caine mix	1	2.0

These reactions generally resolved within an average of 10 days (range, 2 to 42 days) with the following frequencies: 1 to 10 days (22), 11 to 20 days (9), 21 to 30 days (1), 31 to 45 days (1). The time of resolution for three patients is not available. A further breakdown of the positive results obtained with the T.R.U.E. Test nickel sulfate patch, the medallion, and the earring post is presented below.

Table 7: Positive Reactions Observed in the Nickel Use Test

	+	++	+++	Total
T.R.U.E. Test	13	15	3	31
Medallion	10	11	0	21
Earring Post	2	4	0	6

If the results obtained with the medallion were used as the only basis for determining the presence of contact sensitivity to nickel, then the T.R.U.E. Test nickel patch would demonstrate the following characteristics:

Table 8: Medallion vs. T.R.U.E. Test Nickel Patch Comparison

		Medallion		
		+	−	Total
T.R.U.E. Test	+	20	11	31
Nickel Patch	−	1	18	19
	Total	21	29	50

Sensitivity: 95.2%.
Specificity: 62.1%.
Predictive value of a positive test: 64.5%.
Predictive value of a negative test: 94.7%.
Test efficiency: 76.0%.

In addition, 35.4% of the T.R.U.E. Test nickel patch positive results would have been considered false positives and 5.3% would have been considered false negatives.
However, the results obtained in this study should be interpreted with caution. The metal composition of jewelry can vary greatly from manufacturer to manufacturer and thereby alter the bioavailability of the causative allergen. A different medallion could have produced either a greater or lesser correlation with T.R.U.E. Test nickel patch.
Of the 21 medallion positive patients, 20 also demonstrated a positive response to T.R.U.E. Test nickel patch and the one other patient demonstrated a doubtful (?) T.R.U.E. Test response. In addition, 18 of the 21 medallion responders (85.7%) experienced reactions with T.R.U.E. Test greater than or equal to the medallion reaction.
T.R.U.E. Test demonstrated excellent sensitivity in detecting patients who had positive responses to the medallion. The comparatively large number of additional nickel positive results obtained with T.R.U.E. Test may, in fact, be true positives unresponsive to the particular medallion used in this study, although false-positive reactions cannot be ruled out.
Several studies have been conducted to demonstrate the clinical reproducibility of results obtained with three different production runs of representative allergens. These data are summarized below and demonstrate excellent reproducibility of in vivo responses to different production lots of these allergens. No significant safety concerns were noted in these studies, although no safety data was collected after 21 days.

Table 9: Reaction Frequencies Observed in Lot-to-Lot Consistency Studies

Allergen	Lot no.	−	IR/?	+	++	+++
Nickel sulfate	1	1	0	1	11	0
	2	0	0	2	11	0
	3	1	0	2	10	0
Epoxy resin	1	0	0	3	8	2
	2	0	0	3	7	3
	3	0	0	3	7	3
Balsam of Peru	1	1	0	2	7	1
	2	1	0	2	7	1
	3	1	0	2	7	1
Ethylenediamine dihydrochloride	1	0	0	0	7	6
	2	0	0	0	7	6
	3	0	0	0	7	6
Black rubber mix	1	2	1	4	4	2
	2	2	0	4	5	2
	3	2	0	5	4	2
CI+ Me- Isothiazolinone	1	1	0	1	4	6
	2	1	1	0	4	6
	3	1	0	1	4	6
p-Phenylenediamine	1	1	0	3	4	3
	2	1	0	3	4	3
	3	1	0	2	5	3
Thiuram mix	1	2	0	2	7	1
	2	2	1	1	7	1
	3	2	0	2	7	1

INDICATIONS

T.R.U.E. Test™ is indicated primarily as an aid in the diagnosis of allergic contact dermatitis in patients whose histories suggest sensitivity to one or more of the substances included on the T.R.U.E. Test panels. To determine whether sensitization to an allergen may be etiologically important, T.R.U.E. Test may also be used adjunctively to evaluate other eczemas (atopic, seborrheic, venous, palmar, and plantar hyperkeratotic eczema, vesiculosis, or neurodermatitis) and other dermatologic diseases that do not heal, such as leg ulcers and psoriasis, to determine whether there may be a contact hypersensitivity component.[3,7,17]

Table 5: Comparison of Allergen Reactivity Between Allergens in T.R.U.E. Test and Allergens in Petrolatum

	Frequency of Allergen Reactions in Four North American T.R.U.E. Test Multicenter Studies			North American Contact Dermatitis Group (NACDG) Responses to Allergens in Screening Tray		
Allergen	n	Frequency (%)		Allergen (% in petrolatum)	n	Frequency (%)
1. Nickel sulfate	300	19.7		Nickel sulfate, 2.5%	3,968	10.5
2. Wool alcohols	294	1.4		Wool (lanolin) alcohols, 30%	3,977	1.5
3. Neomycin sulfate	300	4.3		Neomycin sulfate, 20%	3,973	7.2
4. Potassium dichromate	300	1.7		Potassium dichromate, 0.25%	3,947	2.4
5. Caine mix	300	2.0		Benzocaine, 5%*	3,977	2.1
6. Fragrance mix	300	7.0		Cinnamic alcohol, 5%†	3,946	4.8
				Cinnamic aldehyde, 1%†	3,959	3.1
7. Colophony	300	2.7		Rosin, 20%‡	3,940	2.2
8. Epoxy resin	300	1.3		Epoxy resin, 1%	3,983	2.1
9. Quinoline mix	294	0.68				
10. Balsam of Peru	300	4.7		Balsam of Peru, 25%	3,953	5.1
11. Ethylenediamine dihydrochloride	300	2.3		Ethylenediamine dihydrochloride, 1%	3,974	3.8
12. Cobalt chloride	300	7.3				
13. p-tert Butylphenol formaldehyde resin	294	3.1		p-tert Butylphenol formaldehyde resin, 1%	3,988	1.6
14. Paraben mix	294	1.7				
15. Carba mix	294	2.0		Carba mix, 3%	3,988	3.1
16. Black rubber mix	294	1.7		Black rubber mix (PPD mix 0.6%)	3,985	2.1
17. CI+ Me- Isothiazolinone	294	2.7				
18. Quaternium-15	294	6.8		Quaternium-15, 2%	3,985	6.2
19. Mercaptobenzothiazole	294	2.7		Mercaptobenzothiazole, 1%	3,968	2.1
20. p-Phenylenediamine	50	4.0		p-Phenylenediamine, 1%	3,980	6.4
21. Formaldehyde	172	5.8		Formaldehyde, 1% aqueous	3,911	6.8
22. Mercapto mix	294	3.1		Mercapto mix, 1%	3,979	2.5
23. Thimerosal	294	10.5		Thimerosal, 0.1%	3,955	8.7
24. Thiuram mix	300	5.3		Thiuram mix, 1%	3,986	5.5

* T.R.U.E. Test contains caine mix, which is a mixture of benzocaine, dibucaine hydrochloride, and tetracaine hydrochloride.
† Compare with fragrance mix in T.R.U.E. Test.
‡ Compare with colophony in T.R.U.E. Test.

CONTRAINDICATIONS

The minor amount of allergen on each T.R.U.E. Test® patch that penetrates the skin will rarely induce a flare-up of dermatitis. In the case of extensive ongoing contact dermatitis, however, the test should not be applied since it may provoke an intensified reaction on both the present and previously affected sites and may also cause a false-positive test result.

WARNINGS

The use of T.R.U.E. Test® in patients with a known history of severe systemic and/or local reactions to any of the allergen components or inactive substances included in the T.R.U.E. Test panels should be carefully evaluated before application.
Patients should be warned that itching and burning sensations are common occurrences with patch testing and may be severe in extremely sensitive patients. The use of medication may be considered necessary to relieve these itching or burning sensations.
Sensitization to a substance included on the test panel may occur with patch testing but is extremely rare. A test reaction that appears 7 days or later with no preceding reaction may be a sign of contact sensitization.[7]
Dermatitis flare-up may occur in some patients.
Occasionally, hyperpigmentation of the test site occurs during healing. Healing with or without medication normally takes place within 5 days to 2 weeks, although reactions in some individuals may persist longer.
Extremely sensitive patients may exhibit extreme (+++) reactions that may be bullous or ulcerative with pronounced erythema, infiltration, and coalescing vesicles.
Excited skin syndrome (angry back) is a state of hyper-reactivity induced by a dermatitis on other parts of the body or by a strong positive skin-test reaction.[18]
Therefore, test results should be evaluated carefully in patients with multiple, positive, concomitant patch test results. To determine which reactions are false positives, retesting at a later date may be considered.
The safety and efficacy of repetitive testing with T.R.U.E. Test is unknown. Sensitization or increased reactivity to one or more of the allergens may occur. The benefits of repeat testing should therefore be carefully evaluated against the possible risks.
On rare occasions, it may be necessary to remove the test strip from the patient because of severe itching or burning sensations. One patient taking part in the clinical studies removed the test tape after 24 hours because of severe itching.
Formaldehyde is a known carcinogen. Nickel sulfate, potassium dichromate, epoxy resin, cobalt dichloride, and thiuram mix are suspected carcinogens. The potential effects associated with using very low concentrations of these sub-

stances for single or multiple applications are currently unknown.[19,20]

PRECAUTIONS

General: T.R.U.E. Test® may be applied throughout the year. However, during the summer months, excessive sweating is to be avoided in order to maintain sufficient adhesion to the skin. In addition, exposure to the sun should be minimized in order to prevent a sun-induced skin reaction that may interfere with interpretation of test results.
T.R.U.E. Test should only be applied to healthy skin that is free of acne, scars, dermatitis, or any other condition that may interfere with interpretation of test results.
Since steroids may suppress a positive test reaction, use of topical steroids on the test site or oral steroids (equivalent to 15 mg of prednisolone) should be discontinued for at least 2 weeks prior to testing. Topical steroids on nontest areas may be appropriate.
If a severe patch test reaction develops, the patient may be treated with a topical corticosteroid or, in rare cases, with a systemic corticosteroid.
Information for Patients: Patients should be instructed to avoid extreme physical activity and/or mechanical action that may result in reduced adhesion or actual loss of patch test material. Use appropriate measures to avoid getting the area around the patch wet.
Patients should also be advised that a strong allergic response to one or more test allergens can be associated with significant itching, burning, erythema, and vesiculation. Patients who experience intense discomfort should contact their physicians concerning possible removal of the test.
Carcinogenesis, Mutagenesis, Impairment of Fertility: Studies of T.R.U.E. Test to evaluate carcinogenic potential, mutagenesis, or impairment of fertility have not been performed. Nickel refinery dust, nickel sulfite, and formaldehyde are known carcinogens. Nickel sulfate, potassium dichromate, cobalt dichloride, epoxy resin, and thiuram mix are suspected carcinogens. The potential effects of using very low concentrations of these substances for single or multiple applications are currently unknown.[19,20] The following components of T.R.U.E. Test have been reviewed as part of the Cosmetic Ingredient Review and found to be safe or safe with qualifications: those found to be safe are hydroxypropyl cellulose, methylcellulose, wool alcohols, paraben mix, Quaternium-15, and p-phenylenediamine and those found to be safe with qualifications are N-phenyl-p-phenylenediamine, Cl+ Me- isothiazolinone, and formaldehyde.[25]
Pregnancy: Pregnancy Category C: Animal reproduction studies have not been conducted with T.R.U.E. Test. It is also not known whether T.R.U.E. Test can cause fetal harm when

Continued on next page

Glaxo Wellcome—Cont.

administered to pregnant women or whether it can affect reproduction capacity. T.R.U.E. Test should be applied to pregnant women only if clearly needed.

Nursing Mothers: No studies have been performed to evaluate absorption of T.R.U.E. Test allergens in nursing mothers. It is not known if T.R.U.E. Test allergens appear in human milk. Because many drugs are excreted in human milk, caution should be exercised when T.R.U.E. Test is administered to a nursing woman.

Pediatric Use: The safety and effectiveness of T.R.U.E. Test in children have not been established.

Geriatric Use: More frequent patch test responses can be expected in geriatric patients. While no conclusive explanation is available, older patients may exhibit an increased frequency of cutaneous allergies.[10,13]

ADVERSE REACTIONS

Adverse reactions reported with the use of T.R.U.E. Test® and patch testing in general are normally mild and usually occur only at the site of the test application. Table 10 summarizes the adverse reactions recorded in the five clinical studies described in the CLINICAL PHARMACOLOGY section. In some cases, allergenic responses may be delayed in onset. One type of delayed reaction is a sensitization, which is not well defined in the literature but is described as a positive reaction observed at 10 to 14 days after application or later and at 2 to 4 days after the test is repeated.[7] The positive reaction should meet the criteria for an allergic reaction (papular or vesicular erythema and infiltration) in order to distinguish between a false-positive result and a sensitization.

In clinical studies conducted with T.R.U.E. Test, there have been three reports of delayed reactions occurring at 21 days or later. None of these patients were retested to verify a sensitization reaction. There is enough data for only two of these patients to indicate probable sensitization. For more details of these reactions, refer to summaries of studies no. 3 and no. 4 in the CLINICAL PHARMACOLOGY section.

There are reports of other adverse reactions associated with patch testing. These include keloids, sarcoid infiltrates, vitiligo spots, edema, crusting, and sensitization.[3,7,21,22]

[See table 10 above.]

Table 11 below shows data on itching and burning events from the five clinical studies described in the CLINICAL PHARMACOLOGY section. A number of patients in the study groups were prescribed medication to either promote healing or to relieve itching and/or burning sensations. Itching and burning sensations are commonly associated with patch testing. Treatment may be required and the more severe reactions can be expected to require longer times to heal.

In addition, the adhesive tape may also cause an irritation at the test site. Reports of tape irritation are infrequent, usually mild in nature, and self-limiting in clinical studies conducted with T.R.U.E. Test, though no data was collected in these studies beyond a day 21 safety visit. In the nickel use test study and in a Panel 2 clinical study (study no. 2), problems with tape adhesion were observed. Twenty-four percent and 11%, respectively, of the patients in these studies reported poor tape adhesion. (See CLINICAL PHARMACOLOGY section for complete descriptions of these studies.) In both studies, the problem was subsequently attributed to the lot of adhesive tape used to produce the clinical test samples. No adhesion problems have been reported in other studies.

[See table 11 above.]

DOSAGE AND ADMINISTRATION

Dosage: A concentration for each allergen has been established that is high enough to evoke a reaction even in weakly sensitive patients, yet low enough to minimize the risk of irritant reactions. Please refer to the DESCRIPTION section for labeled amounts of allergen.

Administration: Please refer to the WARNINGS section prior to administration.

Physicians may either apply T.R.U.E. Test® patches taken directly from the refrigerator or allow them to come to room temperature (15 to 20 minutes) prior to application, as best benefits their practice.

T.R.U.E. Test Application Instructions:

1. Peel open the package and remove test Panel 1 (Figure 1).

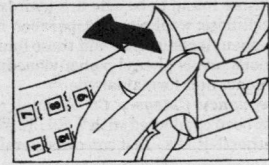

Figure 1

Table 10: Adverse Reactions Reported During Patient Follow-Up*

| | Number of Events Reported | | | | |
Event Reported	Study 1 n†=33	Study 2 n‡=102	Study 3 n‡=104	Study 4 n†=32	Nickel Use n†=31
Erythema	2	2	27	2	—
Hyperpigmentation	9	2	8	6	8
Pruritus	3	1	27	2	—
Scarring	—	—	2	—	—
Urticaria	—	—	—	—	1
Delayed reaction (allergen known)	—	—	1§	—	—
Delayed reaction (allergen unknown)	—	2	2	—	—
Sensitization (potential)	—	—	1¶	—	—
Sensitization (probable)	—	—	1#	1**	—

* Patient follow-up was either via telephone or an office visit; time of follow-up ranged from 4 to 80 days after testing.
† Number of patients with positive test results who took part in clinical follow-up.
‡ Number of total patients who took part in the clinical follow-up.
§ Neomycin sulfate.
¶ Wool alcohols.
# *p*-tert Butylphenol formaldehyde resin.
** Cl+ Me- Isothiazolinone.

Table 11: Incidences of Itching and Burning Sensations Reported by Patients at the Time of Patch Test Removal

| | Number of Events Reported | | | | |
Event Reported	Study 1 n*=128	Study 2 n*=122	Study 3 n*=122	Study 4 n*=50	Nickel Use n*=50
Itching					
Mild	31	23	48	14	30
Moderate	—	—	—	2	—
Strong	21	5	17	—	24
Burning sensations					
Mild	7	4	8	14	4
Moderate	—	—	—	2	—
Strong	5	2	1	—	8
Total events	64	34	74	32	66

* Total number of patients in study.

Note that individual patients may exhibit one or both symptoms.

---

2. Remove the protective plastic covering from the test surface of the panel (Figure 2). Be careful not to touch the test substances.

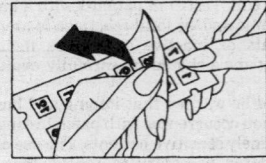

Figure 2

3. Position the test on the upper left side of the patient's back (approximately 5 cm from the midline) so that no. 1 allergen is in the upper left corner. Avoid applying the test on the margin of the scapula. From the center of the panel, smooth outward toward the edges, making sure each allergen makes firm contact with the skin (Figure 3).

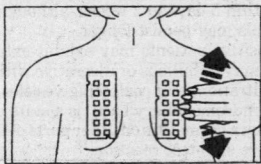

Figure 3

4. With a medical marking pen, indicate on the skin the location of the two notches on the panel (Figure 4).

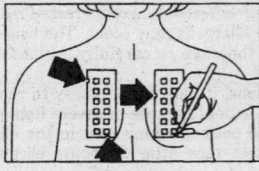

Figure 4

5. Repeat the process with test panel 2. Position the test on the upper right side of the patient's back so that no. 13 allergen is in the upper left corner.

The test should only be applied to healthy skin that is free of acne, scars, dermatitis, or any other condition that might interfere with the interpretation of results (see PRECAUTIONS).

The test is best applied on the upper part of the back, about 5 cm from the midline.

The patient should wear T.R.U.E. Test for a minimum of 48 hours before it is removed.

Interpretation: The reaction should be read at 72 to 96 hours, when allergic reactions are fully developed and mild irritant reactions have faded. If reading at 48 hours is considered, another reading at 72 to 96 hours is recommended. Patients should be advised to report reactions occurring after 7 days to detect potential sensitizations.

It is important to note that *p*-phenylenediamine will turn the patch test area black on all patients. However, this is because the allergen is a dye and does not represent an allergic reaction. This discoloration may remain for up to approximately 2 weeks.

Neomycin sulfate and *p*-phenylenediamine sometimes cause reactions that may not appear until 4 to 5 days (or later) after the application. Patients should be instructed to report this. If appropriate, an additional office visit will verify a late reaction.

An identification template is provided for quick identification of any allergen that causes a reaction. To assure correct positioning, marks on the skin should correlate with the notches on the template.

The interpretation method, similar to the one recommended by the International Contact Dermatitis Research Group, is as follows.[7]

?   Doubtful reaction:
     faint macular erythema only

+   Weak (nonvesicular) positive reaction:
     erythema
     infiltration
     possibly papules

++   Strong (vesicular) positive reaction:
     erythema
     infiltration
     papules
     vesicles

+++   Extreme positive reaction:
     bullous reaction

-   Negative reaction

IR   Irritant reaction of different types:
Pustules as well as patchy follicular or homogeneous erythema without infiltrations are usually signs of irritation and do not indicate allergy.

False Negatives: False-negative results may be due to insufficient patch contact with the skin, sensitization to a substance not present in the test panel, and/or premature evaluation of the test.

Retesting may be indicated. The effect of repetitive testing with T.R.U.E. Test is unknown (see WARNINGS).

False Positives: A false-positive result may occur when an irritant reaction cannot be differentiated from an allergic reaction. Pustules as well as patchy follicular or homogeneous erythema without infiltration are usually signs of irritation and do not indicate allergy.

A positive test reaction should meet the criteria for an allergic reaction (papular or vesicular erythema and infiltration). If an irritant reaction cannot be distinguished from a true positive reaction or if a doubtful reaction is present, a retest may be considered in a few weeks or months.

It is important when evaluating a positive test result not only to consider the intensity of the reaction but also to consider whether it is relevant to the patient's existing condition either as a primary cause or an aggravating factor. Excited skin syndrome (angry back) consists of a hyper-reactive state of the skin in which false-positive patch test reactions concur with dermatitis at a distant body site or with adjacent strong positive skin test reactions.[23] This rare state of hyper-reactivity is not well understood clinically. There has only been one reported case of suspected angry back in a patient that was being tested with T.R.U.E. Test. This patient had the standard screening allergens and a special shoe series on his back and also had T.R.U.E. Test on his thigh. He displayed symptoms of angry back on his back but not on his thigh. This patient was retested 1 month after complete cure and an accurate diagnosis was made using the standard series and T.R.U.E. Test.[24]

There are several publications available that further describe the reading and interpretation of patch test reactions.[3,7,21]

HOW SUPPLIED

T.R.U.E. Test® is supplied in multipack cartons of five units (NDC 0173-0457-01).

Store between 2° and 8°C (36° and 46°F). Refrigeration required. The expiration date is stated on the package; data available currently support a 12-month dating period.

REFERENCES

1. Storrs FJ, Rosenthal LE, Adams RM, et al. Prevalence and relevance of allergic reactions in patients patch tested in North America, 1984-1985. *J Am Acad Dermatol.* 1989;20:1038-1045.
2. Dahlquist I, Fregert S. Contact allergy to atranorin in lichens and perfumes. *Contact Dermatitis.* 1980;6:111-119.
3. Fregert S. *Manual of Contact Dermatitis.* 2nd ed. Chicago, Ill: Year Book Medical Publisher; 1981.
4. Roitt I, Brostoff J, Male D. *Immunology.* New York, NY: Gower Medical Publishing; 1985. Chap 22.
5. Andersen KE, Benzra C, Burrows D, et al. Contact dermatitis—a review. *Contact Dermatitis.* 1987;16:55-78.
6. Adams RM, Fischer AA. Contact allergen alternatives: 1986. *J Am Acad Dermatol.* 1986;14:951-969.
7. Fisher AA. *Contact Dermatitis.* 3rd ed. Philadelphia, Pa: Lea & Febiger; 1986.
8. Nethercott J. The positive predictive accuracy of patch tests. *Immun All Clin N Amer.* 1989;9:549-553.
9. Nethercott JR. Practical problems in the use of patch testing in the evaluation of patients with contact dermatitis. *Curr Probl Dermatol.* 1990;4:95-123.
10. Rietschel R, Rosenthal L, North American Contact Dermatitis Group. Standard patch test screening series used diagnostically in young and elderly patients. *Am J Contact Dermatitis.* 1990;1:53-55.
11. Nethercott J, Holness DL, Adams RM, et al. Patch testing with a routine screening tray in North America, 1985-1989. I: Frequency of Response. *Am J Contact Dermatitis.* 1991;2:122-129.
12. Nethercott J, Holness DL, Adams RM, et al. Patch testing with a routine screening tray in North America, 1985-1989. II: Gender and Response. *Am J Contact Dermatitis.* 1991;2:130-134.
13. Nethercott J, Holness DL, Adams RM, et al. Patch testing with a routine screening tray in North America, 1985–1989. III: Age and Response. *Am J Contact Dermatitis.* 1991;2:198-201.
14. Nethercott J, Holness DL, Adams RM, et al. Patch testing with a routine screening tray in North America, 1985-1989. IV: Occupation and Response. *Am J Contact Dermatitis.* 1991;2:247-254.
15. Data on file, Kabi Pharmacia Service A/S.
16. Emmett EA, Risby TH, Jiang L, Ng SK, Feinam S. Allergic contact dermatitis to nickel: bioavailability from consumer products and provocation threshold. *J Am Acad Dermatol.* 1988;19:314-322.
17. Shupp DL, Winkelmann RK. The role of patch testing in stasis dermatitis. *Cutis.* December 1988;42:528-530.
18. Bruynzeel DP, Maibach HI. Excited skin syndrome (angry back). *Arch Dermatol.* 1986;122:323-328.
19. Sittig M. *Handbook of Toxic and Hazardous Chemicals and Carcinogens.* 2nd ed. Park Ridge, NJ: Noyles Publications; 1985.
20. *Registry of Toxic Effects of Chemical Substances.* Washington, DC: U.S. Department of Health and Human Services; April 1989.
21. Fischer T, Maibach HI. Patch testing in allergic contact dermatitis: an update. *Semin Dermatol.* September 1986;5:214-244.
22. Calnan CD. *The Use and Abuse of Patch Tests in Occupational and Industrial Dermatology.* Maibach HI, Gellin GA, eds. Chicago, Ill: Year Book Medical Publisher Inc; 1982:35-37.
23. Pasche-Koo F, Hauser C. How to better understand the angry back syndrome. *Dermatology.* 1992;184:337.
24. Romaguera C, Grimalt R, Vilaplana J. Allergic contact dermatitis from shoes: "angry back" without "angry thigh". *Contact Dermatitis.* 1989;21:267-281.
25. *CIR Compendium of Abstracts, Discussions, and Conclusions.* Washington, DC: Cosmetic Ingredient Review; December 1993.

U.S. Patents 4,836,217 and 5,182,081
November 1994/RL-159
Shown in Product Identification Guide, page 314

VALTREX® Caplets   ℞
(valacyclovir hydrochloride)
[văl 'trĕks]

DESCRIPTION

VALTREX (valacyclovir hydrochloride) is the hydrochloride salt of L-valyl ester of the antiviral drug acyclovir (ZOVIRAX® Brand, Glaxo Wellcome Inc.).

VALTREX Caplets are for oral administration. Each caplet contains valacyclovir hydrochloride equivalent to 500 mg valacyclovir and the inactive ingredients carnauba wax, colloidal silicon dioxide, crospovidone, FD&C Blue No. 2 Lake, hydroxypropyl methylcellulose, magnesium stearate, microcrystalline cellulose, polyethylene glycol, polysorbate 80, povidone, and titanium dioxide. The blue, film-coated caplets are printed with edible white ink.

The chemical name of valacyclovir hydrochloride is L-valine, 2-[(2-amino-1,6-dihydro-6-oxo-9H-purin-9-yl)methoxy]ethyl ester, monohydrochloride.

Valacyclovir hydrochloride is a white to off-white powder with the molecular formula $C_{13}H_{20}N_6O_4$, HCl and a molecular weight of 360.80. The maximum solubility in water at 25°C is 174 mg/mL. The pk_a's for valacyclovir hydrochloride are 1.90, 7.47, and 9.43.

CLINICAL PHARMACOLOGY

After oral administration, valacyclovir hydrochloride is rapidly absorbed from the gastrointestinal tract. Valacyclovir is rapidly and nearly completely converted to acyclovir and L-valine by first-pass intestinal and/or hepatic metabolism.

Virology:

Mechanism of Antiviral Action: Valacyclovir hydrochloride is rapidly converted to acyclovir, which has in vitro and in vivo inhibitory activity against herpes simplex virus types 1 (HSV-1) and 2 (HSV-2) and varicella-zoster virus (VZV). In cell culture, acyclovir's highest antiviral activity is against HSV-1, followed in decreasing order of potency against HSV-2 and VZV.

The inhibitory activity of acyclovir is highly selective due to its affinity for the enzyme thymidine kinase (TK) encoded by HSV, VZV, and EBV. This viral enzyme converts acyclovir into acyclovir monophosphate, a nucleotide analogue. The monophosphate is further converted into diphosphate by cellular guanylate kinase and into triphosphate by a number of cellular enzymes. In vitro, acyclovir triphosphate stops replication of herpes viral DNA. This is accomplished in three ways: 1) competitive inhibition of viral DNA polymerase, 2) incorporation and termination of the growing viral DNA chain, and 3) inactivation of the viral DNA polymerase. The greater antiviral activity of acyclovir against HSV compared to VZV is due to its more efficient phosphorylation by the viral TK.

Antiviral Activities: The quantitative relationship between the in vitro susceptibility of herpes viruses to antivirals and the clinical response to therapy has not been established in humans, and virus sensitivity testing has not been standardized. Sensitivity testing results, expressed as the concentration of drug required to inhibit by 50% the growth of virus in cell culture (IC_{50}), vary greatly depending upon a number of factors. Using plaque-reduction assays, the IC_{50} against herpes simplex virus isolates ranges from 0.02 to 13.5 µg/mL for HSV-1 and from 0.01 to 9.9 µg/mL for HSV-2. The IC_{50} for acyclovir against most laboratory strains and clinical isolates of VZV ranges from 0.12 to 10.8 µg/mL. Acyclovir also demonstrates activity against the Oka vaccine strain of VZV with a mean IC_{50} of 1.35 µg/mL.

Drug Resistance: Resistance of VZV to antiviral nucleoside analogues can result from qualitative or quantitative changes in the viral TK or DNA polymerase. Clinical isolates of VZV with reduced susceptibility to acyclovir have been recovered from patients with AIDS. In these cases, TK-deficient mutants of VZV have been recovered.

Resistance of HSV to antiviral nucleoside analogues occurs by the same mechanisms as resistance to VZV. While most of the ACV-resistant mutants isolated thus far from immunocompromised patients have been found to be TK-deficient mutants, other mutants involving the viral TK gene (TK partial and TK altered) and DNA polymerase have also been isolated. TK-negative mutants may cause severe disease in immunocompromised patients. The possibility of viral resistance to valacyclovir (and therefore acyclovir) should be considered in patients who show poor clinical response during therapy.

Pharmacokinetics:

The pharmacokinetics of valacyclovir and acyclovir after oral administration of VALTREX have been investigated in 12 volunteer studies involving 253 adults.

Absorption and Bioavailability: The absolute bioavailability of acyclovir after administration of VALTREX is 54.5% ± 9.1% as determined following a 1 g oral dose of VALTREX and a 350 mg intravenous acyclovir dose to 12 healthy volunteers. Acyclovir bioavailability from the administration of VALTREX is not altered by administration with food (30 minutes after an 873 Kcal breakfast, which included 51 grams of fat).

There was a lack of dose proportionality in acyclovir maximum concentration (C_{max}) and area under the acyclovir concentration-time curve (AUC) after single-dose administration of 100 mg, 250 mg, 500 mg, 750 mg, and 1 g of VALTREX to eight healthy volunteers. The mean C_{max} (± S.D.) was 0.83 (± 0.14), 2.15 (± 0.50), 3.28 (± 0.83), 4.17 (± 1.14), and 5.65 (± 2.37) µg/mL, respectively; and the mean AUC (± S.D.) was 2.28 (± 0.40), 5.76 (± 0.60), 11.59 (± 1.79), 14.11 (± 3.54), and 19.52 (± 6.04) hr·µg/mL, respectively. There was also a lack of dose proportionality in acyclovir C_{max} and AUC after the multiple-dose administration of 250 mg, 500 mg, and 1 g of VALTREX administered four times daily for 11 days in parallel groups of eight healthy volunteers. The mean C_{max} (± S.D.) was 2.11 (± 0.33), 3.69 (± 0.87), and 4.96 (± 0.64) µg/mL, respectively, and the mean AUC (± S.D.) was 5.66 (± 1.09), 9.88 (± 2.01), and 15.70 (± 2.27) hr·µg/mL, respectively.

There is no accumulation of acyclovir after the administration of valacyclovir at the recommended dosage regimens in healthy volunteers with normal renal function.

Distribution: The binding of valacyclovir to human plasma proteins ranged from 13.5% to 17.9%.

Metabolism: After oral administration, valacyclovir hydrochloride is rapidly absorbed from the gastrointestinal tract. Valacyclovir is rapidly and nearly completely converted to acyclovir and L-valine by first-pass intestinal and/or hepatic metabolism. Acyclovir is converted to a small extent to inactive metabolites by aldehyde oxidase and by alcohol and aldehyde dehydrogenase. Neither valacyclovir nor acyclovir metabolism is associated with liver microsomal enzymes. Plasma concentrations of unconverted valacyclovir are low and transient, generally becoming non-quantifiable by 3 hours after administration. Peak plasma valacyclovir concentrations are generally less than 0.5 µg/mL at all doses. After single-dose administration of 1 g of VALTREX, average plasma valacyclovir concentrations observed were 0.5, 0.4, and 0.8 µg/mL in patients with hepatic dysfunction, renal insufficiency, and in healthy volunteers who received concomitant cimetidine and probenecid, respectively.

Elimination: The pharmacokinetic disposition of acyclovir delivered by valacyclovir is consistent with previous experience from intravenous and oral acyclovir. Following the oral administration of a single 1 g dose of radiolabeled valacyclovir to four healthy subjects, 45.60% and 47.12% of administered radioactivity was recovered in urine and feces over 96 hours, respectively. Acyclovir accounted for 88.60% of the radioactivity excreted in the urine. Renal clearance of acyclovir following the administration of a single 1 g dose of VALTREX to 12 healthy volunteers was approximately 255 ± 86 mL/min which represents 41.9% of total acyclovir apparent plasma clearance.

The plasma elimination half-life of acyclovir typically averaged 2.5 to 3.3 hours in all studies of VALTREX in volunteers with normal renal function.

End-Stage Renal Disease (ESRD): Following administration of VALTREX to volunteers with ESRD, the average acyclovir half-life is approximately 14 hours. During hemodialysis, the acyclovir half-life is approximately 4 hours. Approximately one-third of acyclovir in the body is removed by dialysis during a 4-hour hemodialysis session. Apparent plasma clearance of acyclovir in dialysis patients was 86.3 ± 21.3

Continued on next page

Glaxo Wellcome—Cont.

mL/min/1.73 m^2, compared to 679.16 ± 162.76 mL/min/1.73 m^2 in healthy volunteers.
Reduction in dosage is recommended in patients with renal impairment (see **DOSAGE AND ADMINISTRATION**).
Geriatrics: After single-dose administration of 1 g of VALTREX in healthy geriatric volunteers (n = 9, mean age ± S.D. = 74.0 ± 5.4 years), the half-life of acyclovir was 3.11 ± 0.51 hours, compared to 2.91 ± 0.63 hours in healthy volunteers (n = 33, mean age ± S.D. = 41.2 ± 10.1 years). Dosage modification may be necessary in geriatric patients with reduced renal function (see **DOSAGE AND ADMINISTRATION**).
Pediatrics: Valacyclovir pharmacokinetics have not been evaluated in pediatric patients.
Liver Disease: Administration of VALTREX to patients with moderate (biopsy-proven cirrhosis) or severe (with and without ascites and biopsy-proven cirrhosis) liver disease indicated that the rate but not the extent of conversion of valacyclovir to acyclovir is reduced, and the acyclovir half-life is not affected. Dosage modification is not recommended for patients with cirrhosis.
HIV Disease: In nine patients with advanced HIV disease (CD4 cell counts < 50 cells/mm^3) who received VALTREX at a dosage of 1 g four times daily for 30 days, the pharmacokinetics of valacyclovir and acyclovir were not different from that observed in healthy volunteers (see **WARNINGS**).
Drug Interactions: The administration of cimetidine and probenecid, separately or together, reduced the rate but not the extent of conversion of valacyclovir to acyclovir. Acyclovir C_{max} was increased 8.4% ± 27.8%, 22.5% ± 25.3%, and 29.6% ± 27.5% by cimetidine, probenecid, and combination treatment (concomitant cimetidine and probenecid administration), respectively. Acyclovir AUC (0 to 24) was increased 31.9% ± 22.9%, 49.0% ± 27.9%, and 77.9% ± 38.6% by cimetidine, probenecid, and combination treatment, respectively. The renal clearance of acyclovir was reduced by approximatley 23.5% ± 9.6%, 33.0% ± 10.4%, and 46% ± 11.2% with cimetidine, probenecid, and combination treatment, respectively, resulting in higher plasma acyclovir concentrations. Thiazide diuretics did not affect acyclovir pharmacokinetics after administration of VALTREX in a geriatric population.
Clinical Trials:
Herpes Zoster Infections: Two randomized double-blind clinical trials in immunocompetent patients with localized herpes zoster were conducted. VALTREX was compared to placebo in patients less than 50 years of age, and to ZOVIRAX in patients greater than 50 years of age. All patients were treated within 72 hours of appearance of zoster rash. In patients less than 50 years of age, the median time to cessation of new lesion formation was two days for those treated with VALTREX compared to three days for those treated with placebo. In patients greater than 50 years of age, the median time to cessation of new lesions was three days in patients treated with either VALTREX or ZOVIRAX. In patients less than 50 years of age, no difference was found with respect to the duration of pain after rash healing (post-herpetic neuralgia) between the recipients of VALTREX and placebo. In patients greater than 50 years of age who reported pain after rash healing (post-herpetic neuralgia), there was a nonsignificant trend toward a shorter median duration of pain after healing in patients treated with VALTREX for 7 to 14 days (40 or 43 days) compared to patients treated with ZOVIRAX for 7 days (59 days).
Recurrent Genital Herpes: Two double-blind placebo-controlled trials in immunocompetent patients with recurrent genital herpes were conducted. Patients self-initiated therapy within 24 hours of the first sign or symptom of a recurrent genital herpes episode.
In one study, patients were randomized to receive five days of treatment with either VALTREX 500 mg bid (n = 360) or placebo (n = 259). The median time to lesion healing was four days in the group receiving VALTREX 500 mg versus six days in the placebo group, and the median time to cessation of viral shedding in patients with at least one positive culture (42% of the overall study population) was two days in the group receiving VALTREX 500 mg versus four days in the placebo group. The median time to cessation of pain was three days in the group receiving VALTREX 500 mg versus four days in the placebo group. Results supporting efficacy were replicated in a second trial.

INDICATIONS AND USAGE

Herpes Zoster: VALTREX is indicated for the treatment of herpes zoster (shingles) in immunocompetent adults.
Recurrent Genital Herpes: VALTREX is indicated for the episodic treatment of recurrent genital herpes in immunocompetent adults.

CONTRAINDICATIONS

VALTREX is contraindicated in patients with known hypersensitivity or intolerance to valacyclovir, acyclovir, or any component of the formulation.

WARNINGS

THROMBOTIC THROMBOCYTOPENIC PURPURA/HEMOLYTIC UREMIC SYNDROME (TTP/HUS), IN SOME CASES RESULTING IN DEATH, HAS BEEN REPORTED IN PATIENTS WITH ADVANCED HIV DISEASE AND ALSO IN BONE MARROW TRANSPLANT AND RENAL TRANSPLANT RECIPIENTS PARTICIPATING IN CLINICAL TRIALS OF VALTREX. VALTREX IS NOT INDICATED FOR THE TREATMENT OF IMMUNOCOMPROMISED PATIENTS. THIS SYNDROME HAS NOT BEEN OBSERVED IN IMMUNOCOMPETENT PATIENTS TREATED WITH VALTREX IN CLINICAL TRIALS.

PRECAUTIONS

The efficacy of VALTREX has not been established in immunocompromised patients or for the treatment of initital genital herpes infection, disseminated herpes zoster, or suppression of recurrent genital herpes.
Dosage adjustment is recommended when administering VALTREX to patients with renal impairment (see DOSAGE AND ADMINISTRATION). Caution should also be exercised when administering VALTREX to patients receiving potentially nephrotoxic agents since this may increase the risk of renal dysfunction and/or the risk of reversible central nervous system symptoms such as those that have been reported in patients treated with intravenous acyclovir.
Information for Patients: *Herpes Zoster:* There are no data on treatment initiated more than 72 hours after onset of the zoster rash. Patients should be advised to inititate treatment as soon as possible after a diagnosis of herpes zoster.
Recurrent Genital Herpes: Patients should be informed that VALTREX is not a cure for genital herpes. There are no data evaluating whether VALTREX will prevent transmission of infection to others. Because genital herpes is a sexually transmitted disease, patients should avoid contact with lesions or intercourse when lesions and/or symptoms are present to avoid infecting partners. Genital herpes can also be transmitted in the absence of symptoms through asymptomatic viral shedding. If medical management of a genital herpes recurrence is indicated, patients should be advised to initiate therapy at the first sign or symptom of an episode. There are no data on the effectiveness of treatment with VALTREX when initiated more than 24 hours after the onset of signs or symptoms.
Drug Interactions: An additive increase in acyclovir AUC and C_{max} was observed when VALTREX was administered to healthy volunteers who were taking cimetidine, probenecid, or a combination of both cimetidine and probenecid (see CLINICAL PHARMACOLOGY: Pharmacokinetics).
Carcinogenesis, Mutagenesis, Impairment of Fertility: The data presented below include references to the steady-state acyclovir AUC observed in humans treated with 1 g VALTREX given orally three times a day to treat herpes zoster. Plasma drug concentrations in animal studies are expressed as multiples of human exposure to acyclovir (see CLINICAL PHARMACOLOGY: Pharmacokinetics).
Valacyclovir was noncarcinogenic in lifetime carcinogenicity bioassays at single daily doses (gavage) of up to 120 mg/kg/day for mice and 100 mg/kg/day for rats. There was no significant difference in the incidence of tumors between treated and control animals, nor did valacyclovir shorten the latency of tumors. Plasma concentrations of acyclovir were equivalent to human levels in the mouse bioassay and 1.4 to 2.3 times human levels in the rat bioassay.
Valacyclovir was tested in five genetic toxicity assays. An Ames assay was negative in the absence or presence of metabolic activation. Also negative were an in vitro cytogenetic study with human lymphocytes and a rat cytogenic study at a single oral dose of 3000 mg/kg (8 to 9 times human plasma levels).
In the mouse lymphoma assay, valacyclovir was negative in the absence of metabolic activation. In the presence of metabolic activation (76% to 88% conversion to acyclovir), valacyclovir was weakly mutagenic.
A mouse micronucleus assay was negative at 250 mg/kg but weakly positive at 500 mg/kg (acyclovir concentrations 26 to 51 times human plasma levels).
Valacyclovir did not impair fertility or reproduction in rats at 200 mg/kg/day (6 times human plasma levels).
Pregnancy: *Teratogenic Effects:* Pregnancy Category B. Valacyclovir was not teratogenic in rats or rabbits given 400 mg/kg (which results in exposures of 10 and 7 times human plasma levels, respectively) during the period of major organogenesis. There are no adequate and well-controlled studies of VALTREX or ZOVIRAX in pregnant women. A prospective epidemiologic registry of acyclovir use during pregnancy has been ongoing since 1984. As of December 1994, outcomes of live births have been documented in 380 women exposed to systemic acyclovir during the first trimester of pregnancy. The occurrence rate of birth defects approximates that found in the general population. However, the small size of the registry is insufficient to evaluate the risk for less common defects or to permit reliable and definitive conclusions regarding the safety of acyclovir in pregnant women and their developing fetuses. VALTREX should be used during pregnancy only if the potential benefit justifies the potential risk to the fetus.
Pregnancy Exposure Registry: To monitor maternal-fetal outcomes of pregnant women exposed to VALTREX, Glaxo Wellcome Inc. maintains a Valacyclovir in Pregnancy Registry. Physicians are encouraged to register their patients by calling (800) 722-9292, ext. 39437.
Nursing Mothers: There is no experience with VALTREX. However, acyclovir concentrations have been documented in breast milk in two women following oral administration of ZOVIRAX and ranged from 0.6 to 4.1 times corresponding plasma levels. These concentrations would potentially expose the nursing infant to a dose of acyclovir as high as 0.3 mg/kg/day. VALTREX should be administered to a nursing mother with caution and only when indicated. Consideration should be given to temporary discontinuation of nursing, as the safety of VALTREX has not been established in infants.
Pediatric Use: Safety and effectiveness of VALTREX in pediatric patients have not been established.
Geriatric Use: Of the total number of patients included in clinical studies of VALTREX, 810 were age 65 or older, and 339 were age 75 or older. A total of 34 volunteers age 65 or older completed a pharmacokinetic trial of VALTREX. The pharmacokinetics of acyclovir following single- and multiple-dose oral administration of VALTREX in geriatric volunteers varied with renal function. Dosage reduction may be required in geriatric patients, depending on the underlying renal status of the patient (see CLINICAL PHARMACOLOGY and DOSAGE AND ADMINISTRATION).

ADVERSE REACTIONS

The adverse events reported by greater than 2% of a given treatment group in clinical trials of VALTREX are listed in Table 1.
[See table at left.]

OVERDOSAGE

There have been no reports of overdosage from the administration of VALTREX. However, it is known that precipitation of acyclovir in renal tubules may occur when the solubility (2.5 mg/mL) is exceeded in the intratubular fluid. In the

Table 1
Incidence (%) of Adverse Events in Herpes Zoster and Genital Herpes Study Populations

	Herpes Zoster				Genital Herpes	
	>50 years Median age = 69		18–50 years Median age = 36		18–79 years Median age = 34	
Adverse Event	VALTREX (n=765) 1 g tid 14 days: n= 381; 7 days: n= 384	ZOVIRAX (n=376) 800 mg 5× daily × 7 days	VALTREX (n=202) 1 g tid × 7 days	Placebo (n=195)	VALTREX (n=1235) 1 g bid × 5 days: n= 876 500 bid × 5 days: n= 359	Placebo (n=439)
Nausea	16	19	10	8	6	8
Headache	13	13	17	12	17	14
Vomiting	7	8	4	3	<1	<1
Diarrhea	5	7	4	6	4	6
Constipation	5	5	1	3	<1	≤1
Asthenia	4	5	3	4	2	4
Dizziness	4	6	2	2	3	3
Abdominal Pain	3	3	2	2	2	3
Anorexia	3	3	<1	2	<1	<1

event of acute renal failure and anuria, the patient may benefit from hemodialysis until renal function is restored (see DOSAGE AND ADMINISTRATION).

DOSAGE AND ADMINISTRATION

VALTREX Caplets may be given without regard to meals.

Herpes Zoster: The recommended dosage of VALTREX for the treatment of herpes zoster is 1 g (two 500 mg caplets) orally three times daily for 7 days. Therapy should be initiated at the earliest sign or symptom of herpes zoster and is most effective when started within 48 hours of onset of zoster rash. No data are available on efficacy of treatment started greater than 72 hours after rash onset.

Recurrent Genital Herpes: The recommended dosage of VALTREX for the treatment of recurrent genital herpes is 500 mg twice daily for 5 days. If medical management of a genital herpes recurrence is indicated, patients should be advised to initiate therapy at the first sign or symptom of an episode. There are no data on the effectiveness of treatment with VALTREX when initiated more than 24 hours after the onset of signs and symptoms.

Patients with Acute or Chronic Renal Impairment: In patients with reduced renal function, reduction in dosage is recommended (see Table 2).

Table 2
Dosages for Patients with Renal Impairment

Creatinine Clearance (mL/min)	Dosage for Herpes Zoster	Dosage for Genital Herpes
≥ 50	1 g every 8 hours	500 mg every 12 hours
30–49	1 g every 12 hours	500 mg every 12 hours
10–29	1 g every 24 hours	500 mg every 24 hours
< 10	500 mg every 24 hours	500 mg every 24 hours

Hemodialysis: During hemodialysis, the half-life of acyclovir after administration of VALTREX is approximately 4 hours. About one-third of acyclovir in the body is removed by dialysis during a 4-hour hemodialysis session. Patients requiring hemodialysis should receive the recommended dose of VALTREX after hemodialysis.

Peritoneal Dialysis: There is no information specific to administration of VALTREX in patients receiving peritoneal dialysis. The effect of chronic ambulatory peritoneal dialysis (CAPD) and continuous arteriovenous hemofiltration/dialysis (CAVHD) on acyclovir pharmacokinetics has been studied. The removal of acyclovir after CAPD and CAVHD is less pronounced than with hemodialysis, and the pharmacokinetic parameters closely resemble those observed in patients with ESRD not receiving hemodialysis. Therefore, supplemental doses of VALTREX should not be required following CAPD or CAVHD.

HOW SUPPLIED

VALTREX Caplets (blue, film-coated, capsule-shaped tablets) containing valacyclovir hydrochloride equivalent to 500 mg valacyclovir and printed with "VALTREX 500 mg"—Bottle of 42 (NDC 0173-0933-03) and unit dose pack of 100 (NDC 0173-0933-56).
Store at 15° to 25°C (59° to 77°F).
U.S. Patent No. 4957924
January 1996/RL-237

Shown in Product Identification Guide, page 314

VASOXYL® Injection
[văz "ox 'ŭl]
(methoxamine hydrochloride)
20 mg in 1 ml

℞

DESCRIPTION

VASOXYL (methoxamine hydrochloride) Injection is a sterile solution for intravenous or intramuscular injection, made isotonic with sodium chloride. Each 1-mL ampul contains 20 mg methoxamine hydrochloride. Citric acid anhydrous 0.3% and sodium citrate 0.3% are added as buffers and potassium metabisulfite 0.1% is added as an antioxidant. Methoxamine hydrochloride is a sympathomimetic amine. It has the empirical formula $C_{11}H_{17}NO_3 \cdot HCl$ and a molecular weight of 247.72. The drug is very soluble in water, soluble in ethanol, but practically insoluble in ether, benzene, or chloroform. It is known chemically as α-(1-aminoethyl)-2,5-dimethoxybenzenemethanol hydrochloride.

CLINICAL PHARMACOLOGY

VASOXYL is an alpha-receptor stimulant which produces a prompt and prolonged rise in blood pressure following parenteral administration. It is especially useful for maintaining blood pressure during operations under spinal anesthesia[1,2,3] and may also be used safely during general anesthesia. VASOXYL does not increase the irritability of the cyclopropane-sensitized heart, making it useful during cyclopropane anesthesia.[4,5] Tachyphylaxis has not been a clinical problem.[1]

The major pharmacological effect of VASOXYL is a potent, prolonged pressor action following parenteral administration. Vasoxyl differs from most other sympathomimetic amines both in animals[4,6,7] and in humans[1,8] by having a predominantly peripheral action and lacking inotropic and chronotropic effects. Vasoxyl has less arrhythmogenic potential than other sympathomimetic amines and rarely causes ventricular tachycardia, fibrillation, or increased sinoatrial rate.[4] On occasion, a decrease in rate occurs as blood pressure increases,[1,9,10] apparently caused by a carotid sinus reflex. This bradycardia can be abolished by atropine.[9] The pressor action appears to be due to peripheral vasoconstriction rather than a centrally mediated effect. Evidence for direct action on blood vessels is provided in part by the observation of intense constriction along the course of a vein into which VASOXYL has been injected.[1] VASOXYL also increases venous pressure.[8]

Following intravenous administration of VASOXYL in dogs[11] and humans,[9,12] the peak pressor effect occurs within 0.5 to 2 minutes. In a group of human surgical patients,[13] the duration of the pressor effect following a single intravenous dose of 2 to 4 mg of VASOXYL was 10 to 15 minutes. No clinical pharmacology studies are available concerning the onset and duration of action after administration of recommended intramuscular doses (10 to 15 mg). With administration of 10 to 40 mg VASOXYL intramuscularly to patients, however, the peak effect occurs within 15 to 20 minutes, and the duration of action is approximately $1^1/_2$ hours.[14]

Data from pharmacokinetic studies of VASOXYL following either intravenous or intramuscular administration are not available.

INDICATIONS AND USAGE

VASOXYL is intended for supporting, restoring, or maintaining blood pressure during anesthesia (including cyclopropane anesthesia). It can be used to terminate some episodes of supraventricular tachycardia.

CONTRAINDICATIONS

VASOXYL is contraindicated in patients with severe hypertension, or in patients who are hypersensitive to methoxamine.

WARNINGS

The use of VASOXYL in patients receiving monoamine oxidase inhibitors, tricyclic antidepressants, or oxytocic agents such as vasopressin or certain ergot alkaloids may result in potentiation of the pressor effect (see PRECAUTIONS: Drug Interactions).

Contains potassium metabisulfite, a sulfite that may cause allergic-type reactions including anaphylactic symptoms and life-threatening or less severe asthmatic episodes in certain susceptible people. The overall prevalence of sulfite sensitivity in the general population is unknown and probably low. Sulfite sensitivity is seen more frequently in asthmatic than in nonasthmatic people.

PRECAUTIONS

General: VASOXYL, like other vasopressor agents, should be used with caution in patients with hyperthyroidism, bradycardia, partial heart block, myocardial disease, or severe arteriosclerosis. Caution should be exercised to avoid overdosage, preventing undesirable high blood pressure and/or bradycardia. Note: Bradycardia may be abolished with atropine (see OVERDOSAGE). Also, caution should be taken when VASOXYL is used closely following the parenteral injection of ergot alkaloids to avoid an excessive rise in bloodpressure.

Drug Interactions: The pressor effect of VASOXYL may be markedly potentiated when VASOXYL is used in conjunction with monoamine oxidase inhibitors, tricyclic antidepressants, vasopressin, or ergot alkaloids such as ergotamine, ergonovine, or methylergonovine. Therefore, when initiating pressor therapy in patients receiving these drugs the initial dose should be small and given with caution (see WARNINGS).

Drug/Laboratory Test Interactions: VASOXYL may increase plasma cortisol and ACTH levels. Caution should be used when interpreting plasma cortisol and ACTH levels in a patient concurrently receiving VASOXYL.[15,16]

Carcinogenesis, Mutagenesis, Impairment of Fertility: No long-term animal studies have been performed to evaluate the potential of VASOXYL in these areas.

Pregnancy: *Teratogenic Effects:* Pregnancy Category C: VASOXYL has been shown to decrease uterine blood flow, decrease fetal heart rate and adversely affect the fetal acid-base status in pregnant ewes and monkeys at doses comparable to those used in humans. There are no adequate and well-controlled studies in pregnant women. There has been one report of a fetal death; the mother received VASOXYL concomitantly with several other drugs. A direct causal relationship to VASOXYL was not established. VASOXYL should be used during pregnancy only if the potential benefit justifies the potential risk to the fetus.

VASOXYL (2.5 mg IV, one to three times over a 45 minute period) given to seven pregnant ewes showed a significant deterioration in fetal acid-base status as evidenced by hypoxia, hypercarbia and metabolic acidosis.[17] An inverse relationship between pressor response to VASOXYL and uteroplacental blood flow has been shown in 16 pregnant ewes studied at doses ranging from 0.025 mg/kg to 0.2 mg/kg.[18] Uterine blood flow was decreased at all doses, but no significant change in fetal blood gas or acid-base status was demonstrated. Administration of VASOXYL to four fetuses (50 mcg/kg/min for 60 minutes) and to four ewes (25 mcg/kg/min for 30 minutes) was associated with a decrease in fetal heart rate and uterine blood flow.[19] Nine monkeys studied at an average dose of VASOXYL of 1.3 mg/kg administered over 57 minutes showed a decrease in uterine blood flow and a possible association with fetal asphyxia.[20]

Labor and Delivery: If vasopressor drugs are used to correct hypotension or added to the local anesthetic solution during labor and delivery, some oxytocic drugs (vasopressin, ergotamine, ergonovine, methylergonovine) may cause severe persistent hypertension (see WARNINGS and PRECAUTIONS: Drug Interactions).

Note: In pregnant animals, VASOXYL has been shown to decrease uterine blood flow, possibly resulting in fetal asphyxia. Uterine hypertonus and fetal bradycardia may also be produced. (See ADVERSE REACTIONS and PRECAUTIONS: Drug Interactions.)

Nursing Mothers: It is not known whether this drug is excreted in human milk. Because many drugs are excreted in human milk, caution should be exercised when VASOXYL is administered to a nursing woman.

Pediatric Use: Safety and effectiveness in pediatric patients have not been established.

ADVERSE REACTIONS

The following adverse reactions have been observed, but there are insufficient data to support an estimate of their frequency:

Cardiovascular: Excessive blood pressure elevations particularly with high dosage, ventricular ectopic beats

Gastrointestinal: Nausea, vomiting (often projectile)

Central Nervous System: Headache (often severe), anxiety

Integumentary: Sweating, pilomotor response

Genitourinary: Uterine hypertonus, fetal bradycardia (see PRECAUTIONS: Labor and Delivery), urinary urgency

OVERDOSAGE

Overdosage of VASOXYL may be manifested as an undesirable elevation in blood pressure and/or bradycardia. Should a clinically significant elevation of blood pressure occur that requires treatment, it may be immediately reversed with an alpha-adrenergic blocking agent (e.g., phentolamine). Bradycardia may be abolished by atropine.

DOSAGE AND ADMINISTRATION

Blood volume depletion should always be corrected before any vasopressor is administered. The usual intravenous dose of VASOXYL for emergencies is 3 to 5 mg, injected slowly. Intravenous injection may be supplemented by intramuscular injections to provide a more prolonged effect. The usual intramuscular dose is 10 to 15 mg given shortly before or at the time of administering spinal anesthesia to prevent a fall in blood pressure. The tendency for the blood pressure to fall is greater with higher levels of spinal anesthesia, hence the dosage may be adjusted accordingly; 10 mg may be adequate at lower spinal levels while 15 to 20 mg may be required at high levels of spinal anesthesia. Repeated doses may be given if necessary, but time should be allowed for the previous dose to act (about 15 minutes, see CLINICAL PHARMACOLOGY). For cases of only moderate hypotension, 5 to 10 mg intramuscularly may be adequate.

For purposes of correcting a fall in blood pressure, an intramuscular injection of 10 to 15 mg of VASOXYL may be given depending upon the degree of fall. In cases where the systolic pressure falls to 60 mmHg or less, or whenever an emergency exists, an intravenous injection of 3 to 5 mg VASOXYL is indicated. This intravenous dose may be accompanied by 10 to 15 mg intramuscularly to provide more prolonged effect.

For termination of episodes of supraventricular tachycardia not responsive to other modes of therapy, the usual dose of VASOXYL is 10 mg intravenously, administered by slow push (i.e., 3 to 5 minutes).

Parenteral drug products should be inspected visually for particulate matter and discoloration prior to administration whenever solution and container permit.

HOW SUPPLIED

1-mL ampuls, containing 20 mg methoxamine hydrochloride. Box of 10 (NDC 0173-0957-10). Store at 15° to 25°C (59° to 77°F) and protect from light.

Continued on next page

Glaxo Wellcome—Cont.

REFERENCES

1. King BD, Dripps RD. The use of methoxamine for maintenance of the circulation during spinal anesthesia. *Surg Gynecol Obstet* 1950;90:659-665.
2. Kistler EM, Ruben JE. Methoxamine in 1 percent procaine as a prophylactic vasopressor in spinal anesthesia. *Arch Surg* 1951;62:64-69.
3. Poe MF. Use of methoxamine hydrochloride as a pressor agent during spinal analgesia. *Anesthesiology* 1952; 13:89-93.
4. Lahti RE, Brill IC, McCawley EL. The effect of methoxamine hydrochloride (VASOXYL) on cardiac rhythm. *J Pharmacol Exp Ther* 1955;115:268-274.
5. Stutzman JW, Pettinga FL, Fruggiero EJ. Cardiac effects of methoxamine (β-[2,5-dimethoxy-phenyl]-β-hydroxyisopropylamine HCl) and desoxyephedrine during cyclopropane anesthesia. *J Pharmacol Exp Ther* 1949; 97:385-387.
6. West JW, Faulk AT, Guzman SV. Comparative study of effects of levarterenol and methoxamine in shock associated with acute myocardial ischemia in dogs. *Circ Res* 1962;10:712-721.
7. Goldberg LI, Cotten M, Darby TD, Howell EV. Comparative heart contractile force effects of equipressor doses of several sympathomimetic amines. *J Pharmacol Exp Ther* 1953;108:177-185.
8. Aviado DM, Wnuck AL. Mechanisms for cardiac slowing by methoxamine. *J Pharmacol Exp Ther* 1957;119:99-106.
9. Nathanson MH, Miller H. Clinical observations on a new epinephrin-like compound, methoxamine. *Am J Med Sci* 1952;223:270-279.
10. Stanfield CA, Yu PN. Hemodynamic effects of methoxamine in mitral valve disease. *Circ Res* 1960;8:859-864.
11. Imai S, Shigei T, Hashimoto K. Cardiac actions of methoxamine with special reference to its antagonist action to epinephrine. *Circ Res* 1961;9:552-560.
12. *The Extra Pharmacopoeia, Martindale* 28th Ed., Reynolds, JEF, ed., Pharmaceutical Press (London), pp. 19.
13. Goldberg LI, Bloodwell RD, Braunwald E, et al. The direct effects of norepinephrine, epinephrine, and methoxamine on myocardial contractile force in man. *Circ.* 1960;22:1125-1132.
14. Data on file, Glaxo Wellcome Inc.
15. Laurian L, Oberman Z, Hoerer E, et al. Low cortisol and growth hormone secretion in response to methoxamine administration in obese subjects. *Isr J Med Sci* 1977;13:477-481.
16. Nakai Y, Imura H, Yoshimi T, Matsukura S. Adrenergic control mechanism for ACTH secretion in man. *Acta Endocrinol* 1973;74:263-270.
17. Shnider SM, DeLorimier AA, Asling JH, Morishima HO. Vasopressors in obstetrics. II. Fetal hazards of methoxamine administration during obstetric spinal anesthesia. *Am J Obstet Gynecol* 1970;106:680-686.
18. Ralston DH, Shnider SM, DeLorimier AA. Effects of equipotent ephedrine, metaraminol, mephentermine and methoxamine on uterine blood flow in the pregnant ewe. *Anesthesiology* 1974;40:354-370.
19. Oakes GK, Ehrenkranz RA, Walker AM, et al. Effect of α-adrenergic agonist and antagonist infusion on the umbilical and uterine circulations of pregnant sheep. *Biol Neonate* 1980;38:229-237.
20. Eng M, Berges PU, Ueland K, et al. The effects of methoxamine and ephedrine in normotensive pregnant primates. *Anesthesiology* 1971;35:354-360.

June 1996/RL-322

Shown in Product Identification Guide, page 315

VENTOLIN® Inhalation Aerosol   ℞
[vent'ō-lin]
(albuterol, USP)
Bronchodilator Aerosol
For Oral Inhalation Only

DESCRIPTION

The active component of Ventolin® (albuterol) Inhalation Aerosol is albuterol, USP, racemic (α^1-[(*tert*-butylamino)methyl]-4-hydroxy-*m*-xylene-α,α'-diol) and a relatively selective beta$_2$-adrenergic bronchodilator.

Albuterol is the official generic name in the United States. The World Health Organization recommended name for the drug is salbutamol. The molecular weight of albuterol is 239.3, and the empirical formula is $C_{13}H_{21}NO_3$. Albuterol is a white to off-white crystalline solid. It is soluble in ethanol, sparingly soluble in water, and very soluble in chloroform. Ventolin Inhalation Aerosol is a metered-dose aerosol unit for oral inhalation. It contains a microcrystalline (95% ≤10 µm) suspension of albuterol in propellants (trichloromonofluoromethane and dichlorodifluoromethane) with oleic acid. Each actuation delivers from the mouthpiece 90 mcg of albuterol. Each 6.8-g canister provides at least 80 inhalations and each 17-g canister provides at least 200 inhalations.

CLINICAL PHARMACOLOGY

In vitro studies and *in vivo* pharmacological studies have demonstrated that albuterol has a preferential effect on beta$_2$-adrenergic receptors compared with isoproterenol. While it is recognized that beta$_2$-adrenergic receptors are the predominant receptors in bronchial smooth muscle, recent data indicate that there is a population of beta$_2$-receptors in the human heart existing in a concentration between 10% and 50%. The precise function of these, however, is not yet established.

The pharmacological effects of beta-adrenergic agonist drugs, including albuterol, are at least in part attributable to stimulation through beta-adrenergic receptors of intracellular adenyl cyclase, the enzyme that catalyzes the conversion of adenosine triphosphate (ATP) to cyclic-3',5'-adenosine monophosphate (cyclic AMP). Increased cyclic AMP levels are associated with relaxation of bronchial smooth muscle and inhibition of release of mediators of immediate hypersensitivity from cells, especially from mast cells.

Albuterol has been shown in most controlled clinical trials to have more effect on the respiratory tract, in the form of bronchial smooth muscle relaxation, than isoproterenol at comparable doses while producing fewer cardiovascular effects. Controlled clinical studies and other clinical experience have shown that inhaled albuterol, like other beta-adrenergic agonist drugs, can produce a significant cardiovascular effect in some patients, as measured by pulse rate, blood pressure, symptoms, and/or electrocardiographic changes. Albuterol is longer acting than isoproterenol in most patients by any route of administration because it is not a substrate for the cellular uptake processes for catecholamines nor for catechol-*O*-methyl transferase.

Because of its gradual absorption from the bronchi, systemic levels of albuterol are low after inhalation of recommended doses. Studies undertaken with four subjects administered tritiated albuterol resulted in maximum plasma concentrations occurring within 2 to 4 hours. Due to the sensitivity of the assay method, the metabolic rate and half-life of elimination of albuterol in plasma could not be determined. However, urinary excretion provided data indicating that albuterol has an elimination half-life of 3.8 hours. Approximately 72% of the inhaled dose is excreted within 24 hours in the urine, and consists of 28% as unchanged drug and 44% as metabolite.

Animal studies show that albuterol does not pass the blood-brain barrier.

Recent studies in laboratory animals (minipigs, rodents, and dogs) recorded the occurrence of cardiac arrhythmias and sudden death (with histologic evidence of myocardial necrosis) when beta-agonists and methylxanthines were administered concurrently. The significance of these findings when applied to humans is currently unknown.

The effects of rising doses of albuterol and isoproterenol aerosols were studied in volunteers and asthmatic patients. Results in normal volunteers indicated that albuterol is one half to one quarter as active as isoproterenol in producing increases in heart rate. In asthmatic patients similar cardiovascular differentiation between the two drugs was also seen.

In controlled clinical trials involving adults with asthma, the onset of improvement in pulmonary function was within 15 minutes, as determined by both MMEF (maximum midexpiratory flow rate) and FEV$_1$ (forced expiratory volume in 1 second). MMEF measurements also showed that near maximum improvement in pulmonary function generally occurs within 60 to 90 minutes following two inhalations of albuterol and that clinically significant improvement generally continues for 3 to 4 hours in most patients. Some patients showed a therapeutic response (defined by maintaining FEV$_1$ values 15% or more above baseline) that was still apparent at 6 hours. Continued effectiveness of albuterol was demonstrated over a 13-week period in these same trials. In controlled clinical trials involving children 4 to 12 years of age, FEV$_1$ measurements showed that maximum improvement in pulmonary function occurs within 30 to 60 minutes. The onset of clinically significant (≥15%) improvement in FEV$_1$ was observed as soon as 5 minutes following 180 mcg of albuterol in 18 of 30 (60%) children in a controlled dose-ranging study. Clinically significant improvement in FEV$_1$ continued in the majority of patients for 2 hours and in 33% to 47% for 4 hours among 56 patients receiving inhalation aerosol in one pediatric study. In a second study among 48 patients receiving inhalation aerosol, clinically significant improvement continued in the majority for up to 1 hour and in 23% to 40% for 4 hours. In addition, at least 50% of the patients in both studies achieved an improvement in FEF$_{25\%-75\%}$ (forced expiratory flow rate between 25% and 75% of the forced vital capacity) of at least 20% for 2 to 5 hours. Continued effectiveness of albuterol was demonstrated over the 12-week study period.

In other clinical studies in adults and children, two inhalations of Ventolin® (albuterol) Inhalation Aerosol taken approximately 15 minutes before exercise prevented exercise-induced bronchospasm, as demonstrated by the maintenance of FEV$_1$ within 80% of baseline values in the majority of patients. One study in adults also evaluated the duration of the prophylactic effect to repeated exercise challenges, which was evident at 4 hours in the majority of patients and at 6 hours in approximately one third of the patients.

INDICATIONS AND USAGE

Ventolin® (albuterol) Inhalation Aerosol is indicated for the prevention and relief of bronchospasm in patients 4 years of age and older with reversible obstructive airway disease and for the prevention of exercise-induced bronchospasm in patients 4 years of age and older.

Ventolin Inhalation Aerosol can be used with or without concomitant steroid therapy.

CONTRAINDICATIONS

Ventolin® (albuterol) Inhalation Aerosol is contraindicated in patients with a history of hypersensitivity to any of its components.

WARNINGS

As with other inhaled beta-adrenergic agonists, Ventolin® (albuterol) Inhalation Aerosol can produce paradoxical bronchospasm that can be life-threatening. If it occurs, the preparation should be discontinued immediately and alternative therapy instituted.

Fatalities have been reported in association with excessive use of inhaled sympathomimetic drugs. The exact cause of death is unknown, but cardiac arrest following the unexpected development of a severe acute asthmatic crisis and subsequent hypoxia is suspected.

Immediate hypersensitivity reactions may occur after administration of albuterol inhalation aerosol, as demonstrated by rare cases of urticaria, angioedema, rash, bronchospasm, anaphylaxis, and oropharyngeal edema.

The contents of Ventolin Inhalation Aerosol are under pressure. Do not puncture. Do not use or store near heat or open flame. Exposure to temperatures above 120°F may cause bursting. Never throw container into fire or incinerator. Keep out of reach of children.

PRECAUTIONS

General: Albuterol, as with all sympathomimetic amines, should be used with caution in patients with cardiovascular disorders, especially coronary insufficiency, cardiac arrhythmias, and hypertension; in patients with convulsive disorders, hyperthyroidism, or diabetes mellitus; and in patients who are unusually responsive to sympathomimetic amines. Large doses of intravenous albuterol have been reported to aggravate pre-existing diabetes mellitus and ketoacidosis. As with other beta-agonists, inhaled and intravenous albuterol may produce significant hypokalemia in some patients, possibly through intracellular shunting, which has the potential to produce adverse cardiovascular effects. The decrease is usually transient, not requiring supplementation.

Although there have been no reports concerning the use of Ventolin® (albuterol) Inhalation Aerosol during labor and delivery, it has been reported that high doses of albuterol administered intravenously inhibit uterine contractions. Although this effect is extremely unlikely as a consequence of aerosol use, it should be kept in mind.

Information for Patients: The action of Ventolin Inhalation Aerosol may last up to 6 hours, and therefore it should not be used more frequently than recommended. Do not increase the number or frequency of doses without medical consultation. If recommended dosage does not provide relief of symptoms or symptoms become worse, seek immediate medical attention. While taking Ventolin Inhalation Aerosol, other inhaled drugs should not be used unless prescribed.

In general, the technique for administering Ventolin Inhalation Aerosol to children is similar to that for adults, since children's smaller ventilatory exchange capacity automatically provides proportionally smaller aerosol intake. Children should use Ventolin Inhalation Aerosol under adult supervision, as instructed by the patient's physician.

See illustrated Patient's Instructions for Use in product package insert.

Drug Interactions: Other sympathomimetic aerosol bronchodilators should not be used concomitantly with albuterol. If additional adrenergic drugs are to be administered by any route, they should be used with caution to avoid deleterious cardiovascular effects.

Albuterol should be administered with extreme caution to patients being treated with monoamine oxidase inhibitors or tricyclic antidepressants because the action of albuterol on the vascular system may be potentiated.

Beta-receptor blocking agents and albuterol inhibit the effect of each other.

Carcinogenesis, Mutagenesis, Impairment of Fertility: Albuterol sulfate caused a significant dose-related increase in the incidence of benign leiomyomas of the mesovarium in a 2-year study in the rat at oral doses of 2, 10, and 50 mg/kg, corresponding to 93, 463, and 2,315 times, respectively, the maximum inhalational dose for a 50-kg human. In another study this effect was blocked by the coadministration of propranolol. The relevance of these findings to humans is not

known. An 18-month study in mice and a lifetime study in hamsters revealed no evidence of tumorigenicity. Studies with albuterol revealed no evidence of mutagenesis. Reproduction studies in rats revealed no evidence of impaired fertility.

Pregnancy: *Teratogenic Effects: Pregnancy Category C:* Albuterol has been shown to be teratogenic in mice when given in doses corresponding to 14 times the human dose. There are no adequate and well-controlled studies in pregnant women. Albuterol should be used during pregnancy only if the potential benefit justifies the potential risk to the fetus. A reproduction study in CD-1 mice given albuterol subcutaneously (0.025, 0.25, and 2.5 mg/kg, corresponding to 1.15, 11.5, and 115 times, respectively, the maximum inhalational dose for a 50-kg human) showed cleft palate formation in 5 of 111 (4.5%) fetuses at 0.25 mg/kg and in 10 of 108 (9.3%) fetuses at 2.5 mg/kg. None was observed at 0.025 mg/kg. Cleft palate also occurred in 22 of 72 (30.5%) fetuses treated with 2.5 mg/kg of isoproterenol (positive control). A reproduction study with oral albuterol in Stride Dutch rabbits revealed cranioschisis in 7 of 19 (37%) fetuses at 50 mg/kg, corresponding to 2,315 times the maximum inhalational dose for a 50-kg human.

During worldwide marketing experience, various congenital anomalies, including cleft palate and limb defects, have been rarely reported in the offspring of patients being treated with albuterol. Some of the mothers were taking multiple medications during their pregnancies. No consistent pattern of defects can be discerned, and a relationship between albuterol use and congenital anomalies has not been established.

Nursing Mothers: It is not known whether this drug is excreted in human milk. Because of the potential for tumorigenicity shown for albuterol in animal studies, a decision should be made whether to discontinue nursing or to discontinue the drug, taking into account the importance of the drug to the mother.

Pediatric Use: Safety and effectiveness in children below 4 years of age have not been established.

ADVERSE REACTIONS

The adverse reactions to albuterol are similar in nature to reactions to other sympathomimetic agents, although the incidence of certain cardiovascular effects is lower with albuterol.

A 13-week, double-blind study compared albuterol and isoproterenol aerosols in 147 asthmatic patients aged 12 years and older. The results of this study showed that the incidence of cardiovascular effects was: palpitations, fewer than 10 per 100 with albuterol and fewer than 15 per 100 with isoproterenol; tachycardia, 10 per 100 with both albuterol and isoproterenol; and increased blood pressure, fewer than 5 per 100 with both albuterol and isoproterenol. In the same study, both drugs caused tremor or nausea in fewer than 15 patients per 100, and dizziness or heartburn in fewer than 5 per 100 patients. Nervousness occurred in fewer than 10 per 100 patients receiving albuterol and in fewer than 15 per 100 patients receiving isoproterenol.

Twelve-week, double-blind studies involving the use of Ventolin® (albuterol) Inhalation Aerosol 180 mcg q.i.d. by 104 asthmatic children aged 4 to 11 years showed the following side effects:

Central Nervous System: Headache, 3 of 104 patients (3%); nervousness, lightheadedness, agitation, nightmares, hyperactivity, and aggressive behavior, each in 1%.
Gastrointestinal: Nausea and/or vomiting, 6 of 104 (6%); stomachache, 3 of 104 (3%); diarrhea in 1%.
Oropharyngeal: Throat irritation, 6 of 104 (6%); discoloration of teeth in 1%.
Respiratory: Epistaxis, 3 of 104 (3%); coughing, 2 of 104 (2%).
Musculoskeletal: Tremor and muscle cramp, each in 1%.
Rare cases of urticaria, angioedema, rash, bronchospasm, hoarseness, and oropharyngeal edema have been reported after the use of inhaled albuterol.

In addition, albuterol, like other sympathomimetic agents, can cause adverse reactions such as hypertension, angina, vertigo, central nervous system stimulation, insomnia, and unusual taste.

OVERDOSAGE

Manifestations of overdosage may include seizures, anginal pain, hypertension, hypokalemia, tachycardia with rates up to 200 beats per minute, and exaggeration of the pharmacologic effects listed in ADVERSE REACTIONS.

As with all sympathomimetic aerosol medications, cardiac arrest and even death may be associated with abuse.

The oral LD_{50} in male and female rats and mice was greater than 2,000 mg/kg. The inhalational LD_{50} could not be determined.

Dialysis is not appropriate treatment for overdosage of Ventolin® (albuterol) Inhalation Aerosol. The judicious use of a cardioselective beta-receptor blocker, such as metoprolol tartrate, is suggested, bearing in mind the danger of inducing an asthmatic attack.

DOSAGE AND ADMINISTRATION

For treatment of acute episodes of bronchospasm or prevention of asthmatic symptoms, the usual dosage for adults and children 4 years of age and older is two inhalations repeated every 4 to 6 hours; in some patients, one inhalation every 4 hours may be sufficient. More frequent administration or a larger number of inhalations are not recommended.

The use of Ventolin® (albuterol) Inhalation Aerosol can be continued as medically indicated to control recurring bouts of bronchospasm. During this time most patients gain optimal benefit from regular use of the inhaler. Safe usage for periods extending over several years has been documented. If a previously effective dosage regimen fails to provide the usual relief, medical advice should be sought immediately as this is often a sign of seriously worsening asthma that would require reassessment of therapy.

Exercise-Induced Bronchospasm Prevention: The usual dosage for adults and children 4 years and older is two inhalations 15 minutes before exercise.

For treatment, see above.

HOW SUPPLIED

Ventolin® (albuterol) Inhalation Aerosol is supplied in 6.8-g canisters containing 80 metered inhalations (NDC 0173-0463-00) and in 17-g canisters containing 200 metered inhalations (NDC 0173-0321-88), each in boxes on one. Each actuation delivers 90 mcg of albuterol from the mouthpiece. Each canister is supplied with an oral adapter and patient's instructions. Also available, Ventolin Inhalation Aerosol Refill 17-g canister only with patient's instructions (NDC 0173-0321-98).

Store between 15° and 30°C (59° and 86°F). As with most inhaled medications in aerosol canisters, the therapeutic effect of this medication may decrease when the canister is cold. Shake well before using.
March 1994/RL-103

Shown in Product Identification Guide, page 315

VENTOLIN®   ℞
(albuterol sulfate, USP)
Inhalation Solution, 0.5%*
*Potency expressed as albuterol.

DESCRIPTION

The active component of Ventolin® (albuterol sulfate, USP) Inhalation Solution is albuterol sulfate, USP, the racemic form of albuterol and a relatively selective beta$_2$-adrenergic bronchodilator (see CLINICAL PHARMACOLOGY). It has the chemical name α^1-[(*tert*-butylamino)methyl]-4-hydroxy-*m*-xylene-α,α'-diol sulfate (2:1)(salt).

Albuterol sulfate has a molecular weight of 576.7, and the empirical formula is $(C_{13}H_{21}NO_3)_2 \cdot H_2SO_4$. Albuterol sulfate is a white crystalline powder, soluble in water and slightly soluble in ethanol.

The World Health Organization recommended name for albuterol base is salbutamol.

Ventolin Inhalation Solution, 0.5% is in concentrated form. Dilute 0.5 mL of the solution with 2.5 mL of sterile normal saline solution before administration.

Each milliliter of Ventolin Inhalation Solution contains 5 mg of albuterol (as 6 mg of albuterol sulfate) in an aqueous solution containing benzalkonium chloride; sulfuric acid is used to adjust the pH to between 3 and 5. Ventolin Inhalation Solution contains no sulfiting agents.

Ventolin Inhalation Solution is a clear, colorless to light yellow solution.

CLINICAL PHARMACOLOGY

The pharmacologic effects of beta-adrenergic agonist drugs, including albuterol, are at least in part attributable to stimulation through beta-adrenergic receptors of intracellular adenyl cyclase, the enzyme that catalyzes the conversion of adenosine triphosphate (ATP) to cyclic-3',5'-adenosine monophosphate (cyclic AMP). Increased cyclic AMP levels are associated with relaxation of bronchial smooth muscle and inhibition of release of mediators of immediate hypersensitivity from cells, especially from mast cells.

In vitro studies and *in vivo* pharmacologic studies have demonstrated that albuterol has a preferential effect on beta$_2$-adrenergic receptors compared with isoproterenol. While it is recognized that beta$_2$-adrenergic receptors are the predominant receptors in bronchial smooth muscle, recent data indicate that there is a population of beta$_2$-receptors in the human heart existing in a concentration between 10% and 50%. The precise function of these, however, is not yet established (see WARNINGS).

Albuterol has been shown in most controlled clinical trials to have more effect on the respiratory tract, in the form of bronchial smooth muscle relaxation, than isoproterenol at comparable doses while producing fewer cardiovascular effects. Controlled clinical studies and other clinical experience have shown that inhaled albuterol, like other beta-adrenergic agonist drugs, can produce a significant cardiovascular

effect in some patients, as measured by pulse rate, blood pressure,, symptoms, and/or electrocardiographic changes. Albuterol is longer acting than isoproterenol in most patients by any route of administration because it is not a substrate for the cellular uptake processes for catecholamines nor for catechol-*O*-methyl transferase.

Studies in asthamtic patients have shown that less than 20% of a single albuterol dose was absorbed following either intermittent positive-pressure breathing (IPPB) or nebulizer administration; the remaining amount was recovered from the nebulizer and apparatus and expired air. Most of the absorbed dose was recovered in the urine 24 hours after drug administration. Following a 3-mg dose of nebulized albuterol, the maximum albuterol plasma levels at 0.5 hours were 2.1 ng/mL (range, 1.4 to 3.2 ng/mL). There was significant dose-related response in FEV$_1$ (forced expiratory volume in 1 second) and peak flow rate. It has been demonstrated that following oral administration of 4 mg of albuterol, the elimination half-life was 5 to 6 hours.

Animal studies show that albuterol does not pass the blood-brain barrier.

Recent studies in laboratory animals (minipigs, rodents, and dogs) recorded the occurrence of cardiac arrhythmias and sudden death (with histologic evidence of myocardial necrosis) when beta-agonists and methylxanthines were administered concurrently. The significance of these findings when applied to humans is currently unknown.

In controlled clinical trials, most patients exhibited an onset of improvement in pulmonary function within 5 minutes as determined by FEV$_1$. FEV$_1$ measurements also showed that the maximum average improvement in pulmonary function usually occurred at approximately 1 hour following inhalation of 2.5 mg of albuterol by compressor-nebulizer and remained close to peak for 2 hours. Clinically significant improvement in pulmonary function (defined as maintenance of a 15% or more increase in FEV$_1$ over baseline values) continued for 3 to 4 hours in most patients, with some patients continuing up to 6 hours.

In repetitive dose studies, continued effectiveness was demonstrated throughout the 3-month period of treatment in some patients.

INDICATIONS AND USAGE

Ventolin® (albuterol sulfate) Inhalation Solution is indicated for the relief of bronchospasm in patients with reversible obstructive airway disease and acute attacks of bronchospasm.

CONTRAINDICATIONS

Ventolin® (albuterol sulfate) Inhalation Solution is contraindicated in patients with a history of hypersensitivity to any of the components.

WARNINGS

As with other inhaled beta-adrenergic agonists, Ventolin® (albuterol sulfate) Inhalation Solution can produce paradoxical bronchospasm that can be life threatening. If it occurs, the preparation should be discontinued immediately and alternative therapy instituted.

Fatalities have been reported in association with excessive use of inhaled sympathomimetic drugs and with the home use of nebulizers. It is therefore essential that the physician instruct the patient in the need for further evaluation if his/her asthma becomes worse. In individual patients, any beta$_2$-adrenergic agonist, including albuterol inhalation solution, may have a clinically significant cardiac effect.

Immediate hypersensitivity reactions may occur after administration of albuterol, as demonstrated by rare cases of urticaria, angioedema, rash, bronchospasm, and oropharyngeal edema.

PRECAUTIONS

General: Albuterol, as with all sympathomimetic amines, should be used with caution in patients with cardiovascular disorders, especially coronary insufficiency, cardiac arrhythmias, and hypertension; in patients with convulsive disorders, hyperthyroidism, or diabetes mellitus; and in patients who are unusually responsive to sympathomimetic amines. Large doses of intravenous albuterol have been reported to aggravate pre-existing diabetes mellitus and ketoacidosis. As with other beta-agonists, inhaled and intravenous albuterol may produce significant hypokalemia in some patients, possibly through intracellular shunting, which has the potential to produce adverse cardiovascular effects. The decrease is usually transient, not requiring supplementation.

Information for Patients: The action of Ventolin® (albuterol sulfate) Inhalation Solution may last up to 6 hours, and therefore it should not be used more frequently than recommended. Do not increase the dose or frequency of medication without medical consultation. If symptoms get worse, medical consultation should be sought promptly. While taking Ventolin Inhalation Solution, other antiasthma medicines should not be used unless prescribed.

Continued on next page

Glaxo Wellcome—Cont.

Drug compatibility (physical and chemical), efficacy, and safety of Ventolin Inhalation Solution when mixed with other drugs in a nebulizer have not been established.
See illustrated Patient's Instructions for Use in product package insert.
Drug Interactions: Other sympathomimetic aerosol bronchodilators or epinephrine should not be used concomitantly with albuterol.
Albuterol should be administered with extreme caution to patients being treated with monoamine oxidase inhibitors or tricyclic antidepressants because the action of albuterol on the vascular system may be potentiated.
Beta-receptor blocking agents and albuterol inhibit the effect of each other.
Carcinogenesis, Mutagenesis, Impairment of Fertility: Albuterol sulfate caused a significant dose-related increase in the incidence of benign leiomyomas of the mesovarium in a 2-year study in the rat, at oral doses of 2, 10, and 50 mg/kg, corresponding to 10, 50, and 250 times, respectively, the maximum nebulization dose for a 50-kg human. In another study, this effect was blocked by the coadministration of propranolol. The relevance of these findings to humans is not known. An 18-month study in mice and a lifetime study in hamsters revealed no evidence of tumorigenicity. Studies with albuterol revealed no evidence of mutagenesis. Reproduction studies in rats revealed no evidence of impaired fertility.
Pregnancy: ***Teratogenic Effects: Pregnancy Category C:*** Albuterol has been shown to be teratogenic in mice when given subcutaneously in doses corresponding to 1.25 times the human nebulization dose (based on a 50-kg human). There are no adequate and well-controlled studies in pregnant women. Albuterol should be used during pregnancy only if the potential benefit justifies the potential risk to the fetus. A reproduction study in CD-1 mice given albuterol subcutaneously (0.025, 0.25, and 2.5 mg/kg, corresponding to 0.125, 1.25, and 12.5 times, respectively, the maximum nebulization dose for a 50-kg human) showed cleft palate formation in 5 of 111 (4.5%) fetuses at 0.25 mg/kg and in 10 of 108 (9.3%) fetuses at 2.5 mg/kg. None was observed at 0.025 mg/kg. Cleft palate also occurred in 22 of 72 (30.5%) fetuses treated with 2.5 mg/kg of isoproterenol (positive control). A reproduction study with oral albuterol in Stride Dutch rabbits revealed cranioschisis in 7 of 19 (37%) fetuses at 50 mg/kg, corresponding to 250 times the maximum nebulization dose for a 50-kg human.
During worldwide marketing experience, various congenital anomalies, including cleft palate and limb defects, have been rarely reported in the offspring of patients being treated with albuterol. Some of the mothers were taking multiple medications during their pregnancies. No consistent pattern of defects can be discerned, and a relationship between albuterol use and congenital anomalies has not been established.
Labor and Delivery: Oral albuterol has been shown to delay preterm labor in some reports. There are presently no well-controlled studies that demonstrate that it will stop preterm labor or prevent labor at term. Therefore, cautious use of Ventolin Inhalation Solution is required in pregnant patients when given for relief of bronchospasm so as to avoid interference with uterine contractility.
Nursing Mothers: It is not known whether this drug is excreted in human milk. Because of the potential for tumorigenicity shown for albuterol in some animal studies, a decision should be made whether to discontinue nursing or to discontinue the drug, taking into account the importance of the drug to the mother.
Pediatric Use: Safety and effectiveness in children below 12 years of age have not been established.

ADVERSE REACTIONS

The results of clinical trials with Ventolin® (albuterol sulfate) Inhalation Solution in 135 patients showed the following side effects that were considered probably or possibly drug related:
Central Nervous System: Tremors (20%), dizziness (7%), nervousness (4%), headache (3%), insomnia (1%).
Gastrointestinal: Nausea (4%), dyspepsia (1%).
Ear, Nose, and Throat: Pharyngitis (<1%), nasal congestion (1%).
Cardiovascular: Tachycardia (1%), hypertension (1%).
Respiratory: Bronchospasm (8%), cough (4%), bronchitis (4%), wheezing (1%).
No clinically relevant laboratory abnormalities related to Ventolin Inhalation Solution administration were determined in these studies.
In comparing the adverse reactions reported for patients treated with Ventolin Inhalation Solution with those of patients treated with isoproterenol during clinical trials of 3 months, the following moderate to severe reactions, as judged by the investigators, were reported. This table does not include mild reactions.

Percent Incidence of Moderate to Severe Adverse Reactions

Reaction	Albuterol n=65	Isoproterenol n=65
Central nervous system		
Tremor	10.7%	13.8%
Headache	3.1%	1.5%
Insomnia	3.1%	1.5%
Cardiovascular		
Hypertension	3.1%	3.1%
Arrhythmias	0%	3.0%
Palpitation*	0%	22.0%
Respiratory		
Bronchospasm†	15.4%	18.0%
Cough	3.1%	5.0%
Bronchitis	1.5%	5.0%
Wheezing	1.5%	1.5%
Sputum increase	1.5%	1.5%
Dyspnea	1.5%	1.5%
Gastrointestinal		
Nausea	3.1%	0%
Dyspepsia	1.5%	0%
Systemic		
Malaise	1.5%	0%

* The finding of no arrhythmias and no palpitations after albuterol administration in this clinical study should not be interpreted as indicating that these adverse effects cannot occur after the administration of inhaled alburterol.
† In most cases of bronchospasm, this term was generally used to describe exacerbations in the underlying pulmonary disease.

Rare cases of urticaria, angioedema, rash, bronchospasm, and oropharyngeal edema have been reported after the use of inhaled albuterol.

OVERDOSAGE

The expected symptoms with overdosage are those of excessive beta-stimulation and/or occurrence or exaggeration of any of the symptoms listed under ADVERSE REACTIONS, e.g., seizures, angina, hyptertension or hypotension, tachycardia with rates up to 200 beats per minute, arrhythmias, nervousness, headache, tremor, dry mouth, palpitation, nausea, dizziness, fatigue, malaise, and insomnia. Hypokalemia may also occur.
Treatment consists of discontinuation of albuterol together with appropriate symptomatic therapy.
The oral LD_{50} in male and female rats and mice was greater than 2,000 mg/kg. The inhalational LD_{50} could not be determined.
There is insufficient evidence to determine if dialysis is beneficial for overdosage of Ventolin® (albuterol sulfate) Inhalation Solution.

DOSAGE AND ADMINISTRATION

To avoid cross contamination, proper aseptic technique should be used.
The usual dosage for adults and children 12 years and older is 2.5 mg of albuterol administered three to four times daily by nebulization. More frequent administration or higher doses are not recommended. To administer 2.5 mg of albuterol, dilute 0.5 mL of the 0.5% inhalation solution with 2.5 mL of sterile normal saline solution. The flow rate is regulated to suit the particular nebulizer so that Ventolin® (albuterol sulfate) Inhalation Solution will be delivered over approximately 5 to 15 minutes.
The use of Ventolin Inhalation Solution can be continued as medically indicated to control recurring bouts of bronchospasm. During this time most patients gain optimal benefit from regular use of the inhalation solution.
If a previously effective dosage regimen fails to provide the usual relief, medical advice should be sought immediately as this is often a sign of seriously worsening asthma that would require reassessment of therapy.
Drug compatibility (physical and chemical), efficacy, and safety of Ventolin Inhalation Solution when mixed with other drugs in a nebulizer have not been established.

HOW SUPPLIED

Ventolin® Inhalation Solution, 0.5% is supplied in bottles of 20 mL (NDC 0173-0385-58) with accompanying calibrated dropper in boxes of one.
Store between 2° and 25°C (36° and 77°F).
May 1995/RL-198
Shown in Product Identification Guide, page 315

VENTOLIN NEBULES® ℞

(albuterol sulfate, USP)
Inhalation Solution, 0.083%*
***Potency expressed as albuterol.**

DESCRIPTION

Ventolin Nebules® (albuterol sulfate, USP) Inhalation Solution is a relatively selective $beta_2$-adrenergic bronchodilator (see CLINICAL PHARMACOLOGY). Albuterol sulfate, USP, the racemic form of albuterol, has the chemical name α^1-[(*tert*-butylamino)methyl] -4- hydroxy-*m*-xylene-α,α'-diol sulfate (2:1)(salt).
Albuterol sulfate has a molecular weight of 576.7, and the empirical formula is $(C_{13}H_{21}NO_3)_2 \cdot H_2SO_4$. Albuterol sulfate is a white crystalline powder, soluble in water and slightly soluble in ethanol.
The World Health Organization recommended name for albuterol base is salbutamol.
Ventolin Nebules Inhalation Solution requires no dilution before administration.
Each milliliter of Ventolin Nebules Inhalation Solution contains 0.83 mg of albuterol (as 1 mg of albuterol sulfate) in an isotonic, sterile, aqueous solution containing sodium chloride; sulfuric acid is used to adjust the pH to between 3 and 5.
Ventolin Nebules Inhalation Solution contains no sulfiting agents or preservatives.
Ventolin Nebules Inhalation Solution is a clear, colorless solution.

CLINICAL PHARMACOLOGY

The prime action of beta-adrenergic drugs is to stimulate adenyl cyclase, the enzyme that catalyzes the formation of cyclic-3',5'-adenosine monophosphate (cyclic AMP) from adenosine triphosphate (ATP). The cyclic AMP thus formed mediates the cellular responses. *In vitro* studies and *in vivo* pharmacologic studies have demonstrated that albuterol has a preferential effect on $beta_2$-adrenergic receptors compared with isoproterenol. While it is recognized that $beta_2$-adrenergic receptors are the predominant receptors in bronchial smooth muscle, recent data indicate that 10% to 50% of the beta-receptors in the human heart may be $beta_2$receptors. The precise function of these, however, is not yet established.
Albuterol has been shown in most controlled clinical trials to have more effect on the respiratory tract, in the form of bronchial smooth muscle relaxation, than isoproterenol at comparable does while producing fewer cardiovascular effects.
Controlled clinical studies and other clinical experience have shown that inhaled albuterol, like other beta-adrenergic agonist drugs, can produce a significant cardiovascular effect in some patients, as measured by pulse rate, blood pressure, symptoms, and/or electrocardiographic changes.
Albuterol is longer acting than isoproterenol in most patients by any route of administration because it is not a substrate for the cellular uptake processes for catecholamines nor for catechol-*O*-methyl transferase.
Studies in asthmatic patients have shown that less than 20% of a single albuterol dose was absorbed following either IPPB (intermittent positive-pressure breathing) or nebulizer administration; the remaining amount was recovered from the nebulizer and apparatus and expired air. Most of the absorbed dose was recovered in the urine 24 hours after drug administration. Following a 3-mg dose of nebulized albuterol, the maximum albuterol plasma levels at 0.5 hours were 2.1 ng/mL (range, 1.4 to 3.2 ng/mL). There was a significant dose-related response in FEV_1 (forced expiratory volume in one second) and peak flow rate. It has been demonstrated that following oral administration of 4 mg of albuterol, the elimination half-life was 5 to 6 hours.
Animal studies show that albuterol does not pass the blood-brain barrier.
Recent studies in laboratory animals (minipigs, rodents, and dogs) recorded the occurrence of cardiac arrhythmias and sudden death (with histologic evidence of myocardial necrosis) when beta-agonists and methylxanthines were administered concurrently. The significance of these findings when applied to humans is currently unknown.
In controlled clinical trials, most patients exhibited an onset of improvement in pulmonary function within 5 minutes as determined by FEV_1. FEV_1 measurements also showed that the maximum average improvement in pulmonary function usually occurred at approximately 1 hour following inhalation of 2.5 mg of albuterol by compressor-nebulizer and remained close to peak for 2 hours. Clinically significant improvement in pulmonary function (defined as maintenance of a 15% or more increase in FEV_1 over baseline values) continued for 3 to 4 hours in most patients, with some patients continuing up to 6 hours.
In repetitive dose studies, continued effectiveness was demonstrated throughout the 3-month period of treatment in some patients.

INDICATIONS AND USAGE

Ventolin Nebules® (albuterol sulfate USP) Inhalation Solution is indicated for the relief of bronchospasm in patients with reversible obstructive airway disease and acute attacks of bronchospasm.

CONTRAINDICATIONS

Ventolin Nebules® (albuterol sulfate, USP) Inhalation Solution is contraindicated in patients with a history of hypersensitivity to any of the components.

WARNINGS

As with other inhaled beta-adrenergic agonists, Ventolin Nebules® (albuterol sulfate, USP) Inhalation Solution can produce paradoxical bronchospasm that can be life threatening. If it occurs, the preparation should be discontinued immediately and alternative therapy instituted.

Fatalities have been reported in association with excessive use of inhaled sympathomimetic drugs and with the home use of nebulizers. It is therefore essential that the physician instruct the patient in the need for further evaluation if his/her asthma becomes worse. In individual patients, any beta$_2$-adrenergic agonist, including albuterol inhalation solution, may have a clinically significant cardiac effect.

Immediate hypersensitivity reactions may occur after administration of albuterol, as demonstrated by rare cases of urticaria, angioedema, rash, bronchospasm, and oropharyngeal edema.

PRECAUTIONS

General: Albuterol, as with all sympathomimetic amines, should be used with caution in patients with cardiovascular disorders, especially coronary insufficiency, cardiac arrhythmias, and hypertension; in patients with convulsive disorders, hyperthyroidism, or diabetes mellitus; and in patients who are unusually responsive to sympathomimetic amines.

Large doses of intravenous albuterol have been reported to aggravate pre-existing diabetes mellitus and ketoacidosis. As with other beta-agonists, inhaled and intravenous albuterol may produce a significant hypokalemia in some patients, possibly through intracellular shunting, which has the potential to produce adverse cardiovascular effects. The decrease is usually transient, not requiring supplementation.

Information for Patients: The action of Ventolin Nebules® (albuterol sulfate, USP) Inhalation Solution may last up to 6 hours, and therefore it should not be used more frequently than recommended. Do not increase the dose or frequency of medication without medical consultation. If symptoms get worse, medical consultation should be sought promptly. While taking Ventolin Nebules Inhalation Solution, other antiasthma medicines should not be used unless prescribed. Drug compatibility (physical and chemical), efficacy, and safety of Ventolin Nebules Inhalation Solution when mixed with other drugs in a nebulizer have not been established. See illustrated Patient's Instructions for Use in product package insert.

Drug Interactions: Other sympathomimetic aerosol bronchodilators or epinephrine should not be used concomitantly with albuterol.

Albuterol should be administered with extreme caution to patients being treated with monoamine oxidase inhibitors or tricyclic antidepressants because the action of albuterol on the vascular system may be potentiated.

Beta-receptor blocking agents and albuterol inhibit the effect of each other.

Carcinogenesis, Mutagenesis, Impairment of Fertility: Albuterol sulfate caused a significant dose-related increase in the incidence of benign leiomyomas of the mesovarium in a 2-year study in the rat at oral doses of 2, 10, and 50 mg/kg, corresponding to 10, 50, and 250 times, respectively, the maximum nebulizaton dose for a 50-kg human. In another study, this effect was blocked by the coadministration of propranolol. The relevance of these findings to humans is not known. An 18-month study in mice and a lifetime study in hamsters revealed no evidence of tumorigenicity. Studies with albuterol revealed no evidence of mutagenesis. Reproduction studies in rats revealed no evidence of impaired fertility.

Pregnancy: ***Teratogenic Effects: Pregnancy Category C:*** Albuterol has been shown to be teratogenic in mice when given subcutaneously in doses corresponding to 1.25 times the human nebulization dose (based on a 50-kg human). There are no adequate and well-controlled studies in pregnant women. Albuterol should be used during pregnancy only if the potential benefit justifies the potential risk to the fetus. A reproduction study in CD-1 mice given albuterol subcutaneously (0.025, 0.25, and 2.5 mg/kg, corresponding to 0.125, 1.25, and 12.5 times, respectively, the maximum nebulization dose for a 50-kg human) showed cleft palate formation in 5 of 111 (4.5%) fetuses at 0.25 mg/kg and in 10 of 108 (9.3%) fetuses at 2.5 mg/kg. None was observed at 0.025 mg/kg. Cleft palate also occurred in 22 of 72 (30.5%) fetuses treated with 2.5 mg/kg of isoproterenol (positive control). A reproduction study with oral albuterol in Stride Dutch rabbits revealed cranioschisis in 7 or 19 (37%) fetuses at 50 mg/kg, corresponding to 250 times the maximum nebulization dose for a 50-kg human.

During worldwide marketing experience, various congenital anomalies, including cleft palate and limb defects, have been rarely reported in the offspring of patients being treated with albuterol. Some of the mothers were taking multiple medications during their pregnancies. No consistent pattern of defects can be discerned, and a relationship between albuterol use and congenital anomalies has not been established.

Labor and Delivery: Oral albuterol has been shown to delay preterm labor in some reports. There are presently no well-controlled studies that demonstrate that it will stop preterm labor or prevent labor at term. Therefore, cautious use of Ventolin Nebules Inhalation Solution is required in pregnant patients when given for relief of bronchospasm so as to avoid interference with uterine contractility.

Nursing Mothers: It is not known whether this drug is excreted in human milk. Because of the potential for tumorigenicity shown for albuterol in some animal studies, a decision should be made whether to discontinue nursing or to discontinue the drug, taking into account the importance of the drug to the mother.

Pediatric Use: Safety and effectiveness in children below 12 years of age have not been established.

ADVERSE REACTIONS

The results of clinical trials with Ventolin® (albuterol sulfate, USP) Inhalation Solution, 0.5% in 135 patients showed the following side effects that were considered probably or possibly drug related:

Central Nervous System: Tremors (20%), dizziness (7%), nervousness (4%), headache (3%), insomnia (1%).

Gastrointestinal: Nausea (4%), dyspepsia (1%).

Ear, Nose, and Throat: Pharyngitis (<1%), nasal congestion (1%).

Cardiovascular: Tachycardia (1%), hypertension (1%).

Respiratory: Bronchospasm (8%), cough (4%), bronchitis (4%), wheezing (1%).

No clinically relevant laboratory abnormalities related to Ventolin Inhalation Solution administration were determined in these studies.

In comparing the adverse reactions reported for patients treated with Ventolin Inhalation Solution with those of patients treated with isoproterenol during clinical trials of 3 months, the following moderate to severe reactions, as judged by the investigators, were reported. This table does not include mild reactions.

Percent Incidence of Moderate to Severe Adverse Reactions

Reaction	Albuterol n=65	Isoproterenol n=65
Central nervous system		
Tremor	10.7%	13.8%
Headache	3.1%	1.5%
Insomnia	3.1%	1.5%
Cardiovascular		
Hypertension	3.1%	3.1%
Arrhythmias	0%	3.0%
Palpitation*	0%	22.0%
Respiratory		
Bronchospasm†	15.4%	18.0%
Cough	3.1%	5.0%
Bronchitis	1.5%	5.0%
Wheezing	1.5%	1.5%
Sputum increase	1.5%	1.5%
Dyspnea	1.5%	1.5%
Gastrointestinal		
Nausea	3.1%	0%
Dyspepsia	1.5%	0%
Systemic		
Malaise	1.5%	0%

* The finding of no arrhythmias and no palpitations after albuterol administration in this clinical study should not be interpreted as indicating that these adverse effects cannot occur after the administration of inhaled albuterol.

† In most cases of bronchospasm, this term was generally used to describe exacerbations in the underlying pulmonary diease.

Rare cases of urticaria, angioedema, rash, bronchospasm, and oropharyngeal edema have been reported after the use of inhaled albuterol.

OVERDOSAGE

Manifestations of overdosage may include seizures, anginal pain, hypertension, hypokalemia, tachycardia with rates up to 200 beats per minute, and exaggeration of the pharmacologic effects listed in ADVERSE REACTIONS.

The oral LD_{50} in rats and mice was greater than 2,000 mg/kg. The inhalational LD_{50} could not be determined.

There is insufficient evidence to determine if dialysis is beneficial for overdosage of Ventolin Nebules® (albuterol sulfate, USP) Inhalation Solution.

DOSAGE AND ADMINISTRATION

The usual dosage for adults and children 12 years and older is 2.5 mg of albuterol administered three to four times daily by nebulization. More frequent administration or higher doses are not recommended. To administer 2.5 mg of albuterol, administer the contents of one sterile unit dose Nebule® (3 mL of 0.083% inhalation solution) by nebulization. The flow rate is regulated to suit the particular nebulizer so that Ventolin Nebules® (albuterol sulfate, USP) Inhalation Solution will be delivered over approximately 5 to 15 minutes.

The use of Ventolin Nebules Inhalation Solution can be continued as medically indicated to control recurring bouts of bronchospasm. During this time most patients gain optimal benefit from regular use of the inhalation solution.

If a previously effective dosage regimen fails to provide the usual relief, medical advice should be sought immediately as this is often a sign of seriously worsening asthma that would require reassessment of therapy.

Drug compatibility (physical and chemical), efficacy, and safety of Ventolin Nebules Inhalation Solution when mixed with other drugs in a nebulizer have not been established.

HOW SUPPLIED

Ventolin Nebules® (albuterol sulfate USP) Inhalation Solution, 0.083% is supplied in sterile unit dose nebules of 3 mL each in boxes of 25 (NDC 0173-0419-00).

Protect from light. Store in a refrigerator between 2° and 8°C (36° and 46°F). Ventolin Nebules Inhalation Solution may be held at room temperature for up to 2 weeks before use. (Nebules must be used within 2 weeks of removal from refrigerator; record date the nebules are removed from the refrigerator in the space provided on the product carton). Discard if solution becomes discolored. (Note: Ventolin Nebules Inhalation Solution is colorless.)

May 1995/RL-199

Shown in Product Identification Guide, page 315

VENTOLIN ROTACAPS® ℞

(albuterol sulfate, USP)
for Inhalation
FOR INHALATION ONLY
For Use With the Rotahaler® Inhalation Device

DESCRIPTION

Ventolin Rotacaps® (albuterol sulfate, USP) for Inhalation contain a dry powder presentation of albuterol sulfate intended for oral inhalation only. Each light blue and clear, hard gelatin capsule contains a mixture of 200 mcg of microfine (95% ≤10 µm) albuterol (as the sulfate) with 25 mg of lactose.

The contents of each capsule are inhaled using a specially designed plastic device for inhaling powder called the Rotahaler®. When turned, this device opens the capsule and facilitates dispersion of the albuterol sulfate into the airstream created when the patient inhales through the mouthpiece.

Ventolin Rotacaps for Inhalation are an alternative inhalation form of albuterol to the metered-dose pressurized inhaler.

The active component of Ventolin Rotacaps for Inhalation is albuterol sulfate, USP, the racemic form of albuterol and a relatively selective beta$_2$-adrenergic bronchodilator. It has the chemical name α^1-[(*tert*-butylamino)methyl]-4-hydroxy-*m*-xylene -α,α'-diol sulfate (2:1)(salt).

Albuterol sulfate has a molecular weight of 576.7, and the empirical formula is $(C_{13}H_{21}NO_3)_2 \cdot H_2SO_4$. Albuterol sulfate is a white crystalline powder, soluble in water and slightly soluble in ethanol.

The World Health Organization recommended name for albuterol base is salbutamol.

CLINICAL PHARMACOLOGY: The pharmacologic effects of beta-adrenergic agonist drugs, including albuterol, are at least in part attributable to stimulation through beta-adrenergic receptors of intracellular adenyl cyclase, the enzyme that catalyzes the conversion of adenosine triphosphate (ATP) to cyclic-3′,5′-adenosine monophosphate (cyclic AMP). Increased cyclic AMP levels are associated with relaxation of bronchial smooth muscle and inhibition of release of mediators of immediate hypersensitivity from cells, especially from mast cells.

In vitro studies and *in vivo* pharmacologic studies have demonstrated that albuterol has a preferential effect on beta$_2$-adrenergic receptors compared with isoproterenol. While it is recognized that beta$_2$-adrenergic receptors are the predominant receptors in bronchial smooth muscle, recent data indicate that there is a population of beta$_2$-receptors in the human heart existing in a concentration between 10% and 50%. The precise function of these, however, is not yet established (see WARNINGS).

Albuterol has been shown in most controlled clinical trials to have more effect on the respiratory tract, in the form of bronchial smooth muscle relaxation, than isoproterenol at comparable doses while producing fewer cardiovascular effects. Controlled clinical studies and other clinical experience have shown that inhaled albuterol, like other beta-adrenergic agonist drugs, can produce a significant cardiovascular effect in some patients, as measured by pulse rate, blood pressure, symptoms, and/or electrocardiographic changes.

Continued on next page

Glaxo Wellcome—Cont.

Albuterol is longer acting than isoproterenol in most patients by any route of administration because it is not a substrate for the normal cellular uptake processes for catecholamines nor for catechol-*O*-methyl transferase.
Studies undertaken with four subjects administered tritiated albuterol from a metered-dose aerosol inhaler resulted in maximum plasma concentrations occurring within 2 to 4 hours. Due to the sensitivity of the assay method, the metabolic rate and half-life elimination of albuterol in plasma could not be determined. However, urinary excretion provided data indicating that albuterol has an elimination half-life of 3.8 hours. Approximately 72% of the inhaled dose is excreted within 24 hours in the urine, and consists of 28% as unchanged drug and 44% as metabolite.
Animal studies show that albuterol does not pass the blood-brain barrier.
Recent studies in laboratory animals (minipigs, rodents, and dogs) recorded the occurrence of cardiac arrthythmias and sudden death (with histologic evidence of myocardial necrosis) when beta-agonists and methylxanthines were administered concurrently. The significance of these findings when applied to humans is currently unknown.
In single, dose-range, crossover trials with Ventolin Rotacaps® (albuterol sulfate) for Inhalation in patients 12 years of age and older, the onset of improvement in pulmonary function was within 5 minutes as determined by a 15% increase in FEV_1 (forced expiratory volume in 1 second) following administration of either a 200- or 400-mcg dose. Maximum increases in FEV_1 occurred within 60 minutes following inhalation of either dose. The duration of effect (defined as an increase in $FEV_1$of 15% or greater in a single-dose study) was 1 to 2 hours after the 200-mcg dose and 3 to 4 hours after the 400-mcg dose. In a single-dose study, an increase in $FEF_{25\%-75\%}$ (forced expiratory flow rate between 25% and 75% of the forced vital capacity) of 20% or greater continued for 3 to 4 hours after the 200-mcg dose and for 3 to 6 hours following the 400-mcg dose. A therapeutic response continued for 4 hours in the majority of patients and for 6 hours in 38% of the patients following the 400-mcg dose. Twenty-two percent of the patients receiving the 200-mcg dose had a duration of effect of 8 hours.
In 12-week, double-blind, comparative evaluations in patients 12 years of age and older of one 200-mcg Ventolin Rotacaps for Inhalation capsule versus two inhalations of Ventolin® (albuterol, USP) Inhalation Aerosol, the two dosage regimens were found to be equivalent. Based on a 15% or more increase in FEV_1 determinations, both provided a therapeutic response that persisted for 2 or 3 hours in 50% of 231 patients aged 12 years and older. Similar results were found in two controlled, 12-week clinical trials involving 204 children aged 4 to 11 years. Both formulations produced a therapeutic response (defined as maintenance of mean increase over baseline of at least 15% in FEV_1, or 20% in $FEF_{25\%-75\%}$). Therapeutic improvement of $FEF_{25\%-75\%}$ persisted for 3 to 5 hours in over 50% of the children throughout the study. Continued effectiveness and safety of Ventolin Rotacaps for Inhalation was demonstrated over the 12-week study periods in both adults and children.
In other clinical studies in adults and children, one 200-mcg Ventolin Rotacaps for Inhalation capsule taken approximately 15 minutes before exercise prevented exercise-induced bronchospasm, as demonstrated by the maintenance of FEV_1 within 80% of baseline values in the majority of patients. One study in adults also evaluated the duration of the prophylactic effect to repeated exercise challenges, which was evident at 4 hours in the majority of patients and at 6 hours in approximately one third of the patients.

INDICATIONS AND USAGE

Ventolin Rotacaps® (albuterol sulfate) for Inhalation are indicated for the prevention and relief of bronchospasm in patients 4 years of age and older with reversible obstructive airway disease and for the prevention of exercise-induced brochospasm in patients 4 years of age and older. The Ventolin Rotacaps for Inhalation formulation is particularly useful in patients who are unable to properly use the pressurized aerosol form of albuterol or who prefer an alternative formulation. Ventolin Rotacaps for Inhalation can be used with or without concomitant steroid therapy.

CONTRAINDICATIONS

Ventolin Rotacaps® (albuterol sulfate) for Inhalation are contraindicated in patients with a history of hypersensitivity to any of the components.

WARNINGS

As with other inhaled beta-adrenergic agonists, Ventolin Rotacaps® (albuterol sulfate) for Inhalation can produce paradoxical bronchospasm that can be life threatening. If it occurs, the preparation should be discontinued immediately and alternative therapy instituted.
Fatalities have been reported in association with excessive use of inhaled sympathomimetic drugs. The exact cause of death is unknown, but cardiac arrest following unexpected development of severe acute asthmatic crisis and subsequent hypoxia is suspected.
Immediate hypersensitivity reactions may occur after administration of albuterol, as demonstrated by rare cases of urticaria, angioedema, rash, bronchospasm, anaphylaxis, and oropharyngeal edema.
Inhalation of capsule particles may result if damage to the capsule has occurred from handling by the patient.

PRECAUTIONS

General: Although no effect on the cardiovascular system is usually seen after the administration of inhaled albuterol at recommended doses, cardiovascular and central nervous system (CNS) effects seen with all sympathomimetic drugs can occur after use of inhaled albuterol and may require discontinuation of the drug. As with all sympathomimetic amines, albuterol should be used with caution in patients with cardiovascular disorders, including coronary insufficiency, hypertension, and cardiac arrhythmia; in patients with hyperthyroidism or diabetes mellitus; in patients who are unusually responsive to sympathomimetic amines; and in patients with convulsive disorders. Clinically significant changes in systolic and diastolic blood pressure have been seen in individual patients and could be expected to occur in some patients after use of any beta-adrenergic bronchodilator. As with other beta-agonists, inhaled and intravenous albuterol may produce significant hypokalemia in some patients, possibly through intracellular shunting, which has the potential to produce adverse cardiovascular effects. The decrease is usually transient, not requiring supplementation.
Although there have been no reports concerning the use of Ventolin Rotacaps® (albuterol sulfate) for Inhalation during labor and delivery, it has been reported that high doses of albuterol administered intravenously inhibit uterine contractions. Although this effect is extremely unlikely as a consequence of Ventolin Rotacaps for Inhalation use, it should be kept in mind.
Information for Patients: The action of Ventolin Rotacaps for Inhalation may last for 6 hours or longer, and therefore they should not be used more frequently than recommended. Do not increase the frequency of doses without medical consultation. If the recommended dosage does not provide relief of symptoms or symptoms become worse, seek immediate medical attention. While using Ventolin Rotacaps for Inhalation, other inhaled drugs should not be used unless prescribed.
Children should use Ventolin Rotacaps for Inhalation under adult supervision, as instructed by the patient's physician. See illustrated Patient's Instructions for Use in product package insert.
Drug Interactions: Other sympathomimetic aerosol bronchodilators should not used concomitantly with albuterol. If additional adrenergic drugs are to be administered by any route, they should be used with caution to avoid deleterious cardiovascular effects.
Albuterol should be administered with extreme caution to patients being treated with monoamine oxidase inhibitors or tricyclic antidepressants because the action of albuterol on the vascular system may be potentiated.
Beta-receptor blocking agents and albuterol inhibit the effect of each other.
Carcinogenesis, Mutagenesis, Impairment of Fertility: Albuterol sulfate caused a significant dose-related increase in the incidence of benign leiomyomas of the mesovarium in a 2-year oral study in the rat at doses of 2, 10, and 50 mg/kg, corresponding to 42, 208, and 1,042 times, respectively, the maximum inhalational dose for a 50-kg human. In another study this effect was blocked by the coadministration of propranolol. The relevance of these findings to humans is not known. An 18-month oral study in mice, at doses corresponding to 10,417 times the human inhalational dose, and a lifetime oral study in hamsters, at doses corresponding to 1,042 times the human inhalational dose, showed no evidence of tumorigenicity. Studies with albuterol showed no evidence of mutagenesis. Oral reproduction studies in rats, at doses corresponding to 1,042 times the human inhalational dose, showed no evidence of impairment of fertility.
Pregnancy: ***Teratogenic Effects: Pregnancy Category C:*** Albuterol has been shown to be teratogenic in mice when given in doses corresponding to five times the human inhalational dose. There are no adequate and well-controlled studies in pregnant women. Albuterol should be used during pregnancy only if the potential benefit justifies the potential risk to the fetus. A reproduction study in CD-1 mice given albuterol subcutaneously (0.025, 0.25, and 2.5 mg/kg, corresponding to 0.52, 5.2, and 52 times, respectively, the maximum inhalational dose for a 50-kg human) showed cleft palate formation in 5 of 111 (4.5%) fetuses at 0.25 mg/kg and in 10 of 108 (9.3%) fetuses at 2.5 mg/kg. None was observed at 0.025 mg/kg. Cleft palate also occurred in 22 of 72 (30.5%) fetuses treated with 2.5 mg/kg of isoproterenol (positive control). A reproduction study with oral albuterol in Stride Dutch rabbits revealed cranioschisis in 7 of 19 (37%) fetuses at 50 mg/kg, corresponding to 1,042 times the maximum inhalational dose for a 50-kg human.
During worldwide marketing experience, various congenital anomalies, including cleft palate and limb defects, have been rarely reported in the offspring of patients being treated with albuterol. Some of the mothers were taking multiple medications during their pregnancies. No consistent pattern of defects can be discerned, and a relationship between albuterol use and congenital anomalies has not been established.
Labor and Delivery: Oral albuterol has been shown to delay preterm labor in some reports. There are presently no well-controlled studies that demonstrate that it will stop preterm labor or prevent labor at term. Therefore, cautious use of Ventolin Rotacaps for Inhalation is required in pregnant patients when given for relief of bronchospasm so as to avoid interference with uterine contractility.
Nursing Mothers: It is not known whether this drug is excreted in human milk after inhalation of recommended doses. Because of the potential for tumorigenicity shown for albuterol in animal studies, a decision should be made whether to discontinue nursing or to discontinue the drug, taking into account the importance of the drug to the mother.
Pediatric Use: Safety and effectiveness in children below 4 years of age have not been established.

ADVERSE REACTIONS

The adverse reactions to albuterol are similar in nature to reactions to other sympathomimetic agents, although the incidence of certain cardiovascular effects is lower with albuterol. Results of clinical trials with Ventolin Rotacaps® (albuterol sulfate) for Inhalation 200 mcg in 172 patients aged 12 years and older (adults) and 129 patients aged 4 to 12 years (children) showed the following side effects:
CNS: ***Adults:*** Headache in 4 of 172 patients (2%); nervousness in 2 of 172 (1%); dizziness, insomnia, lightheadedness, each in <1%. ***Children:*** Headache in 6 of 129 (5%); dizziness and hyperactivity, each in <1%.
Gastrointestinal: ***Adults:*** Burning in stomach in <1%. ***Children:*** Nausea and/or vomiting in 5 of 129 (4%), stomachache in 2 of 129 (2%), diarrhea in <1%.
Oropharyngeal: ***Adults:*** Throat irritation in 3 of 172 (2%); dry mouth and voice changes, each in <1%. ***Children:*** Throat irritation in 3 of 129 (2%), unusual taste in 2 of 129 (2%).
Respiratory: ***Adults:*** Cough in 8 of 172 (5%), bronchospasm in 2 of 172 (1%). ***Children:*** Cough and nasal congestion, each in 3 of 129 (2%); hoarseness and epistaxis, each in 2 of 129 (2%).
Musculoskeletal: ***Adults:*** Tremor in 2 of 172 (1%). ***Children:*** None reported.
Rare cases of urticaria, angioedema, rash, hoarseness, and oropharyngeal edema have been reported after the use of inhaled albuterol.
In addition, albuterol, like other sympathomimetic agents, can cause adverse reactions such as hypertension, angina, vertigo, and CNS stimulation.

OVERDOSAGE

Overdosage with albuterol may be expected to result in exaggeration of those drug effects listed in the ADVERSE REACTIONS section, such as seizures, anginal pain, hypertension, tachycardia with rates up to 200 beats per minute, and hypokalemia. In these cases, therapy with albuterol and all beta-adrenergic-stimulating drugs should be stopped, supportive therapy provided, and judicious use of a cardioselective beta-adrenergic blocking agent should be considered, bearing in mind the possibility that such agents can produce profound bronchospasm.
The oral LD_{50} in male and female rats and mice was greater than 2,000 mg/kg. The inhalational LD_{50} could not be determined.
Dialysis is not appropriate treatment for overdosage of Ventolin Rotacaps® (albuterol sulfate) for Inhalation.

DOSAGE AND ADMINISTRATION

The usual dosage of Ventolin Rotacaps® (albuterol sulfate) for Inhalation for adults and children 4 years of age and older is the contents of one 200-mcg capsule inhaled every 4 to 6 hours using a Rotahaler® inhalation device. In some patients, the contents of two 200-mcg capsules inhaled every 4 to 6 hours may be required. Larger doses or more frequent administration is not recommended.
The use of Ventolin Rotacaps for Inhalation can be continued as medically indicated to control recurring bouts of bronchospasm. During this time most patients gain optimal benefit from regular use of the Ventolin Rotacaps for Inhalation formulation.
If a previously effective dosage regimen fails to provide the usual relief, medical advice should be sought immediately as this is often a sign of seriously worsening asthma that would require reassessment of therapy.
Exercise-Induced Bronchospasm Prevention: The usual dosage of Ventolin Rotacaps for Inhalation for adults and children 4 years of age and older is the contents of one 200-mcg capsule inhaled using a Rotahaler 15 minutes before exercise.

HOW SUPPLIED

Ventolin Rotacaps® (albuterol sulfate) for Inhalation, 200 mcg, are light blue and clear, with "VENTOLIN 200" printed on the blue cap and "GLAXO" printed on the clear body.

Ventolin Rotacaps for Inhalation are supplied in a kit containing one bottle of 100 capsules and one Rotahaler® inhalation device with patient's instructions (NDC 0173-0389-01). Also available, Ventolin Rotacaps for Inhalation Refill bottle of 100 capsules with patient's instructions (NDC 0173-0389-02).

Ventolin Rotacaps for Inhalation are also supplied in a hospital unit dose kit containing one unit dose pack of 24 capsules and one Rotahaler inhalation device (NDC 0173-0389-03).

Store between 2° and 30°C (36° and 86°F). Replace cap securely after each opening.

July 1995/RL-211

Shown in Product Identification Guide, page 315

VENTOLIN® ℞

(albuterol sulfate, USP)
Syrup

DESCRIPTION

VENTOLIN Syrup contains albuterol sulfate, USP, the racemic form of albuterol and a relatively selective beta$_2$-adrenergic bronchodilator. Albuterol sulfate has the chemical name α^1-[(*tert*-Butylamino) methyl]-4-hydroxy-*m*-xylene-α,α'-diol sulfate (2:1)(salt).

Albuterol sulfate has a molecular weight of 576.7 and the empirical formula $(C_{13}H_{21}NO_3)_2 \cdot H_2SO_4$. Albuterol sulfate is a white crystalline powder, soluble in water and slightly soluble in ethanol.

The World Health Organization recommended name for albuterol base is salbutamol.

VENTOLIN Syrup contains 2 mg of albuterol as 2.4 mg of albuterol sulfate in each teaspoonful (5 mL).

The inactive ingredients for VENTOLIN Syrup include: citric acid, FD&C Yellow No. 6, flavor, hydroxypropyl methylcellulose, saccharin, sodium benzoate, sodium citrate, and water.

CLINICAL PHARMACOLOGY

The prime action of beta-adrenergic drugs is to stimulate adenyl cyclase, the enzyme which catalyzes the formation of cyclic-3′,5′-adenosine monophosphate (cyclic AMP) from adenosine triphosphate (ATP). The cyclic AMP thus formed mediates the cellular responses. Based on pharmacologic studies in animals, albuterol appears to exert direct and preferential action on beta$_2$-adrenoceptors, including those of the bronchial tree and uterus, and may have less cardiac stimulant effect than isoproterenol when given in the usual recommended dose.

Albuterol is longer acting than isoproterenol in most patients by any route of administration because it is not a substrate for the cellular uptake processes for catecholamines nor for catechol-*O*-methyl transferase.

After oral administration of 10 mL VENTOLIN Syrup (4 mg albuterol) in normal volunteers, albuterol is rapidly absorbed. Maximum plasma albuterol concentrations of about 18 ng/mL are achieved within 2 hours, and the drug is eliminated with a half-life of about 5 hours. In other studies, the analysis of urine samples of patients given 8 mg tritiated albuterol orally showed that 76% of the dose was excreted over 3 days, with the majority of the dose being excreted within the first 24 hours. Sixty percent of this radioactivity was shown to be the metabolite. Feces collected over this period contained 4% of the administered dose.

Animal studies show that albuterol does not pass the blood-brain barrier.

INDICATIONS AND USAGE

VENTOLIN Syrup is indicated for the relief of bronchospasm in adults and children 2 years of age and older with reversible obstructive airway disease.

In controlled clinical trials in patients with asthma, the onset of improvement in pulmonary function, as measured by maximum midexpiratory flow rate (MMEF) and forced expiratory volume in one second (FEV$_1$), was within 30 minutes after a dose of VENTOLIN Syrup. Peak improvement of pulmonary function occurred between 2 and 3 hours. In a controlled clinical trial involving 55 children, clinically significant improvement (defined as maintenance of mean values over baseline of 15% to 20% or more in the FEV$_1$ and MMEF, respectively) continued to be recorded up to 6 hours. No decrease in the effectiveness was reported in one uncontrolled study of 32 children who took VENTOLIN Syrup for a 3-month period.

CONTRAINDICATIONS

VENTOLIN Syrup is contraindicated in patients with a history of hypersensitivity to any of its components.

WARNINGS

Immediate hypersensitivity reactions may occur after administration of albuterol, as demonstrated by rare cases of anaphylaxis, angioedema, oropharyngeal edema, bronchospasm, urticaria, and rash.

Rarely, erythema multiforme and Stevens-Johnson syndrome have been associated with the administration of albuterol sulfate syrup in children.

PRECAUTIONS:

General: Although albuterol usually has minimal effects on the beta$_1$-adrenoceptors of the cardiovascular system at the recommended dosage, occasionally the usual cardiovascular and CNS stimulatory effects common to all sympathomimetic agents have been seen with patients treated with albuterol, necessitating discontinuation. Therefore, albuterol, as with all sympathomimetic amines, should be used with caution in patients with cardiovascular disorders, including coronary insufficiency, cardiac arrhythmias, and hypertension; in patients with convulsive disorders, hyperthyroidism, or diabetes mellitus; and in patients who are unusually responsive to sympathomimetic amines.

Large doses of intravenous albuterol have been reported to aggravate preexisting diabetes mellitus and ketoacidosis. Additionally, albuterol and other beta-agonists, when given intravenously, may cause a decrease in serum potassium, possibly through intracellular shunting. The decrease is usually transient, not requiring supplementation. The relevance of these observations to the use of VENTOLIN Syrup is unknown.

Information for Patients: The action of VENTOLIN Syrup may last up to 6 hours and therefore it should not be taken more frequently than recommended. Do not increase the dose or frequency of medication without medical consultation. If symptoms get worse, medical consultation should be sought promptly. If pregnant or nursing, consult with your physician.

Drug Interactions: The concomitant use of VENTOLIN Syrup and other oral sympathomimetic agents is not recommended since such combined use may lead to deleterious cardiovascular effects. This recommendation does not preclude the judicious use of an aerosol bronchodilator of the adrenergic stimulant type in patients receiving VENTOLIN Syrup. Such concomitant use, however, should be individualized and not given on a routine basis. If regular coadministration is required, then alternative therapy should be considered.

Albuterol should be administered with extreme caution to patients being treated with monoamine oxidase inhibitors or tricyclic antidepressants, since the action of albuterol on the vascular system may be potentiated.

Beta-receptor blocking agents and albuterol inhibit the effect of each other.

Since albuterol may lower serum potassium, care should be taken in patients also using other drugs which lower serum potassium as the effects may be additive.

After single-dose administration of albuterol to normal volunteers who had received digoxin for 10 days, a 16%-22% decrease in serum digoxin levels was demonstrated. The clinical significance of these findings for patients with obstructive airway disease who are receiving albuterol and digoxin on a chronic basis is unclear. Nevertheless, it would be prudent to carefully evaluate the serum digoxin levels in patients who are concurrently receiving digoxin and albuterol.

Carcinogenesis, Mutagenesis, Impairment of Fertility: Albuterol sulfate, like other agents in its class, caused a significant dose-related increase in the incidence of benign leiomyomas of the mesovarium in a 2-year study in the rat, at doses corresponding to 2, 9, and 46 times the maximum human (child weighing 21 kg) oral dose. In another study this effect was blocked by the coadministration of propranolol. The relevance of these findings to humans is not known. An 18-month study in mice and a lifetime study in hamsters revealed no evidence of tumorigenicity. Studies with albuterol revealed no evidence of mutagenesis. Reproduction studies in rats revealed no evidence of impaired fertility.

Teratogenic Effects-Pregnancy Category C: Albuterol has been shown to be teratogenic in mice when given subcutaneously in doses corresponding to 0.2 times the maximum human (child weighing 21 kg) oral dose. There are no adequate and well-controlled studies in pregnant women. Albuterol should be used during pregnancy only if the potential benefit justifies the potential risk to the fetus. A reproduction study in CD-1 mice with albuterol showed cleft palate formation in 5 of 111 (4.5%) fetuses at 0.25 mg/kg and in 10 of 108 (9.3%) fetuses at 2.5 mg/kg; none was observed at 0.025 mg/kg. Cleft palate also occurred in 22 of 72 (30.5%) fetuses treated with 2.5 mg/kg of isoproterenol (positive control). A reproduction study in Stride Dutch rabbits revealed cranioschisis in 7 of 19 (37%) fetuses at 50 mg/kg, corresponding to 46 times the maximum human (child weighing 21 kg) oral dose of albuterol sulfate. During marketing, various congenital anomalies, including cleft palate and limb defects, have been reported in the offspring of patients being treated with albuterol. Some of the mothers were taking multiple medications during their pregnancies. Because no consistent pattern of defects can be discerned, a relationship between albuterol use and congenital anomalies cannot be established.

Labor and Delivery: Oral albuterol has been shown to delay preterm labor in some reports. There are presently no well-controlled studies which demonstrate that it will stop preterm labor or prevent labor at term. Therefore, cautious use of VENTOLIN Syrup is required in pregnant patients when given for relief of bronchospasm so as to avoid interference with uterine contractility. Use in such patients should be restricted to those patients in whom the benefits clearly outweigh the risks.

Nursing Mothers: It is not known whether this drug is excreted in human milk. Because of the potential for tumorigenicity shown for albuterol in animal studies, a decision should be made whether to discontinue nursing or to discontinue the drug, taking into account the importance of the drug to the mother.

Pediatric Use: Safety and effectiveness in children below 2 years of age have not yet been adequately demonstrated.

ADVERSE REACTIONS

The adverse reactions to albuterol are similar in nature to those of other sympathomimetic agents. The most frequent adverse reactions to VENTOLIN Syrup in adults and older children were tremor, 10 of 100 patients; nervousness and shakiness, each 9 of 100 patients. Other reported adverse reactions were headache, 4 of 100 patients; dizziness and increased appetite, each 3 of 100 patients; hyperactivity and excitement, each 2 of 100 patients; tachycardia, epistaxis, irritable behavior, and sleeplessness, each 1 of 100 patients. The following adverse effects occurred in less than 1 of 100 patients each: muscle spasm; disturbed sleep; epigastric pain; cough; palpitations; stomach ache; irritable behavior; dilated pupils; sweating; chest pain; weakness.

In young children 2 to 6 years of age, some adverse reactions were noted more frequently than in adults and older children. Excitement was noted in approximately 20% of patients; and nervousness in 15%. Hyperkinesia occurred in 4% of patients; insomnia, tachycardia, and gastrointestinal symptoms in 2% each. Anorexia, emotional lability, pallor, fatigue, and conjunctivitis were seen in 1%.

In addition, albuterol, like other sympathomimetic agents, can cause adverse reactions such as hypertension, angina, vomiting, vertigo, central nervous system stimulation, unusual taste, and drying or irritation of the oropharynx.

The reactions are generally transient in nature, and it is usually not necessary to discontinue treatment with VENTOLIN Syrup. In selected cases, however, dosage may be reduced temporarily; after the reaction has subsided, dosage should be increased in small increments to the optimal dosage.

OVERDOSAGE

Manifestations of overdosage include anginal pain, hypertension, hypokalemia, and exaggeration of the effects listed in ADVERSE REACTIONS.

The oral LD_{50} in rats and mice was greater than 2,000 mg/kg. Dialysis is not appropriate treatment for overdosage of VENTOLIN Syrup. The judicious use of a cardioselective beta-receptor blocker, such as metoprolol tartrate, is suggested, bearing in mind the danger of inducing an asthmatic attack.

DOSAGE AND ADMINISTRATION

The following dosages of VENTOLIN Syrup are expressed in terms of albuterol base.

Usual Dose: The usual starting dosage for adults and children over 14 years of age is 2 mg (1 teaspoonful) or 4 mg (2 teaspoonfuls) three or four times a day.

The usual starting dosage for children 6 to 14 years of age is 2 mg (1 teaspoonful) three or four times a day.

For children 2 to 6 years of age, dosing should be initiated at 0.1 mg/kg of body weight three times a day. This starting dosage should not exceed 2 mg (1 teaspoonful) three times a day.

Dosage Adjustment: For adults and children over age 14, a dosage above 4 mg four times a day should be used *only* when the patient fails to respond. If a favorable response does not occur, the dosage may be cautiously increased stepwise, but the dosage should not exceed 8 mg four times a day.

For children from 6 to 14 years of age who fail to respond to the initial starting dosage of 2 mg four times a day, the dosage may be cautiously increased stepwise, but not to exceed 24 mg per day (given in divided doses).

For children 2 to 6 years of age who do not respond satisfactorily to the initial dosage, the dosage may be increased stepwise to 0.2 mg/kg of body weight three times a day, but not to exceed a maximum of 4 mg (2 teaspoonfuls) given three times a day.

For elderly patients and those sensitive to beta-adrenergic stimulation, the initial dosage should be restricted to 2 mg three or four times a day and individually adjusted thereafter.

Continued on next page

Glaxo Wellcome—Cont.

HOW SUPPLIED

VENTOLIN Syrup, a clear, orange-yellow liquid with a strawberry flavor, contains 2 mg albuterol as the sulfate per 5 mL; bottles of 16 fluid ounces (NDC 0173-0351-54).

Store between 2° and 30°C (36° and 86°F).

July 1996/RL-334

Shown in Product Identification Guide, page 315

VENTOLIN® ℞

(albuterol sulfate, USP)
Tablets

DESCRIPTION

Ventolin® (albuterol sulfate, USP) Tablets contain albuterol sulfate, USP, the racemic form of albuterol and a relatively selective $beta_2$-adrenergic bronchodilator. Albuterol sulfate has the chemical name (±) α^1-[(*tert*-butylamino)methyl]-4-hydroxy-*m*-xylene-α,α'-diol sulfate (2:1)(salt).

Albuterol sulfate has a molecular weight of 576.7, and the empirical formula is $(C_{13}H_{21}NO_3)_2 \cdot H_2SO_4$. Albuterol sulfate is a white crystalline powder, soluble in water and slightly soluble in ethanol.

The World Health Organization recommended name for albuterol base is salbutamol.

Each Ventolin Tablet contains 2 or 4 mg of albuterol as 2.4 or 4.8 mg, respectively, of albuterol sulfate. Each tablet also contains the inactive ingredients corn starch, lactose, and magnesium stearate.

CLINICAL PHARMACOLOGY

In vitro studies and *in vivo* pharmacologic studies have demonstrated that albuterol has a preferential effect on $beta_2$-adrenergic receptors compared with isoproterenol. While it is recognized that $beta_2$-adrenergic receptors are the predominant receptors in bronchial smooth muscle, recent data indicate that there is a population of $beta_2$-receptors in the human heart existing in a concentration between 10% and 50%. The precise function of these, however, is not yet established (see WARNINGS).

The pharmacologic effects of beta-adrenergic agonist drugs, including albuterol, are at least in part attributable to stimulation through beta-adrenergic receptors of intracellular adenyl cyclase, the enzyme that catalyzes the conversion of adenosine triphosphate (ATP) to cyclic-3',5'-adenosine monophosphate (cyclic AMP). Increased cyclic AMP levels are associated with relaxation of bronchial smooth muscle and inhibition of release of mediators of immediate hypersensitivity from cells, especially from mast cells.

Albuterol has been shown in most controlled clinical trials to have more effect on the respiratory tract, in the form of bronchial smooth muscle relaxation, than isoproterenol at comparable doses while producing fewer cardiovascular effects.

Albuterol is longer acting than isoproterenol in most patients by any route of administration because it is not a substrate to the cellular uptake processes for catecholamines nor for catechol-*O*-methyl transferase.

Animal studies show that albuterol does not pass the blood-brain barrier.

Recent studies in laboratory animals (minipigs, rodents, and dogs) recorded the occurrence of cardiac arrhythmias and sudden death (with histologic evidence of myocardial necrosis) when beta-agonists and methylxanthines were administered concurrently. The significance of these findings when applied to humans is currently unknown.

Albuterol is rapidly absorbed after oral administration of 4-mg Ventolin® (albuterol sulfate) Tablets in normal volunteers. Maximum plasma concentrations of about 18 ng/mL of albuterol are achieved within 2 hours, and the drug is eliminated with a half-life of about 5 hours.

In other studies, the analysis of urine samples of patients given 8 mg of tritiated albuterol orally showed that 76% of the dose was excreted over 3 days, with the majority of the dose being excreted within the first 24 hours. Sixty percent of this radioactivity was shown to be the metabolite. Feces collected over this period contained 4% of the administered dose.

INDICATIONS AND USAGE

Ventolin® (albuterol sulfate) Tablets are indicated for the relief of bronchospasm in patients with reversible obstructive airway disease.

In controlled clinical trials in patients with asthma, the onset of improvement in pulmonary function, as measured by maximum midexpiratory flow rate (MMEF), was within 30 minutes after a dose of Ventolin Tablets, with peak improvement occurring between 2 and 3 hours. In controlled clinical trials in which measurements were conducted for 6 hours, clinically significant improvement (defined as maintaining a 15% or more increase in forced expiratory volume in 1 second $[FEV_1]$ and a 20% or more increase in MMEF over baseline values) was observed in 60% of patients at 4 hours and in 40% at 6 hours. In other single-dose, controlled clinical trials, clinically significant improvement was observed in at least 40% of the patients at 8 hours. No decrease in the effectiveness of Ventolin Tablets has been reported in patients who received long-term treatment with the drug in uncontrolled studies for periods up to 6 months.

CONTRAINDICATIONS

Ventolin® (albuterol sulfate) Tablets are contraindicated in patients with a history of hypersensitivity to any of the components.

WARNINGS

Immediate hypersensitivity reactions may occur after administration of albuterol, as demonstrated by rare cases of urticaria, angioedema, rash, bronchospasm, and oropharyngeal edema. Albuterol, like other beta-adrenergic agonists, can produce a significant cardiovascular effect in some patients, as measured by pulse rate, blood pressure, symptoms, and/or electrocardiographic changes.

PRECAUTIONS

General: Albuterol, as with all sympathomimetic amines, should be used with caution in patients with cardiovascular disorders, especially coronary insufficiency, cardiac arrhythmias, and hypertension; in patients with convulsive disorders, hyperthyroidism, or diabetes mellitus; and in patients who are unusually responsive to sympathomimetic amines. Clinically significant changes in systolic and diastolic blood pressure have been seen in individual patients and could be expected to occur in some patients after use of any beta-adrenergic bronchodilator.

Large doses of intravenous albuterol have been reported to aggravate pre-existing diabetes mellitus and ketoacidosis. As with other beta-agonists, inhaled and intravenous albuterol may produce significant hypokalemia in some patients, possibly through intracellular shunting, which has the potential to produce adverse cardiovascular effects. The decrease is usually transient, not requiring supplementation.

Information for Patients: The action of Ventolin® (albuterol sulfate) Tablets may last for 8 hours or longer, and therefore they should not be taken more frequently than recommended. Do not increase the dose or frequency of medication without medical consultation. If symptoms get worse, medical consultation should be sought promptly.

Drug Interactions: The concomitant use of Ventolin Tablets and other oral sympathomimetic agents is not recommended since such combined use may lead to deleterious cardiovascular effects. This recommendation does not preclude the judicious use of an aerosol bronchodilator of the adrenergic stimulant type in patients receiving Ventolin Tablets. Such concomitant use, however, should be individualized and not given on a routine basis. If regular coadministration is required, then alternative therapy should be considered.

Albuterol should be administered with extreme caution to patients being treated with monoamine oxidase inhibitors or tricyclic antidepressants because the action of albuterol on the vascular system may be potentiated.

Beta-receptor blocking agents and albuterol inhibit the effect of each other.

Carcinogenesis, Mutagenesis, Impairment of Fertility: Albuterol sulfate caused a significant dose-related increase in the incidence of benign leiomyomas of the mesovarium in a 2-year study in the rat, at oral doses of 2, 10, and 50 mg/kg, corresponding to 3, 16, and 78 times, respectively, the maximum oral dose for a 50-kg human. In another study this effect was blocked by the coadministration of propranolol. The relevance of these findings to humans is not known. An 18-month study in mice and a lifetime study in hamsters revealed no evidence of tumorigenicity. Studies with albuterol revealed no evidence of mutagenesis. Reproduction studies in rats revealed no evidence of impaired fertility.

Pregnancy: ***Teratogenic Effects: Pregnancy Category C:*** Albuterol has been shown to be teratogenic in mice when given subcutaneously in doses corresponding to 0.4 times the maximum human oral dose. There are no adequate and well-controlled studies in pregnant women. Albuterol should be used during pregnancy only if the potential benefit justifies the potential risk to the fetus. A reproduction study in CD-1 mice given albuterol subcutaneously (0.025, 0.25, and 2.5 mg/kg, corresponding to 0.04, 0.4, and 3.9 times, respectively, the maximum oral dose for a 50-kg human) showed cleft palate formation in 5 of 111 (4.5%) fetuses at 0.25 mg/kg and in 10 of 108 (9.3%) fetuses at 2.5 mg/kg. None was observed at 0.025 mg/kg. Cleft palate also occurred in 22 of 72 (30.5%) fetuses treated with 2.5 mg/kg of isoproterenol (positive control). A reproduction study with oral albuterol in Stride Dutch rabbits revealed cranioschisis in 7 of 19 (37%) fetuses at 50 mg/kg, 78 times the maximum oral dose for a 50-kg human.

During worldwide marketing experience, various congenital anomalies, including cleft palate and limb defects, have been rarely reported in the offspring of patients being treated with albuterol. Some of the mothers were taking multiple medications during their pregnancies. No consistent pattern of defects can be discerned, and a relationship between albuterol use and congenital anomalies has not been established.

Labor and Delivery: Oral albuterol has been shown to delay preterm labor in some reports. There are presently no well-controlled studies that demonstrate that it will stop preterm labor or prevent labor at term. Therefore, cautious use of Ventolin Tablets is required in pregnant patients when given for relief of bronchospasm so as to avoid interference with uterine contractility. Use in such patients should be restricted to those patients in whom the benefits clearly outweigh the risks.

Nursing Mothers: It is not known whether this drug is excreted in human milk. Because of the potential for tumorigenicity shown for albuterol in animal studies, a decision should be made whether to discontinue nursing or to discontinue the drug, taking into account the importance of the drug to the mother.

Pediatric Use: Safety and effectiveness in children below 6 years of age have not been established.

ADVERSE REACTIONS

The adverse reactions to albuterol are similar in nature to reactions to other sympathomimetic agents, although the incidence of certain cardiovascular effects is lower with albuterol. The most frequent adverse reactions to Ventolin® (albuterol sulfate) Tablets were nervousness and tremor, with each occurring in approximately 20 of 100 patients. Other reported reactions were headache, 7 of 100 patients; tachycardia and palpitations, 5 of 100 patients; muscle cramps, 3 of 100 patients; and insomnia, nausea, weakness, and dizziness, each in 2 of 100 patients. Drowsiness, flushing, restlessness, irritability, chest discomfort, and difficulty in micturition each occurred in fewer than 1 of 100 patients. Rare cases of urticaria, angioedema, rash, bronchospasm, and oropharyngeal edema have been reported after the use of albuterol.

In addition, albuterol, like other sympathomimetic agents, can cause adverse reactions such as hypertension, angina, vomiting, vertigo, central nervous system stimulation, unusual taste, and drying or irritation of the oropharynx.

The reactions are generally transient in nature, and it is usually not necessary to discontinue treatment with Ventolin Tablets. In selected cases, however, dosage may be reduced temporarily; after the reaction has subsided, dosage should be increased in small increments to the optimal dosage.

OVERDOSAGE

The expected symptoms with overdosage are those of excessive beta-stimulation and/or occurrence or exaggeration of any of the symptoms listed under ADVERSE REACTIONS, e.g., seizures, angina, hypertension or hypotension, tachycardia with rates up to 200 beats per minute, arrhythmias, nervousness, headache, tremor, dry mouth, palpitation, nausea, dizziness, fatigue, malaise, and insomnia. Hypokalemia may also occur.

Treatment consists of discontinuation of albuterol together with appropriate symptomatic therapy.

The oral LD_{50} in male and female rats and mice was greater than 2,000 mg/kg.

There is insufficient evidence to determine if dialysis is beneficial for overdosage of Ventolin® (albuterol sulfate) Tablets.

DOSAGE AND ADMINISTRATION

The following dosages of Ventolin® (albuterol sulfate) Tablets are expressed in terms of albuterol base.

Usual Dosage: The usual starting dosage for adults and children 12 years and older is 2 or 4 mg three or four times a day.

The usual starting dosage for children 6 to 12 years of age is 2 mg three or four times a day.

Dosage Adjustment: For adults and children 12 years and older, a dosage above 4 mg four times a day should be used *only* when the patient fails to respond. If a favorable response does not occur with the 4-mg initial dosage, it should be cautiously increased stepwise up to a maximum of 8 mg four times a day as tolerated.

For children from 6 to 12 years of age who fail to respond to the initial starting dosage of 2 mg four times a day, the dosage may be cautiously increased stepwise, but not to exceed 24 mg per day (given in divided doses).

Elderly Patients and Those Sensitive to Beta-adrenergic Stimulators: An initial dosage of 2 mg three or four times a day is recommended for elderly patients and for those with a history of unusual sensitivity to beta-adrenergic stimulators. If adequate bronchodilatation is not obtained, dosage may be increased gradually to as much as 8 mg three or four times a day.

The total daily dose should not exceed 32 mg in adults and children 12 years and older.

HOW SUPPLIED

Ventolin® (albuterol sulfate) Tablets, 2 mg of albuterol as the sulfate, are white, round compressed tablets impressed with the product name (VENTOLIN) and the number 2 on

one side and scored on the other with "GLAXO" impressed on each side of the score in bottles of 100 (NDC 0173-0341-43) and 500 (NDC 0173-0341-44).
Ventolin Tablets, 4 mg of albuterol as the sulfate, are white, round, compressed tablets impressed with the product name (VENTOLIN) and the number 4 on one side and scored on the other with "GLAXO" impressed on each side of the score in bottles of 100 (NDC 0173-0342-43) and 500 (NDC 0173-0342-44).

Store between 2° and 25°C (36° and 77°F). Replace cap securely after each opening.

March 1994/RL-082

Shown in Product Identification Guide, page 315

VIROPTIC® ℞
[*vī-rŏp'tĭk"*]
(trifluridine)
Ophthalmic Solution, 1% Sterile

DESCRIPTION

VIROPTIC is the brand name for trifluridine (also known as trifluorothymidine, F_3TdR, F_3T), an antiviral drug for topical treatment of epithelial keratitis caused by Herpes simplex virus. The chemical name of trifluridine is α-α-α-trifluorothymidine.
VIROPTIC sterile ophthalmic solution contains 1% trifluridine in an aqueous solution with acetic acid and sodium acetate (buffers), sodium chloride, and thimerosal 0.001% (added as a preservative).

CLINICAL PHARMACOLOGY

Trifluridine is a fluorinated pyrimidine nucleoside with *in vitro* and *in vivo* activity against Herpes simplex virus, types 1 and 2 and vacciniavirus. Some strains of Adenovirus are also inhibited *in vitro*.
Trifluridine interferes with DNA synthesis in cultured mammalian cells. However, its antiviral mechanism of action is not completely known.
In vitro perfusion studies on excised rabbit corneas have shown that trifluridine penetrates the intact cornea as evidenced by recovery of parental drug and its major metabolite, 5-carboxy-2′-deoxyuridine, on the endothelial side of the cornea. Absence of the corneal epithelium enhances the penetration of trifluridine approximately two-fold.
Intraocular penetration of trifluridine occurs after topical instillation of VIROPTIC into human eyes. Decreased corneal integrity or stromal or uveal inflammation may enhance the penetration of trifluridine into the aqueous humor. Unlike the results of ocular penetration of trifluridine *in vitro*, 5-carboxy-2′-deoxyuridine was not found in detectable concentrations within the aqueous humor of the human eye.
Systemic absorption of trifluridine following therapeutic dosing with VIROPTIC appears to be negligible. No detectable concentrations of trifluridine or 5-carboxy-2′-deoxyuridine were found in the sera of adult healthy normal subjects who had VIROPTIC instilled into their eyes seven times daily for 14 consecutive days.

INDICATIONS AND USAGE

VIROPTIC (trifluridine) Ophthalmic Solution, 1% is indicated for the treatment of primary keratoconjunctivitis and recurrent epithelial keratitis due to Herpes simplex virus, types 1 and 2. VIROPTIC is also effective in the treatment of epithelial keratitis that has not responded clinically to the topical administration of idoxuridine or when ocular toxicity or hypersensitivity to idoxuridine has occurred. In a smaller number of patients found to be resistant to topical vidarabine, VIROPTIC was also effective.
The clinical efficacy of VIROPTIC in the treatment of stromal keratitis and uveitis due to Herpes simplex virus or ophthalmic infections caused by vacciniavirus and Adenovirus has not been established by well-controlled clinical trials. VIROPTIC has not been shown to be effective in the prophylaxis of Herpes simplex virus keratoconjunctivitis and epithelial keratitis by well-controlled clinical trials. VIROPTIC isnot effective against bacterial, fungal, or chlamydial infections of the cornea or nonviral trophic lesions.
During controlled multicenter clinical trials, 92 of 97 (95%) patients (78 of 81 with dendritic and 14 of 16 with geographic ulcers) responded to therapy with VIROPTIC as evidenced by complete corneal re-epithelialization within the 14-day therapy period. In these controlled studies, 56 of 75 (75%) patients (49 of 58 with dendritic and 7 of 17 with geographic ulcers) responded to idoxuridine therapy. The mean time to corneal re-epithelialization for dendritic ulcers (6 days) and geographic ulcers (7 days) was similar for both therapies. In other clinical studies, VIROPTIC was evaluated in the treatment of Herpes simplex virus keratitis in patients who were unresponsive or intolerant to the topical administration of idoxuridine or vidarabine. VIROPTIC was effective in 138 of 150 (92%) patients (109 of 114 with dendritic and 29 of 36 with geographic ulcers) as evidenced by corneal re-epithelialization. The mean time to corneal re-epithelialization was 6 days for patients with dendritic ulcers and 12 days for patients with geographic ulcers.

CONTRAINDICATIONS

VIROPTIC (trifluridine) Ophthalmic Solution, 1%, is contraindicated for patients who develop hypersensitivity reactions or chemical intolerance to trifluridine.

WARNINGS

The recommended dosage and frequency of administration should not be exceeded (see DOSAGE AND ADMINISTRATION).

PRECAUTIONS

General: VIROPTIC (trifluridine) Ophthalmic Solution, 1% should be prescribed only for patients who have a clinical diagnosis of herpetic keratitis.
VIROPTIC may cause mild local irritation of the conjunctiva and cornea when instilled, but these effects are usually transient.
Although documented *in vitro* viral resistance to trifluridine has not been reported following multiple exposure to VIROPTIC, the possibility exists of viral resistance development.
Drug Interactions: The following drugs have been administered topically to the eye and concurrently with VIROPTIC in a limited number of patients without apparent evidence of adverse interaction: antibiotics—chloramphenicol, erythromycin, polymyxin B sulfate, bacitracin, gentamicin sulfate, tetracycline HCl, sodium sulfacetamide, neomycin sulfate; steroids—dexamethasone, dexamethasone sodium phosphate, prednisolone acetate, prednisolone sodium phosphate, hydrocortisone, fluorometholone; and other ophthalmic drugs—atropine sulfate, scopolamine hydrobromide, naphazoline hydrochloride, cyclopentolate hydrochloride, homatropine hydrobromide, pilocarpine, l-epinephrine hydrochloride, sodium chloride.
Carcinogenesis, Mutagenesis, Impairment of Fertility: ***Mutagenic Potential:*** Trifluridine has been shown to exert mutagenic, DNA-damaging, and cell-transforming activities in various standard *in vitro* test systems, and clastogenic activity in *Vicia faba* cells. It did not induce chromosome aberrations in bone marrow cells of male or female rats following a single subcutaneous dose of 100 mg/kg, but was weakly positive in female, but not in male, rats following daily subcutaneous administration at 700 mg/kg/day for 5 days.
Although the significance of these test results is not clear or fully understood, there exists the possibility that mutagenic agents may cause genetic damage in humans.
Oncogenic Potential: Lifetime carcinogenicity bioassays in rats and mice given daily subcutaneous doses of trifluridine have been performed. Rats tested at 1.5, 7.5, and 15 mg/kg/day had increased incidences of adenocarcinomas of the intestinal tract and mammary glands, hemangiosarcomas of the spleen and liver, carcinosarcomas of the prostate gland, and granulosa-thecal cell tumors of the ovary. Mice were tested at 1, 5, and 10 mg/kg/day; those given 10 mg/kg/day trifluridine had significantly increased incidences of adenocarcinomas of the intestinal tract and uterus. Those given 10 mg/kg/day also had a significantly increased incidence of testicular atrophy as compared to vehicle control mice.
Pregnancy: ***Teratogenic Effects:*** Pregnancy Category C. Trifluridine was not teratogenic at doses up to 5.0 mg/kg/day (23 times the estimated human exposure) when given subcutaneously to rats and rabbits. However, fetal toxicity consisting of delayed ossification of portions of the skeleton occurred at dose levels of 2.5 and 5.0 mg/kg/day in rats and at 2.5 mg/kg/day in rabbits. In addition, both 2.5 and 5.0 mg/kg/day produced fetal death and resorption in rabbits. In both rats and rabbits, 1.0 mg/kg/day (5 times the estimated human exposure) was a no-effect level. There were no teratogenic or fetotoxic effects after topical application of VIROPTIC Ophthalmic Solution 1% (approximately 5 times the estimated human exposure) to the eyes of rabbits on the 6th through the 18th days of pregnancy.[1] In a non-standard test, trifluridine solution has been shown to be teratogenic when injected directly into the yolk sac of chicken eggs.[2] There are no adequate and well-controlled studies in pregnant women. VIROPTIC Ophthalmic Solution 1% should be used during pregnancy only if the potential benefit justifies the potential risk to the fetus.
Nursing Mothers: It is unlikely that trifluridine is excreted in human milk after ophthalmic instillation of VIROPTIC because of the relatively small dosage (≤ 5.0 mg/day), its dilution in body fluids, and its extremely short half-life (approximately 12 minutes). The drug should not be prescribed for nursing mothers unless the potential benefits outweigh the potential risks.

ADVERSE REACTIONS

The most frequent adverse reactions reported during controlled clinical trials were mild, transient burning or stinging upon instillation (4.6%) and palpebral edema (2.8%). Other adverse reactions in decreasing order of reported frequency were superficial punctate keratopathy, epithelial keratopathy, hypersensitivity reaction, stromal edema, irritation, keratitis sicca, hyperemia, and increased intraocular pressure.

OVERDOSAGE

Overdosage by ocular instillation is unlikely because any excess solution should be quickly expelled from the conjunctival sac.
Acute overdosage by accidental oral ingestion of VIROPTIC has not occurred. However, should such ingestion occur, the 75 mg dosage of trifluridine in a 7.5 mL bottle of VIROPTIC is not likely to produce adverse effects. Single intravenous doses of 1.5 to 30 mg/kg/day in children and adults with neoplastic disease produce reversible bone marrow depression as the only potentially serious toxic effect and only after 3 to 5 courses of therapy.[3] The acute oral LD_{50} in the mouse and rat was 4379 mg/kg or higher.

DOSAGE AND ADMINISTRATION

Instill one drop of VIROPTIC Ophthalmic Solution, 1% onto the cornea of the affected eye every 2 hours while awake for a maximum daily dosage of nine drops until the corneal ulcer has completely re-epithelialized. Following re-epithelialization, treatment for an additional 7 days of one drop every 4 hours while awake for a minimum daily dosage of five drops is recommended.
If there are no signs of improvement after seven days of therapy or complete re-epithelialization has not occurred after 14 days of therapy, other forms of therapy should be considered. Continuous administration of VIROPTIC for periods exceeding 21 days should be avoided because of potential ocular toxicity.

HOW SUPPLIED

VIROPTIC Ophthalmic Solution, 1% is supplied as a sterile ophthalmic solution in a plastic Drop Dose® dispenser bottle of 7.5 mL. (NDC 0173-0968-02)
Store under refrigeration 2° to 8°C (36° to 46°F).

ANIMAL PHARMACOLOGY AND ANIMAL TOXICOLOGY

Corneal wound healing studies in rabbits showed that VIROPTIC did not significantly retard closure of epithelial wounds. However, mild toxic changes such as intracellular edema of the basal cell layer, mild thinning of the overlying epithelium, and reduced strength of stromal wounds were observed.
Whereas instillation of VIROPTIC into rabbit eyes during a subchronic toxicity study produced some degree of corneal epithelial thinning, a 12-month chronic toxicity study in rabbits in which VIROPTIC was instilled into eyes in intermittent, multiple, full-therapy courses showed no drug-related changes in the cornea.

REFERENCES

1. Itoi M, Getter JW, Kaneko N, et al. Teratogenicities of ophthalmic drugs. I. Antiviral ophthalmic drugs. *Arch Ophthalmol.*1975;93:46-51.
2. Kury G, Crosby RJ. The teratogenic effect of 5-trifluoromethyl-2′-deoxyuridine in chicken embryos. *Toxicol Appl Pharmacol.* 1967;11:72-80.
3. Ansfield FJ, Ramirez G. Phase I and II studies of 2′-deoxy-5-(trifluoromethyl)-uridine (NSC-75520). *Cancer Chemother Rep.* 1971;55(pt 1):205-208.

January 1996/RL-258

Shown in Product Identification Guide, page 315

WELLBUTRIN® ℞
[*wel 'byü-trin*]
(bupropion hydrochloride)
Tablets

DESCRIPTION

Wellbutrin (bupropion hydrochloride), an antidepressant of the aminoketone class, is chemically unrelated to tricyclic, tetracyclic, or other known antidepressant agents. Its structure closely resembles that of diethylpropion; it is related to phenylethylamines. It is designated as (±)-1-(3-chlorophenyl)-2-[(1,1-dimethylethyl)amino]-1-propanone hydrochloride. The molecular weight is 276.2. The empirical formula is $C_{13}H_{18}ClNO \cdot HCl$. Bupropion powder is white, crystalline, and highly soluble in water. It has a bitter taste and produces the sensation of local anesthesia on the oral mucosa.
Wellbutrin is supplied for oral administration as 75 mg (yellow-gold) and 100 mg (red) film-coated tablets. Each tablet contains the labeled amount of bupropion hydrochloride and the inactive ingredients: 75 mg tablet—D&C Yellow No. 10 Lake, FD&C Yellow No. 6 Lake, hydroxypropyl cellulose, hydroxypropyl methylcellulose, microcrystalline cellulose, polyethylene glycol, talc, and titanium dioxide; 100 mg tablet—FD&C Red No. 40 Lake, FD&C Yellow No. 6 Lake, hydroxypropyl cellulose, hydroxypropyl methylcellulose, microcrystalline cellulose, polyethylene glycol, talc, and titanium dioxide.

Continued on next page

Glaxo Wellcome—Cont.

CLINICAL PHARMACOLOGY

Pharmacodynamics and Pharmacological Actions: The neurochemical mechanism of the antidepressant effect of bupropion is not known. Bupropion does not inhibit monoamine oxidase. Compared to classical tricyclic antidepressants, it is a weak blocker of the neuronal uptake of serotonin and norepinephrine; it also inhibits the neuronal re-uptake of dopamine to some extent.

Bupropion produces dose-related CNS stimulant effects in animals, as evidenced by increased locomotor activity, increased rates of responding in various schedule-controlled operant behavior tasks, and, at high doses, induction of mild stereotyped behavior.

Bupropion causes convulsions in rodents and dogs at doses approximately tenfold the dose recommended as the human antidepressant dose.

Absorption, Distribution, Pharmacokinetics, Metabolism, and Elimination:

Oral bioavailability and single-dose pharmacokinetics: In humans, following oral administration of WELLBUTRIN, peak plasma bupropion concentrations are usually achieved within 2 hours, followed by a biphasic decline. The average half-life of the second (post-distributional) phase is approximately 14 hours, with a range of 8 to 24 hours. Six hours after a single dose, plasma bupropion concentrations are approximately 30% of peak concentrations. Plasma bupropion concentrations are dose-proportional following single doses of 100 to 250 mg; however, it is not known if the proportionality between dose and plasma level is maintained in chronic use.

The absolute bioavailability of WELLBUTRIN tablets in humans has not been determined because an intravenous formulation for human use is not available.

However, it appears likely that only a small proportion of any orally administered dose reaches the systemic circulation intact. For example, the absolute bioavailability of bupropion in animals (rats and dogs) ranges from 5% to 20%.

Metabolism: Following oral administration of 200 mg of ^{14}C-bupropion, 87% and 10% of the radioactive dose were recovered in the urine and feces, respectively. However, the fraction of the oral dose of WELLBUTRIN excreted unchanged was only 0.5%, a finding documenting the extensive metabolism of bupropion.

Several of the known metabolites of bupropion are pharmacologically active, but their potency and toxicity relative to bupropion have not been fully characterized. However, because of their longer elimination half-lives, the plasma concentrations of at least two of the known metabolites can be expected, especially in chronic use, to be very much higher than the plasma concentration of bupropion. This is of potential clinical importance because factors or conditions altering metabolic capacity (e.g., liver disease, congestive heart failure, age, concomitant medications, etc.) or elimination may be expected to influence the degree and extent of accumulation of these active metabolites.

Furthermore, bupropion has been shown to induce its own metabolism in three animal species (mice, rats, and dogs) following subchronic administration. If induction also occurs in humans, the relative contribution of bupropion and its metabolites to the clinical effects of WELLBUTRIN may be changed in chronic use.

Plasma and urinary metabolites so far identified include biotransformation products formed via reduction of the carbonyl group and/or hydroxylation of the *tert-* butyl group of bupropion. Four basic metabolites have been identified. They are the *erythro-* and *threo-* amino alcohols of bupropion, the *erythro-* amino diol of bupropion, and a morpholinol metabolite (formed from hydroxylation of the *tert-* butyl group of bupropion).

The morpholinol metabolite appears in the systemic circulation almost as rapidly as the parent drug following a single oral dose. Its peak level is three times the peak level of the parent drug; it has a half-life on the order of 24 hours; and its AUC 0 to 60 hours is about 15 times that of bupropion.

The *threo-* amino alcohol metabolite has a plasma concentration-time profile similar to that of the morpholinol metabolite. The *erythro*-amino alcohol and the *erythro-* amino diol metabolites generally cannot be detected in the systemic circulation following a single oral dose of the parent drug. The morpholinol and the *threo-* amino alcohol metabolites have been found to be half as potent as bupropion in animal screening tests for antidepressant drugs.

During a chronic dosing study in 14 depressed patients with left ventricular dysfunction, it was found that there was substantial interpatient variability (two- to fivefold) in the trough steady-state concentrations of bupropion and the morpholinol and *threo-* amino alcohol metabolites. In addition, the steady-state plasma concentrations of these metabolites were 10 to 100 times the steady-state concentrations of the parent drug.

The effect of other disease states and altered organ function on the metabolism and/or elimination of bupropion has not

been studied in detail. However, the elimination of the major metabolites of bupropion may be affected by reduced renal or hepatic function because they are moderately polar compounds and are likely to undergo conjugation in the liver prior to urinary excretion. The preliminary results of a comparative single-dose pharmacokinetic study in normal versus cirrhotic patients indicated that half-lives of the metabolites were prolonged by cirrhosis and that the metabolites accumulated to levels two to three times those in normals. The effect of age on plasma concentrations of bupropion and its metabolites has not been characterized.

In vitro tests show that bupropion is 80% or more bound to human albumin at plasma concentrations up to 800 micromolar (200 μg/mL).

INDICATIONS AND USAGE

WELLBUTRIN is indicated for the treatment of depression. A physician considering WELLBUTRIN for the management of a patient's first episode of depression should be aware that the drug may cause generalized seizures with an approximate incidence of 0.4% (4/1000). This incidence of seizures may exceed that of other marketed antidepressants by as much as fourfold. This relative risk is only an approximate estimate because no direct comparative studies have been conducted.

The efficacy of WELLBUTRIN has been established in three placebo-controlled trials, including two of approximately 3 weeks duration in depressed inpatients, and one of approximately 6 weeks duration in depressed outpatients. The depressive disorder of the patients studied corresponds most closely to the Major Depression category of the APA Diagnostic and Statistical Manual III.

Major Depression implies a prominent and relatively persistent depressed or dysphoric mood that usually interferes with daily functioning (nearly every day for at least 2 weeks); it should include at least four of the following eight symptoms: change in appetite, change in sleep, psychomotor agitation or retardation, loss of interest in usual activities or decrease in sexual drive, increased fatigability, feelings of guilt or worthlessness, slowed thinking or impaired concentration, and suicidal ideation or attempts.

Effectiveness of WELLBUTRIN in long-term use, that is, for more than 6 weeks, has not been systematically evaluated in controlled trials. Therefore, the physician who elects to use WELLBUTRIN for extended periods should periodically re-evaluate the long-term usefulness of the drug for the individual patient.

CONTRAINDICATIONS

WELLBUTRIN is contraindicated in patients with a seizure disorder. WELLBUTRIN is also contraindicated in patients with a current or prior diagnosis of bulimia or anorexia nervosa because of a higher incidence of seizures noted in such patients treated with WELLBUTRIN. The concurrent administration of WELLBUTRIN and a monoamine oxidase (MAO) inhibitor is contraindicated. At least 14 days should elapse between discontinuation of an MAO inhibitor and initiation of treatment with WELLBUTRIN. WELLBUTRIN is contraindicated in patients who have shown an allergic response to it.

WARNINGS

SEIZURES: WELLBUTRIN is associated with seizures in approximately 0.4% (4/1000) of patients treated at doses up to 450 mg/day. This incidence of seizures may exceed that of other marketed antidepressants by as much as fourfold. This relative risk is only an approximate estimate because no direct comparative studies have been conducted. The estimated seizure incidence for WELLBUTRIN increases almost tenfold between 450 and 600 mg/day, which is twice the usually required daily dose (300 mg) and one and one-third the maximum recommended daily dose (450 mg). Given the wide variability among individuals and their capacity to metabolize and eliminate drugs, this disproportionate increase in seizure incidence with dose incrementation calls for caution in dosing.

During the initial development, 25 among approximately 2400 patients treated with WELLBUTRIN experienced seizures. At the time of seizure, seven patients were receiving daily doses of 450 mg or below for an incidence of 0.33% (3/1000) within the recommended dose range. Twelve patients experienced seizures at 600 mg per day (2.3% incidence); six additional patients had seizures at daily doses between 600 and 900 mg (2.8% incidence).

A separate, prospective study was conducted to determine the incidence of seizure during an 8-week treatment exposure in approximately 3200 additional patients who received daily doses of up to 450 mg. Patients were permitted to continue treatment beyond 8 weeks if clinically indicated. Eight seizures occurred during the initial 8-week treatment period and five seizures were reported in patients continuing treatment beyond 8 weeks, resulting in a total seizure incidence of 0.4%.

The risk of seizure appears to be strongly associated with dose and the presence of predisposing factors. A significant predisposing factor (e.g., history of head trauma or prior seizure, CNS tumor, concomitant medications that lower sei-

zure threshold, etc.) was present in approximately one-half of the patients experiencing a seizure. Sudden and large increments in dose may contribute to increased risk. While many seizures occurred early in the course of treatment, some seizures did occur after several weeks at fixed dose.

Recommendations for reducing the risk of seizure: Retrospective analysis of clinical experience gained during the development of WELLBUTRIN suggests that the risk of seizure may be minimized if (1) the total daily dose of WELLBUTRIN does *not* exceed 450 mg, (2) the daily dose is administered t.i.d., with each single dose *not* to exceed 150 mg to avoid high peak concentrations of bupropion and/or its metabolites, and (3) the rate of incrementation of dose is very gradual. Extreme caution should be used when WELLBUTRIN is (1) administered to patients with a history of seizure, cranial trauma, or other predisposition(s) toward seizure, or (2) prescribed with other agents (e.g., antipsychotics, other antidepressants, etc.) or treatment regimens (e.g., abrupt discontinuation of a benzodiazepine) that lower seizure threshold.

Potential for Hepatotoxicity: In rats receiving large doses of bupropion chronically, there was an increase in incidence of hepatic hyperplastic nodules and hepatocellular hypertrophy. In dogs receiving large doses of bupropion chronically, various histologic changes were seen in the liver, and laboratory tests suggesting mild hepatocellular injury were noted. Although scattered abnormalities in liver function tests were detected in patients participating in clinical trials, there is no clinical evidence that bupropion acts as a hepatotoxin in humans.

PRECAUTIONS

General:

Agitation and Insomnia: A substantial proportion of patients treated with WELLBUTRIN experience some degree of increased restlessness, agitation, anxiety, and insomnia, especially shortly after initiation of treatment. In clinical studies, these symptoms were sometimes of sufficient magnitude to require treatment with sedative/hypnotic drugs. In approximately 2% of patients, symptoms were sufficiently severe to require discontinuation of treatment with WELLBUTRIN.

Psychosis, Confusion, and Other Neuropsychiatric Phenomena: Patients treated with WELLBUTRIN have been reported to show a variety of neuropsychiatric signs and symptoms including delusions, hallucinations, psychotic episodes, confusion, and paranoia. Because of the uncontrolled nature of many studies, it is impossible to provide a precise estimate of the extent of risk imposed by treatment with WELLBUTRIN. In several cases, neuropsychiatric phenomena abated upon dose reduction and/or withdrawal of treatment.

Activation of Psychosis and/or Mania: Antidepressants can precipitate manic episodes in Bipolar Manic Depressive patients during the depressed phase of their illness and may activate latent psychosis in other susceptible patients. WELLBUTRIN is expected to pose similar risks.

Altered Appetite and Weight: A weight loss of greater than 5 pounds occurred in 28% of patients receiving WELLBUTRIN. This incidence is approximately double that seen in comparable patients treated with tricyclics or placebo. Furthermore, while 34.5% of patients receiving tricyclic antidepressants gained weight, only 9.4% of patients treated with WELLBUTRIN did. Consequently, if weight loss is a major presenting sign of a patient's depressive illness, the anorectic and/or weight reducing potential of WELLBUTRIN should be considered.

Suicide: The possibility of a suicide attempt is inherent in depression and may persist until significant remission occurs. Accordingly, prescriptions for WELLBUTRIN should be written for the smallest number of tablets consistent with good patient management.

Use in Patients with Systemic Illness: There is no clinical experience establishing the safety of WELLBUTRIN in patients with a recent history of myocardial infarction or unstable heart disease. Therefore, care should be exercised if it is used in these groups. WELLBUTRIN was well tolerated in patients who had previously developed orthostatic hypotension while receiving tricyclic antidepressants.

Because bupropion HCl and its metabolites are almost completely excreted through the kidney and metabolites are likely to undergo conjugation in the liver prior to urinary excretion, treatment of patients with renal or hepatic impairment should be initiated at reduced dosage as bupropion and its metabolites may accumulate in such patients beyond concentrations expected in patients without renal or hepatic impairment. The patient should be closely monitored for possible toxic effects of elevated blood and tissue levels of drug and metabolites.

Information for Patients: Physicians are advised to discuss the following issues with patients:

Patients should be instructed to take WELLBUTRIN in equally divided doses three or four times a day to minimize the risk of seizure.

Patients should be told that any CNS-active drug like WELLBUTRIN may impair their ability to perform tasks

requiring judgment or motor and cognitive skills. Consequently, until they are reasonably certain that WELLBUTRIN does not adversely affect their performance, they should refrain from driving an automobile or operating complex, hazardous machinery.

Patients should be told that the use and cessation of use of alcohol may alter the seizure threshold, and, therefore, that the consumption of alcohol should be minimized, and, if possible, avoided completely.

Patients should be advised to inform their physician if they are taking or plan to take any prescription or over-the-counter drugs. Concern is warranted because WELLBUTRIN and other drugs may affect each other's metabolism.

Patients should be advised to notify their physician if they become pregnant or intend to become pregnant during therapy.

Drug Interactions: No systematic data have been collected on the consequences of the concomitant administration of WELLBUTRIN and other drugs.

However, animal data suggest that WELLBUTRIN may be an inducer of drug metabolizing enzymes. This may be of potential clinical importance because the blood levels of co-administered drugs may be altered.

Alternatively, because bupropion is extensively metabolized, the co-administration of other drugs may affect its clinical activity. In particular, care should be exercised when administering drugs known to affect hepatic drug-metabolizing enzyme systems (e.g., carbamazepine, cimetidine, phenobarbital, phenytoin).

Studies in animals demonstrate that the acute toxicity of bupropion is enhanced by the MAO inhibitor phenelzine (see CONTRAINDICATIONS).

Limited clinical data suggest a higher incidence of adverse experiences in patients receiving concurrent administration of WELLBUTRIN and L-dopa. Administration of WELLBUTRIN to patients receiving L-dopa concurrently should be undertaken with caution, using small initial doses and small gradual dose increases.

Concurrent administration of WELLBUTRIN and agents which lower seizure threshold should be undertaken only with extreme caution (see WARNINGS). Low initial dosing and small gradual dose increases should be employed.

Carcinogenesis, Mutagenesis, Impairment of Fertility: Lifetime carcinogenicity studies were performed in rats and mice at doses up to 300 and 150 mg/kg/day, respectively. In the rat study there was an increase in nodular proliferative lesions of the liver at doses of 100 to 300 mg/kg/day; lower doses were not tested. The question of whether or not such lesions may be precursors of neoplasms of the liver is currently unresolved. Similar liver lesions were not seen in the mouse study, and no increase in malignant tumors of the liver and other organs was seen in either study.

Bupropion produced a borderline positive response (2 to 3 times control mutation rate) in some strains in the Ames bacterial mutagenicity test, and a high oral dose (300, but not 100 or 200 mg/kg) produced a low incidence of chromosomal aberrations in rats. The relevance of these results in estimating the risk of human exposure to therapeutic doses is unknown.

A fertility study was performed in rats; no evidence of impairment of fertility was encountered at oral doses up to 300 mg/kg/day.

Pregnancy: ***Teratogenic Effects:*** Pregnancy Category B: Reproduction studies have been performed in rabbits and rats at doses up to 15 to 45 times the human daily dose and have revealed no definitive evidence of impaired fertility or harm to the fetus due to bupropion. (In rabbits, a slightly increased incidence of fetal abnormalities was seen in two studies, but there was no increase in any specific abnormality). There are no adequate and well-controlled studies in pregnant women. Because animal reproduction studies are not always predictive of human response, this drug should be used during pregnancy only if clearly needed.

Labor and Delivery: The effect of WELLBUTRIN on labor and delivery in humans is unknown.

Nursing Mothers: Because of the potential for serious adverse reactions in nursing infants from WELLBUTRIN, a decision should be made whether to discontinue nursing or to discontinue the drug, taking into account the importance of the drug to the mother.

Pediatric Use: The safety and effectiveness of WELLBUTRIN in individuals under 18 years old have not been established.

Use in the Elderly: WELLBUTRIN has not been systematically evaluated in older patients.

ADVERSE REACTIONS

(See also WARNINGS and PRECAUTIONS) Adverse events commonly encountered in patients treated with WELLBUTRIN are agitation, dry mouth, insomnia, headache/migraine, nausea/vomiting, constipation, and tremor.

Adverse events were sufficiently troublesome to cause discontinuation of treatment with WELLBUTRIN in approximately 10% of the 2400 patients and volunteers who participated in clinical trials during the product's initial development. The more common events causing discontinuation include neuropsychiatric disturbances (3.0%), primarily agitation and abnormalities in mental status; gastrointestinal disturbances (2.1%), primarily nausea and vomiting; neurological disturbances (1.7%), primarily seizures, headaches, and sleep disturbances; and dermatologic problems (1.4%), primarily rashes. It is important to note, however, that many of these events occurred at doses that exceed the recommended daily dose.

Accurate estimates of the incidence of adverse events associated with the use of any drug are difficult to obtain. Estimates are influenced by drug dose, detection technique, setting, physician judgments, etc. Consequently, the table below is presented solely to indicate the relative frequency of adverse events reported in representative controlled clinical studies conducted to evaluate the safety and efficacy of WELLBUTRIN under relatively similar conditions of daily dosage (300 to 600 mg), setting, and duration (3 to 4 weeks). The figures cited cannot be used to predict precisely the incidence of untoward events in the course of usual medical practice where patient characteristics and other factors must differ from those which prevailed in the clinical trials. These incidence figures also cannot be compared with those obtained from other clinical studies involving related drug products as each group of drug trials is conducted under a different set of conditions.

Finally, it is important to emphasize that the tabulation does not reflect the relative severity and/or clinical importance of the events. A better perspective on the serious adverse events associated with the use of WELLBUTRIN is provided in WARNINGS and PRECAUTIONS.

[See table above.]

TREATMENT EMERGENT ADVERSE EXPERIENCE INCIDENCE IN PLACEBO-CONTROLLED CLINICAL TRIALS*
(Percent of Patients Reporting)

Adverse Experience	WELLBUTRIN Patients (n = 323)	Placebo Patients (n = 185)
CARDIOVASCULAR		
Cardiac Arrhythmias	5.3	4.3
Dizziness	22.3	16.2
Hypertension	4.3	1.6
Hypotension	2.5	2.2
Palpitations	3.7	2.2
Syncope	1.2	0.5
Tachycardia	10.8	8.6
DERMATOLOGIC		
Pruritus	2.2	0.0
Rash	8.0	6.5
GASTROINTESTINAL		
Anorexia	18.3	18.4
Appetite Increase	3.7	2.2
Constipation	26.0	17.3
Diarrhea	6.8	8.6
Dyspepsia	3.1	2.2
Nausea/Vomiting	22.9	18.9
Weight Gain	13.6	22.7
Weight Loss	23.2	23.2
GENITOURINARY		
Impotence	3.4	3.1
Menstrual Complaints	4.7	1.1
Urinary Frequency	2.5	2.2
Urinary Retention	1.9	2.2
MUSCULOSKELETAL		
Arthritis	3.1	2.7
NEUROLOGICAL		
Akathisia	1.5	1.1
Akinesia/Bradykinesia	8.0	8.6
Cutaneous Temperature Disturbance	1.9	1.6
Dry Mouth	27.6	18.4
Excessive Sweating	22.3	14.6
Headache/Migraine	25.7	22.2
Impaired Sleep Quality	4.0	1.6
Increased Salivary Flow	3.4	3.8
Insomnia	18.6	15.7
Muscle Spasms	1.9	3.2
Pseudoparkinsonism	1.5	1.6
Sedation	19.8	19.5
Sensory Disturbance	4.0	3.2
Tremor	21.1	7.6
NEUROPSYCHIATRIC		
Agitation	31.9	22.2
Anxiety	3.1	1.1
Confusion	8.4	4.9
Decreased Libido	3.1	1.6
Delusions	1.2	1.1
Disturbed Concentration	3.1	3.8
Euphoria	1.2	0.5
Hostility	5.6	3.8
NONSPECIFIC		
Fatigue	5.0	8.6
Fever/Chills	1.2	0.5
RESPIRATORY		
Upper Respiratory Complaints	5.0	11.4
SPECIAL SENSES		
Auditory Disturbance	5.3	3.2
Blurred Vision	14.6	10.3
Gustatory Disturbance	3.1	1.1

*Events reported by at least 1% of Wellbutrin patients are included.

Other Events Observed During the Development of WELLBUTRIN: The conditions and duration of exposure to Wellbutrin varied greatly and a substantial proportion of the experience was gained in open and uncontrolled clinical settings. During this experience, numerous adverse events were reported; however, without appropriate controls, it is impossible to determine with certainty which events were or were not caused by WELLBUTRIN. The following enumeration is organized by organ system and describes events in terms of their relative frequency of reporting in the data base. Events of major clinical importance are also described in WARNINGS and PRECAUTIONS.

The following definitions of frequency are used: Frequent adverse events are defined as those occurring in at least 1/100 patients. Infrequent adverse events are those occurring in 1/100 to 1/1000 patients, while rare events are those occurring in less than 1/1000 patients.

Cardiovascular: Frequent was edema; infrequent were chest pain, EKG abnormalities (premature beats and nonspecific ST-T changes), and shortness of breath/dyspnea; rare were flushing, pallor, phlebitis, and myocardial infarction.

Dermatologic: Frequent were nonspecific rashes; infrequent were alopecia and dry skin; rare were change in hair color, hirsutism, and acne.

Endocrine: Infrequent was gynecomastia; rare were glycosuria and hormone level change.

Gastrointestinal: Infrequent were dysphagia, thirst disturbance, and liver damage/jaundice; rare were rectal complaints, colitis, G.I. bleeding, intestinal perforation, and stomach ulcer.

Genitourinary: Frequent was nocturia; infrequent were vaginal irritation, testicular swelling, urinary tract infection, painful erection, and retarded ejaculation; rare were dysuria, enuresis, urinary incontinence, menopause, ovarian disorder, pelvic infection, cystitis, dyspareunia, and painful ejaculation.

Hematologic/Oncologic: Rare were lymphadenopathy, anemia, and pancytopenia.

Musculosketetal: Rare was musculosketetal chest pain.

Neurological: (see WARNINGS) Frequent were ataxia/incoordination, seizure, myoclonus, dyskinesia, and dystonia; infrequent were mydriasis, vertigo, and dysarthria; rare were EEG abnormality, abnormal neurological exam, impaired attention, sciatica, and aphasia.

Neuropsychiatric: (see PRECAUTIONS) Frequent were mania/hypomania, increased libido, hallucinations, decrease in sexual function, and depression; infrequent were memory impairment, depersonalization, psychosis, dysphoria, mood instability, paranoia, formal thought disorder, and frigidity; rare was suicidal ideation.

Oral Complaints: Frequent was stomatitis; infrequent were toothache, bruxism, gum irritation, and oral edema; rare was glossitis.

Respiratory: Infrequent were bronchitis and shortness of breath/dyspnea; rare were epistaxis, rate or rhythm disorder, pneumonia, and pulmonary embolism.

Special Senses: Infrequent was visual disturbance; rare was diplopia.

Nonspecific: Frequent were flu-like symptoms; infrequent was nonspecific pain; rare were body odor, surgically related pain, infection, medication reaction, and overdose.

Postintroduction Reports: Voluntary reports of adverse events temporally associated with WELLBUTRIN that have been received since market introduction and which may have no causal relationship with the drug include the following:

Cardiovascular: orthostatic hypotension, third degree heart block

Endocrine: syndrome of inappropriate antidiuretic hormone secretion

Gastrointestinal: esophagitis, hepatitis

Hemic and Lymphatic: ecchymosis, leukocytosis, leukopenia

Continued on next page

Glaxo Wellcome—Cont.

Dosing Regimen

Treatment Day	Total Daily Dose	Tablet Strength	Number of Tablets: Morning	Midday	Evening
1	200 mg	100 mg	1	0	1
4	300 mg	100 mg	1	1	1

Musculoskeletal: arthralgia, myalgia, muscle rigidity/fever/rhabdomyolysis
Nervous: coma, delirium, dream abnormalities, paresthesia, unmasking of tardive dyskinesia
Skin and Appendages: Stevens-Johnson syndrome, angioedema, exfoliative dermatitis, urticaria
Special Senses: tinnitus

DRUG ABUSE AND DEPENDENCE

Humans: Controlled clinical studies conducted in normal volunteers, in subjects with a history of multiple drug abuse, and in depressed patients showed some increase in motor activity and agitation/excitement.

In a population of individuals experienced with drugs of abuse, a single dose of 400 mg WELLBUTRIN produced mild amphetamine-like activity as compared to placebo on the morphine-benzedrine subscale of the Addiction Research Center Index (ARCI) and a score intermediate between placebo and amphetamine on the Liking Scale of the ARCI. These scales measure general feelings of euphoria and drug desirability.

Findings in clinical trials, however, are not known to predict the abuse potential of drugs reliably. Nonetheless, evidence from single-dose studies does suggest that the recommended daily dosage of bupropion when administered in divided doses is not likely to be especially reinforcing to amphetamine or stimulant abusers. However, higher doses, which could not be tested because of the risk of seizure, might be modestly attractive to those who abuse stimulant drugs.

Animals: Studies in rodents have shown that bupropion exhibits some pharmacologic actions common to psychostimulants, including increases in locomotor activity and the production of a mild stereotyped behavior and increases in rates of responding in several schedule-controlled behavior paradigms. Drug discrimination studies in rats showed stimulus generalization between bupropion and amphetamine and other psychostimulants. Rhesus monkeys have been shown to self-administer bupropion intravenously.

OVERDOSAGE

Lethal Doses in Animals: In rats, the acute oral LD_{50} values were 607 mg/kg (males) and 482 mg/kg (females). Respective values for mice were 544 mg/kg and 636 mg/kg. Signs of acute toxicity included labored breathing, salivation, arched back, ptosis, ataxia, and convulsions.

Human Overdose Experience: There has been limited clinical experience with overdosage of WELLBUTRIN. Thirteen overdoses occurred during clinical trials. Twelve patients ingested 850 to 4200 mg and recovered without significant sequelae. Another patient who ingested 9000 mg of WELLBUTRIN and 300 mg of tranylcypromine experienced a grand mal seizure and recovered without further sequelae.

Since introduction, WELLBUTRIN overdoses up to 17,500 mg have been reported. Seizure was reported in approximately one-third of all cases. Other serious reactions reported with overdoses of WELLBUTRIN alone included hallucinations, loss of consciousness, and tachycardia. Fever, muscle rigidity, rhabdomyolysis, hypotension, stupor, coma, and respiratory failure have been reported when WELLBUTRIN was part of multiple drug overdoses.

Although most patients recovered without sequelae, deaths associated with overdoses of WELLBUTRIN alone have been reported rarely in patients ingesting massive doses of WELLBUTRIN. Multiple uncontrolled seizures, bradycardia, cardiac failure, and cardiac arrest prior to death were reported in these patients.

Management of Overdose: Following suspected overdose, hospitalization is advised. If the patient is conscious, vomiting should be induced by syrup of ipecac. Activated charcoal also may be administered every 6 hours during the first 12 hours after ingestion. Baseline laboratory values should be obtained. Electrocardiogram and EEG monitoring also are recommended for the next 48 hours. Adequate fluid intake should be provided.

If the patient is stuporous, comatose, or convulsing, airway intubation is recommended prior to undertaking gastric lavage. Although there is little clinical experience with lavage following an overdose of WELLBUTRIN, it is likely to be of benefit within the first 12 hours after ingestion since absorption of the drug may not yet be complete.

While diuresis, dialysis, or hemoperfusion are sometimes used to treat drug overdosage, there is no experience with their use in the management of overdoses of WELLBUTRIN. Because diffusion of WELLBUTRIN from tissue to plasma may be slow, dialysis may be of minimal benefit several hours after overdose.

Based on studies in animals, it is recommended that seizures be treated with an intravenous benzodiazepine preparation and other supportive measures, as appropriate.

Further information about the treatment of overdoses may be available from a poison control center.

DOSAGE AND ADMINISTRATION

General Dosing Considerations: It is particularly important to administer WELLBUTRIN in a manner most likely to minimize the risk of seizure (see WARNINGS). Increases in dose should not exceed 100 mg/day in a 3-day period. Gradual escalation in dosage is also important if agitation, motor restlessness, and insomnia, often seen during the initial days of treatment, are to be minimized. If necessary, these effects may be managed by temporary reduction of dose or the short-term administration of an intermediate to long-acting sedative hypnotic. A sedative hypnotic usually is not required beyond the first week of treatment. Insomnia may also be minimized by avoiding bedtime doses. If distressing, untoward effects supervene, dose escalation should be stopped.

No single dose of WELLBUTRIN should exceed 150 mg. WELLBUTRIN should be administered t.i.d., preferably with at least 6 hours between successive doses.

Usual Dosage for Adults: The usual adult dose is 300 mg/day, given t.i.d. Dosing should begin at 200 mg/day, given as 100 mg b.i.d. Based on clinical response, this dose may be increased to 300 mg/day, given as 100 mg t.i.d., no sooner than 3 days after beginning therapy. [See table above.]

Increasing the Dosage Above 300 mg/Day: As with other antidepressants, the full antidepressant effect of WELLBUTRIN may not be evident until 4 weeks of treatment or longer. An increase in dosage, up to a maximum of 450 mg/day, given in divided doses of not more than 150 mg each, may be considered for patients in whom no clinical improvement is noted after several weeks of treatment at 300 mg/day. Dosing above 300 mg/day may be accomplished using the 75 or 100 mg tablets. The 100 mg tablet must be administered q.i.d. with at least 4 hours between successive doses, in order not to exceed the limit of 150 mg in a single dose. WELLBUTRIN should be discontinued in patients who do not demonstrate an adequate response after an appropriate period of treatment at 450 mg/day.

Elderly Patients: In general, older patients are known to metabolize drugs more slowly and to be more sensitive to the anticholinergic, sedative, and cardiovascular side effects of antidepressant drugs. Clinical trials enrolled several hundred patients 60 years of age and older. The experience with these patients and younger ones was similar.

Maintenance: The lowest dose that maintains remission is recommended. Although it is not known how long the patient should remain on Wellbutrin, it is generally recognized that acute episodes of depression require several months or longer of antidepressant drug treatment.

HOW SUPPLIED

WELLBUTRIN (bupropion hydrochloride) Tablets are supplied as 75 mg (yellow-gold) round, biconvex tablets printed "WELLBUTRIN" and "75," bottles of 100 (NDC 0173-0177-55); and 100 mg (red) round, biconvex tablets printed "WELLBUTRIN" and "100," bottles of 100 (NDC 0173-0178-55).

Store at 15° to 25°C (59° to 77°F). Protect from light and moisture.

January 1996RL-249

Shown in Product Identification Guide, page 315

ZANTAC® Injection ℞
[zan'tak]
(ranitidine hydrochloride)

ZANTAC® Injection Premixed ℞
(ranitidine hydrochloride)

DESCRIPTION

The active ingredient in ZANTAC Injection and ZANTAC Injection Premixed is ranitidine hydrochloride (HCl), a histamine H_2-receptor antagonist. Chemically it is N[2-[[[5-[(dimethylamino)methyl]-2-furanyl]methyl]thio] ethyl]-N′-methyl-2-nitro-1,1-ethenediamine, hydrochloride. The empirical formula is $C_{13}H_{22}N_4O_3S \cdot HCl$, representing a molecular weight of 350.87.

Ranitidine HCl is a white to pale yellow, granular substance that is soluble in water.

ZANTAC Injection is a clear, colorless to yellow, nonpyrogenic liquid. The yellow color of the liquid tends to intensify without adversely affecting potency. The pH of the injection solution is 6.7 to 7.3.

Sterile Injection for Intramuscular or Intravenous Administration: Each 1 mL of aqueous solution contains ranitidine 25 mg (as the hydrochloride); phenol 5 mg as preservative; and 0.96 mg of monobasic potassium phosphate and 2.4 mg of dibasic sodium phosphate as buffers.

A pharmacy bulk package is a container of a sterile preparation for parenteral use that contains many single doses. The contents are intended for use in a pharmacy admixture program and are restricted to the preparation of admixtures for intravenous (IV) infusion.

Sterile, Premixed Solution for Intravenous Administration in Single-Dose, Flexible Plastic Containers: Each 50 mL contains ranitidine HCl equivalent to 50 mg of ranitidine, sodium chloride 225 mg, and citric acid 15 mg and dibasic sodium phosphate 90 mg as buffers in water for injection. It contains no preservatives. The osmolarity of this solution is 180 mOsm/L (approx.), and the pH is 6.7 to 7.3.

The flexible plastic container is fabricated from a specially formulated, nonplasticized, thermoplastic co-polyester (CR3). Water can permeate from inside the container into the overwrap but not in amounts sufficient to affect the solution significantly. Solutions inside the plastic container also can leach out certain of the chemical components in very small amounts before the expiration period is attained. However, the safety of the plastic has been confirmed by tests in animals according to USP biological standards for plastic containers.

CLINICAL PHARMACOLOGY

ZANTAC is a competitive, reversible inhibitor of the action of histamine at the histamine H_2-receptors, including receptors on the gastric cells. ZANTAC does not lower serum Ca^{++} in hypercalcemic states. ZANTAC is not an anticholinergic agent.

Antisecretory Activity: ***1. Effects on Acid Secretion:***
ZANTAC Injection inhibits basal gastric acid secretion as well as gastric acid secretion stimulated by betazole and pentagastrin, as shown in the following table:

[See first table on top of next page.]

In a group of 10 known hypersecretors, ranitidine plasma levels of 71, 180, and 376 ng/mL inhibited basal acid secretion by 76%, 90%, and 99.5%, respectively.

It appears that basal- and betazole-stimulated secretions are most sensitive to inhibition by ZANTAC, while pentagastrin-stimulated secretion is more difficult to suppress.

2. Effects on Other Gastrointestinal Secretions:
Pepsin: ZANTAC does not affect pepsin secretion. Total pepsin output is reduced in proportion to the decrease in volume of gastric juice.
Intrinsic Factor: ZANTAC has no significant effect on pentagastrin-stimulated intrinsic factor secretion.
Serum Gastrin: ZANTAC has little or no effect on fasting or postprandial serum gastrin.

Other Pharmacologic Actions:
a. Gastric bacterial flora—increase in nitrate-reducing organisms, significance not known.
b. Prolactin levels—no effect in recommended oral or IV dosage, but small, transient, dose-related increases in serum prolactin have been reported after IV bolus injections of 100 mg or more.
c. Other pituitary hormones—no effect on serum gonadotropins, TSH, or GH. Possible impairment of vasopressin release.
d. No change in cortisol, aldosterone, androgen, or estrogen levels.
e. No antiandrogenic action.
f. No effect on count, motility, or morphology of sperm.

Pharmacokinetics: Serum concentrations necessary to inhibit 50% of stimulated gastric acid secretion are estimated to be 36 to 94 ng/mL. Following single IV or intramuscular (IM) 50-mg doses, serum concentrations of ZANTAC are in this range for 6 to 8 hours.

Following IV injection, approximately 70% of the dose is recovered in the urine as unchanged drug. Renal clearance averages 530 mL/min, with a total clearance of 760 mL/min. The volume of distribution is 1.4 L/kg, and the elimination half-life is 2 to 2.5 hours.

Four patients with clinically significant renal function impairment (creatinine clearance 25 to 35 mL/min) administered 50 mg of ranitidine intravenously had an average plasma half-life of 4.8 hours, a ranitidine clearance of 29 mL/min, and a volume of distribution of 1.76 L/kg. In general, these parameters appear to be altered in propor-

tion to creatinine clearance (see DOSAGE AND ADMINISTRATION).

ZANTAC is absorbed very rapidly after IM injection. Mean peak levels of 576 ng/mL occur within 15 minutes or less following a 50-mg IM dose. Absorption from IM sites is virtually complete, with a bioavailability of 90% to 100% compared with IV administration. Following oral administration, the relative bioavailability of ZANTAC® (ranitidine HCl) Tablets is 50%.

In man, the N-oxide is the principal metabolite in the urine; however, this amounts to <4% of the dose. Other metabolites are the S-oxide (1%) and the desmethyl ranitidine (1%). The remainder of the administered dose is found in the stool. Studies in patients with hepatic dysfunction (compensated cirrhosis) indicate that there are minor, but clinically insignificant, alterations in ranitidine half-life, distribution, clearance, and bioavailability.

Serum protein binding averages 15%.

Clinical Trials: ***Active Duodenal Ulcer:*** In a multicenter, double-blind, controlled, US study of endoscopically diagnosed duodenal ulcers, earlier healing was seen in the patients treated with oral ZANTAC as shown in the following table:

[See second table above.]

In these studies, patients treated with oral ZANTAC reported a reduction in both daytime and nocturnal pain, and they also consumed less antacid than the placebo-treated patients.

[See third table at right.]

Pathological Hypersecretory Conditions (such as Zollinger-Ellison syndrome): ZANTAC inhibits gastric acid secretion and reduces occurrence of diarrhea, anorexia, and pain in patients with pathological hypersecretion associated with Zollinger-Ellison syndrome, systemic mastocytosis, and other pathological hypersecretory conditions (e.g., postoperative, "short-gut" syndrome, idiopathic). Use of oral ZANTAC was followed by healing of ulcers in 8 of 19 (42%) patients who were intractable to previous therapy.

In a retrospective review of 52 Zollinger-Ellison patients given ZANTAC as a continuous IV infusion for up to 15 days, no patients developed complications of acid-peptic disease such as bleeding or perforation. Acid output was controlled to $\leq$10 mEq/h.

Effect of Intravenous ZANTAC on Gastric Acid Secretion

	Time After Dose, h	% Inhibition of Gastric Acid Output by Intravenous Dose, mg		
		20 mg	60 mg	100 mg
Betazole	Up to 2	93	99	99
Pentagastrin	Up to 3	47	66	77

	Oral ZANTAC*		Oral Placebo*	
	Number Entered	Healed/ Evaluable	Number Entered	Healed/ Evaluable
Outpatients				
Week 2	195	69/182 (38%)†	188	31/164 (19%)
Week 4		137/187 (73%)†		76/168 (45%)

*All patients were permitted p.r.n. antacids for relief of pain.
†P<0.0001.

Mean Daily Doses of Antacid

	Ulcer Healed	Ulcer Not Healed
Oral ZANTAC	0.06	0.71
Oral placebo	0.71	1.43

INDICATIONS AND USAGE

ZANTAC Injection and ZANTAC Injection Premixed are indicated in some hospitalized patients with pathological hypersecretory conditions or intractable duodenal ulcers, or as an alternative to the oral dosage form for short-term use in patients who are unable to take oral medication.

CONTRAINDICATIONS

ZANTAC Injection and ZANTAC Injection Premixed are contraindicated for patients known to have hypersensitivity to the drug.

PRECAUTIONS

General: 1. Symptomatic response to ZANTAC therapy does not preclude the presence of gastric malignancy.

2. Since ZANTAC is excreted primarily by the kidney, dosage should be adjusted in patients with impaired renal function (see DOSAGE AND ADMINISTRATION). Caution should be observed in patients with hepatic dysfunction since ZANTAC is metabolized in the liver.

3. In controlled studies in normal volunteers, elevations in SGPT have been observed when H_2-antagonists have been administered intravenously at greater than recommended dosages for 5 days or longer. Therefore, it seems prudent in patients receiving IV ranitidine at dosages $\geq$100 mg q.i.d. for periods of 5 days or longer to monitor SGPT daily (from day 5) for the remainder of IV therapy.

4. Bradycardia in association with rapid administration of ZANTAC Injection has been reported rarely, usually in patients with factors predisposing to cardiac rhythm disturbances. Recommended rates of administration should not be exceeded (see DOSAGE AND ADMINISTRATION).

5. Rare reports suggest that ZANTAC may precipitate acute porphyria attacks in patients with acute porphyria. ZANTAC should therefore be avoided in patients with a history of acute porphyria.

Laboratory Tests: False-positive tests for urine protein with MULTISTIX® may occur during ZANTAC therapy, and therefore testing with sulfosalicylic acid is recommended.

Drug Interactions: Although ZANTAC has been reported to bind weakly to cytochrome P-450 *in vitro,* recommended doses of the drug do not inhibit the action of the cytochrome P-450–linked oxygenase enzymes in the liver. However, there have been isolated reports of drug interactions that suggest that ZANTAC may affect the bioavailability of certain drugs by some mechanism as yet unidentified (e.g., a pH-dependent effect on absorption or a change in volume of distribution).

Increased or decreased prothrombin times have been reported during concurrent use of ranitidine and warfarin. However, in human pharmacokinetic studies with dosages of ranitidine up to 400 mg/d, no interaction occurred; ranitidine had no effect on warfarin clearance or prothrombin time. The possibility of an interaction with warfarin at dosages of ranitidine higher than 400 mg/d has not been investigated.

Carcinogenesis, Mutagenesis, Impairment of Fertility: There was no indication of tumorigenic or carcinogenic effects in life-span studies in mice and rats at oral dosages up to 2,000 mg/kg per day.

Ranitidine was not mutagenic in standard bacterial tests *(Salmonella, Escherichia coli)* for mutagenicity at concentrations up to the maximum recommended for these assays.

In a dominant lethal assay, a single oral dose of 1,000 mg/kg to male rats was without effect on the outcome of two matings per week for the next 9 weeks.

Pregnancy: ***Teratogenic Effects: Pregnancy Category B:*** Reproduction studies have been performed in rats and rabbits at oral doses up to 160 times the human oral dose and have revealed no evidence of impaired fertility or harm to the fetus due to ZANTAC. There are, however, no adequate and well-controlled studies in pregnant women. Because animal reproduction studies are not always predictive of human response, this drug should be used during pregnancy only if clearly needed.

Nursing Mothers: ZANTAC is secreted in human milk. Caution should be exercised when ZANTAC is administered to a nursing mother.

Pediatric Use: Safety and effectiveness in pediatric patients have not been established.

Use in Elderly Patients: Ulcer healing rates in elderly patients (65 to 82 years of age) treated with oral ZANTAC were no different from those in younger age-groups. The incidence rates for adverse events and laboratory abnormalities were also not different from those seen in other age-groups.

ADVERSE REACTIONS

Transient pain at the site of IM injection has been reported. Transient local burning or itching has been reported with IV administration of ZANTAC.

The following have been reported as events in clinical trials or in the routine management of patients treated with oral or parenteral ZANTAC. The relationship to ZANTAC therapy has been unclear in many cases. Headache, sometimes severe, seems to be related to ZANTAC administration.

Central Nervous System: Rarely, malaise, dizziness, somnolence, insomnia, and vertigo. Rare cases of reversible mental confusion, agitation, depression, and hallucinations have been reported, predominantly in severely ill elderly patients. Rare cases of reversible blurred vision suggestive of a change in accommodation have been reported. Rare reports of reversible involuntary motor disturbances have been received.

Cardiovascular: As with other H_2-blockers, rare reports of arrhythmias such as tachycardia, bradycardia, asystole, atrioventricular block, and premature ventricular beats.

Gastrointestinal: Constipation, diarrhea, nausea/vomiting, abdominal discomfort/pain, and rare reports of pancreatitis.

Hepatic: In normal volunteers, SGPT values were increased to at least twice the pretreatment levels in 6 of 12 subjects receiving 100 mg q.i.d. intravenously for 7 days, and in 4 of 24 subjects receiving 50 mg q.i.d. intravenously for 5 days. There have been occasional reports of hepatitis, hepatocellular or hepatocanalicular or mixed, with or without jaundice. In such circumstances, ranitidine should be immediately discontinued. These events are usually reversible, but in exceedingly rare circumstances death has occurred.

Musculoskeletal: Rare reports of arthralgias and myalgias.

Hematologic: Blood count changes (leukopenia, granulocytopenia, and thrombocytopenia) have occurred in a few patients. These were usually reversible. Rare cases of agranulocytosis, pancytopenia, sometimes with marrow hypoplasia, and aplastic anemia and exceedingly rare cases of acquired immune hemolytic anemia have been reported.

Endocrine: Controlled studies in animals and man have shown no stimulation of any pituitary hormone by ZANTAC and no antiandrogenic activity, and cimetidine-induced gynecomastia and impotence in hypersecretory patients have resolved when ZANTAC has been substituted. However, occasional cases of gynecomastia, impotence, and loss of libido have been reported in male patients receiving ZANTAC, but the incidence did not differ from that in the general population.

Integumentary: Rash, including rare cases of erythema multiforme, and, rarely, alopecia.

Other: Rare cases of hypersensitivity reactions (e.g., bronchospasm, fever, rash, eosinophilia), anaphylaxis, angioneurotic edema, and small increases in serum creatinine.

OVERDOSAGE

There has been virtually no experience with overdosage with ZANTAC Injection and limited experience with oral doses of ranitidine. Reported acute ingestions of up to 18 g orally have been associated with transient adverse effects similar to those encountered in normal clinical experience (see ADVERSE REACTIONS). In addition, abnormalities of gait and hypotension have been reported.

When overdosage occurs, clinical monitoring and supportive therapy should be employed.

Studies in dogs receiving dosages of ZANTAC in excess of 225 mg/kg per day have shown muscular tremors, vomiting, and rapid respiration. Single oral doses of 1,000 mg/kg in mice and rats were not lethal. Intravenous LD_{50} values in mice and rats were 77 and 83 mg/kg, respectively.

DOSAGE AND ADMINISTRATION

Parenteral Administration: In some hospitalized patients with pathological hypersecretory conditions or intractable duodenal ulcers, or in patients who are unable to take oral medication, ZANTAC may be administered parenterally according to the following recommendations:

Intramuscular Injection: 50 mg (2 mL) every 6 to 8 hours. (No dilution necessary.)

Intermittent Intravenous Injection:

a. Intermittent Bolus: 50 mg (2 mL) every 6 to 8 hours. Dilute ZANTAC Injection, 50 mg, in 0.9% sodium chloride injection or other compatible IV solution (see Stability) to a concentration no greater than 2.5 mg/mL (20 mL). Inject at a rate no greater than 4 mL/min (5 minutes).

b. Intermittent Infusion: 50 mg (2 mL) every 6 to 8 hours. Dilute ZANTAC Injection, 50 mg, in 5% dextrose injection or other compatible IV solution (see Stability) to a concentration no greater than 0.5 mg/mL (100 mL). Infuse at a rate no greater than 5 to 7 mL/min (15 to 20 minutes).

ZANTAC Injection Premixed solution, 50 mg, in 0.45% sodium chloride, 50 mL, requires no dilution and should be infused over 15 to 20 minutes.

In some patients it may be necessary to increase dosage. When this is necessary, the increases should be made by more frequent administration of the dose, but generally should not exceed 400 mg/d.

Continuous Intravenous Infusion: Add ZANTAC Injection to 5% dextrose injection or other compatible IV solution (see

Continued on next page

Glaxo Wellcome—Cont.

Stability). Deliver at a rate of 6.25 mg/h (e.g., 150 mg [6 mL] of ZANTAC Injection in 250 mL of 5% dextrose injection at 10.7 mL/h).

For Zollinger-Ellison patients, dilute ZANTAC Injection in 5% dextrose injection or other compatible IV solution (see Stability) to a concentration no greater than 2.5 mg/mL. Start the infusion at a rate of 1.0 mg/kg per hour. If after 4 hours either a measured gastric acid output is >10 mEq/h or the patient becomes symptomatic, the dose should be adjusted upward in 0.5-mg/kg per hour increments, and the acid output should be remeasured. Dosages up to 2.5 mg/kg per hour and infusion rates as high as 220 mg/h have been used.

ZANTAC Injection Premixed in Flexible Plastic Containers: Instructions for Use: ***To Open:*** Tear outer wrap at notch and remove solution container. Check for minute leaks by squeezing container firmly. If leaks are found, discard unit as sterility may be impaired.

Preparation for Administration: Use aseptic technique.

1. Close flow control clamp of administration set.
2. Remove cover from outlet port at bottom of container.
3. Insert piercing pin of administration set into port with a twisting motion until the pin is firmly seated. NOTE: See full directions on administration set carton.
4. Suspend container from hanger.
5. Squeeze and release drip chamber to establish proper fluid level in chamber during infusion of ZANTAC Injection Premixed.
6. Open flow control clamp to expel air from set. Close clamp.
7. Attach set to venipuncture device. If device is not indwelling, prime and make venipuncture.
8. Perform venipuncture.
9. Regulate rate of administration with flow control clamp.

Caution: ZANTAC Injection Premixed in flexible plastic containers is to be administered by slow IV drip infusion only. **Additives should not be introduced into this solution.** If used with a primary IV fluid system, the primary solution should be discontinued during ZANTAC Injection Premixed infusion.

Do not administer unless solution is clear and container is undamaged.

Warning: Do not use flexible plastic container in series connections.

Dosage Adjustment for Patients With Impaired Renal Function: The administration of ranitidine as a continuous infusion has not been evaluated in patients with impaired renal function. On the basis of experience with a group of subjects with severely impaired renal function treated with ZANTAC, the recommended dosage in patients with a creatinine clearance <50 mL/min is 50 mg every 18 to 24 hours. Should the patient's condition require, the frequency of dosing may be increased to every 12 hours or even further with caution. Hemodialysis reduces the level of circulating ranitidine. Ideally, the dosing schedule should be adjusted so that the timing of a scheduled dose coincides with the end of hemodialysis.

Stability: Undiluted, ZANTAC Injection tends to exhibit a yellow color that may intensify over time without adversely affecting potency. ZANTAC Injection is stable for 48 hours at room temperature when added to or diluted with most commonly used IV solutions, e.g., 0.9% sodium chloride injection, 5% dextrose injection, 10% dextrose injection, lactated ringer's injection, or 5% sodium bicarbonate injection. ZANTAC Injection Premixed in flexible plastic containers is sterile through the expiration date on the label when stored under recommended conditions.

Note: Parenteral drug products should be inspected visually for particulate matter and discoloration before administration whenever solution and container permit.

Directions for Dispensing: ***Pharmacy Bulk Package—Not for Direct Infusion:*** The pharmacy bulk package is for use in a pharmacy admixture service only under a laminar flow hood. The closure should be penetrated only once with a sterile transfer set or other sterile dispensing device, which allows measured distribution of the contents, and the contents dispensed in aliquots using aseptic technique. CONTENTS SHOULD BE USED AS SOON AS POSSIBLE FOLLOWING INITIAL CLOSURE PUNCTURE. DISCARD ANY UNUSED PORTION WITHIN 24 HOURS OF FIRST ENTRY. Following closure puncture, container should be maintained below 30°C (86°F) under a laminar flow hood until contents are dispensed.

HOW SUPPLIED

ZANTAC Injection, 25 mg/mL, containing phenol 0.5% as preservative, is available as follows:

NDC 0173-0362-38 2-mL single-dose vials (Tray of 10)
NDC 0173-0363-01 6-mL multidose vials (Singles)
NDC 0173-0363-00 40-mL pharmacy bulk packages (Singles)

Store between 4° and 30°C (39° and 86°F). Protect from light. Store the 40-mL pharmacy bulk vial in carton until time of use.

ZANTAC Injection Premixed, 50 mg/50 mL, in 0.45% sodium chloride, is available as a sterile, premixed solution for IV administration in single-dose, flexible plastic containers (NDC 0173-0441-00) (case of 24). It contains no preservatives.

Store between 2° and 25°C (36° and 77°F). Protect from light. Exposure of pharmaceutical products to heat should be minimized. Avoid excessive heat; however, brief exposure up to 40°C does not adversely affect the product. Protect from freezing.

June 1996/RL-324

Shown in Product Identification Guide, page 315

ZANTAC® 150 Tablets, USP ℞
[zan'tak]
(ranitidine hydrochloride)

ZANTAC® 300 Tablets, USP ℞
(ranitidine hydrochloride)

ZANTAC® 150 ℞
(ranitidine hydrochloride)
GELdose® Capsules

ZANTAC® 300 ℞
(ranitidine hydrochloride)
GELdose® Capsules

ZANTAC® 150 ℞
(ranitidine hydrochloride)
EFFERdose® Tablets

ZANTAC® 150 ℞
(ranitidine hydrochloride)
EFFERdose® Granules

ZANTAC® Syrup, USP ℞
(ranitidine hydrochloride)

DESCRIPTION

The active ingredient in ZANTAC 150 Tablets, ZANTAC 300 Tablets, ZANTAC 150 GELdose Capsules, ZANTAC 300 GELdose Capsules, ZANTAC 150 EFFERdose Tablets, ZANTAC 150 EFFERdose Granules, and ZANTAC Syrup is ranitidine hydrochloride (HCl), a histamine H_2-receptor antagonist. Chemically it is N[2-[[[5-[(dimethylamino) methyl]-2-furanyl]methyl]thio]ethyl]-N'-methyl-2-nitro-1,1-ethenediamine, HCl.

The empirical formula is $C_{13}H_{22}N_4O_3S \cdot HCl$, representing a molecular weight of 350.87.

Ranitidine HCl is a white to pale yellow, granular substance that is soluble in water. It has a slightly bitter taste and sulfurlike odor.

Each ZANTAC 150 Tablet for oral administration contains 168 mg of ranitidine HCl equivalent to 150 mg of ranitidine. Each tablet also contains the inactive ingredients FD&C Yellow No. 6 Aluminum Lake, hydroxypropyl methylcellulose, magnesium stearate, microcrystalline cellulose, titanium dioxide, triacetin and yellow iron oxide.

Each ZANTAC 300 Tablet for oral administration contains 336 mg of ranitidine HCl equivalent to 300 mg of ranitidine. Each tablet also contains the inactive ingredients croscarmellose sodium, D&C Yellow No. 10 Aluminum Lake, hydroxypropyl methylcellulose, magnesium stearate, microcrystalline cellulose, titanium dioxide, and triacetin.

ZANTAC 150 GELdose Capsules and ZANTAC 300 GELdose Capsules for oral administration are soft gelatin capsules containing 168 mg of ranitidine HCl equivalent to 150 mg of ranitidine and 336 mg of ranitidine HCl equivalent to 300 mg of ranitidine, respectively, in a nonaqueous matrix of synthetic coconut oil and synthetic triglycerides. The soft gelatin capsule shell contains gelatin, Sorbitol Special™ (sorbitol and sorbitol anhydrides), glycerin, purified water, titanium dioxide, FD&C Yellow No. 6, FD&C Blue No. 1, and FD&C Red No. 40. The capsule shell may also contain mineral oil and soybean lecithin. The capsules are printed with edible ink.

ZANTAC 150 EFFERdose Tablets and ZANTAC 150 EFFERdose Granules for oral administration are effervescent formulations of ranitidine that must be dissolved in water before use. Each individual tablet or the contents of a packet contain 168 mg of ranitidine HCl equivalent to 150 mg of ranitidine and the following inactive ingredients: aspartame, monosodium citrate anhydrous, povidone, and sodium bicarbonate. Each tablet also contains sodium benzoate. The total sodium content of each tablet is 183.12 mg (7.96 mEq) per 150 mg of ranitidine, and the total sodium content of each packet of granules is 173.54 mg (7.55 mEq) per 150 mg of ranitidine.

Each 1 mL of ZANTAC Syrup contains 16.8 mg of ranitidine HCl equivalent to 15 mg of ranitidine. ZANTAC Syrup also contains the inactive ingredients alcohol (7.5%), butylparaben, dibasic sodium phosphate, hydroxypropyl methylcellulose, peppermint flavor, monobasic potassium phosphate, propylparaben, purified water, saccharin sodium, sodium chloride, and sorbitol.

CLINICAL PHARMACOLOGY

ZANTAC is a competitive, reversible inhibitor of the action of histamine at the histamine H_2-receptors, including receptors on the gastric cells. ZANTAC does not lower serum Ca^{++} in hypercalcemic states. ZANTAC is not an anticholinergic agent.

Antisecretory Activity: ***1. Effects on Acid Secretion:*** ZANTAC inhibits both daytime and nocturnal basal gastric acid secretions as well as gastric acid secretion stimulated by food, betazole, and pentagastrin, as shown in the following table:

[See table below.]

It appears that basal-, nocturnal-, and betazole-stimulated secretions are most sensitive to inhibition by ZANTAC, responding almost completely to doses of 100 mg or less, while pentagastrin- and food-stimulated secretions are more difficult to suppress.

2. Effects on Other Gastrointestinal Secretions:

Pepsin: Oral ZANTAC does not affect pepsin secretion. Total pepsin output is reduced in proportion to the decrease in volume of gastric juice.

Intrinsic Factor: Oral ZANTAC has no significant effect on pentagastrin-stimulated intrinsic factor secretion.

Serum Gastrin: ZANTAC has little or no effect on fasting or postprandial serum gastrin.

Other Pharmacologic Actions:

a. Gastric bacterial flora—increase in nitrate-reducing organisms, significance not known.

b. Prolactin levels—no effect in recommended oral or intravenous (IV) dosage, but small, transient, dose-related increases in serum prolactin have been reported after IV bolus injections of 100 mg or more.

c. Other pituitary hormones—no effect on serum gonadotropins, TSH, or GH. Possible impairment of vasopressin release.

d. No change in cortisol, aldosterone, androgen, or estrogen levels.

e. No antiandrogenic action.

f. No effect on count, motility, or morphology of sperm.

Pharmacokinetics: ZANTAC is 50% absorbed after oral administration, compared to an IV injection with mean peak levels of 440 to 545 ng/mL occurring at 2 to 3 hours after a 150-mg dose. The syrup, GELdose, and EFFERdose formulations are bioequivalent to the tablets. In a pharmacodynamic comparison of the EFFERdose with the ZANTAC Tablets, during the first hour after administration, the EFFERdose tablet formulation gave a significantly higher intragastric pH, by approximately 1 pH unit, compared to the ZANTAC Tablets. The elimination half-life is 2.5 to 3 hours.

Absorption is not significantly impaired by the administration of food or antacids. Propantheline slightly delays and increases peak blood levels of ZANTAC, probably by delaying gastric emptying and transit time. In one study, simultaneous administration of high-potency antacid (150 mmol) in fasting subjects has been reported to decrease the absorption of ZANTAC.

Serum concentrations necessary to inhibit 50% of stimulated gastric acid secretion are estimated to be 36 to 94 ng/mL. Following a single oral dose of 150 mg, serum concentrations of ZANTAC are in this range up to 12 hours. However, blood levels bear no consistent relationship to dose or degree of acid inhibition.

The principal route of excretion is the urine, with approximately 30% of the orally administered dose collected in the urine as unchanged drug in 24 hours. Renal clearance is about 410 mL per minute, indicating active tubular excretion. Four patients with clinically significant renal function impairment (creatinine clearance 25 to 35 mL per minute) administered 50 mg of ranitidine intravenously had an average plasma half-life of 4.8 hours, a ranitidine clearance of 29 mL per minute, and a volume of distribution of 1.76 L/kg. In general, these parameters appear to be altered in proportion

Effect of Oral ZANTAC on Gastric Acid Secretion

	Time After Dose, h	% Inhibition of Gastric Acid Output by Dose, mg			
		75–80	100	150	200
Basal	Up to 4		99	95	
Nocturnal	Up to 13	95	96	92	
Betazole	Up to 3		97	99	
Pentagastrin	Up to 5	58	72	72	80
Meal	Up to 3		73	79	95

to creatinine clearance (see DOSAGE AND ADMINISTRATION).

In man, the N-oxide is the principal metabolite in the urine; however, this amounts to <4% of the dose. Other metabolites are the S-oxide (1%) and the desmethyl ranitidine (1%). The remainder of the administered dose is found in the stool. Studies in patients with hepatic dysfunction (compensated cirrhosis) indicate that there are minor, but clinically insignificant, alterations in ranitidine half-life, distribution, clearance, and bioavailability.

The volume of distribution is about 1.4 L/kg. Serum protein binding averages 15%.

Clinical Trials: *Active Duodenal Ulcer:* In a multicenter, double-blind, controlled, US study of endoscopically diagnosed duodenal ulcers, earlier healing was seen in the patients treated with ZANTAC as shown in Table I:
[See Table I above.]

In these studies, patients treated with ZANTAC reported a reduction in both daytime and nocturnal pain, and they also consumed less antacid than the placebo-treated patients.
[See Table II above.]

Foreign studies have shown that patients heal equally well with 150 mg b.i.d. and 300 mg h.s. (85% versus 84%, respectively) during a usual 4-week course of therapy. If patients require extended therapy of 8 weeks, the healing rate may be higher for 150 mg b.i.d. as compared to 300 mg h.s. (92% versus 87%, respectively).

Studies have been limited to short-term treatment of acute duodenal ulcer. Patients whose ulcers healed during therapy had recurrences of ulcers at the usual rates.

Maintenance Therapy in Duodenal Ulcer: Ranitidine has been found to be effective as maintenance therapy for patients following healing of acute duodenal ulcers. In two independent, double-blind, multicenter, controlled trials, the number of duodenal ulcers observed was significantly less in patients treated with ZANTAC (150 mg h.s.) than in patients treated with placebo over a 12-month period.

Duodenal Ulcer Prevalence

Double-blind, Multicenter, Placebo-Controlled Trials

Multicenter Trial	Drug	Duodenal Ulcer Prevalence 0–4 Months	0–8 Months	0–12 Months	No. of Patients
USA	RAN	20%*	24%*	35%*	138
	PLC	44%	54%	59%	139
Foreign	RAN	12%*	21%*	28%*	174
	PLC	56%	64%	68%	165

% = Life table estimate.
* = *p* <0.05 (ZANTAC versus comparator).
RAN = ranitidine (ZANTAC).
PLC = placebo.

As with other H_2-antagonists, the factors responsible for the significant reduction in the prevalence of duodenal ulcers include prevention of recurrence of ulcers, more rapid healing of ulcers that may occur during maintenance therapy, or both.

Gastric Ulcer: In a multicenter, double-blind, controlled, US study of endoscopically diagnosed gastric ulcers, earlier healing was seen in the patients treated with ZANTAC as shown in the following table:

	ZANTAC* Number Entered	Healed/ Evaluable	Placebo* Number Entered	Healed/ Evaluable
Outpatients				
Week 2		16/83 (19%)		10/83 (12%)
	92		94	
Week 6		50/73 (68%)†		35/69 (51%)

* All patients were permitted p.r.n. antacids for relief of pain.
† *p* = 0.009.

In this multicenter trial, significantly more patients treated with ZANTAC became pain free during therapy.

Maintenance of Healing of Gastric Ulcers: In two multicenter, double-blind, randomized, placebo-controlled, 12-month trials conducted in patients whose gastric ulcers had been previously healed, ZANTAC 150 mg h.s. was significantly more effective than placebo in maintaining healing of gastric ulcers.

Pathological Hypersecretory Conditions (such as Zollinger-Ellison syndrome): ZANTAC inhibits gastric acid secretion and reduces occurrence of diarrhea, anorexia, and pain in patients with pathological hypersecretion associated with Zollinger-Ellison syndrome, systemic mastocytosis, and other pathological hypersecretory conditions (e.g., postoper-

Table I

	ZANTAC* Number Entered	Healed/ Evaluable	Placebo* Number Entered	Healed/ Evaluable
Outpatients				
Week 2	195	69/182 (38%)†	188	31/164 (19%)
Week 4		137/187 (73%)†		76/168 (45%)

*All patients were permitted p.r.n. antacids for relief of pain.   †*p* <0.0001.

Table II

	Mean Daily Doses of Antacid Ulcer Healed	Ulcer Not Healed
ZANTAC	0.06	0.71
Placebo	0.71	1.43

ative, "short-gut" syndrome, idiopathic). Use of ZANTAC was followed by healing of ulcers in 8 of 19 (42%) patients who were intractable to previous therapy.

Gastroesophageal Reflux Disease (GERD): In two multicenter, double-blind, placebo-controlled, 6-week trials performed in the United States and Europe, ZANTIC 150 mg b.i.d. was more effective than placebo for the relief of heartburn and other symptoms associated with GERD. Ranitidine-treated patients consumed significantly less antacid than did placebo-treated patients.

The US trial indicated that ZANTAC 150 mg b.i.d. significantly reduced the frequency of heartburn attacks and severity of heartburn pain within 1 to 2 weeks after starting therapy. The improvement was maintained throughout the 6-week trial period. Moreover, patient response rates demonstrated that the effect on heartburn extends through both the day and night time periods.

Erosive Esophagitis: In two multicenter, double-blind, randomized, placebo-controlled, 12-week trials performed in the United States, ZANTAC 150 mg q.i.d. was significantly more effective than placebo in healing endoscopically diagnosed erosive esophagitis and in relieving associated heartburn. The erosive esophagitis healing rates were as follows:

Erosive Esophagitis Patient Healing Rates

	Healed/Evaluable Placebo* n = 229	ZANTAC 150 mg q.i.d.* n = 215
Week 4	43/198 (22%)	96/206 (47%)†
Week 8	63/176 (36%)	142/200 (71%)†
Week 12	92/159 (58%)	162/192 (84%)†

* All patients were permitted p.r.n. antacids for relief of pain.
† *p* <0.001 versus placebo.

No additional benefit in healing of esophagitis or in relief of heartburn was seen with a ranitidine dose of 300 mg q.i.d.

Maintenance of Healing of Erosive Esophagitis: In two multicenter, double-blind, randomized, placebo-controlled, 48-week trials conducted in patients whose erosive esophagitis had been previously healed, ZANTAC 150 mg b.i.d. was significantly more effective than placebo in maintaining healing of erosive esophagitis.

INDICATIONS AND USAGE

ZANTAC is indicated in:

1. Short-term treatment of active duodenal ulcer. Most patients heal within 4 weeks. Studies available to date have not assessed the safety of ranitidine in uncomplicated duodenal ulcer for periods of more than 8 weeks.
2. Maintenance therapy for duodenal ulcer patients at reduced dosage after healing of acute ulcers. No placebo-controlled comparative studies have been carried out for periods of longer than 1 year.
3. The treatment of pathological hypersecretory conditions (e.g., Zollinger-Ellison syndrome and systemic mastocytosis).
4. Short-term treatment of active, benign gastric ulcer. Most patients heal within 6 weeks and the usefulness of further treatment has not been demonstrated. Studies available to date have not assessed the safety of ranitidine in uncomplicated, benign gastric ulcer for periods of more than 6 weeks.
5. Maintenance therapy for gastric ulcer patients at reduced dosage after healing of acute ulcers. Placebo-controlled studies have been carried out for 1 year.
6. Treatment of GERD. Symptomatic relief commonly occurs within 1 or 2 weeks after starting therapy with ZANTAC 150 mg b.i.d.
7. Treatment of endoscopically diagnosed erosive esophagitis. Symptomatic relief of heartburn commonly occurs

within 24 hours of therapy initiation with ZANTAC 150 mg q.i.d.
8. Maintenance of healing of erosive esophagitis. Placebo-controlled trials have been carried out for 48 weeks.

Concomitant antacids should be given as needed for pain relief to patients with active duodenal ulcer; active, benign gastric ulcer; hypersecretory states; GERD; and erosive esophagitis.

CONTRAINDICATIONS

ZANTAC is contraindicated for patients known to have hypersensitivity to the drug or any of the ingredients (see PRECAUTIONS).

PRECAUTIONS

General: 1. Symptomatic response to ZANTAC therapy does not preclude the presence of gastric malignancy.

2. Since ZANTAC is excreted primarily by the kidney, dosage should be adjusted in patients with impaired renal function (see DOSAGE AND ADMINISTRATION). Caution should be observed in patients with hepatic dysfunction since ZANTAC is metabolized in the liver.

3. Rare reports suggest that ZANTAC may precipitate acute porphyria attacks in patients with acute porphyria. ZANTAC should therefore be avoided in patients with a history of acute porphyria.

Information for Patients: *Phenylketonurics:* ZANTAC 150 EFFERdose Tablets and ZANTAC 150 EFFERdose Granules contain phenylalanine 16.84 mg per 150 mg of ranitidine.

Laboratory Tests: False-positive tests for urine protein with MULTISTIX® may occur during ZANTAC therapy, and therefore testing with sulfosalicylic acid is recommended.

Drug Interactions: Although ZANTAC has been reported to bind weakly to cytochrome P-450 *in vitro*, recommended doses of the drug do not inhibit the action of the cytochrome P-450–linked oxygenase enzymes in the liver. However, there have been isolated reports of drug interactions that suggest that ZANTAC may affect the bioavailability of certain drugs by some mechanism as yet unidentified (e.g., a pH-dependent effect on absorption or a change in volume of distribution).

Increased or decreased prothrombin times have been reported during concurrent use of ranitidine and warfarin. However, in human pharmacokinetic studies with dosages of ranitidine up to 400 mg per day, no interaction occurred; ranitidine had no effect on warfarin clearance or prothrombin time. The possibility of an interaction with warfarin at dosages of ranitidine higher than 400 mg per day has not been investigated.

Carcinogenesis, Mutagenesis, Impairment of Fertility: There was no indication of tumorigenic or carcinogenic effects in life-span studies in mice and rats at dosages up to 2,000 mg/kg per day.

Ranitidine was not mutagenic in standard bacterial tests (*Salmonella, Escherichia coli*) for mutagenicity at concentrations up to the maximum recommended for these assays.

In a dominant lethal assay, a single oral dose of 1,000 mg/kg to male rats was without effect on the outcome of two matings per week for the next 9 weeks.

Pregnancy: *Teratogenic Effects: Pregnancy Category B:* Reproduction studies have been performed in rats and rabbits at doses up to 160 times the human dose and have revealed no evidence of impaired fertility or harm to the fetus due to ZANTAC. There are, however, no adequate and well-controlled studies in pregnant women. Because animal reproduction studies are not always predictive of human response, this drug should be used during pregnancy only if clearly needed.

Nursing Mothers: ZANTAC is secreted in human milk. Caution should be exercised when ZANTAC is administered to a nursing mother.

Pediatric Use: Safety and effectiveness in children have not been established.

Continued on next page

Glaxo Wellcome—Cont.

Use in Elderly Patients: Ulcer healing rates in elderly patients (65 to 82 years of age) were no different from those in younger age-groups. The incidence rates for adverse events and laboratory abnormalities were also not different from those seen in other age-groups.

ADVERSE REACTIONS

The following have been reported as events in clinical trials or in the routine management of patients treated with ZANTAC. The relationship to ZANTAC therapy has been unclear in many cases. Headache, sometimes severe, seems to be related to ZANTAC administration.

Central Nervous System: Rarely, malaise, dizziness, somnolence, insomnia, and vertigo. Rare cases of reversible mental confusion, agitation, depression, and hallucinations have been reported, predominantly in severely ill elderly patients. Rare cases of reversible blurred vision suggestive of a change in accommodation have been reported. Rare reports of reversible involuntary motor disturbances have been received.

Cardiovascular: As with other H_2-blockers, rare reports of arrhythmias such as tachycardia, bradycardia, atrioventricular block, and premature ventricular beats.

Gastrointestinal: Constipation, diarrhea, nausea/vomiting, abdominal discomfort/pain, and rare reports of pancreatitis.

Hepatic: In normal volunteers, SGPT values were increased to at least twice the pretreatment levels in 6 of 12 subjects receiving 100 mg q.i.d. intravenously for 7 days, and in 4 of 24 subjects receiving 50 mg q.i.d. intravenously for 5 days. There have been occasional reports of hepatitis, hepatocellular or hepatocanalicular or mixed, with or without jaundice. In such circumstances, ranitidine should be immediately discontinued. These events are usually reversible, but in exceedingly rare circumstances death has occurred.

Musculoskeletal: Rare reports of arthralgias and myalgias.

Hematologic: Blood count changes (leukopenia, granulocytopenia, and thrombocytopenia) have occurred in a few patients. These were usually reversible. Rare cases of agranulocytosis, pancytopenia, sometimes with marrow hypoplasia, and aplastic anemia and exceedingly rare cases of acquired immune hemolytic anemia have been reported.

Endocrine: Controlled studies in animals and man have shown no stimulation of any pituitary hormone by ZANTAC and no antiandrogenic activity, and cimetidine-induced gynecomastia and impotence in hypersecretory patients have resolved when ZANTAC has been substituted. However, occasional cases of gynecomastia, impotence, and loss of libido have been reported in male patients receiving ZANTAC, but the incidence did not differ from that in the general population.

Integumentary: Rash, including rare cases of erythema multiforme, and, rarely, alopecia.

Other: Rare cases of hypersensitivity reactions (e.g., bronchospasm, fever, rash, eosinophilia), anaphylaxis, angioneurotic edema, and small increases in serum creatinine.

OVERDOSAGE

There has been limited experience with overdosage. Reported acute ingestions of up to 18 g orally have been associated with transient adverse effects similar to those encountered in normal clinical experience (see ADVERSE REACTIONS). In addition, abnormalities of gait and hypotension have been reported.

When overdosage occurs, the usual measures to remove unabsorbed material from the gastrointestinal tract, clinical monitoring, and supportive therapy should be employed. Studies in dogs receiving dosages of ZANTAC in excess of 225 mg/kg per day have shown muscular tremors, vomiting, and rapid respiration. Single oral doses of 1,000 mg/kg in mice and rats were not lethal. Intravenous LD_{50} values in mice and rats were 77 and 83 mg/kg, respectively.

DOSAGE AND ADMINISTRATION

Active Duodenal Ulcer: The current recommended adult oral dosage of ZANTAC for duodenal ulcer is 150 mg or 10 mL (2 teaspoonfuls equivalent to 150 mg of ranitidine) twice daily. An alternative dosage of 300 mg or 20 mL (4 teaspoonfuls equivalent to 300 mg of ranitidine) once daily after the evening meal or at bedtime can be used for patients in whom dosing convenience is important. The advantages of one treatment regimen compared to the other in a particular patient population have yet to be demonstrated (see Clinical Trials: *Active Duodenal Ulcer*). Smaller doses have been shown to be equally effective in inhibiting gastric acid secretion in US studies, and several foreign trials have shown that 100 mg b.i.d. is as effective as the 150-mg dose.

Antacid should be given as needed for relief of pain (see CLINICAL PHARMACOLOGY: Pharmacokinetics).

Maintenance of Healing of Duodenal Ulcers: The current recommended adult oral dosage is 150 mg or 10 mL (2 teaspoonfuls equivalent to 150 mg of ranitidine) at bedtime.

Pathological Hypersecretory Conditions (such as Zollinger-Ellison syndrome): The current recommended adult oral dosage is 150 mg or 10 mL (2 teaspoonfuls equivalent to

150 mg of ranitidine) twice a day. In some patients it may be necessary to administer ZANTAC 150-mg doses more frequently. Dosages should be adjusted to individual patient needs, and should continue as long as clinically indicated. Dosages up to 6 g per day have been employed in patients with severe disease.

Benign Gastric Ulcer: The current recommended adult oral dosage is 150 mg or 10 mL (2 teaspoonfuls equivalent to 150 mg of ranitidine) twice a day.

Maintenance of Healing of Gastric Ulcers: The current recommended adult oral dosage is 150 mg or 10 mL (2 teaspoonfuls equivalent to 150 mg of ranitidine) at bedtime.

GERD: The current recommended adult oral dosage is 150 mg or 10 mL (2 teaspoonfuls equivalent to 150 mg of ranitidine) twice a day.

Erosive Esophagitis: The current recommended adult oral dosage is 150 mg or 10 mL (2 teaspoonfuls equivalent to 150 mg of ranitidine) four times a day.

Maintenance of Healing of Erosive Esophagitis: The current recommended adult oral dosage is 150 mg or 10 mL (2 teaspoonfuls equivalent to 150 mg of ranitidine) twice a day.

Dosage Adjustment for Patients With Impaired Renal Function: On the basis of experience with a group of subjects with severely impaired renal function treated with ZANTAC, the recommended dosage in patients with a creatinine clearance <50 mL per minute is 150 mg or 10 mL (2 teaspoonfuls equivalent to 150 mg of ranitidine) every 24 hours. Should the patient's condition require, the frequency of dosing may be increased to every 12 hours or even further with caution. Hemodialysis reduces the level of circulating ranitidine. Ideally, the dosing schedule should be adjusted so that the timing of a scheduled dose coincides with the end of hemodialysis.

Preparation of ZANTAC 150 EFFERdose Tablets and ZANTAC 150 EFFERdose Granules: Dissolve each dose in approximately 6 to 8 oz of water before drinking.

HOW SUPPLIED

ZANTAC 150 Tablets (ranitidine HCl equivalent to 150 mg of ranitidine) are peach, film-coated, five-sided tablets embossed with "ZANTAC 150" on one side and "Glaxo" on the other. They are available in bottles of 60 (NDC 0173-0344-42), 180 (NDC 0173-0344-17), 500 (NDC 0173-0344-14), and 1,000 (NDC 0173-0344-12) tablets and unit dose packs of 100 (NDC 0173-0344-47) tablets.

ZANTAC 300 Tablets (ranitidine HCl equivalent to 300 mg of ranitidine) are yellow, film-coated, capsule-shaped tablets embossed with "ZANTAC 300" on one side and "Glaxo" on the other. They are available in bottles of 30 (NDC 0173-0393-40) and 250 (NDC 0173-0393-06) tablets and unit dose packs of 100 (NDC 0173-0393-47) tablets.

Store between 15° and 30°C (59° and 86°F) in a dry place. Protect from light. Replace cap securely after each opening.

ZANTAC 150 GELdose Capsules (ranitidine HCl equivalent to 150 mg of ranitidine) are beige, soft gelatin capsules imprinted with "ZANTAC 150" on one side and "GLAXO" on the other. They are available in bottles of 60 (NDC 0173-0428-00) capsules and unit dose packs of 60 (NDC 0173-0428-02) capsules.

ZANTAC 300 GELdose Capsules (ranitidine HCl equivalent to 300 mg of ranitidine) are beige, soft gelatin capsules imprinted with "ZANTAC 300" on one side and "GLAXO" on the other. They are available in bottles of 30 (NDC 0173-0429-00) capsules and unit dose packs of 30 (NDC 0173-0429-02) capsules.

Store between 2° and 25°C (36° and 77°F) in a dry place. Protect from light. Replace cap securely after each opening.

ZANTAC 150 EFFERdose Tablets (ranitidine HCl equivalent to 150 mg of ranitidine) are white to pale yellow, round, flat-faced, bevel-edged tablets embossed with "ZANTAC 150" on one side and "427" on the other. They are packaged individually in foil and are available in cartons of 30 (NDC 0173-0427-00) and 60 (NDC 0173-0427-02) tablets.

ZANTAC 150 EFFERdose Granules (ranitidine HCl equivalent to 150 mg of ranitidine) are white to pale yellow granules. Each 150-mg dose of granules (approximately 1.44 g) is packaged in individual foil packets and is available in cartons of 30 (NDC 0173-0451-00) and 60 (NDC 0173-0451-01) packets.

Store between 2° and 30°C (36° and 86°F).

ZANTAC Syrup, a clear, peppermint-flavored liquid, contains 16.8 mg of ranitidine HCl equivalent to 15 mg of ranitidine per 1 mL in bottles of 16 fluid ounces (one pint) (NDC 0173-0383-54).

Store between 4° and 25°C (39° and 77°F). Dispense in tight, light-resistant containers as defined in the USP/NF.

© Copyright 1996 Glaxo Wellcome Inc. All rights reserved. February 1996/RL-283

Shown in Product Identification Guide, page 315

ZINACEF®
[zin'ah-sef]
(sterile cefuroxime sodium)

ZINACEF®
(cefuroxime sodium injection)

DESCRIPTION

Cefuroxime is a semisynthetic, broad-spectrum, cephalosporin antibiotic for parenteral administration. It is the sodium salt of (6R, 7R)-3-carbamoyloxymethyl-7-[Z-2-methoxyimino-2-(fur-2-yl) acetamido]ceph-3-em-4-carboxylate.

The empirical formula is $C_{16}H_{15}N_4NaO_8S$, representing a molecular weight of 446.4.

ZINACEF contains approximately 54.2 mg (2.4 mEq) of sodium per gram of cefuroxime activity.

ZINACEF in sterile crystalline form is supplied in vials equivalent to 750 mg, 1.5 g, or 7.5 g of cefuroxime as cefuroxime sodium and in ADD-Vantage® vials equivalent to 750 mg or 1.5 g of cefuroxime as cefuroxime sodium. Solutions of ZINACEF range in color from light yellow to amber, depending on the concentration and diluent used. The pH of freshly constituted solutions usually ranges from 6 to 8.5.

ZINACEF is available as a frozen, iso-osmotic, sterile, nonpyrogenic solution with 750 mg or 1.5 g of cefuroxime as cefuroxime sodium. Approximately 1.4 g of dextrose hydrous, USP has been added to the 750-mg dose to adjust the osmolality. Sodium citrate hydrous, USP has been added as a buffer (300 mg and 600 mg to the 750-mg and 1.5-g doses, respectively). ZINACEF contains approximately 111 mg (4.8 mEq) and 222 mg (9.7 mEq) of sodium in the 750-mg and 1.5-g doses, respectively. The pH has been adjusted with hydrochloric acid and may have been adjusted with sodium hydroxide. Solutions of premixed ZINACEF range in color from light yellow to amber. The solution is intended for intravenous (IV) use after thawing to room temperature. The osmolality of the solution is approximately 300 mOsmol/kg, and the pH of thawed solutions ranges from 5 to 7.5.

The plastic container for the frozen solution is fabricated from a specially designed multilayer plastic, PL 2040. Solutions are in contact with the polyethylene layer of this container and can leach out certain chemical components of the plastic in very small amounts within the expiration period. The suitability of the plastic has been confirmed in tests in animals according to USP biological tests for plastic containers as well as by tissue culture toxicity studies.

CLINICAL PHARMACOLOGY

After intramuscular (IM) injection of a 750-mg dose of cefuroxime to normal volunteers, the mean peak serum concentration was 27 mcg/mL. The peak occurred at approximately 45 minutes (range, 15 to 60 minutes). Following IV doses of 750 mg and 1.5 g, serum concentrations were approximately 50 and 100 mcg/mL, respectively, at 15 minutes. Therapeutic serum concentrations of approximately 2 mcg/mL or more were maintained for 5.3 hours and 8 hours or more, respectively. There was no evidence of accumulation of cefuroxime in the serum following IV administration of 1.5-g doses every 8 hours to normal volunteers. The serum half-life after either IM or IV injections is approximately 80 minutes.

Approximately 89% of a dose of cefuroxime is excreted by the kidneys over an 8-hour period, resulting in high urinary concentrations.

Following the IM administration of a 750-mg single dose, urinary concentrations averaged 1,300 mcg/mL during the first 8 hours. Intravenous doses of 750 mg and 1.5 g produced urinary levels averaging 1,150 and 2,500 mcg/mL, respectively, during the first 8-hour period. The concomitant oral administration of probenecid with cefuroxime slows tubular secretion, decreases renal clearance by approximately 40%, increases the peak serum level by approximately 30%, and increases the serum half-life by approximately 30%. Cefuroxime is detectable in therapeutic concentrations in pleural fluid, joint fluid, bile, sputum, bone, cerebrospinal fluid (in patients with meningitis), and aqueous humor.

Cefuroxime is approximately 50% bound to serum protein.

Microbiology: Cefuroxime has *in vitro* activity against a wide range of gram-positive and gram-negative organisms, and it is highly stable in the presence of beta-lactamases of certain gram-negative bacteria. The bactericidal action of cefuroxime results from inhibition of cell-wall synthesis. Cefuroxime is usually active against the following organisms *in vitro*.

Aerobes, Gram-positive: *Staphylococcus aureus, Staphylococcus epidermidis, Streptococcus pneumoniae,* and *Streptococcus pyogenes* (and other streptococci).

NOTE: Most strains of enterococci, e.g., *Enterococcus faecalis* (formerly *Streptococcus faecalis*), are resistant to cefuroxime. Methicillin-resistant staphylococci and *Listeria monocytogenes* are resistant to cefuroxime.

Aerobes, Gram-negative: *Citrobacter* spp., *Enterobacter* spp., *Escherichia coli, Haemophilus influenzae* (including ampicillin-resistant strains), *Haemophilus parainfluenzae, Klebsiella* spp. (including *Klebsiella pneumoniae*), *Moraxella*

(Branhamella) catarrhalis (including ampicillin- and cephalothin-resistant strains), *Morganella morganii* (formerly *Proteus morganii*), *Neisseria gonorrhoeae* (including penicillinase- and non-penicillinase-producing strains), *Neisseria meningitidis, Proteus mirabilis, Providencia rettgeri* (formerly *Proteus rettgeri*), *Salmonella* spp., and *Shigella* spp. NOTE: Some strains of *Morganella morganii, Enterobacter cloacae,* and *Citrobacter* spp. have been shown by *in vitro* tests to be resistant to cefuroxime and other cephalosporins. *Pseudomonas* and *Campylobacter* spp., *Acinetobacter calcoaceticus,* and most strains of *Serratia* spp. and *Proteus vulgaris* are resistant to most first- and second-generation cephalosporins.

Anaerobes: Gram-positive and gram-negative cocci (including *Peptococcus* and *Peptostreptococcus* spp.), gram-positive bacilli (including *Clostridium* spp.), and gram-negative bacilli (including *Bacteroides* and *Fusobacterium* spp.). NOTE: *Clostridium difficile* and most strains of *Bacteroides fragilis* are resistant to cefuroxime.

Susceptibility Tests: *Diffusion Techniques:* Quantitative methods that require measurement of zone diameters give an estimate of antibiotic susceptibility. One such standard procedure[1] that has been recommended for use with disks to test susceptibility of organisms to cefuroxime uses the 30-mcg cefuroxime disk. Interpretation involves the correlation of the diameters obtained in the disk test with the minimum inhibitory concentration (MIC) for cefuroxime.

A report of "Susceptible" indicates that the pathogen is likely to be inhibited by generally achievable blood levels. A report of "Moderately Susceptible" suggests that the organism would be susceptible if high dosage is used or if the infection is confined to tissues and fluids in which high antibiotic levels are attained. A report of "Intermediate" suggests an equivocable or indeterminate result. A report of "Resistant" indicates that achievable concentrations of the antibiotic are unlikely to be inhibitory and other therapy should be selected.

Reports from the laboratory giving results of the standard single-disk susceptibility test for organisms other than *Haemophilus* spp. and *Neisseria gonorrhoeae* with a 30-mcg cefuroxime disk should be interpreted according to the following criteria:

Zone Diameter (mm)	Interpretation
≥ 18	(S) Susceptible
15–17	(MS) Moderately Susceptible
≤ 14	(R) Resistant

Results for *Haemophilus* spp. should be interpreted according to the following criteria:

Zone Diameter (mm)	Interpretation
≥ 24	(S) Susceptible
21–23	(I) Intermediate
≤ 20	(R) Resistant

Results for *Neisseria gonorrhoeae* should be interpreted according to the following criteria:

Zone Diameter (mm)	Interpretation
≥ 31	(S) Susceptible
26–30	(MS) Moderately Susceptible
≤ 25	(R) Resistant

Organisms should be tested with the cefuroxime disk since cefuroxime has been shown by *in vitro* tests to be active against certain strains found resistant when other beta-lactam disks are used. The cefuroxime disk should not be used for testing susceptibility to other cephalosporins.

Standardized procedures require the use of laboratory control organisms. The 30-mcg cefuroxime disk should give the following zone diameters.

1. Testing for organisms other than *Haemophilus* spp. and *Neisseria gonorrhoeae:*

Organism	Zone Diameter (mm)
Staphylococcus aureus ATCC 25923	27–35
Escherichia coli ATCC 25922	20–26

2. Testing for *Haemophilus* spp.:

Organism	Zone Diameter (mm)
Haemophilus influenzae ATCC 49766	28–36

3. Testing for *Neisseria gonorrhoeae:*

Organism	Zone Diameter (mm)
Neisseria gonorrhoeae ATCC 49226	33–41
Staphylococcus aureus ATCC 25923	29–33

Dilution Techniques: Use a standardized dilution method[1] (broth, agar, microdilution) or equivalent with cefuroxime powder. The MIC values obtained for bacterial isolates other than *Haemophilus* spp. and *Neisseria gonorrhoeae* should be interpreted according to the following criteria:

MIC (mcg/mL)	Interpretation
≤ 8	(S) Susceptible
16	(MS) Moderately Susceptible
≥ 32	(R) Resistant

MIC values obtained for *Haemophilus* spp. should be interpreted according to the following criteria:

MIC (mcg/mL)	Interpretation
≤ 4	(S) Susceptible
8	(I) Intermediate
≥ 16	(R) Resistant

MIC values obtained for *Neisseria gonorrhoeae* should be interpreted according to the following criteria:

MIC (mcg/mL)	Interpretation
≤ 1	(S) Susceptible
2	(MS) Moderately Susceptible
≥ 4	(R) Resistant

As with standard diffusion techniques, dilution methods require the use of laboratory control organisms. Standard cefuroxime powder should provide the following MIC values.
1. For organisms other than *Haemophilus* spp. and *Neisseria gonorrhoeae:*

Organism	MIC (mcg/mL)
Staphylococcus aureus ATCC 29213	0.5–2.0
Escherichia coli ATCC 25922	2.0–8.0

2. For *Haemophilus* spp.:

Organism	MIC (mcg/mL)
Haemophilus influenzae ATCC 49766	0.25–1.0

3. For *Neisseria gonorrhoeae:*

Organism	MIC (mcg/mL)
Neisseria gonorrhoeae ATCC 49226	0.25–1.0
Staphylococcus aureus ATCC 29213	0.25–1.0

INDICATIONS AND USAGE

ZINACEF is indicated for the treatment of patients with infections caused by susceptible strains of the designated organisms in the following diseases:

1. **Lower Respiratory Tract Infections,** including pneumonia, caused by *Streptococcus pneumoniae, Haemophilus influenzae* (including ampicillin-resistant strains), *Klebsiella* spp., *Staphylococcus aureus* (penicillinase- and non-penicillinase-producing strains), *Streptococcus pyogenes,* and *Escherichia coli.*

2. **Urinary Tract Infections** caused by *Escherichia coli* and *Klebsiella* spp.

3. **Skin and Skin-Structure Infections** caused by *Staphylococcus aureus* (penicillinase- and non-penicillinase-producing strains), *Streptococcus pyogenes, Escherichia coli, Klebsiella* spp., and *Enterobacter* spp.

4. **Septicemia** caused by *Staphylococcus aureus* (penicillinase- and non-penicillinase-producing strains), *Streptococcus pneumoniae, Escherichia coli, Haemophilus influenzae* (including ampicillin-resistant strains), and *Klebsiella* spp.

5. **Meningitis** caused by *Streptococcus pneumoniae, Haemophilus influenzae* (including ampicillin-resistant strains), *Neisseria meningitidis,* and *Staphylococcus aureus* (penicillinase- and non-penicillinase-producing strains).

6. **Gonorrhea:** Uncomplicated and disseminated gonococcal infections due to *Neisseria gonorrhoeae* (penicillinase- and non-penicillinase-producing strains) in both males and females.

7. **Bone and Joint Infections** caused by *Staphylococcus aureus* (penicillinase- and non-penicillinase-producing strains).

Clinical microbiological studies in skin and skin-structure infections frequently reveal the growth of susceptible strains of both aerobic and anaerobic organisms. ZINACEF has been used successfully in these mixed infections in which several organisms have been isolated. Appropriate cultures and susceptibility studies should be performed to determine the susceptibility of the causative organisms to ZINACEF.

Therapy may be started while awaiting the results of these studies; however, once these results become available, the antibiotic treatment should be adjusted accordingly. In certain cases of confirmed or suspected gram-positive or gram-negative sepsis or in patients with other serious infections in which the causative organism has not been identified, ZINACEF may be used concomitantly with an aminoglycoside (see PRECAUTIONS). The recommended doses of both antibiotics may be given depending on the severity of the infection and the patient's condition.

Prevention: The preoperative prophylactic administration of ZINACEF may prevent the growth of susceptible disease-causing bacteria and thereby may reduce the incidence of certain postoperative infections in patients undergoing surgical procedures (e.g., vaginal hysterectomy) that are classified as clean-contaminated or potentially contaminated procedures. Effective prophylactic use of antibiotics in surgery depends on the time of administration. ZINACEF should usually be given one-half to 1 hour before the operation to allow sufficient time to achieve effective antibiotic concentrations in the wound tissues during the procedure. The dose should be repeated intraoperatively if the surgical procedure is lengthy.

Prophylactic administration is usually not required after the surgical procedure ends and should be stopped within 24 hours. In the majority of surgical procedures, continuing prophylactic administration of any antibiotic does not reduce the incidence of subsequent infections but will increase the possibility of adverse reactions and the development of bacterial resistance.

The perioperative use of ZINACEF has also been effective during open heart surgery for surgical patients in whom infections at the operative site would present a serious risk. For these patients it is recommended that ZINACEF therapy be continued for at least 48 hours after the surgical procedure ends. If an infection is present, specimens for culture should be obtained for the identification of the causative

organism, and appropriate antimicrobial therapy should be instituted.

CONTRAINDICATIONS

ZINACEF is contraindicated in patients with known allergy to the cephalosporin group of antibiotics.

WARNINGS

BEFORE THERAPY WITH ZINACEF IS INSTITUTED, CAREFUL INQUIRY SHOULD BE MADE TO DETERMINE WHETHER THE PATIENT HAS HAD PREVIOUS HYPERSENSITIVITY REACTIONS TO CEPHALOSPORINS, PENICILLINS, OR OTHER DRUGS. THIS PRODUCT SHOULD BE GIVEN CAUTIOUSLY TO PENICILLIN-SENSITIVE PATIENTS. ANTIBIOTICS SHOULD BE ADMINISTERED WITH CAUTION TO ANY PATIENT WHO HAS DEMONSTRATED SOME FORM OF ALLERGY, PARTICULARLY TO DRUGS. IF AN ALLERGIC REACTION TO ZINACEF OCCURS, DISCONTINUE THE DRUG. SERIOUS ACUTE HYPERSENSITIVITY REACTIONS MAY REQUIRE EPINEPHRINE AND OTHER EMERGENCY MEASURES.

Pseudomembranous colitis has been reported with nearly all antibacterial agents, including cefuroxime, and may range in severity from mild to life threatening. Therefore, it is important to consider this diagnosis in patients who present with diarrhea subsequent to the administration of antibacterial agents.

Treatment with antibacterial agents alters the normal flora of the colon and may permit overgrowth of clostridia. Studies indicate that a toxin produced by *Clostridium difficile* is one primary cause of "antibiotic-associated colitis."

After the diagnosis of pseudomembranous colitis has been established, appropriate therapeutic measures should be initiated. Mild cases of pseudomembranous colitis usually respond to drug discontinuation alone. In moderate to severe cases, consideration should be given to management with fluids and electrolytes, protein supplementation, and treatment with an antibacterial drug clinically effective against *Clostridium difficile* colitis.

When the colitis is not relieved by drug discontinuation or when it is severe, oral vancomycin is the treatment of choice for antibiotic-associated pseudomembranous colitis produced by *Clostridium difficile.* Other causes of colitis should also be considered.

PRECAUTIONS

Although ZINACEF rarely produces alterations in kidney function, evaluation of renal status during therapy is recommended, especially in seriously ill patients receiving the maximum doses. Cephalosporins should be given with caution to patients receiving concurrent treatment with potent diuretics as these regimens are suspected of adversely affecting renal function.

The total daily dose of ZINACEF should be reduced in patients with transient or persistent renal insufficiency (see DOSAGE AND ADMINISTRATION), because high and prolonged serum antibiotic concentrations can occur in such individuals from usual doses.

As with other antibiotics, prolonged use of ZINACEF may result in overgrowth of nonsusceptible organisms. Careful observation of the patient is essential. If superinfection occurs during therapy, appropriate measures should be taken. Broad-spectrum antibiotics should be prescribed with caution in individuals with a history of gastrointestinal disease, particularly colitis.

Nephrotoxicity has been reported following concomitant administration of aminoglycoside antibiotics and cephalosporins.

As with other therapeutic regimens used in the treatment of meningitis, mild-to-moderate hearing loss has been reported in a few pediatric patients treated with cefuroxime sodium. Persistence of positive CSF (cerebrospinal fluid) cultures at 18 to 36 hours has also been noted with cefuroxime sodium injection, as well as with other antibiotic therapies; however, the precise relevance of this is unknown.

Drug/Laboratory Test Interactions: A false-positive reaction for glucose in the urine may occur with copper reduction tests (Benedict's or Fehling's solution or with CLINITEST® tablets) but not with enzyme-based tests for glycosuria (e.g., TES-TAPE®). As a false-negative result may occur in the ferricyanide test, it is recommended that either the glucose oxidase or hexokinase method be used to determine blood plasma glucose levels in patients receiving ZINACEF.

Cefuroxime does not interfere with the assay of serum and urine creatinine by the alkaline picrate method.

Carcinogenesis, Mutagenesis, Impairment of Fertility: Although no long-term studies in animals have been performed to evaluate carcinogenic potential, no mutagenic potential of cefuroxime was found in standard laboratory tests.

Reproductive studies revealed no impairment of fertility in animals.

Pregnancy: *Teratogenic Effects: Pregnancy Category B:* Reproduction studies have been performed in mice and rabbits at doses up to 60 times the human dose and have re-

Continued on next page

Glaxo Wellcome—Cont.

vealed no evidence of impaired fertility or harm to the fetus due to cefuroxime. There are, however, no adequate and well-controlled studies in pregnant women. Because animal reproduction studies are not always predictive of human response, this drug should be used during pregnancy only if clearly needed.

Nursing Mothers: Since cefuroxime is excreted in human milk, caution should be exercised when ZINACEF is administered to a nursing woman.

Pediatric Use: Safety and effectiveness in children below 3 months of age have not been established. Accumulation of other members of the cephalosporin class in newborn infants (with resulting prolongation of drug half-life) has been reported.

ADVERSE REACTIONS

ZINACEF is generally well tolerated. The most common adverse effects have been local reactions following IV administration. Other adverse reactions have been encountered only rarely.

Local Reactions: Thrombophlebitis has occurred with IV administration in 1 in 60 patients.

Gastrointestinal: Gastrointestinal symptoms occurred in 1 in 150 patients and included diarrhea (1 in 220 patients) and nausea (1 in 440 patients). Onset of pseudomembranous colitis symptoms may occur during or after treatment (see WARNINGS).

Hypersensitivity Reactions: Hypersensitivity reactions have been reported in fewer than 1% of the patients treated with ZINACEF and include rash (1 in 125). Pruritus, urticaria, and positive Coombs' test each occurred in fewer than 1 in 250 patients, and, as with other cephalosporins, rare cases of anaphylaxis, drug fever, erythema multiforme, interstitial nephritis, toxic epidermal necrolysis, and Stevens-Johnson syndrome have occurred.

Blood: A decrease in hemoglobin and hematocrit has been observed in 1 in 10 patients and transient eosinophilia in 1 in 14 patients. Less common reactions seen were transient neutropenia (fewer than 1 in 100 patients) and leukopenia (1 in 750 patients). A similar pattern and incidence were seen with other cephalosporins used in controlled studies. As with other cephalosporins, there have been rare reports of thrombocytopenia.

Hepatic: Transient rise in SGOT and SGPT (1 in 25 patients), alkaline phosphatase (1 in 50 patients), LDH (1 in 75 patients), and bilirubin (1 in 500 patients) levels has been noted.

Kidney: Elevations in serum creatinine and/or blood urea nitrogen and a decreased creatinine clearance have been observed, but their relationship to cefuroxime is unknown.

In addition to the adverse reactions listed above that have been observed in patients treated with cefuroxime, the following adverse reactions and altered laboratory tests have been reported for cephalosporin-class antibiotics:

Adverse Reactions: Vomiting, abdominal pain, colitis, vaginitis including vaginal candidiasis, toxic nephropathy, hepatic dysfunction including cholestasis, aplastic anemia, hemolytic anemia, hemorrhage.

Several cephalosporins have been implicated in triggering seizures, particularly in patients with renal impairment when the dosage was not reduced (see DOSAGE AND ADMINISTRATION). If seizures associated with drug therapy should occur, the drug should be discontinued. Anticonvulsant therapy can be given if clinically indicated.

Altered Laboratory Tests: Prolonged prothrombin time, pancytopenia, agranulocytosis.

OVERDOSAGE

Overdosage of cephalosporins can cause cerebral irritation leading to convulsions. Serum levels of cefuroxime can be reduced by hemodialysis and peritoneal dialysis.

DOSAGE AND ADMINISTRATION

Dosage: *Adults:* The usual adult dosage range for ZINACEF is 750 mg to 1.5 grams every 8 hours, usually for 5 to 10 days. In uncomplicated urinary tract infections, skin and skin-structure infections, disseminated gonococcal infec-

tions, and uncomplicated pneumonia, a 750-mg dose every 8 hours is recommended. In severe or complicated infections, a 1.5-gram dose every 8 hours is recommended.

In bone and joint infections, a 1.5-gram dose every 8 hours is recommended. In clinical trials, surgical intervention was performed when indicated as an adjunct to ZINACEF therapy. A course of oral antibiotics was administered when appropriate following the completion of parenteral administration of ZINACEF.

In life-threatening infections or infections due to less susceptible organisms, 1.5 grams every 6 hours may be required. In bacterial meningitis, the dosage should not exceed 3 grams every 8 hours. The recommended dosage for uncomplicated gonococcal infection is 1.5 grams given intramuscularly as a single dosage at two different sites together with 1 gram of oral probenecid. For preventive use for clean-contaminated or potentially contaminated surgical procedures, a 1.5-gram dose administered intravenously just before surgery (approximately one-half to 1 hour before the initial incision) is recommended. Thereafter, give 750 mg intravenously or intramuscularly every 8 hours when the procedure is prolonged.

For preventive use during open heart surgery, a 1.5-gram dose administered intravenously at the induction of anesthesia and every 12 hours thereafter for a total of 6 grams is recommended.

Impaired Renal Function: A reduced dosage must be employed when renal function is impaired. Dosage should be determined by the degree of renal impairment and the susceptibility of the causative organism (see Table 1).

Table 1: Dosage of ZINACEF in Adults with Reduced Renal Function

Creatinine Clearance (mL/min)	Dose	Frequency
> 20	750 mg–1.5 grams	q8h
10–20	750 mg	q12h
< 10	750 mg	q24h*

* Since ZINACEF is dialyzable, patients on hemodialysis should be given a further dose at the end of the dialysis.

When only serum creatinine is available, the following formula[2] (based on sex, weight, and age of the patient) may be used to convert this value into creatinine clearance. The serum creatinine should represent a steady state of renal function.

Males: $\text{Creatinine Clearance (mL/min)} = \dfrac{\text{Weight (kg)} \times (140 - \text{age})}{72 \times \text{serum creatinine (mg/dL)}}$

Females: $0.85 \times \text{male value}$

Note: As with antibiotic therapy in general, administration of ZINACEF should be continued for a minimum of 48 to 72 hours after the patient becomes asymptomatic or after evidence of bacterial eradication has been obtained; a minimum of 10 days of treatment is recommended in infections caused by *Streptococcus pyogenes* in order to guard against the risk of rheumatic fever or glomerulonephritis; frequent bacteriologic and clinical appraisal is necessary during therapy of chronic urinary tract infection and may be required for several months after therapy has been completed; persistent infections may require treatment for several weeks; and doses smaller than those indicated above should not be used. In staphylococcal and other infections involving a collection of pus, surgical drainage should be carried out where indicated.

Pediatric Patients Above 3 Months of Age: Administration of 50 to 100 mg/kg per day in equally divided doses every 6 to 8 hours has been successful for most infections susceptible to cefuroxime. The higher dosage of 100 mg/kg per day (not to exceed the maximum adult dosage) should be used for the more severe or serious infections.

In bone and joint infections, 150 mg/kg per day (not to exceed the maximum adult dosage) is recommended in equally divided doses every 8 hours. In clinical trials, a course of oral antibiotics was administered to children following the completion of parenteral administration of ZINACEF.

In cases of bacterial meningitis, a larger dosage of ZINACEF is recommended, 200 to 240 mg/kg per day intravenously in divided doses every 6 to 8 hours.

In children with renal insufficiency, the frequency of dosing should be modified consistent with the recommendations for adults.

Preparation of Solution and Suspension: The directions for preparing ZINACEF for both IV and IM use are summarized in Table 2.

For Intramuscular Use: Each 750-mg vial of ZINACEF should be constituted with 3.0 mL of sterile water for injection. Shake gently to disperse and withdraw completely the resulting suspension for injection.

For Intravenous Use: Each 750-mg vial should be constituted with 8.0 mL of sterile water for injection. Withdraw completely the resulting solution for injection.

Each 1.5-gram vial should be constituted with 16.0 mL of sterile water for injection, and the solution should be completely withdrawn for injection.

The 7.5-gram pharmacy bulk vial should be constituted with 77 mL of sterile water for injection; each 8 mL of the resulting solution contains 750 mg of cefuroxime.

Each 750-mg and 1.5-gram infusion pack should be constituted with 100 mL of sterile water for injection, 5% dextrose injection, 0.9% sodium chloride injection, or any of the solutions listed under the Intravenous portion of the COMPATIBILITY AND STABILITY section. [See Table 2 below.]

Administration: After constitution, ZINACEF may be given intravenously or by deep IM injection into a large muscle mass (such as the gluteus or lateral part of the thigh). Before injecting intramuscularly, aspiration is necessary to avoid inadvertent injection into a blood vessel.

Intravenous Administration: The IV route may be preferable for patients with bacterial septicemia or other severe or life-threatening infections or for patients who may be poor risks because of lowered resistance, particularly if shock is present or impending.

For direct intermittent IV administration, slowly inject the solution into a vein over a period of 3 to 5 minutes or give it through the tubing system by which the patient is also receiving other IV solutions.

For intermittent IV infusion with a Y-type administration set, dosing can be accomplished through the tubing system by which the patient may be receiving other IV solutions. However, during infusion of the solution containing ZINACEF, it is advisable to temporarily discontinue administration of any other solutions at the same site.

ADD-Vantage® vials are to be constituted only with 50 or 100 mL of 5% dextrose injection, 0.9% sodium chloride injection, or 0.45% sodium chloride injection in Abbott ADD-Vantage flexible diluent containers (see Instructions for Constitution section of the product package insert). ADD-Vantage vials that have been joined to Abbott ADD-Vantage diluent containers and activated to dissolve the drug are stable for 24 hours at room temperature or for 7 days under refrigeration. Joined vials that have not been activated may be used within a 14-day period; this period corresponds to that for use of Abbott ADD-Vantage containers following removal of the outer packaging (overwrap). Freezing solutions of ZINACEF in the ADD-Vantage system is not recommended.

For continuous IV infusion, a solution of ZINACEF may be added to an IV infusion pack containing one of the following fluids: 0.9% sodium chloride injection; 5% dextrose injection; 10% dextrose injection; 5% dextrose and 0.9% sodium chloride injection; 5% dextrose and 0.45% sodium chloride injection; or 1/6 M sodium lactate injection.

Solutions of ZINACEF, like those of most beta-lactam antibiotics, should not be added to solutions of aminoglycoside antibiotics because of potential interaction.

However, if concurrent therapy with ZINACEF and an aminoglycoside is indicated, each of these antibiotics can be administered separately to the same patient.

Directions for Use of ZINACEF Frozen in GALAXY® Plastic Containers: ZINACEF supplied as a frozen, sterile, iso-osmotic, nonpyrogenic solution in plastic containers is to be administered after thawing either as a continuous or intermittent IV infusion. The thawed solution of the premixed product is stable for 28 days if stored under refrigeration (5° C) or for 24 hours if stored at room temperature (25° C).

Do not Refreeze.

Thaw container at room temperature (25°C) or under refrigeration (5°C). Do not force thaw by immersion in water baths or by microwave irradiation. Components of the solution may precipitate in the frozen state and will dissolve upon reaching room temperature with little or no agitation. Potency is not affected. Mix after solution has reached room temperature. Check for minute leaks by squeezing bag firmly. Discard bag if leaks are found as sterility may be impaired. Do not add supplementary medication. Do not use unless solution is clear and seal is intact.

Use sterile equipment.

Caution: Do not use plastic containers in series connections. Such use could result in air embolism due to residual air being drawn from the primary container before administration of the fluid from the secondary container is complete.

Table 2: Preparation of Solution and Suspension

Strength	Amount of Diluent to Be Added (mL)	Volume to Be Withdrawn	Approximate Cefuroxime Concentration (mg/mL)
750-mg Vial	3.0 (IM)	Total*	220
750-mg Vial	8.0 (IV)	Total	90
1.5-gram Vial	16.0 (IV)	Total	90
750-mg Infusion pack	100 (IV)	—	7.5
1.5-gram Infusion pack	100 (IV)	—	15
7.5-gram Pharmacy bulk package	77 (IV)	Amount Needed†	95

*Note: ZINACEF is a suspension at IM concentrations.

†8 mL of solution contains 750 mg of cefuroxime; 16 mL of solution contains 1.5 grams of cefuroxime.

Preparation for Administration:
1. Suspend container from eyelet support.
2. Remove protector from outlet port at bottom of container.
3. Attach administration set. Refer to complete directions accompanying set.

COMPATIBILITY AND STABILITY

Intramuscular: When constituted as directed with sterile water for injection, suspensions of ZINACEF for IM injection maintain satisfactory potency for 24 hours at room temperature and for 48 hours under refrigeration (5°C).
After the periods mentioned above any unused suspensions should be discarded.
Intravenous: When the 750-mg, 1.5-g, and 7.5-g pharmacy bulk vials are constituted as directed with sterile water for injection, the ZINACEF solutions for IV administration maintain satisfactory potency for 24 hours at room temperature and for 48 hours (750-mg and 1.5-g vials) or for 7 days (7.5-g pharmacy bulk vial) under refrigeration (5°C). More dilute solutions, such as 750 mg or 1.5 g plus 100 mL of sterile water for injection, 5% dextrose injection, or 0.9% sodium chloride injection, also maintain satisfactory potency for 24 hours at room temperature and for 7 days under refrigeration.
These solutions may be further diluted to concentrations of between 1 and 30 mg/mL in the following solutions and will lose not more than 10% activity for 24 hours at room temperature or for at least 7 days under refrigeration: 0.9% sodium chloride injection; 1/6 M sodium lactate injection; ringer's injection, USP; lactated ringer's injection, USP; 5% dextrose and 0.9% sodium chloride injection; 5% dextrose injection; 5% dextrose and 0.45% sodium chloride injection; 5% dextrose and 0.225% sodium chloride injection; 10% dextrose injection; and 10% invert sugar in water for injection. Unused solutions should be discarded after the time periods mentioned above.
ZINACEF has also been found compatible for 24 hours at room temperature when admixed in IV infusion with heparin (10 and 50 U/mL) in 0.9% sodium chloride injection and potassium chloride (10 and 40 mEq/L) in 0.9% sodium chloride injection. Sodium bicarbonate injection, USP is not recommended for the dilution of ZINACEF.
The 750-mg and 1.5-g ZINACEF ADD-Vantage vials, when diluted in 50 or 100 mL of 5% dextrose injection, 0.9% sodium chloride injection, or 0.45% sodium chloride injection, may be stored for up to 24 hours at room temperature or for 7 days under refrigeration.
Frozen Stability: Constitute the 750-mg, 1.5-g, or 7.5-g vial as directed for IV administration in Table 2. Immediately withdraw the total contents of the 750-mg or 1.5-g vial or 8 or 16 mL from the 7.5-g bulk vial and add to a Baxter VIAFLEX® MINI-BAG™ containing 50 or 100 mL of 0.9% sodium chloride injection or 5% dextrose injection and freeze. Frozen solutions are stable for 6 months when stored at −20°C. Frozen solutions should be thawed at room temperature and not refrozen. Do not force thaw by immersion in water baths or by microwave irradiation. Thawed solutions may be stored for up to 24 hours at room temperature or for 7 days in a refrigerator.
Note: Parenteral drug products should be inspected visually for particulate matter and discoloration before administration whenever solution and container permit.
As with other cephalosporins, ZINACEF powder as well as solutions and suspensions tend to darken, depending on storage conditions, without adversely affecting product potency.
Directions for Dispensing: ***Pharmacy Bulk Package—Not for Direct Infusion:*** The pharmacy bulk package is for use in a pharmacy admixture service only under a laminar flow hood. Entry into the vial must be made with a sterile transfer set or other sterile dispensing device, and the contents dispensed in aliquots using aseptic technique. The use of syringe and needle is not recommended as it may cause leakage (see DOSAGE AND ADMINISTRATION). AFTER INITIAL WITHDRAWAL USE ENTIRE CONTENTS OF VIAL PROMPTLY. ANY UNUSED PORTION MUST BE DISCARDED WITHIN 24 HOURS.

HOW SUPPLIED

ZINACEF in the dry state should be stored between 15° and 30°C (59° and 86°F) and protected from light. ZINACEF is a dry, white to off-white powder supplied in vials and infusion packs as follows:
NDC 0173-0352-31 750-mg* Vial (Tray of 25)
NDC 0173-0354-35 1.5-g* Vial (Tray of 25)
NDC 0173-0353-32 750-mg* Infusion Pack (Tray of 10)
NDC 0173-0356-32 1.5-g* Infusion Pack (Tray of 10)
NDC 0173-0400-00 7.5-g* Pharmacy Bulk Package (Tray of 6)
NDC 0173-0436-00 750-mg ADD-Vantage® Vial (Tray of 25)
NDC 0173-0437-00 1.5-g ADD-Vantage® Vial (Tray of 10)
(The above ADD-Vantage vials are to be used only with Abbott ADD-Vantage diluent containers).
ZINACEF frozen as a premixed solution of cefuroxime sodium should not be stored above −20° C. ZINACEF is supplied frozen in 50-mL, single-dose, plastic containers as follows:
NDC 0173-0424-00 750-mg* Plastic Container (Carton of 24)
NDC 0173-0425-00 1.5-g* Plastic Container (Carton of 24)
*Equivalent to cefuroxime.

REFERENCES

1. National Committee for Clinical Laboratory Standards. *Performance Standards for Antimicrobial Susceptibility Testing.* Third Informational Supplement. NCCLS Document M100-S3, Vol. 11, No. 17. Villanova, Pa: NCCLS; 1991.
2. Cockcroft DW, Gault MH: Prediction of creatinine clearance from serum creatinine. *Nephron.* 1976;16:31-41.
ZINACEF is a registered trademark of Glaxo.
ADD-Vantage is a registered trademark of Abbott Laboratories.
CLINITEST is a registered trademark of Ames Division, Miles Laboratories, Inc.
TES-TAPE is a registered trademark of Eli Lilly and Company.
GALAXY and VIAFLEX are registered trademarks of Baxter International Inc.
February 1996/RL-229
Shown in Product Identification Guide, page 315

ZOVIRAX® Capsules ℞
ZOVIRAX® Tablets ℞
ZOVIRAX® Suspension ℞
[*zō″vī′răx*]
(acyclovir)

DESCRIPTION

ZOVIRAX is the brand name for acyclovir, an antiviral drug. ZOVIRAX Capsules, Tablets, and Suspension are formulations for oral administration. Each capsule of ZOVIRAX contains 200 mg of acyclovir and the inactive ingredients corn starch, lactose, magnesium stearate, and sodium lauryl sulfate. The capsule shell consists of gelatin, FD&C Blue No. 2, and titanium dioxide. May contain one or more parabens. Printed with edible black ink.
Each 800 mg tablet of ZOVIRAX contains 800 mg of acyclovir and the inactive ingredients FD&C Blue No. 2, magnesium stearate, microcrystalline cellulose, povidone, and sodium starch glycolate.
Each 400 mg tablet of ZOVIRAX contains 400 mg of acyclovir and the inactive ingredients magnesium stearate, microcrystalline cellulose, povidone, and sodium starch glycolate.
Each teaspoonful (5 mL) of ZOVIRAX Suspension contains 200 mg of acyclovir and the inactive ingredients methylparaben 0.1% and propylparaben 0.02% (added as preservatives), carboxymethylcellulose sodium, flavor, glycerin, microcrystalline cellulose, and sorbitol.
The chemical name of acyclovir is 2-amino-1,9-dihydro-9-[(2-hydroxyethoxy)methyl]-6*H*-purin-6-one.
Acyclovir is a white, crystalline powder with a molecular weight of 225 daltons, and a maximum solubility in water of 2.5 mg/mL at 37°C.

CLINICAL PHARMACOLOGY

Mechanism of Antiviral Effects: Acyclovir is a synthetic purine nucleoside analogue with in vitro and in vivo inhibitory activity against human herpes viruses including herpes simplex types 1 (HSV-1) and 2 (HSV-2), varicella-zoster virus (VZV), Epstein-Barr virus (EBV), and cytomegalovirus (CMV). In cell culture, acyclovir has the highest antiviral activity against HSV-1, followed in decreasing order of potency against HSV-2, VZV, EBV, and CMV.[1]
The inhibitory activity of acyclovir for HSV-1, HSV-2, VZV, and EBV is highly selective. The enzyme thymidine kinase (TK) of normal uninfected cells does not effectively use acyclovir as a substrate. However, TK encoded by HSV, VZV, and EBV[2] converts acyclovir into acyclovir monophosphate, a nucleotide analogue. The monophosphate is further converted into diphosphate by cellular guanylate kinase and into triphosphate by a number of cellular enzymes.[3] Acyclovir triphosphate interferes with herpes simplex virus DNA polymerase and inhibits viral DNA replication. Acyclovir triphosphate also inhibits cellular α-DNA polymerase, but to a lesser degree. In vitro, acyclovir triphosphate can be incorporated into growing chains of DNA by viral DNA polymerase and to a much smaller extent by cellular α-DNA polymerase.[4] When incorporation occurs, the DNA chain is terminated.[5,6] Acyclovir is preferentially taken up and selectively converted to the active triphosphate form by herpesvirus-infected cells. Thus, acyclovir is much less toxic in vitro for normal uninfected cells because: 1) less is taken up; 2) less is converted to the active form; 3) cellular α-DNA polymerase is less sensitive to the effects of the active form. The mode of acyclovir phosphorylation in cytomegalovirus-infected cells is not clearly established, but may involve virally induced cell kinases or an unidentified viral enzyme. Acyclovir is not efficiently activated in cytomegalovirus-infected cells, which may account for the reduced susceptibility of cytomegalovirus to acyclovir in vitro.
Microbiology: The quantitative relationship between the in vitro susceptibility of herpes simplex and varicella-zoster viruses to acyclovir and the clinical response to therapy has not been established in humans, and virus sensitivity testing has not been standardized. Sensitivity testing results, expressed as the concentration of drug required to inhibit by 50% the growth of virus in cell culture (ID_{50}), vary greatly depending upon the particular assay used,[7] the cell type employed,[8] and the laboratory performing the test.[1] The ID_{50} of acyclovir against HSV-1 isolates may range from 0.02 μg/mL (plaque reduction in Vero cells) to 5.9 to 13.5 μg/mL (plaque reduction in green monkey kidney [GMK] cells).[1] The ID_{50} against HSV-2 ranges from 0.01 μg/mL to 9.9 μg/mL (plaque reduction in Vero and GMK cells, respectively).[1] Using a dye-uptake method in Vero cells,[9] which gives ID_{50} values approximately 5- to 10-fold higher than plaque reduction assays, 1417 HSV isolates (553 HSV-1 and 864 HSV-2) from approximately 500 patients were examined over a 5-year period.[10] These assays found that 90% of HSV-1 isolates were sensitive to $\leq$ 0.9 μg/mL acyclovir and 50% of all isolates were sensitive to $\leq$ 0.2 μg/mL acyclovir. For HSV-2 isolates, 90% were sensitive to $\leq$ 2.2 μg/mL and 50% of all isolates were sensitive to $\leq$ 0.7 μg/mL of acyclovir. Isolates with significantly diminished sensitivity were found in 44 patients. It must be emphasized that neither the patients nor the isolates were randomly selected and, therefore, do not represent the general population.
Most of the less sensitive HSV clinical isolates have been relatively deficient in the viral TK.[11-19] Strains with alterations in viral TK[20] or viral DNA polymerase[21] have also been reported. Prolonged exposure to low concentrations (0.1 μg/mL) of acyclovir in cell culture has resulted in the emergence of a variety of acyclovir-resistant strains.[22]
The ID_{50} against VZV ranges from 0.17 to 1.53 μg/mL (yield reduction, human foreskin fibroblasts) to 1.85 to 3.98 μg/mL (foci reduction, human embryo fibroblasts [HEF]). Reproduction of EBV genome is suppressed by 50% in superinfected Raji cells or P3HR-1 lymphoblastoid cells by 1.5 μg/mL acyclovir. CMV is relatively resistant to acyclovir with ID_{50} values ranging from 2.3 to 17.6 μg/mL (plaque reduction, HEF cells) to 1.82 to 56.8 μg/mL (DNA hybridization, HEF cells). The latent state of the genome of any of the human herpesviruses is not known to be sensitive to acyclovir.[1]
Pharmacokinetics: The pharmacokinetics of acyclovir after oral administration have been evaluated in 6 clinical studies involving 110 adult patients. In one uncontrolled study of 35 immunocompromised patients with herpes simplex or varicella-zoster infection, ZOVIRAX Capsules were administered in doses of 200 to 1000 mg every 4 hours, 6 times daily for 5 days, and steady-state plasma levels were reached by the second day of dosing. Mean steady-state peak and trough concentrations following the final 200 mg dose were 0.49 μg/mL (0.47 to 0.54 μg/mL) and 0.31 μg/mL (0.18 to 0.41 μg/mL), respectively, and following the final 800 mg dose were 2.8 μg/mL (2.3 to 3.1 μg/mL) and 1.8 μg/mL (1.3 to 2.5 μg/mL), respectively. In another uncontrolled study of 20 younger immunocompetent patients with recurrent genital herpes simplex infections, ZOVIRAX Capsules were administered in doses of 800 mg every 6 hours, 4 times daily for 5 days; the mean steady-state peak and trough concentrations were 1.4 μg/mL (0.66 to 1.8 μg/mL) and 0.55 μg/mL (0.14 to 1.1 μg/mL), respectively.
In general, the pharmacokinetics of acyclovir in children is similar to adults. Mean half-life after oral doses of 300 mg/m^2 and 600 mg/m^2, in children ages 7 months to 7 years, was 2.6 hours (range 1.59 to 3.74 hours).
A single oral dose bioavailability study in 23 normal volunteers showed that ZOVIRAX Capsules 200 mg are bioequivalent to 200 mg acyclovir in aqueous solution; and in a separate study in 20 volunteers, it was shown that ZOVIRAX Suspension is bioequivalent to ZOVIRAX Capsules. In a different single-dose bioavailability/bioequivalence study in 24 volunteers, one ZOVIRAX 800 mg Tablet was demonstrated to be bioequivalent to four ZOVIRAX 200 mg Capsules.
In a multiple-dose crossover study where 23 volunteers received ZOVIRAX as one 200 mg capsule, one 400 mg tablet, and one 800 mg tablet 6 times daily, absorption decreased with increasing dose and the estimated bioavailabilities of acyclovir were 20%, 15%, and 10%, respectively. The decrease in bioavailability is believed to be a function of the dose and not the dosage form. It was demonstrated that acyclovir is not dose proportional over the dosing range 200 mg to 800 mg. In this study, steady-state peak and trough concentrations of acyclovir were 0.83 and 0.46 μg/mL, 1.21 and 0.63 μg/mL, and 1.61 and 0.83 μg/mL for the 200, 400, and 800 mg dosage regimens, respectively.
In another study in 6 volunteers, the influence of food on the absorption of acyclovir was not apparent.
Following oral administration, the mean plasma half-life of acyclovir in volunteers and patients with normal renal function ranged from 2.5 to 3.3 hours. The mean renal excretion of unchanged drug accounts for 14.4% (8.6% to 19.8%) of the orally administered dose. The only urinary metabolite (iden-

Continued on next page

Glaxo Wellcome—Cont.

tified by high performance liquid chromatography) is 9-[(carboxymethoxy)methyl]guanine. The half-life and total body clearance of acyclovir are dependent on renal function. A dosage adjustment is recommended for patients with reduced renal function (see DOSAGE AND ADMINISTRATION).

Orally administered acyclovir in children less than 2 years of age has not yet been fully studied.

INDICATIONS AND USAGE

ZOVIRAX Capsules, Tablets, and Suspension are indicated for the treatment of initial episodes and the management of recurrent episodes of genital herpes in certain patients.

ZOVIRAX Capsules, Tablets, and Suspension are indicated for the acute treatment of herpes zoster (shingles) and chickenpox (varicella).

Genital Herpes Infections: The severity of disease is variable depending upon the immune status of the patient, the frequency and duration of episodes, and the degree of cutaneous or systemic involvement. These factors should determine patient management, which may include symptomatic support and counseling only, or the institution of specific therapy. The physical, emotional, and psychosocial difficulties posed by herpes infections as well as the degree of debilitation, particularly in immunocompromised patients, are unique for each patient, and the physician should determine therapeutic alternatives based on his or her understanding of the individual patient's needs. Thus, orally administered ZOVIRAX is not appropriate in treating all genital herpes infections. The following guidelines may be useful in weighing the benefit/risk considerations in specific disease categories:

First Episodes (primary and nonprimary infections—commonly known as initial genital herpes):

Double-blind, placebo-controlled studies[23,24,25] have demonstrated that orally administered ZOVIRAX significantly reduced the duration of acute infection (detection of virus in lesions by tissue culture) and lesion healing. The duration of pain and new lesion formation was decreased in some patient groups. The promptness of initiation of therapy and/or the patient's prior exposure to herpes simplex virus may influence the degree of benefit from therapy. Patients with mild disease may derive less benefit than those with more severe episodes. In patients with extremely severe episodes, in which prostration, central nervous system involvement, urinary retention, or inability to take oral medication require hospitalization and more aggressive management, therapy may be best initiated with intravenous ZOVIRAX.

Recurrent Episodes:

Double-blind, placebo-controlled studies[16,26-32] in patients with frequent recurrences (6 or more episodes per year) have shown that orally administered ZOVIRAX given daily for 4 months to 3 years prevented or reduced the frequency and/or severity of recurrences in greater than 95% of patients. In a study of 283 patients who received ZOVIRAX 400 mg (two 200 mg capsules) twice daily for 3 years, 45%, 52%, and 63% of patients remained free of recurrences in the first, second, and third years, respectively. Serial analyses of the 3-month recurrence rates for the 283 patients showed that 71% to 87% were recurrence-free in each quarter, indicating that the effects are consistent over time.

The frequency and severity of episodes of untreated genital herpes may change over time. After 1 year of therapy, the frequency and severity of the patient's genital herpes infection should be re-evaluated to assess the need for continuation of therapy with ZOVIRAX. Re-evaluation will usually require a trial off ZOVIRAX to assess the need for reinstitution of suppressive therapy. Some patients, such as those with very frequent or severe episodes before treatment, may warrant uninterrupted suppression for more than a year.

Chronic suppressive therapy is most appropriate when, in the judgement of the physician, the benefits of such a regimen outweigh known or potential adverse effects. In general, orally administered ZOVIRAX should not be used for the suppression of recurrent disease in mildly affected patients. Unanswered questions concerning the relevance to humans of in vitro mutagenicity studies and reproductive toxicity studies in animals given high parenteral doses of acyclovir for short periods (see PRECAUTIONS: Carcinogenesis, Mutagenesis, Impairment of Fertility) should be borne in mind when designing long-term management for individual patients. Discussion of these issues with patients will provide them the opportunity to weigh the potential for toxicity against the severity of their disease. Thus, this regimen should be considered only for appropriate patients with annual re-evaluation.

Limited studies[31,32] have shown that there are certain patients for whom intermittent short-term treatment of recurrent episodes is effective. This approach may be more appropriate than a suppressive regimen in patients with infrequent recurrences.

Immunocompromised patients with recurrent herpes infections can be treated with either intermittent or chronic sup-

pressive therapy. Clinically significant resistance, although rare, is more likely to be seen with prolonged or repeated therapy in severely immunocompromised patients with active lesions.

Herpes Zoster Infections: In a double-blind, placebo-controlled study of 187 normal patients with localized cutaneous zoster infection (93 randomized to ZOVIRAX and 94 to placebo), ZOVIRAX (800 mg 5 times daily for 10 days) shortened the times to lesion scabbing, healing, and complete cessation of pain, and reduced the duration of viral shedding and the duration of new lesion formation.[33]

In a similar double-blind, placebo-controlled study in 83 normal patients with herpes zoster (40 randomized to ZOVIRAX and 43 to placebo), ZOVIRAX (800 mg 5 times daily for 7 days) shortened the times to complete lesion scabbing, healing, and cessation of pain, reduced the duration of new lesion formation, and reduced the prevalence of localized zoster-associated neurologic symptoms (paresthesia, dysesthesia, or hyperesthesia).[34]

Chickenpox: In a double-blind, placebo-controlled efficacy study in 110 normal patients, ages 5 to 16 years, who presented **within 24 hours** of the onset of a typical chickenpox rash, ZOVIRAX was administered orally 4 times daily for 5 to 7 days at doses of 10, 15, or 20 mg/kg depending on the age group. Treatment with ZOVIRAX reduced the maximum number of lesions (336 vs. greater than 500; lesions beyond 500 were not counted). Treatment with ZOVIRAX also shortened the mean time to 50% healing (7.1 days vs. 8.7 days), reduced the number of vesicular lesions by the second day of treatment (49 vs. 113), and decreased the proportion of patients with fever (temperature greater than 100°F) by the second day (19% vs. 57%). Treatment with ZOVIRAX did not affect the antibody response to varicella-zoster virus measured 1 month and 1 year following the treatment.[35]

In two concurrent double-blind, placebo-controlled studies, a total of 883 normal patients, ages 2 to 18 years, were enrolled **within 24 hours** of the onset of a typical chickenpox rash, and ZOVIRAX was administered at 20 mg/kg orally up to 800 mg 4 times daily for 5 days. In the larger study of 815 children ages 2 to 12 years, treatment with ZOVIRAX reduced the median maximum number of lesions (277 vs. 386), reduced the median number of vesicular lesions by the second day of treatment (26 vs. 40), and reduced the proportion of patients with moderate to severe itching by the third day of treatment (15% vs. 34%).[36] In addition, in both studies (883 patients, ages 2 to 18 years), treatment with ZOVIRAX also decreased the proportion of patients with fever (temperature greater than 100°F), anorexia, and lethargy by the second day of treatment, and decreased the mean number of residual lesions on Day 28.[36,37] There were no substantial differences in VZV-specific humoral or cellular immune responses measured at 1 month following treatment in patients receiving ZOVIRAX compared to patients receiving placebo.[38]

Diagnosis: Diagnosis is confirmed by virus isolation. Accelerated viral culture assays or immunocytology allow more rapid diagnosis than standard viral culture. For patients with initial episodes of genital herpes, appropriate examinations should be performed to rule out other sexually transmitted diseases. While cutaneous lesions associated with herpes simplex and varicella-zoster infections are often characteristic, the finding of multinucleated giant cells in smears prepared from lesion exudate or scrapings may provide additional support to the clinical diagnosis.[39]

Multinucleated giant cells in smears do not distinguish varicella-zoster from herpes simplex infections.

CONTRAINDICATIONS

ZOVIRAX Capsules, Tablets, and Suspension are contraindicated for patients who develop hypersensitivity or intolerance to the components of the formulations.

WARNINGS

ZOVIRAX Capsules, Tablets, and Suspension are intended for oral ingestion only.

PRECAUTIONS

General: ZOVIRAX has caused decreased spermatogenesis at high parenteral doses in some animals and mutagenesis in some acute studies at high concentrations of drug (see PRECAUTIONS: Carcinogenesis, Mutagenesis, Impairment of Fertility). The recommended dosage should not be exceeded (see DOSAGE AND ADMINISTRATION).

Exposure of herpes simplex and varicella-zoster isolates to acyclovir in vitro can lead to the emergence of less sensitive viruses. The possibility of the appearance of less sensitive viruses in humans must be borne in mind when treating patients. The relationship between the in vitro sensitivity of herpes simplex or varicella-zoster virus to acyclovir and clinical response to therapy has yet to be established (see CLINICAL PHARMACOLOGY: Microbiology).

Because of the possibility that less sensitive virus may be selected in patients who are receiving acyclovir, all patients should be advised to take particular care to avoid potential transmission of virus if active lesions are present while they are on therapy. In severely immunocompromised patients, the physician should be aware that prolonged or repeated

courses of acyclovir may result in selection of resistant viruses which may not fully respond to continued acyclovir therapy.

Caution should be exercised when administering ZOVIRAX to patients receiving potentially nephrotoxic agents since this may increase the risk of renal dysfunction.

Information for Patients: Patients are instructed to consult with their physician if they experience severe or troublesome adverse reactions, they become pregnant or intend to become pregnant, they intend to breastfeed while taking orally administered ZOVIRAX, or they have any other questions.

Genital Herpes Infections: Genital herpes is a sexually transmitted disease and patients should avoid intercourse when visible lesions are present because of the risk of infecting intimate partners. ZOVIRAX Capsules, Tablets, and Suspension are for oral ingestion only. Medication should not be shared with others. The prescribed dosage should not be exceeded. ZOVIRAX does not eliminate latent viruses. Patients are instructed to consult with their physician if they do not receive sufficient relief in the frequency and severity of their genital herpes recurrences.

There are still unanswered questions concerning reproductive/gonadal toxicity and mutagenesis; long-term studies are continuing. Decreased sperm production has been seen at high doses in some animals; a placebo-controlled clinical study using 400 mg or 1000 mg of ZOVIRAX per day for 6 months in humans did not show similar findings.[40] Chromosomal breaks were seen in vitro after brief exposure to high concentrations. Some other currently marketed medications also cause chromosomal breaks, and the significance of this finding is unknown. A placebo-controlled clinical study using 800 mg of ZOVIRAX per day for 1 year in humans did not show any abnormalities in structure or number of chromosomes.[28]

Herpes Zoster Infections: Adults age 50 or older tend to have more severe shingles, and treatment with ZOVIRAX showed more significant benefit for older patients. Treatment was begun within 72 hours of rash onset in these studies, and was more useful if started within the first 48 hours.

Chickenpox: Although chickenpox in otherwise healthy children is usually a self-limited disease of mild to moderate severity, adolescents and adults tend to have more severe disease. Treatment was initiated within 24 hours of the typical chickenpox rash in the controlled studies, and there is no information regarding the effects of treatment begun later in the disease course. It is unknown whether the treatment of chickenpox in childhood has any effect on long-term immunity. However, there is no evidence to indicate that treatment of chickenpox with ZOVIRAX would have any effect on either decreasing or increasing the incidence or severity of subsequent recurrences of herpes zoster (shingles) later in life. Intravenous ZOVIRAX is indicated for the treatment of varicella-zoster infections in immunocompromised patients.

Drug Interactions: Co-administration of probenecid with intravenous acyclovir has been shown to increase the mean half-life and the area under the concentration-time curve. Urinary excretion and renal clearance were correspondingly reduced.[41] The clinical effects of this combination have not been studied.

Carcinogenesis, Mutagenesis, Impairment of Fertility: The data presented below include references to peak steady-state plasma acyclovir concentrations observed in humans treated with 800 mg given orally 6 times a day (dosing appropriate for treatment of herpes zoster) or 200 mg given orally 6 times a day (dosing appropriate for treatment of genital herpes). Plasma drug concentrations in animal studies are expressed as multiples of human exposure to acyclovir at the higher and lower dosing schedules (see Pharmacokinetics).

Acyclovir was tested in lifetime bioassays in rats and mice at single daily doses of up to 450 mg/kg administered by gavage. There was no statistically significant difference in the incidence of tumors between treated and control animals, nor did acyclovir shorten the latency of tumors. At 450 mg/kg/day, plasma concentrations were 3 to 6 times human levels in the mouse bioassay and 1 to 2 times human levels in the rat bioassay.

Acyclovir was tested in two in vitro cell transformation assays. Positive results were observed at the highest concentration tested (31 to 63 times human levels) in one system and the resulting morphologically transformed cells formed tumors when inoculated into immunosuppressed, syngeneic, weanling mice. Acyclovir was negative (40 to 80 times human levels) in the other, possibly less sensitive, transformation assay.

In acute cytogenetic studies, there was an increase, though not statistically significant, in the incidence of chromosomal damage at maximum tolerated parenteral doses of acyclovir (100 mg/kg) in rats (62 to 125 times human levels) but not in Chinese hamsters; higher doses of 500 and 1000 mg/kg were clastogenic in Chinese hamsters (380 to 760 times human levels). In addition, no activity was found after 5 days dosing in a dominant lethal study in mice (36 to 73 times human levels). In all 4 microbial assays, no evidence of mutagenicity was observed. Positive results were obtained in 2 of 7 genetic

toxicity assays using mammalian cells in vitro. In human lymphocytes, a positive response for chromosomal damage was seen at concentrations 150 to 300 times the acyclovir plasma levels achieved in humans. At one locus in mouse lymphoma cells, mutagenicity was observed at concentrations 250 to 500 times human plasma levels. Results in the other five mammalian cell loci follow: at 3 loci in a Chinese hamster ovary cell line, the results were inconclusive at concentrations at least 1850 times human levels; at 2 other loci in mouse lymphoma cells, no evidence of mutagenicity was observed at concentrations at least 1500 times human levels.

Acyclovir has not been shown to impair fertility or reproduction in mice (450 mg/kg/day, p.o.) or in rats (25 mg/kg/day, s.c.). In the mouse study, plasma levels were 9 to 18 times human levels, while in the rat study they were 8 to 15 times human levels. At a higher dose in the rat (50 mg/kg/day, s.c.), there was a statistically significant increase in postimplantation loss, but no concomitant decrease in litter size. In female rabbits treated subcutaneously with acyclovir subsequent to mating, there was a statistically significant decrease in implantation efficiency but no concomitant decrease in litter size at a dose of 50 mg/kg/day (16 to 31 times human levels). No effect upon implantation efficiency was observed when the same dose was administered intravenously (53 to 106 times human levels). In a rat peri- and postnatal study at 50 mg/kg/day s.c. (11 to 22 times human levels), there was a statistically significant decrease in the group mean numbers of corpora lutea, total implantation sites, and live fetuses in the F1 generation. Although not statistically significant, there was also a dose-related decrease in group mean numbers of live fetuses and implantation sites at 12.5 mg/kg/day and 25 mg/kg/day, s.c. The intravenous administration of 100 mg/kg/day, a dose known to cause obstructive nephropathy in rabbits, caused a significant increase in fetal resorptions and a corresponding decrease in litter size (plasma levels were not measured). However, at a maximum tolerated intravenous dose of 50 mg/kg/day in rabbits (53 to 106 times human levels), no drug-related reproductive effects were observed.

Intraperitoneal doses of 80 or 320 mg/kg/day acyclovir given to rats for 6 and 1 months, respectively, caused testicular atrophy. Plasma levels were not measured in the 1-month study and were 24 to 48 times human levels in the 6-month study. Testicular atrophy was persistent through the 4-week postdose recovery phase after 320 mg/kg/day; some evidence of recovery of sperm production was evident 30 days postdose. Intravenous doses of 100 and 200 mg/kg/day acyclovir given to dogs for 31 days caused aspermatogenesis. At 100 mg/kg/day plasma levels were 47 to 94 times human levels, while at 200 mg/kg/day they were 159 to 317 times human levels. No testicular abnormalities were seen in dogs given 50 mg/kg/day i.v. for one month (21 to 41 times human levels) and in dogs given 60 mg/kg/day orally for 1 year (6 to 12 times human levels).

Pregnancy: ***Teratogenic Effects:*** Pregnancy Category C. Acyclovir was not teratogenic in the mouse (450 mg/kg/day, p.o.), rabbit (50 mg/kg/day, s.c. and i.v.), or in standard tests in the rat (50 mg/kg/day, s.c.). These exposures resulted in plasma levels 9 and 18, 16 and 106, and 11 and 22 times, respectively, human levels. In a non-standard test in rats, there were fetal abnormalities, such as head and tail anomalies, and maternal toxicity.[42] In this test, rats were given 3 s.c. doses of 100 mg/kg acyclovir on gestation day 10, resulting in plasma levels 63 and 125 times human levels. There are no adequate and well-controlled studies in pregnant women. Acyclovir should not be used during pregnancy unless the potential benefit justifies the potential risk to the fetus. Although acyclovir was not teratogenic in standard animal studies, the drug's potential for causing chromosome breaks at high concentration should be taken into consideration in making this determination.

Pregnancy Exposure Registry: To monitor maternal-fetal outcomes of pregnant women exposed to systemic acyclovir, Glaxo Wellcome Inc. maintains an Acyclovir in Pregnancy Registry. Physicians are encouraged to register patients by calling (800) 722-9292, ext. 58465.

Nursing Mothers: Acyclovir concentrations have been documented in breast milk in two women following oral administration of ZOVIRAX and ranged from 0.6 to 4.1 times corresponding plasma levels.[43,44] These concentrations would potentially expose the nursing infant to a dose of acyclovir up to 0.3 mg/kg/day. Caution should be exercised when ZOVIRAX is administered to a nursing woman.

Pediatric Use: Safety and effectiveness in pediatric patients less than 2 years of age have not been adequately studied.

ADVERSE REACTIONS

Herpes Simplex: ***Short-Term Administration:*** The most frequent adverse events reported during clinical trials of treatment of genital herpes with orally administered ZOVIRAX were nausea and/or vomiting in 8 of 298 patient treatments (2.7%) and headache in 2 of 298 (0.6%). Nausea and/or vomiting occurred in 2 of 287 (0.7%) patients who received placebo.

Less frequent adverse events, each of which occurred in 1 of 298 patient treatments with orally administered ZOVIRAX

Normal Dosage Regimen	Creatinine Clearance (mL/min/1.73 m²)	Adjusted Dosage Regimen: Dose (mg)	Adjusted Dosage Regimen: Dosing Interval
200 mg every 4 hours	>10	200	every 4 hours, 5x daily
	0-10	200	every 12 hours
400 mg every 12 hours	>10	400	every 12 hours
	0–10	200	every 12 hours
800 mg every 4 hours	>25	800	every 4 hours, 5x daily
	10–25	800	every 8 hours
	0–10	800	every 12 hours

(0.3%), included diarrhea, dizziness, anorexia, fatigue, edema, skin rash, leg pain, inguinal adenopathy, medication taste, and sore throat.

Long-Term Administration: The most frequent adverse events reported in a clinical trial for the prevention of recurrences with continuous administration of 400 mg (two 200 mg capsules) 2 times daily for 1 year in 586 patients treated with ZOVIRAX were: nausea (4.8%), diarrhea (2.4%), headache (1.9%), and rash (1.7%). The 589 control patients receiving intermittent treatment of recurrences with ZOVIRAX for 1 year reported diarrhea (2.7%), nausea (2.4%), headache (2.2%), and rash (1.5%).

The most frequent adverse events reported during the second year by 390 patients who elected to continue daily administration of 400 mg (two 200 mg capsules) 2 times daily for 2 years were headache (1.5%), rash (1.3%), and paresthesia (0.8%). Adverse events reported by 329 patients during the third year included asthenia (1.2%), paresthesia (1.2%), and headache (0.9%).

Herpes Zoster: The most frequent adverse events reported during three clinical trials of treatment of herpes zoster (shingles) with 800 mg of oral ZOVIRAX 5 times daily for 7 to 10 days in 323 patients were: malaise (11.5%), nausea (8.0%), headache (5.9%), vomiting (2.5%), diarrhea (1.5%), and constipation (0.9%). The 323 placebo recipients reported malaise (11.1%), nausea (11.5%), headache (11.1%), vomiting (2.5%), diarrhea (0.3%), and constipation (2.4%).

Chickenpox: The most frequent adverse events reported during three clinical trials of treatment of chickenpox with oral ZOVIRAX in 495 patients were: diarrhea (3.2%), abdominal pain (0.6%), rash (0.6%), vomiting (0.6%), and flatulence (0.4%). The 498 patients receiving placebo reported: diarrhea (2.2%), flatulence (0.8%), and insomnia (0.4%).

Observed During Clinical Practice: Based on clinical practice experience in patients treated with oral ZOVIRAX in the U.S., spontaneously reported adverse events are uncommon. Data are insufficient to support an estimate of their incidence or to establish causation. These events may also occur as part of the underlying disease process. Voluntary reports of adverse events which have been received since market introduction include:

General: fever, headache, pain, peripheral edema, and rarely, anaphylaxis

Nervous: confusion, dizziness, hallucinations, paresthesia, seizure, somnolence (These symptoms may be marked, particularly in older adults.)

Digestive: diarrhea, elevated liver function tests, gastrointestinal distress, nausea

Hemic and Lymphatic: leukopenia, lymphadenopathy

Musculoskeletal: myalgia

Skin: alopecia, pruritus, rash, urticaria

Special Senses: visual abnormalities

Urogenital: elevated creatinine

OVERDOSAGE

Patients have ingested intentional overdoses of up to 100 capsules (20 g) of ZOVIRAX, with no unexpected adverse effects.

Precipitation of acyclovir in renal tubules may occur when the solubility (2.5 mg/mL) in the intratubular fluid is exceeded. Renal lesions considered to be related to obstruction of renal tubules by precipitated drug crystals occurred in the following species: rats treated with i.v. and i.p. doses of 20 mg/kg/day for 21 and 31 days, respectively, and at s.c. doses of 100 mg/kg/day for 10 days; rabbits at s.c. and i.v. doses of 50 mg/kg/day for 13 days; and dogs at i.v. doses of 100 mg/kg/day for 31 days. A 6-hour hemodialysis results in a 60% decrease in plasma acyclovir concentration. Data concerning peritoneal dialysis are incomplete but indicate that this method may be significantly less efficient in removing acyclovir from the blood. In the event of acute renal failure and anuria, the patient may benefit from hemodialysis until renal function is restored (see DOSAGE AND ADMINISTRATION).

DOSAGE AND ADMINISTRATION

Treatment of Initial Genital Herpes: 200 mg (one 200 mg capsule or one teaspoonful [5 mL] suspension) every 4 hours, 5 times daily for 10 days.

Chronic Suppressive Therapy for Recurrent Disease: 400 mg (two 200 mg capsules, one 400 mg tablet, or two teaspoonfuls [10 mL] suspension) 2 times daily for up to 12 months, followed by re-evaluation. See INDICATIONS AND USAGE and PRECAUTIONS for considerations on continuation of suppressive therapy beyond 12 months. Alternative regimens have included doses ranging from 200 mg 3 times daily to 200 mg 5 times daily.

Intermittent Therapy: 200 mg (one 200 mg capsule or one teaspoonful [5 mL] suspension) every 4 hours, 5 times daily for 5 days. Therapy should be initiated at the earliest sign or symptom (prodrome) of recurrence.

Acute Treatment of Herpes Zoster: 800 mg (four 200 mg capsules, two 400 mg tablets, one 800 mg tablet, or four teaspoonfuls [20 mL] suspension) every 4 hours orally, 5 times daily for 7 to 10 days.

Treatment of Chickenpox: ***Children (2 years of age and older):*** 20 mg/kg **per dose** orally four times daily (80 mg/kg/day) for 5 days. Children over 40 kg should receive the adult dose for chickenpox.

Adults and children over 40 kg: 800 mg four times daily for 5 days.

Therapy should be initiated at the earliest sign or symptom of chickenpox to derive the maximal benefits of therapy.

Patients With Acute or Chronic Renal Impairment: Comprehensive pharmacokinetic studies have been completed following intravenous acyclovir infusions in patients with renal impairment. Based on these studies, dosage adjustments are recommended in the following chart for genital herpes and herpes zoster indications:

[See table above.]

Hemodialysis: For patients who require hemodialysis, the mean plasma half-life of acyclovir during hemodialysis is approximately 5 hours. This results in a 60% decrease in plasma concentrations following a 6-hour dialysis period. Therefore, the patient's dosing schedule should be adjusted so that an additional dose is administered after each dialysis.[45,46]

Peritoneal Dialysis: No supplemental dose appears to be necessary after adjustment of the dosing interval.[47,48]

HOW SUPPLIED

ZOVIRAX Capsules (blue, opaque cap and body) containing 200 mg acyclovir and printed with "Wellcome ZOVIRAX 200"—Bottle of 100 (NDC 0173-0991-55), and unit dose pack of 100 (NDC 0173-0991-56). Store at 15° to 25°C (59° to 77°F) and protect from moisture.

ZOVIRAX Tablets (light blue, oval) containing 800 mg acyclovir and engraved with "ZOVIRAX 800"—Bottle of 100 (NDC 0173-0945-55) and unit dose pack of 100 (NDC 0173-0945-56). Store at 15° to 25°C (59° to 77°F) and protect from moisture.

ZOVIRAX Tablets (white, shield-shaped) containing 400 mg acyclovir and engraved with "ZOVIRAX" on one side and a triangle on the other side—Bottle of 100 (NDC 0173-0949-55). Store at 15° to 25°C (59° to 77°F) and protect from moisture.

ZOVIRAX Suspension (off-white, banana-flavored) containing 200 mg acyclovir in each teaspoonful (5 mL)—Bottle of 1 pint (473 mL) (NDC 0173-0953-96). Store at 15° to 25°C (59° to 77°F).

REFERENCES

1. O'Brien JJ, Campoli-Richards DM. Acyclovir—an updated review of its antiviral activity, pharmacokinetic properties, and therapeutic efficacy. *Drugs.* 1989;37:233-309.
2. Littler E, Zeuthen J, McBride AA, et al. Identification of an Epstein-Barr virus-coded thymidine kinase. *EMBO J.* 1986;5:1959-1966.
3. Miller WH, Miller RL. Phosphorylation of acyclovir (acycloguanosine) monophosphate by GMP kinase. *J Biol Chem.* 1980;255:7204-7207.
4. Furman PA, St Clair MH, Fyfe JA, et al. Inhibition of herpes simplex virus-induced DNA polymerase activity and viral DNA replication by 9-(2-hydroxyethoxymethyl)guanine and its triphosphate. *J Virol.* 1979;32:72-77.
5. Derse D, Cheng YC, Furman PA, et al. Inhibition of purified human and herpes simplex virus-induced DNA

Continued on next page

Glaxo Wellcome—Cont.

polymerases by 9-(2-hydroxyethoxymethyl)guanine triphosphate: effects on primer-template function. *J Biol Chem.* 1981;256:11447-11451.
6. McGuirt PV, Shaw JE, Elion GB, et al. Identification of small DNA fragments synthesized in herpes simplex virus-infected cells in the presence of acyclovir. *Antimicrob Agents Chemother.* 1984;25:507-509.
7. Barry DW, Blum MR: Antiviral drugs: acyclovir. In: Turner P, Shand DG, eds: *Recent Advances in Clinical Pharmacology,* ed 3. New York: Churchill Livingstone; 1983: chap 4.
8. DeClercq E. Comparative efficacy of antiherpes drugs in different cell lines. *Antimicrob Agents Chemother.* 1982; 21:661–663.
9. McLaren C, Ellis MN, Hunter GA. A colorimetric assay for the measurement of the sensitivity of herpes simplex viruses to antiviral agents. *Antiviral Res.* 1983;3:223–234.
10. Barry DW, Nusinoff-Lehrman S. Viral resistance in clinical practice: summary of five years experience with acyclovir. In: Kono R, Nakajima A eds. *Herpes Viruses and Virus Chemotherapy (Ex Med Int Congr Ser 667).* New York: *Excerpta Medica;* 1985;269–270.
11. Dekker C. Ellis MN, McLaren C, et al. Virus resistance in clinical practice. *J Antimicrob Chemother.* 1983;12 (suppl B):137–152.
12. Sibrack CD, Gutman LT, Wilfert CM, et al. Pathogenicity of acyclovir-resistant herpes simplex virus type 1 from an immunodeficient child. *J Infect Dis.* 1982;146: 673–682.
13. Crumpacker CS, Schnipper LE, Marlowe SI, et al. Resistance to antiviral drugs of herpes simplex virus isolated from a patient treated with acyclovir. *N Engl J Med.* 1982;306:343–346.
14. Wade JC, Newton B, McLaren C, et al. Intravenous acyclovir to treat mucocutaneous herpes simplex virus infection after marrow transplantation: a double-blind trial. *Ann Intern Med.* 1982;96:265–269.
15. Burns WH, Saral R, Santos GW, et al. Isolation and characterization of resistant herpes simplex virus after acyclovir therapy. *Lancet.* 1982;1:421–423.
16. Straus SE, Takiff HE, Seidlin M, et al. Suppression of frequently recurring genital herpes: a placebo-controlled double-blind trial of oral acyclovir. *N Engl J Med.* 1984;310:1545–1550.
17. Collins P. Viral sensitivity following the introduction of acyclovir. *Am J Med.* 1988;85:129–134.
18. Erlich KS, Mills J, Chatis P, et al. Acyclovir-resistant herpes simplex virus infections in patients with the acquired immunodeficiency syndrome. *N Engl J Med.* 1989;320:293–296.
19. Hill EL, Ellis MN, Barry DW. In: *28th Intersci Conf on Antimicrob Agents Chemother.* Los Angeles: 1988, Abst. No. 0840:260.
20. Ellis MN, Keller PM, Fyfe JA, et al. Clinical isolates of herpes simplex virus type 2 that induces thymidine kinase with altered substrate specificity. *Antimicrob Agents Chemother.* 1987;31:1117–1125.
21. Collins P, Larder BA, Oliver NM, et al. Characterization of a DNA polymerase mutant of herpes simplex virus from a severely immunocompromised patient receiving acyclovir. *J Gen Virol.* 1989;70:375–382.
22. Field HJ, Darby G, Wildy P. Isolation and characterization of acyclovir-resistant mutants of herpes simplex virus. *J Gen Virol.* 1980;49:115–124.
23. Bryson YJ, Dillon M, Lovett M, et al. Treatment of first episodes of genital herpes simplex virus infection with oral acyclovir: a randomized double-blind controlled trial in normal subjects. *N Engl J Med.* 1983;308:916–921.
24. Mertz GJ, Critchlow CW, Benedetti J, et al. Double-blind placebo-controlled trial of oral acyclovir in first-episode genital herpes simplex virus infection. *JAMA.* 1984; 252:1147–1151.
25. Nilsen AE, Aasen T, Halsos AM, et al. Efficacy of oral acyclovir in the treatment of initial and recurrent genital herpes. *Lancet.* 1982;2:571–573.
26. Douglas JM, Critchlow C, Benedetti J, et al. A double-blind study of oral acyclovir for suppression of recurrences of genital herpes simplex virus infection. *N Engl J Med.* 1984;310:1551–1556.
27. Mindel A, Weller IV, Faherty A, et al. Prophylactic oral acyclovir in recurrent genital herpes. *Lancet.* 1984;2: 57–59.
28. Mattison HR, Reichman RC, Benedetti J, et al. Double-blind, placebo-controlled trial comparing long-term suppressive with short-term oral acyclovir therapy for management of recurrent genital herpes. *Am J Med.* 1988;85(suppl 2A):20–25.
29. Straus SE, Croen KD, Sawyer MH, et al. Acyclovir suppression of frequently recurring genital herpes. *JAMA.* 1988;260:2227–2230.
30. Mertz GJ, Eron L, Kaufman R, et al. The Acyclovir Study Group. Prolonged continuous versus intermittent oral acyclovir treatment in normal adults with frequently recurring genital herpes simplex virus infection. *Am J Med.* 1988;85(suppl 2A):14–19.
31. Goldberg LH, Kaufman R, Conant MA, et al. Episodic twice daily treatment for recurrent genital herpes. *Am J Med.* 1988;85:10–13.
32. Reichman RC, Badger GJ, Mertz GJ, et al. Treatment of recurrent genital herpes simplex infections with oral acyclovir: a controlled trial. *JAMA.* 1984;251:2103–2107.
33. Huff JC, Bean B, Balfour HH Jr, et al. Therapy of herpes zoster with oral acyclovir. *Am J Med.* 1988;85(suppl 2A):85–89.
34. Morton P, Thompson AN. Oral acyclovir in the treatment of herpes zoster in general practice. *NZ Med J.* 1989;102:93–95.
35. Balfour HH Jr, Kelly JM, Suarez CS, et al. Acyclovir treatment of varicella in otherwise healthy children. *J Pediatr.* 1990;116:633–639.
36. Dunkle LM, Arvin AM, Whitley RJ, et al. A controlled trial of acyclovir for chickenpox in normal children. *N Engl J Med.* 1991;325:1539–1544.
37. Balfour HH Jr, Rotbart HA, Feldman S, et al. Acyclovir treatment of varicella in otherwise healthy adolescents. *J Pediatr.* 1992;120:627–633.
38. Rotbart HA, Levin MJ, Hayward AR. Immune responses to varicella zoster virus infections in healthy children. *J Infect Dis.* 1993;167:195–199.
39. Naib ZM, Nahmias AJ, Josey WE, et al. Relation of cytohistopathology of genital herpesvirus infection to cervical anaplasia. *Cancer Res.* 1973;33:1452–1463.
40. Douglas JM, David LG, Remington ML, et al. A double-blind, placebo-controlled trial of the effect of chronically administered oral acyclovir on sperm production in man with frequently recurrent genital herpes. *J Infect Dis.* 1988;157:588–593.
41. Laskin OL, deMiranda P, King DH, et al. Effects of probenecid on the pharmacokinetics and elimination of acyclovir in humans. *Antimicrob Agents Chemother.* 1982;21:804–807.
42. Stahlmann R, Klug S, Lewandowski C, et al. Teratogenicity of acyclovir in rats. *Infection.* 1987;15:261–262.
43. Lau RJ, Emery MG, Galinsky RE, et al. Unexpected accumulation of acyclovir in breast milk with estimate of infant exposure. *Obstet Gynecol.* 1987;69:468–471.
44. Meyer LJ, deMiranda P, Sheth N, et al. Acyclovir in human breast milk. *Am J Obstet Gynecol.* 1988;158:586–588.
45. Laskin OL, Longstreth JA, Whelton A, et al. Effect of renal failure on the pharmacokinetics of acyclovir. *Am J Med.* 1982;73:197–201.
46. Krasny HC, Liao SH, deMiranda P, et al. Influence of hemodialysis on acyclovir pharmacokinetics in patients with chronic renal failure. *Am J Med.* 1982;73:202–204.
47. Boelart J, Schurgers M, Daneels R, et al. Multiple dose pharmacokinetics of intravenous acyclovir in patients on continuous ambulatory peritoneal dialysis. *J Antimicrob Chemother.* 1987;20:69–76.
48. Shah GM, Winer RL, Krasny HC. Acyclovir pharmacokinetics in a patient on continuous ambulatory peritoneal dialysis. *Am J Kidney Dis.* 1986;7:507–510.

U.S. Patent No. 4,199,574
May 1996/RL-316

Shown in Product Identification Guide, page 315

ZOVIRAX® Ointment 5% ℞

[zō″vī′răx]
(acyclovir)

DESCRIPTION

ZOVIRAX is the brand name for acyclovir, an antiviral drug active against herpes viruses. ZOVIRAX Ointment 5% is a formulation for topical administration. Each gram of ZOVIRAX Ointment 5% contains 50 mg of acyclovir in a polyethylene glycol (PEG) base.

The chemical name of acyclovir is 2-amino-1,9-dihydro-9-[(2-hydroxyethoxy)methyl]-6*H*-purin-6-one.

Acyclovir is a white, crystalline powder with a molecular weight of 225 daltons, and a maximum solubility in water of 1.3 mg/mL.

CLINICAL PHARMACOLOGY

Acyclovir is a synthetic acyclic purine nucleoside analogue with in vitro inhibitory activity against Herpes simplex types 1 and 2 (HSV-1 and HSV-2), varicella-zoster, Epstein-Barr, and cytomegalovirus. In cell cultures, the inhibitory activity of acyclovir for Herpes simplex virus is highly selective. Cellular thymidine kinase does not effectively utilize acyclovir as a substrate. Herpes simplex virus-coded thymidine kinase, however, converts acyclovir into acyclovir monophosphate, a nucleotide. The monophosphate is further converted into diphosphate by cellular guanylate kinase and into triphosphate by a number of cellular enzymes.[1] Acyclovir triphosphate interferes with Herpes simplex virus DNA polymerase and inhibits viral DNA replication. Acyclovir triphosphate also inhibits cellular α-DNA polymerase but to a lesser degree. In vitro, acyclovir triphosphate can be incorporated into growing chains of DNA by viral DNA polymerase and to a much smaller extent by cellular α-DNA polymerase.[2] When incorporation occurs, the DNA chain is terminated.[3] Acyclovir is preferentially taken up and selectively converted to the active triphosphate form by herpesvirus-infected cells. Thus, acyclovir is much less toxic in vitro for normal uninfected cells because: 1) less is taken up; 2) less is converted to the active form; 3) cellular α-DNA polymerase is less sensitive to the effects of the active form.

The relationship between in vitro susceptibility of Herpes simplex virus to antiviral drugs and clinical response has not been established. The techniques and cell culture types used for determining in vitro susceptibility may influence the results obtained. Using a quantitative assay to determine the acyclovir concentration producing 50% inhibition of viral cytopathic effect (ID_{50}), 28 HSV-1 clinical isolates had a mean ID_{50} of 0.17 μg/mL and 32 HSV-2 clinical isolates had a mean ID_{50} of 0.46 μg/mL.* Results from other studies using different assays have yielded mean ID_{50} values for clinical HSV-1 isolates of 0.018, 0.03, and 0.043 μg/mL and for clinical HSV-2 isolates of 0.027, 0.36, and 0.03 μg/mL, respectively.[4,5,6]

Two clinical pharmacology studies were performed with ZOVIRAX Ointment 5% in adult immunocompromised patients at risk of developing mucocutaneous Herpes simplex virus infections or with localized varicella-zoster infections. These studies were designed to evaluate the dermal tolerance, systemic toxicity, and percutaneous absorption of acyclovir.

In one of these studies, which included 16 inpatients, the complete ointment or its vehicle were randomly administered in a dose of 1 cm strips (25 mg acyclovir) four times a day for 7 days to an intact skin surface area of 4.5 square inches. No local intolerance, systemic toxicity, or contact dermatitis were observed. In addition, no drug was detected in blood and urine by radioimmunoassay (sensitivity, 0.01 μg/mL).

The other study included 11 patients with localized varicella-zoster. In this uncontrolled study, acyclovir was detected in the blood of nine patients and in the urine of all patients tested. Acyclovir levels in plasma ranged from <0.01 to 0.28 μg/mL in eight patients with normal renal function, and from <0.01 to 0.78 μg/mL in one patient with impaired renal function. Acyclovir excreted in the urine ranged from <0.02% to 9.4% of the daily dose. Therefore, systemic absorption of acyclovir after topical application is minimal.

INDICATIONS AND USAGE

ZOVIRAX (acyclovir) Ointment 5% is indicated in the management of initial herpes genitalis and in limited nonlife-threatening mucocutaneous Herpes simplex virus infections in immunocompromised patients. In clinical trials of initial herpes genitalis, ZOVIRAX Ointment 5% has shown a decrease in healing time and, in some cases, a decrease in duration of viral shedding and duration of pain. In studies in immunocompromised patients with mainly herpes labialis, there was a decrease in duration of viral shedding and a slight decrease in duration of pain.

By contrast, in studies of recurrent herpes genitalis and of herpes labialis in nonimmunocompromised patients, there was no evidence of clinical benefit; there was some decrease in duration of viral shedding.

Diagnosis: Whereas cutaneous lesions associated with Herpes simplex infections are often characteristic, the finding of multinucleated giant cells in smears prepared from lesion exudate or scrapings may assist in the diagnosis.[7] Positive cultures for Herpes simplex virus offer a reliable means for confirmation of the diagnosis. In genital herpes, appropriate examinations should be performed to rule out other sexually transmitted diseases.

CONTRAINDICATIONS

ZOVIRAX Ointment 5% is contraindicated for patients who develop hypersensitivity or chemical intolerance to the components of the formulation.

WARNINGS

ZOVIRAX Ointment 5% is intended for cutaneous use only and should not be used in the eye.

PRECAUTIONS

General: The recommended dosage, frequency of applications, and length of treatment should not be exceeded (see DOSAGE AND ADMINISTRATION). There exist no data which demonstrate that the use of ZOVIRAX Ointment 5% will either prevent transmission of infection to other persons or prevent recurrent infections when applied in the absence of signs and symptoms. ZOVIRAX Ointment 5% should not be used for the prevention of recurrent HSV infections. Although clinically significant viral resistance associated with the use of ZOVIRAX Ointment 5% has not been observed, this possibility exists.

Drug Interactions: Clinical experience has identified no interactions resulting from topical or systemic admin-

istration of other drugs concomitantly with ZOVIRAX Ointment 5%.

Carcinogenesis, Mutagenesis, Impairment of Fertility: Acyclovir was tested in lifetime bioassays in rats and mice at single daily doses of 50, 150, and 450 mg/kg/day given by gavage. These studies showed no statistically significant difference in the incidence of benign and malignant tumors produced in drug-treated as compared to control animals, nor did acyclovir induce the occurrence of tumors earlier in drug-treated animals as compared to controls. In two in vitro cell transformation assays, used to provide preliminary assessment of potential oncogenicity in advance of these more definitive lifetime bioassays in rodents, conflicting results were obtained. Acyclovir was positive at the highest dose used in one system and the resulting morphologically transformed cells formed tumors when inoculated into immunosuppressed, syngeneic, weanling mice. Acyclovir was negative in another transformation system.

No chromosome damage was observed at maximum tolerated parenteral doses of 100 mg/kg acyclovir in rats or Chinese hamsters; higher doses of 500 and 1000 mg/kg were clastogenic in Chinese hamsters. In addition, no activity was found in a dominant lethal study in mice. In nine of 11 microbial and mammalian cell assays, no evidence of mutagenicity was observed. In two mammalian cell assays (human lymphocytes and L5178Y mouse lymphoma cells in vitro), positive response for mutagenicity and chromosomal damage occurred, but only at concentrations at least 1000 times the plasma levels achieved in humans following topical application.

Acyclovir does not impair fertility or reproduction in mice at oral doses up to 450 mg/kg/day or in rats at subcutaneous doses up to 25 mg/kg/day. In rabbits given a high dose of acyclovir (50 mg/kg/day, s.c.), there was a statistically significant decrease in implantation efficiency.

Pregnancy: *Teratogenic Effects.* Pregnancy Category C. Acyclovir was not teratogenic in the mouse (450 mg/kg/day, p.o.), rabbit (50 mg/kg/day, s.c. and i.v.) or in standard tests in the rat (50 mg/kg/day, s.c.). In a non-standard test in rats, fetal abnormalities, such as head and tail anomalies, were observed following subcutaneous administration of acyclovir at very high doses associated with toxicity to the maternal rat. The clinical relevance of these findings is uncertain.[8] There are no adequate and well-controlled studies in pregnant women. Acyclovir should not be used during pregnancy unless the potential benefit justifies the potential risk to the fetus.

Nursing Mothers: It is not known whether topically applied acyclovir is excreted in breast milk. After oral administration of ZOVIRAX, acyclovir concentrations have been documented in breast milk in two women and ranged from 0.6 to 4.1 times the corresponding plasma levels.[9,10] Caution should be exercised when ZOVIRAX Ointment is administered to a nursing woman.

ADVERSE REACTIONS

Because ulcerated genital lesions are characteristically tender and sensitive to any contact or manipulation, patients may experience discomfort upon application of ointment. In the controlled clinical trials, mild pain (including transient burning and stinging) was reported by 103 (28.3%) of 364 patients treated with acyclovir and by 115 (31.1%) of 370 patients treated with placebo; treatment was discontinued in 2 of these patients. Other local reactions among acyclovir-treated patients included pruritus in 15 (4.1%), rash in 1 (0.3%), and vulvitis in 1 (0.3%). Among the placebo-treated patients, pruritus was reported by 17 (4.6%) and rash by 1 (0.3%).

In all studies, there was no significant difference between the drug and placebo group in the rate or type of reported adverse reactions nor were there any differences in abnormal clinical laboratory findings.

Observed During Clinical Practice: Based on clinical practice experience in patients treated with ZOVIRAX Ointment in the U.S., spontaneously reported adverse events are uncommon. Data are insufficient to support an estimate of their incidence or to establish causation. These events may also occur as part of the underlying disease process. Voluntary reports of adverse events which have been received since market introduction include:

General: edema and/or pain at the application site
Skin: pruritus, rash

OVERDOSAGE

Overdosage by topical application of ZOVIRAX Ointment 5% is unlikely because of limited transcutaneous absorption (see CLINICAL PHARMACOLOGY).

DOSAGE AND ADMINISTRATION

Apply sufficient quantity to adequately cover all lesions every 3 hours 6 times per day for 7 days. The dose size per application will vary depending upon the total lesion area but should approximate a one-half inch ribbon of ointment per 4 square inches of surface area. A finger cot or rubber glove should be used when applying ZOVIRAX to prevent autoinoculation of other body sites and transmission of infection to other persons. **Therapy should be initiated as early as possible following onset of signs and symptoms.**

HOW SUPPLIED

ZOVIRAX Ointment 5% is supplied in 15 g tubes (NDC 0173-0993-94) and 3 g tubes (NDC 0173-0993-41). Each gram contains 50 mg acyclovir in a polyethylene glycol base.
Store at 15° to 25°C (59° to 77°F) in a dry place.

ANIMAL PHARMACOLOGY AND ANIMAL TOXICOLOGY

Topical treatment of guinea pigs with 10% acyclovir in polyethylene glycol ointment for 3 weeks did not result in cutaneous irritation or systemic toxicity. Also, a wide variety of animal tests by parenteral routes demonstrated that acyclovir has a low order of toxicity.
Acyclovir did not cause dermal sensitization in guinea pigs.

REFERENCES

1. Miller WH, Miller RL. Phosphorylation of acyclovir (acycloguanosine) monophosphate by GMP kinase. *J Biol Chem.* 1980;255:7204-7207.
2. Furman PA, St. Clair MH, Fyfe JA, et al. Inhibition of herpes simplex virus-induced DNA polymerase activity and viral DNA replication by 9-(2-hydroxyethoxymethyl)guanine and its triphosphate. *J Virol.* 1979; 32:72-77.
3. Derse D, Cheng YC, Furman PA, et al. Inhibition of purified human and herpes simplex virus-induced DNA polymerases by 9-(2-hydroxyethoxymethyl)guanine triphosphate: effects on primer-template function. *J Biol Chem.* 1981;256:11447-11451.
4. Collins P, Bauer DJ. The activity in vitro against herpes virus of 9-(2-hydroxyethoxymethyl)guanine (acycloguanosine), a new antiviral agent. *J Antimicrob Chemother.* 1979;5:431-436.
5. Crumpacker CS, Schnipper LE, Zaia JA, et al. Growth inhibition of acycloguanosine of herpesviruses isolated from human infections. *Antimicrob Agents Chemother.* 1979;15:642-645.
6. DeClercq E, Descamps J, Verhelst G, et al. Comparative efficacy of antiherpes drugs against different strains of herpes simplex virus. *J Infect Dis.* 1980;141:563-574.
7. Naib ZM, Nahmias AJ, Josey WE, et al. Relation of cytohistopathology of genital herpesvirus infection to cervical anaplasia. *Cancer Res.* 1973;33:1452-1463.
8. Stahlmann R, Klug S, Lewandowski C, et al. Teratogenicity of acyclovir in rats. *Infection.* 1987;15:261-262.
9. Lau RJ, Emery MG, Galinsky RE, et al. Unexpected accumulation of acyclovir in breast milk with estimate of infant exposure. *Obstet Gynecol.* 1987;69:468-471.
10. Meyer LJ, deMiranda P, Sheth N, et al. Acyclovir in human breast milk. *Am J Obstet Gynecol.* 1988;158: 586-588.

*Data on file at Glaxo Wellcome Inc.
U.S. Patent No. 4199574
February 1996/RL-269

Shown in Product Identification Guide, page 315

ZOVIRAX® Sterile Powder ℞

[zō″vī′răx]
(acyclovir sodium)
FOR INTRAVENOUS INFUSION ONLY

DESCRIPTION

ZOVIRAX is the brand name for acyclovir, an antiviral drug active against herpesviruses. ZOVIRAX Sterile Powder is a formulation for intravenous administration. Each 5.49 mg of sterile lyophilized acyclovir sodium is equivalent to 5 mg acyclovir.

The chemical name of acyclovir sodium is 2-amino-1,9-dihydro-9-[(2-hydroxyethoxy)methyl]-6*H*-purin-6-one monosodium salt.

Acyclovir sodium is a white, crystalline powder with a molecular weight of 247 daltons, and a solubility in water exceeding 100 mg/mL. Each 500 mg or 1000 mg vial of ZOVIRAX Sterile Powder when reconstituted with 10 mL or 20 mL, respectively, sterile diluent yields 50 mg/mL acyclovir (pH approximately 11). Further dilution in any appropriate intravenous solution must be performed before infusion (see Method of Preparation). At physiologic pH, acyclovir exists as the un-ionized form with a molecular weight of 225 daltons and a maximum solubility of 2.5 mg/mL at 37°C.

CLINICAL PHARMACOLOGY

Mechanism of Antiviral Effects: Acyclovir is a synthetic purine nucleoside analogue with in vitro and in vivo inhibitory activity against human herpes viruses including herpes simplex types 1 (HSV-1) and 2 (HSV-2), varicella-zoster virus (VZV), Epstein-Barr virus (EBV), and cytomegalovirus (CMV). In cell culture, acyclovir has the highest antiviral activity against HSV-1, followed in decreasing order of potency against HSV-2, VZV, EBV, and CMV.[1]

The inhibitory activity of acyclovir for HSV-1, HSV-2, VZV, and EBV is highly selective. The enzyme thymidine kinase (TK) of normal uninfected cells does not effectively use acyclovir as a substrate. However, TK encoded by HSV, VZV, and EBV[2] converts acyclovir into acyclovir monophosphate, a nucleotide analogue. The monophosphate is further converted into diphosphate by cellular guanylate kinase and into triphosphate by a number of cellular enzymes.[3] Acyclovir triphosphate interferes with Herpes simplex virus DNA polymerase and inhibits viral DNA replication. Acyclovir triphosphate also inhibits cellular α-DNA polymerase but to a lesser degree. In vitro, acyclovir triphosphate can be incorporated into growing chains of DNA by viral DNA polymerase and to a much smaller extent by cellular α-DNA polymerase.[4] When incorporation occurs, the DNA chain is terminated.[5,6] Acyclovir is preferentially taken up and selectively converted to the active triphosphate form by herpesvirus-infected cells. Thus, acyclovir is much less toxic in vitro for normal uninfected cells because: 1) less is taken up; 2) less is converted to the active form; 3) cellular α-DNA polymerase is less sensitive to the effects of the active form. The mode of acyclovir phosphorylation in cytomegalovirus-infected cells is not clearly established, but may involve virally induced cell kinases or an unidentified viral enzyme. Acyclovir is not efficiently activated in cytomegalovirus infected cells, which may account for the reduced susceptibility of cytomegalovirus to acyclovir in vitro.

Microbiology: The quantitative relationship between the in vitro susceptibility of herpes simplex virus to acyclovir and the clinical response to therapy has not been established in humans, and virus sensitivity testing has not been standardized. Sensitivity testing results, expressed as the concentration of drug required to inhibit by 50% the growth of virus in cell culture (ID_{50}), vary greatly depending upon the particular assay used,[7] the cell type employed,[8] and the laboratory performing the test.[1] The ID_{50} of acyclovir against HSV-1 isolates may range from 0.02 μg/mL (plaque reduction in Vero cells) to 5.9 to 13.5 μg/mL (plaque reduction in green monkey kidney [GMK] cells).[1] The ID_{50} against HSV-2 ranges from 0.01 μg/mL to 9.9 μg/mL (plaque reduction in Vero and GMK cells, respectively).[1]

Using a dye-uptake method in Vero cells,[9] which gives ID_{50} values approximately 5- to 10-fold higher than plaque reduction assays, 1417 isolates (553 HSV-1 and 864 HSV-2) from approximately 500 patients were examined over a 5-year period.[10] These assays found that 90% of HSV-1 isolates were sensitive to $\leq$ 0.9 μg/mL acyclovir and 50% of all isolates were sensitive to $\leq$ 0.2 μg/mL acyclovir. For HSV-2 isolates, 90% were sensitive to $\leq$ 2.2 μg/mL and 50% of all isolates were sensitive to $\leq$ 0.7 μg/mL of acyclovir. Isolates with significantly diminished sensitivity were found in 44 patients. It must be emphasized that neither the patients nor the isolates were randomly selected and, therefore, do not represent the general population.

Most of the less sensitive clinical isolates have been relatively deficient in the viral TK.[11-19] Strains with alterations in viral TK[20] or viral DNA polymerase[21] have also been reported. Prolonged exposure to low concentrations (0.1 μg/mL) of acyclovir in cell culture has resulted in the emergence of a variety of acyclovir-resistant strains.[22]

The ID_{50} against VZV ranges from 0.17 to 1.53 μg/mL (yield reduction, human foreskin fibroblasts) to 1.85 to 3.98 μg/mL (foci reduction, human embryo fibroblasts [HEF]). Reproduction of EBV genome is suppressed by 50% in superinfected Raji cells or P3HR-1 lymphoblastoid cells by 1.5 μg/mL acyclovir. CMV is relatively resistant to acyclovir with ID_{50} values ranging from 2.3 to 17.6 μg/mL (plaque reduction, HEF cells) to 1.82 to 56.8 μg/mL (DNA hybridization, HEF cells). The latent state of the genome of any of the human herpesviruses is not known to be sensitive to acyclovir.[1]

Pharmacokinetics: The pharmacokinetics of acyclovir has been evaluated in 95 patients (nine studies). Results were obtained in adult patients with normal renal function during Phase 1/2 studies after single doses ranging from 0.5 to 15 mg/kg and after multiple doses ranging from 2.5 to 15 mg/kg every 8 hours. Pharmacokinetics was also determined in pediatric patients with normal renal function ranging in age from 1 to 17 years at doses of 250 mg/m^2 or 500 mg/m^2 every 8 hours. In these studies, dose-independent pharmacokinetics is observed in the range of 0.5 to 15 mg/kg. Proportionality between dose and plasma levels is seen after single doses or at steady state after multiple dosing.[23] When ZOVIRAX was administered to adults at 5 mg/kg (approximately 250 mg/ m^2) by 1-hour infusions every 8 hours, mean steady-state peak and trough concentrations of 9.8 μg/mL (5.5 to 13.8 μg/mL) and 0.7 μg/mL (0.2 to 1.0 μg/mL), respectively, were achieved. Similar concentrations are achieved in children over 1 year of age when doses of 250 mg/m^2 are given by 1-hour infusions every 8 hours. At a dose of 10 mg/kg given by 1-hour infusion every 8 hours, mean steady-state peak and trough concentrations were 22.9 μg/mL (14.1 to 44.1 μg/mL) and 1.9 μg/mL (0.5 to 2.9 μg/mL). Similar concentrations were achieved in children dosed at 500 mg/m^2 given by 1-hour infusion every 8 hours. Concentrations achieved in the cerebrospinal fluid are approximately 50% of plasma values. Plasma protein binding is relatively low (9% to 33%)

Continued on next page

Glaxo Wellcome—Cont.

and drug interactions involving binding site displacement are not anticipated.[23]

Renal excretion of unchanged drug by glomerular filtration and tubular secretion is the major route of acyclovir elimination accounting for 62% to 91% of the dose as determined by ^{14}C-labelled drug. The only major urinary metabolite detected is 9-carboxymethoxymethylguanine. This may account for up to 14.1% of the dose in patients with normal renal function. An insignificant amount of drug is recovered in feces and expired CO_2 and there is no evidence to suggest tissue retention.[23] However, postmortem examinations have shown that acyclovir is widely distributed in tissues and body fluids including brain, kidney, lung, liver, muscle, spleen, uterus, vaginal mucosa, vaginal secretions, cerebrospinal fluid, and herpetic vesicular fluid.

The half-life and total body clearance of acyclovir is dependent on renal function as shown below.[23]

Creatinine Clearance (mL/min/1.73m²)	Half-Life (hr)	Total Body Clearance (mL/min/1.73m²)
>80	2.5	327
50–80	3.0	248
15–50	3.5	190
0 (Anuric)	19.5	29

ZOVIRAX was administered at a dose of 2.5 mg/kg to six adult patients with severe renal failure. The peak and trough plasma levels during the 47 hours preceding hemodialysis were 8.5 µg/mL and 0.7 µg/mL, respectively.[24,25] Consult DOSAGE AND ADMINISTRATION section for recommended adjustments in dosing based upon creatinine clearance. The half-life and total body clearance of acyclovir in pediatric patients over 1 year of age is similar to those in adults with normal renal function (see DOSAGE AND ADMINISTRATION).

INDICATIONS AND USAGE

ZOVIRAX Sterile Powder is indicated for the treatment of initial and recurrent mucosal and cutaneous Herpes simplex (HSV-1 and HSV-2) and varicella-zoster (shingles) infections in immunocompromised patients. It is also indicated for herpes simplex encephalitis in patients over 6 months of age and for severe initial clinical episodes of herpes genitalis in patients who are not immunocompromised.

Herpes Simplex Infections in Immunocompromised Patients

A multicenter trial of ZOVIRAX Sterile Powder at a dose of 250 mg/m² every 8 hours (750 mg/m²/day) for 7 days was conducted in 98 immunocompromised patients (73 adults and 25 children) with oro-facial, esophageal, genital, and other localized infections (52 treated with ZOVIRAX and 46 with placebo). ZOVIRAX significantly decreased virus excretion, reduced pain, and promoted scabbing and rapid healing of lesions.[14,26,27,28]

Initial Episodes of Herpes Genitalis

In placebo-controlled trials, 58 patients with initial genital herpes were treated with intravenous ZOVIRAX 5 mg/kg or placebo (27 patients treated with ZOVIRAX and 31 treated with placebo) every 8 hours for 5 days. ZOVIRAX decreased the duration of viral excretion, new lesion formation, and duration of vesicles, and promoted healing of lesions.[28,29,30]

Herpes Simplex Encephalitis

Sixty-two patients ages 6 months to 79 years with brain biopsy-proven herpes simplex encephalitis were randomized to receive either ZOVIRAX (30 mg/kg/day) or adenine arabinoside (Vira-A) (15 mg/kg/day) for 10 days (28 were treated with ZOVIRAX and 34 with Vira-A).[31] Overall mortality at 6 months for patients treated with ZOVIRAX was 18% compared to 59% for patients treated with Vira-A ($P = 0.003$). The proportion of patients treated with ZOVIRAX functioning normally or with only mild sequelae (e.g., decreased attention span) was 39% compared to 9% of patients treated with Vira-A ($P = 0.01$). The remaining patients in both groups had moderate (e.g., hemiparesis, speech impediment, or seizure) or severe (continuous supportive care required) neurologic sequelae.

After 12 months of follow-up, two additional patients treated with ZOVIRAX had died, resulting in an overall mortality of 25% compared to 59% for patients treated with Vira-A ($P = 0.02$). Morbidity assessments at that time indicated that 32% of patients treated with ZOVIRAX were functioning normally, or with only mild sequelae compared to 12% of patients treated with Vira-A ($P = 0.06$). Moderate to severe impairment was noted in all remaining patients in both groups who were available for evaluation. Patients less than 30 years of age and those who had the least severe neurologic involvement at time of entry into study had the best outcome with treatment with ZOVIRAX. An additional controlled study performed in Europe[32] demonstrated similar findings. The superiority of ZOVIRAX over Vira-A for neonatal herpes encephalitis has not been demonstrated.

Varicella-Zoster Infections in Immunocompromised Patients

A multicenter trial of ZOVIRAX Sterile Powder at a dose of 500 mg/m² every 8 hours for 7 days was conducted in immunocompromised patients with zoster infections (shingles). Ninety-four (94) patients were evaluated (52 patients were treated with ZOVIRAX and 42 with placebo). ZOVIRAX halted progression of infection as determined by significant reductions in cutaneous dissemination, visceral dissemination, or the proportion of patients deemed treatment failures.[28,33]

A comparative trial of ZOVIRAX and vidarabine was conducted in 22 severely immunocompromised patients with zoster infections. ZOVIRAX was shown to be superior to vidarabine as demonstrated by significant differences in the time of new lesion formation, the time to pain reduction, the time to lesion crusting, the time to complete healing, the incidence of fever, and the duration of positive viral cultures. In addition, cutaneous dissemination occurred in none of the 10 patients treated with ZOVIRAX compared to 5 of the 10 vidarabine recipients who presented with localized dermatomal disease.[34]

Diagnosis

Diagnosis is confirmed by virus isolation. Accelerated viral culture assays or immunocytology allow more rapid diagnosis than standard viral culture. In initial episodes of genital herpes, appropriate examinations should be performed to rule out other sexually transmitted diseases. Whereas cutaneous lesions associated with Herpes simplex and varicella-zoster infections are often characteristic, the finding of multinucleated giant cells in smears prepared from lesion exudate or scrapings may assist in the diagnosis.[35]

The Tzanck smear does not distinguish varicella-zoster from herpes simplex infections. Culture of varicella-zoster is not widely available.

Herpes encephalitis should be confirmed by brain biopsy to obtain tissue for histologic examination and viral culture and to exclude other causes of neurologic disease. A presumptive diagnosis of herpes encephalitis may be made on the basis of focal changes in the temporal lobe visualized with various diagnostic methods including magnetic resonance imaging, computerized tomography, radionuclide scans, or electroencephalography. Culture of the cerebrospinal fluid for herpes simplex virus is unreliable.

CONTRAINDICATIONS

ZOVIRAX Sterile Powder is contraindicated for patients who develop hypersensitivity to the drug.

WARNINGS

ZOVIRAX Sterile Powder is intended for intravenous infusion only, and should not be administered topically, intramuscularly, orally, subcutaneously, or in the eye. Intravenous infusions must be given over a period of at least 1 (one) hour to reduce the risk of renal tubular damage (see PRECAUTIONS and DOSAGE AND ADMINISTRATION).

PRECAUTIONS

General: The recommended dosage, frequency, and length of treatment should not be exceeded (see DOSAGE AND ADMINISTRATION).

Although the aqueous solubility of acyclovir sodium (for infusion) is >100 mg/mL, precipitation of acyclovir crystals in renal tubules can occur if the maximum solubility of free acyclovir (2.5 mg/mL at 37°C in water) is exceeded or if the drug is administered by bolus injection. This complication causes a rise in serum creatinine and blood urea nitrogen (BUN), and a decrease in renal creatinine clearance. Ensuing renal tubular damage can produce acute renal failure.

Abnormal renal function (decreased creatinine clearance) can occur as a result of acyclovir administration and depends on the state of the patient's hydration, other treatments, and the rate of drug administration. Bolus administration of the drug leads to a 10% incidence of renal dysfunction, while in controlled studies, infusion of 5 mg/kg (250 mg/m²) and 10 mg/kg (500 mg/m²) over an hour was associated with a lower frequency—3.8%. Concomitant use of other nephrotoxic drugs, pre-existing renal disease, and dehydration make further renal impairment with acyclovir more likely. In most instances, alterations of renal function were transient and resolved spontaneously or with improvement of water and electrolyte balance, drug dosage adjustment, or discontinuation of drug administration. However, in some instances, these changes may progress to acute renal failure. Administration of ZOVIRAX by intravenous infusion must be accompanied by adequate hydration. Since maximum urine concentration occurs within the first 2 hours following infusion, particular attention should be given to establishing sufficient urine flow during that period in order to prevent precipitation in renal tubules. Recommended urine output is ≥ 500 mL per gram of drug infused. In patients with encephalitis, the recommended hydration should be balanced by the risk of cerebral edema.

When dosage adjustments are required, they should be based on estimated creatinine clearance (see DOSAGE AND ADMINISTRATION).

Approximately 1% of patients receiving intravenous acyclovir have manifested encephalopathic changes character-

ized by either lethargy, obtundation, tremors, confusion, hallucinations, agitation, seizures, or coma. ZOVIRAX should be used with caution in those patients who have underlying neurologic abnormalities and those with serious renal, hepatic, or electrolyte abnormalities or significant hypoxia. It should also be used with caution in patients who have manifested prior neurologic reactions to cytotoxic drugs or those receiving concomitant intrathecal methotrexate or interferon.

Exposure of HSV isolates to acyclovir in vitro can lead to the emergence of less sensitive viruses. These viruses usually are deficient in thymidine kinase (required for acyclovir activation) and are less pathogenic in animals. Similar isolates have been observed in severely immunocompromised patients during the course of controlled and uncontrolled studies of intravenously administered ZOVIRAX. These occurred in patients with severe combined immunodeficiencies or following bone marrow transplantation. The presence of these viruses was not associated with a worsening of clinical illness and, in some instances, the virus disappeared spontaneously. The possibility of the appearance of less sensitive viruses must be recognized when treating such patients.[11-19] The relationship between the in vitro sensitivity of herpes simplex or varicella-zoster virus to acyclovir and clinical response to therapy has not been established.

Drug Interactions: Co-administration of probenecid with acyclovir has been shown to increase the mean half-life and the area under the concentration-time curve. Urinary excretion and renal clearance were correspondingly reduced.[36] The clinical effects of this combination have not been studied.

Carcinogenesis, Mutagenesis, Impairment of Fertility: The data presented below include references to peak steady-state plasma acyclovir concentrations observed in humans treated with 30 mg/kg/day (10 mg/kg/every 8 hours, dosing appropriate for treatment of herpes zoster or herpes encephalitis), or 15 mg/kg/day (5 mg/kg/every 8 hours, dosing appropriate for treatment of primary genital herpes or herpes simplex infections in immunocompromised patients). Plasma drug concentrations in animal studies are expressed as multiples of human exposure to acyclovir at the higher and lower dosing schedules (see CLINICAL PHARMACOLOGY: Pharmacokinetics).

Acyclovir was tested in lifetime bioassays in rats and mice at single daily doses of up to 450 mg/kg administered by gavage. There was no statistically significant difference in the incidence of tumors between treated and control animals, nor did acyclovir shorten the latency of tumors. At 450 mg/kg/day, plasma concentrations in both the mouse and rat bioassay were lower than concentrations in humans.

Acyclovir was tested in two in vitro cell transformation assays. Positive results were observed at the highest concentration tested (3 to 5 times human levels) in one system and the resulting morphologically transformed cells formed tumors when inoculated into immunosuppressed, syngeneic, weanling mice. Acyclovir was negative (3 to 6 times human levels) in the other, possibly less sensitive, transformation assay. In acute cytogenetic studies, there was an increase, though not statistically significant, in the incidence of chromosomal damage at maximum tolerated parenteral doses of acyclovir (100 mg/kg) in rats (5 to 10 times human levels) but not in Chinese hamsters; higher doses of 500 and 1000 mg/kg were clastogenic in Chinese hamsters (31 to 61 times human levels). In addition, no activity was found after 5 days dosing in a dominant lethal study in mice (3 to 6 times human levels). In all four microbial assays, no evidence of mutagenicity was observed. Positive results were obtained in two of seven genetic toxicity assays using mammalian cells in vitro. In human lymphocytes, a positive response for chromosomal damage was seen at concentrations 13 to 25 times the acyclovir plasma levels achieved in humans. At one locus in mouse lymphoma cells, mutagenicity was observed at concentrations 20 to 40 times human plasma levels. Results in the other five mammalian cell loci follow: at three loci in a Chinese hamster ovary cell line, the results were inconclusive at concentrations at least 150 times human levels; at two other loci in mouse lymphoma cells, no evidence of mutagenicity was observed at concentrations at least 120 times human levels.

Acyclovir has not been shown to impair fertility or reproduction in mice (450 mg/kg/day, p.o.) or in rats (25 mg/kg/day, s.c.). In the mouse study, plasma levels were the same as human levels. At 50 mg/kg/day, s.c. in the rat (1 to 2 times human levels), there was a statistically significant increase in post-implantation loss, but no concomitant decrease in litter size. In female rabbits treated subcutaneously with acyclovir subsequent to mating, there was a statistically significant decrease in implantation efficiency but no concomitant decrease in litter size at a dose of 50 mg/kg/day (1 to 3 times human levels). No effect upon implantation efficiency was observed when the same dose was administered intravenously (4 to 9 times human levels). In a rat peri- and postnatal study at 50 mg/kg/day, s.c., (1 to 2 times human levels), there was a statistically significant decrease in the group mean numbers of corpora lutea, total implantation sites and live fetuses in the F_1 generation. Although not statistically

significant, there was also a dose-related decrease in group mean numbers of live fetuses and implantation sites, at 12.5 mg/kg/day and 25 mg/kg/day, s.c. The intravenous administration of 100 mg/kg/day, a dose known to cause obstructive nephropathy in rabbits, caused a significant increase in fetal resorptions and a corresponding decrease in litter size (plasma levels were not measured). However, at a maximum tolerated intravenous dose of 50 mg/kg/day in rabbits (4 to 9 times human levels), no drug-related reproductive effects were observed.

Intraperitoneal doses of 80 or 320 mg/kg/day acyclovir given to rats for 6 and 1 months, respectively, caused testicular atrophy. Plasma levels were not measured in the 1-month study and were 2 to 4 times human levels in the 6-month study. Testicular atrophy was persistent through the 4-week postdose recovery phase after 320 mg/kg/day; some evidence of recovery of sperm production was evident 30 days postdose. Intravenous doses of 100 and 200 mg/kg/day acyclovir given to dogs for 31 days caused aspermatogenesis. At 100 mg/kg/day, plasma levels were 4 to 8 times human levels, while at 200 mg/kg/day, they were 13 to 25 times human levels. No testicular abnormalities were seen in dogs given 50 mg/kg/day i.v. for 1 month (2 to 3 times human levels) and in dogs given 60 mg/kg/day orally for 1 year (the same as human levels).

Pregnancy: *Teratogenic Effects:* Pregnancy Category C. Acyclovir was not teratogenic in the mouse (450 mg/kg/day, p.o.), rabbit (50 mg/kg/day, s.c. and i.v.) or in standard tests in the rat (50 mg/kg/day, s.c.). These exposures resulted in plasma levels the same as, 4 and 9, and 1 and 2 times, respectively, human levels. In a non-standard test in rats, there were fetal abnormalities, such as head and tail anomalies, and maternal toxicity.[37] In this test, rats were given three s.c. doses of 100 mg/kg acyclovir on gestation day 10, resulting in plasma levels 5 and 10 times human levels. There are no adequate and well-controlled studies in pregnant women. Acyclovir should not be used during pregnancy unless the potential benefit justifies the potential risk to the fetus. Although acyclovir was not teratogenic in standard animal studies, the drug's potential for causing chromosome breaks at high concentration should be taken into consideration in making this determination.

Pregnancy Exposure Registry: To monitor maternal-fetal outcomes of pregnant women exposed to systemic acyclovir. Glaxo Wellcome Inc. maintains an Acyclovir in Pregnancy Registry. Physicians are encouraged to register patients by calling (800) 722-9292, ext. 58465.

Nursing Mothers: Acyclovir concentrations have been documented in breast milk in two women following oral administration of ZOVIRAX and ranged from 0.6 to 4.1 times corresponding plasma levels.[38,39] These concentrations would potentially expose the nursing infant to a dose of acyclovir up to 0.3 mg/kg/day. Caution should be exercised when ZOVIRAX is administered to a nursing woman.

ADVERSE REACTIONS

The adverse reactions listed below have been observed in controlled and uncontrolled clinical trials in approximately 700 patients who received ZOVIRAX at ~ 5 mg/kg (250 mg/m²) three times daily, and approximately 300 patients who received ~ 10 mg/kg (500 mg/m²) three times daily.

The most frequent adverse reactions reported during administration of ZOVIRAX were inflammation or phlebitis at the injection site in approximately 9% of the patients, and transient elevations of serum creatinine or BUN in 5% to 10% (the higher incidence occurred usually following rapid [less than 10 minutes] intravenous infusion). Nausea and/or vomiting occurred in approximately 7% of the patients (the majority occurring in nonhospitalized patients who received 10 mg/kg). Itching, rash, or hives occurred in approximately 2% of patients. Elevation of transaminases occurred in 1% to 2% of patients.

Approximately 1% of patients receiving intravenous acyclovir have manifested encephalopathic changes characterized by either lethargy, obtundation, tremors, confusion, hallucinations, agitation, seizures, or coma (see PRECAUTIONS).

Adverse reactions which occurred at a frequency of less than 1% and which were probably or possibly related to intravenous administration of ZOVIRAX were: anemia, anuria, hematuria, hypotension, edema, anorexia, lightheadedness, thirst, headache, diaphoresis, fever, neutropenia, thrombocytopenia, abnormal urinalysis (characterized by an increase in formed elements in urine sediment), and pain on urination.

Other reactions have been reported with a frequency of less than 1 % in patients receiving ZOVIRAX, but a causal relationship between ZOVIRAX and the reaction could not be determined. These include pulmonary edema with cardiac tamponade, abdominal pain, chest pain, thrombocytosis, leukocytosis, neutrophilia, ischemia of digits, hypokalemia, purpura fulminans, pressure on urination, hemoglobinemia, and rigors.

Observed During Clinical Practice: Based on clinical practice experience in patients treated with ZOVIRAX Sterile Powder in the U.S., spontaneously reported adverse events are uncommon. Data are insufficient to support an estimate of their incidence or to establish causation. These events may also occur as part of the underlying disease process. Voluntary reports of adverse events which have been received since market introduction include:

General: fever, pain, and rarely, anaphylaxis
Digestive: elevated liver function tests, nausea
Hemic and Lymphatic: leukopenia
Nervous: agitation, coma, confusion, convulsions, delirium, hallucinations, obtundation, psychosis
Skin: rash
Urogenital: elevated blood urea nitrogen, elevated creatinine, renal failure

OVERDOSAGE

Overdosage has been reported following administration of bolus injections, or inappropriately high doses, and in patients whose fluid and electrolyte balance was not properly monitored. This has resulted in elevations in BUN, serum creatinine, and subsequent renal failure. Lethargy, convulsions, and coma have been reported rarely.

Precipitation of acyclovir in renal tubules may occur when the solubility (2.5 mg/mL) in the intratubular fluid is exceeded (see PRECAUTIONS). Renal lesions related to obstruction of renal tubules by precipitated drug crystals occurred in the following species: rats treated with i.v. and i.p. doses of 20 mg/kg/day for 21 and 31 days, respectively, and at s.c. doses of 100 mg/kg/day for 10 days; rabbits at s.c. and i.v. doses of 50 mg/kg/day for 13 days; and dogs at i.v. doses of 100 mg/kg/day for 31 days. In the event of overdosage, sufficient urine flow must be maintained to prevent precipitation of drug in renal tubules. Recommended urine output is ≥ 500 mL per gram of drug infused. A 6-hour hemodialysis results in a 60% decrease in plasma acyclovir concentration. Data concerning peritoneal dialysis are incomplete but indicate that this method may be significantly less efficient in removing acyclovir from the blood. In the event of acute renal failure and anuria, the patient may benefit from hemodialysis until renal function is restored (see DOSAGE AND ADMINISTRATION).

DOSAGE AND ADMINISTRATION

CAUTION— RAPID OR BOLUS INTRAVENOUS AND INTRAMUSCULAR OR SUBCUTANEOUS INJECTION MUST BE AVOIDED. Therapy should be initiated as early as possible following onset of signs and symptoms. For diagnosis— see INDICATIONS.

Dosage:

Herpes Simplex Infections
Mucosal and Cutaneous Herpes Simplex (HSV-1 and HSV-2) Infections in Immunocompromised Patients: 5 mg/kg infused at a constant rate over 1 hour, every 8 hours (15 mg/kg/day) for 7 days in adult patients with normal renal function. In children under 12 years of age, more accurate dosing can be attained by infusing 250 mg/m² at a constant rate over 1 hour, every 8 hours (750 mg/m²/day) for 7 days.
Severe Initial Clinical Episodes of Herpes Genitalis: The same dose given above—administered for 5 days.
Herpes Simplex Encephalitis: 10 mg/kg infused at a constant rate over at least 1 hour, every 8 hours for 10 days. In children between 6 months and 12 years of age, more accurate dosing is achieved by infusing 500 mg/m², at a constant rate over at least one hour, every 8 hours for 10 days.
Varicella Zoster Infections
Zoster in Immunocompromised Patients: 10 mg/kg infused at a constant rate over 1 hour, every 8 hours for 7 days in adult patients with normal renal function. In children under 12 years of age, equivalent plasma concentrations are attained by infusing 500 mg/m² at a constant rate over at least 1 hour, every 8 hours for 7 days. Obese patients should be dosed at 10 mg/kg (Ideal Body Weight). A maximum dose equivalent to 500 mg/m² every 8 hours should not be exceeded for any patient.

PATIENTS WITH ACUTE OR CHRONIC RENAL IMPAIRMENT: Refer to DOSAGE AND ADMINISTRATION section for recommended doses, and adjust the dosing interval as indicated in the table below.

Creatinine Clearance (mL/min/1.73 m²)	Percent of Recommended Dose	Dosing Interval (hours)
>50	100%	8
25–50	100%	12
10–25	100%	24
0–10	50%	24

Hemodialysis: For patients who require dialysis, the mean plasma half-life of acyclovir during hemodialysis is approximately 5 hours. This results in a 60% decrease in plasma concentrations following a 6-hour dialysis period. Therefore, the patient's dosing schedule should be adjusted so that an additional dose is administered after each dialysis.[24,25]
Peritoneal Dialysis: No supplemental dose appears to be necessary after adjustment of the dosing interval.[40,41]

Method of Preparation: Each 10 mL vial contains acyclovir sodium equivalent to 500 mg of acyclovir. Each 20 mL vial contains acyclovir sodium equivalent to 1000 mg of acyclovir. The contents of the vial should be dissolved in Sterile Water for Injection as follows:

Contents of Vial	Amount of Diluent
500 mg	10 mL
1000 mg	20 mL

The resulting solution in each case contains 50 mg acyclovir per mL (pH approximately 11). Shake the vial well to assure complete dissolution before measuring and transferring each individual dose. DO NOT USE BACTERIOSTATIC WATER FOR INJECTION CONTAINING BENZYL ALCOHOL OR PARABENS.

Administration: The calculated dose should then be removed and added to any appropriate intravenous solution at a volume selected for administration during each 1-hour infusion. Infusion concentrations of approximately 7 mg/mL or lower are recommended. In clinical studies, the average 70 kg adult received between 60 and 150 mL of fluid per dose. Higher concentrations (e.g., 10 mg/mL) may produce phlebitis or inflammation at the injection site upon inadvertent extravasation. Standard, commercially available electrolyte and glucose solutions are suitable for intravenous administration; biologic or colloidal fluids (e.g., blood products, protein solutions, etc.) are not recommended.

Once in solution in the vial at a concentration of 50 mg/mL, the drug should be used within 12 hours. Once diluted for administration, each dose should be used within 24 hours. Refrigeration of reconstituted solutions may result in formation of a precipitate which will redissolve at room temperature.

HOW SUPPLIED

10 mL sterile vials, each containing acyclovir sodium equivalent to 500 mg of acyclovir, tray of 10 (NDC 0173-0995-01). 20 mL sterile vials, each containing acyclovir sodium equivalent to 1000 mg of acyclovir, tray of 10 (NDC 0173-0952-01). Store at 15° to 25°C (59° to 77°F).

Also available: ZOVIRAX Ointment, 5% in 3 g and 15 g tubes (each gram contains 50 mg acyclovir in a polyethylene glycol base), ZOVIRAX Capsules in bottles of 100 and unit dose pack of 100 (each capsule contains 200 mg acyclovir); ZOVIRAX Tablets in bottles of 100 and unit dose pack of 100 (each tablet contains 800 mg acyclovir); ZOVIRAX Tablets in bottles of 100 (each tablet contains 400 mg acyclovir); and ZOVIRAX Suspension in 1 pint bottles (each 5 mL contains 200 mg acyclovir).

REFERENCES

1. O'Brien JJ, Campoli-Richards DM. Acyclovir—an updated review of its antiviral activity, pharmacokinetic properties and therapeutic efficacy. *Drugs* 1989; 37:233-309.
2. Littler E, Zeuthen J, McBride AA, et al. Identification of an Epstein-Barr virus-coded thymidine kinase. *EMBO J.* 1986;5:1959-1966.
3. Miller WH, Miller RL. Phosphorylation of acyclovir (acycloguanosine) monophosphate by GMP kinase. *J Biol Chem.* 1980;255:7204-7207.
4. Furman PA, St Clair MH, Fyfe JA, et al. Inhibition of herpes simplex virus-induced DNA polymerase activity and viral DNA replication by 9-(2-hydroxyethoxymethyl)guanine and its triphosphate. *J Virol.* 1979;32:72-77.
5. Derse D, Cheng YC, Furman PA, et al. Inhibition of purified human and herpes simplex virus-induced DNA polymerases by 9-(2-hydroxyethoxymethyl)guanine triphosphate: effects on primer-template function. *J Biol Chem.* 1981;256:11447-11451.
6. McGuirt PV, Shaw JE, Elion GB, et al. Identification of small DNA fragments synthesized in herpes simplex virus-infected cells in the presence of acyclovir. *Antimicrob Agents Chemother.* 1984;25:507-509.
7. Barry DW, Blum MR. Antiviral drugs: acyclovir. In: Turner P, Shand DG, eds. *Recent Advances in Clinical Pharmacology.* ed 3. New York: Churchill Livingstone, 1983: chap 4.
8. DeClercq E. Comparative efficacy of antiherpes drugs in different cell lines. *Antimicrob Agents Chemother.* 1982;21:661-663.
9. McLaren C, Ellis MN, Hunter GA. A colorimetric assay for the measurement of the sensitivity of herpes simplex viruses to antiviral agents. *Antiviral Res.* 1983; 3:223-234.
10. Barry DW, Nusinoff-Lehrman S. Viral resistance in clinical practice: summary of five years experience with acyclovir. In: Kono R, Nakajima A, eds. *Herpes Viruses*

Continued on next page

Glaxo Wellcome—Cont.

and Virus Chemotherapy (Ex Med Int Congr Ser 667). New York: Excerpta Medica, 1985;269-270.

11. Dekker C, Ellis MN, McLaren C, et al. Virus resistance in clinical practice. *J Antimicrob Chemother.* 1983;12 (suppl B):137-152.
12. Sibrack CD, Gutman LT, Wilfert CM, et al. Pathogenicity of acyclovir-resistant herpes simplex virus type 1 from an immunodeficient child. *J Infect Dis.* 1982; 146:673-682.
13. Crumpacker CS, Schnipper LE, Marlowe Sl, et al. Resistance to antiviral drugs of herpes simplex virus isolated from a patient treated with acyclovir. *N Engl J Med.* 1982;306:343-346.
14. Wade JC, Newton B, McLaren C, et al. Intravenous acyclovir to treat mucocutaneous herpes simplex virus infection after marrow transplantation: a double-blind trial. *Ann Intern Med.* 1982;96:265-269.
15. Burns WH, Saral R, Santos GW, et al. Isolation and characterization of resistant herpes simplex virus after acyclovir therapy. *Lancet.* 1982;1:421-423.
16. Straus SE, Takiff HE, Seidlin M, et al. Suppression of frequently recurring genital herpes: a placebo-controlled double-blind trial of oral acyclovir. *N Engl J Med.* 1984;310:1545-1550.
17. Collins P. Viral sensitivity following the introduction of acyclovir. *Am J Med.* 1988;85(suppl 2A):129-134.
18. Erlich KS, Mills J, Chatis P, et al. Acyclovir-resistant herpes simplex virus infections in patients with the acquired immunodeficiency syndrome. *N Engl J Med.* 1989;320:293-296.
19. Hill EL, Ellis MN, Barry DW. In: *28th Intersci Conf on Antimicrob Agents Chemother.* Los Angeles, 1988, Abst. No. 0840:260.
20. Ellis MN, Keller PM, Fyfe JA, et al. Clinical isolates of herpes simplex virus type 2 that induces a thymidine kinase with altered substrate specificity. *Antimicrob Agents Chemother.* 1987;31:1117-1125.
21. Collins P, Larder BA, Oliver NM, et al. Characterization of a DNA polymerase mutant of herpes simplex virus from a severely immunocompromised patient receiving acyclovir. *J Gen Virol.* 1989;70:375-382.
22. Field HJ, Darby G, Wildy P. Isolation and characterization of acyclovir-resistant mutants of herpes simplex virus. *J Gen Virol.* 1980;49:115-124.
23. Blum MR, Liao SH, deMiranda P. Overview of acyclovir pharmacokinetic disposition in adults and children. *Am J Med.* 1982;73:186-192.
24. Laskin OL, Longstreth JA, Whelton A, et al. Effect of renal failure on the pharmacokinetics of acyclovir. *Am J Med.* 1982;73:197-201.
25. Krasny HC, Liao SH, deMiranda P, et al. Influence of hemodialysis on acyclovir pharmacokinetics in patients with chronic renal failure. *Am J Med.* 1982;73:202-204.
26. Mitchell CD, Bean B, Gentry SR, et al. Acyclovir therapy for mucocutaneous herpes simplex infections in immunocompromised patients. *Lancet.* 1981;1:1389-1392.
27. Meyers JD, Wade JC, Mitchell CD, et al. Multicenter collaborative trial of intravenous acyclovir for treatment of mucocutaneous herpes simplex virus infection in the immunocompromised host. *Am J Med.* 1982:73: 229-235.
28. Data on file, Glaxo Wellcome Inc.
29. Corey L, Fife KH, Benedetti JK, et al. Intravenous acyclovir for the treatment of primary genital herpes. *Ann Intern Med.* 1983;98:914-921.
30. Mindel A, Adler MW, Sutherland S, et al. Intravenous acyclovir treatment for primary genital herpes. *Lancet.* 1982;1:697-700.
31. Whitley RJ, Alford CA, Hirsch MS, et al. Vidarabine versus acyclovir therapy in herpes simplex encephalitis. *N Engl J Med.* 1986;314:144-149.
32. Sköldenberg B, Forsgren M, Alestig K, et al. Acyclovir versus vidarabine in herpes simplex encephalitis: randomized multicenter study in consecutive Swedish patients. *Lancet.* 1984;2:707-711.
33. Balfour HH Jr, Bean B, Laskin OL, et al. Acyclovir halts progression of herpes zoster in immunocompromised patients. *N Engl J Med.* 1983;308:1448-1453.
34. Shepp DH, Danliker PS, Meyers JD. Treatment of varicella-zoster virus infection in severely immunocompromised patients. *N Engl J Med.* 1986;314:208-212.
35. Naib ZM, Nahmias AJ, Josey WE, et al. Relation of cytohistopathology of genital herpesvirus infection to cervical anaplasia. *Cancer Res.* 1973;33:1452-1463.
36. Laskin OL, deMiranda P, King DH, et al. Effects of probenecid on the pharmacokinetics and elimination of acyclovir in humans. *Antimicrob Agents Chemother.* 1982;21:804-807.
37. Stahlmann R, Klug S, Lewandowski C, et al. Teratogenicity of acyclovir in rats. *Infection.* 1987;15:261-262.
38. Lau RJ, Emery MG, Galinsky RE, et al. Unexpected accumulation of acyclovir in breast milk with estimate of infant exposure. *Obstet Gynecol.* 1987;69:468-471.
39. Meyer LJ, deMiranda P, Sheth N, et al. Acyclovir in human breast milk. *Am J Obstet Gynecol.* 1988; 158:586-588.
40. Boelart J, Schurgers M, Daneels R, et al. Multiple dose pharmacokinetics of intravenous acyclovir in patients on continuous ambulatory peritoneal dialysis. *J Antimicrob Chemother.* 1987;20:69-76.
41. Shah GM, Winer RL, Krasny HC. Acyclovir pharmacokinetics in a patient on continuous ambulatory peritoneal dialysis. *Am J Kidney Dis.* 1986;7:507-510.

U.S. Patent No. 4199574.
February 1996/RL-270

Shown in Product Identification Guide, page 316

ZYLOPRIM ® ℞

[zī'lō-prĭm]
(allopurinol)
100 mg Scored Tablets and
300 mg Scored Tablets

DESCRIPTION

ZYLOPRIM (allopurinol) is known chemically as 1,5-dihydro-4*H*-pyrazolo[3,4-*d*]pyrimidin-4-one. It is a xanthine oxidase inhibitor which is administered orally. Each scored white tablet contains 100 mg allopurinol and the inactive ingredients lactose, magnesium stearate, potato starch, and povidone. Each scored peach tablet contains 300 mg allopurinol and the inactive ingredients corn starch, FD&C Yellow No. 6 Lake, lactose, magnesium stearate, and povidone. Its solubility in water at 37°C is 80.0 mg/dL and is greater in an alkaline solution.

CLINICAL PHARMACOLOGY

ZYLOPRIM (allopurinol) acts on purine catabolism, without disrupting the biosynthesis of purines. It reduces the production of uric acid by inhibiting the biochemical reactions immediately preceding its formation.

ZYLOPRIM is a structural analogue of the natural purine base, hypoxanthine. It is an inhibitor of xanthine oxidase, the enzyme responsible for the conversion of hypoxanthine to xanthine and of xanthine to uric acid, the end product of purine metabolism in man. ZYLOPRIM is metabolized to the corresponding xanthine analogue, oxipurinol (alloxanthine), which also is an inhibitor of xanthine oxidase.

It has been shown that reutilization of both hypoxanthine and xanthine for nucleotide and nucleic acid synthesis is markedly enhanced when their oxidations are inhibited by ZYLOPRIM and oxipurinol. This reutilization does not disrupt normal nucleic acid anabolism, however, because feedback inhibition is an integral part of purine biosynthesis. As a result of xanthine oxidase inhibition, the serum concentration of hypoxanthine plus xanthine in patients receiving ZYLOPRIM for treatment of hyperuricemia is usually in the range of 0.3 to 0.4 mg/dL compared to a normal level of approximately 0.15 mg/dL. A maximum of 0.9 mg/dL of these oxypurines has been reported when the serum urate was lowered to less than 2 mg/dL by high doses of ZYLOPRIM. These values are far below the saturation levels at which point their precipitation would be expected to occur (above 7 mg/dL).

The renal clearance of hypoxanthine and xanthine is at least 10 times greater than that of uric acid. The increased xanthine and hypoxanthine in the urine have not been accompanied by problems of nephrolithiasis. Xanthine crystalluria has been reported in only three patients. Two of the patients had Lesch-Nyhan syndrome, which is characterized by excessive uric acid production combined with a deficiency of the enzyme, hypoxanthineguanine phosphoribosyltransferase (HGPRTase). This enzyme is required for the conversion of hypoxanthine, xanthine, and guanine to their respective nucleotides. The third patient had lymphosarcoma and produced an extremely large amount of uric acid because of rapid cell lysis during chemotherapy.

ZYLOPRIM is approximately 90% absorbed from the gastrointestinal tract. Peak plasma levels generally occur at 1.5 hours and 4.5 hours for ZYLOPRIM and oxipurinol respectively, and after a single oral dose of 300 mg ZYLOPRIM, maximum plasma levels of about 3 μg/mL of ZYLOPRIM and 6.5 μg/mL of oxipurinol are produced.

Approximately 20% of the ingested ZYLOPRIM is excreted in the feces. Because of its rapid oxidation to oxipurinol and a renal clearance rate approximately that of glomerular filtration rate, ZYLOPRIM has a plasma half-life of about 1 to 2 hours. Oxipurinol, however, has a longer plasma half-life (approximately 15.0 hours) and therefore effective xanthine oxidase inhibition is maintained over a 24-hour period with single daily doses of ZYLOPRIM. Whereas ZYLOPRIM is cleared essentially by glomerular filtration, oxipurinol is reabsorbed in the kidney tubules in a manner similar to the reabsorption of uric acid.

The clearance of oxipurinol is increased by uricosuric drugs, and as a consequence, the addition of a uricosuric agent reduces to some degree the inhibition of xanthine oxidase by oxipurinol and increases to some degree the urinary excretion of uric acid. In practice, the net effect of such combined therapy may be useful in some patients in achieving minimum serum uric acid levels provided the total urinary uric acid load does not exceed the competence of the patient's renal function.

Hyperuricemia may be primary, as in gout, or secondary to diseases such as acute and chronic leukemia, polycythemia vera, multiple myeloma, and psoriasis. It may occur with the use of diuretic agents, during renal dialysis, in the presence of renal damage, during starvation or reducing diets, and in the treatment of neoplastic disease where rapid resolution of tissue masses may occur. Asymptomatic hyperuricemia is not an indication for treatment with ZYLOPRIM (see INDICATIONS AND USAGE).

Gout is a metabolic disorder which is characterized by hyperuricemia and resultant deposition of monosodium urate in the tissues, particularly the joints and kidneys. The etiology of this hyperuricemia is the overproduction of uric acid in relation to the patient's ability to excrete it. If progressive deposition of urates is to be arrested or reversed, it is necessary to reduce the serum uric acid level below the saturation point to suppress urate precipitation.

Administration of ZYLOPRIM generally results in a fall in both serum and urinary uric acid within two to three days. The degree of this decrease can be manipulated almost at will since it is dose-dependent. A week or more of treatment with ZYLOPRIM may be required before its full effects are manifested; likewise, uric acid may return to pretreatment levels slowly (usually after a period of seven to ten days following cessation of therapy). This reflects primarily the accumulation and slow clearance of oxipurinol. In some patients a dramatic fall in urinary uric acid excretion may not occur, particularly in those with severe tophaceous gout. It has been postulated that this may be due to the mobilization of urate from tissue deposits as the serum uric acid level begins to fall.

The action of ZYLOPRIM differs from that of uricosuric agents, which lower the serum uric acid level by increasing urinary excretion of uric acid. ZYLOPRIM reduces both the serum and urinary uric acid levels by inhibiting the formation of uric acid. The use of ZYLOPRIM to block the formation of urates avoids the hazard of increased renal excretion of uric acid posed by uricosuric drugs.

ZYLOPRIM can substantially reduce serum and urinary uric acid levels in previously refractory patients even in the presence of renal damage serious enough to render uricosuric drugs virtually ineffective. Salicylates may be given conjointly for their antirheumatic effect without compromising the action of ZYLOPRIM. This is in contrast to the nullifying effect of salicylates on uricosuric drugs.

ZYLOPRIM also inhibits the enzymatic oxidation of mercaptopurine, the sulfur-containing analogue of hypoxanthine, to 6-thiouric acid. This oxidation, which is catalyzed by xanthine oxidase, inactivates mercaptopurine. Hence, the inhibition of such oxidation by ZYLOPRIM may result in as much as a 75% reduction in the therapeutic dose requirement of mercaptopurine when the two compounds are given together.

INDICATIONS AND USAGE

THIS IS NOT AN INNOCUOUS DRUG. IT IS NOT RECOMMENDED FOR THE TREATMENT OF ASYMPTOMATIC HYPERURICEMIA.

ZYLOPRIM (allopurinol) reduces serum and urinary uric acid concentrations. Its use should be individualized for each patient and requires an understanding of its mode of action and pharmacokinetics (see CLINICAL PHARMACOLOGY, CONTRAINDICATIONS, WARNINGS and PRECAUTIONS).

ZYLOPRIM is indicated in:

(1) the management of patients with signs and symptoms of primary or secondary gout (acute attacks, tophi, joint destruction, uric acid lithiasis and/or nephropathy).

(2) the management of patients with leukemia, lymphoma, and malignancies who are receiving cancer therapy which causes elevations of serum and urinary uric acid levels. Treatment with ZYLOPRIM should be discontinued when the potential for overproduction of uric acid is no longer present.

(3) the management of patients with recurrent calcium oxalate calculi whose daily uric acid excretion exceeds 800 mg/day in male patients and 750 mg/day in female patients. Therapy in such patients should be carefully assessed initially and reassessed periodically to determine in each case that treatment is beneficial and that the benefits outweigh the risks.

CONTRAINDICATIONS

Patients who have developed a severe reaction to ZYLOPRIM (allopurinol) should not be restarted on the drug.

WARNINGS

ZYLOPRIM (ALLOPURINOL) SHOULD BE DISCONTINUED AT THE FIRST APPEARANCE OF SKIN RASH OR

OTHER SIGNS WHICH MAY INDICATE AN ALLERGIC REACTION. In some instances a skin rash may be followed by more severe hypersensitivity reactions such as exfoliative, urticarial, and purpuric lesions as well as Stevens-Johnson syndrome (erythema multiforme exudativum), and/or generalized vasculitis, irreversible hepatotoxicity, and on rare occasions death.

In patients receiving PURINETHOL® (mercaptopurine) or IMURAN® (azathioprine), the concomitant administration of 300 to 600 mg of ZYLOPRIM per day will require a reduction in dose to approximately one-third to one-fourth of the usual dose of mercaptopurine or azathioprine. Subsequent adjustment of doses of mercaptopurine or azathioprine should be made on the basis of therapeutic response and the appearance of toxic effects (see CLINICAL PHARMACOLOGY).

A few cases of reversible clinical hepatotoxicity have been noted in patients taking ZYLOPRIM, and in some patients asymptomatic rises in serum alkaline phosphatase or serum transaminase have been observed. If anorexia, weight loss, or pruritus develop in patients on ZYLOPRIM, evaluation of liver function should be part of their diagnostic workup. In patients with pre-existing liver disease, periodic liver function tests are recommended during the early stages of therapy.

Due to the occasional occurrence of drowsiness, patients should be alerted to the need for due precaution when engaging in activities where alertness is mandatory.

The occurrence of hypersensitivity reactions to ZYLOPRIM may be increased in patients with decreased renal function receiving thiazides and ZYLOPRIM concurrently. For this reason, in this clinical setting, such combinations should be administered with caution and patients should be observed closely.

PRECAUTIONS

General: An increase in acute attacks of gout has been reported during the early stages of ZYLOPRIM (allopurinol) administration, even when normal or subnormal serum uric acid levels have been attained. Accordingly, maintenance doses of colchicine generally should be given prophylactically when ZYLOPRIM is begun. In addition, it is recommended that the patient start with a low dose of ZYLOPRIM (100 mg daily) and increase at weekly intervals by 100 mg until a serum uric acid level of 6 mg/dL or less is attained but without exceeding the maximum recommended dose (800 mg per day). The use of colchicine or anti-inflammatory agents may be required to suppress gouty attacks in some cases. The attacks usually become shorter and less severe after several months of therapy. The mobilization of urates from tissue deposits which cause fluctuations in the serum uric acid levels may be a possible explanation for these episodes. Even with adequate therapy with ZYLOPRIM, it may require several months to deplete the uric acid pool sufficiently to achieve control of the acute attacks.

A fluid intake sufficient to yield a daily urinary output of at least two liters and the maintenance of a neutral or, preferably, slightly alkaline urine are desirable to (1) avoid the theoretical possibility of formation of xanthine calculi under the influence of ZYLOPRIM therapy and (2) help prevent renal precipitation of urates in patients receiving concomitant uricosuric agents.

Some patients with pre-existing renal disease or poor urate clearance have shown a rise in BUN during administration with ZYLOPRIM . Although the mechanism responsible for this has not been established, patients with impaired renal function should be carefully observed during the early stages of administration of ZYLOPRIM and dosage decreased or the drug withdrawn if increased abnormalities in renal function appear and persist.

Renal failure in association with administration of ZYLOPRIM has been observed among patients with hyperuricemia secondary to neoplastic diseases. Concurrent conditions such as multiple myeloma and congestive myocardial disease were present among those patients whose renal dysfunction increased after ZYLOPRIM was begun. Renal failure is also frequently associated with gouty nephropathy and rarely with hypersensitivity reactions associated with ZYLOPRIM. Albuminuria has been observed among patients who developed clinical gout following chronic glomerulonephritis and chronic pyelonephritis.

Patients with decreased renal function require lower doses of ZYLOPRIM than those with normal renal function. Lower than recommended doses should be used to initiate therapy in any patients with decreased renal function and they should be observed closely during the early stages of administration of ZYLOPRIM. In patients with severely impaired renal function or decreased urate clearance, the half-life of oxipurinol in the plasma is greatly prolonged. Therefore, a dose of 100 mg per day or 300 mg twice a week, or perhaps less, may be sufficient to maintain adequate xanthine oxidase inhibition to reduce serum urate levels.

Bone marrow depression has been reported in patients receiving ZYLOPRIM, most of whom received concomitant drugs with the potential for causing this reaction. This has

occurred as early as six weeks to as long as six years after the initiation of therapy of ZYLOPRIM. Rarely a patient may develop varying degrees of bone marrow depression, affecting one or more cell lines, while receiving ZYLOPRIM alone.

Information for Patients: Patients should be informed of the following:

(1) They should be cautioned to discontinue ZYLOPRIM (allopurinol) and to consult their physician immediately at the first sign of a skin rash, painful urination, blood in the urine, irritation of the eyes, or swelling of the lips or mouth. (2) They should be reminded to continue drug therapy prescribed for gouty attacks since optimal benefit of ZYLOPRIM may be delayed for two to six weeks. (3) They should be encouraged to increase fluid intake during therapy to prevent renal stones. (4) If a single dose of ZYLOPRIM is occasionally forgotten, there is no need to double the dose at the next scheduled time. (5) There may be certain risks associated with the concomitant use of ZYLOPRIM and dicumarol, sulfinpyrazone, mercaptopurine, azathioprine, ampicillin, amoxicillin, and thiazide diuretics, and they should follow the instructions of their physician. (6) Due to the occasional occurrence of drowsiness, patients should take precautions when engaging in activities where alertness is mandatory. (7) Patients may wish to take ZYLOPRIM after meals to minimize gastric irritation.

Laboratory Tests: The correct dosage and schedule for maintaining the serum uric acid within the normal range is best determined by using the serum uric acid as an index. In patients with pre-existing liver disease, periodic liver function tests are recommended during the early stages of therapy (see WARNINGS).

ZYLOPRIM (allopurinol) and its primary active metabolite oxipurinol are eliminated by the kidneys; therefore, changes in renal function have a profound effect on dosage. In patients with decreased renal function or who have concurrent illnesses which can affect renal function such as hypertension and diabetes mellitus, periodic laboratory parameters of renal function, particularly BUN and serum creatinine or creatinine clearance, should be performed and the patient's dosage of ZYLOPRIM reassessed.

The prothrombin time should be reassessed periodically in the patients receiving dicumarol who are given ZYLOPRIM.

Drug Interactions: In patients receiving PURINETHOL (mercaptopurine) or IMURAN (azathioprine), the concomitant administration of 300 to 600 mg of ZYLOPRIM (allopurinol) per day will require a reduction in dose to approximately one-third to one-fourth of the usual dose of mercaptopurine or azathioprine. Subsequent adjustment of doses of mercaptopurine or azathioprine should be made on the basis of therapeutic response and the appearance of toxic effects (see CLINICAL PHARMACOLOGY).

It has been reported that ZYLOPRIM prolongs the half-life of the anticoagulant, dicumarol. The clinical basis of this drug interaction has not been established but should be noted when ZYLOPRIM is given to patients already on dicumarol therapy.

Since the excretion of oxipurinol is similar to that of urate, uricosuric agents, which increase the excretion of urate, are also likely to increase the excretion of oxipurinol and thus lower the degree of inhibition of xanthine oxidase. The concomitant administration of uricosuric agents and ZYLOPRIM has been associated with a decrease in the excretion of oxypurines (hypoxanthine and xanthine) and an increase in urinary uric acid excretion compared with that observed with ZYLOPRIM alone. Although clinical evidence to date has not demonstrated renal precipitation of oxypurines in patients either on ZYLOPRIM alone or in combination with uricosuric agents, the possibility should be kept in mind.

The reports that the concomitant use of ZYLOPRIM and thiazide diuretics may contribute to the enhancement of allopurinol toxicity in some patients have been reviewed in an attempt to establish a cause-and-effect relationship and a mechanism of causation. Review of these case reports indicates that the patients were mainly receiving thiazide diuretics for hypertension and that tests to rule out decreased renal function secondary to hypertensive nephropathy were not often performed. In those patients in whom renal insufficiency was documented, however, the recommendation to lower the dose of ZYLOPRIM was not followed. Although a causal mechanism and a cause-and-effect relationship have not been established, current evidence suggests that renal function should be monitored in patients on thiazide diuretics and ZYLOPRIM even in the absence of renal failure, and dosage levels should be even more conservatively adjusted in those patients on such combined therapy if diminished renal function is detected.

An increase in the frequency of skin rash has been reported among patients receiving ampicillin or amoxicillin concurrently with ZYLOPRIM compared to patients who are not receiving both drugs. The cause of the reported association has not been established.

Enhanced bone marrow suppression by cyclophosphamide and other cytotoxic agents has been reported among patients with neoplastic disease, except leukemia, in the presence of

ZYLOPRIM. However, in a well-controlled study of patients with lymphoma on combination therapy, ZYLOPRIM did not increase the marrow toxicity of patients treated with cyclophosphamide, doxorubicin, bleomycin, procarbazine, and/or mechlorethamine.

Tolbutamide's conversion to inactive metabolites has been shown to be catalyzed by xanthine oxidase from rat liver. The clinical significance, if any, of these observations is unknown.

Chlorpropamide's plasma half-life may be prolonged by ZYLOPRIM, since ZYLOPRIM and chlorpropamide may compete for excretion in the renal tubule. The risk of hypoglycemia secondary to this mechanism may be increased if ZYLOPRIM and chlorpropamide are given concomitantly in the presence of renal insufficiency.

Rare reports indicate that cyclosporine levels may be increased during concomitant treatment with ZYLOPRIM. Monitoring of cyclosporine levels and possible adjustment of cyclosporine dosage should be considered when these drugs are co-administered.

Drug/Laboratory Test Interactions: ZYLOPRIM (allopurinol) is not known to alter the accuracy of laboratory tests.

Pregnancy: *Teratogenic Effects:* Pregnancy Category C. Reproductive studies have been performed in rats and rabbits at doses up to twenty times the usual human dose (5 mg/kg/day), and it was concluded that there was no impaired fertility or harm to the fetus due to ZYLOPRIM (allopurinol). There is a published report of a study in pregnant mice given 50 or 100 mg/kg allopurinol intraperitoneally on gestation days 10 or 13. There were increased numbers of dead fetuses in dams given 100 mg/kg allopurinol but not in those given 50 mg/kg. There were increased numbers of external malformations in fetuses at both doses of allopurinol on gestation day 10 and increased numbers of skeletal malformations in fetuses at both doses on gestation day 13. It cannot be determined whether this represented a fetal effect or an effect secondary to maternal toxicity. There are, however, no adequate or well-controlled studies in pregnant women. Because animal reproduction studies are not always predictive of human response, this drug should be used during pregnancy only if clearly needed.

Experience with ZYLOPRIM during human pregnancy has been limited partly because women of reproductive age rarely require treatment with ZYLOPRIM. There are two unpublished reports and one published paper of women giving birth to normal offspring after receiving ZYLOPRIM during pregnancy.

Nursing Mothers: ZYLOPRIM (allopurinol) and oxipurinol have been found in the milk of a mother who was receiving ZYLOPRIM. Since the effect of ZYLOPRIM on the nursing infant is unknown, caution should be exercised when ZYLOPRIM is administered to a nursing woman.

Pediatric Use: ZYLOPRIM (allopurinol) is rarely indicated for use in children with the exception of those with hyperuricemia secondary to malignancy or to certain rare inborn errors of purine metabolism (see INDICATIONS and DOSAGE AND ADMINISTRATION).

ADVERSE REACTIONS

Data upon which the following estimates of incidence of adverse reactions are made are derived from experiences reported in the literature, unpublished clinical trials, and voluntary reports since marketing of ZYLOPRIM (allopurinol) began. Past experience suggested that the most frequent event following the initiation of allopurinol treatment was an increase in acute attacks of gout (average 6% in early studies). An analysis of current usage suggests that the incidence of acute gouty attacks has diminished to less than 1%. The explanation for this decrease has not been determined but may be due in part to initiating therapy more gradually (see PRECAUTIONS and DOSAGE AND ADMINISTRATION).

The most frequent adverse reaction to ZYLOPRIM is skin rash. Skin reactions can be severe and sometimes fatal. Therefore, treatment with ZYLOPRIM should be discontinued immediately if a rash develops (see WARNINGS). Some patients with the most severe reaction also had fever, chills, arthralgias, cholestatic jaundice, eosinophilia, and mild leukocytosis or leukopenia. Among 55 patients with gout treated with ZYLOPRIM for 3 to 34 months (average greater than 1 year) and followed prospectively, Rundles observed that 3% of patients developed a type of drug reaction which was predominantly a pruritic maculopapular skin eruption, sometimes scaly or exfoliative. However, with current usage, skin reactions have been observed less frequently than 1%. The explanation for this decrease is not obvious. The incidence of skin rash may be increased in the presence of renal insufficiency. The frequency of skin rash among patients receiving ampicillin or amoxicillin concurrently with ZYLOPRIM has been reported to be increased (see PRECAUTIONS).

Continued on next page

Glaxo Wellcome—Cont.

Most Common Reactions*
Probably Causally Related

Gastrointestinal: diarrhea, nausea, alkaline phosphatase increase, SGOT/SGPT increase
Metabolic and Nutritional: acute attacks of gout
Skin and Appendages: rash, maculopapular rash
*Early clinical studies and incidence rates from early clinical experience with ZYLOPRIM suggested that these adverse reactions were found to occur at a rate of greater than 1%. The most frequent event observed was acute attacks of gout following the initiation of therapy. Analyses of current usage suggest that the incidence of these adverse reactions is now less than 1%. The explanation for this decrease has not been determined, but it may be due to following recommended usage (see ADVERSE REACTIONS introduction, INDICATIONS, PRECAUTIONS and DOSAGE AND ADMINISTRATION).

Incidence Less Than 1%
Probably Causally Related

Body as a whole: ecchymosis, fever, headache
Cardiovascular: necrotizing angiitis, vasculitis
Gastrointestinal: hepatic necrosis, granulomatous hepatitis, hepatomegaly, hyperbilirubinemia, cholestatic jaundice, vomiting intermittent abdominal pain, gastritis, dyspepsia
Hemic and Lymphatic: thrombocytopenia, eosinophilia, leukocytosis, leukopenia
Musculoskeletal: myopathy, arthralgias
Nervous: peripheral neuropathy, neuritis, paresthesia, somnolence
Respiratory: epistaxis
Skin and Appendages: erythema multiforme exudativum (Stevens-Johnson syndrome), toxic epidermal necrolysis (Lyell's syndrome), hypersensitivity vasculitis, purpura, vesicular bullous dermatitis, exfoliative dermatitis, eczematoid dermatitis, pruritus, urticaria, alopecia, onycholysis, lichen planus
Special Senses: taste loss/perversion
Urogenital: renal failure, uremia (see PRECAUTIONS)

Incidence Less Than 1%
Causal Relationship Unknown

Body as a whole: malaise
Cardiovascular: pericarditis, peripheral vascular disease, thrombophlebitis, bradycardia, vasodilation
Endocrine: infertility (male), hypercalcemia, gynecomastia (male)
Gastrointestinal: hemorrhagic pancreatitis, gastrointestinal bleeding, stomatitis, salivary gland swelling, hyperlipidemia, tongue edema, anorexia
Hemic and Lymphatic: aplastic anemia, agranulocytosis, eosinophilic fibrohistiocytic lesion of bone marrow, pancytopenia, prothrombin decrease, anemia, hemolytic anemia, reticulocytosis, lymphadenopathy, lymphocytosis
Musculoskeletal: myalgia
Nervous: optic neuritis, confusion, dizziness, vertigo, foot drop, decrease in libido, depression, amnesia, tinnitus, asthenia, insomnia
Respiratory: bronchospasm, asthma, pharyngitis, rhinitis
Skin and Appendages: furunculosis, facial edema, sweating, skin edema
Special Senses: cataracts, macular retinitis, iritis, conjunctivitis, amblyopia
Urogenital: nephritis, impotence, primary hematuria, albuminuria

OVERDOSAGE

Massive overdosing or acute poisoning by ZYLOPRIM (allopurinol) has not been reported.
In mice the 50% lethal dose (LD$_{50}$) is 160 mg/kg given intraperitoneally (i.p.) with deaths delayed up to five days and 700 mg/kg orally (p.o.) (approximately 140 times the usual human dose) with deaths delayed up to three days. In rats the acute LD$_{50}$ is 750 mg/kg i.p. and 6000 mg/kg p.o. (approximately 1200 times the human dose).
In the management of overdosage there is no specific antidote for ZYLOPRIM. There has been no clinical experience in the management of a patient who has taken massive amounts of ZYLOPRIM.
Both ZYLOPRIM and oxipurinol are dialyzable; however, the usefulness of hemodialysis or peritoneal dialysis in the management of an overdose of ZYLOPRIM is unknown.

DOSAGE AND ADMINISTRATION

The dosage of ZYLOPRIM (allopurinol) to accomplish full control of gout and to lower serum uric acid to normal or near-normal levels varies with the severity of the disease. The average is 200 to 300 mg per day for patients with mild gout and 400 to 600 mg per day for those with moderately severe tophaceous gout. The appropriate dosage may be administered in divided doses or as a single equivalent dose with the 300 mg tablet. Dosage requirements in excess of 300 mg should be administered in divided doses. The minimal effective dosage is 100 to 200 mg daily and the maximal recommended dosage is 800 mg daily. To reduce the possibility of flare-up of acute gouty attacks, it is recommended that the patient start with a low dose of ZYLOPRIM (100 mg daily) and increase at weekly intervals by 100 mg until a serum uric acid level of 6 mg/dL or less is attained but without exceeding the maximal recommended dosage.
Normal serum urate levels are usually achieved in one to three weeks. The upper limit of normal is about 7 mg/dL for men and postmenopausal women and 6 mg/dL for premenopausal women. Too much reliance should not be placed on a single serum uric acid determination since, for technical reasons, estimation of uric acid may be difficult. By selecting the appropriate dosage and, in certain patients, using uricosuric agents concurrently, it is possible to reduce serum uric acid to normal or, if desired, to as low as 2 to 3 mg/dL and keep it there indefinitely.
While adjusting the dosage of ZYLOPRIM in patients who are being treated with colchicine and/or anti-inflammatory agents, it is wise to continue the latter therapy until serum uric acid has been normalized and there has been freedom from acute gouty attacks for several months.
In transferring a patient from a uricosuric agent to ZYLOPRIM, the dose of the uricosuric agent should be gradually reduced over a period of several weeks and the dose of ZYLOPRIM gradually increased to the required dose needed to maintain a normal serum uric acid level.
It should also be noted that ZYLOPRIM is generally better tolerated if taken following meals. A fluid intake sufficient to yield a daily urinary output of at least two liters and the maintenance of a neutral or, preferably, slightly alkaline urine are desirable.
Since ZYLOPRIM and its metabolites are primarily eliminated only by the kidney, accumulation of the drug can occur in renal failure, and the dose of ZYLOPRIM should consequently be reduced. With a creatinine clearance of 10 to 20 mL/min, a daily dosage of 200 mg of ZYLOPRIM is suitable. When the creatinine clearance is less than 10 mL/min the daily dosage should not exceed 100 mg. With extreme renal impairment (creatinine clearance less than 3 mL/min) the interval between doses may also need to be lengthened.
The correct size and frequency of dosage for maintaining the serum uric acid just within the normal range is best determined by using the serum uric acid level as an index.
For the prevention of uric acid nephropathy during the vigorous therapy of neoplastic disease, treatment with 600 to 800 mg daily for two or three days is advisable together with a high fluid intake. Otherwise similar considerations to the above recommendations for treating patients with gout govern the regulation of dosage for maintenance purposes in secondary hyperuricemia.
The dose of ZYLOPRIM recommended for management of recurrent calcium oxalate stones in hyperuricosuric patients is 200 to 300 mg/day in divided doses or as the single equivalent. This dose may be adjusted up or down depending upon the resultant control of the hyperuricosuria based upon subsequent 24 hour urinary urate determinations. Clinical experience suggests that patients with recurrent calcium oxalate stones may also benefit from dietary changes such as the reduction of animal protein, sodium, refined sugars, oxalate-rich foods, and excessive calcium intake as well as an increase in oral fluids and dietary fiber.
Children, 6 to 10 years of age, with secondary hyperuricemia associated with malignancies may be given 300 mg ZYLOPRIM daily while those under 6 years are generally given 150 mg daily. The response is evaluated after approximately 48 hours of therapy and a dosage adjustment is made if necessary.

HOW SUPPLIED

100 mg (white) scored, flat cylindrical tablets imprinted with "ZYLOPRIM 100" on a raised hexagon.
Bottles of 100 (NDC 0173-0996-55).
Store at 15° to 25°C (59° to 77°F) in a dry place.
300 mg (peach) scored, flat, cylindrical tablets imprinted with "ZYLOPRIM 300" on a raised hexagon.
Bottles of 100 (NDC 0173-0998-55) and 500 (NDC 0173-0998-70).
Store at 15° to 25°C (59° to 77°F) in a dry place and protect from light.
January 1996/RL-251

Shown in Product Identification Guide, page 316

Glaxo Wellcome Oncology/HIV
A DIVISION OF GLAXO
WELLCOME INC.
FIVE MOORE DRIVE
RESEARCH TRIANGLE PARK, NC 27709

For Medical Information Contact:
Generally:
Medical Services Department
1-800-334-0089

In Emergencies:
Medical Services Department
1-800-334-0089

For Consumer Inquiries Contact:
1-800-722-9292

ALKERAN®   ℞
[ăl'kur-ăn]
(melphalan hydrochloride)
for Injection

> **WARNING:** Melphalan should be administered under the supervision of a qualified physician experienced in the use of cancer chemotherapeutic agents. Severe bone marrow suppression with resulting infection or bleeding may occur. Controlled trials comparing intravenous to oral melphalan have shown more myelosuppression with the intravenous formulation. Hypersensitivity reactions, including anaphylaxis, have occurred in approximately 2% of patients who received the intravenous formulation. Melphalan is leukemogenic in humans. Melphalan produces chromosomal aberrations in vitro and in vivo and, therefore, should be considered potentially mutagenic in humans.

DESCRIPTION

Melphalan, also known as L-phenylalanine mustard, phenylalanine mustard, L-PAM, or L-sarcolysin, is a phenylalanine derivative of nitrogen mustard. Melphalan is a bifunctional alkylating agent which is active against selected human neoplastic diseases. It is known chemically as 4-[bis(2-chloroethyl)amino]-L-phenylalanine. The molecular formula is $C_{13}H_{18}Cl_2N_2O_2$ and the molecular weight is 305.20.
Melphalan is the active L-isomer of the compound and was first synthesized in 1953 by Bergel and Stock; the D-isomer, known as medphalan, is less active against certain animal tumors, and the dose needed to produce effects on chromosomes is larger than that required with the L-isomer. The racemic (DL-) form is known as merphalan or sarcolysin.
Melphalan is practically insoluble in water and has a pKa$_1$ of ~2.5.
ALKERAN for Injection is supplied as a sterile, non-pyrogenic, freeze-dried powder. Each single-use vial contains melphalan hydrochloride equivalent to 50 mg melphalan and 20 mg povidone. ALKERAN for Injection is reconstituted using the sterile diluent provided. Each vial of sterile diluent contains sodium citrate 0.2 g, propylene glycol 6.0 mL, ethanol (96%) 0.52 mL, and Water for Injection to a total of 10 mL. ALKERAN for Injection is administered intravenously.

CLINICAL PHARMACOLOGY

Melphalan is an alkylating agent of the bischloroethylamine type. As a result, its cytotoxicity appears to be related to the extent of its interstrand cross-linking with DNA, probably by binding at the N^7 position of guanine. Like other bifunctional alkylating agents, it is active against both resting and rapidly dividing tumor cells.
Pharmacokinetics: The pharmacokinetics of melphalan after intravenous administration has been extensively studied in adult patients. Following injection, drug plasma concentrations declined rapidly in a biexponential manner with distribution phase and terminal elimination phase half-lives of approximately 10 and 75 minutes, respectively. Estimates of average total body clearance varied among studies, but typical values of approximately 7 to 9 mL/min/kg (250 to 325 mL/min/m^2) were observed. One study has reported that on repeat dosing of 0.5 mg/kg every 6 weeks, the clearance of melphalan decreased from 8.1 mL/min/kg after the first course, to 5.5 mL/min/kg after the third course, but did not decrease appreciably after the third course. Mean (±SD) peak melphalan plasma concentrations in myeloma patients given melphalan intravenously at doses of 10 or 20 mg/m^2 were 1.2±0.4 and 2.8±1.9 ng/mL, respectively.
The steady-state volume of distribution of melphalan is 0.5 L/kg. Penetration into cerebrospinal fluid (CSF) is low. The extent of melphalan binding to plasma proteins ranges from 60% to 90%. Serum albumin is the major binding protein,

while α_1-acid glycoprotein appears to account for about 20% of the plasma protein binding. Approximately 30% of the drug is (covalently) irreversibly bound to plasma proteins. Interactions with immunoglobulins have been found to be negligible.

Melphalan is eliminated from plasma primarily by chemical hydrolysis to monohydroxy- and dihydroxymelphalan. Aside from these hydrolysis products, no other melphalan metabolites have been observed in humans. Although the contribution of renal elimination to melphalan clearance appears to be low, one study noted an increase in the occurrence of severe leukopenia in patients with elevated BUN after 10 weeks of therapy.

Clinical Trial: A randomized trial compared prednisone plus intravenous melphalan to prednisone plus oral melphalan in the treatment of myeloma. As discussed below, overall response rates at week 22 were comparable; however, because of changes in trial design, conclusions as to the relative activity of the two formulations after week 22 are impossible to make.

Both arms received oral prednisone starting at 0.8 mg/kg/day with doses tapered over 6 weeks. Melphalan doses in each arm were:

Arm 1   Oral melphalan 0.15 mg/kg/day × 7 followed by 0.05 mg/kg/day when WBC began to rise.

Arm 2   Intravenous melphalan 16 mg/m² q 2 weeks × 4 (over 6 weeks) followed by the same dose every 4 weeks.

Doses of melphalan were adjusted according to the following criteria:

WBC/mm³	Platelets	% of full dose
≥ 4000	≥ 100,000	100
≥ 3000	≥ 75,000	75
≥ 2000	≥ 50,000	50
< 2000	< 50,000	0

One hundred seven patients were randomized to the oral melphalan arm and 203 patients to the intravenous melphalan arm. More patients had a poor-risk classification (58% vs 44%) and high tumor load (51% vs 34%) on the oral compared to the I.V. arm ($P < 0.04$). Response rates at week 22 are shown in the following table:

Initial arm	Evaluable patients	Responders n(%)	P
Oral melphalan	100	44 (44%)	P > 0.2
I.V. melphalan	195	74 (38%)	P > 0.2

Because of changes in protocol design after week 22, other efficacy parameters such as response duration and survival cannot be compared.

Severe myelotoxicity (WBC ≤ 1000 and/or platelets ≤ 25,000) was more common in the intravenous melphalan arm (28%) than in the oral melphalan arm (11%).

An association was noted between poor renal function and myelosuppression; consequently, an amendment to the protocol required a 50% reduction in I.V. melphalan dose if the BUN was ≥ 30 mg/dL. The rate of severe leukopenia in the I.V. arm in the patients with BUN over 30 mg/dL decreased from 50% (8/16) before protocol amendment to 11% (3/28) ($P = .01$) after the amendment.

Before the dosing amendment, there was a 10% (8/77) incidence of drug-related death in the I.V. arm. After the dosing amendment, this incidence was 3% (3/108). This compares to an overall 1% (1/100) incidence of drug-related death in the oral arm.

INDICATIONS AND USAGE

ALKERAN (melphalan hydrochloride) for Injection is indicated for the palliative treatment of patients with multiple myeloma for whom oral therapy is not appropriate.

CONTRAINDICATIONS

Melphalan should not be used in patients whose disease has demonstrated prior resistance to this agent. Patients who have demonstrated hypersensitivity to melphalan should not be given the drug.

WARNINGS

Melphalan should be administered in carefully adjusted dosage by or under the supervision of experienced physicians who are familiar with the drug's actions and the possible complications of its use.

As with other nitrogen mustard drugs, excessive dosage will produce marked bone marrow suppression. Bone marrow suppression is the most significant toxicity associated with ALKERAN for Injection in most patients. Therefore, the following tests should be performed at the start of therapy and prior to each subsequent dose of ALKERAN: platelet

count, hemoglobin, white blood cell count, and differential. Thrombocytopenia and/or leukopenia are indications to withhold further therapy until the blood counts have sufficiently recovered. Frequent blood counts are essential to determine optimal dosage and to avoid toxicity. Dose adjustment on the basis of blood counts at the nadir and day of treatment should be considered.

Hypersensitivity reactions including anaphylaxis have occurred in approximately 2% of patients who received the intravenous formulation (see ADVERSE REACTIONS). These reactions usually occur after multiple courses of treatment. Treatment is symptomatic. The infusion should be terminated immediately, followed by the administration of volume expanders, pressor agents, corticosteroids, or antihistamines at the discretion of the physician. If a hypersensitivity reaction occurs, intravenous or oral melphalan should not be readministered since hypersensitivity reactions have also been reported with oral melphalan.

Carcinogenesis: Secondary malignancies, including acute nonlymphocytic leukemia, myeloproliferative syndrome, and carcinoma, have been reported in patients with cancer treated with alkylating agents (including melphalan). Some patients also received other chemotherapeutic agents or radiation therapy. Precise quantitation of the risk of acute leukemia, myeloproliferative syndrome, or carcinoma is not possible. Published reports of leukemia in patients who have received melphalan (and other alkylating agents) suggest that the risk of leukemogenesis increases with chronicity of treatment and with cumulative dose. In one study, the 10-year cumulative risk of developing acute leukemia or myeloproliferative syndrome after oral melphalan therapy was 19.5% for cumulative doses ranging from 730 mg to 9652 mg. In this same study, as well as in an additional study, the 10-year cumulative risk of developing acute leukemia or myeloproliferative syndrome after oral melphalan therapy was less than 2% for cumulative doses under 600 mg. This does not mean that there is a cumulative dose below which there is no risk of the induction of secondary malignancy. The potential benefits from melphalan therapy must be weighed on an individual basis against the possible risk of the induction of a second malignancy.

Adequate and well-controlled carcinogenicity studies have not been conducted in animals. However, i.p. administration of melphalan in rats (5.4 to 10.8 mg/m²) and in mice (2.25 to 4.5 mg/m²) 3 times per week for 6 months followed by 12 months post-dose observation produced peritoneal sarcoma and lung tumors, respectively.

Mutagenesis: Melphalan has been shown to cause chromatid or chromosome damage in man. Intramuscular administration of melphalan at 6 and 60 mg/m² produced structural aberrations of the chromatid and chromosomes in bone marrow cells of Wistar rats.

Impairment of Fertility: Melphalan causes suppression of ovarian function in premenopausal women, resulting in amenorrhea in a significant number of patients. Reversible and irreversible testicular suppression have also been reported.

Pregnancy: Pregnancy Category D. Melphalan may cause fetal harm when administered to a pregnant woman. While adequate animal studies have not been conducted with intravenous melphalan, oral (6 to 18 mg/m²/day for 10 days) and i.p. (18 mg/m²/kg single dose) administration in rats was embryolethal and teratogenic. Malformations resulting from melphalan included alterations of the brain (underdevelopment, deformation, meningocele, and encephalocele) and eye (anophthalmia and microphthalmos), reduction of the mandible and tail, as well as hepatocele (exomphaly). There are no adequate and well-controlled studies in pregnant women. If this drug is used during pregnancy, or if the patient becomes pregnant while taking this drug, the patient should be apprised of the potential hazard to the fetus. Women of childbearing potential should be advised to avoid becoming pregnant.

PRECAUTIONS

General: In all instances where the use of ALKERAN for Injection is considered for chemotherapy, the physician must evaluate the need and usefulness of the drug against the risk of adverse events. Melphalan should be used with extreme caution in patients whose bone marrow reserve may have been compromised by prior irradiation or chemotherapy or whose marrow function is recovering from previous cytotoxic therapy.

Dose reduction should be considered in patients with renal insufficiency receiving I.V. melphalan. In one trial, increased bone marrow suppression was observed in patients with BUN levels ≥ 30 mg/dL. A 50% reduction in the I.V. melphalan dose decreased the incidence of severe bone marrow suppression in the latter portion of this study.

Information for Patients: Patients should be informed that the major acute toxicities of melphalan are related to bone marrow suppression, hypersensitivity reactions, gastrointestinal toxicity, and pulmonary toxicity. The major long-term toxicities are related to infertility and secondary malignancies. Patients should never be allowed to take the drug without close medical supervision and should be advised to con-

sult their physicians if they experience skin rash, signs or symptoms of vasculitis, bleeding, fever, persistent cough, nausea, vomiting, amenorrhea, weight loss, or unusual lumps/masses. Women of childbearing potential should be advised to avoid becoming pregnant.

Laboratory Tests: Periodic complete blood counts with differentials should be performed during the course of treatment with melphalan. At least one determination should be obtained prior to each dose. Patients should be observed closely for consequences of bone marrow suppression, which include severe infections, bleeding, and symptomatic anemia (see WARNINGS).

Drug Interactions: The development of severe renal failure has been reported in patients treated with a single dose of intravenous melphalan followed by standard oral doses of cyclosporine. Cisplatin may affect melphalan kinetics by inducing renal dysfunction and subsequently altering melphalan clearance. Intravenous melphalan may also reduce the threshold for BCNU lung toxicity. When nalidixic acid and intravenous melphalan are given simultaneously, the incidence of severe hemorrhagic necrotic enterocolitis has been reported to increase in pediatric patients.

Carcinogenesis, Mutagenesis, Impairment of Fertility: See WARNINGS section.

Pregnancy: *Teratogenic Effects:* Pregnancy Category D: See WARNINGS section.

Nursing Mothers: It is not known whether this drug is excreted in human milk. Intravenous melphalan should not be given to nursing mothers.

Pediatric Use: The safety and effectiveness in pediatric patients have not been established.

Geriatric Use: Clinical experience with ALKERAN has not identified differences in responses between the elderly and younger patients. In general, dose selection for an elderly patient should be cautious, reflecting the greater frequency of decreased hepatic, renal, or cardiac function, and of concomitant disease or other drug therapy.

ADVERSE REACTIONS (see OVERDOSAGE):

The following information on adverse reactions is based on data from both oral and intravenous administration of melphalan as a single agent, using several different dose schedules for treatment of a wide variety of malignancies.

Hematologic: The most common side effect is bone marrow suppression. White blood cell count and platelet count nadirs usually occur 2 to 3 weeks after treatment, with recovery in 4 to 5 weeks after treatment. Irreversible bone marrow failure has been reported.

Gastrointestinal: Gastrointestinal disturbances such as nausea and vomiting, diarrhea, and oral ulceration occur infrequently. Hepatic toxicity, including veno-occlusive disease, has been reported.

Hypersensitivity: Acute hypersensitivity reactions including anaphylaxis were reported in 2.4% of 425 patients receiving ALKERAN for Injection for myeloma (see WARNINGS). These reactions were characterized by urticaria, pruritus, edema, and in some patients, tachycardia, bronchospasm, dyspnea, and hypotension. These patients appeared to respond to antihistamine and corticosteroid therapy. If a hypersensitivity reaction occurs, intravenous or oral melphalan should not be readministered since hypersensitivity reactions have also been reported with oral melphalan.

Miscellaneous: Other reported adverse reactions include skin hypersensitivity, skin ulceration at injection site, skin necrosis rarely requiring skin grafting, vasculitis, alopecia, hemolytic anemia, allergic reaction, pulmonary fibrosis, and interstitial pneumonitis.

OVERDOSAGE

Overdoses resulting in death have been reported. Overdoses, including doses up to 290 mg/m², have produced the following symptoms: severe nausea and vomiting, decreased consciousness, convulsions, muscular paralysis, and cholinomimetic effects. Severe mucositis, stomatitis, colitis, diarrhea, and hemorrhage of the gastrointestinal tract occur at high doses (> 100 mg/m²). Elevations in liver enzymes and veno-occlusive disease occur infrequently. Significant hyponatremia caused by an associated inappropriate secretion of ADH syndrome has been observed. Nephrotoxicity and adult respiratory distress syndrome have been reported rarely. The principal toxic effect is bone marrow suppression. Hematologic parameters should be closely followed for three to six weeks. An uncontrolled study suggests that administration of autologous bone marrow or hematopoietic growth factors (i.e., sargramostim, filgrastim) may shorten the period of pancytopenia. General supportive measures together with appropriate blood transfusions and antibiotics should be instituted as deemed necessary by the physician. This drug is not removed from plasma to any significant degree by hemodialysis or hemoperfusion. A pediatric patient survived a 254 mg/m² overdose treated with standard supportive care.

DOSAGE AND ADMINISTRATION

The usual intravenous dose is 16 mg/m². Dosage reduction of up to 50% should be considered in patients with renal insuf-

Continued on next page

Glaxo Wellcome Onc.—Cont.

ficiency (BUN ≥30 mg/dL) (see PRECAUTIONS: General). The drug is administered as a single infusion over 15 to 20 minutes. Melphalan is administered at 2-week intervals for four doses, then, after adequate recovery from toxicity, at 4-week intervals. Available evidence suggests about one-third to one-half of the patients with multiple myeloma show a favorable response to the drug. Experience with oral melphalan suggests that repeated courses should be given since improvement may continue slowly over many months, and the maximum benefit may be missed if treatment is abandoned prematurely. Dose adjustment on the basis of blood cell counts at the nadir and day of treatment should be considered.

Administration Precautions: As with other toxic compounds, caution should be exercised in handling and preparing the solution of ALKERAN. Skin reactions associated with accidental exposure may occur. The use of gloves is recommended. If the solution of ALKERAN contacts the skin or mucosa, immediately wash the skin or mucosa thoroughly with soap and water.

Procedures for proper handling and disposal of anticancer drugs should be considered. Several guidelines on this subject have been published.[1–7] There is no general agreement that all of the procedures recommended in the guidelines are necessary or appropriate.

Parenteral drug products should be visually inspected for particulate matter and discoloration prior to administration whenever solution and container permit. If either occurs, do not use this product.

Preparation for Administration/Stability:

1. ALKERAN for Injection must be reconstituted by rapidly injecting 10 mL of the supplied diluent directly into the vial of lyophilized powder using a sterile needle (20 gauge or larger needle diameter) and syringe. Immediately shake vial vigorously until a clear solution is obtained. This provides a 5 mg/mL solution of melphalan. Rapid addition of the diluent followed by immediate vigorous shaking is important for proper dissolution.
2. **Immediately** dilute the dose to be administered in 0.9% sodium chloride injection, U.S.P., to a concentration not greater than 0.45 mg/mL.
3. Administer the diluted product over a minimum of 15 minutes.
4. Complete administration within 60 minutes of reconstitution.

The time between reconstitution/dilution and administration of ALKERAN should be kept to a minimum because reconstituted and diluted solutions of ALKERAN are unstable. Over as short a time as 30 minutes, a citrate derivative of melphalan has been detected in reconstituted material from the reaction of ALKERAN with Sterile Diluent for ALKERAN. Upon further dilution with saline, nearly 1% label strength of melphalan hydrolyzes every 10 minutes.

A precipitate forms if the reconstituted solution is stored at 5°C. DO NOT REFRIGERATE THE RECONSTITUTED PRODUCT.

HOW SUPPLIED

ALKERAN for Injection is supplied in a carton containing one single-use clear glass vial of freeze-dried melphalan hydrochloride equivalent to 50 mg melphalan and one 10 mL clear glass vial of sterile diluent (NDC 0173-0130-93).

Store at controlled room temperature 15° to 30°C (59° to 86°F) and protect from light.

REFERENCES

1. Recommendations for the safe handling of parenteral antineoplastic drugs. Washington, DC: Division of Safety, National Institutes of Health; 1983. US Dept of Health and Human Services, Public Health Service publication NIH 83-2621.
2. AMA Council on Scientific Affairs. Guidelines for handling parenteral antineoplastics. *JAMA.* 1987; 253:1590–1591.
3. National Study Commission on Cytotoxic Exposure. Recommendations for handling cytotoxic agents. 1987. Available from Louis P. Jeffrey, Chairman, National Study Commission on Cytotoxic Exposure, Massachusetts College of Pharmacy and Allied Health Sciences, 179 Longwood Avenue, Boston, MA 02115.
4. Clinical Oncological Society of Australia. Guidelines and recommendations for safe handling of antineoplastic agents. *Med J Australia.* 1983;1:426–428.
5. Jones RB, Frank R, Mass T. Safe handling of chemotherapeutic agents: a report from the Mount Sinai Medical Center. *CA-A Cancer J for Clin.* 1983;33:258–263.
6. American Society of Hospital Pharmacists. ASHP technical assistance bulletin on handling cytotoxic and hazardous drugs. *Am J Hosp Pharm.* 1990;47:1033–1049.
7. Yodaiken RE, Bennett D. OSHA work-practice guidelines for personnel dealing with cytotoxic (antineoplastic) drugs. *Am J Hosp Pharm.* 1986;43:1193–1204.

U.S. Patent No. 4997651
January 1996/RL-262

Shown in Product Identification Guide, page 316

ALKERAN® ℞

[*ăl-kur 'ăn*]
(melphalan)
2 mg Scored Tablets

> **WARNING:** ALKERAN (melphalan) should be administered under the supervision of a qualified physician experienced in the use of cancer chemotherapeutic agents. Severe bone marrow suppression with resulting infection or bleeding may occur. Melphalan is leukemogenic in humans.
> Melphalan produces chromosomal aberrations in vitro and in vivo and, therefore, should be considered potentially mutagenic in humans.

DESCRIPTION

ALKERAN (melphalan), also known as L-phenylalanine mustard, phenylalanine mustard, L-PAM, or L-sarcolysin, is a phenylalanine derivative of nitrogen mustard. Melphalan is a bifunctional alkylating agent which is active against selective human neoplastic diseases. It is known chemically as 4-[bis(2-chloroethyl)amino]-*L*-phenylalanine. The molecular formula is $C_{13}H_{18}Cl_2N_2O_2$ and the molecular weight is 305.20.

Melphalan is the active L-isomer of the compound and was first synthesized in 1953 by Bergel and Stock; the D-isomer, known as medphalan, is less active against certain animal tumors, and the dose needed to produce effects on chromosomes is larger than that required with the L-isomer. The racemic (DL–) form is known as merphalan or sarcolysin.

Melphalan is practically insoluble in water and has a pKa_1 of ~2.5.

ALKERAN (melphalan) is available in tablet form for oral administration. Each scored tablet contains 2 mg melphalan and the inactive ingredients lactose, magnesium stearate, potato starch, povidone, and sucrose.

CLINICAL PHARMACOLOGY

Melphalan is an alkylating agent of the bischloroethylamine type. As a result, its cytotoxicity appears to be related to the extent of its interstrand cross-linking with DNA, probably by binding at the N^7 position of guanine. Like other bifunctional alkylating agents, it is active against both resting and rapidly dividing tumor cells.

Pharmacokinetics: The pharmacokinetics of ALKERAN after oral administration has been extensively studied in adult patients. Plasma melphalan levels are highly variable after oral dosing, both with respect to the time of the first appearance of melphalan in plasma (range 0 to 336 minutes) and to the peak plasma concentration (range 0.166 to 3.741 μg/mL) achieved. These results may be due to incomplete intestinal absorption, a variable "first pass" hepatic metabolism, or to rapid hydrolysis. Five patients were studied after both oral and intravenous dosing with 0.6 mg/kg as a single bolus dose by each route. The areas under the plasma concentration-time curves after oral administration averaged 61% ± 26% (± standard deviation; range 25% to 89%) of those following intravenous administration. In 18 patients given a single oral dose of 0.6 mg/kg of ALKERAN, the terminal plasma half-disappearance time of parent drug was 89.5 ± 50 minutes. The 24-hour urinary excretion of parent drug in these patients was 10% ± 4.5%, suggesting that renal clearance is not a major route of elimination of parent drug.

One study using universally labeled ^{14}C-melphalan, found substantially less radioactivity in the urine of patients given the drug by mouth (30% of administered dose in 9 days) than in the urine of those given it intravenously (35% to 65% in 7 days). Following either oral or intravenous administration, the pattern of label recovery was similar, with the majority being recovered in the first 24 hours. Following oral administration, peak radioactivity occurred in plasma at 2 hours and then disappeared with a half-life of approximately 160 hours. In one patient where parent drug (rather than just radiolabel) was determined, the melphalan half-disappearance time was 67 minutes.

The steady-state volume of distribution of melphalan is 0.5 L/kg. Penetration into cerebrospinal fluid (CSF) is low. The extent of melphalan binding to plasma proteins ranges from 60% to 90%. Serum albumin is the major binding protein, while α_1-acid glycoprotein appears to account for about 20% of the plasma protein binding. Approximately 30% of melphalan is (covalently) irreversibly bound to plasma proteins. Interactions with immunoglobulins have been found to be negligible.

Melphalan is eliminated from plasma primarily by chemical hydrolysis to monohydroxy- and dihydroxymelphalan. Aside from these hydrolysis products, no other melphalan metabolites have been observed in humans. Although the contribution of renal elimination to melphalan clearance appears to be low, one pharmacokinetic study showed a significant positive correlation between the elimination rate constant for melphalan and renal function and a significant negative correlation between renal function and the area under the plasma melphalan concentration/time curve.

INDICATIONS AND USAGE

ALKERAN (melphalan) Tablets are indicated for the palliative treatment of multiple myeloma and for the palliation of non-resectable epithelial carcinoma of the ovary.

CONTRAINDICATIONS

ALKERAN should not be used in patients whose disease has demonstrated a prior resistance to this agent. Patients who have demonstrated hypersensitivity to melphalan should not be given the drug.

WARNINGS

ALKERAN should be administered in carefully adjusted dosage by or under the supervision of experienced physicians who are familiar with the drug's actions and the possible complications of its use.

As with other nitrogen mustard drugs, excessive dosage will produce marked bone marrow suppression. Bone marrow suppression is the most significant toxicity associated with ALKERAN in most patients. Therefore, the following tests should be performed at the start of therapy and prior to each subsequent course of ALKERAN: platelet count, hemoglobin, white blood cell count, and differential. Thrombocytopenia and/or leukopenia are indications to withhold further therapy until the blood counts have sufficiently recovered. Frequent blood counts are essential to determine optimal dosage and to avoid toxicity (see PRECAUTIONS: Laboratory Tests). Dose adjustment on the basis of blood counts at the nadir and day of treatment should be considered.

Hypersensitivity reactions, including anaphylaxis, have occurred rarely (see ADVERSE REACTIONS). These reactions have occurred after multiple courses of treatment and have recurred in patients who experienced a hypersensitivity reaction to intravenous ALKERAN. If a hypersensitivity reaction occurs, oral or intravenous ALKERAN should not be readministered.

Carcinogenesis: Secondary malignancies, including acute nonlymphocytic leukemia, myeloproliferative syndrome, and carcinoma have been reported in patients with cancer treated with alkylating agents (including melphalan). Some patients also received other chemotherapeutic agents or radiation therapy. Precise quantitation of the risk of acute leukemia, myeloproliferative syndrome, or carcinoma is not possible. Published reports of leukemia in patients who have received melphalan (and other alkylating agents) suggest that the risk of leukemogenesis increases with chronicity of treatment and with cumulative dose. In one study, the 10-year cumulative risk of developing acute leukemia or myeloproliferative syndrome after melphalan therapy was 19.5% for cumulative doses ranging from 730 mg to 9652 mg. In this same study, as well as in an additional study, the 10-year cumulative risk of developing acute leukemia or myeloproliferative syndrome after melphalan therapy was less than 2% for cumulative doses under 600 mg. This does not mean that there is a cumulative dose below which there is no risk of the induction of secondary malignancy. The potential benefits from melphalan therapy must be weighed on an individual basis against the possible risk of the induction of a second malignancy.

Adequate and well-controlled carcinogenicity studies have not been conducted in animals. However, i.p. administration of melphalan in rats (5.4 to 10.8 mg/m²) and in mice (2.25 to 4.5 mg/m²) three times per week for 6 months followed by 12 months post-dose observation produced peritoneal sarcoma and lung tumors, respectively.

Mutagenesis: ALKERAN has been shown to cause chromatid or chromosome damage in humans. Intramuscular administration of ALKERAN at 6 and 60 mg/m² produced structural aberrations of the chromatid and chromosomes in bone marrow cells of Wistar rats.

Impairment of Fertility: ALKERAN causes suppression of ovarian function in pre-menopausal women, resulting in amenorrhea in a significant number of patients. Reversible and irreversible testicular suppression have also been reported.

Pregnancy: Pregnancy Category D. ALKERAN may cause fetal harm when administered to a pregnant woman. Melphalan was embryolethal and teratogenic in rats following oral (6 to 18 mg/m²/day for 10 days) and intraperitoneal (18 mg/m²/kg single dose) administration. Malformations resulting from melphalan included alterations of the brain (underdevelopment, deformation, meningocele, and encephalocele) and eye (anophthalmia and microphthalmos), reduction of the mandible and tail, as well as hepatocele (exomphalyl).

There are no adequate and well-controlled studies in pregnant women. If this drug is used during pregnancy, or if the patient becomes pregnant while taking this drug, the patient should be apprised of the potential hazard to the fetus.

Women of childbearing potential should be advised to avoid becoming pregnant.

PRECAUTIONS

General: In all instances where the use of ALKERAN is considered for chemotherapy, the physician must evaluate the need and usefulness of the drug against the risk of adverse events. ALKERAN should be used with extreme caution in patients whose bone marrow reserve may have been compromised by prior irradiation or chemotherapy, or whose marrow function is recovering from previous cytotoxic therapy. If the leukocyte count falls below 3,000 cells/μL, or the platelet count below 100,000 cells/μL, ALKERAN should be discontinued until the peripheral blood cell counts have recovered.

A recommendation as to whether or not dosage reduction should be made routinely in patients with renal insufficiency cannot be made because:

(a) There is considerable inherent patient-to-patient variability in the systemic availability of melphalan in patients with normal renal function.

(b) Only a small amount of the administered dose appears as parent drug in the urine of patients with normal renal function.

Patients with azotemia should be closely observed, however, in order to make dosage reductions, if required, at the earliest possible time.

Information for Patients: Patients should be informed that the major toxicities of ALKERAN are related to bone marrow suppression, hypersensitivity reactions, gastrointestinal toxicity, and pulmonary toxicity. The major long-term toxicities are related to infertility and secondary malignancies. Patients should never be allowed to take the drug without close medical supervision and should be advised to consult their physician if they experience skin rash, vasculitis, bleeding, fever, persistent cough, nausea, vomiting, amenorrhea, weight loss, or unusual lumps/masses. Women of childbearing potential should be advised to avoid becoming pregnant.

Laboratory Tests: Periodic complete blood counts with differentials should be performed during the course of treatment with ALKERAN. At least one determination should be obtained prior to each treatment course. Patients should be observed closely for consequences of bone marrow suppression, which include severe infections, bleeding, and symptomatic anemia (see WARNINGS).

Drug Interactions: There are no known drug/drug interactions with oral ALKERAN.

Carcinogenesis, Mutagenesis, Impairment of Fertility: See WARNINGS section.

Pregnancy: ***Teratogenic Effects:*** Pregnancy Category D: See WARNINGS section.

Nursing Mothers: It is not known whether this drug is excreted in human milk. ALKERAN should not be given to nursing mothers.

Pediatric Use: The safety and effectiveness of ALKERAN in pediatric patients have not been established.

Geriatric Use: Clinical experience with ALKERAN has not identified differences in responses between the elderly and younger patients. In general, dose selection for an elderly patient should be cautious, reflecting the greater frequency of decreased hepatic, renal, or cardiac function, and of concomitant disease or other drug therapy.

ADVERSE REACTIONS

Hematologic: The most common side effect is bone marrow suppression. Although bone marrow suppression frequently occurs, it is usually reversible if melphalan is withdrawn early enough. However, irreversible bone marrow failure has been reported.

Gastrointestinal: Gastrointestinal disturbances such as nausea and vomiting, diarrhea, and oral ulceration occur infrequently. Hepatic toxicity has been reported rarely.

Miscellaneous: Other reported adverse reactions include: pulmonary fibrosis and interstitial pneumonitis, skin hypersensitivity, vasculitis, alopecia, and hemolytic anemia. Allergic reactions, including rare anaphylaxis, have occurred after multiple courses of treatment.

OVERDOSAGE

Overdoses, including doses up to 50 mg/day for 16 days, have been reported. Immediate effects are likely to be vomiting, ulceration of the mouth, diarrhea, and hemorrhage of the gastrointestinal tract. The principal toxic effect is bone marrow suppression. Hematologic parameters should be closely followed for 3 to 6 weeks. An uncontrolled study suggests that administration of autologous bone marrow or hematopoietic growth factors (i.e., sargramostim, filgrastim) may shorten the period of pancytopenia. General supportive measures, together with appropriate blood transfusions and antibiotics, should be instituted as deemed necessary by the physician. This drug is not removed from plasma to any significant degree by hemodialysis.[1]

DOSAGE AND ADMINISTRATION

Multiple Myeloma: The usual oral dose is 6 mg (3 tablets) daily. The entire daily dose may be given at one time. The dose is adjusted, as required, on the basis of blood counts done at approximately weekly intervals. After 2 to 3 weeks of treatment, the drug should be discontinued for up to 4 weeks during which time the blood count should be followed carefully. When the white blood cell and platelet counts are rising, a maintenance dose of 2 mg daily may be instituted. Because of the patient-to-patient variation in melphalan plasma levels following oral administration of the drug, several investigators have recommended that the dosage of ALKERAN be cautiously escalated until some myelosuppression is observed in order to assure that potentially therapeutic levels of the drug have been reached.

Other dosage regimens have been used by various investigators. Osserman and Takatsuki have used an initial course of 10 mg/day for 7 to 10 days.[2,3] They report that maximal suppression of the leukocyte and platelet counts occurs within 3 to 5 weeks and recovery within 4 to 8 weeks. Continuous maintenance therapy with 2 mg/day is instituted when the white blood cell count is greater than 4,000 cells/μL and the platelet count is greater than 100,000 cells/μL. Dosage is adjusted to between 1 and 3 mg/day depending upon the hematological response. It is desirable to try to maintain a significant degree of bone marrow depression so as to keep the leukocyte count in the range of 3,000 to 3,500 cells/μL. Hoogstraten *et al.* have started treatment with 0.15 mg/kg/day for 7 days.[4] This is followed by a rest period of at least 14 days, but it may be as long as 5 to 6 weeks. Maintenance therapy is started when the white blood cell and platelet counts are rising. The maintenance dose is 0.05 mg/kg/day or less and is adjusted according to the blood count.

Available evidence suggests that about one-third to one-half of the patients with multiple myeloma show a favorable response to oral administration of the drug.

One study by Alexanian *et al.* has shown that the use of ALKERAN in combination with prednisone significantly improves the percentage of patients with multiple myeloma who achieve palliation.[5] One regimen has been to administer courses of ALKERAN at 0.25 mg/kg/day for 4 consecutive days (or, 0.20 mg/kg/day for 5 consecutive days) for a total dose of 1 mg/kg per course. These 4- to 5-day courses are then repeated every 4 to 6 weeks if the granulocyte count and the platelet count have returned to normal levels.

It is to be emphasized that response may be very gradual over many months; it is important that repeated courses or continuous therapy be given since improvement may continue slowly over many months, and the maximum benefit may be missed if treatment is abandoned too soon.

In patients with moderate to severe renal impairment, currently available pharmacokinetic data do not justify an absolute recommendation on dosage reduction to those patients, but it may be prudent to use a reduced dose initially.

Epithelial Ovarian Cancer: One commonly employed regimen for the treatment of ovarian carcinoma has been to administer ALKERAN at a dose of 0.2 mg/kg daily for 5 days as a single course. Courses are repeated every 4 to 5 weeks depending upon hematologic tolerance.[6,7]

Administration Precautions:

Procedures for proper handling and disposal of anticancer drugs should be considered. Several guidelines on this subject have been published.[8–14]

There is no general agreement that all of the procedures recommended in the guidelines are necessary or appropriate.

HOW SUPPLIED

ALKERAN (melphalan) is supplied as white, scored tablets containing 2 mg melphalan, imprinted with "ALKERAN" and "A2A"; in bottles of 50 (NDC 0173-0045-35).

Store at 15° to 25°C (59° to 77°F) in a dry place, protect from light, and dispense in glass.

Also Available:

ALKERAN for Injection, carton containing one single-use vial of freeze-dried melphalan hydrochloride equivalent to 50 mg melphalan and one 10 mL vial of sterile diluent.

REFERENCES

1. Pallante SL, Fenselau C, Mennel RG, et al. Quantitation by gas chromatography-chemical ionization-mass spectrometry of phenylalanine mustard in plasma of patients. *Cancer Res.* 1980;40:2268–2272.
2. Osserman EF. Therapy of plasma cell myeloma with melphalan (1-phenylalanine mustard). *Proc Am Assoc Cancer Res.* 1963;4:50. Abstract.
3. Osserman EF, Takatsuki K. Plasma cell myeloma: gamma globulin synthesis and structure. A review of biochemical and clinical data, with the description of a newly-recognized and related syndrome, "H-gamma-2-chain" (Franklin's) disease. *Medicine* (Balt). 1963;42:357–384.
4. Hoogstraten B, Sheehe PR, Cuttner J, et al. Melphalan in multiple myeloma. *Blood.* 1967;30:74–83.
5. Alexanian R, Haut A, Khan AU, et al. Treatment for multiple myeloma; combination chemotherapy with different melphalan dose regimens. *JAMA.* 1969;208:1680–1685.
6. Smith JP, Rutledge FN: Chemotherapy in advanced ovarian cancer. *Natl Cancer Inst Monogr.* 1975; 42:141–143.
7. Young RC, Chabner BA, Hubbard SP, et al. Advanced ovarian adenocarcinoma: a prospective clinical trial of melphalan (L-PAM) versus combination chemotherapy. *N Engl J Med.* 1978;299:1261–1266.
8. Recommendations for the safe handling of parenteral antineoplastic drugs. Washington, DC: Division of Safety, National Institutes of Health; 1983. US Dept of Health and Human Services, Public Health Service publication NIH 83-2621.
9. AMA Council on Scientific Affairs. Guidelines for handling parenteral antineoplastics. *JAMA.* 1985; 253:1590–1591.
10. National Study Commission on Cytotoxic Exposure. Recommendations for handling cytotoxic agents. 1987. Available from Louis P. Jeffrey, Chairman, National Study Commission on Cytotoxic Exposure, Massachusetts College of Pharmacy and Allied Health Sciences, 179 Longwood Avenue, Boston, MA 02115.
11. Clinical Oncological Society of Australia. Guidelines and recommendations for safe handling of antineoplastic agents. *Med J Australia.* 1983;1:426–428.
12. Jones RB, Frank R, Mass T. Safe handling of chemotherapeutic agents: a report from the Mount Sinai Medical Center. *CA-A Cancer J for Clin.* 1983;33:258–263.
13. American Society of Hospital Pharmacists. ASHP technical assistance bulletin on handling cytotoxic and hazardous drugs. *Am J Hosp Pharm.* 1990;47:1033–1049.
14. Yodaiken RE, Bennett D. OSHA work-practice guidelines for personnel dealing with cytotoxic (antineoplastic) drugs. *Am J Hosp Pharm.* 1986;43:1193–1204.

February 1996/RL-265

Shown in Product Identification Guide, page 316

DARAPRIM® ℞

[dair 'ah-prĭm ʺ]

(pyrimethamine)

25 mg Scored Tablets

DESCRIPTION

DARAPRIM (pyrimethamine) is an antiparasitic available in tablet form for oral administration. Each scored tablet contains 25 mg pyrimethamine and the inactive ingredients corn and potato starch, lactose, and magnesium stearate. Pyrimethamine is known chemically as 5-(4-chlorophenyl)-6-ethyl-2,4-pyrimidinediamine.

CLINICAL PHARMACOLOGY

Pyrimethamine is well absorbed, with peak levels occurring between 2 to 6 hours following administration. It is eliminated slowly and has a plasma half-life of approximately 96 hours. Pyrimethamine is 87% bound to human plasma proteins.

Microbiology: Pyrimethamine is a folic acid antagonist and the rationale for its therapeutic action is based on the differential requirement between host and parasite for nucleic acid precursors involved in growth. This activity is highly selective against plasmodia and *Toxoplasma gondii.*

Pyrimethamine possesses blood schizonticidal and some tissue schizonticidal activity against malaria parasites of humans. However, its blood schizonticidal activity may be slower than that of 4-aminoquinoline compounds. It does not destroy gametocytes but arrests sporogony in the mosquito.

The action of DARAPRIM against *Toxoplasma gondii* is greatly enhanced when used in conjunction with sulfonamides. This was demonstrated by Eyles and Coleman[1] in the treatment of experimental toxoplasmosis in the mouse. Jacobs et al[2] demonstrated that combination of the two drugs effectively prevented the development of severe uveitis in most rabbits following the inoculation of the anterior chamber of the eye with toxoplasma.

INDICATIONS AND USAGE

DARAPRIM (pyrimethamine) is indicated for the chemoprophylaxis of malaria due to susceptible strains of plasmodia. It should not be used alone to treat an acute attack of malaria. Fast-acting schizonticides such as chloroquine or quinine are indicated and preferable for the treatment of acute attacks. However, conjoint use of DARAPRIM will initiate *transmission control* and *suppressive cure* for susceptible strains of plasmodia.

DARAPRIM is also indicated for the treatment of toxoplasmosis. For this purpose the drug should be used conjointly with a sulfonamide since synergism exists with this combination.

CONTRAINDICATIONS

Use of DARAPRIM is contraindicated in patients with known hypersensitivity to pyrimethamine. Use of the drug is

Continued on next page

Glaxo Wellcome Onc.—Cont.

also contraindicated in patients with documented megaloblastic anemia due to folate deficiency.

WARNINGS

The dosage of pyrimethamine required for the treatment of toxoplasmosis is 10 to 20 times the recommended antimalaria dosage and approaches the toxic level. If signs of folate deficiency develop (see ADVERSE REACTIONS), reduce the dosage or discontinue the drug according to the response of the patient. Folinic acid (leucovorin) should be administered in a dosage of 5 to 15 mg daily (orally, I.V., or I.M.) until normal hematopoiesis is restored.

Daraprim should be kept out of the reach of children as children and infants are extremely susceptible to adverse effects from an overdose. Deaths in children have been reported after accidental ingestion.

PRECAUTIONS

General: The recommended dosage for chemoprophylaxis of malaria should not be exceeded. A small "starting" dose for toxoplasmosis is recommended in patients with convulsive disorders to avoid the potential nervous system toxicity of pyrimethamine. DARAPRIM should be used with caution in patients with impaired renal or hepatic function or in patients with possible folate deficiency, such as individuals with malabsorption syndrome, alcoholism, or pregnancy, and those receiving therapy, such as phenytoin, affecting folate levels (see Pregnancy subsection).

Information for Patients: Patients should be warned that at the first appearance of a skin rash they should stop use of DARAPRIM and seek medical attention immediately. Patients should also be warned that the appearance of sore throat, pallor, purpura, or glossitis may be early indications of serious disorders which require prophylactic treatment to be stopped and medical treatment to be sought. Patients should be warned to keep DARAPRIM out of the reach of children. Patients should be warned that if anorexia and vomiting occur, they may be minimized by taking the drug with meals.

Laboratory Tests: In patients receiving high dosage, as for the treatment of toxoplasmosis, semiweekly blood counts, including platelet counts should be done.

Drug Interactions: Pyrimethamine may be used with sulfonamides, quinine, and other antimalarials, and with other antibiotics. However, the concomitant use of other antifolic drugs, such as sulfonamides or trimethoprim-sulfamethoxazole combinations, while the patient is receiving pyrimethamine for antimalarial prophylaxis, may increase the risk of bone marrow suppression. If signs of folate deficiency develop, pyrimethamine should be discontinued. Folinic acid (leucovorin) should be administered until normal hematopoiesis is restored (see WARNINGS). Mild hepatotoxicity has been reported in some patients when lorazepam and pyrimethamine were administered concomitantly.

Carcinogenesis, Mutagenesis, Impairment of Fertility:

Carcinogenesis: Pyrimethamine has been reported to produce a significant increase in the number of lung tumors per mouse when given intraperitoneally at high doses (0.025 g/kg).[3] There have been two reports of cancer associated with pyrimethamine administration: a 51-year-old female who developed chronic granulocytic leukemia after taking pyrimethamine for two years for toxoplasmosis,[4] and a 56-year-old patient who developed reticulum cell sarcoma after 14 months of pyrimethamine for toxoplasmosis.[5]

Mutagenesis: Pyrimethamine has been shown to be nonmutagenic in the following in vitro assays: the Ames point mutation assay, the Rec assay, and the *E. coli* WP2 assay. It was positive in the L5178Y/TK +/− mouse lymphoma assay in the absence of exogenous metabolic activation.[6] Human blood lymphocytes cultured in vitro had structural chromosome aberrations induced by pyrimethamine.

In vivo, chromosomes analyzed from the bone marrow of rats dosed with pyrimethamine showed an increased number of structural and numerical aberrations.

Impairment of Fertility: The effects of pyrimethamine on rat pregnancy seem to indicate that the fertility index of rats treated with pyrimethamine is lowered only when the higher dosage is used, suggesting a possible toxic effect upon the whole organism and/or the conceptuses.[7]

Pregnancy: *Teratogenic Effects:* Pregnancy Category C. Pyrimethamine has been shown to be teratogenic in rats, hamsters, and Goettingen miniature pigs. There are no adequate and well-controlled studies in pregnant women. DARAPRIM should be used during pregnancy only if the potential benefit justifies the potential risk to the fetus. Concurrent administration of folinic acid is strongly recommended when used for the treatment of toxoplasmosis during pregnancy.

Thiersch[8] reported that when rats were given an oral dose of pyrimethamine of 12.5 mg/kg from day 7 to 9 of the gestation period, there was 66.2% resorption and 32.8% of the live fetuses were stunted. When lower doses of 1 mg/kg and 0.5 mg/kg were given for 10 days (days 4 to 13 of gestation), there was 15% and 8.5% resorption, respectively, and 16.6% and 6.9% of the live fetuses were stunted. A daily oral dose as low as 0.3 mg/kg given for days 7 to 16 of gestation still resulted in 2.7% of the fetuses being stunted.

Sullivan and Takacs[9] found that less than 10% of hamster fetuses died or were malformed following single doses of 20 mg to the mother, which on a mg/kg basis was eight to nine times greater than that given to rats.

Hayama and Kokue[10] reported on the administration of pyrimethamine to pregnant female Goettingen miniature pigs. Sows given 0.9 mg/kg/day, during days 11 to 35 of pregnancy (i.e., the period of organogenesis in the pig) delivered normal offspring. Sows administered a high dose 3.6 mg/kg/day during the same gestational period delivered offspring with a high incidence of malformations including cleft palate, club foot, and micrognathia.

Nursing Mothers: Pyrimethamine is excreted in human milk. Milk samples obtained from lactating mothers after treatment with pyrimethamine were found to have measurable concentrations of the drug, with peak concentration at 6 hours postadministration. It is estimated that after a single 75 mg dose of oral pyrimethamine, approximately 3 to 4 mg of the drug would be passed on to the feeding child over a 48-hour period.

Because of the potential for serious adverse reactions in nursing infants from DARAPRIM, a decision should be made whether to discontinue nursing or to discontinue the drug, taking into account the importance of the drug to the mother (see Carcinogenesis, Mutagenesis, Impairment of Fertility and Pregnancy subsections).

Pediatric Use: See DOSAGE AND ADMINISTRATION section.

ADVERSE REACTIONS

Hypersensitivity reactions, occasionally severe, can occur at any dose, particularly when pyrimethamine is administered concomitantly with a sulfonamide. With large doses of pyrimethamine, anorexia and vomiting may occur. Vomiting may be minimized by giving the medication with meals; it usually disappears promptly upon reduction of dosage. Doses used in toxoplasmosis may produce megaloblastic anemia, leukopenia, thrombocytopenia, pancytopenia, atrophic glossitis, hematuria, and disorders of cardiac rhythm. Hematologic effects, however, may also occur at low doses in certain individuals (see PRECAUTIONS—General).

Insomnia, diarrhea, headache, light-headedness, dryness of the mouth or throat, fever, malaise, dermatitis, abnormal skin pigmentation, depression, seizures, pulmonary eosinophilia, and hyperphenylalaninemia have been reported rarely.

OVERDOSAGE

Acute intoxication may follow the ingestion of an excessive amount of pyrimethamine. Gastrointestinal and/or central nervous system signs may be present, including convulsions. The initial symptoms are usually gastrointestinal and may include abdominal pain, nausea, severe and repeated vomiting, possibly including hematemesis. Central nervous system toxicity may be manifest by initial excitability, generalized and prolonged convulsions which may be followed by respiratory depression, circulatory collapse, and death within a few hours. Neurological symptoms appear rapidly (30 minutes to 2 hours after drug ingestion), suggesting that in gross overdosage pyrimethamine has a direct toxic effect on the central nervous system.

The fatal dose is variable, with the smallest reported fatal single dose being 250 mg to 300 mg. There are, however, reports of children who have recovered after taking 375 mg to 625 mg.

There is no specific antidote to acute pyrimethamine poisoning. Gastric lavage is recommended and is effective if carried out very soon after drug ingestion. A parenteral barbiturate may be indicated to control convulsions. Folinic acid may also be given to counteract effects on the hematopoietic system (see WARNINGS).

DOSAGE AND ADMINISTRATION

For Chemoprophylaxis of Malaria:

Adults and children over 10 years—25 mg (1 tablet) once weekly

Children 4 through 10 years—12.5 mg (1/2 tablet) once weekly

Infants and children under 4 years—6.25 mg (1/4 tablet) once weekly

Regimens planned to include *suppressive cure* should be extended through any characteristic periods of early recrudescence and late relapse for at least 10 weeks in each case.

For Treatment of Acute Attacks: DARAPRIM is recommended in areas where only susceptible plasmodia exist. This drug is not recommended alone in the treatment of acute attacks of malaria in nonimmune persons. Fast-acting schizonticides such as chloroquine or quinine are indicated for treatment of acute attacks. However, conjoint DARAPRIM dosage of 25 mg daily for 2 days will initiate *transmission control* and *suppressive cure.* Should circumstances arise wherein DARAPRIM must be used alone in semi-immune persons, the adult dosage for an acute attack is 50 mg for 2 days; children 4 through 10 years old may be given 25 mg daily for 2 days. In any event, clinical cure should be followed by the once-weekly regimen described above.

For Toxoplasmosis: The dosage of DARAPRIM for the treatment of toxoplasmosis must be carefully adjusted so as to provide maximum therapeutic effect and a minimum of side effects. At the high dosage required, there is a marked variation in the tolerance to the drug. Young patients may tolerate higher doses than older individuals.

The adult *starting* dose is 50 to 75 mg of the drug daily, together with 1 to 4 g daily of a sulfonamide of the sulfapyrimidine type, e.g., sulfadiazine. This dosage is ordinarily continued for 1 to 3 weeks, depending on the response of the patient and his tolerance of the therapy. The dosage may then be reduced to about one-half that previously given for each drug and continued for an additional 4 to 5 weeks.

The pediatric dosage of DARAPRIM is 1 mg/kg per day divided into 2 equal daily doses; after 2 to 4 days this dose may be reduced to one-half and continued for approximately one month. The usual pediatric sulfonamide dosage is used in conjunction with DARAPRIM.

HOW SUPPLIED

White, scored tablets containing 25 mg pyrimethamine, imprinted with "DARAPRIM" and "A3A" in bottles of 100 (NDC 0173-0201-55).

Store at 15° to 25°C (59° to 77°F) in a dry place and protect from light.

REFERENCES

1. Eyles DE, Coleman N. Synergistic effect of sulfadiazine and DARAPRIM against experimental toxoplasmosis in the mouse. *Antibiot Chemother.* 1953;3:483–490.
2. Jacobs L, Melton ML, Kaufman HE. Treatment of experimental ocular toxoplasmosis, *Arch Ophthalmol.* 1964;71:111–118.
3. Bahna L. Pyrimethamine. *LARC Monogr Eval Carcinog Risk Chem.* 1977; 13:233–242.
4. Jim RTS, Elizaga FV. Development of chronic granulocytic leukemia in a patient treated with pyrimethamine. *Hawaii Med J.* 1977;36:173–176.
5. Sadoff L. Antimalarial drugs and Burkitt's lymphoma. *Lancet.* 1973; 2:1262–1263.
6. Clive D, Johnson KO, Spector JKS, et al. Validation and characterization of the L5178Y/TK +/− mouse lymphoma mutagen assay system. *Mut Res.* 1979;59:61–108.
7. Andrade ATL, Guerra MO, Silva NOG, et al. Antifertility effects of pyrimethamine. *Excerpta Med Int Cong Ser.* 1976;370:317–321.
8. Thiersch JB. Effects of certain 2,4-diaminopyrimidine antagonists of folic acid on pregnancy and rat fetus. *Proc Soc Exp Biol Med.* 1954;87:571–577.
9. Sullivan GE, Takacs E. Comparative teratogenicity of pyrimethamine in rats and hamsters. *Teratology.* 1971;4:205–210.
10. Hayama T, Kokue E. Use of Goettingen miniature pigs for studying pyrimethamine teratogenesis, *CRC Crit Rev Toxicol.* 1985;14:403–421.

April 1994

Shown in Product Identification Guide, page 316

EPIVIR® Tablets ℞

[ep'ə-vir]

(lamivudine tablets)

EPIVIR® Oral Solution

(lamivudine oral solution)

WARNING: EPIVIR is indicated for use in combination with RETROVIR® (zidovudine) for the treatment of human immunodeficiency virus (HIV) infection when antiretrovial therapy is warranted based on clinical and/or immunological evidence of disease progression. This indication is based on analyses of surrogate endpoints. At present, there are no results from controlled clinical trials evaluating the effect of therapy with EPIVIR plus RETROVIR on the clinical progression of HIV infection, such as the incidence of opportunistic infections or survival.

Patients receiving EPIVIR plus RETROVIR may continue to develop opportunistic infections and other complications of HIV infection, and therefore should remain under close observation by physicians experienced in the treatment of patients with HIV-associated diseases.

DESCRIPTION

EPIVIR (formerly known as 3TC) is the brand name for lamivudine, a synthetic nucleoside analogue with activity against HIV. The chemical name of lamivudine is (2R,cis)-4-amino-1-(2-hydroxymethyl-1,3-oxathiolan-5-yl)-(1H)-pyrimidin-2-one. Lamivudine is the (−)enantiomer of a dideoxy

analogue of cytidine. Lamivudine has also been referred to as $(-)2',3'$-dideoxy, $3'$-thiacytidine. It has a molecular formula of $C_8H_{11}N_3O_3S$ and a molecular weight of 229.3. It has the following structural formula:

$$\text{[chemical structure]}$$

Lamivudine is a white to off-white crystalline solid with a solubility of approximately 70 mg/mL in water at 20°C.

EPIVIR Tablets are for oral administration. Each tablet contains 150 mg of lamivudine and the inactive ingredients magnesium stearate, microcrystalline cellulose, and sodium starch glycolate. Opadry YS-1-7706-G White is the coloring agent in the tablet coating.

EPIVIR Oral Solution is for oral administration. One milliliter (1 mL) of EPIVIR Oral Solution contains 10 mg of lamivudine (10 mg/mL) in an aqueous solution and the inactive ingredients artificial strawberry and banana flavors, citric acid (anhydrous), edetate disodium, ethanol (6% v/v), methylparaben, propylene glycol, propylparaben, and sucrose.

CLINICAL PHARMACOLOGY

Mechanism of Action: Lamivudine is a synthetic nucleoside analogue. *In vitro* studies have shown that, intracellularly, lamivudine is phosphorylated to its active $5'$-triphosphate metabolite (L-TP), which has an intracellular half-life of 10.5 to 15.5 hours. The principal mode of action of L-TP is inhibition of HIV reverse transcription via viral DNA chain termination. L-TP also inhibits the RNA- and DNA-dependent DNA polymerase activities of reverse transcriptase (RT). L-TP is a weak inhibitor of mammalian α-, β-, and γ-DNA polymerases.

Microbiology: *Antiviral Activity In Vitro:* The relationship between *in vitro* susceptibility of HIV to lamivudine and the inhibition of HIV replication in humans has not been established. *In vitro* activity of lamivudine against HIV-1 was assessed in a number of cell lines (including monocytes and fresh human peripheral blood lymphocytes) using standard susceptibility assays. IC_{50} values (50% inhibitory concentrations) were in the range of 2 nM to 15 μM. Lamivudine had anti–HIV-1 activity in all acute virus-cell infections tested. In HIV-1–infected MT-4 cells, lamivudine in combination with zidovudine had synergistic antiretroviral activity. Synergistic activity of lamivudine/zidovudine was also shown in a variable-ratio study.

Drug Resistance: Lamivudine-resistant isolates of HIV-1 have been studied *in vitro*. The resistant isolates showed reduced susceptibility to lamivudine and genotypic analysis showed that the resistance was due to specific substitution mutations in the HIV-1 reverse transcriptase at codon 184 from methionine to either isoleucine or valine. HIV-1 strains resistant to both lamivudine and zidovudine have been isolated.

Susceptibility of clinical isolates to lamivudine and zidovudine was monitored in controlled clinical trials. In patients receiving lamivudine monotherapy or combination therapy with lamivudine plus zidovudine, HIV-1 isolates from most patients became phenotypically and genotypically resistant to lamivudine within 12 weeks. In some patients harboring zidovudine-resistant virus, phenotypic sensitivity to zidovudine by 12 weeks of treatment was restored. Combination therapy with lamivudine plus zidovudine delayed the emergence of mutations conferring resistance to zidovudine.

Pharmacokinetics in Adults: The pharmacokinetic properties of lamivudine have been studied in asymptomatic, HIV-infected adult patients after administration of single intravenous (IV) doses ranging from 0.25 to 8 mg/kg, as well as single and multiple (b.i.d. regimen) oral doses ranging from 0.25 to 10 mg/kg.

Absorption and Bioavailability: Lamivudine was rapidly absorbed after oral administration in HIV-infected patients. Absolute bioavailability in 12 adult patients was 86% $\pm$ 16% (mean $\pm$ S.D.) for the tablet and 87% $\pm$ 13% for the oral solution. After oral administration of 2 mg/kg twice a day to nine adults with HIV, the peak serum lamivudine concentration (C_{max}) was 1.5 $\pm$ 0.5 μg/mL (mean $\pm$ S.D.). The area under the plasma concentration versus time curve (AUC) and C_{max} increased in proportion to oral dose over the range from 0.25 to 10 mg/kg.

An investigational 25-mg dosage form of lamivudine was administered orally to 12 asymptomatic, HIV-infected patients on two occasions, once in the fasted state and once with food (1,099 kcal; 75 grams fat, 34 grams protein, 72 grams carbohydrate). Absorption of lamivudine was slower in the fed state (T_{max}: 3.2 $\pm$ 1.3 hours) compared with the fasted state (T_{max}: 0.9 $\pm$ 0.3 hours); C_{max} in the fed state was

Table 1: Pharmacokinetic Parameters (Mean $\pm$ S.D.) After a Single 300-mg Oral Dose of Lamivudine in Three Groups of Adults With Varying Degrees of Renal Function (CrCl > 60 mL/min, CrCl = 10–30 mL/min, and CrCl < 10 mL/min)

Number of subjects	6	4	6
Creatinine clearance criterion	> 60 mL/min	10–30 mL/min	< 10 mL/min
Creatinine clearance (mL/min)	111 $\pm$ 14	28 $\pm$ 8	6 $\pm$ 2
C_{max} (μg/mL)	2.6 $\pm$ 0.5	3.6 $\pm$ 0.8	5.8 $\pm$ 1.2
AUC_∞ (μg·h/mL)	11.0 $\pm$ 1.7	48.0 $\pm$ 19	157 $\pm$ 74
Cl/F (mL/min)	464 $\pm$ 76	114 $\pm$ 34	36 $\pm$ 11

40% $\pm$ 23% (mean $\pm$ S.D.) lower than in the fasted state. There was no significant difference in systemic exposure (AUC_∞) in the fed and fasted states; therefore, EPIVIR Tablets and Oral Solution may be administered with or without food.

The accumulation ratio of lamivudine in HIV-positive asymptomatic adults with normal renal function was 1.50 following 15 days of oral administration of 2 mg/kg b.i.d.

Distribution: The apparent volume of distribution after IV administration of lamivudine to 20 patients was 1.3 $\pm$ 0.4 L/kg, suggesting that lamivudine distributes into extravascular spaces. Volume of distribution was independent of dose and did not correlate with body weight.

Binding of lamivudine to human plasma proteins is low (< 36%). *In vitro* studies showed that, over the concentration range of 0.1 to 100 μg/mL, the amount of lamivudine associated with erythrocytes ranged from 53% to 57% and was independent of concentration.

Metabolism: Metabolism of lamivudine is a minor route of elimination. In man, the only known metabolite of lamivudine is the trans-sulfoxide metabolite. Within 12 hours after a single oral dose of lamivudine in six HIV-infected adults, 5.2% $\pm$ 1.4% (mean $\pm$ S.D.) of the dose was excreted as the trans-sulfoxide metabolite in the urine. Serum concentrations of this metabolite have not been determined.

Elimination: The majority of lamivudine is eliminated unchanged in the urine. In 20 patients given a single IV dose, renal clearance was 0.22 $\pm$ 0.06 L/hr*kg (mean $\pm$ S.D.), representing 71% $\pm$ 16% (mean $\pm$ S.D.) of total clearance of lamivudine.

In most single-dose studies in HIV-infected patients with serum sampling for 24 hours after dosing, the observed mean elimination half-life ($T^1/_2$) ranged from 5 to 7 hours. Total clearance was 0.37 $\pm$ 0.05 L/hr*kg (mean $\pm$ S.D.), Oral clearance and elimination half-life were independent of dose and body weight over an oral dosing range from 0.25 to 10 mg/kg.

Special Populations: *Adults With Impaired Renal Function:* The pharmacokinetic properties of lamivudine have been determined in a small group of HIV-infected adults with impaired renal function, as summarized in Table 1. [See table above.]

Exposure (AUC_∞), C_{max}, and half-life increased with diminishing renal function (as expressed by creatinine clearance). Apparent total oral clearance (Cl/F) of lamivudine decreased as creatinine clearance decreased. T_{max} was not significantly affected by renal function. Based on these observations, it is recommended that the dosage of lamivudine be modified in patients with renal impairment (see DOSAGE AND ADMINISTRATION). The effects of renal impairment on lamivudine pharmacokinetics in pediatric patients are not known.

Pediatric Patients: For pharmacokinetic properties of lamivudine in pediatric patients, see PRECAUTIONS: Pediatric Use.

Geriatric Patients: Lamivudine pharmacokinetics have not been specifically studied in patients over 65 years of age.

Gender: The pharmacokinetics of lamivudine with respect to gender have not been evaluated.

Race: The pharmacokinetics of lamivudine with respect to race have not been evaluated.

Drug Interactions: Lamivudine and zidovudine were coadministered to 12 asymptomatic HIV-positive adult patients in a single-center, open-label, randomized, crossover study. No significant differences were observed in AUC_∞ or total clearance for lamivudine or zidovudine when the two drugs were administered together. Coadministration of lamivudine with zidovudine resulted in an increase of 39% $\pm$ 62% (mean $\pm$ S.D.) in C_{max} of zidovudine.

Lamivudine and trimethoprim/sulfamethoxazole (TMP/SMX) were coadministered to 14 HIV-positive patients in a single-center, open-label, randomized, crossover study. Each patient received treatment with a single 300-mg dose of lamivudine and TMP 160 mg/SMX 800 mg once a day for 5 days with concomitant administration of lamivudine 300 mg with the fifth dose in a crossover design. Coadministration of TMP/SMX with lamivudine resulted in an increase of 44% $\pm$ 23% (mean $\pm$ S.D.) in lamivudine AUC_∞, a decrease of 29% $\pm$ 13% in lamivudine oral clearance, and a decrease of 30% $\pm$ 36% in lamivudine renal clearance. The pharmacokinetic properties of TMP and SMX were not altered by coadministration with lamivudine.

INDICATIONS AND USAGE

EPIVIR in combination with RETROVIR is indicated for the treatment of HIV infection when therapy is warranted based on clinical and/or immunological evidence of disease progression. This indication is based on analyses of surrogate endpoints. At present, there are no results from controlled trials evaluating the effect of EPIVIR plus RETROVIR on clinical progression of HIV infection, such as the incidence of opportunistic infections or survival.

Description of Clinical Studies: *Adults Without Prior Antiretroviral Therapy:* Two studies were conducted in patients who received up to 4 weeks of prior antiretroviral therapy. A3001 was a randomized, double-blind study comparing EPIVIR 150 mg b.i.d. plus RETROVIR 200 mg t.i.d.; EPIVIR 300 mg b.i.d. plus RETROVIR; EPIVIR 300 mg b.i.d.; and RETROVIR. 366 adults enrolled with the following demographics: male (87%), Caucasian (61%), median age of 34 years, asymptomatic HIV infection (80%), and baseline CD4 cell counts of 200 to 500 cells/mm³ (median = 352 cells/mm³). B3001 was a randomized, double-blind study comparing EPIVIR 300 mg b.i.d. plus RETROVIR 200 mg t.i.d. versus RETROVIR. 129 adults enrolled with the following demographics: male (74%), Caucasian (82%), median age of 33 years, asymptomatic HIV infection (64%), and baseline CD4 cell counts of 100 to 400 cells/mm³ (median = 260 cells/mm³). Mean changes in CD4 counts through 24 weeks of treatment for studies A3001 and B3001 are summarized in Figures 1 and 2, respectively.

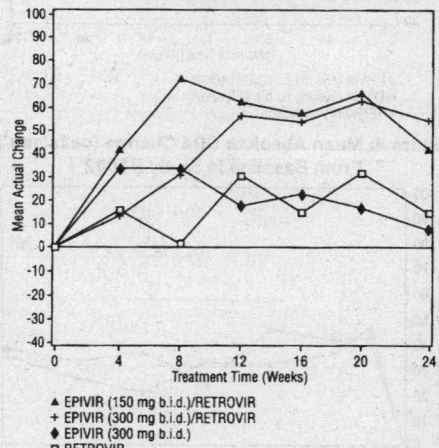

Figure 1: Mean Absolute CD4 Change (cells/mm³) From Baseline in Study A3001

▲ EPIVIR (150 mg b.i.d.)/RETROVIR
+ EPIVIR (300 mg b.i.d.)/RETROVIR
♦ EPIVIR (300 mg b.i.d.)
□ RETROVIR

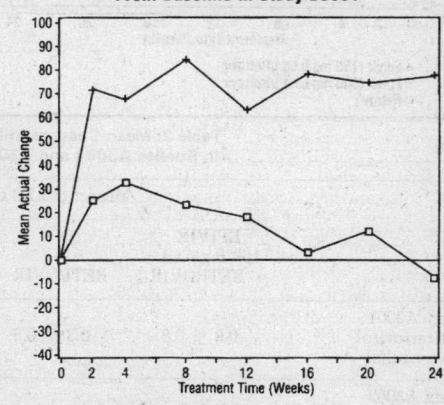

Figure 2: Mean Absolute CD4 Change (cells/mm³) From Baseline in Study B3001

+ EPIVIR (300 mg b.i.d.)/RETROVIR
□ RETROVIR

Continued on next page

Glaxo Wellcome Onc.—Cont.

Adults With Prior Zidovudine Therapy: Two studies were conducted in patients who received at least 24 weeks of prior zidovudine therapy. A3002 was a randomized, double-blind study comparing EPIVIR 150 mg b.i.d. plus RETROVIR 200 mg t.i.d.; EPIVIR 300 mg b.i.d. plus RETROVIR; and RETROVIR plus zalcitabine 0.75 mg t.i.d. 254 adults enrolled with the following demographics: male (83%), Caucasian (63%), median age of 37 years, asymptomatic HIV infection (58%), median duration of prior zidovudine use of 24 months, and baseline CD4 cell counts of 100 to 300 cells/mm^3 (median = 211 cells/mm^3). B3002 was a randomized, double-blind study comparing EPIVIR 150 mg b.i.d. plus RETROVIR, EPIVIR 300 mg b.i.d. plus RETROVIR, and RETROVIR. 223 adults enrolled with the following demographics: male (83%), Caucasian (96%), median age of 36 years, asymptomatic HIV infection (53%), median duration of prior zidovudine use of 23 months, and baseline CD4 cell counts of 100 to 400 cells/mm^3 (median = 241 cells/mm^3). Mean changes in CD4 counts through 24 weeks of treatment in studies A3002 and B3002 are summarized in Figures 3 and 4, respectively.

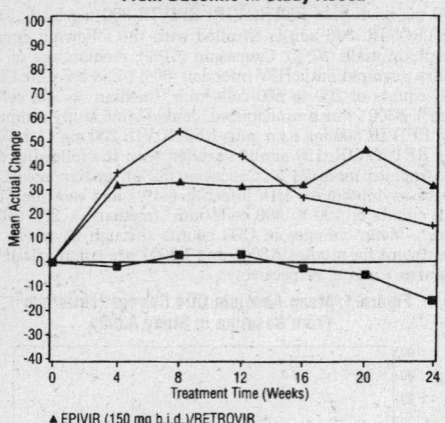

Figure 3: Mean Absolute CD4 Change (cells/mm^3) From Baseline in Study A3002

▲ EPIVIR (150 mg b.i.d.)/RETROVIR
+ EPIVIR (300 mg b.i.d.)/RETROVIR
■ RETROVIR/zalcitabine

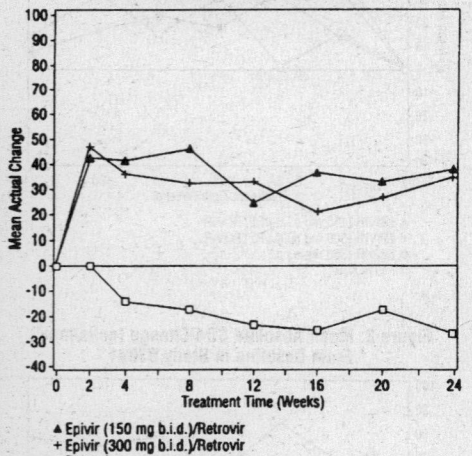

Figure 4: Mean Absolute CD4 Change (cells/mm^3) From Baseline in Study B3002

▲ Epivir (150 mg b.i.d.)/Retrovir
+ Epivir (300 mg b.i.d.)/Retrovir
□ Retrovir

HIV RNA: Mean changes from baseline HIV RNA are summarized in Table 2.
[See table below.]

CONTRAINDICATIONS

EPIVIR Tablets and Oral Solution are contraindicated in patients with previously demonstrated clinically significant hypersensitivity to any of the components of the products.

WARNINGS

PANCREATITIS IN PEDIATRIC PATIENTS: IN PEDIATRIC PATIENTS WITH A HISTORY OF PANCREATITIS OR OTHER SIGNIFICANT RISK FACTORS FOR THE DEVELOPMENT OF PANCREATITIS, THE COMBINATION OF EPIVIR AND RETROVIR SHOULD BE USED WITH EXTREME CAUTION AND ONLY IF THERE IS NO SATISFACTORY ALTERNATIVE THERAPY. TREATMENT WITH EPIVIR SHOULD BE STOPPED IMMEDIATELY IF CLINICAL SIGNS, SYMPTOMS, OR LABORATORY ABNORMALITIES SUGGESTIVE OF PANCREATITIS OCCUR (SEE ADVERSE REACTIONS).

The complete prescribing information for RETROVIR should be consulted before combination therapy with EPIVIR and RETROVIR is initiated.

PRECAUTIONS

Patients With Impaired Renal Function: Reduction of the dosage of EPIVIR is recommended for patients with impaired renal function (see CLINICAL PHARMACOLOGY and DOSAGE AND ADMINISTRATION).

Information for Patients: EPIVIR is not a cure for HIV infection and patients may continue to experience illnesses associated with HIV infection, including opportunistic infections. Treatment with EPIVIR has not been shown to reduce the frequency of such illnesses and patients should remain under the care of a physician when using EPIVIR. Patients should be advised that the use of EPIVIR has not been shown to reduce the risk of transmission of HIV to others through sexual contact or blood contamination.

Patients should be advised that the long-term effects of EPIVIR are unknown at this time.

EPIVIR Tablets and Oral Solution are for oral ingestion only.

Patients should be advised of the importance of taking EPIVIR exactly as it is prescribed.

Parents or guardians should be advised to monitor pediatric patients for signs and symptoms of pancreatitis.

Drug Interaction: TMP 160 mg/SMX 800 mg once daily has been shown to increase lamivudine exposure (AUC). The effect of higher doses of TMP/SMX on lamivudine pharmacokinetics has not been investigated (see CLINICAL PHARMACOLOGY).

Carcinogenesis, Mutagenesis, and Impairment of Fertility: Long-term carcinogenicity studies of lamivudine in animals have not yet been completed. Lamivudine was not active in a microbial mutagenicity screen or an *in vitro* cell transformation assay, but showed weak *in vitro* mutagenic activity in a cytogenetic assay using cultured human lymphocytes and in the mouse lymphoma assay. However, lamivudine showed no evidence of *in vivo* genotoxic activity in the rat at oral doses of up to 2,000 mg/kg (approximately 65 times the recommended human dose based on body surface area comparisons). In a study of reproductive performance, lamivudine, administered to rats at doses up to 130 times the usual adult dose based on body surface area comparisons, revealed no evidence of impaired fertility and no effect on the survival, growth, and development to weaning of the offspring.

Pregnancy: *Pregnancy Category C:* Reproduction studies have been performed in rats and rabbits at orally administered doses up to approximately 130 and 60 times, respectively, the usual adult dose and have revealed no evidence of harm to the fetus due to lamivudine. Some evidence of early embryolethality was seen in the rabbit at doses similar to those produced by the usual adult dose and higher, but there was no indication of this effect in the rat at orally administered doses up to 130 times the usual adult dose. Studies in

pregnant rats and rabbits showed that lamivudine is transferred to the fetus through the placenta. There are no adequate and well-controlled studies in pregnant women. Because animal reproductive toxicity studies are not always predictive of human response, lamivudine should be used during pregnancy only if the potential benefits outweigh the risks.

Antiretroviral Pregnancy Registry: To monitor maternal-fetal outcomes of pregnant women exposed to EPIVIR, an Antiretroviral Pregnancy Registry has been established. Physicians are encouraged to register patients by calling (800) 722-9292, ext.38465.

Nursing Mothers: A study in which lactating rats were administered 45 mg/kg of lamivudine showed that lamivudine concentrations in milk were slightly greater than those in plasma. Although it is not known if lamivudine is excreted in human milk, there is a potential for adverse effects from lamivudine in nursing infants. Mothers should be instructed to discontinue nursing if they are receiving lamivudine. This instruction is consistent with the Centers for Disease Control recommendation that HIV-infected mothers not breast-feed their infants to avoid risking postnatal transmission of HIV infection.

Pediatric Use: THERE ARE NO DATA ON THE USE OF EPIVIR IN COMBINATION WITH RETROVIR IN PEDIATRIC PATIENTS.

Lamivudine monotherapy was studied in one open-label, uncontrolled trial (study A2002) in 97 pediatric patients with the following demographics: male (56%), Caucasian (57%), median age of 7.7 years (range: 0.4 to 17.3 years), symptomatic HIV (84%), median duration of prior antiretroviral therapy (148 weeks), and median baseline CD4 of 132 cells/mm^3. Pharmacokinetic properties of lamivudine were assessed in a subset of 57 patients (age range: 4.8 months to 16 years, weight range: 5 to 66 kg) after oral and IV administration of 1, 2, 4, 8, 12, and 20 mg/kg per day. In the 9 infants and children receiving 8 mg/kg per day (the usual recommended pediatric dose), absolute bioavailability was $66\% \pm 26\%$ (mean ± S.D.), which is less than the $86\% \pm 16\%$ (mean ± S.D.) observed in adolescents and adults. The mechanism for the diminished absolute bioavailability of lamivudine in infants and children is unknown.

Systemic clearance decreased with increasing age in pediatric patients, as shown in Figure 5.

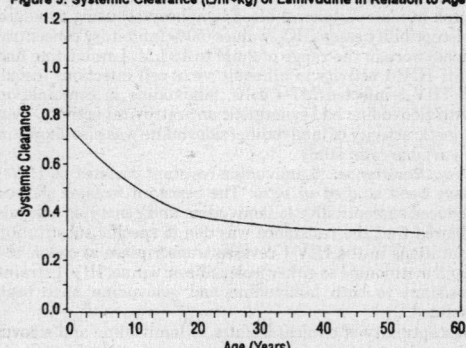

Figure 5: Systemic Clearance (L/hr•kg) of Lamivudine in Relation to Age

After oral administration of 8 mg/kg per day of lamivudine to 11 pediatric patients ranging from 4 months to 14 years of age, C_{max} was 1.1 ± 0.6 μg/mL and half-life was 2.0 ± 0.6 hours. (In adults with similar blood sampling, the half-life was 3.7 ± 1 hours.) Total exposure to lamivudine, as reflected by mean AUC values, was comparable between pediatric patients receiving an 8 mg/kg/day dose and adults receiving a 4 mg/kg/day dose.

Distribution of lamivudine into cerebrospinal fluid (CSF) was assessed in 38 pediatric patients after multiple oral dosing with lamivudine. CSF samples were collected between 2 and 4 hours postdose. At the dose of 8 mg/kg/day, CSF lamivudine concentrations in eight patients ranged from 5.6% to 30.9% (mean ± S.D. for 14.2% ± 7.9%) of the concentration in a simultaneous serum sample, with CSF lamivudine concentrations ranging from 0.04 to 0.3 μg/mL. See INDICATIONS AND USAGE: Description of Clinical Studies, WARNINGS, ADVERSE REACTIONS, and DOSAGE AND ADMINISTRATION sections.

ADVERSE REACTIONS

Adults: Selected clinical adverse events with a ≥5% frequency during therapy with EPIVIR 150 mg b.i.d. plus RETROVIR 200 mg t.i.d. compared with zidovudine are listed in Table 3.
[See Table 3 at top of next column.]

Pancreatitis was observed in 3 of the 656 adult patients (<0.5%) who received EPIVIR in controlled clinical trials. Selected laboratory abnormalities observed during therapy are listed in Table 4.
[See Table 4 in next column.]

Table 2: Mean Changes in log 10 HIV RNA From Baseline in Studies A3001 and A3002 at 24 Weeks of Treatment

	EPIVIR 150 mg b.i.d. + RETROVIR	RETROVIR	EPIVIR 300 mg b.i.d.	EPIVIR 300 mg b.i.d. + RETROVIR	RETROVIR + Zalcitabine
Mean (± S.D.) Changes in log 10 HIV RNA From Baseline*					
Study A3001 (antiretroviral-naive adults)	−0.9 ± 0.8	−0.3 ± 0.8	−0.4 ± 0.8	−1.0 ± 0.8	not applicable
Study A3002 (antiretroviral-experienced adults)	−0.7 ± 0.8	not applicable	not applicable	−0.7 ± 0.8	−0.7 ± 0.8

*THE CLINICAL SIGNIFICANCE OF CHANGES IN HIV RNA DURING THERAPY IS UNKNOWN.

Table 3: Selected Clinical Adverse Events (≥ 5% Frequency) in Four Controlled Clinical Trials (A3001, A3002, B3001, B3002)

Adverse Event	EPIVIR 150 mg b.i.d. plus RETROVIR (n = 251)	RETROVIR (n = 230)
Body as a whole		
Headache	35%	27%
Malaise & fatigue	27%	23%
Fever or chills	10%	12%
Digestive		
Nausea	33%	29%
Diarrhea	18%	22%
Nausea & vomiting	13%	12%
Anorexia and/or decreased appetite	10%	7%
Abdominal pain	9%	11%
Abdominal cramps	6%	3%
Dyspepsia	5%	5%
Nervous system		
Neuropathy	12%	10%
Insomnia & other sleep disorders	11%	7%
Depressive disorders	9%	4%
Dizziness	10%	4%
Respiratory		
Nasal signs & symptoms	20%	11%
Cough	18%	13%
Skin		
Skin rashes	9%	6%
Musculoskeletal		
Musculoskeletal pain	12%	10%
Myalgia	8%	6%
Arthralgia	5%	5%

Table 4: Frequencies of Selected Laboratory Abnormalities Among Adults in Four Controlled Clinical Trials (A3001, A3002, B3001, B3002)*

Test (Abnormal Level)	EPIVIR 150 mg b.i.d. Plus RETROVIR % (n)	RETROVIR % (n)
Neutropenia (ANC < 750/mm^3)	7.2% (237)	5.4% (222)
Anemia (Hgb < 8.0 g/dL)	2.9% (241)	1.8% (218)
Thrombocytopenia (platelets < 50,000/mm^3)	0.4% (240)	1.3% (223)
ALT (> 5.0 × ULN)	3.7% (241)	3.6% (224)
AST (> 5.0 × ULN)	1.7% (241)	1.8% (223)
Bilirubin (> 2.5 ULN)	0.8% (241)	0.4% (220)
Amylase (> 2.0 ULN)	4.2% (72)	1.5% (133)

ULN = Upper limit of normal.
ANC = Absolute neutrophil count.
n = Number of patients assessed.
* Frequencies of these laboratory abnormalities were higher in patients with mild laboratory abnormalities at baseline.

Pediatric Patients: Limited information on the incidence of adverse events in children receiving lamivudine monotherapy is available from one open-label, uncontrolled study (see PRECAUTIONS: Pediatric Use section for description of study A2002). Of 97 pediatric patients, 14 patients (14%) developed pancreatitis while receiving monotherapy with EPIVIR. In a second ongoing study in 47 pediatric patients (age range: 3 months to 18 years) enrolled in an open-label evaluation of EPIVIR/didanosine, EPIVIR/RETROVIR, and EPIVIR/RETROVIR/didanosine, 7 patients (15%) developed pancreatitis (see WARNINGS).
Paresthesias and peripheral neuropathies were reported in 13 patients (13%) in study A2002 and resulted in treatment discontinuation in 3 patients.
Selected laboratory abnormalities during lamivudine therapy in children are listed in Table 5.
[See Table 5 at top of next column.]

OVERDOSAGE

There is no known antidote for EPIVIR. One case of an adult ingesting 6 g of EPIVIR was reported; there were no clinical signs or symptoms noted and hematologic tests remained normal. It is not known whether lamivudine can be removed by peritoneal dialysis or hemodialysis.

DOSAGE AND ADMINISTRATION

Adults and Adolescents (12 to 16 years): The recommended oral dose of EPIVIR for adults and adolescents is 150 mg twice daily administered in combination with RETROVIR. The complete prescribing information for RETROVIR should be consulted for information on its dosage and administration.

Table 5: Frequencies of Selected Laboratory Abnormalities in an Uncontrolled Phase I/II Clinical Trial of EPIVIR in 97 Pediatric Patients

Test (Abnormal Level)	Patients With Normal Baselines % (n)	Patients With Abnormal Baselines % (n)
Neutropenia (ANC < 750/mm^3)	22% (55)	45% (33)
Anemia (Hgb < 8.0 g/dL)	2% (50)	24% (46)
Thrombocytopenia (platelets < 40,000/mm^3)	0% (68)	25% (12)
ALT (> 5.0 × ULN)	4% (51)	29% (42)
AST (> 5.0 × ULN)	0% (29)	19% (57)
Amylase (> 2.0 ULN)	3% (69)	23% (13)

ULN = Upper limit of normal.
ANC = Absolute neutrophil count.
n = Number of patients assessed.

For adults with low body weights (less than 50 kg or 110 lbs), the recommended oral dose of EPIVIR is 2 mg/kg twice daily administered in combination with RETROVIR. No data are available to support a dosage recommendation for adolescents with low body weight (less than 50 kg).
Pediatric Patients: The recommended oral dose of EPIVIR for pediatric patients 3 months to up to 12 years of age 4 mg/kg twice daily (up to a maximum of 150 mg twice a day) administered in combination with RETROVIR. The complete prescribing information for RETROVIR should be consulted for information on its dosage and administration.
Dose Adjustment: It is recommended that doses of EPIVIR be adjusted in accordance with renal function in patients older than age 16 years (see Table 6). (See CLINICAL PHARMACOLOGY section.)

Table 6: Adjustment of Dosage of EPIVIR in Accordance With Creatinine Clearance

Creatinine Clearance (mL/min)	Recommended Dosage of EPIVIR
≥ 50	150 mg twice daily
30–49	150 mg once daily
15–29	150 mg first dose, then 100 mg once daily
5–14	150 mg first dose, then 50 mg once daily
< 5	50 mg first dose, then 25 mg once daily

Insufficient data are available to recommend a dosage of EPIVIR in patients undergoing dialysis.

HOW SUPPLIED

EPIVIR Tablets, 150 mg, are white, modified diamond-shaped, film-coated tablets imprinted with "150" on one side and "GXCJ7" on the reverse side. They are available in bottles of 60 tablets (NDC 0173-0470-01) with child-resistant closures. **Store between 2° and 30°C (36° and 86°F) in tightly closed bottles.**
EPIVIR Oral Solution, a clear, colorless to pale yellow, strawberry-banana flavored liquid, contains 10 mg of lamivudine in each 1 mL in plastic bottles of 240 mL (NDC 0173-0471-00) with child-resistant closures. This product does not require reconstitution. **Store between 2° and 25°C (36° and 77°F) in tightly closed bottles.**
U.S. Patent 5,047,407
©Copyright 1996 Glaxo Wellcome Inc. All rights reserved.
January 1996/RL-277

Shown in Product Identification Guide, page 316

LEUCOVORIN CALCIUM FOR INJECTION ℞
WELLCOVORIN® brand STERILE POWDER
100 mg per vial

DESCRIPTION

Wellcovorin brand Leucovorin Calcium For Injection Sterile Powder is a sterile preparation containing leucovorin present as the calcium salt pentahydrate of N-[4-[[(2-amino-5-for-myl-1, 4, 5, 6, 7, 8-hexahydro-4-oxo-6-pteridinyl)methyl]amino]benzoyl]-L-glutamic acid. Each 5 mg of leucovorin is equivalent to 5.40 mg of anhydrous leucovorin calcium.
Leucovorin is a water soluble vitamin in the folate group; it is useful as an antidote to drugs which act as folic acid antagonists.
Each 100 mg vial of Wellcovorin brand Leucovorin Calcium For Injection Sterile Powder, when reconstituted with 10 mL of sterile diluent, contains leucovorin (as the calcium salt) 10 mg/mL. The inactive ingredients are sodium chloride 80 mg per vial and sodium hydroxide and/or hydrochloric acid added to adjust the pH to approximately 8.1. The dry product contains no preservative. Dilute with Bacteriostatic Water

for Injection, USP, which contains benzyl alcohol (see WARNINGS), or with Sterile Water for Injection, USP. Wellcovorin brand Leucovorin Calcium For Injection Sterile Powder, when reconstituted as directed, is suitable for IM or IV administration.
There is 0.004 mEq of calcium per mg leucovorin.

CLINICAL PHARMACOLOGY

Leucovorin is a mixture of the diastereoisomers of the 5-formyl derivative of tetrahydrofolic acid. The biologically active compound of the mixture is the (-)-L-isomer, known as Citrovorum factor or (-)-folinic acid. Leucovorin does not require reduction by the enzyme dihydrofolate reductase in order to participate in reactions utilizing folates as a source of "one-carbon" moieties. After intravenous administration of 25 mg calcium leucovorin, total reduced folate (as measured by *Lactobacillus casei* assay) reached a mean peak of 1259 ng/mL (range 897 to 1625).
The mean time to peak was 10 minutes. This initial rise in total reduced folate was primarily due to the parent compound 5-formyl THF (measured by S. *faecalis* assay) which rose to 1206 ng/mL at 10 minutes. A sharp drop in parent compound follows and coincides with the appearance of the metabolite (also active) 5-CH$_3$-THF which becomes the predominant circulating form of the drug. The mean peak of 5-CH$_3$-THF was 258 ng/mL occurring at 1.3 hours. The t$^1/_2$ was 6.2 hours for total reduced folates. After intramuscular injection of 25 mg the mean peak total THF was 436 ng/mL (range 240 to 725) which occurred at a mean time of 52 minutes. Similar to IV administration, the initial sharp rise was due to the parent compound (5-CHO-THF) 360 ng/mL at 28 minutes, and the level of the metabolite 5-CH$_3$-THF increased subsequently over time until at 1.5 hours it represented 50% of the circulating total folate. The mean peak of 5-CH$_3$-THF was 226 ng/mL at 2.8 hours. The t$^1/_2$ of total reduced folate was 6.2 hours. There was no difference of statistical significance between IM and IV administration in the AUC for the total THF, 5-CHO-THF, or 5-CH$_3$-THF.

INDICATIONS AND USAGE

Wellcovorin brand Leucovorin Calcium For Injection Sterile Powder is indicated (a) to diminish the toxicity and counteract the effect of inadvertently administered overdosages of folic acid antagonists and (b) in the treatment of the megaloblastic anemias due to sprue, nutritional deficiency, pregnancy, and infancy when oral therapy is not feasible.

CONTRAINDICATIONS

Leucovorin is improper therapy for pernicious anemia and other megaloblastic anemias secondary to the lack of vitamin B$_{12}$. A hematologic remission may occur while neurologic manifestations remain progressive.

WARNINGS

In the treatment of accidental overdosage of folic acid antagonists, leucovorin should be administered as promptly as possible. As the time interval between antifolate administration (e.g., methotrexate [MTX]) and leucovorin rescue increases, leucovorin's effectiveness in counteracting hematologic toxicity diminishes.
Monitoring of serum MTX concentration is essential in determining the optimal dose and duration of treatment with leucovorin which should be such that the resulting levels of tetrahydrofolate are equal to or greater than that of MTX. In determining the dose and duration of leucovorin therapy, it should be remembered that there may be a delay of MTX excretion in the presence of a third space (i.e., ascites, pleural effusion) or if renal insufficiency or inadequate hydration exists. Under such circumstances, high doses of leucovorin are recommended. These doses are higher than those recommended for oral use and must be given intravenously.
If MTX is administered intrathecally as local therapy and leucovorin is administered concurrently, the presence of tetrahydrofolate which diffuses readily into the cerebrospinal fluid may negate the antineoplastic effect of MTX.
Leucovorin may enhance the toxicity of fluorouracil. Deaths from severe enterocolitis, diarrhea, and dehydration have been reported in elderly patients receiving leucovorin and fluorouracil. Concomitant granulocytopenia and fever were present in some but not all of patients.
There have been rare reports of seizures and/or syncope associated with the use of leucovorin, particularly high doses, in combination with fluorouracil for treatment of malignancies in patients with a history of prior seizures or in patients with central nervous system abnormalities.
The concomitant use of leucovorin with trimethoprim-sulfamethoxazole for the acute treatment of *Pneumocystis carinii* pneumonia in patients with HIV infection was associated with increased rates of treatment failure and morbidity in a placebo-controlled study.
Because of the preservative contained in Bacteriostatic Water for Injection, USP (benzyl alcohol preserved), doses greater than 10 mg/m^2 with this diluent are not recommended. If greater doses are required (see DOSAGE AND ADMINISTRATION) the desiccated powder should be recon-

Continued on next page

Glaxo Wellcome Onc.—Cont.

stituted with Sterile Water for Injection, USP, and used immediately.

PRECAUTIONS

General: Following chemotherapy with folic acid antagonists, parenteral administration of leucovorin is preferable to oral dosing if there is a possibility that the patient may vomit and not absorb the leucovorin. In the presence of pernicious anemia, a hematologic remission may occur while neurologic manifestations remain progressive. Leucovorin has no effect on other established toxicities of MTX such as the nephrotoxicity resulting from drug precipitation in the kidney.

Drug Interactions: Folic acid in large amounts may counteract the antiepileptic effect of phenobarbital, phenytoin, and primidone, and increase the frequency of seizures in susceptible pediatric patients.

Leucovorin may enhance the toxicity of fluorouracil (see WARNINGS).

Pregnancy: ***Teratogenic Effects:*** Pregnancy Category C. Animal reproduction studies have not been conducted with leucovorin. It is also not known whether leucovorin can cause fetal harm when administered to a pregnant woman or can affect reproduction capacity. Leucovorin should be given to a pregnant woman only if clearly needed.

Nursing Mothers: It is not known whether this drug is excreted in human milk. Because many drugs are excreted in human milk, caution should be exercised when leucovorin is administered to a nursing mother.

Pediatric Use: See Drug Interactions.

ADVERSE REACTIONS

Allergic sensitization has been reported following both oral and parenteral administration of folic acid.

OVERDOSAGE

Excessive amounts of leucovorin may nullify the chemotherapeutic effect of folic acid antagonists.

DOSAGE AND ADMINISTRATION

Inadvertent Overdosage of Antifol: As soon as possible after an inadvertent overdosage of the antifol, MTX, leucovorin should be given in a dosage regimen of 10 mg/m^2 every 6 hours IV or IM until the serum MTX levels are below 10^{-8} M. If there is adequate gastrointestinal function, doses subsequent to the initial dose may be given orally (see labeling of oral product). Concomitant hydration (3 L/d) and urinary alkalinization with sodium bicarbonate should be employed. The bicarbonate dose should be adjusted to maintain a urinary pH at 7 or greater.

Serum samples should be assayed for creatinine levels and MTX levels at 24-hour intervals. If the 24-hour serum creatinine level has increased 50% over baseline or if the 24-hour MTX level is $> 5 \times 10^{-6}$ M or the 48-hour MTX level is $> 9 \times 10^{-7}$ M, the doses of leucovorin should be increased to 100 mg/m^2 q 3 hours IV until the MTX level is $< 10^{-8}$ M. When such doses are administered, a non-preserved diluent should be used (see WARNINGS). The rate of injection of leucovorin calcium should not exceed 17.5 mL (175 mg leucovorin) per minute.

Megaloblastic Anemia: No more than or up to 1 mg daily. There is no evidence that doses > 1 mg daily have greater efficacy than those of 1 mg; additionally, loss of folate in urine becomes roughly logarithmic as the amount administered exceeds 1 mg.

Instructions for Reconstitution: Read WARNINGS for considerations in choice of diluent. The contents of each vial should be reconstituted with Bacteriostatic Water for Injection, USP (benzyl alcohol preserved) or with Sterile Water for Injection.

The 100 mg vial should be diluted with 10 mL, resulting in a solution containing 10 mg leucovorin per mL.

When reconstituted with Bacteriostatic Water for Injection, the resulting solution must be used within 7 days. If reconstituted with Sterile Water for Injection, use immediately and discard any unused portion.

Parenteral drug products should be inspected visually for particulate matter and discoloration prior to administration, whenever solution and container permit.

HOW SUPPLIED

100 mg/vial, Box of 1 (NDC 0173-0638-93).

Store dry powder and reconstituted solution at controlled room temperature 15° to 30°C (59° to 86°F). Protect from light.

April 1996/RL-304

Shown in Product Identification Guide, page 316

LEUCOVORIN CALCIUM TABLETS ℞
WELLCOVORIN® brand

DESCRIPTION

WELLCOVORIN brand Leucovorin Calcium Tablets contain either 5 mg or 25 mg leucovorin as the calcium salt of *N*-[4-[[(2-amino-5-formyl-1, 4, 5, 6, 7, 8-hexahydro-4-oxo-6-pteridinyl)-methyl]amino]benzoyl]-*L*-glutamic acid and the inactive ingredients corn starch, FD&C Yellow No. 6 Lake (25 mg tablet only), lactose, povidone, and magnesium stearate. This is equivalent to 5.40 mg or 27.01 mg of anhydrous leucovorin calcium.

Leucovorin is a water soluble form of reduced folate in the folate group; it is useful as an antidote to drugs which act as folic acid antagonists. These tablets are intended for oral administration only.

CLINICAL PHARMACOLOGY

Leucovorin is a racemic mixture of the diastereoisomers of the 5-formyl derivative of tetrahydrofolic acid. The biologically active compound of the mixture is the (-)-*L*-isomer, known as *Citrovorum factor,* or (-)-folinic acid. Leucovorin does *not* require reduction by the enzyme dihydrofolate reductase in order to participate in reactions utilizing folates as a source of "one-carbon" moieties. Following oral administration, leucovorin is rapidly absorbed and enters the general body pool of reduced folates. The increase in plasma and serum folate activity (determined microbiologically with *Lactobacillus casei*) seen after oral administration of leucovorin is predominantly due to 5-methyltetrahydrofolate.

Twenty normal men were given a single oral 15 mg dose (7.5 mg/m^2) of leucovorin calcium and serum folate concentrations were assayed with *L casei.* Mean values observed (± one standard error) were:

a) Time to peak serum folate concentration: 1.72 ± 0.08 hours,
b) Peak serum folate concentration achieved: 268 ± 18 ng/mL,
c) Serum folate half-disappearance time: 3.5 hours.

Oral tablets yielded areas under the serum folate concentration-time curves (AUCs) that were 12% greater than equal amounts of leucovorin given intramuscularly and equal to the same amounts given intravenously. Oral absorption of leucovorin is saturable at doses above 25 mg. The apparent bioavailability of leucovorin was 97% for 25 mg, 75% for 50 mg, and 37% for 100 mg.

INDICATIONS AND USAGE

WELLCOVORIN brand Leucovorin Calcium Tablets are indicated to diminish the toxicity and counteract the effects of impaired methotrexate elimination and of inadvertent overdosages of folic acid antagonists.

CONTRAINDICATIONS

Leucovorin is improper therapy for pernicious anemia and other megaloblastic anemias secondary to the lack of vitamin B_{12}. A hematologic remission may occur while neurological manifestations continue to progress.

WARNINGS

In the treatment of accidental overdosage of folic acid antagonists, leucovorin should be administered as promptly as possible. As the time interval between antifolate administration (e.g., methotrexate [MTX]) and leucovorin rescue increases, leucovorin's effectiveness in counteracting hematologic toxicity decreases.

Monitoring of the serum MTX concentration is essential in determining the optimal dose and duration of treatment with leucovorin.

Delayed MTX excretion may be caused by a third space fluid accumulation (i.e., ascites, pleural effusion), renal insufficiency, or inadequate hydration. Under such circumstances, higher doses of leucovorin or prolonged administration may be indicated. Doses higher than those recommended for oral use must be given intravenously.

Leucovorin may enhance the toxicity of fluorouracil. Deaths from severe enterocolitis, diarrhea, and dehydration have been reported in elderly patients receiving weekly leucovorin and fluorouracil.[1] Concomitant granulocytopenia and fever were present in some but not all of the patients.

The concomitant use of leucovorin with trimethoprim-sulfamethoxazole for the acute treatment of *Pneumocystis carinii* pneumonia in patients with HIV infection was associated with increased rates of treatment failure and morbidity in a placebo-controlled study.

PRECAUTIONS

General: Parenteral administration of leucovorin is preferable to oral dosing if there is a possibility that the patient may vomit or not absorb the leucovorin. Leucovorin has no effect on other established toxicities of MTX, such as the nephrotoxicity resulting from drug and/or metabolite precipitation in the kidney.

Drug Interactions: Folic acid in large amounts may counteract the antiepileptic effect of phenobarbital, phenytoin, and primidone, and increase the frequency of seizures in susceptible children.

Preliminary animal and human studies have shown that small quantities of systemically administered leucovorin enter the CSF primarily as 5-methyltetrahydrofolate and, in humans, remain one to three orders of magnitude lower than the usual MTX concentrations following intrathecal administration. However, high doses of leucovorin may reduce the efficacy of intrathecally administered MTX.

Leucovorin may enhance the toxicity of fluorouracil (see WARNINGS).

Pregnancy: ***Teratogenic Effects:*** Pregnancy Category C. Animal reproduction studies have not been conducted with leucovorin. It is also not known whether leucovorin can cause fetal harm when administered to a pregnant woman or can affect reproduction capacity. Leucovorin should be given to a pregnant woman only if clearly needed.

Nursing Mothers: It is not known whether this drug is excreted in human milk. Because many drugs are excreted in human milk, caution should be exercised when leucovorin is administered to a nursing mother.

Pediatric Use: See Drug Interactions subsection.

ADVERSE REACTIONS

Allergic sensitization has been reported following both oral and parenteral administration of folic acid.

OVERDOSAGE

Excessive amounts of leucovorin may nullify the chemotherapeutic effect of folic acid antagonists.

DOSAGE AND ADMINISTRATION

Leucovorin calcium tablets are intended for oral administration. Because absorption is saturable, oral administration of doses greater than 25 mg is not recommended.

Impaired Methotrexate Elimination or Inadvertent Overdosage: Leucovorin rescue should begin as soon as possible after an inadvertent overdosage and within 24 hours of methotrexate administration when there is delayed excretion (see WARNINGS). Leucovorin 15 mg (10 mg/m^2) should be administered I.M., I.V., or P.O. every 6 hours until the serum methotrexate level is less than 10^{-8}M. In the presence of gastrointestinal toxicity, nausea or vomiting, leucovorin should be administered parenterally.

Serum creatinine and methotrexate levels should be determined at 24-hour intervals. If the 24-hour serum creatinine has increased 50% over baseline or if the 24-hour methotrexate level is greater than 5×10^{-6}M or the 48-hour level is greater than 9×10^{-7}M, the dose of leucovorin should be increased by 150 mg (100 mg/m^2) I.V. every 3 hours until the methotrexate level is less than 10^{-8}M. Doses greater than 25 mg should be given parenterally (see CLINICAL PHARMACOLOGY).

Hydration (3L/d) and urinary alkalinization with sodium bicarbonate should be employed concomitantly. The bicarbonate dose should be adjusted to maintain the urine pH at 7.0 or greater.

The recommended dose of leucovorin to counteract hematologic toxicity from folic acid antagonists with less affinity for mammalian dihydrofolate reductase than methotrexate (i.e., trimethoprim, pyrimethamine) is substantially less, and 5 to 15 mg of leucovorin per day has been recommended by some investigators.

Patients who experience delayed early methotrexate elimination are likely to develop reversible non-oliguric renal failure. In addition to appropriate leucovorin therapy, these patients require continuing hydration and urinary alkalinization, and close monitoring of fluid and electrolyte status, until the serum methotrexate level has fallen to below 0.05 micromolar and the renal failure has resolved.

Some patients will have abnormalities in methotrexate elimination or renal function following methotrexate administration, which are significant but less severe. These abnormalities may or may not be associated with significant clinical toxicity. If significant clinical toxicity is observed, leucovorin rescue should be extended for an additional 24 hours (total of 14 doses over 84 hours) in subsequent courses of therapy. The possibility that the patient is taking other medications which interact with methotrexate (e.g., medications which may interfere with methotrexate elimination or binding to serum albumin) should always be reconsidered when laboratory abnormalities or clinical toxicities are observed.

HOW SUPPLIED

5 mg (off-white) scored tablets containing 5 mg leucovorin as the calcium salt imprinted with "WELLCOVORIN" and "5"; bottles of 20 (NDC 0081-0631-20) and 100 (NDC 0173-0631-55); unit dose pack of 50 (NDC 0081-0631-35).

25 mg (peach) scored tablets containing 25 mg leucovorin as the calcium salt imprinted with "WELLCOVORIN" and "25"; bottle of 25 (NDC 0173-0632-25); and Unit Dose Rescue Pak® of 10 (NDC 0173-0632-13).

Store at 15° to 25°C (59° to 77°F). Protect from light and moisture.

REFERENCES

1. Grem JL, Shoemaker DD, Petrelli NJ, Douglass HO Jr. Severe and fatal toxic effects observed in treatment with high- and low-dose leucovorin plus 5-fluorouracil for colorectal carcinoma. *Cancer Treat Rep* 1987;71:1122.
2. Link MP, Goorin AM, Miser AW, et al. The effect of adjuvant chemotherapy on relapse-free survival patients with osteosarcoma of the extremity. *N Engl J Med.* 1986;314:1600–1606.

March 1996/RL-299

Shown in Product Identification Guide, page 316

LEUKERAN®
[lū 'kŭh-răn]
(chlorambucil)
2 mg Sugar-coated Tablets

℞

> **WARNING:** LEUKERAN (chlorambucil) can severely suppress bone marrow function. Chlorambucil is a carcinogen in humans. Chlorambucil is probably mutagenic and teratogenic in humans. Chlorambucil produces human infertility (see WARNINGS and PRECAUTIONS).

DESCRIPTION

LEUKERAN (chlorambucil) was first synthesized by Everett et al.[1] It is a bifunctional alkylating agent of the nitrogen mustard type that has been found active against selected human neoplastic diseases. Chlorambucil is known chemically as 4-[bis(2-chlorethyl)amino]benzenebutanoic acid. Chlorambucil hydrolyzes in water and has a pKa of 5.8. LEUKERAN (chlorambucil) is available in tablet form for oral administration. Each sugar-coated tablet contains 2 mg chlorambucil and the inactive ingredients acacia, corn and wheat starch, lactose, magnesium stearate, pharmaceutical glaze, polysorbate 60, sucrose, and talc. Printed with edible black ink.

CLINICAL PHARMACOLOGY

Chlorambucil is rapidly and completely absorbed from the gastrointestinal tract. After single oral doses of 0.6 to 1.2 mg/kg, peak plasma chlorambucil levels are reached within 1 hour and the terminal half-life of the parent drug is estimated at 1.5 hours. Chlorambucil undergoes rapid metabolism to phenylacetic acid mustard, the major metabolite, and the combined chlorambucil and phenylacetic acid mustard urinary excretion is extremely low—less than 1% in 24 hours. The peak plasma levels of chlorambucil and phenylacetic acid mustard are similar, approximating 1 μg/mL; however, the metabolite's half-life is 1.6 times greater than the parent drug.[2,3]

Chlorambucil and its metabolites are extensively bound to plasma and tissue proteins. In vitro, chlorambucil is 99% bound to plasma proteins, specifically albumin.[4] Cerebrospinal fluid levels of chlorambucil have not been determined. Evidence of human teratogenicity suggests that the drug crosses the placenta.[5,6]

Chlorambucil is extensively metabolized in the liver primarily to phenylacetic acid mustard which has antineoplastic activity.[2,3] Chlorambucil and its major metabolite spontaneously degrade in vivo forming monohydroxy and dihydroxy derivatives.[2] After a single dose of radiolabeled chlorambucil (^{14}C) approximately 15% to 60% of the radioactivity appears in the urine after 24 hours. Again, less than 1% of the urinary radioactivity is in the form of chlorambucil or phenylacetic acid mustard.[2] In summary, the pharmacokinetic data suggest that oral chlorambucil undergoes rapid gastrointestinal absorption and plasma clearance and that it is almost completely metabolized, having extremely low urinary excretion.

INDICATIONS AND USAGE

LEUKERAN (chlorambucil) is indicated in the treatment of chronic lymphatic (lymphocytic) leukemia, malignant lymphomas including lymphosarcoma, giant follicular lymphoma, and Hodgkin's disease. It is not curative in any of these disorders but may produce clinically useful palliation.

CONTRAINDICATIONS

Chlorambucil should not be used in patients whose disease has demonstrated a prior resistance to the agent. Patients who have demonstrated hypersensitivity to chlorambucil should not be given the drug.[7-9] There may be cross-hypersensitivity (skin rash) between chlorambucil and other alkylating agents.[10]

WARNINGS

Because of its carcinogenic properties, chlorambucil should not be given to patients with conditions other than chronic lymphatic leukemia or malignant lymphomas. Convulsions,[11] infertility,[12] leukemia[13,14] and secondary malignancies[15] have been observed when chlorambucil was employed in the therapy of malignant and non-malignant diseases. There are many reports of acute leukemia arising in patients with both malignant[16] and non-malignant[17] diseases following chlorambucil treatment. In many instances, these patients also received other chemotherapeutic agents or some form of radiation therapy. The quantitation of the risk of chlorambucil-induction of leukemia or carcinoma in humans is not possible. Evaluation of published reports of leukemia developing in patients who have received chlorambucil (and other alkylating agents) suggests that the risk of leukemogenesis increases with both chronicity of treatment and large cumulative doses. However, it has proved impossible to define a cumulative dose below which there is no risk of the induction of secondary malignancy. The potential benefits from chlorambucil therapy must be weighed on an individual basis against the possible risk of the induction of a secondary malignancy.

Chlorambucil has been shown to cause chromatid or chromosome damage in man.[18,19] Both reversible and permanent sterility have been observed in both sexes receiving chlorambucil.

A high incidence of sterility has been documented when chlorambucil is administered to prepubertal and pubertal males.[20] Prolonged or permanent azoospermia has also been observed in adult males.[21] While most reports of gonadal dysfunction secondary to chlorambucil have related to males, the induction of amenorrhea in females with alkylating agents is well documented, and chlorambucil is capable of producing amenorrhea. Autopsy studies of the ovaries from women with malignant lymphoma treated with combination chemotherapy including chlorambucil have shown varying degrees of fibrosis, vasculitis, and depletion of primordial follicles.[22,23]

Rare instances of skin rash, progressing to erythema multiforme, toxic epidermal necrolysis, or Stevens-Johnson syndrome have been reported.[8-9] Chlorambucil should be discontinued promptly in patients who develop skin reactions.

Pregnancy: Pregnancy Category D. Chlorambucil can cause fetal harm when administered to a pregnant woman. Unilateral renal agenesis has been observed in two offspring whose mothers received chlorambucil during the first trimester.[5,6] Urogenital malformations, including absence of a kidney, were found in fetuses of rats given chlorambucil.[24] There are no adequate and well-controlled studies in pregnant women. If this drug is used during pregnancy, or if the patient becomes pregnant while taking this drug, the patient should be apprised of the potential hazard to the fetus. Women of childbearing potential should be advised to avoid becoming pregnant.

PRECAUTIONS

General: Many patients develop a slowly progressive lymphopenia during treatment. The lymphocyte count usually rapidly returns to normal levels upon completion of drug therapy. Most patients have some neutropenia after the third week of treatment, and this may continue for up to 10 days after the last dose. Subsequently, the neutrophil count usually rapidly returns to normal. Severe neutropenia appears to be related to dosage and usually occurs only in patients who have received a total dosage of 6.5 mg/kg or more in one course of therapy with continuous dosing. About one-quarter of all patients receiving the continuous-dose schedule, and one-third of those receiving this dosage in 8 weeks or less may be expected to develop severe neutropenia.[25]

While it is not necessary to discontinue chlorambucil at the first evidence of a fall in neutrophil count, it must be remembered that the fall may continue for 10 days after the last dose and that as the total dose approaches 6.5 mg/kg there is a risk of causing irreversible bone marrow damage. The dose of chlorambucil should be decreased if leukocyte or platelet counts fall below normal values and should be discontinued for more severe depression.

Chlorambucil should **not** be given at full dosages before 4 weeks after a full course of radiation therapy or chemotherapy because of the vulnerability of the bone marrow to damage under these conditions. If the pretherapy leukocyte or platelet counts are depressed from bone marrow disease process prior to institution of therapy, the treatment should be instituted at a reduced dosage.

Persistently low neutrophil and platelet counts or peripheral lymphocytosis suggest bone marrow infiltration. If confirmed by bone marrow examination, the daily dosage of chlorambucil should not exceed 0.1 mg/kg. Chlorambucil appears to be relatively free from gastrointestinal side effects or other evidence of toxicity apart from the bone marrow depressant action. In humans, single oral doses of 20 mg or more may produce nausea and vomiting.

Children with nephrotic syndrome[11] and patients receiving high pulse doses of chlorambucil[26] may have an increased risk of seizures. As with any potentially epileptogenic drug, caution should be exercised when administering chlorambucil to patients with a history of seizure disorder, head trauma, or receiving other potentially epileptogenic drugs.

Information for Patients: Patients should be informed that the major toxicities of chlorambucil are related to hypersensitivity, drug fever, myelosuppression, hepatotoxicity, infertility, seizures, gastrointestinal toxicity, and secondary malignancies. Patients should never be allowed to take the drug without medical supervision and should consult their physician if they experience skin rash, bleeding, fever, jaundice, persistent cough, seizures, nausea, vomiting, amenorrhea, or unusual lumps/masses. Women of childbearing potential should be advised to avoid becoming pregnant.

Laboratory Tests: Patients must be followed carefully to avoid life-endangering damage to the bone marrow during treatment. Weekly examination of the blood should be made to determine hemoglobin levels, total and differential leukocyte counts, and quantitative platelet counts. Also, during the first 3 to 6 weeks of therapy, it is recommended that white blood cell counts be made 3 or 4 days after each of the weekly complete blood counts. Galton et al[25] have suggested that in following patients it is helpful to plot the blood counts on a chart at the same time that body weight, temperature, spleen size, etc., are recorded. It is considered dangerous to allow a patient to go more than 2 weeks without hematological and clinical examination during treatment.

Drug Interactions: There are no known drug/drug interactions with chlorambucil.

Carcinogenesis, Mutagenesis, Impairment of Fertility: See WARNINGS section for information on carcinogenesis, mutagenesis, and impairment of fertility.

Pregnancy: *Teratogenic Effects:* Pregnancy Category D: See WARNINGS section.

Nursing Mothers: It is not known whether this drug is excreted in human milk. Because many drugs are excreted in human milk and because of the potential for serious adverse reactions in nursing infants from chlorambucil, a decision should be made whether to discontinue nursing or to discontinue the drug, taking into account the importance of the drug to the mother.

Pediatric Use: The safety and effectiveness in pediatric patients have not been established.

ADVERSE REACTIONS

Hematologic: The most common side effect is bone marrow suppression.[27] Although bone marrow suppression frequently occurs, it is usually reversible if the chlorambucil is withdrawn early enough. However, irreversible bone marrow failure has been reported.[28,29]

Gastrointestinal: Gastrointestinal disturbances such as nausea and vomiting, diarrhea, and oral ulceration occur infrequently.

CNS: Tremors, muscular twitching, confusion, agitation, ataxia, flaccid paresis, and hallucinations have been reported as rare adverse experiences to chlorambucil which resolve upon discontinuation of drug. Rare, focal and/or generalized seizures have been reported to occur in both children[11,30,31] and adults[26,32-35] at both therapeutic daily doses pulse dosing regimens, and in acute overdose (see PRECAUTIONS: General).

Dermatologic: Skin hypersensitivity (including rare reports of skin rash progressing to erythema multiforme,[9] toxic epidermal necrolysis,[8] and Stevens-Johnson syndrome) has been reported (see WARNINGS).

Miscellaneous: Other reported adverse reactions include: pulmonary fibrosis, hepatotoxicity and jaundice, drug fever, peripheral neuropathy, interstitial pneumonia, sterile cystitis, infertility, leukemia, and secondary malignancies (see WARNINGS).

OVERDOSAGE

Reversible pancytopenia was the main finding of inadvertent overdoses of chlorambucil.[36,37] Neurological toxicity ranging from agitated behavior and ataxia to multiple grand mal seizures has also occurred.[30,36] As there is no known antidote, the blood picture should be closely monitored and general supportive measures should be instituted, together with appropriate blood transfusions, if necessary. Chlorambucil is not dialyzable.

Oral LD$_{50}$ single doses in mice are 123 mg/kg. In rats, a single intraperitoneal dose of 12.5 mg/kg of chlorambucil produces typical nitrogen-mustard effects; these include atrophy of the intestinal mucous membrane and lymphoid tissues, severe lymphopenia becoming maximal in 4 days, anemia, and thrombocytopenia. After this dose, the animals begin to recover within 3 days and appear normal in about a week although the bone marrow may not become completely normal for about 3 weeks. An intraperitoneal dose of 18.5 mg/kg kills about 50% of the rats with development of convulsions. As much as 50 mg/kg has been given orally to rats as a single dose, with recovery. Such a dose causes bradycardia, excessive salivation, hematuria, convulsions, and respiratory dysfunction.

DOSAGE AND ADMINISTRATION

The usual oral dosage is 0.1 to 0.2 mg/kg body weight daily for 3 to 6 weeks as required. This usually amounts to 4 to 10 mg a day for the average patient. The entire daily dose may be given at one time. These dosages are for initiation of therapy or for short courses of treatment. The dosage must be carefully adjusted according to the response of the patient and must be reduced as soon as there is an abrupt fall in the white blood cell count. Patients with Hodgkin's disease usually require 0.2 mg/kg daily whereas patients with other lymphomas or chronic lymphocytic leukemia usually require only 0.1 mg/kg daily. When lymphocytic infiltration of the bone marrow is present, or when the bone marrow is hypoplastic, the daily dose should not exceed 0.1 mg/kg (about 6 mg for the average patient).

Alternate schedules for the treatment of chronic lymphocytic leukemia employing intermittent, biweekly, or once monthly pulse doses of chlorambucil have been reported.[38,39] Intermittent schedules of chlorambucil begin with an initial single dose of 0.4 mg/kg. Doses are generally increased by 0.1 mg/kg until control of lymphocytosis or toxicity is observed.

Continued on next page

Glaxo Wellcome Onc.—Cont.

Subsequent doses are modified to produce mild hematologic toxicity. It is felt that the response rate of chronic lymphocytic leukemia to the biweekly or once monthly schedule of chlorambucil administration is similar or better to that previously reported with daily administration and that hematologic toxicity was less than or equal to that encountered in studies using daily chlorambucil.

Radiation and cytotoxic drugs render the bone marrow more vulnerable to damage, and chlorambucil should be used with particular caution within 4 weeks of a full course of radiation therapy or chemotherapy. However, small doses of palliative radiation over isolated foci remote from the bone marrow will not usually depress the neutrophil and platelet count. In these cases chlorambucil may be given in the customary dosage.

It is presently felt that short courses of treatment are safer than continuous maintenance therapy, although both methods have been effective. It must be recognized that continuous therapy may give the appearance of "maintenance" in patients who are actually in remission and have no immediate need for further drug. If maintenance dosage is used, it should not exceed 0.1 mg/kg daily and may well be as low as 0.03 mg/kg daily. A typical maintenance dose is 2 mg to 4 mg daily, or less, depending on the status of the blood counts. It may, therefore, be desirable to withdraw the drug after maximal control has been achieved since intermittent therapy reinstituted at time of relapse may be as effective as continuous treatment.

Procedures for proper handling and disposal of anticancer drugs should be considered. Several guidelines on this subject have been published.[40–46]

There is no general agreement that all of the procedures recommended in the guidelines are necessary or appropriate.

HOW SUPPLIED

White sugar-coated tablet containing 2 mg chlorambucil and printed with "635"; bottle of 50 (NDC 0173-0635-35).

Store at 15° to 25°C (59° to 77°F) in a dry place.

REFERENCES

1. Everett JL, Roberts JJ, Ross WCJ. Aryl-2-halogenoalkylamines. Pt. XII. Some carboxylic derivatives of NN-Di-2-chloroethylaniline. *J Chem Soc.* 1953;3:2386–2392.
2. Alberts DS, Chang SY, Chen H-SG, Larcom BJ, Jones SE. Pharmacokinetics and metabolism of chlorambucil in man. *Cancer Treat Rev.* 1979;6 (suppl):9–17.
3. McLean A, Woods RL, Catovsky D, Farmer P. Pharmacokinetics and metabolism of chlorambucil in patients with malignant disease. *Cancer Treat Rev.* 1979; 6(suppl):33–42.
4. Ehrsson H, Lönroth U, Wallin I, Ehrnebo M, Nilsson SO. Degradation of chlorambucil in aqueous solution: influence of human albumin binding. *J Pharm Pharmacol.* 1981;33:313–315. Communications.
5. Shotton D, Monie IW. Possible teratogenic effect of chlorambucil on a human fetus. *JAMA.* 1963;186:74–75.
6. Steege JF, Caldwell DS. Renal agenesis after first trimester exposure to chlorambucil. *South Med J.* 1980;73:1414–1415.
7. Knisley RE, Settipane GA, Albala MM. Unusual reaction to chlorambucil in a patient with chronic lymphocytic leukemia. *Arch Dermatol.* 1971;104:77–79.
8. Pietrantonio F. Moriconi L, Torino F, Romano A, Gangovich A. Unusual reaction to chlorambucil: a case report. *Cancer Lett.* 1990;54:109–111.
9. Hitchins RN, Hocker GA, Thomson DB. Chlorambucil allergy—a series of three cases. *Aust NZ J Med.* 1987;17:600–602.
10. Weiss RB, Bruno S. Hypersensitivity reactions to cancer chemotherapeutic agents. *Ann Intern Med.* 1981; 94:66–72.
11. Williams SA, Makker SP, Grupe WE. Seizures: a significant side effect of chlorambucil therapy in children. *J Pediatr.* 1978;93:516–518.
12. Freckman HA, Fry HL, Mendez FL, Maurer ER. Chlorambucil-prednisolone therapy for disseminated breast carcinoma. *JAMA.* 1964;189:23–26.
13. Aymard JP, Frustin J, Witz F, Colomb JN, Lederlin P, Herbeuval R. Acute leukemia after prolonged chlorambucil treatment for non-malignant disease: a report of a new case and literature survey. *Acta Haematol (Basel).* 1980;63:283–285.
14. Berk PD, Goldberg JD, Silverstein MN, et al. Increased incidence of acute leukemia in polycythemia vera associated with chlorambucil therapy. *N Engl J Med.* 1981;304:441–447.
15. Lerner HJ. Acute myelogenous leukemia in patients receiving chlorambucil as long-term adjuvant chemotherapy for stage II breast cancer. *Cancer Treat Rep.* 1978;62:1135–1138.
16. Zarrabi MH, Grünwald HW, Rosner F. Chronic lymphocytic leukemia terminating in acute leukemia. *Arch Intern Med.* 1977;137:1059–1064.
17. Cameron S: Chlorambucil and leukemia. *N Eng J Med.* 1977;296:1065.
18. Lawler SD, Lele KP. Chromosomal damage induced by chlorambucil in chronic lymphocytic leukemia. *Scand J Haematol* 1972;9:603–612.
19. Stevenson AC, Patel C. Effects of chlorambucil on human chromosomes. *Mutat Res.* 1973;18:333–351.
20. Guesry P, Lenoir G, Broyer M. Gonadal effects of chlorambucil given to prepubertal and pubertal boys for nephrotic syndrome. *J Pediatr.* 1978;92:299–303.
21. Richter P, Calamera JC, Morgenfeld MC, Kierszenbaum AL, Lavieri JC, Mancini RE. Effect of chlorambucil on spermatogenesis in the human with malignant lymphoma. *Cancer.* 1970;25:1026–1030.
22. Morgenfeld MC, Goldberg V, Parisier H, Bugnard SC, Bur GE. Ovarian lesions due to cytostatic agents during the treatment of Hodgkin's disease. *Surg Gynecol Obstet.* 1972;134:826–828.
23. Sobrinho LG, Levine RA, DeConti RC. Amenorrhea in patients with Hodgkin's disease treated with antineoplastic agents. *Am J Obstet Gynecol.* 1971;109:135–139.
24. Monie IW. Chlorambucil-induced abnormalities of the urogenital system of rat fetuses. *Anat Rec.* 1961;139:145–153.
25. Galton DAG, Israels LG, Nabarro JDN, Till M. Clinical trials of p-(DI-2-chloroethylamino)-phenylbutyric acid (CB 1348) in malignant lymphoma. *Br Med J.* 1955;2:1172–1176.
26. Ciobanu N, Runowicz C, Gucalp R, et al. Reversible central nervous system toxicity associated with high-dose chlorambucil in autologous bone marrow transplantation for ovarian carcinoma. *Cancer Treat Rep.* 1987;71:1324–1325.
27. Moore GE, Bross ID, Ausman R, et al. Effects of chlorambucil (NSC-3088) in 374 patients with advanced cancer. Eastern Clinical Drug Evaluation Program. *Cancer Chemother Rep.* 1968;52(pt 1):661–666.
28. Galton DA, Wiltshaw E, Szur L, Dacie JV. The use of chlorambucil and steroids in the treatment of chronic lymphocytic leukemia. *Br J Haematol.* 1961;7:73–98.
29. Rudd P, Fries JF, Epstein WV. Irreversible bone marrow failure with chlorambucil. *J Rheumatol.* 1975;2:421–429.
30. Wolfson S, Olney MB. Accidental ingestion of a toxic dose of chlorambucil: report of a case in a child. *JAMA.* 1957;165:239–240.
31. Byrne TN, Moseley TAE, Finer MA. Myoclonic seizures following chlorambucil overdose. *Ann Neurol.* 1981;9:191–194.
32. LaDelfa I, Bayer N, Myers R, Hoffstein V. Chlorambucil-induced myoclonic seizures in an adult. *J Clin Oncol.* 1985;3:1691–1692.
33. Naysmith A, Robson RH: Focal fits during chlorambucil therapy. *Postgrad Med J.* 1979;55:806–807.
34. Blank DW, Nanji AA, Schreiber DH, Hudman C, Sanders HD. Acute renal failure and seizures associated with chlorambucil overdose. *J Toxicol Clin Toxicol.* 1983;20:361–365.
35. Ammenti A, Reitter B, Muller-Wiefel DE. Chlorambucil neurotoxicity: report of two cases. *Helv Paediatr Acta.* 1980;35:281–287.
36. Green AA, Naiman JL. Chlorambucil poisoning. *Am J Dis Child.* 1968;116:190–191.
37. Enck RE, Bennett JM. Inadvertent chlorambucil overdose in adults. *NY State J Med.* 1977;77:1480–1481.
38. Knospe WH, Loeb V Jr, Huguley CM. Bi-weekly chlorambucil treatment of chronic lymphocytic leukemia. *Cancer.* 1974;33:555–562.
39. Sawitsky A, Rai KR, Glidewell O, et al. Comparison of daily versus intermittent chlorambucil and prednisone therapy in the treatment of patients with chronic lymphocytic leukemia. *Blood.* 1977;50:1049–1059.
40. Recommendations for the safe handling of parenteral antineoplastic drugs. Washington, DC: Division of Safety; National Institutes of Health; 1983. US Dept of Health and Human Services, Public Health Service publication NIH 83-2621.
41. AMA Council on Scientific Affairs. Guidelines for handling parenteral antineoplastics. *JAMA.* 1985;253: 1590–1591.
42. National Study Commission on Cytotoxic Exposure. Recommendations for handling cytotoxic agents. 1987. Available from Louis P. Jeffrey, Chairman, National Study Commission on Cytotoxic Exposure. Massachusetts College of Pharmacy and Allied Health Sciences, 179 Longwood Avenue, Boston, MA, 02115.
43. Clinical Oncological Society of Australia. Guidelines and recommendations for safe handling of antineoplastic agents. *Med J Australia.* 1983;1:426–428.
44. Jones RB, Frank R, Mass T. Safe handling of chemotherapeutic agents: a report from the Mount Sinai Medical Center. *CA-A Cancer J for Clin.* 1983;33:258–263.
45. American Society of Hospital Pharmacists. ASHP technical assistance bulletin on handling cytotoxic and hazardous drugs. *Am J Hosp Pharm.* 1990;47:1033–1049.
46. Yodaiken RE, Bennett D. OSHA work-practice guidelines for personnel dealing with cytotoxic (antineoplastic) drugs. *Am J Hosp Pharm.* 1986;43:1193–1204.

April 1996/RL-307

Shown in Product Identification Guide, page 316

MEPRON® ℞
[mĕ'prŏn]
(atovaquone)
Suspension

DESCRIPTION

MEPRON (atovaquone) is an antiprotozoal agent. The chemical name of atovaquone is *trans*-2-[4-(4-chlorophenyl)cyclohexyl]-3-hydroxy-1,4-naphthalenedione. Atovaquone is a yellow crystalline solid that is practically insoluble in water. It has a molecular weight of 366.84 and the molecular formula $C_{22}H_{19}ClO_3$.

MEPRON Suspension is a formulation of micro-fine particles of atovaquone. The atovaquone particles, which were reduced in size to facilitate absorption, are significantly smaller than those in the previously marketed tablet formulation. MEPRON Suspension is for oral administration and is bright yellow with a citrus flavor. Each teaspoonful (5 mL) contains 750 mg of atovaquone and the inactive ingredients benzyl alcohol, flavor, poloxamer 188, purified water, saccharin sodium, and xanthan gum.

CLINICAL PHARMACOLOGY

Mechanism of Action: Atovaquone is a hydroxy-1,4-naphthoquinone, an analog of ubiquinone, with antipneumocystis activity. The mechanism of action against *Pneumocystis carinii* has not been fully elucidated. In *Plasmodium* species, the site of action appears to be the cytochrome bc_1 complex (Complex III). Several metabolic enzymes are linked to the mitochondrial electron transport chain via ubiquinone. Inhibition of electron transport by atovaquone will result in indirect inhibition of these enzymes. The ultimate metabolic effects of such blockade may include inhibition of nucleic acid and ATP synthesis.

Microbiology:

Pneumocystis carinii: Several laboratories, using different in vitro methodologies, have shown the IC_{50} (50% Inhibitory Concentration) of atovaquone against rat *P. carinii* to be in the range of 0.1 to 3.0 µg/mL.

Pharmacokinetics:

Absorption: Atovaquone is a highly lipophilic compound with low aqueous solubility. The bioavailability of atovaquone is highly dependent on formulation and diet. The suspension formulation provides an approximately two-fold increase in atovaquone bioavailability in the fasting or fed state compared to the previously marketed tablet formulation. The absolute bioavailability of a 750 mg dose of MEPRON Suspension administered under fed conditions in nine HIV-infected (CD4 > 100 cells/mm³) volunteers was 47% ± 15%. In the same study, the bioavailability of a 750 mg dose of the previously marketed tablet formulation was 23% ± 11%.

Administering atovaquone with food enhances its absorption by approximately two-fold. In one study, 16 healthy volunteers received a single dose of 750 mg MEPRON Suspension after an overnight fast and following a standard breakfast (23 g fat: 610 kCal). The mean (±SD) area under the concentration-time curve (AUC) values were 324±115 and 801±320 hr·µg/mL under fasting and fed conditions, respectively, representing a 2.6±1.0 fold increase. The effect of food (23 g fat: 400 kCal) on plasma atovaquone concentrations was also evaluated in a multiple-dose, randomized, crossover study in 19 HIV-infected volunteers (CD4 < 200 cells/mm³) receiving daily doses of 500 mg MEPRON Suspension. AUC was 280±114 hr·µg/mL when atovaquone was administered with food as compared to 169±77 hr·µg/mL under fasting conditions. Maximum plasma atovaquone concentration (C_{max}) was 15.1±6.1 and 8.8±3.7 µg/mL when atovaquone was administered with food and under fasting conditions, respectively.

Dose Proportionality: Plasma atovaquone concentrations do not increase proportionally with dose. When MEPRON Suspension was administered with food at dosage regimens of 500 mg once daily, 750 mg once daily, and 1000 mg once daily, average steady-state plasma atovaquone concentrations were 11.7±4.8, 12.5±5.8, and 13.5±5.1 µg/mL, respectively. The corresponding C_{max} concentrations were 15.1±6.1, 15.3±7.6, and 16.8±6.4 µg/mL. When MEPRON Suspension was administered to five HIV-infected volunteers at a dose of 750 mg twice daily, the average steady-state plasma atovaquone concentration was 21.0±4.9 µg/mL and C_{max} was 24.0±5.7 µg/mL. The minimum plasma atovaquone concentration (C_{min}) associated with the 750 mg twice daily regimen was 16.7±4.6 µg/mL.

Distribution: Following the intravenous administration of atovaquone, the volume of distribution at steady state (Vd_{ss})

was 0.60±0.17 L/kg (n=9). Atovaquone is extensively bound to plasma proteins (99.9%) over the concentration range of 1 to 90 μg/mL. In three HIV-infected children who received 750 mg atovaquone as the tablet formulation four times daily for 2 weeks, the cerebrospinal fluid concentrations of atovaquone were 0.04 μg/mL, 0.14 μg/mL, and 0.26 μg/mL, representing less than 1% of the plasma concentration.

Elimination: The plasma clearance of atovaquone following intravenous administration in nine HIV-infected volunteers was 10.4±5.5 mL/min (0.15±0.09 mL/min/kg). The half-life of atovaquone was 62.5±35.3 hours after I.V. administration and ranged from 67.0±33.4 to 77.6±23.1 hours across studies following administration of MEPRON Suspension. The half-life of atovaquone is long due to presumed enterohepatic cycling and eventual fecal elimination. In a study where ^{14}C-labelled atovaquone was administered to healthy volunteers, greater than 94% of the dose was recovered as unchanged atovaquone in the feces over 21 days. There was little or no excretion of atovaquone in the urine (less than 0.6%). There is indirect evidence that atovaquone may undergo limited metabolism; however, a specific metabolite has not been identified.

Special Populations:

Pediatrics: Preliminary analysis of an ongoing study of MEPRON Suspension in 15 HIV-infected, asymptomatic infants and children between 1 month and 13 years of age suggests that the pharmacokinetics of atovaquone is age dependent. Those between 2 and 13 years of age achieved average steady-state plasma atovaquone concentrations of 16.8±6.4 μg/mL and 37.1±10.9 μg/mL when given doses of 10 and 30 mg/kg, respectively. Those between 3 and 24 months of age achieved average steady-state plasma atovaquone concentrations of 5.7±5.1 μg/mL and 8.9±3.1 μg/mL when given doses of 10 and 30 mg/kg, respectively.

Hepatic/Renal Impairment: The pharmacokinetics of atovaquone has not been studied in patients with hepatic or renal impairment.

Drug Interactions:

Rifampin: In a study with 13 HIV-infected volunteers, the oral administration of rifampin 600 mg every 24 hours with MEPRON Suspension 750 mg every 12 hours resulted in a 52%±13% decrease in the average steady-state plasma atovaquone concentration and a 37%±42% increase in the average steady-state plasma rifampin concentration. The half-life of atovaquone decreased from 82±36 hours when administered without rifampin to 50±16 hours with rifampin.

Rifabutin, another rifamycin, is structurally similar to rifampin and may possibly have some of the same drug interactions as rifampin. No interaction trials have been conducted with MEPRON and rifabutin.

Trimethoprim/Sulfamethoxazole (TMP-SMX): The possible interaction between atovaquone and TMP-SMX was evaluated in six HIV-infected adult volunteers as part of a larger multiple-dose, dose-escalation, and chronic dosing study of MEPRON Suspension. In this cross-over study, MEPRON Suspension 500 mg once daily, or SEPTRA® DS Tablets (160 mg trimethoprim and 800 mg sulfamethoxazole) twice daily, or the combination were administered with food to achieve steady state. No difference was observed in the average steady-state plasma atovaquone concentration after co-administration with TMP-SMX. Co-administration of MEPRON with TMP-SMX resulted in a 17% and 8% decrease in average steady-state concentrations of trimethoprim and sulfamethoxazole in plasma, respectively. This effect is minor and would not be expected to produce clinically significant events.

Zidovudine: Data from 14 HIV-infected volunteers who were given atovaquone tablets 750 mg every 12 hours with zidovudine 200 mg every 8 hours showed a 24%±12% decrease in zidovudine apparent oral clearance, leading to a 35%±23% increase in plasma zidovudine AUC. The glucuronide metabolite:parent ratio decreased from a mean of 4.5 when zidovudine was administered alone to 3.1 when zidovudine was administered with atovaquone tablets. This effect is minor and would not be expected to produce clinically significant events. Zidovudine had no effect on atovaquone pharmacokinetics.

Relationship Between Plasma Atovaquone Concentration and Clinical Outcome: In a comparative study of atovaquone tablets with trimethoprim-sulfamethoxazole (TMP-SMX) for oral treatment of mild to moderate *Pneumocystis carinii* pneumonia (PCP) (see INDICATIONS AND USAGE), where AIDS patients received 750 mg atovaquone tablets three times daily for 21 days, the mean steady-state atovaquone concentration was 13.9±6.9 μg/mL (n=133). Analysis of these data established a relationship between plasma atovaquone concentration and successful treatment. This is shown in Table 1.

Table 1
Relationship Between Plasma Atovaquone Concentration and Successful Treatment

Steady-State Plasma Atovaquone Concentrations (μg/mL)	Successful Treatment* (No. Successes/No. in Group) (%) Observed		Predicted †	
0 to <5	0/6	(0%)	1.5/6	(25%)
5 to <10	18/26	(69%)	14.7/26	(57%)
10 to <15	30/38	(79%)	31.9/38	(84%)
15 to <20	18/19	(95%)	18.1/19	(95%)
20 to <25	18/18	(100%)	17.8/18	(99%)
25+	6/6	(100%)	6/6	(100%)

*Successful treatment was defined as improvement in clinical and respiratory measures persisting at least 4 weeks after cessation of therapy. This was based on data from patients for which both outcome and steady-state plasma atovaquone concentration data are available.

†Based on logistic regression analysis.

[See table above.]

A dosing regimen of MEPRON Suspension for the treatment of mild to moderate PCP has been selected to achieve average plasma atovaquone concentrations of approximately 20 μg/mL, because this plasma concentration was previously shown to be well tolerated and associated with the highest treatment success rates (Table 1). In an open-label PCP treatment study with MEPRON Suspension, dosing regimens of 1000 mg once daily, 750 mg twice daily, 1500 mg once daily, and 1000 mg twice daily were explored. The average steady-state plasma atovaquone concentration achieved at the 750 mg twice daily dose given with meals was 22.0±10.1 μg/mL (n=18).

INDICATIONS AND USAGE

MEPRON Suspension is indicated for the acute oral treatment of mild to moderate *Pneumocystis carinii* pneumonia (PCP) in patients who are intolerant to trimethoprim-sulfamethoxazole (TMP-SMX).

This indication is based on the results of comparative pharmacokinetic studies of the suspension and tablet formulations (see CLINICAL PHARMACOLOGY) and clinical efficacy studies of the tablet formulation which established a relationship between plasma atovaquone concentration and successful treatment. The results of a randomized, double-blind trial comparing MEPRON to TMP-SMX in AIDS patients with mild to moderate PCP (defined in the study protocol as an alveolar-arterial oxygen diffusion gradient $[(A\text{-}a)DO_2]^1 \leq 45$ mm Hg and $PaO_2 \geq 60$ mm Hg on room air) and a randomized trial comparing MEPRON to intravenous pentamidine isethionate in patients with mild to moderate PCP intolerant to trimethoprim or sulfa-antimicrobials are summarized below:

TMP-SMX Comparative Study: This double-blind, randomized trial initiated in 1990 was designed to compare the safety and efficacy of MEPRON to that of TMP-SMX for the treatment of AIDS patients with histologically confirmed PCP. Only patients with mild to moderate PCP were eligible for enrollment.

A total of 408 patients were enrolled into the trial at 37 study centers. Eighty-six patients without histologic confirmation of PCP were excluded from the efficacy analyses. Of the 322 patients with histologically confirmed PCP, 160 were randomized to receive MEPRON and 162 to TMP-SMX.

Study participants randomized to treatment with MEPRON were to receive 750 mg MEPRON (three 250 mg tablets) three times daily for 21 days and those randomized to TMP-SMX were to receive 320 mg TMP plus 1600 mg SMX three times daily for 21 days.

Therapy success was defined as improvement in clinical and respiratory measures persisting at least 4 weeks after cessation of therapy. Therapy failures included lack of response, treatment discontinuation due to an adverse experience, and unevaluable.

There was a significant difference (P =0.03) in mortality rates between the treatment groups. Among the 322 patients with confirmed PCP, 13 of 160 (8%) patients treated with MEPRON and four of 162 (2.5%) patients receiving TMP-SMX died during the 21-day treatment course or 8-week follow-up period. In the intent-to-treat analysis for all 408 randomized patients, there were 16 (8%) deaths in the arm treated with MEPRON and seven (3.4%) deaths in the TMP-SMX arm (P =0.051). Of the 13 patients treated with MEPRON who died, four died of PCP and five died with a combination of bacterial infections and PCP; bacterial infections did not appear to be a factor in any of the four deaths among TMP-SMX-treated patients.

A correlation between plasma atovaquone concentrations and death was demonstrated; in general, patients with lower plasma concentrations were more likely to die. For those patients for whom day 4 plasma atovaquone concentration data are available, five (63%) of the eight patients with concentrations <5 μg/mL died during participation in the study. However, only one (2.0%) of the 49 patients with day 4 plasma atovaquone concentrations ≥5 μg/mL died.

Sixty-two percent of patients on MEPRON and 64% of patients on TMP-SMX were classified as protocol-defined therapy successes (Table 2).

Table 2
Outcome of Treatment for PCP-Positive Patients Enrolled in the TMP-SMX Comparative Study

Outcome of Therapy*	Number of patients (% of Total) MEPRON® (n=160)		TMP-SMX (n=162)		P Value
Therapy Success	99	(62%)	103	(64%)	0.75
Therapy Failure					
–Lack of Response	28	(17%)	10	(6%)	<0.01
–Adverse Experience	11	(7%)	33	(20%)	<0.01
–Unevaluable	22	(14%)	16	(10%)	0.28
Required Alternate PCP Therapy During Study	55	(34%)	55	(34%)	0.95

*As defined by the protocol and described in study description above.

The failure rate due to lack of response was significantly larger for patients receiving MEPRON while the failure rate due to adverse experiences was significantly larger for patients receiving TMP-SMX .

There were no significant differences in the effect of either treatment on additional indicators of response (i.e., arterial blood gas measurements, vital signs, serum LDH levels, clinical symptoms, and chest radiographs).

Pentamidine Comparative Study: This unblinded, randomized trial initiated in 1991 was designed to compare the safety and efficacy of MEPRON to that of pentamidine for the treatment of histologically confirmed mild or moderate PCP in AIDS patients. Approximately 80% of the patients either had a history of intolerance to trimethoprim or sulfa-antimicrobials (the primary therapy group) or were experiencing intolerance to TMP-SMX with treatment of an episode of PCP at the time of enrollment in the study (the salvage treatment group).

Patients randomized to MEPRON were to receive 750 mg atovaquone (three 250 mg tablets) three times daily for 21 days and those randomized to pentamidine isethionate were to receive a 3 to 4 mg/kg single intravenous infusion daily for 21 days.

A total of 174 patients were enrolled into the trial at 22 study centers. Thirty-nine patients without histologic confirmation of PCP were excluded from the efficacy analyses. Of the 135 patients with histologically confirmed PCP, 70 were randomized to receive MEPRON and 65 to pentamidine. One hundred and ten (110) of these were in the primary therapy group and 25 were in the salvage therapy group. One patient in the primary therapy group randomized to receive pentamidine did not receive study medication.

There was no difference in mortality rates between the treatment groups. Among the 135 patients with confirmed PCP, 10 of 70 (14%) patients randomized to MEPRON and nine of 65 (14%) patients randomized to pentamidine died during the 21-day treatment course or 8-week follow-up period. In the intent-to-treat analysis for all randomized patients, there were 11 (12.5%) deaths in the arm treated with MEPRON and 12 (14%) deaths in the pentamidine arm. For those patients for whom day 4 plasma atovaquone concentrations are available, three of five (60%) patients with concentrations <5 μg/mL died during participation in the study. However, only two of 21 (9%) patients with day 4 plasma concentrations ≥5 μg/mL died.

Continued on next page

Glaxo Wellcome Onc.—Cont.

Table 3
Outcome of Treatment for PCP-Positive Patients Enrolled in the Pentamidine Comparative Study

	Primary Treatment			Salvage Treatment		
Outcome of Therapy	MEPRON® (n=56)	Pentamidine (n=53)	P Value	MEPRON (n=14)	Pentamidine (n=11)	P Value
Therapy Success	32 (57%)	21 (40%)	0.09	13 (93%)	7 (64%)	0.14
Therapy Failure						
—Lack of Response	16 (29%)	9 (17%)	0.18	0	0	—
—Adverse Experience	2 (3.6%)	19 (36%)	<0.01	0	3 (27%)	0.07
—Unevaluable	6 (11%)	4 (8%)	0.75	1 (7%)	1 (9%)	1.00
Required Alternate PCP Therapy During Study	19 (34%)	29 (55%)	0.04	0	4 (36%)	0.03

The therapeutic outcomes for the 134 patients who received study medication in this trial are presented in Table 3. [See table above.]

Data on Chronic Use: MEPRON has not been systematically evaluated as a chronic suppressive agent to prevent the development of PCP in patients at high risk for *Pneumocystis carinii* disease.

CONTRAINDICATIONS

MEPRON Suspension is contraindicated for patients who develop or have a history of potentially life-threatening allergic reactions to any of the components of the formulation.

WARNINGS

Clinical experience with MEPRON has been limited to patients with mild to moderate PCP [(A-a)DO₂ ≤ 45 mm Hg]. Treatment of more severe episodes of PCP has not been systematically studied with this agent. Also, the efficacy of MEPRON in patients who are failing therapy with TMP-SMX has not been systematically studied. MEPRON has not been evaluated as an agent for PCP prophylaxis.

PRECAUTIONS

General: Absorption of orally administered MEPRON is limited but can be significantly increased when the drug is taken with food. Plasma atovaquone concentrations have been shown to correlate with the likelihood of successful treatment and survival. Therefore, parenteral therapy with other agents should be considered for patients who have difficulty taking MEPRON with food (see CLINICAL PHARMACOLOGY). Gastrointestinal disorders may limit absorption of orally administered drugs. Patients with these disorders also may not achieve plasma concentrations of atovaquone associated with response to therapy in controlled trials.

Based upon the spectrum of in vitro antimicrobial activity, atovaquone is not effective therapy for concurrent pulmonary conditions such as bacterial, viral or fungal pneumonia or mycobacterial diseases. Clinical deterioration in patients may be due to infections with other pathogens, as well as progressive PCP. All patients with acute PCP should be carefully evaluated for other possible causes of pulmonary disease and treated with additional agents as appropriate.

Information for Patients: The importance of taking the prescribed dose of MEPRON should be stressed. Patients should be instructed to take their daily doses of MEPRON with meals, as the presence of food will significantly improve the absorption of the drug.

Drug Interactions: Atovaquone is highly bound to plasma protein (>99.9%). Therefore, caution should be used when administering MEPRON concurrently with other highly plasma protein-bound drugs with narrow therapeutic indices, as competition for binding sites may occur. The extent of plasma protein binding of atovaquone in human plasma is not affected by the presence of therapeutic concentrations of phenytoin (15 μg/mL), nor is the binding of phenytoin affected by the presence of atovaquone.

Rifampin: Co-administration of rifampin and MEPRON Suspension results in a significant decrease in average steady-state plasma atovaquone concentration (see CLINICAL PHARMACOLOGY: Drug Interactions). Alternatives to rifampin should be considered during the course of PCP treatment with MEPRON.

Rifabutin, another rifamycin, is structurally similar to rifampin and may possibly have some of the same drug interactions as rifampin. No interaction trials have been conducted with MEPRON and rifabutin.

Drug/Laboratory Test Interactions: It is not known if MEPRON interferes with clinical laboratory test or assay results.

Carcinogenesis, Mutagenesis, Impairment of Fertility: Carcinogenicity studies in rats were negative; 24-month studies in mice showed treatment-related increases in incidence of hepatocellular adenoma and hepatocellular carcinoma at all doses tested which ranged from 1.4 to 3.6 times the average steady-state plasma concentrations in humans during acute treatment of *Pneumocystis carinii* and pneumonia. Atovaq-

uone was negative with or without metabolic activation in the Ames *Salmonella* mutagenicity assay, the Mouse Lymphoma mutagenesis assay, and the Cultured Human Lymphocyte cytogenetic assay. No evidence of genotoxicity was observed in the in vivo Mouse Micronucleus assay.

Pregnancy: Pregnancy Category C. Atovaquone was not teratogenic and did not cause reproductive toxicity in rats at plasma concentrations up to two to three times the estimated human exposure. Atovaquone caused maternal toxicity in rabbits at plasma concentrations that were approximately one-half the estimated human exposure. Mean fetal body lengths and weights were decreased and there were higher numbers of early resorption and post-implantation loss per dam. It is not clear whether these effects were caused by atovaquone directly or were secondary to maternal toxicity. Concentrations of atovaquone in rabbit fetuses averaged 30% of the concurrent maternal plasma concentrations. In a separate study in rats given a single ¹⁴C-radiolabelled dose, concentrations of radiocarbon in rat fetuses were 18% (middle gestation) and 60% (late gestation) of concurrent maternal plasma concentrations. There are no adequate and well-controlled studies in pregnant women. MEPRON should be used during pregnancy only if the potential benefit justifies the potential risk to the fetus.

Nursing Mothers: It is not known whether atovaquone is excreted into human milk. Because many drugs are excreted into human milk, caution should be exercised when MEPRON is administered to a nursing woman. In a rat study, atovaquone concentrations in the milk were 30% of the concurrent atovaquone concentrations in the maternal plasma.

Pediatric Use: Safety and effectiveness in pediatric patients have not been established. Clinical experience with MEPRON Suspension in the pediatric population is limited to a pharmacokinetic study in children who were at risk of developing PCP. Preliminary analysis of a study of MEPRON Suspension in 15 HIV-infected, asymptomatic infants and children between 1 month and 13 years of age suggests that the pharmacokinetics of atovaquone is age dependent (see CLINICAL PHARMACOLOGY; Special Populations). No treatment-limiting adverse events were observed.

Geriatric Use: MEPRON has not been systematically evaluated in patients greater than 65 years of age. Caution should be exercised when treating elderly patients reflecting the greater frequency of decreased hepatic, renal, and cardiac function in this population.

ADVERSE REACTIONS

Because many patients who participated in clinical trials with MEPRON had complications of advanced HIV disease, it was often difficult to distinguish adverse events caused by MEPRON from those caused by underlying medical conditions. There were no life-threatening or fatal adverse experiences caused by MEPRON.

Table 4 summarizes all the clinical adverse experiences reported by ≥5% of the study population during the TMP-SMX comparative study of MEPRON (n=408), regardless of attribution. The incidence of adverse experiences with MEPRON Suspension at the recommended dose was similar to that seen with the tablet formulation of atovaquone.

Table 4
Treatment-Emergent Adverse Experiences in the TMP-SMX Comparative PCP Treatment Study

Treatment-Emergent Adverse Experience	Number of Patients with Treatment-Emergent Adverse Experience (% of Total)	
	MEPRON® (n=203)	TMP-SMX (n=205)
Rash (including maculopapular)	47 (23%)	69 (34%)*
Nausea	43 (21%)	90 (44%)*
Diarrhea	39 (19%)*	15 (7%)
Headache	33 (16%)	44 (22%)
Vomiting	29 (14%)	72 (35%)*
Fever	28 (14%)	52 (25%)*
Insomnia	20 (10%)	18 (9%)
Asthenia	17 (8%)	16 (8%)
Pruritus	11 (5%)	18 (9%)
Monilia, Oral	11 (5%)	21 (10%)
Abdominal Pain	9 (4%)	15 (7%)
Constipation	7 (3%)	35 (17%)*
Dizziness	7 (3%)	17 (8%)*
No. Patients Discontinuing Therapy due to an Adverse Experience	19 (9%)	50 (24%)*
No. Patients Reporting at least one Adverse Experience	127 (63%)	134 (65%)

*P<0.05.

Although an equal percentage of patients receiving MEPRON and TMP-SMX reported at least one adverse experience, more patients receiving TMP-SMX required discontinuation of therapy due to an adverse event. Twenty-four percent of patients receiving TMP-SMX were prematurely discontinued from therapy due to an adverse experience versus 9% of patients receiving MEPRON. Four percent of patients receiving MEPRON had therapy discontinued due to development of rash. The majority of cases of rash among patients receiving MEPRON were mild and did not require the discontinuation of dosing. The only other clinical adverse experience that led to premature discontinuation of dosing of MEPRON by more than one patient was vomiting (<1%). The most common adverse experience requiring discontinuation of dosing in the TMP-SMX group was rash (8%).

Laboratory test abnormalities reported for ≥5% of the study population during the treatment period are summarized in Table 5. Two percent of patients treated with MEPRON and 7% of patients treated with TMP-SMX had therapy prematurely discontinued due to elevations in ALT/AST. In general, patients treated with MEPRON developed fewer abnormalities in measures of hepatocellular function (ALT, AST, alkaline phosphatase) or amylase values than patients treated with TMP-SMX.

Table 5
Treatment-Emergent Laboratory Test Abnormalities in the TMP-SMX Comparative PCP Treatment Study

Laboratory Test Abnormality	Patients Developing a Laboratory Test Abnormality (% of Total)	
	MEPRON®	TMP-SMX
Anemia (Hgb<8.0 g/dL)	6%	7%
Neutropenia (ANC<750 cells/mm³)	3%	9%
Elevated ALT (>5 × ULN)	6%	16%
Elevated AST (>5 × ULN)	4%	14%
Elevated Alkaline Phosphatase (>2.5 × ULN)	8%	6%
Elevated Amylase (>1.5 × ULN)	7%	12%
Hyponatremia (<0.96 × LLN)	7%	26%

ULN=upper limit of normal range
LLN=lower limit of normal range

Table 6 summarizes the clinical adverse experiences reported by ≥5% of the primary therapy study 000population (n=144) during the comparative trial of MEPRON and intravenous pentamidine, regardless of attribution. A slightly lower percentage of patients who received MEPRON reported occurrence of adverse events than did those who received pentamidine (63% vs 72%). However, only 7% of patients discontinued treatment with MEPRON due to adverse events, while 41% of patients who received pentamidine discontinued treatment for this reason (P<0.001). Of the five patients who discontinued therapy with MEPRON, three reported rash (4%). Rash was not severe in any patient. No other reason for discontinuation of MEPRON was cited more than once. The most frequently cited reasons for discontinuation of pentamidine therapy were hypoglycemia (11%) and vomiting (9%).

Table 6
Treatment-Emergent Adverse Experiences in the Pentamidine Comparative PCP Treatment Study (Primary Therapy Group)

Treatment-Emergent Adverse Experience	Number of Patients with Treatment-Emergent Adverse Experience (% of Total)	
	MEPRON® (n=73)	Pentamidine (n=71)
Fever	29 (40%)	18 (25%)
Nausea	16 (22%)	26 (37%)
Rash	16 (22%)	9 (13%)
Diarrhea	15 (21%)	22 (31%)
Insomnia	14 (19%)	10 (14%)
Headache	13 (18%)	20 (28%)
Vomiting	10 (14%)	12 (17%)
Cough	10 (14%)*	1 (1%)
Abdominal Pain	7 (10%)	8 (11%)
Pain	7 (10%)	7 (10%)
Sweat	7 (10%)	2 (3%)
Monilia, Oral	7 (10%)	2 (3%)
Asthenia	6 (8%)	10 (14%)
Dizziness	6 (8%)	10 (14%)
Anxiety	5 (7%)	7 (10%)
Anorexia	5 (7%)	7 (10%)
Sinusitis	5 (7%)	4 (6%)
Dyspepsia	4 (5%)	7 (10%)
Rhinitis	4 (5%)	5 (7%)
Taste Perversion	2 (3%)	9 (13%)*
Hypoglycemia	1 (1%)	11 (15%)*
Hypotension	1 (1%)	7 (10%)*
No. Patients Discontinuing Therapy due to an Adverse Experience	5 (7%)	29 (41%)†
No. Patients Reporting at least one Adverse Experience	46 (63%)	51 (72%)

* P<0.05.
† P<0.001.

Laboratory test abnormalities reported in ≥5% of patients in the pentamidine comparative study are presented in Table 7. Laboratory abnormality was reported as the reason for discontinuation of treatment in two of 73 patients who received MEPRON. One patient (1%) had elevated creatinine and BUN levels and one patient (1%) had elevated amylase levels. Laboratory abnormalities were the sole or contributing factor in 14 patients who prematurely discontinued pentamidine therapy. In the 71 patients who received

pentamidine, laboratory parameters most frequently reported as reasons for discontinuation were hypoglycemia (11%), elevated creatinine levels (6%), and leukopenia (4%).

Table 7
Treatment-Emergent Laboratory Test Abnormalities in the Pentamidine Comparative PCP Treatment Study

Laboratory Test Abnormality	Patients Developing a Laboratory Test Abnormality (% of Total)	
	MEPRON®	Pentamidine
Anemia (Hgb<8.0 g/dL)	4%	9%
Neutropenia (ANC<750 cells/mm³)	5%	9%
Hyponatremia (<0.96 × LLN)	10%	10%
Hyperkalemia (>1.18 × ULN)	0%	5%
Alkaline Phosphatase (>2.5 × ULN)	5%	2%
Hyperglycemia (>1.8 × ULN)	9%	13%
Elevated AST (>5 × ULN)	0%	5%
Elevated Amylase (>1.5 × ULN)	8%	4%
Elevated Creatinine (>1.5 × ULN)	0%	7%

ULN=upper limit of normal range
LLN=lower limit of normal range

OVERDOSAGE

There have been no reports of overdosage from the administration of MEPRON.

DOSAGE AND ADMINISTRATION

The recommended oral dose is 750 mg (5 mL) administered with meals twice daily for 21 days (total daily dose 1500 mg). Failure to administer MEPRON Suspension with meals may result in lower plasma atovaquone concentrations and may limit response to therapy (see CLINICAL PHARMACOLOGY and PRECAUTIONS).
SHAKE GENTLY BEFORE USING.

HOW SUPPLIED

MEPRON Suspension (bright yellow, citrus flavored) containing 750 mg atovaquone in each teaspoonful (5 mL).
Bottle of 210 mL with child-resistant cap (NDC 0173-0665-18).
Store at 15° to 25°C (59° to 77°F). DO NOT FREEZE. Dispense in tight container as defined in U.S.P.
^{1}(A-a)DO$_2$=[(713 × FiO$_2$) - (PaCO$_2$/0.8)] - PaO$_2$ (mmHg)
U.S. Patent No. 5053432
U.S. Patent No. 4981874 (Use Patent)
June 1996/RL-330

Shown in Product Identification Guide, page 316

MYLERAN® ℞
[mǐ'lə-răn"]
(busulfan)
2 mg Scored Tablets

DESCRIPTION

MYLERAN (busulfan) is a bifunctional alkylating agent. Busulfan is known chemically as 1,4-butanediol dimethanesulfonate.
Busulfan is *not* a structural analog of the nitrogen mustards.
MYLERAN is available in tablet form for oral administration. Each scored tablet contains 2 mg busulfan and the inactive ingredients magnesium stearate and sodium chloride.
The activity of busulfan in chronic myelogenous leukemia was first reported by D.A.G. Galton in 1953.[1]

CLINICAL PHARMACOLOGY

No analytical method has been found which permits the quantitation of non-radiolabeled busulfan or its metabolites in biological tissues or plasma. All studies of the pharmacokinetics of busulfan in humans have employed radiolabeled drug using either sulfur-35 (labeling the "carrier" portion of the molecule) or carbon-14 or tritium in the alkane portion of the 4-carbon chain (labels in the "alkylating" portion of the molecule).
Studies with ^{35}S-busulfan.[2] Following the intravenous administration of a single therapeutic dose of ^{35}S-busulfan, there was rapid disappearance of radioactivity from the blood; 90% to 95% of the ^{35}S-label disappeared within 3 to 5 minutes after injection. Thereafter, a constant, low level of radioactivity (1% to 3% of the injected dose) was maintained during the subsequent 48-hour period of observation. Following the oral administration of ^{35}S-busulfan, there was a lag period of $^1/_2$ to 2 hours prior to the detection of radioactivity in the blood. However, at 4 hours the (low) level of circulating radioactivity was comparable to that obtained following intravenous administration.
After either oral or intravenous administration of ^{35}S-busulfan to humans, 45% to 60% of the radioactivity was recovered in the urine in the 48 hours after administration; the majority of the total urinary excretion occurred in the first 24 hours. In man, over 95% of the urinary sulfur-35 occurs as ^{35}S-methanesulfonic acid.
The fact that urinary recovery of sulfur-35 was equivalent, irrespective of whether the drug was given intravenously or orally, suggests virtually complete absorption by the oral route.
Studies with ^{14}C-busulfan.[2] Oral and intravenous administration of 1,4-^{14}C-busulfan showed the same rapid initial disappearance of plasma radioactivity with a subsequent low-level plateau as observed following the administration of ^{35}S-labeled drug. Cumulative radioactivity in the urine after 48 hours was 25% to 30% of the administered dose (contrasting with 45% to 60% for ^{35}S-busulfan) and suggests a slower excretion of the alkylating portion of the molecule and its metabolites than for the sulfonoxymethyl moieties. Regardless of the route of administration, 1,4-^{14}C-busulfan yielded a complex mixture of at least 12 radiolabeled metabolites in urine; the main metabolite being 3-hydroxytetrahydrothiophene-1, 1-dioxide.
Studies with ^{3}H-busulfan.[3] Human pharmacokinetic studies have been conducted employing busulfan labeled with tritium on the tetramethylene chain. These experiments confirmed a rapid initial clearance of the radioactivity from plasma, irrespective of whether the drug was given orally or intravenously, and showed a gradual accumulation of radioactivity in the plasma after repeated doses. Urinary excretion of less than 50% of the total dose given suggested a slow elimination of the metabolic products from the body.
There is no experience with the use of dialysis in an attempt to modify the clinical toxicity of busulfan. One technical difficulty would derive from the extremely poor water solubility of busulfan. Additionally, all studies of the metabolism of busulfan employing radiolabeled materials indicate rapid chemical reactivity of the parent compound with prolonged retention of some of the metabolites (particularly the metabolites arising from the "alkylating" portion of the molecule). The effectiveness of dialysis at removing significant quantities of unreacted drug would be expected to be minimal in such a situation.
No information is available regarding the penetration of busulfan into brain or cerebrospinal fluid.
Biochemical Pharmacology: In aqueous media, busulfan undergoes a wide range of nucleophilic substitution reactions. While this chemical reactivity is relatively non-specific, alkylation of the DNA is felt to be an important biological mechanism for its cytotoxic effect.[4] Coliphage T7 exposed to busulfan was found to have the DNA crosslinked by intrastrand crosslinkages, but no interstrand linkages were found.
The metabolic fate of busulfan has been studied in rats and humans using ^{14}C- and ^{35}S-labeled materials.[2,5,6] In humans,[2] as in the rat,[6] almost all of the radioactivity in ^{35}S-labeled busulfan is excreted in the urine in the form of ^{35}S-methanesulfonic acid. No unchanged drug was found in human urine,[2] although a small amount has been reported in rat urine.[6] Roberts and Warwick demonstrated that the for-

Continued on next page

Glaxo Wellcome Onc.—Cont.

mation of methanesulfonic acid in vivo in the rat is not due to a simple hydrolysis of busulfan to 1,4-butanediol, since only about 4% of 2,3-^{14}C-busulfan was excreted as carbon dioxide whereas 2,3-^{14}C-1,4-butanediol was converted almost exclusively to carbon dioxide.[5] The predominant reaction of busulfan in the rat is the alkylation of sulfhydryl groups (particularly cysteine and cysteine-containing compounds) to produce a cyclic sulfonium compound which is the precursor of the major urinary metabolite of the 4-carbon portion of the molecule, 3-hydroxytetrahydrothiophene-1, 1-dioxide.[5] This has been termed a "sulfur-stripping" action of busulfan and it may modify the function of certain sulfur-containing amino acids, polypeptides, and proteins; whether this action makes an important contribution to the cytotoxicity of busulfan is unknown.

The biochemical basis for acquired resistance to busulfan is largely a matter of speculation. Although altered transport of busulfan into the cell is one possibility, increased intracellular inactivation of the drug before it reaches the DNA is also possible. Experiments with other alkylating agents have shown that resistance to this class of compounds may reflect an acquired ability of the resistant cell to repair alkylation damage more effectively.[4]

INDICATIONS AND USAGE

MYLERAN (busulfan) is indicated for the palliative treatment of chronic myelogenous (myeloid, myelocytic, granulocytic) leukemia. Although not curative, busulfan reduces the total granulocyte mass, relieves symptoms of the disease, and improves the clinical state of the patient. Approximately 90% of adults with previously untreated chronic myelogenous leukemia will obtain hematologic remission with regression or stabilization of organomegaly following the use of busulfan. It has been shown to be superior to splenic irradiation with respect to survival times and maintenance of hemoglobin levels, and to be equivalent to irradiation at controlling splenomegaly.[7]

It is not clear whether busulfan unequivocally prolongs the survival of responding patients beyond the 31 months experienced by an untreated group of historical controls.[8] Median survival figures of 31 to 42 months have been reported for several groups of patients treated with busulfan, but concurrent control groups of comparable, untreated patients are not available.[7,9,10,11] The median survival figures reported from different studies will be influenced by the percentage of "poor risk" patients initially entered into the particular study. Patients who are alive 2 years following the diagnosis of chronic myelogenous leukemia, and who have been treated during that period with busulfan, are estimated to have a mean annual mortality rate during the second to fifth year which is approximately two-thirds that of patients who received either no treatment, conventional x-ray or ^{32}P-irradiation, or chemotherapy with minimally active drugs.[12] Busulfan is clearly less effective in patients with chronic myelogenous leukemia who lack the Philadelphia (Ph^1) chromosome.[13] Also, the so-called "juvenile" type of chronic myelogenous leukemia, typically occurring in young children and associated with the absence of a Philadelphia chromosome, responds poorly to busulfan.[14] The drug is of no benefit in patients whose chronic myelogenous leukemia has entered a "blastic" phase.

CONTRAINDICATIONS

MYLERAN should not be used unless a diagnosis of chronic myelogenous leukemia has been adequately established and the responsible physician is knowledgeable in assessing response to chemotherapy.

MYLERAN should not be used in patients whose chronic myelogenous leukemia has demonstrated prior resistance to this drug.

MYLERAN is of no value in chronic lymphocytic leukemia, acute leukemia, or in the "blastic crisis" of chronic myelogenous leukemia.

WARNINGS

The most frequent, serious side effect of treatment with busulfan is the induction of bone marrow failure (which may or may not be anatomically hypoplastic) resulting in severe pancytopenia. The pancytopenia caused by busulfan may be more prolonged than that induced with other alkylating agents. It is generally felt that the usual cause of busulfan-induced pancytopenia is the failure to stop administration of the drug soon enough; individual idiosyncrasy to the drug does not seem to be an important factor. *MYLERAN should be used with extreme caution and exceptional vigilance in patients whose bone marrow reserve may have been compromised by prior irradiation or chemotherapy, or whose marrow function is recovering from previous cytotoxic therapy.* Although recovery from busulfan-induced pancytopenia may take from 1 month to 2 years, this complication is potentially reversible, and the patient should be vigorously supported through any period of severe pancytopenia.[15]

A rare, important complication of busulfan therapy is the development of bronchopulmonary dysplasia with pulmonary fibrosis.[16] Symptoms have been reported to occur within 8 months to 10 years after initiation of therapy—the average duration of therapy being 4 years. The histologic findings associated with "busulfan lung" mimic those seen following pulmonary irradiation. Clinically, patients have reported the insidious onset of cough, dyspnea, and low-grade fever. Pulmonary function studies have revealed diminished diffusion capacity and decreased pulmonary compliance. It is important to exclude more common conditions (such as opportunistic infections or leukemic infiltration of the lungs) with appropriate diagnostic techniques. If measures such as sputum cultures, virologic studies, and exfoliative cytology fail to establish an etiology for the pulmonary infiltrates, lung biopsy may be necessary to establish the diagnosis. Treatment of established busulfan-induced pulmonary fibrosis is unsatisfactory; in most cases the patients have died within 6 months after the diagnosis was established. There is no specific therapy for this complication other than the immediate discontinuation of busulfan. The administration of corticosteroids has been suggested, but the results have not been impressive or uniformly successful.

Busulfan may cause cellular dysplasia in many organs in addition to the lung. Cytologic abnormalities characterized by giant, hyperchromatic nuclei have been reported in lymph nodes, pancreas, thyroid, adrenal glands, liver, and bone marrow. This cytologic dysplasia may be severe enough to cause difficulty in interpretation of exfoliative cytologic examinations from the lung, bladder, breast, and the uterine cervix.

In addition to the widespread epithelial dysplasia that has been observed during busulfan therapy, chromosome aberrations have been reported in cells from patients receiving busulfan.

Busulfan is mutagenic in mice and, possibly, in humans.

A number of malignant tumors have been reported in patients on busulfan therapy and this drug may be a human carcinogen. Four cases of acute leukemia occurred among 243 patients treated with busulfan as adjuvant chemotherapy following surgical resection of bronchogenic carcinoma. All four cases were from a subgroup of 19 of these 243 patients who developed pancytopenia while taking busulfan 5 to 8 years before leukemia became clinically apparent. These findings suggest that busulfan is leukemogenic, although its mode of action is uncertain.[17]

Ovarian suppression and amenorrhea with menopausal symptoms commonly occur during busulfan therapy in premenopausal patients. Busulfan interferes with spermatogenesis in experimental animals, and there have been clinical reports of sterility, azoospermia, and testicular atrophy in male patients.

Hepatic veno-occlusive disease, which may be life-threatening, has been reported following the investigational use of very high doses of busulfan in combination with cyclophosphamide or other chemotherapeutic agents prior to bone marrow transplantation.[18-24] Possible risk factors for the development of hepatic veno-occlusive disease include: total busulfan dose exceeding 16 mg/kg based on ideal body weight, and concurrent use of multiple alkylating agents. A clear cause and effect relationship with busulfan has not been demonstrated. Periodic measurement of serum transaminases, alkaline phosphatase, and bilirubin is indicated for early detection of hepatotoxicity.

Cardiac tamponade has been reported in a small number of patients with thalassemia (2% in one series) who received high doses of busulfan and cyclophosphamide as the preparatory regimen for bone marrow transplantation. In this series, the cardiac tamponade was often fatal. Abdominal pain and vomiting preceded the tamponade in most patients.

Pregnancy: Pregnancy Category D. Busulfan may cause fetal harm when administered to a pregnant woman. Although there have been a number of cases reported where apparently normal children have been born after busulfan treatment during pregnancy,[25] one case has been cited where a malformed baby was delivered by a mother treated with busulfan. During the pregnancy that resulted in the malformed infant, the mother received x-ray therapy early in the first trimester, mercaptopurine until the third month, then busulfan until delivery.[26] In pregnant rats, busulfan produces sterility in both male and female offspring due to the absence of germinal cells in testes and ovaries.[27] Germinal cell aplasia or sterility in offspring of mothers receiving busulfan during pregnancy has not been reported in humans. There are no adequate and well-controlled studies in pregnant women. If this drug is used during pregnancy, or if the patient becomes pregnant while taking this drug, the patient should be apprised of the potential hazard to the fetus. Women of childbearing potential should be advised to avoid becoming pregnant.

PRECAUTIONS

General: The most consistent, dose-related toxicity is bone marrow suppression. This may be manifest by anemia, leukopenia, thrombocytopenia, or any combination of these. It is imperative that patients be instructed to report promptly the development of fever, sore throat, signs of local infection, bleeding from any site, or symptoms suggestive of anemia.

Any one of these findings may indicate busulfan toxicity; however, they may also indicate transformation of the disease to an acute "blastic" form. Since busulfan may have a delayed effect, it is important to withdraw the medication temporarily at the first sign of an abnormally large or exceptionally rapid fall in any of the formed elements of the blood. *Patients should never be allowed to take the drug without close medical supervision.*

Seizures have been reported in patients receiving very high, investigational doses of busulfan.[18,28-32] As with any potentially epileptogenic drug, caution should be exercised when administering very high doses of busulfan to patients with a history of seizure disorder, head trauma, or receiving other potentially epileptogenic drugs. Some investigators have used prophylactic anticonvulsant therapy in this setting.

Information for Patients: Patients beginning therapy with busulfan should be informed of the importance of having periodic blood counts and to immediately report any unusual fever or bleeding. Aside from the major toxicity of myelosuppression, patients should be instructed to report any difficulty in breathing, persistent cough, or congestion. They should be told that diffuse pulmonary fibrosis is an infrequent, but serious and potentially life-threatening, complication of long-term busulfan therapy. Patients should be alerted to report any signs of abrupt weakness, unusual fatigue, anorexia, weight loss, nausea and vomiting, and melanoderma that could be associated with a syndrome resembling adrenal insufficiency. Patients should never be allowed to take the drug without medical supervision and they should be informed that other encountered toxicities to busulfan include infertility, amenorrhea, skin hyperpigmentation, drug hypersensitivity, dryness of the mucous membranes, and, rarely, cataract formation. Women of childbearing potential should be advised to avoid becoming pregnant. The increased risk of a second malignancy should be explained to the patient.

Laboratory Tests: It is recommended that evaluation of the hemoglobin or hematocrit, total white blood cell count and differential count, and quantitative platelet count be obtained weekly while the patient is on busulfan therapy. In cases where the cause of fluctuation in the formed elements of the peripheral blood is obscure, bone marrow examination may be useful for evaluation of marrow status. A decision to increase, decrease, continue, or discontinue a given dose of busulfan must be based not only on the absolute hematologic values, but also on the rapidity with which changes are occurring. The dosage of busulfan may need to be reduced if this agent is combined with other drugs whose primary toxicity is myelosuppression. Occasional patients may be unusually sensitive to busulfan administered at standard dosage and suffer neutropenia or thrombocytopenia after a relatively short exposure to the drug. Busulfan should not be used where facilities for complete blood counts, including quantitative platelet counts, are not available at weekly (or more frequent) intervals.

Drug Interactions: Busulfan may cause additive myelosuppression when used with other myelosuppressive drugs.

In one study, 12 of approximately 330 patients receiving continuous busulfan and thioguanine therapy for treatment of chronic myelogenous leukemia were found to have esophageal varices associated with abnormal liver function tests.[33] Subsequent liver biopsies were performed in four of these patients, all of which showed evidence of nodular regenerative hyperplasia. Duration of combination therapy prior to the appearance of esophageal varices ranged from 6 to 45 months. With the present analysis of the data, no cases of hepatotoxicity have appeared in the busulfan alone arm of the study. Long-term continuous therapy with thioguanine and busulfan should be used with caution.

Carcinogenesis, Mutagenesis, Impairment of Fertility: See WARNINGS section.

Pregnancy: *Teratogenic effects:* Pregnancy Category D. See WARNINGS section.

Nonteratogenic Effects: There have been reports in the literature of small infants being born after the mothers received busulfan during pregnancy, in particular, during the third trimester.[34] One case was reported where an infant had mild anemia and neutropenia at birth after busulfan was administered to the mother from the eighth week of pregnancy to term.[25]

Nursing Mothers: It is not known whether this drug is excreted in human milk. Because of the potential for tumorigenicity shown for busulfan in animal and human studies, a decision should be made whether to discontinue nursing or to discontinue the drug, taking into account the importance of the drug to the mother.

ADVERSE REACTIONS

Hematological Effects: The most frequent, serious, toxic effect of busulfan is myelosuppression resulting in leukopenia, thrombocytopenia, and anemia. Myelosuppression is most frequently the result of a failure to discontinue dosage in the face of an undetected decrease in leukocyte or platelet counts.[15]

Pulmonary: Interstitial pulmonary fibrosis has been reported rarely, but it is a clinically significant adverse effect

when observed and calls for immediate discontinuation of further administration of the drug. The role of corticosteroids in arresting or reversing the fibrosis has been reported to be beneficial in some cases and without effect in others.[16]

Cardiac: Cardiac tamponade has been reported in a small number of patients with thalassemia who received high doses of busulfan and cyclophosphamide as the preparatory regimen for bone marrow transplantation (see WARNINGS).

One case of endocardial fibrosis has been reported in a 79-year-old woman who received a total dose of 7,200 mg of busulfan over a period of 9 years for the management of chronic myelogenous leukemia.[35] At autopsy, she was found to have endocardial fibrosis of the left ventricle in addition to interstitial pulmonary fibrosis.

Ocular: Busulfan is capable of inducing cataracts in rats and there have been several reports indicating that this is a rare complication in humans. In the few cases reported in humans, cataracts have occurred only after prolonged administration of busulfan.[36]

Dermatologic: Hyperpigmentation is the most common adverse skin reaction and occurs in 5% to 10% of patients, particularly those with a dark complexion.

Metabolic: In a few cases, a clinical syndrome closely resembling adrenal insufficiency and characterized by weakness, severe fatigue, anorexia, weight loss, nausea and vomiting, and melanoderma has developed after prolonged busulfan therapy. The symptoms have sometimes been reversible when busulfan was withdrawn. Adrenal responsiveness to exogenously administered ACTH has usually been normal. However, pituitary function testing with metyrapone revealed a blunted urinary 17-hydroxycorticosteroid excretion in two patients.[37] Following the discontinuation of busulfan (which was associated with clinical improvement), rechallenge with metyrapone revealed normal pituitary-adrenal function.

Hyperuricemia and/or hyperuricosuria are not uncommon in patients with chronic myelogenous leukemia. Additional rapid destruction of granulocytes may accompany the initiation of chemotherapy and increase the urate pool. Adverse effects can be minimized by increased hydration, urine alkalinization, and the prophylactic administration of a xanthine oxidase inhibitor such as ZYLOPRIM® (allopurinol).

Hepatic Effects: Esophageal varices have been reported in patients receiving continuous busulfan and thioguanine therapy for treatment of chronic myelogenous leukemia (see PRECAUTIONS: Drug Interactions). Hepatic veno-occlusive disease has been observed in patients receiving higher than recommended doses of busulfan (see WARNINGS).

Miscellaneous: Other reported adverse reactions include: urticaria, erythema multiforme, erythema nodosum, alopecia, porphyria cutanea tarda, excessive dryness and fragility of the skin with anhidrosis, dryness of the oral mucous membranes and cheilosis, gynecomastia, cholestatic jaundice, and myasthenia gravis. Most of these are single case reports, and in many, a clear cause and effect relationship with busulfan has not been demonstrated.

Seizures (see PRECAUTIONS: General) have been observed in patients receiving higher than recommended doses of busulfan.

OVERDOSAGE

There is no known antidote to busulfan. The principal toxic effect is on the bone marrow. Survival after a single 140 mg dose has been reported in an 18 kg, 4-year-old child,[38] but hematologic toxicity is likely to be more profound with chronic overdosage. The hematologic status should be closely monitored and vigorous supportive measures instituted if necessary. Induction of vomiting or gastric lavage followed by administration of charcoal would be indicated if ingestion were recent. It is not known whether busulfan is dialyzable (see CLINICAL PHARMACOLOGY).

Oral LD_{50} single doses in mice are 120 mg/kg. Two distinct types of toxic response are seen at median lethal doses given intraperitoneally. Within a matter of hours there are signs of stimulation of the central nervous system with convulsions and death on the first day. Mice are more sensitive to this effect than are rats. With doses at the LD_{50} there is also delayed death due to damage to the bone marrow. At three times the LD_{50}, atrophy of the mucosa of the large intestine is found after a week, whereas that of the small intestine is little affected.[39] After doses in the order of 10 times those used therapeutically were added to the diet of rats, irreversible cataracts were produced after several weeks. Small doses had no such effect.[40]

DOSAGE AND ADMINISTRATION

Busulfan is administered orally. The usual adult dose range for *remission induction* is 4 to 8 mg, total dose, daily. Dosing on a weight basis is the same for both children and adults, approximately 60 μg/kg of body weight or 1.8 mg/m² of body surface, daily. Since the rate of fall of the leukocyte count is dose related, daily doses exceeding 4 mg per day should be reserved for patients with the most compelling symptoms; the greater the total daily dose, the greater is the possibility of inducing bone marrow aplasia.

A decrease in the leukocyte count is not usually seen during the first 10 to 15 days of treatment; the leukocyte count may actually increase during this period and it should not be interpreted as resistance to the drug, nor should the dose be increased.[41] Since the leukocyte count may continue to fall for more than 1 month after discontinuing the drug, it is important that busulfan be discontinued *prior* to the total leukocyte count falling into the normal range. When the total leukocyte count has declined to approximately 15,000/μL the drug should be withheld.

With a constant dose of busulfan, the total leukocyte count declines exponentially; a weekly plot of the leukocyte count on semi-logarithmic graph paper aids in predicting the time when therapy should be discontinued.[42] With the recommended dose of busulfan, a normal leukocyte count is usually achieved in 12 to 20 weeks.

During remission, the patient is examined at monthly intervals and treatment resumed with the induction dosage when the total leukocyte count reaches approximately 50,000/μL. When remission is shorter than 3 months, maintenance therapy of 1 to 3 mg daily may be advisable in order to keep the hematological status under control and prevent rapid relapse.

Procedures for proper handling and disposal of anticancer drugs should be considered. Several guidelines on this subject have been published.[43–49]

There is no general agreement that all of the procedures recommended in the guidelines are necessary or appropriate.

HOW SUPPLIED

White, scored tablets containing 2 mg busulfan, imprinted with "MYLERAN" and "K2A" on each tablet; bottle of 25 (NDC 0173-0713-25).

Store at 15° to 25°C (59° to 77°F) in a dry place.

REFERENCES

1. Galton DAG. Myleran in chronic myeloid leukemia: results of treatment. *Lancet.* 1953;1:208–213.
2. Nadkarni MV, Trams EG, Smith PK. Preliminary studies on the distribution and fate of TEM, TEPA, and MYLERAN in the human. *Cancer Res.* 1959;19:713–718.
3. Vodopick H, Hamilton HE, Jackson HL, Peng C-T, Sheets RF. Metabolic fate of tritiated busulfan in man. *J Lab Clin Med.* 1969;73:266–276.
4. Fox BW. Mechanism of action of methane sulfonates. In: Sartorelli AC, Johns DG, eds. *Antineoplastic and Immunosuppressive Agents,* Part II. Berlin: Springer Verlag; 1975:35–46.
5. Roberts JJ, Warwick GP. The mode of action of alkylating agents, III: the formation of 3-hydroxytetrahydrothiophene-1:1-dioxide from 1:4-dimethanesulphonyloxybutane (Myleran), S-β-L-alanyltetrahydrothiophenium mesylate, tetrahydrothiophene and tetrahydrothiophene-1:1-dioxide in the rat, rabbit and mouse. *Biochem Pharmacol.* 1961;6:217–227.
6. Peng C-T. Distribution and metabolic fate of S^{35}-labeled Myleran (busulfan) in normal and tumor-bearing rats. *J Pharmacol Exp Ther.* 1957;120:229–238.
7. Medical Research Council's Working Party for Therapeutic Trials in Leukemia. Chronic granulocytic leukaemia: comparison of radiotherapy and busulfan therapy. *Br Med J.* 1968;1:201–208.
8. Minot GR, Buckman TE, Isaacs R. Chronic myelogenous leukemia: age incidence, duration, and benefit derived from irradiation. *JAMA.* 1924;82:1489–1494.
9. Haut A, Abbott WS, Wintrobe MM, Cartwright GE. Busulfan in the treatment of chronic myelocytic leukemia: the effect of long term intermittent therapy. *Blood.* 1961;17:1–19.
10. Monfardini S, Gee T, Fried J, Clarkson B. Survival in chronic myelogenous leukemia: influence of treatment and extent of disease at diagnosis. *Cancer.* 1973;31:492–501.
11. Conrad FG. Survival in granulocytic leukemia. *Arch Intern Med.* 1973;131:684–685.
12. Sokal JE. Evaluation of survival data for chronic myelocytic leukemia. *Am J Hematol.* 1976;1:493–500.
13. Ezdinli EZ, Sokal JE, Crosswhite L, Sandberg AA. Philadelphia chromosome-positive and -negative chronic myelocytic leukemia. *Ann Intern Med.* 1970;72:175–182.
14. Smith KL, Johnson W. Classification of chronic myelocytic leukemia in children. *Cancer.* 1974; 34:670–679.
15. Stuart JJ, Crocker DL, Roberts HR. Treatment of busulfan-induced pancytopenia. *Arch Intern Med.* 1977; 136:1181–1183.
16. Sostman HD, Matthay RA, Putman CE. Cytotoxic drug-induced lung disease. *Am J Med.* 1977;62:608–615.
17. Stott H, Fox W, Girling DJ, Stephens RJ, Galton DAG. Acute leukaemia after busulfan. *Br Med J.* 1977;2:1513–1517.
18. Hartmann O, et al. High-dose busulfan and cyclophosphamide with autologous bone marrow transplantation support in advanced malignancies in children: A Phase II study. *J Clin Oncol.* 1986;4:1804–1810.
19. Copelan EA, et al. Marrow transplantation following busulfan and cyclophosphamide for chronic myelogenous leukemia in accelerated or blastic phase. *Br J Haematol.* 1989; 71:487–491.
20. Kirchner H, et al. Allogeneic and autologous bone marrow transplanation (BMT) after high-dose busulfan and cyclophosphamide treatment. *Blut.* 1988;57:198. Abstract.
21. Thompson J, et al. Allogeneic bone marrow transplantation (BMT) following transplant preparation with cyclophosphamide (CTX) and busulfan (BU). *Proc ASCO.* 1989; 8:18. Abstract.
22. Geller RB, et al. Allogeneic bone marrow transplantation after high-dose busulfan and cyclophosphamide in patients with acute non-lymphocytic leukemia. *Blood.* 1989; 73:2209–2218.
23. Lu C, et al. Preliminary results of high-dose busulfan and cyclophosphamide with syngeneic or autologous bone marrow rescue. *Cancer Treat Rep.* 1984; 68:711–717.
24. Groshow LB, et al. Pharmacokinetics of busulfan: correlation with veno-occlusive disease in patients undergoing bone marrow transplantation. *Cancer Chemother Pharmacol.* 1989; 25:55–61.
25. Dugdale M, Fort AT. Busulfan treatment of leukemia during pregnancy: case report and review of the literature. *JAMA.* 1967;199:131–133.
26. Diamond I, Anderson MM, McCreadie SR. Transplacental transmission of busulfan (Myleran) in a mother with leukemia: production of fetal malformation and cytomegaly. *Pediatrics.* 1960;25:85–90.
27. Bollag W. Cytostatica in der Schwangerschaft. *Schweiz Med Wochenschr.* 1954;84:393–395.
28. Marcus RE, et al. Convulsions due to high-dose busulfan. *Lancet.* 1984;2:1463. Letter.
29. Martell RW, et al. High-dose busulfan and myoclonic epilepsy. *Ann Intern Med.* 1987; 106:173. Letter.
30. Sureda A, et al. High-dose busulfan and seizures. *Ann Intern Med.* 1989; 111:543–544. Letter.
31. Grigg AP, et al. Busulfan and phenytoin. *Ann Intern Med.* 1989; 111:1049–1050. Letter.
32. Beelen DW, et al. Acute toxicity and first clinical results of intensive post-induction therapy using a modified busulfan and cyclophosphamide regimen with autologous bone marrow rescue in first remission of acute myeloid leukemia. *Blood.* 1989; 74:1507–1516.
33. Key NS, Kelly PMA, Emerson PM, Chapman RWG, Allan NC, McGee JO'D. Oesophageal varices associated with busulfan-thioguanine combination therapy for chronic myeloid leukaemia. *Lancet.* 1987;2:1050–1052.
34. Boros SJ, Reynolds JW. Intrauterine growth retardation following third-trimester exposure to busulfan. *Am J Obstet Gynecol.* 1977;129:111–112.
35. Weinberger A, Pinkhas J, Sandbank U, Shaklai M, deVries A. Endocardial fibrosis following busulfan treatment. *JAMA.* 1975;231:495.
36. Ravindranathan MP, Paul VJ, Kuriakose ET. Cataract after busulfan treatment. *Br Med J.* 1972;1:218–219.
37. Vivacqua RJ, Haurani Fl, Erslev AJ. "Selective" pituitary insufficiency secondary to busulfan. *Ann Intern Med.* 1967;67:380–387.
38. DeOliveira HP, Cruz E, Fonseca A de S, Medeiros M. Accidental ingestion of a toxic dose of Myleran by a child. *Acta Haematol* (Basel). 1963;29:249–255.
39. Sternberg SS, Phillips FS, Scholler J. Pharmacological and pathological effects of alkylating agents. *Ann NY Acad Sci.* 1958;68:811–825.
40. Solomon C, Light AE, deBeer EJ. Cataracts produced in rats by 1,4-dimethanesulfonoxybutane (MYLERAN). *AMA Arch Ophthal.* 1955;54:850–852.
41. Stryckmans PA: Current concepts in chronic myelogenous leukemia. *Semin Hematol.* 1974;11:101–127.
42. Galton DAG. Chemotherapy of chronic myelocytic leukemia. *Semin Hematol.* 1969;6:323–343.
43. Recommendations for the safe handling of parenteral antineoplastic drugs. Washington, DC: Division of Safety, National Institutes of Health; 1983. US Dept of Health and Human Services, Public Health Service publication NIH 83–2621.
44. AMA Council on Scientific Affairs. Guidelines for handling parenteral antineoplastics. *JAMA.* 1985;253: 1590–1591.
45. National Study Commission on Cytotoxic Exposure. Recommendations for handling cytotoxic agents. 1987. Available from Louis P. Jeffrey, Chairman, National Study Commission on Cytotoxic Exposure. Massachusetts College of Pharmacy and Allied Health Sciences, 179 Longwood Avenue, Boston, Massachusetts, 02115.
46. Clinical Oncological Society of Australia. Guidelines and recommendations for safe handling of antineoplastic agents. *Med J Australia.* 1983;1:426–428.
47. Jones RB, Frank R, Mass T. Safe handling of chemotherapeutic agents: a report from the Mount Sinai Medical Center. *CA-A Cancer J for Clin.* 1983;33:258–263.

Continued on next page

Glaxo Wellcome Onc.—Cont.

48. American Society of Hospital Pharmacists. ASHP technical assistance bulletin on handling cytotoxic and hazardous drugs. *AM J Hosp Pharm.* 1990;47:1033–1049.
49. Yodaiken RE, Bennett D. OSHA work-practice guidelines for personnel dealing with cytotoxic (antineoplastic) drugs. *Am J Hosp Pharm.* 1986;43:1193–1204.

April 1996/RL-308

Shown in Product Identification Guide, page 316

NAVELBINE® ℞

[na ′vəl-bēn]
(vinorelbine tartrate)
Injection

> **WARNING:** NAVELBINE (vinorelbine tartrate) Injection should be administered under the supervision of a physician experienced in the use of cancer chemotherapeutic agents. This product is for intravenous use only. Intrathecal administration of other vinca alkaloids has resulted in death. Syringes containing this product should be labeled "WARNING—NAVELBINE FOR INTRAVENOUS USE ONLY."
>
> Severe granulocytopenia resulting in increased susceptibility to infection may occur. Granulocyte counts should be ≥ 1000 cells/mm^3 prior to the administration of NAVELBINE. The dosage should be adjusted according to complete blood counts with differentials obtained on the day of treatment.
>
> Caution—It is extremely important that the intravenous needle or catheter be properly positioned before NAVELBINE is injected. Improper administration of NAVELBINE may result in extravasation causing local tissue necrosis and/or thrombophlebitis (see DOSAGE AND ADMINISTRATION: Administration Precautions).

DESCRIPTION

NAVELBINE (vinorelbine tartrate) Injection is for intravenous administration. Each vial contains vinorelbine tartrate equivalent to 10 mg (1 mL vial) or 50 mg (5 mL vial) vinorelbine in Water for Injection. No preservatives or other additives are present. The aqueous solution is sterile and non-pyrogenic.

Vinorelbine tartrate is a semi-synthetic vinca alkaloid with antitumor activity. The chemical name is 3′,4′-didehydro-4′-deoxy-C′-norvincaleukoblastine [R-(R*,R*)-2,3-dihydroxybutanedioate (1:2)(salt)].

Vinorelbine tartrate is a white to yellow or light brown amorphous powder with the molecular formula $C_{45}H_{54}N_4O_8 \cdot 2C_4H_6O_6$ and molecular weight of 1079.12. The aqueous solubility is >1000 mg/mL in distilled water. The pH of NAVELBINE Injection is approximately 3.5.

CLINICAL PHARMACOLOGY

Vinorelbine is a vinca alkaloid that interferes with microtubule assembly. The vinca alkaloids are structurally similar compounds comprised of two multiringed units, vindoline and catharanthine. Unlike other vinca alkaloids, the catharanthine unit is the site of structural modification for vinorelbine. The antitumor activity of vinorelbine is thought to be due primarily to inhibition of mitosis at metaphase through its interaction with tubulin. Like other vinca alkaloids, vinorelbine may also interfere with: 1) amino acid, cyclic AMP, and glutathione metabolism, 2) calmodulin-dependent Ca^{++}-transport ATPase activity, 3) cellular respiration, and 4) nucleic acid and lipid biosynthesis. In intact tectal plates from mouse embryos, vinorelbine, vincristine, and vinblastine inhibited mitotic microtubule formation at the same concentration (2 µM), inducing a blockade of cells at metaphase. Vincristine produced depolymerization of axonal microtubules at 5 µM, but vinblastine and vinorelbine did not have this effect until concentrations of 30 µM and 40 µM, respectively. These data suggest relative selectivity of vinorelbine for mitotic microtubules.

Pharmacokinetics: The pharmacokinetics of vinorelbine were studied in 49 patients who received doses of 30 mg/m^2 in four clinical trials. Doses were administered by 15- to 20-minute constant rate infusions. Following intravenous administration, vinorelbine concentration in plasma decays in a triphasic manner. The initial rapid decline primarily represents distribution of drug to peripheral compartments followed by metabolism and excretion of the drug during subsequent phases. The prolonged terminal phase is due to relatively slow efflux of vinorelbine from peripheral compartments. The terminal phase half-life averages 27.7 to 43.6 hours, and the mean plasma clearance ranges from 0.97 to 1.26 L/hr/kg. Steady-state volume of distribution (V_{SS}) values range from 25.4 to 40.1 L/kg.

Vinorelbine demonstrated high binding to human platelets and lymphocytes. The free fraction was approximately 0.11 in pooled human plasma over a concentration range of 234 to 1169 ng/mL. The binding to plasma constituents in cancer patients ranged from 79.6% to 91.2%. Vinorelbine binding was not altered in the presence of cisplatin, 5-fluorouracil, or doxorubicin.

Vinorelbine undergoes substantial hepatic elimination in humans, with large amounts recovered in feces after intravenous administration to humans. One metabolite, deacetylvinorelbine, has been shown to possess antitumor activity. This metabolite has been detected but not quantified in human plasma. The effects of renal or hepatic dysfunction on the disposition of vinorelbine have not been assessed, but based on experience with other anticancer vinca alkaloids, dose adjustments are recommended for patients with impaired hepatic function (see DOSAGE AND ADMINISTRATION).

The disposition of radiolabeled vinorelbine given intravenously was studied in a limited number of patients. Approximately 18% of the administered dose was recovered in the urine and 46% in the feces. Incomplete recovery in humans is consistent with results in animals where recovery is incomplete, even after prolonged sampling times. A separate study of the urinary excretion of vinorelbine using specific chromatographic analytical methodology showed that 10.9% $\pm$ 0.7% of a 30 mg/m^2 intravenous dose was excreted unchanged in the urine.

The pharmacokinetics of vinorelbine are not influenced by the concurrent administration of cisplatin with NAVELBINE (see PRECAUTIONS: Drug Interactions).

Clinical Trials: Data from two controlled clinical studies (823 patients), as well as additional data from more than 100 patients enrolled in two uncontrolled clinical trials, support the use of NAVELBINE in patients with advanced non-small cell lung cancer (NSCLC). In a large European clinical trial, 612 patients with Stage III or IV NSCLC, no prior chemotherapy, and WHO Performance Status of 0, 1, or 2 were randomized to treatment with single-agent NAVELBINE (30 mg/m^2/week), NAVELBINE (30 mg/m^2/week) plus cisplatin (120 mg/m^2 days 1 and 29, then every 6 weeks), and vindesine (3 mg/m^2/week for 7 weeks, then every other week) plus cisplatin (120 mg/m^2 days 1 and 29, then every 6 weeks). NAVELBINE plus cisplatin produced longer survival times than vindesine plus cisplatin (median survival 40 weeks vs. 32 weeks, $P=0.03$). The median survival time for patients receiving single-agent NAVELBINE was similar to that observed with vindesine plus cisplatin (31 weeks vs. 32 weeks). The 1-year survival rates were 35% for NAVELBINE plus cisplatin, 27% for vindesine plus cisplatin, and 30% for single-agent NAVELBINE. The overall objective response rate (all partial responses) was significantly higher in the patients treated with NAVELBINE plus cisplatin (28%) than in those treated with vindesine plus cisplatin (19%, $P=0.03$) and in those treated with single-agent NAVELBINE (14%, $P<0.001$). The response rates reported for vindesine plus cisplatin and single-agent NAVELBINE were not significantly different. Significantly less nausea, vomiting, alopecia, and neurotoxicity were observed in patients receiving single-agent NAVELBINE compared to those receiving the combination of vindesine and cisplatin.

Single-agent NAVELBINE was studied in a North American, randomized clinical trial in which patients with Stage IV NSCLC, no prior chemotherapy, and Karnofsky Performance Status ≥ 70 were treated with NAVELBINE (30 mg/m^2) weekly or 5-fluorouracil (5-FU) (425 mg/m^2 I.V. bolus) plus leucovorin (LV) (20 mg/m^2 I.V. bolus) daily for 5 days every 4 weeks. A total of 211 patients were randomized at a 2:1 ratio to NAVELBINE (143) or 5-FU/LV (68). NAVELBINE showed improved survival time compared to 5-FU/LV. In an intent-to-treat analysis, the median survival time for patients receiving NAVELBINE was 30 weeks and for those receiving 5-FU/LV was 22 weeks ($P=0.06$). The 1-year survival rates were 24% ($\pm 4\%$ S.E.) for NAVELBINE and 16% ($\pm 5\%$ S.E.) for the 5-FU/LV group, using the Kaplan-Meier product-limit estimates. The median survival time with 5-FU/LV was similar to, or slightly better than, that usually observed in untreated patients with advanced NSCLC, suggesting that the difference was not related to some unknown detrimental effect of 5-FU/LV therapy. The response rates (all partial responses) for NAVELBINE and 5-FU/LV were 12% and 3%, respectively. Quality-of-life (QOL) was also an endpoint in this study. Patients completed a modified Southwest Oncology Group QOL questionnaire which assessed the domains of role functioning, physical functioning, symptom distress, and global QOL. Quality-of-life was not adversely affected by NAVELBINE when compared to control.

A dose-ranging study of NAVELBINE (20, 25, or 30 mg/m^2/week) plus cisplatin (120 mg/m^2 days 1 and 29, then every 6 weeks) in 32 patients with NSCLC demonstrated a median survival of 44 weeks. There were no responses at the lowest dose level; the response rate was 33% in the 21 patients treated at the two highest dose levels.

INDICATIONS AND USAGE

NAVELBINE is indicated as a single agent or in combination with cisplatin for the first-line treatment of ambulatory patients with unresectable, advanced non-small cell lung cancer (NSCLC). In patients with Stage IV NSCLC, NAVELBINE is indicated as a single agent or in combination with cisplatin. In Stage III NSCLC, NAVELBINE is indicated in combination with cisplatin.

CONTRAINDICATIONS

Administration of NAVELBINE is contraindicated in patients with pretreatment granulocyte counts <1000 cells/mm^3 (see WARNINGS).

WARNINGS

NAVELBINE should be administered in carefully adjusted doses by or under the supervision of a physician experienced in the use of cancer chemotherapeutic agents.

Patients treated with NAVELBINE should be frequently monitored for myelosuppression both during and after therapy. Granulocytopenia is dose-limiting. Granulocyte nadirs occur between 7 and 10 days after dosing with granulocyte count recovery usually within the following 7 to 14 days. Complete blood counts with differentials should be performed and results reviewed prior to administering each dose of NAVELBINE. NAVELBINE should not be administered to patients with granulocyte counts <1000 cells/mm^3. Patients developing severe granulocytopenia should be monitored carefully for evidence of infection and/or fever. See DOSAGE AND ADMINISTRATION for recommended dose adjustments for granulocytopenia.

Pregnancy: Pregnancy Category D. NAVELBINE may cause fetal harm if administered to a pregnant woman. A single dose of vinorelbine has been shown to be embryo- and/or fetotoxic in mice and rabbits at doses of 9 mg/m^2 and 5.5 mg/m^2, respectively (one-third and one-sixth the human dose). At nonmaternotoxic doses, fetal weight was reduced and ossification was delayed. There are no studies in pregnant women. If NAVELBINE is used during pregnancy, or if the patient becomes pregnant while receiving this drug, the patient should be apprised of the potential hazard to the fetus. Women of childbearing potential should be advised to avoid becoming pregnant during therapy with NAVELBINE.

PRECAUTIONS

General: Most drug-related adverse events of NAVELBINE are reversible. If severe adverse events occur, NAVELBINE should be reduced in dosage or discontinued and appropriate corrective measures taken. Reinstitution of therapy with NAVELBINE should be carried out with caution and alertness as to possible recurrence of toxicity.

NAVELBINE should be used with extreme caution in patients whose bone marrow reserve may have been compromised by prior irradiation or chemotherapy, or whose marrow function is recovering from the effects of previous chemotherapy (see DOSAGE AND ADMINISTRATION).

Acute shortness of breath and severe bronchospasm have been reported infrequently following the administration of NAVELBINE and other vinca alkaloids, most commonly when the vinca alkaloid was used in combination with mitomycin. These adverse events may require treatment with supplemental oxygen, bronchodilators, and/or corticosteroids, particularly when there is pre-existing pulmonary dysfunction.

Care must be taken to avoid contamination of the eye with concentrations of NAVELBINE used clinically. Severe irritation of the eye has been reported with accidental exposure to another vinca alkaloid. If exposure occurs, the eye should immediately be thoroughly flushed with water.

Information for Patients: Patients should be informed that the major acute toxicities of NAVELBINE are related to bone marrow toxicity, specifically granulocytopenia with increased susceptibility to infection. They should be advised to report fever or chills immediately. Women of childbearing potential should be advised to avoid becoming pregnant during treatment.

Laboratory Tests: Since dose-limiting clinical toxicity is the result of depression of the white blood cell count, it is imperative that complete blood counts with differentials be obtained and reviewed on the day of treatment prior to each dose of NAVELBINE (see ADVERSE REACTIONS: Hematologic).

Hepatic: There is no evidence that the toxicity of NAVELBINE is enhanced in patients with elevated liver enzymes. No data are available for patients with severe baseline cholestasis, but the liver plays an important role in the metabolism of NAVELBINE. Because clinical experience in patients with severe liver disease is limited, caution should be exercised when administering NAVELBINE to patients with severe hepatic injury or impairment (see DOSAGE AND ADMINISTRATION).

Drug Interactions: Acute pulmonary reactions have been reported with NAVELBINE and other anticancer vinca alkaloids used in conjunction with mitomycin. Although the pharmacokinetics of vinorelbine are not influenced by the

concurrent administration of cisplatin, the incidence of granulocytopenia with NAVELBINE used in combination with cisplatin is significantly higher than with single-agent NAVELBINE.

Carcinogenesis, Mutagenesis, Impairment of Fertility: The carcinogenic potential of NAVELBINE has not been studied. Vinorelbine has been shown to affect chromosome number and possibly structure in vivo (polyploidy in bone marrow cells from Chinese hamsters and a positive micronucleus test in mice). It was not mutagenic in the Ames test and gave inconclusive results in the mouse lymphoma TK Locus assay. The significance of these or other short term test results for human risk is unknown. Vinorelbine did not affect fertility to a statistically significant extent when administered to rats on either a once weekly (9 mg/m^2, approximately one-third the human dose) or alternate day schedule (4.2 mg/m^2, approximately one-seventh the human dose) prior to and during mating. However, biweekly administration for 13 or 26 weeks in the rat at 2.1 and 7.2 mg/m^2 (approximately one-fifteenth and one-fourth the human dose) resulted in decreased spermatogenesis and prostate/seminal vesicle secretion.

Pregnancy: Pregnancy Category D. See WARNINGS section.

Nursing Mothers: It is not known whether the drug is excreted in human milk. Because many drugs are excreted in human milk and because of the potential for serious adverse reactions in nursing infants from NAVELBINE, it is recommended that nursing be discontinued in women who are receiving therapy with NAVELBINE.

Pediatric Use: Safety and effectiveness in pediatric patients have not been established.

Geriatric Use: Of the total number of patients in North American clinical studies of I.V. NAVELBINE, approximately one-third were 65 years of age or greater. No overall differences in effectiveness or safety were observed between these patients and younger patients. Other reported clinical experience has not identified differences in responses between the elderly and younger patients, but greater sensitivity of some older individuals cannot be ruled out.

ADVERSE REACTIONS

Granulocytopenia is the major dose-limiting toxicity with NAVELBINE. Dose adjustments are required for hematologic toxicity and hepatic insufficiency (see DOSAGE AND ADMINISTRATION).

Data in the following table are based on the experience of 365 patients (143 patients with NSCLC; 222 patients with advanced breast cancer) treated with I.V. NAVELBINE as a single agent in three clinical studies. The dosing schedule in each study was 30 mg/m^2 NAVELBINE on a weekly basis. [See table 1 above.]

Hematologic: Granulocytopenia was the major dose-limiting toxicity with NAVELBINE; it was generally reversible and not cumulative over time. Granulocyte nadirs occurred 7 to 10 days after the dose, with granulocyte recovery usually within the following 7 to 14 days. Granulocytopenia resulted in hospitalizations for fever and/or sepsis in 8% of patients. Septic deaths occurred in approximately 1% of patients. Prophylactic hematologic growth factors have not been routinely used with NAVELBINE. If medically necessary, growth factors may be administered at recommended doses no earlier than 24 hours after the administration of cytotoxic chemotherapy. Growth factors should not be administered in the period 24 hours before the administration of chemotherapy.

Grade 3 or 4 anemia occurred in 1% of patients, although blood products were administered to 18% of patients who received NAVELBINE. Grade 3 or 4 thrombocytopenia was reported in 1% of patients.

Neurologic: Mild to moderate peripheral neuropathy manifested by paresthesia and hypesthesia were the most frequently reported neurologic toxicities. Loss of deep tendon reflexes occurred in less than 5% of patients. The development of severe peripheral neuropathy was infrequent (1%) and generally reversible.

Skin: Alopecia was reported in 12% of patients and was usually mild.

Like other anticancer vinca alkaloids, NAVELBINE is a moderate vesicant. Injection site reactions, including erythema, pain at injection site, and vein discoloration occurred in approximately one-third of patients; 5% were severe. Chemical phlebitis along the vein proximal to the site of injection was reported in 10% of patients.

Gastrointestinal: Mild or moderate nausea occurred in 34% of patients treated with NAVELBINE; severe nausea was infrequent (<2%). Prophylactic administration of antiemetics was not routine in patients treated with single-agent NAVELBINE. Due to the low incidence of severe nausea and vomiting with single-agent NAVELBINE, the use of serotonin antagonists is generally not required. Constipation occurred in 29% of patients, with paralytic ileus occurring in 1%. Vomiting, diarrhea, anorexia, and stomatitis were usually mild or moderate, and each occurred in less than 20% of patients.

Table 1

Summary of Adverse Events in 365 Patients Receiving Single-Agent NAVELBINE®*†

Adverse Event		All Patients (n=365) (% Incidence)	NSCLC (n=143) (% Incidence)
Bone Marrow			
Granulocytopenia	<2,000 cells/mm^3	90	80
	<500 cells/mm^3	36	29
Leukopenia	<4,000 cells/mm^3	92	81
	<1,000 cells/mm^3	15	12
Thrombocytopenia	<100,000 cells/mm^3	5	4
	<50,000 cells/mm^3	1	1
Anemia	<11 g/dL	83	77
	<8 g/dL	9	1
Hospitalizations due to granulocytopenic complications		9	8

Adverse Event	All Grades (% Incidence)		Grade 3 (% Incidence)		Grade 4 (% Incidence)	
	All Patients	NSCLC	All Patients	NSCLC	All Patients	NSCLC
Clinical Chemistry Elevations						
Total Bilirubin (n=351)	13	9	4	3	3	2
SGOT (n=346)	67	54	5	2	1	1
General						
Asthenia	36	27	7	5	0	0
Injection Site Reactions	28	38	2	5	0	0
Injection Site Pain	16	13	2	1	0	0
Phlebitis	7	10	<1	1	0	0
Digestive						
Nausea	44	34	2	1	0	0
Vomiting	20	15	2	1	0	0
Constipation	35	29	3	2	0	0
Diarrhea	17	13	1	1	0	0
Peripheral Neuropathy‡	25	20	1	1	<1	0
Dyspnea	7	3	2	2	1	0
Alopecia	12	12	≤1	1	0	0

*None of the reported toxicities were influenced by age. Grade based on modified criteria from the National Cancer Institute.

†Patients with NSCLC had not received prior chemotherapy. The majority of the remaining patients had received prior chemotherapy.

‡Incidence of paresthesia plus hypesthesia.

Hepatic: Transient elevations of liver enzymes were reported without clinical symptoms.

Cardiovascular: Chest pain was reported in 5% of patients. Most reports of chest pain were in patients who had either a history of cardiovascular disease or tumor within the chest. There have been rare reports of myocardial infarction.

Pulmonary: Shortness of breath was reported in 3% of patients; it was severe in 2% (see PRECAUTIONS: General). Interstitial pulmonary changes were documented in a few patients.

Other: Fatigue occurred in 27% of patients. It was usually mild or moderate but tended to increase with cumulative dosing.

Other toxicities that have been reported in less than 5% of patients include jaw pain, myalgia, arthralgia, and rash. Hemorrhagic cystitis and the syndrome of inappropriate ADH secretion were each reported in <1% of patients.

Combination Use: In a randomized study, 206 patients received treatment with NAVELBINE plus cisplatin and 206 patients received single-agent NAVELBINE. The toxicity profile of cisplatin is known (see full prescribing information for cisplatin). The incidence of severe nausea and vomiting was 30% for NAVELBINE/cisplatin compared to <2% for single-agent NAVELBINE. Cisplatin did not appear to increase the incidence of neurotoxicity observed with single-agent NAVELBINE. However, myelosuppression, specifically Grade 3 and 4 granulocytopenia, was greater with the combination of NAVELBINE/cisplatin (79%) than with single-agent NAVELBINE (53%). The incidence of fever and infection may be increased with the combination.

Observed During Clinical Practice: In addition to the adverse experiences reported during clinical trials, the following adverse events have been reported in patients receiving marketed NAVELBINE. For these events the frequency and causality for NAVELBINE has not been established.

Events include systemic allergic reactions reported as anaphylaxis, pruritus, urticaria, and angioedema. Localized rash and urticaria at the injection site have also been reported. Pain in tumor-containing tissue and back pain have been reported.

OVERDOSAGE

There is no known antidote for overdoses of NAVELBINE. The primary anticipated complications of overdosage would consist of bone marrow suppression and peripheral neurotoxicity. If overdosage occurs, general supportive measures together with appropriate blood transfusions and antibiotics should be instituted as deemed necessary by the physician.

DOSAGE AND ADMINISTRATION

The usual initial dose of NAVELBINE is 30 mg/m^2 administered weekly. The recommended method of administration is an intravenous injection over 6 to 10 minutes. In controlled trials, single-agent NAVELBINE was given weekly until progression or dose-limiting toxicity. NAVELBINE was used at the same dose in combination with 120 mg/m^2 of cisplatin, given on days 1 and 29, then every 6 weeks.

No dose adjustments are required for renal insufficiency. If moderate or severe neurotoxicity develops, NAVELBINE should be discontinued. The dosage should be adjusted according to hematologic toxicity or hepatic insufficiency, whichever results in the lower dose.

Dose Modifications for Hematologic Toxicity: Granulocyte counts should be ≥1000 cells/mm^3 prior to the administration of NAVELBINE. Adjustments in the dosage of NAVELBINE should be based on granulocyte counts obtained on the day of treatment according to Table 2.

Table 2

Dose Adjustments Based on Granulocyte Counts

Granulocytes (cells/mm^3) on Days of Treatment	Dose of NAVELBINE® (mg/m^2)
≥1500	30
1000 to 1499	15

Continued on next page

Consult 1997 supplements and future editions for revisions

Glaxo Wellcome Onc.—Cont.

<1000	Do not administer. Repeat granulocyte count in 1 week. If three consecutive weekly doses are held because granulocyte count is <1000 cells/mm^3, discontinue NAVELBINE.

Note: For patients who, during treatment with NAVELBINE, have experienced fever and/or sepsis while granulocytopenic or had two consecutive weekly doses held due to granulocytopenia, subsequent doses of NAVELBINE should be:

22.5 mg/m^2 for granulocytes ≥1500 cells/mm^3
11.25 mg/m^2 for granulocytes 1000 to 1499 cells/mm^3

Dose Modification for Hepatic Insufficiency: NAVELBINE should be administered with caution to patients with hepatic insufficiency. In patients who develop hyperbilirubinemia during treatment with NAVELBINE, the dose should be adjusted for total bilirubin according to Table 3.

Table 3
Dose Modification Based on Total Bilirubin

Total Bilirubin (mg/dL)	Dose of NAVELBINE® (mg/m^2)
≤2.0	30
2.1 to 3.0	15
>3.0	7.5

Dose Modification for Concurrent Hematologic Toxicity and Hepatic Insufficiency: In patients with both hematologic toxicity and hepatic insufficiency, the lower of the doses determined from Table 2 and Table 3 should be administered.

Administration Precautions: Caution—NAVELBINE must be administered intravenously. It is extremely important that the intravenous needle or catheter be properly positioned before any NAVELBINE is injected. Leakage into surrounding tissue during intravenous administration of NAVELBINE may cause considerable irritation, local tissue necrosis, and/or thrombophlebitis. If extravasation occurs, the injection should be discontinued immediately, and any remaining portion of the dose should then be introduced into another vein. Since there are no established guidelines for the treatment of extravasation injuries with NAVELBINE, institutional guidelines may be used. The *ONS Chemotherapy Guidelines* provide additional recommendations for the prevention of extravasation injuries.[1]

As with other toxic compounds, caution should be exercised in handling and preparing the solution of NAVELBINE. Skin reactions may occur with accidental exposure. The use of gloves is recommended. If the solution of NAVELBINE contacts the skin or mucosa, immediately wash the skin or mucosa thoroughly with soap and water. Severe irritation of the eye has been reported with accidental contamination of the eye with another vinca alkaloid. If this happens with NAVELBINE, the eye should be flushed with water immediately and thoroughly.

Procedures for proper handling and disposal of anticancer drugs should be used. Several guidelines on this subject have been published.[2-8] There is no general agreement that all of the procedures recommended in the guidelines are necessary or appropriate.

NAVELBINE Injection is a clear, colorless to pale yellow solution. Parenteral drug products should be visually inspected for particulate matter and discoloration prior to administration whenever solution and container permit. If particulate matter is seen, NAVELBINE should not be administered.

Preparation for Administration: NAVELBINE Injection must be diluted in either a syringe or I.V. bag using one of the recommended solutions. The diluted NAVELBINE should be administered over 6 to 10 minutes into the side port of a free-flowing I.V. **closest to the I.V. bag** followed by flushing with at least 75 to 125 mL of one of the solutions. Diluted NAVELBINE may be used for up to 24 hours under normal room light when stored in polypropylene syringes or polyvinyl chloride bags at 5° to 30°C (41° to 86°F).

Syringe: The calculated dose of NAVELBINE should be diluted to a concentration between 1.5 and 3.0 mg/mL. The following solutions may be used for dilution:

5% Dextrose Injection, USP
0.9% Sodium Chloride Injection, USP

I.V. Bag: The calculated dose of NAVELBINE should be diluted to a concentration between 0.5 and 2 mg/mL. The following solutions may be used for dilution:

5% Dextrose Injection, USP
0.9% Sodium Chloride Injection, USP
0.45% Sodium Chloride Injection, USP
5% Dextrose and 0.45% Sodium Chloride Injection, USP
Ringer's Injection, USP
Lactated Ringer's Injection, USP

Stability: Unopened vials of NAVELBINE are stable until the date indicated on the package when stored under refrigeration at 2° to 8°C (36° to 46°F) and protected from light in the carton. Unopened vials of NAVELBINE are stable at temperatures up to 25°C (77°F) for up to 72 hours. This product should not be frozen.

HOW SUPPLIED

NAVELBINE Injection is a clear, colorless to pale yellow solution in Water for Injection, containing 10 mg vinorelbine per mL. NAVELBINE Injection is available in single-use, clear glass vials with black elastomeric stoppers and royal blue caps, individually packaged in a carton in the following vial sizes:

10 mg/1 mL Single-Use Vial, Carton of 1 (NDC 0173-0656-01).
50 mg/5 mL Single-Use Vial, Carton of 1 (NDC 0173-0656-44).

Store the vials under refrigeration at 2° to 8°C (36° to 46°F) in the carton. Protect from light. DO NOT FREEZE.

REFERENCES

1. ONS Clinical Practice Committee. Cancer Chemotherapy Guidelines: Recommendations for the management of vesicant extravasation, hypersensitivity, and anaphylaxis. Pittsburgh, Pa: Oncology Nursing Society; 1992:1-4.
2. Recommendations for the safe handling of parenteral antineoplastic drugs. Washington, DC: Division of Safety, National Institutes of Health; 1983. US Dept of Health and Human Services, Public Health Service publication NIH 83-2621.
3. AMA Council on Scientific Affairs. Guidelines for handling parenteral antineoplastics. *JAMA.* 1985;253:1590-1591.
4. National Study Commission on Cytotoxic Exposure. Recommendations for handling cytotoxic agents. 1987. Available from Louis P. Jeffrey, Chairman, National Study Commission on Cytotoxic Exposure. Massachusetts College of Pharmacy and Allied Health Sciences, 179 Longwood Avenue, Boston, MA 02115.
5. Clinical Oncological Society of Australia. Guidelines and recommendations for safe handling of antineoplastic agents. *Med J Australia* 1983;1:426-428.
6. Jones RB, Frank R, Mass T. Safe handling of chemotherapeutic agents: a report from the Mount Sinai Medical Center. *CA-A Cancer J for Clin.* 1983;33:258-263.
7. American Society of Hospital Pharmacists. ASHP technical assistance bulletin on handling cytotoxic and hazardous drugs. *Am J Hosp Pharm.* 1990;47:1033-1049.
8. Yodaiken RE, Bennet D. OSHA work-practice guidelines for personnel dealing with cytotoxic (antineoplastic) drugs. *Am J Hosp Pharm.* 1986;43:1193-1204.

U.S. Patent No. 4307100
Under license of Pierre Fabre Médicament–Centre National de la Recherche Scientifique-France
March 1996/RL298

Shown in Product Identification Guide, page 316

PURINETHOL® ℞

[*pur 'in-eth-awl*]
(mercaptopurine)
50 mg Scored Tablets

CAUTION: PURINETHOL (mercaptopurine) is a potent drug. It should not be used unless a diagnosis of acute lymphatic leukemia has been adequately established and the responsible physician is knowledgeable in assessing response to chemotherapy.

DESCRIPTION

PURINETHOL was synthesized and developed by Hitchings, Elion, and associates at the Wellcome Research Laboratories.[1] It is one of a large series of purine analogues which interfere with nucleic acid biosynthesis and has been found active against human leukemias.

Mercaptopurine, known chemically as 1,7-dihydro-6*H*-purine-6-thione monohydrate, is an analogue of the purine bases adenine and hypoxanthine.

PURINETHOL is available in tablet form for oral administration. Each scored tablet contains 50 mg mercaptopurine and the inactive ingredients corn and potato starch, lactose, magnesium stearate, and stearic acid.

CLINICAL PHARMACOLOGY

Clinical studies have shown that the absorption of an oral dose of mercaptopurine in man is incomplete and variable, averaging approximately 50% of the administered dose.[2] The factors influencing absorption are unknown. Intravenous administration of an investigational preparation of mercaptopurine revealed a plasma half-disappearance time of 21 minutes in children and 47 minutes in adults. The volume of distribution usually exceeded that of the total body water.[2]

Following the oral administration of ^{35}S-6-mercaptopurine in one subject, a total of 46% of the dose could be accounted for in the urine (as parent drug and metabolites) in the first 24 hours. Metabolites of mercaptopurine were found in urine within the first 2 hours after administration. Radioactivity (in the form of sulfate) could be found in the urine for weeks afterwards.[3]

There is negligible entry of mercaptopurine into cerebrospinal fluid.

Plasma protein binding averages 19% over the concentration range 10 to 50 μg/mL (a concentration only achieved by intravenous administration of mercaptopurine at doses exceeding 5 to 10 mg/kg).[2]

Monitoring of plasma levels of mercaptopurine during therapy is of questionable value.[3] There is technical difficulty in determining plasma concentrations which are seldom greater than 1 to 2 μg/mL after a therapeutic oral dose. More significantly, mercaptopurine enters rapidly into the anabolic and catabolic pathways for purines, and the active intracellular metabolites have appreciably longer half-lives than the parent drug. The biochemical effects of a single dose of mercaptopurine are evident long after the parent drug has disappeared from plasma. Because of this rapid metabolism of mercaptopurine to active intracellular derivatives, hemodialysis would not be expected to appreciably reduce toxicity of the drug. There is no known pharmacologic antagonist to the biochemical actions of mercaptopurine in vivo.

Mercaptopurine competes with hypoxanthine and guanine for the enzyme hypoxanthine-guanine phosphoribosyltransferase (HGPRTase) and is itself converted to thioinosinic acid (TIMP). This intracellular nucleotide inhibits several reactions involving inosinic acid (IMP), including the conversion of IMP to xanthylic acid (XMP) and the conversion of IMP to adenylic acid (AMP) via adenylosuccinate (SAMP). In addition, 6-methylthioinosinate (MTIMP) is formed by the methylation of TIMP. Both TIMP and MTIMP have been reported to inhibit glutamine-5-phosphoribosylpyrophosphate amidotransferase, the first enzyme unique to the de novo pathway for purine ribonucleotide synthesis.[3]

Experiments indicate that radiolabeled mercaptopurine may be recovered from the DNA in the form of deoxythioguanosine.[4] Some mercaptopurine is converted to nucleotide derivatives of 6-thioguanine (6-TG) by the sequential actions of inosinate (IMP) dehydrogenase and xanthylate (XMP) aminase, converting TIMP to thioguanylic acid (TGMP).

Animal tumors that are resistant to mercaptopurine often have lost the ability to convert mercaptopurine to TIMP. However, it is clear that resistance to mercaptopurine may be acquired by other means as well, particularly in human leukemias.

It is not known exactly which of any one or more of the biochemical effects of mercaptopurine and its metabolites are directly or predominantly responsible for cell death.[5]

The catabolism of mercaptopurine and its metabolites is complex. In man, after oral administration of ^{35}S-6-mercaptopurine, urine contains intact mercaptopurine, thiouric acid (formed by direct oxidation by xanthine oxidase, probably via 6-mercapto-8-hydroxypurine), and a number of 6-methylated thiopurines. The methylthiopurines yield appreciable amounts of inorganic sulfate.[3] The importance of the metabolism by xanthine oxidase relates to the fact that ZYLOPRIM® (allopurinol) inhibits this enzyme and retards the catabolism of mercaptopurine and its active metabolites. A significant reduction in mercaptopurine dosage is mandatory if a potent xanthine oxidase inhibitor and mercaptopurine are used simultaneously in a patient (see PRECAUTIONS).

INDICATIONS AND USAGE

PURINETHOL (mercaptopurine) is indicated for remission induction and maintenance therapy of acute lymphatic leukemia. The response to this agent depends upon the particular subclassification of acute lymphatic leukemia and the age of the patient (child or adult).

Acute Lymphatic (Lymphocytic, Lymphoblastic) Leukemia: Given as a single agent for remission induction, PURINETHOL induces complete remission in approximately 25% of children and 10% of adults. However, reliance upon PURINETHOL alone is not justified for initial remission induction of acute lymphatic leukemia since combination chemotherapy with vincristine, prednisone, and L-asparaginase results in more frequent complete remission induction than with PURINETHOL alone or in combination. The duration of complete remission induced in acute lymphatic leukemia is so brief without the use of maintenance therapy that some form of drug therapy is considered essential. PURINETHOL as a single agent, is capable of significantly prolonging complete remission duration; however, combination therapy has produced remission duration longer than that achieved with PURINETHOL alone.

Acute Myelogenous (and Acute Myelomonocytic) Leukemia: As a single agent, PURINETHOL will induce complete remission in approximately 10% of children and adults with acute myelogenous leukemia or its subclassifications. These

results are inferior to those achieved with combination chemotherapy employing optimum treatment schedules.

Central Nervous System Leukemia: PURINETHOL is not effective for prophylaxis or treatment of central nervous system leukemia.

Other Neoplasms: PURINETHOL is not effective in chronic lymphatic leukemia, the lymphomas (including Hodgkin's Disease), or solid tumors.

CONTRAINDICATIONS

PURINETHOL should not be used unless a diagnosis of acute lymphatic leukemia has been adequately established and the responsible physician is knowledgeable in assessing response to chemotherapy.

PURINETHOL should not be used in patients whose disease has demonstrated prior resistance to this drug. In animals and man, there is usually complete cross-resistance between mercaptopurine and thioguanine.

WARNINGS

SINCE DRUGS USED IN CANCER CHEMOTHERAPY ARE POTENTIALLY HAZARDOUS, IT IS RECOMMENDED THAT ONLY PHYSICIANS EXPERIENCED WITH THE RISKS OF PURINETHOL AND KNOWLEDGEABLE IN THE NATURAL HISTORY OF ACUTE LEUKEMIAS ADMINISTER THIS DRUG.

Bone Marrow Toxicity: The most consistent, dose-related toxicity is bone marrow suppression. This may be manifest by anemia, leukopenia, thrombocytopenia, or any combination of these. Any of these findings may also reflect progression of the underlying disease. Since mercaptopurine may have a delayed effect, it is important to withdraw the medication temporarily at the first sign of an abnormally large fall in any of the formed elements of the blood.

There are rare individuals with an inherited deficiency of the enzyme thiopurine methyltransferase (TPMT) who may be unusually sensitive to the myelosuppressive effects of mercaptopurine and prone to developing rapid bone marrow suppression following the initiation of treatment.[6,7] Substantial dosage reductions may be required to avoid the development of life-threatening bone marrow suppression in these patients. This toxicity may be more profound in patients treated with concomitant allopurinol (see PRECAUTIONS: Drug Interactions).

Hepatotoxicity: Mercaptopurine is hepatotoxic in animals and man. A small number of deaths have been reported which may have been attributed to hepatic necrosis due to administration of mercaptopurine. Hepatic injury can occur with any dosage, but seems to occur with more frequency when doses of 2.5 mg/kg/day are exceeded. The histologic pattern of mercaptopurine hepatotoxicity includes features of both intrahepatic cholestasis and parenchymal cell necrosis, either of which may predominate. It is not clear how much of the hepatic damage is due to direct toxicity from the drug and how much may be due to a hypersensitivity reaction. In some patients jaundice has cleared following withdrawal of mercaptopurine and reappeared with its reintroduction.[8]

Published reports have cited widely varying incidences of overt hepatotoxicity. In a large series of patients with various neoplastic diseases, mercaptopurine was administered orally in doses ranging from 2.5 mg/kg to 5.0 mg/kg without any evidence of hepatotoxicity. It was noted by the authors that no definite clinical evidence of liver damage could be ascribed to the drug, although an occasional case of serum hepatitis did occur in patients receiving 6-MP who previously had transfusions.[8] In reports of smaller cohorts of adult and pediatric leukemic patients, the incidence of hepatotoxicity ranged from 0 to 6%.[9-11] In an isolated report by Einhorn and Davidsohn, jaundice was observed more frequently (40%), especially when doses exceeded 2.5 mg/kg.[12] Usually, clinically detectable jaundice appears early in the course of treatment (1 to 2 months). However, jaundice has been reported as early as 1 week and as late as 8 years after the start of treatment with mercaptopurine.[13]

Monitoring of serum transaminase levels, alkaline phosphatase, and bilirubin levels may allow early detection of hepatotoxicity. It is advisable to monitor these liver function tests at weekly intervals when first beginning therapy and at monthly intervals thereafter. Liver function tests may be advisable more frequently in patients who are receiving mercaptopurine with other hepatotoxic drugs or with known pre-existing liver disease.

The concomitant administration of mercaptopurine with other hepatotoxic agents requires especially careful clinical and biochemical monitoring of hepatic function. Combination therapy involving mercaptopurine with other drugs not felt to be hepatotoxic should nevertheless be approached with caution. The combination of mercaptopurine with doxorubicin was reported to be hepatotoxic in 19 of 20 patients undergoing remission-induction therapy for leukemia resistant to previous therapy.[14]

The hepatotoxicity has been associated in some cases with anorexia, diarrhea, jaundice, and ascites. Hepatic encephalopathy has occurred.

The onset of clinical jaundice, hepatomegaly, or anorexia with tenderness in the right hypochondrium are immediate indications for withholding mercaptopurine until the exact etiology can be identified. Likewise, any evidence of deterioration in liver function studies, toxic hepatitis, or biliary stasis should prompt discontinuation of the drug and a search for an etiology of the hepatotoxicity.

Immunosuppression: Mercaptopurine recipients may manifest decreased cellular hypersensitivities and impaired allograft rejection. Induction of immunity to infectious agents or vaccines will be subnormal in these patients; the degree of immunosuppression will depend on antigen dose and temporal relationship to drug. This immunosuppressive effect should be carefully considered with regard to intercurrent infections and risk of subsequent neoplasia.

Pregnancy: Pregnancy Category D. Mercaptopurine can cause fetal harm when administered to a pregnant woman. Women receiving mercaptopurine in the first trimester of pregnancy have an increased incidence of abortion; the risk of malformation in offspring surviving first trimester exposure is not accurately known.[15] In a series of twenty-eight women receiving mercaptopurine after the first trimester of pregnancy, three mothers died undelivered, one delivered a stillborn child, and one aborted; there were no cases of macroscopically abnormal fetuses.[16] Since such experience cannot exclude the possibility of fetal damage, mercaptopurine should be used during pregnancy only if the benefit clearly justifies the possible risk to the fetus, and particular caution should be given to the use of mercaptopurine in the first trimester of pregnancy.

There are no adequate and well controlled studies in pregnant women. If this drug is used during pregnancy or if the patient becomes pregnant while taking the drug, the patient should be apprised of the potential hazard to the fetus. Women of childbearing potential should be advised to avoid becoming pregnant.

PRECAUTIONS

General: The safe and effective use of PURINETHOL demands a thorough knowledge of the natural history of the condition being treated. After selection of an initial dosage schedule, therapy will frequently need to be modified depending upon the patient's response and manifestations of toxicity.

The most frequent, serious, toxic effect of PURINETHOL is myelosuppression resulting in leukopenia, thrombocytopenia, and anemia. These toxic effects are often unavoidable during the induction phase of adult acute leukemia if remission induction is to be successful. Whether or not these manifestations demand modification or cessation of dosage depends both upon the response of the underlying disease and a careful consideration of supportive facilities (granulocyte and platelet transfusions) which may be available. Life-threatening infections and bleeding have been observed as a consequence of mercaptopurine-induced granulocytopenia and thrombocytopenia. Severe hematologic toxicity may require supportive therapy with platelet transfusions for bleeding, and antibiotics and granulocyte transfusions if sepsis is documented.

If it is not the intent to deliberately induce bone marrow hypoplasia, it is important to discontinue the drug temporarily at the first evidence of an abnormally large fall in white blood cell count, platelet count, or hemoglobin concentration. In many patients with severe depression of the formed elements of the blood due to PURINETHOL, the bone marrow appears hypoplastic on aspiration or biopsy, whereas in other cases it may appear normocellular. The qualitative changes in the erythroid elements toward the megaloblastic series, characteristically seen with the folic acid antagonists and some other antimetabolites, are not seen with this drug. It is probably advisable to start with smaller dosages in patients with impaired renal function, since the latter might result in slower elimination of the drug and metabolites and a greater cumulative effect.

Information for Patients: Patients should be informed that the major toxicities of PURINETHOL are related to myelosuppression, hepatotoxicity, and gastrointestinal toxicity. Patients should never be allowed to take the drug without medical supervision and should be advised to consult their physician if they experience fever, sore throat, jaundice, nausea, vomiting, signs of local infection, bleeding from any site, or symptoms suggestive of anemia. Women of childbearing potential should be advised to avoid becoming pregnant.

Laboratory Tests: It is recommended that evaluation of the hemoglobin or hematocrit, total white blood cell count and differential count, and quantitative platelet count be obtained weekly while the patient is on therapy with PURINETHOL. In cases where the cause of fluctuations in the formed elements in the peripheral blood is obscure, bone marrow examination may be useful for the evaluation of marrow status. The decision to increase, decrease, continue, or discontinue a given dosage of PURINETHOL must be based not only on the absolute hematologic values, but also upon the rapidity with which changes are occurring. In many instances, particularly during the induction phase of acute

leukemia, complete blood counts will need to be done more frequently than once weekly in order to evaluate the effect of the therapy.

Drug Interactions:

Interaction with allopurinol: When allopurinol and mercaptopurine are administered concomitantly, it is imperative that the dose of mercaptopurine be reduced to one-third to one-quarter of the usual dose. Failure to observe this dosage reduction will result in a delayed catabolism of mercaptopurine and the strong likelihood of inducing severe toxicity.

There is usually complete cross-resistance between mercaptopurine and thioguanine.

The dosage of mercaptopurine may need to be reduced when this agent is combined with other drugs whose primary or secondary toxicity is myelosuppression. Enhanced marrow suppression has been noted in some patients also receiving trimethoprim-sulfamethoxazole.[17,18]

Carcinogenesis, Mutagenesis, Impairment of Fertility: Mercaptopurine causes chromosomal aberrations in animals and man and induces dominant-lethal mutations in male mice. In mice, surviving female offspring of mothers who received chronic low doses of mercaptopurine during pregnancy were found sterile or if they became pregnant had smaller litters and more dead fetuses as compared to control animals.[19] Carcinogenic potential exists in man, but the extent of the risk is unknown.

The effect of mercaptopurine on human fertility is unknown for either males or females.

Pregnancy: *Teratogenic Effects:* Pregnancy Category D. See WARNINGS section.

Nursing Mothers: It is not known whether this drug is excreted in human milk. Because many drugs are excreted in human milk, and because of the potential for serious adverse reactions in nursing infants from mercaptopurine, a decision should be made whether to discontinue nursing or to discontinue the drug, taking into account the importance of the drug to the mother.

ADVERSE REACTIONS

The principal and potentially serious toxic effects of PURINETHOL are bone marrow toxicity and hepatotoxicity (see WARNINGS).

Hematologic: The most frequent adverse reaction to PURINETHOL is myelosuppression. The induction of complete remission of acute lymphatic leukemia frequently is associated with marrow hypoplasia. Maintenance of remission generally involves multiple drug regimens whose component agents cause myelosuppression. Anemia, leukopenia, and thrombocytopenia are frequently observed. Dosages and schedules are adjusted to prevent life-threatening cytopenias.

Renal: Hyperuricemia may occur in patients receiving PURINETHOL as a consequence of rapid cell lysis accompanying the antineoplastic effect. Adverse effects can be minimized by increased hydration, urine alkalinization, and the prophylactic administration of a xanthine oxidase inhibitor such as allopurinol. The dosage of PURINETHOL should be reduced to one-third to one-quarter of the usual dose if allopurinol is given concurrently.

Gastrointestinal: Intestinal ulceration has been reported.[20] Nausea, vomiting and anorexia are uncommon during initial administration. Mild diarrhea and sprue-like symptoms have been noted occasionally, but it is difficult at present to attribute these to the medication. Oral lesions are rarely seen, and when they occur they resemble thrush rather than antifolic ulcerations.

An increased risk of pancreatitis may be associated with the investigational use of PURINETHOL in inflammatory bowel disease.[21-23]

Miscellaneous: While dermatologic reactions can occur as a consequence of disease, the administration of PURINETHOL has been associated with skin rashes and hyperpigmentation.[24]

Drug fever has been very rarely reported with PURINETHOL. Before attributing fever to PURINETHOL, every attempt should be made to exclude more common causes of pyrexia, such as sepsis, in patients with acute leukemia.

OVERDOSAGE

Signs and symptoms of overdosage may be immediate such as anorexia, nausea, vomiting, and diarrhea; or delayed such as myelosuppression, liver dysfunction, and gastroenteritis. Dialysis cannot be expected to clear mercaptopurine. Hemodialysis is thought to be of marginal use due to the rapid intracellular incorporation of mercaptopurine into active metabolites with long persistence. The oral LD$_{50}$ of mercaptopurine was determined to be 480 mg/kg in the mouse and 425 mg/kg in the rat.[25]

There is no known pharmacologic antagonist of mercaptopurine. The drug should be discontinued immediately if unintended toxicity occurs during treatment. If a patient is seen immediately following an accidental overdosage of the drug, it may be useful to induce emesis.

Continued on next page

Glaxo Wellcome Onc.—Cont.

DOSAGE AND ADMINISTRATION

Induction Therapy: PURINETHOL is administered orally. The dosage which will be tolerated and be effective varies from patient to patient, and therefore careful titration is necessary to obtain the optimum therapeutic effect without incurring excessive, unintended toxicity. The usual initial dosage for children and adults is 2.5 mg/kg of body weight per day (100 to 200 mg in the average adult and 50 mg in an average 5-year-old child). Children with acute leukemia have tolerated this dose without difficulty in most cases; it may be continued daily for several weeks or more in some patients. If, after 4 weeks at this dosage, there is no clinical improvement and no definite evidence of leukocyte or platelet depression, the dosage may be increased up to 5 mg/kg daily. A dosage of 2.5 mg/kg per day may result in a rapid fall in leukocyte count within 1 to 2 weeks in some adults with acute lymphatic leukemia and high total leukocyte counts.

The total daily dosage may be given at one time. It is calculated to the nearest multiple of 25 mg. The dosage of PURINETHOL should be reduced to one-third to one-quarter of the usual dose if allopurinol is given concurrently. Because the drug may have a delayed action, it should be discontinued at the first sign of an abnormally large or rapid fall in the leukocyte or platelet count. If subsequently the leukocyte count or platelet count remains constant for 2 or 3 days, or rises, treatment may be resumed.

Maintenance Therapy: Once a complete hematologic remission is obtained, maintenance therapy is considered essential. Maintenance doses will vary from patient to patient. A usual daily maintenance dose of PURINETHOL is 1.5 to 2.5 mg/kg/day as a single dose. It is to be emphasized that in children with acute lymphatic leukemia in remission, superior results have been obtained when PURINETHOL has been combined with other agents (most frequently with methotrexate) for remission maintenance. PURINETHOL should rarely be relied upon as a single agent for the maintenance of remissions induced in acute leukemia.

Procedures for proper handling and disposal of anticancer drugs should be considered. Several guidelines on this subject have been published.[26–32]

There is no general agreement that all of the procedures recommended in the guidelines are necessary or appropriate.

HOW SUPPLIED

Pale yellow to buff, scored tablets containing 50 mg mercaptopurine, imprinted with "PURINETHOL" and "04A"; bottles of 25 (NDC 0173-0807-25) and 250 (NDC 0173-0807-65). Store at 15° to 25°C (59°to 77°F) in a dry place.

REFERENCES

1. Hitchings GH, Elion GB. The chemistry and biochemistry of purine analogs. *Ann NY Acad Sci.* 1954; 60:195–199.
2. Loo TL, Luce JK, Sullivan MP, Frei E III. Clinical pharmacologic observations on 6-mercaptopurine and 6-methylthiopurine ribonucleoside. *Clin Pharmacol Ther.* 1968; 9:180–194.
3. Elion GB. Biochemistry and pharmacology of purine analogs. *Fed Proc.* 1967; 26:898–904.
4. Scannell JP, Hitchings GH. Thioguanine in deoxyribonucleic acid from tumors of 6-mercaptopurine-treated mice. *Proc Soc Exp Biol Med.* 1966; 122:627–629.
5. Paterson ARP, Tidd DM. 6-thiopurines. In Sartorelli AC, Johns DG eds. *Antineoplastic and Immunosuppressive Agents,* Part II. Berlin, Springer-Verlag; 1975; 384–403.
6. Lennard L, Gibson BES, Nicole T, Lilleyman JS. Congenital thiopurine methyltransferase deficiency and 6-mercaptopurine toxicity during treatment for acute lymphoblastic leukemia. *Arch Dis Child.* 1993:69:577–579.
7. Evans WE, Homer M, Chu YQ, Kalwinsky D, Roberts WM. Altered mercaptopurine metabolism, toxic effects, and dosage requirement in a thiopurine methyltransferase-deficient child with acute lymphocylic leukemia. *J Pediatr.* 1991; 119:985–989.
8. Burchenal JH, Ellison RR, Murphy ML, et al. Clinical studies on 6-mercaptopurine. *Ann NY Acad Sc.* 1954; 60:359–368.
9. Farber S. Summary of experience with 6-mercaptopurine. *Ann NY Acad Sc.* 1954; 60:412–414.
10. Fountain JR. Clinical observations of the treatment of leukemia and allied disorders with 6-mercaptopurine. *Ann NY Acad Sc.* 1954; 60:439–446.
11. Hyman GA, Gellhorn A, Wolff JA. The therapeutic effect of mercaptopurine in a variety of human neoplastic diseases. *Ann NY Acad Sc.* 1954; 60:430–435.
12. Einhorn M, Davidsohn I. Hepatotoxicity of mercaptopurine. *JAMA.* 1964; 188:802–806.
13. Schein PS, Winokur SH. Immunosuppressive and cytotoxic chemotherapy: long-term complications. *Ann Intern Med.* 1975; 82:84–95.
14. Stern MH, Minow RA, Casey JH, Luna MA. Hepatotoxicity in patients treated with adriamycin and 6-mercaptopurine for refractory leukemia. *Am J Clin Pathol.* 1975; 63:758–759. Abstract.
15. Blatt J, Mulvihill JJ, Ziegler JL, Young RC, Poplack DG. Pregnancy outcome following cancer chemotherapy. *Am J Med.* 1980; 69:828–832.
16. Nicholson HO. Cytotoxic drugs in pregnancy: review of reported cases. *J Obstet Gynaecol Br Commonw.* 1968; 75:307–312.
17. Woods WG, Daigle AE, Hutchinson RJ, Robison LL. Myelosuppression associated with cotrimoxazole as a prophylactic antibiotic in the maintenance phase of childhood acute lymphocytic leukemia. *J Pediatr.* 1984; 105:639–644.
18. Rees CA, Lennard L, Lilleyman JS, Maddocks JL. Disturbance of 6-mercaptopurine metabolism by cotrimoxazole in childhood lymphoblastic leukemia. *Cancer Chemother Pharmacol.* 1984;12:87–89.
19. Reimers TJ, Sluss PM. 6-mercaptopurine treatment of pregnant mice: effects on second and third generations. *Science.* 1978;201:65–67.
20. Clark PA, Hsia YE, Huntsman RG. Toxic complications of treatment with 6-mercaptopurine. *Br Med J [Clin Res].* 1960;1:393–395.
21. Present DH, Meltzer SJ, Wolke A, Korelitz BI. Short and long term toxicity to 6-mercaptopurine in the management of inflammatory bowel disease. *Gastroenterology.* 1985;88:1545. Abstract.
22. Bank L, Wright JP. 6-mercaptopurine-related pancreatitis in 2 patients with inflammatory bowel disease. *Dig Dis Sci.* 1984;29:357–359.
23. Singleton JW, Law DH, Kelley ML Jr, Mekhjian HS, Sturdevant RAL. National Cooperative Crohn's disease study: adverse reactions to study drugs. *Gastroenterology.* 1979;77:870–882.
24. Dreizen S, Bodey GP, Rodriguez V, McCredie KB. Cutaneous complications of cancer chemotherapy. *Postgrad Med.* 1975;58(Nov):150–158.
25. Unpublished data on file with Glaxo Wellcome Inc.
26. Recommendations for the safe handling of parenteral antineoplastic drugs. Washington, DC: Division of Safety: National Institutes of Health; 1983. US Dept of Health and Human Services. Public Health Service publication NIH 83-2621.
27. AMA Council Report on Scientific Affairs. Guidelines for handling parenteral antineoplastics. *JAMA.* 1985; 253:1590–1591.
28. National Study Commission on Cytotoxic Exposure. Recommendations for handling cytotoxic agents. 1987. Available from Louis P. Jeffrey, Chairman, National Study Commission on Cytotoxic Exposure. Massachusetts College of Pharmacy and Allied Health Sciences, 179 Longwood Avenue, Boston, MA 02115.
29. Clinical Oncological Society of Australia. Guidelines and recommendations for safe handling of antineoplastic agents. *Med J Australia.* 1983;1:426–428.
30. Jones RB, Frank R, Mass T. Safe handling of chemotherapeutic agents: a report from the Mount Sinai Medical Center. *CA—A Cancer J for Clinicians.* 1983;33:258–263.
31. American Society of Hospital Pharmacists. ASHP technical assistance bulletin on handling cytotoxic and hazardous drugs. *Am J Hosp Pharm.* 1990;47:1033–1049.
32. Yodaiken RE, Bennett D. OSHA work-practice guidelines for personnel dealing with cytotoxic (antineoplastic) drugs. *Am J Hosp Pharm.* 1986;43:1193–1204.

May 1996/RL-313

Shown in Product Identification Guide, page 316

RETROVIR® ℞
[*ré trō-vir*]
(zidovudine)
Capsules

RETROVIR® ℞
(zidovudine)
Syrup

WARNING: RETROVIR (ZIDOVUDINE) MAY BE ASSOCIATED WITH HEMATOLOGIC TOXICITY INCLUDING GRANULOCYTOPENIA AND SEVERE ANEMIA PARTICULARLY IN PATIENTS WITH ADVANCED HIV DISEASE (SEE WARNINGS). PROLONGED USE OF RETROVIR HAS BEEN ASSOCIATED WITH SYMPTOMATIC MYOPATHY SIMILAR TO THAT PRODUCED BY HUMAN IMMUNODEFICIENCY VIRUS. RARE OCCURRENCES OF LACTIC ACIDOSIS IN THE ABSENCE OF HYPOXEMIA, AND SEVERE HEPATOMEGALY WITH STEATOSIS HAVE BEEN REPORTED WITH THE USE OF ANTIRETROVIRAL NUCLEOSIDE ANALOGUES, INCLUDING RETROVIR AND ZALCITABINE, AND ARE POTENTIALLY FATAL (SEE WARNINGS).

DESCRIPTION

RETROVIR is the brand name for zidovudine (formerly called azidothymidine [AZT]), a pyrimidine nucleoside analogue active against human immunodeficiency virus (HIV).

Capsules: RETROVIR Capsules are for oral administration. Each capsule contains 100 mg of zidovudine and the inactive ingredients corn starch, magnesium stearate, microcrystalline cellulose, and sodium starch glycolate. The 100 mg empty hard gelatin capsule, printed with edible black ink, consists of black iron oxide, dimethylpolysiloxane, gelatin, pharmaceutical shellac, soya lecithin, and titanium dioxide. The blue band around the capsule consists of gelatin and FD&C Blue No. 2.

Syrup: RETROVIR Syrup is for oral administration. Each teaspoonful (5 mL) of RETROVIR Syrup contains 50 mg of zidovudine and the inactive ingredients sodium benzoate 0.2% (added as a preservative), citric acid, flavors, glycerin, and liquid sucrose. Sodium hydroxide may be added to adjust pH.

The chemical name of zidovudine is 3′-azido-3′-deoxythymidine.

Zidovudine is a white to beige, odorless, crystalline solid with a molecular weight of 267.24 and a solubility of 20.1 mg/mL in water at 25°C. The molecular formula $C_{10}H_{13}N_5O_4$.

CLINICAL PHARMACOLOGY

Zidovudine is an inhibitor of the in vitro replication of some retroviruses including HIV. This drug is a thymidine analogue in which the 3′-hydroxy (-OH) group is replaced by an azido ($-N_3$) group. Cellular thymidine kinase converts zidovudine into zidovudine monophosphate. The monophosphate is further converted into the diphosphate by cellular thymidylate kinase and to the triphosphate derivative by other cellular enzymes. Zidovudine triphosphate interferes with the HIV viral RNA dependent DNA polymerase (reverse transcriptase) and thus, inhibits viral replication. Zidovudine triphosphate also inhibits cellular α-DNA polymerase, but at concentrations 100-fold higher than those required to inhibit reverse transcriptase. In vitro, zidovudine triphosphate has been shown to be incorporated into growing chains of DNA by viral reverse transcriptase. When incorporation by the viral enzyme occurs, the DNA chain is terminated. Studies in cell culture suggest that zidovudine incorporation by cellular α-DNA polymerase may occur, but only to a very small extent and not in all test systems. Cellular γ-DNA polymerase shows some sensitivity to inhibition by the zidovudine triphosphate with 50% inhibitory concentration (IC_{50}) values 400 to 900 times greater than that for HIV reverse transcriptase.

Microbiology: The relationship between in vitro susceptibility of HIV to zidovudine and the inhibition of HIV replication in humans or clinical response to therapy has not been established. In vitro sensitivity results vary greatly depending upon the time between virus infection and zidovudine treatment of cell cultures, the particular assay used, the cell type employed, and the laboratory performing the test.

Zidovudine blocked 90% of detectable HIV replication in vitro at concentrations of ≤ 0.13 μg/mL (ID_{90}) when added shortly after laboratory infection of susceptible cells. This level of antiviral effect was observed in experiments measuring reverse transcriptase activity in HIV-infected H9 cells, PHA stimulated peripheral blood lymphocytes, and unstimulated peripheral blood lymphocytes. The concentration of drug required to produce a 50% decrease in supernatant reverse transcriptase was 0.013 μg/mL (ID_{50}) in both HIV-infected H9 cells and peripheral blood lymphocytes. Zidovudine at concentrations of 0.13 μg/mL also provided $>90\%$ protection from a strain of HIV (HTLV IIIB) induced cytopathic effects in two tetanus-specific T4 cell lines. HIV-p24 antigen expression was also undetectable at the same concentration in these cells. Partial inhibition of viral activity in cells with chronic HIV infection (presumed to carry integrated HIV DNA) required concentrations of zidovudine (8.8 μg/mL in one laboratory to 13.3 μg/mL in another) which are approximately 100 times as high as those necessary to block HIV replication in acutely infected cells. HIV isolates from 18 untreated individuals with AIDS or ARC had ID_{50} sensitivity values between 0.003 to 0.013 μg/mL and ID_{95} sensitivity values between 0.03 to 0.3 μg/mL.

Zidovudine has been shown to act additively or synergistically with a number of anti-HIV agents, including zalcitabine, didanosine, and interferon-alpha, in inhibiting the replication of HIV in cell culture.

The development of resistance to zidovudine has been studied extensively. The emergence of resistance is a function of both duration of zidovudine therapy and stage of disease. Asymptomatic patients developed resistance at significantly slower rates than patients with advanced disease. In contrast, virus isolates from patients with AIDS who received a year or more of zidovudine may show more than 100-fold increases in ID_{50} compared to isolates pre-therapy.

In vitro resistance to zidovudine is due to the accumulation of specific mutations in the HIV reverse transcriptase coding region. Five amino acid substitutions (Met41 → Leu, A67 → Asn, Lys70 → Arg, Thr215 → Tyr or Phe, and Lys219 → Gln)

have been described in viruses with decreased in vitro susceptibility to zidovudine inhibition. The extent of resistance appears to be correlated with number of mutations in reverse transcriptase.

A significant correlation between zidovudine resistance and poor clinical outcome in children with advanced disease has been reported; in addition, a correlation between reduced sensitivity to zidovudine and lower CD4 cell counts in symptom-free adults treated with zidovudine for up to 3 years has also been reported. However, the specific relationship between emergence of zidovudine resistance and clinical progression of disease in adults has not yet been defined.

Combination therapy of zidovudine plus zalcitabine does not appear to prevent the emergence of zidovudine-resistant isolates. In vitro studies with zidovudine-resistant virus isolates indicate zidovudine-resistant strains are usually sensitive to zalcitabine and didanosine.

The major metabolite of zidovudine, 3'-azido-3'-deoxy-5'-O-β-D-glucopyranuronosylthymidine (GZDV, formerly called GAZT), does not inhibit HIV replication in vitro. GZDV does not antagonize the antiviral effect of zidovudine in vitro nor does GZDV compete with zidovudine triphosphate as an inhibitor of HIV reverse transcriptase.

The cytotoxicity of zidovudine for various cell lines was determined using a cell growth inhibition assay. ID_{50} values for several human cell lines showed little growth inhibition by zidovudine except at concentrations >50 µg/mL. However, one human T-lymphocyte cell line was sensitive to the cytotoxic effect of zidovudine with an ID_{50} of 5 µg/mL. Moreover, in a colony-forming unit assay designed to assess the toxicity of zidovudine for human bone marrow, an ID_{50} value of <1.25 µg/mL was estimated. Two of ten human lymphocyte cultures tested were found to be sensitive to zidovudine at 5 µg/mL or less.

Zidovudine has antiviral activity against some other mammalian retroviruses in addition to HIV. Human immunodeficiency virus-2 (HIV-2) replication in vitro is inhibited by zidovudine with an ID_{50} of 0.015 µg/mL, while HTLV-1 transmission to susceptible cells is inhibited by 1 to 3 µg/mL of drug.

Several strains of simian immunodeficiency virus (SIV) are also inhibited by zidovudine with ID_{50} values ranging from 0.13 to 6.5 µg/mL, depending upon species of origin and assay method used. No significant inhibitory activity was exhibited against a variety of other human and animal viruses, except an ID_{50} of 1.4 to 2.7 µg/mL against the Epstein-Barr virus, the clinical significance of which is unknown.

The following microbiological activities of zidovudine have been observed in vitro, but the clinical significance is unknown. Many *Enterobacteriaceae*, including strains of *Shigella, Salmonella, Klebsiella, Enterobacter, Citrobacter,* and *Escherichia coli* are inhibited in vitro by low concentrations of zidovudine (0.005 to 0.5 µg/mL). Synergy of zidovudine with trimethoprim has been observed against some of these bacteria in vitro. Limited data suggest that bacterial resistance to zidovudine develops rapidly. Zidovudine has no activity against gram positive organisms, anaerobes, mycobacteria, or fungal pathogens including *Candida albicans* and *Cryptococcus neoformans*. Although *Giardia lamblia* is inhibited by 1.9 µg/mL of zidovudine, no activity was observed against other protozoal pathogens.

Pharmacokinetics:

Adults: The pharmacokinetics of zidovudine has been evaluated in 22 adult HIV-infected patients in a Phase 1 dose-escalation study. After oral dosing, zidovudine was rapidly absorbed from the gastrointestinal tract with peak serum concentrations occurring within 0.5 to 1.5 hours. Dose-independent kinetics was observed over the range of 2 mg/kg every 8 hours to 10 mg/kg every 4 hours. The mean zidovudine half-life was approximately 1 hour and ranged from 0.78 to 1.93 hours following oral dosing.

Zidovudine is rapidly metabolized to 3'-azido-3'-deoxy-5'-O-β-D-glucopyranuronosylthymidine (GZDV) which has an apparent elimination half-life of 1 hour (range 0.61 to 1.73 hours). Following oral administration, urinary recovery of zidovudine and GZDV accounted for 14% and 74% of the dose, respectively, and the total urinary recovery averaged 90% (range 63% to 95%), indicating a high degree of absorption. However, as a result of first-pass metabolism, the average oral capsule bioavailability of zidovudine is 65% (range 52% to 75%). A second metabolite, 3'-amino-3'-deoxythymidine (AMT), has been identified in the plasma following single dose intravenous administration of zidovudine. AMT area-under-the-curve (AUC) was one-fifth of the AUC of zidovudine and had a half-life of 2.7 ± 0.7 hours. In comparison, GZDV AUC was about 3-fold greater than the AUC of zidovudine.

Additional pharmacokinetic data following intravenous dosing indicated dose-independent kinetics over the range of 1 to 5 mg/kg with a mean zidovudine half-life of 1.1 hours (range 0.48 to 2.86 hours). Total body clearance averaged 1900 mL/min/70 kg and the apparent volume of distribution was 1.6 L/kg. Renal clearance is estimated to be 400 mL/min/70 kg, indicating glomerular filtration and active tubular secretion by the kidneys. Zidovudine plasma protein

binding is 34% to 38%, indicating that drug interactions involving binding site displacement are not anticipated. The zidovudine cerebrospinal fluid (CSF)/plasma concentration ratio determined in 39 patients receiving chronic therapy with RETROVIR. The median ratio measured in 50 paired samples drawn 1 to 8 hours after the last dose of RETROVIR WAS 0.6.

Adults with Impaired Renal Function: The pharmacokinetics of zidovudine has been evaluated in patients with impaired renal function following a single 200 mg oral dose. In 14 patients (mean creatinine clearance 18±2 mL/min, the half-life of zidovudine was 1.4 hours compared to 1.0 hour for control subjects with normal renal function: AUC values were approximately twice those of controls. Additionally, GZDV half-life in these patients was 8.0 hours (vs 0.9 hours for control) and AUC was 17 times higher than for control subjects. The pharmacokinetics and tolerance was evaluated in a multiple-dose study in patients undergoing hemodialysis (n=5) or peritoneal dialysis (n=6). Patients received escalating doses of zidovudine up to 200 mg 5 times daily for 8 weeks. Daily doses of 500 mg or less were well tolerated despite significantly elevated plasma levels of GZDV. Apparent oral clearance of zidovudine was approximately 50% of that reported in patients with normal renal function. The plasma concentrations of AMT are not known in patients with renal insufficiency. Daily doses of 300 to 400 mg should be appropriate in HIV-infected patients with severe renal dysfunction (see DOSAGE AND ADMINISTRATION: Dose Adjustment). Hemodialysis and peritoneal dialysis appear to have a negligible effect on the removal of zidovudine, whereas GZDV elimination is enhanced.

Children and Infants: The pharmacokinetics and bioavailability of zidovudine have been evaluated in 21 HIV-infected children, aged 6 months through 12 years, following intravenous doses administered over the range of 80 to 160 mg/m² every 6 hours, and following oral doses of the intravenous solution administered over the range of 90 to 240 mg/m² every 6 hours. After discontinuation of the I.V. infusion, zidovudine plasma concentrations decayed biexponentially, consistent with two-compartment pharmacokinetics. Proportional increases in AUC and in zidovudine concentrations were observed with increasing dose, consistent with dose-independent kinetics over the dose range studied. The mean terminal half-life and total body clearance across all dose levels administered were 1.5 hours and 30.9 mL/min/kg, respectively. These values compare to mean half-life and total body clearance in adults of 1.1 hours and 27.1 mL/min/kg.

The mean oral bioavailability of 65% was independent of dose. This value is the same as the bioavailability in adults. Doses of 180 mg/m² four times daily in pediatric patients produced similar systemic exposure (24-hour AUC 10.7 hr · µg/mL) as doses of 200 mg six times daily in adult patients (10.9 hr · µg/mL).

The pharmacokinetics of zidovudine has been studied in neonates from birth to 3 months of life. In one study of the pharmacokinetics of zidovudine in women during the last trimester of pregnancy, zidovudine elimination was determined immediately after birth in eight infants who were exposed to zidovudine *in utero*. The half-life was 13.0 ± 5.8 hours. In another study, the pharmacokinetics of zidovudine was evaluated in infants (ranging in age of 1 day to 3 months) of normal birth weight for gestational age and with normal renal and hepatic function. In infants less than or equal to 14 days old, mean ± SD total body clearance was 10.9 ± 4.8 mL/min/kg (n=18) and half-life was 3.1 ± 1.2 hours (n=21). In infants greater than 14 days, total body clearance was 19.0 ± 4.0 mL/min/kg (n=16) and half-life was 1.9 ± 0.7 hours (n=18). Bioavailability was 89% ± 19% (n=15) in the younger age group and decreased to 61% ± 19% (n=17) in infants older than 14 days.

Concentrations of zidovudine in cerebrospinal fluid were measured after both intermittent oral and I.V. drug administration in 21 children during Phase 1 and Phase 2 studies. The mean zidovudine CSF/plasma concentration ratio measured at an average time of 2.2 hours postdose at oral doses of 120 to 240 mg/m² was 0.52 ± 0.44 (n=28): after an I.V. infusion of doses of 80 to 160 mg/m² over 1 hour, the mean CSF/plasma concentration ratio was 0.87 ± 0.66 (n=23) at 3.2 hours after the start of the infusion. During continuous I.V. infusion, mean steady-state CSF/plasma ratio was 0.26 ± 0.17 (n=28).

As in adult patients, the major route of elimination in children was by metabolism to GZDV. After I.V. dosing, about 29% of the dose was excreted in the urine unchanged and about 45% of the dose was excreted as GZDV. Overall, the pharmacokinetics of zidovudine in pediatric patients greater than 3 months of age is similar to that of zidovudine in adult patients.

Pregnancy: The pharmacokinetics of zidovudine has been studied in a Phase 1 study of eight women during the last trimester of pregnancy. As pregnancy progressed, there was no evidence of drug accumulation. The pharmacokinetics of zidovudine was similar to that of nonpregnant adults. Consistent with passive transmission of the drug across the placenta, zidovudine concentrations in infant plasma at birth

were essentially equal to those in maternal plasma at delivery. Although data are limited, methadone maintenance therapy in five pregnant women did not appear to alter zidovudine pharmacokinetics. However, in another patient population, a potential for interaction has been identified (see PRECAUTIONS).

Capsules: Steady-state serum concentrations of zidovudine following chronic oral administration of 250 mg every 4 hours were determined in 21 adult patients in a controlled trial. Mean steady-state predose and 1.5 hours postdose zidovudine concentrations were 0.16 µg/mL (range 0 to 0.84 µg/mL) and 0.62 µg/mL (range 0.05 to 1.46 µg/mL), respectively.

Syrup: In a multiple dose bioavailability study conducted in 12 HIV-infected adults receiving doses of 100 or 200 mg every 4 hours, RETROVIR Syrup was demonstrated to be bioequivalent to RETROVIR Capsules with respect to area under the zidovudine plasma concentration-time curve (AUC). The rate of absorption of RETROVIR Syrup was greater than that of RETROVIR Capsules, as indicated by mean times to peak concentration of 0.5 and 0.8 hours, respectively. Mean values for steady-state peak concentration (dose-normalized to 200 mg) were 1.5 and 1.2 µg/mL for syrup and capsules, respectively.

Effect of Food on Absorption: Administration of RETROVIR Capsules with food decreased peak plasma concentrations by greater than 50%; however, bioavailability as determined by AUC may not be affected.

Description of Clinical Studies:

Monotherapy-Adults:
Randomized double-blind studies have demonstrated clinical benefit of initial treatment with RETROVIR compared to placebo, didanosine, or zalcitabine. Therapy with RETROVIR has been shown to prolong survival and decrease the incidence of opportunistic infections in patients with advanced HIV disease at the initiation of therapy and to delay disease progression in asymptomatic HIV-infected patients.

Other randomized studies suggest that the duration of the clinical benefit of monotherapy with RETROVIR is time-limited. Patients randomized to other antiviral regimens after initial therapy with RETROVIR had fewer AIDS progression end-points than those randomized to continue monotherapy with RETROVIR. The design of those studies did not define optimally when and how the antiviral regimen should be modified. Factors which may contribute to the development of disease progression while on therapy with RETROVIR are under clinical investigation and may include incomplete suppression of viral replication and development of decreased viral susceptibility to RETROVIR.

Advanced HIV Disease: A randomized, double-blind, placebo-controlled trial (BW 02) of oral RETROVIR (1500 mg/day) was conducted in 281 adults with advanced HIV disease which included 160 patients with AIDS and 121 patients with ARC.[1,2]

There were 19 deaths (12 in patients with AIDS, 7 in patients with ARC) in the placebo group and 1 death (patient with AIDS) in the group receiving RETROVIR. Treatment with RETROVIR significantly improved the probability of survival for 24 weeks in both the AIDS and ARC subgroups. During a follow-up protocol with open-label treatment with RETROVIR, patients who were initially randomized to receive RETROVIR continued to have better overall survival than did patients initially randomized to placebo. Survival rates in the group of patients originally randomized to receive RETROVIR declined to 85% after 1 year, 41% after 2 years, and 23% after 3 years. These survival rates may be lower than currently observed due to the absence of opportunistic infection prophylaxis in this study. RETROVIR also significantly reduced the risk of acquiring an AIDS-defining opportunistic infection, and patients who received RETROVIR generally did better than the placebo group in terms of several other measures of efficacy including performance level, neuropsychiatric function, maintenance of body weight, and the number and severity of symptoms associated with HIV disease.

In separate studies, initial therapy with RETROVIR was compared to initial therapy with either didanosine or zalcitabine. Survival rates in patients with no prior exposure to RETROVIR were significantly better for patients treated with RETROVIR than for patients treated with alternative monotherapy.

Asymptomatic HIV Infection and Early HIV Disease (CD4 between 200 to 500 cells/mm³): The population indicated for monotherapy with RETROVIR was extended to asymptomatic or symptomatic adults with CD4 cell counts of 500 cells/mm³ or less based on the results of two randomized double-blind placebo-controlled trials (ACTG 019[3], ACTG 016[4]) of 2051 adults. Treatment with RETROVIR reduced the risk of progression to advanced HIV disease (advanced AIDS Related Complex [ARC], AIDS or death) and significantly improved CD4 cell count. Survival benefit could not be assessed due to limited duration of follow-up at the time the

Continued on next page

Glaxo Wellcome Onc.—Cont.

placebo arms were discontinued. Other large studies of longer duration have not shown additional survival benefit of early versus delayed therapy with RETROVIR above that seen for patients with advanced HIV disease.

Monotherapy-Pediatrics:

Pediatric HIV Disease: Two open-label studies (n=36; mean follow-up 465 days, and n=88: mean follow-up 186 days) have evaluated the pharmacokinetics, safety, and efficacy of RETROVIR in children with advanced HIV disease (84 with AIDS and 40 with other clinical and laboratory evidence of advanced HIV disease). The median age at entry was 3.3 years (range: 3.5 months to 12 years) with 17 subjects younger than 12 months of age. In 73% of the cases, HIV was acquired by vertical transmission from an HIV-infected mother.

Clinical, immunologic, and virologic improvements were observed among some of the children receiving RETROVIR in these open-label studies. Clinical improvements included reductions in hepatosplenomegaly and increases in weight percentiles in children with delayed growth. The probability of remaining free of opportunistic infections through 12 months of follow-up was 0.76 and the probability of survival at 12 months was 0.87 for these patients.

Improvements in CD4 cell counts and normalization of immunoglobulin concentration were observed among the patients receiving RETROVIR. An antiretroviral effect was demonstrated by reductions in serum and CSF p24 antigen concentrations, as well as by a reduction in the number of patients with positive CSF HIV cultures.

Pregnant Women and Their Newborn Infants:

The utility of RETROVIR for the prevention of maternal-fetal HIV transmission was demonstrated in a randomized, double-blind, placebo-controlled trial (ACTG 076) conducted in HIV-infected pregnant women with CD4 cell counts of 200 to 1818 cells/mm^3 (median in the treated group: 560 cells/mm^3) who had little or no previous exposure to RETROVIR. Oral RETROVIR was initiated between 14 and 34 weeks of gestation (median 11 weeks of therapy) followed by intravenous administration of RETROVIR during labor and delivery. After birth, infants received oral RETROVIR Syrup for 6 weeks. The study showed a statistically significant difference in the incidence of HIV infection in the infants (based on viral culture from peripheral blood) between the group receiving RETROVIR and the group receiving placebo. Of 363 infants evaluated in the study, the estimated risk of HIV infection was 8.3% in the group receiving RETROVIR and 25.5% in the placebo group, a relative reduction in transmission risk of 67.5%.

RETROVIR was well-tolerated by mothers and infants. There was no difference in pregnancy-related adverse events between the treatment groups. The mean difference in hemoglobin values was less than 1.0 g/dL for infants receiving RETROVIR compared to infants receiving placebo. Infants did not require transfusion and hemoglobin values spontaneously returned to normal within 6 weeks after completion of therapy with RETROVIR. The long-term consequences of *in utero* and infant exposure to RETROVIR are unknown.

Combination Therapy with RETROVIR and Zalcitabine:

Patients with Prior Exposure to RETROVIR: The use of RETROVIR in combination with zalcitabine in patients who have previously received RETROVIR is based on the results from a subgroup analysis of a Phase 3, randomized, double-blind clinical trial (ACTG 155). ACTG 155 was a comparative study (n=1001) of zalcitabine alone or in combination with RETROVIR versus RETROVIR alone in patients with an entry CD4 cell count ≤300 cells/mm^3 who had previously received RETROVIR for 6 months or more (median 18 months).

Overall, there were no significant differences in disease progression or death for the three study groups. However, for those patients on combination RETROVIR and zalcitabine with baseline CD4 cell counts between 150 to 300 cells/mm^3 at entry, there were fewer study endpoints of disease progression when compared to the group receiving monotherapy with RETROVIR but not the zalcitabine monotherapy group. There were too few deaths in the ≥150 cells/mm^3 subgroup for an effect on survival alone to be assessed. All treatment arms eventually showed decline in CD4 cell count despite treatment, although for the combination arm there was an initial increase for patients with CD4 cell counts ≥150 cells/mm^3. Further studies are ongoing to confirm clinical benefit from combination therapy.

Patients without Prior Exposure to RETROVIR: The use of RETROVIR in combination with zalcitabine in patients without prior exposure to RETROVIR (<4 weeks prior therapy) is based on two small clinical studies (ACTG 106 and BW 34,225-02) showing a greater rise in CD4 cell counts, which was maintained longer with combination therapy when compared to monotherapy with RETROVIR.[5,6]

There have been no results from controlled studies of combination therapy with primary clinical endpoints of disease progression or death in patients who were naive to antiretroviral therapy when combination therapy was initiated.

INDICATIONS AND USAGE

Monotherapy:

Adults: RETROVIR is indicated for the initial treatment of HIV-infected adults with CD4 cell counts of 500 cells/mm^3 or less (see CLINICAL PHARMACOLOGY: Description of Clinical Studies). Therapy with RETROVIR has been shown to prolong survival and decrease the incidence of opportunistic infections in patients with advanced HIV disease at the time of initiation of therapy and to delay disease progression in asymptomatic HIV-infected patients.

Studies in adults found monotherapy with RETROVIR to be clinically superior to didanosine or zalcitabine monotherapy for the initial management of HIV-infected patients who have not received previous antiretroviral treatment. However, randomized studies have shown that for some patients with advanced disease on prolonged therapy with RETROVIR, modifying the antiviral regimen may be more effective in delaying disease progression than remaining on monotherapy with RETROVIR.

Pediatrics: RETROVIR is indicated for HIV-infected children over 3 months of age who have HIV-related symptoms or who are asymptomatic with abnormal laboratory values indicating significant HIV-related immunosuppression (see CLINICAL PHARMACOLOGY: Description of Clinical Studies).

Maternal-Fetal HIV Transmission: RETROVIR is also indicated for the prevention of maternal-fetal HIV transmission as part of a regimen that includes oral RETROVIR beginning between 14 and 34 weeks of gestation, intravenous RETROVIR during labor, and administration of RETROVIR Syrup to the newborn after birth. However, transmission to infants may still occur in some cases despite the use of this regimen. The efficacy of this regimen for preventing HIV transmission in women who have received RETROVIR for a prolonged period before pregnancy has not been evaluated. The safety of RETROVIR for the mother or fetus during the first trimester of pregnancy has not been assessed (see CLINICAL PHARMACOLOGY: Description of Clinical Studies).

Combination Therapy with RETROVIR and Zalcitabine:

RETROVIR in combination with zalcitabine is indicated for the treatment of selected patients with advanced HIV disease (CD4 cell count ≤300 cells/mm^3). In patients without prior exposure to RETROVIR, this indication is based on greater increases in CD4 cell counts that were maintained longer for patients treated with combination therapy as compared to monotherapy with RETROVIR. In patients with no prior exposure to RETROVIR, there have been no studies showing clinical benefit from combination therapy compared to RETROVIR alone. For patients with prior exposure to RETROVIR, this indication is based on a subgroup analysis of clinical data that showed a clinical benefit only for those patients with a CD4 cell count ≥150 cells/mm^3 at the time of initiation of therapy. No benefit from combination therapy has been observed in a study of patients with extensive prior exposure to RETROVIR (median 18 months) and CD4 cell counts <150 cell/mm^3; combination therapy is therefore not recommended for these patients (see CLINICAL PHARMACOLOGY: Description of Clinical Studies).

CONTRAINDICATIONS

RETROVIR Capsules and Syrup are contraindicated for patients who have potentially life-threatening allergic reactions to any of the components of the formulations.

WARNINGS

Note: The full safety and efficacy profile of RETROVIR has not been defined, particularly in regard to prolonged use in HIV-infected individuals who have less advanced disease (see INDICATIONS AND USAGE, CLINICAL PHARMACOLOGY: Microbiology, and PRECAUTIONS: Carcinogenesis, Mutagenesis, Impairment of Fertility). The incidence of adverse reactions appears to increase with disease progression, and patients should be monitored carefully, especially as disease progression occurs.

The safety profile of combination therapy with RETROVIR and zalcitabine reflects the individual safety profiles of each component. The complete prescribing information for zalcitabine should be consulted before combination therapy with RETROVIR and zalcitabine is initiated.

Bone Marrow Suppression: RETROVIR should be used with extreme caution in patients who have bone marrow compromise evidenced by granulocyte count <1000 cells/mm^3 or hemoglobin <9.5 g/dL. In all of the placebo-controlled studies, but most frequently in patients with advanced symptomatic HIV disease, anemia and granulocytopenia were the most significant adverse events observed (see ADVERSE REACTIONS). There have been reports of pancytopenia associated with the use of RETROVIR, which was reversible in most instances after discontinuance of the drug.

Significant anemia most commonly occurred after 4 to 6 weeks of therapy and in many cases required dose adjustment, discontinuation of RETROVIR, and/or blood transfusions. Frequent blood counts are strongly recommended in patients with advanced HIV disease taking RETROVIR. For asymptomatic HIV-infected individuals and patients with early HIV disease, most of whom have better marrow reserve, blood counts may be obtained less frequently, depending upon the patient's overall status. If anemia or granulocytopenia develops, dosage adjustments may be necessary (see DOSAGE AND ADMINISTRATION).

Myopathy: Myopathy and myositis with pathological changes, similar to that produced by HIV disease, have been associated with prolonged use of RETROVIR.

Lactic Acidosis/Severe Hepatomegaly with Steatosis: Rare occurrences of lactic acidosis in the absence of hypoxemia, and severe hepatomegaly with steatosis have been reported with the use of antiretroviral nucleoside analogues, including RETROVIR and zalcitabine, and are potentially fatal; it is not known whether these events are causally related to the use of thesse drugs. Lactic acidosis should be considered whenever a patient receiving therapy with RETROVIR develops unexplained tachypnea, dyspnea, or fall in serum bicarbonate level. Under these circumstances, therapy with RETROVIR should be suspended until the diagnosis of lactic acidosis has been excluded. Caution should be exercised when administering RETROVIR to any patient, particularly obese women, with hepatomegaly, hepatitis, or other known risk factor for liver disease. These patients should be followed closely while on therapy with RETROVIR. The significance of elevated aminotransferase levels suggesting hepatic injury in HIV-infected patients prior to starting RETROVIR or while on RETROVIR is unclear. Treatment with RETROVIR should be suspended in the setting of rapidly elevating aminotransferase levels, progressive hepatomegaly, or metabolic/lactic acidosis of unknown etiology.

Other Serious Adverse Reactions: Several serious adverse events have been reported with use of RETROVIR in clinical practice. Reports of pancreatitis, sensitization reactions (including anaphylaxis in one patient), vasculitis, and seizures have been rare. These adverse events, except for sensitization, have also been associated with HIV disease. Changes in skin and nail pigmentation have been associated with the use of RETROVIR.

Use in Infancy: A positive test for HIV-antibody in children under 15 months of age may represent passively acquired maternal antibodies, rather than an active antibody response to infection in the infant. Thus, the presence of HIV antibody in a child less than 15 months of age must be interpreted with caution, especially in the asymptomatic infant. Confirmatory tests such as serum p24 antigen or viral culture should be pursued in such children.

PRECAUTIONS

General: Zidovudine is eliminated from the body primarily by renal excretion following metabolism in the liver (glucuronidation). In patients with severely impaired renal function, dosage reduction is recommended (see CLINICAL PHARMACOLOGY: Pharmacokinetics and DOSAGE AND ADMINISTRATION). Although very little data are available, patients with severely impaired hepatic function may be at greater risk of toxicity.

Information for Patients: RETROVIR is not a cure for HIV infections, and patients may continue to acquire illnesses associated with HIV infection, including opportunistic infections. Therefore, patients should be advised to seek medical care for any significant change in their health status.

The safety and efficacy of RETROVIR in women, intravenous drug users, and racial minorities[7–9] is not significantly different than that observed in white males.

Patients should be informed that the major toxicities of RETROVIR are granulocytopenia and/or anemia. The frequency and severity of these toxicities are greater in patients with more advanced disease and in those who initiate therapy later in the course of their infection. They should be told that if toxicity develops, they may require transfusions or dose modifications including possible discontinuation. They should be told of the extreme importance of having their blood counts followed closely while on therapy, especially for patients with advanced symptomatic HIV disease. They should be cautioned about the use of other medications, including ganciclovir and interferon-alpha, that may exacerbate the toxicity of RETROVIR (see PRECAUTIONS: Drug Interactions). Patients should be informed that other adverse effects of RETROVIR include nausea and vomiting. Patients should also be encouraged to contact their physician if they experience muscle weakness, shortness of breath, symptoms of hepatitis or pancreatitis, or any other unexpected adverse events while being treated with RETROVIR.

RETROVIR Capsules and Syrup are for oral ingestion only. Patients should be told of the importance of taking RETROVIR exactly as prescribed. They should be told not to share medication and not to exceed the recommended dose. Patients should be told that the long-term effects of RETROVIR are unknown at this time.

Pregnant women considering the use of RETROVIR during pregnancy for prevention of HIV-transmission to their infants should be advised that transmission may still occur in

some cases despite therapy. The long-term consequences of *in utero* and infant exsporue to RETROVIR are unknown. HIV-infected pregnant women should be advised not to breast-feed to avoid postnatal transmission of HIV to a child who may not yet be infected.

Patients should be advised that therapy with RETROVIR has not been shown to reduce the risk of transmission of HIV to others through sexual contact or blood contamination.

Drug Interactions:

Ganciclovir: Use of RETROVIR in combination with ganciclovir increases the risk of hematologic toxicities in some patients with advanced HIV disease. Should the use of this combination become necessary in the treatment of patients with HIV disease, dose reduction or interruption of one or both agents may be necessary to minimize hematologic toxicity. Hematologic parameters, including hemoglobin, hematocrit, and white blood cell count with differential, should be monitored frequently in all patients receiving this combination.

Interferon-alpha: Hematologic toxicities have also been seen when RETROVIR is used concomitantly with interferon-alpha. As with the concomitant use of RETROVIR and ganciclovir, dose reduction or interruption of one or both agents may be necessary, and hematologic parameters should be monitored frequently.

Bone Marrow Suppressive Agents/Cytotoxic Agents: Coadministration of RETROVIR with drugs that are cytotoxic or which interfere with RBC/WBC number or function (e.g., dapsone, flucytosine, vincristine, vinblastine, or adriamycin) may increase the risk of hematologic toxicity.

Probenecid: Limited data suggest that probenecid may increase zidovudine levels by inhibiting glucuronidation and/or by reducing renal excretion of zidovudine. Some patients who have used RETROVIR concomitantly with probenecid have developed flu-like symptoms consisting of myalgia, malaise, and/or fever and maculopapular rash.

Phenytoin: Phenytoin plasma levels have been reported to be low in some patients receiving RETROVIR, while in one case a high level was documented. However, in a pharmacokinetic interaction study in which 12 HIV-positive volunteers received a single 300 mg phenytoin dose alone and during steady-state zidovudine conditions (200 mg every 4 hours), no change in phenytoin kinetics was observed. Although not designed to optimally assess the effect of phenytoin on zidovudine kinetics, a 30% decrease in oral zidovudine clearance was observed with phenytoin.

Methadone: In a pharmacokinetic study of nine HIV-positive patients receiving methadone-maintenance (30 to 90 mg daily) concurrent with 200 mg of RETROVIR every 4 hours, no changes were observed in the pharmacokinetics of methadone upon initiation of therapy with RETROVIR and after 14 days of treatment with RETROVIR. No adjustments in methadone-maintenance requirements were reported. For four patients, the mean zidovudine AUC was elevated twofold, while for five patients, the value was equal to that of control patients. The exact mechanism and clinical significance of these data are unknown.

Fluconazole: The coadministration of fluconazole with RETROVIR has been reported to interfere with the oral clearance and metabolism of RETROVIR. In a pharmacokinetic interaction study in which 12 HIV-positive men received RETROVIR 200 mg every 8 hours alone and in combination with fluconazole 400 mg daily, fluconazole increased th zidovudine AUC (74%; range 28% to 173%) and the zidovudine half-life (128%; range −4% to 189%) at steady state. The clinical significance of this interaction is unknown.

Atovaquone: Data from 14 HIV-infected volunteers who were given atovaquone tablets 750 mg every 12 hours with zidovudine 200 mg every 8 hours showed a $24\% \pm 12\%$ decrease in zidovudine oral clearance, leading to a $35\% \pm 23\%$ increase in plasma zidovudine AUC. The glucuronide metabolite:parent ratio decreased from a mean of 4.5 when zidovudine was administered alone to 3.1 when zidovudine was administered with atovaquone tablets. This effect is minor and would not be expected to produce clinically significant events. Zidovudine had no effect on atovaquone pharmacokinetics.

Valproic Acid: The concomitant administration of valproic acid 250 mg (n = 5) or 500 mg (n = 1) every 8 hours and zidovudine 100 mg orally every 8 hours for 4 days to six HIV-infected, asymptomatic male volunteers resulted in a $79\% \pm 61\%$ (mean ± SD) increase in the plasma zidovudine AUC and a $22\% \pm 10\%$ decrease in the plasma GZDV AUC as compared to the administration of zidovudine in the absence of valproic acid. The GZDV/zidovudine urinary excretion ratio decreased $58\% \pm 12\%$. Because no change in the zidovudine plasma half-life occurred, these results suggest that valproic acid may increase the oral bioavailability of zidovudine through inhibition of first-pass metabolism. Although the clinical significance of this interaction is unknown, patients should be monitored more closely for a possible increase in zidovudine-related adverse effects. The effect of zidovudine on the pharmacokinetics of valproic acid was not evaluated.

Other Nucleoside Analogues: Some experimental nucleoside analogues which are being evaluated in HIV-infected patients may affect RBC/WBC number or function and may increase the potential for hematologic toxicity of RETROVIR. Some experimental nucleoside analogues affecting DNA replication such as ribavirin, antagonize the in vitro antiviral activity of RETROVIR against HIV and thus, concomitant use of such drugs should be avoided.

Other Agents: Some drugs such as trimethoprim-sulfamethoxazole, pyrimethamine, and acyclovir may be necessary for the management or prevention of opportunistic infections. In the placebo-controlled trial in patients with advanced HIV disease, increased toxicity was not detected with limited exposure to these drugs. However, there is one published report of neurotoxicity (profound lethargy) associated with concomitant use of RETROVIR and acyclovir. Preliminary data from a drug interaction study (n = 10) suggest that coadministration of 200 mg RETROVIR and 600 mg rifampin decreases the area under the plasma concentration curve by an average of $48\% \pm 34\%$. However, the effect of once daily dosing of rifampin on multiple daily doses of RETROVIR is unknown.

Carcinogenesis, Mutagenesis, Impairment of Fertility: Zidovudine was administered orally at three dosage levels to separate groups of mice and rats (60 females and 60 males in each group). Initial single daily doses were 30, 60, and 120 mg/kg/day in mice and 80, 220, and 600 mg/kg/day in rats. The doses in mice were reduced to 20, 30, and 40 mg/kg/day after day 90 because of treatment-related anemia, whereas in rats only the high dose was reduced to 450 mg/kg/day on day 91 and then to 300 mg/kg/day on day 279.

In mice, seven late-appearing (after 19 months) vaginal neoplasms (five non-metastasizing squamous cell carcinomas, one squamous cell papilloma, and one squamous polyp) occurred in animals given the highest dose. One late-appearing squamous cell papilloma occurred in the vagina of a middle dose animal. No vaginal tumors were found at the lowest dose.

In rats, two late-appearing (after 20 months), non-metastasizing vaginal squamous cell carcinomas occurred in animals given the highest dose. No vaginal tumors occurred at the low or middle dose in rats. No other drug-related tumors were observed in either sex of either species.

It is not known how predictive the results of rodent carcinogenicity studies may be for humans. At doses that produced tumors in mice and rats, the estimated drug exposure (as measured by AUC) was approximately 3 times (mouse) and 24 times (rat) the estimated human exposure at the recommended therapeutic dose of 100 mg every 4 hours.

No evidence of mutagenicity (with or without metabolic activation) was observed in the Ames *Salmonella* mutagenicity assay at concentrations up to 10 μg per plate, which was the maximum concentration that could be tested because of the antimicrobial activity of zidovudine against the *Salmonella* species. In a mutagenicity assay conducted in L5178Y/TK$^{+/-}$ mouse lymphoma cells, zidovudine was weakly mutagenic in the absence of metabolic activation only at the highest concentrations tested (4000 and 5000 μg/mL). In the presence of metabolic activation, the drug was weakly mutagenic at concentrations of 1000 μg/mL and higher. In an in vitro mammalian cell transformation assay, zidovudine was positive at concentrations of 0.5 μg/mL and higher. In an in vitro cytogenetic study performed in cultured human lymphocytes, zidovudine induced dose-related structural chromosomal abnormalities at concentrations of 3 μg/mL and higher. No such effects were noted at the two lowest concentrations tested, 0.3 and 1 μg/mL. In an in vivo cytogenetic study in rats given a single intravenous injection of zidovudine at doses of 37.5 to 300 mg/kg, there were no treatment-related structural or numerical chromosomal alterations in spite of plasma levels that were as high as 453 μg/mL 5 minutes after dosing.

In two in vivo micronucleus studies (designed to measure chromosome breakage or mitotic spindle apparatus damage) in male mice, oral doses of zidovudine 100 to 1000 mg/kg/day administered once daily for approximately 4 weeks induced dose-related increases in micronucleated erythrocytes. Similar results were also seen after 4 or 7 days of dosing at 500 mg/kg/day in rats and mice.

In a study involving 11 AIDS patients, it was reported that the seven patients who were receiving RETROVIR (1200 mg/day) as their only medication for 4 weeks to 7 months showed a chromosome breakage frequency of 8.29 ± 2.65 breaks per 100 peripheral lymphocytes. This was significantly ($P < 0.05$) higher than the incidence of 0.5 ± 0.29 breaks per 100 cells that was observed in the four AIDS patients who had not received RETROVIR.

No effect on male or female fertility (judged by conception rates) was seen in rats given zidovudine orally at doses up to 450 mg/kg/day.

Pregnancy: Pregnancy Category C. Oral teratology studies in the rat and in the rabbit at doses up to 500 mg/kg/day revealed no evidence of teratogenicity with zidovudine. Zidovudine treatment resulted in embryo/fetal toxicity as evidenced by an increase in the incidence of fetal resorptions in rats given 150 or 450 mg/kg/day and rabbits given 500 mg/kg/day. The doses used in the teratology studies resulted in peak zidovudine plasma concentrations (after one-half of the daily dose) in rats 66 to 226 times, and in rabbits 12 to 87 times, mean steady-state peak human plasma concentrations (after one-sixth of the daily dose) achieved with the recommended daily dose (100 mg every 4 hours). In an in vitro experiment with fertilized mouse oocytes, zidovudine exposure resulted in a dose-dependent reduction in blastocyst formation. In an additional teratology study in rats, a dose of 3000 mg/kg/day (very near the oral median lethal dose in rats of 3683 mg/kg) caused marked maternal toxicity and an increase in the incidence of fetal malformations. This dose resulted in peak zidovudine plasma concentrations 350 times peak human plasma concentrations. (Estimated area-under-the-curve [AUC] in rats at this dose level was 300 times the daily AUC in humans given 600 mg per day.) No evidence of teratogenicity was seen in this experiment at doses of 600 mg/kg/day or less.

A randomized, double-blind, placebo-controlled trial was conducted in HIV-infected pregnant women to determine the utility of RETROVIR for the prevention of maternal-fetal HIV-transmission (see CLINICAL PHARMACOLOGY: Clinical Studies). Congenital abnormalities occurred with similar frequency between infants born to mothers who received RETROVIR and infants born to mothers who received placebo. Abnormalities were either problems in embryogenesis (prior to 14 weeks) or were recognized on ultrasound before or immediately after initation of study drug.

Antiretroviral Pregnancy Registry: To monitor maternal-fetal outcomes of pregnant women exposed to RETROVIR, an Antiretroviral Pregnancy Registry has been established. Physicians are encouraged to register patients by calling (800) 722-9292, ext. 38465.

Nursing Mothers: The U.S. Public Health Service Centers for Disease Control and Prevention advises HIV-infected women not to breast-feed to avoid postnatal transmission of HIV to a child who may not yet be infected.

It is not known whether zidovudine is excreted in human milk or whether RETROVIR reduces the potential for transmission of HIV in breast milk. Lactating mice administered zidovudine (200 mg/kg intraperitoneally) were found to have milk concentrations of zidovudine five times the corresponding serum zidovudine concentration. Milk concentrations of zidovudine declined at a slower rate than serum zidovudine concentrations.

Pediatric Use: See INDICATIONS, ADVERSE REACTIONS, and DOSAGE AND ADMINISTRATION sections.

ADVERSE REACTIONS

Monotherapy: *Adults:* The frequency and severity of adverse events associated with the use of RETROVIR in adults are greater in patients with more advanced infection at the time of initiation of therapy. The following table summarizes the relative incidence of hematologic adverse events ob-

Table 1

Stage of Disease	RETROVIR® Daily Dose* (mg)	Granulocytopenia (<750 cells/mm³)	Anemia (Hgb < 8.0 g/dL)
Asymptomatic			
ACTG 019[3]	500	1.8%†	1.1%†
Early HIV Disease			
(CD4 > 200 cells/mm³)			
ACTG 016[4]	1200	4%	4%
Advanced HIV Disease			
(CD4 > 200 cells/mm³)			
BW 02[1]	1500	10%†	3%†‡
(CD4 ≤ 200 cells/mm³)			
ACTG 002[10]	600	37%	29%
BW 02[1]	1500	47%	29%‡

*The currently recommended dose is 500 to 600 mg daily.
†Not statistically significant compared to placebo.
‡Anemia = Hgb <7.5 g/dL.

Continued on next page

Glaxo Wellcome Onc.—Cont.

served in clinical studies by severity of HIV disease present at the start of treatment.
[See table at bottom of preceding page.]

The anemia reported in patients with advanced HIV disease receiving RETROVIR appeared to be the result of impaired erythrocyte maturation as evidenced by macrocytosis while on drug. Although mean platelet counts in patients receiving RETROVIR were significantly increased compared to mean baseline values, thrombocytopenia did occur in some of these patients with advanced disease.[1] Twelve percent of patients receiving RETROVIR compared to 5% of patients receiving placebo had >50% decreases from baseline platelet count. Mild drug-associated elevations in total bilirubin levels have been reported as an uncommon occurrence in patients treated for asymptomatic HIV infection.

The HIV-infected adults participating in these clinical trials often had baseline symptoms and signs of HIV disease and/or experienced adverse events at some time during study. It was often difficult to distinguish adverse events possibly associated with administration of RETROVIR from underlying signs of HIV disease or intercurrent illness. The following table summarizes clinical adverse events or symptoms which occurred in at least 5% of all patients with advanced HIV disease treated with 1500 mg/day of RETROVIR in the original placebo-controlled study.[2] Of the items listed in the table, only severe headache, nausea, insomnia, and myalgia were reported at a significantly greater rate in patients receiving RETROVIR.

Table 2

Percentage (%) of Patients with Clinical Events in Advanced HIV Disease (BW 02)

Adverse Event	RETROVIR® 1500 mg/day* (n = 144)%	Placebo (n = 137)%
BODY AS A WHOLE		
Asthenia	19	18
Diaphoresis	5	4
Fever	16	12
Headache	42	37
Malaise	8	7
GASTROINTESTINAL		
Anorexia	11	8
Diarrhea	12	18
Dyspepsia	5	4
GI Pain	20	19
Nausea	46	18
Vomiting	6	3
MUSCULOSKELETAL		
Myalgia	8	2
NERVOUS		
Dizziness	6	4
Insomnia	5	1
Paresthesia	6	3
Somnolence	8	9
RESPIRATORY		
Dyspnea	5	3
SKIN		
Rash	17	15
SPECIAL SENSES		
Taste Perversion	5	8

*The currently recommended dose is 500 to 600 mg/daily.

All events of a severe or life-threatening nature were monitored for adults in the placebo-controlled studies in early HIV disease and asymptomatic HIV infection. Data concerning the occurrence of additional signs or symptoms were also collected. No distinction was made in reporting events between those possibly associated with the administration of the study medication and those due to the underlying disease. The following tables summarize all those events reported at a statistically significant greater incidence for patients receiving RETROVIR in these studies:

Table 3

Percentage (%) of Patients with Adverse Events in Early HIV Disease (ACTG 016)

Adverse Event	RETROVIR® 1200 mg/day* (n = 361)%	Placebo (n = 352)%
BODY AS A WHOLE		
Asthenia	69	62
GASTROINTESTINAL		
Dyspepsia	6	1
Nausea	61	41
Vomiting	25	13

*The currently recommended dose is 500 to 600 mg/daily.

Table 4

Percentage (%) of Patients with Adverse Events* in Asymptomatic HIV Infection (ACTG 019)

Adverse Event	RETROVIR® 500 mg/day (n = 453)%	Placebo (n = 428)%
BODY AS A WHOLE		
Asthenia	8.6†	5.8
Headache	62.5	52.6
Malaise	53.2	44.9
GASTROINTESTINAL		
Anorexia	20.1	10.5
Constipation	6.4†	3.5
Nausea	51.4	29.9
Vomiting	17.2	9.8
NERVOUS		
Dizziness	17.9†	15.2

*Reported in ≥5% of study population.
†Not statistically significant verus placebo.

Several serious adverse events have been reported with the use of RETROVIR in clinical practice. Myopathy and myositis with pathological changes, similar to that produced by HIV disease, have been associated with prolonged use of RETROVIR. Reports of hepatomegaly with steatosis, hepatitis, pancreatitis, lactic acidosis, sensitization reactions (including anaphylaxis in one patient), hyperbilirubinemia, vasculitis, and seizures have been rare. These adverse events, except for sensitization, have also been associated with HIV disease. A single case of macular edema has been reported with the use of RETROVIR.

Additional adverse events reported in clinical trials at a rate not significantly different from placebo are listed below. Selected events from post-marketing clinical experience with RETROVIR are also included. Many of these events may occur as part of HIV disease. The clinical significance of the association between treatment with RETROVIR and these events is unknown.

Body as a Whole: abdominal pain, back pain, body odor, chest pain, chills, edema of the lip, fever, flu syndrome, hyperalgesia.
Cardiovascular: syncope, vasodilation.
Gastrointestinal: bleeding gums, constipation, diarrhea, dysphagia, edema of the tongue, eructation, flatulence, mouth ulcer, rectal hemorrhage.
Hemic and Lymphatic: lymphadenopathy.
Musculoskeletal: arthralgia, muscle spasm, tremor, twitch.
Nervous: anxiety, confusion, depression, dizziness, emotional lability, loss of mental acuity, nervousness, paresthesia, somnolence, vertigo.
Respiratory: cough, dyspnea, epistaxis, hoarseness, pharyngitis, rhinitis, sinusitis.
Skin: acne, changes in skin and nail pigmentation, pruritus, rash, sweat, urticaria.
Special senses: amblyopia, hearing loss, photophobia, taste perversion.
Urogenital: dysuria, polyuria, urinary frequency, urinary hesitancy.

Pediatrics: Anemia and granulocytopenia among children with advanced HIV disease receiving RETROVIR occurred with similar incidence to that reported for adults with AIDS or advanced ARC (see above). Management of neutropenia and anemia included, in some cases, dose modification and/or blood product transfusions. In the open-label studies, 17% had their dose modified (generally a reduction in dose by 30%) due to anemia and 25% had their dose modified (temporary discontinuation or dose reduction by 30%) for neutropenia. Four children had RETROVIR permanently discontinued for neutropenia. The following table summarizes the occurrence of anemia (Hgb <7.5 g/dL) and granulocytopenia (<750 cells/mm³) among 124 children receiving RETROVIR for a mean of 267 days (range 3 to 855 days):

Table 5

Advanced Pediatric HIV disease (n= 124)	Granulocytopenia (<750 cells/mm³)		Anemia (Hgb <7.5 g/dL)	
	n	%	n	%
	48	39	28*	23

*Twenty-two children received one or more transfusions due to a decline in hemoglobin to <7.5 g/dL; an additional 15 children were transfused for hemoglobin levels >7.5 g/dL. Fifty-nine percent of the patients transfused had a pre-study history of anemia or transfusion requirement.

Macrocytosis was observed among the majority of children enrolled in the studies.

In the open-label studies involving 124 children, 16 clinical adverse events were reported by 24 children. No event was

reported by more than 5.6% of the study populations. Due to the open-label design of the studies, it was difficult to determine possible events related to use of RETROVIR versus disease-related events. Therefore, all clinical events reported as associated with therapy with RETROVIR or of unknown relationship to therapy with RETROVIR are presented in the following table:

Table 6

Percentage (%) of Pediatric Patients with Clinical Events in Open-Label Studies

Adverse Event	n	%
BODY AS A WHOLE		
Fever	4	3.2
Phlebitis*/Bacteremia	2	1.6
Headache	2	1.6
GASTROINTESTINAL		
Nausea	1	0.8
Vomiting	6	4.8
Abdominal Pain	4	3.2
Diarrhea	1	0.8
Weight Loss	1	0.8
NERVOUS		
Insomnia	3	2.4
Nervousness/Irritability	2	1.6
Decreased Reflexes	7	5.6
Seizure	1	0.8
CARDIOVASCULAR		
Left Ventricular Dilation	1	0.8
Cardiomyopathy	1	0.8
S₃ Gallop	1	0.8
Congestive Heart Failure	1	0.8
Generalized Edema	1	0.8
ECG Abnormality	3	2.4
UROGENITAL		
Hematuria/Viral Cystitis	1	0.8

*Peripheral vein I.V. catheter site.

The clinical adverse events reported among adult recipients of RETROVIR may also occur in children.

Use for the Prevention of Maternal-Fetal Transmission of HIV: In a randomized, double-blind, placebo-controlled trial in HIV-infected women and their infants conducted to determine the utility of RETROVIR for the prevention of maternal-fetal HIV transmission, RETROVIR Syrup at 2 mg/kg was administered every 6 hours for 6 weeks to infants beginning within 12 hours after birth. The most commonly reported adverse experiences were anemia (hemoglobin <9.0 g/dL) and neutropenia (<1000 cells/mm³). Anemia occurred in 22% of the infants who received RETROVIR and in 12% of the infants who received placebo. The mean difference in hemoglobin values was less than 1.0 g/dL for infants receiving RETROVIR compared to infants receiving placebo. No infants with anemia required transfusion and all hemoglobin values spontaneously returned to normal within 6 weeks after completion of therapy with RETROVIR. Neutropenia was reported with similar frequency in the group that received RETROVIR (21%) and in the group that received placebo (27%). The long-term consequences of *in utero* and infant exposure to RETROVIR are unknown.

Combination Therapy with RETROVIR and Zalcitabine: The safety profile of combination therapy with RETROVIR and zalcitabine reflects the individual safety profile of each component. The complete prescribing information for zalcitabine should be consulted before combination therapy with RETROVIR and zalcitabine is initiated.

OVERDOSAGE

Cases of acute overdoses in both children and adults have been reported with doses up to 50 grams. None were fatal. The only consistent finding in these cases of overdose was spontaneous or induced nausea and vomiting. Hematologic changes were transient and not severe. Some patients experienced nonspecific CNS symptoms such as headache, dizziness, drowsiness, lethargy, and confusion. One report of a grand mal seizure possibly attributable to RETROVIR occurred in a 35-year-old male 3 hours after ingesting 36 grams of RETROVIR. No other cause could be identified. All patients recovered without permanent sequelae. Hemodialysis and peritoneal dialysis appear to have a negligible effect on the removal of zidovudine while elimination of its primary metabolite, GZDV, is enhanced.

DOSAGE AND ADMINISTRATION

Monotherapy:
Adults: For adults with symptomatic HIV infection, including AIDS, the recommended oral dose is 100 mg (one 100 mg

capsule or 2 teaspoonsful [10 mL] syrup) every 4 hours (600 mg total daily dose). The effectiveness of this dose compared to higher dosing regimens in improving the neurologic dysfunction associated with HIV disease is unknown. A small randomized study found a greater effect of higher doses of RETROVIR on improvement of neurological symptoms in patients with pre-existing neurological disease.

For asymptomatic HIV infection, the recommended dose for adults is 100 mg administered orally every 4 hours while awake (500 mg/day).

Pediatrics: The recommended dose in children 3 months to 12 years of age is 180 mg/m^2 every 6 hours (720 mg/m^2 per day), not to exceed 200 mg every 6 hours.

Maternal-Fetal HIV Transmission: The recommended dosing regimen for administration to pregnant women (>14 weeks of pregnancy) and their newborn infants is:

Maternal Dosing: 100 mg orally 5 times per day until the start of labor. During labor and delivery, intravenous RETROVIR should be administered at 2 mg/kg (total body weight) over 1 hour followed by a continuous intravenous infusion of 1 mg/kg/h (total body weight) until clamping of the umbilical cord.

Infant Dosing: 2 mg/kg orally every 6 hours starting within 12 hours after birth and continuing through 6 weeks of age. Infants unable to receive oral dosing may be administered RETROVIR intravenously at 1.5 mg/kg, infused over 30 minutes, every 6 hours. (See PRECAUTIONS if hepatic disease or renal insufficiency is present.)

Combination Therapy with RETROVIR and Zalcitabine: The recommended dosage regimen consists of RETROVIR 200 mg taken orally with zalcitabine 0.75 mg every 8 hours.

Monitoring of Patients: Hematologic toxicities appear to be related to pretreatment bone marrow reserve and to dose and duration of therapy. In patients with poor bone marrow reserve, particularly in patients with advanced symptomatic HIV disease, frequent monitoring of hematologic indices is recommended to detect serious anemia or granulocytopenia (see WARNINGS). In patients who experience hematologic toxicity, reduction in hemoglobin may occur as early as 2 to 4 weeks, and granulocytopenia usually occurs after 6 to 8 weeks.

Dose Adjustment: Significant anemia (hemoglobin of <7.5 g/dL or reduction of >25% of baseline) and/or significant granulocytopenia (granulocyte count of <750 cells/mm^3 or reduction of >50% from baseline) may require a dose interruption until evidence of marrow recovery is observed (see WARNINGS). For less severe anemia or granulocytopenia, a reduction in daily dose may be adequate. In patients who develop significant anemia, dose modification does not necessarily eliminate the need for transfusion. If marrow recovery occurs following dose modification, gradual increases in dose may be appropriate depending on hematologic indices and patient tolerance.

In end-stage renal disease patients maintained on hemodialysis or peritoneal dialysis, recommended dosing is 100 mg every 6 to 8 hours (see CLINICAL PHARMACOLOGY; Pharmacokinetics).

There are insufficient data to recommend dose adjustment of RETROVIR in patients with impaired hepatic function.

HOW SUPPLIED

RETROVIR Capsules 100 mg (white, opaque cap and body with a dark blue band) containing 100 mg zidovudine and printed with "Wellcome" and unicorn logo on cap and "Y9C" and "100" on body. Bottles of 100 (NDC 0173-0108-55) and Unit Dose Pack of 100 (NDC 0173-0108-56).

Store at 15° to 25°C (59° to 77°F) and protect from moisture.

RETROVIR Syrup (colorless to pale yellow, strawberry-flavored) containing 50 mg zidovudine in each teaspoonful (5 mL). Bottle of 240 mL (NDC 0173-0113-18) with child-resistant cap.

Store at 15° to 25°C (59° to 77°F).

REFERENCES

1. Fischl MA, Richman DD, Grieco MH, et al. The efficacy of azidothymidine (AZT) in the treatment of patients with AIDS and AIDS-related complex. A double-blind, placebo-controlled trial. *N Engl J Med.* 1987;317:185–191.
2. Richman DD, Fischl MA, Grieco MH, et al. The toxicity of azidothymidine (AZT) in the treatment of patients with AIDS and AIDS-related complex. A double-blind, placebo-controlled trial. *N Engl J Med.* 1987;317:192–197.
3. Volberding PA, Lagakos SW, Koch MA, et al. Zidovudine in asymptomatic human immunodeficiency virus infection. A controlled trial in persons with fewer than 500 CD4-positive cells per cubic millimeter. *N Engl J Med.* 1990:322:941–949.
4. Fischl MA, Richman DD, Hansen N, et al. The safety and efficacy of zidovudine in the treatment of patients with mildly symptomatic HIV infection. A double-blind, placebo-controlled trial. *Ann Intern Med.* 1990; 112:727–737.
5. Meng T-C, Fischi MA, Boota AM, et al. Combination therapy with zidovudine and dideoxycytidine in patients with advanced human immunodeficiency virus infection. *Ann Intern Med.* 1992;116:13–20.
6. Schooley R and the Wellcome Resistance Study Collaborative Group. Trial of ZDV/ddI vs ZDV/ddC vs ZDV in HIV-infected patients with CD4 cell counts less than 300: Preliminary Results. Fourth European Conference on Clinical Aspects and Treatment of HIV infection, Milan, Italy, March 16–18, 1994, 052.
7. Creagh-Kirk T, Doi P, Andrews E, et al. Survival experience among patients with AIDS receiving zidovudine. Follow-up of patients in a compassionate plea program. *JAMA.* 1988;260:3009–3015.
8. Lagakos S, Fischl MA, Stein DS, Lim L, Volberding P. Effects of zidovudine therapy in minority and other subpopulations with early HIV infection. *JAMA.* 1991;266:2709–2712.
9. Easterbrook PJ, Keruly JC, Creagh-Kirk T. et al. Racial and ethnic differences in outcome in zidovudine-treated patients with advanced HIV disease, *JAMA.* 1991;266:2713–2718.
10. Fischl M, Parker C, Pettinelli C, Wulfsohn M, Hirsch M, Collier A, et al. A randomized controlled trial of a reduced daily dose of zidovudine in patients with the acquired immunodeficiency syndrome. *N Engl J Med.* 1990;323:1009–1014.

U.S. Patent Nos. 4818538 and 4828838 (Product Patents); 4724232, 4833130, and 4837208 (Use Patents)

February 1996/RL-271

Shown in Product Identification Guide, page 316

RETROVIR® ℞

[re 'trō-vir]

(zidovudine)

I.V. Infusion

FOR INTRAVENOUS INFUSION ONLY

WARNING: RETROVIR (ZIDOVUDINE) MAY BE ASSOCIATED WITH HEMATOLOGIC TOXICITY INCLUDING GRANULOCYTOPENIA AND SEVERE ANEMIA PARTICULARLY IN PATIENTS WITH ADVANCED HIV DISEASE (SEE WARNINGS). PROLONGED USE OF RETROVIR HAS ALSO BEEN ASSOCIATED WITH SYMPTOMATIC MYOPATHY SIMILAR TO THAT PRODUCED BY HUMAN IMMUNODEFICIENCY VIRUS.

RARE OCCURRENCES OF LACTIC ACIDOSIS IN THE ABSENCE OF HYPOXEMIA, AND SEVERE HEPATOMEGALY WITH STEATOSIS HAVE BEEN REPORTED WITH USE OF ANTIRETROVIRAL NUCLEOSIDE ANALOGUES, INCLUDING RETROVIR AND ZALCITABINE, AND ARE POTENTIALLY FATAL (SEE WARNINGS).

DESCRIPTION

RETROVIR is the brand name for zidovudine (formerly called azidothymidine [AZT]), a pyrimidine nucleoside analogue active against human immunodeficiency virus (HIV). RETROVIR I.V. Infusion is a sterile solution for intravenous infusion only. Each mL contains 10 mg zidovudine in Water for Injection. Hydrochloric acid and/or sodium hydroxide may have been added to adjust the pH to approximately 5.5. RETROVIR I.V. Infusion contains no preservatives.

The chemical name of zidovudine is 3′-azido-3′-deoxythymidine.

Zidovudine is a white to beige, odorless, crystalline solid with a molecular weight of 267.24 and a solubility of 20.1 mg/mL in water at 25°C. The molecular formula is $C_{10}H_{13}N_5O_4$.

CLINICAL PHARMACOLOGY

Zidovudine is an inhibitor of the in vitro replication of some retroviruses including HIV. This drug is a thymidine analogue in which the 3′-hydroxy (-OH) group is replaced by an azido (-N_3) group. Cellular thymidine kinase converts zidovudine into zidovudine monophosphate. The monophosphate is further converted into the diphosphate by cellular thymidylate kinase and to the triphosphate derivative by other cellular enzymes. Zidovudine triphosphate interferes with the HIV viral RNA dependent DNA polymerase (reverse transcriptase) and thus, inhibits viral replication. Zidovudine triphosphate also inhibits cellular α-DNA polymerase, but at concentrations 100-fold higher than those required to inhibit reverse transcriptase. In vitro, zidovudine triphosphate has been shown to be incorporated into growing chains of DNA by viral reverse transcriptase. When incorporation by the viral enzyme occurs, the DNA chain is terminated. Studies in cell culture suggest that zidovudine incorporation by cellular α-DNA polymerase may occur, but only to a very small extent and not in all test systems. Cellular γ-DNA polymerase shows some sensitivity to inhibition by the zidovudine triphosphate with 50% inhibitory concentration (IC_{50}) values 400 to 900 times greater than that for HIV reverse transcriptase.

Microbiology: The relationship between in vitro susceptibility of HIV to zidovudine and the inhibition of HIV replication in humans or clinical response to therapy has not been established. In vitro sensitivity results vary greatly depending upon the time between virus infection and zidovudine treatment of cell cultures, the particular assay used, the cell type employed, and the laboratory performing the test.

Zidovudine blocked 90% of detectable HIV replication in vitro at concentrations of ≤ 0.13 μg/mL (ID_{90}) when added shortly after laboratory infection of susceptible cells. This level of antiviral effect was observed in experiments measuring reverse transcriptase activity in HIV-infected H9 cells, PHA stimulated peripheral blood lymphocytes, and unstimulated peripheral blood lymphocytes. The concentration of drug required to produce a 50% decrease in supernatant reverse transcriptase was 0.013 μg/mL (ID_{50}) in both HIV-infected H9 cells and peripheral blood lymphocytes. Zidovudine at concentrations of 0.13 μg/mL also provided >90% protection from a strain of HIV (HTLV IIIB) induced cytopathic effects in two tetanus-specific T4 cell lines. HIV-p24 antigen expression was also undetectable at the same concentration in these cells. Partial inhibition of viral activity in cells with chronic HIV infection (presumed to carry integrated HIV DNA) required concentrations of zidovudine (8.8 μg/mL in one laboratory to 13.3 μg/mL in another) which are approximately 100 times as high as those necessary to block HIV replication in acutely infected cells. HIV isolates from 18 untreated individuals with AIDS or ARC had ID_{50} sensitivity values between 0.003 to 0.013 μg/mL and ID_{95} sensitivity values between 0.03 to 0.3 μg/mL.

Zidovudine has been shown to act additively or synergistically with a number of anti-HIV agents, including zalcitabine, didanosine, and interferon-alpha, in inhibiting the replication of HIV in cell culture.

The development of resistance to zidovudine has been studied extensively. The emergence of resistance is a function of both duration of zidovudine therapy and stage of disease. Asymptomatic patients developed resistance at significantly slower rates than patients with advanced disease. In contrast, virus isolates from patients with AIDS who received a year or more of zidovudine may show more than 100-fold increases in ID_{50} compared to isolates pre-therapy. In vitro resistance to zidovudine is due to the accumulation of specific mutations in the HIV reverse transcriptase coding region. Five amino acid substitutions (Met41→Leu, A67→Asn, Lys70→Arg, Thr215→Tyr or Phe, and Lys219→Gin) have been described in viruses with decreased in vitro susceptibility to zidovudine inhibition. The extent of resistance appears to be correlated with number of mutations in reverse transcriptase.

A significant correlation between zidovudine resistance and poor clinical outcome in pediatric patients with advanced disease has been reported; in addition, a correlation between reduced sensitivity to zidovudine and lower CD4 cell counts in symptom-free adults treated with zidovudine for up to 3 years has also been reported. However, the specific relationship between emergence of zidovudine resistance and clinical progression of disease in adults has not yet been defined.

Combination therapy of zidovudine plus zalcitabine does not appear to prevent the emergence of zidovudine-resistant isolates. In vitro studies with zidovudine-resistant virus isolates indicate zidovudine-resistant strains are usually sensitive to zalcitabine and didanosine.

The major metabolite of zidovudine, 3′-azido-3′-deoxy-5′-*O*-β-*D*-glucopyranuronosylthymidine (GZDV, formerly called GAZT), does not inhibit HIV replication in vitro. GZDV does not antagonize the antiviral effect of zidovudine in vitro nor does GZDV compete with zidovudine triphosphate as an inhibitor of HIV reverse transcriptase.

The cytotoxicity of zidovudine for various cell lines was determined using a cell growth inhibition assay. ID_{50} values for several human cell lines showed little growth inhibition by zidovudine except at concentrations >50 μg/mL. However, one human T-lymphocyte cell line was sensitive to the cytotoxic effect of zidovudine with an ID_{50} of 5 μg/mL. Moreover, in a colony-forming unit assay designed to assess the toxicity of zidovudine for human bone marrow, an ID_{50} value of <1.25 μg/mL was estimated. Two of ten human lymphocyte cultures tested were found to be sensitive to zidovudine at 5 μg/mL or less.

Zidovudine has antiviral activity against some other mammalian retroviruses in addition to HIV. Human immunodeficiency virus-2 (HIV-2) replication in vitro is inhibited by zidovudine with an ID_{50} of 0.015 μg/mL, while HTLV-1 transmission to susceptible cells is inhibited by 1 to 3 μg/mL concentrations of drug. Several strains of simian immunodeficiency virus (SIV) are also inhibited by zidovudine with ID_{50} values ranging from 0.13 to 6.5 μg/mL, depending upon species of origin and assay method used. No significant inhibitory activity was exhibited against a variety of other human and animal viruses, except an ID_{50} of 1.4 to 2.7 μg/mL against the Epstein-Barr virus, the clinical significance of which is unknown.

Continued on next page

Glaxo Wellcome Onc.—Cont.

The following microbiological activities of zidovudine have been observed in vitro, but the clinical significance is unknown. Many *Enterobacteriaceae,* including strains of *Shigella, Salmonella, Klebsiella, Enterobacter, Citrobacter,* and *Escherichia coli* are inhibited in vitro by low concentrations of zidovudine (0.005 to 0.5 μg/mL). Synergy of zidovudine with trimethoprim has been observed against some of these bacteria in vitro. Limited data suggest that bacterial resistance to zidovudine develops rapidly. Zidovudine has no activity against gram-positive organisms, anaerobes, mycobacteria, or fungal pathogens including *Candida albicans* and *Cryptococcus neoformans.* Although *Giardia lamblia* is inhibited by 1.9 μg/mL of zidovudine, no activity was observed against other protozoal pathogens.

Pharmacokinetics: ***Adults:*** The pharmacokinetics of zidovudine has been evaluated in 22 adult HIV-infected patients in a Phase I dose-escalation study. Following intravenous dosing, dose-independent kinetics was observed over the range of 1 to 5 mg/kg with a mean zidovudine half-life of 1.1 hours (range 0.48 to 2.86 hours). Total body clearance averaged 1900 mL/min/70 kg, and the apparent volume of distribution was 1.6 L/kg. At a dose of 7.5 mg/kg every 4 hours, total body clearance was calculated to be about 1200 mL/min/70 kg, with no change in half-life. Renal clearance is estimated to be 400 mL/min/70 kg, indicating glomerular filtration and active tubular secretion by the kidneys. Zidovudine plasma protein binding is 34% to 38%, indicating that drug interactions involving binding site displacement are not anticipated.

The mean steady-state peak and trough concentrations of zidovudine at 2.5 mg/kg every 4 hours were 1.06 and 0.12 μg/mL, respectively.

The zidovudine cerebrospinal fluid (CSF)/plasma concentration ratio was determined in 39 patients receiving chronic therapy with RETROVIR. The median ratio measured in 50 paired samples drawn 1 to 8 hours after the last dose of RETROVIR was 0.6.

Zidovudine is rapidly metabolized to 3′-azido-3′-deoxy-5′-*O*-*β-D*-glucopyranuronosylthymidine (GZDV) which has an apparent elimination half-life of 1 hour (range 0.61 to 1.73 hours). A second metabolite, 3′-amino-3′-deoxythymidine (AMT), has been identified in the plasma following single-dose intravenous administration of zidovudine. AMT area-under-the-curve (AUC) was one-fifth of the AUC of zidovudine and had a half-life of 2.7±0.7 hours. In comparison, GZDV AUC was about 3-fold greater than the AUC of zidovudine. Following intravenous administration, urinary recoveries of zidovudine and GZDV accounted for 18% and 60% of the dose, respectively, and the total urinary recovery averaged 77% (range 64% to 98%).

Adults with Impaired Renal Function: The pharmacokinetics of zidovudine has been evaluated in patients with impaired renal function following a single 200 mg oral dose. In 14 patients (mean creatinine clearance 18±2 mL/min) the half-life of zidovudine was 1.4 hours compared to 1.0 hour for control subjects with normal renal function; AUC values were approximately twice those of controls. Additionally, GZDV half-life in these patients was 8.0 hours (vs 0.9 hours for control) and AUC was 17 times higher than for control subjects. The pharmacokinetics and tolerance were evaluated in a multiple-dose study in patients undergoing hemodialysis (n=5) or peritoneal dialysis (n=6). Patients received escalating oral doses of zidovudine up to 200 mg five times daily for 8 weeks. Daily oral doses of 500 mg or less were well tolerated despite significantly elevated plasma levels of GZDV. Apparent oral clearance of zidovudine was approximately 50% of that reported in patients with normal renal function. The plasma concentrations of AMT are not known in patients with renal insufficiency. Daily oral doses of 300 to 400 mg should be appropriate in HIV-infected patients with severe renal dysfunction (see DOSAGE AND ADMINISTRATION: Dose Adjustment). Hemodialysis and peritoneal dialysis appear to have a negligible effect on the removal of zidovudine, whereas GZDV elimination is enhanced.

Pediatrics: The pharmacokinetics and bioavailability of zidovudine have been evaluated in 21 HIV-infected pediatric patients, aged 6 months through 12 years, following intravenous doses administered over the range of 80 to 160 mg/m² every 6 hours, and following oral doses of the intravenous solution administered over the range of 90 to 240 mg/m² every 6 hours. After discontinuation of the I.V. infusion, zidovudine plasma concentrations decayed biexponentially, consistent with two-compartment pharmacokinetics. Proportional increases in AUC and in zidovudine concentrations were observed with increasing dose, consistent with dose-independent kinetics over the dose range studied. The mean terminal half-life and total body clearance across all dose levels administered were 1.5 hours and 30.9 mL/min/kg, respectively. These values compare to mean half-life and total body clearance in adults of 1.1 hours and 27.1 mL/min/kg.

The pharmacokinetics of zidovudine has been studied in pediatric patients from birth to 3 months of life. In one study of the pharmacokinetics of zidovudine in women during the last trimester of pregnancy, zidovudine elimination was determined immediately after birth in eight neonates who were exposed to zidovudine *in utero.* The half-life was 13.0 ± 5.8 hours. In another study, the pharmacokinetics of zidovudine was evaluated in pediatric patients (ranging in age of 1 day to 3 months) of normal birth weight for gestational age and with normal renal and hepatic function. In neonates less than or equal to 14 days old, mean ± SD total body clearance was 10.9 ± 4.8 mL/min/kg (n=18) and half-life was 3.1 ± 1.2 hours (n=21). In neonates and infants greater than 14 days, total body clearance was 19.0 ± 4.0 mL/min/kg (n=16) and half-life was 1.9 ± 0.7 hours (n=18).

Concentrations of zidovudine in cerebrospinal fluid were measured after both intermittent oral and I.V. drug administration in 21 pediatric patients during Phase 1 and Phase 2 studies. The mean zidovudine CSF/plasma concentration ratio measured at an average time of 2.2 hours postdose at oral doses of 120 to 240 mg/m² was 0.52 ± 0.44 (n=28); after an I.V. infusion of doses of 80 to 160 mg/m² over 1 hour, the mean CSF/plasma concentration ratio was 0.87 ± 0.66 (n=23) at 3.2 hours after the start of the infusion. During continuous I.V. infusion, mean steady-state CSF/plasma ratio was 0.26 ± 0.17 (n=28).

As in adult patients, the major route of elimination in pediatric patients was by metabolism to GZDV. After I.V. dosing, about 29% of the dose was excreted in the urine unchanged and about 45% of the dose was excreted as GZDV. Overall, the pharmacokinetics of zidovudine in pediatric patients greater than 3 months of age is similar to that of zidovudine in adult patients.

Pregnancy: The pharmacokinetics of zidovudine has been studied in a Phase 1 study of eight women during the last trimester of pregnancy. As pregnancy progressed, there was no evidence of drug accumulation. The pharmacokinetics of zidovudine was similar to that of nonpregnant adults. Consistent with passive transmission of the drug across the placenta, zidovudine concentrations in infant plasma at birth were essentially equal to those in maternal plasma at delivery. Although data are limited, methadone maintenance therapy in five pregnant women did not appear to alter zidovudine pharmacokinetics. However, in another patient population, a potential for interaction has been identified (see PRECAUTIONS).

Nursing Mothers: After administration of a single dose of 200 mg zidovudine to 13 HIV-infected women, zidovudine was detected in human milk in concentrations similar to those achieved in serum (see PRECAUTIONS section).

Description of Clinical Studies:

Adults:

Randomized double-blind studies have demonstrated clinical benefit of initial treatment with RETROVIR compared to placebo, didanosine, or zalcitabine. Therapy with RETROVIR has been shown to prolong survival and decrease the incidence of opportunistic infections in patients with advanced HIV disease at the time of initiation of therapy and to delay disease progression in asymptomatic HIV-infected patients.

Other randomized studies suggest that the duration of the clinical benefit of monotherapy with RETROVIR is time-limited. Patients randomized to other antiviral regimens after initial therapy with RETROVIR had fewer AIDS progression end-points than those randomized to continue monotherapy with RETROVIR. The design of those studies did not define optimally when and how the antiviral regimen should be modified. Factors which may contribute to the development of disease progression while on therapy with RETROVIR are under clinical investigation and may include incomplete suppression of viral replication and development of decreased viral susceptibility to RETROVIR.

Advanced HIV Disease: A randomized, double-blind, placebo-controlled trial (BW 02) of oral RETROVIR (1500 mg/day) was conducted in 281 adults with advanced HIV disease which included 160 patients with AIDS and 121 patients with ARC.[1,2]

There were 19 deaths (12 in patients with AIDS, 7 in patients with ARC) in the placebo group and 1 death (patient with AIDS) in the group receiving RETROVIR. Treatment with RETROVIR significantly improved the probability of survival for 24 weeks in both the AIDS and ARC subgroups. During a follow-up protocol with open-label treatment with RETROVIR, patients who were initially randomized to receive RETROVIR continued to have better overall survival than did patients initially randomized to placebo. Survival rates in the group of patients initially randomized to receive RETROVIR declined to 85% after 1 year, 41% after 2 years, and 23% after 3 years. These survival rates may be lower than currently observed due to the absence of opportunistic infection (OI) prophylaxis in this study. RETROVIR also significantly reduced the risk of acquiring an AIDS-defining opportunistic infection, and patients who received RETROVIR generally did better than the placebo group in terms of several other measures of efficacy including performance level, neuropsychiatric function, maintenance of body weight, and the number and severity of symptoms associated with HIV disease.

In separate studies, initial therapy with RETROVIR was compared to initial therapy with either didanosine or zalcitabine. Survival rates in patients with no prior exposure to RETROVIR were significantly better for patients treated with RETROVIR than for patients treated with alternative monotherapy.

Asymptomatic HIV Infection and Early HIV Disease (CD4 between 200 to 500 cells/mm³): The population indicated for monotherapy with RETROVIR was extended to asymptomatic or symptomatic adults with CD4 cell counts of 500 cells/mm³ or less based on the results of two randomized double-blind placebo-controlled trials (ACTG 019[3], ACTG 016[4]) of 2051 adults. Treatment with RETROVIR reduced the risk of progression to advanced HIV disease (advanced AIDS Related Complex [ARC], AIDS, or death) and significantly improved CD4 cell count. Survival benefit could not be assessed due to limited duration of follow-up at the time the placebo arms were discontinued. Other large studies of longer duration have not shown additional survival benefit of early versus delayed therapy with RETROVIR above that seen for patients with advanced HIV disease.

Pediatrics:

Pediatric HIV Disease: Two open-label studies (n=36: mean follow-up 465 days, and n=88; mean follow-up 186 days) have evaluated the pharmacokinetics, safety, and efficacy of RETROVIR in pediatric patients with advanced HIV disease (84 with AIDS and 40 with other clinical and laboratory evidence of advanced HIV disease). The median age at entry was 3.3 years (range: 3.5 months to 12 years) with 17 subjects younger than 12 months of age. In 73% of the cases, HIV was acquired by vertical transmission from an HIV-infected mother.

Clinical, immunologic, and virologic improvements were observed among some of the pediatric patients receiving RETROVIR in these open-label studies. Clinical improvements included reductions in hepatosplenomegaly and increases in weight percentiles in patients with delayed growth. The probability of remaining free of opportunistic infections through 12 months of follow-up was 0.76 and the probability of survival at 12 months was 0.87 for these patients.

Improvements in CD4 cell counts and normalization of immunoglobulin concentration were observed among the patients receiving RETROVIR. An antiretroviral effect was demonstrated by reductions in serum and CSF p24 antigen concentrations, as well as by a reduction in the number of patients with positive CSF HIV cultures.

Pregnant Women and Their Neonates:

The utility of RETROVIR for the prevention of maternal-fetal HIV transmission was demonstrated in a randomized, double-blind, placebo-controlled trial (ACTG 076) conducted in HIV-infected pregnant women with CD4 cell counts of 200 to 1818 cells/mm³ (median in the treated group: 560 cells/mm³) who had little or no previous exposure to RETROVIR. Oral RETROVIR was initiated between 14 and 34 weeks of gestation (median 11 weeks of therapy) followed by intravenous administration of RETROVIR during labor and delivery. After birth, neonates received oral RETROVIR Syrup for 6 weeks. The study showed a statistically significant difference in the incidence of HIV infection in the neonates (based on viral culture from peripheral blood) between the group receiving RETROVIR and the group receiving placebo. Of 363 neonates evaluated in the study, the estimated risk of HIV infection was 8.3% in the group receiving RETROVIR and 25.5% in the placebo group, a relative reduction in transmission risk of 67.5%.

RETROVIR was well tolerated by mothers and neonates. There was no difference in pregnancy-related adverse events between the treatment groups. The mean difference in hemoglobin values was less than 1.0 g/dL for neonates receiving RETROVIR compared to neonates receiving placebo. Neonates did not require transfusion, and hemoglobin values spontaneously returned to normal within 6 weeks after completion of therapy with RETROVIR. The long-term consequences of *in utero* and neonatal exposure to RETROVIR are unknown.

INDICATIONS AND USAGE

Adults: RETROVIR I.V. Infusion is indicated for the initial treatment of HIV-infected adults with CD4 cell counts of 500 cells/mm³ or less (see CLINICAL PHARMACOLOGY: Description of Clinical Studies). Therapy with RETROVIR has been shown to prolong survival and decrease the incidence of opportunistic infections in patients with advanced HIV disease at the time of initiation of therapy and to delay disease progression in asymptomatic HIV-infected patients.

Studies in adults found monotherapy with RETROVIR to be clinically superior to didanosine or zalcitabine monotherapy for the initial management of HIV-infected patients who have not received previous antiretroviral treatment. However, randomized studies have shown that for some patients with advanced disease on prolonged therapy with RETROVIR, modifying the antiviral regimen may be more

effective in delaying disease progression than remaining on monotherapy with RETROVIR.

Pediatrics: RETROVIR is indicated for HIV-infected pediatric patients over 3 months of age who have HIV-related symptoms or who are asymptomatic with abnormal laboratory values indicating significant HIV-related immunosuppression (see CLINICAL PHARMACOLOGY: Description of Clinical Studies).

Maternal-Fetal HIV Transmission: RETROVIR is also indicated for the prevention of maternal-fetal HIV transmission as part of a regimen that includes oral RETROVIR beginning between 14 and 34 weeks of gestation, intravenous RETROVIR during labor, and administration of RETROVIR Syrup to the neonate after birth. However, transmission to neonates may still occur in some cases despite the use of this regimen. The efficacy of this regimen for preventing HIV transmission in women who have received RETROVIR for a prolonged period before pregnancy has not been evaluated. The safety of RETROVIR for the mother or fetus during the first trimester of pregnancy has not been assessed (see CLINICAL PHARMACOLOGY: Description of Clinical Studies).

CONTRAINDICATIONS

RETROVIR I.V. Infusion is contraindicated for patients who have potentially life-threatening allergic reactions to any of the components of the formulation.

WARNINGS

Note: The full safety and efficacy profile of RETROVIR has not been defined, particularly in regard to prolonged use in HIV-infected individuals who have less advanced disease (see INDICATIONS AND USAGE, CLINICAL PHARMACOLOGY: Microbiology, and PRECAUTIONS: Carcinogenesis, Mutagenesis, Impairment of Fertility). The incidence of adverse reactions appears to increase with disease progression, and patients should be monitored carefully, especially as disease progression occurs.

Bone Marrow Suppression: RETROVIR should be used with extreme caution in patients who have bone marrow compromise evidenced by granulocyte count <1000 cells/mm^3 or hemoglobin <9.5 g/dL. In all of the placebo-controlled studies, but most frequently in patients with advanced symptomatic HIV disease, anemia and granulocytopenia were the most significant adverse events observed (see ADVERSE REACTIONS). There have been reports of pancytopenia associated with the use of RETROVIR, which was reversible in most instances after discontinuance of the drug.

Significant anemia most commonly occurred after 4 to 6 weeks of therapy and in many cases required dose adjustment, discontinuation of RETROVIR, and/or blood transfusions. Frequent blood counts are strongly recommended in patients with advanced HIV disease taking RETROVIR. For asymptomatic HIV-infected individuals and patients with early HIV disease, most of whom have better marrow reserve, blood counts may be obtained less frequently, depending upon the patient's overall status. If anemia or granulocytopenia develops, dosage adjustments may be necessary (see DOSAGE AND ADMINISTRATION).

Myopathy: Myopathy and myositis with pathological changes, similar to that produced by HIV disease, have been associated with prolonged use of RETROVIR.

Lactic Acidosis/Severe Hepatomegaly with Steatosis: Rare occurrences of lactic acidosis in the absence of hypoxemia, and severe hepatomegaly with steatosis have been reported with the use of antiretroviral nucleoside analogues, including RETROVIR and zalcitabine, and are potentially fatal; it is not known whether these events are causally related to the use of these drugs. Lactic acidosis should be considered whenever a patient receiving therapy with RETROVIR develops unexplained tachypnea, dyspnea, or fall in serum bicarbonate level. Under these circumstances, therapy with RETROVIR should be suspended until the diagnosis of lactic acidosis has been excluded. Caution should be exercised when administering RETROVIR to any patient, particularly obese women, with hepatomegaly, hepatitis, or other known risk factor for liver disease. These patients should be followed closely while on therapy with RETROVIR. The significance of elevated aminotransferase levels suggesting hepatic injury in HIV-infected patients prior to starting RETROVIR or while on RETROVIR is unclear. Treatment with RETROVIR should be suspended in the setting of rapidly elevating aminotransferase levels, progressive hepatomegaly, or metabolic/lactic acidosis of unknown etiology.

Other Serious Adverse Reactions: Several serious adverse events have been reported with use of RETROVIR in clinical practice. Reports of pancreatitis, sensitization reactions (including anaphylaxis in one patient), vasculitis, and seizures have been rare. These adverse events, except for sensitization, have also been associated with HIV disease. Changes in skin and nail pigmentation have been associated with the use of RETROVIR.

Use in Pediatric Patients: A positive test for HIV-antibody in pediatric patients under 15 months of age may represent passively acquired maternal antibodies, rather than an active antibody response to infection in the patient. Thus, the presence of HIV antibody in a pediatric patient less than 15 months of age must be interpreted with caution, especially in the asymptomatic pediatric patient. Confirmatory tests such as serum p24 antigen or viral culture should be pursued in such patients.

PRECAUTIONS

General: Zidovudine is eliminated from the body primarily by renal excretion following metabolism in the liver (glucuronidation). In patients with severely impaired renal function, dosage reduction is recommended (see CLINICAL PHARMACOLOGY: Pharmacokinetics and DOSAGE AND ADMINISTRATION). Although very little data are available, patients with severely impaired hepatic function may be at greater risk of toxicity.

Information for Patients: RETROVIR is not a cure for HIV infections, and patients may continue to acquire illnesses associated with HIV infection, including opportunistic infections. Therefore, patients should be advised to seek medical care for any significant change in their health status.

The safety and efficacy of RETROVIR in treating women, intravenous drug users, and racial minorities[5–7] is not significantly different than that observed in white males.

Patients should be informed that major toxicities of RETROVIR are granulocytopenia and/or anemia. The frequency and severity of these toxicities are greater in patients with more advanced disease and in those who initiate therapy later in the course of their infection. They should be told that if toxicity develops, they may require transfusions or dose modifications including possible discontinuation. They should be told of the extreme importance of having their blood counts followed closely while on therapy, especially for patients with advanced symptomatic HIV disease. They should be cautioned about the use of other medications, including ganciclovir and interferon-alpha, that may exacerbate the toxicity of RETROVIR (see PRECAUTIONS: Drug Interactions). Patients should be informed that other adverse effects of RETROVIR include nausea and vomiting. Patients should also be encouraged to contact their physician if they experience muscle weakness, shortness of breath, symptoms of hepatitis or pancreatitis, or any other unexpected adverse events while being treated with RETROVIR.

Pregnant women considering the use of RETROVIR during pregnancy for prevention of HIV-transmission to their infants should be advised that transmission may still occur in some cases despite therapy. The long-term consequences of *in utero* and infant exposure to RETROVIR are unknown.

HIV-infected pregnant women should be advised not to breast-feed to avoid postnatal transmission of HIV to a child who may not yet be infected.

Patients should be advised that therapy with RETROVIR has not been shown to reduce the risk of transmission of HIV to others through sexual contact or blood contamination.

Drug Interactions:

Ganciclovir: Use of RETROVIR in combination with ganciclovir increases the risk of hematologic toxicities in some patients with advanced HIV disease. Should the use of this combination become necessary in the treatment of patients with HIV disease, dose reduction or interruption of one or both agents may be necessary to minimize hematologic toxicity. Hematologic parameters, including hemoglobin, hematocrit, and white blood cell count with differential, should be monitored frequently in all patients receiving this combination.

Interferon-alpha: Hematologic toxicities have also been seen when RETROVIR is used concomitantly with interferon-alpha. As with the concomitant use of RETROVIR and ganciclovir, dose reduction or interruption of one or both agents may be necessary, and hematologic parameters should be monitored frequently.

Bone Marrow Suppressive Agents/Cytotoxic Agents: Coadministration of RETROVIR with drugs that are cytotoxic or which interfere with RBC/WBC number or function (e.g., dapsone, flucytosine, vincristine, vinblastine, or adriamycin) may increase the risk of hematologic toxicity.

Probenecid: Limited data suggest that probenecid may increase zidovudine levels by inhibiting glucuronidation and/or by reducing renal excretion of zidovudine. Some patients who have used RETROVIR concomitantly with probenecid have developed flu-like symptoms consisting of myalgia, malaise, and/or fever and maculopapular rash.

Phenytoin: Phenytoin plasma levels have been reported to be low in some patients receiving RETROVIR, while in one case a high level was documented. However, in a pharmacokinetic interaction study in which 12 HIV-positive volunteers received a single 300 mg phenytoin dose alone and during steady-state zidovudine conditions (200 mg every 4 hours), no change in phenytoin kinetics was observed. Although not designed to optimally assess the effect of phenytoin on zidovudine kinetics, a 30% decrease in oral zidovudine clearance was observed with phenytoin.

Methadone: In a pharmacokinetic study of nine HIV-positive patients receiving methadone-maintenance (30 to 90 mg daily) concurrent with 200 mg of RETROVIR every 4 hours, no changes were observed in the pharmacokinetics of methadone upon initiation of therapy with RETROVIR and after 14 days of treatment with RETROVIR. No adjustments in methadone-maintenance requirements were reported. For four patients, the mean zidovudine AUC was elevated twofold, while for five patients, the value was equal to that of control patients. The exact mechanism and clinical significance of these data are unknown.

Fluconazole: The coadministration of fluconazole with RETROVIR has been reported to interfere with the oral clearance and metabolism of RETROVIR. In a pharmacokinetic interaction study in which 12 HIV-positive men received RETROVIR 200 mg every 8 hours alone and in combination with fluconazole 400 mg daily, fluconazole increased the zidovudine AUC (74%; range 28% to 173%) and the zidovudine half-life (128%; range −4% to 189%) at steady state. The clinical significance of this interaction is unknown.

Atovaquone: Data from 14 HIV-infected volunteers who were given atovaquone tablets 750 mg every 12 hours with zidovudine 200 mg every 8 hours showed a 24% ± 12% decrease in zidovudine oral clearance, leading to a 35% ± 23% increase in plasma zidovudine AUC. The glucuronide metabolite:parent ratio decreased from a mean of 4.5 when zidovudine was administered alone to 3.1 when zidovudine was administered with atovaquone tablets. This effect is minor and would not be expected to produce clinically significant events. Zidovudine had no effect on atovaquone pharmacokinetics.

Valproic Acid: The concomitant administration of valproic acid 250 mg (n=5) or 500 mg (n=1) every 8 hours and zidovudine 100 mg orally every 8 hours for 4 days to six HIV-infected, asymptomatic male volunteers resulted in a 79% ± 61% (mean ± SD) increase in the plasma zidovudine AUC and a 22% ± 10% decrease in the plasma GZDV AUC as compared to the administration of zidovudine in the absence of valproic acid. The GZDV zidovudine urinary excretion ratio decreased 58% ± 12%. Because no change in the zidovudine plasma half-life occurred, these results suggest that valproic acid may increase the oral bioavailability of zidovudine through inhibition of first-pass metabolism. Although the clinical significance of this interaction is unknown, patients should be monitored more closely for a possible increase in zidovudine-related adverse effects. The effect of zidovudine on the pharmacokinetics of valproic acid was not evaluated.

Other Nucleoside Analogues: Some experimental nucleoside analogues which are being evaluated in HIV-infected patients may affect RBC/WBC number or function and may increase the potential for hematologic toxicity of RETROVIR. Some experimental nucleoside analogues affecting DNA replication, such as ribavirin, antagonize the in vitro antiviral activity of RETROVIR against HIV and thus, concomitant use of such drugs should be avoided.

Other Agents: Some drugs such as trimethoprim-sulfamethoxazole, pyrimethamine, and acyclovir may be necessary for the management or prevention of opportunistic infections. In the placebo-controlled trial in patients with advanced HIV disease, increased toxicity was not detected with limited exposure to these drugs. However, there is one published report of neurotoxicity (profound lethargy) associated with concomitant use of RETROVIR and acyclovir. Preliminary data from a drug interaction study (n=10) suggest that coadministration of 200 mg RETROVIR and 600 mg rifampin decreases the area under the plasma concentration curve by an average of 48%±34%. However, the effect of once daily dosing of rifampin on multiple daily doses of RETROVIR is unknown.

Carcinogenesis, Mutagenesis, Impairment of Fertility: Zidovudine was administered orally at three dosage levels to separate groups of mice and rats (60 females and 60 males in each group). Initial single daily doses were 30, 60, and 120 mg/kg/day in mice and 80, 220, and 600 mg/kg/day in rats. The doses in mice were reduced to 20, 30, and 40 mg/kg/day after day 90 because of treatment-related anemia, whereas in rats only the high dose was reduced to 450 mg/kg/day on day 91, and then to 300 mg/kg/day on day 279.

In mice, seven late-appearing (after 19 months) vaginal neoplasms (5 non-metastasizing squamous cell carcinomas, one squamous cell papilloma, and one squamous polyp) occurred in animals given the highest dose. One late-appearing squamous cell papilloma occurred in the vagina of a middle dose animal. No vaginal tumors were found at the lowest dose.

In rats, two late-appearing (after 20 months), non-metastasizing vaginal squamous cell carcinomas occurred in animals given the highest dose. No vaginal tumors occurred at the low or middle dose in rats. No other drug-related tumors were observed in either sex of either species.

It is not known how predictive the results of rodent carcinogenicity studies may be for humans. At doses that produced tumors in mice and rats, the estimated drug exposure (as measured by AUC) was approximately 3 times (mouse) and 24 times (rat) the estimated human exposure at the recommended therapeutic dose of 100 mg every 4 hours.

Continued on next page

Glaxo Wellcome Onc.—Cont.

Table 1

Stage of Disease	RETROVIR® Daily Dose* (mg)	Granulocytopenia (<750 cells/mm³)	Anemia (Hgb < 8.0 g/dL)
Asymptomatic			
ACTG 019[3]	500	1.8%†	1.1%†
Early HIV Disease (CD4 > 200 cells/mm³)			
ACTG 016[4]	1200	4%	4%
Advanced HIV Disease (CD4 > 200 cells/mm³)			
BW 02[1]	1500	10%†	3%†‡
(CD4 ≤ 200 cells/mm³)			
ACTG 002[8]	600	37%	29%
BW 02[1]	1500	47%	29%‡

* The currently recommended oral dose is 500 to 600 mg daily.
† Not statistically significant compared to placebo.
‡ Anemia = Hgb <7.5 g/dL.

No evidence of mutagenicity (with or without metabolic activation) was observed in the Ames *Salmonella* mutagenicity assay at concentrations up to 10 μg per plate, which was the maximum concentration that could be tested because of the antimicrobial activity of zidovudine against the *Salmonella* species. In a mutagenicity assay conducted in L5178Y/TK$^{+/-}$ mouse lymphoma cells, zidovudine was weakly mutagenic in the absence of metabolic activation only at the highest concentrations tested (4000 and 5000 μg/mL). In the presence of metabolic activation, the drug was weakly mutagenic at concentrations of 1000 μg/mL and higher. In an in vitro mammalian cell transformation assay, zidovudine was positive at concentrations of 0.5 μg/mL and higher. In an in vitro cytogenetic study performed in cultured human lymphocytes, zidovudine induced dose-related structural chromosomal abnormalities at concentrations of 3 μg/mL and higher. No such effects were noted at the two lowest concentrations tested, 0.3 and 1 μg/mL. In an in vivo cytogenetic study in rats given a single intravenous injection of zidovudine at doses of 37.5 to 300 mg/kg, there were no treatment-related structural or numerical chromosomal alterations in spite of plasma levels that were as high as 453 μg/mL 5 minutes after dosing.

In two in vivo micronucleus studies (designed to measure chromosome breakage or mitotic spindle apparatus damage) in male mice, oral doses of zidovudine 100 to 1000 mg/kg/day administered once daily for approximately 4 weeks induced dose-related increases in micronucleated erythrocytes. Similar results were also seen after 4 or 7 days of dosing at 500 mg/kg/day in rats and mice.

In a study involving 11 AIDS patients, it was reported that the seven patients who were receiving RETROVIR (1200 mg/day) as their only medication for 4 weeks to 7 months showed a chromosome breakage frequency of 8.29 ± 2.65 breaks per 100 peripheral lymphocytes. This was significantly ($P<0.05$) higher than the incidence of 0.5 ± 0.29 breaks per 100 cells that was observed in the four AIDS patients who had not received RETROVIR. No effect on male or female fertility (judged by conception rates) was seen in rats given zidovudine orally at doses up to 450 mg/kg/day.

Pregnancy: Pregnancy Category C. Oral teratology studies in the rat and in the rabbit at doses up to 500 mg/kg/day revealed no evidence of teratogenicity with zidovudine. Zidovudine treatment resulted in embryo/fetal toxicity as evidenced by an increase in the incidence of fetal resorptions in rats given 150 or 450 mg/kg/day and rabbits given 500 mg/kg/day. The doses used in the teratology studies resulted in peak zidovudine plasma concentrations (after one-half of the daily dose) in rats 66 to 226 times, and in rabbits 12 to 87 times, mean steady-state peak human plasma concentrations (after one-sixth of the daily dose) achieved with the recommended daily dose (100 mg every 4 hours). In an in vitro experiment with fertilized mouse oocytes, zidovudine exposure resulted in a dose-dependent reduction in blastocyst formation. In an additional teratology study in rats, a dose of 3000 mg/kg/day (very near the oral median lethal dose in rats of 3683 mg/kg) caused marked maternal toxicity and an increase in the incidence of fetal malformations. This dose resulted in peak zidovudine plasma concentrations 350 times peak human plasma concentrations. (Estimated area-under-the-curve [AUC] in rats at this dose level was 300 times the daily AUC in humans given 600 mg per day.) No evidence of teratogenicity was seen in this experiment at doses of 600 mg/kg/day or less.

A randomized, double-blind, placebo-controlled trial was conducted in HIV-infected pregnant women to determine the utility of RETROVIR for the prevention of maternal-fetal HIV-transmission (see CLINICAL PHARMACOLOGY: Description of Clinical Studies). Congenital abnormalities occurred with similar frequency between neonates born to mothers who received RETROVIR and neonates born to mothers who received placebo. Abnormalities were either

problems in embryogenesis (prior to 14 weeks) or were recognized on ultrasound before or immediately after initation of study drug.

Antiretroviral Pregnancy Registry: To monitor maternal-fetal outcomes of pregnant women exposed to RETROVIR, an Antiretroviral Pregnancy Registry has been established. Physicians are encouraged to register patients by calling (800) 722-9292, ext. 38465.

Nursing Mothers: The U.S. Public Health Service Centers for Disease Control and Prevention advises HIV-infected women not to breast-feed to avoid postnatal transmission of HIV to a child who may not yet be infected.

Zidovudine is excreted in human milk (see CLINICAL PHARMACOLOGY: Pharmacokinetics).

Pediatric Use: See INDICATIONS, ADVERSE REACTIONS, and DOSAGE AND ADMINISTRATION

ADVERSE REACTIONS

The adverse events reported during intravenous administration of RETROVIR I.V. Infusion are similar to those reported with oral administration; granulocytopenia and anemia were reported most frequently. Long-term intravenous administration beyond 2 to 4 weeks has not been studied in adults and may enhance hematologic adverse events. Local reaction, pain, and slight irritation during intravenous administration occur infrequently.

Adults: The frequency and severity of adverse events associated with the use of oral RETROVIR in adults are greater in patients with more advanced infection at the time of initiation of therapy. The following table summarizes the relative incidence of hematologic adverse events observed in clinical studies by severity of HIV disease present at the start of treatment with oral RETROVIR.
[See Table 1 above.]

The anemia reported in patients with advanced HIV disease receiving RETROVIR appeared to be the result of impaired erythrocyte maturation as evidenced by macrocytosis while on drug. Although mean platelet counts in patients receiving RETROVIR were significantly increased compared to mean baseline values, thrombocytopenia did occur in some of these patients with advanced disease.[1] Twelve percent of patients receiving RETROVIR compared to 5% of patients receiving placebo had >50% decreases from baseline platelet count. Mild drug-associated elevations in total bilirubin levels have been reported as an uncommon occurrence in patients treated for asymptomatic HIV infection.

The HIV-infected adults participating in these clinical trials often had baseline symptoms and signs of HIV disease and/or experienced adverse events at some time during study. It was often difficult to distinguish adverse events possibly associated with administration of RETROVIR from underlying signs of HIV disease or intercurrent illnesses. The following table summarizes clinical adverse events or symptoms which occurred in at least 5% of all patients with advanced HIV disease treated with 1500 mg/day of oral RETROVIR in the original placebo-controlled study.[2] Of the items listed in the table, only severe headache, nausea, insomnia, and myalgia were reported at a significantly greater rate in patients receiving RETROVIR.

Table 2
Percentage (%) of Patients with Adverse Events in Advanced HIV Disease (BW 02)

Adverse Event	RETROVIR® 1500 mg/day* (n = 144)%	Placebo (n = 137)%
BODY AS A WHOLE		
Asthenia	19	18
Diaphoresis	5	4
Fever	16	12
Headache	42	37
Malaise	8	7
GASTROINTESTINAL		
Anorexia	11	8
Diarrhea	12	18
Dyspepsia	5	4
GI Pain	20	19
Nausea	46	18
Vomiting	6	3
MUSCULOSKELETAL		
Myalgia	8	2
NERVOUS		
Dizziness	6	4
Insomnia	5	1
Paresthesia	6	3
Somnolence	8	9
RESPIRATORY		
Dyspnea	5	3
SKIN		
Rash	17	15
SPECIAL SENSES		
Taste Perversion	5	8

*The currently recommended oral dose is 500 to 600 mg daily.

All events of a severe or life-threatening nature were monitored for adults in the placebo-controlled studies in early HIV disease and asymptomatic HIV infection. Data concerning the occurrence of additional signs or symptoms were also collected. No distinction was made in reporting events between those possibly associated with the administration of the study medication and those due to the underlying disease. The following tables summarize all those events reported at a statistically significant greater incidence for patients receiving RETROVIR in these studies:

Table 3
Percentage (%) of Patients with Adverse Events in Early HIV Disease (ACTG 016)

Adverse Event	RETROVIR® 1200 mg/day* (n = 361)%	Placebo (n = 352)%
BODY AS A WHOLE		
Asthenia	69	62
GASTROINTESTINAL		
Dyspepsia	6	1
Nausea	61	41
Vomiting	25	13

*The currently recommended dose is 500 to 600 mg daily.

Table 4
Percentage (%) of Patients with Adverse Events* in Asymptomatic HIV Infection (ACTG 019)

Adverse Event	RETROVIR® 500 mg/day* (n = 453)%	Placebo (n = 428)%
BODY AS A WHOLE		
Asthenia	8.6†	5.8
Headache	62.5	52.6
Malaise	53.2	44.9
GASTROINTESTINAL		
Anorexia	20.1	10.5
Constipation	6.4†	3.5
Nausea	51.4	29.9
Vomiting	17.2	9.8
NERVOUS		
Dizziness	17.9†	15.2

*Reported in ≥5% of study population.
†Not statistically significant versus placebo.

Several serious adverse events have been reported with the use of RETROVIR in clinical practice. Myopathy and myositis with pathological changes, similar to that produced by HIV disease, have been associated with prolonged use of RETROVIR. Reports of hepatomegaly with steatosis, hepatitis, pancreatitis, lactic acidosis, sensitization reactions (including anaphylaxis in one patient), hyperbilirubinemia, vasculitis, and seizures have been rare. These adverse events, except for sensitization, have also been associated with HIV disease. A single case of macular edema has been reported with the use of RETROVIR.

Additional adverse events reported in clinical trials at a rate not significantly different from placebo are listed below. Selected events from post-marketing clinical experience with RETROVIR are also included. Many of these events may also occur as part of HIV disease. The clinical significance of the association between treatment with RETROVIR and these events is unknown.

Body as a Whole: abdominal pain, back pain, body odor, chest pain, chills, edema of the lip, fever, flu syndrome, hyperalgesia.

Cardiovascular: syncope, vasodilation.
Gastrointestinal: bleeding gums, constipation, diarrhea, dysphagia, edema of the tongue, eructation, flatulence, mouth ulcer, rectal hemorrhage.
Hemic and Lymphatic: lymphadenopathy.
Musculoskeletal: arthralgia, muscle spasm, tremor, twitch.
Nervous: anxiety, confusion, depression, dizziness, emotional lability, loss of mental acuity, nervousness, paresthesia, somnolence, vertigo.
Respiratory: cough, dyspnea, epistaxis, hoarseness, pharyngitis, rhinitis, sinusitis.
Skin: acne, changes in skin and nail pigmentation, pruritus, rash, sweat, urticaria.
Special senses: amblyopia, hearing loss, photophobia, taste perversion.
Urogenital: dysuria, polyuria, urinary frequency, urinary hesitancy.

Pediatrics: Anemia and granulocytopenia among pediatric patients with advanced HIV disease receiving RETROVIR occurred with similar incidence to that reported for adults with AIDS or advanced ARC (see above). Management of neutropenia and anemia included, in some cases, dose modification and/or blood product transfusions. In the open-label studies, 17% had their dose modified (generally a reduction in dose by 30%) due to anemia and 25% had their dose modified (temporary discontinuation or dose reduction by 30%) for neutropenia. Four pediatric patients had RETROVIR permanently discontinued for neutropenia. The following table summarizes the occurrence of anemia (Hgb <7.5 g/dL) and granulocytopenia (<750 cells/mm^3) among 124 pediatric patients receiving oral RETROVIR for a mean of 267 days (range 3 to 855 days):

Table 5

Advanced Pediatric HIV disease (n=124)	Granulocytopenia (<750 cells/mm^3)		Anemia (Hgb <7.5 g/dL)	
	n	%	n	%
	48	39	28*	23

*Twenty-two pediatric patients received one or more transfusions due to a decline in hemoglobin to <7.5 g/dL; an additional 15 pediatric patients were transfused for hemoglobin levels >7.5 g/dL. Fifty-nine percent of the patients transfused had a pre-study history of anemia or transfusion requirement.

Macrocytosis was observed among the majority of pediatric patients enrolled in the studies.
In the open-label studies involving 124 pediatric patients, 16 clinical adverse events were reported by 24 pediatric patients. No event was reported by more than 5.6% of the study populations. Due to the open-label design of the studies, it was difficult to determine possible events related to the use of RETROVIR versus disease-related events. Therefore, all clinical events reported as associated with therapy with RETROVIR or of unknown relationship to therapy with RETROVIR are presented in the following table:

Table 6
Percentage (%) of Pediatric Patients with Clinical Events in Open-Label Studies

Adverse Event	n	%
BODY AS A WHOLE		
Fever	4	3.2
Phlebitis*/Bacteremia	2	1.6
Headache	2	1.6
GASTROINTESTINAL		
Nausea	1	0.8
Vomiting	6	4.8
Abdominal Pain	4	3.2
Diarrhea	1	0.8
Weight Loss	1	0.8
NERVOUS		
Insomnia	3	2.4
Nervousness/Irritability	2	1.6
Decreased Reflexes	7	5.6
Seizure	1	0.8
CARDIOVASCULAR		
Left Ventricular Dilation	1	0.8
Cardiomyopathy	1	0.8
S_3 Gallop	1	0.8
Congestive Heart Failure	1	0.8
Generalized Edema	1	0.8
ECG Abnormality	3	2.4
UROGENITAL		
Hematuria/Viral Cystitis	1	0.8

*Peripheral vein I.V. catheter site.

The clinical adverse events reported among adult recipients of RETROVIR may also occur in pediatric patients.

Use for the Prevention of Maternal-Fetal Transmission of HIV: In a randomized, double-blind, placebo-controlled trial in HIV-infected women and their neonates conducted to determine the utility of RETROVIR for the prevention of maternal-fetal HIV transmission, RETROVIR Syrup at 2 mg/kg was administered every 6 hours for 6 weeks to neonates beginning within 12 hours after birth. The most commonly reported adverse experiences were anemia (hemoglobin <9.0 g/dL) and neutropenia (<1000 cells/mm^3). Anemia occurred in 22% of the neonates who received RETROVIR and in 12% of the neonates who received placebo. The mean difference in hemoglobin values was less than 1.0 g/dL for neonates receiving RETROVIR compared to infants receiving placebo. No neonates with anemia required transfusion, and all hemoglobin values spontaneously returned to normal within 6 weeks after completion of therapy with RETROVIR. Neutropenia was reported with similar frequency in the group that received RETROVIR (21%) and in the group that received placebo (27%). The long-term consequences of *in utero* and neonatal exposure to RETROVIR are unknown.

OVERDOSAGE

Cases of acute overdoses in both pediatric patients and adults have been reported with doses up to 50 grams. None were fatal. The only consistent finding in these cases of overdose was spontaneous or induced nausea and vomiting. Hematologic changes were transient and not severe. Some patients experienced nonspecific CNS symptoms such as headache, dizziness, drowsiness, lethargy, and confusion. One report of a grand mal seizure possibly attributable to RETROVIR occurred in a 35-year-old male 3 hours after ingesting 36 grams of RETROVIR. No other cause could be identified. All patients recovered without permanent sequelae. Hemodialysis appears to have a negligible effect on the removal of zidovudine while elimination of its primary metabolite, GZDV, is enhanced.

DOSAGE AND ADMINISTRATION

Adults: For adults with symptomatic HIV infection, including AIDS, the recommended intravenous dose is 1 mg/kg infused over 1 hour. This dose should be administered every 4 hours around the clock (6 mg/kg daily).The effectiveness of this dose compared to higher dosing regimens in improving the neurologic dysfunction associated with HIV disease is unknown. A small randomized study found a greater effect of higher doses of RETROVIR on improvement of neurological symptoms in patients with pre-existing neurological disease. For asymptomatic HIV infection, the recommended intravenous dose for adults is 1 mg/kg every 4 hours while awake (5 mg/kg daily).
Patients should receive RETROVIR I.V. Infusion only until oral therapy can be administered. The intravenous dosing regimen equivalent to the oral administration of 100 mg every 4 hours is approximately 1 mg/kg intravenously every 4 hours.

Maternal-Fetal HIV Transmission: The recommended dosing regimen for administration to pregnant women (>14 weeks of pregnancy) and their newborn infants is:
Maternal Dosing: 100 mg orally five times per day until the start of labor. During labor and delivery, intravenous RETROVIR should be administered at 2 mg/kg (total body weight) over 1 hour followed by a continuous intravenous infusion of 1 mg/kg/h (total body weight) until clamping of the umbilical cord.
Neonatal Dosing: 2 mg/kg orally every 6 hours starting within 12 hours after birth and continuing through 6 weeks of age. Neonates unable to receive oral dosing may be administered RETROVIR intravenously at 1.5 mg/kg, infused over 30 minutes, every 6 hours. (See PRECAUTIONS if hepatic disease or renal insufficiency is present.)

Monitoring of Patients: Hematologic toxicities appear to be related to pretreatment bone marrow reserve and to dose and duration of therapy. In patients with poor bone marrow reserve, particularly in patients with advanced symptomatic HIV disease, frequent monitoring of hematologic indices is recommended to detect serious anemia or granulocytopenia (see WARNINGS). In patients who experience hematologic toxicity, reduction in hemoglobin may occur as early as 2 to 4 weeks, and granulocytopenia usually occurs after 6 to 8 weeks.

Dose Adjustment: Significant anemia (hemoglobin of <7.5 g/dL or reduction of >25% of baseline) and/or significant granulocytopenia (granulocyte count of <750/mm^3 or reduction of >50% from baseline) may require a dose interruption until some evidence of marrow recovery is observed. For less severe anemia or granulocytopenia, a reduction in daily dose may be adequate. In patients who develop significant anemia, dose modification does not necessarily eliminate the need for transfusion. If marrow recovery occurs following dose modification, gradual increases in dose may be appropriate depending on hematologic indices and patient tolerance.
In end-stage renal disease patients maintained on hemodialysis or peritoneal dialysis, recommended dosing is 1 mg/kg every 6 to 8 hours (see CLINICAL PHARMACOLOGY; Pharmacokinetics).
There are insufficient data to recommend dose adjustment of zidovudine in patients with impaired hepatic function.

Method of Preparation: RETROVIR I.V. Infusion must be diluted prior to administration. The calculated dose should be removed from the 20 mL vial and added to 5% Dextrose Injection solution to achieve a concentration no greater than 4 mg/mL. Admixture in biologic or colloidal fluids (e.g., blood products, protein solutions, etc.) is not recommended.
After dilution, the solution is physically and chemically stable for 24 hours at room temperature and 48 hours if refrigerated at 2° to 8°C (36° to 46°F). Care should be taken during admixture to prevent inadvertent contamination. As an additional precaution, the diluted solution should be administered within 8 hours if stored at 25°C (77°F) or 24 hours if refrigerated at 2° to 8°C to minimize potential administration of a microbially contaminated solution.
Parenteral drug products should be inspected visually for particulate matter and discoloration prior to administration whenever solution and container permit. Should either be observed, the solution should be discarded and fresh solution prepared.

Administration: RETROVIR I.V. Infusion is administered intravenously at a constant rate over one hour. Rapid infusion or bolus injection should be avoided. RETROVIR I.V. Infusion should not be given intramuscularly.

HOW SUPPLIED

RETROVIR I.V. Infusion, 10 mg zidovudine in each mL. 20 mL Single-Use Vial, Tray of 10 (NDC 0173-0107-93).
Store vials at 15° to 25°C (59° to 77°F) and protect from light.
Also Available: RETROVIR Capsules 100 mg, bottle of 100; RETROVIR Syrup, bottle of 240 mL.

REFERENCES

1. Fischl MA, Richman DD, Grieco MH, et al. The efficacy of azidothymidine (AZT) in the treatment of patients with AIDS and AIDS-related complex. A double-blind, placebo-controlled trial. *N Engl J Med.* 1987;317:185–191.
2. Richman DD, Fischl MA, Grieco MH, et al. The toxicity of azidothymidine (AZT) in the treatment of patients with AIDS and AIDS-related complex. A double-blind, placebo-controlled trial. *N Engl J Med.* 1987;317:192–197.
3. Volberding PA, Lagakos SW, Koch MA, et al. Zidovudine in asymptomatic human immunodeficiency virus infection. A controlled trial in persons with fewer than 500 CD4-positive cells per cubic millimeter. *N Engl J Med.* 1990:322:941–949.
4. Fischl MA, Richman DD, Hansen N, et al. The safety and efficacy of zidovudine in the treatment of patients with mildly symptomatic HIV infection. A double-blind, placebo-controlled trial. *Ann Intern Med.* 1990; 112:727–737.
5. Creagh-Kirk T, Doi P, Andrews E, et al. Survival experience among patients with AIDS receiving zidovudine. Follow-up of patients in a compassionate plea program. *JAMA.* 1988;260:3009–3015.
6. Lagakos S, Fischl MA, Stein DS, Lim L, Volberding P. Effects of zidovudine therapy in minority and other subpopulations with early HIV infection. *JAMA.* 1991:266:2709–2712.
7. Easterbrook PJ, Keruly JC, Creagh-Kirk T. et al. Racial and ethnic differences in outcome in zidovudine-treated patients with advanced HIV disease, *JAMA.* 1991:266:2713–2718.
8. Fischl M, Parker C, Pettinelli C, Wulfsohn M, Hirsch M, Collier A, et al. A randomized controlled trial of a reduced daily dose of zidovudine in patients with the acquired immunodeficiency syndrome. *N Engl J Med.* 1990;323:1009–1014.

U.S. Patent Nos. 4818538 (Product Patent) 4724232, 4833130, and 4837208 (Use Patents)
April 1996/RL-301
Shown in Product Identification Guide, page 316

TABLOID® brand Thioguanine ℞
[*tab 'loid*]
40 mg Scored Tablets

CAUTION: TABLOID brand Thioguanine is a potent drug. It should not be used unless a diagnosis of acute nonlymphocytic leukemia has been adequately established and the responsible physician is knowledgeable in assessing response to chemotherapy.

DESCRIPTION

TABLOID brand Thioguanine was synthesized and developed by Hitchings, Elion and associates at the Wellcome Research Laboratories. It is one of a large series of purine analogues which interfere with nucleic acid biosynthesis, and has been found active against selected human neoplastic diseases.[1]

Continued on next page

Glaxo Wellcome Onc.—Cont.

Thioguanine, known chemically as 2-amino-1,7-dihydro-6H-purine-6-thione, is an analogue of the nucleic acid constituent guanine, and is closely related structurally and functionally to PURINETHOL® (mercaptopurine).

TABLOID brand Thioguanine is available in tablets for oral administration. Each scored tablet contains 40 mg thioguanine and the inactive ingredients gum acacia, lactose, magnesium stearate, potato starch, and stearic acid.

CLINICAL PHARMACOLOGY

Clinical studies have shown that the absorption of an oral dose of thioguanine in man is incomplete and variable, averaging approximately 30% of the administered dose (range: 14% to 46%).[2,3] Following oral administration of ^{35}S-6-thioguanine, total plasma radioactivity reached a maximum at 8 hours and declined slowly thereafter. Parent drug represented only a very small fraction of the total plasma radioactivity at any time, being virtually undetectable throughout the period of measurements.

The oral administration of radiolabeled thioguanine revealed only trace quantities of parent drug in the urine. However, a methylated metabolite, 2-amino-6-methylthiopurine (MTG), appeared very early, rose to a maximum 6 to 8 hours after drug administration, and was still being excreted after 12 to 22 hours. Radiolabeled sulfate appeared somewhat later than MTG but was the principal metabolite after 8 hours. Thiouric acid and some unidentified products were found in the urine in small amounts.[3] Intravenous administration of ^{35}S-6-thioguanine disclosed a median plasma half-disappearance time of 80 minutes (range: 25 to 240 minutes) when the compound was given in single doses of 65 to 300 mg/m^2. Although initial plasma levels of thioguanine did correlate with the dose level, there was no correlation between the plasma half-disappearance time and the dose.[2] Thioguanine is incorporated into the DNA and the RNA of human bone marrow cells. Studies with intravenous ^{35}S-6-thioguanine have shown that the amount of thioguanine incorporated into nucleic acids is more than 100 times higher after five daily doses than after a single dose. With the 5-dose schedule, from one-half to virtually all of the guanine in the residual DNA was replaced by thioguanine.[2] Tissue distribution studies of ^{35}S-6-thioguanine in mice showed only traces of radioactivity in brain after oral administration. No measurements have been made of thioguanine concentrations in human cerebrospinal fluid, but observations on tissue distribution in animals, together with the lack of CNS penetration by the closely related compound, mercaptopurine, suggest that thioguanine does not reach therapeutic concentrations in the CSF.

Monitoring of plasma levels of thioguanine during therapy is of questionable value.[3] There is technical difficulty in determining plasma concentrations, which are seldom greater than 1 to 2 µg/mL after a therapeutic oral dose. More significantly, thioguanine enters rapidly into the anabolic and catabolic pathways for purines, and the active intracellular metabolites have appreciably longer half-lives than the parent drug. The biochemical effects of a single dose of thioguanine are evident long after the parent drug has disappeared from plasma. Because of this rapid metabolism of thioguanine to active intracellular derivatives, hemodialysis would not be expected to appreciably reduce toxicity of the drug.

Thioguanine competes with hypoxanthine and guanine for the enzyme hypoxanthine-guanine phosphoribosyltransferase (HGPRTase) and is itself converted to 6-thioguanylic acid (TGMP). This nucleotide reaches high intracellular concentrations at therapeutic doses. TGMP interferes at several points with the synthesis of guanine nucleotides. It inhibits de novo purine biosynthesis by pseudo-feedback inhibition of glutamine-5-phosphoribosylpyrophosphate amidotransferase—the first enzyme unique to the de novo pathway for purine ribonucleotide synthesis. TGMP also inhibits the conversion of inosinic acid (IMP) to xanthylic acid (XMP) by competition for the enzyme IMP dehydrogenase. At one time TGMP was felt to be a significant inhibitor of ATP:GMP phosphotransferase (guanylate kinase),[4] but recent results have shown this not to be so.[5]

Thioguanylic acid is further converted to the di- and tri-phosphates, thioguanosine diphosphate (TGDP) and thioguanosine triphosphate (TGTP) (as well as their 2'-deoxyribosyl analogues) by the same enzymes which metabolize guanine nucleotides.[6] Thioguanine nucleotides are incorporated into both the RNA and the DNA by phosphodiester linkages[2] and it has been argued that incorporation of such fraudulent bases contributes to the cytotoxicity of thioguanine.

Thus, thioguanine has multiple metabolic effects and at present it is not possible to designate one major site of action. Its tumor inhibitory properties may be due to one or more of its effects on (a) feedback inhibition of de novo purine synthesis; (b) inhibition of purine nucleotide interconversions; or (c) incorporation into the DNA and the RNA. The net consequence of its actions is a sequential blockade of the synthesis and utilization of the purine nucleotides.[4,6,7]

The catabolism of thioguanine and its metabolites is complex and shows significant differences between man and the mouse.[2,3] In both humans and mice, after oral administration of ^{35}S-6-thioguanine, urine contains virtually no detectable intact thioguanine. While deamination and subsequent oxidation to thiouric acid occurs only to a small extent in man, it is the main pathway in mice. The product of deamination by guanase, 6-thioxanthine is inactive, having negligible antitumor activity. This pathway of thioguanine inactivation is not dependent on the action of xanthine oxidase, and an inhibitor of that enzyme (such as allopurinol), will not block the detoxification of thioguanine even though the inactive 6-thioxanthine is normally further oxidized by xanthine oxidase to thiouric acid before it is eliminated. In man, methylation of thioguanine is much more extensive than in the mouse. The product of methylation, 2-amino-6-methylthiopurine, is also substantially less active and less toxic than thioguanine and its formation is likewise unaffected by the presence of allopurinol. Appreciable amounts of inorganic sulfate are also found in both murine and human urine, presumably arising from further metabolism of the methylated derivatives.

In some animal tumors, resistance to the effect of thioguanine correlates with the loss of HGPRTase activity and the resulting inability to convert thioguanine to thioguanylic acid. However, other resistance mechanisms, such as increased catabolism of TGMP by a nonspecific phosphatase, may be operative. Although not invariable, it is usual to find cross-resistance between thioguanine and its close analogue, PURINETHOL (mercaptopurine).

INDICATIONS AND USAGE

a) Acute Nonlymphocytic Leukemias: TABLOID brand Thioguanine is indicated for remission induction, remission consolidation, and maintenance therapy of acute nonlymphocytic leukemias.[8,9] The response to this agent depends upon the age of the patient (younger patients faring better than older) and whether thioguanine is used in previously treated or previously untreated patients. Reliance upon thioguanine alone is seldom justified for initial remission induction of acute nonlymphocytic leukemias because combination chemotherapy including thioguanine results in more frequent remission induction and longer duration of remission than thioguanine alone.

b) Other Neoplasms: TABLOID brand Thioguanine is not effective in chronic lymphocytic leukemia, Hodgkin's lymphoma, multiple myeloma, or solid tumors. Although thioguanine is one of several agents with activity in the treatment of the chronic phase of chronic myelogenous leukemia, more objective responses are observed with MYLERAN® (busulfan), and therefore busulfan is usually regarded as the preferred drug.

CONTRAINDICATIONS

Thioguanine should not be used in patients whose disease has demonstrated prior resistance to this drug. In animals and man, there is usually complete cross-resistance between PURINETHOL (mercaptopurine) and TABLOID brand Thioguanine.

WARNINGS

SINCE DRUGS USED IN CANCER CHEMOTHERAPY ARE POTENTIALLY HAZARDOUS, IT IS RECOMMENDED THAT ONLY PHYSICIANS EXPERIENCED WITH THE RISKS OF THIOGUANINE AND KNOWLEDGEABLE IN THE NATURAL HISTORY OF ACUTE NONLYMPHOCYTIC LEUKEMIAS ADMINISTER THIS DRUG.

The most consistent, dose-related toxicity is bone marrow suppression. This may be manifested by anemia, leukopenia, thrombocytopenia, or any combination of these. Any one of these findings may also reflect progression of the underlying disease. Since thioguanine may have a delayed effect, it is important to withdraw the medication temporarily at the first sign of an abnormally large fall in any of the formed elements of the blood.

It is recommended that evaluation of the hemoglobin concentration or hematocrit, total white blood cell count and differential count, and quantitative platelet count be obtained frequently while the patient is on thioguanine therapy. In cases where the cause of fluctuations in the formed elements in the peripheral blood is obscure, bone marrow examination may be useful for the evaluation of marrow status. The decision to increase, decrease, continue, or discontinue a given dosage of thioguanine must be based not only on the absolute hematologic values, but also upon the rapidity with which changes are occurring. In many instances, particularly during the induction phase of acute leukemia, complete blood counts will need to be done more frequently in order to evaluate the effect of the therapy. The dosage of thioguanine may need to be reduced when this agent is combined with other drugs whose primary toxicity is myelosuppression.

Myelosuppression is often unavoidable during the induction phase of adult acute nonlymphocytic leukemias if remission induction is to be successful. Whether or not this demands modification or cessation of dosage depends both upon the response of the underlying disease and a careful consider-

ation of supportive facilities (granulocyte and platelet transfusions) which may be available. Life-threatening infections and bleeding have been observed as consequences of thioguanine-induced granulocytopenia and thrombocytopenia.

The effect of thioguanine on the immunocompetence of patients is unknown.

Pregnancy: Pregnancy Category D. Drugs such as thioguanine are potential mutagens and teratogens. Thioguanine may cause fetal harm when administered to a pregnant woman. Thioguanine has been shown to be teratogenic in rats when given in doses five (5) times the human dose. When given to the rat on the 4th and 5th days of gestation, 13% of surviving placentas did not contain fetuses, and 19% of offspring were malformed or stunted. The malformations noted included generalized edema, cranial defects, and general skeletal hypoplasia, hydrocephalus, ventral hernia, situs inversus, and incomplete development of the limbs.[10] There are no adequate and well-controlled studies in pregnant women. If this drug is used during pregnancy, or if the patient becomes pregnant while taking the drug, the patient should be apprised of the potential hazard to the fetus. Women of childbearing potential should be advised to avoid becoming pregnant.

PRECAUTIONS

General: Although the primary toxicity of thioguanine is myelosuppression, other toxicities have occasionally been observed, particularly when thioguanine is used in combination with other cancer chemotherapeutic agents.

A few cases of jaundice have been reported in patients with leukemia receiving thioguanine. Among these were two adult male patients and four children with acute myelogenous leukemia and an adult male with acute lymphocytic leukemia who developed veno-occlusive hepatic disease while receiving chemotherapy for their leukemia.[11,12] Six patients had received cytarabine prior to treatment with thioguanine, and some were receiving other chemotherapy in addition to thioguanine when they became symptomatic. While veno-occlusive hepatic disease has not been reported in patients treated with thioguanine alone, it is recommended that thioguanine be withheld if there is evidence of toxic hepatitis or biliary stasis, and that appropriate clinical and laboratory investigations be initiated to establish the etiology of the hepatic dysfunction. Deterioration in liver function studies during thioguanine therapy should prompt discontinuation of treatment and a search for an explanation of the hepatotoxicity.

Information for Patients: Patients should be informed that the major toxicities of thioguanine are related to myelosuppression, hepatotoxicity, and gastrointestinal toxicity. Patients should never be allowed to take the drug without medical supervision and should be advised to consult their physician if they experience fever, sore throat, jaundice, nausea, vomiting, signs of local infection, bleeding from any site, or symptoms suggestive of anemia. Women of childbearing potential should be advised to avoid becoming pregnant.

Laboratory Tests: It is advisable to monitor liver function tests (serum transaminases, alkaline phosphatase, bilirubin) at weekly intervals when first beginning therapy and at monthly intervals thereafter. It may be advisable to perform liver function tests more frequently in patients with known pre-existing liver disease or in patients who are receiving thioguanine and other hepatotoxic drugs. Patients should be instructed to discontinue thioguanine immediately if clinical jaundice is detected (see WARNINGS).

Drug Interactions: There is usually complete cross-resistance between PURINETHOL (mercaptopurine) and TABLOID brand Thioguanine.

In one study, 12 of approximately 330 patients receiving continuous busulfan and thioguanine therapy for treatment of chronic myelogenous leukemia were found to have esophageal varices associated with abnormal liver function tests.[13] Subsequent liver biopsies were performed in four of these patients, all of which showed evidence of nodular regenerative hyperplasia. Duration of combination therapy prior to the appearance of esophageal varices ranged from 6 to 45 months. With the present analysis of the data, no cases of hepatotoxicity have appeared in the busulfan alone arm of the study. Long-term continuous therapy with thioguanine and busulfan should be used with caution.

Carcinogenesis, Mutagenesis, Impairment of Fertility: In view of its action on cellular DNA, thioguanine is potentially mutagenic and carcinogenic, and consideration should be given to the theoretical risk of carcinogenesis when thioguanine is administered (see WARNINGS).

Pregnancy: *Teratogenic Effects:* Pregnancy Category D. See WARNINGS section.

Nursing Mothers: It is not known whether this drug is excreted in human milk. Because of the potential for tumorigenicity shown for thioguanine, a decision should be made whether to discontinue nursing or to discontinue the drug, taking into account the importance of the drug to the mother.

ADVERSE REACTIONS

The most frequent adverse reaction to thioguanine is myelosuppression. The induction of complete remission of acute myelogenous leukemia usually requires combination chemotherapy in dosages which produce marrow hypoplasia.[14] Since consolidation and maintenance of remission are also effected by multiple drug regimens whose component agents cause myelosuppression, pancytopenia is observed in nearly all patients. Dosages and schedules must be adjusted to prevent life-threatening cytopenias whenever these adverse reactions are observed.

Hyperuricemia frequently occurs in patients receiving thioguanine as a consequence of rapid cell lysis accompanying the antineoplastic effect. Adverse effects can be minimized by increased hydration, urine alkalinization, and the prophylactic administration of a xanthine oxidase inhibitor such as ZYLOPRIM® (allopurinol). Unlike PURINETHOL (mercaptopurine) and IMURAN® (azathioprine), thioguanine may be continued in the usual dosage when allopurinol is used conjointly to inhibit uric acid formation.

Less frequent adverse reactions include nausea, vomiting, anorexia, and stomatitis. Intestinal necrosis and perforation have been reported in patients who received multiple drug chemotherapy including thioguanine.

Hepatic Effects: Liver enzyme and other liver function studies are occasionally abnormal. If jaundice, hepatomegaly, or anorexia with tenderness in the right hypochondrium occurs, thioguanine should be withheld until the exact etiology can be determined. There have been reports of veno-occlusive liver disease occurring in patients who received combination chemotherapy including thioguanine.[11,12] Esophageal varices have been reported in patients receiving continuous busulfan and thioguanine therapy for treatment of chronic myelogenous leukemia (see PRECAUTIONS: Drug Interactions).

OVERDOSAGE

Signs and symptoms of overdosage may be immediate, such as nausea, vomiting, malaise, hypertension, and diaphoresis; or delayed, such as myelosuppression and azotemia.[15] It is not known whether thioguanine is dialyzable. Hemodialysis is thought to be of marginal use due to the rapid intracellular incorporation of thioguanine into active metabolites with long persistence. The oral LD_{50} of thioguanine was determined to be 823 mg/kg ± 50.73 mg/kg and 740 mg/kg ± 45.24 mg/kg for male and female rats, respectively.[16] Symptoms of overdosage may occur after a single dose of as little as 2.0 to 3.0 mg/kg thioguanine. As much as 35 mg/kg has been given in a single oral dose with reversible myelosuppression observed. There is no known pharmacologic antagonist of thioguanine. The drug should be discontinued immediately if unintended toxicity occurs during treatment. Severe hematologic toxicity may require supportive therapy with platelet transfusions for bleeding, and granulocyte transfusions and antibiotics if sepsis is documented. If a patient is seen immediately following an accidental overdosage of the drug, it may be useful to induce emesis.

DOSAGE AND ADMINISTRATION

TABLOID brand Thioguanine is administered orally. The dosage which will be tolerated and effective varies according to the stage and type of neoplastic process being treated. Because the usual therapies for adult and childhood acute nonlymphocytic leukemias involve the use of thioguanine with other agents in combination, physicians responsible for administering these therapies should be experienced in the use of cancer chemotherapy and in the chosen protocol.

Ninety-six (59%) of one hundred sixty-three children with previously untreated acute nonlymphocytic leukemia obtained complete remission with a multiple drug protocol including thioguanine, prednisone, cytarabine, cyclophosphamide, and vincristine. Remission was maintained with daily thioguanine, 4-day pulses of cytarabine and cyclophosphamide, and a single dose of vincristine every 28 days. The median duration of remission was 11.5 months.[8]

Fifty-three percent of previously untreated adults with acute nonlymphocytic leukemias attained remission following use of the combination of thioguanine and cytarabine according to a protocol developed at The Memorial Sloan-Kettering Cancer Center. A median duration of remission of 8.8 months was achieved with the multiple drug maintenance regimen which included thioguanine.[9]

On those occasions when single agent chemotherapy with thioguanine may be appropriate, the usual initial dosage for children and adults is approximately 2 mg/kg of body weight per day. If, after 4 weeks on this dosage, there is no clinical improvement and no leukocyte or platelet depression, the dosage may be cautiously increased to 3 mg/kg per day. The total daily dose may be given at one time.

The dosage of thioguanine used does not depend on whether or not the patient is receiving ZYLOPRIM (allopurinol); **this is in contradistinction to the dosage reduction which is mandatory when PURINETHOL (mercaptopurine) or IMURAN (azathioprine) is given simultaneously with allopurinol.**

Procedures for proper handling and disposal of anticancer drugs should be considered. Several guidelines on this subject have been published.[17-23]

There is no general agreement that all of the procedures recommended in the guidelines are necessary or appropriate.

HOW SUPPLIED

Greenish-yellow, scored tablets containing 40 mg thioguanine, imprinted with "WELLCOME" and "U3B" on each tablet; in bottle of 25 (NDC 0173-0880-25). Store at 15° to 25°C (59° to 77°F) in a dry place.

REFERENCES

1. Hitchings GH, Elion GB. The chemistry and biochemistry of purine analogs. *Ann NY Acad Sci.* 1954;60:195-199.
2. LePage GA, Whitecar JP Jr. Pharmacology of 6-thioguanine in man. *Cancer Res.* 1971;31:1627-1631.
3. Elion GB. Biochemistry and pharmacology of purine analogues. *Fed Proc.* 1967;26:898-904.
4. Miech RP, Parks RE Jr, Anderson JH Jr, Sartorelli AC. An hypothesis on the mechanism of action of 6-thioguanine. *Biochem Pharmacol.* 1967;16:2222-2227.
5. Miller RL, Adamczyk DL, Spector T, Agarwal KC, Miech RP, Panks RE Jr. Reassessment of the interactions of guanylate kinase and 6-thioguanine 5′-phosphate. *Biochem Pharmacol.* 1977;26:1573-1576.
6. Paterson ARP, Tidd DN. 6-Thiopurines. In: Sartorelli AC, Johns DG, eds. *Antineoplastic and Immunosuppressive Agents,* Part II. Berlin: Springer Verlag; 1975:384-403.
7. Nelson JA, Carpenter JW, Rose LM, Adamson DJ. Mechanisms of action of 6-thioguanine, 6-mercaptopurine, and 8-azaguanine. *Cancer Res.* 1975;35:2872-2878.
8. Chard RL Jr, Finklestein JZ, Sonley MJ, et al. Increased survival in childhood acute nonlymphocytic leukemia after treatment with prednisone, cytosine arabinoside, 6-thioguanine, cyclophosphamide, and oncovin (PATCO) combination therapy. *Med Ped Oncol.* 1978;4:263-273.
9. Mertelsmann R, Drapkin RL, Gee TS, et al. Treatment of acute nonlymphocytic leukemia in adults: response to 2,2-anhydro-1-B-D-arabinofuranosyl-5-fluorocytosine and thioguanine on the L-12 protocol. *Cancer.* 1981;48:2136-2142.
10. Thiersch JB: Effect of 2-6 diaminopurine (2-6DP): 6 chlorpurine (CIP) and thioguanine (ThG) on rat litter *in utero. Proc Soc Exp Biol Med.* 1957;94:40-43.
11. Griner PF, Elbadawi A, Packman CH. Veno-occlusive disease of the liver after chemotherapy of acute leukemia: report of two cases. *Ann Intern Med.* 1976;85:578-582.
12. Gill RA, Onstad GR, Cardamone JM, Maneval DC, Sumner HW. Hepatic veno-occlusive disease caused by 6-thioguanine. *Ann Intern Med.* 1982;96:58-60.
13. Key NS, Kelly PMA, Emerson PM, Chapman RWG, Allan NC, McGee JO'D. Oesophageal varices associated with busulfan-thioguanine combination therapy for chronic myeloid leukaemia. *Lancet.* 1987;2:1050-1052.
14. Clarkson BD, Dowling MD, Gee TS, Cunningham IB, Burchenal JH. Treatment of acute leukemia in adults. *Cancer.* 1975;36:775-795.
15. Presant CA, Denes AE, Klein L, Garrett S, Metter GE. Phase I and preliminary phase II observations of high-dose intermittent 6-thioguanine. *Cancer Treat Rep.* 1980;64:1109-1113.
16. Unpublished data on file with Glaxo Wellcome Inc.
17. Recommendations for the safe handling of parenteral antineoplastic drugs. Washington, DC: Division of Safety, National Institutes of Health; 1983. US Dept. of Health and Human Services, Public Health Service publication NIH 83-2621.
18. AMA Council on Scientific Affairs. Guidelines for handling parenteral antineoplastics. *JAMA.* 1985;253:1590-1591.
19. National Study Commission on Cytotoxic Exposure. Recommendations for handling cytotoxic agents. 1987. Available from Louis P. Jeffrey, Chairman, National Study Commission on Cytotoxic Exposure. Massachusetts College of Pharmacy and Allied Health Services, 179 Longwood Avenue, Boston, MA 02115.
20. Clinical Oncological Society of Australia. Guidelines and recommendations for safe handling of antineoplastic agents. *Med J Australia.* 1983;1:426-428.
21. Jones RB, Frank R, Mass T. Safe handling of chemotherapeutic agents: A report from the Mount Sinai Medical Center. *CA—A Cancer J for Clin.* 1983;33:258-263.
22. American Society of Hospital Pharmacists. ASHP technical assistance bulletin on handling cytotoxic and hazardous drugs. *Am J Hosp Pharm.* 1990;47:1033-1049.
23. Yodaiken RE, Bennett D. OSHA work-practice guidelines for personnel dealing with cytotoxic (antineoplastic) drugs. *Am. J Hosp Pharm.* 1986;43:1193-1204.

January 1996/RL-256

Shown in Product Identification Guide, page 316

ZOFRAN® Injection ℞
[*zō'fran*]
(ondansetron hydrochloride)

ZOFRAN® Injection Premixed ℞
[*zō'fran*]
(ondansetron hydrochloride)

DESCRIPTION

The active ingredient in ZOFRAN Injection and ZOFRAN Injection Premixed is ondansetron hydrochloride (HCl), the racemic form of ondansetron and a selective blocking agent of the serotonin 5-HT_3 receptor type. Chemically it is (±) 1, 2, 3, 9-tetrahydro-9-methyl-3-[(2-methyl-1H-imidazol-1-yl) methyl]-4H-carbazol-4-one, monohydrochloride, dihydrate. The empirical formula is $C_{18}H_{19}N_3O \cdot HCl \cdot 2H_2O$, representing a molecular weight of 365.9.

Ondansetron HCl is a white to off-white powder that is soluble in water and normal saline.

Sterile Injection for Intravenous Administration: Each 1 mL of aqueous solution in the 2-mL single-dose vial contains 2 mg of ondansetron as the hydrochloride dihydrate; 9.0 mg of sodium chloride, USP; and 0.5 mg of citric acid monohydrate, USP and 0.25 mg of sodium citrate dihydrate, USP as buffers in Water for Injection, USP.

Each 1 mL of aqueous solution in the 20-mL multidose vial contains 2 mg of ondansetron as the hydrochloride dihydrate; 8.3 mg of sodium chloride, USP; 0.5 mg of citric acid monohydrate, USP and 0.25 mg of sodium citrate dihydrate, USP as buffers; and 1.2 mg of methylparaben, NF and 0.15 mg of propylparaben, NF as preservatives in Water for Injection, USP.

ZOFRAN Injection is a clear, colorless, nonpyrogenic, sterile solution for intravenous (IV) injection. The pH of the injection solution is 3.3 to 4.0.

Sterile, Premixed Solution for Intravenous Administration in Single-Dose, Flexible Plastic Containers: Each 50 mL contains ondansetron 32 mg (as the hydrochloride dihydrate); dextrose 2,500 mg; and citric acid 26 mg and sodium citrate 11.5 mg as buffers in Water for Injection, USP. It contains no preservatives. The osmolarity of this solution is 270 mOsm/L (approx.), and the pH is 3.0 to 4.0.

The flexible plastic container is fabricated from a specially formulated, nonplasticized, thermoplastic co-polyester (CR3). Water can permeate from inside the container into the overwrap but not in amounts sufficient to affect the solution significantly. Solutions inside the container also can leach out certain of the chemical components in very small amounts before the expiration period is attained. However, the safety of the plastic has been confirmed by tests in animals according to USP biological standards for plastic containers.

CLINICAL PHARMACOLOGY

Pharmacodynamics: Ondansetron is a selective 5-HT_3 receptor antagonist. While ondansetron's mechanism of action has not been fully characterized, it is not a dopamine-receptor antagonist. Serotonin receptors of the 5-HT_3 type are present both peripherally on vagal nerve terminals and centrally in the chemoreceptor trigger zone of the area postrema. It is not certain whether ondansetron's antiemetic action in chemotherapy-induced emesis is mediated centrally, peripherally, or in both sites. However, cytotoxic chemotherapy appears to be associated with release of serotonin from the enterochromaffin cells of the small intestine. In humans, urinary 5-HIAA (5-hydroxyindoleacetic acid) excretion increases after cisplatin administration in parallel with the onset of emesis. The released serotonin may stimulate the vagal afferents through the 5-HT_3 receptors and initiate the vomiting reflex.

In animals, the emetic response to cisplatin can be prevented by pretreatment with an inhibitor of serotonin synthesis, bilateral abdominal vagotomy and greater splanchnic nerve section, or pretreatment with a serotonin 5-HT_3 receptor antagonist.

In normal volunteers, single IV doses of 0.15 mg/kg of ondansetron had no effect on esophageal motility, gastric motility, lower esophageal sphincter pressure, or small intestinal transit time. In another study in six normal male volunteers, a 16-mg dose infused over 5 minutes showed no effect of the drug on cardiac output, heart rate, stroke volume, blood pressure, or electrocardiogram (ECG). Multiday administration of ondansetron has been shown to slow colonic transit in normal volunteers. Ondansetron has no effect on plasma prolactin concentrations.

Ondansetron does not alter the respiratory depressant effects produced by alfentanil or the degree of neuromuscular blockade produced by atracurium. Interactions with general or local anesthetics have not been studied.

Pharmacokinetics: Ondansetron is extensively metabolized in humans, with approximately 5% of a radiolabeled dose recovered as the parent compound from the urine. The primary metabolic pathway is hydroxylation on the indole ring followed by glucuronide or sulfate conjugation.

Continued on next page

Glaxo Wellcome Onc.—Cont.

In normal volunteers, the following mean pharmacokinetic data have been determined following a single 0.15-mg/kg IV dose.

Pharmacokinetics in Normal Volunteers

Age-group	n	Peak Plasma Concentration (ng/mL)	Mean Elimination Half-life (h)	Plasma Clearance (L/h/kg)
19-40	11	102	3.5	0.381
61-74	12	106	4.7	0.319
≥ 75	11	170	5.5	0.262

From a single-dose infusion study, patients with severe hepatic impairment showed a fivefold and those with mild-to-moderate liver impairment a twofold reduction in mean plasma clearance, with increases in the mean apparent volume of distribution of less than twofold, as compared to normals. The mean half-life of 3.6 hours in normals increased to 9.2 hours in patients with mild-to-moderate hepatic impairment and was prolonged to 20.6 hours in patients with severe hepatic insufficiency.

A reduction in clearance and increase in elimination half-life are seen in patients over 75 years old. In clinical trials with patients with cancer, there was neither a difference in safety nor efficacy between patients over 65 years of age and those under 65 years of age; there was an insufficient number of patients over 75 years of age to permit conclusions in that age-group. No adjustment in dosage is recommended in the elderly.

In adult cancer patients, the mean elimination half-life was 4.0 hours, and there was no difference in the multidose pharmacokinetics over a 4-day period. In a study of 21 pediatric cancer patients (aged 4 to 18 years) who received three IV doses of 0.15 mg/kg of ondansetron at 4-hour intervals, patients older than 15 years of age exhibited ondansetron pharmacokinetic parameters similar to those of adults. Patients aged 4 to 12 years generally showed higher clearance and somewhat larger volume of distribution than adults. Most pediatric patients younger than 15 years of age with cancer had a shorter (2.4 hours) ondansetron plasma half-life than patients older than 15 years of age. It is not known whether these differences in ondansetron plasma half-life may result in differences in efficacy between adults and some young children (see CLINICAL TRIALS: Pediatric Studies).

In a study of 21 pediatric patients (aged 3 to 12 years) who were undergoing surgery requiring anesthesia for a duration of 45 minutes to 2 hours, a single IV dose of ondansetron, 2 mg (3 to 7 years) or 4 mg (8 to 12 years), was administered immediately prior to anesthesia induction. Mean weight-normalized clearance and volume of distribution values in these pediatric surgical patients were similar to those previously reported for young adults. Mean terminal half-life was slightly reduced in pediatric patients (range, 2.5 to 3 hours) in comparison with adults (range, 3 to 3.5 hours).

In normal volunteers (19 to 39 years old, n=23), the peak plasma concentration was 264 ng/mL following a single 32-mg dose administered as a 15-minute IV infusion. The mean elimination half-life was 4.1 hours. Systemic exposure to 32 mg of ondansetron was not proportional to dose as measured by comparing dose-normalized AUC values to an 8-mg dose. This is consistent with a small decrease in systemic clearance with increasing plasma concentrations.

Plasma protein binding of ondansetron as measured in vitro was 70% to 76%, with binding constant over the pharmacologic concentration range (10 to 500 ng/mL). Circulating drug also distributes into erythrocytes.

A positive lymphoblast transformation test to ondansetron has been reported, which suggests immunologic sensitivity to ondansetron.

CLINICAL TRIALS

Chemotherapy-Induced Nausea and Vomiting: In a double-blind study of three different dosing regimens of ZOFRAN Injection, 0.015 mg/kg, 0.15 mg/kg, and 0.30 mg/kg, each given three times during the course of cancer chemotherapy, the 0.15-mg/kg dosing regimen was more effective than the 0.015-mg/kg dosing regimen. The 0.30-mg/kg dosing regimen was not shown to be more effective than the 0.15-mg/kg dosing regimen.

Cisplatin-Based Chemotherapy: In a double-blind study in 28 patients, ZOFRAN Injection (three 0.15-mg/kg doses) was significantly more effective than placebo in preventing nausea and vomiting induced by cisplatin-based chemotherapy. Treatment response was as follows:
[See first table above.]

Ondansetron was compared with metoclopramide in a single-blind trial in 307 patients receiving cisplatin ≥ 100 mg/m² with or without other chemotherapeutic agents. Patients received the first dose of ondansetron or metoclopramide 30 minutes before cisplatin. Two additional ondansetron doses were administered 4 and 8 hours later, or five additional

---

Prevention of Chemotherapy-Induced Nausea and Emesis in Single-Day Cisplatin Therapy*

	ZOFRAN Injection	Placebo	p Value†
Number of patients	14	14	
Treatment response			
0 Emetic episodes	2 (14%)	0 (0%)	
1–2 Emetic episodes	8 (57%)	0 (0%)	
3–5 Emetic episodes	2 (14%)	1 (7%)	
More than 5 emetic episodes/rescued	2 (14%)	13 (93%)	0.001
Median number of emetic episodes	1.5	Undefined‡	
Median time to first emetic episode (h)	11.6	2.8	0.001
Median nausea scores (0–100)§	3	59	0.034
Global satisfaction with control of nausea and vomiting (0–100)‖	96	10.5	0.009

* Chemotherapy was high dose (100 and 120 mg/m²; ZOFRAN Injection n=6, placebo n=5) or moderate dose (50 and 80 mg/m²; ZOFRAN Injection n=8, placebo n=9). Other chemotherapeutic agents included fluorouracil, doxorubicin, and cyclophosphamide. There was no difference between treatments in the types of chemotherapy that would account for differences in response.
†Efficacy based on "all patients treated" analysis.
‡Median undefined since at least 50% of the patients were rescued or had more than five emetic episodes.
§ Visual analog scale assessment of nausea: 0=no nausea, 100=nausea as bad as it can be.
‖Visual analog scale assessment of satisfaction: 0=not at all satisfied, 100=totally satisfied.

Prevention of Emesis Induced by Cisplatin (≥ 100 mg/m²) Single-Day Therapy*

	ZOFRAN Injection	Metoclopramide	p Value
Dose	0.15 mg/kg × 3	2 mg/kg × 6	
Number of patients in efficacy population	136	138	
Treatment response			
0 Emetic episodes	54 (40%)	41 (30%)	
1–2 Emetic episodes	34 (25%)	30 (22%)	
3–5 Emetic episodes	19 (14%)	18 (13%)	
More than 5 emetic episodes/rescued	29 (21%)	49 (36%)	
Comparison of treatments with respect to			
0 Emetic episodes	54/136	41/138	0.083
More than 5 emetic episodes/rescued	29/136	49/138	0.009
Median number of emetic episodes	1	2	0.005
Median time to first emetic episode (h)	20.5	4.3	< 0.001
Global satisfaction with control of nausea and vomiting (0–100)†	85	63	0.001
Acute dystonic reactions	0	8	0.005
Akathisia	0	10	0.002

* In addition to cisplatin, 68% of patients received other chemotherapeutic agents, including cyclophosphamide, etoposide, and fluorouracil. There was no difference between treatments in the types of chemotherapy that would account for differences in response.
†Visual analog scale assessment: 0=not at all satisfied, 100=totally satisfied.

Prevention of Chemotherapy-Induced Nausea and Emesis in Single-Dose Therapy

	Ondansetron Dose		
	0.15 mg/kg x 3	32 mg x 1	P Value
High-dose cisplatin (≥ 100 mg/m²)			
Number of patients	100	102	
Treatment response			
0 Emetic episodes	41 (41%)	49 (48%)	0.315
1–2 Emetic episodes	19 (19%)	25 (25%)	
3–5 Emetic episodes	4 (4%)	8 (8%)	
More than 5 emetic episodes/rescued	36 (36%)	20 (20%)	0.009
Median time to first emetic episode (h)	21.7	23	0.173
Median nausea scores (0–100)*	28	13	0.004
Medium-dose cisplatin (50–70 mg/m²)			
Number of patients	101	93	
Treatment response			
0 Emetic episodes	62 (61%)	68 (73%)	0.083
1–2 Emetic episodes	11 (11%)	14 (15%)	
3–5 Emetic episodes	6 (6%)	3 (3%)	
More than 5 emetic episodes/rescued	22 (22%)	8 (9%)	0.011
Median time to first emetic episode (h)	Undefined†	Undefined	0.084
Median nausea scores (0–100)*	9	3	0.131

* Visual analog scale assessment: 0=no nausea, 100=nausea as bad as it can be.
†Median undefined since at least 50% of patients did not have any emetic episodes.

---

metoclopramide doses were administered 2, 4, 7, 10, and 13 hours later. Cisplatin was administered over a period of 3 hours or less. Episodes of vomiting and retching were tabulated over the period of 24 hours after cisplatin. The results of this study are summarized below:
[See second table above.]

Forty-one of the ondansetron patients were over 65 years of age. The complete response rate (zero emetic episodes) was 41% in this group compared with 40% in those 65 years old or younger.

In a stratified, randomized, double-blind, parallel-group, multicenter study, a single 32-mg dose of ondansetron was compared with three 0.15-mg/kg doses in patients receiving cisplatin doses of either 50 to 70 mg/m² or ≥ 100 mg/m². Patients received the first ondansetron dose 30 minutes before cisplatin. Two additional ondansetron doses were administered 4 and 8 hours later to the group receiving three 0.15–mg/kg doses. In both strata, significantly fewer patients on the single 32-mg dose than those receiving the three-dose regimen failed.
[See third table on preceding page.]

Cyclophosphamide-Based Chemotherapy: In a double-blind, placebo-controlled study of ZOFRAN Injection (three 0.15-mg/kg doses) in 20 patients receiving cyclophosphamide (500 to 600 mg/m²) chemotherapy, ZOFRAN Injection was significantly more effective than placebo in preventing nausea and vomiting. The results are summarized below:
[See first table at right.]

Re-treatment: In uncontrolled trials, 127 patients receiving cisplatin (median dose, 100 mg/m²) and ondansetron who had two or fewer emetic episodes were re-treated with ondansetron and chemotherapy, mainly cisplatin, for a total of 269 re-treatment courses (median, 2; range, 1 to 10). No emetic episodes occurred in 160 (59%), and two or fewer emetic episodes occurred in 217 (81%) re-treatment courses.

Pediatric Studies: Four open-label, noncomparative (one US, three foreign) trials have been performed with 209 pediatric cancer patients aged 4 to 18 years given a variety of cisplatin or noncisplatin regimens. In the three foreign trials, the initial ZOFRAN Injection dose ranged from 0.04 to 0.87 mg/kg for a total dose of 2.16 to 12 mg. This was followed by the oral administration of ondansetron ranging from 4 to 24 mg daily for 3 days. In the US trial, ZOFRAN was administered intravenously (only) in three doses of 0.15 mg/kg each for a total daily dose of 7.2 to 39 mg. In these studies, 58% of the 196 evaluable patients had a complete response (no emetic episodes) on day 1. Thus, prevention of emesis in these children was essentially the same as for patients older than 18 years of age. Overall, ZOFRAN Injection was well tolerated in these pediatric patients.

Postoperative Nausea and Vomiting: Prevention of Postoperative Nausea and Vomiting: Surgical patients who received ondansetron immediately before the induction of general balanced anesthesia (barbiturate: thiopental, methohexital or thiamylal; opioid: alfentanil or fentanyl; nitrous oxide; neuromuscular blockade: succinylcholine/curare and/or vecuronium or atracurium; and supplemental isoflurane) were evaluated in two double-blind US studies involving 554 patients. ZOFRAN Injection (4 mg) IV given over 2 to 5 minutes was significantly more effective than placebo. The results of these studies are summarized below:
[See second table at right.]

**The study populations in all trials thus far consisted of mainly women undergoing laparoscopic procedures.
While some men were included in some trials with similar results, clearance of the drug is more rapid in men and sufficient numbers of men have not been clinically studied to be certain that efficacy and safety have been established. Few patients undergoing major abdominal surgery have been studied.**

Pediatric Studies: Three double-blind, placebo-controlled studies have been performed (one US, two foreign) in 1,049 male and female patients (2 to 12 years of age) undergoing general anesthesia with nitrous oxide. The surgical procedures included tonsillectomy with or without adenoidectomy, strabismus surgery, herniorrhaphy, and orchidopexy. Patients were randomized to either single IV doses of ondansetron (0.1 mg/kg for children weighing 40 kg or less, a single 4-mg dose for children weighing more than 40 kg) or placebo. Study drug was administered over at least 30 seconds, immediately prior to or following anesthesia induction. Ondansetron was significantly more effective than placebo in preventing nausea and vomiting. The results of these studies are summarized below:
[See third table at right.]

Prevention of Further Postoperative Nausea and Vomiting: Surgical patients receiving general balanced anesthesia (barbiturate: thiopental, methohexital, or thiamylal; opioid: alfentanil or fentanyl; nitrous oxide; neuromuscular blockade: succinylcholine/curare and/or vecuronium or atracurium; and supplemental isoflurane) who received no prophylactic antiemetics and who experienced nausea and/or vomiting within 2 hours postoperatively were evaluated in two double-blind US studies involving 441 patients. Patients who experienced an episode of postoperative nausea and/or vomiting were given ZOFRAN Injection (4 mg) IV over 2 to 5 minutes, and this was significantly more effective than placebo. The results of these studies are summarized below: [See table at top of next page.]

Prevention of Chemotherapy-Induced Nausea and Emesis in Single-Day Cyclophosphamide Therapy*			
	ZOFRAN Injection	Placebo	P Value†
Number of patients	10	10	
Treatment response			
0 Emetic episodes	7 (70%)	0 (0%)	0.001
1–2 Emetic episodes	0 (0%)	2 (20%)	
3–5 Emetic episodes	2 (20%)	4 (40%)	
More than 5 emetic episodes/rescued	1 (10%)	4 (40%)	0.131
Median number of emetic episodes	0	4	0.008
Median time to first emetic episode (h)	Undefined‡	8.79	
Median nausea scores (0–100)§	0	60	0.001
Global satisfaction with control of nausea and vomiting (0–100)ǁ	100	52	0.008

*Chemotherapy consisted of cyclophosphamide in all patients, plus other agents, including fluorouracil, doxorubicin, methotrexate, and vincristine. There was no difference between treatments in the type of chemotherapy that would account for differences in response.
†Efficacy based on "all patients treated" analysis.
‡Median undefined since at least 50% of patients did not have any emetic episodes.
§Visual analog scale assessment of nausea: 0=no nausea, 100=nausea as bad as it can be.
ǁVisual analog scale assessment of satisfaction: 0=not at all satisfied, 100=totally satisfied.

Prevention of Postoperative Nausea and Vomiting			
	Ondansetron 4 mg IV	Placebo	P Value
Study 1			
Emetic episodes:			
Number of patients	136	139	
Treatment response over 24-hr postoperative period			
0 Emetic episodes	103 (76%)	64 (46%)	< 0.001
1 Emetic episode	13 (10%)	17 (12%)	
More than 1 emetic episode/rescued	20 (15%)	58 (42%)	
Nausea assessments:			
Number of patients	134	136	
No nausea over 24-hr postoperative period	56 (42%)	39 (29%)	
Study 2			
Emetic episodes:			
Number of patients	136	143	
Treatment response over 24-hr postoperative period			
0 Emetic episodes	85 (63%)	63 (44%)	0.002
1 Emetic episode	16 (12%)	29 (20%)	
More than 1 emetic episode/rescued	35 (26%)	51 (36%)	
Nausea assessments:			
Number of patients	125	133	
No nausea over 24-hr postoperative period	48 (38%)	42 (32%)	

Prevention of Postoperative Nausea and Vomiting			
Treatment Response Over 24 Hours	Ondansetron n (%)	Placebo n (%)	P Value
Study 1			
Number of patients	205	210	
0 Emetic episodes	140 (68%)	82 (39%)	≤ 0.001
Failure*	65 (32%)	128 (61%)	
Study 2			
Number of patients	112	110	
0 Emetic episodes	68 (61%)	38 (35%)	≤ 0.001
Failure*	44 (39%)	72 (65%)	
Study 3			
Number of patients	206	206	
0 Emetic episodes	123 (60%)	96 (47%)	≤ 0.01
Failure*	83 (40%)	110 (53%)	
Nausea assessments†:			
Number of patients	185	191	
None	119 (64%)	99 (52%)	≤ 0.01

* Failure was one or more emetic episodes, rescued, or withdrawn.
† Nausea measured as none, mild, or severe.

**The study populations in all trials thus far consisted of mainly women undergoing laparoscopic procedures.
While some men were included in some trials with similar results, clearance of the drug is more rapid in men and sufficient numbers of men have not been clinically studied to be certain that efficacy and safety have been established. Few patients undergoing major abdominal surgery have been studied.**
Pediatric Studies: One double-blind, placebo-controlled, U.S. study was performed in 351 male and female outpatients (2 to 12 years of age) who received general anesthesia with nitrous oxide and no prophylactic antiemetics. Surgical procedures were unrestricted. Patients who experienced two or more emetic episodes within 2 hours following discontinuation of nitrous oxide were randomized to a single IV dose of ondansetron (0.1 mg/kg for children weighing 40 kg or less, a single 4-mg dose for children weighing more than 40 kg) or placebo administered over at least 30 seconds.

Continued on next page

Glaxo Wellcome Onc.—Cont.

Ondansetron was significantly more effective than placebo in preventing further episodes of nausea and vomiting. The results of the study are summarized below:
[See second table at right.]

INDICATIONS AND USAGE

1. Prevention of nausea and vomiting associated with initial and repeat courses of emetogenic cancer chemotherapy, including high-dose cisplatin. Efficacy of the 32-mg single dose beyond 24 hours in these patients has not been established.

2. Prevention of postoperative nausea and/or vomiting. As with other antiemetics, routine prophylaxis is not recommended for patients in whom there is little expectation that nausea and/or vomiting will occur postoperatively. In patients where nausea and/or vomiting must be avoided postoperatively, ZOFRAN Injection is recommended even where the incidence of postoperative nausea and/or vomiting is low. For patients who have nausea and/or vomiting postoperatively, ZOFRAN Injection may be given to prevent further episodes (see CLINICAL TRIALS).

CONTRAINDICATIONS

ZOFRAN Injection and ZOFRAN Injection Premixed are contraindicated for patients known to have hypersensitivity to the drug.

PRECAUTIONS

Ondansetron is not a drug that stimulates gastric or intestinal peristalsis. It should not be used instead of nasogastric suction. The use of ondansetron in patients following abdominal surgery or in patients with chemotherapy-induced nausea and vomiting may mask a progressive ileus and/or gastric distention.

Drug Interactions: Ondansetron does not itself appear to induce or inhibit the cytochrome P-450 drug-metabolizing enzyme system of the liver. Because ondansetron is metabolized by hepatic cytochrome P-450 drug-metabolizing enzymes, inducers or inhibitors of these enzymes may change the clearance and, hence, the half-life of ondansetron. On the basis of limited available data, no dosage adjustment is recommended for patients on these drugs. Tumor response to chemotherapy in the P 388 mouse leukemia model is not affected by ondansetron. In humans, carmustine, etoposide, and cisplatin do not affect the pharmacokinetics of ondansetron.

Carcinogenesis, Mutagenesis, Impairment of Fertility: Carcinogenic effects were not seen in 2-year studies in rats and mice with oral ondansetron doses up to 10 and 30 mg/kg per day, respectively. Ondansetron was not mutagenic in standard tests for mutagenicity. Oral administration of ondansetron up to 15 mg/kg per day did not affect fertility or general reproductive performance of male and female rats.

Pregnancy: *Teratogenic Effects: Pregnancy Category B:* Reproduction studies have been performed in pregnant rats and rabbits at IV doses up to 4 mg/kg per day and have revealed no evidence of impaired fertility or harm to the fetus due to ondansetron. There are, however, no adequate and well-controlled studies in pregnant women. Because animal reproduction studies are not always predictive of human response, this drug should be used during pregnancy only if clearly needed.

Nursing Mothers: Ondansetron is excreted in the breast milk of rats. It is not known whether ondansetron is excreted in human milk. Because many drugs are excreted in human milk, caution should be exercised when ondansetron is administered to a nursing woman.

Pediatric Use: Little information is available about dosage in children under 2 years of age (see DOSAGE AND ADMINISTRATION section for use in children 4 to 18 years of age receiving cancer chemotherapy or for use in pediatric patients 2 to 12 years of age receiving general anesthesia).

Use in Elderly Patients: Dosage adjustment is not needed in patients over the age of 65 (see CLINICAL PHARMACOLOGY). Prevention of nausea and vomiting in elderly patients was no different than in younger age-groups.

ADVERSE REACTIONS

Chemotherapy-Induced Nausea and Vomiting: The following adverse events have been reported in individuals receiving ondansetron at a dosage of three 0.15-mg/kg doses or as a single 32-mg dose in clinical trials. These patients were receiving concomitant chemotherapy, primarily cisplatin, and IV fluids. Most were receiving a diuretic.
[See third table above.]
The following have been reported during controlled clinical trials or in the routine management of patients. The percentage figures are based on clinical trial experience.

Gastrointestinal: Constipation has been reported in 11% of chemotherapy patients receiving multiday ondansetron.

Hepatic: In comparative trials in cisplatin chemotherapy patients with normal baseline values of aspartate transaminase (AST) and alanine transaminase (ALT), these enzymes have been reported to exceed twice the upper limit of normal in approximately 5% of patients. The increases were transient and did not appear to be related to dose or duration of therapy. On repeat exposure, similar transient elevations in transaminase values occurred in some courses, but symptomatic hepatic disease did not occur.

There have been reports of liver failure and death in patients with cancer receiving concurrent medications including potentially hepatotoxic cytotoxic chemotherapy and antibiotics. The etiology of the liver failure is unclear.

Integumentary: Rash has occurred in approximately 1% of patients receiving ondansetron.

Central Nervous System: There have been rare reports consistent with, but not diagnostic of, extrapyramidal reactions in patients receiving ondansetron.

Cardiovascular: Rare instances of tachycardia, angina (chest pain), bradycardia, hypotension, syncope, and electrocardiographic alterations, including second degree heart block. In many cases the relationship to ZOFRAN Injection was unclear.

Special Senses: Transient blurred vision, in some cases associated with abnormalities of accommodation, and transient dizziness during or shortly after IV infusion.

Local Reactions: Pain, redness, and burning at site of injection.

Other: Rare cases of hypokalemia and grand mal seizures have been reported. The relationship to ZOFRAN Injection was unclear. Rare cases of hypersensitivity reactions, sometimes severe (e.g., anaphylaxis, bronchospasm, shortness of breath, hypotension, shock, angioedema, urticaria), have also been reported.

Postoperative Nausea and Vomiting: The following adverse events have been reported in ≥2% of adults receiving ondansetron at a dosage of 4 mg IV over 2 to 5 minutes in clinical trials. Rates of these events were not significantly different in the ondansetron and placebo groups. These patients were receiving multiple concomitant perioperative and postoperative medications.

Prevention of Further Postoperative Nausea and Vomiting

	Ondansetron 4 mg IV	Placebo	P Value
Study 1			
Emetic episodes:			
Number of patients	104	117	
Treatment response 24 h after study drug			
0 Emetic episodes	49 (47%)	19 (16%)	< 0.001
1 Emetic episode	12 (12%)	9 (8%)	
More than 1 emetic episode/rescued	43 (41%)	89 (76%)	
Median time to first emetic episode (min)*	55.0	43.0	
Nausea assessments:			
Number of patients	98	102	
Mean nausea score over 24-h postoperative period†	1.7	3.1	
Study 2			
Emetic episodes:			
Number of patients	112	108	
Treatment response 24 h after study drug			
0 Emetic episodes	49 (44%)	28 (26%)	0.006
1 Emetic episode	14 (13%)	3 (3%)	
More than 1 emetic episode/rescued	49 (44%)	77 (71%)	
Median time to first emetic episode (min)*	60.5	34.0	
Nausea assessments:			
Number of patients	105	85	
Mean nausea score over 24-h postoperative period†	1.9	2.9	

* After administration of study drug.
† Nausea measured on a scale of 0–10 with 0=no nausea, 10=nausea as bad as it can be.

Prevention of Further Postoperative Nausea and Vomiting

Treatment Response Over 24 Hours	Ondansetron n (%)	Placebo n (%)	P Value
Study 1			
Number of patients	180	171	
0 Emetic episodes	96 (53%)	29 (17%)	≤ 0.001
Failure*	84 (47%)	142 (83%)	

* Failure was one or more emetic episodes, rescued, or withdrawn.

Principal Adverse Events in Comparative Trials

	ZOFRAN Injection 0.15 mg/kg × 3 n=419	ZOFRAN Injection 32 mg × 1 n=220	Metoclopramide n=156	Placebo n=34
Diarrhea	16%	8%	44%	18%
Headache	17%	25%	7%	15%
Fever	8%	7%	5%	3%
Akathisia	0%	0%	6%	0%
Acute dystonic reactions*	0%	0%	5%	0%

*See Central Nervous System below.

	ZOFRAN Injection 4 mg IV n=547 patients	Placebo n=547 patients
Headache	92 (17%)	77 (14%)
Dizziness	67 (12%)	88 (16%)
Musculoskeletal pain	57 (10%)	59 (11%)
Drowsiness/sedation	44 (8%)	37 (7%)
Shivers	38 (7%)	39 (7%)
Malaise/fatigue	25 (5%)	30 (5%)
Injection site reaction	21 (4%)	18 (3%)
Urinary retention	17 (3%)	15 (3%)

Postoperative CO$_2$-related pain*	12 (2%)	16 (3%)
Chest pain (unspecified)	12 (2%)	15 (3%)
Anxiety/ agitation	11 (2%)	16 (3%)
Dysuria	11 (2%)	9 (2%)
Hypotension	10 (2%)	12 (2%)
Fever	10 (2%)	6 (1%)
Cold sensation	9 (2%)	8 (1%)
Pruritus	9 (2%)	3 (<1%)
Paresthesia	9 (2%)	2 (<1%)

* Sites of pain included abdomen, stomach, joints, rib cage, shoulder.

Pediatric Use: The following were the most commonly reported adverse events in pediatric patients receiving ondansetron (0.1 mg/kg for children weighing 40 kg or less, a single 4-mg dose for children weighing more than 40 kg) administered intravenously over at least 30 seconds. Rates of these events were not significantly different in the ondansetron and placebo groups. These patients were receiving multiple concomitant perioperative and postoperative medications.

Frequency of Adverse Events From Controlled Studies

Adverse Event	Odansetron n=755 Patients	Placebo n=731 Patients
Wound problem	80 (11%)	86 (12%)
Anxiety/agitation	49 (6%)	47 (6%)
Headache	44 (6%)	43 (6%)
Drowsiness/sedation	41 (5%)	56 (8%)
Pyrexia	32 (4%)	41 (6%)

Drug Abuse and Dependence: Animal studies have shown that ondansetron is not discriminated as a benzodiazepine nor does it substitute for benzodiazepines in direct addiction studies.

OVERDOSAGE

There is no specific antidote for ondansetron overdose. Patients should be managed with appropriate supportive therapy. Individual doses as large as 145 mg and total daily dosages (three doses) as large as 252 mg have been administered intravenously without significant adverse events. These doses are more than 10 times the recommended daily dose.

"Sudden blindness" (amaurosis) of 2 to 3 minutes' duration plus severe constipation occurred in one patient that was administered 72 mg of ondansetron intravenously as a single dose. Hypotension (and faintness) occurred in another patient that took 48 mg of oral ondansetron. Following infusion of 32 mg over only a 4-minute period, a vasovagal episode with transient second degree heart block was observed. In all instances, the events resolved completely.

DOSAGE AND ADMINISTRATION

Prevention of Chemotherapy-Induced Nausea and Vomiting: The recommended IV dosage of ZOFRAN is a single 32-mg dose or three 0.15-mg/kg doses. A single 32-mg dose is infused over 15 minutes beginning 30 minutes before the start of emetogenic chemotherapy. The recommended infusion rate should not be exceeded (see OVERDOSAGE). With the three-dose (0.15-mg/kg) regimen, the first dose is infused over 15 minutes beginning 30 minutes before the start of emetogenic chemotherapy. Subsequent doses (0.15 mg/kg) are administered 4 and 8 hours after the first dose of ZOFRAN.
ZOFRAN Injection should not be mixed with solutions for which physical and chemical compatibility have not been established. In particular, this applies to alkaline solutions as a precipitate may form.
Vial: DILUTE BEFORE USE. ZOFRAN Injection should be diluted in 50 mL of 5% dextrose injection or 0.9% sodium chloride injection before administration.
Flexible Plastic Container. ZOFRAN Injection Premixed, 32 mg in 5% dextrose, 50 mL **REQUIRES NO DILUTION.**
Pediatric Use: DILUTE BEFORE USE. On the basis of the limited available information (see CLINICAL TRIALS: Pediatric Studies and CLINICAL PHARMACOLOGY: Pharmacokinetics), the dosage in children 4 to 18 years of age should be three 0.15-mg/kg doses (see above). Little information is available about dosage in children 3 years of age or younger.
Use in the Elderly: The dosage recommendation is the same as for the general population.

ZOFRAN Injection Premixed in Flexible Plastic Containers: Instructions for Use: To Open: Tear outer wrap at notch and remove solution container. Check for minute leaks by squeezing container firmly. If leaks are found, discard unit as sterility may be impaired.
Preparation for Administration: Use aseptic technique.
1. Close flow control clamp of administration set.
2. Remove cover from outlet port at bottom of container.
3. Insert piercing pin of administration set into port with a twisting motion until the pin is firmly seated. NOTE: See full directions on administration set carton.
4. Suspend container from hanger.
5. Squeeze and release drip chamber to establish proper fluid level in chamber during infusion of ZOFRAN Injection Premixed.
6. Open flow control clamp to expel air from set. Close clamp.
7. Attach set to venipuncture device. If device is not indwelling, prime and make venipuncture.
8. Perform venipuncture.
9. Regulate rate of administration with flow control clamp.
Caution: ZOFRAN Injection Premixed in flexible plastic containers is to be administered by IV drip infusion only. ZOFRAN Injection Premixed should not be mixed with solutions for which physical and chemical compatibility have not been established. In particular, this applies to alkaline solutions as a precipitate may form. If used with a primary IV fluid system, the primary solution should be discontinued during ZOFRAN Injection Premixed infusion.
Do not administer unless solution is clear and container is undamaged.
Warning: Do not use flexible plastic container in series connections.
Prevention of Postoperative Nausea and Vomiting: The recommended IV dosage of ZOFRAN for adults is 4 mg administered intravenously in not less than 30 seconds, preferably over 2 to 5 minutes, immediately before induction of anesthesia, or postoperatively if the patient experiences nausea and/or vomiting occurring shortly after surgery.
Vial: ZOFRAN Injection **REQUIRES NO DILUTION.**
Repeat dosing for patients who continue to experience nausea and/or vomiting postoperatively has not been studied. While recommended as a fixed dose for patients weighing more than 40 kg, few patients above 80 kg have been studied.
Pediatric Use: The recommended IV dosage of ZOFRAN for pediatric patients 2 to 12 years of age is 0.1 mg/kg for children weighing 40 kg or less, or a single 4-mg dose for children weighing more than 40 kg. The rate of administration should not be less than 30 seconds, preferably over 2 to 5 minutes.
Use in the Elderly: NO DILUTION NECESSARY. The dosage recommendation is the same as for the general population.
Dosage Adjustment for Patients With Impaired Renal Function: No specific studies have been conducted in patients with renal insufficiency.
Dosage Adjustment for Patients With Impaired Hepatic Function: In patients with severe hepatic impairment according to Child-Pugh[1] criteria, a single maximal daily dose of 8 mg to be infused over 15 minutes beginning 30 minutes before the start of the emetogenic chemotherapy is recommended. There is no experience beyond first-day administration of ondansetron.
Stability: ZOFRAN Injection is stable at room temperature under normal lighting conditions for 48 hours after dilution with the following IV fluids: 0.9% Sodium Chloride Injection, 5% Dextrose Injection, 5% Dextrose and 0.9% Sodium Chloride Injection, 5% Dextrose and 0.45% Sodium Chloride Injection, and 3% Sodium Chloride Injection.
Although ZOFRAN Injection is chemically and physically stable when diluted as recommended, sterile precautions should be observed because diluents generally do not contain preservative. After dilution, do not use beyond 24 hours.
Note: Parenteral drug products should be inspected visually for particulate matter and discoloration before administration whenever solution and container permit.
Precaution: Occasionally, ondansetron precipitates at the stopper/vial interface in vials stored upright. Potency and safety are not affected. If a precipitate is observed, resolubilize by shaking the vial vigorously.

HOW SUPPLIED

ZOFRAN Injection, 2 mg/mL, is supplied as follows:
NDC 0173-0442-02 2-mL single-dose vials (Carton of 5)
NDC 0173-0442-00 20-mL multidose vials (Singles)
Store between 2° and 30°C (36° and 86°F). Protect from light.
ZOFRAN Injection Premixed, 32 mg/50 mL, in 5% Dextrose, contains no preservatives and is supplied as a sterile, premixed solution for IV administration in single-dose, flexible plastic containers (NDC 0173-0461-00) (case of 6).
Store between 2° and 30°C (36° and 86°F). Protect from light. Avoid excessive heat. Protect from freezing.
REFERENCE: 1. Pugh RNH, Murray-Lyon IM, Dawson JL, Pietroni MC, Williams R. Transection of the oesophagus for bleeding oesophageal varices. *Brit J Surg.* 1973; 60:646-649.
© Copyright 1996 Glaxo Wellcome Inc. All rights reserved.
June 1996/RL-317

Shown in Product Identification Guide, page 316

ZOFRAN® Tablets
[zō'-frăn]
(ondansetron hydrochloride)

℞

DESCRIPTION

The active ingredient in ZOFRAN Tablets is ondansetron hydrochloride (HCl) as the dihydrate, the racemic form of ondansetron and a selective blocking agent of the serotonin 5-HT$_3$ receptor type. Chemically it is (±) 1, 2, 3, 9-tetrahydro-9-methyl-3-[(2-methyl-1H-imidazol-1-yl)methyl]-4H-carbazol-4-one, monohydrochloride, dihydrate.
The empirical formula is $C_{18}H_{19}N_3O \cdot HCl \cdot 2H_2O$, representing a molecular weight of 365.9.
Ondansetron HCl dihydrate is a white to off-white powder that is soluble in water and normal saline.
Each 4-mg ZOFRAN Tablet for oral administration contains ondansetron HCl dihydrate equivalent to 4 mg of ondansetron. Each 8-mg ZOFRAN Tablet for oral administration contains ondansetron HCl dihydrate equivalent to 8 mg of ondansetron. Each tablet also contains the inactive ingredients lactose, microcrystalline cellulose, pregelatinized starch, hydroxypropyl methylcellulose, magnesium stearate, titanium dioxide, iron oxide yellow (8-mg tablet only), and sodium benzoate (4-mg tablet only).

CLINICAL PHARMACOLOGY

Pharmacodynamics: Ondansetron is a selective 5-HT$_3$ receptor antagonist. While its mechanism of action has not been fully characterized, ondansetron is not a dopamine-receptor antagonist. Serotonin receptors of the 5-HT$_3$ type are present both peripherally on vagal nerve terminals and centrally in the chemoreceptor trigger zone of the area postrema. It is not certain whether ondansetron's antiemetic action is mediated centrally, peripherally, or in both sites. However, cytotoxic chemotherapy appears to be associated with release of serotonin from the enterochromaffin cells of the small intestine. In humans, urinary 5-HIAA (5-hydroxyindoleacetic acid) excretion increases after cisplatin administration in parallel with the onset of emesis. The released serotonin may stimulate the vagal afferents through the 5-HT$_3$ receptors and initiate the vomiting reflex.
In animals, the emetic response to cisplatin can be prevented by pretreatment with an inhibitor of serotonin synthesis, bilateral abdominal vagotomy and greater splanchnic nerve section, or pretreatment with a serotonin 5-HT$_3$ receptor antagonist.
In normal volunteers, single intravenous doses of 0.15 mg/kg of ondansetron had no effect on esophageal motility, gastric motility, lower esophageal sphincter pressure, or small intestinal transit time. Multiday administration of ondansetron has been shown to slow colonic transit in normal volunteers. Ondansetron has no effect on plasma prolactin concentrations.
Pharmacokinetics: Ondansetron is extensively metabolized in humans, with approximately 5% of a radiolabeled dose recovered from the urine as the parent compound. The primary metabolic pathway is hydroxylation on the indole ring followed by subsequent glucuronide or sulfate conjugation. Although some nonconjugated metabolites have pharmacologic activity, these are not found in plasma concentrations likely to significantly contribute to the biological activity of ondansetron.
Oral ondansetron is well absorbed and undergoes limited first-pass metabolism. Following the administration of a single 8-mg ondansetron tablet to healthy, young, male volunteers and from pooled studies, the time to peak plasma ondansetron concentration is approximately 1.7 hours, the terminal elimination half-life is approximately 3 hours, and bioavailability is approximately 56%. Gender differences were shown in the disposition of ondansetron given as a single dose. The extent and rate of ondansetron's absorption is greater in women than men. Slower clearance in women, a smaller apparent volume of distribution (adjusted for weight), and higher absolute bioavailability resulted in higher plasma ondansetron levels. These higher plasma levels may in part be explained by differences in body weight between men and women. It is not known whether these gender-related differences were clinically important. More detailed pharmacokinetic information is contained in the following table taken from one study.
[See table at top of next page.]
Both AUC and C_{max} more than double on increasing the tablet dose from 8 to 16 mg (123% and 118%, respectively). This may result from saturation of first-pass metabolism leading to greater oral bioavailability at 16 mg than 8 mg.
The administration of oral ondansetron with food increases significantly (about 17%) the extent of absorption of ondansetron. The peak plasma concentration and time to peak plasma concentration are not significantly affected. This change in the extent of absorption is not believed to be of any clinical relevance.

Continued on next page

Glaxo Wellcome Onc.—Cont.

There was no significant effect of antacid administration on the pharmacokinetics of orally administered ondansetron. Because ondansetron undergoes extensive metabolism, the modest reduction in clearance in the over-75 age-group was not unexpected. However, since there was a difference in neither safety nor efficacy between patients over 65 years of age and those under 65 years of age, no adjustment in dosage is required in the elderly.

Plasma protein binding of ondansetron as measured in vitro was 70% to 76% over the concentration range of 10 to 500 ng/mL. Circulating drug also distributes into erythrocytes.

CLINICAL TRIALS

Chemotherapy-Induced Nausea and Vomiting: In one double-blind US study in 67 patients, ZOFRAN Tablets were significantly more effective than placebo in preventing vomiting induced by cyclophosphamide-based chemotherapy containing doxorubicin. Treatment response is based on the total number of emetic episodes over the 3-day study period. The results of this study are summarized below:

[See second table at right.]

In one double-blind US study in 336 patients, ZOFRAN Tablets 8 mg administered twice a day were as effective as ZOFRAN Tablets 8 mg administered three times a day in preventing nausea and vomiting induced by cyclophosphamide-based chemotherapy containing either methotrexate or doxorubicin. Treatment response is based on the total number of emetic episodes over the 3-day study period. The results of this study are summarized below:

[See third table at right.]

Re-treatment: In uncontrolled trials, 148 patients receiving cyclophosphamide-based chemotherapy were re-treated with 8 mg t.i.d. of oral ondansetron during subsequent chemotherapy for a total of 396 re-treatment courses. No emetic episodes occurred in 314 (79%) of the re-treatment courses, and only one to two emetic episodes occurred in 43 (11%) of the re-treatment courses.

Pediatric Studies: Three open-label, uncontrolled, foreign trials have been performed with 182 patients 4 to 18 years old with cancer who were given a variety of cisplatin or non-cisplatin regimens. In these foreign trials, the initial dose of ZOFRAN® (ondansetron HCl) Injection ranged from 0.04 to 0.87 mg/kg for a total dose of 2.16 to 12 mg. This was followed by the oral administration of ondansetron ranging from 4 to 24 mg daily for 3 days. In these studies, 58% of the 170 evaluable patients had a complete response (no emetic episodes) on day 1. Two studies showed the response rates for patients less than 12 years of age who received 4 mg of ondansetron three times a day to be similar to those in patients 12 to 18 years of age who received 8 mg of ondansetron three times daily. Thus, prevention of emesis in these children was essentially the same as for patients older than 18 years of age. Overall, ZOFRAN Tablets were well tolerated in these pediatric patients.

Elderly Patients: One hundred thirty-seven (137) patients 65 years of age or older have received oral ondansetron. Prevention of emesis was similar to that in patients younger than 65 years of age and adverse reactions were not seen in increased frequency.

Radiation-Induced Nausea and Vomiting: *Total Body Irradiation:* In a randomized, double-blind study in 20 patients, ZOFRAN Tablets (8 mg given 1.5 hours before each fraction of radiotherapy for 4 days) was significantly more effective than placebo in preventing vomiting induced by total body irradiation. Total body irradiation consisted of 11 fractions (120 cGy per fraction) over 4 days for a total of 1,320 cGy. Patients received three fractions for 3 days, then two fractions on day 4.

Single High-Dose Fraction Radiotherapy: Ondansetron was significantly more effective than metoclopramide with respect to complete control of emesis (0 emetic episodes) in a double-blind trial in 105 patients receiving single high-dose radiotherapy (800 to 1,000 cGy) over an anterior or posterior field size of ≥ 80 cm^2 to the abdomen. Patients received the first dose of ondansetron (8 mg) or metoclopramide (10 mg) 1 to 2 hours before radiotherapy. If radiotherapy was given in the morning, two additional doses of study treatment were given (one tablet late afternoon and one tablet before bedtime). If radiotherapy was given in the afternoon, patients took only one further tablet that day before bedtime. Patients continued the oral medication on a t.i.d. basis for 3 days.

Daily Fractionated Radiotherapy: Ondansetron was significantly more effective than prochlorperazine with respect to complete control of emesis (0 emetic episodes) in a double-blind trial in 135 patients receiving a 1- to 4-week course of fractionated radiotherapy (180 cGy doses) over a field size of ≥ 100 cm^2 to the abdomen. Patients received the first dose of ondansetron (8 mg) or prochlorperazine (10 mg) 1 to 2 hours before the patient received the first daily radiotherapy fraction, with two subsequent doses on a t.i.d. basis. Patients continued the oral medication on a t.i.d. basis on each day of radiotherapy.

Pharmacokinetics in Normal Volunteers: Single 8-mg Oral Dose

Age-group (years)	Mean Weight (kg)	n	Peak Plasma Concentration (ng/mL)	Time of Peak Plasma Concentration (h)	Mean Elimination Half-life (h)	Systemic Plasma Clearance L/h/kg	Absolute Bioavailability
18-40 M	69.0	6	26.2	2.0	3.1	0.403	0.483
F	62.7	5	42.7	1.7	3.5	0.354	0.663
61-74 M	77.5	6	24.1	2.1	4.1	0.384	0.585
F	60.2	6	52.4	1.9	4.9	0.255	0.643
≥75 M	78.0	5	37.0	2.2	4.5	0.277	0.619
F	67.6	6	46.1	2.1	6.2	0.249	0.747

Emetic Episodes: Treatment Response

	Ondansetron 8 mg b.i.d. Oral*	Placebo	p Value
Number of patients	33	34	
Treatment response			
0 Emetic episodes	20 (61%)	2 (6%)	< 0.001
1–2 Emetic episodes	6 (18%)	8 (24%)	
More than 2 emetic episodes/withdrawn	7 (21%)	24 (71%)	< 0.001
Median number of emetic episodes	0.0	Undefined†	
Median time to first emetic episode (h)	Undefined‡	6.5	

*The first dose was administered 30 minutes before the start of emetogenic chemotherapy, with a subsequent dose 8 hours after the first dose. An 8-mg tablet was administered twice a day for 2 days after completion of chemotherapy.
†Median undefined since at least 50% of the patients were withdrawn or had more than two emetic episodes.
‡Median undefined since at least 50% of the patients did not have any emetic episodes.

Emetic Episodes: Treatment Response

	Ondansetron	
	8 mg b.i.d. Oral*	8 mg t.i.d. Oral†
Number of patients	165	171
Treatment response		
0 Emetic episodes	101 (61%)	99 (58%)
1–2 Emetic episodes	16 (10%)	17 (10%)
More than 2 emetic episodes/withdrawn	48 (29%)	55 (32%)
Median number of emetic episodes	0.0	0.0
Median time to first emetic episode (h)	Undefined‡	Undefined‡
Median nausea scores (0–100)§	6	6

*The first dose was administered 30 minutes before the start of emetogenic chemotherapy, with a subsequent dose 8 hours after the first dose. An 8-mg tablet was administered twice a day for 2 days after completion of chemotherapy.
†The first dose was administered 30 minutes before the start of emetogenic chemotherapy, with subsequent doses 4 and 8 hours after the first dose. An 8-mg tablet was administered three times a day for 2 days after completion of chemotherapy.
‡Median undefined since at least 50% of patients did not have any emetic episodes.
§Visual analog scale assessment: 0=no nausea, 100=nausea as bad as it can be.

Postoperative Nausea and Vomiting: Surgical patients who received ondansetron 1 hour before the induction of general balanced anesthesia (barbiturate: thiopental, methohexital, or thiamylal; opioid: alfentanil, sufentanil, morphine, or fentanyl; nitrous oxide; neuromuscular blockade: succinylcholine/curare or gallamine and/or vecuronium, pancuronium, or atracurium; and supplemental isoflurane or enflurane) were evaluated in two double-blind studies (one US, one foreign) involving 865 patients. ZOFRAN Tablets (16 mg) were significantly more effective than placebo in preventing postoperative nausea and vomiting.

The study populations in all trials thus far consisted of women undergoing inpatient surgical procedures. No studies have been performed in males. No controlled clinical study comparing ZOFRAN Tablets to ZOFRAN Injection has been performed.

INDICATIONS AND USAGE

1. Prevention of nausea and vomiting associated with initial and repeat courses of moderately emetogenic cancer chemotherapy.
2. Prevention of nausea and vomiting associated with radiotherapy in patients receiving either total body irradiation, single high-dose fraction to the abdomen, or daily fractions to the abdomen.
3. Prevention of postoperative nausea and/or vomiting. As with other antiemetics, routine prophylaxis is not recommended for patients in whom there is little expectation that nausea and/or vomiting will occur postoperatively. In patients where nausea and/or vomiting must be avoided postoperatively, ZOFRAN Tablets are recommended even where the incidence of postoperative nausea and/or vomiting is low.

CONTRAINDICATIONS

ZOFRAN Tablets are contraindicated for patients known to have hypersensitivity to the drug.

PRECAUTIONS

Drug Interactions: Ondansetron does not itself appear to induce or inhibit the cytochrome P-450 drug-metabolizing enzyme system of the liver. Because ondansetron is metabolized by hepatic cytochrome P-450 drug-metabolizing enzymes, inducers or inhibitors of these enzymes may change the clearance and, hence, the half-life of ondansetron. On the basis of available data, no dosage adjustment is recommended for patients on these drugs. Tumor response to chemotherapy in the P 388 mouse leukemia model is not affected by ondansetron. In humans, carmustine, etoposide, and cisplatin do not affect the pharmacokinetics of ondansetron.

Use in Surgical Patients: The coadministration of ondansetron had no effect on the pharmacokinetics and pharmacodynamics of temazepam.

Carcinogenesis, Mutagenesis, Impairment of Fertility: Carcinogenic effects were not seen in 2-year studies in rats and mice with oral ondansetron doses up to 10 and 30 mg/kg per day, respectively. Ondansetron was not mutagenic in standard tests for mutagenicity. Oral administration of ondansetron up to 15 mg/kg per day did not affect fertility or general reproductive performance of male and female rats.

Pregnancy: *Teratogenic Effects: Pregnancy Category B:* Reproduction studies have been performed in pregnant rats and rabbits at daily oral doses up to 15 and 30 mg/kg per day, respectively, and have revealed no evidence of impaired fertility or harm to the fetus due to ondansetron. There are, however, no adequate and well-controlled studies in pregnant women. Because animal reproduction studies are not

always predictive of human response, this drug should be used during pregnancy only if clearly needed.

Nursing Mothers: Ondansetron is excreted in the breast milk of rats. It is not known whether ondansetron is excreted in human milk. Because many drugs are excreted in human milk, caution should be exercised when ondansetron is administered to a nursing woman.

Pediatric Use: Little information is available about dosage in children 4 years of age or younger (see CLINICAL PHARMACOLOGY and DOSAGE AND ADMINISTRATION sections for use in children 4 to 18 years of age).

Use in Elderly Patients: Dosage adjustment is not needed in patients over the age of 65 (see CLINICAL PHARMACOLOGY). Prevention of nausea and vomiting in elderly patients was no different than in younger age-groups.

ADVERSE REACTIONS

Chemotherapy-Induced Nausea and Vomiting: The following adverse events have been reported in adults receiving either 8 mg of ondansetron two or three times a day for 3 days or placebo in four trials. These patients were receiving concurrent chemotherapy, primarily cyclophosphamide-based regimens.

Principal Adverse Events in US Trials: 3 Days of Oral Therapy

Event	Ondansetron 8 mg b.i.d. n=242	Ondansetron 8 mg t.i.d. n=415	Placebo n=262
Headache	58 (24%)	113 (27%)	34 (13%)
Malaise/fatigue	32 (13%)	37 (9%)	6 (2%)
Constipation	22 (9%)	26 (6%)	1 (<1%)
Diarrhea	15 (6%)	16 (4%)	10 (4%)
Dizziness	13 (5%)	18 (4%)	12 (5%)
Abdominal pain	3 (1%)	13 (3%)	1 (<1%)
Xerostomia	5 (2%)	6 (1%)	1 (<1%)
Weakness	0 (0%)	7 (2%)	1 (<1%)

Central Nervous System: There have been rare reports consistent with, but not diagnostic of, extrapyramidal reactions in patients receiving ondansetron.

Hepatic: In 723 patients receiving cyclophosphamide-based chemotherapy in US clinical trials, AST and/or ALT values have been reported to exceed twice the upper limit of normal in approximately 1% to 2% of patients receiving oral ondansetron. The increases were transient and did not appear to be related to dose or duration of therapy. On repeat exposure, similar transient elevations in transaminase values occurred in some courses, but symptomatic hepatic disease did not occur. The role of cancer chemotherapy in these biochemical changes cannot be clearly determined.

There have been reports of liver failure and death in patients with cancer receiving concurrent medications including potentially hepatotoxic cytotoxic chemotherapy and antibiotics. The etiology of the liver failure is unclear.

Integumentary: Rash has occurred in approximately 1% of patients receiving ondansetron.

Other: Rare cases of anaphylaxis, bronchospasm, tachycardia, angina (chest pain), hypokalemia, electrocardiographic alterations, vascular occlusive events, and grand mal seizures have been reported. Except for bronchospasm and anaphylaxis, the relationship to ZOFRAN was unclear.

Radiation-Induced Nausea and Vomiting: The adverse events reported in patients receiving ondansetron and concurrent radiotherapy were similar to those reported in patients receiving ondansetron and concurrent chemotherapy. The most frequently reported adverse events were headache, constipation, and diarrhea.

Postoperative Nausea and Vomiting: The following adverse events have been reported in ≥5% of patients receiving ondansetron at a dosage of 16 mg orally in clinical trials. With the exception of headache, rates of these events were not significantly different in the ondansetron and placebo groups. These patients were receiving multiple concomitant perioperative and postoperative medications.

Frequency of Adverse Events From Controlled Studies

Adverse Event	Ondansetron 16 mg (n=550)	Placebo (n=531)
Wound problem	152 (28%)	162 (31%)
Drowsiness/sedation	112 (20%)	122 (23%)
Headache	49 (9%)	27 (5%)
Hypoxia	49 (9%)	35 (7%)
Pyrexia	45 (8%)	34 (6%)
Dizziness	36 (7%)	34 (6%)
Gynecological disorder	36 (7%)	33 (6%)
Anxiety/agitation	33 (6%)	29 (5%)
Bradycardia	32 (6%)	30 (6%)
Shiver(s)	28 (5%)	30 (6%)
Urinary retention	28 (5%)	18 (3%)
Hypotension	27 (5%)	32 (6%)
Pruritus	27 (5%)	20 (4%)

DRUG ABUSE AND DEPENDENCE

Animal studies have shown that ondansetron is not discriminated as a benzodiazepine nor does it substitute for benzodiazepines in direct addiction studies.

OVERDOSAGE

There is no specific antidote for ondansetron overdose. Patients should be managed with appropriate supportive therapy. Individual intravenous doses as large as 145 mg and total daily intravenous doses as large as 252 mg have been inadvertently administered without significant adverse events. These doses are more than 10 times the recommended daily dose.

Hypotension (and faintness) occurred in a patient that took 48 mg of oral ondansetron. The events resolved completely.

DOSAGE AND ADMINISTRATION

Prevention of Nausea and Vomiting Associated With Moderately Emetogenic Cancer Chemotherapy: The recommended adult oral dosage of ZOFRAN Tablets is one 8-mg tablet given twice a day. The first dose should be administered 30 minutes before the start of emetogenic chemotherapy, with a subsequent dose 8 hours after the first dose. One 8-mg ZOFRAN Tablet should be administered twice a day (every 12 hours) for 1 to 2 days after completion of chemotherapy.

Pediatric Use: For patients 12 years of age and older, the dosage is the same as for adults. For patients 4 through 11 years of age, the dosage is one 4-mg tablet given three times a day. The first dose should be administered 30 minutes before the start of emetogenic chemotherapy, with subsequent doses 4 and 8 hours after the first dose. One 4-mg ZOFRAN Tablet should be administered three times a day (every 8 hours) for 1 to 2 days after completion of chemotherapy.

Use in the Elderly: The dosage is the same as for the general population.

Prevention of Nausea and Vomiting Associated With Radiotherapy, Either Total Body Irradiation, or Single High-Dose Fraction or Daily Fractions to the Abdomen: The recommended oral dosage of ZOFRAN Tablets is one 8-mg tablet given three times a day.

For total body irradiation, an 8-mg dose should be administered 1 to 2 hours before each fraction of radiotherapy administered each day.

For single high-dose fraction radiotherapy to the abdomen, an 8-mg dose should be administered 1 to 2 hours before radiotherapy, with subsequent doses every 8 hours after the first dose for 1 to 2 days after completion of radiotherapy.

For daily fractionated radiotherapy to the abdomen, an 8-mg dose should be administered 1 to 2 hours before radiotherapy, with subsequent doses every 8 hours after the first dose for each day radiotherapy is given.

Pediatric Use: There is no experience with the use of ZOFRAN Tablets in the prevention of radiation-induced nausea and vomiting in children.

Use in the Elderly: The dosage recommendation is the same as for the general population.

Postoperative Nausea and Vomiting: The recommended oral dosage is 16 mg given as a single dose (2 8-mg tablets) 1 hour before induction of anesthesia.

Pediatric Use: There is no experience with the use of ZOFRAN Tablets in the prevention of postoperative nausea and vomiting in children.

Use in the Elderly: The dosage is the same as for the general population.

Dosage Adjustment for Patients With Impaired Renal Function: No specific studies have been conducted in patients with renal insufficiency.

Dosage Adjustment for Patients With Impaired Hepatic Function: In patients with severe hepatic insufficiency, clearance is reduced, apparent volume of distribution is increased with a resultant increase in plasma half-life, and bioavailability approaches 100%. In such patients, a total daily dose of 8 mg should not be exceeded.

HOW SUPPLIED

ZOFRAN Tablets, 4 mg (ondansetron HCl dihydrate equivalent to 4 mg of ondansetron), are white, oval, film-coated tablets engraved with "ZOFRAN" on one side and "4" on the other in daily unit dose packs of 3 tablets (NDC 0173-0446-04), bottles of 30 tablets (NDC 0173-0446-00), and unit dose packs of 100 tablets (NDC 0173-0446-02).

ZOFRAN Tablets, 8 mg (ondansetron HCl dihydrate equivalent to 8 mg of ondansetron), are yellow, oval, film-coated tablets engraved with "ZOFRAN" on one side and "8" on the other in daily unit dose packs of 3 tablets (NDC 0173-0447-04), bottles of 30 tablets (NDC 0173-0447-00), and unit dose packs of 100 tablets (NDC 0173-0447-02).

Store between 2° and 30°C (36° and 86°F). Protect from light. Store blisters and bottles in carton.

©Copyright 1996 Glaxo Wellcome Inc. All rights reserved.
March 1996/RL-289

Shown in Product Identification Guide, page 316

Glenwood-Palisades
**82 N. SUMMIT STREET
TENAFLY, NJ 07670**

Direct Inquiries to:
Professional Services Department
201-569-0050
(800) 237-9083

**For Medical Information Contact:
In Emergencies:**
Professional Services Department
201-569-0050
(800) 237-9083

BICHLORACETIC ACID® KAHLENBERG ℞
Dichloroacetic Acid—Topical

DESCRIPTION
BICHLORACETIC ACID (dichloroacetic acid) Kahlenberg ($CHCl_2COOH$) is a clear, colorless liquid (sp. gr. 1.56) supplied full strength ready to use. It does not contain or require a solvent or diluent, is always uniform in potency. BICHLORACETIC ACID (dichloroacetic acid) remains colorless and retains its potency if kept in a tightly closed bottle and not contaminated with dissolved keratin or wooden applicators.

ACTIONS
BICHLORACETIC ACID (dichloroacetic acid) rapidly penetrates and cauterizes skin, keratin and other tissues. Its cauterizing effect is comparable to that obtained with such methods as electrocautery or freezing.

INDICATIONS
The lesions for which therapy with BICHLORACETIC ACID (dichloroacetic acid) is indicated are: calluses; hard and soft corns; xanthoma palpebrarum; seborrheic keratoses; ingrown nails; cysts and benign erosion of the cervix including endocervicitis and epistaxis.

CONTRAINDICATION
Topically applied chemical cauterant-keratolytics should not be used for the treatment of malignant or premalignant lesions.

WARNING
BICHLORACETIC ACID (dichloroacetic acid) is an extremely powerful keratolytic and cauterant. It should be restricted to those areas where these effects are desired.

ADMINISTRATION AND DOSAGE
The amount of BICHLORACETIC ACID (dichloroacetic acid) which should be applied varies with the nature of the lesion. Dense horny lesions such as corns and calluses require repeated extensive treatment. Lesions of light density such as xanthoma palpebrarum, soft corns, and seborrheic keratoses, should receive lighter applications.

Similarly, the number of treatments necessary will vary depending on the particular lesion being treated.

[See Figure at top of next column.]

The treatment kit provides 10 ml. BICHLORACETIC ACID KAHLENBERG, 16 grams of petrolatum in a bottle, approximately 100 applicators, and a product insert with directions. Also included are a microdropper and holder and two sealed-stem acid receptacles of differing capacity.

HOW SUPPLIED
Bichloracetic Acid® Kahlenberg
Complete Treatment Kit, NDC 0516-1004-11

Continued on next page

Glenwood-Palisades—Cont.

COMPLETE TREATMENT KIT

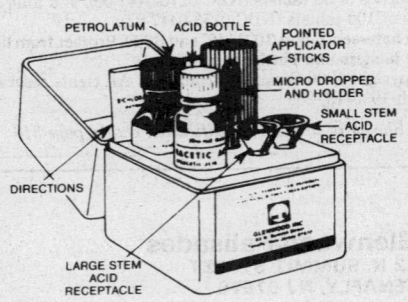

Restocking Unit, NDC 0516-1006-77, 75 ml. bottle
Replenishment Unit, NDC 0516-1007-11, 10 ml. bottle
Unit-Kit, NDC 0516-1010-05, 0.5 ml. single-use, disposable
ampule

CALPHOSAN®   ℞
(calcium glycerophosphate/calcium lactate)
calcium/phosphorus solution in metabolic disorders involving low calcium

COMPOSITION
CALPHOSAN is a specially processed solution containing calcium glycerophosphate and calcium lactate. CALPHOSAN is isotonic, with a pH of about 7 or somewhat above. (Other calcium solutions are usually quite acid, with pH values of 4.5 to 5.5). Each 10 ml. CALPHOSAN contains calcium glycerophosphate 50 mg. and calcium lactate 50 mg. in a physiological solution of sodium chloride, with 0.25% phenol as a preservative.

ADVANTAGES
Intramuscular injections of CALPHOSAN raise blood serum calcium levels, do not raise the calcium levels above normal. Of conspicuous importance, intramuscular injections of CALPHOSAN are without pain, inflammatory reactions or sloughing.

INDICATIONS
Wherever calcium is indicated or in conditions associated with hypocalcemia.

ADMINISTRATION
10 ml. 1 to 4 times weekly or as determined by the physician.

USE IN PREGNANCY
Safety for use in pregnancy or during lactation has not been established.

CONTRAINDICATIONS
Hypercalcemia, and in view of the fact that hypercalcemia is associated with sarcoidosis and bone metastasis of neoplastic processes, it should not be used in those conditions. As there is a similarity in the actions of calcium and digitalis on the contractility and excitability of the heart muscle, CALPHOSAN is contraindicated in fully digitalized patients. **Do not use intramuscularly in infants and young children.**

AVAILABILITY
60 ml. multiple dose vials—NDC 0516-0060-60.

PALS™   OTC
[*pals*]
Internal Deodorant
Chlorophyllin Copper Complex

POTABA®   ℞
Systemic ANTIFIBROSIS THERAPY

PRODUCT OVERVIEW
KEY FACTS
Potaba® (Aminobenzoate Potassium) is considered a member of the vitamin B complex. It has been suggested that the antifibrotic action of Potaba® is due to its mediation of increased oxygen uptake at the tissue level.

MAJOR USES
Potaba® offers a means of treatment of serious and often chronic entities, such as scleroderma and Peyronie's Disease.

SAFETY INFORMATION
Contraindicated in patients taking sulfonamides. Anorexia, nausea, fever and rash have occurred infrequently and subside with omission of the drug. Often, desensitization can be accomplished and treatment resumed.

PRESCRIBING INFORMATION

POTABA®   ℞
Systemic ANTIFIBROSIS THERAPY

FORMULA
POTABA is chemically Aminobenzoate Potassium, U.S.P.

> ### INDICATIONS
> Based on a review of this drug by the National Academy of Sciences-National Research Council and/or other information, FDA has classified the indications as follows:
> "Possibly" effective: Potassium aminobenzoate is possibly effective in the treatment of scleroderma, dermatomyositis, morphea, linear scleroderma, pemphigus, and Peyronie's disease.
> Final classification of the less-than-effective indications requires further investigation.

ADVANTAGES
POTABA offers a means of treatment of serious and often chronic entities involving fibrosis and nonsuppurative inflammation.

PHARMACOLOGY
P-Aminobenzoate is considered a member of the vitamin B complex. Small amounts are found in cereal, eggs, milk and meats. Detectable amounts are normally present in human blood, spinal fluid, urine, and sweat. PABA is a component of several biologically important systems, and it participates in a number of fundamental biological processes. It has been suggested that the antifibrosis action of POTABA is due to its mediation of increased oxygen uptake at the tissue level. Fibrosis is believed to occur from either too much serotonin or too little monoamine oxidase activity over a period of time. Monoamine oxidase requires an adequate supply of oxygen to function properly. By increasing oxygen supply at the tissue level POTABA may enhance MAO activity and prevent or bring about regression of fibrosis.

CLINICAL USES
PEYRONIE'S DISEASE: 21 patients with Peyronie's disease were placed on POTABA therapy for periods ranging from 3 months to 2 years. Pain disappeared from 16 of 16 cases in which it had been present. There was objective improvement in penile deformity in 10 of 17 patients, and decrease in plaque size in 16 of 21. The authors suggest that this medication offers no hazard of further local injury as may result from other therapy. There were no significant untoward effects encountered on long term POTABA therapy.
SCLERODERMA: Of 135 patients with diffuse systemic sclerosis treated with POTABA every patient but one has shown softening of the involved skin if treatment has been continued for 3 months or longer. The responses have been reported in a number of publications. The treatment program consists of systemic antifibrosis therapy with POTABA, physical therapy, including deep breathing exercises and dynamic traction splints where indicated, and bethanechol chloride (MYOTONACHOL, Glenwood) for relief of dysphagia as well as small doses of reserpine for amelioration of Raynaud's phenomena.
DERMATOMYOSITIS: Five patients with scleroderma and 2 with dermatomyositis were treated with POTABA. There was striking clinical improvement in each patient. Doses of 15-20 grams per day were well tolerated, and patients were easily able to take these doses.
MORPHEA and LINEAR SCLERODERMA: All 14 patients with localized forms of scleroderma placed on longterm POTABA treatment showed softening of the sclerotic component of their disorder. Treatment is particularly indicated in patients where persistent compressive sclerosis may contribute even greater disfigurement or functional embarrassment from secondary pressure atrophy.

DOSAGE AND ADMINISTRATION
The average adult daily dose of POTABA is 12 grams, usually given in four to six divided doses. Tablets and capsules 0.5 gram are given at the rate of 4 tablets or capsules 6 times daily, or 6 given four times daily, usually with meals, and at bed-time with a snack. Tablets must be dissolved in an adequate amount of liquid to prevent gastrointestinal upset. POTABA Envules contain 2 grams pure drug each, and 6 Envules are given for a total of 12 grams POTABA daily. POTABA Powder is used to prepare solutions, which are kept refrigerated, but for no longer than one week. 100 grams POTABA powder make 1 quart of 10% solution when dissolved in potable tap water. Children are given 1 gram POTABA daily in divided doses for each 10 lbs. of body weight.

SIDE EFFECTS
Anorexia, nausea, fever and rash have occurred infrequently and subside with omission of the drug. Often, desensitization can be accomplished and treatment resumed.

USAGE IN PREGNANCY
Safety for use in pregnancy or during lactation has not been established.

PRECAUTIONS
Should anorexia or nausea occur, therapy is interrupted until the patient is eating normally again. This permits prompt subsidence of symptoms and also avoids the possible development of hypoglycemia. Give cautiously to patients with renal disease. If a hypersensitivity reaction should occur, POTABA should be stopped.

CONTRAINDICATIONS
POTABA should not be administered to patients taking sulfonamides.

HOW SUPPLIED
POTABA Capsules—0.5 gm.
NDC 0516-0051-25 Bottle of 250
NDC 0516-0051-10 Bottle of 1000
POTABA Tablets—0.5 gm.
NDC 0516-0054-01 Bottle of 100
NDC 0516-0054-10 Bottle of 1000
POTABA Envules—2 gm.
NDC 0516-0052-50 Box of 50
POTABA Powder, pure
NDC 0516-0053-01 Bottle of 100 gms.
NDC 0516-0053-16 Bottle of 1 lb.
Shown in Product Identification Guide, page 316

SCLEROMATE™   ℞
[*skle "ro-māt*]
MORRHUATE SODIUM INJECTION U.S.P.

DESCRIPTION
Morrhuate Sodium Injection, U.S.P. is a mixture of the sodium salts of the saturated and unsaturated fatty acids of Cod Liver Oil. SCLEROMATE Morrhuate Sodium Injection, U.S.P. is prepared by the saponification of selected Cod Liver Oils, it is overlaid with filtered Nitrogen to prevent discoloration that occurs on exposure to oxygen. Morrhuate Sodium occurs as a pale-yellowish, granular powder with a slight fishy odor and is soluble in water and in alcohol. NOTE: Solid matter may develop a hazy appearance on standing and the injection should not be used if the solid matter does not dissolve completely on warming. The pH of the injection is adjusted to approximately 9.5.

CLINICAL PHARMACOLOGY
Morrhuate Sodium, when injected into the vein, causes inflammation of the intima and formation of a thrombus. This blood clot occludes the injected vein and fibrous tissue develops, resulting in the obliteration of the vein.

INDICATIONS AND USAGE
Morrhuate Sodium Injection is used for the obliteration of primary varicosed veins that consist of simple dilation with competent valves.
Sclerotherapy should not be used in patients with significant valvular or deep vein incompetence. (See Precautions.)
Although Morrhuate Sodium has been used as a sclerosing agent for the treatment of internal hemorrhoids, there is no substantial evidence that the drug is useful for this purpose. Most patients with symptomatic primary varicosed veins should be treated initially with compression stockings. If this treatment is inadequate, surgery may be required. Sclerosing agents may be useful as a supplement to venous ligation to obliterate residual varicosed veins or in patients who have conditions which increase the risk of surgery. However, many clinicians consider sclerotherapy if not effective may decrease the potential success of later surgery, should this be required.

CONTRAINDICATIONS
Morrhuate Sodium is contraindicated in patients who have shown a previous hypersensitivity reaction to the drug or to the fatty acids of cod liver oil. Continued administration of the drug is contraindicated when an unusual local reaction at the injection site or a systemic reaction occurs.
Thrombosis induced by Morrhuate Sodium may extend into the deep venous system in patients with significant valvular incompetence, therefore, valvular competency, deep vein patency, and deep vein competency should be determined by angiography and/or by tests such as the Trendelenberg and Perthes before injection of sclerosing agents. The drug is contraindicated for obliterations of superficial veins in patients with persistent occlusion of the deep veins. Morrhuate Sodium is also contraindicated in patients with acute superficial thrombophlebitis; underlying arterial disease; varicosi-

ties caused by abdominal and pelvic tumors, uncontrolled diabetes mellitus, thyrotoxicosis, tuberculosis, neoplasms, asthma, sepsis, blood dyscrasias, acute respiratory or skin disease; and in bedridden patients. Treatment with Morrhuate Sodium should be delayed in patients with acute local or systemic infections (including infected ulcers). Extensive therapy with the drug is inadvisable in patients who are severely debilitated or senile.

PRECAUTIONS

Burning or cramping sensations indicate local reactions. Urticaria may result. Sloughing and necrosis of tissue may occur with extravasation of the drug. Technique development is essential for optimal success in sclerotherapy, therefore the drug should be administered only by a physician familiar with proper injection technique. Drowsiness and headache may occur rarely. Pulmonary embolism has been reported.

Rarely, patients may have, or may develop hypersensitivity to Morrhuate Sodium, characterized by dizziness, weakness, vascular collapse, asthma, respiratory depression, gastrointestinal disturbances (i.e., nausea, vomiting), and urticaria. Anaphylactic reactions may occur within a few minutes after injection of the drug and are most likely to occur when therapy is reinstituted after an interval of several weeks. Morrhuate Sodium should only be administered when adequate facilities, drugs (i.e., epinephrine, antihistamines, corticosteroids), and personnel are available for the treatment of anaphylactic reactions.

PREGNANCY

Safety in use of Morrhuate Sodium during pregnancy has not been established.

DOSAGE

Morrhuate Sodium is administered only by INTRAVENOUS Injection. Care must be taken to avoid extravasation. (See Precautions.) Specialized references should be consulted for specific procedures and techniques of administration. When small veins are injected, or the injection solution is cold, or if solid matter has separated in the solution, the vial should be warmed by immersing in hot water. The solution should become clear on warming; only a clear solution should be used. Because the solution froths easily, a large bore needle should be used to fill the syringe, however, a small bore needle should be used for the injection.

To determine possible sensitivity to the drug, some clinicians recommend injection of 0.25–1 ml of 5% Morrhuate Sodium injection into a varicosity 24 hours before administration of a large dose.

Dosage of Morrhuate Sodium depends on the size and degree of varicosity. The usual adult dose for obliteration of small or medium veins is 50–100mg (1–2ml of the 5% injection). For large veins, 150–250 mg (3–5ml of the injection) is used. The drug may be given as multiple injections at one time or in single doses. Therapy may be repeated at 5–7 day intervals, according to the patient's response. Following injection of Morrhuate Sodium, the vein promptly becomes hard and swollen for 2–4 inches, depending on the size and response of the vein. After 24 hours, the vein is hard and slightly tender to the touch (with little or no periphlebitis). The skin around the injection becomes light-bronze; this color usually disappears shortly. An aching sensation and feeling of stiffness usually occur and last approximately 48 hours.

HOW SUPPLIED

MORRHUATE SODIUM INJECTION 5%
NDC-53159-003-01   30ml multiple use vials

STORAGE

Store below 40 degrees C. (104 degrees F.) preferably in a refrigerator, or between 15–30 degrees C. (59–86 degrees F.). Rev. July 1985

Shown in Product Identification Guide, page 316

YOCON®
[yō′kon]
(brand of yohimbine hydrochloride)

DESCRIPTION

Yohimbine is a 3α-15α-20β-17α-hydroxy Yohimbine-16α-carboxylic acid methyl ester. The alkaloid is found in Rubaceae and related trees. Also in Rauwolfia Serpentina (L) Benth.

Yohimbine is an indolalkylamine alkaloid with chemical similarity to reserpine. It is a crystalline powder, odorless. Each compressed tablet contains (1/12 gr.) 5.4 mg of Yohimbine Hydrochloride.

ACTION

Yohimbine blocks presynaptic alpha-2 adrenergic receptors. Its action on peripheral blood vessels resembles that of reserpine, though it is weaker and of short duration. Yohimbine's peripheral autonomic nervous system effect is to increase parasympathetic (cholinergic) and decrease sympathetic (adrenergic) activity. It is to be noted that in male sexual performance, erection is linked to cholinergic activity and to alpha-2 adrenergic blockade which may theoretically result in increased penile inflow, decreased penile outflow or both. Yohimbine exerts a stimulating action on the mood and may increase anxiety. Such actions have not been adequately studied or related to dosage although they appear to require high doses of the drug. Yohimbine has a mild anti-diuretic action, probably via stimulation of hypothalamic centers and release of posterior pituitary hormone.

Reportedly, Yohimbine exerts no significant influence on cardiac stimulation and other effects mediated by β-adrenergic receptors, its effect on blood pressure, if any, would be to lower it; however, no adequate studies are at hand to quantitate this effect in terms of Yohimbine dosage.

INDICATIONS

YOCON is indicated as a sympatholytic and mydriatic. It may have activity as an aphrodisiac.

CONTRAINDICATIONS

Renal diseases, and patients sensitive to the drug. In view of the limited and inadequate information at hand, no precise tabulation can be offered of additional contraindications.

WARNING

Generally, this drug is not proposed for use in females and certainly must not be used during pregnancy. Neither is this drug proposed for use in pediatric, geriatric or cardio-renal patients with gastric or duodenal ulcer history. Nor should it be used in conjunction with mood-modifying drugs such as antidepressants, or in psychiatric patients in general.

ADVERSE REACTIONS

Yohimbine readily penetrates the (CNS) and produces a complex pattern of responses in lower doses than required to produce peripheral α-adrenergic blockade. These include anti-diuresis, a general picture of central excitation including elevation of blood pressure and heart rate, increased motor activity, irritability and tremor. Sweating, nausea and vomiting are common after parenteral administration of the drug.[1,2] Also dizziness, headache, skin flushing reported when used orally[1,3].

DOSAGE AND ADMINISTRATION

Experimental dosage reported in treatment of erectile impotence:[1,3,4] 1 tablet (5.4 mg) 3 times a day, to adult males taken orally. Occasional side effects reported with this dosage are nausea, dizziness or nervousness. In the event of side effects dosage is to be reduced to $1/2$ tablet 3 times a day, followed by gradual increases to 1 tablet 3 times a day. Reported therapy not more than 10 weeks[3].

HOW SUPPLIED

Oral tablets of Yocon® 1/12 gr 5.4 mg in bottles of 100's **NDC 53159-001-01**, 1000's **NDC 53159-001-10**, and blister-paks of 30's **NDC 53159-001-30**.

REFERENCES

1. A. Morales et al., New England Journal of Medicine: 1221. November 12, 1981.
2. Goodman, Gilman —The Pharmacological Basis of Therapeutics 6th ed., p. 176-188, McMillan
3. Weekly Urological Clinical letter, 27:2, July 4, 1983.
4. A. Morales et al., The Journal of Urology *128* : 45-47, 1982.
Rev. January 1985

Shown in Product Identification Guide, page 316

YODOXIN®
210 mg. & 650 mg. Tablets
(IODOQUINOL TABLETS U.S.P.)

PRODUCT OVERVIEW

KEY FACTS

Yodoxin (Iodoquinol) is amebicidal against the cyst and trophozoite forms of Entaemeoba histolytica. Yodoxin® contains 64% organically bound iodine.

MAJOR USES

Yodoxin® is used in the treatment of intestinal amebiasis.

SAFETY INFORMATION

Contraindicated in patients with hepatic damage and in patients with known hypersensitivity to iodine and 8-hydroxyquinolines. Long term use of this drug should be avoided as optic neuritis, optic atrophy and peripheral neuropathy have been reported following prolonged high dosage with halogenated 8-hydroxyquinolines.

PRODUCT ILLUSTRATION

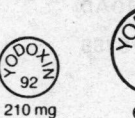
210 mg

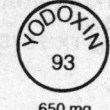
650 mg

PRESCRIBING INFORMATION

YODOXIN®
210 mg. & 650 mg. Tablets
(IODOQUINOL TABLETS U.S.P.)

℞

DESCRIPTION

Iodoquinol is of a light yellowish to tan color, nearly odorless and stable in air. The compound is practically insoluble in water, and sparingly soluble in most other solvents. It contains 64 per cent organically bound iodine.

ACTION

Iodoquinol is amebicidal against Entamoeba histolytica and is considered effective against the trophozoite and cyst forms.

INDICATIONS

Iodoquinol is used in the treatment of intestinal amebiasis. Iodoquinol is not recommended for the treatment of non-specific diarrhea.

CONTRAINDICATIONS

Known hypersensitivity to iodine and 8-hydroxyquinolines. Contraindicated in patients with hepatic damage.

WARNINGS

Optic neuritis, optic atrophy, and peripheral neuropathy have been reported following prolonged high dosage therapy with halogenated 8-hydroxyquinolines. Long term use of this drug should be avoided.

USE IN PREGNANCY

Safety for use in pregnancy or during lactation has not been established.

PRECAUTIONS

Iodoquinol should be used with caution in patients with thyroid disease.

Protein-bound serum iodine levels may be increased during treatment with iodoquinol and therefore interfere with certain thyroid function tests. These effects may persist for as long as six months after discontinuation of therapy. Discontinue the drug if hypersensitivity reactions occur.

ADVERSE REACTIONS

Skin: various forms of skin eruptions (acneiform papular and pustular; bullae; vegetating of tuberous iododerma), urticaria and pruritus. Gastrointestinal: nausea, vomiting, abdominal cramps, diarrhea, and pruritus ani.

Fever, chills, headache, vertigo and enlargement of thyroid have been reported. Optic neuritis, optic atrophy and peripheral neuropathy have been reported in association with prolonged high-dosage 8-hydroxyquinoline therapy.

DOSAGE AND ADMINISTRATION

Usual adult dose: (210 mg. each) 3 tablets three times daily, after meals for 20 days. Children 6 to 12 years: (210 mg. each) 2 tablets, t.i.d. Children under 6: (210 mg. each) one tablet per 15 pounds of body weight. Usual adult dose: (650 mg. each) one tablet three times a day for twenty days, to be taken after meals. Children (650 mg. each): For twenty days, 40 mg. per Kg. of body weight daily divided into 3 doses, not to exceed 1.95 grams in 24 hours, for 20 days.

HOW SUPPLIED

YODOXIN Tablets—210 mg.
NDC-0516-0092-01 Bottle of 100
NDC-0516-0092-10 Bottle of 1000
YODOXIN Tablets—650 mg.
NDC-0516-0093-01 Bottle of 100
NDC-0516-0093-10 Bottle of 1000

STORAGE

Store at Controlled Room Temperature 15–30°C. (59–86°F.)

CAUTION

Federal law prohibits dispensing without prescription.

For EMERGENCY telephone numbers,
consult the **Manufacturers' Index.**

A.C. Grace Co.
1100 QUITMAN ROAD
P.O. BOX 570
BIG SANDY, TX 75755

Direct Inquiries to:
Roy Erickson
(903) 636-4368
FAX: (903) 636-4051

For Medical Emergencies Contact:
Roy Erickson
(903) 636-4368
FAX: (903) 636-4051

UNIQUE E™ Vitamin E   OTC

DESCRIPTION
Each beef gelatin 400 I.U. Softgel Capsule contains All-Natural _Un_esterified Extra-High Antioxidant Concentrated Mixed Tocopherols. Not esterified acetate, succinate, _ordinary_ Mixed Tocopherols nor d_l_ synthetic. Contains _NO_ SOY OIL, WHEAT GERM OIL or _ANY_ OTHER OIL _DILUENT_ which will turn rancid causing harmful free radical pathology. NO ALLERGENS, PRESERVATIVES, COLORS OR FLAVORS. Minimum shelf life FIVE YEARS.
All known natural related tocopherols for _extra-high_ antioxidant function _PLUS_ full biological activity and synergistic benefits of the complete all-natural Vitamin E Complex. The _ONLY_ form providing all known vital functions of Vitamin E.
Unlike _ordinary_ Mixed Tocopherols which can vary in the important d-alpha tocopherol potency, UNIQUE E Softgel capsules are stabilized and Certified by Assay to provide 400 I.U. (International Units) of d-alpha tocopherol _PLUS_ all vital antioxidant factors.

DOSAGE
One or more capsules as directed by physician. Take _ENTIRE_ daily dosage just before or with morning meal.

HOW SUPPLIED
Bottles of 180 and 90 Softgel Capsules in safety-sealed, light protected plastic bottles.

Gray Pharmaceutical Co.
affiliate, The Purdue Frederick Company
100 CONNECTICUT AVENUE
NORWALK, CT 06850-3590

For Medical Information Contact:
Medical Department
(203) 853-0123

Senna
X-PREP® BOWEL EVACUANT LIQUID   OTC
[ěx 'prep]
(extract of senna concentrate)

INDICATIONS
An easy-to-administer, palatable, highly effective bowel evacuant for cleansing the colon prior to x-ray, endoscopic examination or surgery. Permits excellent visualization without residual oil droplets. "Senna" X-PREP Liquid is fully prepared in a single dose container—all the patient has to do is drink the contents of one small bottle ($2^1/_2$ fl. oz.). Good patient cooperation is ensured because of highly pleasant taste. Predictable effectiveness helps reduce or eliminate the need for enemas prior to radiography.

DESCRIPTION
Each bottle contains 130 mg sennosides. Active Ingredient: Extract of Senna Concentrate. Inactive Ingredients: Alcohol 7%, by volume, Methyl paraben, Potassium sorbate, Propylparaben, Sodium lauryl sulfate, Sucrose, Water, Natural and Artificial Flavors and other ingredients.

CONTRAINDICATIONS
Acute surgical abdomen.

WARNINGS
Do not use this product unless directed by a physician. Do not use when abdominal pain, nausea or vomiting is present, unless directed by a physician. As with any drug, if you are pregnant or nursing a baby, seek the advice of a health professional before using this product. In case of accidental overdose, seek professional assistance or contact a Poison Control Center immediately. Keep out of children's reach.

CAUTION
In diabetic patients, the physician should be aware of the sugar content of "Senna" X-PREP Liquid (50 grams per $2^1/_2$ fl. oz. dose).

ADMINISTRATION AND DOSAGE
Recommended Dosage (or as directed by physician):
Adults and children 12 years of age and older: Take one bottle between 2 and 4 p.m. on day prior to x-ray or other diagnostic procedures. Drink entire contents. For children under 12 years of age, consult a doctor. A strong bowel action can be expected approximately 6 hours after drinking. After "Senna" X-PREP Liquid is taken, diet should be confined to clear fluids.

HOW SUPPLIED
$2^1/_2$ fl. oz. bottles (alcohol 7% by volume), each providing a single, complete adult dose.
Also Available—Two X-PREP® Bowel Evacuant Kits.
Kit #1 contains: Two SENOKOT-S® Tablets (standardized senna concentrate and docusate sodium), one bottle of X-PREP Liquid $2^1/_2$ fl. oz., and one RECTOLAX® Suppository (bisacodyl 10 mg), plus easy-to-follow patient instructions for hydration, clear liquid diet, and the correct time-sequence for administering the above laxatives.
Kit #2 contains: One dose CITRALAX® Granules 1.06 oz. (effervescent citrate/sulfate of magnesia), one bottle of X-PREP Liquid $2^1/_2$ fl. oz., and one RECTOLAX Suppository (bisacodyl 10 mg), plus easy-to-follow patient instructions.
Copyright © 1991, 1996, Gray Pharmaceutical Co., Norwalk, CT 06850-3590.

Guardian Laboratories
a division of United-Guardian, Inc.
P.O. Box 18050
HAUPPAUGE, N.Y. 11788

For Medical Information Contact:
Director of Medical Research
(516) 273-0900
(800) 645-5566

CLORPACTIN® WCS-90   OTC
[klor-pak 'tin]
(brand of sodium oxychlorosene)

COMPOSITION
Stabilized organic derivative of hypochlorous acid. A white, water soluble powder with a characteristic smell of hypochlorous acid. Active chlorine derived from calcium hypochlorite: 3–4%.

ACTION AND USES
For use as a topical antiseptic for treating localized infections, particularly when resistant organisms are present. Complete spectrum (bacteria, fungi, viruses, mold, yeast and spores); effective in cases of antibiotic resistance; nontoxic and non-allergenic in use concentrations.

ADMINISTRATION AND DOSAGE
Applied by irrigation, instillations, spray, soaks or wet compresses, preferably thoroughly cleansing with gravity flow irrigation or syringe to provide copious quantities of fresh solution to remove the organic wastes and debris from the site of the involvement. Also for preoperative skin preparation and postoperative protection. Generally applied as the 0.4% solution in water, or isotonic saline, but as the 0.1% to 0.2% in Urology and Ophthalmology.

CONTRAINDICATIONS
The use of this product is contraindicated where the site of the infection is not exposed to the direct contact with the solution. Not for systemic use.

HOW SUPPLIED
In boxes containing 5 x 2 gram bottles.

RENACIDIN® (Citric Acid,   ℞
Glucono-delta-lactone, and Magnesium Carbonate)
Irrigation

DESCRIPTION
Renacidin® (Citric Acid, Glucono-delta-lactone, and Magnesium Carbonate) Irrigation is a sterile, non-pyrogenic irrigation for use within the urinary tract in the prevention and dissolution of calculi.
Each 100 ml. of Renacidin Irrigation contains:
Active ingredients:
Citric Acid (anhydrous), U.S.P.   6.602 grams
  $C_6H_8O_7$

Glucono-delta-lactone   0.198 grams
  $C_6H_{10}O_6$
Magnesium Carbonate, U.S.P.   3.177 grams
  $(MgCO_3)_4 \cdot Mg(OH)_2 \cdot 3H_2O$

Citric Acid	Glucono-delta-lactone
CH_2COOH	
$HOCCOOH$	
CH_2COOH	

Magnesium Carbonate
  $(MgCO_3)_4 \cdot Mg(OH)_2 \cdot 3H_2O$
Inert ingredients:
Benzoic Acid, U.S.P.   0.023 grams
Solution pH: 3.85 (3.50–4.20)

HOW SUPPLIED
Renacidin Irrigation is available as a sterile, non-pyrogenic solution in 500 ml containers, packaged in cartons of six. Exposure of Renacidin Irrigation to heat or cold should be minimized. Renacidin Irrigation should be stored at controlled room temperature, 59° to 86°F (15° to 30°C). Avoid excessive heat or cold (keep from freezing). Brief exposure to temperatures of up to 40°C or temperatures down to 5°C does not adversely affect the product.
NDC: 0327-0011-05
PRODUCT CODE: RN500

RENACIDIN® Powder   ℞
[ren "a-sē 'din]

Healthpoint Medical
2400 HANDLEY-EDERVILLE ROAD
FORT WORTH, TX 76118

Direct Inquiries to:
800-441-8227

ACCUZYME™   ℞
PAPAIN-UREA DEBRIDING OINTMENT

DESCRIPTION
Each gram of Accuzyme enzymatic debriding ointment contains papain (1.1×10^6 USP units of activity) and 100mg urea in a hydrophilic ointment base composed of purified water, emulsifying wax, glycerin, isopropyl palmitate, potassium phosphate monobasic, fragrance, methylparaben and propylparaben.

CLINICAL PHARMACOLOGY
Papain, the proteolytic enzyme from the fruit of carica papaya, is a potent digestant of nonviable protein matter but is harmless to viable tissue. It is active over a pH range of 3 to 12. Papain is relatively ineffective when used alone as a debriding agent and requires the presence of activators to stimulate its digestive potency. In Accuzyme, papain is combined with urea, a denaturant of proteins, to bring about two supplemental chemical actions: (1) to expose by solvent action the activators of papain, and (2) to denature the nonviable protein matter in lesions and thereby render it more susceptible to enzymatic digestion. Pharmacologic studies have shown that the combination of papain and urea result in twice as much digestive activity as papain alone.

INDICATIONS AND USAGE
Accuzyme is indicated for debridement of necrotic tissue and liquefaction of pus in acute and chronic lesions such as pressure ulcers, varicose and diabetic ulcers, burns, postoperative wounds, pilonidal cyst wounds, carbuncles and miscellaneous traumatic or infected wounds.

CONTRAINDICATIONS
Accuzyme is contraindicated in patients who have shown sensitivity to papain or any other components of this preparation.

PRECAUTIONS
See Dosage and Administration. Not to be used in eyes.

ADVERSE REACTIONS
Accuzyme is generally well-tolerated and non-irritating. A transient "burning" sensation may be experienced by a small percentage of patients upon applying Accuzyme. Occasionally, the profuse exudate from enzymatic digestion may irritate the skin. In such cases, more frequent dressing changes will alleviate discomfort until exudate decreases.

DOSAGE AND ADMINISTRATION

Cleanse the wound with Curasol™ Wound Cleanser or saline. Avoid cleansing with hydrogen peroxide solution as it may inactivate the papain. Apply Accuzyme directly to the wound, cover with appropriate dressing, secure into place and change once per day. Irrigate the wound at each redressing to remove any accumulation of liquefied necrotic material. NOTE: Papain may also be inactivated by the salts of heavy metals such as lead, silver and mercury. Contact with medications containing these metals should be avoided.

HOW SUPPLIED

30g tubes. Store in a cool place.
CAUTION: Federal law prohibits dispensing without prescription.
NDC–0064-1000-01
HEALTHPOINT®
Healthpoint Medical, San Antonio, Texas 78215
1-800-441-8227
REORDER NO. 1000-01   126959-1195
Shown in Product Identification Guide, page 316

Heel/BHI, Inc.
11600 COCHITI SE
ALBUQUERQUE, NM 87123

Direct Inquiries to:
Medical Department
800–621–7644
(505) 293–3843
Fax: (505) 275–1672

TRAUMEEL® Tablets   OTC
Anti-inflammatory/Analgesic

TRAUMEEL® Ointment   OTC
Anti-inflammatory/Analgesic

TRAUMEEL® Oral Drops   OTC
Anti-inflammatory/Analgesic

TRAUMEEL® Oral Liquid in Vials   OTC
Anti-inflammatory/Analgesic

TRAUMEEL® Injection Solution   ℞
Anti-inflammatory/Analgesic

DESCRIPTION

TRAUMEEL® Injection Solution is an anti-inflammatory, analgesic, anti-edematous, anti-exudative combination formulation of 12 botanical substances and 1 mineral substance.
TRAUMEEL® Injection Solution is officially classified as a homeopathic combination remedy (1).
1. Botanical ingredients:
   Arnica montana, radix (mountain arnica)
   Calendula officinalis (calendula)
   Hamamelis virginiana (witch hazel)
   Millefolium (milfoil)
   Belladonna (deadly nightshade)
   Aconitum napellus (monkshood)
   Chamomilla (chamomile)
   Symphytum officinale (comfrey)
   Bellis perennis (daisy)
   Echinacea angustifolia (narrow-leafed cone flower)
   Echinacea purpurea (purple cone flower)
   Hypericum perforatum (St John's wort)
2. Mineral ingredient:
   Hepar sulphuris calcareum (calcium sulfide)
Injection Solution: Each 2.0 ml ampule contains as active ingredients: Hepar sulphuris calcareum 8 X 200.0 μl; Belladonna 3 X 20.0 μl; Calendula officinalis 3 X 20.0 μl; Chamomilla 4 X 20.0 μl; Millefolium 4 X 20.0 μl; Aconitum napellus 3 X 12.0 μl; Bellis perennis 3 X 10.0 μl; Hypericum perforatum 3 X 6.0 μl; Echinacea angustifolia 3 X 5.0 μl; Echinacea purpurea 3 X 5.0 μl; Arnica montana, radix 2 X 2.0 μl; Hamamelis virginiana 2 X 2.0 μl; Symphytum officinale 6 X 2.0 μl. Each 2.0 ml ampule contains as inactive ingredients; Sterile isotonic sodium chloride solution.

CLINICAL PHARMACOLOGY

The exact mechanism of action of TRAUMEEL® Injection Solution is not fully understood. Various cellular and biochemical pathways appear to be modulated by the product ingredients. The mechanism of action of TRAUMEEL® Injection Solution does not appear to be the result of cyclooxygenase or lipoxygenase enzyme inhibition, as is the case with nonsteroidal anti-inflammatory drugs (NSAIDs). TRAUMEEL® Injection Solution does not inhibit the arachidonic acid pathway of prostaglandin synthesis. Instead, the mechanism of action of TRAUMEEL® Injection Solution appears to be the result of modulation of the release of oxygen radicals from activated neutrophils, and inhibition of release of inflammatory mediators (possibly interleukin 1 from activated macrophages) and neuropeptides (2).
In vitro studies show that the ingredients of TRAUMEEL® Injection Solution are noncytotoxic to granulocytes, lymphocytes, platelets and endothelia, which indicates that the defensive functions of these cells are preserved during treatment with TRAUMEEL® Injection Solution (3).
The anti-inflammatory, analgesic, anti-edematous and anti-exudative effects of TRAUMEEL® Injection Solution have been demonstrated in clinical trials as well as in a number of *in vivo* experimental models including the carrageenin-induced edema test and the adjuvant arthritis test (3).

INDICATIONS AND USAGE

TRAUMEEL® Injection Solution is indicated for the treatment of symptoms associated with inflammatory, exudative and degenerative processes due to acute trauma (such as contusions, lacerations, fractures, sprains, post-operative wounds, etc.), repetitive or overuse injuries (such as tendonitis, bursitis, epicondylitis, etc.), and for minor aches and pains associated with such conditions. TRAUMEEL® Injection Solution is also indicated for the treatment of minor aches and pains associated with backache, muscular aches and the minor pain from rheumatoid arthritis, osteoarthritis, gouty arthritis and ankylosing spondylitis.

CONTRAINDICATIONS

TRAUMEEL® Injection Solution is contraindicated in patients with a known hypersensitivity to TRAUMEEL® Injection Solution or any of its ingredients (see **ADVERSE REACTIONS**).

WARNINGS

TRAUMEEL® Injection Solution should not be administered for pain for more than 10 days for adults or 5 days for children. If pain persists or worsens, if new symptoms occur, or if redness or swelling is present, the patient should be carefully evaluated because these could be signs of a serious condition. TRAUMEEL® Injection Solution should not be administered to children for the pain of arthritis unless directed by a physician.

PRECAUTIONS

General:
Adverse effects with TRAUMEEL® Injection Solution are extremely rare. TRAUMEEL® Injection Solution exhibits no known adverse renal, hepatic, cardiovascular, gastrointestinal or central nervous system effects.
Information for Patients:
No harmful or potentially hazardous side effects such as central nervous system depression are known. TRAUMEEL® Injection Solution is generally well-tolerated.
Drug Interactions:
TRAUMEEL® Injection Solution is not known to interact with other medications. Furthermore, the administration of TRAUMEEL® Injection Solution can be safely augmented by the application of a topical dosage form of TRAUMEEL®.
Drug/Laboratory Test Interactions:
TRAUMEEL® Injection Solution is not known to interact with any laboratory tests.
Carcinogenesis:
No studies have been performed to evaluate the carcinogenicity of TRAUMEEL® Injection Solution. In world-wide post-marketing surveillance no evidence of carcinogenicity has been found (2).
Pregnancy:
Pregnancy Category C. In general, medications such as TRAUMEEL® Injection Solution that are classified as homeopathic are not known to cause direct or indirect harm to the fetus. However, animal reproduction studies have not been performed and there are no well-controlled studies in pregnant women. In cases of pregnancy or suspected pregnancy, TRAUMEEL® Injection Solution should be used only if potential benefits justify potential risks to the fetus.
Nursing Mothers:
It is not known whether any of the ingredients in TRAUMEEL® Injection Solution are excreted in human milk. However, because many drugs are excreted in human milk, TRAUMEEL® Injection Solution should be administered with caution to nursing mothers.
Pediatric Use:
TRAUMEEL® Injection Solution can be safely administered to children as young as 2 years (see **DOSAGE AND ADMINISTRATION**). A physician should be consulted before administering TRAUMEEL® Injection Solution to children below the age of 2 years.

ADVERSE REACTIONS

In rare cases, patients with hypersensitivity to botanicals of the Compositae family may experience an allergic reaction after administration of TRAUMEEL® Injection Solution, including anaphylactic reaction. TRAUMEEL® Injection Solution ingredients of the Compositae family are:
   Arnica montana, radix (mountain arnica)
   Calendula oifficinalis (calendula)
   Millefolium (milfoil)
   Chamomilla (chamomile)
   Bellis perennis (daisy)
   Echinacea angustifolia (narrow-leafed cone flower)
   Echinacea purpurea (purple cone flower)

OVERDOSAGE

Due to the low concentration of active ingredients in homeopathic preparations such as TRAUMEEL® Injection Solution, adverse reactions following overdosage are extremely unlikely. However, care must be taken not to exceed the recommended dosage.

DOSAGE AND ADMINISTRATION

The dosage schedules listed below can be used as a general guide for the administration of TRAUMEEL® Injection Solution. TRAUMEEL® Injection Solution shows individual differences in clinical response. Therefore, the dosage for each patient should be individualized according to the patient's response to therapy. For best results, treatment with TRAUMEEL® Injection Solution should be initiated immediately following injury or at the first sign of symptoms. TRAUMEEL® Injection Solution may be administered until symptoms disappear. However, if symptoms persist or worsen, a physician should be consulted (see **WARNINGS**).
TRAUMEEL® Injection Solution:
Adults: 1 ampule daily for acute disorders, or 1 or 2 ampules 1 to 3 times weekly.
Children (2 to 6 years): Half the adult dosage.
TRAUMEEL® Injection Solution may be administered either intravenously, intramuscularly, subcutaneously or intradermally. TRAUMEEL® Injection Solution is indicated for peri-articular administration. However, it is **NOT FOR INTRA-ARTICULAR USE. Note:** Parenteral drug products like TRAUMEEL® Injection Solution should be inspected visually for particulate matter and discoloration prior to administration whenever solution and container permit. Discolored solutions should be discarded.

HOW SUPPLIED

TRAUMEEL® Injection Solution in 2.0 ml ampules: Packs of 10: NDC 50114-7000-1.
Avoid freezing and excessive heat. Store at controlled room temperature between 15°C and 30°C (59°F and 86°F). Protect from light.

CAUTION:

Federal law prohibits dispensing without a prescription.

REFERENCES

(1) The Homeopathic Pharmacopoeia of the United Stated (HPUS), 8th edition, Falls Church, Virginia, 1979; and the Homeopathic Pharmacopoeia of the United States Revision Service (HPRS), 1988.
(2) Data on file, Heel GmbH, Baden-Baden, Germany.
(3) Conforti A, et al: In Vitro and In vivo Studies on the Anti-inflammatory Activity of Traumee S. Unpublished report on file, 1995. Heel GmbH, Baden-Baden, Germany.

High Chemical Co.
3901-A NEBRASKA ST.
LEVITTOWN, PA 19056

Direct Inquiries to:
800-447-8792

SARAPIN®   ℞

DESCRIPTION

A sterile aqueous solution of soluble salts of the volatile bases from Sarraceniaceae (Pitcher Plant). Benzyl Alcohol 0.75%.

ACTIONS

The painful syndromes most commonly encountered in general practice which are relieved by SARAPIN® treatment are as follows:
Sciatic Pain
Intercostal Neuralgia
Alcoholic Neuritis
Occipital Neuritis
Brachial Plexus Neuralgia
Meralgia Paresthetica
Lumbar Neuralgia
Trigeminal Neuralgia

ADMINISTRATION

These and allied conditions may be treated with success in a majority of cases by nerve block or local infiltration:

Continued on next page

High Chemical—Cont.

Paravertebral—Careful localization of the zone of tenderness permits a determination of the corresponding trunk levels to be injected.

Perineural—In some instances, as in sciatica, the affected nerve can be injected at a site distant from its origin.

Local Infiltration—Multiple injections throughout an area of tenderness provide for diffusion into all the affected parts.

DOSAGE

Paravertebral Injections

Cervical	2–3 ml
Dorsal	5–10 ml
Lumbar	5–10 ml
Sacral	3–5 ml
Caudal Canal	10 ml
Sciatic Nerve	10 ml
Local Infiltration	5–10 ml

WARNINGS

Withdraw plunger of syringe to make sure the needle point is not in a blood vessel.

PRECAUTIONS

Procedure should be gentle and unhurried.
SARAPIN® is intended only for professional use. Its successful employment depends upon a thorough knowledge of the anatomy involved.

ADVERSE REACTIONS

Patients should be maintained in a recumbent position for 10 to 15 minutes following injection. A local sensation is to be expected, limited to the distribution of the nerve injected, and usually appearing as a temporary feeling of heaviness, although some cases will feel heat or a transitory aggravation of symptoms.

CONTRAINDICATIONS

SARAPIN® is non-toxic, has no side effects other than above and is contraindicated only in areas of local inflammation.

HOW SUPPLIED

50 ml Multiple Dose Vial.
NDC-10541-492-50

CAUTION: Federal law prohibits dispensing without prescription.

HIGH CHEMICAL COMPANY
3901-A Nebraska Street
Levittown, PA 19056-3333
800-447-8792

Hill Dermaceuticals, Inc.
505 WEST ROBINSON STREET
ORLANDO, FL 32801

Direct Inquiries to:
Rosario G. Ramirez
(407) 896-8280
FAX: (407) 246-1520

DERMA-SMOOTHE/FS TOPICAL OIL   ℞
Fluocinolone acetonide, 0.01%, Topical Oil

FS SHAMPOO, 0.01%   ℞
Fluocinolone acetonide, 0.01%, Shampoo

HOECHST MARION ROUSSEL
10236 MARION PARK DRIVE
MAIL: P.O. BOX 9627
KANSAS CITY, MO 64134-0627

Direct Inquiries to:
Customer Information Center, Kl-M0928
P.O. Box 9627
Kansas City, MO 64134-0627
(800) 552-3656

For Medical Information Contact:
Generally:
Medical Informatics
P.O. Box 9627
Kansas City, MO 64134-0627
(800) 633-1610
After Hours and Weekend Emergencies:
(816) 966-5000

PRODUCT IDENTIFICATION
NUMERICAL SUMMARY
SOLID ORAL DOSAGE FORMS

Hoechst Marion Roussel
Kansas City, MO 64134
To provide quick and positive identification of Hoechst Marion Roussel prescription drug products, we have imprinted an identifying number and the name MARION on the following tablets or capsules.

1555   PAVABID® Capsules, 150 mg (papaverine hydrochloride)

1771   CARDIZEM® Tablets, 30 mg (diltiazem hydrochloride)

1772   CARDIZEM® Tablets, 60 mg (diltiazem hydrochloride)

ALTACE® (ramipril) Capsules 1.25 mg are imprinted with "ALTACE 1.25 MG" on one end and "HOECHST" on the other.
ALTACE® (ramipril) Capsules 2.5 mg are imprinted with "ALTACE 2.5 MG" on one end and "HOECHST" on the other.
ALTACE® (ramipril) Capsules 5 mg are imprinted with "ALTACE 5 MG" on one end and "HOECHST" on the other.
ALTACE® (ramipril) Capsules 10 mg are imprinted with "ALTACE 10 MG" on one end and "HOECHST" on the other.
AMARYL® (glimepiride) Tablets 1 mg, 2 mg, and 4 mg are imprinted with "AMARYL" on one side and the Hoechst logo on both sides of the bisect on the other side.
BENTYL® Capsules, 10 mg (dicyclomine hydrochloride USP) is imprinted BENTYL 10.
BENTYL® Tablets, 20 mg (dicyclomine hydrochloride USP) is debossed BENTYL 20.
BRICANYL® Tablets, 2.5 mg (terbutaline sulfate USP) is debossed BRICANYL 2$^{1}/_{2}$.
BRICANYL® Tablets, 5 mg (terbutaline sulfate USP) is debossed BRICANYL 5.
CANTIL® Tablets, 25 mg (mepenzolate bromide USP) is debossed MERRELL 37.
CARAFATE® Tablets, 1 g (sucralfate) is identified by the brand name CARAFATE embossed on one side and 1712 on the reverse side.
CARDIZEM® Tablets, 90 mg (diltiazem hydrochloride) is imprinted with the brand name CARDIZEM on one side and 90 mg on the reverse side.
CARDIZEM® Tablets, 120 mg (diltiazem hydrochloride) is imprinted with the brand name CARDIZEM on one side and 120 mg on the reverse side.
CARDIZEM® SR Capsules, 60 mg (diltiazem hydrochloride) is imprinted with the Cardizem logo on one end and Cardizem SR 60 mg on the other.
CARDIZEM® SR Capsules, 90 mg (diltiazem hydrochloride) is imprinted with the Cardizem logo on one end and Cardizem SR 90 mg on the other.
CARDIZEM® SR Capsules, 120 mg (diltiazem hydrochloride) is imprinted with the Cardizem logo on one end and Cardizem SR 120 mg on the other.
CARDIZEM® CD Capsules, 120 mg (diltiazem hydrochloride) is imprinted with the Marion Merrell Dow Inc. logo on one end and Cardizem CD and 120 mg on the other.
CARDIZEM® CD Capsules, 180 mg (diltiazem hydrochloride) is imprinted with the Marion Merrell Dow Inc. logo on one end and CARDIZEM CD and 180 mg on the other.
CARDIZEM® CD Capsules, 240 mg (diltiazem hydrochloride) is imprinted with the Marion Merrell Dow Inc. logo on one end and CARDIZEM CD and 240 mg on the other.
CARDIZEM® CD Capsules, 300 mg (diltiazem hydrochloride) is imprinted with the Marion Merrell Dow Inc. logo on one end and CARDIZEM CD and 300 mg on the other.
CLOMID® Tablets, 50 mg (clomiphene citrate) is debossed CLOMID 50.
DIAβETA® (glyburide) Tablets 1.25 mg, 2.5 mg, and 5 mg are monogrammed "Diaβ".
DITROPAN® (oxybutynin chloride) Tablets are engraved with DITROPAN on one side and 13 and 75, separated by a horizontal score, on the other side.
HIPREX® Tablets, 1 g (methenamine hippurate) is debossed MERRELL 277.
LASIX® (furosemide) Tablets 20 mg are imprinted with "Lasix® " on one side and "HOECHST" on the other.
LASIX® (furosemide) Tablets 40 mg are imprinted with "Lasix® 40" on one side and the Hoechst logo on the other.

LASIX® (furosemide) Tablets 80 mg are imprinted with "Lasix® 80" on one side and the Hoechst logo on the other.
NORPRAMIN® Tablets, 10 mg (desipramine hydrochloride USP) is imprinted 68-7.
NORPRAMIN® Tablets, 25 mg (desipramine hydrochloride USP) is imprinted NORPRAMIN 25.
NORPRAMIN® Tablets, 50 mg (desipramine hydrochloride USP) is imprinted NORPRAMIN 50.
NORPRAMIN® Tablets, 75 mg (desipramine hydrochloride USP) is imprinted NORPRAMIN 75.
NORPRAMIN® Tablets, 100 mg (desipramine hydrochloride USP) is imprinted NORPRAMIN 100.
NORPRAMIN® Tablets, 150 mg (desipramine hydrochloride USP) is imprinted NORPRAMIN 150.
NOVAFED® A Capsules, 120 mg pseudoephedrine hydrochloride and 8 mg chlorpheniramine maleate is imprinted NOVAFED A.
RIFADIN® Capsules, 150 mg (rifampin) is imprinted RIFADIN 150.
RIFADIN® Capsules, 300 mg (rifampin) is imprinted RIFADIN 300.
RIFAMATE® Capsules, 300 mg rifampin and 150 mg isoniazid is imprinted RIFAMATE.
RIFATER® Tablets, 120 mg rifampin, 50 mg isoniazid, and 300 mg pyrazinamide is imprinted RIFATER.
SELDANE® Tablets, 60 mg (terfenadine) is debossed SELDANE.
SELDANE-D® Tablets, 60 mg terfenadine and 120 mg pseudoephedrine hydrochloride is debossed SELDANE-D.
TACE® Capsules, 12 mg (chlorotrianisene USP) is imprinted MERRELL 690.
TENUATE® Tablets, 25 mg (diethylpropion hydrochloride USP) is debossed TENUATE 25.
TENUATE® DOSPAN® Controlled-Release Tablets, 75 mg (diethylpropion hydrochloride USP) is debossed TENUATE 75.
TRENTAL® (pentoxifylline) Tablets are imprinted "TRENTAL".

ALTACE®   ℞
[ôl'tās]
(ramipril)*

> **USE IN PREGNANCY**
> When used in pregnancy during the second and third trimesters, ACE Inhibitors can cause injury and even death to the developing fetus. When pregnancy is detected, ALTACE® should be discontinued as soon as possible. See WARNINGS: Fetal/neonatal morbidity and mortality.

DESCRIPTION

Ramipril is a 2-aza-bicyclo [3.3.0]-octane-3-carboxylic acid derivative. It is a white, crystalline substance soluble in polar organic solvents and buffered aqueous solutions. Ramipril melts between 105° C and 112° C.
The CAS Registry Number is 87333-19-5. Ramipril's chemical name is (2*S*,3a*S*,6a*S*)-1-[(*S*)-*N*-[(*S*)-1-Carboxy-3-phenylpropyl]alanyl]octahydrocyclopenta[*b*]pyrrole-2-carboxylic acid, 1-ethyl ester, its structural formula is:

Its empiric formula is $C_{23}H_{32}N_2O_5$, and its molecular weight is 416.5.
Ramiprilat, the diacid metabolite of ramipril, is a non-sulfhydryl angiotensin converting enzyme inhibitor. Ramipril is converted to ramiprilat by hepatic cleavage of the ester group.
ALTACE® (ramipril) is supplied as hard shell capsules for oral administration containing 1.25 mg, 2.5 mg, 5 mg, and 10 mg of ramipril. The inactive ingredients present are pregelatinized starch NF, gelatin, and titanium dioxide. The 1.25 mg capsule shell contains yellow iron oxide, the 2.5 mg capsule shell contains D&C yellow #10 and FD&C red #40, the 5 mg capsule shell contains FD&C blue #1 and FD&C red #40, and the 10 mg capsule shell contains FD&C blue #1.

CLINICAL PHARMACOLOGY

Mechanism of Action

Ramipril and ramiprilat inhibit angiotensin-converting enzyme (ACE) in human subjects and animals. ACE is a peptidyl dipeptidase that catalyzes the conversion of angiotensin I to the vasoconstrictor substance, angiotensin II. Angiotensin II also stimulates aldosterone secretion by the adrenal cortex. Inhibition of ACE results in decreased plasma angiotensin II, which leads to decreased vasopressor activity and to decreased aldosterone secretion. The latter decrease may result in a small increase of serum potassium. In hypertensive patients with normal renal function treated with ALTACE® alone for up to 56 weeks, approximately 4% of patients during the trial had an abnormally high serum potassium and an increase from baseline greater than 0.75 mEq/L, and none of the patients had an abnormally low potassium and a decrease from baseline greater than 0.75 mEq/L. In the same study, approximately 2% of patients treated with ALTACE® and hydrochlorothiazide for up to 56 weeks had abnormally high potassium values and an increase from baseline of 0.75 mEq/L or greater, and approximately 2% had abnormally low values and decreases from baseline of 0.75 mEq/L or greater. (See PRECAUTIONS.)

Removal of angiotensin II negative feedback on renin secretion leads to increased plasma renin activity.

The effect of ramipril on hypertension appears to result at least in part from inhibition of both issue and circulating ACE activity, thereby reducing antiotensin II formation in tissue and plasma.

ACE is identical to kininase, an enzyme that degrades bradykinin. Whether increased levels of bradykinin, a potent vasodepressor peptide, play a role in the therapeutic effects of ALTACE® remains to be elucidated.

While the mechanism through which ALTACE® lowers blood pressure is believed to be primarily suppression of the renin-angiotensin-aldosterone system, ALTACE® has an antihypertensive effect even in patients with low-renin hypertension. Although ALTACE® was antihypertensive in all races studied, black hypertensive patients (usually a low-renin hypertensive population) had a smaller average response to monotherapy than non-black patients.

Pharmacokinetics and Metabolism

Following oral administration of ALTACE®, peak plasma concentrations of ramipril are reached within one hour. The extent of absorption is at least 50–60% and is not significantly influenced by the presence of food in the GI tract, although the rate of absorption is reduced.

In a trial in which subjects received ALTACE® capsules or the contents of identical capsules dissolved in water, dissolved in apple juice, or suspended in apple sauce, serum ramiprilat levels were essentially unrelated to the use or nonuse of the concomitant liquid or food.

Cleavage of the ester group (primarily in the liver) converts ramipril to its active diacid metabolite, ramiprilat. Peak plasma concentrations of ramiprilat are reached 2–4 hours after drug intake. The serum protein binding of ramipril is about 73% and that of ramiprilat about 56%; *in vitro*, these percentages are independent of concentration over the range of 0.01 to 10μg/mL.

Ramipril is almost completely metabolized to ramiprilat, which has about 6 times the ACE inhibitory activity of ramipril, and to the diketopiperazine ester, the diketopiperazine acid, and the glucuronides of ramipril and ramiprilat, all of which are inactive. After oral administration of ramipril, about 60% of the parent drug and its metabolites are eliminated in the urine, and about 40% is found in the feces. Drug recovered in the feces may represent both biliary excretion of metabolites and/or unabsorbed drug, however the proportion of a dose eliminated by the bile has not been determined. Less than 2% of the administered dose is recovered in urine as unchanged ramipril.

Blood concentrations of ramipril and ramiprilat increase with increased dose, but are not strictly dose-proportional. The 24-hour AUC for ramiprilat, however, is dose-proportional over the 2.5–20 mg dose range. The absolute bioavailabilities of ramipril and ramiprilat were 28% and 44%, respectively, when 5 mg of oral ramipril was compared with the same dose of ramipril given intravenously.

Plasma concentrations of ramiprilat decline in a triphasic manner (initial rapid decline, apparent elimination phase, terminal elimination phase). The initial rapid decline, which represents distribution of the drug into a large peripheral compartment and subsequent binding to both plasma and tissue ACE, has a half-life of 2–4 hours. Because of its potent binding to ACE and slow dissociation from the enzyme, ramiprilat shows two elimination phases. The apparent elimination phase corresponds to the clearance of free ramiprilat and has a half-life of 9–18 hours. The terminal elimination phase has a prolonged half-life (>50 hours) and probably represents the binding/dissociation kinetics of the ramiprilat/ACE complex. It does not contribute to the accumulation of the drug. After multiple daily doses of ramipril 5–10 mg, the half-life of ramiprilat concentrations within the therapeutic range was 13–17 hours.

After once-daily dosing, steady-state plasma concentrations of ramiprilat are reached by the fourth dose. Steady-state concentrations of ramiprilat are somewhat higher than those seen after the first dose of ALTACE®, especially at low doses (2.5 mg), but the difference is clinically insignificant.

In patients with creatinine clearance less than 40 ml/min/1.73m², peak levels of ramiprilat are approximately doubled, and trough levels may be as much as quintupled. In multiple-dose regimens, the total exposure to ramiprilat (AUC) in these patients is 3–4 times as large as it is in patients with normal renal function who receive similar doses.

The urinary excretion of ramipril, ramiprilat, and their metabolites is reduced in patients with impaired renal function. Compared to normal subjects, patients with creatinine clearance less than 40 ml/min/1.73m² had higher peak and trough ramiprilat levels and slightly longer times to peak concentrations. (See DOSAGE AND ADMINISTRATION.)

In patients with impaired liver function, the metabolism of ramipril to ramiprilat appears to be slowed, possibly because of diminished activity of hepatic esterases, and plasma ramipril levels in these patients are increased about 3-fold. Peak concentrations of ramiprilat in these patients, however, are not different from those seen in subjects with normal hepatic function, and the effect of a given dose of plasma ACE activity does not vary with hepatic function.

Pharmacodynamics

Single doses of ramipril of 2.5–20 mg produce approximately 60–80% inhibition of ACE activity 4 hours after dosing with approximately 40–60% inhibition after 24 hours. Multiple oral doses of ramipril of 2.0 mg or more cause plasma ACE activity to fall by more than 90% 4 hours after dosing, with over 80% inhibition of ACE activity remaining 24 hours after dosing. The more prolonged effect of even small multiple doses presumably reflects saturation of ACE binding sites by ramiprilat and relatively slow release from those sites.

Pharmacodynamics and Clinical Effects

Hypertension

Administration of ALTACE® to patients with mild to moderate hypertension results in a reduction of both supine and standing blood pressure to about the same extent with no compensatory tachycardia. Symptomatic postural hypotension is infrequent, although it can occur in patients who are salt- and/or volume-depleted. (See WARNINGS.) Use of ALTACE® in combination with thiazide diuretics gives a blood pressure lowering effect greater than that seen with either agent alone.

In single-dose studies, doses of 5–20 mg of ALTACE® lowered blood pressure within 1–2 hours, with peak reductions achieved 3–6 hours after dosing. The antihypertensive effect of a single dose persisted for 24 hours. In longer term (4–12 weeks) controlled studies, once-daily doses of 2.5–10 mg were similar in their effect, lowering supine or standing systolic and diastolic blood pressures 24 hours after dosing by about 6/4 mm Hg more than placebo. In comparisons of peak vs. trough effect, the trough effect represented about 50–60% of the peak response. In a titration study comparing divided (bid) vs. qd treatment, the divided regimen was superior, indicating that for some patients the antihypertensive effect with once-daily dosing is not adequately maintained. (See DOSAGE AND ADMINISTRATION).

In most trials, the antihypertensive effect of ALTACE® increased during the first several weeks of repeated measurements. The antihypertensive effect of ALTACE® has been shown to continue during long-term therapy for at least 2 years. Abrupt withdrawal of ALTACE® has not resulted in a rapid increase in blood pressure.

ALTACE® has been compared with other ACE inhibitors, beta-blockers, and thiazide diuretics. It was approximately as effective as other ACE inhibitors and as atenolol. In both caucasians and blacks, hydrochlorothiazide (25 or 50 mg) was significantly more effective than ramipril.

Except for thiazides, no formal interaction studies of ramipril with other antihypertensive agents have been carried out. Limited experience in controlled and uncontrolled trials combining ramipril with a calcium channel blocker, a loop diuretic, or triple therapy (beta-blocker, vasodilator, and a diuretic) indicate no unusual drug-drug interactions. Other ACE inhibitors have had less than additive effects with beta adrenergic blockers, presumably because both drugs lower blood pressure by inhibiting parts of the renin-angiotensin system.

ALTACE® was less effective in blacks than in caucasians. The effectiveness of ALTACE® was not influenced by age, sex, or weight.

In a baseline controlled study of 10 patients with mild essential hypertension, blood pressure reduction was accompanied by a 15% increase in renal blood flow. In healthy volunteers, glomerular filtration rate was unchanged.

Heart Failure post myocardial infarction

ALTACE® was studied in the Acute Infarction Ramipril Efficacy (AIRE) trial. This was a multinational (mainly European) 161-center, 2006-patient, double-blind, randomized, parallel-group study comparing ALTACE® to placebo in stable patients, 2-9 days after an acute myocardial infarction (MI), who had shown clinical signs of congestive heart failure (CHF) at any time after the MI. Patients in severe (NYHA class IV) heart failure, patients with unstable angina, patients with heart failure of congenital or valvular etiology, and patients with contraindications to ACE inhibitors were all excluded. The majority of patients had received thrombolytic therapy at the time of the index infarction, and the average time between infarction and initiation of treatment was 5 days.

Patients randomized to ramipril treatment were given an initial dose of 2.5 mg twice daily. If the initial regimen caused undue hypotension, the dose was reduced to 1.25 mg, but in either event doses were titrated upward (as tolerated) to a target regimen (achieved in 77% of patients randomized to ramipril) of 5 mg twice daily. Patients were then followed for an average of 15 months (range 6–46).

The use of ALTACE® was associated with a 27% reduction ($p=0.002$), in the risk of death from any cause; about 90% of the deaths that occurred were cardiovascular, mainly sudden death. The risks of progression to severe heart failure and of CHF-related hospitalization were also reduced, by 23% ($p=0.017$) and 26% ($p=0.011$), respectively. The benefits of ALTACE® therapy were seen in both genders, and they were not affected by the exact timing of the initiation of therapy, but older patients may have had a greater benefit than those under 65. The benefits were seen in patients on, and not on, various concomitant medications; at the time of randomization these included aspirin (about 80% of patients), diuretics (about 60%), organic nitrates (about 55%), beta-blockers (about 20%), calcium channel blockers (about 15%), and digoxin (about 12%).

INDICATIONS AND USAGE

Hypertension

ALTACE® is indicated for the treatment of hypertension. It may be used alone or in combination with thiazide diuretics.

In using ALTACE®, consideration should be given to the fact that another angiotensin converting enzyme inhibitor, captopril, has caused agranulocytosis, particularly in patients with renal impairment or collagen-vascular disease. Available data are insufficient to show that ALTACE® does not have a similar risk. (See WARNINGS.)

In considering use of ALTACE®, it should be noted that in controlled trials ACE inhibitors have an effect on blood pressure that is less in black patients than in non-blacks. In addition, ACE inhibitors (for which adequate data are available) cause a higher rate of angioedema in black than in non-black patients. (See WARNINGS, Angioedema.)

Heart Failure post myocardial infarction

Ramipril is indicated in stable patients who have demonstrated clinical signs of congestive heart failure within the first few days after sustaining acute myocardial infarction. Administration of ramipril to such patients has been shown to decrease the risk of death (principally cardiovascular death) and to decrease the risks of failure-related hospitalization and progression to severe/resistant heart failure. (See CLINICAL PHARMACOLOGY, Heart Failure post myocardial infarction for details and limitations of the survival trial.)

CONTRAINDICATIONS

ALTACE® is contraindicated in patients who are hypersensitive to this product and in patients with a history of angioedema related to previous treatment with an angiotensin converting enzyme inhibitor.

WARNINGS

Anaphylactoid and Possibly Related Reactions

Presumably because angiotensin-converting enzyme inhibitors affect the metabolism of eicosanoids and polypeptides, including endogenous bradykinin, patients receiving ACE inhibitors (including ALTACE®) may be subject to a variety of adverse reactions, some of them serious.

Angioedema

Patients with a history of angioedema unrelated to ACE inhibitor therapy may be at increased risk of angioedema while receiving an ACE inhibitor. (See also CONTRAINDICATIONS.)

Angioedema of the face, extremeties, lips, tongue, glottis, and larynx has been reported in patients treated with angiotensin converting enzyme inhibitors. Angioedema associated with laryngeal edema can be fatal. If laryngeal stridor or angioedema of the face, tongue, or glottis occurs, treatment with ALTACE® should be discontinued and appropriate therapy instituted immediately. Where there is involvement of the tongue, glottis, or larynx, likely to cause airway obstruction, appropriate therapy, e.g., subcutaneous epinephrine solution 1:1,000 (0.3 ml to 0.5 ml) should be promptly administered. (See ADVERSE REACTIONS.)

In a large U.S. postmarketing study, angioedema (defined as reports of angio, face, larynx, tongue, or throat edema) was reported in 3/1523 (0.20%) of black patients and in 8/8680 (0.09%) of white patients. These rates were not different statistically. Anaphylactoid reactions during desensitization: Two patients undergoing desensitizing treatment with hymenoptera venom while receiving ACE inhibitors sus-

Continued on next page

Hoechst Marion Roussel—Cont.

tained life-threatening anaphylactoid reactions. In the same patients, these reactions were avoided when ACE inhibitors were temporarily withheld, but they reappeared upon inadvertent rechallenge.

Anaphylactoid reactions during membrane exposure: Anaphylactoid reactions have been reported in patients dialyzed with high-flux membranes and treated concomitantly with an ACE inhibitor. Anaphylactoid reactions have also been reported in patients undergoing low-density lipoprotein apheresis with dextran sulfate absorption (a procedure dependent upon devises not approved in the United States).

Hypotension

ALTACE® can cause symptomatic hypotension, after either the initial dose or a later dose when the dosage has been increased. Like other ACE inhibitors, ramipril has been only rarely associated with hypotension in uncomplicated hypertensive patients. Symptomatic hypotension is most likely to occur in patients who have been volume- and/or salt-depleted as a result of prolonged diuretic therapy, dietary salt restriction, dialysis, diarrhea, or vomiting. Volume and/or salt depletion should be corrected before initiating therapy with ALTACE®.

In patients with congestive heart failure, with or without associated renal insufficiency, ACE inhibitor therapy may cause excessive hypotension, which may be associated with oliguria or azotemia and, rarely, with acute renal failure and death. In such patients, ALTACE® therapy should be started under close medical supervision; they should be followed closely for the first 2 weeks of treatment and whenever the dose of ramipril or diuretic is increased.

If hypotension occurs, the patient should be placed in a supine position and, if necessary, treated with intravenous infusion of physiological saline. ALTACE® treatment usually can be continued following restoration of blood pressure and volume.

Hepatic Failure

Rarely, ACE inhibitors have been associated with a syndrome that starts with cholestatic jaundice and progresses to fulminant hepatic necrosis and (sometimes) death. The mechanism of this syndrome is not understood. Patients receiving ACE inhibitors who develop jaundice or marked elevations of hepatic enzymes should discontinue the ACE inhibitor and receive appropriate medical follow-up.

Neutropenia/Agranulocytosis

Another angiotensin converting enzyme inhibitor, captopril, has been shown to cause agranulocytosis and bone marrow depression, rarely in uncomplicated patients, but more frequently in patients with renal impairment, especially if they also have a collagen-vascular disease such as systemic lupus erythematosus or scleroderma. Available data from clinical trials of ramipril are insufficient to show that ramipril does not cause agranulocytosis at similar rates. Monitoring of white blood cell counts should be considered in patients with collagen-vascular disease, especially if the disease is associated with impaired renal function.

Fetal/neonatal morbidity and mortality

ACE inhibitors can cause fetal and neonatal morbidity and death when administered to pregnant women. Several dozen cases have been reported in the world literature. When pregnancy is detected, ACE inhibitors should be discontinued as soon as possible.

The use of ACE inhibitors during the second and third trimesters of pregnancy has been associated with fetal and neonatal injury, including hypotension, neonatal skull hypoplasia, anuria, reversible or irreversible renal failure, and death. Oligohydramnios has also been reported, presumably resulting from decreased fetal renal function; oligohydramnios in this setting has been associated with fetal limb contractures, craniofacial deformation, and hypoplastic lung development. Prematurity, intrauterine growth retardation, and patent ductus arteriosus have also been reported, although it is not clear whether these occurrences were due to the ACE inhibitor exposure.

These adverse effects do not appear to have resulted from intrauterine ACE inhibitor exposure that has been limited to the first trimester. Mothers whose embryos and fetuses are exposed to ACE inhibitors only during the first trimester should be so informed. Nonetheless, when patients become pregnant, physicians should make every effort to discontinue the use of ALTACE® as soon as possible. Rarely (probably less often than once in every thousand pregnancies), no alternative to ACE inhibitors will be found. In these rare cases, the mothers should be apprised of the potential hazards to their fetuses, and serial ultrasound examinations should be performed to assess the intraamniotic environment.

If oligohydramnios is observed, ALTACE® should be discontinued unless it is considered life-saving for the mother. Contraction stress testing (CST), a nonstress test (NST), or biophysical profiling (BPP) may be appropriate, depending upon the week of pregnancy. Patients and physicians should

be aware, however, that oligohydramnios may not appear until after the fetus has sustained irreversible injury.

Infants with histories of *in utero* exposure to ACE inhibitors should be closely observed for hypotension, oliguria, and hyperkalemia. If oliguria occurs, attention should be directed toward support of blood pressure and renal perfusion. Exchange transfusion or dialysis may be required as means of reversing hypotension and/or substituting for disordered renal function. ALTACE® which crosses the placenta can be removed from the neonatal circulation by these means, but limited experience has not shown that such removal is central to the treatment of these infants.

No teratogenic effects of ALTACE® were seen in studies of pregnant rats, rabbits, and cynomolgus monkeys. On a body surface area basis, the doses used were up to approximately 400 times (in rats and monkeys) and 2 times (in rabbits) the recommended human dose.

PRECAUTIONS

Impaired Renal Function: As a consequence of inhibiting the renin-angiotensin-aldosterone system, changes in renal function may be anticipated in susceptible individuals. In patients with severe congestive heart failure whose renal function may depend on the activity of the renin-angiotensin-aldosterone system, treatment with angiotensin converting enzyme inhibitors, including ALTACE®, may be associated with oliguria and/or progressive azotemia and (rarely) with acute renal failure and/or death.

In hypertensive patients with unilateral or bilateral renal artery stenosis, increases in blood urea nitrogen and serum creatinine may occur. Experience with another angiotensin converting enzyme inhibitor suggests that these increases are usually reversible upon discontinuation of ALTACE® and/or diuretic therapy. In such patients renal function should be monitored during the first few weeks of therapy. Some hypertensive patients with no apparent pre-existing renal vascular disease have developed increases in blood urea nitrogen and serum creatinine, usually minor and transient, especially when ALTACE® has been given concomitantly with a diuretic. This is more likely to occur in patients with pre-existing renal impairment. Dosage reduction of ALTACE® and/or discontinuation of the diuretic may be required.

Evaluation of the hypertensive patient should always include assessment of renal function. (See DOSAGE AND ADMINISTRATION.)

Hyperkalemia: In clinical trials, hyperkalemia (serum potassium greater than 5.7 mEq/L) occurred in approximately 1% of hypertensive patients receiving ALTACE® (ramipril). In most cases, these were isolated values, which resolved despite continued therapy. None of these patients was discontinued from the trials because of hyperkalemia. Risk factors for the development of hyperkalemia include renal insufficiency, diabetes mellitus, and the concomitant use of potassium-sparing diuretics, potassium supplements, and/or potassium-containing salt substitutes which should be used cautiously, if at all, with ALTACE®. (See DRUG INTERACTIONS.)

Cough: Presumably due to the inhibition of the degradation of endogenous bradykinin, persistent nonproductive cough has been reported with all ACE inhibitors, always resolving after discontinuation of therapy. ACE inhibitor-induced cough should be considered in the differential diagnosis of cough.

Impaired Liver Function: Since ramipril is primarily metabolized by hepatic esterases to its active moiety, ramiprilat, patients with impaired liver function could develop markedly elevated plasma levels of ramipril. No formal pharmacokinetic studies have been carried out in hypertensive patients with impaired liver function.

Surgery/Anesthesia: In patients undergoing surgery or during anesthesia with agents that produce hypotension, ramipril may block angiotensin. If formation that would otherwise occur secondary to compensatory renin release. Hypotension that occurs as a result of this mechanism can be corrected by volume expansion.

Information for Patients

Pregnancy: Female patients of childbearing age should be told about the consequences of second- and third-trimester exposure to ACE inhibitors, and they should also be told that these consequences do not appear to have resulted from intrauterine ACE inhibitor exposure that has been limited to the first trimester. These patients should be asked to report pregnancies to their physicians as soon as possible.

Angioedema: Angioedema, including laryngeal edema, can occur with treatment with ACE inhibitors, especially following the first dose. Patients should be so advised and told to report immediately any signs or symptoms suggesting angioedema (swelling of face, eyes, lips, or tongue, or difficulty in breathing) and to take no more drug until they have consulted with the prescribing physician.

Symptomatic Hypotension: Patients should be cautioned that lightheadedness can occur, especially during the first days of therapy, and it should be reported. Patients should be told that if syncope occurs, ALTACE® should be discontinued until the physician has been consulted.

All patients should be cautioned that inadequate fluid intake or excessive perspiration, diarrhea, or vomiting can lead to an excessive fall in blood pressure, with the same consequences of lightheadedness and possible syncope.

Hyperkalemia: Patients should be told not to use salt substitutes containing potassium without consulting their physician.

Neutropenia: Patients should be told to promply report any indication of infection (e.g., sore throat, fever), which could be a sign of neutropenia.

Drug Interactions

With diuretics: Patients on diuretics, especially those in whom diuretic therapy was recently instituted, may occasionally experience an excessive reduction of blood pressure after initiation of therapy with ALTACE®. The possibility of hypotensive effects with ALTACE® can be minimized by either discontinuing the diuretic or increasing the salt intake prior to initiation of treatment with ALTACE®. If this is not possible, the starting dose should be reduced. (See DOSAGE AND ADMINISTRATION.)

With potassium supplements and potassium-sparing diuretics: ALTACE® can attenuate potassium loss caused by thiazide diuretics. Potassium-sparing diuretics (spironolactone, amiloride, triamterene, and others) or potassium supplements can increase the risk of hyperkalemia. Therefore, if concomitant use of such agents is indicated, they should be given with caution, and the patient's serum potassium should be monitored frequently.

With lithium: Increased serum lithium levels and symptoms of lithium toxicity have been reported in patients receiving ACE inhibitors during therapy with lithium. These drugs should be coadministred with caution, and frequent monitoring of serum lithium levels is recommended. If a diuretic is also used, the risk of lithium toxicity may be increased.

Other: Neither ALTACE® nor its metabolites have been found to interact with food, digoxin, antacid, furosemide, cimetidine, indomethacin, and simvastatin. The combination of ALTACE® and propranolol showed no adverse effects on dynamic parameters (blood pressure and heart rate). The co-administration of ALTACE® and warfarin did not adversely affect the anticoagulant effects of the latter drug. Additionally, co-administration of ALTACE® with phenprocoumon did not affect minimum phenprocoumon levels or interfere with the subjects' state of anti-coagulation.

Carcinogenesis, Mutagenesis, Impairment of Fertility

No evidence of a tumorigenic effect was found when ramipril was given by gavage to rats for up to 24 months at doses of up to 500 mg/kg/day or to mice for up to 18 months at doses of up to 1000 mg/kg/day. (For either species, these doses are about 200 times the maximum recommended human dose when compared on the basis of body surface area.) No mutagenic activity was detected in the Ames test in bacteria, the micronucleus test in mice, unscheduled DNA synthesis in a hyman cell line, or a forward gene-mutation assay in a Chinese hamster ovary cell line. Several metabolites and degradation products of ramipril were also negative in the Ames test. A study in rats with dosages as great as 500 mg/kg/day did not produce adverse effects on fertility.

Pregnancy

Pregnancy Category C (first trimester) and D (second and third trimesters). See WARNINGS: Fetal/neonatal morbidity and mortality.

Nursing Mothers

Ingestion of single 10 mg oral dose of ALTACE® resulted in undetectable amounts of ramipril and its metabolites in breast milk. However, because multiple doses may produce low mild concentrations that are not predictable from single doses, women receiving ALTACE® should not breast feed.

Geriatric Use

Of the total number of patients who received ramipril in US clinical studies of ALTACE® 11.0% were 65 and over while 0.2% were 75 and over. No overall differences in effectiveness or safety were observed between these patients and younger patients, and other reported clinical experience has not identified differences in responses between the elderly and younger patients, but greater sensitivity of some older individuals cannot be ruled out.

One pharmacokinetic study conducted in hospitalized elderly patients indicated that peak ramiprilat levels and area under the plasma concentration time curve (AUC) for ramiprilat are higher in older patients.

Pediatric Use

Safety and effectiveness in pediatric patients have not been established.

ADVERSE REACTIONS

Hypertension

ALTACE® has been evaluated for safety in over 4,000 patients with hypertension; of these, 1,230 patients were studied in US controlled trials, and 1,107 were studied in foreign controlled trials. Almost 700 of these patients were treated for at least one year. The overall incidence of reported adverse events was similar in ALTACE® and placebo patients. The most frequent clinical side effects (possibly or probably related to study drug) reported by patients receiving

ALTACE® in US placebo-controlled trials were: headache (5.4%), "dizziness" (2.2%) and fatigue or asthenia (2.0%), but only the last was more common in ALTACE® patients than in patients given placebo. Generally, the side effects were mild and transient, and there was no relation to total dosage within the range of 1.25 to 20 mg. Discontinuation of therapy because of a side effect was required in approximately 3% of US patients treated with ALTACE®. The most common reasons for discontinuation were: cough (1.0%), "dizziness" (0.5%), and impotence (0.4%).

The side effects considered possibly or probably related to study drug that occurred in US placebo-controlled trials in more than 1% of patients treated with ALTACE® are shown below.

PATIENTS IN US PLACEBO CONTROLLED STUDIES

	Altace® (N=651) n	%	Placebo (N=286) n	%
Headache	35	5.4	17	5.9
"Dizziness"	14	2.2	9	3.1
Asthenia (Fatigue)	13	2.0	2	0.7
Nausea/Vomiting	7	1.1	3	1.0

In placebo-controlled trials, there was also an excess of upper respiratory infection and flu symptoms in the ramipril group. As these studies were carried out before the relationship of cough to ACE inhibitors was recognized, some of these events may represent ramipril-induced cough. In a later 1-year study, increased cough was seen in almost 12% of ramipril patients, with about 4% of these patients requiring discontinuation of treatment.

Heart Failure post myocardial infarction

Adverse reactions (except laboratory abnormalities) considered possibly/probably related to study drug that occurred in more than one percent of patients with heart failure treated with ALTACE® are shown below. The incidences represent the experiences from the AIRE study. The follow-up time was between 6 and 46 months for this study.

Percentage of Patients with Adverse Events Possibly/Probably Related to Study Drug

Placebo-Controlled (AIRE) Mortality Study

Adverse Event	Ramipril (N=1004)	Placebo (N=982)
Hypotension	10.7	4.7
Cough Increased	7.6	3.7
Dizziness	4.1	3.2
Angina Pectoris	2.9	2.0
Nausea	2.2	1.4
Postural Hypotension	2.2	1.4
Syncope	2.1	1.4
Heart Failure	2.0	2.2
Severe/Resistance Heart Failure	2.0	3.0
Myocardial Infarct	1.7	1.7
Vomiting	1.6	0.5
Vertigo	1.5	0.7
Headache	1.2	0.8
Kidney Function	1.2	0.5
Abnormal Chest Pain	1.1	0.9
Diarrhea	1.1	0.4
Asthenia	0.3	0.8

Other adverse experiences reported in controlled clinical trials (in less than 1% of ramipril patients), or rarer events seen in postmarketing experience, include the following (in some, a causal relationship to drug use is uncertain):

Body As a Whole: Anaphylactoid reactions. (See WARNINGS.)

Cardiovascular: Symptomatic hypotension (reported in 0.5% of patients in US trials) (See WARNINGS and PRECAUTIONS), syncope (not reported in US trials), angina pectoris, arrhythmia, chest pain, palpitations, myocardial infarction, and cerebrovascular events.

Hematologic: Pancytopenia, hemolytic anemia and thrombocytopenia.

Renal: Some hypertensive patients with no apparent preexisting renal disease have developed minor, usually transient, increases in blood urea nitrogen and serum creatinine when taking ALTACE®, particularly when ALTACE® was given concomitantly with a diuretic. (See WARNINGS.)

Angioneurotic Edema: Angioneurotic edema has been reported in 0.3% of patients in US clinical trials. (See WARNINGS.)

Cough: A tickling, dry, persistent, nonproductive cough has been reported with the use of ACE inhibitors. Approximately 1% of patients treated with ALTACE® have required discontinuation because of cough. The cough disappears shortly after discontinuation of treatment. (See PRECAUTIONS, Cough subsection.)

Gastrointestinal Pancreatitis, abdominal pain (sometimes with enzyme changes suggesting pancreatitis), anorexia, constipation, diarrhea, dry mouth, dyspepsia, dysphagia, gastroenteritis, hepatitis, nausea, increased salivation, taste disturbance, and vomiting.

Dermatologic: Apparent hypersensitivity reactions (manifested by urticaria, pruritis, or rash, with or without fever), erythema multiforme, photosensitivity, and purpura.

Neurologic and Psychiatric: Anxiety, amnesia, convulsions, depression, hearing loss, insomnia, nervousness, neuralgia, neuropathy, paresthesia, somnolence, tinnitus, tremor, vertigo, and vision disturbances.

Miscellaneous: As with other ACE inhibitors, a symptom complex has been reported which may include a positive ANA, an elevated erythrocyte sedimentation rate, arthralgia/arthritis, myalgia, fever, vasculitis, eosinophilia, photosensitivity, rash and other dermatologic manifestations.

Fetal/neonatal morbidity and mortality. See WARNINGS: Fetal/neonatal morbidity and mortality.

Other: arthralgia, arthritis, dyspnea, edema, epistaxis, impotence, increased sweating, malaise, myalgia, and weight gain.

Clinical Laboratory Test Findings:

Creatinine and Blood Urea Nitrogen: Increases in creatinine levels occurred in 1.2% of patients receiving ALTACE® alone, and in 1.5% of patients receiving ALTACE® and a diuretic. Increases in blood urea nitrogen levels occurred in 0.5% of patients receiving ALTACE® alone and in 3% of patients receiving ALTACE® with a diuretic. None of these increases required discontinuation of treatment. Increases in these laboratory values are more likely to occur in patients with renal insufficiency or those pretreated with a diuretic and, based on experience with other ACE inhibitors, would be expected to be especially likely in patients with renal artery stenosis. (See WARNINGS and PRECAUTIONS.) Since ramipril decreases aldosterone secretion, elevation of serum potassium can occur. Potassium supplements and potassium-sparing diuretics should be given with caution, and the patient's serum potassium should be monitored frequently. (See WARNINGS and PRECAUTIONS.)

Hemoglobin and Hematocrit: Decreases in hemoglobin or hematocrit (a low value and a decrease of 5 g/dl or 5% respectively) were rare, occurring in 0.4% of patients receiving ALTACE® alone and in 1.5% of patients receiving ALTACE® plus a diuretic. No US patients discontinued treatment because of decreases in hemoglobin or hematocrit.

Other (causal relationships unknown): Clinically important changes in standard laboratory tests were rarely associated with ALTACE® administration. Elevations of liver enzymes, serum bilirubin, uric acid, and blood glucose have been reported, as have cases of hyponatremia and scattered incidents of leukopenia, eosinophilia, and proteinuria. In US trials, less than 0.2% of patients discontinued treatment for laboratory abnormalities: all of these were cases of proteinuria or abnormal liver-function tests.

OVERDOSAGE

Single oral doses in rats and mice of 10–11 g/kg resulted in significant lethality. In dogs, oral doses as high as 1 g/kg induced only mild gastrointestinal distress. Limited data on human overdosage are available. The most likely clinical manifestations would be symptoms attributable to hypotension.

Laboratory determinations of serum levels of ramipril and its metabolites are not widely available, and such determinations have, in any event, no established role in the management of ramipril overdose.

No data are available to suggest physiological maneuvers (e.g., maneuvers to change the pH of the urine) that might accelerate elimination of ramipril and its metabolites. Similarly, it is not known which, if any, of these substances can be usefully removed from the body by hemodialysis.

Angiotensin II could presumably serve as a specific antagonist-antidote in the setting of ramipril overdose, but angiotensin II is essentially unavailable outside of scattered research facilities. Because the hypotensive effect of ramipril is achieved through vasodilation and effective hypovolemia, it is reasonable to treat ramipril overdose by infusion of normal saline solution.

DOSAGE AND ADMINISTRATION

Hypertension

The recommended initial dose for patients not receiving a diuretic is 2.5 mg once a day. Dosage should be adjusted according to the blood pressure response. The usual maintenance dosage range is 2.5 to 20 mg per day administered as a single dose or in two equally divided doses. In some patients treated once daily, the antihypertensive effect may diminish toward the end of the dosing interval. In such patients, an increase in dosage or twice daily administration should be considered. If blood pressure is not controlled with ALTACE® alone, a diuretic can be added.

Heart Failure post myocardial infarction

For the treatment of post-infarction patients who have shown signs of congestive failure, the recommended starting dose of ALTACE® is 2.5 mg twice daily. A patient who becomes hypotensive at this dose may be switched to 1.25 mg twice daily, but all patients should then be titrated (as tolerated) toward a target dose of 5 mg twice daily.

After the initial dose of ALTACE®, the patient should be observed under medical supervision for at least two hours and until blood pressure has stabilized for at least an additional hour. (See WARNINGS and PRECAUTIONS, Drug Interactions.) If possible, the dose of any concomitant diuretic should be reduced which may diminish the likelihood of hypotension. The appearance of hypotension after the initial dose of ALTACE® does not preclude subsequent careful dose titration with the drug, following effective management of the hypotension.

The ALTACE® Capsule is usually swallowed whole. The ALTACE® Capsule can also be opened and the contents sprinkled on a small amount (about 4 oz.) of apple sauce or mixed in 4 oz. (120 ml) of water or apple juice. To be sure that ramipril is not lost when such a mixture is used, the mixture should be consumed in its entirety. The described mixtures can be pre-prepared and stored for up to 24 hours at room temperature or up to 48 hours under refrigeration.

Concomitant administration of ALTACE® with potassium supplements, potassium salt substitutes, or potassium-sparing diuretics can lead to increases of serum potassium (See PRECAUTIONS.)

In patients who are currently being treated with a diuretic, symptomatic hypotension occasionally can occur following the initial dose of ALTACE®. To reduce the likelihood of hypotension, the diuretic should, if possible, be discontinued two to three days prior to beginning therapy with ALTACE®. (See WARNINGS.) Then, if blood pressure is not controlled with ALTACE® alone, diuretic therapy should be resumed.

If the diuretic cannot be discontinued, an initial dose of 1.25 mg ALTACE® should be used to avoid excess hypotension.

Dosage Adjustment in Renal Impairment

In patients with creatinine clearance <40 ml/min/1.73m^2 (serum creatinine approximately >2.5 mg/dl) doses only 25% of those normally used should be expected to induce full therapeutic levels of ramiprilat. (See CLINICAL PHARMACOLOGY.)

Hypertension: For patients with hypertension and renal impairment, the recommended initial dose is 1.25 mg ALTACE® once daily. Dosage may be titrated upward until blood pressure is controlled or to a maximum total daily dose of 5 mg.

Heart Failure post myocardial infarction: For patients with heart failure and renal impairment, the recommended initial dose is 1.25 mg ALTACE® once daily. The dose may be increased to 1.25 mg b.i.d. and up to a maximum dose of 2.5 mg b.i.d. depending upon clinical response and tolerability.

HOW SUPPLIED

ALTACE® is available in potencies of 1.25 mg, 2.5 mg, 5 mg, and 10 mg in hard gelatin capsules, packaged in bottles of 100 capsules. ALTACE® is also supplied in blister packages (10 capsules/blister card).

ALTACE® capsules are supplied as follows:

Dose (mg)	Color	Bottle of 100	Unit Dose Carton of 100
1.25	yellow	NDC 0039-0103-10	NDC 0039-0103-11
2.5	orange	NDC 0039-0104-10	NDC 0039-0104-11
5	red	NDC 0039-0105-10	NDC 0039-0105-11
10	Process Blue	NDC 0039-0106-10	

Dispense in well-closed container with safety closure.

Store at controlled room temperature (59 to 86° F).

Caution: Federal law prohibits dispensing without prescription.

*US Patent 4,587,258

ALTACE REG TM HOECHST AG — Made in USA

Hoechst-Roussel Pharmaceuticals
Division of Hoechst Marion Roussel, Inc.
Kansas City, MO 64137
7/95

Shown in Product Identification Guide, page 316

AMARYL® ℞

glimepiride* TABLETS
1, 2, and 4 mg

DESCRIPTION

AMARYL® (glimepiride tablets) is an oral blood-glucose-lowering drug of the sulfonylurea class. Glimepiride is a white to yellowish-white, crystalline, odorless to practically odorless powder formulated into tablets of 1-mg, 2-mg, and 4-mg strengths for oral administration. AMARYL® tablets contain the active ingredient glimepiride and the following inactive ingredients: lactose (hydrous), sodium starch glycolate, povidone, microcrystalline cellulose, and magnesium stearate. In addition, AMARYL® 1-mg tablets contain Ferric Oxide Red, AMARYL® 2-mg tablets contain Ferric Oxide Yellow and FD&C Blue #2 Aluminum Lake, and AMARYL® 4-mg tablets contain FD&C Blue #2 Aluminum Lake.

Continued on next page

Hoechst Marion Roussel—Cont.

Chemically, glimepiride is identified as 1-[[p-[2-(3-ethyl-4-methyl-2-oxo-3-pyrroline-1-carboxamido) ethyl]phenyl]-sulfonyl]-3-(trans-4-methylcyclohexyl)urea. The structural formula is:

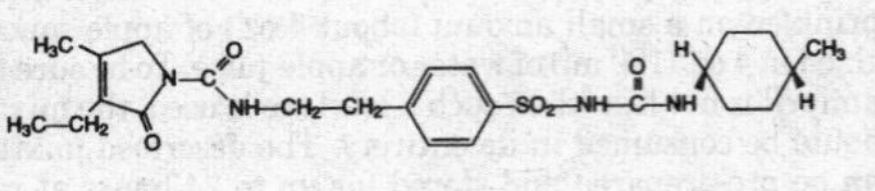

Molecular Formula: $C_{24}H_{34}N_4O_5S$
Molecular Weight: 490.62

Glimepiride is practically insoluble in water.

CLINICAL PHARMACOLOGY

Mechanism Of Action

The primary mechanism of action of glimepiride in lowering blood glucose appears to be dependent on stimulating the release of insulin from functioning pancreatic beta cells. In addition, extrapancreatic effects may also play a role in the activity of sulfonylureas such as glimepiride. This is supported by both preclinical and clinical studies demonstrating that glimepiride administration can lead to increased sensitivity of peripheral tissues to insulin. These findings are consistent with the results of a long-term, randomized, placebo-controlled trial in which AMARYL® therapy improved postprandial insulin/C-peptide responses and overall glycemic control without producing clinically meaningful increases in fasting insulin/C-peptide levels. However, as with other sulfonylureas, the mechanism by which glimepiride lowers blood glucose during long-term administration has not been clearly established.

Pharmacodynamics

A mild glucose-lowering effect first appeared following single oral doses as low as 0.5–0.6 mg in healthy subjects. The time required to reach the maximum effect (i.e., minimum blood glucose level [T_{min}]) was about 2 to 3 hours. In noninsulin-dependent (Type II) diabetes mellitus (NIDDM) patients, both fasting and 2-hour postprandial glucose levels were significantly lower with glimepiride (1, 2, 4, and 8 mg once daily) than with placebo after 14 days of oral dosing. The glucose-lowering effect in all active treatment groups was maintained over 24 hours.

In larger dose-ranging studies, blood glucose and HbA1c were found to respond in a dose-dependent manner over the range of 1 to 4 mg/day of AMARYL®. Some patients, particularly those with higher fasting plasma glucose (FPG) levels, may benefit from doses of AMARYL® up to 8 mg once daily. No difference in response was found when AMARYL® was administered once or twice daily.

In two 14-week, placebo-controlled studies in 720 subjects, the average net reduction in HbA1c for AMARYL® patients treated with 8 mg once daily was 2.0% in absolute units compared with placebo-treated patients. In a long-term, randomized, placebo-controlled study of NIDDM patients unresponsive to dietary management, AMARYL® therapy improved postprandial insulin/C-peptide responses, and 75% of patients achieved and maintained control of blood glucose and HbA1c. Efficacy results were not affected by age, gender, weight, or race.

In long-term extension trials with previously-treated patients, no meaningful deterioration in mean fasting blood glucose (FBG) or HbA1c levels was seen after 2½ years of AMARYL® therapy.

Combination therapy with AMARYL® and insulin (70% NPH/30% regular) was compared to placebo/insulin in secondary failure patients whose body weight was >130% of their ideal body weight. Initially, 5–10 units of insulin were administered with the main evening meal and titrated upward weekly to achieve predefined FPG values. Both groups in this double-blind study achieved similar reductions in FPG levels but the AMARYL®/insulin therapy group used approximately 38% less insulin.

AMARYL® therapy is effective in controlling blood glucose without deleterious changes in the plasma lipoprotein profiles of patients treated for NIDDM.

Pharmacokinetics

Absorption. After oral administration, glimepiride is completely (100%) absorbed from the GI tract. Studies with single oral doses in normal subjects and with multiple oral doses in patients with NIDDM have shown significant absorption of glimepiride within 1 hour after administration and peak drug levels (C_{max}) at 2 to 3 hours. When glimepiride was given with meals, the mean T_{max} (time to reach C_{max}) was slightly increased (12%) and the mean C_{max} and AUC (area under the curve) were slightly decreased (8% and 9%, respectively).

Distribution. After intravenous (IV) dosing in normal subjects, the volume of distribution (Vd) was 8.8 L (113 mL/kg), and the total body clearance (CL) was 47.8 mL/min. Protein binding was greater than 99.5%.

Metabolism. Glimepiride is completely metabolized by oxidative biotransformation after either an IV or oral dose. The major metabolites are the cyclohexyl hydroxy methyl derivative (M1) and the carboxyl derivative (M2). Cytochrome P450 II C9 has been shown to be involved in the biotransformation of glimepiride to M1. M1 is further metabolized to M2 by one or several cytosolic enzymes. M1, but not M2, possesses about ⅓ of the pharmacological activity as compared to its parent in an animal model; however, whether the glucose-lowering effect of M1 is clinically meaningful is not clear.

Excretion. When ^{14}C-glimepiride was given orally, approximately 60% of the total radioactivity was recovered in the urine in 7 days and M1 (predominant) and M2 accounted for 80–90% of that recovered in the urine. Approximately 40% of the total radioactivity was recovered in feces and M1 and M2 (predominant) accounted for about 70% of that recovered in feces. No parent drug was recovered from urine or feces. After IV dosing in patients, no significant biliary excretion of glimepiride or its M1 metabolite has been observed.

Pharmacokinetic Parameters. The pharmacokinetic parameters of glimepiride obtained from a single-dose, crossover, dose-proportionality (1, 2, 4, and 8 mg) study in normal subjects and from a single- and multiple-dose, parallel, dose-proportionality (4 and 8 mg) study in patients with NIDDM are summarized below.

[See table below.]

These data indicate that glimepiride did not accumulate in serum, and the pharmacokinetics of glimepiride were not different in healthy volunteers and in NIDDM patients. Oral clearance of glimepiride did not change over the 1–8-mg dose range, indicating linear pharmacokinetics.

Variability. In normal healthy volunteers, the intra-individual variabilities of C_{max}, AUC, and CL/f for glimepiride were 23%, 17%, and 15%, respectively, and the inter-individual variabilities were 25%, 29%, and 24%, respectively.

Special Populations

Geriatric. Comparison of glimepiride pharmacokinetics in NIDDM patients ≤ 65 years and those > 65 years was performed in a study using a dosing regimen of 6 mg daily. There were no significant differences in glimepiride pharmacokinetics between the two age groups. The mean AUC at steady state for the older patients was about 13% lower than that for the younger patients; the mean weight-adjusted clearance for the older patients was about 11% higher than that for the younger patients.

Pediatric. No studies were performed in pediatric patients.

Gender. There were no differences between males and females in the pharmacokinetics of glimepiride when adjustment was made for differences in body weight.

Race. No pharmacokinetic studies to assess the effects of race have been performed, but in placebo-controlled studies of AMARYL® in patients with NIDDM, the antihyperglycemic effect was comparable in whites (n=536), blacks (n=63), and Hispanics (n=63).

	Volunteers	Patients with NIDDM	
	Single Dose Mean ± SD	Single Dose (Day 1) Mean ± SD	Multiple Dose (Day 10) Mean ± SD
C_{max} (ng/mL)			
1 mg	103 ± 34 (12)	—	—
2 mg	177 ± 44 (12)	—	—
4 mg	308 ± 69 (12)	352 ± 222 (12)	309 ± 134 (12)
8 mg	557 ± 152 (12)	591 ± 232 (14)	578 ± 265 (11)
T_{max} (h)	2.4 ± 0.8 (48)	2.5 ± 1.2 (26)	2.8 ± 2.2 (23)
CL/f (mL/min)	52.1 ± 16.0 (48)	48.5 ± 29.3 (26)	52.7 ± 40.3 (23)
Vd/f (L)	21.8 ± 13.9 (48)	19.8 ± 12.7 (26)	37.1 ± 18.2 (23)
T½ (h)	5.3 ± 4.1 (48)	5.0 ± 2.5 (26)	9.2 ± 3.6 (23)

( ) = No. of subjects
CL/f = Total body clearance after oral dosing
Vd/f = Volume of distribution calculated after oral dosing

Renal Insufficiency. A single-dose, open-label study was conducted in 15 patients with renal impairment. AMARYL® (3 mg) was administered to 3 groups of patients with different levels of mean creatinine clearance (CLcr); (Group I, CLcr = 77.7 mL/min, n=5), (Group II, CLcr = 27.7 mL/min, n=3), and (Group III, CLcr = 9.4 mL/min, n=7). AMARYL® was found to be well tolerated in all 3 groups. The results showed that glimepiride serum levels decreased as renal function decreased. However, M1 and M2 serum levels (mean AUC values) increased 2.3 and 8.6 times from Group I to Group III. The apparent terminal half-life ($T_{1/2}$) for glimepiride did not change, while the half-lives for M1 and M2 increased as renal function decreased. Mean urinary excretion of M1 plus M2 as percent of dose, however, decreased (44.4%, 21.9%, and 9.3% for Groups I to III).

A multiple-dose titration study was also conducted in 16 NIDDM patients with renal impairment using doses ranging from 1–8 mg daily for 3 months. The results were consistent with those observed after single doses. All patients with a CLcr less than 22 mL/min had adequate control of their glucose levels with a dosage regimen of only 1 mg daily. The results from this study suggested that a starting dose of 1 mg AMARYL® may be given to NIDDM patients with kidney disease, and the dose may be titrated based on fasting blood glucose levels.

Hepatic Insufficiency. No studies were performed in patients with hepatic insufficiency.

Other Populations. There were no important differences in glimepiride metabolism in subjects identified as phenotypically different drug-metabolizers by their metabolism of sparteine.

The pharmacokinetics of glimepiride in morbidly obese patients were similar to those in the normal weight group, except for a lower C_{max} and AUC. However, since neither C_{max} nor AUC values were normalized for body surface area, the lower values of C_{max} and AUC for the obese patients were likely the result of their excess weight and not due to a difference in the kinetics of glimepiride.

Drug Interactions. The hypoglycemic action of sulfonylureas may be potentiated by certain drugs, including nonsteroidal anti-inflammatory drugs and other drugs that are highly protein bound, such as salicylates, sulfonamides, chloramphenicol, coumarins, probenecid, monoamine oxidase inhibitors, and beta adrenergic blocking agents. When these drugs are administered to a patient receiving AMARYL®, the patient should be observed closely for hypoglycemia. When these drugs are withdrawn from a patient receiving AMARYL®, the patient should be observed closely for loss of glycemic control.

Certain drugs tend to produce hyperglycemia and may lead to loss of control. These drugs include the thiazides and other diuretics, corticosteroids, phenothiazines, thyroid products, estrogens, oral contraceptives, phenytoin, nicotinic acid, sympathomimetics, and isoniazid. When these drugs are administered to a patient receiving AMARYL®, the patient should be closely observed for loss of control. When these drugs are withdrawn from a patient receiving AMARYL®, the patient should be observed closely for hypoglycemia.

Coadministration of aspirin (1 g tid) and AMARYL® led to a 34% decrease in the mean glimepiride AUC and, therefore, a 34% increase in the mean CL/f. The mean C_{max} had a decrease of 4%. Blood glucose and serum C-peptide concentrations were unaffected and no hypoglycemic symptoms were reported. Pooled data from clinical trials showed no evidence of clinically significant adverse interactions with uncontrolled concurrent administration of aspirin and other salicylates.

Coadministration of either cimetidine (800 mg once daily) or ranitidine (150 mg bid) with a single 4-mg oral dose of AMARYL® did not significantly alter the absorption and disposition of glimepiride, and no differences were seen in hypoglycemic symptomatology. Pooled data from clinical trials showed no evidence of clinicallly significant adverse interactions with uncontrolled concurrent administration of H2-receptor antagonists.

Concomitant administration of propranolol (40 mg tid) and AMARYL® significantly increased C_{max}, AUC, and $T_{1/2}$ of glimepiride by 23%, 22%, and 15%, respectively, and it decreased CL/f by 18%. The recovery of M1 and M2 from urine, however, did not change. The pharmacodynamic responses to glimepiride were nearly identical in normal subjects receiving propranolol and placebo. Pooled data from clinical trials in patients with NIDDM showed no evidence of clinically significant adverse interactions with uncontrolled concurrent administration of beta-blockers. However, if beta-blockers are used, caution should be exercised and patients should be warned about the potential for hypoglycemia.

Concomitant administration of AMARYL® (4 mg once daily) did not alter the pharmacokinetic characteristics of R- and S-warfarin enantiomers following administration of a single dose (25 mg) of racemic warfarin to healthy subjects. No changes were observed in warfarin plasma protein binding. AMARYL® treatment did result in a slight, but statistically significant, decrease in the pharmacodynamic response

to warfarin. The reductions in mean area under the prothrombin time (PT) curve and maximum PT values during AMARYL® treatment were very small (3.3% and 9.9%, respectively) and are unlikely to be clinically important.

The responses of serum glucose, insulin, C-peptide, and plasma glucagon to 2 mg AMARYL® were unaffected by coadministration of ramipril (an ACE inhibitor) 5 mg once daily in normal subjects. No hypoglycemic symptoms were reported. Pooled data from clinical trials in patients with NIDDM showed no evidence of clinically significant adverse interactions with uncontrolled concurrent administration of ACE inhibitors.

A potential interaction between oral miconazole and oral hypoglycemic agents leading to severe hypoglycemia has been reported. Whether this interaction also occurs with the intravenous, topical, or vaginal preparations of miconazole is not known. Potential interactions of glimepiride with other drugs metabolized by cytochrome P450 II C9 also include phenytoin, diclofenac, ibuprofen, naproxen, and mefenamic acid.

Although no specific interaction studies were performed, pooled data from clinical trials showed no evidence of clinically significant adverse interactions with uncontrolled concurrent administration of calcium-channel blockers, estrogens, fibrates, NSAIDS, HMG CoA reductase inhibitors, sulfonamides, or thyroid hormone.

INDICATIONS AND USAGE

AMARYL® is indicated as an adjunct to diet and exercise to lower the blood glucose in patients with noninsulin-dependent (Type II) diabetes mellitus (NIDDM) whose hyperglycemia cannot be controlled by diet and exercise alone.

AMARYL® is also indicated for use in combination with insulin to lower blood glucose in patients whose hyperglycemia cannot be controlled by diet and exercise in conjunction with an oral hypoglycemic agent. Combined use of glimepiride and insulin may increase the potential for hypoglycemia.

In initiating treatment for noninsulin-dependent diabetes, diet and exercise should be emphasized as the primary form of treatment. Caloric restriction, weight loss, and exercise are essential in the obese diabetic patient. Proper dietary management and exercise alone may be effective in controlling the blood glucose and symptoms of hyperglycemia. In addition to regular physical activity, cardiovascular risk factors should be identified and corrective measures taken where possible.

If this treatment program fails to reduce symptoms and/or blood glucose, the use of an oral sulfonylurea or insulin should be considered. Use of AMARYL® must be viewed by both the physician and patient as a treatment in addition to diet and exercise and not as a substitute for diet and exercise or as a convenient mechanism for avoiding dietary restraint. Furthermore, loss of blood glucose control on diet and exercise alone may be transient, thus requiring only short-term administration of AMARYL®.

During maintenance programs, AMARYL® monotherapy should be discontinued if satisfactory lowering of blood glucose is no longer achieved. Judgments should be based on regular clinical and laboratory evaluations. Secondary failures to AMARYL® monotherapy can be treated with AMARYL®-insulin combination therapy.

In considering the use of AMARYL® in asymptomatic patients, it should be recognized that blood glucose control in NIDDM has not definitely been established to be effective in preventing the long-term cardiovascular and neural complications of diabetes. However, the Diabetes Control and Complications Trial (DCCT) demonstrated that control of HbA1c and glucose was associated with a decrease in retinopathy, neuropathy, and nephropathy for insulin-dependent diabetic (IDDM) patients.

CONTRAINDICATIONS

AMARYL® is contraindicated in patients with
1. Known hypersensitivity to the drug.
2. Diabetic ketoacidosis, with or without coma. This condition should be treated with insulin.

WARNINGS

SPECIAL WARNING ON INCREASED RISK OF CARDIOVASCULAR MORTALITY

The administration of oral hypoglycemic drugs has been reported to be associated with increased cardiovascular mortality as compared to treatment with diet alone or diet plus insulin. This warning is based on the study conducted by the University Group Diabetes Program (UGDP), a long-term, prospective clinical trial designed to evaluate the effectiveness of glucose-lowering drugs in preventing or delaying vascular complications in patients with non-insulin-dependent diabetes. The study involved 823 patients who were randomly assigned to one of four treatment groups (Diabetes, 19 supp. 2: 747–830, 1970).

UGDP reported that patients treated for 5 to 8 years with diet plus a fixed dose of tolbutamide (1.5 grams per day) had a rate of cardiovascular mortality approximately 2½ times that of patients treated with diet alone. A significant increase in total mortality was not observed, but the use of

tolbutamide was discontinued based on the increase in cardiovascular mortality, thus limiting the opportunity for the study to show an increase in overall mortality. Despite controversy regarding the interpretation of these results, the findings of the UGDP study provide an adequate basis for this warning. The patient should be informed of the potential risks and advantages of AMARYL® (glimepiride tablets) and of alternative modes of therapy.

Although only one drug in the sulfonylurea class (tolbutamide) was included in this study, it is prudent from a safety standpoint to consider that this warning may also apply to other oral hypoglycemic drugs in this class, in view of their close similarities in mode of action and chemical structure.

PRECAUTIONS

General

Hypoglycemia: All sulfonylurea drugs are capable of producing severe hypoglycemia. Proper patient selection, dosage, and instructions are important to avoid hypoglycemic episodes. Patients with impaired renal function may be more sensitive to the glucose-lowering effect of AMARYL®. A starting dose of 1 mg once daily followed by appropriate dose titration is recommended in those patients. Debilitated or malnourished patients, and those with adrenal, pituitary, or hepatic insufficiency are particularly susceptible to the hypoglycemic action of glucose-lowering drugs. Hypoglycemia may be difficult to recognize in the elderly and in people who are taking beta-adrenergic blocking drugs or other sympatholytic agents. Hypoglycemia is more likely to occur when caloric intake is deficient, after severe or prolonged exercise, when alcohol is ingested, or when more than one glucose-lowering drug is used.

Loss of control of blood glucose: When a patient stabilized on any diabetic regimen is exposed to stress such as fever, trauma, infection, or surgery, a loss of control may occur. At such times, it may be necessary to add insulin in combination with AMARYL® or even use insulin monotherapy. The effectiveness of any oral hypoglycemic drug, including AMARYL®, in lowering blood glucose to a desired level decreases in many patients over a period of time, which may be due to progression of the severity of the diabetes or to diminished responsiveness to the drug. This phenomenon is known as secondary failure, to distinguish it from primary failure in which the drug is ineffective in an individual patient when first given. Should secondary failure occur with AMARYL® monotherapy, AMARYL®-insulin combination therapy may be instituted. Combined use of glimepiride and insulin may increase the potential for hypoglycemia.

Information for Patients

Patients should be informed of the potential risks and advantages of AMARYL® and of alternative modes of therapy. They should also be informed about the importance of adherence to dietary instructions, of a regular exercise program, and of regular testing of blood glucose.

The risks of hypoglycemia, its symptoms and treatment, and conditions that predispose to its development should be explained to patients and responsible family members. The potential for primary and secondary failure should also be explained.

Laboratory Tests

Fasting blood glucose should be monitored periodically to determine therapeutic response. Glycosylated hemoglobin should also be monitored, usually every 3 to 6 months, to more precisely assess long-term glycemic control.

Drug Interactions

(See CLINICAL PHARMACOLOGY, Drug Interactions.)

Carcinogenesis, Mutagenesis, and Impairment of Fertility

Studies in rats at doses of up to 5000 ppm in complete feed (approximately 340 times the maximum recommended human dose, based on surface area) for 30 months showed no evidence of carcinogenesis. In mice, administration of glimepiride for 24 months resulted in an increase in benign pancreatic adenoma formation which was dose related and is thought to be the result of chronic pancreatic stimulation. The no-effect dose for adenoma formation in mice in this study was 320 ppm in complete feed, or 46-54 mg/kg body weight/day. This is about 35 times the maximum human recommended dose of 8 mg once daily based on surface area. Glimepiride was non-mutagenic in a battery of in vitro and in vivo mutagenicity studies (Ames test, somatic cell mutation, chromosomal aberration, unscheduled DNA synthesis, mouse micronucleus test).

There was no effect of glimepiride on male mouse fertility in animals exposed up to 2500 mg/kg body weight (>1,700 times the maximum recommended human dose based on surface area). Glimepiride had no effect on the fertility of male and female rats administered up to 4000 mg/kg body weight (approximately 4,000 times the maximum recommended human dose based on surface area).

Pregnancy

Teratogenic Effects. Pregnancy Category C. Glimepiride did not produce teratogenic effects in rats exposed orally up to 4000 mg/kg body weight (approximately 4,000 times the maximum recommended human dose based on surface area) or in rabbits exposed up to 32 mg/kg body weight (approxi-

mately 60 times the maximum recommended human dose based on surface area). Glimepiride has been shown to be associated with intrauterine fetal death in rats when given in doses as low as 50 times the human dose based on surface area and in rabbits when given in doses as low as 0.1 times the human dose based on surface area. This fetotoxicity, observed only at doses inducing maternal hypoglycemia, has been similarly noted with other sulfonylureas, and is believed to be directly related to the pharmacologic (hypoglycemic) action of glimepiride.

There are no adequate and well-controlled studies in pregnant women. On the basis of results from animal studies, AMARYL® should not be used during pregnancy. Because recent information suggests that abnormal blood glucose levels during pregnancy are associated with a higher incidence of congenital abnormalities, many experts recommend that insulin be used during pregnancy to maintain glucose levels as close to normal as possible.

Nonteratogenic Effects. In some studies in rats, offspring of dams exposed to high levels of glimepiride during pregnancy and lactation developed skeletal deformities consisting of shortening, thickening, and bending of the humerus during the postnatal period. Significant concentrations of glimepiride were observed in the serum and breast milk of the dams as well as in the serum of the pups. These skeletal deformations were determined to be the result of nursing from mothers exposed to glimepiride.

Prolonged severe hypoglycemia (4 to 10 days) has been reported in neonates born to mothers who were receiving a sulfonylurea drug at the time of delivery. This has been reported more frequently with the use of agents with prolonged half-lives. Patients who are planning a pregnancy should consult their physician, and it is recommended that they change over to insulin for the entire course of pregnancy and lactation.

Nursing Mothers

In rat reproduction studies, significant concentrations of glimepiride were observed in the serum and breast milk of the dams, as well as in the serum of the pups. Although it is not known whether AMARYL® is excreted in human milk, other sulfonylureas are excreted in human milk. Because the potential for hypoglycemia in nursing infants may exist, and because of the effects on nursing animals, AMARYL® should be discontinued in nursing mothers. If AMARYL® is discontinued, and if diet and exercise alone are inadequate for controlling blood glucose, insulin therapy should be considered. (See above Pregnancy, Nonteratogenic Effects.)

Pediatric Use

Safety and effectiveness in pediatric patients have not been established.

ADVERSE REACTIONS

The incidence of hypoglycemia with AMARYL®, as documented by blood glucose values <60 mg/dL, ranged from 0.9–1.7% in two large, well-controlled, 1-year studies. (See WARNINGS and PRECAUTIONS.)

AMARYL® has been evaluated for safety in 2,013 patients in US controlled trials, and in 1,551 patients in foreign controlled trials. More than 1,650 of these patients were treated for at least 1 year.

Adverse events, other than hypoglycemia, considered to be possibly or probably related to study drug that occurred in US placebo-controlled trials in more than 1% of patients treated with AMARYL® are shown below.

Adverse Events Occurring in ≥1%
AMARYL® Patients

	AMARYL®		Placebo	
	No.	%	No.	%
Total Treated	746	100	294	100
Dizziness	13	1.7	1	0.3
Asthenia	12	1.6	3	1.0
Headache	11	1.5	4	1.4
Nausea	8	1.1	0	0.0

Gastrointestinal Reactions

Vomiting, gastrointestinal pain, and diarrhea have been reported, but the incidence in placebo-controlled trials was less than 1%. Isolated transaminase elevations have been reported. Cholestatic jaundice has been reported to occur rarely with sulfonylureas.

Dermatologic Reactions

Allergic skin reactions, e.g., pruritus, erythema, urticaria, and morbilliform or maculopapular eruptions, occur in less than 1% of treated patients. These may be transient and may disappear despite continued use of AMARYL®; if skin reactions persist, the drug should be discontinued. Porphyria cutanea tarda and photosensitivity reactions have been reported with sulfonylureas.

Hematologic Reactions

Leukopenia, agranulocytosis, thrombocytopenia, hemolytic anemia, aplastic anemia, and pancytopenia have been reported with sulfonylureas.

Continued on next page

Hoechst Marion Roussel—Cont.

Metabolic Reactions

Hepatic porphyria reactions and disulfiram-like reactions have been reported with sulfonylureas; however, no cases have yet been reported with AMARYL®. Cases of hyponatremia have been reported with glimepiride and all other sulfonylureas, most often in patients who are on other medications or have medical conditions known to cause hyponatremia or increase release of antidiuretic hormone. The syndrome of inappropriate antidiuretic hormone (SIADH) secretion has been reported with certain other sulfonylureas, and it has been suggested that these sulfonylureas may augment the peripheral (antidiuretic) action of ADH and/or increase release of ADH.

Other Reactions

Changes in accommodation and/or blurred vision may occur with the use of AMARYL®. This is thought to be due to changes in blood glucose, and may be more pronounced when treatment is initiated. This condition is also seen in untreated diabetic patients, and may actually be reduced by treatment. In placebo-controlled trials of AMARYL®, the incidence of blurred vision was placebo, 0.7%, and AMARYL®, 0.4%.

OVERDOSAGE

Overdosage of sulfonylureas, including AMARYL®, can produce hypoglycemia. Mild hypoglycemic symptoms without loss of consciousness or neurologic findings should be treated aggressively with oral glucose and adjustments in drug dosage and/or meal patterns. Close monitoring should continue until the physician is assured that the patient is out of danger. Severe hypoglycemic reactions with coma, seizure, or other neurological impairment occur infrequently, but constitute medical emergencies requiring immediate hospitalization. If hypoglycemic coma is diagnosed or suspected, the patient should be given a rapid intravenous injection of concentrated (50%) glucose solution. This should be followed by a continuous infusion of a more dilute (10%) glucose solution at a rate that will maintain the blood glucose at a level above 100 mg/dL. Patients should be closely monitored for a minimum of 24 to 48 hours, because hypoglycemia may recur after apparent clinical recovery.

DOSAGE AND ADMINISTRATION

There is no fixed dosage regimen for the management of diabetes mellitus with AMARYL® or any other hypoglycemic agent. The patient's fasting blood glucose and HbA1c must be measured periodically to determine the minimum effective dose for the patient; to detect primary failure, i.e., inadequate lowering of blood glucose at the maximum recommended dose of medication; and to detect secondary failure, i.e., loss of adequate blood glucose lowering response after an initial period of effectiveness. Glycosylated hemoglobin levels should be performed to monitor the patient's response to therapy.

Short-term administration of AMARYL® may be sufficient during periods of transient loss of control in patients usually controlled well on diet and exercise.

Usual Starting Dose

The usual starting dose of AMARYL® as initial therapy is 1–2 mg once daily, administered with breakfast or the first main meal. Those patients who may be more sensitive to hypoglycemic drugs should be started at 1 mg once daily, and should be titrated carefully. (See **PRECAUTIONS** Section for patients at increased risk.)

No exact dosage relationship exists between AMARYL® and the other oral hypoglycemic agents. The maximum starting dose of AMARYL® should be no more than 2 mg.

Failure to follow an appropriate dosage regimen may precipitate hypoglycemia. Patients who do not adhere to their prescribed dietary and drug regimen are more prone to exhibit unsatisfactory response to therapy.

Usual Maintenance Dose

The usual maintenance dose is 1 to 4 mg once daily. The maximum recommended dose is 8 mg once daily. After reaching a dose of 2 mg, dosage increases should be made in increments of no more than 2 mg at 1–2 week intervals based upon the patient's blood glucose response. Long-term efficacy should be monitored by measurement of HbA1c levels, for example, every 3 to 6 months.

AMARYL®-Insulin Combination Therapy

Combination therapy with AMARYL® and insulin may be used in secondary failure patients. The fasting glucose level for instituting combination therapy is in the range of > 150 mg/dL in plasma or serum depending on the patient. The recommended AMARYL® dose is 8 mg once daily administered with the first main meal. After starting with low-dose insulin, upward adjustments of insulin can be done approximately weekly as guided by frequent measurements of fasting blood glucose. Once stable, combination-therapy patients should monitor their capillary blood glucose on an ongoing basis, preferably daily. Periodic adjustments of insulin may also be necessary during maintenance as guided by glucose and HbA1c levels.

Specific Patient Populations

AMARYL® is not recommended for use in pregnancy, nursing mothers, or children. In elderly, debilitated, or malnourished patients, or in patients with renal or hepatic insufficiency, the initial dosing, dose increments, and maintenance dosage should be conservative to avoid hypoglycemic reactions (See **CLINICAL PHARMACOLOGY**, Special Populations and **PRECAUTIONS**, General).

Patients Receiving Other Oral Hypoglycemic Agents

As with other sulfonylurea hypoglycemic agents, no transition period is necessary when transferring patients to AMARYL®. Patients should be observed carefully (1–2 weeks) for hypoglycemia when being transferred from longer half-life sulfonylureas (e.g., chlorpropamide) to AMARYL® due to potential overlapping of drug effect.

HOW SUPPLIED

AMARYL® tablets are available in the following strengths and package sizes:

1 mg (pink, flat-faced, oblong with notched sides at double bisect, imprinted with "AMA RYL" on one side and the Hoechst logo on both sides of the bisect on the other side)
Bottles of 100   (NDC 0039-0221-10)
Unit Dose Cartons (100)   (NDC 0039-0221-11)

2 mg (green, flat-faced, oblong with notched sides at double bisect, imprinted with "AMA RYL" on one side and the Hoechst logo on both sides of the bisect on the other side)
Bottles of 100   (NDC 0039-0222-10)
Unit Dose Cartons (100)   (NDC 0039-0222-11)

4 mg (blue, flat-faced, oblong with notched sides at double bisect, imprinted with "AMA RYL" on one side and the Hoechst logo on both sides of the bisect on the other side)
Bottles of 100   (NDC 0039-0223-10)
Unit Dose Cartons (100)   (NDC 0039-0223-11)

Store between 59°and 86° F (15° to 30° C).
Dispense in well-closed containers with safety closures.
Caution: Federal law prohibits dispensing without a prescription.
AMARYL® REG TM HOECHST AG
*US Patent 4,379,785

ANIMAL TOXICOLOGY

Reduced serum glucose values and degranulation of the pancreatic beta cells were observed in beagle dogs exposed to 320 mg glimepiride/kg/day for 12 months (approximately 1,000 times the recommended human dose based on surface area). No evidence of tumor formation was observed in any organ. One female and one male dog developed bilateral subcapsular cataracts. Non-GLP studies indicated that glimepiride was unlikely to exacerbate cataract formation. Evaluation of the co-cataractogenic potential of glimepiride in several diabetic and cataract rat models was negative and there was no adverse effect of glimepiride on bovine ocular lens metabolism in organ culture.

HUMAN OPHTHALMOLOGY DATA

Ophthalmic examinations were carried out in over 500 subjects during long-term studies using the methodology of Taylor and West and Laties et al. No significant differences were seen between AMARYL® and glyburide in the number of subjects with clinically important changes in visual acuity, intra-ocular tension, or in any of the five lens-related variables examined.

Ophthalmic examinations were carried out during long-term studies using the method of Chylack et al. No significant or clinically meaningful differences were seen between AMARYL® and glipizide with respect to cataract progression by subjective LOCS II grading and objective image analysis systems, visual acuity, intraocular pressure, and general ophthalmic examination.

Hoechst-Roussel Pharmaceuticals
Division of Hoechst Marion Roussel, Inc.
Kansas City, MO 64137   722200-10/95
REG TM HOECHST AG
Shown in Product Identification Guide, page 316

A/T/S®
(erythromycin)
2% ACNE TOPICAL SOLUTION
FOR DERMATOLOGIC USE ONLY.
NOT FOR USE IN EYES.

℞

DESCRIPTION

A/T/S® (erythromycin) is an antibiotic produced from a strain of *Streptomyces erythraeus*. It is basic and readily forms salts with acids. Each mL of A/T/S® Topical Solution contains 20 mg of erythromycin base in a vehicle consisting of alcohol USP (66%), propylene glycol USP, and citric acid USP to adjust pH. The CAS Registry Number is 114-07-8.

ACTIONS

Although the mechanism of action by which A/T/S® Topical Solution acts in reducing inflammatory lesions of acne vulgaris is unknown, it is presumably due to its antibiotic action.

INDICATIONS

A/T/S® is indicated for the topical control of acne vulgaris.

CONTRAINDICATIONS

A/T/S® is contraindicated in persons who have shown hypersensitivity to any of its ingredients.

WARNING

The safe use of A/T/S® Topical Solution during pregnancy or lactation has not been established.

PRECAUTIONS

General: The use of antibiotic agents may be associated with the overgrowth of antibiotic-resistant organisms. If this occurs, administration of the drug should be discontinued and appropriate measures taken.

Information for Patients: A/T/S® (erythromycin) is for external use only and should be kept away from the eye, nose, mouth, and other mucous membranes. Concomitant topical acne therapy should be used with caution because a cumulative irritant effect may occur, especially with the use of peeling, desquamating, or abrasive agents.

Carcinogenesis, Mutagenesis, Impairment of Fertility: Long-term animal studies to evaluate carcinogenic potential, or the effect on fertility of erythromycin have not been performed.

Pregnancy: Pregnancy Category C. Animal reproduction studies have not been conducted with erythromycin. It is also not known whether erythromycin can cause fetal harm when administered to a pregnant women or can affect reproduction capacity. Erythromycin should be given to a pregnant women only if clearly needed.

Nursing Mothers: Erythromycin is excreted in breast milk. Caution should be exercised when erythromycin is administered to a nursing woman.

ADVERSE REACTIONS

Adverse conditions reported with the use of erythromycin topical solutions include dryness, tenderness, pruritus, desquamation, erythema, oiliness, and burning sensation. Irritation of the eye has also been reported. A case of generalized urticarial reaction, possibly related to the drug, which required the use of systemic steroid therapy has been reported. Of a total of 90 patients exposed to A/T/S® during clinical effectiveness studies, 17 experienced some type of adverse effect. These included dry skin, scaly skin, pruritis, irritation of the eye, and burning sensation.

DOSAGE AND ADMINISTRATION

A/T/S® Topical Solution should be applied to the affected area twice a day after the skin is thoroughly washed with warm water and soap and patted dry. Moisten the applicator or a pad with A/T/S®, then rub over the affected area. Acne lesions on the face, neck, shoulder, chest, and back may be treated in this manner.

HOW SUPPLIED

A/T/S® 2% Acne Topical Solution—60 mL
Store at controlled room temperature (59–86°F).
Distributed by:
Hoechst-Roussel Pharmaceuticals
Division of Hoechst Marion Roussel, Inc.
Kansas City, MO 64137
Rev. 8/91
716000
Shown in Product Identification Guide, page 316

A/T/S®
(Erythromycin Topical Gel USP) 2%
FOR DERMATOLOGIC USE ONLY
NOT FOR OPTHALMIC USE

℞

DESCRIPTION

A/T/S® Topical Gel contains erythromycin. Erythromycin is a macrolide antibiotic obtained from cultures of *Streptomyces erythraeus*.

Structural Formula

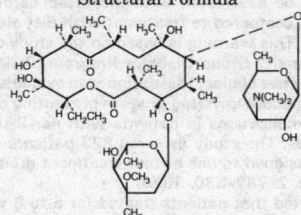

Erythromycin
Empirical Formula: $C_{37}H_{67}NO_{13}$
Molecular Weight: 733.94

Contains: erythromycin, USP .... 2% (20 mg/g)
with: alcohol 92% and hydroxypropyl cellulose.

CLINICAL PHARMACOLOGY

The exact mechanism by which erythromycin reduces lesions of acne vulgaris is not fully known; however, the effect appears to be due in part to the antibacterial activity of the drug.

MICROBIOLOGY

Erythromycin appears to inhibit protein synthesis in susceptible organisms by reversibly binding to ribosomal subunits, thereby inhibiting translocation of aminoacyl transfer-RNA and inhibiting polypeptide synthesis. Antagonism has been demonstrated between erythromycin, lincomycin, chloramphenicol, and clindamycin.

INDICATIONS AND USAGE

A/T/S® is indicated for the topical treatment of acne vulgaris.

CONTRAINDICATIONS

A/T/S® is contraindicated in those individuals who have shown hypersensitivity to any of its components.

PRECAUTIONS

General: For topical use only; not for ophthalmic use. Concomitant topical acne therapy should be used with caution since a possible cumulative irritancy effect may occur, especially with the use of peeling, desquamating or abrasive agents.
Avoid contact with eyes and all mucous membranes. The use of antibiotic agents may be associated with the overgrowth of antibiotic-resistant organisms. If this occurs, discontinue use and take appropriate measures.
Carcionesis, mutagenesis, impairment of fertility:
Animal studies to evaluate carcinogenic and mutagenic potential, or effects, on fertility have not been performed with erythromycin.
Pregnancy Category B:
There was no evidence of teratogenicity or any other adverse effect on reproduction in female rats fed erythromycin base (up to 0.25% of diet) prior to and during mating, during gestation and through weaning of two successive litters. There are, however, no adequate and well-controlled studies in pregnant women. Because animal reproduction studies are not always predictive of human response, this drug should be used in pregnancy only if clearly needed. Erythromycin has been reported to cross the placental barrier in humans, but fetal plasma levels are generally low.
Nursing Mothers:
It is not known whether topically applied erythromycin is excreted in human milk. A decision should be made whether to discontinue nursing or to discontinue the drug, taking into account the importance of the drug to the mother.
Pediatric Use:
Safety and effectiveness in children have not been established.

ADVERSE REACTIONS

The most common adverse reaction reported with A/T/S® (Erythromycin Topical Gel USP) 2% was burning. The following have been reported occasionally: peeling, dryness, itching, erythema, and oiliness, irritation of the eyes and tenderness of the skin have also been reported with the topical use of erythromycin. A generalized urticerial reaction, possibly related to the use of erythromycin, which required systemic steroid therapy has been reported.

DOSAGE AND ADMINISTRATION

Apply sparingly as a thin film once or twice a day to the affected area(s) after the skin is thoroughly cleansed and patted dry. If there has been no improvement after 6 to 8 weeks, or if the condition becomes worse, treatment should be discontinued, and the physician should be consulted. Spread the medication lightly rather than rubbing it in. The hands should be washed after application. There are no data directly comparing the safety and efficacy of b.i.d. versus q.d. dosing.

HOW SUPPLIED

A/T/S® (Erythromycin Topical Gel USP) 2% - 30 gram plastic tubes (NDC0039-0116-30).
Note: FLAMMABLE. Keep away from heat and flame. Keep tube tightly closed. Store between 15° and 25°C (59° and 77°F).
CAUTION: Federal law prohibits dispensing without prescription.
Manufactured by:
ALLERGAN Herbert
Skin Care Division of ALLERGAN, INC.
Irvine, CA 92715
Distributed by:
Hoechst-Roussel Pharmaceuticals
Division of Hoechst Marion Roussel, Inc.
Kansas City, MO 64137
711600-12/93

Shown in Product Identification Guide, page 316

AVC™   ℞
(sulfanilamide)
Cream/Suppositories
Prescribing information as of January 1995

DESCRIPTION

AVC™ is a preparation for vaginal administration for the treatment of *Candida albicans* infections and available in the following forms:
AVC Cream
Each tube contains:
Sulfanilamide 15.0%
in a water-miscible, non-staining base made from lactose, propylene glycol, stearic acid, diglycol stearate, methylparaben, propylparaben, trolamine, and water; buffered with lactic acid to an acid pH of approximately 4.3.
AVC Suppositories
Each suppository contains:
Sulfanilamide .... 1.05 g
with lactose, in a base made from polyethylene glycol 400, polysorbate 80, polyethylene glycol 3350, and glycerin, buffered with lactic acid to an acid pH of approximately 4.5. AVC Suppositories have an inert, white, non-staining covering, which dissolves promptly in the vagina. The covering is composed of gelatin, glycerin, water, methylparaben, propylparaben, and coloring.
Sulfanilamide is an anti-infective agent. It is *p*-amino-benzenesulfonamide with the chemical structure:

$$H_2N\!-\!\!\bigcirc\!\!-\!SO_2NH_2$$

Sulfanilamide occurs as a white odorless crystalline powder with a slightly bitter taste and sweet aftertaste. It is slightly soluble in water, alcohol, acetone, glycerin, propylene glycol, hydrochloric acid, and solutions of potassium and sodium hydroxide. It is practically insoluble in chloroform, ether, benzene, and petroleum ether.

CLINICAL PHARMACOLOGY

Sulfanilamide has been a useful ingredient of vaginal formulations for about four decades. It blocks certain metabolic processes essential for the growth of susceptible bacteria. In AVC, the sulfanilamide is in a specially compounded base buffered to the pH (about 4.3) of the normal vagina to encourage the presence of the normally occurring Döderlein's bacilli of the vagina.
The use of AVC for the treatment of vulvovaginitis caused by *Candida albicans* is supported by three clinical investigations. The three studies show AVC with sulfanilamide to be significantly more effective (p ≤ 0.01) than placebo as follows:
In Study I, the ratio of effectiveness was 71% for the AVC with sulfanilamide versus 49% for placebo with 30 days of treatment;
In Study II, the percentages were 48% and 24%, respectively, with 15 days of treatment;
In Study III, the percentages were 66% versus 33%, respectively, with 30 days of treatment.

INDICATIONS AND USAGE

For the treatment of vulvovaginitis caused by *Candida albicans*. (See CLINICAL PHARMACOLOGY.)

CONTRAINDICATIONS

AVC should not be used in patients known to be sensitive to this product or to the sulfonamides.

PRECAUTIONS

General
Because sulfonamides are absorbed from the vaginal mucosa, the usual precautions for oral sulfonamides apply. Patients should be observed for skin rash or evidence of systemic toxicity, and if these develop, the medications should be discontinued.
Deaths associated with administration of oral sulfonamides have reportedly occurred from hypersensitivity reactions, agranulocytosis, aplastic anemia, and other blood dyscrasias. Goiter production, diuresis, and hypoglycemia have reportedly occurred rarely in patients receiving oral sulfonamides. Cross-sensitivity may exist with these agents. Rats appear to be especially susceptible to the goitrogenic effects of sulfonamides, and long-term administration has reportedly produced thyroid malignancies in this species.
Vaginal applicators or inserters should be used with caution after the seventh month of pregnancy.
Information For Patients
The doctor should advise the patient that in the event unusual local itching and burning occur, or other unusual symptoms develop, medication should be discontinued and not restarted without further consultation.
Drug Interactions
Drug interactions have not been documented with AVC.

Carcinogenesis, Mutagenesis, Impairment of Fertility
No data are available on long-term potential of AVC for carcinogenicity, mutagenicity, or impairment of fertility in animals or humans.
Pregnancy
Teratogenic Effects. Pregnancy Category C: Animal reproductive studies have been conducted with sulfonamides, including sulfanilamide (see below). It is not known whether AVC can cause fetal harm when administered to a pregnant woman or can affect reproductive capacity. AVC should be given to a pregnant woman only if clearly needed.
Sulfonamides, including sulfanilamide, readily pass through the placenta and reach fetal circulation. The concentration in the fetus is from 50–90% of that in the maternal blood and if high enough, can cause toxic effects. The safe use of sulfonamides, including sulfanilamide, in pregnancy has not been established. The teratogenic potential of most sulfonamides has not been thoroughly investigated in either animals or humans. However, a significant increase in the incidence of cleft palate and other bony abnormalities of offspring has been observed with certain sulfonamides of the short-, intermediate-, and long-acting types (including sulfanilamide) when given to pregnant rats and mice at high oral doses (seven to 25 times the human therapeutic oral dose).
Nursing Mothers
Sulfanilamide should be avoided in nursing mothers because absorbed sulfonamides will appear in maternal milk, and have caused kernicterus in the newborn. Because of the potential for serious adverse reactions in nursing infants from sulfonamides, a decision should be made whether to discontinue nursing or to discontinue the drug.
Pediatric Use
Safety and effectiveness of AVC in pediatric patients have not been established.

ADVERSE REACTIONS

Local sensitivity reactions such as increased discomfort or a burning sensation have occasionally been reported following the use of topical sulfonamides. With the use of AVC Cream, sensitivity reactions (only local) were reported for 0.2% of the investigational patients.
Treatment should be discontinued if either local or systemic manifestations of sulfonamide toxicity or sensitivity occur.

DRUG ABUSE AND DEPENDENCE

Tolerance, abuse, or dependence with AVC have not been reported.

OVERDOSAGE

There have been no reports of accidental overdosage with AVC.
The acute oral LD$_{50}$ of sulfanilamide is 3700–4200 mg/kg in mice.
The minimum human lethal dose of AVC has not been established.
It is not known if AVC is dialyzable.

DOSAGE AND ADMINISTRATION

One applicatorful (about 6 g) or one suppository intravaginally once or twice daily. Improvements in symptoms should occur within a few days, but treatment should be continued for a period of 30 days.
Douching with a suitable solution before insertion may be recommended for hygienic purposes.

HOW SUPPLIED

AVC Cream
NDC 0068-0099-04 4 oz tube with applicator
Store at room temperature, below 86°F. Protect from cold. Product darkens with age. Potency is maintained throughout labeled shelf life when stored as directed.
AVC Suppositories
NDC 0068-0098-16 Box of 16 white gelatin suppositories with inserter
Store at room temperature, below 86°F. Protect from excessive cold and moisture.
Prescribing information as of January 1995
Suppositories Manufactured by
R.P. Scherer, North America
Saint Petersburg, Florida 33716
for
Merrell Pharmaceuticals Inc.
Subsidiary of Hoechst Marion Roussel, Inc.
Kansas City, MO 64137

Continued on next page

Hoechst Marion Roussel—Cont.

BENTYL® ℞

[*běn'tĭl*]

(dicyclomine hydrochloride USP)

Prescribing Information as of April 1995

DESCRIPTION

BENTYL is an antispasmodic and anticholinergic (antimuscarinic) agent available in the following forms:

1. BENTYL capsules for oral use contain 10 mg dicyclomine hydrochloride USP. BENTYL 10 mg capsules also contain inactive ingredients: calcium sulfate, corn starch, FD&C Blue No. 1, FD&C Red No. 40, gelatin, lactose, magnesium stearate, pregelatinized corn starch, and titanium dioxide.
2. BENTYL tablets for oral use contain 20 mg dicyclomine hydrochloride USP. BENTYL 20 mg tablets also contain inactive ingredients: acacia, dibasic calcium phosphate, corn starch, FD&C Blue No. 1, lactose, magnesium stearate, pregelatinized corn starch, and sucrose.
3. BENTYL syrup for oral use contains 10 mg dicyclomine hydrochloride USP in each 5 mL (1 teaspoonful). BENTYL syrup also contains inactive ingredients: citric acid, D&C Red No. 33, FD&C Blue No. 1, FD&C Red No. 40, FD&C Yellow No. 6, flavors, glucose, methylparaben, propylene glycol, propylparaben, saccharin sodium, and water.
4. BENTYL Injection is a sterile, pyrogen-free, aqueous solution for intramuscular injection (NOT FOR INTRAVENOUS USE).

Ampul. 2 mL—Each mL contains 10 mg dicyclomine hydrochloride USP in sterile water for injection, made isotonic with sodium chloride.

Vial. 10 mL—Each mL contains 10 mg dicyclomine hydrochloride USP in sterile water for injection, made isotonic with sodium chloride. A preservative containing 0.5% chlorobutanol hydrous (chloral derivative) has been added.

Chemically, BENTYL (dicyclomine hydrochloride) is [bicyclohexyl]-1-carboxylic acid, 2-(diethylamino)ethylester, hydrochloride with the chemical structure:

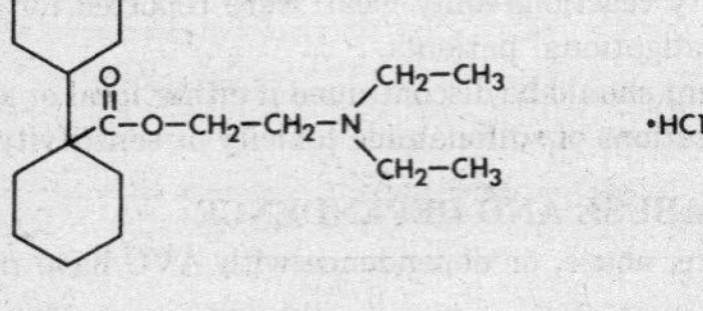

Dicyclomine hydrochloride occurs as a fine, white, crystalline, practically odorless powder with a bitter taste. It is soluble in water, freely soluble in alcohol and chloroform, and very slightly soluble in ether.

CLINICAL PHARMACOLOGY

Dicyclomine relieves smooth muscle spasm of the gastrointestinal tract. Animal studies indicate that this action is achieved via a dual mechanism: (1) a specific anticholinergic effect (antimuscarinic) at the acetylcholine-receptor sites with approximately $^1/_8$ the milligram potency of atropine (in vitro, guinea pig ileum); and (2) a direct effect upon smooth muscle (musculotropic) as evidenced by dicyclomine's antagonism of bradykinin- and histamine-induced spasms of the isolated guinea pig ileum. Atropine did not affect responses to these two agonists. In vivo studies in cats and dogs showed dicyclomine to be equally potent against acetylcholine (ACh)-or barium chloride ($BaCl_2$)-induced intestinal spasm while atropine was at least 200 times more potent against effects of ACh than $BaCl_2$. Tests for mydriatic effects in mice showed that dicyclomine was approximately 1/500 as potent as atropine; antisialagogue tests in rabbits showed dicyclomine to be 1/300 as potent as atropine.

In man, dicyclomine is rapidly absorbed after oral administration, reaching peak values within 60–90 minutes. The principal route of elimination is via the urine (79.5% of the dose). Excretion also occurs in the feces, but to a lesser extent (8.4%). Mean half-life of plasma elimination in one study was determined to be approximately 1.8 hours when plasma concentrations were measured for 9 hours after a single dose. In subsequent studies, plasma concentrations were followed for up to 24 hours after a single dose, showing a secondary phase of elimination with a somewhat longer half-life. Mean volume of distribution for a 20 mg oral dose is approximately 3.65 L/kg suggesting extensive distribution in tissues.

In controlled clinical trials involving over 100 patients who received drug, 82% of patients treated for functional bowel/irritable bowel syndrome with dicyclomine hydrochloride at initial doses of 160 mg daily (40 mg q.i.d.) demonstrated a favorable clinical response compared with 55% treated with placebo. ($P < .05$). In these trials, most of the side effects were typically anticholinergic in nature (see table) and were reported by 61% of the patients.

Side Effect	Dicyclomine Hydrochloride (40 mg q.i.d.) %	Placebo %
Dry Mouth	33	5
Dizziness	29	2
Blurred Vision	27	2
Nausea	14	6
Light-Headedness	11	3
Drowsiness	9	1
Weakness	7	1
Nervousness	6	2

Nine percent (9%) of patients were discontinued from the drug because of one or more of these side effects (compared with 2% in the placebo group). In 41% of the patients with side effects, side effects disappeared or were tolerated at the 160 mg daily dose without reduction. A dose reduction from 160 mg daily to an average daily dose of 90 mg was required in 46% of the patients with side effects who then continued to experience a favorable clinical response; their side effects either disappeared or were tolerated. (See ADVERSE REACTIONS.)

INDICATIONS AND USAGE

For the treatment of functional bowel/irritable bowel syndrome.

CONTRAINDICATIONS

1. Obstructive uropathy
2. Obstructive disease of the gastrointestinal tract
3. Severe ulcerative colitis (See PRECAUTIONS)
4. Reflux esophagitis
5. Unstable cardiovascular status in acute hemorrhage
6. Glaucoma
7. Myasthenia gravis
8. Evidence of prior hypersensitivity to dicyclomine hydrochloride or other ingredients of these formulations
9. Infants less than 6 months of age (See WARNINGS and PRECAUTIONS: Information for Patients.)
10. Nursing Mothers (See WARNINGS and PRECAUTIONS: Information for Patients.)

WARNINGS

In the presence of a high environmental temperature, heat prostration can occur with drug use (fever and heat stroke due to decreased sweating). If symptoms occur, the drug should be discontinued and supportive measures instituted.

Diarrhea may be an early symptom of incomplete intestinal obstruction, especially in patients with ileostomy or colostomy. In this instance, treatment with this drug would be inappropriate and possibly harmful.

BENTYL may produce drowsiness or blurred vision. The patient should be warned not to engage in activities requiring mental alertness, such as operating a motor vehicle or other machinery or performing hazardous work while taking this drug.

Psychosis has been reported in sensitive individuals given anticholinergic drugs. CNS signs and symptoms include confusion, disorientation, short-term memory loss, hallucinations, dysarthria, ataxia, coma, euphoria, decreased anxiety, fatigue, insomnia, agitation and mannerisms, and inappropriate affect.

These CNS signs and symptoms usually resolve within 12 to 24 hours after discontinuation of the drug.

There are reports that administration of dicyclomine hydrochloride syrup to infants has been followed by serious respiratory symptoms (dyspnea, shortness of breath, breathlessness, respiratory collapse, apnea, asphyxia), seizures, syncope, pulse rate fluctuations, muscular hypotonia, and coma. Death has been reported. No causal relationship between these effects observed in infants and dicyclomine administration has been established. BENTYL IS CONTRAINDICATED IN INFANTS LESS THAN 6 MONTHS OF AGE AND IN NURSING MOTHERS. (See CONTRAINDICATIONS and PRECAUTIONS: Nursing Mothers and Pediatric Use.)

Safety and efficacy of dicyclomine hydrochloride in pediatric patients have not been established.

PRECAUTIONS

General

Use with caution in patients with:

1. Autonomic neuropathy
2. Hepatic or renal disease
3. Ulcerative colitis-large doses may suppress intestinal motility to the point of producing a paralytic ileus and the use of this drug may precipitate or aggravate the serious complication of toxic megacolon (see CONTRAINDICATIONS)
4. Hyperthyroidism
5. Hypertension
6. Coronary heart disease
7. Congestive heart failure
8. Cardiac tachyarrhythmia
9. Hiatal hernia (see CONTRAINDICATIONS: reflux esophagitis)
10. Known or suspected prostatic hypertrophy.

Investigate any tachycardia before administration of dicyclomine hydrochloride since it may increase the heart rate.

With overdosage, a curare-like action may occur (i.e., neuromuscular blockade leading to muscular weakness and possible paralysis).

Information For Patients

BENTYL may produce drowsiness or blurred vision. The patient should be warned not to engage in activities requiring mental alertness, such as operating a motor vehicle or other machinery or to perform hazardous work while taking this drug.

BENTYL is contraindicated in infants less than 6 months of age and in nursing mothers. (See CONTRAINDICATIONS, WARNINGS, and PRECAUTIONS: Nursing Mothers and Pediatric Use.)

In the presence of a high environmental temperature, heat prostration can occur with drug use (fever and heat stroke due to decreased sweating). If symptoms occur, the drug should be discontinued and a physician contacted.

Drug Interactions

The following agents may increase certain actions or side effects of anticholinergic drugs: amantadine, antiarrhythmic agents of class I (e.g., quinidine), antihistamines, antipsychotic agents (e.g., phenothiazines), benzodiazepines, MAO inhibitors, narcotic analgesics (e.g., meperidine), nitrates and nitrites, sympathomimetic agents, tricyclic antidepressants, and other drugs having anticholinergic activity.

Anticholinergics antagonize the effects of antiglaucoma agents. Anticholinergic drugs in the presence of increased intraocular pressure may be hazardous when taken concurrently with agents such as corticosteroids. (See also CONTRAINDICATIONS.)

Anticholinergic agents may affect gastrointestinal absorption of various drugs, such as slowly dissolving dosage forms of digoxin; increased serum digoxin concentrations may result. Anticholinergic drugs may antagonize the effects of drugs that alter gastrointestinal motility, such as metoclopramide. Because antacids may interfere with the absorption of anticholinergic agents, simultaneous use of these drugs should be avoided.

The inhibiting effects of anticholinergic drugs on gastric hydrochloric acid secretion are antagonized by agents used to treat achlorhydria and those used to test gastric secretion.

Carcinogenesis, Mutagenesis, Impairment of Fertility

There are no known human data on long-term potential for carcinogenicity or mutagenicity.

Long-term studies in animals to determine carcinogenic potential are not known to have been conducted.

In studies in rats at doses of up to 100 mg/kg/day, BENTYL produced no deleterious effects on breeding, conception, or parturition.

Pregnancy

Teratogenic Effects. Pregnancy Category B. Reproduction studies have been performed in rats and rabbits at doses up to 33 times the maximum recommended human dose based on 160 mg/day (3 mg/kg) and have revealed no evidence of impaired fertility or harm to the fetus due to dicyclomine. Epidemiologic studies in pregnant women with products containing dicyclomine hydrochloride (at doses up to 40 mg/day) have not shown that dicyclomine increases the risk of fetal abnormalities if administered during the first trimester of pregnancy. There are, however, no adequate and well-controlled studies in pregnant women at the recommended doses (80–160 mg/day). Because animal reproduction studies are not always predictive of human response, BENTYL as indicated for functional bowel/irritable bowel syndrome should be used during pregnancy only if clearly needed.

Nursing Mothers

Since dicyclomine hydrochloride has been reported to be excreted in human milk, BENTYL IS CONTRAINDICATED IN NURSING MOTHERS. (See CONTRAINDICATIONS WARNINGS, PRECAUTIONS: Pediatric Use and ADVERSE REACTIONS.)

Pediatric Use

(See CONTRAINDICATIONS, WARNINGS, and PRECAUTIONS: Nursing Mothers.) BENTYL IS CONTRAINDICATED IN INFANTS LESS THAN 6 MONTHS OF AGE. Safety and effectiveness in pediatric patients have not been established.

ADVERSE REACTIONS

Controlled clinical trials have provided frequency information for reported adverse effects of dicyclomine hydrochloride listed in a decreasing order of frequency. (See CLINICAL PHARMACOLOGY.)

Not all of the following adverse reactions have been reported with dicyclomine hydrochloride. Adverse reactions are included here that have been reported for pharmacologically similar drugs with anticholinergic/antispasmodic action.

Gastrointestinal: dry mouth, nausea, vomiting, constipation, bloated feeling, abdominal pain, taste loss, anorexia

Central Nervous System: dizziness, light-headedness, tingling, headache, drowsiness, weakness, nervousness, numbness, mental confusion and/or excitement (especially in elderly persons), dyskinesia, lethargy, syncope, speech disturbance, insomnia
Ophthalmologic: blurred vision, diplopia, mydriasis, cycloplegia, increased ocular tension
Dermatologic/Allergic: rash, urticaria, itching, and other dermal manifestations; severe allergic reaction or drug idiosyncrasies including anaphylaxis
Genitourinary: urinary hesitancy, urinary retention
Cardiovascular: tachycardia, palpitations
Respiratory: Dyspnea, apnea, asphyxia (see WARNINGS)
Other: decreased sweating, nasal stuffiness or congestion, sneezing, throat congestion, impotence, suppression of lactation (see PRECAUTIONS: Nursing Mothers.)
With the injectable form, there may be temporary sensation of light-headedness. Some local irritation and focal coagulation necrosis may occur following the I.M. injection of the drug.

DRUG ABUSE AND DEPENDENCE

Tolerance, abuse, or dependence with BENTYL has not been reported.

OVERDOSAGE

Signs and Symptoms

The signs and symptoms of overdosage are headache; nausea; vomiting; blurred vision; dilated pupils; hot, dry skin; dizziness; dryness of the mouth; difficulty in swallowing; and CNS stimulation. A curare-like action may occur (i.e., neuromuscular blockade leading to muscular weakness and possible paralysis).

Oral LD_{50}

The acute oral LD_{50} of the drug is 625 mg/kg in mice.

Minimum Human Lethal Dose/Maximum Human Dose Recorded

The amount of drug in a single dose that is ordinarily associated with symptoms of overdosage or that is likely to be life-threatening, has not been defined. The maximum human oral dose recorded was 600 mg by mouth in a 10–month-old child and approximately 1500 mg in an adult, each of whom survived.

In three of the infants who died following administration of dicyclomine hydrochloride (see WARNINGS), the blood concentrations of drug were 200, 220, and 505 ng/mL, respectively.

Dialysis

It is not known if BENTYL is dialyzable.

Treatment

Treatment should consist of gastric lavage, emetics, and activated charcoal. Sedatives (e.g., short-acting barbiturates, benzodiazepines) may be used for management of overt signs of excitement. If indicated, an appropriate parenteral cholinergic agent may be used as an antidote.

DOSAGE AND ADMINISTRATION

DOSAGE MUST BE ADJUSTED TO INDIVIDUAL PATIENT NEEDS. (See CLINICAL PHARMACOLOGY.)

Adults—Oral. The only oral dose clearly shown to be effective is 160 mg per day (in equally divided doses). Since this dose is associated with a significant incidence of side effects, it is prudent to begin with 80 mg per day (in 4 equally divided doses). Depending upon the patient's response during the first week of therapy, the dose should be increased to 160 mg per day unless side effects limit dosage escalation.

If efficacy is not achieved within 2 weeks or side effects require doses below 80 mg per day, the drug should be discontinued. Documented safety data are not available for doses above 80 mg daily for periods longer than 2 weeks.

Adults—Intramuscular Injection. NOT FOR INTRAVENOUS USE.

The intramuscular dosage form is to be used temporarily when the patient cannot take oral medication. Intramuscular injection is about twice as bioavailable as oral dosage forms; consequently, the recommended intramuscular dose is 80 mg daily (in 4 equally divided doses).

Oral dicyclomine hydrochloride should be started as soon as possible and the intramuscular form should not be used for periods longer than 1 or 2 days.

ASPIRATE THE SYRINGE BEFORE INJECTING TO AVOID INTRAVASCULAR INJECTION, SINCE THROMBOSIS MAY OCCUR IF THE DRUG IS INADVERTENTLY INJECTED INTRAVASCULARLY. Parenteral drug products should be inspected visually for particulate matter and discoloration prior to administration, whenever solution and container permit.

HOW SUPPLIED

10 mg blue capsules, imprinted BENTYL 10
NDC 0068–0120–61: bottles of 100
Store at room temperature, preferably below 86°F (30°C).
20 mg compressed, light blue, round tablets, debossed BENTYL 20
NDC 0068–0123–61: bottles of 100
To prevent fading, avoid exposure to direct sunlight. Store at room temperature, preferably below 86°F (30°C).
10 mg/5mL pink syrup
NDC 0068–0125–16: 16 ounce bottle
Store at room temperature, preferably below 86°F (30°C). Protect from excessive heat.
10 mg/mL injection (for intramuscular use only, NOT FOR INTRAVENOUS USE)
NDC 0068–0810–61: 10 mL multiple dose vials
Store at room temperature, preferably below 86°F (30°C). Protect from freezing.
NDC 0068–0809–23: boxes of five 2 mL ampuls
Store at room temperature, preferably below 86°F (30°C). Protect from freezing.

Prescribing information as of April 1995
Merrell Pharmaceuticals Inc.
Subsidiary of Hoechst Marion Roussel, Inc.
Kansas City, MO 64137 USA

Shown in Product Identification Guide, page 316

BRICANYL® ℞
[*brĭk'ă-nĭl*]
(terbutaline sulfate USP)
Subcutaneous Injection

DESCRIPTION

Bricanyl (terbutaline sulfate USP) Subcutaneous Injection is a sterile isotonic solution. Each mL of solution contains 1 mg terbutaline sulfate (equivalent to 0.82 mg free base) and 8.9 mg sodium chloride in water for injection. Hydrochloric acid is used to adjust pH to 3–5. Filled under nitrogen.

Terbutaline sulfate (5-[2-[(1,1-dimethylethyl)amino]-1-hydroxyethyl]-1,3-benzenediol sulfate) is a β-adrenergic agonist bronchodilator having the chemical structure:

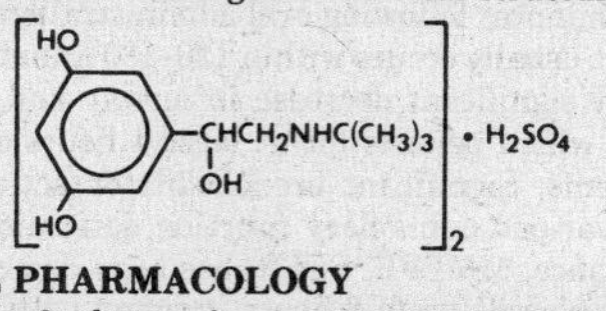

CLINICAL PHARMACOLOGY

Bricanyl is a β-adrenergic receptor agonist which has been shown by *in vitro* and *in vivo* pharmacologic studies in animals to exert a preferential effect on β_2-adrenergic receptors, such as those located in bronchial smooth muscle. However, controlled clinical studies of patients who were administered the drug have not revealed a preferential β_2-adrenergic effect.

It has been postulated that β-adrenergic agonists produce many of their pharmacologic effects by activation of adenyl cyclase, the enzyme which catalyzes the conversion of adenosine triphosphate to cyclic adenosine monophosphate.

Bricanyl Injection has been shown in controlled clinical studies to relieve acute bronchospasm in acute and chronic obstructive pulmonary disease, resulting in a clinically significant increase in pulmonary flow rates, e.g., an increase of 15% or greater in FEV_1 in some patients. Following administration of 0.25 mg by subcutaneous injection, a measurable change in flow rate is usually observed within five minutes, and a clinically significant increase in FEV_1 occurs by 15 minutes following the injection. The maximum effect usually occurs within 30–60 minutes and clinically significant bronchodilator activity has been observed to persist for 90 minutes to four hours in most patients. The duration of clinically significant improvement is comparable to that found with equimilligram doses of epinephrine.

Subcutaneously administered Bricanyl shows peak plasma concentrations 15–30 minutes after injection (0.5 mg dose, mean peak plasma level 7.6 μg/L). Approximately one-third is metabolized (inactive), the majority of the dose being excreted in urine unchanged. A half-life of 3–4 hours has been reported.

Terbutaline crosses the placenta. After single dose IV administration of terbutaline to 22 women in late pregnancy who were delivered by elective Caesarean section due to clinical reasons, umbilical blood levels of terbutaline were found to range from 11 to 48% of the maternal blood levels.

Recent studies in laboratory animals (minipigs, rodents, and dogs) recorded the occurrence of cardiac arrhythmias and sudden death (with histologic evidence of myocardial necrosis) when β agonists and methylxanthines were administered concurrently. The significance of these findings when applied to humans is currently unknown.

INDICATIONS AND USAGE

Bricanyl is indicated as a bronchodilator for the relief of reversible bronchospasm in patients with obstructive airway diseases such as asthma, bronchitis and emphysema.

CONTRAINDICATIONS

Bricanyl is contraindicated in patients with a history of hypersensitivity to any of its components or sympathomimetic amines.

WARNINGS

Usage in Labor and Delivery: Bricanyl is not indicated and should not be used for the management of preterm labor. Serious adverse reactions have been reported following administration of terbutaline sulfate to women in labor. These reports have included transient hypokalemia, pulmonary edema (sometimes after delivery) and hypoglycemia in the mother and/or the neonatal child. Maternal death has been reported with terbutaline sulfate and other drugs of this class.

There have been rare reports of seizures occurring in patients receiving terbutaline, which do not recur when the drug is discontinued and have not been explained on any other basis.

PRECAUTIONS

General

Terbutaline sulfate is a sympathomimetic amine and as such should be used with caution in patients with cardiovascular disorders (including arrhythmias, coronary insufficiency and hypertension), in patients with hyperthyroidism or diabetes mellitus, history of seizures, or in patients who are unusually responsive to sympathomimetic amines. Age-related differences in the hemodynamic response to β-adrenergic receptor stimulation have been reported.

Patients susceptible to hypokalemia should be monitored because transient early falls in serum potassium levels have been reported with β agonists.

Immediate hypersensitivity reactions and exacerbation of bronchospasm have been reported after terbutaline administration.

Preparation of Other Dosage Forms: Use of the subcutaneous injection for preparation of other dosage forms, e.g., IV infusion, is not appropriate. Sterility, stability, and accurate dosing cannot be assured if the ampuls are not used in accordance with information in DOSAGE AND ADMINISTRATION.

Large doses of intravenous terbutaline sulfate have been reported to aggravate preexisting diabetes and ketoacidosis.

Information for Patients

Patients should be advised regarding the potential adverse reactions associated with Bricanyl.

Drug Interactions

Other sympathomimetic bronchodilators or epinephrine should not be used concomitantly with terbutaline sulfate since their combined effect on the cardiovascular system may be deleterious to the patient.

Terbutaline sulfate should be administered with caution in patients being treated with monoamine oxidase (MAO) inhibitors or tricyclic antidepressants, since the action of terbutaline sulfate on the vascular system may be potentiated.

β-adrenergic receptor blocking agents not only block the pulmonary effect of terbutaline but may produce severe asthmatic attacks in asthmatic patients. Therefore, patients requiring treatment for both bronchospastic disease and hypertension should be treated with medication other than β-adrenergic blocking agents for hypertension.

Carcinogenesis, Mutagenesis, Impairment of Fertility

A 2 year, oral carcinogenesis bioassay of terbutaline sulfate (50, 500, 1000, and 2000 mg/kg, corresponding to 5,000, 50,000, 100,000, and 200,000 times the recommended daily adult subcutaneous dose, respectively) in the Sprague-Dawley rat revealed drug-related changes in the female genital system. Females showed dose-related increases in leiomyomas of the mesovarium: 3 (5%) at 50 mg/kg, 17 (28%) at 500 mg/kg, 21 (35%) at 1000 mg/kg, and 23 (38%) at 2000 mg/kg, which were significant at the three highest levels. None occurred in female controls. The incidence of ovarian cysts was significantly elevated at all dose levels except at 2000 mg/kg and hyperplasia of the mesovarium was increased significantly at 500 and 2000 mg/kg. A 21-month oral study of terbutaline sulfate (5, 50 and 200 mg/kg, corresponding to 500, 5,000 and 20,000 times the recommended daily adult subcutaneous dose, respectively) in the mouse revealed no evidence of carcinogenicity.

Studies of terbutaline sulfate have not been conducted to determine mutagenic potential.

An oral reproduction study of terbutaline sulfate up to 50 mg/kg (corresponding to 5,000 times the human subcutaneous dose) in the rat revealed no adverse effects on fertility.

Pregnancy

Teratogenic Effects

Pregnancy Category B: Reproduction studies in mice (up to 1.1 mg/kg subcutaneously, corresponding to 110 times the human subcutaneous dose) and in rats and rabbits (up to 50 mg/kg orally, corresponding to 5,000 times the human subcutaneous dose) have revealed no evidence of impaired fertility or harm to the fetus due to terbutaline. There are, however, no adequate and well-controlled studies in pregnant women. Because animal reproduction studies are not always predictive of human response, this drug should be used during pregnancy only if clearly needed.

Continued on next page

Hoechst Marion Roussel—Cont.

Labor and Delivery
Usage in Labor and Delivery: The safe use of Bricanyl for the management of preterm labor or for other uses during labor and delivery has not been established and the drug should not be used. (See WARNINGS.)
Nursing Mothers
Terbutaline is excreted in breast milk. Caution should be exercised when Bricanyl is administered to a nursing woman.
Pediatric Use
Safety and effectiveness in children below the age of 12 have not been established.

ADVERSE REACTIONS

The adverse reactions of terbutaline sulfate are similar to those of other sympathomimetic agents.
The most commonly observed side effects are tremor and nervousness. These occur more frequently at doses in excess of 0.25 mg. Other commonly reported reactions include increased heart rate, palpitations and dizziness. Other reported reactions include headache, drowsiness, vomiting, nausea, sweating, and muscle cramps. These reactions are generally transient and usually do not require treatment. There have been rare reports of elevations in liver enzymes and of hypersensitivity vasculitis.

OVERDOSAGE

Overdosage information is limited. Excessive adrenergic-receptor stimulation may augment the signs and symptoms listed under ADVERSE REACTIONS and may be accompanied by other adrenergic effects.
Signs and symptoms of overdosage may include the following—
CARDIOVASCULAR: tachycardia of varying degrees, transient arrhythmias, and extrasystoles. A significant drop in blood pressure may occur due to peripheral vasodilation.
NEUROMUSCULAR: tremors of varying degrees, nervousness, drowsiness, muscle cramps, headache, and sweating.
GASTROINTESTINAL: nausea and vomiting.
ENDOCRINE: varying degrees of hyperglycemia and rise in insulin levels which could be followed by rebound hypoglycemia. Hypokalemia in the early stages may occur. The duration of these signs and symptoms will be dependent on the degree of overdosage.
In the case of terbutaline overdosage, the patient should be treated symptomatically for sympathomimetic overdosage with careful consideration to the appropriateness of any chosen therapy and possible effect on the patient's underlying disease state. (See also WARNINGS.)
Studies in mice, rats, rabbits, and dogs have established the LD_{50} of terbutaline to be 1–9 g/kg orally and 0.3–1.6 g/kg subcutaneously.
It is not known whether terbutaline is dialyzable.

DOSAGE AND ADMINISTRATION

Parenteral drug products should be inspected visually for particulate matter and discoloration prior to administration, whenever solution and container permit.
The usual subcutaneous dose of Bricanyl is 0.25 mg (0.25 mL, ¼ ampul contents) injected into the lateral deltoid area. If significant clinical improvement does not occur by 15–30 minutes, a second dose of 0.25 mg may be administered. A total dose of 0.5 mg should not be exceeded within a four-hour period. If a patient fails to respond to a second 0.25 mg (0.25 mL) dose within 15–30 minutes, other therapeutic measures should be considered.

HOW SUPPLIED

Each 2 mL size ampul contains 1 mL of solution (1 mg terbutaline sulfate). Note: 0.25 mL of solution will provide the usual clinical dose of 0.25 mg.
NDC 0068-0702-20: package of 10 ampuls
Solutions of terbutaline sulfate are sensitive to excessive heat and light. Ampuls should, therefore, be stored at controlled room temperature 15°–30°C (59°–86°F) in their original carton to provide protection from light until dispensed. Solutions should not be used if discolored.

Product Information as of August, 1992

Manufactured for
Merrell Pharmaceuticals Inc.
Subsidiary of Hoechst Marion Roussel, Inc.
Kansas City, MO 64137

Shown in Product Identification Guide, page 317

BRICANYL® ℞

[brĭk'ă-nĭl]
(terbutaline sulfate USP)
Tablets

DESCRIPTION

BRICANYL (terbutaline sulfate USP) Tablets for oral administration contain 2.5 or 5 mg of terbutaline sulfate (equivalent to 2.05 and 4.1 mg free base, respectively). Both the 2.5 and 5 mg tablets contain the following inactive ingredients: corn starch (or pregelatinized corn starch), lactose, magnesium stearate, microcrystalline cellulose, and povidone.
Terbutaline sulfate (5-[2-[(1,1-dimethylethyl)amino]-1-hydroxyethyl]-1,3-benzenediol sulfate) is a β-adrenergic agonist bronchodilator having the chemical structure:

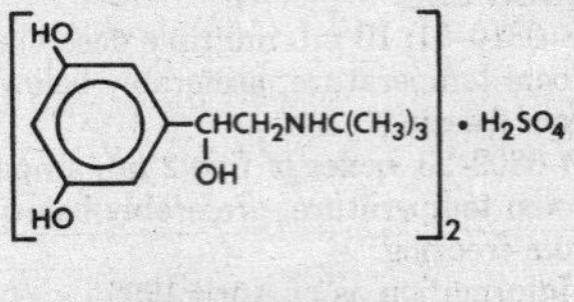

CLINICAL PHARMACOLOGY

BRICANYL is a β-adrenergic receptor agonist which has been shown by *in vitro* and *in vivo* pharmacologic studies in animals to exert a preferential effect on β_2-adrenergic receptors, such as those located in bronchial smooth muscle. However, controlled clinical studies on patients who were administered the drug have not revealed a preferential β_2-adrenergic effect.
It has been postulated that β-adrenergic agonists produce many of their pharmacologic effects by activation of adenyl cyclase, the enzyme which catalyzes the conversion of adenosine triphosphate to cyclic adenosine monophosphate.
BRICANYL Tablets have been shown in controlled clinical studies to relieve bronchospasm in chronic obstructive pulmonary disease, such as asthma, chronic bronchitis, and emphysema. This action was manifested by a clinically significant increase in pulmonary function as demonstrated by an increase of 15% or greater in FEV_1 in some patients. A measurable change in pulmonary function usually occurs within 30 minutes following oral administration. The maximum effect usually occurs within 120–180 minutes. There is a clinically significant decrease in airway and pulmonary resistance which persists for at least 4 hours or longer in most patients. Significant bronchodilator action, as measured by various pulmonary function determinations (airway resistance, MMEFR, PEFR) has been demonstrated in studies for periods up to 8 hours in many patients.
Clinical studies have evaluated the effectiveness of oral BRICANYL for periods up to 12 months and the drug continued to produce significant improvement of pulmonary function throughout the period of treatment.
Orally administered terbutaline sulfate is 30–70% absorbed in the GI tract (food reduces bioavailability by one-third). Sixty percent of the absorbed oral dose is metabolized via first pass conjugation in the gut wall and liver. There are no known active metabolites. After single oral doses, peak concentrations are found 30 minutes to 5 hours after administration. Each mg of orally administered terbutaline sulfate (in fasting adults) produces an average peak serum concentration of approximately 1 μg/L. Terbutaline has a half-life of 3–4 hours and is excreted in the urine.
Terbutaline crosses the placenta. After single dose IV administration of terbutaline to 22 women in late pregnancy who were delivered by elective Caesarean section due to clinical reasons, umbilical blood levels of terbutaline were found to range from 11 to 48% of the maternal blood levels.
Recent studies in laboratory animals (minipigs, rodents, and dogs) recorded the occurrence of cardiac arrhythmias and sudden death (with histologic evidence of myocardial necrosis) when β agonists and methylxanthines were administered concurrently. The significance of these findings when applied to humans is currently unknown.

INDICATIONS AND USAGE

BRICANYL is indicated as a bronchodilator for the relief of reversible bronchospasm in patients with obstructive airway diseases, such as asthma, bronchitis, and emphysema.

CONTRAINDICATIONS

BRICANYL is contraindicated in patients with a history of hypersensitivity to any of its components or sympathomimetic amines.

WARNINGS

Usage in Labor and Delivery. BRICANYL is not indicated and should not be used for the management of preterm labor. Serious adverse reactions have been reported following administration of terbutaline sulfate to women in labor. These reports have included transient hypokalemia, pulmonary edema (sometimes after delivery), and hypoglycemia in the mother and/or the neonatal child. Maternal death has been reported with terbutaline sulfate and other drugs of this class.
There have been rare reports of seizures occurring in patients receiving terbutaline, which do not recur when the drug is discontinued and have not been explained on any other basis.

PRECAUTIONS

General
Terbutaline sulfate is a sympathomimetic amine and as such should be used with caution in patients with cardiovascular disorders (including arrhythmias, coronary insufficiency, and hypertension), in patients with hyperthyroidism or diabetes mellitus, history of seizures, or in patients who are unusually responsive to sympathomimetic amines. Age-related differences in the hemodynamic response to β-adrenergic receptor stimulation have been reported.
Patients susceptible to hypokalemia should be monitored because transient early falls in serum potassium levels have been reported with β agonists.
Large doses of intravenous terbutaline sulfate have been reported to aggravate preexisting diabetes and ketoacidosis. The relevance of this observation to the use of BRICANYL Tablets is unknown.
Immediate hypersensitivity reactions and exacerbation of bronchospasm have been reported after terbutaline administration.

Information for Patients
The patient should be advised regarding the potential adverse reactions associated with BRICANYL and that: (1) the action of BRICANYL Tablets may last up to 8 hours and, therefore, should not be used more frequently than recommended, (2) the number or frequency of doses should not be increased without medical consultation, (3) medical consultation should be sought promptly if symptoms get worse, and (4) other medicines should not be used while taking BRICANYL without consulting the physician.

Drug Interactions
Other sympathomimetic bronchodilators or epinephrine should not be used concomitantly with terbutaline sulfate, since their combined effect on the cardiovascular system may be deleterious to the patient. This recommendation does not preclude the judicious use of an aerosol bronchodilator of the adrenergic stimulant type in patients receiving BRICANYL Tablets.
Such concomitant use, however, should be individualized and not given on a routine basis. If regular coadministration is required, alternative therapy should be considered. Terbutaline sulfate should be administered with caution in patients being treated with monoamine oxidase (MAO) inhibitors or tricyclic antidepressants, since the action of terbutaline sulfate on the vascular system may be potentiated.
β-Adrenergic receptor blocking agents not only block the pulmonary effect of terbutaline, but may produce severe asthmatic attacks in asthmatic patients. Therefore, patients requiring treatment for both bronchospastic disease and hypertension should be treated with medication other than β-adrenergic blocking agents for hypertension.

Carcinogenesis, Mutagenesis, Impairment of Fertility
A 2-year, oral carcinogenesis bioassay of terbutaline sulfate (50, 500, 1000 and 2000 mg/kg, corresponding to 167, 1667, 3333, and 6667 times the recommended daily adult oral dose, respectively) in the Sprague-Dawley rat revealed drug-related changes in the female genital system. Females showed dose-related increases in leiomyomas of the mesovarium: 3 (5%) at 50 mg/kg, 17 (28%) at 500 mg/kg, 21 (35%) at 1000 mg/kg, and 23 (38%) at 2000 mg/kg, which were significant at the three highest levels. None occurred in female controls. The incidence of ovarian cysts was significantly elevated at all dose levels except at 2000 mg/kg and hyperplasia of the mesovarium was increased significantly at 500 and 2000 mg/kg. A 21-month oral study of terbutaline sulfate (5, 50 and 200 mg/kg, corresponding to 17, 167 and 667 times the recommended daily adult oral dose, respectively) in the mouse revealed no evidence of carcinogenicity.
Studies of terbutaline sulfate have not been conducted to determine mutagenic potential.
An oral reproduction study of terbutaline sulfate up to 50 mg/kg (corresponding to 167 times the human oral dose) in the rat revealed no adverse effects on fertility.

Pregnancy
Teratogenic Effects. Pregnancy Category B: Reproduction studies in mice (up to 1.1 mg/kg subcutaneously, corresponding to four times the human oral dose) and in rats and rabbits (up to 50 mg/kg orally, corresponding to 167 times the human oral dose) have revealed no evidence of impaired fertility or harm to the fetus due to terbutaline. There are, however, no adequate and well-controlled studies in pregnant women. Because animal reproduction studies are not always predictive of human response, this drug should be used during pregnancy only if clearly needed.

Labor and Delivery
Usage in Labor and Delivery. The safe use of BRICANYL for the mangement of preterm labor or for other uses during labor and delivery has not been established and the drug should not be used. (See WARNINGS.)

Nursing Mothers
Terbutaline is excreted in breast milk. Caution should be exercised when BRICANYL is administered to a nursing woman.

Pediatric Use

Safety and effectiveness in children below the age of 12 have not been established.

ADVERSE REACTIONS

The adverse reactions of terbutaline sulfate are similar to those of other sympathomimetic agents.

The most commonly observed side effects are tremor and nervousness. The frequency of these side effects appear to diminish with continued therapy. Other commonly reported reactions include increased heart rate, palpitations, and dizziness. Other reported reactions include headache, drowsiness, vomiting, nausea, sweating, and muscle cramps. These reactions are generally transient and usually do not require treatment.

There have been rare reports of elevations in liver enzymes and of hypersensitivity vasculitis.

OVERDOSAGE

Overdosage information is limited. Excessive adrenergic-receptor stimulation may augment the signs and symptoms listed under ADVERSE REACTIONS and may be accompanied by other adrenergic effects.

Signs and symptoms of overdosage may include the following:

Cardiovascular: tachycardia of varying degrees, transient arrhythmias, and extrasystoles. A significant drop in blood pressure may occur due to peripheral vasodilation.
Neuromuscular: tremors of varying degrees, nervousness, drowsiness, muscle cramps, headache, and sweating.
Gastrointestinal: nausea and vomiting.
Endocrine: varying degrees of hyperglycemia and rise in insulin levels which could be followed by rebound hypoglycemia. Hypokalemia in the early stages may occur. The duration of these sign and symptoms will be dependent on the degree of overdosage.

Treat the alert patient who has taken excessive oral medication by emptying the stomach by means of induced emesis, followed by gastric lavage. In the unconscious patient, secure the airway with a cuffed endotracheal tube before beginning lavage (do not induce emesis). Instillation of activated charcoal slurry may help reduce absorption of terbutaline sulfate. Maintain adequate respiratory exchange. Provide cardiac and respiratory support as needed. Continue observation until symptom-free.

Careful consideration should be given to the appropriateness of any chosen therapy and possible effect on the patient's underlying disease state. (See also WARNINGS.) Studies in mice, rats, rabbits, and dogs have established the LD_{50} of terbutaline to be 1–9 g/kg orally and 0.3–1.6 g/kg subcutaneously.

It is not known whether terbutaline is dialyzable.

DOSAGE AND ADMINISTRATION

Adults. Usual dose is 5 mg three times daily. Dosing may be initiated at 2.5 mg three or four times daily and titrated upward depending on clinical response. A total dose of 15 mg in a 24-hour period should not be exceeded.

Children. (12–15 yrs). 2.5 mg three times daily.

If a previously effective dosage regimen fails to provide the usual relief, medical advice should be sought immediately as this is often a sign of seriously worsening asthma which would require reassessment of therapy.

HOW SUPPLIED

2.5 mg tablets (*round, white, debossed "BRICANYL 2½"*):
NDC 0068-0725-61: Bottle of 100
5.0 mg tablets (*square, white, scored, debossed "BRICANYL 5"*):
NDC 0068-0750-61: Bottle of 100
Store at controlled room temperature 15°–30°C (59°–86°F).
Prescribing Information as of August 1992
Merrell Pharmaceuticals Inc.
Subsidiary of Hoechst Marion Roussel, Inc.
Kansas City, MO 64137
Shown in Product Identification Guide, page 317

CARAFATE® Tablets
[kär'afāt]
(sucralfate)
Prescribing Information as of January 1996

DESCRIPTION

CARAFATE (sucralfate) is an α-D-glucopyranoside, β-D-fructofuranosyl-, octakis-(hydrogen sulfate), aluminum complex.
[See chemical structure at top of next column.]

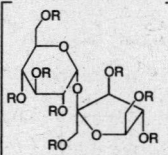

$[Al(OH)_3]_x [H_2O]_y$
(x = 8 to 10 and y = 22 to 31)

$R = SO_3Al(OH)_2$

Tablets for oral administration contain 1 g of sucralfate. Also contain: D&C Red #30 Lake, FD&C Blue #1 Lake, magnesium stearate, microcrystalline cellulose, and starch. Therapeutic category: antiulcer.

CLINICAL PHARMACOLOGY

Sucralfate is only minimally absorbed from the gastrointestinal tract. The small amounts of the sulfated disaccharide that are absorbed are excreted primarily in the urine. Although the mechanism of sucralfate's ability to accelerate healing of duodenal ulcers remains to be fully defined, it is known that it exerts its effect through a local, rather than systemic, action. The following observations also appear pertinent:

1. Studies in human subjects and with animal models of ulcer disease have shown that sucralfate forms an ulcer-adherent complex with proteinaceous exudate at the ulcer site.
2. In vitro, a sucralfate-albumin film provides a barrier to diffusion of hydrogen ions.
3. In human subjects, sucralfate given in doses recommended for ulcer therapy inhibits pepsin activity in gastric juice by 32%.
4. In vitro, sucralfate adsorbs bile salts.

These observations suggest that sucralfate's antiulcer activity is the result of formation of an ulcer-adherent complex that covers the ulcer site and protects it against further attack by acid, pepsin, and bile salts. There are approximately 14 to 16 mEq of acid-neutralizing capacity per 1-g dose of sucralfate.

CLINICAL TRIALS

Acute Duodenal Ulcer
Over 600 patients have participated in well-controlled clinical trials worldwide. Multicenter trials conducted in the United States, both of them placebo-controlled studies with endoscopic evaluation at 2 and 4 weeks, showed:

STUDY 1

Treatment Groups	Ulcer Healing/No. Patients	
	2 wk	4 wk (Overall)
Sucralfate	37/105 (35.2%)	82/109 (75.2%)
Placebo	26/106 (24.5%)	68/107 (63.6%)

STUDY 2

Treatment Groups	Ulcer Healing/No. Patients	
	2 wk	4 wk (Overall)
Sucralfate	8/24 (33%)	22/24 (92%)
Placebo	4/31 (13%)	18/31 (58%)

The sucralfate-placebo differences were statistically significant in both studies at 4 weeks but not at 2 weeks. The poorer result in the first study may have occurred because sucralfate was given 2 hours after meals and at bedtime rather than 1 hour before meals and at bedtime, the regimen used in international studies and in the second United States study. In addition, in the first study liquid antacid was utilized as needed, whereas in the second study antacid tablets were used.

Maintenance Therapy After Healing of Duodenal Ulcer
Two double-blind randomized placebo-controlled U.S. multicenter trials have demonstrated that sucralfate (1 g bid) is effective as maintenance therapy following healing of duodenal ulcers.

In one study, endoscopies were performed monthly for 4 months. Of the 254 patients who enrolled, 239 were analyzed in the intention-to-treat life table analysis presented below.

Duodenal Ulcer Recurrence Rate (%)

Drug	n	Months of Therapy			
		1	2	3	4
CARAFATE	122	20*	30*	38†	42†
Placebo	117	33	46	55	63

*P < 0.05, †P < 0.01
In this study, prn antacids were not permitted.

In the other study, scheduled endoscopies were performed at 6 and 12 months, but for–cause endoscopies were permitted as symptoms dictated. Median symptom scores between the sucralfate and placebo groups were not significantly differ-

---

ent. A life table intention-to-treat analysis for the 94 patients enrolled in the trial had the following results:

Duodenal Ulcer Recurrence Rate (%)

Drug	n	6 months	12 months
CARAFATE	48	19*	27*
Placebo	46	54	65

*P < 0.002
In this study, prn antacids were permitted.

Data from placebo-controlled studies longer than 1 year are not available.

INDICATIONS AND USAGE

CARAFATE® (sucralfate) is indicated in:
• Short-term treatment (up to 8 weeks) of active duodenal ulcer. While healing with sucralfate may occur during the first week or two, treatment should be continued for 4 to 8 weeks unless healing has been demonstrated by x-ray or endoscopic examination.
• Maintenance therapy for duodenal ulcer patients at reduced dosage after healing of acute ulcers.

CONTRAINDICATIONS

There are no known contraindications to the use of sucralfate.

PRECAUTIONS

Duodenal ulcer is a chronic, recurrent disease. While short-term treatment with sucralfate can result in complete healing of the ulcer, a successful course of treatment with sucralfate should not be expected to alter the posthealing frequency or severity of duodenal ulceration.
Special Populations: Chronic Renal Failure and Dialysis Patients
When sucralfate is administered orally, small amounts of aluminum are absorbed from the gastrointestinal tract. Concomitant use of sucralfate with other products that contain aluminum, such as aluminum-containing antacids, may increase the total body burden of aluminum. Patients with normal renal function receiving the recommended doses of sucralfate and aluminum-containing products adequately excrete aluminum in the urine. Patients with chronic renal failure or those receiving dialysis have impaired excretion of absorbed aluminum. In addition, aluminum does not cross dialysis membranes because it is bound to albumin and transferrin plasma proteins. Aluminum accumulation and toxicity (aluminum osteodystrophy, osteomalacia, encephalopathy) have been described in patients with renal impairment. Sucralfate should be used with caution in patients with chronic renal failure.
Drug Interactions
Some studies have shown that simultaneous sucralfate administration in healthy volunteers reduced the extent of absorption (bioavailability) of single doses of the following: cimetidine, digoxin, fluoroquinolone antibiotics, ketoconazole, l-thyroxine, phenytoin, quinidine, ranitidine, tetracycline, and theophylline. Subtherapeutic prothrombin times with concomitant warfarin and sucralfate therapy have been reported in spontaneous and published case reports. However, two clinical studies have demonstrated no change in either serum warfarin concentration or prothrombin time with the addition of sucralfate to chronic warfarin therapy. The mechanism of these interactions appears to be nonsystemic in nature, presumably resulting from sucralfate binding to the concomitant agent in the gastrointestinal tract. In all cases studied to date (cimetidine, ciprofloxacin, digoxin, norfloxacin, ofloxacin, and ranitidine), dosing the concomitant medication 2 hours before sucralfate eliminated the interaction. Because of the potential of CARAFATE to alter the absorption of some drugs, CARAFATE should be administered separately from other drugs when alterations in bioavailability are felt to be critical. In these cases, patients should be monitored appropriately.
Carcinogenesis, Mutagenesis, Impairment of Fertility
Chronic oral toxicity studies of 24 months' duration were conducted in mice and rats at doses up to 1 g/kg (12 times the human dose). There was no evidence of drug-related tumorigenicity. A reproduction study in rats at doses up to 38 times the human dose did not reveal any indication of fertility impairment. Mutagenicity studies were not conducted.
Pregnancy
Teratogenic effects. Pregnancy Category B. Teratogenicity studies have been performed in mice, rats, and rabbits at doses up to 50 times the human dose and have revealed no evidence of harm to the fetus due to sucralfate. There are, however, no adequate and well-controlled studies in pregnant women. Because animal reproduction studies are not always predictive of human response, this drug should be used during pregnancy only if clearly needed.

Continued on next page

Hoechst Marion Roussel—Cont.

Nursing Mothers
It is not known whether this drug is excreted in human milk. Because many drugs are excreted in human milk, caution should be exercised when sucralfate is administered to a nursing woman.

Pediatric Use
Safety and effectiveness in pediatric patients have not been established.

ADVERSE REACTIONS
Adverse reactions to sucralfate in clinical trials were minor and only rarely led to discontinuation of the drug. In studies involving over 2700 patients treated with sucralfate tablets, adverse effects were reported in 129 (4.7%).
Constipation was the most frequent complaint (2%). Other adverse effects reported in less than 0.5% of the patients are listed below by body system:
Gastrointestinal: diarrhea, nausea, vomiting, gastric discomfort, indigestion, flatulence, dry mouth
Dermatological: pruritus, rash
Nervous System: dizziness, insomnia, sleepiness, vertigo
Other: back pain, headache
Postmarketing reports of hypersensitivity reactions, including urticaria (hives), angioedema, respiratory difficulty, rhinitis laryngospasm, and facial swelling have been reported in patients receiving sucralfate tablets. Similar events were reported with sucralfate suspension. However, a causal relationship has not been established.
Bezoars have been reported in patients treated with sucralfate. The majority of patients had underlying medical conditions that may predispose to bezoar formation (such as delayed gastric emptying) or were receiving concomitant enteral tube feedings.
Inadvertent injection of insoluble sucralfate and its insoluble excipients has led to fatal complications, including pulmonary and cerebral emboli. Sucralfate is not intended for intravenous administration.

OVERDOSAGE
Due to limited experience in humans with overdosage of sucralfate, no specific treatment recommendations can be given. Acute oral toxicity studies in animals, however, using doses up to 12 g/kg body weight, could not find a lethal dose. Sucralfate is only minimally absorbed from the gastrointestinal tract. Risks associated with acute overdosage should, therefore, be minimal. In rare reports describing sucralfate overdose, most patients remained asymptomatic. Those few reports where adverse events were described included symptoms of dyspepsia, abdominal pain, nausea, and vomiting.

DOSAGE AND ADMINISTRATION
Active Duodenal Ulcer: The recommended adult oral dosage for duodenal ulcer is 1 g four times a day on an empty stomach.
Antacids may be prescribed as needed for relief of pain but should not be taken within one-half hour before or after sucralfate.
While healing with sucralfate may occur during the first week or two, treatment should be continued for 4 to 8 weeks unless healing has been demonstrated by x-ray or endoscopic examination.
Maintenance Therapy: The recommended adult oral dosage is 1 g twice a day.

HOW SUPPLIED
CARAFATE (sucralfate) 1g tablets are supplied in bottles of 100 (NDC 0088-1712-47), 120 (NDC 0088-1712-53), and 500 (NDC 0088-1712-55) and in Unit Dose Identification Paks of 100 (NDC 0088-1712-49). Light pink scored oblong tablets are embossed with CARAFATE on one side and 1712 on the other.
Hoechst Marion Roussel, Inc.
Kansas City, MO 64137 USA
Shown in Product Identification Guide, page 317

CARAFATE® ℞
[*kär'afāt*]
(sucralfate)
Suspension
Prescribing Information as of January 1995

DESCRIPTION
CARAFATE (sucralfate) is an α-D-glucopyranoside, β-D-fructofuranosyl-, octakis-(hydrogen sulfate), aluminum complex.
[See chemical structure at top of next column.]

CARAFATE Suspension for oral administration contains 1 g of sucralfate per 10 mL.
CARAFATE Suspension also contains: colloidal silicon dioxide NF, FD&C Red #40, flavor, glycerin USP, methylcellulose USP, methylparaben NF, microcrystalline cellulose NF,

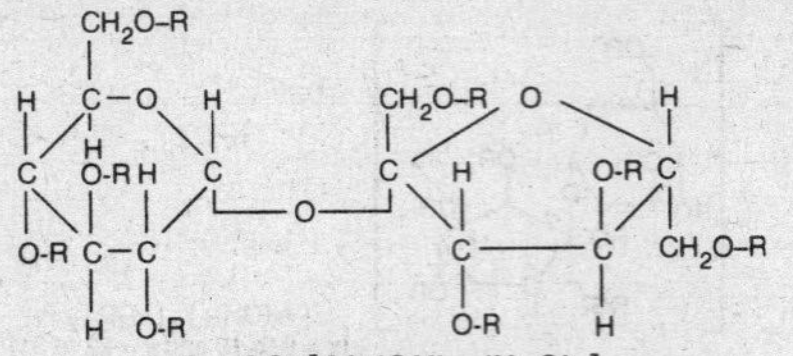

$R = SO_3[Al_2(OH)_5 \cdot (H_2O)_2]$

purified water USP, simethicone USP, and sorbitol solution USP.
Therapeutic category: antiulcer.

CLINICAL PHARMACOLOGY
Sucralfate is only minimally absorbed from the gastrointestinal tract. The small amounts of the sulfated disaccharide that are absorbed are excreted primarily in the urine.
Although the mechanism of sucralfate's ability to accelerate healing of duodenal ulcers remains to be fully defined, it is known that it exerts its effect through a local, rather than systemic, action. The following observations also appear pertinent:
1. Studies in human subjects and with animal models of ulcer disease have shown that sucralfate forms an ulcer-adherent complex with proteinaceous exudate at the ulcer site.
2. In vitro, a sucralfate-albumin film provides a barrier to diffusion of hydrogen ions.
3. In human subjects, sucralfate given in doses recommended for ulcer therapy inhibits pepsin activity in gastric juice by 32%.
4. In vitro, sucralfate adsorbs bile salts.

These observations suggest that sucralfate's antiulcer activity is the result of formation of an ulcer-adherent complex that covers the ulcer site and protects it against further attack by acid, pepsin, and bile salts. There are approximately 14–16 mEq of acid-neutralizing capacity per 1-g dose of sucralfate.

CLINICAL TRIALS
In a multicenter, double-blind, placebo-controlled study of CARAFATE Suspension, a dosage regimen of 1 g (10 mL) four times daily was demonstrated to be superior to placebo in ulcer healing.

Results From Clinical Trials
Healing Rates for Acute Duodenal Ulcer

Treatment	n	Week 2 Healing Rates	Week 4 Healing Rates	Week 8 Healing Rates
CARAFATE Suspension	145	23(16%)*	66(46%)†	95(66%)‡
Placebo	147	10(7%)	39(27%)	58(39%)

* $P = 0.016$ †$P = 0.001$ ‡$P = 0.0001$

Equivalence of sucralfate suspension to sucralfate tablets has not been demonstrated.

INDICATIONS AND USAGE
CARAFATE (sucralfate) Suspension is indicated in the short-term (up to 8 weeks) treatment of active duodenal ulcer.

CONTRAINDICATIONS
There are no known contraindications to the use of sucralfate.

PRECAUTIONS
Duodenal ulcer is a chronic, recurrent disease. While short-term treatment with sucralfate can result in complete healing of the ulcer, a successful course of treatment with sucralfate should not be expected to alter the posthealing frequency or severity of duodenal ulceration.

Special Populations: Chronic Renal Failure and Dialysis Patients
When sucralfate is administered orally, small amounts of aluminum are absorbed from the gastrointestinal tract. Concomitant use of sucralfate with other products that contain aluminum, such as aluminum-containing antacids, may increase the total body burden of aluminum. Patients with normal renal function receiving the recommended doses of sucralfate and aluminum-containing products adequately excrete aluminum in the urine. Patients with chronic renal failure or those receiving dialysis have impaired excretion of absorbed aluminum. In addition, aluminum does not cross dialysis membranes because it is bound to albumin and transferrin plasma proteins. Aluminum accumulation and toxicity (aluminum osteodystrophy, osteomalacia, encephalopathy) have been described in patients with renal impairment. Sucralfate should be used with caution in patients with chronic renal failure.

Drug Interactions
Some studies have shown that simultaneous sucralfate administration in healthy volunteers reduced the extent of absorption (bioavailability) of single doses of the following: cimetidine, digoxin, fluoroquinolone antibiotics, ketoconazole, l-thyroxine, phenytoin, quinidine, ranitidine, tetracycline, and theophylline. Subtherapeutic prothrombin times with concomitant warfarin and sucralfate therapy have been reported in spontaneous and published case reports. However, two clinical studies have demonstrated no change in either serum warfarin concentration or prothrombin time with the addition of sucralfate to chronic warfarin therapy.
The mechanism of these interactions appears to be nonsystemic in nature, presumably resulting from sucralfate binding to the concomitant agent in the gastrointestinal tract. In all cases studied to date (cimetidine, ciprofloxacin, digoxin, norfloxacin, ofloxacin, and ranitidine), dosing the concomitant medication 2 hours before sucralfate eliminated the interaction. Because of the potential of CARAFATE to alter the absorption of some drugs, CARAFATE should be administered separately from other drugs when alterations in bioavailability are felt to be critical. In these cases, patients should be monitored appropriately.

Carcinogenesis, Mutagenesis, Impairment of Fertility
Chronic oral toxicity studies of 24 months' duration were conducted in mice and rats at doses up to 1 g/kg (12 times the human dose). There was no evidence of drug-related tumorigenicity. A reproduction study in rats at doses up to 38 times the human dose did not reveal any indication of fertility impairment. Mutagenicity studies were not conducted.

Pregnancy
Teratogenic effects. Pregnancy Category B. Teratogenicity studies have been performed in mice, rats, and rabbits at doses up to 50 times the human dose and have revealed no evidence of harm to the fetus due to sulcralfate. There are, however, no adequate and well-controlled studies in pregnant women. Because animal reproduction studies are not always predictive of human response, this drug should be used during pregnancy only if clearly needed.

Nursing Mothers
It is not known whether this drug is excreted in human milk. Because many drugs are excreted in human milk, caution should be exercised when sucralfate is administered to a nursing woman.

Pediatric Use
Safety and effectiveness in pediatric patients have not been established.

ADVERSE REACTIONS
Adverse reactions to sucralfate tablets in clinical trials were minor and only rarely led to discontinuation of the drug. In studies involving over 2700 patients treated with sucralfate, adverse effects were reported in 129 (4.7%).
Constipation was the most frequent complaint (2%). Other adverse effects reported in less than 0.5% of the patients are listed below by body system:
Gastrointestinal: diarrhea, dry mouth, flatulence, gastric discomfort, indigestion, nausea, vomiting
Dermatological: pruritus, rash
Nervous System: dizziness, insomnia, sleepiness, vertigo
Other: back pain, headache
Postmarketing reports of hypersensitivity reactions, including urticaria (hives), angioedema, respiratory difficulty, rhinitis, laryngospasm, and facial swelling have been reported in patients receiving sucralfate tablets. Similar events were reported with sucralfate suspension. However, a causal relationship has not been established.
Bezoars have been reported in patients treated with sucralfate. The majority of patients had underlying medical conditions that may predispose to bezoar formation (such as delayed gastric emptying) or were receiving concomitant enteral tube feedings.
Inadvertent injection of insoluble sucralfate and its insoluble excipients has led to fatal complications, including pulmonary and cerebral emboli. Sucralfate is not intended for intravenous administration.

OVERDOSAGE
Due to limited experience in humans with overdosage of sucralfate, no specific treatment recommendations can be given. Acute oral studies in animals, however, using doses up to 12 g/kg body weight, could not find a lethal dose. Sucralfate is only minimally absorbed from the gastrointestinal tract. Risks associated with acute overdosage should, therefore, be minimal. In rare reports describing sucralfate overdose, most patients remained asymptomatic. Those few reports where adverse events were described included symptoms of dyspepsia, abdominal pain, nausea, and vomiting.

DOSAGE AND ADMINISTRATION
Active Duodenal Ulcer. The recommended adult oral dosage for duodenal ulcer is 1 g (10 mL/2 teaspoonfuls) four times per day. CARAFATE should be administered on an empty stomach.
Antacids may be prescribed as needed for relief of pain but should not be taken within one-half hour before or after sucralfate.

While healing with sucralfate may occur during the first week or two, treatment should be continued for 4 to 8 weeks unless healing has been demonstrated by x-ray or endoscopic examination.

HOW SUPPLIED

CARAFATE (sucralfate) Suspension 1 g/10 mL is a pink suspension supplied in bottles of 14 fl oz (NDC 0088-1700-15).

SHAKE WELL BEFORE USING

Store at controlled room temperature 59–86°F (15–30°C). Avoid freezing.

Prescribing Information as of January 1995
Hoechst Marion Roussel, Inc.
Kansas City, MO 64137

CARDIZEM® CD ℞

[kar'diz-em]
(diltiazem HCl)
Capsules
Prescribing Information as of July 1995

DESCRIPTION

CARDIZEM® (diltiazem hydrochloride) is a calcium ion influx inhibitor (slow channel blocker or calcium antagonist). Chemically, diltiazem hydrochloride is 1,5-benzothiazepin-4(5H)one,3-(acetyloxy)-5-[2-(dimethylamino)ethyl]-2,3-dihydro-2-(4-methoxyphenyl)-, monohydrochloride,(+)-cis. The chemical structure is:

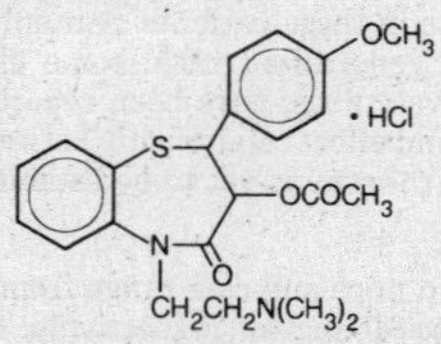

Diltiazem hydrochloride is a white to off-white crystalline powder with a bitter taste. It is soluble in water, methanol, and chloroform. It has a molecular weight of 450.98. CARDIZEM CD is formulated as a once-a-day extended release capsule containing either 120 mg, 180 mg, 240 mg, or 300 mg diltiazem hydrochloride.

Also contains: black iron oxide, ethylcellulose, FD&C Blue #1, fumaric acid, gelatin-NF, sucrose, starch, talc, titanium dioxide, white wax, and other ingredients.

For oral administration.

CLINICAL PHARMACOLOGY

The therapeutic effects of CARDIZEM CD are believed to be related to its ability to inhibit the influx of calcium ions during membrane depolarization of cardiac and vascular smooth muscle.

Mechanisms of Action

Hypertension. CARDIZEM CD produces its antihypertensive effect primarily by relaxation of vascular smooth muscle and the resultant decrease in peripheral vascular resistance. The magnitude of blood pressure reduction is related to the degree of hypertension; thus hypertensive individuals experience an antihypertensive effect, whereas there is only a modest fall in blood pressure in normotensives.

Angina. CARDIZEM CD has been shown to produce increases in exercise tolerance, probably due to its ability to reduce myocardial oxygen demand. This is accomplished via reductions in heart rate and systemic blood pressure at submaximal and maximal work loads. Diltiazem has been shown to be a potent dilator of coronary arteries, both epicardial and subendocardial. Spontaneous and ergonovine-induced coronary artery spasm are inhibited by diltiazem.

In animal models, diltiazem interferes with the slow inward (depolarizing) current in excitable tissue. It causes excitation-contraction uncoupling in various myocardial tissues without changes in the configuration of the action potential. Diltiazem produces relaxation of coronary vascular smooth muscle and dilation of both large and small coronary arteries at drug levels which cause little or no negative inotropic effect. The resultant increases in coronary blood flow (epicardial and subendocardial) occur in ischemic and nonischemic models and are accompanied by dose-dependent decreases in systemic blood pressure and decreases in peripheral resistance.

Hemodynamic and Electrophysiologic Effects

Like other calcium channel antagonists, diltiazem decreases sinotrial and atrioventricular conduction in isolated tissues and has a negative inotropic effect in isolated preparations. In the intact animal, prolongation of the AH interval can be seen at higher doses.

In man, diltiazem prevents spontaneous and ergonovine-provoked coronary artery spasm. It causes a decrease in peripheral vascular resistance and a modest fall in blood pressure in normotensive individuals and, in exercise tolerance studies in patients with ischemic heart disease, reduces the heart rate-blood pressure product for any given work load. Studies to date, primarily in patients with good ventricular function, have not revealed evidence of a negative inotropic effect; cardiac output, ejection fraction, and left ventricular end diastolic pressure have not been affected. Such data have no predictive value with respect to effects in patients with poor ventricular function, and increased heart failure has been reported in patients with preexisting impairment of ventricular function. There are as yet few data on the interaction of diltiazem and beta-blockers in patients with poor ventricular function. Resting heart rate is usually slightly reduced by diltiazem.

In hypertensive patients, CARDIZEM CD produces antihypertensive effects both in the supine and standing positions. In a double-blind, parallel, dose-response study utilizing doses ranging from 90 to 540 mg once daily, CARDIZEM CD lowered supine diastolic blood pressure in an apparent linear manner over the entire dose range studied. The changes in diastolic blood pressure, measured at trough, for placebo, 90 mg, 180 mg, 360 mg, and 540 mg were −2.9, −4.5, −6.1, −9.5, and −10.5 mm Hg, respectively. Postural hypotension is infrequently noted upon suddenly assuming an upright position. No reflex tachycardia is associated with the chronic antihypertensive effects. CARDIZEM CD decreases vascular resistance, increases cardiac output (by increasing stroke volume), and produces a slight decrease or no change in heart rate. During dynamic exercise, increases in diastolic pressure are inhibited, while maximum achievable systolic pressure is usually reduced. Chronic therapy with CARDIZEM CD produces no change or an increase in plasma catecholamines. No increased activity of the renin-angiotensin-aldosterone axis has been observed. CARDIZEM CD reduces the renal and peripheral effects of angiotensin II. Hypertensive animal models respond to diltiazem with reductions in blood pressure and increased urinary output and natriuresis without a change in urinary sodium/potassium ratio.

In a double-blind, parallel dose-response study of doses from 60 mg to 480 mg once daily, CARDIZEM CD increased time to termination of exercise in a linear manner over the entire dose range studied. The improvement in time to termination of exercise utilizing a Bruce exercise protocol, measured at trough, for placebo, 60 mg, 120 mg, 240 mg, 360 mg, and 480 mg was 29, 40, 56, 51, 69, and 68 seconds, respectively. As doses of CARDIZEM CD were increased, overall angina frequency was decreased. CARDIZEM CD, 180 mg once daily, or placebo was administered in a double-blind study to patients receiving concomitant treatment with long-acting nitrates and/or beta-blockers. A significant increase in time to termination of exercise and a significant decrease in overall angina frequency was observed. In this trial the overall frequency of adverse events in the CARDIZEM CD treatment group was the same as the placebo group.

Intravenous diltiazem in doses of 20 mg prolongs AH conduction time and AV node functional and effective refractory periods by approximately 20%. In a study involving single oral doses of 300 mg of CARDIZEM in six normal volunteers, the average maximum PR prolongation was 14% with no instances of greater than first-degree AV block. Diltiazem-associated prolongation of the AH interval is not more pronounced in patients with first-degree heart block. In patients with sick sinus syndrome, diltiazem significantly prolongs sinus cycle length (up to 50% in some cases).

Chronic oral administration of CARDIZEM to patients in doses of up to 540 mg/day has resulted in small increases in PR interval, and on occasion produces abnormal prolongation. (See WARNINGS.)

Pharmacokinetics and Metabolism

Diltiazem is well absorbed from the gastrointestinal tract and is subject to an extensive first-pass effect, giving an absolute bioavailability (compared to intravenous administration) of about 40%. CARDIZEM undergoes extensive metabolism in which only 2% to 4% of the unchanged drug appears in the urine. Drugs which induce or inhibit hepatic microsomal enzymes may alter diltiazem disposition.

Total radioactivity measurement following short IV administration in healthy volunteers suggests the presence of other unidentified metabolites, which attain higher concentrations than those of diltiazem and are more slowly eliminated; half-life of total radioactivity is about 20 hours compared to 2 to 5 hours for diltiazem.

In vitro binding studies show CARDIZEM is 70% to 80% bound to plasma proteins. Competitive in vitro ligand binding studies have also shown CARDIZEM binding is not altered by therapeutic concentrations of digoxin, hydrochlorothiazide, phenylbutazone, propranolol, salicylic acid, or warafin. The plasma elimination half-life following single or multiple drug administration is approximately 3.0 to 4.5 hours. Desacetyl diltiazem is also present in the plasma at levels of 10% to 20% of the parent drug and is 25% to 50% as potent as a coronary vasodilator as diltiazem. Minimum therapeutic plasma diltiazem concentrations appear to be in the range of 50 to 200 ng/mL. There is a departure from linearity when dose strengths are increased; the half-life is slightly increased with dose. A study that compared patients with normal hepatic function to patients with cirrhosis found an increase in half-life and a 69% increase in bioavailability in the hepatically impaired patients. A single study in nine patients with severely impaired renal function showed no difference in the pharmacokinetic profile of diltiazem compared to patients with normal renal function.

CARDIZEM CD Capsules. When compared to a regimen of CARDIZEM tablets at steady-state, more than 95% of drug is absorbed from the CARDIZEM CD formulation. A single 360-mg dose of the capsule results in detectable plasma levels within 2 hours and peak plasma levels between 10 and 14 hours; absorption occurs throughout the dosing interval. When CARDIZEM CD was coadministered with a high fat content breakfast, the extent of diltiazem absorption was not affected. Dose-dumping does not occur. The apparent elimination half-life after single or multiple dosing is 5 to 8 hours. A departure from linearity similar to that seen with CARDIZEM tablets and CARDIZEM SR capsules is observed. As the dose of CARDIZEM CD capsules is increased from a daily dose of 120 mg to 240 mg, there is an increase in the area-under-the-curve of 2.7 times. When the dose is increased from 240 mg to 360 mg there is an increase in the area-under-the-curve of 1.6 times.

INDICATIONS AND USAGE

CARDIZEM CD is indicated for the treatment of hypertension. It may be used alone or in combination with other antihypertensive medications.

CARDIZEM CD is indicated for the management of chronic stable angina and angina due to coronary artery spasm.

CONTRAINDICATIONS

CARDIZEM is contraindicated in (1) patients with sick sinus syndrome except in the presence of a functioning ventricular pacemaker, (2) patients with second- or third-degree AV block except in the presence of a functioning ventricular pacemaker, (3) patients with hypotension (less than 90 mm Hg systolic), (4) patients who have demonstrated hypersensitivity to the drug, and (5) patients with acute myocardial infarction and pulmonary congestion documented by x-ray on admission.

WARNINGS

1. **Cardiac Conduction.** CARDIZEM prolongs AV node refractory periods without significantly prolonging sinus node recovery time, except in patients with sick sinus syndrome. This effect may rarely result in abnormally slow heart rates (particularly in patients with sick sinus syndrome) or second- or third-degree AV block (13 of 3290 patients or 0.40%). Concomitant use of diltiazem with beta-blockers or digitalis may result in additive effects on cardiac conduction. A patient with Prinzmetal's angina developed periods of asystole (2 to 5 seconds) after a single dose of 60 mg of diltiazem. (See ADVERSE REACTIONS section.)
2. **Congestive Heart Failure.** Although diltiazem has a negative inotropic effect in isolated animal tissue preparations, hemodynamic studies in humans with normal ventricular function have not shown a reduction in cardiac index nor consistent negative effects on contractility (dp/dt). An acute study of oral diltiazem in patients with impaired ventricular function (ejection fraction 24% ± 6%) showed improvement in indices of ventricular function without significant decrease in contractile function (dp/dt). Worsening of congestive heart failure has been reported in patients with preexisting impairment of ventricular function. Experience with the use of CARDIZEM (diltiazem hydrochloride) in combination with beta-blockers in patients with impaired ventricular function is limited. Caution should be exercised when using this combination.
3. **Hypotension.** Decreases in blood pressure associated with CARDIZEM therapy may occasionally result in symptomatic hypotension.
4. **Acute Hepatic Injury.** Mild elevations of transaminases with and without concomitant elevation in alkaline phosphatase and bilirubin have been observed in clinical studies. Such elevations were usually transient and frequently resolved even with continued diltiazem treatment. In rare instances, significant elevations in enzymes such as alkaline phosphatase, LDH, SGOT, SGPT, and other phenomena consistent with acute hepatic injury have been noted. These reactions tended to occur early after therapy initiation (1 to 8 weeks) and have been reversible upon discontinuation of drug therapy. The relationship to CARDIZEM is uncertain in some cases, but probable in some. (See PRECAUTIONS.)

PRECAUTIONS

General

CARDIZEM (diltiazem hydrochloride) is extensively metabolized by the liver and excreted by the kidneys and in bile. As with any drug given over prolonged periods, laboratory parameters of renal and hepatic function should be monitored at regular intervals. The drug should be used with caution in patients with impaired renal or hepatic function. In subacute and chronic dog and rat studies designed to produce toxicity, high doses of diltiazem were associated with hepatic damage. In special subacute hepatic studies, oral doses of 125 mg/kg and higher in rats were associated with histological

Continued on next page

Hoechst Marion Roussel—Cont.

changes in the liver which were reversible when the drug was discontinued. In dogs, doses of 20 mg/kg were also associated with hepatic changes; however, these changes were reversible with continued dosing.

Dermatological events (see ADVERSE REACTIONS section) may be transient and may disappear despite continued use of CARDIZEM. However, skin eruptions progressing to erythema multiforme and/or exfoliative dermatitis have also been infrequently reported. Should a dermatologic reaction persist, the drug should be discontinued.

Drug Interactions

Due to the potential for additive effects, caution and careful titration are warranted in patients receiving CARDIZEM concomitantly with other agents known to affect cardiac contractility and/or conduction. (See WARNINGS.) Pharmacologic studies indicate that there may be additive effects in prolonging AV conduction when using beta-blockers or digitalis concomitantly with CARDIZEM. (See WARNINGS.)

As with all drugs, care should be exercised when treating patients with multiple medications. CARDIZEM undergoes biotransformation by cytochrome P-450 mixed function oxidase. Coadministration of CARDIZEM with other agents which follow the same route of biotransformation may result in the competitive inhibition of metabolism. Especially in patients with renal and/or hepatic impairment, dosage of similarly metabolized drugs, particularly those of low therapeutic ratio, may require adjustment when starting or stopping concomitantly administered diltiazem to maintain optimum therapeutic blood levels.

Beta-blockers. Controlled and uncontrolled domestic studies suggest that concomitant use of CARDIZEM and beta-blockers is usually well tolerated, but available data are not sufficient to predict the effects of concomitant treatment in patients with left ventricular dysfunction or cardiac conduction abnormalities.

Administration of CARDIZEM (diltiazem hydrochloride) concomitantly with propranolol in five normal volunteers resulted in increased propranolol levels in all subjects and bioavailability of propranolol was increased approximately 50%. In vitro, propranolol appears to be displaced from its binding sites by diltiazem. If combination therapy is initiated or withdrawn in conjunction with propranolol, an adjustment in the propranolol dose may be warranted. (See WARNINGS.)

Cimetidine. A study in six healthy volunteers has shown a significant increase in peak diltiazem plasma levels (58%) and area-under-the-curve (53%) after a 1-week course of cimetidine at 1200 mg per day and a single dose of diltiazem 60 mg. Ranitidine produced smaller, nonsignificant increases. The effect may be mediated by cimetidine's known inhibition of hepatic cytochrome P-450, the enzyme system responsible for the first-pass metabolism of diltiazem. Patients currently receiving diltiazem therapy should be carefully monitored for a change in pharmacological effect when initiating and discontinuing therapy with cimetidine. An adjustment in the diltiazem dose may be warranted.

Digitalis. Administration of CARDIZEM with digoxin in 24 healthy male subjects increased plasma digoxin concentrations approximately 20%. Another investigator found no increase in digoxin levels in 12 patients with coronary artery disease. Since there have been conflicting results regarding the effect of digoxin levels, it is recommended that digoxin levels be monitored when initiating, adjusting, and discontinuing CARDIZEM therapy to avoid possible over- or under-digitalization. (See WARNINGS.)

Anesthetics. The depression of cardiac contractility, conductivity, and automaticity as well as the vascular dilation associated with anesthetics may be potentiated by calcium channel blockers. When used concomitantly, anesthetics and calcium blockers should be titrated carefully.

Cyclosporine. A pharmacokinetic interaction between diltiazem and cyclosporine has been observed during studies involving renal and cardiac transplant patients. In renal and cardiac transplant recipients, a reduction of cyclosporine dose ranging from 15% to 48% was necessary to maintain cyclosporine through concentrations similar to those seen prior to the addition of diltiazem. If these agents are to be administered concurrently, cyclosporine concentrations should be monitored, especially when diltiazem therapy is initiated, adjusted, or discontinued.

The effect of cyclosporine diltiazem plasma concentrations has not been evaluated.

Carbamazepine. Concomitant administration of diltiazem with carbamazepine has been reported to result in elevated serum levels of carbamazepine (40% to 72% increase), resulting in toxicity in some cases. Patients receiving these drugs concurrently should be monitored for a potential drug interaction.

Carcinogenesis, Mutagenesis, Impairment of Fertility

A 24-month study in rats at oral dosage levels of up to 100 mg/kg/day and a 21-month study in mice at oral dosage levels of up to 30 mg/kg/day showed no evidence of carcinogenicity. There was also no mutagenic response in vitro or in vivo in mammalian cell assays or in vitro in bacteria. No evidence of impaired fertility was observed in a study performed in male and female rats at oral dosages of up to 100 mg/kg/day.

Pregnancy

Category C. Reproduction studies have been conducted in mice, rats and rabbits. Administration of doses ranging from five to ten times greater (on a mg/kg basis) than the daily recommended therapeutic dose has resulted in embryo and fetal lethality. These doses, in some studies, have been reported to cause skeletal abnormalities. In the perinatal/postnatal studies, there was an increased incidence of still-births at doses of 20 times the human dose or greater.

There are no well-controlled studies in pregnant women; therefore, use CARDIZEM in pregnant women only if the potential benefit justifies the potential risk to the fetus.

Nursing Mothers

Diltiazem is excreted in human milk. One report suggests that concentrations in breast milk may approximate serum levels. If use of CARDIZEM is deemed essential, an alternative method of infant feeding should be instituted.

Pediatric Use

Safety and effectiveness in pediatric patients have not been established.

ADVERSE REACTIONS

Serious adverse reactions have been rare in studies carried out to date, but it should be recognized that patients with impaired ventricular function and cardiac conduction abnormalities have usually been excluded from these studies.

The following table presents the most common adverse reactions reported in placebo-controlled angina and hypertension trials in patients receiving CARDIZEM CD up to 360 mg with rates in placebo patients shown for comparison.

CARDIZEM CD Capsule Placebo-Controlled Angina and Hypertension Trials Combined

Adverse Reactions	Cardizem CD (n=607)	Placebo (n=301)
Headache	5.4%	5.0%
Dizziness	3.0%	3.0%
Bradycardia	3.3%	1.3%
AV Block First Degree	3.3%	0.0%
Edema	2.6%	1.3%
ECG Abnormality	1.6%	2.3%
Asthenia	1.8%	1.7%

In clinical trials of CARDIZEM CD capsules, CARDIZEM tablets, and CARDIZEM SR capsules involving over 3200 patients, the most common events (ie, greater than 1%) were edema (4.6%), headache (4.6%), dizziness (3.5%), asthenia (2.6%), first-degree AV block (2.4%), bradycardia (1.7%), flushing (1.4%), nausea (1.4%), and rash (1.2%).

In addition, the following events were reported infrequently (less than 1%) in angina or hypertension trials:

Cardiovascular: Angina, arrhythmia, AV block (second- or third-degree), bundle branch block, congestive heart failure, ECG abnormalities, hypotension, palpitations, syncope, tachycardia, ventricular extrasystoles.

Nervous System: Abnormal dreams, amnesia, depression, gait abnormality, hallucinations, insomnia, nervousness, paresthesia, personality change, somnolence, tinnitus, tremor.

Gastrointestinal: Anorexia, constipation, diarrhea, dry mouth, dysgeusia, dyspepsia, mild elevations of SGOT, SGPT, LDH, and alkaline phosphatase (see hepatic warnings), thirst, vomiting, weight increase.

Dermatological: Petechiae, photosensitivity, pruritus, urticaria.

Other: Amblyopia, CPK increase, dyspnea, epistaxis, eye irritation, hyperglycemia, hyperuricemia, impotence, muscle cramps, nasal congestion, nocturia, osteoarticular pain, polyuria, sexual difficulties.

The following postmarketing events have been reported infrequently in patients receiving CARDIZEM: allergic reactions, alopecia, angioedema (including facial or periorbital edema), asystole, erythema multiforme (including Stevens-Johnson syndrome, toxic epidermal necrolysis), exfoliative dermatitis, extrapyramidal symptoms, gingival hyperplasia, hemolytic anemia, increased bleeding time, leukopenia, purpura, retinopathy, and thrombocytopenia. In addition, events such as myocardial infarction have been observed which are not readily distinguishable from the natural history of the disease in these patients. A number of well-documented cases of generalized rash, some characterized as leukocytoclastic vasculitis, have been reported. However, a definitive cause and effect relationship between these events and CARDIZEM therapy is yet to be established.

OVERDOSAGE

The oral LD_{50}'s in mice and rats range from 415 to 740 mg/kg and from 560 to 810 mg/kg, respectively. The intravenous LD_{50}'s in these species were 60 and 38 mg/kg, respectively. The oral LD_{50} in dogs is considered to be in excess of 50 mg/kg, while lethality was seen in monkeys at 360 mg/kg.

The toxic dose in man is not known. Due to extensive metabolism, blood levels after a standard dose of diltiazem can vary over tenfold, limiting the usefulness of blood levels in overdose cases. There have been 29 reports of diltiazem overdose in doses ranging from less than 1 g to 10.8 g. Sixteen of these reports involved multiple drug ingestions.

Twenty-two reports indicated patients had recovered from diltiazem overdose ranging from less than 1 g to 10.8 g. There were seven reports with a fatal outcome; although the amount of diltiazem ingested was unknown, multiple drug ingestions were confirmed in six of the seven reports.

Events observed following diltiazem overdose included bradycardia, hypotension, heart block, and cardiac failure. Most reports of overdose described some supportive medical measure and/or drug treatment. Bradycardia frequently responded favorably to atropine as did heart block, although cardiac pacing was also frequently utilized to treat heart block. Fluids and vasopressors were used to maintain blood pressure, and in cases of cardiac failure, inotropic agents were administered. In addition, some patients received treat-

CARDIZEM® CD
(diltiazem hydrochloride)
Capsules

Strength	Quantity	NDC Number	Description
120 mg	30 btl 90 btl 100 UDIP®	0088-1795-30 0088-1795-42 0088-1795-49	Light turquoise blue/light turquoise blue capsule imprinted with the Marion Merrell Dow Inc. logo on one end and CARDIZEM CD and 120 mg on the other.
180 mg	30 btl 90 btl 100 UDIP®	0088-1796-30 0088-1796-42 0088-1796-49	Light turquoise blue/blue capsule imprinted with the Marion Merrell Dow Inc. logo on one end and CARDIZEM CD and 180 mg on the other.
240 mg	30 btl 90 btl 100 UDIP®	0088-1797-30 0088-1797-42 0088-1797-49	Blue/blue capsule imprinted with the Marion Merrell Dow Inc. logo on one end and CARDIZEM CD and 240 mg on the other.
300 mg	30 btl 90 btl 100 UDIP®	0088-1798-30 0088-1798-42 0088-1798-49	Light gray/blue capsule imprinted with the Marion Merrell Dow Inc. logo on one end and CARDIZEM CD and 300 mg on the other.

ment with ventilatory support, gastric lavage, activated charcoal and/or intravenous calcium. Evidence of the effectiveness of intravenous calcium administration to reverse the pharmacological effects of diltiazem overdose was conflicting.

In the event of overdose or exaggerated response, appropriate supportive measures should be employed in addition to gastrointestinal decontamination. Diltiazem does not appear to be removed by peritoneal or hemodialysis. Limited data suggest that plasmapheresis or charcoal hemoperfusion may hasten diltiazem elimination following overdose. Based on the known pharmacological effects of diltiazem and/or reported clinical experiences, the following measures may be considered:

Bradycardia: Administer atropine (0.60 to 1.0 mg). If there is no response to vagal blockade, administer isoproterenol cautiously.

High-degree AV Block: Treat as for bradycardia above. Fixed high-degree AV block should be treated with cardiac pacing.

Cardiac Failure: Administer inotropic agents (isoproterenol, dopamine, or dobutamine) and diuretics.

Hypotension: Vasopressors (eg, dopamine or levarterenol bitartrate).

Actual treatment and dosage should depend on the severity of the clinical situation and the judgment and experience of the treating physician.

DOSAGE AND ADMINISTRATION

Patients controlled on diltiazem alone or in combination with other medications may be switched to CARDIZEM CD capsules at the nearest equivalent total daily dose. Higher doses of CARDIZEM CD may be needed in some patients. Patients should be closely monitored. Subsequent titration to higher or lower doses may be necessary and should be initiated as clinically warranted. There is limited general clinical experience with doses above 360 mg, but doses to 540 mg have been studied in clinical trials. The incidence of side effects increases as the dose increases with first-degree AV block, dizziness, and sinus bradycardia bearing the strongest relationship to dose.

Hypertension. Dosage needs to be adjusted by titration to individual patient needs. When used as monotherapy, reasonable starting doses are 180 to 240 mg once daily, although some patients may respond to lower doses. Maximum antihypertensive effect is usually observed by 14 days of chronic therapy; therefore, dosage adjustments should be scheduled accordingly. The usual dosage range studied in clinical trials was 240 to 360 mg once daily. Individual patients may respond to higher doses of up to 480 mg once daily.

Angina. Dosages for the treatment of angina should be adjusted to each patient's needs, starting with a dose of 120 or 180 mg once daily. Individual patients may respond to higher doses of up to 480 mg once daily. When necessary, titration may be carried out over a 7- to 14-day period.

Concomitant Use With Other Cardiovascular Agents.

1. **Sublingual NTG.** May be taken as required to abort acute anginal attacks during CARDIZEM CD (diltiazem hydrochloride) therapy.
2. **Prophylactic Nitrate Therapy.** CARDIZEM CD may be safely coadministered with short- and long-acting nitrates.
3. **Beta-blockers.** (See WARNINGS and PRECAUTIONS.)
4. **Antihypertensives.** CARDIZEM CD has an additive antihypertensive effect when used with other antihypertensive agents. Therefore, the dosage of CARDIZEM CD or the concomitant antihypertensives may need to be adjusted when adding one to the other.

HOW SUPPLIED

[See table on bottom of preceding page.]

Storage Conditions: Store at controlled room temperature 59–86°F (15–30°C). Avoid excessive humidity.

Prescribing Information as of July 1995

Hoechst Marion Roussel, Inc.
Kansas City, MO 64137 USA

Shown in Product Identification Guide, page 317

CARDIZEM® Injectable ℞
(diltiazem HCl)

CARDIZEM® Lyo-Ject Syringe
(diltiazem HCl)

DESCRIPTION

CARDIZEM® (diltiazem hydrochloride) is a calcium ion influx inhibitor (slow channel blocker or calcium channel antagonist). Chemically, diltiazem hydrochloride is 1,5-benzothiazepin-4(5H)one,3-(acetyloxy)-5-[2-(dimethylamino)-ethyl]-2, 3-dihydro-2-(4-methoxyphenyl)-, monohydrochloride,(+)-cis-. The chemical structure is:

[See structure at top of next column.]

Diltiazem hydrochloride is a white to off-white crystalline powder with a bitter taste. It is soluble in water, methanol, and chloroform. It has a molecular weight of 450.98.

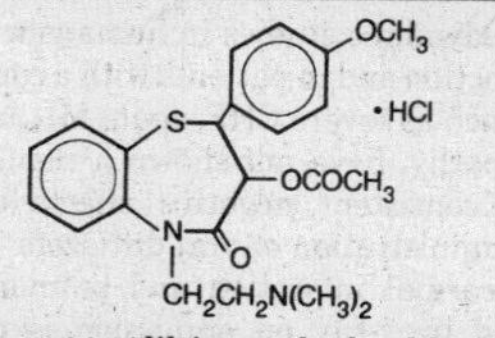

CARDIZEM Injectable (diltiazem hydrochloride) is a clear, colorless, sterile, nonpyrogenic solution. It has a pH range of 3.7 to 4.1.

CARDIZEM Injectable is for direct intravenous bolus injection and continuous intravenous infusion.

25-mg, 5-mL vial–each sterile vial contains 25 mg diltiazem hydrochloride, 3.75 mg citric acid USP, 3.25 mg sodium citrate dihydrate USP, 357 mg sorbitol solution USP, and water for injection USP up to 5 mL. Sodium hydroxide or hydrochloric acid is used for pH adjustment.

50-mg, 10-mL vial–each sterile vial contains 50 mg diltiazem hydrochloride, 7.5 mg citric acid USP, 6.5 mg sodium citrate dihydrate USP, 714 mg sorbitol solution USP, and water for injection USP up to 10 mL. Sodium hydroxide or hydrochloric acid is used for pH adjustment.

CARDIZEM Lyo-Ject Syringe (diltiazem hydrochloride) after reconstitution contains a clear, colorless, sterile, nonpyrogenic solution. It has a pH range of 4.0 to 7.0.

CARDIZEM Lyo-Ject Syringe after reconstitution is for direct intravenous bolus injection and continuous intravenous infusion.

CARDIZEM Lyo-Ject Syringe 25-mg syringe is available in a dual chamber, disposable syringe. Chamber 1 contains lyophilized powder comprised of diltiazem hydrochloride 25 mg and mannitol USP 37.5 mg. Chamber 2 contains sterile diluent composed of 5 mL water for injection with 0.5% benzyl alcohol NF, and 0.6% sodium chloride USP.

CLINICAL PHARMACOLOGY

Mechanisms of Action.

CARDIZEM inhibits the influx of calcium (Ca^{2+}) ions during membrane depolarization of cardiac and vascular smooth muscle. The therapeutic benefits of CARDIZEM in supraventricular tachycardias are related to its ability to slow AV nodal conduction time and prolong AV nodal refractoriness. CARDIZEM exhibits frequency (use) dependent effects on AV nodal conduction such that it may selectively reduce the heart rate during trachycardias involving the AV node with little or no effect on normal AV nodal conduction at normal heart rates.

CARDIZEM slows the ventricular rate in patients with a rapid ventricular response during atrial fibrillation or atrial flutter. CARDIZEM converts paroxysmal supraventricular tachycardia (PSVT) to normal sinus rhythm by interrupting the reentry circuit in AV nodal reentrant tachycardias and reciprocating tachycardias, eg, Wolff-Parkinson-White syndrome (WPW).

CARDIZEM prolongs the sinus cycle length. It has no effect on the sinus node recovery time or on the sinoatrial conduction time in patients without SA nodal dysfunction.

CARDIZEM has no significant electrophysiologic effects on tissues in the heart that are fast sodium channel dependent, eg, His-Purkinje tissue, atrial and ventricular muscle, and extranodal accessory pathways.

Like other calcium channel antagonists, because of its effect on vascular smooth muscle, CARDIZEM decreases total peripheral resistance resulting in a decrease in both systolic and diastolic blood pressure.

Hemodynamics.

In patients with cardiovascular disease, CARDIZEM Injectable (diltiazem hydrochloride) administered intravenously in single bolus doses, followed in some cases by a continuous infusion, reduced blood pressure, systemic vascular resistance, the rate-pressure product, and coronary vascular resistance and increased coronary blood flow. In a limited number of studies of patients with compromised myocardium (severe congestive heart failure, acute myocardial infarction, hypertrophic cardiomyopathy), administration of intravenous diltiazem produced no significant effect on contractility, left ventricular end diastolic pressure, or pulmonary capillary wedge pressure. The mean ejection fraction and cardiac output/index remained unchanged or increased. Maximal hemodynamic effects usually occurred within 2 to 5 minutes of an injection. However, in rare instances, worsening of congestive heart failure has been reported in patients with preexisting impaired ventricular function.

Pharmacodynamics.

The prolongation of PR interval correlated significantly with plasma diltiazem concentration in normal volunteers using the Sigmoidal E_{max} model. Changes in heart rate, systolic blood pressure, and diastolic blood pressure did not correlate with diltiazem plasma concentrations in normal volunteers. Reduction in mean arterial pressure correlated linearly with diltiazem plasma concentration in a group of hypertensive patients.

In patients with atrial fibrillation and atrial flutter, a significant correlation was observed between the percent reduction in HR and plasma diltiazem concentration using the Sigmoidal E_{max} model. Based on this relationship, the mean plasma diltiazem concentration required to produce a 20% decrease in heart rate was determined to be 80 ng/mL. Mean plasma diltiazem concentrations of 130 ng/mL and 300 ng/mL were determined to produce reductions in heart rate of 30% and 40%.

Pharmacokinetics and Metabolism.

Following a single intravenous injection in healthy male volunteers, CARDIZEM appears to obey linear pharmacokinetics over a dose range of 10.5 to 21.0 mg. The plasma elimination half-life is approximately 3.4 hours. The apparent volume of distribution of CARDIZEM is approximately 305 L. CARDIZEM is extensively metabolized in the liver with a systemic clearance of approximately 65 L/h.

After constant rate intravenous infusion to healthy male volunteers, diltiazem exhibits nonlinear pharmacokinetics over an infusion range of 4.8 to 13.2 mg/h for 24 hours. Over this infusion range, as the dose is increased, systemic clearance decreases from 64 to 48 L/h while the plasma elimination half-life increases from 4.1 to 4.9 hours. The apparent volume of distribution remains unchanged (360 to 391 L). In patients with atrial fibrillation or atrial flutter, diltiazem systemic clearance has been found to be decreased compared to healthy volunteers. In patients administered bolus doses ranging from 2.5 mg to 38.5 mg, systemic clearance averaged 36 L/h. In patients administered continuous infusions at 10 mg/h or 15 mg/h for 24 hours, diltiazem systemic clearance averaged 42 L/h and 31 L/h, respectively.

Based on the results of pharmacokinetic studies in healthy volunteers administered different ***oral*** CARDIZEM formulations, constant rate intravenous infusions of CARDIZEM at 3, 5, 7, and 11 mg/h are predicted to produce steady-state plasma diltiazem concentrations equivalent to 120-, 180-, 240-, and 360-mg total daily oral doses of CARDIZEM tablets or CARDIZEM SR capsules.

After oral administration, CARDIZEM undergoes extensive metabolism in man by deacetylation, N-demethylation, and O-demethylation via cytochrome P-450 (oxidative metabolism) in addition to conjugation. Metabolites N-monodesmethyldiltiazem, desacetyldiltiazem, desacetyl-N-monodesmethyldiltiazem, desacetyl-O-desmethyldiltiazem, and desacetyl-N, O-desmethyldiltiazem have been identified in human urine. Following oral administration, 2% to 4% of the unchanged CARDIZEM appears in the urine. Drugs which induce or inhibit hepatic microsomal enzymes may alter diltiazem disposition.

Following single intravenous injection of CARDIZEM, however, plasma concentrations of N-monodesmethyldiltiazem and desacetyldiltiazem, two principal metabolites found in plasma after oral administration, are typically not detected. These metabolites are observed, however, following 24 hour constant rate intravenous infusion. Total radioactivity measurement following short IV administration in healthy volunteers suggests the presence of other unidentified metabolites which attain higher concentrations than those of diltiazem and are more slowly eliminated; half-life of total radioactivity is about 20 hours compared to 2 to 5 hours for diltiazem.

CARDIZEM is 70% to 80% bound to plasma proteins. In vitro studies suggest $alpha_1$-acid glycoprotein binds approximately 40% of the drug at clinically significant concentrations. Albumin appears to bind approximately 30% of the drug, while other constituents bind the remaining bound fraction. Competitive in vitro ligand binding studies have shown that CARDIZEM binding is not altered by therapeutic concentrations of digoxin, phenytoin, hydrochlorothiazide, indomethacin, phenylbutazone, propranolol, salicylic acid, tolbutamide, or warfarin.

Renal insufficiency, or even end-stage renal disease, does not appear to influence diltiazem disposition following ***oral*** administration. Liver cirrhosis was shown to reduce diltiazem's apparent ***oral*** clearance and prolong its half-life.

INDICATIONS AND USAGE

CARDIZEM Injectable or CARDIZEM Lyo-Ject Syringe (diltiazem hydrochloride) are indicated for the following:

1. **Atrial Fibrillation or Atrial Flutter.** Temporary control of rapid ventricular rate in atrial fibrillation or atrial flutter. It should not be used in patients with atrial fibrillation or atrial flutter associated with an accessory bypass tract such as in Wolff-Parkinson-White (WPW) syndrome or short PR syndrome.
2. **Paroxysmal Supraventricular Tachycardia.** Rapid conversion of paroxysmal supraventricular tachycardias (PSVT) to sinus rhythm. This includes AV nodal reentrant tachycardias and reciprocating tachycardias associated with an extranodal accessory pathway such as the WPW syndrome or short PR syndrome. Unless otherwise contraindicated, appropriate vagal maneuvers should be attempted prior to administration of CARDIZEM Injectable or Lyo-Ject Syringe.

The use of CARDIZEM Injectable or Lyo-Ject Syringe for control of ventricular response in patients with atrial fibrillation or atrial flutter or conversion to sinus rhythm in pa-

Continued on next page

Hoechst Marion Roussel—Cont.

tients with PSVT should be undertaken with caution when the patient is compromised hemodynamically or is taking other drugs that decrease any or all of the following: peripheral resistance, myocardial filling, myocardial contractility, or electrical impulse propagation in the myocardium.

For either indication and particularly when employing continuous intravenous infusion, the setting should include continuous monitoring of the ECG and frequent measurement of blood pressure. A defibrillator and emergency equipment should be readily available.

In domestic controlled trials in patients with atrial fibrillation or atrial flutter, bolus administration of CARDIZEM Injectable was effective in reducing heart rate by at least 20% in 95% of patients. CARDIZEM Injectable rarely converts atrial fibrillation or atrial flutter to normal sinus rhythm. Following administration of one or two intravenous bolus doses of CARDIZEM Injectable, response usually occurs within 3 minutes and maximal heart rate reduction generally occurs in 2 to 7 minutes. Heart rate reduction may last from 1 to 3 hours. If hypotension occurs, it is generally short-lived, but may last from 1 to 3 hours.

A 24-hour continuous infusion of CARDIZEM Injectable in the treatment of atrial fibrillation or atrial flutter maintained at least a 20% heart rate reduction during the infusion in 83% of patients. Upon discontinuation of infusion, heart rate reduction may last from 0.5 hours to more than 10 hours (median duration 7 hours). Hypotension, if it occurs, may be similarly persistent.

In the controlled clinical trials, 3.2% of patients required some form of intervention (typically, use of intravenous fluids or the Trendelenburg position) for blood pressure support following CARDIZEM Injectable.

In domestic controlled trials, bolus administration of CARDIZEM Injectable was effective in converting PSVT to normal sinus rhythm in 88% of patients within 3 minutes of the first or second bolus dose.

Symptoms associated with the arrhythmia were improved in conjunction with decreased heart rate or conversion to normal sinus rhythm following administration of CARDIZEM Injectable.

CONTRAINDICATIONS

CARDIZEM Injectable and CARDIZEM Lyo-Ject Syringe are contraindicated in:

1. Patients with sick sinus syndrome except in the presence of a functioning ventricular pacemaker.
2. Patients with second- or third-degree AV block except in the presence of a functioning ventricular pacemaker.
3. Patients with severe hypotension or cardiogenic shock.
4. Patients who have demonstrated hypersensitivity to the drug.
5. Intravenous diltiazem and intravenous beta-blockers should not be administered together or in close proximity (within a few hours).
6. Patients with atrial fibrillation or atrial flutter associated with an accessory bypass tract such as in WPW syndrome or short PR syndrome.

   As with other agents which slow AV nodal conduction and do not prolong the refractoriness of the accessory pathway (eg, verapamil, digoxin), in rare instances patients in atrial fibrillation or atrial flutter associated with an accessory bypass tract may experience a potentially life-threatening increase in heart rate accompanied by hypotension when treated with CARDIZEM Injectable or Lyo-Ject Syringe. As such, the initial use of CARDIZEM Injectable or Lyo-Ject Syringe should be, if possible, in a setting where monitoring and resuscitation capabilities, including DC cardioversion/defibrillation, are present (see OVERDOSAGE). Once familiarity of the patient's response is established, use in an office setting may be acceptable.
7. Patients with ventricular tachycardia. Administration of other calcium channel blockers to patients with wide complex tachycardia (QRS ≥ 0.12 seconds) has resulted in hemodynamic deterioration and ventricular fibrillation. It is important that an accurate pretreatment diagnosis distinguish wide complex QRS tachycardia of supraventricular origin from that of ventricular origin prior to administration of CARDIZEM Injectable.
8. In newborns, due to the presence of benzyl alcohol as a preservative (CARDIZEM Lyo-Ject only).

WARNINGS

1. **Cardiac Conduction.** Diltiazem prolongs AV nodal conduction and refractoriness that may rarely result in second- or third-degree AV block in sinus rhythm. Concomitant use of diltiazem with agents known to affect cardiac conduction may result in additive effects (see Drug Interactions). If high-degree AV block occurs in sinus rhythm, intravenous diltiazem should be discontinued and appropriate supportive measures instituted (see OVERDOSAGE).
2. **Congestive Heart Failure.** Although diltiazem has a negative inotropic effect in isolated animal tissue prepara-

tions, hemodynamic studies in humans with normal ventricular function and in patients with a compromised myocardium, such as severe CHF, acute MI, and hypertrophic cardiomyopathy, have not shown a reduction in cardiac index nor consistent negative effects on contractility (dp/dt). Administration of oral diltiazem in patients with acute myocardial infarction and pulmonary congestion documented by x-ray on admission is contraindicated. Experience with the use of CARDIZEM Injectable in patients with impaired ventricular function is limited. Caution should be exercised when using the drug in such patients.

3. **Hypotension.** Decreases in blood pressure associated with CARDIZEM Injectable therapy may occasionally result in symptomatic hypotension (3.2%). The use of intravenous diltiazem for control of ventricular response in patients with supraventricular arrhythmias should be undertaken with caution when the patient is compromised hemodynamically. In addition, caution should be used in patients taking other drugs that decrease peripheral resistance, intravascular volume, myocardial contractility or conduction.
4. **Acute Hepatic Injury.** In rare instances, significant elevations in enzymes such as alkaline phosphatase, LDH, SGOT, SGPT, and other phenomena consistent with acute hepatic injury have been noted following oral diltiazem. Therefore, the potential for acute hepatic injury exists following administration of intravenous diltiazem.
5. **Ventricular Premature Beats (VPBs).** VPBs may be present on conversion of PSVT to sinus rhythm with CARDIZEM Injectable. These VPBs are transient, are typically considered to be benign, and appear to have no clinical significance. Similar ventricular complexes have been noted during cardioversion, other pharmacologic therapy, and during spontaneous conversion of PSVT to sinus rhythm.

PRECAUTIONS

General

CARDIZEM (diltiazem hydrochloride) is extensively metabolized by the liver and excreted by the kidneys and in bile. The drug should be used with caution in patients with impaired renal or hepatic function (see WARNINGS). High intravenous dosages (4.5 mg/kg tid) administered to dogs resulted in significant bradycardia and alterations in AV conduction. In subacute and chronic dog and rat studies designed to produce toxicity, high oral doses of diltiazem were associated with hepatic damage. In special subacute hepatic studies, oral doses of 125 mg/kg and higher in rats were associated with histological changes in the liver, which were reversible when the drug was discontinued. In dogs, oral doses of 20 mg/kg were also associated with hepatic changes; however, these changes were reversible with continued dosing.

Dermatologic events progressing to erythema multiforme and/or exfoliative dermatitis have been infrequently reported following oral diltiazem. Therefore, the potential for these dermatologic reactions exists following exposure to intravenous diltiazem. Should a dermatologic reaction persist, the drug should be discontinued.

Drug Interactions

Due to potential for additive effects, caution is warranted in patients receiving CARDIZEM Injectable or CARDIZEM Lyo-Ject Syringe concomitantly with other agent(s) known to affect cardiac contractility and/or SA or AV node conduction (see WARNINGS).

As with all drugs, care should be exercised when treating patients with multiple medications. CARDIZEM undergoes extensive metabolism by the cytochrome P-450 mixed function oxidase system. Although specific pharmacokinetic drug-drug interaction studies have not been conducted with single intravenous injection or constant rate intravenous infusion, coadministration of CARDIZEM Injectable or Lyo-Ject Syringe with other agents which primarily undergo the same route of biotransformation may result in competitive inhibition of metabolism.

Digitalis. Intravenous diltiazem has been administered to patients receiving either intravenous or oral digitalis therapy. The combination of the two drugs was well tolerated without serious adverse effects. However, since both drugs affect AV nodal conduction, patients should be monitored for excessive slowing of the heart rate and/or AV block.

Beta-blockers. Intravenous diltiazem has been administered to patients on chronic oral beta-blocker therapy. The combination of the two drugs was generally well tolerated without serious adverse effects. If intravenous diltiazem is administered to patients receiving chronic oral beta-blocker therapy, the possibility for bradycardia, AV block, and/or depression of contractility should be considered (see CONTRAINDICATIONS). *Oral* administration of diltiazem with propranolol in five normal volunteers resulted in increased propranolol levels in all subjects and bioavailability of propranolol was increased approximately 50%. In vitro, propranolol appears to be displaced from its binding sites by diltiazem.

Anesthetics. The depression of cardiac contractility, conductivity, and automaticity as well as the vascular dilation associated with anesthetics may be potentiated by calcium channel blockers. When used concomitantly, anesthetics and calcium blockers should be titrated carefully.

Cyclosporine. A pharmacokinetic interaction between diltiazem and cyclosporine has been observed during studies involving renal and cardiac transplant patients. In renal and cardiac transplant recipients, a reduction of cyclosporine dose ranging from 15% to 48% was necessary to maintain cyclosporine trough concentrations similar to those seen prior to the addition of diltiazem. If these agents are to be administered concurrently, cyclosporine concentrations should be monitored, especially when diltiazem therapy is initiated, adjusted or discontinued.

The effect of cyclosporine on diltiazem plasma concentrations has not been evaluated.

Carbamazepine. Concomitant administration of *oral* diltiazem with carbamazepine has been reported to result in elevated plasma levels of carbamazepine (by 40 to 72%), resulting in toxicity in some cases. Patients receiving these drugs concurrently should be monitored for a potential drug interaction.

Carcinogenesis, Mutagenesis, Impairment of Fertility

A 24-month study in rats at oral dosage levels of up to 100 mg/kg/day, and a 21-month study in mice at oral dosage levels of up to 30 mg/kg/day showed no evidence of carcinogenicity. There was also no mutagenic response in vitro or in vivo in mammalian cell assays or in vitro in bacteria. No evidence of impaired fertility was observed in a study performed in male and female rats at oral dosages of up to 100 mg/kg/day.

Pregnancy

Category C. Reproduction studies have been conducted in mice, rats, and rabbits. Administration of oral doses ranging from five to ten times greater (on a mg/kg basis) than the daily recommended oral antianginal therapeutic dose has resulted in embryo and fetal lethality. These doses, in some studies, have been reported to cause skeletal abnormalities. In the perinatal/postnatal studies there was some reduction in early individual pup weights and survival rates. There was an increased incidence of stillbirths at doses of 20 times the human oral antianginal dose or greater.

There are no well-controlled studies in pregnant women; therefore, use CARDIZEM in pregnant women only if the potential benefit justifies the potential risk to the fetus.

Nursing Mothers

Diltiazem is excreted in human milk. One report with oral diltiazem suggests that concentrations in breast milk may approximate serum levels. If use of CARDIZEM is deemed essential, an alternative method of infant feeding should be instituted.

Pediatric Use

Safety and effectiveness in pediatric patients have not been established.

ADVERSE REACTIONS

The following adverse reaction rates are based on the use of CARDIZEM Injectable in over 400 domestic clinical trial patients with atrial fibrillation/flutter or PSVT under double-blind or open-label conditions. Worldwide experience in over 1300 patients was similar.

Adverse events reported in controlled and uncontrolled clinical trials were generally mild and transient. Hypotension was the most commonly reported adverse event during clinical trials. Asymptomatic hypotension occurred in 4.3% of patients. Symptomatic hypotension occurred in 3.2% of patients. When treatment for hypotension was required, it generally consisted of administration of saline or placing the patient in the Trendelenburg position. Other events reported in at least 1% of the diltiazem-treated patients were injection site reactions (eg, itching, burning)–3.9%, vasodilation (flushing)–1.7%, and arrhythmia (junctional rhythm or isorhythmic dissociation)–1.0%

In addition, the following events were reported infrequently (less than 1%):

Cardiovascular: Asystole, atrial flutter, AV block first degree, AV block second degree, bradycardia, chest pain, congestive heart failure, sinus pause, sinus node dysfunction, syncope, ventricular arrhythmia, ventricular fibrillation, ventricular tachycardia

Dermatologic: Pruritus, sweating

Gastrointestinal: Constipation, elevated SGOT or alkaline phosphatase, nausea, vomiting

Nervous System: Dizziness, paresthesia

Other: Amblyopia, asthenia, dry mouth, dyspnea, edema, headache, hyperuricemia

Although not observed in clinical trials with CARDIZEM Injectable, the following events associated with oral diltiazem may occur:

Cardiovascular: AV block (third degree), bundle branch block, ECG abnormality, palpitations, syncope, tachycardia, ventricular extrasystoles

Dermatologic: Alopecia, erythema multiforme (including Stevens-Johnson syndrome, toxic epidermal necrolysis),

Diluent Volume	Quantity of CARDIZEM Injectable or Lyo-Ject to Add	Final Concentration	Administration	
			Dose*	Infusion Rate
100 mL	125 mg (25 mL) Final Volume 125 mL	1.0 mg/mL	10 mg/h 15 mg/h	10 mL/h 15 mL/h
250 mL	250 mg (50 mL) Final Volume 300 mL	0.83 mg/mL	10 mg/h 15 mg/h	12 mL/h 18 mL/h
500 mL	250 mg (50 mL) Final Volume 550 mL	0.45 mg/mL	10 mg/h 15 mg/h	22 mL/h 33 mL/h

* 5 mg/h may be appropriate for some patients

exfoliative dermatitis, leukocytoclastic vasculitis, petechiae, photosensitivity, purpura, rash, urticaria

Gastrointestinal: Anorexia, diarrhea, dysgeusia, dyspepsia, mild elevations of SGPT and LDH, thirst, weight increase

Nervous System: Abnormal dreams, amnesia, depression, extrapyramidal symptoms, gait abnormality, hallucinations, insomnia, nervousness, personality change, somnolence, tremor

Other: Allergic reactions, angioedema (including facial or periorbital edema), CPK elevation, epistaxis, eye irritation, gingival hyperplasia, hemolytic anemia, hyperglycemia, impotence, increased bleeding time, leukopenia, muscle cramps, nasal congestion, nocturia, osteoarticular pain, polyuria, retinopathy, sexual difficulties, thrombocytopenia, tinnitus

Events such as myocardial infarction have been observed which are not readily distinguishable from the natural history of the disease for the patient.

OVERDOSAGE

Overdosage experience is limited. In the event of overdosage or an exaggerated response, appropriate supportive measures should be employed. The following measures may be considered:

Bradycardia: Administer atropine (0.60 to 1.0 mg). If there is no response to vagal blockade administer isoproterenol cautiously.

High-degree AV Block: Treat as for bradycardia above. Fixed high-degree AV block should be treated with cardiac pacing.

Cardiac Failure: Administer inotropic agents (isoproterenol, dopamine, or dobutamine) and diuretics.

Hypotension: Vasopressors (eg, dopamine or levarterenol bitartrate).

Actual treatment and dosage should depend on the severity of the clinical situation and the judgment and experience of the treating physician.

Diltiazem does not appear to be removed by peritoneal or hemodialysis. Limited data suggest that plasmapheresis or charcoal hemoperfusion may hasten diltiazem elimination following overdose.

The intravenous LD$_{50}$'s in mice and rats were 60 and 38 mg/kg, respectively. The toxic dose in man is not known.

DOSAGE AND ADMINISTRATION

Direct Intravenous Single Injections (Bolus)

The initial dose of CARDIZEM Injectable or CARDIZEM Lyo-Ject Syringe (see instructions for reconstitution of Lyo-Ject syringe in blister pack) should be 0.25 mg/kg actual body weight as a bolus administered over 2 minutes (20 mg is a reasonable dose for the average patient). If response is inadequate, a second dose may be administered after 15 minutes. The second bolus dose of CARDIZEM Injectable or Lyo-Ject should be 0.35 mg/kg actual body weight administered over 2 minutes (25 mg is a reasonable dose for the average patient). Subsequent intravenous bolus doses should be individualized for each patient. Patients with low body weights should be dosed on a mg/kg basis. Some patients may respond to an initial dose of 0.15 mg/kg, although duration of action may be shorter. Experience with this dose is limited.

Continuous Intravenous Infusion

For continued reduction of the heart rate (up to 24 hours) in patients with atrial fibrillation or atrial flutter, an intravenous infusion of CARDIZEM Injectable or Lyo-Ject may be administered. Immediately following bolus administration of 20 mg (0.25 mg/kg) or 25 mg (0.35 mg/kg) CARDIZEM Injectable or Lyo-Ject and reduction of heart rate, begin an intravenous infusion of CARDIZEM Injectable or Lyo-Ject. The recommended initial infusion rate of CARDIZEM Injectable or Lyo-Ject is 10 mg/h. Some patients may maintain response to an initial rate of 5 mg/h. The infusion rate may be increased in 5 mg/h increments up to 15 mg/h as needed, if further reduction in heart rate is required. The infusion may be maintained for up to 24 hours.

Diltiazem shows dose-dependent, non-linear pharmacokinetics. Duration of infusion longer than 24 hours and infusion rates greater than 15 mg/h have not been studied. Therefore, infusion duration exceeding 24 hours and infusion rates exceeding 15 mg/h are not recommended.

Dilution: To prepare CARDIZEM Injectable or Lyo-Ject for continuous intravenous infusion aseptically transfer the appropriate quantity (see chart) of CARDIZEM Injectable or Lyo-Ject to the desired volume of either Normal Saline, D5W, or D5W/0.45% NaCl. Mix thoroughly. Use within 24 hours. Keep refrigerated until use.

[See table above.]

CARDIZEM Injectable and CARDIZEM Lyo-Ject Syringe were tested for compatibility with three commonly used intravenous fluids at a maximal concentration of 1 mg diltiazem hydrochloride per milliliter. CARDIZEM Injectable and Lyo-Ject were found to be physically compatible and chemically stable in the following parenteral solutions for at least 24 hours when stored in glass or polyvinylchloride (PVC) bags at controlled room temperature 15–30°C (59–86°F) or under refrigeration 2–8°C (36–46°F).

- dextrose (5%) injection USP
- sodium chloride (0.9%) injection USP
- dextrose (5%) and sodium chloride (0.45%) injection USP.

Because of potential physical incompatibilities, it is recommended that CARDIZEM Injectable and Lyo-Ject not be mixed with any other drugs in the same container. If possible, it is recommended that CARDIZEM Injectable or Lyo-Ject Syringe not be co-infused in the same intravenous line.

Physical incompatibilities (precipitate formation or cloudiness) were observed when CARDIZEM Injectable or Lyo-Ject was infused in the same intravenous line with the following drugs: acetazolamide, acyclovir, aminophylline, ampicillin, ampicillin sodium/sulbactam sodium, cefamandole, cefoperazone, diazepam, furosemide, hydrocortisone sodium succinate, insulin, (regular: 100 units/mL), methylprednisolone sodium succinate, mezlocillin, nafcillin, phenytoin, rifampin, and sodium bicarbonate.

NOTE: CARDIZEM Lyo-Ject was found to be compatible with insulin (regular, 100 units/mL).

Parenteral drug products should be inspected visually for particulate matter and discoloration prior to administration whenever solution and container permit.

Transition to Further Antiarrhythmic Therapy.

Transition to other antiarrhythmic agents following administration of CARDIZEM Injectable is generally safe. However, reference should be made to the respective agent manufacturer's package insert for information relative to dosage and administration.

In controlled clinical trials, therapy with antiarrhythmic agents to maintain reduced heart rate in atrial fibrillation or atrial flutter or for prophylaxis of PSVT was generally started within 3 hours after bolus administration of CARDIZEM Injectable. These antiarrhythmic agents were intravenous or oral digoxin, Class 1 antiarrhythmics (eg, quinidine, procainamide), calcium channel blockers, and oral beta-blockers.

Experience in the use of antiarrhythmic agents following maintenance infusion of CARDIZEM Injectable is limited. Patients should be dosed on an individual basis and reference should be made to the respective manufacturer's package insert for information relative to dosage and administration.

HOW SUPPLIED

CARDIZEM® Injectable (diltiazem hydrochloride injection) is supplied in boxes of six 5-mL vials with each vial containing 25 mg of diltiazem hydrochloride (5 mg/mL) (NDC 0088-1790-32) and boxes of six 10-mL vials with each vial containing 50 mg diltiazem hydrochloride (5 mg/mL) (NDC 0088-1790-33).

SINGLE-USE CONTAINERS. DISCARD UNUSED PORTION.

STORE PRODUCT UNDER REFRIGERATION 2–8°C (36–46°F). DO NOT FREEZE. MAY BE STORED AT ROOM TEMPERATURE FOR UP TO 1 MONTH. DESTROY AFTER 1 MONTH AT ROOM TEMPERATURE.

CARDIZEM Lyo-Ject 25-mg syringe is supplied in a single molded nonsterile tray in cartons of 6 syringes (NDC 0088-1790-17). PRODUCT IS TO BE STORED AT ROOM TEMPERATURE 15–30°C (59–86°F). DO NOT FREEZE. RECONSTITUTED MATERIAL IS STABLE FOR 24 HOURS AT CONTROLLED ROOM TEMPERATURE. SINGLE-USE CONTAINERS. DISCARD UNUSED PORTION.

Prescribing Information as of September 1995
Mfd for;
Hoechst Marion Roussel, Inc.
Kansas City, MO 64137 USA

Shown in Product Identification Guide, page 317

CARDIZEM® SR ℞

[kar'diz-em]
(diltiazem HCl)
Sustained Release Capsules
Prescribing Information as of July 1995

DESCRIPTION

CARDIZEM® (diltiazem hydrochloride) is a calcium ion influx inhibitor (slow channel blocker or calcium antagonist). Chemically, diltiazem hydrochloride is 1,5-Benzothiazepin-4(5H)one,3-acetyloxy)-5-[2-(dimethylamino)ethyl]-2, 3-dihydro-2-(4-methoxyphenyl)-,monohydrochloride,(+-cis-. The chemical structure is:

Diltiazem hydrochloride is a white to off-white crystalline powder with a bitter taste. It is soluble in water, methanol, and chloroform. It has a molecular weight of 450.98. Each CARDIZEM SR capsule contains either 60 mg, 90 mg, or 120 mg diltiazem hydrochloride. Also contains: D&C Yellow #10, FD&C Blue #1, FD&C Red #40, FD&C Yellow #6, fumaric acid, povidone, starch, sucrose, talc, titanium dioxide, and other ingredients.

For oral administration.

CLINICAL PHARMACOLOGY

The therapeutic effects of CARDIZEM are believed to be related to its ability to inhibit the influx of calcium ions during membrane depolarization of cardiac and vascular smooth muscle.

Mechanisms of Action

CARDIZEM SR produces its antihypertensive effect primarily by relaxation of vascular smooth muscle and the resultant decrease in peripheral vascular resistance. The magnitude of blood pressure reduction is related to the degree of hypertension; thus hypertensive individuals experience an antihypertensive effect, whereas there is only a modest fall in blood pressure in normotensives.

Hemodynamic and Electrophysiologic Effects

Like other calcium antagonists, diltiazem decreases sinoatrial and atrioventricular conduction in isolated tissues and has a negative inotropic effect in isolated preparations. In the intact animal, prolongation of the AH interval can be seen at higher doses.

In man, diltiazem prevents spontaneous and ergonovine-provoked coronary artery spasm. It causes a decrease in peripheral vascular resistance and a modest fall in blood pressure in normotensive individuals and, in exercise tolerance studies in patients with ischemic heart disease, reduces the heart rate-blood pressure product for any given work load. Studies to date, primarily in patients with good ventricular function, have not revealed evidence of a negative inotropic effect, cardiac output, ejection fraction, and left ventricular and diastolic pressure have not been affected. Increased heart failure has, however, been reported in occasional patients with preexisting impairment of ventricular function. There are as yet few data on the interaction of diltiazem and beta-blockers in patients with poor ventricular function. Resting heart rate is usually slightly reduced by diltiazem. CARDIZEM SR produces antihypertensive effects both in the supine and standing positions. Postural hypotension is infrequently noted upon suddenly assuming an upright position. No reflex tachycardia is associated with the chronic antihypertensive effects. CARDIZEM SR decreases vascular resistance, increases cardiac output (by increasing stroke volume), and produces a slight decrease or no change in heart rate. During dynamic exercise, increases in diastolic pressure are inhibited while maximum achievable systolic pressure is usually reduced. Heart rate at maximum exercise does not change or is slightly reduced. Chronic therapy with

Continued on next page

Hoechst Marion Roussel—Cont.

CARDIZEM produces no change or an increase in plasma catecholamines. No increased activity of the renin-angiotensin-aldosterone axis has been observed. CARDIZEM SR antagonizes the renal and peripheral effects of angiotensin II. Hypertensive animal models respond to diltiazem with reductions in blood pressure and increased urinary output and natriuresis without a change in urinary sodium/potassium ratio.

Intravenous diltiazem in doses of 20 mg prolongs AH conduction time and AV node functional and effective refractory periods by approximately 20%. In a study involving single oral doses of 300 mg of CARDIZEM in six normal volunteers, the average maximum PR prolongation was 14% with no instances of greater than first-degree AV block. Diltiazem-associated prolongation of the AH interval is not more pronounced in patients with first-degree heart block. In patients with sick sinus syndrome, diltiazem significantly prolongs sinus cycle length (up to 50% in some cases).

Chronic oral administration of CARDIZEM in doses of up to 360 mg/day has resulted in small increases in PR interval, and on occasion produces abnormal prolongation. (See WARNINGS.)

Pharmacokinetics and Metabolism

Diltiazem is well absorbed from the gastrointestinal tract and is subject to an extensive first-pass effect, giving an absolute bioavailability (compared to intravenous administration) of about 40%. CARDIZEM undergoes extensive metabolism in which 2% to 4% of the unchanged drug appears in the urine. In vitro binding studies show CARDIZEM is 70% to 80% bound to plasma proteins. Competitive in vitro ligand binding studies have also shown CARDIZEM binding is not altered by therapeutic concentrations of digoxin, hydrochlorothi-azide, phenylbutazone, propranolol, salicylic acid, or warfarin. The plasma elimination half-life following single or multiple drug administration is approximately 3.0 to 4.5 hours. Desacetyl diltiazem is also present in the plasma at levels of 10% to 20% of the parent drug and is 25% to 50% as potent a coronary vasodilator as diltiazem. Minimum therapeutic plasma levels of CARDIZEM appear to be in the range of 50–200 ng/mL. There is a departure from linearity when dose strengths are increased; the half-life is slightly increased with dose. A study that compared patients with normal hepatic function to patients with cirrhosis found an increase in half-life and a 69% increase in bioavailability in the hepatically impaired patients. A single study in nine patients with severely impaired renal function showed no difference in the pharmacokinetic profile of diltiazem compared to patients with normal renal function.

CARDIZEM SR Capsules. Diltiazem is absorbed from the capsule formulation to about 92% of a reference solution at steady-state. A single 120-mg dose of the capsule results in detectable plasma levels within two to three hours and peak plasma levels at six to 11 hours. The apparent elimination half-life after single or multiple dosing is five to seven hours. A departure from linearity similar to that observed with the CARDIZEM tablet is observed. As the dose of CARDIZEM SR capsules is increased from a daily dose of 120 mg (60 mg bid) to 240 mg (120 mg bid) daily, there is an increase in area-under-the-curve of 2.6 times. When the dose is increased from 240 mg to 360 mg daily, there is an increase in area-under-the-curve of 1.8 times. The average plasma levels of the capsule dosed twice daily at steady-state are equivalent to the tablet dosed four times daily when the same total daily dose is administered.

INDICATIONS AND USAGE

CARDIZEM SR is indicated for the treatment of hypertension. It may be used alone or in combination with other antihypertensive medications, such as diuretics.

CONTRAINDICATIONS

CARDIZEM is contraindicated in (1) patients with sick sinus syndrome except in the presence of a functioning ventricular pacemaker, (2) patients with second- or third-degree AV block except in the presence of a functioning ventricular pacemarker, (3) patients with hypotension (less than 90 mm Hg systolic), (4) patients who have demonstrated hypersensitivity to the drug, and (5) patients with acute myocardial infarction and pulmonary congestion documented by x-ray on admission.

WARNINGS

1. **Cardiac Conduction.** CARDIZEM prolongs AV node refractory periods without significantly prolonging sinus node recovery time, except in patients with sick sinus syndrome. This effect may rarely result in abnormally slow heart rates (particularly in patients with sick sinus syndrome) or second- or third-degree AV block (nine of 2,111 patients or 0.43%). Concomitant use of diltiazem with beta-blockers or digitalis may result in additive effects on cardiac conduction. A patient with Prinzmetal's angina developed periods of asystole (2 to 5 seconds) after a single dose of 60 mg of diltiazem. (See ADVERSE REACTIONS section.)
2. **Congestive Heart Failure.** Although diltiazem has a negative inotropic effect in isolated animal tissue preparations, hemodynamic studies in humans with normal ventricular function have not shown a reduction in cardiac index nor consistent negative effects on contractility (dp/dt). An acute study of oral diltiazem in patients with impaired ventricular function (ejection fraction 24% $\pm$ 6%) showed improvement in indices of ventricular function without significant decrease in contractile function (dp/dt). Experience with the use of CARDIZEM (diltiazem hydrochloride) in combination with beta-blockers in patients with impaired ventricular function is limited. Caution should be exercised when using this combination.
3. **Hypotension.** Decreases in blood pressure associated with CARDIZEM therapy may occasionally result in symptomatic hypotension.
4. **Acute Hepatic Injury.** Mild elevations of transaminases with and without concomitant elevation in alkaline phosphatase and bilirubin have been observed in clinical studies. Such elevations were usually transient and frequently resolved even with continued diltiazem treatment. In rare instances, significant elevations in enzymes such as alkaline phosphatase, LDH, SGOT, SGPT, and other phenomena consistent with acute hepatic injury have been noted. These reactions tended to occur early after therapy initiation (1 to 8 weeks) and have been reversible upon discontinuation of drug therapy. The relationship to CARDIZEM is uncertain in some cases, but probable in some. (See PRECAUTIONS.)

PRECAUTIONS

General

CARDIZEM (diltiazem hydrochloride) is extensively metabolized by the liver and excreted by the kidneys and in bile. As with any drug given over prolonged periods, laboratory parameters of renal and hepatic function should be monitored at regular intervals. The drug should be used with caution in patients with impaired renal or hepatic function. In subacute and chronic dog and rat studies designed to produce toxicity, high doses of diltiazem were associated with hepatic damage. In special subacute hepatic studies, oral doses of 125 mg/kg and higher in rats were associated with histological changes in the liver which were reversible when the drug was discontinued. In dogs, doses of 20 mg/kg were also associated with hepatic changes; however, these changes were reversible with continued dosing.

Dermatological events (see ADVERSE REACTIONS section) may be transient and may disappear despite continued use of CARDIZEM. However, skin eruptions progressing to erythema multiforme and/or exfoliative dermatitis have also been infrequently reported. Should a dermatologic reaction persist, the drug should be discontinued.

Drug Interactions

Due to the potential for additive effects, caution and careful titration are warranted in patients receiving CARDIZEM concomitantly with any agents known to affect cardiac contractility and/or conduction. (See WARNINGS.) Pharmacologic studies indicate that there may be additive effects in prolonging AV conduction when using beta-blockers or digitalis concomitantly with CARDIZEM. (See WARNINGS.)

As with all drugs, care should be exercised when treating patients with multiple medications. CARDIZEM undergoes biotransformation by cytochrome P-450 mixed function oxidase. Coadministration of CARDIZEM with other agents which follow the same route of biotransformation may result in the competitive inhibition of metabolism. Especially in patients with renal and/or hepatic impairment, dosages of similarly metabolized drugs, particularly those of low therapeutic ratio may require adjustment when starting or stopping concomitantly administered diltiazem to maintain optimum therapeutic blood levels.

Beta-blockers. Controlled and uncontrolled domestic studies suggest that concomitant use of CARDIZEM and beta-blockers is usually well tolerated, but available data are not sufficient to predict the effects of concomitant treatment in patients with left ventricular dysfunction or cardiac conduction abnormalities.

Administration of CARDIZEM (diltiazem hydrochloride) concomitantly with propranolol in five normal volunteers resulted in increased propranolol levels in all subjects and bioavailability of propranolol was increased approximately 50%. In vitro, propranolol appears to be displaced from its binding sites by diltiazem. If combination therapy is initiated or withdrawn in conjunction with propranolol, an adjustment in the propranolol dose may be warranted. (See WARNINGS.)

Cimetidine. A study in six healthy volunteers has shown a significant increase in peak diltiazem plasma levels (58%) and area-under-the-curve (53%) after a 1-week course of cimetidine at 1,200 mg per day and a single dose of diltiazem 60 mg. Ranitidine produced smaller, nonsignificant increases. The effect may be mediated by cimetidine's known inhibition of hepatic cytochrome P-450, the enzyme system responsible for the first-pass metabolism of diltiazem. Patients currently receiving diltiazem therapy should be carefully monitored for a change in pharmacological effect when initiating and discontinuing therapy with cimetidine. An adjustment in the diltiazem dose may be warranted.

Digitalis. Administration of CARDIZEM with digoxin in 24 healthy male subjects increased plasma digoxin concentrations approximately 20%. Another investigator found no increase in digoxin levels in 12 patients with coronary artery disease. Since there have been conflicting results regarding the effect of digoxin levels, it is recommended that digoxin levels be monitored when initiating, adjusting, and discontinuing CARDIZEM therapy to avoid possible over- or under-digitalization. (See WARNINGS.)

Anesthetics. The depression of cardiac contractility, conductivity, and automaticity as well as the vascular dilation associated with anesthetics may be potentiated by calcium channel blockers. When used concomitantly, anesthetics and calcium blockers should be titrated carefully.

Cyclosporine. A pharmacokinetic interaction between diltiazem and cyclosporine has been observed during studies involving renal and cardiac transplant patients. In renal and cardiac transplant recipients, a reduction of cyclosporine dose ranging from 15% to 48% was necessary to maintain cyclosporine trough concentrations similar to those seen prior to the addition of diltiazem. If these agents are to be administered concurrently, cyclosporine concentrations should be monitored, especially when diltiazem therapy is initiated, adjusted or discontinued. The effect of cyclosporine on diltiazem plasma concentrations has not been evaluated.

Carbamazepine. Concomitant administration of diltiazem with carbamazepine has been reported to result in elevated serum levels of carbamazepine (40 to 72% increase), resulting in toxicity in some cases. Patients receiving these drugs concurrently should be monitored for a potential drug interaction.

Carcinogenesis, Mutagenesis, Impairment of Fertility

A 24-month study in rats and a 21-month study in mice showed no evidence of carcinogenicity. There was also no mutagenic response in in vitro bacterial tests. No intrinsic effect on fertility was observed in rats.

Pregnancy

Category C. Reproduction studies have been conducted in mice, rats, and rabbits. Administration of doses ranging from five to ten times greater (on a mg/kg basis) than the daily recommended therapeutic dose has resulted in embryo and fetal lethality. These doses, in some studies, have been reported to cause skeletal abnormalities. In the perinatal/postnatal studies, there was some reduction in early individual pup weights and survival rates. There was an increased incidence of stillbirths at doses of 20 times the human dose or greater.

There are no well-controlled studies in pregnant women; therefore, use CARDIZEM in pregnant women only if the potential benefit justifies the potential risk to the fetus.

Nursing Mothers

Diltiazem is excreted in human milk. One report suggests that concentrations in breast milk may approximate serum levels. If use of CARDIZEM is deemed essential, an alternative method of infant feeding should be instituted.

CARDIZEM® SR
(diltiazem hydrochloride)
Sustained Release Capsules

Strength	Quantity	NDC Number	Description
60 mg	100 btl 100 UDIP®	0088-1777-47 0088-1777-49	Ivory/brown capsule imprinted with CARDIZEM logo on one end and CARDIZEM SR 60 mg on the other
90 mg	100 btl 100 UDIP®	0088-1778-47 0088-1778-49	Gold/brown capsule imprinted with CARDIZEM logo on one end and CARDIZEM SR 90 mg on the other
120 mg	100 btl 100 UDIP®	0088-1779-47 0088-1779-49	Caramel/brown capsule imprinted with CARDIZEM logo on one end and CARDIZEM SR 120 mg on the other

Pediatric Use

Safety and effectiveness in pediatric patients have not been established.

ADVERSE REACTIONS

Serious adverse reactions have been rare in studies carried out to date, but it should be recognized that patients with impaired ventricular function and cardiac conduction abnormalities have usually been excluded from these studies.

The adverse events described below represent events observed in clinical studies of hypertensive patients receiving either CARDIZEM Tablets or CARDIZEM SR Capsules as well as experiences observed in studies of angina and during marketing. The most common events in hypertension studies are shown in a table with rates in placebo patients shown for comparison. Less common events are listed by body system; these include any adverse reactions seen in angina studies that were not observed in hypertension studies. In all hypertensive patients studied (over 900), the most common adverse events were edema (9%), headache (8%), dizziness (6%), asthenia (5%), sinus bradycardia (3%), flushing (3%), and first-degree AV block (3%). Only edema and perhaps bradycardia and dizziness were dose related. The most common events observed in clinical studies (over 2,100 patients) of angina and hypertensive patients receiving CARDIZEM Tablets or CARDIZEM SR Capsules were (ie, greater than 1%) edema (5.4%), headache (4.5%), dizziness (3.4%), asthenia (2.8%), first-degree AV block (1.8%), flushing (1.7%), nausea (1.6%), bradycardia (1.5%), and rash (1.5%).

Double Blind Placebo Controlled Hypertension Trials

Adverse	Diltiazem n = 315 # pts (%)	Placebo n = 211 # pts (%)
headache	38 (12%)	17 (8%)
AV block first degree	24 (7.6%)	4 (1.9%)
dizziness	22 (7%)	6 (2.8%)
edema	19 (6%)	2 (0.9%)
bradycardia	19 (6%)	3 (1.4%)
ECG abnormality	13 (4.1%)	3 (1.4%)
asthenia	10 (3.2%)	1 (0.5%)
constipation	5 (1.6%)	2 (0.9%)
dyspepsia	4 (1.3%)	1 (0.5%)
nausea	4 (1.3%)	2 (0.9%)
palpitations	4 (1.3%)	2 (0.9%)
polyuria	4 (1.3%)	2 (0.9%)
somnolence	4 (1.3%)	—
alk phos increase	3 (1%)	1 (0.5%)
hypotension	3 (1%)	1 (0.5%)
insomnia	3 (1%)	1 (0.5%)
rash	3 (1%)	1 (0.5%)
AV block second degree	2 (0.6%)	—

In addition, the following events were reported infrequently (less than 1%) with CARDIZEM SR Capsules or CARDIZEM Tablets or have been observed in angina or hypertension trials.

Cardiovascular: Angina, arrhythmia, second- or third-degree AV block (see conduction warning), bundle branch block, congestive heart failure, syncope, tachycardia, ventricular extrasystoles.

Nervous System: Abnormal dreams, amnesia, depression, gait abnormality, hallucinations, nervousness, paresthesia, personality change, tremor.

Gastrointestinal: Anorexia, diarrhea, dry mouth, dysgeusia, mild elevations of SGOT, SGPT, and LDH (see hepatic warnings), thirst, vomiting, weight increase.

Dermatological: Petechiae, photosensitivity, pruritus, urticaria

Other: Amblyopia, CPK increase, dyspnea, epistaxis, eye irritation, hyperglycemia, hyperuricemia, impotence, muscle cramps, nasal congestion, nocturia, osteoarticular pain, sexual difficulties, tinnitus. The following postmarketing events have been reported infrequently in patients receiving CARDIZEM: allergic reactions, alopecia, angioedema (including facial or periorbital edema), asystole, erythema multiforme (including Stevens-Johnson syndrome, toxic epidermal necrolysis), extrapyramidal symptoms, gingival hyperplasia, hemolytic anemia, increased bleeding time, leukopenia, purpura, retinopathy, and thrombocytopenia. There have been observed cases of a generalized rash, some characterized as leukocytoclastic vasculitis. In addition, events such as myocardial infarction have been observed which are not readily distinguishable from the natural history of the disease in these patients. A definitive cause and effect relationship between these events and CARDIZEM therapy cannot yet be established. Exfoliative dermatitis (proven by rechallenge) has also been reported.

OVERDOSAGE OR EXAGGERATED RESPONSE

The oral LD_{50} 's in mice and rats range from 415 to 740 mg/kg and from 560 to 810 mg/kg, respectively. The intravenous LD_{50} 's in these species were 60 and 38 mg/kg, respectively. The oral LD_{50} in dogs is considered to be in excess of 50 mg/kg, while lethality was seen in monkeys at 360 mg/kg.

The toxic dose in man is not known. Due to extensive metabolism, blood levels after a standard dose of diltiazem can vary over tenfold, limiting the usefulness of blood levels in overdose cases.

There have been 29 reports of diltiazem overdose in doses ranging from less than 1 g to 10.8 g. Sixteen of these reports involved multiple drug ingestions.

Twenty-two reports indicated patients had recovered from diltiazem overdose ranging from less than 1 g to 10.8 g. There were seven reports with a fatal outcome; although the amount of diltiazem ingested was unknown, multiple drug ingestions were confirmed in six of the seven reports.

Events observed following diltiazem overdose included bradycardia, hypotension, heart block, and cardiac failure. Most reports of overdose described some supportive medical measure and/or drug treatment. Bradycardia frequently responded favorably to atropine, as did heart block, although cardiac pacing was also frequently utilized to treat heart block. Fluids and vasopressors were used to maintain blood pressure and in cases of cardiac failure inotropic agents were administered. In addition, some patients received treatment with ventilatory support, gastric lavage, activated charcoal, and/or intravenous calcium. Evidence of the effectiveness of intravenous calcium administration to reverse the pharmacological effects of diltiazem overdose was conflicting.

In the event of overdose or exaggerated response, appropriate supportive measures should be employed in addition to gastrointestinal decontamination. Diltiazem does not appear to be removed by peritoneal or hemodialysis. Limited data suggest that plasmapheresis or charcoal hemoperfusion may hasten diltiazem elimination following overdose. Based on the known pharmacological effects of diltiazem and/or reported clinical experiences the following measures may be considered.

Bradycardia: Administer atropine (0.60 to 1.0 mg). If there is no response to vagal blockade, administer isoproterenol cautiously.

High-Degree AV Block: Treat as for bradycardia above. Fixed high-degree AV block should be treated with cardiac pacing.

Cardiac Failure: Administer inotropic agents (isoproterenol, dopamine, or dobutamine) and diuretics.

Hypotension: Vasopressors (eg, dopamine or levarterenol bitartrate).

Actual treatment and dosage should depend on the severity of the clinical situation and the judgment and experience of the treating physician.

DOSAGE AND ADMINISTRATION

Dosages must be adjusted to each patient's needs, starting with 60 to 120 mg twice daily. Maximum antihypertensive effect is usually observed by 14 days of chronic therapy: therefore, dosage adjustments should be scheduled accordingly. Although individual patients may respond to lower doses, the usual optimum dosage range in clinical trials was 240 to 360 mg/day.

CARDIZEM SR has an additive antihypertensive effect when used with other antihypertensive agents. Therefore, the dosage of CARDIZEM SR or the concomitant antihypertensives may need to be adjusted when adding one to the other. See WARNINGS and PRECAUTIONS regarding use with beta-blockers.

HOW SUPPLIED

[See table on bottom of preceding page.]

Storage Conditions: Store at controlled room temperature 59–86°F (15–30°C)

Prescribing Information as of July 1995

Hoechst Marion Roussel, Inc.

Kansas City, MO 64137 USA

Shown in Product Identification Guide, page 317

CARDIZEM® ℞

[*kar'diz-em*]

(diltiazem hydrochloride)

Prescribing Information as of July 1995

DESCRIPTION

Diltiazem hydrochloride is a calcium ion influx inhibitor (slow channel blocker or calcium antagonist). Chemically, diltiazem hydrochloride is 1,5-benzothiazepin-4(5H) one,3-(acetyloxy)-5-[2-(dimethylamino)ethyl]-2, 3-dihydro-2-(4-methoxyphenyl)-,monohydrochloride,(+)-cis-. The chemical structure is.

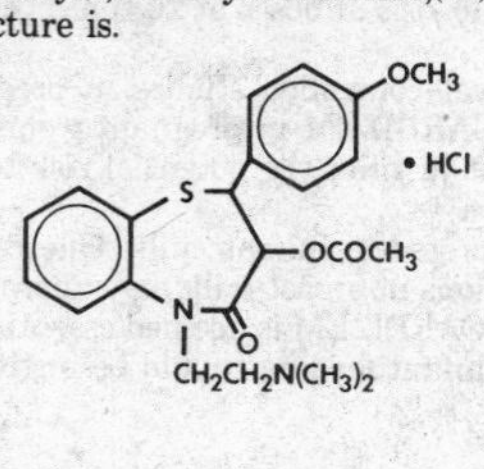

Diltiazem hydrochloride is a white to off-white crystalline powder with a bitter taste. It is soluble in water, methanol, and chloroform. It has a molecular weight of 450.98. Each tablet of CARDIZEM contains 30 mg, 60 mg, 90 mg, or 120 mg diltiazem hydrochloride.

Also contains: D&C Yellow #10, FD&C Yellow #6 (60 mg and 120 mg), or FD&C Blue #1 (30 mg and 90 mg), hydroxypropylcellulose, hydroxypropyl methylcellulose, lactose, magnesium stearaate, methylparaben, polyethylene glycol, talc, and other ingredients.

For oral administration.

CLINICAL PHARMACOLOGY

The therapeutic benefits achieved with CARDIZEM are believed to be related to its ability to inhibit the influx of calcium ions during membrane depolarization of cardiac and vascular smooth muscle.

Mechanisms of Action

Although precise mechanisms of its antianginal actions are still being delineated, CARDIZEM is believed to act in the following ways:

1. **Angina Due to Coronary Artery Spasm.** CARDIZEM has been shown to be a potent dilator of coronary arteries both epicardial and subendocardial. Spontaneous and ergonovine-induced coronary artery spasm are inhibited by CARDIZEM.
2. **Exertional Angina.** CARDIZEM has been shown to produce increases in exercise tolerance, probably due to its ability to reduce myocardial oxygen demand. This is accomplished via reductions in heart rate and systemic blood pressure at submaximal and maximal exercise workloads.

In animal models, diltiazem interferes with the slow inward (depolarizing) current in excitable tissue. It causes excitation-contraction uncoupling in various myocardial tissues without changes in the configuration of the action potential. Diltiazem produces relaxation of coronary vascular smooth muscle and diation of both large and small coronary arteries at drug levels which cause little or no negative inotropic effect. The resultant increases in coronary blood flow (epicardial and subendocardial) occur in ischemic, and nonischemic models and are accompanied by dose-dependent decreases in systemic blood pressure and decreases in peripheral resistance.

Hemodynamic and Electrophysiologic Effects

Like other calcium antagonists, diltiazem decreases sinoatrial and atrioventicular conduction in isolaated tissues and has a negative inotropic effect in isolated preparations. In the intact animal, prolongation of the AH interval can be seen at higher doses.

In man, diltiazem prevents spontaneous and ergonovine-provoked coronary artery spasm. It causes a decrease in peripheral vascular resistance and a modest fall in blood pressure and, in exercise tolerance studies in patients with ischemic heart disease, reduces the heart rate-blood pressure product for any given workload. Studies to date, primarily in patients with good ventricular function, have not revealed evidence of a negative inotropic effect; cardiac output, ejection fraction, and left ventricular end-diastolic pressure have not been affected. There are as yet few data on the interaction of diltiazem and beta-blockers. Resting heart rate is usually unchanged or slightly reduced by diltiazem.

Intravenous diltiazem in doses of 20 mg prolongs AH conduction time and AV node functional and effective refractory periods approximately 20%. In a study involving single oral doses of 300 mg of CARDIZEM in six normal volunteers, the average maximum PR prolongation was 14% with no instances of greater than first-degree AV block. Diltiazem-associated prolongation of the AH interval is not more pronounced in patients with first-degree heart block. In patients with sick sinus syndrome, diltiazem significantly prolongs sinus cycle length (up to 50% in some cases).

Chronic oral administration of CARDIZEM in doses of up to 240 mg/day has resulted in small increases in PR interval, but has not usually produced abnormal prolongation.

Pharmacokinetics and Metabolism

Diltiazem is well absorbed from the gastrointestinal tract and is subject to an extensive first-pass effect, giving an absolute bioavailability (compared to intravenous dosing) of about 40%. CARDIZEM undergoes extensive metabolism in which 2% to 4% of the unchanged drug appears in the urine. In vitro binding studies show CARDIZEM is 70% to 80% bound to plasma proteins. Competitive in vitro ligand binding studies have also shown CARDIZEM binding is not altered by therapeutic concentrations of digoxin, hydrochlorothiazide, phenylbutazone, propranolol, salicylic acid, or warfarin. The plasma elimination half-life following single or multiple drug administration is approximately 3.0 to 4.5 hours. Desacetyl diltiazem is also present in the plasma at levels of 10% to 20% of the parent drug and is 25% to 50% as potent as a coronary vasodilator as diltiazem. Minimum therapeutic plasma levels of CARDIZEM appear to be in the range of 50-200 ng/mL. There is a departure from linearity when dose strengths are increased. A study that compared

Continued on next page

Hoechst Marion Roussel—Cont.

patients with normal hepatic function to patients with cirrhosis found an increase in half-life and a 69% increase in AUC (area-under-the-plasma concentration vs time curve) in the hepatically impaired patients. A single study in nine patients with severely impaired renal functions showed no difference in the pharmacokinetic profile of diltiazem as compared to patients with normal renal function.

CARDIZEM Tablets. Diltiazem is absorbed from the tablet formulation to about 98% of a reference solution. Single oral doses of 30 to 120 mg of CARDIZEM tablets result in detectable plasma levels within 30 to 60 minutes and peak plasma levels 2 to 4 hours after drug administration. As the dose of CARDIZEM tablets is increased from a daily dose of 120 mg (30 mg qid) to 240 mg (660 mg qid) daily, there is an increase in area-under-the-curve of 2.3 times. When the dose is increased from 240 mg to 360 mg daily, there is an increase in area-under-the-curve of 1.8 times.

INDICATIONS AND USAGE

CARDIZEM is indicated for the management of chronic stable angina and angina due to coronary artery spasm.

CONTRAINDICATIONS

CARDIZEM is contraindicated in (1) patients with sick sinus syndrome except in the presence of a functioning ventricular pacemaker, (2) patients with second- or third-degree AV block except in the presence of a functioning ventricular pacemaker, (3) patients with hypotension (less than 90 mm Hg systolic), (4) patients who have demonstrated hypersensitivity to the drug, and (5) patients with acute myocardial infarction and pulmonary congestion documented by x-ray on admission.

WARNINGS

1. Cardiac Conduction. CARDIZEM prolongs AV node refractory periods without significantly prolonging sinus node recovery time, except in patients with sick sinus syndrome. This effect may rarely result in abnormally slow heart rates (particularly in patients with sick sinus syndrome) or second- or third-degree AV block (six of 1243 patients for 0.48%). Concomitant use of diltiazem with betablockers or digitalis may result in additive effects on cardiac conduction. A patient with Prinzmetal's angina developed periods of asystole (2 to 5 seconds) after a single dose of 60 mg of diltiazem. (See ADVERSE REACTIONS section.)

2. Congestive Heart Failure. Although diltiazem has a negative inotropic, effect in isolated animal tissue, preparations, hemodynamic studies in humans with normal ventricular function have not shown a reduction in cardiac index nor consistent negative effects on contractility (dp/dt). Experience with the use of CARDIZEM alone or in combination with beta-blockers in patients with impaired ventricular function is very limited. Caution should be exercised when using the drug in such patients.

3. Hypotension. Decreases in blood pressure associated with CARDIZEM therapy may occasionally result in symptomatic hypotension.

4. Acute Hepatic Injury. In rare instances, significant elevations in enzymes such as alkaline phosphatase, LDH, SGOT, SGPT, and other phenomena consistent with acute hepatic injury have been noted. These reactions have been reversible upon discontinuation of drug therapy. The relationship to CARDIZEM is uncertain in most cases, but probable in some. (See PRECAUTIONS.)

PRECAUTIONS

General

CARDIZEM (diltiazem hydrochloride) is extensively metabolized by the liver and excreted by the kidneys and in bile. As with any drug given over prolonged periods, laboratory parameters of renal and hepatic function should be monitored at regular intervals. The drug should be used with caution in patients with impaired renal or hepatic function. In subacute and chronic dog and rat studies designed to produce toxicity, high doses of diltiazem were associated with hepatic damage. In special subacute hepatic studies, oral doses of 125 mg/kg and higher in rats were associated with histological changes in the liver, which were reversible when the drug was discontinued. In dogs, doses of 20 mg/kg were also associated with hepatic changes; however, these changes were reversible with continued dosing.

Dermatological events (see ADVERSE REACTIONS section) may be transient and may disappear despite continued use of CARDIZEM. However, skin eruptions progressing to erythema multiforme and/or exfoliative dermatitis have also been infrequently reported. Should a dermatologic reaction persist, the drug should be discontinued.

Drug Interactions

Due to the potential for additive effects, caution and careful titration are warranted in patients receiving CARDIZEM concomitantly with any agents known to affect cardiac contractility and/or conduction. (See WARNINGS.)

Phamacologic studies indicate that there may be additive effects in prolonging AV conduction when using beta-block-

ers or digitalis concomitantly with CARDIZEM, (See WARNINGS.)

As with all drugs, care should be exercised when treating patients with multiple medications. CARDIZEM undergoes biotransformation by cytochrome P-450 mixed function oxidase. Coadministration of CARDIZEM with other agents which follow the same route of biotransformation may result in the competitive inhibition of metabolism. Especially in patients with renal and/or hepatic impairment, dosages of similarly metabolized drugs, particularly those of low therapeutic ratio, may require adjustment when starting or stopping concomitantly administered diltiazem to maintain optimum therapeutic blood levels.

Beta-blockers. Controlled and uncontrolled domestic studies suggest that concomitant use of CARDIZEM and beta-blockers is usually well tolerated. Available data are not sufficient, however, to predict the effects of concomitant treatment, particularly in patients with left ventricular dysfunction or cardiac conduction abnormalities.

Administration of CARDIZEM (diltiazem hydrochloride) concomitantly with propranolol in five normal volunteers resulted in increased propranolol levels in all subjects, and bioavailability of propranolol was increased approximately 50%. In vitro, propranolol appears to be displaced from its binding sites by diltiazem. If combination therapy is initiated or withdrawn in conjunction with propranolol, an adjustment in the propranolol dose may be warranted. (See WARNINGS.)

Cimetidine. A study in six healthy volunteers has shown a significant increase in peak diltiazem plasma levels (58%) and area-under-the-curve (53%) after a 1-week course of cimetidine at 1200 mg per day and a single dose of diltiazem 60 mg. Ranitidine produced smaller, nonsignificant increases. The effect may be mediated by cimetidine's known inhibition of hepatic cytochrome P-450, the enzyme system responsible for the first-pass metabolism of diltiazem. Patients currently receiving diltiazem therapy should be carefully monitored for a change in phamacological effect when initiating and discontinuing therapy with cimetidine. An adjustment in the diltiazem dose may be warranted.

Digitalis. Administration of CARDIZEM with digoxin in 24 healthy male subjects increased plasma digoxin concentrations approximately 20%. Another investigator found no increase in digoxin levels in 12 patients with coronary artery disease. Since there have been conflicting results regarding the effect of digoxin levels, it is recommended that digoxin levels be monitored when initiating, adjusting, and discontinuing CARDIZEM therapy to avoid possible over- or underdigitalization. (See WARNINGS.)

Anesthetics. The depression of cardiac contractility, conductivity, and automaticity, as well as the vascular dilation associated with anesthetics, may be potentiated by calcium channel blockers. When used concomitantly, anesthetics and calcium blockers should be titrated carefully.

Cyclosporine. A pharmacokinetic interaction between diltiazem and cyclosporine has been observed during studies involving renal and cardiac transplant patients. In renal and cardiac transplant recipients, a reduction of cyclosporine trough dose ranging from 15% to 48% was necessary to maintain concentrations similar to those seen prior to the addition of diltiazem. If these agents are to be administered concurrently, cyclosporine concentrations should be monitored, especially when diltiazem therapy is initiated, adjusted, or discontinued. The effect of cyclosporine on diltiazem plasma concentrations has not been evaluated.

Carbamazepine. Concomitant administration of diltiazem with carbamazepine has been reported to result in evaluated serum levels of carbamazepine (40% to 72% increase) resulting in toxicity in some cases. Patients receiving these drugs concurrently should be monitored for a potential drug interaction.

Carcinogenesis, Mutagenesis, Impairment of Fertility

A 24-month study in rats and a 21-month study in mice showed no evidence of carcinogenicity. There was also no mutagenic response in in vitro bacterial tests. No intrinsic effect on fertility was observed in rats.

Pregnancy

Category C. Reproduction studies have been conducted in mice, rats, and rabbits. Administration of doses ranging from five to ten times greater (on a mg/kg basis) than the daily recommended therapeutic dose has resulted in embryo and fetal lethality. These doses, in some studies, have been reported to cause skeletal abnormalities. In the perinatal/postnatal studies, there was some reduction in early individual pup weights and survival rates. There was an increased incidence of stillbirths at doses at 20 times the human dose or greater.

There are no well-controlled studies in pregnant women; therefore, use CARDIZEM in pregnant woman only if the potential benefit justifies the potential risk to the fetus.

Nursing Mothers

Diltiazem is excreted in human milk. One report suggests that concentrations in breast milk may approximate serum levels. If use of CARDIZEM is deemed essential, an alternative method of infant feeding should be instituted.

Pediatric Use

Safety and effectiveness in pediatric patients have not been established.

ADVERSE REACTIONS

Serious adverse reactions have been rare in studies carried out to date, but it should be recognized that patients with impaired ventricular function and cardiac conduction abnormalities usually have been excluded.

In domestic placebo-controlled angina trials, the incidence of adverse reactions report during CARDIZEM therapy was not greater than reported during placebo therapy.

The following represent occurrences observed in clinical studies of angina patients. In many cases, the relationship to CARDIZEM has not been established. The most common occurrences from these studies, as well as their frequency of presentation, are edema (2.4%), headache (2.1%), nausea (1.9%), dizziness (1.5%), rash (1.3%), and asthenia (1.2%). In addition, the following events were reported infrequently (less than 1%):

Cardiovascular: Angina, arrhythmia, AV block (first degree), AV block (second or third degree—see conduction warning), bradycardia, bundle branch block, congestive heart failure, ECG abnormality, flushing, hypotension, palpitations, syncope, tachycardia, ventricular extrasystoles

Nervous System: Abnormal dreams, amnesia, depression, gait abnormality, hallucinations, insomnia, nervousness, paresthesia, personality change, somnolence, tremor

Gastrointestinal: Anorexia, constipation, diarrhea, dysgeusia, dyspepsia, mild elevations of alkaline phosphatase, SGOT, SGPT, and LDH (see hepatic warnings), thirst, vomiting, weight increase

Dermatological: Petechiae, photosensitivity, pruritus, urticaria

Other: Amblyopia, CPK elevation, dry mouth, dyspnea, epistaxis, eye irritation, hyperglycemia, hyperuricemia, impotence, muscle cramps, nasal congestion, nocturia, osteoarticular pain, polyuria, sexual difficulties, tinnitus

The following postmarketing events have been reported infrequently in patients receiving CARDIZEM: allergic reactions, alopecia, angioedema (including facial or periorbital edema), asystole, erythema multiforme (including Stevens-Johnson syndrome, toxic epidermal necrolysis), extrapyramidal symptoms, gingival hyperplasia, hemolytic anemia, increased bleeding time, leukopenia, purpura, retinopathy, and thrombocytopenia. There have been observed cases of a generalized rash, some characterized as leukocytoclastic vasculitis. In addition, events such as myocardial infarction have been observed, which are not readily distinguishable from the natural history of the disease in these patients. A definitive cause and effect relationship between these events and CARDIZEM therapy cannot yet be established. Exfoliative dermatitis (proven by rechallenge) has also been reported.

OVERDOSAGE OR EXAGGERATED RESPONSE

The oral LD_{50}s in mice and rats range from 415 to 740 mg/kg and from 560 to 810 mg/kg, respectively. The intravenous LD_{50}s in these species were 60 and 38 mg/kg, respectively. The oral LD_{50}s in dogs is considered to be in excess of 50 mg/kg, while lethality was seen in monkeys at 360 mg/kg.

The toxic dose in man is not known. Due to extensive metabolism, blood levels after a standard dose of diltiazem can vary over tenfold, limiting the usefulness of blood levels in overdose cases.

There have been 29 reports of diltiazem overdose in doses ranging from less than 1 g to 10.8 g. Sixteen of these reports involving multiple drug ingestions.

Twenty-two reports indicated patients had recovered from diltiazem overdose ranging from less than 1 g to 10.8 g. There were seven reports with a fatal outcome; although the amount of diltiazem ingested was unknown, multiple drug ingestions were confirmed in six of the seven reports.

Events observed following diltiazem overdose included bradycardia, hypotension, heart block, and cardiac failure. Most reports of overdose described some supportive medical measure and/or drug treatment. Bradycardia frequently responded favorably to atropine, as did heart block, although cardiac pacing was also frequently utilized to treat heart block. Fluids and vasopressors were used to maintain blood pressure, and in cases of cardiac failure, inotropic agents were administrated. In addition, some patients received treatment with ventilatory support, gastric lavage, activated charcoal, and/or intravenous calcium. Evidence of the effectiveness of intravenous calcium administration to reverse the pharmacological effects of diltiazem overdose was conflicting.

In the event of overdose or exaggerated response, appropriate supportive measure should be employed in addition to gastrointestinal decontamination. Diltiazem does not appear to be removed by pertioneal or hemodialysis. Limited data suggest that plasmapheresis or charcoal hemoperfusion may hasten diltiazem elimination following overdose. Based on the known pharmacological effects of diltiazem and/or reported clinical experiences, the following measure may be considered:

Bradycardia: Administer atropine (0.06 to 1.0 mg). If there is not response to vagal blockade, administer isoproterenol cautiously.
High-Degree AV Block: Treat as for bradycardia above. Fixed high-degree AV block should be treated with cardiac pacing.
Cardiac Failure: Administer inotropic agents (isoproterenol, dopamine, or dobutamine) and diuretics.
Hypotension: Vasopressors (eg, dopamine or levarterenol bitartrate).
Actual treatment and dosage should depend on the severity of the clinical situation and the judgment and experience of the treating physician.

DOSAGE AND ADMINISTRATION

Exertional Angina Pectoris Due to Atherosclerotic Coronary Artery Disease or Angina Pectoris at Rest Due to Coronary Artery Spasm. Dosage must be adjusted to reach patient's needs. Starting with 30 mg four times daily, before meals, and at bedtime, dosage should be increased gradually (given in divided doses three or four times daily) at 1- to 2-day intervals until optimum response is obtained. Although individual patients may respond to any dosage level, the average optimum dosage range appears to be 180 to 360 mg/day. There are no available data concerning dosage requirements in patients with impaired renal or hepatic function. If the drug must be used in such patients, titration should be carried out with particular caution.

Concomitant Use With Other Cardiovascular Agents

1. **Sublingual MTG** may be taken as required to abort acute anginal attacks during CARDIZEM (diltiazem hydrochloride) therapy.
2. **Prophylactic Nitrate Therapy.** CARDIZEM may be safely coadministered with short- and long-acting nitrates, but there have been no controlled studies to evaluate the antianginal effectiveness of this combination.
3. **Beta-blockers.** (See WARNINGS and PRECAUTIONS.)

HOW SUPPLIED

CARDIZEM 30-mg tablets are supplied in bottles of 100 (NDC 0088-1771-47) and 500 (NDC 0088-1771-55) and in Unit Dose Identification Paks of 100 (NDC 0088-1771-49). Each green tablet is engraved with MARION on one side and 1771 on the other.
CARDIZEM 60-mg scored tablets are supplied in bottles of 100 (NDC 0088-1772-47) and 500 (NDC 0088-1772-55) and in Unit Dose Identification Paks of 100 (NDC 0088-1772-49). Each yellow tablet is engraved with MARION on one side and 1772 on the other.
CARDIZEM 90-mg scored tablets are supplied in bottles of 100 (NDC 0088-1791-47) and in Unit Dose Identification Paks of 100 (NDC 0088-1791-49). Each green oblong tablet is engraved with CARDIZEM on one side and 90 mg on the other.
CARDIZEM 120-mg scored tablets are supplied in bottles of 100 (NDC 0088-1792-47) and in Unit Dose Identification Paks of 100 (NDC 0088-1792-49). Each yellow oblong tablet is engraved with CARDIZEM on one side and 120 mg on the other.
Store at controlled room temperature 59–86°F (15–30°C).
Prescribing Information as of July 1995
Hoechst Marion Roussel, Inc.
Kansas City, MO 64137 USA

Shown in Product Identification Section, page 317

CLAFORAN® ℞

[kla'fər-an]
Sterile (sterile cefotaxime sodium)
and
Injection (cefotaxime sodium injection)

DESCRIPTION

Sterile Claforan® (cefotaxime sodium) is a semisynthetic, broad spectrum cephalosporin antibiotic for parenteral administration. It is the sodium salt of 7-[2-(2-amino-4-thiazolyl) glyoxylamido]-3-(hydroxymethyl)-8-oxo-5-thia-1-azabicyclo [4.2.0] oct-2-ene-2-carboxylate 7^2-(Z)-(o-methyloxime), acetate (ester). Claforan® contains approximately 50.5 mg (2.2 mEq) of sodium per gram of cefotaxime activity. Solutions of Claforan® range from very pale yellow to light amber depending on the concentration and the diluent used. The pH of the injectable solutions usually ranges from 5.0 to 7.5. The CAS Registry Number is 64485-93-4.

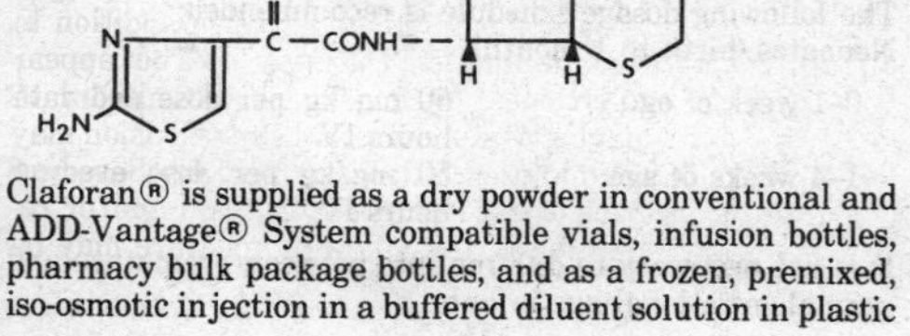

Claforan® is supplied as a dry powder in conventional and ADD-Vantage® System compatible vials, infusion bottles, pharmacy bulk package bottles, and as a frozen, premixed, iso-osmotic injection in a buffered diluent solution in plastic containers. Claforan®, equivalent to 1 gram and 2 grams cefotaxime, is supplied as frozen, premixed iso-osmotic injections in plastic containers. Solutions range from very pale yellow to light amber. Dextrose Hydrous, USP has been added to adjust osmolality (approximately 1.7 g and 700 mg to the 1 g and 2 g cefotaxime dosages, respectively). The injections are buffered with sodium citrate hydrous, USP. The pH is adjusted with hydrochloric acid and may be adjusted with sodium hydroxide.
The plastic container is fabricated from a specially designed multilayer plastic (PL2040). Solutions are in contact with the polyethylene layer of this container and can leach out certain chemical components of the plastic in very small amounts within the expiration period. The suitability of the plastic has been confirmed in tests in animals according to the USP biological tests for plastic containers, as well as by tissue culture toxicity studies.

CLINICAL PHARMACOLOGY

Following IM administration of a single 500 mg or 1 g dose of Claforan® to normal volunteers, mean peak serum concentrations of 11.7 and 20.5 μg/mL respectively were attained within 30 minutes and declined with an elimination half-life of approximately 1 hour. There was a dose-dependent increase in serum levels after the IV administration of 500 mg, 1 g, and 2 g of Claforan® (38.9, 101.7, and 214.4 μg/mL respectively) without alteration in the elimination half-life. There is no evidence of accumulation following repetitive IV infusion of 1 g doses every 6 hours for 14 days as there are no alterations of serum or renal clearance. About 60% of the administered dose was recovered from urine during the first 6 hours following the start of the infusion.
Approximately 20–36% of an intravenously administered dose of ^{14}C-cefotaxime is excreted by the kidney as unchanged cefotaxime and 15–25% as the desacetyl derivative, the major metabolite. The desacetyl metabolite has been shown to contribute to the bactericidal activity. Two other urinary metabolites (M_2 and M_3) account for about 20–25%. They lack bactericidal activity.
A single 50 mg/kg dose of Claforan® was administered as an intravenous infusion over a 10- to 15-minute period to 29 newborn infants grouped according to birth weight and age. The mean half-life of cefotaxime in infants with lower birth weights (≤ 1500 grams), regardless of age, was longer (4.6 hours) than the mean half-life (3.4 hours) in infants whose birth weight was greater than 1500 grams. Mean serum clearance was also smaller in the lower birth weight infants. Although the differences in mean half-life values are statistically significant for weight, they are not clinically important. Therefore, dosage should be based solely on age. (See **DOSAGE AND ADMINISTRATION** section.)
Additionally, no disulfiram-like reactions were reported in a study conducted in 22 healthy volunteers administered Claforan® and ethanol.

Microbiology

The bactericidal activity of cefotaxime sodium results from inhibition of cell wall synthesis. Cefotaxime sodium has *in vitro* activity against a wide range of gram-positive and gram-negative organisms. Claforan® has a high degree of stability in the presence of beta-lactamases, both penicillinases and cephalosporinases, of gram-negative and gram-positive bacteria. Cefotaxime sodium has been shown to be a potent inhibitor of β-lactamases produced by certain gram-negative bacteria. Cefotaxime sodium is usually active against the following microorganisms both *in vitro* and in clinical infections (see **INDICATIONS AND USAGE** section.)
Aerobes, Gram-positive: *Staphylococcus aureus,* including penicillinase and non-penicillinase producing strains, *Staphylococcus epidermidis, Enterococcus* species, *Streptococcus pyogenes* (Group A beta-hemolytic streptococci), *Streptococcus agalactiae* (Group B streptococci), *Streptococcus pneumoniae* (formerly *Diplococcus pneumoniae*).
Aerobes, Gram-negative: *Citrobacter* species, *Enterobacter* species, *Escherichia coli, Haemophilus influenzae* (including ampicillin-resistant *H. influenzae*), *Haemophilus parainfluenzae, Klebsiella* species (including *K. pneumoniae*), *Neisseria gonorrhoeae* (including penicillinase and non-penicillinase producing strains), *Neisseria meningitidis, Proteus mirabilis, Proteus vulgaris, Proteus inconstans,* Group B, *Morganella morganii, Providencia rettgeri, Serratia* species, and *Acinetobacter* species.
NOTE: Many strains of the above organisms that are multiply resistant to other antibiotics, e.g., penicillins, cephalosporins, and aminoglycosides, are susceptible to cefotaxime sodium.
Cefotaxime sodium is active against some strains of *Pseudomonas aeruginosa.*
Anaerobes: *Bacteroides* species, including some strains of *B. fragilis, Clostridium* species (NOTE: Most strains of *C. difficile* are resistant.), *Peptococcus* species, *Peptostreptococcus* species, and *Fusobacterium* species (including *F. nucleatum*).
Cefotaxime sodium is highly stable *in vitro* to four of the five major classes of β-lactamases described by Richmond et al., including type IIIa (TEM) which is produced by many gram-negative bacteria. The drug is also stable to β-lactamase (penicillinase) produced by staphylococci. In addition, cefotaxime sodium shows high affinity for penicillin-binding proteins in the cell wall, including PBP, Ib and III.
Cefotaxime sodium also demonstrates *in vitro* activity against the following microorganisms although clinical significance is unknown: *Salmonella* species (including *S. typhi*), *Providencia* species, and *Shigella* species.
Cefotaxime sodium and aminoglycosides have been shown to be synergistic *in vitro* against some strains of *Pseudomonas aeruginosa.*

Susceptibility Tests

Quantitative methods that require measurement of zone diameters give the most precise estimate of antibiotic susceptibility. One such procedure[1] has been recommended for use with discs to test susceptibility to cefotaxime sodium. Interpretation involves correlation of the diameters obtained in the disc test with minimum inhibitory concentration (MIC) values for cefotaxime sodium.
Reports from the laboratory giving results of the standardized single-disc susceptibility test using a 30 μg cefotaxime sodium disc should be interpreted according to the following criteria:

Susceptible organisms produce zones of 20 mm or greater, indicating that the tested organism is likely to respond to therapy.

Organisms that produce zones of 15 to 19 mm are expected to be susceptible if high dosage is used or if the infection is confined to tissues and fluids (e.g., urine) in which high antibiotic levels are attained.

Resistant organisms produce zones of 14 mm or less, indicating that other therapy should be selected.

Organisms should be tested with the cefotaxime sodium disc, since cefotaxime sodium has been shown by *in vitro* tests to be active against certain strains found resistant when other beta lactam discs are used. The cefotaxime sodium disc should not be used for testing susceptibility to other cephalosporins. Organisms having zones of less than 18 mm around the cephalothin disc are not necessarily of intermediate susceptibility or resistant to cefotaxime sodium.
A bacterial isolate may be considered susceptible if the MIC value for cefotaxime sodium is not more than 16 μg/mL. Organisms are considered resistant to cefotaxime sodium if the MIC is equal to or greater than 64 μg/mL. Organisms having an MIC value of less than 64 μg/mL but greater than 16 μg/mL are expected to be susceptible if high dosage is used or if the infection is confined to tissues and fluids (e.g., urine) in which high antibiotic levels are attained.

INDICATIONS AND USAGE

Treatment

Claforan® is indicated for the treatment of patients with serious infections caused by susceptible strains of the designated microorganisms in the diseases listed below.
(1) **Lower respiratory tract infections,** including pneumonia, caused by *Streptococcus pneumoniae* (formerly *Diplococcus pneumoniae*), *Streptococcus pyogenes** (Group A streptococci) and other streptococci (excluding enterococci, e.g., *Streptococcus faecalis*), *Staphylococcus aureus* (penicillinase and non-penicillinase producing), *Escherichia coli, Klebsiella* species, *Haemophilus influenzae* (including ampicillin resistant strains), *Haemophilus parainfluenzae, Proteus mirabilis, Serratia marcescens,* Enterobacter* species, indole positive *Proteus* and *Pseudomonas* species (including *P. aeruginosa*).
(2) **Genitourinary infections.** Urinary tract infections caused by *Enterococcus* species, *Staphylococcus epidermidis, Staphylococcus aureus** (penicillinase and non-penicillinase producing), *Citrobacter* species, *Enterobacter* species, *Escherichia coli, Klebsiella* species, *Proteus mirabilis, Proteus vulgaris,* Proteus inconstans* Group B, *Morganella morganii,* Providencia rettgeri,** and *Serratia marcescens,* and *Pseudomonas* species (including *P. aeruginosa*). Also, uncomplicated gonorrhea of single or multiple sites caused by *Neisseria gonorrhoeae,* including penicillinase producing strains.
(3) **Gynecologic infections,** including pelvic inflammatory disease, endometritis and pelvic cellulitis caused by *Staphylococcus epidermidis, Streptococcus* species, *Enterococcus* species, *Enterobacter* species,* *Klebsiella* species,* *Escherichia coli, Proteus mirabilis, Bacteroides* species (including *Bacteroides fragilis**), *Clostridium* species, and anaerobic cocci (including *Peptostreptococcus* species and *Peptococcus* species) and *Fusobacterium* species (including *F. nucleatum**).
Claforan®, like other cephalosporins, has no activity against *Chlamydia trachomatis.* Therefore, when cephalosporins are used in the treatment of patients with pelvic inflammatory disease and *C. trachomatis* is one of the suspected pathogens, appropriate anti-chlamydial coverage should be added.
(4) **Bacteremia/Septicemia** caused by *Escherichia coli, Klebsiella* species, *Serratia marcescens, Staphylococcus aureus,* and *Streptococcus* species (including *S. pneumoniae*).
(5) **Skin and skin structure infections** caused by *Staphylococcus aureus* (penicillinase and non-penicillinase producing),

Continued on next page

Hoechst Marion Roussel—Cont.

Staphylococcus epidermidis, Streptococcus pyogenes (Group A streptococci) and other streptococci, *Enterococcus* species, *Acinetobacter* species,* *Escherichia coli, Citrobacter* species (including *C. freundii**). *Enterobacter* species, *Klebsiella* species, *Proteus mirabilis, Proteus vulgaris,* Morganella morganii, Providencia rettgeri,* Pseudomonas* species, *Serratia marcescens, Bacteroides* species, and anaerobic cocci (including *Peptostreptococcus** species and *Peptococcus* species).

(6) **Intra-abdominal infections** including peritonitis caused by *Streptococcus* species,* *Escherichia coli, Klebsiella* species, *Bacteroides* species, and anaerobic cocci (including *Peptostreptococcus** species and *Peptococcus** species), *Proteus mirabilis,** and *Clostridium* species.*

(7) **Bone and/or joint infections** caused by *Staphylococcus aureus* (penicillinase and non-penicillinase producing strains), *Streptococcus* species (including *S. pyogenes**), *Pseudomonas* species (including *P. aeruginosa**), and *Proteus mirabilis.**

(8) **Central nervous system infections,** e.g., meningitis and ventriculitis, caused by *Neisseria meningitidis, Haemophilus influenzae, Streptococcus pneumoniae, Klebsiella pneumoniae,** and *Escherichia coli.**

(*) Efficacy for this organism, in this organ system, has been studied in fewer than 10 infections.

Although many strains of enterococci (e.g., *S. faecalis*) and *Pseudomonas* species are resistant to cefotaxime sodium *in vitro,* Claforan® has been used successfully in treating patients with infections caused by susceptible organisms.

Specimens for bacteriologic culture should be obtained prior to therapy in order to isolate and identify causative organisms and to determine their susceptibilities to Claforan®. Therapy may be instituted before results of susceptibility studies are known; however, once these results become available, the antibiotic treatment should be adjusted accordingly.

In certain cases of confirmed or suspected gram-positive or gram-negative sepsis or in patients with other serious infections in which the causative organism has not been identified, Claforan® may be used concomitantly with an aminoglycoside. The dosage recommended in the labeling of both antibiotics may be given and depends on the severity of the infection and the patient's condition. Renal function should be carefully monitored, especially if higher dosages of the aminoglycosides are to be administered or if therapy is prolonged, because of the potential nephrotoxicity and ototoxicity of aminoglycoside antibiotics. It is possible that nephrotoxicity may be potentiated if Claforan® is used concomitantly with an aminoglycoside.

Prevention

The administration of Claforan® preoperatively reduces the incidence of certain infections in patients undergoing surgical procedures (e.g., abdominal or vaginal hysterectomy, gastrointestinal and genitourinary tract surgery) that may be classified as contaminated or potentially contaminated.

In patients undergoing cesarean section, intraoperative (after clamping the umbilical cord) and postoperative use of Claforan® may also reduce the incidence of certain postoperative infections. (See **DOSAGE AND ADMINISTRATION** section.)

Effective use for elective surgery depends on the time of administration. To achieve effective tissue levels, Claforan® should be given ½ to 1½ hours before surgery. (See **DOSAGE AND ADMINISTRATION** section.)

For patients undergoing gastrointestinal surgery, preoperative bowel preparation by mechanical cleansing as well as with a non-absorbable antibiotic (e.g., neomycin) is recommended.

If there are signs of infection, specimens for culture should be obtained for identification of the causative organism so that appropriate therapy may be instituted.

CONTRAINDICATIONS

Claforan® is contraindicated in patients who have shown hypersensitivity to cefotaxime sodium or the cephalosporin group of antibiotics.

WARNINGS

BEFORE THERAPY WITH CLAFORAN® IS INSTITUTED, CAREFUL INQUIRY SHOULD BE MADE TO DETERMINE WHETHER THE PATIENT HAS HAD PREVIOUS HYPERSENSITIVITY REACTIONS TO CEFOTAXIME SODIUM, CEPHALOSPORINS, PENICILLINS, OR OTHER DRUGS. THIS PRODUCT SHOULD BE GIVEN WITH CAUTION TO PATIENTS WITH TYPE I HYPERSENSITIVITY REACTIONS TO PENICILLIN. ANTIBIOTICS SHOULD BE ADMINISTERED WITH CAUTION TO ANY PATIENT WHO HAS DEMONSTRATED SOME FORM OF ALLERGY, PARTICULARLY TO DRUGS. IF AN ALLERGIC REACTION TO CLAFORAN® OCCURS, DISCONTINUE TREATMENT WITH THE DRUG. SERIOUS HYPERSENSITIVITY REACTIONS MAY REQUIRE EPINEPHRINE AND OTHER EMERGENCY MEASURES.

During post-marketing surveillance, a potentially life-threatening arrhythmia was reported in each of six patients who received a rapid (less than 60 seconds) bolus injection of cefotaxime through a central venous catheter. Therefore, cefotaxime should only be administered as instructed in the DOSAGE AND ADMINISTRATION section.

Pseudomembranous colitis has been reported with nearly all antibacterial agents, including cefotaxime, and may range from mild to life threatening. Therefore, it is important to consider its diagnosis in patients with diarrhea subsequent to the administration of antibacterial agents.

Treatment with antibacterial agents alters the normal flora of the colon and may permit overgrowth of Clostridia. Studies indicate that a toxin produced by *Clostridium difficile* is one primary cause of antibiotic-associated colitis.

After the diagnosis of pseudomembranous colitis has been established, appropriate therapeutic measures should be initiated. Mild cases of colitis may respond to drug discontinuance alone. In moderate to severe cases, consideration should be given to management with fluids and electrolytes, protein supplementation, and treatment with an antibacterial drug clinically effective against *Clostridium difficile* colitis.

When the colitis is not relieved by drug discontinuance or when it is severe, oral vancomycin is the treatment of choice for antibiotic-associated pseudomembranous colitis produced by *C. difficile.* Other causes of colitis should also be considered.

PRECAUTIONS

Claforan® should be prescribed with caution in individuals with a history of gastrointestinal disease, particularly colitis.

Because high and prolonged serum antibiotic concentrations can occur from usual doses in patients with transient or persistent reduction of urinary output because of renal insufficiency, the total daily dosage should be reduced when Claforan® is administered to such patients. Continued dosage should be determined by degree of renal impairment, severity of infection, and susceptibility of the causative organism.

Although there is no clinical evidence supporting the necessity of changing the dosage of cefotaxime sodium in patients with even profound renal dysfunction, it is suggested that, until further data are obtained, the dose of cefotaxime sodium be halved in patients with estimated creatinine clearances of less than 20 mL/min/1.73 m^2.

When only serum creatinine is available, the following formula[2] (based on sex, weight, and age of the patient) may be used to convert this value into creatinine clearance. The serum creatinine should represent a steady state of renal function.

Males: $\dfrac{\text{Weight (kg)} \times (140 - \text{age})}{72 \times \text{serum creatinine}}$

Females: $0.85 \times$ above value

As with other antibiotics, prolonged use of Claforan® may result in overgrowth of nonsusceptible organisms. Repeated evaluation of the patient's condition is essential. If superinfection occurs during therapy, appropriate measures should be taken.

As with other beta-lactam antibiotics, granulocytopenia and, more rarely, agranulocytosis may develop during treatment with Claforan®, particularly if given over long periods. For courses of treatment lasting longer than 10 days, blood counts should therefore be monitored.

Claforan®, like other parenteral anti-infective drugs, may be locally irritating to tissues. In most cases, perivascular extravasation of Claforan®, responds to changing of the infusion site. In rare instances, extensive perivascular extravasation of Claforan® may result in tissue damage and require surgical treatment. To minimize the potential for tissue inflammation, infusion sites should be monitored regularly and changed when appropriate.

Drug Interactions: Increased nephrotoxicity has been reported following concomitant administration of cephalosporins and aminoglycoside antibiotics.

Carcinogenesis, Mutagenesis: Long-term studies in animals have not been performed to evaluate carcinogenic potential. Mutagenic tests included a micronucleus and an Ames test. Both tests were negative for mutagenic effects.

Pregnancy (Category B): Reproduction studies have been performed in mice and rats at doses up to 30 times the usual human dose and have revealed no evidence of impaired fertility or harm to the fetus because of cefotaxime sodium. However, there are no well-controlled studies in pregnant women. Because animal reproductive studies are not always predictive of human response, this drug should be used during pregnancy only if clearly needed.

Nonteratogenic Effects: Use of the drug in women of child-bearing potential requires that the anticipated benefit be weighed against the possible risks.

In perinatal and postnatal studies with rats, the pups in the group given 1200 mg/kg of Claforan® were significantly lighter in weight at birth and remained smaller than pups in the control group during the 21 days of nursing.

Nursing Mothers: Claforan® is excreted in human milk in low concentrations. Caution should be exercised when Claforan® is administered to a nursing woman.

Pediatric Use: Se Precautions above regarding perivascular extravasation. The potential for toxic effects in pediatric patients from chemicals that may leach from the plastic in single dose Galaxy® containers (premixed Claforan® Injection) has not been determined.

ADVERSE REACTIONS

Claforan® is generally well tolerated. The most common adverse reactions have been local reactions following IM or IV injection. Other adverse reactions have been encountered infrequently.

The most frequent adverse reactions (greater than 1%) are:

Local (4.3%)—Injection site inflammation with IV administration. Pain, induration, and tenderness after IM injection.

Hypersensitivity (2.4%)—Rash, pruritus, fever, and eosinophilia and less frequently urticaria and anaphylaxis.

Gastrointestinal (1.4%)—Colitis, diarrhea, nausea, and vomiting.

Symptoms of pseudomembranous colitis can appear during or after antibiotic treatment.

Nausea and vomiting have been reported rarely.

Less frequent adverse reactions (less than 1%) are:

Cardiovascular System—Potentially life-threatening arrhythmias following rapid (less than 60 seconds) bolus administration via central venous catheter have been observed.

Hematologic System—Neutropenia, transient leukopenia, eosinophilia, thrombocytopenia and agranulocytosis have been reported. Some individuals have developed positive direct Coombs Tests during treatment with Claforan® (cefotaxime sodium) and other cephalosporin antibiotics. Rare cases of hemolytic anemia have been reported.

Genitourinary System—Moniliasis, vaginitis.

Central Nervous System—Headache.

Liver—Transient elevations in SGOT, SGPT, serum LDH, and serum alkaline phosphatase levels have been reported.

Kidney—As with some other cephalosporins, interstitial nephritis and transient elevations of BUN and creatinine have been occasionally observed with Claforan®.

DOSAGE AND ADMINISTRATION

Adults

Dosage and route of administration should be determined by susceptibility of the causative organisms, severity of the infection, and the condition of the patient (see table for dosage guidelines). Claforan® may be administered IM or IV after reconstitution. Premixed Claforan® Injection is intended for IV administration after thawing. The maximum daily dosage should not exceed 12 grams.

[See table below.]

If *C. trachomatis* is a suspected pathogen, appropriate anti-chlamydial coverage should be added, because cefotaxime sodium has no activity against this organism.

To prevent postoperative infection in contaminated or potentially contaminated surgery, the recommended dose is a single 1 gram IM or IV administered 30 to 90 minutes prior to start of surgery.

Cesarean Section Patients

The first dose of 1 gram is administered intravenously as soon as the umbilical cord is clamped. The second and third doses should be given as 1 gram intravenously or intramuscularly at 6 and 12 hours after the first dose.

Neonates, Infants, and Children

The following dosage schedule is recommended:

Neonates (birth to 1 month):

0–1 week of age	50 mg/kg per dose every 12 hours IV
1–4 weeks of age	50 mg/kg per dose every 8 hours IV

It is not necessary to differentiate between premature and normal-gestational age infants.

GUIDELINES FOR DOSAGE OF CLAFORAN®

Type of Infection	Daily Dose (grams)	Frequency and Route
Gonorrhea	1	1 gram IM (single dose)
Uncomplicated infections	2	1 gram every 12 hours IM or IV
Moderate to severe infections	3–6	1–2 grams every 8 hours IM or IV
Infections commonly needing antibiotics in higher dosage (e.g., septicemia)	6–8	2 grams every 6–8 hours IV
Life-threatening infections	up to 12	2 grams every 4 hours IV

Infants and Children (1 month to 12 years): For body weights less than 50 kg, the recommended daily dose is 50 to 180 mg/kg IM or IV of body weight divided into four to six equal doses. The higher dosages should be used for more severe or serious infections, including meningitis. For body weights 50 kg or more, the usual adult dosage should be used; the maximum daily dosage should not exceed 12 grams.

Impaired Renal Function —see **PRECAUTIONS** section.

NOTE: As with antibiotic therapy in general, administration of Claforan® should be continued for a minimum of 48 to 72 hours after the patient defervesces or after evidence of bacterial eradication has been obtained; a minimum of 10 days of treatment is recommended for infections caused by Group A beta-hemolytic streptococci in order to guard against the risk of rheumatic fever or glomerulonephritis; frequent bacteriologic and clinical appraisal is necessary during therapy of chronic urinary tract infection and may be required for several months after therapy has been completed; persistent infections may require treatment of several weeks and doses smaller than those indicated above should not be used.

PREPARATION OF CLAFORAN® STERILE

Claforan® for IM or IV administration should be reconstituted as follows:

Strength	Diluent (mL)	Withdrawable Volume (mL)	Approximate Concentration (mg/mL)
500 mg vial* (IM)	2	2.2	230
1g vial* (IM)	3	3.4	300
2g vial* (IM)	5	6.0	330
500 mg vial* (IV)	10	10.2	50
1g vial* (IV)	10	10.4	95
2g vial* (IV)	10	11.0	180
1g infusion	50–100	50–100	20–10
2g infusion	50–100	50–100	40–20
10g bottle	47	52.0	200
10g bottle	97	102.0	100

*In conventional vials

Shake to dissolve; inspect for particulate matter and discoloration prior to use. Solutions of Claforan® range from very pale yellow to light amber, depending on concentration, diluent used, and length and condition of storage.

For intramuscular use: Reconstitute VIALS with Sterile Water for Injection or Bacteriostatic Water for Injection as described above.

For intravenous use: Reconstitute VIALS with at least 10 mL of Sterile Water for Injection. Reconstitute INFUSION BOTTLES with 50 or 100 mL of 0.9% Sodium Chloride Injection or 5% Dextrose Injection. For other diluents, see **COMPATIBILITY AND STABILITY** section.

Pharmacy Bulk Package: Reconstitute with 47 mL of diluent for an approximate concentration of 200 mg/mL or 97 mL of diluent for an approximate concentration of 100 mg/mL. Stock solutions may be further diluted for IV infusion with diluents as listed in **COMPATIBILITY AND STABILITY** section.

NOTE: Solutions of Claforan® must not be admixed with aminoglycoside solutions. If Claforan® and aminoglycosides are to be administered to the same patient, they must be administered separately and not as mixed injection.

A SOLUTION OF 1 G CLAFORAN® IN 14 ML OF STERILE WATER FOR INJECTION IS ISOTONIC.

IM Administration: As with all IM preparations, Claforan® should be injected well within the body of a relatively large muscle such as the upper outer quadrant of the buttock (i.e., gluteus maximus); aspiration is necessary to avoid inadvertent injection into a blood vessel. Individual IM doses of 2 grams may be given if the dose is divided and is administered in different intramuscular sites.

IV Administration: The IV route is preferable for patients with bacteremia, bacterial septicemia, peritonitis, meningitis, or other severe or life-threatening infections, or for patients who may be poor risks because of lowered resistance resulting from such debilitating conditions as malnutrition, trauma, surgery, diabetes, heart failure, or malignancy, particularly if shock is present or impending.

For intermittent IV administration, a solution containing 1 gram or 2 grams in 10 mL of Sterile Water for Injection can be injected over a period of three to five minutes. Cefotaxime should not be administered over a period of less than three minutes. (See WARNINGS.) With an infusion system, it may also be given over a longer period of time through the tubing system by which the patient may be receiving other IV solutions. However, during infusion of the solution containing Claforan®, it is advisable to discontinue temporarily the administration of other solutions at the same site.

For the administration of higher doses by continuous IV infusion, a solution of Claforan® may be added to IV bottles containing the solutions discussed below.

Strength	Reconstituted Concentration mg/mL	Stability at or below 22°C	Stability under Refrigeration (at or below 5°C) Original Containers	Plastic Syringes
500 mg vial IM	200	12 hours	7 days	5 days
1g vial IM	300	12 hours	7 days	5 days
2g vial IM	330	12 hours	7 days	5 days
500 mg vial IV	50	24 hours	7 days	5 days
1g vial IV	95	24 hours	7 days	5 days
2g vial IV	180	12 hours	7 days	5 days
1g infusion bottle	10–20	24 hours	10 days	
2g infusion bottle	20–40	24 hours	10 days	

DIRECTIONS FOR USE OF CLAFORAN® (cefotaxime sodium) INJECTION IN GALAXY® CONTAINER (PL 2040 PLASTIC)

Claforan® (cefotaxime sodium) Injection in Galaxy® containers (PL 2040 plastic) is for continuous or intermittent infusion using sterile equipment.

Storage

Store in a freezer capable of maintaining a temperature of −20°C/−4°F.

Thawing of Plastic Container

Thaw frozen container at room temperature or under refrigeration (5°C/41°F). [DO NOT FORCE THAW BY IMMERSION IN WATER BATHS OR BY MICROWAVE IRRADIATION.]

Check for minute leaks by squeezing container firmly. If leaks are detected, discard solution as sterility may be impaired.

DO NOT ADD SUPPLEMENTARY MEDICATION.

The container should be visually inspected. Components of the solution may precipitate in the frozen state and will dissolve upon reaching room temperature with little or no agitation. Potency is not affected. Agitate after solution has reached room temperature. If after visual inspection the solution remains cloudy or if an insoluble precipitate is noted or if any seals or outlet ports are not intact, the container should be discarded.

The thawed solution is stable for 10 days under refrigeration (at or below 5°C) or 24 hours at or below 22°C. Do not refreeze thawed antibiotics.

CAUTION: Do not use plastic containers in series connections. Such use could result in air embolism due to residual air being drawn from the primary container before administration of the fluid from the secondary container is complete.

Preparation for Intravenous Administration:
1. Suspend container from eyelet support.
2. Remove protector from outlet port at bottom of container.
3. Attach administration set. Refer to complete directions accompanying set.

PREPARATION OF CLAFORAN® STERILE IN ADD-VANTAGE® SYSTEM

Claforan® Sterile 1 g or 2 g may be reconstituted in 50 mL or 100 mL of 5% Dextrose or 0.9% Sodium Chloride in the ADD-Vantage® diluent container. Refer to enclosed, separate INSTRUCTIONS FOR ADD-VANTAGE® SYSTEM.

COMPATIBILITY AND STABILITY

Solutions of Claforan® Sterile reconstituted as described above (**Preparation of Claforan® Sterile**) remain chemically stable (potency remains above 90%) as follows when stored in original containers and disposable plastic syringes:

[See table on top of page.]

Reconstituted solutions stored in original containers and plastic syringes remain stable for 13 weeks frozen.

For the 10g bottle withdraw reconstituted contents immediately. However, if it is not possible, aliquoting operations must be completed within four hours of reconstitution. Discard the reconstituted stock solution 4 hours after initial entry.

Reconstituted solutions may be further diluted up to 1000 mL with the following solutions and maintain satisfactory potency for 24 hours at or below 22°C, and at least 5 days under refrigeration (at or below 5°C); 0.9% Sodium Chloride Injection; 5 or 10% Dextrose Injection; 5% Dextrose and 0.9% Sodium Chloride Injection; 5% Dextrose and 0.45% Sodium Chloride Injection; 5% Dextrose and 0.2% Sodium Chloride Injection; Lactated Ringer's Solution; Sodium Lactate Injection (M/6); 10% Invert Sugar Injection, 8.5% TRAVASOL® (Amino Acid) Injection without Electrolytes.

Solutions of Claforan® Sterile reconstituted in 0.9% Sodium Chloride Injection or 5% Dextrose Injection in Viaflex® plastic containers maintain satisfactory potency for 24 hours at or below 22°C, 5 days under refrigeration (at or below 5°C) and 13 weeks frozen. Solutions of Claforan® Sterile reconstituted in 0.9% Sodium Chloride Injection or 5% Dextrose Injection in the ADD-Vantage® flexible containers maintain satisfactory potency for 24 hours at or below 22°C. DO NOT FREEZE.

NOTE: Claforan® solutions exhibit maximum stability in the pH 5–7 range. Solutions of Claforan® should not be prepared with diluents having a pH above 7.5, such as Sodium Bicarbonate Injection.

HOW SUPPLIED

Sterile Claforan® is a dry off-white to pale yellow crystalline powder supplied in vials and bottles containing cefotaxime sodium as follows:

500 mg cefotaxime (free acid equivalent) in vials in packages of 10 (NDC 0039-0017-10).

1 g cefotaxime (free acid equivalent) in vials in packages of 10 (NDC 0039-0018-10), packages of 25 (NDC 0039-0018-25), packages of 50 (NDC 0039-0018-50); infusion bottles in packages of 10 (NDC 0039-0018-11).

2 g cefotaxime (free acid equivalent) in vials in packages of 10 (NDC 0039-0019-10), packages of 25 (NDC 0039-0019-25), packages of 50 (NDC 0039-0019-50); infusion bottles in packages of 10 (NDC 0039-0019-11).

10 g cefotaxime (free acid equivalent) in bottles (NDC 0039-0020-01).

1 g cefotaxime (free acid equivalent) in ADD-Vantage® System vials in packages of 25 (NDC 0039-0023-25) and 50 (NDC 0039-0023-50).

2 g cefotaxime (free acid equivalent) in ADD-Vantage® System vials in packages of 25 (NDC 0039-0024-25) and 50 (NDC 0039-0024-50).

ADD-Vantage® System diluents (5% Dextrose or 0.9% Sodium Chloride) are available from Abbott Laboratories.

NOTE: Claforan® in the dry state should be stored below 30°C. The dry material as well as solutions tend to darken depending on storage conditions and should be protected from elevated temperatures and excessive light.

Premixed Claforan® Injection is supplied as a frozen, iso-osmotic, sterile, nonpyrogenic solution in 50 mL single dose Galaxy® containers (PL 2040 plastic) as follows:

1 g cefotaxime (free acid equivalent) in packages of 12 (NDC 0039-0037-05) 2G3518.

2 g cefotaxime (free acid equivalent) in packages of 12 (NDC 0039-0038-05) 2G3519.

NOTE: Store Premixed Claforan® Injection at or below −20°C/−4°F. [See DIRECTIONS FOR USE OF CLAFORAN® (cefotaxime sodium) INJECTION IN GALAXY® CONTAINERS (PL 2040 PLASTIC)].

Claforan® Injection supplied as a frozen, iso-osmotic, sterile, nonpyrogenic solution in Galaxy® containers (PL 2040 plastic) is manufactured for Hoechst-Roussel Pharmaceuticals Inc., by Baxter Healthcare Corporation.

REFERENCES

1) Bauer, A.W.; Kirby, W.M.M.; Sherris, J.C.; and Turck, M.: Antibiotic Susceptibility Testing by a Standardized Single Disk Method, *Am J Clin Pathol*. 1966;45:493. Standardized Disc Susceptibility Test, Federal Register, 39:19182-4, 1974. National Committee for Clinical Laboratory Standards, Approved Standard: ASM-2, Performance Standards for Antimicrobial Disc Susceptibility Tests, July, 1975.

2) Cockcroft, D.W. and Gault, M.H.: Prediction of Creatinine Clearance from Serum Creatinine. *Nephron*. 1976;16:31-41.

Sterile cefotaxime sodium US Patents 4,152,432; 4,224,371; 4,298,606; cefotaxime sodium injection US Patents 4,152,432; 4,298,606. Claforan REG TM ROUSSEL-UCLAF. Galaxy and PL 2040 REG TM Baxter International Inc. ADD-Vantage REG TM Abbott Laboratories
US Patent ADD-Vantage System: 4,614,267; 4,614,515; 4,757,911; 4,703,864; 4,784,658; 4,784,259; 4,948,000; 4,936,445.

Revised 2/95
C14

Hoechst-Roussel Pharmaceuticals
Division of Hoechst Marion Roussel, Inc.
Kansas City, MO 64137

Shown in Product Identification Guide, page 317

Continued on next page

Hoechst Marion Roussel—Cont.

CLOMID® ℞
(clomiphene citrate tablets USP)
Prescribing Information as of June 1995

DESCRIPTION

CLOMID (clomiphene citrate tablets USP) is an orally administered, nonsteroidal, ovulatory stimulant designated chemically as 2-[p-(2-chloro-1,2-diphenylvinyl)phenoxyl] triethylamine citrate (1:1). It has the molecular formula of $C_{26}H_{28}ClNO \cdot C_6H_8O_7$ and a molecular weight of 598.09. It is represented structurally as:

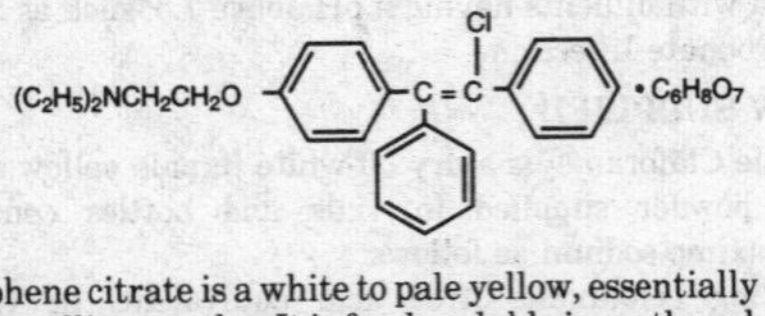
Cl
(C2H5)2NCH2CH2O
C = C
• C6H8O7

Clomiphene citrate is a white to pale yellow, essentially odorless, crystalline powder. It is freely soluble in methanol; soluble in ethanol; slight soluble in acetone, water, and chloroform; and insoluble in ether.
CLOMID is a mixture of two geometric isomers [cis (zuclomiphene) and trans (enclomiphene)] containing between 30% and 50% of the cis-isomer.
Each white scored tablet contains 50 mg clomiphene citrate USP. The tablet also contains the following inactive ingredients: corn starch, lactose, magnesium stearate, pregelatinized corn starch, and sucrose.

CLINICAL PHARMACOLOGY

Action
CLOMID is a drug of considerable pharmacologic potency. With careful selection and proper management of the patient, CLOMID has been demonstrated to be a useful therapy for the anovulatory patient desiring pregnancy.
Clomiphene citrate is capable of interacting with estrogen-receptor-containing tissues, including the hypothalamus, pituitary, ovary, endometrium, vagina, and cervix. It may compete with estrogen for estrogen-receptor-binding sites and may delay replenishment of intracellular estrogen receptors. Clomiphene citrate initiates a series of endocrine events culminating in a preovulatory gonadotropin surge and subsequent follicular rupture. The first endocrine event in response to a course of clomiphene therapy is an increase in the release of pituitary gonadotropins. This initiates steroidogenesis and folliculogenesis, resulting in growth of the ovarian follicle and an increase in the circulating level of estradiol. Following ovulation, plasma progesterone and estradiol rise and fall as they would in a normal ovulatory cycle.
Available data suggest that both the estrogenic and antiestrogenic properties of clomiphene may participate in the initiation of ovulation. The two clomiphene isomers have been found to have mixed estrogenic and antiestrogenic effects, which may vary from one species to another. Some data suggest that zuclomiphene has greater estrogenic activity then enclomiphene.
Clomiphene citrate has no apparent progestational, androgenic, or antiandrogenic effects and does not appear to interfere with pituitary-adrenal or pituitary-thyroid function.
Although there is no evidence of a "carryover effect" of CLOMID, spontaneous ovulatory menses have been noted in some patients after CLOMID therapy.
Pharmacokinetics
Based on early studies with ^{14}C-labeled clomiphene citrate, the drug was shown to be readily absorbed orally in humans and excreted principally in the feces. Cumulative urinary and fecal excretion of the ^{14}C averaged about 50% of the oral dose and 37% of an intravenous dose after 5 days. Mean urinary excretion was approximately 8% with fecal excretion of about 42%.
Some ^{14}C label was still present in the feces 6 weeks after administration. Subsequent single-dose studies in normal volunteers showed that zuclomiphene (cis) has a longer half-life than enclomiphene (trans). Detectable levels of zuclomiphene persisted for longer than a month in these subjects. This may be suggestive of stereo-specific enterohepatic recycling or sequestering of the zuclomiphene. Thus, it is possible that some active drug may remain in the body during early pregnancy in women who conceive in the menstrual cycle during CLOMID therapy.

CLINICAL STUDIES

During clinical investigations, 7578 patients received CLOMID, some of whom had impediments to ovulation other than ovulatory dysfunction (see INDICATIONS AND USAGE). In those clinical trials, successful therapy characterized by pregnancy occurred in approximately 30% of these patients.
There were a total of 2635 pregnancies reported during the clinical trial period. Of those pregnancies, information on outcome was only available for 2369 of the cases. Table 1 summarizes the outcome of these cases.
Of the reported pregnancies, the incidence of multiple pregnancies was 7.98%: 6.9% twin, 0.5% triplet, 0.3% quadruplet, and 0.1% quintuplet. Of the 165 twin pregnancies for which sufficient information was available, the ratio of monozygotic to dizygotic twins was about 1:5. Table 1 reports the survival rate of the live multiple births.
A sextuplet birth was reported after completion of original clinical studies; none of the sextuplets survived (each weighed less than 400 g), although each appeared grossly normal.

Table 1. Outcome of Reported Pregnancies in Clinical Trials (n = 2369)

Outcome	Total Number of Pregnancies	Survival Rate
Pregnancy Wastage		
Spontaneous Abortions	483*	
Stillbirths	24	
Live Births		
Single Births	1697	98.16%†
Multiple Births	165	83.26%†

*Includes 28 ectopic pregnancies, 4 hydatiform moles, and 1 fetus papyraceous.
†Indicates percentage of surviving infants from these pregnancies.

The overall survival of infants from multiple pregnancies including spontaneous abortions, stillbirths, and neonatal deaths is 73%.

INDICATIONS AND USAGE

CLOMID is indicated for the treatment of ovulatory dysfunction in women desiring pregnancy. Impediments to achieving pregnancy must be excluded or adequately treated before beginning CLOMID therapy. Those patients most likely to achieve success with clomiphene therapy include patients with polycystic ovary syndrome (see WARNINGS: Ovarian Hyperstimulation Syndrome), amenorrhea-galactorrhea syndrome, psychogenic amenorrhea, post-oral-contraceptive amenorrhea, and certain cases of secondary amenorrhea of undetermined etiology.
Properly timed colitus in relationship to ovulation is important. A basal body temperature graph or other appropriate tests may help the patient and her physician determine if ovulation occurred. Once ovulation has been established, each course of CLOMID should be started on or about the 5th day of the cycle. Long-term cyclic therapy is not recommended beyond a total of about six cycles (including three ovulatory cycles). See DOSAGE AND ADMINISTRATION and PRECAUTIONS.)
CLOMID is indicated only in patients with demonstrated ovulatory dysfunction who meet the conditions described below (see CONTRAINDICATIONS):
1. Patients who are not pregnant.
2. Patients without ovarian cysts. CLOMID should not be used in patients with ovarian enlargement except those with polycystic ovary syndrome. Pelvic examination is necessary prior to the first and each subsequent course of CLOMID treatment.
3. Patients without abnormal vaginal bleeding. If abnormal vaginal bleeding is present, the patient should be carefully evaluated to ensure that neoplastic lesions are not present.
4. Patients with normal liver function.

In addition, patients selected for CLOMID therapy should be evaluated in regard to the following:
1. **Estrogen Levels.** Patients should have adequate levels of endogenous estrogen (as estimated from vaginal smears, endometrial biopsy, assay of urinary estrogen, or from bleeding in response to progesterone). Reduced estrogen levels, while less favorable, do not preclude successful therapy.
2. **Primary Pituitary or Ovarian Failure.** CLOMID therapy cannot be expected to substitute for specific treatment of other causes of ovulatory failure.
3. **Endometriosis and Endometrial Carcinoma.** The incidence of endometriosis and endometrial carcinoma increases with age as does the incidence of ovulatory disorders. Endometrial biopsy should always be performed prior to CLOMID therapy in this population.
4. **Other Impediments to Pregnancy.** Impediments to pregnancy can include thyroid disorders, adrenal disorders, hyperprolactinemia, and male factor infertility.
5. **Uterine Fibroids.** Caution should be exercised when using CLOMID in patients with uterine fibroids due to the potential for further enlargement of the fibroids.

There are no adequate or well-controlled studies that demonstrate the effectiveness of CLOMID in the treatment of male infertility. In addition, testicular tumors and gynecomastia have been reported in males using clomiphene. The cause and effect relationship between reports of testicular tumors and the administration of CLOMID is not known.
Although the medical literature suggests various methods, there is no universally accepted standard regimen for combined therapy (ie, CLOMID in conjunction with other ovulation-inducing drugs). Similarly, there is no standard CLOMID regimen for ovulation-induction in *in vitro* fertilization programs to produce ova for fertilization and reintroduction. Therefore, CLOMID is not recommended for these uses.

CONTRAINDICATIONS

Hypersensitivity
CLOMID is contraindicated in patients with a known hypersensitivity or allergy to clomiphene citrate or to any of its ingredients.
Pregnancy
CLOMID should not be administered during pregnancy. CLOMID may cause fetal harm in animals (see Animal Fetotoxicity). Although no causative evidence of a deleterious effect of CLOMID therapy on the human fetus has been established, there have been reports of birth anomalies which, during clinical studies, occurred at an incidence within the range reported for the general population (see Fetal/Neonatal Anomalies and Mortality: ADVERSE REACTIONS).
To avoid inadvertent CLOMID administration during early pregnancy, appropriate tests should be utilized during each treatment cycle to determine whether ovulation occurs. The patient should be evaluated carefully to exclude pregnancy, ovarian enlargement, or ovarian cyst formation between each treatment cycle. The next course of CLOMID therapy should be delayed until these conditions have been excluded.
Fetal/Neonatal Anomalies and Mortality. The following fetal abnormalities have been reported subsequent to pregnancies following ovulation induction therapy with CLOMID during clinical trials. Each of the following fetal abnormalities were reported at a rate of <1% (experiences are listed in order of decreasing frequency): Congenital heart lesions, Down syndrome, club foot, congenital gut lesions, hypospadias, microcephaly, harelip and cleft palate, congenital hip, hemangioma, undescended testicles, polydactyly, conjoined twins and teratomatous malformation, patent ductus arteriosus, amaurosis, arteriovenous fistula, inguinal hernia, umbilical hernia, syndactyly, pectus excavatum, myopathy, dermoid cyst of scalp, omphalocele, spina bifida occulta, ichthyosis, and persistent lingual frenulum. Neonatal death and fetal death/stillbirth in infants with birth defects have also been reported at a rate of <1%. The overall incidence of reported birth anomalies from pregnancies associated with maternal CLOMID ingestion during clinical studies was within the range of that reported for the general population.
In addition, reports of birth anomalies have been received during postmarketing surveillance of CLOMID (see ADVERSE REACTIONS).
Animal Fetotoxicity. Oral administration of clomiphene citrate to pregnant rats during organogenesis at doses of 1 to 2 mg/kg/day resulted in hydramnion and weak, edematous fetuses with wavy ribs and other temporary bone changes. Doses of 8 mg/kg/day or more also caused increased resorptions and dead fetuses, dystocia, and delayed parturition, and 40 mg/kg/day resulted in increased maternal mortality. Single doses of 50 mg/kg caused fetal cataracts, while 200 mg/kg caused cleft palate.
Following injection of clomiphene citrate 2 mg/kg to mice and rats during pregnancy, the offspring exhibited metaplastic changes of the reproduction tract. Newborn mice and rats injected during the first few days of life also developed metaplastic changes in uterine and vaginal mucosa, as well as premature vaginal opening and anovulatory ovaries. These findings are similar to the abnormal reproductive behavior and sterility described with other estrogens and antiestrogens.
In rabbits, some temporary bone alterations were seen in fetuses from dams given oral doses of 20 or 40 mg/kg/day during pregnancy, but not following 8 mg/kg/day. No permanent malformations were observed in those studies. Also, rhesus monkeys given oral doses of 1.5 to 4.5 mg/kg/day for various periods during pregnancy did not have any abnormal offspring.
Liver Disease. CLOMID therapy is contraindicated in patients with liver disease or a history of liver dysfunction (see also INDICATIONS AND USAGE and ADVERSE REACTIONS).
Abnormal Uterine Bleeding. CLOMID is contraindicated in patients with abnormal uterine bleeding of undetermined origin (see INDICATIONS AND USAGE).
Ovarian Cysts. CLOMID is contraindicated in patients with ovarian cysts or enlargement not due to polycystic ovarian syndrome (see INDICATIONS AND USAGE and WARNINGS).
Other. CLOMID is contraindicated in patients with uncontrolled thyroid or adrenal dysfunction or in the presence of an organic intracranial lesion such as pituitary tumor (see INDICATIONS AND USAGE).

WARNINGS

Visual Symptoms

Patients should be advised that blurring or other visual symptoms such as spots or flashes (scintillating scotomata) may occasionally occur during therapy with CLOMID. These visual symptoms increase in incidence with increasing total dose or therapy duration and generally disappear within a few days or weeks after CLOMID is discontinued. Patients should be warned that these visual symptoms may render such activities as driving a car or operating machinery more hazardous than usual, particularly under conditions of variable lighting.

These visual symptoms appear to be due to intensification and prolongation of afterimages. Symptoms often first appear or are accentuated with exposure to a brightly lit environment. While measured visual acuity usually has not been affected, a study patient taking 200 mg CLOMID daily developed visual blurring on the 7th day of treatment, which progressed to severe diminution of visual acuity by the 10th day. No other abnormaltiy was found, and the visual acuity returned to normal on the 3rd day after treatment was stopped.

Ophthalmologically definable scotomata and retinal cell function (electroretinographic) changes have also been reported. A patient treated during clinical studies developed phosphenes and scotomata during prolonged CLOMID administration, which disappeared by the 32nd day after stopping therapy.

Postmarketing surveillance of adverse events has also revealed other visual signs and symptoms during CLOMID therapy (see ADVERSE REACTIONS).

While the etiology of these visual symptoms is not yet understood, patients with any visual symptoms should discontinue treatment and have a complete ophthalmological evaluation carried out promptly.

Ovarian Hyperstimulation Syndrome

The ovarian hyperstimulation syndrome (OHSS) has been reported to occur in patients receiving clomiphene citrate therapy for ovulation induction. In some cases, OHSS occurred following cyclic use of clomiphene citrate therapy or when clomiphene citrate was used in combination with gonadotropins. Transient liver function test abnormalities suggestive of hepatic dysfunction, which may be accompanied by morphlogic changes on liver biopsy, have been reported in association with ovarian hyperstimulation syndrome (OHSS).

OHSS is a medical event distinct from uncomplicated ovarian enlargement. The clinical signs of this syndrome in severe cases can include gross ovarian enlargement, gastrointestinal symptoms, ascites, dyspnea, oliguria, and pleural effusion. In addition, the following symptoms have been reported in association with this syndrome: pericardial effusion, anasarca, hydrothorax, acute abdomen, hypotension, renal failure, pulmonary edema, intraperitoneal and ovarian hemorrhage, deep venous thrombosis, torsion of the ovary, and acute respiratory distress. The early warning signs of OHSS are abdominal pain and distention, nausea, vomiting, diarrhea, and weight gain. Elevated urinary steroid levels, varying degrees of electrolyte imbalance, hypovolemia, hemoconcentration, and hypoproteinemia may occur. Death due to hypovolemic shock, hemoconcentration, or thromboembolism has occurred. Due to fragility of enlarged ovaries in severe cases, abdominal and pelvic examination should be performed very cautiously. If conception results, rapid progression to the severe form of the syndrome may occur.

To minimize the hazard associated with occasional abnormal ovarian enlargement associated with CLOMID therapy, the lowest dose consistent with expected clinical results should be used. Maximal enlargement of the ovary, whether physiologic or abnormal, may not occur until several days after discontinuation of the recommended dose of CLOMID. Some patients with polycystic ovary syndrome who are unusually sensitive to gonadotropin may have an exaggerated response to usual doses of CLOMID. Therefore, patients with polycystic ovary syndrome should be started on the lowest recommended dose and shortest treatment duration for the first course of therapy (see DOSAGE AND ADMINISTRATION). If enlargement of the ovary occurs, additional CLOMID therapy should not be given until the ovaries have returned to pretreatment size, and the dosage or duration of the next course should be reduced. Ovarian enlargement and cyst formation associated with CLOMID therapy usually regress spontaneously within a few days or weeks after discontinuing treatment. The potential benefit of subsequent CLOMID therapy in these cases should exceed the risk. Unless surgical indication for laparotomy exists, such cystic enlargement should always be managed conservatively.

A causal relationship between ovarian hyperstimulation and ovarian cancer has not been determined. However, because a correlation between ovarian cancer and nulliparity, infertility, and age has been suggested, if ovarian cysts do not regress spontaneously, a thorough evaluation should be performed to rule out the presence of ovarian neoplasia.

PRECAUTIONS

General

Careful attention should be given to the selection of candidates for CLOMID therapy. Pelvic examination is necessary prior to CLOMID treatment and before each subsequent course (see CONTRAINDICATIONS and WARNINGS).

Information for Patients

The purpose and risks of CLOMID therapy should be presented to the patient before starting treatment. It should be emphasized that the goal of CLOMID therapy is ovulation for subsequent pregnancy. The physician should counsel the patient with special regard to the following potential risks:

Visual Symptoms: Advise that blurring or other visual symptoms occasionally may occur during or shortly after CLOMID therapy. Warn that visual symptoms may render such activities as driving a car or operating machinery more hazardous than usual, particularly under conditions of variable lighting (see WARNINGS).

The patient should be instructed to inform the physician whenever any unusual visual symptoms occur. If the patient has any visual symptoms, treatment should be discontinued and complete ophthalmologic evaluation performed.

Abdominal/Pelvic Pain or Distention: Ovarian enlargement may occur during or shortly after therapy with CLOMID. To minimize the risks associated with ovarian enlargement, the patient should be instructed to inform the physician of any abdominal or pelvic pain, weight gain, discomfort, or distention after taking CLOMID (see WARNINGS).

Multiple Pregnancy: Inform the patient that there is an increased chance of multiple pregnancy, including bilateral tubal pregnancy and coexisting tubal and intrauterine pregnancy, when conception occurs in relation to CLOMID therapy. The potential complications and hazards of multiple pregnancy should be explained.

Pregnancy Wastage and Birth Anomalies: The physician should explain the assumed risk of any pregnancy, whether ovulation is induced with the aid of CLOMID or occurs naturally. The patient should be informed of the greater risks associated with certain characteristics or conditions of any pregnant woman, eg, age of female and male partner, history of spontaneous abortions, Rh genotype, abnormal menstrual history, infertility history, organic heart disease, diabetes, exposure to infectious agents such as rubella, familial history of birth anomaly, that may be pertinent to the patient for whom CLOMID is being considered. Based upon the evaluation of the patient, genetic counseling may be indicated. The overall incidence of reported birth anomalies from pregnancies associated with maternal CLOMID ingestion during the investigational studies was within the range of that reported in published references for the general population. (See CONTRAINDICATIONS: Pregnancy.)

During clinical investigation, the experience from patients with known pregnancy outcome (Table 1) shows a spontaneous abortion rate of 20.4% and stillbirth rate of 1.0%. (See CLINICAL PHARMACOLOGY.)

Drug Interactions

Drug interactions with CLOMID have not been documented.

Carcinogenesis, Mutagenesis, Impairment of Fertility

Long-term toxicity studies in animals have not been performed to evaluate the carcinogenic or mutagenic potential of clomiphene citrate.

Oral administration of CLOMID to male rats at doses of 0.3 or 1 mg/kg/day caused decreased fertility, while higher doses caused temporary infertility. Oral doses of 0.1 mg/kg/day in female rats temporarily interrupted the normal cyclic vaginal smear pattern and prevented conception. Doses of 0.3 mg/kg/day slightly reduced the number of ovulated ova and corpora lutea, while 3 mg/kg/day inhibited ovulation.

Pregnancy

Pregnancy Category X. (See CONTRAINDICATIONS.)

Nursing Mothers

It is not known whether CLOMID is excreted in human milk. Because many drugs are excreted in human milk, caution should be exercised if CLOMID is administered to a nursing woman. In some patients, CLOMID may reduce lactation.

Ovarian Cancer

Prolonged use of clomiphene citrate tablets USP may increase the risk of a borderline or invasive ovarian tumor (see ADVERSE REACTIONS).

ADVERSE REACTIONS

Clinical Trial Adverse Events. CLOMID, at recommended dosages, is generally well tolerated. Adverse reactions usually have been mild and transient and most have disappeared promptly after treatment has been discontinued. Adverse experiences reported in patients treated with clomiphene citrate during clinical studies are shown in Table 2.

Table 2. Incidence of Adverse Events In Clinical Studies (Events Greater than 1%)
(n = 8029*)

Adverse Event	%
Ovarian Enlargement	13.6
Vasomotor Flushes	10.4
Abdominal-Pelvic Discomfort/ Distention/Bloating	5.5
Nausea and Vomiting	2.2
Breast Discomfort	2.1
Visual Symptoms Blurred vision, lights, floaters, waves, unspecified visual complaints, photophobia, diplopia, scotomata, phosphenes	1.5
Headache	1.3
Abnormal Uterine Bleeding Intermenstrual spotting, menorrhagia	1.3

* Includes 498 patients whose reports may have been duplicated in the event totals and could not be distinguished as such. Also, excludes 47 patients who did not report symptom data.

The following adverse events have been reported in fewer than 1% of patients in clinical trials: Acute abdomen, appetite increase, constipation, dermatitis or rash, depression, diarrhea, dizziness, fatigue, hair loss/dry hair, increased urinary frequency/volume, insomnia, light-headedness, nervous tension, vaginal dryness, vertigo, weight gain/loss. Patients on prolonged CLOMID therapy may show elevated serum levels of desmosterol. This is most likely due to a direct interference with cholesterol synthesis. However, the serum sterols in patients receiving the recommended dose of CLOMID are not significantly altered. Ovarian cancer has been infrequently reported in patients who have received fertility drugs. Infertility is a primary risk factor for ovarian cancer; however, epidemiology data suggest that prolonged use of clomiphene may increase the risk of a borderline or invasive ovarian tumor.

Postmarketing Adverse Events

The following adverse experiences were reported spontaneously with CLOMID: The cause and effect relationship of the listed events to the administration of CLOMID is not known.

Dermatologic: Acne, allergic reaction, erythema, erythema multiforme, erythema nodosum, hypertrichosis, pruritus

Central Nervous System: Migraine headache, paresthesia, seizure, stroke, syncope

Psychiatric: Anxiety, irritability, mood changes, pschosis

Visual Disorders: Abnormal accommodation, cataract, eye pain, macular edema, optic neuritis, photopsia, posterior vitreous detachment, retinal hemorrhage, retinal thrombosis, retinal vascular spasm, temporary loss of vision

Cardiovascular: Arrhythmia, chest pain, edema, hypertension, palpitation, phlebitis, pulmonary embolism, shortness of breath, tachycardia, thrombophlebitis

Musculoskeletal: Arthralgia, back pain, myalgia

Hepatic: Transaminases increased, hepatitis

Neoplasms: Liver (hepatic hemanglosarcoma, liver cell adenoma, hepatocellular carcinoma); breast (fibrocystic disease, breast carcinoma); endometrium (endometrial carcinoma); nervous system (astrocytoma, pituitary tumor, prolactinoma, neurofibromatosis, glioblastoma, multiforme, brain abcess); ovary (luteoma of pregnancy, dermoid cyst of the ovary, ovarian carcinoma); trophoblastic (hydatiform mole, choriocarcinoma); miscellaneous (melanoma, myeloma, perianal cysts, renal cell carcinoma, Hodgkin's lymphoma, tongue carcinoma, bladder carcinoma); and neoplasms of offspring (neuroectodermal tumor, thyroid tumor, hepatoblastoma, lymphocytic leukemia)

Genitourinary: Endometriosis, ovarian cyst (ovarian enlargement or cysts could, as such, be complicated by adnexal torsion), ovarian hemorrhage, tubal pregnancy, uterine hemorrhage

Body as a Whole: Fever, tinnitus, weakness

Other: Leukocytosis, thyroid disorder

Fetal/Neonatal anomalies. The following fetal abnormalities have also been reported during postmarketing surveillance: delayed development; abnormal bone development including skeletal malformations of the skull, face, nasal passages, jaw, hand, limb (ectromelia including amelia, hemimelia, and phocomelia), foot, and joints; tissue malformations including imperforate anus, tracheoesophageal fistula, diaphragmatic hernia, renal agenesis and dysgenesis, and malformations of the eye and lens (cataract), ear, lung, heart (ventricular septal defect and tetralogy of Fallot), and genitalia; as well as dwarfism, deafness, mental retardation, chromosomal disorders, and neural tube defects (including anencephaly).

DRUG ABUSE AND DEPENDENCE

Tolerance, abuse, or dependence with CLOMID has not been reported.

OVERDOSAGE

Signs and Symptoms

Toxic effects accompanying acute overdosage of CLOMID have not been reported. Signs and symptoms of overdosage as a result of the use of more than the recommended dose

Continued on next page

Hoechst Marion Roussel—Cont.

during CLOMID therapy include nausea, vomiting, vasomotor flushes, visual blurring, spots or flashes, scotomata, ovarian enlargement with pelvic or abdominal pain. (See CONTRAINDICATIONS: Ovarian Cyst.)

Oral LD_{50}. The acute oral LD_{50} of CLOMID is 1700 mg/kg in mice and 5750 mg/kg in rats. The toxic dose in humans is not known.

Dialysis: It is not known if CLOMID is dialyzable.

Treatment

In the event of overdose, appropriate supportive measures should be employed in addition to gastrointestinal decontamination.

DOSAGE AND ADMINISTRATION

General Considerations

The workup and treatment of candidates for CLOMID therapy should be supervised by physicians experienced in management of gynecologic or endocrine disorders. Patients should be chosen for therapy with CLOMID only after careful diagnostic evaluation (see INDICATIONS AND USAGE). The plan of therapy should be outlined in advance. Impediments to achieving the goal of therapy must be excluded or adequately treated before beginning CLOMID. The therapeutic objective should be balanced with potential risks and discussed with the patient and others involved in the achievement of a pregnancy.

Ovulation most often occurs from 5 to 10 days after a course of CLOMID. Coitus should be timed to coincide with the expected time of ovulation. Appropriate tests to determine ovulation may be useful during this time.

Recommended Dosage

Treatment of the selected patient should begin with a low dose, 50 mg daily (1 tablet) for 5 days. The dose should be increased only in those patients who do not ovulate in response to cyclic 50 mg CLOMID. A low dosage or duration of treatment course is particularly recommended if unusual sensitivity to pituitary gonadotropin is suspected, such as in patients with polycystic ovary syndrome (see WARNINGS: Ovarian Hyperstimulation Syndrome).

The patient should be evaluated carefully to exclude pregnancy, ovarian enlargement, or ovarian cyst formation between each treatment cycle.

If progestin-induced bleeding is planned, or if spontaneous uterine bleeding occurs prior to therapy, the regimen of 50 mg daily for 5 days should be started on or about the 5th day of the cycle. Therapy may be started at any time in the patient who has had no recent uterine bleeding. when ovulation occurs at this dosage, there is no advantage to increasing the dose in subsequent cycles of treatment. If ovulation does not appear to occur after the first course of therapy, a second course of 100 mg daily (two 50 mg tablets given as a single daily dose) for 5 days should be given. This course may be started as early as 30 days after the previous one after precautions are taken to exclude the presence of pregnancy. Increasing the dosage or duration of therapy beyond 100 mg/day for 5 days is not recommended.

The majority of patients who are going to ovulate will do so after the first course of therapy. If ovulation does not occur after three courses of therapy, further treatment with CLOMID is not recommended and the patient should be reevaluated. If three ovulatory responses occur, but pregnancy has not been achieved, further treatment is not recommended. If menses does not occur after an ovulatory response, the patient should be reevaluated. Long-term cyclic therapy is not recommended beyond a total of about six cycles (see PRECAUTIONS).

HOW SUPPLIED

NDC 0068-0226-30: 50 mg tablets in cartons of 30

Tablets are round, white, scored, and debossed CLOMID 50.

Store tablets at controlled room temperature 59–86°F (15–30°C).

Protect from heat, light, and excessive humidity, and store in closed containers.

Prescribing Information as of June 1995

Merrell Pharmaceuticals Inc.

Subsidiary of Hoechst Marion Roussel, Inc.

Kansas City, MO 64137

clop0695p

Shown in Product Identification Guide, page 317

DERMATOP® ℞

[dur 'mə-täp]

EMOLLIENT CREAM

(prednicarbate emollient cream) 0.1%

FOR DERMATOLOGIC USE ONLY.

NOT FOR USE IN EYES.

DESCRIPTION

Dermatop® Emollient Cream (prednicarbate emollient cream) 0.1% contains the nonhalogenated prednisolone derivative prednicarbate. Topical corticosteroids constitute a class of primarily synthetic steroids used topically as anti-inflammatory and antipruritic agents.

Each gram of Dermatop® Emollient Cream 0.1% contains 1.0 mg of prednicarbate in a base consisting of white petrolatum USP, purified water USP, isopropyl myristate NF, lanolin alcohols NF, mineral oil USP, cetostearyl alcohol NF, aluminum stearate, edetate disodium USP, lactic acid USP, and magnesium stearate DAB 9.

The chemical name of prednicarbate is 11β, 17, 21-trihydroxypregna-1,4-diene-3,20-dione 17-(ethyl carbonate) 21-propionate. Prednicarbate has the empirical formula $C_{27}H_{36}O_8$ and a molecular weight of 488.58. The CAS Registry Number is 73771-04-7. The chemical structure is:

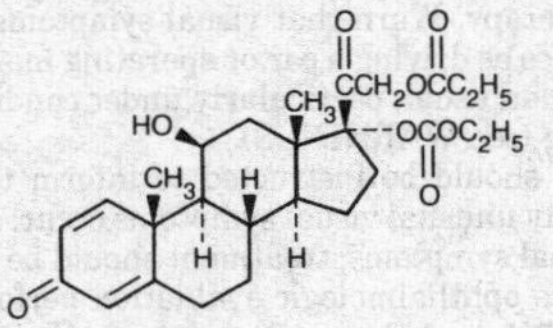

CLINICAL PHARMACOLOGY

In common with other topical corticosteroids, prednicarbate has anti-inflammatory, antipruritic and vasoconstrictive properties. In general, the mechanism of the anti-inflammatory activity of topical steroids is unclear. However, corticosteroids are thought to act by the induction of phospholipase A_2 inhibitory proteins, collectively called lipocortins. It is postulated that these proteins control the biosynthesis of potent mediators of inflammation such as prostaglandins and leukotrienes by inhibiting the release of their common precursor arachidonic acid. Arachidonic acid is released from membrane phospholipids by phospholipase A_2.

Pharmacokinetics

The extent of percutaneous absorption of topical corticosteroids is determined by many factors, including the vehicle and the integrity of the epidermal barrier. Use of occlusive dressings with hydrocortisone for up to 24 hours has not been shown to increase penetration; however, occlusion of hydrocortisone for 96 hours does markedly enhance penetration. Topical corticosteroids can be absorbed from normal intact skin, whereas inflammation and/or other disease processes in the skin increase percutaneous absorption.

Studies performed with Dermatop® Emollient Cream 0.1% indicate that the drug is in the medium range of potency compared with other topical corticosteroids.

INDICATIONS AND USAGE

Dermatop® Emollient Cream 0.1% is a medium-potency corticosteroid indicated for the relief of the inflammatory and pruritic manifestations of corticosteroid-responsive dermatoses.

CONTRAINDICATIONS

Dermatop® Emollient Cream 0.1% is contraindicated in those patients with a history of hypersensitivity to any of the components of the preparations.

PRECAUTIONS

General

Systemic absorption of topical corticosteroids can produce reversible hypothalamic-pituitary-adrenal (HPA) axis suppression with the potential for glucocorticosteroid insufficiency after withdrawal of treatment. Manifestations of Cushing's syndrome, hyperglycemia, and glucosuria can also be produced in some patients by systemic absorption of topical corticosteroids while on treatment.

Patients receiving a large dose of a higher-potency topical steroid applied to a large surface area or under occlusion should be evaluated periodically for evidence of HPA-axis suppression. This may be done by using the ACTH stimulation, AM plasma cortisol, and urinary free cortisol tests.

Dermatop® Emollient Cream 0.1% did not produce significant HPA-axis suppression when used at a dose of 30 g/day for a week in 10 patients with extensive psoriasis or atopic dermatitis.

If HPA-axis suppression is noted, an attempt should be made to withdraw the drug, to reduce the frequency of application, or to substitute a less potent corticosteroid. Recovery of HPA-axis function is generally prompt and complete upon discontinuation of topical corticosteroids. Infrequently, signs and symptoms of glucocorticosteroid insufficiency may occur, requiring supplemental systemic corticosteroids. For information on systemic supplementation, see prescribing information for those products.

Pediatric patients may be more susceptible to systemic toxicity from equivalent doses due to their larger skin surface to body mass ratios. (See **PRECAUTIONS—Pediatric Use**).

If irritation develops, Dermatop® Emollient Cream 0.1% should be discontinued and appropriate therapy instituted. Allergic contact dermatitis with corticosteroids is usually diagnosed by observing failure to heal rather than noting a clinical exacerbation, as observed with most topical products not containing corticosteroids. Such an observation should be corroborated with appropriate diagnostic patch testing.

If concomitant skin infections are present or develop, an appropriate antifungal or antibacterial agent should be used. If a favorable response does not occur promptly, use of Dermatop® Emollient Cream 0.1% should be discontinued until the infection has been adequately controlled.

Information for Patients

Patients using topical corticosteroids should receive the following information and instructions:

1. This medication is to be used as directed by the physician. It is for external use only. Avoid contact with the eyes.
2. This medication should not be used for any disorder other than that for which it was prescribed.
3. The treated skin area should not be bandaged or otherwise covered or wrapped so as to be occlusive, unless directed by the physician.
4. Patients should report any signs of local adverse reactions to their physician.

Laboratory Tests

The following tests may be helpful in evaluating patients for HPA-axis suppression:

ACTH stimulation test
AM plasma cortisol test
Urinary free cortisol test

Carcinogenesis, Mutagenesis, and Impairment of Fertility

In a study of the effect of prednicarbate on fertility, pregnancy, and postnatal development in rats, no effect was noted on the fertility or pregnancy of the parent animals or postnatal development of the offspring after administration of up to 0.80 mg/kg of prednicarbate subcutaneously.

Prednicarbate has been evaluated in the Salmonella reversion test (Ames test) over a wide range of concentrations in the presence and absence of an S-9 liver microsomal fraction, and did not demonstrate mutagenic activity. Similarly, prednicarbate did not produce any significant changes in the numbers of micronuclei seen in erythrocytes when mice were given doses ranging from 1 to 160 mg/kg of the drug.

Pregnancy: Teratogenic Effects: Pregnancy Category C.

Corticosteroids have been shown to be teratogenic in laboratory animals when administered systemically at relatively low dosage levels. Some corticosteroids have been shown to be teratogenic after dermal application in laboratory animals.

Prednicarbate has been shown to be teratogenic and embryotoxic in Wistar rats and Himalayan rabbits when given subcutaneously during gestation at doses 1900x and 45x the recommended topical human dose, assuming a percutaneous absorption of approximately 3%.

In the rats, slightly retarded fetal development and an incidence of thickened and wavy ribs higher than the spontaneous rate were noted.

In rabbits, increased liver weights and slight increase in the fetal intrauterine death rate were observed. The fetuses that were delivered exhibited reduced placental weight, increased frequency of cleft palate, ossification disorders in the sternum, omphalocele, and anomalous posture of the forelimbs.

There are no adequate and well-controlled studies in pregnant women on teratogenic effects of prednicarbate. Therefore, Dermatop® Emollient Cream (prednicarbate emollient cream) 0.1% should be used during pregnancy only if the potential benefit justifies the potential risk to the fetus.

Nursing Mothers

Systemically administered corticosteroids appear in human milk and could suppress growth, interfere with endogenous corticosteroid production, or cause other untoward effects. It is not known whether topical administration of corticosteroids could result in sufficient systemic absorption to produce detectable quantities in human milk. Because many drugs are excreted in human milk, caution should be exercised when Dermatop® Emollient Cream 0.1% is administered to a nursing woman.

Pediatric Use

Safety and effectiveness of Dermatop® Emollient Cream 0.1% in persons below the age of 18 years have not been established. Because of a higher ratio of skin surface area to body mass, pediatric patients are at a greater risk than adults of HPA-axis suppression when they are treated with topical corticosteroids. They are therefore also at greater risk of glucocorticosteroid insufficiency after withdrawal of treatment and at greater risk of Cushing's syndrome while on treatment. Adverse effects including striae have been reported with inappropriate use of topical corticosteroids in pediatric patients (see **PRECAUTIONS**).

HPA-axis suppression, Cushing's syndrome, and intracranial hypertension have been reported in pediatric patients receiving topical corticosteroids. Manifestations of adrenal suppression in pediatric patients include linear growth retardation, delayed weight gain, low plasma cortisol levels, and absence of response to ACTH stimulation. Manifestations of intracranial hypertension include bulging fontanelles, headaches, and bilateral papilledema.

ADVERSE REACTIONS

In controlled clinical studies, the incidence of adverse reactions probably or possibly associated with the use of Dermatop® Emollient Cream 0.1%, was approximately 4%. Reported reactions included mild signs of skin atrophy in 1% of treated patients, as well as the following reactions which were reported in less than 1% of patients: pruritus, edema, paresthesia, urticaria, burning, allergic contact dermatitis and rash.
The following additional local adverse reactions are reported infrequently with topical corticosteroids, but may occur more frequently with the use of occlusive dressings and especially with higher-potency corticosteroids. These reactions are listed in an approximate decreasing order of occurrence: dryness, folliculitis, acneiform eruptions, hypopigmentation, perioral dermatitis, secondary infection, striae, and milaria.

OVERDOSAGE

Topically applied corticosteroids can be absorbed in sufficient amounts to produce systemic effects (see **PRECAUTIONS**).

DOSAGE AND ADMINISTRATION

Apply a thin film of Dermatop® Emollient Cream 0.1% to the affected skin areas twice daily. Rub in gently.

HOW SUPPLIED

Dermatop® Emollient Cream 0.1% is supplied in 15 g (NDC 0039-0088-15) and 60 g (NDC 0039-0088-60) tubes.
Store between 41° and 77° F (5° and 25° C).

CLINICAL STUDIES

Dermatop® Emollient Cream 0.1% was studied in vehicle controlled clinical trials in psoriasis and atopic dermatitis. In both studies, patients were to be treated twice daily for 21 days. Improvement in erythema, induration and scaling were studied in the psoriasis protocol. At Endpoint (i.e., patient's last visit), the mean total sign scores for patients had decreased from baseline (i.e., improved) by 37% and were significantly better than vehicle ($p < 0.001$).
Improvement in erythema, induration and pruritus were studied in the atopic dermatitis protocol. At Endpoint (i.e., patient's last visit), the mean total sign/symptom scores for patients had decreased from baseline (i.e., improved) by 76% and were significantly better than vehicle ($p < 0.001$).
The evaluations were performed in separate protocols by different panels of investigators. Different sets of signs/symptoms were evaluated in each protocol. These data are presented for comparison purposes only.

Overall Improvement of Disease at Endpoint—% of Patients

	Scale Number					
Indication	0	1	2	3	4	5
Psoriasis (n=105)	1%	16%	17%	51%	13%	1%
Atopic Dermatitis (n=98)	31%	42%	9%	12%	2%	4%

Scale:
0=Cleared; 100% clearance of signs except for residual discoloration
1=Excellent improvement; at least 75%, but less than 100% clearance of signs monitored
2=Moderate improvement; at least 50%, but less than 75% clearance of signs monitored
3=Slight improvement; less than 50% clearance of signs monitored
4=No change; no detectable improvement from baseline condition
5=Exacerbation; flare of sites under study

Prednicarbate US Patent 4,242,334 has been extended.
Dermatop REG TM HOECHST AG
Hoechst-Roussel Pharmaceuticals
Division of Hoechst Marion Roussel, Inc.
Kansas City, MO 64137
REG TM HOECHST AG

908800-3/95

Shown in Product Identification Guide, page 317

DIAβETA® ℞

[dī″ə-bū′ta]
(glyburide)
Tablets 1.25, 2.5 and 5 mg

DESCRIPTION

Diaβeta® (glyburide) is an oral blood-glucose-lowering drug of the sulfonylurea class. It is a white, crystalline compound, formulated as tablets of 1.25 mg, 2.5 mg, and 5 mg strengths for oral administration. Diaβeta® tablets contain the active ingredient glyburide and the following inactive ingredients: dibasic calcium phosphate USP, magnesium stearate NF, microcrystalline cellulose NF, sodium alginate NF, talc USP. Diaβeta® 1.25 mg tablets also contain D&C Yellow #10 Aluminum Lake and FD&C Red #40 Aluminum Lake. Diaβeta® 2.5 mg tablets also contain FD&C Red #40 Aluminum Lake. Diaβeta® 5 mg tablets also contain D&C Yellow #10 Aluminum Lake, and FD&C Blue #1. Chemically, Diaβeta® is identified as 1-[[p-[2-(5-Chloro-*o*-anisamido) ethyl] phenyl] sulfonyl]-3-cyclohexylurea.
The CAS Registry Number is 10238-21-8.
The structural formula is:

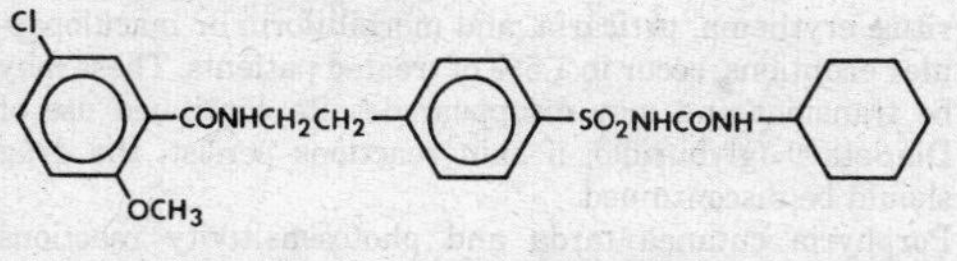

The molecular weight is 493.99. The aqueous solubility of Diaβeta® increases with pH as a result of salt formation.

CLINICAL PHARMACOLOGY

Diaβeta® appears to lower the blood glucose acutely by stimulating the release of insulin from the pancreas, an effect dependent upon functioning beta cells in the pancreatic islets. The mechanism by which Diaβeta® lowers blood glucose during long-term administration has not been clearly established.
With chronic administration in Type II diabetic patients, the blood glucose lowering effect persists despite a gradual decline in the insulin secretory response to the drug. Extrapancreatic effects may play a part in the mechanism of action of oral sulfonylurea hypoglycemic drugs.
In addition to its blood glucose lowering actions, Diaβeta® produces a mild diuresis by enhancement of renal free water clearance. Clinical experience to date indicates an extremely low incidence of disulfiram-like reactions in patients while taking Diaβeta®.

Pharmacokinetics

Single-dose studies with Diaβeta® in normal subjects demonstrate significant absorption within one hour, peak drug levels at about four hours, and low but detectable levels at twenty-four hours. Mean serum levels of glyburide, as reflected by areas under the serum concentration-time curve, increase in proportion to corresponding increases in dose. Multiple-dose studies with Diaβeta® in diabetic patients demonstrate drug level concentration-time curves similar to single-dose studies, indicating no build-up of drug in tissue depots. The decrease of glyburide in the serum of normal healthy individuals is biphasic, the terminal half-life being about 10 hours. In single-dose studies in fasting normal subjects, the degree and duration of blood glucose lowering is proportional to the dose administered and to the area under the drug level concentration-time curve. The blood glucose lowering effect persists for 24 hours following single morning doses in non-fasting diabetic patients. Under conditions of repeated administration in diabetic patients, however, there is no reliable correlation between blood drug levels and fasting blood glucose levels. A one-year study of diabetic patients treated with Diaβeta® showed no reliable correlation between administered dose and serum drug level.
The major metabolite of Diaβeta® is the 4-trans-hydroxy derivative. A second metabolite, the 3-cis-hydroxy derivative, also occurs. These metabolites contribute no significant hypoglycemic action since they are only weakly active (1/400th and 1/40th, respectively, as glyburide) in rabbits.
Diaβeta® is excreted as metabolites in the bile and urine, approximately 50% by each route. This dual excretory pathway is qualitatively different from that of other sulfonylureas, which are excreted primarily in the urine.
Sulfonylurea drugs are extensively bound to serum proteins. Displacement from protein binding sites by other drugs may lead to enhanced hypoglycemic action. *In vitro*, the protein binding exhibited by Diaβeta® is predominantly non-ionic, whereas that of other sulfonylureas (chlorpropamide, tolbutamide, tolazamide) is predominantly ionic. Acidic drugs such as phenylbutazone, warfarin, and salicylates displace the ionic-binding sulfonylureas from serum proteins to a far greater extent than the non-ionic binding Diaβeta®. It has not been shown that this difference in protein binding will result in fewer drug-drug interactions with Diaβeta® in clinical use.

INDICATIONS AND USAGE

Diaβeta® is indicated as an adjunct to diet to lower the blood glucose in patients with non-insulin-dependent diabetes mellitus (Type II) whose hyperglycemia cannot be controlled by diet alone.
In initiating treatment for non-insulin-dependent diabetes, diet should be emphasized as the primary form of treatment. Caloric restriction and weight loss are essential in the obese diabetic patient. Proper dietary management alone may be effective in controlling the blood glucose and symptoms of hyperglycemia. The importance of regular physical activity should also be stressed, and cardiovascular risk factors should be identified and corrective measures taken where possible.
If this treatment program fails to reduce symptoms and/or blood glucose, the use of an oral sulfonylurea or insulin should be considered. Use of Diaβeta® must be viewed by both the physician and patient as a treatment in addition to diet, and not as a substitute for diet or as a convenient mechanism for avoiding dietary restraint. Furthermore, loss of blood glucose control on diet alone may be transient, thus requiring only short-term administration of Diaβeta®.
During maintenance programs, Diaβeta® should be discontinued if satisfactory lowering of blood glucose is no longer achieved. Judgments should be based on regular clinical and laboratory evaluations.
In considering the use of Diaβeta® in asymptomatic patients, it should be recognized that controlling the blood glucose in non-insulin dependent diabetes has not been definitely established to be effective in preventing the long-term cardiovascular or neural complications of diabetes.

CONTRAINDICATIONS

Diaβeta® is contraindicated in patients with:
1. Known hypersensitivity to the drug.
2. Diabetic ketoacidosis, with or without coma.
   This condition should be treated with insulin.

WARNINGS

SPECIAL WARNING ON INCREASED RISK OF CARDIOVASCULAR MORTALITY

The administration of oral hypoglycemic drugs has been reported to be associated with increased cardiovascular mortality as compared to treatment with diet alone or diet plus insulin. This warning is based on the study conducted by the University Group Diabetes Program (UGDP), a long-term prospective clinical trial designed to evaluate the effectiveness of glucose-lowering drugs in preventing or delaying vascular complications in patients with non-insulin-dependent diabetes. The study involved 823 patients who were randomly assigned to one of four treatment groups (Diabetes 19 (supp. 2): 747-830, 1970).
UGDP reported that patients treated for 5 to 8 years with diet plus a fixed dose of tolbutamide (1.5 grams per day) had a rate of cardiovascular mortality approximately 2 $^{1}/_{2}$ times that of patients treated with diet alone. A significant increase in total mortality was not observed, but the use of tolbutamide was discontinued based on the increase in cardiovascular mortality, thus limiting the opportunity for the study to show an increase in overall mortality. Despite controversy regarding the interpretation of these results, the findings of the UGDP study provide an adequate basis for this warning. The patient should be informed that the potential risks and advantages of Diaβeta® and of alternative modes of therapy.
Although only one drug in the sulfonylurea class (tolbutamide) was included in this study, it is prudent from a safety standpoint to consider that this warning may also apply to other oral hypoglycemic drugs in this class, in view of their close similarities in mode of action and chemical structure.

PRECAUTIONS

General

Hypoglycemia: All sulfonylurea drugs are capable of producing severe hypoglycemia. Proper patient selection, dosage, and instructions are important to avoid hypoglycemic episodes. Renal or hepatic insufficiency may cause elevated blood levels of Diaβeta® and the latter may also diminish gluconeogenic capacity, both of which increase the risk of serious hypoglycemic reactions. Elderly, debilitated or malnourished patients, and those with adrenal or pituitary insufficiency are particularly susceptible to the hypoglycemic action of glucose-lowering drugs. Hypoglycemia may be difficult to recognize in the elderly, and in people who are taking beta-adrenergic blocking drugs or other sympatholytic agents. Hypoglycemia is more likely to occur when caloric intake is deficient, after severe or prolonged exercise, when alcohol is ingested, or when more than one glucose-lowering drug is used. Loss of control of blood glucose: When a patient stabilized on any diabetic regimen is exposed to stress such as fever, trauma, infection, or surgery, a loss of control may occur. At such times, it may be necessary to discontinue Diaβeta® and administer insulin.
The effectiveness of any oral hypoglycemic drug, including Diaβeta®, in lowering blood glucose to a desired level decreases in many patients over a period of time, which may be due to progression of the severity of the diabetes or to diminish responsiveness to the drug. This phenomenon is known as secondary failure, to distinguish it from primary failure in which the drug is ineffective in an individual patient when first given.

Information for Patients

Patients should be informed of the potential risks and advantages of Diaβeta® and of alternative modes of therapy. They should also be informed about the importance of adherence to dietary instructions, of a regular exercise program, and of regular testing of blood glucose.

Continued on next page

Hoechst Marion Roussel—Cont.

The risks of hypoglycemia, its symptoms and treatment, and conditions that predipose to its development should be explained to patients and responsible family members. Primary and secondary failure should also be explained.

Laboratory Tests

Periodic fasting blood glucose measurements should be performed to monitor therapeutic response. A glycosylated hemoglobin determination should also be performed periodically.

Drug Interactions

The hypoglycemic action of sulfonylureas may be potentiated by certain drugs including nonsteroidal anti-inflammatory agents and other drugs that are highly protein bound, salicylates, sulfonamides, chloramphenicol, probenecid, monoamine oxidase inhibitors and beta adrenergic blocking agents. When such drugs are administered to a patient receiving Diaβeta®, the patient should be observed closely for hypoglycemia. When such drugs are withdrawn from a patient receiving Diaβeta®, the patient should be observed closely for loss of control.

A possible interaction between glyburide and fluoroquinolone antibiotics has been reported resulting in a potentiation of the hypoglycemic action of glyburide. The mechanism for this interaction is not known.

Possible interactions between glyburide and coumarin derivatives have been reported that may either potentiate or weaken the effects of coumarin derivatives. The mechanism of these interactions is not known.

Certain drugs tend to produce hyperglycemia and may lead to loss of control. These drugs include the thiazides and other diuretics, corticosteroids, phenothiazines, thyroid products, estrogens, oral contraceptives, phenytoin, nicotinic acid, sympathomimetics, calcium channel blocking drugs, and isoniazid. When such drugs are administered to a patient receiving Diaβeta®, the patient should be closely observed for loss of control. When such drugs are withdrawn from a patient receiving Diaβeta®, the patient should be observed closely for hypoglycemia. A potential interaction between oral miconazole and oral hypoglycemic agents leading to severe hypoglycemia has been reported. Whether this interaction also occurs with the intravenous, topical or vaginal preparations of miconazole is not known.

Carcinogenesis, Mutagenesis, and Impairment of Fertility

Diaβeta® is non-mutagenic when studied in the Salmonella microsome test (Ames test) and in the DNA damage/alkaline elution assay. Studies in rats at doses up to 300 mg/kg/day for 18 months showed no carcinogenic effects.

No drug related effects were noted in any of the criteria evaluated in the two year oncogenicity study of glyburide in mice.

Pregnancy

Teratogenic Effects: Pregnancy Category C

Diaβeta® has been shown to effect the maturation of the long bones (humerus and femur) in rat pups when given in doses 6250 times the maximum recommended human dose. These effects, which were seen during the period of lactation and not during organogenesis, are a shortening of the bones with effects to various structures of the long bones, especially in humerus and femur.

There are no adequate and well-controlled studies in pregnant women. Because animal reproduction studies are not always predictive of human response, Diaβeta® should be used during pregnancy only if the potential benefit justifies the risk to the fetus. Because recent information suggests that abnormal blood glucose levels during pregnancy are associated with a higher incidence of congenital abnormalities, many experts recommend that insulin be used during pregnancy to maintain blood glucose levels as close to normal as possible.

Nonteratogenic Effects

Prolonged severe hypoglycemia (4 to 10 days) has been reported in neonates born to mothers who were receiving a sulfonylurea drug at the time of delivery. This has been reported more frequently with the use of agents with prolonged half-lives. If Diaβeta® is used during pregnancy, it should be discontinued at least two weeks before the expected delivery date.

Nursing Mothers

Although it is not known whether Diaβeta® is excreted in human milk, some sulfonylureas are known to be excreted in human milk. Because of the potential for hypoglycemia in nursing infants may exist, a decision should be made whether to discontinue nursing or to discontinue administering the drug, taking into account the importance of the drug to the mother. If Diaβeta® is discontinued and if diet alone is inadequate for controlling blood glucose, insulin therapy should be considered.

PEDIATRIC USE

Safety and effectiveness in pediatric patients have not been established.

ADVERSE REACTIONS

Hypoglycemia: See PRECAUTIONS and OVERDOSAGE Sections.

Gastrointestinal Reactions: Cholestatic jaundice and hepatitis may occur rarely; Diaβeta® should be discontinued if this occurs. Liver function abnormalities, including isolated transaminase elevations, have been reported. Gastrointestinal disturbances, e.g., nausea, epigastric fullness, and heartburn, are the most common reactions and occur in 1.8% of treated patients. They tend to be dose-related and may disappear when dosage is reduced.

Dermatologic Reactions: Allergic skin reactions, e.g., pruritus, erythema, urticaria, and morbilliform or maculopapular eruptions, occur in 1.5% of treated patients. These may be transient and may disappear despite continued use of Diaβeta® (glyburide); if skin reactions persist, the drug should be discontinued.

Porphyria cutanea tarda and photosensitivity reactions have been reported with sulfonylureas.

Hematologic Reactions: Leukopenia, agranulocytosis, thrombocytopenia, which occasionally may present as purpura, hemolytic anemia, aplastic anemia, and pancytopenia have been reported with sulfonylureas.

Metabolic Reactions: Hepatic porphyria reactions have been reported with sulfonylureas; however, these have not been reported with Diaβeta®. Disulfiram-like reactions have been reported very rarely with Diaβeta®. Cases of hyponatremia have been reported with glyburide and all other sulfonylureas, most often in patients who are on other medications or have medical conditions known to cause hyponatremia or increase release of antidiuretic hormone. The syndrome of inappropriate antidiuretic hormone (SIADH) secretion has been reported with certain other sulfonylureas, and it has been suggested that these sulfonylureas may augment the peripheral (antidiuretic) action of ADH and/or increase release of ADH.

Other Reactions: Changes in accommodation and/or blurred vision have been reported with glyburide and other sulfonylureas. These are thought to be related to fluctuation in glucose levels.

In addition to dermatologic reactions, allergic reactions such as angioedema, arthralgia, myalgia and vasculitis have been reported.

OVERDOSAGE

Overdosage of sulfonylureas, including Diaβeta®, can produce hypoglycemia. Mild hypoglycemic symptoms without loss of consciousness or neurologic findings should be treated aggressively with oral glucose and adjustments in drug dosage and/or meal patterns. Close monitoring should continue until the physician is assured that the patient is out of danger. Severe hypoglycemic reactions with coma, seizures, or other neurological impairment occur infrequently, but constitute medical emergencies requiring immediate hospitalization. If hypoglycemic coma is diagnosed or suspected, the patient should be given a rapid intravenous injection of concentrated (50%) glucose solution. This should be followed by a continuous infusion of a more dilute (10%) glucose solution at a rate that will maintain the blood glucose at a level above 100 mg/mL. Patients should be closely monitored for a minimum of 24 to 48 hours, since hypoglycemia may recur after apparent clinical recovery.

DOSAGE AND ADMINISTRATION

There is no fixed dosage regimen for the management of diabetes mellitus with Diaβeta® or any other hypoglycemic agent. The patient's fasting blood glucose must be measured periodically to determine the minimum effective dose for the patient; to detect primary failure, i.e., inadequate lowering of blood glucose at the maximum recommended dose of medication; and to detect secondary failure, i.e., loss of adequate blood glucose lowering response after an initial period of effectiveness. Periodic glycosylated hemoglobin determinations should be performed.

Short-term administration of Diaβeta® may be sufficient during periods of transient loss of control in patients usually controlled well on diet.

1. Usual Starting Dose

   The usual starting dose of Diaβeta® as initial therapy is 2.5 to 5 mg daily, administered with breakfast or the first main meal. Those patients who may be more sensitive to hypoglycemic drugs should be started at 1.25 mg daily. (See **PRECAUTIONS** Section for patients at increased risk). Failure to follow an appropriate dosage regimen may precipitate hypoglycemia. Patients who do not adhere to their prescribed dietary and drug regimen are more prone to exhibit unsatisfactory response to therapy. Transfer of patients from other oral antidiabetic regimens to Diaβeta® should be done conservatively and the initial daily dose should be 2.5 to 5 mg. When transferring patients from oral hypoglycemic agents other than chlorpropamide, to Diaβeta®, no transition period and no initial priming dose is necessary. When transferring patients from chlorpropamide, particular care should be exercised during the first two weeks because the prolonged retention of chlorpropamide in the body and subsequent overlapping drug effects may provoke hypoglycemia.

   Bioavailability studies have demonstrated that Glynase® PresTab® Tablets 3 mg are not bioequivalent to Diaβeta® Tablets 5 mg. Therefore, these products are not substituted and patients should be retitrated if transferred.

   Some Type II diabetic patients being treated with insulin may respond satisfactorily to Diaβeta®. If the insulin dose is less than 20 units daily, substitution of Diaβeta® 2.5 to 5 mg as a single daily dose may be tried. If the insulin dose is between 20 and 40 units daily, the patient may be placed directly on Diaβeta® 5 mg daily as a single dose. If the insulin dose is more than 40 units daily, a transition period is required for conversion to Diaβeta®. In these patients, insulin dosage is decreased by 50% and Diaβeta® 5 mg daily is started. Please refer to Usual Maintenance Dose for further explanation.

2. **Usual Maintenance Dose**

   The usual maintenance dose is in the range of 1.25 to 20 mg daily, which may be given as a single dose or in divided doses (See Dosage Interval Section). Dosage increases should be made in increments of no more than 2.5 mg at weekly intervals based upon the patient's blood glucose response.

   No exact dosage relationship exists between Diaβeta® and the other oral hypoglycemic agents. Although patients may be transferred from the maximum dose of other sulfonylureas, the maximum starting dose of 5 mg of Diaβeta® should be observed. A maintenance dose of 5 mg Diaβeta® provides approximately the same degree of blood glucose control as 250 to 375 mg chlorpropamide, 250 to 375 mg tolazamide, 500 to 750 mg acetohexamide, or 1000 to 1500 mg tolbutamide.

   When transferring patients receiving more than 40 units of insulin daily, they may be started on a daily dose of Diaβeta® 5 mg concomitantly with a 50% reduction in insulin dose. Progressive withdrawal of insulin and increase of Diaβeta® in increments of 1.25 to 2.5 mg every 2 to 10 days is then carried out. During this conversion period when both insulin and Diaβeta® are being used, hypoglycemia may rarely occur. During insulin withdrawal, patients should self-test their blood for glucose and their urine for acetone at least 3 times daily and report results to their physician. Self-testing of urinary glucose is a less desirable alternative. The appearance of persistent acetonuria with glycosuria indicates that the patient is a Type I diabetic who requires insulin therapy.

3. **Maximum Dose**

   Daily doses of more than 20 mg are not recommended.

4. **Dosage Interval**

   Once-a-day therapy is usually satisfactory, based upon usual meal patterns and a 10 hour half-life of Diaβeta®. Some patients, particularly those receiving more than 10 mg daily, may have a more satisfactory response with twice-a-day dosage.

In elderly patients, debilitated or malnourished patients, and patients with impaired renal or hepatic function, the initial and maintenance dosing should be conservative to avoid hypoglycemic reactions. (See PRECAUTIONS Section.)

HOW SUPPLIED

Diaβeta® tablets are supplied as peach, oblong, monogrammed, scored tablets of 1.25 mg in bottles of 50 (NDC 0039-0053-005, NSN 6505-01-187-6584); pink, oblong, monogrammed, scored tablets of 2.5 mg in bottles of 30 (NDC 0039-0051-03, NSN 6505-01-312-1256); bottles of 60 (NDC 0039-0051-06, NSN 6505-01-312-1255); bottles of 100 (NDC 0039-0051-10, NSN 6505-01-187-6586); bottles of 500 (NDC 0039-0051-50, NSN 6505-01-313-3707); and in Unit Dose Cartons of 100 (NDC 0039-0051-11, NSN 6505-01-204-5416); and light green, oblong, monogrammed, scored tablets of 5 mg in bottles of 30 (NDC 0039-0052-03, NSN 6505-01-259-1553); bottles of 60 (NDC 0039-0052-06, NSN 6505-01-258-7132); bottles of 100 (NDC 0039-0052-10, NSN 6505-01-187-6585; bottles of 500 (NDC 0039-0052-50, NSN 6505-01-190-4388; bottles of 1000 (NDC 0039-0052-70, NSN 6505-01-277-2804), and in Unit Dose Cartons of 100 (NDC 0039-0052-11, NSN 6505-01-203-6280).

Store at controlled room temperature (59 to 86° F).

Dispense in well-closed containers with safety closures.

Caution: Federal law prohibits dispensing without a prescription.

Glynase and PresTab are registered trademarks of The Upjohn Company

Made in USA 4/95

Hoechst-Roussel Pharmaceuticals
Division of Hoechst Marion Roussel
Kansas City, MO 64137

Shown in Product Identification Guide, page 317

DITROPAN® ℞
[di 'trō-pan]
(oxybutynin chloride)
Tablets and Syrup

Prescribing Information as of January 1995

DESCRIPTION

Each scored biconvex, engraved blue DITROPAN® Tablet contains 5 mg of oxybutynin chloride. Each 5 mL of DITROPAN® Syrup contains 5 mg of oxybutynin chloride. Chemically, oxybutynin chloride is d,l (racemic) 4-diethylamino-2-butynyl phenylcyclohexylglycolate hydrochloride. The empirical formula of oxybutynin chloride is $C_{22}H_{31}NO_3 \cdot HCl$. The structural formula appears below:

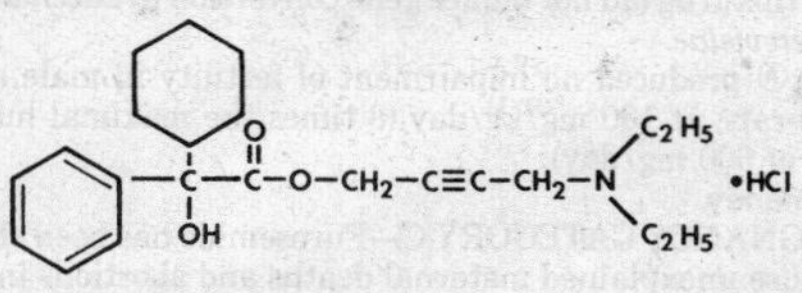

Oxybutynin chloride is a white crystalline solid with a molecular weight of 393.9. It is soluble in water and acids, but relatively insoluble in alkalis.
DITROPAN® Tablets
Also contains: calcium stearate, FD&C Blue #1 Lake, lactose, and microcrystalline cellulose.
DITROPAN® Syrup
Also contains: citric acid, FD&C Green #3, glycerin, methylparaben, flavor, sodium citrate, sorbitol, sucrose, and water.
DITROPAN® Tablets and Syrup are for oral administration.
Therapeutic Category: Antispasmodic, anticholinergic.

CLINICAL PHARMACOLOGY

DITROPAN® (oxybutynin chloride) exerts direct antispasmodic effect on smooth muscle and inhibits the muscarinic action of acetylcholine on smooth muscle. DITROPAN exhibits only one fifth of the anticholinergic activity of atropine on the rabbit detrusor muscle, but four to ten times the antispasmodic activity. No blocking effects occur at skeletal neuromuscular junctions or autonomic ganglia (antinicotinic effects).
DITROPAN relaxes bladder smooth muscle. In patients with conditions characterized by involuntary bladder contractions, cystometric studies have demonstrated that DITROPAN increases bladder (vesical) capacity, diminishes the frequency of uninhibited contractions of the detrusor muscle, and delays the initial desire to void. DITROPAN thus decreases urgency and the frequency of both incontinent episodes and voluntary urination.
DITROPAN was well tolerated in patients administered the drug in controlled studies of 30 days' duration and in uncontrolled studies in which some of the patients received the drug for 2 years. Pharmacokinetic information is not currently available.

INDICATIONS AND USAGE

DITROPAN is indicated for the relief of symptoms of bladder instability associated with voiding in patients with uninhibited neurogenic or reflex neurogenic bladder (ie, urgency, frequency, urinary leakage, urge incontinence, dysuria).

CONTRAINDICATIONS

DISTROPAN® (oxybutynin chloride) is contraindicated in patients with untreated angle closure glaucoma and in patients with untreated narrow anterior chamber angles since anticholinergic drugs may aggravate these conditions. It is also contraindicated in partial or complete obstruction of the gastrointestinal tract, paralytic ileus, intestinal atony of the elderly or debilitated patient, megacolon, toxic megacolon complicating ulcerative colitis, severe colitis, and myasthenia gravis. It is contraindicated in patients with obstructive uropathy and in patients with unstable cardiovascular status in acute hemorrhage.
DITROPAN is contraindicated in patients who have demonstrated hypersensitivity to the product.

WARNINGS

DITROPAN® (oxybutynin chloride), when administered in the presence of high environmental temperature, can cause heat prostration (fever and heat stroke due to decreased sweating).
Diarrhea may be an early symptom of incomplete intestinal obstruction, especially in patients with ileostomy or colostomy. In this instance treatment with DITROPAN would be inappropriate and possibly harmful.
DITROPAN may produce drowsiness or blurred vision. The patient should be cautioned regarding activities requiring mental alertness such as operating a motor vehicle or other machinery or performing hazardous work while taking this drug.
Alcohol or other sedative drugs may enhance the drowsiness caused by DITROPAN.

PRECAUTIONS

DITROPAN® (oxybutynin chloride) should be used with caution in the elderly and in all patients with autonomic neuropathy, hepatic or renal disease. DITROPAN may aggravate the symptoms of hyperthyroidism, coronary heart disease, congestive heart failure, cardiac arrhythmias, hiatal hernia, tachycardia, hypertension, and prostatic hypertrophy. Administration of DITROPAN® (oxybutynin chloride) to patients with ulcerative colitis may suppress intestinal motility to the point of producing a paralytic ileus and precipitate or aggravate toxic megacolon, a serious complication of the disease.
Carcinogenesis, Mutagenesis, Impairment of Fertility. A 24–month study in rats at dosages up to approximately 400 times the recommended human dosage showed no evidence of carcinogenicity.
DITROPAN showed no increase of mutagenic activity when treated in *Schizosaccharomyces pompholiciformis, Saccharomyces cerevisiae* and *Salmonella typhimurium* test systems. Reproduction studies in the hamster, rabbit, rat, and mouse have shown no definite evidence of impaired fertility.
Pregnancy. Category B. Reproduction studies in the hamster, rabbit, rat, and mouse have shown no definite evidence of impaired fertility or harm to the animal fetus. The safety of DITROPAN administered to women who are or who may become pregnant has not been established. Therefore, DITROPAN should not be given to pregnant women unless, in the judgment of the physician, the probable clinical benefits outweigh the possible hazards.
Nursing Mothers. It is not known whether this drug is excreted in human milk. Because many drugs are excreted in human milk, caution should be exercised when DITROPAN is administered to a nursing woman.
Pediatric Use. The safety and efficacy of DITROPAN administration have been demonstrated for pediatric patients 5 years of age and older (see DOSAGE AND ADMINISTRATION). However, as there is insufficient clinical data for pediatric populations under age 5, DITROPAN is not recommended for this age group.

ADVERSE REACTIONS

Following administration of DITROPAN® (oxybutynin chloride), the symptoms that can be associated with the use of other anticholinergic drugs may occur.
Cardiovascular: Palpitations tachycardia, vasodilatation
Dermatologic: Decreased sweating, rash
Gastrointestinal/Genitourinary: Constipation, decreased gastrointestinal motility, dry mouth, nausea, urinary hesitance and retention
Nervous System: Asthenia, dizziness, drowsiness, hallucinations, insomnia, restlessness
Ophthalmic: Amblyopia, cycloplegia, decreased lacrimation, mydriasis
Other: Impotence, suppression of lactation

OVERDOSAGE

The symptoms of overdosage with DITROPAN® (oxybutynin chloride) may be any of those seen with other anticholinergic agents. Symptoms may include signs of central nervous system excitation (eg, restlessness, tremor irritability, convulsions, delirium, hallucinations), flushing, fever, nausea, vomiting, tachycardia, hypotension or hypertension, respiratory failure, paralysis, and coma.
In the event of an overdose or exaggerated response, treatment should be symptomatic and supportive. Maintain respiration and induce emesis or perform gastric lavage (emesis is contraindicated in precomatose, convulsive, or psychotic state). Activated charcoal may be administered as well as a cathartic. Physostigmine may be considered to reverse symptoms of anticholinergic intoxication. Hyperpyrexia may be treated symptomatically with ice bags or other cold applications and alcohol sponges.

DOSAGE AND ADMINISTRATION

Tablets
Adults: The usual dose is one 5-mg tablet two to three times a day. The maximum recommended dose is one 5-mg tablet four times a day.
Pediatric patients over 5 years of age: The usual dose is one 5-mg tablet two times a day. The maximum recommended dose is one 5-mg tablet three times a day.
Syrup
Adults: The usual dose is one teaspoon (5 mg/5 mL) syrup two to three times a day. The maximum recommended dose is one teaspoon (5 mg/5 mL) syrup four times a day.
Pediatric patients over 5 years of age: The usual dose is one teaspoon (5 mg/5 mL) two times a day. The maximum recommended dose is one teaspoon (5 mg/5 mL) three times a day.

HOW SUPPLIED

DITROPAN® (oxybutynin chloride) Tablets are supplied in bottles of 100 tablets (NDC 0088-1375-47) and 1000 tablets (NDC 0088-1375-58) and in Unit Dose Identification Paks of 100 tablets (NDC 0088-1375-49).
Blue scored tablets (5 mg) are engraved with DITROPAN on one side with 13 and 75, separated by a horizontal score, on the other side.
DITROPAN® Syrup (5 mg/5 mL) is supplied in bottles of 16 fluid ounces (473 mL) (NDC 0088-1373-18).
Pharmacist: Dispense in tight, light-resistant container as defined in the USP.
Store at controlled room temperature (59–86°F).
Prescribing Information as of January 1995
Hoechst Marion Roussel, Inc.
Kansas City, MO 64137 USA
Shown in Product Identification Guide, page 317

LASIX® ℞
[la' siks]
(furosemide)
Injection (10 mg/mL)
Oral Solution (10 mg/mL)
Tablets (20, 40, and 80 mg)

WARNING

Lasix® (furosemide) is a potent diuretic which, if given in excessive amounts, can lead to a profound diuresis with water and electrolyte depletion. Therefore, careful medical supervision is required and dose and dose schedule must be adjusted to the individual patient's needs. (See "DOSAGE AND ADMINISTRATION".)

DESCRIPTION

Lasix® is a diuretic which is an anthranilic acid derivative, Lasix® Injection is composed of 4-chloro-N-furfuryl-5-sulfamoylanthranilic acid, sodium chloride for isotonicity and sodium hydroxide to adjust pH.
Lasix® Injection 10 mg/mL is a sterile, non-pyrogenic solution in ampules, disposable syringes and single dose vials for intravenous and intramuscular injection.
Furosemide is a white to off-white odorless crystalline powder. It is practically insoluble in water, sparingly soluble in alcohol, freely soluble in dilute alkali solutions and insoluble in dilute acids.
Lasix® Oral Solution contains furosemide as the active ingredient and the following inactive ingredients: alcohol USP 11.5%, D&C yellow #10, FD&C yellow #6 as color additives, flavors, glycerin USP, parabens NF, purified water USP, sorbitol NF; sodium hydroxide NF added to adjust pH. Chemically, it is 4-chloro-N-furfuryl-5-sulfamoylanthranilic acid. Lasix® Oral Solution 10 mg/mL is an orange flavored liquid for oral administration.
Lasix® tablets for oral administration contain furosemide as the active ingredient and the following inactive ingredients: lactose USP, magnesium stearate NF, starch NF and talc USP. Chemically, it is 4-chloro-N-furfuryl-5-sulfamoylanthranilic acid. Lasix® is available as white tablets for oral administration in dosage strengths of 20, 40 and 80 mg. Furosemide is a white to off-white odorless crystalline powder. It is practically insoluble in water, sparingly soluble in alcohol, freely soluble in dilute alkali solutions and insoluble in dilute acids.
The CAS Registry Number is 54-31-9.
The structural formula is as follows:

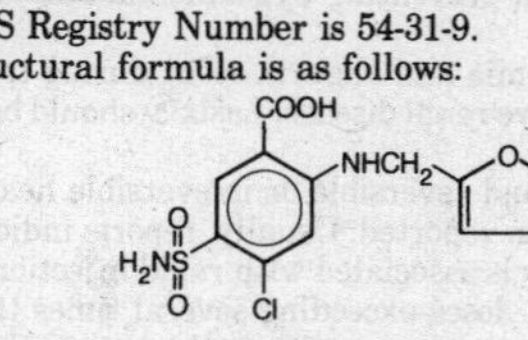

CLINICAL PHARMACOLOGY

Investigations into the mode of action of Lasix® have utilized micropuncture studies in rats, stop flow experiments in dogs and various clearance studies in both humans and experimental animals. It has been demonstrated that Lasix® inhibits primarily the absorption of sodium and chloride not only in the proximal and distal tubules but also in the loop of Henle. The high degree of efficacy is largely due to the unique site of action. The action on the distal tubule is independent of any inhibitory effect on carbonic anhydrase and aldosterone.
Recent evidence suggests that furosemide glucuronide is the only or at least the major biotransformation product of furosemide in man. Furosemide is extensively bound to plasma proteins, mainly to albumin. Plasma concentrations ranging from 1 to 400 μg/mL are 91 to 99% bound in healthy individuals. The unbound fraction averages 2.3 to 4.1% at therapeutic concentrations.
The onset of diuresis following oral administration is within 1 hour. The peak effect occurs within the first or second hour. The duration of diuretic effect is 6 to 8 hours.
In fasted normal men, the mean bioavailability of furosemide from Lasix® Tablets and Lasix® Oral Solution is 64% and 60%, respectively, of that from an intravenous injection of the drug. Although furosemide is more rapidly absorbed from the oral solution (50 minutes) than from the tablet (87 minutes), peak plasma levels and area under the plasma

Continued on next page

Hoechst Marion Roussel—Cont.

concentration-time curves do not differ significantly. Peak plasma concentrations increase with increasing dose but times-to-peak do not differ among doses. The terminal half-life of furosemide is approximately 2 hours.

Significantly more furosemide is excreted in urine following the IV injection than after the tablet or oral solution. There are no significant differences between the two oral formulations in the amount of unchanged drug excreted in urine.

INDICATIONS AND USAGE

Lasix® (furosemide) Injection (10mg/mL)

Parenteral therapy should be reserved for patients unable to take oral medication or for patients in emergency clinical situations.

Edema

Lasix® is indicated in adults, infants, and children for the treatment of edema associated with congestive heart failure, cirrhosis of the liver, and renal disease, including the nephrotic syndrome. Lasix® is particularly useful when an agent with greater diuretic potential is desired.

Lasix® is indicated as adjunctive therapy in acute pulmonary edema. The intravenous administration of Lasix® is indicated when a rapid onset of diuresis is desired, eg, in acute pulmonary edema.

If gastrointestinal absorption is impaired or oral medication is not practical for any reason, Lasix® (furosemide) is indicated by the intravenous or intramuscular route. Parenteral use should be replaced with oral Lasix® as soon as practical.

Lasix® (furosemide) Oral Solution (10 mg/mL)

Lasix® (furosemide) tablets

Edema

Lasix® is indicated in adults and pediatric patients for the treatment of edema associated with congestive heart failure, cirrhosis of the liver, and renal disease, including the nephrotic syndrome. Lasix® is particularly useful when an agent with greater diuretic potential is desired.

Hypertension

Oral Lasix® may be used in adults for the treatment of hypertension alone or in combination with other antihypertensive agents. Hypertensive patients who cannot be adequately controlled with thiazides will probably also not be adequately controlled with Lasix® alone.

CONTRAINDICATIONS

Lasix® is contraindicated in patients with anuria and in patients with a history of hypersensitivity to furosemide.

WARNINGS

In patients with hepatic cirrhosis and ascites, Lasix® therapy is best initiated in the hospital. In hepatic coma and in states of electrolyte depletion, therapy should not be instituted until the basic condition is improved. Sudden alterations of fluid and electrolyte balance in patients with cirrhosis may precipitate hepatic coma; therefore, strict observation is necessary during the period of diuresis. Supplemental potassium chloride and, if required, an aldosterone antagonist are helpful in preventing hypokalemia and metabolic alkalosis.

If increasing azotemia and oliguria occur during treatment of severe progressive renal disease, Lasix® should be discontinued.

Cases of tinnitus and reversible or irreversible hearing impairment have been reported. Usually, reports indicate that Lasix® ototoxicity is associated with rapid injection, severe renal impairment, doses exceeding several times the usual recommended dose, or concomitant therapy with aminoglycoside antibiotics, ethacrynic acid, or other ototoxic drugs. If the physician elects to use high dose parenteral therapy, controlled intravenous infusion is advisable (for adults, an infusion rate not exceeding 4 mg Lasix® per minute has been used).

Lasix® (furosemide) Injection (10mg/mL)

Pediatric Use

In premature neonates with respiratory distress syndrome, diuretic treatment with furosemide in the first few weeks of life may increase the risk of persistent patent ductus arteriosus (PDA), possibly through a prostaglandin-E-mediated process.

Hearing loss in neonates has been associated with the use of furosemide injection (see WARNINGS, above).

PRECAUTIONS

General

Excessive diuresis may cause dehydration and blood volume reduction with circulatory collapse and possibly vascular thrombosis and embolism, particularly in elderly patients. As with any effective diuretic, electrolyte depletion may occur during Lasix® therapy, especially in patients receiving higher doses and a restricted salt intake. Hypokalemia may develop with Lasix®, especially with brisk diuresis, inadequate oral electrolyte intake, when cirrhosis is present, or during concomitant use of corticosteroids or ACTH. Digitalis therapy may exaggerate metabolic effects of hypokalemia, especially myocardial effects.

All patients receiving Lasix® therapy should be observed for these signs or symptoms of fluid or electrolyte imbalance (hyponatremia, hypochloremic alkalosis, hypokalemia, hypomagnesemia or hypocalcemia): dryness of mouth, thirst, weakness, lethargy, drowsiness, restlessness, muscle pains or cramps, muscular fatigue, hypotension, oliguria, tachycardia, arrhythmia, or gastrointestinal disturbances such as nausea and vomiting. Increases in blood glucose and alterations in glucose tolerance tests (with abnormalities of the fasting and 2-hour postprandial surgar) have been observed, and rarely, precipitation of diabetes mellitus has been reported. Asymptomatic hyperuricemia can occur and gout may rarely be precipitated.

The sorbitol present in the vehicle may cause diarrhea (especially in children) when higher doses of Lasix® (furosemide) Oral Solution are given.

Patients allergic to sulfonamides may also be allergic to Lasix®. The possibility exists of exacerbation or activation of systemic lupus erythematosus.

As with many other drugs, patients should be observed regularly for the possible occurrence of blood dyscrasias, liver or kidney damage, or other idiosyncratic reactions.

Information for Patients

Patients receiving Lasix® should be advised that they may experience symptoms from excessive fluid and/or electrolyte losses. The postural hypotension that sometimes occurs can usually be managed by getting up slowly. Potassium supplements and/or dietary measures may be needed to control or avoid hypokalemia.

Patients with diabetes mellitus should be told that furosemide may increase blood glucose levels and thereby affect urine glucose tests. The skin of some patients may be more sensitive to the effects of sunlight while taking furosemide.

Hypertensive patients should avoid medications that may increase blood pressure, including over-the-counter products for appetite suppression and cold symptoms.

Laboratory Tests

Serum electrolytes (particularly potassium), CO_2 creatinine and BUN should be determined frequently during the first few months of Lasix® therapy and periodically thereafter. Serum and urine electrolyte determinations are particularly important when the patient is vomiting profusely or receiving parenteral fluids. Abnormalities should be corrected or the drug temporarily withdrawn. Other medications may also influence serum electrolytes.

Reversible elevations of BUN may occur and are associated with dehydration, which should be avoided, particularly in patients with renal insufficiency.

Urine and blood glucose should be checked periodically in diabetics receiving Lasix®, even in those suspected of latent diabetes.

Lasix® may lower serum levels of calcium (rarely cases of tetany have been reported) and magnesium. Accordingly, serum levels of these electrolytes should be determined periodically.

Drug Interactions

Lasix® may increase the ototoxic potential of aminoglycoside antibiotics, especially in the presence of impaired renal function. Except in life-threatening situations, avoid this combination.

Lasix® should not be used concomitantly with ethacrynic acid because of the possibility of ototoxicity. Patients receiving high doses of salicylates concomitantly with Lasix®, as in rheumatic disease, may experience salicylate toxicity at lower doses because of competitive renal excretory sites.

Lasix® has a tendency to antagonize the skeletal muscle relaxing effect of tubocurarine and may potentiate the action of succinylcholine.

Lithium generally should not be given with diuretics because they reduce lithium's renal clearance and add a high risk of lithium toxicity.

Lasix® (furosemide) may add to or potentiate the therapeutic effect of other antihypertensive drugs. Potentiation occurs with ganglionic or peripheral adrenergic blocking drugs.

Lasix® may decrease arterial responsiveness to norepinephrine. However, norepinephrine may still be used effectively.

One study in six subjects demonstrated that the combination of furosemide and acetylsalicylic acid temporarily reduced creatinine clearance in patients with chronic renal insufficiency. There are case reports of patients who developed increased BUN, serum creatinine and serum potassium levels, and weight gain when furosemide was used in conjunction with NSAIDs.

Literature reports indicate that coadministration of indomethacin may reduce the natriuretic and antihypertensive effects of Lasix® in some patients by inhibiting prostaglandin synthesis. Indomethacin may also affect plasma renin levels, aldosterone excretion, and renin profile evaluation. Patients receiving both indomethacin and Lasix® should be observed closely to determine if the desired diuretic and/or antihypertensive effect of Lasix® is achieved.

Carcinogenesis, Mutagenesis, Impairment of Fertility

Furosemide was tested for carcinogenicity by oral administration in one strain of mice and one strain of rats. A small but significantly increased incidence of mammary gland carcinomas occurred in female mice at a dose 17.5 times the maximum human dose of 600 mg. There were marginal increases in uncommon tumors in male rats at a dose of 15 mg/kg (slightly greater than the maximum human dose) but not at 30 mg/kg.

Furosemide was devoid of mutagenic activity in various strains of *Salmonella typhimurium* when tested in the presence or absence of an *in vitro* metabolic activation system, and questionably positive for gene mutation in mouse lymphoma cells in the presence of rat liver S9 at the highest dose tested. Furosemide did not induce sister chromatid exchange in human cells *in vitro*, but other studies on chromosomal aberrations in human cells *in vitro* gave conflicting results. In Chinese hamster cells it induced chromosomal damage but was questionably positive for sister chromatid exchange. Studies on the induction by furosemide of chromosomal aberrations in mice were inconclusive. The urine of rats treated with this drug did not induce gene conversion in *Saccharomyces cerevisiae*.

Lasix® produced no impairment of fertility in male or female rats, at 100 mg/kg/day (8 times the maximal human dose of 600 mg/day).

Pregnancy

PREGNANCY CATEGORY C—Furosemide has been shown to cause unexplained maternal deaths and abortions in rabbits at 2, 4, and 8 times the maximal recommended human oral dose. There are no adequate and well-controlled studies in pregnant women. Lasix® should be used during pregnancy only if the potential benefit justifies the potential risk to the fetus.

The effects of furosemide on embryonic and fetal development and on pregnant dams were studied in mice, rats and rabbits.

Furosemide caused unexplained maternal deaths and abortions in the rabbit at the lowest dose of 25 mg/kg (2 times the maximal recommended human oral dose of 600 mg/day). In another study, a dose of 50 mg/kg (4 times the maximal recommended human oral dose of 600 mg/day) also caused maternal deaths and abortions when administered to rabbits between Days 12 and 17 of gestation. In a third study, none of the pregnant rabbits survived an oral dose of 100 mg/kg. Data from the above studies indicate fetal lethality that can precede maternal deaths.

The results of the mouse study and one of the three rabbit studies also showed an increased incidence and severity of hydronephrosis (distention of the renal pelvis and, in some cases, of the ureters) in fetuses derived from treated dams as compared with the incidence in fetuses from the control group.

Nursing Mothers

Because it appears in breast milk, caution should be exercised when Lasix® (furosemide) is administered to a nursing mother.

Pediatric Use

Renal calcifications (from barely visible on x-ray to staghorn) have occurred in some severely premature infants treated with intravenous Lasix® for edema due to patent ductus arteriosus and hyaline membrane disease. The concurrent use of chlorothiazide has been reported to decrease hypercalciuria and dissolve some calculi.

ADVERSE REACTIONS

Adverse reactions are categorized below by organ system and listed by decreasing severity.

Gastrointestinal System Reactions

1. pancreatitis	5. cramping
2. jaundice (intrahepatic cholestatic jaundice)	6. diarrhea
3. anorexia	7. constipation
4. oral and gastric irritation	8. nausea
	9. vomiting

Systemic Hypersensitivity Reactions

1. systemic vasculitis
2. interstitial nephritis
3. necrotizing angiitis

Central Nervous System Reactions

1. tinnitus and hearing loss	4. dizziness
	5. headache
2. paresthesias	6. blurred vision
3. vertigo	7. xanthopsia

Hematologic Reactions

1. aplastic anemia (rare)	4. hemolytic anemia
2. thrombocytopenia	5. leukopenia
3. agranulocytosis (rare)	6. anemia

Dermatologic-Hypersensitivity Reactions

1. exfoliative dermatitis	5. urticaria
2. erythema multiforme	6. rash
3. purpura	7. pruritus
4. photosensitivity	

Cardiovascular Reaction

Orthostatic hypotension may occur and be aggravated by alcohol, barbiturates or narcotics.

Other Reactions

1. hyperglycemia	6. restlessness
2. glycosuria	7. urinary bladder spasm
3. hyperuricemia	8. thrombophlebitis
4. muscle spasm	9. fever
5. weakness	

Whenever adverse reactions are moderate or severe, Lasix® dosage should be reduced or therapy withdrawn.

OVERDOSAGE

The principal signs and symptoms of overdose with Lasix® are dehydration, blood volume reduction, hypotension, electrolyte imbalance, hypokalemia and hypochloremic alkalosis, and are extensions of its diuretic action.
The acute toxicity of Lasix® has been determined in mice, rats and dogs. In all three, the oral LD_{50} exceeded 1000 mg/kg body weight, while the intravenous LD_{50} ranged from 300 to 680 mg/kg. The acute intragastric toxicity in neonatal rats is 7 to 10 times that of adult rats.
The concentration of Lasix® in biological fluids associated with toxicity or death is not known.
Treatment of overdosage is supportive and consists of replacement of excessive fluid and electrolyte losses. Serum electrolytes, carbon dioxide level and blood pressure should be determined frequently. Adequate drainage must be assured in patients with urinary bladder outlet obstruction (such as prostatic hypertrophy).
Hemodialysis does not accelerate furosemide elimination.

DOSAGE AND ADMINISTRATION

Adults – Parenteral therapy with Lasix® Injection should be used only in patients unable to take oral medication or in emergency situations and should be replaced with oral therapy as soon as practical.
Edema
The usual initial dose of Lasix® is 20 to 40 mg given as a single dose, injected intramuscularly or intravenously. The intravenous dose should be given slowly (1 to 2 minutes). Ordinarily a prompt diuresis ensues. If needed, another dose may be administered in the same manner 2 hours later or the dose may be increased. The dose may be raised by 20 mg and given not sooner than 2 hours after the previous dose until the desired diuretic effect has been obtained. This individually determined single dose should then be given once or twice daily.
Therapy should be individualized according to patient response to gain maximal therapeutic response and to determine the minimal dose needed to maintain that response. Close medical supervision is necessary.
If the physician elects to use high dose parenteral therapy, add the Lasix® (furosemide) to either Sodium Chloride Injection USP, Lactated Ringer's Injection USP, or Dextrose (5%) Injection USP after pH has been adjusted to above 5.5, and administer as a controlled intravenous infusion at a rate not greater than 4 mg/min. Lasix® Injection is a buffered alkaline solution with a pH of about 9 and the drug may precipitate at pH values below 7. Care must be taken to ensure that the pH of the prepared infusion solution is in the weakly alkaline to neutral range. Acid solutions, including other parenteral medications (e.g., labetalol, ciprofloxacin, amrinone, and milrinone) must not be administered concurrently in the same infusion because they may cause precipitation of the furosemide. In addition, furosemide injection should not be added to a running intravenous line containing any of these acidic products.
Acute Pulmonary Edema
The usual initial dose of Lasix® is 40 mg injected slowly intravenously (over 1 to 2 minutes). If a satisfactory response does not occur within 1 hour, the dose may be increased to 80 mg injected slowly intravenously (over 1 to 2 minutes).
If necessary, additional therapy (eg, digitalis, oxygen) may be administered concomitantly.

Infants and Children – Parenteral therapy should be used only in patients unable to take oral medication or in emergency situations and should be replaced with oral therapy as soon as practical.
The usual initial dose of Lasix® Injection (intravenously or intramuscularly) in infants and children is 1 mg/kg body weight and should be given slowly under close medical supervision. If the diuretic response to the initial dose is not satisfactory, dosage may be increased by 1 mg/kg not sooner than 2 hours after the previous dose, until the desired diuretic effect has been obtained. Doses greater than 6 mg/kg body weight are not recommended.
Lasix® (furosemide) Injection should be inspected visually for particulate matter and discoloration before administration. Do not use if solution is discolored.
Lasix® (furosemide) Oral Solution (10 mg/mL)
Lasix® (furosemide) tablets
Edema
Therapy should be individualized according to patient response to gain maximal therapeutic response and to determine the minimal dose needed to maintain that response.

Adults – The usual initial dose of Lasix® is 20 to 80 mg given as a single dose. Ordinarily a prompt diuresis ensues. If needed, the same dose can be administered 6 to 8 hours later or the dose may be increased. The dose may be raised by 20 or 40 mg and given not sooner than 6 to 8 hours after the previous dose until the desired diuretic effect has been obtained. The individually determined single dose should then be given once or twice daily (eg. at 8 am and 2 pm). The dose of Lasix® may be carefully titrated up to 600 mg/day in patients with clinically severe edematous states.
Edema may be most efficiently and safely mobilized by giving Lasix® on 2 to 4 consecutive days each week.
When doses exceeding 80 mg/day are given for prolonged periods, careful clinical observation and laboratory monitoring are particularly advisable. (See **PRECAUTIONS: Laboratory Tests.**)
Pediatric patients – The usual initial dose of oral Lasix® in pediatric patients is 2 mg/kg body weight, given as a single dose. If the diuretic response is not satisfactory after the initial dose, dosage may be increased by 1 or 2 mg/kg no sooner than 6 to 8 hours after the previous dose. Doses greater than 6 mg/kg body weight are not recommended. For maintenance therapy in pediatric patients, the dose should be adjusted to the minimum effective level.
Hypertension
Therapy should be individualized according to the patient's response to gain maximal therapeutic response and to determine the minimal dose needed to maintain the therapeutic response.
Adults – The usual initial dose of Lasix® for hypertension is 80 mg, usually divided into 40 mg twice a day. Dosage should then be adjusted according to response. If response is not satisfactory add other antihypertensive agents.
Changes in blood pressure must be carefully monitored when Lasix® is used with other antihypertensive drugs, especially during initial therapy. To prevent excessive drop in blood pressure, the dosage of other agents should be reduced by at least 50 percent when Lasix® is added to the regimen. As the blood pressure falls under the potentiating effect of Lasix®, a further reduction in dosage or even discontinuation of other antihypertensive drugs may be necessary.

HOW SUPPLIED

Lasix® Injection, brand of furosemide, (10 mg/mL), is supplied as a sterile solution in 2 mL, 4 mL, and 10 mL amber ampules, single use vials, and in syringes.
Ampules:
2 mL 5's (NDC 0039-0061-15); 50's (NDC 0039-0061-05)
4 mL 5's (NDC 0039-0061-45); 25's (NDC 0039-0061-65)
10 mL 5's (NDC 0039-0061-08); 25's (NDC 0039-0061-25)
Syringes:
2 mL 5's (NDC 0039-0062-08); 4 mL 5's (NDC 0039-0064-08), and 10 mL 5's (NDC 0039-0065-08)
Single Use Vials:
2 mL 25's (NDC 0039-0162-25); 4 mL 25's (NDC 0039-0163-25), and 10 mL 25's (NDC 0039-0164-25)
Syringes supplied with 22 gauge x $1^1/_4$" needle.
To insure patient safety, this needle should be handled with care and should be destroyed and discarded if damaged in any manner. If cannula is bent, no attempt should be made to straighten.
To prevent needle-stick injuries, needles should not be recapped, purposely bent, or broken by hand.
Store at controlled room temperature (59 to 86° F).
Do not use if solution is discolored.
Protect syringes from light. Do not remove syringe from individual package until time of use.
Lasix® Oral Solution 10 mg/mL is supplied as orange-flavored liquid in bottles of 60 mL (NDC 0039-0063-06) and 120 mL (NDC 0039-0063-40). Each bottle size is accompanied by a graduated dropper.
Note: Store at controlled room temperature (59 to 86° F). Dispense in light-resistant containers. Discard opened bottle after 60 days.
Lasix® Tablets 20 mg are supplied as white, oval, monogrammed tablets in Bottles of 100 (NDC 0039-0067-10), 500 (NDC 0039-0067-50), 1000 (NDC 0039-0067-70), and in Unit Dose Packs of 100 (NDC 0039-0067-11). The 20 mg tablets are imprinted with "Lasix®" on one side and "HOECHST" on the other.
Lasix® Tablets 40 mg are supplied as white, round, monogrammed, scored tablets in Bottles of 100 (NDC 0039-0060-13), 500 (NDC 0039-0060-50), 1000 (NDC 0039-0060-70), and Unit Dose Packs of 100 (NDC 0039-0060-11). The 40 mg tablets are imprinted with "Lasix® 40" on one side and the Hoechst logo on the other.
Lasix® Tablets 80 mg are supplied as white, round, monogrammed, facetted edge tablets in Bottles of 50 (NDC 0039-0066-05), 500 (NDC 0039-0066-50), and in Unit Dose Packs of 100 (NDC 0039-0066-11). The 80 mg tablets are imprinted with "Lasix® 80" on one side and the Hoechst logo on the other.
Note: Dispense in well-closed, light-resistant containers. Exposure to light might cause a slight discoloration. Discolored tablets should not be dispensed.
Tested by USP Dissolution Test 2
Manufactured for:
Hoechst-Roussel Pharmaceuticals
Division of Hoechst Marion Roussel, Inc.
Kansas City, MO 64137
763000–10/94
705060–11/94

Shown in Product Identification Guide, page 317

LOPROX® ℞

[*lō'prŏks*]
(ciclopirox olamine)
Cream 1% & Lotion 1%

FOR DERMATOLOGIC USE ONLY. NOT FOR USE IN EYES.

DESCRIPTION

Loprox® (ciclopirox olamine) Cream 1% is for topical use.
Each gram of Loprox® Cream 1% contains 10 mg ciclopirox olamine in a water miscible vanishing cream base consisting of purified water USP, octyldodecanol NF, mineral oil USP, stearyl alcohol NF, cetyl alcohol NF, cocamide DEA, polysorbate 60 NF, myristyle alcohol NF, sorbitan monostearate NF, lactic acid USP, and benzyl alcohol NF (1%) as preservative.
Loprox® Cream 1% contains a synthetic, broad-spectrum, antifungal agent ciclopirox olamine. The chemical name is 6-cyclohexyl-1-hydroxy-4-methyl-2(1*H*)-pyridone, 2-aminoethanol salt.
Loprox® (ciclopirox olamine) Lotion 1% is for topical use.
Each gram of Loprox® Lotion 1% contains 10 mg of ciclopirox olamine in a water miscible lotion base consisting of purified water USP, cocamide DEA, octyldodecanol NF, mineral oil USP, stearyl alcohol NF, cetyl alcohol NF, polysorbate 60 NF, myristyl alcohol NF, sorbitan monostearate NF, lactic acid USP, and benzyl alcohol NF (1%) as preservative.
Loprox® Lotion contains a synthetic, broad-spectrum, antifungal agent ciclopirox olamine. The chemical name is 6-cyclohexyl-1-hydroxy-4-methyl-2(1*H*)-pyridone, 2-aminoethanol salt.
The CAS Registry Number is 41621-49-2.
The chemical structure is:

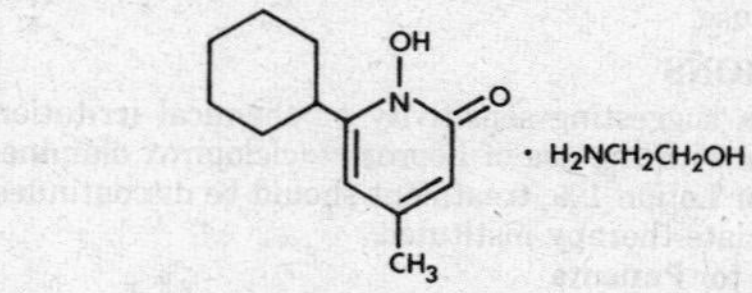

Loprox® (ciclopirox olamine) Cream 1% and Lotion 1% have a pH of 7.

CLINICAL PHARMACOLOGY

Loprox (ciclopirox olamine) Cream 1%
Ciclopirox olamine is a broad-spectrum, antifungal agent that inhibits the growth of pathogenic dermatophytes, yeasts, and *Malassezia furfur*. Ciclopirox olamine exhibits fungicidal activity *in vitro* against isolates of *Trichophyton rubrum, Trichophyton mentagrophytes, Epidermophyton floccosum, Microsporum canis,* and *Candida albicans.*
Pharmacokinetic studies in men with tagged 1% ciclopirox olamine solution in polyethylene glycol 400 showed an average of 1.3% absorption of the dose when it was applied topically to 750 cm^2 on the back followed by occlusion for 6 hours. The biological half-life was 1.7 hours and excretion occurred via the kidney. Two days after application only 0.01% of the dose applied could be found in the urine. Fecal excretion was negligible.
Penetration studies in human cadaverous skin from the back, with Loprox® (ciclopirox olamine) Cream 1% with tagged ciclopirox olamine showed the presence of 0.8 to 1.6% of the dose in the stratum corneum 1.5 to 6 hours after application. The levels in the dermis were still 10 to 15 times above the minimum inhibitory concentrations. Autoradiographic studies with human cadaverous skin showed that ciclopirox olamine penetrates into the hair and through the epidermis and hair follicles into the sebaceous glands and dermis, while a portion of the drug remains in the stratum corneum.
Draize Human Sensitization Assay, 21-Day Cumulative Irritancy study, Phototoxicity study, and Photo-Draize study conducted in a total of 142 healthy male subjects showed no contact sensitization of the delayed hypersensitivity type, no irritation, no phototoxicity, and no photo-contact sensitization due to Loprox® Cream 1%.
Loprox (ciclopirox olamine) Lotion 1%
Ciclopirox olamine is a broad-spectrum, antifungal agent that inhibits the growth of pathogenic dermatophytes, yeasts, and *Malassezia furfur*. Ciclopirox olamine exhibits fungicidal activity *in vitro* against isolates of *Trichophyton rubrum, Trichophyton mentagrophytes, Epidermophyton floccosum, Microsporum canis,* and *Candida albicans.*
Pharmacokinetic studies in men with radiolabeled 1% ciclopirox olamine solution in polyethylene glycol 400 showed an average of 1.3% absorption of the dose when it was applied topically to 750 cm^2 on the back followed by occlusion for 6 hours. The biological half-life was 1.7 hours and excretion occurred via the kidney. Two days after application, only 0.01% of the dose applied could be found in the urine. Fecal excretion was negligible. Autoradiographic studies with human cadaver skin showed that ciclopirox olamine

Continued on next page

Hoechst Marion Roussel—Cont.

penetrates into the hair and through the epidermis and hair follicles into the sebaceous glands and dermis, while a portion of the drug remains in the stratum corneum.

In vitro penetration studies in frozen or fresh excised human cadaver and pig skin indicated that the penetration of Loprox® (ciclopirox olamine) Lotion 1% is equivalent to that of Loprox® Cream 1%. Therapeutic equivalence of cream and lotion formulations also was indicated by studies of experimentally induced guinea pig and human trichophytosis.

INDICATIONS AND USAGE

Loprox® Cream 1% is indicated for the topical treatment of the following dermal infections: tinea pedis, tinea cruris and tinea corporis due to *Trichophyton rubrum, Trichophyton mentagrophytes, Epidermophyton floccosum,* and *Microsporum canis; candidiasis* (moniliasis) due to *Candida albicans*; and tinea (pityriasis) versicolor due to *Malassezia furfur.*
Loprox® (ciclopirox olamine) Lotion 1% is indicated for the topical treatment of the following dermal infections: tinea pedis, tinea cruris and tinea corporis due to *Trichophyton rubrum, Trichophyton mentagrophytes, Epidermophyton floccosum,* and *Microsporum canis*; cutaneous candidiasis (moniliasis) due to *Candida albicans*; and tinea (pityriasis) versicolor due to *Malassezia furfur.*

CONTRAINDICATIONS

Loprox® Lotion 1% is contraindicated in individuals who have shown hypersensitivity to any of its components.

WARNINGS

General: Loprox® Cream 1% and Lotion 1% are not for ophthalmic use.

PRECAUTIONS

If a reaction suggesting sensitivity or chemical irritation should occur with the use of Loprox® (ciclopirox olamine) Cream 1% or Lotion 1%, treatment should be discontinued and appropriate therapy instituted.

Information for Patients
The patient should be told to:
1. Use the medication for the full treatment time even though symptoms may have improved and notify the physician if there is no improvement after four weeks.
2. Inform the physician if the area of application shows signs of increased irritation (redness, itching, burning, blistering, swelling, oozing) indicative of possible sensitization.
3. Avoid the use of occlusive wrappings or dressings.

Carcinogenesis, Mutagenesis, Impairment of Fertility
A carcinogenicity study in female mice dosed cutaneously twice per week for 50 weeks followed by a 6-month drug-free observation period prior to necropsy revealed no evidence of tumors at the application site.
The following *in vitro* and *in vivo* genotoxicity tests have been conducted with ciclopirox olamine: studies to evaluate gene mutation in the Ames *Salmonella*/Mammalian Microsome Assay (negative) and Yeast Saccharomyces Cerevisiae Assay (negative) and studies to evaluate chromosome aberrations *in vivo* in the Mouse Dominant Lethal Assay and in the Mouse Micronucleus Assay at 500 mg/kg (negative).
The following battery of *in vitro* genotoxicity tests were conducted with *ciclopirox*: a chromosome aberration assay in V79 Chinese Hamster Cells, with and without metabolic activation (positive); a gene mutation assay in the HGPRT-test with V79 Chinese Hamster Cells (negative); and a primary DNA damage assay (i.e., unscheduled DNA Synthesis Assay in A549 Human Cells (negative)). An *in vitro* Cell Transformation Assay in BALB/C 3T3 Cells was negative for cell transformation. In an *in vivo* Chinese Hamster Bone Marrow Cytogenetic Assay, ciclopirox was negative for chromosome aberrations at 5000 mg/kg.

Pregnancy Category B
Reproduction studies have been performed in the mouse, rat, rabbit, and monkey, (via various routes of administration) at doses 10 times or more the topical human dose and have revealed no significant evidence of impaired fertility or harm to the fetus due to ciclopirox olamine. There are, however, no adequate or well-controlled studies in pregnant women. Because animal reproduction studies are not alwas predictive of human response this drug should be used during pregnancy only if clearly needed.

Nursing Mothers
It is not known whether this drug is excreted in human milk. Because many drugs are excreted in human milk, caution should be exercised when Loprox® (ciclopirox olamine) Cream 1% is administered to a nursing woman.

Pediatric Use
Safety and effectiveness in pediatric patients below the age of 10 years have not been established.

ADVERSE REACTIONS

In all controlled clinical studies with 514 patients using Loprox® Cream 1% and in 296 patients using the vehicle cream, the incidence of adverse reactions was low. This included pruritus at the site of application in one patient and

worsening of the clinical signs and symptoms in another patient using ciclopirox olamine cream 1% and burning in one patient and worsening of the clinical signs and symptoms in another patient using the vehicle cream.
In the controlled clinical trial with 89 patients using Loprox® Lotion 1% and 89 patients using the vehicle, the incidence of adverse reactions was low. Those considered possibly related to treatment or occurring in more than one patient were pruritus, which occurred in two patients using ciclopirox olamine lotion 1% and one patient using the lotion vehicle, and burning, which occurred in one patient using ciclopirox olamine lotion 1%.

DOSAGE AND ADMINISTRATION

Gently massage Loprox® Cream 1% into the affected and surrounding skin areas twice daily, in the morning and evening. Clinical improvement with relief of pruritus and other symptoms usually occurs within the first week of treatment. If a patient shows no clinical improvement after four weeks of treatment with Loprox® Cream 1%, the diagnosis should be redetermined. Patients with tinea versicolor usually exhibit clinical and mycological clearing after two weeks of treatment.
Gently massage Loprox® (ciclopirox olamine) Lotion 1% into the affected and surrounding skin areas twice daily, in the morning and evening. Clinical improvement with relief of pruritus and other symptoms usually occurs within the first week of treatment. If a patient shows no clinical improvement after four weeks of treatment with Loprox® Lotion 1% the diagnosis should be redetermined. Patients with tinea versicolor usually exhibit clinical and mycological clearing after two weeks of treatment.

HOW SUPPLIED

Loprox® Cream 1% is supplied in 15 gram (NDC 0039-0009-15), 30 gram (NDC 0039-0009-30), and 90 gram (NDC 0039-0009-90) tubes.
Store between 59 and 86° F.
Caution: Federal law prohibits dispensing without prescription.
Loprox® Lotion 1% is supplied in 30 mL bottles (NDC 0039-0008-30) and 60 mL bottles (NDC 0039-0008-06).
Bottle space provided to allow for vigorous shaking before each use.
Store between 41 and 77° F (5 and 25° C).
Caution: Federal law prohibits dispensing without prescription.
Loprox REG TM HOECHST AG
Hoechst-Roussel Pharmaceuticals
Division of Hoechst Marion Roussel, Inc.
Kansas City, MO 64137
Shown in Product Identification Guide, page 317

NITRO-BID® IV   ℞
[ni 'tro-bid]
Prescribing Information as of April 1995
(nitroglycerin injection USP)

FOR INTRAVENOUS USE ONLY. NOT FOR DIRECT INTRAVENOUS INJECTION. NITRO-BID® MUST BE DILUTED IN DEXTROSE (5%) INJECTION USP OR SODIUM CHLORIDE (0.9%) INJECTION USP PRIOR TO ITS INFUSION (SEE DOSAGE AND ADMINISTRATION SECTION). THE ADMINISTRATION SET USED FOR INFUSION WILL AFFECT THE AMOUNT OF NITRO-BID IV DELIVERED TO THE PATIENT. (SEE WARNINGS AND DOSAGE AND ADMINISTRATION SECTIONS.)

CAUTION

SEVERAL PREPARATIONS OF NITROGLYCERIN FOR INJECTION ARE AVAILABLE. THEY DIFFER IN CONCENTRATION AND/OR VOLUME PER VIAL. WHEN SWITCHING FROM ONE PRODUCT TO ANOTHER ATTENTION MUST BE PAID TO THE DILUTION AND DOSAGE AND ADMINISTRATION INSTRUCTIONS.

DESCRIPTION

Nitroglycerin is 1,2,3-propanetriol trinitrate, an organic nitrate whose structural formula is:

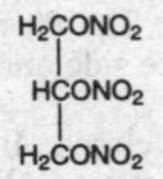

$$H_2CONO_2$$
$$HCONO_2$$
$$H_2CONO_2$$

Whose molecular formula is $C_3H_5N_3O_9$, and whose molecular weight is 227.09. The organic nitrates are vasodilators, active on both arteries and veins.
NITRO-BID IV (nitroglycerin injection USP) is a clear, practically colorless additive solution or intravenous infusion after dilution. Each milliliter contains 5 mg nitroglycerin and 45 mg propylene glycol dissolved in 70% ethanol.
The solution is sterile, nonpyrogenic, and nonexplosive.

CLINICAL PHARMACOLOGY

The principal pharmacological action of NITRO-BID IV (nitroglycerin) is relaxation of vascular smooth muscle and consequent dilatation of peripheral arteries and veins, especially the latter. Dilatation of the veins promotes peripheral pooling of blood and decreases venous return to the heart, thereby reducing left ventricular end diastolic pressure and pulmonary capillary wedge pressure (preload). Arteriolar relaxation reduces systemic vascular resistance, systolic arterial pressure, and mean arterial pressure (after-load). Dilatation of the coronary arteries also occurs. The relative importance of preload reduction, afterload reduction, and coronary dilatation remains undefined.
Dosing regimens for most chronically used drugs are designed to provide plasma concentrations that are continuously greater than a minimally effective concentration. This strategy is inappropriate for organic nitrates. Several well-controlled clinical trials have used exercise testing to assess the antianginal efficacy of continuously delivered nitrates. In the large majority of these trials, active agents were indistinguishable from placebo after 24 hours (or less) of continuous therapy. Attempts to overcome nitrate tolerance by dose escalation, even to doses far in excess of those used acutely, have consistently failed. Only after nitrates have been absent from the body for several hours has their antianginal efficacy been restored.

Pharmacokinetics
The volume of distribution of nitroglycerin is about 3 L/kg, and nitroglycerin is cleared from this volume at extremely rapid rates, with a resulting serum half-life of about 3 minutes. The observed clearance rates (close to 1 L/kg/min) greatly exceed hepatic blood flow; known sites of extrahepatic metabolism include red blood cells and vascular walls. The first products in the metabolism of nitroglycerin are inorganic nitrate and the 1,2- and 1,3-dinitroglycerols. The dinitrates are less effective vasodilators than nitroglycerin, but they are longer lived in the serum, and their net contribution to the overall effect of chronic nitroglycerin regimens is not known. The dinitrates are further metabolized to (nonvasoactive) mononitrates and, ultimately, to glycerol and carbon dioxide.
To avoid development of tolerance to nitroglycerin, drug-free intervals of 10 to 12 hours are known to be sufficient; shorter intervals have not been well studied. In one well-controlled clinical trial, subjects receiving nitroglycerin appeared to exhibit a rebound or withdrawal effect, so that their exercise tolerance at the end of the daily drug-free interval was *less* than that exhibited by the parallel group receiving placebo.

Clinical Trials
Blinded, placebo-controlled trials of intravenous nitroglycerin have not been reported, but multiple investigators have reported open-label studies, and there are scattered reports of studies in which intravenous nitroglycerin was tested in blinded fashion against sodium nitroprusside.
In each of these studies, therapeutic doses of intravenous nitroglycerin were found to reduce systolic and diastolic arterial blood pressure. The heart rate was usually increased, presumably as a reflexive response to the fall in blood pressure. Coronary perfusion pressure was usually, but not always, maintained.
Intravenous nitroglycerin reduced central venous pressure (CVP), right atrial pressure (RAP), pulmonary arterial pressure (PAP), pulmonary capillary wedge pressure (PCWP), pulmonary vascular resistance (PVR), and systemic vascular resistance (SVR). When these parameters were elevated, reducing them toward normal usually caused a rise in cardiac output. Conversely, intravenous nitroglycerin usually *reduced* cardiac output when it was given to patients whose CVP, RAP, PAP, PCWP, PVR, and SVR were all normal. Most clinical trials of intravenous nitroglycerin have been brief; they have typically followed hemodynamic parameters during a single surgical procedure. In one careful study, one of the few that lasted more than a few hours, continuous intravenous nitroglycerin had lost almost all of its hemodynamic effect after 48 hours. In the same study, patients who received nitroglycerin infusions for only 12 hours out of each 24 demonstrated no similar attenuation of effect. These results are consistent with those seen in multiple large, double-blind, placebo-controlled trials of other formulations of nitroglycerin and other nitrates.

INDICATIONS AND USAGE

NITRO-BID IV (nitroglycerin) is indicated for treatment of perioperative hypertension, for control of congestive heart failure in the setting of acute myocardial infarction, for treatment of angina pectoris in patients who have not responded to sublingual nitroglycerin and beta-blockers, and for induction of intraoperative hypotension.

CONTRAINDICATIONS

Allergic reactions to organic nitrates are extremely rare, but they do occur. NITRO-BID IV is contraindicated in patients who are allergic to it.
In patients with pericardial tamponade, restrictive cardiomyopathy, or constrictive pericarditis, cardiac output is

dependent upon venous return. Intravenous nitroglycerin is contraindicated in patients with these conditions.

WARNINGS

Nitroglycerin readily migrates into many plastics, including the polyvinyl chloride (PVC) plastics commonly used for intravenous administration sets. Nitroglycerin absorption by PVC tubing is increased when the tubing is long, the flow rates are low, and the nitroglycerin concentration of the solution is high. The delivered fraction of the solution's original nitroglycerin content has been 20% to 60% in published studies using PVC tubing; the fraction varies with time during a single infusion, and no simple correction factor can be used. PVC tubing has been used in most published studies of intravenous nitroglycerin, but the reported doses have been calculated by simply multiplying the flow rate of the solution by the solution's original concentration of nitroglycerin. *The actual doses delivered have been less, sometimes much less, than those reported.*

Some in-line intravenous filters also absorb nitroglycerin; these filters should be avoided. Because of the absorption problem, Marion Merrell Dow Inc. recommends the use of the least absorptive infusion tubing available (i.e., non-PVC tubing) for infusions of NITRO-BID IV (see DOSAGE AND ADMINISTRATION).

DOSING INSTRUCTIONS MUST BE FOLLOWED WITH CARE. WHEN THE APPROPRIATE INFUSION SETS ARE USED, THE CALCULATED DOSE WILL BE DELIVERED TO THE PATIENT, BECAUSE THE LOSS OF NITRO-BID IV SEEN WITH STANDARD PVC TUBING WILL BE AVOIDED. THE DOSAGES REPORTED IN PUBLISHED STUDIES UTILIZED GENERAL-USE PVC ADMINISTRATION SETS, AND RECOMMENDED DOSES BASED ON THIS EXPERIENCE WILL BE TOO HIGH IF THE LOW-ABSORBING INFUSION SETS ARE USED.

PRECAUTIONS

General

Severe hypotension and shock may occur with even small doses of NITRO-BID IV (nitroglycerin). This drug should, therefore, be used with caution in patients who may be volume-depleted; who, for whatever reason, are already hypotensive; or who, because of inadequate circulation to the brain or to other vital organs, would be unusually compromised by undue hypotension. Hypotension induced by nitroglycerin may be accompanied by paradoxical bradycardia and increased angina pectoris.

Nitrate therapy may aggravate the angina caused by hypertrophic cardiomyopathy.

As tolerance to other forms of nitroglycerin develops, the effect of sublingual nitroglycerin on exercise tolerance, although still observable, is somewhat blunted.

In industrial workers who have had long-term exposure to unknown (presumably high) doses of organic nitrates, tolerance clearly occurs. Chest pain, acute myocardial infarction, and even sudden death have occurred during temporary withdrawal of nitrates from these workers, demonstrating the existence of true physical dependence.

Some clinical trials in angina patients have provided nitroglycerin for about 12 continuous hours of every 24-hour day. During the nitrate-free intervals in some of the trials, angina attacks have been more easily provoked than before treatment, and patients have demonstrated hemodynamic rebound and *decreased* exercise tolerance. The importance of these observations to the routine, clinical use of intravenous nitroglycerin is not known.

Lower concentrations of nitroglycerin increase the potential precision of dosing, but these concentrations increase the total fluid volume that must be delivered to the patient. Total fluid load may be a dominant consideration in patients with compromised function of the heart, liver, and/or kidneys.

Nitroglycerin infusions should be administered only via a pump that can maintain a constant infusion rate.

Intracoronary injection of nitroglycerin infusions has not been studied.

Laboratory Tests

Because of propylene glycol content of intravenous nitroglycerin, serum triglyceride assays that rely on glycerol oxidase may give falsely elevated results in patients receiving this medication.

Drug Interactions

The vasodilating effects of nitroglycerin may be additive with those of other vasodilators. Administration of nitroglycerin infusions through the same infusion set as blood can result in pseudoagglutination and hemolysis. More generally, nitroglycerin in 5% dextrose or sodium chloride 0.9% should not be mixed with any other medication of any kind.

Intravenous nitroglycerin interferes, at least in some patients, with the anticoagulant effect of heparin. In patients receiving intravenous nitroglycerin, concomitant heparin therapy should be guided by frequent measurement of the activated partial thromboplastin time.

Carcinogenesis, Mutagenesis, Impairment of Fertility

Animal carcinogenesis studies with injectable nitroglycerin have not been performed. Rats receiving up to 434 mg/kg/day of dietary nitroglycerin for 2 years developed dose-related fibrotic and neoplastic changes in liver, including carcinomas, and intersitial cell tumors in testes. At high dose, the incidences of hepatocellular carcinomas in both sexes were 52% vs. 0% in controls, and incidences of testicular tumors were 52% vs. 8% in controls. Incidences of pituitary adenomas and female mammary tumors normally seen in aged rats were significantly reduced, consistent with treatment-related decrease in food intake and body weight; increased life span was also seen in high dose females. Lifetime dietary administration of up to 1058 mg/kg/day of nitroglycerin was not tumorigenic in mice. Nitroglycerin was weakly mutagenic in Ames tests performed in two different laboratories. There was no evidence of mutagenicity in an *in vivo* dominant lethal assay with male rats treated with doses up to about 363 mg/kg/day, p.o. or *in vitro* cytogenetic tests in rat and dog tissues.

In a three-generation reproduction study, rats received dietary nitroglycerin at doses up to about 434 mg/kg/day for six months prior to mating of the F_0 generation with treatment continuing through successive F_1 and F_2 generations. The high-dose was associated with decreased feed intake and body weight gain in both sexes at all matings. No specific effect on the fertility of the F_0 generation was seen. Infertility noted in subsequent generations, however, was attributed to increased interstitial cell tissue and aspematogenesis in the high dose males. In this three-generation study there was no clear evidence of teratogenicity.

Pregnancy

Pregnancy Category C. Animal teratology studies have not been conducted with nitroglycerin injection. Teratology studies in rats and rabbits, however, were conducted with topically applied nitroglycerin ointment at doses up to 80 mg/kg/day and 240 mg/kg/day, respectively. No toxic effects on dams or fetuses were seen at any dose tested. There are no adequate and well-controlled studies in pregnant women. Nitroglycerin should be given to a pregnant woman only if clearly needed.

Nursing Mothers

It is now known whether nitroglycerin is excreted in human milk. Because many drugs are excreted in human milk, caution should be exercised when NITRO-BID IV is administered to a nursing woman.

Pediatric Use

Safety and effectiveness in pediatric patients have not been established.

ADVERSE REACTIONS

Adverse reactions to NITRO-BID IV (nitroglycerin) are generally dose related, and almost all of these reactions are the result of nitroglycerin's activity as a vasodilator. Headache, which may be severe, is the most commonly reported side effect. Headache may be recurrent with each daily dose, especially at higher doses. Transient episodes of light-headedness, occasionally related to blood pressure changes, may also occur. Hypotension occurs infrequently, but in some patients, it may be severe enough to warrant discontinuation of therapy. Syncope, crescendo angina, and rebound hypertension have been reported but are uncommon.

Allergic reactions to nitroglycerin are also uncommon, and the great majority of those reported have been cases of contact dermatitis or fixed drug eruptions in patients receiving nitroglycerin in ointments or patches. There have been a few reports of genuine anaphylactoid reactions, and these reactions can probably occur in patients receiving nitroglycerin by any route.

Extremely rarely, ordinary doses of organic nitrates have caused methemoglobinemia in normal-seeming patients; for further discussion of its diagnosis and treatment, see OVERDOSAGE.

Data are not available to allow estimation of the frequency of adverse reactions during treatment with nitroglycerin injection.

OVERDOSAGE

Hemodynamic Effects

The ill effects of NITRO-BID IV (nitroglycerin) overdose are generally the results of nitroglycerin's capacity to induce vasodilatation, venous pooling, reduced cardiac output, and hypotension. These hemodynamic changes may have protean manifestations, including increased intracranial pressure, with any or all of the following: persistent throbbing headache, confusion, and moderate fever; vertigo; palpitation; visual disturbances; nausea and vomiting (possibly with colic and even bloody diarrhea); syncope (especially in the upright posture); air hunger and dyspnea, later followed by reduced ventilatory effort; diaphoresis, with the skin either flushed or cold and clammy; heart block and bradycardia; paralysis; coma; seizures; and death.

Laboratory determinations of serum levels of NITRO-BID IV and its metabolites are not widely available, and such determinations have, in any event, no established role in the management of NITRO-BID IV overdose.

No data are available to suggest physiological maneuvers (e.g., maneuvers to change the pH of the urine) that might accelerate elimination of nitroglycerin and its active metabolites. Similarly, it is not known which, if any, of these substances can usefully be removed from the body by hemodialysis.

No specific antagonist to the vasodilator effects of NITRO-BID IV is known, and no intervention has been subject to controlled study as a therapy of nitroglycerin overdose. Because the hypotension associated with nitroglycerin overdose is the result of venodilatation and arterial hypovolemia, prudent therapy in this situation should be directed toward increase in central fluid volume. Passive elevation of the patient's legs may be sufficient, but intravenous infusion of normal saline or similar fluid may also be necessary.

The use of epinephrine or other arterial vasoconstrictors in this setting is likely to do more harm than good.

In patients with renal disease or congestive heart failure, therapy resulting in central volume expression is not without hazard. Treatment of NITRO-BID IV overdose in these patients may be subtle and difficult, and invasive monitoring may be required.

Methemoglobinemia

Nitrate ions liberated during metabolism of nitroglycerin can oxidize hemoglobin into methemoglobin. Even in patients totally without cytochrome b_5 reductase activity, however, and even assuming that the nitrate moieties of nitroglycerin are quantitatively applied to oxidation of hemoglobin, about 1 mg/kg of nitroglycerin should be required before any of these patients manifests clinically significant ($\geq 10\%$) methemoglobinemia. In patients with normal reductase function, significant production of methemoglobin should require even larger doses of nitroglycerin. In one study in which 36 patients received 2 to 4 weeks of continuous nitroglycerin therapy at 3.1 to 4.4 mg/hr, the average methemoglobin level measured was 0.2%; this was comparable to that observed in parallel patients who received placebo.

Notwithstanding these observations, there are case reports of significant methemoglobinemia in association with moderate overdoses of organic nitrates. None of the affected patients had been thought to be unusually susceptible.

Methemoglobin levels are available from most clinical laboratories. The diagnosis should be suspected in patients who exhibit signs of impaired oxygen delivery despite adequate cardiac output and adequate arterial pO_2. Classically, methemoglobinemic blood is described as chocolate brown, without color change on exposure to air.

When methemoglobinemia is diagnosed, the treatment of choice is methylene blue, 1 to 2 mg/kg intravenously.

DOSAGE AND ADMINISTRATION

NOT FOR DIRECT INTRAVENOUS INJECTION.

NITRO-BID IV (NITROGLYCERIN) IS A CONCENTRATED, POTENT DRUG, WHICH MUST BE DILUTED IN DEXTROSE (5%) INJECTION USP OR SODIUM CHLORIDE (0.9%) INJECTION USP PRIOR TO ITS INFUSION. NITRO-BID IV SHOULD NOT BE MIXED WITH OTHER DRUGS.

1. **Initial Dilution.**
   Aseptically transfer the contents of one NITRO-BID IV vial (containing 25 or 50 mg of nitroglycerin) into a 500 mL *glass* bottle of either dextrose (5%) injection USP or sodium chloride (0.9%) injection USP. This yields a final concentration of 50 mcg/mL or 100 mcg/mL. Diluting 5 mg NITRO-BID IV into 100 mL will also yield a final concentration of 50 mcg/mL.
2. **Maintenance Dilution.**
   It is important to consider the fluid requirements of the patient as well as the expected duration of infusion in selecting the appropriate dilution of NITRO-BID IV (nitroglycerin).
   After the initial dosage titration, the concentration of the solution may be increased, if necessary, to limit fluids given to the patient. The NITRO-BID IV concentration should not exceed 400 mcg/mL. (See chart).

NOTE:
If the concentration is adjusted, it is imperative to flush or replace the infusion set before a new concentration is utilized. If the set is not flushed or replaced, it could take minutes to hours, depending upon the flow rate and the dead space of the set, for the new concentration to reach the patient.

Invert the glass parenteral bottle several times to assure uniform dilution of NITRO-BID IV.

Dosage is affected by the type of container and administration set used. (See WARNINGS.)

Although the usual starting adult dose range reported in clinical studies was 25 mcg/min or more, these studies used PVC administration sets. THE USE OF NONABSORBING TUBING WILL RESULT IN THE NEED FOR REDUCED DOSES.

Continued on next page

Hoechst Marion Roussel—Cont.

If a peristaltic action infusion pump is used, an appropriate administration set should be selected with a drip chamber that delivers approximately 60 microdrops/mL. The NITRO-BID IV Dilution and Administration tables below may be used to calculate NITRO-BID dilution and flow rate in microdrops/minute to achieve the desired NITRO-BID IV administration rate.

If a volumetric infusion pump is used, the NITRO-BID IV Dilution and Administration table below may still be used; however, flow rate will be determined directly by the infusion pump, independent of the drop size of the drip chambers. Thus, the reference to "MICRODROPS/MIN" is not applicable, and the corresponding flow rate in mL/hr should be used to determine pump settings.

When using a nonabsorbing infusion set, initial dosage should be 5 mcg/min delivered through an infusion pump capable of exact and constant delivery of the drug. Subsequent titration must be adjusted to the clinical situation, with dose increments becoming more cautious as partial response is seen. Initial titration should be in 5 mcg/min increments, with increases every 3 to 5 minutes until some response is noted. If no response is seen at 20 mcg/min, increments of 10 and later 20 mcg/min can be used. Once a partial blood pressure response is observed, the dose increase should be reduced and the interval between increases should be lengthened.

Some patients with normal or low left ventricular filling pressures or pulmonary capillary wedge pressure (e.g., angina patients without other complications) may be hypersensitive to the effects of NITRO-BID IV and may respond fully to doses as small as 5 mcg/min. These patients require especially careful titrating and monitoring.

There is no fixed optimum dose of NITRO-BID IV. Due to variations in the responsiveness of individual patients to the drug, each patient must be titrated to the desired level of hemodynamic function. Therefore, continuous monitoring of physiologic parameters (i.e., blood pressure and heart rate in all patients and other measurements such as pulmonary capillary wedge pressure, as appropriate) MUST be performed to achieve the correct dose. Adequate systemic blood pressure and coronary perfusion pressure must be maintained.

As with all parenteral drug products, NITRO-BID IV should be inspected visually for particulate matter and discoloration prior to administration, whenever solution and container permit.

HOW SUPPLIED

NITRO-BID® IV is supplied in boxes of ten 1-mL vials (NDC 0088-1800-31), each vial containing 5 mg of nitroglycerin (5 mg/mL); ten 5-mL vials (NDC 0088-1800-32), each vial containing 25 mg nitroglycerin (5 mg/mL); and five 10-mL vials (NDC 0088-1800-33), each vial containing 50 mg nitroglycerin (5 mg/mL).

PROTECT FROM LIGHT BY RETAINING PRODUCT IN CARTON UNTIL READY TO USE.
NITRO-BID IV VIALS ARE INTENDED FOR SINGLE-DOSE USE ONLY. PROPERLY DISCARD ANY UNUSED PORTION.
Protect from freezing.
Store at controlled room temperature 15-30°C (59-86°F).

Dilution Table

Diluent Volume	Quantity of NITRO-BID IV (5 mg/mL)	Approximate Final Concentration
100 mL	10 mg (2 mL)	100 mcg/mL
100 mL	20 mg (4 mL)	200 mcg/mL
100 mL	40 mg (8 mL)	400 mcg/mL
250 mL	25 mg (5 mL)	100 mcg/mL
250 mL	50 mg (10 mL)	200 mcg/mL
250 mL	100 mg (20 mL)	400 mcg/mL
500 mL	50 mg (10 mL)	100 mcg/mL
500 mL	100 mg (20 mL)	200 mcg/mL
500 mL	200 mg (40 mL)	400 mcg/mL

Administration Table
(60 microdrops = 1 milliliter)

Concentration (mg/mL)	100	200	400
Dose (mg/min)	Flow Rate (microdrops/min = mL/h)		
5	3	—	—
10	6	3	—
15	9	—	—
20	12	6	3
30	18	9	—
40	24	12	6
60	36	18	9
80	48	24	12
120	72	36	18
160	96	48	24
240	—	72	36
320	—	96	48
480	—	—	72
640	—	—	96

Prescribing Information as of April 1995
Manufactured for:
Hoechst Marion Roussel, Inc.
Kansas City, MO 64137 USA

NITRO-BID® OINTMENT 2% ℞
[ni 'trō-bid]
(nitroglycerin ointment USP)
Prescribing Information as of February 1996

DESCRIPTION
Nitroglycerin is 1,2,3,-propanetriol trinitrate, an organic nitrate whose structural formula is:

$$CH_2-ONO_2$$
$$|$$
$$CH-ONO_2$$
$$|$$
$$CH_2-ONO_2$$

and whose molecular weight is 227.09. The organic nitrates are vasodilators, active on both arteries and veins.
NITRO-BID Ointment contains lactose and 2% nitroglycerin in a base of lanolin and white petrolatum. Each inch (2.5 cm), as squeezed from the tube, contains approximately 15 mg of nitroglycerin.

CLINICAL PHARMACOLOGY
The principal pharmacological action of nitroglycerin is relaxation of vascular smooth muscle and consequent dilatation of peripheral arteries and veins, especially the latter. Dilatation of the veins promotes peripheral pooling of blood and decreases venous return to the heart, thereby reducing left ventricular end-diastolic pressure and pulmonary capillary wedge pressure (preload). Arteriolar relaxation reduces systemic vascular resistance, systolic arterial pressure, and mean arterial pressure (afterload). Dilatation of the coronary arteries also occurs. The relative importance of preload reduction, afterload reduction, and coronary dilatation remains undefined.
Dosing regimens for most chronically used drugs are designed to provide plasma concentrations that are continuously greater than a minimally effective concentration. This strategy is inappropriate for organic nitrates. Several well-controlled clinical trials have used exercise testing to assess the antianginal efficacy of continuously delivered nitrates. In the large majority of these trials, active agents were indistinguishable from placebo after 24 hours (or less) of continuous therapy. Attempts to overcome nitrate tolerance by dose escalation, even to doses far in excess of those used acutely, have consistently failed. Only after nitrates had been absent from the body for several hours was their antianginal efficacy restored.

Pharmacokinetics
The volume of distribution of nitroglycerin is about 3 L/kg, and nitroglycerin is cleared from this volume at extremely rapid rates, with a resulting serum half-life of about 3 minutes. The observed clearance rates (close to 1 L/kg/min) greatly exceed hepatic blood flow; known sites of extrahepatic metabolism include red blood cells and vascular walls. The first products in the metabolism of nitroglycerin are inorganic nitrate and the 1,2- and 1,3-dinitroglycerols. The dinitrates are less effective vasodilators than nitroglycerin but they are longer-lived in the serum, and their net contribution to the overall effect of chronic nitroglycerin regimens is not known. The dinitrates are further metabolized to (nonvasoactive) mononitrates and, ultimately, to glycerol and carbon dioxide.
To avoid development of tolerance to nitrolglycerin, drug-free intervals of 10 to 12 hours are known to be sufficient; shorter intervals have not been well studied. In one well-controlled clinical trial, subjects receiving nitroglycerin appeared to exhibit a rebound or withdrawal effect, so that

their exercise tolerance at the end of the daily drug-free interval was less than that exhibited by the parallel group receiving placebo.
Reliable assay techniques for plasma nitroglycerin levels have only recently become available, and studies using these techniques to define the pharmacokinetics of nitroglycerin ointment have not been reported. Published studies using older techniques provide results that often differ, in similar experimental settings, by an order of magnitude. The data are consistent, however, in suggesting that nitroglycerin levels rise to a steady state within an hour or so of application of ointment, and that after removal of nitroglycerin ointment, levels wane with a half-life of about half an hour. The onset of action of transdermal nitroglycerin is not sufficiently rapid for this product to be useful in aborting an acute anginal episode.
The maximal achievable daily duration of antianginal activity provided by nitroglycerin ointment therapy has not been studied. Recent studies of other formulations of nitroglycerin suggest that the maximal achievable daily duration of anti-anginal effect from nitroglcerin ointment will be about 12 hours.
It is reasonable to believe that the rate and extent of nitroglycerin absorption from ointment may vary with the site and square measure of the skin over which a given dose of ointment is spread, but these relationships have not been adequately studied.

Clinical Trials
Controlled trials have demonstrated that nitroglycerin ointment can effectively reduce exercise-related angina for up to 7 hours after a single application. Doses used in clinical trials have ranged from ½ inch (1.3 cm; 7.5 mg) to 2 inches (5.1 cm; 30 mg), typically applied to 36 square inches (232 square centimeters) of truncal skin.
In some controlled trials of other organic nitrate formulations, efficacy has declined with time. Because controlled, long-term trials of nitroglycerin ointment have not been reported, it is not known how the efficacy of NITRO-BID Ointment may vary during extended therapy.

INDICATIONS AND USAGE
Nitroglycerin ointment is indicated for the prevention of angina pectoris due to coronary artery disease. The onset of action of transdermal nitroglycerin is not sufficiently rapid for this product to be useful in aborting an acute anginal episode.

CONTRAINDICATIONS
Allergic reactions to organic nitrates are extremely rare, but they do occur. Nitroglycerin is contraindicated in patients who are allergic to it.

WARNINGS
The benefits of transdermal nitroglycerin in patients with acute myocardial infarction or congestive heart failure have not been established. If one elects to use nitroglycerin in these conditions, careful clinical or hemodynamic monitoring must be used to avoid the hazards of hypotension and tachycardia.

PRECAUTIONS
General
Severe hypotension, particularly with upright posture, may occur with even small doses of nitroglycerin. This drug should, therefore, be used with caution in patients who may be volume depleted or who, for whatever reason, are already hypotensive. Hypotension induced by nitroglycerin may be accompanied by paradoxical bradycardia and increased angina pectoris.
Nitrate therapy may aggravate the angina caused by hypertrophic cardiomyopathy.
As tolerance to other forms of nitroglycerin develops, the effect of sublingual nitroglycerin on exercise tolerance, although still observable, is somewhat blunted.
In industrial workers who have had long-term exposure to unknown (presumably high) doses of organic nitrates, tolerance clearly occurs.
Chest pain, acute myocardial infarction, and even sudden death have occurred during temporary withdrawal of nitrates from these workers, demonstrating the existence of true physical dependence.
Some clinical trials in angina patients have provided nitroglycerin for about 12 continuous hours of every 24-hour day. During the nitrate-free intervals in some of these trials, anginal attacks have been more easily provoked than before treatment, and patients have demonstrated hemodynamic rebound and decreased exercise tolerance. The importance of these observations to the routine clinical use of transdermal nitroglycerin is not known.

Information for Patients
Daily headaches sometimes accompany treatment with nitroglycerin. In patients who get these headaches, the headaches are a marker of the activity of the drug. Patients should resist the temptation to avoid headaches by altering the schedule of their treatment with nitroglycerin since loss of headache is likely to be associated with simultaneous loss of antianginal efficacy.

Treatment with nitroglycerin may be associated with lightheadedness on standing, especially just after rising from a recumbent or seated position.
This effect may be more frequent in patients who have also consumed alcohol.

Drug Interactions

The vasodilating effects of nitroglycerin may be additive with those of other vasodilators. Alcohol, in particular, has been found to exhibit additive effects of this variety.
Marked symptomatic orthostatic hypotension has been reported when calcium channel blockers and organic nitrates were used in combination. Dose adjustments of either class of agents may be necessary.

Carcinogenesis, Mutagenesis, and Impairment of Fertility

Studies to evaluate the carcinogenic or mutagenic potential of nitroglycerin have not been performed. Nitroglycerin's effect upon reproductive capacity is similarly unknown.

Pregnancy

Category C. Animal reproduction studies have not been conducted with nitroglycerin. It is also not known whether nitroglycerin can cause fetal harm when administered to a pregnant woman or whether it can affect reproductive capacity. Nitroglycerin should be given to a pregnant woman only if clearly needed.

Nursing Mothers

It is not known whether nitroglycerin is excreted in human milk. Because many drugs are excreted in human milk, caution should be exercised when nitroglycerin is administered to a nursing woman.

Pediatric Use

Safety and effectiveness in pediatric patients have not been established.

ADVERSE REACTIONS

Adverse reactions to nitroglycerin are generally dose-related, and almost all of these reactions are the result of nitroglycerin's activity as a vasodilator. Headache, which may be severe, is the most commonly reported side effect. Headache may be recurrent with each daily dose, especially at higher doses. Transient episodes of light-headedness, occasionally related to blood pressure changes, also may occur. Hypotension occurs infrequently, but in some patients it may be severe enough to warrant discontinuation of therapy. Snycope, crescendo angina, and rebound hypertension have been reported but are uncommon.
Allergic reactions to nitroglycerin are also uncommon, and the great majority of those reported have been cases of contact dermatitis or fixed drug eruptions in patients receiving nitroglycerin in ointments of patches. There have been a few reports of genuine anaphylactoid reactions, and these reactions can probably occur in patients receiving nitroglycerin by any route.
Extremely rarely, ordinary doses of organic nitrates have caused methemoglobinemia in normal-seeming patients; for further discussion of its diagnosis and treatment, see OVERDOSAGE.
Data are not available to allow estimation of the frequency of adverse reactions during treatment with NITRO-BID Ointment.

OVERDOSAGE

Hemodynamic Effects

The ill effects of nitroglycerin overdose are generally the result of nitroglycerin's capacity to induce vasodilation, venous pooling, reduced cardiac output, and hypotension. These hemodynamic changes may have protean manifestations, including increased intracranial pressure, with any or all of the following: persistent throbbing headache, confusion, and moderate fever; vertigo; palpitations; visual disturbances; nausea and vomiting (possibly with colic and even bloody diarrhea); syncope (especially in the upright posture); air hunger and dyspnea, later followed by reduced ventilatory effort: diaphoresis, with the skin either flushed or cold and clammy; heart block and bradycardia; paralysis; coma; seizures; and death.
Laboratory determinations of serum levels of nitroglycerin and its metabolites are not widely available, and such determinations, in any event, have no established role in the management of nitroglycerin overdose.
No data are available to suggest physiological maneuvers (eg, maneuvers to change the pH of the urine) that might accelerate elimination of nitroglycerin and its active metabolites. Similarly, it is not known which, if any, of these substances can usefully be removed from the body by hemodialysis.
No specific antagonist to the vasodilator effects of nitroglycerin is known, and no intervention has been subject to controlled study as a therapy for nitroglycerin overdose. Because the hypotension associated with nitroglycerin overdose is the result of venodilatation and arterial hypovolemia, prudent therapy in this situation should be directed toward increase in central fluid volume. Passive elevation of the patient's legs may be sufficient, but intravenous infusion of normal saline or similar fluid may also be necessary.
The use of epinephrine or other arterial vasoconstrictors in this setting is likely to do more harm than good.
In patients with renal disease or congestive heart failure, therapy resulting in central volume expansion is not without hazard. Treatment of nitroglycerin overdose in these patients may be subtle and difficult, and invasive monitoring may be required.

Methemoglobinemia

Nitrate ions liberated during metabolism of nitroglycerin can oxidize hemoglobin into methemoglobin. Even in patients totally without cytochrome b_5 reductase activity, however, and even assuming that the nitrate moieties of nitroglycerin are quantitatively applied to oxidation of hemoglobin, about 1 mg/kg of nitroglycerin should be required before any of these patients manifests clinically significant ($\geq 10\%$) methemoglobinemia. In patients with normal reductase function, significant production of methemoglobin should require even larger doses of nitroglycerin. In one study in which 36 patients received 2 to 4 weeks of continuous nitroglycerin therapy at 3.1 to 4.4 mg/hr, the average methemoglobin level measured was 0.2%; this was comparable to that observed in parallel patients who received placebo.
Notwithstanding these observations, there are case reports of significant methemoglobinemia in association with moderate overdoses of organic nitrates. None of the affected patients had been thought to be unusually susceptible.
Methemoglobin levels are available from most clinical laboratories. The diagnosis should be suspected in patients who exhibit signs of impaired oxygen delivery despite adequate cardiac output and adequate arterial pO_2. Classically, methemoglobinemic blood is described as chocolate brown without color change on exposure to air.
When methemoglobinemia is diagnosed, the treatment of choice is methylene blue, 1 to 2 mg/kg intravenously.

DOSAGE AND ADMINISTRATION

As noted above (CLINICAL PHARMACOLOGY), controlled trials have demonstrated that nitroglycerin ointment can effectively reduce exercise-related angina for up to 7 hours after a single application. Doses used in clinical trials have ranged from ½ inch (1.3 cm; 7.5 mg) to 2 inches (5.1 cm; 30 mg), typically applied to 36 square inches (232 square centimeters) of truncal skin.
It is reasonable to believe that the rate and extent of nitroglycerin absorption from ointment may vary with the site and square measure of the skin over which a given dose of ointment is spread, but these relationships have not been adequately studied.
Controlled trials with other formulations of nitroglycerin have demonstrated that, if plasma levels are maintained continuously, all antianginal efficacy is lost within 24 hours. This tolerance cannot be overcome by increasing the dose of nitroglycerin. As a result, any regimen of NITRO-BID Ointment administration should include a daily nitrate-free interval. The minimum necessary length of such an interval has not been defined, but studies with other nitroglycerin formulations have shown that 10 to 12 hours is sufficient.
Thus, one appropriate dosing schedule for NITRO-BID Ointment would begin with two daily ½-inch (7.5-mg) doses, one applied on rising in the morning and one applied 6 hours later. The dose could be doubled, and even doubled again, in patients tolerating this dose but failing to respond to it.
Each tube of ointment is supplied with a pad of ruled, impermeable paper applicators. These applicators allow ointment to be absorbed through a much smaller area of skin that used in any of the reported clinical trials, and the significance of this difference is not known. To apply the ointment using one of the applicators, place the applicator on a flat surface, printed side down. Squeeze the necessary amount of ointment from the tube onto the applicator, place the applicator (ointment side down) on the desired area of skin, and tape the applicator into place.

HOW SUPPLIED

NITRO-BID® Ointment 2% (nitroglycerin ointment USP) is available in 20-g (NDC 0088-1552-20) and 60-g (NDC 0088-1552-60) tubes and in Unit Dose Identification Paks of 100 1-g foil pouches (NDC 0088-1552-49).
Prescribing Information as of February 1996
Hoechst Marion Roussel, Inc.
Kansas City, MO 64137 USA

NORPRAMIN® ℞

[nor·pram 'in]
(desipramine hydrochloride tablets UPS)

Prescribing information as of January 1996

DESCRIPTION

NORPRAMIN (desipramine hydrochloride USP) is an antidepressant drug of the tricyclic type, and is chemically: 5*H*-Dibenz[*bf*]azepine-5-propanamine, 10,11- dihydro-*N*-methyl-, monohydrochloride.
[See chemical structure at top of next column.]

Inactive Ingredients

The following inactive ingredients are contained in all dosage strengths: acacia, calcium carbonate, corn starch, D&C Red No. 30 and D&C Yellow No. 10 (except 10 mg and 150 mg), FD&C Blue No. 1 (except 50 mg, 75 mg, and 100 mg), hydrogenated soy oil, iron oxide, light mineral oil, magne-

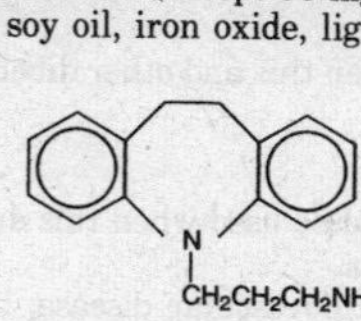

sium stearate, mannitol, polyethylene glycol 8000, pregelatinized corn starch, sodium benzoate (except 150 mg), sucrose, talc, titanium dioxide, and other ingredients.

CLINICAL PHARMACOLOGY

Mechanism of Action

Available evidence suggests that many depressions have a biochemical basis in the form of a relative deficiency of neurotransmitters such as norepinephrine and serotonin. Norepinephrine deficiency may be associated with relatively low urinary 3-methoxy-4-hydroxyphenyl glycol (MHPG) levels, while serotonin deficiencies may be associated with low spinal fluid levels of 5-hydroxyindoleacetic acid.
While the precise mechanism of action of the tricyclic antidepressants is unknown, a leading theory suggests that they restore normal levels of neurotransmitters by blocking the re-uptake of these substances from the synapse in the central nervous system. Evidence indicates that the secondary amine tricyclic antidepressants, including NORPRAMIN, may have greater activity in blocking the re-uptake of norepinephrine. Tertiary amine tricyclic antidepressants, such as amitriptyline, may have greater effect on serotonin re-uptake.
NORPRAMIN (desipramine hydrochloride) is not a monoamine oxidase (MAO) inhibitor and does not act primarily as a central nervous system stimulant. It has been found in some studies to have a more rapid onset of action than imipramine. Earliest therapeutic effects may occasionally be seen in 2 to 5 days, but full treatment benefit usually requires 2 to 3 weeks to obtain.

Metabolism

Tricyclic antidepressants, such as desipramine hydrochloride, are rapidly absorbed from the gastrointestinal tract. Tricyclic antidepressants or their metabolites are to some extent excreted through the gastric mucosa and reabsorbed from the gastrointestinal tract. Desipramine is metabolized in the liver, and approximately 70% is excreted in the urine.
The rate of metabolism of tricyclic antidepressants varies widely from individual to individual, chiefly on a genetically determined basis. Up to a 36-fold difference in plasma level may be noted among individuals taking the same oral dose of desipramine. In general, the elderly metabolize tricyclic antidepressants more slowly than do younger adults.
Certain drugs, particularly the psychostimulants and the phenothiazines, increase plasma levels of concomitantly administered tricyclic antidepressants through competition for the same metabolic enzyme systems. Concurrent administration of cimetidine and tricyclic antidepressants can produce clinically significant increases in the plasma concentrations of the tricyclic antidepressants. Conversely, decreases in plasma levels of the tricyclic antidepressants have been reported upon discontinuation of cimetidine, which may result in the loss of the therapeutic efficacy of the tricyclic antidepressant. Other substances, particularly barbiturates and alcohol, induce liver enzyme activity and thereby reduce tricyclic antidepressant plasma levels. Similar effects have been reported with tobacco smoke.
Research on the relationship of plasma level to therapeutic response with the tricyclic antidepressants has produced conflicting results. While some studies report no correlation, many studies cite therapeutic levels for most tricyclics in the range of 50 to 300 nanograms per milliliter. The therapeutic range is different for each tricyclic antidepressant. For desipramine, an optimal range of therapeutic plasma levels has not been established.

INDICATIONS AND USAGE

NORPRAMIN (desipramine hydrochloride) is indicated for the treatment of depression.

CONTRAINDICATIONS

Desipramine hydrochloride should not be given in conjunction with, or within 2 weeks of, treatment with an MAO inhibitor drug; hyperpyretic crises, severe convulsions, and death have occurred in patients taking MAO inhibitors and tricyclic antidepressants. When NORPRAMIN (desipramie hydrochloride) is substituted for an MAO inhibitor, at least 2 weeks should elapse between treatments. NORPRAMIN should then be started cautiously and should be increased gradually.
The drug is contraindicated in the acute recovery period following myocardial infarction. It should not be used in those who have shown prior hypersensitivity to the drug.

Continued on next page

Hoechst Marion Roussel—Cont.

Cross-sensitivity between this and other dibenzazepines is a possibility.

WARNINGS

Extreme caution should be used when this drug is given in the following situations:

a. In patients with cardiovascular disease, because of the possibility of conduction defects, arrhythmias, tachycardias, strokes, and acute myocardial infarction.

b. In patients with a history of urinary retention or glaucoma, because of the anticholinergic properties of the drug.

c. In patients with thyroid disease or those taking thyroid medication, because of the possibility of cardiovascular toxicity, including arrhythmias.

d. In patients with a history of seizure disorder, because this drug has been shown to lower the seizure threshold.

This drug is capable of blocking the antihypertensive effect of guanethidine and similarly acting compounds.

The patient should be cautioned that this drug may impair the mental and/or physical abilities required for the performance of potentially hazardous tasks such as driving a car or operating machinery.

In patients who may use alcohol excessively, it should be borne in mind that the potentiation may increase the danger inherent in any suicide attempt or overdosage.

Use in Pregnancy

Safe use of desipramine hydrochloride during pregnancy and lactation has not been established; therefore, if it is to be given to pregnant patients, nursing mothers, or women of childbearing potential, the possible benefits must be weighed against the possible hazards to mother and child. Animal reproductive studies have been inconclusive.

Use in Children

NORPRAMIN (desipramine hydrochloride) is not recommended for use in children since safety and effectiveness in the pediatric age group have not been established. (See ADVERSE REACTIONS, Cardiovascular.)

PRECAUTIONS

General

It is important that this drug be dispensed in the least possible quantities to depressed outpatients, since suicide has been accomplished with this class of drug. Ordinary prudence requires that children not have access to this drug or to potent drugs of any kind; if possible, this drug should be dispensed in containers with child-resistant safety closures. Storage of this drug in the home must be supervised responsibly.

If serious adverse effects occur, dosage should be reduced or treatment should be altered.

NORPRAMIN (desipramine hydrochloride) therapy in patients with manic-depressive illness may induce a hypomanic state after the depressive phase terminates.

The drug may cause exacerbation of psychosis in schizophrenic patients.

Both elevation and lowering of blood sugar levels have been reported.

Leukocyte and differential counts should be performed in any patient who develops fever and sore throat during therapy; the drug should be discontinued if there is evidence of pathologic neutrophil depression.

Clinical experience in the concurrent administration of ECT and antidepressant drugs is limited. Thus, if such treatment is essential, the possibility of increased risk relative to benefits should be considered.

This drug should be discontinued as soon as possible prior to elective surgery because of possible cardiovascular effects. Hypertensive episodes have been observed during surgery in patients taking desipramine hydrochloride.

Drug Interactions

Drugs Metabolized by P450 2D6. The biochemical activity of the drug metabolizing isozyme cytochrome P450 2D6 (debrisoquin hydroxylase) is reduced in a subset of the Caucasian population (about 7% to 10% of Caucasians are so called "poor metabolizers"); reliable estimates of the prevalence of reduced P450 2D5 isozyme activity among Asian, African and other populations are not yet available. Poor metabolizers have higher than expected plasma concentrations of tricyclic antidepressants (TCAs) when given usual doses. Depending on the fraction of drug metabolized by P450 2D6, the increase in plasma concentration may be small, or quite large (8 fold increase in plasma AUC of the TCA).

In addition, certain drugs inhibit the activity of this isozyme and make normal metabolizers resemble poor metabolizers. An individual who is stable on a given dose of TCA may become abruptly toxic when given one of these inhibiting drugs as concomitant therapy. The drugs that inhibit cytochrome P450 2D6 include some that are not metabolized by the enzyme (quinidine; cimetidine) and many that are substrates for P450 2D6 (many other antidepressants, phenothiazines, and the Type 1C antiarrhythmics propafenone and flecainide). While all the selective serotonin reuptake inhibitors (SSRIs), e.g., fluoxetine, sertraline, paroxetine, inhibit P450 2D6, they may vary in the extent of inhibition. The extent to which SSRI TCA interactions may pose clinical problems will depend on the degree of inhibition and the pharmacokinetics of the SSRI involved. Nevertheless, caution is indicated in the co-administration of TCAs with any of the SSRIs and also in switching from one class to the other. Of particular importance, sufficient time must elapse before initiating TCA treatment in a patient withdrawn from fluoxetine, given the long half-life of the parent and active metabolite (at least 5 weeks may be necessary).

Concomitant use of tricyclic antidepressants with drugs that can inhibit cytochrome P450 2D6 may require lower doses than usually prescribed for either the tricyclic antidepressant or the other drug. Furthermore, whenever one of these other drugs is withdrawn from co-therapy, an increased dose of tricyclic antidepressant may be required. It is desirable to monitor TCA plasma levels whenever a TCA is going to be co-administered with another drug known to be an inhibitor of P450 2D6.

Close supervision and careful adjustment of dosage are required when this drug is given concomitantly with anticholinergic or sympathomimetic drugs.

Patients should be warned that while taking this drug their response to alcoholic beverages may be exaggerated.

If NORPRAMIN (desipramine hydrochloride) is to be combined with other psychotropic agents such as tranquilizers or sedative/hypnotics, careful consideration should be given to the pharmacology of the agents employed since the sedative effects of NORPRAMIN and benzodiazepines (e.g., chlordiazepoxide or diazepam) are additive. Both the sedative and anticholinergic effects of the major tranquilizers are also additive to those of NORPRAMIN.

ADVERSE REACTIONS

Included in the following listing are a few adverse reactions that have not been reported with this specific drug. However, the pharmacologic similarities among the tricyclic antidepressant drugs require that each of the reactions be considered when NORPRAMIN (desipramine hydrochloride) is given.

Cardiovascular: hypotension, hypertension, palpitations, heart block, myocardial infarction, stroke, arrhythmias, premature ventricular contractions, tachycardia, ventricular tachycardia, ventricular fibrillation, sudden death

There has been a report of an "acute collapse" and "sudden death" in an 8-year-old (18 kg) male, treated for 2 years for hyperactivity.

There have been additional reports of sudden death in children. (See WARNINGS, Use in Children.)

Psychiatric: confusional states (especially in the elderly) with hallucinations, disorientation, delusions; anxiety, restlessness, agitation; insomnia and nightmares; hypomania; exacerbation of psychosis

Neurologic: numbness, tingling, paresthesias of extremities; incoordination, ataxia, tremors; peripheral neuropathy; extrapyramidal symptoms; seizures; alterations in EEG patterns; tinnitus

Symptoms attributed to Neuroleptic Malignant Syndrome have been reported during desipramine use with and without concomitant neuroleptic therapy.

Anticholinergic: dry mouth, and rarely associated sublingual adenitis; blurred vision, disturbance of accommodation, mydriasis, increased intraocular pressure; constipation, paralytic ileus; urinary retention, delayed micturition, dilation of urinary tract

Allergic: skin rash, petechiae, urticaria, itching, photosensitization (avoid excessive exposure to sunlight), edema (of face and tongue or general), drug fever, cross-sensitivity with other tricyclic drugs

Hematologic: bone marrow depressions including agranulocytosis, eosinophilia, purpura, thrombocytopenia

Gastrointestinal: anorexia, nausea and vomiting, epigastric distress, peculiar taste, abdominal cramps, diarrhea, stomatitis, black tongue, hepatitis, jaundice (simulating obstructive), altered liver function, elevated liver function tests, increased pancreatic enzymes

Endocrine: gynecomastia in the male, breast enlargement and galactorrhea in the female; increased or decreased libido, impotence, painful ejaculation, testicular swelling; elevation or depression of blood sugar levels; syndrome of inappropriate antidiuretic hormone secretion (SIADH)

Other: weight gain or loss; perspiration, flushing; urinary frequency, nocturia; parotid swelling; drowsiness, dizziness, weakness and fatigue; headache; fever; alopecia; elevated alkaline phosphatase

Withdrawal Symptoms: Though not indicative of addiction, abrupt cessation of treatment after prolonged therapy may produce nausea, headache, and malaise.

OVERDOSAGE*

Deaths may occur from overdosage with this class of drugs. Multiple drug ingestion (including alcohol) is common in deliberate tricyclic antidepressant overdose. As the management is complex and changing, it is recommended that the physician contact a poison control center for current information on treatment. Signs and symptoms of toxicity develop rapidly after tricyclic antidepressant overdose; therefore, hospital monitoring is required as soon as possible. There is no specific antidote for desipramine overdosage.

*Poisindex®: Toxicologic Management
Topic: Antidepressants, Tricyclic
Micromedex Inc. Vol. 85

Oral LD$_{50}$

The oral LD$_{50}$ of desipramine is 290 mg/kg in male mice and 320 mg/kg in female rats.

Manifestations of Overdosage

Critical manifestations of overdose include: cardiac dysrhythmias, severe hypotension, convulsions, and CNS depression, including coma. Changes in the electrocardiogram, particularly in QRS axis or width, are clinically significant indicators or tricyclic antidepressant toxicity.

Other signs of overdose may include: confusion, disturbed concentration, transient visual hallucinations, dilated pupils, agitation, hyperactive reflexes, stupor, drowsiness, muscle rigidity, vomiting, hypothermia, hyperpyrexia, or any of the symptoms listed under ADVERSE REACTIONS.

Management

Aggressive supportive care and serum alkalinization are the mainstays of therapy.

General. Obtain an ECG and immediately initiate cardiac monitoring. Protect the patient's airway, establish an intravenous line, and initiate gastric decontamination. A minimum of 6 hours of observation with cardiac monitoring and observation for signs of CNS or respirator depression, hypotension, cardiac dysrhythmias and/or conduction blocks, and seizures is necessary. If signs of toxicity occur at any time during this period, extended monitoring is required. Follow ECG, renal function, CPK, and arterial blood gasses as clinically indicated. There are case reports of patients succumbing to fatal dysrhythmias late after overdose; these patients had clinical evidence of significant poisoning prior to death, and most received inadequate gastrointestinal decontamination. Monitoring of plasma drug levels should not guide management of the patient.

Gastrointestinal Decontamination. All patients suspected of tricyclic antidepressant overdose should receive gastrointestinal decontamination. This should include large volume gastric lavage followed by activated charcoal. If consciousness is impaired, the airway should be secured prior to lavage. Emesis is contraindicated.

Cardiovascular. A maximal limb-lead QRS duration of ≥0.10 seconds may be the best indication of the severity of the overdose. Serum alkalinization, to a pH of 7.45 to 7.55, using intravenous sodium bicarbonate and hyperventilation (as needed) should be instituted for patients with dysrhythmias and/or QRS widening. A pH > 7.60 or a pCO$_2$ < 20mm Hg is undesirable. Dysrhythmias unresponsive to sodium bicarbonate therapy/hyperventilation may respond to lidocaine, bretylium or phenytoin. Type IA and IC antiarrhythmics are generally contraindicated (eg, quinidine, disopyramide, and procainamide).

In rare instances, hemoperfusion may be beneficial in acute refractory cardiovascular instability in patients with acute toxicity. However, hemodialysis, peritoneal dialysis, exchange transfusions, and forced diuresis generally have been reported as ineffective in tricyclic antidepressant poisoning.

CNS. In patients with CNS depression, early intubation is advised because of the potential for abrupt deterioration. Seizures should be controlled with benzodiazepines. If these are ineffective or seizures recur, other anticonvulsants (eg, phenobarbital, phenytoin) may be used. Physostigmine is not recommended except to treat life-threatening symptoms that have been unresponsive to other therapies, and then only in consultation with a poison control center.

Psychiatric Follow-up. Since overdosage is often deliberate, patients may attempt suicide by other means during the recovery phase. Psychiatric referral may be appropriate.

Pediatric Management. The principles of management of child and adult overdosages are similar. It is strongly recommended that the physician contact the local poison control center for specific pediatric treatment.

DOSAGE AND ADMINISTRATION

Not recommended for use in children (see WARNINGS). Lower dosages are recommended for elderly patients and adolescents. Lower dosages are also recommended for outpatients compared to hospitalized patients, who are closely supervised. Dosage should be initiated at a low level and increased according to clinical response and any evidence of intolerance. Following remission, maintenance medication may be required for a period of time and should be at the lowest dose that will maintain remission.

Usual Adult Dose

The usual adult dose is 100 to 200 mg per day. In more severely ill patients, dosage may be further increased gradually to 300 mg/day if necessary. Dosages above 300 mg/day are not recommended.

Dosage should be initiated at a lower level and increased according to tolerance and clinical response.

Treatment of patients requiring as much as 300 mg should generally be initiated in hospitals, where regular visits by

the physician, skilled nursing care, and frequent electrocardiograms (ECGs) are available.
The best available evidence of impending toxicit from very high doses of NORPRAMIN is prolongation of the QRS or QT intervals on the ECG. Prolongation of the PR interval is also significant, but less closely correlated with plasma levels. Clinical symptoms of intolerance, especially drowsiness, dizziness, and postural hypotension, should also alert the physician to the need for reduction in dosage. Plasma desipramine measurement would constitute the optimal guide to dosage monitoring.
Initial therapy may be administered in divided doses or a single daily dose.
Maintenance therapy may be given on a once-daily schedule for patient convenience and compliance.

Adolescent and Geriatric Dose

The usual adolescent and geriatric dose is 25 to 100 mg daily. Dosage should be initiated at a lower level and increased according to tolerance and clinical response to a usual maximum of 100 mg daily. In more severely ill patients, dosage may be further increased to 150 mg/day. Doses above 150 mg/day are not recommended in these age groups.
Initial therapy may be administered in divided doses or a single daily dose.
Maintenance therapy may be given on a once-daily schedule for patient convenience and compliance.

HOW SUPPLIED

10 mg blue coated tablets imprinted 68-7
NDC 0068-0007-01: bottles of 100
25 mg yellow coated tablets imprinted NORPRAMIN 25
NDC 0068-0011-01: bottles of 100
NDC 0068-0011-61: unit dose dispenser of 100
50 mg green coated tablets imprinted NORPRAMIN 50
NDC 0068-0015-01: bottles of 100
NDC 0068-0015-61: unit dose dispenser of 100
75 mg orange coated tablets imprinted NORPRAMIN 75
NDC 0068-0019-01: bottles of 100
100 mg peach coated tablets imprinted NORPRAMIN 100
NDC 0068-0020-01: bottles of 100
150 mg white coated tablets imprinted NORPRAMIN 150
NDC 0068-0021-50: bottles of 50
NORPRAMIN tablets should be stored at room temperature, preferably below 86°F (30°C). Protect from excessive heat.
Prescribing Information as of January 1996
Merrell Pharmaceuticals Inc.
Subsidiary of Hoechst Marion Roussel, Inc.
Kansas City, MO 64137 USA
Shown in Product Identification Guide, page 317

PENTASA® ℞
[pen-tas'a]
(mesalamine)
Controlled-Release Capsules 250 mg
Prescribing information as of August 1995

DESCRIPTION

PENTASA (mesalamine) for oral administration is a controlled-release formulation of mesalamine, an aminosalicylate anti-inflammatory agent for gastrointestinal use.
Chemically, mesalamine is 5-amino-2-hydroxybenzoic acid. It has a molecular weight of 153.14.
The structural formula is:

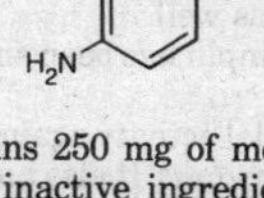

Each capsule contains 250 mg of mesalamine. It also contains the following inactive ingredients: acetylated monoglyceride, castor oil, colloidal silicon dioxide, ethylcellulose, hydroxypropyl methylcellulose, starch, stearic acid, sugar, talc, and white wax. The capsule shell contains D&C Yellow #10, FD&C Blue #1, FD&C Green #3, gelatin, titanium dioxide, and other ingredients.

CLINICAL PHARMACOLOGY

Sulfasalazine is split by bacterial action in the colon into sulfapyridine (SP) and mesalamine (5-ASA). It is thought that the mesalamine component is therapeutically active in ulcerative colitis. The usual oral dose of sulfasalazine for active ulcerative colitis in adults is 2 to 4 g per day in divided doses. Four grams of sulfasalazine provide 1.6 g of free mesalamine to the colon.
The mechanism of action of mesalamine (and sulfasalazine) is unknown, but appears to be topical rather than systemic. Mucosal production of arachidonic acid (AA) metabolites, both through the cyclooxygenase pathways, ie, prostanoids, and through the lipoxygenase pathways, ie, leukotnenes (LTs) and hydroxyeicosatetraenoic acids (HETEs), is increased in patients with chronic inflammatory bowel disease, and it is possible that mesalamine diminishes inflammation by blocking cycloxygenase and inhibiting prostaglandin (PG) production in the colon.

Human Pharmacokinetics and Metabolism

Absorption. PENTASA is an ethylcellulose-coated, controlled-release formulation of mesalamine designed to release therapeutic quantities of mesalamine throughout the gastrointestinal tract. Based on urinary excretion data, 20% to 30% of the mesalamine in PENTASA is absorbed. In contrast, when mesalamine is administered orally as an unformulated 1-g aqueous suspension, mesalamine is approximately 80% absorbed.
Plasma mesalamine concentration peaked at approximately 1 μg/mL 3 hours following a 1-g PENTASA dose and declined in a biphasic manner. The literature describes a mean terminal half-life of 42 minutes for mesalamine following intravenous administration. Because of the continuous release and absorption of mesalamine from PENTASA throughout the gastrointestinal tract, the true elimination half-life cannot be determined after oral administration. N-acetylmesalamine, the major metabolite of mesalamine, peaked at approximately 3 hours at 1.8 μg/mL, and its concentration followed a biphasic decline. Phamacological activities of N-acetylmesalamine are unknown, and other metabolites have not been identified.
Oral mesalamine pharmacokinetics were nonlinear when PENTASA capsules were dosed from 250 mg to 1 g four times daily, with steadystate mesalamine plasma concentrations increasing about nine times, from 0.14 μg/mL to 1.21 μg/mL, suggesting saturable first-pass metabolism. N-acetylmesalamine pharmacokinetics were linear.
Elimination. About 130 mg free mesalamine was recovered in the feces following a single 1-g PENTASA dose, which was comparable to the 140 mg of mesalamine recovered from the molar equivalent sulfasalazine tablet dose of 2.5 g. Elimination of free mesalamine and salicylates in feces increased proportionately with PENTASA dose. N-acetylmesalamine was the primary compound excreted in the urine (19% to 30%) following PENTASA dosing.

CLINICAL TRIALS

In two randomized, double-blind, placebo-controlled, dose-response trials (UC-1 and UC-2) of 625 patients with active mild to moderate ulcerative colitis, PENTASA, at an oral dose of 4 g/day given 1 g four times daily, produced consistent improvement in prospectively identified primary efficacy parameters, PGA, Tx F, and Sl as shown in the table below.
The 4-g dose of PENTASA also gave consistent improvement in secondary efficacy parameters, namely the frequency of trips to the toilet, stool consistency, rectal bleeding, abdominal/rectal pain, and urgency. The 4-g dose of PENTASA induced remission as assessed by endoscopic and symptomatic endpoints.
In some patients, the 2-g dose of PENTASA was observed to improve efficacy parameters measured. However, the 2-g dose gave inconsistent results in primary efficacy parameters across the two adequate and well-controlled trials.

	Clinical Trial UC-1			Clinical Trial UC-2		
		PENTASA			PENTASA	
Parameter Evaluated	PL (n=90)	4 g/day (n=95)	2 g/day (n=97)	PL (n=83)	4 g/day (n=85)	2 g/day (n=83)
PGA	36%	59%*	57%*	31%	55%*	41%
Tx F	22%	9%*	18%	31%	9%*	17%*
SI	−2.5	−5.0*	−4.3*	−1.6	−3.8*	−2.6
Remission†	12%	26%*	24%*	12%	27%*	12%

* p <0.05 vs placebo.
PGA: Physician Global Assessment: proportion of patients with complete or marked improvement.
Tx F: Treatment Failure: proportion of patients developing severe or fulminant UC requiring steroid therapy or hospitalization or worsening of the disease at 7 days of therapy, or lack of significant improvement by 14 days of therapy.
SI: Sigmoidoscopic Index: an objective measure of disease activity rated by a standard (15-point) scale that includes mucosal vascular pattern, erythema, friability, granularity/ulcerations, and mucopus: improvement over baseline.
† Defined as complete resolution of symptoms plus improvement of endoscopic endpoints. To be considered in remission, patients had a "1" score for one of the endoscopic components (mucosal vascular pattern, erythema, granularity, or friability) and "0" for the others.

INDICATIONS AND USAGE

PENTASA is indicated for the induction of remission and for the treatment of patients with mildly to moderately active ulcerative colitis.

CONTRAINDICATIONS

PENTASA is contraindicated in patients who have demonstrated hypersensitivity to mesalamine, any other components of this medication, or salicylates.

PRECAUTIONS

General

Caution should be exercised if PENTASA is administered to patients with impaired hepatic function.
Mesalamine has been associated with an acute intolerance syndrome that may be difficult to distinguish from a flare of inflammatory bowel disease. Although the exact frequency of occurrence cannot be ascertained, it has occurred in 3% of patients in controlled clinical trials of mesalamine or sulfasalazine. Symptoms include cramping, acute abdominal pain and bloody diarrhea, sometimes fever, headache, and rash. If acute intolerance syndrome is suspected, prompt withdrawal is required. If a rechallenge is performed later in order to validate the hypersensitivity, it should be carried out under close medical supervision at reduced dose and only if clearly needed.

Renal

Caution should be exercised if PENTASA is administered to patients with impaired renal function. Single reports of nephrotic syndrome and interstitial nephritis associated with mesalamine therapy have been described in the foreign literature. There have been rare reports of interstitial nephritis in patients receiving PENTASA. In animal studies, a 13-week oral toxicity study in mice and 13-week and 52-week oral toxicity studies in rats and cynomolgus monkeys have shown the kidney to be the major target organ of mesalamine toxicity. Oral daily doses of 2400 mg/kg in mice and 1150 mg/kg in rats produced renal lesions including granular and hyaline casts, tubular degeneration, tubular dilation, renal infarct, papillary necrosis, tubular necrosis, and interstitial nephritis. In cynomolgus monkeys, oral daily doses of 250 mg/kg or higher produced nephrosis, papillary edema, and interstitial fibrosis. Patients with preexisting renal disease, increased BUN or serum creatinine, or proteinuria should be carefully monitored.

Carcinogenesis, Mutagenesis, Impairment of Fertility

Long-term studies of the carcinogenic potential of mesalamine in mice and rats are ongoing. No evidence of mutagenicity was observed in an in vitro Ames test and in an in vivo mouse micronucleus test. No effects on fertility or reproductive performance were observed in male or female rats at doses up to 400 mg/kg/day (2360 mg/M^2). For a 50-kg person (1.3 M^2 body surface area), this represents five times the recommended clinical dose (80 mg/kg/day) on a mg/kg basis and 0.8 times the clinical dose (2960 mg/M^2) on body surface area basis.
Semen abnomalities and infertility in men, which have been reported in association with sulfasalazine, have not been seen with PENTASA capsules during controlled clinical trials.

Pregnancy

Category B. Reproduction studies have been performed in rats at doses up to 1000 mg/kg/day (5900 mg/M^2) and rabbits at doses of 800 mg/kg/day (6856 mg/M^2) and have revealed no evidence of teratogenic effects or harm to the fetus due to mesalamine. There are, however, no adequate and well-controlled studies in pregnant women. Because animal reproduction studies are not always predictive of human response, PENTASA should be used during pregnancy only if clearly needed.
Mesalamine is known to cross the placental barrier.

Nursing Mothers

Minute quantities of mesalamine were distributed to breast milk and amniotic fluid of pregnant women following sulfasalazine therapy. When treated with sulfasalazine at a dose equivalent to 1.25 g/day of mesalamine, 0.02 μg/mL to 0.08 μg/mL and trace amounts of mesalamine were measured in amniotic fluid and breast milk, respectively. N-acetylmesalamine, in quantities of 0.07 μg/mL to 0.77 μg/mL and 1.13 μg/mL to 3.44 μg/mL, was identified in the same fluids, respectively.
Caution should be exercised when PENTASA is administered to a nursing woman.

Pediatric Use

Safety and efficacy of PENTASA in pediatric patients have not been established.

ADVERSE REACTIONS

In combined domestic and foreign clinical trials, more than 2100 patients with ulcerative colitis or Crohn's disease received PENTASA therapy. Generally, PENTASA therapy was well tolerated. The most common events (ie, greater than or equal to 1%) were diarrhea (3.4%), headache (2.0%),

Continued on next page

Hoechst Marion Roussel—Cont.

nausea (1.8%), abdominal pain (1.7%), dyspepsia (1.6%), vomiting (1.5%), and rash (1.0%).

In two domestic placebo-controlled trials involving over 600 ulcerative colitis patients, adverse events were fewer in PENTASA-treated patients than in the placebo group (PENTASA 14% vs placebo 18%) and were not dose-related. Events occurring at 1% or more are shown in the table below. Of these, only nausea and vomiting were more frequent in the PENTASA group. Withdrawal from therapy due to adverse events was more common on placebo than PENTASA (7% vs 4%).

Table 1. Adverse Events Occurring In More Than 1% of Either Placebo or PENTASA Patients in Domestic Placebo-controlled Ulcerative Colitis Trials. (PENTASA Comparison to Placebo)

Event	PENTASA n=451	Placebo n=173
Diarrhea	16 (3.5%)	13 (7.5%)
Headache	10 (2.2%)	6 (3.5%)
Nausea	14 (3.1%)	—
Abdominal Pain	5 (1.1%)	7 (4.0%)
Melena (Bloody Diarrhea)	4 (0.9%)	6 (3.5%)
Rash	6 (1.3%)	2 (1.2%)
Anorexia	5 (1.1%)	2 (1.2%)
Fever	4 (0.9%)	2 (1.2%)
Rectal Urgency	1 (0.2%)	4 (2.3%)
Nausea and Vomiting	5 (1.1%)	—
Worsening of Ulcerative Colitis	2 (0.4%)	2 (1.2%)
Acne	1 (0.2%)	2 (1.2%)

Clinical laboratory measurements showed no significant abnormal trends for any test, including measurement of hematologic, liver, and kidney function.

The following adverse events, presented by body system, were reported infrequently (ie, less than 1%) during domestic ulcerative colitis and Crohn's disease trials. In many cases, the relationship to PENTASA has not been established.

Gastrointestinal: abdominal distention, anorexia, constipation, duodenal ulcer, dysphagia, eructation, esophageal ulcer, fecal incontinence, GGTP increase, GI bleeding, increased alkaline phosphatase, LDH increase, mouth ulcer, oral moniliases, pancreatitis, rectal bleeding, SGOT increase, SGPT increase, stool abnormalities (color or texture change), thirst

Dermatological: acne, alopecia, dry skin, eczema, erythema nodosum, nail disorder, photosensitivity, pruritus, sweating, urticaria

Nervous System: depression, dizziness, insomnia, somnolence, paresthesia

Cardiovascular: palpitations, pericarditis, vasodilation

Other: albuminuria, amenorrhea, amylase increase, arthralgia, astheria, breast pain, conjunctivitis, ecchymosis, edema, fever, hematuria, hypomenorrhea, Kawasaki-like syndrome, leg cramps, lichen planus, lipase increase, malaise, menorrhagia, metrorrhagia, myalgia, pulmonary infiltrates, thrombocythemia, thrombocytopenia, urinary frequency

One week after completion of an 8-week ulcerative colitis study, a 72-year-old male, with no previous history of pulmonary problems, developed dyspnea. The patient was subsequently diagnosed with interstitial pulmonary fibrosis without eosinophilia by one physician and bronchiolitis obliterans with organizing pneumonitis by a second physician. A causal relationship between this event and mesalamine therapy has not been established.

Published case reports and/or spontaneous postmarketing surveillance have described infrequent instances of pericarditis, fatal myocarditis, chest pain and T-wave abnormalities, hypersensitivity pneumonitis, pancreatitis, nephrotic syndrome, intersititial nephritis, hepatitis, aplastic anemia, pancytopenia, leukopenia, or anemia while receiving mesalamine therapy. Anemia can be a part of the clinical presentation of inflammatory bowel disease.

OVERDOSAGE

Single oral doses of mesalamine up to 5 g/kg in pigs or a single intravenous dose of mesalamine at 920 mg/kg in rats were not lethal.

There is no clinical experience with PENTASA overdosage. PENTASA is an aminosalicylate, and symptoms of salicylate toxicity may be possible, such as: tinnitus, vertigo, headache, confusion, drowsiness, sweating, hyperventilation, vomiting, and diarrhea. Severe intoxication with salicylates can lead to disruption of electrolyte balance and blood pH, hyperthermia, and dehydration.

Treatment of Overdosage. Since PENTASA is an aminosalicylate, conventional therapy for salicylate toxicity may be beneficial in the event of acute overdosage. This includes prevention of further gastrointestinal tract absorption by emesis and, if necessary, by gastric lavage. Fluid and electrolyte imbalance should be corrected by the administration of appropriate intravenous therapy. Adequate renal function should be maintained.

DOSAGE AND ADMINISTRATION

The recommended dosage for the induction of remission and the symptomatic treatment of mildly to moderately active ulcerative colitis is 1 g (4 PENTASA capsules) four times a day for a total daily dose of 4 g. Treatment duration in controlled trials was up to 8 weeks.

HOW SUPPLIED

PENTASA controlled-release capsules are supplied in bottles of 240 capsules (NDC 0088-2010-46); and blister packs of 80 capsules (NDC 0088-2010-80). Each green and blue capsule contains 250 mg of mesalamine in controlled-release beads. PENTASA controlled-release capsules are identified with a pentagonal starburst logo and the number 2010 on the green portion and PENTASA 250 mg and the Marion Merrell Dow Inc. logo on the blue portion of the capsules.

Store at room temperature 59–86°F (15–30°C).

Prescribing Information as of August 1995.

Hoechst Marion Roussel, Inc.
Kansas City, MO 64137 USA

Licensed U.S. Patent Nos. B1 4,496,553 and 4,980,173

Shown in Product Identification Guide, page 317

RIFADIN® ℞
[rif 'uh-din]
(rifampin capsules)
and
RIFADIN® I.V.
(rifampin for injection)

Prescribing information as of May 1995

DESCRIPTION

RIFADIN (rifampin) capsules for oral administration contain 150 mg or 300 mg rifampin per capsule. The 150 mg and 300 mg capsules also contain, as inactive ingredients: corn starch, D&C Red No. 28, FD&C Blue No. 1, FD&C Red No. 40, gelatin, magnesium stearate, and titanium dioxide.

RIFADIN I.V. (rifampin for injection) contains rifampin 600 mg, sodium formaldehyde sulfoxylate 10 mg, and sodium hydroxide to adjust pH.

Rifampin is a semisynthetic antibiotic derivative of rifamycin B. The chemical name for rifampin is 3-(4-methyl-1piperazinyl-iminomethyl)-rifamycin SV. Its chemical structure is:

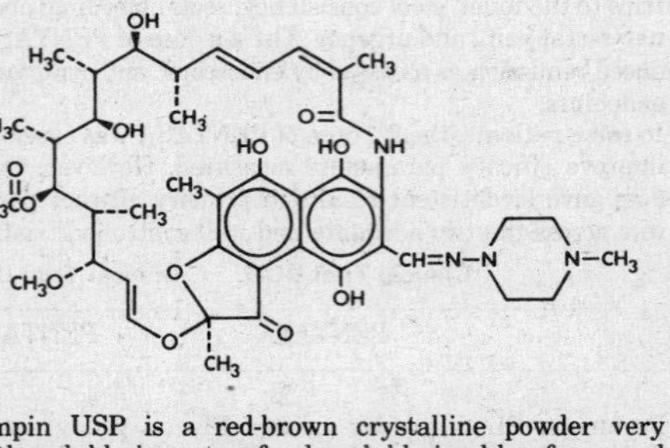

Rifampin USP is a red-brown crystalline powder very slightly soluble in water, freely soluble in chloroform, and soluble in ethyl acetate and in methanol. Its molecular weight is 822.95.

CLINICAL PHARMACOLOGY

Human Pharmacology—Oral. Rifampin is readily absorbed from the gastrointestinal tract. Peak blood levels in normal adults vary widely from individual to individual. The peak level averages 7 μg/mL but may vary from 4 to 32 μg/mL. Absorption of rifampin is reduced when the drug is ingested with food.

In normal subjects, the biological half-life of rifampin in serum averages about 3 hours after a 600 mg oral dose, with increases up to 5.1 hours reported after a 900 mg dose. With repeated administration, the half-life decreases and reaches average values of approximately 2–3 hours. It does not differ in patients with renal failure at doses not exceeding 600 mg daily and, consequently, no dosage adjustment is required. Refer to WARNINGS for information regarding patients with hepatic insufficiency.

After absorption, rifampin is rapidly eliminated in the bile, and an enterohepatic circulation ensues. During this process, rifampin undergoes progressive deacetylation so that nearly all the drug in the bile is in this form in about 6 hours. This metabolite is microbiologically active. Intestinal reabsorption is reduced by deacetylation, and elimination is facilitated. Up to 30% of a dose is excreted in the urine, with about half of this being unchanged drug.

Rifampin is widely distributed throughout the body. It is present in effective concentrations in many organs and body fluids, including cerebrospinal fluid. Rifampin is about 80% protein bound. Most of the unbound fraction is not ionized and therefore diffuses freely into tissues.

Serum Levels in Pediatric Patients. In one recent study, pediatric patients 6–58 months old were given rifampin suspended in simple syrup or as dry powder mixed with applesauce at a dose of 10 mg/kg body weight. Peak serum levels of 10.7 and 11.5 μg/mL were obtained 1 hour after preprandial ingestion of the drug suspension and the applesauce mixture, respectively. The calculated $t_{1/2}$ for both preparations was 2.9 hrs. It should be noted that in other studies in pediatric populations, at doses of 10 mg/kg body weight, mean peak serum levels of 3.5 μg/mL to 15 μg/mL have been reported.

Human Pharmacology—I.V. After intravenous administration of a 300 or 600 mg dose of rifampin infused over 30 minutes to healthy male volunteers (n=11), mean peak plasma concentrations were 9.0 and 17.5 μg/mL, respectively. The average plasma concentrations in these volunteers remained detectable for 8 and 12 hours, respectively (see table).

Plasma Concentrations (μg/mL) Rifampin Dosage I.V.	30 min	1 hr	2 hr	4 hr	8 hr	12 hr
300 mg	8.9	4.9	4.0	2.5	<2	<2
600 mg	17.4	11.7	9.4	6.4	3.5	<2

Plasma concentrations after the 600 mg dose, which were disproportionately higher (up to 50% greater than expected) than those found after the 300 mg dose, indicated that the elimination of larger doses was not as rapid.

After repeated once-a-day infusions (3 hr duration) of 600 mg in patients (n=5) for 7 days, concentrations of I.V. rifampin decreased from 5.8 μg/mL 8 hours after the infusion on day 1 to 2.6 μg/mL 8 hours after the infusion on day 7.

The rifampin dose is widely distributed throughout the body. It is present in effective concentrations in many organs and body fluids, including cerebrospinal fluid. Rifampin is about 80% protein bound. Most of the unbound fraction is not ionized and therefore diffuses freely into tissues.

Rifampin is rapidly eliminated in the bile and undergoes progressive enterohepatic circulation and deacetylation to the primary metabolite, 25-desacetyl-rifampin. This metabolite is microbiologically active. Less than 30% of the dose is excreted as rifampin or metabolites. Serum concentrations do not differ in patients with renal failure and, consequently, no dosage adjustment is required.

Serum Concentrations of Rifampin in Pediatric Patients. In patients 0.25 to 12.8 years old (n=12), the mean peak serum concentration of rifampin at the end of a 30 minute infusion of approximately 300 mg/m^2 was 26 μg/mL. In these patients, peak concentrations 1 to 4 days after initiation of therapy ranged from 11.7 to 41.5 μg/mL; peak concentrations 5 to 14 days after initiation of therapy were 13.6 to 37.4 μg/mL. The serum half-life of rifampin decreased significantly from 1.34 to 3.24 hours early in therapy to 1.17 to 3.19 hours 5 to 14 days after therapy was initiated.

Microbiology. Rifampin inhibits DNA-dependent RNA polymerase activity in susceptible cells. Specifically, it interacts with bacterial RNA polymerase but does not inhibit the mammalian enzyme. Rifampin is particularly active against rapidly growing extracellular organisms but has been demonstrated to have intracellular bactericidal activity against susceptible organisms as well.

Cross-resistance to rifampin has been shown only with other rifamycins.

Rifampin has bactericidal activity against slow and intermittently growing *M. tuberculosis.* It also has significant activity against *Neisseria meningitidis* (see INDICATIONS AND USAGE).

In the treatment of both tuberculosis and the meningococcal carrier state (see INDICATIONS AND USAGE), the small number of resistant cells present within large populations of susceptible cells can rapidly become predominant. In addition, resistance to rifampin has been determined to occur as single-step mutations of the DNA-dependent RNA polymerase. Since resistance can emerge rapidly, appropriate susceptibility tests should be performed in the event of persistent positive cultures.

Rifampin has been shown to have initial in vitro activity against the following organisms; however, clinical efficacy has not been established (see INDICATIONS AND USAGE): *Mycobacterium leprae, Haemophilus influenzae, Staphylococcus aureus,* and *Staphylococcus epidermidis.* Both penicillinase-producing and non-penicillinase-producing strains, and β-lactam resistant staphylococci (Methicillin Resistant *S. aureus*/MRSA) are initially susceptible to rifampin in vitro.

Susceptibility Testing. Use only diagnostic products and methods approved by the Food and Drug Administration for rifampin susceptibility testing of *Mycobacterium tuberculosis*

and *Neisseria meningitidis*. Consult the Food and Drug Administration-approved labeling of the diagnostic products for interpretation criteria and quality control parameters.

For the other organisms listed in the microbiology subsection of the labeling, in vitro susceptibility testing should be assessed by standardized methods developed by the National Committee for Clinical Laboratory Standards.

INDICATIONS AND USAGE

Tuberculosis: Rifampin is indicated in the treatment of all forms of tuberculosis. Rifadin® (rifampin) must always be used in conjunction with at least one other antituberculosis drug. Frequently used regimens are rifampin and isoniazid; rifampin, isoniazid, and pyrazinamide; rifampin, isoniazid, and ethambutol; and rifampin and ethambutol.

Rifadin I.V. is indicated for the initial treatment and retreatment of tuberculosis when the drug cannot be taken by mouth.

Meningococcal Carriers: Rifampin is indicated for the treatment of asymptomatic carriers of *N. meningitidis* to eliminate meningococci from the nasopharynx. *Rifampin is not indicated for the treatment of meningococcal infection because of the possibility of the rapid emergence of resistant organisms.* (See WARNINGS.)

Rifampin should not be used indiscriminately, and therefore diagnostic laboratory procedures, including serotyping and susceptibility testing, should be performed for establishment of the carrier state and the correct treatment. So that the usefulness of rifampin in the treatment of asymptomatic meningococcal carriers is preserved, the drug should be used only when the risk of meningococcal disease is high.

In the treatment of both tuberculosis and the meningococcal carrier state, the small number of resistant cells present within large populations of susceptible cells can rapidly become predominant. Since resistance can emerge rapidly, susceptibility tests should be performed in the event of persistent positive cultures.

CONTRAINDICATIONS

Rifampin is contraindicated in patients with a history of hypersensitivity to any of the rifamycins. (See WARNINGS.)

WARNINGS

Rifampin has been shown to produce liver dysfunction. Fatalities associated with jaundice have occurred in patients with liver disease and in patients taking rifampin with other hepatotoxic agents. Patients with impaired liver function should only be given rifampin in cases of necessity and then with caution and under strict medical supervision.

In these patients, careful monitoring of liver function, especially serum glutamic pyruvic transaminase (SGPT) and serum glutamic oxaloacetic transaminase (SGOT) should be carried out prior to therapy and then every two to four weeks during therapy. If signs of hepatocellular damage occur, rifampin should be withdrawn.

In some cases, hyperbilirubinemia resulting from competition between rifampin and bilirubin for excretory pathways of the liver at the cell level can occur in the early days of treatment. An isolated report showing a moderate rise in bilirubin and/or transaminase level is not in itself an indication for interrupting treatment; rather, the decision should be made after repeating the tests, noting trends in the levels, and considering them in conjunction with the patient's clinical condition.

Rifampin has enzyme-inducing properties, including induction of delta amino levulinic acid synthetase. Isolated reports have associated porphyria exacerbation with rifampin administration.

The possibility of rapid emergence of resistant meningococci restricts the use of RIFADIN to short-term treatment of the asymptomatic carrier state. *RIFADIN is not to be used for the treatment of meningococcal disease.*

PRECAUTIONS

General. For the treatment of tuberculosis, rifampin is usually administered on a daily basis. High doses of rifampin (greater than 600 mg) given once or twice weekly have resulted in a high incidence of adverse reactions, including the "flu syndrome" (fever, chills and malaise), hematopoietic reactions (leukopenia, thrombocytopenia, or acute hemolytic anemia), cutaneous, gastrointestinal, and hepatic reactions, shortness of breath, shock, and renal failure. Recent studies indicate that regimens using twice-weekly doses of rifampin 600 mg plus isoniazid 15 mg/kg are much better tolerated.

Intermittent therapy may be used if the patient cannot or will not self-administer drugs on a daily basis. Patients on intermittent therapy should be closely monitored for compliance and cautioned against intentional or accidental interruption of prescribed therapy because of the increased risk of serious adverse reactions.

RIFADIN I.V.

For intravenous infusion only. Must not be administered by intramuscular or subcutaneous route. Avoid extravasation during injection; local irritation and inflammation due to extravascular infiltration of the infusion have been observed. If these occur, the infusion should be discontinued and restarted at another site.

Information for Patients. The patient should be told that this medication may cause the urine, feces, saliva, sputum, sweat, and tears to turn red-orange. Permanent discoloration of soft contact lenses may occur.

The patient should be advised that the reliability of oral contraceptives may be affected; consideration should be given to using alternative contraceptive measures.

Laboratory Tests. A complete blood count (CBC) should be obtained prior to instituting therapy and periodically throughout the course of therapy. Because of a possible transient rise in transaminase and bilirubin values, blood for baseline clinical chemistries should be obtained before rifampin dosing.

Drug Interactions. Rifampin has liver enzyme-inducing properties and may reduce the activity of a number of drugs, including anticoagulants, corticosteroids, cyclosporine, cardiac glycoside preparations, quinidine, oral contraceptives, oral hypoglycemic agents (sulfonylureas), dapsone, narcotics, and analgesics. Rifampin also has been reported to diminish the effects of concurrently administered methadone, barbiturates, diazepam, verapamil, beta-adrenergic blockers, clofibrate, progestins, disopyramide, mexiletine, theophylline, chloramphenicol, and anticonvulsants. It may be necessary to adjust the dosages of these drugs if they are given concurrently with rifampin.

Patients using oral contraceptives should be advised to change to nonhormonal methods of birth control during rifampin therapy. Also, diabetes may become more difficult to control.

When rifampin is taken with paraaminosalicylic acid (PAS), rifampin levels in the serum may decrease. Therefore, the drugs should be taken at least 8 hours apart.

Probenecid has been reported to increase rifampin blood levels. Halothane, when given concomitantly with rifampin, has been reported to increase the hepatotoxicity of both drugs.

Ketoconazole, when given concomitantly with rifampin, has been reported to diminish the serum concentrations of both drugs. Dosage should be adjusted if indicated by the patient's clinical condition. An interaction has also been reported with rifampin-isoniazid and Vitamin D.

Drug/Laboratory Interactions. Therapeutic levels of rifampin have been shown to inhibit standard microbiological assays for serum folate and Vitamin B_{12}. Thus, alternate assay methods should be considered. Transient abnormalities in liver function tests (e.g., elevation in serum bilirubin, abnormal bromsulphalein (BSP) excretion, alkaline phosphatase, and serum transaminases), and reduced biliary excretion of contrast media used for visualization of the gallbladder have also been observed. Therefore, these tests should be performed before the morning dose of rifampin.

Carcinogenesis, Mutagenesis, Impairment of Fertility. There are no known human data on long-term potential for carcinogenicity, mutagenicity, or impairment of fertility. A few cases of accelerated growth of lung carcinoma have been reported in man, but a causal relationship with the drug has not been established. An increase in the incidence of hepatomas in female mice (of a strain known to be particularly susceptible to the spontaneous development of hepatomas) was observed when rifampin was administered in doses 2 to 10 times the average daily human dose for 60 weeks followed by an observation period of 46 weeks. No evidence of carcinogenity was found in male mice of the same strain, mice of a different strain, or rats, under similar experimental conditions.

Rifampin has been reported to possess immunosuppressive potential in rabbits, mice, rats, guinea pigs, human lymphocytes in vitro, and humans. Antitumor activity in vitro has also been shown with rifampin.

There was no evidence of mutagenicity in bacteria, *Drosophila melanogaster*, or mice, nor did rifampin induce chromosome aberrations in human lymphocytes treated in vitro. However, an increase in chromatid breaks was noted when whole-blood cell cultures were treated with rifampin.

Pregnancy—Teratogenic Effects. Pregnancy—Category C: Rifampin has been shown to be teratogenic in rodents given oral doses of rifampin 15 to 25 times the human dose. Although rifampin has been reported to cross the placental barrier and appear in cord blood, the effect of RIFADIN, alone or in combination with other antituberculosis drugs, on the human fetus is not known. Neonates of rifampin-treated mothers should be carefully observed for any evidence of adverse effects. Isolated cases of fetal malformations have been reported; however, there are no adequate and well-controlled studies in pregnant women. Rifampin should be used during pregnancy only if the potential benefit justifies the potential risk to the fetus. Rifampin in oral doses of 150 to 250 mg/kg produced teratogenic effects in mice and rats. Malformations were primarily cleft palate in the mouse and spina bifida in the rat. The incidence of these anomalies was dose-dependent. When rifampin was given to pregnant rabbits in doses up to 20 times the usual daily human dose, imperfect osteogenesis and embryotoxicity were reported.

When administered during the last few weeks of pregnancy, rifampin can cause post-natal hemorrhages in the mother and infant for which treatment with Vitamin K may be indicated.

Nursing Mothers. Because of the potential for tumorigenicity shown for rifampin in animal studies, a decision should be made whether to discontinue nursing or discontinue the drug, taking into account the importance of the drug to the mother.

Pediatric Use—See CLINICAL PHARMACOLOGY—Serum Levels in Pediatric Patients; see also DOSAGE AND ADMINISTRATION.

ADVERSE REACTIONS

Gastrointestinal. Heartburn, epigastric distress, anorexia, nausea, vomiting, jaundice, flatulence, cramps, and diarrhea have been noted in some patients. Although *C. difficile* has been shown in vitro to be sensitive to rifampin, pseudomembranous colitis has been reported with the use of rifampin (and other broad spectrum antibiotics). Therefore, it is important to consider this diagnosis in patients who develop diarrhea in association with antibiotic use. Rarely, hepatitis or a shock-like syndrome with hepatic involvement and abnormal liver function tests has been reported.

Hematologic. Thrombocytopenia has occurred primarily with high dose intermittent therapy, but has also been noted after resumption of interrupted treatment. It rarely occurs during well supervised daily therapy. This effect is reversible if the drug is discontinued as soon as purpura occurs. Cerebral hemorrhage and fatalities have been reported when rifampin administration has been continued or resumed after the appearance of purpura.

Transient leukopenia, hemolytic anemia, and decreased hemoglobin have been observed.

Central Nervous System. Headache, fever, drowsiness, fatigue, ataxia, dizziness, inability to concentrate, mental confusion, behavioral changes, muscular weakness, pains in extremities, and generalized numbness have been observed. Rare reports of myopathy have also been observed.

Ocular. Visual disturbances have been observed.

Endocrine. Menstrual disturbances have been observed.

Renal. Elevations in BUN and serum uric acid have been reported. Rarely, hemolysis, hemoglobinuria, hematuria, interstitial nephritis, renal insufficiency, and acute renal failure have been noted. These are generally considered to be hypersensitivity reactions. They usually occur during intermittent therapy or when treatment is resumed following intentional or accidental interruption of a daily dosage regimen, and are reversible when rifampin is discontinued and appropriate therapy instituted.

Dermatologic. Cutaneous reactions are mild and self-limiting and do not appear to be hypersensitivity reactions. Typically, they consist of flushing and itching with or without a rash. More serious cutaneous reactions which may be due to hypersensitivity occur but are uncommon.

Hypersensitivity Reactions. Occasionally, pruritus, urticaria, rash, pemphigoid reaction, eosinophilia, sore mouth, sore tongue, and conjunctivitis have been observed.

Miscellaneous. Edema of the face and extremities has been reported. Other reactions reported to have occurred with intermittent dosage regimens include "flu" syndrome (such as episodes of fever, chills, headache, dizziness, and bone pain), shortness of breath, wheezing, decrease in blood pressure, and shock. The "flu" syndrome may also appear if rifampin is taken irregularly by the patient or if daily administration is resumed after a drug free interval.

OVERDOSAGE

Signs and Symptoms. Nausea, vomiting, and increasing lethargy will probably occur within a short time after ingestion; unconsciousness may occur when there is severe hepatic disease. Brownish-red or orange discoloration of the skin, urine, sweat, saliva, tears, and feces will occur, and its intensity is proportional to the amount ingested.

Liver enlargement, possibly with tenderness, may develop within a few hours after severe overdosage; jaundice may develop rapidly. Hepatic involvement may be more marked in patients with prior impairment of hepatic function. Other physical findings remain essentially normal.

Bilirubin levels may increase rapidly with severe overdosage; hepatic enzyme levels may be affected, especially with prior impairment of hepatic function. A direct effect upon the hematopoietic system, electrolyte levels, or acid-base balance is unlikely.

Acute Toxicity. In animal studies, the LD_{50} of rifampin is approximately 885 mg/kg in the mouse, 1720 mg/kg in the rat, and 2120 mg/kg in the rabbit.

Non-fatal overdoses with as high as 12 g of rifampin have been reported. In one patient who swallowed 12 g of rifampin, vomiting occurred four times within 1 hour of ingestion. Gastric lavage with 20 liters of water was initiated 5 hours after ingestion. Twelve hours after ingestion of rifampin, a plasma concentration of 400 μg of rifampin/mL was measured by microbiological assay. The plasma concentration fell to 64 μg/mL on the following day, and to 0.1 μg/mL on the third day. Urinary rifampin concentration was

Continued on next page

Hoechst Marion Roussel—Cont.

313 μg/mL approximately 30 hours after ingestion of the drug, 625 μg/mL after 36 hours, and 78 μg/mL after 40 hours. By the fourth day following the dose, only 0.1 μg/mL rifampin was present in the urine. There was biochemical evidence of mild impairment of liver function. Liver function tests had returned to normal within 5 days, and the patient's recovery was described as uneventful.
One case of fatal overdose is known: a 26-year-old man died after self-administering 60 g of rifampin.
Treatment. Since nausea and vomiting are likely to be present, gastric lavage is probably preferable to induction of emesis. Following evacuation of the gastric contents, the instillation of activated charcoal slurry into the stomach may help absorb any remaining drug from the gastrointestinal tract. Antiemetic medication may be required to control severe nausea and vomiting.
Active diuresis (with measured intake and output) will help promote excretion of the drug. Hemodialysis may be of value in some patients. In patients with previously adequate hepatic function, reversal of liver enlargement and of impaired hepatic excretory function probably will be noted within 72 hours, with a rapid return toward normal thereafter.

DOSAGE AND ADMINISTRATION

Rifampin can be administered by the oral route or by I.V. infusion (see INDICATIONS AND USAGE).

Tuberculosis

Adults: 600 mg in a single daily administration, oral or I.V.
Pediatric Patients: 10–20 mg/kg, not to exceed 600 mg/day, oral or I.V.
It is recommended that oral rifampin be administered once daily, either one hour before or two hours after a meal.
In the treatment of tuberculosis, rifampin should always be administered with at least one other antituberculosis drug.
In general, therapy for tuberculosis should be continued for 6 to 9 months or until at least 6 months have elapsed from conversion of sputum to culture negativity. In patients who cannot be relied on for compliance, intermittent therapy with 600 mg/day two or three times/week under close supervision may be prescribed and substituted for the daily regimen after 1–2 months of an initial daily phase of therapy.
The 9-Month Regimen ordinarily consists of rifampin and isoniazid, usually supplemented during the initial phase by pyrazinamide, streptomycin, or ethambutol.
The 6-Month Regimen ordinarily consists of an initial 2-month phase of rifampin, isoniazid and pyrazinamide, and, if clinically indicated, streptomycin or ethambutol, followed by 4 months of rifampin and isoniazid.
Either of the above regimens is recommended as standard therapy.
The above recommendations apply to patients with drug-susceptible organisms. Patients with drug-resistant organisms may require longer treatment with other drug regimens.

Meningococcal Carriers

Adults: For adults, it is recommended that 600 mg rifampin be administered twice daily for two days.
Pediatric Patients: Pediatric patients 1 month of age or older: 10 mg/kg every 12 hours for two days.
Pediatric patients under 1 month of age: 5 mg/kg every 12 hours for two days.

Preparation of Solution for I.V. Infusion

Reconstitute the lyophilized powder by transferring 10 mL of sterile water for injection to a vial containing 600 mg of rifampin for injection. Swirl vial gently to completely dissolve the antibiotic. The reconstituted solution contains 60 mg rifampin per mL and is stable at room temperature for 24 hours. Immediately prior to administration, withdraw from the reconstituted solution a volume equivalent to the amount of rifampin calculated to be administered and add to 500 mL of infusion medium. Mix well and infuse at a rate allowing for complete infusion in 3 hours. In some cases, the amount of rifampin calculated to be administered may be added to 100 mL of infusion medium and infused in 30 minutes. The 500 mL and 100 mL infusion solutions should be prepared and used within a total 4-hour period. Precipitation of rifampin from the infusion solution may occur beyond this time.

CAUTION: Dextrose 5% for injection is the recommended infusion medium. Sterile saline may be used when dextrose is contraindicated, but the stability of rifampin is slightly reduced. Other infusion media are not recommended.

Preparation of Extemporaneous Oral Suspension

For pediatric and adult patients in whom capsule swallowing is difficult or where lower doses are needed, a liquid suspension may be prepared as follows:

RIFADIN 1% w/v suspension (10 mg/mL) can be compounded using one of five syrups—Simple Syrup (Syrup NF), Simple Syrup (Humco Laboratories), Simple Syrup (Whiteworth Inc.), Wild Cherry Syrup (Eli Lilly and Company), and Syrpalta® Syrup (Emerson Laboratories).

1. Empty contents of four RIFADIN 300 mg capsules or eight RIFADIN 150 mg capsules onto a piece of weighing paper.
2. If necessary, gently crush the capsule contents with a spatula to produce a fine powder.
3. Transfer rifampin powder blend to a 4-ounce amber glass prescription bottle.
4. Rinse the paper and spatula with 20 mL of one of the above-mentioned syrups and add the rinse to the bottle. Shake vigorously.
5. Add 100 mL of syrup to the bottle and shake vigorously.

This compounding procedure results in a 1% w/v suspension containing 10 mg rifampin/mL. Stability studies indicate that the suspension is stable when stored at room temperature (25 ± 3°C) or in a refrigerator (2–8°C) for four weeks. This extemporaneously prepared suspension must be shaken well prior to administration.

HOW SUPPLIED

150 mg maroon and scarlet capsules imprinted "RIFADIN 150".
Bottles of 30 (NDC 0068-0510-30)
300 mg maroon and scarlet capsules imprinted "RIFADIN 300".
Bottles of 30 (NDC 0068-0508-30)
Bottles of 60 (NDC 0068-0508-60)
Bottles of 100 (NDC 0068-0508-61)
Storage: Keep tightly closed. Store in a dry place. Avoid excessive heat.
RIFADIN I.V. (rifampin for injection) is available in glass vials containing 600 mg rifampin (NDC 0068-0597-01).
Storage: Avoid excessive heat (temperatures above 40°C or 104°F). Protect from light.

1. National Committee for Clinical Laboratory Standards, Approved Standard: Performance Standards for Antimicrobial Disk Susceptibility Tests (M2-A2), Fourth Edition: Approved Standard (1990).
2. National Committee for Clinical Laboratory Standards, Approved Standard: Methods for Dilution-Antimicrobial Susceptibility Tests for Bacteria that Grow Aerobically (M7-A4), Second Edition: Approved Standard (1990).

Prescribing Information as of May 1995
Merrell Pharmaceuticals Inc.
Subsidiary of Hoechst Marion Roussel, Inc.
Kansas City, MO 64137
Rifadin I.V. (rifampin for injection) is manufactured by:
GRUPPO LEPETIT S.p.A.
20020 Lainate, Italy for
Merrell Pharmaceuticals Inc.
Subsidiary of Hoechst Marion Roussel, Inc.
Kansas City, MO 64137

Shown in Product Identification Guide, page 317

RIFAMATE® ℞

[*rĭf'uh-māt*]
(rifampin and isoniazid capsules)

> **WARNING**
> Severe and sometimes fatal hepatitis associated with isoniazid therapy may occur and may develop even after many months of treatment. The risk of developing hepatitis is age related. Approximate case rates by age are: 0 per 1,000 for persons under 20 years of age, 3 per 1,000 for persons in the 20–34 year age group, 12 per 1,000 for persons in the 35–49 year age group, 23 per 1,000 for persons in the 50–64 year age group, and 8 per 1,000 for persons over 65 years of age. The risk of hepatitis is increased with daily consumption of alcohol. Precise data to provide a fatality rate for isoniazid-related hepatitis is not available; however, in a U.S. Public Health Service Surveillance Study of 13,838 persons taking isoniazid, there were 8 deaths among 174 cases of hepatitis.
> Therefore, patients given isoniazid should be carefully monitored and interviewed at monthly intervals. Serum transaminase concentration becomes elevated in about 10–20 percent of patients, usually during the first few months of therapy, but it can occur at any time. Usually enzyme levels return to normal despite continuance of drug, but in some cases progressive liver dysfunction occurs. Patients should be instructed to report immediately any of the prodromal symptoms of hepatitis, such as fatigue, weakness, malaise, anorexia, nausea, or vomiting. If these symptoms appear or if signs suggestive of hepatic damage are detected, isoniazid should be discontinued promptly, since continued use of the drug in these cases has been reported to cause a more severe form of liver damage.
> Patients with tuberculosis should be given appropriate treatment with alternative drugs. If isoniazid must be reinstituted, it should be reinstituted only after symptoms and laboratory abnormalities have cleared. The drug should be restarted in very small and gradually increasing doses and should be withdrawn immediately if there is any indication of recurrent liver involvement.
> Treatment should be deferred in persons with acute hepatic diseases.

DESCRIPTION

RIFAMATE is a combination capsule containing 300 mg rifampin and 150 mg isoniazid. The capsules also contain as inactive ingredients: colloidal silicon dioxide, FD&C Blue No. 1, FD&C Red No. 40, gelatin, magnesium stearate, sodium starch glycolate, and titanium dioxide.
Rifampin is a semisynthetic antibiotic derivative of rifamycin B. The chemical name for rifampin is 3-(4-methyl-1-piperazinyl iminomethyl) rifamycin SV.
Isoniazid is the hydrazide of isonicotinic acid. It exists as colorless or white crystals or as a white, crystalline powder that is water soluble, odorless, and slowly affected by exposure to air and light.

ACTIONS

Rifampin

Rifampin inhibits DNA-dependent RNA polymerase activity in susceptible cells. Specifically, it interacts with bacterial RNA polymerase but does not inhibit the mammalian enzyme. This is the mechanism of action by which rifampin exerts its therapeutic effect. Rifampin cross resistance has only been shown with other rifamycins.
In a study of 14 normal human adult males, peak blood levels of rifampin occured 1 ½ to 3 hours following oral administration of two RIFAMATE capsules. The peaks ranged from 6.9 to 14 mcg/ml with an average of 10 mcg/ml.
In normal subjects the $T½$ (biological half-life) of rifampin in blood is approximately 3 hours. Elimination occurs mainly through the bile and, to a much lesser extent, the urine.

Isoniazid

Isoniazid acts against actively growing tubercle bacilli.
After oral administration isoniazid produces peak blood levels within 1 to 2 hours which decline to 50% or less within 6 hours. It diffuses readily into all body fluids (cerebrospinal, pleural, and ascitic fluids), tissues, organs and excreta (saliva, sputum, and feces). The drug also passes through the placental barrier and into milk in concentrations comparable to those in the plasma. From 50 to 70% of a dose of isoniazid is excreted in the urine in 24 hours.
Isoniazid is metabolized primarily by acetylation and dehydrazination. The rate of acetylation is genetically determined. Approximately 50% of Blacks and Caucasians are "slow inactivators"; the majority of Eskimos and Orientals are "rapid inactivators."
The rate of acetylation does not significantly alter the effectiveness of isoniazid. However, slow acetylation may lead to higher blood levels of the drug, and thus an increase in toxic reactions.
Pyridoxine deficiency (B_6) is sometimes observed in adults with high doses of isoniazid and is considered probably due to its competition with pyridoxal phosphate for the enzyme apotryptophanase.

INDICATIONS

For pulmonary tuberculosis in which organisms are susceptible, and when the patient has been titrated on the individual components and it has therefore been established that this fixed dosage is therapeutically effective.
This fixed-dosage combination drug is not recommended for initial therapy of tuberculosis or for preventive therapy.
In the treatment of tuberculosis, small numbers of resistant cells, present within large populations of susceptible cells, can rapidly become the predominating type. Since rapid emergence of resistance can occur, culture and susceptibility tests should be performed in the event of persistent positive cultures.
This drug is not indicated for the treatment of meningococcal infections or asymptomatic carriers of *N. meningitidis* to eliminate meningococci from the nasopharynx.

CONTRAINDICATIONS

Previous isoniazid-associated hepatic injury; severe adverse reactions to isoniazid, such as drug fever, chills, and arthritis; acute liver disease of any etiology, a history of previous hypersensitivity reaction to any of the rifamycins or to isoniazid, including drug-induced hepatitis.

WARNINGS

RIFAMATE (rifampin-isoniazid) is a combination of two drugs, each of which has been associated with liver dysfunction. Liver function tests should be performed prior to therapy with RIFAMATE and periodically during treatment.

Rifampin

Rifampin has been shown to produce liver dysfunction. There have been fatalities associated with jaundice in patients with liver disease or receiving rifampin concomitantly with other hepatoxic agents. Since an increased risk may exist for individuals with liver disease, benefits must be weighed carefully against the risk of further liver damage.
Several studies of tumorigenicity potential have been done in rodents. In one strain of mice known to be particularly susceptible to the spontaneous development of hepatomas, rifampin given at a level 2–10 times the maximum dosage

used clinically resulted in a significant increase in the occurrence of hepatomas in female mice of this strain after one year of administration.

There was no evidence of tumorigenicity in the males of this strain, in males or females of another mouse strain, or in rats.

Isoniazid

See the boxed warning.

PRECAUTIONS

Rifampin

Rifampin is not recommended for intermittent therapy; the patient should be cautioned against intentional or accidental interruption of the daily dosage regimen since rare renal hypersensitivity reactions have been reported when therapy was resumed in such cases.

Rifampin has been observed to increase the requirements for anticoagulant drugs of the coumarin type. The cause of the phenomenon is unknown. In patients receiving anticoagulants and rifampin concurrently, it is recommended that the prothrombin time be performed daily or as frequently as necessary to establish and maintain the required dose of anticoagulant.

Urine, feces, saliva, sputum, sweat and tears may be colored red-orange by rifampin and its metabolites. Soft contact lenses may be permanently stained. Individuals to be treated should be made aware of these possibilities.

It has been reported that the reliability of oral contraceptives may be affected in some patients being treated for tuberculosis with rifampin in combination with at least one other antituberculosis drug. In such cases, alternative contraceptive measures may need to be considered.

It has also been reported that rifampin given in combination with other antituberculosis drugs may decrease the pharmacologic activity of methadone, oral hypoglycemics, digitoxin, quinidine, disopyramide, dapsone and corticosteroids. In these cases, dosage adjustment of the interacting drugs is recommended.

Therapeutic levels of rifampin have been shown to inhibit standard microbiological assays for serum folate and vitamin B_{12}. Alternative methods must be considered when determining folate and vitamin B_{12} concentrations in the presence of rifampin.

Since rifampin has been reported to cross the placental barrier and appear in cord blood and in maternal milk, neonates and newborns of rifampin-treated mothers should be carefully observed for any evidence of untoward effects.

Isoniazid

All drugs should be stopped and an evaluation of the patient should be made at the first sign of a hypersensitivity reaction.

Use of isoniazid should be carefully monitored in the following:

1. Patients who are receiving phenytoin (diphenylhydantoin) concurrently. Isoniazid may decrease the excretion of phenytoin or may enhance its effects. To avoid phenytoin intoxication, appropriate adjustment of the anticonvulsant dose should be made.
2. Daily users of alcohol. Daily ingestion of alcohol may be associated with a higher incidence of isoniazid hepatitis.
3. Patients with current chronic liver disease or severe renal dysfunction.

Periodic ophthalmoscopic examination during isoniazid therapy is recommended when visual symptoms occur.

Usage in Pregnancy and Lactation

Rifampin

Although rifampin has been reported to cross the placental barrier and appear in cord blood, the effect of rifampin, alone or in combination with other antituberculosis drugs, on the human fetus is not known. An increase in congenital malformations, primarily spina bifida and cleft palate, has been reported in the offspring of rodents given oral doses of 150–250 mg/kg/day of rifampin during pregnancy.

The possible teratogenic potential in women capable of bearing children should be carefully weighed against the benefits of therapy.

Isoniazid

It has been reported that in both rats and rabbits, isoniazid may exert an embryocidal effect when administered orally during pregnancy, although no isoniazid-related congenital anomalies have been found in reproduction studies in mammalian species (mice, rats, and rabbits). Isoniazid should be prescribed during pregnancy only when therapeutically necessary. The benefit of preventive therapy should be weighed against a possible risk to the fetus. Preventive treatment generally should be started after delivery because of the increased risk of tuberculosis for new mothers.

Since isoniazid is known to cross the placental barrier and to pass into maternal breast milk, neonates and breast-fed infants of isoniazid treated mothers should be carefully observed for any evidence of adverse effects.

Carcinogenesis: Isoniazid has been reported to induce pulmonary tumors in a number of strains of mice.

ADVERSE REACTIONS

Rifampin

Nervous system reactions: headache, drowsiness, fatigue, ataxia, dizziness, inability to concentrate, mental confusion, visual disturbances, muscular weakness, pain in extremities, and generalized numbness

Gastrointestinal disturbances: in some patients heartburn, epigastric distress, anorexia, nausea, vomiting, gas, cramps, and diarrhea

Hepatic reactions: transient abnormalities in liver function tests (e.g., elevations in serum bilirubin, BSP, alkaline phosphatase, serum transaminases) have been observed. Rarely, hepatitis or a shocklike syndrome with hepatic involvement and abnormal liver function tests

Renal reactions: Elevations in BUN and serum uric acid have been reported. Rarely, hemolysis, hemoglobinuria, hematuria, interstitial nephritis, renal insufficiency and acute renal failure have been noted. These are generally considered to be hypersensitivity reactions. They usually occur during intermittent therapy or when treatment is resumed following intentional or accidental interruption of a daily dosage regimen, and are reversible when rifampin is discontinued and appropriate therapy instituted.

Hematologic reactions: thrombocytopenia, transient leukopenia, hemolytic anemia, eosinophilia and decreased hemoglobin have been observed. Thrombocytopenia has occurred when rifampin and ethambutol were administered concomitantly according to an intermittent dose schedule twice weekly and in high doses.

Allergic and immunological reactions: occasionally pruritus, urticaria, rash, pemphigoid reaction, eosinophilia, sore mouth, sore tongue, and exudative conjunctivitis. Rarely, hemolysis, hemoglobinuria, hematuria, renal insufficiency or acute renal failure have been reported which are generally considered to be hypersensitivity reactions. These have usually occurred during intermittent therapy or when treatment was resumed following intentional or accidental interruption of a daily dosage regimen and were reversible when rifampin was discontinued and appropriate therapy instituted.

Although rifampin has been reported to have an immunosuppressive effect in some animal experiments, available human data indicate that this has no clinical significance.

Metabolic reactions: elevations in BUN and serum uric acid have occurred.

Miscellaneous reactions: fever and menstrual disturbances have been noted.

Isoniazid

The most frequent reactions are those affecting the nervous system and the liver.

Nervous system reactions: peripheral neuropathy is the most common toxic effect. It is dose-related, occurs most often in the malnourished and in those predisposed to neuritis (e.g., alcoholics and diabetics), and is usually preceded by paresthesias of the feet and hands. The incidence is higher in "slow inactivators."

Other neurotoxic effects, which are uncommon with conventional doses, are convulsions, toxic encephalopathy, optic neuritis and atrophy, memory impairment, and toxic psychosis.

Gastrointestinal reactions: nausea, vomiting, and epigastric distress

Hepatic reactions: elevated serum transaminases (SGOT; SGPT), bilirubinemia, bilirubinuria, jaundice, and occasionally severe and sometimes fatal hepatitis. The common prodromal symptoms are anorexia, nausea, vomiting, fatigue, malaise, and weakness. Mild and transient elevations of serum transaminase levels occurs in 10 to 20 percent of persons taking isoniazid. The abnormality usually occurs in the first 4 to 6 months of treatment but can occur at any time during therapy. In most instances, enzyme levels return to normal with no necessity to discontinue medication. In occasional instances, progressive liver damage occurs, with accompanying symptoms. In these cases, the drug should be discontinued immediately. The frequency of progressive liver damage increases with age. It is rare in persons under 20, but occurs in up to 2.3 percent of those over 50 years of age.

Hematologic reactions: agranulocytosis, hemolytic sideroblastic or aplastic anemia, thrombocytopenia and eosinophilia

Hypersensitivity reactions: fever, skin eruptions (morbilliform, maculopapular, purpuric, or exfoliative), lymphadenopathy and vasculitis

Metabolic and endocrine reactions: pyridoxine deficiency, pellagra, hyperglycemia, metabolic acidosis, and gynecomastia

Miscellaneous reactions: rheumatic syndrome and systemic lupus erythematosus-like syndrome

OVERDOSAGE

Rifampin

Signs and Symptoms

Nausea, vomiting, and increasing lethargy will probably occur within a short time after ingestion; actual unconsciousness may occur with severe hepatic involvement. Brownish-red or orange discoloration of the skin, urine, sweat, saliva, tears, and feces is proportional to amount ingested.

Liver enlargement, possibly with tenderness, can develop within a few hours after severe overdosage, and jaundice may develop rapidly. Hepatic involvement may be more marked in patients with prior impairment of hepatic function. Other physical findings remain essentially normal. Direct and total bilirubin levels may increase rapidly with severe overdosage; hepatic enzyme levels may be affected, especially with prior impairment of hepatic function. A direct effect upon hemopoietic system, electrolyte levels, or acid-base balance is unlikely.

Isoniazid

Signs and Symptoms

Isoniazid overdosage produces signs and symptoms within 30 minutes to 3 hours. Nausea, vomiting, dizziness, slurring of speech, blurring of vision, visual hallucinations (including bright colors and strange designs), are among the early manifestations. With marked overdosage, respiratory distress and CNS depression, progressing rapidly from stupor to profound coma, are to be expected, along with severe, intractable seizures. Severe metabolic acidosis, acetonuria, and hyperglycemia are typical laboratory findings.

RIFAMATE (rifampin and isoniazid capsules)

Treatment

The airway should be secured and adequate respiratory exchange established. Only then should gastric emptying (lavage-aspiration) be attempted; this may be difficult because of seizures. Since nausea and vomiting are likely to be present, gastric lavage is probably preferable to induction of emesis.

Activated charcoal slurry instilled into the stomach following evacuation of gastric contents can help absorb any remaining drug in the GI tract. Antiemetic medication may be required to control severe nausea and vomiting.

Blood samples should be obtained for immediate determination of gases, electrolytes, BUN, glucose, etc. Blood should be typed and crossmatched in preparation for possible hemodialysis.

Rapid control of metabolic acidosis is fundamental to management. Intravenous sodium bicarbonate should be given at once and repeated as needed, adjusting subsequent dosage on the basis of laboratory findings (i.e. serum sodium, pH, etc.). At the same time, anticonvulsants should be given intravenously (i.e., barbiturates, diphenylhydantoin, diazepam) as required, and large doses of intravenous pyridoxine. Forced osmotic diuresis must be started early and should be continued for some hours after clinical improvement to hasten renal clearance of drug and help prevent relapse. Fluid intake and output should be monitored.

Bile drainage may be indicated in presence of serious impairment of hepatic function lasting more than 24–48 hours. Under these circumstances and for severe cases, extracorporeal hemodialysis may be required; if this is not available, peritoneal dialysis can be used along with forced diuresis. Along with measures based on initial and repeated determination of blood gases and other laboratory tests as needed, meticulous respiratory and other intensive care should be utilized to protect against hypoxia, hypotension, aspiration, pneumonitis, etc.

In patients with previously adequate hepatic function, reversal of liver enlargement and impaired hepatic excretory function probably will be noted within 72 hours, with rapid return toward normal thereafter.

Untreated or inadequately treated cases of gross isoniazid overdosage can terminate fatally, but good response has been reported in most patients brought under adequate treatment within the first few hours after drug ingestion.

DOSAGE AND ADMINISTRATION

In general, therapy should be continued until bacterial conversion and maximal improvement have occurred.

Adults: Two RIFAMATE (rifampin-isoniazid) capsules (600 mg rifampin, 300 mg isoniazid) once daily, administered one hour before or two hours after a meal.

Concomitant administration of pyridoxine (B_6) is recommended in the malnourished, in those predisposed to neuropathy (e.g., diabetic), and in adolescents.

Susceptibility Testing

Rifampin

Rifampin susceptibility powders are available for both direct and indirect methods of determining the susceptibility of strains of mycobacteria. The MIC's of susceptible clinical isolates when determined in 7H10 or other non-egg-containing media have ranged from 0.1 to 2 mcg/ml.

Quantitative methods that require measurement of zone diameters give the most precise estimates of antibiotic susceptibility. One such procedure has been recommended for use with discs for testing susceptibility to rifampin. Interpretations correlate zone diameters from the disc test with MIC (minimal inhibitory concentration) values for rifampin.

Continued on next page

Hoechst Marion Roussel—Cont.

HOW SUPPLIED

Capsules (opaque red), containing 300 mg rifampin and 150 mg isoniazid; bottles of 60 (NDC 0068-0509-60).
Prescribing Information as of May 1991
Merrell Pharmaceuticals, Inc.
Subsidiary of Hoechst Marion Roussel, Inc.
Kansas City, MO 64137
Shown in Product Identification Guide, page 317

RIFATER®

[*rif 'uh-ter*]
(rifampin, isoniazid
and pyrazinamide)
Tablets

℞

WARNING

Severe and sometimes fatal hepatitis associated with isoniazid therapy may occur and may develop even after many months of treatment. The risk of developing hepatitis is age related. Approximate case rates by age are: 0 per 1,000 for persons under 20 years of age, 3 per 1,000 for persons in the 20 to 34 year age group, 12 per 1,000 for persons in the 35 to 49 year age group, 23 per 1,000 for persons in the 50 to 64 year age group, and 8 per 1,000 for persons over 65 years of age. The risk of hepatitis is increased with daily consumption of alcohol. Precise data to provide a fatality rate for isoniazid-related hepatitis is not available; however, in a U.S. Public Health Service Surveillance Study of 13,838 persons taking isoniazid, there were 8 deaths among 174 cases of hepatitis.

Therefore, patients given isoniazid should be carefully monitored and interviewed at monthly intervals. Serum transaminase concentration becomes elevated in about 10% to 20% of patients, usually during the first few months of therapy, but it can occur at any time. Usually enzyme levels return to normal despite continuance of drug, but in some cases progressive liver dysfunction occurs. Patients should be instructed to report immediately any of the prodromal symptoms of hepatitis, such as fatigue, weakness, malaise, anorexia, nausea, or vomiting. If these symptoms appear or if signs suggestive of hepatic damage are detected, isoniazid should be discontinued promptly since continued use of the drug in these cases has been reported to cause a more severe form of liver damage.

Patients with tuberculosis should be given appropriate treatment with alternative drugs. If isoniazid must be reinstituted, it should be reinstituted only after symptoms and laboratory abnormalities have cleared. The drug should be restarted in very small and gradually increasing doses and should be withdrawn immediately if there is any indication of recurrent liver involvement. Treatment should be deferred in persons with acute hepatic diseases.

DESCRIPTION

RIFATER (rifampin/isoniazid/pyrazinamide) tablets are combination tablets containing 120 mg rifampin, 50 mg isoniazid, and 300 mg pyrazinamide for use in antibacterial therapy. The tablets also contain as inactive ingredients: povidone, carboxymethylcellulose sodium, calcium stearate, sodium lauryl sulfate, sucrose, talc, acacia, titanium dioxide, kaolin, magnesium carbonate, colloidal silicon dioxide, dried aluminum hydroxide gel, ferric oxide, black iron oxide, carnauba wax, white beeswax, colophony, hard paraffin, lecithin, shellac, and propylene glycol. The RIFATER triple therapy combination was developed for dosing convenience.
Rifampin is a semisynthetic antibiotic derivative of rifamycin B. Rifampin is a red-brown crystalline powder very

slightly soluble in water at neutral pH, freely soluble in chloroform, soluble in ethyl acetate and methanol. Its molecular weight is 822.95 and its chemical formula is $C_{43}H_{58}N_4O_{12}$. The chemical name for rifampin is either:

3-[[(4-methyl-1-piperazinyl) imino]-methyl]-rifamycin;

or

5,6,9,17,19,21 -hexahydroxy- 23methoxy -2,4,12,16,18,20,22 heptamethyl-8-[N-(4-methyl-1-piperazinyl) formimidoyl]-2,7-(epoxypentadeca [1,11,13]trienimino)naphthol[2,1-b]furan-1, 11(2H)-dione 21-acetate.

Its structural formula is:

Isoniazid is the hydroxide of isonicotinic acid. It is a colorless or white crystalline powder or white crystals. It is odorless and slowly affected by exposure to air and light. It is freely soluble in water, sparingly soluble in alcohol and slightly soluble in chloroform and in ether. Its molecular weight is 137.14 and its chemical formula is $C_6H_7N_3O$. The chemical name for isoniazid is 4-pyridinecarboxylic acid, hydrazide and its structural formula is:

Pyrazinamide, the pyrazine analogue of nicotinamide, is a white, crystalline powder, stable at room temperature, and sparingly soluble in water. The chemical name for pyrazinamide is pyrazinecarboxamide and its molecular weight is 123.11. Its chemical formula is $C_5H_5N_3O$ and its structural formula is:

CLINICAL PHARMACOLOGY

General

Rifampin. Rifampin is readily absorbed from the gastrointestinal tract. Peak serum levels in normal adults and children vary widely from individual to individual. Following a single 600 mg oral dose of rifampin in healthy adults, the peak serum level averages 7 μg/mL but may vary from 4 to 32 μg/mL. Absorption of rifampin is reduced when the drug is ingested with food.

In normal subjects, the biological half-life of rifampin in serum averages about 3 hours after a 600 mg oral dose, with increases up to 5.1 hours reported after a 900 mg dose. With repeated administration, the half-life decreases and reaches average values of approximately 2 to 3 hours. The half-life does not differ in patients with renal failure at doses not exceeding 600 mg daily and, consequently, no dosage adjustment is required. The half-life of rifampin at a dose of 720 mg daily has not been established in patients with renal failure. Following a single 900 mg oral dose of rifampin in patients with varying degrees of renal insufficiency, the half-life increased from 3.6 hours in normal subjects to 5.0, 7.3 and 11.0 hours in patients with glomerular filtration rates of 30–50 mL/min, less than 30 mL/min, and in anuric patients, respectively. Refer to WARNINGS section for information regarding patients with hepatic insufficiency.

After absorption, rifampin is rapidly eliminated in the bile, and an enterohepatic circulation ensues. During this pro-

cess, rifampin undergoes progressive deacetylation so that nearly all the drug in the bile is in this form in about 6 hours. This metabolite has antibacterial activity. Intestinal reabsorption is reduced by deacetylation, and elimination is facilitated. Up to 30% of a dose is excreted in the urine, with about half as unchanged drug.

Rifampin is widely distributed throughout the body. It is present in effective concentrations in many organs and body fluids, including cerebrospinal fluid. Rifampin is about 80% protein bound. Most of the unbound fraction is not ionized and therefore is diffused freely in tissues.

Isoniazid. After oral administration, isoniazid is readily absorbed from the GI tract and produces peak blood levels within 1 to 2 hours. It diffuses readily into all body fluids (cerebrospinal, pleural, and ascitic fluids), tissues, organs, and excreta (saliva, sputum, and feces). Isoniazid is not substantially bound to plasma proteins. The drug also passes through the placental barrier and into milk in concentrations comparable to those in the plasma. The plasma half-life of isoniazid in patients with normal renal and hepatic function ranges from 1–4 hours, depending on the rate of metabolism. From 50% to 70% of a dose of isoniazid is excreted in the urine within 24 hours, mostly as metabolites.

Isoniazid is metabolized in the liver mainly by acetylation and dehydrazination. The rate of acetylation is genetically determined. Approximately 50% of African Americans and Caucasians are "slow inactivators" and the rest are "rapid inactivators"; the majority of Eskimos and Asians are "rapid inactivators." The rate of acetylation does not significantly alter the effectiveness of Isoniazid. However, slow acetylation may lead to higher blood levels of the drug, and thus, an increase in toxic reactions.

Pyridoxine (B_6) deficiency is sometimes observed in adults with high doses of isoniazid and is probably due to its competition with pyridoxal phosphate for the enzyme apotryptophanase.

Pyrazinamide. Pyrazinamide is well absorbed from the gastrointestinal tract and attains peak plasma concentrations within 2 hours. Plasma concentrations generally range from 30 to 50 μg/mL with doses of 20 to 25 mg/kg. It is widely distributed in body tissues and fluids including the liver, lungs, and cerebrospinal fluid (CSF). The CSF concentration is approximately equal to concurrent steady-state plasma concentrations in patients with inflamed meninges. Pyrazinamide is approximately 10% bound to plasma proteins. The plasma half-life of pyrazinamide is 9 to 10 hours in patients with normal renal and hepatic function. The half-life of the drug may be prolonged in patients with impaired renal or hepatic function. Pyrazinamide is hydrolyzed in the liver to its major active metabolite, pyrazinoic acid. Pyrazinoic acid is hydroxylated to the main excretory product, 5-hydroxypyrazinoic acid.

Within 24 hours, approximately 70% of an oral dose of pyrazinamide is excreted in urine, mainly by glomerular filtration. About 4% to 14% of the dose is excreted as unchanged drug; the remainder is excreted as metabolites.

RIFATER

In a single-dose bioavailability study of five RIFATER tablets (Treatment A, n=23) versus RIFADIN 600 mg, isoniazid 250 mg, and pyrazinamide 1500 mg (Treatment B, n=24) administered concurrently in normal subjects, there was no difference in extent of absorption, as measured by the area under the plasma concentration versus time curve (AUC), of all three components. However, the mean peak plasma concentration of rifampin was approximately 18% lower following the single-dose administration of RIFATER tablets as compared to RIFADIN administered in combination with pyrazinamide and isoniazid. Mean ($\pm$SD) pharmacokinetic parameters are summarized in the following table.
[See table below.]

Microbiology

Rifampin, isoniazid, and pyrazinamide at therapeutic levels have demonstrated bactericidal activity against both intracellular and extracellular *Mycobacterium tuberculosis* organisms.

Mechanism of Action

Rifampin. Rifampin inhibits DNA-dependent RNA polymerase activity in susceptible *Mycobacterium tuberculosis* organisms. Specifically, it interacts with bacterial RNA polymerase, but does not inhibit the mammalian enzyme. Organisms resistant to rifampin are likely to be resistant to other rifamycins.

Isoniazid. Isoniazid kills actively growing tubercle bacilli by inhibiting the biosynthesis of mycolic acids which are major components of the cell wall of *Mycobacterium tuberculosis*.

Pyrazinamide. The exact mechanism of action by which pyrazinamide inhibits the growth of *Mycobacterium tuberculosis* organisms is unknown. *In vitro* and *in vivo* studies have demonstrated that pyrazinamide is only active at a slightly acidic pH (pH 5.5).

Susceptibility Testing

Prior to initiation of therapy, appropriate specimens should be collected for identification of the infecting organism and *in vitro* susceptibility tests.

Parameter	C_{max} (μg/mL)		Half-life (hr)		Apparent Oral Clearance (L/hr)		Bioavailability (%)
Treatment	A	B	A	B	A	B	A
Isoniazid	3.09 $\pm$ 0.88	3.14 $\pm$ 0.92	2.80 $\pm$ 1.02	2.80 $\pm$ 1.11	24.02 $\pm$15.29	25.72 $\pm$18.38	100.6 $\pm$ 16.6
Rifampin	11.04 $\pm$ 3.08	13.61 $\pm$ 3.96	3.19 $\pm$ 0.63	3.41 $\pm$ 0.86	9.62 $\pm$ 3.00	8.30 $\pm$ 2.50	88.8 $\pm$ 16.5
Pyrazinamide	28.02 $\pm$ 4.52	29.21 $\pm$ 4.35	10.04 $\pm$ 1.54	10.08 $\pm$ 1.29	3.82 $\pm$ 0.65	3.70 $\pm$ 0.59	96.8 $\pm$ 7.6

The effect of food on the pharmacokinetics of RIFATER tablets was not studied.

Two standardized *in vitro* susceptibility methods are available for testing isoniazid, rifampin, and pyrazinamide against *Mycobacterium tuberculosis* organisms. The agar proportion method (CDC or NCCLS M24-P) utilizes Middlebrook 7H10 medium impregnated with isoniazid at 0.2 and 1.0 μg/mL and rifampin at 1.0 μg/mL for the final concentrations of drug. The final concentration for pyrazinamide is 25.0 μg/mL at pH 5.5. After 3 weeks of incubation MIC_{99} values are calculated by comparing the quantity of organisms growing in the medium containing drug to the control cultures. Mycobacterial growth in the presence of drug $\geq 1\%$ of the control indicates resistance.

The radiometric broth method employs the BACTEC 460 machine to compare the growth index from untreated control cultures to cultures grown in the presence of 0.2 and 1.0 μg/mL of isoniazid and 2.0 μg/mL of rifampin. Strict adherence to the manufacturer's instructions for sample processing and data interpretation is required for this assay. The radiometric broth method has not been approved for the testing of pyrazinamide.

Susceptibility test results obtained by the two different methods can only be compared if the appropriate rifampin or isoniazid concentrations are used for each test method as indicated above. Both test procedures require the use of *Mycobacterium tuberculosis* H37Rv, ATCC 27294, as a control organism.

The clinical relevance of *in vitro* susceptibility test results for mycobacterial species other than *Mycobacterium tuberculosis* using either the radiometric broth method or the proportion method has not been determined.

CLINICAL TRIALS

A total of 250 patients were enrolled in an open label, prospective, randomized, parallel group, active controlled trial, for the treatment of pulmonary tuberculosis. There were 241 patients evaluable for efficacy, 123 patients received isoniazid, rifampin and pyrazinamide as separate tablets and capsules for 56 days, and 118 patients received 4 to 6 RIFATER tablets based on body weight for 56 days. RIFATER tablets and the drugs dosed as separate tablets and capsules were administered based on body weight during the intensive phase of treatment according to the following table.

[See table above.]

During the continuation phase, both treatment groups received 450 mg of rifampin and 300 mg of isoniazid per day for 4 months if the patient weighed < 50 kg or 600 mg of rifampin and 300 mg of isoniazid per day for 4 months if the patient weighed $\geq$ 50 kg. Patients were followed for occurrence of relapses for up to 30 months after the end of therapy.

There were no significant differences in the negative bacteriological sputum results (available in a subset of patients) between the two treatments at 2 and 6 months during the trial and during the follow-up period. See table below.

[See table below.]

For adverse events, see ADVERSE REACTIONS section.

INDICATIONS AND USAGE

RIFATER is indicated in the initial phase of the short-course treatment of pulmonary tuberculosis. During this phase, which should last 2 months. RIFATER should be administered on a daily, continuous basis (see DOSAGE AND ADMINISTRATION section).

Following the initial phase and treatment with RIFATER, treatment should be continued with rifampin and isoniazid (eg, RIFAMATE) for at least 4 months. Treatment should be continued for a longer period of time if the patient is still sputum or culture postive, if resistant organisms are present, or if the patient is HIV positive.

In the treatment of tuberculosis, the small number of resistant cells present within large populations of susceptible cells can rapidly become the predominant type. Since resistance can emerge rapidly, susceptibility tests should be performed in the event of persistent positive cultures during the course of treatment. Bacteriologic smears or cultures should be obtained before the start of therapy to confirm the susceptibility of the organism to rifampin, isoniazid, and pyrazinamide and they should be repeated throughout therapy to monitor response to the treatment. If test results show resistance to any of the components of RIFATER and the patient is not responding to therapy, the drug regimen should be modified.

Dose of Isoniazid, Rifampin and Pyrazinamide Administered as Separate Drugs

Patient Weight	Isoniazid (mg)	Rifampin (mg)	Pyrazinamide (mg)
< 50 kg	300	450	1500
$\geq$ 50 kg	300	600	2000

Dose of Isoniazid, Rifampin and Pyrazinamide Administered as RIFATER

Patient Weight	Number of Tablets	Isoniazid (mg)	Rifampin (mg)	Pyrazinamide (mg)
$\leq$ 44 kg	4	200	480	1200
45 to 54 kg	5	250	600	1500
$\geq$ 55 kg	6	300	720	1800

CONTRAINDICATIONS

RIFATER is contraindicated in patients with a history of hypersensitivity to rifampin, isoniazid, pyrazinamide, or any of the components. Other contraindications include patients with severe hepatic damage; severe adverse reactions to isoniazid, such as drug fever, chills, and arthritis; patients with acute liver disease of any etiology; and patients with acute gout.

WARNINGS

RIFATER is a combination of the three drugs, rifampin, isoniazid, and pyrazinamide. Each of these individual drugs has been associated with liver dysfunction.

Rifampin. Rifampin has been shown to produce liver dysfunction. Fatalities associated with jaundice have occurred in patients with liver disease and in patients taking rifampin with other hepatoxic agents. Because RIFATER contains both rifampin and isoniazid, it should only be given with caution and under strict medical supervision to patients with impaired liver function. In these patients, careful monitoring of liver function, especially serum glutamic pyruvic transaminase (SGPT) and serum glutamic oxaloacetic transaminase (SGOT) should be carried out prior to therapy and then every 2 to 4 weeks during therapy. If signs of hepatocellular damage occur, RIFATER should be withdrawn.

In some cases, hyperbilirubinemia resulting from competition between rifampin and bilirubin for excretory pathways of the liver at the cell level can occur in the early days of treatment. An isolated report showing a moderate rise in bilirubin and/or transaminase level is not in itself an indication for interrupting treatment; rather, the decision should be made after repeating the tests, noting trends in the levels, and considering them in conjunction with the patient's clinical condition.

Rifampin has enzyme-inducing properties, including induction of delta amino levulinic acid synthetase. Isolated reports have associated porphyria exacerbation with rifampin administration.

Isoniazid. See the boxed WARNING.

Since RIFATER contains isoniazid, ophthalmologic examinations (including ophthalmoscopy) should be done before treatment is started and periodically thereafter, even without occurrence of visual symptoms.

Pyrazinamide. Since RIFATER contains pyrazinamide, patients started on RIFATER should have baseline serum uric acid and liver function determinations. Patients with preexisting liver disease or those patients at increased risk for drug related hepatitis (eg, alcohol abusers) should be followed closely.

Because it contains pyrazinamide, RIFATER should be discontinued and not be resumed if signs of hepatocellular damage or hyperuricemia accompanied by an acute gouty arthritis appear. If hyperuricemia accompanied by an acute gouty arthritis occurs without liver dysfunction, the patient should be transferred to a regimen not containing pyrazinamide.

PRECAUTIONS

General

RIFATER should be used with caution in patients with a history of diabetes mellitus, as diabetes management may be more difficult.

Rifampin. For treatment of tuberculosis, rifampin is usually administered on a daily basis. Doses of rifampin (> 600 mg) given once or twice weekly have resulted in a higher incidence of adverse reactions, including the "flu syndrome" (fever, chills and malaise); hematopoietic reactions (leukopenia, thrombocytopenia, or acute hemolytic anemia); cutaneous, gastrointestinal, and hepatic reactions; shortness of breath; shock and renal failure.

The patient should be advised that the reliability of oral contraceptives may be affected; consideration should be given to using alternative contraceptive measures.

Isoniazid. All drugs should be stopped and an evaluation of the patient should be made at the first sign of a hypersensitivity reaction.

Use of RIFATER, because it contains isoniazid, should be carefully monitored in the following:
1. Patients who are receiving phenytoin (diphenylhydantoin) concurrently. Isoniazid may decrease the excretion of phenytoin or may enhance its effects. To avoid phenytoin intoxication, appropriate adjustment of the anticonvulsant dose should be made.
2. Daily users of alcohol. Daily ingestion of alcohol may be associated with a higher incidence of isoniazid hepatitis.
3. Patients with current chronic liver disease or severe renal dysfunction.

Pyrazinamide. Pyrazinamide inhibits renal excretion of urates, frequently resulting in hyperuricemia which is usually asymptomatic. If hyperuricemia is accompanied by acute gouty arthritis, RIFATER, because it contains pyrazinamide, should be discontinued.

Information for Patients

Food Interactions: Because isoniazid has some monoamine oxidase inhibiting activity, an interaction with tyramine-containing foods (cheese, red wine) may occur. Diamine oxidase may also be inhibited, causing exaggerated response (eg, headache, sweating, palpitations, flushing, hypotension) to foods containing histamine (eg, skipjack, tuna, other tropical fish). Tyramine- and histamine-containing foods should be avoided in patients receiving RIFATER.

RIFATER, because it contains rifampin, may produce a reddish coloration of the urine, sweat, sputum, and tears, and the patient should be forewarned of this. Soft contact lenses may be permanently stained.

Patients should be instructed to take RIFATER either 1 hour before or 2 hours after a meal.

Patients should be instructed to notify their physicians promptly if they experience any of the following: fever, loss of appetite, malaise, nausea and vomiting, darkened urine, yellowish discoloration of the skin and eyes, pain or swelling of the joints.

Compliance with the full course of therapy must be emphasized, and the importance of not missing any doses must be stressed.

Laboratory Tests

A complete blood count (CBC), liver function tests, and blood uric acid determinations should be obtained prior to instituting therapy and periodically throughout the course of therapy. Because of a possible transient rise in transaminase and bilirubin values, blood for baseline clinical chemistries should be obtained before RIFATER dosing.

Drug Interactions

Rifampin. Enzyme Induction: Rifampin is known to induce certain cytochrome P-450 enzymes. Coadministration of RIFATER, because it contains rifampin, with drugs that undergo biotransformation through these metabolic pathways may accelerate elimination. To maintain optimum

Negative Sputums/No. of Patients (Percent Negative)

Treatment	2 Months	6 Months	Follow-up Period*
RIFATER	91/96 (95%)	100/104 (96%)	99/101 (98%)
Separate†	99/108 (92%)	95/96 (99%)	105/106 (99%)

*The median follow-up time for all the RIFATER patients was 756 days with a range of 42 to 1325 days and 745 days with a range of 50 to 1427 days for the patients dosed with separate tablets and capsules.
†Isoniazid, rifampin, and pyrazinamide dosed as separate tablets and capsules.

Continued on next page

Hoechst Marion Roussel—Cont.

therapeutic blood levels, dosages of drugs metabolized by these enzymes may require adjustment when starting or stopping concomitantly administered rifampin.
Rifampin has been reported to accelerate the metabolism of the following drugs: anticonvulsants (eg, phenytoin), antiarrhythmics (eg, disopyramide, mexiletine, quinidine, tocainide), anticoagulants, antifungals (eg, fluconazole, itraconazole, ketoconazole), barbiturates, beta-blockers, calcium channel blockers (eg, diltiazem, nifedipine, verapamil), chloramphenicol, ciprofloxacin, corticosteroids, cyclosporine, cardiac glycoside preparations, clofibrate, oral contraceptives, dapsone, diazepam, haloperidol, oral hypoglycemic agents (sulfonylureas), methadone, narcotic analgesics, nortriptyline, progestins, and theophylline. It may be necessary to adjust dosages of these drugs if they are given concurrently with RIFATER since it contains rifampin.
Rifampin has been observed to increase the requirements for anticoagulant drugs of the coumarin type. In patients receiving anticoagulants and RIFATER concurrently, it is recommended that the prothrombin time be performed daily or as frequently as necessary to establish and maintain the required dose of anticoagulant.
Concurrent use of ketoconazole and rifampin has resulted in decreased serum concentration of both drugs. Concurrent use of rifampin and enalapril has resulted in decreased concentrations of enalaprilat, the active metabolite of enalapril. Since RIFATER contains rifampin, dosage adjustments should be made if RIFATER is concurrently administered with ketoconazole or enalapril if indicated by the patient's clinical condition.
Other Interactions: Concomitant antacid administration may reduce the absorption of rifampin. Daily doses of RIFATER, because it contains rifampin, should be given at least 1 hour before the ingestion of antacids.
Probenecid and cotrimoxazole have been reported to increase the blood level of rifampin.
When rifampin is given concomitantly with either halothane or isoniazid the potential for hepatotoxicity is increased. The concomitant use of RIFATER, because it contains both rifampin and isoniazid, and halothane should be avoided. Patients receiving both rifampin and isoniazid as in RIFATER should be monitored closely for hepatotoxicity. See the boxed WARNING.
Plasma concentrations of sulfapyridine may be reduced following the concomitant administration of sulfasalazine and RIFATER, because it contains rifampin. This finding may be the result of alteration in the colonic bacteria responsible for the reduction of sulfasalazine to sulfapyridine and mesalamine.
Isoniazid. Enzyme Inhibition: Isoniazid is known to inhibit certain cytochrome P-450 enzymes. Coadministration of isoniazid with drugs that undergo biotransformation through these metabolic pathways may decrease elimination. Consequently, dosages of drugs metabolized by these enzymes may require adjustment when starting or stopping concomitantly administered RIFATER, because it contains isoniazid, to maintain optimum therapeutic blood levels.
Isoniazid has been reported to inhibit the metabolism of the following drugs: anticonvulsants (eg, carbamazepine, phenytoin, primidone, valproic acid), benzodiazepines (eg, diazepam), haloperidol, ketoconazole, theophylline, and warfarin. It may be necessary to adjust the dosages of these drugs if they are given concurrently with RIFATER because it contains isoniazid. The impact of the competing effects of rifampin and isoniazid on the metabolism of these drugs is unknown.
Other Interactions: Concomitant antacid administration may reduce the absorption of isoniazid. Ingestion with food may also reduce the absorption of isoniazid. Daily doses of RIFATER, because it contains isoniazid, should be given on an empty stomach at least 1 hour before the ingestion of antacids or food.
Corticosteroids (eg, prednisolone) may decrease the serum concentration of isoniazid by increasing acetylation rate and/or renal clearance. Para-aminosalicylic acid may increase the plasma concentration and elimination half-life of isoniazid by competition of acetylating enzymes.
Pharmacodynamic Interactions: Daily ingestion of alcohol may be associated with a higher incidence of isoniazid hepatitis. Isoniazid, when given concomitantly with rifampin, has been reported to increase the hepatotoxicity of both drugs. Patients receiving both rifampin and isoniazid as in RIFATER should be monitored closely for hepatotoxicity.
The CNS effects of meperidine (drowsiness), cycloserine (dizziness, drowsiness), and disulfiram (acute behavioral and coordination changes) may be exaggerated when concomitant RIFATER, because it contains isoniazid, is given. Concurrent RIFATER, because it contains isoniazid, and levodopa administration may produce symptoms of excess catecholamine stimulation (agitation, flushing, palpitations) or lack of levodopa effect.
Isoniazid may produce hyperglycemia and lead to loss of glucose control in patients on oral hypoglycemics.
Fast acetylation of isoniazid may produce high concentrations of hydrazine which facilitate deflorination of enflurane. Renal function should be monitored in patients receiving both RIFATER and enflurane.
Food Interactions: Because isoniazid has some monoamine oxidase inhibiting activity, an interaction with tyramine-containing foods (cheese, red wine) may occur. Diamine oxidase may also be inhibited, causing exaggerated response (eg, headache, sweating, palpitations, flushing, hypotension) to foods containing histamine (eg, skipjack, tuna, other tropical fish). Tyramine- and histamine-containing foods should be avoided by patients receiving RIFATER.

Drug/Laboratory Tests Interaction

Rifampin. Therapeutic levels of rifampin have been shown to inhibit standard microbiological assays for serum folate and vitamin B_{12}. Therefore, alternative assay methods should be considered. Transient abnormalities in liver function tests (eg, elevation in serum bilirubin, abnormal bromsulphalein [BSP] excretion, alkaline phosphatase and serum transaminases), and reduced biliary excretion of contrast media used for visualization of the gallbladder have also been observed. Therefore, tests should be performed before the morning dose of RIFATER.
Rifampin and isoniazid have been reported to alter vitamin D metabolism. In some cases, reduced levels of circulating 25-hydroxy vitamin D and 1,25-dihydroxy vitamin D have been accompanied by reduced serum calcium and phosphate, and elevated parathyroid hormone.
Pyrazinamide. Pyrazinamide has been reported to interfere with ACETEST® and KETOSTIX® urine tests to produce a pink-brown color.

Carcinogenesis, Mutagenesis, Impairment of Fertility

Increased frequency of chromosomal aberrations was observed *in vitro* in lymphocytes obtained from patients treated with combinations of rifampin, isoniazid, and pyrazinamide and combinations of streptomycin, rifampin, isoniazid, and pyrazinamide.
Rifampin. There are no known human data on long-term potential for carcinogenicity, mutagenicity, or impairment of fertility. A few cases of accelerated growth of lung carcinoma have been reported in man, but a causal relationship with the drug has not been established. An increase in the incidence of hepatomas in female mice (of a strain known to be particularly susceptible to the spontaneous development of hepatomas) was observed when rifampicin was administered in doses two to ten times the average daily human dose for 60 weeks followed by an observation period of 46 weeks. No evidence of carcinogenicity was found in male mice of the same strain, mice of a different strain, or rats under similar experimental conditions.
Rifampin has been reported to possess immunosuppressive potential in rabbits, mice, rats, guinea pigs, human lymphocytes *in vitro,* and humans. Antitumor activity *in vitro* has also been shown with rifampin.
There was no evidence of mutagenicity in bacteria, *Drosophilia melanogaster,* or mice. An increase in chromatid breaks was noted when whole blood cell cultures were treated with rifampin.
Isoniazid. Isoniazid has been reported to induce pulmonary tumors in a number of strains of mice.
Pyrazinamide. In lifetime bioassays in rats and mice, pyrazinamide was administered in the diet at concentrations of up to 10,000 ppm. This resulted in estimated daily doses of 2 g/kg for the mouse, or 40 times the maximum human dose, and 0.5 g/kg for the rat, or 10 times the maximum human dose. Pyrazinamide was not carcinogenic in rats or male mice and no conclusion was possible for female mice.
Pyrazinamide was not mutagenic in the Ames bacterial test, but induced chromosomal aberrations in human lymphocyte cell cultures.

Pregnancy—Teratogenic Effects

Category C. Animal reproduction studies have not been conducted with RIFATER. It is also not known whether RIFATER can cause fetal harm when administered to a pregnant woman. RIFATER should be given to a pregnant woman only if clearly needed.
Rifampin. Although rifampin has been reported to cross the placental barrier and appear in cord blood, the effect of rifampin, alone or in combination with other antituberculosis drugs, on the human fetus is not known. An increase in congenital malformations, primarily spina bifida and cleft palate, has been reported in the offspring of rodents given oral doses of 150 to 250 mg/kg/day of rifampin during pregnancy. The possible teratogenic potential in women capable of bearing children should be carefully weighed against the benefits of RIFATER therapy.
Isoniazid. It has been reported that in both rats and rabbits, isoniazid may exert an embryocidal effect when administered orally during pregnancy, although no isoniazid-related congenital anomalies have been found in reproduction studies in mammalian species (mice, rats, and rabbits). RIFATER, because it contains isoniazid, should be prescribed during pregnancy only when therapeutically necessary. The benefit of preventive therapy should be weighed against a possible risk to the fetus. Preventive treatment generally should be started after delivery because of the increased risk of tuberculosis for new mothers.
Pyrazinamide. Animal reproductive studies have not been conducted with pyrazinamide. It is also not known whether pyrazinamide can cause fetal harm when administered to a pregnant woman. RIFATER, because it contains pyrazinamide, should be given to a pregnant woman only if clearly needed.

Pregnancy—Non-Teratogenic Effects

It is not known whether RIFATER can affect reproduction capacity.
Rifampin. When administered during the last few weeks of pregnancy, rifampin can cause postnatal hemorrhages in the mother and infant. In this case, treatment with vitamin K may be indicated for postnatal hemorrhage.

Nursing Mothers

Since rifampin, isoniazid, and pyrazinamide are known to pass into maternal breast milk, a decision should be made whether to discontinue nursing or to discontinue RIFATER, taking into account the importance of the drug to the mother.

Pediatric Use

Safety and effectiveness in children or adolescents under the age of 15 have not been established.

ADVERSE REACTIONS

Adverse Experiences During the Clinical Trial

Adverse event data reported for the RIFATER and the separate drug treatment groups during the first 2 months of the trial are shown in the table below
[See table at top of next page.]
No serious adverse events were reported in the patients receiving RIFATER tablets. Three serious adverse events were reported in the patients given isoniazid, rifampin, and pyrazinamide as separate tablets and capsules. The three serious adverse events were two general hypersensitivity reactions and one jaundice reaction.
There were no significant differences between the two treatment groups in standard liver function, renal function and hematological laboratory test values measured at baseline and after 8 weeks of treatment. As would be expected for these drugs, there were alterations in liver enzymes (SGOT, SGPT) and serum uric acid levels. The adverse reactions reported during therapy with RIFATER are consistent with those described below for the individual components.

Adverse Reactions Reported for Individual Components

Rifampin. Gastrointestinal: Heatburn, epigastric distress, anorexia, nausea, vomiting, jaundice, flatulence, cramps, and diarrhea have been noted in some patients. Although *Clostridium difficile* has been shown *in vitro* to be sensitive to rifampin, pseudomembranous colitis has been reported with the use of rifampin (and other broad spectrum antibiotics). Therefore, it is important to consider this diagnosis in patients who develop diarrhea in association with antibiotic use. Rarely, hepatitis or a shocklike syndrome with hepatic involvement and abnormal liver function tests has been reported.
Hematologic: Thrombocytopenia has occurred primarily with high dose intermittent therapy, but has also been noted after resumption of interrupted treatment. It rarely occurs during well-supervised daily therapy. This effect is reversible if the drug is discontinued as soon as purpura occurs. Cerebral hemorrhage and fatalities have been reported when rifampin administration has been continued or resumed after the appearance of purpura.
Transient leukopenia, hemolytic anemia, and decreased hemoglobin have been observed.
Central Nervous System: Headache, fever, drowsiness, fatigue, ataxia, dizziness, inability to concentrate, mental confusion, behavioral changes, muscular weakness, pains in extremities, and generalized numbness have been observed. Rare reports of myopathy have also been observed.
Ocular: Visual disturbances have been observed.
Endocrine: Menstrual disturbances have been observed.
Renal: Elevations in BUN and serum uric acid have been reported. Rarely, hemolysis, hemoglobinuria, hematuria, interstitial nephritis, renal insufficiency, and acute renal failure have been noted. These are generally considered to be hypersensitivity reactions. They usually occur during intermittent therapy or when treatment is resumed following intentional or accidental interruption of a daily dosage regimen, and are reversible when rifampin is discontinued and appropriate therapy instituted.
Dermatologic: Cutaneous reactions are mild and self-limiting and do not appear to be hypersensitivity reactions. Typically, they consist of flushing and itching with or without a rash. More serious cutaneous reactions which may be due to hypersensitivity occur but are uncommon.
Hypersensitivity Reactions: Occasionally pruritis, urticaria, rash, pemphigoid reaction, eosinophilia, sore mouth, sore tongue and conjunctivitis have been observed.
Miscellaneous: Edema of the face and extremities have been reported. Other reactions which have occurred with intermittent dosage reigmens include "flu" syndrome (such as episodes of fever, chills, headache, dizziness, and bone pain),

shortness of breath, wheezing, decrease in blood pressure and shock. The "flu" syndrome may also appear if rifampin is taken irregularly by the patient or if daily administration is resumed after a drug free interval.

Isoniazid. The most frequent reactions are those affecting the nervous system and the liver. See the boxed WARNING.

Nervous System: Peripheral neuropathy is the most common toxic effect. It is dose-related, occurs most often in the malnourished and in those predisposed to neuritis (eg, alcoholics and diabetics), and is usually preceded by paresthesias of the feet and hands. The incidence is higher in "slow inactivators."

Other neurotoxic effects, which are uncommon with conventional doses, are convulsions, toxic encephalopathy, optic neuritis and atrophy, memory impairment, and toxic psychosis.

Gastrointestinal: Nausea, vomiting, and epigastric distress.

Hepatic: Elevated serum transaminases (SGOT, SGPT), bilirubinemia, bilirubinuria, jaundice, and occasionally severe and sometimes fatal hepatitis. The common prodromal symptoms are anorexia, nausea, vomiting, fatigue, malaise, and weakness. Mild and transient elevation of serum transaminase levels occurs in 10 to 20% of persons taking isoniazid. The abnormality usually occurs in the first 4 to 6 months of treatment but can occur at any time during therapy. In most instances, enzyme levels return to normal with no necessity to discontinue medication. In occasional instances, progressive liver damage occurs, with accompanying symptoms. In these cases, the drug should be discontinued immediately. The frequency of progressive liver damage increases with age. It is rare in persons under 20, but occurs in up to 2.3% of those over 50 years of age.

Hematologic: Agranulocytosis; hemolytic, sideroblastic, or aplastic anemia, thrombocytopenia; and eosinophilia.

Hypersensitivity Reactions: Fever, skin eruptions (morbilliform, maculopapular, purpuric, or exfoliative), lymphadenopathy, and vasculitis.

Metabolic and Endocrine: Pyridoxine deficiency, pellagra, hyperglycemia, metabolic acidosis, and gynecomastia.

Miscellaneous: Rheumatic syndrome and systemic lupus erythematosus-like syndrome.

Pyrazinamide. The principal adverse effect is a hepatic reaction (see WARNINGS). Hepatotoxicity appears to be dose related and may appear at any time during therapy. Pyrazinamide can cause hyperuricemia and gout (see PRECAUTIONS).

Gastrointestinal: GI disturbances including nausea, vomiting, and anorexia have also been reported.

Hematologic and Lymphatic: Thrombocytopenia and sideroblastic anemia with erythroid hyperplasia, vacuolation of erythrocytes and increased serum concentration have occurred rarely with this drug. Adverse effects on blood clotting mechanisms have also been rarely reported.

Other: Mild arthralgia and myalgia have been reported frequently. Hypersensitivity reactions including rashes, urticaria, and pruritis have been reported. Fever, acne, photosensitivity, porphyria, dysuria, and interstitial nephritis have been reported rarely.

OVERDOSAGE

RIFATER. There is no human experience with RIFATER overdosage.

Rifampin. Non-fatal overdoses with as high as 12 g of rifampin have been reported. One case of fatal overdose is known: A 26-year old man died after self-administering 60 g of rifampin.

Isoniazid. Untreated or inadequately treated cases of gross isoniazid overdosage can be fatal, but good response has been reported in most patients treated within the first few hours after drug ingestion.

Ingested acutely, as little as 1.5 g isoniazid may cause toxicity in adults. Doses of 35 to 40 mg/kg have resulted in seizures. Ingestion of 80 to 150 mg/kg isoniazid has been associated with severe toxicity and, if untreated, significant mortality.

Pyrazinamide. Overdosage experience with pyrazinamide is limited.

Signs and Symptoms

The following signs and symptoms have been seen with each individual component in an overdosage situation.

Rifampin. Nausea, vomiting, and increasing lethargy will probably occur within a short time after rifampin overdosage; unconsciousness may occur when there is severe hepatic disease. Brownish red or orange discoloration of the skin, urine, sweat, saliva, tears, and feces will occur, and its intensity is proportional to the amount ingested.

Liver enlargement, possibly with tenderness, can develop within a few hours after severe overdosage; bilirubin levels may increase and jaundice may develop rapidly. Hepatic involvement may be more marked in patients with prior impairment of hepatic function. Other physical findings remain essentially normal. A direct effect upon the hematopoietic system, electrolyte levels, or acid-base balance is unlikely.

Isoniazid. Isoniazid overdosage produces signs and symptoms within 30 minutes to 3 hours. Nausea, vomiting, dizziness,

---

Adverse Events Reported During the Clinical Study

Adverse Events by Body Systems During First 2 Months of Trial	Number of Patients With Adverse Events*	
	RIFATER n=122‡	Separate† n=123‡
Cutaneous (rash, erythroderma, erythema, exfoliative dermatitis, Lyell syndrome, urticaria, localized skin rash, diffuse skin rash, pruritus, generalized hypersensitivity)	8 (7%)	21 (17%)
Gastrointestinal (nausea, vomiting, digestive pain, diarrhea)	8 (7%)	14 (11%)
Musculoskeletal (arthralgia, long bones pain, phlebitis localized joint pain, diffuse joint pain, edema of the legs)	5 (4%)	8 (7%)
Hearing and Vestibular (tinnitus, vertigo, vertigo with loss of equilibrium)	3 (2%)	6 (5%)
Liver and Biliary (hepatitis with conjunctival jaundice, hepatitis with deep jaundice)	0 (0%)	2 (2%)
Central and Peripheral Nervous System (sweating, headache, insomnia, diffuse paresthesia of the legs, anxiety, diabetic coma)	5 (4%)	4 (3%)
Total Body (spiking fever, persistent fever)	2 (2%)	4 (3%)
Cardiorespiratory (tightness in chest, coughing, diffuse chest pain, hemoptysis, angina, palpitation, total pneumothorax)	8 (7%)	3 (2%)
Total number of patients with one or more adverse events	29	43

* A given patient may have experienced ≥1 adverse event.
† Isoniazid, rifampin and pyrazinamide dosed as separate tablets and capsules.
‡ A total of 250 patients (124 RIFATER; 126 separate) were originally enrolled in the study. Five patients (2 RIFATER; 3 separate) were excluded due to admission errors.

---

slurring of speech, blurring of vision, and visual hallucinations (including bright colors and strange designs) are among the early manifestations. With marked overdosage, respiratory distress and CNS depression, progressing rapidly from stupor to profound coma, are to be expected along with severe, intractable seizures. Severe metabolic acidosis, acetonuria, and hyperglycemia are typical laboratory findings.

Pyrazinamide. In one case of pyrazinamide overdosage, abnormal liver function tests developed. These spontaneously reverted to normal when the drug was stopped.

Treatment

The airway should be secured and adequate respiratory exchange should be established in cases of overdosage with RIFATER.

Obtain blood samples for immediate determination of gases, electrolytes, BUN, glucose, etc; type and cross-match blood in preparation for possible hemodialysis.

Gastric lavage within the first 2 to 3 hours after ingestion is advised, but it should not be attempted until convulsions are under control. To treat convulsions, administer IV diazepam or short-acting barbiturates, and IV pyridoxine (usually 1 mg/1 mg isoniazid ingested). Following evacuation of gastric contents, the instillation of activated charcoal slurry into the stomach may help absorb any remaining drug from the gastrointestinal tract. Antiemetic medication may be required to control severe nausea and vomiting.

RAPID CONTROL OF METABOLIC ACIDOSIS IS FUNDAMENTAL TO MANAGEMENT. Give IV sodium bicarbonate at once and repeat as needed, adjusting subsequent dosage on the basis of laboratory findings (ie, serum sodium, pH, etc).

Forced osmotic diuresis must be started early and should be continued for some hours after clinical improvement to hasten renal clearance of drug and help prevent relapse; monitor fluid intake and output.

Hemodialysis is advised for severe cases; if this is not available, peritoneal dialysis can be used along with forced diuresis.

Along with measures based on initial and repeated determination of blood gases and other laboratory tests as needed, utilize meticulous respiratory and other intensive care to protect against hypoxia, hypotension, aspiration pneumonitis, etc.

DOSAGE AND ADMINISTRATION

Adults: Patients should be given the following single daily dose of RIFATER either 1 hour before or 2 hours after a meal with a full glass of water.

Patients weighing ≤ 44 kg—4 tablets
Patients weighing between 45–54 kg—5 tablets
Patients weighing ≥ 55 kg—6 tablets

Children: The ratio of the drugs in RIFATER may not be appropriate in children or adolescents under the age of 15 (eg, higher mg/kg doses of isoniazid are usually given in children than adults).

RIFATER is recommended in the initial phase of short-course therapy which is usually continued for 2 months. The Advisory Council for the Elimination of Tuberculosis, the American Thoracic Society, and the Centers for Disease Control and Prevention recommend that either streptomycin or ethambutol be added as a fourth drug in a regimen containing isoniazid (INH), rifampin and pyrazinamide for initial treatment of tuberculosis unless the likelihood of INH or rifampin resistance is very low. The need for a fourth drug should be reassessed when the results of susceptibility testing are known. If community rates of INH resistance are currently less than 4%, an initial treatment regimen with less than four drugs may be considered.

Following the initial phase, treatment should be continued with rifampin and isoniazid (eg, RIFAMATE®) for at least 4 months. Treatment should be continued for longer if the patient is still sputum or culture positive, if resistant organisms are present, or if the patient is HIV positive.

Concomitant administration of pyridoxine (B₆) is recommended in the malnourished, in those predisposed to neuropathy (eg, alcoholics and diabetics), and in adolescents.

See CLINICAL PHARMACOLOGY: General for dosing information in patients with renal failure.

HOW SUPPLIED

RIFATER tablets are light beige, smooth, round, and shiny sugar-coated tablets imprinted with "RIFATER" in black ink and contain 120 mg rifampin, 50 mg isoniazid, and 300 mg pyrazinamide, and are supplied as:
Bottles of 60 tablets (NDC 0088-0576-41).
Unit dose blister packages of 100 tablets (NDC 0088-0576-49).

Storage Conditions: Store at controlled room temperature 59–86°F (15–30°C). Protect from excessive humidity.

Reference: 1. National Committee for Clinical Laboratory Standards. 1990. Antimycobacterial Susceptibility Testing (Proposed Standard). Document M24-P.
Prescribing information as of June 1994

Mfd by Gruppo Lepetit, S.p.A.
20020 Lainate, Italy, for
Hoechst Marion Roussel, Inc.
Kansas City, MO 64137

Shown in Product Identification Guide, page 317

Continued on next page

Hoechst Marion Roussel—Cont.

SELDANE® ℞
[*sĕl'dān*]
(terfenadine)
60 mg Tablets

WARNING BOX
QT INTERVAL PROLONGATION/VENTRICULAR ARRHYTHMIA
RARE CASES OF SERIOUS CARDIOVASCULAR ADVERSE EVENTS, INCLUDING DEATH, CARDIAC ARREST, TORSADES DE POINTES, AND OTHER VENTRICULAR ARRHYTHMIAS, HAVE BEEN OBSERVED IN THE FOLLOWING CLINICAL SETTINGS, FREQUENTLY IN ASSOCIATION WITH INCREASED TERFENADINE LEVELS WHICH LEAD TO ELECTROCARDIOGRAPHIC QT PROLONGATION:
1. **CONCOMITANT ADMINISTRATION OF KETOCONAZOLE (NIZORAL) OR ITRACONAZOLE (SPORANOX)**
2. **OVERDOSE, INCLUDING SINGLE DOSES AS LOW AS 360 MG**
3. **CONCOMITANT ADMINISTRATION OF CLARITHROMYCIN, ERYTHROMYCIN, OR TROLEANDOMYCIN**
4. **SIGNIFICANT HEPATIC DYSFUNCTION**

TERFENADINE IS CONTRAINDICATED IN PATIENTS TAKING KETOCONAZOLE, ITRACONAZOLE, ERYTHROMYCIN, CLARITHROMYCIN, OR TROLEANDOMYCIN, AND IN PATIENTS WITH SIGNIFICANT HEPATIC DYSFUNCTION.
DO NOT EXCEED RECOMMENDED DOSE.
IN SOME CASES, SEVERE ARRHYTHMIAS HAVE BEEN PRECEDED BY EPISODES OF SYNCOPE. SYNCOPE IN PATIENTS RECEIVING TERFENADINE SHOULD LEAD TO DISCONTINUATION OF TREATMENT AND FULL EVALUATION OF POTENTIAL ARRHYTHMIAS.
(See CONTRAINDICATIONS, WARNINGS, CLINICAL PHARMACOLOGY, AND PRECAUTIONS: DRUG INTERACTIONS.)

DESCRIPTION

SELDANE (terfenadine) is available as tablets for oral administration. Each tablet contains 60 mg terfenadine. Tablets also contain, as inactive ingredients: corn starch, gelatin, lactose, magnesium stearate, and sodium bicarbonate.
Terfenadine is a histamine H_1-receptor antagonist with the chemical name α-[4-(1,1-Dimethylethyl) phenyl]-4-(hydroxydiphenylmethyl)-1-piperidinebutanol (±). The molecular weight is 471.68. The molecular formula is $C_{32}H_{41}NO_2$.
It has the following chemical structure:

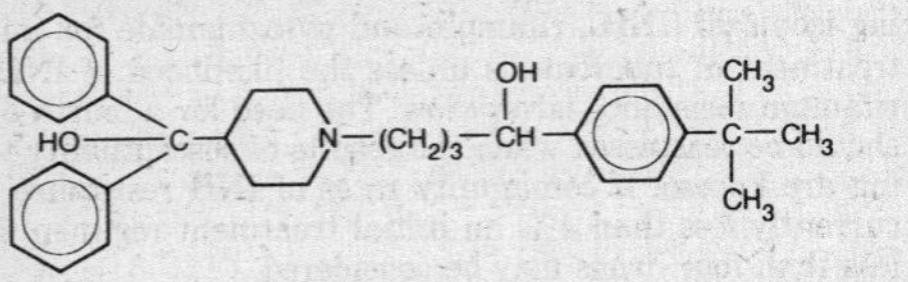

Terfenadine occurs as a white to off-white crystalline powder. It is freely soluble in chloroform, soluble in ethanol, and very slightly soluble in water.

CLINICAL PHARMACOLOGY

Terfenadine is chemically distinct from other antihistamines.
Histamine skin wheal studies have shown that SELDANE in single and repeated doses of 60 mg in 64 subjects has an antihistaminic effect beginning at 1–2 hours, reaching its maximum at 3–4 hours, and lasting in excess of 12 hours. The correlation between response on skin wheal testing and clinical efficacy is unclear. The four best controlled and largest clinical trials each lasted 7 days and involved about 1,000 total patients in comparisons of SELDANE (60 mg b.i.d.) with an active drug (chlorpheniramine, 4 mg t.i.d.; dexchlorpheniramine, 2 mg t.i.d.; or clemastine 1 mg b.i.d.). About 50–70% of SELDANE or other antihistamine recipients had moderate to complete relief of symptoms, compared with 30–50% of placebo recipients. The frequency of drowsiness with SELDANE was similar to the frequency with placebo and less than with other antihistamines. None of these studies showed a difference between SELDANE and other antihistamines in the frequency of anticholinergic effects. In studies which included 52 subjects in whom EEG assessments were made, no depressant effects have been observed.
Animal studies have demonstrated that terfenadine is a histamine H_1-receptor antagonist. In these animal studies, no sedative or anticholinergic effects were observed at effective antihistaminic doses. Radioactive disposition and autoradiographic studies in rats and radioligand binding studies with guinea pig brain H_1-receptors indicate that, at effective antihistamine doses, neither terfenadine nor its metabolites penetrate the blood brain barrier well.
On the basis of a mass balance study using ^{14}C labeled terfenadine the oral absorption of terfenadine was estimated to be at least 70%. Terfenadine itself undergoes extensive (99%) first pass metabolism to two primary metabolites, an active acid metabolite and an inactive dealkylated metabolite. Therefore, systemic availability of terfenadine is low under normal conditions, and parent terfenadine is not normally detectable in plasma at levels >10 ng/mL. Although in rare cases there was measurable plasma terfenadine in apparently normal individuals without identifiable risk factors, the implications of this finding with respect to the variability of terfenadine metabolism in the normal population cannot be assessed without further study. Further studies of terfenadine metabolism in the general population are pending. From information gained in the ^{14}C study it appears that approximately forty percent of the total dose is eliminated renally (40% as acid metabolite, 30% dealkyl metabolite, and 30% minor unidentified metabolites). Sixty percent of the dose is eliminated in the feces (50% as the acid metabolite, 2% unchanged terfenadine, and the remainder as minor unidentified metabolites). Studies investigating the effect of hepatic and renal insufficiency on the metabolism and excretion of terfenadine are incomplete. Preliminary information indicates that in cases of hepatic impairment, significant concentrations of unchanged terfenadine can be detected with the rate of acid metabolite formation being decreased. A single-dose study in patients with hepatic impairment revealed increased parent terfenadine and impaired metabolism, suggesting that additional drug accumulation may occur after repetitive dosing in such patients. Terfenadine is contraindicated for use in patients with significant hepatic dysfunction. (See CONTRAINDICATIONS and WARNINGS.) In subjects with normal hepatic function, unchanged terfenadine plasma concentrations have not been detected. **Elevated levels of parent terfenadine, whether due to significant hepatic dysfunction, concomitant medications, or overdose, have been associated with QT interval prolongation and serious cardiac adverse events.** (See CONTRAINDICATIONS and WARNINGS.) In controlled clinical trials in otherwise normal patients with rhinitis, small increases in QTc interval were observed at doses of 60 mg b.i.d. In studies at 300 mg b.i.d. a mean increase in QTc of 10% (range −4% to +30%) (mean increase of 46 msec) was observed.
Data have been reported demonstrating that compared to young subjects, elderly subjects experience a 25% reduction in clearance of the acid metabolite after single-dose oral administration of 120 mg. Further studies are necessary to fully characterize pharmacokinetics in the elderly.
In vitro studies demonstrate that terfenadine is extensively (97%) bound to human serum protein while the acid metabolite is approximately 70% bound to human serum protein.
Based on data gathered from in vitro models of antihistaminic activity, the acid metabolite of terfenadine has approximately 30% of the H_1 blocking activity of terfenadine. The relative contribution of terfenadine and the acid metabolite to the pharmacodynamic effects have not been clearly defined. Since unchanged terfenadine is usually not detected in plasma, and active acid metabolite concentrations are relatively high, the acid metabolite may be the entity responsible for the majority of efficacy after oral administration of terfenadine.
In a study involving the administration of a single 60 mg SELDANE tablet to 24 subjects, mean peak plasma levels of the acid metabolite were 263 ng/mL (range 133–423 ng/mL) and occurred approximately 2.5 hours after dosing. Plasma concentrations of unchanged terfenadine were not detected. The elimination profile of the acid metabolite was biphasic in nature with an initial mean plasma half-life of 3.5 hours followed by a mean plasma half-life of 6 hours. Ninety percent of the plasma level time curve was associated with these half-lives. Although the elimination profile is somewhat complex, the effective pharmacokinetic half-life can be estimated at approximately 8.5 hours. However, receptor binding and pharmacologic effects, both therapeutic and adverse, may persist well beyond that time.

INDICATIONS AND USAGE

SELDANE is indicated for the relief of symptoms associated with seasonal allergic rhinitis such as sneezing, rhinorrhea, pruritus, and lacrimation.
Clinical studies conducted to date have not demonstrated effectiveness of terfenadine in the common cold.

CONTRAINDICATIONS

CONCOMITANT ADMINISTRATION OF TERFENADINE WITH KETOCONAZOLE (NIZORAL) OR ITRACONAZOLE (SPORANOX) IS CONTRAINDICATED. TERFENADINE IS ALSO CONTRAINDICATED IN PATIENTS WITH DISEASE STATES OR OTHER CONCOMITANT MEDICATIONS KNOWN TO IMPAIR ITS METABOLISM, INCLUDING SIGNIFICANT HEPATIC DYSFUNCTION, AND CONCURRENT USE OF CLARITHROMYCIN, ERYTHROMYCIN, OR TROLEANDOMYCIN. QT PROLONGATION HAS BEEN DEMONSTRATED IN SOME PATIENTS TAKING TERFENADINE IN THESE SETTINGS, AND RARE CASES OF SERIOUS CARDIOVASCULAR EVENTS, INCLUDING DEATH, CARDIAC ARREST, AND TORSADES DE POINTES, HAVE BEEN REPORTED IN THESE PATIENT POPULATIONS. (See WARNINGS and PRECAUTIONS: Drug Interactions.)
SELDANE is contraindicated in patients with a known hypersensitivity to terfenadine or any of its ingredients.

WARNINGS

Terfenadine undergoes extensive metabolism in the liver by a specific cytochrome P-450 isoenzyme. This metabolic pathway may be impaired in patients with hepatic dysfunction (alcoholic cirrhosis, hepatitis) or who are taking drugs such as ketoconazole, itraconazole, or clarithromycin, erythromycin, or troleandomycin (macrolide antibiotics), or other potent inhibitors of this isoenzyme. Interference with this metabolism can lead to elevated terfenadine plasma levels associated with QT prolongation and increased risk of ventricular tachyarrhythmias (such as torsades de pointes, ventricular tachycardia, and ventricular fibrillation) at the recommended dose. SELDANE is contraindicated for use by patients with these conditions (see WARNING BOX, CONTRAINDICATIONS, and PRECAUTIONS: Drug Interactions).
Other patients who may be at risk for these adverse cardiovascular events include patients who may experience new or increased QT prolongation while receiving certain drugs or having conditions which lead to QT prolongation. These include patients taking certain antiarrhythmics, bepridil, certain psychotropics, probucol, or astemizole; patients with electrolyte abnormalities such as hypokalemia or hypomagnesemia, or taking diuretics with potential for inducing electrolyte abnormalities; and patients with congenital QT syndrome. SELDANE is not recommended for use by patients with these conditions.
The relationship of underlying cardiac disease to the development of ventricular tachyarrhythmias while on SELDANE therapy is unclear; nonetheless, SELDANE should also be used with caution in these patients.

PRECAUTIONS

Information for Patients
Patients taking SELDANE should receive the following information and instructions. Antihistamines are prescribed to reduce allergic symptoms. Patients should be advised to take SELDANE only as needed and NOT TO EXCEED THE PRESCRIBED DOSE. Patients should be questioned about use of any other prescription or over-the-counter medication, and should be cautioned regarding the potential for life-threatening arrhythmias with concurrent use of ketoconazole, itraconazole, clarithromycin, erythromycin, or troleandomycin. Patients should be advised to consult the physician before concurrent use of other medications with terfenadine. Patients should be questioned about pregnancy or lactation before starting SELDANE therapy, since the drug should be used in pregnancy or lactation only if the potential benefit justifies the potential risk to fetus or baby. Patients should also be instructed to store this medication in a tightly closed container in a cool, dry place, away from heat or direct sunlight, and away from children.

Drug Interactions
Ketoconazole
Spontaneous adverse reaction reports of patients taking concomitant ketoconazole with recommended doses of terfenadine demonstrate QT interval prolongation and rare serious cardiac events, e.g. death, cardiac arrest, and ventricular arrhythmia including torsades de pointes. Pharmacokinetic data indicate that ketoconazole markedly inhibits the metabolism of terfenadine, resulting in elevated plasma terfenadine levels. Presence of unchanged terfenadine is associated with statistically significant prolongation of the QT and QTc intervals. **Concomitant administration of ketoconazole and terfenadine is contraindicated** (see CONTRAINDICATIONS, WARNINGS, and ADVERSE REACTIONS).
Itraconazole
Torsades de pointes and elevated parent terfenadine levels have been reported during concomitant use of terfenadine and itraconazole in clinical trials of itraconazole and from foreign post-marketing sources. One death has also been reported from foreign post-marketing sources. **Concomitant administration of itraconazole and terfenadine is contraindicated** (see CONTRAINDICATIONS, WARNINGS and ADVERSE REACTIONS).
Due to the chemical similarity of other azole-type antifungal agents (including fluconazole, metronidazole, and miconazole) to ketoconazole and itraconazole, concomitant use of these products with terfenadine is not recommended pending full examination of potential interactions.
Macrolides
Clinical drug interaction studies indicate that erythromycin and clarithromycin can exert an effect on terfenadine metabolism by a mechanism which may be similar to that of ketoconazole, but to lesser extent. Although erythromycin

measurably decreases the clearance of the terfenadine acid metabolite, its influence on terfenadine plasma levels is still under investigation. A few spontaneous accounts of QT interval prolongation with ventricular arrhythmia, including torsades de pointes, have been reported in patients receiving erythromycin or troleandomycin.

Concomitant administration of terfenadine with clarithromycin, erythromycin, or troleandomycin is contraindicated (see CONTRAINDICATIONS, WARNINGS, and ADVERSE REACTIONS). Pending full characterization of potential interactions, concomitant administration of terfenadine with other macrolide antibiotics, including azithromycin, is not recommended. Studies to evaluate the potential interaction of terfenadine with azithromycin are in progress.

Carcinogenesis, Mutagenesis, Impairment of Fertility

Oral doses of terfenadine, corresponding to 63 times the recommended human daily dose, in mice for 18 months or in rats for 24 months, revealed no evidence of tumorigenicity. Microbial and micronucleus test assays with terfendine have revealed no evidence of mutagenesis.

Reproduction and fertility studies in rats showed no effects on male or female fertility at oral doses of up to 21 times the human daily dose. At 63 times the human daily dose there was a small but significant reduction in implants and at 125 times the human daily dose reduced implants and increased post-implantation losses were observed, which were judged to be secondary to maternal toxicity.

Pregnancy Category C

There was no evidence of animal teratogenicity. Reproduction studies have been performed in rats at doses 63 times and 125 times the human daily dose and have revealed decreased pup weight gain and survival when terfenadine was administered throughout pregnancy and lactation. There are no adequate and well-controlled studies in pregnant women. SELDANE should be used during pregnancy only if the potential benefit justifies the potential risk to the fetus.

Nonteratogenic Effects

SELDANE is not recommended for nursing women. The drug has caused decreased pup weight gain and survival in rats given doses 63 times and 125 times the human daily dose throughout pregnancy and lactation. Effects on pups exposed to SELDANE only during lactation are not known, and there are no adequate and well-controlled studies in women during lactation.

Pediatric Use

Safety and effectiveness of SELDANE in pediatric patients below the age of 12 years have not been established.

ADVERSE REACTIONS

Cardiovascular Adverse Events

Rare reports of severe cardiovascular adverse effects have been received which include ventricular tachyarrhythmias (torsades de pointes, ventricular tachycardia, ventricular fibrillation, and cardiac arrest), hypotension, palpitations, syncope, and dizziness. Rare reports of deaths resulting from ventricular tachyarrhythmias have been received (see CONTRAINDICATIONS, WARNINGS, and PRECAUTIONS: Drug Interactions). Hypotension, palpitations, syncope, and dizziness could reflect undetected ventricular arrhythmia. IN SOME PATIENTS, DEATH, CARDIAC ARREST, OR TORSADES DE POINTES HAVE BEEN PRECEDED BY EPISODES OF SYNCOPE. (See WARNING BOX.) Rare reports of serious cardiovascular adverse events have been received, some involving QT prolongation and torsades de pointes, in apparently normal individuals without identifiable risk factors; there is not conclusive evidence of a causal relationship of these events with terfenadine. Although in rare cases there was measurable plasma terfenadine, the implications of this finding with respect to the variability of terfenadine metabolism in the normal population cannot be assessed without further study. In controlled clinical trials in otherwise normal patients with rhinitis, small increases in QTc interval were observed at doses of 60 mg b.i.d. In studies at 300 mg b.i.d. a mean increase in QTc of 10% (range −4% to +30%) (mean increase of 46 msec) was observed.

General Adverse Events

Experience from clinical studies, including both controlled and uncontrolled studies involving more than 2,400 patients who received SELDANE, provides information on adverse experience incidence for periods of a few days up to six months. The usual dose in these studies was 60 mg twice daily, but in a small number of patients, the dose was as low as 20 mg twice a day, or as high as 600 mg daily.

In controlled clinical studies using the recommended dose of 60 mg b.i.d., the incidence of reported adverse effects in patients receiving SELDANE was similar to that reported in patients receiving placebo. (See Table below.)

[See table above.]

In addition to the more frequent side effects reported in clinical trials (See Table), adverse effects have been reported at a lower incidence in clinical trials and/or spontaneously during marketing of SELDANE that warrant listing as possibly associated with drug administration. These include: alopecia (hair loss or thinning), anaphylaxis, angioedema, bronchospasm, confusion, depression, galactorrhea, insomnia, menstrual disorders (including dysmenorrhea), musculoskeletal

symptoms, nightmares, paresthesia, photosensitivity, rapid flare of psoriasis, seizures, sinus tachycardia, sweating, thrombocytopenia, tremor, urinary frequency, and visual disturbances.

In clinical trials, several instances of mild, or in one case, moderate transaminase elevations were seen in patients receiving SELDANE. Mild elevations were also seen in placebo treated patients. Marketing experiences include isolated reports of jaundice, cholestatic hepatitis, and hepatitis. In most cases available information is incomplete.

OVERDOSAGE

Signs and symptoms of overdosage may be absent or mild (e.g. headache, nausea, confusion); but adverse cardiac events including cardiac arrest, ventricular arrhythmias including torsades de pointes and QT prolongation have been reported at overdoses of 360 mg or more and occur more frequently at doses in excess of 600 mg, and QTc prolongations of up to 30% have been observed at a dose of 300 mg b.i.d. Seizures and syncope have also been reported. USE OF DOSES IN EXCESS OF 60 MG B.I.D. IS NOT RECOMMENDED. (See WARNING BOX, CLINICAL PHARMACOLOGY, and ADVERSE REACTIONS.)

In overdose cases, where ventricular arrhythmias are associated with significant QTc prolongation, treatment with antiarrhythmics known to prolong QTc intervals is not recommended.

Therefore, in cases of overdosage, cardiac monitoring for at least 24 hours is recommended and for as long as QTc is prolonged, along with standard measures to remove any unabsorbed drug. Limited experience with the use of hemoperfusion (n = 1) or hemodialysis (n = 3) was not successful in completely removing the acid metabolite of terfenadine from the blood.

Treatment of the signs and symptoms of overdosage should be symptomatic and supportive after the acute stage.

Oral LD$_{50}$ values for terfenadine were greater than 5000 mg/kg in mature mice and rats. The oral LD$_{50}$ was 438 mg/kg in newborn rats.

DOSAGE AND ADMINISTRATION

One tablet (60 mg) twice daily for adults and children 12 years and older.

USE OF DOSES IN EXCESS OF 60 MG B.I.D. IS NOT RECOMMENDED BECAUSE OF THE INCREASED POTENTIAL FOR QT INTERVAL PROLONGATION AND ADVERSE CARDIAC EVENTS. (See WARNING BOX.) USE OF TERFENADINE IN PATIENTS WITH SIGNIFICANT HEPATIC DYSFUNCTION AND IN PATIENTS TAKING KETOCONAZOLE, ITRACONAZOLE, CLARITHROMYCIN, ERYTHROMYCIN, OR TROLEANDOMYCIN IS CONTRAINDICATED. (See CONTRAINDICATIONS, WARNINGS, and PRECAUTIONS: Drug Interactions.)

HOW SUPPLIED

NDC 0068-0723-61
60 mg tablets in bottles of 100.
NDC 0068-0723-65
60 mg tablets in bottles of 500.
Tablets are round, white, and debossed "SELDANE". Store tablets at controlled room temperature (59–86°F) (15–30°C).

Protect from exposure to temperatures above 104°F (40°C) and moisture.

Prescribing information as of January 1995
Merrell Pharmaceuticals Inc.
Subsidiary of Hoechst Marion Roussel, Inc.
Kansas City, MO 64137
U.S. Patent 4,254,129.
Other patent applications pending.

PATIENT INFORMATION

SELDANE®
Generic name
terfenadine (ter-FEN-a-deen)
60 mg Tablets

This leaflet is a summary of important information about SELDANE. Be sure to ask your doctor if you have any questions or want to know more.

What is SELDANE and What is It Used For?

SELDANE is an antihistamine. It is used to relieve symptoms of seasonal allergies or hay fever. These symptoms include runny nose, sneezing, itching of the nose or throat, and itchy, watery eyes.

Clinical studies conducted to date with SELDANE have not demonstrated effectiveness in relieving the symptoms of the common cold.

How Do I Take SELDANE?

* Take SELDANE only as needed when you have symptoms of seasonal allergy or hay fever.
* The recommended dose of SELDANE is one tablet taken twice a day. DO NOT TAKE MORE OFTEN THAN ONE TABLET EVERY TWELVE HOURS.
* Follow any other instructions your doctor gives you.

What Are The Important Warnings About Using SELDANE?

WARNING: DO NOT USE SELDANE IF YOU ARE USING KETOCONAZOLE (NIZORAL), ITRACONAZOLE (SPORANOX), ERYTHROMYCIN, CLARITHROMYCIN (BIAXIN), OR TROLEANDOMYCIN (TAO). IF YOU HAVE ANY LIVER OR HEART PROBLEMS, TALK TO YOUR DOCTOR BEFORE YOU USE SELDANE.

Do not use SELDANE with any other prescription or nonprescription medicines without first talking to your doctor and pharmacist.

If you faint, become dizzy, have any unusual heartbeats, or any other unusual symptoms while using SELDANE, contact your doctor.

If you become pregnant or are nursing a baby, talk to your doctor about whether you should take SELDANE. Your doctor will decide whether you should take SELDANE based on the benefits and the risks.

What Are the Risks of Using SELDANE?

The side effects which occur most often are headaches and mild stomach or intestinal problems.

In rare cases, SELDANE has caused IRREGULAR HEARTBEATS which may cause serious problems like fainting, dizziness, cardiac arrest, or death. In these rare cases, this occurred when SELDANE was taken:

* in more than the recommended dose (remember, do not take more often than one tablet every twelve hours.);
* with the antifungal drugs ketoconazole (Nizoral) or itraconazole (Sporanox);

ADVERSE EVENTS REPORTED IN CLINICAL TRIALS

Adverse Event	Percent of Patients Reporting				
	Controlled Studies*			All Clinical Studies**	
	SELDANE n = 781	Placebo n = 665	Control n = 626***	SELDANE n = 2462	Placebo n = 1478
Central Nervous System					
Drowsiness	9.0	8.1	18.1	8.5	8.2
Headache	6.3	7.4	3.8	15.8	11.2
Fatigue	2.9	0.9	5.8	4.5	3.0
Dizziness	1.4	1.1	1.0	1.5	1.2
Nervousness	0.9	0.2	0.6	1.7	1.0
Weakness	0.9	0.6	0.2	0.6	0.5
Appetite Increase	0.6	0.0	0.0	0.5	0.0
Gastrointestinal System					
Gastrointestinal Distress (Abdominal distress, Nausea, Vomiting, Change in bowel habits)	4.6	3.0	2.7	7.6	5.4
Eye, Ear, Nose, and Throat					
Dry Mouth/Nose/Throat	2.3	1.8	3.5	4.8	3.1
Cough	0.9	0.2	0.5	2.5	1.7
Sore Throat	0.5	0.3	0.5	3.2	1.6
Epistaxis	0.0	0.8	0.2	0.7	0.4
Skin					
Eruption (including rash and urticaria) or itching	1.0	1.7	1.4	1.6	2.0

* Duration of treatment in "CONTROLLED STUDIES" was usually 7–14 days.
** Duration of treatment in "ALL CLINICAL STUDIES" was up to 6 months.
*** CONTROLLED DRUGS: Chlorpheniramine (291 patients), d-Chlorpheniramine (189 patients), Clemastine (146 patients)

Continued on next page

Hoechst Marion Roussel—Cont.

- with the antibiotic drugs erythromycin, clarithromycin (Biaxin), or troleandomycin (TAO);
- by patients with serious liver disease.

How Do I Store SELDANE?
SELDANE should be stored in a tightly closed container, in a cool place, out of direct sunlight. It should be kept away from children.
Patient Information as of January 1995
Shown in Product Identification Guide, page 318

SELDANE-D® ℞

[sĕl'dān dee]
(terfenadine and pseudoephedrine hydrochloride)
Extended-Release Tablets

Prescribing Information as of January 1995a

WARNING BOX
QT INTERVAL PROLONGATION/VENTRICULAR ARRHYTHMIA
RARE CASES OF SERIOUS CARDIOVASCULAR ADVERSE EVENTS, INCLUDING DEATH, CARDIAC ARREST, TORSADES DE POINTES, AND OTHER VENTRICULAR ARRHYTHMIAS, HAVE BEEN OBSERVED IN THE FOLLOWING CLINICAL SETTINGS, FREQUENTLY IN ASSOCIATION WITH INCREASED TERFENADINE LEVELS WHICH LEAD TO ELECTROCARDIOGRAPHIC QT PROLONGATION:
1. **CONCOMITANT ADMINISTRATION OF KETOCONAZOLE (NIZORAL) OR ITRACONAZOLE (SPORANOX)**
2. **OVERDOSE, INCLUDING SINGLE TERFENADINE DOSES AS LOW AS 360 MG**
3. **CONCOMITANT ADMINISTRATION OF CLARITHROMYCIN, ERYTHROMYCIN, OR TROLEANDOMYCIN**
4. **SIGNIFICANT HEPATIC DYSFUNCTION**

TERFENADINE IS CONTRAINDICATED IN PATIENTS TAKING KETOCONAZOLE, ITRACONAZOLE, ERYTHROMYCIN, CLARITHROMYCIN, OR TROLEANDOMYCIN, AND IN PATIENTS WITH SIGNIFICANT HEPATIC DYSFUNCTION.
DO NOT EXCEED RECOMMENDED DOSE.
IN SOME CASES, SEVERE ARRHYTHMIAS HAVE BEEN PRECEDED BY EPISODES OF SYNCOPE. SYNCOPE IN PATIENTS RECEIVING TERFENADINE SHOULD LEAD TO DISCONTINUATION OF TREATMENT AND FULL EVALUATION OF POTENTIAL ARRHYTHMIAS.
(See CONTRAINDICATIONS, WARNINGS, CLINICAL PHARMACOLOGY, AND PRECAUTIONS: DRUG INTERACTIONS.)

DESCRIPTION
SELDANE-D (terfenadine and pseudoephedrine hydrochloride) Extended-Release Tablets are available for oral administration.
Each tablet contains 60 mg terfenadine and 10 mg of pseudoephedrine hydrochloride in an outer press-coat for immediate release and 110 mg pseudoephedrine hydrochloride in an extended-release core. Tablets also contain, as inactive ingredients: colloidal silicon dioxide, hydroxypropyl methylcellulose 2208, hydroxy-propyl methylcellulose 2910, lactose, magnesium stearate, microcrystalline cellulose, polyethylene glycol, polysorbate 80, precipitated calcium carbonate, pregelatinized corn starch, sodium lauryl sulfate, sodium starch glycolate, titanium dioxide, and zinc stearate.
Terfenadine is a histamine H_1-receptor antagonist with the chemical name α-[4-(1,1-Dimethylethyl)phenyl]-4-(hydroxydiphenylmethyl)-1-piperidinebutanol (±). It has the following structure:

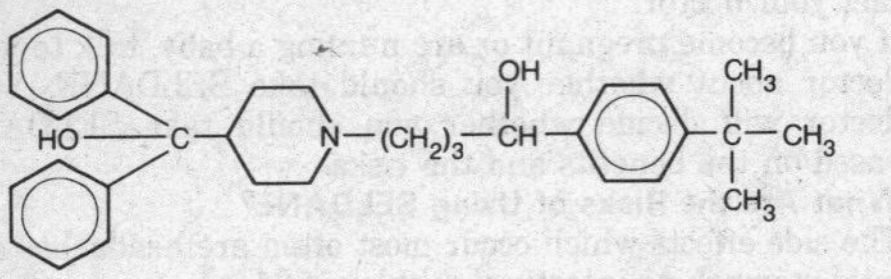

The molecular weight is 471.68. The molecular formula is $C_{32}H_{41}NO_2$.
Terfenadine occurs as a white to off-white crystalline powder. It is freely soluble in chloroform, soluble in ethanol, and very slightly soluble in water.
Pseudoephedrine hydrochloride is an adrenergic (vasoconstrictor) agent with the chemical name [S-R*,R*)]α-[1-(methylamino)ethyl]-benzenemethanol hydrochloride. It has the following chemical structure:
[See chemical structure at top of next column.]

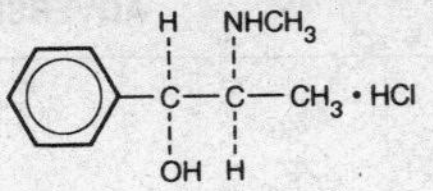

The molecular weight is 201.70. The molecular formula is $C_{10}H_{15}NO \cdot HCl$.
Pseudoephedrine hydrochloride occurs as fine, white to off-white crystals or powder, having a faint characteristic odor. It is very soluble in water, freely soluble in alcohol, and sparingly soluble in chloroform.

CLINICAL PHARMACOLOGY
Terfenadine, a histamine H_1-receptor antagonist, is chemically distinct from other antihistamines.
Histamine skin wheal studies have shown the terfenadine in single and repeated doses of 60 mg in 64 subjects has an antihistaminic effect beginning at 1–2 hours, reaching its maximum at 3–4 hours, and lasting in excess of 12 hours. the correlation between response on skin wheal testing and clinical efficacy is unclear.
The four best controlled and largest clinical trials of SELDANE each lasted 7 days and involved about 1,000 total patients in comparisons of SELDANE (60 mg b.i.d.) with an active drug (chlorpheniramine, 4 mg t.i.d.; dexchlorpheniramine, 2 mg t.i.d.; or clemastine 1 mg b.i.d.). About 50–70% of SELDANE or other antihistamine recipients had moderate to complete relief of symptoms, compared with 30–50% of placebo recipients. The frequency of drowsiness with SELDANE was similar to the frequency with placebo and less than with other antihistamines. In studies which included 52 subjects in whom EEG assessments were made, no depressant effects have been observed. SELDANE-D has not been studied for effectiveness in relieving the symptoms of the common cold.
Animal studies have demonstrated that terfenadine is a histamine H_1-receptor antagonist. In these animal studies, no sedative or anticholinergic effects were observed at effective antihistaminic doses. Radioactive disposition and autoradiographic studies in rats and radioligand binding studies with guinea pig brain H_1-receptors indicate that, at effective antihistamine doses, neither terfenadine nor its metabolites penetrate the blood brain barrier well.
On the basis of a mass balance study using ^{14}C labeled terfenadine the oral absorption of terfenadine was estimated to be at least 70%. Terfenadine itself undergoes extensive (99%) first pass metabolism to two primary metabolities, an active acid metabolite and an inactive dealkylated metabolite. Therefore, systemic availability of terfenadine is low under normal conditions, and parent terfenadine is not normally detectable in plasma at levels > 10 ng/mL. Although in rare cases there was measurable plasma terfenadine in apparently normal individuals without identifiable risk factors, the implications of this finding with respect to the variability of terfenadine metabolism in the normal population cannot be assessed without further study. Further studies of terfenadine metabolism in the general population are pending. From information gained in the ^{14}C study it appears that approximately forty percent of the total dose is eliminated renally (40% as acid metabolite, 30% dealkyl metabolite, and 30% minor unidentified metabolites). Sixty percent of the dose is eliminated in the feces (50% as the acid metabolite, 2% unchanged terfenadine, and the remainder as minor unidentified metabolites). Studies investigating the effect of hepatic and renal insufficiency on the metabolism and excretion of terfenadine are incomplete. Preliminary information indicates that a cases of hepatic impairment, significant concentrations of unchanged terfenadine can be detected with the rate of acid metabolite formation being decreased. A single-dose study in patients with hepatic impairment revealed increased parent terfenadine and impaired metabolism, suggesting that additional drug accumulation may occur after repetitive dosing in such patients. Terfenadine is contraindicated for use in patients with significant hepatic dysfunction. (See CONTRAINDICATIONS and WARNINGS.) In subjects with normal hepatic function unchanged terfenadine plasma concentrations have not been detected. **Elevated levels of parent terfenadine, whether due to significant hepatic dysfunction, concomitant medications, or overdose, have been associated with QT interval prolongation and serious cardiac adverse events.** (See CONTRAINDICATIONS and WARNINGS.) In controlled clinical trials in otherwise normal patients with rhinitis, small increases in QTc interval were observed at doses of 60 mg b.i.d. In studies at 300 mg b.i.d. a mean increase in QTc of 10% (range −4% to +30%) (mean increase of 46 msec) was observed.
Data have been reported demonstrating that compared to young subjects, elderly subjects experience a 25% reduction in clearance of the acid metabolite after single-dose oral administration of 120 mg. Further studies are necessary to fully characterize pharmacokinetics in the elderly.
In vitro studies demonstrate that terfenadine is extensively (97%) bound to human serum protein while the acid metabolite is approximately 70% bound to human serum protein. Based on data gathered from in vitro models of antihistaminic activity, the acid metabolite of terfenadine has approximately 30% of the H_1-blocking activity of terfenadine. The relative contribution of terfenadine and the acid metabolite to the pharmacodynamic effects have not been clearly defined. Since unchanged terfenadine is usually not detected in plasma and active acid metabolite concentrations are relatively high, the acid metabolite may be the entity responsible for the majority of efficacy after oral administration of terfenadine.
In a study involving the administration of a single 60 mg terfenadine tablet to 24 subjects, mean peak plasma levels of the acid metabolite were 263 ng/mL (range 133–423 ng/mL) and occurred approximately 2.5 hours after dosing. Plasma concentrations of unchanged terfenadine were not detected.
The elimination profile of the acid metabolite was biphasic in nature with an initial mean plasma half-life of 3.5 hours followed by a mean plasma half-life of 6 hours. Ninety percent of the plasma level time curve was associated with these half-lives. Although the elimination profile is somewhat complex, the effective pharmacokinetic half-life can be estimated at approximately 8.5 hours. However, receptor binding and pharmacologic effects, both therapeutic and adverse, may persist well beyond that time.
Pseudoephedrine is an orally active sympathomimetic amine and exerts a decongestant action on the nasal mucosa. It is recognized as an effective agent for the relief of nasal congestion due to allergic rhinitis. Pseudoephedrine produces peripheral effects similar to those of epinephrine and central effects similar to, but less intense than, amphetamines. It has the potential for excitatory side effects. At the recommended oral dose it has little or no pressor effect in normotensive adults. The serum half-life of pseudoephedrine is approximately 4 to 6 hours. The serum half-life is decreased with increased excretion of drug at urine pH lower than 6 and may be increased with decreased excretion at urine pH higher than 8.
Ingestion of food was found not to affect the absorption of pseudoephedrine from SELDANE-D. The effect of food on the absorption of terfenadine from SELDANE-D is not known; however, plasma levels of the active metabolite do not appear to be affected by food administered with SELDANE-D.
A bioavailability study comparing SELDANE-D to immediate-release terfenadine and immediate-release pseudoephedrine showed that pseudoephedrine is slowly released from SELDANE-D to permit twice daily dosage.

INDICATIONS AND USAGE
SELDANE-D is indicated for the relief of symptoms associated with seasonal allergic rhinitis such as sneezing, rhinorrhea, pruritus, lacrimation, and nasal congestion. It should be administered when both the antihistaminic properties of SELDANE (terfenadine) and the nasal decongestant activity of pseudoephedrine hydrochloride are desired (see CLINICAL PHARMACOLOGY).
SELDANE-D has not been studied for effectiveness in relieving the symptoms of the common cold.

CONTRAINDICATIONS
CONCOMITANT ADMINISTRATION OF SELDANE-D WITH KETOCONAZOLE (NIZORAL) OR ITRACONAZOLE (SPORANOX) IS CONTRAINDICATED SELDANE-D IS ALSO CONTRAINDICATED IN PATIENTS WITH DISEASE STATES OR OTHER CONCOMITANT MEDICATIONS KNOWN TO IMPAIR ITS METABOLISM, INCLUDING SIGNIFICANT HEPATIC DYSFUNCTION, AND CONCURRENT USE OF CLARITHROMYCIN, ERYTHROMYCIN, OR TROLEANDOMYCIN. QT PROLONGATION HAS BEEN DEMONSTRATED IN SOME PATIENTS TAKING TERFENADINE IN THESE SETTINGS, AND RARE CASES OF SERIOUS CARDIOVASCULAR EVENTS, INCLUDING DEATH, CARDIAC ARREST, AND TORSADES DE POINTES, HAVE BEEN REPORTED IN THESE PATIENT POPULATIONS. (See WARNINGS and PRECAUTIONS: Drug Interactions.)
SELDANE-D is contraindicated in nursing mothers, patients with severe hypertension or severe coronary artery disease, patients receiving monoamine oxidase (MAO) inhibitor therapy, and in patients with a known hypersensitivity to any of its ingredients (see DESCRIPTION section).

WARNINGS
Terfenadine undergoes extensive metabolism in the liver by a specific cytochrome P-450 isoenzyme. The metabolic pathway may be impaired in patients with hepatic dysfunction (alcoholic cirrhosis, hepatitis) or who are taking drugs such as ketoconazole, itraconazole, or clarithromycin, erythromycin, or troleandomycin (macrolide antibiotics), or other potent inhibitors of this isoenzyme. Interference with this metabolism can lead to elevated terfenadine plasma levels associated with QT prolongation and increased risk of ventricular tachyarrhythmias (such as torsades de pointes, ventricular tachycardia, and ventricular fibrillation) at the recommended dose. SELDANE-D is contraindicated for use by patients with these conditions (see WARNING BOX, CONTRAINDICATIONS, and PRECAUTIONS: Drug Interactions.)

Other patients who may be at risk for these adverse cardio-vascular events include patients who may experience new or increased QT prolongation while receiving certain drugs or having conditions which lead to QT prolongation. These include patients taking certain antiarrhythmics, bepridil, certain psychotropics, probucol, astemizole; patients with electrolyte abnormalities such as hypokalemia or hypomagnesemia, or taking diuretics with potential for inducing electrolyte abnormalities; and patients with congenital QT syndrome. SELDANE-D is not recommended for use by patients with these conditions.

The relationship of underlying cardiac disease to the development of ventricular tachyarrhythmias while or SELDANE-D therapy is unclear; nonetheless, SELDANE-D should also be used with caution in these patients.

Sympathomimetic amines should be used judiciously and sparingly in patients with hypertension, diabetes mellitus, ischemic heart disease, increased intraocular pressure, hyperthyroidism, or prostatic hypertrophy (See CONTRAINDICATIONS). Sympathomimetic amines may produce CNS stimulation with convulsions of cardiovascular collapse with accompanying hypotension.

Use in Elderly
The elderly are more likely to have adverse reactions to sympathomimetic amines.

PRECAUTIONS

General
SELDANE-D should be used with caution in patients with diabetes, hypertension, cardiovascular disease, and hyperreactivity to ephedrine.

Information for Patients
Patients taking SELDANE-D should receive the following information and instructions. Patients should be advised to take SELDANE-D only as needed and NOT TO EXCEED THE PRESCRIBED DOSE. Patients should be questioned about use of any other prescription or over-the-counter medication, and should be cautioned regarding the potential for life-threatening arrhythmias with concurrent use of ketoconazole, itraconazole, clarithromycin, erythromycin, or troleandomycin. Patients should be advised to consult the physician before concurrent use of other medications with terfenadine. Patients should be questioned about pregnancy or lactation before starting SELDANE-D therapy, since the drug is contraindicated in nursing women and should be used in pregnancy only if the potential benefit justifies the potential risk to the fetus. Patients should be directed to swallowed the tablet whole. Patients should also be instructed to store this medication in a tightly closed container in a cool, dry place, away from heat, moisture, or direct sunlight, and away from children.

Drug Interactions (see CONTRAINDICATIONS)
Monoamine oxidase (MAO) inhibitors and beta-adrenergic agonists increase the effect of sympathomimetic amines. Sympathomimetic amines may reduce the antihypertensive effects of methyldopa, mecamylamine, and reserpine. MAO inhibitors may prolong and intensify the effects of antihistamines.

Care should be taken in the administration of SELDANE-D concomitantly with other sympathomimetic amines because combined effects on the cardiovascular system may be harmful to the patient.

Ketoconazole
Spontaneous adverse reaction reports of patients taking concomitant ketoconazole with recommended doses of terfenadine demonstrate QT interval prolongation and rare serious cardiac events, e.g., death, cardiac arrest, and ventricular arrhythmia including torsades de pointes. Pharmacokinetic data indicate that ketoconazole markedly inhibits the metabolism of terfenadine, resulting in elevated plasma terfenadine levels. Presence of unchanged terfenadine is associated with statistically significant prolongation of the QT and QTc intervals. Concomitant administration of ketoconazole and SELDANE-D is contraindicated (see CONTRAINDICATIONS, WARNINGS, and ADVERSE REACTIONS).

Itraconazole
Torsades de pointes and elevated parent terfenadine levels have been reported during concomitant use of terfenadine and itraconazole in clinical trials of itraconazole and from foreign post-marketing sources. One death has also been reported from foreign post-marketing sources. Concomitant administration of itraconazole and SELDANE-D is contraindicated (see CONTRAINDICATIONS, WARNINGS, and ADVERSE REACTIONS).

Due to the chemical similarity of other azole-type antifungal agents (including fluconazole, metronidazole, and miconazole) to ketoconazole and itraconazole, concomitant use of these products with SELDANE-D is not recommended pending full examination of potential interactions.

Macrolides
Clinical drug interactions studies indicate that erythromycin and clarithromycin can exert an effect on terfenadine metabolism by a mechanism which may be similar to that of ketoconazole, but to a lesser extent. Although erythromycin measurably decreases the clearance of the terfenadine acid

metabolite, its influence on terfenadine plasma levels is still under investigation. A few spontaneous accounts of QT interval prolongation with ventricular arrhythmia including torsades de pointes have been reported in patients receiving erythromycin and troleandomycin.

Concomitant administration of SELDANE-D with clarithromycin, erythromycia, or troleandomycin is contraindicated (see CONTRAINDICATIONS, WARNINGS, and ADVERSE REACTIONS). Pending full characterization of potential interactions, concomitant administration of SELDANE-D with other macrolide antibiotics, including azithromycin is not recommended. Studies to evaluate potential interaction of terfenadine with azithromycin are in progress.

Carcinogenesis, Mutagenesis, Impairment of Fertility
No studies have been conducted to evaluate the carcinogenic potential of SELDANE-D.

Oral doses of terfenadine, corresponding to 63 times the recommended human daily dose, in mice for 18 months or in rats for 24 months, revealed no evidence of tumorigenicity. Microbial and micronucleus test assays with terfenadine have revealed no evidence of mutagenesis.

Reproduction and fertility studies with terfenadine in rats showed no effects on male or female fertility at oral doses of up to 21 times the human daily dose. At 63 times the human daily dose there was a small but significant reduction in implants and at 125 times the human daily dose reduced implants and increased post-implantation losses were observed, which were judged to be secondary to maternal toxicity. Animal reproduction studies have not been carried out with pseudoephedrine.

Pregnancy Category C
The combination of terfenadine and pseudoephedrine hydrochloride (in a ratio of 1:2 by weight) has been shown to produce reduced fetal weight in rats and rabbits at 42 times the human dose, and delayed ossification with wavy ribs in a few fetuses when given to rats at a dose of 63 times the human daily dose. There are no adequate and well-controlled studies in pregnant women. SELDANE-D should be used during pregnancy only if the potential benefit justifies the potential risk to the fetus.

Nursing Mothers (see CONTRAINDICATIONS)
Terfenadine has caused decreased pup weight gain and survival in rats given doses 63 times and 125 times the human daily dose throughout pregnancy and lactation.

Pediatric Use
Safety and effectiveness of SELDANE-D in pediatric patients below the age of 12 years have not been established.

ADVERSE REACTIONS

Cardiovascular Adverse Events
With terfenadine, rare reports of severe cardiovascular adverse effects have been received which include ventricular tachyarrhythmias (torsades de pointes, ventricular tachycardia, ventricular fibrillation, and cardiac arrest), hypotension, palpitations, syncope, and dizziness. Rare reports of

deaths resulting from ventricular tachyarrhythmias have been received (see CONTRAINDICATIONS, WARNINGS, and PRECAUTIONS; Drug Interactions).

Hypotension, palpitations, syncope, and dizziness could reflect undetected ventricular arrhythmia. IN SOME PATIENTS, DEATH, CARDIAC ARREST, OR TORSADES DE POINTES HAVE BEEN PRECEDED BY EPISODES OF SYNCOPE. (See WARNING BOX.) Rare reports of serious cardiovascular adverse events have been received, some involving QT prolongation and torsades de pointes, in apparently normal individuals without identifiable risk factors; there is not conclusive evidence of a causal relationship of these events with terfenadine. Although in rare cases there was measurable plasma terfenadine, the implications of this finding with respect to the variability of terfenadine metabolism in the normal population cannot be assessed without further study. In controlled clinical trials in otherwise normal patients with rhinitis, small increases in QTc interval were observed at doses of 60 mg b.i.d. in studies at 300 mg b.i.d. a mean increase in QTc of 10% (range −4% to +30%) (mean increase of 46 msec) was observed.

General Adverse Events
In double-blind, parallel, controlled studies in over 300 patients in which SELDANE-D was compared to extend-release pseudoephedrine, adverse reactions reported for greater than 1% of the patients receiving SELDANE-D were not clinically different from those reported for patients receiving pseudoephedrine (see Table below).

[See table above.]

*SELDANE-D B.I.D., pseudoephedrine 120 mg B.I.D.

Pseudoephedrine may cause ephedrine-like reactions such as tachycardia, palpitations, headache, dizziness, or nausea. Sympathomimetic drugs have also been associated with certain untoward reactions including fear, anxiety, tenseness, restlessness, tremor, weakness, pallor, respiratory difficulty, dysuria, insomnia, hallucinations, convulsions, CNS depression, arrhythmias, and cardiovascular collapse with hypotension.

In controlled clinical trials with terfenadine, using the recommended daily dose of 60 mg b.i.d., the incidence of adverse events in patients receiving terfenadine was similar to that reported in patients receiving placebo. These effects included:

Central Nervous System: Drowsiness, headache, fatigue, dizziness, nervousness, weakness, appetite increase.

Gastrointestinal System: Abdominal distress, nausea, vomiting, change in bowel habits.

Eye, Ear, Nose and Throat: Dry mouth/nose/throat, cough, sore throat, epistaxis.

Skin: Eruption (including rash and urticaria) or itching. Also reported spontaneously during the marketing of terfenadine were: alopecia (hair loss or thinning), anaphylaxis,

FREQUENTLY (> 1%) REPORTED ADVERSE EVENTS FOR SELDANE-D IN DOUBLE-BLIND, PARALLEL, CONTROLLED CLINICAL TRIALS*

Adverse Event	Percent of Patients Reporting		
	SELDANE-D (n=374)	Pseudo-ephedrine (n=287)	Placebo (n=193)
Central Nervous System			
Insomnia	25.9	26.8	6.2
Headache	17.4	17.1	22.3
Drowsiness/Sedation	7.2	4.9	11.4
Nervousness	6.7	8.4	1.6
Anorexia	3.7	3.8	0.0
Fatigue	2.1	1.4	2.1
Restlessness	2.1	1.0	0.0
Irritability	1.1	0.0	1.0
Disorientation	1.1	0.0	0.5
Increased Energy	1.1	0.0	0.0
Hyperkinesia	1.1	1.0	0.0
Autonomic			
Dry Mouth/Nose/Throat	21.7	21.3	11.4
Blurring of Vision	1.1	0.3	0.5
Gastrointestinal			
Nausea	4.5	6.6	5.2
Skin			
Rash	1.1	0.0	0.0
Cardiovascular			
Palpitations	2.4	3.8	0.5
Allergy Symptoms			
Sore Throat	1.9	1.7	1.0
Cough	1.6	0.3	1.0
Other			
Infection, Upper Respiratory	1.3	2.4	0.5
Taste Alterations	1.1	1.0	1.0

*SELDANE-D B.I.D., pseudoephedrine 120 mg B.I.D.

Continued on next page

Hoechst Marion Roussel—Cont.

angioedema, bronchospasm, confusion, depression, galactorrhea, insomnia, menstrual disorders (including dysmenorrhea), musculoskeletal symptoms, nightmares, paresthesia, photosensitivity, rapid flare of psoriasis, seizures, sinus tachycardia, sweating, thrombocytopenia, tremor, urinary frequency, and visual disturbances.
Also in clinical trials, several instances of mild or, in one case, moderate transaminase elevations were seen in patients receiving terfenadine. Mild elevations were also seen in placebo treated patients. Marketing experiences include isolated reports of jaundice, cholestatic hepatitis, and hepatitis. In most cases available information is incomplete.

OVERDOSAGE

Acute overdosage with SELDANE-D tablets may produce clinical signs of CNS stimulation or depression and various cardiovascular effects, including cardiac collapse and death. Sympathomimetic amines should be used with great caution in the presence of pseudoephedrine. Patients with signs of stimulation should be treated conservatively.
Adverse cardiac events including cardiac arrest, ventricular arrhythmias including torsades de pointes and QT prolongation have been reported at overdoses of 360 mg or more of terfenadine and occur more frequently at doses in excess of 600 mg, and QTc prolongations of up to 30% have been observed at a dose of 300 mg b.i.d. Seizures and syncope have also been reported. USE OF DOSES IN EXCESS OF ONE TABLET B.I.D. IS NOT RECOMMENDED. (See WARNING BOX, CLINICAL PHARMACOLOGY, and ADVERSE REACTIONS.)
In overdose cases where ventricular arrhythmias are associated with significant QTc prolongation, treatment with antiarrhythmics known to prolong QTc intervals is not recommended.
Therefore, in cases of overdosage, cardiac monitoring for at least 24 hours is recommended and for as long as QTc is prolonged, along with standard measures to remove any unabsorbed drug. Limited experience with the use of hemoperfusion ($n = 1$) and hemodialysis ($n = 3$) was not successful in completely removing the acid metabolite of terfenadine from the blood.
Oral LD_{50} values for terfenadine were greater than 5000 mg/kg in mature mice and rats.
The oral LD_{50} was 438 mg/kg in newborn rats. The LD_{50} of pseudoephedrine hydrochloride alone in male and female rats was 1674 mg/kg, while the LD_{50} of pseudoephedrine hydrochloride administered with terfenadine was 3017 mg/kg.

DOSAGE AND ADMINISTRATION

Adults and pediatric patients 12 years and older: one table swallowed whole, morning and night.
USE OF DOSES IN EXCESS OF ONE TABLET B.I.D. IS NOT RECOMMENDED BECAUSE OF THE INCREASED POTENTIAL FOR QT INTERVAL PROLONGATION AND ADVERSE CARDIAC EVENTS, (See WARNING BOX.) USE OF SELDANE-D IN PATIENTS WITH SIGNIFICANT HEPATIC DYSFUNCTION AND IN PATIENTS TAKING KETOCONAZOLE, ITRACONAZOLE, CLARITHROMYCIN, ERYTHROMYCIN, OR TROLEANDOMYCIN IS CONTRAINDICATED. (See CONTRAINDICATIONS, WARNINGS, and PRECAUTIONS: Drug Interactions.)

HOW SUPPLIED

SELDANE-D Tablets containing 60 mg of terfenadine and 10 mg of pseudoephedrine hydrochloride in an outer press-coat for immediate release and 110 mg of pseudoephedrine hydrochloride in an extended-release core are supplied as follows:
NDC0068-0722-61: Bottles of 100 tablets.
Tablets are white to off-white biconvex capsule-shaped; debossed "SELDANE-D". Store at controlled room temperature (59–86°F) (15–30°C). Protect from moisture.
Merrell Pharmaceuticals Inc.
Subsidiaary of Hoechst Marion Roussel, Inc.
Kansas City, MO 64137
U.S. Patents 4,929,605; 4,996,061; 4,254,129.

PATIENT INFORMATION

SELDANE-D®
Generic names of active Ingredients:
terfenadine (ter-FEN-a-deen) 60 mg and pseudoephedrine HCL (SOO-do-e-FED-rin HCl) 120 mg Tablets
This leaflet is a summary of important information about SELDANE-D. Be sure to ask your doctor if you have any questions or want to know more.
What is SELDANE-D and What Is It Used For?
SELDANE-D is a combination product. Each tablet contains an antihistamine (terfenadine) and a decongestant (pseudoephedrine). It is an extended-release tablet that works for 12 hours.
It is used to relieve symptoms of seasonal allergies or hay fever. These symptoms may include a runny nose, sneezing, itching of the nose or throat, itchy, watery eyes, and stuffy nose.
SELDANE-D has not been studied for effectiveness in relieving the symptoms of the common cold.
How Do I Take SELDANE-D?
- Take SELDANE-D only as needed when you have symptoms of seasonal allergy or hay fever.
- The recommended dose of SELDANE-D is one tablet taken twice a day. **DO NOT TAKE MORE OFTEN THAN ONE TABLET EVERY TWELVE HOURS.**
- Swallow each tablet whole. Do not crush or chew SELDANE-D. Crushing or chewing SELDANE-D destroys the special character of the tablet that allows slow absorption over twelve hours.
- Follow any other instructions your doctor gives you.

What Are the Important Warnings About Using SELDANE-D?
WARNING: DO NOT USE SELDANE-D IF YOU ARE USING KETOCONAZOLE (NIZORAL), ITRACONAZOLE (SPORANOX), ERYTHROMYCIN, CLARITHROMYCIN (BIAXIN), OR TROLEANDOMYCIN (TAO). IF YOU HAVE ANY LIVER OR HEART PROBLEMS, TALK TO YOUR DOCTOR BEFORE YOU USE SELDANE-D.
Do not use SELDANE-D with any other prescription or nonprescription medicines, including those for allergies, weight loss, or colds, without first talking to your doctor and pharmacist.
If you faint, become dizzy, have any unusual heartbeats, or any other unusual symptoms while using SELDANE-D, contact your doctor.
The decongestant (pseudoephedrine) that is in SELDANE-D can have adverse effects in certain medical conditions or situations using other drugs. **WARNING: IF YOU ARE USING CERTAIN MEDICINES THAT TREAT DEPRESSION (MONOAMINE OXIDASE INHIBITOR DRUGS), DO NOT USE SELDANE-D.** Talk to your doctor before taking SELDANE-D if you have:
- heart disease
- high blood pressure
- diabetes
- thyroid disease
- an enlarged prostate gland (difficulty urinating)

If you become pregnant or are nursing a baby, talk to your doctor about whether you should take SELDANE-D. Your doctor will decide whether you should take SELDANE-D based on the benefits and the risks.
What Are the Risks of Using SELDANE-D?
The side effects which occur most often are difficulty falling asleep (insomnia), nervousness, dry mouth, headaches, and mild stomach or intestinal problems.
In rare cases, SELDANE-D has caused **IRREGULAR HEARTBEATS** which may cause serious problems like fainting, dizziness, cardiac arrest, or death. In these rare cases, this occurred when SELDANE-D was taken:
- in more than the recommended dose (remember, do not take more often than one tablet every twelve hours.):
- with the antifungal drugs ketoconazole (Nizoral) or itraconazole (Sporanox);
- with the antibiotic drugs erythromycin, clarithromycin (Biaxin), or troleandomycin (TAO);
- by patients with serious liver disease.

How Do I Store SELDANE-D?
SELDANE-D should be stored in a tightly closed container, in a cool place, out of direct sunlight. It should be kept away from children.
Patient information as of January 1995.
Shown in Product Identification Guide, page 318

SILVADENE® CREAM 1% ℞

[sil'vuh-dēn]
(silver sulfadiazine)

DESCRIPTION

SILVADENE Cream 1% is a soft, white, water-miscible cream containing the antimicrobial agent silver sulfadiazine in micronized form, which has the following structural formula:

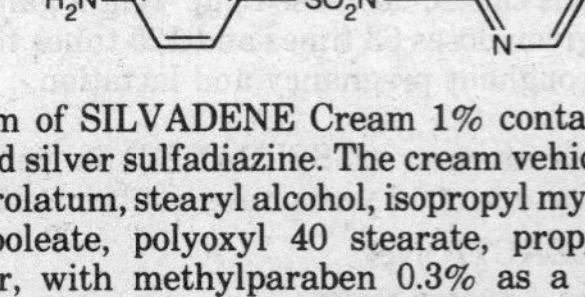

Each gram of SILVADENE Cream 1% contains 10 mg of micronized silver sulfadiazine. The cream vehicle consists of white petrolatum, stearyl alcohol, isopropyl myristate, sorbitan monooleate, polyoxyl 40 stearate, propylene glycol, and water, with methylparaben 0.3% as a preservative. SILVADENE Cream 1% (silver sulfadiazine) spreads easily and can be washed off readily with water.

CLINICAL PHARMACOLOGY

Silver sulfadiazine has broad antimicrobial activity. It is bactericidal for many gram-negative and gram-positive bacteria as well as being effective against yeast. Results from in vitro testing are listed below.
Sufficient data have been obtained to demonstrate that silver sulfadiazine will inhibit bacteria that are resistant to other antimicrobial agents and that the compound is superior to sulfadiazine.
Studies utilizing radioactive micronized silver sulfadiazine, electron microscopy, and biochemical techniques have revealed that the mechanism of action of silver sulfadiazine on bacteria differs from silver nitrate and sodium sulfadiazine. Silver sulfadiazine acts only on the cell membrane and cell wall to produce its bactericidal effect.

Results of In Vitro Testing With SILVADENE® Cream 1% (silver sulfadiazine)
Concentration of Silver Sulfadiazine
Number of Sensitive Strains/Total Number of Strains Tested

Genus & Species	50 μg/mL	100 μg/mL
Pseudomonas aeruginosa	130/130	130/130
Xanthomonas (Pseudomonas) maltophilia	7/7	7/7
Enterobacter species	48/50	50/50
Enterobacter cloacae	24/24	24/24
Klebsiella species	53/54	54/54
Escherichia coli	63/63	63/63
Serratia species	27/28	28/28
Proteus mirabilis	53/53	53/53
Morganella morganii	10/10	10/10
Providencia rettgeri	2/2	2/2
Providencia species	1/1	1/1
Proteus vulgaris	2/2	2/2
Citrobacter species	10/10	10/10
Acinetobacter calcoaceticus	10/11	11/11
Staphylococcus aureus	100/101	100/101
Staphylococcus epidermidis	51/51	51/51
β-Hemolytic *Streptococcus*	4/4	4/4
Enterococcus species	52/53	53/53
Corynebacterium diphtheriae	2/2	2/2
Clostridium perfringens	0/2	2/2
Candida albicans	43/50	50/50

Silver sulfadiazine is not a carbonic anhydrase inhibitor and may be useful in situations where such agents are contraindicated.

INDICATIONS AND USAGE

SILVADENE Cream 1% (silver sulfadiazine) is a topical antimicrobial drug indicated as an adjunct for the prevention and treatment of wound sepsis in patients with second- and third-degree burns.

CONTRAINDICATIONS

SILVADENE Cream 1% (silver sulfadiazine) is contraindicated in patients who are hypersensitive to silver sulfadiazine or any of the other ingredients in the preparation.
Because sulfonamide therapy is known to increase the possibility of kernicterus, SILVADENE Cream 1% should not be used on pregnant women approaching or at term, on premature infants, or on newborn infants during the first 2 months of life.

WARNINGS

There is potential cross-sensitivity between silver sulfadiazine and other sulfonamides. If allergic reactions attributable to treatment with silver sulfadiazine occur, continuation of therapy must be weighed against the potential hazards of the particular allergic reaction.
Fungal proliferation in and below the eschar may occur. However, the incidence of clinically reported fungal superinfection is low.
The use of SILVADENE Cream 1% (silver sulfadiazine) in some cases of glucose-6-phosphate dehydrogenase-deficient individuals may be hazardous, as hemolysis may occur.

PRECAUTIONS

General
If hepatic and renal functions become impaired and elimination of drug decreases, accumulation may occur and discontinuation of SILVADENE Cream 1% (silver sulfadiazine) should be weighed against the therapeutic benefit being achieved.
In considering the use of topical proteolytic enzymes in conjunction with SILVADENE Cream 1%, the possibility should be noted that silver may inactivate such enzymes.
Laboratory Tests
In the treatment of burn wounds involving extensive areas of the body, the serum sulfa concentrations may approach adult therapeutic levels (8 mg% to 12 mg%). Therefore, in these patients it would be advisable to monitor serum sulfa concentrations. Renal function should be carefully monitored, and the urine should be checked for sulfa crystals. Absorption of the propylene glycol vehicle has been reported to affect serum osmolality, which may affect the interpretation of laboratory tests.

Carcinogenesis, Mutagenesis, Impairment of Fertility
Long-term dermal toxicity studies of 24 months' duration in rats and 18 months' in mice with concentrations of silver sulfadiazine three to ten times the concentration in SILVADENE Cream 1% revealed no evidence of carcinogenicity.

Pregnancy
Teratogenic Effects. Pregnancy Category B. A reproductive study has been performed in rabbits at doses up to three to ten times the concentration of silver sulfadiazine in SILVADENE Cream 1% and has revealed no evidence of harm to the fetus due to silver sulfadiazine. There are, however, no adequate and well-controlled studies in pregnant women. Because animal reproduction studies are not always predictive of human response, this drug should be used during pregnancy only if clearly justified, especially in pregnant women approching or at term. (See CONTRAINDICATIONS.)

Nursing Mothers
It is not known whether silver sulfadiazine is excreted in human milk. However, sulfonamides are known to be excreted in human milk, and all sulfonamide derivatives are known to increase the possibility of kernicterus. Because of the possibility for serious adverse reactions in nursing infants from sulfonamides, a decision should be made whether to discontinue nursing or to discontinue the drug, taking into account the importance of the drug to the mother.

Pediatric Use
Safety and effectiveness in pediatric patients have not been established. (See CONTRAINDICATIONS.)

ADVERSE REACTIONS
Several cases of transient leukopenia have been reported in patients receiving silver sulfadiazine therapy.[1,2,3] Leukopenia associated with silver sulfadiazine administration is primarily characterized by decreased neutrophil count. Maximal white blood cell depression occurs within 2 to 4 days of initiation of therapy. Rebound to normal leukocyte levels follows onset within 2 to 3 days. Recovery is not influenced by continuation of silver sulfadiazine therapy. An increased incidence of leukopenia has been reported in patients treated concurrently with cimetidine.
Other infrequently occurring events include skin necrosis, erythema multiforme, skin discoloration, burning sensation, rashes, and intestitial nephritis.
Reduction in bacterial growth after application of topical antibacterial agents has been reported to permit spontaneous healing of deep partial-thickness burns by preventing conversion of the partial thickness to full thickness by sepsis. However, reduction in bacterial colonization has caused delayed separation, in some cases necessitating escharotomy in order to prevent contracture.
Absorption of silver sulfadiazine varies depending upon the percent of body surface area and the extent of the tissue damage. Although few have been reported, it is possible that any adverse reaction associated with sulfonamides may occur. Some of the reactions which have been associated with sulfonamides are as follows: blood dyscrasias, including agranulocytosis, aplastic anemia, thrombocytopenia, leukopenia and hemolytic anemia; dermatologic and allergic reactions, including Stevens-Johnson syndrome and exfoliative dermatitis; gastrointestinal reactions; hepatitis and hepatocellular necrosis; CNS reactions; and toxic nephrosis.

DOSAGE AND ADMINISTRATION
Prompt insitution of appropriate regimens for care of the burned patient is of prime importance and includes the control of shock and pain. The burn wounds are then cleansed and debrided, and SILVADENE Cream 1% (silver sulfadiazine) is applied under sterile conditions. The burn areas should be covered with SILVADENE Cream 1% at all times. The cream should be applied once to twice daily to a thickness of approximately 1/16 inch. Whenever necessary, the cream should be reapplied to any areas from which it has been removed by patient activity. Administration may be accomplished in minimal time because dressings are not required. However if individual patient requirements make dressings necessary, they may be used.
Reapply immediately after hydrotherapy.
Treatment with SILVADENE Cream 1% should be continued until satisfactory healing has occurred, or until the burn site is ready for grafting. The drug should not be withdrawn from the therapeutic regimen while there remains the possibility of infection except if a significant adverse reaction occurs.

HOW SUPPLIED
SILVADENE Cream 1% (silver sulfadiazine) is available in jars containing 50 g (NDC 0088-1050-50), 400 g (NDC 0088-1050-72), and 1000 g (NDC 0088-1050-58) and tubes containing 20 g (NDC 0088-1050-20) and 85 g (NDC 0088-1050-85).

REFERENCES

1. Caffee F, Bingham H. Leukopenia and silver sulfadiazine. *J Trauma.* 1982;22:586–587.
2. Jarret F, Ellerbe S, Demling R. Acute leukopenia during topical burn therapy with silver sulfadiazine. *Amer J Surg.* 1978;135:818–819.
3. Kiker RG, Carvajal HF, Micak RP, Larson, DL. A controlled study of the effects of silver sulfadiazine on white blood cell counts in burned children. *J Trauma.* 1977;17:835–836.

Prescribing Information as of January 1995
Hoechst Marion Roussel, Inc.
Kansas City, MO 64137

Shown in Product Identification Guide, page 318

TOPICORT® (desoximetasone) ℞
Emollient Cream 0.25%
and
TOPICORT® LP (desoximetasone)
Emollient Cream 0.05%

FOR DERMATOLOGIC USE ONLY. NOT FOR USE IN EYES.

DESCRIPTION
Topicort® (desoximetasone) Emollient Cream 0.25% and Topicort® LP (desoximetasone) Emollient Cream 0.05% contain the active synthetic corticosteroid desoximetasone. The topical corticosteroids constitute a class of primarily synthetic steroids used as anti-inflammatory and anti-pruritic agents.
Each gram of Topicort® Emollient Cream 0.25% contains 2.5 mg of desoximetasone in an emollient cream consisting of white petrolatum USP, purified water USP, isopropyl myristate NF, lanolin alcohols NF, mineral oil USP, cetostearyl alcohol NF, aluminum stearate and magnesium stearate.
Each gram of Topicort® LP Emollient Cream 0.05% contains 0.5 mg desoximetasone in an emollient cream consisting of white petrolatum USP, purified water USP, isopropyl myristate NF, lanolin alcohols NF, mineral oil USP, cetostearyl alcohol NF, aluminum stearate, edetate disodium USP, lactic acid USP and magnesium stearate.
The chemical name of desoximetasone is Pregna-1,4-diene-3, 20-dione, 9-fluoro-11, 21-dihydroxy-16-methyl-, (11β, 16α)-.
Desoximetasone has the empirical formula $C_{22}H_{29}FO_4$ and a molecular weight of 376.47.
The CAS Registry Number is 382-67-2. The chemical structure is:

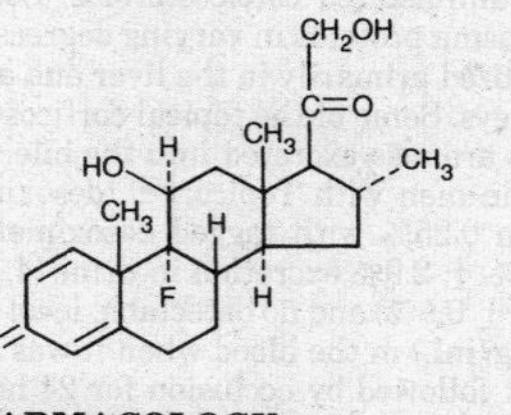

CLINICAL PHARMACOLOGY
Topical corticosteroids share anti-inflammatory, antipruritic and vasoconstrictive actions.
The mechanism of anti-inflammatory activity of the topical corticosteroids is unclear. Various laboratory methods, including vasoconstrictor assays, are used to compare and predict potencies and/or clinical efficacies of the topical corticosteroids. There is some evidence to suggest that a recognizable correlation exists between vasoconstrictor potency and therapeutic efficacy in man.

Pharmacokinetics
The extent of percutaneous absorption of topical corticosteroids is determined by many factors including the vehicle, the integrity of the epidermal barrier, and the use of occlusive dressings.
Topical corticosteroids can be absorbed from normal intact skin. Inflammation and/or other disease processes in the skin increase percutaneous absorption. Occlusive dressings substantially increase the percutaneous absorption of topical corticosteroids. Thus, occlusive dressings may be a valuable therapeutic adjunct for treatment of resistant dermatoses.
Once absorbed through the skin, topical corticosteroids are handled through pharmacokinetic pathways similar to systemically administered corticosteroids. Corticosteroids are bound to plasma proteins in varying degrees. Corticosteroids are metabolized primarily in the liver and are then excreted by the kidneys. Some of the topical corticosteroids and their metabolites are also excreted into the bile.
Pharmacokinetic studies in men with Topicort® (desoximetasone) Emollient Cream 0.25% with tagged desoximetasone showed a total of 5.2% ± 2.9% excretion in urine (4.1% ± 2.3%) and feces (1.1% ± 0.6%) and no detectable level (limit of sensitivity: 0.005 μg/mL) in the blood when it was applied topically on the back followed by occlusion for 24 hours. Seven days after application, no further radioactivity was detected in urine or feces. The half-life of the material was 15 ± 2 hours (for urine) and 17 ± 2 hours (for feces) between the third and fifth trial day. Studies with other similarly structured steroids have shown that predominant metabolite reaction occurs through conjugation to form the glucuronide and sulfate ester.

INDICATIONS AND USAGE
Topicort® Emollient Cream 0.25% and Topicort® LP (desoximetasone) Emollient Cream 0.05% are indicated for the relief of the inflammatory and pruritic manifestations of corticosteroid-responsive dermatoses.

CONTRAINDICATIONS
Topical corticosteroids are contraindicated in those patients with a history of hypersensitivity to any of the components of the preparation.

PRECAUTIONS
General
Systemic absorption of topical corticosteroids has produced reversible hypothalamic-pituitary-adrenal (HPA) axis suppression, manifestations of Cushing's syndrome, hyperglycemia, and glucosuria in some patients.
Conditions which augment systemic absorption include the application of the more potent steroids, use over large surface areas, prolonged use, and the addition of occlusive dressings.
Therefore, patients receiving a large dose of a potent topical steroid applied to a large surface area or under an occlusive dressing should be evaluated periodically for evidence of HPA axis suppression by using the urinary free cortisol and ACTH stimulation tests. If HPA axis suppression is noted, an attempt should be made to withdraw the drug, to reduce the frequency of application, or to substitute a less potent steroid. Recovery of HPA axis function is generally prompt and complete upon discontinuation of the drug. Infrequently, signs and symptoms of steroid withdrawal may occur, requiring supplemental systemic corticosteroids.
Pediatric patients may absorb proportionally larger amounts of topical corticosteroids and thus be more susceptible to systemic toxicity. (See **PRECAUTIONS—Pediatric Use**). If irritation develops, topical corticosteroids should be discontinued and appropriate therapy instituted.
In the presence of dermatological infections, the use of an appropriate antifungal or antibacterial agent should be instituted. If a favorable response does not occur promptly, the corticosteroid should be discontinued until the infection has been adequately controlled.

Information for the Patient
Patients using topical corticosteroids should receive the following information and instructions:
1. This medication is to be used as directed by the physician. It is for external use only. Avoid contact with the eyes.
2. Patients should be advised not to use this medication for any disorder other than for which it was prescribed.
3. The treated skin area should not be bandaged or otherwise covered or wrapped as to be occlusive unless directed by the physician.
4. Patients should report any signs of local adverse reactions especially under occlusive dressing.
5. Parents of pediatric patients should be advised not to use tight-fitting diapers or plastic pants on a child being treated in the diaper area, as these garments may constitute occlusive dressings.

Laboratory Tests
The following tests may be helpful in evaluating the HPA axis suppression: Urinary free cortisol test and ACTH stimulation test.

Carcinogenesis, Mutagenesis, and Impairment of Fertility
Long-term animal studies have not been performed to evaluate the carcinogenic potential or the effect on fertility of topical corticosteroids.
Studies to determine mutagenicity with prednisolone and hydrocortisone have revealed negative results. Desoximetasone did not show potential for mutagenic activity *in vitro* in the Ames microbial mutagent test with or without metabolic activation.

Pregnancy Category C
Corticosteroids are generally teratogenic in laboratory animals when administered systemically at relatively low dosage levels. The more potent corticosteroids have been shown to be teratogenic after dermal application in laboratory animals.
Desoximetasone has been shown to be teratogenic and embryotoxic in mice, rats, and rabbits when given by subcutaneous or dermal routes of administration in doses 3 to 30 times the human dose of Topicort® (desoximetasone) Emollient Cream 0.25% or 15 to 150 times the human dose of Topicort® LP (desoximetasone) Emollient Cream 0.05%.
There are no adequate and well-controlled studies in pregnant women on teratogenic effects from topically applied corticosteroids. Therefore, Topicort® Emollient Cream 0.25% and Topicort® LP Emollient Cream 0.05% should be used during pregnancy only if the potential benefit justifies the potential risk to the fetus. Drugs of this class should not be used extensively on pregnant patients, in large amounts, or for prolonged periods of time.

Continued on next page

Hoechst Marion Roussel—Cont.

Nursing Mothers
It is not known whether topical administration of corticosteroids could result in sufficient systemic absorption to produce detectable quantities in breast milk. Systemically administered corticosteroids are secreted into breast milk in quantities not likely to have a deleterious effect on the infant. Nevertheless, caution should be exercised when topical corticosteroids are administered to a nursing woman.

Pediatric Use
Pediatric patients may demonstrate greater susceptibility to topical corticosteroid-induced HPA axis suppression and Cushing's syndrome than mature patients because of a larger skin surface area to body weight ratio.
Hypothalamic-pituitary-adrenal (HPA) axis suppression, Cushing's syndrome, and intracranial hypertension have been reported in pediatric patients receiving topical corticosteroids. Manifestations of adrenal suppression in pediatric patients include linear growth retardation, delayed weight gain, low plasma cortisol levels, and absence of response to ACTH stimulation. Manifestations of intracranial hypertension include bulging fontanelles, headaches, and bilateral papilledema.
Administration of topical corticosteroids to pediatric patients should be limited to the least amount compatible with an effective therapeutic regimen. Chronic corticosteroid therapy may interfere with the growth and development of pediatric patients.

ADVERSE REACTIONS
The following local adverse reactions are reported infrequently with topical corticosteroids, but may occur more frequently with the use of occlusive dressings. These reactions are listed in an approximate decreasing order of occurrence:

Burning	Hypopigmentation
Itching	Perioral dermatitis
Irritation	Allergic contact dermatitis
Dryness	Maceration of the skin
Folliculitis	Secondary infection
Hypertrichosis	Skin Atrophy
Acneiform	Striae
eruptions	Miliaria

In controlled clinical studies the incidence of adverse reactions was low (0.8%) for Topicort® (desoximetasone) Emollient Cream 0.25% and included burning, folliculitis and folliculo-pustular lesions. The incidence of adverse reactions was also 0.8% for Topicort® LP (desoximetasone) Emollient Cream 0.05% and included pruritus, erythema, vesiculation and burning sensation.

OVERDOSAGE
Topically applied corticosteroids can be absorbed in sufficient amounts to produce systemic effects. (See **PRECAUTIONS**).

DOSAGE AND ADMINISTRATION
Apply a thin film of Topicort® Emollient Cream 0.25% or Topicort® LP Emollient Cream 0.05% to the affected skin areas twice daily. Rub in gently.

HOW SUPPLIED
Topicort® Emollient Cream 0.25% is supplied in 15 gram (NDC 0039-0011-23), 60 gram (NDC 0039-0011-60), and 4 ounce (NDC 0039-0011-04) tubes.
Topicort® LP Emollient Cream 0.05% is supplied in 15 gram (NDC 0039-0012-23) and 60 gram (NDC 0039-0012-60) tubes.

Store at controlled room temperature (59 to 86° F).
CAUTION: FEDERAL LAW PROHIBITS DISPENSING WITHOUT PRESCRIPTION.
Topicort REG TM ROUSSEL UCLAF
HOECHST-ROUSSEL Pharmaceuticals
Division of Hoechst Marion Roussel. Inc.
Kansas City, MO 64137
REG TM HOECHST AG 711000-2/96
Shown in Product Identification Guide, page 318

TOPICORT® Gel ℞
(desoximetasone) 0.05%

FOR DERMATOLOGIC USE ONLY. NOT FOR USE IN EYES.

DESCRIPTION
Topicort® Gel (desoximetasone) 0.05% contains the active synthetic corticosteroid desoximetasone. The topical corticosteroids constitute a class of primarily synthetic steroids used as anti-inflammatory and anti-pruritic agents.
Each gram of Topicort® Gel 0.05% contains 0.5 mg desoximetasone in a gel consisting of purified water USP. SD alcohol 40 (20% w/w), isopropyl myristate NF, carbomer 940, trolamine NF, edetate disodium USP, and docusate sodium USP.
The chemical name of desoximetasone is Pregna-1, 4-diene-3, 20-dione, 9-fluoro-11, 21-dihydroxy-16-methyl-, (11β, 16α)-. Desoximetasone has the empirical formula $C_{22}H_{29}FO_4$ and a molecular weight of 376.47.
The CAS Registry Number is 382-67-2.
The chemical structure is:

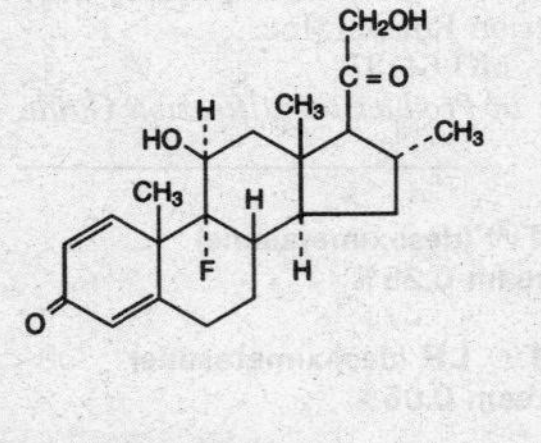

CLINICAL PHARMACOLOGY
Topical corticosteroids share anti-inflammatory, anti-pruritic and vasoconstrictive actions.
The mechanism of anti-inflammatory activity of the topical corticosteroids in unclear. Various laboratory methods, including vasoconstrictor assays, are used to compare and predict potencies and/or clinical efficacies of the topical corticosteroids. There is some evidence to suggest that a recognizable correlation exists between vasoconstrictor potency and therapeutic efficacy in man.

Pharmacokinetics
The extent of percutaneous absorption to topical corticosteroids is determined by many factors including the vehicle, the integrity of the epidermal barrier, and the use of occlusive dressings.
Topical corticosteroids can be absorbed from normal intact skin. Inflammation and/or other disease processes in the skin increase percutaneous absorption. Occlusive dressings substantially increase the percutaneous absorption of topical corticosteroids. Thus, occlusive dressings may be a valuable therapeutic adjunct for treatment of resistant dermatoses.
Once absorbed through the skin, topical corticosteroids are handled through pharmacokinetic pathways similar to systemically administered corticosteroids. Corticosteroids are bound to plasma proteins in varying degrees. Corticosteroids are metabolized primarily in the liver and are then excreted by the kidneys. Some of the topical corticosteroids and their metabolites are also excreted into the bile. Pharmacokinetics studies in men with Topicort® (desoximetasone) Emollient Cream 0.25% with tagged desoximetasone showed a total of 5.2% ± 2.9% excretion in urine (4.1% ± 2.3%) and feces (1.1% ± 0.6%) and no detectable level (limit of sensitivity: 0.005 μg/mL) in the blood when it was applied topically on the back followed by occlusion for 24 hours. Seven days after application, no further radioactivity was detected in urine or feces. The half-life of the material was 15 ± 2 hours (for urine) and 17 ± 2 hours (for feces) between the third and fifth trial day. Studies with other similarly structured steroids have shown that predominant metabolite reaction occurs through conjugation to form the glucuronide and sulfate ester.

INDICATIONS AND USAGE
Topicort® Gel 0.05% is indicated for the relief of the inflammatory and pruritic manifestations of corticosteroid-responsive dermatoses.

CONTRAINDICATIONS
Topical corticosteroids are contraindicated in those patients with a history of hypersensivity to any of the components of the preparation.

PRECAUTIONS
General
Systemic absorption of topical corticosteroids has produced reversible hypothalamic-pituitary-adrenal (HPA) axis suppression, manifestations of Cushing's syndrome, hyperglycemia, and glucosuria in some patients.
Conditions which augment systemic absorption include the application of the more potent steroids, use over large surface areas, prolonged use, and the addition of occlusive dressings.
Therefore, patients receiving a large dose of a potent topical steroid applied to a large surface area or under an occlusive dressing should be evaluated periodically for evidence of HPA axis suppression by using the urinary free cortisol and ACTH stimulation tests. If HPA axis suppression is noted, an attempt should be made to withdraw the drug, to reduce the frequency of application, or to substitute a less potent steroid. Recovery of HPA axis function is generally prompt and complete upon discontinuation of the drug. Infrequently, signs and symptoms of steroid withdrawal may occur, requiring supplemental systemic corticosteroids.
Pediatric patients may absorb proportionally larger amounts of topical corticosteroids and thus be more susceptible to systemic toxicity. (See **PRECAUTIONS—Pediatric Use**). If irritation develops, topical corticosteroids should be discontinued and appropriate therapy instituted.
In the presence of dermatological infections, the use of an appropriate antifungal or antibacterial agent should be instituted. If a favorable response does not occur promptly, the corticosteroid should be discontinued until the infection has been adequately controlled.

Information for the patient
Patients using topical corticosteroids should receive the following information and instructions:
1. This medication is to be used as directed by the physician. It is for external use only. Avoid contact with the eyes.
2. Patients should be advised not to use this medication for any disorder other than for which it was prescribed.
3. The treated skin area should not be bandaged or otherwise covered or wrapped as to be occlusive unless directed by the physician.
4. Patients should report any signs of local adverse reactions especially under occlusive dressing.
5. Parents of pediatric patients should be advised not to use tight-fitting diapers or plastic pants on a child being treated in the diaper area, as these garments may constitute occlusive dressings.

Laboratory Tests
The following tests may be helpful in evaluating the HPA axis suppression:
Urinary free cortisol test
ACTH stimulation test

Carcinogenesis, Mutagenesis, and Impairment of Fertility
Long-term animal studies have not been performed to evaluate the carcinogenic potential or the effect on fertility of topical corticosteroids.
Studies to determine mutagenicity with prednisolone and hydrocortisone have revealed negative results. Desoximetasone did not show potential for mutagenic activity *in vitro* in the Ames microbial mutagen test with or without metabolic activation.

Pregnancy Category C
Corticosteroids are generally teratogenic in laboratory animals when administered systemically at relatively low dosage levels. The more potent corticosteroids have been shown to be teratogenic after dermal application in laboratory animals.
Desoximetasone has been shown to be teratogenic and embryotoxic in mice, rats, and rabbits when given by subcutaneous or dermal routes of administration in doses 15 to 150 times the human dose of Topicort® Gel (desoximetasone) 0.05%.
There are no adequate and well-controlled studies in pregnant women on teratogenic effects from topically applied corticosteroids. Therefore, Topicort® Gel 0.05% should be used during pregnancy only if the potential benefit justifies the potential risk to the fetus. Drugs of this class should not be used extensively on pregnant patients, in large amounts, or for prolonged periods of time.

Nursing Mothers
It is not known whether topical administration of corticosteroids could result in sufficient systemic absorption to produce detectable quantities in breast milk. Systemically administered corticosteroids are secreted into breast milk in quantities not likely to have a deleterious effect on the infant. Nevertheless, caution should be exercised when topical corticosteroids are administered to a nursing woman.

Pediatric Use
Pediatric patients may demonstrate greater susceptibility to topical corticosteroid-induced HPA axis suppression and Cushing's syndrome than mature patients because of a larger skin surface area to body weight ratio.
Hypothalamic-pituitary-adrenal (HPA) axis suppression, Cushing's syndrome, and intracranial hypertension have been reported in pediatric patients receiving topical corticosteroids. Manifestations of adrenal suppression in pediatric patients include linear growth retardation, delayed weight gain, low plasma cortisol levels, and absence of response to ACTH stimulation. Manifestations of intracranial hypertension include bulging fontanelles, headaches, and bifateral papilledema.
Administration of topical corticosteroids to pediatric patients should be limited to the least amount compatible with an effective therapeutic regimen. Chronic corticosteroid therapy may interfere with the growth and development of pediatric patients.

ADVERSE REACTIONS
The following local adverse reactions are reported infrequently with topical corticosteroids, but may occur more frequently with the use of occlusive dressings. These reactions are listed in an approximate decreasing order of occurrence:
Burning
Itching
Irritation
Dryness
Folliculitis
Hypertrichosis
Acneiform eruptions

Hypopigmentation
Perioral dematitis
Allergic contact dermatitis
Maceration of the skin
Secondary infection
Skin Atrophy
Striae
Miliaria

OVERDOSAGE

Topically applied corticosteroids can be absorbed in sufficient amounts to produce systermic effects. (See PRECAUTIONS.)

DOSAGE AND ADMINISTRATION

Apply a thin film of Topicort® Gel (desoxlmetasone) 0.05% to the affected skin areas twice daily. Rub in gently.

HOW SUPPLIED

Topicort® Gel 0.05% is supplied in 15 gram (NDC 0039-0014-23) and 60 gram (NDC 0039-0014-60) tubes.
Store at controlled room temperature (59 to 86°F).
"CAUTION: FEDERAL LAW PROHIBITS DISPENSING WITHOUT PRESCRIPTION."
Topicort REG TM ROUSSEL UCLAF714000-2/95
Hoechst-Roussel Pharmaceuticals
Division of Hoechst Marion Roussel, Inc.
Kansas City, MO 64137
Shown in Product Identification Guide, page 318

TOPICORT® Ointment℞
[tä p' i-kõrt]
(desoximetasone) 0.25%
FOR DERMATOLOGICAL USE ONLY. NOT FOR USE IN EYES

DESCRIPTION

Topicort® Ointment (desoximetasone) 0.25% contains the active synthetic corticosteroid desoximetasone. The topical corticosteroids constitute a class of primarily synthetic steroids used as anti-inflammatory and anti-pruritic agents.
Each gram of Topicort® Ointment 0.25% contains 2.5 mg of desoximetasone in a base consisting of white petrolatum USP, propylene glycol USP, sorbitan sesquioleate, beeswax, fatty alcohol citrate fatty acid pentaerythritol ester, aluminum stearate, citric acid, and butylated hydroxyanisole.
The chemical name of desoximetasone is Pregna-1, 4-diene-3, 20-dione, 9-fluoro-11, 21-dihydroxy-16-methyl-, (11β, 16α)-. Desoximetasone has the empirical formula $C_{22}H_{29}FO_4$ and a molecular weight of 376.47.
The CAS Registry Number is 382-67-2. The chemical structure is:

CLINICAL PHARMACOLOGY

Topical corticosteroids share anti-inflammatory, anti-pruritic and vasoconstrictive actions.
The mechanism of anti-inflammatory activity of the topical corticosteroids is unclear. Various laboratory methods, including vasoconstrictor assays, are used to compare and predict potencies and/or clinical efficacies of the topical corticosteroids. There is some evidence to suggest that a recognizable correlation exists between vasoconstrictor potency and therapeutic efficacy in man.

Pharmacokinetics

The extent of percutaneous absorption of topical corticosteroids is determined by many factors including the vehicle, the itegrity of the epidermal barrier, and the use of occlusive dressings.
Topical corticosteroids can be absorbed from normal intact skin. Inflammation and/or other disease processes in the skin increase percutaneous absorption. Occlusive dressings substantially increase the percutaneous absorption of topical corticosteroids. Thus, occlusive dressings may be a valuable therapeutic adjunct for treatment of resistant dermatoses.
Once absorbed through the skin, topical corticosteroids are handled through pharmacokinetic pathways similar to systemically administered corticosteroids. Corticosteroids are bound to plasma proteins in varying degrees. Corticosteroids are metabolized primarily in the liver and are then excreted by the kidneys. Some of the topical corticosteroids and their metabolites are also excreted into the bile.

Pharmacokinetic studies in men with Topicort® Ointment (desoximetasone) 0.25% with tagged desoximetasone showed no detectable level (limit of sensitivity: 0.003 μg/mL) in 1 subject and 0.004 and 0.006 μg/mL in the remaining 2 subjects in the blood when it was applied topically on the back followed by occlusion for 24 hours. The extent of absorption for the ointment was 7% based on radioactivity recovered from urine and feces. Seven days after application. no further radioactivity was detected in urine or feces. Studies with other similarly structured steroids have shown that predominant metabolite reaction occurs through conjugation to form the glucuronide and sulfate ester.

IMDICATIONS AND USAGE

Topicort® Ointment 0.25% is indicated or the relief of the inflammatory and pruritic manifestations of corticosteroid-responsive dermatoses.

CONTRAINDICATIONS

Topical corticosteroids are contraindicated in those patients with a history of hypersensitivity to any of the components of the preparation.

PRECAUTIONS

General

Systemic absorption of topical corticosteroids has produced reversible hypothalamic-pituitary-adrenal (HPA) axis suppression, manifestations of Cushing's syndrome, hyperglycemia, and glucosuria in some patients.
Conditions which augment systemic absorption include the application of the more potent steroids, use over large surface areas, prolonged use, and the addition of occlusive dressings.
Therefore, patients receiving a large dose of a potent topical steroid applied to a large surface area or under an occlusive dressing should be evaluated periodically for evidence of HPA axis suppression by using the urinary free cortisol and ACTH stimulation tests. If HPA axis suppression is noted, an attempt should be made to withdraw the drug, to reduce the frequency of application, or to substitute a less potent steroid. Recovery of HPA axis function is generally prompt and complete upon discontinuation of the drug. Infrequently, signs and symptoms of steroid withdrawal may occur, requiring supplemental systemic corticosteroids.
Pediatric patients may absorb proportionally larger amounts of topical corticosteroids and thus be more susceptible toxicity. (See **PRECAUTIONS — Pediatric Use**.)
If irritation develops, topical corticosteroids should be discontinued and appropriate therapy instituted.
In the presence of dermatological infections, the use of an appropriate antifungal or antibacterial agent should be instituted. If a favorable response does not occur promptly, the corticosteroid should be discontinued until the infection has been adequately controlled.

Information for the Patient

Patients using topical corticosteroids should receive the following information and instructions:
1. This medication is to be used as directed by the physician. It is for external use only. Avoid contact with the eyes.
2. Patients should be advised not to use this medication for any disorder other than for which it was prescribed.
3. The treated skin area should not be bandaged or otherwise covered or wrapped as to be occlusive unless directed by the physician.
4. Patients should report any signs of local adverse reactions especially under occlusive dressing.
5. Parents of pediatric patients should be advised not to use tight-fitting diapers or plastic pants on a child being treated in the diaper area, as these garments may constitute occlusive dressings.

Laboratory Tests

The following tests may be helpful in evaluating the HPA axis suppression:
    Urinary free cortisol test
    ACTH stimulation test

Carcinogenesis, Mutagenesis, and Impairment of Fertility

Long-term animal studies have not been performed to evaluate the carcinogenic potential or the effect on fertility of topical corticosteroids.
Studies to determine mutagenicity with prednisolone and hydrocortisone have revealed negative results. Desoximetasone did not show potential for mutagenic activity *in vitro* in the Ames microbial mutagen test with or without metabolic activation.

Pregnancy Category C

Corticosteroids are generally teratogenic in laboratory animals when administered systemically at relatively low dosage levels. The more potent corticosteroids have been shown to be teratogenic after dermal application in laboratory animals.
Desoximetasone has been shown to be teratogenic and embryotoxic in mice, rats, and rabbits when given by subcutaneous or dermal routes of administration in doses 3 to 30 times the human dose of Topicort® Ointment (desoximetasone) 0.25%.
There are no adequate and well-controlled studies in pregnant women on teratogenic effects from topically applied

corticosteroids. Therefore, Topicort® Ointment 0.25% should be used during pregnancy only if the potential benefit justifies the potential risk to the fetus. Drugs of this class should not be used extensively on pregnant patients, in large amounts, or for prolonged periods of time.

Nursing Mothers

It is not known whether topical administration of corticosteroids could result in sufficient systemic absorption to produce detectable quantities in breast milk. Systemically administered corticosteroids are secreted into breast milk in quantities not likely to have a deleterious effect on the infant. Nevertheless, caution should be exercised when topical corticosteroids are administered to a nursing woman.

Pediatric Use

Pediatric patients may demonstrate greater susceptibility to topical corticosteroid-induced HPA axis suppression and Cushing's syndrome than mature patients because of a larger skin surface area to body weight ratio.
Hypothalamic-pituitary-adrenal (HPA) axis suppression. Cushing's syndrome, and intracranial hypertension have been reported in pediatric patients receiving topical corticosteroids. Manifestations of adrenal suppression in pediatric patients include linear growth retardation, delayed weight gain, low plasma cortisol levels, and absence of response to ACTH stimulation. Manifestations of intracranial hypertension include bulging fontanelles, headaches, and bilateral papilledema.
Administration of topical corticosteroids to pediatric patients should be limited to the least amount compatible with an effective therapeutic regimen.
Chronic corticosteroid therapy may interfere with the growth and development of pediatric patients. Safety and effectiveness of Topicort® Ointment (desoximetasone) 0.25% in pediatric patients below the age of 10 have not been established.

ADVERSE REACTIONS

The following local adverse reactions are reported infrequently with topical corticosteroids, but may occur more frequently with the use of occlusive dressings. These reactions are listed in an approximate decreasing order of occurrence:

Burning	Perioral dermatitis
Itching	Allergic contact dermatitis
Irritation	Maceration of the skin
Dryness	Secondary infection
Folliculitis	Skin Atrophy
Hypertrichosis	Striae
Acneiform eruptions	Miliaria
Hypopigmentation	

In controlled clinical studies the incidence of adverse reactions was low (0.3%) for Topicort® Ointment 0.25% and consisted of development of comedones at the site of application.

OVERDOSAGE

Topically applied corticosteroids can be absorbed in sufficient amounts to produce systemic effects. (See PRECAUTIONS.)

DOSAGE AND ADMINISTRATION

Apply a thin film of Topicort® Ointment 0.25% to the affected skin areas twice daily. Rub in gently.

HOW SUPPLIED

Topicort® Ointment 0.25% is supplied in 15 gram (NDC 0039-0025-15) and 60 gram (NDC 0039-0025-60) tubes.
Store at controlled room temperature (59 to 86°F).
"CAUTION: FEDERAL LAW PROHIBITS DISPENSING WITHOUT PRESCRIPTION."
Topicort REG TM ROUSSEL UCLAF
Hoechst-Roussel Pharmaceuticals
Division of Hoechst Marion Roussel, Inc.
Kansas City, MO 64137   725000-3/95
Shown in Product Identification Guide, page 318

TRENTAL®℞
[tren 'tal]
(pentoxifylline)*
Tablets, 400 mg

DESCRIPTION

Trental® (pentoxifylline) tablets for oral administration contain 400 mg of the active drug and the following inactive ingredients: benzyl alcohol NF, D&C Red No. 27 Aluminum Lake or FD&C Red No. 3, hydroxypropyl methylcellulose USP, magnesium stearate NF, polyethylene glycol NF, povidone USP, talc USP, titanium dioxide USP, and other ingredients in a controlled-release formulation. Trental® is a tri-substituted xanthine derivative designated chemically as 1-(5-oxohexyl)-3, 7-dimethylxanthine that, unlike theophylline, is a hemorrheologic agent, i.e. and agent that affects

Continued on next page

Hoechst Marion Roussel—Cont.

blood viscosity. Pentoxifylline is soluble in water and ethanol, and sparingly soluble in toluene. The CAS Registry Number is 6493-05-6.
The chemical structure is:

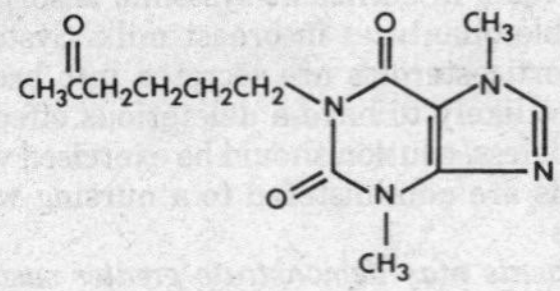

CLINICAL PHARMACOLOGY

Mode of Action
Pentoxifylline and its metabolites improve the flow properties of blood by decreasing its viscosity. In patients with chronic peripheral arterial disease, this increases blood flow to the affected microcirculation and enhances tissue oxygenation. The precise mode of action of pentoxifylline and the sequence of events leading to clinical improvement are still to be defined. Pentoxifylline administration has been shown to produce dose related hemorrheologic effects, lowering blood viscosity, and improving erythrocyte flexibility. Leukocyte properties of hemorrheologic importance have been modified in animal and *in vitro* human studies. Pentoxifylline has been shown to increase leukocyte deformability and to inhibit neutrophil adhesion and activation. Tissue oxygen levels have been shown to be significantly increased by therapeutic doses of pentoxifylline in patients with peripheral arterial disease.

Pharmacokinetics and Metabolism
After oral administration in aqueous solution pentoxifylline is almost completely absorbed. It undergoes a first-pass effect and the various metabolites appear in plasma very soon after dosing. Peak plasma levels of the parent compound and its metabolites are reached within 1 hour. The major metabolites are Metabolite I (1-[5-hydroxyhexyl]-3,7-dimethylxanthine) and Metabolite V (1-[3-carboxypropyl]-3,7-dimethylxanthine), and plasma levels of these metabolites are 5 and 8 times greater, respectively, than pentoxifylline.
Following oral administration of aqueous solutions containing 100 to 400 mg of pentoxifylline, the pharmacokinetics of the parent compound and Metabolite I are dose-related and not proportional (non-linear), with half-life and area under the blood-level time curve (AUC) increasing with dose. The elimination kinetics of Metabolite V are not dose-dependent. The apparent plasma half-life of pentoxifylline varies from 0.4 to 0.8 hours and the apparent plasma half-lives of its metabolites vary from 1 to 1.6 hours. There is no evidence of accumulation or enzyme induction (Cytochrome P450) following multiple oral doses.
Excretion is almost totally urinary; the main biotransformation product is Metabolite V. Essentially no parent drug is found in the urine. Despite large variations in plasma levels of parent compound and its metabolites, the urinary recovery of Metabolite V is consistent and shows dose proportionality. Less than 4% of the administered dose is recovered in feces. Food intake shortly before dosing delays absorption of an immediate-release dosage form but does not affect total absorption. The pharmacokinetics and metabolism of Trental® have not been studied in patients with renal and/or hepatic dysfunction, but AUC was increased and elimination rate decreased in an older population (60–68 years) compared to younger individuals (22–30 years).
After administration of the 400 mg controlled-release Trental® tablet, plasma levels of the parent compound and its metabolites reach their maximum within 2 to 4 hours and remain constant over an extended period of time. The controlled release of pentoxifylline from the tablet eliminates peaks and troughs in plasma levels for improved gastrointestinal tolerance.

INDICATIONS AND USAGE

Trental® is indicated for the treatment of patients with intermittent claudication on the basis of chronic occlusive arterial disease of the limbs. Trental® can improve function and symptoms but is not intended to replace more definitive therapy, such as surgical bypass, or removal of arterial obstructions when treating peripheral vascular disease.

CONTRAINDICATIONS

Trental® should not be used in patients with recent cerebral and/or retinal hemorrhage or in patients who have previously exhibited intolerance to this product or methylxanthines such as caffeine, theophylline, and theobromine.

PRECAUTIONS

General: Patients with chronic occlusive arterial disease of the limbs frequently show other manifestations of arteriosclerotic disease. Trental® has been used safely for treatment of peripheral arterial disease in patients with concurrent coronary artery and cerebrovascular diseases, but there have been occasional reports of angina, hypotension, and arrhythmia. Controlled trials do not show that Trental® causes such adverse effects more often than placebo, but, as it is a methylxanthine derivative, it is possible some individuals will experience such responses. Patients on Warfarin should have more frequent monitoring of prothrombin times, while patients with other risk factors complicated by hemorrhage (e.g. recent surgery, peptic ulceration, cerebral and/or retinal bleeding) should have periodic examinations for bleeding including, hematocrit and/or hemoglobin.

Drug Interactions: Although a causal relationship has not been established, there have been reports of bleeding and/or prolonged prothrombin time in patients treated with Trental® with and without anticoagulants or platelet aggregation inhibitors. Patients on Warfarin should have more frequent monitoring of prothrombin times, while patients with other risk factors complicated by hemorrhage (e.g., recent surgery, peptic ulceration) should have periodic examinations for bleeding including hematocrit and/or hemoglobin. Concomitant administration of Trental® and theophylline-containing drugs leads to increased theophylline levels and theophylline toxicity in some individuals. Such patients should be closely monitored for signs of toxicity and have their theophylline dosage adjusted as necessary. Trental® has been used concurrently with antihypertensive drugs, beta blockers, digitalis, diuretics, antidiabetic agents, and antiarrhythmics, without observed problems. Small decreases in blood pressure have been observed in some patients treated with Trental®; periodic systemic blood pressure monitoring is recommended for patients receiving concomitant antihypertensive therapy. If indicated, dosage of the antihypertensive agents should be reduced.

Carcinogenesis, Mutagenesis and Impairment of Fertility: Long-term studies of the carcinogenic potential of pentoxifylline were conducted in mice and rats by dietary administration of the drug at doses up to 450 mg/kg (approximately 19 times) the maximum recommended human daily dose (MRHD) in both species when based on body weight 1.5 times the MRHD in the mouse and 3.3 times the MRHD in the rat when based on body surface area). In mice, the drug was administered for 18 months, whereas in rats, the drug was administered for 18 months followed by an additional 6 months without drug exposure. In the rat study, there was a statistically significant increase in benign mammary fibroadenomas in females of the 450 mg/kg group. The relevance of this finding to human use is uncertain. Pentoxifylline was devoid of mutagenic activity in various strains of *Salmonella* (Ames test) and in cultured mammalian cells (unscheduled DNA synthesis test) when tested in the presence and absence of metabolic activation. It was also negative in the in vivo mouse micronucleus test.

Pregnancy: Category C. Teratogenic studies have been performed in rats and rabbits using oral doses up to 576 and 264 mg/kg, respectively. On a weight basis, these doses are 24 and 11 times the maximum recommended human daily dose (MRHD); on a body-surface-area basis, they are 4.2 and 3.5 times the MRHD. No evidence of fetal malformation was observed. Increased resorption was seen in rats of the 576 mg/kg group. . There are no adequate and well controlled studies in pregnant women. Trental® (pentoxifylline) should be used during pregnancy only if the potential benefit justifies the potential risk to the fetus.

Nursing Mothers: Pentoxifylline and its metabolites are excreted in human milk. Because of the potential for tumorigenicity shown for pentoxifylline in rats, a decision should be made whether to discontinue nursing or discontinue the drug, taking into account the importance of the drug to the mother.

Pediatric Use: Safety and effectiveness in pediatric patients have not been established.

ADVERSE REACTIONS

Clinical trials were conducted using either controlled-release Trental® tablets for up to 60 weeks or immediate-release Trental® capsules for up to 24 weeks. Dosage ranges in the tablet studies were 400 mg bid to tid and in the capsule studies, 200–400 mg tid. The table summarizes the incidence (in percent) of adverse reactions considered drug related, as well as the numbers of patients who received controlled-release Trental® tablets, immediate-release Trental® capsules, or the corresponding placebos. The incidence of adverse reactions was higher in the capsule studies (where dose related increases were seen in digestive and nervous system side effects) than in the tablet studies. Studies with the capsule include domestic experience, whereas studies with the controlled-release tablets were conducted outside the U.S. The table indicates that in the tablet studies few patients discontinued because of adverse effects.
[See table below.]

INCIDENCE (%) OF SIDE EFFECTS

	Controlled-Release Tablets Commercially Available		Immediate-Release Capsules Used only for Controlled Clinical Trials	
	Trental®	**Placebo**	**Trental®**	**Placebo**
(Numbers of Patients at Risk)	(321)	(128)	(177)	(138)
Discontinued for Side Effect	3.1	0	9.6	7.2
CARDIOVASCULAR SYSTEM				
Angina/Chest pain	0.3	—	1.1	2.2
Arrhythmia/Palpitation	—	—	1.7	0.7
Flushing	—	—	2.3	0.7
DIGESTIVE SYSTEM				
Abdominal Discomfort	—	—	4.0	1.4
Belching/Flatus/Bloating	0.6	—	9.0	3.6
Diarrhea	—	—	3.4	2.9
Dyspepsia	2.8	4.7	9.6	2.9
Nausea	2.2	0.8	28.8	8.7
Vomiting	1.2	—	4.5	0.7
NERVOUS SYSTEM				
Agitation/Nervousness	—	—	1.7	0.7
Dizziness	1.9	3.1	11.9	4.3
Drowsiness	—	—	1.1	5.8
Headache	1.2	1.6	6.2	5.8
Insomnia	—	—	2.3	2.2
Tremor	0.3	0.8	—	—
Blurred Vision	—	—	2.3	1.4

Trental® has been marketed in Europe and elsewhere since 1972. In addition to the above symptoms, the following have been reported spontaneously since marketing or occurred in other clinical trials with an incidence of less than 1%; the causal relationship was uncertain:

- Cardiovascular—dyspnea, edema, hypotension.
- Digestive—anorexia, cholecystitis, constipation, dry mouth/thirst.
- Nervous—anxiety, confusion, depression, seizures.
- Respiratory—epistaxis, flu-like symptoms, laryngitis, nasal congestion.
- Skin and Appendages—brittle fingernails, pruritus, rash, urticaria, angiodema.
- Special Senses—blurred vision, conjunctivitis, earache, scotoma.
- Miscellaneous—bad taste, excessive salivation, leukopenia, malaise, sore throat/swollen neck glands, weight change.

A few rare events have been reported spontaneously worldwide since marketing in 1972. Although they occurred under circumstances in which a causal relationship with pentoxifylline could not be established, they are listed to serve as information for physicians: "Cardiovascular—angina, arrhythmia, tachycardia anaphylactoid reactions." Digestive—hepatitis, jaundice, increased liver enzymes; and Hemic and Lymphatic—decreased serum fibrinogen, pancytopenia, aplastic anemia, leukemia, purpura, thrombocytopenia.

OVERDOSAGE

Overdosage with Trental® has been reported in children and adults. Symptoms appear to be dose related. A report from a poison control center on 44 patients taking overdoses of enteric-coated pentoxifylline tablets noted that symptoms usually occurred 4–5 hours after ingestion and lasted about 12 hours. The highest amount ingested was 80 mg/kg; flushing, hypotension, convulsions, somnolence, loss of consciousness, fever, and agitation occurred. All patients recovered. In addition to symptomatic treatment and gastric lavage, special attention must be given to supporting respiration, maintaining systemic blood pressure, and controlling convulsions.

Activated charcoal has been used to absorb pentoxifylline in patients who have overdosed.

DOSAGE AND ADMINISTRATION

The usual dosage of Trental® in controlled-release tablet form is one tablet (400 mg) three times a day with meals. While the effect of Trental® may be seen within 2 to 4 weeks, it is recommended that treatment be continued for at least 8 weeks. Efficacy has been demonstrated in double-blind clinical studies of 6 months duration.

Digestive and central nervous system side effects are dose related. If patients develop these side effects it is recommended that the dosage be lowered to one tablet twice a day (800 mg/day). If side effects persist at this lower dosage, the administration of Trental® should be discontinued.

HOW SUPPLIED

Trental® is available for oral administration as 400 mg pink film-coated oblong tablets imprinted Trental®; supplied in bottles of 100 (NDC 0039-0078-10), Bulk Pack 5000 (NDC 0039-0078-80, and Unit Dose Packs of 100 (NDC 0039-0078-11).

Store at controlled room temperature (59° to 86° F).
Dispense in well-closed, light-resistant containers.
Protect blisters from light.
*U.S. Patents 3,737,433 & 4,189,469
US Patent 3,737,433 patent term has been extended.
Trental® REG TM HOECHST AG
11/95
Hoechst-Roussel Pharmaceutical
Division of Hoechst Marion Roussel, Inc.
Kansas City, MO 64137

Shown in Product Identification Guide, page 318

Horus Therapeutics, Inc.

2320 BRIGHTON-HENRIETTA TOWN LINE ROAD
ROCHESTER, NY 14623

Direct Inquiries to:
Bernard Ouellette
(716) 292-4820
FAX: (716) 292-4836

THALITONE® ℞
(chlorthalidone tablets, USP)

DESCRIPTION

Thalitone® (chlorthalidone USP) is an antihypertensive/diuretic supplied as 15 or 25 mg tablets for oral use. It is a monosulfamyl diuretic that differs chemically from thiazide diuretics in that a double ring system is incorporated in its structure. It is a racemic mixture of 2-chloro-5-(1-hydroxy-3-oxo-1-isoindolinyl) benzenesulfonamide, with the following structural formula:

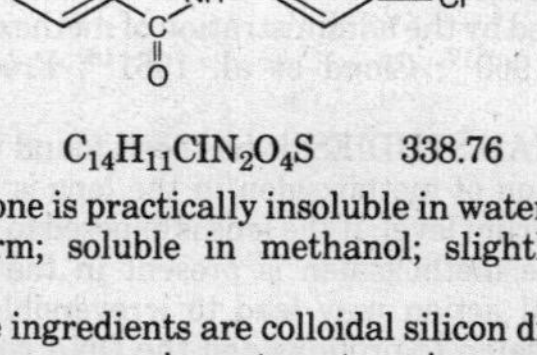

$C_{14}H_{11}ClN_2O_4S$ 338.76

Chlorthalidone is practically insoluble in water, in ether and in chloroform; soluble in methanol; slightly soluble in alcohol.

The inactive ingredients are colloidal silicon dioxide, lactose monohydrate, magnesium stearate, microcrystalline cellulose, povidone, sodium starch glycolate.

CLINICAL PHARMACOLOGY

Chlorthalidone is a long-acting oral diuretic with antihypertensive activity. Its diuretic action commences a mean of 2.6 hours after dosing and continues for up to 72 hours. The drug produces diuresis with increased excretion of sodium and chloride. The diuretic effects of chlorthalidone and the benzothiadiazine (thiazide) diuretics appear to arise from similar mechanisms and the maximal effect of chlorthalidone and the thiazides appear to be similar. The site of the action appears to be the distal convoluted tubule of the nephron. The diuretic effects of chlorthalidone lead to decreased extracellular fluid volume, plasma volume, cardiac output, total exchangeable sodium glomerular filtration rate, and renal plasma flow. Although the mechanism of action of chlorthalidone and related drugs is not wholly clear, sodium and water depletion appear to provide a basis for its antihypertensive effect. Like the thiazide diuretics, chlorthalidone produces dose-related reductions in serum potassium levels, elevations in serum uric acid and blood glucose, and it can lead to decreased sodium and chloride levels.

The mean plasma half-life of chlorthalidone is about 40 to 60 hours. It is eliminated primarily as unchanged drug in the urine. Non-renal routes of elimination have yet to be clarified. In the blood, approximately 75% of the drug is bound to plasma proteins.

Thalitone® (chlorthalidone USP) has been formulated with PVP (povidone polyvinylpyrrolidone), a bioavailability enhancer that provides 104% to 116% bioavailability relative to an oral solution of chlorthalidone. Thalitone cannot be substituted for other formulations of chlorthalidone and likewise, other formulations of chlorthalidone cannot be substituted for Thalitone.

INDICATIONS AND USAGE

Thalitone® (chlorthalidone USP) is indicated in the management of hypertension either alone or in combination with other antihypertensive drugs.

Chlorthalidone is indicated as adjunctive therapy in edema associated with congestive heart failure, hepatic cirrhosis, and corticosteroid and estrogen therapy.

Chlorthalidone has also been found useful in edema due to various forms of renal dysfunction such as nephrotic syndrome, acute glomerulonephritis, and chronic renal failure.

Usage in Pregnancy: The routine use of diuretics in an other wise healthy woman is inappropriate and exposes mother and fetus to unnecessary hazard. Diuretics do not prevent development of toxemia of pregnancy and there is no satisfactory evidence that they are useful in the treatment of developed toxemia.

Edema during pregnancy may arise from pathological causes or from the physiologic and mechanical consequences of pregnancy. Chlorthalidone is indicated in pregnancy when edema is due to pathologic causes just as it is in the absence of pregnancy (however, see WARNINGS below). Dependent edema in pregnancy resulting from restriction of venous return by the expanded uterus is properly treated through elevation of the lower extremities and use of support hose; use of diuretics to lower intravascular volume in this case is illogical and unnecessary. There is hypervolemia during normal pregnancy that is harmful to neither the fetus nor the mother (in the absence of cardiovascular disease) but that is associated with edema, including generalized edema, in the majority of pregnant women. If this edema produces discomfort, increased recumbency will often provide relief. In rare instances, this edema may cause extreme discomfort that is not relieved by rest. In these cases, a short course of diuretics may provide relief and may be appropriate.

CONTRAINDICATIONS

Anuria. Known hypersensitivity to chlorthalidone or other sulfonamide-derived drugs.

WARNINGS

Thalitone® (chlorthalidone USP) should be used with caution in severe renal disease. In patients with renal disease, chlorthalidone or related drugs may precipitate azotemia. Cumulative effects of the drug may develop in patients with impaired renal function.

Chlorthalidone should be used with caution in patients with impaired hepatic function or progressive liver disease, because minor alterations of fluid and electrolyte balance may precipitate hepatic coma.

Sensitivity reactions may occur in patients with a history of allergy or bronchial asthma.

The possibility of exacerbation or activation of systemic lupus erythematosus has been reported with thiazide diuretics which are structurally related to chlorthalidone. However, systemic lupus erythematosus has not been reported following chlorthalidone administration.

PRECAUTIONS

General: Hypokalemia and other electrolyte abnormalities, including hyponatremia and hypochloremic alkalosis, are common in patients receiving chlorthalidone. These abnormalities are dose-related but may occur even at the lowest marketed doses of chlorthalidone. Serum electrolytes should be determined before initiating therapy and at periodic intervals during therapy. Serum and urine electrolyte determinations are particularly important when the patient is vomiting excessively or receiving parenteral fluids. All patients taking chlorthalidone should be observed for clinical signs of electrolyte imbalance, including dryness of mouth, thirst, weakness, lethargy, drowsiness, restlessness, muscle pains or cramps, muscular fatigue, hypotension, oliguria, tachycardia, palpitations and gastrointestinal disturbances, such as nausea and vomiting. Digitalis therapy may exaggerate metabolic effects of hypokalemia especially with reference to myocardial activity.

Any chloride deficit is generally mild and usually does not require specific treatment except under extraordinary circumstances (as in liver disease or renal disease). Dilutional hyponatremia may occur in edematous patients in hot weather; appropriate therapy is water restriction, rather than administration of salt, except in rare instances when the hyponatremia is life-threatening. In cases of actual salt depletion, appropriate replacement is the therapy of choice.

Thiazide-like diuretics have been shown to increase the urinary excretion of magnesium; this may result in hypomagnesemia.

Calcium excretion is decreased by thiazide-like drugs. Pathological changes in the parathyroid gland with hypercalcemia and hypophosphatemia have been observed in a few patients on thiazide therapy. The common complications of hyperparathyroidism such as renal lithiasis, bone resorption and peptic ulceration have not been seen.

Uric Acid: Hyperuricemia may occur or frank gout may be precipitated in certain patients receiving chlorthalidone.

Other: Increase in serum glucose may occur and latent diabetes mellitus may become manifest during chlorthalidone therapy (see PRECAUTIONS Drug Interactions). Chlorthalidone and related drugs may decrease serum PBI levels without signs of thyroid disturbance.

Information For Patients: Patients should inform their doctor if they have: 1) had an allergic reaction to chlorthalidone or other diuretics or have asthma 2) kidney disease 3) liver disease 4) gout 5) systemic lupus erythematosus, or 6) been taking other drugs such as cortisone, digitalis, lithium carbonate, or drugs for diabetes.

Patients should be cautioned to contact their physician if they experience any of the following symptoms of potassium loss; excess thirst, tiredness, drowsiness, restlessness, muscle pains or cramps, nausea, vomiting or increased heart rate or pulse.

Patients should also be cautioned that taking alcohol can increase the chance of dizziness occurring.

Laboratory Tests: Periodic determination of serum electrolytes to detect possible electrolyte imbalance should be performed at appropriate intervals.

All patients receiving chlorthalidone should be observed for clinical signs of fluid or electrolyte imbalance: namely, hyponatremia, hypochloremic alkalosis and hypokalemia. Serum and urine electrolyte determinations are particularly important when the patient is vomiting excessively or receiving parenteral fluids.

Drug Interactions: Chlorthalidone may add to or potentiate the action of other antihypertensive drugs.

Insulin requirements in diabetic patients may be increased, decreased or unchanged. Higher dosage of oral hypoglycemic agents may be required.

Chlorthalidone and related drugs may increase the responsiveness to tubocurarine.

Chlorthalidone and related drugs may decrease arterial responsiveness to norepinephrine. This diminution is not sufficient to preclude effectiveness of the pressor agent for therapeutic use.

Lithium renal clearance is reduced by chlorthalidone, increasing the risk of lithium toxicity.

Drug/Laboratory Test Interactions: Chlorthalidone and related drugs may decrease serum PBI levels without signs of thyroid disturbance.

Carcinogenesis, Mutagenesis, Impairment of Fertility: No information is available.

Pregnancy/Teratogenic Effects: *PREGNANCY CATEGORY B:* Reproduction studies have been performed in the rat and the rabbit at doses up to 420 times the human dose and have revealed no evidence of harm to the fetus due to chlorthalidone. There are, however, no adequate and well-controlled studies in pregnant women. Because animal reproduction studies are not always predictive of human response, this drug should be used during pregnancy only if clearly needed.

Pregnancy/Non-Teratogenic Effects: Thiazides cross the placental barrier and appear in cord blood. The use of chlorthalidone and related drugs in pregnant women requires that the anticipated benefits of the drug be weighed against possible hazards to the fetus. These hazards include fetal or neonatal jaundice, thrombocytopenia, and possibly other adverse reactions that have occurred in the adult.

Nursing Mothers: Thiazides are excreted in human milk. Because of the potential for serious adverse reactions in nursing infants from chlorthalidone, a decision should be made whether to discontinue nursing or to discontinue the drug, taking into account the importance of the drug to the mother.

Pediatric Use: Safety and effectiveness in children have not been established.

ADVERSE REACTIONS

The following adverse reactions have been observed, but there is not enough systematic collection of data to support an estimate of their frequency.

Gastrointestinal System Reactions: anorexia, gastric irritation, nausea, vomiting, cramping, diarrhea, constipation, jaundice (intrahepatic cholestatic jaundice), pancreatitis.

Central Nervous System Reactions: dizziness, vertigo, paresthesias, headache, xanthopsia.

Hematologic Reactions: leukopenia, agranulocytosis, thrombocytopenia, aplastic anemia.

Dermatologic-Hypersensitivity Reactions: purpura, photosensitivity, rash, urticaria, necrotizing angiitis (vasculitis)

Continued on next page

Horus Therapeutics—Cont.

(cutaneous vasculitis)/ Lyell's syndrome (toxic epidermal necrolysis).

Cardiovascular Reaction: Orthostatic hypotension may occur and may be aggravated by alcohol, barbiturates or narcotics.

Other Adverse Reactions: hyperglycemia, glycosuria, hyperuricemia, muscle spasm, weakness, restlessness, impotence. Whenever adverse reactions are moderate or severe, chlorthalidone dosage should be reduced or therapy withdrawn.

OVERDOSAGE

Symptoms of acute overdosage include nausea, weakness, dizziness and disturbances of electrolyte balance. The oral LD_{50} of the drug in the mouse and the rat is more than 25,000 mg/kg body weight. The minimum lethal dose (MLD) in humans has not been established. There is no specific antidote but gastric lavage is recommended, followed by supportive treatment. Where necessary, this may include intravenous dextrose-saline with potassium, administered with caution.

DOSAGE AND ADMINISTRATION

Therapy should be initiated with the lowest possible dose, then titrated according to individual patient response. A single dose given in the morning with food is recommended; divided doses are unnecessary.

Hypertension: Therapy in most patients should be initiated with a single daily dose of 15 mg. If the response is insufficient after a suitable trial, the dosage may be increased to 30 mg and then to a single daily dose of 45–50 mg. If additional control is required, the addition of a second antihypertensive drug is recommended. Increases in serum uric acid and decreases in serum potassium are dose-related over the 15–50 mg/day range and beyond.

Edema: *INITIATION:* Adults, initially 30 to 60 mg daily or 60 mg on alternate days. Some patients may require 90 to 120 mg at these intervals or up to 120 mg daily. Dosages above this level, however, do not usually produce a greater response.

MAINTENANCE: Maintenance doses may often be lower than initial doses and should be adjusted according to the individual patient. Effectiveness is well sustained during continued use.

HOW SUPPLIED

White, kidney-shaped, compressed tablets coded HTI/77 containing 15 mg of chlorthalidone in bottles of 100 (NDC 59229-077-01) and white, kidney-shaped, compressed scored tablets coded HTI/76 containing 25 mg of chlorthalidone in bottles of 100 (NDC 59229-076-01).

Store below 30°C (86°F).

HORUS THERAPEUTICS, INC.
Marketed by:
HORUS THERAPEUTICS, INC.
2320 Brighton-Henrietta Town Line Road
Rochester, NY 14623
Revised 10/94 83032A

ICN Pharmaceuticals, Inc.

ICN PLAZA
3300 HYLAND AVENUE
COSTA MESA, CA 92626

Direct Inquiries to:
Professional Service Department
(800) 556-1937
(714) 545-0100

8-MOP® CAPSULES ℞

(Methoxsalen, 10 mg)

CAUTION: FEDERAL LAW PROHIBITS DISPENSING WITHOUT PRESCRIPTION.
CAUTION: METHOXSALEN IS A POTENT DRUG. READ ENTIRE BROCHURE PRIOR TO PRESCRIBING OR DISPENSING THIS MEDICATION.

> Methoxsalen with UV radiation should be used only by physicians who have special competence in the diagnosis and treatment of psoriasis and vitiligo and who have special training and experience in photochemotherapy. Psoralen and ultraviolet radiation therapy should be under constant supervision of such a physician. For the treatment of patients with psoriasis, photochemotherapy should be restricted to patients with severe, recalcitrant, disabling psoriasis which is not adequately responsive to other forms of therapy, and only when the diagnosis has been supported by biopsy. Because of the possiblities of ocular damage, aging of the skin, and skin cancer (including melanoma), the patient should be fully informed by the physician of the risks inherent in this therapy. When methoxsalen is used in combination with photopheresis, refer to the UVAR* System Operator's Manual for specific warnings, cautions, indications, and instructions related to photopheresis.

I. DESCRIPTION

8-MOP (Methoxsalen, 8-Methoxypsoralen) Capsules, 10mg. Methoxsalen is a naturally occurring photoactive substance found in the seeds of the **Ammi majus** (Umbelliferae) plant. It belongs to a group of compounds known as psoralens, or furocoumarins. The chemical name of methoxsalen is 9-methoxy-7 H-furo[3,2-g][1]-benzopyran-7-one; it has the following structure:

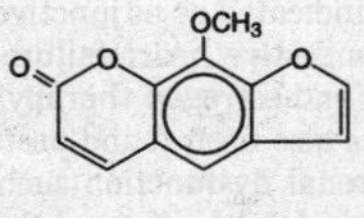

II. CLINICAL PHARMACOLOGY

The combination treatment regimen of psoralen (P) and ultraviolet radiation of 320–400 nm wavelength commonly referred to as UVA is known by the acronym, PUVA. Skin reactivity to UVA (320–400 nm) radiation is markedly enhanced by the ingestion of methoxsalen. The drug reaches its maximum bioavailability 1½–3 hours after oral administration and may last for up to 8 hours (Pathak et al., 1974)[1]. Methoxsalen is reversibly bound to serum albumin and is also preferentially taken up by epidermal cells (Artuc et al. 1979)[2]. At a dose which is six times larger than that used in humans, it induces mixed function oxidases in the liver of mice (Mandula et al. 1978)[3]. In both mice and man, methoxsalen is rapidly metabolized. Approximately 95% of the drug is excreted as a series of metabolites in the urine within 24 hours (Pathak et al. 1977)[4].

The exact mechanism of action of methoxsalen with the epidermal melanocytes and keratinocytes is not known. The best known biochemical reaction of methoxsalen is with DNA. Methoxsalen, upon photoactiviation, conjugates and forms covalent bonds with DNA which leads to the formation of both monofunctional (addition to a single strand of DNA) and bifunctional adducts (crosslinking of psoralen to both strands of DNA) (Dall' Acqua et al., 1971[5]; Cole, 1970[6]; Musajo et al., 1974[7]; Dall' Acqua et al., 1979[8]). Reactions with proteins have also been described (Yoshikawa, et al., 1979[9]).

Methoxsalen acts as a photosensitizer. Administration of the drug and subsequent exposure to UVA can lead to cell injury. Orally administered methoxsalen reaches the skin via the blood and UVA penetrates well into the skin. If sufficient cell injury occurs in the skin, an inflammatory reaction occurs. The most obvious manifestation of this reaction is delayed erythema, which may not begin for several hours and peaks at 48–72 hours. The inflammation is followed, over several days to weeks, by repair which is manifested by increased melanization of the epidermis and thickening of the stratum corneum. The mechanisms of therapy are not known. In the treatment of vitiligo, it has been suggested that melanocytes in the hair follicle are stimulated to move up the follicle and to repopulate the epidermis (Ortonne et al, 1979[10]). In the treatment of psoriasis, the mechanism is most often assumed to be DNA photodamage and resulting decrease in cell proliferation but other vascular, leukocyte, or cell regulatory mechanisms may also be playing some role. Psoriasis is a hyperproliferative disorder and other agents known to be therapeutic for psoriasis are known to inhibit DNA synthesis.

III. INDICATIONS AND USAGE

A. Photochemotherapy (methoxsalen with long wave UVA radiation) is indicated for the symptomatic control of severe, recalcitrant, disabling psoriasis not adequately responsive to other forms of therapy and when the diagnosis has been supported by biopsy. Photochemotherapy is intended to be administered only in conjunction with a schedule of controlled doses of long wave ultraviolet radiation.

B. Photochemotherapy (methoxsalen with long wave ultraviolet radiation) is indicated for the repigmentation of idiopathic vitiligo.

C. Photopheresis (methoxsalen with long wave ultraviolet radiation of white blood cells) is indicated for use with the UVAR* System in the palliative treatment of the skin manifestations of cutaneous T-cell lymphoma (CTCL) in persons who have not been responsive to other forms of treatment. While this dosage form of methoxsalen has been approved for use in combination with photopheresis, Oxsoralen Ultra® Capsules have not been approved for that use.

IV. CONTRAINDICATIONS

A. Patients exhibiting idiosyncratic reactions to psoralen compounds.

B. Patients possessing a specific history of light sensitive disease states should not initiate methoxsalen therapy. Diseases associated with photosensitivity include lupus erythematosus, porphyria cutanea tarda, erythropoietic protoporphyria, variegate porphyria, xeroderma pigmentosum, and albinism.

C. Patients exhibiting melanoma or possessing a history of melanoma.

D. Patients exhibiting invasive squamous cell carcinomas.

E. Patients with aphakia, because of the significantly increased risk of retinal damage due to the absence of lenses.

V. WARNINGS—GENERAL

A. SKIN BURNING: Serious burns from either UVA or sunlight (even through window glass) can result if the recommended dosage of the drug and/or exposure schedules are not maintained.

B. CARCINOGENICITY:

1. ANIMAL STUDIES: Topical or intraperitoneal methoxsalen has been reported to be a potent photocarcinogen in albino mice and hairless mice. However, methoxsalen given by the oral route to albino mice or by any route in pigmented mice is considerably less phototoxic or carcinogenic (Hakim et al. 1960[11]; Pathak et al. 1959[12]).

2. HUMAN STUDIES: A prospective study of 1380 patients over 5 years revealed an approximately ninefold increase in risks of squamous cell carcinoma among PUVA treated patients (Stern et al. 1979[13] and Stern et al. 1980[14]). This increase in risk appears greatest among patients who are fair skinned or had pre-PUVA exposure to 1) prolonged tar and UVB treatment, 2) ionizing radiation, or 3) arsenic.

In addition, an approximately two-fold increase in the risk of basal cell carcinoma was noted in this study. Roenigk et al. 1980[15] studied 690 patients for up to 4 years and found no increase in the risk of non-melanoma skin cancer. However, patients in this cohort had significantly less exposure to PUVA than in the Stern et al study. After 5 years, two of 1380 patients in the Stern et al PUVA study have developed malignant melanoma. In addition, more than 1/5 of patients in this cohort have developed macular pigmented lesions on the buttocks. While there is no evidence that an increased risk of melanoma exists in PUVA treated patients, these observations indicate the need for continued evaluation of melanoma risk in PUVA treated patients.

In a study in Indian patients treated for 4 years for vitiligo, 12 percent developed keratoses, but not cancer, in the depigmented, vitiliginous areas (Mosher, 1980[16]). Clinically, the keratoses were keratotic papules, actinic keratosis-like macules, nonscaling dome-shaped papules, and lichenoid porokeratotic-like papules.

C. CATARACTOGENICITY:

1. ANIMAL STUDIES: Exposure to large doses of UVA causes cataracts in animals, and this effect is enhanced by the administration of methoxsalen (Cloud et al. 1960[17]; Cloud et al. 1961[18]; Freeman et al. 1969[19]).

2. HUMAN STUDIES: It has been found that the concentration of methoxsalen in the lens is proportional to the serum level. If the lens is exposed to UVA during the time methoxsalen is present in the lens, photochemical action may lead to irreversible binding of methoxsalen to proteins and the DNA components of the lens (Lerman et al. 1980[20]). However, if the lens is shielded from UVA, the methoxsalen will diffuse out of the lens in a 24 hour period[20]. Patients should be told emphatically to wear UVA-absorbing, wrap-around sunglasses for the twenty-four (24) hour period following ingestion of methoxsalen, whether exposed to direct or indirect sunlight in the open or through a window glass.

Among patients using proper eye protection, there is no evidence for a significantly increased risk of cataracts in association with PUVA therapy.[13] Thirty-five of 1380 patients have developed cataracts in the five years since their first PUVA treatment. This incidence is comparable to that expected in a population of this size and age distribution. No relationship between PUVA dose and cataract risk in this group has been noted.

D. ACTINIC DEGENERATION: Exposure to sunlight and/or ultraviolet radiation may result in "premature aging" of the skin.

E. BASAL CELL CARCINOMAS: Patients exhibiting multiple basal cell carcinomas or having a history of

basal cell carcinomas should be diligently observed and treated.

F. RADIATION THERAPY: Patients having a history of previous x-ray therapy or grenz ray therapy should be diligently observed for signs of carcinoma.

G. ARSENIC THERAPY: Patients having a history of previous arsenic therapy should be diligently observed for signs of carcinoma.

H. HEPATIC DISEASES: Patients with hepatic insufficiency should be treated with caution since hepatic biotransformation is necessary for drug urinary excretion.

I. CARDIAC DISEASES: Patients with cardiac diseases or others who may be unable to tolerate prolonged standing or exposure to heat stress should not be treated in a vertical UVA chamber.

J. TOTAL DOSAGE: The total cumulative dose of UVA that can be given over long periods of time with safety has not as yet been established.

K. CONCOMITANT THERAPY: Special care should be exercised in treating patients who are receiving concomitant therapy (either topically or systemically) with known photosensitizing agents such as anthralin, coal tar or coal tar derivatives, griseofulvin, phenothiazines, nalidixic acid, halogenated salicylanilides (bacteriostatic soaps), sulfonamides, tetracyclines, thiazides, and certain organic staining dyes such as methylene blue, toluidine blue, rose bengal, and methyl orange.

VI. PRECAUTIONS

This product contains FD&C Yellow No. 5 (tartrazine) which may cause allergic-type reactions (including bronchial asthma) in certain susceptible persons. Although the overall incidence of FD&C Yellow No. 5 (tartrazine) sensitivity in the general population is low, it is frequently seen in patients who also have aspirin hypersensitivity.

A. GENERAL—APPLICABLE TO BOTH VITILIGO AND PSORIASIS TREATMENT:

1. BEFORE METHOXSALEN INGESTION

Patients must not sunbathe during the 24 hours prior to methoxsalen ingestion and UV exposure. The presence of a sunburn may prevent an accurate evaluation of the patient's response to photochemotherapy.

2. AFTER METHOXSALEN INGESTION

a. UVA-absorbing wrap-around sunglasses should be worn during daylight for 24 hours after methoxsalen ingestion. The protective eyewear must be designed to prevent entry of stray radiation to the eyes, including that which may enter from the sides of the eyewear. The protective eyewear is used to prevent the irreversible binding of methoxsalen to the proteins and DNA components of the lens. Cataracts form when enough of the binding occurs. Visual discrimination should be permitted by the eyewear for patient well-being and comfort.

b. Patients must avoid sun exposure, even through window glass or cloud cover, for at least 8 hours after methoxsalen ingestion. If sun exposure cannot be avoided, the patient should wear protective devices such as a hat and gloves, and/or apply sunscreens which contain ingredients that filter out UVA radiation (e.g., sunscreens containing benzophenone and/or PABA esters which exhibit a sun protective factor equal to or greater than 15). These chemical sunscreens should be applied to all areas that might be exposed to the sun (including lips). Sunscreens should not be applied to areas affected by psoriasis until after the patient has been treated in the UVA chamber.

3. DURING PUVA THERAPY

a. Total UVA-absorbing/blocking goggles mechanically designed to give maximal ocular protection must be worn. Failure to do so may increase the risk of cataract formation. A reliable radiometer can be used to verify elimination of UVA transmission through the goggles.

b. Abdominal skin, breasts, genitalia, and other sensitive areas should be protected for approximately ⅓ of the initial exposure time until tanning occur.

c. Unless affected by disease, male genitalia should be shielded.

4. AFTER COMBINED METHOXSALEN/UVA THERAPY

a. UVA-absorbing wrap-around sunglasses should be worn during the daylight for 24 hours after combined methoxsalen/UVA therapy.

b. Patients should not sunbathe for 48 hours after therapy. Erythema and/or burning due to photochemotherapy and sunburn due to sun exposure are additive.

5. VITILIGO THERAPY

a. The dosage of methoxsalen should not be increased above 0.6 mg/kg since overdosage may result in serious burning of the skin.

b. Eye and skin sun protection as described in the Precautions—General section should be observed.

B. INFORMATION FOR PATIENTS: See accompanying Patient Package Insert.

C. LABORATORY TESTS:

1. Patients should have an ophthalmologic examination prior to the start of therapy, and thence yearly.

2. Patients should have the following tests prior to the start of therapy and should be retested 6–12 months subsequently. Additional tests at more extended time periods should be conducted as clinically indicated.

a. Complete Blood Count (Hemoglobin or Hematocrit; White Blood Count—if abnormal, a differential count).

b. Anti-nuclear Antibodies.

c. Liver Function Tests.

d. Renal Function Tests (Creatinine or Blood Urea Nitrogen).

D. DRUG INTERACTIONS: See Warnings Section.

E. CARCINOGENESIS: See Warnings Section.

F. PREGNANCY:

Pregnancy Category C. Animal reproduction studies have not been conducted with methoxsalen. It is also not known whether methoxsalen can cause fetal harm when administered to a pregnant woman or can affect reproduction capacity. Methoxsalen should be given to a woman only if clearly needed.

G. NURSING MOTHERS:

It is not known whether this drug is excreted in human milk. Because many drugs are excreted in human milk, caution should be exercised when methoxsalen is administered to a nursing woman.

H. PEDIATRIC USE:

Safety in children has not been established. Potential hazards of long-term therapy include the possibilities of carcinogenicity and cataractogenicity as described in the Warnings Section as well as the probability of actinic degeneration which is also described in the Warnings Section.

VII. ADVERSE REACTIONS

A. METHOXSALEN:

The most commonly reported side effect of methoxsalen alone is nausea, which occurs with approximately 10% of all patients. This effect may be minimized or avoided by instructing the patient to take methoxsalen with milk or food, or to divide the dose into two portions, taken approximately one-half hour apart. Other effects include nervousness, insomnia, and psychological depression.

B. COMBINED METHOXSALEN/UVA THERAPY:

1. PRURITUS: This adverse reaction occurs with approximately 10% of all patients. In most cases, pruritus can be alleviated with frequent application of bland emollients or other topical agents; severe pruritus may require systemic treatment. If pruritus is unresponsive to these measures, shield pruritic areas from further UVA exposure until the condition resolves. If intractable pruritus is generalized, UVA treatment should be discontinued until the pruritus disappears.

2. ERYTHEMA: Mild, transient erythema at 24–48 hours after PUVA therapy is an expected reaction and indicates that a therapeutic interaction between methoxsalen and UVA occurred. Any area showing moderate erythema (greater than Grade 2—See Table 1 for grades of erythema) should be shielded during subsequent UVA exposures until the erythema has resolved. Erythema greater than Grade 2 which appears within 24 hours after UVA treatment may signal a potentially severe burn. Erythema may become progressively worse over the next 24 hours, since the peak erythemal reaction characteristically occurs 48 hours or later after methoxsalen ingestion. The patient should be protected from further UVA exposures and sunlight, and should be monitored closely.

3. IMPORTANT DIFFERENCES BETWEEN PUVA ERYTHEMA AND SUNBURN: PUVA-induced inflammation differs from sunburn or UVB phototherapy in several ways. The **in situ** depth of photochemistry is deeper within the tissue because UVA is transmitted further into the skin. The DNA lesions induced by PUVA are very different from UV-induced thymine dimers and may lead to a DNA crosslink. This DNA lesion may be more problematic to the cell because crosslinks are more lethal and psoralen-DNA photoproducts may be "new" or unfamiliar substrates for DNA repair enzymes. DNA synthesis is also suppressed longer after PUVA. The time course of delayed erythema is different with PUVA and may not involve the usual mediators seen in sunburn. PUVA-induced redness may be just beginning at 24 hours, when UVB erythema has already passed its peak. The erythema dose-response curve is also steeper for PUVA. Compared to equally erythemogenic doses of UVB, the histologic alterations induced by PUVA show more dermal vessel damage and longer duration of epidermal and dermal abnormalities.

4. OTHER ADVERSE REACTIONS: Those reported include edema, dizziness, headache, malaise, depression, hypopigmentation, vesiculation and bullae formation, non-specific rash, herpes simplex, miliaria, urticaria, folliculitis, gastrointestinal disturbances, cutaneous tenderness, leg cramps, hypotension, and extension of psoriasis.

VIII. OVERDOSAGE

In the event of methoxsalen overdosage, induce emesis and keep the patient in a darkened room for at least 24 hours. Emesis is beneficial only within the first 2 to 3 hours after ingestion of methoxsalen, since maximum blood levels are reached by this time.

IX. DRUG DOSAGE & ADMINISTRATION

A. VITILIGO THERAPY

1. DRUG DOSAGE: Two capsules (10 mg each) in one dose taken with milk or in food two to four hours before ultraviolet light exposure.

2. LIGHT EXPOSURE: The exposure time to sunlight should comply with the following guide:

	Basic Skin Color		
	Light	**Medium**	**Dark**
Initial Exposure	15 min.	20 min.	25 min.
Second Exposure	20 min.	25 min.	30 min.
Third Exposure	25 min.	30 min.	35 min.
Fourth Exposure	30 min.	35 min.	40 min.

Subsequent Exposure: Gradually increase exposure based on erythema and tenderness of the amelanotic skin.

Therapy should be on alternate days and never two consecutive days.

B. PSORIASIS THERAPY

1. DRUG DOSAGE—INITIAL THERAPY: The methoxsalen capsules should be taken 2 hours before UVA exposure with some food or milk according to the following table:

Patient's Weight (kg)	Patient's Weight (lbs)	Dose (mg)
<30	<65	10
30–50	65–100	20
51–65	101–145	30
66–80	146–175	40
81–90	176–200	50
91–115	201–250	60
>115	>250	70

Additional drug dosage directions are as follows:

a. Weight Change: In the event that the weight of a patient changes during treatment such that he/she falls into an adjacent weight range/dose category, no change in the dose of methoxsalen is usually required. If, in the physician's opinion, however, a weight change is sufficiently great to modify the drug dose, then an adjustment in the time of exposure to UVA should be made.

b. Dose/Week: The number of doses per week of methoxsalen capsules will be determined by the patient's schedule of UVA exposures. In no case should treatments be given more often than once every other day because the full extent of phototoxic reactions may not be evident until 48 hours after each exposure.

c. Dosage Increase: Dosage may be increased by 10 mg. after the fifteenth treatment under the conditions outlined in section XI.B.4.b.

X. UVA RADIATION SOURCE SPECIFICATIONS & INFORMATION

A. IRRADIANCE UNIFORMITY: (For photopheresis, refer to the UVAR* System Operator's Manual.)

The following specifications should be met with the window of the detector held in a vertical plane:

1. Vertical variation: For readings taken at any point along the vertical center axis of the chamber (to within 15 cm from the top and bottom), the lowest reading should not be less than 70 percent of the highest reading.

2. Horizontal variation: Throughout any specific horizontal plane, the lowest reading must be at least 80 percent of the highest reading, excluding the peripheral 3 cm of the patient treatment space:

B. PATIENT SAFETY FEATURES:

The following safety features should be present: (1) Protection from electrical hazard: All units should be grounded and conform to applicable electrical codes. The patient or operator should not be able to touch any live electrical parts. There should be ground fault protection. (2) Protective shielding of lamps: The patient should not be able to come in contact with the bare lamps. In the event of lamp breakage, the patient should not be exposed to broken lamp components. (3) Hand rails and hand holds: Appropriate supports should be available to the patient. (4) Patient viewing window: A window which blocks UV should be provided for viewing the patient during treatment. (5) Door and latches: Patients should be able to open the door from the inside with only slight pressure to the

Continued on next page

ICN—Cont.

door. (6) Non-skid floor: The floor should be of a non-skid nature. (7) Thermoregulation: Sufficient air flow should be provided for patient safety and comfort, limiting temperature within the UVA radiator cabinet to approximately less than 100° F. (8) Timer: The irradiator should be equipped with an automatic timer which terminates the exposure at the conclusion of a pre-set time interval. (9) Patient alarm device: An alarm device within the UVA irradiator chamber should be accessible to the patient for emergency activation. (10) Danger label: The unit should have a label prominently displayed which reads as follows:
DANGER—Ultraviolet Radiation—Follow your physician's instructions—Failure to use protective eyewear may result in eye injury.

C. UVA EXPOSURE DOSIMETRY MEASUREMENTS:

The maximum radiant exposure or irradiance (within $\pm$ 15 percent) of UVA (320–400 nm) delivered to the patient should be determined by using an appropriate radiometer calibrated to be read in Joules/cm^2 or mW/cm^2. In the absence of a standard measuring technique approved by the National Bureau of Standards, the system should use a detector corrected to a cosine spatial response. The use and recalibration frequency of such a radiometer for a specific UVA irradiator chamber should be specified by the manufacturer because the UVA dose (exposure) is determined by the design of the irradiator, the number of lamps, and the age of the lamps. If irradiance is measured, the radiometer reading in mW/cm^2 is used to calculate the exposure time in minutes to deliver the required UVA dose in Joules/cm^2 to a patient in the UVA irradiator cabinet. The equation is:

$$\frac{\text{Exposure Time}}{\text{in minutes}} = \frac{\text{Desired UVA Dose (J/cm}^2)}{0.06 \times \text{Irradiance (mW/cm}^2)}$$

Overexposure due to human error should be minimized by using an accurate automatic timing device, which is set by the operator and controlled by energizing and de-energizing the UVA irradiator lamp. The timing device calibration interval should be specified by the manufacturer. Safety systems should be included to minimize the possibility of delivering a UVA exposure which exceeds the prescribed dose, in the event the timer or radiometer should malfunction.

D. UVA SPECTRAL OUTPUT DISTRIBUTION:

The spectral distributions of the lamps should meet the following specifications:

Wavelength Band (Nanometers)	Output[1]
< 310	< 1
310 to 320	1 to 3
320 to 330	4 to 8
330 to 340	11 to 17
340 to 350	18 to 25
350 to 360	19 to 28
360 to 370	15 to 23
370 to 380	8 to 12
380 to 390	3 to 7
390 to 400	1 to 3

[1]As a percentage of total irradiance between 320 and 400 nanometers.

XI. PUVA TREATMENT PROTOCOL

A. INITIAL EXPOSURE: The initial UVA exposure should be conducted according to the guidelines presented previously under IX.B.1 and 2, Psoriasis therapy, Drug dosage-initial Therapy and Exposure.
[See table below.]

B. CLEARING PHASE: Specific recommendations for patient treatment are as follows:
1. SKIN TYPES I, II & III. Patients with skin types I, II and III may be treated 2 or 3 times per week. UVA exposure may be held constant or increased by up to 1.0 Joule/cm^2 at each treatment, according to the patient's response. If erythema occurs, however, do not increase exposure time until erythema resolves. The severity and extent of the patient's erythema may be used to determine whether the next exposure should be shortened, omitted, or maintained at the previous dosage. See Adverse Reactions section for additional information.

2. SKIN TYPES IV, V & VI. Patients with skin types IV, V and VI may be treated 2 or 3 times per week. UVA exposure may be held constant or increased by up to 1.5 Joules/cm^2 at each treatment unless erythema occurs. If erythema occurs, follow instructions outlined above in the procedures for patients with skin types I, II and III.

3. ERYTHRODERMIC PSORIASIS. Patients with erythrodermic psoriasis should be treated with special attention because pre-existing erythema may obscure observations of possible treatment-related phototoxic erythema. These patients may be treated 2 or 3 times per week, as a Type I patient.

4. MISCELLANEOUS SITUATIONS:
a. If there is no response after a total of 10 treatments, the exposure of UVA energy may be increased by an additional 0.5–1.0 Joules/cm^2 above the prior incremental increases for each treatment. (Example: a patient whose exposure dosage is being increased by 1.0 Joule/cm^2 may now have all subsequent doses increased by 1.5–2.0 Joules/cm^2.)
b. If there is no response, or only minimal response, after 15 treatments, the dosage of methoxsalen may be increased by 10 mg. (a one-time increase in dosage). This increased dosage may be continued for the remainder of the course of treatment but should not be exceeded.
c. If a patient misses a treatment, the UVA exposure time of the next treatment should not be increased. If more than one treatment is missed, reduce the exposure by 0.5 Joules/cm^2 for each treatment missed.
d. If the lower extremities are not responding as well as the rest of the body and do not show erythema, cover all other body area and give 25 percent of the present exposure dose as an additional exposure to the lower extremities. This additional exposure to the lower extremities should be terminated if erythema develops on these areas.
e. Non-responsive psoriasis: If a patient's generalized psoriasis is not responding, or if the condition appears to be worsening during treatment, the possibility of a generalized phototoxic reaction should be considered. This may be confirmed by the improvement of the condition following temporary discontinuance of this therapy for two weeks. If no improvement occurs during the interruption of treatment, this patient may be considered a treatment failure.

C. ALTERNATIVE EXPOSURE SCHEDULE:

As an alternative to increasing the UVA exposure at each treatment, the following schedule may be followed; this schedule may reduce the total number of Joules/cm^2 received by the patient over the entire course of therapy.
1. Incremental increases in UVA exposure for all patients may range from 0.5 to 1.5 Joules/cm^2, according to the patient's response to therapy.
2. Once Grade 2 clearing (see Table 2) has been reached and the patient is progressing adequately, UVA dosage is held constant. This dosage is maintained until Grade 4 clearing is reached.
3. If the rate of clearing significantly decreases, exposure dosage may be increased at each treatment (0.1–1.5 Joules/cm^2) until Grade 3 clearing and a satisfactory progress rate is attained. The UVA exposure will be held constant again until Grade 4 clearing is attained. These increases may be used also if the rate of clearing significantly decreases between Grade 3 and Grade 4 response. However, the possibility of a phototoxic reaction should be considered; see Nonresponsive Psoriasis, above.
4. In summary, this schedule raises slightly the increments (Joules/cm^2) of UVA dosage, but limits these increases to those periods when the patient is not responding adequately. Otherwise, the UVA exposure is held at the lowest effective dose.

D. MAINTENANCE PHASE:

The goal of maintenance treatment is to keep the patient as symptom-free as possible with the least amount of UVA exposure.
1. SCHEDULE OF EXPOSURES: When patients have achieved 95 percent clearing, or Grade 4 response (Table 2), they may be placed on the following maintenance schedules (M_1–M_4), in sequence. It is recommended that each maintenance schedule be adhered to for at least 2 treatments (unless erythema or psoriatic flare occurs, in which case see (2a) and (2b) below).

Maintenance Schedules
M_1–once/week
M_2–once/2 week
M_3–once/3 weeks
M_4–p.r.n. (i.e., for flares)

2. LENGTH OF EXPOSURE: The UVA exposure for the first maintenance treatment of any schedule (except M_4 as noted below) is the same as that of the patient's last treatment under the previous schedule. For skin types I-IV, however, it is recommended that the maximum UVA dosage during maintenance treatments not exceed the following:

Skin Types	Joules/cm^2/treatment
I	12
II	14
III	18
IV	22

If the patient develops erythema or new lesions of psoriasis, proceed as follows:
a. Erythema: During maintenance therapy, the patient's tan and threshold dose for erythema may gradually decrease. If maintenance treatments produce significant erythema, the exposure to UVA should be decreased by 25 percent until further treatments no longer produce erythema.
b. Psoriasis: If the patient develops new areas of psoriasis during maintenance therapy (but still is classified as having a Grade 4 response), the exposure to UVA may be increased by 0.5–1.5 Joules/cm^2 at each treatment; this is appropriate for all types of patients. These increases are continued until the psoriasis is brought under control and the patient is again clear. The exposure being administered when this clearing is reached should be used for further maintenance treatment.

3. FLARES DURING MAINTENANCE: If the patient flares during maintenance treatment (i.e., develops psoriasis on more than 5 percent of the originally involved areas of the body) his maintenance treatment schedule may be changed to the preceding maintenance or clearing schedule. The patient may be kept on his schedule until again 95 percent clear. If the original maintenance treatment schedule is unable to control the psoriasis, the schedule may be changed to a more frequent regimen. If a flare occurs less than 6 weeks after the last treatment, 25 percent of the maximum exposure received during the clearing phase, may be used and then proceed with the clearing schedule previously followed for this patient. (At 95 percent clearing follow regular maintenance until the optimum maintenance schedule is determined for the patient.) If more than 6 weeks have elapsed since the last treatment was given, treat patients as if they were beginning therapy insofar as exposure dosages are concerned, since their threshold for erythema may have decreased.

Table 1. Grades of Erythema

Grade	Erythema Level
0	No erythema
1	Minimally perceptible erythema—faint pink
2	Marked erythema but with no edema
3	Fiery erythema with edema
4	Fiery erythema with edema and blistering

[See table 2 at top of next page.]

XII. HOW SUPPLIED

8-MOP Capsules, each containing 10 mg. of methoxsalen (8-methoxypsoralen) packaged in amber glass bottles of 50 (NDC 0187-0651-42).

BIBLIOGRAPHY

1. Pathak, M.A., Kramer, D.M., Fitzpatrick, T.B.: Photobiology and Photochemistry of Furocoumarins (Psoralens), SUNLIGHT AND MAN: Normal and Abnormal Photobiologic Responses. Edited by M.A. Pathak, L.C. Harbor, M. Seiji et al. University of Tokyo Press. 1974, pp. 335–368.
2. Artuc, M., Stuettgen, G., Schalla, W., Schaefer, H., and Gazith, J.: Reversible binding of 5- and 8-methoxypsoralen to human serum proteins (albumin) and to epidermis in vitro: Brit. J. Dermat. 101, pp. 669–677 (1979).

Skin Type	History	Recommended Joules/cm^2
I	Always burn, never tan (Patients with Erythrodermic psoriasis are to be classed as Type I for determination of UVA dosage.)	0.5 J/cm^2
II	Always burn, but sometimes tan	1.0 J/cm^2
III	Sometimes burn, but always tan	1.5 J/cm^2
IV	Never burn, always tan	2.0 J/cm^2
	Physician Examination	
V*	Moderately pigmented	2.5 J/cm^2
VI*	Blacks	3.0 J/cm^2

[*Patients with natural pigmentation of these types should be classified into a lower skin type category if the sunburning history so indicates.]

Table 2. Response to Therapy

Grade	Criteria	Percent Improvement (compared to original extent of disease
−1	Psoriasis worse	0
0	No change	0
1	Minimal improvement—slightly less scale and/or erythema	5–20
2	Definite improvement—partial flattening of all plaques—less scaling and less erythema	20–50
3	Considerable improvement—nearly complete flattening of all plaques but borders of plaques still palpable	50–95
4	Clearing; complete flattening of plaques including borders; plaques may be outlined by pigmentation	95

3. Mandula, B.B., Pathak, M.A., Nakayama, Y., and Davidson, S.J.: Induction of mixed-function oxidases in mouse liver by psoralens., Ibid, 99, pp. 687–692 (1978).
4. Pathak, M.A., Fitzpatrick, T.B., Parrish, J.A.: PSORIASIS, Proceedings of the Second International Symposium. Edited by E.M. Farber, A.J. Cox, Yorke Medical Books, pp. 262–265 (1977).
5. Dall' Acqua, F., Marciani, S., Ciavatta, L, Rodighiero, G.: Formation of interstrand cross-linkings in the photoreactions between furocoumarins and DNA; Z Naturforsch (B), 26, pp. 561–569 (1971).
6. Cole, R.S.: Light-induced cross-linkings of DNA in the presence of a furocoumarin (psoralen), Biochem. Biophys. Acta, 217, pp. 30–39 (1970).
7. Musajo, L., Rodighiero, G., Caporale, G., Dall' Acqua, F., Marciani, S., Bordin, F., Baccichetti, F., Bevilacqua, R.: Photoreactions between Skin-Photosensitizing Furocoumarins and Nucleic Acids, SUNLIGHT AND MAN; Normal and Abnormal Photobiologic Responses. Edited by M.A. Pathak, L.C. Harber, M. Seiji et al. University of Tokyo Press, pp. 369–387 (1974).
8. Dall' Acqua, F., Vedaldi, D., Bordin, F., and Rodighiero, G.: New studies in the interaction between 8-methoxypsoralen and DNA in vitro; J. Investigative Dermat., 73, pp. 191–197 (1979).
9. Yoshikawa, K., Mori, N., Sakakibara, S., Mizuno, N., Song, P.: Photo-Conjugation of 8-methoxypsoralen with Proteins; Photochem. & Photobiol. 29, pp. 1127–1133 (1979).
10. Ortonne, J. P., MacDonald, D.M., Micoud, A., Thivolet, J.: PUVA-induced repigmentation of vitiligo: a histochemical (split-DOPA) and ultra-structural study: Brit. J. of Dermat., 101, pp. 1–12 (1979).
11. Hakim, R.D., Griffin, A.C., Knox, J.M.: Erythema and tumor formation in methoxsalen treated mice exposed to fluorescent light; Arch. Dermatol. 82, 572–577 (1960).
12. Pathak, M.A., Daniels, F., Hopkins, C.E., Fitzpatrick, T.B.: Ultraviolet carcinogenesis in albino and pigmented mice receiving furocoumarins: psoralens and 8-methoxypsoralen, Nature 183, pp. 728–730 (1959).
13. Stern, R.S., Thibodeau, L.A., Kleinerman, R.A., Parrish, J.A., Fitzpatrick, T.B., and 22 Participating Investigators: Risk of Cutaneous Carcinoma in Patients Treated with Oral Methoxsalen Photochemotherapy for Psoriasis: NEJM, 300. No. 15, pp. 809–813 (1979).
14. Stern, R.S., Parrish, J.A., Zierler, S.: Skin Carcinoma in Patients with Psoriasis Treated with Topical Tar and Artificial Ultraviolet Radiation. Lancet, 1, pp. 732–735 (1980).
15. Roenigk, Jr., H.H., and 12 Cooperating Investigators: Skin Cancer in the PUVA-48 Cooperative Study of Psoriasis. Program for Forty-First Annual Meeting for The Society of Investigative Dermatology, Inc., Sheraton Washington Hotel, Washington, D.C., May 12, 13, and 14, 1980. Abstracts JID, 74, No. 4, p. 250 (April, 1980).
16. Mosher, D.B., Pathak, M.A., Harris, T.J., Fitzpatrick, T.B.: Development of Cutaneous Lesions in Vitiligo During Long-Term PUVA Therapy. Program for Forty-First Annual Meeting for The Society for Investigative Dermatology, Inc., Sheraton Washington Hotel, Washington, D.C., May 12, 13, and 14, 1980. Abstracts JID, 74, No. 4, p. 259 (April, 1980).
17. Cloud, T.M., Hakim, R., Griffin, A.C.: Photosensitization of the eye with methoxsalen. I. Acute effects; Arch. Ophthalmol. 64, pp. 346–352 (1960).
18. Cloud, T.M., Hakim, R., Griffen, A.C.: Photosensitization of the eye with methoxsalen. II. Chronic effects, Ibid, 66, pp. 689–694 (1961).
19. Freeman, R.G., Troll, D.: Photosensitization of the eye by 8-methoxypsoralen, JID, 53, pp. 449–453 (1969).
20. Lerman, S., Megaw, J., Willis, I.: Potential ocular complications from PUVA therapy and their prevention; J. Invest. Dermat., 74, pp. 197–199 (1980).

2292-03 EL ICN Pharmaceuticals, Inc. Rev. 6-94
3300 Hyland Ave.
Costa Mesa, CA 92626

Shown in Product Identification Guide, page 318

ANDROID® ℞

Brand of Methyltestosterone Capsules USP, 10 mg

DESCRIPTION

The androgens are steroids that develop and maintain primary and secondary male sex characteristics.

Androgens are derivatives of cyclopentanoperhydrophenanthrene. Endogenous androgens are C-19 steroids with a side chain at C-17, and with two angular methyl groups. Testosterone is the primary endogenous androgen. In their active form, all drugs in the class have a 17-beta hydroxy group. 17-alpha alkylation (methyltestosterone) increases the pharmacologic activity per unit weight compared to testosterone when given orally.

Methyltestosterone, a synthetic derivative of testosterone, is an androgenic preparation given by the oral route in a capsule form. Each capsule contains 10 mg of Methyltestosterone USP. It has the following structural formula:

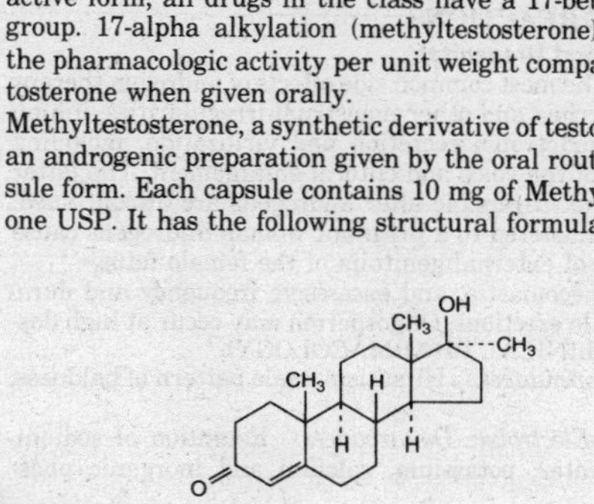

$C_{20}H_{30}O_2$ M.W. 302.46
17-β-hydroxy-17-methylandrost-4-en-3-one

Methyltestosterone occurs as white or creamy white crystals or powder, which is soluble in various organic solvents but is practically insoluble in water.

Each capsule, for oral administration, contains 10 mg of Methyltestosterone. In addition, each capsule contains the following inactive ingredients: Corn starch NF, Gelatin NF, FD&C Blue #1, FD&C Red #40.

CLINICAL PHARMACOLOGY

Endogenous androgens are responsible for the normal growth and development of the male sex organs and for maintenance of secondary sex characteristics. These effects include the growth and maturation of prostate, seminal vesicles, penis, and scrotum. The development of male hair distribution, such as beard, pubic, chest, and axillary hair; laryngeal enlargement, vocal chord thickening, alterations in body musculature, and fat distribution. Drugs in this class also cause retention of nitrogen, sodium, potassium, phosphorus, and decreased urinary excretion of calcium. Androgens have been reported to increase protein anabolism and decrease protein catabolism. Nitrogen balance is improved only when there is sufficient intake of calories and protein.

Androgens are responsible for the growth spurt of adolescence and for the eventual termination of linear growth which is brought about by fusion of the epiphyseal growth centers. In children, exogenous androgens accelerate linear growth rates, but may cause a disproportionate advancement in bone maturation. Use over long periods may result in fusion of the epiphyseal growth centers and termination of growth process. Androgens have been reported to stimulate the production of red blood cells by enhancing the production of erythropoietic stimulating factor.

During exogenous administration of androgens, endogenous testosterone release is inhibited through feedback inhibition of pituitary luteinizing hormone (LH). At large doses of exogenous androgens, spermatogenesis may also be suppressed through feedback inhibition of pituitary follicle stimulating hormone (FSH).

There is a lack of substantial evidence that androgens are effective in fractures, surgery, convalescence and functional uterine bleeding.

Pharmacokinetics

Testosterone given orally is metabolized by the gut and 44 percent is cleared by the liver of the first pass. Oral doses as high as 400 mg per day are needed to achieve clinically effective blood levels for full replacement therapy. The synthetic androgen, methyltestosterone, is less extensively metabolized by the liver and has a longer half-life. It is more suitable than testosterone for oral administration.

Testosterone in plasma is 98 percent bound to a specific testosterone-estradiol binding globulin, and about 2 percent is free. Generally, the amount of this sex-hormone binding globulin in the plasma will determine the distribution of testosterone between free and bound forms, and the free testosterone concentration will determine its half-life.

About 90 percent of a dose of testosterone is excreted in the urine as glucuronic and sulfuric acid conjugates of testosterone and its metabolites: and 6 percent of a dose is excreted in the feces, mostly in the unconjugated form. Inactivation of testosterone occurs primarily in the liver. Testosterone is metabolized to various 17-keto steroids through two different pathways. There are considerable variations of the half-life of testosterone as reported in the literature, ranging from 10 to 100 minutes.

In many tissues the activity of testosterone appears to depend on reduction to dihydrotestosterone, which binds to cytosol receptor proteins. The steroid-receptor complex is transported to the nucleus where it initiates transcription events and cellular changes related to androgen action.

INDICATIONS AND USAGE

1. Males

Androgens are indicated for replacement therapy in conditions associated with a deficiency or absence of endogenous testosterone.

a. Primary hipogonadism (congenital or acquired) — (testicular failure due to cryptorchidism, bilateral torsions, orchitis, vanishing testis syndrome; or orchidectomy.
b. Hypogonadotropic hypogonadism (congenital or acquired) — idiopathic gonadotropin or LHRH deficiency, or pituitary hypothalamic injury from tumors, trauma, or radiation. If the above conditions occur prior to puberty, androgen replacement therapy will be needed during the adolescent years for development of secondary sexual characteristics. Prolonged androgen treatment will be required to maintain sexual characteristics in these and other males who develop testosterone deficiency after puberty.
c. Androgens may be used to stimulate puberty in carefully selected males with clearly delayed puberty. These patients usually have a familial pattern of delayed puberty that is not secondary to a pathological disorder; puberty is expected to occur spontaneously at a relatively late date. Brief treatment with conservative doses may occasionally be justified in these patients if they do not respond to psychological support. The potential adverse effect on bone maturation should be discussed with the patient and parents prior to androgen administration. An X-ray of the hand and wrist to determine bone age should be obtained every 6 months to assess the effect of treatment on the epiphyseal centers (see WARNINGS).

2. Females

Androgens may be used secondarily in women with advancing inoperable metastatic (skeletal) mammary cancer who are 1 to 5 years postmenopausal. Primary goals of therapy in these women include ablation of the ovaries. Other methods of counteracting estrogen activity are adrenalectomy, hypophysectomy, and/or antiestrogen therapy. This treatment has also been used in premenopausal women with breast cancer who have benefited from oophorectomy and are considered to have a hormone-responsive tumor. Judgment concerning androgen therapy should be made by an oncologist with expertise in this field.

CONTRAINDICATIONS

Androgens are contraindicated in men with carcinomas of the breast or with known or suspected carcinomas of the prostate, and in women who are or may become pregnant. When administered to pregnant woman, androgens cause virilization of the external genitalia of the female fetus. This virilization includes clitoromegaly, abnormal vaginal development, and fusion of genital folds to form a scrotal-like structure. The degree of masculinization is related to the amount of drug given and the age of the fetus, and is most likely to occur in the female fetus when the drugs are given in the first trimester. If the patients becomes pregnant while taking these drugs, she should be apprised of the potential hazard to the fetus.

WARNINGS

In patients with breast cancer, androgen therapy may cause hypercalcemia by stimulating osteolysis. In this case, the drug should be discontinued.

Prolonged use of high doses of adrogens has been associated with the development of peliosis hepatis and hepatic neo-

Continued on next page

ICN—Cont.

plasms including hepatocellular carcinoma. (See PRECAUTIONS—Carcinogenesis). Peliosis hepatis can be a life-threatening or fatal complication.
Cholestatic hepatitis and jaundice occur with 17-alpha-alkylandrogens at a relatively low dose. If cholestatic hepatitis with jaundice appears or if liver function tests become abnormal, the androgen should be discontinued and the etiology should be determined. Drug-induced jaundice is reversible when the medication is discontinued.
Geriatric patients treated with androgens may be at an increased risk for the development of prostatic hypertrophy and prostatic carcinoma.
Edema with or without congestive heart failure may be a serious complication in patients with preexisting cardiac, renal, or hepatic disease. In addition to discontinuation of the drug, diuretic therapy may be required.
Gynecomastia frequently develops and occasionally persists in patients being treated for hypogonadism.
Androgen therapy should be used cautiously in healthy males with delayed puberty. The effect on bone maturation should be monitored by assessing bone age of the wrist and hand every 6 months. In children, androgen treatment may accelerate bone maturation without producing compensatory gain in linear growth. This adverse effect may result in compromised adult stature. The younger the child the greater the risk of compromising final mature height.
This drug has not been shown to be safe and effective for the enhancement of athletic performance. Because of the potential risk of serious adverse health effects, this drug should not be used for such purpose.

PRECAUTIONS

General
Women should be observed for signs of virilization (deepening of the voice, hirsutism, acne, clitoromegaly and menstrual irregularities). Discontinuation of drug therapy at the time of evidence of mild virilism is necessary to prevent irreversible virilization. Such virilization is usual following androgen use at high doses. A decision may be made by the patient and the physician that some virilization will be tolerated during treatment for breast carcinoma.

Information for the Patient
The physician should instruct patients to report any of the following side effects of androgens:

Adult or Adolescent Males:	Too frequent or persistent erections of the penis. Any male adolescent patient receiving androgens for delayed puberty should have bone development checked every six months.
Women:	Hoarseness, acne, changes in menstrual periods or more hair on the face.
All Patients:	Any nausea, vomiting, changes in skin color or ankle swelling.

Laboratory Tests
1. Women with disseminated breast carcinoma should have frequent determination of urine and serum calcium levels during the course of androgen therapy (See WARNINGS).
2. Because of the hepatotoxicity associated with the use of 17-alpha-alkylated androgens, liver function tests should be obtained periodically.
3. Periodic (every 6 months) X-ray examinations of bone age should be made during treatment of prepubertal males to determine the rate of bone maturation and the effects of androgen therapy on the epiphyseal centers.
4. Hemoglobin and hematocrit should be checked periodically for polycythemia in patients who are receiving high doses of androgens.

Drug Interactions
1. **Anticoagulants:** C-17 substituted derivatives of testosterone, such as methandrostenolone, have been reported to decrease the anticoagulant requirements of patients receiving oral anticoagulants. Patients receiving oral anticoagulant therapy require close monitoring, especially when androgens are started or stopped.
2. **Oxyphenbutazone:** Concurrent administration of oxyphenbutazone and androgens may result in elevated serum levels of oxyphenbutazone.
3. **Insulin:** In diabetic patients the metabolic effects of androgens may decrease blood glucose and insulin requirements.

Drug/Laboratory Test Interferences
Androgens may decrease levels of thyroxine-binding globulin, resulting in decreased total T4 serum levels and increased resin uptake of T3 and T4. Free thyroid hormone levels remain unchanged, however, and there is no clinical evidence of thyroid dysfunction.

Carcinogenesis
Animal Data
Testosterone has been tested by subcutaneous injection and implantation in mice and rats. The implant induced cervical-uterine tumors in mice, which metastasized in some cases. There is suggestive evidence that injection of testosterone into some strains of female mice increases their susceptibility to hepatoma. Testosterone is also known to increase the number of tumors and decrease the degree of differentiation of chemically induced carcinomas of the liver in rats.

Human Data
There are rare reports of hepatocellular carcinoma in patients receiving long-term therapy with androgens in high doses. Withdrawal of the drugs did not lead to regression of the tumors in all cases.
Geriatric patients treated with androgens may be at an increased risk for the development of prostatic hypertrophy and prostatic carcinoma.

Pregnancy
Teratogenic effects. Pregnancy Category X (See CONTRAINDICATIONS).

Nursing Mothers
It is not known whether androgens are excreted in human milk. Because many drugs are excreted in human milk and because of the potential for serious adverse reactions in nursing infants from androgens, a decision should be made whether to discontinue nursing or to discontinue the drug, taking into account the importance of the drug to the mother.

Pediatric Use
Androgen therapy should be used very cautiously in children and only by specialists who are aware of the adverse effects on bone maturation. Skeletal maturation must be monitored every six months by an X-ray of hand and wrist (See INDICATIONS AND USAGE and WARNINGS).

ADVERSE REACTIONS

Endocrine and Urogenital
Female: The most common side effects of androgen therapy are amenorrhea and other menstrual irregularities, inhibition of gonadotropin secretion and virilization, including deepening of the voice and clitoral enlargement. The latter usually is not reversible after androgens are discontinued. When administered to a pregnant woman androgens cause virilization of external genitalia of the female fetus.
Male: Gynecomastia, and excessive frequency and duration of penile erections. Oligospermia may occur at high dosages (see CLINICAL PHARMACOLOGY).
Skin and appendages: Hirsutism, male pattern of baldness, and acne.
Fluid and Electrolyte Disturbances: Retention of sodium, chloride, water, potassium, calcium and inorganic phosphates.
Gastrointestinal: Nausea, cholestatic jaundice, alterations in liver function tests, rarely hepatocellular neoplasms and peliosis hepatitis (see WARNINGS).
Hematologic: Suppression of clotting factors II, V, VII, and X, bleeding in patients on concomitant anticoagulant therapy and polycythemia.
Nervous System: Increased or decreased libido, headache, anxiety, depression, and generalized paresthesia.
Metabolic: Increased serum cholesterol.
Miscellaneous: Rarely anaphylactoid reactions.

DRUG ABUSE AND DEPENDENCE

Methyltestosterone Capsules are classified as a schedule III Controlled Substance under the Anabolic Steroids Act of 1990.

OVERDOSAGE

There have been no reports of acute overdosage with the androgens.

DOSAGE AND ADMINISTRATION

Methyltestosterone capsules are administered orally. The suggested dosage for androgens varies depending on the age, sex, and diagnosis of the individual patient. Dosage is adjusted according to the patient's response and the appearance of adverse reactions.
Replacement therapy in androgen-deficient males is 10 to 50 mg of methyltestosterone daily. Various dosage regimens have been used to induce pubertal changes in hypogonadal males, some experts have advocated lower dosages initially, gradually increasing the dose as puberty progresses with or without a decrease to maintenance levels. Other experts emphasize that higher dosages are needed to induce pubertal changes and lower dosages can be used for maintenance after puberty. The chronological and skeletal ages must be taken into consideration both in determining the initial dose and in adjusting the dose.
Doses used in delayed puberty generally are in the lower range of that given above, and for a limited duration, for example 4 to 6 months.
Women with metastatic breast carcinoma must be followed closely because androgen therapy occasionally appears to accelerate the disease. Thus, many experts prefer to use the shorter acting androgen preparations rather than those with prolonged activity for treating breast carcinoma, particularly during the early stages of androgen therapy. The dosage of methyltestosterone for androgen therapy in breast carcinoma in females is from 50–200 mg daily.

HOW SUPPLIED

Methyltestosterone capsules USP 10 mg are red capsules imprinted "ICN 0901" on both sections. They are available in bottles of 100.
CAUTION: Federal (USA) law prohibits dispensing without prescription.
ICN
ICN Pharmaceuticals, Inc.
ICN Plaza
3300 Hyland Avenue
Costa Mesa, CA 92626
(714)545-0100
7004821 Rev. 7/94

BENOQUIN® CREAM 20% ℞
(Monobenzone, Cream)
Potent Depigmenting Agent

FEDERAL (U.S.A.) LAW PROHIBITS DISPENSING WITHOUT PRESCRIPTION.
FOR EXTERNAL USE ONLY

DESCRIPTION

Monobenzone is the monobenzyl ether of hydroquinone. Monobenzone occurs as a white, almost tasteless crystalline powder, soluble in alcohol and practically insoluble in water. Chemically, monobenzone is designated as p-(benzyloxy)-phenol; the empirical formula is $C_{13}H_{12}O_2$; molecular weight 200.24. The structural formula is:

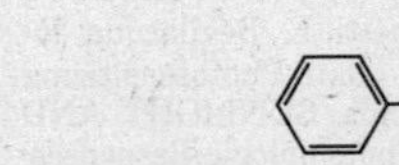

$C_{13}H_{12}O_2$ 200.24

Each gram of Benoquin Cream contains 200 mg of monobenzone USP, in a water-washable base consisting of purified water, cetyl alcohol, propylene glycol, sodium lauryl sulfate and white wax.

CLINICAL PHARMACOLOGY

Benoquin Cream 20% is a depigmenting agent whose mechanism of action is not fully understood.
The topical application of monobenzone in animals, increases the excretion of melanin from the melanocytes. The same action is thought to be responsible for the depigmenting effect of the drug in humans. Monobenzone may cause destruction of melanocytes and permanent depigmentation. This effect is erratic and may take one to four months to occur while existing melanin is lost with normal sloughing of the stratum corneum. Hyperpigmented skin appears to fade more rapidly than does normal skin, and exposure to sunlight reduces the depigmenting effect of the drug. The histology of the skin after depigmentation with topical monobenzone is the same as that seen in vitiligo; the epidermis is normal except for the absence of identifiable melanocytes.

INDICATIONS AND USAGE

Benoquin Cream 20% is indicated for final depigmentation in extensive Vitiligo.
Benoquin Cream 20% is applied topically to permanently depigment normal skin surrounding vitiliginous lesions in patients with disseminated (greater than 50 percent of body surface area) idiopathic vitiligo.
Benoquin Cream 20% is not recommended in freckling; hyperpigmentation caused by photosensitization following the use of certain perfumes (berlock dermatitis); melasma (chloasma) of pregnancy; or hyperpigmentation resulting from inflammation of the skin. Benoquin Cream 20% is not effective for the treatment of cafe-au-lait spots, pigmented nevi, malignant melanoma or pigmentation resulting from pigments other than melanin (e.g.: bile, silver, or artificial pigments).

CONTRAINDICATIONS

Benoquin Cream 20% contains a potent depigmenting agent and is not a cosmetic skin bleach. Use of Benoquin Cream 20% is contraindicated in any conditions other than disseminated vitiligo. Benoquin Cream 20% frequently produces irreversible depigmentation, and it must not be used as a substitute for hydroquinone.
Benoquin Cream 20% is also contraindicated in individuals with a history of sensitivity or allergic reactions to this product, or any of its ingredients.

WARNINGS

Benoquin Cream 20% is a potent depigmenting agent, not a mild cosmetic bleach. Do not use except for final depigmentation in extensive vitiligo.
Keep this, and all medications out of the reach of children. In case of accidental ingestion, call a physician or a Poison Control Center immediately.

PRECAUTIONS (See Warnings)

General. Benoquin Cream 20% is for External Use Only. Following therapy with Benoquin Cream 20%, the skin will be sensitive for the rest of the patient's life. He/she must use sunscreens during exposure to the sun.

Information for the Patient. Benoquin Cream 20% contains a potent depigmenting agent and is not a cosmetic skin bleach. Use of Benoquin Cream 20% is contraindicated in any conditions other than disseminated vitiligo. Use only for final depigmentation in extensive vitiligo. Areas of normal skin distant to the site of Benoquin Cream 20% application may become depigmented, and irregular, excessive, unsightly, and frequently permanent depigmentation may occur.

Carcinogenesis, mutagenesis, impairment of fertility. No long term studies have been performed to evaluate carcinogenic potential.

Pregnancy: Category C. Animal reproduction studies have not been conducted with Benoquin Cream 20%. It is also not known whether Benoquin Cream 20% can cause fetal harm when administered to a pregnant woman, or can affect reproduction capacity. Benoquin Cream 20% should be given to a pregnant woman only if clearly needed.

Nursing Mothers. It is not known whether this drug is excreted in human milk. Because many drugs are excreted in human milk, caution should be exercised when Benoquin Cream 20% is administered to a nursing woman.

Pediatric Use. The safety and effectiveness of Benoquin Cream 20% in pediatric patients below the age of 12 years have not been established.

ADVERSE REACTIONS

Mild, transient skin irritation and sensitization, including erythematous and eczematous reactions have occurred following topical application of Benoquin Cream 20%. Although those reactions are usually transient, treatment with Benoquin Cream 20% should be discontinued if irritation, a burning sensation, or dermatitis occur. Areas of normal skin distant to the site of Benoquin Cream 20% application frequently have become depigmented, and irregular, excessive, unsightly, and frequently permanent depigmentation has occurred.

DOSAGE AND ADMINISTRATION

A thin layer of Benoquin Cream 20% should be applied and rubbed into the pigmented area two or three times daily, or as directed by a physician. Prolonged exposure to sunlight should be avoided during treatment with Benoquin Cream 20%, or a sunscreen should be used.

Depigmentation is usually accomplished after one to four months of Benoquin Cream 20% treatment. If satisfactory results are not obtained after four months of Benoquin Cream 20% treatment, the drug should be discontinued. When the desired degree of depigmentation is obtained, Benoquin Cream 20% should be applied only as often as needed to maintain depigmentation (usually only two times weekly).

HOW SUPPLIED

Benoquin Cream 20% in 1 1/4 oz. tubes (35.4 g) (NDC 0187-0380-34).

Benoquin Cream 20% should be stored at room temperature (15–30°C) (59–86°F)

ICN Pharmaceuticals, Inc.
3300 Hyland Ave.
Costa Mesa, CA 92626
(714) 545-0100
Revised: 1/95

ELDOQUIN FORTE® 4% Cream (Hydroquinone USP, 4%) ℞
(Skin Bleaching Cream)
ELDOPAQUE FORTE® 4% Cream (Hydroquinone USP, 4%)
(Skin Bleaching Cream with Sunblock)
SOLAQUIN FORTE® 4% Cream (Hydroquinone USP, 4%)
(Skin Bleaching Cream with Sunscreens)
SOLAQUIN FORTE® 4% Gel (Hydroquinone USP, 4%)
(Skin Bleaching Gel with Sunscreens)
VIQUIN FORTE® 4% Cream (Hydroquinone USP, 4%)
(Skin Bleaching Moisturizing Cream with Sunscreens, SPF 19)

FOR EXTERNAL USE ONLY

DESCRIPTION

Hydroquinone is 1,4-benzenediol. Hydroquinone is structurally related to monobenzone. Hydroquinone occurs as fine, white needles. The drug is freely soluble in water and in alcohol and has a pK_a of 9.96. Chemically, hydroquinone is designated as p-dihydroxybenzene; the empirical formula is $C_6H_6O_2$; molecular weight 110.1.

The structural formula is:

[See chemical structure at top of next column.]

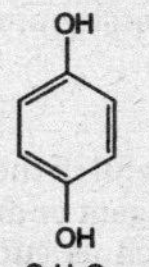

$C_6H_6O_2$

Each gram of Eldoquin Forte 4% Cream contains 40 mg of Hydroquinone USP in a vanishing cream base of purified water USP, stearing acid NF, propylene glycol USP, polyoxyl 40 stearate NF, polyoxyethylene (25) propylene glycol stearate, glycerol monostearate, light mineral oil NF, squalane NF, propylparaben NF and sodium metabisulfite NF.

Each gram of Eldopaque Forte 4% Cream contains 40 mg of Hydroquinone USP in a tinted sunblocking cream base of purified water USP, stearic acid NF, talc USP, polyoxyl 40 stearate NF, polyoxethylene (25) propylene glycol stearate, propylene glycol USP, glycerol monostearate, iron oxides, light mineral oil NF, squalane NF, edetate disodium USP, sodium metabisulfite NF and potassium sorbate NF.

Each gram of Solaquin Forte 4% Cream contains 40 mg of Hydroquinone USP, 80 mg Padimate O USP, 30 mg Dioxybenzone USP and 20 mg Oxybenzone USP in a vanishing cream base of purified water USP, glycerol monostearate, polyoxyethylene stearate, octyldodecyl stearoyl stearate, glyceryl dilaurate, quaternium-26, cetearyl alcohol and ceteareth-20, stearyl alcohol NF, propylene glycol USP, diethylaminoethyl stearate, polydimethylsiloxane, polysorbate 80 NF, lactic acid USP, ascorbic acid USP, hydroxyethyl cellulose, myristalkonium chloride, quaternium-14, edetate disodium USP and sodium metabisulfite NF.

Each gram of Solaquin Forte 4% Gel contains 40 mg of Hydroquinone USP, 50 mg of Padimate O USP and 30 mg Dioxybenzone USP, in a hydro-alcoholic base of alcohol USP, purified water USP, propylene glycol USP, entprol, carbomer 940, edetate disodium USP and sodium metabisulfite NF.

Each gram of Viquin Forte 4% Cream contains 40 mg of Hydroquinone USP, 80 mg Padimate O USP, 30 mg Dioxybenzone USP and 20 mg Oxybenzone USP in a vanishing cream base of purified water USP, glycolic acid, glycerol monostearate, polyoxyethylene stearate, octyldodecyl stearoyl stearate, glyceryl dilaurate, stearyl alcohol NF, cetearyl alcohol and ceteareth-20, quaternium-26, propylene glycol USP, diethylaminoethyl stearate, polydimethylsiloxane, polysorbate 80 NF, lactic acid USP, ascorbic acid USP, hydroxyethyl cellulose, myristalkonium chloride, quaternium-14, edetate disodium USP, sodium metabisulfite NF and sodium hydroxide NF.

CLINICAL PHARMACOLOGY

Topical application of hydroquinone produces a reversible depigmentation of the skin by inhibition of the enzymatic oxidation of tyrosine to 3,4–dihydroxyphenylalanine (dopa) (Denton, C. et al., 1952)[1] and supression of other melanocyte metabolic processes (Jimbow, K. et al., 1974).[2] Exposure to sunlight or ultraviolet light will cause repigmentation of bleached areas which may be prevented by the sunblocking agents contained in Eldopaque Forte 4% Cream and by the broad spectrum sunscreen agents contained in Viquin Forte 4% Cream, Solaquin Forte 4% Cream and Solaquin Forte 4% Gel (Parrish, J. A. et al., 1978).[3]

INDICATIONS AND USAGE

For the gradual bleaching of hyperpigmented skin conditions such as chloasma, melasma, freckles, senile lentigines and other unwanted areas of melanin hyperpigmentation.

CONTRAINDICATIONS

Prior history of sensitivity or allergic reaction to these products or any of the ingredients. The safety of topical hydroquinone use during pregnancy or in children (12 years and under) has not been established.

WARNINGS

Caution: Hydroquinone is a skin bleaching agent which may produce unwanted cosmetic effects if not used as directed. The physician should be familiar with the contents of the package insert before prescribing or dispensing these medications.

Test for skin sensitivity before using by applying a small amount to an unbroken patch of skin and check in 24 hours. Minor redness is not a contraindication, but where there is itching or vesicle formation or excessive inflammatory response, further treatment is not advised. Close patient supervision is recommended. Contact with the eyes should be avoided. If no bleaching or lightening effect is noted after 2 months of treatment use, the medication should be discontinued. Eldoquin Forte 4% Cream, Eldopaque Forte 4% Cream, Viquin Forte 4% Cream, Solaquin Forte 4% Cream and Solaquin Forte 4% Gel are formulated for use as skin bleaching agents and should not be used for the prevention of sunburn. Sunscreen use is an essential aspect of hydroquinone therapy because even minimal sunlight sustains melanocytic activity. The sunblock in Eldopaque Forte 4% Cream and the sunscreens in Solaquin Forte 4% Cream, Solaquin Forte 4% Gel and Viquin Forte 4% Cream provide the necessary sun protection during skin bleaching therapy. After clearing and during maintenance therapy, sun exposure should be avoided on bleached skin by application of a sunscreen or sunblock agent or protective clothing to prevent repigmentation.

Keep this and all medication out of the reach of children. In case of accidental ingestion, call a physician or a poison control center immediately.

Warning: Contains sodium metabisulfite, a sulfite that may cause serious allergic type reactions (e.g, hives, itching, wheezing, anaphylaxis, severe asthma attack) in certain susceptible persons.

PRECAUTIONS (SEE WARNINGS)

General. Treatment should be limited to relatively small areas of the body at one time since some patients experience a transient skin reddening and a mild burning sensation which does not preclude treatment.

Pregnancy Category C. Animal reproduction studies have not been conducted with topical hydroquinone. It is also not known whether hydroquinone can cause fetal harm when used topically on a pregnant woman or affect reproductive capacity. It is not known to what degree, if any, topical hydroquinone is absorbed systemically. Topical hydroquinone should be used in pregnant women only when clearly indicated.

Nursing mothers. It is not known whether topical hydroquinone is absorbed or excreted in human milk. Caution is advised when topical hydroquinone is used by a nursing mother.

Pediatric usage. Safety and effectiveness in pediatric patients below the age of 12 years have not been established.

ADVERSE REACTIONS

No systemic adverse reactions have been reported. Occasional hypersensitivity (localized contact dermatitis) may occur, in which case the medication should be discontinued and the physician notified immediately.

DOSAGE AND ADMINISTRATION

Viquin Forte 4% Cream, Solaquin Forte 4% Cream and Solaquin Forte 4% Gel should be applied to the affected area and rubbed in well twice daily or as directed by a physician.

Eldopaque Forte 4% Cream should be applied to the affected area twice daily or as directed by a physician. Do not rub in.

Eldoquin Forte 4% Cream should be applied to the affected area and rubbed in well twice daily or as directed by a physician. During the day, effective broad spectrum sunscreen should be used and unnecessary solar exposure avoided, or protective clothing should be worn to cover bleached skin in order to prevent repigmentation from occurring.

HOW SUPPLIED

ELDOQUIN FORTE 4% CREAM is available as follows:

SIZE	NDC NUMBER
1.0 ounce tube (28.4 grams)	0187-0394-31

ELDOPAQUE FORTE 4% CREAM is available as follows:

SIZE	NDC NUMBER
1.0 ounce tube (28.4 grams)	0187-0395-31

SOLAQUIN FORTE 4% CREAM is available as follows:

SIZE	NDC NUMBER
1.0 ounce tube (28.4 grams)	0187-0396-31

SOLAQUIN FORTE 4% GEL is available as follows:

SIZE	NDC NUMBER
1.0 ounce tube (28.4 grams)	0187-0523-31

VIQUIN FORTE 4% CREAM is available as follows:

SIZE	NDC NUMBER
1.0 ounce tube (28.4 grams)	0187-0398-31

Store at controlled room temperature (15°–30°C) 59°–86°F.

CAUTION: Federal (U.S.A.) Law Prohibits Dispensing without a Prescription

REFERENCES

1. Denton, C., A. B. Lerner and T. B. Fitzpatrick, "Inhibition of Melanin Formation by Chemical Agents," *Journal of Investigative Dermatology*, 18:119–135, 1952.
2. Jimbow, K., H. Obata, M. Pathak and T. B. Fitzpatrick, "Mechanism of Depigmentation by Hydroquinone," *Journal of Investigative Dermatology*, 62:436–449, 1974.
3. Parrish, J. A., R. R. Anderson, F. Urbach, D. Pitts, "UVA, Biological Effects of Ultraviolet Radiation with Emphasis on Human Responses to Longwave Ultraviolet," *Plenum Press*, New York and London, 1978, p. 151.

ICN PHARMACEUTICALS, INC.
3300 Hyland Avenue
Costa Mesa, CA 92626, U.S.A.
(714) 545-0100
Rev. 5/96.

Continued on next page

ICN—Cont.

FOTOTAR® CREAM ℞
PSORIASIS AND SEBORRHEIC DERMATITIS CREAM

DESCRIPTION
FOTOTAR® Cream contains coal tar extract (equivalent to 2% Coal Tar, USP) in an emollient, moisturizing cream base.

INDICATIONS
For the relief of itching, irritation, and skin flaking associated with psoriasis and seborrheic dermatitis.

CONTRAINDICATIONS
FOTOTAR® Cream is contraindicated in patients with a history of sensitivity to this product or to other coal tar products. FOTOTAR® Cream should not be used on patients who have a disease characterized by photosensitivity, such as lupus erythematosus or allergy to sunlight.

DIRECTIONS FOR USE
Apply to affected areas one to four times daily or as directed by a physician.

WARNINGS
FOR EXTERNAL USE ONLY.
Avoid contact with eyes. If contact occurs, rinse eyes thoroughly with water. If condition worsens or does not improve after regular use of this product as directed, consult a physician. Use caution in exposing skin to sunlight after applying this product. It may increase your tendency to sunburn for up to 24 hours after application. Do not use this product in or around the rectum or in the genital area or groin except on the advice of a physician. Do not use for prolonged periods without consulting a physician. Do not use this product with other forms of psoriasis therapy, such as ultraviolet radiation or prescription drugs, unless directed by a physician. If condition covers a large area of the body, consult your physician before using this product.
Keep out of reach of children. In case of accidental ingestion, seek professional assistance or contact a Poison Control Center immediately.

PRECAUTIONS
Staining of clothing may occur which is normally removed by standard laundry methods. Use on the scalp may cause temporary staining of light colored hair.

HOW SUPPLIED
FOTOTAR® Cream is available as follows:

SIZE	NDC NUMBER
3.0 oz. (85.05g) Tube	0187-0526-03
1 lb. (453g) Jar	0187-0526-05

STORAGE
FOTOTAR® Cream should be stored at controlled room temperature (15°– 30°C) 59°– 86°F.
Manufactured by
ICN PHARMACEUTICALS, INC.
3300 Hyland Ave.
Costa Mesa, CA 92626
U.S.A.
239–03EL Rev. 3/96

MESTINON® INJECTABLE ℞
[*mes 'tin-on*]
(pyridostigmine bromide)

DESCRIPTION
Mestinon (pyridostigmine bromide) Injectable is an active cholinesterase inhibitor. Chemically, pyridostigmine bromide is 3-hydroxy-1-methylpyridinium bromide dimethylcarbamate. Its structural formula is:

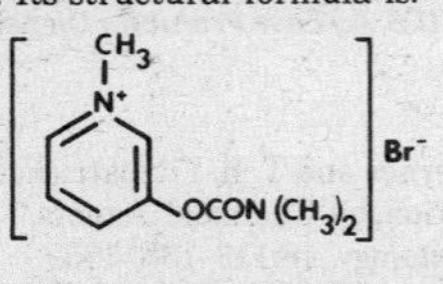

Each ml contains 5 mg pyridostigmine bromide compounded with 0.2% parabens (methyl and propyl) as preservatives, 0.02% sodium citrate and pH adjusted to approximately 5.0 with citric acid and, if necessary, sodium hydroxide.

ACTIONS
Mestinon facilitates the transmission of impulses across the myoneural junction by inhibiting the destruction of acetylcholine by cholinesterase. Pyridostigmine is an analog of neostigmine (Prostigmin®) but differs from it clinically by having fewer side effects. Currently available data indicate that pyridostigmine may have a significantly lower degree and incidence of bradycardia, salivation and gastrointestinal stimulation. Animal studies using the injectable form of pyridostigmine and human studies using the oral preparation have indicated that pyridostigmine has a longer duration of action than does neostigmine measured under similar circumstances.

INDICATIONS
Mestinon Injectable is useful in the treatment of myasthenia gravis and as a reversal agent or antagonist to nondepolarizing muscle relaxants such as curariform drugs and gallamine triethiodide.

CONTRAINDICATIONS
Known hypersensitivity to anticholinesterase agents; intestinal and urinary obstructions of mechanical type.

WARNINGS
Mestinon Injectable should be used with particular caution in patients with bronchial asthma or cardiac dysrhythmias. Transient bradycardia may occur and be relieved by atropine sulfate. Atropine should also be used with caution in patients with cardiac dysrhythmias. When large doses of Mestinon are administered, as during reversal of muscle relaxants, the prior or simultaneous injection of atropine sulfate is advisable. Because of the possibility of hypersensitivity in an occasional patient, atropine and antishock medication should always be readily available.
As is true of all cholinergic drugs, overdosage of Mestinon may result in cholinergic crisis, a state characterized by increasing muscle weakness which, through involvement of the muscles of respiration, may lead to death. Myasthenic crisis due to an increase in the severity of the disease is also accompanied by extreme muscle weakness and thus may be difficult to distinguish from cholinergic crisis on a symptomatic basis. Such differentiation is extremely important, since increases in doses of Mestinon or other drugs in this class in the presence of cholinergic crisis or of a refractory or "insensitive" state could have grave consequences. Osserman and Genkins[1] indicate that the two types of crisis may be differentiated by the use of Tensilon® (edrophonium chloride) as well as by clinical judgment. The treatment of the two conditions obviously differs radically. Whereas the presence of *myasthenic crisis* requires more intensive anticholinesterase therapy, *cholinergic crisis*, according to Osserman and Genkins,[1] calls for the prompt withdrawal of all drugs of this type. The immediate use of atropine in cholinergic crisis is also recommended. A syringe containing 1 mg of atropine sulfate should be immediately available to be given in aliquots intravenously to counteract severe cholinergic reactions.
Atropine may also be used to abolish or obtund gastrointestinal side effects or other muscarinic reactions; but such use, by masking signs of overdosage, can lead to inadvertent induction of cholinergic crisis.
For detailed information on the management of patients with myasthenia gravis, the physician is referred to one of the excellent reviews such as those by Osserman and Genkins,[2] Grob[3] or Schwab.[4,5]
When used as an antagonist to nondepolarizing muscle relaxants, adequate recovery of voluntary respiration and neuromuscular transmission must be obtained prior to discontinuation of respiratory assistance and there should be continuous patient observation. Satisfactory recovery may be defined by a combination of clinical judgment, respiratory measurements and observation of the effects of peripheral nerve stimulation. If there is any doubt concerning the adequacy of recovery from the effects of the nondepolarizing muscle relaxant, artificial ventilation should be continued until all doubt has been removed.
Usage in Pregnancy: The safety of Mestinon during pregnancy or lactation in humans has not been established. Therefore, use of Mestinon in women who may become pregnant requires weighing the drug's potential benefits against its possible hazards to mother and child.

ADVERSE REACTIONS
The side effects of Mestinon are most commonly related to overdosage and generally are of two varieties, muscarinic and nicotinic. Among those in the former group are nausea, vomiting, diarrhea, abdominal cramps, increased peristalsis, increased salivation, increased bronchial secretions, miosis and diaphoresis. Nicotinic side effects are comprised chiefly of muscle cramps, fasciculation and weakness. Muscarinic side effects can usually be counteracted by atropine, but for reasons shown in the preceding section the expedient is not without danger. As with any compound containing the bromide radical, a skin rash may be seen in an occasional patient. Such reactions usually subside promptly upon discontinuance of the medication. Thrombophlebitis has been reported subsequent to intravenous administration.

DOSAGE AND ADMINISTRATION
For Myasthenia Gravis—To supplement oral dosage, pre- and postoperatively, during labor and postpartum, during myasthenic crisis, or whenever oral therapy is impractical, approximately 1/30th of the oral dose of Mestinon may be given parenterally, either by intramuscular or *very slow* intravenous injection. *The patient must be closely observed for cholinergic reactions, particularly if the intravenous route is used.*
For details regarding the management of myasthenic patients who are to undergo major surgical procedures, see the article by Foldes.[6]
Neonates of myasthenic mothers may have transient difficulty in swallowing, sucking and breathing. Injectable Mestinon may be indicated—by symptomatology and use of the Tensilon® (edrophonium chloride) test—until Mestinon Syrup can be taken. To date the world literature consists of less than 100 neonate patients.[7] Of these only 5 were treated with injectable pyridostigmine, with the vast majority of the remaining neonates receiving neostigmine. Dosage requirements of Mestinon Injectable are minute, ranging from 0.05 mg to 0.15 mg/kg of body weight given intramuscularly. It is important to differentiate between cholinergic and myasthenic crises in neonates. (See **WARNINGS.**)
Mestinon given parenterally one hour before completion of second stage labor enables patients to have adequate strength during labor and provides protection to infants in the immediate postnatal state. For further information on the use of Mestinon Injectable in neonates of myasthenic mothers, see the article by Namba.[7]
NOTE: For information on a diagnostic test for myasthenia gravis, and on the evaluation and stabilization of therapy, please see product information on Tensilon® (edrophonium chloride).
For Reversal of Nondepolarizing Muscle Relaxants: When Mestinon Injectable is given intravenously to reverse the action of muscle relaxant drugs, it is recommended that atropine sulfate (0.6 to 1.2 mg) also be given intravenously immediately prior to the Mestinon. Side effects, notably excessive secretions and bradycardia, are thereby minimized. Usually 10 or 20 mg of Mestinon will be sufficient for antagonism of the effects of the nondepolarizing muscle relaxants. Although full recovery may occur within 15 minutes in most patients, others may require a half hour or more. Satisfactory reversal can be evident by adequate voluntary respiration, respiratory measurements and use of a peripheral nerve stimulator device. It is recommended that the patient be well ventilated and a patent airway maintained until complete recovery of normal respiration is assured. Once satisfactory reversal has been attained, recurarization has not been reported. For additional information on the use of Mestinon for antagonism of nondepolarizing muscle relaxants see the article by Katz[8] and McNall.[9]

Failure of Mestinon Injectable to provide prompt (within 30 minutes) reversal may occur, *e.g.*, in the presence of extreme debilitation, carcinomatosis, or with concomitant use of certain broad spectrum antibiotics or anesthetic agents, notably ether. Under these circumstances ventilation must be supported by artificial means until the patient has resumed control of his respiration.

HOW SUPPLIED
Mestinon is available in 2-ml ampuls (boxes of 10) (NDC 0187-3011-10).

REFERENCES

1. K. E. Osserman and G. Genkins, *J.A.M.A., 183:* 97, 1963.
2. K. E. Osserman and G. Genkins, *New York State J. Med., 61:* 2076, 1961.
3. D. Grob, *Arch. Intern. Med., 108:* 615, 1961.
4. R. S. Schwab, *New Eng. J. Med., 268:* 596, 1963.
5. R. S. Schwab, *New Eng. J. Med., 268:* 717, 1963.
6. F. F. Foldes and P. McNall, *Anesthesiology, 23:* 837, 1962.
7. T. Namba *et al., Pediatrics, 45:* 488, 1970.
8. R. L. Katz, *Anesthesiology, 28:* 528, 1967.
9. P. McNall *et al., Anesthesia and Analgesia, 48:* 1026, 1969.

Manufactured for ICN Pharmaceuticals, Inc.
Costa Mesa, CA 92626
by Hoffmann-La Roche Inc.
Nutley, N.J. 07110
Rev. 7/90

MESTINON® ℞
[*mes 'tin-on*]
(pyridostigmine bromide)
TABLETS, SYRUP and TIMESPAN® TABLETS

DESCRIPTION
Mestinon (pyridostigmine bromide) is an orally active cholinesterase inhibitor. Chemically, pyridostigmine bromide is 3-hydroxy-1-methylpyridinium bromide dimethylcarbamate. Its structural formula is:

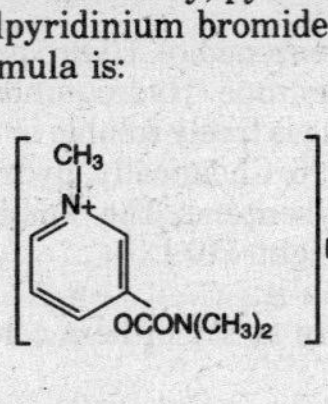

Mestinon is available in the following forms: Syrup containing 60 mg pyridostigmine bromide per teaspoonful in a vehicle containing 5% alcohol, glycerin, lactic acid, sodium benzoate, sorbitol, sucrose, FD&C Red No. 40, FD&C Blue No. 1, flavors and water. *Tablets* containing 60 mg pyridostigmine bromide; each tablet also contains lactose, silicon dioxide and stearic acid. *Timespan Tablets* containing 180 mg pyridostigmine bromide; each tablet also contains carnauba wax, corn-derived proteins, magnesium stearate, silica gel and tribasic calcium phosphate.

ACTIONS

Mestinon inhibits the destruction of acetylcholine by cholinesterase and thereby permits freer transmission of nerve impulses across the neuromuscular junction. Pyridostigmine is an analog of neostigmine (Prostigmin®), but differs from it in certain clinically significant respects; for example, pyridostigmine is characterized by a longer duration of action and fewer gastrointestinal side effects.

INDICATION

Mestinon is useful in the treatment of myasthenia gravis.

CONTRAINDICATIONS

Mestinon is contraindicated in mechanical intestinal or urinary obstruction, and particular caution should be used in its administration to patients with bronchial asthma. Care should be observed in the use of atropine for counteracting side effects, as discussed below.

WARNINGS

Although failure of patients to show clinical improvement may reflect underdosage, it can also be indicative of overdosage. As is true of all cholinergic drugs, overdosage of Mestinon may result in cholinergic crisis, a state characterized by increasing muscle weakness which, through involvement of the muscles of respiration, may lead to death. Myasthenic crisis due to an increase in the severity of the disease is also accompanied by extreme muscle weakness, and thus may be difficult to distinguish from cholinergic crisis on a symptomatic basis. Such differentiation is extremely important, since increases in doses of Mestinon or other drugs of this class in the presence of cholinergic crisis or of a refractory or "insensitive" state could have grave consequences. Osserman and Genkins[1] indicate that the differential diagnosis of the two types of crisis may require the use of Tensilon® (edrophonium chloride) as well as clinical judgment. The treatment of the two conditions obviously differs radically. Whereas the presence of myasthenic crisis suggests the need for more intensive anticholinesterase therapy, the diagnosis of cholinergic crisis, according to Osserman and Genkins,[1] calls for the prompt *withdrawal* of all drugs of this type. The immediate use of atropine in cholinergic crisis is also recommended.

Atropine may also be used to abolish or obtund gastrointestinal side effects or other muscarinic reactions; but such use, by masking signs of overdosage, can lead to inadvertent induction of cholinergic crisis.

For detailed information on the management of patients with myasthenia gravis, the physician is referred to one of the excellent reviews such as those by Osserman and Genkins,[2] Grob[3] or Schwab.[4,5]

Usage in Pregnancy: The safety of Mestinon during pregnancy or lactation in humans has not been established. Therefore, use of Mestinon in women who may become pregnant requires weighing the drug's potential benefits against its possible hazards to mother and child.

PRECAUTION

Pyridostigmine is mainly excreted unchanged by the kidney.[6,7,8] Therefore, lower doses may be required in patients with renal disease, and treatment should be based on titration of drug dosage to effect.[6,7]

ADVERSE REACTIONS

The side effects of Mestinon are most commonly related to overdosage and generally are of two varieties, muscarinic and nicotinic. Among those in the former group are nausea, vomiting, diarrhea, abdominal cramps, increased peristalsis, increased salivation, increased bronchial secretions, miosis and diaphoresis. Nicotinic side effects are comprised chiefly of muscle cramps, fasciculation and weakness. Muscarinic side effects can usually be counteracted by atropine, but for reasons shown in the preceding section the expedient is not without danger. As with any compound containing the bromide radical, a skin rash may be seen in an occasional patient. Such reactions usually subside promptly upon discontinuance of the medication.

DOSAGE AND ADMINISTRATION

Mestinon is available in three dosage forms:

Syrup—raspberry-flavored, containing 60 mg pyridostigmine bromide per teaspoonful (5 ml). This form permits accurate dosage adjustment for children and "brittle" myasthenic patients who require fractions of 60-mg doses. It is more easily swallowed, especially in the morning, by patients with bulbar involvement.

Conventional tablets—each containing 60 mg pyridostigmine bromide.

Timespan tablets—each containing 180 mg pyridostigmine bromide. This form provides uniformly slow release, hence prolonged duration of drug action; it facilitates control of myasthenic symptoms with fewer individual doses daily. The immediate effect of a 180-mg Timespan tablet is about equal to that of a 60-mg conventional tablet; however, its duration of effectiveness, although varying in individual patients, averages 2½ times that of a 60-mg dose.

Dosage: The size and frequency of the dosage must be adjusted to the needs of the individual patient.

Syrup and conventional tablets—The average dose is ten 60-mg tablets or ten 5-ml teaspoonfuls daily, spaced to provide maximum relief when maximum strength is needed. In severe cases as many as 25 tablets or teaspoonfuls a day may be required, while in mild cases one to six tablets or teaspoonfuls a day may suffice.

Timespan tablets—One to three 180-mg tablets, once or twice daily, will usually be sufficient to control symptoms; however, the needs of certain individuals may vary markedly from this average. The interval between doses should be at least six hours. For optimum control, it may be necessary to use the more rapidly acting regular tablets or syrup in conjunction with Timespan therapy.

Note: For information on a diagnostic test for myasthenia gravis, and for the evaluation and stabilization of therapy, please see product literature on Tensilon® (edrophonium chloride).

HOW SUPPLIED

Syrup, 60 mg pyridostigmine bromide per teaspoonful (5 ml) and 5% alcohol—bottles of 16 fluid ounces (1 pint) (NDC 0187-3012-20).

Tablets, scored, 60 mg pyridostigmine bromide each—bottles of 100 (NDC 0187-3010-30) and 500 (NDC 0187-3010-40).

Timespan tablets, scored, 180 mg pyridostigmine bromide each—bottles of 100 (NDC 0187-3013-50).

Note: Because of the hygroscopic nature of the Timespan tablets, mottling may occur. This does not affect their efficacy.

REFERENCES

1. Osserman KE, Genkins G. Studies in myasthenia gravis: Reduction in mortality rate after crisis. *JAMA.* Jan 1963; 183:97–101.
2. Osserman KE, Genkins G. Studies in myasthenia gravis. *NY State J. Med.* June 1961; 61:2076–2085.
3. Grob D. Myasthenia gravis. A review of pathogenesis and treatment. *Arch Intern Med.* Oct 1961; 108:615–638.
4. Schwab RS. Management of myasthenia gravis. *New Eng J Med.* Mar 1963; 268:596–597.
5. Schwab RS.Management of myasthenia gravis. *New Eng J Med.* Mar 1963; 268:717–719.
6. Cronnelly R, Stanski DR, Miller RD, Sheiner LB. Pyridostigmine kinetics with and without renal function. *Clin Pharmacol Ther.* 1980; 28:No. 1, 78–81.
7. Miller RD. Pharmacodynamics and pharmacokinetics of anticholinesterase. In: Ruegheimer E, Zindler M, ed. *Anaesthesiology.* (Hamburg, Germany: Congress; Sep 14–21, 1980; 222–223.) (Int Congr. No. 538), Amsterdam, Netherlands: Excerpta Medica; 1981.
8. Breyer-Pfaff U, Maier U, Brinkmann AM, Schumm F. Pyridostigmine kinetics in healthy subjects and patients with myasthenia gravis. *Clin Pharmacol Ther.* 1985;5:495–501.

Manufactured for ICN Pharmaceuticals, Inc.
Costa Mesa, CA 92626
by Hoffmann-La Roche Inc.
Nutley, N.J. 07110
Rev. 9/95

Shown in Product Identification Guide, page 318

OXSORALEN® LOTION 1% ℞

[ox ′sore ″a-len]

(methoxsalen USP, 1%)

CAUTION: FEDERAL (U.S.A.) LAW PROHIBITS DISPENSING WITHOUT A PRESCRIPTION.

CAUTION: METHOXSALEN LOTION IS A POTENT TOPICAL DRUG. READ ENTIRE BROCHURE BEFORE PRESCRIBING OR USING THIS MEDICATION.

WARNING: METHOXSALEN LOTION IS A POTENT DRUG CAPABLE OF PRODUCING SEVERE BURNS IF IMPROPERLY USED. IT SHOULD BE APPLIED ONLY BY A PHYSICIAN UNDER CONTROLLED CONDITIONS FOR LIGHT EXPOSURE AND SUBSEQUENT LIGHT SHIELDING.

THIS PREPARATION SHOULD NEVER BE DISPENSED TO A PATIENT.

DESCRIPTION

Each ml of Oxsoralen Lotion contains 10 mg methoxsalen in an inert vehicle containing alcohol (71% v/v), propylene glycol, acetone, and purified water.

Methoxsalen is a naturally occurring substance found in the seeds of the Ammi majus (Umbelliferae) plant; it belongs to a group of compounds known as psoralens or furocoumarins. The chemical name of methoxsalen is 9-methoxy-7H-furo(3, 2g) (1)-benzopyran-7-one. It has the following structure:

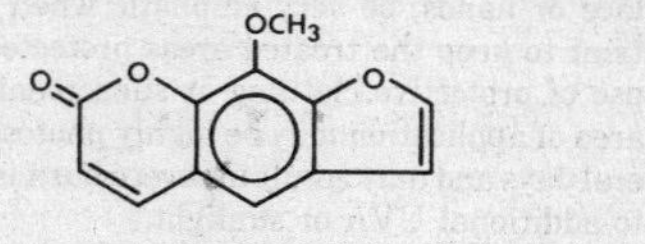

CLINICAL PHARMACOLOGY

The exact mechanism of action of methoxsalen with the epidermal melanocytes and keratinocytes is not known. Psoralens given orally are preferentially taken up by epidermal cells (Artuc et al, 1979).[1] The best known biochemical reaction of methoxsalen is with DNA. Methoxsalen, upon photoactivation, conjugates and forms covalent bonds with DNA which leads to the formation of both monofunctional (addition to a single strand of DNA) and bifunctional adducts (crosslinking of psoralen to both strands of DNA) (Dall'Acqua et al, 1971).[2] Reactions with proteins have also been described (Yoshikawa et al, 1979).[3]

Methoxsalen acts as a photosensitizer. Topical application of this drug and subsequent exposure to UVA, whether artificial or sunlight, can cause cell injury. If sufficient cell injury occurs in the skin an inflammatory reaction will result. The most obvious manifestation of this reaction is delayed erythema which may not begin for several hours and may not peak for 2 to 3 days or longer. It is crucial to realize that the length of time the skin remains sensitized or when the maximum erythema will occur is quite variable from person to person. The erythematous reaction is followed over several days or weeks by repair which is manifested by increased melanization of the epidermis and thickening of the stratum corneum. The exact mechanics are unknown but it has been suggested melanocytes in the hair follicles are stimulated to move up the follicle and to repopulate the epidermis. (Ortonne, et al, 1979).[4]

INDICATIONS AND USAGE

As a topical repigmenting agent in vitiligo in conjunction with controlled doses of ultraviolet A (320–400 nm) or sunlight.

CONTRAINDICATIONS

A. Patients exhibiting idiosyncratic reactions to psoralen compounds or a history of sensitivity reactions to them.
B. Patients exhibiting melanoma or with a history of melanoma.
C. Patients exhibiting invasive skin carcinoma generally.
D. Patients with photosensitivity diseases such as porphyria, acute lupus erythematosus, xeroderma pigmentosum, etc.
E. Children under 12 since clinical studies to determine the efficacy and safety of treatment in this age group have not been done.

WARNINGS

A. **Skin Burns**

Serious skin burns from either UVA or sunlight (even through window glass) can result if recommended exposure schedule is exceeded and/or protective covering or sunscreens are not used. The blistering of the skin sometimes encountered after UVA exposure generally heals without complication or scarring. (Farrington Daniels, Jr, M.D., personal communication). Suitable covering of the area of application or a topical sunblock should follow the therapeutic UVA exposure.

B. **Carcinogenicity**

1. Animal Studies. Topical methoxsalen has been reported to be a potent photocarcinogen in certain strains of mice. (Pathak et al 1959).[5]

2. Human Studies. None of our clinical investigators reported skin cancer as a complication of topical treatment for vitiligo. However, it is recommended that caution be exercised when the patient is fair-skinned or has a history of prior coal tar UVA treatment, or has had ionizing radiation or taken arsenical compounds. Such patients who subsequently have oral psoralen—UVA treatment (PUVA) are at increased risk for developing skin cancer.

C. **Concomitant Therapy**

Special care should be exercised in treating patients who are receiving concomitant therapy (either topically or systemically) with known photosensitizing agents such as anthralin, coal tar or coal tar derivatives, griseofulvin, phenothiazines, nalidixic acid, halogenated salicylanilides (bacteriostatic soaps), sulfonamides, tetracyclines, thiazides, and certain organic staining dyes such as methylene blue, toluidine blue, rose bengal, and methyl orange.

PRECAUTIONS

A. This product should be applied only in small well defined lesions and preferably on lesions which can be protected

Continued on next page

ICN—Cont.

by clothing or a sunscreen from subsequent exposure to radiant UVA. If this product is used to treat vitiligo of face or hands, be very emphatic when instructing patient to keep the treated areas protected from light by use of protective clothing or sunscreening agents. The area of application may be highly photosensitive for several days and may result in severe burn injury if exposed to additional UVA or sunlight.

B. CARCINOGENESIS: See Warning Section

C. Pregnancy Category C. Animal reproduction studies have not been conducted with topical methoxsalen. It is also not known whether methoxsalen can cause fetal harm when used topically on a pregnant woman or affect reproductive capacity. It is not known to what degree, if any, topical methoxsalen is absorbed systemically. Topical methoxsalen should be used in pregnant women only when clearly indicated.

D. Nursing Mothers. It is not known whether topical methoxsalen is absorbed or excreted in human milk. Caution is advised when topical methoxsalen is used in a nursing mother.

E. Pediatric Usage. Safety and effectiveness in children below the age of 12 years have not been established.

ADVERSE REACTIONS

Systemic adverse reactions have not been reported. The most common adverse reaction is severe burns of the treated area from overexposure to UVA, including sunlight. TREATMENT MUST BE INDIVIDUALIZED. Minor blistering of the skin is not a contraindication to further treatment and generally heals without incident. Treatment would be the standard for burn therapy. Since 1953, many studies have demonstrated the safety and effectiveness of topical methoxsalen and UVA for the treatment of vitiligo when used as directed. (Lerner, A.B., et al, 1953)[6] (Fitzpatrick, T.B., et al, 1966)[7] (Fulton, James F. et al, 1969)[8].

OVERDOSAGE

This does not apply to topical usage. In the unlikely event that the lotion is ingested, standard procedures for poisoning should be followed, including gastric lavage. Protection from UVA or daylight for hours or days would also be necessary. The patient should be kept in a darkened room.

ADMINISTRATION

OXSORALEN® Lotion is applied to a well-defined area of vitiligo by the physician and the area is then exposed to a suitable source of UVA. Initial exposure time should be conservative and not exceed that which is predicted to be one-half the minimal erythema dose. Treatment intervals should be regulated by the erythema response; generally once a week is recommended or less often depending on the results. The hands and fingers of the person applying the medication should be protected by gloves or finger cots to avoid photosensitization and possible burns.

Pigmentation may begin after a few weeks but significant repigmentation may require up to 6 to 9 months of treatment. Periodic re-treatment may be necessary to retain all of the new pigment. Idiopathic vitiligo is reversible but not equally reversible in every patient. Treatment must be individualized. Repigmentation will vary in completeness, time of onset, and duration. Repigmentation occurs more rapidly in fleshy areas such as face, abdomen, and buttocks and less rapidly over less fleshy areas such as the dorsum of the hands or feet.

HOW SUPPLIED

Oxsoralen Lotion containing 1% methoxsalen (8-methoxypsoralen) packaged in 1 ounce (30 ml) amber glass bottles (NDC 0187-0402-31).

Oxsoralen Lotion 1% should be stored at controlled room temperature (15–30°C) (59–86°F).

REFERENCES

1. Artuc, M.; Stuettgen, G.; Schalla, W.; Schaefer, H.; Gazith, J.: Reversible binding of 5- and 8-methoxypsoralen to human serum proteins (albumin) and to epidermis **in vitro; Brit. J. Dermat., 101**, pp. 669–677 (1979).
2. Dall'Acqua, F.; Marciani, S.; Ciavatta, L.; Rodighiero, G.: formation of interstrand cross-linkings in the photoreactions between furocoumarins and DNA.; **Z Naturforsch** (B), **26**, pp. 561–569 (1971).
3. Yoshikawa, K; Mori, N.; Sakakibara, S.; Mizuno, N.; Song, P.: Photo-Conjugation of 8-methoxypsoralen with Proteins; **Photochem & Photobiol, 29**, pp. 1127–1133 (1979).
4. Ortonne, J.P.; MacDonald, D.M.; Micoud, A.; Thivolet, J.: PUVA-induced repigmentation of vitiligo: a histochemical (split-DOPA) and ultra-structural study; **Brit. J. Dermat., 101**, pp. 1–12 (1979).
5. Pathak, M.A.; Daniels, F.; Hopkins, C.E.; Fitzpatrick, T.B.: Ultraviolet carcinogenesis in albino and pigmented mice receiving furocoumarins: psoralens and 8-methoxypsoralen, **Nature, 183**, pp. 728–730 (1959).
6. Lerner, A.B.; Denton, C.R.; Fitzpatrick, T.B.: Clinical and experimental studies with 8-methoxypsoralen in vitiligo; **J. Invest. Derm., 20**, pp. 299–314 (April, 1953).
7. Fitzpatrick, T.B.; Arndt, K.A.; El Mofty, A.M.: Hydroquinone and psoralens in the therapy of hypermelanosis and vitiligo; **Arch Derm., 93**, pp. 589–599 (May, 1966).
8. Fulton, James F.; Leyden, James; Papa, Christopher: Treatment of vitiligo with topical methoxsalen and blacklite; **Arch. Derm., 101**, pp. 224–229 (1969).

Rev. 8/93

OXSORALEN-ULTRA® CAPSULES ℞

[ox′-sore″a-len]

(Methoxsalen, 10 mg)

Caution: Federal Law prohibits dispensing without prescription.

CAUTION: METHOXSALEN IS A POTENT DRUG, READ ENTIRE BROCHURE PRIOR TO PRESCRIBING OR DISPENSING THIS MEDICATION.

Methoxsalen with UV radiation should be used only by physicians who have special competence in the diagnosis and treatment of psoriasis and who have special training and experience in photochemotherapy. The use of Psoralen and ultraviolet radiation therapy should be under constant supervision of such a physician. For the treatment of patients with psoriasis, photochemotherapy should be restricted to patients with severe, recalcitrant, disabling psoriasis which is not adequately responsive to other forms of therapy, and only when the diagnosis has been supported by biopsy. Because of the possibilities of ocular damage, aging of the skin, and skin cancer (including melanoma), the patient should be fully informed by the physician of the risks inherent in this therapy.

CAUTION: Oxsoralen-Ultra® should not be used interchangeably with regular Oxsoralen®. This new dosage form of methoxsalen exhibits significantly greater bioavailability and earlier photosensitization onset time than previous methoxsalen dosage forms. Patients should be treated in accordance with the dosimetry specifically recommended for this product. The minimum phototoxic dose (MPD) and phototoxic peak time after drug administration prior to onset of photochemotherapy with this dosage form should be determined.

DESCRIPTION

Oxsoralen-Ultra (methoxsalen, 8-methoxypsoralen) Capsules, 10mg. Methoxsalen is a naturally occurring photoactive substance found in the seeds of the **Ammi majus** (Umbelliferae) plant. It belongs to a group of compounds known as psoralens, or furocoumarins. The chemical name of methoxsalen is 9-methoxy-7H-furo [3,2-g] [1]benzopyran-7-one; it has the following structure:

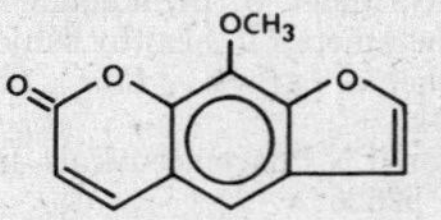

CLINICAL PHARMACOLOGY

The combination treatment regimen of psoralen (P) and ultraviolet radiation of 320–400 nm wavelength commonly referred to as UVA is known by the acronym, PUVA. Skin reactivity to UVA (320–400nm) radiation is markedly enhanced by the ingestion of methoxsalen. In a well controlled bioavailability study, Oxsoralen-Ultra Capsules reached peak drug levels in the blood of test subjects between 0.5 and 4 hours (Mean = 1.8 hours) as compared to between 1.5 and 6 hours (Mean = 3.0 hours) for regular Oxsoralen when administered with 8 ounces of milk. Peak drug levels were 2 to 3 fold greater when the overall extent of drug absorption was approximately two fold greater for Oxsoralen-Ultra Capsules as compared to regular Oxsoralen Capsules. Detectable methoxsalen levels were observed up to 12 hours post dose. The drug half-life is approximately 2 hours. Photosensitivity studies demonstrate a shorter time of peak photosensitivity of 1.5 to 2.1 hours vs. 3.9 to 4.25 hours for regular Oxsoralen capsules. In addition, the mean minimal erythema dose (MED), J/cm^2, for the Oxsoralen-Ultra Capsules is substantially less than that required for regular Oxsoralen Capsules (Levins et al., 1984 and private communication[1]).

Methoxsalen is reversibly bound to serum albumin and is also preferentially taken up by epidermal cells (Artuc et al., 1979[2]). At a dose which is six times larger than that used in humans, it induces mixed function oxidases in the liver of mice (Mandula et al., 1978[3]). In both mice and man, methoxsalen is rapidly metabolized. Approximately 95% of the drug is excreted as a series of metabolites in the urine within 24 hours (Pathak et al., 1977[4]). The exact mechanism of action of methoxsalen with the epidermal melanocytes and keratinocytes is not known. The best known biochemical reaction of methoxsalen is with DNA. Methoxsalen, upon photoactivation, conjugates and forms covalent bonds with DNA which leads to the formation of both monofunctional (addition to a single strand of DNA) and bifunctional (cross-linking of psoralen to both strands of DNA) adducts (Dall' Acqua et al., 1971[5]; Cole, 1970[6]; Musajo et al., 1974[7]; Dall' Acqua et al., 1979[8]). Reactions with proteins have also been described (Yoshikawa, et al., 1979[9]).

Methoxsalen acts as a photosensitizer. Administration of the drug and subsequent exposure to UVA can lead to cell injury. Orally administered methoxsalen reaches the skin via the blood and UVA penetrates well into the skin. If sufficient cell injury occurs in the skin, an inflammatory reaction occurs. The most obvious manifestation of this reaction is delayed erythema, which may not begin for several hours and peaks at 48–72 hours. The inflammation is followed, over several days to weeks, by repair which is manifested by increased melanization of the epidermis and thickening of the stratum corneum. The mechanisms of therapy are not known. In the treatment of psoriasis, the mechanism is most often assumed to be DNA photodamage and resulting decrease in cell proliferation but other vascular, leukocyte, or cell regulatory mechanisms may also be playing some role. Psoriasis is a hyper-proliferative disorder and other agents known to be therapeutic for psoriasis are known to inhibit DNA synthesis.

INDICATIONS AND USAGE

Photochemotherapy (methoxsalen with long wave UVA radiation) is indicated for the symptomatic control of severe, recalcitrant, disabling psoriasis not adequately responsive to other forms of therapy and when the diagnosis has been supported by biopsy. Methoxsalen is intended to be administered only in conjunction with a schedule of controlled doses of long wave ultraviolet radiation.

CONTRAINDICATIONS

A. Patients exhibiting idiosyncratic reactions to psoralen compounds.

B. Patients possessing a specific history of light sensitive disease states should not initiate methoxsalen therapy except under special circumstances. Diseases associated with photosensitivity include lupus erythematosus, porphyria cutanea tarda, erythropoietic protoporphyria, variegate porphyria, xeroderma pigmentosum, and albinism.

C. Patients with melanoma or with a history of melanoma.

D. Patients with invasive squamous cell carcinomas.

E. Patients with aphakia, because of the significantly increased risk of retinal damage due to the absence of lenses.

WARNINGS

—GENERAL

A. SKIN BURNING: Serious burns from either UVA or sunlight (even through window glass) can result if the recommended dosage of the drug and/or exposure schedules are exceeded.

B. CARCINOGENICITY:

1. ANIMAL STUDIES: Topical or intraperitoneal methoxsalen has been reported to be a potent photocarcinogen in albino mice and hairless mice (Hakim et al., 1960[10]). However, methoxsalen given by the oral route to Swiss albino mice suggests this agent exerts a protective effect against ultraviolet carcinogenesis; mice given 8-methoxypsoralen in their diet showed 38% ear tumors 180 days after the start of ultraviolet therapy compared to 62% for controls (O'Neal et al., 1957[11]).

2. HUMAN STUDIES: A 5.7 year prospective study of 1380 psoriasis patients treated with oral methoxsalen and ultraviolet A photochemotherapy (PUVA) demonstrated that the risk of cutaneous squamous-cell carcinoma developing at least 22 months following the first PUVA exposure was approximately 12.8 times higher in the high dose patients than in the low dose patients (Stern et al., 1979[12], Stern et al., 1980[13], and Stern et al., 1984[14]). The substantial dose-dependent increase was observed in patients with neither a prior history of skin cancer nor significant exposure to cutaneous carcinogens. Reduction in PUVA dosage significantly reduces the risk. No substantial dose related increase was noted for basal cell carcinoma according to Stern et al., 1984[14]. Increases appear greatest in patients who have pre-PUVA exposure to 1) prolonged tar and UVB treatment, 2) ionizing radiation, or 3) arsenic.

Roenigk et al., 1980[15], studied 690 patients for up to 4 years and found no increase in the risk of non-melanoma skin cancer, although patients in this cohort had significantly less exposure to PUVA than in the Stern et al. study. After 5 years, two of 1380 patients in the Stern et al. PUVA study have developed malignant melanoma. In addition, more than ⅓ of the patients in this cohort have developed macular pigmented lesions on the buttocks.

While there is no evidence that an increased risk of melanoma exists in PUVA treated patients, these observations indicate the need for continued evaluation of melanoma risk of PUVA treated patients.
In a study in Indian patients treated for 4 years for vitiligo, 12 percent developed keratoses, but not cancer, in the depigmented, vitiliginous areas (Mosher, 1980[16]). Clinically, the keratoses were keratotic papules, actinic keratosis-like macules, nonscaling dome-shaped papules, and lichenoid porokeratotic-like papules.

C. CATARACTOGENICITY:
1. ANIMAL STUDIES: Exposure to large doses of UVA causes cataracts in animals, and this effect is enhanced by the administration of methoxsalen (Cloud et al, 1960[17]; Cloud et al, 1961[18]; Freeman et al, 1969[19]).
2. HUMAN STUDIES: It has been found that the concentration of methoxsalen in the lens is proportional to the serum level. If the lens is exposed to UVA during the time methoxsalen is present in the lens, photochemical action may lead to irreversible binding of methoxsalen to proteins and the DNA components of the lens (Lerman et al, 1980[20]). However, if the lens is shielded from UVA, the methoxsalen will diffuse out of the lens in a 24 hour period (Lerman et al., 1980[20]). Patients should be told emphatically to wear UVA-absorbing, wrap-around sunglasses for the twenty-four (24) hour period following ingestion of methoxsalen, whether exposed to direct or indirect sunlight in the open or through a window glass.
Among patients using proper eye protection, there is no evidence for a significantly increased risk of cataracts in association with PUVA therapy. (Stern et al., 1979[12]). Thirty-five of 1380 patients have developed cataracts in the five years since their first PUVA treatment. This incidence is comparable to that expected in a population of this size and age distribution. No relationship between PUVA dose and cataract risk in this group has been noted.

D. ACTINIC DEGENERATION: Exposure to sunlight and/or ultraviolet radiation may result in "premature aging" of the skin.

E. BASAL CELL CARCINOMAS: Patients exhibiting multiple basal cell carcinomas or having a history of basal cell carcinomas should be diligently observed and treated.

F. RADIATION THERAPY: Patients having a history of previous x-ray therapy or grenz ray therapy should be diligently observed for signs of carcinoma.

G. ARSENIC THERAPY: Patients having a history of previous arsenic therapy should be diligently observed for signs of carcinoma.

H. HEPATIC DISEASES: Patients with hepatic insufficiency should be treated with caution since hepatic biotransformation is necessary for drug urinary excretion.

I. CARDIAC DISEASES: Patients with cardiac diseases or others who may be unable to tolerate prolonged standing or exposure to heat stress should not be treated in a vertical UVA chamber.

J. TOTAL DOSAGE: The total cumulative dose of UVA that can be given over long periods of time with safety has not as yet been established.

K. CONCOMITANT THERAPY: Special care should be exercised in treating patients who are receiving concomitant therapy (either topically or systemically) with known photosensitizing agents such as anthralin, coal tar or coal tar derivatives, griseofulvin, phenothiazines, nalidixic acid, halogenated salicylanilides (bacteriostatic soaps), sulfonamides, tetracyclines, thiazides and certain organic staining dyes such as methylene blue, toluidine blue, rose bengal, and methyl orange.

PRECAUTIONS

A. GENERAL—APPLICABLE TO PSORIASIS TREATMENT
1. BEFORE METHOXSALEN INGESTION
Patients must not sunbathe during the 24 hours prior to methoxsalen ingestion and UV exposure. The presence of a sunburn may prevent an accurate evaluation of the patient's response to photochemotherapy.
2. AFTER METHOXSALEN INGESTION
a. UVA-absorbing wrap-around sunglasses should be worn during daylight for 24 hours after methoxsalen ingestion. The protective eyewear must be designed to prevent entry of stray radiation to the eyes, including that which may enter from the sides of the eyewear. The protective eyewear is used to prevent the irreversible binding of methoxsalen to the proteins and DNA components of the lens. Cataracts form when enough of the binding occurs. Visual discrimination should be permitted by the eyewear for patient well-being and comfort.
b. Patients must avoid sun exposure, even through window glass or cloud cover, for at least 8 hours after methoxsalen ingestion. If sun exposure cannot be avoided, the patient should wear protective devices such as a hat and gloves, and/or apply sunscreens which contain ingredients that filter out UVA radiation (e.g. sunscreens containing benzophenone and/or PABA esters which exhibit a sun protective factor equal to or greater than 15). These chemical sunscreens should be applied to all areas that might be exposed to the sun (including lips). Sunscreens should not be applied to areas affected by psoriasis until after the patient has been treated in the UVA chamber.
3. DURING PUVA THERAPY
a. Total UVA-absorbing/blocking goggles mechanically designed to give maximal ocular protection must be worn. Failure to do so may increase the risk of cataract formation. A reliable radiometer can be used to verify elimination of UVA transmission through the goggles.
b. Abdominal skin, breasts, genitalia, and other sensitive areas should be protected for approximately $\frac{1}{3}$ of the initial exposure time until tanning occurs.
c. Unless affected by disease, male genitalia should be shielded.
4. AFTER COMBINED METHOXSALEN/UVA THERAPY
a. UVA-absorbing wrap-around sunglasses should be worn during daylight for 24 hours after combined methoxsalen/UVA therapy.
b. Patients should not sunbathe for 48 hours after therapy. Erythema and/or burning due to photochemotherapy and sunburn due to sun exposure are additive.

B. INFORMATION FOR PATIENTS: See accompanying Patient Package Insert.

C. LABORATORY TESTS:
1. Patients should have an ophthalmologic examination prior to start of therapy, and thence yearly.
2. Patients should have routine laboratory tests prior to the start of therapy and at regular periods thereafter if patients are on extended treatments.

D. DRUG INTERACTIONS: See Warnings Section.

E. CARCINOGENESIS: See Warnings Section.

F. PREGNANCY:
Pregnancy Category C. Animal reproduction studies have not been conducted with methoxsalen. It is also not known whether methoxsalen can cause fetal harm when administered to a pregnant woman or can affect reproduction capacity. Methoxsalen should be given to a woman with reproductive capacity only if clearly needed.

G. NURSING MOTHERS:
It is not known whether this drug is excreted in human milk. Because many drugs are excreted in human milk, either methoxsalen ingestion or nursing should be discontinued.

H. PEDIATRIC USE:
Safety in children has not been established. Potential hazards of long-term therapy include the possibilities of carcinogenicity and cataractogenicity as described in the Warnings Section as well as the probability of actinic degeneration which is also described in the Warnings Section.

ADVERSE REACTIONS

A. METHOXSALEN:
The most commonly reported side effect of methoxsalen alone is nausea, which occurs with approximately 10% of all patients. This effect may be minimized or avoided by instructing the patient to take methoxsalen in milk or food, or to divide the dose into two portions, taken approximately one-half hour apart. Other effects include nervousness, insomnia, and depression.

B. COMBINED METHOXSALEN/UVA THERAPY:
1. PRURITUS: This adverse reaction occurs with approximately 10% of all patients. In most cases, pruritus can be alleviated with frequent application of bland emollients or other topical agents; severe pruritus may require systemic treatment. If pruritus is unresponsive to these measures, shield pruritic areas from further UVA exposure until the condition resolves. If intractable pruritus is generalized, UVA treatment should be discontinued until the pruritus disappears.
2. ERYTHEMA: Mild, transient erythema at 24–48 hours after PUVA therapy is an expected reaction and indicates that a therapeutic interaction between methoxsalen and UVA occurred. Any area showing moderate erythema (greater than Grade 2—See Table 1 for grades of erythema) should be shielded during subsequent UVA exposures until the erythema has resolved. Erythema greater than Grade 2 which appears within 24 hours after UVA treatment may signal a potentially severe burn. Erythema may become progressively worse over the next 24 hours, since the peak erythemal reaction characteristically occurs 48 hours or later after methoxsalen ingestion. The patient should be protected from further UVA exposures and sunlight, and should be monitored closely.
3. IMPORTANT DIFFERENCES BETWEEN PUVA ERYTHEMA AND SUNBURN: PUVA-induced inflammation differs from sunburn or UVB phototherapy in several ways. The percent transmission of UVB varies between 0% to 34% through skin whereas UVA varies between 1% to 80% transmission; thus, UVA is transmitted to a larger percent through the skin. (Diffey, 1982[21]). The DNA lesions induced by PUVA are very different from UV-induced thymine dimers and may lead to a DNA crosslink. This DNA lesion may be more problematic to the cell because crosslinks are more lethal and psoralen-DNA photoproducts may be "new" or unfamiliar substrates for DNA repair enzymes. DNA synthesis is also suppressed longer after PUVA. The time course of delayed erythema is different with PUVA and may not involve the usual mediators seen in sunburn. PUVA-induced redness may be just beginning at 24 hours, when UVB erythema has already passed its peak. The erythema dose-response curve is also steeper for PUVA. Compared to equally erythemogenic doses of UVB, the histologic alterations induced by PUVA show more dermal vessel damage and longer duration of epidermal and dermal abnormalities.
4. OTHER ADVERSE REACTIONS: Those reported include edema, dizziness, headache, malaise, depression, hypopigmentation, vesiculation and bullae formation, non-specific rash, herpes simplex, miliaria, urticaria, folliculitis, gastrointestinal disturbances, cutaneous tenderness, leg cramps, hypotension, and extension of psoriasis.

OVERDOSAGE

In the event of methoxsalen overdosage, induce emesis and keep the patient in a darkened room for at least 24 hours. Emesis is most beneficial within the first 2 to 3 hours after ingestion of methoxsalen, since maximum blood levels are reached by this time.

DRUG DOSAGE AND ADMINISTRATION

CAUTION: Oxsoralen-Ultra represents a new dose form of methoxsalen. This new dosage form of methoxsalen exhibits significantly greater bioavailability and earlier photosensitization onset time than previous methoxsalen dosage forms. Each patient should be evaluated by determining the minimum phototoxic dose (MPD) and phototoxic peak time after drug administration prior to onset of photochemotherapy with this dosage form. Human bioavailability studies have indicated the following drug dosage and administration directions are to be used as a guideline only.

PSORIASIS THERAPY
1. DRUG DOSAGE-INITIAL THERAPY: The methoxsalen capsules should be taken $1\frac{1}{2}$ to 2 hours before UVA exposure with some low fat food or milk according to the following table:

Patient's Weight		Dose
(kg)	(lbs)	(mg)
<30	<65	10
30–50	65–100	20
51–65	101–145	30
66–80	146–175	40
81–90	176–200	50
91–115	201–250	60
>115	>250	70

2. INITIAL EXPOSURE: The initial UVA exposure energy level and corresponding time of exposure is determined by the patient's skin characteristics for sunburning and tanning as follows:

Skin Type	History	Recommended Joules/cm²
I	Always burn, never tan (patients with erythrodermic psoriasis are to be classed as Type I for determination of UVA dosage.)	0.5 J/cm²
II	Always burn, but sometimes tan	1.0 J/cm²
III	Sometimes burn, but always tan	1.5 J/cm²
IV	Never burn, always tan	2.0 J/cm²
Skin Type	**Physician Examination**	**Joules/cm²**
V*	Moderately pigmented	2.5 J/cm²
VI*	Blacks	3.0 J/cm²

(*Patients with natural pigmentation of these types should be classified into a lower skin type category if the sunburning history so indicates.)
If the MPD is done, start at $\frac{1}{2}$ MPD.
Additional drug dosage directions are as follows:
a. Weight Change: In the event that the weight of a patient changes during treatment such that he/she falls into an adjacent weight range/dose category, no change in the dose of methoxsalen is usually required. If, in the physician's opinion, however, a weight change is sufficiently great to modify the drug dose, then an adjustment in the time of exposure to UVA should be made.
b. Dose/Week: The number of doses per week of methoxsalen capsules will be determined by the patient's schedule of UVA exposures. In no case should treatments be given more often than once every other day because the full extent of

Continued on next page

ICN—Cont.

phototoxic reactions may not be evident until 48 hours after each exposure.

c. Dosage Increase: Dosage may be increased by 10 mg after the fifteenth treatment under the conditions outlined in section XI. B. 4b.

UVA RADIATION SOURCE SPECIFICATIONS & INFORMATION

A. IRRADIANCE UNIFORMITY

The following specifications should be met with the window of the detector held in a vertical plane:

1. Vertical variation: For readings taken at any point along the vertical center axis of the chamber (to within 15 cm from the top and bottom), the lowest reading should not be less than 70 percent of the highest reading.

2. Horizontal variation: Throughout any specific horizontal plane, the lowest reading must be at least 80 percent of the highest reading, excluding the peripheral 3 cm of the patient treatment space.

B. PATIENT SAFETY FEATURES:

The following safety features should be present: (1) Protection from electrical hazard: All units should be grounded and conform to applicable electrical codes. The patient or operator should not be able to touch any live electrical parts. There should be ground fault protection. (2) Protective shielding of lamps: The patient should not be able to come in contact with the bare lamps. In the event of lamp breakage, the patient should not be exposed to broken lamp components. (3) Hand rails and hand holds: Appropriate supports should be available to the patient. (4) Patient viewing window: A window which blocks UV should be provided for viewing the patient during treatment. (5) Door and latches: Patients should be able to open the door from the inside with only slight pressure to the door. (6) Non-skid floor: The floor should be of a non-skid nature. (7) Thermoregulation: Sufficient air flow should be provided for patient safety and comfort, limiting temperature within the UVA radiator cabinet to approximately less than 100°F. (8) Timer: The irradiator should be equipped with an automatic timer which terminates the exposure at the conclusion of a pre-set time interval. (9) Patient alarm device: An alarm device within the UVA irradiator chamber should be accessible to the patient for emergency activation. (10) Danger label: The unit should have a label prominently displayed which reads as follows:

DANGER—Ultraviolet Radiation—Follow your physician's instructions—Failure to use protective eyewear may result in eye injury.

C. UVA EXPOSURE DOSIMETRY MEASUREMENTS:

The maximum radiant exposure or irradiance (within ± 15 percent) of UVA (320–400 nm) delivered to the patient should be determined by using an appropriate radiometer calibrated to be read in Joules/cm² or mW/cm². In the absence of a standard measuring technique approved by the National Bureau of Standards, the system should use a detector corrected to a cosine spatial response. The use and recalibration frequency of such a radiometer for a specific UVA irradiator chamber should be specified by the manufacturer because the UVA dose (exposure) is determined by the design of the irradiator, the number of lamps, and the age of the lamp. If irradiance is measured, the radiometer reading in mW/cm² is used to calculate the exposure time in minutes to deliver the required UVA in Joules/cm² to a patient in the UVA irradiator cabinet. The equation is:

$$\text{Exposure Time (minutes)} = \frac{\text{Desired UVA Dose (J/cm}^2\text{)}}{0.06 \times \text{Irradiance (mW/cm}^2\text{)}}.$$

Overexposure due to human error should be minimized by using an accurate automatic timing device, which is set by the operator and controlled by energizing and deenergizing the UVA irradiator lamp. The timing device calibration interval should be specified by the manufacturer. Safety systems should be included to minimize the possibility of delivering a UVA exposure which exceeds the prescribed dose, in the event the timer or radiometer should malfunction.

D. UVA SPECTRAL OUTPUT DISTRIBUTION:

The spectral distributions of the lamps should meet the following specifications:

Wavelength band (nanometers)	Output[1]
<310	<1
310 to 320	1 to 3
320 to 330	4 to 8
330 to 340	11 to 17
340 to 350	18 to 25
350 to 360	19 to 28
360 to 370	15 to 23
370 to 380	8 to 12
380 to 390	3 to 7
390 to 400	1 to 3

[1] As a percentage of total irradiance between 320 and 400 nanometers.

PUVA TREATMENT PROTOCOL

INTRODUCTION:

The Oxsoralen-Ultra® Capsules reach their maximum bioavailability in 1½ to 2 hours after ingestion.

On average, the serum level achieved with Oxsoralen-Ultra is twice that obtained with 8-MOP (formerly Oxsoralen) and reach their peak concentration in less than ½ the time of the 8-MOP capsules.

As a result the mean MED J/cm² for the Oxsoralen-Ultra Capsules is substantially less than that required for 8-MOP (Levins et al., 1984 and private communication[1]).

Photosensitivity studies demonstrate a shorter time of peak photosensitivity of 1.5 to 2.1 hours vs. 3.9 to 4.25 hours for regular methoxsalen capsules.

A. INITIAL EXPOSURE: The initial UVA exposures should be conducted according to the guidelines presented previously under IX.B.1 and 2, Psoriasis Therapy, Drug Dosage-initial Therapy and Exposure.

B. CLEARING PHASE: Specific recommendations for patient treatment are as follows:

1. SKIN TYPES I, II, & III. Patients with skin types I, II, and III may be treated 2 or 3 times per week. UVA exposure may be held constant or increased by up to 1.0 Joule/cm² at each treatment, according to the patient's response. If erythema occurs, however, do not increase exposure time until erythema resolves. The severity and extent of the patient's erythema may be used to determine whether the next exposure should be shortened, omitted, or maintained at the previous dosage. See Adverse Reactions section for additional information.

2. SKIN TYPES IV, V, & VI. Patients with skin types IV, V, and VI may be treated 2 or 3 times per week. UVA exposure may be held constant or increased by up to 1.5 Joules/cm² at each treatment unless erythema occurs. If erythema occurs, follow instructions outlined above in the procedures for patients with skin types I, II, and III.

3. ERYTHRODERMIC PSORIASIS. Patients with erythrodermic psoriasis should be treated with special attention because pre-existing erythema may obscure observations of possible treatment-related phototoxic erythema. These patients may be treated 2 or 3 times per week, as a Type I patient.

4. MISCELLANEOUS SITUATIONS:

a. If there is no response after a total of 10 treatments, the exposure of UVA energy may be increased by an additional 0.5-1.0 Joules/cm² above the prior incremental increases for each treatment. (Example: a patient whose exposure dose is being increased by 1.0 Joule/cm² may now have all subsequent doses increased by 1.5-2.0 Joules/cm².)

b. If there is no response, or only minimal response, after 15 treatments, the dosage of methoxsalen may be increased by 10 mg (a one-time increase in dosage). This increased dosage may be continued for the remainder of the course of treatment but should not be exceeded.

c. If a patient misses a treatment, the UVA exposure time of the next treatment should not be increased. If more than one treatment is missed, reduce the exposure by 0.5 Joules/cm² for each treatment missed.

d. If the lower extremities are not responding as well as the rest of the body and do not show erythema, cover all other body areas and give 25 percent of the present exposure dose as an additional exposure to the lower extremities. This additional exposure to the lower extremities should be terminated if erythema develops on these areas.

e. Non-responsive psoriasis: If a patient's generalized psoriasis is not responding, or if the condition appears to be worsening during treatment, the possibility of a generalized phototoxic reaction should be considered. This may be confirmed by the improvement of the condition following temporary discontinuance of this therapy for two weeks. If no improvement occurs during the interruption of treatment, this patient may be considered a treatment failure.

C. ALTERNATIVE EXPOSURE SCHEDULE:

As an alternative to increasing the UVA exposure at each treatment, the following schedule may be followed; this schedule may reduce the total number of Joules/cm² received by the patient over the entire course of therapy.

1. Incremental increases in UVA exposure for all patients may range from 0.5 to 1.5 Joules/cm², according to the patient's response to therapy.

2. Once Grade 2 clearing (see Table 2) has been reached and the patient is progressing adequately, UVA dosage is held constant. The dosage is maintained until Grade 4 clearing is reached.

3. If the rate of clearing significantly decreases, exposure dosage may be increased at each treatment (0.1–1.5 Joules/cm²) until Grade 3 clearing and a satisfactory progress rate is attained. The UVA exposure will be held constant again until Grade 4 clearing is attained. These increases may be used also if the rate of clearing significantly decreases between Grade 3 and Grade 4 response. However, the possibility of a phototoxic reaction should be considered; see Non-responsive Psoriasis, above.

4. In summary, this schedule raises slightly the increments (Joules/cm²) of UVA dosage, but limits these increases to those periods when the patient is not responding adequately. Otherwise, the UVA exposure is held at the lowest effective dose.

D. MAINTENANCE PHASE:

The goal of maintenance treatment is to keep the patient as symptom-free as possible with the least amount of UVA exposure.

1. SCHEDULE OF EXPOSURES: When patients have achieved 95 percent clearing, or Grade 4 response (Table 2), they may be placed on the following maintenance schedules (M_1–M_4), in sequence. It is recommended that each maintenance schedule be adhered to for at least 2 treatments (unless erythema or psoriatic flare occurs, in which case see (2a) and (2b) below).

Maintenance Schedules

M_1—once/week
M_2—once/2 weeks
M_3—once/3 weeks
M_4—p.r.n. (i.e. for flares)

2. LENGTH OF EXPOSURE: The UVA exposure for the first maintenance treatment of any schedule (except M_4 as noted below) is the same as that of the patient's last treatment under the previous schedule. For skin types I–IV, however, it is recommended that the maximum UVA dosage during maintenance treatments not exceed the following:

Skin Types	Joules/cm²/treatment
I	12
II	14
III	18
IV	22

If the patient develops erythema or new lesions of psoriasis, proceed as follows:

a. Erythema: During maintenance therapy, the patient's tan and threshold dose for erythema may gradually decrease. If maintenance treatments produce significant erythema, the exposure to UVA should be decreased by 25 percent until further treatments no longer produce erythema.

b. Psoriasis: If the patient develops new areas of psoriasis during maintenance therapy (but still is classified as having a Grade 4 response), the exposure to UVA may be increased by 0.5–1.5 Joules/cm² at each treatment; this is appropriate for all types of patients. These increases are continued until the psoriasis is brought under control and the patient is again clear. The exposure being administered when this clearing is reached should be used for further maintenance treatment.

3. FLARES DURING MAINTENANCE: If the patient flares during maintenance treatment (i.e., develops psoriasis on more than 5 percent of the originally involved areas of the body) his maintenance treatment schedule may be changed to the preceding maintenance or clearing schedule. The patient may be kept on his schedule until again 95 percent clear. If the original maintenance treatment schedule is unable to control the psoriasis, the schedule may be changed to a more frequent regimen. If a flare occurs less than 6 weeks after the last treatment, 25 percent of the maximum exposure received during the clearing phase, with the clearing schedule received during the clearing phase, may be used and then proceed with the clearing schedule previously followed for this patient. (At 95 percent clearing, follow regular maintenance until the optimum maintenance schedule is determined for the patient.) If more than 6 weeks have elapsed since the last treatment was given, treat patients as if they were beginning therapy insofar as exposure dosages are concerned, since their threshold for erythema may have decreased.

Table 1. Grades of Erythema

Grades	Erythema
0	No erythema
1	Minimally perceptible erythema—faint pink
2	Marked erythema but with no edema
3	Fiery erythema with edema
4	Fiery erythema with edema and blistering

Table 2. Response to Therapy

Grade	Criteria	Percent Improvement (compared to original extent of disease)
−1	Psoriasis worse	0
0	No change	0
1	Minimal improvement—slightly less scale and/or erythema	5–20

2	Definite improvement—partial flattening of all plaques—less scaling and less erythema	20–50
3	Considerable improvement—nearly complete flattening of all plaques but borders of plaques still palpable	50–95
4	Clearing; complete flattening of plaques including borders; plaques may be outlined by pigmentation	95

HOW SUPPLIED

Oxsoralen-Ultra Capsules, each containing 10 mg of methoxsalen (8-methoxypsoralen) in a soft gelatin capsule packaged in amber glass bottles are available as follows:

Unit Count	NDC Number
50	0187-0650-42

ICN Pharmaceuticals, Inc. Rev. Jan., 1990
Costa Mesa, Ca 92626

BIBLIOGRAPHY

1. Levins, P.C., Gange, R.W., Momtaz-T.K., Parrish, J.A., and Fitzpatrick, T.B.: A New Liquid Formulation of 8-Methoxypsoralen: Bioactivity and Effect of Diet: JID, *82,* No. 2, pp. 185–187 (1984) and private communication.
2. Artuc, M., Stuettgen, G. Schalla, W., Schaefer, H., and Gazith, J.: Reversible binding of 5- and 8-methoxypsoralen to human serum proteins (albumin) and to epidermis in vitro: Brit. J. Dermat. *101,* pp. 669–677 (1979).
3. Mandula, B.B., Pathak, M.A., Nakayama, T., and Davidson, S.J.: Induction of mixed-function oxidases in mouse liver by psoralens., Ibid, *99,* pp. 687–692 (1978).
4. Pathak, M.A., Fitzpatrick, T.B., Parrish, J.A.: PSORIASIS, Proceedings of the Second International Symposium. Edited by E.M. Farber, A.J. Cox, Yorke Medical Books, pp. 262–265 (1977).
5. Dall'Acqua, F., Marciani, S., Ciavatta, L., Rodighiero, G.: Formation of interstrand cross-linkings in the photoreactions between furocoumarins and DNA; Z Naturforsch (B), *26,* pp. 561–569 (1971).
6. Cole, R.S.: Light-induced cross-linkings of DNA in the presence of a furocoumarin (psoralen), Biochem. Biophys. Acta, *217,* pp. 30–39 (1970).
7. Musajo, L, Rodighiero, G., Caporale, G., Dall'Acqua, F, Marciani, S., Bordin, F., Baccichetti, F., Bevilacqua, R.: Photoreactions between Skin-Photosensitizing Furocoumarins and Nucleic Acids, *Sunlight and Man;* Normal and Abnormal Photobiologic Responses. Edited by M.A. Pathak, LC. Harber, M. Seiji et al. University of Tokyo Press, pp. 369–387 (1974).
8. Dall'Acqua, F., Vedaldi, D., Bordin, F., and Rodighiero, G.: New studies in the interaction between 8-methoxypsoralen and DNA *in vitro:* JID, *73,* pp. 191–197 (1979).
9. Yoshikawa, K., Mori, N., Sakakibara, S., Mizuno, N. Song, P.: Photo Conjugation of 8-methoxypsoralen with Proteins; Photochem. & Photobiol. *29,* pp. 1127–1133 (1979).
10. Hakim, R.D., Griffin, A.C.: Knox, J.M.: Erythema and tumor formation in methoxsalen treated mice exposed to fluorescent light; Arch. Dermatol. *82,* pp. 572–577 (1960).
11. O'Neal, M.A., Griffin, A.C.: The Effect of Oxypsoralen upon Ultraviolet Carcinogenesis in Albino Mice, Cancer Res., *17,* pp. 911–916 (1957).
12. Stern, R.S., Unpublished personal communication.
13. Stern, R.S., Parrish, J.A., Zierler, S.: Skin Carcinoma in Patients with Psoriasis Treated with Topical Tar and Artificial Ultraviolet Radiation. Lancet, *1,* pp. 732–735 (1980).
14. Stern, R.S., Laird, N., Melski, J. Parrish, J.A., Fitzpatrick, T.B., Bleich, H.L.: Cutaneous Squamous-Cell Carcinoma in Patients Treated with PUVA: NEJM, *310,* No. 18, pp. 1156–1161 (1984).
15. Roenigk, Jr., H.H., and 12 Cooperating Investigators: Skin Cancer in the PUVA-48 Cooperative Study of Psoriasis. Program for Forty-First Annual Meeting for The Society of Investigative Dermatology, Inc., Sheraton Washington Hotel, Washington, D.C., May 12, 13, and 14, 1980). Abstracts JID, *74,* No. 4, p. 250 (April, 1980).
16. Mosher, D.B., Pathak, M.A., Harris, T.J., Fitzpatrick, T.B.: Development of Cutaneous Lesions in Vitiligo During Long-Term PUVA Therapy. Program for Forty-First Annual Meeting for the Society for Investigative Dermatology, Inc., Sheraton Washington Hotel, Washington, D.C., May 12, 13, and 14, 1980. Abstracts JID, *74,* No. 4, p 259 (April, 1980).
17. Cloud, T.M. Hakim, R., Griffin, A.C.: Photosensitization of the eye with methoxsalen. I. Acute effects; Arch. Ophthalmol. *64,* pp. 346–352 (1960).
18. Cloud, T.M. Hakim, R., Griffin, A.C.: Photosensitization of the eye with methoxsalen. II. Chronic effects, Ibid, *66,* pp. 689–694 (1961).
19. Freeman, R.G., Troll, D.: Photosensitization of the eye by 8-methoxypsoralen, JID, *53,* pp. 449–453 (1969).
20. Lerman, S., Megaw, J., Willis, I.:Potential ocular complications from PUVA therapy and their prevention; JID, *74,* pp. 197–199 (1980).
21. Diffey, B.L., Medical Physics Handbook 11, Ultraviolet Radiation in Medicine, Adam Hilger, Ltd., Bristol, p. 86 (1982).

Shown in Product Identification Guide, page 318

PROSTIGMIN® ℞

[pro-stig'min]
(neostigmine methylsulfate)
INJECTABLE

DESCRIPTION

Prostigmin (neostigmine methylsulfate) Injectable, an anticholinesterase agent, is a sterile aqueous solution intended for intramuscular, intravenous or subcutaneous administration.

Prostigmin Injectable is available in the following concentrations:

Prostigmin 1:2000 Ampuls — each ml contains 0.5 mg neostigmine methylsulfate compounded with 0.2% parabens (methyl and propyl) as preservatives and sodium hydroxide to adjust pH to approximately 5.9.

Prostigmin 1:1000 Multiple Dose Vials — each ml contains 1 mg neostigmine methylsulfate compounded with 0.45% phenol as preservative, 0.2 mg sodium acetate, and acetic acid and sodium hydroxide to adjust pH to approximately 5.9.

Prostigmin 1:2000 Multiple Dose Vials — each ml contains 0.5 mg neostigmine methylsulfate compounded with 0.45% phenol as preservative, 0.2 mg sodium acetate, and acetic acid and sodium hydroxide to adjust pH to approximately 5.9.

Chemically, neostigmine methylsulfate is (*m*-hydroxyphenyl)trimethylammonium methylsulfate dimethylcarbamate. It has a molecular weight of 334.39 and the following structural formula:

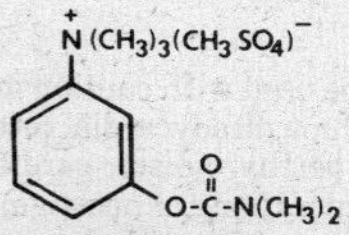

CLINICAL PHARMACOLOGY

Neostigmine inhibits the hydrolysis of acetylcholine by competing with acetylcholine for attachment to acetylcholinesterase at sites of cholinergic transmission. It enhances cholinergic action by facilitating the transmission of impulses across neuromuscular junctions. It also has a direct cholinomimetic effect on skeletal muscle and possibly on autonomic ganglion cells and neurons of the central nervous system. Neostigmine undergoes hydrolysis by cholinesterase and is also metabolized by microsomal enzymes in the liver. Protein binding to human serum albumin ranges from 15 to 25 percent.

Following intramuscular administration, neostigmine is rapidly absorbed and eliminated. In a study of five patients with myasthenia gravis, peak plasma levels were observed at 30 minutes, and the half-life ranged from 51 to 90 minutes. Approximately 80 percent of the drug was eliminated in urine within 24 hours; approximately 50% as the unchanged drug, and 30 percent as metabolites. Following intravenous administration, plasma half-life ranges from 47 to 60 minutes have been reported with a mean half-life of 53 minutes.

The clinical effects of neostigmine usually begin within 20 to 30 minutes after intramuscular injection and last from 2.5 to 4 hours.

INDICATIONS AND USAGE

Prostigmin is indicated for:
—the symptomatic control of myasthenia gravis when oral therapy is impractical.
—the prevention and treatment of postoperative distention and urinary retention after mechanical obstruction has been excluded.
—reversal of effects of nondepolarizing neuromuscular blocking agents (*e.g.,* tubocurarine, metocurine, gallamine, or pancuronium) after surgery.

CONTRAINDICATIONS

Prostigmin is contraindicated in patients with known hypersensitivity to the drug. It is also contraindicated in patients with peritonitis or mechanical obstruction of the intestinal or urinary tract.

WARNINGS

Prostigmin should be used with caution in patients with epilepsy, bronchial asthma, bradycardia, recent coronary occlusion, vagotonia, hyperthyroidism, cardiac arrhythmias or peptic ulcer. When large doses of Prostigmin are administered, the prior or simultaneous injection of atropine sulfate may be advisable. Separate syringes should be used for the Prostigmin and atropine. Because of the possibility of hypersensitivity in an occasional patient, atropine and antishock medication should always be readily available.

PRECAUTIONS

General: It is important to differentiate between myasthenic crisis and cholinergic crisis caused by overdosage of Prostigmin. Both conditions result in extreme muscle weakness but require radically different treatment. (See OVERDOSAGE section.)

Drug Interactions: Prostigmin does not antagonize, and may in fact prolong, the Phase I block of *depolarizing* muscle relaxants such as succinylcholine or decamethonium. Certain antibiotics, especially neomycin, streptomycin and kanamycin, have a mild but definite nondepolarizing blocking action which may accentuate neuromuscular block. These antibiotics should be used in the myasthenic patient only where definitely indicated, and then careful adjustment should be made of the anticholinesterase dosage. Local and some general anesthetics, antiarrhythmic agents and other drugs that interfere with neuromuscular transmission should be used cautiously, if at all, in patients with myasthenia gravis; the dose of Prostigmin may have to be increased accordingly.

Carcinogenesis, Mutagenesis and Impairment of Fertility: There have been no studies with Prostigmin which would permit an evaluation of its carcinogenic or mutagenic potential. Studies on the effect of Prostigmin on fertility and reproduction have not been performed.

Pregnancy:
Teratogenic Effects: Pregnancy Category C. There are no adequate or well-controlled studies of Prostigmin in either laboratory animals or in pregnant women. It is not known whether Prostigmin can cause fetal harm when administered to a pregnant woman or can affect reproductive capacity. Prostigmin should be given to a pregnant woman only if clearly needed.

Nonteratogenic Effects: Anticholinesterase drugs may cause uterine irritability and induce premature labor when given intravenously to pregnant women near term.

Nursing Mothers: It is not known whether Prostigmin is excreted in human milk. Because many drugs are excreted in human milk and because of the potential for serious adverse reactions from Prostigmin in nursing infants, a decision should be made whether to discontinue nursing or to discontinue the drug, taking into account the importance of the drug to the mother.

Pediatric Use: Safety and effectiveness in children have not been established.

ADVERSE REACTIONS

Side effects are generally due to an exaggeration of pharmacological effects of which salivation and fasciculation are the most common. Bowel cramps and diarrhea may also occur. The following additional adverse reactions have been reported following the use of either neostigmine bromide or neostigmine methylsulfate:

Allergic: Allergic reactions and anaphylaxis.
Neurologic: Dizziness, convulsions, loss of consciousness, drowsiness, headache, dysarthria, miosis and visual changes.
Cardiovascular: Cardiac arrhythmias (including bradycardia, tachycardia, A-V block and nodal rhythm) and nonspecific EKG changes have been reported, as well as cardiac arrest, syncope and hypotension. These have been predominantly noted following the use of the injectable form of Prostigmin.
Respiratory: Increased oral, pharyngeal and bronchial secretions, dyspnea, respiratory depression, respiratory arrest and bronchospasm.
Dermatologic: Rash and urticaria.
Gastrointestinal: Nausea, emesis, flatulence and increased peristalsis.
Genitourinary: Urinary frequency.
Musculoskeletal: Muscle cramps and spasms, arthralgia.
Miscellaneous: Diaphoresis, flushing and weakness.

OVERDOSAGE

Overdosage of Prostigmin can cause cholinergic crisis, which is characterized by increasing muscle weakness, and through involvement of the muscles of respiration, may result in death. Myasthenic crisis, due to an increase in the severity of the disease, is also accompanied by extreme muscle weakness and may be difficult to distinguish from cholinergic crisis on a symptomatic basis. However, such differentiation is extremely important because increases in the dose of Prostigmin or other drugs in this class, in the presence of cholinergic crisis or of a refractory or "insensitive" state, could have grave consequences. The two types of crises may be differentiated by the use of Tensilon® (edrophonium chloride) as well as by clinical judgment.

Treatment of the two conditions differs radically. Whereas the presence of *myasthenic crisis* requires more intensive anticholinesterase therapy, *cholinergic crisis* calls for the prompt withdrawal of all drugs of this type. The immediate use of atropine in cholinergic crisis is also recommended.

Continued on next page

ICN—Cont.

Atropine may also be used to abolish or minimize gastrointestinal side effects or other muscarinic reactions; but such use, by masking signs of overdosage, can lead to inadvertent induction of cholinergic crisis.

The LD_{50} of neostigmine methylsulfate in mice is 0.3 ± 0.02 mg/kg intravenously, 0.54 ± 0.03 mg/kg subcutaneously, and 0.395 ± 0.025 mg/kg intramuscularly; in rats the LD_{50} is 0.315 ± 0.019 mg/kg intravenously, 0.445 ± 0.032 mg/kg subcutaneously, and 0.423 ± 0.032 mg/kg intramuscularly.

DOSAGE AND ADMINISTRATION

Symptomatic control of myasthenia gravis: One ml of the 1:2000 solution (0.5 mg) subcutaneously or intramuscularly. Subsequent doses should be based on the individual patient's response. In most patients, however, oral treatment with Prostigmin (neostigmine bromide) tablets, 15 mg each, is adequate for control of symptoms.

Prevention of postoperative distention and urinary retention: One ml of the 1:4000 solution (0.25 mg) subcutaneously or intramuscularly as soon as possible after operation; repeat every 4 to 6 hours for two or three days.

Treatment of postoperative distention: One ml of the 1:2000 solution (0.5 mg) subcutaneously or intramuscularly, as required.

Treatment of urinary retention: One ml of the 1:2000 solution (0.5 mg) subcutaneously or intramuscularly. If urination does not occur within an hour, the patient should be catheterized. After the patient has voided, or the bladder has been emptied, continue the 0.5 mg injections every three hours for at least 5 injections.

Reversal of Effects of Nondepolarizing Neuromuscular Blocking Agents: When Prostigmin is administered intravenously, it is recommended that atropine sulfate (0.6 to 1.2 mg) also be given intravenously using separate syringes. Some authorities have recommended that the atropine be injected several minutes before the Prostigmin rather than concomitantly. The usual dose is 0.5 to 2 mg Prostigmin given by *slow* intravenous injection, repeated as required. Only in exceptional cases should the total dose of Prostigmin exceed 5 mg. It is recommended that the patient be well ventilated and a patent airway maintained until complete recovery of normal respiration is assured. The optimum time for administration of the drug is during hyperventilation when the carbon dioxide level of the blood is low. It should never be administered in the presence of high concentrations of halothane or cyclopropane. In cardiac cases and severely ill patients, it is advisable to titrate the exact dose of Prostigmin required, using a peripheral nerve stimulator device. In the presence of bradycardia, the pulse rate should be increased to about 80/minute with atropine before administering Prostigmin.

Parenteral drug products should be inspected visually for particulate matter and discoloration prior to administration, whenever solution and container permit.

HOW SUPPLIED

Prostigmin 1:2000 (0.5 mg neostigmine methylsulfate/ml), 1-ml ampuls — boxes of 10 (NDC 0187-3101-30).
Prostigmin 1:4000 (0.25 mg neostigmine methylsulfate/mL), 1-mL ampuls — boxes of 10 (NDC 0187-3102-40).
Prostigmin 1:1000 (1 mg neostigmine methylsulfate/ml), 10-ml multiple dose vials — boxes of 10 (NDC 0187-3103-50).
Prostigmin 1:2000 (0.5 mg neostigmine methylsulfate/ml), 10-ml multiple dose vials — boxes of 10 (NDC 0187-3104-60).
Manufactured for ICN Pharmaceuticals, Inc.
Costa Mesa, CA 92626
by Hoffmann-La Roche Inc.
Nutley, N.J. 07110
Rev. 7/90

PROSTIGMIN® ℞
[*pro-stig'min*]
(neostigmine bromide)
TABLETS

DESCRIPTION

Prostigmin (neostigmine bromide), an anticholinesterase agent, is available for oral administration in 15-mg tablets. Each tablet also contains gelatin, lactose, corn starch, stearic acid, sugar and talc.

Chemically, neostigmine bromide is (*m*-hydroxyphenyl) trimethylammonium bromide dimethylcarbamate. It is a white, crystalline, bitter powder, soluble 1:1 in water, with a molecular weight of 303.20 and the following structural formula:

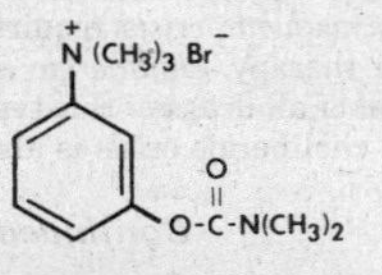

CLINICAL PHARMACOLOGY

Neostigmine inhibits the hydrolysis of acetylcholine by competing with acetylcholine for attachment to acetylcholinesterase at sites of cholinergic transmission. It enhances cholinergic action by facilitating the transmission of impulses across neuromuscular junctions. It also has a direct cholinomimetic effect on skeletal muscle and possibly on autonomic ganglion cells and neurons of the central nervous system. Neostigmine undergoes hydrolysis by cholinesterase and is also metabolized by microsomal enzymes in the liver. Protein binding to human serum albumin ranges from 15 to 25 percent.

Neostigmine bromide is poorly absorbed from the gastrointestinal tract following oral administration. As a rule, 15 mg of neostigmine bromide orally is equivalent to 0.5 mg of neostigmine methylsulfate parenterally, due to poor absorption of the tablet from the intestinal tract. In a study in fasting myasthenic patients, the extent of absorption was estimated to be 1 to 2 percent of the ingested 30-mg single oral dose. Peak concentrations in plasma occurred 1 to 2 hours following drug ingestion, with considerable individual variations. The half-life ranged from 42 to 60 minutes with a mean half-life of 52 minutes.

INDICATIONS AND USAGE

Prostigmin is indicated for the symptomatic treatment of myasthenia gravis. Its greatest usefulness is in prolonged therapy where no difficulty in swallowing is present. In acute myasthenic crisis where difficulty in breathing and swallowing is present, the parenteral form (neostigmine methylsulfate) should be used. The patient can be transferred to the oral form as soon as it can be tolerated.

CONTRAINDICATIONS

Prostigmin is contraindicated in patients with known hypersensitivity to the drug. Because of the presence of the bromide ion, it should not be used in patients with a previous history of reaction to bromides. It is contraindicated in patients with peritonitis or mechanical obstruction of the intestinal or urinary tract.

WARNINGS

Prostigmin should be used with caution in patients with epilepsy, bronchial asthma, bradycardia, recent coronary occlusion, vagotonia, hyperthyroidism, cardiac arrhythmias or peptic ulcer. As a rule, 15 mg of neostigmine bromide orally is equivalent to 0.5 mg of neostigmine methylsulfate parenterally, due to poor absorption of the tablet from the intestinal tract. Large doses should be avoided in situations where there might be an increased absorption rate from the intestinal tract. It should be used with caution when co-administered with anticholinergic drugs, in order to avoid reduction of intestinal motility.

PRECAUTIONS

General: It is important to differentiate between myasthenic crisis and cholinergic crisis caused by overdosage of Prostigmin. Both conditions result in extreme muscle weakness but require radically different treatment. (See OVERDOSAGE section.)

Drug Interactions: Certain antibiotics, especially neomycin, streptomycin and kanamycin, have a mild but definite nondepolarizing blocking action which may accentuate neuromuscular block. These antibiotics should be used in the myasthenic patient only where definitely indicated, and then careful adjustment should be made of adjunctive anticholinesterase dosage.

Local and some general anesthetics, antiarrhythmic agents and other drugs that interfere with neuromuscular transmission should be used cautiously, if at all, in patients with myasthenia gravis; the dose of Prostigmin may have to be increased accordingly.

Carcinogenesis, Mutagenesis and Impairment of Fertility: There have been no studies with Prostigmin which would permit an evaluation of its carcinogenic or mutagenic potential. Studies on the effect of Prostigmin on fertility and reproduction have not been performed.

Pregnancy:

Teratogenic Effects: Pregnancy Category C. There are no adequate or well-controlled studies of Prostigmin in either laboratory animals or in pregnant women. It is not known whether Prostigmin can cause fetal harm when administered to a pregnant woman or can affect reproductive capacity. Prostigmin should be given to a pregnant woman only if clearly needed.

Nonteratogenic Effects: Anticholinesterase drugs may cause uterine irritability and induce premature labor when given intravenously to pregnant women near term.

Nursing Mothers: It is not known whether Prostigmin is excreted in human milk. Because many drugs are excreted in human milk and because of the potential for serious adverse reactions from Prostigmin in nursing infants, a decision should be made whether to discontinue nursing or to discontinue the drug, taking into account the importance of the drug to the mother.

Pediatric Use: Safety and effectiveness in children have not been established.

ADVERSE REACTIONS

Side effects are generally due to an exaggeration of pharmacological effects of which salivation and fasciculation are the most common. Bowel cramps and diarrhea may also occur. The following additional adverse reactions have been reported following the use of either neostigmine bromide or neostigmine methylsulfate:

Allergic: Allergic reactions and anaphylaxis.
Neurologic: Dizziness, convulsions, loss of consciousness, drowsiness, headache, dysarthria, miosis and visual changes.
Cardiovascular: Cardiac arrhythmias (including bradycardia, tachycardia, A-V block and nodal rhythm) and nonspecific EKG changes have been reported, as well as cardiac arrest, syncope and hypotension. These have been predominantly noted following the use of the injectable form of Prostigmin.
Respiratory: Increased oral, pharyngeal and bronchial secretions, and dyspnea. Respiratory depression, respiratory arrest and bronchospasm have been reported following the use of the injectable form of Prostigmin.
Dermatologic: Rash and urticaria.
Gastrointestinal: Nausea, emesis, flatulence and increased peristalsis.
Genitourinary: Urinary frequency.
Musculoskeletal: Muscle cramps and spasms, arthralgia.
Miscellaneous: Diaphoresis, flushing and weakness.

OVERDOSAGE

Overdosage of Prostigmin can cause cholinergic crisis, which is characterized by increasing muscle weakness, and through involvement of the muscles of respiration, may result in death. Myasthenic crisis, due to an increase in the severity of the disease, is also accompanied by extreme muscle weakness and may be difficult to distinguish from cholinergic crisis on a symptomatic basis. However, such differentiation is extremely important because increases in the dose of Prostigmin or other drugs in this class, in the presence of cholinergic crisis or of a refractory or "insensitive" state, could have grave consequences. The two types of crises may be differentiated by the use of Tensilon® (edrophonium chloride) as well as by clinical judgment.

Treatment of the two conditions differs radically. Whereas the presence of *myasthenic crisis* requires more intensive anticholinesterase therapy, *cholinergic crisis* calls for the prompt withdrawal of all drugs of this type. The immediate use of atropine in cholinergic crisis is also recommended.

Atropine may also be used to abolish or minimize gastrointestinal side effects or other muscarinic reactions; but such use, by masking signs of overdosage, can lead to inadvertent induction of cholinergic crisis.

The LD_{50} of neostigmine methylsulfate in mice is 0.3 ± 0.02 mg/kg intravenously, 0.54 ± 0.03 mg/kg subcutaneously, and 0.395 ± 0.025 mg/kg intramuscularly; in rats the LD_{50} is 0.315 ± 0.019 mg/kg intravenously, 0.445 ± 0.032 mg/kg subcutaneously, and 0.423 ± 0.032 mg/kg intramuscularly.

DOSAGE AND ADMINISTRATION

The onset of action of Prostigmin given orally is slower than when given parenterally, but the duration of action is longer and the intensity of action more uniform. Dosage requirements for optimal results vary from 15 mg to 375 mg per day. In some instances it may be necessary to exceed these dosages, but the possibility of cholinergic crisis must be recognized. The average dose is 10 tablets (150 mg) administered over a 24-hour period. The interval between doses is of paramount importance. The dosage schedule should be adjusted for each patient and changed as the need arises. Frequently, therapy is required day and night. Larger portions of the total daily dose may be given at times when the patient is more prone to fatigue (afternoon, mealtimes, etc.). The patient should be encouraged to keep a daily record of his or her condition to assist the physician in determining an optimal therapeutic regimen.

HOW SUPPLIED

Scored, white tablets containing 15 mg neostigmine bromide — bottles of 100 (NDC 0187-3100-10). Imprint on tablets: (front) PROSTIGMIN 15: (back) ICN.
Manufactured for ICN Pharmaceuticals, Inc.
Costa Mesa, CA 92626
by Hoffmann-La Roche Inc.
Nutley, N.J. 07110
Rev. 10/89

Shown in Product Identification Guide, page 318

TENSILON® ℞

[*ten 'sil-on*]

(edrophonium chloride)

Injectable Solution

ampuls • vials

DESCRIPTION

Tensilon is a short and rapid-acting cholinergic drug. Chemically, edrophonium chloride is ethyl (*m*- hydroxyphenyl)-dimethylammonium chloride.

10-ml vials: Each ml contains, in a sterile solution, 10 mg edrophonium chloride compounded with 0.45% phenol and 0.2% sodium sulfite as preservatives, buffered with sodium citrate and citric acid, and pH adjusted to approximately 5.4.

1-ml ampuls: Each ml contains, in a sterile solution, 10 mg edrophonium chloride compounded with 0.2% sodium sulfite, buffered with sodium citrate and citric acid, and pH adjusted to approximately 5.4.

ACTIONS

Tensilon is an anticholinesterase drug. Its pharmacological action is due primarily to the inhibition of acetylcholinesterase at sites of cholinergic transmission. Its effect is manifest within 30 to 60 seconds after injection and lasts an average of 10 minutes.

INDICATIONS

Tensilon is recommended for the differential diagnosis of myasthenia gravis and as an adjunct in the evaluation of treatment requirements in this disease. It may also be used for evaluating emergency treatment in myasthenic crises. Because of its brief duration of action, it is not recommended for maintenance therapy in myasthenia gravis.

Tensilon is also useful whenever a curare antagonist is needed to reverse the neuromuscular block produced by curare, tubocurarine, gallamine triethiodide or dimethyl-tubocurarine. It is *not* effective against decamethonium bromide and succinylcholine chloride. It may be used adjunctively in the treatment of respiratory depression caused by curare overdosage.

CONTRAINDICATIONS

Known hypersensitivity to anticholinesterase agents; intestinal and urinary obstructions of mechanical type.

WARNINGS

Whenever anticholinesterase drugs are used for testing, a syringe containing 1 mg of atropine sulfate should be immediately available to be given in aliquots intravenously to counteract severe cholinergic reactions which may occur in the hypersensitive individual, whether he is normal or myasthenic. Tensilon should be used with caution in patients with bronchial asthma or cardiac dysrhythmias. The transient bradycardia which sometimes occurs can be relieved by atropine sulfate. Isolated instances of cardiac and respiratory arrest following administration of Tensilon have been reported. It is postulated that these are vagotonic effects.

Tensilon solution contains sodium sulfite, a sulfite that may cause allergic-type reactions, including anaphylactic symptoms and life-threatening or less severe asthmatic episodes in certain susceptible people. The overall prevalence of sulfite sensitivity in the general population is unknown and probably low. Sulfite sensitivity is seen more frequently in asthmatic than in nonasthmatic people.

Usage in Pregnancy: The safety of Tensilon during pregnancy or lactation in humans has not been established. Therefore, use of Tensilon in women who may become pregnant requires weighing the drug's potential benefits against its possible hazards to mother and child.

PRECAUTIONS

Patients may develop "anticholinesterase insensitivity" for brief or prolonged periods. During these periods the patients should be carefully monitored and may need respiratory assistance. Dosages of anticholinesterase drugs should be reduced or withheld until patients again become sensitive to them.

ADVERSE REACTIONS

Careful observation should be made for severe cholinergic reactions in the hyperreactive individual. The myasthenic patient in crisis who is being tested with Tensilon should be observed for bradycardia or cardiac standstill and cholinergic reactions if an overdose is given. The following reactions common to anticholinesterase agents may occur, although not all of these reactions have been reported with the administration of Tensilon, probably because of its short duration of action and limited indications: **Eye:** Increased lacrimation, pupillary constriction, spasm of accommodation, diplopia, conjunctival hyperemia. **CNS:** Convulsions, dysarthria, dysphonia, dysphagia. **Respiratory:** Increased tracheobronchial secretions, laryngospasm, bronchiolar constriction, paralysis of muscles of respiration, central respiratory paralysis. **Cardiac:** Arrhythmias (especially bradycardia), fall in cardiac output leading to hypotension. **G.I.:** Increased salivary, gastric and intestinal secretion, nausea, vomiting, increased peristalsis, diarrhea, abdominal cramps. **Skeletal Muscle:** Weakness, fasciculations. **Miscellaneous:** Increased urinary frequency and incontinence, diaphoresis.

	Myasthenic*	Adequate†	Cholinergic‡
Muscle Strength (ptosis, diplopia, dysphonia, dysphagia, dysarthria, respiration, limb strength)	Increased	No change	Decreased
Fasciculations (orbicularis oculi, facial muscles, limb muscles)	Absent	Present or absent	Present or absent
Side reactions (lacrimation, diaphoresis, salivation, abdominal cramps, nausea, vomiting, diarrhea)	Absent	Minimal	Severe

* Myasthenic Response—occurs in untreated myasthenics and may serve to establish diagnosis; in patients under treatment, indicates that therapy is inadequate.

† Adequate Response—observed in treated patients when therapy is stabilized; a typical response in normal individuals. In addition to this response in nonmyasthenics, the phenomenon of forced lid closure is often observed in psychoneurotics.[1]

‡ Cholinergic Response—seen in myasthenics who have been overtreated with anticholinesterase drugs.

DOSAGE AND ADMINISTRATION

Tensilon Test in the Differential Diagnosis of Myasthenia Gravis:[1–8]

Intravenous Dosage (Adults): A tuberculin syringe containing 1 ml (10 mg) of Tensilon is prepared with an intravenous needle, and 0.2 ml (2 mg) is injected intravenously within 15 to 30 seconds. The needle is left *in situ. Only* if no reaction occurs after 45 seconds is the remaining 0.8 ml (8 mg) injected. If a cholinergic reaction (muscarinic side effects, skeletal muscle fasciculations and increased muscle weakness) occurs after injection of 0.2 ml (2 mg), the test is discontinued and atropine sulfate 0.4 mg to 0.5 mg is administered intravenously. After one-half hour the test may be repeated.

Intramuscular Dosage (Adults): In adults with inaccessible veins, dosage for intramuscular injection is 1 ml (10 mg) of Tensilon. Subjects who demonstrate hyperreactivity to this injection (cholinergic reaction), should be retested after one-half hour with 0.2 ml (2 mg) of Tensilon intramuscularly to rule out false-negative reactions.

Dosage (Children): The intravenous testing dose of Tensilon in children weighing up to 75 lbs is 0.1 ml (1 mg); above this weight, the dose is 0.2 ml (2 mg). If there is no response after 45 seconds, it may be titrated up to 0.5 ml (5 mg) in children under 75 lbs, given in increments of 0.1 ml (1 mg) every 30 to 45 seconds and up to 1 ml (10 mg) in heavier children. In infants, the recommended dose is 0.05 ml (0.5 mg). Because of technical difficulty with intravenous injection in children, the intramuscular route may be used. In children weighing up to 75 lbs, 0.2 ml (2 mg) is injected intramuscularly. In children weighing more than 75 lbs, 0.5 ml (5 mg) is injected intramuscularly. All signs which would appear with the intravenous test appear with the intramuscular test except that there is a delay of two to ten minutes before a reaction is noted.

Tensilon Test for Evaluation of Treatment Requirements in Myasthenia Gravis: The recommended dose is 0.1 ml to 0.2 ml (1 mg to 2 mg) of Tensilon, administered intravenously one hour after oral intake of the drug being used in treatment.[1–5] Response will be myasthenic in the undertreated patient, adequate in the controlled patient, and cholinergic in the overtreated patient. Responses to Tensilon in myasthenic and nonmyasthenic individuals are summarized in the following chart:[2]

[See table above.]

Tensilon Test in Crisis: The term *crisis* is applied to the myasthenic whenever severe respiratory distress with objective ventilatory inadequacy occurs and the response to medication is not predictable. This state may be secondary to a sudden increase in severity of myasthenia gravis (myasthenic crisis), or to overtreatment with anticholinesterase drugs (cholinergic crisis).

When a patient is apneic, controlled ventilation must be secured immediately in order to avoid cardiac arrest and irreversible central nervous system damage. No attempt is made to test with Tensilon until respiratory exchange is adequate. *Dosage used at this time is most important:* If the patient is cholinergic, Tensilon will cause increased oropharyngeal secretions and further weakness in the muscles of respiration. If the crisis is myasthenic, the test clearly improves respiration and the patient can be treated with longer-acting intravenous anticholinesterase medication. When the test is performed, there should not be more than 0.2 ml (2 mg) Tensilon in the syringe. An intravenous dose of 0.1 ml (1 mg) is given initially. The patient's heart action is carefully observed. If, after an interval of one minute, this dose does not further impair the patient, the remaining 0.1 ml (1 mg) can be injected. If no clear improvement of respiration occurs after 0.2 ml (2 mg) dose, it is usually wisest to discontinue all anticholinesterase drug therapy and secure controlled ventilation by tracheostomy with assisted respiration.[5]

For Use as a Curare Antagonist: Tensilon should be administered by intravenous injection in 1 ml (10 mg) doses given slowly over a period of 30 to 45 seconds so that the onset of cholinergic reaction can be detected. This dosage may be repeated whenever necessary. The maximal dose for any one patient should be 4 ml (40 mg). Because of its brief effect, Tensilon should not be given prior to the administration of curare, tubocurarine, gallamine triethiodide or dimethyl-tubocurarine; it should be used at the time when its effect is needed. When given to counteract curare overdosage, the effect of each dose on the respiration should be carefully observed before it is repeated, and assisted ventilation should always be employed.

DRUG INTERACTIONS

Care should be given when administering this drug to patients with symptoms of myasthenic weakness who are also on anticholinesterase drugs. Since symptoms of anticholinesterase overdose (cholinergic crisis) may mimic underdosage (myasthenic weakness), their condition may be worsened by the use of this drug. (See OVERDOSAGE section for treatment.)

OVERDOSAGE

With drugs of this type, muscarine-like symptoms (nausea, vomiting, diarrhea, sweating, increased bronchial and salivary secretions and bradycardia) often appear with overdosage (cholinergic crisis). An important complication that can arise is obstruction of the airway by bronchial secretions. These may be managed with suction (especially if tracheostomy has been performed) and by the use of atropine. Many experts have advocated a wide range of dosages of atropine *(for Tensilon, see atropine dosage below)*, but if there are copious secretions, up to 1.2 mg intravenously may be given initially and repeated every 20 minutes until secretions are controlled. Signs of atropine overdosage such as dry mouth, flush and tachycardia should be avoided as tenacious secretions and bronchial plugs may form. A total dose of atropine of 5 to 10 mg or even more may be required. The following steps should be taken in the management of overdosage of Tensilon:

1. Adequate respiratory exchange should be maintained by assuring an open airway, and the use of assisted respiration augmented by oxygen.
2. Cardiac function should be monitored until complete stabilization has been achieved.
3. Atropine sulfate in doses of 0.4 to 0.5 mg should be administered intravenously. This may be repeated every 3 to 10 minutes. Because of the short duration of action of Tensilon the total dose required will seldom exceed 2 mg.
4. If convulsions or shock is present, appropriate measures should be instituted.

HOW SUPPLIED

Multiple Dose Vials, 10 ml, boxes of 10 (NDC 0187-3200-20).

Ampuls, 1 ml, boxes of 10 (NDC 0187-3200-10).

REFERENCES

1. Osserman, K.E. and Kaplan, L.I., *J.A.M.A., 150:* 265, 1952.
2. Osserman, K.E., Kaplan, L.I. and Besson, G., *J. Mt. Sinai Hosp., 20:* 165, 1953.
3. Osserman, K.E. and Kaplan, L.I., *Arch. Neurol. & Psychiat., 70:* 385, 1953.
4. Osserman, K.E. and Teng, P., *J.A.M.A., 160:* 153, 1956.
5. Osserman, K.E. and Genkins, G., *Ann. N.Y. Acad. Sci., 135:* 312, 1966.
6. Tether, J.E., Second International Symposium Proceedings, Myasthenia Gravis, 1961, p. 444.
7. Tether, J.E., in H.F. Conn: *Current Therapy 1960,* Philadelphia, W. B. Saunders Company, p. 551.
8. Tether, J.E., in H.F. Conn: *Current Therapy 1965,* Philadelphia, W. B. Saunders Company, p. 556.
9. Grob, D. and Johns, R.J., *J.A.M.A., 166:* 1855, 1958.

Manufactured for ICN Pharmaceuticals, Inc.
Costa Mesa, CA 92626
by Hoffmann-La Roche Inc.
Nutley, NJ 07110
Rev. 11/93

Continued on next page

ICN—Cont.

TESTRED® Ⓒ℞

Methyltestosterone Capsules, USP 10 mg

DESCRIPTION

The androgens are steroids that develop and maintain primary and secondary male sex characteristics. Androgens are derivatives of cyclopentanoperhydrophenanthrene. Endogenous androgens are C-19 steroids with a side chain at C-17, and with two angular methyl groups. Testosterone is the primary endogenous androgen. In their active form, all drugs in the class have a 17-beta-hydroxy group. 17-alpha alkylation (methyltestosterone) increases the pharmacologic activity per unit weight compared to testosterone when given orally. Methyltestosterone, a synthetic derivative of testosterone, is an androgenic preparation given by the oral route in a capsule form. Each capsule contains 10 mg of methyltestosterone USP. It has the following structural formula:

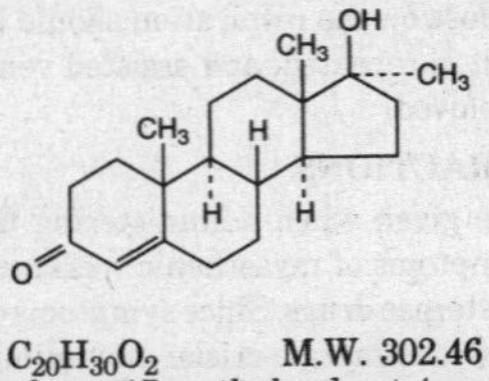

$C_{20}H_{30}O_2$ M.W. 302.46

17β-hydroxy-17-methylandrost-4-en-3-one

Methyltestosterone occurs as white or creamy white crystals or powder, which is soluble in various organic solvents but is practically insoluble in water.

Each capsule, for oral administration, contains 10 mg of methyltestosterone. In addition, each capsule contains the following inactive ingredients: Corn starch NF, Gelatin NF, FD&C Blue #1, FD&C Red #40.

CLINICAL PHARMACOLOGY

Endogenous androgens are responsible for the normal growth and development of the male sex organs and for maintenance of secondary sex characteristics. These effects include the growth and maturation of prostate, seminal vesicles, penis, and scrotum. The development of male hair distribution, such as beard, pubic, chest, and axillary hair; laryngeal enlargement, vocal chord thickening, alterations in body musculature and fat distribution. Drugs in this class also cause retention of nitrogen, sodium, potassium, phosphorus, and decreased urinary excretion of calcium. Androgens have been reported to increase protein anabolism and decrease protein catabolism. Nitrogen balance is improved only when there is sufficient intake of calories and protein.

Androgens are responsible for the growth spurt of adolescence and for the eventual termination of linear growth which is brought about by fusion of the epiphyseal growth centers. In children, exogenous androgens accelerate linear growth rates, but may cause a disproportionate advancement in bone maturation. Use over long periods may result in fusion of the epiphyseal growth centers and termination of growth process. Androgens have been reported to stimulate the production of red blood cells by enhancing the production of erythropoietic stimulating factor.

During exogenous administration of androgens, endogenous testosterone release is inhibited through feedback inhibition of pituitary luteinizing hormone (LH). At large doses of exogenous androgens, spermatogenesis may also be suppressed through feedback inhibition of pituitary follicle stimulating hormone (FSH).

There is a lack of substantial evidence that androgens are effective in fractures, surgery, convalescence and functional uterine bleeding.

Pharmacokinetics

Testosterone given orally is metabolized by the gut and 44 percent is cleared by the liver of the first pass. Oral doses as high as 400 mg per day are needed to achieve clinically effective blood levels for full replacement therapy. The synthetic androgen, methyltestosterone, is less extensively metabolized by the liver and has a longer half-life. It is more suitable than testosterone for oral administration.

Testosterone in plasma is 98 percent bound to a specific testosterone-estradiol binding globulin, and about 2 percent is free. Generally, the amount of this sex-hormone binding globulin in the plasma will determine the distribution of testosterone between free and bound forms, and the free testosterone concentration will determine its half-life.

About 90 percent of a dose of testosterone is excreted in the urine as glucuronic and sulfuric acid conjugates of testosterone and its metabolites; about 6 percent of a dose is excreted in the feces, mostly in the unconjugated form. Inactivation of testosterone occurs primarily in the liver. Testosterone is metabolized to various 17-keto steroids through two different pathways. There are considerable variations of the half-life of testosterone as reported in the literature, ranging from 10 to 100 minutes.

In many tissues the activity of testosterone appears to depend on reduction to dihydrotestosterone, which binds to cytosol receptor proteins. The steroid-receptor complex is transported to the nucleus where it initiates transcription events and cellular changes related to androgen action.

INDICATIONS AND USAGE

1. Males

Androgens are indicated for replacement therapy in conditions associated with a deficiency or absence of endogenous testosterone;

a. Primary hypogonadism (congenital or acquired)—testicular failure due to cryptorchidism, bilateral torsions, orchitis, vanishing testis syndrome; or orchidectomy.
b. Hypogonadotropic hypogonadism (congenital or acquired)—idiopathic gonadotropin or LHRH deficiency, or pituitary-hypothalamic injury from tumors, trauma or radiation.

   If the above conditions occur prior to puberty, androgen replacement therapy will be needed during the adolescent years for development of secondary sexual characteristics. Prolonged androgen treatment will be required to maintain sexual characteristics in these and other males who develop testosterone deficiency after puberty.
c. Androgens may be used to stimulate puberty in carefully selected males with clearly delayed puberty. These patients usually have a familial pattern of delayed puberty that is not secondary to a pathological disorder; puberty is expected to occur spontaneously at a relatively late date. Brief treatment with conservative doses may occasionally be justified in these patients if they do not respond to psychological support. The potential adverse effect on bone maturation should be discussed with the patient and parents prior to androgen adminstration. An X-ray of the hand and wrist to determine bone age should be obtained every 6 months to assess the effect of treatment on the epiphyseal centers (see WARNINGS).

2. Females

Androgens may be used secondarily in women with advancing inoperable metastatic (skeletal) mammary cancer who are 1 to 5 years postmenopausal. Primary goals of therapy in these women include ablation of the ovaries. Other methods of counteracting estrogen activity are adrenalectomy, hypophysectomy, and/or antiestrogen therapy. This treatment has also been used in premenopausal women with breast cancer who have benefited from oophorectomy and are considered to have a hormone-responsive tumor. Judgment concerning androgen therapy should be made by an oncologist with expertise in this field.

CONTRAINDICATIONS

Androgens are contraindicated in men with carcinomas of the breast or with known or suspected carcinomas of the prostate, and in women who are or may become pregnant. When administered to pregnant women, androgens cause virilization of the external genitalia of the female fetus. This virilization includes clitoromegaly, abnormal vaginal development, and fusion of genital folds to form a scrotal-like structure. The degree of masculinization is related to the amount of drug given and the age of the fetus, and is most likely to occur in the female fetus when the drugs are given in the first trimester. If the patient becomes pregnant while taking these drugs, she should be apprised of the potential hazard to the fetus.

WARNINGS

In patients with breast cancer, androgen therapy may cause hypercalcemia by stimulating osteolysis. In this case, the drug should be discontinued.

Prolonged use of high doses of androgens has been associated with the development of peliosis hepatis and hepatic neoplasms including hepatocellular carcinoma. (See PRECAUTIONS-Carcinogenesis). Peliosis hepatis can be a life-threatening or fatal complication.

Cholestatic hepatitis and jaundice occur with 17-alpha-alkylandrogens at a relatively low dose. If cholestatic hepatitis with jaundice appears or if liver function tests become abnormal, the androgen should be discontinued and the etiology should be determined. Drug-induced jaundice is reversible when the medication is discontinued.

Geriatric patients treated with androgens may be at an increased risk for the development of prostatic hypertrophy and prostatic carcinoma.

Edema with or without congestive heart failure may be a serious complication in patients with preexisting cardiac, renal, or hepatic disease. In addition to discontinuation of the drug, diuretic therapy may be required.

Gynecomastia frequently develops and occasionally persists in patients being treated for hypogonadism. Androgen therapy should be used cautiously in healthy males with delayed puberty. The effect on bone maturation should be monitored by assessing bone age of the wrist and hand every 6 months. In children, androgen treatment may accelerate bone maturation without producing compensatory gain in linear growth. This adverse effect may result in compromised adult stature. The younger the child the greater the risk of compromising final mature height.

This drug has not been shown to be safe and effective for the enhancement of athletic performance. Because of the potential risk of serious adverse health effects, this drug should not be used for such purpose.

PRECAUTIONS

General

Women should be observed for signs of virilization (deepening of the voice, hirsutism, acne, clitoromegaly and menstrual irregularities). Discontinuation of drug therapy at the time of evidence of mild virilism is necessary to prevent irreversible virilization. Such virilization is usual following androgen use at high doses. A decision may be made by the patient and the physician that some virilization will be tolerated during treatment for breast carcinoma.

Information for the Patient

The physician should instruct patients to report any of the following side effects of androgens:

Adult or Adolescent Males:	Too frequent or persistent erections of the penis. Any male adolescent patient receiving androgens for delayed puberty should have bone development checked every six months.
Women:	Hoarseness, acne, changes in menstrual periods, or more hair on the face.
All Patients:	Any nausea, vomiting, changes in skin color or ankle swelling.

Laboratory Tests

1. Women with disseminated breast carcinoma should have frequent determination of urine and serum calcium levels during the course of androgen therapy. (See WARNINGS).
2. Because of the hepatotoxicity associated with the use of 17-alpha-alkylated androgens, liver function tests should be obtained periodically.
3. Periodic (every 6 months) x-ray examinations of bone age should be made during treatment of prepubertal males to determine the rate of bone maturation and the effects of androgen therapy on the epiphyseal centers.
4. Hemoglobin and hematocrit should be checked periodically for polycythemia in patients who are receiving high doses of androgens.

Drug Interactions

1. **Anticoagulants:** C-17 substituted derivatives of testosterone, such as methandrostenolone, have been reported to decrease the anticoagulant requirements of patients receiving oral anticoagulants. Patients receiving oral anticoagulant therapy require close monitoring, especially when androgens are started or stopped.
2. **Oxyphenbutazone:** Concurrent administration of oxyphenbutazone and androgens may result in elevated serum levels of oxyphenbutazone.
3. **Insulin:** In diabetic patients the metabolic effects of androgens may decrease blood glucose and insulin requirements.

Drug/Laboratory Test Interferences

Androgens may decrease levels of thyroxine-binding globulin, resulting in decreased total T4 serum levels and increased resin uptake of T3 and T4. Free thyroid hormone levels remain unchanged, however, and there is no clinical evidence of thyroid dysfunction.

Carcinogenesis

Animal Data

Testosterone has been tested by subcutaneous injection and implantation in mice and rats. The implant induced cervical-uterine tumors in mice, which metastasized in some cases. There is suggestive evidence that injection of testosterone into some strains of female mice increases their susceptibility to hepatoma. Testosterone is also known to increase the number of tumors and decrease the degree of differentiation of chemically induced carcinomas of the liver in rats.

Human Data

There are rare reports of hepatocellular carcinoma in patients receiving long-term therapy with androgens in high doses. Withdrawal of the drugs did not lead to regression of the tumors in all cases.

Geriatric patients treated with androgens may be at an increased risk for the development of prostatic hypertrophy and prostatic carcinoma.

Pregnancy

Teratogenic effects. Pregnancy Category X (See CONTRAINDICATIONS).

Nursing Mothers

It is not known whether androgens are excreted in human milk. Because many drugs are excreted in human milk and because of the potential for serious adverse reactions in nursing infants from androgens, a decision should be made whether to discontinue nursing or to discontinue the drug, taking into account the importance of the drug to the mother.

Pediatric Use

Androgen therapy should be used very cautiously in children and only by specialists who are aware of the adverse effects on bone maturation. Skeletal maturation must be monitored every six months by an x-ray of hand and wrist (See INDICATIONS AND USAGE and WARNINGS).

ADVERSE REACTIONS

Endocrine and Urogenital

Female: The most common side effects of androgen therapy are amenorrhea and other menstrual irregularities, inhibition of gonadotropin secretion, and virilization, including deepening of the voice and clitoral enlargement. The latter usually is not reversible after androgens are discontinued. When administered to a pregnant woman androgens cause virilization of external genitalia of the female fetus.

Male: Gynecomastia, and excessive frequency and duration of penile erections. Oligospermia may occur at high dosages (see CLINICAL PHARMACOLOGY).

Skin and appendages: Hirsutism, male pattern of baldness, and acne.

Fluid and Electrolyte Disturbances: Retention of sodium, chloride, water, potassium, calcium, and inorganic phosphates.

Gastrointestinal: Nausea, cholestatic jaundice, alterations in liver function tests, rarely hepatocellular neoplasms and peliosis hepatis (see WARNINGS).

Hematologic: Suppression of clotting factors II, V, VII, and X, bleeding in patients on concomitant anticoagulant therapy, and polycythemia.

Nervous System: Increased or decreased libido, headache, anxiety, depression, and generalized paresthesia.

Metabolic: Increased serum cholesterol.

Miscellaneous: Rarely anaphylactoid reactions.

DRUG ABUSE AND DEPENDENCE

Testred Capsules are classified as a schedule III Controlled Substance under the Anabolic Steroids Act of 1990.

OVERDOSAGE

There have been no reports of acute overdosage with the androgens.

DOSAGE AND ADMINISTRATION

Methyltestosterone capsules are administered orally. The suggested dosage for androgens varies depending on the age, sex, and diagnosis of the individual patient. Dosage is adjusted according to the patient's response and the appearance of adverse reactions.

Replacement therapy in androgen-deficient males is 10 to 50 mg of methyltestosterone daily. Various dosage regimens have been used to induce pubertal changes in hypogonadal males; some experts have advocated lower dosages initially, gradually increasing the dose as puberty progresses, with or without a decrease to maintenance levels. Other experts emphasize that higher dosages are needed to induce pubertal changes and lower dosages can be used for maintenance after puberty. The chronological and skeletal ages must be taken into consideration, both in determining the initial dose and in adjusting the dose.

Doses used in delayed puberty generally are in the range of that given above, and for a limited duration, for example, 4 to 6 months.

Women with metastatic breast carcinoma must be followed closely because androgen therapy occasionally appears to accelerate the disease. Thus, many experts prefer to use the shorter acting androgen preparations rather than those with prolonged activity for treating breast carcinoma, particularly during the early stages of androgen therapy. The dosage of methyltestosterone for androgen therapy in breast carcinoma in females is from 50–200 mg daily.

HOW SUPPLIED

Methyltestosterone capsules USP 10 mg are red capsules imprinted "ICN 0901" on both sections. They are available in bottles of 100.

CAUTION: Federal (U.S.A.) law prohibits dispensing without prescription.

Revision July 1994

ICN Pharmaceuticals, Inc.
ICN Plaza
3300 Hyland Avenue
Costa Mesa, CA 92626
(714) 545-0100

Shown in Product Identification Guide, page 318

TRISORALEN® * ℞

[trī 'sore "a-len]

(Trioxsalen USP, 5 mg)

To facilitate repigmentation in vitiligo, increase tolerance to solar exposure and enhance pigmentation.

CAUTION: THIS IS A POTENT DRUG.

CAUTION: Federal (U.S.A.) law prohibits dispensing without prescription.

DESCRIPTION

Trisoralen Tablets 5 mg.

TRISORALEN (TRIOXSALEN) is the first synthetic psoralen compound made available to the medical profession. It possesses greater activity than Methoxsalen (1) (2) (3) (4), yet the LD 50 of (TRIOXSALEN) is six times that of Methoxsalen.

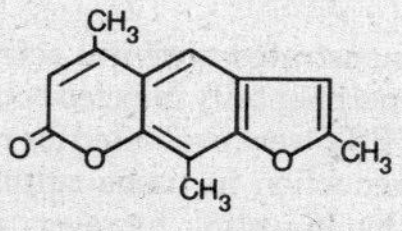

(4, 5′, 8-Trimethylpsoralen)

ACTIONS

Pigment formation with TRISORALEN (TRIOXSALEN)

The normal pigmentation of the skin is due to melanin which is produced in the cytoplasm of the melanocytes located in the basal layers of the epidermis at its junction with the dermis. Melanin is formed by the oxidation of tyrosine to DOPA (Dihydroxyphenylalanine) with tyrosinase as catalyst. This enzymatic reaction, however, must be activated by radiant energy in the form of ultraviolet light, preferably between 2900 and 3800 angstroms (black light) (10).

The exact mechanism of the action of psoralens in the process of melanogenesis is not known. One group of investigators feel that the psoralens have a specific effect on the epidermis or, more specifically, on the melanocytes. Another group feels that the primary response to the psoralens is an inflammatory one and that the process of melanogenesis is secondary.

INDICATIONS

TRISORALEN (TRIOXSALEN), taken approximately two hours before measured periods of exposure to ultraviolet facilitates:

1. **Repigmentation of idiopathic vitiligo.** (12) (13) (14) Repigmentation, not equally reversible in every patient, will vary in completeness, time of onset, and duration. The rate of completeness of pigmentation with respect to locations of lesions, occurs more rapidly on fleshy regions, such as the face, abdomen, and buttocks, and less rapidly over bony areas such as the dorsum of the hands and feet. Repigmentation may begin after a few weeks; however, significant results may take as long as six to nine months, and repigmentation, at the optimum level, may, in some cases, require maintenance dosage to retain the new pigment. If follicular repigmentation is not apparent after three months of daily treatment, treatment should be discontinued as a failure.
2. **Increasing tolerance to sunlight.** (14) In blond persons and those with fair complexions who suffer painful reactions when exposed to sunlight, TRISORALEN (TRIOXSALEN) aids in increasing resistance to solar damage. Certain persons who are allergic to sunlight or exhibit sun sensitivity may be benefited by the protective action of TRISORALEN (TRIOXSALEN) (5). In albinism, TRISORALEN (TRIOXSALEN) will increase the tolerance of the skin to sunlight, although no pigment is formed (6) (7) (8). This protective action seems to be related to the thickening of the horny layer and retention of melanin which produced a thickened, melanized stratum corneum and formation of a stratum lucidum (9) (10).
3. **Enhancing pigmentation** (3) (4). The use of TRISORALEN (TRIOXSALEN) accelerates pigmentation only when the administration of the drug is followed by exposure of the skin to sunlight or ultraviolet irradiation. The increase in pigmentation is not immediate but occurs gradually within a few days of repeated exposure and may become equivalent in a degree to that achieved by a full summer of sun exposure. Since sufficient pigmentation will have been formed within two weeks of continuous therapy, the use of TRISORALEN (TRIOXSALEN) should not be continued beyond this period. Pigmentation can be maintained by periodic exposure to sunlight.

CONTRAINDICATIONS

In those diseases associated with photosensitivity, such as porphyria, acute lupus erythematosus, or leukoderma of infectious origin. To date, the safety of this drug in young persons (12 and under), has not been established and is, therefore contraindicated. No preparation with any photosensitizing capacity, internal or external should be used concomitantly with TRISORALEN (TRIOXSALEN) therapy.

WARNINGS

TRISORALEN IS A POTENT DRUG.

Read entire brochure before prescribing or dispensing this medication. The dosage of this medication should not be increased. The dosage of TRISORALEN (TRIOXSALEN) and exposure time should not be increased. Overdosage and/or overexposure may result in serious burning and blistering. When used to increase tolerance to sunlight or accelerate tanning, TRISORALEN (TRIOXSALEN) total dosage should not exceed 28 tablets, taken in daily single doses of two tablets on a continuous or interrupted regimen. To prevent harmful effects, the physician should carefully instruct the patient to adhere to the prescribed dosage schedule and procedure.

*U.S. Patent 3,201,421

PRECAUTIONS

ACCIDENTAL OVERDOSAGE:

If an overdose of TRISORALEN (TRIOXSALEN) or ultraviolet light has been taken, emesis should be encouraged. The individual should be kept in a darkened room for eight hours or until cutaneous reactions subside. The treatment for severe reactions resulting from overdosage or over-exposure should follow accepted procedures for treatment of severe burns. There have not been any clinical reports or tests to verify that more severe reactions may result from the concomitant ingestion of furocoumarin-containing food while on TRISORALEN (TRIOXSALEN) therapy; but the physician should warn the patient that taking limes, figs, parsley, parsnips, mustard, carrots and celery, might be dangerous.

ADVERSE REACTIONS AND SIDE EFFECTS

Severe burns can result from excessive sunlight or sun lamp ultraviolet exposure. Occasionally, there may occur gastric discomfort; to minimize this gastric effect, the tablets may be taken with milk or after a meal. Some patients who are unable to tolerate 10 mg. will tolerate 5 mg. This dosage produces the same therapeutic effect but more slowly.

DOSAGE

(Adults and children over 12 years of age)

VITILIGO: Two tablets daily, taken two to four hours before measured periods of ultraviolet exposure or fluorescent black light (10). (See suggested sun exposure guide.)

To increase tolerance to sunlight and/or enhance pigmentation: Two tablets daily, taken two hours before measured periods of exposure to sun or ultraviolet irradiation. Not to be continued for longer than 14 days. The dosage should **NOT** be increased, as severe burning may occur. (See suggested sun exposure guide.)

SUGGESTED SUN EXPOSURE GUIDE

The exposure time to sunlight should be limited according to the following plan:

	Basic Skin Color	
	Light	**Medium**
Initial Exposure	15 min.	20 min.
Second Exposure	20 min.	25 min.
Third Exposure	25 min.	30 min.
Fourth Exposure	30 min.	35 min.

Subsequent Exposure: Gradually increase exposure based on erythema and tenderness.

Sunglasses should be worn during exposure and the lips protected with a light-screening lipstick (10).

SUN-LAMP EXPOSURE: Should be initiated according to directions of the sun-lamp manufacturer.

HOW SUPPLIED

TRISORALEN Tablets 5 mg.

UNIT COUNT	NDC NO.
28	0187-0303-28
100	0187-0303-01

Store at controlled room temperature (15°–30°C) 59°–86°F.

REFERENCES

1. Pathak, M.A., and Fitzpatrick, T.B.: Bioassay of Natural and Synthetic Furocoumarins (Psoralens). J. Invest. Dermat. 32, 509–518, 1959.
2. Pathak, M.A.; Fellman, J.H.; and Kaufman, K.D.,: The Effect of Structural Alterations on the Erytheral Activity of Furocoumarins: Psoralens. J. Invest. Dermat. 35, 165–183, 1960.
3. Lerner, R.M., and Lerner, A.B.,: Dermatologic Medications, Second Edition. Year book Publishers, Pages 98–99.
4. Pathak, M.A., and Fitzpatrick, T.B.,: Relationship of Molecular Configuration to the Activity of Furocoumarins Which Increase the Cutaneous Responses Following Long Wave Ultraviolet Radiation. J. Invest. Dermat. 32, No. 2, 255–262, 1959.
5. Becker, S.W., Jr.,: Prevention of Sunburn and Light Allergy with Methoxsalen. G.P. 19, 115–117, 1959.
6. Hu, F.; Fosnaugh, R.P.; and Lesney, P.F.,: Studies on Albinism, Arch. Dermat. 83, 723–729, 1961.
7. Lerner, A.B.,; Denton, C.R.; and Fitzpatrick, T.B.,: Clinical and Experimental Studies on 8-Methoxypsoralen in Vitiligo. J. Invest. Dermat. 20, 878, 1958.
8. Sulzberger, M.B., and Lerner, A.B.,: Suntanning-Potentiation with Oral Medication. J.A.M.A., 167, 2077–2079, 1958.
9. Becker, S.W., Jr.,: Effects of 8-Methoxypsoralen and Ultraviolet Light on Human Skin. Science, 127, 878, 1958.

Continued on next page

ICN—Cont.

10. Stegmaier, O.C.,: The Use of Methoxsalen in Suntanning. J. Invest. Dermat. 32, No. 2, 345–349, 1959.
11. Fitzpatrick, T.B.,: Current Therapy, W.B. Saunders Co., Page 515, 1958.
12. Fitzpatrick, T.B.; Arndt, K.A.; El Mofty, A.M. and Pathak, M.A.: Hydroquinone and Psoralens in Therapy of Hypermelanosis and Vitiligo, ARCH. DERM. 93, 589–600, 1966.
13. Becker, S.W., Jr.,: Psoralen Phototherapeutic Agents, J.A.M.A., 202, 422–424, 1967.
14. El Mofty, A.M.; Vitiligo and Psoralens, PERGAMON PRESS INC., Long Island City, New York, 1st Edition, 1968.

ICN PHARMACEUTICALS, INC.
3300 Hyland Ave.
Costa Mesa, CA 92626 USA

Revised August, 1993

Shown in Product Identification Guide, page 318

VIRAZOLE® ℞

[*vira'zahl'*]

(Ribavirin for Inhalation Solution)

WARNINGS:

USE OF AEROSOLIZED VIRAZOLE IN PATIENTS REQUIRING MECHANICAL VENTILATOR ASSISTANCE SHOULD BE UNDERTAKEN ONLY BY PHYSICIANS AND SUPPORT STAFF FAMILIAR WITH THE SPECIFIC VENTILATOR BEING USED AND THIS MODE OF ADMINISTRATION OF THE DRUG. STRICT ATTENTION MUST BE PAID TO PROCEDURES THAT HAVE BEEN SHOWN TO MINIMIZE THE ACCUMULATION OF DRUG PRECIPITATE, WHICH CAN RESULT IN MECHANICAL VENTILATOR DYSFUNCTION AND ASSOCIATED INCREASED PULMONARY PRESSURES (SEE WARNINGS).

SUDDEN DETERIORATION OF RESPIRATORY FUNCTION HAS BEEN ASSOCIATED WITH INITIATION OF AEROSOLIZED VIRAZOLE USE IN INFANTS. RESPIRATORY FUNCTION SHOULD BE CAREFULLY MONITORED DURING TREATMENT. IF INITIATION OF AEROSOLIZED VIRAZOLE TREATMENT APPEARS TO PRODUCE SUDDEN DETERIORATION OF RESPIRATORY FUNCTION, TREATMENT SHOULD BE STOPPED AND REINSTITUTED ONLY WITH EXTREME CAUTION, CONTINUOUS MONITORING AND CONSIDERATION OF CONCOMITANT ADMINISTRATION OF BRONCHODILATORS (SEE WARNINGS).

VIRAZOLE IS NOT INDICATED FOR USE IN ADULTS. PHYSICIANS AND PATIENTS SHOULD BE AWARE THAT RIBAVIRIN HAS BEEN SHOWN TO PRODUCE TESTICULAR LESIONS IN RODENTS AND TO BE TERATOGENIC IN ALL ANIMAL SPECIES IN WHICH ADEQUATE STUDIES HAVE BEEN CONDUCTED (RODENTS AND RABBITS); (SEE CONTRAINDICATIONS).

DESCRIPTION

Virazole® is a brand name for ribavirin, a synthetic nucleoside with antiviral activity. VIRAZOLE for inhalation solution is a sterile, lyophilized powder to be reconstituted for aerosol administration. Each 100 ml glass vial contains 6 grams of ribavirin, and when reconstituted to the recommended volume of 300 ml with sterile water for injection or sterile water for inhalation (no preservatives added), will contain 20 mg of ribavirin per ml, pH approximately 5.5. Aerosolization is to be carried out in a Small Particle Aerosol Generator (SPAG-2) nebulizer only.

Ribavirin is 1-beta-D-ribofuranosyl-1H-1,2,4-triazole-3-carboxamide, with the following structural formula:

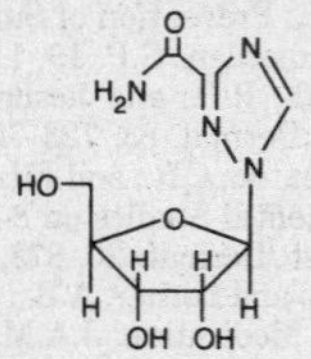

Ribavirin is a stable, white, crystalline compound with a maximum solubility in water of 142 mg/ml at 25°C and with only a slight solubility in ethanol. The empirical formula is $C_8H_{12}N_4O_5$ and the molecular weight is 244.21.

CLINICAL PHARMACOLOGY

Mechanism of Action

In cell cultures the inhibitory activity of ribavirin for respiratory syncytial virus (RSV) is selective. The mechanism of action is unknown. Reversal of the *in vitro* antiviral activity by guanosine or xanthosine suggests ribavirin may act as an analogue of these cellular metabolites.

Microbiology

Ribavirin has demonstrated antiviral activity against RSV *in vitro*[1] and in experimentally infected cotton rats.[2] Several clinical isolates of RSV were evaluated for ribavirin susceptibility by plaque reduction in tissue culture. Plaques were reduced 85–98% by 16 μg/ml; however, results may vary with the test system. The development of resistance has not been evaluated *in vitro* or in clinical trials.

In addition to the above, ribavirin has been shown to have *in vitro* activity against influenza A and B viruses and herpes simplex virus, but the clinical significance of these data is unknown.

Immunologic Effects

Neutralizing antibody responses to RSV were decreased in aerosolized VIRAZOLE treated infants compared to placebo treated infants.[3] One study also showed that RSV-specific IgE antibody in bronchial secretions was decreased in patients treated with aerosolized VIRAZOLE. In rats, ribavirin administration resulted in lymphoid atrophy of the thymus, spleen, and lymph nodes. Humoral immunity was reduced in guinea pigs and ferrets. Cellular immunity was also mildly depressed in animal studies. The clinical significance of these observations is unknown.

Pharmacokinetics

Assay for VIRAZOLE in human materials is by a radioimmunoassay which detects ribavirin and at least one metabolite.

VIRAZOLE brand of ribavirin, when administered by aerosol, is absorbed systemically. Four pediatric patients inhaling VIRAZOLE aerosol administered by face mask for 2.5 hours each day for 3 days had plasma concentrations ranging from 0.44 to 1.55 μM, with a mean concentration of 0.76 μM. The plasma half-life was reported to be 9.5 hours. Three pediatric patients inhaling aerosolized VIRAZOLE administered by face mask or mist tent for 20 hours each day for 5 days had plasma concentrations ranging from 1.5 to 14.3 μM, with a mean concentration of 6.8 μM.

The bioavailability of aerosolized VIRAZOLE is unknown and may depend on the mode of aerosol delivery. After aerosol treatment, peak plasma concentrations of ribavirin are 85% to 98% less than the concentration that reduced RSV plaque formation in tissue culture. After aerosol treatment, respiratory tract secretions are likely to contain ribavirin in concentrations many fold higher than those required to reduce plaque formation. However, RSV is an intracellular virus and it is unknown whether plasma concentrations or respiratory secretion concentrations of the drug better reflect intracellular concentrations in the respiratory tract.

In man, rats, and rhesus monkeys, accumulation of ribavirin and/or metabolites in the red blood cells has been noted, plateauing in red cells in man in about 4 days and gradually declining with an apparent half-life of 40 days (the half-life of erythrocytes). The extent of accumulation of ribavirin following inhalation therapy is not well defined.

Animal Toxicology

Ribavirin, when administered orally or as an aerosol, produced cardiac lesions in mice, rats, and monkeys, when given at doses of 30, 36 and 120 mg/kg or greater for 4 weeks or more (estimated human equivalent doses of 4.8, 12.3 and 111.4 mg/kg for a 5 kg child, or 2.5, 5.1 and 40 mg/kg for a 60 kg adult, based on body surface area adjustment). Aerosolized ribavirin administered to developing ferrets at 60 mg/kg for 10 or 30 days resulted in inflammatory and possibly emphysematous changes in the lungs. Proliferative changes were seen in the lungs following exposure at 131 mg/kg for 30 days. The significance of these findings to human administration is unknown.

INDICATIONS AND USAGE

VIRAZOLE is indicated for the treatment of hospitalized infants and young children with severe lower respiratory tract infections due to respiratory syncytial virus. Treatment early in the course of severe lower respiratory tract infection may be necessary to achieve efficacy.

Only severe RSV lower respiratory tract infection should be treated with VIRAZOLE. The vast majority of infants and children with RSV infection have disease that is mild, self-limited, and does not require hospitalization or antiviral treatment. Many children with mild lower respiratory tract involvement will require shorter hospitalization than would be required for a full course of VIRAZOLE aerosol (3 to 7 days) and should not be treated with the drug. Thus the decision to treat with VIRAZOLE should be based on the severity of the RSV infection.

The presence of an underlying condition such as prematurity, immunosuppression or cardiopulmonary disease may increase the severity of clinical manifestations and complications of RSV infection.

Use of aerosolized VIRAZOLE in patients requiring mechanical ventilator assistance should be undertaken only by physicians and support staff familiar with this mode of administration and the specific ventilator being used (see Warnings, and Dosage and Administration).

Diagnosis

RSV infection should be documented by a rapid diagnostic method such as demonstration of viral antigen in respiratory tract secretions by immunofluorescence[3,4] or ELISA[5] before or during the first 24 hours of treatment. Treatment may be initiated while awaiting rapid diagnostic test results. However, treatment should not be continued without documentation of RSV infection.

Non-culture antigen detection techniques may have false positive or false negative results. Assessment of the clinical situation, the time of year and other parameters may warrant reevaluation of the laboratory diagnosis.

Description of Studies

Non-Mechanically-Ventilated Infants: In two placebo controlled trials in infants hospitalized with RSV lower respiratory tract infection, aerosolized VIRAZOLE treatment had a therapeutic effect, as judged by the reduction in severity of clinical manifestations of disease by treatment day 3.[3,4] Treatment was most effective when instituted within the first 3 days of clinical illness. Virus titers in respiratory secretions were also significantly reduced with VIRAZOLE in one of these original studies.[4] Additional controlled studies conducted since these initial trials of aerosolized VIRAZOLE in the treatment of RSV infection have supported these data.

Mechanically-Ventilated Infants: A randomized, double-blind, placebo controlled evaluation of aerosolized VIRAZOLE at the recommended dose was conducted in 28 infants requiring mechanical ventilation for respiratory failure caused by documented RSV infection.[6] Mean age was 1.4 months (SD, 1.7 months). Seven patients had underlying diseases predisposing them to severe infection and 21 were previously normal. Aerosolized VIRAZOLE treatment significantly decreased the duration of mechanical ventilation required (4.9 vs. 9.9 days, $p=0.01$) and duration of required supplemental oxygen (8.7 vs 13.5 days, $p=0.01$). Intensive patient management and monitoring techniques were employed in this study. These included endotracheal tube suctioning every 1 to 2 hours; recording of proximal airway pressure, ventilatory rate, and F_IO_2 every hour; and arterial blood gas monitoring every 2 to 6 hours. To reduce the risk of VIRAZOLE precipitation and ventilator malfunction, heated wire tubing, two bacterial filters connected in series in the expiratory limb of the ventilator (with filter changes every 4 hours), and water column pressure release valves to monitor internal ventilator pressures were used in connecting ventilator circuits to the SPAG-2.

Employing these techniques, no technical difficulties with VIRAZOLE administration were encountered during the study. Adverse events consisted of bacterial pneumonia in one case, staphyloccus bacteremia in one case and two cases of post-extubation stridor. None were felt to be related to VIRAZOLE administration.

CONTRAINDICATIONS

VIRAZOLE is contraindicated in individuals who have shown hypersensitivity to the drug or its components, and in women who are or may become pregnant during exposure to the drug. Ribavirin has demonstrated significant teratogenic and/or embryocidal potential in all animal species in which adequate studies have been conducted (rodents and rabbits). Therefore, although clinical studies have not been performed, it should be assumed that VIRAZOLE may cause fetal harm in humans. Studies in which the drug has been administered systemically demonstrate that ribavirin is concentrated in the red blood cells and persists for the life of the erythrocyte.

WARNINGS

SUDDEN DETERIORATION OF RESPIRATORY FUNCTION HAS BEEN ASSOCIATED WITH INITIATION OF AEROSOLIZED VIRAZOLE USE IN INFANTS. Respiratory function should be carefully monitored during treatment. If initiation of aerosolized VIRAZOLE treatment appears to produce sudden deterioration of respiratory function, treatment should be stopped and reinstituted only with extreme caution, continuous monitoring, and consideration of concomitant administration of bronchodilators.

Use with Mechanical Ventilators

USE OF AEROSOLIZED VIRAZOLE IN PATIENTS REQUIRING MECHANICAL VENTILATOR ASSISTANCE SHOULD BE UNDERTAKEN ONLY BY PHYSICIANS AND SUPPORT STAFF FAMILIAR WITH THIS MODE OF ADMINISTRATION AND THE SPECIFIC VENTILATOR BEING USED. Strict attention must be paid to procedures that have been shown to minimize the accumulation of drug precipitate, which can result in mechanical ventilator dysfunction and associated increased pulmonary pressures. These procedures include the use of bacteria filters in series in the expiratory limb of the ventilator circuit with frequent changes (every 4 hours), water column pressure release valves to indicate elevated ventilator pressures, frequent

monitoring of these devices and verification that ribavirin crystals have not accumulated within the ventilator circuitry, and frequent suctioning and monitoring of the patient (see Clinical Studies).

Those administering aersolized VIRAZOLE in conjunction with mechanical ventilator use should be thoroughly familiar with detailed descriptions of these procedures as outlined in the SPAG-2 manual.

PRECAUTIONS

General: Patients with severe lower respiratory tract infection due to respiratory syncytial virus require optimum monitoring and attention to respiratory and fluid status (see SPAG-2 manual).

Drug Interactions

Clinical studies of interactions of VIRAZOLE with other drugs commonly used to treat infants with RSV infections, such as digoxin, bronchodilators, other antiviral agents, antibiotics, or anti-metabolites have not been conducted. Interference by VIRAZOLE with laboratory tests has not been evaluated.

Carcinogenesis and Mutagenesis

Ribavirin increased the incidence of cell transformations and mutations in mouse Balb/c 3T3 (fibroblasts) and L5178Y (lymphoma) cells at concentrations of 0.015 and 0.03–5.0 mg/ml, respectively (without metabolic activation.) Modest increases in mutation rates (3–4x) were observed at concentrations between 3.75–10.0 mg/ml in L5178Y cells *in vitro* with the addition of a metabolic activation fraction. In the mouse micronucleus assay, ribavirin was clastogenic at intravenous doses of 20–200 mg/kg, (estimated human equivalent of 1.67–16.7 mg/kg, based on body surface area adjustment for a 60 kg adult). Ribavirin was not mutagenic in a dominant lethal assay in rats at intraperitoneal doses between 50–200 mg/kg when administered for 5 days (estimated human equivalent of 7.14–28.6 mg/kg, based on body surface area adjustment; see Pharmacokinetics).

In vivo carcinogenicity studies with ribavirin are incomplete. However, results of a chronic feeding study with ribavirin in rats, at doses of 16–100 mg/kg/day (estimated human equivalent of 2.3–14.3 mg/kg/day, based on body surface area adjustment for the adult), suggest that ribavirin may induce benign mammary, pancreatic, pituitary and adrenal tumors. Preliminary results of 2 oral gavage oncogenicity studies in the mouse and rat (18–24 months; doses of 20–75 and 10–40 mg/kg/day, respectively [estimated human equivalent of 1.67–6.25 and 1.43–5.71 mg/kg/day, respectively, based on body surface area adjustment for the adult]) are inconclusive as to the carcinogenic potential of ribavirin (see Pharmacokinetics). However, these studies have demonstrated a relationship between chronic ribavirin exposure and increased incidences of vascular lesions (microscopic hemorrhages in mice) and retinal degeneration (in rats).

Impairment of Fertility

The fertility of ribavirin-treated animals (male or female) has not been fully investigated. However, in the mouse, administration of ribavirin at doses between 35–150 mg/kg/day (estimated human equivalent of 2.92–12.5 mg/kg/day, based on body surface area adjustment for the adult) resulted in significant seminiferous tubule atrophy, decreased sperm concentrations, and increased numbers of sperm with abnormal morphology. Partial recovery of sperm production was apparent 3–6 months following dose cessation. In several additional toxicology studies, ribavirin has been shown to cause testicular lesions (tubular atrophy), in adult rats at oral dose levels as low as 16 mg/kg/day (estimated human equivalent of 2.29 mg/kg/day, based on body surface area adjustment; see Pharmacokinetics). Lower doses were not tested. The reproductive capacity of treated male animals has not been studied.

Pregnancy: Category X

Ribavirin has demonstrated significant teratogenic and/or embryocidal potential in all animal species in which adequate studies have been conducted. Teratogenic effects were evident after single oral doses of 2.5 mg/kg or greater in the hamster, and after daily oral doses of 0.3 and 1.0 mg/kg in the rabbit and rat, respectively (estimated human equivalent doses of 0.12 and 0.14 mg/kg, based on body surface area adjustment for the adult). Malformations of the skull, palate, eye, jaw, limbs, skeleton, and gastrointestinal tract were noted. The incidence and severity of teratogenic effects increased with escalation of the drug dose. Survival of fetuses and offspring was reduced. Ribavirin caused embryolethality in the rabbit at daily oral dose levels as low as 1 mg/kg. No teratogenic effects were evident in the rabbit and rat administered daily oral doses of 0.1 and 0.3 mg/kg, respectively with estimated human equivalent doses of 0.01 and 0.04 mg/kg, based on body surface area adjustment (see Pharmacokinetics). These doses are considered to define the "No Observable Teratogenic Effects Level" (NOTEL) for ribavirin in the rabbit and rat.

Following oral administration of ribavirin in the pregnant rat (1.0 mg/kg) and rabbit (0.3 mg/kg), mean plasma levels of drug ranged from 0.10–0.20 μM [0.024–0.049 μg/ml] at 1 hour after dosing, to undetectable levels at 24 hours. At 1 hour following the administration of 0.3 or 0.1 mg/kg in the rat and rabbit (NOTEL), respectively, mean plasma levels of drug in both species were near or below the limit of detection (0.05 μM; see Pharmacokinetics),

Although clinical studies have not been performed, VIRAZOLE may cause fetal harm in humans. As noted previously, ribavirin is concentrated in red blood cells and persists for the life of the cell. Thus the terminal half-life for the systemic elimination of ribavirin is essentially that of the half-life of circulating erythrocytes. The minimum interval following exposure to VIRAZOLE before pregnancy may be safely initiated is unknown (see Contraindications, Warnings, and Information for Health Care Personnel).

Nursing Mothers

VIRAZOLE has been shown to be toxic to lactating animals and their offspring. It is not known if VIRAZOLE is excreted in human milk.

Information for Health Care Personnel

Health care workers directly providing care to patients receiving aerosolized VIRAZOLE should be aware that ribavirin has been shown to be teratogenic in all animal species in which adequate studies have been conducted (rodents and rabbits). Although no reports of teratogenesis in offspring of mothers who were exposed to aerosolized VIRAZOLE during pregnancy have been confirmed, no controlled studies have been conducted in pregnant women. Studies of environmental exposure in treatment settings have shown that the drug can disperse into the immediate bedside area during routine patient care activities with highest ambient levels closest to the patient and extremely low levels outside of the immediate bedside area. Adverse reactions resulting from actual occupational exposure in adults are described below (see Adverse Events in Health Care Workers). Some studies have documented ambient drug concentrations at the bedside that could potentially lead to systemic exposures above those considered safe for exposure during pregnancy (1/1000 of the NOTEL dose in the most sensitive animal species).[7,8,9]

A 1992 study conducted by the National Institute of Occupational Safety and Health (NIOSH) demonstrated measurable urine levels of ribavirin in health care workers exposed to aerosol in the course of direct patient care.[7] Levels were lowest in workers caring for infants receiving aerosolized VIRAZOLE with mechanical ventilation and highest in those caring for patients being administered the drug via an oxygen tent or hood. This study employed a more sensitive assay to evaluate ribavirin levels in urine than was available for several previous studies of environmental exposure that failed to detect measurable ribavirin levels in exposed workers. Creatinine adjusted urine levels in the NIOSH study ranged from less than 0.001 to 0.140 μM of ribavirin per gram of creatinine in exposed workers. However, the relationship between urinary ribavirin levels in exposed workers, plasma levels in animal studies, and the specific risk of teratogenesis in exposed pregnant women is unknown.

It is good practice to avoid unnecessary occupational exposure to chemicals wherever possible. Hospitals are encouraged to conduct training programs to minimize potential occupational exposure to VIRAZOLE. Health care workers who are pregnant should consider avoiding direct care of patients receiving aerosolized VIRAZOLE. If close patient contact cannot be avoided, precautions to limit exposure should be taken. These include administration of VIRAZOLE in negative pressure rooms; adequate room ventilation (at least six air exchanges per hour); the use of VIRAZOLE aerosol scavenging devices; turning off the SPAG-2 device for 5 to 10 minutes prior to prolonged patient contact, and wearing appropriately fitted respirator masks. Surgical masks do not provide adequate filtration of VIRAZOLE particles. Further information is available from NIOSH's Hazard Evaluation and Technical Assistance Branch and additional recommendations have been published in an Aerosol Consensus Statement by the American Respiratory Care Foundation and the American Association for Respiratory Care.[10]

ADVERSE REACTIONS

The description of adverse reactions is based on events from clinical studies (approximately 200 patients) conducted prior to 1986, and the controlled trial of aerosolized VIRAZOLE conducted in 1989–1990. Additional data from spontaneous post-marketing reports of adverse events in individual patients have been available since 1986.

Deaths

Deaths during or shortly after treatment with aerosolized VIRAZOLE have been reported in 20 cases of patients treated with VIRAZOLE (12 of these patients were being treated for RSV infections). Several cases have been characterized as "possibly related" to VIRAZOLE by the treating physician; these were in infants who experienced worsening respiratory status related to bronchospasm while being treated with the drug. Several other cases have been attributed to mechanical ventilator malfunction in which VIRAZOLE precipitation within the ventilator apparatus led to excessively high pulmonary pressures and diminished oxygenation. In these cases the monitoring procedures described in the current package insert were not employed (see Description of Studies, Warnings, and Dosage and Administration).

Pulmonary and Cardiovascular

Pulmonary function significantly deteriorated during aerosolized VIRAZOLE treatment in six of six adults with chronic obstructive lung disease and in four of six asthmatic adults. Dyspnea and chest soreness were also reported in the latter group. Minor abnormalities in pulmonary function were also seen in healthy adult volunteers.

In the original study population of approximately 200 infants who received aerosolized VIRAZOLE, several serious adverse events occurred in severely ill infants with life-threatening underlying diseases, many of whom required assisted ventilation. The role of VIRAZOLE in these events is indeterminate. Since the drug's approval in 1986, additional reports of similar serious, though non-fatal, events have been filed infrequently. Events associated with aerosolized VIRAZOLE use have included the following:

<u>Pulmonary:</u> Worsening of respiratory status, bronchospasm, pulmonary edema, hypoventilation, cyanosis, dyspnea, bacterial pneumonia, pneumothorax, apnea, atelectasis and ventilator dependence.

<u>Cardiovascular:</u> Cardiac arrest, hypotension, bradycardia and digitalis toxicity. Bigeminy, bradycardia and tachycardia have been described in patients with underlying congenital heart disease.

Some subjects requiring assisted ventilation experienced serious difficulties, due to inadequate ventilation and gas exchange. Precipitation of drug within the ventilatory apparatus, including the endotracheal tube, has resulted in increased positive end expiratory pressure and increased positive inspiratory pressure. Accumulation of fluid in tubing ("rain out") has also been noted. Measures to avoid these complications should be followed carefully (see Dosage and Administration).

Hematologic

Although anemia was not reported with use of aerosolized VIRAZOLE in controlled clinical trials, most infants treated with the aerosol have not been evaluated 1 to 2 weeks post-treatment when anemia is likely to occur. Anemia has been shown to occur frequently with experimental oral and intravenous VIRAZOLE in humans. Also, cases of anemia (type unspecified), reticulocytosis and hemolytic anemia associated with aerosolized VIRAZOLE use have been reported through post-marketing reporting systems. All have been reversible with discontinuation of the drug.

Other

Rash and conjunctivitis have been associated with the use of aerosolized VIRAZOLE. These usually resolve within hours of discontinuing therapy. Seizures and asthenia associated with experimental intravenous VIRAZOLE therapy have also been reported.

Adverse Events in Health Care Workers

Studies of environmental exposure to aerosolized VIRAZOLE in health care workers administering care to patients receiving the drug have not detected adverse signs or symptoms related to exposure. However, 152 health care workers have reported experiencing adverse events through post-marketing surveillance. Nearly all were in individuals providing direct care to infants receiving aerosolized VIRAZOLE. Of 358 events from these 152 individual health care worker reports, the most common signs and symptoms were headache (51% of reports), conjunctivitis (32%), and rhinitis, nausea, rash, dizziness, pharyngitis, or lacrimation (10–20% each). Several cases of bronchospasm and/or chest pain were also reported, usually in individuals with known underlying reactive airway disease. Several case reports of damage to contact lenses after prolonged close exposure to aerosolized VIRAZOLE have also been reported. Most signs and symptoms reported as having occurred in exposed health care workers resolved within minutes to hours of discontinuing close exposure to aerosolized VIRAZOLE (also see Information for Health Care Personnel).

The symptoms of RSV in adults can include headache, conjunctivitis, sore throat and/or cough, fever, hoarseness, nasal congestion and wheezing, although RSV infections in adults are typically mild and transient. Such infections represent a potential hazard to uninfected hospital patients. It is unknown whether certain symptoms cited in reports from health care workers were due to exposure to the drug or infection with RSV. Hospitals should implement appropriate infection control procedures.

Overdosage

No overdosage with VIRAZOLE by aerosol administration has been reported in humans. The LD_{50} in mice is 2 gm orally and is associated with hypoactivity and gastrointestinal symptoms (estimated human equivalent dose of 0.17gm/kg, based on body surface area conversion). The mean plasma half-life after administration of aerosolized VIRAZOLE for pediatric patients is 9.5 hours. VIRAZOLE is concentrated and persists in red blood cells for the life of the erythrocyte (see Pharmacokinetics).

Continued on next page

ICN—Cont.

DOSAGE AND ADMINISTRATION

BEFORE USE, READ THOROUGHLY THE VIRATEK SMALL PARTICLE AEROSOL GENERATOR (SPAG) MODEL SPAG-2 OPERATOR'S MANUAL FOR SMALL PARTICLE AEROSOL GENERATOR OPERATING INSTRUCTIONS. AEROSOLIZED VIRAZOLE SHOULD NOT BE ADMINISTERED WITH ANY OTHER AEROSOL GENERATING DEVICE.

The recommended treatment regimen is 20 mg/ml VIRAZOLE as the starting solution in the drug reservoir of the SPAG-2 unit, with continuous aerosol administration for 12–18 hours per day for 3 to 7 days. Using the recommended drug concentration of 20 mg/ml the average aerosol concentration for a 12 hour delivery period would be 190 micrograms/liter of air. Aerosolized VIRAZOLE should not be administered in a mixture for combined aerosolization or simultaneously with other aerosolized medications.

Non-mechanically ventilated infants

VIRAZOLE should be delivered to an infant oxygen hood from the SPAG-2 aerosol generator. Administration by face mask or oxygen tent may be necessary if a hood cannot be employed (see SPAG-2 manual). However, the volume and condensation area are larger in a tent and this may alter delivery dynamics of the drug.

Mechanically ventilated infants

The recommended dose and administration schedule for infants who require mechanical ventilation is the same as for those who do not. Either a pressure or volume cycle ventilator may be used in conjunction with the SPAG-2. In either case, patients should have their endotracheal tubes suctioned every 1–2 hours, and their pulmonary pressures monitored frequently (every 2–4 hours). For both pressure and volume ventilators, heated wire connective tubing and bacteria filters in series in the expiratory limb of the system (which must be changed frequently, i.e., every 4 hours) must be used to minimize the risk of VIRAZOLE precipitation in the system and the subsequent risk of ventilator dysfunction. Water column pressure release valves should be used in the ventilator circuit for pressure cycled ventilators, and may be utilized with volume cycled ventilators (SEE SPAG-2 MANUAL FOR DETAILED INSTRUCTIONS).

Method of Preparation

VIRAZOLE brand of ribavirin is supplied as 6 grams of lyophilized powder per 100 ml vial for aerosol administration only. By sterile technique, reconstitute drug with a minimum of 75 ml of sterile USP water for injection or inhalation in the original 100 ml glass vial. Shake well. Transfer to the clean, sterilized 500 ml SPAG-2 reservoir and further dilute to a final volume of 300 ml with Sterile Water for Injection, USP, or Inhalation. The final concentration should be 20 mg/ml. **Important:** This water should NOT have had any antimicrobial agent or other substance added. The solution should be inspected visually for particulate matter and discoloration prior to administration. Solutions that have been placed in the SPAG-2 unit should be discarded at least every 24 hours and when the liquid level is low before adding newly reconstituted solution.

HOW SUPPLIED

VIRAZOLE (ribavirin for inhalation solution) is supplied in 100 ml glass vials with 6 grams of sterile, lyophilized drug which is to be reconstituted with 300 ml Sterile Water for Injection or Sterile Water for Inhalation (no preservatives added) and administered only by a small particle aerosol generator (SPAG-2). Vials containing the lyophilized drug powder should be stored in a dry place at 15–25°C (59–78°F). Reconstituted solutions may be stored, under sterile conditions, at room temperature (20–30°C, 68–86°F) for 24 hours. Solutions which have been placed in the SPAG-2 unit should be discarded at least every 24 hours.

REFERENCES

1. Hruska JF, Bernstein JM, Douglas Jr., RG, and Hall CB. Effects of Virazole on respiratory syncytial virus in vitro. Antimicrob Agents Chemother 17:770–775, 1 1980.
2. Hruska JF, Morrow PE, Suffin SC, and Douglas Jr., RG. In vivo inhibition of respiratory syncytial virus by Virazole. Antimicrob Agents Chemother 21:125–130, 1982.
3. Taber LH, Knight V, Gilbert BE, McClung HW et al. Virazole aerosol treatment of bronchiolitis associated with respiratory tract infection in infants. Pediatrics 72:613–618, 1983.
4. Hall CB, McBride JT, Walsh EE, Bell DM et al. Aerosolized Virazole treatment of infants with respiratory syncytial viral infection. N Engl J Med 308:1443–7, 1983.
5. Hendry RM, McIntosh K, Fahnestock ML, and Pierik LT. Enzyme-linked immunosorbent assay for detection of respiratory syncytial virus infection. J Clin Microbiol 16:329–33, 1982.
6. Smith, David W., Frankel, Lorry R., Mather, Larry H., Tang, Allen T.S., Ariagno, Ronald L., Prober, Charles G. A Controlled Trial of Aerosolized Ribavirin in Infants Receiving Mechanical Ventilation for Severe Respiratory Syncytial Virus Infection. The New England Journal of Medicine 1991; 325:24–29.
7. Decker, John, Shultz, Ruth A., Health Hazard Evaluation Report: Florida Hospital, Orlando, Florida, Cincinnati OH: U.S. Department of Health and Human Services, Public Health Service, Centers for NIOSH Report No. HETA 91-104-2229.*
8. Barnes, D.J. and Doursew, M. Reference dose: Description and use in health risk assessments. Regul Tox. and Pharm. Vol. 8; p. 471–486, 1988.
9. Federal Register Vol. 53 No. 126 Thurs. June 30, 1988 p. 24834–24847.
10. American Association for Respirtory Care [1991]. Aerosol Consensus Statement-1991. Respiratory Care 36(9):916–921.

* Copies of the Report may be purchased from National Technical Information Service, 5285 Port Royal Road, Springfield, VA 22161; Ask for Publication PB 93119-345.

1957-04
Rev. 5-94
ICN PHARMACEUTICALS, INC.
ICN Plaza
3300 Hyland Avenue
Costa Mesa, California 92626
714-545-0100

Immunex Corporation
51 UNIVERSITY STREET
SEATTLE, WA 98101

For Medical Information Contact:
Generally:
Professional Services
(800) 466-8639
FAX: (800) 221-6820
FAX: (206) 223-5525
In Emergencies:
Professional Services
(800) 466-8639
FAX: (800) 221-6820
FAX: (206) 223-5525

AMICAR® ℞
(Aminocaproic Acid)
Syrup, Tablets, and Injection

DESCRIPTION

AMICAR (aminocaproic acid) is 6-aminohexanoic acid, which acts as an inhibitor of fibrinolysis.
Its chemical structure is:

$$H_2C(CH_2)_3CH_2COOH$$
$$|$$
$$NH_2$$

$C_6H_{13}NO_2$ MW 131.17

AMICAR is soluble in water, acid and alkaline solutions; it is sparingly soluble in methanol and practically insoluble in chloroform.

AMICAR (aminocaproic acid) Injection, for intravenous administration, is a sterile pyrogen-free solution containing 250 mg/mL of aminocaproic acid with benzyl alcohol 0.9% as preservative and Water for Injection. Hydrochloric acid may be added to adjust pH to approximately 6.8 during manufacture.

AMICAR (aminocaproic acid) Syrup, 25%, for oral administration, contains 250 mg/mL of aminocaproic acid with potassium sorbate 0.2% and sodium benzoate 0.1% as preservatives and the following inactive ingredients: citric acid, flavorings, sodium saccharin and sorbitol solution.

Each AMICAR (aminocaproic acid) Tablet, for oral administration, contains 500 mg of aminocaproic acid and the following inactive ingredients: magnesium stearate, stearic acid, and povidone.

CLINICAL PHARMACOLOGY

The fibrinolysis-inhibitory effects of AMICAR appear to be exerted principally via inhibition of plasminogen activators and to a lesser degree through antiplasmin activity.

In adults, oral absorption appears to be a zero-order process with an absorption rate of 5.2 g/hr. The mean lag time in absorption is 10 minutes. After a single oral dose of 5 g, absorption was complete (F=1). Mean ± SD peak plasma concentrations (164 ± 28 mcg/mL) were reached within 1.2 ± 0.45 hours.

After oral administration, the apparent volume of distribution was estimated to be 23.1 ± 6.6 L (mean ± SD). Correspondingly, the volume of distribution after intravenous administration has been reported to be 30.0 ± 8.2 L. After prolonged administration, AMICAR has been found to distribute throughout extravascular and intravascular compartments of the body, penetrating human red blood cells as well as other tissue cells.

Renal excretion is the primary route of elimination, whether AMICAR is administered orally or intravenously. Sixty-five percent of the dose is recovered in the urine as unchanged drug and 11% of the dose appears as the metabolite adipic acid. Renal clearance (116 mL/min) approximates endogenous creatinine clearance. The total body clearance is 169 mL/min. The terminal elimination half-life for AMICAR is approximately 2 hours.

INDICATIONS AND USAGE

AMICAR is useful in enhancing hemostasis when fibrinolysis contributes to bleeding. In life-threatening situations, fresh whole blood transfusions, fibrinogen infusions, and other emergency measures may be required.

Fibrinolytic bleeding may frequently be associated with surgical complications following heart surgery (with or without cardiac bypass procedures) and portacaval shunt; hematological disorders such as aplastic anemia, abruptio placentae, hepatic cirrhosis, neoplastic disease such as carcinoma of the prostate, lung, stomach, and cervix.

Urinary fibrinolysis, usually a normal physiological phenomenon, may frequently be associated with life-threatening complications following severe trauma, anoxia, and shock. Symptomatic of such complications is surgical hematuria (following prostatectomy and nephrectomy) or nonsurgical hematuria (accompanying polycystic or neoplastic diseases of the genitourinary system). (See WARNINGS.)

CONTRAINDICATIONS

AMICAR should not be used when there is evidence of an active intravascular clotting process.

When there is uncertainty as to whether the cause of bleeding is primary fibrinolysis or disseminated intravascular coagulation (DIC), this distinction must be made before administering AMICAR.

The following tests can be applied to differentiate the two conditions:
- Platelet count is usually decreased in DIC but normal in primary fibrinolysis.
- Protamine paracoagulation test is positive in DIC; a precipitate forms when protamine sulphate is dropped into citrated plasma. The test is negative in the presence of primary fibrinolysis.
- The euglobulin clot lysis test is abnormal in primary fibrinolysis but normal in DIC.

AMICAR must not be used in the presence of DIC without concomitant heparin.

WARNINGS

In patients with upper urinary tract bleeding, AMICAR administration has been known to cause intrarenal obstruction in the form of glomerular capillary thrombosis, or clots in the renal pelvis and ureters. For this reason, AMICAR should not be used in hematuria of upper urinary tract origin, unless the possible benefits outweigh the risk.

Subendocardial hemorrhages have been observed in dogs given intravenous infusions of 0.2 times the maximum human therapeutic dose of AMICAR and in monkeys given 8 times the maximum human therapeutic dose of AMICAR.

Fatty degeneration of the myocardium has been reported in dogs given intravenous doses of AMICAR at 0.8 to 3.3 times the maximum human therapeutic dose and in monkeys given intravenous doses of AMICAR at 6 times the maximum human therapeutic dose.

Rarely, skeletal muscle weakness with necrosis of muscle fibers has been reported following prolonged administration. Clinical presentation may range from mild myalgias with weakness and fatigue to a severe proximal myopathy with rhabdomyolysis, myoglobinuria, and acute renal failure. Muscle enzymes, especially creatine phosphokinase (CPK) are elevated. CPK levels should be monitored in patients on long-term therapy. AMICAR administration should be stopped if a rise in CPK is noted. Resolution follows discontinuation of AMICAR; however, the syndrome may recur if AMICAR is restarted.

The possibility of cardiac muscle damage should also be considered when skeletal myopathy occurs. One case of cardiac and hepatic lesions observed in man has been reported. The patient received 2 g of aminocaproic acid every 6 hours for a total dose of 26 g. Death was due to continued cerebrovascular hemorrhage. Necrotic changes in the heart and liver were noted at autopsy.

PRECAUTIONS

General

AMICAR Injection contains benzyl alcohol as a preservative and is not recommended for use in newborns.

AMICAR inhibits both the action of plasminogen activators and to a lesser degree, plasmin activity. The drug should NOT be administered without a definite diagnosis and/or laboratory finding indicative of hyperfibrinolysis (hyperplasminemia).[1]

Rapid intravenous administration of the drug should be avoided since this may induce hypotension, bradycardia, and/or arrhythmia.

Inhibition of fibrinolysis by aminocaproic acid may theoretically result in clotting or thrombosis. However, there is no definite evidence that administration of aminocaproic acid has been responsible for the few reported cases of intravascular clotting which followed this treatment. Rather, it appears that such intravascular clotting was most likely due to the patient's preexisting clinical condition, e.g., the presence of DIC. It has been postulated that extravascular clots formed *in vivo* may not undergo spontaneous lysis as do normal clots.

Reports have appeared in the literature of an increased incidence of certain neurological deficits such as hydrocephalus, cerebral ischemia, or cerebral vasospasm associated with the use of antifibrinolytic agents in the treatment of subarachnoid hemorrhage (SAH). All of these events have also been described as part of the natural course of SAH, or as a consequence of diagnostic procedures such as angiography. Drug relatedness remains unclear.

Thrombophlebitis, a possibility with all intravenous therapy, should be guarded against by strict attention to the proper insertion of the needle and the fixing of its position.

Laboratory Tests

The use of AMICAR should be accompanied by tests designed to determine the amount of fibrinolysis present. There are presently available: (a) general tests such as those for the determination of the lysis of a clot of blood or plasma; and (b) more specific tests for the study of various phases of fibrinolytic mechanisms. These latter tests include both semiquantitative and quantitative techniques for the determination of profibrinolysin, fibrinolysin, and antifibrinolysin.

Drug Laboratory Test Interactions

Prolongation of the template bleeding time has been reported during continuous intravenous infusion of AMICAR at dosages exceeding 24 g/day. Platelet function studies in these patients have not demonstrated any significant platelet dysfunction. However, *in vitro* studies have shown that at high concentrations (7.4 mMol/L or 0.97 mg/mL and greater) EACA inhibits ADP and collagen-induced platelet aggregation, the release of ATP and serotonin, and the binding of fibrinogen to the platelets in a concentration-response manner. Following a 10 g bolus of AMICAR, transient peak plasma concentrations of 4.6 mMol/L or 0.60 mg/mL have been obtained. The concentration of AMICAR necessary to maintain inhibition of fibrinolysis is 0.99 mMol/L or 0.13 mg/mL. Administration of a 5 g bolus followed by 1 to 1.25 g/hr should achieve and sustain plasma levels of 0.13 mg/mL. Thus, concentrations which have been obtained *in vivo* clinically in patients with normal renal function are considerably lower than the *in vitro* concentrations found to induce abnormalities in platelet function tests. However, higher plasma concentrations of AMICAR may occur in patients with severe renal failure.

Carcinogenesis, Mutagenesis, Impairment of Fertility

Long-term studies in animals to evaluate the carcinogenic potential of AMICAR and studies to evaluate its mutagenic potential have not been conducted. Dietary administration of an equivalent of the maximum human therapeutic dose of AMICAR to rats of both sexes impaired fertility as evidenced by decreased implantations, litter sizes and number of pups born.

Pregnancy

Pregnancy Category C. Animal teratological studies have not been conducted with AMICAR. It is also not known whether AMICAR can cause fetal harm when administered to a pregnant woman or can affect reproduction capacity. AMICAR should be given to a pregnant woman only if clearly needed.

Nursing Mothers

It is not known whether this drug is excreted in human milk. Because many drugs are excreted in human milk, caution should be exercised when AMICAR is administered to a nursing woman.

Pediatric Use

Safety and effectiveness in pediatric patients have not been established.

ADVERSE REACTIONS

AMICAR is generally well tolerated. The following adverse experiences have been reported:

General: Edema, fever, headache, hemorrhage, malaise.

Hypersensitivity Reactions: Allergic and anaphylactoid reactions, anaphylaxis.

Local Reactions: Injection site reactions, pain and necrosis.

Cardiovascular: Bradycardia, hypotension, ischemia, thrombosis.

Gastrointestinal: Abdominal pain, diarrhea, nausea, vomiting.

Hematologic: Agranulocytosis, coagulation disorder, leukopenia, thrombocytopenia.

Musculoskeletal: CPK increased, muscle weakness, myalgia, myopathy (see WARNINGS), myositis, rhabdomyolysis.

Neurologic: Confusion, convulsions, delirium, dizziness, hallucinations, intracranial hypertension, stroke, syncope.

Respiratory: Dyspnea, nasal congestion, pulmonary embolism.

Skin: Pruritus rash.

Special Senses: Deafness, glaucoma, tinnitus, vision decreased, watery eyes.

Urogenital: BUN increased, ejaculatory disorder, renal failure.

OVERDOSAGE

A few cases of acute overdosage with AMICAR administered intravenously have been reported. The effects have ranged from no reaction to transient hypotension to severe acute renal failure leading to death. One patient with a history of brain tumor and seizures, experienced seizures after receiving an 8 gram bolus injection of AMICAR. The single dose of AMICAR causing symptoms of overdosage or considered to be life-threatening is unknown. Patients have tolerated doses as high as 100 grams while acute renal failure has been reported following a dose of 12 grams.

The intravenous and oral LD_{50} of AMICAR were 3.0 and 12.0 g/kg respectively in the mouse and 3.2 and 16.4 g/kg, respectively in the rat. An intravenous infusion dose of 2.3 g/kg was lethal in the dog. On intravenous administration, tonic-clonic convulsions were observed in dogs and mice.

No treatment for overdosage is known, although evidence exists that AMICAR is removed by hemodialysis and may be removed by peritoneal dialysis. Pharmacokinetic studies have shown that total body clearance of AMICAR is markedly decreased in patients with severe renal failure.

DOSAGE AND ADMINISTRATION

Intravenous

AMICAR (aminocaproic acid) Injection is administered by infusion, utilizing the usual compatible intravenous vehicles (e.g., Sterile Water for Injection, Sodium Chloride for Injection, 5% Dextrose or Ringer's Injection). Although Sterile Water for Injection is compatible for intravenous injection the resultant solution is hypo-osmolar. RAPID INJECTION OF AMICAR INJECTION UNDILUTED INTO A VEIN IS NOT RECOMMENDED.

For the treatment of acute bleeding syndromes due to elevated fibrinolytic activity, it is suggested that 16 to 20 mL (4 to 5 g) of AMICAR Injection in 250 mL of diluent be administered by infusion during the first hour of treatment, followed by a continuing infusion at the rate of 4 mL (1 g) per hour in 50 mL of diluent. This method of treatment would ordinarily be continued for about 8 hours or until the bleeding situation has been controlled.

Parenteral drug products should be inspected visually for particulate matter and discoloration prior to administration, whenever solution and container permit.

Oral Therapy

If the patient is able to take medication by mouth, an identical dosage regimen may be followed by administering AMICAR Tablets or AMICAR Syrup, 25% as follows: For the treatment of acute bleeding syndromes due to elevated fibrinolytic activity, it is suggested that 10 tablets (5 g) or 4 teaspoonfuls of syrup (5 g) of AMICAR be administered during the first hour of treatment, followed by a continuing rate of 2 tablets (1 g) or 1 teaspoonful of syrup (1.25 g) per hour. This method of treatment would ordinarily be continued for about 8 hours or until the bleeding situation has been controlled.

HOW SUPPLIED

AMICAR® (aminocaproic acid) Injection, supplied as follows:

Each 20 mL vial contains 5 g of aminocaproic acid (250 mg/mL) as an aqueous solution with benzyl alcohol 0.9% as preservative.

20 mL vial—NDC 58406-610-12

Each 96 mL single-use infusion vial contains 24 g of aminocaproic acid (250 mg/mL) as an aqueous solution with benzyl alcohol 0.9% as preservative.

96 mL vial—NDC 58406-610-13

STORE BETWEEN 15°–30°C (59°–86°F).

DO NOT FREEZE.

Manufactured for IMMUNEX CORPORATION, Seattle, WA 98101

by LEDERLE PARENTERALS, INC., Carolina, Puerto Rico 00987

AMICAR® (aminocaproic acid) Syrup, 25%, supplied as follows:

Each mL of raspberry-flavored syrup contains 250 mg of aminocaproic acid.

16 Fl Oz (473 mL) Bottle—NDC 58406-611-90

STORE BETWEEN 15°–30°C (59°–86°F).

Dispense in tight containers.

DO NOT FREEZE.

AMICAR® (aminocaproic acid) Tablets, supplied as follows:

Each round, white tablet, engraved with LL on one side and scored on the other with A to the left of the score and 10 on the right, contains 500 mg of aminocaproic acid.

Bottle of 100—NDC 58406-612-61

STORE BETWEEN 15°–30°C (59°–86°F).

Dispense in tight containers.

Manufactured for
IMMUNEX CORPORATION
Seattle, WA 98101
by
LEDERLE LABORATORIES DIVISION
American Cyanamid Company, Pearl River, NY 10965

REFERENCES

1. Stefanini M, Dameshek, W: The Hemorrhagic Disorders, Ed. 2, New York, Grune and Stratton. 1962; pp. 510–514.

IMMUNEX®

Rev 0162-01 50629-95 (IM4)
Issued 4/95

LEUCOVORIN CALCIUM FOR INJECTION ℞

[*lu-cō-vor-ĭn căl-sēē-um*]

DESCRIPTION

Leucovorin is one of several active, chemically reduced derivatives of folic acid. It is useful as an antidote to drugs which act as folic acid antagonists.

Also known as folinic acid, Citrovorum factor, or 5-formyl-5,6,7,8-tetrahydrofolic acid, this compound has the chemical designation of L-Glutamic acid, *N*-[4-[[(2-amino-5-formyl-1,4,5,6,7,8-hexahydro-4-oxo-6-pteridinyl)methyl]amino] benzoyl]-, calcium salt (1:1). The formula weight is 511.51 and the structural formula of leucovorin calcium is:

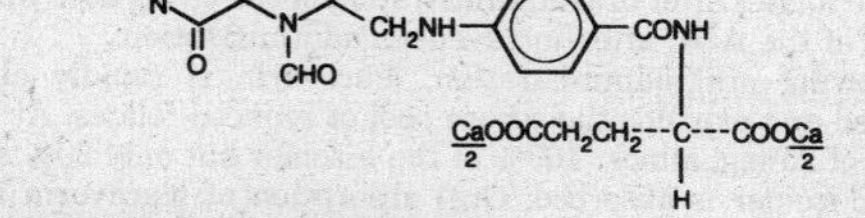

Leucovorin Calcium for Injection

Leucovorin Calcium for Injection is indicated for intravenous or intramuscular administration and is supplied as a sterile lyophilized powder. The 50, 100 and 350 mg vials are preservative free. The inactive ingredient is sodium chloride 40 mg/vial for the 50 mg vial, 80 mg/vial for the 100 mg vial, and 140 mg/vial for the 350 mg vial. Sodium hydroxide and/or hydrochloric acid are used to adjust the pH to approximately 8.1 during manufacture. There is 0.004 mEq of calcium per mg of leucovorin in each dosage form.

CLINICAL PHARMACOLOGY

Leucovorin is a mixture of the diastereoisomers of the 5-formyl derivative of tetrahydrofolic acid (THF). The biologically active compound of the mixture is the (-)-*l*-isomer, known as Citrovorum factor or (-)-folinic acid. Leucovorin does not require reduction by the enzyme dihydrofolate reductase in order to participate in reactions utilizing folates as a source of "one-carbon" moieties. *l*-Leucovorin (*l*-5-formyltetrahydrofolate) is rapidly metabolized (via 5, 10-methenyltetrahydrofolate then 5,10-methylenetetrahydrofolate) to *l*-5-methyltetrahydrofolate. *l*-5-Methyltetrahydrofolate can in turn be metabolized via other pathways back to 5,10-methylenetetrahydrofolate, which is converted to 5-methyltetrahydrofolate by an irreversible, enzyme catalyzed reduction using the cofactors $FADH_2$ and NADPH.

Administration of leucovorin can counteract the therapeutic and toxic effects of folic acid antagonists such as methotrexate, which act by inhibiting dihydrofolate reductase.

In contrast, leucovorin can enhance the therapeutic and toxic effects of fluoropyrimidines used in cancer therapy, such as 5-fluorouracil. Concurrent administration of leucovorin does not appear to alter the plasma pharmacokinetics of 5-fluorouracil. 5-Fluorouracil is metabolized to fluorodeoxyuridylic acid, which binds to and inhibits the enzyme thymidylate synthase (an enzyme important in DNA repair and replication).

Leucovorin is readily converted to another reduced folate, 5,10-methylenetetrahydrofolate, which acts to stabilize the binding of fluorodeoxyuridylic acid to thymidylate synthase and thereby enhances the inhibition of this enzyme.

The pharmacokinetics after intravenous, intramuscular, and oral administration of a 25 mg dose of leucovorin were studied in male volunteers. After intravenous administration, serum total reduced folates (as measured by *Lactobacillus casei* assay) reached a mean peak of 1259 ng/mL (range 897–1625). The mean time to peak was 10 minutes. This initial rise in total reduced folates was primarily due to the parent compound 5-formyl-THF (measured by *Streptococcus faecalis* assay) which rose to 1206 ng/mL at 10 minutes. A sharp drop in parent compound followed and coincided with the appearance of the active metabolite 5-methyl-THF which became the predominant circulating form of the drug.

The mean peak of 5-methyl-THF was 258 ng/mL and occurred at 1.3 hours. The terminal half-life for total reduced folates was 6.2 hours. The area under the concentration ver-

Continued on next page

Immunex—Cont.

sus time curves (AUCs) for *l*-leucovorin, *d*-leucovorin and 5-methyltetrahydrofolate were 28.4 ± 3.5, 956 ± 97 and 129 ± 12 (mg.min/L ± S.E.). When a higher dose of *d,l*-leucovorin (200 mg/m^2) was used, similar results were obtained. The *d*-isomer persisted in plasma at concentrations greatly exceeding those of the *l*-isomer.

After intramuscular injection, the mean peak of serum total reduced folates was 436 ng/mL (range 240–725) and occurred at 52 minutes. Similar to IV administration, the initial sharp rise was due to the parent compound. The mean peak of 5-formyl-THF was 360 ng/mL and occurred at 28 minutes. The level of the metabolite 5-methyl-THF increased subsequently over time until at 1.5 hours it represented 50% of the circulating total folates. The mean peak of 5-methyl-THF was 226 ng/mL at 2.8 hours. The terminal half-life of total reduced folates was 6.2 hours. There was no difference of statistical significance between IM and IV administration in the AUC for total reduced folates, 5-formyl-THF, or 5-methyl-THF.

After oral administration of leucovorin reconstituted with aromatic elixir, the mean peak concentration of serum total reduced folates was 393 ng/mL (range 160–550). The mean time to peak was 2.3 hours and the terminal half-life was 5.7 hours. The major component was the metabolite 5-methyltetrahydrofolate to which leucovorin is primarily converted in the intestinal mucosa. The mean peak of 5-methyl-THF was 367 ng/mL at 2.4 hours. The peak level of the parent compound was 51 ng/mL at 1.2 hours. The AUC of total reduced folates after oral administration of the 25 mg dose was 92% of the AUC after intravenous administration.

Following oral administration, leucovorin is rapidly absorbed and expands the serum pool of reduced folates. At a dose of 25 mg, almost 100% of the *l*-isomer but only 20% of the *d*-isomer is absorbed. Oral absorption of leucovorin is saturable at doses above 25 mg. The apparent bioavailability of leucovorin was 97% for 25 mg, 75% for 50 mg, and 37% for 100 mg.

In a randomized clinical study conducted by the Mayo Clinic and the North Central Cancer Treatment Group (Mayo/NCCTG) in patients with advanced metastatic colorectal cancer three treatment regimens were compared: Leucovorin (LV) 200 mg/m^2 and 5-fluorouracil (5-FU) 370 mg/m^2 versus LV 20 mg/m^2 and 5-FU 425 mg/m^2 versus 5-FU 500 mg/m^2. All drugs were by slow intravenous infusion daily for 5 days repeated every 28–35 days. Response rates were 26% ($p = 0.04$ versus 5-FU alone), 43% ($p = 0.001$ versus 5-FU alone), and 10% for the high dose leucovorin, low-dose leucovorin and 5-FU alone groups respectively. Respective median survival times were 12.2 months ($p = 0.037$), 12 months ($p = 0.050$), and 7.7 months. The low dose LV regimen gave a statistically significant improvement in weight gain of more than 5%, relief of symptoms, and improvement in performance status. The high dose LV regimen gave a statistically significant improvement in performance status and trended toward improvement in weight gain and in relief of symptoms but these were not statistically significant.[1]

In a second Mayo/NCCTG randomized clinical study the 5-FU alone arm was replaced by a regimen of sequentially administered methotrexate (MTX), 5-FU, and LV. Response rates with LV 200 mg/m^2 and 5-FU 370 mg/m^2 versus LV 20 mg/m^2 and 5-FU 425 mg/m^2 versus sequential MTX and 5-FU and LV were respectively 31% ($p = <.01$) 42% ($p = <.01$), and 14%. Respective median survival times were 12.7 months ($p = <.04$), 12.7 months ($p = <.01$), and 8.4 months. No statistically significant difference in weight gain of more than 5% or in improvement in performance status was seen between the treatment arms.[2]

INDICATIONS AND USAGE

Leucovorin calcium rescue is indicated after high-dose methotrexate therapy in osteosarcoma. Leucovorin calcium is also indicated to diminish the toxicity and counteract the effects of impaired methotrexate elimination and of inadvertent overdosages of folic acid antagonists.

Leucovorin calcium is indicated in the treatment of megaloblastic anemias due to folic acid deficiency when oral therapy is not feasible.

Leucovorin is also indicated for use in combination with 5-fluorouracil to prolong survival in the palliative treatment of patients with advanced colorectal cancer. Leucovorin should not be mixed in the same infusion as 5-fluorouracil because a precipitate may form.

CONTRAINDICATIONS

Leucovorin is improper therapy for pernicious anemia and other megaloblastic anemias secondary to the lack of vitamin B_{12}. A hematologic remission may occur while neurologic manifestations continue to progress.

WARNINGS

In the treatment of accidental overdosages of folic acid antagonists, leucovorin should be administered as promptly as possible. As the time interval between antifolate administration [eg, methotrexate (MTX)] and leucovorin rescue increases, leucovorin's effectiveness in counteracting toxicity decreases. Do not administer leucovorin intrathecally.

Monitoring of the serum MTX concentration is essential in determining the optimal dose and duration of treatment with leucovorin.

Delayed MTX excretion may be caused by a third space fluid accumulation (ie, ascites, pleural effusion), renal insufficiency, or inadequate hydration. Under such circumstances, higher doses of leucovorin or prolonged administration may be indicated. Doses higher than those recommended for oral use must be given intravenously.

Because of the benzyl alcohol contained in certain diluents used for Leucovorin Calcium for Injection, when doses greater than 10 mg/m^2 are administered, Leucovorin Calcium for Injection should be reconstituted with Sterile Water for Injection, USP, and used immediately. (See **DOSAGE AND ADMINISTRATION**.)

Because of the calcium content of the leucovorin solution, no more than 160 mg of leucovorin should be injected intravenously per minute (16 mL of a 10 mg/mL, or 8 mL of a 20 mg/mL solution per minute).

Leucovorin enhances the toxicity of 5-fluorouracil. When these drugs are administered concurrently in the palliative therapy of advanced colorectal cancer, the dosage of 5-fluorouracil must be lower than usually administered. Although the toxicities observed in patients treated with the combination of leucovorin plus 5-fluorouracil are qualitatively similar to those observed in patients treated with 5-fluorouracil alone, gastrointestinal toxicities (particularly stomatitis and diarrhea) are observed more commonly and may be more severe and of prolonged duration in patients treated with the combination.

In the first Mayo/NCCTG controlled trial, toxicity, primarily gastrointestinal, resulted in 7% of patients requiring hospitalization when treated with 5-fluorouracil alone or 5-fluorouracil in combination with 200 mg/m^2 of leucovorin and 20% when treated with 5-fluorouracil in combination with 20 mg/m^2 of leucovorin. In the second Mayo/NCCTG trial, hospitalizations related to treatment toxicity also appeared to occur more often in patients treated with the low dose leucovorin/5-fluorouracil combination than in patients treated with the high dose combination—11% versus 3%.

Therapy with leucovorin/5-fluorouracil must not be initiated or continued in patients who have symptoms of gastrointestinal toxicity of any severity, until those symptoms have completely resolved. Patients with diarrhea must be monitored with particular care until the diarrhea has resolved, as rapid clinical deterioration leading to death can occur. In an additional study utilizing higher weekly doses of 5-FU and leucovorin, elderly and/or debilitated patients were found to be at greater risk for severe gastrointestinal toxicity.[3]

Seizures and/or syncope have been reported rarely in cancer patients receiving leucovorin, usually in association with fluropyrimidine administration, and most commonly in those with CNS mestastases or other predisposing factors. however, a causal relationship has not been established.[5]

PRECAUTIONS

General

Parenteral administration is preferable to oral dosing if there is a possibility that the patient may vomit or not absorb the leucovorin. Leucovorin has no effect on non-hematologic toxicities of MTX such as the nephrotoxicity resulting from drug and/or metabolite precipitation in the kidney.

Since leucovorin enhances the toxicity of fluorouracil, leucovorin/5-fluorouracil combination therapy for advanced colorectal cancer should be administered under the supervision of a physician experienced in the use of antimetabolite cancer chemotherapy. Particular care should be taken in the treatment of elderly or debilitated colorectal cancer patients, as these patients may be at increased risk of severe toxicity.

Laboratory Tests

Patients being treated with the leucovorin/5-fluorouracil combination should have a CBC with differential and platelets prior to each treatment. During the first two courses a CBC with differential and platelets has to be repeated weekly and thereafter once each cycle at the time of anticipated WBC nadir. Electrolytes and liver function tests should be performed prior to each treatment for the first three cycles then prior to every other cycle. Dosage modifications of fluorouracil should be instituted as follows, based on the most severe toxicities:

Diarrhea and/or Stomatitis	WBC/mm^3 Nadir	Platelets/mm^3 Nadir	5-FU Dose
Moderate	1,000–1,900	25–75,000	decrease 20%
Severe	<1,000	<25,000	decrease 30%

If no toxicity occurs, the 5-fluorouracil dose may increase 10%.

Treatment should be deferred until WBCs are 4,000/mm^3 and platelets 130,000/mm^3. If blood counts do not reach these levels within two weeks, treatment should be discontinued. Patients should be followed up with physical examination prior to each treatment course and appropriate radiological examination as needed. Treatment should be discontinued when there is clear evidence of tumor progression.

Drug Interactions

Folic acid in large amounts may counteract the antiepileptic effect of phenobarbital, phenytoin and primidone, and increase the frequency of seizures in susceptible children.

Preliminary animal and human studies have shown that small quantities of systemically administered leucovorin enter the CSF primarily as 5-methyltetrahydrofolate and, in humans, remain 1–3 orders of magnitude lower than the usual methotrexate concentrations following intrathecal administration. However, high doses of leucovorin may reduce the efficacy of intrathecally administered methotrexate.

Leucovorin may enhance the toxicity of 5-fluorouracil. (See **WARNINGS**.)

Pregnancy: Teratogenic Effects:

"Pregnancy Category C." Adequate animal reproduction studies have not been conducted with leucovorin. It is also not known whether leucovorin can cause fetal harm when administered to a pregnant woman or can affect reproduction capacity. Leucovorin should be given to a pregnant woman only if clearly needed.

Nursing Mothers: It is not known whether this drug is excreted in human milk. Because many drugs are excreted in human milk, caution should be exercised when leucovorin is administered to a nursing mother.

Pediatric Use: See **Drug Interactions.**

ADVERSE REACTIONS

Allergic sensitization, including anaphylactoid reactions and urticaria, has been reported following administration of both oral and parenteral leucovorin. No other adverse reactions have been attributed to the use of leucovorin *per se*.

The following table summarizes significant adverse events occurring in 316 patients treated with the leucovorin-5-fluorouracil combinations compared against 70 patients treated with 5-fluorouracil alone for advanced colorectal carcinoma. These data are taken from the Mayo/NCCTG large multicenter prospective trial evaluating the efficacy and safety of the combination regimen.

[See first table at top of next page.]

OVERDOSAGE

Excessive amounts of leucovorin may nullify the chemotherapeutic effect of folic acid antagonists.

DOSAGE AND ADMINISTRATION

Advanced Colorectal Cancer: Leucovorin should not be mixed in the same infusion as 5-fluorouracil because a precipitate may form. Either of the following two regimens is recommended:

1. Leucovorin is administered at 200 mg/m^2 by slow intravenous injection over a minimum of 3 minutes, followed by 5-fluorouracil at 370 mg/m^2 by intravenous injection.
2. Leucovorin is administered at 20 mg/m^2 by intravenous injection followed by 5-fluorouracil at 425 mg/m^2 by intravenous injection.

Treatment is repeated daily for five days. This five-day treatment course may be repeated at 4 week (28-day) intervals, for 2 courses and then repeated at 4–5 week (28–35 day) intervals provided that the patient has completely recovered from the toxic effects of the prior treatment course.

In subsequent treatment courses, the dosage of 5-fluorouracil should be adjusted based on patient tolerance of the prior treatment course. The daily dosage of 5-fluorouracil should be reduced by 20% for patients who experienced moderate hematologic or gastrointestinal toxicity in the prior treatment course, and by 30% for patients who experienced severe toxicity (see **PRECAUTIONS: Laboratory Tests**). For patients who experienced no toxicity in the prior treatment course, 5-fluorouracil dosage may be increased by 10%. Leucovorin dosages are not adjusted for toxicity.

Several other doses and schedules of leucovorin/5-fluorouracil therapy have also been evaluated in patients with advanced colorectal cancer; some of these alternative regimens may also have efficacy in the treatment of this disease. However, further clinical research will be required to confirm the safety and effectiveness of these alternative leucovorin/5-fluorouracil treatment regimens.

Leucovorin Rescue After High-Dose Methotrexate Therapy. The recommendations for leucovorin rescue are based on a methotrexate dose of 12–15 grams/m^2 administered by intravenous infusion over 4 hours (see methotrexate package insert for full prescribing information).[4]

Leucovorin rescue at a dose of 15 mg (approximately 10 mg/m^2) every 6 hours for 10 doses starts 24 hours after the beginning of the methotrexate infusion. In the presence of gastrointestinal toxicity, nausea or vomiting, leucovorin should be administered parenterally. Do not administer leucovorin intrathecally.

PERCENTAGE OF PATIENTS TREATED WITH LEUCOVORIN/FLUOROURACIL FOR ADVANCED COLORECTAL CARCINOMA REPORTING ADVERSE EXPERIENCES OR HOSPITALIZED FOR TOXICITY

	High LV/5-FU (N=155)		Low LV/5-FU (N=161)		5-FU Alone (N=70)	
	Any (%)	Grade 3+ (%)	Any (%)	Grade 3+ (%)	Any (%)	Grade 3+ (%)
Leukopenia	69	14	83	23	93	48
Thrombocytopenia	8	2	8	1	18	3
Infection	8	1	3	1	7	2
Nausea	74	10	80	9	60	6
Vomiting	46	8	44	9	40	7
Diarrhea	66	18	67	14	43	11
Stomatitis	75	27	84	29	59	16
Constipation	3	0	4	0	1	—
Lethargy/Malaise/ Fatigue	13	3	12	2	6	3
Alopecia	42	5	43	6	37	7
Dermatitis	21	2	25	1	13	—
Anorexia	14	1	22	4	14	—
Hospitalization for Toxicity	5%		15%		7%	

High LV = Leucovorin 200 mg/m², Low LV = Leucovorin 20 mg/m²
Any = percentage of patients reporting toxicity of any severity
Grade 3 + = percentage of patients reporting toxicity of Grade 3 or higher

GUIDELINES FOR LEUCOVORIN DOSAGE AND ADMINISTRATION
DO NOT ADMINISTER LEUCOVORIN INTRATHECALLY

Clinical Situation	Laboratory Findings	Leucovorin Dosage and Duration
Normal Methotrexate Elimination	Serum methotrexate level approximately 10 micromolar at 24 hours after administration, 1 micromolar at 48 hours, and less than 0.2 micromolar at 72 hours.	15 mg PO, IM, or IV q 6 hours for 60 hours (10 doses starting at 24 hours after start of methotrexate infusion)
Delayed Late Methotrexate Elimination	Serum methotrexate level remaining above 0.2 micromolar at 72 hours, and more than 0.05 micromolar at 96 hours after administration.	Continue 15 mg PO, IM, or IV q 6 hours, until methotrexate level is less than 0.05 micromolar.
Delayed Early Methotrexate Elimination and/or Evidence of Acute Renal Injury	Serum methotrexate level of 50 micromolar or more at 24 hours, or 5 micromolar or more at 48 hours after administration, OR; a 100% or greater increase in serum creatinine level at 24 hours after methotrexate administration (eg, an increase from 0.5 mg/dL to a level of 1 mg/dL or more)	150 mg IV q 3 hours, until methotrexate level is less than 1 micromolar; then 15 mg IV q 3 hours, until methotrexate level is less than 0.05 micromolar.

Serum creatinine and methotrexate levels should be determined at least once daily. Leucovorin administration, hydration, and urinary alkalinization (pH of 7.0 or greater) should be continued until the methotrexate level is below 5×10^{-8} M (0.05 micromolar). The leucovorin dose should be adjusted or leucovorin rescue extended based on the following guidelines:
[See second table above.]
Patients who experience delayed early methotrexate elimination are likely to develop reversible renal failure. In addition to appropriate leucovorin therapy, these patients require continuing hydration and urinary alkalinization, and close monitoring of fluid and electrolyte status, until the serum methotrexate level has fallen to below 0.05 micromolar and the renal failure has resolved.
Some patients will have abnormalities in methotrexate elimination or renal function following methotrexate administration, which are significant but less severe than the abnormalities described in the table above. These abnormalities may or may not be associated with significant clinical toxicity. If significant clinical toxicity is observed, leucovorin rescue should be extended for an additional 24 hours (total of 14 doses over 84 hours) in subsequent courses of therapy. The possibility that the patient is taking other medications which interact with methotrexate (eg, medications which may interfere with methotrexate elimination or binding to serum albumin) should always be reconsidered when laboratory abnormalities or clinical toxicities are observed.

Impaired Methotrexate Elimination or Inadvertent Overdosage: Leucovorin rescue should begin as soon as possible after an inadvertent overdosage and within 24 hours of methotrexate administration when there is delayed excretion (see WARNINGS). Leucovorin 10 mg/m² should be administered IV, IM, or PO every 6 hours until the serum methotrexate level is less than 10^{-8} M. In the presence of gastrointestinal toxicity, nausea, or vomiting, leucovorin should be administered parenterally. Do not administer leucovorin intrathecally.
Serum creatinine and methotrexate levels should be determined at 24 hour intervals. If the 24 hour serum creatinine has increased 50% over baseline or if the 24 hour methotrexate level is greater than 5×10^{-6} M or the 48 hour level is greater than 9×10^{-7} M, the dose of leucovorin should be increased to 100 mg/m² IV every 3 hours until the methotrexate level is less than 10^{-8} M.
Hydration (3 L/d) and urinary alkalinization with sodium bicarbonate solution should be employed concomitantly. The bicarbonate dose should be adjusted to maintain the urine pH at 7.0 or greater.

Megaloblastic Anemia Due to Folic Acid Deficiency: Up to 1 mg daily. There is no evidence that doses greater than 1 mg/day have greater efficacy than those of 1 mg; additionally, loss of folate in urine becomes roughly logarithmic as the amount administered exceeds 1 mg.

Each 50 and 100 mg vial of Leucovorin Calcium for Injection when reconstituted with 5 and 10 mL, respectively, of sterile diluent yields a leucovorin concentration of 10 mg per mL. Each 350 mg vial of Leucovorin Calcium for Injection when reconstituted with 17 mL of sterile diluent yields a leucovorin concentration of 20 mg leucovorin per mL. Leucovorin Calcium for Injection contains no preservative. Reconstitute with Bacteriostatic Water for Injection, USP, which contains benzyl alcohol, or with Sterile Water for Injection, USP. When reconstituted with Bacteriostatic Water for Injection, USP, the resulting solution must be used within 7 days. If the product is reconstituted with Sterile Water for Injection, USP, it must be used immediately. Because of the benzyl alcohol contained in Bacteriostatic Water for Injection, USP, when doses greater than 10 mg/m² are administered Leucovorin Calcium for Injection should be reconstituted with Sterile Water for Injection, USP, and used immediately. (See WARNINGS.) Because of the calcium content of the leucovorin solution, no more than 160 mg of leucovorin should be injected intravenously per minute (16 mL of a 10 mg/mL, or 8 mL of a 20 mg/mL solution per minute).
Parenteral drug products should be inspected visually for particulate matter and discoloration prior to administration, whenever solution and container permit.

HOW SUPPLIED
Leucovorin Calcium for Injection
NDC 58406-621-05-50 mg Vial
NDC 58406-622-06-100 mg Vial
NDC 58406-623-07-350 mg Vial
STORE BETWEEN 15°-25°C (59°-77°F).
PROTECT FROM LIGHT.

REFERENCES
1. Poon MA, et al. Biochemical Modulation of Fluorouracil: Evidence of Significant Improvement of Survival and Quality of Life in patients with Advanced Colorectal Carcinoma, *J Clin Oncol* 1989; 7:1407–1418.
2. Poon MA, et al. Biochemical Modulation of Fluorouracil with Leucovorin: Confirmatory Evidence of Improved Therapeutic Efficacy in Advanced Colorectal Cancer, *J Clin Oncol* 1991; 9, 11:1967–1972.
3. Grem JL, Shoemaker DD, Petrelli NJ, Douglas HO. "Severe and Fatal Toxic Effects Observed in Treatment with High- and Low-Dose Leucovorin Plus 5-Fluorouracil for Colorectal Carcinoma," *Cancer Treat Rep* 1987; 71:1122.
4. Link MP, Goorin AM, Miser AW, et al. "The Effect of Adjuvant Chemotherapy on Relapse-Free Survival in Patients with Osteosarcoma of the Extremity." *N Engl J Med* 1986; 314:1600–1606.
5. Meropol NJ, Creaven PJ, White RM, et al. "Seizures Associated With Leucovorin Administration in Cancer Patients." *J NCI* 1995; 87(1):56–58.

Manufactured for
IMMUNEX CORPORATION,
Seattle, WA 98101
by LEDERLE PARENTERALS, INC.,
Carolina, Puerto Rico 00987
©1995 Immunex Corporation
CI 4820-1
Rev 0163-01   Issued 11/95

LEUCOVORIN CALCIUM TABLETS   R
[lu-cō-vor-ĭn căl-sēē-um]

DESCRIPTION
Leucovorin is one of several active, chemically reduced derivatives of folic acid. It is useful as an antidote to drugs which act as folic acid antagonists. Also known as folinic acid, Citrovorum factor, or 5-formyl-5,6,7,8-tetrahydrofolic acid, this compound has the chemical designation of L-Glutamic acid, N-[4-[[(2-amino-5-formyl-1,4,5,6,7,8-hexahydro -4 -oxo-6-pteridinyl)methyl]amino]benzoyl] -, calcium salt (1:1). The formula weight is 511.51 and the structural formula of leucovorin calcium is:
[See chemical structure at top of next column.]
Leucovorin Calcium Tablets, 5 mg, contain 5 mg of leucovorin (equivalent to 5.40 mg of anhydrous leucovorin calcium) and the following inactive ingredients: Corn Starch, Dibasic Calcium Phosphate, Magnesium Stearate, and Pregelatinized Starch.
Leucovorin Calcium Tablets, 15 mg, contain 15 mg of leucovorin (equivalent to 16.20 mg of anhydrous leucovorin

Continued on next page

Immunex—Cont.

calcium) and the following inactive ingredients: Lactose, Magnesium Stearate, Microcrystalline Cellulose, Pregelatinized Starch, and Sodium Starch Glycolate.
Leucovorin Calcium Tablets are indicated for oral administration only.

CLINICAL PHARMACOLOGY

Leucovorin is a mixture of the diastereoisomers of the 5-formyl derivative of tetrahydrofolic acid. The biologically active component of the mixture is the (-)-L-isomer, known as Citrovorum factor, or (-)-folinic acid. Leucovorin does not require reduction by the enzyme dihydrofolate reductase in order to participate in reactions utilizing folates as a source of "one-carbon" moieties. Following oral administration, leucovorin is rapidly absorbed and enters the general body pool of reduced folates.

The increase in plasma and serum reduced folate activity (determined microbiologically with *Lactobacillus casei*) seen after oral administration of leucovorin is predominantly due to 5-methyltetrahydrofolate.

Following a 20 mg dose of leucovorin calcium, the mean maximum serum total reduced folate concentrations were:

Tablet	364 ± 12.1 ng/mL	at 2.0 ± 0.07 hours
Oral Solution	375 ± 12.8 ng/mL	at 2.1 ± 0.11 hours
Parenteral	355 ± 17.2 ng/mL	at 0.96 ± 0.10 hours

The half-life of plasma 5-formyltetrahydrofolate was 1.5 ± 0.08 hours and that of the 5-methyltetrahydrofolate was 3.0 ± 0.09 hours.

Oral tablets produced equivalent bioavailability (8% difference) when compared to the parenteral administration. The parenteral solution also provided equal bioavailability to the tablets when administered orally (2% difference). Oral absorption of leucovorin is saturable at doses above 25 mg. The apparent bioavailability of leucovorin was 97% for 25 mg, 75% for 50 mg and 37% for 100 mg.

INDICATIONS

Leucovorin calcium rescue is indicated after high-dose methotrexate therapy in osteosarcoma. Leucovorin is also indicated to diminish the toxicity and counteract the effects of impaired methotrexate elimination and of inadvertent overdosages of folic acid antagonists.

CONTRAINDICATIONS

Leucovorin is improper therapy for pernicious anemia and other megaloblastic anemias secondary to the lack of vitamin B_{12}. A hematologic remission may occur while neurologic manifestations remain progressive.

WARNINGS

In the treatment of accidental overdosages of folic acid antagonists, leucovorin should be administered as promptly as possible. As the time interval between antifolate administration [eg, methotrexate (MTX)] and leucovorin rescue increases, leucovorin's effectiveness in counteracting toxicity diminishes.

Monitoring of serum MTX concentration is essential in determining the optimal dose and duration of treatment with leucovorin.

Delayed MTX excretion may be caused by a third space fluid accumulation (ie, ascites, pleural effusion), renal insufficiency, or inadequate hydration. Under such circumstances, higher doses of leucovorin or prolonged administration may be indicated. Doses higher than those recommended for oral use must be given intravenously.

Leucovorin may enhance the toxicity of fluorouracil. Deaths from severe enterocolitis, diarrhea, and dehydration have been reported in elderly patients receiving weekly leucovorin and fluorouracil.[1] Concomitant granulocytopenia and fever were present in some but not all of the patients. Seizures and/or syncope have been reported rarely in cancer patients receiving leucovorin, usually in association with fluoropyrimidine administration, and most commonly in those with CNS metastases or other predisposing factors, however, a causal relationship has not been established.[2]

PRECAUTIONS

General

Parenteral administration is preferable to oral dosing if there is a possibility that the patient may vomit or not absorb the leucovorin. Leucovorin has no effect on other established toxicities of MTX such as the nephrotoxicity resulting from drug and/or metabolite precipitation in the kidney.

Drug Interactions

Folic acid in large amounts may counteract the antiepileptic effect of phenobarbital, phenytoin and primidone, and increase the frequency of seizures in susceptible children. Preliminary animal and human studies have shown that small quantities of systemically administered leucovorin enter the CSF primarily as 5-methyltetrahydrofolate and, in humans, remain 1–3 orders of magnitude lower than the usual methotrexate concentrations following intrathecal administration. However, high doses of leucovorin may reduce the efficacy of intrathecally administered methotrexate.

Leucovorin may enhance the toxicity of fluorouracil (see WARNINGS).

Pregnancy: Teratogenic Effects
"Pregnancy Category C." Animal reproduction studies have not been conducted with leucovorin. It is also not known whether leucovorin can cause fetal harm when administered to a pregnant woman or can affect reproduction capacity. Leucovorin should be given to a pregnant woman only if clearly needed.

Nursing Mothers: It is not known whether this drug is excreted in human milk. Because many drugs are excreted in human milk, caution should be exercised when leucovorin is administered to a nursing mother.

Pediatric Use: see **Drug Interactions.**

ADVERSE REACTIONS

Allergic sensitization, including anaphylactoid reactions and urticaria, has been reported following the administration of both oral and parenteral leucovorin.

OVERDOSAGE

Excessive amounts of leucovorin may nullify the chemotherapeutic effect of folic acid antagonists.

DOSAGE AND ADMINISTRATION

Leucovorin Calcium Tablets are intended for oral administration. Because absorption is saturable, oral administration of doses greater than 25 mg is not recommended.

Leucovorin Rescue After High-Dose Methotrexate Therapy: The recommendations for leucovorin rescue are based on a methotrexate dose of 12–15 grams/m² administered by intravenous infusion over 4 hours (see methotrexate package insert for full prescribing information).[3] Leucovorin rescue at a dose of 15 mg (approximately 10 mg/m²) every 6 hours for 10 doses starts 24 hours after the beginning of the methotrexate infusion. In the presence of gastrointestinal toxicity, nausea or vomiting, leucovorin should be administered parenterally.

Serum creatinine and methotrexate levels should be determined at least once daily. Leucovorin administration, hydration, and urinary alkalinization (pH of 7.0 or greater) should be continued until the methotrexate level is below 5×10^{-8} M (0.05 micromolar). The leucovorin dose should be adjusted or leucovorin rescue extended based on the following guidelines:
[See table at left.]

Patients who experience delayed early methotrexate elimination are likely to develop reversible renal failure. In addition to appropriate leucovorin therapy, these patients require continuing hydration and urinary alkalinization, and close monitoring of fluid and electrolyte status, until the serum methotrexate level has fallen to below 0.05 micromolar and the renal failure has resolved.

Some patients will have abnormalities in methotrexate elimination or renal function following methotrexate administration, which are significant but less severe than the abnormalities described in the table above. These abnormalities may or may not be associated with significant clinical toxicity. If significant clinical toxicity is observed, leucovorin rescue should be extended for an additional 24 hours (total of 14 doses over 84 hours) in subsequent courses of therapy. The possibility that the patient is taking other medications which interact with methotrexate (eg, medications which may interfere with methotrexate elimination or binding to serum albumin) should always be reconsidered when laboratory abnormalities or clinical toxicities are observed.

Impaired Methotrexate Elimination or Inadvertent Overdosage: The same dosage and administration guidelines may be used. However, leucovorin administration should begin as soon as possible after an inadvertent overdosage is recognized.

HOW SUPPLIED

Leucovorin Calcium Tablets, 5 mg are round, convex, yellowish-white, engraved LL above 5 on one side, scored in half on the other side and engraved C above the score and 33 below, each containing 5 mg of leucovorin as the calcium salt, supplied as follows:
NDC 58406-624-62–Bottle of 30 with CRC
NDC 58406-624-67–Bottle of 100
Leucovorin Calcium Tablets, 15 mg are oval, convex, yellowish-white, engraved LL on left and 15 on right on one side, scored in half on the other side and engraved C to the left of the score and 35 to the right, each containing 15 mg of leucovorin as the calcium salt, supplied as follows:

GUIDELINES FOR LEUCOVORIN DOSAGE AND ADMINISTRATION
DO NOT ADMINISTER LEUCOVORIN INTRATHECALLY

Clinical Situation	Laboratory Findings	Leucovorin Dosage and Duration
Normal Methotrexate Elimination	Serum methotrexate level approximately 10 micromolar at 24 hours after administration, 1 micromolar at 48 hours, and less than 0.2 micromolar at 72 hours.	15 mg PO, IM, or IV q 6 hours for 60 hours (10 doses starting at 24 hours after start of methotrexate infusion).
Delayed Late Methotrexate Elimination	Serum methotrexate level remaining above 0.2 micromolar at 72 hours, and more than 0.05 micromolar at 96 hours after administration.	Continue 15 mg PO, IM, or IV q 6 hours, until methotrexate level is less than 0.05 micromolar.
Delayed Early Methotrexate Elimination and/or Evidence of Acute Renal Injury	Serum methotrexate level of 50 micromolar or more at 24 hours, or 5 micromolar or more at 48 hours after administration, OR; a 100% or greater increase in serum creatinine level at 24 hours after methotrexate administration (eg, an increase from 0.5 mg/dL to a level of 1 mg/dL or more).	150 mg IV q 3 hours, until methotrexate level is less than 1 micromolar; then 15 mg IV q 3 hours until methotrexate level is less than 0.05 micromolar.

NDC 58406-626-68–Bottle of 12 with CRC
NDC 58406-626-74–Bottle of 24 with CRC
STORE BETWEEN 15°–30°C (59°–86°F). PROTECT FROM LIGHT.

REFERENCES

1. Grem JL, Shoemaker DD, Petrelli NJ, Douglas HO. "Severe and Fatal Toxic Effects Observed in Treatment with High- and Low-Dose Leucovorin Plus 5-Fluorouracil for Colorectal Carcinoma." *Cancer Treat Rep* 1987; 71:1122.
2. Meropol NJ, Creaven PJ, White RM, et al. "Seizures Associated With Leucovorin Administration in Cancer Patients." *J NCI* 1995; 87(1):56-58.
3. Link MP, Goorin AM, Miser AW, et al. "The Effect of Adjuvant Chemotherapy on Relapse-Free Survival in Patients with Osteosarcoma of the Extremity." *N Engl J Med* 1986; 314:1600-1606.

IMMUNEX®
Manufactured for
IMMUNEX CORPORATION
Seattle, WA 98101
by
LEDERLE LABORATORIES DIVISION
Pearl River, NY 10965
©1996 Immunex Corporation   Rev 0164-01 Issued 3/96
                                 CI 4819-1

LEUKINE®   ℞
[lu-kīne]
Sargramostim
Lyophilized

Caution: Federal law prohibits dispensing without prescription.

DESCRIPTION

LEUKINE® (Sargramostim) is a recombinant human granulocyte-macrophage colony stimulating factor (rhu GM-CSF) produced by recombinant DNA technology in a yeast *(S. cerevisiae)* expression system. GM-CSF is a hematopoietic growth factor which stimulates proliferation and differentiation of hematopoietic progenitor cells. LEUKINE is a glycoprotein of 127 amino acids characterized by 3 primary molecular species having molecular masses of 19,500, 16,800 and 15,500 daltons. The amino acid sequence of LEUKINE differs from the natural human GM-CSF by a substitution of leucine at position 23, and the carbohydrate moiety may be different from the native protein. Sargramostim has been selected as the proper name for yeast-derived rhu GM-CSF. LEUKINE is formulated as a sterile, white, preservative-free, lyophilized powder and is intended for subcutaneous (SC) injection or intravenous (IV) infusion following reconstitution with 1 mL Sterile Water for Injection, USP or 1 mL Bacteriostatic Water for Injection, USP containing 0.9% benzyl alcohol. Each vial of LEUKINE contains either 250 mcg or 500 mcg Sargramostim; 40 mg Mannitol, USP; 10 mg Sucrose, NF; and 1.2 mg Tromethamine, USP. The pH of the reconstituted, isotonic solution is 7.4 ± 0.3. Biological potency is expressed in International Units as tested against the WHO First International Reference Standard. The specific activity of LEUKINE is approximately 5.6×10^6 IU/mg.

CLINICAL PHARMACOLOGY

General GM-CSF belongs to a group of growth factors termed colony stimulating factors which support survival, clonal expansion, and differentiation of hematopoietic progenitor cells. GM-CSF induces partially committed progenitor cells to divide and differentiate in the granulocyte-macrophage pathways.
GM-CSF is also capable of activating mature granulocytes and macrophages. GM-CSF is a multilineage factor and, in addition to dose-dependent effects on the myelomonocytic lineage, can promote the proliferation of megakaryocytic and erythroid progenitors.[1] However, other factors are required to induce complete maturation in these two lineages. The various cellular responses (i.e., division, maturation, activation) are induced through GM-CSF binding to specific receptors expressed on the cell surface of target cells.[2]
In vitro **Studies of LEUKINE in Human Cells** The biological activity of GM-CSF is species-specific. Consequently, *in vitro* studies have been performed on human cells to characterize the pharmacological activity of LEUKINE. *In vitro* exposure of human bone marrow cells to LEUKINE at concentrations ranging from 1–100 ng/mL results in the proliferation of hematopoietic progenitors and in the formation of pure granulocyte, pure macrophage and mixed granulocyte-macrophage colonies.[3] Chemotactic, anti-fungal and anti-parasitic[4] activities of granulocytes and monocytes are increased by exposure to LEUKINE *in vitro*. LEUKINE increases the cytotoxicity of monocytes toward certain neoplastic cell lines[3] and activates polymorphonuclear neutrophils to inhibit the growth of tumor cells.
In vivo **Primate Studies of LEUKINE** Pharmacology/toxicology studies of LEUKINE were performed in cynomolgus monkeys. An acute toxicity study revealed an absence of

treatment-related toxicity following a single IV bolus injection at a dose of 300 mcg/kg. Two subacute studies were performed using IV injection (maximum dose 200 mcg/kg/day × 14 days) and subcutaneous injection (maximum dose 200 mcg/kg/day × 28 days). No major visceral organ toxicity was documented. Notable histopathology findings included increased cellularity in hematologic organs, heart and lung tissues. A dose-dependent increase in leukocyte count occurred during the dosing period which consisted primarily of segmented neutrophils; increases in monocytes, basophils, eosinophils and lymphocytes were also noted. Leukocyte counts decreased to pretreatment values over a 1–2 week recovery period.
Pharmacokinetics Pharmacokinetic profiles have been analyzed in patients with various neoplastic diseases following intravenous administration of LEUKINE. In 8 patients receiving 250 mcg/m² of LEUKINE by 2 hour IV infusion, serum concentration ranged from 120 to 1500 pg/mL (mean ± SEM = 775 ± 210 pg/mL) at the termination of the infusion. Then the serum levels decreased with a mean initial half-life and terminal half-life of approximately 11 minutes and 1.6 hours, respectively, while the mean AUC was 5.35 mcg/mL/hr. When the same patients were treated with 250 mcg/m² of LEUKINE as a subcutaneous injection, serum levels peaked at 3 hours and ranged between 100 and 1500 pg/mL (mean ± SEM = 450 ± 170 pg/mL). The serum levels decreased with a mean terminal half-life and terminal half-life of approximately 2.6 hours, while the mean AUC was 4.65 mcg/mL/hr. The mean serum levels of LEUKINE remained above 100 pg/mL for 12 hours after the subcutaneous injection and 6 hours after the 2 hour IV infusion.[5]
The pharmacokinetic profile, calculated from 5 patients receiving 500–750 mcg/m² of LEUKINE by 2 hour IV infusion, revealed decreased serum levels (initial half-life and terminal half-life of approximately 12–17 minutes and 2 hours, respectively). Four patients with myelodysplastic syndrome treated with 125 mcg/m² of LEUKINE by subcutaneous injection every 12 hours, showed serum levels which ranged from 55–450 pg/mL within 5 minutes of administration. LEUKINE serum levels peaked at 2 hours and ranged from 350–3900 pg/mL and remained at detectable levels for 6 hours following injection (range 150–2700 pg/mL).[6]
Antibody Formation Serum samples collected before and after LEUKINE treatment from 214 patients with a variety of underlying diseases have been examined for the presence of antibodies. Neutralizing antibodies were detected in 5 of 214 patients (2.3%) after receiving LEUKINE by continuous IV infusion (3 patients) or subcutaneous injection (2 patients) for 28 to 84 days in multiple courses. All 5 patients had impaired hematopoiesis before the administration of LEUKINE and consequently the effect of the development of anti-GM-CSF antibodies on normal hematopoiesis could not be assessed. Drug-induced neutropenia, neutralization of endogenous GM-CSF activity and diminution of the therapeutic effect of LEUKINE secondary to formation of neutralizing antibody remain a theoretical possibility.

INDICATIONS AND USAGE

Use Following Induction Chemotherapy in Acute Myelogenous Leukemia LEUKINE is indicated for use following induction chemotherapy in older adult patients with acute myelogenous leukemia (AML) to shorten time to neutrophil recovery and to reduce the incidence of severe and life-threatening infections and infections resulting in death. The safety and efficacy of LEUKINE have not been assessed in patients with AML under 55 years of age.
The term acute myelogenous leukemia, also referred to as acute non-lymphocytic leukemia (ANLL), encompasses a heterogeneous group of leukemias arising from various non-lymphoid cell lines which have been defined morphologically by the French-American-British (FAB) system of classication.

Use in Mobilization and Following Transplantation of Autologous Peripheral Blood Progenitor Cells LEUKINE is indicated for the mobilization of hematopoietic progenitor cells into peripheral blood for collection by leukapheresis. Mobilization allows for the collection of increased numbers of progenitor cells capable of engraftment as compared with collection without mobilization. After myeloablative chemotherapy, the transplantation of an increased number of progenitor cells can lead to more rapid engraftment, which may result in a decreased need for supportive care. Myeloid reconstitution is further accelerated by administration of LEUKINE following peripheral blood progenitor cell transplantation.
Use in Myeloid Reconstitution After Autologous Bone Marrow Transplantation LEUKINE is indicated for acceleration of myeloid recovery in patients with non-Hodgkin's lymphoma (NHL), acute lymphoblastic leukemia (ALL) and Hodgkin's disease undergoing autologous bone marrow transplantation (BMT). After autologous BMT in patients with NHL, ALL, or Hodgkin's disease, LEUKINE has been found to be safe and effective in accelerating myeloid engraftment, decreasing median duration of antibiotic administration, reducing the median duration of infectious episodes and shortening the median duration of hospitalization.

Hematologic response to LEUKINE can be detected by complete blood count (CBC) with differential performed twice per week.
Use in Myeloid Reconstitution After Allogeneic Bone Marrow Transplantation LEUKINE is indicated for acceleration of myeloid recovery in patients undergoing allogeneic BMT from HLA-matched related donors. LEUKINE has been found to be safe and effective in accelerating myeloid engraftment, reducing the incidence of bacteremia and other culture positive infections, and shortening the median duration of hospitalization.
Use in Bone Marrow Transplantation Failure or Engraftment Delay LEUKINE is indicated in patients who have undergone allogeneic or autologous bone marrow transplantation (BMT) in whom engraftment is delayed or has failed. LEUKINE has been found to be safe and effective in prolonging survival of patients who are experiencing graft failure or engraftment delay, in the presence or absence of infection, following autologous or allogeneic BMT. Survival benefit may be relatively greater in those patients who demonstrate one or more of the following characteristics: autologous BMT failure or engraftment delay, no previous total body irradiation, malignancy other than leukemia or a multiple organ failure (MOF) score ≤2 (See CLINICAL EXPERIENCE). Hematologic response to LEUKINE can be detected by complete blood count (CBC) with differential performed twice per week.

CLINICAL EXPERIENCE

Acute Myelogenous Leukemia The safety and efficacy of Sargramostim in patients with AML who are younger than 55 years of age have not been determined. Based on Phase II data suggesting the best therapeutic effects could be achieved in patients at highest risk for severe infections and mortality while neutropenic, the Phase III clinical trial was conducted in older patients. The safety and efficacy of LEUKINE in the treatment of AML were evaluated in a multi-center, randomized, double-blind placebo-controlled trial of 99 newly diagnosed adult patients, 55–70 years of age, receiving induction with or without consolidation.[7] A combination of standard doses of daunorubicin (days 1–3) and ara-C (days 1–7) was administered during induction and high dose ara-C was administered days 1–6 as a single course of consolidation, if given. Bone marrow evaluation was performed on day 10 following induction chemotherapy. If hypoplasia with <5% blasts was not achieved, patients immediately received a second cycle of induction chemotherapy. If the bone marrow was hypoplastic with <5% blasts on day 10 or 4 days following the second cycle of induction chemotherapy, LEUKINE (250 mcg/m²/day) or placebo was given IV over 4 hours each day, starting 4 days after the completion of chemotherapy. Study drug was continued until an ANC ≥1500/mm³ for three consecutive days was attained or a maximum of 42 days. LEUKINE or placebo was also administered after the single course of consolidation chemotherapy if delivered (ara-C 3–6 weeks after induction following neutrophil recovery). Study drug was discontinued immediately if leukemic regrowth occurred.
LEUKINE (Sargramostim) significantly shortened the median duration of ANC <500/mm³ by 4 days and <1000/mm³ by 7 days following induction (see table at right). 75% of patients receiving LEUKINE achieved ANC >500/mm³ by day 16, compared to day 25 for patients receiving placebo. The proportion of patients receiving 1 cycle (70%) or 2 cycles (30%) of induction was similar in both treatment groups; LEUKINE significantly shortened the median times to neutrophil recovery whether one cycle (12 versus 15 days) or two cycles (14 versus 23 days) of induction chemotherapy was administered. Median times to platelet (>20,000/mm³) and RBC transfusion independence were not significantly different between treatment groups.

Hematological Recovery: Induction

Dataset	Sargramostim n=52* Median (25%, 75%)	Placebo n=47 Median (25%, 75%)	p-value**
ANC > 500/mm³ [a]	13 (11, 16)	17 (13, 25)	0.009
ANC > 1000/mm³ [b]	14 (12, 18)	21 (13, 34)	0.003
PLT > 20,000/mm³ [c]	11 (7, 14)	12 (9, >42)	0.10
RBC [d]	12 (9, 24)	14 (9, 42)	0.53

* *Patients with missing data censored.*
[a] *2 patients on Sargramostim and 4 patients on placebo had missing values.*
[b] *2 patients on Sargramostim and 3 patients on placebo had missing values.*
[c] *4 patients on placebo had missing values.*
[d] *3 patients on Sargramostim and 4 patients on placebo had missing values.*
***p = Generalized Wilcoxon*

Continued on next page
Consult 1997 supplements and future editions for revisions

Immunex—Cont.

During the consolidation phase of treatment, LEUKINE did not shorten the median time to recovery of ANC to 500/mm^3 (13 days) or 1000/mm^3 (14.5 days) compared to placebo. There were no significant differences in time to platelet and RBC transfusion independence.

The incidence of severe infections and deaths associated with infections was significantly reduced in patients who received LEUKINE. During induction or consolidation, 27 of 52 patients receiving LEUKINE and 35 of 47 patients receiving placebo had at least one grade 3, 4 or 5 infection (p=0.02). Twenty-five patients receiving LEUKINE and 30 patients receiving placebo experienced severe and fatal infections during induction only. There were significantly fewer deaths from infectious causes in the Sargramostim arm (3 versus 11, p=0.02). The majority of deaths in the placebo group were associated with fungal infections with pneumonia as the primary infection.

Disease outcomes were not adversely affected by the use of LEUKINE. The proportion of patients achieving complete remission (CR) was higher in the LEUKINE group (69% as compared to 55% for the placebo group), but the difference was not significant (p=0.21). There was no significant difference in relapse rates; 12 of 36 patients who received LEUKINE and 5 of 26 patients who received placebo relapsed within 180 days of documented CR (p=0.26). The overall median survival was 378 days for patients receiving LEUKINE and 268 days for those on placebo (p=0.17). The study was not sized to assess the impact of LEUKINE treatment on response or survival.

Mobilization of PBPC and Engraftment A retrospective review was conducted of data from patients with cancer undergoing collection of peripheral blood progenitor cells (PBPC) at a single transplant center. Mobilization of PBPC and myeloid reconstitution post-transplant were compared among four groups of patients (n=196) receiving LEUKINE for mobilization and a historical control group who did not receive any mobilization treatment [progenitor cells collected by leukapheresis without mobilization (n=100)]. Sequential cohorts received LEUKINE. The cohorts differed by dose (125 or 250 mcg/m^2/day), route (IV over 24 hours or SC) and use of post-transplant LEUKINE. Leukaphereses were initiated for all mobilization groups after the WBC reached 10,000/mm^3. Leukaphereses continued until both a minimum number of mononucleated cells (MNC) were collected (6.5 or 8.0 $\times$ 10^8/kg body weight) and a minimum number of phereses (5-8) were performed. Both minimum requirements varied by treatment cohort and planned conditioning regimen. If subjects failed to reach a WBC of 10,000 cells/mm^3 by day 5, another cytokine was substituted for LEUKINE; these subjects were all successfully leukapheresed and transplanted. The most marked mobilization and post-transplant effects were seen in patients administered the higher dose of LEUKINE (250 mcg/m^2) either IV (n=63) or SC (n=41).

PBPCs from patients treated at the 250 mcg/m^2/day dose had significantly higher number of granulocyte-macrophage colony-forming units (CFU-GM) than those collected without mobilization. The mean value after thawing was 11.41 x 10^4 CFU-GM/kg for all LEUKINE-mobilized patients, compared to 0.96 x 10^4/kg for the non-mobilized group. A similar difference was observed in the mean number of erythrocyte burst-forming units (BFU-E) collected (23.96 x 10^4/kg for patients mobilized with 250 mcg/m^2 doses of LEUKINE administered SC vs. 1.63 x 10^4/kg for non-mobilized patients).

After transplantation, mobilized subjects had shorter times to myeloid engraftment, and fewer days between transplantation and the last platelet transfusion compared to non-mobilized subjects. Neutrophil recovery (ANC >500/mm^3) was more rapid in patients administered LEUKINE following PBPC transplantation with LEUKINE-mobilized cells (see table at right). Mobilized patients also had fewer days to the last platelet transfusion and last RBC transfusion, and a shorter duration of hospitalization than did non-mobilized subjects.
[See table below.]

	Route for Mobilization	Post-transplant LEUKINE	ENGRAFTMENT (median value in days) ANC >500/mm^3	Last platelet transfusion
No mobilization	—	no	29	28
LEUKINE 250 mcg/m^2	IV	no	21	24
	IV	yes	12	19
	SC	yes	12	17

Autologous BMT: Combined Analysis from Placebo-Controlled Clinical Trials of Responses in Patients with NHL and ALL

Median Values (days)

	ANC $\geq$500/mm^3	ANC $\geq$1000/mm^3	Duration of Hospitalization	Duration of Infection	Duration of Antibacterial Therapy
LEUKINE (n=54)	18*#	24* #	25*	1*	21*
Placebo (n =50)	24	32	31	4	25

*$p < 0.05$ Wilcoxon or CMH ridit chi-squared # $p < 0.05$ Log rank
Note: The single AML patient was not included.

A second retrospective review of data from patients undergoing PBPC at another single transplant center was also conducted. LEUKINE was given SC at 250 mcg/m^2/day once a day (n=10) or twice a day (n=21) until completion of the aphereses. Aphereses were begun on day 5 of LEUKINE administration and continued until the targeted MNC count of 9 x 10^8/kg or CD34+ cell count of 1 x 10^6/kg was reached. There was no difference in CD34+ cell count in patients receiving LEUKINE once or twice a day. The median time to ANC>500/mm^3 was 12 days and to platelet recovery (>25,000/mm^3) was 23 days.

Survival studies comparing mobilized study patients to the non-mobilized patients and to an autologous historical bone marrow transplant group showed no differences in median survival time.

Autologous Bone Marrow Transplantation[8] Following a dose-ranging Phase I/II trial in patients undergoing autologous BMT for lymphoid malignancies,[9,10] three single-center, randomized, placebo-controlled and double-blinded studies were conducted to evaluate the safety and efficacy of LEUKINE for promoting hematopoietic reconstitution following autologous BMT. A total of 128 patients (65 LEUKINE, 63 placebo) were enrolled in these 3 studies. The majority of the patients had lymphoid malignancy (87 NHL, 17 ALL), 23 patients had Hodgkin's disease, and 1 patient had acute myeloblastic leukemia (AML). In 72 patients with NHL or ALL, the bone marrow harvest was purged prior to storage with one of several monoclonal antibodies. No chemical agent was used for *in vitro* treatment of the bone marrow. Preparative regimens in the 3 studies included cyclophosphamide (total dose 120–150 mg/kg) and total body irradiation (total dose 1,200–1,575 rads). Other regimens used in patients with Hodgkin's disease and NHL without radiotherapy consisted of 3 or more of the following in combination (expressed as total dose): cytosine arabinoside (400 mg/m^2) and carmustine (300 mg/m^2), cyclophosphamide (140–150 mg/kg), hydroxyurea (4.5 gm/m^2) and etoposide (375–450 mg/m^2).

Compared to placebo, administration of LEUKINE in 2 studies (n=44 and 47) significantly improved the following hematologic and clinical endpoints: time to neutrophil engraftment, duration of hospitalization and infection experience or antibacterial usage. In the third study (n=37) there was a positive trend toward earlier myeloid engraftment in favor of LEUKINE. This latter study differed from the other 2 in having enrolled a large number of patients with Hodgkin's disease who had also received extensive radiation and chemotherapy prior to harvest of autologous bone marrow. A subgroup analysis of the data from all 3 studies revealed that the median time to engraftment for patients with Hodgkin's disease, regardless of treatment, was 6 days longer when compared to patients with NHL and ALL, but that the overall beneficial LEUKINE treatment effect was the same. In the following combined analysis of the 3 studies, these 2 subgroups (NHL and ALL vs. Hodgkin's disease) are presented separately.

Patients with Lymphoid Malignancy (Non-Hodgkin's Lymphoma and Acute Lymphoblastic Leukemia): Myeloid engraftment (absolute neutrophil count [ANC] $\geq$ 500 cells/mm^3) in 54 patients receiving LEUKINE was observed 6 days earlier than in 50 patients treated with placebo (see table at right). Accelerated myeloid engraftment was associated with significant clinical benefits. The median duration of hospitalization was 6 days shorter for the LEUKINE group than for the placebo group. Median duration of infectious episodes (defined as fever and neutropenia; or 2 positive cultures of the same organism; or fever >38°C and 1 positive blood culture; or clinical evidence of infection) was 3 days less in the group treated with LEUKINE. The median duration of antibacterial administration in the post-transplantation period was 4 days shorter for the patients treated with LEUKINE than for placebo-treated patients. The study was unable to detect a significant difference between the treatment groups in rate of disease relapse 24 months post-transplantation. As a group, leukemic subjects receiving LEUKINE derived less benefit than NHL subjects. However, both the leukemic and NHL groups receiving LEUKINE engrafted earlier than controls.
[See table above.]

Patients with Hodgkin's Disease: If patients with Hodgkin's disease are analyzed separately, a trend toward earlier myeloid engraftment is noted. LEUKINE-treated patients engrafted earlier (by 5 days) than the placebo-treated patients (p=0.189, Wilcoxon) but the number of patients was small (n=22). Studies are in progress to confirm statistically the trend toward earlier engraftment with LEUKINE in patients with Hodgkin's disease.

Allogeneic Bone Marrow Transplantation A multi-center, randomized, placebo-controlled, and double-blinded study was conducted to evaluate the safety and efficacy of LEUKINE for promoting hematopoietic reconstitution following allogeneic BMT. A total of 109 patients (53 LEUKINE, 56 placebo) were enrolled in the study. Twenty-three patients (11 LEUKINE, 12 placebo) were 18 years old or younger. Sixty-seven patients had myeloid malignancies (33 AML, 34 CML), 17 had lymphoid malignancies (12 ALL, 5 NHL), 3 patients had Hodgkin's disease, 6 had multiple myeloma, 9 had myelodysplastic disease, and 7 patients had aplastic anemia. In 22 patients at one of the seven study sites, bone marrow harvests were depleted of T cells. Preparative regimens included cyclophosphamide, busulfan, cytosine arabinoside, etoposide, methotrexate, corticosteroids, and asparaginase. Some patients also received total body, splenic, or testicular irradiation. Primary graft-versus-host disease (GVHD) prophylaxis was cyclosporine A and a corticosteroid.

Accelerated myeloid engraftment was associated with significant laboratory and clinical benefits. Compared to placebo, administration of LEUKINE significantly improved the following: time to neutrophil engraftment, duration of hospitalization, number of patients with bacteremia and overall incidence of infection (see table at right).

[See table at top of next page.]

Median time to myeloid engraftment (ANC $\geq$ 500 cells/mm^3) in 53 patients receiving LEUKINE (Sargramostim) was 4 days less than in 56 patients treated with placebo (see table at right). The number of patients with bacteremia and infection was significantly lower in the LEUKINE group compared to the placebo group (9/53 versus 19/56 and 30/53 versus 42/56, respectively). There were a number of secondary laboratory and clinical endpoints. Of these, only the incidence of severe (grade 3/4) mucositis was significantly improved in the LEUKINE group (4/53) compared to the placebo group (16/56) at $p < 0.05$. LEUKINE-treated patients also had a shorter median duration of post-transplant IV antibiotic infusions, and shorter median number of days to last platelet and RBC transfusions compared to placebo patients, but none of these differences reached statistical significance.

Bone Marrow Transplantation Failure or Engraftment Delay A historically controlled study was conducted in patients experiencing graft failure following allogeneic or autologous BMT to determine whether LEUKINE improved survival after BMT failure.

Three categories of patients were eligible for this study:
1) patients displaying a delay in engraftment (ANC $\leq$100 cells/mm^3 by day 28 post-transplantation);
2) patients displaying a delay in engraftment (ANC $\leq$100 cells/mm^3 by day 21 post-transplantation) and who had evidence of an active infection; and

3) patients who lost their marrow graft after a transient engraftment (manifested by an average of ANC ≥ 500 cells/mm^3 for at least one week followed by loss of engraftment with ANC < 500 cells/mm^3 for at least one week beyond day 21 post-transplantation).

A total of 140 eligible patients from 35 institutions were treated with LEUKINE and evaluated in comparison to 103 historical control patients from a single institution. One hundred sixty-three patients had lymphoid or myeloid leukemia, 24 patients had non-Hodgkin's lymphoma, 19 patients had Hodgkin's disease and 37 patients had other diseases, such as aplastic anemia, myelodysplasia or non-hematologic malignancy. The majority of patients (223 out of 243) had received prior chemotherapy with or without radiotherapy and/or immunotherapy prior to preparation for transplantation.

One hundred day survival was improved in favor of the patients treated with LEUKINE after graft failure following either autologous or allogeneic BMT. In addition, the median survival was improved by greater than 2-fold. The median survival of patients treated with LEUKINE after autologous failure was 474 days versus 161 days for the historical patients. Similarly, after allogeneic failure, the median survival was 97 days with LEUKINE treatment and 35 days for the historical controls. Improvement in survival was better in patients with fewer impaired organs.

The MOF score is a simple clinical and laboratory assessment of 7 major organ systems: cardiovascular, respiratory, gastrointestinal, hematologic, renal, hepatic and neurologic.[11] Assessment of the MOF score is recommended as an additional method of determining the need to initiate treatment with LEUKINE in patients with graft failure or delay in engraftment following autologous or allogeneic BMT

Factors that Contribute to Survival: The probability of survival was relatively greater for patients with any one of the following characteristics: autologous BMT failure or delay in engraftment, exclusion of total body irradiation from the preparative regimen, a non-leukemic malignancy or MOF score ≤ 2 (0, 1 or 2 dysfunctional organ systems). Leukemic subjects derived less benefit than other subjects.

[See table below.]

Allogeneic BMT: Analysis of Data from Placebo-Controlled Clinical Trial

Median Values (days or number of patients)

	ANC ≥ 500/mm^3	ANC ≥ 1000/mm^3	Number of Patients with Infections	Number of Patients with Bacteremia	Days of Hospitalization
LEUKINE (n=53)	13*	14*	30*	9**	25*
Placebo (n=56)	17	19	42	19	26

*$p < 0.05$ generalized Wilcoxon test **$p < 0.05$ simple chi-square test

CONTRAINDICATIONS

LEUKINE is contraindicated:

1) in patients with excessive leukemic myeloid blasts in the bone marrow or peripheral blood (≥ 10%).
2) in patients with known hypersensitivity to GM-CSF, yeast-derived products or any component of the product.
3) for concomitant use with chemotherapy and radiotherapy. Due to the potential sensitivity of rapidly dividing hematopoietic progenitor cells, LEUKINE should not be administered simultaneously with cytotoxic chemotherapy or radiotherapy or within 24 hours preceding or following chemotherapy or radiotherapy. In one controlled study, patients with small cell lung cancer received LEUKINE and concurrent thoracic radiotherapy and chemotherapy or the identical radiotherapy and chemotherapy without LEUKINE. The patients randomized to LEUKINE had significantly higher adverse events, including higher mortality and a higher incidence of grade 3 and 4 infections and grade 3 and 4 thrombocytopenia.[12]

WARNINGS

Fluid Retention Edema, capillary leak syndrome, pleural and/or pericardial effusion have been reported in patients after LEUKINE administration. In 156 patients enrolled in placebo-controlled studies using LEUKINE at a dose of 250 mcg/m^2/day by 2-hour IV infusion, the reported incidences of fluid retention (LEUKINE vs. placebo) were as follows: peripheral edema, 11% vs. 7%; pleural effusion, 1% vs. 0%; and pericardial effusion, 4% vs. 1%. Capillary leak syndrome was not observed in this limited number of studies; based on other uncontrolled studies and reports from users of marketed LEUKINE, the incidence is estimated to be less than 1%. In patients with preexisting pleural and pericardial effusions, administration of LEUKINE may aggravate fluid retention; however, fluid retention associated with or worsened by LEUKINE has been reversible after interruption or dose reduction of LEUKINE with or without diuretic therapy. LEUKINE should be used with caution in patients with preexisting fluid retention, pulmonary infiltrates or congestive heart failure.

Respiratory Symptoms Sequestration of granulocytes in the pulmonary circulation has been documented following LEUKINE infusion,[13] and dyspnea has been reported occasionally in patients treated with LEUKINE. Special attention should be given to respiratory symptoms during or immediately following LEUKINE infusion, especially in patients with preexisting lung disease. In patients displaying dyspnea during LEUKINE administration, the rate of infusion should be reduced by half. If respiratory symptoms worsen despite infusion rate reduction, the infusion should be discontinued. Subsequent IV infusions may be administered following the standard dose schedule with careful monitoring. LEUKINE should be administered with caution in patients with hypoxia. Benzyl alcohol is a constituent of Bacteriostatic Water for Injection diluent. Benzyl alcohol has been reported to be associated with a fatal "Gasping Syndrome" in premature infants (see DOSAGE AND ADMINISTRATION).

Cardiovascular Symptoms Occasional transient supraventricular arrhythmia has been reported in uncontrolled studies during LEUKINE administration, particularly in patients with a previous history of cardiac arrhythmia. However, these arrhythmias have been reversible after discontinuation of LEUKINE. LEUKINE should be used with caution in patients with preexisting cardiac disease.

Renal and Hepatic Dysfunction In some patients with preexisting renal or hepatic dysfunction enrolled in uncontrolled clinical trials, administration of LEUKINE has induced elevation of serum creatinine or bilirubin and hepatic enzymes. Dose reduction or interruption of LEUKINE administration has resulted in a decrease to pretreatment values. However, in controlled clinical trials the incidences of renal and hepatic dysfunction were comparable between LEUKINE (250 mcg/m^2/day by 2-hour IV infusion) and placebo-treated patients. Monitoring of renal and hepatic function in patients displaying renal or hepatic dysfunction prior to initiation of treatment is recommended at least every other week during LEUKINE administration.

PRECAUTIONS

General Parenteral administration of recombinant proteins should be attended by appropriate precautions in case an allergic or untoward reaction occurs. Serious allergic or anaphylactic reactions have been reported. If any serious allergic or anaphylactic reaction occurs, LEUKINE therapy should immediately be discontinued and appropriate therapy initiated (see WARNINGS).

A syndrome characterized by respiratory distress, hypoxia, flushing, hypotension, syncope, and/or tachycardia has been reported following the first administration of LEUKINE (Sargramostim) in a particular cycle. These signs have resolved with symptomatic treatment and usually do not recur with subsequent doses in the same cycle of treatment.

Stimulation of marrow precursors with LEUKINE may result in a rapid rise in white blood cell (WBC) count. If the ANC exceeds 20,000 cells/mm^3 or if the platelet count exceeds 500,000/mm^3, LEUKINE administration should be interrupted or the dose reduced by half. The decision to reduce the dose or interrupt treatment should be based on the clinical condition of the patient. Excessive blood counts have returned to normal or baseline levels within 3 to 7 days following cessation of LEUKINE therapy. Twice weekly monitoring of CBC with differential (including examination for the presence of blast cells) should be performed to preclude development of excessive counts.

Growth Factor Potential LEUKINE is a growth factor that primarily stimulates normal myeloid precursors. However, the possibility that LEUKINE can act as a growth factor for any tumor type, particularly myeloid malignancies, cannot be excluded. Because of the possibility of tumor growth potentiation, precaution should be exercised when using this drug in any malignancy with myeloid characteristics. Should disease progression be detected during LEUKINE treatment, LEUKINE therapy should be discontinued. LEUKINE has been administered to patients with myelodysplastic syndromes (MDS) in uncontrolled studies without evidence of increased relapse rates.[14,15,16] Controlled studies have not been performed in patients with MDS.

Use in Patients Receiving Purged Bone Marrow LEUKINE is effective in accelerating myeloid recovery in patients receiving bone marrow purged by anti-B lymphocyte monoclonal antibodies. Data obtained from uncontrolled studies suggest that if *in vitro* marrow purging with chemical agents causes a significant decrease in the number of responsive hematopoietic progenitors, the patient may not respond to LEUKINE. When the bone marrow purging process preserves a sufficient number of progenitors (> 1.2×10^4/kg), a beneficial effect of LEUKINE on myeloid engraftment has been reported.[17]

Use in Patients Previously Exposed to Intensive Chemotherapy/Radiotherapy In patients who before autologous BMT, have received extensive radiotherapy to hematopoietic sites for the treatment of primary disease in the abdomen or chest, or have been exposed to multiple myelotoxic agents (alkylating agents, anthracycline antibiotics and antimetabolites), the effect of LEUKINE on myeloid reconstitution may be limited.

Use in Patients with Malignancy Undergoing LEUKINE-Mobilized PBPC Collection When using LEUKINE to mobilize PBPC, the limited *in vitro* data suggest that tumor cells may be released and reinfused into the patient in the leukapheresis product. The effect of reinfusion of tumor cells has not been well studied and the data are inconclusive

Patient Monitoring LEUKINE can induce variable increases in WBC and/or platelet counts. In order to avoid potential complications of excessive leukocytosis (WBC > 50,000 cells/mm^3; ANC > 20,000 cells/mm^3), a CBC is recommended twice per week during LEUKINE therapy. Monitoring of renal and hepatic function in patients displaying renal or hepatic dysfunction prior to initiation of treatment is recommended at least biweekly during LEUKINE administration. Body weight and hydration status should be carefully monitored during LEUKINE administration.

Drug Interaction Interactions between LEUKINE and other drugs have not been fully evaluated. Drugs which may potentiate the myeloproliferative effects of LEUKINE, such as lithium and corticosteroids, should be used with caution.

Carcinogenesis, Mutagenesis, Impairment of Fertility Animal studies have not been conducted with LEUKINE to evaluate the carcinogenic potential or the effect on fertility.

Pregnancy (Category C) Animal reproduction studies have not been conducted with LEUKINE. It is not known whether LEUKINE can cause fetal harm when administered to a pregnant woman or can affect reproductive capability. LEUKINE should be given to a pregnant woman only if clearly needed.

Nursing Mothers It is not known whether LEUKINE is excreted in human milk. Because many drugs are excreted in human milk, LEUKINE should be administered to a nursing woman only if clearly needed.

Pediatric Use Safety and effectiveness in pediatric patients have not been established; however, available safety data indicate that LEUKINE does not exhibit any greater toxicity in pediatric patients than in adults. A total of 124 pediatric subjects between the ages of 4 months and 18 years have been treated with LEUKINE in clinical trials at doses ranging from 60-1,000 mcg/m^2/day intravenously and 4-1,500 mcg/m^2/day subcutaneously. In 53 pediatric patients enrolled in controlled studies at a dose of 250 mcg/m^2/day by 2-hour IV infusion, the type and frequency of adverse events were comparable to those reported for the adult population.

LEUKINE reconstituted with Bacteriostatic Water for Injection, USP (0.9% benzyl alcohol) should not be administered to neonates (see WARNINGS).

Median Survival by Multiple Organ Failure (MOF) Category

Median Survival (days)

	MOF ≤2 Organs	MOF ≥2 Organs	MOF (Composite of Both Groups)
Autologous BMT			
LEUKINE	474 (n=58)	78.5 (n=10)	474 (n=68)
Historical	165 (n=14)	39 (n=3)	161 (n=17)
Allogeneic BMT			
LEUKINE	174 (n=50)	27 (n=22)	97 (n=72)
Historical	52.5 (n=60)	15.5 (n=26)	35 (n=86)

Continued on next page

Immunex—Cont.

ADVERSE REACTIONS

Autologous and Allogeneic Bone Marrow Transplantation LEUKINE is generally well tolerated. In 3 placebo-controlled studies enrolling a total of 156 patients after autologous BMT or peripheral blood progenitor cell transplantation, events reported in at least 10% of patients who received IV LEUKINE or placebo were as reported at right:
[See first table at right.]

No significant differences were observed between LEUKINE and placebo-treated patients in the type or frequency of laboratory abnormalities, including renal and hepatic parameters. In some patients with preexisting renal or hepatic dysfunction enrolled in uncontrolled clinical trials, administration of LEUKINE has induced elevation of serum creatinine or bilirubin and hepatic enzymes (see WARNINGS). In addition, there was no significant difference in relapse rate and 24 month survival between the LEUKINE and placebo-treated patients.

In the placebo-controlled trial of 109 patients after allogeneic BMT, events reported in at least 10% of patients who received IV LEUKINE or placebo were as reported at right:
[See second table at right.]

There were no significant differences in the incidence or severity of GVHD, relapse rates and survival between the LEUKINE and placebo-treated patients.

Adverse events observed for the patients treated with LEUKINE (Sargramostim) in the historically controlled BMT failure study were similar to those reported in the placebo-controlled studies. In addition, headache (26%), pericardial effusion (25%), arthralgia (21%) and myalgia (18%) were also reported in patients treated with LEUKINE in the graft failure study.

In uncontrolled Phase I/II studies with LEUKINE in 215 patients, the most frequent adverse events were fever, asthenia, headache, bone pain, chills and myalgia. These systemic events were generally mild or moderate and were usually prevented or reversed by the administration of analgesics and antipyretics such as acetaminophen. In these uncontrolled trials, other infrequent events reported were dyspnea, peripheral edema, and rash.

Reports of events occurring with marketed LEUKINE include arrhythmia, eosinophilia, hypotension, injection site reactions, pain (including abdominal, back, chest, and joint pain), tachycardia, thrombosis, and transient liver function abnormalities.

In patients with preexisting edema, capillary leak syndrome, pleural and/or pericardial effusion, administration of LEUKINE may aggravate fluid retention (see WARNINGS). Body weight and hydration status should be carefully monitored during LEUKINE administration.

Adverse events observed in pediatric patients in controlled studies were comparable to those observed in adult patients.

Acute Myelogenous Leukemia Adverse events reported in at least 10% of patients who received LEUKINE or placebo were as reported at right:
[See table at top of next page.]

Nearly all patients reported leukopenia, thrombocytopenia and anemia. The frequency and type of adverse events observed following induction were similar between LEUKINE and placebo groups. The only significant difference in the rates of these adverse events was an increase in skin associated events in the LEUKINE group (p=0.002). No significant differences were observed in laboratory results, renal or hepatic toxicity. No significant differences were observed between the LEUKINE and placebo-treated patients for adverse events following consolidation. There was no significant difference in response rate or relapse rate.

In a historically controlled study of 86 patients with acute myelogenous leukemia (AML), the LEUKINE treated group exhibited an increased incidence of weight gain (p=0.007), low serum proteins and prolonged prothrombin time (p=0.02) when compared to the control group. Two LEUKINE treated patients had progressive increase in circulating monocytes and promonocytes and blasts in the marrow which reversed when LEUKINE was discontinued. The historical control group exhibited an increased incidence of cardiac events (p=0.018), liver function abnormalities (p=0.008), and neurocortical hemorrhagic events (p=0.025).[14]

Overdosage The maximum amount of LEUKINE that can be safely administered in single or multiple doses has not been determined. Doses up to 100 mcg/kg/day (4,000 mcg/m²/day or 16 times the recommended dose) were administered to 4 patients in a Phase I uncontrolled clinical study by continuous IV infusion for 7 to 18 days. Increases in WBC up to 200,000 cells/mm³ were observed. Adverse events reported were dyspnea, malaise, nausea, fever, rash, sinus tachycardia, headache and chills. All these events were reversible after discontinuation of LEUKINE.

In case of overdosage, LEUKINE therapy should be discontinued and the patient carefully monitored for WBC increase and respiratory symptoms.

Percent of AuBMT Patients Reporting Events

Events by Body System	LEUKINE (n=79)	Placebo (n=77)	Events by Body System	LEUKINE (n=79)	Placebo (n=77)
Body, General			**Metabolic/Nutritional Disorder**		
Fever	95	96	Edema	34	35
Mucous membrane disorder	75	78	Peripheral edema	11	7
Asthenia	66	51	**Respiratory System**		
Malaise	57	51	Dyspnea	28	31
Sepsis	11	14	Lung disorder	20	23
Digestive System			**Hemic and Lymphatic System**		
Nausea	90	96	Blood dyscrasia	25	27
Diarrhea	89	82	**Cardiovascular System**		
Vomiting	85	90	Hemorrhage	23	30
Anorexia	54	58	**Urogenital System**		
GI disorder	37	47	Urinary tract disorder	14	13
GI hemorrhage	27	33	Kidney function abnormal	8	10
Stomatitis	24	29	**Nervous System**		
Liver damage	13	14	CNS disorder	11	16
Skin and Appendages					
Alopecia	73	74			
Rash	44	38			

Percent of Allogeneic BMT Patients Reporting Events

Events by Body System	LEUKINE (n=53)	Placebo (n=56)	Events by Body System	LEUKINE (n=53)	Placebo (n=56)
Body, General			**Metabolic/Nutritional Disorders**		
Fever	77	80	Bilirubinemia	30	27
Abdominal pain	38	23	Hyperglycemia	25	23
Headache	36	36	Peripheral edema	15	21
Chills	25	20	Increased creatinine	15	14
Pain	17	36	Hypomagnesemia	15	9
Asthenia	17	20	Increased SGPT	13	16
Chest pain	15	9	Edema	13	11
Back pain	9	18	Increased alk. phosphatase	8	14
Digestive System			**Respiratory System**		
Diarrhea	81	66	Pharyngitis	23	13
Nausea	70	66	Epistaxis	17	16
Vomiting	70	57	Dyspnea	15	14
Stomatitis	62	63	Rhinitis	11	14
Anorexia	51	57	**Hemic and Lymphatic System**		
Dyspepsia	17	20	Thrombocytopenia	19	34
Hematemesis	13	7	Leukopenia	17	29
Dysphagia	11	7	Petechia	6	11
GI hemorrhage	11	5	Agranulocytosis	6	11
Constipation	8	11	**Urogenital System**		
Skin and Appendages			Hematuria	9	21
Rash	70	73	**Nervous System**		
Alopecia	45	45	Paresthesia	11	13
Pruritis	23	13	Insomnia	11	9
Musculo-skeletal System			Anxiety	11	2
Bone pain	21	5	**Laboratory Abnormalities** *		
Arthralgia	11	4	High glucose	41	49
Special Senses			Low albumin	27	36
Eye hemorrhage	11	0	High BUN	23	17
Cardiovascular System			Low calcium	2	7
Hypertension	34	32	High cholesterol	17	8
Tachycardia	11	9			

Grade 3 and 4 laboratory abnormalities only. Denominators may vary due to missing laboratory measurements.

DOSAGE AND ADMINISTRATION

Neutrophil Recovery Following Chemotherapy in Acute Myelogenous Leukemia The recommended dose is 250 mcg/m²/day administered intravenously over a 4 hour period starting approximately on day 11 or 4 days following the completion of induction chemotherapy, if the day 10 bone marrow is hypoplastic with <5% blasts. If a second cycle of induction chemotherapy is necessary, LEUKINE should be administered approximately 4 days after the completion of chemotherapy if the bone marrow is hypoplastic with <5% blasts. LEUKINE should be continued until an ANC >1500/mm³ for 3 consecutive days or a maximum of 42 days. LEUKINE should be discontinued immediately if leukemic regrowth occurs. If a severe adverse reaction occurs, the dose can be reduced by 50% or temporarily discontinued until the reaction abates.

In order to avoid potential complications of excessive leukocytosis (WBC > 50,000 cells/mm³ or ANC > 20,000 cells/mm³) a CBC with differential is recommended twice per week during LEUKINE therapy. LEUKINE treatment should be interrupted or the dose reduced by half if the ANC exceeds 20,000 cells/mm³.

Mobilization of Peripheral Blood Progenitor Cells The recommended dose is 250 mcg/m²/day administered IV over 24 hours or SC once daily. Dosing should continue at the same dose through the period of PBPC collection. The optimal schedule for PBPC collection has not been established. In clinical studies, collection of PBPC was usually begun by day 5 and performed daily until protocol specied targets were achieved (see CLINICAL EXPERIENCE, Mobilization of PBPC and Engraftment). If WBC > 50,000 cells/mm³, the LEUKINE dose should be reduced by 50%. If adequate numbers of progenitor cells are not collected, other mobilization therapy should be considered.

Post Peripheral Blood Progenitor Cell Transplantation The recommended dose is 250 mcg/m²/day administered IV over 24 hours or SC once daily beginning immediately following infusion of progenitor cells and continuing until an ANC > 1500 for 3 consecutive days is attained.

Myeloid Reconstitution After Autologous or Allogeneic Bone Marrow Transplantation The recommended dose is 250 mcg/m²/day administered IV over a 2-hour period beginning 2 to 4 hours after bone marrow infusion, and not less than 24 hours after the last dose of chemotherapy and 12 hours after the last dose of radiotherapy. Patients should not receive LEUKINE until the post marrow infusion ANC is less than 500 cells/mm³. LEUKINE should be continued until an ANC > 1500/mm³ for 3 consecutive days is attained. If a severe adverse reaction occurs, the dose can be reduced by 50% or temporarily discontinued until the reaction abates. Leukine should be discontinued immediately if blast cells appear or disease progression occurs. In order to avoid potential complications of excessive leukocytosis (WBC > 50,000 cells/mm³, ANC > 20,000 cells/mm³) a CBC with differential is recommended twice per week during LEUKINE therapy. LEUKINE treatment should be interrupted or the dose reduced by 50% if the ANC exceeds 20,000 cells/mm³.

Bone Marrow Transplantation Failure or Engraftment Delay The recommended dose is 250 mcg/m²/day for 14 days as a 2-hour IV infusion. The dose can be repeated after 7 days off therapy if engraftment has not occurred. If engraftment still has not occurred, a third course of 500 mcg/m²/day for 14 days may be tried after another 7 days of therapy. If there is still no improvement, it is unlikely that further dose escalation will be beneficial. If a severe adverse reaction occurs, the dose can be reduced by 50% or temporarily discontinued until the reaction abates. LEUKINE should be discontinued immediately if blast cells appear or disease progression occurs.

In order to avoid potential complications of excessive leukocytosis (WBC > 50,000 cells/mm³, ANC > 20,000 cells/mm³) a CBC with differential is recommended twice per week during LEUKINE therapy. LEUKINE treatment should be interrupted or the dose reduced by half if the ANC exceeds 20,000 cells/mm³.

Preparation of LEUKINE
1. LEUKINE is a sterile, white, preservative-free, lyophilized powder suitable for SC injection or IV infusion upon reconstitution. LEUKINE (250 mcg or 500 mcg vials) should be reconstituted aseptically with 1.0 mL diluent (see below). The reconstituted LEUKINE solutions are clear, colorless, isotonic with a pH of 7.4 ± 0.3, and contain 250 or 500 mcg/mL of Sargramostim. The contents of vials reconstituted with different diluents should not be mixed together.
Sterile Water for Injection, USP (without preservative): LEUKINE vials contain no antibacterial preservative, and therefore solutions prepared with Sterile Water for Injection, USP should be administered as soon as possible, and within 6 hours following reconstitution and/or dilution for IV infusion. The vial should not be re-entered or reused. Do not save any unused portion for administration more than 6 hours following reconstitution.
Bacteriostatic Water for Injection, USP (0.9% benzyl alcohol): Reconstituted solutions prepared with Bacteriostatic Water for Injection, USP (0.9% benzyl alcohol) may be stored for up to 20 days at 2–8°C prior to use. Discard reconstituted solution after 20 days. Previously reconstituted solutions mixed with freshly reconstituted solutions must be administered within 6 hours following mixing.
Preparations containing benzyl alcohol should not be used in neonates (see WARNINGS).
2. During reconstitution the diluent should be directed at the side of the vial and the contents gently swirled to avoid foaming during dissolution. Avoid excessive or vigorous agitation; do not shake.
3. LEUKINE should be used for SC injection without further dilution. Dilution for IV infusion should be performed in 0.9% Sodium Chloride Injection, USP. If the final concentration of LEUKINE is below 10 mcg/mL, Albumin (Human) at a final concentration of 0.1% should be added to the saline prior to addition of LEUKINE to prevent adsorption to the components of the drug delivery system. To obtain a final concentration of 0.1% Albumin (Human), add 1 mg Albumin (Human) per 1 mL 0.9% Sodium Chloride Injection, USP (e.g., use 1 mL 5% Albumin [Human] in 50 mL 0.9% Sodium Chloride Injection, USP).
4. An in-line membrane filter should not be used for intravenous infusion of LEUKINE.
5. Store LEUKINE solutions under refrigeration at 2–8°C (36°–46°F); do not freeze.
6. In the absence of compatibility and stability information, no other medication should be added to infusion solutions containing LEUKINE. Use only 0.9% Sodium Chloride Injection, USP to prepare IV infusion solutions.
7. Aseptic technique should be employed in the preparation of all LEUKINE solutions. To assure correct concentration following reconstitution, care should be exercised to eliminate any air bubbles from the needle hub of the syringe used to prepare the diluent. Parenteral drug products should be inspected visually for particulate matter and discoloration prior to administration whenever solution and container permit.

HOW SUPPLIED
LEUKINE® is available as a sterile, white, preservative-free, lyophilized powder in vials containing 250 mcg Sargramostim (1.4 x 10⁶ IU) or 500 mcg Sargramostim (2.8 x 10⁶ IU); 40 mg Mannitol, USP; 10 mg Sucrose, NF; and 1.2 mg Tromethamine, USP. Each dosage form is supplied in cartons of 5 vials.
Cartons of 5 vials of 250 mcg LEUKINE® (NDC 58406-002-33)
Cartons of 5 vials of 500 mcg LEUKINE® (NDC 58406-001-35)

STORAGE
The sterile powder, the reconstituted solution and the diluted solution for injection should be refrigerated at 2–8°C (36–46°F). Do not freeze or shake. Do not use beyond the expiration date printed on the vial.

Percent of AML Patients Reporting Events

Events by Body System	LEUKINE (n=52)	Placebo (n=47)
Body, General		
Fever (no infection)	81	74
Infection	65	68
Weight loss	37	28
Weight gain	8	21
Chills	19	26
Allergy	12	15
Sweats	6	13
Digestive System		
Nausea	58	55
Liver	77	83
Diarrhea	52	53
Vomiting	46	34
Stomatitis	42	43
Anorexia	13	11
Abdominal distention	4	13
Skin and Appendages		
Skin	77	45
Alopecia	37	51

Events by Body System	LEUKINE (n=52)	Placebo (n=47)
Metabolic/Nutritional Disorder		
Metabolic	58	49
Edema	25	23
Respiratory System		
Pulmonary	48	64
Hemic and Lymphatic System		
Coagulation	19	21
Cardiovascular System		
Hemorrhage	29	43
Hypertension	25	32
Cardiac	23	32
Hypotension	13	26
Urogenital System		
GU	50	57
Nervous System		
Neuro-clinical	42	53
Neuro-motor	25	26
Neuro-psych	15	26
Neuro-sensory	6	11

REFERENCES
1. Metcalf D. The molecular biology and functions of the granulocyte-macrophage colony-stimulating factors. Blood 1986; 67(2):257-267.
2. Park LS, Friend D, Gillis S, Urdal DL. Characterization of the cell surface receptor for human granulocyte/macrophage colony stimulating factor. J Exp Med 1986; 164:251-262.
3. Grabstein KH, Urdal DL, Tushinski RJ, et al. Induction of macrophage tumoricidal activity by granulocyte-macrophage colony-stimulating factors. Science 1986; 232:506-508.
4. Reed SG, Nathan CF, Pihl DL, et al. Recombinant granulocyte/macrophage colony-stimulating factor activates macrophages to inhibit *Trypanosoma cruzi* and release hydrogen peroxide. J Exp Med 1987; 166:1734-1746.
5. Data on File Immunex Corporation; Seattle, WA.
6. Shadduck RK, Waheed A, Evans C, et al. Serum and urinary levels of recombinant human granulocyte-macrophage colony stimulating factor: Assessment after intravenous infusion and subcutaneous injection. Exp Hem 1990; 18:601.
7. Rowe JM, Andersen JW, Mazza JJ, et al. A randomized placebo-controlled phase III study of granulocyte-macrophage colony-stimulating factor in adult patients (>55 to 70 years of age) with acute myelogenous leukemia: a study of the Eastern Cooperative Oncology Group (E1490). Blood 1995; 86(2):457-462.
8. Nemunaitis J, Rabinowe SN, Singer JW, et al. Recombinant human granulocyte-macrophage colony-stimulating factor after autologous bone marrow transplantation for lymphoid malignancy: Pooled results of a randomized, double-blind, placebo controlled trial. NEJM 1991; 324(25):1773-1778.
9. Nemunaitis J, Singer JW, Buckner CD, et al. Use of recombinant human granulocyte macrophage colony-stimulating factor in autologous bone marrow transplantation for lymphoid malignancies. Blood 1988; 72(2):834-836.
10. Nemunaitis J, Singer JW, Buckner CD, et al. Long-term follow-up of patients who received recombinant human granulocyte-macrophage colony stimulating factor after autologous bone marrow transplantation for lymphoid malignancy. BMT 1991; 7:49-52.
11. Goris RJA, Boekhorst TPA, Nuytinck JKS, et al. Multiple organ failure: Generalized auto-destructive inflammation? Arch Surg 1985; 120:1109-1115.
12. Bunn P, Crowley J, Kelly K, et al. Chemoradiotherapy with or without granulocyte-macrophage colony-stimulating factor in the treatment of limited-stage small-cell lung cancer: a prospective phase III randomized study of the southwest oncology group. JCO 1995; 13(7):1632-1641.
13. Herrmann F, Schulz G, Lindemann A, et al. Yeast-expressed granulocyte-macrophage colony-stimulating factor in cancer patients: A phase Ib clinical study. In Behring Institute Research Communications, Colony Stimulating Factors-CSF. International Symposium, Garmisch-Partenkirchen, West Germany. 1988; 83:107-118.
14. Estey EH, Dixon D, Kantarjian H, et al. Treatment of poor-prognosis, newly diagnosed acute myeloid leukemia with Ara-C and recombinant human granulocyte-macrophage colony-stimulating factor. Blood 1990; 75(9):1766-1769.
15. Vadhan-Raj S, Keating M, LeMaistre A, et al. Effects of recombinant human granulocyte-macrophage colony-stimulating factor in patients with myelodysplastic syndromes. NEJM 1987; 317:1545-1552.
16. Buchner T, Hiddemann W, Koenigsmann M, et al. Recombinant human granulocyte-macrophage colony stimulating factor after chemotherapy in patients with acute myeloid leukemia at higher age or after relapse. Blood 1991; 78(5):1190-1197.
17. Blazar BR, Kersey JH, McGlave PB, et al. In vivo administration of recombinant human granulocyte/macrophage colony-stimulating factor in acute lymphoblastic leukemia patients receiving purged autografts. Blood 1989; 73(3):849-857.

LEVOPROME® ℞
Methotrimeprazine for injection
For Intramuscular Use

CAUTION: Following administration of this drug, orthostatic hypotension, fainting, or dizziness may occur. Ambulation should be avoided or carefully supervised for at least 6 hours following the initial dose. Tolerance to this effect usually develops with continued administration.

DESCRIPTION
LEVOPROME methotrimeprazine is 10H-phenothiazine-10-propanamine, 2-methoxy-N,N,β-trimethyl-, (−) -. It was formerly called levomepromazine. The structural formula is:

$$C_{19}H_{24}N_2OS$$

It is available as a clear transparent solution of the hydrochloride salt containing 20 mg of methotrimeprazine per mL with Benzyl Alcohol (0.9% w/v) as a preservative, and with Disodium Edetate USP (0.065% w/v) and Sodium Metabisulfite (0.3% w/v, see **WARNINGS**) as stabilizers.
It is adjusted to a pH of approximately 4.5 with Sodium Citrate, Citric Acid USP, Anhydrous, and Hydrochloric Acid or Sodium Hydroxide NF. Water for Injection USP qs ad 100%.

ACTIONS
LEVOPROME, a phenothiazine derivative, is a potent central nervous system depressant with sites of action postulated in the thalamus, hypothalamus, reticular and limbic systems, producing suppression of sensory impulses, reduction of motor activity, sedation and tranquilization. It raises the pain threshold and produces amnesia. LEVOPROME also has antihistamine, anticholinergic, and antiadrenalin effects. It is actively metabolized into sulfoxides and glucuronic conjugates and largely excreted into the urine as such. Small amounts of unchanged drug are excreted in the feces and in the urine (1%). Low concentrations of drug occur in the blood serum in man. Elimination into the urine usually continues for several days after intramuscular administration of the drug is discontinued.
LEVOPROME produces an analgesic effect in both animals and man comparable to morphine and meperidine. A sedative effect is produced as well. Its use thus far has not been reported to result in signs of addiction, dependence or withdrawal symptoms even with large doses or with prolonged administration. Maximum analgesic effect usually occurs within 20 to 40 minutes after intramuscular injection and is maintained for about 4 hours.

Continued on next page

Immunex—Cont.

Respiratory depression in the patient or in the newborn during or following preanesthetic or obstetrical use occurs infrequently with LEVOPROME. The drug does not appear to affect the cough reflex.

INDICATIONS

LEVOPROME methotrimeprazine is indicated for the relief of pain of moderate to marked degree of severity in nonambulatory patients.

It is indicated for obstetrical analgesia and sedation where respiratory depression is to be avoided.

LEVOPROME is indicated as a preanesthetic medication for producing sedation, somnolence, and relief of apprehension and anxiety.

CONTRAINDICATIONS

LEVOPROME should not be used:

1. Concurrently with antihypertensive drugs including monoamine oxidase inhibitors.
2. In patients with a history of phenothiazine hypersensitivity.
3. In the presence of overdosage of CNS depressants or comatose states.
4. In the presence of severe myocardial, renal or hepatic disease.
5. In the presence of clinically significant hypotension.
6. In patients under 12 years of age, since safe and effective use has not been established in children under this age.

WARNINGS

LEVOPROME should be used with caution in women of child-bearing potential and during early pregnancy since its safety for the developing embryo has not been clearly established. A possible antifertility effect has been suggested in that successive generations of animals dosed with this drug have shown a diminution of litter size over the controls. There is no evidence of adverse developmental effect when administered during late pregnancy and labor.

LEVOPROME, as with other phenothiazine derivatives, has been found to depress spermatogenesis in experimental animals in doses greatly exceeding the recommended human dose.

LEVOPROME exerts additive effects with central nervous system depressant drugs including narcotics, barbiturates, general anesthetics, and certain drugs such as acetylsalicylic acid, meprobamate, and reserpine. Consequently, the dosage of LEVOPROME methotrimeprazine and of each such drug should be reduced and critically adjusted when used concomitantly or when sequence of use results in overlapping of drug effects.

Contains sodium metabisulfite, a sulfite that may cause allergic-type reactions including anaphylactic symptoms and life-threatening or less severe asthmatic episodes in certain susceptible people. The overall prevalence of sulfite sensitivity in the general population is unknown and probably low. Sulfite sensitivity is seen more frequently in asthmatic than in nonasthmatic people.

PRECAUTIONS

LEVOPROME should be used with caution when given concomitantly with atropine, scopolamine, and succinylcholine in that tachycardia and fall in blood pressure may occur, and undesirable central nervous system effects such as stimulation, delirium, and extrapyramidal symptoms may be aggravated.

Elderly and debilitated patients with heart disease are more sensitive to phenothiazine effects. Therefore, a low initial dose is recommended with adjustment of subsequent doses according to response and tolerance of the patient. The pulse, blood pressure, and general circulatory status should be checked frequently until dosage requirements and response are stabilized.

Continued administration for more than 30 days has usually been unnecessary, and is advised only when narcotic drugs are contraindicated or in terminal illnesses. When long-term use is anticipated, periodic blood counts and liver function studies are recommended.

Patients should remain in bed or be closely supervised for about 6 hours after each of the first several injections, and not be ambulatory because of the possibility of orthostatic hypotension. Once tolerance to this effect is obtained, tolerance will usually be maintained unless more than several days elapse between subsequent doses. Therapy with vasopressor drugs has been required very rarely. Phenylephrine and methoxamine are suitable vasopressor agents; however, epinephrine should not be used, since a paradoxical decrease in blood pressure may result. Levarterenol should be reserved for hypotension not reversed by other vasopressors.

ADVERSE REACTIONS

The most important side effects have been those associated with orthostatic hypotension. These effects, which include fainting or syncope, and weakness, usually can be avoided by keeping the patient in a supine position for about 6 hours (occasionally as much as 12 hours) after injection. A drop in blood pressure (usually within the physiological range) often occurs, beginning generally within 10 to 20 minutes following intramuscular injection, and may last 4 to 6 hours (occasionally up to 12 hours). This effect usually diminishes or disappears with continued or intermittent administration. Occasionally, fall in blood pressure may be profound and require immediate restorative measures.

Adverse reactions sometimes encountered include disorientation, dizziness, excessive sedation, weakness, slurring of speech; abdominal discomfort, nausea, and vomiting; dry mouth, nasal congestion, difficulties in urination; chills; rarely uterine inertia.

Pain at the site of injection is frequently observed following administration of this drug. Local inflammation and swelling have occurred.

Agranulocytosis and jaundice have been reported following long-term, high-dosage use of this drug. Other adverse effects reported following the use of the phenothiazine family of drugs usually during their administration as psychotherapeutic agents have included: blood dyscrasias (agranulocytosis, pancytopenia, leukopenia, eosinophilia, thrombocytopenia); hepatotoxicity (jaundice, biliary stasis); extrapyramidal symptoms (dyskinesia, tilting stance, dystonia, parkinsonism, opisthotonos, hyperreflexia, especially in patients with previous brain damage); grand mal convulsions; potentiation of CNS depressants (opiates, barbiturates, antihistamines, alcohol, analgesics), atropine, phosphorous insecticides, heat; cerebral edema and altered cerebral spinal fluid proteins; reactivation of psychotic processes, catatonia; autonomic reactions (dryness of mouth, constipation) cardiac arrest, tachycardia; hyperpyrexia; endocrine disturbances (menstrual and lactation irregularities); dermatological disorders (photosensitivity, itching, erythema, urticaria, pigmentation, rash, exfoliative dermatitis) ocular changes (lenticular and corneal deposits and pigmentary retinopathy); hypersensitivity reactions (angioneurotic, laryngeal, and peripheral edema, anaphylactoid reactions, and asthma). There is considerable individual variation in type and frequency to these effects and although some are dose-related, many involve individual patient sensitivity. Most of these effects have occurred only on long-term, high-dosage administration and have not necessarily been reported with the recommended analgesic doses of methotrimeprazine.

ADMINISTRATION AND DOSAGE

Adult Administration: LEVOPROME should be administered by deep intramuscular injection into a large muscle mass. As with other intramuscularly administered drugs, proper injection technique is important to prevent inadvertent injection into a blood vessel, into, or in the region of, a peripheral nerve trunk, and to avoid leakage along the needle tract. When multiple injections are used, rotation of the injection sites is advisable. LEVOPROME should not be administered subcutaneously as local irritation may occur. Until more experience is obtained, intravenous administration is not recommended.

LEVOPROME may be given intramuscularly in the same syringe with either Atropine Sulfate USP or Scopolamine Hydrobromide USP. It should NOT be mixed in the same syringe with other drugs.

The usual adult dose for analgesia is 10 to 20 mg (0.5 to 1.0 mL) administered deeply into a large muscle every 4 to 6 hours as required for pain relief. The dose per injection has varied from 5 to 40 mg (0.25 to 2.0 mL) at intervals of from 1 to 24 hours. A flexible dosage schedule and low initial dose of 10 mg are advisable until individual patient response and tolerance have been determined.

In elderly patients who are more sensitive to phenothiazine effects, an initial dose of 5 to 10 mg (0.25 to 0.5 mL) is suggested. If the patient tolerates the drug, and requires greater pain relief, subsequent doses may be slowly increased.

Analgesia for Acute or Intractable Pain: Initial dose of 10 to 20 mg, with adjustment of subsequent doses, at intervals of 4 to 6 hours as required for relief of pain.

Obstetrical Analgesia: During labor, an initial dose of 15 to 20 mg is usually satisfactory. LEVOPROME may be repeated in similar or adjusted amounts at intervals as needed for analgesia and sedation.

Preanesthetic Medication: The preoperative dose has varied from 2 to 20 mg administered 45 minutes to 3 hours before surgery. A dose of 10 mg is often satisfactory, and 15 to 20 mg, may be used when more sedation is desired. Atropine Sulfate USP or Scopolamine Hydrobromide USP may be used concurrently but in lower than usual dosage (see also under **PRECAUTIONS**).

Postoperative Analgesia: In the immediate postoperative period, initial dosage of 2.5 to 7.5 mg is suggested, since residual effects of anesthetic agents and other medications may be additive to the actions of LEVOPROME *methotrimeprazine*. Subsequent doses should be adjusted and administered at intervals of 4 to 6 hours as needed for pain relief. Ambulation must be avoided or carefully supervised (see also under **CAUTION, ADVERSE REACTIONS,** and **PRECAUTIONS**).

HOW SUPPLIED

LEVOPROME® methotrimeprazine for injection is available in 10 mL vials containing 20 mg of methotrimeprazine per mL.

Protect the solutions from light.

Product No. NDC 0205-4534-34

Store at Controlled Room Temperature 15°–30°C (59°–86°F).

LEDERLE PARENTERALS, INC.

Carolina, Puerto Rico 00987

14481
REV. 3/87

METHOTREXATE Sodium Tablets ℞

METHOTREXATE Sodium for Injection ℞

METHOTREXATE LPF® Sodium ℞
(METHOTREXATE Sodium Injection) and

METHOTREXATE Sodium Injection ℞

WARNINGS

METHOTREXATE SHOULD BE USED ONLY BY PHYSICIANS WHOSE KNOWLEDGE AND EXPERIENCE INCLUDE THE USE OF ANTIMETABOLITE THERAPY.

BECAUSE OF THE POSSIBILITY OF SERIOUS TOXIC REACTIONS (WHICH CAN BE FATAL):

METHOTREXATE SHOULD BE USED ONLY IN LIFE THREATENING NEOPLASTIC DISEASES, OR IN PATIENTS WITH PSORIASIS OR RHEUMATOID ARTHRITIS WITH SEVERE, RECALCITRANT, DISABLING DISEASE WHICH IS NOT ADEQUATELY RESPONSIVE TO OTHER FORMS OF THERAPY.

DEATHS HAVE BEEN REPORTED WITH THE USE OF METHOTREXATE IN THE TREATMENT OF MALIGNANCY, PSORIASIS, AND RHEUMATOID ARTHRITIS.

PATIENTS SHOULD BE CLOSELY MONITORED FOR BONE MARROW, LIVER, LUNG AND KIDNEY TOXICITIES. (See PRECAUTIONS.)

PATIENTS SHOULD BE INFORMED BY THEIR PHYSICIAN OF THE RISKS INVOLVED AND BE UNDER A PHYSICIAN'S CARE THROUGHOUT THERAPY.

THE USE OF METHOTREXATE HIGH DOSE REGIMENS RECOMMENDED FOR OSTEOSARCOMA REQUIRES METICULOUS CARE. (See DOSAGE AND ADMINISTRATION.) HIGH DOSE REGIMENS FOR OTHER NEOPLASTIC DISEASES ARE INVESTIGATIONAL AND A THERAPEUTIC ADVANTAGE HAS NOT BEEN ESTABLISHED.

METHOTREXATE FORMULATIONS AND DILUENTS CONTAINING PRESERVATIVES MUST NOT BE USED FOR INTRATHECAL OR HIGH DOSE METHOTREXATE THERAPY.

1. Methotrexate has been reported to cause fetal death and/or congenital anomalies. Therefore, it is not recommended for women of childbearing potential unless there is clear medical evidence that the benefits can be expected to outweigh the considered risks. Pregnant women with psoriasis or rheumatoid arthritis should not receive methotrexate. (See CONTRAINDICATIONS.)

2. Methotrexate elimination is reduced in patients with impaired renal function, ascites, or pleural effusions. Such patients require especially careful monitoring for toxicity, and require dose reduction or, in some cases, discontinuation of methotrexate administration.

3. Unexpectedly severe (sometimes fatal) bone marrow suppression and gastrointestinal toxicity have been reported with concomitant administration of methotrexate (usually in high dosage) along with some nonsteroidal anti-inflammatory drugs (NSAIDs). (See PRECAUTIONS, Drug Interactions.)

4. Methotrexate causes hepatotoxicity, fibrosis and cirrhosis, but generally only after prolonged use. Acutely, liver enzyme elevations are frequently seen. These are usually transient and asymptomatic, and also do not appear predictive of subsequent hepatic disease. Liver biopsy after sustained use often shows histologic changes, and fibrosis and cirrhosis have been reported; these latter lesions may not be preceded by symptoms or abnormal liver function tests in the psoriasis population. For this reason, periodic liver biopsies are usually recommended for psoriatic patients who are under long-term treatment. Persistent abnormalities in liver function tests may precede appearance of fibrosis or cirrhosis in the rheumatoid arthritis population. (See PRECAUTIONS, Organ System Toxicity *Hepatic.)*

5. Methotrexate-induced lung disease is a potentially dangerous lesion, which may occur acutely at any

time during therapy and which has been reported at doses as low as 7.5 mg/week. It is always fully reversible. Pulmonary symptoms (especially a dry, nonproductive cough) may require interruption of treatment and careful investigation.

6. Diarrhea and ulcerative stomatitis require interruption of therapy; otherwise, hemorrhagic enteritis and death from intestinal perforation may occur.
7. Malignant lymphomas, which may regress following withdrawal of methotrexate, may occur in patients receiving low-dose methotrexate and, thus, may not require cytotoxic treatment. Discontinue methotrexate first and, if the lymphoma does not regress, appropriate treatment should be instituted.

DESCRIPTION

Methotrexate (formerly Amethopterin) is an antimetabolite used in the treatment of certain neoplastic diseases, severe psoriasis, and adult rheumatoid arthritis.

Chemically methotrexate is *N*-[4-[[(2,4-diamino-6-pteridinyl)methyl]methylamino]benzoyl]-L-glutamic acid. The structural formula is:

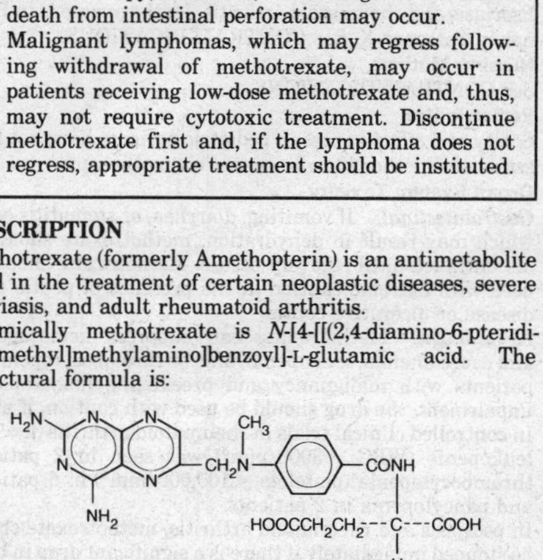

Molecular weight: 454.45 $C_{20}H_{22}N_8O_5$

Methotrexate Sodium Tablets for oral administration are available in bottles of 100 and in a packaging system designated as the RHEUMATREX® Methotrexate Sodium Dose Pack for therapy with a weekly dosing schedule of 5 mg, 7.5 mg, 10 mg, 12.5 mg and 15 mg. Methotrexate Sodium Tablets contain an amount of methotrexate sodium equivalent to 2.5 mg of methotrexate and the following inactive ingredients: Lactose, Magnesium Stearate and Pregelatinized Starch. May also contain Corn Starch.

Methotrexate Sodium Injection and for Injection products are sterile and non-pyrogenic and may be given by the intramuscular, intravenous, intra-arterial or intrathecal route. (See DOSAGE AND ADMINISTRATION.) However, the preservative formulation contains Benzyl Alcohol and must not be used for intrathecal or high dose therapy.

Methotrexate Sodium Injection, Isotonic Liquid, Contains Preservative is available in 25 mg/mL, 2 mL (50 mg) and 10 mL (250 mg) vials.

Each 25 mg/mL, 2 mL and 10 mL vial contains methotrexate sodium equivalent to 50 mg and 250 mg methotrexate respectively, 0.90% w/v of Benzyl Alcohol as a preservative, and the following inactive ingredients: Sodium Chloride 0.260% w/v and Water for Injection qs ad 100% v. Sodium Hydroxide and, if necessary, Hydrochloric Acid are added to adjust the pH to approximately 8.5.

Methotrexate LPF® Sodium (methotrexate sodium injection), Isotonic Liquid, Preservative Free, for single use only, is available in 25 mg/mL, 2 mL (50 mg), 4 mL (100 mg), 8 mL (200 mg) and 10 mL (250 mg) vials.

Each 25 mg/mL, 2 mL, 4 mL, 8 mL and 10 mL vial contains methotrexate sodium equivalent to 50 mg, 100 mg, 200 mg and 250 mg methotrexate respectively, and the following inactive ingredients: Sodium Chloride 0.490% w/v and Water for Injection qs ad 100% v. Sodium Hydroxide and, if necessary, Hydrochloric Acid are added to adjust the pH to approximately 8.5. The 2 mL, 4 mL, 8 mL and 10 mL solutions contain approximately 0.43 mEq, 0.86 mEq, 1.72 mEq and 2.15 mEq of Sodium per vial, respectively, and are isotonic solutions.

Methotrexate Sodium for Injection, Lyophilized, Preservative Free, for single use only, is available in 20 mg, 50 mg and 1 gram vials.

Each 20 mg, 50 mg and 1 g vial of lyophilized powder contains methotrexate sodium equivalent to 20 mg, 50 mg and 1 g methotrexate respectively. Contains no preservative. Sodium Hydroxide and, if necessary, Hydrochloric Acid are added during manufacture to adjust the pH. The 20 mg vial contains approximately 0.14 mEq of Sodium; the 50 mg vial contains approximately 0.33 mEq of Sodium, and the 1 g vial contains approximately 7 mEq Sodium.

CLINICAL PHARMACOLOGY

Methotrexate inhibits dihydrofolic acid reductase. Dihydrofolates must be reduced to tetrahydrofolates by this enzyme before they can be utilized as carriers of one-carbon groups in the synthesis of purine nucleotides and thymidylate. Therefore, methotrexate interferes with DNA synthesis, repair, and cellular replication. Actively proliferating tissues such as malignant cells, bone marrow, fetal cells, buccal and intestinal mucosa, and cells of the urinary bladder are in general more sensitive to this effect of methotrexate. When cellular proliferation in malignant tissues is greater than in most normal tissues, methotrexate may impair malignant growth without irreversible damage to normal tissues.

The mechanism of action in rheumatoid arthritis is unknown; it may affect immune function. Two reports describe *in vitro* methotrexate inhibition of DNA precursor uptake by stimulated mononuclear cells, and another describes in animal polyarthritis partial correction by methotrexate of spleen cell hyporesponsiveness and suppressed IL 2 production. Other laboratories, however, have been unable to demonstrate similar effects. Clarification of methotrexate's effect on immune activity and its relation to rheumatoid immunopathogenesis await further studies.

In patients with rheumatoid arthritis, effects of methotrexate on articular swelling and tenderness can be seen as early as 3 to 6 weeks. Although methotrexate clearly ameliorates symptoms of inflammation (pain, swelling, stiffness), there is no evidence that it induces remission of rheumatoid arthritis nor has a beneficial effect been demonstrated on bone erosions and other radiologic changes which result in impaired joint use, functional disability, and deformity.

Most studies of methotrexate in patients with rheumatoid arthritis are relatively short term (3 to 6 months). Limited data from long-term studies indicate that an initial clinical improvement is maintained for at least two years with continued therapy.

In psoriasis, the rate of production of epithelial cells in the skin is greatly increased over normal skin. This differential in proliferation rates is the basis for the use of methotrexate to control the psoriatic process.

Methotrexate in high doses, followed by leucovorin rescue, is used as a part of the treatment of patients with non-metastatic osteosarcoma. The original rationale for high dose methotrexate therapy was based on the concept of selective rescue of normal tissues by leucovorin. More recent evidence suggests that high dose methotrexate may also overcome methotrexate resistance caused by impaired active transport, decreased affinity of dihydrofolic acid reductase for methotrexate, increased levels of dihydrofolic acid reductase resulting from gene amplification, or decreased polyglutamation of methotrexate. The actual mechanism of action is unknown.

Two Pediatric Oncology Group studies (one randomized and one non-randomized) demonstrated a significant improvement in relapse-free survival in patients with non-metastatic osteosarcoma, when high dose methotrexate with leucovorin rescue was used in combination with other chemotherapeutic agents following surgical resection of the primary tumor. These studies were not designed to demonstrate the specific contribution of high dose methotrexate/leucovorin rescue therapy to the efficacy of the combination. However, a contribution can be inferred from the reports of objective responses to this therapy in patients with metastatic osteosarcoma, and from reports of extensive tumor necrosis following preoperative administration of this therapy to patients with non-metastatic osteosarcoma.

Pharmacokinetics

Absorption—In adults, oral absorption appears to be dose dependent. Peak serum levels are reached within one to two hours. At doses of 30 mg/m^2 or less, methotrexate is generally well absorbed with a mean bioavailability of about 60%. The absorption of doses greater than 80 mg/m^2 is significantly less, possibly due to a saturation effect.

In leukemic pediatric patients, oral absorption has been reported to vary widely (23% to 95%). A twenty fold difference between highest and lowest peak levels (C_{max}: 0.11 to 2.3 micromolar after a 20 mg/m^2 dose) has been reported. Significant interindividual variability has also been noted in time to peak concentration (T_{max}: 0.67 to 4 hrs after a 15 mg/m^2 dose) and fraction of dose absorbed. Food has been shown to delay absorption and reduce peak concentration. Methotrexate is generally completely absorbed from parenteral routes of injection. After intramuscular injection, peak serum concentrations occur in 30 to 60 minutes.

Distribution—After intravenous administration, the initial volume of distribution is approximately 0.18 L/kg (18% of body weight) and steady-state volume of distribution is approximately 0.4 to 0.8 L/kg (40% to 80% of body weight). Methotrexate competes with reduced folates for active transport across cell membranes by means of a single carrier-mediated active transport process. At serum concentrations greater than 100 micromolar, passive diffusion becomes a major pathway by which effective intracellular concentrations can be achieved. Methotrexate in serum is approximately 50% protein bound. Laboratory studies demonstrate that it may be displaced from plasma albumin by various compounds including sulfonamides, salicylates, tetracyclines, chloramphenicol, and phenytoin.

Methotrexate does not penetrate the blood-cerebrospinal fluid barrier in therapeutic amounts when given orally or parenterally. High CSF concentrations of the drug may be attained by intrathecal administration.

In dogs, synovial fluid concentrations after oral dosing were higher in inflamed than uninflamed joints. Although salicylates did not interfere with this penetration, prior prednisone treatment reduced penetration into inflamed joints to the level of normal joints.

Metabolism—After absorption, methotrexate undergoes hepatic and intracellular metabolism to polyglutamated forms which can be converted back to methotrexate by hydrolase enzymes. These polyglutamates act as inhibitors of dihydrofolate reductase and thymidylate synthetase. Small amounts of methotrexate polyglutamates may remain in tissues for extended periods. The retention and prolonged drug action of these active metabolites vary among different cells, tissues and tumors. A small amount of metabolism to 7-hydroxymethotrexate may occur at doses commonly prescribed. Accumulation of this metabolite may become significant at the high doses used in osteogenic sarcoma. The aqueous solubility of 7-hydroxymethotrexate is 3 to 5 fold lower than the parent compound. Methotrexate is partially metabolized by intestinal flora after oral administration.

Half-Life—The terminal half-life reported for methotrexate is approximately three to ten hours for patients receiving treatment for psoriasis, or rheumatoid arthritis or low dose antineoplastic therapy (less than 30 mg/m^2). For patients receiving high doses of methotrexate, the terminal half-life is eight to 15 hours.

Excretion—Renal excretion is the primary route of elimination and is dependent upon dosage and route of administration. With IV administration, 80% to 90% of the administered dose is excreted unchanged in the urine within 24 hours. There is limited biliary excretion amounting to 10% or less of the administered dose. Enterohepatic recirculation of methotrexate has been proposed.

Renal excretion occurs by glomerular filtration and active tubular secretion. Nonlinear elimination due to saturation of renal tubular reabsorption has been observed in psoriatic patients at doses between 7.5 and 30 mg. Impaired renal function, as well as concurrent use of drugs such as weak organic acids that also undergo tubular secretion, can markedly increase methotrexate serum levels. Excellent correlation has been reported between methotrexate clearance and endogenous creatinine clearance.

Methotrexate clearance rates vary widely and are generally decreased at higher doses. Delayed drug clearance has been identified as one of the major factors responsible for methotrexate toxicity. It has been postulated that the toxicity of methotrexate for normal tissues is more dependent upon the duration of exposure to the drug rather than the peak level achieved. When a patient has delayed drug elimination due to compromised renal function, a third space effusion, or other causes, methotrexate serum concentrations may remain elevated for prolonged periods.

The potential for toxicity from high dose regimens or delayed excretion is reduced by the administration of leucovorin calcium during the final phase of methotrexate plasma elimination. Pharmacokinetic monitoring of methotrexate serum concentrations may help identify those patients at high risk for methotrexate toxicity and aid in proper adjustment of leucovorin dosing. Guidelines for monitoring serum methotrexate levels, and for adjustment of leucovorin dosing to reduce the risk of methotrexate toxicity, are provided below in DOSAGE AND ADMINISTRATION.

Methotrexate has been detected in human breast milk. The highest breast milk to plasma concentration ratio reached was 0.08:1.

INDICATIONS AND USAGE

Neoplastic Diseases

Methotrexate is indicated in the treatment of gestational choriocarcinoma, chorioadenoma destruens and hydatidiform mole.

In acute lymphocytic leukemia, methotrexate is indicated in the prophylaxis of meningeal leukemia and is used in maintenance therapy in combination with other chemotherapeutic agents. Methotrexate is also indicated in the treatment of meningeal leukemia.

Methotrexate is used alone or in combination with other anticancer agents in the treatment of breast cancer, epidermoid cancers of the head and neck, advanced mycosis fungoides, and lung cancer, particularly squamous cell and small cell types. Methotrexate is also used in combination with other chemotherapeutic agents in the treatment of advanced stage non-Hodgkin's lymphomas.

Methotrexate in high doses followed by leucovorin rescue in combination with other chemotherapeutic agents is effective in prolonging relapse-free survival in patients with non-metastatic osteosarcoma who have undergone surgical resection or amputation for the primary tumor.

Psoriasis

Methotrexate is indicated in the symptomatic control of severe. recalcitrant, disabling psoriasis that is not adequately responsive to other forms of therapy, *but only when the diagnosis has been established, as by biopsy and/or after dermatologic consultation.* It is important to ensure that a psoriasis "flare" is not due to an undiagnosed concomitant disease affecting immune responses.

Rheumatoid Arthritis

Methotrexate is indicated in the management of selected adults with severe, active, classical or definite rheumatoid

Continued on next page

Immunex—Cont.

arthritis (ARA criteria) who have had an insufficient therapeutic response to, or are intolerant of, an adequate trial of first-line therapy including full dose NSAIDs and usually a trial of at least one or more disease-modifying antirheumatic drugs.

Aspirin, nonsteroidal anti-inflammatory agents, and/or low dose steroids may be continued, although the possibility of increased toxicity with concomitant use of NSAIDs including salicylates has not been fully explored. (See PRECAUTIONS, Drug Interactions.) Steroids may be reduced gradually in patients who respond to methotrexate. Combined use of methotrexate with gold, penicillamine, hydroxychloroquine, sulfasalazine, or cytotoxic agents, has not been studied and may increase the incidence of adverse effects. Rest and physiotherapy as indicated should be continued.

CONTRAINDICATIONS

Methotrexate can cause fetal death or teratogenic effects when administered to a pregnant woman. Methotrexate is contraindicated in pregnant women with psoriasis or rheumatoid arthritis and should be used in the treatment of neoplastic diseases only when the potential benefit outweighs the risk to the fetus. Women of childbearing potential should not be started on methotrexate until pregnancy is excluded and should be fully counseled on the serious risk to the fetus (see PRECAUTIONS) should they become pregnant while undergoing treatment. Pregnancy should be avoided if either partner is receiving methotrexate; during and for a minimum of three months after therapy for male patients, and during and for at least one ovulatory cycle after therapy for female patients. (See Boxed WARNINGS.)

Because of the potential for serious adverse reactions from methotrexate in breast fed infants, it is contraindicated in nursing mothers.

Patients with psoriasis or rheumatoid arthritis with alcoholism, alcoholic liver disease or other chronic liver disease should not receive methotrexate.

Patients with psoriasis or rheumatoid arthritis who have overt or laboratory evidence of immunodeficiency syndromes should not receive methotrexate.

Patients with psoriasis or rheumatoid arthritis who have preexisting blood dyscrasias, such as bone marrow hypoplasia, leukopenia, thrombocytopenia or significant anemia, should not receive methotrexate.

Patients with a known hypersensitivity to methotrexate should not receive the drug.

WARNINGS—SEE BOXED WARNINGS.

PRECAUTIONS

General

Methotrexate has the potential for serious toxicity. (See Boxed WARNINGS.) Toxic effects may be related in frequency and severity to dose or frequency of administration but have been seen at all doses. Because they can occur at any time during therapy, it is necessary to follow patients on methotrexate closely. Most adverse reactions are reversible if detected early. When such reactions do occur, the drug should be reduced in dosage or discontinued and appropriate corrective measures should be taken. If necessary, this could include the use of leucovorin calcium. (See OVERDOSAGE.) If methotrexate therapy is reinstituted, it should be carried out with caution, with adequate consideration of further need for the drug and with increased alertness as to possible recurrence of toxicity.

The clinical pharmacology of methotrexate has not been well studied in older individuals. Due to diminished hepatic and renal function as well as decreased folate stores in this population, relatively low doses should be considered, and these patients should be closely monitored for early signs of toxicity.

Information for Patients

Patients should be informed of the early signs and symptoms of toxicity, of the need to see their physician promptly if they occur, and the need for close follow-up, including periodic laboratory tests to monitor toxicity.

Both the physician and pharmacist should emphasize to the patient that the recommended dose is taken weekly in rheumatoid arthritis and psoriasis, and that mistaken use of the recommended dose has led to fatal toxicity. Patients should be encouraged to read the Patient Instructions sheet within the Dose Pack. Prescriptions should not be written or refilled on a PRN basis.

Patients should be informed of the potential benefit and risk in the use of methotrexate. The risk of effects on reproduction should be discussed with both male and female patients taking methotrexate.

Laboratory Tests

Patients undergoing methotrexate therapy should be closely monitored so that toxic effects are detected promptly. Baseline assessment should include a complete blood count with differential and platelet counts, hepatic enzymes, renal function tests, and a chest X-ray. During therapy of rheumatoid arthritis and psoriasis, monitoring of these parameters is

recommended: hematology at least monthly, renal function and liver function every 1 to 2 months. More frequent monitoring is usually indicated during antineoplastic therapy. *During initial or changing doses*, or during periods of increased risk of elevated methotrexate blood levels (eg, dehydration), more frequent monitoring may also be indicated. Transient liver function test abnormalities are observed frequently after methotrexate administration and are usually not cause for modification of methotrexate therapy. Persistent liver function test abnormalities, and/or depression of serum albumin may be indicators of serious liver toxicity and require evaluation. (See PRECAUTIONS, Organ System Toxicity, *Hepatic*.)

A relationship between abnormal liver function tests and fibrosis or cirrhosis of the liver has not been established for patients with psoriasis. Persistent abnormalities in liver function tests may precede appearance of fibrosis or cirrhosis in the rheumatoid arthritis population.

Pulmonary function tests may be useful if methotrexate-induced lung disease is suspected, especially if baseline measurements are available.

Drug Interactions

Nonsteroidal anti-inflammatory drugs should not be administered prior to or concomitantly with the high doses of methotrexate used in the treatment of osteosarcoma. Concomitant administration of some NSAIDs with high dose methotrexate therapy has been reported to elevate and prolong serum methotrexate levels, resulting in deaths from severe hematologic and gastrointestinal toxicity.

Caution should be used when NSAIDs and salicylates are administered concomitantly with lower doses of methotrexate. These drugs have been reported to reduce the tubular secretion of methotrexate in an animal model and may enhance its toxicity.

Despite the potential interactions, studies of methotrexate in patients with rheumatoid arthritis have usually included concurrent use of constant dosage regimens of NSAIDs, without apparent problems. It should be appreciated, however, that the doses used in rheumatoid arthritis (7.5 to 15 mg/week) are somewhat lower than those used in psoriasis and that larger doses could lead to unexpected toxicity.

Methotrexate is partially bound to serum albumin, and toxicity may be increased because of displacement by certain drugs, such as salicylates, phenylbutazone, phenytoin, and sulfonamides. Renal tubular transport is also diminished by probenecid; use of methotrexate with this drug should be carefully monitored.

In the treatment of patients with osteosarcoma, caution must be exercised if high-dose methotrexate is administered in combination with a potentially nephrotoxic chemotherapeutic agent (eg, cisplatin).

Oral antibiotics such as tetracycline, chloramphenicol, and nonabsorbable broad spectrum antibiotics, may decrease intestinal absorption of methotrexate or interfere with the enterohepatic circulation by inhibiting bowel flora and suppressing metabolism of the drug by bacteria.

Penicillins may reduce the renal clearance of methotrexate; increased serum concentrations of methotrexate with concomitant hematologic and gastrointestinal toxicity have been observed with high and low dose methotrexate. Use of methotrexate with penicillins should be carefully monitored. Patients receiving concomitant therapy with methotrexate and etretinate or other retinoids should be monitored closely for possible increased risk of hepatotoxicity.

Methotrexate may decrease the clearance of theophylline; theophylline levels should be monitored when used concurrently with methotrexate.

Vitamin preparations containing folic acid or its derivatives may decrease responses to systemically administered methotrexate. Preliminary animal and human studies have shown that small quantities of intravenously administered leucovorin enter the CSF primarily as 5-methyltetrahydrofolate and, in humans, remain 1–3 orders of magnitude lower than the usual methotrexate concentrations following intrathecal administration. However, high doses of leucovorin may reduce the efficacy of intrathecally administered methotrexate.

Folate deficiency states may increase methotrexate toxicity. Trimethoprim/sulfamethoxazole has been reported rarely to increase bone marrow suppression in patients receiving methotrexate, probably by an additive antifolate effect.

Carcinogenesis, Mutagenesis, and Impairment of Fertility

No controlled human data exist regarding the risk of neoplasia with methotrexate. Methotrexate has been evaluated in a number of animal studies for carcinogenic potential with inconclusive results. Although there is evidence that methotrexate causes chromosomal damage to animal somatic cells and human bone marrow cells, the clinical significance remains uncertain. Non-Hodgkin's lymphoma and other tumors have been reported in patients receiving low-dose oral methotrexate. However, there have been instances of malignant lymphoma arising during treatment with low-dose oral methotrexate, which have regressed completely following withdrawal of methotrexate, without requiring active anti-lymphoma treatment. Benefits should be weighed against the potential risks before using methotrex-

ate alone or in combination with other drugs, especially in pediatric patients or young adults. Methotrexate causes embryotoxicity, abortion, and fetal defects in humans. It has also been reported to cause impairment of fertility, oligospermia and menstrual dysfunction in humans, during and for a short period after cessation of therapy.

Pregnancy

Psoriasis and rheumatoid arthritis: Methotrexate is in Pregnancy Category X. See CONTRAINDICATIONS.

Nursing Mothers

See CONTRAINDICATIONS.

Pediatric Use

Safety and effectiveness in pediatric patients have not been established, other than in cancer chemotherapy.

Organ System Toxicity

Gastrointestinal: If vomiting, diarrhea, or stomatitis occur, which may result in dehydration, methotrexate should be discontinued until recovery occurs. Methotrexate should be used with extreme caution in the presence of peptic ulcer disease or ulcerative colitis.

Hematologic: Methotrexate can suppress hematopoiesis and cause anemia, leukopenia, and/or thrombocytopenia. In patients with malignancy and preexisting hematopoietic impairment, the drug should be used with caution, if at all. In controlled clinical trials in rheumatoid arthritis (n=128), leukopenia (WBC <3000/mm^3) was seen in 2 patients, thrombocytopenia (platelets <100,000/mm^3) in 6 patients, and pancytopenia in 2 patients.

In psoriasis and rheumatoid arthritis, methotrexate should be stopped immediately if there is a significant drop in blood counts. In the treatment of neoplastic diseases, methotrexate should be continued only if the potential benefit warrants the risk of severe myelosuppression. Patients with profound granulocytopenia and fever should be evaluated immediately and usually require parenteral broad-spectrum antibiotic therapy.

Hepatic: Methotrexate has the potential for acute (elevated transaminases) and chronic (fibrosis and cirrhosis) hepatotoxicity. Chronic toxicity is potentially fatal; it generally has occurred after prolonged use (generally two years or more) and after a total dose of at least 1.5 grams. In studies in psoriatic patients, hepatotoxicity appeared to be a function of total cumulative dose and appeared to be enhanced by alcoholism, obesity, diabetes and advanced age. An accurate incidence rate has not been determined; the rate of progression and reversibility of lesions is not known. Special caution is indicated in the presence of preexisting liver damage or impaired hepatic function.

In psoriasis, liver function tests, including serum albumin, should be performed periodically prior to dosing but are often normal in the face of developing fibrosis or cirrhosis. These lesions may be detectable only by biopsy. The usual recommendation is to obtain a liver biopsy at 1) pretherapy or shortly after initiation of therapy (2–4 months), 2) a total cumulative dose of 1.5 grams, and 3) after each additional 1.0 to 1.5 grams.[1] Moderate fibrosis or cirrhosis normally leads to discontinuation of the drug; mild fibrosis normally suggests a repeat biopsy in 6 months. Milder histologic findings such as fatty change and low grade portal inflammation are relatively common pretherapy. Although these mild changes are usually not a reason to avoid or discontinue methotrexate therapy, the drug should be used with caution.

In rheumatoid arthritis, age at first use of methotrexate and duration of therapy have been reported as risk factors for hepatotoxicity; other risk factors, similar to those observed in psoriasis, may be present in rheumatoid arthritis but have not been confirmed to date. Persistent abnormalities in liver function tests may precede appearance of fibrosis or cirrhosis in this population. There is a combined reported experience in 217 rheumatoid arthritis patients with liver biopsies both before and during treatment (after a cumulative dose of at least 1.5 g) and in 714 patients with a biopsy only during treatment. There are 64 (7%) cases of fibrosis and 1 (0.1%) case of cirrhosis. Of the 64 cases of fibrosis, 60 were deemed mild. The reticulin stain is more sensitive for early fibrosis and its use may increase these figures. It is unknown whether even longer use will increase these risks.

Liver function tests should be performed at baseline and at 4–8 week intervals in patients receiving methotrexate for rheumatoid arthritis. Pretreatment liver biopsy should be performed for patients with a history of excessive alcohol consumption, persistently abnormal baseline liver function test values or chronic hepatitis B or C infection. During therapy, liver biopsy should be performed if there are persistent liver function test abnormalities or there is a decrease in serum albumin below the normal range (in the setting of well controlled rheumatoid arthritis).

If the results of a liver biopsy show mild changes (Roenigk grades I, II, IIIa), methotrexate may be continued and the patient monitored as per recommendations listed above. Methotrexate should be discontinued in any patient who displays persistently abnormal liver function tests and refuses liver biopsy or in any patient whose liver biopsy shows moderate to severe changes (Roenigk grade IIIb or IV).[2]

Infection or Immunologic States: Methotrexate should be used with extreme caution in the presence of active infection, and is usually contraindicated in patients with overt or laboratory evidence of immunodeficiency syndromes. Immunization may be ineffective when given during methotrexate therapy. Immunization with live virus vaccines is generally not recommended. There have been reports of disseminated vaccinia infections after smallpox immunization in patients receiving methotrexate therapy. Hypogammaglobulinemia has been reported rarely.

Opportunistic infections, including *Pneumocystis carinii* infections, have been reported rarely in patients receiving low dose methotrexate. When a patient presents with pulmonary symptoms, the possibility of *Pneumocystis carinii* pneumonia should be considered.

Neurologic: There have been reports of leukoencephalopathy following intravenous administration of methotrexate to patients who have had craniospinal irradiation. Chronic leukoencephalopathy has also been reported in patients who received repeated doses of high-dose methotrexate with leucovorin rescue without cranial irradiation. Discontinuation of methotrexate does not always result in complete recovery. A transient acute neurologic syndrome has been observed in patients treated with high dosage regimens. Manifestations of this stroke-like encephalopathy may include confusion, hemiparesis, seizures and coma. The exact cause is unknown.

After the intrathecal use of methotrexate, the central nervous system toxicity which may occur can be classified as follows: acute chemical arachnoiditis manifested by such symptoms as headache, back pain, nuchal rigidity, and fever; sub-acute myelopathy characterized by paraparesis/paraplegia associated with involvement with one or more spinal nerve roots; chronic leukoencephalopathy manifested by confusion, irritability, somnolence, ataxia, dementia, seizures and coma. This condition can be progressive and even fatal.

Pulmonary: Pulmonary symptoms (especially a dry nonproductive cough) or a nonspecific pneumonitis occurring during methotrexate therapy may be indicative of a potentially dangerous lesion and require interruption of treatment and careful investigation. Although clinically variable, the typical patient with methotrexate induced lung disease presents with fever, cough, dyspnea, hypoxemia, and an infiltrate on chest X-ray; infection needs to be excluded. This lesion can occur at all dosages.

Renal: High doses of methotrexate used in the treatment of osteosarcoma may cause renal damage leading to acute renal failure. Nephrotoxicity is due primarily to the precipitation of methotrexate and 7-hydroxymethotrexate in the renal tubules. Close attention to renal function including adequate hydration, urine alkalinization and measurement of serum methotrexate and creatinine levels are essential for safe administration.

Other Precautions: Methotrexate should be used with extreme caution in the presence of debility.

Methotrexate exits slowly from third space compartments (eg, pleural effusions or ascites). This results in prolonged terminal plasma half-life and unexpected toxicity. In patients with significant third space accumulations, it is advisable to evacuate the fluid before treatment and to monitor plasma methotrexate levels.

Lesions of psoriasis may be aggravated by concomitant exposure to ultraviolet radiation. Radiation dermatitis and sunburn may be "recalled" by the use of methotrexate.

ADVERSE REACTIONS

IN GENERAL, THE INCIDENCE AND SEVERITY OF ACUTE SIDE EFFECTS ARE RELATED TO DOSE AND FREQUENCY OF ADMINISTRATION. THE MOST SERIOUS REACTIONS ARE DISCUSSED ABOVE UNDER ORGAN SYSTEM TOXICITY IN THE PRECAUTION SECTION. THAT SECTION SHOULD ALSO BE CONSULTED WHEN LOOKING FOR INFORMATION ABOUT ADVERSE REACTIONS WITH METHOTREXATE.

The most frequently reported adverse reactions include ulcerative stomatitis, leukopenia, nausea, and abdominal distress. Other frequently reported adverse effects are malaise, undue fatigue, chills and fever, dizziness and decreased resistance to infection.

Other adverse reactions that have been reported with methotrexate are listed below by organ system. In the oncology setting, concomitant treatment and the underlying disease make specific attribution of a reaction to methotrexate difficult.

Alimentary System: gingivitis, pharyngitis, stomatitis, anorexia, nausea, vomiting, diarrhea, hematemesis, melena, gastrointestinal ulceration and bleeding, enteritis, pancreatitis.

Central Nervous System: headaches, drowsiness, blurred vision, Aphasia, hemiparesis, paresis and convulsions have also occurred following administration of methotrexate. Following low doses, occasional patients have reported transient subtle cognitive dysfunction, mood alteration, or unusual cranial sensations.

Ophthalmic: conjunctivitis, serious visual changes of unknown etiology.

Pulmonary System: interstitial pneumonitis deaths have been reported, and chronic interstitial obstructive pulmonary disease has occasionally occurred.

Skin: erythematous rashes, pruritus, urticaria, photosensitivity, pigmentary changes, alopecia, ecchymosis, telangiectasia, acne, furunculosis, erythema multiforme, toxic epidermal necrolysis, Stevens-Johnson syndrome.

Urogenital System: severe nephropathy or renal failure, azotemia, cystitis, hematuria; defective oogenesis or spermatogenesis, transient oligospermia, menstrual dysfunction and vaginal discharge; infertility, abortion, fetal defects.

Other rarer reactions related to or attributed to the use of methotrexate such as nodulosis, vasculitis, opportunistic infection, arthralgia/myalgia, loss of libido/impotence, diabetes, osteoporosis, sudden death, and reversible lymphomas. Anaphylactoid reactions have been reported .

Adverse Reactions in Double-Blind Rheumatoid Arthritis Studies

The approximate incidences of methotrexate attributed (ie, placebo rate subtracted) adverse reactions in 12 to 18 week double-blind studies of patients (n=128) with rheumatoid arthritis treated with low-dose oral (7.5 to 15 mg/week) pulse methotrexate, are listed below. Virtually all of these patients were on concomitant non-steroidal anti-inflammatory drugs and some were also taking low dosages of corticosteroids.

Incidence greater than 10%: Elevated liver function tests 15%, nausea/vomiting 10%.

Incidence 3% to 10%: Stomatitis, thrombocytopenia, (platelet count less than 100,000/mm^3).

Incidence 1% to 3%: Rash/pruritus/dermatitis, diarrhea, alopecia, leukopenia, (WBC less than 3000/mm^3), pancytopenia, dizziness.

No pulmonary toxicity was seen in these two trials. Thus, the incidence is probably less than 2.5% (95% C.L.). Hepatic histology was not examined in these short-term studies (See PRECAUTIONS.)

Other less common reactions included decreased hematocrit, headache, upper respiratory infection, anorexia, arthralgias, chest pain, coughing, dysuria, eye discomfort, epistaxis, fever, infection, sweating, tinnitus, and vaginal discharge.

Adverse Reactions in Psoriasis

There are no recent placebo-controlled trials in patients with psoriasis. There are two literature reports (Roenigk, 1969 and Nyfors, 1978) describing large series (n=204, 248) of psoriasis patients treated with methotrexate. Dosages ranged up to 25 mg per week and treatment was administered for up to four years. With the exception of alopecia, photosensitivity, and "burning of skin lesions" (each 3% to 10%), the adverse reaction rates in these reports were very similar to those in the rheumatoid arthritis studies.

OVERDOSAGE

Leucovorin is indicated to diminish the toxicity and counteract the effect of inadvertently administered overdosages of methotrexate. Leucovorin administration should begin as promptly as possible. As the time interval between methotrexate administration and leucovorin initiation increases, the effectiveness of leucovorin in counteracting toxicity decreases. Monitoring of the serum methotrexate concentration is essential in determining the optimal dose and duration of treatment with leucovorin.

In cases of massive overdosage, hydration and urinary alkalinization may be necessary to prevent the precipitation of methotrexate and/or its metabolites in the renal tubules. Neither hemodialysis nor peritoneal dialysis have been shown to improve methotrexate elimination.

Accidental intrathecal overdosage may require intensive systemic support, high-dose systemic leucovorin, alkaline diuresis and rapid CSF drainage and ventriculolumbar perfusion.

DOSAGE AND ADMINISTRATION

Neoplastic Diseases

Oral administration in tablet form is often preferred when low doses are being administered since absorption is rapid and effective serum levels are obtained. Methotrexate sodium injection and for injection may be given by the intramuscular, intravenous, intra-arterial or intrathecal route. However, the preserved formulation contains Benzyl Alcohol and must not be used for intrathecal or high dose therapy. Parenteral drug products should be inspected visually for particulate matter and discoloration prior to administration, whenever solution and container permit.

Choriocarcinoma and similar trophoblastic diseases: Methotrexate is administered orally or intramuscularly in doses of 15 to 30 mg daily for a five-day course. Such courses are usually repeated for 3 to 5 times as required, with rest periods of one or more weeks interposed between courses, until any manifesting toxic symptoms subside. The effectiveness of therapy is ordinarily evaluated by 24 quantitative analysis of urinary chorionic gonadotropin (hCG), which should return to normal or less than 50 IU/24 hr usually after the third or fourth course and usually be followed by a complete resolution of measurable lesions in 4 to 6 weeks. One to two courses of methotrexate after normalization of hCG is usually recommended. Before each course of the drug careful clinical assessment is essential. Cyclic combination therapy of methotrexate with other antitumor drugs has been reported as being useful.

Since hydatidiform mole may precede choriocarcinoma, prophylactic chemotherapy with methotrexate has been recommended.

Chorioadenoma destruens is considered to be an invasive form of hydratidiform mole. Methotrexate is administered in these disease states in doses similar to those recommended for choriocarcinoma.

Leukemia: Acute lymphoblastic leukemia in pediatric patients and young adolescents is the most responsive to present day chemotherapy. In young adults and older patients, clinical remission is more difficult to obtain and early relapse is more common.

Methotrexate alone or in combination with steroids was used initially for induction of remission in acute lymphoblastic leukemias. More recently corticosteroid therapy, in combination with other antileukemic drugs or in cyclic combinations with methotrexate included, has appeared to produce rapid and effective remissions. When used for induction, methotrexate in doses of 3.3 mg/m^2 in combination with 60 mg/m^2 of prednisone, given daily, produced remissions in 50% of patients treated, usually within a period of 4 to 6 weeks. Methotrexate in combination with other agents appears to be the drug of choice for securing maintenance of drug-induced remissions. When remission is achieved and supportive care has produced general clinical improvement, maintenance therapy is initiated, as follows: Methotrexate is administered 2 times weekly either by mouth or intramuscularly in total weekly doses of 30 mg/m^2. It has also been given in doses of 2.5 mg/kg intravenously every 14 days. If and when relapse does occur, reinduction of remission can again usually be obtained by repeating the initial induction regimen.

A variety of combination chemotherapy regimens have been used for both induction and maintenance therapy in acute lymphoblastic leukemia. The physician should be familiar with the new advances in antileukemic therapy.

Meningeal Leukemia: In the treatment or prophylaxis of meningeal leukemia, methotrexate must be administered intrathecally.

Preservative free methotrexate is diluted to a concentration of 1 mg/mL in an appropriate sterile, preservative free medium such as 0.9% Sodium Chloride Injection, USP.

The cerebrospinal fluid volume is dependent on age and not on body surface area. The CSF is at 40% of the adult volume at birth and reaches the adult volume in several years.

Intrathecal methotrexate administration at a dose of 12 mg/m^2 (maximum 15 mg) has been reported to result in low CSF methotrexate concentrations and reduced efficacy in pediatric patients and high concentrations and neurotoxicity in adults. The following dosage regimen is based on age instead of body surface area:

Age (years)	Dose (mg)
<1	6
1	8
2	10
3 or older	12

In one study in patients under the age of 40, this dosage regimen appeared to result in more consistent CSF methotrexate concentrations and less neurotoxicity. Another study in pediatric patients with acute lymphocytic leukemia compared this regimen to a dose of 12 mg/m^2 (maximum 15 mg), a significant reduction in the rate of CNS relapse was observed in the group whose dose was based on age.

Because the CSF volume and turnover may decrease with age, a dose reduction may be indicated in elderly patients. For the treatment of meningeal leukemia, intrathecal methotrexate may be given at intervals of 2 to 5 days. However, administration at intervals of less than 1 week may result in increased subacute toxicity. Methotrexate is administered until the cell count of the cerebrospinal fluid returns to normal. At this point one additional dose is advisable. For prophylaxis against meningeal leukemia, the dosage is the same as for treatment except for the intervals of administration. On this subject, it is advisable for the physician to consult the medical literature.

Untoward side effects may occur with any given intrathecal injection and are commonly neurological in character. Large doses may cause convulsions. Methotrexate given by the intrathecal route appears significantly in the systemic circulation and may cause systemic methotrexate toxicity. Therefore, systemic antileukemic therapy with the drug should be appropriately adjusted, reduced, or discontinued. Focal leukemic involvement of the central nervous system may not

Continued on next page

Immunex—Cont.

respond to intrathecal chemotherapy and is best treated with radiotherapy.

Lymphomas: In Burkitt's tumor, Stages I–II, methotrexate has produced prolonged remissions in some cases. Recommended dosage is 10 to 25 mg/day orally for 4 to 8 days. In Stage III, methotrexate is commonly given concomitantly with other antitumor agents. Treatment in all stages usually consists of several courses of the drug interposed with 7 to 10 day rest periods. Lymphosarcomas in Stage III may respond to combined drug therapy with methotrexate given in doses of 0.625 to 2.5 mg/kg daily.

Mycosis Fungoides: Therapy with methotrexate appears to produce clinical remissions in one half of the cases treated. Dosage is usually 2.5 to 10 mg daily by mouth for weeks or months. Dose levels of drug and adjustment of dose regimen by reduction or cessation of drug are guided by patient response and hematologic monitoring. Methotrexate has also been given intramuscularly in doses of 50 mg once weekly or 25 mg 2 times weekly.

Osteosarcoma: An effective adjuvant chemotherapy regimen requires the administration of several cytotoxic chemotherapeutic agents. In addition to high-dose methotrexate with leucovorin rescue, these agents may include doxorubicin, cisplatin, and the combination of bleomycin, cyclophosphamide and dactinomycin (BCD) in the doses and schedule shown in the table below. The starting dose for high dose methotrexate treatment is 12 grams/m^2. If this dose is not sufficient to produce peak serum methotrexate concentration of 1,000 micromolar (10^{-3}mol/L) at the end of the methotrexate infusion, the dose may be escalated to 15 grams/m^2 in subsequent treatments. If the patient is vomiting or is unable to tolerate oral medication, leucovorin is given IV or IM at the same dose and schedule.

[See table below.]

When these higher doses of methotrexate are to be administered, the following safety guidelines should be closely observed.

GUIDELINES FOR METHOTREXATE THERAPY WITH LEUCOVORIN RESCUE

1. Administration of methotrexate should be delayed until recovery if:
- the WBC count is less than 1500/microliter
- the neutrophil count is less than 200/microliter
- the platelet count is less than 75,000/microliter
- the serum bilirubin level is greater than 1.2 mg/dL
- the SGPT level is greater than 450 U
- mucositis is present, until there is evidence of healing
- persistent pleural effusion is present; this should be drained dry prior to infusion.

2. Adequate renal function must be documented.

a. Serum creatinine must be normal, and creatinine clearance must be greater than 60 mL/min, before initiation of therapy.

b. Serum creatinine must be measured prior to each subsequent course of therapy. If serum creatinine has increased by 50% or more compared to a prior value, the creatinine clearance must be measured and documented to be greater than 60 mL/min (even if the serum creatinine is still within the normal range).

3. Patients must be well hydrated, and must be treated with sodium bicarbonate for urinary alkalinization.

a. Administer 1,000 mL/m^2 of intravenous fluid over 6 hours prior to initiation of the methotrexate infusion. Continue hydration at 125 mL/m^2hr (3 liters/m^2/day) during the methotrexate infusion, and for 2 days after the infusion has been completed.

b. Alkalinize urine to maintain pH above 7.0 during methotrexate infusion and leucovorin calcium therapy. This can be accomplished by the administration of sodium bicarbonate orally or by incorporation into a separate intravenous solution.

4. Repeat serum creatinine and serum methotrexate 24 hours after starting methotrexate and at least once daily until the methotrexate level is below 5×10^{-8} mol/L (0.05 micromolar).

5. The table below provides guidelines for leucovorin calcium dosage based upon serum methotrexate levels. (See table below.‡)

Patients who experience delayed early methotrexate elimination are likely to develop nonreversible oliguric renal failure. In addition to appropriate leucovorin therapy, these patients require continuing hydration and urinary alkalinization, and close monitoring of fluid and electrolyte status, until the serum methotrexate level has fallen to below 0.05 micromolar and the renal failure has resolved.

6. Some patients will have abnormalities in methotrexate elimination, or abnormalities in renal function following methotrexate administration, which are significant but less severe than the abnormalities described in the table below. These abnormalities may or may not be associated with significant clinical toxicity. If significant clinical toxicity is observed, leucovorin rescue should be extended for an additional 24 hours (total 14 doses over 84 hours) in subsequent courses of therapy. The possibility that the patient is taking other medications which interact with methotrexate (eg, medications which may interfere with methotrexate binding to serum albumin, or elimination) should always be reconsidered when laboratory abnormalities or clinical toxicities are observed.

CAUTION: DO NOT ADMINISTER LEUCOVORIN INTRATHECALLY.

Psoriasis and Rheumatoid Arthritis

The patient should be fully informed of the risks involved and should be under constant supervision of the physician. (See Information for Patients Under PRECAUTIONS.) Assessment of hematologic, hepatic, renal, and pulmonary function should be made by history, physical examination, and laboratory tests before beginning, periodically during, and before reinstituting methotrexate therapy. (See PRECAUTIONS.) Appropriate steps should be taken to avoid conception during methotrexate therapy. (See PRECAUTIONS AND CONTRAINDICATIONS.)

Weekly therapy may be instituted with the RHEUMATREX® Methotrexate Sodium 2.5 mg Tablet Dose Packs which are designed to provide doses over a range of 5 mg to 15 mg administered as a single weekly dose. The dose packs are not recommended for administration of methotrexate in weekly doses greater than 15 mg. All schedules should be continually tailored to the individual patient. An initial test dose may be given prior to the regular dosing schedule to detect any extreme sensitivity to adverse effects. (See ADVERSE REACTIONS.) Maximal myelosuppression usually occurs in seven to ten days.

Psoriasis: Recommended Starting Dose Schedules

1. Weekly single oral, IM or IV dose schedule: 10 to 25 mg per week until adequate response is achieved.
2. Divided oral dose schedule: 2.5 mg at 12-hour intervals for three doses.

Dosages in each schedule may be gradually adjusted to achieve optimal clinical response; 30 mg/week should not ordinarily be exceeded.

Once optimal clinical response has been achieved, each dosage schedule should be reduced to the lowest possible amount of drug and to the longest possible rest period. The use of methotrexate may permit the return to conventional topical therapy. which should be encouraged.

Rheumatoid Arthritis: Recommended Starting Dosage Schedules

1. Single oral doses of 7.5 mg once weekly.
2. Divided oral dosages of 2.5 mg at 12 hour intervals for 3 doses given as a course once weekly.

Dosages in each schedule may be adjusted gradually to achieve an optimal response, but not ordinarily to exceed a total weekly dose of 20 mg. Limited experience shows a significant increase in the incidence and severity of serious toxic reactions, especially bone marrow suppression, at doses greater than 20 mg/wk.

Once response has been achieved, each schedule should be reduced, if possible, to the lowest possible effective dose.

Therapeutic response usually begins within 3 to 6 weeks and the patient may continue to improve for another 12 weeks or more.

The optimal duration of therapy is unknown. Limited data available from long-term studies indicate that the initial clinical improvement is maintained for at least two years with continued therapy. When methotrexate is discontinued, the arthritis usually worsens within 3 to 6 weeks.

HANDLING AND DISPOSAL

Procedures for proper handling and disposal of anticancer drugs should be considered. Several guidelines on this subject have been published.[3–8] There is no general agreement that all of the procedures recommended in the guidelines are necessary or appropriate.

RECONSTITUTION OF LYOPHILIZED POWDERS

Reconstitute immediately prior to use.

Methotrexate Sodium for Injection should be reconstituted with an appropriate sterile, preservative free medium such as 5% Dextrose Solution, USP, or Sodium Chloride Injection, USP. Reconstitute the 20 and 50 mg vials to a concentration no greater than 25 mg/mL. **The 1 gram vial should be reconstituted with 19.4 mL to a concentration of 50 mg/mL.** When high doses of methotrexate are administered by IV infusion, the total dose is diluted in 5% Dextrose Solution. For intrathecal injection, reconstitute to a concentration of 1 mg/mL with an appropriate sterile, preservative free medium such as Sodium Chloride Injection, USP.

DILUTION INSTRUCTIONS FOR LIQUID METHOTREXATE SODIUM INJECTION PRODUCTS

Methotrexate Sodium Injection, Isotonic Liquid, Contains Preservative

If desired, the solution may be further diluted with a compatible medium such as Sodium Chloride Injection, USP. Storage for 24 hours at a temperature of 21 to 25°C results in a product which is within 90% of label potency.

Methotrexate LPF® Sodium (methotrexate sodium injection), Isotonic Liquid, Preservative Free, for Single Use Only

If desired, the solution may be further diluted immediately prior to use with an appropriate sterile, preservative free medium such as 5% Dextrose Solution, USP or Sodium Chloride Injection, USP.

HOW SUPPLIED

Parenteral:

Methotrexate Sodium for Injection, Lyophilized, Preservative Free, for Single Use Only. Each 20 mg, 50 mg and 1 g vial of lyophilized powder contains methotrexate sodium equivalent to 20 mg, 50 mg and 1 g methotrexate respectively.

20 mg Vial—NDC 58406-671-01
50 mg Vial—NDC 58406-671-03
1g Vial—NDC 58406-671-05

Methotrexate LPF® Sodium (methotrexate sodium injection), Isotonic Liquid, Preservative Free, for Single Use Only. Each 25 mg/mL, 2 mL, 4 mL, 8 mL and 10 mL vial contains methotrexate sodium equivalent to 50 mg, 100 mg, 200 mg and 250 mg methotrexate respectively.

50 mg—2 mL Vial—NDC 58406-683-15
100 mg—4 mL Vial—NDC 58406-683-18
200 mg—8 mL Vial—NDC 58406-683-12
250 mg—10 mL Vial—NDC 58406-683-16

Methotrexate Sodium Injection, Isotonic Liquid, Contains Preservative. Each 25 mg/mL, 2 mL and 10 mL vial contains methotrexate sodium equivalent to 50 mg and 250 mg methotrexate respectively.

50 mg—2 mL Vial—NDC 58406-681-14
250 mg—10 mL Vial—NDC 58406-681-17

STORE BETWEEN 15°–25°C (59°–77°F). PROTECT FROM LIGHT.

IMMUNEX®

Manufactured for
IMMUNEX CORPORATION, Seattle, WA 98101
by
LEDERLE PARENTERALS, INC., Carolina, Puerto Rico 00987

Oral:

Description

Methotrexate Sodium Tablets contain an amount of methotrexate sodium equivalent to 2.5 mg of methotrexate and are round, convex, yellow tablets, engraved with LL on

Drug*	Dose*	Treatment Week After Surgery
Methotrexate	12 g/m^2 IV as 4 hour infusion (starting dose)	4, 5, 6, 7, 11, 12, 15, 16, 29, 30, 44, 45
Leucovorin	15 mg orally every six hours for 10 doses starting at 24 hours after start of methotrexate infusion.	
Doxorubicin† as a single drug	30 mg/m^2/day IV × 3 days	8, 17
Doxorubicin†	50 mg/m^2 IV	20, 23, 33, 36
Cisplatin†	100 mg/m^2 IV	20, 23, 33, 36
Bleomycin†	15 units/m^2 IV × 2 days	2, 13, 26, 39, 42
Cyclophosphamide†	600 mg/m^2 IV × 2 days	2, 13, 26, 39, 42
Dactinomycin†	0.6 mg/m^2 IV × 2 days	2, 13, 26, 39, 42

* Link MP, Goorin AM, Miser AW, et al: The effect of adjuvant chemotherapy on relapse-free survival in patients with osteosarcoma of the extremity. *N Engl J Med* 1986; 314 (No.25):1600–1606.

† See each respective package insert for full Prescribing Information. Dosage modifications may be necessary because of drug-induced toxicity.

‡LEUCOVORIN RESCUE SCHEDULES FOLLOWING TREATMENT WITH HIGHER DOSES OF METHOTREXATE

Clinical Situation	Laboratory Findings	Leucovorin Dosage and Duration
Normal Methotrexate Elimination	Serum methotrexate level approximately 10 micromolar at 24 hours after administration, 1 micromolar at 48 hours, and less than 0.2 micromolar at 72 hours.	15 mg PO, IM, or IV q 6 hours for 60 hours (10 doses starting at 24 hours after start of methotrexate infusion).
Delayed Late Methotrexate Elimination	Serum methotrexate level remaining above 0.2 micromolar at 72 hours, and more than 0.05 micromolar at 96 hours after administration.	Continue 15 mg PO, IM, or IV q six hours, until methotrexate level is less than 0.05 micromolar.
Delayed Early Methotrexate Elimination and/or Evidence of Acute Renal Injury	Serum methotrexate level of 50 micromolar or more at 24 hours, or 5 micromolar or more at 48 hours after administration, OR; a 100% or greater increase in serum creatinine level at 24 hours after methotrexate administration (eg, an increase from 0.5 mg/dL to a level of 1.0 mg/dL or more).	150 mg IV q three hours, until methotrexate level is less than 1 micromolar; then 15 mg IV q three hours, until methotrexate level is less than 0.05 micromolar.

one side, scored in half on the other side, and engraved with M above the score, and 1 below.

NDC 0005-4507-23—Bottle of 100

RHEUMATREX® Methotrexate Sodium Tablet 2.5 mg Dose Packs—(each tablet equivalent to 2.5 mg of methotrexate)

NDC 0005-4507-04—RHEUMATREX® Methotrexate Sodium Tablets Dose Pack—4 cards each containing two 2.5 mg tablets, ie, 5 mg per week.

NDC 0005-4507-05—RHEUMATREX® Methotrexate Sodium Tablets Dose Pack—4 cards each containing three 2.5 mg tablets, ie, 7.5 mg per week.

NDC 0005-4507-07—RHEUMATREX® Methotrexate Sodium Tablets Dose Pack—4 cards each containing four 2.5 mg tablets, ie, 10 mg per week.

NDC 0005-4507-09—RHEUMATREX® Methotrexate Sodium Tablets Dose Pack—4 cards each containing five 2.5 mg tablets, ie, 12.5 mg per week.

NDC 0005-4507-91—RHEUMATREX® Methotrexate Sodium Tablets Dose Pack—4 cards each containing six 2.5 mg tablets, ie, 15 mg per week.

STORE AT CONTROLLED ROOM TEMPERATURE 15°–30°C (59°–86°F). PROTECT FROM LIGHT.

LEDERLE LABORATORIES DIVISION
Pearl River, NY 10965
CI 4814-1   Issued 2/96
Rev 0168-02
©1996

REFERENCES

1. Roenigk HH, Auerbach R, Maibach HI, et al. Methotrexate in Psoriasis: Revised Guidelines. *J Am Acad Dermatol* 1988; 19:145–156.
2. Kremer JM, et al. Methotrexate for Rheumatoid Arthritis: Suggested Guidelines for Monitoring Liver Toxicity. *Arth Rheum* 1994; 37:316–328.
3. Recommendations for the Safe Handling of Parenteral Antineoplastic Drugs, NIH Publication No. 83-2621. For sale by the Superintendent of Documents, US Government Printing Office, Washington, DC 20402.
4. AMA Council Report. Guidelines for Handling Parenteral Antineoplastics. *JAMA*, March 15, 1985.
5. National Study Commission on Cytotoxic Exposure— Recommendations for Handling Cytotoxic Agents. Available from Louis P. Jeffrey, ScD, Chairman, National Study Commission on Cytotoxic Exposure, Massachusetts College of Pharmacy and Allied Health Sciences, 179 Longwood Avenue, Boston, Massachusetts 02115.
6. Clinical Oncological Society of Australia: Guidelines and recommendations for safe handling of antineoplastic agents. *Med J Australia* 1983; 1:426–428.
7. Jones RB, et al. Safe handling of chemotherapeutic agents: A report from the Mount Sinai Medical Center. *Ca—A Cancer Journal for Clinicians* Sept/Oct 1983; 258–263.
8. American Society of Hospital Pharmacists technical assistance bulletin on handling cytotoxic and hazardous drugs. *Am J Hosp Pharm* 1990; 47:1033–1049.

[See table above.]

NOVANTRONE®   ℞
[nō-văn-trōne]
Mitoxantrone for Injection Concentrate

DESCRIPTION

NOVANTRONE® (mitoxantrone hydrochloride) is a synthetic antineoplastic anthracenedione for intravenous use. The molecular formula is $C_{22}H_{28}N_4O_6 \cdot 2HCl$ and the molecular weight is 517.41. It is supplied as a concentrate which MUST BE DILUTED PRIOR TO INJECTION. The concentrate is a sterile, nonpyrogenic, dark blue aqueous solution containing mitoxantrone hydrochloride equivalent to 2 mg/mL mitoxantrone free base, with sodium chloride (0.80% w/v), sodium acetate (0.005% w/v), and acetic acid (0.046% w/v) as inactive ingredients. The solution has a pH of 3.0 to 4.5 and contains 0.14 mEq of sodium per mL. The product does not contain preservatives. The chemical name is: 1,4-dihydroxy-5, 8-bis [[2-[(2-hydroxyethyl) amino] ethyl] amino]-9, 10-anthracenedione dihydrochloride and the structural formula is:.

CLINICAL PHARMACOLOGY

Although its mechanism of action is not fully elucidated, NOVANTRONE is a DNA-reactive agent. It has a cytocidal effect on both proliferating and nonproliferating cultured human cells, suggesting lack of cell cycle phase specificity. Pharmacokinetic studies have not been performed in humans receiving multiple daily doses. Pharmacokinetic studies in adult patients following a single intravenous administration of NOVANTRONE have demonstrated multi-exponential plasma clearance. Distribution to tissues is rapid and extensive. Distribution to the brain, spinal cord, eye, and spinal fluid in the monkey is low. The apparent steady-state volume of distribution exceeds 1,000 L/m^2. Elimination of drug is slow with an apparent mean terminal plasma half-life of 5.8 days (range 2.3–13.0). The half-life in tissues may be longer. Multiple intravenous doses in dogs daily for 5 days resulted in significant accumulation in plasma and tissue. The extent of accumulation was fourfold. NOVANTRONE is 78% bound to plasma proteins in the observed concentration range of 26–455 ng/mL. This binding is independent of concentration and was not affected by the presence of phenytoin, doxorubicin, methotrexate, prednisone, prednisolone, heparin, or aspirin.

NOVANTRONE is excreted via the renal and hepatobiliary systems. Renal excretion is limited; only 6%–11% of the dose is recovered in the urine within five days after drug administration. Of the material recovered in the urine, 65% is unchanged drug; the remaining 35% is comprised primarily of two inactive metabolites and their glucuronide conjugates. The metabolites are mono- and dicarboxylic acid derivatives. Hepatobiliary elimination of drug appears to be of greater significance with as much as 25% of the dose recovered in the feces within 5 days of intravenous dosing. No significant difference in the pharmacokinetics of

NOVANTRONE was observed in seven patients with moderately impaired liver function (serum bilirubin 1.3–3.4 mg/dL) as compared with 16 patients without hepatic dysfunction. Results of pharmacokinetic studies in four patients with severe hepatic dysfunction (bilirubin greater than 3.4 mg/dL) suggest that these patients have a lower total body clearance and a larger area under curve than other patients at a comparable NOVANTRONE dose.

In two large randomized multicenter trials, remission induction therapy for acute nonlymphocytic leukemia (ANLL) with NOVANTRONE 12 mg/m² daily for 3 days as a 10-minute intravenous infusion and cytarabine 100 mg/m² for 7 days given as a continuous 24-hour infusion was compared with daunorubicin 45 mg/m² daily by intravenous infusion for 3 days plus the same dose and schedule of cytarabine used with NOVANTRONE. Patients who had an incomplete antileukemic response received a second induction course in which NOVANTRONE or daunorubicin was given for 2 days and cytarabine for 5 days using the same daily dosage schedule. Response rates and median survival information for both the U.S. and international multicenter trials are given in the following table:

Trial	% Complete Response (CR)		Median Time to CR (days)		Median Survival (days)	
	NOV	**DAUN**	**NOV**	**DAUN**	**NOV**	**DAUN**
U.S.	63 (62/98)	53 (54/102)	35	42	312	237
International	50 (56/112)	51 (62/123)	36	42	192	230

NOV = NOVANTRONE® + Cytarabine
DAUN = daunorubicin + Cytarabine

In these studies, two consolidation courses were administered to complete responders on each arm. Consolidation therapy consisted of the same drug and daily dosage used for remission induction, only 5 days of cytarabine and 2 days of NOVANTRONE or daunorubicin were given. The first consolidation course was administered 6 weeks after the start of the final induction course if the patient achieved a complete remission. The second consolidation course was generally administered 4 weeks later. Full hematologic recovery was necessary for patients to receive consolidation therapy. For the U.S. trial, median granulocyte nadirs for patients receiving NOVANTRONE + cytarabine for consolidation courses 1 and 2 were 10/mm³ for both courses, and for those patients receiving daunorubicin + cytarabine were 170/mm³ and 260/mm³, respectively. Median platelet nadirs for patients who received NOVANTRONE + cytarabine for consolidation courses 1 and 2 were 17,000/mm³ and 14,000/mm³, respectively, and were 33,000/mm³ and 22,000/mm³ in courses 1 and 2 for those patients who received daunorubicin + cytarabine. The benefit of consolidation therapy in ANLL patients who achieve a complete remission remains controversial. However, in the only well-controlled prospective, randomized multicenter trials with NOVANTRONE in ANLL, consolidation therapy was given to all patients who achieved a complete remission. During consolidation in the U.S. study, two myelosuppression-related deaths occurred on the NOVANTRONE arm and one on the daunorubicin arm. However, in the international study there were eight deaths on the NOVANTRONE arm during consolidation which were related to the myelosuppression and none on the daunorubicin arm where less myelosuppression occurred.

INDICATIONS AND USAGE

NOVANTRONE in combination with other approved drug(s) is indicated in the initial therapy of acute nonlymphocytic leukemia (ANLL) in adults. This category includes myelogenous, promyelocytic, monocytic, and erythroid acute leukemias.

CONTRAINDICATIONS

NOVANTRONE is contraindicated in patients who have demonstrated prior hypersensitivity to it.

WARNINGS

WHEN NOVANTRONE IS USED IN DOSES INDICATED FOR THE TREATMENT OF LEUKEMIA, SEVERE MYELOSUPPRESSION WILL OCCUR. THEREFORE, IT IS RECOMMENDED THAT NOVANTRONE BE ADMINISTERED ONLY BY PHYSICIANS EXPERIENCED IN THE CHEMOTHERAPY OF THIS DISEASE. LABORATORY AND SUPPORTIVE SERVICES MUST BE AVAILABLE FOR HEMATOLOGIC AND CHEMISTRY MONITORING AND ADJUNCTIVE THERAPIES, INCLUDING ANTIBIOTICS. BLOOD AND BLOOD PRODUCTS MUST BE AVAILABLE TO SUPPORT PATIENTS DURING THE EXPECTED PERIOD OF MEDULLARY HYPOPLASIA AND SEVERE MYELOSUPPRESSION. PARTICULAR CARE SHOULD BE GIVEN TO ASSURING FULL HEMATOLOGIC RECOVERY BEFORE UNDERTAKING CONSOLIDATION THERAPY (IF THIS TREATMENT IS

Continued on next page

Immunex—Cont.

USED) AND PATIENTS SHOULD BE MONITORED CLOSELY DURING THIS PHASE.

Patients with preexisting myelosuppression as the result of prior drug therapy should not receive NOVANTRONE unless it is felt that the possible benefit from such treatment warrants the risk of further medullary suppression.

The safety of NOVANTRONE in patients with hepatic insufficiency is not established. (See **CLINICAL PHARMACOLOGY** section.)

Safety for use by routes other than intravenous administration has not been established.

Pregnancy Category D—NOVANTRONE may cause fetal harm when administered to a pregnant woman. In treated rats, at doses of ≥ 0.1 mg/kg (0.05 fold the recommended human dose on a mg/m^2 basis) low fetal birth weight and retarded development of the fetal kidney were seen in greater frequency. In treated rabbits, an increased incidence of premature delivery was observed at doses ≥ 0.01 mg/kg (0.01 fold the recommended human dose on a mg/m^2 basis). NOVANTRONE was not teratogenic in rabbits. There are no adequate and well-controlled studies in pregnant women. If this drug is used during pregnancy, or if the patient becomes pregnant while taking this drug, the patient should be apprised of the potential hazard to the fetus. Women of childbearing potential should be advised to avoid becoming pregnant.

Cardiac Effects

Because of the possible danger of cardiac effects in patients previously treated with daunorubicin or doxorubicin, the benefit-to-risk ratio of NOVANTRONE therapy in such patients should be determined before starting therapy.

General—Functional cardiac changes including decreases in left ventricular ejection fraction (LVEF) and irreversible congestive heart failure can occur with NOVANTRONE. Cardiac toxicity may be more common in patients with prior treatment with anthracyclines, prior mediastinal radiotherapy, or with preexisting cardiovascular disease. Such patients should have regular cardiac monitoring of LVEF from the initiation of therapy. In investigational trials of intermittent single doses in other tumor types, patients who received up to the cumulative dose of 140 mg/m^2 had a cumulative 2.6% probability of clinical congestive heart failure. The overall cumulative probability rate of moderate or serious decreases in LVEF at this dose was 13% in comparative trials.

Leukemia—Acute congestive heart failure may occasionally occur in patients treated with NOVANTRONE for ANLL. In first-line comparative trials of NOVANTRONE + cytarabine vs daunorubicin + cytarabine in adult patients with previously untreated ANLL, therapy was associated with congestive heart failure in 6.5% of patients on each arm. A causal relationship between drug therapy and cardiac effects is difficult to establish in this setting since myocardial function is frequently depressed by the anemia, fever and infection, and hemorrhage, which often accompany the underlying disease.

PRECAUTIONS

General: Therapy with NOVANTRONE should be accompanied by close and frequent monitoring of hematologic and chemical laboratory parameters, as well as frequent patient observation.

Hyperuricemia may occur as a result of rapid lysis of tumor cells by NOVANTRONE. Serum uric acid levels should be monitored and hypouricemic therapy instituted prior to the initiation of antileukemic therapy.

Systemic infections should be treated concomitantly with or just prior to commencing therapy with NOVANTRONE.

Information for Patients: NOVANTRONE may impart a blue-green color to the urine for 24 hours after administration, and patients should be advised to expect this during therapy. Bluish discoloration of the sclera may also occur. Patients should be advised of the signs and symptoms of myelosuppression.

Laboratory Tests: Serial complete blood counts and liver function tests are necessary for appropriate dose adjustments. (See **DOSAGE AND ADMINISTRATION** section.)

Carcinogenesis, Mutagenesis: NOVANTRONE can result in chromosomal aberrations in animals and it is mutagenic in bacterial systems. NOVANTRONE caused DNA damage and sister chromatid exchanges *in vitro*. Topoisomerase II inhibitors, including NOVANTRONE, in combination with other antineoplastic agents, have been associated with the development of acute leukemia.

Pregnancy Category D: (See **WARNINGS** section.)

Nursing Mothers: It is not known whether NOVANTRONE is excreted in human milk. Because of the potential for serious adverse reactions in infants from NOVANTRONE, breast feeding should be discontinued before starting treatment.

Pediatric Use: Safety and effectiveness in children have not been established.

ADVERSE REACTIONS

NOVANTRONE has been studied in approximately 600 patients with ANLL. The table below represents the adverse reaction experience in the large U.S. comparative study of mitoxantrone + cytarabine vs daunorubicin + cytarabine. Experience in the large international study was similar. A much wider experience in a variety of other tumor types revealed no additional important reactions other than cardiomyopathy (See WARNINGS section.) It should be appreciated that the listed adverse reaction categories include overlapping clinical symptoms related to the same condition, e.g., dyspnea, cough and pneumonia. In addition, the listed adverse reactions cannot all necessarily be attributed to chemotherapy as it is often impossible to distinguish effects of the drug and effects of the underlying disease. It is clear, however, that the combination of NOVANTRONE + cytarabine was responsible for nausea and vomiting, alopecia, mucositis/stomatitis, and myelosuppression.

The following table summarizes adverse reactions occurring in patients treated with NOVANTRONE + cytarabine in comparison with those who received daunorubicin + cytarabine for therapy of ANLL in a large multicenter randomized prospective U.S. trial. Adverse reactions are presented as major categories and selected examples of clinically significant subcategories.

[See table below.]

Allergic Reaction: Hypotension, urticaria, dyspnea, and rashes have been reported occasionally.

Cutaneous: Phlebitis has been reported infrequently at the site of infusion. There have been rare reports of tissue necrosis following extravasation.

Hematologic: Myelosuppression is rapid in onset and is consistent with the requirement to produce significant marrow hypoplasia in order to achieve a response. The incidences of infection and bleeding seen in the U.S. trial are consistent with those reported for other standard induction regimens. Topoisomerase II inhibitors, including NOVANTRONE, in combination with other antineoplastic agents, have been associated with the development of acute leukemia.

Gastrointestinal: Nausea and vomiting occurred acutely in most patients, but were generally mild to moderate and could be controlled through the use of antiemetics. Stomatitis/mucositis occurred within 1 week of therapy.

Cardiovascular: Congestive heart failure, tachycardia, EKG changes including arrhythmias, chest pain, and asymptomatic decreases in left ventricular ejection fraction have occurred (see WARNINGS section).

OVERDOSAGE

There is no known specific antidote for NOVANTRONE. Accidental overdoses have been reported. Four patients receiving 140–180 mg/m^2 as a single bolus injection died as a result of severe leukopenia with infection. Hematologic support and antimicrobial therapy may be required during prolonged periods of medullary hypoplasia.

Although patients with severe renal failure have not been studied, NOVANTRONE is extensively tissue bound and it is unlikely that the therapeutic effect or toxicity would be mitigated by peritoneal or hemodialysis.

DOSAGE AND ADMINISTRATION

(See **WARNINGS** section.)

NOVANTRONE CONCENTRATE MUST BE DILUTED PRIOR TO USE.

Combination Initial Therapy for ANLL in Adults: For induction, the recommended dosage is 12 mg/m^2 of NOVANTRONE daily on days 1–3 given as an intravenous infusion, and 100 mg/m^2 of cytarabine for 7 days given as a continuous 24-hour infusion on days 1–7.

Most complete remissions will occur following the initial course of induction therapy. In the event of an incomplete antileukemic response, a second induction course may be given. NOVANTRONE should be given for 2 days and cytarabine for 5 days using the same daily dosage levels.

If severe or life-threatening nonhematologic toxicity is observed during the first induction course, the second induction course should be withheld until toxicity clears.

Consolidation therapy which was used in 2 large randomized, multicenter trials consisted of NOVANTRONE, 12 mg/m^2 given by intravenous infusion daily on days 1 and 2 and cytarabine, 100 mg/m^2 for 5 days given as a continuous 24-hour infusion on days 1–5. The first course was given approximately 6 weeks after the final induction course, the second was generally administered 4 weeks after the first. Severe myelosuppression occurred. (See CLINICAL PHARMACOLOGY section.)

Parenteral drug products should be inspected visually for particulate matter and discoloration prior to administration whenever solution and container permit.

The dose of NOVANTRONE should be diluted to at least 50 mL with either 0.9% Sodium Chloride Injection (USP) or 5% Dextrose Injection (USP). NOVANTRONE may be further diluted into Dextrose 5% in Water, Normal Saline or Dextrose 5% with Normal Saline and used immediately. DO NOT FREEZE.

NOVANTRONE should not be mixed in the same infusion as heparin since a precipitate may form. Because specific compatibility data are not available, it is recommended that NOVANTRONE not be mixed in the same infusion with other drugs. The diluted solution should be introduced slowly into the tubing as a freely running intravenous infusion of 0.9% Sodium Chloride Injection (USP) or 5% Dextrose Injection (USP) over a period of not less than 3 minutes. Unused infusion solutions should be discarded immediately in an appropriate fashion. In the case of multidose use, after penetration of the stopper, the remaining portion of the undiluted NOVANTRONE concentrate should be stored not longer than 7 days between 15°–25°C (59°–77°F) or 14 days under refrigeration. DO NOT FREEZE. CONTAINS NO PRESERVATIVE.

If extravasation occurs, the administration should be stopped immediately and restarted in another vein. The nonvesicant properties of NOVANTRONE minimize the possibility of severe local reactions following extravasation. However, care should be taken to avoid extravasation at the infu-

	ALL INDUCTION (percentage of pts entering induction)		ALL CONSOLIDATION (percentage of pts entering consolidation)	
	NOV N=102	DAUN N=102	NOV N=55	DAUN N=49
Cardiovascular	26	28	11	24
CHF	5	6	0	0
Arrhythmias	3	3	4	4
Bleeding	37	41	20	6
GI	16	12	2	2
Petechiae/Ecchymoses	7	9	11	2
Gastrointestinal	88	85	58	51
Nausea/Vomiting	72	67	31	31
Diarrhea	47	47	18	8
Abdominal Pain	15	9	9	4
Mucositis/Stomatitis	29	33	18	8
Hepatic	10	11	14	2
Jaundice	3	8	7	0
Infections	66	73	60	43
UTI	7	2	7	2
Pneumonia	9	7	9	0
Sepsis	34	36	31	18
Fungal Infections	15	13	9	6
Renal Failure	8	6	0	2
Fever	78	71	24	18
Alopecia	37	40	22	16
Pulmonary	43	43	24	14
Cough	13	9	9	2
Dyspnea	18	20	6	0
CNS	30	30	34	35
Seizures	4	4	2	8
Headache	10	9	13	6
Eye	7	6	2	4
Conjunctivitis	5	1	0	0

sion site and to avoid contact of NOVANTRONE with the skin, mucous membranes or eyes.

Skin accidentally exposed to NOVANTRONE should be rinsed copiously with warm water and if the eyes are involved, standard irrigation techniques should be used immediately. The use of goggles, gloves, and protective gowns is recommended during preparation and administration of the drug. Spills on equipment and environmental surfaces may be cleaned using an aqueous solution of calcium hypochlorite (5.5 parts calcium hypochlorite in 13 parts by weight of water for each 1 part of NOVANTRONE). Absorb the solution with gauze or towels and dispose of these in a safe manner. Appropriate safety equipment such as goggles and gloves should be worn while working with calcium hypochlorite.

Procedures for proper handling and disposal of anticancer drugs should be considered. Several guidelines on this subject have been published.[1–6] There is no general agreement that all of the procedures recommended in the guidelines are necessary or appropriate.

REFERENCES

1. Recommendations for the Safe Handling of Parenteral Antineoplastic Drugs. NIH Publication No. 83-2621. For sale by the Superintendent of Documents, US Government Printing Office, Washington, DC 20402.
2. AMA Council Report. Guidelines for Handling Parenteral Antineoplastics. *JAMA*. 1985; 253(11):1590–1592.
3. National Study Commission on Cytotoxic Exposure—Recommendations for Handling Cytotoxic Agents. Available from Louis P. Jeffrey, Sc D, Chairman, National Study Commission on Cytotoxic Exposure, Massachusetts College of Pharmacy and Allied Health Sciences, 179 Longwood Avenue, Boston, Massachusetts 02115.
4. Clinical Oncological Society of Australia: Guidelines and recommendations for safe handling of antineoplastic agents. *Med J Australia*. 1983; 1:426–428.
5. Jones RB, et al. Safe handling of chemotherapeutic agents: A report from the Mount Sinai Medical Center. *Ca—A Cancer Journal for Clinicians*. Sept/Oct 1983; 258–263.
6. American Society of Hospital Pharmacists technical assistance bulletin on handling cytotoxic and hazardous drugs. *Am J Hosp Pharm*. 1990; 47:1033–1049.

HOW SUPPLIED

NOVANTRONE (mitoxantrone for injection concentrate) is a sterile aqueous solution containing mitoxantrone hydrochloride at a concentration equivalent to 2 mg mitoxantrone free base per mL supplied in vials for multidose use as follows:

NDC 58406-640-01—5 mL/multidose vial (10 mg)
NDC 58406-640-03–10 mL/multidose vial (20 mg)
NDC 58406-640-05—12.5 mL/multidose vial (25 mg)
NDC 58406-640-07—15 mL/multidose vial (30 mg)

NOVANTRONE (mitoxantrone for injection concentrate) should be stored between 15°-25°C (59°-77°F). DO NOT FREEZE.

IMMUNEX®

Manufactured for IMMUNEX CORPORATION,
Seattle, WA 98101
by LEDERLE PARENTERALS, INC.
Carolina, Puerto Rico 00987

 Rev 0166-02 Issues 11/94
40762-94 (IM2)

THIOPLEX® ℞
(Thiotepa For Injection)
15 mg/Vial

DESCRIPTION

THIOPLEX® (thiotepa for injection) is an ethylenimine-type compound. It is supplied as a non-pyrogenic, sterile lyophilized powder for intravenous, intracavitary or intravesical administration, containing 15 mg of thiotepa. THIOPLEX is a synthetic product with antitumor activity. The chemical name for thiotepa is Azinaine 1.1′.1″-phosphinothioylidynetris-, or Tns (1-aziridinyl) phosphine sulfide.

Thiotepa has the following structural formula:

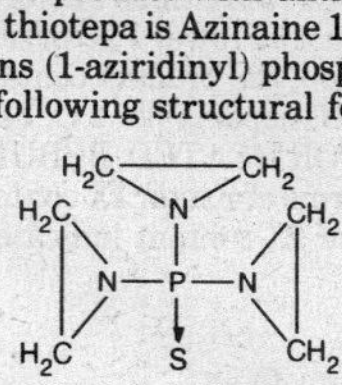

Thiotepa has the empirical formula $C_6H_{12}N_3PS$ and a molecular weight of 189.22. When reconstituted with Sterile Water for Injection, the resulting solution has a pH of approximately 5.5-7.5. Thiotepa is stable in alkaline medium and unstable in acid medium.

CLINICAL PHARMACOLOGY.

Thiotepa is a cytotoxic agent of the polyfunctional type, related chemically and pharmacologically to nitrogen mustard. The radiomimetic action of thiotepa is believed to occur through the release of ethylenimine radicals which, like irridation, disrupt the bonds of DNA. One of the principal bond distruptions is initiated by alkylation of guanine at the N-7 position, which severs the linkage between the purine base and the sugar and liberates alkylated guanines.

The pharmacokinetics of thiotepa and TEPA in thirteen female patients (45–84 years) with advanced stage ovarian cancer receiving 60 mg and 80 mg thiotepa by intravenous infusion on subsequent courses given at 4-week intervals are presented in the following table:

[See table above.]

Pharmacokinetic Parameters (units)	Mean ± SEM Thiotepa 60 mg	80 mg	TEPA 60 mg	30 mg
Peak Serum concentration (ng/mL)	1331 ± 119	1828 ± 135	273 ± 46	353 ± 46
Elimination half-life (h)	2.4 ± 0.3	2.3 ± 0.3	17.6 ± 3.6	15.7 ± 2.7
Area under the curve (ng/h/mL)	2832 ± 412	4127 ± 668	4789 ± 1022	7452 ± 1667
Total body clearance (mL/min)	446 ± 63	419 ± 56		

TEPA, which possesses cytotoxic activity, appears to be the major metabolite of thiotepa found in human serum and urine. Urinary excretion of ^{14}C-labeled thiotepa and metabolites in a 34-year old patient with metastatic carcinoma of the cecum who received a dose of 0.3 mg/kg intravenously was 63%. Thiotepa and TEPA in urine each accounts for less than 2% of the administered dose.

The pharmacokinetics of thiotepa in renal and hepatic dysfunction patients have not been evaluated. Possible pharmacokinetic interactions of thiotepa with any concomitantly administered medications have not been formally investigated.

INDICATIONS AND USAGE

Thiotepa has been tried with varying results in the palliation of a wide variety of neoplastic diseases. However, the most consistent results have been seen in the following tumors:

1. Adenocarcinoma of the breast.
2. Adenocarcinoma of the ovary.
3. For controlling intracavitary effusions secondary to diffuse or localized neoplastic diseases of various serosal cavities.
4. For the treatment of superficial papillary carcinoma of the urinary bladder.

While now largely superseded by other treatments, thiotepa has been effective against other lymphomas, such as lymphosarcoma and Hodgkin's disease.

CONTRAINDICATIONS

THIOPLEX is contraindicated in patients with a known hypersensitivity (allergy) to this preparation.

Therapy is probably contraindicated in cases of existing hepatic, renal, or bone-marrow. However, if the need outweighs the risk in such patients, thiotepa may be used in low dosage, and accompanied by hepatic, renal and hemopoietic function tests.

WARNINGS

Death has occurred after intravesical administration, caused by bone-marrow depression from systematically absorbed drug.

Death from septicemia and hemorrhage has occurred as a direct result of hematopoietic depression by thiotepa.

Thiotepa is highly toxic to the hematopoietic system. A rapidly falling white blood cell or platelet count indicates the necessity for discontinuing or reducing the dosage of thiotepa. Weekly blood and platelet counts are recommended during therapy and for at least 3 weeks after therapy has been discontinued.

Thiotepa can cause fetal harm when administered to a pregnant woman. Thiotepa given by the intraperitoneal (IP) route was teratogenic in mice at doses ≥ 1 mh/kg (3.2 mg/m^2), approximately 8-fold less than the maximum recommended human therapeutic dose (0.8 mg/kg, 27 mg/m^2), based on body-surface area. Thiotepa given by the IP route was teratogenic in rats at doses ≥ 3 mg/kg (21 mg/m^2), approximately equal to the maximum recommended human therapeutic dose, based on body-surface area. Thiotepa was lethal to rabbit fetuses at a dose of 3 mg/kg (41 mg/m^2), approximately two times the maximum recommended human therapeutic dose based on body-surface area.

Effective contraception should be used during thiotepa therapy if either the patient or partner is of childbearing potential. There are no adequate and well-controlled studies in pregnant women. If thiotepa is used during pregnancy, or if pregnancy occurs during thiotepa therapy, the patient and partner should be apprised of the potential hazard to the fetus.

Thiotepa is a polyfunctional alkylating agent, capable of cross-linking the DNA within a cell and changing its nature. The replication of the cell is, therefore, altered, and thiotepa may be described as mutagenic. An *in vitro* study has shown that it causes chromosomal aberrations of the chromatid type and that the frequency of induced aberrations increases with the age of the subject.

Like many alkylating agents, thiotepa has been reported to be carcinogenic when administered to laboratory animals. Carcinogenicity is shown most clearly in studies using mice, but there is some evidence of carcinogenicity in man. In patients treated with thiotepa, cases of myelodysplastic syndromes and acute non-lymphocytic leukemia have been reported.

PRECAUTIONS

General

The serious complication of excessive thiotepa therapy, or sensitivity to the effects of thiotepa, is bone-marrow depression. If proper precautions are not observed thiotepa may cause leukopenia, thrombocytopenia, and anemia.

Information for Patients

The patient should notify the physician in the case of any sign of bleeding (epistaxis, easy bruising, change in color of urine, black stool) or infection (fever, chills) or for possible pregnancy to patient or partner.

Effective contraception should be used during thiotepa therapy if either the patient or the partner is of childbearing potential.

Laboratory Tests

The most reliable guide to thiotepa toxicity is the white blood cell count. If this falls to 3000 or less, the dose should be discontinued. Another good index of thiotepa toxicity is the platelet count: if this falls to 150,000, therapy should be discontinued. Red blood cell count is a less accurate indicator of thiotepa toxicity, if the drug is used in patients with hepatic or renal damage (see **CONTRAINDICATIONS** section), regular assessment of hepatic and renal function tests are indicated.

Drug Interactions

It is not advisable to combine, simultaneously or sequentially, cancer chemotherapeutic agents or a cancer chemotherapeutic agent and a therapeutic modality having the same mechanism of action. Therefore, thiotepa combined with other alkylating agents such as nitrogen mustard or cyclophosphamide or thiotepa combined with irradiation would serve to intensify toxicity rather than to enhance therapeutic response. If these agents must follow each other, it is important that recovery from the first agent, as indicated by white blood cell count, be complete before therapy with the second agent is instituted.

Other drugs which are known to produce bone-marrow depression should be avoided.

Carcinogenesis, Mutagenesis and Impairment of Fertility

Also see **WARNINGS** section.

Carcinogenesis

In mice, repeated IP administration of thiotepa (1.15 or 2.3 mg/kg three times per week for 52 or 43 weeks, respectively) produced a significant increase in the combined incidence of squamous-cell carcinomas of the skin, preputial gland, and ear canal, and combined incidence of lymphoma and lymphocytic leukemia. In other studies in mice repeated IP administration of thiotepa (4 or 8 mg/kg three times per week for 4 weeks followed by a 20-week observation period or 1.8 mg/kg three times per week for 4 weeks followed by a 35-week observation period) resulted in an increased incidence of lung tumors. In rats, repeated IP administration of thiotepa (0.7 or 1.4 mg/kg three times per week for 52 or 34 weeks, respectively) produced significant increases in the incidence of squamous-cell carcinomas of the skin or ear canal, combined hematopoietic neoplasms, and uterine adenocarcinomas. Thiotepa given intravenously (IV) to rats (1 mg/kg once per week for 52 weeks) produced an increased incidence of malignant tumors (abdominal cavity sarcoma, lymphosarcoma, myelosis, seminoma, fibrosarcoma, salivary gland hemangloendothelioma, mammary sarcoma, pheochromocytoma) and benign tumors.

The lowest reported carcinogenic dose in mice (1.15 mg/kg, 3.68 mg/m^2) is approximately 7-fold less than the maximum recommended human therapeutic dose based on body-surface area. The lowest reported carcinogenic dose in rats (0.7 mg/kg, 4.9 mg/m^2) is approximately 6-fold less than the maximum recommended therapeutic dose based on body-surface area.

Mutagenesis

Thiotepa was mutagenic in *in vitro* assays in *Salmonella typhimurium. E. coli.* Chinese hamster lung and human lymphocytes. Chromosomal aberrations and sister chromatid exchanges were observed *in vitro* with thiotepa in bean root tips, human lymphocytes. Chinese hamster lung, and mon-

Continued on next page

Immunex—Cont.

key lymphocytes. Mutations were observed with oral thiotepa in mouse at doses > 2.5 mg/kg (8 mg/m²). The mouse macronucleus test was positive with IP administration of > 1 mg/kg (3.2 mg/m²). Other positive *in vivo* chromosomal aberration or mutation assays included *Drosophila mesanogaster*. Chinese hamster marrow, munne marrow, monkey lymphocyte, and munne germ cell.

Impairment of Fertility
Thiotepa impaired fertility in male mice at PO or IP doses ≥ 0.7 mg/kg (2.24 mg/m²), approximately 12-fold less than the maximum recommended human therapeutic dose based on body-surface area. Thiotepa (0.5 mg) inhibited implantation in female rats when instilled into the uterine cavity. Thiotepa interfered with spermatogenesis in mice at IP doses ≥ 0.5 mg/kg (1.6 mg/m²), approximately 17-fold less than the maximum recommended human therapeutic dose based on body-surface area. Thiotepa interfered with spermatogenesis in hamsters at an IP dose of 1 mg/kg (4.1 mg/m²), approximately 7-fold less than the maximum recommended human therapeutic dose based on body-surface area.

Pregnancy
Category D: See **WARNINGS** section.
Thiotepa can cause fetal harm when administered to a pregnant woman. Thiotepa given by the IP route was teratogenic in mice at doses ≥ 1 mg/kg (3.2 mg/m²), approximately 8-fold less than the maximum recommended human therapeutic dose based on body-surface area. Thiotepa given by the IP route was teratogenic in rats at doses ≥ 3 mg/kg (21 mg/m²), approximately equal to the maximum recommended human therapeutic dose based on body-surface area. Thiotepa was lethal to rabbit fetuses at a dose of 3 mg/kg (41 mg/m²), approximately 2 times the maximum recommended therapeutic dose based on body-surface area. Patients of childbearing potential should be advised to avoid pregnancy. There are no adequate and well-controlled studies in pregnant women. If thiotepa is used during pregnancy, or if pregnancy occurs during thiotepa therapy, the patient and partner should be apprised of the potential hazard to the fetus.

Nursing Mothers
Is is not known whether thiotepa is excreted in human milk. Because many drugs are excreted in human milk and because of the potential for tumorigenicity shown for thiotepa in animal studies, a decision should be made whether to discontinue nursing or to discontinue the drug, taking into account the importance of the drug to the mother.

Pediatric Use
Safety and effectiveness in pediatric patients have not been established.

ADVERSE REACTIONS
In addition to its effect on the blood-forming elements (see **WARNINGS** and **PRECAUTIONS** sections), thiotepa may cause other adverse reactions
General: Fatigue, weakness. Febrile reaction and discharge from a subcutaneous lesion may occur as the result of breakdown of tumor tissue.
Hypersensitivity Reactions: Allergic reactions—rash, urticaria, laryngeal edema, asthma, anaphylactic shock, wheezing.
Local Reactions: Contact dermatitis, pain at the injection site.
Gastrointestinal: Nausea, vomiting, abdominal pain, anorexia.
Renal: Dysuria, urinary retention. There have been rare reports of chemical cystitis or hemorrhagic cystitis following intravesical, but not parenteral administration of thiotepa.
Respiratory: Prolonged apnea has been reported when succinylcholine was administered prior to surgery, following combined use of thiotepa and other anticancer agents. It was theorized that this was caused by decrease of pseudocholinesterase activity caused by the anticancer drugs.
Neurologic: Dizziness, headache, blurred vision.
Skin: Dermatitis. alopecia. Skin depigmentation has been reported following topical use.
Special Senses: Conjunctivitis.
Reproductive: Amenorrhea. interference with spermatogenesis.

OVERDOSAGE
Hematopoietric toxicity can occur following overdose, manifested by a decrease in the white cell count and or platelets. Red blood cell count is a less accurate indicator of thiotepa toxicity. Bleeding manifestations may develop. the patient may become more vulnerable to infection, and less able to combat such infection.

Dosages within and minimally above the recommended therapeutic doses have been associated with potentially life-threatening hematopoietic toxicity. Thiotepa has a toxic effect on the hematopoietic system that is dose related. Thiotepa is dialyzable.
There is no known antidote for overdosage with thiotepa. Transfusion of whole blood or platelets have proven beneficial to the patient in combating hematopoietic toxicity.

DOSAGE AND ADMINISTRATION
Since absorption from the gastrointestinal tract is variable, thiotepa should not be administered orally.
Dosage must be carefully individualized. A slow response to thiotepa does not necessarily indicate a lack of effect. Therefore, increasing the frequency of dosing may only increase toxicity. After maximum benefit is obtained by initial therapy, it is necessary to continue the patient on maintenance therapy (1 to 4 week intervals). In order to continue optimal effect, maintenance doses should not be administered more frequently than weekly in order to preserve correlation between dose and blood counts.

Preparation and Administration Precautions: Thiotepa is a cytotoxic anticancer drug and as with other potentially toxic compounds, caution should be exercised in handing and preparation of thiotepa. Skin reactions associated with accidental exposure to thiotepa may occur. The use of gloves is recommended, if thiotepa solution contacts the skin, immediately wash the skin thoroughly with soap and water. If thiotepa contacts mucous membranes, the membranes should be flushed thoroughly with water.
Preparation of Solution: THIOPLEX (thiotepa for injection) should be reconstituted with 1.5 mL of Sterile Water for injection resulting in a drug concentration of approximately **10 mg/mL.** The actual withdrawable quantities and concentration achieved are illustrated in the following table:
[See table below.]
The reconstituted solution is hypotonic and should be further diluted with Sodium Chloride Injection (0.9% sodium chloride) before use.
When reconstituted with Sterile Water for Injection, solutions of THIOPLEX should be stored in a refrigerator and used within 8 hours. reconstituted solutions further diluted with Sodium Chloride Injection should be used immediately.
In order to eliminate haze, solutions should be filtered through a 0.22 micron filter* prior to administration. Filtering does not alter solution potency. Reconstituted solutions should be clear. Solutions that remain opaque or precipitate after filtration should not be used.
* Polysulfone membrane (Gelman's Sterile Aerodisc®. Single Use) or triton-free mixed ester of cellulose/PVC (Millipore's MILLEX®-GS Filter Unit).
Parenteral drug products should be inspected visually for particulate matter and discoloration prior to administration, whenever solution and container permit.
Initial and Maintenance Doses: Initially the higher dose in the given range is commonly administered. The maintenance dose should be adjusted weekly on the basis of pretreatment control blood counts and subsequent blood counts.
Intravenous Administration: Thiotepa may be given by rapid intravenous administration in doses of 0.3 to 0.4 mg/kg. Doses should be given at 1 to 4 week intervals.
Intracavitary Administration: The dosage recommended is 0.6–0.8 mg/kg. Administration is usualy effected through the same tubing which is used go remove the fluid from the cavity involved.
Intravesical Administration: Patients with papillary carcinoma of the bladder are dehydrated for 8 to 12 hours prior to treatment. then 60 mg of thiotepa in 30–60 mL of Sodium Chloride Injection is instilled into the bladder by catheter. for maximum effect, the solution should be retained for 2 hours. If the patient finds it impossible to retain 60 mL for 2 hours, the dose may be given in a volume of 30 mL. If desired, the patient may be positioned every 15 minutes for maximum area contact. The usual course of treatment is once a week for 4 weeks. The course may be repeated if necessary, but second and third courses must be given with caution since bone-marrow depression may be increased. Deaths have occurred after intravesical administration, caused by bone-marrow depression from systemically absorbed drug.
Handling and Disposal: Follow safe cytotoxic agent hankling procedures. Several guidelines on this subject have been published.[1-6] There is no general agreement that all of the procedures recommended in the guidelines are necessary or appropriate.

HOW SUPPLIED
THIOPLEX® (thiotepa for injection), for single use only, is available in vials containing 15 mg of non-pyrogenic, sterile lyophilized powder, supplied as follows:
NDC 58406-661-31—6 × 15 mg/vial
STORAGE
Store in refrigerator between 2–8°C (36–46°F). PROTECT FROM LIGHT AT ALL TIMES.
REFERENCES
1. Recommendations for the Safe Handling of Parenteral Antineoplastic Drugs. NIH Publication No. 83-2621. For sale by the Superintendent of Documents, US Government Priting Office, Washington, DC 20402.
2. AMA Council Report. Guidelines for Handling Parenteral Antineoplastics. *JAMA.* 1985;253(11):1590-1592.
3. National Study Commission on Cytotoxic Exposure—Recommendations for Handling Cytotoxic Agents. Available from Louis P. Jeffrey, Sc D. Chairman, National Study Commission of Cytotoxic Exposure. Massachusetts College of Pharmacy and allied Health Sciences, 179 Longwood Avenue, Boston, Massachusetts 02115.
4. Clinical Oncological Society of Australia, Guidelines and recommendations for safe handling of antineoplastic agents. *Med J Australia.* 1983: 1:426-428.
5. Jones RB, et al, Safe handling of chemotherapeutic agents: A report from the Mount Sinai Medical Center. *Ca—A Cancer Journal for Clinicians.* Sept/Oct 1983; 258-263.
6. American Society of Hospital Pharmacists technical assistance bulletin on handling cytotoxic and hazarodous drugs. *Am J Hosp Pharm.* 1990; 47:1033-1049.
Manufactured for IMMUNEX CORPORATION. Seattle, WA 98101
by LEDERLE PARENTERALS, INC., Carolina, Puerto Rico 00987
©1994 Immunex Corporation
Rev 0167-00
Issued 12/94
40768-94 (IM1)   LA002-000-THI

Immuno-U.S., Inc.
1200 PARKDALE ROAD
ROCHESTER, MI 48307-1744

Direct Inquiries to:
(810) 652-7872
FAX: (810) 652-6810

ALBUMIN (HUMAN) 5%   ℞

10 bottles per case.
50 mL w/o admin. set	NDC 54129-218-05
250 mL w/admin. set	NDC 54129-218-25
500 mL w/admin. set	NDC 54129-218-50

ALBUMIN (HUMAN) 25%   ℞

10 bottles per case.
20 mL w/o admin. set	NDC 54129-228-02
50 mL w/admin. set	NDC 54129-228-05
100 mL w/admin. set	NDC 54129-228-10

BEBULIN® VH IMMUNO ℞
Factor IX Complex, Vapor Heated

1 Vial   NDC 54129-244-02

A purified, sterile, stable, freeze-dried concentrate of the coagulation Factors IX (Christmas Factor) as well as II (Prothrombin) and X (Stuart Prower Factor) and low amounts of Factor VII. In addition, the product contains small amounts of heparin (≤ 0.15 I.U. heparin per I.U. Factor IX). FACTOR IX COMPLEX, VAPOR HEATED, BEBULIN VH IMMUNO is standardized in terms of Factor IX content and each vial is labeled for the Factor IX content indicated in International Units (I.U.).

FEIBA® VH IMMUNO   ℞
Anti-Inhibitor Coagulant Complex, Vapor Heated

1 Vial   NDC 54129-222-04

A sterile freeze-dried human plasma fraction with Factor VIII inhibitor bypassing activity. In vitro, FEIBA® VH IMMUNO shortens the activated partial thromboplastin time (APTT) of plasma containing Factor VIII inhibitor. Factor VIII inhibitor bypassing activity is expressed in arbitrary units. One IMMUNO Unit of activity is defined as that

Label Claim (mg/vial)	Actual Content (mg/vial)	Amount of Diluent to be Added (mL)	Approximate Withdrawable Volume (mL)	Approximate Withdrawable Amount (mg/vial)	Approximate Reconstituted Concentration (mg/mL)
15.0	15.6	1.5	1.4	14.7	10.4

amount of Anti-Inhibitor Coagulant Complex, Vapor Heated, FEIBA® VH IMMUNO which shortens the APTT of a high titer Factor VIII inhibitor reference plasma to 50% of the blank value. The product is intended for intravenous administration.

IVEEGAM®   ℞
Immune Globulin Intravenous (Human)

1 gm w/20 mL Recon.	NDC 54129-233-10
2.5 gm w/50 mL Recon.	NDC 54129-233-25
5 gm w/100 mL Recon.	NDC 54129-233-50

A sterile freeze-dried concentrate of immunoglobulin G (IgG). Reconstitution of the freeze-dried powder with the accompanying quantity of Sterile Water For Injection U.S.P., gives a 5% protein solution suitable for intravenous administration. This final solution contains, per mL, 50 ±5 mg of IgG, 50 mg of glucose as a stabilizer, and 3 mg of sodium chloride. Trace amounts of IgM and IgA are also present. The reconstituted solution is clear, colorless, and free of detectable aggregates. It contains no preservative.

Interferon Sciences, Inc.
783 JERSEY AVENUE
NEW BRUNSWICK, NJ 08901-3660

Prescribing information for the product Alferon® N Injection is listed under The Purdue Frederick Company.

International Ethical Labs.
AVE. AMERICO MIRANDA # 1021
REPARTO METROPOLITANO
SAN JUAN, PR 00921

Direct Inquiries to:
Mr. Sammy Diaz, President
(787) 765-3510
(787) 763-8414
FAX: (787) 767-1110

AFLAXEN ℞
Naproxen Sodium 550mg Tablets
Boxes of 100 Tablets Unit Dose
White Color Tablets-Dye Free

BIOCEF ℞
CEPHALEXIN Orange Color Capsule
CAPSULES USP
500mg.

BIOCEF Oral Suspension 125mg. ℞

BIOCEF Oral Suspension 250mg. ℞

BIO-TAB ℞ 50 Tabs. in boxes U/D
DOXYCYCLINE HYCLATE 100 mg.

DESPEC SR Bottle of 100 Caplets ℞
Each caplet contains:
Phenylpropanolamine HCl 75mg
Guaifenesin 600mg

DESPEC™ ℞
LIQUID
Each 5ml. (one teaspoonful) contains:
Guaifenesin 100mg.
Phenylpropanolamine HCl 20mg.
Phenylephrine HCl 5mg.
Alcohol 5%

DESPEC SF ℞
Sugar Free-Alcohol Free-Dye Free
Each 5ml (one teaspoonful) contains:
Guaifenesin 100mg
Phenylpropanolamine HCl 20mg
Phenylephrine HCl 5mg

MIO-REL ℞ boxes of 25 amps.
Injectable
Orphenadrine Citrate 60mg. per 2cc ampules

NEUROFORTE-R — Vitamin B-12 ℞
Vial 10cc

NEUROFORTE-SIX — Vitamin B Complex ℞
Monovial 10cc   B-12 and Vitamin C

REDUTEMP 500 mg per 5cc
4 oz Oral suspension
Bottle in a box with calibrated dropper

RELAGESIC (Muscular Relaxant and Analgesic)   ℞
Each tablet contains:
Acetaminophen 650mg
Phenyltoloxamine .... 50 mg

REMULAR-S
(Muscle Relaxant)
Chlorzoxazone 250mg. ℞ bottle of 100

TENCON ℞ bottles of 100
Capsules
Butalbital 50mg.
Acetaminophen 650mg.

TUSS-DA RX 4 oz bottle
Each teaspoonful contains:
Dextromethorphan HBr .... 20 mgs
Pseudoephedrine HCl .... 30 mgs
Alcohol free, Grape Flavor syrup.

Ion Laboratories, Inc.
7431 PEBBLE DR.
FORT WORTH, TEXAS 76118

Direct Inquiries to:
David E. Brown or Judy Martin
(817) 589-7257
FAX: (817) 590-0973

For Medical Information Contact:
In Emergencies:
David E. Brown
(817) 589-7257
FAX: (817) 590-0973

E.N.T.   ℞
Each Sustained-Release (B.I.D.) scored, imprinted tablet contains Phenylpropanolamine HCl 75 mg and Brompheniramine Maleate 12 mg in bottles of 100.

EREX   ℞
Each scored imprinted tablet contains Yohimbine HCl 5.4 mg.
Adult males, orally. 1 tablet three times per day. Bottles of 100.

LIQUIBID (Dye-Free Tablets)   ℞
Each Sustained-Release (B.I.D.) scored, imprinted tablet contains Guaifenesin 600 mg in bottles of 100 and 500.

LIQUIBID-D (Dye-Free Tablets)   ℞
Each Sustained-Release (B.I.D.) scored, imprinted tablet contains Guaifenesin 600 mg and Phenylephrine HCl 40 mg in bottles of 100.

RESCON   ℞
Each Sustained-Release (B.I.D.) imprinted capsule contains Pseudoephedrine HCl 120 mg. and Chlorpheniramine Maleate 12 mg. in bottles of 100.

RESCON Liquid   OTC
(Contains No Sugar, Alcohol, Sodium, Artificial Colors or Flavors).
Each 5 ml (1 tsp.) contains Phenylpropanolamine HCl 12.5 mg and Chlorpheniramine Maleate 2 mg in 4 oz and 16 oz bottles.

RESCON-DM Liquid   OTC
(Sugar, Dye, Alcohol Free)
Each 5 ml (1 tsp.) contains Dextromethorphan Hbr. 10 mg, Pseudoephedrine HCl 30 mg and Chlorpheniramine Maleate 2 mg in 4 oz and 16 oz bottles.

RESCON-ED   ℞
Each Sustained-Release (B.I.D.) imprinted capsule contains Pseudoephedrine HCl 120 mg and Chlorpheniramine Maleate 8 mg in bottles of 100.

RESCON-GG Liquid   OTC
(Contains No Sugar, Alcohol, Sodium, Artificial Colors or Flavors).
Each 5 ml (1 tsp.) contains Phenylephrine HCl 5 mg and Guaifenesin 100 mg in 4 oz bottles.

RESCON JR (Dye-Free)   ℞
Each Sustained-Release (B.I.D.) imprinted capsule contains Pseudoephedrine HCl 60 mg and Chlorpheniramine Maleate 4 mg in bottles of 100.

SINUPAN (Dye-Free)   ℞
Each Sustained-Release (B.I.D.) imprinted capsule contains Phenylephrine HCl 40 mg and Guaifenesin 200 mg in bottles of 100.

ZANTRYL   ℭ ℞
Each Sustained-Release, imprinted black capsule contains Phentermine HCl 30 mg in bottles of 100. Adults one capsule at approximately 2 hours after breakfast.

E.N.T. Plus Treatment Package   ℞

Each ready to dispense treatment package of 60 tablets contains: 30 ENT b.i.d tablets (Phenylpropanolamine Hcl 75 mg./ Brompheniramine maleate 12 mg.) and 30 PLUS b.i.d tablets (Guaifenesin 600 mg.).

Jacobus Pharmaceutical Co., Inc.
37 CLEVELAND LANE
P.O. BOX 5290
PRINCETON, NJ 08540

Direct Inquiries to:
Professional Services
(609) 921-7447
FAX: (609) 799-1176

For Medical Information Contact:
In Emergencies:
Medical Department
(609) 921-7447
FAX: (609) 799-1176

DAPSONE TABLETS USP   ℞
[dap'sōne]
25 mg. & 100 mg.

PRODUCT OVERVIEW

KEY FACTS
Dapsone is a sulfone for the primary treatment of Dermatitis herpetiformis and an antibacterial drug for susceptible cases of leprosy.

MAJOR USES
Dapsone is used to control the dermatologic symptoms of Dermatitis herpetiformis. Dapsone is used alone or in combination with other anti-leprosy drugs for leprosy.

SAFETY INFORMATION
Dapsone is contraindicated in patients with Dapsone hypersensitivity. Complete blood counts and laboratory monitoring should be done frequently. See labeling.

PRODUCT INFORMATION

DAPSONE TABLETS USP   ℞
[dap'sōne]
25 mg. & 100 mg.

DESCRIPTION
Dapsone-USP, 4,4'-diaminodiphenylsulfone (DDS) is a primary treatment for Dermatitis herpetiformis. It is an antibacterial drug for susceptible cases of leprosy. It is a white, odorless crystalline powder, practically insoluble in water and insoluble in fixed and vegetable oils.
Dapsone is issued on prescription in tablets of 25 and 100 mg. for oral use.

$$NH_2 - \!\!\!\!\bigcirc\!\!\!\! - SO_2 - \!\!\!\!\bigcirc\!\!\!\! - NH_2$$

Inactive Ingredients: Colloidal silicone dioxide, magnesium stearate, microcrystalline cellulose, and corn starch.

CLINICAL PHARMACOLOGY
Actions: The mechanism of action in Dermatitis herpetiformis has not been established. By the kinetic method in mice, Dapsone is bactericidal as well as bacteriostatic against *Mycobacterium leprae*.
Absorption and Excretion: Dapsone, when given orally, is rapidly and almost completely absorbed. About 85 percent of the daily intake is recoverable from the urine mainly in the form of water-soluble metabolites. Excretion of the drug is slow and a constant blood level can be maintained with the usual dosage.
Blood Levels: Detected a few minutes after ingestion, the drug reaches peak concentration in 4–8 hours. Daily administration for at least eight days is necessary to achieve a plateau level. With doses of 200 mg. daily, this level averaged 2.3 μg/ml with a range of 0.1–7.0 μg/ml. The half-life in the plasma in different individuals varies from ten hours to fifty hours and averages twenty-eight hours. Repeat tests in the

Continued on next page

Jacobus—Cont.

same individual are constant. Daily administration (50–100 mg.) in leprosy patients will provide blood levels in excess of the usual minimum inhibitory concentration even for patients with a short Dapsone half-life.

INDICATIONS AND USAGE

Dermatitis herpetiformis: (D.H.)
Leprosy: All forms of leprosy except for cases of proven Dapsone resistance.

CONTRAINDICATION

Hypersensitivity to Dapsone and/or its derivatives.

WARNINGS

The patient should be warned to respond to the presence of clinical signs such as sore throat, fever, pallor, purpura or jaundice. Deaths associated with the administration of Dapsone have been reported from agranulocytosis, aplastic anemia and other blood dyscrasias. Complete blood counts should be done frequently in patients receiving Dapsone. The FDA Dermatology Advisory Committee recommended that, when feasible counts should be done weekly for the first month, monthly for six months and semi-annually thereafter. If a significant reduction in leucocytes, platelets or hemopoiesis is noted, Dapsone should be discontinued and the patient followed intensively. Folic acid antagonists have similar effects and may increase the incidence of hematologic reactions; if co-administered with Dapsone the patient should be monitored more frequently. Patients on weekly Pyrimethamine and Dapsone have developed agranulocytosis during the second and third month of therapy.

Severe anemia should be treated prior to initiation of therapy and hemoglobin monitored. Hemolysis and methemoglobin may be poorly tolerated by patients with severe cardio-pulmonary disease.

Cutaneous reactions, especially bullous, include exfoliative dermatitis and are probably one of the most serious, though rare, complications of sulfone therapy. They are directly due to drug sensitization. Such reactions include toxic erythema, erythema multiforme, toxic epidermal necrolysis, morbilliform and scariatiniform reactions, urticaria and erythema nodosum. If new or toxic dermatologic reactions occur, sulfone therapy must be promptly discontinued and appropriate therapy instituted.

Leprosy reactional states, including cutaneous, are not hypersensitivity reactions to Dapsone and do not require discontinuation. See special section.

PRECAUTIONS

General: Hemolysis and Heinz body formation may be exaggerated in individuals with a glucose-6-phosphate dehydrogenase (G6PD) deficiency, or methemoglobin reductase deficiency, or hemoglobin M. This reaction is frequently dose-related. Dapsone should be given with caution to these patients or if the patient is exposed to other agents or conditions such as infection or diabetic ketosis capable of producing hemolysis. Drugs or chemicals which have produced significant hemolysis in G6PD or methemoglobin reductase deficient patients include Dapsone, sulfanilamide, nitrite, aniline, phenylhydrazine, napthalene, niridazole, nitrofurantoin and 8-amino-antimalarials such as primaquine.

Toxic hepatitis and cholestatic jaundice have been reported early in therapy. Hyperbilirubinemia may occur more often in G6PD deficient patients. When feasible, baseline and subsequent monitoring of liver function is recommended. If abnormal, Dapsone should be discontinued until the source of the abnormality is established.

Drug Interactions: Rifampin lowers Dapsone levels 7 to 10-fold by accelerating plasma clearance; in leprosy this reduction has not required a change in dosage.

Folic acid antagonists such as pyrimethamine may increase the likelihood of hematologic reactions.

A modest interaction has been reported for patients receiving 100 mg Dapsone od in combination with trimethoprim 5 mg/kg q6h. On Day 7, the serum Dapsone levels averaged 2.1 $\pm$ 1.0 μg/mL in comparison to 1.5 $\pm$ 0.5 μg/mL for Dapsone alone. On Day 7, trimethoprim levels averaged 18.4 $\pm$ 5.2 μg/mL in comparison to 12.4 $\pm$ 4.5 μg/mL for patients not receiving Dapsone. Thus, there is a mutual interaction between Dapsone and trimethoprim in which each raises the level of the other about 1.5 times.

Carcinogenesis, mutagenesis: Dapsone has been found carcinogenic (sarcomagenic) for male rats and female mice causing mesenchymal tumors in the spleen and peritoneum, and thyroid carcinoma in female rats. Dapsone is not mutagenic with or without microsomal activation in *S. typhimurium* tester strains 1535, 1537, 1538, 98, or 100.

Pregnancy Category C: Animal reproduction studies have not been conducted with Dapsone. Extensive, but uncontrolled experience and two published surveys on the use of Dapsone in pregnant women have not shown that Dapsone increases the risk of fetal abnormalities if administered during all trimesters of pregnancy or can affect reproduction capacity. Because of the lack of animal studies or controlled human experience, Dapsone should be given to a pregnant woman only if clearly needed. In general, for leprosy, USPHS at Carville recommends maintenance of Dapsone. Dapsone has been important for the management of some pregnant D.H. patients.

Nursing Mothers: Dapsone is excreted in breast milk in substantial amounts. Hemolytic reactions can occur in neonates. See section on hemolysis. Because of the potential for tumorgenicity shown for Dapsone in animal studies a decision should be made whether to discontinue nursing or discontinue the drug taking into account the importance of the drug to the mother.

Pediatric Use: Children are treated on the same schedule as adults but with correspondingly smaller doses. Dapsone is generally not considered to have an effect on the later growth, development and functional development of the child.

ADVERSE REACTIONS

In addition to the warnings listed above, the following syndromes and serious reactions have been reported in patients on Dapsone.

Hematologic Effects: Dose-related hemolysis is the most common adverse effect and is seen in patients with or without G6PD deficiency. Almost all patients demonstrate the interrelated changes of a loss of 1–2g of HB, an increase in the reticulocytes (2–12%), a shortened red cell life span and a rise in methemoglobin. G6PD deficient patients have greater responses.

Nervous System Effects: Peripheral neuropathy is a definite but unusual complication of Dapsone therapy in non-leprosy patients. Motor loss is predominent. If muscle weakness appears, Dapsone should be withdrawn. Recovery on withdrawal is usually substantially complete. The mechanism of recovery is reportedly by axonal regeneration. Some recovered patients have tolerated retreatment at reduced dosage. In leprosy this complication may be difficult to distinguish from a leprosy reactional state.

Body As A Whole: In addition to the warnings and adverse effects reported above, additional adverse reactions include: nausea, vomiting, abdominal pains, pancreatitis, vertigo, blurred vision, tinnitus, insomnia, fever, headache, psychosis, phototoxicity, pulmonary eosinophilia, tachycardia, albuminuria, the nephrotic syndrome, hypoalbuminemia without proteinuria, renal papillary necrosis, male infertility, drug-induced Lupus erythematosus and an infectious mononucleosis-like syndrome. In general, with the exception of the complications of severe anoxia from overdosage (retinal and optic nerve damage, etc.) these adverse reactions have regressed off drug.

OVERDOSAGE

Nausea, vomiting, hyperexcitability can appear a few minutes up to 24 hours after ingestion of an overdose. Methemoglobin induced depression, convulsions and severe cyanosis requires prompt treatment. In normal and methemoglobin reductase deficient patients, methylene blue, 1–2 mg/kg of body weight, given slowly intravenously is the treatment of choice. The effect is complete in 30 minutes, but may have to be repeated if methemoglobin reaccumulates. For non-emergencies, if treatment is needed, methylene blue may be given orally in doses of 3–5 mg/kg every 4–6 hours.

Methylene blue reduction depends on G6PD and should not be given to fully expressed G6PD deficient patients.

DOSAGE AND ADMINISTRATION

Dermatitis herpetiformis: The dosage should be individually titrated starting in adults with 50 mg. daily and correspondingly smaller doses in children. If full control is not achieved within the range of 50–300 mg. daily, higher doses may be tried. Dosage should be reduced to a minimum maintenance level as soon as possible. In responsive patients there is a prompt reduction in pruritus followed by clearance of skin lesions. There is no effect on the gastro-intestinal component of the disease.

Dapsone levels are influenced by acetylation rates. Patients with high acetylation rates, or who are receiving treatment affecting acetylation may require an adjustment in dosage.

A strict gluten free diet is an option for the patient to elect, permitting many to reduce or eliminate the need for Dapsone; the average time for dosage reduction is 8 months with a range of 4 months to 2½ years and for dosage elimination 29 months with a range of 6 months to 9 years.

Leprosy: In order to reduce secondary Dapsone resistance, the WHO Expert Committee on Leprosy and the USPHS at Carville, LA, recommend that Dapsone should be commenced in combination with one or more anti-leprosy drugs. In the multi-drug program Dapsone should be maintained at the full dosage of 100 mg. daily without interruption (with correspondingly smaller doses for children) and provided to all patients who have sensitive organisms with new or recrudescent disease or who have not yet completed a two year course of Dapsone monotherapy. For advice and other drugs, the USPHS at Carville, LA, (1 800-642-2477) should be contacted. Before using other drugs consult appropriate product labeling.

In bacteriologically negative tuberculoid and indeterminate disease, the recommendation is the coadministration of Dapsone 100 mg. daily with six months of Rifampin 600 mg. daily. Under WHO, daily Rifampin may be replaced by 600 mg. Rifampin monthly, if supervised. The Dapsone is continued until all signs of clinical activity are controlled—usually after an additional six months. Then Dapsone should be continued for an additional three years for tuberculoid and indeterminate patients and for five years for borderline tuberculoid patients.

In lepromatous and borderline lepromatous patients, the recommendation is the coadministration of Dapsone 100 mg. daily with two years of Rifampin 600 mg. daily. Under WHO, daily Rifampin may be replaced by 600 mg. Rifampin monthly, if supervised. One may elect the concurrent administration of a third anti-leprosy drug, usually either Clofazamine 50–100mg. daily or Ethionamide 250–500 mg. daily. Dapsone 100 mg. daily is continued 3–10 years until all signs of clinical activity are controlled with skin scrapings and biopsies negative for one year. Dapsone should then be continued for an additional 10 years for borderline patients and for life for lepromatous patients.

Secondary Dapsone resistance should be suspected whenever a lepromatous or borderline lepromatous patient receiving Dapsone treatment relapses clinically and bacteriologically, solid staining bacilli being found in the smears taken from the new active lesions. If such cases show no response to regular and supervised Dapsone therapy within three to six months or good compliance for the past 3–6 months can be assured, Dapsone resistance should be considered confirmed clinically. Determination of drug sensitivity using the mouse footpad method is recommended and, after prior arrangement, is available without charge from the USPHS, Carville, LA. Patients with proven Dapsone resistance should be treated with other drugs.

LEPROSY REACTIONAL STATES

Abrupt changes in clinical activity occur in leprosy with any effective treatment and are known as reactional states. The majority can be classified into two groups.

The "Reversal" reaction (Type 1) may occur in borderline or tuberculoid leprosy patients often soon after chemotherapy is started. The mechanism is presumed to result from a reduction in the antigenic load: the patient is able to mount an enhanced delayed hypersensitivity response to residual infection leading to swelling ("Reversal") of existing skin and nerve lesions. If severe, or if neuritis is present, large doses of steroids should always be used. If severe, the patient should be hospitalized. In general anti-leprosy treatment is continued and therapy to suppress the reaction is indicated such as analgesics, steroids, or surgical decompression of swollen nerve trunks. USPHS at Carville, LA should be contacted for advice in management.

Erythema nodosum leprosum (ENL) (lepromatous reaction) (Type 2 reaction) occurs mainly in lepromatous patients and small numbers of borderline patients. Approximately 50% of treated patients show this reaction in the first year. The principal clinical features are fever and tender erythematous skin nodules sometimes associated with malaise, neuritis, orchitis, albuminuria, joint swelling, iritis, epistaxis or depression. Skin lesions can become pustular and/or ulcerate. Histologically there is a vasculitis with an intense polymorphonuclear infiltrate. Elevated circulating immune complexes are considered to be the mechanism of reaction. If severe, patients should be hospitalized. In general, anti-leprosy treatment is continued. Analgesics, steroids, and other agents available from USPHS, Carville, LA, are used to suppress the reaction.

HOW SUPPLIED

Rx: Dapsone 25 mg, round white scored tablet, debossed "25" above and "102" below the score and on the obverse "Jacobus" in light and child-resistant bottles, of 100, NDC 49938-102-01.

Dapsone 100 mg, round white scored tablet, debossed "100" above and "101" below the score and on the obverse "Jacobus" in light and child-resistant bottles of 100, NDC 49938-101-01.

Store at controlled room temperature, (59–86°F).

Protect from light.

CAUTION: Federal law prohibits dispensing without prescription.

Dispense this product in a well-closed child-resistant container.

JACOBUS PHARMACEUTICAL CO., INC.
P.O. Box 5290
Princeton, NJ 08540

9H MAY, 1996

PASER® GRANULES ℞
(aminosalicylic acid granules)

DESCRIPTION

PASER granules are a delayed release granule preparation of aminosalicylic acid (p-aminosalicylic acid: 4–aminosalicylic acid) for use with other anti-tuberculosis drugs for the treatment of all forms of active tuberculosis due to susceptible strains of tubercle bacilli. The granules are designed for gradual release to avoid high peak levels not useful (and perhaps toxic) with bacteriostatic drugs. Aminosalicylic acid is rapidly degraded in acid media; the protective acid-resistant outer coating is rapidly dissolved in neutral media so a mildly acidic food such as orange, apple or tomato juice, yogurt or apple sauce should be used.

Aminosalicylic acid (p-aminosalicylic acid) is 4–Amino-2hydrozybenzoid acid. PASER granules are the free base of aminosalicylic acid and do NOT contain sodium or a sugar. The molecular formula is $C_7H_7NO_3$ with a molecular weight of 153.14. With heat p-aminosalicylic acid is decarboxylated to produce CO_2 and m-aminophenol. If the airtight packets are swollen, storage has been improper. DO NOT USE if packets are swollen or the granules have lost their tan color and are dark brown or purple.

The structural formula is:

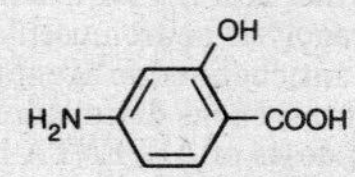

PASAR granules are supplied as off-white tan colored granules with an average diameter of 1.5 mm and an average content of 60% aminosalicylic acid by weight. The acid resistant outer coating will be completely removed by a few minutes at a neutral pH. The inert ingredients are:

colloidal silicon dioxide
dibutyl sebacate
hydroxypropyl methyl cellulose
methacrylic acid copolymer
microcystalline cellulose
talc

The packets contain 4 grams of aminosalicylic acid for oral administration three times a day by sprinkling an apple sauce or yogurt to be eaten without chewing. Suspension in an acidic fruit drink such as orange juice or tomato juice will protect the coating for at least 2 hours. Swirling the juice in the glass will help resuspend the granules if they sink.

CLINICAL PHARMACOLOGY

Mechanism of Action: Aminosalicylic acid is bacteriostatic against Mycobacterium tuberculosis. It inhibits the onset of bacterial resistance to streptomycin and isoniazid. The mechanism of action has been postulated to be inhibition of folic acid synthesis (but without potentiation with antifolic compounds) and/or inhibition of synthesis of the cell wall component, mycobactin, thus reducing iron uptake by M. tuberculosis.

Characteristics: The two major considerations in the clinical pharmacology of aminosalicylic acid are the prompt production of a toxic inactive metabolite under acid conditions and the short serum half life of one hour for the free drug. Both are discussed below.

After two hours in simulated gastric fluid, 10% of unprotected aminosalicylic acid is decarboxylated to form meta-aminophenol, a known hepatotoxin. The acid-resistant coating of the PASER granules protects against degradation in the stomach. The small granules are designed to escape the usual restriction on gastric emptying of large particles. Under neutral conditions such as are found in the small intestine or in neutral foods, the acid-resistant coating is dissolved within one minute. Care must be taken in the administration of these granules to protect the acid-resistant coating by maintaining the granules in an acidic food during dosage administration. Patients who have neutralized gastric acid with antacids will not need to protect the acid resistant coating with an acidic food since no acid is present to spoil the drug. Antacids may influence the absorption of other medications and are not necessary for PASER consumed with an acidic food.

Because PASER granules are protected by an enteric coating absorption does not commence until they leave the stomach; the soft skeletons of the granules remain and may be seen in the stool.

Absorption and excretion: In a single 4 gram pharmacokinetic study with food in normal volunteers the initial time to a 2 µg/mL serum level of aminosalicylic acid was 2 hours with a range of 45 minutes to 24 hours; the median time to peak was 6 hours with a range of 1.5 to 24 hours; the mean peak level was 20 µg/mL with a range of 9 to 35 µg/mL; a level of 2 µg/mL was maintained for an average of 7.9 hours with a range of 5 to 9; a level of 1 µg/mL was maintained for an average of 8.8 hours with a range of 6 to 11.5 hours. The recommended schedule is 4 grams every 8 hours.

80% of aminosalicylic acid is excreted in the urine, with 50% or more of the dosage excreted in acetylated form. The acetylation process is not genetically determined as is the case for isoniazid. Aminosalicylic acid is excreted by glomerular filtration; although previously reported otherwise, probenecid, a tubular blocking agent, does not enhance plasma concentration. In a 1954 study thyroxine synthesis but not iodide uptake was reported reduced about 40% when the sodium salt (not PASER granules) of aminosalicylic acid was administered one hour before radio-iodine; the sodium salt typically produces a serum level over 120 µg/mL at one hour lasting one hour. Occasional goiter development can be prevented by the administration of thyroxine but not iodide. Penetration into the cerebrospinal fluid occurs only if the meninges are inflamed.

Approximately 50–60% of aminosalicylic acid is protein bound; binding is reported to be reduced 50% in kwashiorkor.

Microbiology: The aminosalicylic acid MIC for M. tuberculosis in 7H11 agar was less than 1.0 µg/mL for nine strains including three multidrug resistant strains, but 4 and 8 µg/mL for two other multidrug resistant strains. The 90% inhibition in 7H12 broth (Bactec) showed little dose response but was interpreted as being less than or equal to 0.12–0.25 µg/mL for eight strains of which three were multi-resistant, 0.50 µg/mL for one resistant strain, questionable for four nonresistant strains and greater than 1 µg/mL for one non-resistant and three resistant strains. Aminosalicylic acid is not active in vitro against M. avium.

INDICATIONS AND USAGE

PASER is indicated for the treatment of tuberculosis in combination with other active agents. It is most commonly used in patients with Multi-drug Resistant TB (MDR-TB) or in situations when therapy with isoniazid and rifampin is not possible due to a combination of resistance and/or intolerance. When PASER is added to the treatment regimen in patients with proven or suspected drug resistance, it should be accompanied by at least one and preferably two other new agents to which the patient's organism is known or expected to be susceptible.

CONTRAINDICATIONS

Hypersensitivity to any component of this medication.
Severe renal disease.

Patients with severe renal disease will accumulate aminosalicylic acid and its acetyl metabolite but will continue to acetylate, thus leading exclusively to the inactive acetylated form; deacetylation, if any, is not significant.

The half life of free aminosalicylic acid in renal disease is 30.8 minutes in comparison to 26.4 minutes in normal volunteers, but the half life of the inactive metabolite is 309 minutes in uremic patients in comparison to 51 minutes in normal volunteers. Although aminosalicylic acid passes dialysis membranes, the frequency of dialysis usually is not comparable to the half-life of 50 minutes for the free acid. Patients with end stage renal disease should not receive aminosalicylic acid.

WARNINGS

Liver Function

In one retrospective study of 7492 patients on rapidly absorbed aminosalicylic acid preparations, drug-induced hepatitis occurred in 38 patients (0.5%); in these 38 the first symptom usually appeared within three months of the start of therapy with a rash as the most common event followed by fever and much less frequently by GI disturbances of anorexia, nausea or diarrhea. Only one patient was diagnosed on routine biochemistry.

Premonitory symptoms in 90% of these 38 patients preceded jaundice by a few days to several weeks with the mean time of onset 33 days with a range of 7–90 days. Half of the adverse reactions occurred during the third, fourth or fifth weeks. When aminosalicylic acid-induced hepatitis was diagnosed, hepatomegaly was invariably present with lymphadenopathy in 46%, leucocytosis in 79%, and eosinophilia in 55%. Prompt recognition with discontinuation led to the recovery of all 38 patients. If recognized in the premonitory stage, the reaction is reported to "settle" in 24 hours and no jaundice ensues. From other reported studies failure to recognize the reaction can result in a mortality of up to 21%. The patient must be monitored carefully during the first three months of therapy and treatment must be discontinued immediately at the first sign of a rash, fever or other premonitory signs of intolerance.

PRECAUTIONS

(1) General:

All drugs should be stopped at the first sign suggesting a hypersensitivity reaction. They may be restarted one at a time in very small but gradually increasing doses to determine whether the manifestations are drug-induced and, if so, which drug is responsible.

Desensitization has been accomplished successfully in 15 of 17 patients starting with 10 mg aminosalicylic acid given as a single dose. The dosage is doubled every 2 days until reaching a total of 1 gram after which the dosage is divided to follow the regular schedule of administration. If a mild temperature rise or skin reaction develops, the increment is to be dropped back one level or the progression held for one cycle. Reactions are rare after a total dosage of 1.5 grams.

Patients with hepatic disease may not tolerate aminosalicylic acid as well as normal patients, even though the metabolism in patients with hepatic disease has been reported to be comparable to that in normal volunteers.

(2) Information for Patients:

The patient should be advised that the first signs of hypersensitivity include a rash, often followed by fever, and much less frequently, GI disturbances of anorexia, nausea or diarrhea. If such symptoms develop, the patient should immediately cease taking the medication and arrange for a prompt clinical visit.

Patients should be advised that poor compliance in taking anti-TB medication often leads to treatment failure, and, not infrequently, to the development of resistance of the organisms in the individual patient.

Patients should be advised that the skeleton of the granules may be seen in the stool.

The coating to protect the PASER granules dissolves promptly under neutral conditions; the granules therefore should be administered by sprinkling on acidic foods such as apple sauce or yogurt or by suspension in a fruit drink which will protect the coating, but the granules sink and will have to be swirled. The coating will last at least 2 hours in either system. All juices tested to date have been satisfactory; tested are: tomato, orange, grapefruit, grape, cranberry, apple, "fruit punch".

Patients should be advised to store PASER in a refrigerator or freezer. PASER packets may be stored at room temperature for short periods of time.

Patients should be advised NOT to use if the packets are swollen or the granules have lost their tan color and are dark brown or purple. The patient should inform the pharmacist or physician immediately and return the medication.

(3) Laboratory Tests:

Aminosalicylic acid has been reported to interfere technically with the serum determinations of albumin by dye-binding. SGOT by the azoene dye method and with qualitative urine tests for ketones, bilirubin, urobilinogen or porphobilinogen.

(4) Drug Interactions:

Aminosalicytic acid at a dosage of 12 grams in a rapidly available form has been reported to produce a 20 percent reduction in the acetylation of isoniazid, especially in patients who are rapid acetylators; INH serum levels, half lives and excretions in fast acetylators still remain half of the levels seen in slow acetylators with or without p-aminosalicylic acid. The effect is dose related and, while it has not been studied with the current delayed release preparation, the lower serum levels with this preparation will result in a reduced effect on the acetylation of INH.

Aminosalicylic acid has previously been reported to block the absorption of rifampin. A subsequent report has shown that this blockade was due to an excipient not included in PASER granules. Oral administration of a solution containing both aminosalicylic acid and rifampin showed full absorption of each product.

As a result of competition, Vitamin B_{12} absorption has been reduced 55% by 5 grams of aminosalicylic acid with clinically significant erythrocyte abnormalities developing after depletion; patients on therapy of more than one month should be considered for maintenance B_{12}.

A malabsorption syndrome can develop in patients on aminosalicylic acid but is usually not complete. The complete syndrome includes steatorrhea, an abnormal small bowel pattern on x-ray, villus atrophy, depressed cholesterol, reduced D-xylose and iron absorption. Triglyceride absorption always is normal.

In one literature report 8 hours after the last dosage of aminosalicylic acid at 2 gm qid serum digoxin levels were reduced 40% in two of ten patients but not changed in the remaining eight.

(5) Carcinogenesis, mutagenesis, impairment of fertility: Sodium aminosalicylate produced an occipital bone defect, probably with a dose response, when administered to ten pregnant Wistar rats at five doses from 3.85 to 385 mg/kg from days 6 to 14. There were no significant changes from controls in any group in corpora lutea, early resorptions, total resorptions, fetal death, litter size, or hematomas. For all except the 77 mg/kg group, fetal weights were significantly greater than controls. Chinchilla rabbits on 5 mg/kg from days 7 to 14 did not show any significant differences as compared to controls for the same parameters studied.

Sodium aminosalicylic acid was not mutagenic in Ames tester strain TA 100. In human lymphocyte cultures in-vitro clastogenic effects of achromatic, chromatid, isochromatic breaks or chromatid translocations were not seen at 153 or 600 µg/mL. At 1500 and 3000 µg/mL there was a dose related increase in chromatid aberrations.

Patients on isoniazid and aminosalicylic acid have been reported to have an increased number of chromosomal aberrations as compared to controls.

Continued on next page

Jacobus—Cont.

(6) Pregnancy: Pregnancy Category C:
Aminosalicylic acid has been reported to produce occipital malformations in rats when given at doses within the human dose range. Although there probably is a dose response, the frequency of abnormalities was comparable to controls at the highest level tested (two times the human dosage). When administered to rabbits at 5 mg/kg, throughout all three trimesters, no teratologic embryocidal effects were seen. Literature reports on aminosalicylic acid in pregnant women always report coadministration of other medications. Because there are no adequate and well controlled studies of aminosalicylic acid in humans, PASER granules should be given to a pregnant woman only if clearly needed.
(8) Nursing mothers:
After administration of a different preparation of aminosalicylic acid to one patient, the maximum concentration in the milk was 1 μg/mL at 3 hours with a half-life of 2.5 hours; the maximum maternal plasma concentration was 70 μg/mL at two hours.

ADVERSE EFFECTS

The most common side effect is gastrointestinal intolerance manifested by nausea, vomiting, diarrhea, and abdominal pain.
Hypersensitivity reactions: Fever, skin eruptions of various types, including exfoliative dermatitis, infectious mononucleosis-like, or lymphoma-like syndrome, leucopenia, agranulocytosis, thrombocytopenia, Coombs' positive hemolytic anemia, jaundice, hepatitis, pericarditis, hypoglycemia, optic neuritis, encephalopathy, Leoffler's syndrome, and vasculitis and a reduction in prothrombin.
Crystalluria may be prevented by the maintenance of urine at a neutral or an alkaline pH.

OVERDOSAGE

Overdosage has not been reported.

DOSAGE AND ADMINISTRATION

PASER granules should be administered with other drugs to which the organism is known or expected to be susceptible. It is most commonly administered to patients with Multi-drug Resistant TB (MDR-TB) or in other situations in which therapy with isoniazid or rifampin is not possible due to a combination of resistance and/or tolerance. The adult dosage of four grams (one packet) three times per day or correspondingly smaller doses in children should be given by sprinking on apple sauce or yogurt or by swirling in the glass to suspend the granules in an acidic drink such as tomato or orange juice.
DO NOT USE if the packet is swollen or the granules have lost their tan color, turning dark brown or purple.

HOW SUPPLIED

Carton of 30 PASER packets (NDC 49938-107-04).
Each packet contains four grams aminosalicylic acid.
PASER granules are supplied in packets containing 4 grams of aminosalicylic acid for administration three times a day by suspension in an acidic drink or food with a pH less than 5. Examples include apple sauce, yogurt, tomato or orange juice.
Distributors and Pharmacists: Store below 59°F (15°C) (in a refrigerator or freezer).
Patients are urged to store PASER in a refrigerator or freezer. PASER packets may be stored at room temperature for short periods of time.
AVOID EXCESSIVE HEAT. DO NOT USE if packet is swollen or the granules have lost their tan color, turning dark brown or purple.
Caution: Federal, law prohibits dispensing without prescription.

JACOBUS PHARMACEUTICAL CO. INC.
P.O. Box 5290
Princeton, NJ 08540

2A JULY, 1996

IDENTIFICATION PROBLEM?
Turn to the **Product Identification Guide**,
where you'll find more than
1600 products pictured in actual
size and full color.

Janssen Pharmaceutica Inc.

1125 TRENTON-HARBOURTON ROAD
P.O. BOX 200
TITUSVILLE, NJ 08560-0200

For Medical Information Contact:
Generally:
Professional Services
(800) JANSSEN
(609) 730-2000
FAX: (609) 730-3138
After Hours and Weekends:
(800) JANSSEN

ALFENTA® Ⓒ℞

[ăl-fĕn 'tä]
(alfentanil hydrochloride)
Injection

CAUTION: Federal Law Prohibits Dispensing Without Prescription

DESCRIPTION

ALFENTA (alfentanil hydrochloride) Injection is an opioid analgesic chemically designated as N-[1-[2-(4-ethyl-4, 5-dihydro-5-oxo-1H-tetrazol-1-yl) ethyl]-4-(methoxymethyl)-4-piperidinyl]-N-phenylpropanamide monohydrochloride (1:1) with a molecular weight of 452.98 and an n-octanol: water partition coefficient of 128:1 at pH 7.4.
ALFENTA is a sterile, non-pyrogenic, preservative free aqueous solution containing alfentanil hydrochloride equivalent to 500 μg per mL of alfentanil base for intravenous injection. The solution, which contains sodium chloride for isotonicity, has a pH range of 4–6.

CLINICAL PHARMACOLOGY

ALFENTA (alfentanil hydrochloride) is an opioid analgesic with a rapid onset of action.
At doses of 8–40 mcg/kg for surgical procedures lasting up to 30 minutes, ALFENTA provides analgesic protection against hemodynamic responses to surgical stress with recovery times generally comparable to those seen with equipotent fentanyl dosages.
For longer procedures, doses of up to 75 mcg/kg attenuate hemodynamic responses to laryngoscopy, intubation and incision, with recovery time comparable to fentanyl. At doses of 50–75 mcg/kg followed by a continuous infusion of 0.5–3 mcg/kg/min, ALFENTA attenuates the catecholamine response with more rapid recovery and reduced need for postoperative analgesics as compared to patients administered enflurane. At doses of 5 mcg/kg, ALFENTA provides analgesia for the conscious but sedated patient. Based on patient response, doses higher than 5 mcg/kg may be needed. Elderly or debilitated patients may require lower doses.
High intrasubject and intersubject variability in the pharmacokinetic disposition of ALFENTA has been reported.
The pharmacokinetics of ALFENTA can be described as a three-compartment model with sequential distribution half-lives of 1 and 14 minutes; and a terminal elimination half-life of 90–111 minutes (as compared to a terminal elimination half-life of approximately 475 minutes for fentanyl and approximately 265 minutes for sufentanil at doses of 250 mcg). The liver is the major site of biotransformation.
ALFENTA has an apparent volume of distribution of 0.4–1 L/kg, which is approximately one-fourth to one-tenth that of fentanyl, with an average plasma clearance of 5 mL/kg/min as compared to approximately 8 mL/kg/min for fentanyl.
Only 1.0% of the dose is excreted as unchanged drug; urinary excretion is the major route of elimination of metabolites. Plasma protein binding of ALFENTA is approximately 92%.
In one study involving 15 patients administered ALFENTA with nitrous oxide/oxygen, a narrow range of plasma ALFENTA concentrations, approximately 310–340 ng/mL, was shown to provide adequate anesthesia for intra-abdominal surgery, while lower concentrations, approximately 190 ng/mL, blocked responses to skin closure. Plasma concentrations between 100–200 ng/mL provided adequate anesthesia for superficial surgery.
ALFENTA has an immediate onset of action. At dosages of approximately 105 mcg/kg, ALFENTA produces hypnosis as determined by EEG patterns; an anesthetic ED_{90} of 182 mcg/kg for ALFENTA in unpremedicated patients has been determined, based upon the ability to block response to placement of a nasopharyngeal airway. Based on clinical trials, induction dosage requirements range from 130–245 mcg/kg. For procedures lasting 30–60 minutes, loading dosages of up to 50 mcg/kg produce the hemodynamic responses to endotracheal intubation and skin incision as comparable to those from fentanyl. A pre-intubation loading dose of 50–75 mcg/kg prior to a continuous infusion attenuates the response to laryngoscopy, intubation and incision. Subsequent administration of ALFENTA infusion administered at a rate of 0.5–3.0 mcg/kg/min with nitrous oxide/oxygen attenuates sympathetic responses to surgical stress with more rapid recovery than enflurane.
Requirements for volatile inhalation anesthetics were reduced by thirty to fifty percent during the first 60 minutes of maintenance in patients administered anesthetic doses (above 130 mcg/kg) of ALFENTA as compared to patients given doses of 4–5 mg/kg thiopental for anesthetic induction.
At anesthetic induction dosages, ALFENTA provides a deep level of anesthesia during the first hour of anesthetic maintenance and provides attenuation of the hemodynamic response during intubation and incision.
Following an anesthetic induction dose of ALFENTA, requirements for ALFENTA infusion are reduced by 30 to 50% for the first hour of maintenance.
Patients with compromised liver function and those over 65 years of age have been found to have reduced plasma clearance and extended terminal elimination for ALFENTA, which may prolong postoperative recovery. Repeated or continuous administration of ALFENTA produces increasing plasma concentrations and an accumulation of the drug, particularly in patients with reduced plasma clearance.
Bradycardia may be seen in patients administered ALFENTA. The incidence and degree of bradycardia may be more pronounced when ALFENTA is administered in conjunction with non-vagolytic neuromuscular blocking agents or in the absence of anticholinergic agents such as atropine.
Administration of intravenous diazepam immediately prior to or following high doses of ALFENTA has been shown to produce decreases in blood pressure that may be secondary to vasodilation; recovery may also be prolonged.
Patients administered doses up to 200 mcg/kg of ALFENTA have shown no significant increase in histamine levels and no clinical evidence of histamine release.
Skeletal muscle rigidity is related to the dose and speed of administration of ALFENTA. Muscular rigidity will occur with an immediate onset following anesthetic induction dosages. Preventative measures (see WARNINGS) may reduce the rate and severity.
The duration and degree of respiratory depression and increased airway resistance usually increase with dose, but have also been observed at lower doses. Although higher doses may produce apnea and a longer duration of respiratory depression, apnea may also occur at low doses.
During monitored anesthesia care (MAC), attention must be given to the respiratory effects of ALFENTA Injection. Decreased oxygen saturation, apnea, decreased respiratory rate, and upper airway obstruction can occur. (See WARNINGS)

INDICATIONS AND USAGE

ALFENTA (alfentanil hydrochloride) is indicated:
- as an analgesic adjunct given in incremental doses in the maintenance of anesthesia with barbiturate/nitrous oxide/oxygen.
- as an analgesic administered by continuous infusion with nitrous oxide/oxygen in the maintenance of general anesthesia.
- as a primary anesthetic agent for the induction of anesthesia in patients undergoing general surgery in which endotracheal intubation and mechanical ventilation are required.
- as the analgesic component for monitored anesthesia care (MAC).

SEE DOSAGE CHART FOR MORE COMPLETE INFORMATION ON THE USE OF ALFENTA.

CONTRAINDICATIONS

ALFENTA (alfentanil hydrochloride) is contraindicated in patients with known hypersensitivity to the drug or known intolerance to other opioid agonists.

WARNINGS

ALFENTA SHOULD BE ADMINISTERED ONLY BY PERSONS SPECIFICALLY TRAINED IN THE USE OF INTRAVENOUS AND GENERAL ANESTHETIC AGENTS AND IN THE MANAGEMENT OF RESPIRATORY EFFECTS OF POTENT OPIOIDS.
AN OPIOID ANTAGONIST, RESUSCITATIVE AND INTUBATION EQUIPMENT AND OXYGEN SHOULD BE READILY AVAILABLE.
BECAUSE OF THE POSSIBILITY OF DELAYED RESPIRATORY DEPRESSION, MONITORING OF THE PATIENT MUST CONTINUE WELL AFTER SURGERY.
ALFENTA (alfentanil hydrochloride) administered in initial dosages up to 20 mcg/kg may cause skeletal muscle rigidity, particularly of the truncal muscles. The incidence and severity of muscle rigidity is usually dose-related. Administration of ALFENTA at anesthetic induction dosages (above 130 mcg/kg) will consistently produce muscular rigidity with an immediate onset. The onset of muscular rigidity occurs earlier than with other opioids. ALFENTA may produce muscular rigidity that involves all skeletal muscles, including those of the neck and extremities. The incidence may be reduced by: 1) routine methods of administration of neuromuscular blocking agents for balanced opioid anesthesia; 2) ad-

ministration of up to 1/4 of the full paralyzing dose of a neuromuscular blocking agent just prior to administration of ALFENTA at dosages up to 130 mcg/kg; following loss of consciousness, a full paralyzing dose of a neuromuscular blocking agent should be administered; or 3) simultaneous administration of ALFENTA and a full paralyzing dose of a neuromuscular blocking agent when ALFENTA is used in rapidly administered anesthetic dosages (above 130 mcg/kg). The neuromuscular blocking agent used should be appropriate for the patient's cardiovascular status. Adequate facilities should be available for postoperative monitoring and ventilation of patients administered ALFENTA. It is essential that these facilities be fully equipped to handle all degrees of respiratory depression.

PATIENTS RECEIVING MONITORED ANESTHESIA CARE (MAC) SHOULD BE CONTINUOUSLY MONITORED BY PERSONS NOT INVOLVED IN THE CONDUCT OF THE SURGICAL OR DIAGNOSTIC PROCEDURE; OXYGEN SUPPLEMENTATION SHOULD BE IMMEDIATELY AVAILABLE AND PROVIDED WHERE CLINICALLY INDICATED; OXYGEN SATURATION SHOULD BE CONTINUOUSLY MONITORED; THE PATIENT SHOULD BE OBSERVED FOR EARLY SIGNS OF HYPOTENSION, APNEA, UPPER AIRWAY OBSTRUCTION AND/OR OXYGEN DESATURATION.

Severe and unpredictable potentiation of monoamine oxidose (MAO) inhibitors has been reported for other opioid analgesics, and rarely with alfentanil. Therefore when alfentanil is administered to patients who have received MAO inhibitors within 14 days, appropriate monitoring and ready availability of vasodilators and betablockers for the treatment of hypertension is recommended.

PRECAUTIONS

DELAYED RESPIRATORY DEPRESSION, RESPIRATORY ARREST, BRADYCARDIA, ASYSTOLE, ARRHYTHMIAS AND HYPOTENSION HAVE ALSO BEEN REPORTED. THEREFORE, VITAL SIGNS MUST BE MONITORED CONTINUOUSLY.

General: The initial dose of ALFENTA (alfentanil hydrochloride) should be appropriately reduced in elderly and debilitated patients. The effect of the initial dose should be considered in determining supplemental doses. In obese patients (more than 20% above ideal total body weight), the dosage of ALFENTA should be determined on the basis of lean body weight.

In one clinical trial, the dose of ALFENTA required to produce anesthesia, as determined by appearance of delta waves in EEG, was 40% lower in geriatric patients than that needed in healthy young patients.

In patients with compromised liver function and in geriatric patients, the plasma clearance of ALFENTA may be reduced and postoperative recovery may be prolonged.

Induction doses of ALFENTA should be administered slowly (over three minutes). Administration may produce loss of vascular tone and hypotension. Consideration should be given to fluid replacement prior to induction.

Diazepam administered immediately prior to or in conjunction with high doses of ALFENTA may produce vasodilation, hypotension and result in delayed recovery.

Bradycardia produced by ALFENTA may be treated with atropine. Severe bradycardia and asystole have been successfully treated with atropine and conventional resuscitative methods.

The hemodynamic effects of a particular muscle relaxant and the degree of skeletal muscle relaxation required should be considered in the selection of a neuromuscular blocking agent.

Following an anesthetic induction dose of ALFENTA, requirements for volatile inhalation anesthetics or ALFENTA infusion are reduced by 30 to 50% for the first hour of maintenance.

ALFENTA infusions should be discontinued at least 10–15 minutes prior to the end of surgery during general anesthesia. During administration of ALFENTA for Monitored Anesthesia Care (MAC), infusions may be continued to the end of the procedure.

Respiratory depression caused by opioid analgesics can be reversed by opioid antagonists such as naloxone. Because the duration of respiratory depression produced by ALFENTA may last longer than the duration of the opioid antagonist action, appropriate surveillance should be maintained. As with all potent opioids, profound analgesia is accompanied by respiratory depression and diminished sensitivity to CO_2 stimulation which may persist into or recur in the postoperative period. Intraoperative hyperventilation may further alter postoperative response to CO_2. Appropriate postoperative monitoring should be employed, particularly after infusions and large doses of ALFENTA, to ensure that adequate spontaneous breathing is established and maintained in the absence of stimulation prior to discharging the patient from the recovery area.

Head Injuries: ALFENTA should be used with caution in patients with head injury or increased intracranial pressure, due to the risk of respiratory depression. As with all opioids, ALFENTA may obscure the clinical course of patients with head injuries and should be used only if clinically indicated.

Impaired Respiration: ALFENTA should be used with caution in patients with pulmonary disease, decreased respiratory reserve or potentially compromised respiration. In such patients, opioids may additionally decrease respiratory drive and increase airway resistance. During anesthesia, this can be managed by assisted or controlled respiration.

Impaired Hepatic or Renal Fuction: In patients with liver or kidney dysfunction, ALFENTA should be administered with caution due to the importance of these organs in the metabolism and excretion of ALFENTA.

Drug Interactions: Both the magnitude and duration of central nervous system and cardiovascular effects may be enhanced when ALFENTA is administered in combination with other CNS depressants such as barbiturates, tranquilizers, opioids, or inhalation general anesthetics. Postoperative respiratory depression may be enhanced or prolonged by these agents. In such cases of combined treatment, the dose of one or both agents should be reduced. Limited clinical experience indicates that requirements for volatile inhalation anesthetics are reduced by 30 to 50% for the first sixty (60) minutes following ALFENTA induction.

The concomitant use of erythromycin with ALFENTA can significantly inhibit ALFENTA clearance and may increase the risk of prolonged or delayed respiratory depression.

Cimetidine reduces the clearance of ALFENTA. Therefore smaller ALFENTA doses will be required with prolonged administration and the duration of action of ALFENTA may be extended.

Perioperative administration of drugs affecting hepatic blood flow or enzyme function may reduce plasma clearance and prolong recovery.

Carcinogenesis, Mutagenesis and Impairment of Fertility: No long-term animal studies of ALFENTA have been performed to evaluate carcinogenic potential. No structural chromosome mutations were produced in the *in vivo* micronucleus test in female rats at single intravenous doses of ALFENTA as high as 20 mg/kg body weight (approximately 40 times the upper human dose), equivalent to a dose of 103 mg/m^2 body surface area. No dominant lethal mutations were produced in the *in vivo* dominant lethal test in male and female mice at the maximum intravenous dose of 20 mg/kg (60 mg/m^2). No mutagenic activity was revealed in the *in vitro* Ames *Salmonella typhimurium* test, with and without metabolic activation.

Pregnancy Category C: ALFENTA has been shown to have an embryocidal effect in rats and rabbits when given in doses 2.5 times the upper human dose for a period of 10 days to over 30 days. These effects could have been due to maternal toxicity (decreased food consumption with increased mortality) following prolonged administration of the drug.

No evidence of teratogenic effects has been observed after administration of ALFENTA in rats or rabbits.

There are no adequate and well-controlled studies in pregnant women. ALFENTA should be used during pregnancy only if the potential benefit justifies the potential risk to the fetus.

Labor and Delivery: There are insufficient data to support the use of ALFENTA in labor and delivery. Placental transfer of the drug has been reported; therefore, use in labor and delivery is not recommended.

Nursing Mothers: In one study of nine women undergoing postpartum tubal ligation, significant levels of ALFENTA were detected in colostrum four hours after adminstration of 60 μg/kg of ALFENTA, with no detectable levels present after 28 hours. Caution should be exercised when ALFENTA is administered to a nursing woman.

Pediatric Use: Adequate data to support the use of ALFENTA in children under 12 years of age are not presently available.

ADVERSE REACTIONS

The most common adverse reactions of opioids are respiratory depression and skeletal muscle rigidity, particularly of the truncal muscles. ALFENTA may produce muscular rigidity that involves the skeletal muscles of the neck and extremities. See CLINICAL PHARMACOLOGY, WARNINGS, and PRECAUTIONS on the management of respiratory depression and skeletal muscle rigidity.

The adverse experience profile from 696 patients receiving ALFENTA for Monitored Anesthesia Care (MAC) is similar to the profile established with ALFENTA during general anesthesia. Respiratory events reported during MAC included hypoxia, apnea, and bradypnea. Other adverse events reported by patients receiving ALFENTA for MAC, in order of decreasing frequency, were nausea, hypotension, vomiting, pruritus, confusion, somnolence and agitation.

The following adverse reaction information is derived from controlled and open clinical trials in 785 patients who received intravenous ALFENTA during induction and maintenance of general anesthesia. The controlled trials included treatment comparisons with fentanyl, thiopental sodium, enflurane, saline placebo and halothane. The incidence of certain side effects is influenced by the type of use, e.g., chest wall rigidity has a higher reported incidence in clinical trials of alfentanil induction, and by the type of surgery, e.g., nausea and vomiting have a higher reported incidence in patients undergoing gynecologic surgery. The overall reports of nausea and vomiting with ALFENTA were comparable to fentanyl.

Incidence Greater than 1%—Probably Causally Related
(Derived from clinical trials)

Gastrointestinal:	nausea (28%), vomiting (18%)
Cardiovascular:	arrhythmia, bradycardia (14%), hypertension (18%), hypotension (10%), tachycardia (12%)
Musculoskeletal:	chest wall rigidity (17%), skeletal muscle movements*
Respiratory:	apnea*, postoperative respiratory depression
Central Nervous System:	blurred vision, dizziness*, sleepiness/postoperative sedation

*Incidence 3% to 9%
All others 1% to 3%

Incidence Less than 1%—Probably Causally Related
(Derived from clinical trials)
Adverse events reported in post-marketing surveillance, not seen in clinical trials, are *italicized.*

Body as a whole:	*anaphylaxis*
Central Nervous System:	headache*, *myoclonic movements,* postoperative confusion*, postoperative euphoria*, shivering*
Dermatological:	itching*, urticaria*
Injection Site:	pain*
Musculoskeletal:	*skeletal muscle rigidity of neck and extremities*
Respiratory:	bronchospasm, hypercarbia*, laryngospasm*

*Incidence 0.3% to 1%

DRUG ABUSE AND DEPENDENCE

ALFENTA (alfentanil hydrochloride) is a Schedule II controlled drug substance that can produce drug dependence of the morphine type and therefore has the potential for being abused.

Opioid analgesics have been associated with abuse and dependence in healthcare providers and others with ready access to such drugs. ALFENTA should be handled accordingly.

OVERDOSAGE

Overdosage would be manifested by extension of the pharmacological actions of ALFENTA (alfentanil hydrochloride) (see CLINICAL PHARMACOLOGY) as with other potent opioid analgesics. No experience of overdosage with ALFENTA was reported during clinical trials. The intravenous LD_{50} of ALFENTA is 43–51 mg/kg in rats, 72–74 mg/kg in mice, 72–82 mg/kg in guinea pigs and 60–88 mg/kg in dogs. Intravenous administration of an opioid antagonist such as naloxone should be employed as a specific antidote to manage respiratory depression.

The duration of respiratory depression following overdosage with ALFENTA may be longer than the duration of action of the opioid antagonist. Administration of an opioid antagonist should not preclude immediate establishment of a patent airway, administration of oxygen, and assisted or controlled ventilation as indicated for hypoventilation or apnea. If respiratory depression is associated with muscular rigidity, a neuromuscular blocking agent may be required to facilitate assisted or controlled ventilation. Intravenous fluids and vasoactive agents may be required to manage hemodynamic instability.

DOSAGE AND ADMINISTRATION

The dosage of ALFENTA (alfentanil hydrochloride) should be individualized and titrated to the desired effect in each patient according to body weight, physical status, underlying pathological condition, use of other drugs, and type and duration of surgical procedure and anesthesia. In obese patients (more than 20% above ideal total body weight), the dosage of ALFENTA should be determined on the basis of lean body weight. The dose of ALFENTA should be reduced in elderly or debilitated patients (see PRECAUTIONS).

Vital signs should be monitored routinely.

See Dosage Guidelines for the use of ALFENTA: 1) by incremental injection as an analgesic adjunct to anesthesia with barbiturate/nitrous oxide/oxygen for short surgical procedures (expected duration of less than one hour); 2) by continuous infusion as a maintenance analgesic with nitrous oxide/oxygen for general surgical procedures; and 3) by intravenous injection in anesthetic doses for the induction of anesthesia for general surgical procedures with a minimum expected duration of 45 minutes; and 4) by intravenous injec-

Continued on next page

Janssen Pharmaceutica—Cont.

DOSAGE GUIDELINES
DOSAGE SHOULD BE INDIVIDUALIZED AND TITRATED

FOR USE DURING GENERAL ANESTHESIA

SPONTANEOUSLY BREATHING/ ASSISTED VENTILATION	**Induction of Analgesia:** 8–20 mcg/kg **Maintenance of Analgesia:** 3–5 mcg/kg q 5–20 min or 0.5 to 1 mcg/kg/min **Total dose:** 8–40 mcg/kg
ASSISTED OR CONTROLLED VENTILATION	
Incremental Injection *(To attenuate response to laryngoscopy and intubation)*	**Induction of Analgesia:** 20–50 mcg/kg **Maintenance of Analgesia:** 5–15 mcg/kg q 5–20 min **Total dose:** Up to 75 mcg/kg
Continuous Infusion *(To provide attenuation of response to intubation and incision)*	Infusion rates are variable and should be titrated to the desired clinical effect. SEE INFUSION DOSAGE GUIDELINES BELOW. **Induction of Analgesia:** 50–75 mcg/kg **Maintenance of Analgesia:** 0.5 to 3 mcg/kg/min (Average rate 1 to 1.5 mcg/kg/min) **Total dose:** Dependent on duration of procedure
Anesthetic Induction	**Induction of Anesthesia:** 130–245 mcg/kg **Maintenance of Anesthesia:** 0.5 to 1.5 mcg/kg/min or general anesthetic **Total dose:** Dependent on duration of procedure *At these doses, truncal rigidity should be expected and a muscle relaxant should be utilized.* *Administer slowly (over 3 minutes).* Concentration of inhalation agents reduced by 30–50% for initial hour.
MONITORED ANESTHESIA CARE (MAC) *(For sedated and responsive, spontaneously breathing patients)*	**Induction of MAC:** 3–8 mcg/kg **Maintenance of MAC:** 3–5 mcg/kg q 5–20 min or 0.25 to 1 mcg/kg/min **Total dose:** 3–40 mcg/kg

INFUSION DOSAGE

Continuous Infusion: 0.5–3mcg/kg/min administered with nitrous oxide/oxygen in patients undergoing general surgery. Following an anesthetic induction dose of ALFENTA, infusion rate requirements are reduced by 30–50% for the first hour of maintenance.

Changes in vital signs that indicate a response to surgical stress or lightening of anesthesia may be controlled by increasing the alfentanil to a maximum of 4 mcg/kg/min and/or administration of bolus doses of 7 mcg/kg. If changes are not controlled after three bolus doses given over a five minute period, a barbiturate, vasodilator, and/or inhalation agent should be used. Infusion rates should always be adjusted downward in the absence of these signs until there is some response to surgical stimulation.

Rather than an increase in infusion rate, 7 mcg/kg bolus doses of ALFENTA or a potent inhalation agent should be administered in response to signs of lightening of anesthesia within the last 15 minutes of surgery. ALFENTA infusion should be discontinued at least 10–15 minutes prior to the end of surgery.

tion as the analgesic component for monitored anesthesia care (MAC).
[See table above.]

Usage in Children: Clinical data to support the use of ALFENTA in patients under 12 years of age are not presently available. Therefore, such use is not recommended.

Premedication: The selection of preanesthetic medications should be based upon the needs of the individual patient.

Neuromuscular Blocking Agents: The neuromuscular blocking agent selected should be compatible with the patient's condition, taking into account the hemodynamic effects of a particular muscle relaxant and the degree of skeletal muscle relaxation required (see CLINICAL PHARMACOLOGY, WARNINGS and PRECAUTIONS sections).
In patients administered anesthetic (induction) dosages of ALFENTA, it is essential that qualified personnel and adequate facilities are available for the management of intraoperative and postoperative respiratory depression.
Also see WARNINGS and PRECAUTIONS sections.
For purposes of administering small volumes of ALFENTA accurately, the use of a tuberculin syringe or equivalent is recommended.
The physical and chemical compatibility of ALFENTA have been demonstrated in solution with normal saline, 5% dextrose in normal saline, 5% dextrose in water and Lactated Ringers. Clinical studies of ALFENTA infusion have been conducted with ALFENTA diluted to a concentration range of 25 mcg/mL to 80 mcg/ml.
As an example of the preparation of ALFENTA for infusion, 20 mL of ALFENTA added to 230 mL of diluent provides a 40 μg/mL solution of ALFENTA.
Parenteral drug products should be inspected visually for particulate matter and discoloration prior to administration, whenever solution and container permit.

SAFETY AND HANDLING
ALFENTA (alfentanil hydrochloride) is supplied in individually sealed dosage forms which pose no known risk to healthcare providers having incidental contact. Accidental dermal exposure to ALFENTA should be treated by rinsing the affected area with water.
Protect from light. Store at room temperature 15°–30°C (59°–86°F).

HOW SUPPLIED
Each mL of ALFENTA (alfentanil hydrochloride) Injection for intravenous use contains alfentanil hydrochloride equivalent to 500 μg of alfentanil base. ALFENTA Injection is available as:
NDC 50458-060-02, 2 mL ampoules in packages of 10
NDC 50458-060-05, 5 mL ampoules in packages of 10
NDC 50458-060-10, 10 mL ampoules in packages of 5
NDC 50458-060-20, 20 mL ampoules in packages of 5
U.S. Patent No. 4,167,574
April 1995, May 1995
JANSSEN PHARMACEUTICA INC.
Titusville, NJ 08560-0200
Shown in Product Identification Guide, page 318

DURAGESIC®   Ⓒ℞
[*dūr-a-jē'sik*]
(fentanyl transdermal system)

Full Prescribing Information

> BECAUSE SERIOUS OR LIFE-THREATENING HYPOVENTILATION COULD OCCUR, DURAGESIC IS CONTRAINDICATED:
> - In the management of acute or post-operative pain, including use in out-patient surgeries
> - In the management of mild or intermittent pain responsive to PRN or non–opioid therapy
> - In doses exceeding 25 mcg/hour at the initiation of opioid therapy
> (See CONTRAINDICATIONS for further information.)
> DURAGESIC SHOULD NOT BE ADMINISTERED TO CHILDREN UNDER 12 YEARS OF AGE OR PATIENTS UNDER 18 YEARS OF AGE WHO WEIGH LESS THAN 50 KG (110 LBS) EXCEPT IN AN AUTHORIZED INVESTIGATIONAL RESEARCH SETTING. (See PRECAUTIONS - Pediatric Use.)
> *DURAGESIC is indicated for treatment of chronic pain (such as that of malignancy) that:*
> - cannot be managed by lesser means such as acetaminophen-opioid combinations, non-steroidal analgesics, or PRN dosing with short-acting opioids and

- requires continuous opioid administration.
The 50, 75, and 100 mcg/hour dosages should ONLY be used in patients who are already on and are tolerant to opioid therapy.

WARNING: May be habit forming.

DESCRIPTION
DURAGESIC is a transdermal system providing continuous systemic delivery of fentanyl, a potent opioid analgesic, for 72 hours. The chemical name is N-Phenyl-N-(1-2-phenyl-ethyl-4-piperidyl) propanamide. The structural formula is

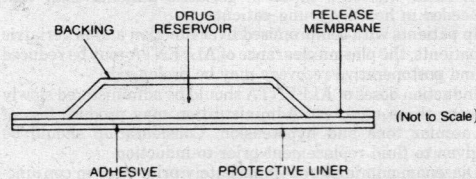

The molecular weight of fentanyl base is 336.5, and the empirical formula is $C_{22}H_{28}N_2O$. The n-octanol:water partition coefficient is 860:1. The pKa is 8.4.

System Components and Structure
The amount of fentanyl released from each system per hour is proportional to the surface area (25 μg/h per 10 cm²). The composition per unit area of all system sizes is identical. Each system also contains 0.1 mL of alcohol USP per 10 cm².

Dose* (μg/h)	Size (cm²)	Fentanyl Content (mg)
25	10	2.5
50**	20	5
75**	30	7.5
100**	40	10

*Nominal delivery rate per hour
**FOR USE ONLY IN OPIOID TOLERANT PATIENTS

DURAGESIC is a rectangular transparent unit comprising a protective liner and four functional layers. Proceeding from the outer surface toward the surface adhering to skin, these layers are:
1) a backing layer of polyester film; 2) a drug reservoir of fentanyl and alcohol USP gelled with hydroxyethyl cellulose; 3) an ethylene-vinyl acetate copolymer membrane that controls the rate of fentanyl delivery to the skin surface; and 4) a fentanyl containing silicone adhesive. Before use, a protective liner covering the adhesive layer is removed and discarded.

The active component of the system is fentanyl. The remaining components are pharmacologically inactive. Less than 0.2 mL of alcohol is also released from the system during use. Do not cut or damage DURAGESIC. If the DURAGESIC system is cut or damaged, controlled drug delivery will not be possible.

CLINICAL PHARMACOLOGY
Pharmacology
Fentanyl is an opioid analgesic. Fentanyl interacts predominately with the opioid μ-receptor. These μ-binding sites are discretely distributed in the human brain, spinal cord, and other tissues.
In clinical settings, fentanyl exerts its principal pharmacologic effects on the central nervous system. Its primary actions of therapeutic value are analgesia and sedation. Fentanyl may increase the patient's tolerance for pain and decrease the perception of suffering, although the presence of the pain itself may still be recognized.
In addition to analgesia, alterations in mood, euphoria and dysphoria, and drowsiness commonly occur. Fentanyl depresses the respiratory centers, depresses the cough reflex, and constricts the pupils. Analgesic blood levels of fentanyl may cause nausea and vomiting directly by stimulating the chemoreceptor trigger zone, but nausea and vomiting are significantly more common in ambulatory than in recumbent patients, as is postural syncope.
Opioids increase the tone and decrease the propulsive contractions of the smooth muscle of the gastrointestinal tract. The resultant prolongation in gastrointestinal transit time may be responsible for the constipating effect of fentanyl. Because opioids may increase biliary tract pressure, some patients with biliary colic may experience worsening rather than relief of pain.
While opioids generally increase the tone of urinary tract smooth muscle, the net effect tends to be variable, in some

cases producing urinary urgency, in others, difficulty in urination.

At therapeutic dosages, fentanyl usually does not exert major effects on the cardiovascular system. However, some patients may exhibit orthostatic hypotension and fainting. Histamine assays and skin wheal testing in man indicate that clinically significant histamine release rarely occurs with fentanyl administration. Assays in man show no clinically significant histamine release in dosages up to 50 µg/kg.

Pharmacokinetics (see table and graph)

DURAGESIC releases fentanyl from the reservoir at a nearly constant amount per unit time. The concentration gradient existing between the saturated solution of drug in the reservoir and the lower concentration in the skin drives drug release. Fentanyl moves in the direction of the lower concentration at a rate determined by the copolymer release membrane and the diffusion of fentanyl through the skin layers. While the actual rate of fentanyl delivery to the skin varies over the 72 hour application period, each system is labeled with a nominal flux which represents the average amount of drug delivered to the systemic circulation per hour across average skin.

While there is variation in dose delivered among patients, the nominal flux of the systems (25, 50, 75, and 100 µg of fentanyl per hour) are sufficiently accurate as to allow individual titration of dosage for a given patient. The small amount of alcohol which has been incorporated into the system enhances the rate of drug flux through the rate-limiting copolymer membrane and increases the permeability of the skin to fentanyl.

Following DURAGESIC application, the skin under the system absorbs fentanyl, and a depot of fentanyl concentrates in the upper skin layers. Fentanyl then becomes available to the systemic circulation. Serum fentanyl concentrations increase gradually following initial DURAGESIC application, generally leveling off between 12 and 24 hours and remaining relatively constant, with some fluctuation, for the remainder of the 72 hour application period. Peak serum levels of fentanyl generally occurred between 24 and 72 hours after initial application. Serum fentanyl concentrations achieved are proportional to the DURAGESIC delivery rate. With continuous use, serum fentanyl concentrations continue to rise for the first few system applications. After several sequential 72-hour applications, patients reach and maintain a steady state serum concentration that is determined by individual variation in skin permeability and body clearance of fentanyl (see graph and Table A).

After system removal, serum fentanyl concentrations decline gradually, falling about 50% in approximately 17 (range 13–22) hours. Continued absorption of fentanyl from the skin accounts for a slower disappearance of the drug from the serum than is seen after an IV infusion, where the apparent half-life ranges from 3–12 hours.

[See graph above.]
[See table A below.]

Fentanyl plasma protein binding capacity decreases with increasing ionization of the drug. Alterations in pH may affect its distribution between plasma and the central nervous system. Fentanyl accumulates in the skeletal muscle and fat and is released slowly into the blood.

The average volume of distribution for fentanyl is 6 L/kg (range 3–8, N=8). The average clearance in patients undergoing various surgical procedures is 46 L/h (range 27–75, N=8). The kinetics of fentanyl in geriatric patients has not been well studied, but in geriatric patients the clearance of IV fentanyl may be reduced and the terminal half-life greatly prolonged (see PRECAUTIONS).

Fentanyl is metabolized primarily in the liver. In humans the drug appears to be metabolized primarily by N-dealkylation to norfentanyl and other inactive metabolites that do not contribute materially to the observed activity of the drug. Within 72 hours of IV fentanyl administration, approx-

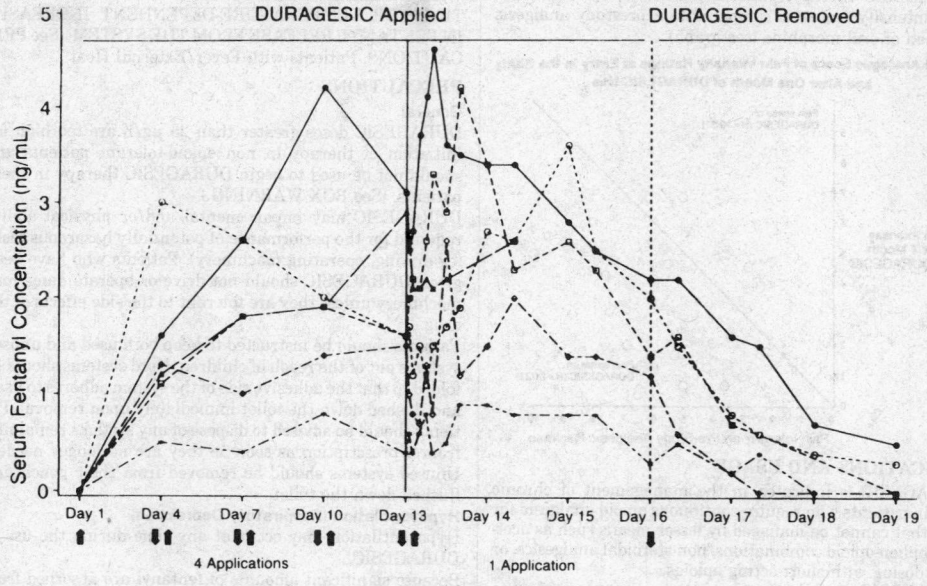

Serum Fentanyl Concentrations Following Multiple Applications of DURAGESIC 100 µg/h

imately 75% of the dose is excreted in urine, mostly as metabolites with less than 10% representing unchanged drug. Approximately 9% of the dose is recovered in the feces, primarily as metabolites. Mean values for unbound fractions of fentanyl in plasma are estimated to be between 13 and 21%. Skin does not appear to metabolize fentanyl delivered transdermally. This was determined in a human keratinocyte cell assay and in clinical studies in which 92% of the dose delivered from the system was accounted for as unchanged fentanyl that appeared in the systemic circulation.

Pharmacodynamics

Analgesia

DURAGESIC is a strong opioid analgesic. In controlled clinical trials in non-opioid tolerant patients, 60 mg/day IM morphine was considered to provide analgesia approximately equivalent to DURAGESIC 100 µg/h in an acute pain model. Minimum effective analgesic serum concentrations of fentanyl in opioid naive patients range from 0.2 to 1.2 ng/mL; side effects increase in frequency at serum levels above 2 ng/mL. Both the minimum effective concentration and the concentration at which toxicity occurs rise with increasing tolerance. The rate of development of tolerance varies widely among individuals.

Ventilatory Effects

At equivalent analgesic serum concentrations, fentanyl and morphine produce a similar degree of hypoventilation. A small number of patients have experienced clinically significant hypoventilation with DURAGESIC. Hypoventilation was manifest by respiratory rates of less than 8 breaths/minute or a pCO_2 greater than 55 mm Hg. In clinical trials of 357 postoperative (acute pain) patients treated with DURAGESIC, 13 patients experienced hypoventilation. As a consequence, 10 of these 13 patients received naloxone, two patients had their dose reduced and one patient required no treatment beyond verbal stimulation. Of the 13 events, seven

were associated with DURAGESIC 100 µg/h and six were associated with DURAGESIC 75 µg/h. In these studies the incidence of hypoventilation was higher in nontolerant women (10) than in men (3) and in patients weighing less than 63 kg (9 of 13). Although patients with impaired respiration were not common in the trials, they had higher rates of hypoventilation.

While most patients using DURAGESIC chronically develop tolerance to fentanyl induced hypoventilation, episodes of slowed respirations may occur at any time during therapy; medical intervention generally was not required in these instances.

Hypoventilation can occur throughout the therapeutic range of fentanyl serum concentrations. However, the risk of hypoventilation increases at serum fentanyl concentrations greater than 2 ng/mL in non opioid-tolerant patients, especially for patients who have an underlying pulmonary condition or who receive usual doses of opioids or other CNS drugs associated with hypoventilation in addition to DURAGESIC. The use of DURAGESIC should be monitored by clinical evaluation. As with other drug level measurements, serum fentanyl concentrations may be useful clinically, although they do not reflect patient sensitivity to fentanyl and should not be used by physicians as a sole indicator of effectiveness or toxicity.

See BOX WARNING, CONTRAINDICATIONS, WARNINGS, PRECAUTIONS, ADVERSE REACTIONS, and OVERDOSAGE for additional information on hypoventilation.

Cardiovascular Effects

Intravenous fentanyl may infrequently produce bradycardia. The incidence of bradycardia in clinical trials with DURAGESIC was less than 1%.

CNS Effects

In opioid naive patients, central nervous system effects increase when serum fentanyl concentrations are greater than 3 ng/mL.

CLINICAL TRIALS

DURAGESIC was studied in patients with acute and chronic pain (postoperative and cancer pain models).

The analgesic efficacy of DURAGESIC was demonstrated in an acute pain model with surgical procedures expected to produce various intensities of pain (eg hysterectomy, major orthopedic surgery). Clinical use and safety was evaluated in patients experiencing chronic pain due to malignancy. Based on the results of these trials, DURAGESIC was determined to be effective in both populations, but safe only for use in patients with chronic pain. Because of the risk of hypoventilation (4% incidence) in postoperative patients with acute pain, DURAGESIC is contraindicated for postoperative analgesia. (See BOX WARNING and CONTRAINDICATIONS.)

DURAGESIC as therapy for pain due to cancer has been studied in 153 patients. In this patient population, DURAGESIC has been administered in doses of 25 µg/h to 600 µg/h. Individual patients have used DURAGESIC continuously for up to 866 days. At one month after initiation of

TABLE A
RANGE OF PHARMACOKINETIC PARAMETERS OF FENTANYL IN PATIENTS

	Clearance (L/h) Range (70 kg)	Volume of Distribution V_{SS} (L/kg) Range	Half Life $t_{1/2}$ (h) Range	Maximal Concentration C_{max} (ng/mL) Range	Time to Maximal Concentration (h) Range
IV Fentanyl					
Surgical Patients	27–75	3–8	3–12		
Hepatically Impaired Patients	3–80†	0.8–8†	4–12†		
Renally Impaired Patients	30–78				
DURAGESIC 25 µg/h			*	0.3–1.2	26–78
DURAGESIC 50 µg/h			*	0.6–1.8†	24–72†
DURAGESIC 75 µg/h			*	1.1–2.6	24–48
DURAGESIC 100 µg/h			*	1.9–3.8	25–72

†Estimated
* After system removal there is continued systemic absorption from residual fentanyl in the skin so that serum concentrations fall 50%, on average, in 17 hours.

Continued on next page

Janssen Pharmaceutica—Cont.

DURAGESIC therapy, patients generally reported lower pain intensity scores as compared to a prestudy analgesic regimen of oral morphine (see graph)

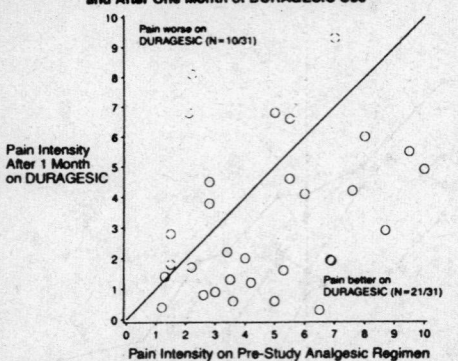

Visual Analogue Score of Pain Intensity Ratings at Entry in the Study and After One Month of DURAGESIC Use

INDICATIONS AND USAGE

DURAGESIC is indicated in the management of chronic pain in patients who require continuous opioid analgesia for pain that cannot be managed by lesser means such as acetaminophen-opioid combinations, non-steroidal analgesics, or PRN dosing with short-acting opioids.

DURAGESIC should not be used in the management of acute or postoperative pain because serious or life-threatening hypoventilation could result. (See BOX WARNING and CONTRAINDICATIONS.)

In patients with chronic pain, it is possible to individually titrate the dose of the transdermal system to minimize the risk of adverse effects while providing analgesia. In properly selected patients, DURAGESIC is a safe and effective alternative to other opioid regimens. (See DOSAGE AND ADMINISTRATION.)

CONTRAINDICATIONS

BECAUSE SERIOUS OR LIFE-THREATENING HYPOVENTILATION COULD OCCUR, DURAGESIC IS CONTRAINDICATED:

- in the management of acute or post-operative pain, including use in out-patient surgeries because there is no opportunity for proper dose titration (See CLINICAL PHARMACOLOGY and DOSAGE AND ADMINISTRATION),
- in the management of mild or intermittent pain that can otherwise be managed by lesser means such as acetaminophen-opioid combinations, non-steriodal analgesics, or PRN dosing with short-acting opioids, and
- in doses exceeding 25 mcg/hour at the initiation of opioid therapy because of the need to individualize dosing by titrating to the desired analgesic effect.

DURAGESIC is also contraindicated in patients with known hypersensitivity to fentanyl or adhesives.

WARNINGS

DURAGESIC SHOULD NOT BE ADMINISTERED TO CHILDREN UNDER 12 YEARS OF AGE OR PATIENTS UNDER 18 YEARS OF AGE WHO WEIGH LESS THAN 50 KG (110 LBS) EXCEPT IN AN AUTHORIZED INVESTIGATIONAL RESEARCH SETTING. (See PRECAUTIONS-Pediatric Use.) PATIENTS WHO HAVE EXPERIENCED ADVERSE EVENTS SHOULD BE MONITORED FOR AT LEAST 12 HOURS AFTER DURAGESIC REMOVAL SINCE SERUM FENTANYL CONCENTRATIONS DECLINE GRADUALLY AND REACH AN APPROXIMATE 50% REDUCTION IN SERUM CONCENTRATIONS 17 HOURS AFTER SYSTEM REMOVAL.

DURAGESIC SHOULD BE PRESCRIBED ONLY BY PERSONS KNOWLEDGEABLE IN THE CONTINUOUS ADMINISTRATION OF POTENT OPIOIDS, IN THE MANAGEMENT OF PATIENTS RECEIVING POTENT OPIOIDS FOR TREATMENT OF PAIN, AND IN THE DETECTION AND MANAGEMENT OF HYPOVENTILATION INCLUDING THE USE OF OPIOID ANTAGONISTS.

THE CONCOMITANT USE OF OTHER CENTRAL NERVOUS SYSTEM DEPRESSANTS, INCLUDING OTHER OPIOIDS, SEDATIVES OR HYPNOTICS, GENERAL ANESTHETICS, PHENOTHIAZINES, TRANQUILIZERS, SKELETAL MUSCLE RELAXANTS, SEDATING ANTIHISTAMINES, AND ALCOHOLIC BEVERAGES MAY PRODUCE ADDITIVE DEPRESSANT EFFECTS. HYPOVENTILATION, HYPOTENSION AND PROFOUND SEDATION OR COMA MAY OCCUR. WHEN SUCH COMBINED THERAPY IS CONTEMPLATED, THE DOSE OF ONE OR BOTH AGENTS SHOULD BE REDUCED BY AT LEAST 50%.

ALL PATIENTS SHOULD BE ADVISED TO AVOID EXPOSING THE DURAGESIC APPLICATION SITE TO DIRECT EXTERNAL HEAT SOURCES, SUCH AS HEATING PADS OR ELECTRIC BLANKETS, HEAT LAMPS, SUANAS, HOT TUBS, AND HEATED WATER BEDS, ETC. WHILE WEARING THE SYSTEM. THERE IS A POTENTIAL FOR TEMPERATURE-DEPENDENT INCREASES IN FENTANYL RELEASE FROM THE SYSTEM. (See PRECAUTIONS, Patients with Fever/External Heat.)

PRECAUTIONS

General

DURAGESIC doses greater than 25 µg/h are too high for initiation of therapy in non opioid-tolerant patients and should not be used to begin DURAGESIC therapy in these patients. (See BOX WARNING.)

DURAGESIC may impair mental and/or physical ability required for the performance of potentially hazardous tasks (eg driving, operating machinery). Patients who have been given DURAGESIC should not drive or operate dangerous machinery unless they are tolerant to the side effects of the drug.

Patients should be instructed to keep both used and unused systems out of the reach of children. Used systems should be folded so that the adhesive side of the system adheres to itself and flushed down the toilet immediately upon removal. Patients should be advised to dispose of any systems remaining from a prescription as soon as they are no longer needed. Unused systems should be removed from their pouch and flushed down the toilet.

Hypoventilation (Respiratory Depression)

Hypoventilation may occur at any time during the use of DURAGESIC.

Because significant amounts of fentanyl are absorbed from the skin for 17 hours or more after the system is removed, hypoventilation may persist beyond the removal of DURAGESIC. Consequently, patients with hypoventilation should be carefully observed for degree of sedation and their respiratory rate monitored until respiration has stabilized. The use of concomitant CNS active drugs requires special patient care and observation. See WARNINGS.

Chronic Pulmonary Disease

Because potent opioids can cause hypoventilation, DURAGESIC® (fentanyl transdermal system) should be administered with caution to patients with preexisting medical conditions predisposing them to hypoventilation. In such patients, normal analgesic doses of opioids may further decrease respiratory drive to the point of respiratory failure.

Head Injuries and Increased Intracranial Pressure

DURAGESIC should not be used in patients who may be particularly susceptible to the intracranial effects of CO_2 retention such as those with evidence of increased intracranial pressure, impaired consciousness, or coma. Opioids may obscure the clinical course of patients with head injury. DURAGESIC should be used with caution in patients with brain tumors.

Cardiac Disease

Intravenous fentanyl may produce bradycardia. Fentanyl should be administered with caution to patients with bradyarrhythmias.

Hepatic or Renal Disease

At the present time insufficient information exists to make recommendations regarding the use of DURAGESIC in patients with impaired renal or hepatic function. If the drug is used in these patients, it should be used with caution because of the hepatic metabolism and renal excretion of fentanyl.

Patients with Fever/External Heat

Based on a pharmacokinetic model, serum fentanyl concentrations could theoretically increase by approximately one third for patients with a body temperature of 40°C (102°F) due to temperature-dependent increases in fentanyl release from the system and increased skin permeability. Therefore, patients wearing DURAGESIC systems who develop fever should be monitored for opioid side effects and the DURAGESIC dose should be adjusted if necessary.

ALL PATIENTS SHOULD BE ADVISED TO AVOID EXPOSING THE DURAGESIC APPLICATION SITE TO DIRECT EXTERNAL HEAT SOURCES, SUCH AS HEATING PADS OR ELECTRIC BLANKETS, HEAT LAMPS, SAUNAS, HOT TUBS, AND HEATED WATER BEDS, ETC. WHILE WEARING THE SYSTEM. THERE IS A POTENTIAL FOR TEMPERATURE-DEPENDENT INCREASES IN FENTANYL RELEASE FROM THE SYSTEM.

Central Nervous System Depressants

When patients are receiving DURAGESIC, the dose of additional opioids or other CNS depressant drugs (including benzodiazepines) should be reduced by at least 50%. With the concomitant use of CNS depressants, hypotension may occur.

Drug or Alcohol Dependence

Use of DURAGESIC in combination with alcoholic beverages and/or other CNS depressants can result in increased risk to the patient. DURAGESIC should be used with caution in individuals who have a history of drug or alcohol abuse, especially if they are outside a medically controlled environment.

Ambulatory Patients

Strong opioid analgesics impair the mental or physical abilities required for the performance of potentially dangerous tasks such as driving a car or operating machinery. Patients who have been given DURAGESIC should not drive or operate dangerous machinery unless they are tolerant to the effects of the drug.

Carcinogenesis, Mutagenesis, and Impairment of Fertility

Because long-term animal studies have not been conducted, the potential carcinogenic effects of DURAGESIC are unknown. There was no evidence of mutagenicity in the Ames Salmonella mutagenicity assay, the primary rat hepatocyte unscheduled DNA synthesis assay, the BALB/c-3T3 transformation test, and the human lymphocyte and CHO chromosomal aberration in-vitro assays.

In the mouse lymphoma assay, fentanyl concentrations 2000 times greater than those seen with chronic DURAGESIC use were only mutagenic in the presence of metabolic activation.

Pregnancy—Pregnancy Category C

Fentanyl has been shown to impair fertility and to have an embryocidal effect in rats when given in intravenous doses 0.3 times the human dose for a period of 12 days. No evidence of teratogenic effects has been observed after administration of fentanyl to rats. There are no adequate and well-controlled studies in pregnant women. DURAGESIC should be used during pregnancy only if the potential benefit justifies the potential risk to the fetus.

Labor and Delivery

DURAGESIC is not recommended for analgesia during labor and delivery.

Nursing Mothers

Fentanyl is excreted in human milk; therefore DURAGESIC is not recommended for use in nursing women because of the possibility of effects in their infants.

Pediatric Use

The safety and efficacy of DURAGESIC in children has not been established. (See BOX WARNING and CONTRAINDICATIONS.)

DURAGESIC SHOULD NOT BE ADMINISTERED TO CHILDREN UNDER 12 YEARS OF AGE OR PATIENTS UNDER 18 YEARS OF AGE WHO WEIGH LESS THAN 50 KG (110 LBS) EXCEPT IN AN AUTHORIZED INVESTIGATIONAL RESEARCH SETTING.

Geriatric Use

Information from a pilot study of the pharmacokinetics of IV fentanyl in geriatric patients indicates that the clearance of fentanyl may be greatly decreased in the population above the age of 60. The relevance of these findings to transdermal fentanyl is unknown at this time.

Since elderly, cachectic, or debilitated patients may have altered pharmacokinetics due to poor fat stores, muscle wasting, or altered clearance, they should not be started on DURAGESIC doses higher than 25 µg/h unless they are already taking more than 135 mg of oral morphine a day or an equivalent dose of another opioid (see DOSAGE AND ADMINISTRATION).

Information for Patients

Instructions for the application, removal, and disposal of DURAGESIC are provided in each carton.

Disposal of DURAGESIC

DURAGESIC should be kept out of the reach of children. DURAGESIC systems should be folded so that the adhesive side of the system adheres to itself, then the system should be flushed down the toilet immediately upon removal. Patients should dispose of any systems remaining from a prescription as soon as they are no longer needed. Unused systems should be removed from their pouch and flushed down the toilet. If the gel from the drug reservoir accidentally contacts the skin, the area should be washed with clear water.

ADVERSE REACTIONS

In post-marketing experience, deaths from hypoventilation due to inappropriate use of DURAGESIC have been reported. (See BOX WARNING and CONTRAINDICATIONS.)

Pre-marketing Clinical Trial Experience:

The safety of DURAGESIC has been evaluated in 357 postoperative patients and 153 cancer patients for a total of 510 patients. Patients with acute pain used DURAGESIC for 1 to 3 days. The duration of DURAGESIC use varied in cancer patients; 56% of patients used DURAGESIC for over 30 days, 28% continued treatment for more than 4 months, and 10% used DURAGESIC for more than 1 year.

Hypoventilation was the most serious adverse reaction observed in 13 (4%) postoperative patients and in 3 (2%) of the cancer patients. Hypotension and hypertension were observed in 11 (3%) and 4 (1%) of the opioid-naive patients. Various adverse events were reported; a causal relationship to DURAGESIC was not always determined. The frequencies presented here reflect the actual frequency of each adverse effect in patients who received DURAGESIC. There has been no attempt to correct for a placebo effect, concomitant use of other opioids, or to subtract the frequencies reported by placebo-treated patients in controlled trials.

The following adverse reactions were reported in 153 cancer patients at a frequency of 1% or greater; similar reactions were seen in the 357 postoperative patients studied.

Body as a Whole: abdominal pain*, headache*
Cardiovascular: arrhythmia, chest pain
Digestive: nausea**, vomiting**, constipation**, dry mouth**, anorexia*, diarrhea*, dyspepsia*, flatulence
Nervous: somnolence**, confusion**, asthenia**, dizziness*, nervousness*, hallucinations*, anxiety*, depression*, euphoria*, tremor, abnormal coordination, speech disorder, abnormal thinking, abnormal gait, abnormal dreams, agitation, paresthesia, amnesia, syncope, paranoid reaction
Respiratory: dyspnea*, hypoventilation*, apnea*, hemoptysis, pharyngitis, hiccups
Skin and Appendages: sweating**, pruritus*, rash, application site reaction - erythema, papules, itching, edema
Urogenital: urinary retention*
*Reactions occurring in 3%–10% of DURAGESIC patients
**Reactions occurring in 10% or more of DURAGESIC patients

The following adverse effects have been reported in less than 1% of the 510 postoperative and cancer patients studied; the association between these events and DURAGESIC administration is unknown. This information is listed to serve as alerting information for the physician.
Digestive: abdominal distention
Nervous: aphasia, hypertonia, vertigo, stupor, hypotonia, depersonalization, hostility
Respiratory: stertorous breathing, asthma, respiratory disorder
Skin and Appendages, General: exfoliative dermatitis, pustules
Special Senses: amblyopia
Urogenital: bladder pain, oliguria, urinary frequency

DRUG ABUSE AND DEPENDENCE

Fentanyl is a Schedule II controlled substance and can produce drug dependence similar to that produced by morphine. DURAGESIC therefore has the potential for abuse. Tolerance, physical and psychological dependence may develop upon repeated administration of opioids. Iatrogenic addiction following opioid administration is relatively rare. Physicians should not let concerns of physical dependence deter them from using adequate amounts of opioids in the management of severe pain when such use is indicated.

OVERDOSAGE

Clinical Presentation

The manifestations of fentanyl overdosage are an extension of its pharmacologic actions with the most serious significant effect being hypoventilation.

Treatment

For the management of hypoventilation immediate countermeasures include removing the DURAGESIC system and physically or verbally stimulating the patient. These actions can be followed by administration of a specific narcotic antagonist such as naloxone. The duration of hypoventilation following an overdose may be longer than the effects of the narcotic antagonist's action (the half-life of naloxone ranges from 30 to 81 minutes). The interval between IV antagonist doses should be carefully chosen because of the possibility of re-narcotization after system removal; repeated administration of naloxone may be necessary. Reversal of the narcotic effect may result in acute onset of pain and the release of catecholamines.
If the clinical situation warrants, ensure a patent airway is established and maintained, administer oxygen and assist or control respiration as indicated and use an oropharyngeal airway or endotracheal tube if necessary. Adequate body temperature and fluid intake should be maintained.
If severe or persistent hypotension occurs, the possibility of hypovolemia should be considered and managed with appropriate parenteral fluid therapy.

DOSAGE AND ADMINISTRATION

With all opioids, the safety of patients using the products is dependent on health care practitioners prescribing them in strict conformity with their approved labeling with respect to patient selection, dosing, and proper conditions for use.
As with all opioids, dosage should be individualized. The most important factor to be considered in determining the appropriate dose is the extent of preexisting opioid tolerance. (See BOX WARNING and CONTRAINDICATIONS.) Initial doses should be reduced in elderly or debilitated patients (see PRECAUTIONS).
DURAGESIC should be applied to non-irritated and non-irradiated skin on a flat surface such as chest, back, flank or upper arm. Hair at the application site should be clipped (not shaved) prior to system application. If the site of DURAGESIC application must be cleansed prior to application of the system, do so with clear water. Do not use soaps, oils, lotions, alcohol, or any other agents that might irritate the skin or alter its characteristics. Allow the skin to dry completely prior to system application.
DURAGESIC should be applied immediately upon removal from the sealed package. Do not alter the system, e.g., cut, in any way prior to application.
The transdermal system should be pressed firmly in place with the palm of the hand for 30 seconds, making sure the contact is complete, especially around the edges.
Each DURAGESIC may be worn continuously for 72 hours. If analgesia for more than 72 hours is required, a new system should be applied to a different skin site after removal of the previous transdermal system.
DURAGESIC should be kept out of the reach of children. Used systems should be folded so that the adhesive side of the system adheres to itself, then the system should be flushed down the toilet immediately upon removal. Patients should dispose of any systems remaining from a prescription as soon as they are no longer needed. Unused systems should be removed from their pouch and flushed down the toilet.

Dose Selection

DOSES MUST BE INDIVIDUALIZED BASED UPON THE STATUS OF EACH PATIENT AND SHOULD BE ASSESSED AT REGULAR INTERVALS AFTER DURAGESIC APPLICATION. REDUCED DOSES OF DURAGESIC ARE SUGGESTED FOR THE ELDERLY AND OTHER GROUPS DISCUSSED IN PRECAUTIONS.
DURAGESIC DOSES GREATER THAN 25 μG/H SHOULD NOT BE USED FOR INITIATION OF DURAGESIC THERAPY IN NON-OPIOID TOLERANT PATIENTS.
In selecting an initial DURAGESIC dose, attention should be given to 1) the daily dose, potency, and characteristics of the opioid the patient has been taking previously (eg whether it is a pure agonist or mixed agonist-antagonist), 2) the reliability of the relative potency estimates used to calculate the DURAGESIC dose needed (potency estimates may vary with the route of administration), 3) the degree of opioid tolerance, if any, and 4) the general condition and medical status of the patient. Each patient should be maintained at the lowest dose providing acceptable pain control.

Initial DURAGESIC Dose Selection

There has been no systematic evaluation of DURAGESIC as an initial opioid analgesic in the management of chronic pain, since most patients in the clinical trials were converted to DURAGESIC from other narcotics. Therefore, unless the patient has pre-existing opioid tolerance, the lowest DURAGESIC dose, 25 μg/h, should be used as the initial dose.
To convert patients from oral or parenteral opioids to DURAGESIC use the following methodology:

1. Calculate the previous 24-hour analgesic requirement.
2. Convert this amount to the equianalgesic oral morphine dose using Table B.
3. Table C displays the range of 24-hour oral morphine doses that are recommended for conversion to each DURAGESIC dose. Use this table to find the calculated 24-hour morphine dose and the corresponding DURAGESIC dose. Initiate DURAGESIC treatment using the recommended dose and titrate patients upwards (no more frequently than every 3 days after the initial dose or than every 6 days thereafter) until analgesic efficacy is attained. For delivery rates in excess of 100 μg/h, multiple systems may be used.

TABLE B
EQUIANALGESIC POTENCY CONVERSION

Name	Equianalgesic Dose (mg) IM[a]	PO
morphine	10	60 (30)[b]
hydromorphone (Dilaudid®)	1.5	7.5
methadone (Dolophine®)	10	20
oxycodone (Percocet®)	15	30
levorphanol (Levo-Dromoran®)	2	4
oxymorphone (Numorphan®)	1	10 (PR)
heroin	5	60
meperidine (Demerol®)	75	—
codeine	130	200

Note: All IM and PO doses in this chart are considered equivalent to 10 mg of IM morphine in analgesic effect. IM denotes intramuscular, PO oral, and PR rectal.
[a] Based on single-dose studies in which an intramuscular dose of each drug listed was compared with morphine to establish the relative potency. Oral doses are those recommended when changing from parenteral to an oral route.
[b] The conversion ratio of 10 mg parenteral morphine = 30 mg oral morphine is based on clinical experience in patients with chronic pain.

Reference:
[a] Foley, K.M. (1985) The treatment of cancer pain. NEJM 313(2):84-95.
[b] Ashburn and Lipman (1993) Management of pain in the cancer patient. Anesth Analg 76: 402–416.

TABLE C
RECOMMENDED DURAGESIC DOSE BASED UPON DAILY ORAL MORPHINE DOSE

Oral 24-hour Morphine (mg/day)	DURAGESIC Dose (μg/hr)
45–134	25
135–224	50
225–314	75
315–404	100
405–494	125
495–584	150
585–674	175
675–764	200
765–854	225
855–944	250
945–1034	275
1035–1124	300

NOTE: In clinical trials these ranges of daily oral morphine doses were used as a basis for conversion to DURAGESIC. Although controlled studies are not available, in clinical practice it is customary to consider the doses of opioid given IM, IV or subcutaneously to be equivalent. There may be some differences in pharmacokinetic parameters such as C_{max} and T_{max}.
The majority of patients are adequately maintained with DURAGESIC administered every 72 hours. A small number of patients may not achieve adequate analgesia using this dosing interval and may require systems to be applied every 48 hours rather than every 72 hours. An increase in the DURAGESIC dose should be evaluated before changing dosing intervals in order to maintain patients on a 72-hour regimen.
Because of the increase in serum fentanyl concentration over the first 24 hours following initial system application, the initial evaluation of the maximum analgesic effect of DURAGESIC cannot be made before 24 hours of wearing. The initial DURAGESIC dosage may be increased after 3 days (see Dose Titration).
During the initial application of DURAGESIC, patients should use short-acting analgesics for the first 24 hours as needed until analgesic efficacy with DURAGESIC is attained. Thereafter, some patients still may require periodic supplemental doses of other short-acting analgesics for 'breakthrough' pain.

Dose Titration

The conversion ratio from oral morphine to DURAGESIC is conservative, and 50% of patients are likely to require a dose increase after initial application of DURAGESIC. The initial DURAGESIC dosage may be increased after 3 days, based on the daily dose of supplemental analgesics required by the patient in the second or third day of the initial application.
Physicians are advised that it may take up to 6 days after increasing the dose of DURAGESIC for the patient to reach equilibrium on the new dose (see graph in CLINICAL PHARMACOLOGY). Therefore, patients should wear a higher dose through two applications before any further increase in dosage is made on the basis of the average daily use of a supplemental analgesic.
Appropriate dosage increments should be based on the daily dose of supplementary opioids, using the ratio of 90 mg/24 hours of oral morphine to a 25 μg/h increase in DURAGESIC dose.

Discontinuation of DURAGESIC

To convert patients to another opioid, remove DURAGESIC and titrate the dose of the new analgesic based upon the patient's report of pain until adequate analgesia has been attained. Upon system removal, 17 hours or more are required for a 50% decrease in serum fentanyl concentrations. For patients requiring discontinuation of opioids, a gradual downward titration is recommended since it is not known what dose level the opioid may be discontinued without producing the signs and symptoms of abrupt withdrawal.

HOW SUPPLIED

DURAGESIC® is supplied in cartons containing 5 individually packaged systems. See chart for information regarding individual systems.

DURAGESIC Dose (μg/h)	System Size (cm²)	Fentanyl Content (mg)	NDC Number
DURAGESIC®-25	10	2.5	50458-033-05
DURAGESIC®-50*	20	5	50458-034-05
DURAGESIC®-75*	30	7.5	50458-035-05
DURAGESIC®-100*	40	10	50458-036-05

*FOR USE ONLY IN OPIOID TOLERANT PATIENTS.

Safety and Handling

DURAGESIC is supplied in sealed transdermal systems which pose little risk of exposure to health care workers. If the gel from the drug reservoir accidentally contacts the

Continued on next page

Janssen Pharmaceutica—Cont.

skin, the area should be washed with copious amounts of water. Do not use soap, alcohol, or other solvents to remove the gel because they may enhance the drug's ability to penetrate the skin. Do not cut or damage DURAGESIC. If the DURAGESIC system is cut or damaged, controlled drug delivery will not be possible.

Do not store above 77°F (25°C). Apply immediately after removal from individual sealed package. Do not use if the seal is broken. **For transdermal use only.**

CAUTION: Federal law prohibits dispensing without prescription

DEA order form required. A schedule CII narcotic.

Manufactured by:
ALZA Corporation
Palo Alto, CA 94304
Distributed by:
JANSSEN PHARMACEUTICA
Titusville, NJ 08560
January 1994 June 1994 7500309

Shown in Product Identification Guide, page 318

ERGAMISOL® ℞

[*ər-gam ′ə-, sōl*]
(levamisole hydrochlorid)
Tablets

DESCRIPTION

ERGAMISOL (levamisole hydrochloride) is an immunomodulator available in tablets for oral administration containing the equivalent of 50 mg as levamisole base. Fifty-nine (59) mg of levamisole HCl is equivalent to 50 mg of levamisole base. Inactive ingredients are colloidal silicon dioxide, hydrogenated vegetable oil, hydroxypropyl methylcellulose, lactose, microcystalline cellulose, polyethylene glycol 6000, polysorbate 80, and talc.

Levamisole hydrochloride is (-)-(S)-2,3,5,6-tetrahydro-6-phenylimidazo [2,1-b] thiazole monohydrochloride.

Levamisole hydrochloride is a white to pale cream colored crystalline powder which is almost odorless and is freely soluble in water. It is quite stable in acid aqueous media but hydrolyzes in alkaline or neutral solutions. It has a molecular weight of 240.75.

CLINICAL PHARMACOLOGY

Two clinical trials having essentially the same design have demonstrated an increase in survival and a reduction in recurrence rate in the subset of patients with resected Dukes' C colon cancer treated with a regimen of ERGAMISOL (levamisole hydrochloride) plus fluorouracil[1,2]. After surgery, patients were randomized to no further therapy, ERGAMISOL alone, or ERGAMISOL plus fluorouracil.

In one clinical trial in which 408 Dukes' B and C colorectal cancer patients were studied, 262 Dukes' C patients were evaluated for a minimum follow-up of five years[1]. A subset analysis of these Dukes' C patients showed the estimated reduction in death rate was 27% for ERGAMISOL plus fluorouracil ($p = 0.11$) and 28% for ERGAMISOL alone ($p = 0.11$)[3]. The estimated reduction in recurrence rate was 36% for ERGAMISOL plus fluorouracil ($p = 0.025$) and 28% for ERGAMISOL alone ($p = 0.11$)[3]. In another clinical trial designed to confirm the above results, 929 Dukes' C colon cancer patients were evaluated for a minimum follow-up of 2 years[2]. The estimated reduction in death rate was 33% for ERGAMISOL plus fluorouracil ($p = 0.006$). The estimated reduction in recurrence rate was 41% for ERGAMISOL plus fluorouracil ($p < 0.0001$). The ERGAMISOL alone group did not show advantage over no treatment on improving recurrence or survival rates. There are presently insufficient data to evaluate the effect of the combination of ERGAMISOL plus fluorouracil in Dukes' B patients. There are also insufficient data to evaluate the effect of ERGAMISOL plus fluorouracil in patients with rectal cancer because only 12 patients with rectal cancer were treated with the combination in the first study and none in the second study.

The mechanism of action of ERGAMISOL in combination with fluorouracil is unknown. The effects of levamisole on the immune system are complex. The drug appears to restore depressed immune function rather than to stimulate response to above-normal levels. Levamisole can stimulate formation of antibodies to various antigens, enhance T-cell responses by stimulating T-cell activation and proliferation, potentiate monocyte and macrophage functions including phagocytosis and chemotaxis, and increase neutrophil mobility, adherence, and chemotaxis. Other drugs have similar short-term effects and the clinical relevance is unclear.

Besides its immunomodulatory function, levamisole has other mammalian pharmacologic activities, including inhibition of alkaline phosphatase, and cholinergic activity.

The pharmacokinetics of ERGAMISOL have not been studied in the dosage regimen recommended with fluorouracil nor in patients with hepatic insufficiency. After administration of a single oral dose of 50 mg of a research formulation of ERGAMISOL, it appears that levamisole is rapidly absorbed from the gastrointestinal tract. Mean peak plasma concentrations of 0.13 mcg/ml are attained within 1.5 to 2 hours. The plasma elimination half-life of levamisole is between 3-4 hours. Following a 150-mg radio-labelled dose, levamisole is extensively metabolized by the liver in humans and the metabolities excreted mainly by the kidneys (70% over 3 days). The elimination half-life of metabolite excretion is 16 hours. Approximately 5% is excreted in the feces. Less than 5% is excreted unchanged in the urine and less than 0.2% in the feces. Approximately 12% is recovered in the urine as the glucuronide of p-hydroxy-levamisole. The clinical significance of these data are unknown since a 150-mg dose may not be proportional to a 50-mg dose.

INDICATIONS AND USAGE

ERGAMISOL (levamisole hydrochloride) is only indicated as adjuvant treatment in combination with fluorouracil after surgical resection in patients with Dukes' stage C colon cancer.

CONTRAINDICATIONS

ERGAMISOL (levamisole hydrochloride) is contraindicated in patients with a known hypersensitivity to the drug or its components.

WARNINGS

ERGAMISOL (levamisole hydrochloride) has been associated with agranulocytosis, sometimes fatal. The onset of agranulocytosis is frequently accompanied by a flu-like syndrome (fever, chills, etc.); however, in a small number of patients it is asymptomatic. A flu-like syndrome may also occur in the absence of agranulocytosis. It is essential that appropriate hematological monitoring be done routinely during therapy with ERGAMISOL and fluorouracil. Neutropenia is usually reversible following discontinuation of therapy. Patients should be instructed to report immediately any flu-like symptoms.

Higher than recommended doses of ERGAMISOL may be associated with an increased incidence of agranulocytosis, so the recommended dose should not be exceeded.

The combination of ERGAMISOL and fluorouracil has been associated with frequent neutropenia, anemia and thrombocytopenia.

PRECAUTIONS

Before beginning this combination adjuvant treatment, the physician should become familiar with the labeling for fluorouracil.

Information for Patients: The patient should be informed that if flu-like symptoms or malaise occurs, the physician should be notified immediately.

Drug Interactions: ERGAMISOL (levamisole hydrochloride) has been reported to produce "ANTABUSE®"-like side effects when given concomitantly with alcohol. Concomitant administration of phenytoin and ERGAMISOL plus fluorouracil has led to increased plasma levels of phenytoin. The physician is advised to monitor plasma levels of phenytoin and to decrease the dose if necessary.

Because of reports of prolongation of the prothrombin time beyond the therapeutic range in patients taking concurrent levamisole and warfarin sodium, it is suggested that the prothrombin time be monitored carefully, and the dose of warfarin sodium or other coumarin-like drugs should be adjusted accordingly, in patients taking both drugs.

Laboratory Tests: On the first day of therapy with ERGAMISOL/fluorouracil, patients should have a CBC with differential and platelets, electrolytes and liver function tests performed. Thereafter, a CBC with differential and platelets should be performed weekly prior to each treatment with fluorouracil with electrolytes and liver function tests peformed every 3 months for a total of one year. Dosage modifications should be instituted as follows: If WBC is 2500-3500/mm^3 defer the fluorouracil dose until WBC is > 3500/mm^3. If WBC is < 2500/mm^3, defer the fluorouracil dose until WBC is > 3500/mm^3; then resume the fluorouracil dose reduced by 20%. If WBC remains < 2500/mm^3 for over 10 days despite deferring fluorouracil, discontinue administration of ERGAMISOL. Both drugs should be deferred unless enough platelets are present (≥ 100,000/mm^3).

Carcinogensis, Mutagenesis, Impairment of Fertility: Adequate animal carcinogenicity studies have not been conducted with levamisole. Studies of levamisole administered in drinking water at 5, 20, and 80 mg/kg/day to mice for up to 18 months or adminstered to rats in the diet at 5, 20, and 80 mg/kg/day for 24 months showed no evidence of neoplastic effects. These studies were not conducted at the maximum tolerated dose, therefore the animals may not have been exposed to a reasonable drug challenge. No mutagenic effects were demonstrated in dominant lethal studies in male and female mice, in an Ames test, and in a study to detect chromosomal aberrations in cultured peripheral human lymphocytes.

Adverse effects were not observed on male or female fertility when levamisole was administered to rats in the diet at doses of 2.5, 10, 40, and 160 mg/kg. In a rat gavage study at doses of 20, 60, and 180 mg/kg, the copulation period was increased, the duration of pregnancy was slightly increased, and fertility, pup viability and weight, lactation index, and number of fetuses were decreased at 60 mg/kg. No negative reproductive effects were present when the offspring were allowed to mate and litter.

Pregnancy: Pregnancy Category C: Teratogenicity studies have been performed in rats and rabbits at oral doses up to 180 mg/kg. Fetal malformations were not observed. In rats, embryotoxicity was present at 160 mg/kg and in rabbits, significant embryotoxicity was observed at 180 mg/kg. There are no adequate and well-controlled studies in pregnant women and ERGAMISOL should not be administered unless the potential benefits outweigh the risks. Women taking the combination of ERGAMISOL and fluorouracil should be advised not to become pregnant.

Nursing Mothers: It is not known whether ERGAMISOL is excreted in human milk; it is excreted in cows' milk. Because of the potential for serious adverse reactions in nursing infants from ERGAMISOL, a decision should be made whether to discontinue nursing or to discontinue the drug, taking into account the importance of the drug to the mother.

Pediatric Use: Safety and effectiveness of ERGAMISOL in children have not been established.

ADVERSE REACTIONS

Almost all patients receiving ERGAMISOL (levamisole hydrochloride) and fluorouracil reported adverse experiences. Tabulated below is the incidence of adverse experiences that occurred in at least 1% of patients enrolled in two clinical trials who were adjuvantly treated with either ERGAMISOL or ERGAMISOL plus fluorouracil following colon surgery. In the larger clinical trial, 66 of 463 patients (14%) discontinued the combination of ERGAMISOL plus fluorouracil because of adverse reactions. Forty-three of these patients (9%) developed isolated or a combination of gastrointestinal toxicities. (e.g., nausea, vomiting, diarrhea, stomatitis and anorexia). Ten patients developed rash and/or pruritus. Five patients discontinued therapy because of flu-like symptoms or fever with chills; ten patients developed central nervous system symptoms such as dizziness, ataxia, depression, confusion, memory loss, weakness, inability to concentrate, and headache; two patients developed reversible neutropenia and sepsis; one patient because of thrombocytopenia; one patient because of hyperbilirubinemia. One patient in the ERGAMISOL plus fluorouracil group developed agranulocytosis and sepsis and died.

In the ERGAMISOL alone arm of the trial, 15 of 310 patients (4.8%) discontinued therapy because of adverse experiences. Six of these (2%) discontinued because of rash, six because of arthralgia/myalgia, and one each for fever and neutropenia, urinary infection, and cough.

[See table at top of next page.]

In worldwide experience with ERGAMISOL, less frequent adverse experiences included exfoliative dermatitis, fixed drug eruptions, periorbital edema, vaginal bleeding, anaphylaxis, confusion, convulsions, hallucinations, impaired concentration, renal failure, pancreatitis, elevated serum creatinine, and increased alkaline phosphatase.

Reports of hyperlipidema have been observed in patients receiving combination therapy of ERGAMISOL and fluorouracil; elevations in triglyceride levels have been greater than increases in cholesterol levels. In worldwide postmarketing experience with the combination therapy, there have been rare cases of elevated hepatic enzymes and hepatosteatosis in patients.

Cases of an encephalopathy—like syndrome associated with demyelination have been reported in patients treated with ERGAMISOL. Worldwide postmarketing experience with the combination therapy of ERGAMISOL and fluorouracil has also included reports of peripheral neuropathy and multifocal inflammatory leukoencephalopathy. The onset of symptoms and the clinical presentation in these cases are quite varied. Symptoms may include coma, confusion, lethargy, memory loss, muscle weakness, parathesia, and speech disturbances. This condition has been associated with MRI and CT scan findings of demyelinating lesions in the white matter. If an acute neurological syndrome occurs, immediate discontinuation of ERGAMISOL and fluorouracil therapy should be discontinued immediately. Patients have generally recovered/improved with drug discontinuation and corticosteroid therapy.

The following additional adverse experiences have been reported for fluorouracil alone: esophagopharyngitis, pancytopenia, myocardial ischemia, angina, gastrointestinal ulceration and bleeding, anaphylaxis and generalized allergic reactions, acute cerebellar syndrome, nystagmus, dry skin, fissuring, photosensitivity, lacrimal duct stenosis, photophobia, euphoria, thrombophlebitis, and nail changes.

OVERDOSAGE

Fatalities have been reported in a three-year-old child who ingested 15 mg/kg and in an adult who ingested 32 mg/kg. No further clinical information is available. In cases of over-

Adverse experience	ERGAMISOL N = 440 %	ERGAMISOL plus fluorouracil N = 599 %
Gastrointestinal		
Nausea	22	65
Diarrhea	13	52
Stomatitis	3	39
Vomiting	6	20
Anorexia	2	6
Abdominal pain	2	5
Constipation	2	4
Flatulence	<1	2
Dyspepsia	<1	1
Hematological		
Leukopenia		
<2000/mm³	<1	1
≥2000 to <4000/mm³	4	19
≥4000/mm³	2	33
unscored category	0	<1
Thrombocytopenia		
<50,000/mm³	0	0
≥50,000 to <130,000/mm³	1	8
≥130,000/mm³	1	10
Anemia	0	6
Granulocytopenia	<1	4
Epistaxis	0	1
Skin and Appendages		
Dermatitis	8	23
Alopecia	3	22
Pruritus	1	2
Skin discoloration	0	2
Urticaria	<1	1
Body as a Whole		
Fatigue	6	11
Fever	3	5
Rigors	3	5
Chest pain	<1	1
Edema	1	1
Resistance Mechanisms		
Infection	5	12
Special Senses		
Taste Perversion	8	8
Altered sense of smell	1	
Musculoskeletal System		
Arthralgia	5	
Myalgia	3	
Central and peripheral nervous system		
Dizziness	3	4
Headache	3	4
Paresthesia	2	
Ataxia	0	4
Psychiatric		
Somnolence	3	4
Depression	1	
Nervousness	1	
Insomnia	1	
Anxiety	1	
Forgetfulness	0	
Vision		
Abnormal tearing	0	4
Blurred vision	1	
Conjunctivitis	<1	2
Liver and biliary system		
Hyperbilirubinemia	<1	1

dosage, gastric lavage is recommended together with symptomatic and supportive measures.

DOSAGE AND ADMINISTRATION

The adjuvant use of ERGAMISOL (levamisole hydrochloride) and fluorouracil is limited to the following dosage schedule:

Initial Therapy:

ERGAMISOL: 50 mg p.o. q8h for 3 days (starting 7–30 days post-surgery)

fluorouracil: 450 mg/m²/day IV for 5 days (starting 21–34 days post-surgery) concomitant with a 3-day course of ERGAMISOL

Maintenance:

ERGAMISOL: 50 mg p.o. q8h for 3 days every 2 weeks.

fluorouracil: 450 mg/m²/day IV once a week beginning 28 days after the initiation of the 5-day course.

Treatment: ERGAMISOL, administered orally, should be initiated no earlier than 7 and no later than 30 days post surgery at a dose of 50 mg q8h × 3 days repeated every 14 days for 1 year. Fluorouracil therapy should be initiated no earlier than 21 days and no later than 35 days after surgery providing the patient is out of the hospital, ambulatory, maintaining normal oral nutrition, has well-healed wounds, and is fully recovered from any postoperative complications.

If ERGAMISOL has been initiated from 7 to 20 days after surgery, initiation of fluorouracil therapy should be coincident with the second course of ERGAMISOL, i.e., at 21 to 34 days. If ERGAMISOL is initiated from 21 to 30 days after surgery, fluorouracil should be initiated simultaneously with the first course of ERGAMISOL.

Fluorouracil should be administered by rapid IV push at a dosage of 450 mg/m²/day for 5 consecutive days. Dosage calculation is based on actual weight (estimated dry weight if there is evidence of fluid retention). *This course should be discontinued before the full 5 doses are administered if the patient develops any stomatitis or diarrhea* (5 or more loose stools). Twenty-eight days after initiation of this course, weekly fluorouracil should be instituted at a dosage of 450 mg/m²/week and continued for a total treatment time of 1 year. If stomatitis or diarrhea develop during weekly therapy, the next dose of fluorouracil should be deferred until these side effects have subsided. If these side effects are moderate to severe, the fluorouracil dose should be reduced 20% when it is resumed.

Dosage modifications should be instituted as follows: If WBC is 2500-3500/mm³ defer the fluorouracil dose until WBC is >3500/mm³. If WBC is <2500/mm³, defer the fluorouracil dose until WBC is >3500/mm³; then resume the fluorouracil dose reduced by 20%. If WBC remains <2500/mm³ for over 10 days despite deferring fluorouracil, discontinue administration of ERGAMISOL. Both drugs should be deferred unless platelets are adequate (≥100,000/mm³).

ERGAMISOL should not be used at doses exceeding the recommended dose or frequency. Clinical studies suggest a relationship between ERGAMISOL adverse experiences and increasing dose, and since some of these, e.g. agranulocytosis, may be life-threatening, the recommended dosage regimen should not be exceeded (see "WARNINGS").

Before beginning this combination adjuvant treatment, the physician should become familiar with the labeling for fluorouracil.

HOW SUPPLIED

ERGAMISOL (levamisole hydrochloride) is available in white, coated tablets containing the equivalent of 50 mg of levamisole base, debossed "JANSSEN"and "L"/"50".

They are supplied in blister packages of 36 tablets (NDC 50458-270-36).

Store at room temperature, 15°–30°C (59°–86°F).

Protect from moisture.

REFERENCES

1. Laurie JA, Moertel CG, Fleming TR, et al. Surgical adjuvant therapy of large-bowel carcinoma: An evaluation of levamisole and the combination of levamisole and fluorouracil. *J Clin Oncol.* 1989; 7:1447–1456.
2. Moertel CG, Fleming TR, Macdonald JS, et al. Levamisole and fluorouracil for adjuvant therapy of resected colon carcinoma. *New Engl J Med.* 1990; 322:352–358.
3. Data on file, Janssen Pharmaceutica Inc.

Manufactured by:
Janssen Pharmaceutica, nv
Beerse, Belgium
Distributed by:
Janssen Pharmaceutica Inc.
Titusville, NJ 08560
Edition March 1994, August 1995
U.S. Patent Number 4,584,305

Shown in Product Identification Guide, page 318

HISMANAL® ℞

[his'ma-nal]
(astemizole) Tablets

DESCRIPTION

HISMANAL® (astemizole) is a histamine H_1-receptor antagonist available in scored white tablets for oral use. Each tablet contains 10 mg of astemizole, and, as inactive ingredients: lactose, cornstarch, microcrystalline cellulose, pregelatinized starch, povidone K90, magnesium stearate, colloidal silicon dioxide, and sodium lauryl sulfate. Astemizole is chemically designated as 1-[(4-fluorophenyl)methyl]-N-[1-[2-(4-methoxyphenyl)ethyl]-4-piperidinyl]-1H-benzimidazol-2-amine, with a molecular weight of 458.58. The empirical formula is $C_{28}H_{31}FN_4O$.

Astemizole is a white to slightly off-white powder; it is insoluble in water, slightly soluble in ethanol and soluble in chloroform and methanol.

CLINICAL PHARMACOLOGY

HISMANAL is a long-acting, selective histamine H_1-receptor antagonist. Receptor binding studies in animals demonstrated that at pharmacological doses, HISMANAL occupies peripheral H_1-receptors but does not reach H_1-receptors in the brain. Whole body autoradiographic studies in rats, radiolabel tissue distribution studies in dogs and radioligand binding studies of guinea pig brain H_1-receptors have shown that HISMANAL does not readily cross the blood-brain barrier. Screening studies in rats at effective antihistaminic doses showed no anticholinergic effects. Studies in humans using the recommended dosage regimens have not been performed to determine whether HISMANAL is associated with a different frequency of anticholinergic effects than therapeutic doses of other antihistamines.

The absorption of HISMANAL is reduced by 60% when taken with meals. In single oral dose studies, HISMANAL was rapidly absorbed from the gastrointestinal tract; peak plasma concentrations of unchanged HISMANAL were reached within one hour. Due to extensive first pass metabolism and significant tissue distribution, plasma concentrations of unchanged drug were low. Elimination of unchanged HISMANAL occurred with a half-life of approximately one day. Elimination of HISMANAL plus hydroxylated metabolites, considered together to represent the pharmacologically active fraction in plasma, was biphasic with half-lives of 20 hours for the distribution phase and 7–11 days for the elimination phase. The pharmacokinetics of HISMANAL plus hydroxylated metabolites are dose proportional following single doses of 10 to 30 mg.

Following chronic administration, steady state plasma concentrations of HISMANAL plus hydroxylated metabolites (mainly desmethylastemizole) were reached within four

Continued on next page

Janssen Pharmaceutica—Cont.

to eight weeks; concentrations of the metabolites are substantially higher than those of unchanged HISMANAL. HISMANAL plus hydroxylated metabolites decayed biphasically with an initial half-life of 7–9 days, with plasma concentrations being reduced by 75% within this phase, and with a terminal half-life of about 19 days. The initial phase ($t_{1/2}$ = 7–9 days) appears to determine the time to reach steady state plasma concentrations of HISMANAL plus hydroxylated metabolites. Steady state plasma concentrations of unchanged HISMANAL were reached by 6 days (with a range of 6–9 days); unchanged HISMANAL was eliminated from plasma with a half-life of approximately 2 days (with a range of 1–2.5 days).

Excretion and metabolism studies with ^{14}C-labeled HISMANAL in volunteers demonstrated that the drug is almost completely metabolized in the liver and primarily excreted in the feces.

Interpatient variability in pharmacokinetic parameters may be greater in patients with liver disease as compared to normal subjects. Systematic evaluation of the pharmacokinetics in patients with hepatic or renal dysfunction has not been performed.

The in-vitro plasma protein binding of unchanged HISMANAL (100 ng/mL) was 96.7% with 2.3% being found as free drug in the plasma water. In human blood with an astemizole concentration of 100 ng/mL, 61.5% of astemizole was bound to the plasma proteins, with 36.2% being distributed to the blood cell fraction. The concentration of astemizole found in the blood was the same as that found in the plasma fraction of the blood. Binding studies for the astemizole metabolite(s) which achieve much higher concentrations than astemizole under chronic dosing conditions have not been conducted.

INDICATIONS AND USAGE

HISMANAL tablets are indicated for the relief of symptoms associated with seasonal allergic rhinitis and chronic idiopathic urticaria. HISMANAL should not be used as a p r n product for immediate relief of symptoms. Patients should be advised not to increase the dose in an attempt to accelerate the onset of action.

Clinical studies have not been conducted to evaluate the effectiveness of HISMANAL in the common cold.

CONTRAINDICATIONS

CONCOMITANT ADMINISTRATION OF ASTEMIZOLE WITH ERYTHROMYCIN IS CONTRAINDICATED BECAUSE ERYTHROMYCIN IS KNOWN TO IMPAIR THE CYTOCHROME P450 ENZYME SYSTEM WHICH ALSO INFLUENCES ASTEMIZOLE METABOLISM. THERE HAVE BEEN TWO REPORTS TO DATE OF SYNCOPE WITH TORSADES DE POINTES, REQUIRING HOSPITALIZATION, IN PATIENTS TAKING COMBINATIONS OF HISMANAL 10 MG DAILY WITH ERYTHROMYCIN. IN EACH CASE THE QT INTERVALS WERE PROLONGED BEYOND 650 MILLISECONDS AT THE TIME OF THE EVENT; ONE PATIENT ALSO RECEIVED KETOCONAZOLE AND THE OTHER PATIENT ALSO HAD HYPOKALEMIA.

CONCOMITANT ADMINISTRATION OF ASTEMIZOLE WITH KETOCONAZOLE TABLETS IS CONTRAINDICATED BECAUSE AVAILABLE HUMAN PHARMACOKINETIC DATA INDICATE THAT ORAL KETOCONAZOLE SIGNIFICANTLY INHIBITS THE METABOLISM OF ASTEMIZOLE, RESULTING IN ELEVATED PLASMA LEVELS OF ASTEMIZOLE AND DESMETHYLASTEMIZOLE. DATA SUGGEST THAT CARDIOVASCULAR EVENTS ARE ASSOCIATED WITH ELEVATION OF ASTEMIZOLE AND/OR ASTEMIZOLE METABOLITE LEVELS, RESULTING IN ELECTROCARDIOGRAPHIC QT PROLONGATION.

CONCOMITANT ADMINISTRATION OF ASTEMIZOLE WITH ITRACONAZOLE IS ALSO CONTRAINDICATED BASED ON THE CHEMICAL RESEMBLANCE OF ITRACONAZOLE AND KETOCONAZOLE. IN-VITRO DATA SUGGEST THAT ITRACONAZOLE HAS A LESS PRONOUNCED EFFECT ON THE BIOTRANSFORMATION SYSTEM RESPONSIBLE FOR THE METABOLISM OF ASTEMIZOLE COMPARED TO KETOCONAZOLE.

CONCOMITANT ADMINISTRATION OF ASTEMIZOLE WITH QUININE IS CONTRAINDICATED BECAUSE HUMAN DATA INDICATE THAT ADMINISTRATION OF QUININE (SINGLE DOSE OF 430MG) WITH ASTEMIZOLE RESULTS IN ELEVATED PLASMA LEVELS OF ASTEMIZOLE AND DESMETHYLASTEMIZOLE WHICH IS ACCOMPANIED BY ELECTROCARDIOGRAPHIC QT PROLONGATION. THESE DATA ALSO INDICATE THAT, ALTHOUGH BEVERAGES CONTAINING QUININE (UP TO 80 MG/DAY OR ABOUT 32 OUNCES OF TONIC WATER) MAY ELEVATE PLASMA LEVELS OF ASTEMIZOLE AND DESMETHYLASTEMIZOLE, THIS EFFECT IS SMALL AND IS NOT AC-COMPANIED BY SIGNIFICANT PROLONGATION OF THE QT INTERVAL.

(See **WARNINGS** and **PRECAUTIONS**: Drug Interactions.)

HISMANAL is contraindicated in patients with known hypersensitivity to astemizole or any of the inactive ingredients.

WARNINGS

> **QT PROLONGATION/VENTRICULAR ARRHYTHMIAS**
>
> RARE CASES OF SERIOUS CARDIOVASCULAR ADVERSE EVENTS INCLUDING DEATH, CARDIAC ARREST, QT PROLONGATION, TORSADES DE POINTES, AND OTHER VENTRICULAR ARRHYTHMIAS HAVE BEEN OBSERVED IN PATIENTS EXCEEDING RECOMMENDED DOSES OF ASTEMIZOLE. WHILE THE MAJORITY OF SUCH EVENTS HAVE OCCURRED FOLLOWING SUBSTANTIAL OVERDOSES OF ASTEMIZOLE, TORSADES DE POINTES (ARRHYTHMIAS) HAVE VERY RARELY OCCURRED AT REPORTED DOSES AS LOW AS 20–30 MG DAILY (2–3 TIMES THE RECOMMENDED DAILY DOSE). DATA SUGGEST THAT THESE EVENTS ARE ASSOCIATED WITH ELEVATION OF ASTEMIZOLE AND/OR ASTEMIZOLE METABOLITE LEVELS, RESULTING IN ELECTROCARDIOGRAPHIC QT PROLONGATION. THESE EVENTS HAVE ALSO OCCURRED AT 10 MG DAILY IN A FEW PATIENTS WITH POSSIBLE AUGMENTING CIRCUMSTANCES (SEE CONTRAINDICATIONS, AND WARNING PARAGRAPHS BELOW WARNINGS BOX). IN VIEW OF THE POTENTIAL FOR CARDIAC ARRHYTHMIAS, ADHERENCE TO THE RECOMMENDED DOSE SHOULD BE EMPHASIZED.
>
> DO NOT EXCEED THE RECOMMENDED DOSE OF 10 MG (ONE TABLET) DAILY.
>
> SOME PATIENTS APPEAR TO INCREASE THE DOSE OF HISMANAL IN AN ATTEMPT TO ACCELERATE THE ONSET OF ACTION. PATIENTS SHOULD BE ADVISED NOT TO DO THIS AND NOT TO USE HISMANAL AS A P R N PRODUCT FOR IMMEDIATE RELIEF OF SYMPTOMS.
>
> CONCOMITANT ADMINISTRATION OF ASTEMIZOLE WITH KETOCONAZOLE TABLETS, ITRACONAZOLE, ERYTHROMYCIN, OR QUININE IS CONTRAINDICATED. (SEE CONTRAINDICATIONS AND PRECAUTIONS: DRUG INTERACTIONS.)
>
> SINCE ASTEMIZOLE IS EXTENSIVELY METABOLIZED BY THE LIVER, THE USE OF ASTEMIZOLE IN PATIENTS WITH SIGNIFICANT HEPATIC DYSFUNCTION SHOULD GENERALLY BE AVOIDED.
>
> IN SOME CASES, SEVERE ARRHYTHMIAS HAVE BEEN PRECEDED BY EPISODES OF SYNCOPE. SYNCOPE IN PATIENTS RECEIVING ASTEMIZOLE SHOULD LEAD TO IMMEDIATE DISCONTINUATION OF TREATMENT AND APPROPRIATE CLINICAL EVALUATION, INCLUDING ELECTROCARDIOGRAPHIC TESTING (LOOKING FOR QT PROLONGATION AND VENTRICULAR ARRHYTHMIA).
>
> (SEE CLINICAL PHARMACOLOGY, CONTRAINDICATIONS, WARNINGS, PRECAUTIONS, AND DOSAGE AND ADMINISTRATION.)

Patients known to have conditions leading to QT prolongation may experience QT prolongation and/or ventricular arrhythmia with astemizole at recommended doses. The effect of astemizole in patients who are receiving agents which alter the QT interval is unknown. However, in view of astemizole's known potential for QT prolongation, it is advisable to avoid its use in patients with QT prolongation syndrome or who are taking medications which are reported to prolong QT intervals (including probucol, certain antiarrhythmics, certain tricyclic antidepressants, certain phenothiazines, certain calcium channel blockers such as bepridil, and terfenadine), patients with electrolyte abnormalities such as hypokalemia or hypomagnesemia, or those taking diuretics with potential for inducing electrolyte abnormalities.

Rare cases of cardiovascular events have been observed in patients with hepatic dysfunction. Systematic evaluation of the pharmacokinetics of astemizole in patients with hepatic dysfunction has not been performed. Since astemizole is extensively metabolized by the liver, the use of HISMANAL in patients with significant hepatic dysfunction should generally be avoided.

PRECAUTIONS

General:
Caution should be given to potential anticholinergic (drying effects) in patients with lower airway diseases.
Caution should be used in patients with cirrhosis or other liver diseases. (See CLINICAL PHARMACOLOGY section.)
HISMANAL does not appear to be dialyzable.
Caution should also be used when treating patients with renal impairment.

Drug Interactions:
See **CONTRAINDICATIONS** and **WARNINGS** sections for discussion of information regarding potential drug interactions.

Ketoconazole/Itraconazole
Concomitant administration of ketoconazole tablets or itraconazole with astemizole is contraindicated. (See CONTRAINDICATIONS and WARNINGS BOX.)
Due to the chemical similarity of fluconazole, metronidazole, and miconazole i.v. to ketoconazole, concomitant use of these products with astemizole is not recommended.

Macrolides (including erythromycin)
Concomitant administration of erythromycin with astemizole is contraindicated. (See CONTRAINDICATIONS and WARNINGS BOX.) Concomitant administration of astemizole with other macrolide antibiotics, including troleandomycin, azithromycin, and clarithromycin, is not recommended.

Quinine
Concomitant administration of astemizole with quinine is contraindicated. (See **CONTRAINDICATIONS** and **WARNINGS BOX**.)

Information for Patients:
Patients taking HISMANAL should receive the following information and instructions. Antihistamines are prescribed to reduce allergic symptoms. Patients taking HISMANAL should be advised 1) to adhere to the recommended dose, and 2) that the use of excessive doses may lead to serious cardiovascular events. Some patients appear to increase the dose of HISMANAL in an attempt to accelerate the onset of action. PATIENTS SHOULD BE ADVISED NOT TO DO THIS and not to use HISMANAL as a p r n product for immediate relief of symptoms. Patients should be questioned about use of any other prescription or over-the-counter medication, and should be cautioned regarding the potential for life-threatening arrhythmias with concurrent use of ketoconazole, itraconazole, erythromycin or quinine. Human data indicate that although beverages containing quinine (up to 80 mg/day or about 32 ounces of tonic water) may elevate plasma levels of astemizole and desmethylastemizole, this effect is small and is not accompanied by significant prolongation of the QT interval. Patients should be advised to consult the physician before concurrent use of other medications with astemizole. Patients should be questioned about pregnancy or lactation before starting HISMANAL therapy, since the drug should be used in pregnancy or lactation only if the potential benefit justifies the potential risk to fetus or baby. (See Pregnancy subsection.) In addition, patients should be instructed to take HISMANAL on an empty stomach, e.g., at least 2 hours after a meal. No additional food should be taken for at least 1 hour after dosing. Patients should also be instructed to store this medication in a tightly closed container in a cool, dry place, away from heat or direct sunlight, and away from children.

Carcinogenesis, Mutagenesis, Impairment of Fertility:
Carcinogenic potential has not been revealed in rats given 260× the recommended human dose of astemizole for 24 months, or in mice given 400× the recommended human dose for 18 months. Micronucleus, dominant lethal, sister chromatid exchange and Ames tests of astemizole have not revealed mutagenic activity.
Impairment of fertility was not observed in male or female rats given 200× the recommended human dose.

Pregnancy: Pregnancy Category C:
Teratogenic effects were not observed in rats administered 200× the recommended human dose or in rabbits given 200× the recommended human dose. Maternal toxicity was seen in rabbits administered 200× the recommended human dose. Embryocidal effects accompanied by maternal toxicity were observed at 100× the recommended human dose in rats. Embryotoxicity or maternal toxicity was not observed in rats or rabbits administered 50× the recommended human dose. There are no adequate and well controlled studies in pregnant women. HISMANAL should be used during pregnancy only if the potential benefit justifies the potential risk to the fetus. Metabolites may remain in the body for as long as 4 months after the end of dosing, calculated on the basis of 6 times the terminal half-life. (See CLINICAL PHARMACOLOGY section.)

Nursing Mothers:
It is not known whether this drug is excreted in human milk. Because certain drugs are known to be excreted in human milk, caution should be exercised when HISMANAL is administered to a nursing woman. HISMANAL is excreted in the milk of dogs.

Pediatric Use:
Safety and efficacy in children under 12 years of age has not been demonstrated.

ADVERSE REACTIONS

For information regarding cardiovascular adverse events (e.g. cardiac arrest, ventricular arrhythmias), please see CONTRAINDICATIONS and WARNINGS BOX. In some cases, recognition of severe arrhythmias has been preceded by episodes of syncope. Similarly, rare cases of hypotension, palpitations, and dizziness have also been reported with

| | Percent of Patients Reporting | | |
| | Controlled Studies* | | |
ADVERSE EVENT	HISMANAL (N=1630) %	PLACEBO (N=1109) %	CLASSICAL** (N=304) %
Central Nervous System			
Drowsiness	7.1	6.4	22.0
Headache	6.7	9.2	3.3
Fatigue	4.2	1.6	11.8
Appetite increase	3.9	1.4	0.0
Weight increase	3.6	0.7	1.0
Nervousness	2.1	1.2	0.3
Dizzy	2.0	1.8	1.0
Gastrointestinal System			
Nausea	2.5	2.9	1.3
Diarrhea	1.8	2.0	0.7
Abdominal pain	1.4	1.2	0.7
Eye, Ear, Nose, and Throat			
Mouth dry	5.2	3.8	7.9
Pharyngitis	1.7	2.3	0.3
Conjunctivitis	1.2	1.2	0.7
Other			
Arthralgia	1.2	1.6	0.0

*Duration of treatment in Controlled Studies ranged from 7 to 182 Days

**Classical Drugs: Clemastine (N=137); Chlorpheniramine (N=100); Pheniramine Maleate (N=47); d-Chlorpheniramine (N=20)

HISMANAL use, which may reflect undetected ventricular arrhythmia.

The reported incidences of adverse reactions listed in the following table are derived from controlled clinical studies in adults. In these studies the usual maintenance dose of HISMANAL was 10 mg once daily.

[See table above.]

Adverse reaction information has been obtained from more than 7500 patients in all clinical trials. Weight gain has been reported in 3.6% of astemizole treated patients involved in controlled studies, with an average treatment duration of 53 days. In 46 of the 59 patients for whom actual weight gain data was available, the average weight gain was 3.2 kg.

Less frequently occurring adverse experiences reported in clinical trials or spontaneously from marketing experience with HISMANAL include: angioedema, asymptomatic liver enzyme elevations, bronchospasm, depression, edema, epistaxis, hepatitis, myalgia, palpitation, paresthesia, photosensitivity, pruritus, and rash.

Marketing experiences include isolated cases of convulsions. A causal relationship with HISMANAL has not been established.

OVERDOSAGE

In the event of overdosage, supportive measures including gastric lavage and emesis should be employed. Substantial overdoses of HISMANAL can cause death, cardiac arrest, QT prolongation, torsades de pointes, and other ventricular arrhythmias. These events can also occur, although rarely, at doses (20–30 mg) close to the recommended dose (10 mg/daily). (See WARNINGS BOX and DOSAGE AND ADMINISTRATION.)

Seizures and syncope have also been reported with overdose and may be associated with a cardiac event.

Overdose patients should be carefully monitored as long as the QT interval is prolonged or arrhythmias are present. In some cases, this has been up to six days. In overdose cases in which ventricular arrhythmias are associated with significant QT prolongation, treatment with antiarrhythmics known to prolong QT intervals is not recommended. HISMANAL does not appear to be dialyzable.

Oral LD_{50} values for HISMANAL were 2052 mg/kg in mice and 3154 mg/kg in rats. In neonatal rats, the oral LD_{50} was 905 mg/kg in males and 1235 mg/kg in females.

DOSAGE AND ADMINISTRATION

The recommended dosage for adults and children 12 years of age and older is 10 mg (1 tablet) once daily.

DO NOT EXCEED THE RECOMMENDED DOSE. Patients should be advised not to increase the dose of HISMANAL in an attempt to accelerate the onset of action. (See WARNINGS BOX.) USE OF HISMANAL IN PATIENTS TAKING KETOCONAZOLE, ITRACONAZOLE, ERYTHROMYCIN, OR QUININE IS CONTRAINDICATED. (See CONTRAINDICATIONS, WARNINGS, and PRECAUTIONS: Drug Interactions.)

Studies evaluating the need for dosage adjustments for patients with hepatic or renal dysfunction have not been performed. Since astemizole is extensively metabolized by the liver, use of HISMANAL in patients with significant hepatic dysfunction should generally be avoided.

HISMANAL should be taken on an empty stomach, e.g., at least two hours after a meal. There should be no additional food intake for at least one hour post-dosing.

HOW SUPPLIED

HISMANAL is available as white, scored tablets containing 10 mg of astemizole debossed "JANSSEN" and on the reverse side debossed "AST"/10.

NDC 50458-510-10 (HDPE bottles of 100 tablets)

NDC 50458-510-13 (HDPE bottles of 30 tablets with a child-resistant closure)

Store tablets at room temperature (59°–86°F) (15°–30°C). Protect from moisture.

U.S. Patent 4,219,559

Revised July 1993, February 1996

JANSSEN PHARMACEUTICA INC.

Titusville, New Jersey 08560-0200

Shown in Product Identification Guide, page 318

IMODIUM®
(loperamide HCl) Capsules

℞

DESCRIPTION

IMODIUM (loperamide hydrochloride), 4-(p-chlorophenyl)-4-hydroxy-N, N-dimethyl-α,α-diphenyl-1-piperidinebutyramide monohydrochloride, is a synthetic antidiarrheal for oral use.

IMODIUM is available in 2 mg capsules.

The inactive ingredients are:

Lactose, cornstarch, talc, and magnesium stearate.

IMODIUM capsules contain F D & C Yellow No. 6.

CLINICAL PHARMACOLOGY

In vitro and animal studies show that IMODIUM acts by slowing intestinal motility and by affecting water and electrolyte movement through the bowel. IMODIUM inhibits peristaltic activity by a direct effect on the circular and longitudinal muscles of the intestinal wall.

In man, IMODIUM prolongs the transit time of the intestinal contents. It reduces the daily fecal volume, increases the viscosity and bulk density, and diminishes the loss of fluid and electrolytes. Tolerance to the antidiarrheal effect has not been observed.

Clinical studies have indicated that the apparent elimination half-life of loperamide in man is 10.8 hours with a range of 9.1–14.4 hours. Plasma levels of unchanged drug remain below 2 nanograms per ml after the intake of a 2 mg capsule of IMODIUM. Plasma levels are highest approximately five hours after administration of the capsule and 2.5 hours after the liquid. The peak plasma levels of loperamide were similar for both formulations. Of the total excreted in urine and feces, most of the administered drug was excreted in feces.

In those patients in whom biochemical and hematological parameters were monitored during clinical trials, no trends toward abnormality during IMODIUM therapy were noted. Similarly, urinalyses, EKG and clinical ophthalmological examinations did not show trends toward abnormality.

INDICATIONS AND USAGE

IMODIUM is indicated for the control and symptomatic relief of acute nonspecific diarrhea and of chronic diarrhea associated with inflammatory bowel disease. IMODIUM is also indicated for reducing the volume of discharge from ileostomies.

CONTRAINDICATIONS

IMODIUM is contraindicated in patients with known hypersensitivity to the drug and in those in whom constipation must be avoided.

WARNINGS

IMODIUM should not be used in the case of acute dysentery, which is characterized by blood in stools and high fever.

Fluid and electrolyte depletion often occur in patients who have diarrhea. In such cases, administration of appropriate fluid and electrolytes is very important. The use of IMODIUM does not preclude the need for appropriate fluid and electrolyte therapy.

In some patients with acute ulcerative colitis, and in pseudomembranous colitis associated with broad-spectrum antibiotics, agents which inhibit intestinal motility or delay intestinal transit time have been reported to induce toxic megacolon. IMODIUM therapy should be discontinued promptly if abdominal distention, constipation, or ileus occurs.

IMODIUM should be used with special caution in young children because of the greater variability of response in this age group. Dehydration, particularly in younger children, may further influence the variability of response to IMODIUM.

PRECAUTIONS

General: In acute diarrhea, if clinical improvement is not observed in 48 hours, the administration of IMODIUM should be discontinued.

Patients with hepatic dysfunction should be monitored closely for signs of CNS toxicity because of the apparent large first pass biotransformation.

Information for Patients: Patients should be advised to check with their physician if their diarrhea does not improve after a couple of days or if they note blood in their stools or develop a fever.

Drug Interactions: There was no evidence in clinical trials of drug interactions with concurrent medications.

Carcinogenesis, mutagenesis, impairment of fertility: In an 18-month rat study with doses up to 133 times the maximum human dose (on a mg/kg basis), there was no evidence of carcinogenesis. Mutagenicity studies were not conducted. Reproduction studies in rats indicated that high doses (150–200 times the human dose) could cause marked female infertility and reduced male fertility.

Pregnancy

Teratogenic Effects

Pregnancy Category B: Reproduction studies in rats and rabbits have revealed no evidence of impaired fertility or harm to the fetus at doses up to 30 times the human dose. Higher doses impaired the survival of mothers and nursing young. The studies offered no evidence of teratogenic activity. There are, however, no adequate and well controlled studies in pregnant women. Because animal reproduction studies are not always predictive of human response, this drug should be used during pregnancy only if clearly needed.

Nursing Mothers: It is not known whether this drug is excreted in human milk. Because many drugs are excreted in human milk, caution should be exercised when IMODIUM is administered to a nursing woman.

Pediatric Use: See the "Warnings" Section for information on the greater variability of response in this age group.

In case of accidental overdosage of IMODIUM by children, see "Overdosage" Section for suggested treatment.

ADVERSE REACTIONS

The adverse effects reported during clinical investigations of IMODIUM are difficult to distinguish from symptoms associated with the diarrheal syndrome. Adverse experiences recorded during clinical studies with IMODIUM were generally of a minor and self-limiting nature. They were more commonly observed during the treatment of chronic diarrhea.

The following patient complaints have been reported and are listed in decreasing order of frequency with the exception of hypersensitivity reactions which is listed first since it may be the most serious.

- Hypersensitivity reactions (including skin rash) have been reported with IMODIUM use.
- Abdominal pain, distention or discomfort
- Nausea and vomiting
- Constipation
- Tiredness
- Drowsiness or dizziness
- Dry mouth

In postmarketing experiences, there have been rare reports of paralytic ileus associated with abdominal distention. Most of these reports occurred in the setting of acute dysentery, overdose, and with very young children of less than two years of age.

DRUG ABUSE AND DEPENDENCE

Abuse: A specific clinical study designed to assess the abuse potential of loperamide at high doses resulted in a finding of extremely low abuse potential.

Continued on next page

Janssen Pharmaceutica—Cont.

Dependence: Studies in morphine-dependent monkeys demonstrated that loperamide hydrochloride at doses above those recommended for humans prevented signs of morphine withdrawal. However, in humans, the naloxone challenge pupil test, which when positive indicates opiate-like effects, performed after a single high dose, or after more than two years of therapeutic use of IMODIUM, was negative. Orally administered IMODIUM (loperamide formulated with magnesium stearate) is both highly insoluble and penetrates the CNS poorly.

OVERDOSAGE

In cases of overdosage, paralytic ileus and CNS depression may occur. Children may be more sensitive to CNS effects than adults. Clinical trials have demonstrated that a slurry of activated charcoal administered promptly after ingestion of loperamide hydrochloride can reduce the amount of drug which is absorbed into the systemic circulation by as much as ninefold. If vomiting occurs spontaneously upon ingestion, a slurry of 100 gms of activated charcoal should be administered orally as soon as fluids can be retained.

If vomiting has not occurred, gastric lavage should be performed followed by administration of 100 gms of the activated charcoal slurry through the gastric tube. In the event of overdosage, patients should be monitored for signs of CNS depression for at least 24 hours. Children may be more sensitive to central nervous system effects than adults. If CNS depression is observed, naloxone may be administered. If responsive to naloxone, vital signs must be monitored carefully for recurrence of symptoms of drug overdose for at least 24 hours after the last dose of naloxone.

In view of the prolonged action of loperamide and the short duration (one to three hours) of naloxone, the patient must be monitored closely and treated repeatedly with naloxone as indicated. Since relatively little drug is excreted in the urine, forced diuresis is not expected to be effective for IMODIUM overdosage.

In clinical trials an adult who took three 20 mg doses within a 24 hour period was nauseated after the second dose and vomited after the third dose. In studies designed to examine the potential for side effects, intentional ingestion of up to 60 mg of loperamide hydrochloride in a single dose to healthy subjects resulted in no significant adverse effects.

DOSAGE AND ADMINISTRATION (1 capsule = 2 mg)

Patients should receive appropriate fluid and electrolyte replacement as needed.

Acute Diarrhea

Adults: The recommended initial dose is 4 mg (two capsules) followed by 2 mg (one capsule) after each unformed stool. Daily dosage should not exceed 16 mg (eight capsules). Clinical improvement is usually observed within 48 hours.

Children: IMODIUM use is not recommended for children under 2 years of age. In children 2 to 5 years of age (20 kg or less), the non-prescription liquid formulation (IMODIUM A-D 1 mg/5 ml) should be used; for ages 6 to 12, either IMODIUM Capsules or IMODIUM A-D Liquid may be used. For children 2 to 12 years of age, the following schedule for capsules or liquid will usually fulfill initial dosage requirements:

Recommended First Day Dosage Schedule

Two to five years:	1 mg t.i.d.
(13 to 20 kg)	(3 mg daily dose)
Six to eight years:	2 mg b.i.d.
(20 to 30 kg)	(4 mg daily dose)
Eight to twelve years:	2 mg t.i.d.
(greater than 30 kg)	(6 mg daily dose)

Recommended Subsequent Daily Dosage

Following the first treatment day, it is recommended that subsequent IMODIUM doses (1 mg/10 kg body weight) be administered only after a loose stool. Total daily dosage should not exceed recommended dosages for the first day.

Chronic Diarrhea

Children: Although IMODIUM has been studied in a limited number of children with chronic diarrhea, the therapeutic dose for the treatment of chronic diarrhea in a pediatric population has not been established.

Adults: The recommended initial dose is 4 mg (two capsules) followed by 2 mg (one capsule) after each unformed stool until diarrhea is controlled, after which the dosage of IMODIUM should be reduced to meet individual requirements. When the optimal daily dosage has been established, this amount may then be administered as a single dose or in divided doses.

The average daily maintenance dosage in clinical trials was 4 to 8 mg (two to four capsules). A dosage of 16 mg (eight capsules) was rarely exceeded. If clinical improvement is not observed after treatment with 16 mg per day for at least 10 days, symptoms are unlikely to be controlled by further administration. IMODIUM administration may be continued if diarrhea cannot be adequately controlled with diet or specific treatment.

HOW SUPPLIED

Capsules—each capsule contains 2 mg of loperamide hydrochloride. The capsules have a light green body and a dark green cap with "JANSSEN" imprinted on one segment and "IMODIUM" on the other segment. IMODIUM capsules are supplied in bottles of 100 and 500 and in blister packs of 10 × 10 capsules.
NDC 50458-400-01
(10 × 10 capsules—blister)
NDC 50458-400-10
(100 capsules)
NDC 50458-400-50
(500 capsules)
Store at controlled room temperature 15°–30°C (59°–86°F)
Revised January 1993, May 1993
CAUTION: FEDERAL LAW PROHIBITS DISPENSING WITHOUT A PRESCRIPTION
JANSSEN PHARMACEUTICA INC.
Titusville, New Jersey 08560-0200
Printed in USA
U.S. Patent 3,714,159
Shown in Product Identification Guide, page 318

NIZORAL® ℞
[nī'zōr-ăl]
(ketoconazole) 2% Cream

DESCRIPTION

NIZORAL® (ketoconazole) 2% Cream contains the broad-spectrum synthetic antifungal agent, ketoconazole 2%, formulated in an aqueous cream vehicle consisting of propylene glycol, stearyl and cetyl alcohols, sorbitan monostearate, polysorbate 60, isopropyl myristate, sodium sulfite anhydrous, polysorbate 80 and purified water.

Ketoconazole is cis-1-acetyl-4-[4-[[2-(2,4-dichlorophenyl)-2-(1H-imidazol-1-ylmethyl)-1,3-dioxolan-4-yl]methoxy]phenyl]piperazine.

CLINICAL PHARMACOLOGY

When NIZORAL® (ketoconazole) 2% Cream was applied dermally to intact or abraded skin of Beagle dogs for 28 consecutive days at a dose of 80 mg, there were no detectable plasma levels using an assay method having a lower detection limit of 2 ng/ml.

After a single topical application to the chest, back and arms of normal volunteers, systemic absorption of ketoconazole was not detected at the 5 ng/ml level in blood over a 72-hour period.

Two dermal irritancy studies, a human sensitization test, a phototoxicity study and a photoallergy study conducted in 38 male and 62 female volunteers showed no contact sensitization of the delayed hypersensitivity type, no irritation, no phototoxicity and no photoallergenic potential due to NIZORAL® (ketoconazole) 2% Cream.

Microbiology: Ketoconazole is a broad spectrum synthetic antifungal agent which inhibits the in vitro growth of the following common dermatophytes and yeasts by altering the permeability of the cell membrane: dermatophytes: *Trichophyton rubrum, T. mentagrophytes, T. tonsurans, Microsporum canis, M. audouini, M. gypseum* and *Epidermophyton floccosum;* yeasts: *Candida albicans, Malassezia ovale (Pityrosporum ovale)* and *C. tropicalis;* and the organism responsible for tinea versicolor, *Malassezia furfur (Pityrosporum orbiculare).* Only those organisms listed in the INDICATIONS AND USAGE Section have been proven to be clinically affected. Development of resistance to ketoconazole has not been reported.

Mode of Action: In vitro studies suggest that ketoconazole impairs the synthesis of ergosterol, which is a vital component of fungal cell membranes. It is postulated that the therapeutic effect of ketoconazole in seborrheic dermatitis is due to the reduction of M. ovale, but this has not been proven.

INDICATIONS AND USAGE

NIZORAL® (ketoconazole) 2% Cream is indicated for the topical treatment of tinea corporis, tinea cruris and tinea pedis caused by *Trichophyton rubrum, T. mentagrophytes* and *Epidermophyton floccosum;* in the treatment of tinea (pityriasis) versicolor caused by *Malassezia furfur (Pityrosporum orbiculare);* in the treatment of cutaneous candidiasis caused by *Candida spp.* and in the treatment of seborrheic dermatitis.

CONTRAINDICATIONS

NIZORAL® (ketoconazole) 2% Cream is contraindicated in persons who have shown hypersensitivity to the active or excipient ingredients of this formulation.

WARNINGS

NIZORAL® (ketoconazole) 2% Cream is not for ophthalmic use.

NIZORAL® (ketoconazole) 2% Cream contains sodium sulfite anhydrous, a sulfite that may cause allergic-type reactions including anaphylactic symptoms and life-threatening or less severe asthmatic episodes in certain susceptible peo-

ple. The overall prevalence of sulfite sensitivity in the general population is unknown and probably low. Sulfite sensitivity is seen more frequently in asthmatic than in nonasthmatic people.

PRECAUTIONS

General: If a reaction suggesting sensitivity or chemical irritation should occur, use of the medication should be discontinued. Hepatitis (1:10,000 reported incidence) and, at high doses, lowered testosterone and ACTH induced corticosteroid serum levels have been seen with orally administered ketoconazole; these effects have not been seen with topical ketoconazole.

Carcinogenesis, Mutagenesis, Impairment of Fertility: A long-term feeding study in Swiss Albino mice and in Wistar rats showed no evidence of oncogenic activity. The dominant lethal mutation test in male and female mice revealed that single oral doses of ketoconazole as high as 80 mg/kg produced no mutation in any stage of germ cell development. The Ames' *Salmonella* microsomal activator assay was also negative.

Pregnancy: Teratogenic effects: Pregnancy Category C: Ketoconazole has been shown to be teratogenic (syndactylia and oligodactylia) in the rat when given orally in the diet at 80 mg/kg/day, (10 times the maximum recommended human oral dose). However, these effects may be related to maternal toxicity, which was seen at this and higher dose levels.

There are no adequate and well-controlled studies in pregnant women. Ketoconazole should be used during pregnancy only if the potential benefit justifies the potential risk to the fetus.

Nursing Mothers: It is not known whether NIZORAL® (ketoconazole) 2% Cream administered topically could result in sufficient systemic absorption to produce detectable quantities in breast milk. Nevertheless, a decision should be made whether to discontinue nursing or discontinue the drug, taking into account the importance of the drug to the mother.

Pediatric Use: Safety and effectiveness in children have not been established.

ADVERSE REACTIONS

During clinical trials 45 (5.0%) of 905 patients treated with NIZORAL® (ketoconazole) 2% Cream and 5 (2.4%) of 208 patients treated with placebo reported side effects consisting mainly of severe irritation, pruritus and stinging. One of the patients treated with NIZORAL® Cream developed a painful allergic reaction.

In worldwide postmarketing experience, rare reports of contact dermatitis have been associated in NIZORAL Cream or one of its excipients, namely sodium sulfite or propylene glycol.

DOSAGE AND ADMINISTRATION

Cutaneous candidiasis, tinea corporis, tinea cruris, tinea pedis and tinea (pityriasis) versicolor: It is recommended that NIZORAL® (ketoconazole) 2% Cream be applied once daily to cover the affected and immediate surrounding area. Clinical improvement may be seen fairly soon after treatment is begun; however, candidal infections and tinea cruris and corporis should be treated for two weeks in order to reduce the possibility of recurrence. Patients with tinea versicolor usually require two weeks of treatment. Patients with tinea pedis require six weeks of treatment.

Seborrheic dermatitis: NIZORAL® (ketoconazole) 2% Cream should be applied to the affected area twice daily for four weeks or until clinical clearing.

If a patient shows no clinical improvement after the treatment period, the diagnosis should be redetermined.

HOW SUPPLIED

NIZORAL® (ketoconazole) 2% Cream is supplied in 15 (NDC 50458-221-15), 30 (NDC 50458-221-30) and 60 (NDC 50458-221-60) gm tubes.
Store below 77°F (25°C)
Revised July 1994, April 1995
U.S. Patent No. 4,335,125
JANSSEN PHARMACEUTICA
Titusville, NJ 08560
Shown in Product Identification Guide, page 318

NIZORAL® ℞
[nī'zōr-ăl]
(ketoconazole) 2% Shampoo

DESCRIPTION

NIZORAL® (ketoconazole) 2% Shampoo is a red-orange liquid for topical application, containing the broad-spectrum synthetic antifungal agent ketoconazole in a concentration of 2% in an aqueous suspension. It also contains: coconut fatty acid diethanolamide, disodium monolauryl ether sulfosuccinate, F.D. & C. Red No. 40, hydrochloric acid, imidurea, laurdimonium hydrolyzed animal collagen, macrogol 120 methyl-glucose dioleate, perfume bouquet, sodium chloride,

sodium hydroxide, sodium lauryl ether sulfate, and purified water.

Ketoconazole is cis-1-acetyl-4-[4-[[2-(2,4-di-chlorophenyl)-2-(1H-imidazol-1-ylmethyl)-1,3-dioxolan-4-yl] methoxy]phenyl]piperazine.

CLINICAL PHARMACOLOGY

When ketoconazole 2% shampoo was applied dermally to intact or abraded skin of rabbits for 28 days at doses up to 50 mg/kg and allowed to remain one hour before being washed away, there were no detectable plasma ketoconazole levels using an assay method having a lower detection limit of 5 ng/mL. NIZORAL® (ketoconazole) was not detected in plasma in 39 patients who shampooed 4–10 times per week for 6 months or in 33 patients who shampooed 2–3 times per week for 3–26 months (mean: 16 months).

Twelve hours after a single shampoo, hair samples taken from six patients showed that high amounts of ketoconazole were present on the hair but only about 5% had penetrated into the hair keratin. Chronic shampooing (twice weekly for two months) increased the ketoconazole levels in the hair keratin to 20%, but did not increase levels on the hair. There were no detectable plasma levels.

An exaggerated use washing test on the sensitive antecubital skin of 10 subjects twice daily for five consecutive days showed that the irritancy potential of ketoconazole 2% shampoo was significantly less than that of 2.5% selenium sulfide shampoo.

A human sensitization test, a phototoxicity study, and a photoallergy study conducted in 38 male and 22 female volunteers showed no contact sensitization of the delayed hypersensitivity type, no phototoxicity and no photoallergenic potential due to NIZORAL® (ketoconazole) 2% Shampoo.

Mode of Action: Interpretations of in vivo studies suggest that ketoconazole impairs the synthesis of ergosterol, which is a vital component of fungal cell membranes. It is postulated that the therapeutic effect of ketoconazole in dandruff is due to the reduction of Pityrosporum ovale (Malassezia ovale), but this has not been proven. Support for this hypothesis comes from a 4-week double-blind, placebo-controlled clinical trial, in which the decrease in P. ovale on the scalp was significantly greater with ketoconazole (36 patients) than with placebo (20 patients) and was comparable to that with selenium sulfide (42 patients). In the same study, ketoconazole and selenium sulfide reduced the severity of adherent dandruff significantly more than the placebo did. Ketoconazole produced significantly higher proportions of patients with at least 50% reductions in adherent dandruff (50% vs. 15%) and in loose dandruff (67% vs. 15%) than did the placebo.

Microbiology: NIZORAL® (ketoconazole) is a broad-spectrum synthetic antifungal agent which inhibits the growth of the following common dermatophytes and yeasts by altering the permeability of the cell membrane: dermatophytes: Trichophyton rubrum, T. mentagrophytes, T. tonsurans, Microsporum canis, M. audouini, M. gypseum and Epidermophyton floccosum; yeasts: Candida albicans, C. tropicalis, Pityrosporum ovale (Malassezia ovale) and Pityrosporum orbiculare (M. furfur). Development of resistance by these microorganisms to ketoconazole has not been reported.

INDICATIONS AND USAGE

NIZORAL® (ketoconazole) 2% Shampoo is indicated for the reduction of scaling due to dandruff.

CONTRAINDICATIONS

NIZORAL® (ketoconazole) 2% Shampoo is contraindicated in persons who have shown hypersensitivity to the active ingredient or excipients of this formulation.

PRECAUTIONS

General: If a reaction suggesting sensitivity or chemical irritation should occur, use of the medication should be discontinued.

Information for Patients: May be irritating to mucous membranes of the eyes and contact with this area should be avoided.

There have been reports that use of the shampoo resulted in removal of the curl from permanently waved hair.

Carcinogenesis, Mutagenesis, Impairment of Fertility: The dominant lethal mutation test in male and female mice revealed that single oral doses of ketoconazole as high as 80 mg/kg produced no mutation in any stage of germ cell development. The Ames Salmonella microsomal activator assay was also negative. A long-term feeding study of ketoconazole in Swiss Albino mice and in Wistar rats showed no evidence of oncogenic activity.

Pregnancy: Teratogenic effects: Pregnancy Category C: Ketoconazole is not detected in plasma after chronic shampooing. Ketoconazole has been shown to be teratogenic (syndactylia and oligodactylia) in the rat when given orally in the diet at 80 mg/kg/day (10 times the maximum recommended human oral dose). However, these effects may be related to maternal toxicity, which was seen at this and higher dose levels.

There are no adequate and well-controlled studies in pregnant women. Ketoconazole should be used during pregnancy only if the potential benefit justifies the potential risk to the fetus.

Nursing mothers: Ketoconazole is not detected in plasma after chronic shampooing. Nevertheless, caution should be exercised when NIZORAL® (ketoconazole) 2% Shampoo is administered to a nursing woman.

Pediatric Use: Safety and effectiveness in children have not been established.

ADVERSE REACTIONS

In 11 double-blind trials in 264 patients using ketoconazole 2% shampoo, an increase in normal hair loss and irritation occurred in less than 1% of patients. In three open-label safety trials in which 41 patients shampooed 4–10 times weekly for six months, the following adverse experiences each occurred once: abnormal hair texture, scalp pustules, mild dryness of the skin, and itching. As with other shampoos, oiliness and dryness of hair and scalp have been reported.

OVERDOSAGE

NIZORAL® (ketoconazole) 2% Shampoo is intended for external use only. In the event of accidental ingestion, supportive measures should be employed. Induced emesis and gastric lavage should usually be avoided.

DOSAGE AND ADMINISTRATION

1. Moisten hair and scalp thoroughly with water.
2. Apply sufficient shampoo to produce enough lather to wash the scalp and hair and gently massage it over the entire scalp area for approximately 1 minute.
3. Rinse the hair thoroughly with warm water.
4. Repeat, leaving the shampoo on the scalp for an additional 3 minutes.
5. After the second thorough rinse, dry the hair with a towel or warm air flow.

Shampoo twice a week for four weeks with at least three days between each shampooing and then intermittently as needed to maintain control.

HOW SUPPLIED

NIZORAL® (ketoconazole) 2% Shampoo is a red-orange liquid supplied in a 4-fluid ounce nonbreakable plastic bottle (NDC 50458-223-04).

Storage conditions: Store at a temperature not above 25°C (77°F). Protect from light.

Manufactured by:
Janssen Pharmaceutica n.v.
Beerse, Belgium
Distributed by:
Janssen Pharmaceutica Inc.
Titusville, NJ 08560
Revised November 1991, November 1992, August 1995
U.S. Patent No. 4,335,125
Shown in Product Identification Guide, page 318

NIZORAL® ℞
[nī 'zōr-ăl]
(ketoconazole)
Tablets

> **WARNING:** When used orally, ketoconazole has been associated with hepatic toxicity, including some fatalities. Patients receiving this drug should be informed by the physician of the risk and should be closely monitored. See WARNINGS and PRECAUTIONS sections.
> Coadministration of terfenadine with ketoconazole tablets is contraindicated. Rare cases of serious cardiovascular adverse events, including death, ventricular tachycardia and torsades de pointes have been observed in patients taking ketoconazole tablets concomitantly with terfenadine, due to increased terfenadine concentrations induced by ketoconazole tablets. See CONTRAINDICATIONS, WARNINGS, and PRECAUTIONS sections.
> Pharmacokinetic data indicate that oral ketoconazole inhibits the metabolism of astemizole, resulting in elevated plasma levels of astemizole and its active metabolite desmethylastemizole which may prolong QT intervals. Coadministration of astemizole with ketoconazole tablets is therefore contraindicated. See CONTRAINDICATIONS, WARNINGS, and PRECAUTIONS sections.
> Coadministration of cisapride with ketoconazole is contraindicated. Serious cardiovascular adverse events including ventricular tachycardia, ventricular fibrillation and torsades de pointes have occurred in patients taking ketoconazole concomitantly with cisapride. See CONTRAINDICATIONS, WARNINGS, and PRECAUTIONS sections.

DESCRIPTION

NIZORAL® (ketoconazole) is a synthetic broad-spectrum antifungal agent available in scored white tablets, each containing 200 mg ketoconazole base for oral administration. Inactive ingredients are colloidal silicon dioxide, corn starch, lactose, magnesium stearate, microcrystalline cellulose, and povidone. Ketoconazole is cis-1-acetyl-4-[4-[[2-(2,4-dichlorophenyl)-2- (1H-imidazol-1-ylmethyl)-1,3-dioxolan-4-yl] methoxyl]phenyl] piperazine.

Ketoconazole is a white to slightly beige, odorless powder, soluble in acids, with a molecular weight of 531.44.

CLINICAL PHARMACOLOGY

Mean peak plasma levels of approximately 3.5 µg/mL are reached within 1 to 2 hours, following oral administration of a single 200 mg dose taken with a meal. Subsequent plasma elimination is biphasic with a half-life of 2 hours during the first 10 hours and 8 hours thereafter. Following absorption from the gastrointestinal tract, NIZORAL (ketoconazole) is converted into several inactive metabolites. The major identified metabolic pathways are oxidation and degradation of the imidazole and piperazine rings, oxidative O-dealkylation and aromatic hydroxylation. About 13% of the dose is excreted in the urine, of which 2 to 4% is unchanged drug. The major route of excretion is through the bile into the intestinal tract. In vitro, the plasma protein binding is about 99% mainly to the albumin fraction. Only a negligible proportion of ketoconazole reaches the cerebral-spinal fluid. Ketoconazole is a weak dibasic agent and thus requires acidity for dissolution and absorption.

NIZORAL Tablets are active against clinical infections with Blastomyces dermatitidis, Candida spp., Coccidioides immitis, Histoplasma capsulatum, Paracoccidioides brasiliensis, and Phialophora spp. NIZORAL Tablets are also active against Trichophyton spp., Epidermophyton spp., and Microsporum spp. Ketoconazole is also active in vitro against a variety of fungi and yeast. In animal models, activity has been demonstrated against Candida spp., Blastomyces dermatitidis, Histoplasma capsulatum, Malassezia furfur, Coccidioides immitis, and Cryptococcus neoformans.

Mode of Action: In vitro studies suggest that ketoconazole impairs the synthesis of ergosterol, which is a vital component of fungal cell membranes.

INDICATIONS AND USAGE

NIZORAL (ketoconazole) Tablets are indicated for the treatment of the following systemic fungal infections: candidiasis, chronic mucocutaneous candidiasis, oral thrush, candiduria, blastomycosis, coccidioidomycosis, histoplasmosis, chromomycosis, and paracoccidioidomycosis. NIZORAL Tablets should not be used for fungal meningitis because it penetrates poorly into the cerebral-spinal fluid.

NIZORAL Tablets are also indicated for the treatment of patients with severe recalcitrant cutaneous dermatophyte infections who have not responded to topical therapy or oral griseofulvin, or who are unable to take griseofulvin.

CONTRAINDICATIONS

Coadministration of terfenadine or astemizole with ketoconazole tablets is contraindicated. (See BOX WARNING, WARNINGS, and PRECAUTIONS sections.)
Concomitant administration of NIZORAL Tablets with cisapride (PROPULSID) is contraindicated. (See BOX WARNING, WARNINGS, and PRECAUTIONS sections.)
Concomitant administration of NIZORAL Tablets with oral triazolam is contraindicated. (See PRECAUTIONS sections.)
NIZORAL is contraindicated in patients who have shown hypersensitivity to the drug.

WARNINGS

Hepatotoxicity, primarily of the hepatocellular type, has been associated with the use of NIZORAL (ketoconazole) Tablets, including rare fatalities. The reported incidence of hepatotoxicity has been about 1:10,000 exposed patients, but this probably represents some degree of under-reporting, as is the case for most reported adverse reactions to drugs. The median duration of NIZORAL Tablet therapy in patients who developed symptomatic hepatotoxicity was about 28 days, although the range extended to as low as 3 days. The hepatic injury has usually, but not always, been reversible upon discontinuation of NIZORAL Tablet treatment. Several cases of hepatitis have been reported in children. Prompt recognition of liver injury is essential. Liver function tests (such as SGGT, alkaline phosphatase, SGPT, SGOT and bilirubin) should be measured before starting treatment and at frequent intervals during treatment. Patients receiving NIZORAL Tablets concurrently with other potentially hepatotoxic drugs should be carefully monitored, particularly those patients requiring prolonged therapy or those who have had a history of liver disease.

Most of the reported cases of hepatic toxicity have to date been in patients treated for onychomycosis. Of 180 patients worldwide developing idiosyncratic liver dysfunction during NIZORAL Tablet therapy, 61.3% had onychomycosis and 16.8% had chronic recalcitrant dermatophytoses.

Transient minor elevations in liver enzymes have occurred during treatment with NIZORAL Tablets. The drug should be discontinued if these persist, if the abnormalities worsen,

Continued on next page

Janssen Pharmaceutica—Cont.

or if the abnormalities become accompanied by symptoms of possible liver injury.

In rare cases anaphylaxis has been reported after the first dose. Several cases of hypersensitivity reactions including urticaria have also been reported.

Coadministration of ketoconazole tablets and terfenadine has led to elevated plasma concentrations of terfenadine which may prolong QT intervals, sometimes resulting in life-threatening cardiac dysrhythmias. Cases of torsades de pointes and other serious ventricular dysrhythmias, in rare cases leading to fatality, have been reported among patients taking terfenadine concurrently with ketoconazole tablets. Coadministration of ketoconazole tablets and terfenadine is contraindicated.

Coadministration of astemizole with ketoconazole tablets is contraindicated. (See BOX WARNING, CONTRAINDICATIONS, and PRECAUTIONS sections.)

Concomitant administration of NIZORAL Tablets with cisapride is contraindicated because it has resulted in markedly elevated cisapride plasma concentrations and prolonged QT interval, and has rarely been associated with ventricular arrhythmias and torsades de pointes. (See BOX WARNINGS, CONTRAINDICATIONS and PRECAUTIONS sections.)

In European clinical trials involving 350 patients with metastatic prostatic cancer, eleven deaths were reported within two weeks of starting treatment with high doses of ketoconazole tablets (1200 mg/day). It is not possible to ascertain from the information available whether death was related to ketoconazole therapy in these patients with serious underlying disease. However, high doses of ketoconazole tablets are known to suppress adrenal corticosteroid secretion.

In female rats treated three to six months with ketoconazole at dose levels of 80 mg/kg and higher, increased fragility of long bones, in some cases leading to fracture, was seen. The maximum "no-effect" dose level in these studies was 20 mg/kg (2.5 times the maximum recommended human dose). The mechanism responsible for this phenomenon is obscure. Limited studies in dogs failed to demonstrate such an effect on the metacarpals and ribs.

PRECAUTIONS

General: NIZORAL (ketoconazole) Tablets have been demonstrated to lower serum testosterone. Once therapy with NIZORAL has been discontinued, serum testosterone levels return to baseline values. Testosterone levels are impaired with doses of 800 mg per day and abolished by 1600 mg per day. NIZORAL Tablets also decrease ACTH induced corticosteroid serum levels at similar high doses. The recommended dose of 200 mg–400 mg daily should be followed closely.

In four subjects with drug-induced achlorhydria, a marked reduction in ketoconazole absorption was observed. NIZORAL Tablets require acidity for dissolution. If concomitant antacids, anticholinergics, and H_2-blockers are needed, they should be given at least two hours after administration of NIZORAL Tablets. In cases of achlorhydria, the patients should be instructed to dissolve each tablet in 4 mL aqueous solution of 0.2 N HCl. For ingesting the resulting mixture, they should use a drinking straw so as to avoid contact with the teeth. This administration should be followed with a cup of tap water.

Information for Patients: Patients should be instructed to report any signs and symptoms which may suggest liver dysfunction so that appropriate biochemical testing can be done. Such signs and symptoms may include unusual fatigue, anorexia, nausea and/or vomiting, jaundice, dark urine or pale stools (see WARNINGS section).

Drug Interactions: Ketoconazole is a potent inhibitor of the cytochrome P450 3A4 enzyme system. Coadministration of NIZORAL Tablets and drugs primarily metabolized by the cytochrome P450 3A4 enzyme system may result in increased plasma concentrations of the drugs that could increase or prolong both therapeutic and adverse effects. Therefore, unless otherwise specified, appropriate dosage adjustments may be necessary. The following drug interactions have been identified involving NIZORAL Tablets and other drugs metabolized by the cytochrome P450 enzyme system.

Ketoconazole tablets inhibit the metabolism of terfenadine, resulting in an increased plasma concentration of terfenadine and a delay in the elimination of its acid metabolite. The increased plasma concentration of terfenadine or its metabolite may result in prolonged QT intervals. (See BOX WARNING, CONTRAINDICATIONS, and WARNINGS sections.)

Pharmacokinetic data indicate that oral ketoconazole inhibits the metabolism of astemizole, resulting in elevated plasma levels of astemizole and its active metabolite desmethylastemizole which may prolong QT intervals. Coadministration of astemizole with ketoconazole tablets is therefore contraindicated. (See BOX WARNING, CONTRAINDICATIONS, and WARNINGS sections.)

Human pharmacokinetics data indicate that oral ketoconazole potently inhibits the metabolism of cisapride resulting in a mean eight-fold increase in AUC of cisapride. Data suggest that coadministration of oral ketoconazole and PROPULSID can result in prolongation of the QT interval on the ECG. Therefore concomitant administration of ketoconazole tablets with PROPULSID is contraindicated. (See BOX WARNING, CONTRAINDICATIONS and WARNINGS sections.)

Ketoconazole tablets may alter the metabolism of cyclosporine, tacrolimus, and methylprednisolone, resulting in elevated plasma concentrations of the latter drugs. Dosage adjustment may be required if cyclosporine, tacrolimus, methylprednisolone are given concomitantly with NIZORAL Tablets.

Coadministration of NIZORAL Tablets with midazolam or triazolam has resulted in elevated plasma concentrations of the latter two drugs. This may potentiate and prolong hypnotic and sedative effects, especially with repeated dosing or chronic administration of these agents. These agents should not be used in patients treated with NIZORAL Tablets. If midazolam is administered parenterally, special precaution is required since the sedative effect may be prolonged.

Rare cases of elevated plasma concentrations of digoxin have been reported. It is not clear whether this was due to the combination of therapy. It is, therefore, advisable to monitor digoxin concentrations in patients receiving ketoconazole.

When taken orally, imidazole compounds like ketoconazole may enhance the anticoagulant effect of coumarin-like drugs. In simultaneous treatment with imidazole drugs and coumarin drugs, the anticoagulant effect should be carefully titrated and monitored.

Because severe hypoglycemia has been reported in patients concomitantly receiving oral miconazole (an imidazole) and oral hypoglycemic agents, such a potential interaction involving the latter agents when used concomitantly with ketoconazole tablets (an imidazole) can not be ruled out.

Concomitant administration of ketoconazole tablets with phenytoin may alter the metabolism of one or both of the drugs. It is suggested to monitor both ketoconazole and phenytoin.

Concomitant administration of rifampin with ketoconazole tablets reduces the blood levels of the latter. INH (Isoniazid) is also reported to affect ketoconazole concentrations adversely. These drugs should not be given concomitantly.

After the coadministration of 200 mg oral ketoconazole twice daily and one 20 mg dose of loratadine to 11 subjects, the AUC and C_{max} of loratadine averaged 302% (± 142 S.D.) and 251% (± 68 S.D.), respectively, of those obtained after cotreatment with placebo. The AUC and C_{max} of descarboethoxyloratadine, an active metabolite, averaged 155% (± 27 S.D.) and 141% (± 35 S.D.), respectively. However, no related changes were noted in the QT_c on ECG taken at 2, 6, and 24 hours after the coadministration. Also, there were no clincally significant differences in adverse events when loratadine was administered with or without ketoconazole.

Rare cases of disulfiram-like reaction to alcohol have been reported. These experiences have been characterized by flushing, rash, peripheral edema, nausea, and headache. Symptoms resolved within a few hours.

Carcinogenesis, Mutagenesis, Impairment of Fertility: The dominant lethal mutation test in male and female mice revealed that single oral doses of ketoconazole as high as 80 mg/kg produced no mutation in any stage of germ cell development. The *Ames Salmonella* microsomal activator assay was also negative. A long term feeding study in Swiss Albino mice and in Wistar rats showed no evidence of oncogenic activity.

Pregnancy: Teratogenic effects: *Pregnancy Category C:* Ketoconazole has been shown to be teratogenic (syndactylia and oligodactylia) in the rat when given in the diet at 80 mg/kg/day (10 times the maximum recommended human dose). However, these effects may be related to maternal toxicity, evidence of which also was seen at this and higher dose levels.

There are no adequate and well controlled studies in pregnant women. NIZORAL should be used during pregnancy only if the potential benefit justifies the potential risk to the fetus.

Nonteratogenic Effects: Ketoconazole has also been found to be embryotoxic in the rat when given in the diet at doses higher than 80 mg/kg during the first trimester of gestation. In addition, dystocia (difficult labor) was noted in rats administered oral ketoconazole during the third trimester of gestation. This occurred when ketoconazole was administered at doses higher than 10 mg/kg (higher than 1.25 times the maximum human dose).

It is likely that both the malformations and the embryotoxicity resulting from the administration of oral ketoconazole during gestation are a reflection of the particular sensitivity of the female rat to this drug. For example, the oral LD_{50} of ketoconazole given by gavage to the female rat is 166 mg/kg whereas in the male rat the oral LD_{50} is 287 mg/kg.

Nursing Mothers: Since ketoconazole is probably excreted in the milk, mothers who are under treatment should not breast feed.

Pediatric Use: NIZORAL (ketoconazole) Tablets have not been systematically studied in children of any age, and essentially no information is available on children under 2 years. NIZORAL should not be used in pediatric patients unless the potential benefit outweighs the risks.

ADVERSE REACTIONS

In rare cases, anaphylaxis has been reported after the first dose. Several cases of hypersensitivity reactions including urticaria have also been reported. However, the most frequent adverse reactions were nausea and/or vomiting in approximately 3%, abdominal pain in 1.2%, pruritus in 1.5%, and the following in less than 1% of the patients: headache, dizziness, somnolence, fever and chills, photophobia, diarrhea, gynecomastia, impotence, thrombocytopenia, leukopenia, hemolytic anemia, and bulging fontanelles. Oligospermia has been reported in investigational studies with the drug at dosages above those currently approved. Oligospermia has not been reported at dosages up to 400 mg daily, however sperm counts have been obtained infrequently in patients treated with these dosages. Most of these reactions were mild and transient and rarely required discontinuation of NIZORAL (ketoconazole) Tablets. In contrast, the rare occurrences of hepatic dysfunction require special attention (see WARNINGS section).

In worldwide postmarketing experience with NIZORAL Tablets there have been rare reports of alopecia, paresthesia, and signs of increased intracranial pressure including bulging fontanelles and papilledema. Hypertriglyceridemia has also been reported but a causal association with NIZORAL is uncertain.

Neuropsychiatric disturbances, including suicidal tendencies and severe depression, have occurred rarely in patients using NIZORAL Tablets.

Ventricular dysrhythmias (prolonged QT intervals) have occurred with the concomitant use of terfenadine with ketoconazole tablets. (See BOX WARNING, CONTRAINDICATIONS, and WARNINGS sections.) Data suggest that coadministration of ketoconazole tablets and cisapride can result in prolongation of the QT interval and has rarely been associated with ventricular arrhythmias. (See CONTRAINDICATIONS, WARNINGS, and PRECAUTIONS sections.)

OVERDOSAGE

In the event of accidental overdosage, supportive measures, including gastric lavage with sodium bicarbonate, should be employed.

DOSAGE AND ADMINISTRATION

Adults: The recommended starting dose of NIZORAL (ketoconazole) Tablets is a single daily administration of 200 mg (one tablet). In very serious infections or if clinical responsiveness is insufficient within the expected time, the dose of NIZORAL may be increased to 400 mg (two tablets) once daily.

Children: In small numbers of children over 2 years of age, a single daily dose of 3.3 to 6.6 mg/kg has been used. NIZORAL Tablets have not been studied in children under 2 years of age.

There should be laboratory as well as clinical documentation of infection prior to starting ketoconazole therapy. Treatment should be continued until tests indicate that active fungal infection has subsided. Inadequate periods of treatment may yield poor response and lead to early recurrence of clinical symptoms. Minimum treatment for candidiasis is one or two weeks. Patients with chronic mucocutaneous candidiasis usually require maintenance therapy. Minimum treatment for the other indicated systemic mycoses is six months.

Minimum treatment for recalcitrant dermatophyte infections is four weeks in cases involving glabrous skin. Palmar and plantar infections may respond more slowly. Apparent cures may subsequently recur after discontinuation of therapy in some cases.

HOW SUPPLIED

NIZORAL (ketoconazole) is available as white, scored tablets containing 200 mg of ketoconazole debossed "JANSSEN" and on the reverse side debossed "NIZORAL". They are supplied in bottles of 100 tablets (NDC 50458-220-10) and in blister packs of 10 × 10 tablets (NDC 50458-220-01).

Store at controlled room temperature
(59°–77°F/15°–25°C). Protect from moisture
U.S. Patent 4,335,125
Rev. October 1995, November 1995
JANSSEN PHARMACEUTICA
Titusville, NJ 08560-0200

Shown in Product Identification Guide, page 318

PROPULSID® ℞

[prō-pəl ′sid]

(cisapride) Tablets/Suspension

> **Warning:** Serious cardiac arrhythmias including ventricular tachycardia, ventricular fibrillation, torsades de pointes, and QT prolongation have been reported in

patients taking PROPULSID® with other drugs that inhibit cytochrome P450 3A4, such as ketoconazole, itraconazole, miconazole, troleandomycin, erythromycin, fluconazole, and clarithromycin. Some of these events have been fatal. PROPULSID® is contraindicated in patients taking any of these drugs. (See CONTRAINDICATIONS, WARNINGS AND PRECAUTIONS, and DRUG INTERACTIONS).

DESCRIPTION

PROPULSID® (cisapride) Tablets and Suspension contain cisapride as the monohydrate, which is an oral gastrointestinal prokinetic agent chemically designated as (+_)-cis-4-amino-5-chloro-N-[1-[3-(4-fluorophenoxy)propyl]-3-methoxy-4-piperidinyl]-2-methoxybenzamide monohydrate. Its empirical formula is $C_{23}H_{29}ClFN_3O_4 \cdot H_2O$. The molecular weight is 483.97 and the structural formula is:

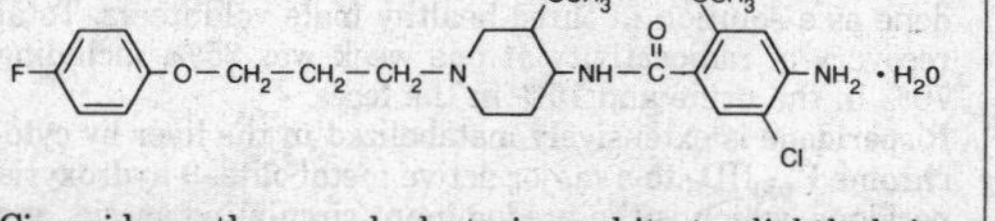

Cisapride as the monohydrate is a white to slightly beige odorless powder. It is practically insoluble in water, sparingly soluble in methanol, and soluble in acetone. Each 1.04 mg of cisapride as the monohydrate is equivalent to one mg of cisapride.

PROPULSID® is available for oral use in tablets containing cisapride as the monohydrate equivalent to 10 mg or 20 mg of cisapride and as a suspension containing 1 mg/mL of cisapride. Inactive ingredients in the tablets are colloidal silicon dioxide, lactose monohydrate, magnesium stearate, microcrystalline cellulose, polysorbate 20, povidone, and starch (corn). The 20 mg tablets also contain FD&C Blue No. 2 aluminum lake. The inactive ingredients in the suspension are hydroxypropyl methylcellulose, methylparaben, microcrystalline cellulose and carboxymethylcellulose sodium, polysorbate 20, propylparaben, sodium chloride, sorbitol, and water. The 1 mg/mL suspension also contains artificial cherry cream flavor and FD&C Red No. 40.

CLINICAL PHARMACOLOGY

Pharmacokinetics

PROPULSID® is rapidly absorbed after oral administration; peak plasma concentrations are reached 1 to 1.5 hours after dosing. The absolute bioavailability of PROPULSID® is 35-40%. When gastric acidity was reduced by high dose histamine H_2 receptor blocker and sodium bicarbonate in fasting subjects, there was a decrease in the rate, and to a lesser degree the extent, of PROPULSID® tablet absorption. (This has not been established for the suspension.) PROPULSID® binds to an extent of 97.5-98% to plasma proteins, mainly to albumin. The volume of distribution of PROPULSID® is about 180 L, indicating extensive tissue distribution.

The plasma clearance of PROPULSID® is about 100 mL/min. The mean terminal half-life reported for PROPULSID® ranges from 6 to 12 hours; longer half-lives, up to 20 hours, have been reported following intravenous (IV) administration. Cisapride is metabolized mainly via the cytochrome P 450 3A4 enzyme. PROPULSID® is extensively metabolized; unchanged drug accounts for less than 10% of urinary and fecal recovery following oral administration. Norcisapride, formed by N-dealkylation, is the principal metabolite in plasma, feces and urine.

There was no unusual drug accumulation due to time-dependent or non-linear changes in PK. After cessation of the repeated dosing, the elimination half-lives (8 to 10 hr) were in the same order as after single dosing. There is some evidence that the degree of accumulation of PROPULSID® and/or its metabolites may be somewhat higher in patients with hepatic or renal impairment and in elderly patients compared to young healthy volunteers, but the differences are not consistent and do not require dosage adjustment.

Pharmacodynamics

The onset of pharmacological action if cisapride is approximately 30 to 60 minutes after oral administration.

The mechanism of action of cisapride is thought to be primarily enhancement of release of acetylcholine at the myenteric plexus. Cisapride does not induce muscarinic or nicotinic receptor stimulation, nor does it inhibit acetylcholinesterase activity. It is less potent than metoclopramide in dopamine receptor-blocking effects in rats. It does not increase or decrease basal or pentagastrin-induced gastric acid secretion.

In vitro studies have shown that cisapride is a serotonin-4 (5-HT_4) receptor agonist. This agonistic action may result in increased gastrointestinal motility and cardiac rate.

Esophagus: Single doses of cisapride (4 to 10 mg IV) increased the lower esophageal sphincter pressure (LESP) and lower esophageal peristalsis compared to placebo and/or metoclopramide. In patients with gastroesophageal reflux disease (GERD) and a LESP of <10 mm Hg, cisapride dose-dependently increased the strength of esophageal peristalsis and more than doubled LESP, raising it to normal values. The increase in LESP was partially reversed by atropine, suggesting that the effect is partly, but not exclusively, cholinergically-mediated. Twenty mg oral cisapride given once to healthy volunteers similarly increased LESP, starting 45 minutes after dosing, with a peak response at 75 minutes. The full duration of the effect was not monitored, and doses smaller than 20 mg were ineffective. Ten mg oral cisapride, administered 3 times daily for several days to patients with GERD, resulted in a significant increase in LESP, and an increased esophageal acid clearance.

Stomach: Cisapride (single 10 mg doses IV or oral or 10 mg given orally 3 times daily up to six weeks) significantly accelerated gastric emptying of both liquids and solids. Acceleration of gastric emptying, measured over a four hour period following a radio-labeled test meal given at lunch time, was greatest when 10 mg cisapride was given both in the morning and again before the test meal, intermediate when 20 mg was given as a single administration in the morning and least when only 10 mg was given on the morning of the test meal. The increases in gastric emptying were proportional to the plasma levels of cisapride measured in these subjects over the same 4 hours that the gastric emptying test was conducted.

Clinical Trials

Clinical trials have shown that cisapride can reduce the symptoms of nocturnal heartburn associated with gastroesophageal reflux disease. Two placebo-controlled studies, one using a dose of 10 mg QID, the other both 10 and 20 mg QID, showed effects on nighttime heartburn, although the 10 mg dose in the second study was only marginally effective. There were no consistent effects on daytime heartburn, symptoms of regurgitation, or histopathology of the esophagus. Use of antacids was only infrequently affected and slightly decreased. In a third controlled trial of similar design to the others, neither 10 mg nor 20 mg taken 4 times was superior to placebo.

These clinical trials did not show a significant effect on LESP, perhaps because the majority of these patients had normal LESP's at the beginning and end of the study period. In a clinical trial comparing 10 mg cisapride to placebo, pH probe evaluation, in a relatively small number of patients, did not reveal a significant difference in pH.

INDICATIONS

PROPULSID® (cisapride) is indicated for the symptomatic treatment of patients with nocturnal heartburn due to gastroesophageal reflux disease.

CONTRAINDICATIONS

Concomitant administration of NIZORAL® (ketoconazole) tablets, SPORANOX® (itraconazole) capsules, MONISTAT i.v.™ (miconazole), fluconazole, erythromycin, clarithromycin, or TAO® (troleandomycin) capsules with PROPULSID® is contraindicated (See WARNINGS and PRECAUTIONS: Drug Interactions).

PROPULSID® (cisapride) should not be used in patients in whom an increase in gastrointestinal motility could be harmful, e.g., in the presence of gastrointestinal hemorrhage, mechanical obstruction, or perforation. PROPULSID® is contraindicated in patients with known sensitivity or intolerance to the drug.

WARNINGS

PROPULSID® undergoes metabolism mainly by the hepatic cytochrome P450 3A4 isoenzyme. Drugs which inhibit this enzyme such as ketoconazole, itraconazole, miconazole, clarithromycin, erythromycin, fluconazole, or troleandomycin can lead to elevated cisapride blood levels.

Rare cases of serious cardiac arrhythmias, including ventricular arrhythmias and torsades de pointes associated with QT prolongation, have been reported in patients taking cisapride with ketoconazole, itraconazole, miconazole, erythromycin, clarithromycin, or fluconazole. Some of these patients did not have known cardiac histories; however, most had been receiving multiple other medications, and had preexisting cardiac disease or risk factors for arrhythmias. Some of these cases have been fatal.

PRECAUTIONS

General: Potential benefits should be weighed against risks prior to administration of cisapride to patients with conditions associated with QT prolongation, such as congenital prolonged QT syndrome, uncorrected electrolyte disturbances or in patients who are taking other medications known to prolong QT interval.

Information for Patients: Patients should be warned against concomitant use of oral ketoconazole, itraconazole, miconazole, erythromycin, clarithromycin, fluconazole, or troleandomycin with PROPULSID®.

Although PROPULSID® (cisapride) does not affect psycomotor function nor does it induce sedation or drowsiness when used alone, patients should be advised that the sedative effects of benzodiazepines and of alcohol may be accelerated by PROPULSID®.

Drug Interactions: Cisapride is metabolized mainly via the cytochrome P450 3A4 enzyme. Human pharmacokinetic data indicate that oral ketoconazole potently inhibits the metabolism of cisapride, resulting in a mean eight-fold increase in AUC of cisapride. A study in 14 normal male and female volunteers suggest that coadministration of PROPULSID® and ketoconazole can result in prolongation of the QT interval on the ECG.

In vitro data indicate that itraconazole, miconazole, fluconazole, erythromycin, clarithromycin, and troleandomycin also markedly inhibit cytochrome P450 3A4 mainly responsible for the metabolism of cisapride.

In some cases where serious ventricular arrhythmias, QT prolongation, and torsades de pointes have occurred when cisapride was taken in conjunction with one of the cytochrome P450 3A4 inhibitors, elevated blood cisapride levels were noted at the time of the QT prolongation. Normalization of the QT interval after cisapride was discontinued has been observed.

Concurrent administration of anticholinergic compounds would be expected to compromise the beneficial effects of PROPULSID®.

The acceleration of gastric emptying by PROPULSID® could affect the rate of absorption of other drugs. Patients receiving narrow therapeutic ratio drugs or other drugs that require careful titration should be followed closely; if plasma levels are being monitored, they should be reassessed.

In patients receiving oral anticoagulants, the coagulation times were increased in some cases. It is advisable to check coagulation time within the first few days after the start and discontinuation of PROPULSID® therapy, with an appropriate adjustment of the anticoagulant dose, if necessary.

Cimetidine coadministration leads to an increased peak plasma concentration and AUC of PROPULSID®; there is no effect on PROPULSID® absorption when it is coadministered with ranitidine. The gastrointestinal absorption of cimetidine and ranitidine is accelerated when they are coadministered with PROPULSID®.

Carcinogenesis, mutagenesis, impairment of fertility: In a twenty-five month oral carcinogenicity study in rats, cisapride at daily doses up to 80 mg/kg was not tumorigenic. For a 50 kg person of average height (1.46 m^2 body surface area), this dose represents 50 times the maximum recommended human dose (1.6 mg/kg/day) on a mg/kg basis and 7 times the maximum recommended human dose (54.4 mg/m^2) on a body surface area basis. In a nineteen month oral carcinogenicity study in mice, cisapride at daily doses up to 80 mg/kg was not tumorigenic. This dose represents 50 times the maximum recommended human dose on a mg/kg basis and about 4 times the maximum recommended human dose on a body surface area basis.

Cisapride was not mutagenic in the *in vitro* Ames test, human lymphocyte chromosomal aberration test, mouse lymphoma cell forward mutation test, and rat hepatocyte UDS test and *in vitro* rat micronucleus test, male and female mouse dominant lethal mutations tests, and sex linked recessive lethal test in male *Drosophila melanogaster.*

Fertility and reproductive performance studies were conducted in male and female rats. Cisapride was found to have no effect on fertility and reproductive performance of male rats at oral doses up to 160 mg/kg/day (100 times the maximum recommended human dose on a mg/kg basis and 14 times the maximum recommended human dose on a mg/m^2 basis). In the female rats, cisapride at oral doses of 40 mg/kg/day and higher prolonged the breeding interval required for impregnation. Similar effects were also observed at maturity in the female offspring (F_1) of the female rats (F_0) treated with oral doses of cisapride at 10 mg/kg/day or higher. Cisapride at an oral dose of 160 mg/kg/day also exerted contragestational/pregnancy disrupting effects in female rats (F_0).

Pregnancy: Teratogenic effects: Pregnancy category C: Oral teratology studies have been conducted in rats (doses up to 160 mg/kg/day) and rabbits (doses up to 40 mg/kg/day). There was no evidence of a teratogenic potential of cisapride in rats or rabbits. Cisapride was embryotoxic and fetotoxic in rats at a dose of 160 mg/kg/day (100 times the maximum recommended human dose on a mg/kg basis and 14 times the maximum recommended human dose on a mg/m^2 basis) and in rabbits at a dose of 20 mg/kg/day (approximately 12 times the maximum recommended human dose on a mg/kg basis) or higher. It also produced reduced birth weights of pups in rats at 40 and 160 mg/kg/day and adversely affected the pup survival. There are no adequate and well-controlled studies in pregnant women. Cisapride should be used during pregnancy only if the potential benefit justifies the potential risk to the fetus.

Nursing Mothers: Cisapride is excreted in human milk at concentrations approximately one twentieth of those observed in plasma. Caution should be exercised when PROPULSID® is administered to a nursing woman, and particular care must be taken if the nursing infant or the mother is taking a drug that might alter PROPULSID®'s metabolism in the infant. (See CONTRAINDICATIONS, WARNINGS, PRECAUTIONS, AND DRUG INTERACTIONS).

Continued on next page

Janssen Pharmaceutica—Cont.

Pediatric Use: Safety and effectiveness in children have not been established.
Geriatric Use: Steady-state plasma levels are generally higher in older than in younger patients, due to a moderate prolongation of the elimination half-life. Therapeutic doses, however, are similar to those used in younger adults.
The rate of adverse experiences in patients greater than 65 years of age was similar to that in younger adults.

ADVERSE REACTIONS

In the U.S. clinical trial population of 1728 patients (comprising 506 with gastroesophageal reflux disorders, and the remainder with other motility disorders) the following adverse experiences were reported in more than 1% of patients treated with PROPULSID® (cisapride) and at least as often on PROPULSID® as on placebo. The percent of patients who discontinued treatment is displayed in parenthesis.

System/Adverse Event	PROPULSID® N=1042	Placebo N=686
Central & Peripheral Nervous Systems		
Headache	19.3% (1.1%)	17.1% (0.4%)
Gastrointestinal		
Diarrhea	14.2 (0.7)	10.3 (0.1)
Abdominal pain	10.2 (1.2)	7.7 (0.9)
Nausea	7.6 (1.0)	7.6 (0.3)
Constipation	6.7 (0.1)	3.4 (0.0)
Flatulence	3.5 (0.4)	3.1 (0.4)
Dyspepsia	2.7 (0.1)	1.0 (0.0)
Respiratory System		
Rhinitis	7.3 (0.1)	5.7 (0.1)
Sinusitis	3.6 (0.0)	3.5 (0.0)
Coughing	1.5 (0.2)	1.2 (0.0)
Resistance Mechanism		
Viral infection	3.6 (0.2)	3.2 (0.0)
Upper respiratory tract infection	3.1 (0.0)	2.8 (0.0)
Body as a Whole		
Pain	3.4 (0.0)	2.3 (0.0)
Fever	2.2 (0.1)	1.5 (0.0)
Urinary System		
Urinary tract infection	2.4 (0.0)	1.9 (0.0)
Micturition frequency	1.2 (0.1)	0.6 (0.0)
Psychiatric		
Insomnia	1.9 (0.3)	1.3 (0.4)
Anxiety	1.4 (0.1)	1.0 (0.1)
Nervousness	1.4 (0.2)	0.7 (0.0)
Skin & Appendages		
Rash	1.6 (0.0)	1.6 (0.3)
Pruritus	1.2 (0.1)	1.0 (0.0)
Musculoskeletal System		
Arthralgia	1.4 (0.1)	1.2 (0.0)
Vision		
Abnormal vision	1.4 (0.2)	0.3 (0.0)
Reproductive, Female		
Vaginitis	1.2 (0.0)	0.9 (0.0)

The following adverse events also reported in more than 1% of PROPULSID® patients were more frequently reported on placebo: dizziness, vomiting, pharyngitis, chest pain, fatigue, back pain, depression, dehydration, and myalgia.
Diarrhea, abdominal pain, constipation, flatulence, and rhinitis all occurred more frequently in patients using 20 mg of PROPULSID® than in patients using 10 mg.
Additional adverse experiences reported to occur in 1% or less of patients in the U.S. clinical studies are: dry mouth, somnolence, palpitation, migraine, tremor, and edema.
In other U.S. and international trials and in foreign marketing experience, there have been rare reports of seizures and extrapyramidal effects, tachycardia, elevated liver enzymes, hepatitis, thrombocytopenia, leukopenia, aplastic anemia, pancytopenia, and granulocytopenia. The relationship of PROPULSID® to the event was not clear in these cases.
There have been rare cases of sinus tachycardia reported. Rechallenge precipitated relapse in some of those patients.
Rare cases of cardiac arrhythmias, including ventricular tachycardia, ventricular fibrillation, torsades de pointes, and QT prolongation, in some cases resulting in death, have been reported. Most of these patients had been receiving multiple other medications and had pre-existing cardiac disease or risk factors for arrhythmias. A causal relationship to PROPULSID® has not been established.

OVERDOSAGE

Reports of overdosage with PROPULSID® (cisapride) include an adult who took 540 mg and for 2 hours experienced retching, borborygmi, flatulence, stool frequency and urinary frequency. A one-month-old male infant received 2 mg/kg of cisapride, 10 times the prescribed dose, four times per day for 5 days. The patient developed third degree heart block and subsequently died of right ventricular perforation caused by pacemaker wire insertion.
Treatment should include gastric lavage and/or activated charcoal, close observation and general supportive measures.
In instances of overdose, patients should be evaluated for possible QT prolongation and for factors that can predispose to the occurrence of ventricular arrhythmias, including torsades de pointes.
Single oral doses of cisapride at 4000 mg/kg, 160 mg/kg, 1280 mg/kg and 640 mg/kg were lethal in adult rats, neonatal rats, mice, and dogs, respectively. Symptoms of acute toxicity were ptosis, tremors, convulsions, dyspnea, loss of righting reflex, catalepsy, catatonia, hypotonia and diarrhea.

DOSAGE AND ADMINISTRATION

5 mL (1 teaspoon) suspension = 5 mg.
Adults: Initiate therapy with one 10 mg tablet of PROPULSID® (cisapride) or 10 mL of the suspension 4 times daily at least 15 minutes before meals and at bedtime. In some patients the dosage will need to be increased to 20 mg, given as above, to obtain a satisfactory result.
In elderly patients, steady-state plasma levels are generally higher due to a moderate prolongation of the elimination half-life. Therapeutic doses, however, are similar to those used in younger adults.

HOW SUPPLIED

PROPULSID® tablets are provided as scored white tablets debossed "Janssen" and P/10 containing the equivalent of 10 mg of cisapride in blister packages of 100 (NDC 50458-430-01) and in bottles of 100 (NDC 50458-430-10) and 500 (NDC 50458-430-50).
PROPULSID® is also provided as blue tablets, debossed "Janssen" and P/20, containing the equivalent of 20 mg cisapride in blister packages of 100 (NDC 50458-440-01) and in bottles of 100 (NDC 50458-440-10) and bottles of 250 (NDC 50458-440-25).
PROPULSID® Suspension is provided as a bright pink homogeneous suspension containing 1 mg/mL of cisapride in 16 oz. bottles containing 450 mL (NDC 50458-450-45).
Store at 15°-25°C (59°-77°F). Protect the tablets from moisture. The 20 mg tablets should also be protected from light.

JANSSEN
PHARMACEUTICA
Titusville, NJ 08560
Revised August 1994, September 1995, February 1996
U.S. Patent No. 4,962,115

Shown in Product Identification Guide, page 318

RISPERDAL® ℞

[ris 'pər dăl]
(risperidone) Tablets

DESCRIPTION

RISPERDAL® (risperidone) is an antipsychotic agent belonging to a new chemical class, the benzisoxazole derivatives. The chemical designation is 3-[2-[4-(6-fluoro-1,2-benzisoxazol-3-yl)-1-piperidinyl]ethyl]-6,7,8,9-tetrahydro-2-methyl-4*H*-pyrido[1,2-a]pyrimidin-4-one. Its molecular formula is $C_{23}H_{27}FN_4O_2$ and its molecular weight is 410.49. The structural formula is:

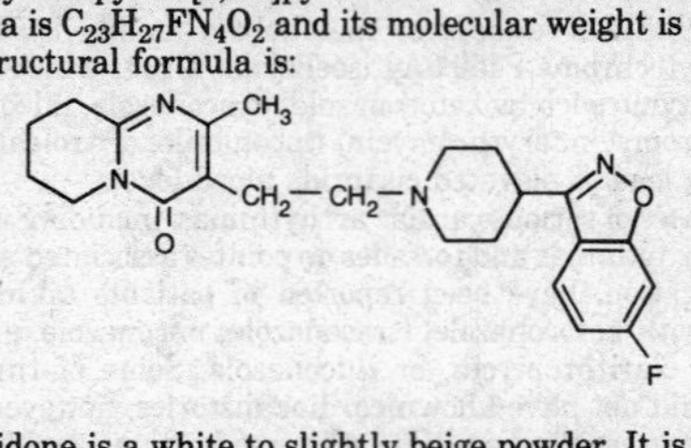

Risperidone is a white to slightly beige powder. It is practically insoluble in water, freely soluble in methylene chloride, and soluble in methanol and 0.1 N HCl.
RISPERDAL® for oral use is available in tablets of 1 mg (white, scored), 2 mg (orange), 3 mg (yellow), and 4 mg (green). Inactive ingredients are colloidal silicon dioxide, hydroxypropyl methylcellulose, lactose, magnesium stearate, microcrystalline cellulose, propylene glycol, sodium lauryl sulfate, and starch (corn). Tablets of 2, 3, and 4 mg also contain talc and titanium dioxide. The 2 mg tablets contain FD&C Yellow No. 6 Aluminum Lake; the 3 mg and 4 mg tablets contain D&C Yellow No. 10; the 4 mg tablets contain FD&C Blue No. 2 Aluminum Lake.
RISPERDAL is also available as a 1 mg/mL oral solution. The inactive ingredients for this solution are; tartaric acid, benzoic acid, sodium hydroxide and purified water (formulation F68).

CLINICAL PHARMACOLOGY

Pharmacodynamics
The mechanism of action of RISPERDAL® (risperidone), as with other antipsychotic drugs, is unknown. However, it has been proposed that this drug's antipsychotic activity is mediated through a combination of dopamine type 2 (D_2) and serotonin type 2 ($5HT_2$) antagonism. Antagonism at receptors other than D_2 and $5HT_2$ may explain some of the other effects of RISPERDAL®.
RISPERDAL® is a selective monoaminergic antagonist with high affinity (Ki of 0.12 to 7.3 nM) for the serotonin type 2 ($5HT_2$), dopamine type 2 (D_2), α_1 and α_2 adrenergic, and H_1 histaminergic receptors. RISPERDAL® antagonizes other receptors, but with lower potency. RISPERDAL® has low to moderate affinity (Ki of 47 to 253 nM) for the serotonin $5HT_{1C}$, $5HT_{1D}$, and $5HT_{1A}$ receptors, weak affinity (Ki of 620 to 800 nM) for the dopamine D_1 and haloperidol-sensitive sigma site, and no affinity (when tested at concentrations $> 10^{-5}$ M) for cholinergic muscarinic or β_1 and β_2 adrenergic receptors.

Pharmacokinetics
Risperidone is well absorbed, as illustrated by a mass balance study involving a single 1 mg oral dose of ^{14}C-risperidone as a solution in three healthy male volunteers. Total recovery of radioactivity at one week was 85%, including 70% in the urine and 15% in the feces.
Risperidone is extensively metabolized in the liver by cytochrome $P_{450}IID_6$ to a major active metabolite, 9-hydroxyrisperidone, which is the predominant circulating specie, and appears approximately equi-effective with risperidone with respect to receptor binding activity and some effects in animals. (A second minor pathway is *N*-dealkylation). Consequently, the clinical effect of the drug likely results from the combined concentrations of risperidone plus 9-hyydroxyrisperidone are dose proportional over the dosing range of 1 to 16 mg daily (0.5 to 8 mg BID). The relative oral bioavailability of risperidone from a tablet was 94% (CV=10%) when compared to a solution. Food does not affect either the rate or extent of absorption of risperidone. Thus, risperidone can be given with or without meals. The absolute oral bioavailability of risperidone was 70% (CV=25%).
The enzyme catalyzing hydroxylation of risperidone to 9-hydroxyrisperidone is cytochrome $P_{450}IID_6$, also called debrisoquin hydroxylase, the enzyme responsible for metabolism of many neuroleptics, antidepressants, antiarrhythmics, and other drugs. Cytochrome $P_{450}IID_6$ is subject to genetic polymorphism (about 6-8% of caucasians, and a very low percent of Asians have little or no activity and are "poor metabolizers") and to inhibition by a variety of substrates and some non-substrates, notably quinidine. Extensive metabolizers convert risperidone rapidly into 9-hydroxyrisperidone, while poor metabolizers convert it much more slowly. Extensive metabolizers, therefore, have lower risperidone and higher 9-hydroxyrisperidone concentrations than poor metabolizers. Following oral administration of solution or tablet, mean peak plasma concentrations occurred at about 1 hour. Peak 9-hydroxyrisperidone occurred at about 3 hours in extensive metabolizers, and 17 hours in poor metabolizers. The apparent half-life of risperidone was three hours (CV=30%) in extensive metabolizers and 20 hours (CV=40%) in poor metabolizers. The apparent half-life of 9-hydroxyrisperidone was about 21 hours (CV=20%) in extensive metabolizers and 30 hours (CV=25%) in poor metabolizers. Steady-state concentrations of risperidone are reached in 1 day in extensive metabolizers and would be expected to reach steady state in about 5 days in poor metabolizers. Steady-state concentrations of 9-hydroxyrisperidone are reached in 5-6 days (measured in extensive metabolizers). Because risperidone and 9-hydroxyrisperidone are approximately equi-effective, the sum of their concentrations is pertinent. The pharmacokinetics of the sum of risperidone and 9-hydroxyrisperidone, after single and multiple doses, were similar in extensive and poor metabolizers, with an overall mean elimination half-life of about 20 hours. In analyses comparing adverse reaction rates in extensive and poor metabolizers in controlled and open studies, no important differences were seen.
Risperidone could be subject to two kinds of drug-drug interactions. First, inhibitors of cytochrome $P_{450}IID_6$ could interfere with conversion of risperidone to 9-hydroxyrisperidone. This in fact occurs with quinidine, giving essentially all recipients a risperidone pharmacokinetic profile typical of poor metabolizers. The favorable and adverse effects of risperidone in patients receiving quinidine have not been evaluated, but observations in a modest number (n is approximately equal to 70) of poor metabolizers given risperidone do not suggest important differences between poor and extensive metabolizers. It would also be possible for risperidone to interfere with metabolism of other drugs metabolized by cytochrome $P_{450}IID_6$. Relatively weak binding of risperidone to the enzyme suggests this is unlikely (See PRECAUTIONS and DRUG INTERACTIONS).
The plasma protein binding of risperidone was about 90% over the in vitro concentration range of 0.5 to 200 ng/mL and increased with increasing concentrations of α_1-acid glycoprotein. The plasma binding of 9-hydroxyrisperidone was 77%. Neither the parent nor the metabolite displaced each other from the plasma binding sites. High therapeutic concentrations of sulfamethazine (100 μg/mL), warfarin (10 μg/mL) and carbamazepine (10 μg/mL) caused only a slight increase

in the free fraction of risperidone at 10 ng/mL and 9-hydroxyrisperidone at 50 ng/mL, changes of unknown clinical significance.

Special Populations

Renal Impairment: In patients with moderate to severe renal disease, clearance of the sum of risperidone and its active metabolite decreased by 60% compared to young healthy subjects. RISPERDAL® doses should be reduced in patients with renal disease (See PRECAUTIONS and DOSAGE AND ADMINISTRATION).

Hepatic Impairment: While the pharmacokinetics of risperidone in subjects with liver disease were comparable to those in young healthy subjects, the mean free fraction of risperidone in plasma was increased by about 35% because of the diminished concentration of both albumin and α_1-acid glycoprotein. RISPERDAL® doses should be reduced in patients with liver disease (See PRECAUTIONS and DOSAGE AND ADMINISTRATION).

Elderly: In healthy elderly subjects renal clearance of both risperidone and 9-hydroxyrisperidone was decreased, and elimination half-lives were prolonged compared to young healthy subjects. Dosing should be modified accordingly in the elderly patients (See DOSAGE AND ADMINISTRATION).

Race and Gender Effects: No specific pharmacokinetic study was conducted to investigate race and gender effects, but a population pharmacokinetic analysis did not identify important differences in the disposition of risperidone due to gender (whether corrected for body weight or not) or race.

Clinical Trials

The efficacy of RISPERDAL® in the management of the manifestations of psychotic disorders was established in three short-term (6- to 8-week) controlled trials of psychotic inpatients who met DSM III-R criteria for schizophrenia. Several instruments were used for assessing psychiatric signs and symptoms in these studies, among them the Brief Psychiatric Rating Scale (BPRS), a multi-item inventory of general psychopathology traditionally used to evaluate the effects of drug treatment in psychosis. The BPRS psychosis cluster (conceptual disorganization, hallucinatory behavior, suspiciousness, and unusual thought content) is considered a particularly useful subset for assessing actively psychotic schizophrenic patients. A second traditional assessment, the Clinical Global Impression (CGI), reflects the impression of a skilled observer, fully familiar with the manifestations of schizophrenia, about the overall clinical state of the patient. In addition, two more recently developed, but less well evaluated scales, were employed; these included the Positive and Negative Syndrome Scale (PANSS) and the Scale for Assessing Negative Symptoms (SANS). The results of the trials follow:

(1) In a 6-week, placebo-controlled trial (n=160) involving titration of RISPERDAL® in doses up to 10 mg/day (BID schedule), RISPERDAL® was generally superior to placebo on the BPRS total score, on the BPRS psychosis cluster, and marginally superior to placebo on the SANS.

(2) In an 8-week, placebo-controlled trial (n=513) involving 4 fixed doses of RISPERDAL® (2, 6, 10, and 16 mg/day, on a BID schedule), all 4 RISPERDAL® groups were generally superior to placebo on the BPRS total score, BPRS psychosis cluster, and CGI severity score; the 3 highest RISPERDAL® dose groups were generally superior to placebo on the PANSS negative subscale. The most consistently positive responses on all measures were seen for the 6 mg dose group, and there was no suggestion of increased benefit from larger doses.

(3) In an 8-week, dose comparison trial (n=1356) involving 5 fixed doses of RISPERDAL® (1, 4, 8, 12, and 16 mg/day, on a BID schedule), the four highest RISPERDAL® dose groups were generally superior to the 1 mg RISPERDAL® dose group on BPRS total score, BPRS psychosis cluster, and CGI severity score. None of the dose groups were superior to the 1 mg group on the PANSS negative subscale. The most consistently positive responses were seen for the 4 mg dose group.

INDICATIONS AND USAGE

RISPERDAL® (risperidone) is indicated for the management of the manifestations of psychotic disorders.

The antipsychotic efficacy of RISPERDAL® was established in short-term (6 to 8 weeks) controlled trials of schizophrenic inpatients (See CLINICAL PHARMACOLOGY).

The effectiveness of RISPERDAL® in long-term use, that is, more than 6 to 8 weeks, has not been systematically evaluated in controlled trials. Therefore, the physician who elects to use RISPERDAL® for extended periods should periodically re-evaluate the long-term usefulness of the drug for the individual patient. (See DOSAGE AND ADMINISTRATION).

CONTRAINDICATIONS

RISPERDAL® (risperidone) is contraindicated in patients with a known hypersensitivity to the product.

WARNINGS

Neuroleptic Malignant Syndrome (NMS)

A potentially fatal symptom complex sometimes referred to as Neuroleptic Malignant Syndrome (NMS) has been reported in association with antipsychotic drugs. Clinical manifestations of NMS are hyperpyrexia, muscle rigidity, altered mental status and evidence of autonomic instability (irregular pulse or blood pressure, tachycardia, diaphoresis and cardiac dysrhythmia). Additional signs may include elevated creatine phosphokinase, myoglobinuria (rhabdomyolysis), and acute renal failure.

The diagnostic evaluation of patients with this syndrome is complicated. In arriving at a diagnosis, it is important to identify cases where the clinical presentation includes both serious medical illness (e.g., pneumonia, systemic infection, etc.) and untreated or inadequately treated extrapyramidal signs and symptoms (EPS). Other important considerations in the differential diagnosis include central anticholinergic toxicity, heat stroke, drug fever, and primary central nervous system pathology.

The management of NMS should include: 1) immediate discontinuation of antipsychotic drugs and other drugs not essential to concurrent therapy; 2) intensive symptomatic treatment and medical monitoring; and 3) treatment of any concomitant serious medical problems for which specific treatments are available. There is no general agreement about specific pharmacological treatment regimens for uncomplicated NMS.

If a patient requires antipsychotic drug treatment after recovery from NMS, the potential reintroduction of drug therapy should be carefully considered. The patient should be carefully monitored, since recurrences of NMS have been reported.

Tardive Dyskinesia

A syndrome of potentially irreversible, involuntary, dyskinetic movements may develop in patients treated with antipsychotic drugs. Although the prevalence of the syndrome appears to be highest among the elderly, especially elderly women, it is impossible to rely upon prevalence estimates to predict, at the inception of antipsychotic treatment, which patients are likely to develop the syndrome. Whether antipsychotic drug products differ in their potential to cause tardive dyskinesia is unknown.

The risk of developing tardive dyskinesia and the likelihood that it will become irreversible are believed to increase as the duration of treatment and the total cumulative dose of antipsychotic drugs administered to the patient increase. However, the syndrome can develop, although much less commonly, after relatively brief treatment periods at low doses.

There is no known treatment for established cases of tardive dyskinesia, although the syndrome may remit, partially or completely, if antipsychotic treatment is withdrawn. Antipsychotic treatment, itself, however, may suppress (or partially suppress) the signs and symptoms of the syndrome and thereby may possibly mask the underlying process. The effect that symptomatic suppression has upon the long-term course of the syndrome is unknown.

Given these considerations, RISPERDAL® (risperidone) should be prescribed in a manner that is most likely to minimize the occurrence of tardive dyskinesia. Chronic antipsychotic treatment should generally be reserved for patients who suffer from a chronic illness that (1) is known to respond to antipsychotic drugs, and (2) for whom alternative, equally effective, but potentially less harmful treatments are not available or appropriate. In patients who do require chronic treatment, the smallest dose and the shortest duration of treatment producing a satisfactory clinical response should be sought. The need for continued treatment should be reassessed periodically.

If signs and symptoms of tardive dyskinesia appear in a patient on RISPERDAL®, drug discontinuation should be considered. However, some patients may require treatment with RISPERDAL® despite the presence of the syndrome.

Potential for Proarrhythmic Effects: Risperidone and/or 9-hydroxyrisperidone appears to lengthen the QT interval in some patients, although there is no average increase in treated patients, even at 12–16 mg/day, well above the recommended dose. Other drugs that prolong the QT interval have been associated with the occurrence of torsades de pointes, a life-threatening arrhythmia. Bradycardia, electrolyte imbalance, concomitant use with other drugs that prolong QT, or the presence of congenital prolongation in QT can increase the risk for occurrence of this arrhythmia.

PRECAUTIONS

General

Orthostatic Hypotension: RISPERDAL® (risperidone) may induce orthostatic hypotension associated with dizziness, tachycardia, and in some patients, syncope, especially during the initial dose-titration period, probably reflecting its alpha-adrenergic antagonistic properties. Syncope was reported in 0.2% (6/2607) of RISPERDAL® treated patients in phase 2–3 studies. The risk of orthostatic hypotension and syncope may be minimized by limiting the initial dose to 1 mg BID in normal adults and 0.5 mg BID in the elderly and patients with renal or hepatic impairment (See DOSAGE AND ADMINISTRATION). A dose reduction should be considered if hypotension occurs. RISPERDAL® should be used with particular caution in patients with known

cardiovascular disease (history of myocardial infarction or ischemia, heart failure, or conduction abnormalities), cerebrovascular disease, and conditions which would predispose patients to hypotension e.g., (dehydration and hypovolemia. Clinically significant hypotension has been observed with concomitant use of RISPERDAL® and antihypertensive medication.

Seizures: During premarketing testing, seizures occurred in 0.3% (9/2607) of RISPERDAL® treated patients, two in association with hyponatremia. RISPERDAL® should be used cautiously in patients with a history of seizures.

Hyperprolactinemia: As with other drugs that antagonize dopamine D_2 receptors, risperidone elevates prolactin levels and the elevation persists during chronic administration. Tissue culture experiments indicate that approximately one-third of human breast cancers are prolactin dependent in vitro, a factor of potential importance if the prescription of these drugs is contemplated in a patient with previously detected breast cancer. Although disturbances such as galactorrhea, amenorrhea, gynecomastia, and impotence have been reported with prolactin-elevating compounds, the clinical significance of elevated serum prolactin levels is unknown for most patients. As is common with compounds which increase prolactin release, an increase in pituitary gland, mammary gland, and pancreatic islet cell hyperplasia and/or neoplasia was observed in the risperidone carcinogenicity studies conducted in mice and rats (See CARCINOGENESIS). However, neither clinical studies nor epidemiologic studies conducted to date have shown an association between chronic administration of this class of drugs and tumorigenesis in humans; the available evidence is considered too limited to be conclusive at this time.

Potential for Cognitive and Motor Impairment: Somnolence was a commonly reported adverse event associated with RISPERDAL® treatment, especially when ascertained by direct questioning of patients. This adverse event is dose related, and in a study utilizing a checklist to detect adverse events, 41% of the high dose patients (RISPERDAL® 16 mg/day) reported somnolence compared to 16% of placebo patients. Direct questioning is more sensitive for detecting adverse events than spontaneous reporting, by which 8% of RISPERDAL® 16 mg/day patients and 1% of placebo patients reported somnolence as an adverse event. Since RISPERDAL® has the potential to impair judgment, thinking, or motor skills, patients should be cautioned about operating hazardous machinery, including automobiles, until they are reasonably certain that RISPERDAL® therapy does not affect them adversely.

Priapism: Rare cases of priapism have been reported. While the relationship of the events to RISPERDAL® use has not been established, other drugs with alpha-adrenergic blocking effects have been reported to induce priapism, and it is possible that RISPERDAL® may share this capacity. Severe priapism may require surgical intervention.

Thrombotic Thrombocytopenic Purpura (TTP): A single case of TTP was reported in a 28 year-old female patient receiving RISPERDAL® in a large, open premarketing experience (approximately 1300 patients). She experienced jaundice, fever, and bruising, but eventually recovered after receiving plasmapheresis. The relationship to RISPERDAL® therapy is unknown.

Antiemetic effect: Risperidone has an antiemetic effect in animals; this effect may also occur in humans, and may mask signs and symptoms of overdosage with certain drugs or of conditions such as intestinal obstruction, Reye's syndrome, and brain tumor.

Body Temperature Regulation: Disruption of body temperature regulation has been attributed to other antipsychotic agents. Caution is advised when prescribing for patients who will be exposed to temperature extremes.

Suicide: The possibility of a suicide attempt is inherent in schizophrenia, and close supervision of high risk patients should accompany drug therapy. Prescriptions for RISPERDAL® should be written for the smallest quantity of tablets consistent with good patient management, in order to reduce the risk of overdose.

Use in Patients with Concomitant Illness: Clinical experience with RISPERDAL® in patients with certain concomitant systemic illnesses is limited. Caution is advisable in using RISPERDAL® in patients with diseases or conditions that could affect metabolism or hemodynamic responses. RISPERDAL® has not been evaluated or used to any appreciable extent in patients with a recent history of myocardial infarction or unstable heart disease. Patients with these diagnoses were excluded from clinical studies during the product's premarket testing. The electrocardiograms of approximately 380 patients who received RISPERDAL® and 120 patients who received placebo in two double-blind, placebo-controlled trials were evaluated and the data revealed one finding of potential concern, i.e., 8 patients taking RISPERDAL® whose baseline QTc interval was less than 450 msec were observed to have QTc intervals greater than 450 msec during treatment; no such prolongations were seen

Continued on next page

Janssen Pharmaceutica—Cont.

in the smaller placebo group. There were 3 such episodes in the approximately 125 patients who received haloperidol. Because of the risks of orthostatic hypotension and QT prolongation, caution should be observed in cardiac patients (See WARNINGS AND PRECAUTIONS).

Increased plasma concentrations of risperidone and 9-hydroxyrisperidone occur in patients with severe renal impairment (creatinine clearance < 30 mL/min/1.73 m²), and an increase in the free fraction of the risperidone is seen in patients with severe hepatic impairment. A lower starting dose should be used in such patients (See DOSAGE AND ADMINISTRATION).

Information for Patients

Physicians are advised to discuss the following issues with patients for whom they prescribe RISPERDAL®:

Orthostatic Hypotension: Patients should be advised of the risk of orthostatic hypotension, especially during the period of initial dose titration.

Interference With Cognitive and Motor Performance: Since RISPERDAL® has the potential to impair judgment, thinking, or motor skills, patients should be cautioned about operating hazardous machinery, including automobiles, until they are reasonably certain that RISPERDAL® therapy does not affect them adversely.

Pregnancy: Patients should be advised to notify their physician if they become pregnant or intend to become pregnant during therapy.

Nursing: Patients should be advised not to breast feed an infant if they are taking RISPERDAL®.

Concomitant Medication: Patients should be advised to inform their physicians if they are taking, or plan to take, any prescription or over-the-counter drugs, since there is a potential for interactions.

Alcohol: Patients should be advised to avoid alcohol while taking RISPERDAL®.

Laboratory Tests

No specific laboratory tests are recommended.

Drug Interactions

The interactions of RISPERDAL® and other drugs have not been systematically evaluated. Given the primary CNS effects of risperidone, caution should be used when RISPERDAL® is taken in combination with other centrally acting drugs and alcohol.

Because of its potential for inducing hypotension, RISPERDAL® may enhance the hypotensive effects of other therapeutic agents with this potential.

RISPERDAL® may antagonize the effects of levodopa and dopamine agonists.

Chronic administration of carbamazepine with risperidone may increase the clearance of risperidone.

Chronic administration of clozapine with risperidone may decrease the clearance of risperidone.

Drugs that Inhibit Cytochrome $P_{450}IID_6$ and Other P_{450} Isozymes: Risperidone is metabolized to 9-hydroxyrisperidone by cytochrome $P_{450}IID_6$, an enzyme that is polymorphic in the population and that can be inhibited by a variety of psychotropic and other drugs (See CLINICAL PHARMACOLOGY). Drug interactions that reduce the metabolism of risperidone to 9-hydroxyrisperidone would increase the plasma concentrations of risperidone and lower the concentrations of 9-hydroxyrisperidone. Analysis of clinical studies involving a modest number of poor metabolizers (n is approximately equal to 70) does not suggest that poor and extensive metabolizers have different rates of adverse effects. No comparison of effectiveness in the two groups has been made. In vitro studies showed that drugs metabolized by other P_{450} isozymes, including 1A1, 1A2, IIC9, MP, and IIIA4, are only weak inhibitors of risperidone metabolism.

Drugs Metabolized by Cytochrome $P_{450}IID_6$: In vitro studies indicate that risperidone is a relatively weak inhibitor of cytochrome $P_{450}IID_6$. Therefore, RISPERDAL® is not expected to substantially inhibit the clearance of drugs that are metabolized by this enzymatic pathway. However, clinical data to confirm this expectation are not available.

Carcinogenesis, Mutagenesis, Impairment of Fertility

Carcinogenesis: Carcinogenicity studies were conducted in Swiss albino mice and Wistar rats. Risperidone was administered in the diet at doses of 0.63, 2.5, and 10 mg/kg for 18 months to mice and for 25 months to rats. These doses are equivalent to 2.4, 9.4 and 37.5 times the maximum human dose (16 mg/day) on a mg/kg basis or 0.2, 0.75 and 3 times the maximum human dose (mice) or 0.4, 1.5, and 6 times the maximum human dose (rats) on a mg/m² basis. A maximum tolerated dose was not achieved in male mice. There were statistically significant increases in pituitary gland adenomas, endocrine pancreas adenomas and mammary gland adenocarcinomas. The following table summarizes the multiples of the human dose on a mg/m² (mg/kg) basis at which these tumors occurred.

TUMOR TYPE	SPECIES	SEX	MULTIPLE OF MAXIMUM HUMAN DOSE in mg/m² (mg/kg): LOWEST EFFECT LEVEL	HIGHEST NO EFFECT LEVEL
Pituitary adenomas	mouse	female	0.75 (*9.4*)	0.2 (*2.4*)
Endocrine pancreas adenomas	rat	male	1.5 (*9.4*)	0.4 (*2.4*)
Mammary gland adeno-carcinomas	mouse	female	0.2 (*2.4*)	none
	rat	female	0.4 (*2.4*)	none
	rat	male	6 (*37.5*)	1.5 (*9.4*)
Mammary gland neoplasms, Total	rat	male	1.5 (*9.4*)	0.4 (*2.4*)

Antipsychotic drugs have been shown to chronically elevate prolactin levels in rodents. Serum prolactin levels were not measured during the risperidone carcinogenicity studies; however, measurements during subchronic toxicity studies showed that risperidone elevated serum prolactin levels 5 to 6 fold in mice and rats at the same doses used in the carcinogenicity studies. An increase in mammary, pituitary, and endocrine pancreas neoplasms has been found in rodents after chronic administration of other antipsychotic drugs and is considered to be prolactin mediated. The relevance for human risk of the findings of prolactin-mediated endocrine tumors in rodents is unknown (See Hyperprolactinemia under PRECAUTIONS, GENERAL).

Mutagenesis: No evidence of mutagenic potential for risperidone was found in the Ames reverse mutation test, mouse lymphoma assay, in vitro rat hepatocyte DNA-repair assay, in vivo micronucleus test in mice, the sex-linked recessive lethal test in Drosophila, or the chromosomal aberration test in human lymphocytes or Chinese hamster cells.

Impairment of Fertility: Risperidone (0.16 to 5 mg/kg) was shown to impair mating, but not fertility, in Wistar rats in three reproductive studies (two Segment I and a multigenerational study) at doses 0.1 to 3 times the maximum recommended human dose on a mg/m² basis. The effect appeared to be in females since impaired mating behavior was not noted in the Segment I study in which males only were treated. In a subchronic study in Beagle dogs in which risperidone was administered at doses of 0.31 to 5 mg/kg, sperm motility and concentration were decreased at doses 0.6 to 10 times the human dose on a mg/m² basis. Dose-related decreases were also noted in serum testosterone at the same doses. Serum testosterone and sperm parameters partially recovered but remained decreased after treatment was discontinued. No no-effect doses were noted in either rat or dog.

Pregnancy

Pregnancy Category C: The teratogenic potential of risperidone was studied in three Segment II studies in Sprague-Dawley and Wistar rats and in one Segment II study in New Zealand rabbits. The incidence of malformations was not increased compared to control in offspring of rats or rabbits given 0.4 to 6 times the human dose on a mg/m² basis. In three reproductive studies in rats (two Segment III and a multigenerational study), there was an increase in pup deaths during the first 4 days of lactation at doses 0.1 to 3 times the human dose on a mg/m² basis. It is not known whether these deaths were due to a direct effect on the fetuses or pups or to effects on the dams. There was no no-effect dose for increased rat pup mortality. In one Segment III study, there was an increase in stillborn rat pups at a dose 1.5 times higher than the human dose on a mg/m² basis.

Placental transfer of risperidone occurs in rat pups. There are no adequate and well-controlled studies in pregnant women. However, there was one report of a case of agenesis of the corpus callosum in an infant exposed to risperidone in utero. The causal relationship to RISPERDAL® therapy is unknown.

RISPERDAL® should be used during pregnancy only if the potential benefit justifies the potential risk to the fetus.

Labor and Delivery

The effect of RISPERDAL® on labor and delivery in humans is unknown.

Nursing Mothers

It is not known whether or not risperidone is excreted in human milk. In animal studies, risperidone and 9-hydroxyrisperidone were excreted in breast milk. Therefore, women receiving RISPERDAL® should not breast feed.

Pediatric Use

Safety and effectiveness in children have not been established.

Geriatric Use

Clinical studies of RISPERDAL® did not include sufficient numbers of patients aged 65 and over to determine whether they respond differently from younger patients. In general, a lower starting dose is recommended for an elderly patient, reflecting a decreased pharmacokinetic clearance in the elderly, as well as a greater frequency of decreased hepatic, renal, or cardiac function, and a greater tendency to postural hypotension (See CLINICAL PHARMACOLOGY and DOSAGE AND ADMINISTRATION).

ADVERSE REACTIONS

Associated with Discontinuation of Treatment

Approximately 9% percent (244/2607) of RISPERDAL® (risperidone)-treated patients in phase 2–3 studies discontinued treatment due to an adverse event, compared with about 7% on placebo and 10% on active control drugs. The more common events (≥0.3%) associated with discontinuation and considered to be possibly or probably drug-related included:

Adverse Event	RISPERDAL®	Placebo
Extrapyramidal symptoms	2.1%	0%
Dizziness	0.7%	0%
Hyperkinesia	0.6%	0%
Somnolence	0.5%	0%
Nausea	0.3%	0%

Suicide attempt was associated with discontinuation in 1.2% of RISPERDAL® treated patients compared to 0.6% of placebo patients, but, given the almost 40-fold greater exposure time in RISPERDAL® compared to placebo patients, it is unlikely that suicide attempt is a RISPERDAL® related adverse event (See PRECAUTIONS). Discontinuation for extrapyramidal symptoms was 0% in placebo patients but 3.8% in active-control patients in the phase 2–3 trials.

Incidence in Controlled Trials

Commonly Observed Adverse Events in Controlled Clinical Trials: In two 6- to 8-week placebo-controlled trials, spontaneously-reported, treatment-emergent adverse events with an incidence of 5% or greater in at least one of the RISPERDAL® groups and at least twice that of placebo were: anxiety, somnolence, extrapyramidal symptoms, dizziness, constipation, nausea, dyspepsia, rhinitis, rash, and tachycardia.

Adverse events were also elicited in one of these two trials (i.e., in the fixed-dose trial comparing RISPERDAL® at doses of 2, 6, 10, and 16 mg/day with placebo) utilizing a checklist for detecting adverse events, a method that is more sensitive than spontaneous reporting. By this method, the following additional common and drug-related adverse events were present at at least 5% and twice the rate of placebo: increased dream activity, increased duration of sleep, accommodation disturbances, reduced salivation, micturition disturbances, diarrhea, weight gain, menorrhagia, diminished sexual desire, erectile dysfunction, ejaculatory dysfunction, and orgastic dysfunction.

Adverse Events Occurring at an Incidence of 1% or More Among RISPERDAL® Treated Patients: The table that follows enumerates adverse events that occurred at an incidence of 1% or more, and were at least as frequent among RISPERDAL® treated patients treated at doses of ≤10 mg/day than among placebo-treated patients in the pooled results of two 6- to 8-week controlled trials. Patients received RISPERDAL® doses of 2, 6, 10, or 16 mg/day in the dose comparison trial, or up to a maximum dose of 10 mg/day in the titration study. This table shows the percentage of patients in each dose group (≤10 mg/day or 16 mg/day) who spontaneously reported at least one episode of an event at some time during their treatment. Patients given doses of 2, 6, or 10 mg did not differ materially in these rates. Reported adverse events were classified using the World Health Organization preferred terms.

The prescriber should be aware that these figures cannot be used to predict the incidence of side effects in the course of usual medical practice where patient characteristics and other factors differ from those which prevailed in this clinical trial. Similarly, the cited frequencies cannot be compared with figures obtained from other clinical investigations involving different treatments, uses and investigators. The cited figures, however, do provide the prescribing physician with some basis for estimating the relative contribution of drug and nondrug factors to the side effect incidence rate in the population studied.

Table 1: Treatment-Emergent Adverse Experience Incidence in 6- to 8-Week Controlled Clinical Trials[1]

Body System/ Preferred Term	RISPERDAL® ≤10 mg/day (N=324)	RISPERDAL® 16 mg/day (N=77)	Placebo (N=142)
Psychiatric Disorders			
Insomnia	26%	23%	19%
Agitation	22%	26%	20%

Anxiety	12%	20%	9%
Somnolence	3%	8%	1%
Aggressive reaction	1%	3%	1%
Nervous System			
Extrapyramidal symptoms[2]	17%	34%	16%
Headache	14%	12%	12%
Dizziness	4%	7%	1%
Gastrointestinal System			
Constipation	7%	13%	3%
Nausea	6%	4%	3%
Dyspepsia	5%	10%	4%
Vomiting	5%	7%	4%
Abdominal pain	4%	1%	0%
Saliva increased	2%	0%	1%
Toothache	2%	0%	0%
Respiratory System			
Rhinitis	10%	8%	4%
Coughing	3%	3%	1%
Sinusitis	2%	1%	1%
Pharyngitis	2%	3%	0%
Dyspnea	1%	0%	0%
Body as a Whole			
Back pain	2%	0%	1%
Chest pain	2%	3%	1%
Fever	2%	3%	0%
Dermatological			
Rash	2%	5%	1%
Dry skin	2%	4%	0%
Seborrhea	1%	0%	0%
Infections			
Upper respiratory	3%	3%	1%
Visual			
Abnormal vision	2%	1%	1%
Musculo-Skeletal			
Arthralgia	2%	3%	0%
Cardiovascular			
Tachycardia	3%	5%	0%

[1] Events reported by at least 1% of patients treated with RISPERDAL® ≤ 10 mg/day are included, and are rounded to the nearest %. Comparative rates for RISPERDAL® 16 mg/day and placebo are provided as well. Events for which the RISPERDAL® incidence (in both dose groups) was equal to or less than placebo are not listed in the table, but included the following: nervousness, injury, and fungal infection.

[2] Includes tremor, dystonia, hypokinesia, hypertonia, hyperkinesia, oculogyric crisis, ataxia, abnormal gait, involuntary muscle contractions, hyporeflexia, akathisia and extrapyramidal disorders. Although the incidence of 'extrapyramidal symptoms' does not appear to differ for the '≤10 mg/day' group and placebo, the data for individual dose groups in fixed dose trials do suggest a dose/response relationship (See DOSE DEPENDENCY OF ADVERSE EVENTS).

Dose Dependency of Adverse Events:

Extrapyramidal symptoms: Data from two fixed dose trials provided evidence of dose-relatedness for extrapyramidal symptoms associated with risperidone treatment.

Two methods were used to measure extrapyramidal symptoms (EPS) in an 8-week trial comparing four fixed doses of risperidone (2, 6, 10, and 16 mg/day), including (1) a parkinsonism score (mean change from baseline) from the Extrapyramidal Symptom Rating Scale and (2) incidence of spontaneous complaints of EPS:

Dose Groups	Placebo	Ris 2	Ris 6	Ris 10	Ris 16
Parkinsonism	1.2	0.9	1.8	2.4	2.6
EPS Incidence	13%	13%	16%	20%	31%

Similar methods were used to measure extrapyramidal symptoms (EPS) in an 8-week trial comparing five fixed doses of risperidone (1, 4, 8, 12, and 16 mg/day):

Dose Groups	Ris 1	Ris 4	Ris 8	Ris 12	Ris 16
Parkinsonism	0.6	1.7	2.4	2.9	4.1
EPS Incidence	7%	12%	18%	18%	21%

Other Adverse Events: Adverse event data elicited by a checklist for side effects from a large study comparing 5 fixed doses of RISPERDAL® (1, 4, 8, 12, and 16 mg/day) were explored for dose-relatedness of adverse events. A Cochran-Armitage Test for trend in these data revealed a positive trend ($\rho < 0.05$) for the following adverse events: sleepiness, increased duration of sleep, accommodation disturbances, orthostatic dizziness, palpitations, weight gain, erectile dysfunction, ejaculatory dysfunction, orgastic dysfunction, asthenia/lassitude/increased fatiguability, and increased pigmentation.

Vital Sign Changes: RISPERDAL® is associated with orthostatic hypotension and tachycardia (See PRECAUTIONS).

Weight changes: The proportions of RISPERDAL® and placebo-treated patients meeting a weight gain criterion of ≥ 7% of body weight were compared in a pool of 6- to 8-week placebo-controlled trials, revealing a statistically significantly greater incidence of weight gain for RISPERDAL® (18%) compared to placebo (9%).

Laboratory Changes: A between group comparison for 6- to 8-week placebo-controlled trials revealed no statistically significant RISPERDAL®/placebo differences in the proportions of patients experiencing potentially important changes in routine serum chemistry, hematology, or urinalysis parameters. Similarly, there were no RISPERDAL®/placebo differences in the incidence of discontinuations for changes in serum chemistry, hematology, or urinalysis. However, RISPERDAL® administration was associated with increases in serum prolactin (See PRECAUTIONS).

ECG Changes: The electrocardiograms of approximately 380 patients who received RISPERDAL® and 120 patients who received placebo in two double-blind, placebo-controlled trials were evaluated and revealed one finding of potential concern; i.e., 8 patients taking RISPERDAL® whose baseline QTc interval was less than 450 msec were observed to have QTc intervals greater than 450 msec during treatment (See WARNINGS). Changes of this type were not seen among about 120 placebo patients, but were seen in patients receiving haloperidol (3/126).

Other Events Observed During the Pre-Marketing Evaluation of RISPERDAL®

During its premarketing assessment, multiple doses of RISPERDAL® (risperidone) were administered to 2607 patients in phase 2 and 3 studies. The conditions and duration of exposure to RISPERDAL® varied greatly, and included (in overlapping categories) open and double-blind studies, uncontrolled and controlled studies, inpatient and outpatient studies, fixed-dose and titration studies, and short-term or longer-term exposure. In most studies, untoward events associated with this exposure were obtained by spontaneous report and recorded by clinical investigators using terminology of their own choosing. Consequently, it is not possible to provide a meaningful estimate of the proportion of individuals experiencing adverse events without first grouping similar types of untoward events into a smaller number of standardized event categories. In two large studies, adverse events were also elicited utilizing the UKU (direct questioning) side effect rating scale, and these events were not further categorized using standard terminology (Note: These events are marked with an asterisk in the listings that follow).

In the listings that follow, spontaneously reported adverse events were classified using World Health Organization (WHO) preferred terms. The frequencies presented, therefore, represent the proportion of the 2607 patients exposed to multiple doses of RISPERDAL® who experienced an event of the type cited on at least one occasion while receiving RISPERDAL®. All reported events are included except those already listed in Table 1, those events for which a drug cause was remote, and those event terms which were so general as to be uninformative. It is important to emphasize that, although the events reported occurred during treatment with RISPERDAL®, they were not necessarily caused by it.

Events are further categorized by body system and listed in order of decreasing frequency according to the following definitions: frequent adverse events are those occurring in at least 1/100 patients (only those not already listed in the tabulated results from placebo controlled trials appear in this listing); infrequent adverse events are those occurring in 1/100 to 1/1000 patients; rare events are those occurring in fewer than 1/1000 patients.

Psychiatric Disorders: *Frequent:* increased dream activity*, diminished sexual desire*, nervousness. *Infrequent:* impaired concentration, depression, apathy, catatonic reaction, euphoria, increased libido, amnesia. *Rare:* emotional lability, nightmares, delirium, withdrawal syndrome, yawning.

Central and Peripheral Nervous System Disorders: *Frequent:* increased sleep duration*. *Infrequent:* dysarthria, vertigo, stupor, paraesthesia, confusion. *Rare:* aphasia, cholinergic syndrome, hypoesthesia, tongue paralysis, leg cramps, torticollis, hypotonia, coma, migraine, hyperreflexia, choreoathetosis.

Gastro-intestinal Disorders: *Frequent:* anorexia, reduced salivation*. *Infrequent:* flatulence, diarrhea, increased appetite, stomatitis, melena, dysphagia, hemorrhoids, gastritis. *Rare:* fecal incontinence, eructation, gastroesophageal reflux, gastroenteritis, esophagitis, tongue discoloration, cholelithiasis, tongue edema, diverticulitis, gingivitis, discolored feces, GI hemorrhage, hematemesis.

Body as a Whole/General Disorders: *Frequent:* fatigue. *Infrequent:* edema, rigors, malaise, influenza-like symptoms. *Rare:* pallor, enlarged abdomen, allergic reaction, ascites, sarcoidosis, flushing.

Respiratory System Disorders: *Infrequent:* hyperventilation, bronchospasm, pneumonia, stridor. *Rare:* asthma, increased sputum, aspiration.

Skin and Appendage Disorders: *Frequent:* increased pigmentation*, photosensitivity*. *Infrequent:* increased sweating, acne, decreased sweating, alopecia, hyperkeratosis, pruritus, skin exfoliation. *Rare:* bullous eruption, skin ulceration, aggravated psoriasis, furunculosis, verruca, dermatitis lichenoid, hypertrichosis, genital pruritus, urticaria.

Cardiovascular Disorders: *Infrequent:* palpitation, hypertension, hypotension, AV block, myocardial infarction. *Rare:* ventricular tachycardia, angina pectoris, premature atrial contractions, T wave inversions, ventricular extrasystoles, ST depression, myocarditis.

Vision Disorders: *Infrequent:* abnormal accommodation, xerophthalmia. *Rare:* diplopia, eye pain, blepharitis, photopsia, photophobia, abnormal lacrimation.

Metabolic and Nutritional Disorders: *Infrequent:* hyponatremia, weight increase, creatine phosphokinase increase, thirst, weight decrease, diabetes mellitus. *Rare:* decreased serum iron, cachexia, dehydration, hypokalemia, hypoproteinemia, hyperphosphatemia, hypertriglyceridemia, hyperuricemia, hypoglycemia.

Urinary System Disorders: *Frequent:* polyuria/polydipsia*. *Infrequent:* urinary incontinence, hematuria, dysuria. *Rare:* urinary retention, cystitis, renal insufficiency.

Musculo-skeletal System Disorders: *Infrequent:* myalgia. *Rare:* arthrosis, synostosis, bursitis, arthritis, skeletal pain.

Reproductive Disorders, Female: *Frequent:* menorrhagia*, orgastic dysfunction*, dry vagina*. *Infrequent:* nonpuerperal lactation, amenorrhea, female breast pain, leukorrhea, mastitis, dysmenorrhea, female perineal pain, intermenstrual bleeding, vaginal hemorrhage.

Liver and Biliary System Disorders: *Infrequent:* increased SGOT, increased SGPT. *Rare:* hepatic failure, cholestatic hepatitis, cholecystitis, cholelithiasis, hepatitis, hepatocellular damage.

Platelet, Bleeding and Clotting Disorders: *Infrequent:* epistaxis, purpura. *Rare:* hemorrhage, superficial phlebitis, thrombophlebitis, thrombocytopenia.

Hearing and Vestibular Disorders: *Rare:* tinnitus, hyperacusis, decreased hearing.

Red Blood Cell Disorders: *Infrequent:* anemia, hypochromic anemia. *Rare:* normocytic anemia.

Reproductive Disorders, Male: *Frequent:* erectile dysfunction*. *Infrequent:* ejaculation failure.

White Cell and Resistance Disorders: *Rare:* leukocytosis, lymphadenopathy, leucopenia, Pelger-Huet anomaly.

Endocrine Disorders: *Rare:* gynecomastia, male breast pain, antidiuretic hormone disorder.

Special Senses: *Rare:* bitter taste.

* Incidence based on elicited reports.

Post introduction Reports: Adverse events reported since market introduction which were temporally (but not necessarily causally) related to RISPERDAL® therapy, include the following: anaphylactic reaction, angioedema, apnea, atrial fibrillation, cerebrovascular disorder, diabetes mellitus aggravated, including diabetic ketoacidosis intestinal obstruction, jaundice, mania, pancreatitis Parkinson's disease aggravated, pulmonary embolism. There have been rare reports of sudden death and/or cardiopulmonary arrest in patients receiving RISPERDAL. A causal relationship with RISPERDAL has not been established. It is important to note that sudden and unexpected death may occur in psychotic patients whether they remain untreated or whether they are treated with other antipsychotic drugs.

DRUG ABUSE AND DEPENDENCE

Controlled Substance Class: RISPERDAL® (risperidone) is not a controlled substance.

Physical and Psychologic Dependence: RISPERDAL® has not been systematically studied in animals or humans for its potential for abuse, tolerance or physical dependence. While the clinical trials did not reveal any tendency for any drug-seeking behavior, these observations were not systematic and it is not possible to predict on the basis of this limited experience the extent to which a CNS-active drug will be misused, diverted and/or abused once marketed. Consequently, patients should be evaluated carefully for a history of drug abuse, and such patients should be observed closely for signs of RISPERDAL® misuse or abuse (e.g., development of tolerance, increases in dose, drug-seeking behavior).

OVERDOSAGE

Human Experience: Premarketing experience included eight reports of acute RISPERDAL® overdosage with estimated doses ranging from 20 to 300 mg and no fatalities. In general, reported signs and symptoms were those resulting from an exaggeration of the drug's known pharmacological effects, i.e., drowsiness and sedation, tachycardia and hypotension, and extrapyramidal symptoms. One case, involving an estimated overdose of 240 mg, was associated with hyponatremia, hypokalemia, prolonged QT, and widened QRS. Another case, involving an estimated overdose of 36 mg, was

Continued on next page

Janssen Pharmaceutica—Cont.

associated with a seizure. Postmarketing experience includes reports of acute RISPERDAL® overdosage, with estimated doses of up to 360 mg. In general, the most frequently reported signs and symptoms are those resulting from an exaggeration of the drug's known pharmacological effects, i.e., drowsiness, sedation, tachycardia and hypotension. Other adverse events reported since market introduction which were temporally, (but not necessarily causally) related to RISPERDAL® overdose, include prolonged QT interval, convulsions, cardiopulmonary arrest, and rare fatality associated with multiple drug overdose.

Management of Overdosage: In case of acute overdosage, establish and maintain an airway and ensure adequate oxygenation and ventilation. Gastric lavage (after intubation, if patient is unconscious) and administration of activated charcoal together with a laxative should be considered. The possibility of obtundation, seizures or dystonic reaction of the head and neck following overdose may create a risk of aspiration with induced emesis. Cardiovascular monitoring should commence immediately and should include continuous electrocardiographic monitoring to detect possible arrhythmias. If antiarrhythmic therapy is administered, disopyramide, procainamide and quinidine carry a theoretical hazard of QT-prolonging effects that might be additive to those of risperidone. Similarly, it is reasonable to expect that the alpha-blocking properties of bretylium might be additive to those of risperidone, resulting in problematic hypotension.

There is no specific antidote to RISPERDAL®. Therefore appropriate supportive measures should be instituted. The possibility of multiple drug involvement should be considered. Hypotension and circulatory collapse should be treated with appropriate measures such as intravenous fluids and/or sympathomimetic agents (epinephrine and dopamine should not be used, since beta stimulation may worsen hypotension in the setting of risperidone-induced alpha blockade). In cases of severe extrapyramidal symptoms, anticholinergic medication should be administered. Close medical supervision and monitoring should continue until the patient recovers.

DOSAGE AND ADMINISTRATION

Usual Initial Dose: RISPERDAL® (risperidone) should be administered on a BID schedule, generally beginning with 1 mg BID initially, with increases in increments of 1 mg BID on the second and third day, as tolerated, to a target dose of 3 mg BID by the third day. In some patients, slower titration may be medically appropriate. Further dosage adjustments, if indicated, should generally occur at intervals of not less than 1 week, since steady state for the active metabolite would not be achieved for approximately 1 week in the typical patient. When dosage adjustments are necessary, small dose increments/decrements of 1 mg BID are recommended.

Antipsychotic efficacy was demonstrated in a dose range of 4 to 16 mg/day in the clinical trials supporting effectiveness of RISPERDAL®, however, maximal effect was generally seen in a range of 4 to 6 mg/day. Doses above 6 mg/day were not demonstrated to be more efficacious than lower doses, were associated with more extrapyramidal symptoms and other adverse effects, and are not generally recommended. The safety of doses above 16 mg/day has not been evaluated in clinical trials.

Dosage in Special Populations: The recommended initial dose is 0.5 mg BID in patients who are elderly or debilitated, patients with severe renal or hepatic impairment, and patients either predisposed to hypotension or for whom hypotension would pose a risk. Dosage increases in these patients should be in increments of no more than 0.5 mg BID. Increases to dosages above 1.5 mg BID should generally occur at intervals of at least 1 week. In some patients, slower titration may be medically appropriate.

Elderly or debilitated patients, and patients with renal impairment, may have less ability to eliminate RISPERDAL® than normal adults. Patients with impaired hepatic function may have increases in the free fraction of the risperidone, possibly resulting in an enhanced effect (See CLINICAL PHARMACOLOGY). Patients with a predisposition to hypotensive reactions or for whom such reactions would pose a particular risk likewise need to be titrated cautiously and carefully monitored (See PRECAUTIONS).

Maintenance Therapy: While there is no body of evidence available to answer the question of how long the patient treated with RISPERDAL® should remain on it, the effectiveness of maintenance treatment is well established for many other antipsychotic drugs. It is recommended that responding patients be continued on RISPERDAL®, but at the lowest dose needed to maintain remission. Patients should be periodically reassessed to determine the need for maintenance treatment.

Reinitiation of Treatment in Patients Previously Discontinued: Although there are no data to specifically address reinitiation of treatment, it is recommended that when restarting patients who have had an interval off RISPERDAL®, the initial titration schedule should be followed.

Switching from Other Antipsychotics: There are no systematically collected data to specifically address switching from other antipsychotics to RISPERDAL®, or concerning concomitant administration with other antipsychotics. While immediate discontinuation of the previous antipsychotic treatment may be acceptable for some patients, more gradual discontinuation may be most appropriate for other patients. In all cases, the period of overlapping antipsychotic administration should be minimized. When switching patients from depot antipsychotics, if medically appropriate, initiate RISPERDAL® therapy in place of the next scheduled injection. The need for continuing existing EPS medication should be reevaluated periodically.

HOW SUPPLIED

RISPERDAL® (risperidone) tablets are imprinted "JANSSEN", and "R" and the strength "1", "2", "3", or "4".
1 mg white, scored, tablet: bottles of 60 NDC 50458-300-06, blister pack of 100 NDC 50458-300-01. bottles of 500 NDC 50458-300-50
2 mg orange tablet: bottles of 60 NDC 50458-320-06, blister pack of 100 NDC 50458-320-01. bottles of 500 NDC 50458-320-50
3 mg yellow tablet: bottles of 60 NDC 50458-330-06, blister pack of 100 NDC 50458-330-01. bottles of 500 NDC 50458-330-50
4 mg green tablet: bottles of 60 NDC 50458-350-06, blister pack of 100 NDC 50458-350-01.
RISPERDAL® (risperidone) 1 mg/mL oral solution (NDC 50458-305-10) is supplied in 100mL bottles with a calibrated (in milligrams and milliliters) pipette. The minimum calibrated volume is 0.25 mL, while the maximum calibrated volume is 3 mL.
Patient Instructions (including illustrations) for using the RISPERDAL® (risperidone) calibrated dispensing-pipette are provided. Tests indicate that RISPERDAL® (risperidone) oral solution is compatible in the following beverages: water, coffee, orange juice and low-fat milk; it is NOT compatible with either cola or tea, however.

STORAGE AND HANDLING - RISPERDAL® tablets should be stored at controlled room temperature (59°–77°F/15°–25°C) away from children, and should be protected from light and moisture.
RISPERDAL® 1 mg/mL oral solution should be stored at controlled room temperature (59°–77°F/15°–25°C) away from children, and should be protected from light and freezing.
US Patent 4,804,663
July 1995, February 1996
JANSSEN
PHARMACEUTICA
Titusville, NJ 08560
Shown in Product Identification Guide, page 318

SPORANOX ℞

[*spər 'ah-näks"*]
(Itraconazole)
100 mg capsules

> **WARNING:** Coadministration of terfenadine with itraconazole is contraindicated. Serious cardiovascular adverse events, including death, ventricular tachycardia, and torsades de pointes have occurred in patients taking itraconazole concomitantly with terfenadine. This is due to elevated terfenadine concentrations caused by itraconazole. See CONTRAINDICATIONS, WARNINGS, and PRECAUTIONS sections.
> Another oral azole antifungal, ketoconazole, inhibits the metabolism of astemizole, resulting in elevated plasma concentrations of astemizole and its active metabolite desmethylastemizole, which may prolong QT intervals. Based on results of an *in vitro* study and the chemical resemblance of itraconazole and ketoconazole, coadministration of astemizole and itraconazole is contraindicated. See CONTRAINDICATIONS, WARNINGS, and PRECAUTIONS sections.
> Coadministration of cisapride with itraconazole is contraindicated. Serious cardiovascular adverse events including death, ventricular tachycardia, and torsades de pointes have occurred in patients taking itraconazole concomitantly with cisapride. See CONTRAINDICATIONS, WARNINGS, and PRECAUTIONS sections.

DESCRIPTION

SPORANOX is the brand name for itraconazole, a synthetic triazole antifungal agent. Itraconazole is a 1:1:1:1 racemic mixture of four diastereomers (two enantiomeric pairs), each possessing three chiral centers. It may be represented by the following nomenclature:
(±)-1-[(R*)-sec-butyl]-4-[p-[4-[p-[[(2R*,4S*)-2- (2,4-dichlorophenyl)-2-(1H-1,2,4-triazol-1-ylmethyl)- 1,3-dioxolan-4-yl]methoxy]phenyl] -1- piperazinyl]phenyl] -Δ^{2}-1,2,4-triazolin-5-one mixture with (±)-1 -[(R*)-sec-butyl]-4-[p-[4- [p- [[(2S*,4R*)-2-(2,4-dichlorophenyl)-2-(1H-1,2,4-triazol-1-ylmethyl)-1,3-dioxolan-4-yl]methoxy]phenyl]-1- piperazinyl]phenyl]-Δ^{2}-1,2,4-triazolin-5-one

or

(±)-1-[(RS)-sec-butyl]-4-[p-[4-[p-[[(2R,4S)-2-(2,4-dichlorophenyl)-2-(1H-1,2,4-triazol-1-ylmethyl)-1,3-dioxolan-4-yl]methoxy]phenyl]-1-piperazinyl]phenyl]-Δ^{2}-1,2,4-triazolin-5-one

Itraconazole has a molecular formula of $C_{35}H_{30}Cl_2N_8O_4$ and a molecular weight of 705.64. It is a white to slightly yellowish powder. It is insoluble in water, very slightly soluble in alcohols, and freely soluble in dichloromethane. It has a pKa of 3.70 (based on extrapolation of values obtained from methanolic solutions) and a log (n-octanol/water) partition coefficient of 5.66 at pH 8.1.

SPORANOX contains 100 mg of itraconazole coated on sugar spheres. Inactive ingredients are gelatin, hydroxypropyl methylcellulose, polyethylene glycol (PEG) 20,000, starch, sucrose, titanium dioxide, FD&C Blue No. 1, FD&C Blue No. 2, D&C Red No. 22 and D&C Red No. 28.

CLINICAL PHARMACOLOGY

Mode of Action: *In vitro* studies have demonstrated that itraconazole inhibits the cytochrome P-450-dependent synthesis of ergosterol, which is a vital component of fungal cell membranes.

Pharmacokinetics and Metabolism: NOTE: The plasma concentrations reported below were measured by high performance liquid chromatography (HPLC) specific for itraconazole. When itraconazole in plasma is measured by a bioassay, values reported are approximately 3.3 times higher than those obtained by HPLC due to the presence of the bioactive metabolite, hydroxyitraconazole. (See *Microbiology* section.)

The pharmacokinetics of itraconazole after intravenous administration and its absolute oral bioavailability from an oral solution were studied in a randomized cross-over study using six healthy male volunteers. The total plasma clearance averaged 381 ± 95 mL/min and the apparent volume of distribution averaged 796 ± 185 L. The observed absolute oral bioavailability of itraconazole was 55%.

The oral bioavailability of itraconazole is maximal when SPORANOX (itraconazole capsules) is taken with a full meal. The pharmacokinetics of itraconazole were studied using six healthy male volunteers who received, in a cross-over design, single 100 mg doses of itraconazole as a polyethylene glycol capsule, with or without a full meal. The same six volunteers also received 50 mg or 200 mg with a full meal in a cross-over design. In this study, only itraconazole plasma concentrations were measured. Presented in the table below are the respective pharmacokinetic parameters for itraconazole:

	50 mg (fed)	100 mg (fed)	100 mg (fasted)	200 mg (fed)
C_{max} (ng/mL)	45 ± 16	132 ± 67	38 ± 20	289 ± 100
T_{max} (hours)	3.2 ± 1.3	4.0 ± 1.1	3.3 ± 1.0	4.7 ± 1.4
$AUC_{0-\infty}$ (ng·h/mL)	567 ± 264	1899 ± 838	722 ± 289	5211 ± 2116

Values are means ± standard deviation

Doubling the SPORANOX dose results in approximately a three-fold increase in the itraconazole plasma concentrations.

Values given in the table below represent data from a crossover pharmacokinetics study in which 27 healthy male volunteers each took a single 200 mg dose of SPORANOX with or without a full meal:

	Itraconazole		Hydroxyitraconazole	
	Fed	Fasted	Fed	Fasted
C_{max} (ng/mL)	239 ± 85	140 ± 65	397 ± 103	286 ± 101
T_{max} (hours)	4.5 ± 1.1	3.9 ± 1.0	5.1 ± 1.6	4.5 ± 1.1
AUC_{∞} (ng·h/mL)	3423 ± 1154	2094 ± 905	7978 ± 2648	5191 ± 2489
$t_{1/2}$ (hours)	21 ± 5	21 ± 7	12 ± 3	12 ± 3

Values are means ± standard deviation

Absorption of itraconazole under fasted conditions in individuals with relative or absolute achlorhydria, such as patients with AIDS or volunteers taking gastric acid secretion suppressors (e.g. H_2 inhibitors), was increased when SPORANOX was administered with a cola beverage. Eighteen males with AIDS received single 200 mg doses of SPORANOX under fasted conditions with 8 ounces of water or 8 ounces of a cola beverage in a crossover design. The ab-

sorption of itraconazole was increased when SPORANOX was coadministered with a cola beverage with AUC_{0-24} and C_{max} increasing 75 ± 121% and 95 ± 128%, respectively. Thirty healthy males received single 200 mg doses of SPORANOX under fasted conditions either 1) with water; 2) with water, after ranitidine 150 mg b.i.d. for 3 days; or 3) with cola, after ranitidine 150 mg b.i.d. for 3 days. When SPORANOX was administered after ranitidine pretreatment, itraconazole was absorbed to a lesser extent than when SPORANOX was administered alone, with decreases in AUC_{0-24} and C_{max} of 39 ±37% and 42 ± 39%, respectively. When SPORANOX was administered with cola after ranitidine pretreatment, itraconazole absorption was comparable to that observed when SPORANOX was administered alone.

Steady-state concentrations were reached within 15 days following oral doses of 50–400 mg daily. Values given in the table below are data at steady-state from a pharmacokinetics study in which 27 healthy male volunteers took 200 mg SPORANOX b.i.d. (with a full meal) for 15 days:

	Itraconazole	Hydroxyitraconazole
C_{max} (ng/mL)	2282 ± 514	3488 ± 742
C_{min} (ng/mL)	1855 ± 535	3349 ± 761
T_{max} (hours)	4.6 ± 1.8	3.4 ± 3.4
AUC_{0-12h} (ng·h/mL)	22569 ± 5375	38572 ± 8450
$t_{1/2}$ (hours)	64 ± 32	56 ± 24

Values are means ± standard deviation

Results of the pharmacokinetics study suggest that itraconazole may undergo saturation metabolism with multiple dosing.

Itraconazole is extensively metabolized by the liver into a large number of metabolites, including hydroxyitraconazole, the major metabolite. Fecal excretion of the parent drug varies between 3–18% of the dose. Renal excretion of the parent drug is less than 0.03% of the dose. About 40% of the dose is excreted as inactive metabolites in the urine. No single excreted metabolite represents more than 5% of a dose. The main metabolic pathways are oxidative scission of the dioxolane ring, aliphatic oxidation at the 1-methylpropyl substituent, N-dealkylation of this 1-methylpropyl substituent, oxidative degradation of the piperazine ring and triazolone scission.

Plasma concentrations of itraconazole in subjects with renal insufficiency were comparable to those obtained in healthy subjects. The effect of hepatic impairment on the plasma concentration of itraconazole is unknown. It is recommended that plasma concentrations of itraconazole in patients with hepatic impairment be carefully monitored.

The plasma protein binding of itraconazole is 99.8% and that of hydroxyitraconazole is 99.5%. Itraconazole is not removed by hemodialysis.

In animal studies, itraconazole is extensively distributed into lipophilic tissues. Concentrations of itraconazole in fatty tissues, omentum, liver, kidney and skin tissues are 2–20 times the corresponding plasma concentrations. Aqueous fluids such as cerebrospinal fluid and saliva contain negligible amounts of the drug.

Microbiology: Itraconazole exhibits *in vitro* activity against *Blastomyces dermatitidis, Histoplasma capsulatum, Histoplasma duboisii, Aspergillus flavus, Aspergillus fumigatus* and *Cryptococcus neoformans.* Itraconazole also exhibits varying *in vitro* activity against *Sporothrix schenckii*, Trichophyton spp., *Candida albicans* and Candida spp. The bioactive metabolite, hydroxyitraconazole, has not been evaluated against *Histoplasma capsulatum* and *Blastomyces dermatitidis.* Correlation between *in vitro* minimum inhibitory concentration (MIC) results and clinical outcome has yet to be established for azole antifungal agents.

Itraconazole administered orally was active in a variety of animal models of fungal infection using standard laboratory strains of fungi. Fungistatic activity has been demonstrated against disseminated fungal infections caused by *Blastomyces dermatitidis, Histoplasma duboisii, Aspergillus fumigatus, Coccidioides immitis, Cryptococcus neoformans, Paracoccidioides brasiliensis, Sporothrix schenckii, Trichophyton rubrum* and *Trichophyton mentagrophytes.* Itraconazole administered at 2.5 mg/kg and 5.0 mg/kg via the oral and parenteral routes increased survival rates and sterilized organ systems in normal and immunosuppressed guinea pigs with disseminated *Aspergillus fumigatus* infections. Oral itraconazole administered daily at 40 mg/kg and 80 mg/kg increased survival rates in normal rabbits with disseminated disease and immunosuppressed rats with pulmonary *Aspergillus fumigatus* infection, respectively. Itraconazole has demonstrated antifungal activity in a variety of animal models infected with *Candida albicans* and other Candida species.

In vivo studies suggest that the activity of amphotericin B may be suppressed by azole antifungal therapy. As with other azoles, ketoconazole and itraconazole inhibit the ^{14}C-demethylation step in the synthesis of ergosterol, a cell wall component of fungi. Ergosterol is the active site for amphotericin B. In one study the antifungal activity of amphotericin B against *Aspergillus fumigatus* infections in mice was inhibited by ketoconazole therapy. The clinical significance of test results obtained in this study is unknown.

INDICATIONS AND USAGE

SPORANOX (itraconazole capsules) is indicated for the treatment of the following fungal infections in immunocompromised and non-immunocompromised patients:

1. Blastomycosis, pulmonary and extrapulmonary;
2. Histoplasmosis, including chronic cavitary pulmonary disease and disseminated, non-meningeal histoplasmosis;
3. Aspergillosis, pulmonary and extrapulmonary, in patients who are intolerant of or who are refractory to amphotericin B therapy; and
4. Onychomycosis due to dermatophytes (tinea unguium) of the toenail with or without fingernail involvement.

Specimens for fungal cultures and other relevant laboratory studies (wet mount, histopathology, serology) should be obtained prior to therapy to isolate and identify causative organisms. Therapy may be instituted before the results of the cultures and other laboratory studies are known; however, once these results become available, anti-infective therapy should be adjusted accordingly.

Blastomycosis: Analyses were conducted on data from two open-label, non-concurrently controlled studies (n=73 combined) in patients with normal or abnormal immune status. The median dose was 200 mg/day. A response for most signs and symptoms was observed within the first two weeks, and all cleared between 3 and 6 months. Results of these two studies demonstrated substantial evidence of the effectiveness of itraconazole, for the treatment of blastomycosis, compared to the natural history of untreated cases.

Histoplasmosis: Analyses were conducted on data from two open-label, non-concurrently controlled studies (n=34 combined) in patients with normal or abnormal immune status (not including HIV-infected patients). The median dose was 200 mg/day. A response for most signs and symptoms was observed within the first 2 weeks, and all cleared between 3 and 12 months. Results of these two studies demonstrated substantial evidence of the effectiveness of itraconazole, for the treatment of histoplasmosis, compared to the natural history of untreated cases.

Histoplasmosis in HIV-infected patients: Data from a small number of HIV-infected patients suggested that the response rate of histoplasmosis in HIV-infected patients is similar to non-HIV-infected patients. The clinical course of histoplasmosis in HIV-infected patients is more severe and usually requires maintenance therapy to prevent relapse. Studies to investigate the efficacy and safety of itraconazole in HIV-infected patients, including optimal dosage regimens for treatment and maintenance therapies, are ongoing.

Aspergillosis: Analyses were conducted on data from an open-label, "single-patient-use" protocol designed to make itraconazole available in the U.S. for patients who either failed or were intolerant to amphotericin B therapy (n=190). The findings were corroborated by two smaller open-label studies (n=31 combined) in the same patient population. Most adult patients were treated with a daily dose of 200 to 400 mg with a median duration of 3 months. Results of these studies demonstrated substantial evidence of effectiveness of itraconazole, as a second-line therapy for the treatment of aspergillosis, compared to the natural history of the disease in patients who either failed or were intolerant to amphotericin B therapy.

Onychomycosis: Analyses were conducted on data from three double-blind, placebo-controlled studies (n=214 total) in which patients with onychomycosis of the toenails received 200 mg once daily for 12 consecutive weeks. Results of these studies demonstrated mycological cure in 54% of patients, defined as simultaneous occurrence of negative KOH plus negative culture. Thirty-five (35) percent of patients were considered an overall success (mycological cure plus clear or minimal nail involvement with significantly decreased signs); 14% of patients demonstrated mycological cure plus clinical cure (clearance of all signs, with or without residual nail deformity). The mean time to overall success was approximately 10 months. Twenty-one (21) percent of the overall success group had a relapse (worsening of the global score or conversion of KOH or culture from negative to positive).

CONTRAINDICATIONS

Coadministration of terfenadine, astemizole or cisapride with SPORANOX (itraconazole capsules) is contraindicated. (See BOX WARNING, WARNINGS, and PRECAUTIONS sections.)

Concomitant administration of SPORANOX with oral triazolam or with oral midazolam is contraindicated. (See PRECAUTIONS section.)

SPORANOX should not be administered for the treatment of onychomycosis to pregnant patients or to women contemplating pregnancy.

SPORANOX is contraindicated in patients who have shown hypersensitivity to the drug or its excipients. There is no information regarding cross hypersensitivity between itraconazole and other azole antifungal agents. Caution should be used in prescribing SPORANOX to patients with hypersensitivity to other azoles.

WARNINGS

In U.S. clinical trials prior to marketing, there have been three cases of reversible idiosyncratic hepatitis reported among more than 2500 patients taking SPORANOX (itraconazole capsules). One patient outside the U.S. developed fulminant hepatitis and died during SPORANOX administration. Since this patient was on multiple medications, the causal association with SPORANOX is uncertain. If clinical signs and symptoms consistent with liver disease develop that may be attributable to itraconazole, SPORANOX should be discontinued.

Prior to U.S. marketing, there have been three cases of life-threatening cardiac dysrhythmias and one death reported in patients receiving terfenadine and itraconazole. (See BOX WARNING, CONTRAINDICATIONS, and PRECAUTIONS sections.)

Coadministration of astemizole with SPORANOX is contraindicated. (See BOX WARNING, CONTRAINDICATIONS, and PRECAUTIONS sections.)

Concomitant administration of oral ketoconazole with cisapride has resulted in markedly elevated cisapride plasma concentrations, prolonged QT intervals, and has rarely been associated with ventricular arrhythmias and torsades de pointes. Due to potent *in vitro* inhibition of the hepatic enzyme system mainly responsible for the metabolism of cisapride (cytochrome P450 3A4), itraconazole is also expected to markedly raise cisapride plasma concentrations; therefore, concomitant use of cisapride with SPORANOX is contraindicated. (See BOX WARNING, CONTRAINDICATIONS, and PRECAUTIONS sections.)

PRECAUTIONS

General: Hepatic enzyme test values should be monitored in patients with preexisting hepatic function abnormalities. Hepatic enzyme test values should be monitored periodically in all patients receiving continuous treatment for more than one month or at any time a patient develops signs or symptoms suggestive of liver dysfunction.

SPORANOX (itraconazole capsules) should be administered after a full meal. (See *Pharmacokinetics and Metabolism* section.)

Under fasted conditions, intraconzole absorption was decreased in the presence of decreased gastric acidity. The absorption of itraconazole may be decreased with the concomitant administration of antacids or gastric acid secretion suppressors. Studies conducted under fasted conditions demonstrated that administration with 8 ounces of a cola beverage resulted in increased absorption of itraconazole in AIDS patients with relative or absolute achlorhydria. This increase relative to the effects of a full meal is unknown. (See *Pharmacokinetics and Metabolism* sectiom.)

Information for patients: Patients should be instructed to take SPORANOX with a full meal.

Patients should be instructed to report any signs and symptoms that may suggest liver dysfunction so that the appropriate laboratory testing can be done. Such signs and symptoms may include ususual fatigue, anorexia, nausea and/or vomiting, jaundice, dark urine or pale stool.

Drug Interactions: Both itraconazole and its major metabolite, hydroxyitraconazole, are inhibitors of the cytochrome P450 3A4 enzyme system. Coadministration of SPORANOX and drugs primarily metabolized by the cytochrome P450 3A4 enzyme system may result in increased plasma concentrations of the drugs that could increase or prolong both therapeutic and adverse effects. Therefore, unless otherwise specified, appropriate dosage adjustments may be necessary.

Coadministration of terfenadine with SPORANOX has led to elevated plasma concentrations of terfenadine, resulting in rare instances of life-threatening cardiac dysrhythmias and one death. (See BOX WARNING, CONTRAINDICATIONS, and WARNINGS sections.)

Another oral azole antifungal, ketoconazole, inhibits the metabolism of astemizole, resulting in elevated plasma concentrations of astemizole and its active metabolite desmethylastemizole which may prolong QT intervals. *In vitro* data suggest that itraconazole, when compared to ketoconazole, has a less pronounced effect on the biotransformation system responsible for the metabolism of astemizole. Based on the chemical resemblance of itraconazole and ketoconazole, coadministration of astemizole with itraconazole is contraindicated. (See BOX WARNING, CONTRAINDICATIONS, and WARNINGS sections.)

Human pharmacokinetics data indicate that oral ketoconazole potently inhibits the metabolism of cisapride resulting in an eight-fold increase in the mean AUC of cisapride. Data suggest that coadministration of oral ketoconazole and cisapride can result in prolongation of the QT interval on the ECG. *In vitro* data suggest that intraconazole also markedly inhibits the biotransformation system mainly responsible for the metabolism of cisapride; therefore concomitant ad-

Continued on next page

Janssen Pharmaceutica—Cont.

ministration of SPORANOX with cisapride is contraindicated. (See BOX WARNING, CONTRAINDICATIONS, and WARNINGS sections.)

Coadministration of SPORANOX with oral midazolam or triazolam has resulted in elevated plasma concentrations of the latter two drugs. This may potentiate and prolong hypnotic and sedative effects. These agents should not be used in patients treated with SPORANOX. If midazolam is administered parenterally, special precaution is required since the sedative effect may be prolonged. (See CONTRAINDICATIONS section.)

Coadministration of SPORANOX and cyclosporine, tacrolimus or digoxin has led to increased plasma concentrations of the latter three drugs. Cyclosporine, tacrolimus and digoxin concentrations should be monitored at the initiation of SPORANOX therapy and frequently thereafter, and the dose of these three drug products adjusted appropriately.

There have been rare reports of rhabdomyolysis involving renal transplant patients receiving the combination of SPORANOX, cyclosporine, and the HMG-CoA reductase inhibitors lovastatin or simvastatin. Rhabdomyolysis has been observed in patients receiving HMG-CoA reductase inhibitors administered alone (at recommended dosages) or concomitantly with immunosuppressive drugs including cyclosporine.

When SPORANOX was coadministered with phenytoin, rifampin, or H$_2$ antagonists, reduced plasma concentrations of itraconazole were reported. The physician is advised to monitor the plasma concentrations of itraconazole when any of these drugs is taken concurrently, and to increase the dose of SPORANOX if necessary. Although no studies have been conducted, concomitant administration of SPORANOX and phenytoin may alter the metabolism of phenytoin; therefore, plasma concentrations of phenytoin should also be monitored when it is given concurrently with SPORANOX.

It has been reported that SPORANOX enhances the anticoagulant effect of coumarin-like drugs. Therefore, prothrombin time should be carefully monitored in patients receiving SPORANOX and coumarin-like drugs simultaneously.

Plasma concentrations of azole antifungal agents are reduced when given concurrently with isoniazid. Itraconazole plasma concentrations should be monitored when SPORANOX and isoniazid are coadministered.

Severe hypoglycemia has been reported in patients concomitantly receiving azole antifungal agents and oral hypoglycemic agents. Blood glucose concentrations should be carefully monitored when SPORANOX and oral hypoglycemic agents are coadministered.

Tinnitus and decreased hearing have been reported in patients concomitantly receiving SPORANOX and quinidine. Edema has been reported in patients concomitantly receiving SPORANOX and dihydropyridine calcium channel blockers. Appropriate dosage adjustments may be necessary. The results from a study in which eight HIV-infected individuals were treated with zidovudine, 8 ± 0.4 mg/kg/day, showed that the pharmacokinetics of zidovudine were not affected during concomitant administration of SPORANOX, 100 mg b.i.d.

Carcinogenesis, Mutagenesis, and Impairment of Fertility: Itraconazole showed no evidence of carcinogenicity potential in mice treated orally for 23 months at dosage levels up to 80 mg/kg/day [approximately 10× the maximum recommended human dose (MRHD)]. Male rats treated with 25 mg/kg/day (3.1× MRHD) had a slightly increased incidence of soft tissue sarcoma. These sarcomas may have been a consequence of hypercholesterolemia, which is a response of rats, but not dogs or humans, to chronic itraconazole administration. Female rats treated with 50 mg/kg/day (6.25× MRHD) had an increased incidence of squamous cell carcinoma of the lung (2/50) as compared to the untreated group. Although the occurrence of squamous cell carcinoma in the lung is extremely uncommon in untreated rats, the increase in this study was not statistically significant.

Itraconazole produced no mutagenic effects when assayed in appropriate bacterial, non-mammalian and mammalian test systems.

Itraconazole did not affect the fertility of male or female rats treated orally with dosage levels of up to 40 mg/kg/day (5×MRHD) even though parental toxicity was present at this dosage level. More severe signs of parental toxicity, including death, were present in the next higher dosage level, 160 mg/kg/day (20× MRHD).

Pregnancy: Teratogenic Effects. Pregnancy Category C: Itraconazole was found to cause a dose-related increase in maternal toxicity, embryotoxicity and teratogenicity in rats at dosage levels of approximately 40–160 mg/kg/day (5–20×MRHD) and in mice at dosage levels of approximately 80 mg/kg/day (10× MRHD). In rats, the teratogenicity consisted of major skeletal defects; in mice it consisted of encephaloceles and/or macroglossia.

There are no studies in pregnant women. SPORANOX should be used for the treatment of systemic fungal infections in pregnancy only if the benefit outweighs the potential

risk. SPORANOX should not be administered for the treatment of onychomycosis to pregnant patients or to women contemplating pregnancy. SPORANOX should not be administered to women of child-bearing potential for the treatment of onychomycosis unless they are taking effective measures to prevent pregnancy and the patient begins therapy on the second or third day of the next normal menstrual period. Effective contraception should be continued throughout SPORANOX therapy and for 2 months following treatment.

Nursing Mothers: Itraconazole is excreted in human milk; therefore, SPORANOX should not be administered to nursing women.

Pediatric Use: The efficacy and safety of SPORANOX have not been established in pediatric patients. No pharmacokinetic data are available in children. A small number of patients age 3 to 16 years have been treated with 100 mg/day of itraconazole for systemic fungal infections and no serious unexpected adverse effects have been reported.

In three toxicology studies using rats, itraconazole induced bone defects at dosage levels as low as 20 mg/kg/day (2.5×MRHD). The induced defects included reduced bone plate activity, thinning of the zona compacta of the large bones and increased bone fragility. At a dosage level of 80 mg/kg/day (10× MRHD) over one year or 160 mg/kg/day (20× MRHD) for six months, itraconazole induced small tooth pulp with hypocellular appearance in some rats.

While no such bone toxicity has been reported in adult patients, the long term effect of itraconazole in pediatric patients is unknown.

HIV-infected Patients: Because hypochlorhydria has been reported in HIV-infected individuals, the absorption of itraconazole in these patients may be decreased.

The results from a study in which eight HIV-infected individuals were treated with zidovudine, 8 ± 0.4 mg/kg/day, showed that the pharmacokinetics of zidovudine were not affected during concomitant administration of SPORANOX, 100 mg b.i.d.

ADVERSE REACTIONS

In U.S. clinical trials prior to marketing, there have been three cases of reversible idiosyncratic hepatitis reported among more than 2500 patients. One patient outside the U.S. developed fulminant hepatitis and died during SPORANOX (itraconazole capsules) administration. Because this patient was on multiple medications, the causal association with SPORANOX is uncertain. (See WARNINGS section.)

ONYCHOMYCOSIS:

Adverse events in the following table led to either temporary or permanent discontinuation of treatment:

Body System/Adverse Event	Incidence (%) (n=112)
Elevated Liver Enzymes (>2× normal range)	4%
Gastrointestinal Disorders	4%
Rash	3%
Hypertension	2%
Orthostatic Hypotension	1%
Headache	1%
Malaise	1%
Myalgia	1%
Vasculitis	1%
Vertigo	1%

SYSTEMIC FUNGAL INFECTIONS:

Adverse experience data in the following table are derived from 602 patients treated for systemic fungal disease in U.S. clinical trials, who were immunocompromised or receiving multiple concomitant medications. Of these patients, treatment was discontinued in 10.5% of patients due to adverse events. The median duration before discontinuation of therapy was 81 days, with a range of 2–776 days. The table lists adverse events reported by at least 1% of patients.

Body System/Adverse Event (Incidence ≥ 1%)	Incidence (%)
Gastrointestinal Disorders	
Nausea	10.6
Vomiting	5.1
Diarrhea	3.3
Abdominal Pain	1.5
Anorexia	1.2
Body as a Whole	
Edema	3.5
Fatigue	2.8
Fever	2.5
Malaise	1.2
Skin and Appendages	
Rash	8.6*
Pruritus	2.5
Central and Peripheral Nervous System	
Headache	3.8
Dizziness	1.7
Psychiatric Disorders	
Libido decreased	1.2
Somnolence	1.2
Cardiovascular Disorders	
Hypertension	3.2
Metabolic and Nutritional Disorders	
Hypokalemia	2.0
Urinary System Disorders	
Albuminuria	1.2
Liver and Biliary System Disorders	
Hepatic function abnormal	2.7
Reproductive Disorders, Male	
Impotence	1.2

*Rash tends to occur more frequently in immunocompromised patients receiving immunosuppressive medications.

Adverse events infrequently reported in all studies included: constipation, gastritis, depression, insomnia, tinnitus, menstrual disorder, adrenal insufficiency, gynecomastia and male breast pain.

In worldwide postmarketing experiencce with SPORANOX, allergic reactions including rash, pruritus, urticaria, angioedema and in rare instances, anaphylaxis and Stevens-Johnson syndrome, have been reported. Marketing experiences have also included reports of elevated liver enzymes and rare hepatitis. Although the causal association with SPORANOX is uncertain, rare hypertriglyceridemia and isolated cases of neuropathy have also been reported.

OVERDOSAGE

Itraconazole is not removed by dialysis. In the event of accidental overdosage, supportive measures, including gastric lavage with sodium bicarbonate, should be employed.

No significant lethality was observed when itraconazole was administered orally to mice and rats at dosage levels of 320 mg/kg or to dogs at 200 mg/kg.

DOSAGE AND ADMINISTRATION

SPORANOX (itraconazole capsules) should be taken with a full meal to ensure maximal absorption.

Treatment of blastomycosis and histoplasmosis: The recommended dose is 200 mg once daily (2 capsules). If there is no obvious improvement or there is evidence of progressive fungal disease, the dose should be increased in 100 mg increments to a maximum of 400 mg daily. Doses above 200 mg per day should be given in two divided doses. **Treatment of aspergillosis:** A daily dose of 200 to 400 mg of itraconazole is recommended.

In life-threatening situations: Although these studies did not provide for a loading dose, it is recommended, based on pharmacokinetic data, that a loading dose of 200 mg (2 capsules) t.i.d. (600 mg/day) be given for the first three days. Treatment should be continued for a minimum of three months and until clinical parameters and laboratory tests indicate that the active fungal infection has subsided. An inadequate period of treatment may lead to recurrence of active infection. The above recommendations for the treatment of blastomycosis and histoplasmosis are based on the results of two open-label studies of patients with blastomycosis (n=73) and histoplasmosis (n=34) where results were compared to the expected outcome for untreated patients from historical controls. The recommendation for the treatment of aspergillosis is based primarily on the results of an open-label, single-patient use protocol designed to make itraconazole available in the U.S. for patients who either failed or were intolerant to amphotericin B therapy (n=190), and is supported by two smaller open-label studies (n=31 combined) in the same patient population.

Onychomycosis: The recommended dose is 200 mg once daily for 12 consecutive weeks.

HOW SUPPLIED

SPORANOX (itraconazole capsules) is available as capsules containing 100 mg of itraconazole, with a blue opaque cap and pink transparent body, imprinted with "JANSSEN" and "SPORANOX 100". They are supplied in unit-dose blister packs of 3 × 10 capsules (NDC 50458-290-01) and bottles of 30 capsules (NDC 50458-290-04).

Store at room temperature (59°–86°F/15°–30°C). Protect from light and moisture.

U.S. Patent No. 4,267,179

Rev. April 1995, September 1995

JANSSEN PHARMACEUTICA RESEARCH FOUNDATION Titusville, NJ 08560-0200

Shown in Product Identification Guide, page 318

SUFENTA® ©Ⅱ ℞
[su-fĕn'ta]
(sufentanil citrate)
Injection

CAUTION: Federal Law Prohibits Dispensing Without Prescription

DESCRIPTION

SUFENTA® (sufentanil citrate) is a potent opioid analgesic chemically designated as N-[-4-(methyoxymethyl)-1-[2-(2-thienyl) ethyl]-4-piperidinyl]-N-phenylpropanamide: 2-hydroxy-1,2,3-propanetricarboxylate (1:1) with a molecular weight of 578.68.

SUFENTA is a sterile, preservative free, aqueous solution containing sufentanil citrate equivalent to 50 μg per mL of sufentanil base for intravenous and epidural injection. The solution has a pH range of 3.5–6.0.

CLINICAL PHARMACOLOGY

Pharmacology

SUFENTA is an opioid analgesic. When used in balanced general anesthesia, SUFENTA has been reported to be as much as 10 times as potent as fentanyl. When administered intravenously as a primary anesthetic agent with 100% oxygen, SUFENTA is approximately 5 to 7 times as potent as fentanyl. Assays of histamine in patients administered SUFENTA have shown no elevation in plasma histamine levels and no indication of histamine release. (See dosage chart for more complete information on the intravenous use of SUFENTA).

Pharmacodynamics

Intravenous use

At intravenous doses of up to 8 μg/kg, SUFENTA is an analgesic component of general anesthesia; at intravenous doses ≥ 8 μg/kg, SUFENTA produces a deep level of anesthesia. SUFENTA produces a dose related attenuation of catecholamine release, particularly norepinephrine.

At intravenous dosages of ≥ 8 μg/kg, SUFENTA produces hypnosis and anesthesia without the use of additional anesthetic agents. A deep level of anesthesia is maintained at these dosages, as demonstrated by EEG patterns. Dosages of up to 25 μg/kg attenuate the sympathetic response to surgical stress. The catecholamine response, particularly norepinephrine, is further attenuated at doses of SUFENTA of 25–30 μg/kg, with hemodynamic stability and preservation of favorable myocardial oxygen balance.

SUFENTA has an immediate onset of action, with relatively limited accumulation. Rapid elimination from tissue storage sites allows for relatively more rapid recovery as compared with equipotent dosages of fentanyl. At dosages of 1–2 μg/kg, recovery times are comparable to those observed with fentanyl; at dosages of > 2–6 μg/kg, recovery times are comparable to enflurane, isoflurane and fentanyl. Within the anesthetic dosage range of 8–30 μg/kg of SUFENTA, recovery times are more rapid compared to equipotent fentanyl dosages.

The vagolytic effects of pancuronium may produce a dose dependent elevation in heart rate during SUFENTA-oxygen anesthesia. The use of moderate doses of pancuronium or of a less vagolytic neuromuscular blocking agent may be used to maintain a stable lower heart rate and blood pressure during SUFENTA-oxygen anesthesia. The vagolytic effects of pancuronium may be reduced in patients administered nitrous oxide with SUFENTA.

Preliminary data suggest that in patients administered high doses of SUFENTA, initial dosage requirements for neuromuscular blocking agents are generally lower as compared to patients given fentanyl or halothane, and comparable to patients given enflurane.

Bradycardia is infrequently seen in patients administered SUFENTA-oxygen anesthesia. The use of nitrous oxide with high doses of SUFENTA may decrease mean arterial pressure, heart rate and cardiac output.

SUFENTA at 20 μg/kg has been shown to provide more adequate reduction in intracranial volume than equivalent doses of fentanyl, based upon requirements for furosemide and anesthesia supplementation in one study of patients undergoing craniotomy. During carotid endarterectomy, SUFENTA-nitrous oxide/oxygen produced reductions in cerebral blood flow comparable to those of enflurane-nitrous oxide/oxygen. During cardiovascular surgery, SUFENTA-oxygen produced EEG patterns similar to fentanyl-oxygen; these EEG changes were judged to be compatible with adequate general anesthesia.

The intraoperative use of SUFENTA at anesthetic dosages maintains cardiac output, with a slight reduction in systemic vascular resistance during the initial postoperative period. The incidence of postoperative hypertension, need for vasoactive agents and requirements for postoperative analgesics are generally reduced in patients administered moderate or high doses of SUFENTA as compared to patients given inhalation agents.

Skeletal muscle rigidity is related to the dose and speed of administration of SUFENTA. This muscular rigidity may occur unless preventative measures are taken (see WARNINGS).

Decreased respiratory drive and increased airway resistance occur with SUFENTA. The duration and degree of respiratory depression are dose related when SUFENTA is used at sub-anesthetic dosages. At high doses, a pronounced decrease in pulmonary exchange and apnea may be produced.

Epidural use in Labor and Delivery

Onset of analgesic effect occurs within approximately 10 minutes of administration of epidural doses of SUFENTA and bupivacaine. Duration of analgesia following a single epidural injection of 10–15 μg SUFENTA and bupivacaine 0.125% averaged 1.7 hours.

During labor and vaginal delivery, the addition of 10–15 μg SUFENTA to 10 mL 0.125% bupivacaine provides an increase in the duration of analgesia compared to bupivacaine without an opioid. Analgesia from 15 μg SUFENTA plus 10 mL 0.125% bupivacaine is comparable to analgesia from 10 mL of 0.25% bupivacaine alone. Apgar scores of neonates following epidural administration of both drugs to women in labor were comparable to neonates whose mothers received bupivacaine without an opioid epidurally.

Pharmacokinetics

Intravenous use

The pharmacokinetics of intravenous SUFENTA can be described as a three-compartment model, with a distribution time of 1.4 minutes, redistribution of 17.1 minutes and an elimination half-life of 164 minutes. The liver and small intestine are the major sites of biotransformation. Approximately 80% of the administered dose is excreted within 24 hours and only 2% of the dose is eliminated as unchanged drug. Plasma protein binding of sufentanil, related to the alpha₁ acid glycoprotein concentration, was approximately 93% in healthy males, 91% in mothers and 79% in neonates.

Epidural use in Labor and Delivery

After epidural administration of incremental doses totaling 5–40 μg SUFENTA during labor and delivery, maternal and neonatal sufentanil plasma concentrations were at or near the 0.05–0.1 ng/mL limit of detection, and were slightly higher in mothers than in their infants.

CLINICAL STUDIES

Epidural use in Labor and Delivery

Epidural sufentanil was tested in 340 patients in two (one single-center and one multicenter) double-blind, parallel studies. Doses ranged from 10 to 15 μg sufentanil and were delivered in a 10 mL volume of 0.125% bupivacaine with and without epinephrine 1:200,000. In all cases sufentanil was administered following a dose of local anesthetic to test proper catheter placement. Since epidural opioids and local anesthetics potentiate each other, these results may not reflect the dose or efficacy of epidural sufentanil by itself.

Individual doses of 10–15 μg SUFENTA plus bupivacaine 0.125% with epinephrine provided analgesia during the first stage of labor with a duration of 1–2 hours. Onset was rapid (within 10 minutes). Subsequent doses (equal dose) tended to have shorter duration. Analgesia was profound (complete pain relief) in 80% to 100% of patients and a 25% incidence of pruritus was observed. The duration of initial doses of SUFENTA plus bupivacaine with epinephrine is approximately 95 minutes, and of subsequent doses, 70 minutes.

There are insufficient data to critically evaluate neonatal neuromuscular and adaptive capacity following recommended doses of maternally administered epidural sufentanil with bupivacaine. However, if larger than recommended doses are used for combined local and systemic analgesia, e.g. after administration of a single dose of 50 μg epidural sufentanil during delivery, then impaired neonatal adaption to sound and light can be detected for 1 to 4 hours and if a dose of 80 μg is used impaired neuromuscular coordination can be detected for more than 4 hours.

INDICATIONS AND USAGE

SUFENTA (sufentanil citrate) is indicated for intravenous administration:

as an analgesic adjunct in the maintenance of balanced general anesthesia in patients who are intubated and ventilated.

as a primary anesthetic agent for the induction and maintenance of anesthesia with 100% oxygen in patients undergoing major surgical procedures, in patients who are intubated and ventilated, such as cardiovascular surgery or neurosurgical procedures in the sitting position, to provide favorable myocardial and cerebral oxygen balance or when extended postoperative ventilation is anticipated.

SUFENTA (sufentanil citrate) is indicated for epidural administration as an analgesic combined with low dose bupivacaine, usually 12.5 mg per administration, during labor and vaginal delivery.

SEE DOSAGE AND ADMINISTRATION SECTION FOR MORE COMPLETE INFORMATION ON THE USE OF SUFENTA.

CONTRAINDICATIONS

SUFENTA is contraindicated in patients with known hypersensitivity to the drug or known intolerance to other opioid agonists.

WARNINGS

SUFENTA SHOULD BE ADMINISTERED ONLY BY PERSONS SPECIFICALLY TRAINED IN THE USE OF INTRAVENOUS AND EPIDURAL ANESTHETICS AND MANAGEMENT OF THE RESPIRATORY EFFECTS OF POTENT OPIOIDS.

AN OPIOID ANTAGONIST, RESUSCITATIVE AND INTUBATION EQUIPMENT AND OXYGEN SHOULD BE READILY AVAILABLE.

PRIOR TO CATHETER INSERTION, THE PHYSICIAN SHOULD BE FAMILIAR WITH PATIENT CONDITIONS (SUCH AS INFECTION AT THE INJECTION SITE, BLEEDING DIATHESIS, ANTICOAGULANT THERAPY, ETC.) WHICH CALL FOR SPECIAL EVALUATION OF THE BENEFIT VERSUS RISK POTENTIAL.

Intravenous use

Intravenous administration or unintentional intravascular injection during epidural administration of SUFENTA may cause skeletal muscle rigidity, particularly of the truncal muscles. The incidence and severity of muscle rigidity is dose related. Administration of SUFENTA may produce muscular rigidity with a more rapid onset of action than that seen with fentanyl. SUFENTA may produce muscular rigidity that involves the skeletal muscles of the neck and extremities. As with fentanyl, muscular rigidity has been reported to occur or recur infrequently in the extended postoperative period. The incidence of muscular rigidity associated with intravenous SUFENTA can be reduced by: 1) administration of up to ¼ of the full paralyzing dose of a non-depolarizing neuromuscular blocking agent just prior to administration of SUFENTA at dosages of up to 8 μg/kg, 2) administration of a full paralyzing dose of a neuromuscular blocking agent following loss of consciousness when SUFENTA is used in anesthetic dosages (above 8 μg/kg) titrated by slow intravenous infusion, or, 3) simultaneous administration of SUFENTA and a full paralyzing dose of a neuromuscular blocking agent when SUFENTA is used in rapidly administered anesthetic dosages (above 8 μg/kg).

The neuromuscular blocking agents used should be compatible with the patient's cardiovascular status. Adequate facilities should be available for post-operative monitoring and ventilation of patients administered SUFENTA. It is essential that these facilities be fully equipped to handle all degrees of respiratory depression.

PRECAUTIONS

General: The initial dose of SUFENTA should be appropriately reduced in elderly and debilitated patients. The effect of the initial dose should be considered in determining supplemental doses.

Vital signs should be monitored routinely.

Nitrous oxide may produce cardiovascular depression when given with high doses of SUFENTA (see CLINICAL PHARMACOLOGY).

Bradycardia has been reported infrequently with SUFENTA-oxygen anesthesia and has been responsive to atropine.

Respiratory depression caused by opioid analgesics can be reversed by opioid antagonists such as naloxone. Because the duration of respiratory depression produced by SUFENTA may last longer than the duration of the opioid antagonist action, appropriate surveillance should be maintained. As with all potent opioids, profound analgesia is accompanied by respiratory depression and diminished sensitivity to CO₂ stimulation which may persist into or recur in the postoperative period. Respiratory depression may be enhanced when SUFENTA is administered in combination with volatile inhalational agents and/or other central nervous system depressants such as barbiturates, tranquilizers, and other opioids. Appropriate postoperative monitoring should be employed to ensure that adequate spontaneous breathing is established and maintained prior to discharging the patient from the recovery area. Respiration should be closely monitored following each administration of an epidural injection of SUFENTA.

Proper placement of the needle or catheter in the epidural space should be verified before SUFENTA is injected to assure that unintentional intravascular or intrathecal administration does not occur. Unintentional intravascular injection of SUFENTA could result in a potentially serious overdose, including acute truncal muscular rigidity and apnea. Unintentional intrathecal injection of the full sufentanil/bupivacaine epidural doses and volume could produce effects of high spinal anesthesia including prolonged paralysis and delayed recovery. If analgesia is inadequate, the placement and integrity of the catheter should be verified prior to the administration of any additional epidural medications. SUFENTA should be administered epidurally by slow injection.

Neuromuscular Blocking Agents: The hemodynamic effects and degree of skeletal muscle relaxation required should be considered in the selection of a neuromuscular blocking agent. High doses of pancuronium may produce increases in

Continued on next page

Janssen Pharmaceutica—Cont.

heart rate during SUFENTA-oxygen anesthesia. Bradycardia and hypotension have been reported with other muscle relaxants during SUFENTA-oxygen anesthesia; this effect may be more pronounced in the presence of calcium channel and/or beta-blockers. Muscle relaxants with no clinically significant effect on heart rate (at recommended doses) would not counteract the vagotonic effect of SUFENTA, therefore a lower heart rate would be expected. Rare reports of bradycardia associated with the concomitant use of succinylcholine and SUFENTA have been reported.

Interaction with Calcium Channel and Beta Blockers: The incidence and degree of bradycardia and hypotension during induction with SUFENTA may be greater in patients on chronic calcium channel and beta blocker therapy. (See Neuromuscular Blocking Agents).

Interaction with Other Central Nervous System Depressants: Both the magnitude and duration of central nervous system and cardiovascular effects may be enhanced when SUFENTA is administered to patients receiving barbiturates, tranquilizers, other opioids, general anesthetics or other CNS depressants. In such cases of combined treatment, the dose of SUFENTA and/or these agents should be reduced.

The use of benzodiazepines with SUFENTA during induction may result in a decrease in mean arterial pressure and systemic vascular resistance.

Head Injuries: SUFENTA may obscure the clinical course of patients with head injuries.

Impaired Respiration: SUFENTA should be used with caution in patients with pulmonary disease, decreased respiratory reserve or potentially compromised respiration. In such patients, opioids may additionally decrease respiratory drive and increase airway resistance. During anesthesia, this can be managed by assisted or controlled respiration.

Impaired Hepatic or Renal Function: In patients with liver or kidney dysfunction, SUFENTA should be administered with caution due to the importance of these organs in the metabolism and excretion of SUFENTA.

Carcinogenesis, Mutagenesis and Impairment of Fertility: No long-term animal studies of SUFENTA have been performed to evaluate carcinogenic potential. The micronucleus test in female rats revealed that single intravenous doses of SUFENTA as high as 80 μg/kg (approximately 2.5 times the upper human dose) produced no structural chromosome mutations. The Ames *Salmonella typhimurium* metabolic activating test also revealed no mutagenic activity. See ANIMAL TOXICOLOGY for reproduction studies in rats and rabbits.

Pregnancy Category C: SUFENTA has been shown to have an embryocidal effect in rats and rabbits when given in doses 2.5 times the upper human intravenous dose for a period of 10 days to over 30 days. These effects were most probably due to maternal toxicity (decreased food consumption with increased mortality) following prolonged administration of the drug.

No evidence of teratogenic effects have been observed after administration of SUFENTA in rats or rabbits.

Labor and Delivery: The use of epidurally administered SUFENTA in combination with bupivacaine 0.125% with or without epinephrine is indicated for labor and delivery. (See INDICATIONS AND USAGE and DOSAGE AND ADMINISTRATION sections.) SUFENTA is not recommended for intravenous use or for use of larger epidural doses during labor and delivery because of potential risks to the newborn infant after delivery. In clinical trials, one case of severe fetal bradycardia associated with maternal hypotension was reported within 8 minutes of maternal administration of sufentanil 15 μg plus bupivacaine 0.125% (10 mL total volume).

Nursing Mothers: It is not known whether sufentanil is excreted in human milk. Because fentanyl analogs are excreted in human milk, caution should be exercised when SUFENTA is administered to a nursing woman.

Pediatric Use: The safety and efficacy of intravenous SUFENTA in children under two years of age undergoing cardiovascular surgery has been documented in a limited number of cases.

Animal Toxicology: The intravenous LD_{50} of SUFENTA is 16.8 to 18.0 mg/kg in mice, 11.8 to 13.0 mg/kg in guinea pigs and 10.1 to 19.5 mg/kg in dogs. Reproduction studies performed in rats and rabbits given doses of up to 2.5 times the upper human intravenous dose for a period of 10 to over 30 days revealed high maternal mortality rates due to decreased food consumption and anoxia, which preclude any meaningful interpretation of the results. Epidural and intrathecal injections of sufentanil in dogs and epidural injections in rats were not associated with neurotoxicity.

ADVERSE REACTIONS

The most common adverse reactions of opioids are respiratory depression and skeletal muscle rigidity, particularly of the truncal muscles. SUFENTA may produce muscular rigidity that involves the skeletal muscles of the neck and extremities. See CLINICAL PHARMACOLOGY, WARNINGS and PRECAUTIONS on the management of respiratory depression and skeletal muscle rigidity.

ADULT DOSAGE RANGE CHART for intravenous use

ANALGESIC COMPONENT TO GENERAL ANESTHESIA
•TOTAL DOSAGE REQUIREMENTS OF 1 μG/KG/HR OR LESS ARE RECOMMENDED

ANALGESIC DOSAGES

TOTAL DOSAGE	MAINTENANCE DOSAGE
Incremental or Infusion: 1–2 μg/kg (expected duration of anesthesia 1–2 hours). Approximately 75% or more of total SUFENTA dosage may be administered prior to intubation by either slow injection or infusion titrated to individual patient response. Dosages in this range are generally administered with nitrous oxide/oxygen in patients undergoing general surgery in which endotracheal intubation and mechanical ventilation are required.	**Incremental:** 10–25 μg (0.2–0.5 mL) may be administered in increments as needed when movement and/or changes in vital signs indicate surgical stress or lightening of analgesia. Supplemental dosages should be individualized and adjusted to remaining operative time anticipated. **Infusion:** SUFENTA may be administered as an intermittent or continuous infusion as needed in response to signs of lightening of analgesia. In absence of signs of lightening of analgesia, infusion rates should always be adjusted downward until there is some response to surgical stimulation. Maintenance infusion rates should be adjusted based upon the induction dose of SUFENTA so that the total dose does not exceed 1 μg/kg/hr of expected surgical time. Dosage should be individualized and adjusted to remaining operative time anticipated.
Incremental or infusion: 2–8 μg/kg (expected duration of anesthesia 2–8 hours). Approximately 75% or less of the total calculated SUFENTA dosage may be administered by slow injection or infusion prior to intubation, titrated to individual patient response. Dosages in this range are generally administered with nitrous oxide/oxygen in patients undergoing more complicated major surgical procedures in which endotracheal intubation and mechanical ventilation are required. At dosages in this range, SUFENTA has been shown to provide some attenuation of sympathetic reflex activity in response to surgical stimuli, provide hemodynamic stability, and provide relatively rapid recovery.	**Incremental:** 10–50 μg (0.2–1 mL) may be administered in increments as needed when movement and/or changes in vital signs indicate surgical stress or lightening of analgesia. Supplemental dosages should be individualized and adjusted to the remaining operative time anticipated. **Infusion:** SUFENTA may be administered as an intermittent or continuous infusion as needed in response to signs of lightening of analgesia. In the absence of signs of lightening of analgesia, infusion rates should always be adjusted downward until there is some response to surgical stimulation. Maintenance infusion rates should be adjusted based upon the induction dose of SUFENTA so that the total dose does not exceed 1 μg/kg/hr of expected surgical time. Dosage should be individualized and adjusted to remaining operative time anticipated.

Urinary retention has been associated with the use of epidural opioids but was not reported in the clinical trials of epidurally administered sufentanil due to the use of indwelling catheters. The incidence of urinary retention in patients without urinary catheters receiving epidural sufentanil is unknown; return of normal bladder activity may be delayed.

The following adverse reaction information is derived from controlled clinical trials in 320 patients who received intravenous sufentanil during surgical anesthesia and in 340 patients who received epidural sufentanil plus bupivacaine 0.125% for analgesia during labor and is presented below. Based on the observed frequency, none of the reactions occurring with an incidence less than 1% were observed during clinical trials of epidural sufentanil used during labor and delivery (N=340).

In general cardiovascular and musculoskeletal adverse experiences were not observed in clinical trials of epidural sufentanil. Hypotension was observed 7 times more frequently in intravenous trials than in epidural trials. The incidence of central nervous system, dermatological and gastrointestinal adverse experiences was approximately 4 to 25 times higher in studies of epidural use in labor and delivery.

Probably Causally Related: Incidence Greater than 1%—Derived from clinical trials (See preceding paragraph)
Cardiovascular: bradycardia*, hypertension*, hypotension*.
Musculoskeletal: chest wall rigidty*.
Central Nervous System: somnolence*.
Dermatological: pruritus (25%).
Gastrointestinal: nausea*, vomiting*.
*Incidence 3% to 9%

Probably Causally Related: Incidence Less Than 1%—Derived from clinical trials (Adverse events reported in post-marketing surveillance, not seen in clinical trials, are *italicized.*)

Body as a whole: anaphylaxis.
Cardiovascular: arrhythmia*, tachycardia*, *cardiac arrest*
Central Nervous System: chills*.
Dermatological: erythema*.
Musculoskeletal: skeletal muscle rigidity of neck and extremities.
Respiratory: apnea*, bronchospasm*, postoperative respiratory depression*.
Miscellaneous: intraoperative muscle movement*.
*0.3% to 1%

DRUG ABUSE AND DEPENDENCE

SUFENTA (sufentanil citrate) is a Schedule II controlled drug substance that can produce drug dependence of the morphine type and therefore has the potential for being abused.

OVERDOSAGE

Overdosage is manifested by an extension of the pharmacological actions of SUFENTA (see CLINICAL PHARMACOLOGY) as with other potent opioid analgesics. The most serious and significant effect of overdose for both intravenous and epidural administration of SUFENTA is respiratory depression. Intravenous administration of an opioid antagonist such as naloxone should be employed as a specific antidote to manage respiratory depression. The duration of respiratory depression following overdosage with SUFENTA may be longer than the duration of action of the opioid antagonist. Administration of an opioid antagonist should not preclude more immediate countermeasures. In the event of overdosage, oxygen should be administered and ventilation assisted or controlled as indicated for hypoventilation or apnea. A patent airway must be maintained, and a nasopharyngeal airway or endotracheal tube may be indicated. If depressed respiration is associated with muscular rigidity, a neuromuscular blocking agent may be required to facilitate assisted or controlled respiration. Intravenous fluids and vasopressors for the treatment of hypotension and other supportive measures may be employed.

DOSAGE AND ADMINISTRATION

The dosage of SUFENTA should be individualized in each case according to body weight, physical status, underlying pathological condition, use of other drugs, and type of surgical procedure and anesthesia. In obese patients (more than 20% above ideal total body weight), the dosage of SUFENTA should be determined on the basis of lean body weight. Dosage should be reduced in elderly and debilitated patients (see PRECAUTIONS).

Vital signs should be monitored routinely.

Parenteral drug products should be inspected visually for particulate matter and discoloration prior to administration, whenever solution and container permit.

<u>Intravenous use</u>

SUFENTA may be administered intravenously by slow injection or infusion 1) in doses of up to 8 μg/kg as an analgesic adjunct to general anesthesia, and 2) in doses ≥ 8 μg/kg as a primary anesthetic agent for induction and maintenance of anesthesia (see Dosage Range Chart). If benzodiazepines, barbiturates, inhalation agents, other opioids or other central nervous system depressants are used concomitantly, the

ANESTHETIC DOSAGES

Incremental or Infusion: 8–30 µg/kg (anesthetic doses). At this anesthetic dosage range SUFENTA is generally administered as a slow injection, as an infusion, or as an injection followed by an infusion. SUFENTA with 100% oxygen and a muscle relaxant has been found to produce sleep at dosages ≥ 8 µg/kg and to maintain a deep level of anesthesia without the use of additional anesthetic agents. The addition of N_2O to these dosages will reduce systolic blood pressure. At dosages in this range of up to 25 µg/kg, catecholamine release is attenuated. Dosages of 25–30 µg/kg have been shown to block sympathetic response including catecholamine release. High doses are indicated in patients undergoing major surgical procedures, in which endotracheal intubation and mechanical ventilation are required, such as cardiovascular surgery and neurosurgery in the sitting position with maintenance of favorable myocardial and cerebral oxygen balance. Postoperative observation is essential and postoperative mechanical ventilation may be required at the higher dosage range due to extended postoperative respiratory depression. Dosage should be titrated to individual patient response.

dose of SUFENTA and/or these agents should be reduced (see PRECAUTIONS). In all cases dosage should be titrated to individual patient response.
Usage in Children: For induction and maintenance of anesthesia in children less than 12 years of age undergoing cardiovascular surgery, an anesthetic dose of 10–25 µg/kg administered with 100% oxygen is generally recommended. Supplemental dosages of up to 25–50 µg are recommended for maintenance, based on response to initial dose and as determined by changes in vital signs indicating surgical stress or lightening of anesthesia.
Premedication: The selection of preanesthetic medications should be based upon the needs of the individual patient.
Neuromuscular Blocking Agents: The neuromuscular blocking agent selected should be compatible with the patient's condition, taking into account the hemodynamic effects of a particular muscle relaxant and the degree of skeletal muscle relaxation required (see CLINICAL PHARMACOLOGY, WARNINGS and PRECAUTIONS).
[See table at top of preceding page.]
[See table above.]
In patients administered high doses of SUFENTA, it is essential that qualified personnel and adequate facilities are available for the management of postoperative respiratory depression.
Also see WARNINGS and PRECAUTIONS sections.
For purposes of administering small volumes of SUFENTA accurately, the use of a tuberculin syringe or equivalent is recommended.

Epidural use in Labor and Delivery
Proper placement of the needle or catheter in the epidural space should be verified before SUFENTA is injected to assure that unintentional intravascular or intrathecal administration does not occur. Unintentional intravascular injection of SUFENTA could result in a potentially serious overdose, including acute truncal muscular rigidity and apnea. Unintentional intrathecal injection of the full sufentanil, bupivacaine epidural doses and volume could produce effects of high spinal anesthesia including prolonged paralysis and delayed recovery. If analgesia is inadequate, the placement and integrity of the catheter should be verified prior to the administration of any additional epidural medications. SUFENTA should be administered by slow injection. Respiration should be closely monitored following each administration of an epidural injection of SUFENTA.
Dosage for Labor and Delivery: The recommended dosage is SUFENTA 10–15 µg administered with 10 mL bupivacaine 0.125% with or without epinephrine. SUFENTA and bupivacaine should be mixed together before administration. Doses can be repeated twice (for a total of three doses) at not less than one-hour intervals until delivery.

HOW SUPPLIED
SUFENTA (sufentanil citrate) Injection is supplied as a sterile aqueous preservative-free solution for intravenous and epidural use as:
NDC 50458-050-01 50 µg/mL sufentanil base, 1 mL ampoules in packages of 10
NDC 50458-050-02 50 µg/mL sufentanil base, 2 mL ampoules in packages of 10
NDC 50458-050-05 50 µg/mL sufentanil base, 5 mL ampoules in packages of 10

Incremental: Depending on the initial dose, maintenance doses of 0.5–10 µg/kg may be administered by slow injection in anticipation of surgical stress such as incision, sternotomy or cardiopulmonary bypass.

Infusion: SUFENTA may be administered by continuous or intermittent infusion as needed in response to signs of lightening of anesthesia. In the absence of lightening of anesthesia, infusion rates should always be adjusted downward until there is some response to surgical stimulation. The maintenance infusion rate for SUFENTA should be based upon the induction dose so that the total dose for the procedure does not exceed 30 µg/kg.

Protect from light. Store at room temperature 15°–30°C (59°–86°F).
U.S. Patent No. 3,998,834
May 1995, September 1995
Shown in Product Identification Guide, page 318

VERMOX®   ℞
[vĕr'mŏx]
(mebendazole)
Chewable Tablets

DESCRIPTION
VERMOX® (mebendazole) is a (synthetic) broad-spectrum anthelmintic available as chewable tablets, each containing 100 mg of mebendazole. Inactive ingredients are: colloidal silicon dioxide, corn starch, hydrogenated vegetable oil, magnesium stearate, microcrystalline cellulose, sodium lauryl sulfate, sodium saccharin, sodium starch glycolate, talc, tetrarome orange, and FD&C yellow No. 6.
Mebendazole is methyl 5-benzoylbenzimidazole-2-carbamate.
Mebendazole is a white to slightly yellow powder with a molecular weight of 295.29. It is less than 0.05% soluble in water, dilute mineral acid solutions, alcohol, ether and chloroform, but is soluble in formic acid.

CLINICAL PHARMACOLOGY
Following administration of 100 mg twice daily for three consecutive days, plasma levels of VERMOX® (mebendazole) and its primary metabolite, the 2-amine, do not exceed 0.03 µg/ml and 0.09 µg/ml, respectively. All metabolites are devoid of anthelmintic activity. In man, approximately 2% of administered VERMOX® is excreted in urine and the remainder in the feces as unchanged drug or a primary metabolite.
Mode of Action: VERMOX® inhibits the formation of the worms' microtubules and causes the worms' glucose depletion.

INDICATIONS AND USAGE
VERMOX® (mebendazole) is indicated for the treatment of *Enterobius vermicularis* (pinworm), *Trichuris trichiura* (whipworm), *Ascaris lumbricoides* (common roundworm),

Ancylostoma duodenale (common hookworm), *Necator americanus* (American hookworm) in single or mixed infections. Efficacy varies as a function of such factors as pre-existing diarrhea and gastrointestinal transit time, degree of infection, and helminth strains. Efficacy rates derived from various studies are shown in the table below:
[See first table below.]

CONTRAINDICATIONS
VERMOX® (mebendazole) is contraindicated in persons who have shown hypersensitivity to the drug.

WARNINGS
There is no evidence that VERMOX® (mebendazole), even at high doses, is effective for hydatid disease. There have been rare reports of neutropenia and liver function elevations, including hepatitis, when VERMOX® is taken for prolonged periods and at dosages substantially above those recommended.

PRECAUTIONS
Information for Patients: Patients should be informed of the potential risk to the fetus in women taking VERMOX® (mebendazole) during pregnancy, especially during the first trimester (see Use in Pregnancy).
Patients should also be informed that cleanliness is important to prevent reinfection and transmission of the infection.
Drug Interactions: Preliminary evidence suggests that cimetidine inhibits mebendazole metabolism and may result in an increase in plasma concentrations of mebendazole.
Carcinogenesis, Mutagenesis: In carcinogenicity tests of mebendazole in mice and rats, no carcinogenic effects were seen at doses as high as 40 mg/kg given daily over two years. Dominant lethal mutation tests in mice showed no mutagenicity at single doses as high as 640 mg/kg. Neither the spermatocyte test, the F_1 translocation test, nor the Ames test indicated mutagenic properties.
Impairment of Fertility: Doses up to 40 mg/kg in mice, given to males for 60 days and to females for 14 days prior to gestation, had no effect upon fetuses and offspring, though there was slight maternal toxicity.
Use in Pregnancy: Pregnancy Category C. Mebendazole has shown embryotoxic and teratogenic activity in pregnant rats at single oral doses as low as 10 mg/kg. In view of these findings the use of VERMOX® is not recommended in pregnant women. In humans, a post-marketing survey has been done of a limited number of women who inadvertently had consumed VERMOX® during the first trimester of pregnancy. The incidence of spontaneous abortion and malformation did not exceed that in the general population. In 170 deliveries on term, no teratogenic risk of VERMOX® was identified. During pregnancy, especially during the first trimester, VERMOX® should be used only if the potential benefit justifies the potential risk to the fetus.
Nursing Mothers: It is not known whether VERMOX® is excreted in human milk. Because many drugs are excreted in human milk, caution should be exercised when VERMOX® is administered to a nursing woman.
Pediatric Use: The drug has not been extensively studied in children under two years; therefore, in the treatment of children under two years the relative benefit/risk should be considered.

ADVERSE REACTIONS
Transient symptoms of abdominal pain and diarrhea have occurred in cases of massive infection and expulsion of worms. Hypersensitivity reactions such as rash urticaria and angioedema have been observed on rare occasions. Very rare cases of convulsions have been reported.

OVERDOSAGE
In the event of accidental overdosage gastrointestinal complaints lasting up to a few hours may occur. Vomiting and purging should be induced. Activated charcoal may be given.

Vermox®	Pinworm (enterobiasis)	Whipworm (trichuriasis)	Common Roundworm (ascariasis)	Hookworm
Cure rates mean	95%	68%	98%	96%
Egg reduction mean	—	93%	99%	99%

Vermox®				
	Pinworm (enterobiasis)	Whipworm (trichuriasis)	Common Roundworm (ascariasis)	Hookworm
Dose	1 tablet, once	1 tablet morning and evening for 3 consecutive days.	1 tablet morning and evening for 3 consecutive days.	1 tablet morning and evening for 3 consecutive days.

Consult 1997 supplements and future editions for revisions

Janssen Pharmaceutica—Cont.

DOSAGE AND ADMINISTRATION

The same dosage schedule applies to children and adults. The tablet may be chewed, swallowed, or crushed and mixed with food.

[See table at bottom of preceding page.]

If the patient is not cured three weeks after treatment, a second course of treatment is advised. No special procedures, such as fasting or purging, are required.

HOW SUPPLIED

VERMOX® (mebendazole) is available as chewable tablets, each containing 100 mg of mebendazole, and is supplied in boxes of twelve tablets.
Store at controlled room temperature 15°–30°C (59°–86°F).
JANSSEN PHARMACEUTICA INC.
Titusville, NJ 08560-0200
Rev. October 1992, October 1993
NDC 50458-110-01 (blister package of 12)
U.S. Patent 3,657,267
Shown in Product Identification Guide, page 318

Johnson & Johnson ● MERCK
Consumer Pharmaceuticals Co.
CAMP HILL ROAD
FORT WASHINGTON, PA 19034

Direct Inquiries to:
Consumer Affairs Department
Fort Washington, PA 19034
(215) 233-7000
For Medical Information Contact:
In Emergencies:
(215) 233-7000

ALternaGEL™   OTC
[al-tern 'a-jel]
Liquid
High-Potency Aluminum Hydroxide Antacid

DESCRIPTION

ALternaGEL is available as a white, pleasant-tasting, high-potency aluminum hydroxide liquid antacid.

INGREDIENTS

Each 5 mL teaspoonful contains: Active: 600 mg aluminum hydroxide (equivalent to dried gel, USP) providing 16 milliequivalents (mEq) of acid-neutralizing capacity (ANC), and less than 2.5 mg (0.109 mEq) of sodium and no sugar. Inactive: butylparaben, flavors, propylparaben, purified water, simethicone, and other ingredients.

INDICATIONS

ALternaGEL is indicated for the symptomatic relief of hyperacidity associated with peptic ulcer, gastritis, peptic esophagitis, gastric hyperacidity, hiatal hernia, and heartburn.
ALternaGEL will be of special value to those patients for whom magnesium-containing antacids are undesirable, such as patients with renal insufficiency, patients requiring control of attendant GI complications resulting from steroid or other drug therapy, and patients experiencing the laxation which may result from magnesium or combination antacid regimens.

DIRECTIONS

One to two teaspoonfuls, as needed, between meals and at bedtime, or as directed by a physician: May be followed by a sip of water if desired. Concentrated product. Shake well before using. Keep tightly closed.

WARNINGS

Keep this and all drugs out of the reach of children. ALternaGEL may cause constipation.
Except under the advice and supervision of a physician: do not take more than 18 teaspoonfuls in a 24-hour period, or use the maximum dose of ALternaGEL for more than two weeks. ALternaGEL may cause constipation.
Prolonged use of aluminum-containing antacids in patients with renal failure may result in or worsen dialysis osteomalacia. Elevated tissue aluminum levels contribute to the development of the dialysis encephalopathy and osteomalacia syndromes. Small amounts of aluminum are absorbed from the gastrointestinal tract and renal excretion of aluminum is impaired in renal failure. Aluminum is not well removed by dialysis because it is bound to albumin and transferrin, which do not cross dialysis membranes. As a result, aluminum is deposited in bone, and dialysis osteomalacia may develop when large amounts of aluminum are ingested orally by patients with imparied renal function.
Aluminum forms insoluble complexes with phosphate in the gastrointestinal tract, thus decreasing phosphate absorption. Prolonged use of aluminum-containing antacids by normophosphatemic patients may result in hypophosphatemia if phosphate intake is not adequate. In its more severe forms, hypophosphatemia can lead to anorexia, malaise, muscle weakness, and osteomalacia.

DRUG INTERACTION PRECAUTION

Antacids may interact with certain prescription drugs. If you are presently taking a prescription drug, do not take this product without checking with your physician or other health professional.

HOW SUPPLIED

ALternaGEL is available in bottles of 12 fluid ounces and 1 fluid ounce hospital unit doses. NDC 16837-860.
Shown in Product Identification Guide, page 318

DIALOSE® Tablets   OTC
[di 'a-lose]
Stool Softener Laxative

DESCRIPTION

DIALOSE is a very low sodium, nonhabit forming, stool softener containing 100 mg docusate sodium per tablet. The docusate in DIALOSE is a highly efficient surfactant which facilitates absorption of water by the stool to form a soft, easily evacuated mass. Unlike stimulant laxatives, DIALOSE does not interfere with normal peristalsis, neither does it cause griping nor sensations of urgency.

INGREDIENTS

Active: Docusate Sodium, 100 mg per tablet
Inactive: Colloidal Silicone Dioxide, Dextrates, Flavors, Hydroxypropyl Methylcellulose, Magnesium Stearate, Microcrystalline Cellulose, Polyethylene Glycol, Polysorbate 80, Pregelatinized Starch, Propylene Glycol, Sodium Starch Glycolate, Titanium Dioxide, D&C Red No. 28, D&C Red No. 27 Aluminum Lake, FD&C Blue No. 1, FD&C Blue No. 1 Aluminum Lake, FD&C Red No. 40.

INDICATIONS

DIALOSE is indicated for the relief of occasional constipation (irregularity).
DIALOSE is an effective aid to soften or prevent formation of hard stools in a wide range of conditions that may lead to constipation. DIALOSE helps to eliminate straining associated with obstetric, geriatric, cardiac, surgical, anorectal, or proctologic conditions. In cases of mild constipation, the fecal softening action of DIALOSE can prevent constipation from progressing and relieve painful defecation.

DIRECTIONS

Adults: One tablet, one to three times daily; adjust dosage as needed.
Children 6 to under 12 years: One tablet daily as needed.
Children under 6 years: As directed by physician.
It is helpful to increase the daily intake of fluids by taking a glass of water with each dose.

WARNINGS

Unless directed by a physician: Do not use when abdominal pain, nausea, or vomiting are present. Do not use for a period longer than one week. Do not take this product if you are presently taking a prescription drug or mineral oil.
As with any drug, if you are pregnant or nursing a baby, seek the advice of a health professional before using this product. Keep out of the reach of children.

HOW SUPPLIED

Bottles of 100 pink tablets. Also available in 100 tablet unit dose boxes (10 strips of 10 tablets each). NDC-16837-870.
Shown in Product Identification Guide, page 318

DIALOSE® PLUS Tablets   OTC
[di 'a-lose Plus]
Stool Softener/Stimulant Laxative

DESCRIPTION

DIALOSE PLUS provides a very low sodium tablet formulation of 100 mg docusate sodium and 65 mg yellow phenolphthalein.

INGREDIENTS

Each tablet contains: Actives: Docusate Sodium, 100 mg., yellow phenolphthalein, 65 mg.
Inactive: Dextrates, Dibasic Calcium Phosphate Dihydrate, Flavors, Hydroxypropyl Methylcellulose, Magnesium Stearate, Microcrystalline Cellulose, Polydextrose, Polyethylene Glycol, Polysorbate 80, Propylene Glycol, Sodium Starch Glycolate, Titanium Dioxide, Triacetin, D&C Yellow NO. 10 Aluminum Lake, D&C Red NO. 28, FD&C Blue NO. 1, FD&C Red NO. 40, FD&C Red NO. 40 Aluminum Lake.

INDICATIONS

DIALOSE PLUS is indicated for the treatment of constipation characterized by lack of moisture in the intestinal contents, resulting in hardness of stool and decreased intestinal motility.
DIALOSE PLUS combines the advantages of the stool softener, docusate sodium, with the peristaltic activating effect of yellow phenolphthalein.

DIRECTIONS

Adults: One or two tablets daily as needed, at bedtime or on arising
Children 6 to under 12 years: One tablet daily as needed
Children under 6 years: As directed by physician.
It is helpful to increase the daily intake of fluids by taking a glass of water with each dose.

WARNINGS

Unless directed by a physician: Do not use when abdominal pain, nausea, or vomiting are present. Do not use for a period longer than one week. If skin rash appears do not use this product or any other preparation containing phenolphthalein. Frequent or prolonged use may result in dependence on laxatives. Do not take this product if you are presently taking a prescription drug or mineral oil.
As with any drug, if you are pregnant or nursing a baby, seek the advice of a health professional before using this Keep out of the reach of children.

HOW SUPPLIED

Bottles of 100 yellow tablets. Also available in 100 tablet unit dose boxes (10 strips of 10 tablets each). NDC 16837-871.
Shown in Product Identification Guide, page 318

INFANTS' MYLICON® Drops   OTC
[my 'li-con]
Antiflatulent

INGREDIENTS

Each 0.6 mL of drops contains: Active: simethicone, 40 mg.
Inactive: carbomer 934P, citric acid, flavors, hydroxypropyl methylcellulose, purified water, Red 3, saccharin calcium, sodium benzoate, sodium citrate.

INDICATIONS

For relief of the symptoms of excess gas in the digestive tract. Such gas is frequently caused by excessive swallowing of air or by eating foods that disagree. The defoaming action of INFANTS' MYLICON® Drops relieves flatulence by dispersing and preventing the formation of mucus-surrounded gas pockets in the gastrointestinal tract. INFANTS' MYLICON® Drops act in the stomach and intestines to change the surface tension of gas bubbles enabling them to coalesce, thereby freeing and eliminating the gas more easily by belching or passing flatus.

DIRECTIONS

Infants (under 2 years): 0.3 ml four times daily after meals and at bedtime, or as directed by a physician. The dosage can also be mixed with 1 oz of cool water, infant formula or other suitable liquids to ease administration.
Adults and children: 0.6 ml four times daily, after meals and at bedtime, or as directed by a physician.

WARNINGS

Do not exceed 12 doses per day except under the advice and supervision of a physician. Keep this and all drugs out of the reach of chldren.

HOW SUPPLIED

INFANTS' MYLICON® Drops are available in bottles of 15 ml (0.5 fl oz) and 30 ml (1.0 fl oz) pink, pleasant tasting liquid. NDC 16837-630.
Shown in Product Identification Guide, page 319

FAST-ACTING MYLANTA® AND MAXIMUM-STRENGTH FAST-ACTING MYLANTA®   OTC

[my-lan'ta]

Aluminum, Magnesium and Simethicone
Liquid
Antacid/Anti-Gas

DESCRIPTION

Fast-acting MYLANTA® and Maximum Strength Fast-Acting MYLANTA® are well-balanced, pleasant-tasting, antacid/anti-gas medications that provide consistent, effective relief of symptoms associated with gastric hyperacidity and excess gas. Non-constipating and very low sodium Fast-Acting MYLANTA® and Maximum Strength Fast-Acting MYLANTA® contain two proven antacids, aluminum hydroxide and magnesium hydroxide, plus simethicone for gas relief.

ACTIVE INGREDIENTS

Each 5 mL teaspoon contains:

	MYLANTA®	MYLANTA® Double Strength
Aluminum Hydroxide	200 mg	400 mg
Magnesium Hydroxide	200 mg	400 mg
Simethicone	20 mg	40 mg

INACTIVE INGREDIENTS

LIQUIDS:
Butylparaben, carboxymethylcellulose sodium, flavors, hydroxypropyl methylcellulose, microcrystalline cellulose, propylparaben, purified water, saccharin sodium, and sorbitol.

SODIUM CONTENT

Each 5 mL teaspoon contains the following amount of sodium:

	MYLANTA®	MYLANTA® Double Strength
Liquid	0.68 mg (0.03 mEq)	1.14 mg (0.05 mEq)

ACID NEUTRALIZING CAPACITY

Two teaspoonfuls have the following acid neutralizing capacity:

	Fast Acting MYLANTA®	Maximum Strength Fast Acting MYLANTA®
Liquid	25.4 mEq	50.8 mEq

INDICATIONS

Fast-Acting MYLANTA® and Maximum Strength Fast-Acting MYLANTA® are indicated for the relief of acid indigestion, heartburn, sour stomach, and symptoms of gas and upset stomach associated with those conditions. Fast-Acting MYLANTA® and Maximum Strength Fast-Acting MYLANTA® are also indicated as antacids for the symptomatic relief of hyperacidity associated with the diagnosis of peptic ulcer, gastritis, peptic esophagitis, heartburn and hiatal hernia and as antiflatulents to alleviate the symptoms of mucus-entrapped gas, including postoperative gas pain.

ADVANTAGES

Fast-Acting MYLANTA and Maximum Strength Fast-Acting MYLANTA are homogenized for a smooth, creamy taste. The choice of three pleasant-tasting liquid flavors and the non-constipating formula encourage patient acceptance, thereby minimizing the skipping of prescribed doses. Fast-Acting MYLANTA and Maximum Strength Fast-Acting MYLANTA are also available in tablets, and both the liquid and tablet forms are very low in sodium. Fast-Acting MYLANTA and Maximum Strength Fast-Acting MYLANTA provide consistent relief in patients suffering from distress associated with hyperacidity, mucus-entrapped gas, or swallowed air.

DIRECTIONS

Liquid:
Shake well. 2-4 teaspoonfuls between meals and at bedtime, or as directed by a physician.

WARNINGS

Keep this and all drugs out of the reach of children. Do not take more than 24 tsps of Fast-Acting MYLANTA® or 12 tsps of Maximum Strength Fast-Acting MYLANTA® in a 24-hour period or use the maximum dose of this product for more than two weeks, except under the advice and supervision of a physician. Do not use this product if you have kidney disease.

Prolonged use of aluminum-containing antacids in patients with renal failure may result in or worsen dialysis osteomalacia. Elevated tissue aluminum levels contribute to the development of the dialysis encephalopathy and osteomalacia syndromes. Small amounts of aluminum are absorbed from the gastrointestinal tract and renal excretion of aluminum is impaired in renal failure. Aluminum is not well removed by dialysis because it is bound to albumin and transferrin, which do not cross dialysis membranes. As a result, aluminum is deposited in bone, and dialysis osteomalacia may develop when large amounts of aluminum are ingested orally by patients with impaired renal function.

Aluminum forms insoluble complexes with phosphate in the gastrointestinal tract, thus decreasing phosphate absorption. Prolonged use of aluminum-containing antacids by normophosphatemic patients may result in hypophosphatemia if phosphate intake is not adequate. In its more severe forms, hypophosphatemia can lead to anorexia, malaise, muscle weakness, and osteomalacia.

DRUG INTERACTION PRECAUTION

Antacids may interact with certain prescription drugs. If you are presently taking a prescription drug, do not take this product without checking with your physician or other health professional.

HOW SUPPLIED

Fast-Acting MYLANTA® and Maximum Strength Fast-Acting MYLANTA® are available as white liquid suspensions in pleasant-tasting flavors, Original, Cherry Creme and Cool Mint Creme. Liquids are supplied in bottles of 5 oz, 12 oz, and 24 oz. Also available for hospital use in liquid unit dose bottles of 1 oz and bottles of 5 oz.

MYLANTA®
NDC 16837-610 ORIGINAL LIQUID
NDC 16837-629 COOL MINT CREME LIQUID
NDC 16837-621 CHERRY CREME LIQUID
MYLANTA® Double Strength
NDC 16837-652 ORIGINAL LIQUID
NDC 16837-624 COOL MINT CREME LIQUID
NDC 16837-622 CHERRY CREME LIQUID
Professional Labeling

INDICATIONS

Stress-induced upper gastrointestinal hemorrhage: Maximum Strength Fast-Acting MYLANTA® is indicated for the prevention of stress-induced upper gastrointestinal hemorrhage. Hyperacidic conditions: As an antacid, for the symptomatic relief of hyperacidity associated with the diagnosis of peptic ulcer and other gastrointestinal conditions where a high degree of acid neutralization is desired.

DIRECTIONS

Prevention of stress-induced upper gastrointestinal hemorrhage: 1) Aspirate stomach via nasogastric tube* and record pH. 2) Instill 10 mL of Maximum Strength Fast-Acting MYLANTA® followed by 30 mL of water via nasogastric tube. Clamp tube. 3) Wait one hour. Aspirate stomach and record pH. 4a) If pH equals or exceeds 4.0, apply drainage or intermittent suction for one hour, then repeat the cycle. 4b) If pH is less than 4.0, instill double (20 mL) Maximum Strength Fast-Acting MYLANTA® followed by 30 mL of water. Clamp tube. 5) Wait one hour. If pH equals or exceeds 4.0, see number 7, if pH is still less than 4.0, instill double (40 mL) Maximum Strength Fast-Acting MYLANTA® followed by 30 mL of water. Clamp tube. 6) Wait one hour. If pH equals or exceeds 4.0, see number 7. If pH is still less than 4.0, instill double (80 mL)† Maximum Strength Fast-Acting MYLANTA® followed by 30 mL of water. 7) Drain for one hour and repeat cycle with the effective dosage of Maximum Strength Fast-Acting MYLANTA®.
* If nasogastric tube is not in place, administer 20 mL of Maximum Strength Fast-Acting MYLANTA® orally q2h.
† In a recent clinical study[1] 20 mL of Maximum Strength Fast-Acting MYLANTA®, q2h, was sufficient in more than 85 percent of the patients. No patient studied required more than 80 mL of Maximum Strength Fast-Acting MYLANTA® q2h.
In hyperacid states for symptomatic relief: One or two teaspoonfuls as needed between meals and at bedtime or as directed by a physician. Higher dosage regimens may be employed under the direct supervision of a physician in the treatment of active peptic ulcer disease.

PRECAUTIONS

Aluminum-magnesium hydroxide containing antacids should be used with caution in patients with renal impairment.

ADVERSE EFFECTS

Occasional regurgitation and mild diarrhea have been reported with the dosage recommended for the prevention of stress-induced upper gastrointestinal hemorrhage:

References: 1. Zinner MJ, Zuidema GD, Smigh PL, Mignosa M: The prevention of upper gastrointestinal tract bleeding in patients in an intensive care unit. *Surg Gynecol Obster* 153:214–220, 1981. 2. Lucas CE, Sugawa C, Riddle J, et al.: Natural history and surgical dilemma of "stress" gastric bleeding. *Arch Surg* 102:266–273, 1971. 3. Hastings PR, Skillman JJ, Bushnell LS, Silen W: Antacid titration in the prevention of acute gastrointestinal bleeding: a controlled, randomized trial in 100 critically ill patients. *N Engl J Med* 298:1042–1045, 1978. 4. Day SB, MacMillan BG, Altemeier WA: *Curling's Ulcer, An Experience of Nature.* Springfield, IL, Charles C Thomas Co., 1972, p. 205. 5. Skillman JJ, Bushnell LS, Goldman H, Silen W: Respiratory failure, hypotension, sepsis, and jaundice. A clinical syndrome associated with lethal hemorrhage from acute stress ulceration of the stomach. *Am J Surg* 117:523–530, 1969. 6. Priebe HJ, Skillman J, Bushnell LS, et al. Antacid versus cimetidine in preventing acute gastrointestinal bleeding. *N Engl J Med* 302:426–430, 1980. 7. Silen W: The prevention and management of stress ulcers. *Hosp Pract* 15:93–97, 1980. 8. Herrmann V, Kaminski DL: Evaluation of intragastric pH in acutely ill patients. *Arch Surg* 114:511–514, 1979. 9. Martin LF, Staloch DK, Simonowitz DA, et al.: Failure of cimetidine prophylaxis in the critically ill. *Arch Surg* 114:492–496, 1979. 10. Zinner MJ, Turtinen L, Gurll NJ, Reynolds DG: The effect of metiamide on gastric mucosal injury in rat restraint. *Clin Res* 23:484A, 1975. 11. Zinner M, Turtinen BA, Gurll NJ: The role of acid and ischemia in production of stress ulcers during canine hemorrhagic shock. *Surgery* 77:807–816, 1975. 12. Winans CS: Prevention and treatment of stress ulcer bleeding: Antacids or cimetidine? *Drug Ther Bull* (hospital) 12:37–45, 1981.

Shown in Product Identification Guide, page 318

FAST-ACTING MYLANTA AND MAXIMUM STRENGTH FAST ACTING MYLANTA   OTC

[mylan'ta]

Calcium Carbonate and Magnesium Hydroxide Tablets
Antacid

DESCRIPTION

Fast-Acting MYLANTA and Maximum Strength Fast-Acting MYLANTA are well balanced, pleasant tasting antacid medications that provide consistent, effective relief of symptoms associated with gastric hyperacidity. Non-constipating and very low in sodium, Fast-Acting MYLANTA and Maximum Strength Fast-Acting MYLANTA contain two proven antacids, calcium carbonate and magnesium hydroxide.

Active Ingredients
Each tablet contains:

	Fast-Acting MYLANTA	Maximum Strength Fast-Acting MYLANTA
Calcium Carbonate	350mg	700mg
Magnesium Hydroxide	150mg	300mg

Inactive Ingredients
Citric acid, confectioner's sugar, flavors, magnesium stearate, sorbitol, FD&C Blue 1 or D&C Yellow 10 or D&C Red 27

Sodium Content
Each chewable tablet contains the following amount of sodium:

Fast-Acting MYLANTA	Maximum Strength Fast-Acting MYLANTA
0.3mg	0.6mg

Acid Neutralizing Capacity
Two chewable tablets have the following acid neutralizing capacity:

Fast-Acting MYLANTA	Maximum Strength Fast-Acting MYLANTA
24.0mEq	48.0mEq

INDICATIONS

Fast-Acting MYLANTA and Maximum Strength Fast-Acting MYLANTA are indicated for the relief of heartburn, acid indigestion, sour stomach and upset stomach associated with these conditions. Fast-Acting MYLANTA and Maximum Strength Fast-Acting MYLANTA are also indicated as antacids for the symptomatic relief of hyperacidity associated with the diagnosis of peptic ulcer, gastritis, peptic esophagitis, heartburn and hiatal hernia.

Continued on next page

Johnson & Johnson o Merck—Cont.

DIRECTIONS
Thoroughly chew 2–4 tablets between meals, at bedtime or as directed by a physician.

WARNINGS
Keep this and all drugs out of the reach of children. Do not take more than 10 tablets of Fast-Acting MYLANTA or 20 tablets of MYLANTA Maximum Strength Fast-Acting in a 24-hour period, or use the maximum dosage for more than two weeks. Do not use this product if you have kidney disease, except under the advise and supervision of a physician.

DRUG INTERACTION PRECAUTION
Antacids may interact with certain prescription drugs. If you are presently taking a prescription drug, do not take this product without checking with your physician or other health professional.

HOW SUPPLIED
Fast-Acting MYLANTA is available as a green Cool Mint Creme chewable tablet. Maximum Strength Fast-Acting MYLANTA is available as a green Cool Mint Creme Chewable tablet and pink Cherry Creme chewable tablet.

Fast-Acting Mylanta
NDC 16837-848 Cool Mint Creme
Maximum Strength Fast-Acting MYLANTA
NDC 16837-869 Cherry Creme
NDC 16837-849 Cool Mint Creme

MYLANTA® GAS Relief Tablets   OTC
Maximum Strength MYLANTA® GAS
Relief Tablets
MYLANTA® Gas Relief Gelcaps
[*My-lan'-ta*]
Antiflatulent

ACTIVE INGREDIENTS
Each chewable tablet contains:

	Simethicone
MYLANTA® GAS Relief	80 mg
Maximum Strength	
MYLANTA® GAS Relief	125 mg
MYLANTA® GAS Relief Gelcaps	62.5 mg

INACTIVE INGREDIENTS
TABLETS: Dextrates, flavor, sorbitol, stearic acid, tricalcium phosphate. Cherry: Red 7.
GELCAPS: Benzyl alcohol, butylparaben, castor oil, croscarmellose sodium, D&C Red 28, D&C Yellow 10, dextrose, dibasic calcium phosphate dihydrate, edetate calcium disodium, FD&C Blue 1, FD&C Red 28, gelatin, hydroxypropyl methylcellulose, maltodextrin, methylparaben, microcrystalline cellulose, propylene glycol, propylparaben, silicon dioxide, sodium lauryl sulfate, sodium propionate, sorbitol, stearic acid, titanium dioxide, tribasic calcium phosphate.

INDICATIONS
For relief of the symptoms of excess gas in the digestive tract. Such gas is frequently caused by excessive swallowing of air or by eating foods that disagree. MYLANTA® GAS Relief Gelcaps, MYLANTA® GAS Relief, and Maximum Strength MYLANTA® GAS Relief Tablets are high capacity antiflatulents for adjunctive treatment of many conditions in which the retention of gas is a problem, such as the following: air swallowing, postoperative gaseous distention, peptic ulcer, spastic or irritable colon, diverticulosis. If condition persists, consult your physician.
MYLANTA® GAS Relief Gelcap, MYLANTA® GAS Relief, and Maximum Strength MYLANTA® GAS Relief Tablets have a defoaming action that relieves flatulence by dispersing and preventing the formation of mucus-surrounded gas pockets in the gastrointestinal tract. MYLANTA® GAS Relief Gelcaps, MYLANTA® GAS Relief, and Maximum Strength MYLANTA® GAS Relief Tablets act in the stomach and intestines to change the surface tension of gas bubbles enabling them to coalesce, thereby freeing and eliminating the gas more easily by belching or passing flatus.

DIRECTIONS
MYLANTA® GAS Relief Tablets
One tablet four times daily after meals and at bedtime. May also be taken as needed up to six tablets daily or as directed by a physician.
Maximum Strength MYLANTA® GAS Relief Tablets
One tablet four times daily after meals and at bedtime or as directed by a physician.
TABLETS SHOULD BE CHEWED THOROUGHLY
MYLANTA® GAS Relief Gelcaps
Swallow 2-4 gelcaps as needed after meals and at bedtime. Do not exceed 8 gelcaps per day unless directed by a physician.

WARNINGS
Keep this and all drugs out of the reach of children.

HOW SUPPLIED
MYLANTA® GAS Relief Tablets are available as white (mint) or pink (cherry) scored, chewable tablets identified "MYL GAS 80." Mint flavor is available in bottles of 60 and 100 tablets and individually wrapped 12 and 30 tablet packages. Cherry flavor is available in packages of 12 individually wrapped tablets. Mint NDC 16837-858. Cherry NDC 16837-859.
Maximum Strength MYLANTA® GAS Relief Tablets are available as white, scored, chewable tablets identified "MYL GAS 125" in individually wrapped 12 and 24 tablet packages and economical 48 tablet bottles. NDC 16837-455.
MYLANTA® Gas Relief Gelcaps are available as blue and yellow gelcaps identified as 'MYLANTA GAS' in individually wrapped 24 tablet packages. NDC 16837-626.
Shown in Product Identification Guide, page 319

MYLANTA® SOOTHING LOZENGES   OTC
[*mi-lan'ta*]
ANTACID

DESCRIPTION
MYLANTA® SOOTHING LOZENGES are a dietically sodium free calcium rich antacid which dissolve in your mouth to quickly soothe your heartburn pain or acid indigestion.

INGREDIENTS
Each MYLANTA® SOOTHING LOZENGE contains:

ACTIVE
Calcium Carbonate, 600 mg

INACTIVE
Citric Acid, Corn Syrup, FD&C Red 40, Flavor, Propylene Glycol, Soybean Oil, Sucrose, Titanium Dioxide

INDICATIONS
For the relief of heartburn, acid indigestion, sour stomach and upset stomach associated with these symptoms.

ACID NEUTRALIZING CAPACITY
Each MYLANTA® SOOTHING LOZENGE has an acid neutralizing capacity of 11.4 mEq.

DIRECTIONS
Allow 1 lozenge to dissolve in your mouth and if necessary, follow with a second. Repeat as needed or as directed by a physician.

WARNINGS
Keep this and all other drugs out of the reach of children. Do not take more than 12 lozenges in a 24-hour period or use the maximum dosage for more than two weeks, except under the advice and supervision of a physician.

DRUG INTERACTION PRECAUTION
Antacids may interact with certain prescription drugs. If you are presently taking a prescription drug, do not take this product without checking with your physician or other health professional.

HOW SUPPLIED
MYLANTA® SOOTHING LOZENGES are available as green Cool Mint Creme flavored lozenges, and as pink Cherry Creme flavored lozenges identified as "M". Lozenges supplied in 18 count boxes and 50 count bottles.
NDC 16837-876 (Cherry Creme)
NDC 16837-875 (Cool Mint Creme)
Shown in Product Identification Guide, page 319

PEPCID AC® ACID CONTROLLER™   OTC

DESCRIPTION
ACTIVE INGREDIENT: Famotidine 10 mg per tablet.
INACTIVE INGREDIENTS: Hydroxypropyl cellulose, hydroxypropyl methylcellulose, red iron oxide, magnesium stearate, microcrystalline cellulose, starch, talc, titanium dioxide.

Product Benefits:
- 1 tablet relieves heartburn and acid indigestion.
- Pepcid AC Acid Controller prevents heartburn and acid indigestion brought on by consuming food and beverages.
It contains famotidine, a prescription-proven medicine.
The ingredient in PEPCID AC Acid Controller, famotidine, has been prescribed by doctors for years to treat millions of patients safely and effectively. The active ingredient in PEPCID AC Acid Controller has been taken safely with many frequently prescribed medications.
Action: It is normal for the stomach to produce acid, especially after consuming food and beverages. However, acid in the wrong place (the esophagus), or too much acid, can cause burning pain and discomfort that interfere with everyday activities.

- **Heartburn—Caused by acid in the esophagus**

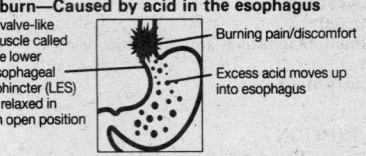

A valve-like muscle called the lower esophageal sphincter (LES) is relaxed in an open position — Burning pain/discomfort — Excess acid moves up into esophagus

In clinical studies, PEPCID AC Acid Controller was significantly better than placebo pills in relieving and preventing heartburn.

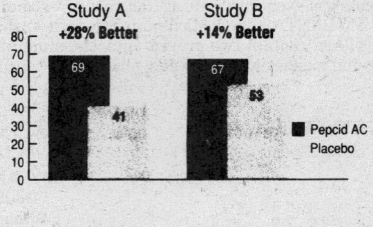

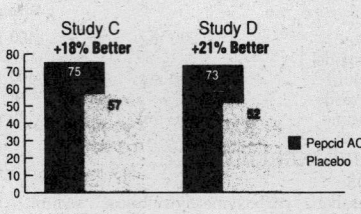

Study A +28% Better — Study B +14% Better — Study C +18% Better — Study D +21% Better — Pepcid AC / Placebo

Uses:
- **For Relief** of heartburn, acid indigestion, and sour stomach;
- **For Prevention** of these symptoms brought on by consuming food and beverages
How to help avoid symptoms
- Do not lie down soon after eating.
- If your are overweight, lose weight.
- If you smoke, stop or cut down.
- Avoid or limit foods such as caffeine, chocolate, fatty foods and alcohol.
- Do not eat just before bedtime.

WARNINGS
- Do not take the maximum daily dosage for more than 2 weeks continuously except under the advice and supervision of a doctor.
- As with any drug, if you are pregnant or nursing a baby, seek the advice of a health professional before using this product.
- If you have trouble swallowing, or persistent abdominal pain, see your doctor promptly. You may have a serious condition that may need different treatment.
- Keep this and all drugs out of the reach of children.
- In case of accidental overdose, seek professional assistance or contact a poison control center immediately.
Caution:
Heartburn and acid indigestion are common, but you should see your doctor promptly if:
- You have trouble swallowing or persistent abdominal pain. You may have a serious condition that may need different treatment.
- You have used the maximum dosage every day for two weeks continously.
Important: As with any drug, if you are pregnant or nursing a baby, seek the advice of a health professional before using this product. This product should not be given to children under 12 years old, unless directed by a doctor. Keep this and all drugs out of the reach of children. In case of accidental overdose, seek professional assistance or contact a poison control center immediately.

DIRECTIONS
- For **Relief** of symptoms **swallow 1 tablet with water.**
- For **Prevention** of symptoms brought on by consuming food and beverages **swallow 1 tablet 1 hour before eating a meal you expect to cause symptoms.**
- Can be used up to twice daily (up to 2 tablets in 24 hours).
- This product should not be given to children under 12 years old unless directed by a doctor.

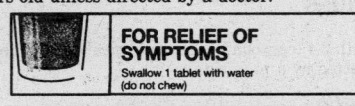

FOR RELIEF OF SYMPTOMS
Swallow 1 tablet with water (do not chew)

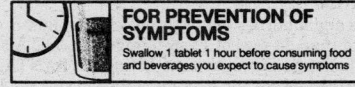

FOR PREVENTION OF SYMPTOMS
Swallow 1 tablet 1 hour before consuming food and beverages you expect to cause symptoms

HOW SUPPLIED

Pepcid AC Acid Controller is available as a rose-colored tablet identified as 'PEPCID AC'.

Pepcid AC is available in blister packs in boxes of 6, 12, 18, 30, 50, and 80 tablets. NDC 16837-872

- Read the directions and warnings before use.
- Keep the carton. It contains important information.

Store at temperatures up to 30°C (86°F).

Protect from moisture.

DO NOT USE IF THE INDIVIDUAL BLISTER UNIT IS OPEN OR BROKEN.

Shown in Product Identification Guide, page 319

Jones Medical Industries, Inc.

**1945 CRAIG ROAD
PO BOX 46903
ST LOUIS, MO 63146**

Direct Inquiries to:
Customer Service:
314-576-6100
Fax:
314-469-5749

BREVITAL® SODIUM
METHOHEXITAL SODIUM
FOR INJECTION, USP
For Intravenous Use

℞

WARNING

This drug should be administered by persons qualified in the use of intravenous anesthetics. Cardiac life support equipment must be immediately available during use of methohexital.

DESCRIPTION

Brevital® Sodium (Methohexital Sodium for Injection, USP) is 2,4,6 (1*H*, 3*H*, 5*H*)-Pyrimidinetrione, 1-methyl-5-(1-methyl-2-pentynyl)-5-(2-propenyl)-, ($\pm$)-, monosodium salt and has the empirical formula $C_{14}H_{17}N_2NaO_3$. Its molecular weight is 284.29.

Methohexital sodium for injection is a freeze-dried, sterile, nonpyrogenic mixture of methohexital sodium with 6% anhydrous sodium carbonate added as a buffer. It contains not less than 90% and not more than 110% of the labeled amount of methohexital sodium. This mixture is ordinarily intended to be reconstituted so as to contain 1% methohexital sodium in Sterile Water for Injection for direct intravenous injection or 0.2% methohexital sodium in 5% dextrose injection (or 0.9% sodium chloride injection) for administration by continuous intravenous drip. This product is oxygen sensitive. The pH of the 1% solution is between 10 and 11; the pH of the 0.2% solution in 5% dextrose is between 9.5 and 10.5.

Methohexital sodium is a rapid, ultrashort-acting barbiturate anesthetic. It occurs as a white, crystalline powder that is freely soluble in water.

The structural formula is as follows:

HOW SUPPLIED

The vials may be stored at room temperature (25°C or below). The expiration period for the vials is 2 years.

Vials*:

500 mg (with 30 mg anhydrous sodium carbonate), 50-mL size, multiple dose (No. 660)—(1s) NDC 0002-1446-01; (25s) NDC 0002-1446-25

500 mg (with 30 mg anhydrous sodium carbonate), 50-mL size, multiple dose, with one 50-mL vial Sterile Water for Injection (No. 760)—(1s) NDC 0002-1465-01

2.5 g (with 150 mg anhydrous sodium carbonate) (No. 663)—(25s) NDC 0002-1448-25

5 g (with 300 mg anhydrous sodium carbonate) (No. 659)—(1s) NDC 0002-1445-01

---

*In crystalline form.

NDC	Product Code	Strength	Embossing	Size
52604-3299-1	NT-1/2	32.4 mg. (1/2 gr.)	JMI NT-1/2	Bottles of 100
52604-3300-1	NT-1	64.8 mg. (1 gr.)	JMI NT-1	Bottles of 100
52604-3308-1	NT-2	129.6 mg. (2 gr.)	JMI NT-2	Bottles of 100

NATURE-THROID
Thyroid Tablets, USP

℞

DESCRIPTION

Thyroid tablets for oral use are prepared from fresh, desiccated animal thyroid glands. Thus, the active thyroid hormones L-thyroxine (T_4) and L-triiodothyronine (T_3) are available in their natural state and ratio attached to a carrier protein and are available for full therapeutic availability. The structural formulas of L-thyroxine (T_4) and L-triiodothyronine (T_3) are as follows:

L-3, 3', 5, 5' tetraiodothyronine (T_4)

L-3, 3', 5 triiodothyronine (T_3)

HOW SUPPLIED

[See table above.]

TABLETS
TAPAZOLE®
METHIMAZOLE TABLETS, USP

℞

DESCRIPTION

Tapazole® (Methimazole Tablets, USP) (1–methylimidazole-2-thiol) is a white, crystalline substance that is freely soluble in water. It differs chemically from the drugs of the thiouracil series primarily because it has a 5-instead of a 6-membered ring.

Each tablet contains 5 or 10 mg (43.8 or 87.6 μmol) methimazole, an orally administered antithyroid drug.

Each tablet also contains lactose, magnesium stearate, starch, and talc.

The molecular weight is 114.16, and the empirical formula is $C_4H_6N_2S$. The structural formula is as follows:

CLINICAL PHARMACOLOGY

Methimazole inhibits the synthesis of thyroid hormones and thus is effective in the treatment of hyperthyroidism. The drug does not inactivate existing thyroxine and triiodothyronine that are stored in the thyroid or circulating in the blood nor does it interfere with the effectiveness of thyroid hormones given by mouth or by injection.

The actions and use of methimazole are similar to those of propylthiouracil. On a weight basis, the drug is at least 10 times as potent as propylthiouracil, but methimazole, may be less consistent in action.

Methimazole is readily absorbed from the gastrointestinal tract. It is metabolized rapidly and requires frequent administration. Methimazole is excreted in the urine.

In laboratory animals, various regimens that continuously suppress thyroid function and thereby increase TSH secretion result in thyroid tissue hypertrophy. Under such conditions, the appearance of thyroid and pituitary neoplasms has also been reported. Regimens that have been studied in this regard include antithyroid agents, as well as dietary iodine deficiency, subtotal thyroidectomy, implantation of autonomous thyrotropic hormone-secreting pituitary tumors, and administration of chemical goitrogens.

INDICATIONS AND USAGE

Tapazole is indicated in the medical treatment of hyperthyroidism. Long-term therapy may lead to remission of the disease. Tapazole may be used to ameliorate hyperthyroi-

dism in preparation for subtotal thyroidectomy or radioactive iodine therapy. Tapazole is also used when thyroidectomy is contraindicated or not advisable.

CONTRAINDICATIONS

Tapazole is contraindicated in the presence of hypersensitivity to the drug and in nursing mothers because the drug is excreted in milk.

WARNINGS

Agranulocytosis is potentially a serious side effect. Patients should be instructed to report to their physicians any symptoms of agranulocytosis, such as fever or sore throat. Leukopenia, thrombocytopenia, and aplastic anemia (pancytopenia) may also occur. The drug should be discontinued in the presence of agranulocytosis, aplastic anemia (pancytopenia), hepatitis, or exfoliative dermatitis. The patient's bone marrow function should be monitored.

Due to the similar hepatic toxicity profiles of Tapazole and propylthiouracil, attention is drawn to the severe hepatic reactions which have occurred with both drugs. There have been rare reports of fulminant hepatitis, hepatic necrosis, encephalopathy, and death. Symptoms suggestive of hepatic dysfunction (anorexia, pruritus, right upper quadrant pain, etc) should prompt evaluation of liver function. Drug treatment should be discontinued promptly in the event of clinically significant evidence of liver abnormality including hepatic transaminase values exceeding 3 times the upper limit of normal.

Tapazole can cause fetal harm when administered to a pregnant woman. Tapazole readily crosses the placental membranes and can induce goiter and even cretinism in the developing fetus. In addition, rare instances of aplasia cutis, as manifested by scalp defects, have occurred in infants born to mothers who received Tapazole during pregnancy. If Tapazole is used during pregnancy or if the patient becomes pregnant while taking this drug, the patient should be warned of the potential hazard to the fetus.

Since scalp defects have not been reported in offspring of patients treated with propylthiouracil, that agent may be preferable to Tapazole in pregnant women requiring treatment with antithyroid drugs.

Postpartum patients receiving Tapazole should not nurse their babies.

PRECAUTIONS

General—Patients who receive Tapazole should be under close surveillance and should be cautioned to report immediately any evidence of illness, particularly sore throat, skin eruptions, fever, headache, or general malaise. In such cases, white-blood-cell and differential counts should be made to determine whether agranulocytosis has developed. Particular care should be exercised with patients who are receiving additional drugs known to cause agranulocytosis.

Laboratory Tests—Because Tapazole may cause hypoprothrombinemia and bleeding, prothrombin time should be monitored during therapy with the drug, especially before surgical procedures (*see* General *under* Precautions).

Periodic monitoring thyroid function is warranted, and the finding of an elevated TSH warrants a decrease in the dosage of Tapazole.

Drug Interactions—The activity of anticoagulants may be potentiated by anti-vitamin-K activity attributed to Tapazole.

Carcinogenesis, Mutagenesis, Impairment of Fertility—In a 2 year study, rats were given methimazole at doses of 0.5, 3, and 18 mg/kg/day. These doses were 0.3, 2, and 12 times the 15 mg/day maximum human maintenance dose (when calculated on the basis of surface area). Thyroid hyperplasia, adenoma, and carcinoma developed in rats at the two higher doses. The clinical significance of these findings is unclear.

Pregnancy Category D—See Warnings—Tapazole used judiciously is an effective drug in hyperthyroidism complicated by pregnancy. In many pregnant women, the thyroid dysfunction diminishes as the pregnancy proceeds; consequently, a reduction in dosage may be possible. In some instances, use of Tapazole can be discontinued 2 or 3 weeks before delivery.

Nursing Mothers—The drug appears in human breast milk and its use is contraindicated in nursing mothers (*see* Warnings).

Usage in Children—See Dosage and Administration.

Continued on next page

Jones Medical—Cont.

ADVERSE REACTIONS

Major adverse reactions (which occur with much less frequency than the minor adverse reactions) include inhibition of myelopoiesis (agranulocytosis, granulocytopenia, and thrombocytopenia), aplastic anemia, drug fever, a lupuslike syndrome, insulin autoimmune syndrome (which can result in hypoglycemia coma), hepatitis (jaundice may persist for several weeks after discontinuation of the drug), periarteritis, and hypoprothrombinemia. Nephritis occurs very rarely.
Minor adverse reactions include skin rash, urticaria, nausea, vomiting, epigastric distress, arthralgia, paresthesia, loss of taste, abnormal loss of hair, myalgia, headache, pruritus, drowsiness, neuritis, edema, vertigo, skin pigmentation, jaundice, sialadenopathy, and lymphadenopathy.
It should be noted that about 10% of patients with untreated hyperthyroidism have leukopenia (white-blood-cell count of less than 4,000/mm^3), often with relative granulopenia.

OVERDOSAGE

Signs and Symptoms—Symptoms may include nausea, vomiting, epigastric distress, headache, fever, joint pain, pruritus, and edema. Aplastic anemia (pancytopenia) or agranulocytosis may be manifested in hours to days. Less frequent events are hepatitis, nephrotic syndrome, exfoliative dermatitis, neuropathies, and CNS stimulation or depression. Although not well studied, methimazole-induced agranulocytosis is generally associated with doses of 40 mg or more in patients older than 40 years of age.
No information is available on the median lethal dose of the drug or the concentration of methimazole in biologic fluids associated with toxicity and/or death.
Treatment—To obtain up-to-date information about the treatment of overdose, a good resource is your certified Regional Poison Control Center. Telephone numbers of certified poison control centers are listed in the *Physicians' Desk Reference* (*PDR*). In managing overdosage, consider the possibility of multiple drug overdoses, interaction among drugs, and unusual drug kinetics in your patient.
Protect the patient's airway and support ventilation and perfusion. Meticulously monitor and maintain, within acceptable limits, the patient's vital signs, blood gases, serum electrolytes, etc. The patient's bone marrow function should be monitored. Absorption of drugs from the gastrointestinal tract may be decreased by giving activated charcoal, which, in many cases, is more effective than emesis or lavage; consider charcoal instead of or in addition to gastric emptying. Repeated doses of charcoal over time may hasten elimination of some drugs that have been absorbed. Safeguard the patient's airway when employing gastric emptying or charcoal.
Forced diuresis, peritoneal dialysis, hemodialysis, or charcoal hemoperfusion have not been established as beneficial for an overdose of methimazole.

DOSAGE AND ADMINISTRATION

Tapazole is administered orally. It is usually given in 3 equal doses at approximately 8-hour intervals.
Adult—The initial daily dosage is 15 mg for mild hyperthyroidism, 30 to 40 mg for moderately severe hyperthyroidism, and 60 mg for severe hyperthyroidism, divided into 3 doses at 8-hour intervals. The maintenance dosage is 5 to 15 mg daily.
Pediatric—Initially, the daily dosage is 0.4 mg/kg of body weight divided into 3 doses and given at 8-hour intervals. The maintenance dosage is approximately ½ of the initial dose.

HOW SUPPLIED

Tapazole® Tablets, are available in:
The 5-mg tablets (UC5385) are white in color, round, beveled, scored, and debossed with "J94".
They are available as follows:

Bottles of 100 (No. 1765)	NDC 52604-1094-1

The 10-mg tablets (UC5386) are white in color, round, beveled, scored, and debossed with "J95".
They are available as follows:

Bottles of 100 (No. 1770)	NDC 52604-1095-1

Store at controlled room temperature, 59° to 86°F (15° to 30°C).
CAUTION—Federal (USA) law prohibits dispensing without prescription.
Literature issued May 1, 1996
Distributed Exclusively by
Jones Medical Industries, Inc.
St. Louis, MO 63146
Mfd. by Eli Lilly and Company
Indianapolis, IN 46285
PV 0370 UCP

THROMBIN, TOPICAL U.S.P. (BOVINE ORIGIN) THROMBIN-JMI™ ℞

Thrombin, Topical (Bovine) must not be injected! Apply on the surface of bleeding tissue.

DESCRIPTION

The thrombin in Thrombin, Topical (Bovine Origin) THROMBIN-JMI™ is a protein substance produced through a conversion reaction in which prothrombin of bovine origin is activated by tissue thromboplastin of bovine origin in the presence of calcium chloride. It is supplied as a sterile powder that has been freeze-dried in the final container. Also contained in the preparation are mannitol, and sodium chloride. Mannitol is included to make the dried product friable and more readily soluble. The material contains no preservative.

HOW SUPPLIED

THROMBIN-JMI™ is supplied in the following packages:
NDC 052604–7100–1
1,000 U.S. unit vial.
NDC 052604–7102–1
5,000 U.S. unit vial with 5 mL diluent.
NDC 052604–7104–3
10,000 U.S. unit vial with 10 mL diluent.
NDC 052604–7105–3
20,000 U.S. unit vial with 20 mL diluent.
NDC 052604–7106–1
50,000 U.S. unit vial.
THROMBIN-JMI™ Spray Kit is supplied in the following packages:
NDC 052604–7104–2
10,000 U.S. unit vial with 10 mL diluent, spray pump and actuator.
NDC 052604–7105–2
20,000 U.S. unit vial with 20 mL diluent, spray pump and actuator.

Key Pharmaceuticals, Inc.

GALLOPING HILL ROAD
KENILWORTH, NJ 07033

For Medical Information Contact:
Generally:
Professional Services Department
(800) 526-4099
(9:00 AM to 5:00 PM EST)
After Hours and Weekends:
(908) 298-4000

Product Identification Codes

To provide quick and positive identification of Key Products, we have imprinted the product identification number of the National Drug Code on most tablets and capsules. In some cases, identification letters also appear.
Additionally: the following telephone numbers are provided for inquiries:

Professional Services Department
9:00 AM to 5:00 PM EST
1-800-526-4099

After regular hours and on weekends (908) 298-4000

IMDUR® ℞
(isosorbide mononitrate)
Extended Release Tablets

DESCRIPTION

Isosorbide mononitrate (ISMN), an organic nitrate and the major biologically active metabolite of isosorbide dinitrate (ISDN), is a vasodilator with effects on both arteries and veins.
IMDUR Tablets contain 30 mg, 60 mg, or 120 mg of isosorbide mononitrate in an extended-release formulation. The inactive ingredients are aluminum silicate, colloidal silicon dioxide, hydroxypropyl cellulose, hydroxypropyl methylcellulose, iron oxide, magnesium stearate, paraffin wax, polyethylene glycol, titanium dioxide, and trace amounts of ethanol.
The chemical name for ISMN is 1,4:3,6-dianhydro-,D-glucitol 5-nitrate; the compound has the following structural formula:
[See chemical structure at top of next column.]
ISMN is a white, crystalline, odorless compound which is stable in air and in solution, has a melting point of about 90°C, and an optical rotation of +144° (2% in water, 20°C).

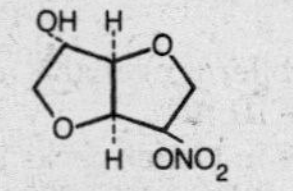

Isosorbide mononitrate is freely soluble in water, ethanol, methanol, chloroform, ethyl acetate, and dichloromethane.

CLINICAL PHARMACOLOGY

Mechanism of Action The IMDUR® product is an oral extended-release formulation of ISMN, the major active metabolite of isosorbide dinitrate; most of the clinical activity of the dinitrate is attributable to the mononitrate.
The principal pharmacological action of ISMN and all organic nitrates in general is relaxation of vascular smooth muscle, producing dilatation of peripheral arteries and veins, especially the latter. Dilatation of the veins promotes peripheral pooling of blood, decreases venous return to the heart, thereby reducing left ventricular end-diastolic pressure and pulmonary capillary wedge pressure (preload). Arteriolar relaxation reduces systemic vascular resistance, and systolic arterial pressure and mean arterial pressure (afterload). Dilatation of the coronary arteries also occurs. The relative importance of preload reduction, afterload reduction, and coronary dilatation remains undefined.
Pharmacodynamics Dosing regimens for most chronically used drugs are designed to provide plasma concentrations that are continuously greater than a minimally effective concentration. This strategy is inappropriate for organic nitrates. Several well-controlled clinical trials have used exercise testing to assess the antianginal efficacy of continuously delivered nitrates. In the large majority of these trials, active agents were indistinguishable from placebo after 24 hours (or less) of continuous therapy. Attempts to overcome tolerance by dose escalation, even to doses far in excess of those used acutely, have consistently failed. Only after nitrates have been absent from the body for several hours has their antianginal efficacy been restored. IMDUR Tablets during long-term use over 42 days dosed at 120 mg once daily continued to improve exercise performance at 4 hours and at 12 hours after dosing but its effects (although better than placebo) are less than or at best equal to the effects of the first dose of 60 mg.
Pharmacokinetics and Metabolism After oral administration of ISMN as a solution or immediate-release tablets, maximum plasma concentrations of ISMN are achieved in 30 to 60 minutes, with an absolute bioavailability of approximately 100%. After intravenous administration, ISMN is distributed into total body water in about 9 minutes with a volume of distribution of approximately 0.6–0.7 L/kg. Isosorbide mononitrate is approximately 5% bound to human plasma proteins and is distributed into blood cells and saliva. Isosorbide mononitrate is primarily metabolized by the liver, but unlike oral isosorbide dinitrate, it is not subject to first-pass metabolism. Isosorbide mononitrate is cleared by denitration to isosorbide and glucuronidation as the mononitrate, with 96% of the administered dose excreted in the urine within 5 days and only about 1% eliminated in the feces. At least six different compounds have been detected in urine, with about 2% of the dose excreted as the unchanged drug and at least five metabolites. The metabolites are not pharmacologically active. Renal clearance accounts for only about 4% of total body clearance. The mean plasma elimination half-life of ISMN is approximately 5 hours.
The disposition of ISMN in patients with various degrees of renal insufficiency, liver cirrhosis, or cardiac dysfunction was evaluated and found to be similar to that observed in healthy subjects. The elimination half-life of ISMN was not prolonged, and there was no drug accumulation in patients with chronic renal failure after multiple oral dosing.
The pharmacokinetics and/or bioavailability of IMDUR Tablets have been studied in both normal volunteers and patients following single- and multiple-dose administration. Data from these studies suggest that the pharmacokinetics of ISMN administered as IMDUR Tablets are similar between normal healthy volunteers and patients with angina pectoris. In single- and multiple-dose studies, the pharmacokinetics of ISMN were dose proportional between 30 mg and 240 mg.
In a multiple-dose study, the effect of age on the pharmacokinetic profile of IMDUR 60 mg and 120 mg (2×60 mg) Tablets was evaluated in subjects ≥45 years. The results of that study indicate that there are no significant differences in any of the pharmacokinetic variables of ISMN between elderly (≥65 years) and younger individuals (45–64 years) for the IMDUR 60 mg dose. The administration of IMDUR Tablets 120 mg (2×60 mg tablets every 24 hours for 7 days) produced a dose-proportional increase in C_{max} and AUC, without changes in T_{max} or the terminal half-life. The older group (65–74 years) showed 30% lower apparent oral clearance (Cl/F) following the higher dose, ie, 120 mg, compared to the younger group (45–64 years); Cl/F was not different between the two groups following the 60 mg regimen. While

Cl/F was independent of dose in the younger group, the older group showed slightly lower Cl/F following the 120 mg regimen compared to the 60 mg regimen. Differences between the two age groups, however, were not statistically significant. In the same study, females showed a slight (15%) reduction in clearance when the dose was increased. Females showed higher AUCs and C_{max} compared to males, but these differences were accounted for by differences in body weight between the two groups. When the data were analyzed using age as a variable, the results indicated that there were no significant differences in any of the pharmacokinetic variables of ISMN between older (≥ 65 years) and younger individuals (45–64 years). The results of this study, however, should be viewed with caution due to the small numbers of subjects in each age subgroup and consequently the lack of sufficient statistical power.

The following table summarizes key pharmacokinetic parameters of ISMN after single- and multiple-dose administration of ISMN as an oral solution or IMDUR Tablets:

[See table above.]

	SINGLE-DOSE STUDIES		MULTIPLE-DOSE STUDIES	
PARAMETER	ISMN 60 mg	IMDUR 60 mg	IMDUR 60 mg	IMDUR 120 mg
C_{max} (ng/mL)	1242–1534	424–541	557–572	1151–1180
T_{max} (hr)	0.6–0.7	3.1–4.5	2.9–4.2	3.1–3.2
AUC (ng·hr/mL)	8189–8313	5990–7452	6625–7555	14241–16800
$t_{1/2}$ (hr)	4.8–5.1	6.3–6.6	6.2–6.3	6.2–6.4
Cl/F (mL/min)	120–122	151–187	132–151	119–140

Food Effects The influence of food on the bioavailability of ISMN after single-dose administration of IMDUR Tablets 60 mg was evaluated in three different studies involving either a "light" breakfast or a high-calorie, high-fat breakfast. Results of these studies indicate that concomitant food intake may decrease the rate (increase in T_{max}) but not the extent (AUC) of absorption of ISMN.

CLINICAL TRIALS

Controlled trials with IMDUR Tablets have demonstrated antianginal activity following acute and chronic dosing. Administration of IMDUR Tablets once daily, taken early in the morning on arising, provided at least 12 hours of antianginal activity.

In a placebo control parallel study, 30, 60, 120, and 240 mg of IMDUR Tablets were administered once daily for up to 6 weeks. Prior to randomization, all patients completed a 1- to 3-week single-blind placebo phase to demonstrate nitrate responsiveness and total exercise treadmill time reproducibility. Exercise tolerance tests using the Bruce Protocol were conducted prior to and at 4 and 12 hours after the morning dose on days 1, 7, 14, 28, and 42 of the double-blind period. IMDUR Tablets 30 and 60 mg (only doses evaluated acutely) demonstrated a significant increase from baseline in total treadmill time relative to placebo at 4 and 12 hours after the administration of the first dose. At day 42, the 120 and 240 mg dose of IMDUR Tablets demonstrated a significant increase in total treadmill time at 4 and 12 hours post dosing, but by day 42 the 30 and 60 mg doses no longer were differentiable from placebo. Throughout chronic dosing rebound was not observed in any IMDUR treatment group.

Pooled data from two other trials, comparing IMDUR Tablets 60 mg once daily, ISDN 30 mg QID, and placebo QID in patients with chronic stable angina using a randomized, double-blind, three-way crossover design found statistically significant increases in exercise tolerance times for IMDUR Tablets compared to placebo at hours 4, 8, and 12 and to ISDN at hour 4. The increases in exercise tolerance on day 14, although statistically significant compared to placebo, were about half of that seen on day 1 of the trial.

INDICATIONS AND USAGE

IMDUR Tablets are indicated for the prevention of angina pectoris due to coronary artery disease. The onset of action of oral isosorbide mononitrate is not sufficiently rapid for this product to be useful in aborting an acute anginal episode.

CONTRAINDICATIONS

IMDUR Tablets are contraindicated in patients who have shown hypersensitivity or idiosyncratic reactions to other nitrates or nitrites.

WARNINGS

The benefits of ISMN in patients with acute myocardial infarction or congestive heart failure have not been established; because the effects of isosorbide mononitrate are difficult to terminate rapidly, this drug is not recommended in these settings.

If isosorbide mononitrate is used in these conditions, careful clinical or hemodynamic monitoring must be used to avoid the hazards of hypotension and tachycardia.

PRECAUTIONS

General Severe hypotension, particularly with upright posture, may occur with even small doses of isosorbide mononitrate. This drug should therefore be used with caution in patients who may be volume depleted or who, for whatever reason, are already hypotensive. Hypotension induced by isosorbide mononitrate may be accompanied by paradoxical bradycardia and increased angina pectoris.

Nitrate therapy may aggravate the angina caused by hypertrophic cardiomyopathy.

In industrial workers who have had long-term exposure to unknown (presumably high) doses of organic nitrates, tolerance clearly occurs. Chest pain, acute myocardial infarction, and even sudden death have occurred during temporary withdrawal of nitrates from these workers, demonstrating the existence of true physical dependence. The importance of these observations to the routine, clinical use of oral isosorbide mononitrate is not known.

Information for Patients Patients should be told that the antianginal efficacy of IMDUR Tablets can be maintained by carefully following the prescribed schedule of dosing. For most patients, this can be accomplished by taking the dose on arising.

As with other nitrates, daily headaches sometimes accompany treatment with isosorbide mononitrate. In patients who get these headaches, the headaches are a marker of the activity of the drug. Patients should resist the temptation to avoid headaches by altering the schedule of their treatment with isosorbide mononitrate, since loss of headache may be associated with simultaneous loss of antianginal efficacy. Aspirin or acetaminophen often successfully relieves isosorbide mononitrate-induced headaches with no deleterious effect on isosorbide mononitrate's antianginal efficacy.

Treatment with isosorbide mononitrate may be associated with light-headedness on standing, especially just after rising from a recumbent or seated position. This effect may be more frequent in patients who have also consumed alcohol.

Drug Interactions The vasodilating effects of isosorbide mononitrate may be additive with those of other vasodilators. Alcohol, in particular, has been found to exhibit additive effects of this variety.

Marked symptomatic orthostatic hypotension has been reported when calcium channel blockers and organic nitrates were used in combination. Dose adjustments of either class of agents may be necessary.

Drug/Laboratory Test Interactions Nitrates and nitrites may interfere with the Zlatkis-Zak color reaction, causing falsely low readings in serum cholesterol determinations.

Carcinogenesis, Mutagenesis, Impairment of Fertility No evidence of carcinogenicity was observed in rats exposed to isosorbide mononitrate in their diets at doses of up to 900 mg/kg/day for the first 6 months and 500 mg/kg/day for the remaining duration of a study in which males were dosed for up to 121 weeks and females were dosed for up to 137 weeks. Isosorbide mononitrate did not produce gene mutations (Ames test, mouse lymphoma test) or chromosome aberrations (human lymphocyte and mouse micronucleus tests) at biologically relevant concentrations.

No effects on fertility were observed in a study in which male and female rats were administered doses of up to 750 mg/kg/day beginning, in males, 9 weeks prior to mating, and in females, 2 weeks prior to mating.

PREGNANCY

Teratogenic Effects *Pregnancy Category B.* In studies designed to detect effects of isosorbide mononitrate on embryo-fetal development, doses of up to 240 or 248 mg/kg/day, administered to pregnant rats and rabbits, were unassociated with evidence of such effects. These animal doses are about 100 times the maximum recommended human dose (120 mg in a 50 kg woman) when comparison is based on body weight; when comparison is based on body surface area, the rat dose is about 17 times the human dose and the rabbit dose is about 38 times the human dose. There are, however, no adequate and well-controlled studies in pregnant women. Because animal reproduction studies are not always predictive of human response, IMDUR Tablets should be used during pregnancy only if clearly needed.

Nonteratogenic Effects Neonatal survival and development and incidence of stillbirths were adversely affected when pregnant rats were administered oral doses of 750 (but not 300) mg isosorbide mononitrate/kg/day during late gestation and lactation. This dose (about 312 times the human dose when comparison is based on body weight and 54 times the human dose when comparison is based on body surface area) was associated with decreases in maternal weight gain and motor activity and evidence of impaired lactation.

Nursing Mothers It is not known whether this drug is excreted in human milk. Because many drugs are excreted in human milk, caution should be exercised when ISMN is administered to a nursing mother.

Pediatric Use The safety and effectiveness of ISMN in children have not been established.

ADVERSE REACTIONS

The table below shows the frequencies of the adverse events that occurred in $>5\%$ of the subjects in three placebo-controlled North American studies, in which patients in the active treatment arm received 30 mg, 60 mg, 120 mg, or 240 mg of isosorbide mononitrate as IMDUR Tablets once daily. In parentheses, the same table shows the frequencies with which these adverse events were associated with the discontinuation of treatment. Overall, 8% of the patients who received 30 mg, 60 mg, 120 mg, or 240 mg of isosorbide mononitrate in the three placebo-controlled North American studies discontinued treatment because of adverse events. Most of these discontinued because of headache. Dizziness was rarely associated with withdrawal from these studies. Since headache appears to be a dose-related adverse effect and tends to disappear with continued treatment, it is recommended that IMDUR treatment be initiated at low doses for several days before being increased to desired levels.

[See table below.]

FREQUENCY AND ADVERSE EVENTS (DISCONTINUED)*

Three Controlled North American Studies					
Dose	Placebo	30 mg	60 mg	120 mg**	240 mg**
Patients	96	60	102	65	65
Headache	15% (0%)	38% (5%)	51% (8%)	42% (5%)	57% (8%)
Dizziness	4% (0%)	8% (0%)	11% (1%)	9% (2%)	9% (2%)

* Some individuals discontinued for multiple reasons.

** Patients were started on 60 mg and titrated to their final dose.

In addition, the three North American trials were pooled with 11 controlled trials conducted in Europe. Among the 14 controlled trials, a total of 711 patients were randomized to IMDUR Tablets. When the pooled data were reviewed, headache and dizziness were the only adverse events that were reported by $>5\%$ of patients. Other adverse events, each reported by $\leq 5\%$ of exposed patients, and in many cases of uncertain relation to drug treatment, were:

Autonomic Nervous System Disorders: Dry mouth, hot flushes.

Body as a Whole: Asthenia, back pain, chest pain, edema, fatigue, fever, flu-like symptoms, malaise, rigors.

Cardiovascular Disorders, General: Cardiac failure, hypertension, hypotension.

Central and Peripheral Nervous System Disorders: Dizziness, headache, hypoesthesia, migraine, neuritis, paresis, paresthesia, ptosis, tremor, vertigo.

Gastrointestinal System Disorders: Abdominal pain, constipation, diarrhea, dyspepsia, flatulence, gastric ulcer, gastritis, glossitis, hemorrhagic gastric ulcer, hemorrhoids, loose stools, melena, nausea, vomiting.

Hearing and Vestibular Disorders: Earache, tinnitus, tympanic membrane perforation.

Heart Rate and Rhythm Disorders: Arrhythmia, arrhythmia atrial, atrial fibrillation, bradycardia, bundle branch

Continued on next page

Key—Cont.

block, extrasystole, palpitation, tachycardia, ventricular tachycardia.

Liver and Biliary System Disorders: SGOT increase, SGPT increase.

Metabolic and Nutritional Disorders: Hyperuricemia, hypokalemia.

Musculoskeletal System Disorders: Arthralgia, frozen shoulder, muscle weakness, musculoskeletal pain, myalgia, myositis, tendon disorder, torticollis.

Myo-, Endo-, Pericardial and Valve Disorders: Angina pectoris aggravated, heart murmur, heart sound abnormal, myocardial infarction, Q-Wave abnormality.

Platelet, Bleeding, and Clotting Disorders: Purpura, thrombocytopenia.

Psychiatric Disorders: Anxiety, concentration impaired, confusion, decreased libido, depression, impotence, insomnia, nervousness, paroniria, somnolence.

Red Blood Cell Disorder: Hypochromic anemia.

Reproductive Disorders, Female: Atrophic vaginitis, breast pain.

Resistance Mechanism Disorders: Bacterial infection, moniliasis, viral infection.

Respiratory System Disorders: Bronchitis, bronchospasm, coughing, dyspnea, increased sputum, nasal congestion, pharyngitis, pneumonia, pulmonary infiltration, rales, rhinitis, sinusitis.

Skin and Appendages Disorders: Acne, hair texture abnormal, increased sweating, pruritus, rash, skin nodule.

Urinary System Disorders: Polyuria, renal calculus, urinary tract infection.

Vascular (Extracardiac) Disorders: Flushing, intermittent claudication, leg ulcer, varicose vein.

Vision Disorders: Conjunctivitis, photophobia, vision abnormal.

In addition, the following spontaneous adverse event has been reported during the marketing of isosorbide mononitrate: syncope.

OVERDOSAGE

Hemodynamic Effects The ill effects of isosorbide mononitrate overdose are generally the results of isosorbide mononitrate's capacity to induce vasodilatation, venous pooling, reduced cardiac output, and hypotension. These hemodynamic changes may have protean manifestations, including increased intracranial pressure, with any or all of persistent throbbing headache, confusion, and moderate fever; vertigo; palpitations; visual disturbances; nausea and vomiting (possibly with colic and even bloody diarrhea); syncope (especially in the upright posture); air hunger and dyspnea, later followed by reduced ventilatory effort; diaphoresis, with the skin either flushed or cold and clammy; heart block and bradycardia; paralysis; coma; seizures and death.

Laboratory determinations of serum levels of isosorbide mononitrate and its metabolites have, in any event, no established role in the management of isosorbide mononitrate overdose. There are no data suggesting what dose of isosorbide mononitrate is likely to be life threatening in humans. In rats and mice, there is significant lethality at doses of 2000 mg/kg and 3000 mg/kg, respectively.

No data are available to suggest physiological maneuvers (eg, maneuvers to change the pH of the urine) that might accelerate elimination of isosorbide mononitrate. In particular, dialysis is known to be ineffective in removing isosorbide mononitrate from the body.

No specific antagonist to the vasodilator effects of isosorbide mononitrate is known, and no intervention has been subject to controlled study as a therapy of isosorbide mononitrate overdose. Because the hypotension associated with isosorbide mononitrate overdose is the result of venodilatation and arterial hypovolemia, prudent therapy in this situation should be directed toward an increase in central fluid volume. Passive elevation of the patient's legs may be sufficient, but intravenous infusion of normal saline or similar fluid may also be necessary.

The use of epinephrine or other arterial vasoconstrictors in this setting is likely to do more harm than good.

In patients with renal disease or congestive heart failure, therapy resulting in central volume expansion is not without hazard. Treatment of isosorbide mononitrate overdose in these patients may be subtle and difficult, and invasive monitoring may be required.

Methemoglobinemia Methemoglobinemia has been reported in patients receiving other organic nitrates, and it probably could also occur as a side effect of isosorbide mononitrate. Certainly nitrate ions liberated during metabolism of isosorbide mononitrate can oxidize hemoglobin into methemoglobin. Even in patients totally without cytochrome b₅ reductase activity, however, and even assuming that the nitrate moiety of isosorbide mononitrate is quantitatively applied to oxidation of hemoglobin, about 2 mg/kg of isosorbide mononitrate should be required before any of these pa-

tients manifest clinically significant (≥10%) methemoglobinemia. In patients with normal reductase function, significant production of methemoglobin should require even larger doses of isosorbide mononitrate. In one study in which 36 patients received 2–4 weeks of continuous nitroglycerin therapy at 3.1 to 4.4 mg/hr (equivalent, in total administered dose of nitrate ions, to 7.8–11.1 mg of isosorbide mononitrate per hour), the average methemoglobin level measured was 0.2%; this was comparable to that observed in parallel patients who received placebo.

Notwithstanding these observations, there are case reports of significant methemoglobinemia in association with moderate overdoses of organic nitrates. None of the affected patients had been thought to be unusually susceptible.

Methemoglobin levels are available from most clinical laboratories. The diagnosis should be suspected in patients who exhibit signs of impaired oxygen delivery despite adequate cardiac output and adequate arterial pO₂. Classically, methemoglobinemic blood is described as chocolate brown, without color change on exposure to air.

When methemoglobinemia is diagnosed, the treatment of choice is methylene blue, 1–2 mg/kg intravenously.

DOSAGE AND ADMINISTRATION

The recommended starting dose of IMDUR Tablets is 30 mg (given as a single 30 mg tablet or as ¹/₂ of a 60 mg tablet) or 60 mg (given as a single tablet) once daily. After several days the dosage may be increased to 120 mg (given as a single 120 mg tablet or as two 60 mg tablets) once daily. Rarely, 240 mg may be required. The daily dose of IMDUR Tablets should be taken in the morning on arising. IMDUR Extended Release Tablets should not be chewed or crushed and should be swallowed together with a half-glassful of fluid.

HOW SUPPLIED

IMDUR Extended Release Tablets (30 mg): rose-colored tablets, scored on both sides and branded with the tradename ("IMDUR") on one side and the strength on the other; bottles of 30 (NDC 0085-3306-02) and 100 (NDC 0085-3306-03); unit-dose packaging of 100 (10 × 10 blister strips) (NDC 0085-3306-01).

IMDUR Extended Release Tablets (60 mg): yellow-colored tablets, scored on both sides and branded with the tradename ("IMDUR") on one side and the strength on the other, repeated on both sides of the score; bottles of 30 (NDC 0085-4110-02) and 100 (NDC 0085-4110-03); unit-dose packaging of 100 (10 × 10 blister strips) (NDC 0085-4110-01).

IMDUR Extended Release Tablets (120 mg): white-colored tablets, branded with the tradename ("IMDUR") on one side and the strength on the other; bottles of 30 (NDC 0085-1153-02) and 100 (NDC 0085-1153-03); unit-dose packaging of 100 (10 × 10 blister strips) (NDC 0085-1153-04).

Store between 2° and 30°C (36° and 86°F).

Protect unit dose from excessive moisture.

IMDUR®

(isosorbide mononitrate)

Extended Release Tablets

Manufactured for Key Pharmaceuticals, Inc., Kenilworth, NJ 07033 by A.B. ASTRA, Sweden.
Copyright © 1993, 1995, Key Pharmaceuticals, Inc.
All rights reserved.
Rev. 8/95

18692902T

Shown in Product Identification Guide, page 319

K-DUR® ℞

Microburst Release System®

(Potassium Chloride) USP

Extended Release Tablets

DESCRIPTION

K-DUR® 20 is an immediately dispersing extended release oral dosage form of potassium chloride containing 1500 mg of microencapsulated potassium chloride USP equivalent to 20 mEq of potassium in a tablet.

K-DUR® 10 is an immediately dispersing extended release oral dosage form of potassium chloride containing 750 mg of microencapsulated potassium chloride USP equivalent to 10 mEq of potassium in a tablet.

These formulations are intended to slow the release of potassium so that the likelihood of a high localized concentration of potassium chloride within the gastrointestinal tract is reduced.

K-DUR is an electrolyte replenisher. The chemical name of the active ingredient is potassium chloride, and the structural formula is KCl. Potassium chloride USP occurs as a white, granular powder or as colorless crystals. It is odorless and has a saline taste. Its solutions are neutral to litmus. It is freely soluble in water and insoluble in alcohol.

K-DUR is a tablet formulation (not enteric coated or wax matrix) containing individually microencapsulated potassium chloride crystals which disperse upon tablet disintegration. In simulated gastric fluid at 37°C and in the absence of outside agitation, K-DUR begins disintegrating into micro-

encapsulated crystals within seconds and completely disintegrates within one minute. The microencapsulated crystals are formulated to provide an extended release of potassium chloride.

Inactive Ingredients: Crospovidone, Ethylcellulose, Hydroxypropyl Cellulose, Magnesium Stearate, and Microcrystalline Cellulose.

CLINICAL PHARMACOLOGY

The potassium ion is the principal intracellular cation of most body tissues. Potassium ions participate in a number of essential physiological processes including the maintenance of intracellular tonicity, the transmission of nerve impulses, the contraction of cardiac, skeletal and smooth muscle and the maintenance of normal renal function.

The intracellular concentration of potassium is approximately 150 to 160 mEq per liter. The normal adult plasma concentration is 3.5 to 5 mEq per liter. An active ion transport system maintains this gradient across the plasma membrane.

Potassium is a normal dietary constituent and under steady state conditions the amount of potassium absorbed from the gastrointestinal tract is equal to the amount excreted in the urine. The usual dietary intake of potassium is 50 to 100 mEq per day.

Potassium depletion will occur whenever the rate of potassium loss through renal excretion and/or loss from the gastrointestinal tract exceeds the rate of potassium intake. Such depletion usually develops as a consequence of therapy with diuretics, primary or secondary hyperaldosteronism, diabetic ketoacidosis, or inadequate replacement of potassium in patients on prolonged parenteral nutrition. Depletion can develop rapidly with severe diarrhea, especially if associated with vomiting. Potassium depletion due to these causes is usually accompanied by a concomitant loss of chloride and is manifested by hypokalemia and metabolic alkalosis. Potassium depletion may produce weakness, fatigue, disturbances of cardiac rhythm (primarily ectopic beats), prominent U-waves in the electrocardiogram, and in advanced cases, flaccid paralysis and/or impaired ability to concentrate urine.

If potassium depletion associated with metabolic alkalosis cannot be managed by correcting the fundamental cause of the deficiency, e.g., where the patient requires long term diuretic therapy, supplemental potassium in the form of high potassium food or potassium chloride may be able to restore normal potassium levels.

In rare circumstances (e.g., patients with renal tubular acidosis) potassium depletion may be associated with metabolic acidosis and hyperchloremia. In such patients potassium replacement should be accomplished with potassium salts other than the chloride, such as potassium bicarbonate, potassium citrate, potassium acetate, or potassium gluconate.

INDICATIONS AND USAGE

BECAUSE OF REPORTS OF INTESTINAL AND GASTRIC ULCERATION AND BLEEDING WITH CONTROLLED RELEASE POTASSIUM CHLORIDE PREPARATIONS, THESE DRUGS SHOULD BE RESERVED FOR THOSE PATIENTS WHO CANNOT TOLERATE OR REFUSE TO TAKE LIQUID OR EFFERVESCENT POTASSIUM PREPARATIONS OR FOR PATIENTS IN WHOM THERE IS A PROBLEM OF COMPLIANCE WITH THESE PREPARATIONS.

1. For the treatment of patients with hypokalemia with or without metabolic alkalosis, in digitalis intoxication and in patients with hypokalemic familial periodic paralysis. If hypokalemia is the result of diuretic therapy, consideration should be given to the use of a lower dose of diuretic, which may be sufficient without leading to hypokalemia.

2. For the prevention of hypokalemia in patients who would be at particular risk if hypokalemia were to develop, e.g., digitalized patients or patients with significant cardiac arrhythmias.

The use of potassium salts in patients receiving diuretics for uncomplicated essential hypertension is often unnecessary when such patients have a normal dietary pattern and when low doses of the diuretic are used. Serum potassium should be checked periodically, however, and if hypokalemia occurs, dietary supplementation with potassium-containing foods may be adequate to control milder cases. In more severe cases, and if dose adjustment of the diuretic is ineffective or unwarranted, supplementation with potassium salts may be indicated.

CONTRAINDICATIONS

Potassium supplements are contraindicated in patients with hyperkalemia since a further increase in serum potassium concentration in such patients can produce cardiac arrest. Hyperkalemia may complicate any of the following conditions: chronic renal failure, systemic acidosis such as diabetic acidosis, acute dehydration, extensive tissue breakdown as in severe burns, adrenal insufficiency, or the administration of a potassium-sparing diuretic (e.g., spironolactone, triamterene, amiloride) (see **OVERDOSAGE**).

Controlled release formulations of potassium chloride have produced esophageal ulceration in certain cardiac patients

with esophageal compression due to enlarged left atrium. Potassium supplementation, when indicated in such patients, should be given as a liquid preparation or as an aqueous (water) suspension of K-DUR (see PRECAUTIONS; Information for Patients, and DOSAGE AND ADMINISTRATION sections).

All solid oral dosage forms of potassium chloride are contraindicated in any patient in whom there is structural, pathological (e.g., diabetic gastroparesis) or pharmacologic (use of anticholinergic agents or other agents with anticholinergic properties at sufficient doses to exert anticholinergic effects) cause for arrest or delay in tablet passage through the gastrointestinal tract.

WARNINGS

Hyperkalemia (see OVERDOSAGE)—In patients with impaired mechanisms for excreting potassium, the administration of potassium salts can produce hyperkalemia and cardiac arrest. This occurs most commonly in patients given potassium by the intravenous route but may also occur in patients given potassium orally. Potentially fatal hyperkalemia can develop rapidly and be asymptomatic. The use of potassium salts in patients with chronic renal disease, or any other condition which impairs potassium excretion, requires particularly careful monitoring of the serum potassium concentration and appropriate dosage adjustment.

Interaction with Potassium Sparing Diuretics—Hypokalemia should not be treated by the concomitant administration of potassium salts and a potassium-sparing diuretic (e.g., spironolactone, triamterene or amiloride) since the simultaneous administration of these agents can produce severe hyperkalemia.

Interaction with Angiotensin Converting Enzyme Inhibitors—Angiotensin converting enzyme (ACE) inhibitors (e.g., captopril, enalapril) will produce some potassium retention by inhibiting aldosterone production. Potassium supplements should be given to patients receiving ACE inhibitors only with close monitoring.

Gastrointestinal Lesions—Solid oral dosage forms of potassium chloride can produce ulcerative and/or stenotic lesions of the gastrointestinal tract. Based on spontaneous adverse reaction reports, enteric coated preparations of potassium chloride are associated with an increased frequency of small bowel lesions (40–50 per 100,000 patient years) compared to sustained release wax matrix formulations (less than one per 100,000 patient years). Because of the lack of extensive marketing experience with microencapsulated products, a comparison between such products and wax matrix or enteric coated products is not available. K-DUR is a tablet formulated to provide a controlled rate of release of microencapsulated potassium chloride and thus to minimize the possibility of a high local concentration of potassium near the gastrointestinal wall.

Prospective trials have been conducted in normal human volunteers in which the upper gastrointestinal tract was evaluated by endoscopic inspection before and after one week of solid oral potassium chloride therapy. The ability of this model to predict events occurring in usual clinical practice is unknown. Trials which approximated usual clinical practice did not reveal any clear differences between the wax matrix and microencapsulated dosage forms. In contrast, there was a higher incidence of gastric and duodenal lesions in subjects receiving a high dose of a wax matrix controlled release formulation under conditions which did not resemble usual or recommended clinical practice (i.e., 96 mEq per day in divided doses of potassium chloride administered to fasted patients, in the presence of an anticholinergic drug to delay gastric emptying). The upper gastrointestinal lesions observed by endoscopy were asymptomatic and were not accompanied by evidence of bleeding (Hemoccult testing). The relevance of these findings to the usual conditions (i.e., nonfasting, no anticholinergic agent, smaller doses) under which controlled release potassium chloride products are used is uncertain; epidemiologic studies have not identified an elevated risk, compared to microencapsulated products, for upper gastrointestinal lesions in patients receiving wax matrix formulations. K-DUR should be discontinued immediately and the possibility of ulceration, obstruction or perforation considered if severe vomiting, abdominal pain, distention, or gastrointestinal bleeding occurs.

Metabolic Acidosis—Hypokalemia in patients with metabolic acidosis should be treated with an alkalinizing potassium salt such as potassium bicarbonate, potassium citrate, potassium acetate, or potassium gluconate.

PRECAUTIONS

General: The diagnosis of potassium depletion is ordinarily made by demonstrating hypokalemia in a patient with a clinical history suggesting some cause for potassium depletion. In interpreting the serum potassium level, the physician should bear in mind that acute alkalosis per se can produce hypokalemia in the absence of a deficit in total body potassium while acute acidosis per se can increase the serum potassium concentration into the normal range even in the presence of a reduced total body potassium. The treatment of potassium depletion, particularly in the presence of cardiac disease, renal disease, or acidosis requires careful attention to acid-base balance and appropriate monitoring of serum electrolytes, the electrocardiogram, and the clinical status of the patient.

Information for Patients: Physicians should consider reminding the patient of the following:
To take each dose with meals and with a full glass of water or other liquid.
To take each dose without crushing, chewing, or sucking the tablets. If those patients are having difficulty swallowing whole tablets, they may try one of the following alternate methods of administration:
a. Break the tablet in half, and take each half separately with a glass of water.
b. Prepare an aqueous (water) suspension as follows:
1. Place the whole tablet(s) in approximately one-half glass of water (4 fluid ounces).
2. Allow approximately 2 minutes for the tablet(s) to disintegrate.
3. Stir for about half a minute after the tablet(s) has disintegrated.
4. Swirl the suspension and consume the entire contents of the glass immediately by drinking or by the use of a straw.
5. Add another one fluid ounce of water, swirl, and consume immediately.
6. Then, add an additional one fluid ounce of water, swirl, and consume immediately.
Aqueous suspension of K-DUR tablets that is not taken immediately should be discarded. The use of other liquids for suspending K-DUR tablets is not recommended.
To take this medicine following the frequency and amount prescribed by the physician. This is especially important if the patient is also taking diuretics and/or digitalis preparations.
To check with the physician at once if tarry stools or other evidence of gastrointestinal bleeding is noticed.

Laboratory Tests: When blood is drawn for analysis of plasma potassium it is important to recognize that artifactual elevations can occur after improper venipuncture technique or as a result of in-vitro hemolysis of the sample.

Drug Interactions: Potassium-sparing diuretics, angiotensin converting enzyme inhibitors (see WARNINGS).

Carcinogenesis, Mutagenesis, Impairment of Fertility: Carcinogenicity, mutagenicity and fertility studies in animals have not been performed. Potassium is a normal dietary constituent.

Pregnancy Category C: Animal reproduction studies have not been conducted with K-DUR. It is unlikely that potassium supplementation that does not lead to hyperkalemia would have an adverse effect on the fetus or would affect reproductive capacity.

Nursing Mothers: The normal potassium ion content of human milk is about 13 mEq per liter. Since oral potassium becomes part of the body potassium pool, so long as body potassium is not excessive, the contribution of potassium chloride supplementation should have little or no effect on the level in human milk.

Pediatric Use: Safety and effectiveness in children have not been established.

ADVERSE REACTIONS

One of the most severe adverse effects is hyperkalemia (see CONTRAINDICATIONS, WARNINGS, and OVERDOSAGE). There have also been reports of upper and lower gastrointestinal conditions including obstruction, bleeding, ulceration, and perforation (see CONTRAINDICATIONS and WARNINGS).

The most common adverse reactions to oral potassium salts are nausea, vomiting, flatulence, abdominal pain/discomfort, and diarrhea. These symptoms are due to irritation of the gastrointestinal tract and are best managed by diluting the preparation further, taking the dose with meals or reducing the amount taken at one time.

OVERDOSAGE

The administration of oral potassium salts to persons with normal excretory mechanisms for potassium rarely causes serious hyperkalemia. However, if excretory mechanisms are impaired or if potassium is administered too rapidly intravenously, potentially fatal hyperkalemia can result (see CONTRAINDICATIONS and WARNINGS). It is important to recognize that hyperkalemia is usually asymptomatic and may be manifested only by an increased serum potassium concentration (6.5–8.0 mEq/L) and characteristic electrocardiographic changes (peaking of T-waves, loss of P-waves, depression of S-T segment, and prolongation of the QT-interval). Late manifestations include muscle-paralysis and cardiovascular collapse from cardiac arrest. (9–12 mEq/L).
Treatment measures for hyperkalemia include the following:
1. Elimination of foods and medications containing potassium and of any agents with potassium-sparing properties.
2. Intravenous administration of 300 to 500 mL/hr of 10% dextrose solution containing 10–20 units of crystalline insulin per 1,000 mL.
3. Correction of acidosis, if present, with intravenous sodium bicarbonate.
4. Use of exchange resins, hemodialysis, or peritoneal dialysis.
In treating hyperkalemia, it should be recalled that in patients who have been stabilized on digitalis, too rapid a lowering of the serum potassium concentration can produce digitalis toxicity.

DOSAGE AND ADMINISTRATION

The usual dietary intake of potassium by the average adult is 50 to 100 mEq per day. Potassium depletion sufficient to cause hypokalemia usually requires the loss of 200 or more mEq of potassium from the total body store.

Dosage must be adjusted to the individual needs of each patient. The dose for the prevention of hypokalemia is typically in the range of 20 mEq per day. Doses of 40–100 mEq per day or more are used for the treatment of potassium depletion. Dosage should be divided if more than 20 mEq per day is given such that no more than 20 mEq is given in a single dose.

Each K-DUR 20 tablet provides 20 mEq of potassium chloride.
Each K-DUR 10 tablet provides 10 mEq of potassium chloride.

K-DUR tablets should be taken with meals and with a glass of water or other liquid. This product should not be taken on an empty stomach because of its potential for gastric irritation (see WARNINGS).

Patients having difficulty swallowing whole tablets may try one of the following alternate methods of administration:
a. Break the tablet in half, and take each half separately with a glass of water.
b. Prepare an aqueous (water) suspension as follows:
1. Place the whole tablet(s) in approximately one-half glass of water (4 fluid ounces).
2. Allow approximately 2 minutes for the tablet(s) to disintegrate.
3. Stir for about half a minute after the tablet(s) has disintegrated.
4. Swirl the suspension and consume the entire contents of the glass immediately by drinking or by the use of a straw.
5. Add another one fluid ounce of water, swirl, and consume immediately.
6. Then, add an additional one fluid ounce of water, swirl, and consume immediately.
Aqueous suspension of K-DUR tablets that is not taken immediately should be discarded. The use of other liquids for suspending K-DUR tablets is not recommended.

HOW SUPPLIED

K-DUR 20 mEq Extended Release Tablets are available in bottles of 100 (NDC 0085-0787-01); bottles of 500 (NDC 0085-0787-06); bottles of 1000 (NDC 0085-0787-10) and boxes of 100 for unit dose dispensing (NDC 0085-0787-81). K-DUR 20 mEq tablets are white, oblong, imprinted K-DUR 20 and scored for flexibility of dosing.
K-DUR 10 mEq Extended Release Tablets are available in bottles of 100 (NDC 0085-0263-01) and boxes of 100 for unit dose dispensing (NDC 0085-0263-81). K-DUR 10 mEq tablets are white, oblong, imprinted K-DUR 10.

STORAGE CONDITIONS

Keep tightly closed. Store at controlled room temperature 15–30°C (59–86°F).

CAUTION

Federal law prohibits dispensing without prescription.
Rev. 4/90   14274766
Copyright © 1986, 1989, 1990,
Key Pharmaceuticals, Inc.
All rights reserved.

Shown in Product Identification Guide, page 319

NITRO–DUR®   ℞
(nitroglycerin)
Transdermal Infusion System

DESCRIPTION

Nitroglycerin is 1,2,3-propanetriol trinitrate, an organic nitrate whose structural formula is:

$$\begin{array}{l} H_2CONO_2 \\ | \\ HCONO_2 \\ | \\ H_2CONO_2 \end{array}$$

and whose molecular weight is 227.09. The organic nitrates are vasodilators, active on both arteries and veins.
The NITRO-DUR (nitroglycerin) Transdermal Infusion System is a flat unit designed to provide continuous controlled release of nitroglycerin through intact skin. The rate of release of nitroglycerin is linearly dependent upon the area of the applied system; each cm² of applied system delivers ap-

Continued on next page

Key—Cont.

proximately 0.02 mg of nitroglycerin per hour. Thus, the 5-, 10-, 15-, 20-, 30-, and 40-cm^2 systems deliver approximately 0.1, 0.2, 0.3, 0.4, 0.6, and 0.8 mg of nitroglycerin per hour, respectively.

The remainder of the nitroglycerin in each system serves as a reservoir and is not delivered in normal use. After 12 hours, for example, each system has delivered approximately 6% of its original content of nitroglycerin.

The NITRO-DUR transdermal system contains nitroglycerin in acrylic-based polymer adhesives with a resinous cross-linking agent to provide a continuous source of active ingredient. Each unit is sealed in a paper polyethylene-foil pouch.

Cross section of the system.

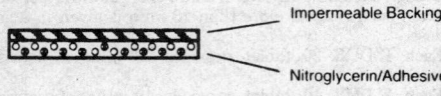

Impermeable Backing

Nitroglycerin/Adhesive

CLINICAL PHARMACOLOGY

The principal pharmacological action of nitroglycerin is relaxation of vascular smooth muscle and consequent dilatation of peripheral arteries and veins, especially the latter. Dilatation of the veins promotes peripheral pooling of blood and decreases venous return to the heart, thereby reducing left ventricular end-diastolic pressure and pulmonary capillary wedge pressure (preload). Arteriolar relaxation reduces systemic vascular resistance, systolic arterial pressure, and mean arterial pressure (afterload). Dilatation of the coronary arteries also occurs. The relative importance of preload reduction, afterload reduction, and coronary dilatation remains undefined.

Dosing regimens for most chronically used drugs are designed to provide plasma concentrations that are continuously greater than a minimally effective concentration. This strategy is inappropriate for organic nitrates. Several well-controlled clinical trials have used exercise testing to assess the antianginal efficacy of continuously delivered nitrates. In the large majority of these trials, active agents were indistinguishable from placebo after 24 hours (or less) of continuous therapy. Attempts to overcome nitrate tolerance by dose escalation, even to doses far in excess of those used acutely, have consistently failed. Only after nitrates have been absent from the body for several hours has their antianginal efficacy been restored.

Pharmacokinetics: The volume of distribution of nitroglycerin is about 3 L/kg, and nitroglycerin is cleared from this volume at extremely rapid rates, with a resulting serum half-life of about 3 minutes. The observed clearance rates (close to 1 L/kg/min) greatly exceed hepatic blood flow; known sites of extrahepatic metabolism include red blood cells and vascular walls.

The first products in the metabolism of nitroglycerin are inorganic nitrate and the 1,2- and 1,3-dinitroglycerols. The dinitrates are less effective vasodilators than nitroglycerin, but they are longer-lived in the serum, and their net contribution to the overall effect of chronic nitroglycerin regimens is not known. The dinitrates are further metabolized to (non-vasoactive) mononitrates and, ultimately, to glycerol and carbon dioxide.

To avoid development of tolerance to nitroglycerin, drug-free intervals of 10–12 hours are known to be sufficient; shorter intervals have not been well studied. In one well-controlled clinical trial, subjects receiving nitroglycerin appeared to exhibit a rebound or withdrawal effect, so that their exercise tolerance at the end of the daily drug-free interval was *less* than that exhibited by the parallel group receiving placebo. In healthy volunteers, steady-state plasma concentrations of nitroglycerin are reached by about 2 hours after application of a patch and are maintained for the duration of wearing the system (observations have been limited to 24 hours). Upon removal of the patch, the plasma concentration declines with a half-life of about an hour.

Clinical Trials: Regimens in which nitroglycerin patches were worn for 12 hours daily have been studied in well-controlled trials up to 4 weeks in duration. Starting about 2 hours after application and continuing until 10–12 hours after application, patches that deliver at least 0.4 mg of nitroglycerin per hour have consistently demonstrated greater antianginal activity than placebo. Lower-dose patches have not been as well studied, but in one large, well-controlled trial in which higher-dose patches were also studied, patches delivering 0.2 mg/hr had significantly *less* antianginal activity than placebo.

It is reasonable to believe that the rate of nitroglycerin absorption from patches may vary with the site of application, but this relationship has not been adequately studied.

INDICATIONS AND USAGE

Transdermal nitroglycerin is indicated for the prevention of angina pectoris due to coronary artery disease. The onset of action of transdermal nitroglycerin is not sufficiently rapid for this product to be useful in aborting an acute attack.

CONTRAINDICATIONS

Allergic reactions to organic nitrates are extremely rare, but they do occur. Nitroglycerin is contraindicated in patients who are allergic to it. Allergy to the adhesives used in nitroglycerin patches has also been reported, and it similarly constitutes a contraindication to the use of this product.

WARNINGS

The benefits of transdermal nitroglycerin in patients with acute myocardial infarction or congestive heart failure have not been established. If one elects to use nitroglycerin in these conditions, careful clinical or hemodynamic monitoring must be used to avoid the hazards of hypotension and tachycardia.

A cardioverter/defibrillator should not be discharged through a paddle electrode that overlies a NITRO-DUR patch. The arcing that may be seen in this situation is harmless in itself, but it may be associated with local current concentration that can cause damage to the paddles and burns to the patient.

PRECAUTIONS

General: Severe hypotension, particularly with upright posture, may occur with even small doses of nitroglycerin. This drug should therefore be used with caution in patients who may be volume depleted or who, for whatever reason, are already hypotensive. Hypotension induced by nitroglycerin may be accompanied by paradoxical bradycardia and increased angina pectoris.

Nitrate therapy may aggravate the angina caused by hypertrophic cardiomyopathy.

As tolerance to other forms of nitroglycerin develops, the effects of sublingual nitroglycerin on exercise tolerance, although still observable, is somewhat blunted.

In industrial workers who have had long-term exposure to unknown (presumably high) doses of organic nitrates, tolerance clearly occurs. Chest pain, acute myocardial infarction, and even sudden death have occurred during temporary withdrawal of nitrates from these workers, demonstrating the existence of true physical dependence.

Several clinical trials in patients with angina pectoris have evaluated nitroglycerin regimens which incorporated a 10- to 12-hour, nitrate-free interval. In some of these trials, an increase in the frequency of anginal attacks during the nitrate-free interval was observed in a small number of patients. In one trial, patients had decreased exercise tolerance at the end of the nitrate-free interval. Hemodynamic rebound has been observed only rarely; on the other hand, few studies were so designed that rebound, if it had occurred, would have been detected. The importance of these observations to the routine, clinical use of transdermal nitroglycerin is unknown.

Information for Patients: Daily headaches sometimes accompany treatment with nitroglycerin. In patients who get these headaches, the headaches may be a marker of the activity of the drug. Patients should resist the temptation to avoid headaches by altering the schedule of their treatment with nitroglycerin, since loss of headache may be associated with simultaneous loss of antianginal efficacy.

Treatment with nitroglycerin may be associated with lightheadedness on standing, especially just after rising from a recumbent or seated position. This effect may be more frequent in patients who have also consumed alcohol.

After normal use, there is enough residual nitroglycerin in discarded patches that they are a potential hazard to children and pets.

A patient leaflet is supplied with the systems.

Drug Interactions: The vasodilating effects of nitroglycerin may be additive with those of other vasodilators. Alcohol, in particular, has been found to exhibit additive effects of this variety.

Carcinogenesis, Mutagenesis, Impairment of Fertility: Animal carcinogenesis studies with topically applied nitroglycerin have not been performed.

Rats receiving up to 434 mg/kg/day of dietary nitroglycerin for 2 years developed dose-related fibrotic and neoplastic changes in liver, including carcinomas, and interstitial cell tumors in testes. At high dose, the incidences of hepatocellular carcinomas in both sexes were 52% vs. 0% in controls, and incidences of testicular tumors were 52% vs. 8% in controls. Lifetime dietary administration of up to 1058 mg/kg/day of nitroglycerin was not tumorigenic in mice.

Nitroglycerin was weakly mutagenic in Ames tests performed in two different laboratories. Nevertheless, there was no evidence of mutagenicity in an *in vivo* dominant lethal assay with male rats treated with doses up to about 363 mg/kg/day, p.o., or in *in vitro* cytogenetic tests in rat and dog tissues.

In a three-generation reproduction study, rats received dietary nitroglycerin at doses up to about 434 mg/kg/day for 6 months prior to mating of the F_0 generation with treatment continuing through successive F_1 and F_2 generations. The high dose was associated with decreased feed intake and body weight gain in both sexes at all matings. No specific effect on the fertility of the F_0 generation was seen. Infertility noted in subsequent generations, however, was attributed to increased interstitial cell tissue and aspermatogenesis in the high-dose males. In this three-generation study there was no clear evidence of teratogenicity.

Pregnancy: Pregnancy Category C:
Animal teratology studies have not been conducted with nitroglycerin transdermal systems. Teratology studies in rats and rabbits, however, were conducted with topically applied nitroglycerin ointment at doses up to 80 mg/kg/day and 240 mg/kg/day, respectively. No toxic effects on dams or fetuses were seen at any dose tested. There are no adequate and well-controlled studies in pregnant women. Nitroglycerin should be given to a pregnant woman only if clearly needed.

Nursing Mothers: It is not known whether nitroglycerin is excreted in human milk. Because many drugs are excreted in human milk, caution should be exercised when nitroglycerin is administered to a nursing woman.

Pediatric Use: Safety and effectiveness in children have not been established.

ADVERSE REACTIONS

Adverse reactions to nitroglycerin are generally dose related, and almost all of these reactions are the result of nitroglycerin's activity as a vasodilator. Headache, which may be severe, is the most commonly reported side effect. Headache may be recurrent with each daily dose, especially at higher doses. Transient episodes of lightheadedness, occasionally related to blood pressure changes, may also occur. Hypotension occurs infrequently, but in some patients it may be severe enough to warrant discontinuation of therapy. Syncope, crescendo angina, and rebound hypertension have been reported but are uncommon.

Allergic reactions to nitroglycerin are also uncommon, and the great majority of those reported have been cases of contact dermatitis or fixed drug eruptions in patients receiving nitroglycerin in ointments or patches. There have been few reports of genuine anaphylactoid reactions, and these reactions can probably occur in patients receiving nitroglycerin by any route.

Extremely rarely, ordinary doses of organic nitrates have caused methemoglobinemia in normal-seeming patients. Methemoglobinemia is so infrequent at these doses that further discussion of its diagnosis and treatment is deferred (see **OVERDOSAGE**).

Application-site irritation may occur but is rarely severe.

In two placebo-controlled trials of intermittent therapy with nitroglycerin patches at 0.2 to 0.8 mg/hr, the most frequent adverse reactions among 307 subjects were as follows:

	Placebo	Patch
Headache	18%	63%
Lightheadedness	4%	6%
Hypotension, and/or Syncope	0%	4%
Increased Angina	2%	2%

OVERDOSAGE

Hemodynamic Effects: The ill effects of nitroglycerin overdose are generally the results of nitroglycerin's capacity to induce vasodilatation, venous pooling, reduced cardiac output, and hypotension. These hemodynamic changes may have protean manifestations, including increased intracranial pressure, with any or all of persistent throbbing headache, confusion, and moderate fever; vertigo; palpitations; visual disturbances; nausea and vomiting (possibly with colic and even bloody diarrhea); syncope (especially in the upright posture); air hunger and dyspnea, later followed by reduced ventilatory effort; diaphoresis, with the skin either flushed or cold and clammy; heart block and bradycardia; paralysis; coma; seizures; and death.

Laboratory determinations of serum levels of nitroglycerin and its metabolites are not widely available, and such determinations have, in any event, no established role in the management of nitroglycerin overdose.

No data are available to suggest physiological maneuvers (eg, maneuvers to change the pH of the urine) that might accelerate elimination of nitroglycerin and its active metabolites. Similarly, it is not known which—if any—of these substances can usefully be removed from the body by hemodialysis.

No specific antagonist to the vasodilator effects of nitroglycerin is known, and no intervention has been subject to controlled study as a therapy of nitroglycerin overdose. Because the hypotension associated with nitroglycerin overdose is the result of venodilatation and arterial hypovolemia, prudent therapy in this situation should be directed toward increase in central fluid volume. Passive elevation of the patient's legs may be sufficient, but intravenous infusion of normal saline or similar fluid may also be necessary.

The use of epinephrine or other arterial vasoconstrictors in this setting is likely to do more harm than good.

In patients with renal disease or congestive heart failure, therapy resulting in central volume expansion is not without hazard. Treatment of nitroglycerin overdose in these patients may be subtle and difficult, and invasive monitoring may be required.

NITRO-DUR System Rated Release In Vivo*	Total Nitroglycerin Content	System Size	Package Size
0.1 mg/hr	20 mg	5 cm²	Unit Dose 30 (NDC 0085-3305-30) Hospital Unit Dose 100 (NDC 0085-3305-01) Institutional Package 30 (NDC 0085-3305-35)
0.2 mg/hr	40 mg	10 cm²	Unit Dose 30 (NDC 0085-3310-30) Hospital Unit Dose 100 (NDC 0085-3310-01) Institutional Package 30 (NDC 0085-3310-35)
0.3 mg/hr	60 mg	15 cm²	Unit Dose 30 (NDC 0085-3315-30) Hospital Unit Dose 100 (NDC 0085-3315-01) Institutional Package 30 (NDC 0085-3315-35)
0.4 mg/hr	80 mg	20 cm²	Unit Dose 30 (NDC 0085-3320-30) Hospital Unit Dose 100 (NDC 0085-3320-01) Institutional Package 30 (NDC 0085-3320-35)
0.6 mg/hr	120 mg	30 cm²	Unit Dose 30 (NDC 0085-3330-30) Hospital Unit Dose 100 (NDC 0085-3330-01) Institutional Package 30 (NDC 0085-3330-35)
0.8 mg/hr	160 mg	40 cm²	Unit Dose 30 (NDC 0085-0819-30) Hospital Unit Dose 100 (NDC 0085-0819-01) Institutional Package 30 (NDC 0085-0819-35)

* Release rates were formerly described in terms of drug delivered per 24 hours. In these terms, the supplied NITRO-DUR systems would be rated at 2.5 mg/24 hours (0.1 mg/hour), 5 mg/24 hours (0.2 mg/hour), 7.5 mg/24 hours (0.3 mg/hour), 10 mg/24 hours (0.4 mg/hour), and 15 mg/24 hours (0.6 mg/hour).

Methemoglobinemia: Nitrate ions liberated during metabolism of nitroglycerin can oxidize hemoglobin into methemoglobin. Even in patients totally without cytochrome b_5 reductase activity, however, and even assuming that the nitrate moieties of nitroglycerin are quantitatively applied to oxidation of hemoglobin, about 1 mg/kg of nitroglycerin should be required before any of these patients manifests clinically significant ($\geq 10\%$) methemoglobinemia. In patients with normal reductase function, significant production of methemoglobin should require even larger doses of nitroglycerin. In one study in which 36 patients received 2–4 weeks of continuous nitroglycerin therapy at 3.1 to 4.4 mg/hr, the average methemoglobin level measured was 0.2%; this was comparable to that observed in parallel patients who received placebo.

Notwithstanding these observations, there are case reports of significant methemoglobinemia in association with moderate overdoses of organic nitrates. None of the affected patients had been thought to be unusually susceptible.

Methemoglobin levels are available from most clinical laboratories. The diagnosis should be suspected in patients who exhibit signs of impaired oxygen delivery despite adequate cardiac output and adequate arterial PO_2. Classically, methemoglobinemic blood is described as chocolate brown, without color change on exposure to air.

When methemoglobinemia is diagnosed, the treatment of choice is methylene blue, 1–2 mg/kg intravenously.

DOSAGE AND ADMINISTRATION

The suggested starting dose is between 0.2 mg/hr* and 0.4 mg/hr*. Doses between 0.4 mg/hr* and 0.8 mg/hr* have shown continued effectiveness for 10–12 hours daily for at least 1 month (the longest period studied) of intermittent administration. Although the minimum nitrate-free interval has not been defined, data show that a nitrate-free interval of 10–12 hours is sufficient (see CLINICAL PHARMACOLOGY). Thus, an appropriate dosing schedule for nitroglycerin patches would include a daily patch-on period of 12–14 hours and a daily patch-off period of 10–12 hours.
* Release rates were formerly described in terms of drug delivered per 24 hours. In these terms, the supplied NITRO-DUR systems would be rated at 2.5 mg/24 hours (0.1 mg/hour), 5 mg/24 hours (0.2 mg/hour), 7.5 mg/24 hours (0.3 mg/hour), 10 mg/24 hours (0.4 mg/hour), and 15 mg/24 hours (0.6 mg/hour).

Although some well-controlled clinical trials using exercise tolerance testing have shown maintenance of effectiveness when patches are worn continuously, the large majority of such controlled trials have shown the development of tolerance (ie, complete loss of effect) within the first 24 hours after therapy was initiated. Dose adjustment, even to levels much higher than generally used, did not restore efficacy.

HOW SUPPLIED
[See table above.]

Store between 15° and 30°C (59° and 86°F). Do not refrigerate.

CAUTION: Federal law prohibits dispensing without prescription.
Key Pharmaceuticals, Inc.
Kenilworth, NJ 07033 USA
Rev. 7/95   18143615
Copyright © 1987, 1994, 1995, Key Pharmaceuticals, Inc. All rights reserved.
U. S. Patent No. 5,186,938
Shown in Product Identification Guide, page 319

THEO-DUR®
(theophylline)
Extended-Release Tablets   ℞

DESCRIPTION
THEO-DUR® Extended-Release Tablets contain anhydrous theophylline in an extended-release formulation for oral administration which allows a 12–hour dosing interval for a majority of patients and a 24–hour dosing interval for selected patients (see **DOSAGE AND ADMINISTRATION** for a description of appropriate patient populations).

Theophylline:
Theophylline is a bronchodilator, structurally classified as a methylxanthine. It occurs as a white, odorless, crystalline powder with a bitter taste. Anhydrous theophylline has the chemical name 1H-Purine-2,6–dione,3,7–dihydro-1,3–dimethyl-, and is represented by the following structural formula:

The molecular formula of anhydrous theophylline is $C_7H_8N_4O_2$ with a molecular weight of 180.17.
THEO-DUR Extended-Release Tablets contain no color additives and are available in four strengths: 100 mg, 200 mg, 300 mg, and 450 mg.
The inactive ingredients for THEO-DUR 100 mg Extended-Release Tablets include: Acacia NF, Acetone USP, Alcohol, Cellulose Acetate Phthalate NF, Cetyl Alcohol NF, Chloroform NF, Confectioner's Sugar 6X NF, Corn Starch NF, Diethyl Phthalate (Ethyl Phthalate), Ethyl Acetate NF, Glyceryl Monostearate NF (Atmul 84), Isopropyl Alcohol USP, Lactose Monohydrate USP, Magnesium Stearate NF, Myristyl Alcohol, Non-Pareil Seeds 18–20 Mesh, Purified Water USP, Sodium Lauryl Sulfate NF (Dupanol C), Talc USP, and White Wax NF.
The inactive ingredients for THEO-DUR 200 mg, 300 mg, and 450 mg Extended-Release Tablets include: Acetone USP, Cellulose Acetate Phthalate NF, Cetyl Alcohol NF, Diethyl Phthalate (Ethyl Phthalate), Glyceryl Monostearate NF (Atmul 84), Hydroxypropyl Methylcellulose 2910 USP (Methocel E-50), Isopropyl Alcohol USP, Anhydrous Lactose USP, Magnesium Stearate NF, Myristyl Alcohol, Non-Pareil Seeds 18–20 Mesh, Purified Water USP, and White Wax NF.

CLINICAL PHARMACOLOGY
Mechanism of Action:
Theophylline has two distinct actions in the airways of patients with reversible obstruction; smooth muscle relaxation (ie, bronchodilation) and suppression of the response of the airways to stimuli (ie, non-bronchodilator prophylactic effects). While the mechanisms of action of theophylline are not known with certainty, studies in animals suggest that bronchodilatation is mediated by the inhibition of two isozymes of phosphodiesterase (PDE III and, to a lesser extent,

PDE IV) while non-bronchodilator prophylactic actions are probably mediated through one or more different molecular mechanisms that do not involve inhibition of PDE III or antagonism of adenosine receptors. Some of the adverse effects associated with theophylline appear to be mediated by inhibition of PDE III (eg, hypotension, tachycardia, headache, and emesis) and adenosine receptor antagonism (eg, alterations in cerebral blood flow).
Theophylline increases the force of contraction of diaphragmatic muscles. This action appears to be due to enhancement of calcium uptake through an adenosine-mediated channel.

Serum Concentration-Effect Relationship:
Bronchodilation occurs over the serum theophylline concentration range of 5–20 mcg/mL. Clinically important improvement in symptom control has been found in most studies to require peak serum theophylline concentrations > 10 mcg/mL, but patients with mild disease may benefit from lower concentrations. At serum theophylline concentrations > 20 mcg/mL, both the frequency and severity of adverse reactions increase. In general, maintaining peak serum theophylline concentrations between 10 and 15 mcg/mL will achieve most of the drug's potential therapeutic benefit while minimizing the risk of serious adverse events.

Pharmacokinetics:
Overview Theophylline is rapidly and completely absorbed after oral administration in solution or immediate-release solid oral dosage form. Theophylline does not undergo any appreciable pre-systemic elimination, distributes freely into fat-free tissues, and is extensively metabolized in the liver. The pharmacokinetics of theophylline vary widely among similar patients and cannot be predicted by age, sex, body weight, or other demographic characteristics. In addition, certain concurrent illnesses and alterations in normal physiology (see **Table I**) and coadministration of other drugs (see **Table II**) can significantly alter the pharmacokinetic characteristics of theophylline. Within-subject variability in metabolism has also been reported in some studies, especially in acutely ill patients. It is, therefore, recommended that serum theophylline concentrations be measured frequently in acutely ill patients (eg, at 24–hr intervals) and periodically in patients receiving long-term therapy (eg, at 6–12 month intervals). More frequent measurements should be made in the presence of any condition that may significantly alter theophylline clearance (see **PRECAUTIONS, Laboratory Tests** and **DOSAGE AND ADMINISTRATION**).
[See table 1 at bottom of next page.]

Absorption Theophylline is rapidly and completely absorbed after oral administration in solution or immediate-release solid oral dosage form. After a single dose of 5 mg/kg in adults, a mean peak serum concentration of about 10 mcg/mL (range 5–15 mcg/mL) can be expected 1–2 hours after the dose. Co-administration of theophylline with food or antacids does not cause clinically significant changes in the absorption of theophylline from immediate-release dosage forms.

Continued on next page

Key—Cont.

Distribution Once theophylline enters the systemic circulation, about 40% is bound to plasma protein, primarily albumin. Unbound theophylline distributes throughout body water, but distributes poorly into body fat. The apparent volume of distribution of theophylline is approximately 0.45 L/kg (range 0.3–0.7 L/kg) based on ideal body weight. Theophylline passes freely across the placenta, into breast milk, and into the cerebrospinal fluid (CSF). Saliva theophylline concentrations approximate unbound serum concentrations, but are not reliable for routine or therapeutic monitoring unless special techniques are used. An increase in the volume of distribution of theophylline, primarily due to reduction in plasma protein binding, occurs in patients with hepatic cirrhosis, uncorrected acidemia, the elderly, and in women during the third trimester of pregnancy. In such cases, the patient may show signs of toxicity at total (bound +unbound) serum concentrations of theophylline in the therapeutic range (10–20 mcg/mL) due to elevated concentrations of the pharmacologically active unbound drug. Similarly, a patient with decreased theophylline binding may have a sub-therapeutic total drug concentration while the pharmacologically active unbound concentration is in the therapeutic range. If only total serum theophylline concentration is measured, this may lead to an unnecessary and potentially dangerous dose increase. In patients with reduced protein binding, measurement of unbound serum theophylline concentration provides a more reliable means of dosage adjustment than measurement of total serum theophylline concentration. Generally, concentrations of unbound theophylline should be maintained in the range of 6–12 mcg/mL.

Metabolism Following oral dosing, theophylline does not undergo any measurable first-pass elimination. Approximately 90% of the dose is metabolized in the liver. Biotransformation takes place through demethylation to 1–methylxanthine and 3-methylxanthine and hydroxylation to 1,3–dimethyluric acid. 1–methylxanthine is further hydroxylated, by xanthine oxidase, to 1–methyluric acid. About 6% of a theophylline dose is N-methylated to caffeine. Theophylline demethylation to 3–methylxanthine is catalyzed by cytochrome P450 1A2, while cytochromes P450 2E1 and P450 3A3 catalyze the hydroxylation to 1,3–dimethyluric acid. Demethylation to 1–methylxanthine appears to be catalyzed either by cytochrome P450 1A2 or a closely related cytochrome.

Caffeine and 3–methylxanthine are the only theophylline metabolites with pharmacologic activity. 3-methylxanthine has approximately one tenth the pharmacologic activity of theophylline and serum concentrations in adults with normal renal function are <1 mcg/mL. In patients with end-stage renal disease, 3–methylxanthine may accumulate to concentrations that approximate the unmetabolized theophylline concentration. Caffeine concentrations are usually undetectable in adults regardless of renal function.

Both the N-demethylation and hydroxylation pathways of theophylline biotransformation are capacity-limited. Due to the wide intersubject variability of the rate of theophylline metabolism and the possibility of intrasubject variability, nonlinearity of elimination may begin in some patients at serum theophylline concentrations <10 mcg/mL. This nonlinearity, also referred to as "saturation kinetics", results in more than proportional changes in serum theophylline concentrations with changes in dose; therefore, it is advisable to titrate the dose in small increments or decrements in order to achieve desired changes in serum theophylline concentrations (see **DOSAGE AND ADMINISTRATION**). Accurate prediction of dose-dependency of theophylline metabolism in patients *a priori* is not possible, but patients with very high initial clearance rates (ie, low steady-state serum theophylline concentrations at above average doses) have the greatest likelihood of experiencing large changes in serum theophylline concentration in response to dosage changes.

Excretion Approximately 10% of the theophylline dose is excreted unchanged in the urine. The remainder is excreted in the urine mainly as 1,3–dimethyluric acid (35–40%), 1-methyluric acid (20–25%), and 3-methylxanthine (15–20%). Since little theophylline is excreted unchanged in the urine and since active metabolites of theophylline (ie, caffeine, 3–methylxanthine) do not accumulate to clinically significant levels even in the face of end-stage renal disease, no dosage adjustment for renal insufficiency is necessary (see **WARNINGS**).

Serum Concentrations at Steady State After multiple doses of theophylline, steady state is reached in 30–65 hours (average 40 hours) in adults. At steady state, on a dosage regimen with 6–hour intervals, the expected mean trough concentration is approximately 60% of the mean peak concentration, assuming a mean theophylline half-life of 8 hours. The difference between peak and trough concentrations is larger in patients with more rapid theophylline clearance. In patients with high theophylline clearance and half-lives of about 4–5 hours, the trough serum theophylline concentration may be only 30% of peak with a 6-hour dosing interval. In these patients a slow-release formulation would allow a longer dosing interval (8–12 hours) with a smaller peak/trough difference.

Special Populations (see Table I for mean clearance and half-life values)

Geriatric: The clearance of theophylline is decreased by an average of 30% in healthy elderly adults (>60 yrs) compared to healthy young adults. Careful attention to dose reduction and frequent monitoring of serum theophylline concentrations are required in elderly patients (see **WARNINGS**).

Children 6 to 16: Theophylline clearance decreases slowly to adult values at about age 16. Careful attention to dosage selection and monitoring of serum theophylline concentrations are required (see **WARNINGS and DOSAGE AND ADMINISTRATION**).

Gender: Gender differences in theophylline clearance are relatively small and unlikely to be of clinical significance. Significant reduction in theophylline clearance, however, has been reported in women on the 20th day of the menstrual cycle and during the third trimester of pregnancy.

Race: Pharmacokinetic differences in theophylline clearance due to race have not been studied.

Renal Insufficiency: Only a small fraction, eg, about 10%, of the administered theophylline dose is excreted unchanged in the urine. Since little theophylline is excreted unchanged in the urine and since active metabolites of theophylline (ie, caffeine, 3–methylxanthine) do not accumulate to clinically significant levels even in the face of end-stage renal disease, no dosage adjustment for renal insufficiency is necessary.

Hepatic Insufficiency: Theophylline clearance is decreased by 50% or more in patients with hepatic insufficiency (eg, cirrhosis, acute hepatitis, cholestasis). Careful attention to dose reduction and frequent monitoring of serum theophylline concentrations are required in patients with reduced hepatic function (see **WARNINGS**).

Congestive Heart Failure (CHF): Theophylline clearance is decreased by 50% or more in patients with CHF. The extent of reduction in theophylline clearance in patients with CHF appears to be directly correlated to the severity of the cardiac disease. Since theophylline clearance is independent of liver blood flow, the reduction in clearance appears to be due to impaired hepatocyte function rather than reduced perfusion. Careful attention to dose reduction and frequent monitoring of serum theophylline concentrations are required in patients with CHF (see **WARNINGS**).

Smokers: Tobacco and marijuana smoking appear to increase the clearance of theophylline by induction of metabolic pathways. The duration of this effect after cessation of smoking is unknown but may require 6 months to 2 years before the rate approaches that of a nonsmoker. Theophylline clearance has been shown to increase by approximately 50% in young adult tobacco smokers and by approximately 80% in elderly tobacco smokers compared to nonsmoking subjects. Passive smoke exposure has also been shown to increase theophylline clearance by up to 50%. Abstinence from tobacco smoking for one week causes a reduction of approximately 40% in theophylline clearance. Careful attention to dose reduction and frequent monitoring of serum theophylline concentrations are required in patients who stop smoking (see **WARNINGS**). Use of nicotine gum has been shown to have no effect on theophylline clearance.

Fever: Fever, regardless of its underlying cause, can decrease the clearance of theophylline. The magnitude and duration of the fever appear to be directly correlated to the degree of decrease of theophylline clearance. Precise data are lacking, but a temperature of 39°C (102°F) for at least 24 hours or lesser temperature elevations (>100°F) for longer periods, are probably required to produce a clinically significant increase in serum theophylline concentrations. Patients with rapid rates of theophylline clearance (ie, those who require a dose that is substantially larger than average [eg, >22 mg/kg/day] to achieve a therapeutic peak serum theophylline concentration when afebrile) may be at greater risk of toxic effects from decreased clearance during sustained fever. Careful attention to dose reduction and frequent monitoring of serum theophylline concentrations are required in patients with sustained fever (see **WARNINGS**).

Miscellaneous: Other factors associated with decreased theophylline clearance include the third trimester of pregnancy, sepsis with multiple organ failure, and hypothyroidism. Careful attention to dose reduction and frequent monitoring of serum thoephylline concentrations are required in patients with any of these conditions (see **WARNINGS**). Other factors associated with increased theophylline clearance include hyperthyroidism and cystic fibrosis.

Table I. Mean and range of total body clearance and half-life of theophylline related to age and altered physiological states.¶

Population characteristics	Total body clearance* mean (range)†† (mL/kg/min)	Half-life mean (range)†† (hr)
Age		
Children		
4–12 years	1.6 (0.8–2.4)	NR†
13–15 years	0.9 (0.48–1.3)	NR†
6–17 years	1.4 (0.2–2.6)	3.7 (1.5–5.9)
Adults (16–60 years) otherwise healthy nonsmoking asthmatics	0.65 (0.27–1.03)	8.7 (6.1–12.8)
Elderly (>60 years) nonsmokers with normal cardiac, liver, and renal function	0.41 (0.21–0.61)	9.8 (1.6–18)
Concurrent illness or altered physiological state		
Acute pulmonary edema	0.33** (0.07–2.45)	19** (3.1–82)
COPD->60 years, stable nonsmoker >1 year	0.54 (0.44–0.64)	11 (9.4–12.6)
COPD with cor pulmonale	0.48 (0.08–0.88)	NR†
Cystic fibrosis (14–28 years)	1.25 (0.31–2.2)	6.0 (1.8–10.2)
Liver disease -cirrhosis	0.31** (0.1–0.7)	32** (10–56)
acute hepatitis	0.35 (0.25–0.45)	19.2 (16.6–21.8)
cholestatis	0.65 (0.25–1.45)	14.4 (5.7–31.8)
Pregnancy -1st trimester	NR†	8.5 (3.1–13.9)
2nd trimester	NR†	8.8 (3.8–13.8)
3rd trimester	NR†	13.0 (8.4–17.6)
Sepsis with multi-organ failure	0.47 (0.19–1.9)	18.8 (6.3–24.1)
Thyroid disease -hypothyroid	0.38 (0.13–0.57)	11.6 (8.2–25)
hyperthyroid	0.8 (0.68–0.97)	4.5 (3.7–5.6)

¶ For various North American patient populations from literature reports. Different rates of elimination and consequent dosage requirements have been observed among other peoples.

* Clearance represents the volume of blood completely cleared of theophylline by the liver in one minute. Values listed were generally determined at serum theophylline concentrations <20 mcg/mL; clearance may decrease and half-life may increase at higher serum concentrations due to nonlinear pharmacokinetics.

†† Reported range or estimated range (mean ±2 S.D.) where actual range not reported.

† NR = not reported or not reported in a comparable format.

** Median

Note: In addition to the factors listed above, theophylline clearance is increased and half-life decreased by low-carbohydrate/high-protein diets, parenteral nutrition, and daily consumption of charcoal-broiled beef. A high-carbohydrate/low-protein diet can decrease the clearance and prolong the half-life of theophylline.

THEO-DUR Product Pharmacokinetics

THEO-DUR (100, 200, 300, and 450 mg) Extended-Release Tablets:

In single-dose studies with 18 normal fasting subjects, the THEO-DUR product at 8 mg/kg body weight (300–700) mg/dose) produced mean peak theophylline plasma levels of 7.5 ± 1.9 mcg/mL at 9.2 ± 1.9 hours following administration. In multiple-dose, steady-state, 3– and 5–day studies with 12 normal subjects, THEO-DUR administered at 8 mg/kg (300–600 mg/dose) twice daily, achieved an average peak-trough difference of 4 mcg/mL. The C_{max} and C_{min} were 13.9 ± 6.9 and 9.9 ± 6.0, respectively. The mean % fluctuation ± S.D. of the plasma concentration at steady state [% fluctuation = 100 $(C_{max} - C_{min})/C_{min}$] was 54.2 ± 45.7%. These pharmacokinetic parameters were measured under fasting conditions.

THEO-DUR (200, 300, and 450 mg) Extended-Release Tablets:

In a multiple-dose (300–500 mg BID) steady-state, 5–day study involving 14 normal, nonfasting subjects with theo-

phylline half-lives between 5.8 and 12.3 hours (mean 8.0 ± 1.8 hours), THEO-DUR dosed twice daily, produced mean C_{max} and C_{min} levels of 12.2 ± 2.0 and 10.2 ± 1.6 mcg/mL, respectively, over the AM dosing interval and C_{max} and C_{min} of 11.6 ± 1.6 and 8.7 ± 1.8 mcg/mL, respectively, over the PM dosing interval. The mean % fluctuation ± S.D. over the AM dosing interval was 30.4 ± 12.9% and 33.7 ± 13.1% over the PM dosing interval. In the same subjects, the THEO-DUR product given once daily, in the morning, in doses ranging from 60–1000 mg (same daily dose as for BID above) produced a mean C_{max} and C_{min} of 14.4 ± 2.2 and 5.5 ± 2.0, respectively, and a mean % fluctuation ± S.D. of 195.8 ± 106.0%. Average peak-trough differences over 24 hours were 8.9 ± 1.3 and 3.7 ± 1.2 mcg/mL when THEO-DUR was given once or twice daily, respectively. In both the twice-daily and once-daily dosing regimens, THEO-DUR exhibited complete bioavailability when compared to an immediate-release product.

THEO-DUR (200, 300, and 450 mg) Extended-Release Tablets:

In a single-dose bioavailability study in eleven subjects, 1000 mg of the THEO-DUR product was administered under fasting conditions and immediately following a high-fat content (62 g) breakfast of approximately 1100 kcal. The rate and extent of absorption of theophylline from THEO-DUR administered in fasting and fed conditions were similar.

Clinical Studies:

In patients with chronic asthma, including patients with severe asthma requiring inhaled corticosteroids or alternate-day oral corticosteroids, many clinical studies have shown that theophylline decreases the frequency and severity of symptoms, including nocturnal exacerbations, and decreases the "as needed" use of inhaled $beta_2$-agonists. Theophylline has also been shown to reduce the need for short courses of daily oral prednisone to relieve exacerbations of airway obstruction that are unresponsive to bronchodilators in asthmatics.

In patients with chronic obstructive pulmonary disease (COPD), clinical studies have shown that theophylline decreases dyspnea, air trapping, the work of breathing, and improves contractility of diaphragmatic muscles with little or no improvement in pulmonary function measurements.

INDICATIONS AND USAGE

THEO-DUR Extended-Release Tablets are indicated for the treatment of the symptoms and reversible airflow obstruction associated with chronic asthma and other chronic lung diseases, eg, emphysema and chronic bronchitis.

CONTRAINDICATIONS

THEO-DUR Extended-Release Tablets are contraindicated in patients with a history of hypersensitivity to theophylline or other components in the product. The product is contraindicated in patients with active peptic ulcer disease and in individuals with underlying seizure disorders.

WARNINGS

Serious side effects such as ventricular arrhythmias, convulsions, or even death may appear as the first sign of toxicity without any previous warning. Less serious signs of theophylline toxicity (ie, nausea and restlessness) may occur frequently when initiating therapy but are usually transient. When such signs are persistent during maintenance therapy, they are often associated with serum concentrations above 20 mcg/mL. Stated differently, serious toxicity is not reliably preceded by less severe side effects. A serum concentration measurement is the only reliable method of predicting potentially life-threatening toxicity.

Concurrent Illness:

Theophylline should be used with extreme caution in patients with cardiac arrhythmias due to the increased risk of exacerbation of the concurrent arrhythmia.

Conditions That Reduce Theophylline Clearance:

There are several readily identifiable causes of reduced theophylline clearance. ***If the total daily dose is not appropriately reduced so as to lower serum theophylline levels to within the therapeutic range in the presence of these risk factors, severe and potentially fatal theophylline toxicity can occur.***

Careful consideration must be given to the benefits and risks of theophylline use and the need for more intensive monitoring of serum theophylline concentrations in patients with the following risk factors:

Age:
Elderly (>60 years)
Concurrent diseases:
Acute pulmonary edema
Congestive heart failure
Cor pulmonale
Fever, ≥102° for 24 hours or more; or lesser temperature elevations for longer periods
Hypothyroidism
Influenza and other viral illnesses
Liver disease; cirrhosis, acute hepatitis
Sepsis with multi-organ failure
Shock

Cessation of Smoking:
(See "*Special Populations — Smokers.*")
Drug Interactions:
Adding a drug that inhibits theophylline metabolism (eg, cimetidine, erythromycin, tacrine) or stopping a concurrently administered drug that enhances theophylline metabolism (eg, carbamazepine, rifampin). (See **PRECAUTIONS, Drug Interactions, Table II.**)

When Signs or Symptoms of Theophylline Toxicity Are Present:

Some of the signs of theophylline toxicity mimic other illnesses. Whenever a patient receiving theophylline develops nausea or vomiting, particularly repetitive vomiting, or other signs or symtoms consistent with theophylline toxicity as noted in the ADVERSE REACTIONS section (even if another cause may be suspected), a serum theophylline concentration should be measured immediately and additional doses of theophylline should be withheld until the diagnosis is confirmed. Patients should be instructed not to continue any dosage that causes adverse effects and to withhold subsequent doses until the symptoms have resolved, at which time the clinician may instruct the patient to resume the drug at a lower dosage (see **DOSAGE AND ADMINISTRATION, Dosage Guidelines**).

Dosage Increases:

Increases in the dose of theophylline should not be made in response to an acute exacerbation of symptoms of chronic lung disease since theophylline provides little added benefit to inhaled $beta_2$-selective agonists and systemically administered corticosteroids in this circumstance and increases the risk of adverse effects. A *peak* steady-state serum theophylline concentration should be measured before increasing the dose in response to persistent chronic symptoms to ascertain whether an increase in dose is safe. Before increasing the theophylline dose on the basis of a low serum concentration, the clinician should consider whether the blood sample was obtained at an appropriate time in relationship to the dose and whether the patient has adhered to the prescribed regimen (see **PRECAUTIONS, Laboratory Tests**).

As the rate of theophylline clearance may be dose-dependent (ie, steady-state serum concentrations may increase disproportionately to the increase in dose), an increase in dose based upon a sub-therapeutic serum concentration measurement should be conservative. In general, limiting dose increases to about 25% of the previous total daily dose will reduce the risk of unintended excessive increases in serum theophylline concentration (see **DOSAGE AND ADMINISTRATION**).

PRECAUTIONS

THEO-DUR TABLETS SHOULD *NOT* BE CHEWED OR CRUSHED AND SHOULD BE BROKEN *ONLY AT THE SCORE.*

General:

Careful consideration of the various interacting drugs (including recently discontinued medications), physiologic conditions, and other factors such as smoking that can alter theophylline clearance and require dosage adjustment should occur prior to initiation of theophylline therapy, prior to increases in theophylline dose, and during follow up (see **WARNINGS**). The dose of theophylline selected for initiation of therapy should be low and, ***if tolerated***, increased slowly over a period of a week or longer with the final dose guided by monitoring serum theophylline concentrations and the patient's clinical response (see **DOSAGE AND ADMINISTRATION**).

Information for Patients:

This information is intended to aid in the safe and effective use of this medication. It is not a disclosure of all possible adverse or intended effects. The physician should reinforce the importance of taking only the prescribed dose, as well as the time interval between prescribed doses. THEO-DUR *should not be chewed or crushed.* When dosing THEO-DUR Extended-Release Tablets on a once-daily (q24h) basis, tablets should be taken whole and not split. As with any extended-release theophylline product, the patient should alert the physician if symptoms occur repeatedly, especially near the end of the dosing interval.

The patient (or parent/caregiver) should be instructed to seek medical advice whenever such symptoms as nausea, vomiting, persistent headache, insomnia, restlessness, or rapid heartbeat occurs during treatment with theophylline, even if another cause is suspected. Patients should be instructed to contact their clinician if they develop a new illness, especially if accompanied by a fever, if they experience worsening of a chronic illness, if they start or stop smoking cigarettes or marijuana, or if another clinician adds a new medication or discontinues a previously prescribed medication. Patients should be informed that theophylline interacts with a wide variety of drugs (see **Table II**). They should be instructed to inform all clinicians involved in their care that they are taking theophylline, especially when a medication is being added or deleted from their treatment. Patients should be instructed to not alter the dose, timing of the dose, or frequency of administration without first consulting their clinician. If a dose is missed, the patient should be instructed to take the next dose at the usually scheduled time and to not attempt to make up for the missed dose.

Laboratory Tests–Monitoring Serum Theophylline Concentrations:

Serum theophylline concentration measurements are readily available and should be used to determine whether the dosage is appropriate. Specifically, the serum theophylline concentration should be measued as follows:

1. When initiating therapy to guide final dosage adjustment after titration.
2. Before making a dose increase to determine whether the serum concentration is sub-therapeutic in a patient who continues to be symptomatic.
3. Whenever signs or symptoms of theophylline toxicity are present.
4. Whenever there is a new illness, worsening of a chronic illness, or a change in the patient's treatment regimen that may alter theophylline clearance [eg, fever (see **CLINICAL PHARMACOLOGY,** *Fever*), hepatitis, or drugs listed in **Table II** are added or discontinued].

To guide a dose increase, the blood sample should be obtained at the time of the expected peak serum theophylline concentration; 4 to 8 hours when medication is taken every 12 hours or 8 hours when taken once daily. It is important that the patient has not missed or taken additional doses during the previous 48 hours and that the dosing intervals were reasonably equally spaced. A trough concentration (ie, at the end of the dosing interval) provides no additional useful information and may lead to an inappropriate dose increase since the peak serum theophylline concentration can be two or more times greater than the trough concentration with an immediate-release formulation. If the serum sample is drawn more than 8 hours after the dose, the results must be interpreted with caution since the concentration may not be reflective of the expected peak concentration. In contrast, when signs or symptoms of theophylline toxicity are present, the serum sample should be obtained as soon as possible, analyzed immediately, and the result reported to the clinician without delay. In patients in whom decreased serum protein binding is suspected (eg, cirrhosis, women during the third trimester of pregnancy), the concentration of unbound theophylline should be measured and the dosage adjusted to achieve an unbound concentration of 6-12 mcg/mL.

Saliva concentrations of theophylline cannot be used reliably to adjust dosage without special techniques.

Effects on Laboratory Tests:

As a result of its pharmacological effects, theophylline at serum concentrations within the 10–20 mcg/mL range modestly increases plasma glucose (from a mean of 88 mg% to 98 mg%), uric acid (from a mean of 4 mg/dL to 6 mg/dL), free fatty acids (from a mean of 451 μeg/dL to 800 μeg/dL), total cholesterol (from a mean of 140 vs 160 mg/dL), HDL (from a mean of 36 to 50 mg/dL), HDL/LDL ratio (from a mean of 0.5 to 0.7), and urinary free cortisol excretion (from a mean of 44 to 63 mcg/24 hr). Theophylline at serum concentrations within the 10-20 mcg/mL range may also transiently decrease serum concentrations of triiodothyronine (144 before, 131 after 1 week and 142 ng/dL after 4 weeks of theophylline). The clinical importance of these changes should be weighed against the potential therapeutic benefit of theophylline in individual patients.

The Effect of Other Drugs on Theophylline Serum Concentration Measurements:

Most serum theophylline assays in clinical use are immunoassays which are specific for theophylline. Other xanthines such as caffeine, dyphylline, and pentoxifylline are not detected by these assays. Some drugs (eg, cefazolin, cephalothin), however, may interfere with certain HPLC techniques. Caffeine and xanthine metabolites in patients with renal dysfunction may cause the reading from some dry reagent office methods to be higher than the actual serum theophylline concentration.

Drug Interactions:

Theophylline interacts with a wide variety of drugs. The interaction may be pharmacodynamic, ie, alterations in the therapeutic response to theophylline or another drug or occurrence of adverse effects without a change in serum theophylline concentration. More frequently, however, the interaction is pharmacokinetic, ie, the rate of theophylline clearance is altered by another drug resulting in increased or decreased serum theophylline concentrations. Theophylline only rarely alters the pharmacokinetics of other drugs.

The drugs listed in **Table II** have the potential to produce clinically significant pharmacodynamic or pharmacokinetic interactions with theophylline. The information in the "**Effect**" column of Table II assumes that the interacting drug is being added to a steady-state theophylline regimen. If theophylline is being initiated in a patient who is already taking a drug that inhibits theophylline clearance (eg, cimetidine, erythromycin), the dose of theophylline required to achieve a therapeutic serum theophylline concentration will be smaller. Conversely, if theophylline is being initiated in a patient who is already taking a drug that enhances theophyl-

Continued on next page

Key—Cont.

line clearance (eg, rifampin), the dose of theophylline required to achieve a therapeutic serum theophylline concentration will be larger. Discontinuation of a concomitant drug that increases theophylline clearance will result in accumulation of theophylline to potentially toxic levels, unless the theophylline dose is appropriately reduced. Discontinuation of a concomitant drug that inhibits theophylline clearance will result in decreased serum theophylline concentrations, unless the theophylline dose is appropriately increased.

The listing of drugs in **Table II** is current as of June 27, 1995. New interactions are continuously being reported for theophylline, especially with new chemical entities. **The clinician should not assume that a drug does not interact with theophylline if it is not listed in Table II.** Before addition of a newly available drug in a patient receiving theophylline, the package insert of the new drug and/or the medical literature should be consulted to determine if an interaction between the new drug and theophylline has been reported.
[See Table II at right and at top of next page.]

Caution should be exercised in the administration of all quinolones to patients receiving concomitant theophylline therapy since it has been shown that some quinolones increase the plasma levels of theophylline by affecting the rate of theophylline clearance.

Drug/Food Interactions:
THEO-DUR 100 mg Extended-Release Tablets have not been adequately studied to determine whether their bioavailability is altered when given with food. Available data suggest that drug administration at the time of food ingestion may influence the absorption characteristics of theophylline controlled-release products resulting in serum values different from those found after administration in the fasting state. A drug-food effect, if any, would likely have its greatest clinical significance when high theophylline serum levels are being maintained and/or when large single doses (greater than 13 mg/kg or 900 mg) of a controlled-release theophylline product are given.

THEO-DUR (200, 300, and 450 mg) Extended-Release Tablets: The rate and extent of absorption of theophylline from THEO-DUR 200 mg, 300 mg, and 450 mg tablets are similar when administered fasting or immediately after a high-fat content breakfast such as 8 oz. whole milk, egg/cheese/bacon on muffin, 1 blueberry muffin with margarine, and 1 serving of hash brown potatoes (about 1100 kcal, including approximately 62 g of fat) (see **CLINICAL PHARMACOLOGY, Pharmacokinetics**).

Carcinogenesis, Mutagenesis, and Impairment of Fertility:
Long-term carcinogenicity studies have been carried out in mice (oral doses 30–150 mg/kg) and rats (oral doses 5–75 mg/kg). Results are pending. Theophylline has been studied in Ames salmonella, *in vivo* and *in vitro* cytogenetics, micronucleus, and Chinese hamster ovary test systems and has not been shown to be genotoxic.
In a 14-week continuous breeding study, theophylline, administered to mating pairs of B6C3F$_1$ mice at oral doses of 120, 270, and 500 mg/kg (approximately 1.0-3.0 times the human dose on a mg/m^2 basis) impaired fertility, as evidenced by decreases in the number of live pups per litter, decreases in the mean number of litters per fertile pair, and increases in the gestation period at the high dose as well as decreases in the proportion of pups born alive at the mid and high dose. In 13-week toxicity studies, theophylline was administered to F344 rats and B6C3F$_1$ mice at oral doses at 40-300 mg/kg (approximately 2.0 times the human dose on a mg/m^2 basis). At the high dose, systemic toxicity was observed in both species including decreases in testicular weight.

Pregnancy:
Category C There are no adequate and well-controlled studies in pregnant women. Additionally, there are no teratogenicity studies in nonrodents (eg, rabbits). Theophylline was not shown to be teratogenic in CD-1 mice at oral doses up to 400 mg/kg, approximately 2.0 times the human dose on a mg/m^2 basis or in CD-1 rats at oral doses up to 260 mg/kg, approximately 3.0 times the recommended human dose on a mg/m^2 basis. At a dose of 220 mg/kg, embryotoxicity was observed in rats in the absence of maternal toxicity.

Nursing Mothers:
Theophylline is excreted into breast milk and may cause irritability or other signs of mild toxicity in nursing human infants. The concentration of theophylline in breast milk is about equivalent to the maternal serum concentration. An infant ingesting a liter of breast milk containing 10-20 mcg/mL of theophylline a day is likely to receive 10-20 mg of theophylline per day. Serious adverse effects in the infant are unlikely unless the mother has toxic serum theophylline concentrations.

Table II.	Clinically significant drug interactions with theophylline*.	
Drug	Type of Interaction	Effect**
Adenosine	Theophylline blocks adenosine receptors.	Higher doses of adenosine may be required to achieve desired effect.
Alcohol	A single large dose of alcohol (eg, 3 mL/kg of whiskey) decreases theophylline clearance for up to 24 hours.	30% increase
Allopurinol	Decreases theophylline clearance at allopurinol doses ≥ 600 mg/day.	25% increase
Aminoglutethimide	Increases theophylline clearance by induction of microsomal enzyme activity.	25% decrease
Carbamazepine	Similar to aminoglutethimide.	30% decrease
Cimetidine	Decreases theophylline clearance by inhibiting cytochrome P450 1A2.	70% increase
Ciprofloxacin	Similar to cimetidine.	40% increase
Clarithromycin	Similar to erythromycin.	25% increase
Diazepam	Benzodiazepines increase CNS concentrations of adenosine, a potent CNS depressant, while theophylline blocks adenosine receptors.	Larger diazepam doses may be required to produce desired level of sedation. Discontinuation of theophylline without reduction of diazepam dose may result in respiratory depression.
Disulfiram	Decreases theophylline clearance by inhibiting hydroxylation and demethylation.	50% increase
Enoxacin	Similar to cimetidine.	300% increase
Ephedrine	Synergistic CNS effects.	Increased frequency of nausea, nervousness, and insomnia.
Erythromycin	Erythromycin metabolite decreases theophylline clearance by inhibiting cytochrome P450 3A3.	35% increase. Erythromycin steady-state serum concentrations decrease by a similar amount.
Estrogen	Estrogen containing oral contraceptives decrease theophylline clearance in a dose-dependent fashion. The effect of progesterone on theophylline clearance is unknown.	30% increase
Flurazepam	Similar to diazepam.	Similar to diazepam.
Fluvoxamine	Similar to cimetidine.	Similar to cimetidine.
Halothane	Halothane sensitizes the myocardium to catecholamines; theophylline increases release of endogenous catecholamines.	Increased risk of ventricular arrhythmias.
Interferon, human recombinant alpha-A	Decreases theophylline clearance.	100% increase
Isoproterenol (IV)	Increases theophylline clearance.	20% decrease
Ketamine	Pharmacologic.	May lower theophylline seizure threshold.
Lithium	Theophylline increases renal lithium clearance.	Lithium dose required to achieve a therapeutic serum concentration increased an average of 60%.
Lorazepam	Similar to diazepam.	Similar to diazepam.
Methotrexate (MTX)	Decreases theophylline clearance.	20% increase after low dose MTX, higher dose MTX may have a greater effect.
Mexiletine	Similar to disulfiram.	80% increase
Midazolam	Similar to diazepam.	Similar to diazepam.
Moricizine	Increases theophylline clearance.	25% decrease
Norfloxacin	Increases serum theophylline levels.	
Ofloxacin	Increases serum theophylline levels.	
Pancuronium	Theophylline may antagonize nondepolarizing neuromuscular blocking effects; possibly due to phosphodiesterase inhibition.	Larger dose of pancuronium may be required to achieve neuromuscular blockade.
Pentoxifylline	Decreases theophylline clearance.	30% increase
Phenobarbital (PB)	Similar to aminoglutethimide.	25% decrease after 2 weeks of concurrent PB.
Phenytoin	Phenytoin increases theophylline clearance by increasing microsomal enzyme activity. Theophylline decreases phenytoin absorption.	Serum theophylline *and* phenytoin concentrations decrease about 40%.
Propafenone	Decreases theophylline clearance and pharmacologic interaction.	40% increase. Beta$_2$-blocking effect may decrease efficacy of theophylline.
Propranolol	Similar to cimetidine and pharmacologic interaction.	100% increase. Beta$_2$-blocking effect may decrease efficacy of theophylline.
Rifampin	Increases theophylline clearance by increasing cytochrome P450 1A2 and 3A3 activity.	20–40% decrease
Sucralfate	Reduces absorption of theophylline.	
Sulfinpyrazone	Increases theophylline clearance by increasing demethylation and hydroxylation. Decreases renal clearance of theophylline.	20% decrease

Table II. Clinically significant drug interactions with theophylline*. (Continued)

Drug	Type of Interaction	Effect**
Tacrine	Similar to cimetidine, also increases renal clearance of theophylline.	90% increase
Thiabendazole	Decreases theophylline clearance.	190% increase
Ticlopidine	Decreases theophylline clearance.	60% increase
Troleandomycin	Similar to erythromycin.	33–100% increase depending on troleandomycin dose.
Verapamil	Similar to disulfiram.	20% increase

*Refer to **PRECAUTIONS, Drug Interactions** for further information regarding table.
**Average effect on steady-state theophylline concentration or other clinical effect for pharmacologic interactions. Individual patients may experience larger changes in serum theophylline concentration than the value listed.

Pediatric Use:

Safety and effectiveness of THEO-DUR Extended-Release Tablets administered:

1. Every 24 hours in children under 12 years of age have not been established.
2. Every 12 hours in children under 6 years of age have not been established.

Geriatric Use:

Elderly patients are at significantly greater risk of experiencing serious toxicity from theophylline than younger patients due to pharmacokinetic and pharmacodynamic changes associated with aging. Theophylline clearance is reduced in patients greater than 60 years of age, resulting in increased serum theophylline concentrations in response to a given theophylline dose. Protein binding may be decreased in the elderly resulting in a larger proportion of the total serum theophylline concentration in the pharmacologically active unbound form. Elderly patients also appear to be more sensitive to the toxic effects of theophylline after chronic overdosage than younger patients. For these reasons, the maximum daily dose of theophylline in patients greater than 60 years of age ordinarily should not exceed 400 mg/day unless the patient continues to be symptomatic and the peak steady-state serum theophylline concentration is < 10 mcg/mL (see **DOSAGE AND ADMINISTRATION**). Theophylline doses greater than 400 mg/day should be prescribed with caution in elderly patients.

ADVERSE REACTIONS

Adverse reactions associated with theophylline are generally mild when peak serum theophylline concentrations are < 20 mcg/mL and mainly consist of transient caffeine-like adverse effects such as nausea, vomiting, headache, and insomnia. When peak serum theophylline concentrations exceed 20 mcg/mL, however, theophylline produces a wide range of adverse reactions including persistent vomiting, cardiac arrhythmias, and intractable seizures which can be lethal (see **OVERDOSAGE**). The transient caffeine-like adverse reactions occur in about 50% of patients when theophylline therapy is initiated at doses higher than recommended initial doses (eg, > 300 mg/day in adults). During the initiation of theophylline therapy, caffeine-like adverse effects may transiently alter patient behavior, especially in school age children, but this response rarely persists. Initiation of theophylline therapy at a low dose with subsequent slow titration to a predetermined age-related maximum dose will significantly reduce the frequency of these transient adverse effects (see **DOSAGE AND ADMINISTRATION**). In a small percentage of patients (< 3% of children and < 10% of adults), the caffeine-like adverse effects persist during maintenance therapy, even at peak serum theophylline concentrations within the therapeutic range (ie, 10-20 mcg/mL). Dosage reduction may alleviate the caffeine-like adverse effects in these patients; however, persistent adverse effects should result in a re-evaluation of the need for continued theophylline therapy and the potential therapeutic benefit of alternative treatment.

Other adverse reactions that have been reported at serum theophylline concentrations < 20 mcg/mL include diarrhea, irritability, restlessness, fine skeletal muscle tremors, epigastric pain, hematemesis, reflex hyperexcitability, muscle twitching, palpitation, extrasystoles, flushing, hypotension, circulatory failure, ventricular arrhythmia, tachypnea, alopecia, hyperglycemia, inappropriate ADH syndrome, rash, and transient diuresis. In patients with hypoxia secondary to COPD, multifocal atrial tachycardia and flutter have been reported at serum theophylline concentrations ≥ 15 mcg/mL. There have been a few isolated reports of seizures at serum theophylline concentrations < 20 mcg/mL in patients with and without underlying neurological disease or in elderly patients. The occurrence of seizures in elderly patients with serum theophylline concentrations < 20 mcg/mL may be secondary to decreased protein binding resulting in a larger proportion of the total serum theophylline concentration in the pharmacologically active unbound form. The clinical characteristics of the seizures reported in patients with serum theophylline concentrations < 20 mcg/mL have generally been milder than seizures associated with excessive serum theophylline concentrations resulting from an overdose (ie, they have generally been transient, often stopped without anticonvulsant therapy, and did not result in neurological residua). However, irreversible brain injury can occur following seizures due to theophylline.

Table III. Manifestations of theophylline toxicity.*

	Percentage of patients reported with sign or symptom			
	Acute Overdose (Large Single Ingestion)		Chronic Overdosage (Multiple Excessive Doses)	
Sign/Symptom	Study 1 (n=157)	Study 2 (n=14)	Study 1 (n=92)	Study 2 (n=102)
Asymptomatic	NR**	0	NR**	6
Gastrointestinal				
Vomiting	73	93	30	61
Abdominal Pain	NR**	21	NR**	12
Diarrhea	NR**	0	NR**	14
Hematemesis	NR**	0	NR**	2
Metabolic/Other				
Hypokalemia	85	79	44	43
Hyperglycemia	98	NR**	18	NR**
Acid/base disturbance	34	21	9	5
Rhabdomyolysis	NR**	7	NR**	0
Cardiovascular				
Sinus tachycardia	100	86	100	62
Other supraventricular tachycardias	2	21	12	14
Ventricular premature beats	3	21	10	19
Atrial fibrillation or flutter	1	NR**	12	NR**
Multifocal atrial tachycardia	0	NR**	2	NR**
Ventricular arrhythmias with hemodynamic instability	7	14	40	0
Hypotension/shock	NR**	21	NR**	8
Neurologic				
Nervousness	NR**	64	NR**	21
Tremors	38	29	16	14
Disorientation	NR**	7	NR**	11
Seizures	5	14	14	5
Death	3	21	10	4

*These data are derived from two studies in patients with serum theophylline concentrations > 30 mcg/mL. In the first study (Study #1-Shanon, *Ann Intern Med.* 1993; 119:1161-67), data were prospectively collected from 249 consecutive cases of theophylline toxicity referred to a regional poison center for consultation. In the second study (Study #2-Sessler, *Am J Med.* 1990;88:567-76), data were retrospectively collected from 116 cases with serum theophylline concentrations > 30 mcg/mL among 6000 blood samples obtained for measurement of serum theophylline concentrations in three emergency departments. Differences in the incidence of manifestations of theophylline toxicity between the two studies may reflect sample selection as a result of study design (eg, in Study #1, 48% of the patients had acute intoxications versus only 10% in Study #2) and different methods of reporting results.

**NR = Not reported in a comparable manner.

OVERDOSAGE

General:

The chronicity and pattern of theophylline overdosage significantly influences clinical manifestations of toxicity, management, and outcome. There are two common presentations: (1) *acute overdose*, ie, ingestion of a single large excessive dose (> 10 mg/kg) as occurs in the context of an attempted suicide or isolated medication error, and (2) *chronic overdosage*, ie, ingestion of repeated doses that are excessive for the patient's rate of theophylline clearance. The most common causes of chronic theophylline overdosage include patient or caregiver error in dosing, clinician prescribing of an excessive dose or a normal dose in the presence of factors known to decrease the rate of theophylline clearance, and increasing the dose in response to an exacerbation of symptoms without first measuring the serum theophylline concentration to determine whether a dose increase is safe.

Severe toxicity from theophylline overdose is a relatively rare event. In one health maintenance organization, the frequency of hospital admissions for chronic overdosage of theophylline was about 1 per 1000 person-years exposure. In another study, among 6000 blood samples obtained for measurement of serum theophylline concentration, for any reason, from patients treated in an emergency department, 7% were in the 20-30 mcg/mL range and 3% were > 30 mcg/mL. Approximately two thirds of the patients with serum theophylline concentrations in the 20-30 mcg/mL range had one or more manifestations of toxicity, while > 90% of patients with serum theophylline concentrations > 30 mcg/mL were clinically intoxicated. Similarly, in other reports, serious toxicity from theophylline is seen principally at serum concentrations > 30 mcg/mL.

Several studies have described the clinical manifestations of theophylline overdose and attempted to determine the factors that predict life-threatening toxicity. In general, patients who experience an acute overdose are less likely to experience seizures than patients who have experienced a chronic overdosage, unless the peak serum theophylline concentration is > 100 mcg/mL. After a chronic overdosage, generalized seizures, life-threatening cardiac arrhythmias, and death may occur at serum theophylline concentrations > 30 mcg/mL. The severity of toxicity after chronic overdosage is more strongly correlated with the patient's age than the peak serum theophylline concentration; patients > 60 years are at the greatest risk for severe toxicity and mortality after a chronic overdosage. Pre-existing or concurrent disease may also significantly increase the susceptibility of a patient to a particular toxic manifestation, eg, patients with neurologic disorders have an increased risk of seizures and patients with cardiac disease have an increased risk of cardiac arrhythmias for a given serum theophylline concentration compared to patients without the underlying disease.

The frequency of various reported manifestations of theophylline overdose according to the mode of overdose are listed in Table III.

Other manifestations of theophylline toxicity include increases in serum calcium, creatine kinase, myoglobin, and leukocyte count, decreases in serum phosphate and magnesium, acute myocardial infarction, and urinary retention in men with obstructive uropathy.

Seizures associated with serum theophylline concentrations > 30 mcg/mL are often resistant to anticonvulsant therapy and may result in irreversible brain injury if not rapidly controlled. Death from theophylline toxicity is most often secondary to cardiorespiratory arrest and/or hypoxic encephalopathy following prolonged generalized seizures or intractable cardiac arrhythmias causing hemodynamic compromise.

Overdose Management:

General Recommendations for Patients with Symptoms of Theophylline Overdose or Serum Theophylline Concentrations > 30 mcg/mL (Note: Serum theophylline concentrations may continue to increase after presentation of the patient for medical care).

1. While simultaneously instituting treatment, contact a regional poison center to obtain updated information and advice on individualizing the recommendations that follow.
2. Institute supportive care, including establishment of intravenous access, maintenance of the airway, and electrocardiographic monitoring.
3. *Treatment of seizures:* Because of the high morbidity and mortality associated with theophylline-induced seizures, treatment should be rapid and aggressive. Anticonvulsant therapy should be initiated with an intravenous benzodiazepine, eg, diazepam, in increments of 0.1–0.2 mg/kg every 1–3 minutes until seizures are terminated. Repetitive seizures should be treated with a loading dose of phenobarbital (20 mg/kg infused over 30–60 minutes). Animal studies and case reports of theophylline overdose in humans suggest that phenytoin is ineffective in terminating theophylline-induced seizures. The doses of benzodiazepines and phenobarbital required to terminate theophylline-induced seizures are close to the doses that may cause severe respiratory depression or respiratory arrest; the clinician should therefore be prepared to provide assisted ventilation. Elderly patients and patients with COPD may be more susceptible to the respiratory depressant effects of anticonvulsants. Barbiturate-induced coma or administration of general anesthesia may be required to terminate repetitive seizures or status epilepticus. General anesthesia should be used with caution in patients with theophylline overdose because fluorinated volatile anesthetics may

Continued on next page

Key—Cont.

sensitize the myocardium to endogenous catecholamines released by theophylline. Enflurane appears less likely to be associated with this effect than halothane and may, therefore, be safer. Neuromuscular blocking agents alone should not be used to terminate seizures since they abolish the musculoskeletal manifestations without terminating seizure activity in the brain.

4. *Anticipate need for anticonvulsants:* In patients with theophylline overdose who are at high risk for theophylline-induced seizures, eg, patients with acute overdoses and serum theophylline concentrations >100 mcg/mL or chronic overdosage in patients >60 years of age with serum theophylline concentrations >30 mcg/mL, the need for anticonvulsant therapy should be anticipated. A benzodiazepine such as diazepam should be drawn into a syringe and kept at the patient's bedside and medical personnel qualified to treat seizures should be immediately available. In selected patients at high risk for theophylline-induced seizures, consideration should be given to the administration of prophylactic anticonvulsant therapy. Situations where prophylactic anticonvulsant therapy should be considered in high-risk patients include anticipated delays in instituting methods for extracorporeal removal of theophylline (eg, transfer of a high-risk patient from one healthcare facility to another for extracorporeal removal) and clinical circumstances that significantly interfere with efforts to enhance theophylline clearance (eg, where dialysis may not be technically feasible or a patient with vomiting unresponsive to antiemetics who is unable to tolerate multiple-dose oral activated charcoal). In animal studies, prophylactic administration of phenobarbital, *but not phenytoin,* has been shown to delay the onset of theophylline-induced generalized seizures and to increase the dose of theophylline required to induce seizures (ie, markedly increases the LD$_{50}$). Although there are no controlled studies in humans, a loading dose of intravenous phenobarbital (20 mg/kg infused over 60 minutes) may delay or prevent life-threatening seizures in high-risk patients while efforts to enhance theophylline clearance are continued. Phenobarbital may cause respiratory depression, particularly in elderly patients and patients with COPD.

5. *Treatment of cardiac arrhythmias:* Sinus tachycardia and simple ventricular premature beats are not harbingers of life-threatening arrhythmias, they do not require treatment in the absence of hemodynamic compromise, and they resolve with declining serum theophylline concentrations. Other arrhythmias, especially those associated with hemodynamic compromise, should be treated with antiarrhythmic therapy appropriate for the type of arrhythmia.

6. *Gastrointestinal decontamination:* Oral activated charcoal (0.5 g/kg up to 20 g and repeat at least once 1–2 hours after the first dose) is extremely effective in blocking the absorption of theophylline throughout the gastrointestinal tract, even when administered several hours after ingestion. If the patient is vomiting, the charcoal should be administered through a nasogastric tube or after administration of an antiemetic. Phenothiazine antiemetics such as prochlorperazine or perphenazine should be avoided since they can lower the seizure threshold and frequently cause dystonic reactions. A single dose of sorbitol may be used to promote stooling to facilitate removal of theophylline bound to charcoal from the gastrointestinal tract. Sorbitol, however, should be dosed with caution since it is a potent purgative which can cause profound fluid and electrolyte abnormalities, particularly after multiple doses. Commercially available fixed combinations of liquid charcoal and sorbitol should be avoided in young children and after the first dose in adolescents and adults since they do not allow for individualization of charcoal and sorbitol dosing. Ipecac syrup should be avoided in theophylline overdoses. Although ipecac induces emesis, it does not reduce the absorption of theophylline unless administered within 5 minutes of ingestion and even then is less effective than oral activated charcoal. Moreover, ipecac-induced emesis may persist for several hours after a single dose and significantly decrease the retention and the effectiveness of oral activated charcoal.

7. *Serum theophylline concentration monitoring:* The serum theophylline concentration should be measured immediately upon presentation, 2–4 hours later, and then at sufficient intervals, eg, every 4 hours, to guide treatment decisions and to assess the effectiveness of therapy. Serum theophylline concentrations may continue to increase after presentation of the patient for medical care as a result of continued absorption of theophylline from the gastrointestinal tract. Serial monitoring of serum theophylline serum concentrations should be continued until it is clear that the concentration is no longer rising and has returned to non-toxic levels.

8. *General monitoring procedures:* Electrocardiographic monitoring should be initiated on presentation and continued until the serum theophylline level has returned to a nontoxic level. Serum electrolytes and glucose should be measured on presentation and at appropriate intervals as indicated by clinical circumstances. Fluid and electrolyte abnormalities should be promptly corrected. **Monitoring and treatment should be continued until the serum concentration decreases below 20 mcg/mL.**

9. *Enhance clearance of theophylline:* Multiple-dose oral activated charcoal (eg, 0.5 mg/kg up to 20 g, every 2 hours) increases the clearance of theophylline at least twofold by adsorption of theophylline secreted into gastrointestinal fluids. Charcoal must be retained in, and pass through, the gastrointestinal tract to be effective; emesis should therefore be controlled by administration of appropriate antiemetics. Alternatively, the charcoal can be administered continuously through a nasogastric tube in conjunction with appropriate antiemetics. A single dose of sorbitol may be administered with the activated charcoal to promote stooling to facilitate clearance of the adsorbed theophylline from the gastrointestinal tract. Sorbitol alone does not enhance clearance of theophylline and should be dosed with caution to prevent excessive stooling which can result in severe fluid and electrolyte imbalances. Commercially available fixed combinations of liquid charcoal and sorbitol should be avoided in young children and after the first dose in adolescents and adults since they do not allow for individualization of charcoal and sorbitol dosing. In patients with intractable vomiting, extracorporeal methods of theophylline removal should be instituted (see **OVERDOSAGE, Extracorporeal Removal**).

Specific Recommendations:

Acute Overdose

A. Serum Concentration >20 <30 mcg/mL
  1. Administer a single dose of oral activated charcoal.
  2. Monitor the patient and obtain a serum theophylline concentration in 2–4 hours to ensure that the concentration is not increasing.

B. Serum Concentration >30 <100 mcg/mL
  1. Administer multiple-dose oral activated charcoal and measures to control emesis.
  2. Monitor the patient and obtain serial theophylline concentrations every 2–4 hours to gauge the effectiveness of therapy and to guide further treatment decisions.
  3. Institute extracorporeal removal if emesis, seizures, or cardiac arrhythmias cannot be adequately controlled (see **OVERDOSAGE, Extracorporeal Removal**).

C. Serum Concentration >100 mcg/mL
  1. Consider prophylactic anticonvulsant therapy.
  2. Administer multiple-dose oral activated charcoal and measures to control emesis.
  3. Consider extracorporeal removal, even if the patient has not experienced a seizure (see **OVERDOSAGE, Extracorporeal Removal**).
  4. Monitor the patient and obtain serial theophylline concentrations every 2–4 hours to gauge the effectiveness of therapy and to guide further treatment decisions.

Chronic Overdosage

A. Serum Concentration >20 <30 mcg/mL (with manifestations of theophylline toxicity)
  1. Administer a single dose of oral activated charcoal.
  2. Monitor the patient and obtain a serum theophylline concentration in 2–4 hours to ensure that the concentration is not increasing.

B. Serum Concentration >30 mcg/mL in patients <60 years of age
  1. Administer multiple-dose oral activated charcoal and measures to control emesis.
  2. Monitor the patient and obtain serial theophylline concentrations every 2–4 hours to gauge the effectiveness of therapy and to guide further treatment decisions.
  3. Institute extracorporeal removal if emesis, seizures, or cardiac arrhythmias cannot be adequately controlled (see **OVERDOSAGE, Extracorporeal Removal**).

C. Serum Concentration >30 mcg/mL in patients ≥60 years of age
  1. Consider prophylactic anticonvulsant therapy.
  2. Administer multiple-dose oral activated charcoal and measures to control emesis.
  3. Consider extracorporeal removal, even if the patient has not experienced a seizure (see **OVERDOSAGE, Extracorporeal Removal**).
  4. Monitor the patient and obtain serial theophylline concentrations every 2–4 hours to gauge the effectiveness of therapy and to guide further treatment decisions.

Extracorporeal Removal:

Increasing the rate of theophylline clearance by extracorporeal methods may rapidly decrease serum concentrations, but the risks of the procedure must be weighed against the potential benefit. Charcoal hemoperfusion is the most effective method of extracorporeal removal, increasing theophylline clearance up to sixfold, but serious complications, including hypotension, hypocalcemia, platelet consumption, and bleeding diatheses may occur. Hemodialysis is about as efficient as multiple-dose oral activated charcoal and has a lower risk of serious complications than charcoal hemoperfusion. Hemodialysis should be considered as an alternative when charcoal hemoperfusion is not feasible and multiple-dose oral charcoal is ineffective because of intractable emesis. Serum theophylline concentrations may rebound 5–10 mcg/mL after discontinuation of charcoal hemoperfusion or hemodialysis due to redistribution of theophylline from the tissue compartment. Peritoneal dialysis is ineffective for theophylline removal; exchange transfusions in neonates have been minimally effective.

DOSAGE AND ADMINISTRATION

General Considerations:

The steady-state peak serum theophylline concentration is a function of the dose, the dosing interval, and the rate of theophylline absorption and clearance in the individual patient. Because of marked individual differences in the rate of theophylline clearance, the dose required to achieve a peak serum theophylline concentration in the 10–20 mcg/mL range varies fourfold among otherwise similar patients in the absence of factors known to alter theophylline clearance (eg, 400–1600 mg/day in adults <60 years old). For a given population there is no simple theophylline dose that will provide both safe and effective serum concentrations for all patients. Administration of the medium theophylline dose required to achieve a therapeutic serum theophylline concentration in a given population may result in either subtherapeutic or potentially toxic serum theophylline concentrations in individual patients. For example, at a dose of 900 mg/day in adults <60 years, the steady-state peak serum theophylline concentration will be <10 mcg/mL in about 30% of patients, 10–20 mcg/mL in about 50%, and 20–30 mcg/mL in about 20% of patients. **The dose of theophylline must be individualized on the basis of peak serum theophylline concentration measurements in order to achieve a dose that will provide maximum potential benefit with minimal risk of adverse effects.**

Transient caffeine-like adverse effects and excessive serum concentrations in slow metabolizers can be avoided in most patients by starting with a sufficiently low dose and slowly increasing the dose, *if judged to be clinically indicated,* in small increments. Dose increases should only be made if the previous dosage is well tolerated and at intervals of no less than 3 days to allow serum theophylline concentrations to reach the new steady state. Final dosage adjustment should be guided by serum theophylline concentration measurement (see **PRECAUTIONS, Laboratory Tests** and **DOSAGE AND ADMINISTRATION**). Healthcare providers should instruct patients and caregivers to discontinue any dosage that causes adverse effects, to withhold the medication until these symptoms are gone, and to then resume therapy at a lower, previously tolerated dosage (see **WARNINGS**).

If the patient's symptoms are well controlled, there are no apparent adverse effects, and no intervening factors that might alter dosage requirements (see **WARNINGS** and **PRECAUTIONS**), serum theophylline concentrations should be monitored at 6-month intervals for rapidly growing children and at yearly intervals for all others. In acutely ill patients, serum theophylline concentrations should be monitored at frequent intervals, eg, every 24 hours.

THEO-DUR (200, 300, and 450 mg) Extended-Release Tablets: The rate and extent of absorption of theophylline from THEO-DUR 200, 300, and 450 mg tablets when administered fasting or immediately after a high-fat content breakfast are similar (see **CLINICAL PHARMACOLOGY, Pharmacokinetics**).

THEO-DUR 100 mg Extended-Release Tablets have not been adequately studied for their bioavailability when administered with food (see **PRECAUTIONS, Drug/Food Interactions**).

Effective use of theophylline (ie, the concentration of drug in the serum associated with optimal benefit and minimal risk of toxicity) is considered to occur when the theophylline concentration is maintained from 10 to 15 mcg/mL.

If it is not possible to obtain serum level determinations, restriction of the daily dose (in otherwise healthy adults) to not greater than 13 mg/kg/day, to a maximum of 900 mg of theophylline will result in relatively few patients exceeding serum levels of 20 mcg/mL and the resultant greater risk of toxicity.

Caution should be exercised for younger children who cannot complain of minor side effects. Older adults, particularly those with cor pulmonale, congestive heart failure, and/or liver disease may have unusually low dosage requirements and thus may experience toxicity at the maximal dosage recommended below.

Theophylline does not distribute into fatty tissue. Dosage should be calculated on the basis of lean (ideal) body weight where mg/kg doses are presented.

Frequency of Dosing:

When immediate-release products with rapid absorption are used, dosing to maintain serum levels generally requires administration every 6 hours. This is particularly true in children, but dosing intervals up to 8 hours may be satisfactory in adults since they eliminate the drug at a slower rate. Adults and some children requiring higher than average doses (those having rapid rates of clearance, eg, half-lives of

under 6 hours) may benefit and be more effectively controlled during chronic therapy when given products with extended-release characteristics since these provide longer dosing intervals and/or less fluctuation in serum concentration between dosing.

DOSAGE GUIDLINES

WARNING: DO NOT ATTEMPT TO MAINTAIN ANY DOSE THAT IS NOT WELL TOLERATED.

Dosage guidelines are approximations only and the wide range of theophylline clearance between individuals (particularly those with concomitant disease) makes indiscriminate usage hazardous. It is recommended that dosing be considered in two stages: initiation of therapy with THEO-DUR, then titration, adjustment, and chronic maintenance.

Initiation of Therapy:

It is recommended that the appropriate dosage be established using an immediate-release preparation. Slow clinical titration is generally preferred to help assure acceptance and safety of the medication, and to allow the patient to develop tolerance to the transient caffeine-like side effects. Then, if the total 24-hour dose can be given by use of the available strengths of this product, the patient can usually be switched to THEO-DUR Extended-Release Tablets giving one half of the daily dose at 12-hour intervals. However, certain patients, such as the young, smokers, and some nonsmoking adults are likely to metabolize theophylline rapidly and require dosing at 8-hour intervals. Such patients can generally be identified as having trough serum concentrations lower than desired or repeatedly exhibiting symptoms near the end of a dosing interval.

Alternatively, therapy can be initiated with THEO-DUR since it is available in dosage forms/strengths which permit titration and adjustment of dosage as outlined in the following dosing guidelines. It is recommended that for children under 25 kg, proper dosage be established with a liquid preparation to permit titration in small increments.

THE AVERAGE INITIAL ADULT AND CHILDREN'S (over 25 kg) DOSE IS ONE THEO-DUR 200 mg TABLET q12h.

Titration, Adjustment, and Chronic Maintenance:

If the desired response is not achieved with the above AVERAGE INITIAL DOSE recommendations, there are no adverse reactions, and the serum theophylline level cannot be measured, dosage adjustment should proceed by increasing the dose in approximately 25% increments at 3-day intervals. Following each adjustment, the clinical response should be assessed. If the response is satisfactory then that dosage level should be maintained. Dosage increases may be made in this manner up to the following:

MAXIMUM DOSE WITHOUT MEASUREMENT OF SERUM CONCENTRATION

	Dose Per Interval
Children (25-35 kg)	250 mg q12h
Adults and Children (35-70 kg)	300 mg q12h
Adults (over 70 kg)	450 mg q12h

It is important that **no patient be maintained on any dosage that is not tolerated.** When increasing dosage according to the schedule above, patients should be instructed not to take a subsequent dose if apparent side effects occur and to resume therapy at a lower dose once adverse effects have disappeared.

If an increased dose is not tolerated because of headache or stomach upset (nausea, vomiting, diarrhea, etc.), decrease dose to previous tolerated level. Do not exceed the above recommended doses unless serum theophylline levels can be measured.

If serum theophylline levels can be measured and the concentration is between 10 and 15 mcg/mL, maintain dose if tolerated. CHECK SERUM CONCENTRATION AT APPROXIMATELY 8 HOURS AFTER A DOSE WHEN NONE HAS BEEN MISSED OR ADDED FOR AT LEAST 3 DAYS. RECHECK SERUM THEOPHYLLINE CONCENTRATION AT 6- TO 12-MONTH INTERVALS. This interval may need to be more frequent in some individuals.

Table IV contains recommendations for final theophylline dosage adjustment based upon serum theophylline concentrations. Application of these general dosing recommendations to individual patients must take into account the unique clinical characteristics of each patient. In general, these recommendations should serve as the upper limit for dosage adjustments in order to decrease the risk of potentially serious adverse events associated with unexpected large increases in serum theophylline concentrations.

Table IV.   Final dosage adjustment guided by serum theophylline concentration.

Peak Serum Concentration	Dosage Adjustment
<9.9 mcg/mL	If symptoms are not controlled and current dosage is tolerated, increase dose about 25%. Recheck serum concentration after 3 days for further dosage adjustment.
10 to 14.9 mcg/mL	If symptoms are controlled and current dosage is tolerated, maintain dose and recheck serum concentration at 6–12 month intervals.¶ If symptoms are not controlled and current dosage is tolerated, consider adding additional medication(s) to treatment regimen.
15–19.9 mcg/mL	Consider 10% decrease in dose to provide greater margin of safety even if current dosage is tolerated.¶
20–24.9 mcg/mL	Decrease dose by 25% even if no adverse effects are present. Recheck serum concentration after 3 days to guide further dosage adjustment.
25–30 mcg/mL	Skip next dose and decrease subsequent doses at least 25% even if no adverse effects are present. Recheck serum concentration after 3 days to guide further dosage adjustment. If symptomatic, consider whether overdose treatment is indicated (see recommendations for chronic overdosage).
> 30 mcg/mL	Treat overdose as indicated (see recommendations for chronic overdosage). If theophylline is subsequently resumed, decrease dose by at least 50% and recheck serum concentration after 3 days to guide further dosage adjustment.

¶ Dose reduction and/or serum theophylline concentration measurement is indicated whenever adverse effects are present, physiologic abnormalities that can reduce theophylline clearance occur (eg, sustained fever), or a drug that interacts with theophylline is added or discontinued (see **WARNINGS**).

DOSAGE ADJUSTMENT BASED ON SERUM THEOPHYLLINE CONCENTRATION MEASUREMENTS WHEN THESE INSTRUCTIONS HAVE NOT BEEN FOLLOWED MAY RESULT IN RECOMMENDATIONS THAT PRESENT RISK OF TOXICITY TO THE PATIENT.

Once-Daily Dose:

The slow absorption rate of this preparation may allow once-daily administration in adult nonsmokers with appropriate total body clearance and other patients with low dosage requirements. Once-daily dosing should be considered only after the patient has been gradually and satisfactorily titrated to therapeutic levels with q12h dosing. Once-daily dosing should be based on twice the q12h dose and should be initiated at the end of the last q12h dosing interval. The trough concentration (C_{min}) obtained following conversion to once-daily dosing may be lower (especially in high-clearance patients) and the peak concentration (C_{max}) may be higher (especially in low-clearance patients) than that obtained with q12h dosing. If symptoms recur, or signs of toxicity appear during the once-daily dosing interval, dosing on the q12h basis should be reinstituted.

It is essential that serum theophylline concentrations be monitored before and after transfer to once-daily dosing. Food and posture, along with changes associated with circadian rhythm, may influence the rate of absorption and/or clearance rates of theophylline from controlled-release dosage forms administered at night. The exact relationship of these and other factors to nighttime serum concentrations and the clinical significance of such findings require additional study. Therefore, it is not recommended that THEO-DUR, when used as a once-a-day product, be administered at night. THEO-DUR, when used as a once-a-day product, must be taken whole and not broken.

HOW SUPPLIED

THEO-DUR 100 mg, 200 mg, and 300 mg Extended-Release Tablets are available in bottles of 100, 500, 1000, and 5000, and in unit-dose packages of 100. THEO-DUR 450 mg Extended-Release Tablets are available in bottles of 100, and unit-dose packages of 100.

100 mg tablet: NDC 0085-0487; round, white to off-white, debossed THEO-DUR 100 on one side and scored on the other side.

200 mg tablet: NDC 0085-0933; oval, white to off-white, debossed THEO-DUR 200 on one side and scored on the other side.

300 mg tablet: NDC 0085-0584; capsule shaped, white to off-white, debossed THEO-DUR 300 on one side and scored on the other side.

450 mg tablet: NDC 0085-0806; capsule shaped, white to off-white, scored, debossed THEO-DUR 450 on one side.

STORAGE CONDITIONS

Keep tightly closed. Store at controlled room temperature 15°–30°C (59°–86°F).

CAUTION: Federal law prohibits dispensing without prescription.

Key Pharmaceuticals, Inc.
Kenilworth, NJ 07033 USA
Copyright © 1987, 1995, 1996, Key Pharmaceuticals, Inc.
All rights reserved.   19042006
Rev. 11/95

Shown in Product Identification Guide, page 319

TRINALIN®   ℞
brand of azatadine maleate, USP and pseudoephedrine sulfate, USP
Long-Acting Antihistamine/Decongestant
REPETABS® Tablets

DESCRIPTION

TRINALIN Long-Acting Antihistamine/Decongestant REPETABS (brand of repeat-action tablets) Tablets contain 1 mg azatadine maleate, USP in the tablet coating and 120 mg pseudoephedrine sulfate, USP, equally distributed between the tablet coating and the barrier-coated core. Following ingestion, the two active components in the coating are quickly liberated; release of the decongestant in the core is delayed for several hours.

Azatadine maleate is an antihistamine having the empirical formula, $C_{20}H_{22}N_2 \cdot 2C_4H_4O_4$, the chemical name, 6,11-Dihydro-11-(-methyl-4-piperidylidene)-5H-benzo [5,6] cyclo-hepta [1,2-b]pyridine maleate (1:2), and the chemical structure:

The molecular weight of azatadine maleate is 522.54. Azatadine maleate is a white to off-white powder and is very soluble in water and soluble in alcohol.

Pseudoephedrine sulfate, a sympathomimetic amine, is a salt of pseudoephedrine, one of the naturally occurring alkaloids obtained from various species of the plant *Ephedra*. The empirical formula for pseudoephedrine sulfate is $(C_{10}H_{15}NO)_2 \cdot H_2SO_4$; the chemical name is Benzenemethanol, α-[1-(methylamino)ethyl]-, [S-(R*, R*)]-, sulfate (2:1) (salt), and the chemical structure:

The molecular weight of pseudoephedrine sulfate is 428.56. It is a white to off-white crystal or powder, very soluble in water, freely soluble in alcohol, and sparingly soluble in chloroform.

The inactive ingredients for TRINALIN REPETABS Tablets are: Acacia, Butylparaben, Calcium Sulfate, Carnauba Wax, Corn Starch, D&C Red No. 30 Al Lake, FD&C Yellow No. 6 Al Lake, Gelatin, Lactose, Magnesium Stearate, Neutral Soap, Oleic Acid, Povidone, Rosin, Sugar, Talc, White Wax, and Zein.

CLINICAL PHARMACOLOGY

Azatadine maleate is an antihistamine, related to cyproheptadine, with antiserotonin, anticholinergic (drying), and sedative effects. Antihistamines appear to compete with histamine for histamine H_1-receptor sites on effector cells. The antihistamines antagonize those pharmacological effects of histamine which are mediated through activation of H_1-receptor sites and thereby reduce the intensity of allergic reactions and tissue injury response involving histamine release. Antihistamines antagonize the vasodilator effect of endogenously released histamine, especially in small vessels, and mitigate the effect of histamine which results in increased capillary permeability and edema formation. As consequences of these actions, antihistamines antagonize the physiological manifestations of histamine release in the nose following antigen-antibody interaction, such as congestion related to vascular engorgement, mucosal edema, and profuse, watery secretion, and irritation and sneezing resulting from histamine action on afferent nerve terminals.

Continued on next page

Key—Cont.

Pseudoephedrine sulfate (d-isoephedrine sulfate) is an orally effective nasal decongestant which appears to exert its sympathomimetic effect indirectly, predominantly through release of adrenergic mediators from post-ganglionic nerve terminals. In effective recommended oral dosage, pseudoephedrine sulfate produces minimal other sympathomimetic effects, such as pressor activity and CNS stimulation. Use of an orally administered vasoconstrictor for shrinkage of congested nasal mucosa has several advantages: a) it produces a gradual but sustained decongestant effect, causing little, if any "rebound" congestion; b) it facilitates shrinkage of swollen mucosa in upper respiratory areas that are relatively inaccessible to topically applied sprays or drops; c) it relieves nasal obstruction without the additional irritation that may result from local medication.

Pseudoephedrine passes through the blood-brain and placental barriers. While the antihistamines have not been studied systematically for passage through these barriers, the occurrence of pharmacologic effects in the central nervous system and in newborns indicate presence of the drug.

Following administration of the two drugs to normal volunteers in either a single TRINALIN REPETABS Tablet or similar doses in two conventional pseudoephedrine sulfate tablets and a conventional tablet of azatadine maleate, the blood levels of pseudoephedrine and the urinary excretion of azatadine showed that the TRINALIN REPETABS Tablets are bioequivalent to the conventional dosage forms. The apparent elimination half-life of pseudoephedrine in TRINALIN REPETABS Tablets was approximately $6^1/_2$ hours. The apparent elimination of half-life of azatadine maleate (available from the outer layer of the TRINALIN REPETABS Tablets or from the conventional azatadine maleate tablet) was approximately 12 hours.

INDICATIONS AND USAGE

TRINALIN Long-Acting Antihistamine/Decongestant REPETABS Tablets are indicated for the relief of the symptoms of upper respiratory mucosal congestion in perennial and allergic rhinitis, and for the relief of nasal congestion and eustachian tube congestion. Analgesics, antibiotics, or both may be administered concurrently, when indicated.

CONTRAINDICATIONS

Antihistamines should not be used to treat lower respiratory tract symptoms, including asthma.

This product is contraindicated in patients with narrow-angle glaucoma or urinary retention, and in patients receiving monoamine oxidase (MAO) inhibitor therapy or within ten days of stopping such treatment. (See **Drug Interactions** section.) It is also contraindicated in patients with severe hypertension, severe coronary artery disease, hyperthyroidism, and in those who have shown hypersensitivity or idiosyncrasy to its components, to adrenergic agents, or to other drugs of similar chemical structures. Manifestations of patient idiosyncrasy to adrenergic agents include: insomnia, dizziness, weakness, tremor, or arrhythmias.

WARNINGS

TRINALIN REPETABS Tablets should be used with considerable caution in patients with: stenosing peptic ulcer, pyloroduodenal obstruction, urinary bladder obstruction due to symptomatic prostatic hypertrophy, or narrowing of the bladder neck. It should also be administered with caution to patients with: cardiovascular disease, including hypertension or ischemic heart disease; increased intraocular pressure (see **CONTRAINDICATIONS**); diabetes mellitus, or in patients receiving digitalis or oral anticoagulants.

Central nervous system stimulation and convulsions or cardiovascular collapse with accompanying hypotension may be produced by sympathomimetics.

Do not exceed recommended dosage.

Use in Activities Requiring Mental Alertness: Patients should be warned about engaging in activities requiring mental alertness, such as driving a car or operating appliances, machinery, etc.

Use in Patients Approximately 60 Years and Older: Antihistamines are more likely to cause dizziness, sedation, and hypotension in patients over 60 years of age. In these patients, sympathomimetics are also more likely to cause adverse reactions, such as confusion, hallucinations, convulsions, CNS depression, and death. For this reason, before considering the use of a repeat-action formulation, the safe use of a short-acting sympathomimetic in that particular patient should be demonstrated.

PRECAUTIONS

General: Because of the atropine-like action of antihistamines, this product should be used with caution in patients with a history of bronchial asthma.

Information for Patients:

1. Products containing antihistamines may cause drowsiness.
2. Patients should not engage in activities requiring mental alertness, such as driving or operating machinery or appliances.

3. Alcohol or other sedative drugs may enhance the drowsiness caused by antihistamines.
4. Patients should not take TRINALIN REPETABS Tablets if they are receiving a monoamine oxidase inhibitor or within 10 days of stopping such treatment, or if they are receiving oral anticoagulants.
5. This medication should not be given to children less than 12 years of age.

Drug Interactions: MAO inhibitors prolong and intensify the effects of antihistamines. Concomitant use of antihistamines with alcohol, tricyclic antidepressants, barbiturates, or other central nervous system depressants may have an additive effect.

When sympathomimetic drugs are given to patients receiving monoamine oxidase inhibitors, hypertensive reactions, including hypertensive crises, may occur. The antihypertensive effects of methyldopa, mecamylamine, reserpine, and veratrum alkaloids may be reduced by sympathomimetics. Beta-adrenergic blocking agents may also interact with sympathomimetics. Increased ectopic pacemaker activity can occur when pseudoephedrine is used concomitantly with digitalis. Antacids increase the rate of absorption of pseudoephedrine, while kaolin decreases it.

Drug/Laboratory Test Interactions: The *in vitro* addition of pseudoephedrine to sera containing the cardiac isoenzyme MB of serum creatine phosphokinase progressively inhibits the activity of the enzyme. The inhibition becomes complete over six hours.

Carcinogenesis, Mutagenesis, and Impairment of Fertility: There is no animal or laboratory study of the mixture of azatadine maleate and pseudoephedrine sulfate to evaluate carcinogenesis or mutagenesis. Reproduction studies of this mixture in rats showed no evidence of impaired fertility.

Pregnancy Category C: Retarded fetal development and the presence of angulated hyoid wings were seen in the offspring of pregnant rabbits administered TRINALIN REPETABS Tablets at about 12.5 times and 5 times the recommended human dosage, respectively; increased resorption was noted at about 25 times the human dosage. A decreased survival rate at day 21 was seen in rat pups born of mothers given TRINALIN during pregnancy at a dose about 12.5 times the human dosage. There are no adequate and well-controlled studies in pregnant women. TRINALIN REPETABS Tablets should be used during pregnancy only if the potential benefits to the mother justify the potential risks to the infant. (See **Nonteratogenic Effects.**)

Nonteratogenic Effects: Antihistamines should not be used in the third trimester of pregnancy because newborns and premature infants may have severe reactions to them, such as convulsions.

Nursing Mothers: It is not known whether these drugs are excreted in human milk. However, certain antihistamines and sympathomimetics are known to be excreted in human milk. Because of the higher risks of antihistamines for infants generally and for newborns and prematures in particular, a decision should be made whether to discontinue nursing or to discontinue the drug, taking into account the importance of the drug to the mother.

There is a report of irritability, excessive crying, and disturbed sleeping patterns in a nursing infant whose mother had taken a product containing an antihistamine and pseudoephedrine.

Pediatric Use: Safety and effectiveness in children below the age of 12 years have not been established.

ADVERSE REACTIONS

The following adverse reactions are associated with antihistamine and sympathomimetic drugs. (Those adverse reactions which occur most frequently with the antihistamines are underlined.)

General: Urticaria, drug rash, anaphylactic shock, photosensitivity, excessive perspiration, chills, dryness of mouth, nose, and throat.

Cardiovascular: Hypertension (see **CONTRAINDICATIONS** and **WARNINGS**), hypotension, arrhythmias and cardiovascular collapse, headache, palpitations, extrasystoles, tachycardia, angina.

Hematologic: Hemolytic anemia, hypoplastic anemia, thrombocytopenia, agranulocytosis.

Central Nervous System: Sedation, sleepiness, dizziness, vertigo, tinnitus, acute labyrinthitis, disturbed coordination, fatigue, mydriasis, confusion, restlessness, excitation, nervousness, tension, tremor, irritability, insomnia, euphoria, paresthesias, blurred vision, hysteria, neuritis, convulsions, fear, anxiety, hallucinations, CNS depression, weakness, pallor.

Gastrointestinal: Epigastric distress, anorexia, nausea, vomiting, diarrhea, constipation, abdominal cramps.

Genitourinary: Urinary frequency, urinary retention, dysuria, early menses.

Respiratory: Thickening of bronchial secretions, tightness of chest and wheezing, nasal stuffiness, respiratory difficulty.

DRUG ABUSE AND DEPENDENCE

There is no information to indicate that abuse or dependency occurs with azatadine maleate.

Pseudoephedrine, like other central nervous system stimulants, has been abused. At high doses, subjects commonly experience an elevation of mood, a sense of increased energy and alertness, and decreased appetite. Some individuals become anxious, irritable, and loquacious. In addition to the marked euphoria, the user experiences a sense of markedly enhanced physical strength and mental capacity. With continued use, tolerance develops, the user increases the dose, and toxic signs and symptoms appear. Depression may follow rapid withdrawal.

OVERDOSAGE

In the event of overdosage, emergency treatment should be started immediately.

Manifestations of overdosage may vary from central nervous system depression (sedation, apnea, diminished mental alertness, cyanosis, coma, cardiovascular collapse) to stimulation (insomnia, hallucinations, tremors, or convulsions) to death. Other signs and symptoms may be euphoria, excitement, tachycardia, palpitations, thirst, perspiration, nausea, dizziness, tinnitus, ataxia, blurred vision, and hypertension or hypotension. Stimulation is particularly likely in children, as are atropine-like signs and symptoms (dry mouth; fixed, dilated pupils; flushing; hyperthermia; and gastrointestinal symptoms).

In large doses sympathomimetics may give rise to giddiness, headache, nausea, vomiting, sweating, thirst, tachycardia, precordial pain, palpitations, difficulty in micturition, muscular weakness and tenseness, anxiety, restlessness, and insomnia. Many patients can present a toxic psychosis with delusions and hallucinations. Some may develop cardiac arrhythmias, circulatory collapse, convulsions, coma, and respiratory failure.

The oral LD_{50} of the mixture of the two drugs in mature rats and mice was greater than 1700 mg/kg and 600 mg/kg, respectively.

Treatment—The patient should be induced to vomit, even if emesis has occurred spontaneously. Pharmacologically induced vomiting by the administration of ipecac syrup is a preferred method. However, vomiting should not be induced in patients with impaired consciousness. The action of ipecac is facilitated by physical activity and by the administration of eight to twelve fluid ounces of water. If emesis does not occur within fifteen minutes, the dose of ipecac should be repeated. Precautions against aspiration must be taken, especially in infants and children. Following emesis, any drug remaining in the stomach may be adsorbed by activated charcoal administered as a slurry with water. If vomiting is unsuccessful or contraindicated, gastric lavage should be performed. Isotonic and one-half isotonic saline are the lavage solutions of choice. Saline cathartics, such as milk of magnesia, draw water into the bowel by osmosis and therefore may be valuable for their action in rapid dilution of bowel content. Dialysis is of little value in antihistamine poisoning. After emergency treatment the patient should continue to be medically monitored.

Treatment of the signs and symptoms of overdosage is symptomatic and supportive. Stimulants (analeptic agents) should not be used. Vasopressors may be used to treat hypotension. Short-acting barbiturates, diazepam, or paraldehyde, may be administered to control seizures. Hyperpyrexia, especially in children, may require treatment with tepid water sponge baths or a hypothermic blanket. Apnea is treated with ventilatory support.

DOSAGE AND ADMINISTRATION

TRINALIN REPETABS Tablets ARE NOT INTENDED FOR USE IN CHILDREN UNDER 12 YEARS OF AGE. The usual adult dosage is one tablet twice a day.

HOW SUPPLIED

TRINALIN REPETABS Tablets contain 1 mg azatadine maleate and 120 mg pseudoephedrine sulfate. TRINALIN REPETABS Tablets are coral-colored, sugar-coated tablets branded in black with the product name TRINALIN and product identification numbers, 703; bottle of 100 (NDC-0085-0703-04).

Store between 2° and 30°C (36° and 86°F).

Copyright © 1981, 1991, Key Pharmaceuticals, Inc. All rights reserved.

Revised 6/91   17070908

Shown in Product Identification Guide, page 319

UNI-DUR®   ℞
(theophylline)
Extended-release Tablets

DESCRIPTION

UNI-DUR® Extended-release Tablets for oral administration contain 400 or 600 mg anhydrous theophylline in an

extended-release system which allows a 24-hour dosing interval for appropriate patients.

Theophylline

Theophylline is a bronchodilator, structurally classified as a methylxanthine. It occurs as a white, odorless, crystalline powder with a bitter taste. Anhydrous theophylline has the chemical name, 1*H*-Purine-2,6-dione,3,7-dihydro-1,3-dimethyl-, and is represented by the following structural formula:

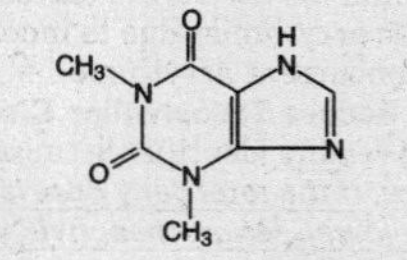

The molecular formula of anhydrous theophylline is $C_7H_8N_4O_2$ with a molecular weight of 180.17.

The inactive ingredients for UNI-DUR 400 and 600 mg Extended-release Tablets include: acacia; cellulose acetate phthalate; cetyl alcohol; confectioner's sugar; corn starch; diethyl phthalate; glyceryl monostearate; lactose monohydrate USP; magnesium stearate; myristyl alcohol; non-pareil seeds (sugar spheres); and white wax.

CLINICAL PHARMACOLOGY

Mechanism of Action:

Theophylline has two distinct actions in the airways of patients with reversible obstruction; smooth muscle relaxation (ie, bronchodilation) and suppression of the response of the airways to stimuli (ie, non-bronchodilator prophylactic effects). While the mechanisms of action of theophylline are not known with certainty, studies in animals suggest that bronchodilatation is mediated by the inhibition of two isozymes of phosphodiesterase (PDE III and, to a lesser extent, PDE IV) while non-bronchodilator prophylactic actions are probably mediated through one or more different molecular mechanisms that do not involve inhibition of PDE III or antagonism of adenosine receptors. Some of the adverse effects associated with theophylline appear to be mediated by inhibition of PDE III (eg, hypotension, tachycardia, headache, and emesis) and adenosine receptor antagonism (eg, alterations in cerebral blood flow).

Theophylline increases the force of contraction of diaphragmatic muscles. This action appears to be due to enhancement of calcium uptake through an adenosine-mediated channel.

Serum Concentration-Effect Relationship:

Bronchodilation occurs over the serum theophylline concentration range of 5–20 mcg/mL. Clinically important improvement in symptom control has been found in most studies to require peak serum theophylline concentrations >10 mcg/mL, but patients with mild disease may benefit from lower concentrations. At serum theophylline concentrations >20 mcg/mL, both the frequency and severity of adverse reactions increase. In general, maintaining peak serum theophylline concentrations between 10 and 15 mcg/mL will achieve most of the drug's potential therapeutic benefit while minimizing the risk of serious adverse events.

Pharmacokinetics:

Overview Theophylline is rapidly and completely absorbed after oral administration in solution or immediate-release solid oral dosage form. Theophylline does not undergo any appreciable pre-systemic elimination, distributes freely into fat-free tissues, and is extensively metabolized in the liver.

The pharmacokinetics of theophylline vary widely among similar patients and cannot be predicted by age, sex, body weight, or other demographic characteristics. In addition, certain concurrent illnesses and alterations in normal physiology (see **Table I**) and coadministration of other drugs (see **Table II**) can significantly alter the pharmacokinetic characteristics of theophylline. Within-subject variability in metabolism has also been reported in some studies, especially in acutely ill patients. It is, therefore, recommended that serum theophylline concentrations be measured frequently in acutely ill patients (eg, at 24-hr intervals) and periodically in patients receiving long-term therapy (eg, at 6–12 month intervals). More frequent measurements should be made in the presence of any condition that may significantly alter theophylline clearance (see **PRECAUTIONS, Laboratory Tests** and **DOSAGE AND ADMINISTRATION**).

[See table I above.]

Absorption Theophylline is rapidly and completely absorbed after oral administration in solution or immediate-release solid oral dosage form. After a single dose of 5 mg/kg in adults, a mean peak serum concentration of about 10 mcg/mL (range 5–15 mcg/mL) can be expected 1–2 hours after the dose. Co-administration of theophylline with food or antacids does not cause clinically significant changes in the absorption of theophylline from immediate-release dosage forms.

Distribution Once theophylline enters the systemic circulation, about 40% is bound to plasma protein, primarily albumin. Unbound theophylline distributes throughout body water, but distributes poorly into body fat. The apparent volume of distribution of theophylline is approximately 0.45 L/kg (range 0.3–0.7 L/kg) based on ideal body weight. Theophylline passes freely across the placenta, into breast milk, and into the cerebrospinal fluid (CSF). Saliva theophylline concentrations approximate unbound serum concentrations, but are not reliable for routine or therapeutic monitoring unless special techniques are used. An increase in the volume of distribution of theophylline, primarily due to reduction in plasma protein binding, occurs in patients with hepatic cirrhosis, uncorrected acidemia, the elderly, and in women during the third trimester of pregnancy. In such cases, the patient may show signs of toxicity at total (bound +unbound) serum concentrations of theophylline in the therapeutic range (10–20 mcg/mL) due to elevated concentrations of the pharmacologically active unbound drug. Similarly, a patient with decreased theophylline binding may have a sub-therapeutic total drug concentration while the pharmacologically active unbound concentration is in the therapeutic range. If only total serum theophylline concentration is measured, this may lead to an unnecessary and potentially dangerous dose increase. In patients with reduced protein binding, measurement of unbound serum theophylline concentration provides a more reliable means of dosage adjustment than measurement of total serum theophylline concentration. Generally, concentrations of unbound theophylline should be maintained in the range of 6–12 mcg/mL.

Table I. Mean and range of total body clearance and half-life of theophylline related to age and altered physiological states.¶

Population characteristics	Total body clearance* mean (range)†† (mL/kg/min)	Half-life mean (range)†† (hr)
Age		
13–15 years	0.9 (0.48–1.3)	NR†
6–17 years	1.4 (0.2–2.6)	3.7 (1.5–5.9)
Adults (16–60 years) otherwise healthy nonsmoking asthmatics	0.65 (0.27–1.03)	8.7 (6.1–12.8)
Elderly (>60 years) nonsmokers with normal cardiac, liver, and renal function	0.41 (0.21–0.61)	9.8 (1.6–18)
Concurrent illness or altered physiological state		
Acute pulmonary edema	0.33** (0.07–2.45)	19** (3.1–82)
COPD- >60 years, stable nonsmoker >1 year	0.54 (0.44–0.64)	11 (9.4–12.6)
COPD with cor pulmonale	0.48 (0.08–0.88)	NR†
Cystic fibrosis (14–28 years)	1.25 (0.31–2.2)	6.0 (1.8–10.2)
Liver disease - cirrhosis	0.31** (0.1–0.7)	32** (10–56)
acute hepatitis	0.35 (0.25–0.45)	19.2 (16.6–21.8)
cholestasis	0.65 (0.25–1.45)	14.4 (5.7–31.8)
Pregnancy - 1st trimester	NR†	8.5 (3.1–13.9)
2nd trimester	NR†	8.8 (3.8–13.8)
3rd trimester	NR†	13.0 (8.4–17.6)
Sepsis with multi-organ failure	0.47 (0.19–1.9)	18.8 (6.3–24.1)
Thyroid disease - hypothyroid	0.38 (0.13–0.57)	11.6 (8.2–25)
hyperthyroid	0.8 (0.68–0.97)	4.5 (3.7–5.6)

¶ For various North American patient populations from literature reports. Different rates of elimination and consequent dosage requirements have been observed among other peoples.

* Clearance represents the volume of blood completely cleared of theophylline by the liver in one minute. Values listed were generally determined at serum theophylline concentrations <20 mcg/mL; clearance may decrease and half-life may increase at higher serum concentrations due to nonlinear pharmacokinetics.

†† Reported range or estimated range (mean ±2 S.D.) where actual range not reported.

† NR = not reported or not reported in a comparable format.

** Median

Note: In addition to the factors listed above, theophylline clearance is increased and half-life decreased by low-carbohydrate/high-protein diets, parenteral nutrition, and daily consumption of charcoal-broiled beef. A high-carbohydrate/low-protein diet can decrease the clearance and prolong the half-life of theophylline.

Metabolism Following oral dosing, theophylline does not undergo any measurable first-pass elimination. Approximately 90% of the dose is metabolized in the liver. Biotransformation takes place through demethylation to 1-methylxanthine and 3-methylxanthine and hydroxylation to 1,3-dimethyluric acid. 1-methylxanthine is further hydroxylated, by xanthine oxidase, to 1-methyluric acid. About 6% of a theophylline dose is N-methylated to caffeine. Theophylline demethylation to 3-methylxanthine is catalyzed by cytochrome P450 1A2, while cytochromes P450 2E1 and P450 3A3 catalyze the hydroxylation to 1,3–dimethyluric acid. Demethylation to 1-methylxanthine appears to be catalyzed either by cytochrome P450 1A2 or a closely related cytochrome.

Caffeine and 3-methylxanthine are the only theophylline metabolites with pharmacologic activity. 3-methylxanthine has approximately one tenth the pharmacologic activity of theophylline and serum concentrations in adults with normal renal function are <1 mcg/mL. In patients with end-stage renal disease, 3-methylxanthine may accumulate to concentrations that approximate the unmetabolized theophylline concentration. Caffeine concentrations are usually undetectable in adults regardless of renal function.

Both the N-demethylation and hydroxylation pathways of theophylline biotransformation are capacity-limited. Due to the wide intersubject variability of the rate of theophylline metabolism and the possibility of intrasubject variability, nonlinearity of elimination may begin in some patients at serum theophylline concentrations <10 mcg/mL. This nonlinearity, also referred to as "saturation kinetics", results in more than proportional changes in serum theophylline concentrations with changes in dose; therefore, it is advisable to titrate the dose in small increments or decrements in order to achieve desired changes in serum theophylline concentrations (see **DOSAGE AND ADMINISTRATION**). Accurate prediction of dose-dependency of theophylline metabolism in patients *a priori* is not possible, but patients with very high initial clearance rates (ie, low steady-state serum theophylline concentrations at above average doses) have the greatest likelihood of experiencing large changes in serum theophylline concentration in response to dosage changes.

Excretion Approximately 10% of the theophylline dose is excreted unchanged in the urine. The remainder is excreted in the urine mainly as 1,3-dimethyluric acid (35–40%), 1-methyluric acid (20–25%), and 3-methylxanthine (15–20%). Since little theophylline is excreted unchanged in the urine and since active metabolites of theophylline (ie, caffeine, 3-methylxanthine) do not accumulate to clinically significant levels even in the face of end-stage renal disease, no dosage adjustment for renal insufficiency is necessary (see **WARNINGS**).

Serum Concentrations at Steady State After multiple doses of theophylline, steady state is reached in 30–65 hours (average 40 hours) in adults. At steady state, on a dosage regimen with 6-hour intervals, the expected mean trough concentration is approximately 60% of the mean peak concentration, assuming a mean theophylline half-life of 8 hours. The difference between peak and trough concentrations is larger in patients with more rapid theophylline clearance. In patients with high theophylline clearance and half-lives of about 4–5 hours, the trough serum theophylline concentration may be only 30% of peak with a 6-hour dosing interval. In these patients a slow-release formulation would allow a longer dosing interval (8–12 hours) with a smaller peak/trough difference.

Special Populations (see Table I for mean clearance and half-life values)

Geriatric: The clearance of theophylline is decreased by an average of 30% in healthy elderly adults (>60 yrs) compared to healthy young adults. Careful attention to dose reduction and frequent monitoring of serum theophylline concentrations are required in elderly patients (see **WARNINGS**).

Children 12 to 16: Theophylline clearance decreases slowly to adult values at about age 16. Careful attention to dosage selection and monitoring of serum theophylline concentrations are required (see **WARNINGS** and **DOSAGE AND ADMINISTRATION**).

Continued on next page

Key—Cont.

Gender: Gender differences in theophylline clearance are relatively small and unlikely to be of clinical significance. Significant reduction in theophylline clearance, however, has been reported in women on the 20th day of the menstrual cycle and during the third trimester of pregnancy.
Race: Pharmacokinetic differences in theophylline clearance due to race have not been studied.
Renal Insufficiency: Only a small fraction, eg, about 10%, of the administered theophylline dose is excreted unchanged in the urine. Since little theophylline is excreted unchanged in the urine and since active metabolites of theophylline (ie, caffeine, 3-methylxanthine) do not accumulate to clinically significant levels even in the face of end-stage renal disease, no dosage adjustment for renal insufficiency is necessary.
Hepatic Insufficiency: Theophylline clearance is decreased by 50% or more in patients with hepatic insufficiency (eg, cirrhosis, acute hepatitis, cholestasis). Careful attention to dose reduction and frequent monitoring of serum theophylline concentrations are required in patients with reduced hepatic function (see **WARNINGS**).
Congestive Heart Failure (CHF): Theophylline clearance is decreased by 50% or more in patients with CHF. The extent of reduction in theophylline clearance in patients with CHF appears to be directly correlated to the severity of the cardiac disease. Since theophylline clearance is independent of liver blood flow, the reduction in clearance appears to be due to impaired hepatocyte function rather than reduced perfusion. Careful attention to dose reduction and frequent monitoring of serum theophylline concentrations are required in patients with CHF (see **WARNINGS**).
Smokers: Tobacco and marijuana smoking appear to increase the clearance of theophylline by induction of metabolic pathways. The duration of this effect after cessation of smoking is unkown but may require 6 months to 2 years before the rate approaches that of a nonsmoker. Theophylline clearance has been shown to increase by approximately 50% in young adult tobacco smokers and by approximately 80% in elderly tobacco smokers compared to nonsmoking subjects. Passive smoke exposure has also been shown to increase theophylline clearance by up to 50%. Abstinence from tobacco smoking for one week causes a reduction of approximately 40% in theophylline clearance. Careful attention to dose reduction and frequent monitoring of serum theophylline concentrations are required in patients who stop smoking (see **WARNINGS**). Use of nicotine gum has been shown to have no effect on theophylline clearance.
Fever: Fever, regardless of its underlying cause, can decrease the clearance of theophylline. The magnitude and duration of the fever appear to be directly correlated to the degree of decrease of theophylline clearance. Precise data are lacking, but a temperature of 39°C (102°F) for at least 24 hours or lesser temperature elevations (>100°F) for longer periods, are probably required to produce a clinically significant increase in serum theophylline concentrations. Patients with rapid rates of theophylline clearance (ie, those who require a dose that is substantially larger than average [eg, >22 mg/kg/day] to achieve a therapeutic peak serum theophylline concentration when afebrile) may be at greater risk of toxic effects from decreased clearance during sustained fever. Careful attention to dose reduction and frequent monitoring of serum theophylline concentrations are required in patients with sustained fever (see **WARNINGS**).
Miscellaneous: Other factors associated with decreased theophylline clearance include the third trimester of pregnancy, sepsis with multiple organ failure, and hypothyroidism. Careful attention to dose reduction and frequent monitoring of serum theophylline concentrations are required in patients with any of these conditions (see **WARNINGS**). Other factors associated with increased theophylline clearance include hyperthyroidism and cystic fibrosis.

UNI-DUR Pharmacokinetics
Following the single-dose crossover administration of a 600 mg UNI-DUR Tablet to 20 healthy male subjects after an overnight fast, a peak serum theophylline concentration of 5.3 ±1.3 mcg/mL was obtained at 13.6 ±3.7 hours and the mean area under the curve extrapolated to infinity (AUC_{inf}) was 132.7 ±45.1 mcg hr/mL. When taken immediately after a high-fat breakfast, the mean AUC_{inf} was 136.0 ±36.7 mcg hr/mL with a mean peak theophylline serum level of 52 ±1.5 mcg/mL at 17.1 ±6.3 hours. While food did not affect the extent of absorption as evidenced by the similar AUC_{inf} values, food did prolong the time to peak concentration. The absorption from half tablets of the 600 mg product was also evaluated and found to be bioequivalent to that of the whole tablets. The relative extent of absorption of theophylline from the 600 mg UNI-DUR Tablet, fasting, when compared to an immediate-release theophylline tablet, was 84.3%; and for the non-fasting treatment was 88.7%.
In a separate multiple-dose study, two 400 mg UNI-DUR Tablets were compared to one 600 mg UNI-DUR Tablet. This study was a two-way, randomized, crossover multiple-dose study in 17 nonsmoking healthy males. Both products were dosed once-a-day in the morning after an overnight fast and 1 hour prior to a meal for 5 days. There was no significant difference in any of the pharmacokinetic parameters when corrected for dose.
The mean dose AUCss (corrected to the 600 mg dose) for the two 400 mg UNI-DUR Tablets was 179.7 ±62.9 mcg hr/mL and for the 600 mg UNI-DUR Tablet was 170.9 ±75.2 mcg hr/mL. The two 400 mg UNI-DUR Tablets reached dose corrected maximum serum concentration of 9.8 ±2.6 mcg/mL and the 600 mg UNI-DUR Tablet reached a maximum of 9.7 ±3.5 mcg/mL. The minimum concentrations were 4.9 ±2.6 mcg/mL and 4.4 ±2.6 mcg/mL for the two 400 mg and 600 mg UNI-DUR Tablets, respectively.
Steady-state pharmacokinetics were determined in a multiple-dose, crossover study with 24 healthy nonsmoking male subjects having an average theophylline clearance of 5.70 ±2.36 (S.D.) liters per hour. Following an overnight fast, a UNI-DUR 600 mg Extended-release Tablet was administered once daily in the morning for 5 consecutive days. The UNI-DUR Tablet exhibited better extended-release characteristics compared with a reference extended-release q12h product (2 ×300 mg) administered once daily in the morning following an overnight fast for 5 consecutive days. The results are noted as follows (mean values ±S.D.):

	AUCss (mcg hr/mL)	C_{max} (mcg/mL)	C_{min} (mcg/mL)	T_{max} (hr)
UNI-DUR	119 ± 36	6.9 ± 2.4	3.7 ± 1.3	11.5 ± 5.7
Reference	154 ± 37	10.5 ± 2.3	2.5 ± 1.1	7.6 ± 1.7

The mean percent fluctuation $[(C_{max}-C_{min}/C_{min}) \times 100]$ was 130% for the once-daily UNI-DUR regimen and 389% for the reference q12h product administered once daily. The extent of theophylline absorption from UNI-DUR Tablets relative to the reference q12h product was 74.9% (95% C.I. =67–84).
Steady-state pharmacokinetics comparing UNI-DUR Tablets once-daily administration with twice-daily administration were determined in a multiple-dose, crossover study with 24 healthy, nonsmoking male subjects having an average theophylline clearance of 4.53 ±1.21 (S.D.) liters per hour. Using UNI-DUR 400 mg Extended-release Tablets, a total daily theophylline dose of 800 mg was administered for 5 consecutive days either once daily as two tablets in the morning (8 AM) with a standardized breakfast or twice daily as one tablet in the morning (8 AM) with a standardized breakfast and one tablet in the evening (8 PM). The once-daily UNI-DUR regimen was bioequivalent to the twice-daily UNI-DUR regimen. The results are noted as follows (mean values ±S.D.):

	AUCss (mcg hr/mL)	C_{max} (mcg/mL)	C_{min} (mcg/mL)	T_{max} (hr)
QD Regimen	187 ± 45	10.4 ± 2.9	6.0 ±1.3	12.0 ± 3.7
q12h Regimen	187 ± 43	9.4 ± 2.2	8.4 ± 2.6	14.5 ± 6.6

The mean percent fluctuation $[(C_{max}-C_{min}/C_{min}) \times 100]$ was 78% for the once-daily UNI-DUR regimen and 17% for the twice-daily UNI-DUR regimen. The extent of theophylline absorption from the once-daily UNI-DUR regimen relative to the twice-daily UNI-DUR regimen was 100% (95% C.I. =95–105).

Clinical Studies:
In patients with chronic asthma, including patients with severe asthma requiring inhaled corticosteroids or alternate-day oral corticosteroids, many clinical studies have shown that theophylline decreases the frequency and severity of symptoms, including nocturnal exacerbations, and decreases the "as needed" use of inhaled $beta_2$-agonists. Theophylline has also been shown to reduce the need for short courses of daily oral prednisone to relieve exacerbations of airway obstruction that are unresponsive to bronchodilators in asthmatics.
In patients with chronic obstructive pulmonary disease (COPD), clinical studies have shown that theophylline decreases dyspnea, air trapping, the work of breathing, and improves contractility of diaphragmatic muscles with little or no improvement in pulmonary function measurements.

INDICATIONS AND USAGE
UNI-DUR Extended-release Tablets are indicated for the treatment of the symptoms and reversible airflow obstruction associated with chronic asthma and other chronic lung diseases, eg, emphysema and chronic bronchitis (see **DOSAGE AND ADMINISTRATION** section for initiation of therapy).

CONTRAINDICATIONS
UNI-DUR Extended-release Tablets are contraindicated in patients with a history of hypersensitivity to theophylline or other components in the product. The product is contraindicated in patients with active peptic ulcer disease and in individuals with underlying seizure disorders.

WARNINGS
Serious side effects such as ventricular arrhythmias, convulsions, or even death may appear as the first sign of toxicity without any previous warning. Less serious signs of theophylline toxicity (ie, nausea and restlessness) may occur frequently when initiating therapy but are usually transient. When such signs are persistent during maintenance therapy, they are often associated with serum concentrations above 20 mcg/mL. Stated differently, serious toxicity is not reliably preceded by less severe side effects. A serum concentration measurement is the only reliable method of predicting potentially life-threatening toxicity.

Concurrent Illness:
Theophylline should be used with extreme caution in patients with cardiac arrythmias due to increased risk of exacerbation of the concurrent arrythmia.

Conditions That Reduce Theophylline Clearance:
There are several readily identifiable causes of reduced theophylline clearance. ***If the total daily dose is not appropriately reduced so as to lower serum theophylline levels to within the therapeutic range in the presence of these risk factors, severe and potentially fatal theophylline toxicity can occur.***
Careful consideration must be given to the benefits and risks of theophylline use and the need for more intensive monitoring of serum theophylline concentrations in patients with the following risk factors:

Age:
Elderly (>60 years)

Concurrent Diseases:
Acute pulmonary edema
Congestive heart failure
Cor pulmonale
Fever; ≥102° for 24 hours or more; or lesser temperature elevations for longer periods
Hypothyroidism
Influenza and other viral illnesses
Liver disease; cirrhosis, acute hepatitis
Sepsis with multi-organ failure
Shock

Cessation of Smoking:
(See "*Special Populations—Smokers*".)

Drug Interactions:
Adding a drug that inhibits theophylline metabolism (eg, cimetidine, erythromycin, tacrine) or stopping a concurrently administered drug that enhances theophylline metabolism (eg, carbamazepine, rifampin). (See **PRECAUTIONS, Drug Interactions, Table II.**)

When Signs or Symptoms of Theophylline Toxicity Are Present:
Some of the signs of theophylline toxicity mimic other illnesses. Whenever a patient receiving theophylline develops nausea or vomiting, particularly repetitive vomiting, or other signs or symptoms consistent with theophylline toxicity as noted in the ADVERSE REACTIONS sections (even if another cause may be suspected), a serum theophylline concentration should be measured immediately and additional doses of theophylline should be withheld until the diagnosis is confirmed. Patients should be instructed not to continue any dosage that causes adverse effects and to withhold subsequent doses until the symptoms have resolved, at which time the clinician may instruct the patient to resume the drug at a lower dosage (see **DOSAGE AND ADMINISTRATION, Dosage Guidelines**).

Dosage Increases:
Increases in the dose of theophylline should not be made in response to an acute exacerbation of symptoms of chronic lung disease since theophylline provides little added benefit to inhaled $beta_2$-selective agonists and systemically administered corticosteroids in this circumstance and increases the risk of adverse effects. A *peak* steady-state serum theophylline concentration should be measured before increasing the dose in response to persistent chronic symptoms to ascertain whether an increase in dose is safe. Before increasing the theophylline dose on the basis of a low serum concentration, the clinician should consider whether the blood sample was obtained at an appropriate time in relationship to the dose and whether the patient has adhered to the prescribed regimen (see **PRECAUTIONS, Laboratory Tests**).
As the rate of theophylline clearance may be dose-dependent (ie, steady-state serum concentrations may increase disproportionately to the increase in dose), an increase in dose based upon a sub-therapeutic serum concentration measurement should be conservative. In general, limiting dose increases to about 25% of the previous total daily dose will reduce the risk of unintended excessive increases in serum theophylline concentration (see **DOSAGE AND ADMINISTRATION**).

PRECAUTIONS
UNI-DUR TABLETS SHOULD *NOT* BE CHEWED OR CRUSHED, AND SHOULD *BE BROKEN ONLY AT THE SCORE.*

General:
Careful consideration of the various interacting drugs (including recently discontinued medications), physiologic conditions, and other factors such as smoking that can alter theophylline clearance and require dosage adjustment should occur prior to initiation of theophylline therapy, prior to increases in theophylline dose, and during follow up (see

WARNINGS). The dose of theophylline selected for initiation of therapy should be low and, *if tolerated*, increased slowly over a period of a week or longer with the final dose guided by monitoring serum theophylline concentrations and the patient's clinical response (see **DOSAGE AND ADMINISTRATION**).

Information for Patients: This information is intended to aid in the safe and effective use of this medication. It is not a disclosure of all possible adverse or intended effects. The physician should reinforce the importance of taking only the prescribed dose, as well as the time interval between prescribed doses. UNI-DUR Tablets *should not be chewed or crushed.* Information relating to taking UNI-DUR Tablets in relation to meals or fasting should be provided. All patients should be asked to report side effects which occur at any time or recurrence of symptoms, especially toward the end of a 24-hour dosing interval.

The patient (or parent/caregiver) should be instructed to seek medical advice whenever such symptoms as nausea, vomiting, persistent headache, insomnia, restlessness, or rapid heartbeat occurs during treatment with theophylline, even if another cause is suspected. Patients should be instructed to contact their clinician if they develop a new illness, especially if accompanied by a fever, if they experience worsening of a chronic illness, if they start or stop smoking cigarettes or marijuana, or if another clinician adds a new medication adds a new medication or discontinues a previously prescribed medication. Patients should be informed that theophylline interacts with a wide variety of drug (see **Table II**). They should be instructed to inform all clinicians involved in their care that they are taking theophylline, especially when a medication is being added or deleted from their treatment. Patients should be instructed to not alter the dose, timing of the dose, or frequency of administration without first consulting their clinician. If a dose is missed, the patient should be instructed to take the next dose at the usually scheduled time and to not attempt to make up for the missed dose.

Laboratory Tests–Monitoring Serum Theophylline Concentrations:

Serum theophylline concentration measurements are readily available and should be used to determine whether the dosage is appropriate. Specifically, the serum theophylline concentration should be measured as follows:

1. When initiating therapy to guide final dosage adjustment after titration.

2. Before making a dose increase to determine whether the serum concentration is sub-therapeutic in a patient who continues to be symptomatic.

3. Whenever signs or symptoms of theophylline toxicity are present.

4. Whenever there is a new illness, worsening of a chronic illness, or a change in the patient's treatment regimen that may alter theophylline clearance [eg, fever (see **CLINICAL PHARMACOLOGY**, *Fever*), hepatitis, or drugs listed in **Table II** are added or discontinued].

To guide a dose increase, the blood sample should be obtained at the time of the expected peak serum theophylline concentration; 8 to 12 hours after a UNI-DUR dose at steady-state. For most patients, steady-state will be reached after 4 days of dosing with UNI-DUR Tablets when no doses have been missed, no extra doses have been added, and none of the doses have been taken at unequal intervals. A trough concentration (ie, at the end of the dosing interval) provides no additional useful information and may lead to an inappropriate dose increase since the peak serum theophylline concentration can be two or more times greater than the trough concentration with an immediate-release formulation. If the serum sample is drawn more than 12 hours after the dose, the results must be interpreted with caution since the concentration may not be reflective of the peak concentration. In contrast, when signs or symptoms of theophylline toxicity are present, the serum sample should be obtained as soon as possible, analyzed immediately, and the result reported to the clinician without delay. In patients in whom decreased serum protein binding is suspected (eg, cirrhosis, women during the third trimester of pregnancy), the concentration of unbound theophylline should be measured and the dosage adjusted to achieve an unbound concentration of 6-12 mcg/mL.

Saliva concentrations of theophylline cannot be used reliably to adjust dosage without special techniques.

Effects on Laboratory Tests:

As a result of its pharmacological effects, theophylline at serum concentration within the 10-20 mcg/mL range modestly increases plasma glucose (from a mean of 88 mg% to 98 mg%), uric acid (from a mean of 4 mg/dL to 6 mg/dL), free fatty acids (from a mean of 451 µEq/dL to 800 µEq/dL), total cholesterol (from a mean of 140 vs 160 mg/dL), HDL (from a mean of 36 to 50 mg/dL), HDL/LDL ratio (from a mean of 0.5 to 0.7), and urinary free cortisol excretion (from a mean of 44 to 63 mcg/24 hr). Theophylline at serum concentrations within the 10-20 mcg/mL range may also transiently decrease serum concentrations of triiodothyronine (144 before, 131 after 1 week and 142 ng/dL after 4 weeks of theophylline). The clinical importance of these changes should be

Table II. Clinically significant drug interactions with theophylline*.

Drug	Type of Interaction	Effect**
Adenosine	Theophylline blocks adenosine receptors.	Higher doses of adenosine may be required to achieve desired effect.
Alcohol	A single large dose of alcohol (eg, 3 mL/kg of whiskey) decreases theophylline clearance for up to 24 hours.	30% increase
Allopurinol	Decreases theophylline clearance at allopurinol doses ≥600 mg/day.	25% increase
Aminoglutethimide	Increases theophylline clearance by induction of microsomal enzyme activity.	25% decrease
Carbamazepine	Similar to aminoglutethimide.	30% decrease
Cimetidine	Decreases theophylline clearance by inhibiting cytochrome P450 1A2.	70% increase
Ciprofloxacin	Similar to cimetidine.	40% increase
Clarithromycin	Similar to erythromycin.	25% increase
Diazepam	Benzodiazepines increase CNS concentrations of adenosine, a potent CNS depressant, while theophylline blocks adenosine receptors.	Larger diazepam doses may be required to produce desired level of sedation. Discontinuation of theophylline without reduction of diazepam dose may result in respiratory depression.
Disulfiram	Decreases theophylline clearance by inhibiting hydroxylation and demethylation.	50% increase
Enoxacin	Similar to cimetidine.	300% increase
Ephedrine	Synergistic CNS effects.	Increased frequency of nausea, nervousness, and insomnia.
Erythromycin	Erythromycin metabolite decreases theophylline clearance by inhibiting cytochrome P450 3A3.	35% increase. Erythromycin steady-state serum concentrations decrease by a similar amount.
Estrogen	Estrogen-containing oral contraceptives decrease theophylline clearance in a dose-dependent fashion. The effect of progesterone on theophylline clearance is unknown.	30% increase
Flurazepam	Similar to diazepam.	Similar to diazepam.
Fluvoxamine	Similar to cimetidine.	Similar to cimetidine.
Halothane	Halothane sensitizes the myocardium to catecholamines; theophylline increases release of endogenous catecholamines.	Increased risk of ventricular arrhythmias.
Interferon, human recombinant alpha-A	Decreases theophylline clearance.	100% increase
Isoproterenol (IV)	Increases theophylline clearance.	20% decrease
Ketamine	Pharmacologic.	May lower theophylline seizure threshold.
Lithium	Theophylline increases renal lithium clearance.	Lithium dose required to achieve a therapeutic serum concentration increased an average of 60%.
Lorazepam	Similar to diazepam.	Similar to diazepam.
Methotrexate (MTX)	Decreases theophylline clearance.	20% increase after low dose MTX, higher dose MTX may have a greater effect.
Mexiletine	Similar to disulfiram.	80% increase
Midazolam	Similar to diazepam.	Similar to diazepam.
Moricizine	Increases theophylline clearance.	25% decrease
Norfloxacin	Increases serum theophylline levels.	
Ofloxacin	Increases serum theophylline levels.	
Pancuronium	Theophylline may antagonize nondepolarizing neuromuscular blocking effects; possibly due to phosphodiesterase inhibition.	Larger dose of pancuronium may be required to achieve neuromuscular blockade.
Pentoxifylline	Decreases theophylline clearance.	30% increase
Phenobarbital (PB)	Similar to aminoglutethimide.	25% decrease after 2 weeks of concurrent PB.
Phenytoin	Phenytoin increases theophylline clearance by increasing microsomal enzyme activity. Theophylline decreases phenytoin absorption.	Serum theophylline *and* phenytoin concentrations decrease about 40%.
Propafenone	Decreases theophylline clearance and pharmacologic interaction.	40% increase. Beta$_2$-blocking effect may decrease efficacy of theophylline.
Propranolol	Similar to cimetidine and pharmacologic interaction.	100% increase. Beta$_2$-blocking effect may decrease efficacy of theophylline.
Rifampin	Increases theophylline clearance by increasing cytochrome P450 1A2 and 3A3 activity.	20–40% decrease
Sucralfate	Reduces absorption of theophylline.	
Sulfinpyrazone	Increases theophylline clearance by increasing demethylation and hydroxylation. Decreases renal clearance of theophylline.	20% decrease

Continued on next page

Key—Cont.

Table II. Clinically significant drug interactions with theophylline*. (Continued)

Drug	Type of Interaction	Effect**
Tacrine	Similar to cimetidine, also increases renal clearance of theophylline.	90% increase
Thiabendazole	Decreases theophylline clearance.	190% increase
Ticlopidine	Decreases theophylline clearance.	60% increase
Troleandomycin	Similar to erythromycin.	33–100% increase depending on troleandomycin dose.
Verapamil	Similar to disulfiram.	20% increase

*Refer to **PRECAUTIONS, Drug Interactions** for further information regarding table.
**Average effect on steady-state theophylline concentration or other clinical effect for pharmacologic interactions. Individual patients may experience larger changes in serum theophylline concentration than the value listed.

weighed against the potential therapeutic benefit of theophylline in individual patients.

The Effect of Other Drugs on Theophylline Serum Concentration Measurements:
Most serum theophylline assays in clinical use are immunoassays which are specific for theophylline. Other xanthines such as caffeine, dyphylline, and pentoxifylline are not detected by these assays. Some drugs (eg, cefazolin, cephalothin), however, may interfere with certain HPLC techniques. Caffeine and xanthine metabolites in patients with renal dysfunction may cause the reading from some dry reagent office methods to be higher than the actual serum theophylline concentration.

Drug Interactions:
Theophylline interacts with a wide variety of drugs. The interaction may be pharmacodynamic, ie, alterations in the therapeutic response to theophylline or another drug or occurrence of adverse effects without a change in serum theophylline concentration. More frequently, however, the interaction is pharmacokinetic, ie, the rate of theophylline clearance is altered by another drug resulting in increased or decreased serum theophylline concentrations. Theophylline only rarely alters the pharmacokinetics of other drugs.
The drugs listed in **Table II** have potential to produce clinically significant pharmacodynamic or pharmacokinetic interactions with theophylline. The information in the "**Effect**" column of Table II assumes that the interacting drug is being added to a steady-state theophylline regimen. If theophylline is being initiated in a patient who is already taking a drug that inhibits theophylline clearance (eg, cimetidine, erythromycin), the dose of theophylline required to achieve a therapeutic serum theophylline concentration will be smaller. Conversely, if theophylline is being initiated in a patient who is already taking a drug that enhances theophylline clearance (eg, rifampin), the dose of theophylline required to achieve a therapeutic serum theophylline concentration will be larger. Discontinuation of a concomitant drug that increases theophylline clearance will result in accumulation of theophylline to potentially toxic levels, unless the theophylline dose is appropriately reduced. Discontinuation of a concomitant drug that inhibits theophylline clearance will result in decreased serum theophylline concentrations, unless the theophylline dose is appropriately increased.
The listing of drugs in **Table II** is current as of June 8, 1995. New interactions are continuously being reported for theophylline, especially with new chemical entities. **The clinician should not assume that a drug does not interact with theophylline if it is not listed in Table II.** Before addition of a newly available drug in a patient receiving theophylline, the package insert of the new drug and/or the medical literature should be consulted to determine if an interaction between the new drug and theophylline has been reported.
[See Table II on preceding page and above.]

Caution should be exercised in the administration of all quinolones to patients receiving concomitant theophylline therapy since it has been shown that some quinolones increase the plasma levels of theophylline by affecting the rate of theophylline clearance.

Drug/Food Interactions:
The extent of theophylline absorption from UNI-DUR Tablets is similar when administered fasting or immediately after a high-fat content breakfast. However, the time to peak concentration was delayed following the high-fat content breakfast (see **CLINICAL PHARMACOLOGY, Pharmacokinetics**). This breakfast contained 729 total kilocalories of which 55% were derived from 45 g of fat; and it consisted of two scrambled eggs, two strips of bacon, one slice of toast with 1 pat of butter, 3 oz. of hash brown potatoes, and 180 mL of whole milk. The influence of the type and amount of other foods, as well as the time interval between drug and food has not been studied.

Carcinogenesis, Mutagenesis, and Impairment of Fertility:
Long-term carcinogenicity studies have been carried out in mice (oral doses 30-150 mg/kg) and rats (oral doses 5-75 mg/kg). Results are pending.
Theophylline has been studied in Ames salmonella, *in vivo* and *in vitro* cytogenetics, micronucleus, and Chinese hamster ovary test systems and has not been shown to be genotoxic.
In a 14-week continuous breeding study, theophylline, administered to mating pairs of $B6C3F_1$ mice at oral doses of 120, 270, and 500 mg/kg (approximately 1.0-3.0 times the human dose on a mg/m^2 basis) impaired fertility, as evidenced by decreases in the number of live pups per litter, decreases in the mean number of litters per fertile pair, and increases in the gestation period at the high dose as well as decreases in the proportion of pups born alive at the mid and high dose. In 13-week toxicity studies, theophylline was administered to F344 rats and $B6C3F_1$ mice at oral doses of 40-300 mg/kg (approximately 2.0 times the human dose on a mg/m^2 basis). At the high dose, systemic toxicity was observed in both species including decreases in testicular weight.

Pregnancy:
Category C There are no adequate and well-controlled studies in pregnant women. Additionally, there are no teratogenicity studies in nonrodents (eg, rabbits). Theophylline was not shown to be teratogenic in CD-1 mice at oral doses up to 400 mg/kg, approximately 2.0 times the human dose on a mg/m^2 basis or in CD-1 rats at oral doses up to 260 mg/kg, approximately 3.0 times the recommended human dose on a mg/m^2 basis. At a dose of 220 mg/kg, embryotoxicity was observed in rats in the absence of maternal toxicity.

Nursing Mothers:
Theophylline is excreted into breast milk and may cause irritablility or other signs of mild toxicity in nursing human infants. The concentration of theophylline in breast milk is about equivalent to the maternal serum concentration. An infant ingesting a liter of breast milk containing 10–20 mcg/mL of theophylline a day is likely too receive 10-20 mg of theophylline per day. Serious adverse effects in the infant are unlikely unless the mother has toxic serum theophylline concentrations.

Pediatric Use:
Safety and effectiveness of UNI-DUR Extended-release Tablets in children under 12 years of age have not been established.

Geriatric Use:
Elderly patients are at significantly greater risk of experiencing serious toxicity from theophylline than younger patients due to pharmacokinetic and pharmacodynamic changes associated with aging. Theophylline clearance is reduced in patients greater than 60 years of age, resulting in increased serum theophylline concentrations in response to a given theophylline dose. Protein binding may be decreased in the elderly resulting in a larger proportion of the total serum theophylline concentration in the pharmacologically active unbound form. Elderly patients also appear to be more sensitive to the toxic effects of theophylline after chronic overdosage than younger patients. For these reasons, the maximum daily dose of theophylline in patients greater than 60 years of age ordinarily should not exceed 400 mg/day unless the patient continues to be symptomatic and the peak steady-state serum theophylline concentration is <10 mcg/mL (see **DOSAGE AND ADMINISTRATION**). Theophylline doses greater than 400 mg/day should be prescribed with caution in elderly patients.

ADVERSE REACTIONS

Adverse reactions associated with theophylline are generally mild when peak serum theophylline concentrations are <20 mcg/mL and mainly consist of transient caffeine-like adverse effects such as nausea, vomiting, headache, and insomnia. When peak serum theophylline concentrations exceed 20 mcg/mL, however, theophylline produces a wide range of adverse reactions including persistent vomiting, cardiac arrhythmias, and intractable seizures which can be lethal (see **OVERDOSAGE**). The transient caffeine-like adverse reactions occur in about 50% of patients when theophylline therapy is initiated at doses higher than recommended initial doses (eg, >300 mg/day in adults). During the initiation of theophylline therapy, caffeine-like adverse effects may transiently alter patient behavior, especially in school age children, but this response rarely persists. Initiation of theophylline therapy at a low dose with subsequent slow titration to a predetermined age-related maximum dose will significantly reduce the frequency of these transient adverse effects (see **DOSAGE AND ADMINISTRATION**). In a small percentage of patients ($<3\%$ of children and $<10\%$ of adults), the caffeine-like adverse effects persist during maintenance therapy, even at peak serum theophylline concentrations within the therapeutic range (ie, 10-20 mcg/mL). Dosage reduction may alleviate the caffeine-like adverse effects in these patients; however, persistent adverse effects should result in a re-evaluation of the need for continued theophylline therapy and the potential therapeutic benefit of alternative treatment.
Other adverse reactions that have been reported at serum theophylline concentrations <20 mcg/mL include diarrhea, irritability, restlessness, fine skeletal muscle tremors, epigastric pain, hematemesis, reflex hyperexcitability, muscle twitching, palpitation, extrasystoles, flushing, hypotension, circulatory failure, ventricular arrhythmia, tachypnea, alopecia, hyperglycemia, inappropriate ADH syndrome, rash, and transient diuresis. In patients with hypoxia secondary to COPD, multifocal atrial tachycardia and flutter have been reported at serum theophylline concentrations ≥ 15 mcg/mL. There have been a few isolated reports of seizures at serum theophylline concentrations <20 mcg/mL in patients with and without underlying neurological disease or in elderly patients. The occurrence of seizures in elderly patients with serum theophylline concentrations <20 mcg/mL may be secondary to decreased protein binding resulting in a larger proportion of the total serum theophylline concentration in the pharmacologically active unbound form. The clinical characteristics of the seizures reported in patients with serum theophylline concentrations <20 mcg/mL have generally been milder than seizures associated with excessive serum theophylline concentrations resulting from an overdose (ie, they have generally been transient, often stopped without anticonvulsant therapy, and did not result in neurological residua). However, irreversible brain injury can occur following seizures due to theophylline.

Table III. Manifestations of theophylline toxicity.*

	Percentage of patients reported with sign or symptom			
	Acute Overdose (Large Single Ingestion)		Chronic Overdosage (Multiple Excessive Doses)	
Sign/Symptom	Study 1 (n=157)	Study 2 (n=14)	Study 1 (n=92)	Study 2 (n=102)
Asymptomatic	NR**	0	NR**	6
Gastrointestinal				
Vomiting	73	93	30	61
Abdominal Pain	NR**	21	NR**	12
Diarrhea	NR**	0	NR**	14
Hematemesis	NR**	0	NR**	2
Metabolic/Other				
Hypokalemia	85	79	44	43
Hyperglycemia	98	NR**	18	NR**
Acid/base disturbance	34	21	9	5
Rhabdomyolysis	NR**	7	NR**	0
Cardiovascular				
Sinus tachycardia	100	86	100	62
Other supraventricular tachycardias	2	21	12	14
Ventricular premature beats	3	21	10	19
Atrial fibrillation or flutter	1	NR**	12	NR**
Multifocal atrial tachycardia	0	NR**	2	NR**
Ventricular arrhythmias with hemodynamic instability	7	14	40	0
Hypotension/shock	NR**	21	NR**	8
Neurologic				
Nervousness	NR**	64	NR**	21
Tremors	38	29	16	14
Disorientation	NR**	7	NR**	11
Seizures	5	14	14	5
Death	3	21	10	4

*These data are derived from two studies in patients with serum theophylline concentrations >30 mcg/mL. In the first study (Study #1-Shanon, *Ann Intern Med.* 1993; 119:1161-67), data were prospectively collected from 249 consecutive cases of theophylline toxicity referred to a regional poison center for consultation. In the second study (Study #2-Sessler, *Am J Med.* 1990;88:567-76), data were retrospectively collected from 116 cases with serum

theophylline concentrations > 30 mcg/mL among 6000 blood samples obtained for measurement of serum theophylline concentrations in three emergency departments. Differences in the incidence of manifestations of theophylline toxicity between the two studies may reflect sample selection as a result of study design (eg, in Study #1, 48% of the patients had acute intoxications versus only 10% in Study #2) and different methods of reporting results.

**NR = Not reported in a comparable manner.

OVERDOSAGE

General:

The chronicity and pattern of theophylline overdosage significantly influences clinical manifestations of toxicity, management, and outcome. There are two common presentations: (1) *acute overdose*, ie, ingestion of a single large excessive dose (> 10 mg/kg) as occurs in the context of an attempted suicide or isolated medication error, and (2) *chronic overdosage*, ie, ingestion of repeated doses that are excessive for the patient's rate of theophylline clearance. The most common causes of chronic theophylline overdosage include patient or caregiver error in dosing, clinician prescribing of an excessive dose or a normal dose in the presence of factors known to decrease the rate of theophylline clearance, and increasing the dose in response to an exacerbation of symptoms without first measuring the serum theophylline concentration to determine whether a dose increase is safe.

Severe toxicity from theophylline overdose is a relatively rare event. In one health maintenance organization, the frequency of hospital admissions for chronic overdosage of theophylline was about 1 per 1000 person-years exposure. In another study, among 6000 blood samples obtained for measurement of serum theophylline concentration, for any reason, from patients treated in an emergency department, 7% were in the 20–30 mcg/mL range and 3% were > 30 mcg/mL. Approximately two thirds of the patients with serum theophylline concentrations in the 20–30 mcg/mL range had one or more manifestations of toxicity while > 90% of patients with serum theophylline concentrations > 30 mcg/mL were clinically intoxicated. Similarly, in other reports, serious toxicity from theophylline is seen principally at serum concentrations > 30 mcg/mL.

Several studies have described the clinical manifestations of theophylline overdose and attempted to determine the factors that predict life-threatening toxicity. In general, patients who experience an acute overdose are less likely to experience seizures than patients who have experienced a chronic overdosage, unless the peak serum theophylline concentration is > 100 mcg/mL. After a chronic overdosage, generalized seizures, life-threatening cardiac arrhythmias, and death may occur at serum theophylline concentrations > 30 mcg/mL. The severity of toxicity after chronic overdosage is more strongly correlated with the patient's age than the peak serum theophylline concentration; patients > 60 years are at the greatest risk for severe toxicity and mortality after a chronic overdosage. Pre-existing or concurrent disease may also significantly increase the susceptibility of a patient to a particular toxic manifestation, eg, patients with neurologic disorders have an increased risk of seizures and patients with cardiac disease have an increased risk of cardiac arrhythmias for a given serum theophylline concentration compared to patients without the underlying disease. The frequency of various reported manifestations of theophylline overdose according to the mode of overdose are listed in Table III.

Other manifestations of theophylline toxicity include increases in serum calcium, creatine kinase, myoglobin, and leukocyte count, decreases in serum phosphate and magnesium, acute myocardial infarction, and urinary retention in men with obstructive uropathy.

Seizures associated with serum theophylline concentrations > 30 mcg/mL are often resistant to anticonvulsant therapy and may result in irreversible brain injury if not rapidly controlled. Death from theophylline toxicity is most often secondary to cardiorespiratory arrest and/or hypoxic encephalopathy following prolonged generalized seizures or intractable cardiac arrhythmias causing hemodynamic compromise.

Overdose Management:

General Recommendations for Patients with Symptoms of Theophylline Overdose or Serum Theophylline Concentrations > 30 mcg/mL (Note: Serum theophylline concentrations may continue to increase after presentation of the patient for medical care).

1. While simultaneously instituting treatment, contact a regional poison center to obtain updated information and advice on individualizing the recommendations that follow.
2. Institute supportive care, including establishment of intravenous access, maintenance of the airway, and electrocardiographic monitoring.
3. *Treatment of seizures:* Because of the high morbidity and mortality associated with theophylline-induced seizures, treatment should be rapid and aggressive. Anticonvulsant therapy should be initiated with an intravenous benzodiazepine, eg, diazepam, in increments of 0.1–0.2 mg/kg every 1–3

minutes until seizures are terminated. Repetitive seizures should be treated with a loading dose of phenobarbital (20 mg/kg infused over 30–60 minutes). Animal studies and case reports of theophylline overdose in humans suggest that phenytoin is ineffective in terminating theophylline-induced seizures. The doses of benzodiazepines and phenobarbital required to terminate theophylline-induced seizures are close to the doses that may cause severe respiratory depression or respiratory arrest; the clinician should therefore be prepared to provide assisted ventilation. Elderly patients and patients with COPD may be more susceptible to the respiratory depressant effects of anticonvulsants. Barbiturate-induced coma or administration of general anesthesia may be required to terminate repetitive seizures or status epilepticus. General anesthesia should be used with caution in patients with theophylline overdose because fluorinated volatile anesthetics may sensitize the myocardium to endogenous catecholamines released by theophylline. Enflurane appears less likely to be associated with this effect than halothane and may, therefore, be safer. Neuromuscular blocking agents alone should not be used to terminate seizures since they abolish the musculoskeletal manifestations without terminating seizure activity in the brain.

4. *Anticipate need for anticonvulsants:* In patients with theophylline overdose who are at high risk for theophylline-induced seizures, eg, patients with acute overdoses and serum theophylline concentrations > 100 mcg/mL or chronic overdosage in patients > 60 years of age with serum theophylline concentrations > 30 mcg/mL, the need for anticonvulsant therapy should be anticipated. A benzodiazepine such as diazepam should be drawn into a syringe and kept at the patient's bedside and medical personnel qualified to treat seizures should be immediately available. In selected patients at high risk for theophylline-induced seizures, consideration should be given to the administration of prophylactic anticonvulsant therapy. Situations where prophylactic anticonvulsant therapy should be considered in high-risk patients include anticipated delays in instituting methods for extracorporeal removal of theophylline (eg, transfer of a high-risk patient from one healthcare facility to another for extracorporeal removal) and clinical circumstances that significantly interfere with efforts to enhance theophylline clearance (eg, where dialysis may not be technically feasible or a patient with vomiting unresponsive to antiemetics who is unable to tolerate multiple-dose oral activated charcoal). In animal studies, prophylactic administration of phenobarbital, *but not phenytoin*, has been shown to delay the onset of theophylline-induced generalized seizures and to increase the dose of theophylline required to induce seizures (ie, markedly increases the LD_{50}). Although there are no controlled studies in humans, a loading dose of intravenous phenobarbital (20 mg/kg infused over 60 minutes) may delay or prevent life-threatening seizures in high-risk patients while efforts to enhance theophylline clearance are continued. Phenobarbital may cause respiratory depression, particularly in elderly patients and patients with COPD.

5. *Treatment of cardiac arrhythmias:* Sinus tachycardia and simple ventricular premature beats are not harbingers of life-threatening arrhythmias, they do not require treatment in the absence of hemodynamic compromise, and they resolve with declining serum theophylline concentrations. Other arrhythmias, especially those associated with hemodynamic compromise, should be treated with antiarrhythmic therapy appropriate for the type of arrhythmia.

6. *Gastrointestinal decontamination:* Oral activated charcoal (0.5 g/kg up to 20 g and repeat at least once 1–2 hours after the first dose) is extremely effective in blocking the absorption of theophylline throughout the gastrointestinal tract, even when administered several hours after ingestion. If the patient is vomiting, the charcoal should be administered through a nasogastric tube or after administration of an antiemetic. Phenothiazine antiemetics such as prochlorperazine or perphenazine should be avoided since they can lower the seizure threshold and frequently cause dystonic reactions. A single dose of sorbitol may be used to promote stooling to facilitate removal of theophylline bound to charcoal from the gastrointestinal tract. Sorbitol, however, should be dosed with caution since it is a potent purgative which can cause profound fluid and electrolyte abnormalities, particularly after multiple doses. Commercially available fixed combinations of liquid charcoal and sorbitol should be avoided in young children and after the first dose in adolescents and adults since they do not allow for individualization of charcoal and sorbitol dosing. Ipecac syrup should be avoided in theophylline overdoses. Although ipecac induces emesis, it does not reduce the absorption of theophylline unless administered within 5 minutes of ingestion and even then is less effective than oral activated charcoal. Moreover, ipecac-induced emesis may persist for several hours after a single dose and significantly decrease the retention and the effectiveness of oral activated charcoal.

7. *Serum theophylline concentration monitoring:* The serum theophylline concentration should be measured immediately upon presentation, 2–4 hours later, and then at sufficient intervals, eg, every 4 hours, to guide treatment decisions and to assess the effectiveness of therapy. Serum theo-

phylline concentrations may continue to increase after presentation of the patient for medical care as a result of continued absorption of theophylline from the gastrointestinal tract. Serious monitoring of serum theophylline serum concentrations should be continued until it is clear that the concentration is no longer rising and has returned to non-toxic levels.

8. *General monitoring procedures:* Electrocardiographic monitoring should be initiated on presentation and continued until the serum theophylline level has returned to a non-toxic level. Serum electrolytes and glucose should be measured on presentation and at appropriate intervals indicated by clinical circumstances. Fluid and electrolyte abnormalities should be promptly corrected. **Monitoring and treatment should be continued until the serum concentration decreases below 20 mcg/mL.**

9. *Enhance clearance of theophylline:* Multiple-dose oral activated charcoal (eg, 0.5 mg/kg up to 20 g, every 2 hours) increases the clearance of theophylline at least twofold by adsorption of theophylline secreted into gastrointestinal fluids. Charcoal must be retained in, and pass through, the gastrointestinal tract to be effective; emesis should therefore be controlled by administration of appropriate antiemetics. Alternatively, the charcoal can be administered continuously through a nasogastric tube in conjunction with appropriate antiemetics. A single dose of sorbitol may be administered with the activated charcoal to promote stooling to facilitate clearance of the adsorbed theophylline from the gastrointestinal tract. Sorbitol alone does not enhance clearance of theophylline and should be dosed with caution to prevent excessive stooling which can result in severe fluid and electrolyte imbalances. Commercially available fixed combinations of liquid charcoal and sorbitol should be avoided in young children and after the first dose in adolescents and adults since they do not allow for individualization of charcoal and sorbitol dosing. In patients with intractable vomiting, extracorporeal methods of theophylline removal should be instituted (see OVERDOSAGE, Extracorporeal Removal).

Specific Recommendations:

Acute Overdose
A. Serum Concentration > 20 < 30 mcg/mL
1. Administer a single dose of oral activated charcoal.
2. Monitor the patient and obtain a serum theophylline concentration in 2–4 hours to ensure that the concentration is not increasing.
B. Serum Concentration > 30 < 100 mcg/mL
1. Administer multiple-dose oral activated charcoal and measures to control emesis.
2. Monitor the patient and obtain serial theophylline concentrations every 2–4 hours to gauge the effectiveness of therapy and to guide further treatment decisions.
3. Institute extracorporeal removal if emesis, seizures, or cardiac arrhythmias cannot be adequately controlled (see OVERDOSAGE, Extracorporeal Removal).
C. Serum Concentration > 100 mcg/mL
1. Consider prophylactic anticonvulsant therapy.
2. Administer multiple-dose oral activated charcoal and measures to control emesis.
3. Consider extracorporeal removal, even if the patient has not experienced a seizure (see OVERDOSAGE, Extracorporeal Removal).
4. Monitor the patient and obtain serial theophylline concentrations every 2–4 hours to gauge the effectiveness of therapy and to guide further treatment decisions.

Chronic Overdosage
A. Serum Concentration > 20 < 30 mcg/mL (with manifestations of theophylline toxicity)
1. Administer a single dose of oral activated charcoal.
2. Monitor the patient and obtain a serum theophylline concentration in 2–4 hours to ensure that the concentration is not increasing.
B. Serum Concentration > 30 mcg/mL in patients < 60 years of age
1. Administer multiple-dose oral activated charcoal and measures to control emesis.
2. Monitor the patient and obtain serial theophylline concentrations every 2–4 hours to gauge the effectiveness of therapy and to guide further treatment decisions.
3. Institute extracorporeal removal if emesis, seizures, or cardiac arrhythmias cannot be adequately controlled (see OVERDOSAGE, Extracorporeal Removal).
C. Serum Concentration > 30 mcg/mL in patients ≥ 60 years of age
1. Consider prophylactic anticonvulsant therapy.
2. Administer multiple-dose oral activated charcoal and measures to control emesis.
3. Consider extracorporeal removal even if the patient has not experienced a seizure (see OVERDOSAGE, Extracorporeal Removal).
4. Monitor the patient and obtain serial theophylline concentrations every 2–4 hours to gauge the effectiveness of therapy and to guide further treatment decisions.

Continued on next page

Consult 1997 supplements and future editions for revisions

Key—Cont.

Extracorporeal Removal:
Increasing the rate of theophylline clearance by extracorporeal methods may rapidly decrease serum concentrations, but the risks of the procedure must be weighed against the potential benefit. Charcoal hemoperfusion is the most effective method of extracorporeal removal, increasing theophylline clearance up to sixfold, but serious complications, including hypotension, hypocalcemia, platelet consumption, and bleeding diatheses may occur. Hemodialysis is about as efficient as multiple-dose oral activated charcoal and has a lower risk of serious complications than charcoal hemoperfusion. Hemodialysis should be considered as an alternative when charcoal hemoperfusion is not feasible and multiple-dose oral charcoal is ineffective because of intractable emesis. Serum theophylline concentrations may rebound 5–10 mcg/mL after discontinuation of charcoal hemoperfusion or hemodialysis due to redistribution of theophylline from the tissue compartment. Peritoneal dialysis is ineffective for theophylline removal; exchange transfusions in neonates have been minimally effective.

DOSAGE AND ADMINISTRATION

General Considerations:
The steady-state peak serum theophylline concentration is a function of the dose, the dosing interval, and the rate of theophylline absorption and clearance in the individual patient. Because of marked individual differences in the rate of theophylline clearance, the dose required to achieve a peak serum theophylline concentration in the 10–20 mcg/mL range varies fourfold among otherwise similar patients in the absence of factors known to alter theophylline clearance (eg, 400–1600 mg/day in adults <60 years old). For a given population there is no single theophylline dose that will provide both safe and effective serum concentrations for all patients. Administration of the medium theophylline dose required to achieve a therapeutic serum theophylline concentration in a given population may result in either sub-therapeutic or potentially toxic serum theophylline concentrations in individual patients. For example, at a dose of 900 mg/day in adults <60 years, the steady-state peak serum theophylline concentration will be <10 mcg/mL in about 30% of patients, 10–20 mcg/mL in about 50%, and 20–30 mcg/mL in about 20% of patients. **The dose of theophylline must be individualized on the basis of peak serum theophylline concentration measurements in order to achieve a dose that will provide maximum potential benefit with minimal risk of adverse effects.**
Transient caffeine-like adverse effects and excessive serum concentrations in slow metabolizers can be avoided in most patients by starting with a sufficiently low dose and slowly increasing the dose, *if judged to be clinically indicated,* in small increments. Dose increases should only be made if the previous dosage is well tolerated and at intervals of no less than 3 days to allow serum theophylline concentrations to reach the new steady state. Final dosage adjustment should be guided by serum theophylline concentration measurement (see **PRECAUTIONS, Laboratory Tests** and **DOSAGE AND ADMINISTRATION**). Healthcare providers should instruct patients and caregivers to discontinue any dosage that causes adverse effects, to withhold the medication until these symptoms are gone, and to then resume therapy at a lower, previously tolerated dosage (see **WARNINGS**).
If the patient's symptoms are well controlled, there are no apparent adverse effects, and no intervening factors that might alter dosage requirements (see **WARNINGS** and **PRECAUTIONS**), serum theophylline concentrations should be monitored at 6-month intervals for rapidly growing children and at yearly intervals for all others. In acutely ill patients, serum theophylline concentrations should be monitored at frequent intervals, eg, every 24 hours.
The extent of absorption of theophylline from UNI-DUR Tablets when administered fasting or immediately after a high-fat content breakfast is similar. However, the time to peak concentration is delayed (see **PRECAUTIONS, Drug/Food Interactions**).
Effective use of theophylline (ie, the concentration of drug in the serum associated with optimal benefit and minimal risk of toxicity) is considered to occur when the theophylline concentration is maintained from 10 to 15 mcg/mL.

Frequency of Dosing:
Patients who clear theophylline normally or relatively slowly, eg, nonsmokers, may be reasonable candidates for taking UNI-DUR Tablets once daily. However, certain patients, such as the young, smokers, and some nonsmoking adults are likely to metabolize theophylline more rapidly and may require dosing at 12-hour intervals. Such patients may experience symptoms of bronchospasm toward the end of a once-daily dosing interval and/or require a higher daily dose (higher than those recommended in labeling) and are more likely to experience relatively wide peak to trough differences in serum theophylline concentrations.

DOSAGE GUIDELINES
WARNING: DO NOT ATTEMPT TO MAINTAIN ANY DOSE THAT IS NOT WELL TOLERATED.
Dosage guidelines are approximations only and the wide range of theophylline clearance between individuals (particularly those with concomitant disease) makes indiscriminate usage hazardous. When appropriate, dosing should be calculated on the basis of lean body weight where mg/kg doses are to be prescribed since theophylline does not distribute into fatty tissue.

I. INITIATION OF THERAPY WITH UNI-DUR TABLETS
a. *Stabilized Patients (12 years of age or older)*
Individuals who are taking an immediate-release or extended-release theophylline product may be transferred to once-daily administration of 400 mg or 600 mg UNI-DUR Tablets on a mg-for-mg basis. For example, a patient stabilized on 400 mg twice daily (800 mg total daily dose) should be given two 400 mg UNI-DUR Tablets as a single daily dose of 800 mg in the morning.
It must be recognized that the peak and trough serum theophylline levels produced by the once-daily dosing may vary from those produced by the previous product and/or regimen.
b. *Initiation of Theophylline Dosing*
Adult patients and children 12 years of age and over not currently receiving theophylline may be titrated using an immediate- or extended-release theophylline product, which can be adjusted in small dosage increments. Once patients have been titrated and stabilized, they may be transferred to once-daily dosage with equivalent doses of UNI-DUR Extended-release Tablets as described in (a) above.

II. TITRATION AND DOSE ADJUSTMENT
a. *When Serum Levels Are Measured*
After 4 days therapy with UNI-DUR Tablets, steady state should have been achieved, and approximate peak serum theophylline concentration samples should be obtained 8 to 12 hours after administration in the morning. Trough concentration should be taken just prior to the administration of the next dose. It is important that the patient not have missed or added any dose during the previous 72 hours, and that the dosing intervals remain relatively constant.
DOSAGE ADJUSTMENTS BASED ON MEASUREMENTS WHEN THESE INSTRUCTIONS HAVE NOT BEEN FOLLOWED MAY RESULT IN TOXICITY.
b. *When Serum Levels Are Not Measured*
In the absence of laboratory facilities for determining serum theophylline concentration levels, clinical judgment should be followed.
- The original total once-daily dose should continue if it is well tolerated and the clinical response is satisfactory.
- If adverse reactions occur, decrease the dose as stated below.

If a patient is better controlled on another regimen than on the once-daily regimen, the patient should be maintained on the more effective regimen.
c. *Increasing or Decreasing the Dose of UNI-DUR Tablets*
If the observed serum theophylline concentration range is too low, or if serum theophylline values are too high, the patient should be transferred to an immediate- or extended-release (BID) theophylline product and dosage adjustments should be made as described in Table IV. **Application of these general dosing recommendations to individual patients must take into account the unique clinical characteristics of each patient. In general, these recommendations should serve as the upper limit for dosage adjustments in order to decrease the risk of potentially serious adverse events associated with unexpected large increases in serum theophylline concentration.**

III. MAINTENANCE THERAPY
Careful clinical titration is important to assure patient acceptance and safety of the medication. When stabilized as established by serum theophylline concentration or respiratory function, patients usually remain controlled without further dosage adjustment. It should be borne in mind, however, that for reasons stated in the **PRECAUTIONS** and **WARNINGS** sections, dosage adjustments may be necessary. Serum theophylline levels should be measured periodically (at 6- to 12-month intervals) even in clinically controlled patients.
The elderly as well as patients with congestive heart failure, cor pulmonale, and/or liver disease may have unusually low dosage requirements and thus may experience toxicity even at the dosage recommendations above.
WARNING: DO NOT MAINTAIN ANY DOSE THAT IS NOT WELL TOLERATED.

Table IV. Final dosage adjustment guided by serum theophylline concentration.

Peak Serum Concentration	Dosage Adjustment
<9.9 mcg/mL	If symptoms are not controlled and current dosage is tolerated, increase dose about 25%. Recheck serum concentration after 3 days for further dosage adjustment.
10 to 14.9 mcg/mL	If symptoms are controlled and current dosage is tolerated, maintain dose and recheck serum concentration at 6–12 month intervals.¶ If symptoms are not controlled and current dosage is tolerated, consider adding additional medication(s) to treatment regimen.
15–19.9 mcg/mL	Consider 10% decrease in dose to provide greater margin of safety even if current dosage is tolerated.¶
20–24.9 mcg/mL	Decrease dose by 25% even if no adverse effects are present. Recheck serum concentration after 3 days to guide further dosage adjustment.
25–30 mcg/mL	Skip next dose and decrease subsequent doses at least 25% even if no adverse effects are present. Recheck serum concentration after 3 days to guide further dosage adjustment. If symptomatic, consider whether overdose treatment is indicated (see recommendations for chronic overdosage).
>30 mcg/mL	Treat overdose as indicated (see recommendations for chronic overdosage). If theophylline is subsequently resumed, decrease dose by at least 50% and recheck serum concentration after 3 days to guide further dosage adjustment.

¶ Dose reduction and/or serum theophylline concentration measurement is indicated whenever adverse effects are present, physiologic abnormalities that can reduce theophylline clearance occur (eg, sustained fever), or a drug that interacts with theophylline is added or discontinued (see **WARNINGS**).

DOSAGE ADJUSTMENT BASED ON SERUM THEOPHYLLINE CONCENTRATION MEASUREMENTS WHEN THESE INSTRUCTIONS HAVE NOT BEEN FOLLOWED MAY RESULT IN RECOMMENDATIONS THAT PRESENT RISK OF TOXICITY TO THE PATIENT.

HOW SUPPLIED

UNI-DUR Extended-release Tablets are supplied as controlled-release tablets containing either 400 mg or 600 mg of theophylline anhydrous. They are mottled white, capsule-shaped tablets; scored on one side and debossed with the product name and strength on the other.
UNI-DUR Extended-release Tablets 400 mg are available in bottles of 100's (NDC 0085-0694-01).
UNI-DUR Extended-release Tablets 600 mg are available in bottles of 100's (NDC 0085-0814-01).

STORAGE CONDITIONS
Keep bottles tightly closed. Store between 15° and 25°C (59° and 77°F).
CAUTION: Federal law prohibits dispensing without prescription.
Key Pharmaceuticals, Inc.
Kenilworth, NJ 07033 USA
Copyright © 1995, 1996, Key Pharmaceuticals, Inc. All rights reserved.
Rev. 2/96 19042200
Shown in Product Identification Guide, page 319

Knoll Laboratories
A Division of
Knoll Pharmaceutical Company
3000 CONTINENTAL DRIVE NORTH
MOUNT OLIVE, NJ 07828

Direct Inquiries to:
Knoll Pharmaceutical Company
(201) 426-2600
Customer Service:
(800) 526-0710

For Medical Information Contact:
(800) 526-0221

AKINETON® TABLETS AND AMPULES ℞
[*ā-kĭn 'ĕ-ton*]
biperiden hydrochloride and biperiden lactate

DESCRIPTION
Each AKINETON® Tablet for oral administration contains 2 mg biperiden hydrochloride. Other ingredients may include corn syrup, lactose, magnesium stearate, potato starch and talc. Each 1 mL AKINETON Ampule for intramuscular

or intravenous administration contains 5 mg biperiden lactate in an aqueous 1.4 percent sodium lactate solution. No added preservative. AKINETON is an anticholinergic agent. Biperiden is α-5-Norbornen-2-yl-α-phenyl-1-piperidinepropanol. It is a white, crystalline, odorless powder, slightly soluble in water and alcohol. It is stable in air at normal temperatures. Biperiden may be represented by the following structural formula:

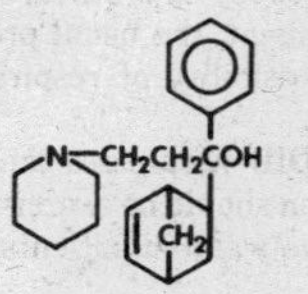

CLINICAL PHARMACOLOGY

AKINETON is a weak peripheral anticholinergic agent. It has, therefore, some antisecretory, antispasmodic and mydriatic effects. In addition, AKINETON possesses nicotinolytic activity. Parkinsonism is thought to result from an imbalance between the excitatory (cholinergic) and inhibitory (dopaminergic) systems in the corpus striatum. The mechanism of action of centrally active anticholinergic drugs such as AKINETON is considered to relate to competitive antagonism of acetylcholine at cholinergic receptors in the corpus striatum, which then restores the balance.

The parenteral form of AKINETON is an effective and reliable agent for the treatment of acute episodes of extrapyramidal disturbances sometimes seen during treatment with neuroleptic agents. Akathisia, akinesia, dyskinetic tremors, rigor, oculogyric crisis, spasmodic torticollis, and profuse sweating are markedly reduced or eliminated. With parenteral AKINETON, these drug-induced disturbances are rapidly brought under control. Subsequently, this can usually be maintained with oral doses which may be given with tranquilizer therapy in psychotic and other conditions requiring an uninterrupted therapeutic program.

Pharmacokinetics and Metabolism: Only limited pharmacokinetic studies of biperiden in humans are available The serum concentration at 1 to 1.5 hours following a single, 4 mg oral dose was 4–5 ng/mL. Plasma levels (0.1–0.2 ng/mL) could be determined up to 48 hours after dosing. Six hours after an oral dose of 250 mg/kg in rats, 87% of the drug had been absorbed. The metabolism of AKINETON is also incompletely understood, but does involve hydroxylation. In normal volunteers a single 10 mg intravenous dose of biperiden seemed to cause a transient rise in plasma cortisol and prolactin. No change in GH, LH, FSH, or TSH levels were seen. Biperiden lactate (10 mg/mL) was not irritating to the tissue of rabbits when injected intramuscularly (1.0 mL) into the sacrospinalis muscles and intradermally (0.25 mL) and subcutaneously (0.5 mL) into the shaved abdominal skin.

INDICATIONS AND USAGE

- As an adjunct in the therapy of all forms of parkinsonism (idiopathic, postencephalitic, arteriosclerotic)
- Control of extrapyramidal disorders secondary to neuroleptic drug therapy (e.g., phenothiazines)

CONTRAINDICATIONS

1) Hypersensitivity to biperiden 2) Narrow angle glaucoma 3) Bowel obstruction 4) Megacolon

WARNINGS

Isolated instances of mental confusion, euphoria, agitation and disturbed behavior have been reported in susceptible patients. Also, the central anticholinergic syndrome can occur as an adverse reaction to properly prescribed anticholinergic medication, although it is more frequently due to overdosage. It may also result from concomitant administration of an anticholinergic agent and a drug that has secondary anticholinergic actions (see Drug Interactions and Overdosage sections). Caution should be observed in patients with manifest glaucoma, though no prohibitive rise in intraocular pressure has been noted following either oral or parenteral administration. Patients with prostatism, epilepsy or cardiac arrhythmia should be given this drug with caution. Occasionally, drowsiness may occur, and patients who drive a car or operate any other potentially dangerous machinery should be warned of this possibility. As with other drugs acting on the central nervous system, the consumption of alcohol should be avoided during AKINETON therapy.

PRECAUTIONS

Drug Interactions: The central anticholinergic syndrome can occur when anticholinergic agents such as AKINETON are administered concomitantly with drugs that have secondary anticholinergic actions, e.g., certain narcotic analgesics such as meperidine, the phenothiazines and other antipsychotics, tricyclic antidepressants, certain antiarrhythmics such as the quinidine salts, and antihistamines. See Overdosage section for signs and symptoms of the central anticholinergic syndrome, and for treatment.

Pregnancy: Pregnancy Category C. Animal reproduction studies have not been conducted with AKINETON. It is also not known whether AKINETON can cause fetal harm when administered to a pregnant woman or can affect reproduction capacity. AKINETON should be given to a pregnant woman only if clearly needed.

Nursing Mothers: It is not known whether this drug is excreted in human milk. Because many drugs are excreted in human milk, caution should be exercised when AKINETON is administered to a nursing woman.

Pediatric Use: Safety and effectiveness in children have not been established.

ADVERSE REACTIONS

Atropine-like side effects such as dry mouth; blurred vision; drowsiness; euphoria or disorientation; urinary retention; postural hypotension; constipation; agitation; disturbed behavior may be seen. There usually are no significant changes in blood pressure or heart rate in patients who have been given the parenteral form of AKINETON. Mild transient postural hypotension and bradycardia may occur. These side effects can be minimized or avoided by slow intravenous administration. No local tissue reactions have been reported following intramuscular injection. If gastric irritation occurs following oral administration, it can be avoided by administering the drug during or after meals.

The central anticholinergic syndrome can occur as an adverse reaction to properly prescribed anticholinergic medication. See Overdosage section for signs and symptoms of the central anticholinergic syndrome, and for treatment.

OVERDOSAGE

Signs and Symptoms: Overdosage with AKINETON produces typical central symptoms of atropine intoxication (the central anticholinergic syndrome). Correct diagnosis depends upon recognition of the peripheral signs of parasympathetic blockade including dilated and sluggish pupils; warm, dry skin; facial flushing; decreased secretions of the mouth, pharynx, nose, and bronchi; foul-smelling breath; elevated temperature, tachycardia, cardiac arrhythmias, decreased bowel sounds, and urinary retention. Neuropsychiatric signs such as delirium, disorientation, anxiety, hallucinations, illusions, confusion, incoherence, agitation, hyperactivity, ataxia, loss of memory, paranoia, combativeness, and seizures may be present. The condition can progress to stupor, coma, paralysis, and cardiac and respiratory arrest and death.

Treatment: Treatment of acute overdose revolves around symptomatic and supportive therapy. If AKINETON was administered orally, gastric lavage or other measures to limit absorption should be instituted. A small dose of diazepam or a short acting barbiturate may be administered if CNS excitation is observed. Phenothiazines are contraindicated because the toxicity may be intensified due to their antimuscarinic action, causing coma. Respiratory support, artificial respiration or vasopressor agents may be necessary. Hyperpyrexia must be reversed, fluid volume replaced and acid-base balance maintained. Urinary catheterization may be necessary.

Routine use of physostigmine for overdose is controversial. Delirium, hallucinations, coma, and supraventricular tachycardia (not ventricular tachycardias or conduction defects) seem to respond. If indicated, 1 mg (half this amount for children or the elderly) may be given intramuscularly or by slow intravenous infusion. If there is no response within 20 minutes, an additional 1 mg dose may be given; this may be repeated until a total of 4 mg has been administered, a reversal of the toxic effects occur or excessive cholinergic signs are seen. Frequent monitoring of clinical signs should be done. Since physostigmine is rapidly destroyed, additional injections may be required every one or two hours to maintain control. The relapse intervals tend to lengthen as the toxic anticholinergic agent is metabolized, so the patient should be carefully observed for 8 to 12 hours following the last relapse.

Toxicity in Animals: The LD_{50} of biperiden in the white mouse is 545 mg/kg orally, 195 mg/kg subcutaneously, and 56 mg/kg intravenously. The acute oral toxicity (LD_{50}) in rats is 750 mg/kg. The intraperitoneal toxicity (LD_{50}) of biperiden lactate in rats was 270 mg/kg and the intravenous toxicity (LD_{50}) in dogs is 222 mg/kg. In dogs under general anesthesia, respiratory arrest occurred at 33 mg/kg (intravenous) and circulatory standstill at 45 mg/kg (intravenous). The oral LD_{50} in dogs was 340 mg/kg. Chronic toxicity studies in both rat and dog have been reported.

DOSAGE AND ADMINISTRATION

Drug-Induced Extrapyramidal Symptoms:

Parenteral: The average adult dose is 2 mg intramuscularly or intravenously. May be repeated every half-hour until there is resolution of symptoms, but not more than four consecutive doses should be given in a 24-hour period.

Note: Parenteral drug products should be inspected visually for particulate matter and discoloration prior to administration, whenever solution and container permit.

Oral: One tablet one to three times daily.

Parkinson's Disease: Oral: The usual beginning dose is one tablet three or four times daily. The dosage should be individualized with the dose titrated upward to a maximum of 8 tablets (16 mg) per 24 hours.

HOW SUPPLIED

AKINETON Tablets, 2 mg each, white, embossed on one face with a triangle, bisected on the reverse and imprinted with the number "11."

Bottles of 100—NDC #0044-0120-02.

Bottles of 1000—NDC #0044-0120-04.

AKINETON Ampules, 1 mL each containing 5 mg biperiden lactate per mL.

Boxes of 10—NDC #0044-0110-01.

Storage: All dosage forms of AKINETON should be stored at 59°–86°F (15°–30°C).

Dispense in tight, light-resistant container as defined in USP.

MR 1987/5427

Revised June, 1987 5427

Shown in Product Identification Guide, page 319

COLLAGENASE SANTYL® Ointment ℞

[săn ′tĭl]

(collagenase)

DESCRIPTION

SANTYL® OINTMENT is a sterile enzymatic debriding ointment which contains 250 collagenase units per gram of white petrolatum USP. The enzyme collagenase is derived from the fermentation by *Clostridium histolyticum.* It possesses the unique ability to digest native and denatured collagen in necrotic tissue.

CLINICAL PHARMACOLOGY

Since collagen accounts for 75% of the dry weight of skin tissue, the ability of collagenase to digest collagen in the physiological pH range and temperature makes it particularly effective in the removal of detritus.[1] Collagenase thus contributes towards the formation of granulation tissue and subsequent epithelization of dermal ulcers and severely burned areas.[2,3,4,5,6] Collagen in healthy tissue or in newly formed granulation tissue is not attacked.[2,3,4,5,6,7,8]

INDICATIONS

Santyl Ointment is indicated for debriding chronic dermal ulcers[2,3,4,5,6,8,9,10,11,12,13,14,15,16,17,18] and severely burned areas.[3,4,5,7,16,19,20,21]

CONTRAINDICATIONS

Santyl Ointment is contraindicated in patients who have shown local or systemic hypersensitivity to collagenase.

PRECAUTIONS

The optimal pH range of collagenase is 6 to 8. Higher or lower pH conditions will decrease the enzyme's activity and appropriate precautions should be taken. The enzymatic activity is also adversely affected by detergents, hexachlorophene and heavy metal ions such as mercury and silver which are used in some antiseptics. When it is suspected such materials have been used, the site should be carefully cleansed by repeated washings with normal saline before Santyl Ointment is applied. Soaks containing metal ions or acidic solutions such as Burow's solution should be avoided because of the metal ion and low pH. Cleansing materials such as hydrogen peroxide, Dakin's solution, and sterile saline are compatible with Santyl Ointment.

Debilitated patients should be closely monitored for systemic bacterial infections because of the theoretical possibility that debriding enzymes may increase the risk of bacteremia.

A slight transient erythema has been noted occasionally in the surrounding tissue, particularly when Santyl Ointment was not confined to the lesion. Therefore, the ointment should be applied carefully within the area of the lesion.

ADVERSE REACTIONS

No allergic sensitivity or toxic reactions have been noted in the recorded clinical investigations. However, one case of systemic manifestations of hypersensitivity to collagenase in a patient treated for more than one year with a combination of collagenase and cortisone has been reported to us.

OVERDOSAGE

Action of the enzyme may be stopped, should this be desired, by the application of Burow's solution USP (pH 3.6–4.4) to the lesion.

DOSAGE AND ADMINISTRATION

Santyl Ointment should be applied once daily (or more frequently if the dressing becomes soiled, as from incontinence) in the following manner:

(1) Prior to application the lesion should be cleansed of debris and digested material by gently rubbing with a gauze pad saturated with hydrogen peroxide or Dakin's solution followed by sterile normal saline.

(2) Whenever infection is present it is desirable to use an appropriate topical antibiotic powder. The antibiotic

Continued on next page

Knoll Laboratories—Cont.

should be applied to the lesion prior to the application of Santyl Ointment. Should the infection not respond, therapy with Santyl Ointment should be discontinued until remission of the infection.

(3) Santyl Ointment should be applied directly to deep lesions with a wooden tongue depressor or spatula. For shallow lesions, Santyl Ointment may be applied to a sterile gauze pad which is then applied to the wound and properly secured.

(4) Crosshatching thick eschar with a #10 blade allows collagenase more surface contact with necrotic debris. It is also desirable to remove, with forceps and scissors, as much loosened detritus as can be done readily.

(5) All excess ointment should be removed each time dressing is changed.

(6) Use of Santyl Ointment should be terminated when debridement of necrotic tissue is complete and granulation tissue is well established.

HOW SUPPLIED

Santyl Ointment contains 250 units of collagenase enzyme per gram of white petrolatum USP. The potency assay of collagenase is based on the digestion of undenatured collagen (from bovine Achilles tendon) at pH 7.2 and 37°C for 24 hours. The number of peptide bonds cleaved are measured by reaction with ninhydrin. Amino groups released by a trypsin digestion control are subtracted. One net collagenase unit will solubilize ninhydrin reactive material equivalent to 4 micromoles of leucine.

Collagenase Santyl Ointment 15g
NDC# 0044-5270-02
Collagenase Santyl Ointment 30g
NDC# 0044-5270-03

REFERENCES

1—Mandl, I., Adv. Enzymol. 23:163, 1961.
2—Boxer, A.M., Gottesman, N., Bernstein, H., & Mandl, I., Geriatrics 24:75, 1969.
3—Mazurek, I., Med. Welt 22:150, 1971.
4—Zimmerman, W.E., in "Collagenase," I. Mandl, ed., Gordon & Breach, Science Publishers, New York, 1971, p. 131, p. 185.
5—Vetra, H., & Whittaker, D., Geriatrics 30:53, 1975.
6—Rao, D.B., Sane, P.G., & Georgiev, E.L., J. Am. Geriatrics Soc. 23:22, 1975.
7—Vrabec, R., Moserova, J., Konickova, Z., Behounkova, E., & Blaha, J., J. Hyg. Epidemiol. Microbiol. Immunol. 18:496, 1974.
8—Lippmann, H.I., Arch. Phys. Med. Rehabil. 54:588, 1973.
9—German, F.M., in "Collagenase," I. Mandl, ed. Gordon & Breach, Science Publishers, New York, 1971, p. 165.
10—Haimovici, H. & Strauch, B., in "Collagenase," I. Mandl, ed., Gordon & Breach, Science Publishers, New York, 1971, p. 177.
11—Lee, L.K., & Ambrus, J.L., Geriatrics 30:91, 1975.
12—Locke, R.K., & Heifitz, N.M., J. Am. Pod. Assoc. 65:242, 1975.
13—Varma, A.O., Bugatch, E., & German, F.M., Surg. Gynecol. Obstet. 136:281, 1973.
14—Barrett, D., Jr., & Klibanski, A., Am. J. Nurs. 73:849, 1973.
15—Bardfeld, L.A., J. Pod. Ed. 1:41, 1970.
16—Blum, G., Schweiz. Rundschau Med. Praxis 62:820, 1973. Abstr. in Dermatology Digest, Feb. 1974, p. 36.
17—Zaruba, F., Lettl, A., Brozkova, L., Skrdlantova, H., & Krs, V., J. Hyg. Epidemiol. Microbiol. Immunol. 18:499, 1974.
18—Altman, M.I., Goldstein, L., Horowitz, S., J. Am. Pod. Assoc. 68:11, 1978.
19—Rehn, V.J., Med. Klin. 58:799, 1963.
20—Krauss, H., Koslowski, L., & Zimmermann, W.E., Langenbecks Arch. Klin. Chir. 303:23, 1963.
21—Gruenagel, H.H., Med. Klin. 58:442, 1963.

Manufactured by
ADVANCE BIOFACTURES CORP.
35 Wilbur Street
Lynbrook, New York 11563

6103

Shown in Product Identification Guide, page 320

DILAUDID® Ⓒ℞

[dī″law′dĭd]
(hydromorphone hydrochloride)

DESCRIPTION

DILAUDID (hydromorphone hydrochloride) (**WARNING:** May be habit forming), a hydrogenated ketone of morphine, is a narcotic analgesic. It is available in:

Ampules (for parenteral administration) containing: 1 mg, 2 mg, and 4 mg hydromorphone hydrochloride per mL with 0.2% sodium citrate, 0.2% citric acid solution. DILAUDID ampules are sterile.

Multiple Dose Vials (for parenteral administration) containing 20 mL of solution. Each mL contains 2 mg hydromorphone hydrochloride and 0.5 mg edetate disodium with 1.8 mg methylparaben and 0.2 mg propylparaben as preservatives. Sodium hydroxide or hydrochloric acid is used for pH adjustment. DILAUDID multiple dose vials are sterile.

Color Coded Tablets (for oral administration) containing:
2 mg hydromorphone hydrochloride (orange tablet) and D&C red #30 Lake dye, D&C yellow #10 Lake dye, lactose, and magnesium stearate.
4 mg hydromorphone hydrochloride (yellow tablet) and D&C yellow #10 Lake dye, lactose, and magnesium stearate.

Suppositories (for rectal administration) containing 3 mg hydromorphone hydrochloride in a cocoa butter base with silicon dioxide.

Non-Sterile Powder (for prescription compounding) containing hydromorphone hydrochloride.

The structural formula of DILAUDID (hydromorphone hydrochloride) is:

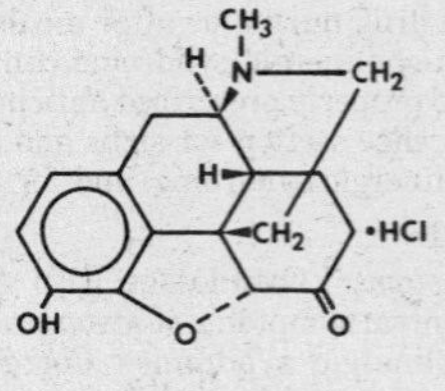

M.W. 321.8

CLINICAL PHARMACOLOGY

DILAUDID is a narcotic analgesic; its principal therapeutic effect is relief of pain. The precise mechanism of action of DILAUDID and other opiates is not known, although it is believed to relate to the existence of opiate receptors in the central nervous system. There is no intrinsic limit to the analgesic effect of DILAUDID; like morphine, adequate doses will relieve even the most severe pain. Clinically, however, dosage limitations are imposed by the adverse effects, primarily respiratory depression, nausea, and vomiting, which can result from high doses.

DILAUDID has diverse additional actions. It may produce drowsiness, changes in mood and mental clouding, depress the respiratory center and the cough center, stimulate the vomiting center, produce pinpoint constriction of the pupil, enhance parasympathetic activity, elevate cerebrospinal fluid pressure, increase biliary pressure, produce transient hyperglycemia.

Generally, the analgesic action of parenterally administered DILAUDID is apparent within 15 minutes and usually remains in effect for more than five hours. The onset of action of oral DILAUDID is somewhat slower, with measurable analgesia occurring within 30 minutes.

In human plasma the half-life of a DILAUDID 4 mg tablet is 2.6 hours. In a random crossover study in six subjects, 4 mg of *oral* DILAUDID produced a mean concentration/time curve similar to that of 2 mg DILAUDID I.V., after the first hour.

INDICATIONS AND USAGE

DILAUDID is indicated for the relief of moderate to severe pain such as that due to:
Surgery
Cancer
Trauma (soft tissue & bone)
Biliary Colic
Myocardial Infarction
Burns
Renal Colic

CONTRAINDICATIONS

DILAUDID is contraindicated in patients with a known hypersensitivity to hydromorphone; in the presence of an intracranial lesion associated with increased intracranial pressure; and whenever ventilatory function is depressed (chronic obstructive pulmonary disease, cor pulmonale, emphysema, kyphoscoliosis, status asthmaticus).

WARNINGS

Respiratory Depression: DILAUDID produces dose-related respiratory depression by acting directly on brain stem respiratory centers. DILAUDID also affects centers that control respiratory rhythm, and may produce irregular and periodic breathing.

Head Injury and Increased Intracranial Pressure: The respiratory depressant effects of narcotics and their capacity to elevate cerebrospinal fluid pressure may be markedly exaggerated in the presence of head injury, other intracranial lesions or a preexisting increase in intracranial pressure. Furthermore, narcotics produce effects which may obscure the clinical course of patients with head injuries.

Acute Abdominal Conditions: The administration of narcotics may obscure the diagnosis or clinical course of patients with acute abdominal conditions.

PRECAUTIONS

Special Risk Patients: DILAUDID should be used with caution in elderly or debilitated patients and those with impaired renal or hepatic function, hypothyroidism, Addison's disease, prostatic hypertrophy or urethral stricture. As with any narcotic analgesic agent, the usual precautions should be observed and the possibility of respiratory depression should be kept in mind.

Cough Reflex: DILAUDID suppresses the cough reflex; as with all narcotics, caution should be exercised when DILAUDID is used postoperatively and in patients with pulmonary disease.

Usage in Ambulatory Patients: Narcotics may impair the mental and/or physical abilities required for the performance of potentially hazardous tasks such as driving a car or operating machinery; patients should be cautioned accordingly.

Drug Interactions: Patients receiving other narcotic analgesics, general anesthetics, phenothiazines, tranquilizers, sedative-hypnotics, tricyclic antidepressants or other CNS depressants (including alcohol) concomitantly with DILAUDID may exhibit an additive CNS depression. When such combined therapy is contemplated, the dose of one or both agents should be reduced.

Parenteral Administration: The parenteral form of DILAUDID may be given intravenously, but the injection should be given very slowly. Rapid intravenous injection of narcotic analgesics increases the possibility of side effects such as hypotension and respiratory depression.

Pregnancy: Pregnancy Category C. DILAUDID has been shown to be teratogenic in hamsters when given in doses 600 times the human dose. There are no adequate and well-controlled studies in pregnant women. DILAUDID should be used during pregnancy only if the potential benefit justifies the potential risk to the fetus.

Nonteratogenic effects: Babies born to mothers who have been taking opioids regularly prior to delivery will be physically dependent. The withdrawal signs include irritability and excessive crying, tremors, hyperactive reflexes, increased respiratory rate, increased stools, sneezing, yawning, vomiting, and fever. The intensity of the syndrome does not always correlate with the duration of maternal opioid use or dose. There is no consensus on the best method of managing withdrawal. Chlorpromazine 0.7 to 1.0 mg/kg q6h, phenobarbital 2 mg/kg q6h, and paregoric 2 to 4 drops/kg q4h, have been used to treat withdrawal symptoms in infants. The duration of therapy is 4 to 28 days, with the dosages decreased as tolerated.

Labor and Delivery: As with all narcotics, administration of DILAUDID to the mother shortly before delivery may result in some degree of respiratory depression in the newborn, especially if higher doses are used.

Nursing Mothers: It is not known whether this drug is excreted in human milk. Because many drugs are excreted in human milk and because of the potential for serious adverse reactions in nursing infants from DILAUDID, a decision should be made whether to discontinue nursing or to discontinue the drug, taking into account the importance of the drug to the mother.

Pediatric Use: Safety and effectiveness in children have not been established.

ADVERSE REACTIONS

Central Nervous System: Sedation, drowsiness, mental clouding, lethargy, impairment of mental and physical performance, anxiety, fear, dysphoria, dizziness, psychic dependence, mood changes.

Gastrointestinal System: Nausea and vomiting occur infrequently; they are more frequent in ambulatory than in recumbent patients. The antiemetic phenothiazines are useful in suppressing these effects; however, some phenothiazine derivatives seem to be antianalgesic and to increase the amount of narcotic required to produce pain relief, while other phenothiazines reduce the amount of narcotic required to produce a given level of analgesia. Prolonged administration of DILAUDID may produce constipation. Opiate agonist-induced increase in intraluminal pressure may endanger surgical anastomosis.

Cardiovascular System: Circulatory depression, peripheral circulatory collapse and cardiac arrest have occurred after rapid intravenous injection. Orthostatic hypotension and fainting may occur if a patient stands up suddenly after receiving an injection of DILAUDID.

Genitourinary System: Ureteral spasm, spasm of vesical sphincters and urinary retention have been reported.

Respiratory Depression: DILAUDID produces dose-related respiratory depression by acting directly on brain stem respiratory centers. DILAUDID also affects centers that control respiratory rhythm, and may produce irregular and periodic breathing. If significant respiratory depression occurs, it may be antagonized by the use of naloxone hydrochloride. The usual adult dose of 0.4 to 0.8 mg given *intramuscularly* or

intravenously, promptly reverses the effects of morphine-like opioid agonists such as DILAUDID. In patients who are physically dependent, small doses of naloxone may be sufficient not only to antagonize respiratory depression, but also to precipitate withdrawal phenomena. The dose of naloxone should therefore be adjusted accordingly in such patients. Since the duration of action of DILAUDID may exceed that of the antagonist, the patient should be kept under continued surveillance; repeated doses of the antagonist may be required to maintain adequate respiration. Apply other supportive measures when indicated.

DRUG ABUSE AND DEPENDENCE

DILAUDID is a Schedule C-II narcotic. Psychic dependence, physical dependence, and tolerance may develop upon repeated administration of narcotics; therefore, DILAUDID should be prescribed and administered with caution. However, psychic dependence is unlikely to develop when DILAUDID is used for a short time for the treatment of pain. Physical dependence, the condition in which continued administration of the drug is required to prevent the appearance of a withdrawal syndrome, usually assumes clinically significant proportions only after several weeks of continued narcotic use, although some mild degree of physical dependence may develop after a few days of narcotic therapy. Tolerance, in which increasingly large doses are required in order to produce the same degree of analgesia, is manifested initially by a shortened duration of analgesic effect, and subsequently by decreases in the intensity of analgesia. The rate of development of tolerance varies among patients.

OVERDOSAGE

Signs and Symptoms: Serious overdosage with DILAUDID is characterized by respiratory depression (a decrease in respiratory rate and/or tidal volume, Cheyne-Stokes respiration, cyanosis), extreme somnolence progressing to stupor or coma, skeletal muscle flaccidity, cold and clammy skin, and sometimes bradycardia and hypotension. In severe overdosage, particularly by the intravenous route, apnea, circulatory collapse, cardiac arrest, and death may occur.

Treatment: Primary attention should be given to the reestablishment of adequate respiratory exchange through provision of a patent airway and institution of assisted or controlled ventilation. The narcotic antagonist naloxone hydrochloride is a specific antidote against respiratory depression which may result from overdosage or unusual sensitivity to narcotics, including DILAUDID. Therefore, naloxone hydrochloride should be administered as described under *Adverse Reactions* (see *Respiratory Depression*) in conjunction with ventilatory assistance.

Since the duration of action of DILAUDID may exceed that of the antagonist, the patient should be kept under continued surveillance; repeated doses of the antagonist may be required to maintain adequate respiration. An antagonist should not be administered in the absence of clinically significant respiratory or cardiovascular depression. Oxygen, intravenous fluids, vasopressors, and other supportive measures should be employed as indicated.

In cases of overdosage with oral DILAUDID, gastric lavage or induced emesis may be useful in removing unabsorbed drug from conscious patients.

DOSAGE AND ADMINISTRATION

Parenteral: The usual starting dose is 1–2 mg *subcutaneously* or *intramuscularly* every 4 to 6 hours as necessary for pain control. The dose should be adjusted according to the severity of pain, as well as the patient's underlying disease, age, and size. Patients with terminal cancer may be tolerant to narcotic analgesics and may, therefore, require higher doses for adequate pain relief. Intravenous or subcutaneous administration is usually not painful. Should intravenous administration be necessary, the injection should be given *slowly,* over at least 2 to 3 minutes, depending on the dose. A gradual increase in dose may be required if analgesia is inadequate, tolerance occurs, or if pain severity increases. The first sign of tolerance is usually a reduced duration of effect.

NOTE: Parenteral drug products should be inspected visually for particulate matter and discoloration prior to administration, whenever solution and container permit. A slight yellowish discoloration may develop in DILAUDID ampules and multiple dose vials. No loss of potency has been demonstrated.

Oral: The usual oral dose is 2 mg every 4 to 6 hours as necessary. The dose must be individually adjusted according to severity of pain, patient response and patient size. More severe pain may require 4 mg or more every 4 to 6 hours. If the pain increases in severity, analgesia is not adequate or tolerance occurs, a gradual increase in dosage may be required. If pain is exceedingly severe, or if prompt response is desired, parenteral DILAUDID should be used initially in adequate amounts to control the pain.

Rectal: DILAUDID suppositories (3 mg) may provide longer duration of relief which could obviate additional medication during the sleeping hours. The usual adult dose is one (1) suppository inserted rectally every 6 to 8 hours or as directed by physician.

HOW SUPPLIED

Ampules: (One mL sterile solution for parenteral administration)

1 mg/mL ampules—Boxes of 10—
NDC# 0044-1011-01.

2 mg/mL ampules—Boxes of 10—
NDC# 0044-1012-01.
Boxes of 25—NDC# 0044-1012-09.

4 mg/mL ampules—Boxes of 10—
NDC# 0044-1014-01.

Multiple Dose Vials: (20 mL sterile solution for parenteral administration)

2 mg/mL—20 mL multiple dose vials
NDC# 0044-1062-05.

Oral Color Coded Tablets: (NOT FOR INJECTION)

2 mg tablet (orange)—Bottles of 100—
NDC# 0044-1022-02.
Unit Dose of 100 (4 × 25)—
NDC# 0044-1022-45
Bottles of 500—NDC# 0044-1022-03.

4 mg tablet (yellow)—Bottles of 100—
NDC# 0044-1024-02.
Unit Dose of 100 (4 × 25)—
NDC# 0044-1024-45
Bottles of 500—NDC# 0044-1024-03.

Rectal Suppositories: 3 mg suppositories—
Boxes of 6—NDC# 0044-1053-01.

Non-Sterile Powder: For prescription compounding.
15 grain vial—NDC# 0044-1040-01.

Storage: Parenteral and oral dosage forms of DILAUDID should be stored at 59°–86°F (15°–30°C).

Protect from light. DILAUDID suppositories should be stored in a refrigerator.

A Schedule C-II Narcotic.

DEA order form required.

Parenteral Products
Manufactured
by Sterling Drug, Inc.
McPherson, KS 67460
RE-1m/Dil6738D/1-9-92
Revised January 1992 6738D

Please see prescribing information for Dilaudid® Oral Liquid and Dilaudid 8 mg Tablets.

Shown in Product Identification Guide, page 319

DILAUDID® COUGH SYRUP C-II ℞
[*dī"law'dĭd*]
(hydromorphone hydrochloride)

DESCRIPTION

Each 5 mL (1 teaspoonful) contains 1 mg DILAUDID (hydromorphone HCl) (**WARNING:** May be habit forming) and 100 mg guaifenesin in a peach-flavored syrup containing 5% alcohol. DILAUDID is a hydrogenated ketone of morphine; it is a narcotic analgesic and antitussive.

The structural formula of DILAUDID (hydromorphone hydrochloride) is:

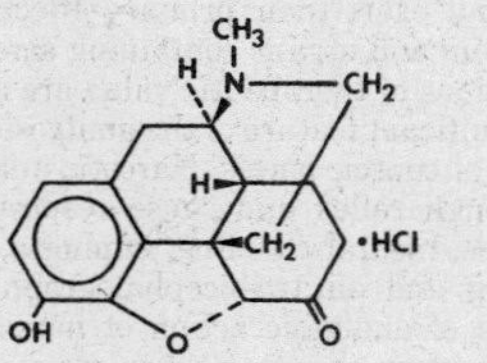

M.W. 321.8

CLINICAL PHARMACOLOGY

DILAUDID (hydromorphone HCl) is a centrally acting narcotic antitussive which acts directly on the cough reflex center.

DILAUDID is also a narcotic analgesic; its principal therapeutic effect is relief of pain. The precise mechanism of action of DILAUDID and other opiates is not known, although it is believed to relate to the existence of opiate receptors in the central nervous system. There is no intrinsic limit to the analgesic effect of DILAUDID; like morphine, adequate doses will relieve even the most severe pain. Clinically, however, dosage limitations are imposed by the adverse effects, primarily respiratory depression, nausea, and vomiting, which can result from high doses.

DILAUDID has diverse additional actions. It produces drowsiness, changes in mood and mental clouding, depresses the respiratory center and the cough center, stimulates the vomiting center, produces pinpoint constriction of the pupil, enhances parasympathetic activity, elevates cerebrospinal fluid pressure, increases biliary pressure, produces transient hyperglycemia.

Generally, the analgesic action of parenterally administered DILAUDID is apparent within 15 minutes and usually remains in effect for more than five hours. The onset of action of oral DILAUDID is somewhat slower, with measurable analgesia occurring within 30 minutes.

Radioimmunoassay techniques have recently been developed for the analysis of DILAUDID in human plasma. In humans the half-life of a DILAUDID 4 mg tablet is 2.6 hours. In a random crossover study in six subjects, 4 mg of oral DILAUDID produced a mean concentration/time curve similar to that of 2 mg DILAUDID I.V., after the first hour.

Guaifenesin (glyceryl guaiacolate) reduces the viscosity of secretions, thereby increasing the efficiency of the cough reflex and of ciliary action in removing accumulated secretions from the trachea and bronchi. Unlike many other expectorants, guaifenesin rarely causes gastric irritation.

INDICATIONS AND USAGE

DILAUDID Cough Syrup is indicated for the control of persistent, exhausting cough or dry, non-productive cough.

CONTRAINDICATIONS

DILAUDID Cough Syrup is contraindicated in patients known to have a hypersensitivity to hydromorphone; in the presence of an intracranial lesion associated with increased intracranial pressure; and whenever ventilatory function is depressed (chronic obstructive pulmonary disease, cor pulmonale, emphysema, kyphoscoliosis, status asthmaticus).

WARNINGS

Respiratory Depression: DILAUDID produces dose-related respiratory depression by acting directly on brain stem respiratory centers. DILAUDID also affects centers that control respiratory rhythm and may produce irregular and periodic breathing.

Head Injury and Increased Intracranial Pressure: The respiratory depressant effects of narcotics and their capacity to elevate cerebrospinal fluid pressure may be markedly exaggerated in the presence of head injury, other intracranial lesions or a preexisting increase in intracranial pressure. Furthermore, narcotics produce adverse effects which may obscure the clinical course of patients with head injuries.

Acute Abdominal Conditions: The administration of narcotics may obscure the diagnosis or clinical course of patients with acute abdominal conditions.

PRECAUTIONS

Special Risk Patients: DILAUDID Cough Syrup should be used with caution in elderly or debilitated patients and those with impaired renal or hepatic function, hypothyroidism, Addison's disease, prostatic hypertrophy or urethral stricture. As with any narcotic analgesic agent, the usual precautions should be observed and the possibility of respiratory depression should be kept in mind.

Cough Reflex: DILAUDID Cough Syrup suppresses the cough reflex; as with all narcotics, caution should be exercised when DILAUDID Cough Syrup is used postoperatively and in patients with pulmonary disease.

Usage in Ambulatory Patients: Narcotics may impair the mental and/or physical abilities required for the performance of potentially hazardous tasks such as driving a car or operating machinery; patients should be cautioned accordingly.

Drug Interactions: Patients receiving other narcotic analgesics, general anesthetics, phenothiazines, tranquilizers, sedative-hypnotics, tricyclic antidepressants or other CNS depressants (including alcohol) concomitantly with DILAUDID Cough Syrup may exhibit an additive CNS depression. When such combined therapy is contemplated, the dose of one or both agents should be reduced.

Usage in Pregnancy: Pregnancy Category C. DILAUDID has been shown to be teratogenic in hamsters when given in doses 600 times the human dose. There are no adequate and well-controlled studies in pregnant women. DILAUDID Cough Syrup should be used during pregnancy only if the potential benefit justifies the potential risk to the fetus.

Nonteratogenic effects: Babies born to mothers who have been taking opioids regularly prior to delivery will be physically dependent. The withdrawal signs include irritability and excessive crying, tremors, hyperactive reflexes, increased respiratory rate, increased stools, sneezing, yawning, vomiting, and fever. The intensity of the syndrome does not always correlate with the duration of maternal opioid use or dose. There is no consensus on the best method of managing withdrawal. Chlorpromazine 0.7 to 1.0 mg/kg q6h, phenobarbital 2 mg/kg q6h, and paregoric 2 to 4 drops/kg q4h, have been used to treat withdrawal symptoms in infants. The duration of therapy is 4 to 28 days, with the dosage decreased as tolerated.

Labor and Delivery: As with all narcotics, administration of DILAUDID Cough Syrup to the mother shortly before delivery may result in some degree of respiratory depression in the newborn, especially if higher doses are used.

Nursing Mothers: It is not known whether this drug is excreted in human milk. Because many drugs are excreted in human milk and because of the potential for serious adverse reactions in nursing infants from DILAUDID Cough Syrup, a decision should be made whether to discontinue nursing or

Continued on next page

Knoll Laboratories—Cont.

to discontinue the drug, taking into account the importance of the drug to the mother.
Pediatric Use: Safety and effectiveness in children have not been established.
FD&C Yellow No. 5: DILAUDID Cough Syrup contains FD&C Yellow No. 5 (tartrazine) dye which may cause allergic-type reactions (including bronchial asthma) in certain susceptible individuals. Although the overall incidence of FD&C Yellow No. 5 (tartrazine) dye sensitivity in the general population is low, it is frequently seen in patients who also have aspirin hypersensitivity.

ADVERSE REACTIONS

Central Nervous System: Sedation, drowsiness, mental clouding, lethargy, impairment of mental and physical performance, anxiety, fear, dysphoria, dizziness, psychic dependence, mood changes.
Gastrointestinal System: Nausea and vomiting occur more frequently in ambulatory than in recumbent patients. The antiemetic phenothiazines are useful in suppressing these effects. Prolonged administration of DILAUDID may produce constipation. Opiate agonist-induced increase in intraluminal pressure may endanger surgical anastomosis.
Genitourinary System: Ureteral spasm, spasm of vesical sphincters and urinary retention have been reported.
Respiratory Depression: DILAUDID produces dose-related respiratory depression by acting directly on brain stem respiratory centers. DILAUDID also affects centers that control respiratory rhythm, and may produce irregular and periodic breathing. If significant respiratory depression occurs, it may be antagonized by the use of naloxone hydrochloride. The usual adult dose of 0.4 to 0.8 mg given intramuscularly or intravenously, promptly reverses the effects of morphine-like opioid agonists such as DILAUDID. In patients who are physically dependent, small doses of naloxone may be sufficient not only to antagonize respiratory depression, but also to precipitate withdrawal phenomena. The dose of naloxone should therefore be adjusted accordingly in such patients. Since the duration of action of DILAUDID may exceed that of the antagonist, the patient should be kept under continued surveillance; repeated doses of the antagonist may be required to maintain adequate respiration. Apply other supportive measures when indicated.

DRUG ABUSE AND DEPENDENCE

DILAUDID is a Schedule Ⓒ II narcotic. Psychic dependence, physical dependence, and tolerance may develop upon repeated administration of narcotics; therefore, DILAUDID should be prescribed and administered with caution. However, psychic dependence is unlikely to develop when DILAUDID Cough Syrup is used for a short time as indicated. Physical dependence, the condition in which continued administration of the drug is required to prevent the appearance of a withdrawal syndrome, usually assumes clinically significant proportions only after several weeks of continued narcotic use, although some mild degree of physical dependence may develop after few days of narcotic therapy.

OVERDOSAGE

Signs and Symptoms: Serious overdosage with DILAUDID is characterized by respiratory depression (a decrease in respiratory rate and/or tidal volume, Cheyne-Stokes respiration, cyanosis), extreme somnolence progressing to stupor or coma, skeletal muscle flaccidity, cold and clammy skin, and sometimes bradycardia and hypotension. In severe overdosage particularly by the intravenous route, apnea, circulatory collapse, cardiac arrest and death may occur.
Treatment: Primary attention should be given to the reestablishment of adequate respiratory exchange through provision of a patent airway and the institution of assisted or controlled ventilation. The narcotic antagonist naloxone hydrochloride is a specific antidote against respiratory depression which may result from overdosage or unusual sensitivity to narcotics, including DILAUDID. Therefore, naloxone hydrochloride should be administered as described under ADVERSE REACTIONS (see Respiratory Depression) in conjunction with ventilatory assistance.
Since the duration of action of Dilaudid may exceed that of the antagonist, the patient should be kept under continued surveillance; repeated doses of the antagonist may be required to maintain adequate respiration. An antagonist should not be administered in the absence of clinically significant respiratory or cardiovascular depression. Oxygen, intravenous fluids, vasopressors and other supportive measures should be employed as indicated.
In cases of overdosage with oral DILAUDID, gastric lavage or induced emesis may be useful in removing unabsorbed drug from conscious patients.

DOSAGE AND ADMINISTRATION

The usual adult dose of DILAUDID Cough Syrup is one teaspoonful (5 mL) every 3 to 4 hours.

HOW SUPPLIED

Bottles of 1 pint (473 mL)—NDC #0044-1080-01.
Storage: Store at 59°–86°F (15°–30°C).
A Schedule Ⓒ II Narcotic.
DEA order form required.
Revised September 1986 8074

DILAUDID-HP® INJECTION Ⓒ II

[*dī"law'dĭd*]
10mg/mL
(hydromorphone hydrochloride)

WARNING: DILAUDID-HP® (HIGH POTENCY) IS A HIGHLY CONCENTRATED SOLUTION OF HYDROMORPHONE INTENDED FOR USE IN NARCOTIC-TOLERANT PATIENTS. DO NOT CONFUSE DILAUDID-HP WITH STANDARD PARENTERAL FORMULATIONS OF DILAUDID OR OTHER NARCOTICS. OVERDOSE AND DEATH COULD RESULT.

DESCRIPTION

DILAUDID (hydromorphone hydrochloride) (WARNING: May be habit forming), a hydrogenated ketone of morphine, is a narcotic analgesic. HIGH POTENCY DILAUDID is available in AMBER ampules or single dose vials for intravenous (IV), subcutaneous (SC), or intramuscular (IM) administration. Each 1 mL of sterile solution contains 10 mg hydromorphone hydrochloride with 0.2% sodium citrate, and 0.2% citric acid solution.
It is also available as lyophilized Dilaudid for intravenous (IV), subcutaneous (SC), or intramuscular (IM) administration. Each single dose vial contains 250mg sterile, lyophilized hydromorphone HCl to be reconstituted with 25mL of Sterile Water for Injection USP to provide a solution containing 10mg/mL.
The structural formula of DILAUDID (hydromorphone hydrochloride) is:

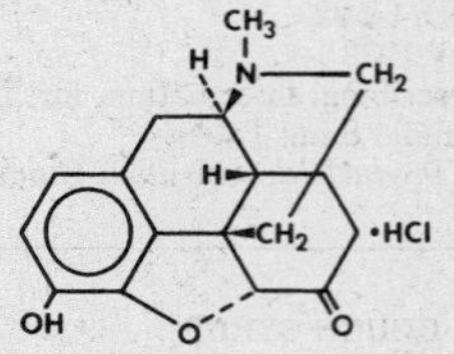

MW 321.8

CLINICAL PHARMACOLOGY

Many of the effects described below are common to the class of narcotic analgesics. In some instances, data may not exist to demonstrate that DILAUDID-HP possesses similar or different effects than those observed with other narcotic analgesics. However, in the absence of data to the contrary, it is assumed that DILAUDID-HP would possess these effects.
Central Nervous System: Narcotic analgesics have multiple actions but exert their primary effects on the central nervous system and organs containing smooth muscle. The principal actions of therapeutic value are analgesia and sedation. A significant feature of the analgesia is that it occurs without loss of consciousness. Narcotic analgesics also suppress the cough reflex and cause respiratory depression, mood changes, mental clouding, euphoria, dysphoria, nausea, vomiting and electroencephalographic changes. The precise mode of analgesic action of narcotic analgesics is unknown. However, specific CNS opiate receptors have been identified. Narcotics are believed to express their pharmacological effects by combining with these receptors.
Narcotics depress the cough reflex by direct effect on the cough center in the medulla.
Narcotics produce respiratory depression by direct effect on brain stem respiratory centers. The mechanism of respiratory depression also involves a reduction in the responsiveness of the brain stem respiratory centers to increases in carbon dioxide tension.
Narcotics cause miosis. Pinpoint pupils are a common sign of narcotic overdose but are not pathognomonic (e.g., pontine lesions of hemorrhagic or ischemic origin may produce similar findings) and marked mydriasis occurs when asphyxia intervenes.
Gastrointestinal Tract and Other Smooth Muscle: Gastric, biliary and pancreatic secretions are decreased by narcotics. Narcotics cause a reduction in motility associated with an increase in tone in the antrum portion of the stomach and duodenum. Digestion of food in the small intestine is delayed and propulsive contractions are decreased. Propulsive peristaltic waves in the colon are decreased, and tone may be increased to the point of spasm. The end result is constipation. Narcotics can cause a marked increase in biliary tract pressure as a result of spasm of the sphincter of Oddi.
Cardiovascular System: Certain narcotics produce peripheral vasodilation which may result in orthostatic hypotension. Release of histamine may occur with narcotics and may contribute to narcotic-induced hypotension. Other manifestations of histamine release and/or peripheral vasodilation may include pruritis, flushing, and red eyes.
Effects on the myocardium after i.v. administration of narcotics are not significant in normal persons, vary with different narcotic analgesic agents and vary with the hemodynamic state of the patient, state of hydration and sympathetic drive.
Pharmacokinetics: In normal human volunteers hydromorphone is metabolized primarily in the liver. It is excreted primarily as the glucuronidated conjugate, with small amounts of parent drug and minor amounts of 6-hydroxy reduction metabolites.
Following intravenous administration of DILAUDID to normal volunteers, the mean half-life of elimination was 2.64 ± 0.88 hours. The mean volume of distribution was 91.5 liters, suggesting extensive tissue uptake. DILAUDID is rapidly removed from the blood stream and distributed to skeletal muscle, kidneys, liver, intestinal tract, lungs, spleen and brain. DILAUDID also crosses the placental membranes.
In terms of area under the analgesic time-effect curve, hydromorphone is approximately 8 times more potent than morphine (i.e., 1.3 mg of hydromorphone produces analgesia equal to that produced by 10 mg of morphine). After intramuscular administration, hydromorphone has a slightly more rapid onset and slightly shorter duration of action than morphine. The duration of DILAUDID analgesia in the non-tolerant patient with usual doses may be up to 4–5 hours. However, in tolerant subjects, duration will vary substantially depending on tolerance and dose. Dose should be adjusted so that 3–4 hours of pain relief may be achieved.

INDICATIONS AND USAGE

DILAUDID-HP is indicated for the relief of moderate-to-severe pain in narcotic-tolerant patients who require larger than usual doses of narcotics to provide adequate pain relief. Because DILAUDID-HP contains 10 mg of hydromorphone per mL, a smaller injection volume can be used than with other parenteral narcotic formulations. Discomfort associated with the intramuscular or subcutaneous injection of an unusually large volume of solution can therefore be avoided.

CONTRAINDICATIONS

DILAUDID-HP is contraindicated in: patients who are not already receiving large amounts of parenteral narcotics, patients with known hypersensitivity to the drug, patients with respiratory depression in the absence of resuscitative equipment, and in patients with status asthmaticus. DILAUDID-HP is also contraindicated for use in obstetrical analgesia.

WARNINGS—DRUG DEPENDENCE

DILAUDID-HP can produce drug dependence of the morphine type and therefore has the potential for being abused. Psychic dependence, physical dependence and tolerance may develop upon repeated administration of DILAUDID-HP, and it should be prescribed and administered with the same degree of caution appropriate for the use of morphine. Since DILAUDID-HP is indicated for use in patients who are already tolerant to and hence physically dependent on narcotics, abrupt discontinuance in the administration of DILAUDID-HP is likely to result in a withdrawal syndrome. (See **Drug Abuse and Dependence**).
Infants born to mothers physically dependent on DILAUDID-HP will also be physically dependent and may exhibit respiratory difficulties and withdrawal symptoms (See **Drug Abuse and Dependence**).
Impaired Respiration: Respiratory depression is the chief hazard of DILAUDID-HP. Respiratory depression occurs most frequently in the elderly, in the debilitated, and in those suffering from conditions accompanied by hypoxia or hypercapnia when even moderate therapeutic doses may dangerously decrease pulmonary ventilation.
DILAUDID-HP should be used with extreme caution in patients with chronic obstructive pulmonary disease or cor pulmonale, patients having a substantially decreased respiratory reserve, hypoxia, hypercapnia, or preexisting respiratory depression. In such patients even usual therapeutic doses of narcotic analgesics may decrease respiratory drive while simultaneously increasing airway resistance to the point of apnea.
Head Injury and Increased Intracranial Pressure: The respiratory depressant effects of DILAUDID-HP with carbon dioxide retention and secondary elevation of cerebrospinal fluid pressure may be markedly exaggerated in the presence of head injury, other intracranial lesions, or preexisting increase in intracranial pressure. Narcotic analgesics including DILAUDID-HP may produce effects which can obscure the clinical course and neurologic signs of further increase in pressure in patients with head injuries.
Hypotensive Effect: Narcotic analgesics, including DILAUDID-HP, may cause severe hypotension in an individual whose ability to maintain his blood pressure has already been compromised by a depleted blood volume, or a concurrent administration of drugs such as phenothiazines or gen-

eral anesthetics (see also **Precautions —Drug Interactions**). DILAUDID-HP may produce orthostatic hypotension in ambulatory patients.

DILAUDID-HP should be administered with caution to patients in circulatory shock, since vasodilation produced by the drug may further reduce cardiac output and blood pressure.

PRECAUTIONS

General: Because of its high concentration, the delivery of precise doses of DILAUDID-HP may be difficult if low doses of hydromorphone are required. Therefore, DILAUDID-HP should be used only if the amount of hydromorphone required can be delivered accurately with this formulation.

In general, narcotics should be given with caution and the initial dose should be reduced in the elderly or debilitated and those with severe impairment of hepatic, pulmonary or renal function; myxedema or hypothyroidism; adrenocortical insufficiency (e.g., Addison's Disease); CNS depression or coma; toxic psychoses; prostatic hypertrophy or urethral stricture; gall bladder disease; acute alcoholism; delirium tremens; or kyphoscoliosis.

In the case of DILAUDID-HP, however, the patient is presumed to be receiving a narcotic to which he or she exhibits tolerance and the initial dose of DILAUDID-HP selected should be estimated based on the relative potency of hydromorphone and the narcotic previously used by the patient. See **(Dosage and Administration)** section.

The administration of narcotic analgesics including DILAUDID-HP may obscure the diagnosis or clinical course in patients with acute abdominal conditions and may aggravate preexisting convulsions in patients with convulsive disorders.

Narcotic analgesics including DILAUDID-HP should also be used with caution in patients about to undergo surgery of the biliary tract since it may cause spasm of the sphincter of Oddi.

Drug Interactions: The concomitant use of other central nervous system depressants including sedatives or hypnotics, general anesthetics, phenothiazines, tranquilizers and alcohol may produce additive depressant effects. Respiratory depression, hypotension and profound sedation or coma may occur. When such combined therapy is contemplated, the dose of one or both agents should be reduced. Narcotic analgesics, including DILAUDID-HP may enhance the action of neuromuscular blocking agents and produce an increased degree of respiratory depression.

PREGNANCY—CATEGORY C:

Human: Adequate animal studies on reproduction have not been performed to determine whether hydromorphone affects fertility in males or females. There are no well-controlled studies in women. Reports based on marketing experience do not identify any specific teratogenic risks following routine (short-term) clinical use. Although there is no clearly defined risk, such reports do not exclude the possibility of infrequent or subtle damage to the human fetus. DILAUDID-HP should be used in pregnant women only when clearly needed (see ***Labor and Delivery*** and ***Drug Abuse and Dependence***).

Animal: Literature reports of hydromorphone hydrochloride administration to pregnant Syrian hamsters show that DILAUDID is teratogenic at a dose of 20 mg/kg which is 600 times the human dose. A maximal teratogenic effect (50% of fetuses affected) in the Syrian hamster was observed at a dose of 125 mg/kg.

Labor and Delivery: DILAUDID-HP is contraindicated in Labor and Delivery (see **Contraindications** section).

Nursing Mothers: Low levels of narcotic analgesics have been detected in human milk. As a general rule, nursing should not be undertaken while a patient is receiving DILAUDID-HP since it, and other drugs in this class, may be excreted in the milk.

Pediatric Use: Safety and effectiveness in children have not been established.

ADVERSE REACTIONS

The adverse effects of DILAUDID-HP are similar to those of other narcotic analgesics, and represent established pharmacological effects of the drug class. The major hazards include respiratory depression and apnea. To a lesser degree, circulatory depression, respiratory arrest, shock and cardiac arrest have occurred.

The most frequently observed adverse effects are lightheadedness, dizziness, sedation, nausea, vomiting, and sweating. These effects seem to be more prominent in ambulatory patients and in those not experiencing severe pain. Some adverse reactions in ambulatory patients may be alleviated if the patient lies down.

Less Frequently Observed with Narcotic Analgesics:

General and CNS: Dysphoria, euphoria, weakness, headache, agitation, tremor, uncoordinated muscle movements, alterations of mood (nervousness, apprehension, depression, floating feelings, dreams), muscle rigidity, paresthesia, muscle tremor, blurred vision, nystagmus, diplopia and miosis, transient hallucinations* and disorientation, visual disturbances, insomnia and increased intracranial pressure may occur.

*Hallucinations, although unusual with pure agonist narcotics, have been observed in one patient following both a 6 mg and a 4 mg DILAUDID-HP dose. However, the patient was receiving several concomitant medications during the second episode and a causal relationship cannot be established.

Cardiovascular: Flushing of the face, chills, tachycardia, bradycardia, palpitation, faintness, syncope, hypotension and hypertension have been reported.

Respiratory: Bronchospasm and laryngospasm have been known to occur.

Gastrointestinal: Dry mouth, constipation, biliary tract spasm, anorexia, diarrhea, cramps and taste alterations have been reported.

Genitourinary: Urinary retention or hesitancy, and antidiuretic effects have been reported.

Dermatologic: Pruritis, urticaria, other skin rashes, wheal and flare over the vein with intravenous injection, and diaphoresis have been reported with narcotic analgesics.

Other: In clinical trials, neither local tissue irritation nor induration was observed at the site of subcutaneous injection of DILAUDID-HP; pain at the injection site was rarely observed. However, local irritation and induration have been seen following parenteral injection of other narcotic drug products.

DRUG ABUSE AND DEPENDENCE

Narcotic analgesics may cause psychological and physical dependence (see ***Warnings***). Physical dependence results in withdrawal symptoms in patients who abruptly discontinue the drug. Withdrawal symptoms also may be precipitated in the patient with physical dependence by the administration of a drug with narcotic antagonist activity, e.g., naloxone (see also ***Overdosage***). Physical dependence usually does not occur to a clinically significant degree until after several weeks of continued narcotic usage. Tolerance, in which increasingly large doses are required in order to produce the same degree of analgesia, is initially manifested by a shortened duration of analgesic effect, and subsequently, by decreases in the intensity of analgesia. In chronic pain patients, and in narcotic-tolerant cancer patients, the dose of DILAUDID-HP should be guided by the degree of tolerance manifested.

In chronic pain patients in whom narcotic analgesics including DILAUDID-HP are abruptly discontinued, a severe abstinence syndrome should be anticipated. This may be similar to the abstinence syndrome noted in patients who withdraw from heroin. The latter abstinence syndrome may be characterized by restlessness, lacrimation, rhinorrhea, yawning, perspiration, gooseflesh, restless sleep or "yen" and mydriasis during the first 24 hours. These symptoms may increase in severity and over the next 72 hours may be accompanied by increasing irritability, anxiety, weakness, twitching and spasms of muscles, kicking movements, severe backache, abdominal and leg pains, abdominal and muscle cramps, hot and cold flashes, insomnia, nausea, anorexia, vomiting, intestinal spasm, diarrhea, coryza and repetitive sneezing, increase in body temperature, blood pressure, respiratory rate and heart rate.

Because of excessive loss of fluids through sweating, or vomiting and diarrhea, there is usually marked weight loss, dehydration, ketosis, and disturbances in acid-base balance. Cardiovascular collapse can occur. Without treatment most observable symptoms disappear in 5–14 days; however, there appears to be a phase of secondary or chronic abstinence which may last for 2–6 months characterized by insomnia, irritability, muscular aches, and autonomic instability.

In the treatment of physical dependence on DILAUDID-HP, the patient may be detoxified by gradual reduction of the dosage, although this is unlikely to be necessary in the terminal cancer patient. If abstinence symptoms become severe, the patient may be given methadone. Temporary administration of tranquilizers and sedatives may aid in reducing patient anxiety. Gastrointestinal disturbances or dehydration should be treated accordingly.

OVERDOSAGE

Serious overdosage with DILAUDID-HP is characterized by respiratory depression, somnolence progressing to stupor or coma, skeletal muscle flaccidity, cold and clammy skin, constricted pupils, and sometimes bradycardia and hypotension. In serious overdosage, particularly following intravenous injection, apnea, circulatory collapse, cardiac arrest and death may occur.

In the treatment of overdosage primary attention should be given to the reestablishment of adequate respiratory exchange through provision of a patent airway and institution of assisted or controlled ventilation.

NARCOTIC-TOLERANT PATIENT: Since tolerance to the respiratory and CNS depressant effects of narcotics develops concomitantly with tolerance to their analgesic effects, serious respiratory depression due to an acute overdose is unlikely to be seen in narcotic-tolerant patients receiving DILAUDID-HP for chronic pain.

NOTE: In such an individual who is physically dependent on narcotics, administration of the usual dose of the antagonist will precipitate an acute withdrawal syndrome. The severity will depend on the degree of physical dependence and the dose of the antagonist administered. Use of a narcotic antagonist in such a person should be avoided. If necessary to treat serious respiratory depression in the physically dependent patient, the antagonist should be administered with extreme care and by titration with smaller than usual doses of the antagonist.

NON-TOLERANT PATIENT: The narcotic antagonist, naloxone, is a specific antidote against respiratory depression which may result from overdosage, or unusual sensitivity to DILAUDID-HP. A dose of naloxone (usually 0.4 to 2.0 mg) should be administered intravenously, if possible, simultaneously with respiratory resuscitation. The dose can be repeated in 3 minutes. Naloxone should not be administered in the absence of clinically significant respiratory or circulatory depression. Naloxone should be administered cautiously to persons who are known, or suspected to be physically dependent on DILAUDID-HP. In such cases, an abrupt or complete reversal of narcotic effects may precipitate an acute abstinence syndrome.

Since the duration of action of DILAUDID-HP may exceed that of the antagonist, the patient should be kept under continued surveillance; repeated doses of the antagonist may be required to maintain adequate respiration. Apply other supportive measures when indicated.

STRONG ANALGESICS AND STRUCTURALLY RELATED DRUGS USED IN THE TREATMENT OF CANCER PAIN*

IM OR SC ADMINISTRATION

Nonproprietary (Trade) Names	Dose, mg Equianalgesic to 10 mg of IM Morphine†	Duration Compared With Morphine
Morphine sulfate	10	Same
Papaveretum (Pantopon)	20	Same
Hydromorphone (DILAUDID) hydrochloride	1.3	Slightly Shorter
Oxymorphone (Numorphan) hydrochloride	1.1	Slightly Shorter
Nalbuphine (Nubain) hydrochloride	12	Same
Heroin, diamorphine hydrochloride (NA in U.S.)	4–5	Slightly Shorter
Levorphanol (Levo-Dromoran) tartrate	2.3	Same
Butorphanol (Stadol) tartrate	1.5–2.5	Same
Pentazocine (Talwin) lactate or hydrochloride	60	Shorter
Meperidine, pethidine (Demerol) hydrochloride	80	Shorter
Methadone (Dolophine) hydrochloride	10	Same

*From Beaver WT. Management of cancer pain with parenteral medication. J. Am. Med. Assoc. 244:2653–2657 (1980).
†(In terms of the area under the analgesic time-effect curve.)

Continued on next page

Knoll Laboratories—Cont.

Supportive measures (including oxygen, vasopressors) should be employed in the management of circulatory shock and pulmonary edema accompanying overdose as indicated. Cardiac arrest or arrhythmias may require cardiac massage or defibrillation.

DOSAGE AND ADMINISTRATION

Parenteral: DILAUDID-HP SHOULD BE GIVEN ONLY TO PATIENTS WHO ARE ALREADY RECEIVING LARGE DOSES OF NARCOTICS. DILAUDID-HP is indicated for relief of moderate-to-severe pain in narcotic-tolerant patients. Thus, these patients will already have been treated with other narcotic analgesics. If the patient is being changed from regular DILAUDID to DILAUDID-HP, similar doses should be used, depending on the patient's clinical response to the drug. If DILAUDID-HP is substituted for a different narcotic analgesic, the following equivalency table should be used as a guide to determine the appropriate dose of DILAUDID-HP (hydromorphone hydrochloride).

[See table on bottom of preceding page.]

In open clinical trials with DILAUDID-HP in patients with terminal cancer, doses ranged from 1–14 mg subcutaneously or intramuscularly; one patient received 30 mg subcutaneously on two occasions. In these trials, both subcutaneous and intramuscular injections of DILAUDID-HP were well-tolerated, with minimal pain and/or burning at the injection site. Mild erythema was rarely noted after intramuscular injection. There was no induration after either intramuscular or subcutaneous administration of DILAUDID-HP. Subcutaneous injections of DILAUDID-HP were particularly well accepted when administered with a short, 30 gauge needle.

Experience with administration of DILAUDID-HP by the intravenous route is limited. Should intravenous administration be necessary, the injection should be given slowly, over at least 2 to 3 minutes. The intravenous route is usually painless.

A gradual increase in dose may be required if analgesia is inadequate, tolerance occurs, or if pain severity increases. The first sign of tolerance is usually a reduced duration of effect.

NOTE: Parenteral drug products should be inspected visually for particulate matter and discoloration prior to administration, whenever solution and container permit. A slight yellowish discoloration may develop in DILAUDID-HP ampules. No loss of potency has been demonstrated. Dilaudid injection is physically compatible and chemically stable for at least 24 hours at 25°C protected from light in most common large volume parenteral solutions.

500mg/50mL Vial: To use this single dose presentation, do not penetrate the stopper with a syringe. Instead, remove both the aluminum flipseal and rubber stopper in a suitable work area such as under a laminar flow hood (or equivalent clean air compounding area). The contents may then be withdrawn for preparation of a single, large volume parenteral solution. Any unused portion should be discarded in an appropriate manner.

Reconstitution of sterile lyophilized Dilaudid HP 250mg: Reconstitution immediately prior to use with 25mL of sterile Water for Injection USP to provide a sterile solution containing 10mg/mL.

HOW SUPPLIED

DILAUDID-HP amber ampules and single dose vials contain 10 mg hydromorphone hydrochloride per mL with 0.2% sodium citrate and 0.2% citric acid solution. No added preservative.

NOTE: DILAUDID-HP ampules are amber in color.

The lyophilized Dilaudid HP Single Dose Vial contains 250mg of sterile, lyophilized hydromorphone HCl.

HIGH POTENCY:
10 mg/1 mL
Box of 10 ampules
NDC 0044-1017-10
*50 mg/5mL
Box of 10 ampules
NDC 0044-1017-25
*500 mg/50 mL
Single dose vial
NDC 0044-1017-06
*lyophilized 250mg
Single Dose Vial
NDC 0044-1911-01
*FOR USE IN THE PREPARATION OF LARGE VOLUME PARENTERAL SOLUTIONS

STORAGE: Parenteral forms of DILAUDID-HP should be stored at 59°–86°F (15°–30°C). Protect from light.

A Schedule Ⓒ Narcotic DEA Order Form Required.

Manufactured by Sanofi Winthrop, Inc.
McPherson, KS 67460

Shown in Product Identification Guide, page 319

DILAUDID® ORAL LIQUID and DILAUDID 8 mg Tablets Ⓒ ℞

(hydromorphone hydrochloride)

WARNING: May be habit forming

DESCRIPTION

DILAUDID (hydromorphone hydrochloride), a hydrogenated ketone of morphine, is a narcotic analgesic.

The structural formula of DILAUDID (hydromorphone hydrochloride) is:

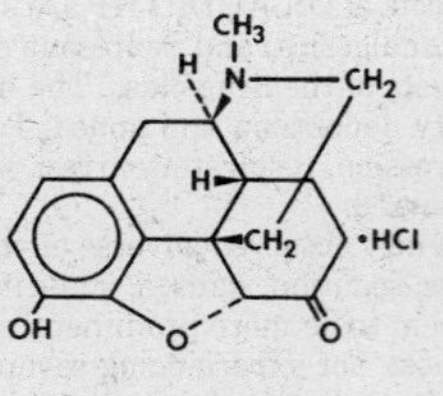

M.W.—321.8

Each 5 mL (1 teaspoon) of DILAUDID ORAL LIQUID contains 5 mg of DILAUDID (hydromorphone hydrochloride). In addition, other ingredients include purified water, methylparaben, propylparaben, sucrose, and glycerin. DILAUDID ORAL LIQUID may contain traces of sodium bisulfite.

Each DILAUDID 8 mg TABLET contains DILAUDID (hydromorphone hydrochloride). In addition, the tablets include lactose anhydrous, and magnesium stearate. DILAUDID 8 mg TABLET may contain traces of sodium bisulfite.

CLINICAL PHARMACOLOGY

Many of the effects described below are common to this class of mu opioid agonist analgesics. In some instances, data may not exist to distinguish the effects of DILAUDID ORAL LIQUID and DILAUDID 8 mg TABLETS from those observed with other opioid analgesics. However, in the absence of data to the contrary, it is assumed that DILAUDID ORAL LIQUID and DILAUDID 8 mg TABLETS would possess all the actions of mu-agonist opioids.

Opioid analgesics exert their primary effects on the central nervous system and organs containing smooth muscle. The principal actions of therapeutic value are analgesia and sedation. A significant feature of the analgesia is that it can occur without loss of consciousness. Opioid analgesics also suppress the cough reflex and may cause respiratory depression, mood changes, mental clouding, euphoria, dysphoria, nausea, vomiting and electroencephalographic changes.

The precise mode of analgesic action of opioid analgesics is unknown. However, specific CNS opiate receptors have been identified. Opioids are believed to express their pharmacological effects by combining with these receptors.

Opioids depress the cough reflex by direct effect on the cough center in the medulla.

Opioids depress the respiratory reflex by a direct effect on brain stem respiratory centers. The mechanism of respiratory depression also involves a reduction in the responsiveness of the brain stem respiratory centers to increases in carbon dioxide tension.

Opioids cause miosis. Pinpoint pupils are a common sign of opioid overdose but are not pathognomonic (e.g., pontine lesions of hemorrhagic or ischemic origin may produce similar findings) and marked mydriasis occurs with asphyxia.

Gastric, biliary and pancreatic secretions are decreased by opioids. Opioids cause a reduction in motility associated with an increase in tone in the gastric antrum and duodenum. Digestion of food in the small intestine is delayed and propulsive contractions are decreased. Propulsive peristaltic waves in the colon are decreased, and tone may be increased to the point of spasm. The end result is constipation. Opioids can cause a marked increase in biliary tract pressure as a result of spasm of the sphincter of Oddi.

Certain opioids produce peripheral vasodilation which may result in orthostatic hypotension. Release of histamine may occur with opioids and may contribute to drug-induced hypotension. Other manifestations of histamine release may include pruritus, flushing, and red eyes.

The dosage of opioid analgesics like hydromorphone should be individualized for any given patient, since adverse events can occur at doses that may not provide complete freedom from pain (see **INDIVIDUALIZATION OF DOSAGE**).

PHARMACOKINETICS

In a single-dose crossover study in 27 normal subjects the pharmacokinetics of Dilaudid 8 mg tablets was compared to that of 8 mL of Dilaudid Oral Liquid (1 mg/mL). Plasma hydromorphone concentration was determined using a sensitive and specific assay. The pharmacokinetic parameters from this study are outlined below.

Parameter Mean & (CV)	8 mg Tablet	8 mg Oral Liquid (1 mg/mL)
C_{max} (ng/mL)	5.5 (33%)	5.7 (31%)
T_{max} (hr)	0.74 (34%)	0.73 (71%)
$AUC_{0-\infty}$ (ng*hr/mL)	23.7 (28%)	24.6 (29%)
T1/2 (hr)	2.6 (18%)	2.8 (20%)

Dose proportionality between the 8 mg Dilaudid tablets and other strengths of Dilaudid tablets has not been established.

In normal human volunteers hydromorphone is metabolized primarily in the liver. It is excreted in the urine primarily as the glucuronidated conjugate, with small amounts of parent drug and minor amounts of 6-hydroxy reduction metabolites. The effects of renal disease on the clearance of hydromorphone are unknown, but caution should be taken to guard against unanticipated accumulation if renal and/or hepatic functions are seriously impaired. Hydromorphone has been shown to cross placental membranes.

CLINICAL TRIALS

Analgesic effects of single doses of DILAUDID oral liquid administered to patients with post-surgical pain have been studied in double-blind controlled trials. In one study with 61 patients, both 5 mg and 10 mg of DILAUDID provided significantly more analgesia than placebo. In another trial with 80 patients, 5 mg and 10 mg of DILAUDID Oral Liquid were compared to 30 mg and 60 mg of morphine sulfate oral liquid. The pain relief provided by 5 mg and 10 mg DILAUDID was comparable to 30 mg and 60 mg oral morphine sulfate, respectively.

INDIVIDUALIZATION OF DOSAGE

Safe and effective administration of opioid analgesics to patients with acute or chronic pain depends upon a comprehensive assessment of the patient. The nature of the pain (severity, frequency, etiology, and pathophysiology) as well as the concurrent medical status of the patient will affect selection of the starting dosage.

In non opioid-tolerant patients, therapy with hydromorphone is typically initiated at an oral dose of 2–4 mg every four hours, but elderly patients may require lower doses (see **PRECAUTIONS**—Geriatric Use).

In patients receiving opioids, both the dose and duration of analgesia will vary substantially depending on the patient's opioid tolerance. The dose should be selected and adjusted so that at least 3–4 hours of pain relief may be achieved.

In patients taking opioid analgesics, the starting dose of DILAUDID should be based on the prior opioid usage. This should be done by converting the total daily usage of the previous opioid to an equivalent total daily dosage of oral DILAUDID using an equianalgesic table (see below). For opioids not in the table, first estimate the equivalent total daily usage of oral morphine, then use the table to find the equivalent total daily dosage of Dilaudid.

Once the total daily dosage of DILAUDID has been estimated, it should be divided into the desired number of doses. Since there is individual variation in response to different opioid drugs, only ½ to ⅔ of the estimated dose of DILAUDID calculated from equivalence tables should be given for the first few doses, then increased as needed according to the patient's response.

In chronic pain, doses should be administered around-the-clock. A supplemental dose of 5–15% of the total daily usage may be administered every two hours on an "as-needed" basis.

Periodic reassessment after the initial dosing is always required. If pain management is not satisfactory and in the absence of significant opioid-induced adverse events, the hydromorphone dose may be increased gradually. If excessive opioid side effects are observed early in the dosing interval, the hydromorphone dose should be reduced. If this results in breakthrough pain at the end of the dosing interval, the dosing interval may need to be shortened. Dose titration should be guided more by the need for analgesia than the absolute dose of opioid employed.

[See table at top of next page.]

Dosages, and ranges of dosages represented, are a compilation of estimated equipotent dosages from published references comparing opioid analgesics in cancer and severe pain.

INDICATIONS AND USAGE

DILAUDID ORAL LIQUID and DILAUDID 8 mg TABLETS are indicated for the management of pain in patients where an opioid analgesic is appropriate.

CONTRAINDICATIONS

DILAUDID ORAL LIQUID and DILAUDID 8 mg TABLETS are contraindicated in: patients with known hypersensitivity to hydromorphone, patients with respiratory depression in the absence of resuscitative equipment, and in patients with status asthmaticus. DILAUDID ORAL LIQUID and

DILAUDID 8 mg TABLETS are also contraindicated for use in obstetrical analgesia.

WARNINGS

Impaired Respiration: Respiratory depression is the chief hazard of DILAUDID ORAL LIQUID and DILAUDID 8 mg TABLETS. Respiratory depression occurs most frequently in overdose situations, in the elderly, in the debilitated, and in those suffering from conditions accompanied by hypoxia or hypercapnia when even moderate therapeutic doses may dangerously decrease pulmonary ventilation.

DILAUDID ORAL LIQUID and DILAUDID 8 mg TABLETS should be used with extreme caution in patients with chronic obstructive pulmonary disease or cor pulmonale, patients having a substantially decreased respiratory reserve, hypoxia, hypercapnia, or in patients with preexisting respiratory depression. In such patients even usual therapeutic doses of opioid analgesics may decrease respiratory drive while simultaneously increasing airway resistance to the point of apnea.

Drug Dependence: DILAUDID is a Schedule II narcotic. DILAUDID ORAL LIQUID and DILAUDID 8 mg TABLETS can produce drug dependence of the morphine type and therefore have the potential for being abused. Psychic dependence, physical dependence and tolerance may develop upon repeated administration of DILAUDID, which should be prescribed and administered with the degree of caution appropriate to the use of morphine. Abrupt discontinuance in the administration of DILAUDID ORAL LIQUID and DILAUDID 8 mg TABLETS in patients who are physically dependent on opioids is likely to result in a withdrawal syndrome (see **DRUG ABUSE AND DEPENDENCE**).

Sulfites: Contains sodium bisulfite, a sulfite that may cause allergic-type reactions including anaphylactic symptoms and life-threatening or less severe asthmatic episodes in certain susceptible people. The overall prevalence of sulfite sensitivity in the general population is unknown and probably low. Sulfite sensitivity is seen more frequently in asthmatic than in nonasthmatic people.

PRECAUTIONS

Special Risk Patients: In general, opioids should be given with caution and the initial dose should be reduced in the elderly or debilitated and those with severe impairment of hepatic, pulmonary or renal functions; myxedema or hypothyroidism; adrenocortical insufficiency (e.g., Addison's Disease); CNS depression or coma; toxic psychoses; prostatic hypertrophy or urethral stricture; gall bladder disease; acute alcoholism; delirium tremens; kyphoscoliosis or following gastrointestinal surgery.

The administration of opioid analgesics including DILAUDID ORAL LIQUID and DILAUDID 8 mg TABLETS may obscure the diagnoses or clinical course in patients with acute abdominal conditions and may aggravate preexisting convulsions in patients with convulsive disorders.

Head Injury and Increased Intracranial Pressure: The respiratory depressant effects of DILAUDID ORAL LIQUID and DILAUDID 8 mg TABLETS with carbon dioxide retention and secondary elevation of cerebrospinal fluid pressure may be markedly exaggerated in the presence of head injury, other intracranial lesions, or preexisting increase in intracranial pressure. Opioid analgesics including DILAUDID ORAL LIQUID and DILAUDID 8 mg TABLETS may produce effects which can obscure the clinical course and neurologic signs of further increase in intracranial pressure in patients with head injuries.

Hypotensive Effect: Opioid analgesics, including DILAUDID ORAL LIQUID and DILAUDID 8 mg TABLETS, may cause severe hypotension in an individual whose ability to maintain blood pressure has already been compromised by a depleted blood volume, or a concurrent administration of drugs such as phenothiazines or general anesthetics (see also **PRECAUTIONS—**Drug Interactions). Therefore, DILAUDID ORAL LIQUID and DILAUDID 8 mg TABLETS should be administered with caution to patients in circulatory shock, since vasodilation produced by the drug may further reduce cardiac output and blood pressure.

Use in Ambulatory Patients: DILAUDID ORAL LIQUID and DILAUDID 8 mg TABLETS may impair mental and/or physical ability required for the performance of potentially hazardous tasks (e.g. driving, operating machinery). Patients should be cautioned accordingly. DILAUDID may produce orthostatic hypotension in ambulatory patients. The addition of other CNS depressants to DILAUDID therapy may produce additive depressant effects, and DILAUDID should not be taken with alcohol.

Use in Biliary Surgery: Opioid analgesics including DILAUDID ORAL LIQUID and DILAUDID 8 mg TABLETS should also be used with caution in patients about to undergo surgery of the biliary tract since it may cause spasm of the sphincter of Oddi.

Use in Drug and Alcohol Dependent Patients: DILAUDID should be used with caution in patients with alcoholism and other drug dependencies due to the increased frequency of narcotic tolerance, dependence, and the risk of addiction observed in these patient populations. Abuse of DILAUDID in combination with other CNS depressant drugs can result in serious risk to the patient.

Opioid Analgesic Equivalents With Approximately Equianalgesic Potency*

Nonproprietary (Trade) Name	IM or SC Dose	ORAL DOSE
Morphine Sulfate	10 mg	40–60 mg
Hydromorphone HCL (DILAUDID)	1.3–2.0 mg	6.5–7.5 mg
Oxymorphone (Numorphan)	1.0–1.1 mg	6.6 mg
Levorphanol (Levo-Dromoran)	2–2.3 mg	4 mg
Meperidine (Demerol)	75–100 mg	300–400 mg
Methadone (Dolophine)	10 mg	10–20 mg

Drug Interactions: The concomitant use of other central nervous system depressants including sedatives or hypnotics, general anesthetics, phenothiazines, tranquilizers and alcohol may produce additive depressant effects. Respiratory depression, hypotension and profound sedation or coma may occur. When such combined therapy is contemplated, the dose of one or both agents should be reduced. Opioid analgesics, including DILAUDID ORAL LIQUID and DILAUDID 8 mg TABLETS, may enhance the action of neuromuscular blocking agents and produce an excessive degree of respiratory depression.

Carcinogenesis, Mutagenesis, Impairment of Fertility: Studies in animals to evaluate the drug's carcinogenic and mutagenic potential or the effect on fertility, have not been conducted.

Pregnancy—Pregnancy Category C: Literature reports of hydromorphone hydrochloride administration to pregnant Syrian hamsters show that DILAUDID is teratogenic at a dose of 20 mg/kg which is 600 times the human dose. A maximal teratogenic effect (50% of fetuses affected) in the Syrian hamster was observed at a dose of 125 mg/kg (738 mg/m^2). There are no well-controlled studies in women. Hydromorphone is known to cross placental membranes. DILAUDID ORAL LIQUID and DILAUDID 8 mg TABLETS should be used in pregnant women only if the potential benefit justifies the potential risk to the fetus (see Labor and Delivery and **DRUG ABUSE AND DEPENDENCE**).

Labor and Delivery: DILAUDID ORAL LIQUID and DILAUDID 8 mg TABLETS are contraindicated in Labor and Delivery (see **CONTRAINDICATIONS**).

Nursing Mothers: Low levels of opioid analgesics have been detected in human milk. As a general rule, nursing should not be undertaken while a patient is receiving DILAUDID ORAL LIQUID and DILAUDID 8 mg TABLETS since it, and other drugs in this class, may be excreted in the milk.

Pediatric Use: Safety and effectiveness in children have not been established.

Geriatric Use: DILAUDID has not been studied in geriatric patients. Elderly subjects have been shown to have at least twice the sensitivity (as measured by EEG changes) of young adults to some opioids. When administering DILAUDID to the elderly, the initial dose should be reduced (see **INDIVIDUALIZATION OF DOSAGE** and **PRECAUTIONS**).

ADVERSE REACTIONS

The adverse effects of DILAUDID ORAL LIQUID and DILAUDID 8 mg TABLETS are similar to those of other agonist analgesics, and represent established pharmacological effects of the drug class. The major hazards include respiratory depression and apnea. To a lesser degree, circulatory depression, respiratory arrest, shock and cardiac arrest have occurred.

The most frequently observed adverse effects are light-headedness, dizziness, sedation, nausea, vomiting, sweating, dysphoria, euphoria, dry mouth, and pruritus. These effects seem to be more prominent in ambulatory patients and in those not experiencing severe pain. Syncopal reactions and related symptoms in ambulatory patients may be alleviated if the patient lies down.

Less Frequently Observed with Opioid Analgesics:

General and CNS: Weakness, headache, agitation, tremor, uncoordinated muscle movements, alterations of mood (nervousness, apprehension, depression, floating feelings, dreams), muscle rigidity, paresthesia, muscle tremor, blurred vision, nystagmus, diplopia and miosis, transient hallucinations and disorientation, visual disturbances, insomnia and increased intracranial pressure may occur.

Cardiovascular: Chills, tachycardia, bradycardia, palpitation, faintness, syncope, hypotension and hypertension have been reported.

Respiratory: Bronchospasm and laryngospasm have been known to occur.

Gastrointestinal: Constipation biliary tract spasm, ileus, anorexia, diarrhea, cramps and taste alteration have been reported.

Genitourinary: Urinary retention or hesitancy, and antidiuretic effects have been reported.

Dermatologic: Urticaria, other skin rashes, and diaphoresis.

DRUG ABUSE AND DEPENDENCE

DILAUDID is a Schedule II narcotic, similar to morphine. Opioid analgesics may cause psychological and physical dependence (see **WARNINGS**). Physical dependence results in withdrawal symptoms in patients who abruptly discontinue the drug. Withdrawal symptoms also may be precipitated in the patient with physical dependence by the administration of a drug with opioid antagonist activity, e.g., naloxone (see also **OVERDOSAGE**).

Physical dependence usually does not occur to a clinically significant degree until after several weeks of continued opioid usage, but it may become clinically detectable after as little as a week. Tolerance, in which increasingly large doses are required in order to produce the same degree of analgesia, is initially manifested by a shortened duration of analgesic effect, and subsequently, by decreases in the intensity of analgesia. In chronic pain patients, and in opioid- tolerant cancer patients, the dose of DILAUDID ORAL LIQUID and DILAUDID 8 mg TABLETS should be guided by the degree of tolerance manifested.

In chronic pain patients in whom opioid analgesics including DILAUDID ORAL LIQUID and DILAUDID 8 mg TABLETS are abruptly discontinued, a severe abstinence syndrome should be anticipated. This may be similar to the abstinence syndrome noted in patients who withdraw from heroin. Because of excessive loss of fluids through sweating, or vomiting and diarrhea, patients experiencing the syndrome usually exhibit marked weight loss, dehydration, ketosis, and disturbances in acid-base balance. Cardiovascular collapse can occur. Without treatment most observable symptoms disappear in 5–14 days; however, there appears to be a phase of secondary or chornic abstinence which may last for 2–6 months characterized by insomnia, irritability, muscular aches, and autonomic instability.

In the treatment of physical dependence on DILAUDID ORAL LIQUID and DILAUDID 8 mg TABLETS, the patient may be detoxified by gradual reduction of the dosage, although this is unlikely to be necessary in the terminal cancer patient. If abstinence symptoms become severe, the patient may be detoxified with methadone. Temporary administration of tranquilizers and sedatives may aid in reducing patient anxiety. Gastrointestinal disturbances or dehydration should be treated accordingly.

OVERDOSAGE

Serious overdosage with DILAUDID ORAL LIQUID and DILAUDID 8 mg TABLETS is characterized by respiratory depression, somnolence progressing to stupor or coma, skeletal muscle flaccidity, cold and clammy skin, constricted pupils, and sometimes bradycardia and hypotension. In serious overdosage, particularly following intravenous injection, apnea, circulatory collapse, cardiac arrest and death may occur.

In the treatment of overdosage, primary attention should be given to the reestablishment of adequate respiratory exchange through provision of a patent airway and institution of assisted or controlled ventilation. A potentially serious oral ingestion, if recent, should be managed with gut decontamination. In unconscious patients with a secure airway, instill activated charcoal (30–100 g in adults, 1–2 g/kg in infants) via a nasogastric tube. A saline cathartic or sorbitol may be added to the first dose of activated charcoal.

Opioid-tolerant patient: Since tolerance to the respiratory and CNS depressant effects of opioids develops concomitantly with tolerance to their analgesic effects, serious respiratory depression due to an acute overdose is unlikely to be seen in opioid-tolerant patients receiving the usual therapeutic dosage of DILAUDID ORAL LIQUID and DILAUDID 8 mg TABLETS for chronic pain.

Note: In an individual who is physically dependent on opioids, administration of the usual dose of an opioid antagonist will precipitate an acute withdrawal syndrome. The severity will depend on the degree of physical dependence and the dose of the antagonist administered. If necessary to treat serious respiratory depression in the physically-dependent patient, the opioid antagonist should be administered with care and by titration, using fractional (one fifth to one tenth) doses of the antagonist.

Non-tolerant patient: The opioid antagonist, naloxone, is a specific antidote against respiratory depression which may result from overdosage, or unusual sensitivity to DILAUDID ORAL LIQUID and DILAUDID 8 mg TABLETS. A dose of naloxone (usually given as a test dose of 0.4 mg, followed by up to 2.0 mg if needed) should be administered intravenously, if possible, simultaneously with respiratory resuscitation. The dose can be repeated in 3 minutes. Naloxone should not be administered in the absence of clinically significant respiratory or circulatory depression. Naloxone should

Continued on next page

Knoll Laboratories—Cont.

be administered cautiously to persons who are known, or suspected to be physically dependent on DILAUDID ORAL LIQUID and DILAUDID 8 mg TABLETS (see The Opioid Tolerant patient, above).
Since the duration of action of DILAUDID ORAL LIQUID and DILAUDID 8 mg TABLETS may exceed that of the antagonist, the patient should be kept under continued surveillance; repeated doses of the antagonist may be required to maintain adequate respiration. Apply other supportive measures when indicated.
Supportive measures (including oxygen, vasopressors) should be employed in the management of circulatory shock and pulmonary edema accompanying overdose as indicated. Cardiac arrest or arrhythmias may require cardiac massage or defibrillation.

DOSAGE AND ADMINISTRATION

DILAUDID ORAL LIQUID: The usual adult oral dosage of DILAUDID ORAL LIQUID is one-half (2.5 mL) to two teaspoonfuls (10 mL) (2.5 mg–10 mg) every 3 to 6 hours as directed by the clinical situation. Oral dosages higher than the usual dosages may be required in some patients.
DILAUDID 8 mg TABLET: The usual starting dose for DILAUDID tablets is 2 mg to 4 mg, orally, every 4 to 6 hours. Appropriate use of the DILAUDID 8 mg TABLET must be decided by careful evaluation of each clinical situation.
A gradual increase in dose may be required if analgesia is inadequate, as tolerance develops, or if pain severity increases. The first sign of tolerance is usually a reduced duration of effect.
SAFETY AND HANDLING INSTRUCTIONS
DILAUDID ORAL LIQUID and DILAUDID 8 mg TABLETS pose little risk of direct exposure to health care personnel and should be handled and disposed of prudently in accordance with hospital or institutional policy. Significant absorption from dermal exposure is unlikely; accidental dermal exposure to DILAUDID ORAL LIQUID should be treated by removal of any contaminated clothing and rinsing the affected area with cool water. Patients and their families should be instructed to flush any DILAUDID ORAL LIQUID and DILAUDID 8 mg TABLETS that are no longer needed.
Access to abuseable drugs such as DILAUDID ORAL LIQUID and DILAUDID tablets presents an occupational hazard for addiction in the health care industry. Routine procedures for handling controlled substances developed to protect the public may not be adequate to protect health care workers. Implementation of more effective accounting procedures and measures to restrict access to drugs of this class (appropriate to the practice setting) may minimize the risk of self-administration by health care providers.

HOW SUPPLIED

DILAUDID ORAL LIQUID is a colorless, sweet, slightly viscous liquid. It is available in:
Bottles of 1 pint (473 mL)—NDC# 0044-1085-01
DILAUDID 8 mg TABLETS are white and triangular shaped, embossed with the number 8 on one side and bisected and embossed with a double "Knoll" triangle on the other side. They are available in:
Bottles of 100—NDC# 0044-1028-02
Storage: DILAUDID ORAL LIQUID and 8 mg TABLETS should be stored at 59–77°F (15–25°C). Protect from light.
A schedule II Narcotic DEA Order Form is Required. D100-1094

Shown in Product Identification Guide, page 319

E-MYCIN® Tablets ℞

(Erythromycin Delayed-Release Tablets, USP)
250 mg/333 mg

E-MYCIN® Tablets (Erythromycin Delayed-Release Tablets, USP) contain erythromycin as the base.

DESCRIPTION

Erythromycin is produced by a strain of *Streptomyces erythreaus* and belongs to the macrolide group of antibiotics. It is basic and readily forms salts with acids. The base is white to off-white crystal or powder slightly soluble in water, soluble in alcohol, in chloroform, and in ether. The chemical name for erythromycin is (3*R**, 4*S**, 5*S**, 6*R**, 7*R**, 9*R**, 11*R**, 12*R**, 13*S**, 14*R**)-4-[(2,6-Dideoxy-3-*C*-methyl-3-*O*-methyl-α-L-*ribo*- hexopyranosyl)-oxy] -14 -ethyl -7, 12, 13-trihydroxy- 3, 5, 7, 9, 11, 13-hexamethyl-6-[[3,4,6 -trideoxy-3-(dimethylamino) -β-D-*xylo*-hexopyranosyl] oxy] oxacyclotetradecane-2, 10-dione and the molecular weight is 733.94. The structural formula is represented below:
[See chemical structure at top of next column.]
E-MYCIN Tablets, available in 250 mg and 333 mg strengths, are specially coated to protect the contents from the inactivating effects of gastric acidity and to permit efficient absorption of the antibiotic in the small intestine.

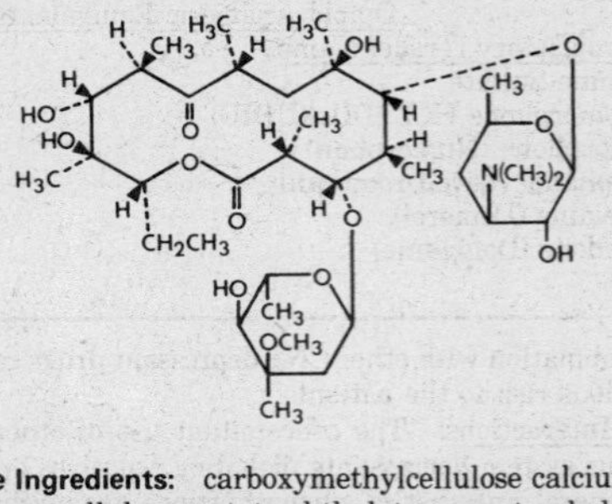

Inactive Ingredients: carboxymethylcellulose calcium, carnauba wax, cellulose acetate phthalate, corn starch, hydroxypropyl cellulose, lactose, magnesium stearate, mineral oil, propylene glycol, sorbic acid, sorbitan monooleate, sucrose, talc, titanium dioxide. **250 mg**—FD&C Yellow No. 6.

CLINICAL PHARMACOLOGY

Microbiology: The mode of action of erythromycin is by inhibition of protein synthesis without affecting nucleic acid synthesis. Many strains of *Haemophilus influenzae* are resistant to erythromycin alone, but are susceptible to erythromycin and sulfonamides together.
Erythromycin is usually active against the following organisms *in vitro* (prior to use, refer to **INDICATIONS AND USAGE** section): **Gram-positive Bacteria:** *Staphylococcus aureus* (resistant organisms may emerge during treatment), *Streptococcus pyogenes* (Group A beta-hemolytic streptococci), Alpha-hemolytic streptococci (viridans group), *Streptococcus* (diplococcus) *pneumoniae, Corynebacterium diphtheriae, Corynebacterium minutissimum.*
Gram-negative Bacteria: *Neisseria gonorroeae, Legionella pneumophila* (agent of Legionnaire's Disease), *Bordetella pertussis.*
Mycoplasma: *Mycoplasma pneumoniae* (Eaton's agent), *Ureaplasma urealyticum.*
Other Microorganism: *Chlamydia trachomatis, Entamoeba histolytica, Treponema pallidum, Listeria monocytogenes.*
Antagonism has been demonstrated *in vitro* between clindamycin, lincomycin, chloramphenicol and erythromycin.
Bioavailability data are available from Knoll Pharmaceutical Company.
After absorption, erythromycin diffuses readily into most body fluids. In the absence of meningeal inflammation, low concentrations are normally achieved in the spinal fluid but passage of the drug across the blood-brain barrier increases in meningitis. In the presence of normal hepatic function, erythromycin is concentrated in the liver and excreted in the bile; the effect of hepatic dysfunction on excretion of erythromycin by the liver into the bile is not known. After oral administration, less than 5 percent of the activity of the administered dose can be recovered in the urine.
Erythromycin crosses the placental barrier but fetal plasma levels are low.
Erythromycin serum levels are not appreciably affected by hemodialysis or peritoneal dialysis.
Susceptibility testing: Culture and susceptibility testing should be done. If the Kirby-Bauer method of disk susceptibility is used, a 15 mcg erythromycin disk should give a zone diameter of at least 18 mm when tested against an erythromycin susceptible organism.

INDICATIONS AND USAGE

E-MYCIN Tablets are indicated in the treatment of infections caused by susceptible strains of the designated organisms in the conditions listed below:
Upper respiratory tract infections of mild to moderate severity due to *Streptococcus pyogenes, Streptococcus pneumoniae,* and *Haemophilus influenzae.* (Since many strains of *H. Influenzae* are not susceptible at the erythromycin concentrations ordinarily achieved, concomitant sulfonamide therapy should be prescribed.)
Lower respiratory tract infections of mild to moderate severity due to *S. pyogenes* and *S. pneumoniae.*
Respiratory infections due to *Mycoplasma pneumoniae* (Eaton's agent, PPLO).
Whooping cough (pertussis) caused by *Bordetella pertussis:* Erythromycin is effective in eliminating the organism from the nasopharynx of infected individuals, rendering them noninfectious. Some clinical studies suggest that erythromycin may be helpful in the prophylaxis of pertussis in exposed susceptible individuals.
Legionnaires' disease due to *Legionella pneumophila:* Although no controlled clinical efficacy studies have been conducted, *in vitro*, preliminary clinical data suggest that erythromycin can be effective in treating Legionnaires' disease.
Infections due to *Chlamydia trachomatis:* Erythromycin is indicated in the treatment of conjunctivitis of the newborn, pneumonia of infancy, and urogenital infections during pregnancy. When tetracyclines are contraindicated or not tolerated, erythromycin is indicated for the treatment of uncomplicated urethral, endocervical or rectal infections in adults due to *C. trachomatis.*
Prophylaxis against bacterial endocarditis due to alpha-hemolytic streptococci (viridans group). Although no controlled clinical efficacy trials have been conducted, oral erythromycin has been suggested by the American Heart Association and the American Dental Association for use in a regimen for prophylaxis against bacterial endocarditis in patients allergic to penicillin who have congenital heart disease or rheumatic or other acquired valvular heart disease when they undergo dental procedures and surgical procedures of the upper respiratory tract. Erythromycin is not suitable prior to genitourinary or gastrointestinal tract surgery.
Prophylaxis of rheumatic fever: Injectable benzathine penicillin G is considered by the American Heart Association to be the drug of choice in the treatment and prevention of streptococcal pharyngitis and in long-term prophylaxis of rheumatic fever. When oral medication is preferred for treatment of the above conditions, penicillin G, V or erythromycin are alternate choices.
Skin and soft tissue infections of mild to moderate severity due to *S. pyrogenes* and *Staphylococcus aureus* (staphylococci may become resistant during treatment).
Diphtheria due to *Corynebacterium diphtheriae:* Erythromycin may be beneficial as adjunctive therapy with antitoxin and to prevent the establishment of carriers, and to eradicate the organism in carriers.
Erythrasma due to *Corynebacterium minutissium.*
Intestinal amebiasis due to *Entamoeba histolytica:* Extraintestinal amebiasis requires treatment with other agents.
Infections due to *Listeria monocytogenes.*
Syphillis (primary) due to *Treponema pallidum:* Erythromycin is an alternate choice of treatment for patients allergic to the penicillins. Spinal fluid examinations should be done before therapy and as part of the follow-up after therapy.
Acute pelvic inflammatory disease due to *Neisseria gonorrhea:* Erythromycin lactobionate for infection in conjunction with erythromycin base orally is an alternative treatment for patients allergic to penicillin. Before treatment of gonorrhea, patients who are suspected of also having syphillis should have a microscopic examination for *T. pallidum* before receiving erythromycin. Monthly serologic test should be done for a minimum of four months.

CONTRAINDICATIONS

Erythromycin is contraindicated in patients with known hypersensitivity to this antibiotic.
Erythromycin is contraindicated in patients taking terfenadine. (see **PRECAUTIONS—Drug Interactions.**)

WARNINGS

There have been reports of hepatic dysfunction, with or without jaundice, occurring in patients receiving oral erythromycin products.
Pseudomembranous colitis has been reported with nearly all antibacterial agents, including erythromycin, and may range in severity from mild to life-threatening. Therefore, it is important to consider this diagnosis in patients who present with diarrhea subsequent to the administration of antibacterial agents.
Treatment with antibacterial agents alters the normal flora of the colon and may permit overgrowth of clostridia. Studies indicate that a toxin produced by *Clostridium difficile* is a primary cause of "antibiotic-associated colitis."
After the diagnosis of pseudomembranous colitis has been established, therapeutic measure should be initiated. Mild cases of pseudomembranous colitis usually respond to discontinuation of the drug alone. In moderate to severe cases, consideration should be given to management with fluids and electrolytes, protein supplementation and treatment with an antibacterial drug effective against *Clostridium difficile.*
Rhabdomyolysis with or without renal impairment has been reported in seriously ill patients receiving erythromycin concomitantly with lovastatin. Therefore, patients receiving concomitant lovastatin and erythromycin should be carefully monitored for creatine kinase (CK) and serum transaminase levels. (See package insert for lovastatin.)

PRECAUTIONS

General: Erythromycin is principally excreted by the liver. Caution should be exercised when erythromycin in administered to patients with impaired hepatic function. (See **CLINICAL PHARMACOLOGY** and **WARNINGS** sections).
Prolonged or repeated use of erythromycin may result in an overgrowth of nonsusceptible bacteria or fungi. If superinfection occurs, erythromycin should be discontinued and appropriate therapy instituted.
When indicated, incision and drainage or other surgical procedures should be performed in conjunction with antibiotic therapy.
Drug/Laboratory Test Interactions: Erythromycin may interfere with AST (SGOT) determinations if azonefast violet B or diphenylhydrazine colorimetric determinations are used. Erythromycin interferes with the fluorometric determination of urinary catecholamines.

Drug Interactions: Erythromycin use in patients who are receiving high doses of theophylline may be associated with an increase in serum theophylline levels and potential theophylline toxicity. In case of theophylline toxicity and/or elevated serum theophylline levels, the dose of theophylline should be reduced while the patient is receiving concomitant erythromycin therapy.

Concomitant administration of erythromycin and digoxin has been reported to result in elevated digoxin serum levels.

There have been reports of increased anticoagulant effects when erythromycin and oral anticoagulants were used concomitantly.

Concurrent use of erythromycin and ergotamine or dihydroergotamine has been associated in some patients with acute ergot toxicity characterized by severe peripheral vasospasm and dysesthesia.

Erythromycin has been reported to decrease the clearance of triazolam and midazolam and, thus, may increase the pharmacologic effect of these benzodiazepines.

The use of erythromycin in patients concurrently taking drugs metabolized by the cytochrome P450 system may be associated with elevations in serum levels of these other drugs. There have been reports of interactions of erythromycin with carbamazepine, cyclosporine, hexobarbital, phenytoin, alfentanil, disopyramide, lovastatin and bromocriptine. Serum concentrations of drugs metabolized by the cytochrome P450 system should be monitored closely in patients concurrently receiving erythromycin.

Erythromycin significantly alters the metabolism of terfenadine when taken concomitantly. Rare cases of serious cardiovascular adverse events, including death, cardiac arrest, torsades de pointes, and other ventricular arrhythmias, have been observed (see **CONTRAINDICATIONS**).

Carcinogenesis, mutagenesis, impairment of fertility: Long-term (2-year) oral studies conducted in rats with erythromycin base did not provide evidence of tumorigenicity. Mutagenicity studies have not been conducted. There was no apparent effect on male or female fertility in rats fed erythromycin (base) at levels up to 0.25 percent of diet.

Pregnancy: Teratogenic effects: Pregnancy category B: There is no evidence of teratogenicity or any other adverse effect on reproduction in female rats fed erythromycin base (up to 0.25 percent of diet) prior to and during mating, during gestation, and through weaning of two successive litters. There are, however, no adequate and well-controlled studies in pregnant women. Because animal reproduction studies are not always predictive of human response, this drug should be used during pregnancy only if clearly needed. Erythromycin has been reported to cross the placental barrier in humans, but fetal plasma levels are generally low.

Labor and delivery: The effect of erythromycin on labor and delivery is unknown.

Nursing mothers: Erythromycin is excreted in human milk, therefore, caution should be exercised when erythromycin is administered to a nursing woman.

Pediatric use: See **INDICATIONS AND USAGE** and **DOSAGE AND ADMINISTRATION** sections.

ADVERSE REACTIONS

The most frequent side effects of erythromycin preparations are gastrointestinal, such as abdominal cramping and discomfort, and are dose related. Nausea, vomiting, and diarrhea occur infrequently with usual oral doses.

Mild allergic reactions such as urticaria and other skin rashes have occurred. Serious allergic reactions, including anaphylaxis, have been reported.

There have been isolated reports of reversible hearing loss occurring chiefly in patients with renal insufficiency and in patients receiving high doses of erythromycin.

DOSAGE AND ADMINISTRATION

E-MYCIN® Tablets (Erythromycin Delayed-Release Tablets, USP) are well absorbed and may be given without regard to meals.

Adults: The usual dose is 250 mg four times daily or 333 mg 3 times daily.

If twice a day dosage is desired, the recommended dose is 500 mg every 12 hours.

Dosage may be increased up to 4 or more grams per day according to the severity of the infection. Twice-a-day dosing is not recommended when doses larger than 1 gram daily are administered.

Children: Age, weight, and severity of the infection are important factors in determining the proper dosage. 30 to 50 mg/kg/day, in divided doses, is the usual dose. For more severe infections, this dose may be doubled.

For the treatment of streptococcal infections: A therapeutic dosage of erythromycin should be administered for at least 10 days. In continuous prophylaxis of streptococcal infections in persons with a history of rheumatic heart disease, the dose is 250 mg twice a day.

For prophylaxis against bacterial endocarditis[1]: In patients with congenital heart disease or rheumatic or other acquired valvular heart disease, when undergoing dental procedures or surgical procedures of the upper respiratory tract, give 1.0 gram (20 mg/kg for children) orally 3–4 hours before the procedure and then 500 mg (10 mg/kg for children) orally 6 hours after the first dose.

NOTE: Due to the pharmacokinetic characteristics of E-MYCIN delayed-release tablets, the above indicated timing of the doses differs from the American Heart Association.

For treatment of primary syphilis: 30 to 40 grams given in divided doses over a period of 10 to 15 days.

For treatment of acute pelvic inflammatory disease caused by *N. gonorrhoeae:* After initial treatment with erythromycin lactobionate for injection (500 mg every 6 hours for 3 days), the oral dosage recommendation is 250 mg every 6 hours for 7 days or 333 mg every 8 hours for 7 days.

Urogenital infections during pregnancy due to *Chlamydia trachomatis:* Although the optimal dose and duration of therapy have not been established, the suggested treatment is erythromycin 500 mg, by mouth, four times a day or two 333 mg tablets every eight hours for at least seven days. For women who cannot tolerate this regimen, a decreased dose of 250 mg, by mouth, four times a day or one 333 mg tablet every eight hours should be used for at least 14 days.[2]

For adults with uncomplicated urethral, endocervical, or rectal infections caused by *Chlamydia trachomatis* in whom tetracyclines are contraindicated or not tolerated: 500 mg, by mouth, four times a day or two 333 mg tablets every eight hours for at least seven days.[2]

For dysenteric amebiasis: 250 mg four times daily or 333 mg every 8 hours for 10 to 14 days, for adults; 30 to 50 mg/kg/day in divided doses for 10 to 14 days, for children.

For use in pertussis: Although optimal dosage and duration have not been established, doses of erythromycin utilized in reported clinical studies were 40 to 50 mg/kg/day, given in divided doses for 5 to 14 days.

For treatment of Legionnaires Disease: Although optimal doses have not been established, doses utilized in reported clinical data were those recommended above (1 to 4 grams daily in divided doses).

Preoperative Prophylaxis for Elective Colorectal Surgery: Listed below is an example of a recommended bowel preparation regimen. A proposed surgery time of 8:00 a.m. has been used.

Pre-op Day 3: Minimum residue or clear liquid diet. Bisacodyl, 1 tablet orally at 6:00 p.m.

Pre-op Day 2: Minimum residue or clear liquid diet. Magnesium sulfate, 30 mL, 50% solution (15g) orally at 10:00 a.m., 2:00 p.m. and 6:00 p.m. Enema at 7:00 p.m. and 8:00 p.m.

Pre-op Day 1: Clear liquid diet. Supplemental (IV) fluids as needed. Magnesium sulfate, 30 mL, 50% solution (15g) orally at 10:00 a.m. and 2:00 p.m. Neomycin sulfate (1.0g) and erythromycin base (three 333 mg tablets or four 250 mg tablets) orally at 1:00 p.m., 2:00 p.m. and 11:00 p.m. No enema.

Day of operation: Patient evacuates rectum at 6:30 a.m. for scheduled operation at 8:00 a.m.

HOW SUPPLIED

E-MYCIN® Tablets (Erythromycin Delayed-Release Tablets, USP):

250 mg: round, convex, orange, enteric-coated tablet with "E-MYCIN 250 mg" printed in black on one face.

Bottles of 40	NDC 0044-0207-99
Bottles of 100	NDC 0044-0207-01
Unit Dose Pkg of 100	NDC 0044-0207-21
Bottles of 500	NDC 0044-0207-05

333 mg: round, convex, white, enteric-coated tablet with "E-MYCIN 333 mg" printed in orange on one face.

Bottles of 100	NDC 0044-0208-01
Unit Dose Pkg of 100	NDC 0044-0208-21
Bottles of 500	NDC 0044-0208-05

Store at controlled room temperature, 15°–30°C (59°–86°F).

CAUTION

Federal (USA) law prohibits dispensing without prescription.

[1] American Heart Association 1984. Prevention of Bacterial Endocarditis. Circulation 70:1123A–1127A.

[2] CDC Sexually Transmitted Diseases Treatment Guidelines 1985.

Manufactured
By
The Upjohn Company
Kalamazoo, Michigan 49001 USA

Rev. 5/6/95 813 929 308
691015

Shown in Product Identification Guide, page 319

IBU® ℞

(Ibuprofen Tablets, USP)

400mg/600 mg/800 mg

DESCRIPTION

IBU (Ibuprofen Tablets, USP) is (±)-2-(*p*-isobutylphenyl) propionic acid. It is a white powder with a melting point of 74–77°C and is very slightly soluble in water (<1 mg/mL) and readily soluble in organic solvents such as ethanol and acetone.

Its structural formula is:

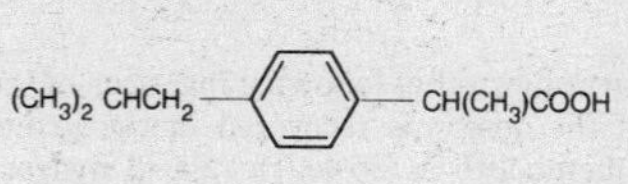
(CH3)2 CHCH2
CH(CH3)COOH

IBU is a nonsteroidal anti-inflammatory agent. It is available in 400, 600 and 800 mg tablets for oral administration.

Inactive Ingredients: 400 mg and 600 mg—colloidal silicon dioxide, hydroxypropyl methylcellulose, Opaspray® M-1-7111-B, pregelatinized starch, starch, stearic acid, talc, 2202C Fine Black Ink (carbon black), or shellac, black iron oxide, lecithin and simethicone. **800 mg**—croscarmellose sodium, hydroxypropyl methylcellulose, hydroxypropyl cellulose, lactose monohydrate, magnesium stearate, propylene glycol, 2202C Fine Black Ink (carbon black) or shellac, black iron oxide, lecithin and simethicone.

CLINICAL PHARMACOLOGY

IBU is a nonsteroidal anti-inflammatory agent that possesses analgesic and antipyretic activities. Its mode of action, like that of other nonsteroidal anti-inflammatory agents, is not completely understood, but may be related to prostaglandin synthetase inhibition.

In clinical studies in patients with rheumatoid arthritis and osteoarthritis, IBU has been shown to be comparable to aspirin in controlling pain and inflammation and to be associated with a statistically significant reduction in the milder gastrointestinal side effects (see **ADVERSE REACTIONS**).

IBU may be well tolerated in some patients who have had gastrointestinal side effects with aspirin, but these patients when treated with IBU should be carefully followed for signs and symptoms of gastrointestinal ulceration and bleeding.

Although it is not definitely known whether ibuprofen causes less peptic ulceration than aspirin, in one study involving 885 patients with rheumatoid arthritis treated for up to one year, there were no reports of gastric ulceration with ibuprofen whereas frank ulceration was reported in 13 patients in the aspirin group (statistically significant $p < .001$).

Gastroscopic studies at varying doses show an increased tendency toward gastric irritation at higher doses. However, at comparable doses, gastric irritation is approximately half that seen with aspirin. Studies using ^{51}Cr-tagged red cells indicate that fecal blood loss associated with ibuprofen in doses up to 2400 mg daily did not exceed the normal range, and was significantly less than that seen in aspirin-treated patients.

In clinical studies in patients with rheumatoid arthritis, ibuprofen has been shown to be comparable to indomethacin in controlling aforementioned signs and symptoms of disease activity and to be associated with a statistically significant reduction of the milder gastrointestinal (see **ADVERSE REACTIONS**) and CNS side effects.

IBU may be used in combination with gold salts and/or corticosteroids.

Controlled studies have demonstrated that ibuprofen is a more effective analgesic than propoxyphene for the relief of episiotomy pain, pain following dental extraction procedures, and for the relief of the symptoms of primary dysmenorrhea.

In patients with primary dysmenorrhea, ibuprofen has been shown to reduce elevated levels of prostaglandin activity in the menstrual fluid and to reduce resting and active intrauterine pressure, as well as the frequency of uterine contractions. The probable mechanism of action is to inhibit prostaglandin synthesis rather than simply to provide analgesia.

Pharmacokinetics:

IBU is rapidly absorbed when administered orally. Peak serum ibuprofen levels are generally attained one to two hours after administration. With single doses up to 800 mg, a linear relationship exists between the amount of drug administered and the integrated area under the serum drug concentration vs time curve. Above 800 mg, however, the area under the curve increases less than proportional to increases in dose. There is no evidence of drug accumulation or enzyme induction.

The administration of IBU tablets either under fasting conditions or immediately before meals yields quite similar serum ibuprofen concentration-time profiles. When IBU is administered immediately after a meal, there is a reduction in the rate of absorption but no appreciable decrease in the extent of absorption. The bioavailability of ibuprofen is minimally altered by the presence of food.

A bioavailability study has shown that there was no interference with the absorption of ibuprofen when given in conjunction with an antacid containing both aluminum hydroxide and magnesium hydroxide.

Ibuprofen is rapidly metabolized and eliminated in the urine. The excretion of ibuprofen is virtually complete 24 hours after the last dose. The serum half-life is 1.8 to 2.0 hours.

Continued on next page

Knoll Laboratories—Cont.

Studies have shown that following ingestion of the drug 45% to 79% of the dose was recovered in the urine within 24 hours as metabolite A (25%), (+)-2-4'-(2 hydroxy-2-methyl-propyl)-phenyl propionic acid and metabolite B (37%), (+)-2-4'-(2 carboxypropyl) phenyl propionic acid; the percentages of free and conjugated ibuprofen were approximately 1% and 14% respectively.

INDICATIONS AND USAGE

IBU is indicated for relief of the signs and symptoms of rheumatoid arthritis and osteoarthritis.

IBU is indicated for the relief of mild to moderate pain.

IBU is also indicated for the treatment of primary dysmenorrhea.

Since there have been no controlled trials to demonstrate whether there is any beneficial effect or harmful interaction with the use of IBU in conjunction with aspirin, the combination cannot be recommended (see **Drug Interactions**). Controlled clinical trials to establish the safety and effectiveness of IBU in children have not been conducted.

CONTRAINDICATIONS

IBU tablets should not be used in patients who have previously exhibited hypersensitivity to it, or in individuals with all or part of the syndrome of nasal polyps, angioedema and bronchospastic reactivity to aspirin or other nonsteroidal anti-inflammatory agents. Anaphylactoid reactions have occurred in such patients.

WARNINGS *Risk of GI Ulceration, Bleeding and Perforation with NSAID Therapy:* Serious gastrointestinal toxicity such as bleeding, ulceration, and perforation can occur at any time, with or without warning symptoms, in patients treated chronically with NSAID therapy. Although minor upper gastrointestinal problems, such as dyspepsia, are common, usually developing early in therapy, physicians should remain alert for ulceration and bleeding in patients treated chronically with NSAIDs even in the absence of previous GI tract symptoms. In patients observed in clinical trials of several months to two years duration, sypmtomatic upper GI ulcers, gross bleeding or perforation appear to occur in approximately 1% of patients treated for 3–6 months, and in about 2–4% of patients treated for one year. Physicians should inform patients about the signs and/or symptoms of serious GI toxicity and what steps to take if they occur.

Studies to date have not identified any subset of patients not at risk of developing peptic ulceration and bleeding. Except for a prior history of serious GI events and other risk factors known to be associated with peptic ulcer disease, such as alcoholism, smoking, etc., no risk factors (e.g., age, sex) have been associated with increased risk. Elderly or debilitated patients seem to tolerate ulceration or bleeding less well than other individuals and most spontaneous reports of fatal GI events are in this population. Studies to date are inconclusive concerning the relative risk of various NSAIDs in causing such reactions. High doses of any NSAID probably carry a greater risk of these reactions, although controlled clinical trials showing this do not exist in most cases. In considering the use of relatively large doses (within the recommended dosage range), sufficient benefit should be anticipated to offset the potential increased risk of GI toxicity.

PRECAUTIONS

General: Blurred and/or diminished vision, scotomata, and/or changes in color vision have been reported. If a patient develops such complaints while receiving IBU, the drug should be discontinued and the patient should have an ophthalmologic examination which includes central visual fields and color vision testing.

Fluid retention and edema have been reported in association with IBU therefore, the drug should be used with caution in patients with a history of cardiac decompensation or hypertension.

IBU, like other nonsteroidal anti-inflammatory agents, can inhibit platelet aggregation but the effect is quantitatively less and of shorter duration than that seen with aspirin. Ibuprofen has been shown to prolong bleeding time (but within the normal range) in normal subjects. Because this prolonged bleeding effect may be exaggerated in patients with underlying hemostatic defects, IBU should be used with caution in persons with intrinsic coagulation defects and those on anticoagulant therapy.

Patients on IBU should report to their physicians signs or symptoms of gastrointestinal ulceration or bleeding, blurred vision or other eye symptoms, skin rash, weight gain, or edema.

In order to avoid exacerbation of disease or adrenal insufficiency, patients who have been on prolonged corticosteroid therapy should have their therapy tapered slowly rather than discontinued abruptly when IBU is added to the treatment program.

The antipyretic and anti-inflammatory activity of ibuprofen may reduce fever and inflammation, thus diminishing their utility as diagnostic signs in detecting complications of presumed noninfectious, noninflammatory painful conditions.

Liver effects: As with other nonsteroidal anti-inflammatory drugs, borderline elevations of one or more liver function tests may occur in up to 15% of patients. These abnormalities may progress, may remain essentially unchanged, or may be transient with continued therapy. The SGPT (ALT) test is probably the most sensitive indicator of liver dysfunction. Meaningful (3 times the upper limit of normal) elevations of SGPT or SGOT (AST) occurred in controlled clinical trials in less than 1% of patients. A patient with symptoms and/or signs suggesting liver dysfunction, or in whom an abnormal liver test has occurred, should be evaluated for evidence of the development of more severe hepatic reactions while on therapy with ibuprofen. Severe hepatic reactions, including jaundice and cases of fatal hepatitis, have been reported with ibuprofen as with other nonsteroidal anti-inflammatory drugs. Although such reactions are rare, if abnormal liver tests persist or worsen, if clinical signs and symptoms consistent with liver disease develop, or if systemic manifestations occur (e.g., eosinophilia, rash, etc.), IBU should be discontinued.

Hemoglobin Levels: In cross-study comparisons with doses ranging from 1200 mg to 3200 mg daily for several weeks, a slight dose-response decrease in hemoglobin/hematocrit was noted. This has been observed with the other nonsteroidal anti-inflammatory drugs; the mechanism is unknown. However, even with daily doses of 3200 mg, the total decrease in hemoglobin usually does not exceed 1 gram; if there are no signs of bleeding, it is probably not clinically important.

In two postmarketing clinical studies the incidence of a decreased hemoglobin level was greater than previously reported. Decrease in hemoglobin of 1 gram or more was observed in 17.1% of 193 patients on 1600 mg ibuprofen daily (osteoarthritis), and in 22.8% of 189 patients taking 2400 mg of ibuprofen daily (rheumatoid arthritis). Positive stool occult blood tests and elevated serum creatinine levels were also observed in these studies.

Aseptic Meningitis: Aseptic meningitis with fever and coma has been observed on rare occasions in patients on ibuprofen therapy. Although it is probably more likely to occur in patients with systemic lupus erythematosus and related connective tissue diseases, it has been reported in patients who do not have an underlying chronic disease. If signs or symptoms of meningitis develop in a patient on IBU, the possibility of its being related to ibuprofen should be considered.

Renal Effects: As with other nonsteroidal anti-inflammatory drugs, long-term administration of ibuprofen to animals has resulted in renal papillary necrosis and other abnormal renal pathology. In humans, there have been reports of acute interstitial nephritis with hematuria, proteinuria, and occasionally nephrotic syndrome.

A second form of renal toxicity has been seen in patients with prerenal conditions leading to a reduction in renal blood flow or blood volume, where the renal prostaglandins have a supportive role in the maintenance of renal perfusion. In these patients administration of a nonsteroidal anti-inflammatory drug may cause a dose dependent reduction in prostaglandin formation and may precipitate overt renal decompensation. Patients at greatest risk of this reaction are those with impaired renal function, heart failure, liver dysfunction, those taking diuretics and the elderly. Discontinuation of nonsteroidal anti-inflammatory drug therapy is typically followed by recovery to the pretreatment state.

Those patients at high risk who chronically take IBU should have renal function monitored if they have signs or symptoms which may be consistent with mild azotemia, such as malaise, fatigue, loss of appetite, etc. Occasional patients may develop some elevation of serum creatinine and BUN levels without signs or symptoms.

Since ibuprofen is eliminated primarily by the kidneys, patients with significantly impaired renal function should be closely monitored and a reduction in dosage should be anticipated to avoid drug accumulation. Prospective studies on the safety of ibuprofen in patients with chronic renal failure have not been conducted.

Information for Patients: Ibuprofen, like other drugs of its class, is not free of side effects. The side effects of these drugs can cause discomfort and, rarely, there are more serious side effects, such as gastrointestinal bleeding, which may result in hospitalization and even fatal outcomes.

NSAIDs (Nonsteroidal Anti-Inflammatory Drugs) are often essential agents in the management of arthritis and have a major role in the treatment of pain, but they also may be commonly employed for conditions which are less serious. Physicians may wish to discuss with their patients the potential risks (see **WARNINGS, PRECAUTIONS,** and **ADVERSE REACTIONS** sections) and likely benefits of NSAID treatment, particularly when the drugs are used for less serious conditions where treatment without NSAIDs may represent an acceptable alternative to both the patient and physician.

Laboratory Tests: Because serious GI tract ulceration and bleeding can occur without warning symptoms, physicians should follow chronically treated patients for the signs and symptoms of ulceration and bleeding and should inform them of the importance of this follow-up (see WARNINGS).

Drug Interactions: *Coumarin-type anticoagulants:* Several short-term controlled studies failed to show that ibuprofen significantly affected prothrombin times or a variety of other clotting factors when administered to individuals on coumarin-type anticoagulants. However, because bleeding has been reported when IBU® (Ibuprofen Tablets, USP) and other nonsteroidal anti-inflammatory agents have been administered to patients on coumarin-type anticoagulants, the physician should be cautious when administering IBU to patients on anticoagulants.

Aspirin: Animal studies show that aspirin given with nonsteroidal anti-inflammatory agents, including ibuprofen, yields a net decrease in anti-inflammatory activity with lowered blood levels of the non-aspirin drug. Single dose bioavailability studies in normal volunteers have failed to show an effect of aspirin on ibuprofen blood levels. Correlative clinical studies have not been done.

Methotrexate: Ibuprofen, as well as other nonsteroidal anti-inflammatory drugs, has been reported to competitively inhibit methotrexate accumulation in rabbit kidney slices. This may indicate that ibuprofen could enhance the toxicity of methotrexate. Caution should be used if IBU is administered concomitantly with methotrexate.

H-2 Antagonists: In studies with human volunteers, coadministration of cimetidine or ranitidine with ibuprofen had no substantive effect on ibuprofen serum concentrations.

Furosemide: Clinical studies, as well as random observations, have shown that ibuprofen can reduce the natriuretic effect of furosemide and thiazides in some patients. This response has been attributed to inhibition of renal prostaglandin synthesis. During concomitant therapy with ibuprofen, the patient should be observed closely for signs of renal failure (see **PRECAUTIONS: Renal Effects**), as well as to assure diuretic efficacy.

Lithium: Ibuprofen produced an elevation of plasma lithium levels and a reduction in renal lithium clearance in a study of eleven normal volunteers. The mean minimum lithium concentration increased 15% and the renal clearance of lithium was decreased by 19% during this period of concomitant drug administration.

This effect has been attributed to inhibition of renal prostaglandin synthesis by ibuprofen. Thus, when ibuprofen and lithium are administered concurrently, subjects should be observed carefully for signs of lithium toxicity. (Read circulars for lithium preparation before use of such concurrent therapy.)

Pregnancy: Reproductive studies conducted in rats and rabbits at doses somewhat less than the maximal clinical dose did not demonstrate evidence of developmental abnormalities. However, animal reproduction studies are not always predictive of human response. As there are no adequate and well-controlled studies in pregnant women, this drug should be used during pregnancy only if clearly needed. Because of the known effects of nonsteroidal anti-inflammatory drugs on the fetal cardiovascular system (closure of ductus arteriosus), use during late pregnancy should be avoided. As with other drugs known to inhibit prostaglandin synthesis, an increased incidence of dystocia and delayed parturition occurred in rats. Administration of IBU is not recommended during pregnancy.

Nursing Mothers: In limited studies, an assay capable of detecting 1 mcg/mL did not demonstrate ibuprofen in the milk of lactating mothers. However, because of the limited nature of the studies and the possible adverse efects of prostaglandin-inhibiting drugs on neonates, IBU is not recommended for use in nursing mothers.

ADVERSE REACTIONS

The most frequent type of adverse reaction occurring with ibuprofen is gastrointestinal. In controlled clinical trials, the percentage of patients reporting one or more gastrointestinal complaints ranged from 4% to 16%

In controlled studies when ibuprofen was compared to aspirin and indomethacin in equally effective doses, the overall incidence of gastrointestinal complaints was about half that seen in either the aspirin-or indomethacin-treated patients. Adverse reactions observed during controlled clinical trials at an incidence greater than 1% are listed in the following paragraphs. Those reactions listed under the heading, Incidence Greater Than 1% (but less than 3%) Probable Causal Relationship, encompass observations in approximately 3,000 patients. More than 500 of these patients were treated for periods of at least 54 weeks.

Still other reactions occurring less frequently than 1 in 100 were reported in controlled clinical trials and from marketing experience. These reactions have been divided into two categories: Precise Incidence Unknown (but less than 1%) Probable Causal Relationship lists reactions with ibuprofen therapy where the probability of a causal relationship exists;

Precise Incidence Unknown (but less than 1%) Causal Relationship Unknown lists reactions with ibuprofen therapy where a causal relationship has not been established.

Reported side effects were higher at doses of 3200 mg/day than at doses of 2400 mg or less per day in clinical trials of patients with rheumatoid arthritis. The increases in incidence were slight and still within the ranges reported in the following paragraphs.

Incidence Greater Then 1%
(but less than 3%)
Probable Causal Relationship

Gastrointestinal: nausea*, epigastric pain*, heartburn*, diarrhea, abdominal distress, nausea and vomiting, indigestion, constipation, abdominal cramps or pain, fullness of GI tract (bloating and flatulence).

Central Nervous System: dizziness*, headache*, nervousness.

Dermatologic: rash* (including maculopapular type), pruritus.

Special Senses: tinnitus.

Metabolic/Endocrine: decreased appetite.

Cardiovascular: edema, fluid retention (generally responds promptly to drug discontinuation) (see **PRECAUTIONS**).

Precise Incidence Unknown
(but less than 1%)
Probable Causal Relationship**

Gastrointestinal: gastric or duodenal ulcer with bleeding and/or perforation, gastrointestinal hemorrhage, pancreatitis, melena, gastritis, hepatitis, jaundice, abnormal liver function tests.

Central Nervous System: depression, insomnia, confusion, emotional lability, somnolence, aseptic meningitis with fever and coma (see **PRECAUTIONS**).

Dermatologic: vesiculobullous eruptions, urticaria, erythema multiforme, Stevens-Johnson syndrome, alopecia.

Special Senses: hearing loss, amblyopia (blurred and/or diminished vision, scotomata and/or changes in color vision) (see **PRECAUTIONS**).

Hematologic: neutropenia, agranulocytosis, aplastic anemia, hemolytic anemia (sometimes Coombs positive), thrombocytopenia with or without purpura, eosinophilia, decrease in hemoglobin and hematocrit (see **PRECAUTIONS**).

Cardiovascular: congestive heart failure in patients with marginal cardiac function, elevated blood pressure, palpitations.

Allergic: syndrome of abdominal pain, fever, chills, nausea and vomiting, anaphylaxis, bronchospasm, (see **CONTRAINDICATIONS**).

Renal: acute renal failure in patients with pre-existing significantly impaired renal function (see **PRECAUTIONS**), decreased creatinine clearance, polyuria, azotemia, cystitis, hematuria.

Miscellaneous: dry eyes and mouth, gingival ulcer, rhinitis.

Precision Incidence Unknown
(but less than 1%)
Causal Relationship Unknown**

Central Nervous System: paresthesias, hallucinations, dream abnormalities, pseudotumor cerebri.

Dermatologic: toxic epidermal necrolysis, photoallergic skin reactions.

Special Senses: conjunctivitis, diplopia, optic neuritis, cataracts.

Hematologic: bleeding episodes (e.g., epistaxis, menorrhagia).

Metabolic/Endocrine: gynecomastia, hypoglycemic reaction, acidosis.

Cardiovascular: arrhythmias (sinus tachycardia, sinus bradycardia).

Allergic: serum sickness, lupus erythematosus syndrome, Henoch-Schonlein vasculitis, angioedema.

Renal: renal papillary necrosis.

* Reactions occurring 3% to 9% of patients treated with ibuprofen. (Those reactions occurring in less than 3% of the patients are unmarked.)

** Reactions are classified under "Probable Causal Relationship (PCR)", if there has been one positive rechallenge or if three or more cases occur which might be causally related. Reactions are classified under "Causal Relationship Unknown" if seven or more events have been reported but the criteria for PCR have not been met.

OVERDOSAGE

Approximately $1^1/_2$ hours after the reported ingestion of from 7 to 10 ibuprofen tablets (400 mg), a 19-month old child weighing 12 kg was seen in the hospital emergency room, apneic and cyanotic, responding only to painful stimuli. This type of stimulus, however, was sufficient to induce respiration. Oxygen and parenteral fluids were given, a greenish-yellow fluid was aspirated from the stomach with no evidence to indicate the presence of ibuprofen. Two hours after ingestion the child's condition seemed stable, she still responded only to painful stimuli and continued to have periods of apnea lasting from 5 to 10 seconds. She was admitted to intensive care and sodium bicarbonate was administered as well as infusions of dextrose and normal saline. By four hours post-ingestion she could be aroused easily, sit by herself and respond to spoken commands. Blood level of ibuprofen was 102.9 mcg/mL approximately $8^1/_2$ hours after accidental ingestion. At 12 hours she appeared to be completely recovered.

In two other reported cases where children (each weighing approximately 10 kg) accidentally, acutely ingested approximately 120 mg/kg, there were no signs of acute intoxication or late sequelae. Blood level in one child 90 minutes after ingestion was 700 mcg/mL, about 10 times the peak levels seen in absorption-excretion studies.

A 19-year old male who had taken 8,000 mg of ibuprofen over a period of a few hours complained of dizziness, and nystagmus was noted. After hospitalization, parenteral hydration and three days bed rest, he recovered with no reported sequelae.

In cases of acute overdosage, the stomach should be emptied by vomiting or lavage, though little drug will likely be recovered if more than an hour has elapsed since ingestion. Because the drug is acidic and is excreted in the urine, it is theoretically beneficial to administer alkali and induce diuresis. In addition to supportive measures, the use of oral activated charcoal may help reduce the absorption and reabsorption of ibuprofen.

DOSAGE AND ADMINISTRATION

Do not exceed 3200 mg total daily dose. If gastrointestinal complaints occur, administer IBU with meals or milk.

Rheumatoid arthritis and osteoarthritis, including flare-ups of chronic disease: ***Suggested Dosage:*** 1200–3200 mg daily (300 mg q.i.d., or 400 mg, 600 mg or 800 mg t.i.d. or q.i.d.). Individual patients may show a better response to 3200 mg daily, as compared with 2400 mg, although in well-controlled clinical trials patients on 3200 mg did not show a better mean response in terms of efficacy. Therefore, when treating patients with 3200 mg/day, the physician should observe sufficient increased clincal benefits to offset potential increased risk.

The dose of ibuprofen should be tailored to each patient, and may be lowered or raised from the suggested doses depending on the severity of symptoms either at time of initiating drug therapy or as the patients responds or fails to respond.

In general, patients with rheumatoid arthritis seem to require higher doses of ibuprofen then do patients with osteoarthritis.

The smallest dose of IBU that yields acceptable control should be employed. A linear blood level dose-response relationship exists with single doses up to 800 mg (see **CLINICAL PHARMACOLOGY**: **Pharmacokinetics** for effects of food on rate of absorption).

The commercial availability of multiple strengths facilitates dosage adjustment.

In chronic conditions, a therapeutic response to IBU therapy is sometimes seen in a few days to a week but most often is observed by two weeks. After a satisfactory response has been achieved, the patient's dose should be reviewed and adjusted as required.

Mild to moderate pain: 400 mg every 4 to 6 hours as necessary for the relief of pain.

In controlled analgesic clinical trials, doses of ibuprofen greater than 400 mg were no more effective than the 400 mg dose.

Dysmenorrhea: For the treatment of dysmenorrhea, beginning with the earliest onset of such pain, IBU should be given in a dose of 400 mg every 4 hours as necessary for the relief of pain.

HOW SUPPLIED

IBU® (Ibuprofen Tablets, USP):

400 mg: elongated, smooth-textured, white, film-coated tablet with "IBU 400" printed in black on one face.

Bottles of 100	NDC 0044-0165-01
Bottles of 500	NDC 0044-0165-05

600 mg: elongated, smooth-textured, white, film-coated tablet with "IBU 600" printed in black on one face.

Bottles of 100	NDC 0044-0162-01
Bottles of 500	NDC 0044-0162-05

800 mg: elongated, smooth-textured, white, film-coated tablet with "IBU 800" printed in black on one face.

Bottles of 100	NDC 0044-0173-01
Bottles of 500	NDC 0044-0173-05

Store at controlled room temperature 15°–30°C (59°–86°F).

CAUTION: Federal (USA) law prohibits dispensing without prescription.

Rev. 5/27/95 9007-00

ISOPTIN® ℞
(verapamil hydrochloride)
Intravenous Injection

DESCRIPTION

ISOPTIN® (verapamil hydrochloride) is a calcium antagonist or slow channel inhibitor. ISOPTIN is available in 5 mg/2 mL and 10 mg/4 mL ampules, 5 mg/2 mL and 10 mg/4 mL single dose vials (for intravenous administration). Each 1 mL of solution contains 2.5 mg verapamil HCl and 8.5 mg sodium chloride in water for injection. Hydrochloric acid and/or sodium hydroxide is used for pH adjustment. The pH of the solution is between 4.1 and 6.0. Protect contents from light. ISOPTIN ampules, and vials are sterile.

The structural formula of verapamil HCl is given below:

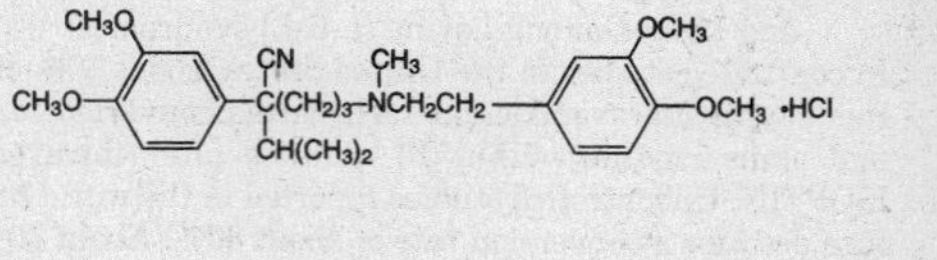

$C_{27}H_{38}N_2O_4 \cdot HCl$ M.W. = 491.08

Benzeneacetonitrile, α-[3-[[2-(3,4-dimethoxyphenyl)ethyl] methylamino]propyl]-3,4-dimethoxy-α-(1-methylethyl) hydrochloride

Verapamil HCl is an almost white, crystalline powder, practically free of odor, with a bitter taste. It is soluble in water, chloroform and methanol. Verapamil HCl is not chemically related to other antiarrhythmic drugs.

CLINICAL PHARMACOLOGY

Mechanism of Action: ISOPTIN (verapamil HCl) inhibits the calcium ion (and possibly sodium ion) influx through slow channels into conductile and contractile myocardial cells and vascular smooth muscle cells. The antiarrhythmic effect of ISOPTIN appears to be due to its effect on the slow channel in cells of the cardiac conduction system. The vasodilatory effect of ISOPTIN appears to be due to its effect on blockade of calcium channels as well as α-receptors.

In the isolated rabbit heart, concentrations of ISOPTIN that markedly affect SA nodal fibers or fibers in the upper and middle regions of the AV node, have very little effect on fibers in the lower AV node (NH region) and no effect on atrial action potentials or His bundle fibers.

Electrical activity in the SA and AV nodes depends, to a large degree, upon calcium influx through the slow channel. By inhibiting this influx, ISOPTIN slows AV conduction and prolongs the effective refractory period within the AV node in a rate-related manner. This effect results in a reduction of the ventricular rate in patients with atrial flutter and/or atrial fibrillation and a rapid ventricular response.

By interrupting reentry at the AV node, ISOPTIN can restore normal sinus rhythm in patients with paroxysmal supraventricular tachycardias (PSVT), including PSVT associated with Wolff-Parkinson-White syndrome.

ISOPTIN does not induce peripheral arterial spasm.

ISOPTIN has a local anesthetic action that is 1.6 times that of procaine on an equimolar basis. It is not known whether this action is important at the doses used in man.

ISOPTIN does not alter total serum calcium levels.

Hemodynamics: ISOPTIN (verapamil HCl) reduces afterload and myocardial contractility. The commonly used intravenous doses of 5–10 mg ISOPTIN produce transient, usually asymptomatic, reduction in normal systemic arterial pressure, systemic vascular resistance and contractility; left ventricular filling pressure is slightly increased. In most patients, including those with organic cardiac disease, the negative inotropic action of ISOPTIN is countered by reduction of afterload, and cardiac index is usually not reduced. However, in patients with moderately severe to severe cardiac dysfunction (pulmonary wedge pressure above 20 mmHg, ejection fraction less than 30%), acute worsening of heart failure may be seen. Peak therapeutic effects occur within 3 to 5 minutes after a bolus injection.

Pharmacokinetics: Intravenously administered ISOPTIN (verapamil HCl) has been shown to be rapidly metabolized. Following intravenous infusion in man, verapamil is eliminated biexponentially, with a rapid early distribution phase (half-life about 4 minutes) and a slower terminal elimination phase (half-life 2–5 hours). In healthy men, orally administered ISOPTIN undergoes extensive metabolism in the liver; 12 metabolites having been identified, most in only trace amounts. The major metabolites have been identified as various N- and O-dealkylated products of ISOPTIN. Approximately 70% of an administered dose is excreted in the urine and 16% or more in the feces within 5 days. About 3–4% is excreted as unchanged drug.

Aging may affect the pharmacokinetics of verapamil given to hypertensive patients. Elimination half-life may be prolonged in the elderly.

INDICATIONS AND USAGE

Intravenous ISOPTIN (verapamil HCl) is indicated for the following:

- Rapid conversion to sinus rhythm of paroxysmal supraventricular tachycardias, including those associated with accessory bypass tracts (Wolff-Parkinson-White [W-P-W] and Lown-Ganong-Levine [L-G-L] syn-

Continued on next page

Knoll Laboratories—Cont.

dromes). When clinically advisable, appropriate vagal maneuvers (e.g. Valsalva maneuver) should be attempted prior to ISOPTIN administration.

- Temporary control of rapid ventricular rate in atrial flutter or atrial fibrillation except when the atrial flutter and/or atrial fibrillation are associated with accessory bypass tracts (Wolff-Parkinson-White [W-P-W] and Lown-Ganong-Levine [L-G-L] syndromes).

In controlled studies in the United States, about 60% of patients with supraventricular tachycardia converted to normal sinus rhythm within 10 minutes after intravenous ISOPTIN. Uncontrolled studies reported in the world literature describe a conversion rate of about 80%. About 70% of patients with atrial flutter and/or fibrillation with a fast ventricular rate respond with a decrease in ventricular rate of at least 20%. Conversion of atrial flutter or fibrillation to sinus rhythm is uncommon (about 10%) after ISOPTIN and may reflect the spontaneous conversion rate, since the conversion rate after placebo was similar. Slowing of the ventricular rate in patients with atrial fibrillation/flutter lasts 30–60 minutes after a single injection.

Because a small fraction (< 1.0%) of patients treated with ISOPTIN respond with life-threatening adverse responses (rapid ventricular rate in atrial flutter/fibrillation and an accessory bypass tract, marked hypotension, or extreme bradycardia/asystole—see Contraindications and Warnings), the initial use of intravenous ISOPTIN should, if possible, be in a treatment setting with monitoring and resuscitation facilities, including DC-cardioversion capability (see Suggested Treatment of Acute Cardiovascular Adverse Reactions). As familiarity with the patient's response is gained, use in an office setting may be acceptable.

Cardioversion has been used safely and effectively after intravenous ISOPTIN.

CONTRAINDICATIONS

Intravenous ISOPTIN (verapamil HCl) is contraindicated in:

1. Severe hypotension or cardiogenic shock.
2. Second- or third-degree AV block (except in patients with a functioning artificial ventricular pacemaker).
3. Sick sinus syndrome (except in patients with a functioning artificial ventricular pacemaker).
4. Severe congestive heart failure (unless secondary to a supraventricular tachycardia amenable to verapamil therapy.)
5. Patients receiving **intravenous** beta adrenergic blocking drugs (e.g., propranolol). **Intravenous** verapamil and **intravenous** beta adrenergic blocking drugs should not be administered in close proximity to each other (within a few hours), since both may have a depressant effect on myocardial contractility and AV conduction.
6. Patients with atrial flutter or atrial fibrillation and an accessory bypass tract (i.e. Wolff-Parkinson-White, Lown-Ganong-Levine syndromes) are at risk to develop ventricular tachyarrhythmia including ventricular fibrillation if verapamil is administered. Therefore the use of verapamil in these patients is contraindicated.
7. Ventricular Tachycardia. Administration of intravenous verapamil to patients with wide-complex ventricular tachycardia (QRS ≥0.12 sec) can result in marked hemodynamic deterioration and ventricular fibrillation. Proper pre-therapy diagnosis and differentiation from wide-complex supraventricular tachycardia is imperative in the emergency room setting.
8. Known hypersensitivity to verapamil hydrochloride.

WARNINGS

ISOPTIN SHOULD BE GIVEN AS A SLOW INTRAVENOUS INJECTION OVER AT LEAST A TWO MINUTE PERIOD OF TIME. (See Dosage and Administration)

Hypotension: Intravenous ISOPTIN (verapamil HCl) often produces a decrease in blood pressure below baseline levels that is usually transient and asymptomatic but may result in dizziness. Administration of intravenous calcium chloride prior to intravenous administration of verapamil may prevent this hemodynamic response. Systolic pressure less than 90 mmHg and/or diastolic pressure less than 60 mmHg was seen in 5–10% of patients in controlled U.S. trials in supraventricular tachycardia and in about 10% of the patients with atrial flutter/fibrillation. The incidence of symptomatic hypotension observed in studies conducted in the U.S. was approximately 1.5%. Three of the five symptomatic patients required intravenous pharmacologic treatment (levarterenol bitartrate, metaraminol bitartrate, or 10% calcium gluconate). All recovered without sequelae.

Extreme Bradycardia/Asystole: ISOPTIN (verapamil HCl) affects the AV and SA nodes and rarely may produce second- or third-degree AV block, bradycardia and, in extreme cases, asystole. This is more likely to occur in patients with a sick sinus syndrome (SA nodal disease), which is more common in older patients. Bradycardia associated with sick sinus syndrome was reported in 0.3% of the patients treated in controlled double-blind trials in the United States. The total incidence of bradycardia (ventricular rate less than 60 beats/min) was 1.2% in these studies. Asystole in patients other than those with sick sinus syndrome is usually of short duration (few seconds or less), with spontaneous return to AV nodal or normal sinus rhythm. If this does not occur promptly, appropriate treatment should be initiated immediately. (See Adverse Reactions and Treatment of Adverse Reactions.)

Heart Failure: When heart failure is not severe or rate related, it should be controlled with digitalis glycosides and diuretics, as appropriate, before ISOPTIN is used. In patients with moderately severe to severe cardiac dysfunction (pulmonary wedge pressure above 20mmHg, ejection fraction less than 30%), acute worsening of heart failure may be seen.

Concomitant Antiarrhythmic Therapy:

Digitalis: Intravenous verapamil has been used concomitantly with digitalis preparations without the occurrence of serious adverse effects. However, since both drugs slow AV conduction, patients should be monitored for AV block or excessive bradycardia.

Procainamide: Intravenous verapamil has been administered to a small number of patients receiving oral procainamide without the occurrence of serious adverse effects.

Quinidine: Intravenous verapamil has been administered to a small number of patients receiving oral quinidine without the occurrence of serious adverse effects. However, three patients have been described in whom the combination resulted in an exaggerated hypotensive response presumably from the combined ability of both drugs to antagonize the effects of catecholamines on α-adrenergic receptors. Caution should therefore be used when employing this combination of drugs.

Beta Adrenergic Blocking Drugs: Intravenous verapamil has been administered to patients receiving oral beta blockers without the development of serious adverse effects. However, since both drugs may depress myocardial contractility and AV conduction, the possibility of detrimental interactions should be considered. The concomitant administration of **intravenous** beta blockers and **intravenous** verapamil has resulted in serious adverse reactions (see Contraindications), especially in patients with severe cardiomyopathy, congestive heart failure or recent myocardial infarction.

Disopyramide: Until data on possible interactions between verapamil and all forms of disopyramide phosphate are obtained, disopyramide should not be administered within 48 hours before or 24 hours after verapamil administration.

Flecainide: A study in healthy volunteers showed that the concomitant administration of flecainide and verapamil may have additive effects reducing myocardial contractility, prolonging AV conduction, and prolonging repolarization.

Heart Block: ISOPTIN (verapamil HCl) prolongs AV conduction time. While high degree AV block has not been observed in controlled clinical trials in the U.S., a low percentage (less than 0.5%) has been reported in the world literature. Development of second- or third-degree AV block or unifascicular, bifascicular or trifascicular bundle branch block requires reduction in subsequent doses or discontinuation of verapamil and institution of appropriate therapy, if needed. (See Treatment of Acute Cardiovascular Adverse Reactions.)

Hepatic and Renal Failure: Significant hepatic and renal failure should not increase the effects of a single intravenous dose of ISOPTIN (verapamil HCl) but may prolong its duration. Repeated injections of intravenous ISOPTIN in such patients may lead to accumulation and an excessive pharmacologic effect of the drug. There is no experience to guide use of multiple doses in such patients and this generally should be avoided. If repeated injections are essential, blood pressure and PR interval should be closely monitored and smaller repeat doses should be utilized. Verapamil cannot be removed by hemodialysis.

Premature Ventricular Contractions: During conversion to normal sinus rhythm, or marked reduction in ventricular rate, a few benign complexes of unusual appearance (sometimes resembling premature ventricular contractions) may be seen after treatment with ISOPTIN (verapamil HCl). Similar complexes are seen during spontaneous conversion of supraventricular tachycardias, after DC-cardioversion and other pharmacologic therapy. These complexes appear to have no clinical significance.

Duchenne's Muscular Dystrophy: Intravenous ISOPTIN (verapamil HCl) can precipitate respiratory muscle failure in these patients and should, therefore, be used with caution.

Increased Intracranial Pressure: Intravenous ISOPTIN (verapamil HCl) has been seen to increase intracranial pressure in patients with supratentorial tumors at the time of anesthesia induction. Caution should be taken and appropriate monitoring performed.

PRECAUTIONS

Drug Interactions: (See Warnings: Concomitant Antiarrhythmic Therapy) Intravenous ISOPTIN (verapamil HCl) has been used concomitantly with other cardioactive drugs (especially digitalis) without evidence of serious negative drug interactions. In rare instances, including when patients with severe cardiomyopathy, congestive heart failure or recent myocardial infarction were given intravenous beta-adrenergic blocking agents or disopyramide concomitantly with **intravenous** verapamil, serious adverse effects have occurred. Concomitant use of ISOPTIN with α-adrenergic blockers may result in an exaggerated hypotensive response. Such an effect was observed in one study following the concomitant administrtation of verapamil and prazosin. It may be necessary to decrease the dose of verapamil and/or dose of the neuromuscular blocking agent when the drugs are used concomitantly. As verapamil is highly bound to plasma proteins, it should be administered with caution to patients receiving other highly protein bound drugs.

OTHER

Cimetidine: The interaction between cimetidine and chronically administered verapamil has not been studied. In acute studies of healthy volunteers, clearance of verapamil was either reduced or unchanged.

Lithium: Increased sensitivity to the effects of lithium (neurotoxicity) has been reported during concomitant verapamil-lithium therapy with either no change or an increase in serum lithium levels. The addition of verapamil, however, has also resulted in the lowering of serum lithium levels in patients receiving chronic stable oral lithium. Patients receiving both drugs must be monitored carefully.

Carbamazepine: Verapamil therapy may increase carbamazepine concentrations during combined therapy. This may produce carbamazepine side effects such as diplopia, headache, ataxia, or dizziness.

Rifampin: Therapy with rifampin may markedly reduce oral verapamil bioavailability.

Phenobarbital: Phenobarbital therapy may increase verapamil clearance.

Cyclosporin: Verapamil therapy may increase serum levels of cyclosporin.

Inhalation Anesthetics: Animal experiments have shown that inhalation anesthetics depress cardiovascular activity by decreasing the inward movement of calcium ions. When used concomitantly, inhalation anesthetics and calcium antagonists (such as verapamil) should be titrated carefully to avoid excessive cardiovascular depression.

Neuromuscular Blocking Agents: Clinical data and animal studies suggest that verapamil may potentiate the activity of depolarizing and nondepolarizing neuromuscular blocking agents. It may be necessary to decrease the dose of verapamil and/or the dose of the neuromuscular blocking agent when the drugs are used concomitantly.

Dantrolene: Two animal studies suggest concomitant intravenous use of verapamil and dantrolene sodium may result in cardiovascular collapse. There has also been one report of hyperkalemia and myocardial depression following the coadministration of oral verapamil and intravenous dantrolene.

Pregnancy: Pregnancy Category C. Reproduction studies have been performed in rabbits and rats at oral verapamil doses up to 1.5 (15 mg/kg/day) and 6 (60 mg/kg/day) times the human oral daily dose, respectively, and have revealed no evidence of teratogenicity. In the rat, however, this multiple of the human dose was embryocidal and retarded fetal growth and development, probably because of adverse maternal effects reflected in reduced weight gains of the dams. This oral dose has also been shown to cause hypotension in rats. There are no adequate and well-controlled studies in pregnant women. Because animal reproduction studies are not always predictive of human response, this drug should be used during pregnancy only if clearly needed.

Labor and Delivery: There have been few controlled studies to determine whether the use of verapamil during labor or delivery has immediate or delayed adverse effects on the fetus, or whether it prolongs the duration of labor or increases the need for forceps delivery or other obstetric intervention. Such adverse experiences have not been reported in the literature, despite a long history of use of intravenous ISOPTIN in Europe in the treatment of cardiac side effects of beta-adrenergic agonist agents used to treat premature labor.

Nursing Mothers: ISOPTIN crosses the placental barrier and can be detected in umbilical vein blood at delivery. Also, ISOPTIN is excreted in human milk. Because of the potential for adverse reactions in nursing infants from verapamil, nursing should be discontinued while verapamil is administered.

Pediatrics: Controlled studies with verapamil have not been conducted in pediatric patients, but uncontrolled experience with intravenous administration in more than 250 patients, about half under 12 months of age and about 25% newborn, indicates that results of treatment are similar to those in adults. **In rare instances, however, severe hemodynamic side effects—some of them fatal—have occurred following the intravenous administration of verapamil to neonates and infants. Caution should therefore be used when administering verapamil to this group of pediatric patients.**

Suggested Treatment of Acute Cardiovascular Adverse Reactions*

The frequency of these adverse reactions was quite low and experience with their treatment has been limited.

Adverse Reaction	Proven Effective Treatment	Supportive Treatment
1. Symptomatic hypotension requiring treatment	Calcium chloride (IV) Levarterenol bitartrate (IV) Metaraminol bitartrate (IV) Isoproterenol HCl (IV) Dopamine (IV)	Intravenous fluids Trendelenburg position
2. Bradycardia, AV block, Asystole	Isoproterenol HCl (IV) Calcium chloride (IV) Cardiac pacing Levarterenol bitartrate (IV) Atropine (IV)	Intravenous fluids (slow drip)
3. Rapid ventricular rate (due to antegrade conduction in flutter/fibrillation with W-P-W or L-G-L syndromes)	DC-cardioversion (high energy may be required) Procainamide (IV) Lidocaine (IV)	Intravenous fluids (slow drip)

Actual treatment and dosage should depend on the severity of the clinical situation and the judgment and experience of the treating physician.

The most commonly used single doses in patients up to 12 months of age have ranged from 0.1 to 0.2 mg/kg of body weight, while in patients aged 1 to 15 years, the most commonly used single doses ranged from 0.1 to 0.3 mg/kg of body weight. Most of the patients received the lower dose of 0.1 mg/kg once but, in some cases, the dose was repeated once or twice every 10 to 30 minutes.

ADVERSE REACTIONS

The following reactions were reported with intravenous ISOPTIN (verapamil HCl) use in controlled U.S. clinical trials involving 324 patients:

Cardiovascular: Symptomatic hypotension (1.5%); bradycardia (1.2%); severe tachycardia (1.0%). The worldwide experience in open clinical trials in more than 7,900 patients was similar.

Central Nervous System Effects: Dizziness (1.2%); headache (1.2%). Occasional cases of seizures during verapamil injection have been reported.

Gastrointestinal: Nausea (0.9%); abdominal discomfort (0.6%).

In rare cases of hypersensitive patients, broncho/laryngeal spasm accompanied by itch and urticaria have been reported.

The following reactions have been reported at low frequency: emotional depression, rotary nystagmus, sleepiness, vertigo, muscle fatigue, diaphoresis and respiratory failure.

[See table above.]

OVERDOSAGE

Treatment of overdosage should be supportive and individualized. Beta-adrenergic stimulation and/or parenteral administration of calcium solutions may increase calcium ion flux across the slow channel, and have been effectively used in treatment of deliberate overdosage with oral ISOPTIN (verapamil HCl). Verapamil cannot be removed by hemodialysis. Clinically significant hypotensive reactions or high degree AV block should be treated with vasopressor agents or cardiac pacing, respectively. Asystole should be handled by the usual measures including isoproterenol hydrochloride, other vasopressor agents or cardiopulmonary resuscitation. (See Treatment of Cardiovascular Adverse Reactions.)

DOSAGE AND ADMINISTRATION

(For Intravenous Use Only): ISOPTIN SHOULD BE GIVEN AS A SLOW INTRAVENOUS INJECTION OVER AT LEAST A TWO MINUTE PERIOD OF TIME UNDER CONTINUOUS ELECTROCARDIOGRAPHIC AND BLOOD PRESSURE MONITORING.

The recommended intravenous doses of ISOPTIN are as follows:

ADULT: Initial dose: 5–10 mg (0.075–0.15 mg/kg body weight) given as an intravenous bolus over at least 2 minutes.

Repeat dose: 10 mg (0.15 mg/kg body weight) 30 minutes after the first dose if the initial response is not adequate. An optimal interval for subsequent I.V. doses has not been determined, and should be individualized for each patient.

Older Patients: The dose should be administered over at least 3 minutes to minimize the risk of untoward drug effects.

PEDIATRIC: Initial dose:

0–1 year: 0.1–0.2 mg/kg body weight (usual single dose range 0.75–2 mg) should be administered as an intravenous bolus over at least 2 minutes **under continuous ECG monitoring.**

1–15 years: 0.1–0.3 mg/kg body weight (usual single dose range 2–5 mg) should be administered as an intravenous bolus over at least 2 minutes. **Do not exceed 5 mg.**

Repeat dose:

0–1 year: 0.1–0.2 mg/kg body weight (usual single dose range 0.75–2 mg) 30 minutes after the first dose if the initial response is not adequate (**under continuous ECG monitoring**). An optimal interval for subsequent I.V. doses has not been determined, and should be individualized for each patient.

1–15 years: 0.1–0.3 mg/kg body weight (usual single dose range 2–5 mg) 30 minutes after the first dose if the initial response is not adequate. **Do not exceed 10 mg as a single dose.** An optimal interval for subsequent I.V. doses has not been determined, and should be individualized for each patient.

NOTE

Parenteral drug products should be inspected visually for particulate matter and discoloration prior to administration, whenever solution and container permit. ISOPTIN is physically compatible and chemically stable for at least 24 hours at 25°C protected from light in most common large volume parenteral solutions. Admixing ISOPTIN with albumin, amphotericin B, hydralazine HCl and trimethoprim with sulfamethoxazole should be avoided. ISOPTIN will precipitate in any solution with a pH above 6.0.

HOW SUPPLIED

Each 1 mL of sterile solution contains 2.5 mg verapamil HCl and 8.5 mg sodium chloride. pH adjusted with hydrochloric acid and/or sodium hydroxide.

5 mg/2 mL ampule—Space saver pack of 10 ampules—NDC 0044-1815-07

5 mg/2 mL vial—Single dose. No preservative. Individual unit carton—NDC 0044-1816-21

10 mg/4 mL ampule—Space saver pack of 10 ampules—NDC 0044-1815-17

10 mg/4 mL vial—Single dose. No preservative. Individual unit carton—NDC 0044-1816-41

Storage: 59°–86°F (15°–30°C). Protect from light.

Manufactured by Sanofi Winthrop
McPherson, Kansas 67460

IIV1502-0894

Shown in Product Identification Guide, page 319

ISOPTIN®

[ĭ-sŏp″tĭn]
(verapamil hydrochloride)
Oral Tablets

℞

DESCRIPTION

ISOPTIN (verapamil hydrochloride) is a calcium ion influx inhibitor (slow channel blocker or calcium ion antagonist). ISOPTIN is available for oral administration as round, scored, film-coated tablets containing 40 mg, 80 mg or 120 mg of verapamil hydrochloride.

The structural formula of verapamil HCl is given below:

$C_{27}H_{38}N_2O_4 \cdot HCl$ M.W. = 491.08

Benzeneacetonitrile,
α-[3-[[2-(3,4-dimethoxyphenyl) ethyl]
methylamino]
propyl]-3,4-dimethoxy-α-(1-methylethyl) hydrochloride

Verapamil HCl is an almost white, crystalline powder, practically free of odor, with a bitter taste. It is soluble in water, chloroform and methanol. Verapamil HCl is not chemically related to other cardioactive drugs.

In addition to verapamil HCl, ISOPTIN tablets may contain: colloidal silicon dioxide, corn starch, dibasic calcium phosphate, lactose, gelatin, microcrystalline cellulose, sodium carboxymethylcellulose, talc, and magnesium stearate. The film coating used for ISOPTIN 40mg, 80mg and 120mg tablets contains hydroxypropyl methylcellulose, polyethylene glycol, propylene glycol, titanium dioxide and polysorbate 80. ISOPTIN 80mg tablets also contain D&C yellow #10 Lake dye. The ISOPTIN 40mg tablet contains FD&C blue #2 Aluminum Lake dye.

CLINICAL PHARMACOLOGY

ISOPTIN is a calcium ion influx inhibitor (slow channel blocker or calcium ion antagonist) that exerts its pharmacologic effects by modulating the influx of ionic calcium across the cell membrane of the arterial smooth muscle as well as in conductile and contractile myocardial cells.

Mechanism of Action

Angina

The precise mechanism of action of ISOPTIN as an antianginal agent remains to be fully determined, but includes the following two mechanisms:

1. **Relaxation and prevention of coronary artery spasm**
   ISOPTIN dilates the main coronary arteries and coronary arterioles, both in normal and ischemic regions, and is a potent inhibitor of coronary artery spasm, whether spontaneous or ergonovine-induced. This property increases myocardial oxygen delivery in patients with coronary artery spasm, and is responsible for the effectiveness of ISOPTIN in vasospastic (Prinzmetal's or variant) as well as unstable angina at rest. Whether this effect plays any role in classical effort angina is not clear, but studies of exercise tolerance have not shown an increase in the maximum exercise rate-pressure product, a widely accepted measure of oxygen utilization. This suggests that, in general, relief of spasm or dilation of coronary arteries is not an important factor in classical angina.

2. **Reduction of oxygen utilization**
   ISOPTIN regularly reduces the total peripheral resistance (afterload) against which the heart works both at rest and at a given level of exercise by dilating peripheral arterioles. This unloading of the heart reduces myocardial energy consumption and oxygen requirements and probably accounts for the effectiveness of ISOPTIN in chronic stable effort angina.

Arrhythmia

Electrical activity through the AV node depends, to a significant degree, upon calcium influx through the slow channel. By decreasing the influx of calcium, ISOPTIN prolongs the effective refractory period within the AV node and slows AV conduction in a rate-related manner. This property accounts for the ability of ISOPTIN to slow the ventricular rate in patients with chronic atrial flutter or atrial fibrillation. Normal sinus rhythm is usually not affected, but in patients with sick sinus syndrome, ISOPTIN may interfere with sinus node impulse generation and may induce sinus arrest, or sinoatrial block. Atrioventricular block can occur in patients without preexisting conduction defects (see WARNINGS). ISOPTIN decreases the frequency of episodes of paroxysmal supraventricular tachycardia.

ISOPTIN does not alter the normal atrial action potential or intraventricular conduction time, but in depressed atrial fibers it decreases amplitude, velocity of depolarization and conduction velocity. ISOPTIN may shorten the antegrade effective refractory period of accessory bypass tracts. Acceleration of ventricular rate and/or ventricular fibrillation has been reported in patients with atrial flutter or atrial fibrillation and a coexisting accessory AV pathway following administration of verapamil (see WARNINGS).

ISOPTIN has a local anesthetic action that is 1.6 times that of procaine on an equimolar basis. It is not known whether this action is important at the doses used in man.

Essential Hypertension

ISOPTIN exerts antihypertensive effects by decreasing systemic vascular resistance usually without orthostatic decreases in blood pressure or reflex tachycardia; bradycardia (rate less than 50 beats/min) is uncommon (1.4%). During isometric or dynamic exercise ISOPTIN does not alter systolic cardiac function in patients with normal ventricular function.

ISOPTIN does not alter total serum calcium levels. However, one report suggested that calcium levels above the normal range may alter the therapeutic effect of ISOPTIN.

Pharmacokinetics and Metabolism: More than 90% of the orally administered dose of ISOPTIN is absorbed. Because of rapid biotransformation of verapamil during its first pass through the portal circulation, bioavailability ranges from 20% to 35%. Peak plasma concentrations are reached be-

Continued on next page

Knoll Laboratories—Cont.

tween 1 and 2 hours after oral administration. Chronic oral administration of 120 mg of ISOPTIN every 6 hours resulted in plasma levels of verapamil ranging from 125 to 400 ng/mL with higher values reported occasionally. A nonlinear correlation between the verapamil dose administered and verapamil plasma levels does exist.

In early dose titration with verapamil a relationship exists between verapamil plasma concentrations and the prolongation of the PR interval. However, during chronic administration this relationship may disappear. The mean elimination half-life in single dose studies ranged from 2.8 to 7.4 hours. In these same studies, after repetitive dosing, the half-life increased to a range from 4.5 to 12.0 hours (after less than 10 consecutive doses given 6 hours apart). Half-life of verapamil may increase during titration. Aging may affect the pharmacokinetics of verapamil. Elimination half-life may be prolonged in the elderly.

In healthy men, orally administered ISOPTIN undergoes extensive metabolism in the liver. Twelve metabolites have been identified in plasma; all except norverapamil are present in trace amounts only. Norverapamil can reach steady-state plasma concentrations approximately equal to those of verapamil itself. The cardiovascular activity of norverapamil appears to be approximately 20% that of verapamil. Approximately 70% of an administered dose is excreted as metabolites in the urine and 16% or more in the feces within 5 days. About 3% to 4% is excreted in the urine as unchanged drug. Approximately 90% is bound to plasma proteins. In patients with hepatic insufficiency, metabolism is delayed and elimination half-life prolonged up to 14 to 16 hours (see PRECAUTIONS); the volume of distribution is increased and plasma clearance reduced to about 30% of normal. Verapamil clearance values suggest that patients with liver dysfunction may attain therapeutic verapamil plasma concentrations with one-third of the oral daily dose required for patients with normal liver function.

After four weeks of oral dosing (120 mg q.i.d.), verapamil and norverapamil levels were noted in the cerebrospinal fluid with estimated partition coefficient of 0.06 for verapamil and 0.04 for norverapamil.

Hemodynamics and Myocardial Metabolism: ISOPTIN reduces afterload and myocardial contractility. Improved left ventricular diastolic function in patients with IHSS and those with coronary heart disease has also been observed with ISOPTIN therapy. In most patients, including those with organic cardiac disease, the negative inotropic action of ISOPTIN is countered by reduction of afterload and cardiac index is usually not reduced. However, in patients with severe left ventricular dysfunction (e.g., pulmonary wedge pressure above 20 mmHg or ejection fraction lower than 30%), or in patients on beta-adrenergic blocking agents or other cardiodepressant drugs, deterioration of ventricular function may occur (see DRUG INTERACTIONS).

Pulmonary Function: ISOPTIN does not induce bronchoconstriction and hence, does not impair ventilatory function.

INDICATIONS AND USAGE

ISOPTIN tablets are indicated for the treatment of the following:

Angina
1. Angina at rest including:
   - Vasospastic (Prinzmetal's, variant) angina
   - Unstable (crescendo, pre-infarction) angina
2. Chronic stable angina (classic effort-associated angina)

Arrhythmias
1. In association with digitalis, for the control of ventricular rate at rest and during stress in patients with chronic atrial flutter and/or atrial fibrillation (see WARNINGS: Accessory Bypass Tract)
2. Prophylaxis of repetitive paroxysmal supraventricular tachycardia

Essential Hypertension

CONTRAINDICATIONS

Verapamil HCl tablets are contraindicated in:
1. Severe left ventricular dysfunction (see WARNINGS)
2. Hypotension (systolic pressure less than 90 mmHg) or cardiogenic shock
3. Sick sinus syndrome (except in patients with a functioning artificial ventricular pacemaker)
4. Second- or third-degree AV block (except in patients with a functioning artificial ventricular pacemaker)
5. Patients with atrial flutter or atrial fibrillation and an accessory bypass tract (e.g., Wolff-Parkinson-White, Lown-Ganong-Levine syndromes) (see Warnings)
6. Patients with known hypersensitivity to verapamil hydrochloride

WARNINGS

Heart Failure: Verapamil has a negative inotropic effect which, in most patients, is compensated by its afterload reduction (decreased systemic vascular resistance) properties without a net impairment of ventricular performance. In clinical experience with 4,954 patients, 87 (1.8%) developed

congestive heart failure or pulmonary edema. Verapamil should be avoided in patients with severe left ventricular dysfunction (e.g., pulmonary wedge pressure above 20 mmHg or ejection fraction less than 30%) or moderate to severe symptoms of cardiac failure and in patients with any degree of ventricular dysfunction if they are receiving a beta adrenergic blocker (see DRUG INTERACTIONS). Patients with milder ventricular dysfunction should, if possible, be controlled with optimum doses of digitalis and/or diuretics before verapamil treatment (Note interactions with digoxin under: PRECAUTIONS).

Hypotension: Occasionally, the pharmacologic action of verapamil may produce a decrease in blood pressure below normal levels which may result in dizziness or symptomatic hypotension. The incidence of hypotension observed in 4,954 patients enrolled in clinical trials was 2.5%. In hypertensive patients, decreases in blood pressure below normal are unusual. Tilt table testing (60 degrees) was not able to induce orthostatic hypotension.

Elevated Liver Enzymes: Elevations of transaminases with and without concomitant elevations in alkaline phosphatase and bilirubin have been reported. Such elevations have sometimes been transient and may disappear even with continued verapamil treatment. Several cases of hepatocellular injury related to verapamil have been proven by rechallenge; half of these cases had clinical symptoms (malaise, fever, and/or right upper quadrant pain) in addition to elevations of SGOT, SGPT and alkaline phosphatase. Periodic monitoring of liver function in patients receiving verapamil is therefore prudent.

Accessory Bypass Tract (Wolff-Parkinson-White or Lown-Ganong-Levine): Some patients with paroxysmal and/or chronic atrial fibrillation or atrial flutter and a coexisting accessory AV pathway have developed increased antegrade conduction across the accessory pathway bypassing the AV node, producing a very rapid ventricular response or ventricular fibrillation after receiving intravenous verapamil (or digitalis). Although a risk of this occurring with oral verapamil has not been established, such patients receiving oral verapamil may be at risk and its use in these patients is contraindicated (see CONTRAINDICATIONS).

Treatment is usually DC-cardioversion. Cardioversion has been used safely and effectively after oral ISOPTIN.

Atrioventricular Block: The effect of verapamil on AV conduction and the SA node may cause asymptomatic first-degree AV block and transient bradycardia, sometimes accompanied by nodal escape rhythms. PR interval prolongation is correlated with verapamil plasma concentrations, especially during the early titration phase of therapy. Higher degrees of AV block, however, were infrequently (0.8%) observed. Marked first-degree block or progressive development to second- or third-degree AV block requires a reduction in dosage or, in rare instances, discontinuation of verapamil HCl and institution of appropriate therapy depending upon the clinical situation.

Patients with Hypertrophic Cardiomyopathy (IHSS): In 120 patients with hypertrophic cardiomyopathy (most of them refractory or intolerant to propranolol) who received therapy with verapamil at doses up to 720 mg/day, a variety of serious adverse effects were seen. Three patients died in pulmonary edema; all had severe left ventricular outflow obstruction and a past history of left ventricular dysfunction. Eight other patients had pulmonary edema and/or severe hypotension; abnormally high (greater than 20 mmHg) pulmonary wedge pressure and a marked left ventricular outflow obstruction were present in most of these patients. Concomitant administration of quinidine (See DRUG INTERACTIONS) preceded the severe hypotension in 3 of the 8 patients (2 of whom developed pulmonary edema). Sinus bradycardia occurred in 11% of the patients, second-degree AV block in 4% and sinus arrest in 2%. It must be appreciated that this group of patients had a serious disease with a high mortality rate. Most adverse effects responded well to dose reduction and only rarely did verapamil have to be discontinued.

PRECAUTIONS

General

Use in Patients with Impaired Hepatic Function: Since verapamil is highly metabolized by the liver, it should be administered cautiously to patients with impaired hepatic function. Severe liver dysfunction prolongs the elimination half-life of verapamil to about 14 to 16 hours; hence, approximately 30% of the dose given to patients with normal liver function should be administered to these patients. Careful monitoring for abnormal prolongation of the PR interval or other signs of excessive pharmacologic effects (See OVERDOSAGE) should be carried out.

Use in Patients with Attenuated (decreased) Neuromuscular Transmission: It has been reported that verapamil decreases neuromuscular transmission in patients with Duchenne's muscular dystrophy, and that verapamil prolongs recovery from the neuromuscular blocking agent vecuronium. It may be necessary to decrease the dosage of verapamil when it is administered to patients with attenuated neuromuscular transmission.

Use in Patients with Impaired Renal Function: About 70% of an administered dose of verapamil is excreted as metabolites in the urine. Verapamil is not removed by hemodialysis. Until further data are available, verapamil should be administered cautiously to patients with impaired renal function. These patients should be carefully monitored for abnormal prolongation of the PR interval or other signs of overdosage (see OVERDOSAGE).

Drug Interactions

Beta Blockers: Controlled studies in small numbers of patients suggest that the concomitant use of ISOPTIN and oral beta-adrenergic blocking agents may be beneficial in certain patients with chronic stable angina or hypertension, but available information is not sufficient to predict with confidence the effects of concurrent treatment in patients with left ventricular dysfunction or cardiac conduction abnormalities. Concomitant therapy with beta-adrenergic blockers and verapamil may result in additive negative effects on heart rate, atrioventricular conduction and/or cardiac contractility.

In one study involving 15 patients treated with high doses of propranolol (median dose: 480 mg/day, range 160 to 1280 mg/day) for severe angina, with preserved left ventricular function (ejection fraction greater than 35%), the hemodynamic effects of additional therapy with verapamil HCl were assessed using invasive methods. The addition of verapamil to high-dose beta blockers induced modest negative inotropic and chronotropic effects which were not severe enough to limit short-term (48 hours) combination therapy in this study. These modest cardiodepressant effects persisted for greater than 6, but less than 30 hours after abrupt withdrawal of beta blockers and were closely related to plasma levels of propranolol. The primary verapamil/beta-blocker interaction in this study appeared to be hemodynamic rather than electrophysiologic.

In other studies, verapamil did not generally induce significant negative inotropic, chronotropic, or dromotropic effects in patients with preserved left ventricular function receiving low or moderate doses of propranolol (less than or equal to 320 mg/day); in some patients, however, combined therapy did produce such effects. Therefore, if combined therapy is used, close surveillance of clinical status should be carried out. Combined therapy should usually be avoided in patients with atrioventricular conduction abnormalities and those with depressed left ventricular function.

Asymptomatic bradycardia (36 beats/min) with a wandering atrial pacemaker has been observed in a patient receiving concomitant timolol (a beta-adrenergic blocker) eyedrops and oral verapamil.

A decrease in metoprolol clearance has been observed when verapamil and metoprolol were administered together. A similar effect has not been seen when verapamil and atenolol were given together.

Digitalis: Clinical use of verapamil in digitalized patients has shown the combination to be well tolerated if digoxin doses are properly adjusted. However, chronic verapamil treatment can increase serum digoxin levels by 50% to 75% during the first week of therapy, and this can result in digitalis toxicity. In patients with hepatic cirrhosis the influence of verapamil on digoxin kinetics is magnified. Verapamil may reduce total body clearance and extrarenal clearance of digitoxin by 27% and 29%, respectively. Maintenance and digitalization doses should be reduced when verapamil is administered, and the patient should be reassessed to avoid over- or underdigitalization. Whenever overdigitalization is suspected, the daily dose of digitalis should be reduced or temporarily discontinued. Upon discontinuation of ISOPTIN (verapamil HCl), the patient should be reassessed to avoid underdigitalization.

Antihypertensive Agents: Verapamil administered concomitantly with oral antihypertensive agents (e.g., vasodilators, angiotensin-converting enzyme inhibitors, diuretics, beta blockers) will usually have an additive effect on lowering blood pressure. Patients receiving these combinations should be appropriately monitored. Concomitant use of agents that attenuate alpha-adrenergic function with verapamil may result in a reduction in blood pressure that is excessive in some patients. Such an effect was observed in one study following the concomitant administration of verapamil and prazosin.

Antiarrhythmic Agents

Disopyramide: Until data on possible interactions between verapamil and disopyramide are obtained, disopyramide should not be administered within 48 hours before or 24 hours after verapamil administration.

Flecainide: A study in healthy volunteers showed that the concomitant administration of flecainide and verapamil may have additive effects on myocardial contractility, AV conduction, and repolarization. Concomitant therapy with flecainide and verapamil may result in additive negative inotropic effect and prolongation of atrioventricular conduction.

Quinidine: In a small number of patients with hypertrophic cardiomyopathy (IHSS), concomitant use of verapamil and quinidine resulted in significant hypotension. Until further data are obtained, combined therapy of verapamil and quini-

dine in patients with hypertrophic cardiomyopathy should probably be avoided.

The electrophysiological effects of quinidine and verapamil on AV conduction were studied in 8 patients. Verapamil significantly counteracted the effects of quinidine on AV conduction. There has been a report of increased quinidine levels during verapamil therapy.

Other

Nitrates: Verapamil has been given concomitantly with short- and long-acting nitrates without any undesirable drug interactions. The pharmacologic profile of both drugs and the clinical experience suggest beneficial interactions.

Cimetidine: The interaction between cimetidine and chronically administered verapamil has not been studied. Variable results on clearance have been obtained in acute studies of healthy volunteers; clearance of verapamil was either reduced or unchanged.

Lithium: Pharmacokinetic and pharmacodynamic interactions between oral verapamil and lithium have been reported. The former may result in a lowering of serum lithium levels in patients receiving chronic stable oral lithium therapy. The latter may result in an increased sensitivity to the effects of lithium. Patients receiving both drugs must be monitored carefully.

Carbamazepine: Verapamil therapy may increase carbamazepine concentrations during combined therapy. This may produce carbamazepine side effects such as diplopia, headache, ataxia, or dizziness.

Rifampin: Therapy with rifampin may markedly reduce oral verapamil bioavailability.

Phenobarbital: Phenobarbital therapy may increase verapamil clearance.

Cyclosporin: Verapamil therapy may increase serum levels of cyclosporin.

Inhalation Anesthetics: Animal experiments have shown that inhalation anesthetics depress cardiovascular activity by decreasing the inward movement of calcium ions. When used concomitantly, inhalation anesthetics and calcium antagonists, such as verapamil, should each be titrated carefully to avoid excessive cardiovascular depression.

Neuromuscular Blocking Agents: Clinical data and animal studies suggest that verapamil may potentiate the activity of neuromuscular blocking agents (curare-like and depolarizing). It may be necessary to decrease the dose of verapamil and/or the dose of the neuromuscular blocking agent when the drugs are used concomitantly.

Carcinogenesis, Mutagenesis, Impairment of Fertility: An 18-month toxicity study in rats, at a low multiple (6 fold) of the maximum recommended human dose, and not the maximum tolerated dose, did not suggest a tumorigenic potential. There was no evidence of a carcinogenic potential of verapamil administered in the diet of rats for two years at doses of 10, 35 and 120 mg/kg per day or approximately 1x, 3.5x and 12x, respectively, the maximum recommended human daily dose (480 mg per day or 9.6 mg/kg/day).

Verapamil was not mutagenic in the Ames test in 5 test strains at 3 mg per plate, with or without metabolic activation.

Studies in female rats at daily dietary doses up to 5.5 times (55 mg/kg/day) the maximum recommended human dose did not show impaired fertility. Effects on male fertility have not been determined.

Pregnancy: Pregnancy Category C. Reproduction studies have been performed in rabbits and rats at oral doses up to 1.5 (15 mg/kg/day) and 6 (60 mg/kg/day) times the human oral daily dose, respectively, and have revealed no evidence of teratogenicity. In the rat, however, this multiple of the human dose was embryocidal and retarded fetal growth and development, probably because of adverse maternal effects reflected in the reduced weight gains of the dams. This oral dose has also been shown to cause hypotension in rats. There are no adequate and well-controlled studies in pregnant women. Because animal reproduction studies are not always predictive of human response, this drug should be used during pregnancy only if clearly needed.

Verapamil crosses the placental barrier and can be detected in umbilical vein blood at delivery.

Labor and Delivery: It is not known whether the use of verapamil during labor or delivery has immediate or delayed adverse effects on the fetus, or whether it prolongs the duration of labor or increases the need for forceps delivery or other obstetric intervention. Such adverse experiences have not been reported in the literature, despite a long history of use of verapamil in Europe in the treatment of cardiac side effects of beta-adrenergic agonist agents used to treat premature labor.

Nursing Mothers: Verapamil is excreted in human milk. Because of the potential for adverse reactions in nursing infants from verapamil, nursing should be discontinued while verapamil is administered.

Pediatric Use: Safety and efficacy of ISOPTIN in children below the age of 18 years have not been established.

Animal Pharmacology and/or Animal Toxicology: In chronic animal toxicology studies verapamil caused lenticular and/or suture line changes at 30 mg/kg/day or greater and frank cataracts at 62.5 mg/kg/day or greater in the beagle dog but not the rat. Development of cataracts due to verapamil has not been reported in man.

ADVERSE REACTIONS

Serious adverse reactions are uncommon when ISOPTIN therapy is initiated with upward dose titration within the recommended single and total daily dose. See WARNINGS for discussion of heart failure, hypotension, elevated liver enzymes, AV block and rapid ventricular response. The following reactions to orally administered verapamil occurred at rates greater than 1.0% or occurred at lower rates but appeared clearly drug-related in clinical trials in 4,954 patients.

Constipation	7.3%	Fatigue	1.7%
Dizziness	3.3%	Dyspnea	1.4%
Nausea	2.7%	Bradycardia (HR < 50/min)	1.4%
Hypotension	2.5%	AV block— total 1°, 2°, 3°	1.2%
Headache	2.2%	2° and 3°	0.8%
Edema	1.9%	Rash	1.2%
CHF, Pulmonary Edema	1.8%	Flushing	0.6%

Elevated Liver Enzymes (see WARNINGS)

In clinical trials related to the control of ventricular response in digitalized patients who had atrial fibrillation or flutter, ventricular rate below 50 at rest occurred in 15% of patients and asymptomatic hypotension occurred in 5% of patients.

The following reactions, reported in 1.0% or less of patients, occurred under conditions (open trials, marketing experience) where a causal relationship is uncertain; they are listed to alert the physician to a possible relationship:

Cardiovascular: angina pectoris, atrioventricular dissociation, chest pain, claudication, myocardial infarction, palpitations, purpura (vasculitis), syncope.

Digestive System: diarrhea, dry mouth, gastrointestinal distress, gingival hyperplasia.

Hemic and Lymphatic: ecchymosis or bruising.

Nervous System: cerebrovascular accident, confusion, equilibrium disorders, insomnia, muscle cramps, paresthesia, psychotic symptoms, shakiness, somnolence.

Skin: arthralgia and rash, exanthema, hair loss, hyperkeratosis, maculae, sweating, urticaria, Stevens-Johnson syndrome, erythema multiforme.

Special Senses: blurred vision.

Urogenital: gynecomastia, increased urination, spotty menstruation, impotence.

Treatment of Acute Cardiovascular Adverse Reactions: The frequency of cardiovascular adverse reactions which require therapy is rare; hence, experience with their treatment is limited. Whenever severe hypotension or complete AV block occur following oral administration of verapamil, the appropriate emergency measures should be applied immediately, e.g., intravenously administered norepinephrine bitartrate, atropine sulfate, isoproterenol HCl (all in the usual doses), or calcium gluconate (10% solution). In patients with hypertrophic cardiomyopathy (IHSS), alpha-adrenergic agents (phenylephrine HCl, metaraminol bitartrate or methoxamine HCl) should be used to maintain blood pressure, and isoproterenol and norepinephrine should be avoided. If further support is necessary, dopamine HCl or dobutamine HCl may be administered. Actual treatment and dosage should depend on the severity and the clinical situation and the judgment and experience of the treating physician.

OVERDOSAGE

Treatment of overdosage should be supportive. Beta-adrenergic stimulation or parenteral administration of calcium solutions may increase calcium ion flux across the slow channel, and have been used effectively in treatment of deliberate overdosage with verapamil. Verapamil cannot be removed by hemodialysis. Clinically significant hypotensive reactions or fixed high degree AV block should be treated with vasopressor agents or cardiac pacing, respectively. Asystole should be handled by the usual measures including cardiopulmonary resuscitation.

DOSAGE AND ADMINISTRATION

The dose of verapamil must be individualized by titration. ISOPTIN is available in 40 mg, 80 mg, and 120 mg tablets. The usefulness and safety of dosages exceeding 480 mg/day have not been established; therefore, this daily dosage should not be exceeded. Since the half-life of verapamil increases during chronic dosing, maximum response may be delayed.

Angina: Clinical trials show that the usual dose is 80 mg to 120 mg three times a day. However, 40 mg three times a day may be warranted in patients who may have an increased response to verapamil (e.g., decreased hepatic function, elderly, etc.). Upward titration should be based on therapeutic efficacy and safety evaluated approximately eight hours after dosing. Dosage may be increased at daily (e.g., patients with unstable angina) or weekly intervals until optimum clinical response is obtained.

Arrhythmias: The dosage in digitalized patients with chronic atrial fibrillation (see PRECAUTIONS) ranges from 240 to 320 mg per day in divided (t.i.d. or q.i.d.) doses. The dosage for prophylaxis of PSVT (non-digitalized patients) ranges from 240 to 480 mg in divided (t.i.d. or q.i.d.) doses. In general, maximum effects for any given dosage will be apparent during the first 48 hours of therapy.

Essential Hypertension: Dose should be individualized by titration. The usual initial monotherapy dose in clinical trials was 80 mg three times a day (240 mg). Daily dosages of 360 and 480 mg have been used but there is no evidence that doses beyond 360 mg provide added effect. Consideration should be given to beginning titration at 40 mg, three times per day in patients who might respond to lower doses, such as the elderly or people of small stature. The antihypertensive effects of ISOPTIN are evident within the first week of therapy. Upward titration should be based on therapeutic efficacy, assessed at the end of the dosing interval.

HOW SUPPLIED

ISOPTIN (verapamil HCl) tablets are supplied as round, scored, film-coated tablets containing either 40 mg, 80 mg or 120 mg of verapamil hydrochloride. The 80 mg and 120 mg tablets are embossed with "ISOPTIN 80" or "ISOPTIN 120" on one side and "Knoll" on the reverse side. The 40 mg tablet is embossed on one side with the number "40" surrounded by the Knoll triangle.

40 mg (lt. blue)—
- Bottle of 100—NDC #0044-1821-02
- Hospital Unit Dose (100 tablets-Strips of 10)—NDC #0044-1821-10

80 mg (yellow)—
- Bottle of 100—NDC #0044-1822-02
- Bottle of 500—NDC #0044-1822-05
- Bottle of 1000—NDC #0044-1822-04
- Hospital Unit Dose (100 tablets—Strips of 10)—NDC #0044-1822-10

120 mg (white)—
- Bottle of 100—NDC #0044-1823-02
- Bottle of 500—NDC #0044-1823-05
- Bottle of 1000—NDC #0044-1823-04
- Hospital Unit Dose (100 tablets—Strips of 10)—NDC #0044-1823-10

Storage: 59° to 86°F (15° to 30°C).

Dispense in a tight, light-resistant container as defined in the USP.

MR 1988/ 2636

Revised September 1988 2659

Shown in Product Identification Guide, page 319

ISOPTIN® SR ℞
(verapamil HCl)
Sustained Release Oral Tablets

DESCRIPTION

ISOPTIN SR (verapamil hydrochloride) is a calcium ion influx inhibitor (slow channel blocker or calcium ion antagonist). ISOPTIN SR is available for oral administration as light green, capsule shaped, scored, film-coated tablets containing 240 mg verapamil hydrochloride, as light pink, oval shaped, scored, film-coated containing 180 mg verapamil hydrochloride, and as light violet, oval shaped, film-coated tablets containing 120 mg verapamil hydrochloride. The tablets are designed for sustained release of the drug in the gastrointestinal tract; sustained release characteristics are not altered when the tablet is divided in half.

The structural formula of verapamil HCl is given below:

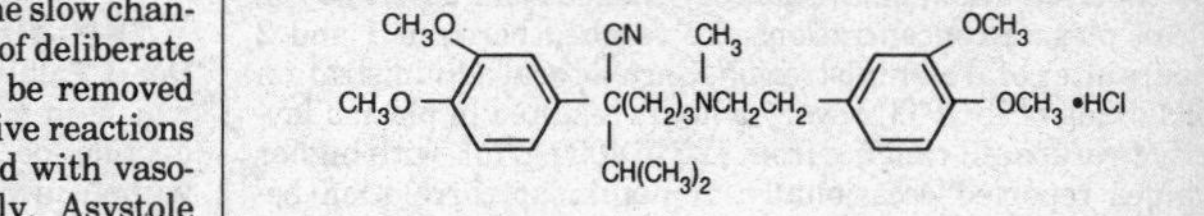

CH3O
CN
CH3
OCH3
CH3O
C(CH2)3NCH2CH2
OCH3 •HCl
CH(CH3)2

$C_{27}H_{38}N_2O_4 \cdot HCl$ M.W. = 491.08

Benzeneacetonitrile,
α-[3-[[2-(3,4-dimethoxyphenyl) ethyl] methylamino]
propyl]-3,4-dimethoxy-α-(1-methylethyl) hydrochloride

Verapamil HCl is an almost white, crystalline powder, practically free of odor, with a bitter taste. It is soluble in water, chloroform and methanol. Verapamil HCL is not chemically related to other cardioactive drugs.

In addition to verapamil HCl, the ISOPTIN SR tablet contains the following ingredients: alginate, hydroxypropyl methylcellulose, magnesium stearate, microcrystalline cellulose, polyethylene glycol, polyvinyl pyrrolidone, talc, and titanium dioxide. The following are the color additives per tablet strength:

Strength (mg)	Color Additive(s)
120	Iron Oxide
180	Iron Oxide
240	D&C yellow #10 Lake dye, and FD&C blue #2 Lake dye

Continued on next page

Knoll Laboratories—Cont.

CLINICAL PHARMACOLOGY

ISOPTIN is a calcium ion influx inhibitor (slow channel blocker or calcium ion antagonist) which exerts its pharmacologic effects by modulating the influx of ionic calcium across the cell membrane of the arterial smooth muscle as well as in conductile and contractile myocardial cells.

Mechanism of Action
Essential Hypertension

ISOPTIN exerts antihypertensive effects by decreasing systemic vascular resistance, usually without orthostatic decreases in blood pressure or reflex tachycardia; bradycardia (rate less than 50 beats/min) is uncommon (1.4%). During isometric or dynamic exercise ISOPTIN does not alter systolic cardiac function in patients with normal ventricular function. ISOPTIN does not alter total serum calcium levels. However, one report suggested that calcium levels above the normal range may alter the therapeutic effect of ISOPTIN.

Other Pharmacologic Acts of ISOPTIN include the Following

ISOPTIN (verapamil HCl) dilates the main coronary arteries and coronary arterioles, both in normal and ischemic regions, and is a potent inhibitor of coronary artery spasm, whether spontaneous or ergonovine-induced. This property increases myocardial oxygen delivery in patients with coronary artery spasm and is responsible for the effectiveness of ISOPTIN in vasospastic (Prinzmetal's or variant) as well as unstable angina at rest. Whether this effect plays any role in classical effort angina is not clear, but studies of exercise tolerance have not shown an increase in the maximum exercise rate-pressure product, a widely accepted measure of oxygen utilization. This suggests that, in general, relief of spasm of dilation of coronary arteries is not an important factor in classical angina.

ISOPTIN regularly reduces the total systemic resistance (afterload) against which the heart works both at rest and at a given level of exercise by dilating peripheral arterioles. Electrical activity through the AV node depends, to a significant degree, upon calcium influx through the slow channel. By decreasing the influx of calcium, ISOPTIN prolongs the effective refractory period within the AV node and slows AV conduction in a rate-related manner.

Normal sinus rhythm is usually not affected, but in patients with sick sinus syndrome, ISOPTIN may interfere with sinus node impulse generation and may induce sinus arrest or sinoatrial block. Atrioventricular block can occur in patients without preexisting conduction defects (see WARNINGS). ISOPTIN does not alter the normal atrial action potential or intraventricular conduction time, but depresses amplitude, velocity of depolarization and conduction in depressed atrial fibers. ISOPTIN may shorten the antegrade effective refractory period of accessory bypass tracts. Acceleration of ventricular rate and/or ventricular fibrillation has been reported in patients with atrial flutter or atrial fibrillation and a coexisting accessory AV pathway following administration of verapamil (see WARNINGS).

ISOPTIN has a local anesthetic action that is 1.6 times that of procaine on an equimolar basis. It is not known whether this action is important at the doses used in man.

Pharmacokinetics and Metabolism: With the immediate release formulation, more than 90% of the orally administered dose of ISOPTIN is absorbed. Because of rapid biotransformation of verapamil during its first pass through the portal circulation, bioavailability ranges from 20% to 35%. Peak plasma concentrations are reached between 1 and 2 hours after oral administration. Chronic oral administration of 120 mg of ISOPTIN every 6 hours resulted in plasma levels of verapamil ranging from 125 to 400 ng/mL with higher values reported occasionally. A nonlinear correlation between the verapamil dose administered and verapamil plasma levels does exist. No relationship has been established between the plasma concentration of verapamil and a reduction in blood pressure.

In early dose titration with verapamil a relationship exists between verapamil plasma concentrations and the prolongation of the PR interval. However, during chronic administration this relationship may disappear. The mean elimination half-life in single dose studies ranged from 2.8 to 7.4 hours. In these same studies, after repetitive dosing, the half-life increased to a range from 4.5 to 12.0 hours (after less than 10 consecutive doses given 6 hours apart). Half-life of verapamil may increase during titration.

Aging may affect the pharmacokinetics of verapamil. Elimination half-life may be prolonged in the elderly.

In multiple dose studies under fasting conditions the bioavailability measured by AUC of ISOPTIN SR was similar to ISOPTIN immediate release; rates of absorption were, of course, different. In a randomized, single-dose, crossover study using healthy volunteers, administration of 240 mg ISOPTIN SR with food produced peak plasma verapamil concentrations of 79 ng/mL, time to peak plasma verapamil concentrations of 7.71 hours, and AUC (0-24 hr) of 841 ng-hr/mL. When ISOPTIN SR was administered to fasting sub-

jects, peak plasma verapamil concentrations was 164 ng/mL; time to peak plasma verapamil concentrations was 5.21 hours; and AUC (0-24 hr) was 1,478 ng-hr/mL. Similar results were demonstrated for plasma norverapamil. Food thus produces decreased bioavailability (AUC) but a narrower peak to trough ratio. Good correlation of dose and response is not available, but controlled studies of ISOPTIN SR have shown effectiveness of doses similar to the effective doses of ISOPTIN (immediate release).

In healthy man, orally administered ISOPTIN undergoes extensive metabolism in the liver. Twelve metabolites have been identified in plasma; all except norverapamil are present in trace amounts only. Norverapamil can reach steady-state plasma concentrations approximately equal to those of verapamil itself. The cardiovascular activity of norverapamil appears to be approximately 20% that of verapamil. Approximately 70% of an administered dose is excreted as metabolites in the urine and 16% or more in the feces within 5 days. About 3% to 4% is excreted in the urine as unchanged drug. Approximately 90% is bound to plasma proteins. In patients with hepatic insufficiency, metabolism of immediate release verapamil is delayed and elimination half-life prolonged up to 14 to 16 hours (see PRECAUTIONS); the volume of distribution is increased and plasma clearance reduced to about 30% of normal. Verapamil clearance values suggest that patients with liver dysfunction may attain therapeutic verapamil plasma concentrations with one-third of the oral daily dose required for patients with normal liver function.

After four weeks of oral dosing (120 mg q.i.d.), verapamil and norverapamil levels were noted in the cerebrospinal fluid with estimated partition coefficient of 0.06 for verapamil and 0.04 for norverapamil.

Hemodynamics and Myocardial Metabolism: ISOPTIN reduces afterload and myocardial contractility. Improved left ventricular diastolic function in patients with IHSS and those with coronary heart disease has also been observed with ISOPTIN therapy. In most patients, including those with organic cardiac disease, the negative inotropic action of ISOPTIN is countered by reduction of afterload and cardiac index is usually not reduced. In patients with severe left ventricular dysfunction however, (e.g., pulmonary wedge pressure above 20 mmHg or ejection fraction lower than 30%), or in patients on beta-adrenergic blocking agents or other cardiodepressant drugs, deterioration of ventricular function may occur (see DRUG INTERACTIONS).

Pulmonary Function: ISOPTIN does not induce bronchoconstriction and hence, does not impair ventilatory function.

INDICATIONS AND USAGE

ISOPTIN SR (verapamil HCl) is indicated for the management of essential hypertension.

CONTRAINDICATIONS

Verapamil HCl is contraindicated in:
1. Severe left ventricular dysfunction (see WARNINGS)
2. Hypotension (less than 90 mmHg systolic pressure) or cardiogenic shock
3. Sick sinus syndrome (except in patients with a functioning artificial ventricular pacemaker)
4. Second- or third-degree AV block (except patients with a functioning artificial ventricular pacemaker).
5. Patients with atrial flutter or atrial fibrillation and an accessory bypass tract (e.g., Wolff-Parkinson-White, Lown-Ganong-Levine syndromes). (see WARNINGS).
6. Patients with known hypersensitivity to verapamil hydrochloride.

WARNINGS

Heart Failure: Verapamil has a negative inotropic effect which, in most patients, is compensated by its afterload reduction (decreased systemic vascular resistance) properties without a net impairment of ventricular performance. In clinical experience with 4,954 patients, 87 (1.8%) developed congestive heart failure or pulmonary edema. Verapamil should be avoided in patients with severe left ventricular dysfunction (e.g., ejection fraction less than 30%, pulmonary wedge pressure above 20mm Hg, or severe symptoms of cardiac failure) and in patients with any degree of ventricular dysfunction if they are receiving a beta adrenergic blocker (see DRUG INTERACTIONS). Patients with milder ventricular dysfunction should, if possible, be controlled with optimum doses of digitalis and/or diuretics before verapamil treatment (Note interactions with digoxin under: PRECAUTIONS).

Hypotension: Occasionally, the pharmacologic action of verapamil may produce a decrease in blood pressure below normal levels which may result in dizziness or symptomatic hypotension. The incidence of hypotension observed in 4,954 patients enrolled in clinical trials was 2.5%. In hypertensive patients, decreases in blood pressure below normal are unusual. Tilt table testing (60 degrees) was not able to induce orthostatic hypotension.

Elevated Liver Enzymes: Elevations of transaminases with and without concomitant elevations in alkaline phosphatase and bilirubin have been reported. Such elevations has sometimes been transient and may disappear even in the face of

continued verapamil treatment. Several cases of hepatocellular injury related to verapamil have been proven by rechallenge: half of these had clinical symptoms (malaise, fever, and/or right upper quadrant pain) in addition to elevations of SGOT, SGPT and alkaline phosphatase. Periodic monitoring of liver function in patients receiving verapamil is therefore prudent.

Accessory Bypass Tract (Wolff-Parkinson-White or Lown-Ganong-Levine): Some patients with paroxysmal and/or chronic atrial fibrillation or atrial flutter and a coexisting accessory AV pathway have developed increased antegrade conduction across the accessory pathway bypassing the AV node, producing a very rapid ventricular response or ventricular fibrillation after receiving intravenous verapamil (or digitalis). Although a risk of this occurring with oral verapamil has not been established, such patients receiving oral verapamil may be at risk and its use in these patients is contraindicated (see CONTRAINDICATIONS).

Treatment is usually DC-cardioversion. Cardioversion has been used safely and effectively after oral ISOPTIN.

Atrioventricular Block: The effect of verapamil on AV conduction and the DA node may lead to asymptomtic first-degree AV block and transient bradycardia, sometimes accompanied by nodal escape rhythms. PR interval prolongation is correlated with verapamil plasma concentrations, especially during the early titration phases of therapy. Higher degrees of AV block, however, were infrequently (0.8%) observed. Marked first-degree block or progressive development to second- or third-degree AV block requires a reduction in dosage or, in rare instances, discontinuation of verapamil HCl and institution of appropriate therapy depending upon the clinical situation.

Patients with Hypertrophic Cardiomyopathy (IHSS): In 120 patients with hypertrophic cardiomyopathy (most of them refractory or intolerant to propranolol) who received therapy with verapamil at doses up to 720 mg/day, a variety of serious adverse effects were seen. Three patients died in pulmonary edema; all had severe left ventricular outflow obstruction and a past history of left ventricular dysfunction. Eight other patients had pulmonary edema and/or severe hypotension; abnormally high (over 20 mmHg) capillary wedge pressure and a marked left ventricular outflow obstruction were present in most of these patients. Concomitant administration of quinidine (see DRUG INTERACTIONS) preceded the severe hypotension in 3 of the 8 patients (2 of whom developed pulmonary edema). Sinus bradycardia occurred in 11% of the patients, second-degree AV block in 4% and sinus arrest in 2%. It must be appreciated that this group of patients had a serious disease with a high mortality rate. Most adverse effects responded well to dose reduction and only rarely did verapamil have to be discontinued.

PRECAUTIONS

General

Use in Patients with Impaired Hepatic Functions: Since verapamil is highly metabolized by the liver, it should be administered cautiously to patients with impaired hepatic function. Severe liver dysfunction prolongs the elimination half-life of immediate release verapamil to about 14 to 16 hours; hence, approximately 30% of the dose given to patients with normal liver function should be administered to these patients. Careful monitoring for abnormal prolongation of the PR interval or other signs of excessive pharmacologic effects (see OVERDOSAGE) should be carried out.

Use in Patients with Attenuated (Decreased) Neuromuscular Transmission: It has been reported that verapamil decreases neuromuscular transmission in patients with Duchenne's muscular dystrophy, and that verapamil prolongs recovery from the neuromuscular blocking agent vecuronium. It may be necessary to decrease the dosage of verapamil when it is administered to patients with attenuated neuromuscular transmission.

Use in Patients with Impaired Renal Function: About 70% of an administered dose of verapamil is excreted as metabolites in the urine. Verapamil is not removed by hemodialysis. Until further data are available, verapamil should be administered cautiously to patients with impaired renal function. These patients should be carefully monitored for abnormal prolongation of the PR interval or other signs of overdosage (see OVERDOSAGE).

Drug Interactions

Beta Blockers: Concomitant therapy with beta-adrenergic blockers and verapamil may result in additive negative effects on heart rate, atrioventricular conduction, and/or cardiac contractility. The combination of sustained-release verapamil and beta-adrenergic blocking agents has not been studied. However, there have been reports of excessive bradycardia and AV block, including complete heart block, when the combination has been used for the treatment of hypertension. For hypertensive patients, the risks of combined therapy may outweigh the potential benefits. The combination should be used only with caution and close monitoring.

Asymptomatic bradycardia (36 beats/min) with an wandering atrial pacemaker has been observed in a patient receiv-

ing concomitant timolol (a beta-adrenergic blocker) eyedrops and oral verapamil.

A decrease in metoprolol and propranolol clearance has been observed when either drug is administered concomitantly with verapamil. A variable effect has been seen when verapamil and atenolol were given together.

Digitalis: Clinical use of verapamil in digitalized patients has shown the combination to be well tolerated if digoxin doses are properly adjusted. Chronic verapamil treatment can increase serum digoxin levels by 50 to 75% during the first week of therapy, and this can result in digitalis toxicity. In patients with hepatic cirrhosis the influence of verapamil on digoxin kinetics is magnified. Verapamil may reduce total body clearance and extrarenal clearance of digitoxin by 27% and 29%, respectively. Maintenance digitalis doses should be reduced when verapamil is administered, and the patient should be carefully monitored to avoid over- or underdigitalization. Whenever overdigitalization is suspected, the daily dose of digitalis should be reduced or temporarily discontinued. Upon discontinuation of ISOPTIN (verapamil HCl), the patient should be reassessed to avoid underdigitalization.

Antihypertensive Agents: Verapamil administered concomitantly with oral antihypertensive agents (e.g., vasodilators, angiotensin-converting enzyme inhibitors, diuretics, beta blockers) will usually have an additive effect on lowering blood pressure. Patients receiving these combinations should be appropriately monitored. Concomitant use of agents that attenuate alpha-adrenergic function with verapamil may result in a reduction in blood pressure that is excessive in some patients. Such an effect was observed in one study following the concomitant administration of verapamil and prazosin.

Antiarrhythmic Agents

Disopyramide: Until data on possible interactions between verapamil and disopyramide phosphate are obtained, disopyramide should not be administered within 48 hours before or 24 hours after verapamil administration.

Flecainide: A study of healthy volunteers showed that the concomitant administration of flecainide and verapamil may have additive effects on myocardial contractility, AV conduction, and repolarization. Concomitant therapy with flecainide and verapamil may result in additive negative inotropic effect and prolongation of atrioventricular conduction.

Quinidine: In a small number of patients with hypertrophic cardiomyopathy (IHSS), concomitant use of verapamil and quinidine resulted in significant hypotension. Until further data are obtained, combined therapy of verapamil and quinidine in patients with hypertrophic cardiomyopathy should probably be avoided.

The electrophysiological effects of quinidine and verapamil on AV conduction were studied in 8 patients. Verapamil significantly counteracted the effects of quinidine on AV conduction. There has been a report of increased quinidine levels during verapamil therapy.

Nitrates: Verapamil has been given concomitantly with short- and long-acting nitrates without any undesirable drug interactions. The pharmacologic profile of both drugs and the clinical experience suggest beneficial interactions.

Other

Cimetidine: The interaction between cimetidine and chronically administered verapamil has not been studied. Variable results on clearance have been obtained in acute studies of healthy volunteers; clearance of verapamil was either reduced or unchanged.

Lithium: Increased sensitivity to the effects of lithium (neurotoxicity) has been reported during concomitant verapamil-lithium therapy with either no change or an increase in serum lithium levels. However, the addition of verapamil has also resulted in the lowering of serum lithium levels in patients receiving chronic stable oral lithium. Patients receiving both drugs must be monitored carefully.

Carbamazepine: Verapamil therapy may increase carbamazepine concentrations during combined therapy. This may produce carbamazepine side effects such as diplopia, headache, ataxia, or dizziness.

Rifampin: Therapy with rifampin may markedly reduce oral verapamil bioavailability.

Phenobarbital: Phenobarbital therapy may increase verapamil clearance.

Cyclosporin: Verapamil therapy may increase serum levels of cyclosporin.

Theophylline: Verapamil may inhibit the clearance and increase the plasma levels of theophylline.

Inhalation Anesthetics: Animal experiments have shown that inhalation anesthetics depress cardiovascular activity by decreasing the inward movement of calcium ions. When used concomitantly, inhalation anesthetics and calcium antagonists, such as verapamil, should be titrated carefully to avoid excessive cardiovascular depression.

Neuromuscular Blocking Agents: Clinical data and animal studies suggest that verapamil may potentiate the activity of neuromuscular blocking agents (curare-like and depolarization). It may be necessary to decrease the dose of verapamil and/or the dose of the neuromuscular blocking agent when the drugs are used concomitantly.

Carcinogenesis, Mutagenesis, Impairment of Fertility: An 18-month toxicity study in rats, at a low multiple (6 fold) of the maximum recommended human dose, and not the maximum tolerated dose, did not suggest a tumorigenic potential. There was no evidence of a carcinogenic potential of verapamil administered in the diet of rats for two years at doses of 10, 35, and 120 mg/kg per day or approximately 1x, 3.5x, and 12x, respectively, the maximum recommended human daily dose (480 mg per day or 9.6 mg/kg/day).

Verapamil was not mutagenic in the Ames test in 5 test strains at 3 mg per plate, with or without metabolic activation.

Studies in female rats at daily dietary doses up to 5.5 times (55 mg/kg/day) the maximum recommended human doses did not show impaired fertility. Effects on male fertility have not been determined.

Pregnancy: Pregnancy Category C. Reproduction studies have been performed in rabbits and rats at oral doses up to 1.5 (15 mg/kg/day) and 6 (60 mg/kg/day) times the human oral daily dose, respectively, and have revealed no evidence of teratogenicity. In the rat, however, this multiple of the human dose was embryocidal and retarded fetal growth and development, probably because of adverse maternal effects reflected in the reduced weight gains of the dams. This oral dose has also been shown to cause hypotension in rats. There are no adequate and well-controlled studies in pregnant women. Because animal reproduction studies are not always predictive of human response, this drug should be used during pregnancy only if clearly needed. ISOPTIN (verapamil HCl) crosses the placental barrier and can be detected in umbilical vein blood at delivery.

Labor and Delivery: It is not known whether the use of verapamil during labor or delivery has immediate or delayed adverse effects on the fetus, or whether it prolongs the duration of labor or increases the need for forceps delivery or other obstetric intervention. Such adverse experiences have not been reported in the literature, despite a long history of use of ISOPTIN in Europe in the treatment of cardiac side effects of beta-adrenergic agonist agents used to treat premature labor.

Nursing Mothers: ISOPTIN is excreted in human milk. Because of the potential for adverse reactions in nursing infants for verapamil, nursing should be discontinued while verapamil is administered.

Pediatric Use: Safety and efficacy of ISOPTIN in children below the age of 18 years have not been established.

Animal Pharmacology and/or Animal Toxicology: In chronic animal toxicology studies verapamil caused lenticular and/or suture line changes at 30 mg/kg/day or greater and frank cataracts at 62.5 mg/kg/day or greater in the beagle dog but not the rat. Development of cataracts due to verapamil has not been reported in man.

ADVERSE REACTIONS

Serious adverse reactions are uncommon when ISOPTIN (verapamil HCl) therapy is initiated with upward dose titration within the recommended single and total daily dose. See WARNINGS for discussion of heart failure, hypotension, elevated liver enzymes, AV block, and rapid ventricular response. Reversible (upon discontinuation of verapamil) non-obstructive, paralytic, ileus has been infrequently reported in association with he use of verapamil. The following reactions to orally administered ISOPTIN occurred at rates greater than 1.0% or occurred at lower rates but appeared clearly drug-related in clinical trials in 4,954 patients.

Constipation	7.3%
Dizziness	3.3%
Nausea	2.7%
Hypotension	2.5%
Headache	2.2%
Edema	1.9%
CHF/Pulmonary Edema	1.8%
Fatigue	1.7%
Dyspnea	1.4%
Bradycardia (HR <50/min)	1.4%
AV Block-total 1°, 2°, 3°	1.2%
2° and 3°	0.8%
Rash	1.2%
Flushing	0.6%
Elevated Liver Enzymes (see WARNINGS)	

In clinical trials related to the control of ventricular response in digitalized patients who had atrial fibrillation or atrial flutter, ventricular rates below 50/min at rest occurred in 15% of patients and asymptomatic hypotension occurred in 5% of patients.

The following reactions, reported in 1.0% or less of patients, occurred under conditions (open trials, marketing experience) where a causal relationship is uncertain; they are listed to alert the physician to a possible relationship:

Cardiovascular: angina pectoris, atrioventricular dissociation, chest pain, claudication, myocardial infarction, palpitations, purpura (vasculitis), syncope.

Digestive System: diarrhea, dry mouth, gastrointestinal distress, gingival hyperplasia.

Hemic and Lymphatic: ecchymosis or bruising.

Nervous System: cerebrovascular accident, confusion, equilibrium disorders, insomnia, muscle cramps, paresthesia, psychotic symptoms, shakiness, somnolence.

Skin: arthralgia and rash, exanthema, hair loss, hyperkeratosis, maculae, sweating, urticaria, Stevens-Johnson syndrome, erythema multiforme.

Special Senses: blurred vision.

Urogenital: gynecomastia, impotence, galactorrhea/hyperprolactinemia, increased urination, spotty menstruation.

Treatment of Acute Cardiovascular Adverse Reactions: The frequency of cardiovascular adverse reactions which require therapy is rare, hence, experience with their treatment is limited. Whenever severe hypotension or complete AV block occur following oral administration of verapamil, the appropriate emergency measures should be applied immediately, e.g., intravenously administered isoproterenol HCl, levarterenol bitartrate, atropine (all in the usual dose), or calcium gluconate (10% solution). In patients with hypertrophic cardiomyopathy (IHSS), alpha-adrenergic agents (phenylephrine, metaraminol bitartrate or methoxamine) should be used to maintain blood pressure, and isoproterenol and levarterenol should be avoided. If further support is necessary, inotropic agents (dopamine or dobutamine) may be administered. Actual treatment and dosage should depend on the severity and the clinical situation and the judgment and experience of the treating physician.

OVERDOSAGE

Treat all verapamil overdoses as serious and maintain observation for at least 48 hours (especially Isoptin SR), preferably under continuous hospital care. Delayed pharmacodynamic consequences may occur with the sustained released formulation. Verapamil is known to decrease gastrointestinal transit time.

Treatment of overdosage should be supportive. Beta adrenergic stimulation or parenteral administration of calcium solutions may increase calcium ion flux across the slow channel, and have been used effectively in treatment of deliberate overdosage with verapamil. Verapamil cannot be removed by hemodialysis. Clinically significant hypotensive reactions or high degree AV block should be treated with vasopressor agents or cardiac pacing, respectively. Asystole should be handled by the usual measures including cardiopulmonary resuscitation.

DOSAGE AND ADMINISTRATION

Essential Hypertension

The dose of ISOPTIN SR should be individualized by titration and the drug should be administered with food. Initiate therapy with 180 mg of sustained-release verapamil HCl, ISOPTIN SR, given in the morning. Lower, initial doses of 120 mg a day may be warranted in patients who may have an increased response to verapamil (e.g., the elderly or small people etc.). Upward titration should be based on therapeutic efficacy and safety evaluated weekly and approximately 24 hours after the previous dose. The antihypertensive effects of ISOPTIN SR are evident within the first week of therapy.

If adequate response is not obtained with 180 mg of ISOPTIN SR, the dose may be titrated upward in the following manner:

a) 240 mg each morning,
b) 180 mg each morning plus 180 mg each evening, or 240 mg each morning plus 120 mg each evening
c) 240 mg every twelve hours.

When switching from immediate release ISOPTIN to ISOPTIN SR, the total daily dose in milligrams may remain the same.

HOW SUPPLIED

ISOPTIN® SR 240 mg tablets are supplied as light green, capsule shaped, scored, film-coated tablets containing 240 mg of verapamil hydrochloride. The tablet is embossed with a double Knoll triangle on one side and "ISOPTIN SR" on the other side. ISOPTIN® SR 180 mg tablets are supplied as light pink, oval shaped, scored, film-coated tablets containing 180 mg of verapamil hydrochloride. The tablet is embossed with "ISOPTIN SR" on one side, and "180 mg" on the other side. The ISOPTIN® SR 120 mg tablets are supplied as light violet, oval shaped, film-coated tablets containing 120 mg of verapamil hydrochloide. The tablet is embossed with "KNOLL" on one side and "120 SR" on the other side.

240 mg (light green)—	Bottle of 30— NDC #0044-1826-93
	Bottle of 100— NDC #0044-1826-02
	Hospital Unit Dose (100 Tablets— Strips of 10)—NDC #0044-1826-10
180 mg (light pink)—	Bottle of 100— NDC #0044-1825-02
	Hospital Unit Dose (100 Tablets— Strips of 10)—NDC #0044-1825-12
120 mg (light violet)—	Bottle of 100— NDC #0044-1827-02
	Hospital Unit Dose (100 Tablets— Strips of 10) —NDC #0044-1827-12

Continued on next page

Knoll Laboratories—Cont.

Storage: 59°–77°F (15°–25°C)
Protect from light and moisture.
Dispense in a light, light-resistant container as defined in the USP.
Revised August 1992   2834
Shown in Product Identification Guide, page 319

QUADRINAL™ Tablets   ℞
[kwă 'drĭ-nawl]

DESCRIPTION

Each QUADRINAL™ Tablet contains ephedrine hydrochloride 24 mg; phenobarbital 24 mg [Warning: May be habit forming]; theophylline calcium salicylate 130 mg (equivalent to 65 mg anhydrous theophylline); potassium iodide 320 mg. Other ingredients include magnesium stearate, potato starch, sodium thiosulfate and talc.
QUADRINAL contains two bronchodilators, theophylline and ephedrine. Phenobarbital serves as a mild sedative to help counteract central nervous system stimulation which may be caused by ephedrine. Wheezing and coughing are relieved by improved bronchodilation while the expectorant action of potassium iodide helps to remove secretions from the bronchial tree. Dyspnea is thus relieved or prevented and acute episodes of bronchospasm are often eliminated with consequent lessening of apprehension and distress.

CLINICAL PHARMACOLOGY

Theophylline directly relaxes the smooth muscle of the bronchial airways and pulmonary blood vessels, thus acting mainly as a bronchodilator, pulmonary vasodilator and smooth muscle relaxant. It also possesses other actions typical of the xanthine derivatives: coronary vasodilator, diuretic, and cardiac, cerebral, and skeletal muscle stimulant. The actions of theophylline may be mediated through inhibition of phosphodiesterase and a resultant increase in intracellular cyclic AMP which could mediate smooth muscle relaxation.
In vitro, theophylline has been shown to react synergistically with beta agonists (such as isoproterenol) that increase intracellular cyclic AMP through the stimulation of adenyl cyclase, but synergism has not been demonstrated in clinical studies and more data are needed to determine if theophylline and beta agonists have clinically important additive effects *in vivo.*
Apparently, tolerance does not develop with chronic use of theophylline.
The half-life is shortened with cigarette smoking. The half-life of theophylline in smokers (1 to 2 packs/day) averaged 4 to 5 hours in various studies, much shorter than the 7 to 9 hour half-life in nonsmokers. The increase in theophylline clearance caused by smoking is probably the result of induction of drug-metabolizing enzymes that do not readily normalize after cessation of smoking. It appears that between 3 months and 2 years may be necessary for normalization of the effect of smoking on theophylline pharmacokinetics. The half-life is prolonged in alcoholism, reduced hepatic or renal function, congestive heart failure, and in patients receiving cimetidine or antibiotics such as troleandomycin (TAO, Cyclamycin), erythromycin, lincomycin and clindamycin. High fever for prolonged periods may decrease theophylline elimination.
Newborn infants have extremely slow clearances with half-lives exceeding 24 hours. These approach those seen for older children after about 3-6 months.
Older adults with chronic obstructive pulmonary disease, patients with cor pulmonale or other causes of heart failure, and patients with liver pathology may have much lower clearances with half-lives that may exceed 24 hours.

Theophylline Elimination Characteristics

	Theophylline Clearance Rates (mean ± S.D.)	Half-life Average (mean ± S.D.)
Children (over 6 months of age)	1.45 ± .58 mL/kg/min	3.7 ± 1.1 hours
Adult non-smokers with uncomplicated asthma	0.65 ± .19 mL/kg/min	8.7 ± 2.2 hours

INDICATIONS

For chronic respiratory disease in which tenacious mucus and bronchospasm are dominant symptoms, such as bronchial asthma, chronic bronchitis and pulmonary emphysema.

CONTRAINDICATIONS

Use of QUADRINAL is contraindicated in patients with enlarged thyroid or goiter or with known sensitivity to theo-

Drug	Effect
Aminophylline with lithium carbonate	Increased excretion of lithium carbonate
Potassium iodide with lithium	Increased hypothyroid and goiterogenic effects
Aminophylline with propranolol	Antagonism of propranolol effect
Theophylline with furosemide	Increased diuresis
Theophylline with hexamethonium	Decreased hexamethonium induced chronotropic effect
Theophylline with reserpine	Reserpine-induced tachycardia
Theophylline with chlordiazepoxide	Chlordiazepoxide-induced fatty acid mobilization
Theophylline with troleandomycin (TAO, Cyclamycin), erythromycin, lincomycin, clindamycin	Increased theophylline plasma levels
Theophylline with phenytoin	Decreased phenytoin levels
Theophylline with cimetidine	Increased theophylline blood levels
Ephedrine with digitalis glycosides or anesthetics	May cause cardiac arrhythmias
Ephedrine with ergonovine, methylergonovine or oxytocin	Hypertension
Ephedrine with guanethidine	Decreased hypotensive effect
Ephedrine with MAO inhibitors	Potentiation of pressor effect of ephedrine
Ephedrine with reserpine	Decreased pressor effect of ephedrine
Ephedrine with other sympathomimetics	Increased effects of either medication
Ephedrine with tricyclic antidepressants	May antagonize the pressor action of ephedrine
Phenobarbital with alcohol, general anesthetics, other CNS depressants, or MAO inhibitors	Increased effects of either medication
Phenobarbital with oral anticoagulants	Decreased anticoagulant effects
Phenobarbital with corticosteroids, digitalis, digitoxin, doxycycline, tricyclic antidepressants, griseofulvin or phenytoin	Decreased effects of these drugs

phylline, potassium iodide, ephedrine or sympathomimetics, or barbiturates.
The iodide in QUADRINAL can cause fetal harm when administered to a pregnant woman. Development of goiter has been reported in infants whose mothers received iodide-containing medications during pregnancy. A few neonatal deaths resulting from tracheal obstruction due to congenital goiters have been reported. Use of barbiturates during pregnancy may cause physical dependence with resulting withdrawal symptoms in the neonate; may cause birth defects; may be associated with neonatal hemorrhage due to reduction in levels of vitamin K-dependent clotting factors in the neonate; may cause respiratory depression in the neonate. QUADRINAL is contraindicated in women who are or may become pregnant. If this drug is used during pregnancy, or if the patient becomes pregnant while taking this drug, the patient should be apprised of the potential hazard to the fetus.

WARNINGS

QUADRINAL contains thiosulfate, a sulfite that may cause allergic-type reactions including anaphylactic symptoms and life-threatening or less severe asthmatic episodes in certain susceptible people. The overall prevalence of sulfite sensitivity in the general population is unknown and probably low. Sulfite sensitivity is seen more frequently in asthmatic than non-asthmatic people.
QUADRINAL contains theophylline calcium salicylate. Salicylates have been reported to be associated with the development of Reye's syndrome in children and teenagers with chicken pox or flu.
Excessive theophylline doses may be associated with toxicity; determination of serum theophylline levels is recommended to assure maximal benefit without excessive risk. Incidence of toxicity increases at serum levels greater than 20 mcg/mL. Because of the theophylline content of QUADRINAL, it is unlikely that toxic levels of theophylline would be reached unless a serious overdosage occurs.
Morphine, curare, and stilbamidine should be used with caution in patients with airflow obstruction since they stimulate histamine release and can induce asthmatic attacks. They may also suppress respiration leading to respiratory failure. Alternative drugs should be chosen whenever possible.
There is an excellent correlation between clinical manifestations of toxicity and high blood levels of theophylline resulting from conventional doses in patients with lowered body plasma clearances (due to transient cardiac decompensation), patients with liver dysfunction or chronic obstructive lung disease, and patients who are older than 55 years of age, particularly males. In about 50% of patients, nausea and restlessness precede more severe manifestations of toxicity. In other patients, ventricular arrhythmias or seizures may be the first signs of toxicity. These more serious side effects

are more likely to occur after intravenous administration of theophylline. Many patients who have high theophylline serum levels exhibit a tachycardia, and theophylline may worsen preexisting arrhythmias.

PRECAUTIONS

Mean half-life in smokers is shorter than in nonsmokers; therefore, smokers may require larger doses of theophylline. QUADRINAL, like all theophylline products, should not be administered concurrently with other xanthine medications. Use with caution in patients with severe cardiac disease, severe hypoxemia, hypertension, hyperthyroidism, acute myocardial injury, cor pulmonale, congestive heart failure, liver disease, peptic ulcer and in the elderly (especially males) and in neonates. Great caution should be used especially in giving theophylline to patients in congestive heart failure; such patients have shown markedly prolonged theophylline blood level curves with theophylline persisting in serum for long periods following discontinuation of the drug. Theophylline may occasionally act as a local irritant to the G.I. tract although gastrointestinal symptoms are more commonly central in origin and associated with serum concentrations over 20 mcg/mL.
Ephedrine-containing medications should be used with caution in patients with cardiovascular disease, diabetes mellitus, predisposition to glaucoma, hypertension, hyperthyroidism, or prostatic hypertrophy.
Potassium iodide may aggravate acne in adolescents and adults.
Phenobarbital should be used with caution in patients with a history of drug abuse or dependence, impaired renal or hepatic function, hyperkinesis, uncontrolled pain, or history of porphyria.
Usage in Pregnancy: Pregnancy Category X. See "Contraindications" section.
Nursing Mothers: Because of the potential for serious adverse reactions in nursing infants from the potassium iodide, ephedrine and phenobarbital in QUADRINAL, a decision should be made whether to discontinue nursing or to discontinue the drug, taking into account the importance of the drug to the mother.
Pediatric Use: QUADRINAL is indicated for use in children on a short term basis. Chronic use should be reserved for patients in whom other expectorants have not been effective. If QUADRINAL is used chronically in children, the patient should be observed for signs of thyroid enlargement and worsening of acne.
Geriatric Patients: Geriatric patients may be more sensitive to the effects of ephedrine.

ADVERSE REACTIONS

The most frequent adverse reactions to theophylline are usually due to overdose (serum levels in excess of 20 mcg/

mL) and are: nausea, vomiting, epigastric pain, hematemesis, diarrhea, headaches, irritability, restlessness, insomnia, reflex hyperexcitability, muscle twitching, clonic and tonic generalized convulsions, palpitations, tachycardia, extra systoles, flushing, hypotension, circulatory failure, ventricular arrhythmias, tachypnea, albuminuria, increased excretion of renal tubular cells and red blood cells, potentiation of diuresis, hyperglycemia and inappropriate ADH syndrome.
Thyroid adenoma, goiter and myxedema are possible side effects of potassium iodide.
Hypersensitivity to iodides may be manifested by angioneurotic edema, cutaneous and mucosal hemorrhages, and symptoms resembling serum sickness, such as fever, arthralgia, lymph node enlargement and eosinophilia.
Chronic ingestion of iodides may result in chronic iodide poisoning, or iodism. Initial symptoms include an unpleasant brassy taste, burning in the mouth and throat, soreness of the teeth and gums, increased salivation, coryza, sneezing, irritation of the eyes with swelling of the eyelids, headache, cough, skin lesions, diarrhea, gastric irritation, anorexia, fever and depression. The symptoms of iodism disappear spontaneously within a few days after stopping the administration of iodide. Therefore, treatment consists of stopping QUADRINAL therapy and providing supportive measures as indicated by the symptoms. Abundant fluid and sodium chloride intake may hasten iodide elimination. In severe cases, the use of mannitol to establish an osmotic diuresis may be appropriate. Potassium iodide may produce hyperkalemia and, if ingested chronically, may lead to goiter.
Adverse reactions to ephedrine include nervousness, restlessness, trouble in sleeping, irregular heartbeat, difficult or painful urination, dizziness or light-headedness, headache, loss of appetite, nausea or vomiting, trembling, troubled breathing, unusual increase in sweating, unusual paleness, feeling of warmth, and weakness. Tolerance to ephedrine may develop with prolonged or excessive use.
Adverse reactions to phenobarbital include mental confusion or depression, shortness of breath or troubled breathing, skin rash, hives, swelling of eyelids, face or lips, wheezing or tightness in chest, sore throat and fever, unusual bleeding or bruising, unusual excitement, tiredness or weakness, unusually slow heartbeat, yellowing of eyes or skin.

DRUG INTERACTIONS

Toxic synergism of theophylline with ephedrine has been documented and may occur with some other sympathomimetic bronchodilators.
[See table on top of preceding page.]

OVERDOSAGE

A. If potential overdose is established and seizure has not occurred and patient is conscious:
   1) Induce vomiting.
   2) Administer a cathartic.
   3) Administer activated charcoal.
B. If patient is having a seizure:
   1) Establish an airway.
   2) Administer O_2.
   3) Treat the seizure with intravenous diazepam, 0.1 to 0.3 mg/kg up to 10 mg.
   4) Monitor vital signs, maintain blood pressure and provide adequate hydration.
C. Post-seizure coma:
   1) Maintain airway and oxygenation.
   2) Following above recommendations to prevent absorption of drug, but intubation and lavage will have to be performed instead of inducing emesis, and introduce the cathartic and charcoal via a large bore gastric lavage tube.
   3) Continue to provide full supportive care and adequate hydration while waiting for drug to be metabolized. In general, the drug is metabolized sufficiently rapidly so as not to require dialysis.

DOSAGE AND ADMINISTRATION

When rapidly absorbed products such as uncoated tablets with rapid dissolution are used, dosing to maintain "around the clock" blood levels generally requires administration every 6 hours in children; dosing intervals up to 8 hours may be satisfactory for adults because of their slower elimination rate.
Pulmonary function measurements before and after a period of treatment permit an objective assessment of response to QUADRINAL.

Usual dose:
Adults—One tablet 3 or 4 times daily; if needed, an additional one tablet upon retiring for nighttime relief. In severe attacks, the usual dose may be increased by one half.
Children 6 to 12 years—one half tablet three times daily.
Children under 6 years—dose is proportionately less.

HOW SUPPLIED

QUADRINAL Tablets— white, round, bi-convex tablets, engraved with a triangle on one side, bisected on the other side and imprinted with the number "14".
Bottles of 100—NDC #0044-4520-02.

STORAGE

Store at 59°–86°F (15°–30°C).
Dispense in tight, light-resistant container as defined in USP.
MR 1987/8448
Revised May, 1987 8449
Shown in Product Identification Guide, page 319

RYTHMOL® TABLETS ℞
(propafenone hydrochloride)

DESCRIPTION

RYTHMOL (propafenone hydrochloride) is an antiarrhythmic drug supplied in scored, film-coated tablets of 150 and 300 mg for oral administration. Propafenone has some structural similarities to beta-blocking agents.
The structural formula of propafenone hydrochloride is given below:

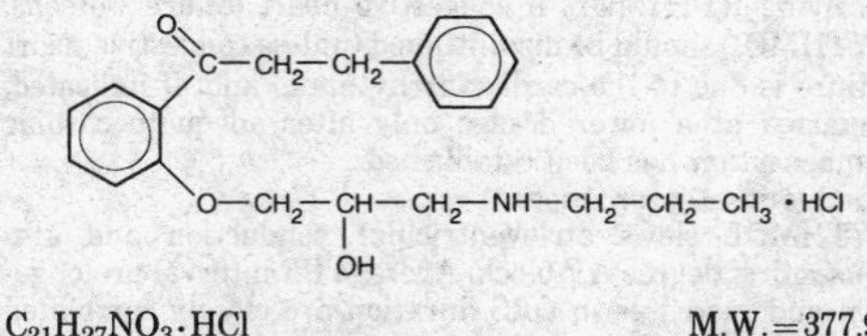

$C_{21}H_{27}NO_3 \cdot HCl$ M.W. = 377.92
2′-[2-Hydroxy-3-(propylamino)-propoxy]-3-phenylpropiophenone hydrochloride

Propafenone hydrochloride occurs as colorless crystals or white crystalline powder with a very bitter taste. It is slightly soluble in water (20°C), chloroform and ethanol. The following inactive ingredients are contained in the tablet: corn starch, hydroxypropyl methyl cellulose, magnesium stearate, polyethylene glycol, polysorbate, povidone, propylene glycol, sodium starch glycolate and titanium dioxide.

CLINICAL PHARMACOLOGY

Mechanism of Action:
RYTHMOL (propafenone HCl) is a Class IC antiarrhythmic drug with local anesthetic effects, and a direct stabilizing action on myocardial membranes. The electrophysiological effect of RYTHMOL manifests itself in a reduction of upstroke velocity (Phase 0) of the monophasic action potential. In Purkinje fibers, and to a lesser extent myocardial fibers, RYTHMOL reduces the fast inward current carried by sodium ions. Diastolic excitability threshold is increased and effective refractory period prolonged. Propafenone reduces spontaneous automaticity and depresses triggered activity.
Studies in anesthetized dogs and isolated organ preparations show that RYTHMOL has beta-sympatholytic activity at about 1/50 the potency of propranolol. Clinical studies employing isoproterenol challenge and exercise testing after single doses of propafenone indicate a beta-adrenergic blocking potency (per mg) about 1/40 that of propranolol in man. In clinical trials, resting heart rate decreases of about 8% were noted at the higher end of the therapeutic plasma concentration range. At very high concentrations in vitro, propafenone can inhibit the slow inward current carried by calcium but this calcium antagonist effect probably does not contribute to antiarrhythmic efficacy. Propafenone has local anesthetic activity approximately equal to procaine.

Electrophysiology:
Electrophysiology studies in patients with ventricular tachycardia have shown that RYTHMOL prolongs atrioventricular conduction while having little or no effect on sinus node function. Both AV nodal conduction time (AH interval) and His-Purkinje conduction time (HV interval) are prolonged. Propafenone has little or no effect on the atrial functional refractory period, but AV nodal functional and effective refractory periods are prolonged. In patients with WPW, RYTHMOL reduces conduction and increases the effective refractory period of the accessory pathway in both directions. Propafenone slows conduction and consequently produces dose-related changes in the PR interval and QRS duration. QT_c interval does not change.
[See table below.]
In any individual patient, the above ECG changes cannot be readily used to predict either efficacy or plasma concentration.
RYTHMOL causes a dose-related and concentration-related decrease in the rate of single and multiple PVCs and can suppress recurrence of ventricular tachycardia. Based on the percent of patients attaining substantial (80–90%) suppression of ventricular ectopic activity, it appears that trough plasma levels of 0.2 to 1.5 μg/mL can provide good suppression, with higher concentrations giving a greater rate of good response.

Hemodynamics:
Sympathetic stimulation may be a vital component supporting circulatory function in patients with congestive heart failure, and its inhibition by the beta blockade produced by RYTHMOL may in itself aggravate congestive heart failure. Additionally, like other Class IC antiarrhythmic drugs, studies in humans have shown that RYTHMOL exerts a negative inotropic effect on the myocardium. Cardiac catheterization studies in patients with moderately impaired ventricular function (mean C.I. = 2.61 L/min/m^2) utilizing intravenous propafenone infusions (2 mg/kg over 10 min + 2 mg/min for 30 min) that gave mean plasma concentrations of 3.0 μg/mL (well above the therapeutic range of 0.2–1.5 μg/mL) showed significant increases in pulmonary capillary wedge pressure, systemic and pulmonary vascular resistances and depression of cardiac output and cardiac index.

Pharmacokinetics and Metabolism:
RYTHMOL is nearly completely absorbed after oral administration with peak plasma levels occurring approximately 3.5 hours after administration in most individuals. Propafenone exhibits extensive saturable presystemic biotransformation (first pass effect) resulting in a dose dependent and dosage form dependent absolute bioavailability; e.g., a 150 mg tablet had absolute bioavailability of 3.4%, while a 300 mg tablet had absolute bioavailability of 10.6%. A 300 mg solution which was rapidly absorbed, had absolute bioavailability of 21.4%. At still larger doses, above those recommended, bioavailability increases still further. Decreased liver function also increases bioavailability; bioavailability is inversely related to indocyanine green clearance reaching 60–70% at clearances of 7 mL/min and below. The clearance of propafenone is reduced and the elimination half-life increased in patients with significant hepatic dysfunction (see PRECAUTIONS).
RYTHMOL follows a nonlinear pharmacokinetic disposition presumably due to saturation of first pass hepatic metabolism as the liver is exposed to higher concentrations of propafenone and shows a very high degree of interindividual variability. For example, for a three-fold increase in daily dose from 300 to 900 mg/day there is a ten-fold increase in steady-state plasma concentration. The top 25% of patients given 375 mg/day, however, had a mean concentration of propafenone larger than the bottom 25%, and about equal to the second 25%, of patients given a dose of 900 mg. Although food increased peak blood level and bioavailability in a single dose study, during multiple dose administration of propafenone to healthy volunteers food did not change bioavailability significantly.
There are two genetically determined patterns of propafenone metabolism. In over 90% of patients, the drug is rapidly and extensively metabolized with an elimination half-life from 2–10 hours. These patients metabolize propafenone into two active metabolites: 5-hydroxypropafenone and N-depropylpropafenone. In vitro preparations have shown these two metabolites to have antiarrhythmic activity comparable to propafenone, but in man they both are usually present in concentrations less than 20% of propafenone. Nine additional metabolites have been identified, most in only trace amounts. It is the saturable hydroxylation pathway that is responsible for the nonlinear pharmacokinetic disposition.

Mean Changes in ECG Intervals*
Total Daily Dose (mg)

	337.5 mg		450 mg		675 mg		900 mg	
Interval	msec	(%)	msec	(%)	msec	(%)	msec	(%)
RR	−14.5	−1.8	30.6	3.8	31.5	3.9	41.7	5.1
PR	3.6	2.1	19.1	11.6	28.9	17.8	35.6	21.9
QRS	5.6	6.4	5.5	6.1	7.7	8.4	15.6	17.3
QT_c	2.7	0.7	−7.5	−1.8	5.0	1.2	14.7	3.7

*Change and percent change based on mean baseline values for each treatment group.

Continued on next page

Knoll Laboratories—Cont.

In less than 10% of patients (and in any patient also receiving quinidine, see PRECAUTIONS), metabolism of propafenone is slower because the 5-hydroxy metabolite is not formed or is minimally formed. The estimated propafenone elimination half-life ranges from 10–32 hours. Decreased ability to form the 5-hydroxy metabolite of propafenone is associated with a diminished ability to metabolize debrisoquine and a variety of other drugs (encainide, metoprolol, dextromethorphan). In these patients, the N-depropylpropafenone occurs in quantities comparable to the levels occurring in extensive metabolizers. In slow metabolizers propafenone pharmacokinetics are linear.

There are significant differences in plasma concentrations of propafenone in slow and extensive metabolizers, the former achieving concentrations 1.5 to 2.0 times those of the extensive metabolizers at daily doses of 675–900 mg/day. At low doses the differences are greater, with slow metabolizers attaining concentrations more than five times that of extensive metabolizers. Because the difference decreases at high doses and is mitigated by the lack of the active 5-hydroxy metabolite in the slow metabolizers, and because steady-state conditions are achieved after 4–5 days of dosing in all patients, the recommended dosing regimen is the same for all patients. The greater variability in blood levels require that the drug be titrated carefully in all patients with close attention to clinical and ECG evidence of toxicity (see DOSAGE AND ADMINISTRATION).

INDICATIONS AND USAGE

RYTHMOL (propafenone HCL) is indicated for the treatment of documented ventricular arrhythmias, such as sustained ventricular tachycardia, that, in the judgment of the physician are life-threatening. Because of the proarrhythmic effects of RYTHMOL, its use with lesser arrhythmias is generally not recommended. Treatment of patients with asymptomatic ventricular premature contractions should be avoided.

Initiation of RYTHMOL treatment, as with other antiarrhythmic agents used to treat life-threatening arrhythmias, should be carried out in the hospital.

Antiarrhythmic drugs have not been shown to enhance survival in patients with ventricular arrhythmias.

CONTRAINDICATIONS

RYTHMOL (propafenone HCl) is contraindicated in the presence of uncontrolled congestive heart failure, cardiogenic shock, sinoatrial, atrioventricular and intraventicular disorders of impulse generation and/or conduction (e.g., sick sinus node syndrome, atrioventricular block) in the absence of an artificial pacemaker, bradycardia, marked hypotension, bronchospastic disorders, manifest electrolyte imbalance, and known hypersensitivity to the drug.

WARNINGS

Mortality:
In the National Heart, Lung and Blood Institute's Cardiac Arrhythmia Suppression Trial (CAST), a long-term, multi-centered, randomized, double-blind study in patients with asymptomatic non-life-threatening arrhythmias who had had myocardial infarctions more than six days but less than two years previously, an excessive mortality or non-fatal cardiac arrest rate was seen in patients treated with encainide or flecainide (56/730) compared with that seen in patients assigned to matched placebo-treated groups (22/725). The average duration of treatment with encainide or flecainide in this study was ten months.

The applicability of these results to other populations (e.g., those without recent myocardial infarctions) or to other antiarrhythmic drugs is uncertain, but at present it is prudent to consider any antiarrhythmic agent to have a significant risk in patients with structural heart disease.

Proarrhythmic Effects
RYTHMOL (propafenone HCl), like other antiarrhythmic agents, may cause new or worsened arrhythmias. Such proarrhythmic effects range from an increase in frequency of PVCs to the development of more severe ventricular tachycardia, ventricular fibrillation or torsade de pointes; i.e., tachycardia that is more sustained or more rapid which may lead to fatal consequences. It is therefore essential that each patient given RYTHMOL be evaluated electrocardiographically and clinically prior to, and during therapy to determine whether the response to RYTHMOL supports continued treatment.

Overall in clinical trials with propafenone, 4.7% of all patients had new or worsened ventricular arrhythmia possibly representing a proarrhythmic event (0.7% was an increase in PVCs; 4.0% a worsening, or new appearance, of VT or VF). Of the patients who had a worsening of VT (4%), 92% had a history of VT and/or VT/VF, 71% had coronary artery disease, and 68% had a prior myocardial infarction. The incidence of proarrhythmia in patients with less serious or benign arrhythmias, which include patients with an increase in frequency of PVCs, was 1.6%. Although most proarrhythmic events occurred during the first week of ther-

apy, late events also were seen and the CAST study (see above) suggests that an increased risk is present throughout treatment.

Nonallergic Bronchospasm (e.g., chronic bronchitis, emphysema):
PATIENTS WITH BRONCHOSPASTIC DISEASE SHOULD IN GENERAL NOT RECEIVE PROPAFENONE or other agents with beta-adrenergic-blocking activity.

Congestive Heart Failure:
During treatment with oral propafenone in patients with depressed baseline function (mean EF=33.5%), no significant decreases in ejection fraction were seen. In clinical trial experience, new or worsened CHF has been reported in 3.7% of patients; of those 0.9% were considered probably or definitely related to RYTHMOL. Of the patients with congestive heart failure probably related to propafenone, 80% had preexisting heart failure and 85% had coronary artery disease. CHF attributable to RYTHMOL developed rarely (<0.2%) in patients who had no previous history of CHF. As RYTHMOL exerts both beta blockade and a (dose-related) negative inotropic effect on cardiac muscle, patients with congestive heart failure should be fully compensated before receiving RYTHMOL. If congestive heart failure worsens, RYTHMOL should be discontinued (unless congestive heart failure is due to the cardiac arrhythmia) and, if indicated, restarted at a lower dosage only after adequate cardiac compensation has been established.

Conduction Disturbances:
RYTHMOL slows atrioventricular conduction and also causes first degree AV block. Average PR interval prolongation and increases in QRS duration are closely correlated with dosage increases and concomitant increases in propafe-

none plasma concentrations. The incidence of first degree, second degree, and third degree AV block observed in 2,127 patients was 2.5%, 0.6%, and 0.2%, respectively. Development of second or third degree AV block requires a reduction in dosage or discontinuation of RYTHMOL. Bundle branch block (1.2%) and intraventricular conduction delay (1.1%) have been reported in patients receiving propafenone. Bradycardia has also been reported (1.5%). Experience in patients with sick sinus node syndrome is limited and these patients should not be treated with propafenone.

Effects on Pacemaker Threshold:
RYTHMOL may alter both pacing and sensing thresholds of artificial pacemakers. Pacemakers should be monitored and programmed accordingly during therapy.

Hematologic Disturbances:
One case of agranulocytosis with fever and sepsis, probably related to the use of propafenone, was seen in U.S. clinical trials. The agranulocytosis appeared after 8 weeks of therapy. Propafenone therapy was stopped and the white count had normalized by 14 days. The patient recovered. In the course of over 800,000 patient years of exposure during marketing outside the U.S. since 1978, seven additional cases have been reported. In one of these, concomitant captopril, a drug known to cause agranulocytosis, was used. Unexplained fever and/or decrease in white cell count, particularly during the first three months of therapy, warrant consideration of possible agranulocytosis/granulocytopenia. Patients should be instructed to promptly report the development of any signs of infection such as fever, sore throat, or chills.

PRECAUTIONS
Hepatic Dysfunction:
Propafenone is highly metabolized by the liver and should, therefore, be administered cautiously to patients with im-

Adverse Reactions Reported for ≥ 1% of the Patients

	Prop./Placebo Trials		Prop./Quinidine Trial	
	Prop. (N=247)	Placebo (N=111)	Prop. (N=53)	Quinidine (N=52)
Unusual Taste	7.3%	0.9%	22.6%	0.0%
Dizziness	6.5%	5.4%	15.1%	9.6%
First Degree AV Block	4.5%	0.9%	1.9%	0.0%
Headache(s)	4.5%	4.5%	1.9%	7.7%
Constipation	4.0%	0.0%	5.7%	1.9%
Intraventricular Conduction Delay	4.0%	0.0%	—	—
Nausea and/or Vomiting	2.8%	0.9%	5.7%	15.4%
Fatigue	—	—	3.8%	1.9%
Palpitations	2.4%	0.9%	—	—
Blurred Vision	2.0%	0.9%	5.7%	1.9%
Dry Mouth	2.0%	0.9%	5.7%	5.8%
Dyspnea	2.0%	2.7%	3.8%	0.0%
Abdominal Pain/Cramps	—	—	1.9%	7.7%
Dyspepsia	—	—	1.9%	7.7%
Congestive Heart Failure	—	—	1.9%	0.0%
Fever	—	—	1.9%	9.6%
Tinnitus	—	—	1.9%	1.9%
Vision Abnormal	—	—	1.9%	1.9%
Esophagitis	—	—	1.9%	0.0%
Gastroenteritis	—	—	1.9%	0.0%
Anxiety	2.0%	1.8%	—	—
Anorexia	1.6%	0.9%	—	1.9%
Proarrhythmia	1.2%	0.0%	1.9%	0.0%
Flatulence	1.2%	0.0%	1.9%	0.0%
Angina	1.2%	0.0%	1.9%	3.8%
Second Degree AV Block	1.2%	0.0%	—	—
Bundle Branch Block	1.2%	0.0%	1.9%	1.9%
Loss of Balance	1.2%	0.0%	—	—
Diarrhea	1.2%	0.9%	5.7%	38.5%

paired hepatic function. Severe liver dysfunction increases the bioavailability of propafenone to approximately 70% compared to 3–40% for patients with normal liver function. In eight patients with moderate to severe liver disease, the mean half-life was approximately 9 hours. As a result, the dose of propafenone given to patients with impaired hepatic function should be approximately 20–30% of the dose given to patients with normal hepatic function (see DOSAGE AND ADMINISTRATION). Careful monitoring for excessive pharmacological effects (see OVERDOSAGE) should be carried out.

Renal Dysfunction:
A considerable percentage of propafenone metabolites (18.5%–38% of the dose/48 hours) are excreted in the urine. Until further data are available, RYTHMOL (propafenone HCl) should be administered cautiously to patients with impaired renal function. These patients should be carefully monitored for signs of overdosage (see OVERDOSAGE).

Elevated ANA Titers:
Positive ANA titers have been reported in patients receiving propafenone. They have been reversible upon cessation of treatment and may disappear even in the face of continued propafenone therapy. These laboratory findings were usually not associated with clinical symptoms, but there is one published case of drug-induced lupus erythematosus (positive rechallenge); it resolved completely upon discontinuation of therapy. Patients who develop an abnormal ANA test should be carefully evaluated and, if persistent or worsening elevation of ANA titers is detected, consideration should be given to discontinuing therapy.

Impaired Spermatogenesis:
Reversible disorders of spermatogenesis have been demonstrated in monkeys, dogs and rabbits after high dose intravenous administration. Evaluation of the effects of short-term propafenone administration on spermatogenesis in 11 normal subjects suggests that propafenone produced a reversible, short-term drop (within normal range) in sperm count. Subsequent evaluation in 11 patients receiving propafenone chronically have suggested no effect of propafenone on sperm count.

DRUG INTERACTIONS

Quinidine: Small doses of quinidine completely inhibit the hydroxylation metabolic pathway, making all patients, in effect, slow metabolizers (see CLINICAL PHARMACOLOGY). There is, as yet, too little information to recommend concomitant use of propafenone and quinidine.

Local Anesthetics: Concomitant use of local anesthetics (i.e., during pacemaker implantations, surgery, or dental use) may increase the risks of central nervous system side effects.

Digitalis: RYTHMOL produces dose-related increases in serum digoxin levels ranging from about 35% at 450 mg/day to 85% at 900 mg/day of propafenone without affecting digoxin renal clearance. These elevations of digoxin levels were maintained for up to 16 months during concomitant administration. Plasma digoxin levels of patients on concomitant therapy should be measured, and digoxin dosage should ordinarily be reduced when propafenone is started, especially if a relatively large digoxin dose is used or if plasma concentrations are relatively high.

Beta-Antagonists: In a study involving healthy subjects, concomitant administration of propafenone and propranolol has resulted in substantial increases in propranolol plasma concentration and elimination half-life with no change in propafenone plasma levels from control values. Similar observations have been reported with metoprolol. Propafenone appears to inhibit the hydroxylation pathway for the two beta-antagonists (just as quinidine inhibits propafenone metabolism). Increased plasma concentrations of metoprolol could overcome its relative cardioselectivity. In propafenone clinical trials, patients who were receiving beta-blockers concurrently did not experience an increased incidence of side effects. While the therapeutic range for beta-blockers is wide, a reduction in dosage may be necessary during concomitant administration with propafenone.

Warfarin: In a study of eight healthy subjects receiving propafenone and warfarin concomitantly, mean steady-state warfarin plasma concentrations increased 39% with a corresponding increase in prothrombin times of approximately 25%. It is therefore recommended that prothrombin times be routinely monitored and the dose of warfarin be adjusted if necessary.

Cimetidine: Concomitant administration of propafenone and cimetidine in 12 healthy subjects resulted in a 20% increase in steady-state plasma concentrations of propafenone with no detectable changes in electrocardiographic parameters beyond that measured on propafenone alone.

Other: Limited experience with propafenone combined with calcium antagonists and diuretics has been reported without evidence of clinically significant adverse reactions.

Carcinogenesis, Mutagenesis, Impairment of Fertility: Lifetime maximally tolerated oral dose studies in mice (up to 360 mg/kg/day) and rats (up to 270 mg/kg/day) provided no evidence of a carcinogenic potential for propafenone.

ADVERSE REACTIONS REPORTED FOR ≥ 1% OF THE PATIENTS
N = 2127

	Incidence by Total Daily Dose			Total Incidence (N=2127)	% of Pts. Who Discont.
	450 mg (N=1430)	600 mg (N=1337)	≥ 900 mg (N=1333)		
Dizziness	3.6%	6.6%	11.0%	12.5%	2.4%
Nausea and/or Vomiting	2.4%	6.1%	8.9%	10.7%	3.4%
Unusual Taste	2.5%	4.9%	6.3%	8.8%	0.7%
Constipation	2.0%	4.1%	5.3%	7.2%	0.5%
Fatigue	1.8%	2.8%	4.1%	6.0%	1.0%
Dyspnea	2.2%	2.3%	3.6%	5.3%	1.6%
Proarrhythmia	2.0%	2.1%	2.9%	4.7%	4.7%
Angina	1.7%	2.1%	3.2%	4.6%	0.5%
Headache(s)	1.5%	2.5%	2.8%	4.5%	1.0%
Blurred Vision	0.6%	2.4%	3.1%	3.8%	0.8%
CHF	0.8%	2.2%	2.6%	3.7%	1.4%
Ventricular Tachycardia	1.4%	1.6%	2.9%	3.4%	1.2%
Dyspepsia	1.3%	1.7%	2.5%	3.4%	0.9%
Palpitations	0.6%	1.6%	2.6%	3.4%	0.5%
Rash	0.6%	1.4%	1.9%	2.6%	0.8%
AV Block, First Degree	0.8%	1.2%	2.1%	2.5%	0.3%
Diarrhea	0.5%	1.6%	1.7%	2.5%	0.6%
Weakness	0.6%	1.6%	1.7%	2.4%	0.7%
Dry Mouth	0.9%	1.0%	1.4%	2.4%	0.2%
Syncope/Near Syncope	0.8%	1.3%	1.4%	2.2%	0.7%
QRS Duration, Increased	0.5%	0.9%	1.7%	1.9%	0.5%
Chest Pain	0.5%	0.7%	1.4%	1.8%	0.2%
Anorexia	0.5%	0.7%	1.6%	1.7%	0.4%
Abdominal Pain/Cramps	0.8%	0.9%	1.1%	1.7%	0.4%
Ataxia	0.3%	0.6%	1.5%	1.6%	0.2%
Insomnia	0.3%	1.3%	0.7%	1.5%	0.3%
Premature Ventricular Contraction(s)	0.6%	0.6%	1.1%	1.5%	0.1%
Bradycardia	0.5%	0.8%	1.1%	1.5%	0.5%
Anxiety	0.7%	0.5%	0.9%	1.5%	0.6%
Edema	0.6%	0.4%	1.0%	1.4%	0.2%
Tremor(s)	0.3%	0.8%	1.1%	1.4%	0.3%
Diaphoresis	0.6%	0.4%	1.1%	1.4%	0.3%
Bundle Branch Block	0.3%	0.7%	1.0%	1.2%	0.5%
Drowsiness	0.6%	0.5%	0.7%	1.2%	0.2%
Atrial Fibrillation	0.7%	0.7%	0.5%	1.2%	0.4%
Flatulence	0.3%	0.7%	0.9%	1.2%	0.1%
Hypotension	0.1%	0.5%	1.0%	1.1%	0.4%
Intraventricular Conduction Delay	0.2%	0.7%	0.9%	1.1%	0.1%
Pain, Joint(s)	0.2%	0.4%	0.9%	1.0%	0.1%

RYTHMOL was not mutagenic when assayed for genotoxicity in 1) mouse Dominant Lethal test, 2) rat bone marrow Chromosome Analysis, 3) Chinese hamster bone marrow and spermatogonia chromosome analysis, 4) Chinese hamster micronucleus test, and 5) Ames bacterial test.
Propafenone administered intravenously to rabbits, dogs, and monkeys has been shown to decrease spermatogenesis. These effects were reversible, were not found following oral dosing of propafenone, were seen only at lethal or sublethal dose levels and were not seen in rats treated either orally or intravenously (see PRECAUTIONS, Impaired Spermatogenesis). Propafenone did not affect either male or female fertility rates when administered intravenously to rats and rabbits at dose levels up to 18 times the maximum recommended daily human dose of 900 mg (based on 60 kg human body weight).

Continued on next page

Consult 1997 supplements and future editions for revisions

Knoll Laboratories—Cont.

Pregnancy-Teratogenic Effects:

Pregnancy Category C:
Propafenone has been shown to be embryotoxic in rabbits and rats when given in doses 10 and 40 times, respectively, the maximum recommended human dose. No teratogenic potential was apparent in either species. There are no adequate and well-controlled studies in pregnant women. Propafenone should be used during pregnancy only if the potential benefit justifies the potential risk to the fetus.

Pregnancy-Nonteratogenic Effects:
In a perinatal and postnatal study in rats, propafenone, at dose levels of 6 or more times the maximum recommended human dose, produced dose dependent increases in maternal and neonatal mortality, decreased maternal and pup body weight gain and reduced neonatal physiologic development.

Labor and Delivery:
It is not known whether the use of propafenone during labor or delivery has immediate or delayed adverse effects on the fetus, or whether it prolongs the duration of labor or increases the need for forceps delivery or other obstetrical intervention.

Nursing Mothers:
It is not known whether this drug is excreted in human milk. Because many drugs are excreted in human milk and because of the potential for serious adverse reactions in nursing infants from RYTHMOL, a decision should be made whether to discontinue nursing or to discontinue the drug, taking into account the importance of the drug to the mother.

Pediatric Use:
The safety and efficacy of RYTHMOL in children has not been established.

Geriatric Use:
There do not appear to be any age-related differences in adverse reaction rates in the most commonly reported adverse reactions. Because of the possible increased risk of impaired hepatic or renal function in this age group, RYTHMOL should be used with caution. The effective dose may be lower in these patients.

Animal Toxicology:
Renal changes have been observed in the rat following 6 months of oral administration of propafenone at doses of 180 and 360 mg/kg/day (12–24 times the maximum recommended human dose) but not 90 mg/kg/day. Both inflammatory and noninflammatory changes in the renal tubules with accompanying interstitial nephritis were observed. These lesions were reversible in that they were not found in rats treated at these dosage levels and allowed to recover for 6 weeks. Fatty degenerative changes of the liver were found in rats following chronic administration of propafenone at dose levels 19 times the maximum recommended human dose.

ADVERSE REACTIONS

Adverse reactions associated with RYTHMOL (propafenone HCl) occur most frequently in the gastrointestinal, cardiovascular, and central nervous systems. About 20% of patients discontinued due to adverse reactions. Results of controlled trials comparing adverse reaction rates on propafenone and placebo, and on propafenone and quinidine are shown in the following table. Adverse reactions appearing in the table were reported for ≥1% of the patients receiving propafenone. The most common events were dizziness, unusual taste, first degree AV block, intraventricular conduction delay, nausea and/or vomiting, and constipation. Headache was relatively common also, but was not increased compared to placebo.

[See table on page 1400.]

Adverse reactions reported for ≥1% of 2127 patients who received propafenone in U.S. clinical trials are presented in the following table by propafenone daily dose. The most common adverse reactions in controlled clinical trials appeared dose related (but note that most patients spent more time at the larger doses), especially dizziness, nausea and/or vomiting, unusual taste, constipation, and blurred vision. Some less common reactions may also have been dose related such as first degree AV block, congestive heart failure, dyspepsia, and weakness. The principal causes of discontinuation were the most common events and are shown in the table.

[See table on preceding page.]

In addition, the following adverse reactions were reported less frequently than 1% either in clinical trials or in marketing experience (*adverse events for marketing experience are given in italics*). Causality and relationship to propafenone therapy cannot necessarily be judged from these events.

Cardiovascular System: Atrial flutter, AV dissociation, cardiac arrest, flushing, hot flashes, sick sinus syndrome, sinus pause or arrest, supraventricular tachycardia.

Nervous System: Abnormal dreams, abnormal speech, abnormal vision, *apnea, coma,* confusion, depression, memory loss, numbness, paresthesias, psychosis/mania, seizures (0.3%), tinnitus, unusual smell sensation, vertigo

Gastrointestinal: A number of patients with liver abnormalities associated with propafenone therapy have been reported in foreign post-marketing experience. Some appeared due to hepatocellular injury, some were cholestatic and some showed a mixed picture. Some of these reports were simply discovered through clinical chemistries, others because of clinical symptoms. One case was rechallenged with a positive outcome.

Cholestasis (0.2%), elevated liver enzymes (alkaline phosphatase, serum transaminases) (0.2%), gastroenteritis, hepatitis (0.03%)

Hematologic: Agranulocytosis, anemia, bruising, granulocytopenia, *increased bleeding time,* leukopenia, purpura, thrombocytopenia

Other: Alopecia, eye irritation, *hyponatremia/inappropriate ADH secretion,* impotence, increased glucose, *kidney failure,* positive ANA (0.7%), *lupus erythematosus,* muscle cramps, muscle weakness, nephrotic syndrome, pain, pruritus

OVERDOSAGE

The symptoms of overdosage, which are usually most severe within 3 hours of ingestion, may include hypotension, somnolence, bradycardia, intra-atrial and intraventricular conduction disturbances, and rarely convulsions and high grade ventricular arrhythmias. Defibrillation as well as infusion of dopamine and isoproterenol have been effective in controlling rhythm and blood pressure. Convulsions have been alleviated with intravenous diazepam. General supportive measures such as mechanical respiratory assistance and external cardiac massage may be necessary.

DOSAGE AND ADMINISTRATION

The dose of RYTHMOL (propafenone HCl) must be individually titrated on the basis of response and tolerance. It is recommended that therapy be initiated with 150 mg propafenone given every eight hours (450 mg/day). Dosage may be increased at a minimum of 3 to 4 day intervals to 225 mg every 8 hours (675 mg/day) and, if necessary, to 300 mg every 8 hours (900 mg/day). The usefulness and safety of dosages exceeding 900 mg per day have not been established. In those patients in whom significant widening of the QRS complex or second or third degree AV block occurs, dose reduction should be considered.

As with other antiarrhythmic agents, in the elderly or in patients with marked previous myocardial damage, the dose of RYTHMOL should be increased more gradually during the initial phase of treatment.

HOW SUPPLIED

RYTHMOL (propafenone HCl) tablets are supplied as scored, round, film-coated tablets containing either 150 mg, 225 mg or 300 mg of propafenone hydrochloride and embossed with 150, 225 or 300 and an arched triangle on the same side.

150 mg (white)

—Bottle of 100—NDC #0044-5022-02

—Hospital Unit Dose (100 tablets-strips of 10)—NDC #0044-5022-10

225 mg (white)

—Bottle of 100—NDC #0044-5024-02

—Hospital Unit Dose (100 tablets-strips of 10)—NDC #0044-5024-10

300 mg (white)

—Bottle of 100—NDC #0044-5023-02

—Hospital Unit Dose (100 tablets-strips of 10)—NDC #0044-5023-10

Storage: Store at controlled room temperature, 59° to 86°F (15°–30°C). Dispense in tight, light-resistant container as defined in U.S.P.

Revised September 1992   4906

Shown in Product Identification Guide, page 320

SSD™   ℞
(1% Silver Sulfadiazine) Cream

SSD AF®*
(1% Silver Sulfadiazine) Cream

DESCRIPTION

SSD (1% Silver Sulfadiazine) Cream and SSD AF (1% Silver Sulfadiazine) Cream are topical antibacterial preparations which have as their active antimicrobial ingredient silver sulfadiazine. The active moiety is contained within an opaque, white, water-miscible cream base.

Each 1000 grams of SSD/SSD AF Cream contains 10 grams of silver sulfadiazine.

Inactive Ingredients: cetyl alcohol (SSD Cream only), isopropyl myristate, polyoxyl 40 stearate, propylene glycol, purified water, stearyl alcohol, sodium hydroxide, sorbitan monooleate, white petrolatum; with 0.3% methylparaben, as a preservative.

Silver sulfadiazine has an empirical formula of $C_{10}H_9AgN_4O_2S$, molecular weight of 357.14, and structural formula as shown:

CLINICAL PHARMACOLOGY

Silver sulfadiazine has broad antimicrobial activity. It is bactericidal for many gram-negative and gram-positive bacteria as well as being effective against yeast. Results from *in vitro* testing are listed below.

Sufficient data have been obtained to demonstrate that silver sulfadiazine will inhibit bacteria that are resistant to other antimicrobial agents and that the compound is superior to sulfadiazine.

Studies utilizing radioactive micronized silver sulfadiazine, electron microscopy, and biochemical techniques have revealed that the mechanism of action of silver sulfadiazine on bacteria differs from silver nitrate and sodium sulfadiazine. Silver sulfadiazine acts only on the cell wall to produce its bactericidal effect.

Results of *In Vitro* Testing With
Concentrations of Silver Sulfadiazine
Number of Sensitive Strains/Total Number of
Strains Tested

Genus & Species	50 μg/mL	100 μg/mL
Pseudomonas aeruginosa	130/130	130/130
Pseudomonas maltophilia	7/7	7/7
Enterobacter species	48/50	50/50
Enterobacter cloacae	24/24	24/24
Klebsiella species	53/54	54/54
Escherichia coli	63/63	63/63
Serratia species	27/28	28/28
Providencia mirabilis	53/53	53/53
Morganella morganii	10/10	10/10
Proteus rettgeri	2/2	2/2
Proteus vulgaris	2/2	2/2
Providencia species	1/1	1/1
Citrobacter species	10/10	10/10
Acinetobacter calcoaceticus	10/11	11/11
Staphylococcus aureus	100/101	101/101
Staphylococcus epidermidis	51/51	51/51
β-Hemolytic Streptococcus	4/4	4/4
Enterococcus species	52/53	53/53
Corynebacterium diphtheriae	2/2	2/2
Clostridium perfringens	0/2	2/2
Candida albicans	43/50	50/50

Silver sulfadiazine is not a carbonic anhydrase inhibitor and may be useful in situations where such agents are contraindicated.

INDICATIONS AND USAGE

Silver Sulfadiazine Cream is a topical antimicrobial drug indicated as an adjunct for the prevention and treatment of wound sepsis in patients with second and third degree burns.

CONTRAINDICATIONS

Silver Sulfadiazine Cream is contraindicated in patients who are hypersensitive to silver sulfadiazine or any of the other ingredients in the preparation.

Because sulfonamide therapy is known to increase the possibility of kernicterus, Silver Sulfadiazine Cream should not be used on pregnant women approaching or at term, on premature infants, or on newborn infants during the first 2 months of life.

WARNINGS

There is potential cross-sensitivity between silver sulfadiazine and other sulfonamides. If allergic reactions attributable to treatment with silver sulfadiazine occur, continuation of therapy must be weighed against the potential hazards of the particular allergic reaction.

Fungal proliferation in and below the eschar may occur. However, the incidence of clinically reported fungal superinfection is low.

The use of Silver Sulfadiazine Cream in some cases of glucose-6-phosphate dehydrogenase-deficient individuals may be hazardous, as hemolysis may occur.

PRECAUTION

General: If hepatic and renal functions become impaired and elimination of drug decreases, accumulation may occur and discontinuation of Silver Sulfadiazine Cream should be weighed against the therapeutic benefit being achieved.

In considering the use of topical proteolytic enzymes in conjunction with Silver Sulfadiazine Cream, the possibility should be noted that silver may inactivate such enzymes.

Laboratory Tests: In the treatment of burn wounds involving extensive areas of the body, the serum sulfa concentrations may approach adult therapeutic levels (8 to 12 mg%). Therefore, in these patients it would be advisable to monitor serum sulfa concentrations. Renal function should be carefully monitored and the urine should be checked for sulfa crystals.

Absorption of the propylene glycol vehicle has been reported to affect serum osmolality, which may affect the interpretation of laboratory tests.

Carcinogenesis, Mutagenesis, Impairment of Fertility: Long-term dermal toxicity studies of 24 months duration in rats and 18 months in mice with concentrations of silver sulfadiazine three to ten times the concentration in Silver Sulfadiazine Cream revealed no evidence of carcinogenicity.

Pregnancy: Pregnancy category B. A reproductive study has been performed in rabbits at doses up to three to ten times the concentration of silver sulfadiazine in Silver Sulfadiazine Cream and has revealed no evidence of harm to the fetus due to silver sulfadiazine. There are, however, no adequate and well-controlled studies in pregnant women. Because animal reproduction studies are not always predictive of human response, this drug should be used during pregnancy only if clearly justified, especially in pregnant women approaching or at term (see **CONTRAINDICATIONS**).

Nursing Mothers: It is not known whether Silver Sulfadiazine Cream is excreted in human milk. However, sulfonamides are known to be excreted in human milk, and all sulfonamide derivatives are known to increase the possibility of kernicterus. Because of the possibility for serious adverse reactions in nursing infants from sulfonamides, a decision should be made whether to discontinue nursing or to discontinue the drug, taking into account the importance of the drug to the mother.

Pediatric Use: Safety and effectiveness in children have not been established (see **CONTRAINDICATIONS**).

ADVERSE REACTIONS

Several cases of transient leukopenia have been reported in patients receiving silver sulfadiazine therapy. Leukopenia associated with silver sulfadiazine administration is primarily characterized by decreased neutrophil count. Maximal white blood cell depression occurs within two to four days of initiation of therapy. Rebound to normal leukocyte levels follows onset within two to three days. Recovery is not influenced by continuation of silver sulfadiazine therapy. The incidence of leukopenia in various reports averages about 20%. A higher incidence has been seen in patients treated concurrently with cimetidine.

Other infrequently occurring events include skin necrosis, erythema multiforme, skin discoloration, burning sensation, rashes, and interstitial nephritis.

Reduction in bacterial growth after application of topical antibacterial agents has been reported to permit spontaneous healing of deep partial-thickness burns by preventing conversion of the partial thickness to full thickness by sepsis. However, reduction in bacterial colonization has caused delayed separation, in some cases necessitating escharotomy in order to prevent contracture.

Absorption of silver sulfadiazine varies depending upon the percent of body surface area and the extent of the tissue damage. Although few have been reported, it is possible that any adverse reaction associated with sulfonamides may occur. Some of the reactions which have been associated with sulfonamides are as follows: blood dyscrasias, including agranulocytosis, aplastic anemia, thrombocytopenia, leukopenia and hemolytic anemia; dermatologic and allergic reactions, including Stevens-Johnson syndrome and exfoliative dermatitis; gastrointestinal reactions; hepatitis and hepatocellular necrosis; CNS reactions; and toxic nephrosis.

DOSAGE AND ADMINISTRATION

FOR TOPICAL USE ONLY – NOT FOR OPHTHALMIC USE.

Prompt institution of appropriate regimens for care of the burned patient is of prime importance and includes the control of shock and pain. The burn wounds are then cleansed and debrided and Silver Sulfadiazine Cream is applied under sterile conditions. The burn areas should be covered with Silver Sulfadiazine Cream at all times. The cream should be applied once to twice daily to a thickness of approximately 1/16 inch. Whenever necessary, the cream should be reapplied to any areas from which it has been removed by patient activity. Administration may be accomplished in minimal time because dressings are not required. However, if individual patient requirements make dressings necessary, they may be used.

Reapply immediately after hydrotherapy.

Treatment with Silver Sulfadiazine Cream should be continued until satisfactory healing has occurred or until the burn site is ready for grafting. The drug should not be withdrawn from the therapeutic regimen while there remains the possibility of infection except if a significant adverse reaction occurs.

HOW SUPPLIED

SSD™ (1% Silver Sulfadiazine) **Cream:** white to off-white cream.

50 gram jar 3P4000	NDC 0044-2100-71
400 gram jar 3P4007	NDC 0044-2100-70
1000 gram jar 3P4009	NDC 0044-2100-73
25 gram tube	NDC 0044-2100-77
50 gram tube	NDC 0044-2100-78
85 gram tube	NDC 0044-2100-79

SSD AF®* (1% Silver Sulfadiazine) **Cream:** white to off-white cream.

50 gram jar 3P4010	NDC 0044-2110-71
400 gram jar 3P4017	NDC 0044-2110-70
1000 gram jar 3P4019	NDC 0044-2110-73

***Alternate Formula**

Store at controlled room temperature 15°–30°C (59°–86°F).

CAUTION: Federal (USA) law prohibits dispensing without prescription.

Rev. 5/13/95 9029-00

VICODIN HP™ Ⓒ℞

[vīkō-dīn]

(hydrocodone bitartrate* and acetaminophen tablets, USP) 10 mg/660 mg

***Warning:** May be habit forming

DESCRIPTION

Hydrocodone bitartrate and acetaminophen is supplied in tablet form for oral administration.

Hydrocodone bitartrate is an opioid analgesic and antitussive and occurs as fine, white crystals or as a crystalline powder. It is affected by light. The chemical name is 4,5α-epoxy-3-methoxy-17-methylmorphinan-6-one tartrate (1:1) hydrate (2:5). It has the following structural formula:

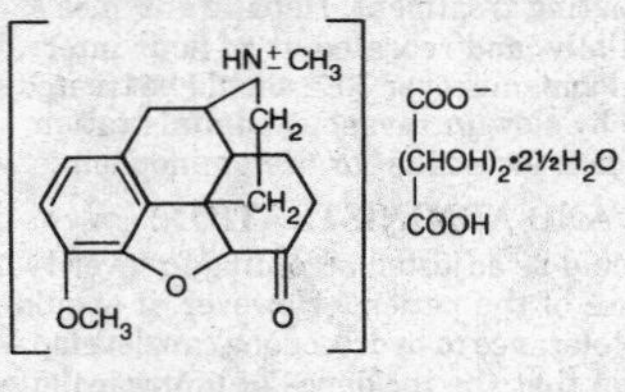

$C_{18}H_{21}NO_3 \cdot C_4H_6O_6 \cdot 2^{1/2}H_2O$ M.W.=494.50

Acetaminophen, 4'-hydroxyacetanilide, a slightly bitter, white, odorless, crystalline powder, is a non-opiate, non-salicylate analgesic and antipyretic. It has the following structural formula:

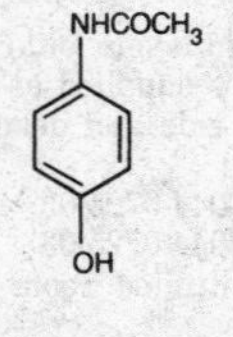

$C_8H_9NO_2$ M.W.=151.17

Each VICODIN HP™ tablet contains:

Hydrocodone Bitartrate	10 mg
(**WARNING:** May be habit forming.)	
Acetaminophen	660 mg

In addition each tablet contains the following inactive ingredients: colloidal silicon dioxide, croscarmellose sodium, magnesium stearate, microcrystalline cellulose, povidone, pregelatinized starch, and stearic acid.

CLINICAL PHARMACOLOGY

Hydrocodone is a semisynthetic narcotic analgesic and antitussive with multiple actions qualitatively similar to those of codeine. Most of these involve the central nervous system and smooth muscle. The precise mechanism of action of hydrocodone and other opiates is not known, although it is believed to relate to the existence of opiate receptors in the central nervous system. In addition to analgesia, narcotics may produce drowsiness, changes in mood and mental clouding.

The analgesic action of acetaminophen involves peripheral influences, but the specific mechanism is as yet undetermined. Antipyretic activity is mediated through hypothalamic heat regulating centers. Acetaminophen inhibits prostaglandin synthetase. Therapeutic doses of acetaminophen have negligible effects on the cardiovascular or respiratory systems; however, toxic doses may cause circulatory failure and rapid, shallow breathing.

Pharmacokinetics: The behavior of the individual components is described below.

Hydrocodone: Following a 10mg oral dose of hydrocodone administered to five adult male subjects, the mean peak concentration was 23.6 ± 5.2ng/mL. Maximum serum levels were achieved at 1.3 ± 0.3 hours and the half-life was determined to be 3.8 ± 0.3 hours. Hydrocodone exhibits a complex pattern of metabolism including O-demethylation, N-demethylation and 6-keto reduction to the corresponding 6-α- and 6-β- hydroxymetabolites. See OVERDOSAGE for toxicity information.

Acetaminophen: Acetaminophen is rapidly absorbed from the gastrointestinal tract and is distributed throughout most body tissues. The plasma half-life is 1.25 to 3 hours, but may be increased by liver damage and following overdosage. Elimination of acetaminophen is principally by liver metabolism (conjugation) and subsequent renal excretion of metabolites. Approximately 85% of an oral dose appears in the urine within 24 hours of administration, most as the glucuronide conjugate, with small amounts of other conjugates and unchanged drug. See OVERDOSAGE for toxicity information.

INDICATIONS AND USAGE

VICODIN HP™ tablets are indicated for the relief of moderate to moderately severe pain.

CONTRAINDICATIONS

This product should not be administered to patients who have previously exhibited hypersensitivity to hydrocodone or acetaminophen.

WARNINGS

Respiratory Depression: At high doses or in sensitive patients, hydrocodone may produce dose-related respiratory depression by acting directly on the brain stem respiratory center. Hydrocodone also affects the center that controls respiratory rhythm, and may produce irregular and periodic breathing.

Head injury and Increased Intracranial Pressure: The respiratory depressant effects of narcotics and their capacity to elevate cerebrospinal fluid pressure may be markedly exaggerated in the presence of head injury, other intracranial lesions or a preexisting increase in intracranial pressure. Furthermore, narcotics produce adverse reactions which may obscure the clinical course of patients with head injuries.

Acute Abdominal Conditions: The administration of narcotics may obscure the diagnosis or clinical course of patients with acute abdominal conditions.

PRECAUTIONS

General

Special Risk Patients: As with any narcotic analgesic agent, VICODIN HP™ Tablets should be used with caution in elderly or debilitated patients, and those with severe impairment of hepatic or renal function, hypothyroidism, Addison's disease, prostatic hypertrophy or urethral stricture. The usual precautions should be observed and the possibility of respiratory depression should be kept in mind.

Cough Reflex: Hydrocodone suppresses the cough reflex; as with all narcotics, caution should be exercised when VICODIN HP™ Tablets are used postoperatively and in patients with pulmonary disease.

Information for Patients: Hydrocodone, like all narcotics, may impair the mental and/or physical abilities required for the performance of potentially hazardous tasks such as driving a car or operating machinery; patients should be cautioned accordingly.

Alcohol and other CNS depressants may produce an additive CNS depression, when taken with this combination product, and should be avoided.

Hydrocodone may be habit forming. Patients should take the drug only for as long as it is prescribed, in the amounts prescribed, and no more frequently than prescribed.

Laboratory Tests: In patients with severe hepatic or renal disease, effects of therapy should be monitored with serial liver and/or renal function tests.

Drug Interactions: Patients receiving narcotics, antihistamines, antipsychotics, antianxiety agents, or other CNS depressants (including alcohol) concomitantly with VICODIN HP™ Tablets may exhibit an additive CNS depression. When combined therapy is contemplated, the dose of one or both agents should be reduced.

The use of MAO inhibitors or tricyclic antidepressant with hydrocodone preparations may increase the effect of either the antidepressant or hydrocodone.

Drug/Laboratory Test Interactions: Acetaminophen may produce false-positive test results for urinary 5-hydroxyindoleacetic acid.

Carcinogenesis, Mutagenesis, Impairment of Fertility: No adequate studies have been conducted in animals to determine whether hydrocodone or acetaminophen have a poten-

Continued on next page

Knoll Laboratories—Cont.

tial for carcinogenesis, mutagenesis, or impairment of fertility.

Pregnancy

Teratogenic Effects: Pregnancy Category C. There are no adequate and well-controlled studies in pregnant women. VICODIN HP™ Tablets should be used during pregnancy only if the potential benefit justifies the potential risk to the fetus.

Nonteratogenic Effects: Babies born to mothers who have been taking opioids regularly prior to delivery will be physically dependent. The withdrawal signs include irritability and excessive crying, tremors, hyperactive reflexes, increased respiratory rate, increased stools, sneezing, yawning, vomiting, and fever. The intensity of the syndrome does not always correlate with the duration of maternal opioid use or dose. There is no consensus on the best method of managing withdrawal.

Labor and Delivery: As with all narcotics, administration of VICODIN HP™ Tablets to the mother shortly before delivery may result in some degree of respiratory depression in the newborn, especially if higher doses are used.

Nursing Mothers: Acetaminophen is excreted in breast milk in small amounts, but the significance of its effects on nursing infants is not known. It is not known whether hydrocodone is excreted in human milk. Because many drugs are excreted in human milk and because of the potential for serious adverse reactions in nursing infants from hydrocodone and acetaminophen, a decision should be made whether to discontinue nursing or to discontinue the drug, taking into account the importance of the drug to the mother.

Pediatric Use: Safety and effectiveness in the pediatric population have not been established.

ADVERSE REACTIONS

The most frequently reported adverse reactions are lightheadedness, dizziness, sedation, nausea and vomiting. These effects seem to be more prominent in ambulatory than in nonambulatory patients, and some of these adverse reactions may be alleviated if the patient lies down.

Other adverse reactions include:

Central Nervous System: Drowsiness, mental clouding, lethargy, impairment of mental and physical performance, anxiety, fear, dysphoria, psychic dependence, mood changes.

Gastrointestinal System: Prolonged administration of VICODIN HP™ Tablets may produce constipation.

Genitourinary System: Ureteral spasm, spasm of vesical sphincters and urinary retention have been reported with opiates.

Respiratory Depression: Hydrocodone bitartrate may produce dose-related respiratory depression by acting directly on the brain stem respiratory centers (see OVERDOSAGE).

Dermatological: Skin rash, pruritus.

The following adverse drug events may be borne in mind as potential effects of acetaminophen: allergic reactions, rash, thrombocytopenia, agranulocytosis.

Potential effects of high dosage are listed in the OVERDOSAGE section.

DRUG ABUSE AND DEPENDENCE

Controlled Substance: VICODIN HP™ Tablets are classified as a Schedule Ⓒ III controlled substance.

Abuse and Dependence: Psychic dependence, physical dependence, and tolerance may develop upon repeated administration of narcotics; therefore, VICODIN HP™ Tablets should be prescribed and administered with caution. However, psychic dependence is unlikely to develop when VICODIN HP™ Tablets are used for a short time for the treatment of pain.

Physical dependence, the condition in which continued administration of the drug is required to prevent the appearance of a withdrawal syndrome, assumes clinically significant proportions only after several weeks of continued narcotic use, although some mild degree of physical dependence may develop after a few days of narcotic therapy. Tolerance, in which increasingly large doses are required in order to produce the same degree of analgesia, is manifested initially by a shortened duration of analgesic effect, and subsequently by decreases in the intensity of analgesia. The rate of development of tolerance varies among patients.

OVERDOSAGE

Following an acute overdosage, toxicity may result from hydrocodone or acetaminophen.

Signs and Symptoms:

Hydrocodone: Serious overdose with hydrocodone is characterized by respiratory depression (a decrease in respiratory rate and/or tidal volume, Cheyne-Stokes respiration, cyanosis), extreme somnolence progressing to stupor or coma, skeletal muscle flaccidity, cold and clammy skin, and sometimes bradycardia and hypotension. In severe overdosage, apnea, circulatory collapse, cardiac arrest and death may occur.

Acetaminophen: In acetaminophen overdosage: dose-dependent, potentially fatal hepatic necrosis is the most serious adverse effect. Renal tubular necrosis, hypoglycemic coma, and thrombocytopenia may also occur.

Early symptoms following a potentially hepatotoxic overdose may include: nausea, vomiting, diaphoresis and general malaise. Clinical and laboratory evidence of hepatic toxicity may not be apparent until 48 to 72 hours post-ingestion.

In adults, hepatic toxicity has rarely been reported with acute overdoses of less than 10 grams, or fatalities with less than 15 grams.

Treatment: A single or multiple overdose with hydrocodone and acetaminophen is a potentially lethal polydrug overdose, and consultation with a regional poison control center is recommended.

Immediate treatment includes support of cardiorespiratory function and measures to reduce drug absorption. Vomiting should be induced mechanically, or with syrup of ipecac, if the patient is alert (adequate pharyngeal and laryngeal reflexes). Oral activated charcoal (1 g/kg) should follow gastric emptying. The first dose should be accompanied by an appropriate cathartic. If repeated doses are used, the cathartic might be included with alternate doses as required. Hypotension is usually hypovolemic and should respond to fluids. Vasopressors and other supportive measures should be employed as indicated. A cuffed endo-tracheal tube should be inserted before gastric lavage of the unconscious patient and, when necessary, to provide assisted respiration.

Meticulous attention should be given to maintaining adequate pulmonary ventilation. In severe cases of intoxication, peritoneal dialysis, or preferably hemodialysis may be considered. If hypoprothrombinemia occurs due to acetaminophen overdose, vitamin K should be administered intravenously.

Naloxone, a narcotic antagonist, can reverse respiratory depression and coma associated with opioid overdose. Naloxone, hydrochloride 0.4 mg to 2 mg is given parenterally. Since the duration of action of hydrocodone may exceed that of the naloxone, the patient should be kept under continuous surveillance and repeated doses of antagonist should be administered as needed to maintain adequate respiration. A narcotic antagonist should not be administered in the absence of clinically significant respiratory or cardiovascular depression.

If the dose of acetaminophen may have exceeded 140 mg/kg, acetylcysteine should be administered as early as possible. Serum acetaminophen levels should be obtained, since levels four or more hours following ingestion help predict acetaminophen toxicity. Do not await acetaminophen assay results before initiating treatment. Hepatic enzymes should be obtained initially, and repeated at 24-hour intervals.

Methemoglobinemia over 30% should be treated with methylene blue by slow intravenous administration.

The toxic dose for adults for acetaminophen is 10 g.

DOSAGE AND ADMINISTRATION:

Dosage should be adjusted according to severity of pain and the response of the patient. However, it should be kept in mind that tolerance to hydrocodone can develop with continued use and that the incidence of untoward effects is dose related.

The usual adult dosage is one tablet every four to six hours as needed for pain. The total daily dosage should not exceed 6 tablets.

HOW SUPPLIED:

VICODIN HP™ (hydrocodone bitartrate and acetaminophen, 10 mg/660 mg) is supplied as a white, oval-shaped, tablet bisected on one side and debossed with "VICODIN HP" on the other side.

Bottles of 100-NDC #0044-0725-02

Bottles of 500-NDC #0044-0725-03

Storage: Store at controlled room temperature 15°-30°C (59°-86°F).

Dispense in a tight, light-resistant container as defined in the USP.

Caution: Federal law prohibits dispensing without prescription.

A Schedule Ⓒ III Narcotic.

Revised: May 1996

Knoll Laboratories
A Division of
Knoll Pharmaceutical Company
Mount Olive, New Jersey 07828

BASF Pharma

0900005-3

Shown in Product Identification Guide, page 320

VICODIN® TABLETS Ⓒ III ℞

[*vī'kō-dĭn*]

DESCRIPTION

Each VICODIN® tablet contains:

Hydrocodone Bitartrate	5 mg
(WARNING: May be habit forming.)	
Acetaminophen	500 mg

Other ingredients include colloidal silicon dioxide, corn starch, croscarmellose sodium, dibasic calcium phosphate, magnesium stearate, microcrystalline cellulose, povidone, and stearic acid.

Hydrocodone bitartrate is an opioid analgesic and antitussive and occurs as fine, white crystals or as a crystalline powder. It is affected by light. The chemical name is: 4,5α epoxy-3-methoxy-17-methylmorphinan-6-one tartrate (1:1) hydrate (2:5).

Its structure is as follows:

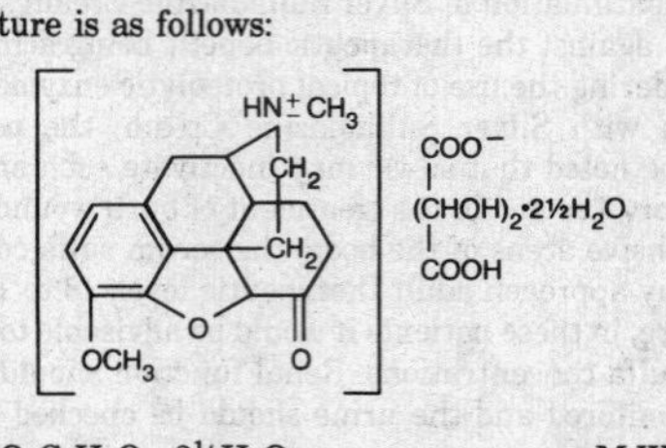

$C_{18}H_{21}NO_3C_4H_6O_6 \cdot 2\frac{1}{2}H_2O$ M.W. 494.50

Acetaminophen, 4′-hydroxyacetanilide, is a non-opiate, non-salicylate analgesic and antipyretic which occurs as a white, odorless crystalline powder possessing a slightly bitter taste.

Its structure is as follows:

$C_8H_9NO_2$ M.W. 151.16

CLINICAL PHARMACOLOGY:

Hydrocodone is a semisynthetic narcotic analgesic and antitussive with multiple actions qualitatively similar to those of codeine. Most of these involve the central nervous system and smooth muscle. The precise mechanism of action of hydrocodone and other opiates is not known, although it is believed to relate to the existence of opiate receptors in the central nervous system. In addition to analgesia, narcotics may produce drowsiness, changes in mood and mental clouding.

Radioimmunoassay techniques have recently been developed for the analysis of hydrocodone in human plasma. After a 10 mg oral dose of hydrocodone bitartrate, a mean peak serum drug level of 23.6 ng/mL and an elimination half-life of 3.8 hours were found.

The analgesic action of acetaminophen involves peripheral and central influences, but the specific mechanism is as yet undetermined. Antipyretic activity is mediated through hypothalmic heat regulating centers. Acetaminophen inhibits prostaglandin synthetase. Therapeutic doses of acetaminophen have negligible effects on the cardiovascular or respiratory systems; however, toxic doses may cause circulatory failure and rapid, shallow breathing. Acetaminophen is rapidly and almost completely absorbed from the gastrointestinal tract, producing maximum serum concentrations within 30 minutes to one hour. The plasma half-life in adults and children ranges from 0.90 hours to 3.25 hours with an average of approximately 2 hours. The drug distributes uniformly in most body fluids and is approximately 25% protein bound. Acetaminophen is conjugated in the liver, with less than 3% of the dose excreted unchanged in 24 hours. The primary metabolic pathway is conjugation to sulfate and glucuronide by-products. A minor oxidative pathway forms cysteine and mercapturic acid. These compounds are subsequently excreted by the kidneys into the urine.

INDICATIONS AND USAGE

For the relief of moderate to moderately severe pain.

CONTRAINDICATIONS

Hypersensitivity to acetaminophen or hydrocodone.

WARNINGS

Respiratory Depression: At high doses or in sensitive patients, hydrocodone may produce dose-related respiratory depression by acting directly on the brain stem respiratory center. Hydrocodone also affects the center that controls respiratory rhythm, and may produce irregular and periodic breathing.

Head Injury and Increased Intracranial Pressure: The respiratory depressant effects of narcotics and their capacity to elevate cerebrospinal fluid pressure may be markedly exaggerated in the presence of head injury, other intracranial lesions or a preexisting increase in intracranial pressure. Furthermore, narcotics produce adverse reactions which may obscure the clinical course of patients with head injuries.

Acute Abdominal Conditions: The administration of narcotics may obscure the diagnosis or clinical course of patients with acute abdominal conditions.

PRECAUTIONS

Special Risk Patients: As with any narcotic analgesic agent, VICODIN Tablets should be used with caution in el-

derly or debilitated patients and those with severe impairment of hepatic or renal function, hypothyroidism, Addison's disease, prostatic hypertrophy or urethral stricture. The usual precautions should be observed and the possibility of respiratory depression should be kept in mind.

Information for Patients: VICODIN Tablets, like all narcotics, may impair the mental and/or physical abilities required for the performance of potentially hazardous tasks such as driving a car or operating machinery; patients should be cautioned accordingly.

Cough Reflex: Hydrocodone suppresses the cough reflex; as with all narcotics, caution should be exercised when VICODIN Tablets are used postoperatively and in patients with pulmonary disease.

Drug Interactions: Patients receiving other narcotic analgesics, antipsychotics, antianxiety agents, or other CNS depressants (including alcohol) concomitantly with VICODIN Tablets may exhibit an additive CNS depression. When combined therapy is contemplated, the dose of one or both agents should be reduced.

The use of MAO inhibitors or tricyclic antidepressants with hydrocodone preparations may increase the effect of either the antidepressant or hydrocodone.

The concurrent use of anticholinergics with hydrocodone may produce paralytic ileus.

Usage in Pregnancy

Teratogenic Effects: Pregnancy Category C. Hydrocodone has been shown to be teratogenic in hamsters when given in doses 700 times the human dose. There are no adequate and well-controlled studies in pregnant women. VICODIN Tablets should be used during pregnancy only if the potential benefit justifies the potential risk to the fetus.

Nonteratogenic Effects: Babies born to mothers who have been taking opioids regularly prior to delivery will be physically dependent. The withdrawal signs include irritability and excessive crying, tremors, hyperactive reflexes, increased respiratory rate, increased stools, sneezing, yawning, vomiting, and fever. The intensity of the syndrome does not always correlate with the duration of maternal opioid use or dose. There is not consensus on the best method of managing withdrawal. Chlorpromazine 0.7 to 1.0 mg/kg q6h, and paregoric 2 to 4 drops/kg q4h, have been used to treat withdrawal symptoms in infants. The duration of therapy is 4 to 28 days, with the dosage decreased as tolerated.

Labor and Delivery: As with all narcotics, administration of VICODIN Tablets to the mother shortly before delivery may result in some degree of respiratory depression in the newborn, especially if higher doses are used.

Nursing Mothers: It is not known whether this drug is excreted in human milk. Because many drugs are excreted in human milk and because of the potential for serious adverse reactions in nursing infants from VICODIN Tablets, a decision should be made whether to discontinue nursing or to discontinue the drug, taking into account the importance of the drug to the mother.

Pediatric Use: Safety and effectiveness in children have not been established.

ADVERSE REACTIONS

The most frequently observed adverse reactions include lightheadedness, dizziness, sedation, nausea and vomiting. These effects seem to be more prominent in ambulatory than in nonambulatory patients and some of these adverse reactions may be alleviated if the patient lies down.

Other adverse reactions include:

Central Nervous System: Drowsiness, mental clouding, lethargy, impairment of mental and physical performance, anxiety, fear, dysphoria, psychic dependence, mood changes.

Gastrointestinal System: The antiemetic phenothiazines are useful in suppressing the nausea and vomiting which may occur (see above); however, some phenothiazine derivatives seem to be antianalgesic and to increase the amount of narcotic required to produce pain relief, while other phenothiazines reduce the amount of narcotic required to produce a given level of analgesia. Prolonged administration of VICODIN Tablets may produce constipation.

Genitourinary System: Ureteral spasm, spasm of vesical sphincters and urinary retention have been reported.

Respiratory Depression: Hydrocodone bitartrate may produce dose-related respiratory depression by acting directly on the brain stem respiratory center. Hydrocodone also affects the center that controls respiratory rhythm, and may produce irregular and periodic breathing. If significant respiratory depression occurs, it may be antagonized by the use of naloxone hydrochloride. Apply other supportive measures when indicated.

DRUG ABUSE AND DEPENDENCE:

VICODIN Tablets are subject to the Federal Controlled Substance Act (Schedule CIII).

Psychic dependence, physical dependence, and tolerance may develop upon repeated administration of narcotics; therefore, VICODIN Tablets should be prescribed and administered with caution. However, psychic dependence is unlikely to develop when VICODIN Tablets are used for a short time for the treatment of pain.

Physical dependence, the condition in which continued administration of the drug is required to prevent the appearance of a withdrawal syndrome, assumes clinically significant proportions only after several weeks of continued narcotic use, although some mild degree of physical dependence may develop after a few days of narcotic therapy. Tolerance, in which increasingly large doses are required in order to produce the same degree of analgesia, is manifested initially by a shortened duration of analgesic effect, and subsequently by decreases in the intensity of analgesia. The rate of development of tolerance varies among patients.

OVERDOSAGE

Acetaminophen:

Signs and Symptoms: In acute acetaminophen overdosage, dose-dependent, potentially fatal hepatic necrosis is the most serious adverse effect. Renal tubular necrosis, hypoglycemic coma, and thrombocytopenia may also occur.

In adults, hepatic toxicity has rarely been reported with acute overdoses of less than 10 grams and fatalities with less than 15 grams. Importantly, young children seem to be more resistant than adults to the hepatotoxic effect of an acetaminophen overdose. Despite this, the measures outlined below should be initiated in any adult or child suspected of having ingested an acetaminophen overdose.

Early symptoms following a potentially hepatotoxic overdose may include: nausea, vomiting, diaphoresis and general malaise. Clinical and laboratory evidence of hepatic toxicity may not be apparent until 48 to 72 hours post-ingestion.

Treatment: The stomach should be emptied promptly by lavage or by induction of emesis with syrup of ipecac. Patients' estimates of the quantity of a drug ingested are notoriously unreliable. Therefore, if an acetaminophen overdose is suspected, a serum acetaminophen assay should be obtained as early as possible, but no sooner than four hours following ingestion. Liver function studies should be obtained initially and repeated at 24-hour intervals.

The antidote, N-acetylcysteine, should be administered as early as possible, preferably within 16 hours of the overdose ingestion for optimal results, but in any case, within 24 hours. Following recovery, there are no residual, structural or functional hepatic abnormalities.

Hydrocodone:

Signs and Symptoms: Serious overdose with hydrocodone is characterized by respiratory depression (a decrease in respiratory rate and/or tidal volume, Cheyne-Stokes respiration, cyanosis), extreme somnolence progressing to stupor or coma, skeletal muscle flaccidity, cold and clammy skin, and sometimes bradycardia and hypotension. In severe overdosage, apnea, circular collapse, cardiac arrest and death may occur.

Treatment: Primary attention should be given to the reestablishment of adequate respiratory exchange through provision of a patent airway and the institution of assisted or controlled ventilation. The narcotic antagonist naloxone is a specific antidote against respiratory depression which may result from overdosage or unusual sensitivity to narcotics, including hydrocodone. Therefore, an appropriate dose of naloxone hydrochloride (see package insert) should be administered, preferably by the intravenous route, and simultaneously with efforts at respiratory resuscitation.

Since the duration of action of hydrocodone may exceed that of the antagonist, the patient should be kept under continued surveillance and repeated doses of the antagonist should be administered as needed to maintain adequate respiration.

An antagonist should not be administered in the absence of clinically significant respiratory or cardiovascular depression. Oxygen, intravenous fluids, vasopressors and other supportive measures should be employed as indicated.

Gastric emptying may be useful in removing unabsorbed drug.

DOSAGE AND ADMINISTRATION

Dosage should be adjusted according to the severity of the pain and the response of the patient. However, it should be kept in mind that tolerance to hydrocodone can develop with continued use and that the incidence of untoward effects is dose related.

The usual adult dosage is one or two tablets every four to six hours as needed for pain. The total 24 hour dose should not exceed 8 tablets.

HOW SUPPLIED

VICODIN is supplied as white, capsule-shaped tablets containing 5 mg hydrocodone bitartrate and 500 mg acetaminophen, bisected on one side and imprinted with "VICODIN" on the other.

Bottles of 100—NDC #0044-0727-02.

Bottles of 500—NDC #0044-0727-03.

Hospital Unit Dose Package—100 tablets (4×25 tablets)—NDC#0044-0727-41.

Storage: Store at controlled room temperature 15°–30°C (59°–86°F).

Dispense in a tight, light-resistant container as defined in the USP.

A Schedule CIII Narcotic.

MR 1987/5809

Vic5883-1092

Revised October, 1992 5883

Shown in Product Identification Guide, page 320

VICODIN ES® TABLETS CIII ℞

(hydrocodone bitartrate 7.5 mg
[Warning: May be habit forming]
and acetaminophen 750 mg)

DESCRIPTION

Each VICODIN ES® tablet contains: Hydrocodone Bitartrate 7.5 mg (**WARNING:** May be habit forming) and Acetaminophen 750 mg

Other ingredients include colloidal silicon dioxide, corn starch, croscarmellose sodium, magnesium stearate, povidone, and stearic acid.

Hydrocodone bitartrate is an opioid analgesic and antitussive and occurs as fine, white crystals or as a crystalline powder. It is affected by light. The chemical name is: 4,5α-epoxy-3-methoxy-17-methylmorphinan-6-one tartrate (1:1) hydrate (2:5). Its structure is as follows:

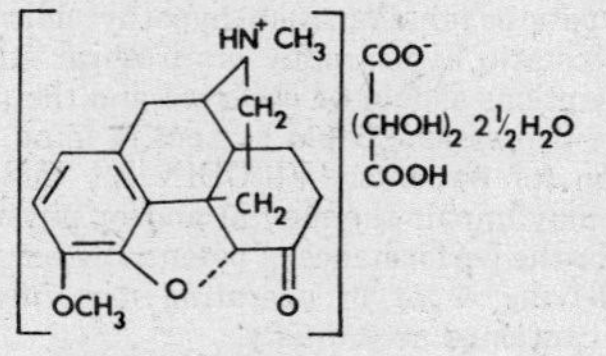

$C_{18}H_{21}NO_3 \cdot C_4H_6O_6 \cdot 2\frac{1}{2} H_2O$ M.W. 494.50

Acetaminophen, 4'-hydroxyacetanilide, is a non-opiate, non-salicylate analgesic and antipyretic which occurs as a white, odorless crystalline powder possessing a slightly bitter taste. Its structure is as follows:

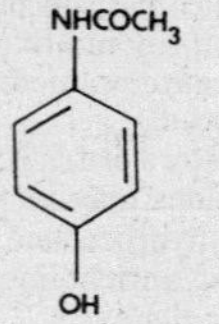

$C_8H_9NO_2$ M.W.151.16

CLINICAL PHARMACOLOGY

Hydrocodone is a semisynthetic narcotic analgesic and antitussive with multiple actions qualitatively similar to those of codeine. Most of these involve the central nervous system and smooth muscle. The precise mechanism of action of hydrocodone and other opiates is not known, although it is believed to relate to the existence of opiate receptors in the central nervous system. In addition to analgesia, narcotics may produce drowsiness, changes in mood and mental clouding.

Radioimmunoassay techniques have recently been developed for the analysis of hydrocodone in human plasma. After a 10 mg oral dose of hydrocodone bitartrate, a mean peak serum drug level of 23.6 ng/mL and an elimination half life of 3.8 hours were found.

The analgesic action of acetaminophen involves peripheral and central influences, but the specific mechanism is as yet undetermined. Antipyretic activity is mediated through hypothalamic heat regulating centers. Acetaminophen inhibits prostaglandin synthetase. Therapeutic doses of acetaminophen have negligible effects on the cardiovascular or respiratory systems; however, toxic doses may cause circulatory failure and rapid, shallow breathing. Acetaminophen is rapidly and almost completely absorbed from the gastrointestinal tract, producing maximum serum concentrations within 30 minutes to one hour. The plasma half-life in adults and children ranges from 0.90 hours to 3.25 hours with an average of approximately 2 hours. The drug distributes uniformly in most body fluids and is approximately 25% protein bound. Acetaminophen is conjugated in the liver, with less than 3% of the dose excreted unchanged in 24 hours. The primary metabolic pathway is conjugation to sulfate and glucuronide by-products. A minor oxidative pathway forms cysteine and mercapturic acid. These compounds are subsequently excreted by the kidneys into the urine.

INDICATIONS AND USAGE

For the relief of moderate to moderately severe pain.

CONTRAINDICATIONS

Hypersensitivity to acetaminophen or hydrocodone.

Continued on next page

Knoll Laboratories—Cont.

WARNINGS

Respiratory Depression: At high doses or in sensitive patients, hydrocodone may produce dose-related respiratory depression by acting directly on the brain stem respiratory center. Hydrocodone also affects the center that controls respiratory rhythm, and may produce irregular and periodic breathing.

Head Injury and Increased Intracranial Pressure: The respiratory depressant effects of narcotics and their capacity to elevate cerebrospinal fluid pressure may be markedly exaggerated in the presence of head injury, other intracranial lesions or a preexisting increase in intracranial pressure. Furthermore, narcotics produce adverse reactions which may obscure the clinical course of patients with head injuries.

Acute Abdominal Conditions: The administration of narcotics may obscure the diagnosis or clinical course of patients with acute abdominal conditions.

PRECAUTIONS

Special Risk Patients: As with any narcotic analgesic agent, VICODIN ES Tablets should be used with caution in elderly or debilitated patients and those with severe impairment of hepatic or renal function, hypothyroidism, Addison's disease, prostatic hypertrophy or urethral stricture. The usual precautions should be observed and the possibility of respiratory depression should be kept in mind.

Information for Patients: VICODIN ES Tablets, like all narcotics, may impair the mental and/or physical abilities required for the performance of potentially hazardous tasks such as driving a car or operating machinery; patients should be cautioned accordingly.

Cough Reflex: Hydrocodone suppresses the cough reflex; as with all narcotics, caution should be exercised when VICODIN ES Tablets are used postoperatively and in patients with pulmonary disease.

Drug Interactions: Patients receiving other narcotic analgesics, antipsychotics, antianxiety agents, or other CNS depressants (including alcohol) concomitantly with VICODIN ES Tablets may exhibit an additive CNS depression. When combined therapy is contemplated, the dose of one or both agents should be reduced.

The use of MAO inhibitors or tricyclic antidepressants with hydrocodone preparations may increase the effect of either the antidepressant or hydrocodone.

The concurrent use of anticholinergics with hydrocodone may produce paralytic ileus.

Usage in Pregnancy:

Teratogenic Effects: Pregnancy Category C. Hydrocodone has been shown to be teratogenic in hamsters when given in doses 700 times the human dose. There are no adequate and well-controlled studies in pregnant women. VICODIN ES Tablets should be used during pregnancy only if the potential benefit justifies the potential risk to the fetus.

Nonteratogenic Effects: Babies born to mothers who have been taking opioids regularly prior to delivery will be physically dependent. The withdrawal signs include irritability and excessive crying, tremors, hyperactive reflexes, increased respiratory rate, increased stools, sneezing, yawning, vomiting, and fever. The intensity of the syndrome does not always correlate with the duration of maternal opioid use or dose. There is no consensus on the best method of managing withdrawal. Chlorpromazine 0.7 to 1 mg/kg q6h, and paregoric 2 to 4 drops/kg q4h, have been used to treat withdrawal symptoms in infants. The duration of therapy is 4 to 28 days, with the dosage decreased as tolerated.

Labor and Delivery: As with all narcotics, administration of VICODIN ES Tablets to the mother shortly before delivery may result in some degree of respiratory depression in the newborn, especially if higher doses are used.

Nursing Mothers: It is not known whether this drug is excreted in human milk. Because many drugs are excreted in human milk and because of the potential for serious adverse reactions in nursing infants from VICODIN ES Tablets, a decision should be made whether to discontinue nursing or to discontinue the drug, taking into account the importance of the drug to the mother.

Pediatric Use: Safety and effectiveness in children have not been established.

ADVERSE REACTIONS

The most frequently observed adverse reactions include lightheadedness, dizziness, sedation, nausea and vomiting. These effects seem to be more prominent in ambulatory than in nonambulatory patients and some of these adverse reactions may be alleviated if the patient lies down.

Other adverse reactions include:

Central Nervous System: Drowsiness, mental clouding, lethargy, impairment of mental and physical performance, anxiety, fear, dysphoria, psychic dependence, mood changes.

Gastrointestinal System: The antiemetic phenothiazines are useful in suppressing the nausea and vomiting which may occur (see above); however, some phenothiazine derivatives seem to be antianalgesic and to increase the amount of narcotic required to produce pain relief, while other phenothiazines reduce the amount of narcotic required to produce a given level of analgesia. Prolonged administration of VICODIN ES Tablets may produce constipation.

Genitourinary System: Ureteral spasm, spasm of vesical sphincters and urinary retention have been reported.

Respiratory Depression: Hydrocodone bitartrate may produce dose-related respiratory depression by acting directly on the brain stem respiratory center. Hydrocodone also affects the center that controls respiratory rhythm, and may produce irregular and periodic breathing.

If significant respiratory depression occurs, it may be antagonized by the use of naloxone hydrochloride. Apply other supportive measures when indicated.

DRUG ABUSE AND DEPENDENCE

VICODIN ES Tablets are subject to the Federal Controlled Substance Act (Schedule CIII)

Psychic dependence, physical dependence, and tolerance may develop upon repeated administration of narcotics; therefore, VICODIN ES Tablets should be prescribed and administered with caution. However, psychic dependence is unlikely to develop when VICODIN ES Tablets are used for a short time for the treatment of pain.

Physical dependence, the condition in which continued administration of the drug is required to prevent the appearance of a withdrawal syndrome, assumes clinically significant proportions only after several weeks of continued narcotic use, although some mild degree of physical dependence may develop after a few days of narcotic therapy. Tolerance, in which increasingly large doses are required in order to produce the same degree of analgesia, is manifested initially by a shortened duration of analgesic effect, and subsequently by decreases in the intensity of analgesia. The rate of development of tolerance varies among patients.

OVERDOSAGE

Acetaminophen:

Signs and Symptoms: In acute acetaminophen overdosage, dose-dependent, potentially fatal hepatic necrosis is the most serious adverse effect. Renal tubular necrosis, hypoglycemic coma, and thrombocytopenia may also occur.

In adults, hepatic toxicity has rarely been reported with acute overdoses of less than 10 grams and fatalities with less than 15 grams. Importantly, young children seem to be more resistant than adults to the hepatotoxic effect of an acetaminophen overdose. Despite this, the measures outlined below should be initiated in any adult or child suspected of having ingested an acetaminophen overdose.

Early symptoms following a potentially hepatotoxic overdose may include: nausea, vomiting, diaphoresis and general malaise. Clinical and laboratory evidence of hepatic toxicity may not be apparent until 48 to 72 hours post-ingestion.

Treatment: The stomach should be emptied promptly by lavage or by induction of emesis with syrup of ipecac. Patients' estimates of the quantity of a drug ingested are notoriously unreliable. Therefore, if an acetaminophen overdose is suspected, a serum acetaminophen assay should be obtained as early as possible, but no sooner than four hours following ingestion. Liver function studies should be obtained initially and repeated at 24-hour intervals.

The antidote, N-acetylcysteine, should be administered as early as possible, preferably within 16 hours of the overdose ingestion for optimal results, but in any case, within 24 hours. Following recovery, there are no residual, structural or functional hepatic abnormalities.

Hydrocodone:

Signs and Symptoms: Serious overdose with hydrocodone is characterized by respiratory depression (a decrease in respiratory rate and/or tidal volume, Cheyne-Stokes respiration, cyanosis), extreme somnolence progressing to stupor or coma, skeletal muscle flaccidity, cold and clammy skin, and sometimes bradycardia and hypotension. In severe overdosage, apnea, circulatory collapse, cardiac arrest and death may occur.

Treatment: Primary attention should be given to the reestablishment of adequate respiratory exchange through provision of a patent airway and the institution of assisted or controlled ventilation. The narcotic antagonist naloxone is a specific antidote against respiratory depression which may result from overdosage or unusual sensitivity to narcotics, including hydrocodone. Therefore, an appropriate dose of naloxone hydrochloride (see package insert) should be administered, preferably by the intravenous route, and simultaneously with efforts at respiratory resuscitation. Since the duration of action of hydrocodone may exceed that of the antagonist, the patient should be kept under continued surveillance and repeated doses of the antagonist should be administered as needed to maintain adequate respiration.

An antagonist should not be administered in the absence of clinically significant respiratory or cardiovascular depression. Oxygen, intravenous fluids, vasopressors and other supportive measures should be employed as indicated.

Gastric emptying may be useful in removing unabsorbed drug.

DOSAGE AND ADMINISTRATION

Dosage should be adjusted according to the severity of the pain and the response of the patient. However, it should be kept in mind that tolerance to hydrocodone can develop with continued use and that the incidence of untoward effects is dose related.

The usual adult dosage is one tablet every four to six hours as needed for pain. The total 24 hour dose should not exceed 5 tablets.

HOW SUPPLIED

VICODIN ES is supplied as a white, oval-shaped, faceted edged tablet containing 7.5 mg hydrocodone bitartrate and 750 mg acetaminophen, bisected on one side and imprinted with "VICODIN ES" on the other side. Bottles of 100—NDC #0044-0728-02. Bottles of 500—NDC #0044-0728-03.

Hospital Unit Dose Package—100 tablets (4×25 tablets)—NDC #0044-0728-41.

Storage: Store at controlled room temperature 15°–30°C (59°–86°F).

Dispense in a tight, light-resistant container as defined in the USP.

A Schedule CIII Narcotic.

Shown in Product Identification Guide, page 320

VICODIN TUSS™ CIII

Expectorant

(hydrocodone bitartrate and guaifenesin)

DESCRIPTION

VICODIN TUSS™ Expectorant Syrup contains hydrocodone (dihydrocodeinone) bitartrate, semi-synthetic centrally-acting narcotic antitussive and guaifenesin, an expectorant for oral administration.

Each teaspoonful (5 mL) contains:

Hydrocodone bitartrate USP .... 5 mg

WARNING: May be habit forming

Guaifenesin USP .... 100 mg

VICODIN TUSS™ Expectorant Syrup also contains: glycerin, L-menthol, methylparaben, propylparaben, propylene glycol, sodium saccharin, sorbitol solution, artificial flavoring, and purified water.

CLINICAL PHARMACOLOGY

Clinical trials have proven hydrocodone bitartrate to be an effective antitussive agent which is pharmacologically 2 to 8 times as potent as codeine. At equi-effective doses, its sedative action is greater than codeine. The precise mechanism of action of hydrocodone and other opiates is not known, however, hydrocodone is believed to act by directly depressing the cough center. In excessive doses hydrocodone, like other opium derivatives, can depress respiration. The effects of hydrocodone in therapeutic doses on the cardiovascular system is insignificant. The constipation effects of hydrocodone are much weaker than that of morphine and no stronger than that of codeine. Hydrocodone can produce miosis, euphoria, physical and psychological dependence. At therapeutic antitussive doses, it does exert analgesic effects. Following a 10 mg oral dose of hydrocodone administered to five male human subjects the mean peak concentration was 23.6 ± 5.2 ng/mL. Maximum serum levels were achieved at 1.3 ± 0.3 hours and half-life was determined to be 3.8 ± 0.3 hours. Hydrocodone exhibits a complex pattern of metabolism including O-demethylation, N-demethylation and 6-ketoreduction to the corresponding 6-α- and 6-β-hydroxymetabolites.

The exact mechanism of action is not established but guaifenesin is believed to act by stimulating receptors in the gastric mucosa that initates a reflex secretion of respiratory tract fluid, thereby increasing the volume and decreasing the viscosity of bronchial secretions. Studies with guaifenesin indicate that it is rapidly absorbed from the gastrointestinal tract and has a half-life of one hour.

INDICATIONS AND USAGE

VICODIN TUSS™ Expectorant is indicated for the symptomatic relief of irritating non-productive cough associated with upper and lower respiratory tract congestion.

CONTRAINDICATIONS

VICODIN TUSS™ Expectorant is contraindicated in patients hypersensitive to hydrocodone or guaifenesin. Patients known to be hypersensitive to other opioids may exhibit cross sensitivity to VICODIN TUSS™ Expectorant. Hydrocodone is contraindicated in the presence of an intracranial lesion associated with increased intracranial pressure; and whenever ventilatory function is depressed.

WARNINGS

May be habit forming. Hydrocodone can produce drug dependence of the morphine type and therefore has the potential for being abused. Psychic dependence, physical dependence and tolerance may develop upon repeated administration of

VICODIN TUSS™ Expectorant and it should be prescribed and administered with the same degree of caution appropriate to the use of other narcotic drugs (see DRUG ABUSE AND DEPENDENCE).

Respiratory Depression: VICODIN TUSS™ Expectorant produces dose-related respiratory depression by directly acting on the brain stem respiratory centers. If respiratory depression occurs, it may be antagonized by the use of naloxone hydrochloride and other supportive measures when indicated.

Head Injury and Increased Intracranial Pressure: The respiratory depressant properties of narcotics and their capacity to elevate cerebrospinal fluid pressure may be markedly exaggerated in the presence of head injury, other intracranial lesions or a pre-existing increase in intracranial pressure. Furthermore, narcotics produce adverse reactions which may obscure the clinical course of patients with head injuries.

Acute Abdominal Conditions: The administration of VICODIN TUSS™ Expectorant or other opioids may obscure the diagnosis or clinical course of patients with acute abdominal conditions.

PRECAUTIONS

Before prescribing medication to suppress or modify cough, it is important to ascertain that the underlying cause of cough is identified, that modification of cough does not increase the risk of clinical or physiologic complications, and that appropriate therapy for the primary disease is provided.

Usage in Ambulatory Patients: Hydrocodone, like all narcotics, may impair the mental and/or physical abilities required for the performance of potentially hazardous tasks such as driving a car or operating machinery, and patients should be warned accordingly.

Drug Interactions: Patients receiving other narcotic analgesics, general anesthetics, phenothiazines, other tranquilizers, sedative hypnotics or other CNS depressants (including alcohol) concomitantly with hydrocodone may exhibit an additive CNS depression. When such combined therapy is contemplated, the dose of one or both agents should be reduced (see WARNINGS).

Laboratory Interactions: The metabolite of guaifenesin has been found to produce an apparent increase in urinary 5-hydroxyindoleacetic acid, and guaifenesin therefore may interfere with the interpretation of this test for the diagnosis of carcinoid syndrome. Guaifenesin administration should be discontinued 24 hours prior to the collection of urine specimens for the determination of 5-hydroxyindoleacetic acid.

Carcinogenesis, mutagenesis, impairment of fertility: Carcinogenicity, mutagenicity and reproduction studies have not been conducted with VICODIN TUSS™ Expectorant.

Usage in Pregnancy: Pregnancy Category C. Animal reproduction studies have not been conducted with VICODIN TUSS™ Expectorant.

It is also not known whether VICODIN TUSS™ Expectorant can cause fetal harm when administered to a pregnant woman or can affect reproductive capacity. VICODIN TUSS™ Expectorant should be given to a pregnant woman only if clearly needed.

Nonteratogenic effects: Babies born to mothers who have been taking opioids regularly prior to delivery will be physically dependent. The withdrawal signs include irritability and excessive crying, tremors, hyperactive reflexes, increased respiratory rate, increased stools, sneezing, yawning, vomiting and fever. The intensity of the syndrome does not always correlate with the duration of maternal opioid use or dose. There is no consensus on the best method of managing withdrawal. Chlorpromazine 0.7–1.0 mg/kg q 6 h, phenobarbital 2 mg/kg q 6 h, and paregoric 2–4 drops/kg q 4 h, have been used to treat withdrawal symptoms in infants. The duration of therapy is 4 to 28 days, with the dosages decreased as tolerated.

Nursing mothers: It is not known whether this drug is excreted in human milk. Because many drugs are excreted in human milk and because of the potential for serious adverse reactions in nursing infants from VICODIN TUSS™ Expectorant, a decision should be made whether to discontinue nursing or discontinue the drug, taking into account the importance of the drug to the mother.

ADVERSE REACTIONS

Respiratory System: Hydrocodone produces dose-related respiratory depression by acting directly on brain stem respiratory centers.

Cardiovascular System: Hypertension, postural hypotension and palpitations.

Genitourinary System: Ureteral spasm, spasm of vesical sphincters and urinary retention have been reported with opiates.

Central Nervous System: Sedation, drowsiness, mental clouding, lethargy, impairment of mental and physical performance, anxiety, fear, dysphoria, dizziness, psychic dependence, mood changes and blurred vision.

Gastrointestinal System: Nausea and vomiting occur more frequently in ambulatory than in recumbent patients.

DRUG ABUSE DEPENDENCE

Special care should be exercised in prescribing hydrocodone for emotionally unstable patients and for those with a history of drug misuse. Such patients should be closely supervised when long-term therapy is contemplated.

VICODIN TUSS™ Expectorant is a Schedule III narcotic. Psychic dependence, physical dependence and tolerance may develop upon repeated administration of narcotics; therefore, VICODIN TUSS™ Expectorant should always be prescribed and administered with caution. Physical dependence is the condition in which continued administration of the drug is required to prevent the appearance of a withdrawal syndrome.

Patients physically dependent on opioids will develop an abstinence syndrome upon abrupt discontinuation of the opioid or following the administration of a narcotic antagonist. The character and severity of the withdrawal symptoms are related to the degree of physical dependence. Manifestations of opioid withdrawal are similar to but milder than that of morphine and include lacrimation, rhinorrhea, yawning, sweating, restlessness, dilated pupils, anorexia, gooseflesh, irritability and tremor. In more severe forms, nausea, vomiting, intestinal spasm and diarrhea, increased heart rate and blood pressure, chills, and pains in bones and muscles of the back and extremities may occur. Peak effects will usually be apparent at 48 to 72 hours.

Treatment of withdrawal is usually managed by providing sufficient quantities of an opioid to suppress **severe** withdrawal symptoms and then gradually reducing the dose of opioid over a period of several days.

OVERDOSAGE

Signs and Symptoms: Serious overdosage with VICODIN TUSS™ Expectorant is characterized by respiratory depression (a decrease in respiratory rate and/or tidal volume, Cheyne-Stokes respiration, cyanosis), extreme somnolence progressing to stupor or coma, skeletal muscle flaccidity, cold and clammy skin, and sometimes bradycardia and hypotension. In severe overdosage apnea, circulatory collapse, cardiac arrest, and death may occur.

Treatment: Primary attention should be given to the reestablishment of adequate respiratory exchange through provision of a patent airway and the institution of assisted or controlled ventilation. The narcotic antagonist naloxone hydrochloride is a specific antidote for respiratory depression which may result from overdosage or unusual sensitivity to narcotics including hydrocodone. Therefore, an appropriate dose of naloxone hydrochloride should be administered, preferably by the intravenous route, simultaneously with efforts at respiratory resuscitation. For further information, see full prescribing information for naloxone hydrochloride. An antagonist should not be administered in the absence of clinically significant respiratory depression. Oxygen, intravenous fluids, vasopressors and other supportive measures should be employed as indicated. Gastric emptying may be useful in removing unabsorbed drug. Activated charcoal may be of benefit.

DOSAGE AND ADMINISTRATION

Usual Adult Dose: One teaspoonful (5 mL) after meals and at bedtime, not less than 4 hours apart (not to exceed 6 teaspoonsful in a 24 hour period). Treatment should be initiated with one teaspoonful and subsequent doses, up to a maximum single dose of 3 teaspoonsful, adjusted if required.

Usual Children's Dose:
Over 12 years: Initial dose 1 teaspoonful; maximum single dose, 2 teaspoonsful.
6 to 12 years: Initial dose ½ teaspoonful; maximum single dose, 1 teaspoonful.

HOW SUPPLIED

VICODIN TUSS™ Expectorant is available in bottles as a colorless, cherry-flavored syrup which contains no sugar, alcohol or dye.
One pint: NDC 0044-0730-16.
Store in a tight, light resistant container as defined in the USP. Keep tightly closed.
Store at controlled room temperature 59°–86°F (15°–30°C).
A Schedule ⒸⒾ Narcotic. Oral prescription where permitted by State Law.

VT100-0493

Shown in Product Identification Guide, page 320

"Cancer Pain Management" (3 credits)
   Home Study Module—Pharmacists

Knoll Pharmaceutical Company
**3000 CONTINENTAL DRIVE NORTH
MOUNT OLIVE, NJ 07828**

BASF Group

Direct Inquiries to:
Knoll Pharmaceutical Company
(201) 426-2600
Customer Service:
(800) 526-0710

For Medical Information Contact:
(800)526-0221

MAVIK®   ℞
[mă′vick]
(Trandolapril) Tablets
PRESCRIBING INFORMATION

> **USE IN PREGNANCY**
> When used in pregnancy during the second and third trimesters, ACE inhibitors can cause injury and even death to the developing fetus. When pregnancy is detected, MAVIK® should be discontinued as soon as possible. See WARNINGS, Fetal/Neonatal Morbidity and Mortality.

DESCRIPTION

Trandolapril is the ethyl ester prodrug of a nonsulfhydryl angiotensin converting enzyme (ACE) inhibitor, trandolaprilat. Trandoapril is chemically described as (2S,3aR,7aS)–1–[(S)–N–[(S)–1–Carboxy–3–phenylpropyl]alanyl]hexahydro–2–indolinecarboxylic acid, 1–ethyl ester. Its empirical formula is $C_{24}H_{34}N_2O_5$ and its structural formula is

R:- C_2H_5: Trandolapril
-H: Trandolaprilat (diacid)

M.W. = 430.54
Melting Point = 125°C

Trandolapril is a colorless, crystalline substance that is soluble (>100 mg/mL) in chloroform, dichloromethane, and methanol. MAVIK® tablets contain 1 mg, 2 mg, or 4 mg of trandolapril for oral administration. Each tablet also contains corn starch, croscarmellose sodium, hydroxypropyl methylcellulose, iron oxide, lactose, povidone, sodium stearyl fumarate.

CLINICAL PHARMACOLOGY

Mechanism of Action:
Trandolapril is deesterified to the diacid metabolite, trandolaprilat, which is approximately eight times more active as an inhibitor of ACE activity. ACE is a peptidyl dipeptidase that catalyzes the conversion of angiotensin I to the vasoconstrictor, angiotensin II. Angiotensin II is a potent peripheral vasoconstrictor that also stimulates secretion of aldosterone by the adrenal cortex and provides negative feedback for renin secretion. The effect of trandolapril in hypertension appears to result primarily from the inhibition of circulating and tissue ACE activity thereby reducing angiotensin II formation, decreasing vasoconstriction, decreasing aldosterone secretion, and increasing plasma renin. Decreased aldosterone secretion leads to diuresis, natriuresis, and a small increase of serum potassium. In controlled clinical trials, treatment with MAVIK® alone resulted in mean increases in potassium of 0.1 mEq/L. (See **PRECAUTIONS**.)

ACE is identical to kininase II, an enzyme that degrades bradykinin, a potent peptide vasodilator; whether increased levels of bradykinin play a role in the therapeutic effect of trandolapril remains to be elucidated.

Continued on next page

Knoll—Cont.

While the principal mechanism of antihypertensive effect is thought to be through the renin–angiotensin–aldosterone system, trandolapril exerts antihypertensive actions even in patients with low–renin hypertension. MAVIK® was an effective antihypertensive in all races studied. Both black patients (usually a predominantly low–renin group) and non–black patients responded to 2 to 4 mg of MAVIK®.

Pharmacokinetics and Metabolism:
Pharmcokinetics Trandolapril's ACE–inhibiting activity is primarily due to its diacid metabolite, trandolaprilat. Cleavage of the ester group of trandolapril, primarily in the liver, is responsible for conversion. Absolute bioavailability after oral administration of trandolapril is about 10% as trandolapril and 70% as trandolaprilat. After oral trandolapril under fasting conditions, peak trandolapril levels occur at about one hour and peak trandolaprilat levels occur between 4 and 10 hours. The elimination half lives of trandolapril and trandolaprilat are about 6 and 10 hours, respectively, but, like all ACE inhibitors, trandolaprilat also has a prolonged terminal elimination phase, involving a small fraction of administered drug, probably representing binding to plasma and tissue ACE. During multiple dosing of trandolapril, there is no significant accumulation of trandolaprilat. Food slows absorption of trandolapril, but does not affect AUC or Cmax of trandolaprilat or Cmax of trandolapril.

Metabolism and Excretion After oral administration of trandolapril, about 33% of parent drug and metabolites are recovered in urine, mostly as trandolaprilat, with about 66% in feces. The extent of the absorbed dose which is biliary excreted has not been determined. Plasma concentrations (Cmax and AUC of trandolapril and Cmax of trandolaprilat) are dose proportional over the 1–4 mg range, but the AUC of trandolaprilat is somewhat less than dose proportional. In addition to trandolaprilat, at least 7 other metabolites have been found, principally glucuronides or deesterificaiton products.

Serum protein binding of trandolapril is about 80%, and is independent of concentration. Binding of trandolaprilat is concentration–dependent, varying from 65% at 1000 ng/mL to 94% at 0.1 ng/mL, indicating saturation of binding with increasing concentration.

The volume of distribution of trandolapril is about 18 liters. Total plasma clearances of trandolapril and trandolaprilat after approximately 2 mg IV doses are about 52 liters/hour and 7 liters/hours respectively. Renal clearance of trandolaprilat varies from 1–4 liters/hour, depending on dose.

Special populations:
Pediatric Trandolapril pharmacokinetics have not been evaluated in patients <18 years of age.
Geriatric and Gender Trandolapril pharmacokinetics have been investigated in the elderly (>65 years) and in both genders. The plasma concentration of trandolapril is increased in elderly hypertensive patients, but the plasma concentration of trandolaprilat and inhibition of ACE activity are similar in elderly and young hypertensive patients. The pharmacokinetics of trandolapril and trandolaprilat and inhibition of ACE activity are similar in male and female elderly hypertensive patients.
Race Pharmacokinetic differences have not been evaluated in different races.
Renal Insufficiency Compared to normal subjects, the plasma concentrations of trandolapril and trandolaprilat are approximately 2–fold greater and renal clearance is reduced by about 85% in patients with creatinine clearence below 30 mL/min and in patients on hemodialysis. Dosage adjustment is recommended in renally impaired patients. (See **DOSAGE** and **ADMINISTRATION**.)
Hepatic Insufficiency Following oral administration in patients with mild to moderate alcoholic cirrhosis, plasma concentrations of trandolapril and trandolaprilat were, respectively, 9–fold and 2–fold greater than in normal subjects, but inhibition of ACE activity was not affected. Lower doses should be considered in patients with hepatic insufficiency. (See **DOSAGE** and **ADMINISTRATION**.)
Drug Interactions Trandolapril did not affect the plasma concentration (pre–dose and 2 hours post–dose) of oral digoxin (0.25 mg). Coadministration of trandolapril and cimetidine led to an increase of about 44% in Cmax for trandolapril, but no difference in the pharmacokinetics of trandolaprilat or in ACE inhibition. Coadministration of trandolapril and furosemide led to an increase of about 25% in the renal clearance of trandolaprilat, but no effect was seen on the pharmacokinetics of furosemide or trandolaprilat or on ACE inhibition.

Pharmacodynamics and Clinical Effects:
A single 2–mg dose of MAVIK® produces 70 to 85% inhibition of plasma ACE activity at 4 hours with about 10% decline at 24 hours and about half the effect manifest at 8 days. Maximum ACE inhibition is achieved with a plasma trandolaprilat concentration of 2 ng/mL. ACE inhibition is a function of trandolaprilat concentration, not trandolapril

concentration. The effect of trandolapril on exogenous angiotensin I was not measured.

Four placebo–controlled dose response studies were conducted using once–daily oral dosing of MAVIK® in doses from 0.25 to 16 mg per day in 827 black and non–black patients with mild to moderate hypertension. The minimal effective once–daily dose was 1 mg in non–black patients and 2 mg in black patients. Further decreases in trough supine diastolic blood pressure were obtained in non–black patients with higher doses, and no further response was seen with doses above 4 mg (up to 16 mg). The antihypertensive effect diminished somewhat at the end of the dosing interval, but trough/peak ratios are well above 50% for all effective doses. There was a slightly greater effect on the diastolic pressure, but no difference on systolic pressure with b.i.d. dosing. During chronic therapy, the maximum reduction in blood pressure with any dose is achieved within one week. Following 6 weeks of monotherapy in placebo–controlled trials in patients with mild to moderate hypertension, once–daily doses of 2 to 4 mg lowered supine or standing systolic/diastolic blood pressure 24 hours after dosing by an average 7–10/4–5 mmHg below placebo responses in non–black patients. Once–daily doses of 2 to 4 mg lowered blood pressure 4–6/3–4 mmHg in black patients. Trough to peak ratios for effective doses ranged from 0.5 to 0.9 . There were no differences in response between men and women, but responses were somewhat greater in patients under 60 than in patients over 60 years old. Abrupt withdrawal of MAVIK® has not been associated with a rapid increase in blood pressure.

Administration of MAVIK® to patients with mild to moderate hypertension results in a reduction of supine, sitting and standing blood pressure to about the same extent without compensatory tachycardia.

Symptomatic hypertension is infrequent, although it can occur in patients who are salt–and/or volume–depleted. (See WARNINGS.) Use of MAVIK® in combination with thiazide diuretics gives a blood pressure lowering effect greater than that seen with either agent alone, and the additional effect of trandolapril is similar to the effect of monotherapy.

INDICATIONS AND USAGE

MAVIK® is indicated for the treatment of hypertension. It may be used alone or in combination with other antihypertensive medication such as hydrochlorothiazide.

In considering the use of MAVIK®, it should be noted that in controlled trials ACE inhibitors (for which adequate data are available) cause a higher rate of angioedema in black than in non–black patients. (See **WARNINGS: Angioedema**.)

When using MAVIK®, consideration should be given to the fact that another angiotensin converting enzyme inhibitor, captopril, has caused agranulocytosis, particularly in patients with renal impairment or collagen–vascular disease. Available data are insufficient to show that MAVIK® does not have a similar risk. (See WARNINGS.)

CONTRAINDICATIONS

MAVIK® is contraindicated in patients who are hypersensitive to this product and in patients with a history of angioedema related to previous treatment with an ACE inhibitor.

WARNINGS

Anaphylactoid and Possibly Related Reactions:
Presumably because angiotensin converting enzyme inhibitors affect the metabolism of eicosanoids and polypeptides, including endogenous bradykinin, patients receiving ACE inhibitors, including MAVIK®, may be subject to a variety of adverse reactions, some of them serious.
Angioedema:
Angioedema of the face, extremities, lips, tongue, glottis, and larynx has been reported in patients treated with ACE inhibitors including MAVIK®. Symptoms suggestive of angioedema or facial edema occurred in 0.13% of MAVIK®–treated patients. Two of the four cases were life–threatening and resolved without treatment or with medication (corticosteroids). Angioedema associated with laryngeal edema can be fatal. If laryngeal stridor or angioedema of the face, tongue or glottis occurs, treatment with MAVIK® should be discontinued immediately, the patient treated in accordance with accepted medical care and carefully observed until the swelling disappears. In instances where swelling is confined to the face and lips, the condition generally resolves without treatment; antihistamines may be useful in relieving symptoms. **Where there is involvement of the tongue, glottis, or larynx, likely to cause airway obstruction, emergency therapy, including but not limited to subcutaneous epinephrine solution 1:1,000 (0.3 to 0.5 mL) should be promptly administered.** (See PRECAUTIONS: Information for Patients and **ADVERSE REACTIONS**.)
Anaphylactoid Reactions During Desensitization Two patients undergoing desensitizing treatment with hymenoptera venom while receiving ACE inhibitors sustained life–threatening anaphylactoid reactions. In the same patients, these reactions did not occur when ACE inhibitors were temporarily withheld, but they reappeared when the ACE inhibitors were inadvertently readministered.

Anaphylactoid Reactions During Membrane Exposure Anaphylactoid reactions have been reported in patients dialyzed with high–flux membranes and treated concomitantly with an ACE inhibitor. Anaphylactoid reactions have also been reported in patients undergoing low–density lipoprotein apheresis with dextran sulfate absorption.
Hypotension:
MAVIK® can cause symptomatic hypotension. Like other ACE inhibitors, MAVIK® has only rarely been associated with symptomatic hypotension in uncomplicated hypertensive patients. Symptomatic hypotension is most likely to occur in patients who have been salt– or volume–depleted as a result of prolonged treatment with diuretics, dietary salt restriction, dialysis, diarrhea, or vomiting. Volume and/or salt depletion should be corrected before initiating treatment with MAVIK®. (See **PRECAUTIONS**, Drug Interactions, and **ADVERSE REACTIONS**.) In controlled and uncontrolled studies, hypotension was reported as an adverse event in 0.6 percent of patients and led to discontinuations in 0.1% of patients.

In patients with concomitant congestive heart failure, with or without associated renal insufficiency, ACE inhibitor therapy may cause excessive hypotension, which may be associated with oliguria or azotemia, and rarely, with acute renal failure and death. In such patients, MAVIK® therapy should be started at the recommended dose under close medical supervision. These patients should be followed closely during the first 2 weeks of treatment and, thereafter, whenever the dosage of MAVIK® or diuretic is increased. (See **DOSAGE** and **ADMINISTRATION**.) Care in avoiding hypotension should also be taken in patients with ischemic heart disease, aortic stenosis, or cerebrovascular disease.

If symptomatic hypotension occurs, the patient should be placed in the supine position and, if necessary, normal saline may be administered intravenously. A transient hypotensive response is not a contraindication to further doses; however, lower doses of MAVIK® or reduced concomitant diuretic therapy should be considered.
Neutropenia/Agranulocytosis:
Another ACE inhibitor, captopril, has been shown to cause agranulocytosis and bone marrow depression rarely in patients with uncomplicated hypertension, but more frequently in patients with renal impairment, especially if they also have a collagen–vascular disease such as systemic lupus erythematosus or scleroderma. Available data from clinical trials of trandolapril are insufficient to show that trandolapril does not cause agranulocytosis at similar rates. As with other ACE inhibitors, periodic monitoring of white blood cell counts in patients with collagen–vascular disease and/or renal disease should be considered.
Hepatic Failure:
ACE inhibitors rarely have been associated with a syndrome of cholestatic jaundice, fulminant hepatic necrosis, and death. The mechanism of this syndrome is not understood. Patients receiving ACE inhibitors who develop jaundice should discontinue the ACE inhibitor and receive appropriate medical follow–up.
Fetal/Neonatal Morbidity and Mortality:
ACE inhibitors can cause fetal and neonatal morbidity and death when administered to pregnant women. Several dozen cases have been reported in the world literature. When pregnancy is detected, ACE inhibitors should be discontinued as soon as possible.

The use of ACE inhibitors during the second and third trimesters of pregnancy has been associated with fetal and neonatal injury, including hypotension, neonatal skull hypoplasia, anuria, reversible or irreversible renal failure, and death. Oligohydramnios has also been reported, presumably resulting from decreased fetal renal function; oligohydramnios in this setting has been associated with fetal limb contractures, craniofacial deformation, and hypoplastic lung development. Prematurity, intrauterine growth retardation, and patent ductus arteriosus have also been reported, although it is not clear whether these occurrences were due to the ACE inhibitor exposure.

These adverse effects do not appear to have resulted from intrauterine ACE–inhibitor exposure that has been limited to the first trimester. Mothers whose embryos and fetuses are exposed to ACE inhibitors only during the first trimester should be so informed. Nonetheless, when patients become pregnant, physicians should make every effort to discontinue the use of trandolapril as soon as possible.

Rarely (probably less often than once in every thousand pregnancies), no alternative to ACE inhibitors will be found. In these rare cases, the mothers should be apprised of the potential hazards to their fetuses, and serial ultrasound examinations should be performed to assess the intra–amniotic environment.

If oligohydramnios is observed, trandolapril should be discontinued unless it is considered life–saving for the mother. Contraction stress testing (CST), a non–stress test (NST), or biophysical profiling (BPP) may be appropriate, depending upon the week of pregnancy.

Patients and physicians should be aware, however, that oligohydramnios may not appear until after the fetus has sustained irreversible injury.

Infants with histories of *in utero* exposure to ACE inhibitors should be closely observed for hypotension, oliguria, and hyperkalemia. If oliguria occurs, attention should be directed toward support of blood pressure and renal perfusion. Exchange transfusions or dialysis may be required as a means of reversing hypotension and/or substituting for disordered renal function.

Doses of 0.8 mg/kg/day (9.4 mg/m^2/day) in rabbits, 1000 mg/kg/day (7000 mg/m^2/day) in rats, and 25 mg/kg/day (295 mg/m^2/day) in cynomolgus monkeys did not produce teratogenic effects. These doses represent 10 and 3 times (rabbits), 1250 and 2564 times (rats), and 312 and 108 times (monkeys) the maximum projected human dose of 4 mg based on body–weight and body–surface–area, respectively assuming a 50 kg woman.

PRECAUTIONS

General

Impaired Renal Function:

As a consequence of inhibiting the renin–angiotensin–aldosterone system, changes in renal function may be anticipated in susceptible individuals. In patients with severe heart failure whose renal function may depend on the activity of the renin–angiotensin–aldosterone system, treatment with ACE inhibitors, including MAVIK®, may be associated with oliguria and/or progressive azotemia and rarely with acute renal failure and/or death.

In hypertensive patients with unilateral or bilateral renal artery stenosis, increases in blood urea nitrogen and serum creatinine have been observed in some patients following ACE inhibitor therapy. These increases were almost always reversible upon discontinuation of the ACE inhibitor and/or diuretic therapy. In such patients, renal function should be monitored during the first few weeks of therapy.

Some hypertensive patients with no apparent preexisting renal vascular disease have developed increases in blood urea and serum creatinine, usually minor and transient, especially when ACE inhibitors have been given concomitantly with a diuretic. This is more likely to occur in patients with preexisting renal impairment. Dosage reduction and/or discontinuation of any diuretic and/or the ACE inhibitor may be required.

Evaluation of hypertensive patients should always include assessment of renal function. (See **DOSAGE** and **ADMINISTRATION.**)

Hyperkalemia and potassium–sparing diuretics:

In clinical trials, hyperkalemia (serum potassium > 6.00 mEq/L) occurred in approximately 0.4 percent of hypertensive patients receiving MAVIK®. In most cases, elevated serum potassium levels were isolated values, which resolved despite continued therapy. None of these patients were discontinued from the trials because of hyperkalemia. Risk factors for the development of hyperkalemia include renal insufficiency, diabetes mellitus, and the concomitant use of potassium–sparing diuretics, potassium supplements, and/or potassium–containing salt substitutes, which should be used cautiously, if at all, with MAVIK®. (See **PRECAUTIONS:** Drug Interactions.)

Cough:

Presumably due to the inhibition of the degradation of endogenous bradykinin, persistent nonproductive cough has been reported with all ACE inhibitors, always resolving after discontinuation of therapy. ACE inhibitor–induced cough should be considered in the differential diagnosis of cough. In controlled trials of trandolapril, cough was present in 2% of tradolapril patients and 0% of patients given placebo. There was no evidence of a relationship to dose.

Surgery/anesthesia:

In patients undergoing major surgery or during anesthesia with agents that produce hypotension, MAVIK® will block angiotensin II formation secondary to compensatory renin release. If hypotension occurs and is considered to be due to this mechanism, it can be corrected by volume expansion.

Information for Patients

Angioedema:

Angioedema, including laryngeal edema, may occur at any time during treatment with ACE inhibitors, including MAVIK®. Patients should be so advised and told to report immediately any signs or symptoms suggesting angioedema (swelling of face, extremities, eyes, lips, tongue, difficulty in swallowing or breathing) and to stop taking the drug until they have consulted with their physician. (See **WARNINGS** and **ADVERSE REACTIONS.**)

Symptomatic Hypotension:

Patients should be cautioned that light–headedness can occur, especially during the first days of MAVIK® therapy, and should be reported to a physician. If actual syncope occurs, patients should be told to stop taking the drug until they have consulted with their physician (See **WARNINGS.**)

All patients should be cautioned that inadequate fluid intake, excessive perspiration, diarrhea, or vomiting, resulting in reduced fluid volume, may precipitate an excessive fall in blood pressure with the same consequences of light–headedness and possible syncope.

Patients planning to undergo any surgery and/or anesthesia should be told to inform their physician that they are taking an ACE inhibitor that has a long duration of action.

Hyperkalemia:

Patients should be told not to use potassium supplements or salt substitutes containing potassium without consulting their physician. (See **PRECAUTIONS.**)

Neutropenia:

Patients should be told to report promptly any indication of infection (e.g., sore throat, fever) which could be a sign of neutropenia.

Pregnancy:

Female patients of childbearing age should be told about the consequences of second– and third–trimester exposure to ACE inhibitors, and they should also be told that these consequences do not appear to have resulted from intrauterine ACE–inhibitor exposure that has been limited to the first trimester. These patients should be asked to report pregnancies to their physicians as soon as possible.

NOTE: As with many other drugs, certain advice to patients being treated with MAVIK® is warranted. This information is intended to aid in the safe and effective use of this medication. It is not a disclosure of all possible adverse or intended effects.

Drug Interactions

Concomitant diuretic therapy:

As with other ACE inhibitors, patients on diuretics, especially those on recently instituted diuretic therapy, may experience an excessive reduction of blood pressure after initiation of therapy with MAVIK®. The possibility of exacerbation of hypotensive effects with MAVIK® may be minimized by either discontinuing the diuretic or cautiously increasing salt intake prior to initiation of treatment with MAVIK®. If it is not possible to discontinue the diuretic, the starting dose of trandolapril should be reduced. (See **DOSAGE** and **ADMINISTRATION.**)

Agents increasing serum potassium:

Trandolapril can attenuate potassium loss caused by thiazide diuretics and increase serum potassium when used alone. Use of potassium–sparing diuretics (spironolactone, triamterene, or amiloride), potassium supplements, or potassium–containing salt substitutes concomitantly with ACE inhibitors can increase the risk of hyperkalemia. If concomitant use of such agents is indicated, they should be used with caution and with appropriate monitoring of serum potassium. (See **PRECAUTIONS.**)

Lithium:

Increased serum lithium levels and symptoms of lithium toxicity have been reported in patients receiving concomitant lithium and ACE inhibitor therapy. These drugs should be coadministered with caution, and frequent monitoring of serum lithium levels is recommended. If a diuretic is also used, the risk of lithium toxicity may be increased.

Other:

No clinically significant interaction has been found between trandolaprilat and food, cimetidine, digoxin, or furosemide. The anticoagulant effect of warfarin was not significantly changed by trandolapril.

Carcinogenesis, Mutagenesis, Impairment of Fertility

Long–term studies were conducted with oral trandolapril administered by gavage to mice (78 weeks) and rats (104 and 106 weeks). No evidence of carcinogenic potential was seen in mice dosed up to 25 mg/kg/day (85 mg/m^2/day) or rats dosed up to 8 mg/kg/day (60 mg/m^2/day). These doses are 313 and 32 times (mice), and 100 and 23 times (rats) the maximum recommended human daily dose (MRHDD) of 4 mg based on body–weight and body–surface–area, respectively assuming a 50 kg individual. The genotoxic potential of trandolapril was evaluated in the microbial mutagenicity (Ames) test, the point mutation and chromosome aberration assays in Chinese hamster V79 cells, and the micronucleus test in mice. There was no evidence of mutagenic or clastogenic potential in these in vitro and in vivo assays.

Reproduction studies in rats did not show any impairment of fertility at doses up to 100 mg/kg/day (710 mg/m^2/day) of trandolapril, or 1250 and 260 times the MRHDD on the basis of body–weight and body–surface–area, respectively.

Pregnancy

Pregnancy Categories C (first trimester) and D (second and third trimesters): See WARNINGS, Fetal/Neonatal Morbidity and mortality.

Nursing Mothers

Radiolabeled trandolapril or its metabolites are secreted in rat milk. MAVIK® (trandolapril) should not be administered to nursing mothers.

Geriatric Use

In placebo–controlled studies of MAVIK®, 31.1% of patients were 60 years and older, 20.1% were 65 years and older, and 2.3% were 75 years and older. No overall differences in effectiveness or safety were observed between these patients and younger patients. (Greater sensitivity of some older individual patients cannot be ruled out).

Pediatric Use

The safety and effectiveness of MAVIK® in pediatric patients have not been established.

ADVERSE REACTIONS

The safety experience in U.S. placebo–controlled trials included 1067 hypertensive patients, of whom 831 received MAVIK®. Nearly 200 hypertensive patients received MAVIK® for over one year in open–label trials. In controlled trials, withdrawals for adverse events were 2.1% on placebo and 1.4% on MAVIK®. Adverse events considered at least possibly related to treatment occurring in 1% of MAVIK®–treated patients and more common on MAVIK® than placebo, pooled for all doses, are shown below, together with the frequency of discontinuation of treatment because of these events.

ADVERSE EVENTS IN PLACEBO–CONTROLLED TRIALS
Occurring at 1% or greater

	MAVIK (N=832) % Incidence (% Discontinuance)	PLACEBO (N=237) % Incidence (% Discontinuance)
Cough	1.9 (0.1)	0.4 (0.4)
Dizziness	1.3 (0.2)	0.4 (0.4)
Diarrhea	1.0 (0.0)	0.4 (0.0)

Headache and fatigue were all seen in more than 1% of MAVIK®–treated patients but were more frequently seen on placebo. Adverse events were not usually persistent or difficult to manage.

Clinical adverse experiences possibly or probably related or of uncertain relationship to therapy occurring in 0.3% to 1.0% (except as noted) of the patients treated with MAVIK® (with or without concomitant calcium ion antagonist or diuretic) in controlled or uncontrolled trials (N=1134) and less frequent, clinically significant events seen in clinical trials or post–marketing experience (the rarer events are in italics) include (listed by body system):

General Body Function: chest pain.

Cardiovascular: AV first degree block, bradycardia, edema, flushing, hypotension, palpitations.

Central Nervous System: drowsiness, insomnia, paresthesia, vertigo.

Dermatologic: pruritus, rash, pemphigus.

Eye, Ear, Nose, Throat: epistaxis, throat inflammation, upper respiratory tract infection.

Emotional, Mental, Sexual States: anxiety, impotence, decreased libido.

Gastrointestinal: abdominal distention, abdominal pain/cramps, constipation, dyspepsia, diarrhea, vomiting, *pancreatitis.*

Hemopoietic: *decreased leukocytes, decreased neutrophils.*

Metabolism and Endocrine: *increased creatinine, increased potassium,* increased SGPT (ALT).

Musculoskeletal System: extremity pain, muscle cramps, gout.

Pulmonary: dyspnea.

Angioedema: Angioedema has been reported in 4 (0.13%) patients receiving MAVIK® in U.S. and foreign studies. Angioedema associated with laryngeal edema may be fatal. If angioedema of the face, extremities, lips, tongue, glottis, and/or larynx occurs, treatment with MAVIK® should be discontinued and appropriate therapy instituted immediately. (See **WARNINGS.**)

Hypotension: In hypertensive patients, symptomatic hypotension occurred in 0.6 percent and near syncope occurred in 0.2 percent. Hypotension or syncope was a cause for discontinuation of therapy in 0.1 percent of hypertensive patients.

Fetal/Neonatal Morbidity and Mortality: See **WARNINGS,** Fetal Neonatal Morbidity and Mortality.

Cough: See **PRECAUTIONS,** Cough.

Clinical Laboratory Test Findings

Hematology: (See **WARNINGS.**) Low white blood cells, low neutrophils, low lymphocytes, thrombocytopenia.

Serum Electrolytes: Hyperkalemia (See **PRECAUTIONS,**) hyponatremia.

Creatinine and Blood Urea Nitrogen: Increases in creatinine levels occurred in 1.1 percent of patients receiving MAVIK® alone and 7.3 percent of patients treated with MAVIK®, a calcium ion antagonist and a diuretic. Increases in blood urea nitrogen levels occurred in 0.6 percent of patients receiving MAVIK® alone and 1.4 percent of patients receiving MAVIK®, a calcium ion antagonist, and a diuretic. None of these increases required discontinuation of treatment. Increases in these laboratory values are more likely to occur in patients with renal insufficiency or those pretreated with a diuretic and, based on experience with other ACE inhibitors, would be expected to be especially likely in patients with renal artery stenosis. (See **PRECAUTIONS** and **WARNINGS.**)

Liver function tests: Occasional elevation of transaminases at the rate of 3X upper normals occurred in 0.8% of patients and persistent increase in bilirubin occurred in 0.2% of patients. Discontinuation for elevated liver enzymes occurred in 0.2 percent of patients.

Continued on next page

Knoll—Cont.

OVERDOSAGE

No date are available with respect to overdosage in humans. The oral LD_{50} of trandolapril in mice was 4875 mg/Kg in males and 3990 mg/Kg in females. In rats, an oral dose of 5000 mg/Kg caused low mortality (1 male out of 5; 0 females). In dogs, an oral dose of 1000 mg/Kg did not cause mortality and abnormal clinical signs were not observed. In humans the most likely clinical manifestation would be symptoms attributable to severe hypotension.

Laboratory determinations of serum levels of trandolapril and its metabolites are not widely available, and such determinations have, in any event, no established role in the management of trandolapril overdose. No data are available to suggest that physiological maneuvers (e.g., maneuvers to change the pH of the urine) might accelerate elimination of trandolapril and its metabolites. Trandolaprilat is removed by hemodialysis. Angiotensin II could presumably serve as a specific antagonist antidote in the setting of trandolapril overdose, but angiotensin II is essentially unavailable outside of scattered research facilities. Because the hypotensive effect of trandolapril is achieved through vasodilation and effective hypovolemia, it is reasonable to treat trandolapril overdose by infusion of normal saline solution.

DOSAGE AND ADMINISTRATION

The recommended initial dosage of MAVIK® for patients not receiving a diuretic is 1 mg once daily in non–black patients and 2 mg in black patients. Dosage should be adjusted according to the blood pressure response. Generally, dosage adjustments should be made at intervals of at least 1 week. Most patients have required dosages of 2 to 4 mg once daily. There is little clinical experience with doses above 8 mg.

Patients inadequately treated with once–daily dosing at 4 mg may be treated with twice–daily dosing. If blood pressure is not adequately controlled with MAVIK® monotherapy, a diuretic may be added.

In patients who are currently being treated with a diuretic, symptomatic hypotension occasionally can occur following the initial dose of MAVIK®. To reduce the likelihood of hypotension, the diuretic should, if possible, be discontinued two to three days prior to beginning therapy with MAVIK®. (See **WARNINGS**.) Then, if blood pressure is not controlled with MAVIK® alone, diuretic therapy should be resumed. If the diuretic cannot be discontinued, an initial dose of 0.5 mg MAVIK® should be used with careful medical supervision for several hours until blood pressure has stabilized. The dosage should subsequently be titrated (as described above) to the optimal response. (See **WARNINGS, PRECAUTIONS,** and **Drug Interactions.**)

Concomitant administration of MAVIK® with potassium supplements, potassium salt substitutes, or potassium–sparing diuretics can lead to increases of serum potassium. (See **PRECAUTIONS**)

Dosage Adjustment in Renal Impairment or Hepatic Cirrhosis:

For patients with a creatinine clearance <30 mL/min. or with hepatic cirrhosis, the recommended starting dose, based on clinical and pharmacokinetic data, is 0.5 mg daily. Patients should subsequently have their dosage titrated (as described above) to the optimal response.

HOW SUPPLIED

MAVIK® tablets are supplied as follows:

1 mg tablet – salmon colored, round shaped, scored, compressed tablets, with code KNOLL 1 on one side.
NDC (0048–5805–01 – bottles of 100)
NDC (0048–5805–41 – unit dose packs of 100)

2 mg tablet – yellow colored, round shaped, compressed tablets, with code KNOLL 2 on one side.
NDC (0048–5806–01 – bottles of 100)
NDC (0048–5806–41 – unit dose packs of 100)

4 mg tablet – rose colored, round shaped, compressed tablets, with code KNOLL 4 on one side.
NDC (0048–5807–01 – bottles of 100)
NDC (0048–5807–41– unit dose packs of 100)

Dispense in well–closed continer with safety closure.

Storage: Store at controlled room temperature: 20–25°C (68–77°F) see USP.

Caution: Federal law prohibits dispensing without prescription.

Revised: April 1996 0983000–1

Knoll Pharmaceutical Company
3000 Continental Drive – North
Mount Olive, New Jersey 07828–1234
BASF Pharma

© 1996 Knoll Pharmaceutical Company
MAVIK is a registered trademark of Knoll AG

Shown in Product Identification Guide, page 320

SYNTHROID® ℞

[sĭn 'throid]

(Levothyroxine Sodium, USP)

SYNTHROID Tablets—for oral administration

SYNTHROID Injection—for parenteral administration

DESCRIPTION

SYNTHROID (Levothyroxine Sodium, USP) Tablets and Injection contain synthetic crystalline L-3,3′,5,5′-tetraiodothyronine sodium salt [levothyroxine (T_4) sodium]. Synthetic T_4 is identical to that produced in the human thyroid gland. Levothyroxine (T_4) Sodium has an empirical formula of $C_{15}H_{10}I_4NNaO_4xH_2O$, molecular weight of 798.86 (anhydrous), and structural formula as shown:

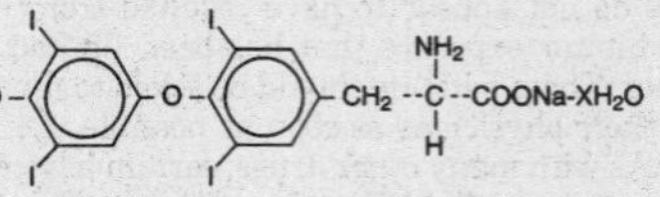

LEVOTHYROXINE SODIUM

Inactive Ingredients (SYNTHROID Tablets): acacia, confectioner's sugar, lactose, magnesium stearate, povidone, talc. The following are the color additives by tablet strength:

Strength (mcg)	Color Additive(s)
25	FD&C Yellow No. 6
50	None
75	FD&C Red No. 40, FD&C Blue No. 2
88	FD&C Blue No. 1, FD&C Yellow No. 6, D&C yellow No. 10
100	D&C Yellow No. 10, FD&C Yellow No. 6
112	D&C Red No. 27 & 30
125	FD&C Yellow No. 6, FD&C Red No. 40, FD&C Blue No. 1
150	FD&C Blue No. 2
175	FD&C Blue No. 1, D&C Red No. 27 & 30
200	FD&C Red No. 40
300	D&C Yellow No. 10, FD&C Yellow No. 6, FD&C Blue No. 1

Inactive Ingredients (SYNTHROID Injection): 10 mg mannitol, USP, sodium hydroxide, 0.7 mg tribasic sodium phosphate, anhydrous dodecahydrate.

Levothyroxine sodium powder for reconstitution for injection is a sterile preparation.

CLINICAL PHARMACOLOGY

The synthesis and secretion of the major thyroid hormones, L-thyroxine (T_4) and L-triiodothyronine (T_3), from the normally functioning thyroid gland are regulated by complex feedback mechanisms of the hypothalamic-pituitary-thyroid axis. The thyroid gland is stimulated to secrete thyroid hormones by the action of thyrotropin (thyroid stimulating hormone, TSH), which is produced in the anterior pituitary gland. TSH secretion is in turn controlled by thyrotropin-releasing hormone (TRH) produced in the hypothalamus, circulating thyroid hormones, and possibly other mechanisms. Thyroid hormones circulating in the blood act as feedback inhibitors of both TSH and TRH secretion. Thus, when serum concentrations of T_3 and T_4 are increased, secretion of TSH and TRH decreases. Conversely, when serum thyroid hormone concentrations are decreased, secretion of TSH and TRH is increased. Administration of exogenous thyroid hormones to euthyroid individuals results in suppression of endogenous thyroid hormone secretion.

The mechanisms by which thyroid hormones exert their physiologic actions have not been completely elucidated. T_4 and T_3 are transported into cells by passive and active mechanisms. T_3 in cell cytoplasm and T_3 generated from T_4 within the cell diffuse into the nucleus and bind to thyroid receptor proteins, which appear to be primarily attached to DNA. Receptor binding leads to activation or repression of DNA transcription, thereby altering the amounts of mRNA and resultant proteins. Changes in protein concentrations are responsible for the metabolic changes observed in organs and tissues.

Thyroid hormones enhance oxygen consumption of most body tissues and increase the basal metabolic rate and metabolism of carbohydrates, lipids, and proteins. Thus, they exert a profound influence on every organ system and are of particular importance in the development of the central nervous system. Thyroid hormones also appear to have direct effects on tissues, such as increased myocardial contractility and decreased systemic vascular resistance.

The physiologic effects of thyroid hormones are produced primarily by T_3, a large portion of which is derived from the deiodination of T_4 in peripheral tissues. About 70 to 90 percent of peripheral T_3 is produced by monodeiodination of T_4 at the 5′ position (outer ring). Peripheral monodeiodination of T_4 at the 5 position (inner ring) results in the formation of reverse triiodothyronine (rT_3), which is calorigenically inactive.

PHARMACOKINETICS

Few clinical studies have evaluated the kinetics of orally administered thyroid hormone. In animals, the most active sites of absorption appear to be the proximal and mid-jejunum. T_4 is not absorbed from the stomach and little, if any, drug is absorbed from the duodenum. There seems to be no absorption of T_4 from the distal colon in animals. A number of human studies have confirmed the importance of an intact jejunum and ileum for T_4 absorption and have shown some absorption from the duodenum. Studies involving radioiodinated T_4 fecal tracer excretion methods, equilibration, and AUC methods have shown that absorption varies from 48 to 80 percent of the administered dose. The extent of absorption is increased in the fasting state and decreased in malabsorption syndromes, such as sprue. Absorption may also decrease with age. The degree of T_4 absorption is dependent on the product formulation as well as on the character of the intestinal contents, including plasma protein and soluble dietary factors, which bind thyroid hormone making it unavailable for diffusion. Decreased absorption may result from administration of infant soybean formula, ferrous sulfate, sodium polystyrene sulfonate, aluminum hydroxide, sucralfate, or bile acid sequestrants. T_4 absorption following intramuscular administration is variable.

Distribution of thyroid hormones in human body tissues and fluids has not been fully elucidated. More than percent of circulating hormones is bound to serum proteins, including thyroxine-binding globulin (TBG), thyroxine-binding prealbumin (TBPA), and albumin (TBA). T_4 is more extensively and firmly bound to serum proteins than is T_3. Only unbound thyroid hormone is metabolically active. The higher affinity of TBG and TBPA for T_4 partly explains the higher serum levels, slower metabolic clearance, and longer serum elimination half-life of this hormone.

Certain drugs and physiologic conditions can alter the binding of thyroid hormones to serum proteins and/or the concentrations of the serum proteins available for thyroid hormone binding. These effects must be considered when interpreting the results of thyroid function tests. (See **Drug Interactions** and **Laboratory Test Interactions.**)

T_4 is eliminated slowly from the body, with a half-life of 6 to 7 days. T_3 has a half-life of 1 to 2 days. The liver is the major site of degradation for both hormones. T_4 and T_3 are conjugated with glucuronic and sulfuric acids and excreted in the bile. There is an enterohepatic circulation of thyroid hormones, as they are liberated by hydrolysis in the intestine and reabsorbed. A portion of the conjugated material reaches the colon unchanged, is hydrolyzed there, and is eliminated as free compounds in the feces. In man, approximately 20 to 40 percent of T_4 is eliminated in the stool. About 70 percent of the T_4 secreted daily is deiodinated to yield equal amounts of T_3 and rT_3 . Subsequent deiodination of T_3 and rT_3 yields multiple forms of diiodothyronine. A number of other minor T_4 metabolites have also been identified. Although some of these metabolites have biologic activity, their overall contribution to the therapeutic effect of T_4 is minimal.

INDICATIONS AND USAGE

SYNTHROID is indicated:

1. As replacement or supplemental therapy in patients of any age or state (including pregnancy) with hypothyroidism of any etiology except transient hypothyroidism during the recovery phase of subacute thyroiditis: primary hypothyroidism resulting from thyroid dysfunction, primary atrophy, or partial or total absence of the thyroid gland, or from the effects of surgery, radiation or drugs, with or without the presence of goiter, including subclinical hypothyroidism; secondary (pituitary) hypothyroidism; and tertiary (hypothalamic) hypothyroidism (see **CONTRAINDICATIONS** and **PRECAUTIONS**). SYNTHROID **Injection** can be used intravenously when rapid repletion is required, and either intravenously or intramuscularly when the oral route is precluded.
2. As a pituitary TSH suppressant in the treatment or prevention of various types of euthyroid goiters, including thyroid nodules, subacute or chronic lymphocytic thyroiditis (Hashimoto's), multinodular goiter, and in conjunction with surgery and radioactive iodine therapy in the management of thyrotropin-dependent well-differentiated papillary or follicular carcinoma of the thyroid.

CONTRAINDICATIONS

SYNTHROID is contraindicated in patients with untreated thyrotoxicosis of any etiology or an apparent hypersensitivity to thyroid hormones or any of the inactive product constituents. (The 50 mcg tablet is formulated without color additives for patients who are sensitive to dyes.) There is no well-documented evidence of true allergic or idiosyncratic reactions to thyroid hormone. SYNTHROID is also contraindicated in the patients with uncorrected adrenal insufficiency, as thyroid hormones increase tissue demands for adrenocortical hormones and may thereby precipitate acute adrenal crisis (see **PRECAUTIONS**).

WARNINGS: Thyroid hormones, either alone or together with other therapeutic agents, should not be used for the treatment of obesity. In euthyroid patients, doses within the range of daily hormonal requirements are ineffective for weight reduction. Larger doses may produce serious or even life threatening manifestations of toxicity, particularly when given in association with sympathomimetic amines such as those used for their anorectic effects.

The use of SYNTHROID in the treatment of obesity, either alone or in combination with other drugs, is unjustified. The use of SYNTHROID is also unjustified in the treatment of male or female infertility unless this condition is associated with hypothroidism.

PRECAUTIONS

General: SYNTHROID should be used with caution in patients with cardiovascular disorders, including angina, coronary artery disease, and hypertension, and in the elderly who have a greater likelihood of occult cardiac disease. Concomitant administration of thyroid hormone and sympathomimetic agents to patients with coronary artery disease may increase the risk of coronary insufficiency.

Use of SNYTHROID in patients with concomitant diabetes mellitus, diabetes insipidus or adrenal cortical insufficiency may aggravate the intensity of their symptoms. Appropriate adjustments of the various therapeutic measures directed at these concomitant endocrine diseases may therefore be required. Treatment of myxedema coma may require simultaneous administration of glucocorticoids (see **DOSAGE AND ADMINISTRATION**).

T_4 enhances the response to anticoagulant therapy. Prothrombin time should be closely monitored in patients taking both SYNTHROID and oral anticoagulants, and the dosage of anticoagulant adjusted accordingly.

Seizures have been reported rarely in association with the initiation of levothyroxine sodium therapy, and may be related to the effect of thyroid hormone on seizure threshold. Lithium blocks the TSH-mediated release of T_4 and T_3. Thyroid function should therefore be carefully monitored during lithium initiation, stabilization, and maintenance. If hypothyroidism occurs during lithium treatment, a higher than usual SYNTHROID dose may be required.

Information for the Patient:

1. SYNTHROID is intended to replace a hormone that is normally produced by your thyroid gland. It is generally taken for life, except in cases of temporary hypothyroidism associated with an inflammation of the thyroid gland.
2. Before or at any time while using SYNTHROID you should tell your doctor if you are allergic to any foods or medicines, are pregnant or intend to become pregnant, are breast-feeding, are taking or start taking any other prescription or nonprescription (OTC) medications, or have any other medical problems (especially hardening of the arteries, heart disease, high blood pressure, or history of thyroid, adrenal or pituitary gland problems).
3. Use SYNTHROID only as prescribed by your doctor. Do not discontinue SYNTHROID or change the amount you take or how often you take it, except as directed by your doctor.
4. SYNTHROID, like all medicines obtained from your doctor, must be used only by you and for the condition determined appropriate by your doctor.
5. It may take a few weeks for SYNTHROID to begin working. Until it begins working, you may not notice any change in your symptoms.
6. You should notify your doctor if you experience any of the following symptoms, or if you experience any other unusual medical event: chest pain, shortness of breath, hives or skin rash, rapid or irregular heartbeat, headache, irritability, nervousness, sleeplessness, diarrhea, excessive sweating, heat intolerance, changes in appetite, vomiting, weight gain or loss, changes in menstrual periods, fever, hand tremors, leg cramps.
7. You should inform your doctor or dentist that you are taking SYNTHROID before having any kind of surgery.
8. You should notify your doctor if you become pregnant while taking SYNTHROID. Your dose of this medicine will likely have to be increased while your are pregnant.
9. If you have diabetes, your dose of insulin or oral antidiabetic agent may need to be changed after starting SYNTHROID. You should monitor your blood or urinary glucose levels as directed by your doctor and report any changes to your doctor immediately.
10. If you are taking an oral anticoagulant drug such as warfarin, your dose may need to be changed after starting SYNTHROID. Your coagulation status should be checked often to determine if a change in dose is required.
11. Partial hair loss may occur rarely during the first few months of SYNTHROID therapy, but it is usually temporary.
12. SYNTHROID is the trade name for tablets containing the thyroid hormone levothyroxine, manufactured by Knoll Pharmaceutical Company. Other manufacturers also make tablets containing levothyroxine. You should not change to another manufacturer's product without discussing that change with your doctor first. Repeat blood tests and a change in the amount of levothyroxine you take may be required.
13. Keep SYNTHROID out of the reach of children. Store SYNTHROID away from heat and moisture.

Laboratory Tests: Treatment of patients with SYNTHROID requires periodic assessment of thyroid status by appropriate laboratory tests and clinical evaluation. Selection of appropriate tests for the diagnosis and management of thyroid disorders depends on patient variables such as presenting signs and symptoms, pregnancy, and concomitant medications. A combination of sensitive TSH assay and free T_4 estimate (free T_4 index, FT_4I) are recommended to confirm a diagnosis of thyroid disease. TSH alone or initially may be useful for thyroid disease screening and for monitoring therapy for primary hypothyroidism as a linear inverse correlation exists between serum TSH and free T_4. Measurement of total serum T_4 and T_3, resin T_3 uptake, and free T_3 concentrations may also be useful. Antithyroid microsomal antibodies are an indicator of autoimmune thyroid disease. The combination of an increased TSH and positive microsomal antibodies in an euthyroid patient is a major risk factor for the future development of clinical hypothyroidism. An elevated serum TSH in the presence of a normal T_4 may indicate subclinical hypothyroidism. Intracellular resistance to thyroid hormone is quite rare, and is suggested by clinical signs and symptoms of hypothyroidism in the presence of high serum T_4 levels. Adequacy of SYNTHROID therapy for hypothyroidism of pituitary or hypothalamic origin should be assessed by measuring FT_4I, which should be maintained in the upper half of the normal range. Measurement of TSH is not a reliable indicator of response to therapy for this condition.

Drug Interactions: The magnitude and relative clinical importance of the effects noted below are likely to be patient-specific and may vary by such factors as age, gender, race, intercurrent illnesses, dose of either agent, additional concomitant medications, and timing of drug administration. Any agent that alters thyroid hormone synthesis, secretion, distribution, effect on target tissues, metabolism, or elimination may alter the optimal therapeutic dose of SYNTHROID.

Levothyroxine sodium absorption—The following agents may bind and decrease absorption of levothyroxine sodium from the gastrointestinal tract: aluminum hydroxide, cholestyramine resin, colestipol hydrochloride, ferrous sulfate, sodium polystyrene sulfonate, soybean flour (e.g., infant formula), sucralfate.

Binding to serum proteins—The following agents may either inhibit levothyroxine sodium binding to serum proteins or alter the concentrations of serum binding proteins: androgens and related anabolic hormones, asparaginase, clofibrate, estrogens and estrogen-containing compounds, 5-fluorouracil, furosemide, glucocorticoids, meclofenamic acid, mefenamic acid, methadone, perphenazine, phenylbutazone, phenytoin, salicylates, tamoxifen.

Thyroid physiology—The following agents may alter thyroid hormone or TSH levels, generally by effects on thyroid hormone synthesis, secretion, distribution, metabolism, hormone action, or elimination, or altered TSH secretion: aminoglutethimide, p-aminosalicylic acid, amiodarone, androgens and related anabolic hormones, complex anions (thiocyanate, perchlorate, pertechnetate), antithyoid drugs, β-adrenergic blocking agents, carbamazepine, chloral hydrate, diazepam, dopamine and dopamine agonists, ethionamide, glucocorticoids, heparin, hepatic enzyme inducers, insulin, iodinated cholestographic agents, iodine-containing compounds, levodopa, lovastatin, lithium, 6-mercaptopurine, metoclopramide, mitotane, nitroprusside, phenobarbital, phenytoin, resorcinol, rifampin, somatostatin analogs, sulfonamides, sulfonylureas, thiazide diuretics.

Adrenocorticoids—Metabolic clearance of adrenocorticoids is decreased in hypothyroid patients and increased in hyperthyroid patients, and may therefore change with changing thyroid status.

Amiodarone—Amiodarone therapy alone can cause hypothyroidism or hyperthyroidism.

Anticoagulants (oral)—The hypoprothrombinemic effect of anticoagulants may be potentiated, apparently by increased catabolism of vitamin K-dependent clotting factors.

Antidiabetic agents (insulin, sulfonylureas)—Requirements for insulin or oral antidiabetic agents may be reduced in hypothyroid patients with diabetes mellitus, and may subsequently increase with the initiation of thyroid hormone replacement therapy.

β-adrenergic blocking agents—Actions of some beta-blocking agents may be impaired when hypothyroid patients become euthyroid.

Cytokines (interferon, interleukin)—Cytokines have been reported to induce both hyperthyroidism and hypothyroidism.

Digitalis glycosides—Therapeutic effects of digitalis glycosides may be reduced. Serum digitalis levels may be decreased in hyperthyroidism or when a hypothyroid patient becomes euthyroid.

Ketamine—Marked hypertension and tachycardia have been reported in association with concomitant administration of levothyroxine sodium and ketamine.

Maprotiline—Risk of cardiac arrhythmias may increase.

Sodium iodide (^{123}I and ^{131}I), sodium pertechnetate Tc99m—Uptake of radiolabeled ions may be decreased.

Somatrem/somatropin—Excessive concurrent use of thyroid hormone may accelerate epiphyseal closure. Untreated hypothyroidism may interfere with the growth response to somatrem or somatropin.

Theophylline—Theophylline clearance may decrease in hypothyroid patients and return toward normal when a euthyroid state is achieved.

Tricyclic antidepressants—Concurrent use may increase the therapeutic and toxic effects of both drugs, possibly due to increased catecholamine sensitivity. Onset of action of tricyclics may be accelerated.

Sympathomimetic agents—Possible increased risk of coronary insufficiency in patients with coronary artery disease.

Laboratory Test Interactions: A number of drugs or moieties are known to alter serum levels of TSH, T_4 and T_3 and may thereby influence the interpretation of laboratory tests of thyroid function (see **Drug Interactions**).

1. Changes in TBG concentration should be taken into consideration when interpreting T_4 and T_3 values. Drugs such as estrogens and estrogen-containing oral contraceptives increase TBG concentrations. TBG concentrations may also be increased during pregnancy and in infectious hepatitis. Decreases in TBG concentrations are observed in nephrosis, acromegaly, and after androgen or corticosteroid therapy. Familial hyper- or hypo-thyroxine-binding-globulinemias have been described. The incidence of TBG deficiency is approximately 1 in 9000. Certain drugs such as salicylates inhibit the protein-binding of T_4. In such cases, the unbound (free) hormone should be measured. Alternatively, an indirect measure of free thyroxine, such as the FT_4I may be used.
2. Medicinal or dietary iodine interferes with *in vivo* tests of radioiodine uptake, producing low uptakes which may not indicate a true decrease in hormone synthesis.
3. Persistent clinical and laboratory evidence of hypothyroidism despite an adequate replacement dose suggests either poor patient compliance, impaired absorption, drug interactions, or decreased potency of the preparation due to improper storage.

Carcinogenesis, Mutagenesis, and Impairment of Fertility: Although animal studies to determine the mutagenic or carcinogenic potential of thyroid hormones have not been performed, synthetic T_4 is identical to that produced by the human thyroid gland. A reported association between prolonged thyroid hormone therapy and breast cancer has not been confirmed and patients receiving levothyroxine sodium for established indications should not discontinue therapy.

Pregnancy: Pregnancy Category A. Studies in pregnant women have not shown that levothyroxine sodium increases the risk of fetal abnormalities if administered during pregnancy. If levothyroxine sodium is used during pregnancy, the possibility of fetal harm appears remote. Because studies cannot rule out the possibility of harm, levothyroxine sodium should be used during pregnancy only if clearly needed.

Thyroid hormones cross the placental barrier to some extent. T_4 levels in the cord blood of athyroid fetuses have been shown to be about one-third of maternal levels. Nevertheless, maternal-fetal transfer of T_4 may not prevent *in utero* hypothyroidism.

Hypothyroidism during pregnancy is associated with a higher rate of complications, including spontaneous abortion and preeclampsia, and has been reported to have an adverse effect on fetal and childhood development. On the basis of current knowledge, SYNTHROID® (Levothyroxine Sodium, USP) should therefore not be discontinued during pregnancy, and hypothyroidism diagnosed during pregnancy should be treated. Studies have shown that during pregnancy T_4 concentrations may decrease and TSH concentrations may increase to values outside normal ranges. Postpartum values are similar to preconception values. Elevations in TSH may occur as early as 4 weeks gestation.

Pregnant women who are maintained on SYNTHROID should have their TSH measured periodically. An elevated TSH should be corrected by an increase in SYNTHROID dose. After pregnancy, the dose can be decreased to the optimal preconception dose.

Nursing Mothers: Minimal amounts of thyroid hormones are excreted in human milk. Thyroid hormones are not associated with serious adverse reactions and do not have known tumorigenic potential. While caution should be exercised when SYNTHROID is administered to a nursing woman, adequate replacement doses of levothyroxine sodium are generally needed to maintain normal lactation.

Pediatric Use: The incidence of congenital hypothyroidism is relatively high (1 in 4,000). Routine determinations of

Continued on next page

Knoll—Cont.

serum T_4 and/or TSH are therefore strongly advised in neonates in view of the deleterious effects of thyroid deficiency on growth and development.

Treatment should be initiated immediately upon diagnosis and generally maintained for life. If, however, transient hypothyroidism is suspected, therapy may be interrupted for 30 days after the age of 3 years to reassess the condition. If T_4 is low and TSH is elevated after that time, permanent hypothyroidism is confirmed and therapy should be reinstituted. If the T_4 and TSH remain in the normal range, a preliminary diagnosis of transient hypothyroidism can be made. Nevertheless, continued close observation with periodic thyroid function testing is warranted.

ADVERSE REACTIONS

Adverse reactions other than those indicative of thyrotoxicosis as a result of therapeutic overdosage, either initially or during the maintenance periods, are rare (see **OVERDOSAGE**). Craniosynostosis has been associated with iatrogenic hyperthyroidism in infants receiving thyroid hormone replacement therapy. Inadequate doses of SYNTHROID may produce or fail to resolve symptoms of hypothyroidism. Hypersensitivity reactions to the product excipients, such as rash and urticaria, may occur. Partial hair loss may occur during the initial months of therapy, but is generally transient. The incidence of continued hair loss is unknown. Pseudotumor cerebri has been reported in pediatric patients receiving thyroid hormone replacement therapy.

OVERDOSAGE

Signs and Symptoms: Excessive doses of SYNTHROID result in a hypermetabolic state indistinguishable from thyrotoxicosis of endogenous origin. Signs and symptoms of thyrotoxicosis include weight loss, increased appetite, palpitations, nervousness, diarrhea, abdominal cramps, sweating, tachycardia, increased pulse and blood pressure, cardiac arrhythmias, tremors, insomnia, heat intolerance, fever, and menstrual irregularities. Symptoms are not always evident or may not appear until several days after ingestion.

Treatment of Overdosage: SYNTHROID should be reduced in dose or temporarily discontinued if signs and symptoms of overdosage appear.

In the treatment of acute massive SYNTHROID overdosage, symptomatic and supportive therapy should be instituted immediately. Treatment is aimed at reducing gastrointestinal absorption and counteracting central and peripheral effects, mainly those of increased sympathetic activity. The stomach should be emptied immediately by emesis or gastric lavage if not otherwise contraindicated (e.g., by coma, convulsions or loss of gag reflex). Cholestyramine and activated charcoal have also been used to decrease levothyroxine sodium absorption. Oxygen should be administered and ventilation maintained as necessary. β-receptor antagonists, particularly propranolol, are useful in counteracting many of the effects of increased sympathetic activity. Propranolol may be administered intravenously at a dosage of 1 to 3 mg over a 10 minute period or orally, 80 to 160 mg/day, especially when no contraindications exist for its use. Cardiac glycosides may be administered if congestive heart failure develops. Measures to control fever, hypoglycemia, or fluid loss should be initiated as necessary. Glucocorticoids may be administered to inhibit the conversion of T_4 to T_3.

Since $T_4$is extensively protein bound, very little drug will be removed by dialysis.

DOSAGE AND ADMINISTRATION

The dosage and rate of administration of SYNTHROID is determined by the indication, and must in every case be individualized according to patient response and laboratory findings.

Hypothyroidism: The goal of therapy for primary hypothyroidism is to achieve and maintain a clinical and biochemical euthyroid state with consequent resolution of hypothyroid signs and symptoms. The starting dose of SYNTHROID, the frequence of dose titration, and the optimal full replacement dose must be individualized for every patient, and will be influenced by such factors as age, weight, cardiovascular status, presence of other illness, and the severity and duration of hypothyroid symptoms.

The usual full replacement dose of SYNTHROID for younger, healthy adults is approximately 1.6 mcg/kg/day administered once daily. In the elderly, the full replacement dose may be altered by decreases in T_4 metabolism and levothyroxine sodium absorption. Older patients may require less than 1 mcg/kg/day. Children generally require higher doses (see **Pediatric Dosage**). Women who are maintained on SYNTHROID during pregnancy may require increased doses (see **Pregnancy**).

Therapy is usually initiated in younger, healthy adults at the anticipated full replacement dose. Clinical and laboratory evaluations should be performed at 6 to 8 week intervals (2 to 3 weeks in severely hypothyroid patients), and the dosage adjusted by 12.5 to 25 mcg increments until the serum TSH concentration is normalized and signs and symptoms resolve. In older patients or in younger patients with a history of cardiovascular disease, the starting dose should be 12.5 to 50 mcg once daily with adjustments of 12.5 to 25 mcg every 3 to 6 weeks until TSH is normalized. If cardiac symptoms develop or worsen, the cardiac disease should be evaluated and the dose of SYNTHROID reduced. Rarely, worsening angina or other signs of cardiac ischemia may prevent achieving a TSH in the normal range.

Treatment of subclinical hypothyroidism, when indicated, may require lower than usual replacement doses, e.g. 1.0 mcg/kg/day. Patients for whom treatment is not initiated should be monitored yearly for changes in clinical status, TSH, and thyroid antibodies.

In patients with hypothyroidism resulting from pituitary or hypothalamic disease, the possibility of secondary adrenal insufficiency should be considered, and if present, treated with glucocorticoids prior to initiation of SYNTHROID. The adequacy of SYNTHROID therapy should be assessed in these patients by measuring FT_4I, which should be maintained in the upper half of the normal range, in addition to clinical assessment. Measurement of TSH is not a reliable indicator of response to therapy for this condition.

Few patients require doses greater than 200 mcg/day. An inadequate response to daily doses of 300 to 400 mcg/day is rare, and may suggest malabsorption, poor patient compliance, and/or drug interactions.

Once optimal replacement is achieved, clinical and laboratory evaluations should be conducted at least annually or whenever warranted by a change in patient status. Levothyroxine sodium products from different manufacturers should not be used interchangeably unless retesting of the patient and retitration of the dosage, as necessary, accompanies the product switch.

SYNTHROID Injection by the intravenous or intramuscular route can be substituted for the oral dosage form when the oral administration is precluded. The initial parenteral dosage should be approxximately one-half the previously established oral dosage of SYNTHROID Tablets. Close observation of the patient is recommended, with adjustment of the dosage as needed. Administration of SYNTHROID Injection by the subcutaneous route is not recommended as studies have shown that the influx of T_4 from the subcutaneous site is very slow, and depends on many factors such as volume of injectate, the anatomic site of injection, ambient temperature, and presence of venospasm.

Myxedema Coma: Myxedema coma represents the extreme expression of severe hypothyroidism and is considered a medical emergency. It is characterized by hypothermia, hypotension, hypoventilation, hyponatremia, and bradycardia. In addition to restoration of normal thyroid hormone levels, therapy should be directed at the correction of electrolyte disturbances and possible infection. Because the mortality rate of patients with untreated myxedema coma is high, treatment must be started immediately, and should include appropriate supportive therapy and corticosteroids to prevent adrenal insufficiency. Possible precipitating factors should also be identified and treated. SYNTHROID may be given via nasogastric tube, but the preferred route of administration is intravenous. A bolus dose of SYNTHROID is given immediately to replete the peripheral pool of T4 , usually 300 to 500 mcg. Although such a dose is usually well-tolerated even in the elderly, the rapid intravenous administration of large doses of levothyroxine sodium to patients with cardiovascular disease is clearly not without risks. Under such circumstances, intravenous therapy should not be undertaken without weighing the alternate risks of myxedema coma and the cardiovascular disease. Clinical judgement in this situation may dictate smaller intravenous doses of SYNTHROID. The initial dose is followed by daily intravenous doses of 75 to 100 mcg until the patient is stable and administration is feasible. Normal T_4 levels are usually achieved in 24 hours, followed by progressive increases in T_3. Improvement in cardiac output, blood pressure, temperature, and mental status generally occur within 24 hours, with improvement in many manifestations of hypothyroidism in 4 to 7 days.

TSH Suppression in Thyroid Cancer and Thyroid Nodules: The rationale for TSH suppression therapy is that a reduction in TSH secretion may decrease the growth and function of abnormal thyroid tissue. Exogeneous thyroid hormone may inhibit recurrence of tumor growth and may produce regression of metastases from well-differentiated (follicular and papillary) carcinoma of the thyroid. It is used as ancillary therapy of these conditions following surgery or radioactive iodine therapy. Medullary and anaplastic carcinoma of the thyroid is unresponsive to TSH suppression therapy. TSH suppression is also used in treating nontoxic solitary nodules and multinodular goiters.

No controlled studies have compared the various degrees of TSH suppression in the treatment of either benign or malignant thyroid nodular disease. Further, the effectiveness of TSH suppression for benign nodular disease is controversial. The dose of SYNTHROID used for TSH suppression should therefore be individualized by the nature of the disease, the patient being treated, and the desired clinical response, weighing the potential benefits of therapy against the risks of iatrogenic thyrotoxicosis. In general, SYNTHROID should be given in the smallest dose that will achieve the desired clinical response.

For well-differentiated thyroid cancer, TSH is generally suppressed to less than 0.1 mU/L. Doses of SYNTHROID greater than 2 mcg/kg/day are usually required. The efficacy of TSH suppression in reducing the size of benign thyroid nodules and in preventing nodule regrowth after surgery are controversial. Nevertheless, when treatment with levothyroxine sodium is considered warranted, TSH is generally suppressed to a higher target range (e.g., 0.1 to 0.3 mU/L) than that employed for the treatment of thyroid cancer. SYNTHROID therapy may also be considered for patients with nontoxic multinodular goiter who have a TSH in the normal range, to moderately suppress TSH (e.g., 0.1 to 0.3 mU/L).

SYNTHROID should be administered with caution to patients in whom there is a suspicion of thyroid gland autonomy, in view of the fact that the effects of exogenous hormone administration will be additive to endogeneous thyroid hormone production.

Pediatric Dosage: The aim of therapy for congential hypothyroidism is to achieve and maintain normal growth and development. During the first three years of life, serum T_4 concentrations should be maintained in the upper half of the normal range with a serum TSH in the normal range (usually less than 10 mU/L). Normalization of TSH may lag significantly behind T_4 in some infants. In general, despite the smaller body size of children, the dosage (on a weight basis) required to sustain full development and general thriving is higher than in adults. See Table 1.

The average initial oral dose of SYNTHROID at the start of treatment is 10 to 15 mcg/kg/day. Infants with very low (less than 5 mU/L) or undetectable serum T_4 levels should be started at 50 mcg daily. A lower dose (e.g., 25 mcg daily) should be considered for premature neonates weighting less than 2 kg and neonates at risk of cardiac failure, increasing to 37.5 or 50 mcg daily after 4 to 6 weeks.

Table I
Recommended Pediatric Dosage
For Congenital Hypothyroidism*

	SYNTHROID (Levothyroxine Sodium Tablets, USP)	
Age	Daily Dose*	Daily dose per kg of body weight
0–6 mos	25–50 mcg	10–15 mcg
6–12 mos	50–75 mcg	6–8 mcg
1–5 yrs	75–100 mcg	5–6 mcg
6–12 yrs	100–150 mcg	4–5 mcg
Older than 12 years	> 150 mcg	2–3 mcg

*To be adjusted on the basis of clinical response and laboratory tests (see **Laboratory Tests**).

Evaluation of the infant's response to SYNTHROID by determination of the serum T_4 and TSH should be performed 2 to 4 weeks after initiation of therapy and after any change in dosage. Additional evaluations should be performed every 1 to 2 months in the first year, every 2 to 3 months between ages 1 and 3, and every 3 to 12 months thereafter until growth is complete. More frequent intervals are indicated when compliance is questioned or abnormal laboratory values are obtained. SYNTHROID may be given to infants and children who cannot swallow intact tablets by crushing the tablet and suspending the freshly crushed tablet in a small amount of water (5 to 10 mL), breast milk or non-soybean based formula. The suspension can be given by spoon or dropper. DO NOT STORE THE SUSPENSION FOR ANY PERIOD OF TIME. The crushed tablet may also be sprinkled over a small amount of food, such as cooked cereal or apple sauce.

HOW SUPPLIED

SYNTHROID* (Levothyroxine Sodium, USP) **Tablets:** round, color coded, scored tablet debossed with 'FLINT' and potency.

25 mcg, orange
Bottles of 100, Code 3P1023 — NDC 0048-1020-03
Bottles of 1000, Code 3P1025 — NDC 0048-1020-05

50 mcg, white
Bottles of 100, Code 3P1043 — NDC 0048-1040-03
Bottles of 1000, Code 3P1045 — NDC 0048-1040-05
Unit Dose Cartons of 100, Code 3P1033 — NDC 0048-1040-13

75 mcg, violet
Bottles of 100, Code 3P1053 — NDC 0048-1050-03
Bottles of 1000, Code 3P1055 — NDC 0048-1050-05
Unit Dose Cartons of 100, Code 3P1003 — NDC 0048-1050-13

88 mcg, olive
Bottles of 100, Code 3P0883 — NDC 0048-1060-03

100 mcg, yellow
Bottles of 100, Code 3P1073 — NDC 0048-1070-03
Bottles of 1000, Code 3P1075 — NDC 0048-1070-05
Unit Dose Cartons of 100, — NDC 0048-1070-13
Code 3P1063
112 mcg, rose
Bottles of 100, Code 3P1183 — NDC 0048-1080-03
Bottles of 1000, Code 3P1185 — NDC 0048-1080-05
125 mcg, brown
Bottles of 100, Code 3P1103 — NDC 0048-1130-03
Bottles of 1000, Code 3P1105 — NDC 0048-1130-05
Unit Dose Cartons of 100, — NDC 0048-1130-13
Code 3P1113
150 mcg, blue
Bottles of 100, Code 3P1093 — NDC 0048-1090-03
Bottles of 1000, Code 3P1095 — NDC 0048-1090-05
Unit Dose Cartons of 100, — NDC 0048-1090-13
Code 3P1083
175 mcg, lilac
Bottles of 100, Code 3P1153 — NDC 0048-1100-03
200 mcg, pink
Bottles of 100, Code 3P1143 — NDC 0048-1140-03
Bottles of 1000, Code 3P1145 — NDC 0048-1140-05
Unit Dose Cartons of 100, — NDC 0048-1140-13
Code 3P1133
300 mcg, green
Bottles of 100, Code 3P1173 — NDC 0048-1170-03
Bottles of 1000, Code 3P1175 — NDC 0048-1170-05

Store at controlled room temperature 15°–30°C (59°–86°F). SYNTHROID Tablets should be protected from light and moisture.

SYNTHROID* (Levothyroxine Sodium, USP) **Injection** is a lyophilized powder. It is supplied in color coded vials as follows:

200 mcg, gray
10 mL Single Dose Vial, Code 3P1312 NDC 0048-1014-99
500 mcg, yellow
10 mL Single Dose Vial, Code 3P1302 NDC 0048-1012-99
Store at controlled room temperature 15°–30°C (59°–86°F).

DIRECTIONS FOR RECONSTITUTION

Reconstitute the lyophilized levothyroxine sodium by aseptically adding 5 mL of 0.9% Sodium Choride Injection, USP or Bacteriostatic Sodium Chloride Injection, USP with Benzyl Alcohol (final volume approximately 5 mL). Shake vial to insure complete mixing. Do not add to other intravenous fluids. Discard any unused portion.
CAUTION: Federal (USA) law prohibits dispensing without a prescription.
Tablets Manufactured by
BASF Pharmaceuticals
A Unit of BASF
Jayuya, Puerto Rico 00664
Injection Manufactured by
Ben Venue Laboratories, Inc.
Bedford, Ohio 44146 USA

7920-07 Rev. 05/24/95
Shown in Product Identification Guide, page 320

EDUCATIONAL MATERIAL

"Treatment of Hypothyroid Disease in the Elderly" (2 credits) Home Study Module-Pharmacists

---

Kramer Laboratories, Inc.
8778 S.W. 8TH STREET
MIAMI, FL 33174

Direct Inquiries to:
8778 S.W. 8th Street
Miami, FL 33174
(800) 824-4894

For Medical Information Contact:
In Emergencies:
Professional Director
(800) 824-4894

CHARCOAL PLUS DS® ENTERIC COATED OTC
250 mg Activated Charcoal Tablets

After every meal

RECOMMENDED CONSUMPTION
Two enteric coated tablets after eating as needed but do not exceed 20 tablets per day. Swallow the tablets whole. Do not chew.

CAUTION
If taking medication allow an interval of 1 hour between ingestion of this product and ingestion of any medication.

HOW SUPPLIED
Bottles of 120 tablets and 36 tablets.

WARNING
Activated Charcoal may cause darkening of the stool.

HALFPRIN® OTC
162 mg. Enteric Coated Aspirin
Aspirin For Suspected Acute MI

DESCRIPTION
Halfprin® is the only 162 mg. enteric coated aspirin available for the indicated use to reduce the risk of vascular mortality in people with a suspected acute myocardial infarction (MI). The Halfprin® 162 mg. aspirin has been determined to be the indicated dose to reduce the risk of fatal and nonfatal cardiovascular and cerebrovascular events in subjects with a suspected acute MI.

INDICATIONS
Suspected Acute MI
The use of aspirin in patients with a suspected acute MI is supported by the results of a large, multicenter 2×2 factorial study of 17,187 subjects with suspected acute MI.(1). Subjects were randomized within 24 hours of the onset of symptoms so that 8,57 subjects received oral aspirin (162.5 milligrams, enteric-coated) daily for 1 month (the first dose crushed, sucked, or chewed) and 8,600 received oral placebo. Of the subjects 8,592 were also randomized to receive a single dose of streptokinase (1.5 million units) infused intravenously for about 1 hour, and 8,595 received a placebo infusion. Thus, 4,295 subject received aspirin plus placebo, 4,300 received streptokinase plus placebo, 4,292 received aspirin plus streptokinase, and 4,300 received double placebo. Vascular mortality (attributed to cardiac, cerebral, hemorrhagic, other vascular, or unknown causes) occurred in 9.4 percent of subjects in the aspirin group and in 11.8 percent of subjects in the oral placebo group in the 35-day follow up. This represents an absolute reduction of 2.4 percent in the mean 35-day vascular mortality attributable to aspirin and a 23 percent reduction in odds of vascular death.
Significant absolute reductions in mortality and corresponding reductions in specific clinical events favoring aspirin were found for reinfarction (1.5 percent absolute reduction, 45 percent odds reduction, $2p < 0.00001$), cardiac arrest (1.2 percent absolute reduction, 14.2 percent odds reduction, $2p < 0.01$), and total stroke (0.4 percent absolute reduction, 41.5 percent odds reduction, $2p < 0.01$). The effect of aspirin over and above its effect on mortality was evidenced by small, but significant, reductions in vascular morbidity in those subjects who were discharged.
The beneficial effects of aspirin on mortality were present with or without streptokinase infusion. Aspirin reduced vascular mortality from 10.4 to 8.0 percent for days 0 to 35 in subjects given streptokinase and reduced vascular mortality from 13.2 to 10.7 percent in the effects of aspirin and thrombolytic therapy with streptokinase in this study were approximately additive. Subjects who received the combination of streptokinase infusion and daily aspirin had significantly lower vascular mortality at 35 days than those who received either active treatment alone (combination 8.0 percent, aspirin 10.7 percent, streptokinase 10.4 percent, and no treatment 13.2 percent. While this study demonstrated that aspirin has an additive benefit in patients given streptokinase, there is no reason to restrict its use to that specific thrombolytic.

ADVERSE REACTIONS
Gastrointestinal Reactions
Doses of 1,000 milligrams per day of aspirin caused gastrointestinal symptoms and bleeding that in some cases were clinically significant. In the Aspirin Myocardial Infarction Study (AMIS) (4) with 4,500 post infarction subjects, the percentage incidences of gastrointestinal symptoms for the aspirin (1,000 milligrams of a standard, solid—tablet formulation) and placebo-treated subjects, respectively, were: Stomach pain (14.5 percent, 4.4 percent); heartburn (11.9 percent, 4.8 percent); nausea and/or vomiting (7.6 percent; 2.1 percent); hospitalization for gastrointestinal disorder (4.8 percent, 3.5 percent). Symptoms and signs of gastrointestinal irritation were not significantly increased in subjects

---

treated for instable angina with 325 milligrams buffered aspirin in solution.
Bleeding
In the AMIS and other trails, aspirin treated subjects had increased rates of gross gastrointestinal bleeding. In the ISIS—2 study (1), there was no significant difference in the incidence of major bleeding (bleeds requiring transfusion) between 8,587 subjects taking 162.5 milligrams aspirin daily and 8,600 subjects taking placebo (31 versus 33 subjects). There were five confirmed cerebral hemorrhage in the aspirin group compared with two in the placebo group, but the incidence of stroke of all causes was significantly reduced from 81 to 47 for the placebo versus aspirin group (0.4 percent absolute change). There was a small and statistically significant excess (0.6 percent) of minor bleeding in people taking aspirin (2.5 percent for aspirin, 1.9 percent for placebo). No other significant adverse effects were reported.
Cardiovascular and Biochemical
In the AMIS trail(4), the dosage of 1,000 milligrams per day of aspirin was associated with small increases in systolic blood pressure (BP) (average 1.5 to 2.1 millimeters Hg) and diastolic BP (0.5 to 0.6 millimeters Hg), depending upon whether maximal or last available readings were used. Blood urea nitrogen and uric acid levels were also increased, but by less than 1.0 milligram percent.
Subjects with marked hypertension or renal insufficiency had been excluded from the trail so that clinical importance of these observations for such subjects or for any subjects treated over more prolonged periods is not known. It is recommended that patients placed on long-term aspirin treatment, even at doses of 160 milligrams per day, be seen at regular intervals to assess changes in these measurements.

DOSAGE AND ADMINISTRATION
The recommended dose of aspirin to treat suspected acute MI is 160 to 162.5 milligrams taken as soon as the first infarct is suspected and then daily for at least 30 days. (One-half of a conventional 325-milligram aspirin tablet or two 80–81 milligram aspirin tablets may be taken.) This use of aspirin applies to both solid, oral dosage forms (buffered, plain, and enteric-coated aspirin) and buffered aspirin in solution. If using a solid dosage form, the first dose should be crushed, sucked, or chewed. After the 30-day treatment, physicians should consider further therapy based on the labeling for dosage and administration of aspirin for prevention of recurrent MI (reinfarction).

REFERENCES
(1) ISIS-2 (Second International Study of Infarct Survival) Collaborative Group. "Randomized Trail of Intravenous Streptokinase, Oral Aspirin, Both, or Neither Among 17,187 Cases of Suspected Acute Myocardial Infarction: ISIS-2," lancet, 2:349–360, August 13, 1988.

HOW SUPPLIED
Halfprin Tablets
162 mg. in bottle of 60* and 200
81 mg. in bottle of 90
*Easy to open bottle/ Not child-resistant caps.

Comments questions or sample request call toll free 1-800-824-4894

SAFE TUSSIN 30 OTC
EXPECTORANT/COUGH SUPPRESSANT

DESCRIPTION
Each 10 cc contains 200 mg Guaifenesin, U.S.P. and 30 mg Dextromethorphan Hydrobromide U.S.P.

INDICATIONS
For temporary relief of cough due to minor throat and bronchial irritation associated with the common cold or inhaled irritants. Helps loosen phlegm (mucus) and thin bronchial secretions to rid the bronchial passageways of bothersome mucus.

DIRECTIONS
Adults and children 12 years of age and over: 2 teaspoonfuls every 6 hours, not to exceed 8 teaspoonfuls in 24 hours. Children 6 to under 12 years of age: 1 teaspoonful every 6 hours not to exceed 4 teaspoonfuls in 24 hours. Children 2 to under 6 years of age: ½ teaspoonful every 6 hours not to exceed 2 teaspoonfuls in 24 hours. Children under 2 years of age consult a physician.

INACTIVE INGREDIENTS
Citric Acid, Benzoic Acid U.S.P., Glycerin U.S.P., Sorbitol, Flavor (Peppermint, Menthol), Water.
Safe Tussin 30 does not contain antihistamines, sugar, alcohol, sodium, dyes, codeine; all of which may pose risks for certain patients. Each dose of Safe Tussin 30 contains .066g sorbitol, a non-nutritive caloric sweetener.

Continued on next page

Kramer Laboratories—Cont.

CONTRAINDICATIONS

Do not take if hypersensitive to Guaifenesin, Dextromethorphan or any of the ingredients listed above.

HOW SUPPLIED

Clear liquid in 4 oz bottles.

YOHIMEX™ Tablets
[yō-him′eks]   ℞

DESCRIPTION

Each tablet for oral administration contains yohimbine hydrochloride, 5.4 mg. ($\frac{1}{12}$ grain). Yohimbine is an indoalkylamine alkaloid with chemical similarity to reserpine. It is the principal alkaloid of the bark of the West African Corynanthe yohimbe tree and is also found in Rauwolfia Serpentina (L) Benth.

ACTIONS

Yohimbine is primarily an alpha-2 adrenergic blocker, which blocks presynaptic alpha-2-adrenoreceptors. PHARMACOLOGY: Its peripheral autonomic nervous system effect is to increase parasympathetic (cholinergic) and decrease sympathetic (adrenergic) activity. In male sexual performance, erection is linked to cholinergic activity which theoretically results in increased penile blood inflow, decreased penile blood outflow or both, causing erectile stimulation without increasing sexual desire. Yohimbine exerts a stimulating action on mood and may increase anxiety. Such actions are not adequately studied, although they appear to require high doses. Yohimbine has a mild antidiuretic action, probably via stimulation of hypothalamic centers and release of posterior pituitary hormone. Its action on peripheral blood vessels resembles that of reserpine, though it is weaker and of short duration. The drug reportedly exerts no significant influence on cardiac stimulation and other effects mediated by beta-adrenergic receptors.

INDICATIONS

Sympathicolytic and mydriatic agent. Impotence has been successfully treated with yohimbine in male patients with vascular or diabetic origins and psychogenic origins (18 mg./day). Urologists have used yohimbine experimentally for the treatment and the diagnostic classification of certain types of male erectile impotence.

CONTRAINDICATIONS

In patients with renal disease; hypersensitivity to any component.

WARNINGS

Not for use in geriatric patients, psychiatric patients or cardio-renal patients with a history of gastric or duodenal ulcer. Generally not for use in females.
USAGE IN PREGNANCY: Do not use during pregnancy.
USAGE IN CHILDREN: Do not use in children.

DRUG INTERACTIONS

Do not use yohimbine with antidepressants and other mood-modifying drugs.

ADVERSE REACTIONS

CNS: Yohimbine readily penetrates the CNS and produces a complex pattern of responses in doses lower than those required to produce peripheral alpha-adrenergic blockade. These include: antidiuresis and central excitation including elevated blood pressure and heart rate, increased motor activity, nervousness, irritability and tremor. Dizziness, headache and skin flushing have been reported.

OVERDOSAGE

Daily doses of 20–30 mg. may produce increases in heart rate and blood pressure, piloerection and rhinorrhea. More severe symptoms may include paresthesias, incoordination, tremulousness and a dissociative state with higher doses.

DOSAGE AND ADMINISTRATION

USUAL ADULT DOSE: One tablet taken 3 times daily. If side effects occur, the dosage is to be reduced to ½ tablet 3 times a day followed by gradual increase to 1 tablet 3 times a day. The therapy reported is not more than 10 weeks.

HOW SUPPLIED

Pink, round tablets in bottles of 100 tablets (NDC 55505-100-15)

Laser, Inc.
2200 W. 97TH PLACE, P.O. BOX 905
CROWN POINT, IN 46307

Direct Inquiries to:
Joseph N. Allegretti, R.Ph.
(219) 663-1165

DALLERGY® CAPLETS, SYRUP, TABLETS   ℞

Each Extended-Release Caplet* (Capsule-shaped tablet) contains: Chlorpheniramine Maleate 8 mg, Phenylephrine Hydrochloride 20 mg, Methscopolamine Nitrate 2.5 mg. Each 5 mL of grape-flavored Syrup contains: Chlorpheniramine Maleate 2 mg, Phenylephrine Hydrochloride 10 mg, Methscopolamine Nitrate 0.625 mg. Each Tablet contains: Chlorpheniramine Maleate 4 mg, Phenylephrine Hydrochloride 10 mg, Methscopolamine Nitrate 1.25 mg.

* In a specially prepared base to provide a prolonged therapeutic effect.

DALLERGY® –JR. CAPSULES   ℞

Each Extended-Release Capsule* contains: Brompheniramine Maleate 6 mg, Pseudoephedrine Hydrochloride 60 mg.

* In a specially prepared base to provide prolonged action.

DONATUSSIN DC SYRUP   ℞

Each 5 mL contains: Hydrocodone* Bitartrate 2.5 mg *(WARNING: May be habit forming), Phenylephrine Hydrochloride 7.5 mg, Guaifenesin 50 mg. Red Syrup.

DONATUSSIN DROPS   ℞

Each mL contains: Chlorpheniramine Maleate 1 mg, Phenylephrine Hydrochloride 2 mg, Guaifenesin 20 mg. Peach-flavored, orange color.

DONATUSSIN SYRUP   ℞

Each 5 mL contains: Dextromethorphan HBr 7.5 mg, Chlorpheniramine Maleate 2 mg, Phenylephrine HCl 10 mg, Guaifenesin 100 mg. Red Syrup.

FUMATINIC® CAPSULES   ℞

Each Extended-Release FUMATINIC Capsule contains: Ferrous Fumarate* 275 mg (equivalent to 90 mg of elemental iron), Vitamin C* (Ascorbic Acid) 100 mg, Vitamin B-12 (Cyanocobalamin) 15 mcg, Folic Acid 1 mg.

* In a specially prepared base to provide prolonged action.

KIE® SYRUP   ℞

Each 5 mL contains: Potassium Iodide 150 mg, Ephedrine Hydrochloride 8 mg. Green Syrup.

LACTOCAL–F TABLETS   ℞

Multivitamin, Multimineral supplement for pregnant or lactating women. White coated dye free tablet.

RESPAIRE®–SR CAPSULES 60 & 120   ℞

Each Extended-Release RESPAIRE-60 SR Capsule contains: Pseudoephedrine Hydrochloride* 60 mg and Guaifenesin† 200 mg. Each Extended-Release RESPAIRE-120 SR Capsule contains: Pseudoephedrine Hydrochloride* 120 mg and Guaifenesin† 250 mg.

* In a specially prepared base to provide prolonged action.
† Designed for immediate release to provide rapid action.

Lederle Piperacillin, Inc.
CAROLINA, PUERTO RICO 00630

Lederle Oncology
A Division of American Cyanamid Co.
ONE CYANAMID PLAZA
WAYNE, NJ 07470

AMICAR® Aminocaproic Acid
Syrup, Tablets, and Injection, USP
LEUCOVORIN CALCIUM FOR INJECTION
LEUCOVORIN CALCIUM TABLETS
LEVOPROME® Methotrimeprazine For Intramuscular Use
METHOTREXATE Sodium for Injection
METHOTREXATE LPF® Sodium (METHOTREXATE Sodium Injection)
METHOTREXATE Sodium Injection
NOVANTRONE® Mitoxantrone for Injection Concentrate
THIOTEPA For Injection Sterile 15 mg/Vial

For more information on these products, please see listings under Immunex on p. 1312 of this 1997 edition of the PDR.

Lederle Parenteral, Inc.
CAROLINA, PUERTO RICO 00630

Lederle Laboratories
A Division of American Cyanamid Co.
ONE CYANAMID PLAZA
WAYNE, NJ 07470

For Medical Information Contact:
MARKETED ONCOLOGY PRODUCTS:
Immunex Corporation
Professional Services Department
51 University Street
Seattle, WA 98101
(800) IMMUNEX

OTHER MARKETED DRUG PRODUCTS:
Lederle Laboratories
Medical Affairs Department
P.O. Box 8299
Philadelphia, PA 19101
Day: (800) 934-5556
8:30 AM to 4:30 PM
(Eastern Standard Time),
Weekdays only
Night: (610) 688-4400 (Emergencies only; non-emergencies should wait until the next day)

MARKETED VACCINES AND TINE TESTS:
Lederle Laboratories
Medical Affairs Department
P.O. Box 8299
Philadelphia, PA 19101
Day: (800) 934-5556
8:30 AM to 4:30 PM
(Eastern Standard Time),
Weekdays only
Night: (610) 688-4400 (Emergencies only; non-emergencies should wait until the next day)

LEDERLE PRODUCTS

The following list of Lederle products includes the alphanumeric LEDERMARK® codes which provide quick and positive identification of Lederle capsules and tablets:

Product Identity Code No.	Product
	ACEL-IMUNE® Diphtheria and Tetanus Toxoids and Acellular Pertussis Vaccine Adsorbed
A11	ARTANE® Tabs., 2mg
A12	ARTANE® Tabs., 5mg
—	ARTANE® Elixir, 2mg/5mL
A13	ASENDIN® Tabs., 25mg
A15	ASENDIN® Tabs., 50mg
A17	ASENDIN® Tabs., 100mg
A18	ASENDIN® Tabs., 150mg
B1	ZEBETA® Tablets, 5mg
B3	ZEBETA® Tablets, 10mg
B12	ZIAC® Tablets, 2.5/6.25mg

B13	ZIAC® Tablets, 5/6.25mg
B14	ZIAC® Tablets, 10/6.25mg
D11	DECLOMYCIN® Tabs., 150mg
D12	DECLOMYCIN® Tabs., 300mg
—	Diphtheria & Tetanus Toxoids Adsorbed PUROGENATED®
—	HibTITER® Haemophilus b Conjugate Vaccine
L1	LOXITANE® Caps., 5mg
L2	LOXITANE® Caps., 10mg
L3	LOXITANE® Caps., 25mg
L4	LOXITANE® Caps., 50mg
—	LOXITANE® IM, 50mg base/mL
—	LOXITANE® C Oral Concentrate, 25mg base/mL
M1	RHEUMATREX® Tabs., 2.5mg
M6	MYAMBUTOL® Tabs., 100mg
M7	MYAMBUTOL® Tabs., 400mg
M45	MINOCIN® Pellet-Filled Caps., 50mg
M46	MINOCIN® Pellet-Filled Caps., 100mg
—	MINOCIN® IV, 100mg vial
—	MINOCIN® Oral Suspension, 50mg/5mL
M77	MATERNA® Tabs.
—	ORIMUNE® Poliovirus Vaccine Live Oral Trivalent
—	PIPRACIL® 2g
—	PIPRACIL® 3g
—	PIPRACIL® 4g
—	PIPRACIL® 40g
—	PNU-IMUNE® 23 Pneumococcal Vaccine Polyvalent
—	PROSTEP® nicotine transdermal system, 11mg
—	PROSTEP® nicotine transdermal system, 22mg
S200	SUPRAX® Tablets, 200mg
S400	SUPRAX® Tablets, 400mg
—	SUPRAX® Powder for oral suspension
—	Tetanus Toxoid Adsorbed PUROGENATED®
—	Tetanus and Diphtheria Toxoids Adsorbed PUROGENATED®
—	TETRAMUNE® Diphtheria and Tetanus Toxoids and Pertussis Vaccine Adsorbed and Haemophilus b Conjugate Vaccine (Diphtheria CRM_{197} Protein Conjugate)
—	TRI-IMMUNOL® Diphtheria and Tetanus Toxoids and Pertussis Vaccine Adsorbed
—	Tuberculin, Old, TINE TEST®
—	Tuberculin, Purified Protein Derivative TINE TEST® PPD
T1	TriHEMIC® 600 Tabs.
V7	VERELAN® Caps., 180mg
V8	VERELAN® Caps., 120mg
V9	VERELAN® Caps., 240mg

DIPHTHERIA and TETANUS TOXOIDS and ACELLULAR PERTUSSIS VACCINE ADSORBED ACEL-IMUNE® ℞

DESCRIPTION

Diphtheria and Tetanus Toxoids and Acellular Pertussis Vaccine Adsorbed, ACEL-IMUNE, is a sterile combination of PUROGENATED® Diphtheria Toxoid, PUROGENATED Tetanus Toxoid, and Acellular Pertussis Vaccine, which is adsorbed to an aluminum salt. ACEL-IMUNE is for intramuscular use only. After shaking, the vaccine is a homogeneous white suspension.

The *Corynebacterium diphtheriae* and *Clostridium tetani* organisms are grown in media according to the method of Mueller and Miller[1,2] and are detoxified by use of formaldehyde. The diphtheria and tetanus toxoids are refined by the Pillemer alcohol fractionation method[3] and are diluted with a solution containing phosphate buffer, glycine, and thimerosal (mercury derivative) as a preservative. The acellular pertussis vaccine component is prepared by growing Phase I *Bordetella pertussis* in Stainer-Scholte defined medium and harvesting the culture fluid. Purification of the acellular pertussis vaccine component is accomplished by ammonium sulfate fractionation steps and a final sucrose density gradient centrifugation. The acellular pertussis vaccine component is detoxified with formaldehyde and thimerosal (mercury derivative) is added as a preservative.

The Diphtheria Toxoid, Tetanus Toxoid, and Acellular Pertussis Vaccine are combined, diluted in phosphate buffered saline (PBS), and adsorbed to aluminum. The aluminum adjuvant content by assay is ≤0.85 mg aluminum per 0.5 mL dose and is present as aluminum hydroxide and aluminum phosphate. The residual free formaldehyde content by assay is ≤0.02%. Thimerosal (mercury derivative) is present in a final concentration of 1:10,000. The final product may also contain gelatin and polysorbate 80 which are used in early stages of the process.

Each 0.5 mL dose is formulated to contain 7.5 Lf of diphtheria toxoid and 5.0 Lf of tetanus toxoid (both toxoids induce not less than 2 units of antitoxin per mL in the guinea pig potency test) and 300 hemagglutinating (HA) units of Acellular Pertussis Vaccine. A hemagglutination unit is that amount of material which completely agglutinates chicken red blood cells as measured by the HA assay.[4] The acellular pertussis vaccine component contains approximately 40 μg (but not more than 60 μg) of pertussis antigens per 0.5 mL dose with approximately 86% filamentous hemagglutinin (FHA), approximately 8% lymphocytosis promoting factor (LPF), approximately 4% per dose 69-kilodalton (69kd) outer membrane protein, and approximately 2% type 2 fimbriae (pertussis-specific agglutinogen).

The potency of the pertussis component is evaluated by measurement of ELISA titers in immunized mice against FHA, LPF, 69kd and fimbriae.

The acellular pertussis vaccine component is produced by Takeda Chemical Industries, Ltd., Osaka, Japan and is combined with diphtheria and tetanus toxoids manufactured by Lederle Laboratories. The bulk vaccine is prepared by Lederle Laboratories. ACEL-IMUNE is filled, labeled, packaged and released by Lederle Laboratories.

CLINICAL PHARMACOLOGY

Simultaneous immunization against diphtheria, tetanus, and pertussis (whooping cough) during infancy and childhood has been a routine practice in the United States since the late 1940s. It has played a major role in markedly reducing the incidence of cases and deaths from each of these diseases.

Diphtheria is primarily a localized and generalized intoxication caused by diphtheria toxin, an extracellular protein metabolite of toxinogenic strains of *C diphtheriae.* While the incidence of diphtheria in the US has decreased from over 200,000 cases reported in 1921, before the general use of diphtheria toxoid, to only 15 cases reported from 1980 to 1983,[5] case fatality rate has remained constant at about 5% to 10%. The highest case fatality rates are in the very young and in the elderly.

Following adequate immunization with diphtheria toxoid, it is thought that protection lasts for at least 10 years.[5] Antitoxin levels of at least 0.01 antitoxin units/mL are generally regarded as protective.[6] This significantly reduces both the risk of developing diphtheria and the severity of clinical illness. It does not, however, eliminate carriage of *C diphtheriae* in the pharynx or on the skin.[5]

Tetanus is an intoxication manifested primarily by neuromuscular dysfunction caused by a potent exotoxin elaborated by *C tetani.* The incidence of tetanus in the US has dropped dramatically with the routine use of tetanus toxoid, remaining relatively constant over the last decade at about 90 cases reported annually. Spores of *C tetani* are ubiquitous, and there is essentially no natural immunity to tetanus toxin.

Thus, universal primary immunization with tetanus toxoid with subsequent maintenance of adequate antitoxin levels, by means of timed boosters, is necessary to protect all age groups.[5] Tetanus toxoid is a highly effective antigen, and a completed primary series generally induces serum antitoxin levels of at least 0.01 antitoxin units, a level which has been reported to be protective.[7] It is thought that protection persists for at least 10 years.[5]

Pertussis (whooping cough) is a highly communicable disease of the respiratory tract that has an attack rate in unimmunized household contacts of over 90%.[5] Since immunization against pertussis (whooping cough) became widespread, the number of reported cases and associated mortality in the US has declined from about 120,000 cases and 1,100 deaths in 1950,[8] to an annual average of about 3,500 cases and 10 fatalities in recent years.[5,9] Precise data do not exist, since bacteriological confirmation of pertussis can be obtained in less than half of the suspected cases. Most reported illness from *B pertussis* occurs in infants and young children; two thirds of reported deaths occur in children less than 1 year old. Older children and adults, in whom classic signs are often absent, may go undiagnosed and serve as reservoirs of disease.[5]

Pertussis disease (whooping cough) is caused by a gram-negative coccobacillus, *B pertussis.* Several antigens that are thought to play a role in protective immunity have been isolated from cultures of *B pertussis.* These include filamentous hemagglutinin (FHA), lymphocytosis promoting factor (LPF), also known as pertussis toxin (PT), a 69-kilodalton (69kd) outer membrane protein, and fimbriae (pertussis-specific agglutinogens).[10–12] Another biologically active component, endotoxin, may contribute to reactogenicity of pertussis vaccines.[13] The Takeda acellular pertussis vaccine component used in ACEL-IMUNE contains inactivated LPF, FHA, 69kd outer membrane protein and type 2 fimbriae (pertussis-specific agglutinogen), with minimal endotoxin compared to that in whole-cell pertussis vaccine. The pertussis component induces immunity against pertussis (whooping cough).

Acellular pertussis vaccines have been used in Japan since 1981, mostly in 2-year-old children. Evidence for the efficacy of these vaccines, as a group, is demonstrated by the decline in pertussis disease with their routine use in that country.[14,15] In addition, a review of epidemiological studies of the Japanese acellular pertussis vaccines estimated that these vaccines, as a group, were 88% efficacious in protecting against clinical pertussis on household exposure, with a 95% confidence interval of 79% to 93%.[16] In three Japanese household contact studies which employed retrospective case ascertainment and non-standard case definitions, the vaccine-specific efficacy of the Takeda vaccine ranged between 89% and 94% but confidence intervals were wide, due to the small number of children in each study.[16–19] Although there were differences in study methods, these estimates of efficacy are quite comparable to that for whole-cell pertussis vaccine in the United States.[20]

Efficacy of the DTP vaccine containing the Takeda acellular pertussis vaccine component was examined, in particular, in a nonblinded household contact study, conducted by Lederle Laboratories, that included both retrospective and prospective case evaluation.[21] As a consequence of the immunization schedule in Japan at the time of study, none of the vaccinated contacts were less than 2 years of age while some of the unvaccinated contacts were less than 2 years of age. When analysis of results was limited to vaccinated and unvaccinated household contacts 2 years of age and over, efficacy was estimated to be 79% (95% confidence interval, 60% to 89%) for physician-diagnosed pertussis disease. This included respiratory illnesses that may have been mild pertussis. When cases were restricted to disease diagnosed as typical pertussis, omitting mild suspect cases, efficacy was estimated to be 97% (95% confidence interval, 82% to 99%). When unvaccinated household contacts under 2 years of age are also included in the analysis, efficacy was estimated to be 81% (95% confidence interval, 64% to 90%) against pertussis disease (including mild suspect cases) and 98% (95% confidence interval, 84% to 99%) against typical pertussis. While there is some uncertainty with regard to the absolute magnitude of these estimates, the data as a whole demonstrate the efficacy of the Takeda Pertussis Vaccine.

Immunogenicity of ACEL-IMUNE compared with whole-cell DTP was studied in approximately 1,000 US children receiving these vaccines as a fourth or fifth dose at 17 to 24 months or 4 to 6 years of age. Antibody response following ACEL-IMUNE was similar to whole-cell DTP for LPF, 69kd protein, and agglutinins, and higher than DTP for FHA (the DTP used in these comparative studies was manufactured by Lederle Laboratories). All children achieved protective antibody levels to diphtheria and tetanus toxoids. A serologic correlate to protection against pertussis disease has not been established.[22] ACEL-IMUNE was less reactogenic than the whole-cell DTP vaccine (manufactured by Lederle Laboratories) in these studies[23–25] with regard to local reactions including less pain/tenderness, erythema, induration and warmth at the injection site. In addition, there was less drowsiness, fretfulness, fever and antipyretic use following ACEL-IMUNE as compared with DTP. The relative frequency of rare events that may be associated with immunization can only be determined in large postmarketing surveillance studies.

INDICATIONS AND USAGE

Diphtheria and Tetanus Toxoids and Acellular Pertussis Vaccine Adsorbed, ACEL-IMUNE, is indicated as a fourth and/or fifth dose for children from 17 months of age up to age 7 years (prior to seventh birthday) who have previously been immunized against diphtheria, tetanus, and pertussis with three or four doses of whole-cell DTP vaccine. The administration of ACEL-IMUNE may be considered for children as young as 15 months of age when it is expected that the child will not return at 18 months to receive the fourth dose in this immunization series although studies in this age group have not been completed.

THIS PRODUCT IS NOT RECOMMENDED FOR USE IN CHILDREN BELOW THE AGE OF 15 MONTHS.

Children who have recovered from culture-confirmed pertussis need not receive further doses of a pertussis-containing vaccine.[5] This vaccine is intended for active immunization against diphtheria, tetanus and pertussis, and is not to be used for treatment of actual infection.

If a contraindication to the pertussis vaccine component occurs, Diphtheria and Tetanus Toxoids, Adsorbed for Pediatric Use (DT) should be substituted for each of the remaining doses.

As with any vaccine, ACEL-IMUNE may not protect 100% of individuals receiving the vaccine.

CONTRAINDICATIONS

HYPERSENSITIVITY TO ANY COMPONENT OF THE VACCINE, INCLUDING THIMEROSAL, A MERCURY DERIVATIVE, IS A CONTRAINDICATION.

IMMUNIZATION SHOULD BE DEFERRED DURING THE COURSE OF ANY FEBRILE ILLNESS OR ACUTE INFEC-

Continued on next page

Lederle—Cont.

TION. A MINOR AFEBRILE ILLNESS SUCH AS A MILD UPPER RESPIRATORY INFECTION IS NOT USUALLY REASON TO DEFER IMMUNIZATION.[5,26]
DATA ON THE USE OF ACEL-IMUNE IN CHILDREN FOR WHOM WHOLE-CELL PERTUSSIS VACCINE IS CONTRAINDICATED ARE NOT AVAILABLE. UNTIL SUCH DATA ARE AVAILABLE, IT WOULD BE PRUDENT TO CONSIDER THE IMMUNIZATION PRACTICES ADVISORY COMMITTEE (ACIP) AND AMERICAN ACADEMY OF PEDIATRICS (AAP) CONTRAINDICATIONS TO WHOLE-CELL PERTUSSIS VACCINE AS CONTRAINDICATIONS TO ACEL-IMUNE.
IMMUNIZATION WITH ACEL-IMUNE IS CONTRAINDICATED IF THE CHILD HAS EXPERIENCED ANY EVENT FOLLOWING PREVIOUS IMMUNIZATION WITH PERTUSSIS VACCINE (DTP or acellular pertussis-containing vaccine), WHICH IS CONSIDERED BY THE AAP OR ACIP TO BE A CONTRAINDICATION TO FURTHER DOSES OF PERTUSSIS VACCINE.
THE ACIP STATES THAT "IF ANY OF THE FOLLOWING EVENTS OCCUR IN TEMPORAL RELATION TO RECEIPT OF DTP, THE DECISION TO GIVE SUBSEQUENT DOSES OF VACCINE CONTAINING THE PERTUSSIS COMPONENT SHOULD BE CAREFULLY CONSIDERED. . .

CONTRAINDICATIONS AND PRECAUTIONS TO FURTHER DTP VACCINATION

CONTRAINDICATIONS
AN IMMEDIATE ANAPHYLACTIC REACTION.
ENCEPHALOPATHY OCCURRING WITHIN 7 DAYS FOLLOWING DTP VACCINATION.

PRECAUTIONS
TEMPERATURE OF ≥ 40.5° C (105° F) WITHIN 48 HOURS NOT DUE TO ANOTHER IDENTIFIABLE CAUSE.
COLLAPSE OR SHOCK-LIKE STATE (HYPOTONIC-HYPORESPONSIVE EPISODE) WITHIN 48 HOURS.
PERSISTENT, INCONSOLABLE CRYING LASTING ≥ 3 HOURS, OCCURRING WITHIN 48 HOURS.
CONVULSIONS WITH OR WITHOUT FEVER OCCURRING WITHIN 3 DAYS.
ALTHOUGH THESE EVENTS WERE CONSIDERED ABSOLUTE CONTRAINDICATIONS IN PREVIOUS ACIP RECOMMENDATIONS, THERE MAY BE CIRCUMSTANCES, SUCH AS A HIGH INCIDENCE OF PERTUSSIS, IN WHICH THE POTENTIAL BENEFITS OUTWEIGH POSSIBLE RISKS, PARTICULARLY BECAUSE THESE EVENTS ARE NOT ASSOCIATED WITH PERMANENT SEQUELAE."[5]
The occurrence of any type of neurological symptoms or signs, including one or more convulsions (seizures) following administration of ACEL-IMUNE or whole-cell DTP vaccine is generally a contraindication to further use. The presence of any evolving or changing disorder affecting the central nervous system is a contraindication to administration of pertussis vaccine regardless of whether the suspected neurological disorder is associated with occurrence of seizure activity of any type.[5,26]
The ACIP and the AAP recognize certain circumstances in which children with stable central nervous system disorders, including well-controlled seizures or satisfactorily explained single seizures, may receive pertussis vaccine. The ACIP and AAP do not consider a family history of seizures to be a contraindication to pertussis vaccine.[5,26,27]
The decision to administer a pertussis-containing vaccine to such children must be made by the physician on an individual basis, with consideration of all relevant factors, and assessment of potential risks and benefits for that individual. The physician should review the full text of ACIP and AAP guidelines prior to considering vaccination for such children.[5,26,27] The parent or guardian should be advised of the potential increased risk involved.
There are no data on whether the prophylactic use of antipyretics can decrease the risk of febrile convulsions. However, data suggest that acetaminophen will reduce the incidence of postvaccination fever. The ACIP and AAP suggest administering acetaminophen at age-appropriate doses at the time of vaccination and every 4 to 6 hours to children at higher risk for seizures than the general population.[5,26,27]
The clinical judgment of the attending physician should prevail at all times.

WARNINGS
THIS PRODUCT IS NOT RECOMMENDED FOR USE IN CHILDREN BELOW THE AGE OF 15 MONTHS. STUDIES IN CHILDREN 15 TO 17 MONTHS OF AGE HAVE NOT BEEN COMPLETED.
NO DETERMINATION OF EFFICACY IN INFANTS HAS BEEN MADE TO DATE. STUDIES DESIGNED TO EVALUATE EFFICACY IN INFANTS ARE ONGOING BUT ARE NOT YET COMPLETE. IN ONE IMMUNOGENICITY STUDY, INFANTS RECEIVING ACEL-IMUNE EXHIBITED REDUCED RESPONSES TO LPF AND AGGLUTINOGENS, SIMILAR RESPONSES TO 69kd PROTEIN AND

HIGHER SEROLOGICAL RESPONSES TO FHA, COMPARED TO THOSE RECEIVING LEDERLE WHOLE-CELL DTP VACCINE.[22] THE ROLE OF SERUM ANTIBODIES TO PERTUSSIS ANTIGENS IN PROTECTION AGAINST PERTUSSIS DISEASE IS UNKNOWN.
THIS PRODUCT IS NOT RECOMMENDED FOR IMMUNIZING PERSONS ON OR AFTER THEIR SEVENTH BIRTHDAY.
DATA ON THE USE OF ACEL-IMUNE IN CHILDREN FOR WHOM WHOLE-CELL PERTUSSIS VACCINE IS CONTRAINDICATED ARE NOT AVAILABLE. UNTIL SUCH DATA ARE AVAILABLE IT WOULD BE PRUDENT TO CONSIDER ACIP AND AAP CONTRAINDICATIONS TO WHOLE-CELL PERTUSSIS VACCINE AS CONTRAINDICATIONS TO ACEL-IMUNE. (See **CONTRAINDICATIONS.**)
ACEL-IMUNE should be given with caution to children with thrombocytopenia or any coagulation disorder that would contraindicate intramuscular injection. (See **Drug Interactions.**)
Routine immunization should be deferred during an outbreak of poliomyelitis, providing the patient has not sustained an injury that increases the risk of tetanus and providing an outbreak of diphtheria or pertussis does not occur simultaneously.

PRECAUTIONS
General
1. PREVIOUS IMMUNIZATION HISTORY SHOULD BE ASCERTAINED TO CONFIRM THAT AT LEAST THREE DOSES OF WHOLE-CELL DTP VACCINE HAVE BEEN GIVEN.
2. PRIOR TO ADMINISTRATION OF ANY DOSE OF ACEL-IMUNE, THE PARENT OR GUARDIAN SHOULD BE ASKED ABOUT THE PERSONAL HISTORY, FAMILY HISTORY, AND RECENT HEALTH STATUS OF THE VACCINE RECIPIENT. THE PHYSICIAN SHOULD ASCERTAIN PREVIOUS IMMUNIZATION HISTORY, CURRENT HEALTH STATUS AND OCCURRENCE OF ANY SYMPTOMS AND/OR SIGNS OF AN ADVERSE EVENT AFTER PREVIOUS IMMUNIZATIONS IN THE CHILD TO BE IMMUNIZED, IN ORDER TO DETERMINE THE EXISTENCE OF ANY CONTRAINDICATION TO IMMUNIZATION WITH ACEL-IMUNE AND TO ALLOW AN ASSESSMENT OF BENEFITS AND RISKS.
3. BEFORE THE INJECTION OF ANY BIOLOGICAL, THE PHYSICIAN SHOULD TAKE ALL PRECAUTIONS KNOWN FOR THE PREVENTION OF ALLERGIC OR ANY OTHER SIDE REACTIONS. This should include: a review of the patient's history regarding possible sensitivity; the ready availability of epinephrine 1:1000 and other appropriate agents used for control of immediate allergic reactions; and a knowledge of the recent literature pertaining to use of the biological concerned, including the nature of side effects and adverse reactions that may follow its use.
4. Children with impaired immune responsiveness, whether due to the use of immunosuppressive therapy (including irradiation, corticosteroids, antimetabolites, alkylating agents, and cytotoxic agents), a genetic defect, human immunodeficiency virus (HIV) infection, or other causes, may have reduced antibody response to active immunization procedures.[5,26,28] Deferral of administration of vaccine may be considered in individuals receiving immunosuppressive therapy.[5,26] Other groups should receive this vaccine according to the usual recommended schedule.[5,26,28,29] (See **Drug Interactions.**)
5. This product is not contraindicated for use in individuals with HIV.
6. Since this product is a suspension containing an adjuvant, shake vigorously to obtain a uniform suspension prior to withdrawing each dose from the multiple dose vial.
7. A separate sterile syringe and needle or a sterile disposable unit should be used for each individual patient to prevent transmission of hepatitis or other infectious agents from one person to another. Needles should be disposed of properly and should not be recapped.
8. Special care should be taken to prevent injection into a blood vessel.

NATIONAL CHILDHOOD VACCINE INJURY ACT
This Act requires that the manufacturer and lot number of the vaccine administered be recorded by the health care provider in the vaccine recipient's permanent medical record, along with the date of administration of the vaccine and the name, address, and title of the person administering the vaccine.
The Act further requires the health care provider to report to a health department or to the FDA the occurrence following immunization of any event set forth in the Vaccine Injury Table including: anaphylaxis or anaphylactic shock within 24 hours, encephalopathy or encephalitis within 7 days, shock-collapse or hypotonic-hyporesponsive collapse within 7 days, residual seizure disorder, any acute complication or sequelae (including death) of above events, or any

event that would contraindicate further doses of vaccine, according to this ACEL-IMUNE package insert.[30]
The US Department of Health and Human Services has established a new Vaccine Adverse Event Reporting System (VAERS) to accept all reports of suspected adverse events after the administration of any vaccine, including but not limited to the reporting of events required by the National Childhood Vaccine Injury Act of 1986.[30] The VAERS toll-free number for VAERS forms and information is 800-822-7967.

INFORMATION FOR PATIENT
PRIOR TO ADMINISTRATION OF THIS VACCINE, HEALTH CARE PERSONNEL SHOULD INFORM THE PARENT, GUARDIAN, OR OTHER RESPONSIBLE ADULT OF THE RECOMMENDED IMMUNIZATION SCHEDULE FOR PROTECTION AGAINST DIPHTHERIA, TETANUS, AND PERTUSSIS AND THE BENEFITS AND RISKS TO THE CHILD RECEIVING A VACCINE CONTAINING AN ACELLULAR PERTUSSIS COMPONENT. GUIDANCE SHOULD BE PROVIDED ON MEASURES TO BE TAKEN SHOULD ADVERSE EVENTS OCCUR, SUCH AS, ANTIPYRETIC MEASURES FOR ELEVATED TEMPERATURES AND THE NEED TO REPORT ADVERSE EVENTS TO THE HEALTH CARE PROVIDER. PARENTS SHOULD BE PROVIDED WITH VACCINE INFORMATION SHEETS (WHEN AVAILABLE FROM THE CENTERS FOR DISEASE CONTROL) AT THE TIME OF EACH VACCINATION, AS STATED IN THE NATIONAL CHILDHOOD VACCINE INJURY ACT.[30]

DRUG INTERACTIONS
Children receiving immunosuppressive therapy may have a reduced response to active immunization procedures.[5,26,28]
As with other intramuscular injections, ACEL-IMUNE should be given with caution to children on anticoagulant therapy.

CARCINOGENESIS, MUTAGENESIS, IMPAIRMENT OF FERTILITY
ACEL-IMUNE has not been evaluated for its carcinogenic, mutagenic potentials, or impairment of fertility.

PEDIATRIC USE
This product is not recommended for use in children below the age of 15 months. Studies in children under 15 to 17 months of age have not been completed.
No determination of efficacy in infants has been made to date. Studies designed to evaluate efficacy in infants are ongoing but are not yet complete. In one immunogenicity study, infants receiving ACEL-IMUNE exhibited reduced responses to LPF and agglutinogens, similar responses to 69kd protein, and higher serological responses to FHA, compared to those receiving Lederle Laboratories' whole-cell DTP vaccine.[22] The role of serum antibodies to pertussis antigens in protection against pertussis disease is unknown. The vaccine is not recommended for use as a primary series in children of any age.
For immunization of children 7 years of age and older, Tetanus and Diphtheria Toxoids Adsorbed for Adult Use (Td) is recommended.[5,26] If a contraindication to the pertussis component exists, Diphtheria and Tetanus Toxoids Adsorbed for Pediatric Use (DT) should be substituted.

ADVERSE REACTIONS
Adverse reactions associated with ACEL-IMUNE have been evaluated in 911 children receiving this vaccine as the fourth or fifth dose in the DTP series. The percent of children experiencing common symptoms at any time within 72 hours following immunization is summarized below.[25]

Symptom	% of children* reporting symptoms within 72 hours of immunization (n=911)
Tenderness	26
Erythema (> 2 cm)	10
Induration (> 2 cm)	7
Injection site temp	17
Fever ≥38°C (100.4°F)	19
>39°C (102.2°F)	1.5
Drowsiness	6
Fretfulness	17
Vomiting	2

* Children age groups 17 to 24 months and 4 to 6 years of age (fourth and fifth doses) are included.

During a 72-hour period following immunization, the most frequently reported adverse events, excluding those listed above, in decreasing order of frequency were: upper respiratory infection/rhinitis (6%), diarrhea/loose stools (3.5%), rash (1.2%). One child experienced a febrile seizure 78 hours after immunization.[25] A cause-and-effect relationship between these latter events and vaccination has not been established.
In investigational studies in 2,041 infants administered a total of 5,719 doses of ACEL-IMUNE the combined frequency of common symptoms, at any time within 72 hours following any dose was as follows: erythema > 2 cm, 4%; induration > 2 cm, 1.5%; fever 38°C (100.4°F), 7%; drowsiness, 12%; fret-

fulness, 20%; vomiting, 3%. During this period, events judged by the investigators to contraindicate further doses of vaccine occurred in the indicated number of children: persistent or unusual cry (11); fever 40.5°C (104.9°F) (1); possible seizure (1); hypotonic-hyporesponsive episode (1); lethargy (1); injection site rash (1). One child died suddenly 6 weeks after immunization following apparent recovery from an enteroviral meningitis[25]; however, a causal relationship with ACEL-IMUNE has not been established.

As with other aluminum-containing vaccines,[31] a nodule may occasionally be palpable at the injection site for several weeks. Although not seen in studies with ACEL-IMUNE, sterile abscess formation or subcutaneous atrophy at the injection site may also occur.

As with any vaccine, there is the possibility that broad use of ACEL-IMUNE could reveal adverse reactions not observed in clinical trials. Events have been reported following administration of other vaccines containing diphtheria, tetanus, and/or pertussis antigens. These include those listed below. Urticaria, erythema multiforme or other rash, arthralgias[32] and more rarely, a severe anaphylactic reaction (eg, urticaria with swelling of the mouth, difficulty breathing, hypotension, or shock) have been reported following administration of preparations containing diphtheria, tetanus, and/or pertussis antigens.

Neurological complications,[33] such as convulsions,[32] encephalopathy[32,34] and various mono- and polyneuropathies,[34–40] including Guillain-Barré syndrome[41,42] have been reported following administration of preparations containing diphtheria, tetanus, and/or pertussis antigens.

Permanent neurological disability and death have been reported rarely in temporal relation to immunization with vaccines containing pertussis antigens.

DOSAGE AND ADMINISTRATION

The dose is 0.5 mL to be given intramuscularly only.

A fourth and/or fifth dose with ACEL-IMUNE is indicated for children who have previously been immunized with at least three doses of whole-cell DTP vaccine.

The fourth dose consists of 0.5 mL of ACEL-IMUNE administered at approximately 18 months of age, and at least 6 months following the third DTP immunization.

A fifth dose consists of 0.5 mL of ACEL-IMUNE and is indicated at 4 to 6 years of age, preferably prior to entrance into kindergarten or elementary school. However, if the fourth dose of the basic immunizing series was administered after the fourth birthday, a booster prior to school entry is not considered necessary.[5]

Shake vigorously to obtain a uniform suspension prior to withdrawing each dose from the multiple dose vial. The vaccine should not be used if it cannot be resuspended.

Parenteral drug products should be inspected visually for particulate matter and discoloration prior to administration whenever solution and container permit. (See **DESCRIPTION.**)

The vaccine should be injected intramuscularly. The preferred sites are the anterolateral aspect of the thigh or the deltoid muscle of the upper arm. The vaccine should not be injected in the gluteal area or areas where there may be a major nerve trunk. Before injection, the skin at the injection site should be cleansed and prepared with a suitable germicide.

After insertion of the needle, aspirate to help avoid inadvertent injection into a blood vessel.

If a contraindication to the pertussis vaccine component occurs, Diphtheria and Tetanus Toxoids, Adsorbed for Pediatric Use (DT) should be substituted for each of the remaining doses.

For either primary or booster immunization against tetanus and diphtheria of individuals 7 years of age or older, the use of Tetanus and Diphtheria Toxoids Adsorbed for Adult Use (Td) is recommended.[5,26]

HOW SUPPLIED

NDC 0005-1950-31 5.0 mL vial

STORAGE

DO NOT FREEZE. STORE REFRIGERATED, AWAY FROM FREEZER COMPARTMENT, AT 2°C TO 8°C (36°F TO 46°F).

REFERENCES

1. Mueller JH, Miller PA. Production of diphtheria toxin of high potency (100 Lf) on a reproducible medium. *J Immunol.* 1941;40:21–32.
2. Mueller JH, Miller PA. Factors influencing the production of tetanus toxin. *J Immunol.* 1947;56:143–147.
3. Pillemer L, Grossberg DB, Wittler RG. The immunochemistry of toxins and toxoids. II. The preparation of immunologic evaluation of purified tetanal toxoid. *J Immunol.* 1946;54:213–224.
4. Arai H, Sato Y. Separation and characterization of two distinct hemagglutinins contained in purified leukocytosis promoter factor from Bordetella pertussis. *Biochimica et Biophysica Acta.* 1976;444:765–782.
5. Diphtheria, tetanus and pertussis: Recommendations for vaccine use and other preventive measures—recommen-

dations of the Immunization Practices Advisory Committee (ACIP). *MMWR.* 1991;Vol. 40/No. RR-10.
6. Ipsen J. Immunization of adults against diphtheria and tetanus. *N Engl J Med.* 1954;251:459–466.
7. *Federal Register Notice.* Friday, December 13, 1985, Vol. 50, No. 240.
8. Reported incidence of notifiable diseases in the United States. *MMWR.* 1970;19(53):44.
9. Pertussis surveillance—United States, 1986–1988. *MMWR.* 1990;39(4);57–66.
10. Cowell JL, Oda M, Burstyn DG, et al. Prospective protective antigens and animal models for pertussis. In: Leive L and Schlessinger D, eds. *Microbiology—1984.* Washington, DC: American Society for Microbiology; 1984:172–175.
11. Shahin RD, Brennan MJ, Li ZM, et al. Characterization of the protective capacity and immunogenicity of the 69 K Da outer membrane protein of *Bordetella pertussis. J Exper Med.* 1990;171(1):63–73.
12. Novotny P, Kobisch M, Cownley K, et al. Evaluation of *Bordetella bronchiseptica* vaccines in specific-pathogen-free piglets with bacterial cell surface antigens in enzyme linked immunosorbent assay. *Infect Immun.* 1985; 50:190–198.
13. Manclark CR, Cowell JL. Pertussis vaccine. In: Germanier R, ed. *Bacterial Vaccines.* New York, NY: Academic Press, Inc.; 1984:69–106.
14. Report of the task force on pertussis and pertussis immunization—1988. *Pediatrics.* 1988;81(6):939–984.
15. Kimura M, Kuno-Sakai H. Developments in pertussis immunisation in Japan. *Lancet.* 1990;336:30–32.
16. Noble GR, Bernier RH, Esber EC, et al. Acellular and whole-cell pertussis vaccines in Japan. *JAMA.* 1987;257:1351–1356.
17. Isomura S, Suzuki S, Sato Y. Clinical efficacy of the Japanese acellular pertussis vaccine after intrafamiliar exposure to pertussis patients. *Dev. Biol. Stand.* 1985;61:531–537.
18. Aoyama T, Murase Y, Gonda T, et al. Type-specific efficacy of acellular pertussis vaccine. *AJDC.* 1988;142:40–42.
19. Kato T, Goshima T, Nakajima N, et al. Protection against pertussis by acellular pertussis vaccines (Takeda, Japan): household contact studies in Kawasaki City, Japan. *Acta Paediatr Jpn.* 1989;31:698–701.
20. Pertussis—United States, 1982 and 1983. *MMWR.* 1984;33(40):573–575.
21. Mortimer EA, Kimura M, Cherry JD, et al. Protective efficacy of the Takeda Acellular Pertussis Vaccine combined with diphtheria and tetanus toxoids following household exposure of Japanese children. *AJDC.* 1990;144:899–904.
22. Blumberg DA, Mink CM, Cherry JD, et al. Comparison of acellular and whole-cell pertussis-component diphtheria-tetanus-pertussis vaccines in infants. *J Pediatr.* 1991;119:194–204.
23. Morgan CM, Blumberg DA, Cherry JD, et al. Comparison of acellular and whole-cell pertussis-component DTP vaccines. *AJDC.* 1990;144:41–45.
24. Blumberg DA, Mink CM, Cherry JD, et al. Comparison of an acellular pertussis-component DTP vaccine with a whole-cell pertussis-component DTP vaccine in 17- to 24-month-old children, with measurement of 69-kilodalton outer membrane protein antibody. *J Pediatr.* 1990;117:46–51.
25. Data on file, Lederle Laboratories, Pearl River, NY.
26. American Academy of Pediatrics. *Report of the Committee on Infectious Diseases.* 22nd ed. Elk Grove Village, IL: American Academy of Pediatrics; 1991.
27. Pertussis immunization: family history of convulsions and use of antipyretics—supplementary ACIP statement. *MMWR.* 1987;36(18):281–282.
28. Recommendation of the ACIP: immunization of children infected with human T-lymphotropic virus type III/lymphadenopathy-associated virus. *MMWR.* 1986; 35(38):595–606.
29. Immunization of children infected with human immunodeficiency virus—supplementary ACIP statement. *MMWR.* 1988;37(12):181–183.
30. National Childhood Vaccine Injury Act: Requirements for permanent vaccination records and for reporting of selected events after vaccination. *MMWR.* 1988; 37(13):197–200.
31. Fawcett HA, Smith NP. Injection-site granuloma due to aluminum. *Arch Dermatol.* 1984;120:1318–1322.
32. Adverse events following immunization. *MMWR.* 1985; 34(3):43–47.
33. Rutledge SL, Snead OC. Neurological complications of immunizations. *J Pediatr.* 1986;109:917–924.
34. Schlenska GK. Unusual neurological complications following tetanus toxoid administration. *J Neurol.* 1977; 215:299–302.
35. Blumstein GI, Kreithen H. Peripheral neuropathy following tetanus toxoid administration. *JAMA.* 1966; 198:1030–1031.

36. Reinstein L, Pargament JM, Goodman JS. Peripheral neuropathy after multiple tetanus toxoid injections. *Arch Phys Med Rehabil.* 1982;63:332–334.
37. Tsairis P, Dyck PJ, Mulder DW. Natural history of brachial plexus neuropathy. *Arch Neurol.* 1972;27:109–117.
38. Quast U, Hennessen W, Widmark RM. Mono- and polyneuritis after tetanus vaccination. *Devel Biol Stand.* 1979;43:25–32.
39. Holliday PL, Bauer RB. Polyradiculoneuritis secondary to immunization with tetanus and diphtheria toxoids. *Arch Neurol.* 1983;40:56–57.
40. Fenichel GM. Neurological complications of tetanus toxoid. *Arch Neurol.* 1983;40:390.
41. Pollard JD, Selby G. Relapsing neuropathy due to tetanus toxoid. *J Neurol Sci.* 1978;37:113–125.
42. Newton N, Janati A. Guillain-Barré syndrome after vaccination with purified tetanus toxoid. *S Med J.* 1987;80:1053–1054.

Manufactured by:
LEDERLE LABORATORIES DIVISION
American Cyanamid Company, Pearl River, NY 10965
Shown in Product Identification Guide, page 320

ACHROMYCIN® V ℞
[a-krō-mī-cin]
tetracycline HCl
for ORAL USE

DESCRIPTION

ACHROMYCIN V is an antibiotic isolated from *Streptomyces aureofaciens.* Chemically it is the monohydrochloride of [4S-(4α,4aα,5aα,6β,12aα,)] -4- (Dimethylamino)-1,4,4a,5,5a,6,11,12a-octahydro-3, 6, 10, 12, 12a-pentahydroxy-6-methyl-1, 11-dioxo-2-naphthacenecarboxamide.

ACHROMYCIN V oral dosage forms contain the following inactive ingredients:

Capsules: Blue 1, FD&C Yellow No. 6, Gelatin, Lactose, Magnesium Stearate, Red 28, Titanium Dioxide, Yellow 10 and other ingredients.

CLINICAL PHARMACOLOGY

The tetracyclines are primarily bacteriostatic and are thought to exert their antimicrobial effect by the inhibition of protein synthesis. Tetracyclines are active against a wide range of gram-negative and gram-positive organisms.

The drugs in the tetracycline class have closely similar antimicrobial spectra, and cross-resistance among them is common. Microorganisms may be considered susceptible if the MIC (minimum inhibitory concentration) is not more than 4 mcg/mL and intermediate if the MIC is 4 to 12.5 mcg/mL. Susceptibility plate testing: A tetracycline disc may be used to determine microbial susceptibility to drugs in the tetracycline class. If the Kirby-Bauer method of disc susceptibility testing is used, a 30 mcg tetracycline HCl disc should give a zone of at least 19 mm when tested against a tetracycline-susceptible bacterial strain.

Tetracyclines are readily absorbed and are bound to plasma proteins in varying degrees. They are concentrated by the liver in the bile and excreted in the urine and feces at high concentrations and in a biologically active form.

INDICATIONS

ACHROMYCIN V is indicated in infections caused by the following microorganisms.

Rickettsiae: (Rocky Mountain spotted fever, typhus fever and the typhus group, Q fever, rickettsialpox, tick fevers).

Mycoplasma pneumoniae (PPLO, Eaton agent).

Agents of psittacosis and ornithosis.

Agents of lymphogranuloma venereum and granuloma inguinale.

The spirochetal agent of relapsing fever (*Borrelia recurrentis*).

The following gram-negative microorganisms:

Haemophilus ducreyi (chancroid),

Yersinia pestis and *Francisella tularensis,* formerly *Pasteurella pestis* and *Pasteurella tularensis,*

Bartonella bacilliformis,

Bacteroides species,

Vibrio comma and *Vibrio fetus,*

Brucella species (in conjunction with streptomycin).

Because many strains of the following groups of microorganisms have been shown to be resistant to tetracyclines, culture and susceptibility testing are recommended.

ACHROMYCIN is indicated for treatment of infections caused by the following gram-negative microorganisms, when bacteriologic testing indicates appropriate susceptibility to the drug:

Escherichia coli,

Enterobacter aerogenes (formerly *Aerobacter aerogenes*),

Shigella species,

Mima species and *Herellea* species,

Continued on next page

Lederle—Cont.

Haemophilus influenzae (respiratory infections),
Klebsiella species (respiratory and urinary infections).
ACHROMYCIN is indicated for treatment of infections caused by the following gram-positive microorganisms, when bacteriologic testing indicates appropriate susceptibility to the drug:
Streptococcus species:
Up to 44% of strains of *Streptococcus pyogenes* and 74% of *Streptococcus faecalis* have been found to be resistant to tetracycline drugs. Therefore, tetracyclines should not be used for streptococcal disease unless the organism has been demonstrated to be sensitive.
For upper respiratory infections due to Group A beta-hemolytic streptococci, penicillin is the usual drug of choice, including prophylaxis of rheumatic fever.
Streptococcus pneumoniae,
Staphylococcus aureus, skin and soft tissue infections.
Tetracyclines are not the drug of choice in the treatment of any type of staphylococcal infection.
When penicillin is contraindicated, tetracyclines are alternative drugs in the treatment of infections due to:
> *Neisseria gonorrhoeae,*
> *Treponema pallidum* and *Treponema pertenue* (syphilis and yaws),
> *Listeria monocytogenes,*
> *Clostridium* species,
> *Bacillus anthracis,*
> *Fusobacterium fusiforme* (Vincent's infection),
> *Actinomyces* species.
In acute intestinal amebiasis, the tetracyclines may be a useful adjunct to amebicides.
In severe acne, the tetracyclines may be useful adjunctive therapy.
ACHROMYCIN V is indicated in the treatment of trachoma, although the infectious agent is not always eliminated, as judged by immunofluorescence.
Inclusion conjunctivitis may be treated with oral tetracyclines or with a combination of oral and topical agents.
ACHROMYCIN is indicated for the treatment of uncomplicated urethral, endocervical or rectal infections in adults caused by *Chlamydia trachomatis*.[1]

CONTRAINDICATIONS
This drug is contraindicated in persons who have shown hypersensitivity to any of the tetracyclines.

WARNINGS
THE USE OF DRUGS OF THE TETRACYCLINE CLASS DURING TOOTH DEVELOPMENT (LAST HALF OF PREGNANCY, INFANCY AND CHILDHOOD TO THE AGE OF 8 YEARS) MAY CAUSE PERMANENT DISCOLORATION OF THE TEETH (YELLOW-GRAY-BROWN). This adverse reaction is more common during long-term use of the drugs but has been observed following repeated short-term courses. Enamel hypoplasia has also been reported. TETRACYCLINE DRUGS, THEREFORE, SHOULD NOT BE USED IN THIS AGE GROUP UNLESS OTHER DRUGS ARE NOT LIKELY TO BE EFFECTIVE OR ARE CONTRAINDICATED.
If renal impairment exists, even usual oral or parenteral doses may lead to excessive systemic accumulation of the drug and possible liver toxicity. Under such conditions, lower than usual total doses are indicated and, if therapy is prolonged, serum level determinations of the drug may be advisable.
Photosensitivity manifested by an exaggerated sunburn reaction has been observed in some individuals taking tetracyclines. Patients apt to be exposed to direct sunlight or ultraviolet light should be advised that this reaction can occur with tetracycline drugs, and treatment should be discontinued at the first evidence of skin erythema.
The anti-anabolic action of the tetracyclines may cause an increase in BUN. While this is not a problem in those with normal renal function, in patients with significantly impaired function, higher serum levels of tetracycline may lead to azotemia, hyperphosphatemia, and acidosis.
Usage in Pregnancy: (See above **WARNINGS** about use during tooth development.) Results of animal studies indicate that tetracyclines cross the placenta, are found in fetal tissues and can have toxic effects on the developing fetus (often related to retardation of skeletal development). Evidence of embryotoxicity has also been noted in animals treated early in pregnancy.
Usage in Newborns, Infants, and Children: (See above **WARNINGS** about use during tooth development.)
All tetracyclines form a stable calcium complex in any bone-forming tissue. A decrease in the fibula growth rate has been observed in prematures given oral tetracycline in doses of 25 mg/kg every six hours. This reaction was shown to be reversible when the drug was discontinued.
Tetracyclines are present in the milk of lactating women who are taking a drug in this class.

PRECAUTIONS
General
Pseudotumor cerebri (benign intracranial hypertension) in adults has been associated with the use of tetracyclines. The usual clinical manifestations are headache and blurred vision. Bulging fontanels have been associated with the use of tetracyclines in infants. While both of these conditions and related symptoms usually resolve soon after discontinuation of the tetracycline, the possibility for permanent sequelae exists.
As with other antibiotics preparations, use of this drug may result in overgrowth of nonsusceptible organisms, including fungi. If superinfection occurs, the antibiotic should be discontinued and appropriate therapy should be instituted.
In venereal diseases when coexistent syphilis is suspected, darkfield examination should be done before treatment is started and the blood serology repeated monthly for at least 4 months.
In long-term therapy, periodic laboratory evaluation of organ systems, including hematopoietic, renal and hepatic studies should be performed.
All infections due to Group A beta-hemolytic streptococci should be treated for at least ten days.

Drug Interactions
Because tetracyclines have been shown to depress plasma prothrombin activity, patients who are on anticoagulant therapy may require downward adjustment of their anticoagulant dosage.
Since bacteriostatic drugs, such as the tetracycline class of antibiotics, may interfere with the bactericidal action of penicillins, it is not advisable to administer these drugs concomitantly.
Concurrent use of tetracyclines with oral contraceptives may render oral contraceptives less effective. Breakthrough bleeding has been reported.

ADVERSE REACTIONS
Gastrointestinal: Anorexia, nausea, vomiting, diarrhea, glossitis, dysphagia, enterocolitis, pancreatitis, and inflammatory lesions (with monilial overgrowth) in the anogenital region, increases in liver enzymes, and hepatic toxicity have been reported rarely. Rare instances of esophagitis and esophageal ulcerations have been reported in patients taking the tetracycline-class antibiotics in capsule and tablet form. Most of these patients took the medication immediately before going to bed (see **DOSAGE AND ADMINISTRATION**).
Skin: Maculopapular and erythematous rashes. Exfoliative dermatitis has been reported but is uncommon. Fixed drug eruptions, including balanitis, have been rarely reported. Photosensitivity is discussed above. (See **WARNINGS.**)
Renal toxicity: Rise in BUN has been reported and is apparently dose related. (See **WARNINGS.**)
Hypersensitivity reactions: Urticaria, angioneurotic edema, anaphylaxis, anaphylactoid purpura, pericarditis and exacerbation of systemic lupus erythematosus.
Blood: Hemolytic anemia, thrombocytopenia, neutropenia and eosinophilia have been reported.
CNS: Pseudotumor cerebri (benign intracranial hypertension) in adults and bulging fontanels in infants. (See **PRECAUTIONS—General**.) Dizziness, tinnitus, and visual disturbances have been reported. Myasthenic syndrome has been reported rarely.
Other: When given over prolonged periods, tetracyclines have been reported to produce brown-black microscopic discoloration of thyroid glands. No abnormalities of thyroid function studies are known to occur.

DOSAGE AND ADMINISTRATION
Therapy should be continued for at least 24 to 48 hours after symptoms and fever have subsided.
Concomitant therapy: Antacids containing aluminum, calcium, or magnesium impair absorption and should not be given to patients taking oral tetracycline.
Foods and some dairy products also interfere with absorption. Oral forms of tetracycline should be given 1 hour before or 2 hours after meals.
In patients with renal impairment: (See **WARNINGS**). Total dosage should be decreased by reduction of recommended individual doses and/or by extending time intervals between doses.
In the treatment of streptococcal infections, a therapeutic dose of tetracycline should be administered for at least ten days.
Adults: Usual daily dose, 1–2 grams divided in two or four equal doses, depending on the severity of the infection.
For children above eight years of age: Usual daily dose, 10 to 20 mg (25 to 50 mg/kg) per pound of body weight divided in two or four equal doses.
For treatment of brucellosis, 500 mg tetracycline four times daily for 3 weeks should be accompanied by streptomycin, 1 gram intramuscularly twice daily the first week and once daily the second week.

For treatment of syphilis, a total of 30–40 grams in equally divided doses over a period of 10–15 days should be given. Close follow-up, including laboratory tests, is recommended. Gonorrhea patients sensitive to pencillin may be treated with tetracycline, administered as an initial oral dose of 1.5 grams followed by 0.5 gram every 6 hours for four days to a total dosage of 9 grams.
Uncomplicated urethral, endocervical, or rectal infection in adults caused by *Chlamydia trachomatis:* 500 mg, by mouth, 4 times a day for at least 7 days.[1]

HOW SUPPLIED
ACHROMYCIN® V tetracycline HCl oral dosage forms are available as follows:
CAPSULES
500 mg - Two-piece, hard shell, elongated, opaque capsules with a blue cap and a yellow body, printed with Lederle over A5 on one half and Lederle over 500 mg on the other in gray ink, supplied as follows:
NDC 0005-4875-23—Bottle of 100
NDC 0005-4875-34—Bottle of 1,000
250 mg - Two-piece, hard shell, opaque capsules with a blue cap and a yellow body, printed with Lederle over A3 on one half and Lederle over 250 mg on the other in gray ink, supplied as follows:
NDC 0005-4880-23—Bottle of 100
NDC 0005-4880-34—Bottle of 1,000
NDC 0005-4880-61—Unit of Issue 12 × 40s
NDC 0005-4880-65—Unit of Issue 12 × 100s
Store at Controlled Room Temperature 15°–30°C (59°–86°F).
Reference: 1. CDC Sexually Transmitted Diseases Treatment Guidelines 1982.

LEDERLE LABORATORIES DIVISION
American Cyanamid Company
Pearl River, NY 10965

ARTANE®   ℞
[ar-tāne]
trihexyphenidyl HCl
For Oral Use

DESCRIPTION
ARTANE trihexyphenidyl HCl is a synthetic antispasmodic drug available in the following forms:
TABLETS: Containing 2 mg and 5 mg ARTANE trihexyphenidyl HCl, each strength also containing as inactive ingredients: Corn Starch, Dibasic Calcium Phosphate, Magnesium Stearate and Pregelatinized Starch.
ELIXIR: Containing 2 mg/5 mL ARTANE trihexyphenidyl HCl in a clear, colorless, lime-mint flavored preparation, also containing as inactive ingredients: Alcohol 5%, Citric Acid, Flavorings, Methylparaben, Propylparaben, Sodium Chloride and Sorbitol Solution.

ACTIONS
ARTANE trihexyphenidyl HCl is the substituted piperidine salt, 3-(1-piperidyl)-1-phenyl-cyclohexyl-1-propanol hydrochloride, which exerts a direct inhibitory effect upon the parasympathetic nervous system. It also has a relaxing effect on smooth musculature; exerted both directly upon the muscle tissue itself and indirectly through an inhibitory effect upon the parasympathetic nervous system. Its therapeutic properties are similar to those of atropine although undesirable side effects are ordinarily less frequent and severe than with the latter.

INDICATIONS
This drug is indicated as an adjunct in the treatment of all forms of parkinsonism (postencephalitic, arteriosclerotic, and idiopathic). It is often useful as adjuvant therapy when treating these forms of parkinsonism with levodopa. Additionally, it is indicated for the control of extrapyramidal disorders caused by central nervous system drugs such as the dibenzoxazepines, phenothiazines, thioxanthenes, and butyrophenones.

WARNING
Patients to be treated with ARTANE should have a gonioscope evaluation and close monitoring of intraocular pressures at regular periodic intervals.

PRECAUTIONS
Although trihexyphenidyl HCl is not contraindicated for patients with cardiac, liver, or kidney disorders, or with hypertension, such patients should be maintained under close observation.
Since the use of trihexyphenidyl HCl may in some cases continue indefinitely and since it has atropine-like properties, patients should be subjected to constant and careful long-term observation to avoid allergic and other untoward reactions. Inasmuch as trihexyphenidyl HCl possesses some parasympatholytic activity, it should be used with caution in patients with glaucoma, obstructive disease of the gastrointestinal or genitourinary tracts, and in elderly males with possible prostatic hypertrophy. Geriatric patients, particu-

larly over the age of 60, frequently develop increased sensitivity to the actions of drugs of this type, and hence, require strict dosage regulation. Incipient glaucoma may be precipitated by parasympatholytic drugs such as trihexyphenidyl HCl.

Tardive dyskinesia may appear in some patients on long-term therapy with antipsychotic drugs or may occur after therapy with these drugs has been discontinued. Antiparkinsonism agents do not alleviate the symptoms of tardive dyskinesia, and in some instances may aggravate them. However, parkinsonism and tardive dyskinesia often coexist in patients receiving chronic neuroleptic treatment, and anticholinergic therapy with ARTANE may relieve some of these parkinsonism symptoms.

ADVERSE REACTIONS

Minor side effects, such as dryness of the mouth, blurring of vision, dizziness, mild nausea or nervousness, will be experienced by 30 to 50 percent of all patients. These sensations, however, are much less troublesome with ARTANE trihexyphenidyl HCl than with belladonna alkaloids and are usually less disturbing than unalleviated parkinsonism. Such reactions tend to become less pronounced, and even to disappear, as treatment continues. Even before these reactions have remitted spontaneously, they may often be controlled by careful adjustment of dosage form, amount of drug, or interval between doses.

Isolated instances of suppurative parotitis secondary to excessive dryness of the mouth, skin rashes, dilatation of the colon, paralytic ileus, and certain psychiatric manifestations such as delusions and hallucinations, plus one doubtful case of paranoia all of which may occur with any of the atropine-like drugs, have been reported rarely with ARTANE.

Patients with arteriosclerosis or with a history of idiosyncrasy to other drugs may exhibit reactions of mental confusion, agitation, disturbed behavior, or nausea and vomiting. Such patients should be allowed to develop a tolerance through the initial administration of a small dose and gradual increase in dose until an effective level is reached. If a severe reaction should occur, administration of the drug should be discontinued for a few days and then resumed at a lower dosage. Psychiatric disturbances can result from indiscriminate use (leading to overdosage) to sustain continued euphoria.

Potential side effects associated with the use of any atropine-like drugs include constipation, drowsiness, urinary hesitancy or retention, tachycardia, dilation of the pupil, increased intraocular tension, weakness, vomiting, and headache.

The occurrence of angle-closure glaucoma due to long-term treatment with trihexyphenidyl hydrochloride has been reported.

DOSAGE AND ADMINISTRATION

Dosage should be individualized. The initial dose should be low and then increased gradually, especially in patients over 60 years of age. Whether ARTANE trihexyphenidyl HCl may best be given before or after meals should be determined by the way the patient reacts. Postencephalitic patients, who are usually more prone to excessive salivation, may prefer to take it after meals and may, in addition, require small amounts of atropine which, under such circumstances, is sometimes an effective adjuvant. If ARTANE tends to dry the mouth excessively, it may be better to take it before meals, unless it causes nausea. If taken after meals, the thirst sometimes induced can be allayed by mint candies, chewing gum or water.

ARTANE Trihexyphenidyl HCl in Idiopathic Parkinsonism
As initial therapy for parkinsonism, 1 mg of ARTANE in tablet or elixir form may be administered the first day. The dose may then be increased by 2 mg increments at intervals of three to five days, until a total of 6 to 10 mg is given daily. The total daily dose will depend upon what is found to be the optimal level. Many patients derive maximum benefit from this daily total of 6 to 10 mg, but some patients, chiefly those in the postencephalitic group, may require a total daily dose of 12 to 15 mg.

ARTANE Trihexyphenidyl HCl in Drug-Induced Parkinsonism
The size and frequency of dose of ARTANE needed to control extrapyramidal reactions to commonly employed tranquilizers, notably the phenothiazines, thioxanthenes, and butyrophenones, must be determined empirically. The total daily dosage usually ranges between 5 and 15 mg although, in some cases, these reactions have been satisfactorily controlled on as little as 1 mg daily. It may be advisable to commence therapy with a single 1 mg dose. If the extrapyramidal manifestations are not controlled in a few hours, the subsequent doses may be progressively increased until satisfactory control is achieved. Satisfactory control may sometimes be more rapidly achieved by temporarily reducing the dosage of the tranquilizer on instituting ARTANE trihexyphenidyl HCl therapy and then adjusting dosage of both drugs until the desired ataractic effect is retained without onset of extrapyramidal reactions.

It is sometimes possible to maintain the patient on a reduced ARTANE dosage after the reactions have remained under control for several days. Instances have been reported in which these reactions have remained in remission for long periods after ARTANE therapy was discontinued.

Concomitant Use of ARTANE trihexyphenidyl HCl with Levodopa
When ARTANE is used concomitantly with levodopa, the usual dose of each may need to be reduced. Careful adjustment is necessary, depending on side effects and degree of symptom control. ARTANE dosage of 3 to 6 mg daily, in divided doses, is usually adequate.

Concomitant Use of ARTANE trihexyphenidyl HCl with Other Parasympathetic Inhibitors
ARTANE trihexyphenidyl HCl may be substituted, in whole or in part, for other parasympathetic inhibitors. The usual technique is partial substitution initially, with progressive reduction in the other medication as the dose of trihexyphenidyl HCl is increased.

ARTANE TABLETS and ELIXIR—The total daily intake of ARTANE tablets or elixir is tolerated best if divided into 3 doses and taken at mealtimes. High doses (> 10 mg daily) may be divided into 4 parts, with 3 doses administered at mealtimes and the fourth at bedtime.

HOW SUPPLIED

ARTANE® trihexyphenidyl HCl is available as follows:
TABLETS
2 mg—round, flat, scored, white tablets; engraved ARTANE above 2 on one side and LL above A11 below the score on the other side, supplied as follows:
  NDC 0005-4434-23—Bottle of 100
  NDC 0005-4434-34—Bottle of 1000
  NDC 0005-4434-60—Unit Dose 10 (2 × 5) Strips
5 mg—round, flat, scored, white tablets; engraved ARTANE above 5 on one side and LL above A12 below the score on the other side, supplied as follows:
  NDC 0005-4436-23—Bottle of 100
  NDC 0005-4436-34—Bottle of 1000
  NDC 0005-4436-60—Unit dose 10 (2×5) Strips
Store at Controlled Room Temperature 15–30°C (59–86°F).
ELIXIR
2mg/5mL—NDC 0005-4440-65—Bottle of 16 fl oz
Store at Controlled Room Temperature 15–30°C (59–86°F).
DO NOT FREEZE.
LEDERLE LABORATORIES DIVISION
American Cyanamid Company
Pearl River, NY 10965
Shown in Product Identification Guide, page 320

ASENDIN®   ℞
[*a-sen-din*]
amoxapine tablets

DESCRIPTION

ASENDIN amoxapine is an antidepressant of the dibenzoxazepine class, chemically distinct from the dibenzazepines, dibenzocycloheptenes, and dibenzoxepines.
It is designated chemically as 2-chloro-11-(1-piperazinyl) dibenz-[*b*,*f*][1,4]oxazepine. The molecular weight is 313.8. The empirical formula is $C_{17}H_{16}ClN_3O$.
ASENDIN is supplied for oral administration as 25 mg, 50 mg, 100 mg, and 150 mg tablets.
Inactive Ingredients: All tablets contain Corn Starch, Dibasic Calcium Phosphate, Magnesium Stearate, Pregelatinized Starch, and Stearic Acid. Additionally, the 50 and 150 mg tablets contain FD&C Yellow No. 6 and the 100 mg tablet contains Blue 2.

CLINICAL PHARMACOLOGY

ASENDIN is an antidepressant with a mild sedative component to its action. The mechanism of its clinical action in man is not well understood. In animals, amoxapine reduced the uptake of norepinephrine and serotonin and blocked the response of dopamine receptors to dopamine. Amoxapine is not a monoamine oxidase inhibitor.
ASENDIN is absorbed rapidly and reaches peak blood levels approximately 90 minutes after ingestion. It is almost completely metabolized. The main route of excretion is the kidney. *In vitro* tests show that amoxapine binding to human serum is approximately 90%.
In man, amoxapine serum concentration declines with a half-life of eight hours. However, the major metabolite, 8-hydroxyamoxapine, has a biologic half-life of 30 hours. Metabolites are excreted in the urine in conjugated form as glucuronides.
Clinical studies have demonstrated that ASENDIN has a more rapid onset of action than either amitriptyline or imipramine. The initial clinical effect may occur within four to seven days and occurs within two weeks in over 80% of responders.

INDICATIONS AND USAGE

ASENDIN is indicated for the relief of symptoms of depression in patients with neurotic or reactive depressive disorders as well as endogenous and psychotic depressions. It is indicated for depression accompanied by anxiety or agitation.

CONTRAINDICATIONS

ASENDIN is contraindicated in patients who have shown prior hypersensitivity to dibenzoxazepine compounds. It should not be given concomitantly with monoamine oxidase inhibitors. Hyperpyretic crises, severe convulsions, and deaths have occurred in patients receiving tricyclic antidepressants and monoamine oxidase inhibitors simultaneously. When it is desired to replace a monoamine oxidase inhibitor with ASENDIN, a minimum of 14 days should be allowed to elapse after the former is discontinued. ASENDIN should then be initiated cautiously with gradual increase in dosage until optimum response is achieved. The drug is not recommended for use during the acute recovery phase following myocardial infarction.

WARNINGS

Tardive Dyskinesia
Tardive dyskinesia, a syndrome consisting of potentially irreversible, involuntary, dyskinetic movements may develop in patients treated with neuroleptic (ie, antipsychotics) drugs. (Amoxapine is not an antipsychotic, but it has substantive neuroleptic activity.) Although the prevalence of the syndrome appears to be highest among the elderly, especially elderly women, it is impossible to rely upon prevalence estimates to predict, at the inception of neuroleptic treatment, which patients are likely to develop the syndrome. Whether neuroleptic drug products differ in their potential to cause tardive dyskinesia is unknown.

Both the risk of developing the syndrome and the likelihood that it will become irreversible are believed to increase as the duration of treatment and the total cumulative dose of neuroleptic drugs administered to the patient increase. However, the syndrome can develop, although much less commonly, after relatively brief treatment periods at low doses. There is no known treatment for established cases of tardive dyskinesia, although the syndrome may remit, partially or completely, if neuroleptic treatment is withdrawn. Neuroleptic treatment itself, however, may suppress (or partially suppress) the signs and symptoms of the syndrome and thereby may possibly mask the underlying disease process. The effect that symptomatic suppression has upon the long-term course of the syndrome is unknown.

Given these considerations, neuroleptics should be prescribed in a manner that is most likely to minimize the occurrence of tardive dyskinesia. Chronic neuroleptic treatment should generally be reserved for patients who suffer from a chronic illness that 1) is known to respond to neuroleptic drugs, and 2) for whom alternative, equally effective, but potentially less harmful treatments are not available or appropriate. In patients who do require chronic treatment, the smallest dose and the shortest duration of treatment producing a satisfactory clinical response should be sought. The need for continued treatment should be reassessed periodically.

If signs and symptoms of tardive dyskinesia appear in a patient on neuroleptics, drug discontinuation should be considered. However, some patients may require treatment despite the presence of the syndrome.

(For further information about the description of tardive dyskinesia and its clinical detection, please refer to **Information for the Patient** and **ADVERSE REACTIONS**.)

Neuroleptic Malignant Syndrome (NMS)
A potentially fatal symptom complex sometimes referred to as Neuroleptic Malignant Syndrome (NMS) has been reported in association with antipsychotic drugs and with amoxapine. Clinical manifestations of NMS are hyperpyrexia, muscle rigidity, altered mental status and evidence of autonomic instability (irregular pulse or blood pressure, tachycardia, diaphoresis, and cardiac dysrhythmias).

The diagnostic evaluation of patients with this syndrome is complicated. In arriving at a diagnosis, it is important to identify cases where the clinical presentation includes both serious medical illness (eg, pneumonia, systemic infection, etc) and untreated or inadequately treated extrapyramidal signs and symptoms (EPS). Other important considerations in the differential diagnosis include central anticholinergic toxicity, heat stroke, drug fever, and primary central nervous system (CNS) pathology.

The management of NMS should include 1) immediate discontinuation of antipsychotic drugs and other drugs not essential to concurrent therapy, 2) intensive symptomatic treatment and medical monitoring, and 3) treatment of any concomitant serious medical problems for which specific treatments are available. There is no general agreement about specific pharmacological treatment regimens for uncomplicated NMS.

If a patient requires antipsychotic drug treatment after recovery from NMS, the potential reintroduction of drug therapy should be carefully considered. The patient should be

Continued on next page

Lederle—Cont.

carefully monitored since recurrences of NMS have been reported.

ASENDIN amoxapine should be used with caution in patients with a history of urinary retention, angle-closure glaucoma, or increased intraocular pressure. Patients with cardiovascular disorders should be watched closely. Tricyclic antidepressant drugs, particularly when given in high doses, can induce sinus tachycardia, changes in conduction time, and arrhythmias. Myocardial infarction and stroke have been reported with drugs of this class.

Extreme caution should be used in treating patients with a history of convulsive disorder or those with overt or latent seizure disorders.

PRECAUTIONS
General:
In prescribing the drug it should be borne in mind that the possibility of suicide is inherent in any severe depression, and persists until a significant remission occurs; the drug should be dispensed in the smallest suitable amount. Manic depressive patients may experience a shift to the manic phase. Schizophrenic patients may develop increased symptoms of psychosis; patients with paranoid symptomatology may have an exaggeration of such symptoms. This may require reduction of dosage or the addition of a major tranquilizer to the therapeutic regimen. Antidepressant drugs can cause skin rashes and/or "drug fever" in susceptible individuals. These allergic reactions may, in rare cases, be severe. They are more likely to occur during the first few days of treatment, but may also occur later. ASENDIN should be discontinued if rash and/or fever develop. Amoxapine possesses a degree of dopamine-blocking activity which may cause extrapyramidal symptoms in <1% of patients. Rarely, symptoms indicative of tardive dyskinesia have been reported.

Information for the Patient:
Given the likelihood that some patients exposed chronically to neuroleptics will develop tardive dyskinesia, it is advised that all patients in whom chronic use is contemplated be given, if possible, full information about this risk. The decision to inform patients and/or their guardians must obviously take into account the clinical circumstances and the competency of the patient to understand the information provided.

Patients should be warned of the possibility of drowsiness that may impair performance of potentially hazardous tasks such as driving an automobile or operating machinery.

Drug Interactions:
See CONTRAINDICATIONS about concurrent usage of tricyclic antidepressants and monoamine oxidase inhibitors. Paralytic ileus may occur in patients taking tricyclic antidepressants in combination with anticholinergic drugs. ASENDIN may enhance the response to alcohol and the effects of barbiturates and other CNS depressants. Serum levels of several tricyclic antidepressants have been reported to be significantly increased when cimetidine is administered concurrently. Although such an interaction has not been reported to date with ASENDIN, specific interaction studies have not been done, and the possibility should be considered.
Drugs Metabolized by P450 2D6: The biochemical activity of the drug metabolizing isozyme cytochrome P450 2D6 (debrisoquin hydroxylase) is reduced in a subset of the caucasian population (about 7–10% of caucasians are so-called "poor metabolizers"); reliable estimates of the prevalence of reduced P450 2D6 isozyme activity among Asian, African and other populations are not yet available. Poor metabolizers have higher than expected plasma concentrations of tricyclic antidepressants (TCAs) when given usual doses. Depending on the fraction of drug metabolized by P450 2D6, the increase in plasma concentration may be small, or quite large (8-fold increase in plasma AUC of the TCA).
In addition, certain drugs inhibit the activity of this isozyme and make normal metabolizers resemble poor metabolizers. An individual who is stable on a given dose of TCA may become abruptly toxic when given one of these inhibiting drugs as concomitant therapy. The drugs that inhibit cytochrome P450 2D6 include some that are not metabolized by the enzyme (quinidine; cimetidine) and many that are substrates for P450 2D6 (many other antidepressants, phenothiazines, and the Type 1C antiarrhythmics propafenone and flecainide). While all the selective serotonin reuptake inhibitors (SSRIs), e.g., fluoxetine, sertraline, and paroxetine, inhibit P450 2D6, they may vary in the extent of inhibition. The extent to which SSRI TCA interactions may pose clinical problems will depend on the degree of inhibition and the pharmacokinetics of the SSRI involved. Nevertheless, caution is indicated in the co-administration of TCAs with any of the SSRIs and also in switching from one class to the other. Of particular importance, sufficient time must elapse before initiating TCA treatment in a patient being withdrawn from fluoxetine, given the long half-life of the parent and active metabolite (at least 5 weeks may be necessary).

Concomitant use of tricyclic antidepressants with drugs that can inhibit cytochrome P450 2D6 may require lower doses than usually prescribed for either the tricyclic antidepressant or the other drug. Furthermore, whenever one of these other drugs is withdrawn from co-therapy, an increased dose of tricyclic antidepressant may be required. It is desirable to monitor TCA plasma levels whenever a TCA is going to be co-administered with another drug known to be an inhibitor of P450 2D6.

Therapeutic Interactions:
Concurrent administration with electroshock therapy may increase the hazards associated with such therapy.

Carcinogenesis, Impairment of Fertility:
In a 21-month toxicity study at three dose levels in rats, pancreatic islet cell hyperplasia occurred with slightly increased incidence at doses 5 to 10 times the human dose. Pancreatic adenocarcinoma was detected in low incidence in the mid-dose group only, and may possibly have resulted from endocrine-mediated organ hyperfunction. The significance of these findings to man is not known.
Treatment of male rats with 5–10 times the human dose resulted in a slight decrease in the number of fertile matings. Female rats receiving oral doses within the therapeutic range displayed a reversible increase in estrous cycle length.

Pregnancy: Pregnancy Category C:
Studies performed in mice, rats, and rabbits have demonstrated no evidence of teratogenic effect due to ASENDIN. Embryotoxicity was seen in rats and rabbits given oral doses approximating the human dose. Fetotoxic effects (intrauterine death, stillbirth, decreased birth weight) were seen in animals studied at oral doses 3–10 times the human dose. Decreased postnatal survival (between days 0–4) was demonstrated in the offspring of rats at 5–10 times the human dose. There are no adequate and well-controlled studies in pregnant women. ASENDIN should be used during pregnancy only if the potential benefit justifies the potential risk to the fetus.

Nursing Mothers:
ASENDIN, like many other systemic drugs, is excreted in human milk. Because effects of the drug on infants are unknown, caution should be exercised when ASENDIN is administered to nursing women.

Pediatric Use:
Safety and effectiveness in children below the age of 16 have not been established.

ADVERSE REACTIONS
Adverse reactions reported in controlled studies in the United States are categorized with respect to incidence below. Following this is a listing of reactions known to occur with other antidepressant drugs of this class but not reported to date with ASENDIN.

INCIDENCE GREATER THAN 1%
The most frequent types of adverse reactions occurring with ASENDIN in controlled clinical trials were sedative and anticholinergic: these included drowsiness (14%), dry mouth (14%), constipation (12%), and blurred vision (7%).
Less frequently reported reactions are:
CNS and Neuromuscular–anxiety, insomnia, restlessness, nervousness, palpitations, tremors, confusion, excitement, nightmares, ataxia, alterations in EEG patterns.
Allergic–edema, skin rash.
Endocrine–elevation of prolactin levels.
Gastrointestinal–nausea.
Other–dizziness, headache, fatigue, weakness, excessive appetite, increased perspiration.
INCIDENCE LESS THAN 1%
Anticholinergic–disturbances of accommodation, mydriasis, delayed micturition, urinary retention, nasal stuffiness.
Cardiovascular–hypotension, hypertension, syncope, tachycardia.
Allergic–drug fever, urticaria, photosensitization, pruritus, rarely vasculitis, hepatitis.
CNS and Neuromuscular–tingling, paresthesias of the extremities, tinnitus, disorientation, seizures, hypomania, numbness, incoordination, disturbed concentration, hyperthermia, extrapyramidal symptoms, including, rarely, tardive dyskinesia. Neuroleptic malignant syndrome has been reported. (See WARNINGS.)
Hematologic–leukopenia, agranulocytosis.
Gastrointestinal–epigastric distress, vomiting, flatulence, abdominal pain, peculiar taste, diarrhea.
Endocrine–increased or decreased libido, impotence, menstrual irregularity, breast enlargement and galactorrhea in the female, syndrome of inappropriate antidiuretic hormone secretion.
Other–lacrimation, weight gain or loss, altered liver function, painful ejaculation.
DRUG RELATIONSHIP UNKNOWN
The following reactions have been reported very rarely, and occurred under uncontrolled circumstances where a drug relationship was difficult to assess. These observations are listed to serve as alerting information to physicians.
Anticholinergic–paralytic ileus.
Cardiovascular–atrial arrhythmias (including atrial fibrillation), myocardial infarction, stroke, heart block.

CNS and Neuromuscular–hallucinations.
Hematologic–thrombocytopenia, eosinophilia, purpura, petechiae.
Gastrointestinal–parotid swelling.
Endocrine–change in blood glucose levels.
Other–pancreatitis, hepatitis, jaundice, urinary frequency, testicular swelling, anorexia, alopecia.
ADDITIONAL ADVERSE REACTIONS
The following reactions have been reported with other antidepressant drugs, but not with ASENDIN.
Anticholinergic–sublingual adenitis, dilation of the urinary tract.
CNS and Neuromuscular–delusions.
Gastrointestinal–stomatitis, black tongue.
Endocrine–gynecomastia.

OVERDOSAGE
Signs and Symptoms:
Toxic manifestations of ASENDIN overdosage differ significantly from those of other tricyclic antidepressants. Serious cardiovascular effects are seldom if ever observed. However, CNS effects—particularly grand mal convulsions—occur frequently, and treatment should be directed primarily toward prevention or control of seizures. Status epilepticus may develop and constitutes a neurologic emergency. Coma and acidosis are other serious complications of substantial ASENDIN overdosage in some cases.
Renal failure may develop two to five days after toxic overdosage in patients who may appear otherwise recovered. Acute tubular necrosis with rhabdomyolysis and myoglobinuria is the most common renal complication in such cases. This reaction probably occurs in less than 5% of overdose cases, and typically in those who have experienced multiple seizures.
Treatment:
Treatment of ASENDIN overdosage should be symptomatic and supportive, but with special attention to prevention or control of seizures. If the patient is conscious, induced emesis followed by gastric lavage with appropriate precautions to prevent pulmonary aspiration should be accomplished as soon as possible. Following lavage, activated charcoal may be administered to reduce absorption, and repeated administrations may facilitate drug elimination. An adequate airway should be established in comatose patients and assisted ventilation instituted if necessary. Seizures may respond to standard anticonvulsant therapy such as intravenous diazepam and/or phenytoin. The value of physostigmine appears less certain. Status epilepticus, should it develop, requires vigorous treatment such as that described by Delgado-Escueta et al (*N Engl J Med* 1982; 306:1337-1340).
Convulsions, when they occur, typically begin within 12 hours after ingestion. Because seizures may occur precipitously in some overdosage patients who appear otherwise relatively asymptomatic, the treating physician may wish to consider prophylactic administration of anticonvulsant medication during this period.
Treatment of renal impairment, should it occur, is the same as that for nondrug-induced renal dysfunction.
Serious cardiovascular effects are remarkably rare following ASENDIN overdosage, and the ECG typically remains within normal limits except for sinus tachycardia. Hence, prolongation of the QRS interval beyond 100 milliseconds within the first 24 hours is *not* a useful guide to the severity of overdosage with this drug.
Fatalities and, rarely, neurologic sequelae have resulted from prolonged status epilepticus in ASENDIN amoxapine overdosage patients. While the lethal dose appears higher than that of other tricyclic antidepressants (80% of lethal ASENDIN overdosages have involved ingestion of 3 grams or more), many factors other than amount ingested are important in assessing probability of survival. These include age and physical condition of the patient, concomitant ingestion of other drugs, and especially the interval between drug ingestion and initiation of emergency treatment.

DOSAGE AND ADMINISTRATION
Effective dosage of ASENDIN may vary from one patient to another. Usual effective dosage is 200 to 300 mg daily. Three weeks constitutes an adequate period of trial providing dosage has reached 300 mg daily (or lower level of tolerance) for at least two weeks. If no response is seen at 300 mg, dosage may be increased, depending upon tolerance, up to 400 mg daily. Hospitalized patients who have been refractory to antidepressant therapy and who have no history of convulsive seizures may have dosage raised cautiously up to 600 mg daily in divided doses.
ASENDIN may be given in a single daily dose, not to exceed 300 mg, preferably at bedtime. If the total daily dosage exceeds 300 mg, it should be given in divided doses.

Initial Dosage for Adults:
Usual starting dosage is 50 mg two or three times daily. Depending upon tolerance, dosage may be increased to 100 mg two or three times daily by the end of the first week. (Initial dosage of 300 mg daily may be given, but notable sedation may occur in some patients during the first few days of therapy at this level.) Increases above 300 mg daily should be

made only if 300 mg daily has been ineffective during a trial period of at least 2 weeks. When effective dosage is established, the drug may be given in a single dose (not to exceed 300 mg) at bedtime.

Elderly Patients:

In general, lower dosages are recommended for these patients. Recommended starting dosage of ASENDIN is 25 mg two or three times daily. If no intolerance is observed, dosage may be increased by the end of the first week to 50 mg two or three times daily. Although 100 to 150 mg daily may be adequate for many elderly patients, some may require higher dosage. Careful increases up to 300 mg daily are indicated in such cases.

Once an effective dosage is established, ASENDIN may conveniently be given in a single bedtime dose, not to exceed 300 mg.

Maintenance

Recommended maintenance dosage of ASENDIN amoxapine is the lowest dose that will maintain remission. If symptoms reappear, dosage should be increased to the earlier level until they are controlled.

For maintenance therapy at dosages of 300 mg or less, a single dose at bedtime is recommended.

HOW SUPPLIED

ASENDIN® amoxapine Tablets are supplied as follows:

25 mg—White, heptagon-shaped tablets, engraved on one side with LL above 25 and with A13 on the other scored side.
NDC 0005-5389-23—Bottle of 100

50 mg—Orange, heptagon-shaped tablets, engraved on one side with LL above 50 and with A15 on the other scored side.
NDC 0005-5390-23—Bottle of 100
NDC 0005-5390-31—Bottle of 500
NDC 0005-5390-60—10 (2 × 5) Strips

100 mg—Blue, heptagon-shaped tablets, engraved on one side with LL above 100 and with A17 on the other scored side.
NDC 0005-5391-23—Bottle of 100
NDC 0005-5391-60—10 (2 × 5) Strips

150 mg—Peach, heptagon-shaped tablets, engraved on one side with LL above 150 and with A18 on the other scored side.
NDC 0005-5392-38—Bottle of 30 with CRC

Store at Controlled Room Temperature 15°–30° C (59°–86° F).

LEDERLE LABORATORIES DIVISION
American Cyanamid Company
Pearl River, NY 10965

Shown in Product Identification Guide, page 320

DECLOMYCIN® ℞

[*dĕk-lō-mī-sĭn*]
Demeclocycline Hydrochloride
For Oral Use

DESCRIPTION

DECLOMYCIN demeclocycline hydrochloride is an antibiotic isolated from a mutant strain of *Streptomyces aureofaciens*. Chemically it is 7-Chloro-4-(dimethylamino)-1,4,4a,5, 5a,6,11,12a-octahydro - 3,6,10,12, 12a- pentahydroxy - 1,11- dioxo -2- naphthacenecarboxamide monohydrochloride.

DECLOMYCIN contains the following inactive ingredients: Tablets: Alginic Acid, Corn Starch, Ethylcellulose, Hydroxypropyl Methylcellulose, Magnesium Stearate, Red 7, Sorbitol, Titanium Dioxide, Yellow 10 and other ingredients. May also contain Sodium Lauryl Sulfate.

CLINICAL PHARMACOLOGY

The tetracyclines are primarily bacteriostatic and are thought to exert their antimicrobial effect by the inhibition of protein synthesis. Tetracyclines are active against a wide range of gram-negative and gram-positive organisms.

The drugs in the tetracycline class have closely similar antimicrobial spectra, and cross-resistance among them is common. Microorganisms may be considered susceptible if the MIC (minimum inhibitory concentration) is not more than 4 mcg/mL and intermediate if the MIC is 4 to 12.5 mcg/mL.

Susceptibility plate testing: A tetracycline disc may be used to determine microbial susceptibility to drugs in the tetracycline class. If the Kirby-Bauer method of disc susceptibility testing is used, a 30 mcg tetracycline disc should give a zone of at least 19 mm when tested against a tetracycline-susceptible bacterial strain.

Tetracyclines are readily absorbed and are bound to plasma proteins in varying degrees. They are concentrated by the liver in the bile and excreted in the urine and feces at high concentrations and in a biologically active form.

INDICATIONS AND USAGE

DECLOMYCIN demeclocycline hydrochloride is indicated in infections caused by the following microorganisms:

Rickettsiae: (Rocky Mountain spotted fever, typhus fever and the typhus group, Q fever, rickettsialpox, tick fevers).

Mycoplasma pneumoniae (PPLO, Eaton agent).

Agents of psittacosis and ornithosis.

Agents of lymphogranuloma venereum and granuloma inguinale.

The spirochetal agent of relapsing fever (*Borrelia recurrentis*).

The following gram-negative microorganisms:

Haemophilus ducreyi (chancroid),
Yersinia pestis and *Francisella tularensis*, formerly *Pasteurella pestis* and *Pasteurella tularensis*,
Bartonella bacilliformis,
Bacteroides species,
Vibrio comma and *Vibrio fetus*.
Brucella species (in conjunction with streptomycin).

Because many strains of the following groups of microorganisms have been shown to be resistant to tetracyclines, culture and susceptibility testing are recommended.

Demeclocycline is indicated for treatment of infections caused by the following gram-negative microorganisms, when bacteriologic testing indicates appropriate susceptibility to the drug:

Escherichia coli,
Enterobacter aerogenes (formerly *Aerobacter aerogenes*),
Shigella species,
Mima species and *Herellea* species,
Haemophilus influenzae (respiratory infections),
Klebsiella species (respiratory and urinary infections).

DECLOMYCIN *demeclocycline hydrochloride* is indicated for treatment of infections caused by the following gram-positive microorganisms when bacteriologic testing indicates appropriate susceptibility to the drug:

Streptococcus species:

Up to 44% of strains of *Streptococcus pyogenes* and 74% of *Streptococcus faecalis* have been found to be resistant to tetracycline drugs. Therefore, tetracyclines should not be used for streptococcal disease unless the organism has been demonstrated to be sensitive.

For upper respiratory infections due to Group A beta-hemolytic streptococci, penicillin is the usual drug of choice, including prophylaxis of rheumatic fever.

Streptococcus pneumoniae,
Staphylococcus aureus, skin and soft tissue infections.

Tetracyclines are not the drugs of choice in the treatment of any type of staphylococcal infection.

When penicillin is contraindicated, tetracyclines are alternative drugs in the treatment of infections due to:

Neisseria gonorrhoeae,
Treponema pallidum and *Treponema pertenue* (syphilis and yaws),
Listeria monocytogenes,
Clostridium species,
Bacillus anthracis,
Fusobacterium fusiforme (Vincent's infection),
Actinomyces species.

In acute intestinal amebiasis, the tetracyclines may be a useful adjunct to amebicides.

DECLOMYCIN is indicated in the treatment of trachoma, although the infectious agent is not always eliminated, as judged by immunofluorescence.

Inclusion conjunctivitis may be treated with oral tetracyclines or with a combination of oral and topical agents.

CONTRAINDICATIONS

This drug is contraindicated in persons who have shown hypersensitivity to any of the tetracyclines.

WARNINGS

THE USE OF DRUGS OF THE TETRACYCLINE CLASS DURING TOOTH DEVELOPMENT (LAST HALF OF PREGNANCY, INFANCY, AND CHILDHOOD TO THE AGE OF 8 YEARS) MAY CAUSE PERMANENT DISCOLORATION OF THE TEETH (YELLOW-GRAY-BROWN).

This adverse reaction is more common during long-term use of the drugs but has been observed following repeated short-term courses. Enamel hypoplasia has also been reported. TETRACYCLINE DRUGS, THEREFORE, SHOULD NOT BE USED IN THIS AGE GROUP UNLESS OTHER DRUGS ARE NOT LIKELY TO BE EFFECTIVE OR ARE CONTRAINDICATED.

If renal impairment exists, even usual oral or parenteral doses may lead to excessive systemic accumulation of the drug and possible liver toxicity. Under such conditions, lower than usual total doses are indicated and, if therapy is prolonged, serum level determinations of the drug may be advisable.

Phototoxic reactions can occur in individuals taking demeclocycline, and are characterized by severe burns of exposed surfaces resulting from direct exposure of patients to sunlight during therapy with moderate or large doses of demeclocycline. Patients apt to be exposed to direct sunlight or ultraviolet light should be advised that this reaction can occur, and treatment should be discontinued at the first evidence of skin erythema.

The anti-anabolic action of the tetracyclines may cause an increase in BUN. While this is not a problem in those with normal renal function, in patients with significantly impaired function, higher serum levels of tetracycline may lead to azotemia, hyperphosphatemia, and acidosis.

Administration of DECLOMYCIN has resulted in appearance of the diabetes insipidus syndrome (polyuria, polydipsia and weakness) in some patients on long-term therapy. The syndrome has been shown to be nephrogenic, dose-dependent and reversible on discontinuance of therapy.

Usage in pregnancy: (See above **WARNINGS** about use during tooth development.) Results of animal studies indicate that tetracyclines cross the placenta, are found in fetal tissues and can have toxic effects on the developing fetus (often related to retardation of skeletal development). Evidence of embryotoxicity has also been noted in animals treated early in pregnancy.

Usage in newborns, infants, and children: (See above **WARNINGS** about use during tooth development.)

All tetracyclines form a stable calcium complex in any bone forming tissue. A decrease in the fibula growth rate has been observed in prematures given oral tetracycline in doses of 25 mg/kg every six hours. This reaction was shown to be reversible when the drug was discontinued.

Tetracyclines are present in the milk of lactating women who are taking a drug in this class.

PRECAUTIONS

General

Pseudotumor cerebri (benign intracranial hypertension) in adults has been associated with the use of tetracyclines. The usual clinical manifestations are headache and blurred vision. Bulging fontanels have been associated with the use of tetracyclines in infants. While both of these conditions and related symptoms usually resolve soon after discontinuation of the tetracycline, the possibility for permanent sequelae exists.

As with other antibiotic preparations, use of this drug may result in overgrowth of nonsusceptible organisms, including fungi. If superinfection occurs, the antibiotic should be discontinued and appropriate therapy should be instituted.

In venereal diseases when coexistent syphilis is suspected, darkfield examination should be done before treatment is started and the blood serology repeated monthly for at least 4 months.

In long-term therapy, periodic laboratory evaluation of organ systems, including hematopoietic, renal and hepatic studies should be performed.

All infections due to Group A beta-hemolytic streptococci should be treated for at least ten days.

Interpretation of Bacteriologic Studies: Following a course of therapy, persistence for several days in both urine and blood of bacterio-suppressive levels of demeclocycline may interfere with culture studies. These levels should not be considered therapeutic.

Drug Interactions

Because the tetracyclines have been shown to depress plasma prothrombin activity, patients who are on anticoagulant therapy may require downward adjustment of their anticoagulant dosage.

Since bacteriostatic drugs, such as the tetracycline class of antibiotics, may interfere with the bactericidal action of penicillins, it is not advisable to administer these drugs concomitantly.

Concurrent use of tetracyclines with oral contraceptives may render oral contraceptives less effective. Breakthrough bleeding has been reported.

ADVERSE REACTIONS

Gastrointestinal: Anorexia, nausea, vomiting, diarrhea, glossitis, dysphagia, enterocolitis, pancreatitis, and inflammatory lesions (with monilial overgrowth) in the anogenital region, increases in liver enzymes, and hepatic toxicity has been reported rarely. Rare instances of esophagitis and esophageal ulcerations have been reported in patients taking the tetracycline-class antibiotics in capsule and tablet form. Most of these patients took the medication immediately before going to bed (see **DOSAGE AND ADMINISTRATION**).

Skin: Maculopapular and erythematous rashes. Exfoliative dermatitis has been reported but is uncommon. Fixed drug eruptions, including balanitis, have been rarely reported. Photosensitivity is discussed above. (See **WARNINGS**.)

Renal Toxicity: Rise in BUN has been reported and is apparently dose related. Nephrogenic diabetes insipidus. (See **WARNINGS.**)

Hypersensitivity Reactions: Urticaria, angioneurotic edema, anaphylaxis, anaphylactoid purpura, pericarditis and exacerbation of systemic lupus erythematosus.

Blood: Hemolytic anemia, thrombocytopenia, neutropenia and eosinophilia have been reported.

CNS: Pseudotumor cerebri (benign intracranial hypertension) in adults and bulging fontanels in infants (see **PRECAUTIONS—General**). Dizziness, tinnitus, and visual disturbances have been reported. Myasthenic syndrome has been reported rarely.

Continued on next page

Lederle—Cont.

Other: When given over prolonged periods, tetracyclines have been reported to produce brown-black microscopic discoloration of thyroid glands. No abnormalities of thyroid function studies are known to occur.

DOSAGE AND ADMINISTRATION

Therapy should be continued for at least 24 to 48 hours after symptoms and fever have subsided.

Concomitant therapy: Antacids containing aluminum, calcium, or magnesium impair absorption and should not be given to patients taking oral tetracycline.

Foods and some dairy products also interfere with absorption. Oral forms of tetracycline should be given one hour before or two hours after meals.

In patients with renal impairment: (See **WARNINGS**.) Total dosage should be decreased by reduction of recommended individual doses and/or by extending time intervals between doses.

In the treatment of streptococcal infections, a therapeutic dose of demeclocycline should be administered for at least ten days.

Adults: Usual daily dose—Four divided doses of 150 mg each or two divided doses of 300 mg each.

For children above eight years of age: Usual daily dose, 3–6 mg per pound body weight per day, depending upon the severity of the disease, divided into two to four doses.

Gonorrhea patients sensitive to penicillin may be treated with demeclocycline administered as an initial oral dose of 600 mg followed by 300 mg every 12 hours for four days to a total of 3 grams.

HOW SUPPLIED

DECLOMYCIN® demeclocycline hydrochloride Tablets, 150 mg are round, convex, red, film coated tablets, engraved with LL on one side and D11 on the other, supplied as follows:

NDC 0005-9218-23—Bottle of 100

DECLOMYCIN® demeclocycline hydrochloride Tablets, 300 mg are round, convex, red, film coated tablets, engraved with LL on one side and D12 on the other, supplied as follows:

NDC 0005-9270-29—Bottle of 48

Store at Controlled Room Temperature 15–30°C (59–86°F).

LEDERLE LABORATORIES DIVISION
American Cyanamid Company
Pearl River, NY 10965

Shown in Product Identification Guide, page 320

DIAMOX®
Acetazolamide Tablets USP
and
DIAMOX®
Sterile Acetazolamide Sodium USP
Intravenous

℞

(For full prescribing information, please refer to the Product Information section for Storz Ophthalmics in the 1997 PDR for Ophthalmology.)

DIAMOX®
Acetazolamide
SEQUELS®
Sustained Release Capsules

℞

(For full prescribing information, please refer to the Product Information section for Storz Ophthalmics in the 1997 PDR for Ophthalmology.)

DIPHTHERIA AND TETANUS TOXOIDS ADSORBED
Aluminum Phosphate-Adsorbed PUROGENATED®
For Pediatric Use

℞

DESCRIPTION

Diphtheria and Tetanus Toxoids Adsorbed, aluminum phosphate-adsorbed PUROGENATED is a sterile combination of refined diphtheria and tetanus toxoids for intramuscular use only. After shaking, the vaccine is a homogeneous white suspension.

The diphtheria and tetanus toxins are produced according to the method of Mueller and Miller[1,2] and are detoxified by use of formaldehyde. The toxoids are refined by the Pillemer alcohol fractionation method[3] and are diluted with a solution containing sodium phosphate monobasic, sodium phosphate dibasic, aluminum phosphate, glycine and thimerosal (mercury derivative) as a preservative. The final concentration of thimerosal in the combined vaccine is

1:10,000. The aluminum content of the final product does not exceed 0.80 mg per 0.5 mL dose.

Each 0.5 mL dose is formulated to contain 12.5 Lf units of diphtheria toxoid, and 5 Lf units of tetanus toxoid.

CLINICAL PHARMACOLOGY

Diphtheria is primarily a localized and generalized intoxication caused by diphtheria toxin, an extracellular protein metabolite of toxinogenic strains of *Corynebacterium diphtheriae*. While the incidence of diphtheria in the U.S. has decreased from over 200,000 cases reported in 1921 before the general use of diphtheria toxoid, to only 15 cases reported from 1980 through 1983, the ratio of fatalities to attack rate has remained constant at about 5% to 10%.[4] The highest case fatality rates are in the very young and the elderly.

Following adequate immunization with diphtheria toxoid, which induces antitoxin, it is thought that protection lasts for at least 10 years.[4] This significantly reduces both the risk of developing diphtheria and the severity of clinical illness. It does not, however, eliminate carriage of *C diphtheriae* in the pharynx or on the skin.[4]

Tetanus is an intoxication manifested primarily by neuromuscular dysfunction, caused by a potent exotoxin elaborated by *Clostridium tetani*. The incidence of tetanus in the U.S. has dropped dramatically with the routine use of tetanus toxoid, remaining relatively constant over the last decade at about 90 cases reported annually.[4] Spores of *C tetani* are ubiquitous, and there is essentially no natural immunity to tetanus toxin. Thus, universal primary immunization with tetanus toxoid, and subsequent maintenance of adequate antitoxin levels by means of timed boosters, is necessary to protect all age groups.[4,6] Tetanus toxoid is a highly effective antigen, and a completed primary series generally induces protective levels of serum antitoxin that persist for at least 10 years.[4]

INDICATIONS AND USAGE

Diphtheria and Tetanus Toxoids Adsorbed is indicated for active immunization of infants and children from 2 months of age up to their seventh birthday both for routine protection and as a preventive measure against diphtheria and tetanus, in circumstances in which the use of a combined triple vaccine containing pertussis antigen is contraindicated.[4,5]

Tetanus or diphtheria infection may not confer immunity; therefore, initiation or completion of active immunization is indicated at the time of recovery from these infections.[4]

CONTRAINDICATIONS

HYPERSENSITIVITY TO ANY COMPONENT OF THE VACCINE, INCLUDING THIMEROSAL, A MERCURY DERIVATIVE, IS A CONTRAINDICATION.

THE OCCURRENCE OF ANY NEUROLOGICAL SYMPTOMS OR SIGNS FOLLOWING ADMINISTRATION OF THIS PRODUCT IS A CONTRAINDICATION TO FURTHER USE.

IMMUNIZATION SHOULD BE DEFERRED DURING THE COURSE OF ANY FEBRILE ILLNESS OR ACUTE INFECTION. A MINOR AFEBRILE ILLNESS SUCH AS A MILD UPPER RESPIRATORY INFECTION IS NOT USUALLY REASON TO DEFER IMMUNIZATION.[4,5]

The clinical judgment of the attending physician should prevail at all times.

Routine immunization should be deferred during an outbreak of poliomyelitis, providing the patient has not sustained an injury that increases the risk of tetanus and providing an outbreak of diphtheria does not occur simultaneously.

WARNINGS

THIS PRODUCT IS NOT RECOMMENDED FOR IMMUNIZING PERSONS ON OR AFTER THEIR SEVENTH BIRTHDAY.

For individuals 7 years of age or older, Tetanus and Diphtheria Toxoids Adsorbed For Adult Use (Td) should be used instead of Diphtheria and Tetanus Toxoids Adsorbed For Pediatric Use (DT). The concentration of diphtheria toxoid in preparations intended for use in persons 7 years of age or older is lower than that of the pediatric formulation; a lower dosage of diphtheria toxoid is recommended for persons 7 years of age or older because adverse reactions to the diphtheria component are thought to be related to both dose and age.[4]

THE OCCURRENCE OF A NEUROLOGICAL OR SEVERE HYPERSENSITIVITY REACTION FOLLOWING A PREVIOUS DOSE IS A CONTRAINDICATION TO FURTHER USE OF THIS PRODUCT.[4]

DT should not be given to infants or children with thrombocytopenia or any coagulation disorder that would contraindicate intramuscular injection unless the potential benefits clearly outweigh the risk of administration.

Patients with impaired immune responsiveness, whether due to the use of immunosuppressive therapy (including irradiation, corticosteroids, antimetabolites, alkylating agents, and cytotoxic agents), a genetic defect, human immunodeficiency virus (HIV) infection, or other causes, may have a reduced antibody response to active immunization

procedures.[4,5,6] Deferral of administration of DT may be considered in individuals receiving immunosuppressive therapy.[4,5] Other groups should generally receive this vaccine according to the usual recommended schedule.[4–7] Special care should be taken to prevent injection into a blood vessel.

PRECAUTIONS

General:

1. THIS PRODUCT SHOULD BE USED FOR THE AGE GROUP BETWEEN 2 MONTHS AND THE SEVENTH BIRTHDAY.
2. PRIOR TO ADMINISTRATION OF ANY DOSE OF DT, THE PARENT OR GUARDIAN SHOULD BE ASKED ABOUT THE RECENT HEALTH STATUS OF THE INFANT OR CHILD TO BE IMMUNIZED IN ORDER TO DETERMINE THE EXISTENCE OF ANY CONTRAINDICATION TO IMMUNIZATION WITH DT (SEE **CONTRAINDICATIONS, WARNINGS**).
3. WHEN AN INFANT OR CHILD RETURNS FOR THE NEXT DOSE IN A SERIES, THE PARENT OR GUARDIAN SHOULD BE QUESTIONED CONCERNING OCCURRENCE OF ANY SYMPTOM AND/OR SIGN OF AN ADVERSE REACTION AFTER THE PREVIOUS DOSE (SEE **CONTRAINDICATIONS, ADVERSE REACTIONS**).
4. BEFORE THE INJECTION OF ANY BIOLOGICAL, THE PHYSICIAN SHOULD TAKE ALL PRECAUTIONS KNOWN FOR PREVENTION OF ALLERGIC OR ANY OTHER SIDE REACTIONS. This should include: a review of the patient's history regarding possible sensitivity; the ready availability of epinephrine 1:1,000 and other appropriate agents used for control of immediate allergic reactions; and a knowledge of the recent literature pertaining to use of the biological concerned, including the nature of side effects and adverse reactions that may follow its use.
5. A separate sterile syringe and needle or a sterile disposable unit should be used for each individual patient to prevent transmission of hepatitis or other infectious agents from one person to another.
6. **Shake vigorously before withdrawing each dose to resuspend the contents of the vial.**
7. NATIONAL CHILDHOOD VACCINE INJURY ACT OF 1986 (AS AMENDED IN 1987)
   This Act requires that the manufacturer and lot number of the vaccine administered be recorded by the health care provider in the vaccine recipient's permanent medical record, along with the date of administration of the vaccine and the name, address and title of the person administering the vaccine.
   The Act further requires the health care provider to report to a health department or to the FDA the occurrence following immunization of any event set forth in the Vaccine Injury Table including: anaphylaxis or anaphylactic shock within 24 hours, encephalopathy or encephalitis within 7 days, residual seizure disorder, any acute complication or sequelae (including death) of above events, or any event that would contraindicate further doses of vaccine, according to this package insert.[8]

Information for the Patient: PRIOR TO THE ADMINISTRATION OF THIS VACCINE, HEALTH CARE PERSONNEL SHOULD INFORM THE PARENT, GUARDIAN, OR OTHER RESPONSIBLE ADULT OF THE BENEFITS AND RISKS TO THE CHILD OF VACCINATION AGAINST DIPHTHERIA AND TETANUS.

Use in Pregnancy: This product is not recommended for administration to females of child-bearing age.

ADVERSE REACTIONS

Local reactions, manifested by varying degrees of erythema, induration, and tenderness, may occur after administration of DT.[9,10] Such local reactions are usually self-limited and require no therapy. Nodule,[11] sterile abscess formation, or subcutaneous atrophy may occur at the site of injection.

Systemic symptoms, including drowsiness, fretfulness, vomiting, anorexia, and persistent crying have been described following DT immunization.[9,10]

In one study, fever ≥ 38°C (100.4°F) was reported in 9.3% of DT recipients, and fever ≥ 39°C (102.2°F) was reported in 0.7% of recipients.[9]

Pallor, coldness, and hyporesponsiveness have been reported in a child receiving a DT vaccine.[10]

NEUROLOGICAL COMPLICATIONS,[12] SUCH AS CONVULSIONS,[13] ENCEPHALOPATHY,[13,14] AND VARIOUS MONO- AND POLYNEUROPATHIES,[14–20] INCLUDING GUILLAIN-BARRE SYNDROME,[21,22] HAVE BEEN REPORTED FOLLOWING ADMINISTRATION OF PREPARATIONS CONTAINING DIPHTHERIA AND/OR TETANUS ANTIGENS.

URTICARIA, ERYTHEMA MULTIFORME OR OTHER RASH, ARTHRALGIAS[13] AND, MORE RARELY, A SEVERE ANAPHYLACTIC REACTION (IE, URTICARIA WITH SWELLING OF THE MOUTH, DIFFICULTY BREATHING, HYPOTENSION, OR SHOCK) HAVE BEEN REPORTED FOLLOWING ADMINISTRATION OF PREP-

ARATIONS CONTAINING DIPHTHERIA, AND/OR TETANUS ANTIGENS.

DOSAGE AND ADMINISTRATION

For Intramuscular Use Only: Shake vigorously before withdrawing each dose to resuspend the contents of the vial.
Parenteral drug products should be inspected visually for particulate matter and discoloration prior to administration. (See **DESCRIPTION**.)

The vaccine should be injected intramuscularly, preferably into the midlateral muscles of the thigh or deltoid, with care to avoid major peripheral nerve trunks.

Before injection, the skin at the injection site should be cleansed and prepared with a suitable germicide.

After insertion of the needle, aspirate to help avoid inadvertent injection into a blood vessel.

This combined preparation against both diphtheria and tetanus is designed particularly to meet the need of children less than 7 years of age for whom the use of a combined triple vaccine containing pertussis antigen is contraindicated.

It is recommended that active immunization against diphtheria and tetanus be started at 2 months of age.

Unimmunized infants and children less than 1 year of age for whom vaccine containing pertussis antigen is contraindicated should receive three doses of 0.5 mL each of DT at 4 to 8 week intervals, followed by a fourth (reinforcing) dose of 0.5 mL, 6 to 12 months after the third dose, for the primary series.

Unimmunized children 1 year of age or older for whom vaccine containing pertussis antigen is contraindicated should receive two doses of 0.5 mL each of DT, 4 to 8 weeks apart, followed by a third (reinforcing) dose 6 to 12 months later, for the primary series.

If after beginning a DTP series, further doses of vaccine containing pertussis antigen become contraindicated, DT should be substituted for each of the remaining doses.[4,5]
The reinforcing dose is an integral part of the primary immunizing series.

Interruption of the recommended schedule with a delay between doses does not interfere with the final immunity achieved, nor does it necessitate starting the series over again, regardless of the length of time elapsed between doses.[4,5]

A booster dose of 0.5 mL is indicated at age 4 to 6 years, preferably prior to entrance into kindergarten or elementary school. However, if the last dose of the primary immunizing series was administered after the fourth birthday, a booster prior to school entry is not considered necessary.[4,5]

For either primary or booster immunization against tetanus and diphtheria of individuals 7 years of age and older, the use of Tetanus and Diphtheria Toxoids Adsorbed For Adult Use is recommended.[4,5]

Diphtheria Prophylaxis for Case Contacts: All case contacts, household and others, who have previously received fewer than three doses of diphtheria toxoid should receive an immediate dose of an appropriate diphtheria toxoid-containing preparation and should complete the series according to schedule. Case contacts who previously received three or more doses, but who have not received a dose of a preparation containing diphtheria toxoid within the previous 5 years, should receive a dose of a diphtheria toxoid-containing preparation appropriate for their age. This combined preparation against both diphtheria and tetanus is designed particularly to meet the need of children less than 7 years of age for whom the use of a combined triple vaccine containing pertussis antigen is contraindicated.

Tetanus Prophylaxis in Wound Management: For routine wound management of children under 7 years of age who are not completely immunized, DT should be used instead of single-antigen tetanus toxoid (if pertussis antigen is contraindicated or individual circumstances are such that potential febrile reactions following DTP might confound the management of the patient).[4] Completion of primary vaccination thereafter should be ensured.

For tetanus-prone wounds in children who have had fewer than three, or an unknown number of immunizations with a tetanus-toxoid containing product, passive immunization with human Tetanus-Immune Globulin (TIG) is also recommended.[4] A separate syringe and site of injection should be used.

HOW SUPPLIED
NDC 0005-1858-31   5.0 mL vial

STORAGE
DO NOT FREEZE. STORE REFRIGERATED, AWAY FROM FREEZER COMPARTMENT, AT 2°C to 8°C (36°F to 46°F).

REFERENCES
1. Mueller JH, Miller PA: Production of diphtheria toxin of high potency (100Lf) on a reproducible medium. *J Immunol* 1941;40:21–32.
2. Mueller JH, Miller PA: Factors influencing the production of tetanal toxin. *J Immunol* 1947;56:143–147.
3. Pillemer L, Grossberg DB, Wittler RG: The immunochemistry of toxins and toxoids. II. The preparation and immunological evaluation of purified tetanal toxoid. *J Immunol* 1946;54:213–224.
4. Recommendation of the Immunization Practices Advisory Committee (ACIP): Diphtheria, tetanus and pertussis: Guidelines for vaccine prophylaxis and other preventive measures. *MMWR* 1985;34:405–426.
5. American Academy of Pediatrics: Report of the Committee on Infectious Diseases, ed 20. Elk Grove Village, IL, American Academy of Pediatrics, 1986.
6. Recommendation of the ACIP: Immunization of children infected with Human T-Lymphotrophic Virus Type III/Lymphadenopathy associated virus. *MMWR* 1986; 35(38):595–606.
7. Immunization of children infected with Human Immunodeficiency Virus—Supplementary ACIP statement. *MMWR* 1988;37(12):181–183.
8. National Childhood Vaccine Injury Act: Requirements for permanent vaccination records and for reporting of selected events after vaccination. *MMWR* 1988;37(13):197–200.
9. Cody C, et al: Nature and rates of adverse reactions associated with DTP and DT immunizations in infants and children. *Pediatrics* 1981;68:650–660.
10. Feery BJ: Incidence and type of reactions to triple antigen (DTP) and DT (CDT) vaccines. *Med Jour of Australia* 1982;2:511–515.
11. Fawcett HA, Smith NP: Injection-site granuloma due to aluminum. *Arch Dermatol* 1984;120:1318–1322.
12. Rutledge SL, Snead OC: Neurological complications of immunizations. *J Pediatr* 1986;109:917–924.
13. Adverse Events Following Immunization. *MMWR* 1985;34(3):43–47.
14. Schlenska GK: Unusual neurological complications following tetanus toxoid administration. *J Neurol* 1977;215:299–302.
15. Blumstein GI, Kreithen H: Peripheral neuropathy following tetanus toxoid administration. *JAMA* 1966;198:1030–1031.
16. Reinstein L, Pargament JM, Goodman JS: Peripheral neuropathy after multiple tetanus toxoid injections. *Arch Phys Med Rehabil* 1982;63:332–334.
17. Tsairis P, Duck PJ, Mulder DW: Natural history of brachial plexus neuropathy. *Arch Neurol* 1972;27:109–117.
18. Quast U, Hennessen W, Widmark RM: Mono- and polyneuritis after tetanus vaccination. *Devel Bio Stand* 1979;43:25–32.
19. Holliday PL, Bauer RB: Polyradiculoneuritis secondary to immunization with tetanus and diphtheria toxoids. *Arch Neurol* 1983;40:56–57.
20. Fenichel GM: Neurological complications of tetanus toxoid. *Arch Neurol* 1983;40:390.
21. Pollard JD, Selby G: Relapsing neuropathy due to tetanus toxoid. *J Neurol Sci* 1978;37:113–125.
22. Newton N, Janati A: Guillain-Barre syndrome after vaccination with purified tetanus toxoid. *S Med J* 1987;80:1053–1054.

Manufactured by:
LEDERLE LABORATORIES DIVISION
American Cyanamid Company
Pearl River, NY 10965

HibTITER® ℞
HAEMOPHILUS b CONJUGATE VACCINE
(Diphtheria CRM₁₉₇ Protein Conjugate)

DESCRIPTION

Haemophilus b Conjugate Vaccine (Diphtheria CRM_{197} Protein Conjugate) HibTITER is a sterile solution of a conjugate of oligosaccharides of the capsular antigen of *Haemophilus influenzae* type b (Haemophilus b) and diphtheria CRM_{197} protein (CRM_{197}) dissolved in 0.9% sodium chloride. The oligosaccharides are derived from highly purified capsular polysaccharide, polyribosylribitol phosphate, isolated from Haemophilus b strain Eagan grown in a chemically defined medium (a mixture of mineral salts, amino acids, and cofactors). The oligosaccharides are purified and sized by diafiltrations through a series of ultrafiltration membranes, and coupled by reductive amination directly to highly purified CRM_{197}.[1,2] CRM_{197} is a nontoxic variant of diphtheria toxin isolated from cultures of *Corynebacterium diphtheriae* C7 (β197) grown in a casamino acids and yeast extract-based medium that is ultrafiltered before use. CRM_{197} is purified through ultrafiltration, ammonium sulfate precipitation, and ion-exchange chromatography to high purity. The conjugate is purified to remove unreacted protein, oligosaccharides, and reagents; sterilized by filtration; and filled into vials. HibTITER is intended for intramuscular use.

The vaccine is a clear, colorless solution. Each single dose of 0.5 mL is formulated to contain 10 µg of purified Haemophilus b saccharide and approximately 25 µg of CRM_{197} protein. Multidose vials contain thimerosal (mercurial derivative) 1:10,000 as a preservative. The potency of HibTITER is determined by chemical assay for polyribosylribitol.

CLINICAL PHARMACOLOGY

For several decades, *Haemophilus influenzae* type b (Haemophilus b) was the most common cause of invasive bacterial disease, including meningitis, in young children in the United States. Although nonencapsulated *H. influenzae* are common and six capsular polysaccharide types are known, strains with the type b capsule caused most of the invasive Haemophilus diseases.[3]

Haemophilus b diseases occurred primarily in children under 5 years of age prior to immunization with *Haemophilus influenzae* type b vaccines. In the US, the cumulative risk of developing invasive Haemophilus b disease during the first 5 years of life was estimated to be about 1 in 200. Approximately 60% of cases were meningitis. Cellulitis, epiglottitis, pericarditis, pneumonia, sepsis, or septic arthritis made up the remaining 40%. An estimated 12,000 cases of Haemophilus b meningitis occurred annually prior to the routine use of conjugate vaccines in toddlers.[3,4] The mortality rate can be 5%, and neurologic sequelae have been observed in up to 38% of survivors.[5]

The incidence of invasive Haemophilus b disease peaks between 6 months and 1 year of age, and approximately 55% of disease occurs between 6 and 18 months of age.[3] Interpersonal transmission of Haemophilus b occurs and risk of invasive disease is increased in children younger than 4 years of age who are exposed in the household to a primary case of disease. Clusters of cases in children in day care have been reported and recent studies suggest that the rate of secondary cases may also be increased among children exposed to a primary case in the day-care setting.[3,6]

The incidence of invasive Haemophilus b disease is increased in certain children, such as those who are native Americans, black, or from lower socioeconomic status, and those with medical conditions such as asplenia, sickle cell disease, malignancies associated with immunosuppression, and antibody deficiency syndromes.[3,4,6]

The protective activity of antibody to Haemophilus b polysaccharide was demonstrated by passive antibody studies in animals and in children with agammaglobulinemia or with Haemophilus b disease[7] and confirmed with the efficacy study of Haemophilus b polysaccharide (HbPs) vaccine.[8] Data from passive antibody studies indicate that a preexisting titer of antibody to HbPs of 0.15 µg/mL correlates with protection.[9] Data from a Finnish field trial in children 18 to 71 months of age indicate that a titer of > 1.0 µg/mL 3 weeks after vaccination is associated with long-term protection.[10,11]

Linkage of Haemophilus b saccharides to a protein such as CRM_{197} converts the saccharide (HbO) to a T-dependent (HbOC) antigen, and results in an enhanced antibody response to the saccharide in young infants that primes for an anamnestic response and is predominantly of the IgG class.[12] Laboratory evidence indicates that the native state of the CRM_{197} protein and the use of oligosaccharides in the formulation of HibTITER enhances its immunogenicity.[13–15] Haemophilus b conjugate vaccines with other carrier proteins will be recognized differently by the immune system.

Prior to licensure, the immunogenicity of HibTITER was evaluated in US infants and children.[15] Infants 1 to 6 months of age at first immunization received three doses at approximately 2-month intervals.[16] Children 7 to 11 and 12 to 14 months of age received 2 doses at the same interval.[15] Children 15 to 23 months of age received a single dose.[17] HibTITER was highly immunogenic in all age groups studied, with 97% to 100% of 1,232 infants attaining titers of ≥ 1 µg/mL and 92% to 100% for bactericidal activity.[15–17] Long-term persistence of the antibody response was observed. More than 80% of the 235 infants who received three doses of vaccine had an anti-HbPs antibody level ≥ 1 µg/mL at 2 years of age.[18]

The vaccine generated an immune response characteristic of a protein antigen. IgG anti-HbPs antibodies of IgG_1 subclass predominated and the immune system was primed for a booster response to HibTITER. There is some evidence suggesting natural increases in antibody levels over time after vaccination, most probably the result of contact with Haemophilus type b organisms or cross-reactive antigens.[18] These studies were carried out at a time when significant levels of Haemophilus b disease were still present in the community. Antibody generated by HibTITER has been found to have high avidity, a measure of the functional affinity of antibody to bind to antigen. High-avidity antibody is more potent than low-avidity antibody in serum bactericidal assays.[19] The contribution to clinical protection is unknown.

Immunogenicity of HibTITER was evaluated in 26 children 22 months to 5 years of age who had not responded to earlier vaccination with Haemophilus b polysaccharide vaccine. One dose of HibTITER was immunogenic in all 26 children and generated titers of ≥ 1 µg/mL in 25 of the 26 infants.[20] HibTITER has been found to be immunogenic in children with sickle cell disease, a condition that may cause increased susceptibility to Haemophilus b disease.[21] HibTITER has also been shown to be immunogenic in native American in-

Continued on next page

Lederle—Cont.

fants, such as the group of 50 studied in Alaska who received three doses at 2, 4, and 6 months of age.[20] Antibody levels achieved were comparable to those seen in healthy US infants who received their first dose at 1 to 2 months of age and subsequent doses at 4 to 6 months of age.[15,16,20]

Postlicensure surveillance of immunogenicity was conducted during the distribution of the first 30 million doses of HibTITER and during the time period over which Haemophilus b disease in children has been decreasing significantly in areas of extensive vaccine usage.[20,22-29] After three doses, titers ranged from 2.37 to 8.45 µg/mL, with 67% to 94% attaining ≥ 1 µg/mL.[20,24,25]

Persistence of antibody was examined in several cohorts of subjects that received either a selected commercial lot or that were part of the initial efficacy trial in northern California. Geometric mean titers for these cohorts were between 0.51 and 1.96 just prior to boosting at 15 to 18 months. These lots not only induced persistent antibody but also provided effective priming for a booster dose with commercial lots, with postboosting titers greater than 1.0 µg/mL in 80% to 97% of subjects.[20]

HibTITER (HbOC) was shown to be effective in a large-scale controlled clinical trial in a multiethnic population in northern California carried out between February 1988 and June 1990.[30,31] There were no (0) vaccine failures in infants who received three doses of HibTITER and 12 cases of Haemophilus b disease (6 cases of meningitis) in the control group. The estimate of efficacy is 100% (P = .0002) with 95% confidence intervals of 68% to 100%. Through the end of 1991, with an additional 49,000 person-years of follow-up, there were still no cases of Haemophilus b disease in fully vaccinated infants less than 2 years of age.[22,23] One case of disease has been reported in a 3½-year-old child who did not receive a booster dose as recommended.

A comparative clinical trial was performed in Finland where approximately 53,000 infants received HibTITER at 4 and 6 months of age and a booster dose at 14 months in a trial conducted from January 1988 through December 1990. Only two children developed Haemophilus b disease after receiving the two-dose primary immunization schedule. One child became ill at 15 months of age and the other at 18 months of age; neither child received the scheduled booster at 14 months of age. No vaccine failure has been reported in children who received the two-dose primary series and the booster dose at 14 months of age. Based on more than 32,000 person-years of follow-up time, the estimate of efficacy is about 95% when compared to historical control groups followed between 1985 and 1988.[20] Historical controls were used since all infants received one of two Haemophilus b conjugate vaccines during the period of the trial.

Evidence of efficacy postlicensure includes significant reductions in Haemophilus b disease that are closely associated with increases in the net doses of Haemophilus b Conjugate Vaccine distributed in the US.[20,22-29] In the northern California Kaiser Permanente there has been a 94% decrease in Haemophilus disease incidence in 1991 for children younger than 18 months of age, compared to 1984–1988, when HibTITER was not available for this age group.[22,23] Furthermore, active surveillance by the Centers for Disease Control and Prevention (CDC) has shown a 71% decrease in Haemophilus b disease in children less than 15 months old, between 1989 and 1991, which corresponds temporally and geographically with increases in net doses of Haemophilus b conjugate vaccine distributed in the US.[26] As with all vaccines, this conjugate vaccine cannot be expected to be 100% effective. There have been rare reports to the Vaccine Adverse Event Reporting System (VAERS) of Haemophilus b disease following full primary immunization.

INDICATIONS AND USAGE

Haemophilus b Conjugate Vaccine (Diphtheria CRM$_{197}$ Protein Conjugate) HibTITER is indicated for the immunization of children 2 months to 71 months of age against invasive diseases caused by *H. influenzae* type b.

As with any vaccine, HibTITER may not protect 100% of individuals receiving the vaccine.

HibTITER may be administered simultaneously but at different sites from other routine pediatric vaccines, eg, Diphtheria and Tetanus Toxoids and Pertussis Vaccine Adsorbed (DTP), Oral Poliovirus Vaccine (OPV), and Measles-Mumps-Rubella Vaccine (MMR).[32,33]

CONTRAINDICATIONS

Hypersensitivity to any component of the vaccine, including diphtheria toxoid, or thimerosal in the multidose presentation, is a contraindication to use of HibTITER.

WARNINGS

HibTITER WILL NOT PROTECT AGAINST *H. INFLUENZAE* OTHER THAN TYPE b STRAINS, NOR WILL HibTITER PROTECT AGAINST OTHER MICROORGAN-

ISMS THAT CAUSE MENINGITIS OR SEPTIC DISEASE. AS WITH ANY INTRAMUSCULAR INJECTION, HibTITER SHOULD BE GIVEN WITH CAUTION TO INFANTS OR CHILDREN WITH THROMBOCYTOPENIA OR ANY COAGULATION DISORDER THAT WOULD CONTRAINDICATE INTRAMUSCULAR INJECTION (SEE **DRUG INTERACTIONS**).

ANTIGENURIA HAS BEEN DETECTED FOLLOWING RECEIPT OF HAEMOPHILUS b CONJUGATE VACCINE[34] AND THEREFORE ANTIGEN DETECTION IN URINE MAY NOT HAVE DIAGNOSTIC VALUE IN SUSPECTED HAEMOPHILUS b DISEASE WITHIN 2 WEEKS OF IMMUNIZATION.

PRECAUTIONS
General

1. CARE IS TO BE TAKEN BY THE HEALTH CARE PROVIDER FOR SAFE AND EFFECTIVE USE OF THIS PRODUCT.
2. PRIOR TO ADMINISTRATION OF ANY DOSE OF HibTITER, THE PARENT OR GUARDIAN SHOULD BE ASKED ABOUT THE PERSONAL HISTORY, FAMILY HISTORY, AND RECENT HEALTH STATUS OF THE VACCINE RECIPIENT. THE HEALTH CARE PROVIDER SHOULD ASCERTAIN PREVIOUS IMMUNIZATION HISTORY, CURRENT HEALTH STATUS, AND OCCURRENCE OF ANY SYMPTOMS AND/OR SIGNS OF AN ADVERSE EVENT AFTER PREVIOUS IMMUNIZATION IN THE CHILD TO BE IMMUNIZED, IN ORDER TO DETERMINE THE EXISTENCE OF ANY CONTRAINDICATION TO IMMUNIZATION WITH HibTITER AND TO ALLOW AN ASSESSMENT OF BENEFITS AND RISKS.
3. BEFORE THE INJECTION OF ANY BIOLOGICAL, THE HEALTH CARE PROVIDER SHOULD TAKE ALL PRECAUTIONS KNOWN FOR THE PREVENTION OF ALLERGIC OR ANY OTHER SIDE REACTIONS. This should include: a review of the patient's history regarding possible sensitivity; the ready availability of epinephrine 1:1,000 and other appropriate agents used for control of immediate allergic reactions; and a knowledge of the recent literature pertaining to use of the biological concerned, including the nature of side effects and adverse reactions that may follow its use.
4. Children with impaired immune responsiveness, whether due to the use of immunosuppressive therapy (including irradiation, corticosteroids, antimetabolites, alkylating agents, and cytotoxic agents), a genetic defect, human immunodeficiency virus (HIV) infection, or other causes, may have reduced antibody response to active immunization procedures.[35,36] Deferral of administration of vaccine may be considered in individuals receiving immunosuppressive therapy.[35] Other groups should receive this vaccine according to the usual recommended schedule.[35-37] (See **DRUG INTERACTIONS**.)
5. This product is not contraindicated based on the presence of human immunodeficiency virus infection.[38]
6. Any acute infection or febrile illness is reason for delaying use of HibTITER except when in the opinion of the physician, withholding the vaccine entails a greater risk. A minor afebrile illness, such as a mild upper respiratory infection, is not usually reason to defer immunization.
7. As reported with Haemophilus b polysaccharide vaccine, cases of Haemophilus b disease may occur prior to the onset of the protective effects of the vaccine.[3,39]
8. The vaccine should not be injected intradermally since the safety and immunogenicity of this route have not been evaluated. The vaccine should be given intramuscularly.
9. A separate sterile syringe and needle or a sterile disposable unit should be used for each individual patient to prevent transmission of infectious agents from one person to another. Needles should be disposed of properly and should not be recapped.
10. Special care should be taken to prevent injection into a blood vessel.

The US Department of Health and Human Services has established a new Vaccine Adverse Event Reporting System (VAERS) to accept all reports of suspected adverse events after the administration of any vaccine, including but not limited to the reporting of events required by the National Childhood Vaccine Injury Act of 1986.[40] The VAERS toll-free number for VAERS forms and information is 800-822-7967.

ALTHOUGH SOME ANTIBODY RESPONSE TO DIPHTHERIA TOXIN OCCURS, IMMUNIZATION WITH HibTITER DOES NOT SUBSTITUTE FOR ROUTINE DIPHTHERIA IMMUNIZATION.

INFORMATION FOR PATIENT

PRIOR TO ADMINISTRATION OF HibTITER, HEALTH CARE PERSONNEL SHOULD INFORM THE PARENT, GUARDIAN, OR OTHER RESPONSIBLE ADULT, OF THE RECOMMENDED IMMUNIZATION SCHEDULE FOR

PROTECTION AGAINST HAEMOPHILUS b DISEASE AND THE BENEFITS AND RISKS TO THE CHILD RECEIVING THIS VACCINE. GUIDANCE SHOULD BE PROVIDED ON MEASURES TO BE TAKEN SHOULD ADVERSE EVENTS OCCUR, SUCH AS, ANTIPYRETIC MEASURES FOR ELEVATED TEMPERATURES AND THE NEED TO REPORT ADVERSE EVENTS TO THE HEALTH CARE PROVIDER. Parents should be provided with vaccine information pamphlets at the time of each vaccination, as stated in the National Childhood Vaccine Injury Act.[40] PATIENTS, PARENTS, OR GUARDIANS SHOULD BE INSTRUCTED TO REPORT ANY SERIOUS ADVERSE REACTIONS TO THEIR HEALTH CARE PROVIDER.

DRUG INTERACTIONS

No impairment of the antibody response to the individual antigens was demonstrated when HibTITER was given at the same time but at separate sites as DTP plus OPV to children 2 to 20 months of age or MMR to children 15 ± 1 month of age.[20,41]

As with other intramuscular injections, HibTITER should be given with caution to children on anticoagulant therapy.

CARCINOGENESIS, MUTAGENESIS, IMPAIRMENT OF FERTILITY

HibTITER has not been evaluated for its carcinogenic, mutagenic potential, or impairment of fertility.

PREGNANCY

REPRODUCTIVE STUDIES—PREGNANCY CATEGORY C

Animal reproduction studies have not been conducted with HibTITER. It is also not known whether HibTITER can cause fetal harm when administered to a pregnant woman or can affect reproduction capability. HibTITER is NOT recommended for use in a pregnant woman.

PEDIATRIC USE

The safety and effectiveness of HibTITER in children below the age of 6 weeks have not been established.

ADVERSE REACTIONS

Adverse reactions associated with HibTITER have been evaluated in 401 infants who were vaccinated initially at 1 to 6 months of age and were given 1,118 doses independent of DTP vaccine. Observations were made during the day of vaccination and days 1 and 2 postvaccination. A temperature > 38.3°C was recorded at least once during the observation period following 2% of the vaccinations. Local erythema, warmth, or swelling (≥ 2 cm) was observed following 3.3% of vaccinations. The incidence of temperature > 38.3°C was greater during the first postvaccination day than during the day of vaccination or the second postvaccination day. The incidence of local erythema, warmth, or swelling was similar during the day of vaccination and the first postvaccination day; it was lower during the second postvaccination day. All side effects have been infrequent, mild, and transient with no serious sequelae (Table 1). No difference in the rates of these complaints was reported after dose 1, 2, or 3.
[See table 1 at top of next page.]

The following complaints were also observed after 1,118 vaccinations with HibTITER: irritability (133), sleepiness (91), prolonged crying (≥ 4 hours) (38), appetite loss (23), vomiting (9), diarrhea (2), and rash (1).

Additional safety data with HibTITER are available from the efficacy studies conducted in young infants.[30] There were 79,483 doses given to 30,844 infants at approximately 2, 4, and 6 months of age in California, usually at the same time as DTP (but at a separate injection site) and OPV; approximately 100,000 doses have been given to 53,000 infants at 4 and 6 months in Finland at the same time as a combined DTP and inactivated polio (IPV) vaccine (but at a separate injection site). The rate and type of reactions associated with the vaccinations were no different from those seen when DTP or DTP-IPV was administered alone. These included fever, local reactions, rash, and one hyporesponsive episode with a single seizure. The safety of HibTITER was also evaluated in the California study by direct phone questioning of the parents or guardians of 6,887 vaccine recipients. The incidence and type of side effects reported within 24 hours of vaccination were similar to those cited in Table 1. In addition, analysis of emergency room (ER) visits within 30 days and hospitalization within 60 days after receipt of 23,800 doses of HibTITER showed no increase in the rates of any type of ER visit or hospitalization.

Table 2 details the side effects associated with a single vaccination of HibTITER given (without DTP) to infants of 15 to 23 months of age.

Similar results have been observed in the analysis of 2,285 subjects of 18 to 60 months of age, vaccinated as part of a postmarketing safety study of HibTITER.[20] These data were collected by telephone survey 24 to 48 hours postvaccination. Additional observations included irritability, restless sleep, and GI symptoms (diarrhea, vomiting, and loss of appetite) in the group that received HibTITER alone. A cause and effect relationship between these observations and the vaccinations has not been established.

TABLE 2
Selected Adverse Reactions* in Children of 15–23 Months of Age Following Vaccination With HibTITER

Adverse Reaction	No. of Subjects	Reaction Within 24 h	% Postvaccination At 48 h
Fever > 38.3°C	354	1.4	0.6
Erythema	354	2.0	—
Swelling	354	1.7	—
Tenderness	354	3.7	0.3

*The following complaints were reported after vaccination of these 354 children in the indicated number of children: diarrhea (9), vomiting (5), prolonged crying [> 4 hours] (4), and rashes (2).

Rash, hives (urticaria), erythema multiforme, convulsions,[42] vomiting/diarrhea,[42] and Guillain-Barré syndrome[43] have been observed following the administration of Haemophilus b polysaccharide and Haemophilus b conjugate vaccines. However, a cause and effect relationship among any of these events and the vaccination has not been established.

DOSAGE AND ADMINISTRATION

HibTITER is for intramuscular use only.

Any parenteral drug product should be inspected visually for extraneous particulate matter and/or discoloration prior to administration whenever solution and container permit. If these conditions exist, HibTITER should not be administered.

Before injection, the skin over the site to be injected should be cleansed with a suitable germicide. After insertion of the needle, aspirate to help avoid inadvertent injection into a blood vessel.

The vaccine should be injected intramuscularly, preferably into the midlateral muscles of the thigh or deltoid, with care to avoid major peripheral nerve trunks.

HibTITER is indicated for children 2 months to 71 months of age for the prevention of invasive Haemophilus b disease. For infants 2 to 6 months of age, the immunizing dose is three separate injections of 0.5 mL given at approximately 2-month intervals. Previously unvaccinated infants from 7 through 11 months of age should receive two separate injections approximately 2 months apart. Children from 12 through 14 months of age who have not been vaccinated previously receive one injection. All vaccinated children receive a single booster dose at 15 months of age or older, but not less than 2 months after the previous dose. Previously unvaccinated children 15 to 71 months of age receive a single injection of HibTITER.[32,33] Preterm infants should be vaccinated with HibTITER according to their chronological age, from birth.[32]

Recommended Immunization Schedule

Age at First Immunization (Mo)	No. of Doses	Booster
2–6	3	Yes
7–11	2	Yes
12 –14	1	Yes
15 and over	1	No

Interruption of the recommended schedules with a delay between doses does not interfere with the final immunity achieved nor does it necessitate starting the series over again, regardless of the length of time elapsed between doses.[32,33]

NO DATA ARE AVAILABLE TO SUPPORT THE INTERCHANGEABILITY OF HibTITER OR OTHER HAEMOPHILUS b CONJUGATE VACCINES WITH ONE ANOTHER FOR THE PRIMARY IMMUNIZATION SERIES. THEREFORE, IT IS RECOMMENDED THAT THE SAME CONJUGATE VACCINE BE USED THROUGHOUT EACH IMMUNIZATION SCHEDULE, CONSISTENT WITH THE DATA SUPPORTING APPROVAL AND LICENSURE OF THE VACCINE.

Each dose of 0.5 mL is formulated to contain 10 μg of purified Haemophilus b saccharide and approximately 25 μg of CRM_{197} protein.

STORAGE

Stability studies indicate that HibTITER can be shipped at ambient temperatures and stored at 2°–8°C (36°–46°F). DO NOT FREEZE.

HOW SUPPLIED

Vial, 1 Dose (4 per package) —Product No. 0005-0104-41
Vial, 10 Dose —Product No. 0005-0201-10

TABLE 1
Number of Subjects (Percent) Manifesting Side Effects Associated with HibTITER Administered Independently from DTP*
(Infants Vaccinated Initially at 1–6 Months of Age)

	Dose 1 n=401			Dose 2 n=383			Dose 3 n=334		
Symptoms	Same Day As Vacc.	+1 Day	+2 Days	Same Day As Vacc.	+1 Day	+2 Days	Same Day As Vacc.	+1 Day	+2 Days
Temp > 38.3°C	0	2	2	2	3	2	2	6	5
	—	<1%	<1%	<1%	<1%	<1%	<1%	1.8%	1.5%
Redness ≥ 2cm	1	0	0	1	6	0	5	4	0
	<1%	—	—	<1%	1.6%	—	1.5%	1.2%	—
Warmth ≥ 2cm	1	1	0	2	1	0	1	6	0
	<1%	<1%	—	<1%	<1%	—	<1%	1.8%	—
Swelling ≥ 2cm	5	1	0	2	2	0	1	0	0
	1.2%	<1%	—	<1%	<1%	—	<1%	—	—

*DTP and HibTITER given 2 weeks apart with DTP having been given first.

REFERENCES

1. United States Patent Number 4,902,506 by Anderson PW, Eby RJ filed May 5, 1986 issued February 20, 1990.
2. Seid RC Jr, Boykins RA, Liu DF, et al. Chemical evidence for covalent linkage of a semi-synthetic glycoconjugate vaccine for *Haemophilus influenzae* type b disease. *Glycoconjugate J.* 1989;6:489–498.
3. Wenger JD, Ward JL, Broome CV. Prevention of *Haemophilus influenzae* type b disease: vaccines and passive prophylaxis. In: Remington JS, Swartz MS, eds. *Current Clinical Topics in Infectious Diseases.* New York, NY: McGraw-Hill Inc; 1989;10:306–339.
4. Recommendation of the Immunization Practices Advisory Committee (ACIP)–polysaccharide vaccine for prevention of *Haemophilus influenzae* type b disease. *MMWR.* 1985;34:201–205.
5. Sell SH. Long term sequelae of bacterial meningitis in children. *Pediatr Infect Dis J.* 1983;2:90–93.
6. Broome CV. Epidemiology of *Haemophilus influenzae* type b infections in the United States. *Pediatr Infect Dis J.* 1987;6:779–782.
7. Alexander HE. The productive or curative element in type b *Haemophilus influenzae* rabbit serum. *Yale J Biol Med.* 1944;16:425–434.
8. Peltola H, Kayhty H, Sivonen A. *Haemophilus influenzae* type b capsular polysaccharide vaccine in children: a double-blind field study of 100,000 vaccinees 3 months to 5 years of age in Finland. *Pediatrics.* 1977;60:730–737.
9. Robbins JB, Parke JC Jr, Schneerson R. Quantitative measurement of "natural" and immunization-induced *Haemophilus influenzae* type b capsular polysaccharide antibodies. *Pediatr Res.* 1973;7:103-110.
10. Kayhty H, Peltola H, Karanko V, et al. The protective level of serum antibodies to the capsular polysaccharide of *Haemophilus influenzae* type b. *J Infect Dis.* 1983;147:1100.
11. Kayhty H, Karanko, V, Peltola H, et al. Serum antibodies after vaccination with *Haemophilus influenzae* type b capsular polysaccharide and responses to reimmunization: no evidence of immunologic tolerance or memory. *Pediatrics.* 1984;74:857–865.
12. Weinberg GA, Granoff DM. Polysaccharide-protein conjugate vaccines for the prevention of *Haemophilus influenzae* type b disease. *J Pediatr.* 1988;113:621–631.
13. Makela O, Péterfy F, Outshoorn IG, et al. Immunogenic properties of a (1–6) dextran, its protein conjugates, and conjugates of its breakdown products in mice. *Scand J Immunol.* 1984;19:541–550.
14. Anderson P, Pichichero ME, Insel RA. Immunogens consisting of oligosaccharides from *Haemophilus influenzae* type b coupled to diphtheria toxoid or the toxin protein CRM_{197}. *J Clin Invest.* 1985;76:52–59.
15. Madore DV, Phipps DC, Eby R, et al. Immune response of young children vaccinated with *Haemophilus influenzae* type b conjugate vaccines. In: Cruse JM, Lewis RE, eds. *Contributions to Microbiology and Immunology: Conjugate Vaccines.* New York, NY: Karger Medical and Scientific Publishers: 1989;10:125–150.
16. Madore DV, Phipps DC, Eby R, et al. Safety and immunologic response to *Haemophilus influenzae* type b oligosaccharide-CRM_{197} conjugate vaccine in 1- to 6-month-old infants. *Pediatrics.* 1990;85:331–337.
17. Madore DV, Johnson CL, Phipps DC, et al. Safety and immunogenicity of *Haemophilus influenzae* type b oligosaccharide-CRM_{197} conjugate vaccine in infants aged 15–23 months. *Pediatrics.* 1990;86:527–534.
18. Rothstein EP, Madore DV, Long S. Antibody persistence four years after primary immunization of infants and toddlers with *Haemophilus influenzae* type b CRM_{197} conjugate vaccine. *J Pediatrics.* 1991;119:655–657.
19. Schlesinger Y, Granoff DM. Avidity and bacteriocidal activity of antibodies elicited by different *Haemophilus influenzae* type b conjugate vaccines. *JAMA.* 1992; 267:1489–1494.
20. Unpublished data available from Lederle Laboratories.
21. Gigliotti F, Feldman S, Wang WC, et al. Immunization of young infants with sickle cell disease with a *Haemophilus influenzae* type b saccharide-diphtheria CRM_{197} protein conjugate vaccine. *J Pediatr.* 1989;114:1006-1010.
22. Black SB, Shinefield HR, The Kaiser Permanente Pediatric Vaccine Study Group. Immunization with oligosaccharide conjugate *Haemophilus influenzae* type b (HbOC) vaccine on a large health maintenance organization population: extended follow-up and impact on *Haemophilus influenzae* disease epidemiology. *Pediatr Infect Dis J.* 1992;11:610–613.
23. Black SB, Shinefield HR, Fireman B, et al. Safety, immunogenicity, and efficacy in infancy of oligosaccharide conjugate *Haemophilus influenzae* type b vaccine in a United States Population: possible implications for optimal use. *J Infect Dis.* 1992;165 (suppl 1):S139–143.
24. Granoff DM, Anderson EL, Osterholm MT, et al. Differences in the immunogenicity of three *Haemophilus influenzae* type b conjugate vaccines in infants. *J Pediatr.* 1992;121:187–194.
25. Decker MD, Edwards KM, Bradley R, et al. Comparative trial in infants of four conjugate *Haemophilus influenzae* type b vaccines. *J Pediatr.* 1992;120:184–189.
26. Adams WG, Deaver KA, Cochi SL, et al. Decline of childhood *Haemophilus influenzae* type b (Hib) disease in the Hib vaccine era. *JAMA.* 1993;269:221–226.
27. Murphy TV, White KE, Pastor P, et al. Declining incidence of *Haemophilus influenzae* type b disease since introduction of vaccination. *JAMA.* 1993;269:246–248.
28. Broadhurst LE, Erickson RL, Kelley PW. Decreases in invasive *Haemophilus influenzae* diseases in US Army children, 1984 through 1991. *JAMA.* 1993;269:227–231.
29. Shapiro ED. Infections caused by *Haemophilus influenzae* type b: the beginning of the end? *JAMA.* 1993;269:264–266.
30. Black SB, Shinefield HR, Lampert D, et al. Safety and immunogenicity of oligosaccharide conjugate *Haemophilus influenzae* type b (HbOC) vaccine in infancy. *Pediatr Infect Dis J.* 1991;10:92–96.
31. Black SB, Shinefield HR, Fireman B, et al. Efficacy in infancy of oligosaccharide conjugate *Haemophilus influenzae* type b (HbOC) vaccine in a United States population of 61,080 children. *Pediatr Infect Dis J.* 1991;10:97–104.
32. Recommendations of the AAP: *Haemophilus influenzae* type b conjugate vaccines: recommendations for immunization of infants and children 2 months of age and older: update. *Pediatrics.* 1991;88:169–172.
33. Recommendation of the ACIP: Haemophilus b conjugate vaccines for prevention of *Haemophilus influenzae* type b disease among infants and children two months of age and older. *MMWR.* 1991;40:1–7.
34. Jones RG, Bass JW, Weisse ME, et al. Antigenuria after immunization with *Haemophilus influenzae* oligosaccharide CRM_{197} conjugate (HbOC) vaccine. *Pediatr Infect Dis J.* 1991;10:557–559.
35. American Academy of Pediatrics: Report of the Committee on Infectious Diseases. 22nd ed. Elk Grove Village, Ill: American Academy of Pediatrics; 1991.
36. Recommendation of the ACIP—immunization of children infected with human T-lymphotrophic virus type III/lymphadenopathy-associated virus. *MMWR.* 1986; 35(38):595–606.
37. Immunization of children infected with human immunodeficiency virus—supplementary ACIP statement. *MMWR.* 1988;37(12):181–183.
38. General Recommendations on Immunization—recommendations of the Immunization Practices Advisory Committee (ACIP). *MMWR.* 1989;38(13):221.
39. Spinola SM, Sheaffer CI, Philbrick KB, et al. Antigenuria after *Haemophilus influenzae* type b polysaccharide immunization: a prospective study. *J Pediatr.* 1986;109:835–837.
40. CDC. Vaccine Adverse Event Reporting System—United States. *MMWR.* 1990;39:730–733.
41. Paradiso PR. Combined childhood immunizations. *JAMA.* 1992;268:1685.
42. Milstein JB, Gross TP, Kuritsky JN. Adverse reactions reported following receipt of *Haemophilus influenzae*

Continued on next page

Lederle—Cont.

type b vaccine: an analysis after one year of marketing. *Pediatrics.* 1987;80:270–274.
43. D'Cruz DF, Shapiro ED, Spiegelman KN, et al. Acute inflammatory demyelinating polyradiculoneuropathy (Guillain-Barré syndrome) after immunization with *Haemophilus influenzae* type b conjugate vaccine. *J Pediatr.* 1989;115:743–746.

Manufactured by:
LEDERLE LABORATORIES
Division of American Cyanamid Company
Pearl River, NY 10965 USA
US Gov't. License No. 17
Marketed by:
WYETH-LEDERLE VACCINES AND PEDIATRICS
Wyeth-Ayerst Laboratories
Philadelphia, PA 19101

Shown in Product Identification Guide, page 320

LOXITANE® ℞
[*lōks-ĭ-tāne*]
Loxapine Succinate
Capsules
LOXITANE® C ℞
Loxapine Hydrochloride
Oral Concentrate
For Oral Use
LOXITANE® IM ℞
Loxapine Hydrochloride
For Intramuscular Use Only

DESCRIPTION
LOXITANE loxapine, a dibenzoxazepine compound, represents a new subclass of tricyclic antipsychotic agent, chemically distinct from the thioxanthenes, butyrophenones, and phenothiazines. Chemically, it is 2-Chloro-11-(4-methyl-1-piperazinyl)-dibenz[*b,f*][1,4]oxazepine. It is present in capsules as the succinate salt, and in the concentrate and parenteral primarily as the hydrochloride salt.
CAPSULES—Each capsule contains loxapine succinate equivalent to 5, 10, 25, or 50 mg of loxapine base and the following inactive ingredients: Blue 1, Gelatin, Lactose, Magnesium Stearate, Titanium Dioxide, and Yellow 10. Additionally, the 5 mg capsule contains Red 33, the 10 mg capsule contains Red 28 and Red 33, and the 25 mg capsule contains FD&C Yellow No. 6.
ORAL CONCENTRATE—Each mL contains loxapine hydrochloride equivalent to 25 mg of loxapine base and propylene glycol as an inactive ingredient.
Hydrochloric acid and, if necessary, sodium hydroxide are used to adjust pH to approximately 5.8 during manufacture.
INTRAMUSCULAR-(Sterile)—Not for Intravenous Use—Each mL contains loxapine hydrochloride equivalent to 50 mg of loxapine base. Inactive Ingredients: Polysorbate 80 NF 5% w/v, Propylene Glycol 70% v/v, and Water for Injection qs ad 100% v.
Hydrochloric acid and, if necessary, sodium hydroxide are used to adjust pH to approximately 5.5 during manufacture.

CLINICAL PHARMACOLOGY
Pharmacodynamics
Pharmacologically, loxapine is a tranquilizer for which the exact mode of action has not been established. However, changes in the level of excitability of subcortical inhibitory areas have been observed in several animal species in association with such manifestations of tranquilization as calming effects and suppression of aggressive behavior.
In normal human volunteers, signs of sedation were seen within 20 to 30 minutes after administration, were most pronounced within $1^1/_2$ to 3 hours, and lasted through 12 hours. Similar timing of primary pharmacologic effects was seen in animals.
Absorption, Distribution, Metabolism, and Excretion
After administration of LOXITANE as an oral solution, systemic bioavailability of the parent drug was only about one third that after an equivalent intramuscular dose (25 mg base) in male volunteers. C_{max} for the parent drug was similar for the IM and oral administrations, whereas T_{max} was significantly longer for the IM administration than the oral administration (approximately 5 *vs* 1 hour). The lower systemic availability of the parent drug after oral administration as compared to the IM administration may be due to first pass metabolism of the oral form. This is supported by the finding that two metabolites found in serum (8-hydroxyloxapine and 8-hydroxydesmethylloxapine) were formed to a lesser extent after IM administration of loxapine as compared to oral administration.
The apparent half-life of loxapine after oral and IM administration is approximately 4 hours (range, 1 to 14 hours) and 12 hours (range, 8 to 23 hours), respectively. The extended half-life for the IM administration as compared to the oral administration may be explained by prolonged absorption of loxapine from the muscle during the concurrent elimination process.
Loxapine is extensively metabolized, and urinary recovery over 48 hours resulted in recoveries of approximately 30% and 40% of an IM and orally administered loxapine dose as five metabolites.

INDICATIONS
LOXITANE is indicated for the management of the manifestations of psychotic disorders. The antipsychotic efficacy of LOXITANE was established in clinical studies which enrolled newly hospitalized and chronically hospitalized acutely ill schizophrenic patients as subjects.

CONTRAINDICATIONS
LOXITANE is contraindicated in comatose or severe drug-induced depressed states (alcohol, barbiturates, narcotics, etc).
LOXITANE is contraindicated in individuals with known hypersensitivity to dibenzoxazepines.

WARNINGS
Tardive Dyskinesia: Tardive dyskinesia, a syndrome consisting of potentially irreversible, involuntary, dyskinetic movements, may develop in patients treated with neuroleptic (antipsychotic) drugs. Although the prevalence of the syndrome appears to be highest among the elderly, especially elderly women, it is impossible to rely upon prevalence estimates to predict, at the inception of neuroleptic treatment, which patients are likely to develop the syndrome. Whether neuroleptic drug products differ in their potential to cause tardive dyskinesia is unknown.
Both the risk of developing the syndrome and the likelihood that it will become irreversible are believed to increase as the duration of treatment and the total cumulative dose of neuroleptic drugs administered to the patient increase. However, the syndrome can develop, although much less commonly, after relatively brief treatment periods at low doses.
There is no known treatment for established cases of tardive dyskinesia, although the syndrome may remit, partially or completely, if neuroleptic treatment is withdrawn. Neuroleptic treatment, itself, however, may suppress (or partially suppress) the signs and symptoms of the syndrome, and thereby may possibly mask the underlying disease process. The effect that symptomatic suppression has upon the long-term course of the syndrome is unknown.
Given these considerations, neuroleptics should be prescribed in a manner that is most likely to minimize the occurrence of tardive dyskinesia. Chronic neuroleptic treatment should generally be reserved for patients who suffer from a chronic illness that, (1) is known to respond to neuroleptic drugs, and (2), for whom alternative, equally effective, but potentially less harmful treatments are *not* available or appropriate. In patients who do require chronic treatment, the smallest dose and the shortest duration of treatment producing a satisfactory clinical response should be sought. The need for continued treatment should be reassessed periodically.
If signs and symptoms of tardive dyskinesia appear in a patient on neuroleptics, drug discontinuation should be considered. However, some patients may require treatment despite the presence of the syndrome. (See **ADVERSE REACTIONS** and *Information for Patients* sections.)
Neuroleptic Malignant Syndrome (NMS)
A potentially fatal symptom complex sometimes referred to as Neuroleptic Malignant Syndrome (NMS) has been reported in association with antipsychotic drugs. Clinical manifestations of NMS are hyperpyrexia, muscle rigidity, altered mental status and evidence of autonomic instability (irregular pulse or blood pressure, tachycardia, diaphoresis, and cardiac dys-rhythmias).
The diagnostic evaluation of patients with this syndrome is complicated. In arriving at a diagnosis, it is important to identify cases where the clinical presentation includes both serious medical illness (eg, pneumonia, systemic infection, etc.) and untreated or inadequately treated extrapyramidal signs and symptoms (EPS). Other important considerations in the differential diagnosis include central anticholinergic toxicity, heat stroke, drug fever and primary central nervous system (CNS) pathology.
The management of NMS should include: (1) immediate discontinuation of antipsychotic drugs and other drugs not essential to concurrent therapy, (2) intensive symptomatic treatment and medical monitoring, and (3) treatment of any concomitant serious medical problems for which specific treatments are available. There is no general agreement about specific pharmacological treatment regimens for uncomplicated NMS.
If a patient requires antipsychotic drug treatment after recovery from NMS, the potential reintroduction of drug therapy should be carefully considered. The patient should be carefully monitored, since recurrences of NMS have been reported.
LOXITANE, like other tranquilizers, may impair mental and/or physical abilities, especially during the first few days of therapy. Therefore, ambulatory patients should be warned about activities requiring alertness (eg, operating vehicles or machinery) and about concomitant use of alcohol and other CNS depressants.
LOXITANE has not been evaluated for the management of behavioral complications in patients with mental retardation, and therefore, it cannot be recommended.

PRECAUTIONS
General
LOXITANE loxapine should be used with extreme caution in patients with a history of convulsive disorders since it lowers the convulsive threshold. Seizures have been reported in patients receiving LOXITANE at antipsychotic dose levels, and may occur in epileptic patients even with maintenance of routine anticonvulsant drug therapy.
LOXITANE has an antiemetic effect in animals. Since this effect may also occur in man, LOXITANE may mask signs of overdosage of toxic drugs and may obscure conditions such as intestinal obstruction and brain tumor.
LOXITANE should be used with caution in patients with cardiovascular disease. Increased pulse rates have been reported in the majority of patients receiving antipsychotic doses; transient hypotension has been reported. In the presence of severe hypotension requiring vasopressor therapy, the preferred drugs may be norepinephrine or angiotensin. Usual doses of epinephrine may be ineffective because of inhibition of its vasopressor effect by LOXITANE.
The possibility of ocular toxicity from loxapine cannot be excluded at this time. Therefore, careful observation should be made for pigmentary retinopathy and lenticular pigmentation, since these have been observed in some patients receiving certain other antipsychotic drugs for prolonged periods.
Because of possible anticholinergic action, the drug should be used cautiously in patients with glaucoma or a tendency to urinary retention, particularly with concomitant administration of anticholinergic-type antiparkinson medication.
Experience to date indicates the possibility of a slightly higher incidence of extrapyramidal effects following intramuscular administration than normally anticipated with oral formulations. The increase may be attributable to higher plasma levels following intramuscular injection.
Neuroleptic drugs elevate prolactin levels; the elevation persists during chronic administration. Tissue culture experiments indicate that approximately one third of human breast cancers are prolactin-dependent *in vitro,* a factor of potential importance if the prescription of these drugs is contemplated in a patient with a previously detected breast cancer. Although disturbances such as galactorrhea, amenorrhea, gynecomastia, and impotence have been reported, the clinical significance of elevated serum prolactin levels is unknown for most patients. An increase in mammary neoplasms has been found in rodents after chronic administration of neuroleptic drugs. Neither clinical studies nor epidemiologic studies conducted to date, however, have shown an association between chronic administration of these drugs and mammary tumorigenesis; the available evidence is considered too limited to be conclusive at this time.
Information for Patients
Given the likelihood that some patients exposed chronically to neuroleptics will develop tardive dyskinesia, it is advised that all patients in whom chronic use is contemplated be given, if possible, full information about this risk. The decision to inform patients and/or their guardians must obviously take into account the clinical circumstances and the competency of the patient to understand the information provided.
Usage in Pregnancy
Safe use of LOXITANE during pregnancy or lactation has not been established; therefore, its use in pregnancy, in nursing mothers, or in women of childbearing potential requires that the benefits of treatment be weighed against the possible risks to mother and child. No embryotoxicity or teratogenicity was observed in studies in rats, rabbits, or dogs, although, with the exception of one rabbit study, the highest dosage was only two times the maximum recommended human dose and in some studies it was below this dose. Perinatal studies have shown renal papillary abnormalities in offspring of rats treated from midpregnancy with doses of 0.6 and 1.8 mg/kg, doses which approximate the usual human dose but which are considerably below the maximum recommended human dose.
Nursing Mothers
The extent of the excretion of LOXITANE or its metabolites in human milk is not known. However, LOXITANE and its metabolites have been shown to be transported into the milk of lactating dogs. LOXITANE administration to nursing women should be avoided if clinically possible.
Usage in Children
Studies have not been performed in children; therefore, this drug is not recommended for use in children below the age of 16.

ADVERSE REACTIONS
CNS Effects: Manifestations of adverse effects on the central nervous system, other than extrapyramidal effects, have been seen infrequently. Drowsiness, usually mild, may occur

at the beginning of therapy or when dosage is increased. It usually subsides with continued LOXITANE therapy. The incidence of sedation has been less than that of certain aliphatic phenothiazines and slightly more than the piperazine phenothiazines. Dizziness, faintness, staggering gait, shuffling gait, muscle twitching, weakness, insomnia, agitation, tension, seizures, akinesia, slurred speech, numbness and confusional states have been reported. Neuroleptic malignant syndrome (NMS) has been reported (see **WARNINGS**).

Extrapyramidal Reactions–Neuromuscular (extrapyramidal) reactions during the administration of LOXITANE *loxapine* have been reported frequently, often during the first few days of treatment. In most patients, these reactions involved parkinsonian-like symptoms such as tremor, rigidity, excessive salivation, and masked facies. Akathisia (motor restlessness) also has been reported relatively frequently. These symptoms are usually not severe and can be controlled by reduction of LOXITANE dosage or by administration of antiparkinson drugs in usual dosage. Dystonic and dyskinetic reactions have occurred less frequently, but may be more severe. Dystonias include spasms of muscles of the neck and face, tongue protrusion, and oculogyric movement. Dyskinetic reactions have been described in the form of choreoathetoid movements. These reactions sometimes require reduction or temporary withdrawal of loxapine dosage in addition to appropriate counteractive drugs.

Persistent Tardive Dyskinesia–As with all antipsychotic agents, tardive dyskinesia may appear in some patients on long-term therapy or may appear after drug therapy has been discontinued. The risk appears to be greater in elderly patients on high-dose therapy, especially females. The symptoms are persistent and in some patients appear to be irreversible. The syndrome is characterized by rhythmical involuntary movement of the tongue, face, mouth, or jaw (eg, protrusion of tongue, puffing of cheeks, puckering of mouth, chewing movements). Sometimes these may be accompanied by involuntary movements of extremities.

There is no known effective treatment for tardive dyskinesia; antiparkinson agents usually do not alleviate the symptoms of this syndrome. It is suggested that all antipsychotic agents be discontinued if these symptoms appear. Should it be necessary to reinstitute treatment, or increase the dosage of the agent, or switch to a different antipsychotic agent, the syndrome may be masked. It has been suggested that fine vermicular movements of the tongue may be an early sign of the syndrome, and if the medication is stopped at that time the syndrome may not develop.

Cardiovascular Effects: Tachycardia, hypotension, hypertension, orthostatic hypotension, light-headedness, and syncope have been reported.

A few cases of ECG changes similar to those seen with phenothiazines have been reported. It is not known whether these were related to LOXITANE administration.

Hematologic: Rarely, agranulocytosis, thrombocytopenia, leukopenia.

Skin: Dermatitis, edema (puffiness of face), pruritus, rash, alopecia and seborrhea have been reported with loxapine.

Anticholinergic Effects: Dry mouth, nasal congestion, constipation, blurred vision, urinary retention and paralytic ileus have occurred.

Gastrointestinal: Nausea and vomiting have been reported in some patients. Hepatocellular injury (ie, SGOT/SGPT elevation) has been reported in association with loxapine administration and, rarely, jaundice and/or hepatitis questionably related to LOXITANE treatment.

Other Adverse Reactions: Weight gain, weight loss, dyspnea, ptosis, hyperpyrexia, flushed facies, headache, paresthesia, and polydipsia have been reported in some patients. Rarely, galactorrhea, amenorrhea, gynecomastia and menstrual irregularity of uncertain etiology have been reported.

DOSAGE AND ADMINISTRATION

LOXITANE is administered, usually in divided doses, two to four times a day. Daily dosage (in terms of base equivalents) should be adjusted to the individual patient's needs as assessed by the severity of symptoms and previous history of response to antipsychotic drugs.

Oral Administration

Initial dosage of 10 mg twice daily is recommended, although in severely disturbed patients initial dosage up to a total of 50 mg daily may be desirable. Dosage should then be increased fairly rapidly over the first seven to ten days until there is effective control of psychotic symptoms. The usual therapeutic and maintenance range is 60 to 100 mg daily. However, as with other antipsychotic drugs, some patients respond to lower dosage and others require higher dosage for optimal benefit. Daily dosage higher than 250 mg is not recommended.

LOXITANE C Oral Concentrate should be mixed with orange or grapefruit juice shortly before administration. Use only the enclosed calibrated (10 mg, 15 mg, 25 mg, 50 mg) dropper for dosage.

Maintenance Therapy

For maintenance therapy, dosage should be reduced to the lowest level compatible with symptom control; many patients have been maintained satisfactorily at dosages in the range of 20 to 60 mg daily.

Intramuscular Administration

LOXITANE IM is utilized for prompt symptomatic control in the acutely agitated patient and in patients whose symptoms render oral medication temporarily impractical. During clinical trial there were only rare reports of significant local tissue reaction.

LOXITANE IM is administered by intramuscular (not intravenous) injection in doses of 12.5 mg ($^1/_4$ mL) to 50 mg (1 mL) at intervals of four to six hours or longer, both dose and interval depending on patient response. Many patients have responded satisfactorily to twice-daily dosage. As described above for oral administration, attention is directed to the necessity for dosage adjustment on an individual basis over the early days of loxapine administration.

Once the desired symptomatic control is achieved and the patient is able to take medication orally, loxapine should be administered in capsule or oral concentrate form. Usually this should occur within 5 days.

OVERDOSAGE

Signs and symptoms of overdosage will depend on the amount ingested and individual patient tolerance. As would be expected from the pharmacologic actions of the drug, the clinical findings may range from mild depression of the CNS and cardiovascular systems to profound hypotension, respiratory depression, and unconsciousness. The possibility of occurrence of extrapyramidal symptoms and/or convulsive seizures should be kept in mind. Renal failure following loxapine overdosage has also been reported.

The treatment of overdosage is essentially symptomatic and supportive. Early gastric lavage and extended dialysis might be expected to be beneficial. Centrally acting emetics may have little effect because of the antiemetic action of loxapine. In addition, emesis should be avoided because of the possibility of aspiration of vomitus. Avoid analeptics, such as pentylenetetrazol, which may cause convulsions. Severe hypotension might be expected to respond to the administration of levarterenol or phenylephrine. EPINEPHRINE SHOULD NOT BE USED SINCE ITS USE IN A PATIENT WITH PARTIAL ADRENERGIC BLOCKADE MAY FURTHER LOWER THE BLOOD PRESSURE. Severe extrapyramidal reactions should be treated with anticholinergic antiparkinson agents or diphenhydramine hydrochloride, and anticonvulsant therapy should be initiated as indicated. Additional measures include oxygen and intravenous fluids.

HOW SUPPLIED

LOXITANE loxapine succinate capsules are available in the following base equivalent strengths:

5 mg—Hard shell, opaque, dark green capsules, printed with Lederle over L1 on one half and 5 mg on the other, are supplied as follows:
- NDC 0005-5359-23—Bottle of 100s
- NDC 0005-5359-60—Unit Dose 10 (2 × 5) Strips

10 mg—Hard shell, opaque, with yellow body and a dark green cap, printed with Lederle over L2 on one half and 10 mg on the other, are supplied as follows:
- NDC 0005-5360-23—Bottle of 100s
- NDC 0005-5360-34—Bottle of 1000s
- NDC 0005-5360-60—Unit Dose 10 (2 × 5) Strips

25 mg—Hard shell, opaque, with a light green body and a dark green cap, printed with Lederle over L3 on one half and 25 mg on the other, are supplied as follows:
- NDC 0005-5361-23—Bottle of 100s
- NDC 0005-5361-34—Bottle of 1000s
- NDC 0005-5361-60—Unit Dose 10 (2 × 5) Strips

50 mg—Hard shell, opaque, with a blue body and a dark green cap, printed with Lederle over L4 on one half and 50 mg on the other, are supplied as follows:
- NDC 0005-5362-23—Bottle of 100s
- NDC 0005-5362-34—Bottle of 1000s
- NDC 0005-5362-60—Unit Dose 10 (2 × 5) Strips

Store at Controlled Room Temperature 15–30° C (59–86° F).

LOXITANE C loxapine hydrochloride Oral Concentrate is supplied as follows:
- NDC 0005-5387-58—4 fl oz (120 mL) with calibrated dropper. Each mL contains loxapine HCl equivalent to 25 mg of loxapine base.

Store at Controlled Room Temperature 15–30° C (59–86° F).
DO NOT FREEZE.

LEDERLE LABORATORIES DIVISION
American Cyanamid Company
Pearl River, NY 10965

LOXITANE IM loxapine hydrochloride for Intramuscular use only is supplied as follows:
- NDC 0205-5385-34—10 mL multi-dose vial

Each mL contains loxapine HCl equivalent to 50 mg of loxapine base.

Keep package closed to protect from light. Intensification of the straw color to a light amber will not alter potency or therapeutic efficacy; if noticeably discolored, ampul or vial should not be used.

Store at Controlled Room Temperature 15-30° C (59-86° F).
DO NOT FREEZE.

LEDERLE PARENTERALS, INC.
Carolina, Puerto Rico 00987

Shown in Product Identification Guide, page 320

MATERNA® ℞

[ma-ter-na]

Prenatal Vitamin and Mineral Tablets
For Use Before, During & After Pregnancy

DESCRIPTION

One tablet daily provides:

VITAMINS	
A*	5,000 IU
D	400 IU
E (*dl*-alpha tocopheryl acetate)	30 IU
C (ascorbic acid)	100 mg
Folic Acid	1 mg
B_1 (thiamine mononitrate)	3 mg
B_2 (riboflavin)	3.4 mg
B_6 (pyridoxine hydrochloride)	10 mg
Niacinamide	20 mg
B_{12} (cyanocobalamin)	12 mcg
Biotin	30 mcg
Pantothenic Acid (calcium pantothenate)	10 mg
MINERALS	
Calcium (calcium carbonate)	250 mg
Iodine (potassium iodide)	150 mcg
Iron (ferrous fumarate)	60 mg
Magnesium (magnesium oxide)	25 mg
Copper (cupric oxide)	2 mg
Zinc (zinc oxide)	25 mg
Chromium (chromium chloride)	25 mcg
Molybdenum (sodium molybdate)	25 mcg
Manganese (manganese sulfate)	5 mg

*Input as vitamin A acetate and beta carotene

MATERNA contains no artificial dyes, flavors or added sweeteners.

INDICATIONS AND USAGE

MATERNA is indicated to provide vitamin and mineral supplementation throughout pregnancy and during the postnatal period for both the lactating and nonlactating mother. It is also useful for improving nutritional status prior to conception.

Each tablet provides essential vitamins and minerals, including 60 mg of elemental iron and 250 mg of elemental calcium and 25 mg zinc. MATERNA also offers 1 mg folic acid to aid in the prevention of megaloblastic anemia.

WARNINGS

As with all medications, keep out of the reach of children. In case of accidental overdose, seek professional assistance or contact a Poison Control Center immediately.

PRECAUTIONS

Folic acid may partially correct the hematological damage due to vitamin B_{12} deficiency of pernicious anemia, while the associated neurological damage progresses. In rare instances, allergic hypersensitivity has been reported following administration of folic acid.

DOSAGE AND ADMINISTRATION

Before, during and after pregnancy, one tablet daily, or as directed by a physician.

HOW SUPPLIED

MATERNA is available as off-white, capsule-shaped tablets identified as "MATERNA" on one side and "M77" on the other side, in bottles of 100, NDC 0005-5573-11.

A child-resistant safety cap is standard as a safeguard against accidental ingestion by children.

NOTICE: Contact with moisture may produce surface discoloration or erosion of the tablet.

Store at room temperature, approximately 25°C; avoid excess heat. Dispense in well-closed, light-resistant container.

Questions or Comments: 1-800-999-9384

LEDERLE LABORATORIES DIVISION
American Cyanamid Company
Pearl River, NY 10965

Shown in Product Identification Guide, page 320

Continued on next page

Lederle—Cont.

MINOCIN® ℞
[mī-nō-sĭn]
Sterile
Minocycline Hydrochloride
Intravenous
100 mg/Vial

DESCRIPTION

MINOCIN minocycline hydrochloride, a semisynthetic derivative of tetracycline, is named [4*S*-(4α,4aα,5aα,12aα)]-4,7-bis(dimethylamino)-1,4,4a,5,5a,6,11,12a-octahydro-3,10,-0 12,12a-tetrahydroxy-1, 11-dioxo-2-naphthacenecarboxamide monohydrochloride.
Each vial, dried by cryodesiccation, contains sterile minocycline HCl equivalent to 100 mg minocycline. When reconstituted with 5 mL of Sterile Water for Injection USP, the pH ranges from 2.0 to 2.8.

ACTIONS

Microbiology
The tetracyclines are primarily bacteriostatic and are thought to exert their antimicrobial effect by the inhibition of protein synthesis. Minocycline HCl is a tetracycline with antibacterial activity comparable to other tetracyclines with activity against a wide range of gram-negative and gram-positive organisms.
Tube dilution testing: Microorganisms may be considered susceptible (likely to respond to minocycline therapy) if the minimum inhibitory concentration (MIC) is not more than 4 mcg/mL. Microorganisms may be considered intermediate (harboring partial resistance) if the MIC is 4 to 12.5 mcg/mL and resistant (not likely to respond to minocycline therapy) if the MIC is greater than 12.5 mcg/mL.
Susceptibility plate testing: If the Kirby-Bauer method of susceptibility testing (using a 30 mcg tetracycline disc) gives a zone of 18 mm or greater, the bacterial strain is considered to be susceptible to any tetracycline. Minocycline shows moderate *in vitro* activity against certain strains of staphylococci which have been found resistant to other tetracyclines. For such strains, minocycline susceptibility powder may be used for additional susceptibility testing.
Human Pharmacology
Following a single dose of 200 mg administered intravenously to 10 healthy male volunteers, serum levels ranged from 2.52 to 6.63 mcg/mL (average 4.18), after 12 hours they ranged from 0.82 to 2.64 mcg/mL (average 1.38). In a group of five healthy male volunteers, serum levels of 1.4 to 1.8 mcg/mL were maintained at 12 and 24 hours with doses of 100 mg every 12 hours for three days. When given 200 mg once daily for three days, the serum levels had fallen to approximately 1 mcg/mL at 24 hours. The serum half-life following I.V. doses of 100 mg every 12 hours or 200 mg once daily did not differ significantly and ranged from 15 to 23 hours. The serum half-life following a single 200 mg oral dose in 12 essentially normal volunteers ranged from 11 to 17 hours, in 7 patients with hepatic dysfunction ranged from 11 to 16 hours, and in 5 patients with renal dysfunction from 18 to 69 hours.
Intravenously administered minocycline appears similar to oral doses in excretion. The urinary and fecal recovery of oral minocycline when administered to 12 normal volunteers is one-half to one-third that of other tetracyclines.

INDICATIONS

MINOCIN is indicated in infections caused by the following microorganisms:
Rickettsiae: (Rocky Mountain spotted fever, typhus fever and the typhus group, Q fever, rickettsialpox, tick fevers).
Mycoplasma pneumoniae (PPLO, Eaton agent).
Agents of psittacosis and ornithosis.
Agents of lymphogranuloma venereum and granuloma inguinale.
The spirochetal agent of relapsing fever (*Borrelia recurrentis*).
The following gram-negative microorganisms:
Haemophilus ducreyi (chancroid),
Yersinia pestis and *Francisella tularensis,* formerly *Pasteurella pestis* and *Pasteurella tularensis,*
Bartonella bacilliformis,
Bacteroides species,
Vibrio comma and *Vibrio fetus,*
Brucella species (in conjunction with streptomycin).
Because many strains of the following groups of microorganisms have been shown to be resistant to tetracyclines, culture and susceptibility testing are recommended.
MINOCIN is indicated for treatment of infections caused by the following gram-negative microorganisms when bacteriologic testing indicates appropriate susceptibility to the drug:
Escherichia coli,
Enterobacter aerogenes (formerly *Aerobacter aerogenes*),
Shigella species,
Mima species and *Herellea* species,
Haemophilus influenzae (respiratory infections),
Klebsiella species (respiratory and urinary infections).
MINOCIN is indicated for treatment of infections caused by the following gram-positive microorganisms when bacteriologic testing indicates appropriate susceptibility to the drug:
Streptococcus species:
Up to 44% of strains of *Streptococcus pyogenes* and 74% of *Streptococcus faecalis* have been found to be resistant to tetracycline drugs. Therefore, tetracyclines should not be used for streptococcal disease unless the organism has been demonstrated to be sensitive.
For upper respiratory infections due to Group A beta-hemolytic streptococci, penicillin is the usual drug of choice, including prophylaxis of rheumatic fever.
Streptococcus pneumoniae,
Staphylococcus aureus, skin and soft tissue infections.
Tetracyclines are not the drugs of choice in the treatment of any type of staphylococcal infection.
When penicillin is contraindicated, tetracyclines are alternative drugs in the treatment of infections due to:
Neisseria gonorrhoeae, and *Neisseria meningitidis,*
Treponema pallidum and *Treponema pertenue* (syphilis and yaws),
Listeria monocytogenes,
Clostridium species,
Bacillus anthracis,
Fusobacterium fusiforme (Vincent's infection),
Actinomyces species.
In acute intestinal amebiasis, the tetracyclines may be a useful adjunct to amebicides.
MINOCIN minocycline HCl is indicated in the treatment of trachoma, although the infectious agent is not always eliminated, as judged by immunofluorescence.
Inclusion conjunctivitis may be treated with oral tetracyclines or with a combination of oral and topical agents.

CONTRAINDICATIONS

This drug is contraindicated in persons who have shown hypersensitivity to any of the tetracyclines.

WARNINGS

In the presence of renal dysfunction, particularly in pregnancy, intravenous tetracycline therapy in daily doses exceeding 2 g has been associated with deaths through liver failure.
When the need for intensive treatment outweighs its potential dangers (mostly during pregnancy or in individuals with known or suspected renal or liver impairment), it is advisable to perform renal and liver function tests before and during therapy. Also, tetracycline serum concentrations should be followed.
If renal impairment exists, even usual oral or parenteral doses may lead to excessive systemic accumulation of the drug and possible liver toxicity. Under such conditions, lower than usual total doses are indicated, and if therapy is prolonged, serum level determinations of the drug may be advisable. This hazard is of particular importance in the parenteral administration of tetracyclines to pregnant or postpartum patients with pyelonephritis. When used under these circumstances, the blood level should not exceed 15 mcg/mL and liver function tests should be made at frequent intervals. Other potentially hepatotoxic drugs should not be prescribed concomitantly.
THE USE OF TETRACYCLINES DURING TOOTH DEVELOPMENT (LAST HALF OF PREGNANCY, INFANCY, AND CHILDHOOD TO THE AGE OF 8 YEARS) MAY CAUSE PERMANENT DISCOLORATION OF THE TEETH (YELLOW-GRAY-BROWN). This adverse reaction is more common during long-term use of the drugs but has been observed following repeated short-term courses. Enamel hypoplasia has also been reported. TETRACYCLINES, THEREFORE, SHOULD NOT BE USED IN THIS AGE GROUP UNLESS OTHER DRUGS ARE NOT LIKELY TO BE EFFECTIVE OR ARE CONTRAINDICATED.
Photosensitivity manifested by an exaggerated sunburn reaction has been observed in some individuals taking tetracyclines. Patients apt to be exposed to direct sunlight or ultraviolet light should be advised that this reaction can occur with tetracycline drugs, and treatment should be discontinued at the first evidence of skin erythema. Studies to date indicate that photosensitivity is rarely reported with MINOCIN minocycline HCl.
The anti-anabolic action of the tetracyclines may cause an increase in BUN. While this is not a problem in those with normal renal function, in patients with significantly impaired function, higher serum levels of tetracycline may lead to azotemia, hyperphosphatemia, and acidosis.
CNS side effects including light-headedness, dizziness or vertigo have been reported. Patients who experience these symptoms should be cautioned about driving vehicles or using hazardous machinery while on minocycline therapy. These symptoms may disappear during therapy and usually disappear rapidly when the drug is discontinued.
Usage in Pregnancy
(See above **WARNINGS** about use during tooth development.)
Results of animal studies indicate that tetracyclines cross the placenta, are found in fetal tissues and can have toxic effects on the developing fetus (often related to retardation of skeletal development). Evidence of embryotoxicity has also been noted in animals treated early in pregnancy.
The safety of MINOCIN for use during pregnancy has not been established.
Usage in Newborns, Infants, and Children
(See above **WARNINGS** about use during tooth development.)
All tetracyclines form a stable calcium complex in any bone-forming tissue. A decrease in the fibula growth rate has been observed in prematures given oral tetracycline in doses of 25 mg/kg every 6 hours. This reaction was shown to be reversible when the drug was discontinued.
Tetracyclines are present in the milk of lactating women who are taking a drug in this class.

PRECAUTIONS

General
Pseudotumor cerebri (benign intracranial hypertension) in adults has been associated with the use of tetracyclines. The usual clinical manifestations are headache and blurred vision. Bulging fontanels have been associated with the use of tetracyclines in infants. While both of these conditions and related symptoms usually resolve soon after discontinuation of the tetracycline, the possibility for permanent sequelae exists.
As with other antibiotic preparations, use of this drug may result in overgrowth of nonsusceptible organisms, including fungi. If superinfection occurs, the antibiotic should be discontinued and appropriate therapy should be instituted.
In venereal diseases when coexistent syphilis is suspected, darkfield examination should be done before treatment is started and the blood serology repeated monthly for at least 4 months.
In long-term therapy, periodic laboratory evaluation of organ systems, including hematopoietic, renal, and hepatic studies should be performed.
All infections due to Group A beta-hemolytic streptococci should be treated for at least ten days.
Drug Interactions
Because tetracyclines have been shown to depress plasma prothrombin activity, patients who are on anticoagulant therapy may require downward adjustment of their anticoagulant dosage.
Since bacteriostatic drugs may interfere with the bactericidal action of penicillin, it is advisable to avoid giving tetracycline in conjunction with penicillin.
Concurrent use of tetracyclines with oral contraceptives may render oral contraceptives less effective.

ADVERSE REACTIONS

Gastrointestinal: Anorexia, nausea, vomiting, diarrhea, glossitis, dysphagia, enterocolitis, pancreatitis, inflammatory lesions (with monilial overgrowth) in the anogenital region, and increases in liver enzymes. Rarely, hepatitis and liver failure have been reported.
These reactions have been caused by both the oral and parenteral administration of tetracyclines.
Skin: Maculopapular and erythematous rashes. Exfoliative dermatitis has been reported but is uncommon. Fixed drug eruptions, including balanitis, have been rarely reported. Erythema multiforme and rarely Stevens-Johnson syndrome have been reported. Photosensitivity is discussed above. (See **WARNINGS.**)
Pigmentation of the skin and mucous membranes has been reported.
Tooth discoloration has been reported, rarely, in adults.
Renal Toxicity: Rise in BUN has been reported and is apparently dose related. (See **WARNINGS.**) Reversible acute renal failure has been rarely reported.
Hypersensitivity Reactions: Urticaria, angioneurotic edema, polyarthralgia, anaphylaxis, anaphylactoid purpura, pericarditis, exacerbation of systemic lupus erythematosus, and rarely, pulmonary infiltrates with eosinophilia have been reported. A transient lupus-like syndrome has also been reported.
Blood: Hemolytic anemia, thrombocytopenia, neutropenia, and eosinophilia have been reported.
CNS: (See **WARNINGS.**) Pseudotumor cerebri (benign intracranial hypertension) in adults and bulging fontanels in infants. (See **PRECAUTIONS—General.**) Headache has also been reported.
Other: When given over prolonged periods, tetracyclines have been reported to produce brown-black microscopic discoloration of the thyroid glands. Very rare cases of abnormal thyroid function have been reported.
Decreased hearing has been rarely reported in patients on MINOCIN.

DOSAGE AND ADMINISTRATION

Note: Rapid administration is to be avoided. Parenteral therapy is indicated only when oral therapy is not adequate or tolerated. Oral therapy should be instituted as soon as possible. If intravenous therapy is given over prolonged periods of time, thrombophlebitis may result.

ADULTS: Usual adult dose: 200 mg followed by 100 mg every 12 hours and should not exceed 400 mg in 24 hours. The cryodesiccated powder should be reconstituted with 5 mL Sterile Water for Injection USP and immediately further diluted to 500 mL to 1,000 mL with Sodium Chloride Injection USP, Dextrose Injection USP, Dextrose and Sodium Chloride Injection USP, Ringer's Injection USP, or Lactated Ringer's Injection USP, but not other solutions containing calcium because a precipitate may form. When further diluted in 500 mL to 1,000 mL compatible solutions (except Lactated Ringers), the pH usually ranges from 2.5 to 4.0. The pH of MINOCIN IV 100 mg in Lactated Ringers 500 mL to 1,000 mL usually ranges from 4.5 to 6.0.

Final dilutions (500 mL to 1,000 mL) should be administered immediately but product and diluents are compatible at room temperature for 24 hours without a significant loss of potency. Any unused portions must be discarded after that period.

For children above eight years of age: Usual pediatric dose: 4 mg/kg followed by 2 mg/kg every 12 hours.

In patients with renal impairment: (See **WARNINGS.**)

Total dosage should be decreased by reduction of recommended individual doses and/or by extending time intervals between doses.

Parenteral drug products should be inspected visually for particulate matter and discoloration prior to administration, whenever solution and container permit.

HOW SUPPLIED

MINOCIN®minocycline HCl Intravenous is supplied as 100 mg vials of sterile cryodesiccated powder.

Product No. NDC 0205-5305-94

Store at Controlled Room Temperature 15–30℃ (59–86°F).

LEDERLE PARENTERALS, INC.

Carolina, Puerto Rico 00987

Shown in Product Identification Guide, page 320

MINOCIN®

Minocycline Hydrochloride
Pellet-Filled Capsules

℞

DESCRIPTION

MINOCIN minocycline hydrochloride, a semisynthetic derivative of tetracycline, is [4S-(4α,4aα,5aα,12aα)]-4,7-bis(dimethylamino)-1,4,4a,5,5a,6,11,12a-octahydro-3,10,12,12a-tetrahydroxy-1,11-dioxo-2-naphthacenecarboxamide monohydrochloride.

MINOCIN minocycline hydrochloride pellet-filled capsules for oral administration contain pellets of minocycline HCl equivalent to 50 mg or 100 mg of minocycline in microcrystalline cellulose.

The capsule shells contain the following inactive ingredients: Blue 1, Gelatin, Titanium Dioxide and Yellow 10. The 50 mg capsule shells also contain Black and Yellow Iron Oxides.

CLINICAL PHARMACOLOGY

MINOCIN minocycline hydrochloride pellet-filled capsules are rapidly absorbed from the gastrointestinal tract following oral administration. Following a single dose of two 100 mg pellet-filled capsules of MINOCIN minocycline HCl administered to 18 normal fasting adult volunteers, maximum serum concentrations were attained in 1 to 4 hours (average 2.1 hours) and ranged from 2.1 to 5.1 mcg/mL (average 3.5 mcg/mL). The serum half-life in the normal volunteers ranged from 11.1 to 22.1 hours (average 15.5 hours).

When MINOCIN minocycline hydrochloride pellet-filled capsules were given concomitantly with a meal which included dairy products, the extent of absorption of MINOCIN minocycline hydrochloride pellet-filled capsules was not noticeably influenced. The peak plasma concentrations were slightly decreased (11.2%) and delayed by one hour when administered with food, compared to dosing under fasting conditions.

In previous studies with other minocycline dosage forms, the minocycline serum half-life ranged from 11 to 16 hours in 7 patients with hepatic dysfunction, and from 18 to 69 hours in 5 patients with renal dysfunction. The urinary and fecal recovery of minocycline when administered to 12 normal volunteers is one-half to one-third that of other tetracyclines.

Microbiology

The tetracyclines are primarily bacteriostatic and are thought to exert their antimicrobial effect by the inhibition of protein synthesis. The tetracyclines, including minocycline, have similar antimicrobial spectra of activity against a wide range of gram-positive and gram-negative organisms. Cross-resistance of these organisms to tetracyclines is common.

While *in vitro* studies have demonstrated the susceptibility of most strains of the following microorganisms, clinical efficacy for infections other than those included in the **INDICATIONS AND USAGE** section has not been documented.

GRAM-NEGATIVE BACTERIA:

Bartonella bacilliformis
Brucella species
Calymmatobacterium granulomatis
Campylobacter fetus
Francisella tularensis
Haemophilus ducreyi
Haemophilus influenzae
Listeria monocytogenes
Neisseria gonorrhoeae
Vibrio cholerae
Yersinia pestis

Because many strains of the following groups of gram-negative microorganisms have been shown to be resistant to tetracyclines, culture and susceptibility tests are especially recommended:

Acinetobacter species
Bacteroides species
Enterobacter aerogenes
Escherichia coli
Klebsiella species
Shigella species

GRAM-POSITIVE BACTERIA:

Because many strains of the following groups of gram-positive microorganisms have been shown to be resistant to tetracyclines, culture and susceptibility testing are especially recommended. Up to 44 percent of *Streptococcus pyogenes* strains have been found to be resistant to tetracycline drugs. Therefore, tetracyclines should not be used for streptococcal disease unless the organism has been demonstrated to be susceptible.

Enterococcus group [*Enterococcus faecalis* (formerly *Streptococcus faecalis*) and *Enterococcus faecium* (formerly *Streptococcus faecium*)]
Streptococcus pneumoniae
Streptococcus pyogenes
Viridans group streptococci

OTHER MICROORGANISMS:

Actinomyces species
Bacillus anthracis
Balantidium coli
Borrelia recurrentis
Chlamydia psittaci
Chlamydia trachomatis
Clostridium species
Entamoeba species
Fusobacterium fusiforme
Mycoplasma pneumoniae
Propionibacterium acnes
Rickettsiae
Treponema pallidum
Treponema pertenue
Ureaplasma urealyticum

Susceptibility Tests

Diffusion Techniques

The use of antibiotic disk susceptibility test methods which measure zone diameter gives an accurate estimation of susceptibility of microorganisms to MINOCIN. One such standard procedure[1] has been recommended for use with disks for testing antimicrobials. Either the 30 mcg tetracycline-class disk or the 30 mcg minocycline disk should be used for the determination of the susceptibility of microorganisms to minocycline.

With this type of procedure a report of "susceptible" from the laboratory indicates that the infecting organism is likely to respond to therapy. A report of "intermediate susceptibility" suggests that the organism would be susceptible if a high dosage is used or if the infection is confined to tissues and fluids (e.g., urine) in which high antibiotic levels are attained. A report of "resistant" indicates that the infecting organism is not likely to respond to therapy. With either the tetracycline-class disk or the minocycline disk, zone sizes of 19 mm or greater indicate susceptibility, zone sizes of 14 mm or less indicate resistance, and zone sizes of 15 to 18 mm indicate intermediate susceptibility.

Standardized procedures require the use of laboratory control organisms. The 30 mcg tetracycline disk should give zone diameters between 19 and 28 mm for *Staphylococcus aureus* ATCC 25923 and between 18 and 25 mm for *Escherichia coli* ATCC 25922. The 30 mcg minocycline disk should give zone diameters between 25 and 30 mm for *S. aureus* ATCC 25923 and between 19 and 25 mm for *E. coli* ATCC 25922.

Dilution Techniques

When using the NCCLS agar dilution or broth dilution (including microdilution) method[2] or equivalent, a bacterial isolate may be considered susceptible if the MIC (minimal inhibitory concentration) of minocycline is 4 mcg/mL or less. Organisms are considered resistant if the MIC is 16 mcg/mL or greater. Organisms with an MIC value of less than 16 mcg/mL but greater than 4 mcg/mL are expected to be susceptible if a high dosage is used or if the infection is confined to tissues and fluids (e.g., urine) in which high antibiotic levels are attained.

As with standard diffusion methods, dilution procedures require the use of laboratory control organisms. Standard tetracycline or minocycline powder should give MIC values of 0.25 mcg/mL to 1.0 mcg/mL for *S. aureus* ATCC 25923, and 1.0 mcg/mL to 4.0 mcg/mL for *E. coli* ATCC 25922.

INDICATIONS AND USAGE

MINOCIN minocycline hydrochloride pellet-filled capsules are indicated in the treatment of the following infections due to susceptible strains of the designated microorganisms:

Rocky Mountain spotted fever, typhus fever and the typhus group, Q fever, rickettsialpox and tick fevers caused by *Rickettsiae*.

Respiratory tract infections caused by *Mycoplasma pneumoniae*.

Lymphogranuloma venereum caused by *Chlamydia trachomatis*.

Psittacosis (Ornithosis) due to *Chlamydia psittaci*.

Trachoma caused by *Chlamydia trachomatis*, although the infectious agent is not always eliminated, as judged by immunofluorescence.

Inclusion conjunctivitis caused by *Chlamydia trachomatis*.

Nongonococcal urethritis in adults caused by *Ureaplasma urealyticum* or *Chlamydia trachomatis*.

Relapsing fever due to *Borrelia recurrentis*.

Chancroid caused by *Haemophilus ducreyi*.

Plague due to *Yersinia pestis*.

Tularemia due to *Francisella tularensis*.

Cholera caused by *Vibrio cholerae*.

Campylobacter fetus infections caused by *Campylobacter fetus*.

Brucellosis due to *Brucella* species (in conjunction with streptomycin).

Bartonellosis due to *Bartonella bacilliformis*.

Granuloma inguinale caused by *Calymmatobacterium granulomatis*.

Minocycline is indicated for treatment of infections caused by the following gram-negative microorganisms, when bacteriologic testing indicates appropriate susceptibility to the drug:

Escherichia coli.
Enterobacter aerogenes.
Shigella species.
Acinetobacter species.

Respiratory tract infections caused by *Haemophilus influenzae*.

Respiratory tract and urinary tract infections caused by *Klebsiella* species.

MINOCIN minocycline hydrochloride pellet-filled capsules are indicated for the treatment of infections caused by the following gram-positive microorganisms when bacteriologic testing indicates appropriate susceptibility to the drug:

Upper respiratory tract infections caused by *Streptococcus pneumoniae*.

Skin and skin structure infections caused by *Staphylococcus aureus*. (Note: Minocycline is not the drug of choice in the treatment of any type of staphylococcal infection.)

Uncomplicated urethritis in men due to *Neisseria gonorrhoeae* and for the treatment of other gonococcal infections when penicillin is contraindicated.

When penicillin is contraindicated, minocycline is an alternative drug in the treatment of the following infections:

Infections in women caused by *Neisseria gonorrhoeae*.

Syphilis caused by *Treponema pallidum*.

Yaws caused by *Treponema pertenue*.

Listeriosis due to *Listeria monocytogenes*.

Anthrax due to *Bacillus anthracis*.

Vincent's infection caused by *Fusobacterium fusiforme*.

Actinomycosis caused by *Actinomyces israelii*.

Infections caused by *Clostridium* species.

In *acute intestinal amebiasis*, minocycline may be a useful adjunct to amebicides.

In severe *acne*, minocycline may be useful adjunctive therapy.

Oral minocycline is indicated in the treatment of asymptomatic carriers of *Neisseria meningitidis* to eliminate meningococci from the nasopharynx. In order to preserve the usefulness of minocycline in the treatment of asymptomatic meningococcal carrier, diagnostic laboratory procedures, including serotyping and susceptibility testing, should be performed to establish the carrier state and the correct treatment. It is recommended that the prophylactic use of minocycline be reserved for situations in which the risk of meningococcal meningitis is high.

Oral minocycline is not indicated for the treatment of meningococcal infection.

Although no controlled clinical efficacy studies have been conducted, limited clinical data show that oral minocycline hydrochloride has been used successfully in the treatment of infections caused by *Mycobacterium marinum*.

CONTRAINDICATIONS

This drug is contraindicated in persons who have shown hypersensitivity to any of the tetracyclines.

Continued on next page

Lederle—Cont.

WARNINGS

MINOCIN PELLET-FILLED CAPSULES, LIKE OTHER TETRACYCLINE-CLASS ANTIBIOTICS, CAN CAUSE FETAL HARM WHEN ADMINISTERED TO A PREGNANT WOMAN. IF ANY TETRACYCLINE IS USED DURING PREGNANCY OR IF THE PATIENT BECOMES PREGNANT WHILE TAKING THESE DRUGS, THE PATIENT SHOULD BE APPRISED OF THE POTENTIAL HAZARD TO THE FETUS. THE USE OF DRUGS OF THE TETRACYCLINE CLASS DURING TOOTH DEVELOPMENT (LAST HALF OF PREGNANCY, INFANCY, AND CHILDHOOD TO THE AGE OF 8 YEARS) MAY CAUSE PERMANENT DISCOLORATION OF THE TEETH (YELLOW-GRAY-BROWN).

This adverse reaction is more common during long-term use of the drug but has been observed following repeated short-term courses. Enamel hypoplasia has also been reported. TETRACYCLINE DRUGS, THEREFORE, SHOULD NOT BE USED DURING TOOTH DEVELOPMENT UNLESS OTHER DRUGS ARE NOT LIKELY TO BE EFFECTIVE OR ARE CONTRAINDICATED.

All tetracyclines form a stable calcium complex in any bone-forming tissue. A decrease in fibula growth rate has been observed in premature human infants given oral tetracycline in doses of 25 mg/kg every six hours. This reaction was shown to be reversible when the drug was discontinued.

Results of animal studies indicate that tetracyclines cross the placenta, are found in fetal tissues, and can have toxic effects on the developing fetus (often related to retardation of skeletal development). Evidence of embryotoxicity has been noted in animals treated early in pregnancy.

The anti-anabolic action of the tetracyclines may cause an increase in BUN. While this is not a problem in those with normal renal function, in patients with significantly impaired function, higher serum levels of tetracycline may lead to azotemia, hyperphosphatemia, and acidosis. If renal impairment exists, even usual oral or parenteral doses may lead to excessive systemic accumulations of the drug and possible liver toxicity. Under such conditions, lower than usual total doses are indicated, and if therapy is prolonged, serum level determinations of the drug may be advisable.

Photosensitivity manifested by an exaggerated sunburn reaction has been observed in some individuals taking tetracyclines. This has been reported rarely with minocycline.

Central nervous system side effects including lightheadedness, dizziness, or vertigo have been reported with minocycline therapy. Patients who experience these symptoms should be cautioned about driving vehicles or using hazardous machinery while on minocycline therapy. These symptoms may disappear during therapy and usually disappear rapidly when the drug is discontinued.

PRECAUTIONS

General

As with other antibiotic preparations, use of this drug may result in overgrowth of non-susceptible organisms, including fungi. If superinfection occurs, the antibiotic should be discontinued and appropriate therapy instituted.

Pseudotumor cerebri (benign intracranial hypertension) in adults has been associated with the use of tetracyclines. The usual clinical manifestations are headache and blurred vision. Bulging fontanels have been associated with the use of tetracyclines in infants. While both of these conditions and related symptoms usually resolve after discontinuation of the tetracycline, the possibility for permanent sequelae exists.

Incision and drainage or other surgical procedures should be performed in conjunction with antibiotic therapy when indicated.

Information for Patients

Photosensitivity manifested by an exaggerated sunburn reaction has been observed in some individuals taking tetracyclines. Patients apt to be exposed to direct sunlight or ultraviolet light should be advised that this reaction can occur with tetracycline drugs, and treatment should be discontinued at the first evidence of skin erythema. This reaction has been reported rarely with use of minocycline.

Patients who experience central nervous system symptoms (see **WARNINGS**) should be cautioned about driving vehicles or using hazardous machinery while on minocycline therapy.

Concurrent use of tetracycline may render oral contraceptives less effective (see **Drug Interactions**).

Laboratory Tests

In venereal disease when coexistent syphilis is suspected, a dark-field examination should be done before treatment is started and the blood serology repeated monthly for at least four months.

In long-term therapy, periodic laboratory evaluations of organ systems, including hematopoietic, renal, and hepatic studies, should be performed.

Drug Interactions

Because tetracyclines have been shown to depress plasma prothrombin activity, patients who are on anticoagulant therapy may require downward adjustment of their anticoagulant dosage.

Since bacteriostatic drugs may interfere with the bactericidal action of penicillin, it is advisable to avoid giving tetracycline-class drugs in conjunction with penicillin.

Absorption of tetracyclines is impaired by antacids containing aluminum, calcium or magnesium, and iron-containing preparations.

The concurrent use of tetracycline and methoxyflurane has been reported to result in fatal renal toxicity.

Concurrent use of tetracyclines with oral contraceptives may render oral contraceptives less effective.

Drug/Laboratory Test Interactions

False elevations of urinary catecholamine levels may occur due to interference with the fluorescence test.

Carcinogenesis, Mutagenesis, Impairment of Fertility

Dietary administration of minocycline in long term tumorigenicity studies in rats resulted in evidence of thyroid tumor production. Minocycline has also been found to produce thyroid hyperplasia in rats and dogs. In addition, there has been evidence of oncogenic activity in rats in studies with a related antibiotic, oxytetracycline (i.e., adrenal and pituitary tumors). Likewise, although mutagenicity studies of minocycline have not been conducted, positive results in *in vitro* mammalian cell assays (i.e., mouse lymphoma and Chinese hamster lung cells) have been reported for related antibiotics (tetracycline hydrochloride and oxytetracycline). Segment I (fertility and general reproduction) studies have provided evidence that minocycline impairs fertility in male rats.

Teratogenic Effects: Pregnancy: *Pregnancy Category D:* (See **WARNINGS**.) Nonteratogenic Effects: (See **WARNINGS**.)

Labor and Delivery

The effect of tetracyclines on labor and delivery is unknown.

Nursing Mothers

Tetracyclines are excreted in human milk. Because of the potential for serious adverse reactions in nursing infants from the tetracyclines, a decision should be made whether to discontinue nursing or discontinue the drug, taking into account the importance of the drug to the mother (see **WARNINGS**).

Pediatric Use: See **WARNINGS.**

ADVERSE REACTIONS

Due to oral minocycline's virtually complete absorption, side effects to the lower bowel, particularly diarrhea, have been infrequent. The following adverse reactions have been observed in patients receiving tetracyclines.

Gastrointestinal: Anorexia, nausea, vomiting, diarrhea, glossitis, dysphagia, enterocolitis, pancreatitis, inflammatory lesions (with monilial overgrowth) in the anogenital region, and increases in liver enzymes. Rarely, hepatitis and liver failure have been reported. Rare instances of esophagitis and esophageal ulcerations have been reported in patients taking the tetracycline-class antibiotics in capsule and tablet form. Most of these patients took the medication immediately before going to bed (see **DOSAGE AND ADMINISTRATION**).

Skin: Maculopapular and erythematous rashes. Exfoliative dermatitis has been reported but is uncommon. Fixed drug eruptions have been rarely reported. Lesions occurring on the glans penis have caused balanitis. Erythema multiforme and rarely Stevens-Johnson syndrome have been reported. Photosensitivity is discussed above (see **WARNINGS**). Pigmentation of the skin and mucous membranes has been reported.

Renal toxicity: Elevations in BUN have been reported and are apparently dose related (see **WARNINGS**). Reversible acute renal failure has been rarely reported.

Hypersensitivity reactions: Urticaria, angioneurotic edema, polyarthralgia, anaphylaxis, anaphylactoid purpura, pericarditis, exacerbation of systemic lupus erythematosus and rarely pulmonary infiltrates with eosinophilia have been reported. A transient lupus-like syndrome has also been reported.

Blood: Hemolytic anemia, thrombocytopenia, neutropenia, and eosinophilia have been reported.

Central nervous system: Bulging fontanels in infants and benign intracranial hypertension (Pseudotumor cerebri) in adults (see **PRECAUTIONS—General**) have been reported. Headache has also been reported.

Other: When given over prolonged periods, tetracyclines have been reported to produce brown-black microscopic discoloration of the thyroid glands. Very rare cases of abnormal thyroid function have been reported.

Decreased hearing has been rarely reported in patients on MINOCIN.

Tooth discoloration in children less than 8 years of age (see **WARNINGS**) and also, rarely, in adults has been reported.

OVERDOSAGE

Minocycline is not removed in significant quantities by hemodialysis or peritoneal dialysis. In one study, four patients received 200 mg oral doses 3 hours prior to hemodialysis, following flow rates of 100 to 200 mL/min there was no consistent difference between venous and arterial minocycline concentrations and no detectable minocycline was found in the dialysate. In another study, four patients were administered IP minocycline over 72 to 96 hours and achieved blood concentrations of 1.5 to 2 mcg/mL, over the following 12 hours drug free dialysate was used. No detectable minocycline was found to transfer from the blood to the dialysate.

In case of overdosage, discontinue medication, treat symptomatically, and institute supportive measures.

DOSAGE AND ADMINISTRATION

THE USUAL DOSAGE AND FREQUENCY OF ADMINISTRATION OF MINOCYCLINE DIFFERS FROM THAT OF THE OTHER TETRACYCLINES. EXCEEDING THE RECOMMENDED DOSAGE MAY RESULT IN AN INCREASED INCIDENCE OF SIDE EFFECTS.

MINOCIN minocycline hydrochloride pellet-filled capsules may be taken with or without food (see **CLINICAL PHARMACOLOGY**).

ADULTS: The usual dosage of MINOCIN minocycline hydrochloride pellet-filled capsules is 200 mg initially followed by 100 mg every 12 hours. Alternatively, if more frequent doses are preferred, two or four 50 mg pellet-filled capsules may be given initially followed by one 50 mg capsule four times daily.

For children above 8 years of age: The usual dosage of MINOCIN minocycline hydrochloride pellet-filled capsules is 4 mg/kg initially followed by 2 mg/kg every 12 hours.

Uncomplicated gonococcal infections other than urethritis and anorectal infections in men: 200 mg initially, followed by 100 mg every 12 hours for a minimum of four days, with post therapy cultures within 2 to 3 days.

In the treatment of uncomplicated gonococcal urethritis in men, 100 mg every 12 hours for five days is recommended.

For the treatment of syphilis, the usual dosage of MINOCIN minocycline hydrochloride pellet-filled capsules should be administered over a period of 10 to 15 days. Close follow-up, including laboratory tests, is recommended.

In the treatment of meningococcal carrier state, the recommended dosage is 100 mg every 12 hours for five days.

Mycobacterium marinum infections: Although optimal doses have not been established, 100 mg every 12 hours for 6 to 8 weeks have been used successfully in a limited number of cases.

Uncomplicated nongonococcal urethral infection in adults caused by *Chlamydia trachomatis* or *Ureaplasma urealyticum:* 100 mg orally, every 12 hours for at least seven days.

Ingestion of adequate amounts of fluids along with capsule and tablet forms of drugs in the tetracycline-class is recommended to reduce the risk of esophageal irritation and ulceration.

In patients with renal impairment (see **WARNINGS**), the total dosage should be decreased by either reducing the recommended individual doses and/or by extending the time intervals between doses.

HOW SUPPLIED

MINOCIN® minocycline hydrochloride pellet-filled capsules are supplied as capsules containing minocycline hydrochloride equivalent to 100 mg and 50 mg minocycline.

100 mg, two-piece, hard-shell capsule with an opaque light green cap and a transparent green body, printed in white ink with Lederle over M46 on one half and Lederle over 100 mg on the other half. Each capsule contains pellets of minocycline HCl equivalent to 100 mg of minocycline, supplied as follows:

NDC 0005-5344-18—Bottle of 50
NDC 0005-5344-27—Bottle of 250

50 mg, two-piece, hard-shell capsule with an opaque yellow cap and a transparent green body, printed in black ink with Lederle over M45 on one half and Lederle over 50 mg on the other half. Each capsule contains pellets of minocycline HCl equivalent to 50 mg of minocycline, supplied as follows:

NDC 0005-5343-23—Bottle of 100
NDC 0005-5343-27—Bottle of 250

Store at Controlled Room Temperature 15°–30°C (59°–86°F). Protect from light, moisture and excessive heat.

ANIMAL PHARMACOLOGY AND TOXICOLOGY

MINOCIN minocycline HCl has been observed to cause a dark discoloration of the thyroid in experimental animals (rats, minipigs, dogs, and monkeys). In the rat, chronic treatment with MINOCIN has resulted in goiter accompanied by elevated radioactive iodine uptake and evidence of thyroid tumor production. MINOCIN has also been found to produce thyroid hyperplasia in rats and dogs.

REFERENCES

1. National Committee for Clinical Laboratory Standards, Approved Standard: *Performance Standards for Antimicrobial Disk Susceptibility Tests,* 3rd Edition, Vol. 4(16):M2-A3, Villanova, PA, December 1984.
2. National Committee for Clinical Laboratory Standards, Approved Standard: *Methods for Dilution Antimicrobial*

Susceptibility Tests for Bacteria that Grow Aerobically, 2nd Edition, Vol. 5(22):M7-A, Villanova, PA, December 1985.

LEDERLE LABORATORIES DIVISION
American Cyanamid Company, Pearl River, NY 10965

Shown in Product Identification Guide, page 320

MINOCIN® ℞
[*mī-nō-sin*]
Minocycline Hydrochloride
Oral Suspension

DESCRIPTION

MINOCIN minocycline hydrochloride, a semisynthetic derivative of tetracycline, is named [4*S*-(4α, 4aα, 5aα, 12aα)]-4,7-bis (dimethylamino)-1,4,4a,5,5a,6,11,12a-octahydro-3,10,12,12a-tetrahydroxy-1,11-dioxo-2-naphthacenecarboxamide monohydrochloride.

Its structural formula is:

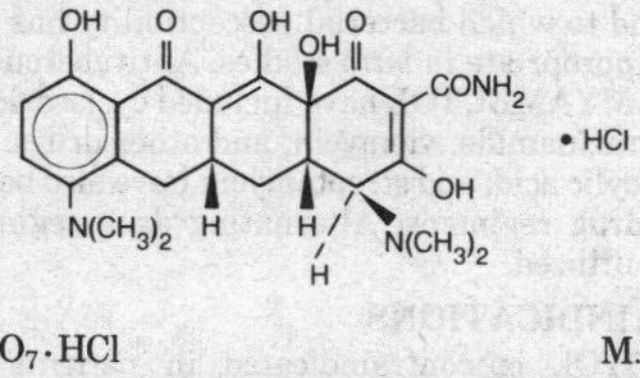

$C_{23}H_{27}N_3O_7 \cdot HCl$ M.W. 493.94

MINOCIN Oral Suspension contains minocycline HCl equivalent to 50 mg of minocycline per 5 mL (10 mg/mL) and the following inactive ingredients: Alcohol, Butylparaben, Calcium Hydroxide, Cellulose, Decaglyceryl Tetraoleate, Edetate Calcium Disodium, Glycol, Guar Gum, Polysorbate 80, Propylparaben, Propylene Glycol, Sodium Saccharin, Sodium Sulfite (see WARNINGS) and Sorbitol.

ACTIONS

Microbiology

The tetracyclines are primarily bacteriostatic and are thought to exert their antimicrobial effect by the inhibition of protein synthesis. Minocycline HCl is a tetracycline with antibacterial activity comparable to other tetracyclines with activity against a wide range of gram-negative and gram-positive organisms.

Tube dilution testing: Microorganisms may be considered susceptible (likely to respond to minocycline therapy) if the minimum inhibitory concentration (MIC) is not more than 4 mcg/mL. Microorganisms may be considered intermediate (harboring partial resistance) if the MIC is 4 to 12.5 mcg/mL and resistant (not likely to respond to minocycline therapy) if the MIC is greater than 12.5 mcg/mL.

Susceptibility plate testing: If the Kirby-Bauer method of susceptibility testing (using a 30 mcg tetracycline disc) gives a zone of 18 mm or greater, the bacterial strain is considered to be susceptible to any tetracycline. Minocycline shows moderate *in vitro* activity against certain strains of staphylococci which have been found resistant to other tetracyclines. For such strains minocycline susceptibility powder may be used for additional susceptibility testing.

Human Pharmacology

Following a single dose of two 100 mg minocycline HCl capsules administered to ten normal adult volunteers, serum levels ranged from 0.74 to 4.45 mcg/mL in one hour (average 2.24), after 12 hours, they ranged from 0.34 to 2.36 mcg/mL (average 1.25). The serum half-life following a single 200 mg dose in 12 essentially normal volunteers ranged from 11 to 17 hours. In seven patients with hepatic dysfunction it ranged from 11 to 16 hours, and in 5 patients with renal dysfunction from 18 to 69 hours. The urinary and fecal recovery of minocycline when administered to 12 normal volunteers is one half to one third that of other tetracyclines.

INDICATIONS

MINOCIN is indicated in infections caused by the following microorganisms:

Rickettsiae: (Rocky Mountain spotted fever, typhus fever and the typhus group, Q fever, rickettsialpox, tick fevers).

Mycoplasma pneumoniae (PPLO, Eaton agent).

Agents of psittacosis and ornithosis.

Agents of lymphogranuloma venereum and granuloma inguinale.

The spirochetal agent of relapsing fever (*Borrelia recurrentis*).

The following gram-negative microorganisms:

Haemophilus ducreyi (chancroid),
Yersinia pestis and *Francisella tularensis* (formerly *Pasteurella pestis* and *Pasteurella tularensis*),
Bartonella bacilliformis,
Bacteroides species,
Vibrio comma and *Vibrio fetus,*
Brucella species (in conjunction with streptomycin).

Because many strains of the following groups of microorganisms have been shown to be resistant to tetracyclines, culture and susceptibility testing are recommended.

MINOCIN is indicated for treatment of infections caused by the following gram-negative microorganisms when bacteriologic testing indicates appropriate susceptibility to the drug:

Escherichia coli,
Enterobacter aerogenes (fomerly *Aerobacter aerogenes*),
Shigella species,
Acinetobacter calcoaceticus (formerly Herellea, Mima),
Haemophilus influenzae (respiratory infections),
Klebsiella species (respiratory and urinary infections).

MINOCIN is indicated for treatment of infections caused by the following gram-positive microorganisms when bacteriologic testing indicates appropriate susceptibility to the drug:

Streptococcus species:

Up to 44% of strains of *Streptococcus pyogenes* and 74% of *Streptococcus faecalis* have been found to be resistant to tetracycline drugs. Therefore, tetracyclines should not be used for streptococcal disease unless the organism has been demonstrated to be sensitive.

For upper respiratory infections due to Group A beta-hemolytic streptococci, penicillin is the usual drug of choice, including prophylaxis of rheumatic fever.

Streptococcus pneumoniae (formerly Diplococcus pneumoniae),
Staphylococcus aureus, skin and soft tissue infections.

Tetracyclines are not the drugs of choice in the treatment of any type of staphylococcal infection.

MINOCIN is indicated for the treatment of uncomplicated gonococcal urethritis in men due to *Neisseria gonorrhoeae.*

When penicillin is contraindicated, tetracyclines are alternative drugs in the treatment of infections due to:

Neisseria gonorrhoeae (in women),
Treponema pallidum and *Treponema pertenue* (syphilis and yaws),
Listeria monocytogenes,
Clostridium species,
Bacillus anthracis,
Fusobacterium fusiforme (Vincent's infection),
Actinomyces species.

In acute intestinal amebiasis, the tetracyclines may be a useful adjunct to amebicides.

In severe acne, the tetracyclines may be useful adjunctive therapy.

MINOCIN minocycline HCl is indicated in the treatment of trachoma, although the infectious agent is not always eliminated, as judged by immunofluorescence.

MINOCIN is indicated for the treatment of uncomplicated urethral, endocervical or rectal infections in adults caused by *Chlamydia trachomatis* or *Ureaplasma urealyticum.*[1]

Inclusion conjunctivitis may be treated with oral tetracyclines or with a combination of oral and topical agents.

MINOCIN is indicated in the treatment of asymptomatic carriers of *Neisseria meningitidis* to eliminate meningococci from the nasopharynx.

In order to preserve the usefulness of MINOCIN in the treatment of asymptomatic meningococcal carriers, diagnostic laboratory procedures, including serotyping and susceptibility testing, should be performed to establish the carrier state and the correct treatment. It is recommended that the drug be reserved for situations in which the risk of meningococcal meningitis is high.

MINOCIN by oral administration is not indicated for the treatment of meningococcal infection.

Although no controlled clinical efficacy studies have been conducted, limited clinical data show that oral MINOCIN has been used successfully in the treatment of infections caused by Mycobacterium marinum.

CONTRAINDICATIONS

This drug is contraindicated in persons who have shown hypersensitivity to any of the tetracyclines.

WARNINGS

THE USE OF DRUGS OF THE TETRACYCLINE CLASS DURING TOOTH DEVELOPMENT (LAST HALF OF PREGNANCY, INFANCY, AND CHILDHOOD TO THE AGE OF 8 YEARS) MAY CAUSE PERMANENT DISCOLORATION OF THE TEETH (YELLOW-GRAY-BROWN). This adverse reaction is more common during long-term use of the drugs but has been observed following repeated short-term courses. Enamel hypoplasia has also been reported. TETRACYCLINE DRUGS, THEREFORE, SHOULD NOT BE USED IN THIS AGE GROUP UNLESS OTHER DRUGS ARE NOT LIKELY TO BE EFFECTIVE OR ARE CONTRAINDICATED.

If renal impairment exists, even usual oral or parenteral doses may lead to excessive systemic accumulations of the drug and possible liver toxicity. Under such conditions, lower than usual total doses are indicated, and if therapy is prolonged, serum level determinations of the drug may be advisable.

Photosensitivity manifested by an exaggerated sunburn reaction has been observed in some individuals taking tetracyclines. Patients apt to be exposed to direct sunlight or ultraviolet light should be advised that this reaction can occur with tetracycline drugs, and treatment should be discontinued at the first evidence of skin erythema. Studies to date indicate that photosensitivity is rarely reported with MINOCIN minocycline HCl.

The anti-anabolic action of the tetracyclines may cause an increase in BUN. While this is not a problem in those with normal renal function, in patients with significantly impaired function, higher serum levels of tetracycline may lead to azotemia, hyperphosphatemia, and acidosis.

CNS side effects including light-headedness, dizziness, or vertigo have been reported. Patients who experience these symptoms should be cautioned about driving vehicles or using hazardous machinery while on minocycline therapy. These symptoms may disappear during therapy and usually disappear rapidly when the drug is discontinued.

MINOCIN Oral Suspension contains sodium sulfite, a sulfite that may cause allergic-type reactions including anaphylactic symptoms and life-threatening or less severe asthmatic episodes in certain susceptible people. The overall prevalence of sulfite sensitivity in the general population is unknown and probably low. Sulfite sensitivity is seen more frequently in asthmatic than in nonasthmatic people.

Usage in Pregnancy (See above **WARNINGS** about use during tooth development.) Results of animal studies indicate that tetracyclines cross the placenta, are found in fetal tissues and can have toxic effects on the developing fetus (often related to retardation of skeletal development). Evidence of embryotoxicity has also been noted in animals treated early in pregnancy.

The safety of MINOCIN for use during pregnancy has not been established.

Usage in Newborns, Infants, and Children (See above **WARNINGS** about use during tooth development.)

All tetracyclines form a stable calcium complex in any bone forming tissue. A decrease in the fibula growth rate has been observed in prematures given oral tetracycline in doses of 25 mg/kg every six hours. This reaction was shown to be reversible when the drug was discontinued.

Tetracyclines are present in the milk of lactating women who are taking a drug in this class.

PRECAUTIONS

General

Pseudotumor cerebri (benign intracranial hypertension) in adults has been associated with the use of tetracyclines. The usual clinical manifestations are headache and blurred vision. Bulging fontanels have been associated with the use of tetracyclines in infants. While both of these conditions and related symptoms usually resolve soon after discontinuation of the tetracycline, the possibility for permanent sequelae exists.

As with other antibiotic preparations, use of this drug may result in overgrowth of non-susceptible organisms, including fungi. If superinfection occurs, the antibiotic should be discontinued and appropriate therapy should be instituted.

In venereal diseases when coexistent syphilis is suspected, darkfield examination should be done before treatment is started and the blood serology repeated monthly for at least 4 months.

In long-term therapy, periodic laboratory evaluation of organ systems, including hematopoietic, renal and hepatic studies should be performed.

All infections due to Group A beta-hemolytic streptococci should be treated for at least ten days.

Drug Interactions

Because tetracyclines have been shown to depress plasma prothrombin activity, patients who are on anticoagulant therapy may require downward adjustment of their anticoagulant dosage.

Since bacteriostatic drugs may interfere with the bactericidal action of penicillin, it is advisable to avoid giving tetracycline in conjunction with penicillin.

Concurrent use of tetracyclines with oral contraceptives may render oral contraceptives less effective.

ADVERSE REACTIONS

Gastrointestinal: Anorexia, nausea, vomiting, diarrhea, glossitis, dysphagia, enterocolitis, pancreatitis, inflammatory lesions (with monilial overgrowth) in the anogenital region and increases in liver enzymes. Rarely, hepatitis and liver failure have been reported.

These reactions have been caused by both the oral and parenteral administration of tetracyclines.

Skin: Maculopapular and erythematous rashes. Exfoliative dermatitis has been reported but is uncommon. Fixed drug eruptions, including balanitis, have been rarely reported. Erythema multiforme and rarely Stevens-Johnson syn-

Continued on next page

Lederle—Cont.

drome have been reported. Photosensitivity is discussed above. (See **WARNINGS.**)
Pigmentation of the skin and mucous membranes has been reported.
Tooth discoloration has been reported rarely in adults.
Renal toxicity: Rise in BUN has been reported and is apparently dose related. (See **WARNINGS.**) Reversible acute renal failure has been rarely reported.
Hypersensitivity reactions: Urticaria, angioneurotic edema, polyarthralgia, anaphylaxis, anaphylactoid purpura, pericarditis, exacerbation of systemic lupus erythematosus and rarely pulmonary infiltrates with eosinophilia have been reported. A transient lupus-like syndrome has also been reported.
Blood: Hemolytic anemia, thrombocytopenia, neutropenia and eosinophilia have been reported.
CNS: (See **WARNINGS.**) Pseudotumor cerebri (benign intracranial hypertension) in adults and bulging fontanels in infants. (See **PRECAUTIONS—General.**) Headache has also been reported.
Other: When given over prolonged periods, tetracyclines have been reported to produce brown-black microscopic discoloration of the thyroid glands. Very rare cases of abnormal thyroid function have been reported.
Decreased hearing has been rarely reported in patients on MINOCIN.

DOSAGE AND ADMINISTRATION

Therapy should be continued for at least 24 to 48 hours after symptoms and fever have subsided.
Concomitant therapy: Antacids containing aluminum, calcium, or magnesium impair absorption and should not be given to patients taking oral tetracycline.
Studies to date have indicated that the absorption of MINOCIN is not notably influenced by foods and dairy products.
In patients with renal impairment: (See **WARNINGS.**) Total dosage should be decreased by reduction of recommended individual doses and/or extending time intervals between doses.
In the treatment of streptococcal infections, a therapeutic dose of tetracycline should be administered for at least ten days.
ADULTS: The usual dosage of MINOCIN is 200 mg initially followed by 100 mg every 12 hours.
For children above eight years of age: The usual dosage of MINOCIN minocycline HCl is 4 mg/kg initially followed by 2 mg/kg every 12 hours.
For treatment of syphilis, the usual dosage of MINOCIN should be administered over a period of 10 to 15 days. Close follow up, including laboratory tests, is recommended.
Gonorrhea patients sensitive to penicillin may be treated with MINOCIN, administered as 200 mg initially followed by 100 mg every twelve hours for a minimum of four days, with post-therapy cultures within 2 to 3 days.
In the treatment of meningococcal carrier state, recommended dosage is 100 mg every 12 hours for five days.
Mycobacterium marinum infections: Although optimal doses have not been established, 100 mg twice a day for 6 to 8 weeks have been used successfully in a limited number of cases.
Uncomplicated urethral, endocervical, or rectal infection in adults caused by *Chlamydia trachomatis* or *Ureaplasma urealyticum:* 100 mg, by mouth, 2 times a day for at least seven days.[1]
In the treatment of uncomplicated gonococcal urethritis in men, 100 mg twice a day orally for five days is recommended.

HOW SUPPLIED

MINOCIN® minocycline hydrochloride Oral Suspension contains minocycline hydrochloride equivalent to 50 mg minocycline per teaspoonful (5 mL). Preserved with propylparaben 0.10% and butylparaben 0.06% with Alcohol USP 5% v/v, Custard-flavored.
NDC 0005-5313-56 Bottle 2 fl. oz. (60 mL)
Store at Controlled Room Temperature 15–30°C (59–86°F).
DO NOT FREEZE.

ANIMAL PHARMACOLOGY AND TOXICOLOGY

MINOCIN has been found to produce high blood concentrations following oral dosage to various animal species and to be extensively distributed to all tissues examined in ^{14}C-labeled drug studies in dogs. MINOCIN has been found experimentally to produce discoloration of the thyroid glands. This finding has been observed in rats and dogs. Changes in thyroid function have also been found in these animal species. However, no change in thyroid function has been observed in humans.

Reference: 1. CDC Sexually Transmitted Diseases Treatment Guidelines 1982.

Shown in Product Identification Guide, page 320

MYAMBUTOL® ℞

[*mī-am-bū-tōl*]
Ethambutol Hydrochloride
Tablets
100 mg and 400 mg

DESCRIPTION

MYAMBUTOL ethambutol hydrochloride is an oral chemotherapeutic agent which is specifically effective against actively growing microorganisms of the genus *Mycobacterium*, including *M. tuberculosis.*
MYAMBUTOL 100 mg and 400 mg tablets contain the following inactive ingredients: Gelatin, Hydroxypropyl Methylcellulose, Magnesium Stearate, Sodium Lauryl Sulfate, Sorbitol, Stearic Acid, Sucrose, Titanium Dioxide, and other ingredients.

ACTION

MYAMBUTOL, following a single oral dose of 25 mg/kg of body weight, attains a peak of 2 to 5 micrograms/mL in serum 2 to 4 hours after administration. When the drug is administered daily for longer periods of time at this dose, serum levels are similar. The serum level of MYAMBUTOL falls to undetectable levels by 24 hours after the last dose except in some patients with abnormal renal function. The intracellular concentrations of erythrocytes reach peak values approximately twice those of plasma and maintain this ratio throughout the 24 hours.
During the 24-hour period following oral administration of MYAMBUTOL, approximately 50% of the initial dose is excreted unchanged in the urine, while an additional 8% to 15% appears in the form of metabolites. The main path of metabolism appears to be an initial oxidation of the alcohol to an aldehydic intermediate, followed by conversion to a dicarboxylic acid. From 20% to 22% of the initial dose is excreted in the feces as unchanged drug. No drug accumulation has been observed with consecutive single daily doses of 25 mg/kg in patients with normal kidney function, although marked accumulation has been demonstrated in patients with renal insufficiency.
MYAMBUTOL diffuses into actively growing *mycobacterium* cells such as tubercle bacilli. MYAMBUTOL appears to inhibit the synthesis of one or more metabolites, thus causing impairment of cell metabolism, arrest of multiplication, and cell death. No cross resistance with other available antimycobacterial agents has been demonstrated.
MYAMBUTOL has been shown to be effective against strains of *Mycobacterium tuberculosis* but does not seem to be active against fungi, viruses, or other bacteria. *Mycobacterium tuberculosis* strains previously unexposed to MYAMBUTOL have been uniformly sensitive to concentrations of 8 or less micrograms/mL, depending on the nature of the culture media. When MYAMBUTOL has been used alone for treatment of tuberculosis, tubercle bacilli from these patients have developed resistance to MYAMBUTOL ethambutol hydrochloride by *in vitro* susceptibility tests; the development of resistance has been unpredictable and appears to occur in a step-like manner. No cross resistance between MYAMBUTOL and other antituberculous drugs has been reported. MYAMBUTOL has reduced the incidence of the emergence of mycobacterial resistance to isoniazid when both drugs have been used concurrently.
An agar diffusion microbiologic assay, based upon inhibition of *Mycobacterium smegmatis* (ATCC 607) may be used to determine concentrations of MYAMBUTOL in serum and urine. This technique has not been published, but further information can be obtained upon inquiry to Lederle Laboratories.

ANIMAL PHARMACOLOGY

Toxicological studies in dogs on high prolonged doses produced evidence of myocardial damage and failure, and depigmentation of the tapetum lucidum of the eyes, the significance of which is not known. Degenerative changes in the central nervous system, apparently not dose-related, have also been noted in dogs receiving ethambutol hydrochloride over a prolonged period.
In the rhesus monkey, neurological signs appeared after treatment with high doses given daily over a period of several months. These were correlated with specific serum levels of ethambutol hydrochloride and with definite neuroanatomical changes in the central nervous system. Focal interstitial carditis was also noted in monkeys which received ethambutol hydrochloride in high doses for a prolonged period.
When pregnant mice or rabbits were treated with high doses of ethambutol hydrochloride, fetal mortality was slightly but not significantly ($P > 0.05$) increased. Female rats treated with ethambutol hydrochloride displayed slight but insignificant ($P > 0.05$) decreases in fertility and litter size.
In fetuses born of mice treated with high doses of MYAMBUTOL during pregnancy, a low incidence of cleft palate, exencephaly and abnormality of the vertebral column were observed. Minor abnormalities of the cervical vertebra were seen in the newborn of rats treated with high doses of ethambutol hydrochloride during pregnancy. Rabbits receiving high doses of MYAMBUTOL during pregnancy gave birth to two fetuses with monophthalmia, one with a shortened right forearm accompanied by bilateral wrist-joint contracture and one with hare lip and cleft palate.

INDICATIONS

MYAMBUTOL is indicated for the treatment of pulmonary tuberculosis. It should not be used as the sole antituberculous drug, but should be used in conjunction with at least one other antituberculous drug. Selection of the companion drug should be based on clinical experience, considerations of comparative safety and appropriate *in vitro* susceptibility studies. In patients who have not received previous antituberculous therapy, ie, initial treatment, the most frequently used regimens have been the following:
MYAMBUTOL plus isoniazid
MYAMBUTOL plus isoniazid plus streptomycin.
In patients who have received previous antituberculous therapy, mycobacterial resistance to other drugs used in initial therapy is frequent. Consequently, in such retreatment patients, MYAMBUTOL should be combined with at least one of the second line drugs not previously administered to the patient and to which bacterial susceptibility has been indicated by appropriate *in vitro* studies. Antituberculous drugs used with MYAMBUTOL have included cycloserine, ethionamide, pyrazinamide, viomycin, and other drugs. Isoniazid, aminosalicylic acid, and streptomycin have also been used in multiple drug regimens. Alternating drug regimens have also been utilized.

CONTRAINDICATIONS

MYAMBUTOL is contraindicated in patients who are known to be hypersensitive to this drug. It is also contraindicated in patients with known optic neuritis unless clinical judgment determines that it may be used.

PRECAUTIONS

The effects of combinations of MYAMBUTOL ethambutol hydrochloride with other antituberculous drugs on the fetus is not known. While administration of this drug to pregnant human patients has produced no detectable effect upon the fetus, the possible teratogenic potential in women capable of bearing children should be weighed carefully against the benefits of therapy. There are published reports of five women who received the drug during pregnancy without apparent adverse effect upon the fetus.
MYAMBUTOL is not recommended for use in children under 13 years of age since safe conditions for use have not been established.
Patients with decreased renal function need the dosage reduced as determined by serum levels of MYAMBUTOL, since the main path of excretion of this drug is by the kidneys.
Because this drug may have adverse effects on vision, physical examination should include ophthalmoscopy, finger perimetry, and testing of color discrimination. In patients with visual defects such as cataracts, recurrent inflammatory conditions of the eye, optic neuritis, and diabetic retinopathy, the evaluation of changes in visual acuity is more difficult, and care should be taken to be sure the variations in vision are not due to the underlying disease conditions. In such patients, consideration should be given to relationship between benefits expected and possible visual deterioration since evaluation of visual changes is difficult. (For recommended procedures, see next paragraphs under **ADVERSE REACTIONS.**)
As with any potent drug, periodic assessment of organ system functions, including renal, hepatic, and hematopoietic, should be made during long-term therapy.

ADVERSE REACTIONS

MYAMBUTOL may produce decreases in visual acuity which appear to be due to optic neuritis and to be related to dose and duration of treatment. The effects are generally reversible when administration of the drug is discontinued promptly. In rare cases recovery may be delayed for up to 1 year or more and the effect may possibly be irreversible in these cases.
Patients should be advised to report promptly to their physician any change of visual acuity.
The change in visual acuity may be unilateral or bilateral and hence *each eye must be tested separately and both eyes tested together.* Testing of visual acuity should be performed before beginning MYAMBUTOL therapy and periodically during drug administration, except that it should be done monthly when a patient is on a dosage of more than 15 mg per kilogram per day. Snellen eye charts are recommended for testing of visual acuity. Studies have shown that there are definite fluctuations of one or two lines of the Snellen chart in the visual acuity of many tuberculous patients *not* receiving MYAMBUTOL.
The following table may be useful in interpreting possible changes in visual acuity attributable to MYAMBUTOL.
[See table at top of next page.]
In general, changes in visual acuity less than those indicated under "Significant Number of Lines" and "Decrease-Num-

Initial Snellen Reading	Reading Indicating Significant Decrease	Significant Number of Lines	Decrease Number of Points
20/13	20/25	3	12
20/15	20/25	2	10
20/20	20/30	2	10
20/25	20/40	2	15
20/30	20/50	2	20
20/40	20/70	2	30
20/50	20/70	1	20

ber of Points," may be due to chance variation, limitations of the testing method or physiologic variability. Conversely, changes in visual acuity equaling or exceeding those under "Significant Number of Lines" and "Decrease-Number of Points" indicate need for retesting and careful evaluation of the patient's visual status. If careful evaluation confirms the magnitude of visual change and fails to reveal another cause, MYAMBUTOL should be discontinued and the patient reevaluated at frequent intervals. Progressive decreases in visual acuity during therapy must be considered to be due to MYAMBUTOL.

If corrective glasses are used prior to treatment, these must be worn during visual acuity testing. During 1 to 2 years of therapy, a refractive error may develop which must be corrected in order to obtain accurate test results. Testing the visual acuity through a pinhole eliminates refractive error. Patients developing visual abnormality during MYAMBUTOL treatment may show subjective visual symptoms before, or simultaneously with, the demonstration of decreases in visual acuity, and all patients receiving MYAMBUTOL should be questioned periodically about blurred vision and other subjective eye symptoms.

Recovery of visual acuity generally occurs over a period of weeks to months after the drug has been discontinued. Patients have then received MYAMBUTOL ethambutol hydrochloride again without recurrence of loss of visual acuity.

Other adverse reactions reported include: anaphylactoid reactions, dermatitis pruritus and joint pain; anorexia, nausea, vomiting, gastrointestinal upset, abdominal pain; fever, malaise, headache, and dizziness; mental confusion, disorientation and possible hallucinations. Numbness and tingling of the extremities due to peripheral neuritis have been reported infrequently.

Elevated serum uric acid levels occur and precipitation of acute gout has been reported. Transient impairment of liver function as indicated by abnormal liver function tests is not an unusual finding. Since MYAMBUTOL is recommended for therapy in conjunction with one or more other antituberculous drugs, these changes may be related to the concurrent therapy.

DOSAGE AND ADMINISTRATION

MYAMBUTOL should not be used alone, in initial treatment or in retreatment. MYAMBUTOL should be administered on a once every 24-hour basis only. Absorption is not significantly altered by administration with food. Therapy, in general, should be continued until bacteriological conversion has become permanent and maximal clinical improvement has occurred.

MYAMBUTOL is not recommended for use in children under thirteen years of age since safe conditions for use have not been established.

Initial Treatment: In patients who have not received previous antituberculous therapy, administer MYAMBUTOL 15 mg per kilogram (7 mg per pound) of body weight, as a single oral dose once every 24 hours. In the more recent studies, isoniazid has been administered concurrently in a single, daily, oral dose.

Retreatment: In patients who have received previous antituberculous therapy, administer MYAMBUTOL 25 mg per kilogram (11 mg per pound) of body weight, as a single oral dose once every 24 hours. Concurrently administer at least one other antituberculous drug to which the organisms have been demonstrated to be susceptible by appropriate *in vitro* tests. Suitable drugs usually consist of those not previously used in the treatment of the patient. After 60 days of MYAMBUTOL administration, decrease the dose to 15 mg per kilogram (7 mg per pound) of body weight, and administer as a single oral dose once every 24 hours.

During the period when a patient is on a daily dose of 25 mg/kg, monthly eye examinations are advised.

See Table for easy selection of proper weight-dose tablet(s).

Weight-Dose Table

Weight Range Pounds	Kilograms	Daily Dose In mg
15 mg/kg (7 mg/lb) Schedule		
Under 85 lbs	Under 37 kg	500
85–94.5	37–43	600
95–109.5	43–50	700
110–124.5	50–57	800
125–139.5	57–64	900
140–154.5	64–71	1000
155–169.5	71–79	1100
170–184.5	79–84	1200
185–199.5	84–90	1300
200–214.5	90–97	1400
215 and Over	Over 97	1500
25 mg/kg (11 mg/lb) Schedule		
Under 85 lbs	Under 38 kg	900
85–92.5	38–42	1000
93–101.5	42–45.5	1100
102–109.5	45.5–50	1200
110–118.5	50–54	1300
119–128.5	54–58	1400
129–136.5	58–62	1500
137–146.5	62–67	1600
147–155.5	67–71	1700
156–164.5	71–75	1800
165–173.5	75–79	1900
174–182.5	79–83	2000
183–191.5	83–87	2100
192–199.5	87–91	2200
200–209.5	91–95	2300
210–218.5	95–99	2400
219 and Over	Over 99	2500

HOW SUPPLIED

MYAMBUTOL® ethambutol hydrochloride Tablets

100 mg—round, convex, white, film coated tablets engraved M6 on one side and LL on the other, are supplied as follows:

NDC 0005-5015-23 - Bottle of 100

400 mg—round, convex, white, scored, film coated tablets engraved with LL on one side and M to the left and 7 to the right of the score on the other side, are supplied as follows:

NDC 0005-5084-62 - Unit-of-Issue 100s with CRC

NDC 0005-5084-34 - Bottle of 1000

NDC 0005-5084-60 - Unit Dose 10 (2 × 5) Strips

Store at Controlled Room Temperature 15–30°C (59–86°F).

LEDERLE LABORATORIES DIVISION
American Cyanamid Company
Pearl River, NY 10965

Shown in Product Identification Guide, page 320

NEPTAZANE® ℞

[nĕp-ta-zāne]
methazolamide
Tablets, USP

(For full prescribing information, please refer to the Product Information section for Storz Ophthalmics in the 1997 PDR for Ophthalmology.)

ORIMUNE® ℞

[or-ĭ-mune]
POLIOVIRUS VACCINE
LIVE ORAL TRIVALENT
0.5 mL Dose Contains Sorbitol
SABIN STRAINS TYPES 1, 2 and 3
FOR ORAL ADMINISTRATION—
NOT FOR INJECTION

DESCRIPTION

Manufacture and Composition: ORIMUNE is a mixture of three types of attenuated polioviruses that have been propagated in monkey kidney cell culture. The cells are grown in the presence of Eagle's basal medium consisting of Earle's balanced salt solution containing amino acids, antibiotics, and calf serum. After cell growth, the medium is removed and replaced with fresh medium containing the inoculating virus but no calf serum. The final vaccine is diluted with a modified cell-culture maintenance medium containing sorbitol. Each dose (0.5 mL) contains less than 25 micrograms of each of the antibiotics, streptomycin and neomycin.

Potency of the vaccine is expressed in terms of the amount of virus (log_{10}) contained in the recommended dose as tissue culture infective doses ($TCID_{50}$). The human dose of vaccine containing all three virus types shall be constituted to have infectivity titers in the final container material of $10^{5.4}$ to $10^{6.4}$ for Type 1, $10^{4.5}$ to $10^{5.5}$ for Type 2, and $10^{5.2}$ to $10^{6.2}$ for Type 3, when the primary monkey kidney tube titration method is used.[1] If the more sensitive Hep-2 microtitration procedure is employed to determine the infectivity titers in each human dose, then equivalent vaccine is achieved with numerical infectivity titers of $10^{6.0}$ to $10^{7.0}$ for Type 1, $10^{5.1}$ to $10^{6.1}$ for Type 2, and $10^{5.8}$ to $10^{6.8}$ for Type 3.[2]

CLINICAL PHARMACOLOGY

Administration of attenuated, live oral poliovirus vaccine (OPV) simulates natural infection, inducing active mucosal and systemic immunity without producing symptoms of disease. For optimal mucosal immunity to occur, it is necessary for the viruses to multiply in the intestinal tract. A primary series of trivalent vaccine is designed to produce an antibody response to poliovirus Types 1, 2, and 3. This response is comparable to the immunity induced by the natural disease. The antibodies thus formed help protect the individual against clinical poliomyelitis infection by any of the three types of poliovirus. Multiple sequential doses of OPV are administered to ensure that immunity to all three types of poliovirus has been achieved.[3] When used in the prescribed manner for immunization, type-specific neutralizing antibodies will be induced in 95% or more of susceptibles.[4]

INDICATIONS AND USAGE

This vaccine is indicated for use in the prevention of poliomyelitis caused by poliovirus Types 1, 2, and 3.

Infants from 6 to 12 weeks of age, *all unimmunized children,* and *adolescents* up to age 18 are the usual candidates for routine prophylaxis.

The Immunization Practices Advisory Committee (ACIP) of the Public Health Service states that trivalent oral poliovirus vaccine (OPV) and inactivated poliovirus vaccine (IPV) are both effective in preventing poliomyelitis.

The choice of OPV as the preferred poliovirus vaccine for primary administration to children in the United States has been made by the ACIP, the Committee on Infectious Diseases of the American Academy of Pediatrics, and a special expert committee of the Institute of Medicine, National Academy of Science.[3–6] OPV is preferred because it induces intestinal immunity, is simple to administer, is well accepted by patients, results in immunization of some contacts of vaccinated persons, and has a record of having essentially eliminated disease associated with wild poliovirus in this country.[4] OPV is also recommended for control of epidemic poliomyelitis.[3,5]

IPV is specifically indicated for use in immunodeficient individuals, their household contacts, or in certain adults (see **CONTRAINDICATIONS** and **INDICATIONS AND USAGE: Use in Adults** for details).[6]

Prior to immunization, the parent, guardian, or adult patient should be informed of the two types of poliovirus vaccines available, the risks and benefits of each to the individual and to the community, and the reasons why recommendations are made for giving specific vaccines under certain circumstances.

Past history of clinical poliomyelitis or prior vaccination with IPV in otherwise healthy individuals does not preclude the administration of OPV when otherwise indicated.

The simultaneous administration of OPV, diphtheria and tetanus toxoids and pertussis vaccine (DTP), and/or measles-mumps-rubella vaccine (MMR), has resulted in seroconversion rates and rates of side effects similar to those observed when the vaccines are administered separately.[7]

Administration of Immune Globulin (IG), if necessary, within 7 days prior to immunization with OPV does not reduce the antibody response to OPV based on a study conducted in Peace Corps volunteers.[8]

Use in Adults: Routine primary poliovirus immunization of adults (generally those 18 years of age or older), residing in the United States, is not recommended by the Immunization Practices Advisory Committee (ACIP). Immunization *is* recommended by the ACIP for certain adults who are at greater risk of exposure to wild polioviruses than the general population, including travelers to areas where poliomyelitis is endemic or epidemic, members of communities or specific population groups with disease caused by wild polioviruses, laboratory workers handling specimens that may contain polioviruses, and health care workers in close contact with patients who might be excreting polioviruses as follows: *Unimmunized adults* - primary immunization with enhanced-potency IPV is recommended. However, if less than 1 month is available before protection is needed, a single dose of either OPV or enhanced-potency IPV is recommended, with the remaining doses given later if the person remains at increased risk. *Incompletely immunized adults* who have had (1) at least one dose of OPV, (2) fewer than three doses of conventional IPV, or (3) a combination of conventional IPV and OPV totaling fewer than three doses, should receive at least one dose of OPV or enhanced-potency IPV. Additional doses needed to complete a primary series should be given prior to exposure, if time permits. *Adults who have completed a primary series* with any one or a combination of polio vaccines may be given a dose of OPV or enhanced-potency IPV.[6]

Immunization with IPV may be undertaken in unimmunized or inadequately immunized adults in households in which children are to be given OPV (see **ADVERSE REACTIONS**).[3,6]

Epidemic Control: Poliovirus Vaccine Live Oral Trivalent has been recommended for epidemic control. Within an epidemic area, OPV should be provided for all persons over 6 weeks of age who have not been completely immunized or

Continued on next page

Lederle—Cont.

whose immunization status is unknown, with the exceptions noted under immunodeficiency.[3,5] (See **CONTRAINDICA-TIONS.**)

In certain tropical endemic areas, where poliomyelitis has been increasing in recent years, the physician may wish to administer OPV to the infant at birth. Because successful immunization is less likely in newborn infants, a complete series of OPV should follow the neonatal dose beginning when the infants are 2 months old.[3] If the physician elects to immunize the infant at birth, it may be prudent to wait until the child is 3 days old, and to recommend abstention from breast-feeding for 2 to 3 hours before and after oral immunization to minimize exposure of the vaccine viruses to colostrum and to permit the establishment of the vaccine viruses in the gut.[9]

CONTRAINDICATIONS

Under no circumstances should this vaccine be administered parenterally.

Poliovirus vaccine live oral trivalent ORIMUNE *must not be* administered to patients with immune deficiency diseases such as combined immunodeficiency, hypogammaglobulinemia, and agammaglobulinemia. Further, ORIMUNE *must not* be administered to patients with altered immune states, such as those occurring in human immunodeficiency virus (HIV) infection, thymic abnormalities, leukemia, lymphoma, generalized malignancy, or advanced debilitating conditions, or by lowered resistance from therapy with corticosteroids, alkylating drugs, antimetabolites, or radiation. Because vaccine viruses are excreted by the vaccinee, and may spread to contacts, ORIMUNE should not be used in families with immunodeficient members.[3,4]

Recipients of the vaccine should avoid close household-type contact with all persons with altered immune status for at least 6 to 8 weeks.

Because of the possibility of immunodeficiency in other children born to a family in which there has been one such case, OPV should not be given to a member of a household in which there is a family history of immunodeficiency until the immune status of the intended recipient and other children in the family is determined to be normal.[4]

Immunization of all persons in the above described circumstances should be with IPV.

WARNINGS

Under no circumstances should this vaccine be administered parenterally.

Immunization should be deferred during the course of any febrile illness or acute infection. In addition, immunization should be deferred in the presence of persistent vomiting or diarrhea, or suspected gastroenteritis infection. Other viruses (including poliovirus and other enteroviruses) may compromise the desired response to this vaccine, since their presence in the intestinal tract may interfere with replication of the attenuated strains of poliovirus.

PRECAUTIONS

The vaccine is not effective in modifying or preventing cases of existing and/or incubating poliomyelitis.

Records Required by the National Childhood Vaccine Injury Act: This Act requires that the manufacturer and lot number of the vaccine administered be recorded by the health care provider in the vaccine recipient's permanent record, along with the date of administration of the vaccine and the name, address, and title of the person administering the vaccine.

The Act further requires that the health care provider report to a health department or to the FDA the occurrence, following immunization, of any event set forth in the Vaccine Injury Table, including: paralytic poliomyelitis—in a nonimmunodeficient recipient within 30 days of vaccination, in an immunodeficient recipient within 6 months of vaccination; any vaccine-associated community case of paralytic poliomyelitis; or any acute complication or sequela (including death) of above events.[10]

Use in Pregnancy: *Pregnancy Category C:* Animal reproduction studies have not been conducted with Poliovirus Vaccine Live Oral Trivalent. It is also not known whether OPV can cause fetal harm when administered to a pregnant woman or can affect reproduction capacity.

Although there is no convincing evidence documenting adverse effects of either OPV or IPV on the developing fetus or pregnant women, it is prudent on theoretical grounds to avoid vaccinating pregnant women. However, if immediate protection against poliomyelitis is needed, OPV is recommended.[3,6] (See **CONTRAINDICATIONS** and **ADVERSE REACTIONS.**)

ADVERSE REACTIONS

Paralytic disease following the ingestion of live poliovirus vaccines has been, on rare occasion, reported in individuals receiving the vaccine, and in persons who were in close contact with vaccinees.[3,4,11,12] The vaccine viruses are shed in the vaccinee's stools up to 6 to 8 weeks as well as via the

pharyngeal route. Most reports of paralytic disease following ingestion of the vaccine or contact with a recent vaccinee are based on epidemiological analysis and temporal association between vaccination or contact and the onset of symptoms, and most authorities believe that a causal relationship exists.[2,5,10,11,12]

A retrospective study of a large population given OPV suggests that this vaccine may also be temporally associated with Guillain-Barré syndrome.[13] A causal relationship has not been established.

Prior to administration of the vaccine, attending physicians should warn or specifically direct personnel acting under their authority to convey the warnings to the vaccinee, parent, guardian, or other responsible person of the possibility of vaccine-associated paralysis, particularly to the recipient, susceptible family members, and other close personal contacts.[3,4]

The Centers for Disease Control and Prevention reports that during the years 1973 through 1984 approximately 274.1 million OPV doses were distributed in the United States. During this same period, 105 vaccine-associated cases were reported (1 case per 2.6 million doses distributed). Of these 105 cases, 35 occurred in vaccine recipients (1 case per 7.8 million doses distributed), 50 occurred in household and nonhousehold contacts of vaccinees (1 case per 5.5 million doses distributed), 14 occurred in immunodeficient recipients or contacts, and 6 occurred in persons with no history of vaccine exposure, from whom vaccine-like viruses were isolated.[11]

Thirty-three (94%) of the recipient cases, 41 (82%) of the contact cases, and 5 (36%) of the immune deficient cases were associated with the recipient's first dose of OPV. Because most cases of vaccine-associated paralysis have occurred in association with the first dose, the CDC has estimated the likelihood of paralysis in association with first *v* subsequent doses of OPV, using the number of births during 1973–1984 to estimate the number of first doses distributed, and subtracting this from the total distribution to estimate the number of subsequent doses distributed. This method estimates a frequency of paralysis for recipients of one case per 1.2 million first doses *v* one case per 116.5 million subsequent doses; for contacts, one case per 1 million first doses *v* one case per 25.9 million subsequent doses; with an overall frequency of 1 case per 520,000 first doses *v* one case per 12.3 million subsequent doses.[11]

Other methods of estimating the likelihood of paralysis in association with OPV have been described. Because the number of susceptible vaccine recipients or contacts of recipients is not known, the true risk of vaccine-associated poliomyelitis is impossible to determine precisely.[10]

When the attenuated vaccine strains are to be introduced into a household with adults who are unimmunized or whose immune status cannot be determined, the risk of vaccine-associated paralysis can be reduced by giving these adults two doses of enhanced potency IPV a month apart before the children receive *poliovirus vaccine live oral trivalent* ORIMUNE. The children may receive the first dose of ORIMUNE at the same visit that the adults receive the second dose of enhanced potency IPV. For partially immunized adult contacts, a booster dose of enhanced potency IPV can be given at the same visit that the first dose of OPV is given to the child.[3]

The responsible adult should also be informed of precautions to be taken such as handwashing after diaper changes.[14]

The ACIP states: "Because of the overriding importance of ensuring prompt and complete immunization of the child and the extreme rarity of OPV-associated disease in contacts, the Committee recommends the administration of OPV to a child regardless of the poliovirus-vaccine status of adult household contacts. This is the usual practice in the United States. The responsible adult should be informed of the small risk involved. An acceptable alternative, if there is a strong assurance that ultimate, full immunization of the child will not be jeopardized or unduly delayed, is to immunize adults. . . [with IPV]. . . before giving OPV to the child.'"[4]

The American Academy of Pediatrics and the American College of Physicians have made similar recommendations.[3,14]

DOSAGE AND ADMINISTRATION

Poliovirus vaccine live oral trivalent ORIMUNE is to be administered *orally, under the supervision of a physician. Under no circumstances should this vaccine be administered parenterally.* For convenience, the vaccine is supplied in a disposable pipette containing a single dose of 0.5 mL which should be administered directly into the mouth of the vaccinee. Breast feeding does not interfere with successful immunization when OPV is administered according to the following schedule.[4]

Primary Series: The primary series consists of three doses. *Infants:* The ACIP and AAP recommend that the first dose of OPV be administered when the infant is approximately 2 months (6 to 12 weeks) of age. The second dose should be given not less than 6 and preferably 8 weeks later, commonly at 4 months of age. A third dose of OPV should be given when the child is approximately 15 to 18 months of age to complete

the primary series, but may be given at any time between 12 and 24 months of age.[3] In endemic areas an additional dose administered 2 months after the second dose is desirable.[3,4]

Older Children and Adolescents (up to 18 years of age): Unimmunized children and adolescents should receive two doses given not less than 6 and preferably 8 weeks apart, followed by a third dose 6 to 12 months after the second dose. If there is substantial risk of exposure to polio, the third dose should be given 6 to 8 weeks after the second dose.[3,4]

Children at any age who are unimmunized or partially immunized should receive the number of doses necessary to complete the required series of three doses. If the schedule has been interrupted, the series does not need to be reinitiated.[3,7]

Adults: See **INDICATIONS** and **ADVERSE REACTIONS.** Where OPV is given to unimmunized adults the dosage regimen is as indicated for older children and adolescents.

Supplemental Doses: *School Entry:* On entering elementary school, all children who have completed the primary series should be given a single follow-up dose of OPV[3,4] (all others should complete the primary series). The fourth supplemental dose is not required in those who received the third primary dose on or after their fourth birthday.[3,4] The ACIP and AAP do not recommend routine booster doses of vaccine beyond that given at the time of entering school.[3,4] It has been shown that over 95% of children studied 5 years after full immunization with oral polio vaccine had protective antibodies to all three types of poliovirus.[15]

Increased Risk: If an individual who has completed a primary series is subjected to a substantially increased risk because of personal contact, travel, or occupation, a single dose of OPV may be given.[3,4]

SIMULTANEOUS ADMINISTRATION WITH OTHER VACCINES

The simultaneous administration of OPV, diphtheria and tetanus toxoids and pertussis vaccine (DTP), and/or measles-mumps-rubella vaccine (MMR), has resulted in seroconversion rates and rates of side effects similar to those observed when the vaccines are administered separately.[7] The AAP states that OPV, DTP, MMR and/or Haemophilus b conjugate vaccines may be given concomitantly.[3,16]

STORAGE

To maintain the potency of *poliovirus vaccine live oral trivalent* ORIMUNE, it is necessary to store this vaccine at a temperature which will maintain ice continuously in a solid state (below 0°C or 32°F). However, since the vaccine contains sorbitol it may remain fluid at temperatures above -14°C (+7°F). Ice cubes that remain frozen continuously when stored in the same freezer compartment will confirm that the temperature is appropriate for storage of ORIMUNE. If frozen, the vaccine must be completely thawed prior to use. A container of vaccine that has been frozen and then is thawed may be carried through a maximum of 10 freeze-thaw cycles, provided the temperature does not exceed 8°C (46°F) during the periods of thaw, and provided the total cumulative duration of thaw does not exceed 24 hours. If the 24-hour period is exceeded, the vaccine must then be used within 30 days, during which time it must be stored at a temperature between 2°C to 8°C (36°F to 46°F). Ideally, an ORIMUNE DISPETTE® should be removed from the freezer and thawed immediately prior to use.

Color Change: This vaccine contains phenol red as a pH indicator. The usual color of the vaccine is pink, although some containers of vaccine, shipped or stored in dry ice, may exhibit a yellow coloration due to the very low temperature or possible absorption of carbon dioxide. The color of the vaccine prior to use (red-pink-yellow) has no effect on the virus or efficacy of the vaccine.

DIRECTIONS FOR USE: Pull off the protective cap and squeeze to expel contents into the vaccinee's mouth.

HOW SUPPLIED

NDC 0005-2084-08—10 (0.5 mL) DISPETTE
NDC 0005-2084-12—50 (0.5 mL) DISPETTE

National Stock Number:
NSN 6505-01-185-8848 50 1-dose DISPETTE

REFERENCES

1. *Code of Federal Regulations.* 21 CFR:630.17[c], page 94, Revised April 1, 1989.
2. Albrecht P, Enterline JC, Boone EJ, et al. Poliovirus and polio antibody assay in Hep-2 and Vero cell cultures. *J Biol Stand.* 1983; 11:91–97.
3. *Report of the Committee on Infectious Diseases. American Academy of Pediatrics.* 21st Edition, 1988; 334–342. Elk Grove Village, IL
4. Recommendations of the Immunization Practices Advisory Committee [ACIP]. Poliomyelitis Prevention. *MMWR.* 1982; 31[3]:22–34.
5. An evaluation of poliomyelitis vaccine policy options. Institute of Medicine, National Academy of Sciences, 1988. Publication No. 10M 88–04.

6. ACIP. Poliomyelitis prevention: Enhanced-Potency Inactivated Poliomyelitis Vaccine—Supplementary Statement. *MMWR.* 1987; 36[48]:795–798.

7. ACIP. General recommendations on immunization. *MMWR.* 1989; 38[13]:206–227.

8. Kaplan JE, Nelson DB, Schonberger LB, et al. The effect of immune globulin on the response to trivalent oral poliovirus and yellow fever vaccinations. *Bull WHO.* 1984; 62[4]:585–590.

9. Welsh JH, et al. Anti-infective properties of breast milk. *J Pediatr.* 1979; 94[1]:1–9.

10. National Childhood Injury Act: Requirements for permanent vaccination records and for reporting of selected events after vaccination. *MMWR.* 1988; 37[13]:197–200.

11. Nkowane BM, Wassilak SGF, Orenstein WA, et al. Vaccine-associated paralytic poliomyelitis. United States: 1973 through 1984. *JAMA.* 1987; 257[10]:1335–1340.

12. Esteves K. Safety of oral poliomyelitis vaccine: results of a WHO enquiry. *Bull WHO.* 1988; 66[6]:739–746.

13. Kinnunen E, Farkkila M, Hovi T, et al. Incidence of Guillain-Barré syndrome during a nationwide oral poliovirus vaccine campaign. *Neurology.* 1989; 39:1034–1036.

14. Guide for Adult Immunization. American College of Physicians, 2nd Edition, 25, 1990. Philadelphia, PA.

15. Krugman RD, et al. Antibody persistence after primary immunization with trivalent oral poliovirus vaccine. *Pediatrics.* 1977; 60[1]:80–82.

16. American Academy of Pediatrics, Haemophilus Influenzae Type B Conjugate Vaccines. Immunization of children 2 to 15 months of age. *PED COMM: AAP MEMBER ALERT,* October 1990.

Manufactured by:

LEDERLE LABORATORIES DIVISION

American Cyanamid Company, Pearl River, NY 10965

Shown in Product Identification Guide, page 320

PIPRACIL® ℞

[pĭp-ra-sĭl]

sterile piperacillin sodium

For Intravenous and Intramuscular Use

DESCRIPTION

PIPRACIL® sterile piperacillin sodium is a semisynthetic broad-spectrum penicillin for parenteral use derived from D(-)-α-aminobenzylpenicillin. The chemical name of piperacillin sodium is 4-Thia-1-azabicyclo [3.2.0] heptane-2-carboxylic acid, 6-[[[[(4-ethyl-2,3-dioxo-1-piperazinyl)carbonyl]amino]-phenylacetyl]amino]-3,3-dimethyl-7-oxo-, monosodium salt, [2S-[2α, 5α, 6β(S*)]].

PIPRACIL is a white to off-white solid having the characteristic appearance of products prepared by freeze-drying. Freely soluble in water and in alcohol. The pH of the aqueous solution is 5.5 to 7.5. One g contains 1.85 mEq (42.5 mg) of sodium (Na^+).

CLINICAL PHARMACOLOGY

Intravenous Administration. In healthy adult volunteers, mean serum levels immediately after a two to three minute intravenous injection of 2, 4, or 6 g were 305, 412, and 775 mcg/mL. Serum levels lack dose proportionality.

[See table below.]

A 30-minute infusion of 6 g every 6 h gave, on the fourth day, a mean peak serum concentration of 420 mcg/mL.

Intramuscular Administration. PIPRACIL is rapidly absorbed after intramuscular injection. In healthy volunteers, the mean peak serum concentration occurs approximately 30 minutes after a single dose of 2 g and is about 36 mcg/mL. The oral administration of 1 g probenecid before injection produces an increase in piperacillin peak serum level of about 30%. The area under the curve (AUC) is increased by approximately 60%.

General: PIPRACIL is not absorbed when given orally. Peak serum concentrations are attained approximately 30 minutes after intramuscular injections and immediately after completion of intravenous injection or infusion. The serum half-life in healthy volunteers ranges from 36 minutes to one hour and 12 minutes. The mean elimination half-life of PIPRACIL in healthy adult volunteers is 54 minutes following administration of 2 g and 63 minutes following 6 g. As with other penicillins, PIPRACIL is eliminated primarily by glomerular filtration and tubular secretion; it is excreted rapidly as unchanged drug in high concentrations in the urine. Approximately 60% to 80% of the administered dose is excreted in the urine in the first 24 hours. Piperacillin urine concentrations, determined by microbioassay, were as high as 14,100 mcg/mL following a 6 g intravenous dose and 8,500 mcg/mL following a 4 g intravenous dose. These urine drug concentrations remained well above 1,000 mcg/mL throughout the dosing interval. The elimination half-life is increased twofold in mild to moderate renal impairment and fivefold to sixfold in severe impairment.

PIPRACIL binding to human serum proteins is 16%. The drug is widely distributed in human tissues and body fluids, including bone, prostate, and heart and reaches high concentrations in bile. After a 4 g bolus, maximum biliary concentrations averaged 3,205 mcg/mL. It penetrates into the cerebrospinal fluid in the presence of inflamed meninges. Because PIPRACIL is excreted by the biliary route as well as by the renal route, it can be used safely in appropriate dosage (see **DOSAGE AND ADMINISTRATION**) in patients with severely restricted kidney function, and can be used effectively in treatment of hepatobiliary infections.

Microbiology: PIPRACIL is an antibiotic which exerts its bactericidal activity by inhibiting both septum and cell wall synthesis. It is active against a variety of gram-positive and gram-negative aerobic and anaerobic bacteria. *In vitro,* piperacillin is active against most strains of clinical isolates of the following microorganisms:

Aerobic and facultatively anaerobic organisms

Gram-negative bacteria:
  Escherichia coli
  Proteus mirabilis
  Proteus vulgaris
  Morganella morganii (formerly *Proteus morganii*)
  Providencia rettgeri (formerly *Proteus rettgeri*)
  Serratia species including *S marcescens* and *S liquefaciens*
  Klebsiella pneumoniae
  Klebsiella species
  Enterobacter species including *E aerogenes* and *E cloacae*
  Citrobacter species including *C freundii* and *C diversus*
  Salmonella species*
  Shigella species*
  Pseudomonas aeruginosa
  Pseudomonas species including *P cepacia,* * *P maltophilia,** and *P fluorescens*
  Acinetobacter species (formerly *Mima-Herellea*)
  Haemophilus influenzae (non-β-lactamase-producing strains)
  Neisseria gonorrhoeae
  *Neisseria meningitidis**
  Moraxella species*
  Yersinia species* (formerly *Pasteurella*)

Gram-positive bacteria:
  Group D streptococci including
    Enterococci (*Streptococcus faecalis, S faecium*)
    Non-enterococci*
  β-hemolytic streptococci including
    Group A *Streptococcus* (*S pyogenes*)
    Group B *Streptococcus* (*S agalactiae*)
  Streptococcus pneumoniae
  Streptococcus viridans
  Staphylococcus aureus (non-penicillinase-producing)*
  Staphylococcus epidermidis (non-penicillinase-producing)*

Anaerobic bacteria:
  Actinomyces species*

Bacteroides species including
  B fragilis group (*B fragilis, B vulgatus*)
  Non-*B fragilis* group (*B melaninogenicus*)
  *B asaccharolyticus**
Clostridium species including
  C perfringens and *C difficile**
Eubacterium species
Fusobacterium species including
  F nucleatum and *F necrophorum*
Peptococcus species
Peptostreptococcus species
Veillonella species

---

*Piperacillin has been shown to be active *in vitro* against these organisms; however, clinical efficacy has not yet been established.

In vitro, PIPRACIL is inactivated by staphylococcal β-lactamases, and β-lactamases produced by gram-negative bacteria. However, it is active against β-lactamase-producing gonococci.

Many strains of gram-negative organisms resistant to certain antibiotics have been found to be susceptible to PIPRACIL.

PIPRACIL has excellent activity against gram-positive organisms, including enterococci (*S faecalis*). It is active against obligate anaerobes such as *Bacteroides* species and also against *C difficile* (which has been associated with pseudomembranous colitis).

Piperacillin is active against many gram-negative bacteria including *Enterobacteriaceae, Klebsiella, Serratia, Pseudomonas, E coli, Proteus,* and *Citrobacter,* and, in addition, it is active against anaerobes and enterococci.

In vitro tests show piperacillin to act synergistically with aminoglycoside antibiotics against most isolates of *P aeruginosa.*

Susceptibility Testing

The use of a 100 mcg piperacillin antibiotic disk with susceptibility test methods which measure zone diameter gives an accurate estimation of susceptibility of organisms to PIPRACIL. The following standard procedure[†] has been recommended for use with disks for testing antimicrobials.

[†] NCCLS Approved Standard; M2-A2 (Formerly ASM-2) Performance Standards for Antimicrobic Disk Susceptibility Tests, Second Edition, available from the National Committee of Clinical Laboratory Standards.

With this type of procedure, a report of "susceptible" from the laboratory indicates that the infecting organism is likely to respond to therapy. A report of "intermediate susceptibility" suggests that the organism would be susceptible if high dosage is used or if the infection is confined to tissue and fluids (eg, urine) in which high antibiotic levels are obtained. A report of "resistant" indicates that the infecting organism is not likely to respond to therapy. With the piperacillin disk, a zone of 18 mm or greater indicates susceptibility, zone sizes of 14 mm or less indicate resistance, and zone sizes of 15 to 17 mm indicate intermediate susceptibility.

Haemophilus and *Neisseria* species which give zones of ≥ 29 mm are susceptible; resistant strains give zones of ≤ 28 mm. The above interpretive criteria are based on the use of the standardized procedure. Antibiotic susceptibility testing requires carefully prescribed procedures. Susceptibility tests are biased to a considerable degree when different methods are used.

The standardized procedure requires the use of control organisms. The 100 mcg piperacillin disk should give zone diameters between 24 and 30 mm for *E coli* ATCC No. 25922 and between 25 and 33 mm for *Pseudomonas aeruginosa* ATCC No. 27853.

PIPERACILLIN SERUM LEVELS IN ADULTS (mcg/mL) AFTER A TWO- TO THREE-MINUTE IV INJECTION

DOSE	0	10 min	20 min	30 min	1 h	1.5 h	2 h	3 h	4 h	6 h	8 h
2	305	202	156	67	40	24	20	8	3	2	—
	(159–615)	(164–225)	(52–165)	(41–88)	(25–57)	(18–31)	(14–24)	(3–11)	(2–4)	(<0.6–3)	
4	412	344	295	117	93	60	36	20	8	4	0.9
	(389–484)	(315–379)	(269–330)	(98–138)	(78–110)	(50–67)	(26–51)	(17–24)	(7–11)	(3.7–4.1)	(0.7–1)
6	775	609	563	325	208	138	90	38	33	8	3.2
	(695–849)	(530–670)	(492–630)	(292–363)	(180–239)	(115–175)	(71–113)	(29–53)	(25–44)	(3–19)	(<2–6)

PIPERACILLIN SERUM LEVELS IN ADULTS (mcg/mL) AFTER A 30-MINUTE IV INFUSION

DOSE	0	5 min	10 min	15 min	30 min	45 min	1 h	1.5 h	2 h	4 h	6 h	7.5 h
4	244	215	186	177	141	146	105	72	53	15	4	2
	(155–298)	(169–247)	(140–209)	(142–213)	(122–156)	(110–265)	(85–133)	(53–105)	(36–69)	(6–24)	(1–9)	(0.5–3)
6	353	298	298	272	229	180	149	104	73	22	16	—
	(324–371)	(242–339)	(232–331)	(219–314)	(185–249)	(144–209)	(117–171)	(89–113)	(66–94)	(12–39)	(5–49)	—

Continued on next page

Lederle—Cont.

Dilution methods such as those described in the International Collaborative Study[‡] have been used to determine susceptibility of organisms to PIPRACIL.

[‡]*Acta Pathol Microbiol Scand* [B] 1971; suppl 217.

Enterobacteriaceae, Pseudomonas species and *Acinetobacter* sp are considered susceptible if the minimal inhibitory concentration (MIC) of piperacillin is no greater than 64 mcg/mL and are considered resistant if the MIC is greater than 128 mcg/mL.

Haemophilus and *Neisseria* species are considered susceptible if the MIC of piperacillin is ≤ to 1 mcg/mL.

When anaerobic organisms are isolated from infection sites, it is recommended that other tests such as the modified Broth-Disk Method[§] be used to determine the antibiotic susceptibility of these slowly growing organisms.

[§] Wilkins TD and Thiel T. *Antimicrob Agents Chemother* 1973;3:350–356.

INDICATIONS AND USAGE

Therapeutic. PIPRACIL is indicated for the treatment of serious infections caused by susceptible strains of the designated organisms in the conditions as listed below.

Intra-Abdominal Infections including hepatobiliary and surgical infections caused by *E coli, P aeruginosa,* enterococci, *Clostridium* sp, anaerobic cocci, and *Bacteroides* sp, including *B fragilis.*

Urinary Tract Infections caused by *E coli, Klebsiella* sp, *P aeruginosa, Proteus* sp, including *P mirabilis,* and enterococci.

Gynecologic Infections including endometritis, pelvic inflammatory disease, pelvic cellulitis caused by *Bacteroides* sp including *B fragilis,* anaerobic cocci, *Neisseria gonorrhoeae,* and enterococci (*S faecalis*).

Septicemia including bacteremia caused by *E coli, Klebsiella* sp, *Enterobacter* sp, *Serratia* sp, *P mirabilis, S pneumoniae,* enterococci, *P aeruginosa, Bacteroides* sp, and anaerobic cocci.

Lower Respiratory Tract Infections caused by *E coli, Klebsiella* sp, *Enterobacter* sp, *Pseudomonas aeruginosa, Serratia* sp, *H influenzae, Bacteroides* sp, and anaerobic cocci. Although improvement has been noted in patients with cystic fibrosis, lasting bacterial eradication may not necessarily be achieved.

Skin and Skin Structure Infections caused by *E coli, Klebsiella* sp, *Serratia* sp, *Acinetobacter* sp, *Enterobacter* sp, *Pseudomonas aeruginosa,* indole-positive *Proteus* sp, *Proteus mirabilis, Bacteroides* sp, including *B fragilis,* anaerobic cocci, and enterococci.

Bone and Joint Infections caused by *P aeruginosa,* enterococci, *Bacteroides* sp, and anaerobic cocci.

Gonococcal Infections. PIPRACIL has been effective in the treatment of uncomplicated gonococcal urethritis.

PIPRACIL has also been shown to be clinically effective for the treatment of infections at various sites caused by *Streptococcus* species including Group A β-hemolytic *Streptococcus* and *S pneumoniae;* however, infections caused by these organisms are ordinarily treated with more narrow spectrum penicillins. Because of its broad spectrum of bactericidal activity against gram-positive and gram-negative aerobic and anaerobic bacteria, PIPRACIL is particularly useful for the treatment of mixed infections and presumptive therapy prior to the identification of the causative organisms.

Also, PIPRACIL may be administered as single drug therapy in some situations where normally two antibiotics might be employed.

Piperacillin has been successfully used with aminoglycosides, especially in patients with impaired host defenses. Both drugs should be used in full therapeutic doses.

Appropriate cultures should be made for susceptibility testing before initiating therapy and therapy adjusted, if appropriate, once the results are known.

Prophylaxis: PIPRACIL is indicated for prophylactic use in surgery including intra-abdominal (gastrointestinal and biliary) procedures, vaginal hysterectomy, abdominal hysterectomy, and cesarean section. Effective prophylactic use depends on the time of administration, and PIPRACIL should be given one-half to one hour before the operation so that effective levels can be achieved in the site prior to the procedure.

The prophylactic use of piperacillin should be stopped within 24 hours, since continuing administration of any antibiotic increases the possibility of adverse reactions, but in the majority of surgical procedures, does not reduce the incidence of subsequent infections. If there are signs of infection, specimens for culture should be obtained for identification of the causative organism so that appropriate therapy can be instituted.

CONTRAINDICATIONS

A history of allergic reactions to any of the penicillins and/or cephalosporins.

WARNINGS

Serious and occasionally fatal hypersensitivity (anaphylactic) reactions have been reported in patients receiving therapy with penicillins. These reactions are more apt to occur in persons with a history of sensitivity to multiple allergens. There have been reports of patients with a history of penicillin hypersensitivity who have experienced severe hypersensitivity reactions when treated with a cephalosporin. Before initiating therapy with PIPRACIL, careful inquiry should be made concerning previous hypersensitivity reactions to penicillins, cephalosporins, and other allergens. If an allergic reaction occurs during therapy with PIPRACIL, the antibiotic should be discontinued. The usual agents (antihistamines, pressor amines, and corticosteroids) should be readily available. SERIOUS ANAPHYLACTOID REACTIONS REQUIRE IMMEDIATE EMERGENCY TREATMENT WITH EPINEPHRINE. OXYGEN AND INTRAVENOUS CORTICOSTEROIDS AND AIRWAY MANAGEMENT INCLUDING INTUBATION SHOULD ALSO BE ADMINISTERED AS NECESSARY.

PRECAUTIONS

General

While piperacillin possesses the characteristic low toxicity of the penicillin group of antibiotics, periodic assessment of organ system functions, including renal, hepatic, and hematopoietic, during prolonged therapy is advisable.

Bleeding manifestations have occurred in some patients receiving β-lactam antibiotics, including piperacillin. These reactions have sometimes been associated with abnormalities of coagulation tests such as clotting time, platelet aggregation and prothrombin time and are more likely to occur in patients with renal failure.

If bleeding manifestations occur, the antibiotic should be discontinued and appropriate therapy instituted.

The possibility of the emergence of resistant organisms which might cause superinfections should be kept in mind, particularly during prolonged treatment. If this occurs, appropriate measures should be taken.

As with other penicillins, patients may experience neuromuscular excitability or convulsions if higher than recommended doses are given intravenously.

PIPRACIL is a monosodium salt containing 1.85 mEq of Na[+] per g. This should be considered when treating patients requiring restricted salt intake. Periodic electrolyte determinations should be made in patients with low potassium reserves, and the possibility of hypokalemia should be kept in mind with patients who have potentially low potassium reserves and who are receiving cytotoxic therapy or diuretics.

Antimicrobials used in high doses for short periods to treat gonorrhea may mask or delay the symptoms of incubating syphilis. Therefore, prior to treatment, patients with gonorrhea should also be evaluated for syphilis. Specimens for darkfield examination should be obtained from patients with any suspected primary lesion, and serologic tests should be performed. In all cases where concomitant syphilis is suspected, monthly serological tests should be made for a minimum of 4 months.

As with other semisynthetic penicillins, PIPRACIL therapy has been associated with an increased incidence of fever and rash in cystic fibrosis patients.

Drug Interactions

The mixing of piperacillin with an aminoglycoside *in vitro* can result in substantial inactivation of the aminoglycosides. Piperacillin when used concomitantly with vecuronium has been implicated in the prolongation of the neuromuscular blockage of vecuronium. Due to their similar mechanism of action, it is expected that the neuromuscular blockade produced by any of the non-depolarizing muscle relaxants could be prolonged in the presence of piperacillin. (See package insert for vecuronium bromide.)

Pregnancy–Pregnancy Category B

Although reproduction studies in mice and rats performed at doses up to 4 times the human dose have shown no evidence of impaired fertility or harm to the fetus, safety of PIPRACIL use in pregnant women has not been determined by adequate and well-controlled studies. Because animal reproduction studies are not always predictive of human response, this drug should be used during pregnancy only if clearly needed. It has been found to cross the placenta in rats.

Nursing Mothers

Caution should be exercised when PIPRACIL is administered to nursing mothers. It is excreted in low concentrations in milk.

Pediatric Use

Dosages for children under the age of 12 have not been established. The safety of PIPRACIL in neonates is not known. In dog neonates, dilated renal tubules and peritubular hyalinization occurred following administration of PIPRACIL.

ADVERSE EFFECTS

PIPRACIL is generally well tolerated. The most common adverse reactions have been local in nature, following intravenous or intramuscular injection. The following adverse reactions may occur.

Local Reactions. In clinical trials thrombophlebitis was noted in 4% of patients. Pain, erythema, and/or induration at the injection site occurred in 2% of patients. Less frequent reactions including ecchymosis, deep vein thrombosis and hematomas have also occurred.

Gastrointestinal. Diarrhea and loose stools were noted in 2% of patients. Other less frequent reactions included vomiting, nausea, increases in liver enzymes (LDH, SGOT, SGPT), hyperbilirubinemia, cholestatic hepatitis, bloody diarrhea and, rarely, pseudomembranous colitis.

Hypersensitivity Reactions: Anaphylactoid Reactions, see **WARNINGS.**

Rash was noted in 1% of patients. Other less frequent findings included pruritus, vesicular eruptions, positive Coombs tests.

Other dermatologic manifestations such as erythema multiforme and Stevens-Johnson syndrome have been reported rarely.

Renal. Elevations of creatinine or BUN, and, rarely, interstitial nephritis.

Central Nervous System. Headache, dizziness, fatigue.

Hemic and Lymphatic. Reversible leukopenia, neutropenia, thrombocytopenia and/or eosinophilia have been reported. As with other β-lactam antibiotics, reversible leukopenia (neutropenia) is more apt to occur in patients receiving prolonged therapy at high dosages or in association with drugs known to cause this reaction.

Serum Electrolytes. Individuals with liver disease or individuals receiving cytotoxic therapy or diuretics were reported rarely to demonstrate a decrease in serum potassium concentrations with high doses of piperacillin.

Skeletal. Rarely, prolonged muscle relaxation.

Other. Superinfection, including candidiasis. Hemorrhagic manifestations.

DOSAGE AND ADMINISTRATION

PIPRACIL may be administered by the intramuscular route (see Note) or intravenously or given in a three- to five-minute intravenous injection. The usual dosage of PIPRACIL for serious infections is 3- to 4-g given every four to six hours as a 20- to 30-minute infusion. For serious infections, the intravenous route should be used.

PIPRACIL should not be mixed with an aminoglycoside in a syringe or infusion bottle since this can result in inactivation of the aminoglycoside.

The maximum daily dose for adults is usually 24 g/day, although higher doses have been used.

Intramuscular injections (See Note) should be limited to 2 g per injection site. This route of administration has been used primarily in the treatment of patients with uncomplicated gonorrhea and urinary tract infections.

NOTE: THE ADD-VANTAGE VIAL IS *NOT* FOR IM USE.

DOSAGE RECOMMENDATIONS

Type of Infection	Usual Total Daily Dose
Serious infections such as septicemia, nosocomial pneumonia, intra-abdominal infections, aerobic and anaerobic gynecologic infections, and skin and soft tissue infections	12–18 g/d IV (200 to 300 mg/kg/d) in divided doses every 4 to 6 h
Complicated urinary tract infections	8–16 g/d IV (125– 200 mg/kg/d) in divided doses every 6 to 8 h
Uncomplicated urinary tract infections and most community-acquired pneumonia	6–8 g/d IM or IV (100 to 125 mg/kg/d) in divided doses every 6 to 12 h
Uncomplicated gonorrhea infections	2 g IM[″] as a one-time dose

[″]One g of probenecid given orally one-half hour prior to injection.

The average duration of PIPRACIL treatment is from seven to 10 days, except in the treatment of gynecologic infections, in which it is from 3 to 10 days; the duration should be guided by the patient's clinical and bacteriological progress. For most acute infections, treatment should be continued for at least 48 to 72 hours after the patient becomes asymptomatic. Antibiotic therapy for Group A β-hemolytic streptococcal infections should be maintained for at least ten days to reduce the risk of rheumatic fever or glomerulonephritis.

When PIPRACIL is given concurrently with aminoglycosides, both drugs should be used in full therapeutic doses.

Renal Impairment:

Dosage in Renal Impairment

Creatinine Clearance mL/min	Urinary Tract Infection (uncomplicated)	Urinary Tract Infection (complicated)	Serious Systemic Infection
>40	No dosage adjustment necessary		
20–40	No dosage adjustment necessary	9 g/day 3 g every 8 h	12 g/day 4 g every 8 h
<20	6 g/day 3 g every 12 h	6 g/day 3 g every 12 h	8 g/day 4 g every 12 h

For patients on hemodialysis the maximum daily dose is 6 g/day (2 g every 8 hours). In addition, because hemodialysis removes 30%–50% of piperacillin in 4 hours, 1 g additional dose should be administered following each dialysis period. For patients with renal failure and hepatic insufficiency, measurement of serum levels of PIPRACIL will provide additional guidance for adjusting dosage.

Prophylaxis
When possible, PIPRACIL should be administered as a 20- to 30-minute infusion just prior to anesthesia. Administration while the patient is awake will facilitate identification of possible adverse reactions during drug infusion.

INDICATION	1st Dose	2nd Dose	3rd Dose
Intra-abdominal Surgery	2 g IV just prior to surgery	2 g during surgery	2 g every 6 h Post-Op for no more than 24 h
Vaginal Hysterectomy	2 g IV just prior to surgery	2 g 6 h after 1st dose	2 g 12 h after 1st dose
Cesarean Section	2 g IV after cord is clamped	2 g 4 h after 1st dose	2 g 8 h after 1st dose
Abdominal Hysterectomy	2 g IV just prior to surgery	2 g on return to recovery room	2 g after 6 h

Infants and Children: Dosages in infants and children under 12 years of age have not been established.

PRODUCT RECONSTITUTION/DOSAGE PREPARATION

Conventional Vials:
Diluents for Reconstitution
Sterile Water for Injection
Bacteriostatic£ Water for Injection
Sodium Chloride Injection
Bacteriostatic£
Sodium Chloride Injection
Dextrose 5% in Water
Dextrose 5% and 0.9% Sodium Chloride
#Lidocaine HCl 0.5% to 1% (without epinephrine)

£ Either Parabens or Benzyl Alcohol
For Intramuscular Use Only. Lidocaine is contraindicated in patients with a known history of hypersensitivity to local anesthetics of the amide type.

Conventional Vials:
Intravenous Solutions
Dextrose 5% in Water
0.9% Sodium Chloride
Dextrose 5% and 0.9% Sodium Chloride
Lactated Ringer's Injection‡
Dextran 6% in 0.9% Sodium Chloride

‡ When PIPRACIL® is further diluted with Lactated Ringer's Injection, the diluted solution must be administered within 2 hours.

Intravenous Admixtures
Normal Saline [+ KCl 40 mEq]
5% Dextrose in Water [+ KCl 40 mEq]
5% Dextrose/Normal Saline [+ KCl 40 mEq]
Ringer's Injection [+ KCl 40 mEq]
Lactated Ringer's Injection [+ KCl 40 mEq]‡

‡ When PIPRACIL® is further diluted with Lactated Ringer's Injection, the diluted solution must be administered within 2 hours.

ADD-Vantage** Vials:
ADD-Vantage System Admixtures
Dextrose 5% in Water (50 or 100 mL)
0.9% Sodium Chloride (50 or 100 mL)

** (ADD-Vantage is the registered trademark of Abbott Laboratories.)

INTRAVENOUS ADMINISTRATION:

Reconstitution Directions for Conventional Vials: Reconstitute each gram of PIPRACIL with at least 5 mL of a suitable diluent (except Lidocaine HCl 0.5% to 1% without epinephrine) listed above. Shake well until dissolved. Reconstituted solution may be further diluted to the desired volume (eg, 50 or 100 mL) in the above listed intravenous solutions and admixtures.

Reconstitution Directions for ADD-Vantage Vials: See Instruction Sheet provided in box.

Reconstitution Directions for PHARMACY BULK VIAL: Reconstitute the 40 g vial with 172 mL of a suitable diluent (except Lidocaine HCl 0.5% to 1% without epinephrine) listed above to achieve a concentration of 1 g per 5 mL.

Directions for Administration:
Intermittent IV Infusion
Infuse diluted solution over a period of about 30 minutes. During infusion it is desirable to discontinue the primary intravenous solution.
Intravenous Injection (Bolus)
Reconstituted solution should be injected slowly over a 3- to 5-minute period to help avoid vein irritation.

INTRAMUSCULAR ADMINISTRATION (CONVENTIONAL VIALS ONLY):
Reconstitution Directions: Reconstitute each gram of PIPRACIL with 2 mL of a suitable diluent listed above to achieve a concentration of 1 g per 2.5 mL. Shake well until dissolved.

Directions for Administration: When indicated by clinical and bacteriological findings, intramuscular administration of 6 to 8 g daily of PIPRACIL, in divided doses, may be utilized for initiation of therapy. In addition, intramuscular administration of the drug may be considered for maintenance therapy after clinical and bacteriologic improvement has been obtained with intravenous piperacillin sodium treatment. Intramuscular administration should not exceed 2 g per injection at any one site.
The preferred site is the upper outer quadrant of the buttock (ie, gluteus maximus).
The deltoid area should be used only if well-developed, and then only with caution to avoid radial nerve injury. Intramuscular injections should not be made into the lower or mid-third of the upper arm.

STABILITY OF PIPRACIL FOLLOWING RECONSTITUTION:
PIPRACIL is stable in both glass and plastic containers when reconstituted with recommended diluents and when diluted with the intravenous solutions and intravenous admixtures indicated above.
Extensive stability studies have demonstrated chemical stability (potency, pH, and clarity) through 24 hours at room temperature, up to one week refrigerated, and up to one month frozen ($-10°$ to $-20°$C). (Note: The 40 g Pharmacy Bulk Vial should not be frozen after reconstitution.) Appropriate consideration of aseptic technique and individual hospital policy, however, may recommend discarding unused portions after storage for 48 hours under refrigeration and discarding after 24 hours storage at room temperature.

ADD-Vantage System:
Stability studies with the ad-mixed ADD-Vantage system have demonstrated chemical stability (potency, pH, and clarity) through 24 hours at room temperature. (Note: The admixed ADD-Vantage should not be refrigerated or frozen after reconstitution.)
Additional stability data available upon request.

HOW SUPPLIED
PIPRACIL® sterile piperacillin sodium is available in vials containing sterile freeze-dried piperacillin sodium powder equivalent to 2, 3, 4 and 40 g of piperacillin. One g of piperacillin (as a monosodium salt) contains 1.85 mEq (42.5 mg) of sodium.

Product Numbers:
2 gram/Vial—10 per box—NDC 0206-3879-16
3 gram/Vial—10 per box—NDC 0206-3882-55
4 gram/Vial—10 per box—NDC 0206-3880-25
3 gram infusion Bottle—10 per box—NDC 0206-3882-65
4 gram infusion Bottle—10 per box—NDC 0206-3880-66
2 gram ADD-Vantage Vial—10 per box—NDC 0206-3879-27
3 gram ADD-Vantage Vial—10 per box—NDC 0206-3882-28
4 gram ADD-Vantage Vial—10 per box—NDC 0206-3880-29
40 gram Pharmacy Bulk Vial—NDC 0206-3877-60
This product should be stored at controlled room temperature 15°–30°C (59°–86°F).

LEDERLE PIPERACILLIN, INC.
Carolina, Puerto Rico 00987
Shown in Product Identification Guide, page 320

PNU-IMUNE® 23 ℞
[new-ĭ-mune]
Pneumococcal Vaccine, Polyvalent

DESCRIPTION
Pneumococcal Vaccine Polyvalent PNU-IMUNE 23 is a sterile preparation intended for intramuscular or subcutaneous use. PNU-IMUNE 23 is indicated for immunization against infections caused by the 23 most prevalent types of *Streptococcus pneumoniae* (pneumococci) which are responsible for approximately 90% of serious pneumococcal disease in the United States and worldwide.[1–5] PNU-IMUNE 23 consists of a mixture of purified capsular polysaccharides from 23 types of *S pneumoniae*. [See table at bottom of next page.]
Each of the pneumococcal polysaccharide types is produced separately to assure a high degree of purity. After an individual pneumococcal type is grown, the polysaccharide is separated from the cell and purified by a series of steps including ethanol fractionation. The vaccine is formulated to contain 25 μg of each of the 23 purified polysaccharide types per 0.5 mL dose of vaccine. Thimerosal (a mercury derivative) at a final concentration of 0.01% is added as a preservative.
The vaccine is a clear, colorless liquid.

CLINICAL PHARMACOLOGY
Disease caused by *S pneumoniae* remains an important cause of morbidity and mortality in the US, particularly in the very young, the elderly, and persons with certain high-risk conditions. Pneumococcal pneumonia accounts for 10% to 25% of all pneumonias and an estimated 40,000 deaths annually.[2]
Studies suggest annual rates of bacteremia of 15 to 19/100,000 for the total population, and 50/100,000 for persons 65 and older. Certain population groups, eg, Native Americans may have considerably higher disease rates.[2]
Mortality from pneumococcal disease is highest in patients with bacteremia or meningitis, patients with underlying medical conditions, and older persons. In some high-risk patients, mortality has been reported to be over 40% for bacteremic disease and 55% for meningitis, despite appropriate antimicrobial therapy.[2]
In addition to the very young and persons 65 years of age or older, patients with certain chronic conditions are at increased risk of developing pneumococcal infection and severe pneumococcal illness. Patients with chronic cardiovascular or pulmonary disease, diabetes mellitus, alcoholism, and cirrhosis are generally immunocompetent but have increased risk. Other patients at greater risk because of decreased responsiveness to polysaccharide antigens or more rapid decline in serum antibody include those with functional or anatomic asplenia (eg, sickle-cell disease or splenectomy), Hodgkin's disease, lymphoma, multiple myeloma, chronic renal failure, nephrotic syndrome, and organ transplantation. Studies indicate that patients with acquired immunodeficiency syndrome (AIDS) are also at increased risk of pneumococcal disease.[6,7] Recurrent pneumococcal meningitis may occur in patients with cerebrospinal fluid leakage that complicates skull fractures or neurologic procedures.
The polysaccharide capsules of pneumococci give these organisms resistance to the phagocytic action of polymorphonuclear leukocytes and monocytes. However, type-specific antibody facilitates their destruction in the body by the mechanism of complement-mediated lysis.
Most healthy adults, including the elderly, demonstrate at least a two-fold rise in type-specific antibodies within two to three weeks of immunization. Similar antibody responses have been reported in patients with alcoholic cirrhosis and diabetes mellitus. In contrast, elderly individuals with chronic pulmonary disease failed to mount a comparable immune response.[8] In immunocompromised patients, the response to immunization may also be lower. Children under two years of age respond poorly to most capsular polysaccharide types. Further, response to some pneumococcal types (eg, 6A and 14) important in pediatric infection is decreased in children less than 5 years of age.[9]
In clinical studies with PNU-IMUNE 23, more than 90% of all adults showed two-fold or greater increase in geometric mean antibody titer for each capsular type contained in the vaccine.[10]
Patients over the age of 2 years, with anatomical or functional asplenia and otherwise intact lymphoid function, generally respond to pneumococcal vaccines with a serological conversion comparable to that observed in healthy individuals of the same age.[11]
Patients with acquired immunodeficiency syndrome (AIDS) may have an impaired antibody response to pneumococcal vaccine.[7,12] However, asymptomatic human immunodeficiency virus (HIV)-infected patients, or those with generalized lymphadenopathy, respond to the 23-valent pneumococcal vaccine.[13]
Following immunization of healthy adults, antibody levels remain elevated for at least 5 years, but in some individuals

Continued on next page

Lederle—Cont.

these may fall to preimmunization levels within 10 years.[14,15] A more rapid decline in antibodies may occur in children, particularly those who have undergone a splenectomy and those with sickle-cell disease, in whom antibodies for some types can fall to preimmunization levels 3 to 5 years after immunization.[16,17] Similar rates of decline can occur in children with nephrotic syndrome.[18]

Controlled clinical trials in South Africa involving 12,000 gold miners have shown a 6-valent and a 13-valent pneumococcal vaccine to be 78.5% effective in preventing type-specific pneumococcal pneumonia and 82.3% effective in preventing pneumococcal bacteremia with the types contained in the vaccine.[19] In a preliminary study of an 8-valent polysaccharide vaccine in a group consisting of 77 patients with sickle-cell disease and 19 asplenic persons, there were no pneumococcal infections in the immunized patients within two years of immunization. There were eight cases of pneumococcal infection in 106 unimmunized, age-matched patients with sickle-cell disease. Antibody response of the asplenic patients was comparable to that of normal controls.[20]

In a study carried out by Austrian and colleagues with 13-valent pneumococcal vaccines prepared for the National Institute of Allergy and Infectious Disease, the reduction in pneumonias caused by the capsular types present in the vaccines was 79%. Reduction in type-specific pneumococcal bacteremia was 82%.[19]

In a double-blind study of a 14-valent pneumococcal vaccine carried out in Papua, New Guinea, pneumococcal infection was 84% lower in the immunized group and mortality from pneumonia 44% lower.[21]

Five case-control studies in the US have evaluated the efficacy of pneumococcal vaccine in the prevention of serious pneumococcal disease. Four of these studies showed the vaccine to be efficacious, with point estimates of efficacy ranging from 61% to 70%.[22–25] One study failed to show efficacy in preventing pneumococcal bacteremia.[26] This study was judged inadequate in determination of vaccination status, and the selection of controls was considered potentially biased.[2]

A prospective study failed to demonstrate efficacy against pneumococcal pneumonia and bronchitis;[8] this study has been criticized for methodological flaws.[2] In contrast, a prospective French study found pneumococcal vaccine to be 77% effective in reducing the incidence of pneumonia among nursing home residents.[27]

Despite conflicting findings, the data continue to support the use of pneumococcal vaccine for certain well-defined groups at risk.[2]

INDICATIONS AND USAGE

PNU-IMUNE 23 is indicated for immunization against pneumococcal disease caused by those pneumococcal types included in the vaccine.

Adults

1. All adults 65 or older,[2] with emphasis on immunization of the older adult while in good health.
2. Immunocompetent adults who are at increased risk of pneumococcal disease or its complications because of chronic illnesses (eg, cardiovascular or pulmonary disease, diabetes mellitus, alcoholism, cirrhosis, or cerebrospinal fluid leaks).[2]
3. Immunocompromised adults at increased risk of pneumococcal disease or its complications (eg, splenic dysfunction or anatomic asplenia, Hodgkin's disease, lymphoma, multiple myeloma, chronic renal failure, nephrotic syndrome, or conditions such as organ transplantation associated with immunosuppression).[2]

Children

1. Children 2 years of age or older with chronic illnesses specifically associated with increased risk of pneumococcal disease or its complications (eg, anatomic or functional asplenia [including sickle-cell disease], nephrotic syndrome, cerebrospinal fluid leaks, and conditions associated with immunosuppression).[2]

Special Groups

1. Persons living in special environments or social settings with an identified increased risk of pneumococcal disease or its complications.[2]
2. Patients with acquired immunodeficiency syndrome (AIDS) have been shown to have an impaired antibody response to pneumococcal vaccine. However, asymptomatic or symptomatic human immunodeficiency virus (HIV)-infected patients or those with persistent generalized lymphadenopathy respond to the 23-valent vaccine.[2]

Timing of Immunization

When elective splenectomy is being considered, pneumococcal vaccine should be given at least two weeks before surgery, if possible.[2]

For planning cancer chemotherapy or other immunosuppressive therapy, the interval between immunization and initiation of chemotherapy or immunosuppression should be at least two weeks.[2]

CONTRAINDICATIONS

HYPERSENSITIVITY TO ANY COMPONENT OF THE VACCINE, INCLUDING THIMEROSAL, A MERCURY DERIVATIVE, IS A CONTRAINDICATION TO THE USE OF THE PRODUCT.

THE OCCURRENCE OF ANY TYPE OF NEUROLOGICAL SYMPTOMS OR SIGNS FOLLOWING ADMINISTRATION OF THIS PRODUCT IS A CONTRAINDICATION TO FURTHER USE.

THE VACCINE SHOULD NOT BE ADMINISTERED TO PERSONS WITH ACUTE FEBRILE ILLNESSES UNTIL THEIR TEMPORARY SYMPTOMS AND/OR SIGNS HAVE ABATED.

The clinical judgment of the attending physician should prevail at all times.

WARNINGS

PNU-IMUNE 23 is not an effective agent for prophylaxis against pneumococcal disease caused by types not present in the vaccine.

PNU-IMUNE 23 is not indicated for children under two years of age, since antibody response to most capsular polysaccharide types is poor in this age group.[2]

Patients with impaired immune responsiveness whether due to the use of immunosuppressive therapy, a genetic defect, human immunodeficiency virus (HIV) infection, or other causes may have a reduced antibody response to active immunization procedures.[2]

Patients who have received extensive chemotherapy and/or splenectomy for the treatment of Hodgkin's disease have been shown to have an impaired serum antibody response to pneumococcal vaccine.[28,29]

In one study, administration of the vaccine to patients on immunosuppressive drugs and/or irradiation for Hodgkin's disease resulted in reduction of preexisting antibody levels in several patients.[28] It is unclear whether this effect was due to the vaccine or to the effects of irradiation and/or chemotherapy.

At least two weeks should elapse between immunization and the initiation of chemotherapy or immunosuppressive therapy.[2]

Routine reimmunization with this vaccine is not recommended. For reimmunization recommendations (including recommendations regarding reimmunization of individuals at highest risk of fatal pneumococcal infection) see **DOSAGE AND ADMINISTRATION.**

In one study, local reactions after reimmunization were more severe than after initial immunization when the interval between immunizations was 13 months.[30]

Patients who have had episodes of pneumococcal pneumonia or other pneumococcal infection may have high levels of preexisting pneumococcal antibodies that may result in increased reactions to PNU-IMUNE 23, mostly local, but occasionally systemic.[31] Caution should be exercised if such patients are considered for immunization with PNU-IMUNE 23.

Do not administer the vaccine intradermally since severe reactions may occur.

PRECAUTIONS

General

1. This product should not be used in children under 2 years of age.
2. PRIOR TO ADMINISTRATION OF ANY DOSE OF PNU-IMUNE 23, THE PARENT, GUARDIAN, OR ADULT PATIENT SHOULD BE ASKED ABOUT THE RECENT HEALTH STATUS, MEDICAL AND IMMUNIZATION HISTORY OF THE PATIENT TO BE IMMUNIZED TO DETERMINE THE EXISTENCE OF ANY CONTRAINDICATION TO IMMUNIZATION WITH PNEUMOCOCCAL VACCINE (SEE **CONTRAINDICATIONS, WARNINGS**).
3. BEFORE ADMINISTRATION OF ANY BIOLOGICAL, THE PHYSICIAN SHOULD TAKE ALL KNOWN PRECAUTIONS FOR PREVENTION OF ALLERGIC OR ANY OTHER REACTIONS. This includes: a review of the patient's history regarding possible sensitivity, the ready availability of epinephrine 1:1,000 and other appropriate agents used for control of immediate allergic reactions, and a knowledge of the recent literature pertaining to use of the biological concerned, including the nature of side effects and adverse reactions that may follow its use.
4. A separate sterile syringe and needle or a sterile disposable unit should be used for each individual patient to prevent transmission of infectious agents from one person to another.

PRIOR TO ADMINISTRATION OF THIS VACCINE, HEALTH CARE PERSONNEL SHOULD INFORM THE PARENT, GUARDIAN, OR ADULT PATIENT OF THE BENEFITS AND RISKS OF IMMUNIZATION WITH PNEUMOCOCCAL VACCINE.

Pregnancy Category C: Animal reproduction studies have not been conducted with PNU-IMUNE 23. It is also not known whether PNU-IMUNE 23 can cause fetal harm when administered to a pregnant woman or affect reproduction capacity. PNU-IMUNE 23 is not recommended for use in pregnant women.

It is not known whether the drug is excreted in human milk. Because many drugs are excreted in human milk, caution should be exercised when PNU-IMUNE 23 is administered to a nursing woman.

ADVERSE REACTIONS

Pneumococcal Vaccine Polyvalent PNU-IMUNE 23 is associated with a relatively low incidence of adverse reactions. The adverse reactivity observed in clinical studies was of short duration and not serious.

In a study of 32 individuals who received PNU-IMUNE 23, 23 (72%) experienced local reaction characterized by soreness at the injection site within 3 days after immunization.[10]

Low grade fever (less than 37.8°C [100°F]) and mild myalgia occur occasionally and are usually confined to the 24-hour period following immunization. Rash and arthralgia have been reported infrequently.

Although rare, fever over 38.9°C (102°F) and marked local swelling have been reported with pneumococcal polysaccharide vaccine. Rash, urticaria, arthritis, arthralgia, and adenitis have been reported rarely.

Patients with otherwise stabilized idiopathic thrombocytopenic purpura have, on rare occasions, experienced a relapse in their thrombocytopenia, occurring 2 to 14 days after immunization, and lasting up to 2 weeks.[32]

Reactions of greater severity, or extent are unusual. Rarely, anaphylactoid reactions have been reported.

Temporal association of neurological disorders such as paresthesias and acute radiculoneuropathy, including Guillain-Barré syndrome, have been reported following parenteral injections of biological products including pneumococcal vaccine.

DOSAGE AND ADMINISTRATION

The immunization schedule consists of a single 0.5 mL dose given intramuscularly or subcutaneously. Intradermal administration should be avoided. *Do not inject intravenously.*

Parenteral drug products should be inspected visually for particulate matter and discoloration prior to administration (see **DESCRIPTION**).

Before injection, the skin at the injection site should be cleansed with a suitable germicide. After insertion of the needle, aspirate to help avoid inadvertent injection into a blood vessel.

Simultaneous Administration with Other Vaccines

Many patients who receive pneumococcal vaccine should also be immunized with influenza vaccine which may be given simultaneously at a different site. In contrast to pneumococcal vaccine, influenza vaccine is recommended annually.[2]

Reimmunization

The incidence of local reactions after reimmunization were found to be more severe than after initial immunization when the interval between immunizations was 13 months.[29]

Reports of reimmunization after longer intervals in children and adults, including a large group of elderly persons reimmunized at least 4 years after primary immunization, suggest a similar incidence of such reactions.[2] The Immunization Practices Advisory Committee (ACIP) recommendations regarding reimmunization are as follows: Persons who receive the 14-valent vaccine should not *routinely* be reimmunized with the 23-valent vaccine. However, reimmunization with 23-valent vaccine should be strongly considered for persons who received the 14-valent vaccine *if they are at highest risk* of fatal pneumococcal infection (eg, asplenic patients). Reimmunization should also be carefully considered for adults at highest risk who received the 23-valent vaccine more than 6 years before and for those shown to have a rapid decline in antibody levels (eg, patients with nephrotic syndrome, renal failure, or transplant patients). Reimmunization should be carefully considered after 3 to 5 years for children with nephrotic syndrome, asplenia, or sickle-cell anemia who would be 10 years old or younger at the time of reimmunization.[2]

HOW SUPPLIED

PNU-IMUNE 23 is supplied as follows:
NDC 0005-2309-31 2.5 mL Vial, for use with syringe only.
NDC 0005-2309-33 5 × One Dose (0.5 mL) LEDERJECT® Disposable Syringes.

STORAGE

DO NOT FREEZE. STORE REFRIGERATED, AWAY FROM FREEZER COMPARTMENT AT 2°C TO 8°C (36°F TO 46°F).

Pneumococcal Types

Nomenclature																							
Danish	1	2	3	4	5	6B	7F	8	9N	9V	10A	11A	12F	14	15B	17F	18C	19F	19A	20	22F	23F	33F
US	1	2	3	4	5	26	51	8	9	68	34	43	12	14	54	17	56	19	57	20	22	23	70

Directions for Use of the LEDERJECT Disposable Syringe:

1. Twist the plunger rod clockwise to be sure the rod is secure to rubber plunger base.
2. Hold needle shield in place with index finger and thumb of one hand while, with the other thumb, exert light pressure on plunger rod until the plunger base has been freed and demonstrates slight movement when pressure is applied.
3. Grasp the rubber needle shield at its base; twist and pull to remove.
4. To prevent needle-stick injuries, needles should not be recapped, purposely bent, or broken by hand.

REFERENCES

1. Austrian R. Surveillance of pneumococcal infection for field trials of polyvalent vaccines. *Annual Contract Prog Report to the Nat Inst of Allerg and Inf Dis* 1975; Update to Dec. 1977, personal communication.
2. Immunization Practices Advisory Committee. Pneumococcal polysaccharide vaccine—recommendations of the ACIP. *MMWR.* 1989;38(5):64–76. Recommendations also published in: *JAMA.* 1989;261(9):1265–1267.
3. Lund E. Distribution of pneumococcal types at different times and different areas. In: Finland M, Marget W, Bartman K eds. *Bayer-Symposium III Bacterial Infections.* New York, NY:Springer-Verlag, 1971:49.
4. Mufson MA, Kruss DM, Wasil RE, et al. Capsular types and outcome of bacteremic pneumococcal disease in the antibiotic era. *Arch Int Med.* 1974;134:505–510.
5. Robbins JB, Austrian R, Lee CJ, et al. Consideration for formulating the second generation pneumococcal capsular polysaccharide vaccine with emphasis on the cross-reactive types within groups. *J Infec Dis.* 1983; 148(6):1136–1159.
6. Lane CH, Masur H, Edgar LC, et al. Abnormalities of B-cell activation and immunoregulation in patients with the acquired immunodeficiency syndrome. *N Engl J Med.* 1983;309:453–458.
7. Ammann AJ, Schiffman G, Abrams D, et al. B-cell immunodeficiency in acquired immune deficiency syndrome. *JAMA.* 1984;251:1447–1449.
8. Simberkoff MS, Cross AP, Al-Ibrahim M, et al. Efficacy of pneumococcal vaccine in high-risk patients: results of a Veterans Administration cooperative study. *N Eng J Med.* 1986;315:1318–1327.
9. Douglas RM, Paton JC, Duncan SJ, et al. Antibody response to pneumococcal vaccination in children younger than five years of age. *J Infect Dis.* 1983;148:131–137.
10. Data on file, Lederle Laboratories.
11. Sullivan JL, Ochs HD, Schiffman G, et al. Immune response after splenectomy. *Lancet.* 1978;1:178–181.
12. Ballet J-J, Sulcebe G, Couderc L-J, et al. Impaired anti-pneumococcal antibody response in patients with AIDS-related persistent generalized lymphadenopathy. *Clin Exp Immunol.* 1987;68:479–487.
13. Huang K-L, Ruben FL, Rinaldo CR Jr, et al. Antibody responses after influenza and pneumococcal immunization in HIV-infected homosexual men. *JAMA.* 1987; 257:2047–2050.
14. Mufson MA, Krause HE, Schiffman G. Long term persistence of antibodies following immunization with pneumococcal polysaccharide vaccine. *Proc Soc Exp Bio Med.* 1983;173:270–275.
15. Mufson MA, Krause HE, Schiffman G, et al. Pneumococcal antibody levels one decade after immunization of healthy adults. *Am J Med Sci.* 1987;293:279–284.
16. Giebiuk GS, Le CT, Schiffman G. Decline of serum antibody in splenectomized children after vaccination with pneumococcal capsular polysaccharides. *J Pediatr.* 1984;105:576–582.
17. Weintrub PS, Schiffman G, Addiego JE Jr, et al. Long-term follow-up and booster immunization with polyvalent pneumococcal polysaccharide in patient with sickle cell anemia. *J Pediatr.* 1984;105:261–263.
18. Spika JS, Halsey NA, Le CT, et al. Decline of vaccine-induced antipneumococcal antibody in children with nephrotic syndrome. *Am J Kidney Dis.* 1986;7:466–470.
19. Austrian R, Douglas RM, Schiffman G, et al. Prevention of pneumococcal pneumonia by vaccination. *Trans Assoc Am Phys.* 1976;89:184–194.
20. Ammann AJ, Addiego K, Wara DW, et al. Polyvalent pneumococcal-polysaccharide immunization of patients with sickle-cell anemia and patients with splenectomy. *N Engl J Med.* 1977;297:897–900.
21. Riley ID, Tarr PI, Andrews M, et al. Immunisation with a polyvalent pneumococcal vaccine: reduction of adult respiratory mortality in a New Guinea Highlands community. *Lancet.* 1977;1:1338–1341.
22. Shapiro ED, Clemens JD. A controlled evaluation of the protective efficacy of pneumococcal vaccine for patients at high risk of serious pneumococcal infections. *Ann Intern Med.* 1984;101:325–330.
23. Shapiro ED, Austrian R, Adair RK, et al. The protective efficacy of pneumococcal vaccine (Abstract). *Clin Res.* 1988;36:470A.
24. Sims RV, Steinmann WC, McConville JH, et al. The clinical effectiveness of pneumococcal vaccine in the elderly. *Ann Intern Med.* 1988;108:653–657.
25. Bolan G, Broome CV, Facklam RR, et al. Pneumococcal vaccine efficacy in selected populations in the United States. *Ann Intern Med.* 1986;104:1–6.
26. Forrester HL, Jahnigen DW, LaForce FM. Inefficacy of pneumococcal vaccine in a high-risk population. *Am J Med.* 1987;83:425–430.
27. Gaillat J, Zmirou D, Mallaret MR, et al. Essai clinique du vaccin antipneumococcique chez des personnes agées vivant en institution. *Rev Epidémiol Santé Publique.* 1985;33:437–444.
28. Siber GR, Weitzman SA, Aisenberg AC, et al. Impaired antibody response to pneumococcal vaccine after treatment for Hodgkin's disease. *N Engl J Med.* 1978;299:442–448.
29. Siber GR, Gorham C, Martin P, et al. Antibody response to pretreatment immunization and post-treatment boosting with bacterial polysaccharide vaccines in patients with Hodgkin's disease. *Ann Intern Med.* 1986;104:467–475.
30. Borgono JM, McLean AA, Vella PP, et al. Vaccination and revaccination with polyvalent pneumococcal polysaccharide vaccines in adults and infants. *Proc Soc Exper Biol Med.* 1978;157:148–154.
31. Ponka A, Leinonen M: Adverse reactions to polyvalent pneumococcal vaccine. *Scand J Infect Dis.* 1982;14:67–71.
32. Kelton JG. Vaccination-associated relapse of immune thrombocytopenia. *JAMA.* 1981;245(4):369–371.

Manufactured by:
LEDERLE LABORATORIES DIVISION
American Cyanamid Company
Pearl River, NY 10965

Shown in Product Identification Guide, page 321

PROSTEP® ℞
(nicotine transdermal system)
Systemic delivery of 22 or 11 mg/day over 24 hours

DESCRIPTION

PROSTEP is a transdermal system that provides systemic delivery of nicotine following its application to intact skin. Nicotine is a tertiary amine composed of a pyridine and a pyrrolidine ring. It is a colorless to pale yellow, freely water-soluble, strongly alkaline, oily, volatile, hygroscopic liquid obtained from the tobacco plant. Nicotine has a characteristic pungent odor and turns brown on exposure to air or light. Of its two stereoisomers, *S* (-)-nicotine is the more active. It is the prevalent form in tobacco, and is the form in the PROSTEP system. The free alkaloid is absorbed rapidly through the skin and respiratory tract.

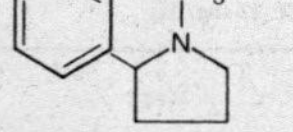

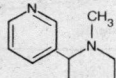

Chemical Name:
S - 3 - (1-methyl-2-pyrrolidinyl) pyridine
Molecular Formula: $C_{10}H_{14}N_2$
Molecular Weight: 162.23
Ionization Constants: $pK_{a1} = 7.84$, $pK_{a2} = 3.04$
Octanol-Water Partition Coefficient: 15.1 at pH 7

The PROSTEP system is a round, flat, adhesive pad with a round well in the center containing nicotine (the active agent) in a hydrogel matrix. Proceeding from the visible outer surface toward the inner surface attached to the skin are: (1) a beige-colored foam tape and pressure-sensitive acrylate adhesive; (2) backing foil, gelatin and low-density polyethylene; (3) nicotine-gel matrix; (4) protective foil with well and (5) release liner which overlies the adhesive layer and must be removed prior to use. PROSTEP systems are packaged in child-resistant pouches.

STICKY SIDE: APPLY TO SKIN — NONSTICKY SIDE: DISCARD

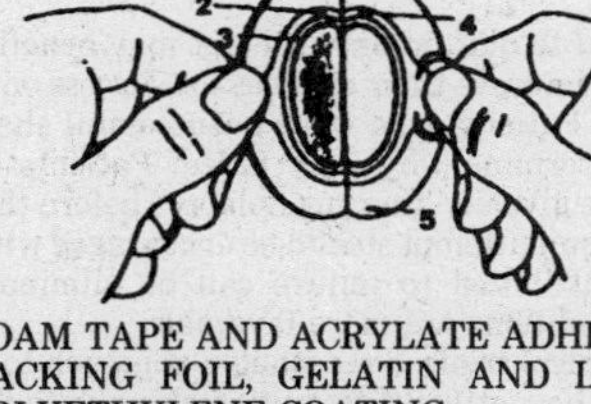

1— FOAM TAPE AND ACRYLATE ADHESIVE
2— BACKING FOIL, GELATIN AND LOW DENSITY POLYETHYLENE COATING
3— NICOTINE-GEL MATRIX
4— PROTECTIVE FOIL WITH WELL
5— RELEASE LINER

Nicotine is the active ingredient; other components of the system are pharmacologically inactive.

The amount of nicotine delivered to the patient from each system (130 mcg/cm²-h) is proportional to the surface area of the nicotine-gel matrix. About 27% of the total amount of nicotine remains in the system 24 hours after application. PROSTEP systems are labelled with the average dose absorbed by the patient. The dose of nicotine absorbed from a PROSTEP system represents 98% of the amount released from the system in 24 hours.

Dose Absorbed in 24 hrs (mg/day)	System Surface Area (cm^2)	Total Nicotine Content (mg)	Residual Nicotine after 24 hrs (mg)
22	7	30	8
11	3.5	15	4

CLINICAL PHARMACOLOGY

Pharmacologic Action

Nicotine, the chief alkaloid in tobacco products, binds stereoselectively to acetylcholine receptors at the autonomic ganglia, in the adrenal medulla, at neuromuscular junctions, and in the brain. Two types of central nervous system effects are believed to be the basis of nicotine's positively reinforcing properties. A stimulating effect, exerted mainly in the cortex via the locus ceruleus, produces increased alertness and cognitive performance. A "reward" effect via the "pleasure system" in the brain is exerted in the limbic system. At low doses the stimulant effects predominate while at high doses the reward effects predominate. Intermittent intravenous administration of nicotine activates neurohormonal pathways, releasing acetylcholine, norepinephrine, dopamine, serotonin, vasopressin, beta-endorphin, growth hormone, and ACTH.

Pharmacodynamics

The cardiovascular effects of nicotine include peripheral vasoconstriction, tachycardia, and elevated blood pressure. Acute and chronic tolerance to nicotine develops from smoking tobacco or ingesting nicotine preparations. Acute tolerance (a reduction in response for a given dose) develops rapidly (less than 1 hour) but not at the same rate for different physiologic effects (skin temperature, heart rate, subjective effects). Withdrawal symptoms, such as cigarette craving, can be reduced in some individuals by plasma nicotine levels lower than those from smoking.

Withdrawal from nicotine in addicted individuals is characterized by craving, nervousness, restlessness, irritability, mood lability, anxiety, drowsiness, sleep disturbances, impaired concentration, increased appetite, minor somatic complaints (headache, myalgia, constipation, fatigue), and weight gain. Nicotine toxicity is characterized by nausea, abdominal pain, vomiting, diarrhea, diaphoresis, flushing, dizziness, disturbed hearing and vision, confusion, weakness, palpitations, altered respirations and hypotension.

The cardiovascular effects of PROSTEP 22 mg/day systems include slight increase in heart rate and blood pressure. The cardiovascular effects of applying one or two PROSTEP 22 mg/day systems used continuously for 24 hours were compared to placebo for 7 days. Changes in heart rate (increased 4 beats/min), systolic blood pressure (increased 4 mmHg) and diastolic blood pressure (increased 3 mmHg) were observed.

Both smoking and nicotine can increase circulating cortisol and catecholamines, and tolerance does not develop to the catecholamine-releasing effects of nicotine. Changes in the response to a concomitantly administered adrenergic agonist or antagonist should be watched for when nicotine intake is altered during nicotine replacement therapy with PROSTEP systems (see **Drug Interactions**).

Pharmacokinetics

Following application of the PROSTEP system to the upper body or upper outer arm, virtually all of the nicotine released from the system enters the systemic circulation. All PROSTEP systems are labelled as to the average amount of nicotine absorbed by patients.

The volume of distribution following IV administration of nicotine is approximately 2 to 3 L/kg and the half-life ranges from 1 to 2 hours. The major eliminating organ is the liver, and average plasma clearance is about 1.2 L/min; the kidney and lung also metabolize nicotine. There is no significant skin metabolism of nicotine. More than 20 metabolites of nicotine have been identified, all of which are believed to be less active than the parent compound. The primary metabolite of nicotine in plasma, cotinine, has a half-life of 15 to 20 hours and concentrations that exceed nicotine by 10-fold.

Plasma protein binding of nicotine is <5%. Therefore changes in nicotine binding from use of concomitant drugs or alterations of plasma proteins by disease states would not be expected to have significant effects on nicotine kinetics.

The primary urinary metabolites are cotinine (15% of the dose) and trans-3-hydroxycotinine (45% of the dose). Usually about 10% of nicotine is excreted unchanged in the urine. As

Continued on next page

Lederle—Cont.

much as 30% may be excreted unchanged in the urine with high urine flow rates and acidification below pH 5.

The pharmacokinetic model which best fits the plasma nicotine concentrations from PROSTEP systems is an open, two compartment model with a skin depot through which nicotine enters the central disposition compartment.

The PROSTEP system gel matrix contacts the skin directly and acts as a reservoir from which nicotine is absorbed slowly over the 24 hours.

Steady-State Plasma Nicotine Concentrations for Two Consecutive Applications of PROSTEP 22 mg/day (Mean ± 2 SD, N = 22)

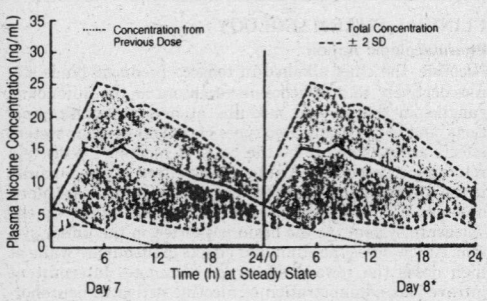

*Day 8 is a reproduction of Day 7 data to represent steady-state dosing.

Following application of a system, nicotine concentrations increase to a peak between 4 and 12 hours and then decrease gradually (see graph). Steady state for nicotine is attained within 2 days of initiating PROSTEP treatment and plasma nicotine concentrations average 23% higher compared to single-dose application. Plasma nicotine concentrations are proportional to dose (i.e., linear kinetics are observed) for the two dosages of PROSTEP systems. Nicotine kinetics are similar for all sites of application on the upper torso and upper outer arm.

Following removal of PROSTEP systems, plasma nicotine concentrations decline in an exponential fashion with an apparent mean half-life of 3 to 4 hours due to continued absorption from the skin depot (see dotted line in figure) in contrast to a half-life of 1–2 hours following IV administration. Most nonsmoking patients will have nondetectable nicotine concentrations in 10 to 12 hours after patch removal.

Steady State Nicotine Pharmacokinetic Parameters for 22 mg/day PROSTEP Systems (mean, std dev, range)

Parameter (units)	22 mg/day (N = 22)		
	Mean	SD	Range
C_{max} (ng/mL)	16	6	7–31
C_{avg} (ng/mL)	11	3	6–17
C_{min} (ng/mL)	5	1	3–9
T_{max} (hrs)	9	5	4–24

C_{max}: maximum observed plasma concentration
C_{avg}: average plasma concentration
C_{min}: minimum observed plasma concentration
T_{max}: time of maximum plasma concentration

CLINICAL TRIALS

The efficacy of PROSTEP treatment as an aid to smoking cessation was demonstrated in two placebo-controlled, double-blind trials in otherwise healthy patients smoking at least one pack per day (N = 516). In one of these trials, PROSTEP therapy was combined with concomitant individual patient counseling (10 minutes each visit) and in the other trial PROSTEP therapy was used with group counseling (1 hour each visit). In both trials, patients were treated for 8 weeks with a fixed dosage of 22 mg/day or placebo followed by abrupt cessation of PROSTEP treatment and decrease in support therapy. Patients in these two trials received prestudy counseling at two visits before beginning treatment. Two earlier trials (N = 409) were carried out without prestudy counseling with treatment for 6 weeks and weaning to the 11 mg/day patch in one of them (N = 329). In all four trials quitting was defined as total abstinence from smoking as measured by patient diary and verified by expired carbon monoxide. The "quit rates" are the proportions of all persons initially enrolled who abstained after week 2.

Quit Rates by Treatment After Week 2 (range by clinics)*

Nicotine Treatment	Number of Patients	After 6 Weeks	After 6 Months
PROSTEP (22 mg/day)	259	10%–57%	0%–37%
Placebo	257	3%–30%	0%–20%

* Trial involved 7 clinics, number of patients per treatment ranged from 29 to 60.

The two trials with prestudy counseling demonstrated that with concomitant support, fixed dosage therapy with PROSTEP therapy was more effective than placebo after 6 weeks and data from these 2 studies are combined in the quit rate table. At 8 weeks, just prior to abrupt termination of PROSTEP treatment (no weaning), quit rates were 6%–50%. At follow-up, three to five days later, quit rates were 3%–50%. In the two other studies without prestudy counseling, quit rates of 0%–46% with PROSTEP 22 mg/day and 3%–31% with placebo were observed at 6 weeks. In each of the four studies, there was a large variation in quit rates among clinics for each treatment.

Patients using PROSTEP systems dropped out of the trials significantly less frequently than did patients receiving placebo (26% vs 34%). The quit rate for 30 patients over age 60 was comparable to the quit rate for 486 patients aged 60 and under.

Patients who used the 22 mg/day PROSTEP treatment in clinical trials had a significant reduction in craving for cigarettes (desire to smoke), a major nicotine withdrawal symptom, as compared to placebo-treated patients (see figure). Reduction in craving, as with quit rate, is quite variable. This variability from clinic to clinic is presumed to be due to inherent differences in patient populations, e.g., patient motivation, concomitant illnesses, number of cigarettes smoked per day, number of years smoking, exposure to other smokers, socioeconomic status, etc., as well as differences among the clinics.

Severity of Craving by Treatment from Clinical Trials (N = 516)

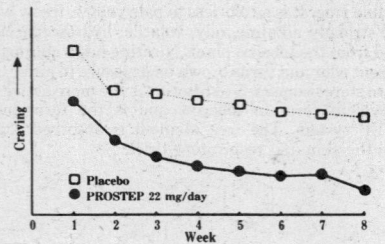

Individualization of Dosage

It is important to make sure that patients read the instructions made available to them and have their questions answered. They should clearly understand the directions for applying and disposing of PROSTEP systems. They should be instructed to stop smoking completely when the first PROSTEP system is applied.

The success or failure of smoking cessation depends heavily on the quality, intensity, and frequency of supportive care. Patients are more likely to quit smoking if they are seen frequently and participate in formal smoking cessation programs.

The goal of PROSTEP therapy is complete abstinence. Significant health benefits have not been demonstrated for reduction of smoking. If a patient is unable to stop smoking by the fourth week of therapy, treatment should probably be discontinued. Patients who have not stopped smoking after four weeks of PROSTEP therapy are unlikely to quit on that attempt.

Patients who fail to quit on any attempt may benefit from interventions to improve their chances for success on subsequent attempts. Patients who were unsuccessful should be counseled to determine why they failed. Patients should then probably be given a "therapy holiday" before the next attempt. A new quit attempt should be encouraged when the factors that contributed to failure can be eliminated or reduced, and conditions are more favorable.

Based on the clinical trials, a reasonable approach to assisting patients in their attempt to quit smoking is to initiate therapy with PROSTEP 22 mg/day except for small patients less than 100 pounds (see **DOSING SCHEDULE** below). The need for dose adjustment should be assessed during the first 2 weeks. The symptoms of nicotine withdrawal and toxicity overlap (see **Pharmacodynamics** and **ADVERSE REACTIONS** sections). Since patients using PROSTEP treatment

may also smoke intermittently, it may be difficult to determine if patients are experiencing nicotine withdrawal or nicotine excess.

The controlled clinical trials using PROSTEP therapy suggest that sweating, abdominal pain, and somnolence are more often symptoms of nicotine excess while irritability is more often a symptom of nicotine withdrawal.

Patients should continue the dose selected with counseling and support over the following month. Those who have successfully stopped smoking during that time can stop PROSTEP treatment or may be weaned (reduction to 11 mg/day) over 4 weeks, after which treatment should be terminated.

DOSING SCHEDULE

	Patients ≥ 100 lbs.	Patients < 100 lbs.
Initial/Starting Dose	22 mg/day	11 mg/day
Duration of Treatment	4–8 weeks	4–8 weeks
Optional Weaning Dose	11 mg/day	off
Duration of Treatment	2–4 weeks	

INDICATIONS AND USAGE

PROSTEP treatment is indicated as an aid to smoking cessation for the relief of nicotine withdrawal symptoms. PROSTEP treatment should be used as a part of a comprehensive behavioral smoking cessation program.

The use of PROSTEP systems for longer than 3 months has not been studied.

CONTRAINDICATIONS

Use of PROSTEP systems is contraindicated in patients with hypersensitivity or allergy to nicotine or to any of the components of the therapeutic system.

WARNINGS

Nicotine from any source can be toxic and addictive. Smoking causes lung cancer, heart disease, emphysema, and may adversely affect the fetus and the pregnant woman. For any smoker, with or without concomitant disease or pregnancy, the risk of nicotine replacement in a smoking-cessation program should be weighed against the hazard of continued smoking while using PROSTEP systems, and the likelihood of achieving cessation of smoking without nicotine replacement.

Pregnancy Warning

Tobacco smoke, which has been shown to be harmful to the fetus, contains nicotine, hydrogen cyanide, and carbon monoxide. Nicotine has been shown in animal studies to cause fetal harm. It is therefore presumed that PROSTEP treatment can cause fetal harm when administered to a pregnant woman. The effect of nicotine delivery by PROSTEP systems has not been examined in pregnancy (see **PRECAUTIONS**). Therefore pregnant smokers should be encouraged to attempt cessation using educational and behavioral interventions before using pharmacological approaches. If PROSTEP therapy is used during pregnancy, or if the patient becomes pregnant while using PROSTEP treatment, the patient should be apprised of the potential hazard to the fetus.

Safety Note Concerning Children

The amounts of nicotine that are tolerated by adult smokers can produce symptoms of poisoning and could prove fatal if PROSTEP systems are applied or ingested by children or pets. Used 22 mg/day systems contain about 27% (8 mg) of their initial drug content. Therefore, patients should be cautioned to keep both used and unused PROSTEP systems out of the reach of children and pets.

PRECAUTIONS

The patient should be urged to stop smoking completely when initiating PROSTEP therapy (see **DOSAGE AND ADMINISTRATION**). Patients should be informed that if they continue to smoke while using PROSTEP systems, they may experience adverse effects due to peak nicotine levels higher than those experienced from smoking alone. If there is a clinically significant increase in cardiovascular or other effects attributable to nicotine, the PROSTEP dose should be reduced or PROSTEP treatment discontinued (see **WARNINGS**). Physicians should anticipate that concomitant medications may need dosage adjustment (see **Drug Interactions**). The use of PROSTEP systems beyond 3 months by patients who stop smoking should be discouraged because the chronic consumption of nicotine by any route can be harmful and addicting.

Allergic Reactions

In a 3-week open-label dermal irritation and sensitization study of PROSTEP systems, 16 of 205 patients (8%) exhibited definite erythema at 24 hours after system removal. None of those patients exhibited contact allergy. In the first 4 weeks of the efficacy trials, moderate erythema following system removal was seen in 22% of patients, some edema in 8%, and dropouts due to skin reactions occurred in 7% of 459 patients using the 22 mg/day system. Patients who develop contact sensitization should be cautioned that a serious reaction

could occur from exposure to other nicotine-containing products or smoking.

Patients should be instructed to promptly discontinue the PROSTEP treatment and contact their physician if they experience severe or persistent local skin reactions at the site of application (e.g., severe erythema, pruritus or edema) or a generalized skin reaction (e.g., urticaria, hives, or generalized rash).

Skin Disease

PROSTEP systems are usually well tolerated by patients with normal skin, but may be irritating for patients with some skin disorders (atopic or eczematous dermatitis).

Cardiovascular or Peripheral Vascular Diseases

The risks of nicotine replacement in patients with certain cardiovascular and peripheral vascular diseases should be weighed against the benefits of including nicotine replacement in a smoking cessation program for them. Specifically, patients with coronary heart disease (history of myocardial infarction and/or angina pectoris), serious cardiac arrhythmias, or vasospastic diseases (Buerger's disease, Prinzmetal's variant angina) should be carefully screened and evaluated before nicotine replacement is prescribed.

Tachycardia occurring in association with the use of PROSTEP treatment was reported occasionally. If serious cardiovascular symptoms occur with PROSTEP treatment, it should be discontinued.

PROSTEP treatment should generally not be used in patients during the immediate post-myocardial infarction period, patients with serious arrhythmias, and patients with severe or worsening angina pectoris.

Renal or Hepatic Insufficiency

The pharmacokinetics of nicotine have not been studied in the elderly or patients with renal or hepatic impairment. However, given that nicotine is extensively metabolized and that its total system clearance is dependent on liver blood flow, some influence of hepatic impairment on drug kinetics (reduced clearance) should be anticipated. Only severe renal impairment would be expected to affect the clearance of nicotine or its metabolites from the circulation (see **Pharmacokinetics**).

Endocrine Diseases

PROSTEP treatment should be used with caution in patients with hyperthyroidism, pheochromocytoma, or insulin-dependent diabetes since nicotine causes the release of catecholamines by the adrenal medulla.

Peptic Ulcer Disease

Nicotine delays healing in peptic ulcer disease; therefore, PROSTEP treatment should be used with caution in patients with active peptic ulcers and only when the benefits of including nicotine replacement in a smoking cessation program outweigh the risks.

Accelerated Hypertension

Nicotine constitutes a risk factor for development of malignant hypertension in patients with accelerated hypertension; therefore, PROSTEP treatment should be used with caution in these patients and only when the benefits of including nicotine replacement in a smoking cessation program outweigh the risks.

Information for Patient

A patient instruction sheet is included in the package of PROSTEP systems dispensed to the patient. It contains important information and instructions on how to use and dispose of PROSTEP systems properly. Patients should be encouraged to ask questions of the physician and pharmacist.

Patients must be advised to keep both used and unused systems out of the reach of children and pets.

Drug Interactions

Smoking cessation, with or without nicotine replacement, may alter the pharmacokinetics of certain concomitant medications.

[See table above.]

May Require a Decrease in Dose at Cessation of Smoking	Possible Mechanism
acetaminophen, caffeine, imipramine, oxazepam, pentazocine, propranolol, theophylline	Deinduction of hepatic enzymes on smoking cessation
insulin	Increase of subcutaneous insulin absorption with smoking cessation
adrenergic antagonists (e.g., prazosin, labetalol)	Decrease in circulating catecholamines with smoking cessation

May Require an Increase in Dose at Cessation of Smoking	Possible Mechanism
adrenergic agonists (e.g., isoproterenol, phenylephrine)	Decrease in circulating catecholamines with smoking cessation

Carcinogenesis, Mutagenesis, Impairment of Fertility

Nicotine itself does not appear to be a carcinogen in laboratory animals. However, nicotine and its metabolites increased the incidences of tumors in the cheek pouches of hamsters and forestomach of F344 rats, respectively, when given in combination with tumor-initiators. One study, which could not be replicated, suggested that cotinine, the primary metabolite of nicotine, may cause lymphoreticular sarcoma in the large intestine in rats.

Neither nicotine nor cotinine were mutagenic in the Ames *Salmonella* test. Nicotine induced repairable DNA damage in an *E. coli* test system. Nicotine was shown to be genotoxic in a test system using Chinese hamster ovary cells. In rats and rabbits, implantation can be delayed or inhibited by a reduction in DNA synthesis that appears to be caused by nicotine. Studies have shown a decrease in litter size in rats treated with nicotine during gestation.

PREGNANCY

Pregnancy Category D (see WARNINGS section)

The harmful effects of cigarette smoking on maternal and fetal health are clearly established. These include low birth weight, an increased risk of spontaneous abortion, and increased perinatal mortality. The specific effects of PROSTEP treatment on fetal development are unknown. Therefore pregnant smokers should be encouraged to attempt cessation using educational and behavioral interventions before using pharmacological approaches.

Spontaneous abortion during nicotine replacement therapy has been reported; as with smoking, nicotine as a contributing factor cannot be excluded.

PROSTEP treatment should be used during pregnancy only if the likelihood of smoking cessation justifies the potential risk of use of nicotine replacement by the patient, who may continue to smoke.

Teratogenicity

Animal Studies: Nicotine was shown to produce skeletal abnormalities in the offspring of mice when given doses toxic to the dams (25 mg/kg IP or SC).

Human Studies: Nicotine teratogenicity has not been studied in humans except as a component of cigarette smoke (each cigarette smoked delivers about 1 mg of nicotine). It has not been possible to conclude whether cigarette smoking is teratogenic to humans.

Other Effects

Animal Studies: A nicotine bolus (up to 2 mg/kg) to pregnant rhesus monkeys caused acidosis, hypercarbia, and hypotension (fetal and maternal concentrations were about 20 times those achieved after smoking one cigarette in 5 minutes). Fetal breathing movements were reduced in the fetal lamb after intravenous injection of 0.25 mg/kg nicotine to the ewe (equivalent to smoking one cigarette every 20 seconds for 5 minutes). Uterine blood flow was reduced about 30% after infusion of 0.1 mg/kg/min nicotine for 20 minutes to pregnant rhesus monkeys (equivalent to smoking about six cigarettes every minute for 20 minutes).

Human Experience: Cigarette smoking during pregnancy is associated with an increased risk of spontaneous abortion, low birth weight infants and perinatal mortality. Nicotine and carbon monoxide are considered the most likely mediators of these outcomes. The effects of cigarette smoking on fetal cardiovascular parameters have been studied near term. Cigarettes increased fetal aortic blood flow and heart rate and decreased uterine blood flow and fetal breathing movements. PROSTEP treatment has not been studied in pregnant humans.

Labor and Delivery

PROSTEP systems are not recommended to be left on during labor and delivery. The effects of nicotine on the mother or the fetus during labor are unknown.

Use in Nursing Mothers

Caution should be exercised when PROSTEP therapy is administered to nursing women. The safety of PROSTEP treatment in nursing infants has not been examined. Nicotine passes freely into breast milk; the milk to plasma ratio averages 2.9. Nicotine is absorbed orally. An infant has the ability to clear nicotine by hepatic first pass clearance; however the efficiency of removal is probably lowest at birth. The nicotine concentrations in milk can be expected to be lower with PROSTEP treatment when used as directed than with cigarette smoking, as maternal plasma nicotine concentrations are generally reduced with nicotine replacement. The risk of exposure of the infant to nicotine from PROSTEP systems should be weighed against the risks associated with the infant's exposure to nicotine from continued smoking by the mother (passive smoke exposure and contamination of breast milk with other components of tobacco smoke) and from PROSTEP systems alone or in combination with continued smoking.

Pediatric Use

PROSTEP systems are not recommended for use in children because the safety and effectiveness of PROSTEP treatment in children and adolescents who smoke have not been evaluated.

Geriatric Use

Thirty patients over the age of 60 participated in clinical trials of PROSTEP therapy. PROSTEP therapy appeared to be as effective in this age group as in younger smokers.

ADVERSE REACTIONS

Assessment of adverse events in the 903 patients who participated in controlled clinical trials is complicated by the occurrence of GI and CNS effects of nicotine withdrawal as well as nicotine excess. The actual incidences of both are confounded by concurrent smoking by many of the patients. In the trials, when reporting adverse events, the investigators did not attempt to identify the cause of the symptom.

Topical Adverse Events

The most common adverse event associated with topical nicotine is a mild short-lived erythema, pruritus, or burning at the application site, which was seen at least once in 54% of patients (N = 459) on PROSTEP treatment in the 6–8 week clinical trials. Local erythema after system removal was noted at least once in 22% of patients and local edema in 8%. Erythema generally resolved within 24 hours. Cutaneous hypersensitivity (contact sensitization) occurred in 3% of patients on PROSTEP treatment (see **PRECAUTIONS, Allergic Reactions**). Skin discoloration at application sites has been rarely reported.

Probably Causally Related

The following adverse events were reported more frequently in PROSTEP-treated patients than in placebo-treated patients or exhibited a dose response in clinical trials. The reports of awakening at night were collected as one of the expected withdrawal symptoms.

Digestive system—Abdominal pain†
Nervous system—Somnolence*
Skin—Rash,† sweating†

Frequencies for 22 mg/day system
* Reported in 3% to 9% of patients
† Reported in 1% to 3% of patients
Unmarked if reported in < 1% of patients

Causal Relationship UNKNOWN

Adverse events reported in PROSTEP and placebo-treated patients at about the same frequency in clinical trials are listed below. The clinical significance of the association between PROSTEP treatment and these events is unknown, but they are reported as alerting information for the clinician.

Body as a Whole—Back pain,† pain*
Digestive system—Constipation,† dyspepsia, nausea†
Musculoskeletal system—Myalgia†
Nervous system—Dizziness,† headache (11%), insomnia*, abnormal dreams‡
Respiratory system—Pharyngitis,* sinusitis*
Urogenital system—Dysmenorrhea†

Frequencies for 22 mg/day system
* Reported in 3% to 9% of patients
† Reported in 1% to 3% of patients
‡ Spontaneous reports only, not seen in clinical trials.
Unmarked if reported in < 1% of patients

DRUG ABUSE AND DEPENDENCE

PROSTEP systems are likely to have a low abuse potential based on differences between it and cigarettes in four characteristics commonly considered important in contributing to abuse: much slower absorption, much smaller fluctuations in blood levels, lower blood levels of nicotine, and less frequent use (i.e., once daily).

Continued on next page

Lederle—Cont.

Nicotine Delivery Rate (in vivo)	Nicotine in System	System Size	Package Size	NDC Number
22 mg/day	30 mg	7.0 cm²	7 systems	0005-2402-90
11 mg/day	15 mg	3.5 cm²	7 systems	0005-2401-90

The abuse potential of PROSTEP systems was examined in a prospective, randomized trial of 10 smokers (5 drug abusers and 5 non-abusers). "Liking" scores for either one (22 mg/day) or two systems (44 mg/day) were no different from placebo. No abuse potential was observed in that study. Dependence on nicotine polacrilex chewing gum replacement therapy has been reported and such dependence might also occur from transference to PROSTEP systems of tobacco-based nicotine dependence. The use of the system beyond 3 months has not been evaluated and should be discouraged.

PROSTEP therapy has been evaluated in both a gradual and abrupt discontinuation of treatment. If gradual withdrawal is desirable, patients using the 22 mg/day PROSTEP treatment should use the 11 mg/day dosage for 2 to 4 weeks (see Individualization of Dosage and **DOSAGE AND ADMINISTRATION**).

OVERDOSAGE

The effects of applying several PROSTEP systems simultaneously or of swallowing unused PROSTEP systems are unknown (see **WARNINGS, Safety Note Concerning Children**). The oral LD$_{50}$ for nicotine in rodents varies with the species but is in excess of 24 mg/kg; death is due to respiratory paralysis. The oral minimum lethal dose of nicotine in dogs is greater than 5 mg/kg. The oral minimum acute lethal dose for nicotine in human adults is reported to be 40 to 60 mg (<1 mg/kg).

PROSTEP gels containing 8 mg of nicotine were ingested by 12 adult smokers with an average weight of 74 kg (range 62–93 kg). Peak nicotine serum levels were 9.5 ng/mL (range 3–18 ng/mL) and occurred at 2 hours (1–2 hours) and declined to baseline levels by 8 hours after ingestion. Some gastrointestinal effects (burning on ingestion and nausea) were reported.

Signs and symptoms of an overdose of PROSTEP systems would be expected to be the same as those of acute nicotine poisoning including: pallor, cold sweat, nausea, salivation, vomiting, abdominal pain, diarrhea, headache, dizziness, disturbed hearing and vision, tremor, mental confusion, and weakness. Prostration, hypotension, and respiratory failure may ensue with large overdoses. Lethal doses produce convulsions quickly and death follows as a result of peripheral or central respiratory paralysis or, less frequently, cardiac failure.

Overdose from Topical Exposure

The PROSTEP system should be removed immediately if the patient shows signs of overdosage and the patient should seek immediate medical care. The skin surface may be flushed with water and dried. No soap should be used since it may increase nicotine absorption. Nicotine will continue to be delivered into the bloodstream for several hours (see **Pharmacokinetics**) after removal of the system because of a depot of nicotine in the skin.

Overdose from Ingestion

Ingestion of a 22 mg/day PROSTEP system containing 30 mg of nicotine is potentially more harmful than ingestion of a used system which contains about 8 mg after 24 hours use. Persons ingesting PROSTEP systems should be referred to a health care facility for management. Due to the possibility of nicotine-induced seizures, activated charcoal should be administered. In unconscious patients with a secure airway, instill activated charcoal via nasogastric tube. A saline cathartic or sorbitol added to the first dose of activated charcoal may speed gastrointestinal passage of the system. Repeated doses of activated charcoal should be administered as long as the system remains in the gastrointestinal tract since it will continue to release nicotine for many hours.

Management of Nicotine Poisoning

Other supportive measures include diazepam or barbiturates for seizures, atropine for excessive bronchial secretions or diarrhea, respiratory support for respiratory failure, and vigorous fluid support for hypotension and cardiovascular collapse.

DOSAGE AND ADMINISTRATION

Patients must desire to stop smoking and should be instructed to *stop smoking immediately* as they begin using PROSTEP therapy. The patient should read the patient instruction sheet on PROSTEP treatment and be encouraged to ask any questions. Treatment should be initiated with PROSTEP 22 mg/day except for patients who weigh less than 100 pounds. They may start with PROSTEP 11 mg/day and the dose increased as appropriate (see **Individualization of Dosage**). Once the appropriate dosage is selected the patient should begin 4–8 weeks of therapy at that dosage. The patient should stop smoking cigarettes completely during this period. If the patient is unable to stop cigarette smoking within 4 weeks, PROSTEP should probably be stopped, since

few additional patients in clinical trials were able to quit after this time.

Those who have successfully stopped smoking during that time may have PROSTEP therapy discontinued. If a gradual reduction is desired, patients may be treated for an additional 2 to 4 weeks, after which treatment should be terminated.

The entire course of nicotine substitution should take 6–12 weeks. The use of PROSTEP systems beyond 3 months has not been studied and should be discouraged.

The PROSTEP system should be applied promptly upon its removal from the protective pouch to prevent evaporative loss of nicotine from the system. PROSTEP systems should be used only when the pouch is intact to assure that the product has not been tampered with.

PROSTEP systems should be applied only once a day to a non-hairy, clean, and dry skin site on the upper trunk or upper outer arm. After 24 hours, the used PROSTEP system should be removed and a new system applied to an alternate skin site. Skin sites should not be reused for at least a week. Patients should be cautioned not to continue to use the same system for more than 24 hours.

SAFETY AND HANDLING

PROSTEP systems can be a dermal irritant and can cause contact sensitization. Although exposure of health care workers to nicotine from PROSTEP systems should be minimal, care should be taken to avoid unnecessary contact with active systems. If you do handle active systems, wash with water alone, since soap may increase nicotine absorption. Do not touch your eyes.

Disposal

When the used system is removed from the skin, it should be folded over with the adhesive sides together and placed in the protective pouch which contained the new system. The used system should be immediately disposed of in such a way as to prevent its access by children or pets. See patient information for further directions for handling and disposal.

HOW SUPPLIED

[See table above.]

How to Store

Do not store above 25°C (77°F) because PROSTEP systems are sensitive to heat. A slight discoloration of the system is not significant.

Do not store unpouched. Once removed from the protective pouch, PROSTEP systems should be applied promptly since nicotine is volatile and the system may lose strength.

CAUTION: Federal law prohibits dispensing without prescription.

© 1992

Manufactured for
LEDERLE LABORATORIES DIVISION
Pearl River, New York 10965
by
élan pharma Ltd.
Athlone, County Westmeath
Ireland
Using Elan's DERMAFLEX® transdermal system.
Shown in Product Identification Guide, page 320

PYRAZINAMIDE TABLETS, USP ℞
500 mg

DESCRIPTION

Pyrazinamide, the pyrazine analogue of nicotinamide, is an antituberculous agent. It is a white crystalline powder, stable at room temperature, and sparingly soluble in water. Pyrazinamide has the following chemical formula: $C_5H_5N_3O$, and the following molecular weight: 123.11.

Each Pyrazinamide tablet for oral administration contains 500 mg of pyrazinamide and the following inactive ingredients: corn starch, magnesium stearate, modified food starch and stearic acid.

CLINICAL PHARMACOLOGY

Pyrazinamide is well absorbed from the GI tract and attains peak plasma concentrations within 2 hours. Plasma concentrations generally range from 30 to 50 mcg/mL with doses of 20 to 25 mg/kg. It is widely distributed in body tissues and fluids including the liver, lungs and cerebrospinal fluid (CSF). The CSF concentration is approximately equal to concurrent steady-state plasma concentrations in patients with inflamed meninges.[1] Pyrazinamide is approximately 10% bound to plasma proteins.[2]

The half-life (t1/2) of pyrazinamide is 9 to 10 hours in patients with normal renal and hepatic function. The plasma half-life may be prolonged in patients with impaired renal or hepatic function. Pyrazinamide is hydrolyzed in the liver to its major active metabolite, pyrazinoic acid. Pyrazinoic acid is hydroxylated to the main excretory product, 5-hydroxypyrazinoic acid.[3]

Approximately 70% of an oral dose is excreted in urine, mainly by glomerular filtration within 24 hours.[3]

Pyrazinamide may be bacteriostatic or bactericidal against *Mycobacterium tuberculosis* depending on the concentration of the drug attained at the site of infection. The mechanism of action is unknown. *In vitro* and *in vivo* the drug is active only at a slightly acidic pH.

INDICATIONS AND USAGE

Pyrazinamide is indicated for the initial treatment of active tuberculosis in adults and children when combined with other antituberculous agents. (The current recommendation of the CDC for drug-susceptible disease is to use a six-month regimen for initial treatment of active tuberculosis, consisting of isoniazid, rifampin and pyrazinamide given for 2 months, followed by isoniazid and rifampin for 4 months.*[4])

(Patients with drug-resistant disease should be treated with regimens individualized to their situation. Pyrazinamide frequently will be an important component of such therapy.)

(In patients with concomitant HIV infection, the physician should be aware of current recommendations of CDC. It is possible these patients may require a longer course of treatment.)

It is also indicated after treatment failure with other primary drugs in any form of active tuberculosis.

Pyrazinamide should only be used in conjunction with other effective antituberculous agents.

*See recommendations of Center for Disease Control (CDC) and American Thoracic Society for complete regimen and dosage recommendations.[4]

CONTRAINDICATIONS

Pyrazinamide is contraindicated in persons:
- with severe hepatic damage.
- who have shown hypersensitivity to it.
- with acute gout.

WARNINGS

Patients started on pyrazinamide should have baseline serum uric acid and liver function determinations. Those patients with preexisting liver disease or those at increased risk for drug related hepatitis (e.g., alcohol abusers) should be followed closely.

Pyrazinamide should be discontinued and not be resumed if signs of hepatocellular damage or hyperuricemia accompanied by an acute gouty arthritis appear.

PRECAUTIONS

General: Pyrazinamide inhibits renal excretion of urates, frequently resulting in hyperuricemia which is usually asymptomatic. If hyperuricemia is accompanied by acute gouty arthritis, pyrazinamide should be discontinued.

Pyrazinamide should be used with caution in patients with a history of diabetes mellitus, as management may be more difficult.

Primary resistance of *M. tuberculosis* to pyrazinamide is uncommon. In cases with known or suspected drug resistance, *in vitro* susceptibility tests with recent cultures of *M. tuberculosis* against pyrazinamide and the usual primary drugs should be performed. There are few reliable *in vitro* tests for pyrazinamide resistance. A reference laboratory capable of performing these studies must be employed.

Information for Patients: Patients should be instructed to notify their physicians promptly if they experience any of the following: fever, loss of appetite, malaise, nausea and vomiting, darkened urine, yellowish discoloration of the skin and eyes, pain or swelling of the joints.

Compliance with the full course of therapy must be emphasized, and the importance of not missing any doses must be stressed.

Laboratory Tests: Baseline liver function studies [especially ALT (SGPT), AST (SGOT) determinations] and uric acid levels should be determined prior to therapy. Appropriate laboratory testing should be performed at periodic intervals and if any clinical signs or symptoms occur during therapy.

Drug/Laboratory Test Interactions: Pyrazinamide has been reported to interfere with ACETEST® and KETOSTIX® urine tests to produce a pink-brown color.[5]

Carcinogenicity, Mutagenicity, Impairment of Fertility[6,7,8]: In lifetime bioassays in rats and mice, pyrazinamide was administered in the diet at concentrations of up to 10,000 ppm. This resulted in estimated daily doses for the mouse of 2 g/kg, or 40 times the maximum human dose, and for the rat of 0.5 g/kg, or 10 times the maximum human dose. Pyrazinamide was not carcinogenic in rats or male mice and no conclusion was possible for female mice due to insufficient numbers of surviving control mice.

Recommended Drugs for the Initial Treatment of Tuberculosis in Children and Adults

Drug	Daily Dose* Children	Daily Dose* Adults	Maximal Daily Dose in Children and Adults	Twice Weekly Dose Children	Twice Weekly Dose Adults
Isoniazid	10 to 20 mg/kg PO or IM	5 mg/kg PO or IM	300 mg	20 to 40 mg/kg Max. 900 mg	15 mg/kg Max. 900 mg
Rifampin	10 to 20 mg/kg PO	10 mg/kg PO	600 mg	10 to 20 mg/kg Max. 600 mg	10 mg/kg Max. 600 mg
Pyrazinamide	15 to 30 mg/kg PO	15 to 30 mg/kg PO	2 g	50 to 70 mg/kg	50 to 70 mg/kg
Streptomycin	20 to 40 mg/kg IM	15 mg/kg** IM	1 g**	25 to 30 mg/kg IM	25 to 30 mg/kg IM
Ethambutol	15 to 25 mg/kg PO	15 to 25 mg/kg PO	2.5 g	50 mg/kg	50 mg/kg

Definition of abbreviations: PO = perorally; IM = intramuscularly.

*Doses based on weight should be adjusted as weight changes.

**In persons older than 60 yrs of age the daily dose of streptomycin should be limited to 10 mg/kg with a maximal dose of 750 mg.

Pyrazinamide was not mutagenic in the Ames bacterial test, but induced chromosomal aberrations in human lymphocyte cell cultures.

Pregnancy: Teratogenic Effects—Pregnancy Category C: Animal reproduction studies have not been conducted with pyrazinamide. It is also not known whether pyrazinamide can cause fetal harm when administered to a pregnant woman or can affect reproduction capacity. Pyrazinamide should be given to a pregnant woman only if clearly needed.

Nursing Mothers: Pyrazinamide has been found in small amounts in breast milk. Therefore, it is advised the pyrazinamide be used with caution in nursing mothers taking into account the risk-benefit of this therapy.[9]

Usage in Children: Pyrazinamide regimens employed in adults are probably equally effective in children.[4,10,11] Pyrazinamide appears to be well tolerated in children.

Geriatric Use[12]: Clinical studies of pyrazinamide did not include sufficient numbers of patients aged 65 and over to determine whether they respond differently from younger patients. Other reported clinical experience has not identified differences in responses between the elderly and younger patients. In general, dose selection for an elderly patient should be cautious, usually starting at the low end of the dosing range, reflecting the greater frequency of decreased hepatic or renal function, and of concomitant disease or other drug therapy.

It does not appear that patients with impaired renal function require a reduction in dose. It may be prudent to select doses at the low end of the dosing range, however.[13]

ADVERSE REACTIONS

General: Fever, porphyria and dysuria have rarely been reported. Gout (see PRECAUTIONS).

Gastrointestinal: The principal adverse effect is a hepatic reaction (see WARNINGS). Hepatotoxicity appears to be dose related, and may appear at any time during therapy. GI disturbances including nausea, vomiting and anorexia have also been reported.

Hematologic and Lymphatic: Thrombocytopenia and sideroblastic anemia with erythroid hyperplasia, vacuolation of erythrocytes and increased serum iron concentration have occurred rarely with this drug. Adverse effects on blood clotting mechanisms have also been rarely reported.

Other: Mild arthralgia and myalgia have been reported frequently. Hypersensitivity reactions including rashes, urticaria, and pruritus have been reported. Fever, acne, photosensitivity, porphyria, dysuria and interstitial nephritis have been reported rarely.

OVERDOSAGE

Overdosage experience is limited. In one case report of overdose, abnormal liver function tests developed. These spontaneously reverted to normal when the drug was stopped. Clinical monitoring and supportive therapy should be employed. Pyrazinamide is dialyzable.[13]

DOSAGE AND ADMINISTRATION

Pyrazinamide should always be administered with other effective antituberculous drugs. It is administered for the initial 2 months of a 6-month or longer treatment regimen for drug-susceptible patients. Patients who are known or suspected to have drug-resistant disease should be treated with regimens individualized to their situation. Pyrazinamide frequently will be an important component of such therapy.

Patients with concomitant HIV infection may require longer courses of therapy. Physicians treating such patients should be alert to any revised recommendations from CDC for this group of patients.

Usual dose: Pyrazinamide is administered orally, 15 to 30 mg/kg once daily. Older regimens employed 3 to 4 divided doses daily, but most current recommendations are for once a day. Three grams per day should not be exceeded. The CDC recommendations do not exceed 2 g per day when given as a daily regimen (see table).

Alternatively, a twice weekly dosing regimen (50 to 70 mg/kg twice weekly based on lean body weight) has been developed to promote patient compliance with a regimen on an outpatient basis. In studies evaluating the twice weekly regimen, doses of pyrazinamide in excess of 3 g twice weekly have been administered. This exceeds the recommended maximum 3 g/daily dose. However, an increased incidence of adverse reactions has not been reported.

The table is taken from the CDC-American Thoracic Society joint recommendations:[4]

[See table above.]

HOW SUPPLIED

Pyrazinamide Tablets, USP 500 mg are round, white, scored tablets, engraved P36 on the scored side, and LL on the other side, supplied as:

NDC 0005-5093-23 - Bottle of 100
NDC 0005-5093-31 - Bottle of 500

Store in a well-closed container at controlled room temperature 15°–30°C (59°–86°F).

Caution: Federal law prohibits dispensing without prescription.

LEDERLE LABORATORIES
A Division of American Cyanamid Company, Pearl River, NY 10965

REFERENCES

1. *Drug Information, American Hospital Formulary Service.* American Society of Hospital Pharmacists. Bethesda, Md. 1991.
2. *USPDI, Drug Information for the Health Care Professional.* United States Pharmacopeial Convention, Inc. Rockville, Md. 1991:1B:2226–2227.
3. Goodman-Gilman A, Rall TW, Nies AS, Taylor P. *The Pharmacological Basis of Therapeutics,* ed 8. New York, Pergamon Press. 1990;1154.
4. Treatment of tuberculosis and tuberculosis infection in adults and children. *Am Rev Respir Dis.* 1986;134:363–368.
5. Reynolds JEF, Parfitt K, Parsons AV, Sweetman SC. *Martindale The Extra Pharmacopoeia,* ed 29. London, The Pharmaceutical Press. 1989;569-570.
6. Bioassay of pyrazinamide for possible carcinogenicity. National Cancer Institute Carcinogenesis Technical Report Series No. 48, 1978.
7. Zerger E, Anderson B, Haworth S, Lawlor T, Mortelmans K, Speck W. Salmonella mutagenicity tests: III. Results from the testing of 255 chemicals. *Environ Mutagen.* 1987;9(Suppl 9):1–109.
8. Roman IC, Georgian L. Cytogenetic effects of some antituberculosis drugs in vitro. *Mutation Research.* 1977;48:215–224.
9. Holdiness M. Antituberculosis drugs and breast-feeding. *Arch Intern Med.* 1984;144:1888.
10. Turcios N, Evans H. Preventing and managing tuberculosis in children. *J Resp Dis.* 1989;10(6)(Jun):23.
11. Starke JR. Multidrug therapy for tuberculosis in children. *Pediatr Infec Dis J.* 1990;9:785–793.
12. Specific requirements on content and format of labeling for human prescription drugs; proposed addition of "geriatric use" subsection in the labeling. *Federal Register.* 1990;55(212) (Nov 1):46134–46137.
13. Stamathakis G, Montes C, Trouvin JH, et al. Pyrazinamide and pyrazinoic acid pharmacokinetics in patients with chronic renal failure. *Clinical Nephrology.* 1988;30:230–234.

RHEUMATREX® Dose Pack ℞
Methotrexate 2.5 mg Tablets

Please see page 1322 for full Prescribing Information for Methotrexate.

Shown in Product Identification Guide, page 321

SUPRAX® ℞
Cefixime
Oral

DESCRIPTION

SUPRAX (cefixime) is a semisynthetic, cephalosporin antibiotic for oral administration. Chemically, it is (6R,7R)-7-[2-(2-Amino-4-thiazolyl)glyoxylamido]-8-oxo-3-vinyl-5-thia-1-azabicyclo[4.2.0]oct-2-ene-2-carboxylic acid, 7^2-(Z)-[O-(carboxymethyl)oxime]trihydrate. Molecular weight = 507.50 as the trihydrate.

SUPRAX is available in scored 200 mg and 400 mg film coated tablets and in a powder for oral suspension which, when reconstituted provides 100 mg/5 mL.

Inactive ingredients contained in the 200 mg and 400 mg tablets are: dibasic calcium phosphate, hydroxypropyl methylcellulose 2910, light mineral oil, magnesium stearate, microcrystalline cellulose, pregelatinized starch, sodium lauryl sulfate, and titanium dioxide. The powder for oral suspension is strawberry flavored and contains sodium benzoate, sucrose, and xanthan gum.

CLINICAL PHARMACOLOGY

SUPRAX, given orally, is about 40% to 50% absorbed whether administered with or without food; however, time to maximal absorption is increased approximately 0.8 hours when administered with food. A single 200 mg tablet of SUPRAX produces an average peak serum concentration of approximately 2 mcg/mL (range 1 to 4 mcg/mL); a single 400 mg tablet produces an average peak concentration of approximately 3.7 mcg/mL (range 1.3 to 7.7 mcg/mL). The oral suspension produces average peak concentrations approximately 25%–50% higher than the tablets, when tested in normal *adult* volunteers. Two hundred and 400 mg doses of oral suspension produce average peak concentrations of 3 mcg/mL (range 1 to 4.5 mcg/mL) and 4.6 mcg/mL (range 1.9 to 7.7 mcg/mL), respectively, when tested in normal *adult* volunteers. The area under the time versus concentration curve is greater by approximately 10%–25% with the oral suspension than with the tablet after doses of 100 to 400 mg, when tested in normal *adult* volunteers. This increased absorption should be taken into consideration if the oral suspension is to be substituted for the tablet. Because of the lack of bioequivalence, tablets should not be substituted for oral suspension in the treatment of otitis media. (See **DOSAGE AND ADMINISTRATION**.) Cross-over studies of tablet versus suspension have not been performed in children.

Peak serum concentrations occur between 2 and 6 hours following oral administration of a single 200 mg tablet, a single 400 mg tablet, or 400 mg of suspension of SUPRAX. Peak serum concentrations occur between 2 and 5 hours following a single administration of 200 mg of suspension.

TABLE

Serum Levels of Cefixime After Administration of Tablets (mcg/mL)

DOSE	1h	2h	4h	6h	8h	12h	24h
100 mg	0.3	0.8	1.0	0.7	0.4	0.2	0.02
200 mg	0.7	1.4	2.0	1.5	1.0	0.4	0.03
400 mg	1.2	2.5	3.5	2.7	1.7	0.6	0.04

Serum Levels of Cefixime After Administration of Oral Suspension (mcg/mL)

DOSE	1h	2h	4h	6h	8h	12h	24h
100 mg	0.7	1.1	1.3	0.9	0.6	0.2	0.02
200 mg	1.2	2.1	2.8	2.0	1.3	0.5	0.07
400 mg	1.8	3.3	4.4	3.3	2.2	0.8	0.07

Approximately 50% of the absorbed dose is excreted unchanged in the urine in 24 hours. In animal studies, it was noted that cefixime is also excreted in the bile in excess of 10% of the administered dose. Serum protein binding is concentration independent with a bound fraction of approximately 65%. In a multiple dose study conducted with a research formulation which is less bioavailable than the tablet or suspension, there was little accumulation of drug in serum or urine after dosing for 14 days.

The serum half-life of cefixime in healthy subjects is independent of dosage form and averages 3.0–4.0 hours but may range up to 9 hours in some normal volunteers. Average AUCs at steady state in elderly patients are approximately 40% higher than average AUCs in other healthy adults.

Continued on next page

Lederle—Cont.

In subjects with moderate impairment of renal function (20 to 40mL/min creatinine clearance), the average serum half-life of cefixime is prolonged to 6.4 hours. In severe renal impairment (5 to 20 mL/min creatinine clearance), the half-life increased to an average of 11.5 hours. The drug is not cleared significantly from the blood by hemodialysis or peritoneal dialysis. However, a study indicated that with doses of 400 mg, patients undergoing hemodialysis have similar blood profiles as subjects with creatinine clearances of 21–60 mL/min. There is no evidence of metabolism of cefixime *in vivo*. Adequate data on CSF levels of cefixime are not available.

Microbiology: As with other cephalosporins, bactericidal action of SUPRAX results from inhibition of cell-wall synthesis. SUPRAX is highly stable in the presence of beta-lactamase enzymes. As a result, many organisms resistant to penicillins and some cephalosporins due to the presence of beta-lactamases, may be susceptible to cefixime. SUPRAX has been shown to be active against most strains of the following organisms both *in vitro* and in clinical infections (see **INDICATIONS AND USAGE**):

Gram-positive Organisms
Streptococcus pneumoniae
Streptococcus pyogenes
Gram-negative Organisms
Haemophilus influenzae (beta-lactamase positive and negative strains)
Moraxella (Branhamella) catarrhalis (most of which are beta-lactamase positive)
Escherichia coli
Proteus mirabilis
Neisseria gonorrhoeae (including penicillinase- and non-penicillinase-producing strains)

SUPRAX has been shown to be active *in vitro* against most strains of the following organisms; however, clinical efficacy has not been established.

Gram-positive Organisms
Streptococcus agalactiae
Gram-negative Organisms
Haemophilus parainfluenzae (beta-lactamase positive and negative strains)
Proteus vulgaris
Klebsiella pneumoniae
Klebsiella oxytoca
Pasteurella multocida
Providencia species
Salmonella species
Shigella species
Citrobacter amalonaticus
Citrobacter diversus
Serratia marcescens

Note: *Pseudomonas* species, strains of group D streptococci (including enterococci), *Listeria monocytogenes*, most strains of staphylococci (including methicillin-resistant strains) and most strains of *Enterobacter* are resistant to SUPRAX. In addition, most strains of *Bacteroides fragilis* and *Clostridia* are resistant to SUPRAX.

SUSCEPTIBILITY TESTING

Susceptibility Tests: *Diffusion Techniques:* Quantitative methods that require measurement of zone diameters give an estimate of antibiotic susceptibility. One such procedure[1–3] has been recommended for use with disks to test susceptibility to cefixime. Interpretation involves correlation of the diameters obtained in the disk test with minimum inhibitory concentration (MIC) for cefixime.

Reports from the laboratory giving results of the standard single-disk susceptibility test with a 5-mcg cefixime disk should be interpreted according to the following criteria:
[See table below.]
A report of "Susceptible" indicates that the pathogen is likely to be inhibited by generally achievable blood levels. A report of "Moderately Susceptible" indicates that inhibitory concentrations of the antibiotic may well be achieved if high dosage is used or if the infection is confined to tissues and fluids (eg, urine) in which high antibiotic levels are attained. A report of "Resistant" indicates that achievable concentrations of the antibiotic are unlikely to be inhibitory and other therapy should be selected.

Standardized procedures require the use of laboratory control organisms. The 5-mcg disk should give the following zone diameter:

MIC Interpretive Standards (µg/mL)

Organisms	Resistant	Moderately Susceptible	Susceptible
Neisseria gonorrhoeae[a]	—	—	≤ 0.25
All other organisms	≥ 4	2	≤ 1

Organism	Zone diameter (mm)
E. coli ATCC 25922	23–27
N. gonorrhoeae ATCC 49226[a]	37–45

[a] Using GC Agar Base with a defined 1% supplement without cysteine.

The class disk for cephalosporin susceptibility testing (the cephalothin disk) is not appropriate because of spectrum differences with cefixime. The 5-mcg cefixime disk should be used for all *in vitro* testing of isolates.

Dilution Techniques: Broth or agar dilution methods can be used to determine the minimum inhibitory concentration (MIC) value for susceptibility of bacterial isolates to cefixime. The recommended susceptibility breakpoints are as follows:
[See table above.]
As with standard diffusion methods, dilution procedures require the use of laboratory control organisms. Standard cefixime powder should give the following MIC ranges in daily testing of quality control organisms:

Organism	MIC Range (µg/mL)
E. coli ATCC 25922	0.25 –1
S. aureus ATCC 29213	8–32
N. gonorrhoeae ATCC 49226[a]	0.008-0.03

[a] Using GC Agar Base with a defined 1% supplement without cysteine.

INDICATIONS AND USAGE

SUPRAX is indicated in the treatment of the following infections when caused by susceptible strains of the designated microorganisms:

Uncomplicated Urinary Tract Infections caused by *Escherichia coli* and *Proteus mirabilis*.

Otitis Media caused by *Haemophilus influenzae* (beta-lactamase positive and negative strains), *Moraxella (Branhamella) catarrhalis*, (most of which are beta-lactamase positive) and *S. pyogenes*.*

Note: For information on otitis media caused by *Streptococcus pneumoniae*, see **CLINICAL STUDIES** section.

Pharyngitis and Tonsillitis, caused by *S. pyogenes*.

Note: Penicillin is the usual drug of choice in the treatment of *S. pyogenes* infections, including the prophylaxis of rheumatic fever. SUPRAX is generally effective in the eradication of *S. pyogenes* from the nasopharynx; however, data establishing the efficacy of SUPRAX in the subsequent prevention of rheumatic fever are not available.

Acute Bronchitis and Acute Exacerbations of Chronic Bronchitis, caused by *Streptococcus pneumoniae* and *Haemophilus influenzae* (beta-lactamase positive and negative strains).

Uncomplicated Gonorrhea (Cervical/Urethral), caused by *Neisseria gonorrhoeae* (penicillinase- and nonpenicillinase-producing strains).

Appropriate cultures and susceptibility studies should be performed to determine the causative organism and its susceptibility to SUPRAX; however, therapy may be started while awaiting the results of these studies. Therapy should be adjusted, if necessary, once these results are known.

*Efficacy for this organism in this organ system was studied in fewer than 10 infections.

CLINICAL STUDIES

In clinical trials of otitis media in nearly 400 children between the ages of 6 months to 10 years, *Streptococcus pneumoniae* was isolated from 47% of the patients, *Haemophilus influenzae* from 34%, *Moraxella (Branhamella) catarrhalis* from 15%, and *S. pyogenes* from 4%.

The overall response rate of *Streptococcus pneumoniae* to cefixime was approximately 10% lower and that of *Haemophilus influenzae* or *Moraxella (Branhamella) catarrhalis* approximately 7% higher (12% when beta-lactamase positive strains of *H. influenzae* are included) than the response rates of these organisms to the active control drugs.

In these studies, patients were randomized and treated with either cefixime at dose regimens of 4 mg/kg BID or 8 mg/kg QD, or with a standard antibiotic regimen. Sixty-nine to 70% of the patients in each group had resolution of signs and symptoms of otitis media when evaluated 2 to 4 weeks post-treatment, but persistent effusion was found in 15% of the patients. When evaluated at the completion of therapy, 17% of patients receiving cefixime and 14% of patients receiving effective comparative drugs (18% including those patients who had *Haemophilus influenzae* resistant to the control drug and who received the control antibiotic) were considered to be treatment failures. By the 2 to 4 week follow-up, a total of 30%–31% of patients had evidence of either treatment failure or recurrent disease.
[See table at top of next page.]

CONTRAINDICATIONS

SUPRAX is contraindicated in patients with known allergy to the cephalosporin group of antibiotics.

WARNINGS

BEFORE THERAPY WITH SUPRAX IS INSTITUTED, CAREFUL INQUIRY SHOULD BE MADE TO DETERMINE WHETHER THE PATIENT HAS HAD PREVIOUS HYPERSENSITIVITY REACTIONS TO CEPHALOSPORINS, PENICILLINS, OR OTHER DRUGS. IF THIS PRODUCT IS TO BE GIVEN TO PENICILLIN-SENSITIVE PATIENTS, CAUTION SHOULD BE EXERCISED BECAUSE CROSS-HYPERSENSITIVITY AMONG BETA-LACTAM ANTIBIOTICS HAS BEEN CLEARLY DOCUMENTED AND MAY OCCUR IN UP TO 10% OF PATIENTS WITH A HISTORY OF PENICILLIN ALLERGY. IF AN ALLERGIC REACTION TO SUPRAX OCCURS, DISCONTINUE THE DRUG. SERIOUS ACUTE HYPERSENSITIVITY REACTIONS MAY REQUIRE TREATMENT WITH EPINEPHRINE AND OTHER EMERGENCY MEASURES, INCLUDING OXYGEN, INTRAVENOUS FLUIDS, INTRAVENOUS ANTIHISTAMINES, CORTICOSTEROIDS, PRESSOR AMINES AND AIRWAY MANAGEMENT, AS CLINICALLY INDICATED.

Antibiotics, including SUPRAX, should be administered cautiously to any patient who has demonstrated some form of allergy, particularly to drugs.

Treatment with broad-spectrum antibiotics, including SUPRAX, alters the normal flora of the colon and may permit overgrowth of clostridia. Studies indicate that a toxin produced by *Clostridium difficile* is a primary cause of severe antibiotic-associated diarrhea, including pseudomembranous colitis.

Pseudomembranous colitis has been reported with the use of SUPRAX and other broad-spectrum antibiotics (including macrolides, semisynthetic penicillins, and cephalosporins); therefore, it is important to consider this diagnosis in patients who develop diarrhea in association with the use of antibiotics. Symptoms of pseudomembranous colitis may occur during or after antibiotic treatment and may range in severity from mild to life- threatening. Mild cases of pseudomembranous colitis usually respond to drug discontinuation alone. In moderate to severe cases, management should include fluids, electrolytes, and protein supplementation. If the colitis does not improve after the drug has been discontinued, or if the symptoms are severe, oral vancomycin is the drug of choice for antibiotic-associated pseudomembranous colitis produced by *C difficile*. Other causes of colitis should be excluded.

PRECAUTIONS

General: The possibility of the emergence of resistant organisms, which might result in overgrowth should be kept in mind, particularly during prolonged treatment. In such use, careful observation of the patient is essential. If superinfection occurs during therapy, appropriate measures should be taken.

The dose of SUPRAX should be adjusted in patients with renal impairment as well as those undergoing continuous ambulatory peritoneal dialysis (CAPD) and hemodialysis (HD). Patients on dialysis should be monitored carefully. (See **DOSAGE AND ADMINISTRATION**.)

SUPRAX should be prescribed with caution in individuals with a history of gastrointestinal disease, particularly colitis.

Drug Interactions: No significant drug interactions have been reported to date.

Drug/Laboratory Test Interactions: A false-positive reaction for ketones in the urine may occur with tests using nitroprusside but not with those using nitroferricyanide. The administration of SUPRAX may result in a false-positive reaction for glucose in the urine using Clinitest®,** Benedict's solution, or Fehling's solution. It is recommended

SUPRAX®	Recommended Susceptibility Ranges: Agar Disk Diffusion		
Organisms	Resistant	Moderately Susceptible	Susceptible
Neisseria gonorrhoeae[a]	—	—	≥ 31 mm
All other organisms	≤ 15 mm	16–18 mm	≥ 19 mm

[a] Using GC Agar Base with a defined 1% supplement without cysteine.

Bacteriological Outcome of Otitis Media at 2 to 4 Weeks Posttherapy
Based on Repeat Middle Ear Fluid Culture or
Extrapolation from Clinical Outcome

Organism	Cefixime[a] 4 mg/kg BID		Cefixime[a] 8 mg/kg QD		Control[a] drugs	
Streptococcus pneumoniae	48/70	(69%)	18/22	(82%)	82/100	(82%)
Haemophilus influenzae beta-lactamase negative	24/34	(71%)	13/17	(76%)	23/34	(68%)
Haemophilus influenzae beta-lactamase positive	17/22	(77%)	9/12	(75%)	1/1[b]	
Moraxella (Branhamella) catarrhalis	26/31	(84%)	5/5		18/24	(75%)
S pyogenes	5/5		3/3		6/7	
All Isolates	120/162	(74%)	48/59	(81%)	130/166	(78%)

[a] Number eradicated/number isolated.
[b] An additional 20 beta-lactamase positive strains of *Haemophilus influenzae* were isolated, but were excluded from this analysis because they were resistant to the control antibiotic. In nineteen of these, the clinical course could be assessed, and a favorable outcome occurred in 10. When these cases are included in the overall bacteriological evaluation of therapy with the control drugs, 140/185 (76%) of pathogens were considered to be eradicated.

that glucose tests based on enzymatic glucose oxidase reactions (such as Clinistix®** or Tes-Tape®**) be used.
A false-positive direct Coombs test has been reported during treatment with other cephalosporin antibiotics; therefore, it should be recognized that a positive Coombs test may be due to the drug.
Carcinogenesis, Mutagenesis, Impairment of Fertility: Lifetime studies in animals to evaluate carcinogenic potential have not been conducted. SUPRAX did not cause point mutations in bacteria or mammalian cells, DNA damage, or chromosome damage *in vitro* and did not exhibit clastogenic potential *in vivo* in the mouse micronucleus test. In rats, fertility and reproductive performance were not affected by cefixime at doses up to 125 times the adult therapeutic dose.
Usage in Pregnancy: *Pregnancy Category B:* Reproduction studies have been performed in mice and rats at doses up to 400 times the human dose and have revealed no evidence of harm to the fetus due to SUPRAX. There are no adequate and well-controlled studies in pregnant women. Because animal reproduction studies are not always predictive of human response, this drug should be used during pregnancy only if clearly needed.
Labor and Delivery: SUPRAX has not been studied for use during labor and delivery. Treatment should only be given if clearly needed.
Nursing Mothers: It is not known whether SUPRAX is excreted in human milk. Consideration should be given to discontinuing nursing temporarily during treatment with this drug.
Pediatric Use: Safety and effectiveness of SUPRAX in children aged less than 6 months old have not been established. The incidence of gastrointestinal adverse reactions, including diarrhea and loose stools, in the pediatric patients receiving the suspension, was comparable to the incidence seen in adult patients receiving tablets.

ADVERSE REACTIONS
Most of the adverse reactions observed in clinical trials were of a mild and transient nature. Five percent (5%) of patients in the US trials discontinued therapy because of drug-related adverse reactions. The most commonly seen adverse reactions in US trials of the tablet formulation were gastrointestinal events, which were reported in 30% of adult patients on either the BID or the QD regimen. Clinically mild gastrointestinal side effects occurred in 20% of all patients, moderate events occurred in 9% of all patients, and severe adverse reactions occurred in 2% of all patients. Individual event rates included diarrhea 16%, loose or frequent stools 6%, abdominal pain 3%, nausea 7%, dyspepsia 3%, and flatulence 4%. The incidence of gastrointestinal adverse reactions, including diarrhea and loose stools, in pediatric patients receiving the suspension was comparable to the incidence seen in adult patients receiving tablets.
These symptoms usually responded to symptomatic therapy or ceased when SUPRAX was discontinued.
Several patients developed severe diarrhea and/or documented pseudomembranous colitis, and a few required hospitalization.
The following adverse reactions have been reported following the use of SUPRAX. Incidence rates were less than 1 in 50 (less than 2%), except as noted above for gastrointestinal events.
Gastrointestinal (SEE ABOVE): Diarrhea, loose stools, abdominal pain, dyspepsia, nausea, and vomiting. Several cases of documented pseudomembranous colitis were identified during the studies. The onset of pseudomembranous colitis symptoms may occur during or after therapy.
Hypersensitivity Reactions: Skin rashes, urticaria, drug fever, and pruritus. Erythema multiforme, Stevens-Johnson syndrome, and serum sickness-like reactions have been reported.

Hepatic: Transient elevations in SGPT, SGOT, and alkaline phosphatase.
Renal: Transient elevations in BUN or creatinine.
Central Nervous System: Headaches or dizziness.
Hemic and Lymphatic Systems: Transient thrombocytopenia, leukopenia, and eosinophilia. Prolongation in prothrombin time was seen rarely.
Other: Genital pruritus, vaginitis, candidiasis.
In addition to the adverse reactions listed above, which have been observed in patients treated with SUPRAX, the following adverse reactions and altered laboratory tests have been reported for cephalosporin-class antibiotics:
Adverse Reactions: Allergic reactions including anaphylaxis, toxic epidermal necrolysis, superinfection, renal dysfunction, toxic nephropathy, hepatic dysfunction including cholestasis, aplastic anemia, hemolytic anemia, hemorrhage, and colitis.
Several cephalosporins have been implicated in triggering seizures, particularly in patients with renal impairment when the dosage was not reduced. (See **DOSAGE AND ADMINISTRATION** and **OVERDOSAGE.**) If seizures associated with drug therapy occur, the drug should be discontinued. Anticonvulsant therapy can be given if clinically indicated.
Abnormal Laboratory Tests: Positive direct Coombs test, elevated bilirubin, elevated LDH, pancytopenia, neutropenia, agranulocytosis.

OVERDOSAGE
Gastric lavage may be indicated; otherwise, no specific antidote exists. Cefixime is not removed in significant quantities from the circulation by hemodialysis or peritoneal dialysis. Adverse reactions in small numbers of healthy adult volunteers receiving single doses up to 2 g of SUPRAX did not differ from the profile seen in patients treated at the recommended doses.

DOSAGE AND ADMINISTRATION
Adults: The recommended dose of SUPRAX is 400 mg daily. This may be given as a 400 mg tablet daily or as 200 mg tablet every 12 hours.
For the treatment of uncomplicated cervical/urethral gonococcal infections, a single oral dose of 400 mg is recommended.
Children: The recommended dose is 8 mg/kg/day of the suspension. This may be administered as a single daily dose or may be given in two divided doses, as 4 mg/kg every 12 hours.

PEDIATRIC DOSAGE CHART

Patient Weight (kg)	Dose/Day mg	Dose/Day mL	Dose/Day tsp of suspension
6.25	50	2.5	0.5
12.5	100	5.0	1.0
18.75	150	7.5	1.5
25.0	200	10.0	2.0
31.25	250	12.5	2.5
37.5	300	15.0	3.0

Children weighing more than 50 kg or older than 12 years should be treated with the recommended adult dose.
Otitis media should be treated with the suspension. Clinical studies of otitis media were conducted with the suspension, and the suspension results in higher peak blood levels than the tablet when administered at the same dose. Therefore, the tablet should not be substituted for the suspension in the treatment of otitis media. (See **CLINICAL PHARMACOLOGY.**)

Efficacy and safety in infants aged less than six months have not been established.
In the treatment of infections due to *S pyogenes,* a therapeutic dosage of SUPRAX should be administered for at least 10 days.
Renal Impairment: SUPRAX may be administered in the presence of impaired renal function. Normal dose and schedule may be employed in patients with creatinine clearances of 60 mL/min or greater. Patients whose clearance is between 21 and 60 mL/min or patients who are on renal hemodialysis may be given 75% of the standard dosage at the standard dosing interval (ie, 300 mg daily). Patients whose clearance is < 20 mL/min, or patients who are on continuous ambulatory peritoneal dialysis may be given half the standard dosage at the standard dosing interval (ie, 200 mg daily). Neither hemodialysis nor peritoneal dialysis removes significant amounts of drug from the body.

Reconstitution Directions for Oral Suspension:

Bottle Size	Reconstitution Directions
100 mL	To reconstitute, suspend with **69 mL water.** Method: Tap the bottle several times to loosen powder contents prior to reconstitution. Add approximately half the total amount of water for reconstitution and shake well. Add the remainder of water and shake well.
75 mL	To reconstitute, suspend with **52 mL water.** Method: Tap the bottle several times to loosen powder contents prior to reconstitution. Add approximately half the total amount of water for reconstitution and shake well. Add the remainder of water and shake well.
50 mL	To reconstitute, suspend with **36 mL water.** Method: Tap the bottle several times to loosen powder contents prior to reconstitution. Add approximately half the total amount of water for reconstitution and shake well. Add the remainder of water and shake well.

After reconstitution, the suspension may be kept for 14 days either at room temperature, or under refrigeration, without significant loss of potency. Keep tightly closed. Shake well before using. Discard unused portion after 14 days.

HOW SUPPLIED
SUPRAX® (cefixime) Tablets, 200 mg, are convex, rectangular, white, film-coated tablets with rounded corners and beveled edges and a divided break line on each side, engraved with SUPRAX across one side and LL to the left and 200 to the right on the other side, supplied as follows:
NDC 0005-3899-23—Bottle of 100
Store at Controlled Room Temperature 15°–30°C (59°–86°F).
SUPRAX® (cefixime) Tablets, 400 mg, are convex, rectangular, white, film-coated tablets with rounded corners and beveled edges and a divided break line on each side, engraved with SUPRAX across one side and LL to the left and 400 to the right on the other side, supplied as follows:
NDC 0005-3897-94—Unit-of-Issue 10s with CRC
NDC 0005-3897-18—Bottle of 50
NDC 0005-3897-23—Bottle of 100
NDC 0005-3897-60—10 (2 × 5) Strips
Store at Controlled Room Temperature 15°–30°C (59°–86°F).
SUPRAX® (cefixime) for Oral Suspension is an off-white to cream-colored powder which when reconstituted as directed contains cefixime 100 mg/5 mL, supplied as follows:
NDC 0005-3898-40—50 mL Bottle
NDC 0005-3898-42—75 mL Bottle
NDC 0005-3898-46—100 mL Bottle
Prior to Reconstitution: Store at Controlled Room Temperature 15°–30°C (59°–86°F).

REFERENCES
1. Bauer AW, Kirby WMM, Sherris JC, et al: Antibiotic susceptibility testing by a standard single disk method. *Am J Clin Pathol* 1966;45:493.
2. National Committee for Clinical Laboratory Standards, Approved Standard: Performance Standards for Antimicrobial Disk Susceptibility Tests (M2-A3), December 1984.
3. Standardized disk susceptibility test. *Federal Register.* 1974;39(May 30): 19182–19184.

**Clinitest® and Clinistix® are registered trademarks of Ames Division, Miles Laboratories, Inc. Tes-Tape® is a registered trademark of Eli Lilly and Company.
Marketed by
ADVANTUS Pharmaceuticals
LEDERLE LABORATORIES DIVISION
American Cyanamid Company, Pearl River, NY 10965

Continued on next page

Lederle—Cont.

Under License of
Fujisawa Pharmaceutical Co., Ltd.
Osaka, Japan
Shown in Product Identification Guide, page 321

**TETANUS AND DIPHTHERIA
TOXOIDS ADSORBED**
FOR ADULT USE
Aluminum Phosphate-Adsorbed
PUROGENATED®   ℞

DESCRIPTION
Tetanus and Diphtheria Toxoids Adsorbed For Adult Use, aluminum phosphate-adsorbed PUROGENATED is a sterile combination of refined tetanus and diphtheria toxoids for intramuscular use only. After shaking, the vaccine is a homogeneous white suspension.
The tetanus and diphtheria toxins are produced according to the method of Mueller and Miller,[1,2] and are detoxified by use of formaldehyde. The toxoids are refined by the Pillemer alcohol fractionation method[3] and are diluted with a solution containing sodium phosphate monobasic, sodium phosphate dibasic, aluminum phosphate, glycine and thimerosal (mercury derivative) as a preservative. The final concentration of thimerosal in the combined vaccine is 1:10,000. The aluminum content of the final product does not exceed 0.80 mg per 0.5 mL dose.
Each 0.5 mL dose is formulated to contain 5 Lf units of tetanus toxoid and 2 Lf units of diphtheria toxoid.

CLINICAL PHARMACOLOGY
Tetanus is an intoxication manifested primarily by neuromuscular dysfunction, caused by a potent exotoxin elaborated by *Clostridium tetani*. The incidence of tetanus in the U.S. has dropped dramatically with the routine use of tetanus toxoid, remaining relatively constant over the last decade at about 90 cases reported annually.[4] Spores of *C tetani* are ubiquitous, and there is essentially no natural immunity to tetanus toxin. Thus, universal primary immunization with tetanus toxoid, and subsequent maintenance of adequate antitoxin levels by means of timed boosters, is necessary to protect all age groups.[4] Tetanus toxoid is a highly effective antigen, and a completed primary series generally induces protective levels of serum antitoxin that persist for at least 10 years.[4]
Diphtheria is primarily a localized and generalized intoxication caused by diphtheria toxin, an extracellular protein metabolite of toxinogenic strains of *Corynebacterium diphtheriae*. While the incidence of diphtheria in the U.S. has decreased from over 200,000 cases reported in 1921 before the general use of diphtheria toxoid to only 15 cases reported from 1980 to 1983, the ratio of fatalities to attack rate has remained constant at about 5% to 10%.[4] The highest case fatality rates are in the very young and the elderly.
Following adequate immunization with diphtheria toxoid, which induces antitoxin, it is thought that protection lasts for at least 10 years.[4] This significantly reduces both the risk of developing diphtheria and the severity of clinical illness. It does not, however, eliminate carriage of *C diphtheriae* in the pharynx or on the skin.[4]

INDICATIONS AND USAGE
Tetanus and Diphtheria Toxoids For Adult Use, aluminum phosphate-adsorbed PUROGENATED (Td) is indicated for active immunization against tetanus and diphtheria in adults and children 7 years of age and older.[4,5]
The Immunization Practices Advisory Committee (ACIP) of the U.S. Public Health Service recommends the use of the combined toxoids vaccine rather than single component vaccines for both primary and booster injections, including active tetanus immunization in wound management.[4]
Persons recovering from tetanus or diphtheria: Tetanus or diphtheria infection may not confer immunity; therefore, initiation or completion of active immunization is indicated at the time of recovery from these infections.[4]
Neonatal tetanus prevention: There is no evidence that tetanus and diphtheria toxoids are teratogenic. A previously unimmunized pregnant woman, who may deliver her child under nonhygienic circumstances and/or surroundings, should receive two properly spaced doses of Td before delivery, preferably during the last two trimesters. Incompletely immunized pregnant women should complete the three-dose series. Those immunized more than 10 years previously should have a booster dose.[4] (See also pregnancy information under **PRECAUTIONS**.)

CONTRAINDICATIONS
HYPERSENSITIVITY TO ANY COMPONENT OF THE VACCINE, INCLUDING THIMEROSAL, A MERCURY DERIVATIVE, IS A CONTRAINDICATION.
THE OCCURRENCE OF ANY NEUROLOGICAL SYMPTOMS OR SIGNS FOLLOWING ADMINISTRATION OF

THIS PRODUCT IS A CONTRAINDICATION TO FURTHER USE.
IMMUNIZATION SHOULD BE DEFERRED DURING THE COURSE OF ANY FEBRILE ILLNESS OR ACUTE INFECTION. A MINOR AFEBRILE ILLNESS SUCH AS A MILD UPPER RESPIRATORY INFECTION IS NOT USUALLY REASON TO DEFER IMMUNIZATION.[4]
The clinical judgment of the attending physician should prevail at all times.
Routine immunization should be deferred during an outbreak of poliomyelitis, providing the patient has not sustained an injury that increases the risk of tetanus and providing an outbreak of diphtheria does not occur simultaneously.

WARNINGS
THIS PRODUCT IS NOT RECOMMENDED FOR IMMUNIZING PERSONS LESS THAN 7 YEARS OF AGE. The concentration of diphtheria toxoid in preparations intended for use in persons 7 years of age or older is lower than that of the pediatric formulation (Diphtheria and Tetanus Toxoids Adsorbed, for pediatric use, [DT]): a lower dosage of diphtheria toxoid is recommended for persons 7 years of age or older because adverse reactions to the diphtheria component are thought to be related to both dose and age.[4]
THE OCCURRENCE OF A NEUROLOGICAL OR SEVERE HYPERSENSITIVITY REACTION FOLLOWING A PREVIOUS DOSE IS A CONTRAINDICATION TO FURTHER USE OF THIS PRODUCT.[4]
THE ADMINISTRATION OF BOOSTER DOSES MORE FREQUENTLY THAN RECOMMENDED (see **DOSAGE AND ADMINISTRATION**) MAY BE ASSOCIATED WITH INCREASED INCIDENCE AND SEVERITY OF REACTIONS.[4]
Persons who experience Arthus-type hypersensitivity reactions or temperature greater than 39.4°C (103°F), after a previous dose of tetanus toxoid usually have very high serum tetanus antitoxin levels and should not be given even emergency doses of Td more frequently than every 10 years, even if they have a wound that is neither clean nor minor.[4]
If a contraindication to using tetanus toxoid-containing preparations exists in a person who has not completed a primary immunizing course of tetanus toxoid, and other than a clean, minor wound is sustained, only passive immunization should be given using human Tetanus Immune Globulin (TIG).[4]
Td should not be given to individuals with thrombocytopenia or any coagulation disorder that would contraindicate intramuscular injection unless the potential benefits clearly outweigh the risk of administration.
Patients with impaired immune responsiveness, whether due to the use of immunosuppressive therapy (including irradiation, corticosteroids, antimetabolites, alkylating agents, and cytotoxic agents), a genetic defect, human immunodeficiency virus (HIV) infection, or other causes, may have a reduced antibody response to active immunization procedures.[4–6] Deferral of administration of vaccine may be considered in individuals receiving immunosuppressive therapy.[4,5]
Special care should be taken to prevent injection into a blood vessel.

PRECAUTIONS
General:
1. **THIS PRODUCT SHOULD BE USED FOR INDIVIDUALS 7 YEARS OF AGE OR OLDER.**
2. PRIOR TO ADMINISTRATION OF ANY DOSE OF Td, THE PARENT, GUARDIAN, OR ADULT PATIENT SHOULD BE ASKED ABOUT THE RECENT HEALTH STATUS AND IMMUNIZATION HISTORY OF THE PATIENT TO BE IMMUNIZED IN ORDER TO DETERMINE THE EXISTENCE OF ANY CONTRAINDICATION TO IMMUNIZATION WITH Td (SEE **CONTRAINDICATIONS, WARNINGS**).
3. WHEN THE PATIENT RETURNS FOR THE NEXT DOSE IN A SERIES, THE PARENT, GUARDIAN, OR ADULT PATIENT SHOULD BE QUESTIONED CONCERNING OCCURRENCE OF ANY SYMPTOM AND/OR SIGN OF AN ADVERSE REACTION AFTER THE PREVIOUS DOSE (SEE **CONTRAINDICATIONS, ADVERSE REACTIONS**).
4. BEFORE THE INJECTION OF ANY BIOLOGICAL, THE PHYSICIAN SHOULD TAKE ALL PRECAUTIONS KNOWN FOR PREVENTION OF ALLERGIC OR ANY OTHER SIDE REACTIONS. This should include: a review of the patient's history regarding possible sensitivity; the ready availability of epinephrine 1:1,000 and other appropriate agents used for control of immediate allergic reactions; and a knowledge of the recent literature pertaining to use of the biological concerned, including the nature of side effects and adverse reactions that may follow its use.
5. A separate sterile syringe and needle or a sterile disposable unit should be used for each individual patient to prevent transmission of hepatitis or other infectious agents from one person to another.

6. **Shake vigorously before withdrawing each dose to resuspend the contents of the vial or syringe.**
7. NATIONAL CHILDHOOD VACCINE INJURY ACT OF 1986 (AS AMENDED IN 1987)
This Act requires that the manufacturer and lot number of the vaccine administered be recorded by the health care provider in the vaccine recipient's permanent medical record, along with the date of administration of the vaccine and the name, address and title of the person administering the vaccine.
The Act further requires the health care provider to report to a health department or to the FDA the occurrence following immunization of any event set forth in the Vaccine Injury Table including: anaphylaxis or anaphylactic shock within 24 hours, encephalopathy or encephalitis within 7 days, residual seizure disorder, any acute complication or sequelae (including death) of above events, or any event that would contraindicate further doses of vaccine, according to this package insert.[7]
Information for the Patient: PRIOR TO ADMINISTRATION OF THIS VACCINE, HEALTH CARE PERSONNEL SHOULD INFORM THE PARENT, GUARDIAN, OR ADULT PATIENT OF THE BENEFITS AND RISKS OF VACCINATION AGAINST TETANUS AND DIPHTHERIA.

Use in Pregnancy: *Pregnancy Category C:* Animal reproductive studies have not been conducted with this product. There is no evidence that tetanus and diphtheria toxoids are teratogenic. Td should be given to inadequately immunized pregnant women because it affords protection against neonatal tetanus.[8] Waiting until the second trimester is a reasonable precaution to minimize any theoretical concern.[4] Maintenance of adequate immunization by routine boosters in nonpregnant women of childbearing age (see **DOSAGE AND ADMINISTRATION**) can obviate the need to vaccinate women during pregnancy.

ADVERSE REACTIONS
Local reactions, such as erythema, induration, and tenderness, are common after the administration of Td.[9–12] Such local reactions are usually self-limited and require no therapy. Nodule,[13] sterile abscess formation, or subcutaneous atrophy may occur at the site of injection. Systemic reactions, such as fever, chills, myalgias, and headaches, also may occur.[9–12]
Arthus-type hypersensitivity reactions, or high fever, may occur in persons who have very high serum antitoxin antibodies due to overly frequent injections of toxoid (see **WARNINGS**).
NEUROLOGICAL COMPLICATIONS,[14] SUCH AS CONVULSIONS,[15] ENCEPHALOPATHY,[15,16] AND VARIOUS MONO- AND POLYNEUROPATHIES,[16–22] INCLUDING GUILLAIN-BARRÉ SYNDROME,[23,24] HAVE BEEN REPORTED FOLLOWING ADMINISTRATION OF PREPARATIONS CONTAINING TETANUS AND/OR DIPHTHERIA ANTIGENS.
URTICARIA, ERYTHEMA MULTIFORME OR OTHER RASH, ARTHRALGIAS,[15] AND, MORE RARELY, A SEVERE ANAPHYLACTIC REACTION (IE, URTICARIA WITH SWELLING OF THE MOUTH, DIFFICULTY BREATHING, HYPOTENSION, OR SHOCK) HAVE BEEN REPORTED FOLLOWING ADMINISTRATION OF PREPARATIONS CONTAINING TETANUS AND/OR DIPHTHERIA ANTIGENS.

DOSAGE AND ADMINISTRATION
For Intramuscular Use Only: Shake vigorously before withdrawing each dose to resuspend the contents of the vial or syringe.
Parenteral drug products should be inspected visually for particulate matter and discoloration prior to administration. (See **DESCRIPTION**.)
The vaccine should be injected intramuscularly, preferably into the deltoid muscle, with care to avoid major peripheral nerve trunks. Before injection, the skin at the injection site should be cleansed and prepared with a suitable germicide. After insertion of the needle, aspirate to help avoid inadvertent injection into a blood vessel.
The primary immunizing course for unimmunized individuals 7 years of age or older consists of two doses of 0.5 mL each, 4 to 8 weeks apart, followed by a third (reinforcing) dose of 0.5 mL 6 to 12 months after the second dose. The reinforcing dose is an integral part of the primary immunizing course.[4] Interruption of the recommended schedule with a delay between doses does not interfere with the final immunity achieved, nor does it necessitate starting the series over again, regardless of the length of time elapsed between doses.[4]
A booster dose of 0.5 mL of Td is given 10 years after completion of primary immunization and every 10 years thereafter. If a dose is given sooner than 10 years, as part of wound management or on exposure to diphtheria, the next booster is not needed for 10 years thereafter. MORE FREQUENT BOOSTER DOSES ARE NOT INDICATED AND MAY BE ASSOCIATED WITH INCREASED INCIDENCE AND SEVERITY OF REACTIONS.[4] (See **WARNINGS**.)

Diphtheria Prophylaxis for Case Contacts: All case contacts, household and others, who have previously received fewer than three doses of diphtheria toxoid, should receive an immediate dose of an appropriate diphtheria toxoid-containing preparation and should complete the series according to schedule. Case contacts who have previously received three or more doses, but who have not received a dose of a preparation containing diphtheria toxoid within the previous 5 years, should receive a booster dose of a diphtheria toxoid-containing preparation appropriate for their age.[4] Td is an appropriate preparation in these circumstances for persons 7 years of age or older.

Tetanus Prophylaxis in Wound Management: The need for active immunization with a tetanus toxoid-containing preparation, with or without passive immunization with human Tetanus Immune Globulin (TIG) depends on both the condition of the wound and the patient's immunization history. Tetanus has rarely occurred among persons with a documented primary series of tetanus toxoid injections. A thorough attempt must be made to determine whether a patient has completed primary immunization.[4]

Individuals who have completed primary immunization against tetanus, and who sustain wounds which are minor and uncontaminated, should receive a booster dose of a tetanus-toxoid preparation only if they have not received tetanus toxoid within the preceding 10 years. For other wounds, a booster is appropriate if the patient has not received tetanus toxoid within the preceding 5 years. Antitoxin antibodies develop rapidly in persons who have previously received at least two doses of tetanus toxoid.[4]

Individuals who have not completed primary immunization against tetanus, or whose immunization history is unknown or uncertain, should be immunized with a tetanus toxoid-containing product. Completion of primary immunization thereafter should be ensured. In addition, if these individuals have sustained a tetanus-prone wound, the use of human Tetanus Immune Globulin (TIG) is recommended. A separate syringe and site of administration should be used.[4]

Summary guide to tetanus prophylaxis in routine wound management[4]*

History of tetanus toxoid (doses)	Clean, minor wounds		All other wounds†	
	Td	TIG	Td	TIG
Unknown < three	Yes	No	Yes	Yes
≥ three‡	No§	No	No"	No

* Important details are in the text.

† Such as, but not limited to, wounds contaminated with dirt, feces, soil, saliva, etc; puncture wounds; avulsions; and wounds resulting from missiles, crushing, burns, and frostbite.

‡ If only three doses of *fluid* toxoid have been received, a fourth dose of toxoid, preferably an adsorbed toxoid, should be given.

§ Yes, if more than 10 years since last dose.

" Yes, if more than 5 years since last dose. (More frequent boosters are not needed and can accentuate side effects.)

Td is the preferred preparation for active tetanus immunization in wound management of patients 7 years of age or older. This is to enhance diphtheria protection, since a large proportion of adults are susceptible. Thus, by taking advantage of acute health care visits for wound management, some patients can be protected who otherwise would remain susceptible.[4]

HOW SUPPLIED

NDC 0005-1875-31 5.0 mL vial

NDC 0005-1875-47 10 (0.5 mL) LEDERJECT® disposable syringes. For directions on use of LEDERJECT® disposable syringe, please see package insert accompanying product.

STORAGE

DO NOT FREEZE. STORE REFRIGERATED, AWAY FROM FREEZER COMPARTMENT, AT 2°C to 8°C (36°F to 46°F).

REFERENCES

1. Mueller JH, Miller PA: Factors influencing the production of tetanal toxin. *J Immunol* 1947;56:143–147.
2. Mueller JH, Miller PA: Production of diphtheria toxin of high potency (100Lf) on a reproducible medium. *J Immunol* 1941;40:21–32.
3. Pillemer L, Grossberg DB, Wittler RG: The immunochemistry of toxins and toxoids. II. The preparation and immunological evaluation of purified tetanal toxoid. *J Immunol* 1946;54:213–224.
4. Recommendation of the Immunization Practices Advisory Committee (ACIP): Diphtheria, tetanus and pertussis: Guidelines for vaccine prophylaxis and other preventive measures. *MMWR* 1985;34:405–426.
5. Committee on Immunization, Council of Medical Societies American College of Physicians: Guide for Adult Immunization, 1st Edition 1985; Philadelphia, PA.
6. Recommendation of the ACIP: Immunization of children infected with Human T-Lymphotrophic Virus Type III/Lymphadenopathy associated virus. *MMWR* 1986;35(38):595–606.
7. National Childhood Vaccine Injury Act: Requirements for permanent vaccination records and for reporting of selected events after vaccination. *MMWR* 1988;37(13):197–200.
8. Recommendations of the ACIP: General recommendations on immunization. *MMWR* 1983;32(1):1–17.
9. Deacon SP, et al: A comparative clinical study of adsorbed tetanus vaccine and adult-type tetanus-diphtheria vaccine. *J Hyg (Cambridge)* 1982;89:513–519.
10. Macko MB, Powell CE: Comparison of the morbidity of tetanus toxoid boosters with tetanus-diphtheria toxoid boosters. *Ann Emerg Med* 1985;14(1):33–35.
11. Myers MG, et al: Primary immunization with tetanus and diphtheria toxoids. *JAMA* 1982;248(19):2478–2480.
12. Sisk CW, et al: Reactions to tetanus-diphtheria toxoid (adult). *Arch Environ Health* 1965;11:34–36.
13. Fawcett HA, Smith NP: Injection-site granuloma due to aluminum. *Arch Dermatol* 1984;120:1318–1322.
14. Rutledge SL, Snead OC: Neurological complications of immunizations. *J Pediatr* 1986;109:917–924.
15. Adverse Events Following Immunization. *MMWR* 1985;34(3):43–47.
16. Schlenska GK: Unusual neurological complications following tetanus toxoid administration. *J Neurol* 1977;215:299–302.
17. Blumstein GI, Kreithen H: Peripheral neuropathy following tetanus toxoid administration. *JAMA* 1966;198:1030–1031.
18. Reinstein L, Pargament JM, Goodman JS: Peripheral neuropathy after multiple tetanus toxoid injections. *Arch Phys Med Rehabil* 1982;63:332–334.
19. Tsairis P, Duck PJ, Mulder DW: Natural history of brachial plexus neuropathy. *Arch Neurol* 1972;27:109–117.
20. Quast U, Hennessen W, Widmark RM: Mono- and polyneuritis after tetanus vaccination. *Devel Bio Stand* 1979;43:25–32.
21. Holliday PL, Bauer RB: Polyradiculoneuritis secondary to immunization with tetanus and diphtheria toxoids. *Arch Neurol* 1983;40:56–67.
22. Fenichel GM: Neurological complications of tetanus toxoid. *Arch Neurol* 1983;40:390.
23. Pollard JD, Selby G: Relapsing neuropathy due to tetanus toxoid. *J Neurol Sci* 1978;37:113–125.
24. Newton N, Janati A: Guillain-Barré syndrome after vaccination with purified tetanus toxoid. *S Med J* 1987;80:1053–1054.

Manufactured by:

LEDERLE LABORATORIES DIVISION
American Cyanamid Company
Pearl River, NY 10965

TETANUS TOXOID ADSORBED   ℞

Tetanus Toxoid Aluminum Phosphate-Adsorbed Purogenated®

DESCRIPTION

Tetanus Toxoid Adsorbed, aluminum phosphate-adsorbed, PUROGENATED is a sterile preparation of refined tetanus toxoid for intramuscular use only. After shaking, the product is a homogeneous white suspension.

The tetanus toxin is produced according to the method of Mueller and Miller[1] and is detoxified by use of formaldehyde. The toxoid is refined by the Pillemer alcohol fractionation method[2] and is diluted with a solution containing sodium phosphate dibasic, sodium phosphate monobasic, glycine, sodium chloride and thimerosal (mercury derivative) in a final concentration of 1:10,000 as a preservative and aluminum phosphate as adjuvant. The aluminum content does not exceed 0.80 mg per 0.5 mL dose.

Each 0.5 mL dose is formulated to contain 5 Lf units of tetanus toxoid.

CLINICAL PHARMACOLOGY

Tetanus is an intoxication manifested primarily by neuromuscular dysfunction caused by a potent exotoxin elaborated by *Clostridium tetani*. The incidence of tetanus in the U.S. has dropped dramatically with the routine use of tetanus toxoid, remaining relatively constant over the last decade at about 90 cases reported annually.[3] Spores of *C tetani* are ubiquitous, and there is essentially no natural immunity to tetanus toxin. Thus, universal primary immunization with tetanus toxoid, and subsequent maintenance of adequate antitoxin levels by means of timed boosters, is necessary to protect all age groups.[3] Tetanus toxoid is a highly effective antigen, and a completed primary series generally induces protective levels of serum antitoxin that persist for at least 10 years.[3]

INDICATIONS AND USAGE

Tetanus Toxoid Adsorbed is indicated for active immunization against tetanus in adults and children 2 months of age or older.

Immunization of persons 7 years of age or older may be accomplished by the use of Tetanus and Diphtheria Toxoids Adsorbed, for Adult Use (Td), Tetanus Toxoid Adsorbed, or Tetanus Toxoid Fluid. The Immunization Practices Advisory Committee (ACIP) of the U.S. Public Health Service recommends the use of the combined toxoids vaccine rather than single component vaccines for both primary and booster injections, including active tetanus immunization in wound management.[3] Individuals for whom the use of a vaccine containing diphtheria toxoid is contraindicated should receive a single-component tetanus toxoid-containing vaccine. Immunization of infants and children 2 months of age up to the seventh birthday is usually accomplished by the use of Diphtheria and Tetanus Toxoids and Pertussis Vaccine Adsorbed (DTP) or Diphtheria and Tetanus Toxoids Adsorbed, for pediatric use (DT). Tetanus Toxoid Adsorbed may be used for immunizing infants and children for whom the use of a vaccine containing diphtheria toxoid and pertussis antigen is contraindicated.

Comparative tests have shown that the adsorbed toxoids are superior to the fluid toxoids in antibody titers produced and in the durability of protection achieved. The promptness of antibody response to booster doses of either fluid or adsorbed toxoid is not sufficiently different to be of clinical importance. When Tetanus Immune Globulin (TIG) is to be administered at the same visit as tetanus toxoid, the adsorbed toxoid should be used.[3,4]

Persons Recovering from Tetanus: Tetanus infection may not confer immunity; therefore, initiation or completion of active immunization is indicated at the time of recovery from this infection.[3]

Neonatal Tetanus Prevention: There is no evidence that tetanus toxoid is teratogenic. A previously unimmunized pregnant woman who may deliver her child under nonhygienic circumstances and/or surroundings should receive two properly spaced doses of a tetanus toxoid-containing preparation before delivery, preferably during the last two trimesters. Incompletely immunized pregnant women should complete the three-dose series. Those immunized more than 10 years previously should have a booster dose.[3] (See also pregnancy information under **PRECAUTIONS**.)

CONTRAINDICATIONS

HYPERSENSITIVITY TO ANY COMPONENT OF THE VACCINE, INCLUDING THIMEROSAL, A MERCURY DERIVATIVE, IS A CONTRAINDICATION.

THE OCCURRENCE OF ANY TYPE OF NEUROLOGICAL SYMPTOMS OR SIGNS FOLLOWING ADMINISTRATION OF THIS PRODUCT IS A CONTRAINDICATION TO FURTHER USE.

IMMUNIZATION SHOULD BE DEFERRED DURING THE COURSE OF ANY FEBRILE ILLNESS OR ACUTE INFECTION. A MINOR AFEBRILE ILLNESS SUCH AS A MILD UPPER RESPIRATORY INFECTION IS NOT USUALLY REASON TO DEFER IMMUNIZATION.[3]

The clinical judgment of the attending physician should prevail at all times.

Routine immunization should be deferred during an outbreak of poliomyelitis, providing the patient has not sustained an injury that increases the risk of tetanus.

WARNINGS

THE OCCURRENCE OF A NEUROLOGICAL OR SEVERE HYPERSENSITIVITY REACTION FOLLOWING A PREVIOUS DOSE IS A CONTRAINDICATION TO FURTHER USE OF THIS PRODUCT.[3]

THE ADMINISTRATION OF BOOSTER DOSES MORE FREQUENTLY THAN RECOMMENDED (see **DOSAGE AND ADMINISTRATION**) MAY BE ASSOCIATED WITH INCREASED INCIDENCE AND SEVERITY OF REACTIONS.[3]

Persons who experience Arthus-type hypersensitivity reactions or temperature greater than 39.4°C (103°F) after a previous dose of tetanus toxoid usually have very high serum tetanus antitoxin levels and should not be given even emergency doses of tetanus toxoid more frequently than every 10 years, even if they have a wound that is neither clean nor minor.[3]

If a contraindication to using tetanus toxoid exists in a person who has not completed a primary immunizing course of tetanus toxoid, and other than a clean, minor wound is sustained, only passive immunization should be given using human Tetanus Immune Globulin (TIG).[3]

Tetanus Toxoid Adsorbed should not be given to individuals with thrombocytopenia or any coagulation disorder that would contraindicate intramuscular injection, unless the potential benefit clearly outweighs the risk of administration.

Patients with impaired immune responsiveness, whether due to the use of immunosuppressive therapy (including

Continued on next page

Lederle—Cont.

irradiation, corticosteroids, antimetabolites, alkylating agents, and cytotoxic agents), a genetic defect, human immunodeficiency virus (HIV) infection, or other causes, may have a reduced antibody response to active immunization procedures.[3–5] Deferral of administration of vaccine may be considered in individuals receiving immunosuppressive therapy.[3,4]

Special care should be taken to prevent injection into a blood vessel.

PRECAUTIONS

General:

1. PRIOR TO ADMINISTRATION OF ANY DOSE OF VACCINE THE PARENT, GUARDIAN, OR ADULT PATIENT SHOULD BE ASKED ABOUT THE RECENT HEALTH STATUS AND IMMUNIZATION HISTORY OF THE PATIENT TO BE IMMUNIZED IN ORDER TO DETERMINE THE EXISTENCE OF ANY CONTRAINDICATIONS TO IMMUNIZATION (SEE **CONTRAINDICATIONS, WARNINGS**).
2. WHEN THE PATIENT RETURNS FOR THE NEXT DOSE IN A SERIES, THE PARENT, GUARDIAN, OR ADULT PATIENT SHOULD BE QUESTIONED CONCERNING OCCURRENCE OF ANY SYMPTOM AND/OR SIGN OF AN ADVERSE REACTION AFTER THE PREVIOUS DOSE (SEE **CONTRAINDICATIONS, ADVERSE REACTIONS**).
3. BEFORE THE INJECTION OF ANY BIOLOGICAL, THE PHYSICIAN SHOULD TAKE ALL PRECAUTIONS KNOWN FOR PREVENTION OF ALLERGIC OR ANY OTHER SIDE REACTIONS. This should include: a review of the patient's history regarding possible sensitivity; the ready availability of epinephrine 1:1,000 and other appropriate agents used for control of immediate allergic reactions; and a knowledge of the recent literature pertaining to use of the biological concerned, including the nature of side effects and adverse reactions that may follow its use.
4. A separate sterile syringe and needle or a sterile disposable unit should be used for each individual patient to prevent transmission of hepatitis or other infectious agents from one person to another.
5. *Shake vigorously before withdrawing each dose to resuspend the contents of the vial.*
6. NATIONAL CHILDHOOD VACCINE INJURY ACT OF 1986 (AS AMENDED IN 1987)

   This Act requires that the manufacturer and lot number of the vaccine administered be recorded by the health care provider in the vaccine recipient's permanent record, along with the date of administration of the vaccine and the name, address and title of the person administering the vaccine.

   The Act further requires the health care provider to report to a health department or to the FDA the occurrence following immunization of any event set forth in the Vaccine Injury Table including: anaphylaxis or anaphylactic shock within 24 hours, encephalopathy or encephalitis within 7 days, residual seizure disorder, any acute complication or sequelae (including death) of above events, or any event that would contraindicate further doses of vaccine, according to this package insert.[6]

Information for the Patient: PRIOR TO ADMINISTRATION OF THIS VACCINE, HEALTH CARE PERSONNEL SHOULD INFORM THE PARENT, GUARDIAN, OR ADULT PATIENT OF THE BENEFITS AND RISKS OF VACCINATION AGAINST TETANUS.

Use in Pregnancy: *Pregnancy Category C:* Animal reproductive studies have not been conducted with this product. There is no evidence that tetanus toxoid is teratogenic. An appropriate tetanus toxoid-containing preparation (usually Td) should be given to inadequately immunized women because it affords protection against neonatal tetanus.[7] Waiting until the second trimester is a reasonable precaution to minimize any theoretical concern.[4] Maintenance of adequate immunization by routine boosters in non-pregnant women of child-bearing age (see **DOSAGE AND ADMINISTRATION**) can obviate the need to vaccinate women during pregnancy.

ADVERSE REACTIONS

Local reactions, such as erythema, induration, and tenderness, are common after the administration of tetanus toxoid.[8–10] Such local reactions are usually self-limiting and require no therapy. Nodule,[11] sterile abscess formation, or subcutaneous atrophy may occur at the site of injection. Systemic reactions, such as fever, chills, myalgia, and headaches also may occur.[8–10]

Arthus-type hypersensitivity reactions, or high fever, may occur in persons who have very high serum antitoxin antibodies due to overly frequent injections of toxoid.[3] (See **WARNINGS**.)

NEUROLOGICAL COMPLICATIONS,[12] SUCH AS CONVULSIONS,[13] ENCEPHALOPATHY,[13,14] AND VARIOUS MONO- AND POLYNEUROPATHIES,[14–20] INCLUDING GUILLAIN-BARRÉ SYNDROME,[21,22] HAVE BEEN REPORTED FOLLOWING ADMINISTRATION OF PREPARATIONS CONTAINING TETANUS ANTIGEN.

URTICARIA, ERYTHEMA MULTIFORME OR OTHER RASH, ARTHRALGIAS,[13] AND, MORE RARELY, A SEVERE ANAPHYLACTIC REACTION (IE, URTICARIA WITH SWELLING OF THE MOUTH, DIFFICULTY BREATHING, HYPOTENSION, OR SHOCK) HAVE BEEN REPORTED FOLLOWING ADMINISTRATION OF PREPARATIONS CONTAINING TETANUS ANTIGEN.

DOSAGE AND ADMINISTRATION

For Intramuscular Use Only: *Shake vigorously before withdrawing each dose to resuspend the contents of the vial or syringe.*

Parenteral drug products should be inspected visually for particulate matter and discoloration prior to administration. (See **DESCRIPTION.**)

Preferred injection sites for intramuscular injection include the anterolateral aspect of the upper thigh and the deltoid area of the upper arm. Care should be taken to avoid major peripheral nerve trunks.

Before injection, the skin at the injection site should be cleansed and prepared with a suitable germicide.

After insertion of the needle, aspirate to help avoid inadvertent injection into a blood vessel.

The primary immunizing course for unimmunized individuals 1 year of age or older consists of **two** doses of 0.5 mL each, 4 to 8 weeks apart, followed by a **third** (reinforcing) dose of 0.5 mL, 6 to 12 months after the second dose. The reinforcing dose is an integral part of the primary immunizing course.

If, after beginning combined immunization against diphtheria, tetanus, and pertussis, further doses of vaccine containing pertussis and diphtheria antigens become contraindicated, Tetanus Toxoid Adsorbed may be substituted for each of the remaining doses.

When immunization with Tetanus Toxoid Adsorbed is begun in the first year of life, the primary series consists of **three** doses of 0.5 mL each, 4 to 8 weeks apart, followed by a **fourth** (reinforcing) dose of 0.5 mL, 6 to 12 months after the third dose.

Interruption of the recommended schedule with a delay between doses does not interfere with the final immunity achieved with Tetanus Toxoid Adsorbed. There is no need to start the series over again, regardless of the length of time elapsed between doses.[3]

Booster Doses: A single injection of 0.5 mL of Tetanus Toxoid Adsorbed is given 10 years after completion of primary immunization and every 10 years thereafter. If a dose is given sooner as part of wound management, the next booster is not needed for 10 years thereafter. MORE FREQUENT BOOSTER DOSES ARE NOT INDICATED AND MAY BE ASSOCIATED WITH INCREASED INCIDENCE AND SEVERITY OF REACTIONS.[3]

Tetanus Prophylaxis in Wound Management: The need for active immunization with a tetanus toxoid-containing preparation, with or without passive immunization with human Tetanus Immune Globulin (TIG) depends on both the condition of the wound and the patient's immunization history. Tetanus has rarely occurred among persons with a documented primary series of toxoid injections. A thorough attempt must be made to determine whether a patient has completed primary immunization.[3]

Individuals who have completed primary immunization against tetanus, and who sustain wounds which are minor and uncontaminated, should receive a booster dose of the appropriate tetanus toxoid-containing preparation (see **INDICATIONS AND USAGE**) only if they have not received tetanus toxoid within the preceding 10 years. For other wounds, a booster is appropriate if the patient has not received tetanus toxoid within the preceding 5 years. Antitoxin antibodies develop rapidly in persons who have previously received at least two doses of tetanus toxoid.[3]

Individuals who have not completed primary immunization against tetanus, or whose immunization history is unknown or uncertain, should be immunized with the appropriate tetanus toxoid-containing product (see **INDICATIONS AND USAGE**). Completion of primary immunization thereafter should be ensured. In addition, if these individuals have sustained a tetanus-prone wound, the use of human Tetanus Immune Globulin (TIG) is recommended. A separate syringe and site of administration should be used. When TIG is to be administered at the same visit as tetanus toxoid, an adsorbed tetanus toxoid-containing preparation should be used.[3]

SUMMARY GUIDE TO TETANUS PROPHYLAXIS IN ROUTINE WOUND MANAGEMENT[3]*

History of tetanus toxoid (doses)	Clean, minor wounds		All other wounds†	
	Td§	TIG	Td§	TIG
Unknown or < three	Yes	No	Yes	Yes
≥ three‖	No**	No	No††	No

* Important details are in the text.

† Such as, but not limited to, wounds contaminated with dirt, feces, soil, saliva, etc; puncture wounds; avulsions; and wounds resulting from missiles, crushing, burns, and frostbite.

§ For children under 7 years old DTP (DT, if pertussis vaccine is contraindicated) is preferred to tetanus toxoid alone. For persons 7 years and older, Td is preferred to tetanus toxoid alone.

‖ If only three doses of **fluid** toxoid have been received, a fourth dose of toxoid, preferably an adsorbed toxoid, should be given.

** Yes, if more than 10 years since last dose.

†† Yes, if more than 5 years since last dose. (More frequent boosters are not needed and can accentuate side effects.)

In order to enhance diphtheria protection in the population, the ACIP recommends Tetanus and Diphtheria Toxoid For Adult Use as the preferred preparation for active tetanus immunization in wound management of patients 7 years of age or older.[3]

HOW SUPPLIED

NDC 0005-1938-31 5.0 mL vial

NDC 0005-1938-47 10×0.5 mL LEDERJECT® disposable syringe. For directions on use of LEDERJECT® disposable syringe, please see package insert accompanying product.

STORAGE

DO NOT FREEZE. STORE REFRIGERATED, AWAY FROM FREEZER COMPARTMENT, AT 2°C to 8°C (36°F to 46°F).

REFERENCES

1. Mueller JH, Miller PA: Factors influencing the production of tetanal toxin. *J Immunol* 1947;56:143–147.
2. Pillemer L, Grossberg DB, Wittler RG: The immunochemistry of toxins and toxoids. II. The preparation and immunological evaluation of purified tetanal toxoid. *J Immunol* 1946;54:213–224.
3. Recommendation of the Immunization Practices Advisory Committee (ACIP): Diphtheria, tetanus and pertussis: Guidelines for vaccine prophylaxis and other preventive measures. *MMWR* 1985;34:405–426.
4. Committee on Immunization, Council of Medical Societies, American College of Physicians: Guide for Adult Immunization, 1st Edition 1985; Philadelphia, PA.
5. Recommendation of the ACIP: Immunization of children infected with Human T-Lymphotrophic Virus Type III/Lymphadenopathy associated virus. *MMWR* 1986;35(38):595–606.
6. National Childhood Vaccine Injury Act: Requirements for permanent vaccination records and for reporting of selected events after vaccination. *MMWR* 1988;37(13):197–200.
7. Recommendations of the ACIP: General recommendations on immunization. *MMWR* 1983;32(1):1–17.
8. Macko MB, Powell CE: Comparison of the morbidity of tetanus toxoid boosters with tetanus-diphtheria toxoid boosters. *Ann Emerg Med* 1985;14:(1)33–35.
9. Deacon SP, et al: A comparative clinical study of adsorbed tetanus vaccine and adult-type tetanus-diphtheria vaccine. *J Hyg (Cambridge)* 1982;89:513–519.
10. Jacobs RL, et al: Adverse reactions to tetanus toxoid. *JAMA* 1982:247(1):40–42.
11. Fawcett HA, Smith N: Injection-site granuloma due to aluminum. *Arch Dermatol* 1984;120:1318–1322.
12. Rutledge SL, Snead OC: Neurologic complications of immunizations. *J Pediatr* 1986;109:917–924.
13. Adverse Events Following Immunization. *MMWR* 1985;34(3):43–47.
14. Schlenska GK: Unusual neurological complications following tetanus toxoid administration. *J Neurol* 1977;215:299–302.
15. Blumstein GI, Kreithen H: Peripheral neuropathy following tetanus toxoid administration. *JAMA* 1966;198:1030–1031.
16. Reinstein L, Pargament JM, Goodman JS: Peripheral neuropathy after multiple tetanus toxoid injections. *Arch Phys Med Rehabil* 1982;63:332–334.
17. Tsairis P, Duck PJ, Mulder DW: Natural history of brachial plexus neuropathy. *Arch Neurol* 1972;27:109–117.
18. Quast U, Hennessen W, Widmark RM: Mono- and polyneuritis after tetanus vaccination. *Devel Bio Stand* 1979;43:25–32.
19. Holliday PL, Bauer RB: Polyradiculoneuritis secondary to immunization with tetanus and diphtheria toxoids. *Arch Neurol* 1983;40:56–57.
20. Fenichel GM: Neurological complications of tetanus toxoid. *Arch Neurol* 1983;40:390.
21. Pollard JD, Selby G: Relapsing neuropathy due to tetanus toxoid. *J Neurol Sci* 1978;37:113–125.
22. Newton N, Janati A: Guillain-Barré syndrome after vaccination with purified tetanus toxoid. *S Med J* 1987;80:1053–1054.

Manufactured by:
LEDERLE LABORATORIES DIVISION
American Cyanamid Company
Pearl River, NY 10965

TETRAMUNE® ℞
[*tet 'rə-myoon*]
Diphtheria and Tetanus Toxoids and Pertussis Vaccine Adsorbed and Haemophilus b Conjugate Vaccine (Diphtheria CRM_{197} Protein Conjugate)

DESCRIPTION

Diphtheria and Tetanus Toxoids and Pertussis Vaccine Adsorbed and Haemophilus b Conjugate Vaccine (Diphtheria CRM^{197} Protein Conjugate) TETRAMUNE, (DTP-HbOC), is a sterile combination of PUROGENATED® Diphtheria Toxoid aluminum phosphate-adsorbed, PUROGENATED® Tetanus Toxoid aluminum phosphate-adsorbed, Pertussis Vaccine (DTP), and a conjugate of oligosaccharides of the capsular antigen of *Haemophilus influenzae* type b and diphtheria CRM_{197} protein (HbOC, HibTITER®, manufactured by Lederle Laboratories. These are antigenic components of TRI-IMMUNOL® and HibTITER®. TETRAMUNE is for intramuscular use only. After shaking, the vaccine is a homogeneous white suspension.

The diphtheria and tetanus toxoids are derived from *Corynebacterium diphtheriae* and *Clostridium tetani*, respectively, which are grown in media according to the method of Mueller and Miller.[1,2] *C. diphtheriae* is grown in a defined medium containing casamino acids and *C. tetani* in a medium containing beef heart infusion. They are detoxified by use of formaldehyde. The toxoids are refined by the Pillemer alcohol fractionation method[3] and are diluted with a solution containing sodium phosphate monobasic, sodium phosphate dibasic, glycine, and thimerosal (mercury derivative) as a preservative.

Pertussis Vaccine is prepared by growing Phase I *Bordetella pertussis* in a modified Cohen-Wheeler broth containing acid hydrolysate of casein. The *B. pertussis* is inactivated with thimerosal, harvested, and then suspended in a solution containing potassium phosphate monobasic, sodium phosphate dibasic, sodium chloride, and thimerosal (mercury derivative) as a preservative.

The oligosaccharides for the Haemophilus b conjugate component are derived from highly purified capsular polysaccharide, polyribosylribitol phosphate, isolated from *Haemophilus influenzae* type b (Haemophilus b) grown in a chemically defined medium (a mixture of mineral salts, amino acids, and cofactors). The oligosaccharides are purified and sized by diafiltrations through a series of ultrafiltration membranes, and coupled by reductive amination directly to highly purified CRM_{197}.[4,5] CRM_{197} is a nontoxic variant of diphtheria toxin isolated from cultures of *C. diphtheriae* C7 (β 197) grown in a casamino acids and yeast extract-based medium. The conjugate is purified through ultrafiltration, ammonium sulfate precipitation, and ion-exchange chromatography to high purity.

The Haemophilus b conjugate component is combined with the diphtheria and tetanus toxoids and pertussis vaccine adsorbed to produce the final vaccine. As a preservative, thimerosal (mercury derivative) is added to the combination vaccine to a final concentration of 1:10,000. The aluminum content (from aluminum phosphate adjuvant) of the final product does not exceed 0.85 mg per 0.5 mL dose as determined by assay. The residual-free formaldehyde content by assay is $\leq$0.02%.

Each single dose of 0.5 mL of TETRAMUNE is formulated to contain 12.5 Lf of diphtheria toxoid, 5 Lf of tetanus toxoid (both toxoids induce not less than 2 units of antitoxin per mL in the guinea pig potency test), 10 μg of purified Haemophilus b saccharide, and approximately 25 μg of CRM_{197} protein. Each 0.5 mL dose of vaccine is formulated to contain less than 16 OPUs of inactivated pertussis cells. The total human immunizing dose (the first three 0.5 mL doses given) contains an estimate of 12 units of pertussis vaccine with an estimate of 4 protective units per single human dose, as determined by the mouse pertussis potency test. The potency for the Haemophilus b conjugate component of TETRAMUNE is determined by gas chromatography assay for total saccharide. Each component of the vaccine—diphtheria, tetanus, pertussis, and Haemophilus b conjugate—meets the required potency standards, and contains no other active ingredients.

CLINICAL PHARMACOLOGY

Simultaneous immunization against diphtheria, tetanus, and pertussis during infancy and childhood has been a routine practice in the United States since the late 1940s, and immunization against Haemophilus b has been a routine practice since 1985. These immunizations have played a major role in markedly reducing the incidence of cases and deaths from each of these diseases.

Diphtheria is primarily a localized and generalized intoxication caused by diphtheria toxin, an extracellular protein metabolite of toxinogenic strains of *C. diphtheriae.* While the incidence of diphtheria in the US has decreased from over 200,000 cases reported in 1921, before the general use of diphtheria toxoid, to only 15 cases reported from 1980 to 1983,[6] the case fatality rate has remained constant at about 5% to 10%. The highest case fatality rates are in the very young and in the elderly.

Following adequate immunization with diphtheria toxoid, it is thought that protection lasts for at least 10 years.[6]

Antitoxin levels of at least 0.01 antitoxin units/mL are generally regarded as protective.[7] This significantly reduces both the risk of developing diphtheria and the severity of clinical illness. It does not, however, eliminate carriage of *C. diphtheriae* in the pharynx or on the skin.[6]

Tetanus is an intoxication manifested primarily by neuromuscular dysfunction caused by a potent exotoxin elaborated by *C. tetani.* The incidence of tetanus in the US has dropped dramatically with the routine use of tetanus toxoid, remaining relatively constant over the last decade at about 90 cases reported annually. Spores of *C. tetani* are ubiquitous, and there is essentially no natural immunity to tetanus toxin.

Thus, universal primary immunization with tetanus toxoid with subsequent maintenance of adequate antitoxin levels, by means of timed boosters, is recommended to protect all age groups.[6] Tetanus toxoid is a highly effective antigen and a completed primary series generally induces serum antitoxin levels of at least 0.01 antitoxin units, a level that has been reported to be protective.[8] It is thought that protection persists for at least 10 years.[6]

The toxoids of tetanus and diphtheria induce neutralizing antibodies to the toxins produced by the infecting organism. In clinical studies with Lederle-produced diphtheria and tetanus toxoids, administered in combination with pertussis vaccine, serum antitoxin levels have been shown to be greater than 0.01 antitoxin units/mL in 97% to 100% of 372 infants following three doses.[9,10] These levels are generally regarded to be protective.[7,8]

Pertussis (whooping cough) is a disease of the respiratory tract caused by *B. pertussis.* This gram-negative coccobacillus produces a variety of active components including endotoxin and a number of other substances that have been defined primarily on the basis of their biological activity in animals. These active components have been associated with a number of effects, such as lymphocytosis, leukocytosis, sensitivity to histamine, changes in glucose and/or insulin levels, possible neurological effects and adjuvant activity.[11] The roles of each of the different components in either the pathogenesis of, or immunity to, pertussis are not well understood.

Pertussis (whooping cough) is a highly communicable disease of the respiratory tract. Attack rates of over 90% have been reported in unimmunized household contacts.[12] Since immunization against pertussis (whooping cough) became widespread, the number of reported cases and associated mortality in the US has declined from about 120,000 cases and 1,100 deaths in 1950,[13] to an annual average of about 3,500 cases and 10 fatalities in recent years.[6,14] Precise data do not exist since bacteriological confirmation of pertussis can be obtained in less than half of the suspected cases. Most reported illness from *B. pertussis* occurs in infants and young children; two thirds of reported deaths occur in children less than 1 year old. Older children and adults, in whom classic signs are often absent, may go undiagnosed and serve as reservoirs of disease.[6,15]

The potency of the pertussis component of the vaccine is measured and shown to be acceptable in the mouse potency test. Previously, serum agglutinin titers of pertussis vaccines have been correlated with clinical protection in the Medical Research Council trials.[8] The pertussis component induces immunity against pertussis disease in humans.

Haemophilus influenzae type b was the most common cause of invasive bacterial disease, including meningitis, in young children in the US prior to licensure of vaccines for this disease. Although nonencapsulated *H. influenzae* are common and six capsular polysaccharide types are known, strains with the type b capsule caused most of the invasive Haemophilus diseases prior to the introduction of Haemophilus b conjugate vaccines.[16]

Prior to routine immunization, Haemophilus b disease occurred primarily in children under 5 years of age. In the US, the incidence of invasive Haemophilus b disease peaked between 6 months and 1 year of age, and approximately 55% of disease occurred between 6 and 18 months of age.[16] The cumulative risk of developing invasive Haemophilus b disease during the first 5 years of life was about 1 in 200 prior to the introduction of Haemophilus b conjugate vaccines. Approximately 60% of cases were meningitis. Cellulitis, epiglottitis, pericarditis, pneumonia, sepsis, or septic arthritis made up the remaining 40%. An estimated 12,000 cases of Haemophilus b meningitis occurred annually prior to the routine use of conjugate vaccines in infants and toddlers.[16,17] The mortality rate can be 5%, and neurologic sequelae have been observed in up to 38% of survivors.[18]

The incidence of invasive Haemophilus b disease is increased in certain children, such as those who are native Americans, black, or from lower socioeconomic status and those with medical conditions such as asplenia, sickle cell disease, malignancies associated with immunosuppression, and antibody deficiency syndromes.[16,17,19]

The protective activity of antibody to Haemophilus b polysaccharide was demonstrated by the efficacy study of Haemophilus b polysaccharide (HbPs) vaccine.[20] Data from passive antibody studies indicate that a preexisting titer of antibody to HbPs of 0.15 μg/mL correlates with protection.[21] Data from a Finnish field trial in children 18 to 71 months of age indicate that a titer of >1.0 μg/mL 3 weeks after vaccination is associated with long-term protection.[22,23]

Linkage of Haemophilus b saccharides to a protein such as CRM_{197} converts the saccharide (HbO) to a T-dependent (HbOC) antigen, and results in an enhanced antibody response to the saccharide in young infants that primes for an anamnestic response and is predominantly of the IgG class.[24]

Laboratory evidence indicates that the native state of the CRM_{197} protein and the use of oligosaccharides in the formulation of HibTITER Haemophilus b Conjugate Vaccine (Diphtheria CRM_{197} Protein Conjugate) (HbOC), enhances its immunogenicity.[25–27] NO PUBLISHED DATA ARE AVAILABLE TO SUPPORT THE INTERCHANGEABILITY OF HbOC AND OTHER HAEMOPHILUS b CONJUGATE VACCINES WITH ONE ANOTHER FOR PRIMARY IMMUNIZATION.

HbOC was shown to be effective in a large-scale controlled clinical trial in a multiethnic population in northern California carried out between February 1988 and June 1990.[28,29] It should be noted that DTP was administered simultaneously with HbOC but at a separate site. There were no (0) vaccine failures in infants who received three doses of HbOC and 12 cases of Haemophilus b disease (6 cases of meningitis) in the control group. The estimate of efficacy is 100% (P=.0002) with 95% confidence intervals of 68% to 100%. Through the end of 1991, with an additional 49,000 person-years of follow-up, there were still no cases of Haemophilus b disease in fully vaccinated infants less than 2 years of age.[10,30] Person-years may be defined as the number of individuals receiving the appropriate number of doses times the average number of years of follow-up for all of the individuals. One case of disease has been reported in a 3½-year-old child who did not receive the recommended booster dose.

Evidence of efficacy postlicensure of Haemophilus b conjugate vaccines in the US is indicated by reports of significant reductions (71% to 94%) in Haemophilus b disease that are closely associated with increases in the net doses of Haemophilus b conjugate vaccines distributed.[30,31] Occasional cases of vaccine failures have, however, been reported to the US Department of Health and Human Services through the Vaccine Adverse Event Reporting System (VAERS) since licensure of Haemophilus b conjugate vaccines.

TETRAMUNE has been given to 6,793 children as part of a series of studies to test the safety and immunogenicity of this combined product when compared to separate administration of DTP and HbOC. The vaccines were given at 2, 4, and 6 months of age or at 15 to 18 months of age. Local reactions and systemic events after vaccination were generally comparable between the groups that received the combination product or separate injections. (It should be noted that comparison of local reactions was done by comparing the combined product to the separate injection site that gave the largest reactions or to the DTP injection site.) Scattered reactions occurred more frequently (P <.05) in the combination group for some doses (swelling and drowsiness after the first dose; irritability and restless sleep after the second dose; injection site warmth and irritability after the third dose; injection site swelling, warmth, tenderness, irritability after the toddler dose). Rash was seen more commonly in the separate group. There was no consistent or identifiable pattern to these group differences across studies or doses. The large trial with 6,497 infants receiving TETRAMUNE allowed analysis of rare adverse events, including SIDS (sudden infant death syndrome), hospitalizations, and emergency room visits, following vaccination. No differences were found between the cohorts (see **ADVERSE REACTIONS**).[10] Taken together, the safety studies conducted in infants and in toddlers indicate that this vaccine is safe and that there was no consistent pattern of enhanced adverse events following combined vaccine (TETRAMUNE) as compared to separate injections.

The antibody response to each of the components of TETRAMUNE was measured (n=189) and compared to separate administration of the DTP and HbOC vaccines (n=189). After three doses, the antibody response to TETRAMUNE was equal to or higher for all four components: tetanus (IU/mL), diphtheria (IU/mL), pertussis (microagglutination), and *H. influenzae* b polysaccharide (μg IgG/mL as per ELISA). In addition, responses to specific pertussis antigens (ie, pertussis toxin, FHA, and 69K protein) were found to be as high or higher in the

Continued on next page

Lederle—Cont.

TETRAMUNE product compared to separate administration of DTP. Therefore, the immunogenicity of the combined vaccine is at least as good as the two vaccines given separately.[10]

INDICATIONS AND USAGE

Diphtheria and Tetanus Toxoids and Pertussis Vaccine Adsorbed and Haemophilus b Conjugate Vaccine (Diphtheria CRM$_{197}$ Protein Conjugate) TETRAMUNE, is indicated for the active immunization of children 2 months of age to 5 years of age for protection against diphtheria, tetanus, pertussis, and Haemophilus b disease when indications for immunization with DTP vaccine and Haemophilus b Conjugate Vaccine coincide. Typically, this is at 2, 4, 6, and 15 months of age.

Children who have recovered from culture-confirmed pertussis need not receive further doses of a vaccine containing pertussis.[6] However, these children should receive additional doses of Diphtheria and Tetanus Toxoids Adsorbed, for Pediatric Use (DT) as well as Haemophilus b Conjugate Vaccine as appropriate to complete the series.

The American Academy of Pediatrics (AAP) has recommended that children who have experienced invasive Haemophilus b disease when < 24 months of age should continue immunization against Haemophilus b, but that children whose disease occurred at ≥ 24 months need not receive further doses of Haemophilus b Conjugate Vaccine.[32] However, these children should receive additional doses of DTP (or if pertussis is contraindicated, DT should be used) as appropriate to complete the series.

TETRAMUNE is intended for active immunization against diphtheria, tetanus, pertussis, and Haemophilus type b diseases and is not to be used for treatment of actual infection. TETRAMUNE is not routinely recommended for immunization of persons older than 5 years of age. Under certain circumstances, TETRAMUNE may be used beyond age 5 years. Because TETRAMUNE contains pediatric DTP vaccine, it is not recommended for use beyond the seventh birthday.

As with any vaccine, TETRAMUNE may not protect 100% of individuals receiving the vaccine.

If passive immunization is needed, Tetanus Immune Globulin (human TIG) and/or Diphtheria Antitoxin are recommended for tetanus and diphtheria, respectively (see **DOSAGE AND ADMINISTRATION**).[6]

CONTRAINDICATIONS

HYPERSENSITIVITY TO ANY COMPONENT OF THE VACCINE, INCLUDING THIMEROSAL, A MERCURY DERIVATIVE, IS A CONTRAINDICATION.

IMMUNIZATION SHOULD BE DEFERRED DURING THE COURSE OF ANY FEBRILE ILLNESS OR ACUTE INFECTION. THE IMMUNIZATION PRACTICES ADVISORY COMMITTEE (ACIP) HAS STATED THAT "... MINOR ILLNESSES SUCH AS MILD UPPER RESPIRATORY INFECTIONS WITH OR WITHOUT LOW GRADE FEVER ARE NOT CONTRAINDICATIONS." [6,33]

IMMUNIZATION WITH TETRAMUNE IS CONTRAINDICATED IF THE CHILD HAS EXPERIENCED ANY EVENT FOLLOWING PREVIOUS IMMUNIZATION WITH A PERTUSSIS-CONTAINING VACCINE, WHICH IS CONSIDERED BY THE AAP OR ACIP TO BE A CONTRAINDICATION TO FURTHER DOSES OF PERTUSSIS VACCINE. THESE EVENTS INCLUDE:

AN IMMEDIATE ANAPHYLACTIC REACTION.
ENCEPHALOPATHY OCCURRING WITHIN 7 DAYS FOLLOWING VACCINATION. THIS IS DEFINED AS AN ACUTE, SEVERE CENTRAL-NERVOUS-SYSTEM DISORDER OCCURRING WITHIN 7 DAYS FOLLOWING VACCINATION, AND GENERALLY CONSISTING OF MAJOR ALTERATIONS IN CONSCIOUSNESS, UNRESPONSIVENESS, GENERALIZED OR FOCAL SEIZURES THAT PERSIST MORE THAN A FEW HOURS, WITH FAILURE TO RECOVER WITHIN 24 HOURS.[6,33]

THE OCCURRENCE OF ANY TYPE OF NEUROLOGICAL SYMPTOMS OR SIGNS, INCLUDING ONE OR MORE CONVULSIONS (SEIZURES) FOLLOWING ADMINISTRATION OF TETRAMUNE, IS GENERALLY A CONTRAINDICATION TO FURTHER USE. ANY DECISION TO ADMINISTER SUBSEQUENT DOSES OF A VACCINE CONTAINING DIPHTHERIA, TETANUS, OR PERTUSSIS ANTIGENS SHOULD BE DELAYED UNTIL THE PATIENT'S NEUROLOGICAL STATUS IS BETTER DEFINED.[6]

THE PRESENCE OF ANY EVOLVING OR CHANGING DISORDER AFFECTING THE CENTRAL NERVOUS SYSTEM IS A CONTRAINDICATION TO ADMINISTRATION OF A PERTUSSIS-CONTAINING VACCINE SUCH AS TETRAMUNE REGARDLESS OF WHETHER THE SUSPECTED NEUROLOGICAL DISORDER IS ASSOCIATED WITH OCCURRENCE OF SEIZURE ACTIVITY OF ANY TYPE.[6,33]

STUDIES HAVE INDICATED THAT A PERSONAL OR FAMILY HISTORY OF SEIZURES IS ASSOCIATED WITH INCREASED FREQUENCY OF SEIZURES FOLLOWING PERTUSSIS IMMUNIZATION.[34–36]

The ACIP and the AAP recognize certain circumstances in which children with stable central nervous system disorders, including well-controlled seizures or satisfactorily explained single seizures, may receive pertussis vaccine. The ACIP and AAP do not consider a family history of seizures to be a contraindication to pertussis vaccine despite the increased risk of seizures in these individuals.[6,33,34]

The decision to administer a pertussis-containing vaccine to children must be made by the physician on an individual basis, with consideration of all relevant factors, and assessment of potential risks and benefits for that individual. The physician should review the full text of ACIP and AAP guidelines prior to considering vaccination for children.[6,33,34] The parent or guardian should be advised of the increased risk involved.

There are no data on whether the prophylactic use of antipyretics can decrease the risk of febrile convulsions. However, data suggest that acetaminophen will reduce the incidence of postvaccination fever.[37] The ACIP and AAP suggest administering acetaminophen at age-appropriate doses at the time of vaccination and every 4 to 6 hours to children at higher risk for seizures than the general population.[6,33,34]

TETRAMUNE is not routinely recommended for immunization of persons older than 5 years of age. Under certain circumstances, TETRAMUNE may be used beyond age 5 years. Because TETRAMUNE contains pediatric DTP vaccine, it is not recommended for use beyond the seventh birthday.

ROUTINE IMMUNIZATION SHOULD BE DEFERRED DURING AN OUTBREAK OF POLIOMYELITIS PROVIDING THE PATIENT HAS NOT SUSTAINED AN INJURY THAT INCREASES THE RISK OF TETANUS AND PROVIDING AN OUTBREAK OF DIPHTHERIA OR PERTUSSIS DOES NOT OCCUR SIMULTANEOUSLY.[38]

The clinical judgment of the attending physician should prevail at all times.

WARNINGS

THE ACIP STATES THAT IF ANY OF THE FOLLOWING EVENTS OCCUR IN TEMPORAL RELATION TO RECEIPT OF DTP, THE DECISION TO GIVE SUBSEQUENT DOSES OF VACCINE CONTAINING THE PERTUSSIS COMPONENT SHOULD BE CAREFULLY CONSIDERED.

TEMPERATURE OF ≥40.5℃ (105°F) WITHIN 48 HOURS NOT DUE TO IDENTIFIABLE CAUSE.
COLLAPSE OR SHOCK-LIKE STATE (HYPOTONIC-HYPORESPONSIVE EPISODE) WITHIN 48 HOURS.
PERSISTENT, INCONSOLABLE CRYING LASTING ≥3 HOURS, OCCURRING WITHIN 48 HOURS.
CONVULSIONS WITH OR WITHOUT FEVER OCCURRING WITHIN 3 DAYS.

"ALTHOUGH THESE EVENTS WERE CONSIDERED ABSOLUTE CONTRAINDICATIONS IN PREVIOUS ACIP RECOMMENDATIONS, THERE MAY BE CIRCUMSTANCES, SUCH AS A HIGH INCIDENCE OF PERTUSSIS, IN WHICH THE POTENTIAL BENEFITS OUTWEIGH POSSIBLE RISKS, PARTICULARLY BECAUSE THESE EVENTS ARE NOT ASSOCIATED WITH PERMANENT SEQUELAE."[6]

IF A CONTRAINDICATION TO ANY OF THE COMPONENTS OF THIS COMBINATION VACCINE EXISTS (SEE **CONTRAINDICATIONS** SECTION), THEN TETRAMUNE SHOULD NOT BE USED. FOR EXAMPLE, IF THERE IS A CONTRAINDICATION AGAINST THE USE OF A PERTUSSIS VACCINE COMPONENT, THEN DIPHTHERIA AND TETANUS TOXOIDS ADSORBED, FOR PEDIATRIC USE (DT), AND HAEMOPHILUS b CONJUGATE VACCINE (DIPHTHERIA CRM$_{197}$ PROTEIN CONJUGATE) HibTITER, AS SEPARATE INJECTIONS, SHOULD BE SUBSTITUTED FOR EACH OF THE REMAINING DOSES.

THE OCCURRENCE OF SUDDEN INFANT DEATH SYNDROME (SIDS) HAS BEEN REPORTED FOLLOWING ADMINISTRATION OF DTP.[39–41] HOWEVER, A LARGE CASE-CONTROL STUDY IN THE US REVEALED NO CAUSAL RELATIONSHIP BETWEEN RECEIPT OF DTP VACCINE AND SIDS.[42] A RECENT STUDY OF 6,497 INFANTS IN NORTHERN CALIFORNIA FOUND NO INCREASE IN THE RATE OF SIDS AMONG TETRAMUNE RECIPIENTS.[10]

AS WITH ANY INTRAMUSCULAR INJECTION, TETRAMUNE SHOULD BE GIVEN WITH CAUTION TO INFANTS OR CHILDREN WITH THROMBOCYTOPENIA OR ANY COAGULATION DISORDER THAT WOULD CONTRAINDICATE INTRAMUSCULAR INJECTION (SEE **DRUG INTERACTIONS**).

As reported with Haemophilus b polysaccharide vaccine, cases of Haemophilus type b disease may occur prior to the onset of the protective effect of this vaccine.[16,43]

TETRAMUNE WILL NOT PROTECT AGAINST H. INFLUENZAE OTHER THAN TYPE b STRAINS.

ANTIGENURIA HAS BEEN DETECTED FOLLOWING RECEIPT OF HAEMOPHILUS b CONJUGATE VACCINE[44] AND, THEREFORE ANTIGEN DETECTION IN URINE MAY NOT HAVE DIAGNOSTIC VALUE IN SUSPECTED HAEMOPHILUS b DISEASE WITHIN 2 WEEKS OF IMMUNIZATION.

PRECAUTIONS

GENERAL

CARE IS TO BE TAKEN BY THE HEALTH CARE PROVIDER FOR SAFE AND EFFECTIVE USE OF THIS PRODUCT.

1. TETRAMUNE is not routinely recommended for immunization of persons older than 5 years of age. Under certain circumstances, TETRAMUNE may be used beyond age 5 years. Because TETRAMUNE contains pediatric DTP vaccine, it is not recommended for use beyond the seventh birthday.

2. PRIOR TO ADMINISTRATION OF ANY DOSE OF TETRAMUNE, THE PARENT OR GUARDIAN SHOULD BE ASKED ABOUT THE PERSONAL HISTORY, FAMILY HISTORY, AND RECENT HEALTH STATUS OF THE VACCINE RECIPIENT. THE HEALTH CARE PROVIDER SHOULD ASCERTAIN PREVIOUS IMMUNIZATION HISTORY, CURRENT HEALTH STATUS, AND OCCURRENCE OF ANY SYMPTOMS AND/OR SIGNS OF AN ADVERSE EVENT AFTER PREVIOUS IMMUNIZATIONS, IN THE CHILD TO BE IMMUNIZED, IN ORDER TO DETERMINE THE EXISTENCE OF ANY CONTRAINDICATION TO IMMUNIZATION WITH TETRAMUNE AND TO ALLOW AN ASSESSMENT OF BENEFITS AND RISKS.

3. BEFORE THE INJECTION OF ANY BIOLOGICAL, THE HEALTH CARE PROVIDER SHOULD TAKE ALL PRECAUTIONS KNOWN FOR THE PREVENTION OF ALLERGIC OR ANY OTHER SIDE REACTIONS. This should include: a review of the patient's history regarding possible sensitivity; the ready availability of epinephrine 1:1,000 and other appropriate agents used for control of immediate allergic reactions; and a knowledge of the recent literature pertaining to use of the biological concerned, including the nature of side effects and adverse reactions that may follow its use.

4. Children with impaired immune responsiveness, whether due to the use of immunosuppressive therapy (including irradiation, corticosteroids, antimetabolites, alkylating agents, and cytotoxic agents), a genetic defect, human immunodeficiency virus (HIV) infection, or other causes, may have reduced antibody response to active immunization procedures.[6,33,45] Deferral of administration of vaccine may be considered in individuals receiving immunosuppressive therapy.[6,33] Other groups should receive this vaccine according to the usual recommended schedule.[6,33,45,46] (See **DRUG INTERACTIONS**.)

5. This product is not contraindicated based on the presence of human immunodeficiency virus infection.[47]

6. *Since this product is a suspension containing an adjuvant, shake vigorously to obtain a uniform suspension prior to withdrawing each dose from the multiple dose vial.*

7. A separate sterile syringe and needle or a sterile disposable unit should be used for each individual patient to prevent transmission of infectious agents from one person to another. Needles should be disposed of properly and should not be recapped.

8. Special care should be taken to prevent injection into a blood vessel.

NATIONAL CHILDHOOD VACCINE INJURY ACT

This Act requires that the manufacturer and lot number of the vaccine administered be recorded by the health care provider in the vaccine recipient's permanent medical record (or in a permanent office log or file), along with the date of administration of the vaccine and the name, address, and title of the person administering the vaccine.

The Act further requires the health care provider to report to the Secretary of the Department of Health and Human Services through the Vaccine Adverse Event Reporting System (VAERS) the occurrence following immunization of any event set forth in the Vaccine Injury Table, including: anaphylaxis or anaphylactic shock within 24 hours; encephalopathy or encephalitis within 7 days; shock-collapse or hypotonic-hyporesponsive collapse within 7 days; residual seizure disorder; any acute complication or sequelae (including death) of above events, or any event that would contraindicate further doses of vaccine, according to this TETRAMUNE package insert.

The US Department of Health and Human Services has established VAERS to accept all reports of suspected adverse events after the administration of any vaccine, including but not limited to the reporting of events required by the National Childhood Vaccine Injury Act of 1986.[48] The VAERS toll-free number for VAERS forms and information is 800-822-7967.

INFORMATION FOR PATIENT

PRIOR TO ADMINISTRATION OF TETRAMUNE, HEALTH CARE PERSONNEL SHOULD INFORM THE PARENT, GUARDIAN, OR OTHER RESPONSIBLE ADULT OF THE RECOMMENDED IMMUNIZATION SCHEDULE FOR PROTECTION AGAINST DIPHTHERIA, TETANUS, PERTUSSIS, AND HAEMOPHILUS b DISEASE AND THE BENEFITS AND RISKS TO THE CHILD

RECEIVING THIS VACCINE. GUIDANCE SHOULD BE PROVIDED ON MEASURES TO BE TAKEN SHOULD ADVERSE EVENTS OCCUR, SUCH AS ANTIPYRETIC MEASURES FOR ELEVATED TEMPERATURES AND THE NEED TO REPORT ADVERSE EVENTS TO THE HEALTH CARE PROVIDER. PARENTS SHOULD BE PROVIDED WITH VACCINE INFORMATION PAMPHLETS AT THE TIME OF EACH VACCINATION, AS STATED IN THE NATIONAL CHILDHOOD VACCINE INJURY ACT.[48]

THE HEALTH CARE PROVIDER SHOULD INFORM THE PATIENT, PARENT, OR GUARDIAN OF THE IMPORTANCE OF COMPLETING THE IMMUNIZATION SERIES.

PATIENTS, PARENTS, OR GUARDIANS SHOULD BE INSTRUCTED TO REPORT ANY SERIOUS ADVERSE REACTIONS TO THEIR HEALTH CARE PROVIDER.

DRUG INTERACTIONS

Children receiving immunosuppressive therapy may have a reduced response to active immunization procedures.[6,33,45]

As with other intramuscular injections, TETRAMUNE should be given with caution to children on anticoagulant therapy.

Tetanus Immune Globulin or Diphtheria Antitoxin, if used, should be given in a separate site with a separate needle and syringe.

The AAP recommends that influenza virus vaccine should not be administered within 3 days of immunization with a pertussis-containing vaccine since both vaccines may cause febrile reactions in young children.[33]

Data are not yet available concerning adverse reactions that may occur when TETRAMUNE is given simultaneously with Oral Poliovirus Vaccine (OPV), Measles-Mumps-Rubella (MMR), or Hepatitis B (HB) vaccine at separate sites. Also, data are not available concerning the effects on immune response of OPV, MMR, or HB vaccine when TETRAMUNE is given simultaneously. Clinical studies with TETRAMUNE did however allow for the administration of OPV according to the routine immunization schedule for OPV.[10]

CARCINOGENESIS, MUTAGENESIS, IMPAIRMENT OF FERTILITY

TETRAMUNE has not been evaluated for its carcinogenic, mutagenic potential, or for impairment of fertility.

PREGNANCY

Pregnancy Category C

Animal reproduction studies have not been conducted with TETRAMUNE. This product is not recommended for use in individuals 7 years of age or older.

PEDIATRIC USE

The safety and effectiveness of TETRAMUNE in children below the age of 6 weeks have not been established.

For immunization of children 7 years of age or older, Tetanus and Diphtheria Toxoids Adsorbed for Adult Use (Td) is recommended.[6,33] If contraindication to the pertussis component exists, Diphtheria and Tetanus Toxoids Adsorbed, for Pediatric Use (DT) should be substituted in children who have not reached their seventh birthday.

Full protection against the indicated diseases (tetanus, diphtheria, pertussis, and Haemophilus type b disease) is based on a full course of immunization.

ADVERSE REACTIONS

The safety of TETRAMUNE has been evaluated in 6,793 children at 2, 4, and 6 months of age or at 15 to 18 months of age in three separate sites. The percent of doses administered associated with injection site reactions within 72 hours, or common systemic symptoms within 4 days, is summarized below:

[See table above.]

Based on review of the Kaiser-Permanente Medical Care Program utilization data base of hospitalizations (within 60 days) and emergency room visits (within 30 days of immunization) in 6,497 infants who received TETRAMUNE, the most common reasons for seeking care include: trauma, viral illness, and respiratory illnesses (eg, upper respiratory infection, otitis media, bronchitis/bronchiolitis, and pneumonia). One child who received TETRAMUNE became transiently pale and tremulous without loss of responsiveness 4 hours after immunization and was hospitalized with a diagnosis of seizure. No other hospital visits for seizure or hypotonic, hyporesponsive episodes were reported within 72 hours of immunization. These results were not different from those observed in 3,935 infants who received DTP and HbOC at separate injection sites.

As with other aluminum-containing vaccines,[49] a nodule may occasionally be palpable at the injection site for several weeks. Although not seen in studies with TETRAMUNE, sterile abscess formation or subcutaneous atrophy at the injection site may also occur.

The following significant adverse events have occurred following administration of DTP vaccines: persistent, inconsolable crying ≥3 hours (1/100 doses), high-pitched, unusual crying (1/1,000 doses), fever ≥40.5°C (105°F) (1/330 doses),

% of Doses Associated with Symptoms[10]

	Infants‡ (542 doses)	Infants§ (7269 doses)	Toddlers (107 doses)
Local*			
Erythema	34	19	40
Pain/Tenderness	21	30	65
Swelling	20	20	43
Warmth	16	—	35
Systemic†			
Fever ≥38.0°C	24	40″	33
Irritability	42	54	49
Drowsiness	26	—	9
Restless Sleep	—	28	—
Loss of Appetite	—	4	—
Vomiting	5	2	1
Diarrhea	9	1	10
Rash	3	—	0

*Within 72 hours of immunization.

†Within 4 days of immunization.

‡A separate multicenter safety and immunogenicity study, not a subset of the 7,269 infant Kaiser study.

§Data for this study all collected within 24 hours of immunization (percentages calculated from a range of 7269 to 7500 doses) in the Kaiser Permanente Safety and Immunogenicity Study.

″Perceived fever.

transient shock-like (hypotonic, hyporesponsive) episode (1/1,750 doses), convulsions (1/1,750 doses).[6,33]

The ACIP states: "Although DTP may rarely produce symptoms that some have classified as acute encephalopathy, a causal relation between DTP vaccine and permanent brain damage has not been demonstrated. If the vaccine ever causes brain damage, the occurrence of such an event must be exceedingly rare. A similar conclusion has been reached by the Committee on Infectious Diseases of the American Academy of Pediatrics, the Child Neurology Society, the Canadian National Advisory Committee on Immunization, the British Joint Committee on Vaccination and Immunization, the British Pediatric Association, and the Institute of Medicine."[6]

The occurrence of sudden infant death syndrome (SIDS) has been reported following administration of DTP.[39–41] However, a large case-control study in the US revealed no causal relationship between receipt of DTP vaccine and SIDS.[42] A recent study of 6,497 infants in northern California found no increase in the rate of SIDS among TETRAMUNE recipients.[10]

Onset of infantile spasms has occurred in infants who have recently received DTP or DT. Analysis of data from the National Childhood Encephalopathy Study on children with infantile spasms showed that receipt of preparations containing diphtheria, tetanus, and/or pertussis antigens was not causally related to infantile spasms.[50] The incidence of onset of infantile spasms increases at 3 to 9 months of age, the time period in which the second and third doses of DTP are generally given. Therefore, some cases of infantile spasms can be expected to be related by chance alone to recent receipt of vaccines containing DTP.[6]

Bulging fontanel[51–53] has been reported after DTP immunization, although no cause and effect relationship has been established.

Cardiac effects[54–56] and respiratory difficulties, including apnea, have been reported rarely following DTP immunization.

Other events that have been reported following administration of vaccines containing diphtheria, tetanus, pertussis, or Haemophilus b antigens include: urticaria, erythema multiforme or other rash, arthralgias,[57] and, more rarely, a severe anaphylactic reaction (eg, urticaria with swelling of the mouth, difficulty breathing, hypotension, or shock) and neurological complications,[58] such as convulsions,[57,59] encephalopathy,[57,60] and various mono- and polyneuropathies,[60–66] including Guillain-Barré syndrome.[67–69] Permanent neurological disability and death have also been reported rarely in temporal relation to immunization although a causal relationship has not been established.

DOSAGE AND ADMINISTRATION

For Intramuscular Use Only

For infants beginning at 2 months of age, the immunization series for TETRAMUNE consists of three doses of 0.5 mL each at approximately 2-month intervals, followed by a fourth dose of 0.5 mL at approximately 15 months of age. TETRAMUNE may be substituted for DTP and HibTITER administered separately, whenever the recommended schedules for use of these two vaccines coincide (see DTP and HibTITER recommended dosage schedules).[6,32,33,70] However, no published data are available to support the interchangeability of the Haemophilus b conjugate vaccine in TETRAMUNE and HibTITER with other Haemophilus b conjugate vaccines for the primary series. Therefore, it is recommended that the same conjugate vaccine be used throughout the primary series, consistent with the data supporting licensure of the vaccine.[32]

RECOMMENDED IMMUNIZATION SCHEDULES

For Previously Unvaccinated *Younger* Children

Dose	Age	Immunization
1	2 months	TETRAMUNE
2	4 months	TETRAMUNE
3	6 months	TETRAMUNE
4	15–18 months	TETRAMUNE*
5	4–6 years	DTP or DTaP

*Children 15 to 18 months of age may receive DTaP plus a Haemophilus b conjugate vaccine as separate injections.

For Previously Unvaccinated *Older* Children[33]

Immunization schedules should be considered on an individual basis for children not vaccinated according to the recommended schedule. Three doses of a product containing DTP, given at approximately 2-month intervals, are required, followed by a fourth dose of a product containing DTP or DTaP approximately 12 months later and a fifth dose of a product containing DTP or DTaP at 4 to 6 years of age. If the fourth dose of a pertussis-containing vaccine is not given until after the fourth birthday, no further doses of a pertussis-containing vaccine are necessary.

The number of doses of an HbOC-containing product indicated depends on the age that immunization is begun. A child 7 to 11 months of age should receive 3 doses of a product containing HbOC. A child 12 to 14 months of age should receive 2 doses of a product containing HbOC. A child 15 to 59 months of age should receive 1 dose of a product containing HbOC.

As indicated previously, TETRAMUNE may be substituted for DTP and HibTITER administered separately, whenever the recommended schedule for use of these two vaccines coincides.

Preterm infants should be vaccinated with TETRAMUNE according to their chronological age, from birth.[6]

Interruption of the recommended schedules with a delay between doses does not interfere with the final immunity achieved; nor does it necessitate starting the series over again, regardless of the length of time elapsed between doses.[6,33]

If a contraindication to the pertussis vaccine component occurs, Diphtheria and Tetanus Toxoids Adsorbed, for Pediatric Use (DT), and Haemophilus b Conjugate Vaccine HibTITER, as separate injections, should be substituted for each of the remaining doses.

The use of reduced volume (fractional doses) is not recommended. The effect of such practices on the frequency of serious adverse events and on protection against disease has not been determined.

Shake vigorously to obtain a uniform suspension prior to withdrawing each dose from the multiple dose vial. The vaccine should not be used if it cannot be resuspended.

Parenteral drug products should be inspected visually for particulate matter and discoloration prior to administration whenever solution and container permit. (See **DESCRIPTION.**)

The vaccine should be injected intramuscularly. The preferred sites are the anterolateral aspect of the thigh or the deltoid muscle of the upper arm. The vaccine should not be injected in the gluteal area or areas where there may be a major nerve trunk. Before injection, the skin at the injection site should be cleansed and prepared with a suitable germicide.

After insertion of the needle, aspirate to help avoid inadvertent injection into a blood vessel.

Continued on next page

Lederle—Cont.

For either primary or booster immunization against tetanus and diphtheria of individuals 7 years of age and older, the use of Tetanus and Diphtheria Toxoids Adsorbed for Adult Use (Td) is recommended.[6,33]

For passive immunization against tetanus and diphtheria, human TIG, and/or Diphtheria Antitoxin are recommended.[6] A separate syringe and site of injection should be used.

HOW SUPPLIED

NDC 0005-1960-31 5.0 mL vial

STORAGE

DO NOT FREEZE. STORE REFRIGERATED, AWAY FROM FREEZER COMPARTMENT, AT 2°C TO 8°C (36°F TO 46°F).

Manufactured by:
LEDERLE LABORATORIES
Division of American Cyanamid Company
Pearl River, NY 10965

REFERENCES

1. Mueller JH, Miller PA. Production of diphtheria toxin of high potency (100 Lf) on a reproducible medium. *J Immunol.* 1941;40:21–32.
2. Mueller JH, Miller PA. Factors influencing the production of tetanal toxin. *J Immunol.* 1947;56:143–147.
3. Pillemer L, Grossberg DB, Wittler RG. The immunochemistry of toxins and toxoids, II. The preparation and immunologic evaluation of purified tetanal toxoid. *J Immunol.* 1946;54:213–224.
4. United States Patent Number 4,902,506 by Anderson PW, Eby RJ filed May 5, 1986 issued February 20, 1990.
5. Seid RC Jr, Boykins RA, Liu DF, et al. Chemical evidence for covalent linkage of a semi-synthetic glycoconjugate vaccine for *Haemophilus influenzae* type b disease. *Glycoconjugate J.* 1989;6:489–498.
6. Diphtheria, tetanus and pertussis: Recommendations for vaccine use and other preventive measures—recommendations of the Immunization Practices Advisory Committee (ACIP). *MMWR.* 1991;40/No. RR-10.
7. Pappenheimer AM Jr. Diphtheria. In: Germanier R, ed. *Bacterial Vaccines.* New York, NY: Academic Press Inc; 1984:1–36.
8. *Federal Register Notice,* Friday, December 13, 1985, Vol. 50, No. 240.
9. Blumberg DA, Mink CM, Cherry JD, et al. Comparison of acellular and whole-cell pertussis-component diphtheria-tetanus-pertussis vaccines in infants. *J Pediatr.* 1991; 119:194–204.
10. Unpublished data available from Lederle Laboratories.
11. Manclark CR, Cowell JL. Pertussis Vaccine. In: Germanier R, ed. *Bacterial Vaccines.* New York, NY: Academic Press Inc; 1984:69–106.
12. Kendrick PL. Secondary familial attack rates from pertussis in vaccinated and unvaccinated children. *Am J Hygiene.* 1940;32:89–91.
13. Reported incidence of notifiable diseases in the United States. *MMWR.* 1970;19(53):44.
14. Pertussis surveillance—United States, 1986–1988. *MMWR.* 1990;39(4):57–66.
15. Mortimer EA Jr. Pertussis and its prevention: a family affair. *J Infect Dis.* 1990;161:437–479.
16. Wenger JD, Ward JL, Broome CV. Prevention of *Haemophilus influenzae* type b disease: vaccines and passive prophylaxis. In: Remington JS, Swartz MS, eds. *Current Clinical Topics in Infectious Diseases.* New York, NY: McGraw-Hill Inc; 1989;10:306–339.
17. Recommendation of the Immunization Practices Advisory Committee (ACIP). Polysaccharide vaccine for prevention of *Haemophilus influenzae* type b disease. *MMWR.* 1985;34:201–205.
18. Sell SH. Long term sequelae of bacterial meningitis in children. *Pediatr Infect Dis J.* 1983;2:90–93.
19. Broome CV. Epidemiology of *Haemophilus influenzae* type b infections in the United States. *Pediatr Infect Dis J.* 1987;6:779–782.
20. Peltola H, Kayhty H, Sivonen A. *Haemophilus influenzae* type b capsular polysaccharide vaccine in children: a double-blind field study of 100,000 vaccines 3 months to 5 years of age in Finland. *Pediatrics.* 1977;60:730–737.
21. Robbins JB, Parke JC, Schneerson R. Quantitative measurement of "natural" and immunization-induced *Haemophilus influenzae* type b capsular polysaccharide antibodies. *Pediatr Res.* 1973;7:103–110.
22. Kayhty H, Peltola H, Karanko V, et al. The protective level of serum antibodies to the capsular polysaccharide of *Haemophilus influenzae* type b. *J Infect Dis.* 1983;147:1100.
23. Kayhty H, Karanko V, Peltola H, et al. Serum antibodies after vaccination with *Haemophilus influenzae* type b capsular polysaccharide and responses to reimmunization: no evidence of immunologic tolerance or memory. *Pediatrics.* 1984;74:857-865.
24. Weinberg GA, Granoff DM. Polysaccharide-protein conjugate vaccines for the prevention of *Haemophilus influenzae* type b disease. *J Pediatr.* 1988;113:621–631.
25. Makela O, Péterfy F, Outshoorn IG, et al. Immunogenic properties of a (1–6) dextran, its protein conjugates, and conjugates of its breakdown products in mice. *Scand J Immunol.* 1984;19:541–550.
26. Anderson P, Pichichero ME, Insel RA. Immunogens consisting of oligosaccharides from *Haemophilus influenzae* type b coupled to diphtheria toxoid or the toxin protein CRM_{197}. *J Clin Invest.* 1985;76:52–59.
27. Madore DV, Phipps DC, Eby R, et al. Immune response of young children vaccinated with *Haemophilus influenzae* type b conjugate vaccines. In: Cruse JM, Lewis RE, eds. *Contributions to Microbiology and Immunology: Conjugate Vaccines.* New York, NY: Karger Medical and Scientific Publishers; 1989;10:125–150.
28. Black SB, Shinefield HR, Lampert D, et al. Safety and immunogenicity of oligosaccharide conjugate *Haemophilus influenzae* type b (HbOC) vaccine in infancy. *Pediatr Infect Dis J.* 1991;10:92–96.
29. Black SB, Shinefield HR, Fireman B, et al. Efficacy in infancy of oligosaccharide conjugate *Haemophilus influenzae* type b (HbOC) vaccine in a United States population of 61,080 children. *Pediatr Infect Dis J.* 1991;10:97–104.
30. Black SB, Shinefield HR, The Kaiser Permanente Pediatric Vaccine Study Group. Immunization with oligosaccharide conjugate *Haemophilus influenzae* type b (HbOC) vaccine on a large health maintenance organization population: extended follow-up and impact on *Haemophilus influenzae* disease epidemiology. *Pediatr Infect Dis J.* 1992;11:610–613.
31. Adams WG, Deaver KA, Cochi SL, et al. Decline of childhood *Haemophilus influenzae* type b (Hib) disease in the Hib vaccine era. *JAMA.* 1993;269:221–226.
32. Recommendations of the AAP: *Haemophilus influenzae* type b conjugate vaccine: recommendations for immunization of infants and children 2 months of age and older: update. *Pediatrics.* 1991;88:169–172.
33. American Academy of Pediatrics: Report of the Committee on Infectious Diseases. 22nd ed. Elk Grove Village, Ill: American Academy of Pediatrics; 1991.
34. Pertussis immunization: family history of convulsions and use of antipyretics—supplementary ACIP statement. *MMWR.* 1987;36(18):281–282.
35. Stetler HC, Orenstein WA, Bart KJ, et al. History of convulsions and use of pertussis vaccine. *J Pediatr.* 1985;107(2):175–179.
36. Hirtz DG, Nelson KB, Ellenberg JH. Seizures following childhood immunizations. *J Pediatr.* 1983; 102(1):14–18.
37. Ipp MM, Gold R, Greenberg S, et al. Acetaminophen prophylaxis of adverse reactions following vaccination of infants with diphtheria-pertussis-tetanus toxoids-polio vaccine. *Pediatr Infect Dis J.* 1987;6:721–725.
38. Sutter RW, Patriarca PA, Suleiman AJM, et al. Attributable risk of DTP (Diphtheria and Tetanus Toxoids and Pertussis Vaccine) injection in provoking paralytic poliomyelitis during a large outbreak in Oman. *J Infect Dis.* 1992;165:444–449.
39. Bernier R, Frank JA, Dondero TJ, et al. Diphtheria-tetanus toxoids, pertussis vaccination and sudden infant deaths in Tennessee. *J Pediatr.* 1982;101:419–421.
40. Baraff L, Ablon WJ, Weiss RC. Possible temporal association between diptheria-tetanus toxoid, pertussis vaccination and sudden infant death syndrome. *Pediatr Inf Dis.* 1983;2:7–11.
41. Walker AM, Jick H, Perera DR, et al. Diphtheria-tetanus-pertussis immunization and sudden infant death. *AJPH.* 1987;77(8):945–951.
42. Hoffman HJ, Hunter JC, Damus K, et al. Diphtheria-tetanus-pertussis immunization and sudden infant death: results of the National Institute of Child Health and Human Development cooperative study of sudden infant death syndrome risk factors. *Pediatrics.* 1987; 79(4):598–611.
43. Mortimer EA. Efficacy of Haemophilus b polysaccharide vaccine: an enigma. *JAMA.* 1988;260:1454–1455.
44. Scheifele D, Bjornsen GLG, Arcand T, et al. Antigenuria after receipt of Haemophilus b Diphtheria Toxoid Conjugate Vaccine. *Pediatr Infect Dis J.* 1989;8:887–888.
45. Recommendation of the ACIP—Immunization of children infected with human T-lymphotrophic virus type III/lymphadenopathy-associated virus. *MMWR.* 1986; 35(38):595–606.
46. Immunization of children infected with human immunodeficiency virus—supplementary ACIP statement. *MMWR.* 1988;37(12):181–183.
47. General Recommendations on Immunization—Recommendations of the Immunization Practices Advisory Committee (ACIP). *MMWR.* 1989;38(13):221.
48. CDC. Vaccine Adverse Event Reporting System—United States. *MMWR.* 1990;39:730–733.
49. Fawcett HA, Smith NP. Injection-site granuloma due to aluminum. *Arch Dermatol.* 1984;120:1318–1322.
50. Bellman MH, Ross EM, Miller DL. Infantile spasms and pertussis immunization. *Lancet.* 1983;1:1031–1034.
51. Mathur R, Kumari S. Bulging fontanel following triple vaccine (letter). *Indian Pediatrics.* 1981;18(6):417–418.
52. Shendurnikar N, Gandhi DJ, Patel J, et al. Bulging fontanel following DTP vaccine (letter). *Indian Pediatrics.* 1986;23(11):960.
53. Jacob J, Mannino F. Increased intracranial pressure after diphtheria, tetanus, and pertussis immunization. *Am J Dis Child.* 1979;133:217–218.
54. Leung A. Congenital heart disease and DTP vaccination. *Can Med Assoc J.* 1984;131:541.
55. Park JM, Ledbetter EO, South MA, et al. Paroxysmal supraventricular tachycardia precipitated by pertussis vaccine. *Pediatrics.* 1983;102(6):883–885.
56. Amsel SG, Hanukoglu A, Fried D, et al. Myocarditis after triple immunization. *Arch Dis Child.* 1986; 61:403–404.
57. CDC. Adverse events following immunization. *MMWR.* 1985;34:43–47.
58. Rutledge SL, Snead OC. Neurologic complications of immunizations. *J Pediatr.* 1986;109:917–924.
59. Milstein JB, Gross TP, Kuritsky JN. Adverse reactions reported following receipt of *Haemophilus influenzae* type b vaccine: an analysis after one year of marketing. *Pediatrics.* 1987;80:270–274.
60. Schlenska GK. Unusual neurological complications following tetanus toxoid administration. *J Neurol.* 1977; 215:299–302.
61. Blumstein GI, Kreithen H. Peripheral neuropathy following tetanus toxoid administration. *JAMA.* 1966; 198:1030–1031.
62. Reinstein L, Pargament JM, Goodman JS. Peripheral neuropathy after multiple tetanus toxoid injections. *Arch Phys Med Rehabil.* 1982;63:332–334.
63. Tsairis P, Dyck PJ, Mulder DW. Natural history of brachial plexus neuropathy. *Arch Neurol.* 1972; 27:109–117.
64. Quast U, Hennessen W, Widmark RM. Mono- and polyneuritis after tetanus vaccination. *Devel Bio Stand.* 1979; 43:25–32.
65. Holliday PL, Bauer RB. Polyradiculoneuritis secondary to immunization with tetanus and diphtheria toxoids. *Arch Neurol.* 1983;40:56–57.
66. Fenichel GM. Neurological complications of tetanus toxoid. *Arch Neurol.* 1983;40:390.
67. Pollard JD, Selby G. Relapsing neuropathy due to tetanus toxoid. *J Neurol Sci.* 1978;37:113–125.
68. Newton N, Janati A. Guillain-Barré syndrome after vaccination with purified tetanus toxoid. *S Med J.* 1987; 80:1053–1054.
69. D'Cruz DF, Shapiro ED, Spiegelman KN, et al. Acute inflammatory demyelinating polyradiculoneuropathy (Guillain-Barré syndrome) after immunization with *Haemophilus influenzae* type b conjugate vaccine. *J Pediatr.* 1989;115:743–746.
70. Recommendation of the ACIP: Haemophilus b conjugate vaccines for prevention of *Haemophilus influenzae* type b disease among infants and children two months of age and older. *MMWR.* 1991;40:1–7.

Shown in Product Identification Guide, page 321

TRI-IMMUNOL® ℞

Diphtheria and Tetanus Toxoids and Pertussis Vaccine Adsorbed

DESCRIPTION

Diphtheria and Tetanus Toxoids and Pertussis Vaccine Adsorbed, (DTP), TRI-IMMUNOL®, is a sterile combination of PUROGENATED® Diphtheria Toxoid aluminum phosphate-adsorbed, PUROGENATED Tetanus Toxoid aluminum phosphate-adsorbed, and Pertussis Vaccine for intramuscular use only. After shaking, the vaccine is a homogeneous white suspension.

The diphtheria and tetanus toxins are produced according to the method of Mueller and Miller[1,2] and are detoxified by use of formaldehyde. The toxoids are refined by the Pillemer alcohol fractionation method[3] and are diluted with a solution containing sodium phosphate monobasic, sodium phosphate dibasic, glycine, and thimerosal (mercury derivative) as a preservative. Pertussis Vaccine is prepared by growing Phase I *Bordetella pertussis* in a modified Cohen-Wheeler broth containing acid hydrolysate of casein. The *B pertussis* culture is harvested, inactivated, and then suspended in a solution containing potassium phosphate monobasic, sodium phosphate dibasic, aluminum phosphate, sodium chloride, and thimerosal as a preservative and is then combined with the refined Diphtheria and Tetanus Toxoids in physiological saline diluent containing thimerosal as a preservative. The final concentration of thimerosal (mercury derivative) in the combined vaccine is 1:10,000. The aluminum content of the final product does not exceed 0.80 mg per 0.5 mL dose.

Each 0.5 mL dose is formulated to contain 12.5 Lf of diphtheria toxoid, and 5 Lf of tetanus toxoid. The total human immunizing dose (the first three 0.5 mL doses given) contains an estimate of 12 units of pertussis vaccine. Each component of the vaccine—diphtheria, tetanus, and pertussis—meets the required potency standards.

The primary immunization against diphtheria, tetanus, and pertussis consists of four 0.5 mL doses when administered as recommended.[4,5]

CLINICAL PHARMACOLOGY

Simultaneous immunization against diphtheria, tetanus, and pertussis during infancy and childhood has been a routine practice in the United States since the late 1940s. It has played a major role in markedly reducing the incidence of cases and deaths from each of these diseases.

Diphtheria is primarily a localized and generalized intoxication caused by diphtheria toxin, an extracellular protein metabolite of toxinogenic strains of *Corynebacterium diphtheriae*. While the incidence of diphtheria in the U.S. has decreased from over 200,000 cases reported in 1921, before the general use of diphtheria toxoid, to only 15 cases reported from 1980 to 1983,[4] the ratio of fatalities to attack rate has remained constant at about 5% to 10%. The highest case fatality rates are in the very young and in the elderly. Following adequate immunization with diphtheria toxoid, which induces antitoxin, it is thought that protection lasts for at least 10 years.[4] This significantly reduces both the risk of developing diphtheria and the severity of clinical illness. It does not, however, eliminate carriage of *C diphtheriae* in the pharynx or on the skin.[4]

Tetanus is an intoxication manifested primarily by neuromuscular dysfunction caused by a potent exotoxin elaborated by *Clostridium tetani*. The incidence of tetanus in the U.S. has dropped dramatically with the routine use of tetanus toxoid, remaining relatively constant over the last decade at about 90 cases reported annually. Spores of *C tetani* are ubiquitous, and there is essentially no natural immunity to tetanus toxin. Thus, universal primary immunization with tetanus toxoid with subsequent maintenance of adequate antitoxin levels, by means of timed boosters, is necessary to protect all age groups.[4] Tetanus toxoid is a highly effective antigen and a completed primary series generally induces protective levels of serum antitoxin that persist for at least 10 years.[4]

Pertussis is a disease of the respiratory tract caused by *B pertussis*. This Gram-negative coccobacillus produces a variety of active components including endotoxin and a number of other substances that have been defined primarily on the basis of their biological activity in animals. These active components have been associated with a number of effects, such as lymphocytosis, leukocytosis, sensitivity to histamine, changes in glucose and/or insulin levels, possible neurological effects and adjuvant activity.[6] The role of each of the different components in either the pathogenesis of, or immunity to, pertussis is not well understood.

Pertussis is a highly communicable disease which has an attack rate in unimmunized populations of over 90%.[4] Since pertussis vaccine has come into widespread use, the number of reported cases and associated mortality in the U.S. has declined from about 120,000 cases and 1,100 deaths in 1950[7] to an annual average of about 2,000 cases and 10 fatalities over the last 10 years.[4] Accurate data do not exist, as bacteriological confirmation of pertussis can be obtained in less than half of the suspected cases. Most reported illnesses from *B pertussis* occur in infants and young children; two thirds of reported deaths occur in children less than 1 year old. Older children and adults, in whom classic signs are often absent, may go undiagnosed and serve as reservoirs of disease.[4]

Evidence of the efficacy of pertussis vaccine can be provided by the British experience, where a reduction in the number of immunized individuals from 79% in 1973, to 31% in 1978 resulted in an epidemic of 102,500 pertussis cases and 36 deaths between late 1977 and 1980, and 1,440 cases per week reported during the winter of 1981 to 1982. A similar situation occurred in Japan.[7]

Because the severity of pertussis decreases with age, and the vaccine may cause side effects and adverse reactions, routine pertussis immunization is not recommended for persons 7 years of age or older.[4]

INDICATIONS AND USAGE

Diphtheria and Tetanus Toxoids and Pertussis Vaccine Adsorbed TRI-IMMUNOL® is indicated for active immunization of infants and children from 2 months of age up to their seventh birthday against diphtheria, tetanus, and pertussis.[4,5]

Children who have recovered from culture-confirmed pertussis need not receive further doses of a vaccine containing pertussis.[4]

CONTRAINDICATIONS

HYPERSENSITIVITY TO ANY COMPONENT OF THE VACCINE, INCLUDING THIMEROSAL, A MERCURY DERIVATIVE, IS A CONTRAINDICATION.

IMMUNIZATION SHOULD BE DEFERRED DURING THE COURSE OF ANY FEBRILE ILLNESS OR ACUTE INFECTION. A MINOR AFEBRILE ILLNESS SUCH AS A MILD UPPER RESPIRATORY INFECTION IS NOT USUALLY REASON TO DEFER IMMUNIZATION.[4,5]

THE OCCURRENCE OF ANY TYPE OF NEUROLOGICAL SYMPTOMS OR SIGNS, INCLUDING ONE OR MORE CONVULSIONS (SEIZURES) FOLLOWING ADMINISTRATION OF THIS PRODUCT IS A CONTRAINDICATION TO FURTHER USE. USE OF THIS PRODUCT IS ALSO CONTRAINDICATED IF THE CHILD HAS A PERSONAL HISTORY OF SEIZURES (SEE FOLLOWING DISCUSSION FOR INFORMATION REGARDING CHILDREN WITH A FAMILY HISTORY OF SEIZURES). THE PRESENCE OF ANY EVOLVING OR CHANGING DISORDER AFFECTING THE CENTRAL NERVOUS SYSTEM IS A CONTRAINDICATION TO ADMINISTRATION OF DTP REGARDLESS OF WHETHER THE SUSPECTED NEUROLOGICAL DISORDER IS ASSOCIATED WITH OCCURRENCE OF SEIZURE ACTIVITY OF ANY TYPE. STUDIES HAVE INDICATED THAT A PERSONAL OR FAMILY HISTORY OF SEIZURES IS ASSOCIATED WITH INCREASED FREQUENCY OF SEIZURES FOLLOWING PERTUSSIS IMMUNIZATION.[8,9,10]

Personal History: THE IMMUNIZATION PRACTICES ADVISORY COMMITTEE (ACIP) OF THE U.S. PUBLIC HEALTH SERVICE STATES: "THE PRESENCE OF A NEUROLOGIC CONDITION CHARACTERIZED BY CHANGING DEVELOPMENTAL OR NEUROLOGIC FINDINGS, REGARDLESS OF WHETHER A DEFINITIVE DIAGNOSIS HAS BEEN MADE, IS ... CONSIDERED A CONTRAINDICATION TO RECEIPT OF PERTUSSIS VACCINE, BECAUSE ADMINISTRATION OF DTP MAY COINCIDE WITH OR POSSIBLY EVEN AGGRAVATE MANIFESTATIONS OF THE DISEASE. SUCH DISORDERS INCLUDE UNCONTROLLED EPILEPSY, INFANTILE SPASMS, AND PROGRESSIVE ENCEPHALOPATHY."[4]

THE IMMUNIZATION PRACTICES ADVISORY COMMITTEE (ACIP) AND THE AMERICAN ACADEMY OF PEDIATRICS (AAP) RECOGNIZE CERTAIN CIRCUMSTANCES IN WHICH CHILDREN WITH STABLE CENTRAL NERVOUS SYSTEM DISORDERS, INCLUDING WELL-CONTROLLED SEIZURES OR SATISFACTORILY EXPLAINED SINGLE SEIZURES, MAY RECEIVE PERTUSSIS VACCINE. THE DECISION TO ADMINISTER VACCINE TO SUCH CHILDREN MUST BE MADE BY THE PHYSICIAN ON AN INDIVIDUAL BASIS, WITH CONSIDERATION OF ALL RELEVANT FACTORS, TO ALLOW AN ACCURATE ASSESSMENT OF RISKS AND BENEFITS FOR THAT INDIVIDUAL. THE PHYSICIAN SHOULD REVIEW THE FULL TEXT OF THE ACIP AND AAP GUIDELINES PRIOR TO CONSIDERING VACCINATION FOR SUCH CHILDREN.[4,5,8] THE PARENT OR GUARDIAN SHOULD BE ADVISED OF THE INCREASED RISK INVOLVED.

Family History: *THE ACIP AND AAP DO NOT CONSIDER A FAMILY HISTORY OF SEIZURES TO BE A CONTRAINDICATION TO PERTUSSIS VACCINE,[4,5,8] DESPITE THE INCREASED RISK OF SEIZURES IN THESE INDIVIDUALS. THE DECISION TO ADMINISTER VACCINE TO SUCH CHILDREN MUST BE MADE BY THE PHYSICIAN ON AN INDIVIDUAL BASIS, WITH CONSIDERATION OF ALL RELEVANT FACTORS, TO ALLOW AN ACCURATE ASSESSMENT OF RISKS AND BENEFITS FOR THAT INDIVIDUAL. THE PARENT OR GUARDIAN SHOULD BE ADVISED OF THE INCREASED RISK INVOLVED.*

THE ACIP STATES: "THERE ARE NO DATA ON WHETHER THE PROPHYLACTIC USE OF ANTIPYRETICS CAN DECREASE THE RISK OF FEBRILE CONVULSIONS. HOWEVER, PRELIMINARY DATA SUGGEST THAT ACETAMINOPHEN... WILL REDUCE THE INCIDENCE OF POSTVACCINATION FEVER. THUS, IT IS REASONABLE TO CONSIDER ADMINISTERING... ACETAMINOPHEN AT AGE-APPROPRIATE DOSES AT THE TIME OF VACCINATION AND EVERY 4 TO 6 HOURS FOR 48 TO 72 HOURS TO CHILDREN AT HIGHER RISK FOR SEIZURES THAN THE GENERAL POPULATION."[8]

Adverse Events Following Previous Immunization: THE ACIP AND AAP CONSIDER THE OCCURRENCE OF ANY OF THE FOLLOWING EVENTS AFTER VACCINATION WITH PERTUSSIS-CONTAINING VACCINE TO BE AN ABSOLUTE CONTRAINDICATION TO FURTHER PERTUSSIS VACCINATION:

1. ALLERGIC HYPERSENSITIVITY TO ANY COMPONENT OF THE VACCINE
2. FEVER OF 40.5°C (105°F) OR GREATER WITHIN 48 HOURS
3. COLLAPSE OR SHOCK-LIKE STATE (HYPOTONIC-HYPORESPONSIVE EPISODE) WITHIN 48 HOURS
4. PERSISTING, INCONSOLABLE CRYING LASTING 3 HOURS OR MORE, OR AN UNUSUAL HIGH-PITCHED CRY OCCURRING WITHIN 48 HOURS
5. CONVULSION(S) WITH OR WITHOUT FEVER OCCURRING WITHIN 3 DAYS. (For convulsions occurring beyond three days, see discussion in **CONTRAINDICATIONS** section and in references 4 and 5 concerning children with a personal history of convulsions).
6. ENCEPHALOPATHY OCCURRING WITHIN 7 DAYS; THIS INCLUDES SEVERE ALTERATIONS IN CONSCIOUSNESS WITH GENERALIZED OR FOCAL NEUROLOGIC SIGNS.[4,5]

The clinical judgment of the attending physician should prevail at all times.

Routine immunization should be deferred during an outbreak of poliomyelitis, providing the patient has not sustained an injury that increases the risk of tetanus and providing an outbreak of diphtheria or pertussis does not occur simultaneously.

WARNINGS

THIS PRODUCT IS NOT RECOMMENDED FOR IMMUNIZING PERSONS ON OR AFTER THEIR SEVENTH BIRTHDAY. DO NOT ATTEMPT IMMUNIZATION IF THE CHILD HAS OR IS SUSPECTED TO HAVE AN EVOLVING NEUROLOGICAL DISORDER. STUDIES HAVE INDICATED THAT A PERSONAL OR FAMILY HISTORY OF SEIZURES IS ASSOCIATED WITH INCREASED FREQUENCY OF SEIZURES FOLLOWING PERTUSSIS IMMUNIZATION.[8,9,10] (SEE DISCUSSION IN **CONTRAINDICATIONS** SECTION.)

SHOULD ANY SYMPTOMATOLOGY RELATED TO NEUROLOGICAL DISORDERS DEVELOP FOLLOWING ADMINISTRATION, DO NOT ATTEMPT FURTHER ADMINISTRATION OF PERTUSSIS VACCINE. THE OCCURRENCE OF ENCEPHALOPATHY (INCLUDING SEVERE ALTERATIONS IN CONSCIOUSNESS WITH GENERALIZED OR FOCAL NEUROLOGICAL SIGNS), CONVULSION, PERSISTING INCONSOLABLE CRYING FOR THREE OR MORE HOURS' DURATION, AN UNUSUAL HIGH-PITCHED CRY, COLLAPSE OR SHOCK-LIKE STATE, FEVER OF 40.5°C (105°F) OR GREATER, AND ALLERGIC REACTIONS AFTER ADMINISTRATION ARE CONTRAINDICATIONS FOR ANY FURTHER USE OF PERTUSSIS-CONTAINING VACCINE. (SEE **CONTRAINDICATIONS** SECTION.)

If a contraindication to pertussis is found, the infant or child should be given Diphtheria and Tetanus Toxoids, Adsorbed, for pediatric use (DT) instead of DTP. **Unimmunized children less than 1 year of age** should receive three doses of DT at 4 to 8 week intervals, followed by a fourth dose 6 to 12 months after the third dose, for the primary series. **Unimmunized children 1 year of age or older** should receive two doses of DT 4 to 8 weeks apart, followed by a third dose 6 to 12 months after the second dose for the primary series. **If, after beginning a DTP series, further doses of vaccine containing pertussis antigen become contraindicated, DT should be substituted for each of the remaining doses.**[4,5]

PARTIAL DOSES OF DTP VACCINE SHOULD NOT BE GIVEN.[4,5] Neither the efficacy of such practice in reducing the frequency of associated serious adverse events, nor the resulting protection against disease has been determined.

The occurrence of sudden infant death syndrome (SIDS) has been reported following administration of DTP.[11,12,13] However, a large case-control study in the U.S. revealed no causal relationship between receipt of DTP vaccine and SIDS.[14]

Onset of infantile spasms has occurred in infants who have recently received DTP or DT. Analysis of data from the National Childhood Encephalopathy Study on children with infantile spasms showed that receipt of DTP or DT was not causally related to infantile spasms.[15] The incidence of onset of infantile spasms increases at 3 to 9 months of age, the time period in which the second and third doses of DTP are generally given. Therefore, some cases of infantile spasms can be expected to be related by chance alone to recent receipt of DTP.[4]

DTP should not be given to infants or children with thrombocytopenia or any coagulation disorder that would contraindicate intramuscular injection unless the potential benefit clearly outweighs the risk of administration.

Patients with impaired immune responsiveness, whether due to the use of immunosuppressive therapy (including irradiation, corticosteroids, antimetabolites, alkylating agents, and cytotoxic agents), a genetic defect, human immunodeficiency virus (HIV) infection, or other causes, may have a reduced antibody response to active immunization procedures.[4,5,16] Deferral of administration of vaccine may be considered in individuals receiving immunosuppressive therapy.[4,5] Other groups should receive this vaccine according to the usual recommended schedule.[4,5,16,17]

Special care should be taken to prevent injection into a blood vessel.

PRECAUTIONS
General
1. THIS PRODUCT SHOULD BE USED FOR THE AGE GROUP BETWEEN 2 MONTHS AND THE SEVENTH BIRTHDAY.

Continued on next page

Lederle—Cont.

2. PRIOR TO ADMINISTRATION OF ANY DOSE OF DTP, THE PARENT OR GUARDIAN SHOULD BE ASKED ABOUT THE PERSONAL AND FAMILY HISTORY AND THE RECENT HEALTH STATUS OF THE INFANT OR CHILD TO BE IMMUNIZED IN ORDER TO DETERMINE THE EXISTENCE OF ANY CONTRAINDICATION TO IMMUNIZATION WITH DTP AND TO ALLOW AN ACCURATE ASSESSMENT OF BENEFITS AND RISKS. (SEE **CONTRAINDICATIONS; WARNINGS**.)

3. WHEN AN INFANT OR CHILD RETURNS FOR THE NEXT DOSE IN THE SERIES, THE PARENT OR GUARDIAN SHOULD BE QUESTIONED CONCERNING OCCURRENCE OF ANY SYMPTOM AND/OR SIGNS OF AN ADVERSE REACTION AFTER THE PREVIOUS DOSE (SEE **CONTRAINDICATIONS, ADVERSE REACTIONS**.)

4. BEFORE THE INJECTION OF ANY BIOLOGICAL, THE PHYSICIAN SHOULD TAKE ALL PRECAUTIONS KNOWN FOR PREVENTION OF ALLERGIC OR ANY OTHER SIDE REACTIONS. This should include: a review of the patient's history regarding possible sensitivity; the ready availability of epinephrine 1:1,000 and other appropriate agents used for control of immediate allergic reactions; and a knowledge of the recent literature pertaining to use of the biological concerned, including the nature of side effects and adverse reactions that may follow its use.

5. *Since this product contains both a bacterial suspension and an adjuvant, shake vigorously before withdrawing each dose from multiple dose vials.*

6. A separate sterile syringe and needle or a sterile disposable unit should be used for each individual patient to prevent transmission of hepatitis or other infectious agents from one person to another.

7. NATIONAL CHILDHOOD VACCINE INJURY ACT OF 1986 (AS AMENDED IN 1987). This Act requires that the manufacturer and lot number of the vaccine administered be recorded by the health care provider in the vaccine recipient's permanent medical record, along with the date of administration of the vaccine and the name, address and title of the person administering the vaccine.

The Act further requires the health care provider to report to a health department or to the FDA the occurrence following immunization of any event set forth in the Vaccine Injury Table including: anaphylaxis or anaphylactic shock within 24 hours, encephalopathy or encephalitis within 7 days, shock-collapse or hypotonic-hyporesponsive collapse within 7 days, residual seizure disorder, any acute complication or sequelae (including death) of above events, or any event that would contraindicate further doses of vaccine, according to this package insert.[18]

Information for Patient: PRIOR TO ADMINISTRATION OF THIS VACCINE, HEALTH CARE PERSONNEL SHOULD INFORM THE PARENT, GUARDIAN, OR OTHER RESPONSIBLE ADULT OF THE BENEFITS AND RISKS TO THE CHILD OF DTP VACCINE. GUIDANCE SHOULD BE PROVIDED ON MEASURES TO BE TAKEN SHOULD ADVERSE EVENTS OCCUR, EG, ANTIPYRETIC MEASURES FOR ELEVATED TEMPERATURES.

ADVERSE REACTIONS

Local reactions are common after administration of DTP, occurring in 35% to 50% of recipients[19] and are manifested by varying degrees of erythema, induration, and tenderness which may occasionally be severe. Such local reactions are usually self-limited and require no therapy. A nodule may be palpable at the injection site for a few weeks. Sterile abscess formation,[20] or subcutaneous atrophy at the site of injection has been reported. Cervical lymphadenopathy has been reported following DTP injections into the arm.[21]

Temperature elevations, fretfulness, drowsiness, vomiting, and anorexia frequently follow DTP administration.[19,22,23] Approximately 50% of DTP recipients will develop temperature elevations > 38°C (100.4°F) after one or more doses of the series; approximately 6% > 39°C (102.2°F);[20] and approximately 0.3% ≥ 40.5°C (105°F).[4] Some data suggest that febrile reactions are more likely to occur in those who have experienced such responses after prior doses.[22]

SIGNIFICANT REACTIONS ATTRIBUTED TO THE PERTUSSIS VACCINE COMPONENT HAVE BEEN: HIGH FEVER OF 40.5°C (105°F), A TRANSIENT SHOCK-LIKE EPISODE, EXCESSIVE SCREAMING (PERSISTENT CRYING OR SCREAMING FOR THREE OR MORE HOURS' DURATION), AN UNUSUAL HIGH-PITCHED CRY, AND CONVULSIONS. ENCEPHALOPATHY HAS BEEN REPORTED FOLLOWING PERTUSSIS VACCINATION; ONE STUDY SUGGESTS THE INCIDENCE OF ENCEPHALOPATHY OCCURRING WITHIN SEVEN DAYS OF VACCINATION MAY BE 1 PER 140,000 DOSES, WITH ENCEPHALOPATHY RESULTING IN DEATH OR PERMANENT DAMAGE TO THE CENTRAL NERVOUS SYSTEM ESTIMATED TO OCCUR IN 1 PER 330,000 DOSES.[24] (SEE **CONTRAINDICATIONS** AND **WARNINGS**.)

THE INCIDENCE OF CONVULSION OR TRANSIENT SHOCK-LIKE EPISODE OCCURRING WITHIN 48 HOURS OF VACCINATION HAS BEEN ESTIMATED TO BE 1 PER 1,750 DOSES.[19]

BULGING FONTANEL[25,26,27] HAS BEEN REPORTED AFTER DTP IMMUNIZATION, ALTHOUGH NO CAUSE AND EFFECT RELATIONSHIP HAS BEEN ESTABLISHED.

CARDIAC EFFECTS[28,29,30] AND RESPIRATORY DIFFICULTIES, INCLUDING APNEA HAVE BEEN REPORTED RARELY.

PERTUSSIS VACCINE HAS BEEN ASSOCIATED WITH A GREATER PROPORTION OF ADVERSE REACTIONS THAN MANY OTHER CHILDHOOD IMMUNIZATIONS.[31] SHOULD SYMPTOMATOLOGY REFERABLE TO THE CENTRAL NERVOUS SYSTEM DEVELOP WITHIN SEVEN DAYS FOLLOWING ADMINISTRATION, FURTHER IMMUNIZATION WITH THIS PRODUCT IS CONTRAINDICATED. (SEE **CONTRAINDICATIONS**.)

NEUROLOGICAL COMPLICATIONS,[32] SUCH AS CONVULSIONS,[19,31] ENCEPHALOPATHY,[24,33] AND VARIOUS MONO- AND POLYNEUROPATHIES,[32–39] INCLUDING GUILLAIN-BARRÉ SYNDROME,[40,41] HAVE BEEN REPORTED FOLLOWING ADMINISTRATION OF PREPARATIONS CONTAINING DIPHTHERIA, TETANUS, AND/OR PERTUSSIS ANTIGENS.

URTICARIA, ERYTHEMA MULTIFORME OR OTHER RASH, ARTHRALGIAS[31] AND RARELY, A SEVERE ANAPHYLACTIC REACTION (EG, URTICARIA WITH SWELLING OF THE MOUTH, DIFFICULTY BREATHING, HYPOTENSION OR SHOCK) HAVE BEEN REPORTED FOLLOWING ADMINISTRATION OF PREPARATIONS CONTAINING DIPHTHERIA, TETANUS, AND/OR PERTUSSIS ANTIGENS.

DOSAGE AND ADMINISTRATION

For Intramuscular Use Only: *Shake vigorously before withdrawing each dose from the multiple dose vials.*

Parenteral drug products should be inspected visually for particulate matter and discoloration prior to administration. (See **DESCRIPTION**.)

The vaccine should be injected intramuscularly. Preferred sites are the anterolateral aspect of the thigh and the deltoid muscle of the upper arm. Care should be taken to avoid major peripheral nerve trunks.

Before injection, the skin at the injection site should be cleansed and prepared with a suitable germicide.

After insertion of the needle, aspirate to help avoid inadvertent injection into a blood vessel.

The primary immunizing course for infants and children from 2 months of age up to their seventh birthday consists of three doses of 0.5 mL each at 4- to 8-week intervals, followed by a fourth dose of 0.5 mL 6 to 12 months after the third dose.[4,5]

If a contraindication to the pertussis component occurs, Diphtheria and Tetanus Toxoids, Adsorbed for pediatric use (DT) should be substituted for the remaining doses, according to the schedule discussed under **WARNINGS**.

The simultaneous administration of DTP, oral poliovirus vaccine (OPV), and/or measles-mumps-rubella vaccine (MMR) has resulted in seroconversion rates and rates of side effects similar to those observed when the vaccines are administered separately.[4]

The simultaneous administration of DTP and Haemophilus b Conjugate Vaccine has resulted in antibody responses to the individual antigens and rates of side effects similar to those observed when the vaccines are administered separately.[42]

The AAP and ACIP recommend that DTP may be administered simultaneously (at separate sites) with other routine childhood vaccines such as Haemophilus b Conjugate Vaccine, OPV, and/or MMR.[43,44]

The American Academy of Pediatrics recommends that Influenza Virus Vaccine should not be administered within 3 days of immunization with a pertussis-containing vaccine.[5]

Premature infants may be immunized with DTP at the usual chronological age.[5]

Interruption of the recommended schedule with a delay between doses does not interfere with the final immunity achieved; nor does it necessitate starting the series over again, regardless of the length of time elapsed between doses.[4,5]

A booster dose of 0.5 mL is indicated at age 4 to 6 years, preferably prior to entrance into kindergarten or elementary school. (Substitute DT when contraindication to pertussis-containing vaccine exists.) (See **CONTRAINDICATIONS** and **WARNINGS** sections.) However, if the fourth dose of the basic immunizing series was administered after the fourth birthday, a booster prior to school entry is not considered necessary.[4]

For either primary or booster immunization against tetanus and diphtheria of individuals 7 years of age and older, the use of Tetanus and Diphtheria Toxoids Adsorbed For Adult Use is recommended.[4,5]

HOW SUPPLIED

NDC 0005-1948-33   7.5 mL vial

STORAGE

DO NOT FREEZE. STORE REFRIGERATED, AWAY FROM FREEZER COMPARTMENT, AT 2°C TO 8°C (36°F TO 46°F).

REFERENCES

1. Mueller JH, Miller PA: Production of diphtheria toxin of high potency (100Lf) on a reproducible medium. *J Immunol.* 1941;40:21–32.
2. Mueller JH, Miller PA: Factors influencing the production of tetanal toxin. *J Immunol.* 1947;56:143–147.
3. Pillemer L, Grossberg DB, Wittler RG: The immunochemistry of toxins and toxoids. II. The preparation and immunological evaluation of purified tetanal toxoid. *J Immunol.* 1946;54:213–224.
4. Diphtheria, tetanus and pertussis: Guidelines for vaccine prophylaxis and other preventive measures—recommendation of the Immunization Practices Advisory Committee (ACIP). *MMWR.* 1985;34(27):405–426.
5. American Academy of Pediatrics: Report of the Committee on Infectious Diseases, ed 21. Elk Grove Village, IL: American Academy of Pediatrics, 1988.
6. Manclark CR, Cowell JL: Pertussis vaccine, in Germanier R. (ed): Bacterial Vaccines. New York: Academic Press Inc, 1984;69–106.
7. Reported incidence of notifiable diseases in the United States. *MMWR.* 1970;19(53):44.
8. Pertussis immunization: family history of convulsions and use of antipyretics—supplementary ACIP statement. *MMWR.* 1987;36(18):281–282.
9. Stetler HC, et al: History of convulsions and use of pertussis vaccine. *J Pediatr.* 1985;107(2):175–179.
10. Hirtz DG, et al: Seizures following childhood immunizations. *J Pediatr.* 1983;102(1):14–18.
11. Bernier R, et al: Diphtheria-tetanus toxoids, pertussis vaccination and sudden infant deaths in Tennessee. *J Pediatr.* 1982;101:419–421.
12. Baraff L, et al: Possible temporal association between diphtheria-tetanus toxoid, pertussis vaccination and sudden infant death syndrome. *Pediatr Inf Dis.* 1983;2:7–11.
13. Walker AM, et al: Diphtheria-tetanus-pertussis immunization and sudden infant death syndrome. *AJPH.* 1987;77(8):945–951.
14. Hoffman HJ, et al: Diphtheria-tetanus-pertussis immunization and sudden infant death; results of the National Institute of Child Health and Human Development cooperative study of sudden infant death syndrome risk factors. *Pediatrics.* 1987;79(4):598–611.
15. Bellman MH, et al: Infantile spasms and pertussis immunization. *Lancet.* 1983;1:1031–1034.
16. Recommendation of the ACIP: Immunization of children infected with Human T-Lymphotrophic Virus Type III/Lymphadenopathy-associated virus. *MMWR.* 1986;35(38):595–606.
17. Immunization of children infected with Human Immunodeficiency Virus—Supplementary ACIP statement. *MMWR.* 1988;37(12):181–183.
18. National Childhood Vaccine Injury Act: Requirements for permanent vaccination records and for reporting of selected events after vaccination. *MMWR.* 1988; 37(13):197–200.
19. Cody C, et al: Nature and rates of adverse reactions associated with DTP and DT immunizations in infants and children. *Pediatrics.* 1981;68:650–660.
20. Bernier R, et al: Abscesses complicating DTP vaccination. *Am J Dis Child.* 1981;135:826–828.
21. Omokoku B, Castells S: Post-DPT inoculation-caused lymphadenitis in children. *NY State J Med.* 1981;81:1667–1668.
22. Baraff L, et al: DTP-associated reactions: An analysis by injection site, manufacturer, prior reactions and dose. *Pediatrics.* 1984;73:31–36.
23. Barkin R, Pichichero M: Diphtheria-pertussis-tetanus vaccine: Reactogenicity of commercial products. *Pediatrics.* 1979;63:256–260.
24. Miller DL, et al: Pertussis vaccine and whooping cough as risk factors in acute neurological illness and death in young children. *Dev Biol Stand.* 1985;61:389–394.
25. Mathur et al: Bulging fontanel following triple vaccine (letter). *Indian Pediatrics.* 1981;18(6):417–418.
26. Shendurnikar et al: Bulging fontanel following DTP vaccine (letter). *Indian Pediatrics.* 1986;23(11):960.
27. Jacob et al: Increased intracranial pressure after diphtheria, tetanus, and pertussis immunization. *Am J Dis Child.* 1979;133:217–218.
28. Leung A: Congenital heart disease and DTP vaccination. *Can Med Assoc J.* 1984;131:541.
29. Park JM, et al: Paroxysmal supraventricular tachycardia precipitated by pertussis vaccine. *Pediatrics.* 1983;102(6):883–885.
30. Amsel SG, et al: Myocarditis after triple immunization. *Arch Dis Child.* 1986;61:403–404.

31. Adverse events following immunization. *MMWR.* 1985;34:43–47.
32. Rutledge SL, Snead OC: Neurologic complications of immunizations. *J Pediatr.* 1986;109:917–924.
33. Schlenska GK: Unusual neurological complications following tetanus toxoid administration. *J Neurol.* 1977;215:299–302.
34. Blumstein GI, Kreithen H: Peripheral neuropathy following tetanus toxoid administration. *JAMA.* 1966;198:1030–1031.
35. Reinstein L, Pargament JM, Goodman JS: Peripheral neuropathy after multiple tetanus toxoid injections. *Arch Phys Med Rehabil.* 1982;63:332–334.
36. Tsairis P, Dyck PJ, Mulder DW: Natural history of brachial plexus neuropathy. *Arch Neurol.* 1972;27:109–117.
37. Quast U, Hennessen W, Widmark RM: Mono- and polyneuritis after tetanus vaccination. *Devel Bio Stand.* 1979;43:25–32.
38. Holliday PL, Bauer RB: Polyradiculoneuritis secondary to immunization with tetanus and diphtheria toxoids. *Arch Neurol.* 1983;40:56–57.
39. Fenichel GM: Neurological complications of tetanus toxoid. *Arch Neurol.* 1983;40:390.
40. Pollard JD, Selby G: Relapsing neuropathy due to tetanus toxoid. *J Neurol Sci.* 1978;37:113–125.
41. Newton N, Janati A: Guillain-Barré syndrome after vaccination with purified tetanus toxoid. *S Med J.* 1987;80:1053–1054.
42. Unpublished data, Praxis Biologics, Inc., Rochester, New York 14623, USA.
43. Recommendation of the AAP: *Haemophilus influenzae* Type b Conjugate Vaccines: Recommendations for Immunization of Infants and Children 2 Months of Age and Older: Update. *Pediatrics.* In Press.
44. Recommendation of the ACIP: *Haemophilus b* Conjugate Vaccines for Prevention of *Haemophilus influenzae* Type b Disease Among Infants and Children Two Months of Age and Older. *MMWR.* 1991;40:1–7.

Manufactured by:
LEDERLE LABORATORIES DIVISION
American Cyanamid Company
Pearl River, NY 10965
Shown in Product Identification Guide, page 321

VERELAN®   ℞
Verapamil HCl
Sustained-Release Pellet Filled Capsules

DESCRIPTION

VERELAN (verapamil hydrochloride capsules) is a calcium ion influx inhibitor (slow channel blocker or calcium ion antagonist). VERELAN is available for oral administration as a 360 mg hard gelatin capsule (lavender cap/yellow body), a 240 mg hard gelatin capsule (dark blue cap/yellow body), a 180 mg hard gelatin capsule (light grey cap/yellow body), and a 120 mg hard gelatin capsule (yellow cap/yellow body). These pellet filled capsules provide a sustained-release of the drug in the gastrointestinal tract.
Chemical name: Benzeneacetonitrile, α-[3-[[2-(3,4-dimethoxyphenyl)-ethyl]methylamino]propyl]-3,4-dimethoxy-α-(1-methylethyl) monohydrochloride.
Verapamil HCl is an almost white, crystalline powder, practically free of odor, with a bitter taste. It is soluble in water, chloroform, and methanol. Verapamil HCl is not structurally related to other cardioactive drugs.
In addition to verapamil HCl the VERELAN capsule contains the following inactive ingredients: fumaric acid, talc, sugar spheres, povidone, shellac, gelatin, FD&C red #40, yellow iron oxide, titanium dioxide, methylparaben, propylparaben, silicon dioxide, and sodium lauryl sulfate. In addition, the VERELAN 240 mg and 360 mg capsules contain FD&C blue #1 and D&C red #28; and the VERELAN 180 mg capsule contains black iron oxide.

CLINICAL PHARMACOLOGY

VERELAN is a calcium ion influx inhibitor (slow channel blocker or calcium ion antagonist) which exerts its pharmacologic effects by modulating the influx of ionic calcium across the cell membrane of the arterial smooth muscle as well as in conductile and contractile myocardial cells.
Normal sinus rhythm is usually not affected by verapamil HCl. However in patients with sick sinus syndrome, verapamil HCl may interfere with sinus node impulse generation and may induce sinus arrest or sinoatrial block. Atrioventricular block can occur in patients without preexisting conduction defects. (See **WARNINGS.**) Verapamil HCl does not alter the normal atrial action potential or intraventricular conduction time, but depresses amplitude, velocity of depolarization and conduction in depressed atrial fibers. Verapamil HCl may shorten the antegrade effective refractory period of accessory bypass tracts. Acceleration of ventricular rate and/or ventricular fibrillation has been reported in patients with atrial flutter or atrial fibrillation

and a coexisting accessory AV pathway following administration of verapamil. (See **WARNINGS.**)
Verapamil HCl has a local anesthetic action that is 1.6 times that of procaine on an equimolar basis. It is not known whether this action is important at the doses used in man.

Mechanism of Action
Essential Hypertension
Verapamil HCl exerts antihypertensive effects by decreasing systemic vascular resistance, usually without orthostatic decreases in blood pressure or reflex tachycardia; bradycardia (rate less than 50 beats/minute is uncommon). Verapamil HCl regularly reduces arterial pressure at rest and at a given level of exercise by dilating peripheral arterioles and reducing the total peripheral resistance (afterload) against which the heart works.

Pharmacokinetics and Metabolism
With the immediate release formulations, more than 90% of the orally administered dose is absorbed, and peak plasma concentrations of verapamil are observed 1 to 2 hours after dosing. Because of rapid biotransformation of verapamil during its first pass through the portal circulation, the absolute bioavailability ranges from 20% to 35%. Chronic oral administration of the highest recommended dose (120 mg every 6 hours) resulted in plasma verapamil levels ranging from 125 to 400 ng/mL with higher values reported occasionally. A nonlinear correlation between the verapamil HCl dose administered and verapamil plasma levels does exist. During initial dose titration with verapamil a relationship exists between verapamil plasma concentrations and the prolongation of the PR interval. However, during chronic administration this relationship may disappear. The quantitative relationship between plasma verapamil concentrations and blood pressure reduction has not been fully characterized.
In a multiple dose pharmacokinetic study, peak concentrations for a single daily dose of VERELAN 240 mg were approximately 65% of those obtained with an 80 mg t.i.d. dose of the conventional immediate-release tablets, and the 24-hour post-dose concentrations were approximately 30% higher. At a total daily dose of 240 mg, VERELAN was shown to have a similar extent of verapamil bioavailability based on the AUC-24 as that obtained with the conventional immediate-release tablets. In this same study VERELAN doses of 120 mg, 240 mg and 360 mg once daily were compared after multiple doses. The ratios of the verapamil and norverapamil AUCs for the VERELAN 120 mg, 240 mg, and 360 mg once daily doses are 1 (565 ng·hr/mL):3 (1660 ng·hr/mL):5 (2729 ng·hr/mL) and 1 (621 ng·hr/mL):3 (1614 ng·hr/mL):4 (2535 ng·hr/mL), respectively, indicating that the AUC increased non-proportionately with increasing doses.
Food does not affect the extent or rate of the absorption of verapamil from the controlled release VERELAN capsule. The VERELAN 240 mg capsule when administered with food had a C_{max} of 77 ng/mL which occurred 9.0 hours after dosing, and an AUC(0-inf) of 1387 ng·hr/mL. VERELAN 240 mg under fasting conditions had a C_{max} of 77 ng/mL which occurred 9.8 hours after dosing, and an AUC(0-inf) of 1541 ng·hr/mL.
The bioequivalence of VERELAN 240 mg, administered as the pellets sprinkled on applesauce and as the intact capsule, was demonstrated in a single-dose, cross-over study in 32 healthy adults. Comparative ratios (sprinkled/intact) of verapamil were 0.95, 1.02, and 1.01 for C_{max}, T_{max}, and AUC (0-inf) respectively. Similar results were observed with norverapamil.
The time to reach maximum verapamil concentrations (T_{max}) with VERELAN has been found to be approximately 7 to 9 hours in each of the single dose (fasting), single dose (fed), the multiple dose (steady state) studies, and dose proportionality pharmacokinetic studies. Similarly the apparent half-life ($t_{1/2}$) has been found to be approximately 12 hours independent of dose. Aging may affect the pharmacokinetics of verapamil. Elimination half-life may be prolonged in the elderly.
In healthy man, orally administered verapamil HCl undergoes extensive metabolism in the liver. Twelve metabolites have been identified in plasma; all except norverapamil are present in trace amounts only. Norverapamil can reach steady-state plasma concentrations approximately equal to those of verapamil itself. The biologic activity of norverapamil appears to be approximately 20% that of verapamil.
Approximately 70% of an administered dose of verapamil HCl is excreted as metabolites in the urine and 16% or more in the feces within 5 days. About 3% to 4% is excreted in the urine as unchanged drug. Approximately 90% is bound to plasma proteins. In patients with hepatic insufficiency, metabolism is delayed and elimination half-life prolonged up to 14 to 16 hours (see **PRECAUTIONS**), the volume of distribution is increased, and plasma clearance reduced to about 30% of normal. Verapamil clearance values suggest that patients with liver dysfunction may attain therapeutic verapamil plasma concentrations with one-third of the oral daily dose required for patients with normal liver function.

After four weeks of oral dosing (120 mg q.i.d.), verapamil and norverapamil levels were noted in the cerebrospinal fluid with estimated partition coefficient of 0.06 for verapamil and 0.04 for norverapamil.
In 10 healthy males, administration of oral verapamil (80 mg every 8 hours for 6 days) and a single oral dose of ethanol (0.8 g/kg), resulted in a 17% increase in mean peak ethanol concentrations (106.45±21.40 to 124.23±24.74 mg/dL) compared with placebo. (See **PRECAUTIONS, Drug Interactions.**)
The area under the blood ethanol concentration versus time curve (AUC over 12 hours) increased by 30% (365.67±93.52 to 475.07±97.24 mg·hr/dL). Verapamil AUCs were positively correlated (r=0.71) to increased ethanol blood AUC values.

Hemodynamics and Myocardial Metabolism
Verapamil HCl reduces afterload and myocardial contractility. Improved left ventricular diastolic function in patients with IHSS and those with coronary heart disease has also been observed with verapamil HCl therapy. In most patients, including those with organic cardiac disease, the negative inotropic action of verapamil HCl is countered by reduction of afterload and cardiac index is usually not reduced. In patients with severe left ventricular dysfuntion however, (e.g., pulmonary wedge pressure above 20 mmHg or ejection fraction lower than 30%), or in patients on beta-adrenergic blocking agents or other cardiodepressant drugs, deterioration of ventricular function may occur. (See **DRUG INTERACTIONS.**)

Pulmonary Function
Verapamil HCl does not induce broncho-constriction and hence, does not impair ventilatory function.

INDICATIONS AND USAGE
VERELAN (verapamil HCl) is indicated for the management of essential hypertension.

CONTRAINDICATIONS
Verapamil HCl is contraindicated in:
1. Severe left ventricular dysfunction. (See **WARNINGS.**)
2. Hypotension (less than 90 mm Hg systolic pressure) or cardiogenic shock.
3. Sick sinus syndrome (except in patients with a functioning artificial ventricular pacemaker).
4. Second- or third-degree AV block (except in patients with a functioning artificial ventricular pacemaker).
5. Patients with atrial flutter or atrial fibrillation and an accessory bypass tract (e.g., Wolff-Parkinson-White, Lown-Ganong-Levine syndromes). (See **WARNINGS.**)
6. Patients with known hypersensitivity to verapamil hydrochloride.

WARNINGS
Heart Failure
Verapamil has a negative inotropic effect which, in most patients, is compensated by its afterload reduction (decreased systemic vascular resistance) properties without a net impairment of ventricular performance. In clinical experience with 4,954 patients, 87 (1.8%) developed congestive heart failure or pulmonary edema. Verapamil should be avoided in patients with severe left ventricular dysfunction (e.g., ejection fraction less than 30% or moderate to severe symptoms of cardiac failure) and in patients with any degree of ventricular dysfunction if they are receiving a beta-adrenergic blocker. (See **Drug Interactions.**) Patients with milder ventricular dysfunction should, if possible, be controlled with optimum doses of digitalis and/or diuretics before verapamil treatment (note interactions with digoxin under: **PRECAUTIONS**).

Hypotension
Occasionally, the pharmacologic action of verapamil may produce a decrease in blood pressure below normal levels which may result in dizziness or symptomatic hypotension. The incidence of hypotension observed in 4,954 patients enrolled in clinical trials was 2.5%. In hypertensive patients, decreases in blood pressure below normal are unusual. Tilt table testing (60 degrees) was not able to induce orthostatic hypotension.

Elevated Liver Enzymes
Elevations of transaminases with and without concomitant elevations in alkaline phosphatase and bilirubin have been reported. Such elevations have sometimes been transient and may disappear even in the face of continued verapamil treatment. Several cases of hepatocellular injury related to verapamil have been proven by rechallenge; half of these had clinical symptoms (malaise, fever, and/or right upper quadrant pain) in addition to elevations of SGOT, SGPT, and alkaline phosphatase. Periodic monitoring of liver function in patients receiving verapamil is therefore prudent.

Accessory Bypass Tract (Wolff-Parkinson-White or Lown-Ganong-Levine)
Some patients with paroxysmal and/or chronic atrial flutter or atrial fibrillation and a coexisting accessory AV pathway have developed increased antegrade conduction across the accessory pathway bypassing the AV node, producing a very

Continued on next page

Lederle—Cont.

rapid ventricular response or ventricular fibrillation after receiving intravenous verapamil (or digitalis). Although a risk of this occurring with oral verapamil has not been established, such patients receiving oral verapamil may be at risk and its use in these patients is contraindicated. (See **CONTRAINDICATIONS.**)

Treatment is usually DC-cardioversion. Cardioversion has been used safely and effectively after oral verapamil.

Atrioventricular Block

The effect of verapamil on AV conduction and the SA node may lead to asymptomatic first-degree AV block and transient bradycardia, sometimes accompanied by nodal escape rhythms. PR interval prolongation is correlated with verapamil plasma concentrations, especially during the early titration phase of therapy. Higher degrees of AV block, however, were infrequently (0.8%) observed.

Marked first-degree block or progressive development to second- or third-degree AV block requires a reduction in dosage or, in rare instances, discontinuation of verapamil HCl and institution of appropriate therapy depending upon the clinical situation.

Patients with Hypertrophic Cardiomyopathy (IHSS)

In 120 patients with hypertrophic cardiomyopathy (most of them refractory or intolerant to propranolol) who received therapy with verapamil at doses up to 720 mg/day, a variety of serious adverse effects were seen. Three patients died in pulmonary edema; all had severe left ventricular outflow obstruction and a past history of left ventricular dysfunction. Eight other patients had pulmonary edema and/or severe hypotension; abnormally high (over 20 mm Hg) capillary wedge pressure and a marked left ventricular outflow obstruction were present in most of these patients. Concomitant administration of quinidine (see **Drug Interactions**) preceded the severe hypotension in 3 of the 8 patients (2 of whom developed pulmonary edema). Sinus bradycardia occurred in 11% of the patients, second-degree AV block in 4% and sinus arrest in 2%. It must be appreciated that this group of patients had a serious disease with a high mortality rate. Most adverse effects responded well to dose reduction and only rarely did verapamil have to be discontinued.

PRECAUTIONS

THE CONTENTS OF THE VERELAN CAPSULE SHOULD NOT BE CRUSHED OR CHEWED.

General

Use in Patients with Impaired Hepatic Function

Since verapamil is highly metabolized by the liver, it should be administered cautiously to patients with impaired hepatic function. Severe liver dysfunction prolongs the elimination half-life of immediate-release verapamil to about 14 to 16 hours; hence, approximately 30% of the dose given to patients with normal liver function should be administered to these patients. Careful monitoring for abnormal prolongation of the PR interval or other signs of excessive pharmacologic effects (see **OVERDOSAGE**) should be carried out.

Use in Patients with Attenuated (Decreased) Neuromuscular Transmission

It has been reported that verapamil decreases neuromuscular transmission in patients with Duchenne's muscular dystrophy, and that verapamil prolongs recovery from the neuromuscular blocking agent, vecuronium. It may be necessary to decrease the dosage of verapamil when it is administered to patients with attenuated neuromuscular transmission.

Use in Patients with Impaired Renal Function

About 70% of an administered dose of verapamil is excreted as metabolites in the urine. Until further data are available, verapamil should be administered cautiously to patients with impaired renal function. These patients should be carefully monitored for abnormal prolongation of the PR interval or other signs of overdosage (see **OVERDOSAGE**).

Information for Patients

When the sprinkle method of administration is prescribed, details of the proper technique should be explained to the patient. (See **DOSAGE AND ADMINISTRATION.**)

Drug Interactions

Beta Blockers

Concomitant therapy with beta-adrenergic blockers and verapamil may result in additive negative effects on heart rate, atrioventricular conduction, and/or cardiac contractility. The combination of sustained-release verapamil and beta-adrenergic blocking agents has not been studied. However, there have been reports of excess bradycardia and AV block, including complete heart block, when the combination has been used for the treatment of hypertension.

For hypertensive patients, the risk of combined therapy may outweigh the potential benefits. The combination should be used only with caution and close monitoring.

Asymptomatic bradycardia (36 beats/min) with a wandering atrial pacemaker has been observed in a patient receiving concomitant timolol (a beta-adrenergic blocker) eyedrops and oral verapamil.

A decrease in metoprolol clearance has been reported when verapamil and metoprolol were administered together. A similar effect has not been observed when verapamil and atenolol are given together.

Digitalis

Clinical use of verapamil in digitalized patients has shown the combination to be well tolerated if digoxin doses are properly adjusted. Chronic verapamil treatment can increase serum digoxin levels by 50% to 75% during the first week of therapy, and this can result in digitalis toxicity. In patients with hepatic cirrhosis the influence of verapamil on digoxin kinetics is magnified. Maintenance digitalis doses should be reduced when verapamil is administered, and the patient should be carefully monitored to avoid over- or underdigitalization. Whenever overdigitalization is suspected, the daily dose of digoxin should be reduced or temporarily discontinued. Upon discontinuation of verapamil HCl, the patient should be reassessed to avoid underdigitalization.

Antihypertensive Agents

Verapamil administered concomitantly with oral antihypertensive agents (e.g., vasodilators, angiotensin-converting enzyme inhibitors, diuretics, beta blockers) will usually have an additive effect on lowering blood pressure. Patients receiving these combinations should be appropriately monitored. Concomitant use of agents that attenuate alpha-adrenergic function with verapamil may result in reduction in blood pressure that is excessive in some patients. Such an effect was observed in one study following the concomitant administration of verapamil and prazosin.

Antiarrhythmic Agents

Disopyramide: Until data on possible interactions between verapamil and disopyramide phosphate are obtained, disopyramide should not be administered within 48 hours before or 24 hours after verapamil administration.

Flecainide: A study in healthy volunteers showed that the concomitant administration of flecainide and verapamil may have additive effects on myocardial contractility, AV conduction, and repolarization. Concomitant therapy with flecainide and verapamil may result in additive negative inotropic effect and prolongation of atrioventricular conduction.

Quinidine: In a small number of patients with hypertrophic cardiomyopathy (IHSS), concomitant use of verapamil and quinidine resulted in significant hypotension. Until further data are obtained, combined therapy of verapamil and quinidine in patients with hypertrophic cardiomyopathy should probably be avoided.

The electrophysiological effects of quinidine and verapamil on AV conduction were studied in 8 patients. Verapamil significantly counteracted the effects of quinidine on AV conduction. There has been a report of increased quinidine levels during verapamil therapy.

Nitrates: Verapamil has been given concomitantly with short- and long-acting nitrates without any undesirable drug interactions. The pharmacologic profile of both drugs and the clinical experience suggest beneficial interactions.

Alcohol: Verapamil has been found to significantly inhibit ethanol elimination resulting in elevated blood ethanol concentrations that may prolong the intoxicating effects of alcohol. (See **CLINICAL PHARMACOLOGY, Pharmacokinetics and Metabolism.**)

Other

Cimetidine: The interaction between cimetidine and chronically administered verapamil has not been studied. Variable results on clearance have been obtained in acute studies of healthy volunteers; clearance of verapamil was either reduced or unchanged.

Lithium: Pharmacokinetic and pharmacodynamic interactions between oral verapamil and lithium have been reported. The former may result in a lowering of serum lithium levels in patients receiving chronic stable oral lithium therapy. The latter may result in an increased sensitivity to the effects of lithium. Patients receiving both drugs must be monitored carefully.

Carbamazepine: Verapamil therapy may increase carbamazepine concentrations during combined therapy. This may produce carbamazepine side effects such as diplopia, headache, ataxia, or dizziness.

Rifampin: Therapy with rifampin may markedly reduce oral verapamil bioavailability.

Phenobarbital: Phenobarbital therapy may increase verapamil clearance.

Cyclosporine: Verapamil therapy may increase serum levels of cyclosporine.

Inhalation Anesthetics: Animal experiments have shown that inhalation anesthetics depress cardiovascular activity by decreasing the inward movement of calcium ions. When used concomitantly, inhalation anesthetics and calcium antagonists, such as verapamil, should be titrated carefully to avoid excessive cardiovascular depression.

Neuromuscular Blocking Agents: Clinical data and animal studies suggest that verapamil may potentiate the activity of neuromuscular blocking agents (curare-like and depolarizing). It may be necessary to decrease the dose of verapamil and/or the dose of the neuromuscular blocking agent when the drugs are used concomitantly.

Carcinogenesis, Mutagenesis, Impairment of Fertility

An 18-month toxicity study in rats, at a low multiple (6-fold)

of the maximum recommended human dose, and not the maximum tolerated dose, did not suggest a tumorigenic potential. There was no evidence of a carcinogenic potential of verapamil administered in the diet of rats for 2 years at doses of 10, 35 and 120 mg/kg per day or approximately 1x, 3.5x, and 12x, respectively, the maximum recommended human daily dose (480 mg per day or 9.6 mg/kg/day).

Verapamil was not mutagenic in the Ames test in 5 test strains at 3 mg per plate, with or without metabolic activation.

Studies in female rats at daily dietary doses up to 5.5 times (55 mg/kg/day) the maximum recommended human dose did not show impaired fertility. Effects on male fertility have not been determined.

Pregnancy

Pregnancy Category C Reproduction studies have been performed in rabbits and rats at oral doses up to 1.5 (15 mg/kg/day) and 6 (60 mg/kg/day) times the maximum recommended human daily dose, respectively, and have revealed no evidence of teratogenicity. In the rat, however, this multiple of the human dose was embryocidal and retarded fetal growth and development, probably because of adverse maternal effects reflected in reduced weight gains of the dams. This oral dose has also been shown to cause hypotension in rats. There are no adequate and well-controlled studies in pregnant women. Because animal reproduction studies are not always predictive of human response, this drug should be used during pregnancy only if clearly needed. Verapamil crosses the placental barrier and can be detected in umbilical vein blood at delivery.

Labor and Delivery

It is not known whether the use of verapamil during labor or delivery has immediate or delayed adverse effects on the fetus, or whether it prolongs the duration of labor or increases the need for forceps delivery or other obstetric intervention. Such adverse experiences have not been reported in the literature, despite a long history of use of verapamil HCl in Europe in the treatment of cardiac side effects of beta-adrenergic agonist agents used to treat premature labor.

Nursing Mothers

Verapamil is excreted in human milk. Because of the potential for adverse reactions in nursing infants from verapamil, nursing should be discontinued while verapamil is administered.

Pediatric Use

Safety and efficacy of verapamil in children below the age of 18 years have not been established.

Animal Pharmacology and/or Animal Toxicology: In chronic animal toxicology studies verapamil causes lenticular and/or suture line changes at 30 mg/kg/day or greater and frank cataracts at 62.5 mg/kg/day or greater in the beagle dog but not the rat. Development of cataracts due to verapamil has not been reported in man.

ADVERSE REACTIONS

Serious adverse reactions are uncommon when verapamil HCl therapy is initiated with upward dose titration within the recommended single and total daily dose. See **WARNINGS** for discussion of heart failure, hypotension, elevated liver enzymes, AV block, and rapid ventricular response. Reversible (upon discontinuation of verapamil) non-obstructive, paralytic ileus has been infrequently reported in association with the use of verapamil.

In clinical trials involving 285 hypertensive patients on VERELAN for greater than 1 week the following adverse reactions were reported in greater than 1.0% of the patients:

Constipation	7.4%
Headache	5.3%
Dizziness	4.2%
Lethargy	3.2%
Dyspepsia	2.5%
Rash	1.4%
Ankle edema	1.4%
Sleep Disturbance	1.4%
Myalgia	1.1%

In clinical trials of other formulations of verapamil HCl (N=4,954) the following reactions have occurred at rates greater than 1.0%:

Constipation	7.3%
Dizziness	3.3%
Nausea	2.7%
Hypotension	2.5%
Edema	1.9%
Headache	2.2%
Rash	1.2%
CHF/Pulmonary Edema	1.8%
Fatigue	1.7%
Bradycardia (HR < 50/min)	1.4%
AV block-total	
1°, 2°, 3°	1.2%
2° and 3°	0.8%
Flushing	0.6%
Elevated Liver Enzyes (see WARNINGS.)	

In clinical trials related to the control of ventricular response in digitalized patients who had atrial fibrillation or atrial flutter, ventricular rate below 50/min at rest occurred in 15% of patients and asymptomatic hypotension occurred in 5% of patients.
The following reactions, reported in 1.0% or less of patients, occurred under conditions (open trials, marketing experience) where a causal relationship is uncertain; they are listed to alert the physician to a possible relationship:
Cardiovascular: angina pectoris, atrioventricular dissociation, chest pain, claudication, myocardial infarction, palpitations, purpura (vasculitis), syncope.
Digestive System: diarrhea, dry mouth, gastrointestinal distress, gingival hyperplasia.
Hemic and Lymphatic: ecchymosis or bruising.
Nervous System: cerebrovascular accident, confusion, equilibrium disorders, insomnia, muscle cramps, paresthesia, psychotic symptoms, shakiness, somnolence.
Respiratory: dyspnea.
Skin: arthralgia and rash, exanthema, hair loss, hyperkeratosis, maculae, sweating, urticaria, Stevens-Johnson syndrome, erythema multiforme.
Special Senses: blurred vision.
Urogenital: gynecomastia, impotence, increased urination, spotty menstruation.

Treatment of Acute Cardiovascular Adverse Reactions
The frequency of cardiovascular adverse reactions which require therapy is rare; hence, experience with their treatment is limited. Whenever severe hypotension or complete AV block occurs following oral administration of verapamil, the appropriate emergency measures should be applied immediately, e.g., intravenously administered isoproterenol HCl, levarterenol bitartrate, atropine (all in the usual doses), or calcium gluconate (10% solution). In patients with hypertrophic cardiomyopathy (IHSS), alpha-adrenergic agents (phenylephrine, metaraminol bitartrate or methoxamine) should be used to maintain blood pressure, and isoproterenol and levarterenol should be avoided. If further support is necessary, inotropic agents (dopamine or dobutamine) may be administered. Actual treatment and dosage should depend on the severity and the clinical situation and the judgment and experience of the treating physician.

OVERDOSAGE

Treatment of overdosage should be supportive. Beta-adrenergic stimulation or parenteral administration of calcium solutions may increase calcium ion flux across the slow channel, and have been used effectively in treatment of deliberate overdosage with verapamil. Verapamil cannot be removed by hemodialysis. Clinically significant hypotensive reactions or high degree AV block should be treated with vasopressor agents or cardiac pacing, respectively. Asystole should be handled by the usual measures including cardiopulmonary resuscitation.

DOSAGE AND ADMINISTRATION

Essential Hypertension: The dose of VERELAN should be individualized by titration. The usual daily dose of sustained-release verapamil, VERELAN, in clinical trials has been 240 mg given by mouth once daily in the morning. However, initial doses of 120 mg a day may be warranted in patients who may have an increased response to verapamil (e.g., elderly, small people, etc). Upward titration should be based on therapeutic efficacy and safety evaluated approximately 24 hours after dosing. The antihypertensive effects of VERELAN are evident within the first week of therapy.
If adequate response is not obtained with 120 mg of VERELAN, the dose may be titrated upward in the following manner: (a) 180 mg in the morning, (b) 240 mg in the morning, (c) 360 mg in the morning, (d) 480 mg in the morning. VERELAN sustained-release capsules are for once-a-day administration. When switching from immediate-release verapamil to VERELAN capsules, the same total daily dose of VERELAN capsules can be used.
As with immediate-release verapamil, dosages of VERELAN capsules should be individualized and titration may be needed in some patients.

Sprinkling the Capsule Contents on Food
VERELAN Pellet Filled Capsules may also be administered by carefully opening the capsule and sprinkling the pellets on a spoonful of applesauce. The applesauce should be swallowed immediately without chewing and followed with a glass of cool water to ensure complete swallowing of the pellets. The applesauce used should not be hot, and it should be soft enough to be swallowed without chewing. Any pellet/applesauce mixture should be used immediately and not stored for future use. Subdividing the contents of a VERELAN capsule is not recommended.

HOW SUPPLIED

VERELAN® verapamil HCl sustained-release pellet filled capsules are supplied in four dosage strengths:
120 mg—Two-piece, size 2 hard gelatin capsule (yellow cap/yellow body), printed with Lederle above V8 on left and VERELAN above 120 mg on right side of the capsule in black ink, supplied as follows:
NDC 0005-2490-23—Bottle of 100s
180 mg—Two-piece, size 1 elongated hard gelatin capsule (light grey cap/yellow body), printed with Lederle above V7 on left and VERELAN above 180 mg on right side of the capsule in black ink, supplied as follows:
NDC 0005-2489-23–Bottle of 100s
240 mg—Two-piece, size 0 hard gelatin capsule (dark blue cap/yellow body), printed with Lederle above V9 on left and VERELAN above 240 mg on right side of the capsule in black ink, supplied as follows:
NDC 0005-2491-23—Bottle of 100s
360 mg—Two-piece, size 00 hard gelatin capsule (lavender cap/yellow body), printed with Lederle above V6 on left and VERELAN above 360 mg on right side of the capsule in black ink, supplied as follows:
NDC 0005-2495-23—Bottle of 100s.
Store at controlled room temperature 20°–25°C (68°–77°F) [See USP]. Avoid excessive heat. Brief digressions above 25°C, while not detrimental, should be avoided. Protect from moisture.
Dispense in tight, light-resistant container as defined in USP.
Manufactured for
LEDERLE LABORATORIES DIVISION
American Cyanamid Company
Pearl River, NY 10965
by
ELAN PHARMA, INC.
Pharmaceutical Division
Gainesville, GA 30504

Shown in Product Identification Guide, page 321

ZEBETA® ℞
[zē-bā-tə]
(Bisoprolol Fumarate)
Tablets

DESCRIPTION

ZEBETA (bisoprolol fumarate) is a synthetic $beta_1$-selective (cardioselective) adrenoceptor blocking agent. The chemical name for bisoprolol fumarate is (±)-1-[4-[[2-(1-Methylethoxy) ethoxy]methyl]phenoxy] -3- [(1-methylethyl)amino] -2- propanol (*E*) -2- butenedioate (2:1) (salt). It possesses an asymmetric carbon atom in its structure and is provided as a racemic mixture. The S(-) enantiomer is responsible for most of the beta-blocking activity. Its empirical formula is $(C_{18}H_{31}NO_4)_2 \cdot C_4H_4O_4$.
Bisoprolol fumarate has a molecular weight of 766.97. It is a white crystalline powder which is approximately equally hydrophilic and lipophilic, and is readily soluble in water, methanol, ethanol, and chloroform.
ZEBETA is available as 5 and 10 mg tablets for oral administration.
Inactive ingredients include Colloidal Silicon Dioxide, Corn Starch, Crospovidone, Diabasic Calcium Phosphate, Hydroxypropyl Methylcellulose, Magnesium Stearate, Microcrystalline Cellulose, Polyethylene Glycol, Polysorbate 80, and Titanium Dioxide. The 5 mg tablets also contain Red and Yellow Iron Oxide.

CLINICAL PHARMACOLOGY

ZEBETA is a $beta_1$-selective (cardioselective) adrenoceptor blocking agent without significant membrane stabilizing activity or intrinsic sympathomimetic activity in its therapeutic dosage range. Cardioselectivity is not absolute, however, and at higher doses (≥ 20 mg) bisoprolol fumarate also inhibits $beta_2$-adrenoceptors, chiefly located in the bronchial and vascular musculature; to retain selectivity, it is therefore important to use the lowest effective dose.

Pharmacokinetics and Metabolism
The absolute bioavailability after a 10 mg oral dose of bisoprolol fumarate is about 80%. Absorption is not affected by the presence of food. The first pass metabolism of bisoprolol fumarate is about 20%.
Binding to serum proteins is approximately 30%. Peak plasma concentrations occur within 2–4 hours of dosing with 5 to 20 mg, and mean peak values range from 16 ng/mL at 5 mg to 70 ng/mL at 20 mg. Once daily dosing with bisoprolol fumarate results in less than twofold intersubject variation in peak plasma levels. The plasma elimination half-life is 9–12 hours and is slightly longer in elderly patients, in part because of decreased renal function in that population. Steady state is attained within 5 days of once daily dosing. In both young and elderly populations, plasma accumulation is low; the accumulation factor ranges from 1.1 to 1.3, and is what would be expected from the first order kinetics and once daily dosing. Plasma concentrations are proportional to the administered dose in the range of 5 to 20 mg. Pharmacokinetic characteristics of the two enantiomers are similar.
Bisoprolol fumarate is eliminated equally by renal and non-renal pathways with about 50% of the dose appearing unchanged in the urine and the remainder appearing in the form of inactive metabolites. In humans, the known metabolites are labile or have no known pharmacologic activity. Less than 2% of the dose is excreted in the feces. Bisoprolol fumarate is not metabolized by cytochrome P450 II D6 (debrisoquin hydroxylase).
In subjects with creatinine clearance less than 40 mL/min, the plasma half-life is increased approximately threefold compared to healthy subjects.
In patients with cirrhosis of the liver, the elimination of ZEBETA (bisoprolol fumarate) is more variable in rate and significantly slower than that in healthy subjects, with plasma half-life ranging from 8.3 to 21.7 hours.

Pharmacodynamics
The most prominent effect of ZEBETA is the negative chronotropic effect, resulting in a reduction in resting and exercise heart rate. There is a fall in resting and exercise cardiac output with little observed change in stroke volume, and only a small increase in right atrial pressure, or pulmonary capillary wedge pressure, at rest or during exercise.
Findings in short-term clinical hemodynamics studies with ZEBETA are similar to those observed with other beta-blocking agents.
The mechanism of action of its antihypertensive effects has not been completely established. Factors which may be involved include:
1) Decreased cardiac output,
2) Inhibition of renin release by the kidneys,
3) Diminution of tonic sympathetic outflow from the vasomotor centers in the brain.

In normal volunteers, ZEBETA therapy resulted in a reduction of exercise- and isoproterenol-induced tachycardia. The maximal effect occurred within 1–4 hours post-dosing. Effects persisted for 24 hours at doses equal to or greater than 5 mg.
Electrophysiology studies in man have demonstrated that ZEBETA significantly decreases heart rate, increases sinus node recovery time, prolongs AV node refractory periods, and, with rapid atrial stimulation, prolongs AV nodal conduction.
$Beta_1$-selectivity of ZEBETA has been demonstrated in both animal and human studies. No effects at therapeutic doses on $beta_2$-adrenoceptor density have been observed. Pulmonary function studies have been conducted in healthy volunteers, asthmatics, and patients with chronic obstructive pulmonary disease (COPD). Doses of ZEBETA ranged from 5 to 60 mg, atenolol from 50 to 200 mg, metoprolol from 100 to 200 mg, and propranolol from 40 to 80 mg. In some studies, slight, asymptomatic increases in airways resistance (AWR) and decreases in forced expiratory volume (FEV_1) were observed with doses of bisoprolol fumarate 20 mg and higher, similar to the small increases in AWR also noted with the other cardioselective beta-blockers. The changes induced by beta-blockade with all agents were reversed by bronchodilator therapy.
ZEBETA had minimal effect on serum lipids during antihypertensive studies. In U.S. placebo-controlled trials, changes in total cholesterol averaged +0.8% for bisoprolol fumarate-treated patients, and +0.7% for placebo. Changes in triglycerides averaged +19% for bisoprolol fumarate-treated patients, and +17% for placebo.
ZEBETA has also been given concomitantly with thiazide diuretics. Even very low doses of hydrochlorothiazide (6.25 mg) were found to be additive with bisoprolol fumarate in lowering blood pressure in patients with mild-to-moderate hypertension.

CLINICAL STUDIES

In two randomized double-blind placebo-controlled trials conducted in the U.S., reductions in systolic and diastolic blood pressure and heart rate 24 hours after dosing in patients with mild-to-moderate hypertension are shown below. In both studies, mean systolic/diastolic blood pressures at baseline were approximately 150/100 mm Hg, and mean heart rate was 76 bpm. Drug effect is calculated by subtracting the placebo effect from the overall change in blood pressure and heart rate.
[See table at bottom of next page.]
Blood pressure responses were seen within one week of treatment and changed little thereafter. They were sustained for 12 weeks and for over a year in studies of longer duration. Blood pressure returned to baseline when bisoprolol fumarate was tapered over two weeks in a long-term study.
Overall, significantly greater blood pressure reductions were observed on bisoprolol fumarate than on placebo, regardless of race, age, or gender. There were no significant differences in response between black and nonblack patients.

INDICATIONS AND USAGE

ZEBETA is indicated in the management of hypertension. It may be used alone or in combination with other antihypertensive agents.

Continued on next page

Lederle—Cont.

CONTRAINDICATIONS

ZEBETA is contraindicated in patients with cardiogenic shock, overt cardiac failure, second or third degree AV block, and marked sinus bradycardia.

WARNINGS

Cardiac Failure

Sympathetic stimulation is a vital component supporting circulatory function in the setting of congestive heart failure, and beta-blockade may result in further depression of myocardial contractility and precipitate more severe failure. In general, beta-blocking agents should be avoided in patients with overt congestive failure. However, in some patients with compensated cardiac failure it may be necessary to utilize them. In such a situation, they must be used cautiously.

In Patients Without a History of Cardiac Failure

Continued depression of the myocardium with beta-blockers can, in some patients, precipitate cardiac failure. At the first signs or symptoms of heart failure, discontinuation of ZEBETA should be considered. In some cases, beta-blocker therapy can be continued while heart failure is treated with other drugs.

Abrupt Cessation of Therapy

Exacerbation of angina pectoris, and, in some instances, myocardial infarction or ventricular arrhythmia, have been observed in patients with coronary artery disease following abrupt cessation of therapy with beta-blockers. Such patients should, therefore, be cautioned against interruption or discontinuation of therapy without the physician's advice. Even in patients without overt coronary artery disease, it may be advisable to taper therapy with ZEBETA over approximately one week with the patient under careful observation. If withdrawal symptoms occur, ZEBETA therapy should be reinstituted, at least temporarily.

Peripheral Vascular Disease

Beta-blockers can precipitate or aggravate symptoms of arterial insufficiency in patients with peripheral vascular disease. Caution should be exercised in such individuals.

Bronchospastic Disease

PATIENTS WITH BRONCHOSPASTIC DISEASE SHOULD, IN GENERAL, NOT RECEIVE BETA-BLOCKERS. Because of its relative $beta_1$-selectivity, however, ZEBETA may be used with caution in patients with bronchospastic disease who do not respond to, or who cannot tolerate other antihypertensive treatment. Since $beta_1$-selectivity is not absolute, the lowest possible dose of ZEBETA should be used, with therapy starting at 2.5 mg. A $beta_2$ agonist (bronchodilator) should be made available.

Anesthesia and Major Surgery

If ZEBETA treatment is to be continued perioperatively, particular care should be taken when anesthetic agents which depress myocardial function, such as ether, cyclopropane, and trichloroethylene, are used. See **OVERDOSAGE** for information on treatment of bradycardia and hypertension.

Diabetes and Hypoglycemia

Beta-blockers may mask some of the manifestations of hypoglycemia, particularly tachycardia. Nonselective beta-blockers may potentiate insulin-induced hypoglycemia and delay recovery of serum glucose levels. Because of its $beta_1$-selectivity, this is less likely with ZEBETA. However, patients subject to spontaneous hypoglycemia, or diabetic patients receiving insulin or oral hypoglycemic agents, should be cautioned about these possibilities and bisoprolol fumarate should be used with caution.

Thyrotoxicosis

Beta-adrenergic blockade may mask clinical signs of hyperthyroidism, such as tachycardia. Abrupt withdrawal of beta-blockade may be followed by an exacerbation of the symptoms of hyperthyroidism or may precipitate thyroid storm.

PRECAUTIONS

Impaired Renal or Hepatic Function

Use caution in adjusting the dose of ZEBETA in patients with renal or hepatic impairment (see **CLINICAL PHARMACOLOGY** and **DOSAGE AND ADMINISTRATION**).

Drug Interactions

ZEBETA should not be combined with other beta-blocking agents. Patients receiving catecholamine-depleting drugs, such as reserpine or guanethidine, should be closely monitored, because the added beta-adrenergic blocking action of ZEBETA may produce excessive reduction of sympathetic activity. In patients receiving concurrent therapy with clonidine, if therapy is to be discontinued, it is suggested that ZEBETA be discontinued for several days before the withdrawal of clonidine.

ZEBETA should be used with care when myocardial depressants or inhibitors of AV conduction, such as certain calcium antagonists [particularly of the phenylalkylamine (verapamil) and benzothiazepine (diltiazem) classes], or antiarrhythmic agents, such as disopyramide, are used concurrently.

Concurrent use of rifampin increases the metabolic clearance of ZEBETA, resulting in a shortened elimination half-life of ZEBETA. However, initial dose modification is generally not necessary. Pharmacokinetic studies document no clinically relevant interactions with other agents given concomitantly, including thiazide diuretics, digoxin and cimetidine. There was no effect of ZEBETA on prothrombin time in patients on stable doses of warfarin.

Risk of Anaphylactic Reaction: While taking beta-blockers, patients with a history of severe anaphylactic reaction to a variety of allergens may be more reactive to repeated challenge, either accidental, diagnostic, or therapeutic. Such patients may be unresponsive to the usual doses of epinephrine used to treat allergic reactions.

Information for Patients

Patients, especially those with coronary artery disease, should be warned about discontinuing use of ZEBETA without a physician's supervision. Patients should also be advised to consult a physician if any difficulty in breathing occurs, or if they develop signs or symptoms of congestive heart failure or excessive bradycardia.

Patients subject to spontaneous hypoglycemia, or diabetic patients receiving insulin or oral hypoglycemic agents, should be cautioned that beta-blockers may mask some of the manifestations of hypoglycemia, particularly tachycardia, and bisoprolol fumarate should be used with caution.

Patients should know how they react to this medicine before they operate automobiles and machinery or engage in other tasks requiring alertness.

Carcinogenesis, Mutagenesis, Impairment of Fertility

Long-term studies were conducted with oral bisoprolol fumarate administered in the feed of mice (20 and 24 months) and rats (26 months). No evidence of carcinogenic potential was seen in mice dosed up to 250 mg/kg/day or rats dosed up to 125 mg/kg/day. On a body-weight basis, these doses are 625 and 312 times, respectively, the maximum recommended human dose (MRHD) of 20 mg, (or 0.4 mg/kg/day based on a 50 kg individual); on a body-surface-area-basis, these doses are 59 times (mice) and 64 times (rats) the MRHD. The mutagenic potential of bisoprolol fumarate was evaluated in the microbial mutagenicity (Ames) test, the point mutation and chromosome aberration assays in Chinese hamster V79 cells, the unscheduled DNA synthesis test, the micronucleus test in mice, and the cytogenetics assay in rats. There was no evidence of mutagenic potential in these *in vitro* and *in vivo* assays.

Reproduction studies in rats did not show any impairment of fertility at doses up to 150 mg/kg/day of bisoprolol fumarate, or 375 and 77 times the MRHD on the basis of body-weight and body-surface-area, respectively.

Pregnancy Category C

In rats, bisoprolol fumarate was not teratogenic at doses up to 150 mg/kg/day which is 375 and 77 times the MRHD on the basis of body-weight and body-surface-area, respectively. Bisoprolol fumarate was fetotoxic (increased late resorptions) at 50 mg/kg/day and maternotoxic (decreased food intake and body-weight gain) at 150 mg/kg/day. The fetotoxicity in rats occurred at 125 times the MRHD on a body-weight-basis and 26 times the MRHD on the basis of body-surface-area. The maternotoxicity occurred at 375 times the MRHD on a body-weight basis and 77 times the MRHD on the basis of body-surface-area. In rabbits, bisoprolol fumarate was not teratogenic at doses up to 12.5 mg/kg/day, which is 31 and 12 times the MRHD based on body-weight and body-surface-area, respectively, but was embryolethal (increased early resorptions) at 12.5 mg/kg/day.

There are no adequate and well-controlled studies in pregnant women. ZEBETA should be used during pregnancy only if the potential benefit justifies the potential risk to the fetus.

Nursing Mothers

Small amounts of bisoprolol fumarate ($<2\%$ of the dose) have been detected in the milk of lactating rats. It is not known whether this drug is excreted in human milk. Because many drugs are excreted in human milk caution should be exercised when bisoprolol fumarate is administered to nursing women.

Use in Elderly Patients

ZEBETA has been used in elderly patients with hypertension. Response rates and mean decreases in systolic and diastolic blood pressure were similar to the decreases in younger patients in the U.S. clinical studies. Although no dose response study was conducted in elderly patients, there was a tendency for older patients to be maintained on higher doses of bisoprolol fumarate.

Observed reductions in heart rate were slightly greater in the elderly than in the young and tended to increase with increasing dose. In general, no disparity in adverse experience reports or dropouts for safety reasons was observed between older and younger patients. Dose adjustment based on age is not necessary.

Pediatric Use

Safety and effectiveness in children have not been established.

ADVERSE REACTIONS

Safety data are available in more than 30,000 patients or volunteers. Frequency estimates and rates of withdrawal of therapy for adverse events were derived from two U.S. placebo-controlled studies.

In Study A, doses of 5, 10 and 20 mg bisoprolol fumarate were administered for 4 weeks. In Study B, doses of 2.5, 10 and 40 mg of bisoprolol fumarate were administered for 12 weeks. A total of 273 patients were treated with 5–20 mg of bisoprolol fumarate; 132 received placebo.

Withdrawal of therapy for adverse events was 3.3% for patients receiving bisoprolol fumarate and 6.8% for patients on placebo. Withdrawals were less than 1% for either bradycardia or fatigue/lack of energy.

The following table presents adverse experiences, whether or not considered drug related, reported in at least 1% of patients in these studies, for all patients studied in placebo controlled clinical trials (2.5–40 mg), as well as for a subgroup that was treated with doses within the recommended dosage range (5–20 mg). Of the adverse events listed in the table, bradycardia, diarrhea, asthenia, fatigue and sinusitis appear to be dose related.

[See table at top of next page.]

The following is a comprehensive list of adverse experiences reported with bisoprolol fumarate in worldwide studies, or in post marketing experience (in italics):

Central Nervous System: Dizziness, vertigo, headache, paresthesia, hypoaesthesia, somnolence, anxiety/restlessness, decreased concentration/memory.

Autonomic Nervous System: Dry mouth.

Cardiovascular: Bradycardia, palpitations and other rhythm disturbances, cold extremities, claudication, hypotension, orthostatic hypotension, chest pain, congestive heart failure, dyspnea on exertion.

Psychiatric: Vivid dreams, insomnia, depression.

Gastrointestinal: Gastric/epigastric/abdominal pain, gastritis, dyspepsia, nausea, vomiting, diarrhea, constipation.

Musculoskeletal: Muscle/joint pain, back/neck pain, muscle cramps, twitching/tremor.

Skin: Rash, acne, eczema, skin irritation, pruritus, flushing, sweating, alopecia, *angioedema, exfoliative dermatitis,* cutaneous vasculitis.

Special Senses: Visual disturbances, ocular pain/pressure, abnormal lacrimation, tinnitus, earache, taste abnormalities.

Metabolic: Gout.

Respiratory: Asthma/bronchospasm, bronchitis, coughing, dyspnea, pharyngitis, rhinitis, sinusitis, URI.

Genito-urinary: Decreased libido/impotence, *Peyronie's disease,* cystitis, renal colic.

Hematologic: Purpura.

General: Fatigue, asthenia, chest pain, malaise, edema, weight gain.

Sitting Systolic/Diastolic Pressure (BP) and Heart Rate (HR)
Mean Decrease (Δ) After 3 to 4 Weeks

Study A

		Bisoprolol Fumarate		
	Placebo	5 mg	10 mg	20 mg
n=	61	61	61	61
Total ΔBP (mm Hg)	5.4/3.2	10.4/8.0	11.2/10.9	12.8/11.9
Drug Effect[a]	—	5.0/4.8	5.8/7.7	7.4/8.7
Total ΔHR (bpm)	0.5	7.2	8.7	11.3
Drug Effect[a]	—	6.7	8.2	10.8

Study B

		Bisoprolol Fumarate	
	Placebo	2.5 mg	10 mg
n=	56	59	62
Total ΔBP (mm Hg)	3.0/3.7	7.6/8.1	13.5/11.2
Drug Effect[a]	—	4.6/4.4	10.5/7.5
Total ΔHR (bpm)	1.6	3.8	10.7
Drug Effect[a]	—	2.2	9.1

[a] Observed total change from baseline minus placebo.

Body System/Adverse Experience	All Adverse Experiences (%[a]) Bisoprolol Fumarate		
	Placebo (n = 132) %	5–20 mg (n = 273) %	2.5–40 mg (n = 404) %
Skin			
increased sweating	1.5	0.7	1.0
Musculo-skeletal			
arthralgia	2.3	2.2	2.7
Central Nervous System			
dizziness	3.8	2.9	3.5
headache	11.4	8.8	10.9
hypoaesthesia	0.8	1.1	1.5
Autonomic Nervous System			
dry mouth	1.5	0.7	1.3
Heart Rate/Rhythm			
bradycardia	0	0.4	0.5
Psychiatric			
vivid dreams	0	0	0
insomnia	2.3	1.5	2.5
depression	0.8	0	0.2
Gastrointestinal			
diarrhea	1.5	2.6	3.5
nausea	1.5	1.5	2.2
vomiting	0	1.1	1.5
Respiratory			
bronchospasm	0	0	0
cough	4.5	2.6	2.5
dyspnea	0.8	1.1	1.5
pharyngitis	2.3	2.2	2.2
rhinitis	3.0	2.9	4.0
sinusitis	1.5	2.2	2.2
URI	3.8	4.8	5.0
Body as a Whole			
asthenia	0	0.4	1.5
chest pain	0.8	1.1	1.5
fatigue	1.5	6.6	8.2
edema (peripheral)	3.8	3.7	3.0

[a] percentage of patients with event.

In addition, a variety of adverse effects have been reported with other beta-adrenergic blocking agents and should be considered potential adverse effects of ZEBETA:

Central Nervous System: Reversible mental depression progressing to catatonia, hallucinations, an acute reversible syndrome characterized by disorientation to time and place, emotional lability, slightly clouded sensorium.

Allergic: Fever, combined with aching and sore throat, laryngospasm, respiratory distress.

Hematologic: Agranulocytosis, thrombocytopenia, thrombocytopenic purpura.

Gastrointestinal: Mesenteric arterial thrombosis, ischemic colitis.

Miscellaneous: The oculomucocutaneous syndrome associated with the beta-blocker practolol has not been reported with ZEBETA during investigational use or extensive foreign marketing experience.

LABORATORY ABNORMALITIES: In clinical trials, the most frequently reported laboratory change was an increase in serum triglycerides, but this was not a consistent finding. Sporadic liver test abnormalities have been reported. In the U.S. controlled trials experience with bisoprolol fumarate treatment for 4–12 weeks, the incidence of concomitant elevations in SGOT and SGPT of between 1–2 times normal was 3.9%, compared to 2.5% for placebo. No patient had concomitant elevations greater than twice normal.

In the long-term, uncontrolled experience with bisoprolol fumarate treatment for 6–18 months, the incidence of one or more concomitant elevations in SGOT and SGPT of between 1–2 times normal was 6.2%. The incidence of multiple occurrences was 1.9%. For concomitant elevations in SGOT and SGPT of greater than twice normal, the incidence was 1.5%. The incidence of multiple occurrences was 0.3%. In many cases these elevations were attributed to underlying disorders, or resolved during continued treatment with bisoprolol fumarate.

Other laboratory changes included small increases in uric acid, creatinine, BUN, serum potassium, glucose, and phosphorus and decreases in WBC and platelets. These were generally not of clinical importance and rarely resulted in discontinuation of bisoprolol fumarate.

As with other beta-blockers, ANA conversions have also been reported on bisoprolol fumarate. About 15% of patients in long-term studies converted to a positive titer, although about one-third of these patients subsequently reconverted to a negative titer while on continued therapy.

OVERDOSAGE

The most common signs expected with overdosage of a beta-blocker are bradycardia, hypotension, congestive heart failure, bronchospasm, and hypoglycemia. To date, a few cases of overdose (maximum: 2000 mg) with bisoprolol fumarate have been reported. Bradycardia and/or hypotension were noted. Sympathomimetic agents were given in some cases, and all patients recovered.

In general, if overdose occurs, ZEBETA therapy should be stopped and supportive and symptomatic treatment should be provided. Limited data suggest that bisoprolol fumarate is not dialyzable. Based on the expected pharmacologic actions and recommendations for other beta-blockers, the following general measures should be considered when clinically warranted:

Bradycardia
Administer IV atropine. If the response is inadequate, isoproterenol or another agent with positive chronotropic properties may be given cautiously. Under some circumstances, transvenous pacemaker insertion may be necessary.

Hypotension
IV fluids and vasopressors should be administered. Intravenous glucagon may be useful.

Heart Block (second or third degree)
Patients should be carefully monitored and treated with isoproterenol infusion or transvenous cardiac pacemaker insertion, as appropriate.

Congestive Heart Failure
Initiate conventional therapy (ie, digitalis, diuretics, inotropic agents, vasodilating agents).

Bronchospasm
Administer bronchodilator therapy such as isoproterenol and/or aminophylline.

Hypoglycemia
Administer IV glucose.

DOSAGE AND ADMINISTRATION

The dose of ZEBETA must be individualized to the needs of the patient. The usual starting dose is 5 mg once daily. In some patients, 2.5 mg may be an appropriate starting dose (see **Bronchospastic Disease** in **WARNINGS**). If the antihypertensive effect of 5 mg is inadequate, the dose may be increased to 10 mg and then, if necessary, to 20 mg once daily.

Patients with Renal or Hepatic Impairment
In patients with hepatic impairment (hepatitis or cirrhosis) or renal dysfunction (creatinine clearance less than 40 mL/min), the initial daily dose should be 2.5 mg and caution should be used in dose-titration. Since limited data suggest that bisoprolol fumarate is not dialyzable, drug replacement is not necessary in patients undergoing dialysis.

Elderly Patients
It is not necessary to adjust the dose in the elderly, unless there is also significant renal or hepatic dysfunction (see above and **Use in Elderly Patients** in **PRECAUTIONS**).

Children
There is no pediatric experience with ZEBETA.

HOW SUPPLIED

ZEBETA® (bisoprolol fumarate) is supplied as 5 mg and 10 mg tablets.

The 5 mg tablet is pink, heart-shaped, biconvex, film-coated, and vertically scored in half on both sides, with an engraved B1 on one side and LL on the reverse side, supplied as follows:

NDC 0005-3816-38—Bottle of 30 with CRC

The 10 mg tablet is white, heart-shaped, biconvex, film-coated, with an engraved B3 on one side and LL on the reverse side, supplied as follows:

NDC 0005-3817-38—Bottle of 30 with CRC

Store at Controlled Room Temperature 15°–30°C (59°– 86°F). Dispense in tight containers as defined in the USP.

LEDERLE LABORATORIES DIVISION
American Cyanamid Company
Pearl River, NY 10965
Under License of E. MERCK
Darmstadt, Germany
Shown in Product Identification Guide, page 321

ZIAC®   ℞
[zī'ăk]
**(Bisoprolol Fumarate and Hydrochlorothiazide)
Tablets**

DESCRIPTION

ZIAC (bisoprolol fumarate and hydrochlorothiazide) is indicated for the treatment of hypertension. It combines two antihypertensive agents in a once-daily dosage: a synthetic beta$_1$-selective (cardioselective) adrenoceptor blocking agent (bisoprolol fumarate) and a benzothiadiazine diuretic (hydrochlorothiazide).

Bisoprolol fumarate is chemically described as (±)-1-[4-[[2-(1-methylethoxy)ethoxy]methyl]phenoxy]-3-[(1-methylethyl)amino]-2-propanol(E)-2-butenedioate (2:1) (salt). It possesses an asymmetric carbon atom in its structure and is provided as a racemic mixture. The S(-) enantiomer is responsible for most of the beta-blocking activity. Its empirical formula is $(C_{18}H_{31}NO_4)_2 \cdot C_4H_4O_4$ and it has a molecular weight of 766.97.

Bisoprolol fumarate is a white crystalline powder, approximately equally hydrophilic and lipophilic, and readily soluble in water, methanol, ethanol, and chloroform.

Hydrochlorothiazide (HCTZ) is 6-Chloro-3,4-dihydro-2H-1,2,4-benzothiadiazine-7-sulfonamide 1,1-dioxide. It is a white, or practically white, practically odorless crystalline powder. It is slightly soluble in water, sparingly soluble in dilute sodium hydroxide solution, freely soluble in n-butylamine and dimethylformamide, soluble in methanol, and insoluble in ether, chloroform, and dilute mineral acids. Its empirical formula is $C_7H_8ClN_3O_4S_2$ and it has a molecular weight of 297.73.

Each ZIAC® 2.5 mg/6.25 mg tablet for oral administration contains:
Bisoprolol fumarate .... 2.5 mg
Hydrochlorothiazide .... 6.25 mg
Each ZIAC® 5 mg/6.25 mg tablet for oral administration contains:
Bisoprolol fumarate .... 5 mg
Hydrochlorothiazide .... 6.25 mg
Each ZIAC® 10 mg/6.25 mg tablet for oral administration contains:
Bisoprolol fumarate .... 10 mg
Hydrochlorothiazide .... 6.25 mg

Inactive ingredients include Colloidal Silicon Dioxide, Corn Starch, Dibasic Calcium Phosphate, Hydroxypropyl Methylcellulose, Magnesium Stearate, Microcrystalline Cellulose, Polyethylene Glycol, Polysorbate 80, and Titanium Dioxide. The 5 mg/6.25 mg tablet also contains Red and Yellow Iron Oxide. The 2.5 mg/6.25 mg tablet also contains Crospovidone, Pregelatinized Starch and Yellow Iron Oxide.

CLINICAL PHARMACOLOGY

Bisoprolol fumarate and HCTZ have been used individually and in combination for the treatment of hypertension. The antihypertensive effects of these agents are additive; HCTZ 6.25 mg significantly increases the antihypertensive effect of bisoprolol fumarate. The incidence of hypokalemia with the bisoprolol fumarate and HCTZ 6.25 mg combination (B/H) is significantly lower than with HCTZ 25 mg. In clinical trials of ZIAC (bisoprolol fumarate and hydrochlorothiazide), mean changes in serum potassium for patients treated with ZIAC 2.5/6.25 mg, 5/6.25 mg or 10/6.25 mg or placebo were less than ± 0.1 mEq/L. Mean changes in serum potassium for patients treated with any dose of bisoprolol in combination with HCTZ 25 mg ranged from –0.1 to –0.3 mEq/L.

Bisoprolol fumarate is a beta$_1$-selective (cardioselective) adrenoceptor blocking agent without significant membrane stabilizing or intrinsic sympathomimetic activities in its therapeutic dose range. At higher doses ($\geq$ 20 mg) bisoprolol fumarate also inhibits beta$_2$-adrenoreceptors located in bronchial and vascular musculature. To retain relative selectivity, it is important to use the lowest effective dose.

Hydrochlorothiazide is a benzothiadiazine diuretic. Thiazides affect renal tubular mechanisms of electrolyte reabsorption and increase excretion of sodium and chloride in

Continued on next page

Lederle—Cont.

approximately equivalent amounts. Natriuresis causes a secondary loss of potassium.

Pharmacokinetics and Metabolism

ZIAC

In healthy volunteers, both bisoprolol fumarate and hydrochlorothiazide are well absorbed following oral administration of ZIAC. No change is observed in the bioavailability of either agent when given together in a single tablet. Absorption is not affected whether ZIAC is taken with or without food. Mean peak bisoprolol fumarate plasma concentrations of about 9.0 ng/mL, 19 ng/mL and 36 ng/mL occur approximately 3 hours after the administration of the 2.5 mg/6.25 mg, 5 mg/6.25 mg and 10 mg/6.25 mg combination tablets, respectively. Mean peak plasma hydrochlorothiazide concentrations of 30 ng/mL occur approximately 2.5 hours following the administration of the combination. Dose proportional increases in plasma bisoprolol concentrations are observed between the 2.5 and 5, as well as between the 5 and 10 mg doses. The elimination of $T_{1/2}$ of bisoprolol ranges from 7 to 15 hours and of hydrochlorothiazide ranges from 4 to 10 hours. The percent of dose excreted unchanged in urine is about 55% for bisoprolol and about 60% for hydrochlorothiazide.

Bisoprolol Fumarate

The absolute bioavailability after a 10 mg oral dose of bisoprolol fumarate is about 80%. The first pass metabolism of bisoprolol fumarate is about 20%.

The pharmacokinetic profile of bisoprolol fumarate has been examined following single doses and at steady state. Binding to serum proteins is approximately 30%. Peak plasma concentrations occur within 2–4 hours of dosing with 2.5 to 20 mg, and mean peak values range from 9.0 ng/mL at 2.5 mg to 70 ng/mL at 20 mg. Once-daily dosing with bisoprolol fumarate results in less than twofold intersubject variation in peak plasma concentrations. Plasma concentrations are proportional to the administered dose in the range of 2.5 to 20 mg. The plasma elimination half-life is 9–12 hours and is slightly longer in elderly patients, in part because of decreased renal function. Steady state is attained within 5 days with once-daily dosing. In both young and elderly populations, plasma accumulation is low; the accumulation factor ranges from 1.1 to 1.3, and is what would be expected from the half-life and once-daily dosing. Bisoprolol is eliminated equally by renal and nonrenal pathways with about 50% of the dose appearing unchanged in the urine and the remainder in the form of inactive metabolites. In humans, the known metabolites are labile or have no known pharmacologic activity. Less than 2% of the dose is excreted in the feces. The pharmacokinetic characteristics of the two enantiomers are similar. Bisoprolol is not metabolized by cytochrome P450 II D6 (debrisoquin hydroxylase).

In subjects with creatinine clearance less than 40 mL/min, the plasma half-life is increased approximately threefold compared to healthy subjects.

In patients with liver cirrhosis, the rate of elimination of bisoprolol is more variable and significantly slower than that in healthy subjects, with a plasma half-life ranging from 8 to 22 hours.

In elderly subjects, mean plasma concentrations at steady state are increased, in part attributed to lower creatinine clearance. However, no significant differences in the degree of bisoprolol accumulation is found between young and elderly populations.

Hydrochlorothiazide

Hydrochlorothiazide is well absorbed (65%–75%) following oral administration. Absorption of hydrochlorothiazide is reduced in patients with congestive heart failure.

Peak plasma concentrations are observed within 1–5 hours of dosing, and range from 70–490 ng/mL following oral doses of 12.5–100 mg. Plasma concentrations are linearly related to the administered dose. Concentrations of hydrochlorothiazide are 1.6–1.8 times higher in whole blood than in plasma. Binding to serum proteins has been reported to be approximately 40% to 68%. The plasma elimination half-life has been reported to be 6–15 hours. Hydrochlorothiazide is elimi-

nated primarily by renal pathways. Following oral doses of 12.5–100 mg, 55%–77% of the administered dose appears in urine and greater than 95% of the absorbed dose is excreted in urine as unchanged drug. Plasma concentrations of hydrochlorothiazide are increased and the elimination half-life is prolonged in patients with renal disease.

Pharmacodynamics

Bisoprolol Fumarate

Findings in clinical hemodynamics studies with bisoprolol fumarate are similar to those observed with other beta-blockers. The most prominent effect is the negative chronotropic effect, giving a reduction in resting and exercise heart rate. There is a fall in resting and exercise cardiac output with little observed change in stroke volume, and only a small increase in right atrial pressure, or pulmonary capillary wedge pressure at rest or during exercise.

In normal volunteers, bisoprolol fumarate therapy resulted in a reduction of exercise- and isoproterenol-induced tachycardia. The maximal effect occurred within 1–4 hours postdosing. Effects generally persisted for 24 hours at doses of 5 mg or greater.

In controlled clinical trials, bisoprolol fumarate given as a single daily dose has been shown to be an effective antihypertensive agent when used alone or concomitantly with thiazide diuretics (see **CLINICAL STUDIES**).

The mechanism of bisoprolol fumarate's antihypertensive effect has not been completely established. Factors that may be involved include:

1) Decreased cardiac output
2) Inhibition of renin release by the kidneys
3) Diminution of tonic sympathetic outflow from vasomotor centers in the brain

Beta$_1$-selectivity of bisoprolol fumarate has been demonstrated in both animal and human studies. No effects at therapeutic doses on beta$_2$-adrenoreceptor density have been observed. Pulmonary function studies have been conducted in healthy volunteers, asthmatics, and patients with chronic obstructive pulmonary disease (COPD). Doses of bisoprolol fumarate ranged from 5 to 60 mg, atenolol from 50 to 200 mg, metoprolol from 100 to 200 mg, and propranolol from 40 to 80 mg. In some studies, slight, asymptomatic increases in airway resistance (AWR) and decreases in forced expiratory volume (FEV$_1$) were observed with doses of bisoprolol fumarate 20 mg and higher, similar to the small increases in AWR noted with other cardioselective beta-blocking agents. The changes induced by beta-blockade with all agents were reversed by bronchodilator therapy.

Electrophysiology studies in man have demonstrated that bisoprolol fumarate significantly decreases heart rate, increases sinus node recovery time, prolongs AV node refractory periods, and, with rapid atrial stimulation, prolongs AV nodal conduction.

Hydrochlorothiazide

Acute effects of thiazides are thought to result from a reduction in blood volume and cardiac output, secondary to a natriuretic effect, although a direct vasodilatory mechanism has also been proposed. With chronic administration, plasma volume returns toward normal, but peripheral vascular resistance is decreased.

Thiazides do not affect normal blood pressure. Onset of action occurs within 2 hours of dosing, peak effect is observed at about 4 hours, and activity persists for up to 24 hours.

CLINICAL STUDIES

In controlled clinical trials, bisoprolol fumarate/hydrochlorothiazide 6.25 mg has been shown to reduce systolic and diastolic blood pressure throughout a 24-hour period when administered once daily. The effects on systolic and diastolic blood pressure reduction of the combination of bisoprolol fumarate and hydrochlorothiazide were additive. Further, treatment effects were consistent across age groups (<60, ≥60 years), racial groups (black, nonblack), and gender (male, female).

In two randomized, double-blind, placebo-controlled trials conducted in the U.S., reductions in systolic and diastolic blood pressure and heart rate 24 hours after dosing in patients with mild-to-moderate hypertension are shown below. In both studies mean systolic/diastolic blood pressure and

heart rate at baseline were approximately 151/101 mm Hg and 77 bpm.
[See table below.]

Blood pressure responses were seen within 1 week of treatment but the maximum effect was apparent after 2 to 3 weeks of treatment. Overall, significantly greater blood pressure reductions were observed on ZIAC than on placebo. Further, blood pressure reductions were significantly greater for each of the bisoprolol fumarate plus hydrochlorothiazide combinations than for either of the components used alone regardless of race, age, or gender. There were no significant differences in response between black and nonblack patients.

INDICATIONS AND USAGE

ZIAC is indicated in the management of hypertension.

CONTRAINDICATIONS

ZIAC is contraindicated in patients in cardiogenic shock, overt cardiac failure (see **WARNINGS**), second or third degree AV block, marked sinus bradycardia, anuria, and hypersensitivity to either component of this product or to other sulfonamide-derived drugs.

WARNINGS

Cardiac Failure: In general, beta-blocking agents should be avoided in patients with overt congestive failure. However, in some patients with compensated cardiac failure, it may be necessary to utilize these agents. In such situations, they must be used cautiously.

Patients Without a History of Cardiac Failure: Continued depression of the myocardium with beta-blockers can, in some patients, precipitate cardiac failure. At the first signs or symptoms of heart failure, discontinuation of ZIAC should be considered. In some cases ZIAC therapy can be continued while heart failure is treated with other drugs.

Abrupt Cessation of Therapy: Exacerbations of angina pectoris and, in some instances, myocardial infarction or ventricular arrhythmia, have been observed in patients with coronary artery disease following abrupt cessation of therapy with beta-blockers. Such patients should, therefore, be cautioned against interruption or discontinuation of therapy without the physician's advice. Even in patients without overt coronary artery disease, it may be advisable to taper therapy with ZIAC over approximately 1 week with the patient under careful observation. If withdrawal symptoms occur, beta-blocking agent therapy should be reinstituted, at least temporarily.

Peripheral Vascular Disease: Beta-blockers can precipitate or aggravate symptoms of arterial insufficiency in patients with peripheral vascular disease. Caution should be exercised in such individuals.

Bronchospastic Disease: PATIENTS WITH BRONCHOSPASTIC PULMONARY DISEASE SHOULD, IN GENERAL, NOT RECEIVE BETA-BLOCKERS. Because of the relative beta$_1$-selectivity of bisoprolol fumarate, ZIAC may be used with caution in patients with bronchospastic disease who do not respond to, or who cannot tolerate other antihypertensive treatment. Since beta$_1$-selectivity is not absolute, the lowest possible dose of ZIAC should be used. A beta$_2$ agonist (bronchodilator) should be made available.

Anesthesia and Major Surgery: If ZIAC treatment is to be continued perioperatively, particular care should be taken when anesthetic agents that depress myocardial function, such as ether, cyclopropane, and trichloroethylene, are used. See OVERDOSAGE for information on treatment of bradycardia and hypotension.

Diabetes and Hypoglycemia: Beta-blockers may mask some of the manifestations of hypoglycemia, particularly tachycardia. Nonselective beta-blockers may potentiate insulin-induced hypoglycemia and delay recovery of serum glucose levels. Because of its beta$_1$-selectivity, this is less likely with bisoprolol fumarate. However, patients subject to spontaneous hypoglycemia, or diabetic patients receiving insulin or oral hypoglycemic agents, should be cautioned about these possibilities. Also, latent diabetes mellitus may become manifest and diabetic patients given thiazides may require adjustment of their insulin dose. Because of the very low dose of HCTZ employed, this may be less likely with ZIAC.

Thyrotoxicosis: Beta-adrenergic blockade may mask clinical signs of hyperthyroidism, such as tachycardia. Abrupt withdrawal of beta-blockade may be followed by an exacerbation of the symptoms of hyperthyroidism or may precipitate thyroid storm.

Renal Disease: Cumulative effects of the thiazides may develop in patients with impaired renal function. In such patients, thiazides may precipitate azotemia. In subjects with creatinine clearance less than 40 mL/min, the plasma half-life of bisoprolol fumarate is increased up to threefold, as compared to healthy subjects. If progressive renal impairment becomes apparent, ZIAC should be discontinued. (See **Pharmacokinetics and Metabolism**.)

Hepatic Disease: ZIAC should be used with caution in patients with impaired hepatic function or progressive liver disease. Thiazides may alter fluid and electrolyte balance, which may precipitate hepatic coma. Also, elimination of bisoprolol fumarate is significantly slower in patients with

Sitting Systolic/Diastolic Pressure (BP) and Heart Rate (HR)
Mean Decrease (Δ) After 3–4 weeks

	Study 1		Study 2			
	Placebo	B5/H6.25 mg	Placebo	H6.25 mg	B2.5/H6.25 mg	B10/H6.25 mg
n=	75	150	56	23	28	25
Total ΔBP (mm Hg)	-2.9/-3.9	-15.8/-12.6	-3.0/-3.7	-6.6/-5.8	-14.1/-10.5	-15.3/-14.3
Drug Effect[a]	—/—	-12.9/-8.7	—/—	-3.6/-2.1	-11.1/-6.8	-12.3/-10.6
Total ΔHR (bpm)	-0.3	-6.9	-1.6	-0.8	-3.7	-9.8
Drug Effect[a]		-6.6		+0.8	-2.1	-8.2

[a] Observed mean change from baseline minus placebo.

cirrhosis than in healthy subjects. (See **Pharmacokinetics and Metabolism**.)

PRECAUTIONS

General: Electrolyte and Fluid Balance Status: Although the probability of developing hypokalemia is reduced with ZIAC because of the very low dose of HCTZ employed, periodic determination of serum electrolytes should be performed, and patients should be observed for signs of fluid or electrolyte disturbances, ie, hyponatremia, hypochloremic alkalosis, and hypokalemia and hypomagnesemia. Thiazides have been shown to increase the urinary excretion of magnesium; this may result in hypomagnesemia.

Warning signs or symptoms of fluid and electrolyte imbalance include dryness of mouth, thirst, weakness, lethargy, drowsiness, restlessness, muscle pains or cramps, muscular fatigue, hypotension, oliguria, tachycardia, and gastrointestinal disturbances such as nausea and vomiting.

Hypokalemia may develop, especially with brisk diuresis when severe cirrhosis is present, during concomitant use of corticosteroids or adrenocorticotropic hormone (ACTH) or after prolonged therapy. Interference with adequate oral electrolyte intake will also contribute to hypokalemia. Hypokalemia and hypomagnesemia can provoke ventricular arrhythmias or sensitize or exaggerate the response of the heart to the toxic effects of digitalis. Hypokalemia may be avoided or treated by potassium supplementation or increased intake of potassium-rich foods.

Dilutional hyponatremia may occur in edematous patients in hot weather; appropriate therapy is water restriction rather than salt administration, except in rare instances when the hyponatremia is life-threatening. In actual salt depletion, appropriate replacement is the therapy of choice.

Parathyroid Disease: Calcium excretion is decreased by thiazides, and pathologic changes in the parathyroid glands, with hypercalcemia and hypophosphatemia, have been observed in a few patients on prolonged thiazide therapy.

Hyperuricemia: Hyperuricemia or acute gout may be precipitated in certain patients receiving thiazide diuretics. Bisoprolol fumarate, alone or in combination with HCTZ, has been associated with increases in uric acid. However, in U.S. clinical trials, the incidence of treatment-related increases in uric acid was higher during therapy with HCTZ 25 mg (25%) than with B/H 6.25 mg (10%). Because of the very low dose of HCTZ employed, hyperuricemia may be less likely with ZIAC.

Drug Interactions: ZIAC may potentiate the action of other antihypertensive agents used concomitantly. ZIAC should not be combined with other beta-blocking agents. Patients receiving catecholamine-depleting drugs, such as reserpine or guanethidine, should be closely monitored because the added beta-adrenergic blocking action of bisoprolol fumarate may produce excessive reduction of sympathetic activity. In patients receiving concurrent therapy with clonidine, if therapy is to be discontinued, it is suggested that ZIAC be discontinued for several days before the withdrawal of clonidine. ZIAC should be used with caution when myocardial depressants or inhibitors of AV conduction, such as certain calcium antagonists (particularly of the phenylalkylamine [verapamil] and benzothiazepine [diltiazem] classes), or antiarrhythmic agents, such as disopyramide, are used concurrently.

Bisoprolol Fumarate: Concurrent use of rifampin increases the metabolic clearance of bisoprolol fumarate, shortening its elimination half-life. However, initial dose modification is generally not necessary. Pharmacokinetic studies document no clinically relevant interactions with other agents given concomitantly, including thiazide diuretics, digoxin and cimetidine. There was no effect of bisoprolol fumarate on prothrombin times in patients on stable doses of warfarin.

Risk of Anaphylactic Reaction: While taking beta-blockers, patients with a history of severe anaphylactic reaction to a variety of allergens may be more reactive to repeated challenge, either accidental, diagnostic, or therapeutic. Such patients may be unresponsive to the usual doses of epinephrine used to treat allergic reactions.

Hydrochlorothiazide: When given concurrently the following drugs may interact with thiazide diuretics.

Alcohol, barbiturates, or narcotics—potentiation of orthostatic hypotension may occur.

Antidiabetic drugs (oral agents and insulin)—dosage adjustment of the antidiabetic drug may be required.

Other antihypertensive drugs—additive effect or potentiation.

Cholestyramine and colestipol resins—absorption of hydrochlorothiazide is impaired in the presence of anionic exchange resins. Single doses of cholestyramine and colestipol resins bind the hydrochlorothiazide and reduce its absorption in the gastrointestinal tract by up to 85 percent and 43 percent, respectively.

Corticosteroids, ACTH—intensified electrolyte depletion, particularly hypokalemia.

Pressor amines (eg, norepinephrine)—possible decreased response to pressor amines but not sufficient to preclude their use.

Skeletal muscle relaxants, nondepolarizing (eg, tubocurarine)—possible increased responsiveness to the muscle relaxant.

Lithium—generally should not be given with diuretics. Diuretic agents reduce the renal clearance of lithium and add a high risk of lithium toxicity. Refer to the package insert for lithium preparations before use of such preparations with ZIAC.

Nonsteroidal anti-inflammatory drugs—in some patients, the administration of a nonsteroidal anti-inflammatory agent can reduce the diuretic, natriuretic, and antihypertensive effects of loop, potassium-sparing and thiazide diuretics. Therefore, when ZIAC and nonsteroidal anti-inflammatory agents are used concomitantly, the patient should be observed closely to determine if the desired effect of the diuretic is obtained.

In patients receiving thiazides, sensitivity reactions may occur with or without a history of allergy or bronchial asthma. Photosensitivity reactions and possible exacerbation or activation of systemic lupus erythematosus have been reported in patients receiving thiazides. The antihypertensive effects of thiazides may be enhanced in the post-sympathectomy patient.

Laboratory Test Interactions: Based on reports involving thiazides, ZIAC may decrease serum levels of protein-bound iodine without signs of thyroid disturbance.

Because it includes a thiazide, ZIAC should be discontinued before carrying out tests for parathyroid function (see **PRECAUTIONS—Parathyroid Disease**).

INFORMATION FOR PATIENTS

Patients, especially those with coronary artery disease, should be warned against discontinuing use of ZIAC without a physician's supervision. Patients should also be advised to consult a physician if any difficulty in breathing occurs, or if they develop other signs or symptoms of congestive heart failure or excessive bradycardia.

Patients subject to spontaneous hypoglycemia, or diabetic patients receiving insulin or oral hypoglycemic agents, should be cautioned that beta-blockers may mask some of the manifestations of hypoglycemia, particularly tachycardia, and bisoprolol fumarate should be used with caution.

Patients should know how they react to this medicine before they operate automobiles and machinery or engage in other tasks requiring alertness. Patients should be advised that photosensitivity reactions have been reported with thiazides.

Carcinogenesis, Mutagenesis, Impairment of Fertility:
Carcinogenesis
ZIAC: Long-term studies have not been conducted with the bisoprolol fumarate/hydrochlorothiazide combination.

Bisoprolol Fumarate: Long-term studies were conducted with oral bisoprolol fumarate administered in the feed of mice (20 and 24 months) and rats (26 months). No evidence of carcinogenic potential was seen in mice dosed up to 250 mg/kg/day or rats dosed up to 125 mg/kg/day. On a body-weight basis, these doses are 625 and 312 times, respectively, the maximum recommended human dose (MRHD) of 20 mg, or 0.4 mg/kg/day, based on 50 kg individuals; on a body-surface-area basis, these doses are 59 times (mice) and 64 times (rats) the MRHD.

Hydrochlorothiazide: Two-year feeding studies in mice and rats, conducted under the auspices of the National Toxicology Program (NTP), treated mice and rats with doses of hydrochlorothiazide up to 600 and 100 mg/kg/day, respectively. On a body-weight basis, these doses are 2400 times (in mice) and 400 times (in rats) the MRHD of hydrochlorothiazide (12.5 mg/day) in ZIAC (bisoprolol fumarate and hydrochlorothiazide). On a body-surface-area basis, these doses are 226 times (in mice) and 82 times (in rats) the MRHD. These studies uncovered no evidence of carcinogenic potential of hydrochlorothiazide in rats or female mice, but there was equivocal evidence of hepatocarcinogenicity in male mice.

Mutagenesis
ZIAC: The mutagenic potential of the bisoprolol fumarate/hydrochlorothiazide combination was evaluated in the microbial mutagenicity (Ames) test, the point mutation and chromosomal aberration assays in Chinese hamster V79 cells, and the micronucleus test in mice. There was no evidence of mutagenic potential in these *in vitro* and *in vivo* assays.

Bisoprolol Fumarate: The mutagenic potential of bisoprolol fumarate was evaluated in the microbial mutagenicity (Ames) test, the point mutation and chromosome aberration assays in Chinese hamster V79 cells, the unscheduled DNA synthesis test, the micronucleus test in mice, and the cytogenetics assay in rats. There was no evidence of mutagenic potential in these *in vitro* and *in vivo* assays.

Hydrochlorothiazide: Hydrochlorothiazide was not genotoxic in *in vitro* assays using strains TA 98, TA 100, TA 1535, TA 1537 and TA 1538 of *Salmonella typhimurium* (the Ames test); in the Chinese Hamster Ovary (CHO) test for chromosomal aberrations; or in *in vivo* assays using mouse germinal cell chromosomes, Chinese hamster bone marrow chromosomes, and the *Drosophila* sex-linked recessive lethal trait gene. Positive test results were obtained in the *in vitro* CHO Sister Chromatid Exchange (clastogenicity) test and in the

mouse Lymphoma Cell (mutagenicity) assays, using concentrations of hydrochlorothiazide of 43 to 1300 µg/mL. Positive test results were also obtained in the *Aspergillus nidulans* nondisjunction assay, using an unspecified concentration of hydrochlorothiazide.

Impairment of Fertility
ZIAC: Reproduction studies in rats did not show any impairment of fertility with the bisoprolol fumarate/hydrochlorothiazide combination doses containing up to 30 mg/kg/day of bisoprolol fumarate in combination with 75 mg/kg/day of hydrochlorothiazide. On a body-weight basis, these doses are 75 and 300 times, respectively, the MRHD of bisoprolol fumarate and hydrochlorothiazide. On a body-surface-area basis, these study doses are 15 and 62 times, respectively, the MRHD.

Bisoprolol Fumarate: Reproduction studies in rats did not show any impairment of fertility at doses up to 150 mg/kg/day of bisoprolol fumarate, or 375 and 77 times the MRHD on the basis of body-weight and body-surface-area, respectively.

Hydrochlorothiazide: Hydrochlorothiazide had no adverse effects on the fertility of mice and rats of either sex in studies wherein these species were exposed, via their diet, to doses of up to 100 and 4 mg/kg/day, respectively, prior to mating and throughout gestation. Corresponding multiples of maximum recommended human doses are 400 (mice) and 16 (rats) on the basis of body-weight and 38 (mice) and 3.3 (rats) on the basis of body-surface-area.

Pregnancy: Teratogenic Effects-Pregnancy Category C:
ZIAC: In rats, the bisoprolol fumarate/hydrochlorothiazide (B/H) combination was not teratogenic at doses up to 51.4 mg/kg/day of bisoprolol fumarate in combination with 128.6 mg/kg/day of hydrochlorothiazide. Bisoprolol fumarate and hydrochlorothiazide doses used in the rat study are, as multiples of the MRHD in the combination, 129 and 514 times greater, respectively, on a body-weight basis, and 26 and 106 times greater, respectively, on the basis of body-surface-area. The drug combination was maternotoxic (decreased body weight and food consumption) at B5.7/H14.3 (mg/kg/day) and higher, and fetotoxic (increased late resorptions) at B17.1/H42.9 (mg/kg/day) and higher. Maternotoxicity was present at 14/57 times the MRHD of B/H, respectively, on a body-weight basis, and 3/12 times the MRHD of B/H doses, respectively, on the basis of body-surface-area. Fetotoxicity was present at 43/172 times the MRHD of B/H, respectively, on a body-weight basis, and 9/35 times the MRHD of B/H doses, respectively, on the basis of body-surface-area. In rabbits, the B/H combination was not teratogenic at doses of B10/H25 (mg/kg/day). Bisoprolol fumarate and hydrochlorothiazide used in the rabbit study were not teratogenic at 25/100 times the B/H MRHD, respectively, on a body-weight basis, and 10/40 times the B/H MRHD, respectively, on the basis of body-surface-area. The drug combination was maternotoxic (decreased body weight) at B1/H2.5 (mg/kg/day) and higher, and fetotoxic (increased resorptions) at B10/H25 (mg/kg/day). The multiples of the MRHD for the B/H combination that were maternotoxic were, respectively, 2.5/10 (on the basis of body-weight) and 1/4 (on the basis of body-surface-area), and for fetotoxicity were, respectively, 25/100 (on the basis of body-weight) and 10/40 (on the basis of body-surface-area).

There are no adequate and well-controlled studies with ZIAC in pregnant women. ZIAC should be used during pregnancy only if the potential benefit justifies the risk to the fetus.

Bisoprolol Fumarate: In rats, bisoprolol fumarate was not teratogenic at doses up to 150 mg/kg/day, which were 375 and 77 times the MRHD on the basis of body-weight and body-surface-area, respectively. Bisoprolol fumarate was fetotoxic (increased late resorptions) at 50 mg/kg/day and maternotoxic (decreased food intake and body-weight gain) at 150 mg/kg/day. The fetotoxicity in rats occurred at 125 times the MRHD on a body-weight basis and 26 times the MRHD on the basis of body-surface-area. The maternotoxicity occurred at 375 times the MRHD on a body-weight basis and 77 times the MRHD on the basis of body-surface-area. In rabbits, bisoprolol fumarate was not teratogenic at doses up to 12.5 mg/kg/day, which is 31 and 12 times the MRHD based on body-weight and body-surface-area, respectively, but was embryolethal (increased early resorptions) at 12.5 mg/kg/day.

Hydrochlorothiazide: Hydrochlorothiazide was orally administered to pregnant mice and rats during respective periods of major organogenesis at doses up to 3000 and 1000 mg/kg/day, respectively. At these doses, which are multiples of the MRHD equal to 12,000 for mice and 4000 for rats, based on body-weight, and equal to 1129 for mice and 824 for rats, based on body-surface-area, there was no evidence of harm to the fetus. There are, however, no adequate and well-controlled studies in pregnant women. Because animal reproduction studies are not always predictive of human response, this drug should be used during pregnancy only if clearly needed.

Nonteratogenic Effects: Thiazides cross the placental barrier and appear in the cord blood. The use of thiazides in

Continued on next page

Lederle—Cont.

pregnant women requires that the anticipated benefit be weighed against possible hazards to the fetus. These hazards include fetal or neonatal jaundice, pancreatitis, thrombocytopenia, and possibly other adverse reactions which have occurred in the adult.

Nursing Mothers: Bisoprolol fumarate alone or in combination with HCTZ has not been studied in nursing mothers. Thiazides are excreted in human breast milk. Small amounts of bisoprolol fumarate (< 2% of the dose) have been detected in the milk of lactating rats. Because of the potential for serious adverse reactions in nursing infants, a decision should be made whether to discontinue nursing or to discontinue the drug, taking into account the importance of the drug to the mother.

Use in Elderly Patients: In clinical trials, at least 270 patients treated with bisoprolol fumarate plus HCTZ were 60 years of age or older. HCTZ added significantly to the antihypertensive effect of bisoprolol in elderly hypertensive patients. No overall differences in effectiveness or safety were observed between these patients and younger patients. Other reported clinical experience has not identified differences in responses between the elderly and younger patients, but greater sensitivity of some older individuals cannot be ruled out.

Pediatric Use: Safety and effectiveness of ZIAC in children have not been established.

ADVERSE REACTIONS

ZIAC:
Bisoprolol fumarate/H6.25 mg is well tolerated in most patients. Most adverse effects (AEs) have been mild and transient. In more than 65,000 patients treated worldwide with bisoprolol fumarate, occurrences of bronchospasm have been rare. Discontinuation rates for AEs were similar for B/H6.25 mg and placebo-treated patients.

In the United States, 252 patients received bisoprolol fumarate (2.5, 5, 10, or 40 mg)/H6.25 mg and 144 patients received placebo in two controlled trials. In Study 1, bisoprolol fumarate 5/H6.25 mg was administered for 4 weeks. In Study 2, bisoprolol fumarate 2.5, 10 or 40/H6.25 mg was administered for 12 weeks. All adverse experiences, whether drug related or not, and drug related adverse experiences in patients treated with B2.5–10/H6.25 mg, reported during comparable, 4 week treatment periods by at least 2% of bisoprolol fumarate/H6.25 mg-treated patients (plus additional selected adverse experiences) are presented in the following table:

[See table below.]

Other adverse experiences that have been reported with the individual components are listed below.

Bisoprolol Fumarate
In clinical trials worldwide, a variety of other AEs, in addition to those listed above, have been reported. While in many cases it is not known whether a causal relationship exists between bisoprolol and these AEs, they are listed to alert the physician to a possible relationship.

Central Nervous System: Unsteadiness, vertigo, syncope, paresthesia, hyperesthesia, sleep disturbance/vivid dreams, depression, anxiety/restlessness, decreased concentration/memory.

Cardiovascular: Palpitations and other rhythm disturbances, cold extremities, claudication, hypotension, orthostatic hypotension, chest pain, congestive heart failure.

Gastrointestinal: Gastric/epigastric/abdominal pain, peptic ulcer, gastritis, vomiting, constipation, dry mouth.

Musculoskeletal: Arthralgia, muscle/joint pain, back/neck pain, twitching/tremor.

Skin: Rash, acne, eczema, psoriasis, skin irritation, pruritus, purpura, flushing, sweating, alopecia, dermatitis, exfoliative dermatitis (very rarely), cutaneous vasculitis.

Special Senses: Visual disturbances, ocular pain/pressure, abnormal lacrimation, tinnitus, decreased hearing, earache, taste abnormalities.

Metabolic: Gout.

Respiratory: Asthma, bronchitis, dyspnea, pharyngitis, sinusitis.

Genito-urinary: Peyronie's disease (very rarely), cystitis, renal colic, polyuria.

General: Malaise, edema, weight gain, angioedema.

In addition, a variety of adverse effects have been reported with other beta-adrenergic blocking agents and should be considered potential adverse effects:

Central Nervous System: Reversible mental depression progressing to catatonia, hallucinations, an acute reversible syndrome characterized by disorientation to time and place, emotional lability, slightly clouded sensorium.

Allergic: Fever, combined with aching and sore throat, laryngospasm, and respiratory distress.

Hematologic: Agranulocytosis, thrombocytopenia.

Gastrointestinal: Mesenteric arterial thrombosis and ischemic colitis.

Miscellaneous: The oculomucocutaneous syndrome associated with the beta-blocker practolol has not been reported with bisoprolol fumarate during investigational use or extensive foreign marketing experience.

Hydrochlorothiazide
The following adverse experiences, in addition to those listed in the above table, have been reported with hydrochlorothiazide (generally with doses of 25 mg or greater).

General: Weakness.

Central Nervous System: Vertigo, paresthesia, restlessness.

Cardiovascular: Orthostatic hypotension (may be potentiated by alcohol, barbiturates, or narcotics).

Gastrointestinal: Anorexia, gastric irritation, cramping, constipation, jaundice (intrahepatic cholestatic jaundice), pancreatitis, cholecystitis, sialadenitis, dry mouth.

Musculoskeletal: Muscle spasm.

Hypersensitive Reactions: Purpura, photosensitivity, rash, urticaria, necrotizing angiitis (vasculitis and cutaneous vasculitis), fever, respiratory distress including pneumonitis and pulmonary edema, anaphylactic reactions.

Special Senses: Transient blurred vision, xanthopsia.

Metabolic: Gout.

Genitourinary: Sexual dysfunction, renal failure, renal dysfunction, interstitial nephritis.

LABORATORY ABNORMALITIES

ZIAC
Because of the low dose of hydrochlorothiazide in ZIAC, adverse metabolic effects with B/H6.25 mg are less frequent and of smaller magnitude than with HCTZ 25 mg. Laboratory data on serum potassium from the U.S. placebo-controlled trials are shown in the following table:

[See table above.]

Treatment with both beta blockers and thiazide diuretics is associated with increases in uric acid. However, the magnitude of the change in patients treated with B/H6.25 mg was smaller than in patients treated with HCTZ 25 mg. Mean increases in serum triglycerides were observed in patients treated with bisoprolol fumarate and hydrochlorothiazide 6.25 mg. Total cholesterol was generally unaffected, but small decreases in HDL cholesterol were noted.

Other laboratory abnormalities that have been reported with the individual components are listed below.

Bisoprolol Fumarate: In clinical trials, the most frequently reported laboratory change was an increase in serum triglycerides, but this was not a consistent finding.

Sporadic liver test abnormalities have been reported. In the U.S. controlled trials experience with bisoprolol fumarate treatment for 4 to 12 weeks, the incidence of concomitant elevations in SGOT and SGPT of between 1 and 2 times normal was 3.9%, compared to 2.5% for placebo. No patient had concomitant elevations greater than twice normal.

In the long-term, uncontrolled experience with bisoprolol fumarate treatment for 6 to 18 months, the incidence of one or more concomitant elevations in SGOT and SGPT of between 1 and 2 times normal was 6.2%. The incidence of multiple occurrence was 1.9%. For concomitant elevations in SGOT and SGPT of greater than twice normal, the incidence was 1.5%. The incidence of multiple occurrences was 0.3%. In many cases these elevations were attributed to underlying disorders, or resolved during continued treatment with bisoprolol fumarate.

Other laboratory changes included small increases in uric acid, creatinine, BUN, serum potassium, glucose, and phosphorus and decreases in WBC and platelets. There have been occasional reports of eosinophilia. These were generally not of clinical importance and rarely resulted in discontinuation of bisoprolol fumarate.

As with other beta-blockers, ANA conversions have also been reported on bisoprolol fumarate. About 15% of patients in long-term studies converted to a positive titer, although about one-third of these patients subsequently reconverted to a negative titer while on continued therapy.

Hydrochlorothiazide: Hyperglycemia, glycosuria, hyperuricemia, hypokalemia and other electrolyte imbalances (see **PRECAUTIONS**), hyperlipidemia, hypercalcemia, leukopenia, agranulocytosis, thrombocytopenia, aplastic anemia, and hemolytic anemia have been associated with HCTZ therapy.

OVERDOSAGE

There are limited data on overdose with ZIAC. However, several cases of overdose with bisoprolol fumarate have been

---

Serum Potassium Data from U.S. Placebo Controlled Studies

	Placebo† (n = 130*)	B2.5/H6.25 mg (n = 28*)	B5/H6.25 mg (n = 149*)	B10/H6.25 mg (n = 28*)	HCTZ25 mg† (n = 142*)
Potassium					
Mean Change[a] (mEq/L)	+0.04	+0.11	–0.08	0.00	–0.30
% Hypokalemia[b]	0.0%	0.0%	0.7%	0.0%	5.5%

*Patients with normal serum potassium at baseline.
[a] Mean change from baseline at Week 4.
[b] Percentage of patients with abnormality at Week 4.
†Combined across studies.

% of Patients With Adverse Experiences*

Body System/ Adverse Experience	All Adverse Experiences		Drug Related Adverse Experiences	
	Placebo† (n=144) %	B2.5–40/H6.25† (n=252) %	Placebo† (n=144) %	B2.5–10/H6.25† (n=221) %
Cardiovascular				
bradycardia	0.7	1.1	0.7	0.9
arrhythmia	1.4	0.4	0.0	0.0
peripheral ischemia	0.9	0.7	0.9	0.4
chest pain	0.7	1.8	0.7	0.9
Respiratory				
bronchospasm	0.0	0.0	0.0	0.0
cough	1.0	2.2	0.7	1.5
rhinitis	2.0	0.7	0.7	0.9
URI	2.3	2.1	0.0	0.0
Body as a Whole				
asthenia	0.0	0.0	0.0	0.0
fatigue	2.7	4.6	1.7	3.0
peripheral edema	0.7	1.1	0.7	0.9
Central Nervous System				
dizziness	1.8	5.1	1.8	3.2
headache	4.7	4.5	2.7	0.4
Musculoskeletal				
muscle cramps	0.7	1.2	0.7	1.1
myalgia	1.4	2.4	0.0	0.0
Psychiatric				
insomnia	2.4	1.1	2.0	1.2
somnolence	0.7	1.1	0.7	0.9
loss of libido	1.2	0.4	1.2	0.4
impotence	0.7	1.1	0.7	1.1
Gastrointestinal				
diarrhea	1.4	4.3	1.2	1.1
nausea	0.9	1.1	0.9	0.9
dyspepsia	0.7	1.2	0.7	0.9

* Averages adjusted to combine across studies.
† Combined across studies.

---

reported (maximum: 2000 mg). Bradycardia and/or hypotension were noted. Sympathomimetic agents were given in some cases, and all patients recovered.

The most frequently observed signs expected with overdosage of a beta-blocker are bradycardia and hypotension. Lethargy is also common, and with severe overdoses, delirium, coma, convulsions, and respiratory arrest have been reported to occur. Congestive heart failure, bronchospasm, and hypoglycemia may occur, particularly in patients with underlying conditions. With thiazide diuretics, acute intoxication is rare. The most prominent feature of overdose is acute loss of fluid and electrolytes. Signs and symptoms include cardiovascular (tachycardia, hypotension, shock), neuromuscular (weakness, confusion, dizziness, cramps of the calf muscles, paresthesia, fatigue, impairment of consciousness), gastrointestinal (nausea, vomiting, thirst), renal (polyuria, oliguria, or anuria [due to hemoconcentration]), and laboratory findings (hypokalemia, hyponatremia, hypochloremia, alkalosis, increased BUN [especially in patients with renal insufficiency]).

If overdosage of ZIAC is suspected, therapy with ZIAC should be discontinued and the patient observed closely. Treatment is symptomatic and supportive; there is no specific antidote. Limited data suggest bisoprolol fumarate is not dialyzable; similarly, there is no indication that hydrochlorothiazide is dialyzable. Suggested general measures include induction of emesis and/or gastric lavage, administration of activated charcoal, respiratory support, correction of fluid and electrolyte imbalance, and treatment of convulsions. Based on the expected pharmacologic actions and recommendations for other beta-blockers and hydrochlorothiazide, the following measures should be considered when clinically warranted:

Bradycardia: Administer IV atropine. If the response is inadequate, isoproterenol or another agent with positive chronotropic properties may be given cautiously. Under some circumstances, transvenous pacemaker insertion may be necessary.

Hypotension, Shock: The patient's legs should be elevated. IV fluids should be administered and lost electrolytes (potassium, sodium) replaced. Intravenous glucagon may be useful. Vasopressors should be considered.

Heart Block (second or third degree): Patients should be carefully monitored and treated with isoproterenol infusion or transvenous cardiac pacemaker insertion, as appropriate.

Congestive Heart Failure: Initiate conventional therapy (ie, digitalis, diuretics, vasodilating agents, inotropic agents).

Bronchospasm: Administer a bronchodilator such as isoproterenol and/or aminophylline.

Hypoglycemia: Administer IV glucose.

Surveillance: Fluid and electrolyte balance (especially serum potassium) and renal function should be monitored until normalized.

DOSAGE AND ADMINISTRATION

Bisoprolol is an effective treatment of hypertension in once-daily doses of 2.5–40 mg, while hydrochlorothiazide is effective in doses of 15–50 mg. In clinical trials of bisoprolol/hydrochlorothiazide combination therapy using bisoprolol doses of 2.5–20 mg and hydrochlorothiazide doses of 6.25–25 mg, the antihypertensive effects increased with increasing doses of either component.

The adverse effects (see **WARNINGS**) of bisoprolol are a mixture of dose-dependent phenomena (primarily bradycardia, diarrhea, asthenia and fatigue) and dose-independent phenomena (eg, occasional rash); those of hydrochlorothiazide are a mixture of dose-dependent phenomena (primarily hypokalemia) and dose-independent phenomena (eg, possibly pancreatitis); the dose-dependent phenomena for each being much more common than the dose-independent phenomena. The latter consist of those few that are truly idiosyncratic in nature or those that occur with such low frequency that a dose relationship may be difficult to discern. Therapy with a combination of bisoprolol and hydrochlorothiazide will be associated with both sets of dose-independent adverse effects, and to minimize these, it may be appropriate to begin combination therapy only after a patient has failed to achieve the desired effect with monotherapy. On the other hand, regimens that combine low doses of bisoprolol and hydrochlorothiazide should produce minimal dose-dependent adverse effects, eg, bradycardia, diarrhea, asthenia and fatigue, and minimal dose-dependent adverse metabolic effects, ie, decreases in serum potassium (see **CLINICAL PHARMACOLOGY**).

Therapy Guided by Clinical Effect: A patient whose blood pressure is not adequately controlled with 2.5–20 mg bisoprolol daily may instead be given ZIAC (bisoprolol fumarate and hydrochlorothiazide). Patients whose blood pressures are adequately controlled with 50 mg of hydrochlorothiazide daily, but who experience significant potassium loss with this regimen, may achieve similar blood pressure control without electrolyte disturbance if they are switched to ZIAC.

Initial Therapy: Antihypertensive therapy may be initiated with the lowest dose of ZIAC, one 2.5/6.25 mg tablet once daily. Subsequent titration (14 day intervals) may be carried out with ZIAC tablets up to the maximum recommended dose 20/12.5 mg (two 10/6.25 mg tablets) once daily, as appropriate.

Replacement Therapy: The combination may be substituted for the titrated individual components.

Cessation of Therapy: If withdrawal of ZIAC therapy is planned, it should be achieved gradually over a period of about 2 weeks. Patients should be carefully observed.

Patients with Renal or Hepatic Impairment: As noted in the **WARNINGS** section, caution must be used in dosing/titrating patients with hepatic impairment or renal dysfunction. Since there is no indication that hydrochlorothiazide is dialyzable, and limited data suggest that bisoprolol is not dialyzable, drug replacement is not necessary in patients undergoing dialysis.

Elderly Patients: Dosage adjustment on the basis of age is not usually necessary, unless there is also significant renal or hepatic dysfunction (see above and **WARNINGS** section).

Children: There is no pediatric experience with ZIAC.

HOW SUPPLIED

ZIAC®-2.5 mg/6.25 mg Tablets (bisoprolol fumarate 2.5 mg and hydrochlorothiazide 6.25 mg) are yellow, round, convex, film coated tablets, engraved with a script "LL" within an engraved heart shape on one side and "B" above "12" on the other; approximately $^1/_4$" in diameter, supplied as follows:
NDC 0005-3238-38—Bottle of 30 with child resistant closure
NDC 0005-3238-23—Bottle of 100

ZIAC®-5 mg/6.25 mg Tablets (bisoprolol fumarate 5 mg and hydrochlorothiazide 6.25 mg) are pink, round, convex, film coated tablets, engraved with a script "LL" within an engraved heart shape on one side and "B" above "13" on the other; approximately $^9/_{32}$" in diameter, supplied as follows:
NDC 0005-3234-38—Bottle of 30 with child resistant closure
NDC 0005-3234-23—Bottle of 100

ZIAC®-10 mg/6.25 mg Tablets (bisoprolol fumarate 10 mg and hydrochlorothiazide 6.25 mg) are white, round, convex, film coated tablets, engraved with a script "LL" within an engraved heart shape on one side and "B" above "14" on the other; approximately $^9/_{32}$" in diameter, supplied as follows:
NDC 0005-3235-38—Bottle of 30 with child resistant closure

Store at Controlled Room Temperature 15°–30°C (59°–86°F) in a well-closed container.

LEDERLE LABORATORIES DIVISION
American Cyanamid Company
Pearl River, NY 10965
Under License of E. MERCK
Darmstadt, Germany

Shown in Product Identification Guide, page 321

ZOSYN® ℞

[zō ′sĭn]

(Sterile Piperacillin Sodium and Tazobactam Sodium)

DESCRIPTION

Zosyn in an injectable antibacterial combination product consisting of the semisynthetic antibiotic piperacillin sodium and the beta-lactamase inhibitor tazobactam sodium for intravenous administration.

Piperacillin sodium is derived from D(-)-α-aminobenzyl-penicillin. The chemical name of piperacillin sodium is sodium (2*S*,5*R*,6*R*)-6-[(*R*)-2-(4-ethyl-2,3-dioxo-1-piperazine-carboxamido) -2- phenylacetamido]-3,3- dimethyl -7- oxo -4- thia-1- azabicyclo(3.2.0) heptane-2- carboxylate. The chemical formula is $C_{23}H_{26}N_5NaO_7S$ and the molecular weight is 539.5.

Tazobactam sodium, a derivative of the penicillin nucleus, is a penicillanic acid sulfone. Its chemical name is sodium (2*S*,3*S*,5*R*)- 3-methyl-7-oxo-3-(1*H*-1,2,3-triazol-1-ylmethyl)-4-thia-1-azabicyclo- (3.2.0)heptane-2-carboxylate-4,4-dioxide. The chemical formula is $C_{10}H_{11}N_4NaO_5S$ and the molecular weight is 322.3.

Zosyn, piperacillin/tazobactam parenteral combination, is a white to off-white sterile, cryodesiccated powder consisting of piperacillin and tazobactam as their sodium salts packaged in glass vials. The product does not contain excipients or preservatives.

Each Zosyn 2.25 g single vial contains an amount of drug sufficient for withdrawal of piperacillin sodium equivalent to 2 grams of piperacillin and tazobactam sodium equivalent to 0.25 g of tazobactam.

Each Zosyn 3.375 g single dose vial contains an amount of drug sufficient for withdrawal of piperacillin sodium equivalent to 3 grams of piperacillin and tazobactam sodium equivalent to 0.375 g of tazobactam.

Each Zosyn 4.5 g single dose vial contains an amount of drug sufficient for withdrawal of piperacillin sodium equivalent to 4 grams of piperacillin and tazobactam sodium equivalent to 0.5 g of tazobactam.

Each Zosyn 4.5 g single dose piggyback infusion vial contains an amount of drug sufficient for withdrawal of piperacillin sodium equivalent to 4 grams of piperacillin and tazobactam sodium equivalent to 0.5 g of tazobactam.

Zosyn is a monosodium salt of piperacillin and a monosodium salt of tazobactam containing a total of 2.35 mEq (54 mg) of Na^+ per gram of piperacillin in the combination product.

CLINICAL PHARMACOLOGY

Peak plasma concentrations of piperacillin and tazobactam are attained immediately after completion of an intravenous infusion of Zosyn. Piperacillin plasma concentrations, following a 30-minute infusion of Zosyn, were similar to those attained when equivalent doses of piperacillin were administered alone, with mean peak plasma concentrations of approximately 134, 242, and 298 μg/mL for the 2.25 g, 3.375 g, and 4.5 g Zosyn (piperacillin/tazobactam) doses, respectively. The corresponding mean peak plasma concentrations of tazobactam were 15, 24, and 34 μg/mL, respectively.

Following a 30-minute I.V. infusion of 3.375 g Zosyn every 6 hours, steady-state plasma concentrations of piperacillin and tazobactam were similar to those attained after the first dose. In like manner, steady-state plasma concentrations were not different from those attained after the first dose when 2.25 g or 4.5 g doses of Zosyn were administered via 30-minute infusions every 6 hours. Steady-state plasma concentrations after 30-minute infusions every 6 hours are provided in Table 1.

Following single or multiple Zosyn doses to healthy subjects, the plasma half-life of piperacillin and of tazobactam ranged from 0.7 to 1.2 hours and was unaffected by dose or duration of infusion.

Piperacillin is metabolized to a minor microbiologically active desethyl metabolite. Tazobactam is metabolized to a single metabolite that lacks pharmacological and antibacterial activities. Both piperacillin and tazobactam are eliminated via the kidney by glomerular filtration and tubular secretion. Piperacillin is excreted rapidly as unchanged drug with 68% of the administered dose excreted in the urine. Tazobactam and its metabolite are eliminated primarily by renal excretion with 80% of the administered dose excreted as unchanged drug and the remainder as the single metabolite. Piperacillin, tazobactam, and desethyl piperacillin are also secreted into the bile.

Both piperacillin and tazobactam are approximately 30% bound to plasma proteins. The protein binding of either piperacillin or tazobactam is unaffected by the presence of the other compound. Protein binding of the tazobactam metabolites is negligible.

Piperacillin and tazobactam are widely distributed into tissues and body fluids including intestinal mucosa, gallbladder, lung, female reproductive tissues (uterus, ovary, and fallopian tube), interstitial fluid, and bile. Mean tissue concentrations are generally 50–100% of those in plasma. Distribution of piperacillin and tazobactam into cerebrospinal fluid is low in subjects with non-inflamed meninges, as with other penicillins.

After the administration of single doses of piperacillin/tazobactam to subjects with renal impairment, the half-life of piperacillin and of tazobactam increases with decreasing creatinine clearance. At creatinine clearance below 20 mL/min, the increase in half-life is twofold for piperacillin and fourfold for tazobactam compared to subjects with normal renal function. Dosage adjustments for Zosyn are recommended when creatinine clearance is below 40 mL/min in patients receiving the usual recommended daily dose of Zosyn. (See **Dosage and Administration** section for specific recommendations for the treatment of patients with renal insufficiency.)

Hemodialysis removes 30–40% of a piperacillin/tazobactam dose with an additional 5% of the tazobactam dose removed as the tazobactam metabolite. Peritoneal dialysis removes approximately 6% and 21% of the piperacillin and tazobactam doses, respectively, with up to 16% of the tazobactam dose removed as the tazobactam metabolite. For dosage recommendations for patients undergoing hemodialysis, see **Dosage and Administration** section.

The half-life of piperacillin and of tazobactam increases by approximately 25% and 18%, respectively, in patients with hepatic cirrhosis compared to healthy subjects. However, this difference does not warrant dosage adjustment of Zosyn due to hepatic cirrhosis.

[See table at bottom of next page.]

MICROBIOLOGY

Piperacillin sodium exerts bactericidal activity by inhibiting septum formation and cell wall synthesis. In vitro, piperacillin is active against a variety of gram-positive and gram-negative aerobic and anaerobic bacteria. Tazobactam sodium has very little intrinsic microbiologic activity due to its very low level binding to penicillin-binding proteins; however, it is a beta-lactamase inhibitor of the Richmond-Sykes class III (Bush class 2b & 2b′) penicillinases and cephalosporinases. It varies in its ability to inhibit class II and IV (2a & 4) penicillinases. Tazobactam does not induce chromosomally-mediated beta-lactamases at tazobactam levels achieved with the recommended dosage regimen.

Piperacillin/tazobactam has been shown to be active against most strains of the following piperacillin resistant, beta-

Continued on next page

Lederle—Cont.

lactamase producing microorganisms both *in vitro* and in clinical infections as described in the **Indications and Usage** section.

Gram-positive aerobes:
Staphylococcus aureus (NOT methicillin/oxacillin-resistant strains)
Gram-negative aerobes:
Escherichia coli
Haemophilus influenzae (NOT β-lactamase negative ampicillin-resistant strains)
Gram-negative anaerobes:
Bacteroides fragilis group (*B. fragilis, B. ovatus, B. thetaiotaomicron* or *B. vulgatus*)

The following *in vitro* data are available; but their clinical significance is unknown.
Piperacillin/tazobactam exhibits *in vitro* minimum inhibitory concentrations (MIC's) of 16.0 μg/mL or less against most (≥ 90%) strains of Enterobacteriaceae, MIC's of 1.0 μg/mL or less against most (≥ 90%) strains of *Haemophilus* species, MIC's of 8.0 μg/mL or less against most (≥ 90%) strains of *Staphylococcus* species, and MIC's of 16.0 μg/mL or less against most (≥ 90%) strains of *Bacteroides* species. Beta-lactamase negative strains should be tested against piperacillin alone; piperacillin break points should be used in evaluation of these results. However, the safey and efficacy of piperacillin/tazobactam in treating clinical infection due to these microorganisms have not been established in adequate and well-controlled clinical trials.
Gram-positive aerobes:
Enterococcus faecalis (piperacillin susceptible)
Staphylococcus epidermidis (NOT methicillin/oxacillin-resistant strains)
Streptococcus agalactiae†
Streptococcus pneumoniae†
Streptococcus pyogenes†
Viridans group streptococci†
Gram-negative aerobes:
Klebsiella oxytoca
Klebsiella pneumoniae
Moraxella catarrhalis
Morganella morganii
Neisseria gonorrhoeae
Neisseria meningitidis†
Proteus mirabilis
Proteus vulgaris
Pseudomonas aeruginosa (piperacillin susceptible)
Serratia marcescens
Gram-positive anaerobes:
Clostridium perfringens
Gram-negative anaerobes:
Bacteroides distasonis
Fusobacterium nucleatum
Prevotella melaninogenica (formerly *Bacteroides melaninogenicus*)

†These are not beta-lactamase producing strains and, therefore, are susceptible to piperacillin alone.

SUSCEPTIBILITY TESTS
Dilution Techniques
Quantitative methods are used to determine minimum inhibitory concentrations (MIC's). These MIC's provide estimates of the susceptibility of bacteria to antimicrobial compounds. The MIC's should be determined using a standardized procedure. Standardized procedures are based on a dilution method[1] (broth or agar) or equivalent with standardized inoculum concentrations and standardized concentrations of piperacillin and tazobactam powders. MIC values should be determined using serial dilutions of piperacillin combined with a fixed concentration of 4 mcg/mL tazobactam. The MIC values obtained should be interpreted according to the following criteria:

For *Enterobacteriaceae*:

MIC (mcg/mL)	Interpretation
≤16	Susceptible (S)
32–64	Intermediate (I)
≥128	Resistant (R)

For *Haemophilus* species:

MIC (mcg/mL)	Interpretation
≤1	Susceptible (S)
≥2	Resistant (R)

For *Staphylococcus* species:

MIC (MCG/ML)	Interpretation
≤8	Susceptible (S)
≥16	Resistant (R)

A report of "Susceptible" indicates that the pathogen is likely to be inhibited if the antimicrobial compound in the blood reaches the concentrations usually achievable. A report of "Intermediate" indicates that the result should be considered equivocal, and, if the microorganism is not fully susceptible to alternative, clinically feasible drugs, the test should be repeated. This category implies possible clinical applicability in body sites where the drug is physiologically concentrated or in situations where high dosage of drug can be used. This category also provides a buffer zone which prevents small uncontrolled technical factors from causing major discrepancies in interpretation. A report of "Resistant" indicates that the pathogen is not likely to be inhibited if the antimicrobial compound in the blood reaches the concentrations usually achievable; other therapy should be selected. Standardized susceptibility test procedures require the use of laboratory control microorganisms to control the technical aspects of the laboratory procedures. Laboratory control microorganisms are specific strains of microbiological assay organisms with intrinsic biological properties relating to resistance mechanisms and their genetic expression within bacteria; the specific strains are not clinically significant in their current microbiological status. Standard piperacillin and tazobactam powders should provide the following MIC values when tested against the designated quality control strains:

Microorganism	MIC (μg/mL)
Escherichia coli ATCC 25922	1–4
Escherichia coli ATCC 35218	0.5–2
Haemophilus influenzae ATCC 49247	0.06–0.5
Staphylococcus aureus ATCC 29213	0.25–2

Anaerobic Techniques
For anaerobic bacteria, the susceptibility to piperacillin/tazobactam can be determined by the reference agar dilution method or by alternate standardized test methods.[2]
For *Bacteroides* species, the dilution values should be interpreted as follows:

MIC (μg/mL)	Interpretation
≤16	Susceptible (S)
≥32	Resistant (R)

Serial dilutions of piperacillin combined with a fixed concentration of 4 μg/mL tazobactam should provide the following MIC values:

Microorganism	MIC (μg/mL)
Bacteroides fragilis ATCC 25285	0.12–0.5
Bacteroides thetaiotaomicron ATCC 29741	4–16

Diffusion Techniques
Quantitative methods that require measurement of zone diameters also provide reproducible estimates of the susceptibility of bacteria to antimicrobial compounds. One such standardized procedure[3] requires the use of standardized inoculum concentrations. This procedure uses paper disks impregnated with 100 μg of piperacillin and 10 μg of tazobactam to test the susceptibility of microorganisms to piperacillin/tazobactam. Interpretation is identical to that stated above for results using dilution techniques. Reports from the laboratory providing results of the standard single-disk susceptibility test with a 100 μg/10 μg piperacillin/tazobactam disk should be interpreted according to the following criteria:

For *Enterobacteriaceae*:

Zone Diameter (mm)	Interpretation
≥21	Susceptible (S)
18–20	Intermediate (I)
≤17	Resistant (R)

For *Staphylococcus* species:

Zone Diameter (mm)	Interpretation
≥20	Susceptible (S)
≤19	Resistant (R)

As with standardized dilution techniques, diffusion methods require the use of laboratory control microorganisms to control the technical aspects of the laboratory procedures. Laboratory control microorganisms are specific strains of microbiological assay organisms with intrinsic biological properties relating to resistance mechanisms and their genetic expression within bacteria; the specific strains are not clinically significant in their current microbiological status. For the diffusion technique, the 100/10-μg piperacillin/tazobactam disk should provide the following zone diameters in these laboratory test quality control strains:

Microorganism	Zone Diameter (mm)
Escherichia coli ATCC 25922	24–30
Escherichia coli ATCC 35218	24–30
Staphylococcus aureus ATCC 25923	27–36
+	

INDICATIONS AND USAGE
Zosyn is indicated for the treatment of patients with moderate to severe infections caused by piperacillin resistant, piperacillin/tazobactam susceptible, β-lactamase producing strains of the designated microorganisms in the specified conditions listed below:
Appendicitis (complicated by rupture or abscess) and peritonitis caused by piperacillin resistant, β-lactamase producing strains of *Escherichia coli* or the following members of the *Bacteroides fragilis* group; B. fragilis, B. ovatus, B. thetaiotamicron, or B. vulgatus. The individual members of this group were studied in less than 10 cases.
Uncomplicated and complicated skin and skin structure infections, including cellulitis, cutaneous abscesses, and ischemic/diabetic foot infections caused by piperacillin resistant, β-lactamase producing strains of *Staphylococcus aureus*.
Postpartum endometritis or pelvic inflammatory disease caused by piperacillin resistant, β-lactamase producing strains of *Escherichia coli*.
Community-acquired pneumonia (moderate severity only) caused by piperacillin resistant, β-lactamase producing strains of *Haemophilius influenzae*.
Nosocomial pneumonia (moderate to severe) caused by piperacillin-resistant, β-lactamase producing strains of *Staphylococcus aureus*.
Initial presumptive treatment of patients with nosocomial pneumonia should start with Zosyn at a dosage of 3.375 g every 4 hours plus an aminoglycoside. Treatment with the aminoglycoside should be continued in patients from whom *Pseudomonas aeruginosa* is isolated. If *Pseudomonas aeruginosa* is not isolated, the aminoglycoside may be discontinued at the discretion of the treating physician. (See **Dosage and Administration**.)

TABLE 1
STEADY STATE MEAN PLASMA CONCENTRATIONS IN ADULTS AFTER 30-MINUTE INTRAVENOUS INFUSION OF PIPERACILLIN/TAZOBACTAM EVERY 6 HOURS

PIPERACILLIN

Piperacillin/[c] Tazobactam Dose	No. of Evaluable Subjects	Plasma Concentrations** (mcg/mL)						AUC** (mcg·hr/mL)
		30 min	1 hr	2 hr	3 hr	4 hr	6 hr	AUC$_{0-6}$
2.25 g	8	134 (14)	57 (14)	17.1 (23)	5.2 (32)	2.5 (35)	0.9 (14)[a]	131 (14)
3.375 g	6	242 (12)	106 (8)	34.6 (20)	11.5 (19)	5.1 (22)	1.0 (10)	242 (10)
4.5 g	8	298 (14)	141 (19)	46.6 (28)	16.4 (29)	6.9 (29)	1.4 (30)	322 (16)

a: N = 4

TAZOBACTAM

Piperacillin/[c] Tazobactam Dose	No. of Evaluable Subjects	Plasma Concentrations** (mcg/mL)						AUC** (mcg·hr/mL)
		30 min	1 hr	2 hr	3 hr	4 hr	6 hr	AUC0-6
2.25 g	8	14.8 (14)	7.2 (22)	2.6 (30)	1.1 (35)	0.7 (6)[b]	<0.5	16.0 (21)
3.375 g	6	24.2 (14)	10.7 (7)	4.0 (18)	1.4 (21)	0.7 (16)[a]	<0.5	25.0 (8)
4.5 g	8	33.8 (15)	17.3 (16)	6.8 (24)	2.8 (25)	1.3 (30)	<0.5	39.8 (15)

** Numbers in parentheses are coefficients of variation (CV%).
a: N = 4
b: N = 3
c: Piperacillin and tazobactam were given in combination.

A study for the treatment of nosocomial lower respiratory tract infection was initiated with Zosyn as monotherapy at 3.375 g every 6 hours. This study was terminated because of an unacceptable level of efficacy at this dosage. However, another multicenter study conducted in North America, used Zosyn at a dosing regimen of 3.375 g every 4 hours in combination with an aminoglycoside in the treatment of patients with nosocomial lower respiratory tract infections. In this study, Zosyn (in combination with varying durations of aminoglycoside therapy) demonstrated acceptable rates of overall clinical and microbiologic success in the treatment of nosocomial pneumonia. There was an insufficient number of nosocomial bronchitis cases to prove efficacy in this condition.

Clinical trial data for the treatment of complicated urinary tract infections demonstrated inadequate efficacy at the dosage regimen of Zosyn studied (i.e., 3.375 g every 8 hours). There are no other adequate and well controlled trial data to support the use of this product in the treatment of complicated urinary tract infections.

As a combination product, Zosyn is indicated only for the specified conditions listed above. Infections caused by piperacillin susceptible organisms, for which piperacillin has been shown to be effective, are also amenable to Zosyn treatment due to its piperacillin content. The tazobactam component of this combination product does not decrease the activity of the piperacillin component against piperacillin-susceptible organisms.

Therefore, the treatment of mixed infections caused by piperacillin-susceptible organisms and piperacillin-resistant, β-lactamase producing organisms susceptible to Zosyn should not require the addition of another antibiotic. An exception is in the treatment of *Pseudomonas aeruginosa* in nosocomial pneumonia which should be in combination with an aminoglycoside.

Zosyn is useful as presumptive therapy in the indicated conditions prior to the identification of causative organisms because of its broad spectrum of bactericidal activity against gram-positive and gram-negative aerobic and anaerobic organisms.

Appropriate cultures should usually be performed before initiating antimicrobial treatment in order to isolate and identify the organisms causing infection and to determine their susceptibility to Zosyn. Antimicrobial therapy should be adjusted, if appropriate, once the results of culture(s) and antimicrobial testing are known.

CONTRAINDICATIONS

Zosyn is contraindicated in patients with a history of allergic reactions to any of the penicillins, cephalosporins, or β-lactamase inhibitors.

WARNINGS

SERIOUS AND OCCASIONALLY FATAL HYPERSENSITIVITY (ANAPHYLACTIC) REACTIONS HAVE BEEN REPORTED IN PATIENTS ON PENICILLIN THERAPY. THESE REACTIONS ARE MORE LIKELY TO OCCUR IN INDIVIDUALS WITH A HISTORY OF PENICILLIN HYPERSENSITIVITY OR A HISTORY OF SENSITIVITY TO MULTIPLE ALLERGENS. THERE HAVE BEEN REPORTS OF INDIVIDUALS WITH A HISTORY OF PENICILLIN HYPERSENSITIVITY WHO HAVE EXPERIENCED SEVERE REACTIONS WHEN TREATED WITH CEPHALOSPORINS. BEFORE INITIATING THERAPY WITH ZOSYN, CAREFUL INQUIRY SHOULD BE MADE CONCERNING PREVIOUS HYPERSENSITIVITY REACTIONS TO PENICILLINS, CEPHALOSPORINS, OR OTHER ALLERGENS. IF AN ALLERGIC REACTION OCCURS, ZOSYN SHOULD BE DISCONTINUED AND APPROPRIATE THERAPY INSTITUTED. SERIOUS ANAPHYLACTIC REACTIONS REQUIRE IMMEDIATE EMERGENCY TREATMENT WITH EPINEPHRINE, OXYGEN, INTRAVENOUS STEROIDS, AND AIRWAY MANAGEMENT, INCLUDING INTUBATION, SHOULD ALSO BE ADMINISTERED AS INDICATED.

Pseudomembranous colitis has been reported with nearly all antibacterial agents, including piperacillin/tazobactam, and may range in severity from mild to life-threatening. Therefore, it is important to consider this diagnosis in patients who present with diarrhea subsequent to the administration of antibacterial agents.

Treatment with antibacterial agents alters the normal flora of the colon and may permit overgrowth of clostridia. Studies indicate that a toxin produced by *Clostridium difficile* is one primary cause of "antibiotic-associated colitis."

After the diagnosis of pseudomembranous colitis has been established, therapeutic measures should be initiated. Mild cases of pseudomembranous colitis usually respond to drug discontinuation alone. In moderate to severe cases, consideration should be given to management with fluids and electrolytes, protein supplementation, and treatment with an antibacterial drug clinically effective against *Clostridium difficile* colitis.

PRECAUTIONS
GENERAL

Bleeding manifestations have occurred in some patients receiving β-lactam antibiotics, including piperacillin. These reactions have sometimes been associated with abnormalities of coagulation tests such as clotting time, platelet aggregation, and prothrombin time and are more likely to occur in patients with renal failure. If bleeding manifestations occur, Zosyn should be discontinued and appropriate therapy instituted.

The possibility of the emergence of resistant organisms that might cause superinfections should be kept in mind. If this occurs, appropriate measures should be taken. As with other penicillins, patients may experience neuromuscular excitability or convulsions if higher than recommended doses are given intravenously (particularly in the presence of renal failure).

Zosyn is a monosodium salt of piperacillin and a monosodium salt of tazobactam and contains a total of 2.35 mEq (54 mg) of NA+ per gram of piperacillin in the combination product. This should be considered when treating patients requiring restricted salt intake. Periodic electrolyte determinations should be performed in patients with low potassium reserves, and the possibility of hypokalemia should be kept in mind with patients who have potentially low potassium reserves and who are receiving cytotoxic therapy or diuretics.

As with other semisynthetic penicillins, piperacillin therapy has been associated with an increased incidence of fever and rash in cystic fibrosis patients.

LABORATORY TESTS

Periodic assessment of hematopoietic function should be performed, especially with prolonged therapy, i.e., ≥ 21 days. (See **Adverse Reactions**—ADVERSE LABORATORY EVENTS)

DRUG INTERACTIONS
Aminoglycosides

The mixing of Zosyn with an aminoglycoside in vitro can result in substantial inactivation of the aminoglycoside. (See COMPATIBLE INTRAVENOUS DILUENT SOLUTIONS, **Dosage and Administration**.)

When Zosyn is co-administered with tobramycin, the area under the curve, renal clearance, and urinary recovery of tobramycin were decreased by 11%, 32%, and 38%, respectively. The alterations in the pharmacokinetics of tobramycin when administered in combination with piperacillin/tazobactam may be due to in vivo and in vitro inactivation of tobramycin in the presence of piperacillin/tazobactam. The inactivation of aminoglycosides in the presence of penicillin class drugs has been recognized. It has been postulated that penicillin-aminoglycoside complexes form; these complexes are microbiologically inactive and of unknown toxicity. In patients with severe renal dysfunction (i.e., chronic hemodialysis patients), the pharmacokinetics of tobramycin are significantly altered when tobramycin is administered in combination with piperacillin.[4] The alteration of tobramycin pharmacokinetics and the potential toxicity of the penicillin-aminoglycoside complexes in patients with mild to moderate renal dysfunction who are administered an aminoglycoside in combination with piperacillin/tazobactam is unknown.

Probenecid

Probenecid administered concomitantly with Zosyn prolongs the half-life of piperacillin by 21% and of tazobactam by 71%.

Vancomycin

No pharmacokinetic interactions have been noted between Zosyn and vancomycin.

Heparin

Coagulation parameters should be tested more frequently and monitored regularly during simultaneous administration of high doses of heparin, oral anticoagulants, or other drugs that may affect the blood coagulation system or the thrombocyte function.

Vecuronium

Piperacillin when used concomitantly with vecuronium has been implicated in the prolongation of the neuromuscular blockade of vecuronium. Zosyn (piperacillin/tazobactam) could produce the same phenomenon if given along with vecuronium. Due to their similar mechanism of action, it is expected that the neuromuscular blockade produced by any of the non-depolarizing muscle relaxants could be prolonged in the presence of piperacillin. (See package insert for vecuronium bromide.)

DRUG/LABORATORY TEST INTERACTIONS

As with other penicillins, the administration of Zosyn may result in a false-positive reaction for glucose in the urine using a copper-reduction method (CLINITEST®§). It is recommended that glucose tests based on enzymatic glucose oxidase reactions (such as DIASTIX®§ or TES-TAPE®§) be used.

CARCINOGENESIS, MUTAGENESIS, IMPAIRMENT OF FERTILITY

Long term carcinogenicity studies in animals have not been conducted with piperacillin/tazobactam, piperacillin, or tazobactam. *Piperacillin/tazobactam* was negative in microbial mutagenicity assays at concentrations up to 14.84/1.86 μg/plate.

Piperacillin/tazobactam was negative in the unscheduled DNA synthesis (UDS) test at concentrations up to 5689/711 μg/mL. Piperacillin/tazobactam was negative in a mammalian point mutation (Chinese hamster ovary cell HPRT) assay at concentrations up to 8000/1000 μg/mL. Piperacillin/tazobactam was negative in a mammalian cell (BALB/c-3T3) transformation assay at concentrations up to 8/1 μg/mL. In vivo, piperacillin/tazobactam did not induce chromosomal aberrations in rats dosed I.V. with 1500/187.5 mg/kg; this dose is similar to the maximum recommended human daily dose on a body-surface-area basis (mg/m²).

Piperacillin was negative in microbial mutagenicity assays at concentrations up to 50 μg/plate. There was no DNA damage in bacteria (Rec assay) exposed to piperacillin at concentrations up to 200 μg/disk. Piperacillin was negative in the UDS test at concentrations up to 10,000 μg/mL. In a mammalian point mutation (mouse lymphoma cells) assay, piperacillin was positive at concentrations ≥ 2500 μg/mL. Piperacillin was negative in a cell (BALB/c-3T3) transformation assay at concentrations up to 3000 μg/mL. In vivo, piperacillin did not induce chromosomal aberrations in mice at I.V. doses up to 2000 mg/kg/day or rats at I.V. doses up to 1500 mg/kg/day. These doses are half (mice) or similar (rats) to the maximum recommended human daily dose based on body-surface area (mg/m²). In another in vivo test, there was no dominant lethal effect when piperacillin was administered to rats at I.V. doses up to 2000 mg/kg/day, which is similar to the maximum recommended human daily dose based on body-surface area (mg/m²). When mice were administered piperacillin at I.V. doses up to 2000 mg/kg/day, which is half the maximum recommended human daily dose based on body-surface area (mg/m²), urine from these animals was not mutagenic when tested in a microbial mutagenicity assay. Bacteria injected into the peritoneal cavity of mice administered piperacillin at I.V. doses up to 2000 mg/kg/day did not show increased mutation frequencies.

Tazobactam was negative in microbial mutagenicity assays at concentrations up to 333 μg/plate. Tazobactam was negative in the UDS test at concentrations up to 2000 μg/mL. Tazobactam was negative in a mammalian point mutation (Chinese hamster ovary cell HPRT) assay at concentrations up to 5000 μg/mL. In another mammalian point mutation (mouse lymphoma cells) assay, tazobactam was positive at concentrations ≥ 3000 μg/mL. Tazobactam was negative in a cell (BALB/c-3T3) transformation assay at concentrations up to 900 μg/mL. In an in vitro cytogenetics (Chinese hamster lung cells) assay, tazobactam was negative at concentrations up to 3000 μg/mL. In vivo, tazobactam did not induce chromosomal aberrations in rats at I.V. doses up to 5000 mg/kg, which is 23 times the maximum recommended human daily dose based on body-surface area (mg/m²).

PREGNANCY
Teratogenic Effects—Pregnancy Category B
Piperacillin/Tazobactam

Reproduction studies have been performed in rats and have revealed no evidence of impaired fertility due to piperacillin/tazobactam administered up to a dose which is similar to the maximum recommended human daily dose based on body-surface area (mg/m²).

Teratology studies have been performed in mice and rats and have revealed no evidence of harm to the fetus due to piperacillin/tazobactam administered up to a dose which is 1 to 2 times and 2 to 3 times the human dose of piperacillin and tazobactam, respectively, based on body-surface area (mg/m²).

Piperacillin

Reproduction and teratology studies have been performed in mice and rats and have revealed no evidence of impaired fertility or harm to the fetus due to piperacillin administered up to a dose which is half (mice) or similar (rats) to the maximum recommended human daily dose based on body-surface area (mg/m²).

Tazobactam

Reproduction studies have been performed in rats and have revealed no evidence of impaired fertility due to tazobactam administered at doses up to 3 times the maximum recommended human daily dose based on body-surface area (mg/m²).

Teratology studies have been performed in mice and rats and have revealed no evidence of harm to the fetus due to tazobactam administered at doses up to 6 and 14 times, respectively, the human dose based on body-surface area (mg/m²). In rats, tazobactam crosses the placenta. Concentrations in the fetus are less than or equal to 10% of those found in maternal plasma.

There are, however, no adequate and well-controlled studies with the piperacillin/tazobactam combination or with piperacillin or tazobactam alone in pregnant women. Because animal reproduction studies are not always predictive of the human response, this drug should be used during pregnancy only if clearly needed.

Continued on next page

Lederle—Cont.

NURSING MOTHERS
Piperacillin is excreted in low concentrations in human milk; tazobactam concentrations in human milk have not been studied. Caution should be exercised when Zosyn is administered to a nursing woman.
PEDIATRIC USE
Safety and efficacy in children below the age of 12 years have not been established.
GERIATRIC USE
Patients over 65 years are not at an increased risk of developing adverse effects solely because of age. However, dosage should be adjusted in the presence of renal insufficiency. (See **Dosage and Administration**.)

ADVERSE REACTIONS

During the initial clinical investigations, 2621 patients worldwide were treated with Zosyn in phase 3 trials. In the key North American clinical trials (n = 830 patients), 90% of the adverse events reported were mild to moderate in severity and transient in nature. However, in 3.2% of the patients treated worldwide, Zosyn was discontinued because of adverse events primarily involving the skin (1.3%), including rash and pruritis; the gastrointestinal system (0.9%), including diarrhea, nausea, and vomiting; and allergic reactions (0.5%).
Adverse local reactions that were reported, irrespective of relationship to therapy with Zosyn, were phlebitis (1.3%), injection site reaction (0.5%), pain (0.2%), inflammation (0.2%), thrombophlebitis (0.2%), and edema (0.1%).
In the completed study of nosocomial lower respiratory tract infections, 155 patients were treated with Zosyn in a dosing regimen of 3.375g every 4 hours in combination with an aminoglycoside. In this trial, 88.5% of the adverse experiences reported were mild to moderate in severity and transient in nature. However, in this trial, therapy with Zosyn was discontinued in four patients (2.6%) due to adverse experiences.
Irrespective of drug relationship or degree of severity, the adverse experiences which led to the discontinuation of Zosyn in these four patients were: thrombocytopenia and pancreatitis in one patient, fever in one patient; fever and eosinophilia in another patient; and diarrhea and elevated liver enzymes in the fourth patient.
ADVERSE CLINICAL EVENTS
Based on patients from the North American trials (n = 1063), the events with the highest incidence in patients, irrespective of relationship to Zosyn therapy, were diarrhea (11.3%); headache (7.7%); constipation (7.7%); nausea (6.9%); insomnia (6.6%); rash (4.2%), including maculopapular, bullous, urticarial, and eczematoid; vomiting (3.3%); dyspepsia (3.3%); pruritis (3.1%); stool changes (2.4%); fever (2.4%); agitation (2.1%); pain (1.7%); moniliasis (1.6%); hypertension (1.6%); dizziness (1.4%); abdominal pain (1.3%); chest pain (1.3%); edema (1.2%); anxiety (1.2%); rhinitis (1.2%); and dyspnea (1.1%).
Based on patients in the completed study of nosocomial lower respiratory tract infections (n = 155), using every 4 hour dosing and aminoglycoside therapy, the events with the highest incidence in patients, irrespective of relationship to Zosyn and aminoglycoside therapy were: diarrhea (20%); constipation (8.4%); agitation (7.1%); nausea (5.8%); headache (4.5%); insomnia (4.5%); oral thrush (3.9%); erythematous rash (3.9%); anxiety (3.2%); fever (3.2%); pain (3.2%); pruritis (3.2%); hiccough (2.6%); vomiting (2.6%); dyspepsia (1.9%); edema (1.9%); fluid overload (1.9%); stool changes (1.9%); anorexia (1.3%); cardiac arrest (1.3%); confusion (1.3%); diaphoresis (1.3%); duodenal ulcer (1.3%); flatulence (1.3%); hypertension (1.3%); hypotension (1.3%); inflammation at injection site (1.3%); pleural effusion (1.3%); pneumothorax (1.3%); rash, not otherwise specified (1.3%); supraventricular tachycardia (1.3%); thrombophlebitis (1.3%); and urinary incontinence (1.3%).
Additional adverse systemic clinical events reported in 1.0% or less of the patients in the initial North American trials and/or in the patients administered Zosyn 3.375g every 4 hours plus an aminoglycoside in the study of nosocomial lower respiratory tract are listed below within each body system (bracketed events occurred only in the nosocomial pneumonia trial);
Autonomic nervous system—hypotension, ileus, syncope
Body as a whole—rigors, back pain, malaise, [asthenia, chest pain]
Cardiovascular—tachycardia, including supraventricular and ventricular; bradycardia; arrhythmia, including atrial fibrillation, ventricular fibrillation, cardiac arrest, cardiac failure, circulatory failure, myocardial infarction, [angina]
Central nervous system—tremor, convulsions, vertigo, [aggressive reaction (combative)]
Gastrointestinal—melena, flatulence, hemorrhage, gastritis, hiccough, ulcerative stomatitis, [fecal incontinence, gastric ulcer, pancreatitis]
Pseudomembranous colitis was reported in one patient during the clinical trials. The onset of pseudomembranous colitis symptoms may occur during or after antibacterial treatment. (See **Warnings.**)
Hearing and Vestibular System—tinnitus, [deafness, earache]
Hypersensitivity—anaphylaxis
Metabolic and Nutritional—symptomatic hypoglycemia, thirst, [gout, vitamin B_{12} deficiency anemia]
Musculoskeletal—myalgia, arthralgia
Platelet, Bleeding, Clotting—mesenteric embolism, purpura, epistaxis, pulmonary embolism, [ecchymosis, hemoptysis] (See **Precautions**—GENERAL.)
Psychiatric—confusion, hallucination, depression
Reproductive, Female—leukorrhea, vaginitis, [perineal irritation/pain]
Reproductive, Male—[balanoposthitis]
Respiratory—pharyngitis, pulmonary edema, bronchospasm, coughing, [atelectasis, dyspnea, hypoxia]
Skin and Appendages—genital pruritus, diaphoresis, [conjunctivitis, xerosis]
Special senses—taste perversion
Urinary—retention, dysuria, oliguria, hematuria, incontinence, [urinary tract infection with trichomonas, yeast in urine]
Vision—photophobia
Vascular (extracardiac)—flushing, [cerebrovascular accident]
ADVERSE LABORATORY EVENTS
Of the studies reported, including that of nosocomial lower respiratory tract infections in which a higher dose of Zosyn was used in combination with an aminoglycoside, changes in laboratory parameters, without regard to drug relationship include:
Hematologic—Decreases in hemoglobin and hematocrit, thrombocytopenia, increases in platelet count, eosinophilia, leukopenia, neutropenia. The leukopenia/neutropenia associated with Zosyn administration appears to be reversible and most frequently associated with prolonged administration, i.e., ≥21 days of therapy. These patients were withdrawn from therapy; some had accompanying systemic symptoms (e.g., fever, rigors, chills).
Coagulation—Positive direct Coombs' test, prolonged prothrombin time, prolonged partial thromboplastin time
Hepatic—Transient elevations of AST (SGOT), ALT (SGPT), alkaline phosphatase, bilirubin
Renal—Increases in serum creatinine, blood urea nitrogen
Urinalysis—Proteinuria, hematuria, pyuria
Additional laboratory events include abnormalities in electrolytes (i.e., increases and decreases in sodium, potassium, and calcium), hyperglycemia, decreases in total protein or albumin.
The following adverse reactions have also been reported for PIPRACIL® (sterile piperacillin sodium):
Skin and Appendages—Erythema multiforme and Stevens-Johnson syndrome, rarely reported
Gastrointestinal—Cholestatic hepatitis
Renal—Rarely, interstitial nephritis
Skeletal—Prolonged muscle relaxation (See **Precautions**—DRUG INTERACTIONS.)

OVERDOSAGE

Information on overdosage of Zosyn in humans is not available.
Excessive serum levels of either piperacillin or tazobactam may be reduced by hemodialysis. (See **Clinical Pharmacology.**) No specific antidote is known. As with other penicillins, neuromuscular excitability or convulsions have occurred following large intravenous doses, primarily in patients with impaired renal function.
In the case of motor excitability or convulsions, general supportive measures, including administration of anticonvulsive agents (e.g., diazepam or barbiturates) may be considered.

DOSAGE AND ADMINISTRATION

Zosyn should be administered by intravenous infusion over 30 minutes
NORMAL RENAL FUNCTION (CREATININE CLEARANCE ≥90 ML/MIN)
The usual total dose of Zosyn for adults is 12g/1.5 g, given 3.375 g every six hours.
Treatment of patients with nosocomial pneumonia should start with Zosyn at a dosage of 3.375 g every four hours plus an aminoglycoside. This gives a total dose of piperacillin/tazobactam of 18g/2.25g in twenty-four hours. Treatment with the aminoglycoside should be continued in patients from whom *Pseudomonas aeruginosa* is isolated. If *Pseudomonas aeruginosa* is not isolated, the aminoglycoside may be discontinued at the discretion of the treating physician as guided by the severity of the infection and the patient's clinical and bacteriological progress.
RENAL INSUFFICIENCY
In patients with renal insufficiency (Creatinine Clearance <90 mL/min), the intravenous dose of Zosyn should be adjusted to the degree of actual renal function impairment. In patients with nosocomial pneumonia receiving concomitant aminoglycoside therapy, the aminoglycoside dosage should be adjusted according to the recommendations of the manufacturer. The recommended daily doses of Zosyn® for patients with renal insufficiency are as follows:

Zosyn Dosage Recommendations For All Indications Including Nosocomial Pneumonia

Creatinine Clearance (mL/min)	Recommended Dosage Regimen
>40–90	12 g/1.5 g/day in divided doses of 3.375 g q6h
20–40	8 g/1.0 g/day in divided doses of 2.25 g q6h
<20	6 g/0.75 g/day in divided doses of 2.25 g q8h

For patients on hemodialysis, irrespective of the condition under treatment, the maximum dose is 2.25 g Zosyn q eight hours. In addition, because hemodialysis removes 30%–40% of a Zosyn dose in four hours, one additional dose of 0.75 g Zosyn should be administered following each dialysis period.
For patients with renal failure, measurement of serum levels of piperacillin and tazobactam will provide additional guidance for adjusting dosage.
DURATION OF THERAPY
The usual duration of Zosyn treatment is from seven to ten days. However, the recommended duration of Zosyn treatment of nosocomial pneumonia is seven to fourteen days. In all conditions, the duration of therapy should be guided by the severity of the infection and the patient's clinical and bacteriological progress.
INTRAVENOUS ADMINISTRATION
For conventional vials, reconstitute Zosyn per gram of piperacillin with 5 mL of a compatible reconstitution diluent from the list provided below. Shake well until dissolved. Single dose vials should be used immediately after reconstitution. Discard any unused portion after 24 hours if stored at room temperature, or after 48 hours if stored at refrigerated temperature (2° to 8°C [36° to 46°]).
COMPATIBLE RECONSTITUTION DILUENTS
0.9% Sodium Chloride for Injection
Sterile Water for Injection
Dextrose 5%
Bacteriostatic Saline/Parabens
Bacteriostatic Water/Parabens
Bacteriostatic Saline/Benzyl Alcohol
Bacteriostatic Water/Benzyl Alcohol
Reconstituted Zosyn solution should be further diluted (recommended volume per dose of 50 mL to 150 mL) in a compatible intravenous diluent solution listed below.
Administer by infusion over a period of at least 30 minutes. During the infusion it is desirable to discontinue the primary infusion solution.
COMPATIBLE INTRAVENOUS DILUENT SOLUTIONS
0.9% Sodium Chloride for Injection
Sterile Water for Injection‡
Dextrose 5%
Dextran 6% in Saline
‡ Maximum recommended volume per dose of Sterile Water for Injection is 50 mL.
For IV infusion: Reconstitute the 4.5-gram piggyback infusion vial with 50 mL of a compatible intravenous diluent solution from the list provided above.
LACTATED RINGERS SOLUTION IS NOT COMPATIBLE WITH ZOSYN.
When concomitant therapy with aminoglycosides is indicated, Zosyn and the aminoglycoside should be reconstituted and administered separately, due to the *in vitro* inactivation of the aminoglycoside by the penicillin. (See Precautions–DRUG INTERACTIONS.)
Zosyn can be used in ambulatory intravenous infusion pumps.
STABILITY OF ZOSYN FOLLOWING RECONSTITUTION
Zosyn in stable in glass and plastic containers (plastic syringes, I.V. bags, and tubing) when used with compatible diluents.
Stability studies in the I.V. bags have demonstrated chemical stability [potency, pH of reconstituted solution, and clarity of solution] for up to 24 hours at room temperature and up to one week at refrigerated temperature. Zosyn contains no preservatives.
Appropriate consideration of aseptic technique should be used.
Stability of Zosyn in an ambulatory intravenous infusion pump has been demonstrated for a period of 12 hours at room temperature. Each dose was reconstituted and diluted to a volume of 37.5 mL or 25 mL. One-day supplies of dosing solution were aseptically transferred into the medication reservoir (I.V. bags or cartridge). The reservoir was fitted to a preprogrammed ambulatory intravenous infusion pump per the manufacturer's instructions. Stability of Zosyn is not affected when administered using an ambulatory intravenous infusion pump.

Parenteral drug products should be inspected visually for particulate matter and discoloration prior to administration, whenever solution and container permit.

HOW SUPPLIED

Zosyn® (sterile piperacillin sodium and tazobactam sodium) is supplied in the following sizes:

Each Zosyn 2.25 g vial provides piperacillin sodium equivalent to 2 grams of piperacillin and tazobactam sodium equivalent to 0.25 gram of tazobactam. Each vial contains 4.69 mEq (108 mg) of sodium.
Supplied 10 per box–NDC 0206-8452-16

Each Zosyn 3.375 g vial provides piperacillin sodium equivalent to 3 grams of piperacillin and tazobactam sodium equivalent to 0.375 gram of tazobactam. Each vial contains 7.04 mEq (162 mg) of sodium.
Supplied 10 per box–NDC 0206-8454-55

Each Zosyn 4.5 g vial provides piperacillin sodium equivalent to 4 grams of piperacillin and tazobactam sodium equivalent to 0.5 gram of tazobactam. Each vial contains 9.39 mEq (216 mg) of sodium.
Supplied 10 per box–NDC 0206-8455-25

Each Zosyn 4.5 g piggyback infusion vial provides piperacillin sodium equivalent to 4 grams of piperacillin and tazobactam sodium equivalent to 0.5 gram of tazobactam.
Each vial contains 9.39 mEq (216 mg) of sodium.
Supplied 10 per box–NDC 0206-8455-29

Zosyn vials should be stored at controlled room temperature 15° to 30°C (59° to 86°F) prior to reconstitution.

REFERENCES

1. National Committee for Clinical Laboratory Standards, Methods for Dilution Antimicrobial Susceptibility Tests for Bacteria that Grow Aerobically–Third Edition. Approved Standard NCCLS Document M7-A3, Vol. 13, No. 25, NCCLS, Villanova, PA, December, 1993.
2. National Committee for Clinical Laboratory Standards, Methods for Antimicrobial Susceptibility Testing for Anaerobic Bacteria–Third Edition. Approved Standard NCCLS Document M11-A3, Vol. 13, No. 26, NCCLS, Villanova, PA, December, 1993.
3. National Committee for Clinical Laboratory Standards. Performance Standard for Antimicrobial Disk Susceptibility Tests–Fifth Edition. Approved Standard NCCLS Document M2-A5, Vol. 13, No. 24, NCCLS, Villanova, PA, December, 1993.
4. Halstenson CE, Hirata CAI, Heim-Duthoy KL, Abraham PA, and Matzke GR. Effect of concomitant administraton of piperacillin on the dispositions of netilmicin and tobramycin in patients with end-stage renal disease. Antimicrob Agents Chemother 34(1):128-133, 1990.
§ CLINITEST® and DIASTIX® are registered trademarks of Ames Division, Miles Laboratories, Inc.
§ TES-TAPE® is a registered trademark of Eli Lilly and Company.

Shown in Product Identification Guide, page 321

ZOSYN® ℞
(Sterile Piperacillin Sodium and Tazobactam Sodium)

```
Pharmacy Bulk Package
Not for Direct Infusion
```

RECONSTITUTED STOCK SOLUTION MUST BE TRANSFERRED AND FURTHER DILUTED FOR I.V. INFUSION

PACKAGE DESCRIPTION

The PHARMACY BULK VIAL is a container of sterile preparation which contains many single doses for parenteral use. The contents are intended for use in a pharmacy admixture program and are restricted to the preparation of admixtures for intravenous infusion.

PRODUCT DESCRIPTION

ZOSYN is an injectable antibacterial combination product consisting of the semisynthetic antibiotic piperacillin sodium and the beta-lactamase inhibitor tazobactam sodium for intravenous administration.
Piperacillin sodium is derived from D(-)-α-aminobenzylpenicillin. The chemical name of piperacillin sodium is sodium (2S, 5R, 6R)-6-[(R)-2-(4-ethyl-2,3-dioxo -1- piperazinecarboxamido) -2- phenylacetamido] -3,3- dimethyl -7- oxo -4- thia-1-azabicyclo[3.2.0]heptane-2-carboxylate. The chemical formula is $C_{23}H_{26}N_5NaO_7S$ and the molecular weight is 539.5.
Tazobactam sodium, a derivative of the penicillin nucleus, is a penicillanic acid sulfone. Its chemical name is sodium (2S, 3S, 5R)-3-methyl-7-oxo-3-(1H-1, 2, 3-triazol-1-ylmethyl)-4-thia-1-azabicyclo[3.2.0]heptane-2-carboxylate-4, 4-dioxide. The chemical formula is $C_{10}H_{11}N_4NaO_5S$ and the molecular weight is 322.3.
ZOSYN, piperacillin/tazobactam parenteral combination, is a white to off-white sterile, cryodesiccated powder consisting of piperacillin and tazobactam as their sodium salts packaged in glass vials. The product does not contain excipients or preservatives.
Each ZOSYN 40.5 g pharmacy bulk vial contains piperacillin sodium equivalent to 36 grams of piperacillin and tazobactam sodium equivalent to 4.5 g of tazobactam sufficient for delivery of multiple doses.
ZOSYN is a monosodium salt of piperacillin and a monosodium salt of tazobactam containing a total of 2.35 mEq (54 mg) of Na$^+$ per gram of piperacillin in the combination product.

HOW SUPPLIED

ZOSYN® (sterile piperacillin sodium and tazobactam sodium) is supplied as a powder in the pharmacy bulk vial as follows:
Each ZOSYN 40.5 g pharmacy bulk vial contains piperacillin sodium equivalent to 36 grams of piperacillin and tazobactam sodium equivalent to 4.5 grams tazobactam. Each pharmacy bulk vial contains 84.5 mEq (1,944 mg) of sodium.
NDC 0206-8620-11
ZOSYN pharmacy bulk vials should be stored at controlled room temperature 15 to 30°C (59 to 86°F) prior to reconstitution.

For Prescribing information write to Professional Service, Wyeth-Ayerst Laboratories, P.O. Box 8299, Philadelphia, PA 19101.

Shown in Product Identification Guide, page 321

Lederle Standard Products
WAYNE, NJ 07470

The following list of Lederle Standard Products includes the alphanumeric LEDERMARK® codes which provide quick and positive identification of Lederle Standard Products capsules and tablets:

Product Identity Code No.	Product
A3	Tetracycline HCl Capsules, 250 mg
A5	Tetracycline HCl Capsules, 500 mg
A7	Atenolol Tablets, 25mg
A31	Ampicillin Trihydrate Capsules, USP, 250mg
A32	Ampicillin Trihydrate Capsules, USP, 500mg
—	Ampicillin Trihydrate for Oral Suspension, USP, 125mg/5mL
—	Ampicillin Trihydrate for Oral Suspension, USP, 250mg/5mL
A33	Amoxicillin Capsules, USP, 250mg
A34	Amoxicillin Capsules, USP, 500mg
—	Amoxicillin for Oral Suspension, USP, 125mg/5mL
—	Amoxicillin for Oral Suspension, USP, 250mg/5mL
A45	Albuterol Sulfate Tablets, 2mg
A46	Albuterol Sulfate Tablets, 4mg
A49	Atenolol Tablets, 50mg
A51	Alprazolam Tablets, USP, 0.25mg
A52	Alprazolam Tablets, USP, 0.5mg
A53	Alprazolam Tablets, USP, 1mg
A54	Alprazolam Tablets, USP, 2mg
A71	Atenolol Tablets, 100mg
—	Clindamycin Phosphate Injection, USP, 125mg/mL, 2mL vial
—	Clindamycin Phosphate Injection, USP, 125mg/mL, 4mL vial
—	Clindamycin Phosphate Injection, USP, 125mg/mL, 6mL vial
—	Clindamycin Phosphate Injection, USP, 125mg/mL, 60mL vial
C42	Clonidine HCl Tablets, USP, 0.1mg
C43	Clonidine HCl Tablets, USP, 0.2mg
C44	Clonidine HCl Tablets, USP, 0.3mg
C61	Cephradine Capsules, USP, 250mg
C62	Cephradine Capsules, USP, 500mg
C64	Cephalexin Capsules, USP, 250mg
C65	Cephalexin Capsules, USP, 500mg
C81	Cephalexin Tablets, USP, 250mg
C82	Cephalexin Tablets, USP, 500mg
—	Cephalexin for Oral Suspension, USP, 125mg/5mL
—	Cephalexin for Oral Suspension, USP, 250mg/5mL
CB300	Cimetidine Tablets, USP, 300mg
CB400	Cimetidine Tablets, USP, 400mg
CB800	Cimetidine Tablets, USP, 800mg
D16	Dicloxacillin Sodium Capsules, USP, 250mg
D17	Dicloxacillin Sodium Capsules, USP, 500mg
D25	Doxycycline Hyclate Capsules, USP, 100mg
D41	Doxycycline Hyclate Tablets, USP, 100mg
D44	Dipyridamole Tablets, 25mg
D45	Dipyridamole Tablets, 50mg
D46	Dipyridamole Tablets, 75mg
D51	Diazepam Tablets, USP, 2mg
D52	Diazepam Tablets, USP, 5mg
D53	Diazepam Tablets, USP, 10mg
D71	Diltiazem HCl Tablets, 30mg
D72	Diltiazem HCl Tablets, 60mg
D75	Diltiazem HCl Tablets, 90mg
D77	Diltiazem HCl Tablets, 120mg
—	Erythromycin Ethylsuccinate/Sulfisoxazole Acetyl for Oral Suspension, 200mg/600mg/5mL
—	Sterile Erythromycin Lactobionate for Injection, USP, 500mg/5 x 10mL vials
—	Sterile Erythromycin Lactobionate for Injection, USP, 1g/5 x 20mL vials
—	Folic Acid Injection, USP, 5mg/mL
F11	Furosemide Tablets, USP, 20mg
F12	Furosemide Tablets, USP 40mg
F13	Furosemide Tablets, USP, 80mg
F22	Fenoprofen Calcium Tablets, USP, 600mg
G17	Gemfibrozil Tablets, USP, 600mg
H11	Hydralazine HCl Tablets, USP, 25mg
H12	Hydralazine HCl Tablets, USP, 50mg
H14	Hydrochlorothiazide Tablets, USP, 25mg
H15	Hydrochlorothiazide Tablets, USP, 50mg
I19	Indomethacin Capsules, USP, 25mg
I20	Indomethacin Capsules, USP, 50mg
K1	Ketoprofen Capsules, 25mg
K2	Ketoprofen Capsules, 50mg
K3	Ketoprofen Capsules, 75mg
L9	Penicillin V Potassium Tablets, USP, 500mg
L10	Penicillin V Potassium Tablets, USP, 250mg
—	Penicillin V Potassium for Oral Solution, 125mg/5mL
—	Penicillin V Potassium for Oral Solution, 250mg/5mL
25/LL	Levothyroxine Sodium Tablets, USP, 25mcg (0.025mg)
50/LL	Levothyroxine Sodium Tablets, USP, 50mcg (0.050mg)
75/LL	Levothyroxine Sodium Tablets, USP, 75mcg (0.075mg)
100/LL	Levothyroxine Sodium Tablets, USP, 100mcg (0.1mg)
125/LL	Levothyroxine Sodium Tablets, USP, 125mcg (0.125mg)
150/LL	Levothyroxine Sodium Tablets, USP, 150mcg (0.15mg)
200/LL	Levothyroxine Sodium Tablets, USP, 200mcg (0.2mg)
300/LL	Levothyroxine Sodium Tablets, USP, 300mcg (0.3mg)
M19	Methocarbamol Tablets, USP, 500mg
M20	Methocarbamol Tablets, USP, 750mg
M22	Methyldopa Tablets, USP, 250mg
M23	Methyldopa Tablets, USP, 500mg
M28	Metoclopramide Tablets, 10mg
M36	Methyldopa and Hydrochlorothiazide Tablets, USP, 250mg/15mg
M37	Methyldopa and Hydrochlorothiazide Tablets, USP, 250mg/25mg
N1	Methazolamide Tablets, USP, 50mg
N2	Methazolamide Tablets, USP, 25mg
N11	Naproxen Tablets, USP, 250mg
N17	Naproxen Tablets, USP, 375mg
N77	Naproxen Tablets, USP, 500mg
—	Nystatin Oral Suspension, 100,000 units/mL
—	Nystatin Powder, USP
P33	Propylthiouracil Tablets, USP, 50mg
P36	Pyrazinamide Tablets, 500mg
P45	Propranolol HCl Tablets, USP, 20mg
P46	Propranolol HCl Tablets, USP, 40mg
P47	Propranolol HCl Tablets, USP, 80mg
P69	Prazosin HCl Capsules, USP, 1mg
P70	Prazosin HCl Capsules, USP, 2mg
P71	Prazosin HCl Capsules, USP, 5mg
Q11	Quinidine Sulfate Tablets, USP, 200mg
S16	Sulindac Tablets, USP, 150mg
S17	Sulindac Tablets, USP, 200mg
SCS 5752	Piroxicam Capsules, USP, 10mg
SCS 5762	Piroxicam Capsules, USP, 20mg
—	Tobramycin Sulfate Injection, USP, 40mg/mL
T13	Sulfamethoxazole and Trimethoprim Tablets, USP, 400mg/80mg
T16	Sulfamethoxazole and Trimethoprim Tablets, USP, 800mg/160mg
—	Vancomycin HCl, USP, 500mg vial
—	Vancomycin HCl, USP, 1g vial
—	Vancomycin HCl, USP, 5g vial

Shown in Product Identification Guide, page 321

LEMMON Company
See TEVA Pharmaceuticals USA

Eli Lilly and Company
LILLY CORPORATE CENTER
INDIANAPOLIS, IN 46285

Direct Inquiries to:
Lilly Corporate Center
Indianapolis, IN 46285
(317) 276-2000
For Medical Information Contact:
Lilly Research Laboratories
Lilly Corporate Center
Indianapolis, IN 46285
(800) 545-5979

LEGEND

ADD-Vantage®—*Vials and Diluent Containers, Abbott*
Disket®—*Dispersible Tablet, Lilly*
Enseal®—*Enteric-Release Tablet, Lilly*
Gelseal®—*Filled Elastic Capsule, Lilly*
Identi-Code®—*Formula Identification Code, Lilly*
Identi-Dose®—*Unit Dose Medication, Lilly*
Pulvule®—*Filled Gelatin Capsule, Lilly*
Redi Vial®—*Dual Compartment Vial, Lilly*
℞Pak—*Prescription Package, Lilly*
Solvet®—*Soluble Tablet, Lilly*
Traypak™—*Multivial Carton, Lilly*

IDENTI-CODE® Index
(formula identification code, Lilly)
Provides Positive Product Identification
A letter-number symbol, a 4-digit number, the name of the product, the strength of the product, or a combination of these appears on each Lilly capsule and most tablets and on each label of pediatric liquids, powders for oral suspension, and suppositories. The letter/number or 4-digit number identifies the product.

Identi-Code®	Product Name

Coated Tablets

C51   **Darvocet-N® 50**
Composition (Each Coated Tablet): Propoxyphene napsylate, 50 mg; acetaminophen, 325 mg (USP)

C53   **Darvon-N®**
Composition (Each Coated Tablet): Propoxyphene Napsylate, USP, 100 mg

C63   **Darvocet-N® 100**
Composition (Each Coated Tablet): Propoxyphene napsylate, 100 mg; acetaminophen, 650 mg (USP)

Pulvules®
F40   **Seconal® Sodium**
Composition (Each Pulvule®): Secobarbital Sodium, USP, 100 mg

F65   **Tuinal®**
Composition (Each Pulvule®): Secobarbital sodium, 50 mg; amobarbital sodium, 50 mg (USP)

F66   **Tuinal®**
Composition (Each Pulvule®): Secobarbital sodium, 100 mg; amobarbital sodium, 100 mg (USP)

H03   **Darvon®**
Composition (Each Pulvule®): Propoxyphene Hydrochloride, USP, 65 mg

H17   **Aventyl® HCl**
Composition (Each Pulvule®): Nortriptyline Hydrochloride, USP, 10 mg (equiv. to base)

H19   **Aventyl® HCl**
Composition (Each Pulvule®): Nortriptyline Hydrochloride, USP, 25 mg (equiv. to base)

3061   **Ceclor®**
Composition (Each Pulvule®): Cefaclor, USP, 250 mg

3062   **Ceclor®**
Composition (Each Pulvule®): Cefaclor, USP, 500 mg

3111   **Darvon® Compound-65**
Composition (Each Pulvule®): Propoxyphene hydrochloride, 65 mg; aspirin, 389 mg; caffeine, 32.4 mg

3125   **Vancocin® HCl**
Composition (Each Pulvule®): Vancomycin hydrochloride, 125 mg

3126   **Vancocin® HCl**
Composition (Each Pulvule®): Vancomycin hydrochloride, 250 mg

3144   **Axid®**
Composition (Each Pulvule®): Nizatidine, 150 mg

3145   **Axid®**
Composition (Each Pulvule®): Nizatidine, 300 mg

3170   **Lorabid®**
Composition (Each Pulvule®): Loracarbef, 200 mg

3171   **Lorabid®**
Composition (Each Pulvule®): Loracarbef, 400 mg

Compressed Tablets

J10   **Codeine Sulfate**
Composition (Each Compressed Tablet): Codeine Sulfate, USP, 30 mg

J11   **Codeine Sulfate**
Composition (Each Compressed Tablet): Codeine Sulfate, USP, 60 mg

J31   **Phenobarbital**
Composition (Each Compressed Tablet): Phenobarbital, USP, 15 mg

J32   **Phenobarbital**
Composition (Each Compressed Tablet): Phenobarbital, USP, 30 mg

J33   **Phenobarbital**
Composition (Each Compressed Tablet): Phenobarbital, USP, 100 mg

J37   **Phenobarbital**
Composition (Each Compressed Tablet): Phenobarbital, USP, 60 mg

J52   **Diethylstilbestrol**
Composition (Each Compressed Tablet): Diethylstilbestrol, USP, 1 mg

J54   **Diethylstilbestrol**
Composition (Each Compressed Tablet): Diethylstilbestrol, USP, 5 mg

J60   **Crystodigin®**
Composition (Each Compressed Tablet): Digitoxin, USP, 0.1 mg

T24   **Sodium Chloride**
Composition (Each Compressed Tablet): Sodium Chloride, USP, 1 g

T29   **Sodium Bicarbonate**
Composition (Each Compressed Tablet): Sodium Bicarbonate, USP, 10 grs (648 mg)

T35   **Calcium Carbonate**
Composition (Each Compressed Tablet): Calcium Carbonate, USP, Aromatic, 10 grs (648 mg)

U03   **Dymelor®**
Composition (Each Compressed Tablet): Acetohexamide, USP, 250 mg

U07   **Dymelor®**
Composition (Each Compressed Tablet): Acetohexamide, USP, 500 mg

UNIT-DOSE PACKAGING

Identi-Dose® (unit dose medication, Lilly)
Reverse-Numbered Package
Closed-circuit control of medication from pharmacy to nurse to patient and return. Simplifies counting and dispensing whether in single-unit or prescription-size quantities. Fits into any dispensing system for ready identification and legibility, better inventory control, protection from contamination, easier handling and recording under Medicare, prevention of drug loss through pilferage or spilling, better control of Federal Controlled Substances, and less chance of medication errors.
The following products are available through normal channels of supply:
Identi-Dose® (ID100)
Pulvules®
No.

℃ 365 Darvon®, 65 mg
℃ 369 Darvon® Compound-65
    387 Aventyl® HCl, 10 mg
    389 Aventyl® HCl, 25 mg
 3061 Ceclor®, 250 mg
 3062 Ceclor®, 500 mg

Tablets
No.
℃ 1883 Darvon-N®, 100 mg
℃ 1890 Darvocet-N® 50
℃ 1893 Darvocet-N® 100
Reverse-Numbered Package (RN500)
Pulvules®
No.
Tablets
No.
℃ 1893 Darvocet-N® 100
Single-Cut Identi-Dose® (ID500)
Tablets
No.
℃ 1893 Darvocet-N® 100

℃, ℃, ℃ Federal Controlled Substances.

AXID®   ℞
[*ak 'sid*]
(nizatidine capsules USP)
PULVULES®

DESCRIPTION

Axid® (Nizatidine, USP) is a histamine H_2-receptor antagonist. Chemically, it is N-[2-[[[2-[(dimethylamino)methyl]-4-thiazolyl]methyl]thio]ethyl]-N'-methyl-2-nitro-1,1-ethenediamine.
The structural formula is as follows:

Nizatidine

Nizatidine has the empirical formula $C_{12}H_{21}N_5O_2S_2$ representing a molecular weight of 331.47. It is an off-white to buff crystalline solid that is soluble in water. Nizatidine has a bitter taste and mild sulfur-like odor. Each Pulvule® (capsule) contains for oral administration gelatin, pregelatinized starch, dimethicone, starch, titanium dioxide, yellow iron oxide, 150 mg (0.45 mmol) or 300 mg (0.91 mmol) of nizatidine, and other inactive ingredients. The 150-mg Pulvule also contains magnesium stearate, and the 300-mg Pulvule also contains croscarmellose sodium, povidone, red iron oxide, and talc.

CLINICAL PHARMACOLOGY

Axid is a competitive, reversible inhibitor of histamine at the histamine H_2-receptors, particularly those in the gastric parietal cells.

Antisecretory Activity—1. Effects on Acid Secretion: Axid significantly inhibited nocturnal gastric acid secretion for up to 12 hours. Axid also significantly inhibited gastric acid secretion stimulated by food, caffeine, betazole, and pentagastrin (Table 1).

Table 1
Effect of Oral Axid on Gastric Acid Secretion

	Time After Dose (h)	% Inhibition of Gastric Acid Output by Dose (mg)				
		20–50	75	100	150	300
Nocturnal	Up to 10	57		73		90
Betazole	Up to 3		93		100	99
Pentagastrin	Up to 6		25		64	67
Meal	Up to 4	41	64		98	97
Caffeine	Up to 3		73		85	96

2. Effects on Other Gastrointestinal Secretions—Pepsin: Oral administration of 75 to 300 mg of Axid did not affect pepsin activity in gastric secretions. Total pepsin output was reduced in proportion to the reduced volume of gastric secretions.
Intrinsic Factor: Oral administration of 75 to 300 mg of Axid increased betazole-stimulated secretion of intrinsic factor.
Serum Gastrin: Axid had no effect on basal serum gastrin. No rebound of gastrin secretion was observed when food was ingested 12 hours after administration of Axid.

3. Other Pharmacologic Actions—
  a. Hormones: Axid was not shown to affect the serum concentrations of gonadotropins, prolactin, growth hormone, antidiuretic hormone, cortisol, triiodothyronine, thyroxin, testosterone, 5α-dihydrotestosterone, androstenedione, or estradiol.

  b. Axid had no demonstrable antiandrogenic action.

Table 2
Healing Response of Ulcers to Axid

	AXID				Placebo	
	300 mg h.s.		150 mg b.i.d.			
	Number Entered	Healed/Evaluable	Number Entered	Healed/Evaluable	Number Entered	Healed/Evaluable
STUDY 1						
Week 2			276	93/265 (35%)*	279	55/260 (21%)
Week 4				198/259 (76%)*		95/243 (39%)
STUDY 2						
Week 2	108	24/103 (23%)*	106	27/101 (27%)*	101	9/93 (10%)
Week 4		65/97 (67%)*		66/97 (68%)*		24/84 (29%)
STUDY 3						
Week 2	92	22/90 (24%)†			98	13/92 (14%)
Week 4		52/85 (61%)*				29/88 (33%)
Week 8		68/83 (82%)*				39/79 (49%)

* $P < 0.01$ as compared with placebo.
† $P < 0.05$ as compared with placebo.

4. Pharmacokinetics—The absolute oral bioavailability of nizatidine exceeds 70%. Peak plasma concentrations (700 to 1,800 μg/L for a 150-mg dose and 1,400 to 3,600 μg/L for a 300-mg dose) occur from 0.5 to 3 hours following the dose. A concentration of 1,000 μg/L is equivalent to 3 μmol/L; a dose of 300 mg is equivalent to 905 μmoles. Plasma concentrations 12 hours after administration are less than 10 μg/L. The elimination half-life is 1 to 2 hours, plasma clearance is 40 to 60 L/h, and the volume of distribution is 0.8 to 1.5 L/kg. Because of the short half-life and rapid clearance of nizatidine, accumulation of the drug would not be expected in individuals with normal renal function who take either 300 mg once daily at bedtime or 150 mg twice daily. Axid exhibits dose proportionality over the recommended dose range.
The oral bioavailability of nizatidine is unaffected by concomitant ingestion of propantheline. Antacids consisting of aluminum and magnesium hydroxides with simethicone decrease the absorption of nizatidine by about 10%. With food, the AUC and C_{max} increase by approximately 10%.
In humans, less than 7% of an oral dose is metabolized as N2-monodesmethylnizatidine, an H_2-receptor antagonist, which is the principal metabolite excreted in the urine. Other likely metabolites are the N2-oxide (less than 5% of the dose) and the S-oxide (less than 6% of the dose).
More than 90% of an oral dose of nizatidine is excreted in the urine within 12 hours. About 60% of an oral dose is excreted as unchanged drug. Renal clearance is about 500 mL/min, which indicates excretion by active tubular secretion. Less than 6% of an administered dose is eliminated in the feces.
Moderate to severe renal impairment significantly prolongs the half-life and decreases the clearance of nizatidine. In individuals who are functionally anephric, the half-life is 3.5 to 11 hours, and the plasma clearance is 7 to 14 L/h. To avoid accumulation of the drug in individuals with clinically significant renal impairment, the amount and/or frequency of doses of Axid should be reduced in proportion to the severity of dysfunction (*see* Dosage and Administration).
Approximately 35% of nizatidine is bound to plasma protein, mainly to α_1-acid glycoprotein. Warfarin, diazepam, acetaminophen, propantheline, phenobarbital, and propranolol did not affect plasma protein binding of nizatidine in vitro.
Clinical Trials—1. Active Duodenal Ulcer: In multicenter, double-blind, placebo-controlled studies in the United States, endoscopically diagnosed duodenal ulcers healed more rapidly following administration of Axid, 300 mg h.s. or 150 mg b.i.d., than with placebo (Table 2). Lower doses, such as 100 mg h.s., had slightly lower effectiveness.
[See table 2 above.]
2. Maintenance of Healed Duodenal Ulcer:
Treatment with a reduced dose of Axid has been shown to be effective as maintenance therapy following healing of active duodenal ulcers. In multicenter, double-blind, placebo-controlled studies conducted in the United States, 150 mg of Axid taken at bedtime resulted in a significantly lower incidence of duodenal ulcer recurrence in patients treated for up to 1 year (Table 3).

Table 3
Percentage of Ulcers Recurring by 3, 6, and 12 Months in Double-Blind Studies Conducted in the United States

Month	Axid, 150 mg h.s.	Placebo
3	13% (28/208)*	40% (82/204)
6	24% (45/188)*	57% (106/187)
12	34% (57/166)*	64% (112/175)

* $P < 0.001$ as compared with placebo.

3. Gastroesophageal Reflux Disease (GERD):
In 2 multicenter, double-blind, placebo-controlled clinical trials performed in the United States and Canada, Axid was more effective than placebo in improving endoscopically diagnosed esophagitis and in healing erosive and ulcerative esophagitis.
In patients with erosive or ulcerative esophagitis, 150 mg b.i.d. of Axid given to 88 patients compared with placebo in 98 patients in Study 1 yielded a higher healing rate at 3 weeks (16% vs 7%) and at 6 weeks (32% vs 16%, $P < 0.05$). Of 99 patients on Axid and 94 patients on placebo, Study 2 at the same dosage yielded similar results at 6 weeks (21% vs 11%, $P < 0.05$) and at 12 weeks (29% vs 13%, $P < 0.01$).
In addition, relief of associated heartburn was greater in patients treated with Axid. Patients treated with Axid consumed fewer antacids than did patients treated with placebo.
4. Active Benign Gastric Ulcer:
In a multicenter, double-blind, placebo-controlled study conducted in the United States and Canada, endoscopically diagnosed benign gastric ulcers healed significantly more rapidly following administration of nizatidine than of placebo (Table 4).

Table 4

Week	Treatment	Healing Rate	vs. Placebo p-value*
4	Niz 300 mg h.s.	52/153 (34%)	0.342
	Niz 150 mg b.i.d.	65/151 (43%)	0.022
	Placebo	48/151 (32%)	
8	Niz 300 mg h.s.	99/153 (65%)	0.011
	Niz 150 mg b.i.d.	105/151 (70%)	<0.001
	Placebo	78/151 (52%)	

* P-values are one-sided, obtained by Chi-square test, and not adjusted for multiple comparisons.

In a multicenter, double-blind, comparator-controlled study in Europe, healing rates for patients receiving nizatidine (300 mg h.s. or 150 mg b.i.d.) were equivalent to rates for patients receiving a comparator drug, and statistically superior to historical placebo control rates.

INDICATIONS AND USAGE

Axid is indicated for up to 8 weeks for the treatment of active duodenal ulcer. In most patients, the ulcer will heal within 4 weeks.
Axid is indicated for maintenance therapy for duodenal ulcer patients, at a reduced dosage of 150 mg h.s. after healing of an active duodenal ulcer. The consequences of continuous therapy with Axid for longer than 1 year are not known.
Axid is indicated for up to 12 weeks for the treatment of endoscopically diagnosed esophagitis, including erosive and ulcerative esophagitis, and associated heartburn due to GERD.
Axid is indicated for up to 8 weeks for the treatment of active benign gastric ulcer. Before initiating therapy, care should be taken to exclude the possibility of malignant gastric ulceration.

CONTRAINDICATION

Axid is contraindicated in patients with known hypersensitivity to the drug. Because cross sensitivity in this class of compounds has been observed, H_2-receptor antagonists, including Axid, should not be administered to patients with a history of hypersensitivity to other H_2-receptor antagonists.

PRECAUTIONS

General—1. Symptomatic response to nizatidine therapy does not preclude the presence of gastric malignancy.
2. Because nizatidine is excreted primarily by the kidney, dosage should be reduced in patients with moderate to severe renal insufficiency (*see* Dosage and Administration).
3. Pharmacokinetic studies in patients with hepatorenal syndrome have not been done. Part of the dose of nizatidine is metabolized in the liver. In patients with normal renal function and uncomplicated hepatic dysfunction, the disposition of nizatidine is similar to that in normal subjects.
Laboratory Tests—False-positive tests for urobilinogen with Multistix® may occur during therapy with nizatidine.
Drug Interactions—No interactions have been observed between Axid and theophylline, chlordiazepoxide, lorazepam, lidocaine, phenytoin, and warfarin. Axid does not inhibit the cytochrome P-450-linked drug-metabolizing enzyme system; therefore, drug interactions mediated by inhibition of hepatic metabolism are not expected to occur. In patients given very high doses (3,900 mg) of aspirin daily, increases in serum salicylate levels were seen when nizatidine, 150 mg b.i.d., was administered concurrently.
Carcinogenesis, Mutagenesis, Impairment of Fertility—A 2-year oral carcinogenicity study in rats with doses as high as 500 mg/kg/day (about 80 times the recommended daily therapeutic dose) showed no evidence of a carcinogenic effect. There was a dose-related increase in the density of enterochromaffin-like (ECL) cells in the gastric oxyntic mucosa. In a 2-year study in mice, there was no evidence of a carcinogenic effect in male mice, although hyperplastic nodules of the liver were increased in the high-dose males as compared with placebo. Female mice given the high dose of Axid (2,000 mg/kg/day, about 330 times the human dose) showed marginally statistically significant increases in hepatic carcinoma and hepatic nodular hyperplasia with no numerical increase seen in any of the other dose groups. The rate of hepatic carcinoma in the high-dose animals was within the historical control limits seen for the strain of mice used. The female mice were given a dose larger than the maximum tolerated dose, as indicated by excessive (30%) weight decrement as compared with concurrent controls and evidence of mild liver injury (transaminase elevations). The occurrence of a marginal finding at high dose only in animals given an excessive and somewhat hepatotoxic dose, with no evidence of a carcinogenic effect in rats, male mice, and female mice (given up to 360 mg/kg/day, about 60 times the human dose), and a negative mutagenicity battery are not considered evidence of a carcinogenic potential for Axid.
Axid was not mutagenic in a battery of tests performed to evaluate its potential genetic toxicity, including bacterial mutation tests, unscheduled DNA synthesis, sister chromatid exchange, the mouse lymphoma assay, chromosome aberration tests, and a micronucleus test.
In a 2-generation, perinatal and postnatal fertility study in rats, doses of nizatidine up to 650 mg/kg/day produced no adverse effects on the reproductive performance of parental animals or their progeny.
Pregnancy—Teratogenic Effects—Pregnancy Category B—Oral reproduction studies in pregnant rats at doses up to 1500 mg/kg/day (9000 mg/m^2/day, 40.5 times the recommended human dose based on body surface area) and in pregnant rabbits at doses up to 275 mg/kg/day (3245 mg/m^2/day, 14.6 times the recommended human dose based on body surface area) have revealed no evidence of impaired fertility or harm to the fetus due to nizatidine. There are, however, no adequate and well-controlled studies in pregnant women. Because animal reproduction studies are not always predictive of human response, this drug should be used during pregnancy only if clearly needed.
Nursing Mothers—Studies conducted in lactating women have shown that 0.1% of the administered oral dose of nizatidine is secreted in human milk in proportion to plasma concentrations. Because of the growth depression in pups reared by lactating rats treated with nizatidine, a decision should be made whether to discontinue nursing or discontinue the drug, taking into account the importance of the drug to the mother.
Pediatric Use—Safety and effectiveness in children have not been established.
Use in Elderly Patients—Ulcer healing rates in elderly patients are similar to those in younger age groups. The incidence rates of adverse events and laboratory test abnormalities are also similar to those seen in other age groups. Age alone may not be an important factor in the disposition of nizatidine. Elderly patients may have reduced renal function (*see* Dosage and Administration).

ADVERSE REACTIONS

Worldwide, controlled clinical trials of nizatidine included over 6,000 patients given nizatidine in studies of varying durations. Placebo-controlled trials in the United States and Canada included over 2,600 patients given nizatidine and over 1,700 given placebo. Among the adverse events in these placebo-controlled trials, anemia (0.2% vs 0%) and urticaria (0.5% vs 0.1%) were significantly more common in the nizatidine group.
Incidence in Placebo-Controlled Clinical Trials in the United States and Canada—Table 5 lists adverse events that occurred at a frequency of 1% or more among nizatidine-treated patients who participated in placebo-controlled trials. The cited figures provide some basis for estimating the relative contribution of drug and nondrug factors to the side effect incidence rate in the population studied.

Continued on next page

• Identi-Code® symbol. This product information was prepared in June 1996. Current information on these and other products of Eli Lilly and Company may be obtained by direct inquiry to Lilly Research Laboratories, Lilly Corporate Center, Indianapolis, Indiana 46285, 800-545-5979.

Lilly—Cont.

Table 5
Incidence of Treatment-Emergent
Adverse Events in Placebo-Controlled
Clinical Trials
In The United States and Canada

Body System/Adverse Event*	Percentage of Patients Reporting Event	
	Nizatidine (N = 2,694)	Placebo (N = 1,729)
Body as a Whole		
Headache	16.6	15.6
Abdominal pain	7.5	12.5
Pain	4.2	3.8
Asthenia	3.1	2.9
Back pain	2.4	2.6
Chest pain	2.3	2.1
Infection	1.7	1.1
Fever	1.6	2.3
Surgical procedure	1.4	1.5
Injury, accident	1.2	0.9
Digestive		
Diarrhea	7.2	6.9
Nausea	5.4	7.4
Flatulence	4.9	5.4
Vomiting	3.6	5.6
Dyspepsia	3.6	4.4
Constipation	2.5	3.8
Dry mouth	1.4	1.3
Nausea and vomiting	1.2	1.9
Anorexia	1.2	1.6
Gastrointestinal disorder	1.1	1.2
Tooth disorder	1.0	0.8
Musculoskeletal		
Myalgia	1.7	1.5
Nervous		
Dizziness	4.6	3.8
Insomnia	2.7	3.4
Abnormal dreams	1.9	1.9
Somnolence	1.9	1.6
Anxiety	1.6	1.4
Nervousness	1.1	0.8
Respiratory		
Rhinitis	9.8	9.6
Pharyngitis	3.3	3.1
Sinusitis	2.4	2.1
Cough, increased	2.0	2.0
Skin and Appendages		
Rash	1.9	2.1
Pruritus	1.7	1.3
Special Senses		
Amblyopia	1.0	0.9

* Events reported by at least 1% of nizatidine-treated patients are included.

A variety of less common events were also reported; it was not possible to determine whether these were caused by nizatidine.

Hepatic—Hepatocellular injury, evidenced by elevated liver enzyme tests (SGOT [AST], SGPT [ALT], or alkaline phosphatase), occurred in some patients and was possibly or probably related to nizatidine. In some cases there was marked elevation of SGOT, SGPT enzymes (greater than 500 IU/L) and, in a single instance, SGPT was greater than 2,000 IU/L. The overall rate of occurrences of elevated liver enzymes and elevations to 3 times the upper limit of normal, however, did not significantly differ from the rate of liver enzyme abnormalities in placebo-treated patients. All abnormalities were reversible after discontinuation of Axid. Since market introduction, hepatitis and jaundice have been reported. Rare cases of cholestatic or mixed hepatocellular and cholestatic injury with jaundice have been reported with reversal of the abnormalities after discontinuation of Axid.

Cardiovascular—In clinical pharmacology studies, short episodes of asymptomatic ventricular tachycardia occurred in 2 individuals administered Axid and in 3 untreated subjects.

CNS—Rare cases of reversible mental confusion have been reported.

Endocrine—Clinical pharmacology studies and controlled clinical trials showed no evidence of antiandrogenic activity due to Axid. Impotence and decreased libido were reported with similar frequency by patients who received Axid and by those given placebo. Rare reports of gynecomastia occurred.

Hematologic—Anemia was reported significantly more frequently in nizatidine- than in placebo-treated patients. Fatal thrombocytopenia was reported in a patient who was treated with Axid and another H$_2$-receptor antagonist. On previous occasions, this patient had experienced thrombocytopenia while taking other drugs. Rare cases of thrombocytopenic purpura have been reported.

Integumental—Sweating and urticaria were reported significantly more frequently in nizatidine- than in placebo-treated patients. Rash and exfoliative dermatitis were also reported. Vasculitis has been reported rarely.

Hypersensitivity—As with other H$_2$-receptor antagonists, rare cases of anaphylaxis following administration of nizatidine have been reported. Rare episodes of hypersensitivity reactions (eg, bronchospasm, laryngeal edema, rash, and eosinophilia) have been reported.

Body as a Whole—Serum sickness-like reactions have occurred rarely in conjunction with nizatidine use.

Genitourinary—Reports of impotence have occurred.

Other—Hyperuricemia unassociated with gout or nephrolithiasis was reported. Eosinophilia, fever, and nausea related to nizatidine administration have been reported.

OVERDOSAGE

Overdoses of Axid have been reported rarely. The following is provided to serve as a guide should such an overdose be encountered.

Signs and Symptoms—There is little clinical experience with overdosage of Axid in humans. Test animals that received large doses of nizatidine have exhibited cholinergic-type effects, including lacrimation, salivation, emesis, miosis, and diarrhea. Single oral doses of 800 mg/kg in dogs and of 1,200 mg/kg in monkeys were not lethal. Intravenous median lethal doses in the rat and mouse were 301 mg/kg and 232 mg/kg respectively.

Treatment—To obtain up-to-date information about the treatment of overdose, a good resource is your certified Regional Poison Control Center. Telephone numbers of certified poison control centers are listed in the *Physicians' Desk Reference (PDR)*. In managing overdosage, consider the possibility of multiple drug overdoses, interaction among drugs, and unusual drug kinetics in your patient.

If overdosage occurs, use of activated charcoal, emesis, or lavage should be considered along with clinical monitoring and supportive therapy. The ability of hemodialysis to remove nizatidine from the body has not been conclusively demonstrated; however, due to its large volume of distribution, nizatidine is not expected to be efficiently removed from the body by this method.

DOSAGE AND ADMINISTRATION

Active Duodenal Ulcer—The recommended oral dosage for adults is 300 mg once daily at bedtime. An alternative dosage regimen is 150 mg twice daily.

Maintenance of Healed Duodenal Ulcer—The recommended oral dosage for adults is 150 mg once daily at bedtime.

Gastroesophageal Reflux Disease—The recommended oral dosage in adults for the treatment of erosions, ulcerations, and associated heartburn is 150 mg twice daily.

Active Benign Gastric Ulcer—The recommended oral dosage is 300 mg given either as 150 mg twice daily or 300 mg once daily at bedtime. Prior to treatment, care should be taken to exclude the possibility of malignant gastric ulceration.

Dosage Adjustment for Patients With Moderate to Severe Renal Insufficiency—The dose for patients with renal dysfunction should be reduced as follows:

Active Duodenal Ulcer, GERD and Benign Gastric Ulcer

C$_{cr}$	Dose
20–50 mL/min	150 mg daily
< 20 mL/min	150 mg every other day

Maintenance Therapy

C$_{cr}$	Dose
20–50 mL/min	150 mg every other day
< 20 mL/min	150 mg every 3 days

Some elderly patients may have creatinine clearances of less than 50 mL/min, and, based on pharmacokinetic data in patients with renal impairment, the dose for such patients should be reduced accordingly. The clinical effects of this dosage reduction in patients with renal failure have not been evaluated.

HOW SUPPLIED

Pulvules*:

Axid® 150 mg (No. 3144) are pale yellow and dark yellow Pulvules with "Lilly 3144" imprinted on one end and "AXID 150 mg" on the other. They are supplied as follows:
NDC 0002-3144-60 RxPak† of 60
NDC 0002-3144-03 RxPak† of 500
NDC 0002-3144-33 ID‡100
NDC 0002-3144-82 FlexPak§ of 20 blister cards of 31
Axid® 300 mg (No. 3145) are pale yellow and brown Pulvules with "Lilly 3145" imprinted on one end and "AXID 300 mg" on the other. They are supplied as follows:
NDC 0002-3145-30 RxPak† of 30

---

* Pulvules® (filled gelatin capsules, Lilly)
† RxPak (prescription package, Lilly)
‡ Identi-Dose® (unit dose medication, Lilly)
§FlexPak (flexible blister card, Lilly)
Store at controlled room temperature-, 20° to 25°C (68° to 77°F) in a tightly closed container [see USP].
The USP defines controlled room temperature as: A temperature maintained thermostatically that encompasses the usual and customary working environment of 20° to 25°C (68° to 77°F); that results in a mean kinetic temperature calculated to be not more than 25°C; and that allows for excursions between 15° and 30°C (59° and 86°F) that are experienced in pharmacies, hospitals, and warehouses.
CAUTION-Federal (USA) law prohibits dispensing without prescription.
Literature revised October 20, 1995
PV 2098

Shown in Product Identification Guide, page 322

CECLOR®
[sē'klŏr]
(cefaclor)
USP

℞

DESCRIPTION

Ceclor® (Cefaclor, USP) is a semisynthetic cephalosporin antibiotic for oral administration. It is chemically designated as 3-chloro-7-D- (2-phenylglycinamido)-3-cephem-4-carboxylic acid monohydrate. The chemical formula for cefaclor is $C_{15}H_{14}ClN_3O_4S \cdot H_2O$ and the molecular weight is 385.82.

Each Pulvule® contains cefaclor monohydrate equivalent to 250 mg (0.68 mmol) or 500 mg (1.36 mmol) anhydrous cefaclor. The Pulvules also contain cornstarch, FD&C Blue No. 1, FD&C Red No. 3, gelatin, magnesium stearate, silicone, titanium dioxide, and other inactive ingredients. The 500-mg Pulvule also contains iron oxide.

After mixing, each 5 mL of Ceclor for Oral Suspension will contain cefaclor monohydrate equivalent to 125 mg (0.34 mmol), 187 mg (0.51 mmol), 250 mg (0.68 mmol), or 375 mg (1.0 mmol) anhydrous cefaclor. The suspensions also contain cellulose, cornstarch, FD&C Red No. 40, flavors, silicone, sodium lauryl sulfate, sucrose, and xanthan gum.

CLINICAL PHARMACOLOGY

Cefaclor is well absorbed after oral administration to fasting subjects. Total absorption is the same whether the drug is given with or without food; however, when it is taken with food, the peak concentration achieved is 50% to 75% of that observed when the drug is administered to fasting subjects and generally appears from three fourths to 1 hour later. Following administration of 250-mg, 500-mg, and 1-g doses to fasting subjects, average peak serum levels of approximately 7, 13, and 23 μg/mL respectively were obtained within 30 to 60 minutes. Approximately 60% to 85% of the drug is excreted unchanged in the urine within 8 hours, the greater portion being excreted within the first 2 hours. During this 8-hour period, peak urine concentrations following the 250-mg, 500-mg, and 1-g doses were approximately 600, 900, and 1,900 μg/mL respectively. The serum half-life in normal subjects is 0.6 to 0.9 hour. In patients with reduced renal function, the serum half-life of cefaclor is slightly prolonged. In those with complete absence of renal function, the plasma half-life of the intact molecule is 2.3 to 2.8 hours. Excretion pathways in patients with markedly impaired renal function have not been determined. Hemodialysis shortens the half-life by 25% to 30%.

Microbiology—In vitro tests demonstrate that the bactericidal action of the cephalosporins results from inhibition of cell-wall synthesis. Cefaclor is active in vitro against most strains of clinical isolates of the following organisms:

Staphylococci, including coagulase-positive, coagulase-negative, and penicillinase-producing strains (when tested by in vitro methods), exhibit cross-resistance between cefaclor and methicillin
Streptococcus pyogenes (group A β-hemolytic streptococci)
Streptococcus pneumoniae
Moraxella (Branhamella) catarrhalis
Haemophilus influenzae, including β-lactamase-producing ampicillin-resistant strains
Escherichia coli
Proteus mirabilis
Klebsiella sp
Citrobacter diversus
Neisseria gonorrhoeae
Propionibacterium acnes and *Bacteroides* sp (excluding *Bacteroides fragilis*)
Peptococci
Peptostreptococci
Note: Pseudomonas sp, *Acinetobacter calcoaceticus* (formerly *Mima* sp and *Herellea* sp), and most strains of enterococci (*Enterococcus faecalis* [formerly *Streptococcus faecalis*], group D streptococci), *Enterobacter* sp, indole-positive *Proteus*, and *Serratia* sp are resistant to cefaclor. When tested by

in vitro methods, staphylococci exhibit cross-resistance between cefaclor and methicillin-type antibiotics.

Disk Susceptibility Tests—Quantitative methods that require measurement of zone diameters give the most precise estimates of antibiotic susceptibility. One such procedure* has been recommended for use with disks for testing susceptibility to cephalothin. The currently accepted zone diameter interpretative criteria for the cephalothin disk are appropriate for determining bacterial susceptibility to cefaclor. With this procedure, a report from the laboratory of "resistant" indicates that the infecting organism is not likely to respond to therapy. A report of "intermediate susceptibility" suggests that the organism would be susceptible if the infection is confined to tissues and fluids (eg, urine) in which high antibiotic levels can be obtained or if high dosage is used.

INDICATIONS AND USAGE

Ceclor is indicated in the treatment of the following infections when caused by susceptible strains of the designated microorganisms:

Otitis media caused by *S. pneumoniae, H. influenzae,* staphylococci, and *S. pyogenes* (group A β-hemolytic streptococci)

Lower respiratory infections, including pneumonia, caused by *S. pneumoniae, H. influenzae,* and *S. pyogenes* (group A β-hemolytic streptococci)

Upper respiratory infections, including pharyngitis and tonsillitis, caused by *S. pyogenes* (group A β-hemolytic streptococci)

Note: Penicillin is the usual drug of choice in the treatment and prevention of streptococcal infections, including the prophylaxis of rheumatic fever. Ceclor is generally effective in the eradication of streptococci from the nasopharynx; however, substantial data establishing the efficacy of Ceclor in the subsequent prevention of rheumatic fever are not available at present.

Urinary tract infections, including pyelonephritis and cystitis, caused by *E. coli, P. mirabilis, Klebsiella* sp, and coagulase-negative staphylococci

Skin and skin structure infections caused by *Staphylococcus aureus* and *S. pyogenes* (group A β-hemolytic streptococci)

Appropriate culture and susceptibility studies should be performed to determine susceptibility of the causative organism to Ceclor.

CONTRAINDICATION

Ceclor is contraindicated in patients with known allergy to the cephalosporin group of antibiotics.

WARNINGS

IN PENICILLIN-SENSITIVE PATIENTS, CEPHALOSPORIN ANTIBIOTICS SHOULD BE ADMINISTERED CAUTIOUSLY. THERE IS CLINICAL AND LABORATORY EVIDENCE OF PARTIAL CROSS-ALLERGENICITY OF THE PENICILLINS AND THE CEPHALOSPORINS AND THERE ARE INSTANCES IN WHICH PATIENTS HAVE HAD REACTIONS, INCLUDING ANAPHYLAXIS, TO BOTH DRUG CLASSES.

Antibiotics, including Ceclor, should be administered cautiously to any patient who has demonstrated some form of allergy, particularly to drugs.

Pseudomembranous colitis has been reported with virtually all broad-spectrum antibiotics (including macrolides, semisynthetic penicillins, and cephalosporins); therefore, it is important to consider its diagnosis in patients who develop diarrhea in association with the use of antibiotics. Such colitis may range in severity from mild to life threatening.

Treatment with broad-spectrum antibiotics alters the normal flora of the colon and may permit overgrowth of clostridia. Studies indicate that a toxin produced by *Clostridium difficile* is a primary cause of antibiotic-associated colitis.

Mild cases of pseudomembranous colitis usually respond to drug discontinuance alone. In moderate to severe cases, management should include sigmoidoscopy, appropriate bacteriologic studies, and fluid, electrolyte, and protein supplementation. When the colitis does not improve after the drug has been discontinued, or when it is severe, oral vancomycin is the drug of choice for antibiotic-associated pseudomembranous colitis produced by *C. difficile.* Other causes of colitis should be ruled out.

PRECAUTIONS

General—If an allergic reaction to Ceclor occurs, the drug should be discontinued, and, if necessary, the patient should be treated with appropriate agents, eg, pressor amines, antihistamines, or corticosteroids.

Prolonged use of Ceclor may result in the overgrowth of nonsusceptible organisms. Careful observation of the patient is essential. If superinfection occurs during therapy, appropriate measures should be taken.

Positive direct Coombs' tests have been reported during treatment with the cephalosporin antibiotics. In hematologic studies or in transfusion cross-matching procedures when antiglobulin tests are performed on the minor side or in Coombs' testing of newborns whose mothers have received cephalosporin antibiotics before parturition, it should be recognized that a positive Coombs' test may be due to the drug.

Ceclor should be administered with caution in the presence of markedly impaired renal function. Since the half-life of cefaclor in anuria is 2.3 to 2.8 hours, dosage adjustments for patients with moderate or severe renal impairment are usually not required. Clinical experience with cefaclor under such conditions is limited; therefore, careful clinical observation and laboratory studies should be made.

As with other β-lactam antibiotics, the renal excretion of cefaclor is inhibited by probenecid.

As a result of administration of Ceclor, a false-positive reaction for glucose in the urine may occur. This has been observed with Benedict's and Fehling's solutions and also with Clinitest® tablets but not with Tes-Tape® (Glucose Enzymatic Test Strip, USP, Lilly).

Broad-spectrum antibiotics should be prescribed with caution in individuals with a history of gastrointestinal disease, particularly colitis.

Pregnancy—Pregnancy Category B—Reproduction studies have been performed in mice and rats at doses up to 12 times the human dose and in ferrets given 3 times the maximum human dose and have revealed no evidence of impaired fertility or harm to the fetus due to Ceclor. There are, however, no adequate and well-controlled studies in pregnant women. Because animal reproduction studies are not always predictive of human response, this drug should be used during pregnancy only if clearly needed.

Nursing Mothers—Small amounts of Ceclor have been detected in mother's milk following administration of single 500-mg doses. Average levels were 0.18, 0.20, 0.21, and 0.16 μg/mL at 2, 3, 4, and 5 hours respectively. Trace amounts were detected at 1 hour. The effect on nursing infants is not known. Caution should be exercised when Ceclor is administered to a nursing woman.

Pediatric Use—Safety and effectiveness of this product for use in infants less than 1 month of age have not been established.

ADVERSE REACTIONS

Adverse effects considered related to therapy with Ceclor are listed below:

Hypersensitivity reactions have been reported in about 1.5% of patients and include morbilliform eruptions (1 in 100). Pruritus, urticaria, and positive Coombs' tests each occur in less than 1 in 200 patients.

Cases of **serum-sickness-like** reactions have been reported with the use of Ceclor. These are characterized by findings of erythema multiforme, rashes, and other skin manifestations accompanied by arthritis/arthralgia, with or without fever, and differ from classic serum sickness in that there is infrequently associated lymphadenopathy and proteinuria, no circulating immune complexes, and no evidence to date of sequelae of the reaction. Occasionally, solitary symptoms may occur, but do not represent a **serum-sickness-like reaction.** While further investigation is ongoing, **serum-sickness-like** reactions appear to be due to hypersensitivity and more often occur during or following a second (or subsequent) course of therapy with Ceclor. Such reactions have been reported more frequently in children than in adults with an overall occurrence ranging from 1 in 200 (0.5%) in one focused trial to 2 in 8,346 (0.024%) in overall clinical trials (with an incidence in children in clinical trials of 0.055%) to 1 in 38,000 (0.003%) in spontaneous event reports. Signs and symptoms usually occur a few days after initiation of therapy and subside within a few days after cessation of therapy; occasionally these reactions have resulted in hospitalization, usually of short duration (median hospitalization = 2 to 3 days, based on postmarketing surveillance studies). In those requiring hospitalization, the symptoms have ranged from mild to severe at the time of admission with more of the severe reactions occurring in children. Antihistamines and glucocorticoids appear to enhance resolution of the signs and symptoms. No serious sequelae have been reported.

More severe hypersensitivity reactions, including Stevens-Johnson syndrome, toxic epidermal necrolysis, and anaphylaxis, have been reported rarely. Anaphylactoid events may be manifested by solitary symptoms, including angioedema, asthenia, edema (including face and limbs), dyspnea, paresthesias, syncope, or vasodilatation. Anaphylaxis may be more common in patients with a history of penicillin allergy.

Rarely, hypersensitivity symptoms may persist for several months.

Gastrointestinal symptoms occur in about 2.5% of patients and include diarrhea (1 in 70).

Symptoms of pseudomembranous colitis may appear either during or after antibiotic treatment. Nausea and vomiting have been reported rarely. As with some penicillins and some other cephalosporins, transient hepatitis and cholestatic jaundice have been reported rarely.

Other effects considered related to therapy included eosinophilia (1 in 50 patients), genital pruritus or vaginitis (less than 1 in 100 patients), and, rarely, thrombocytopenia or reversible interstitial nephritis.

Causal Relationship Uncertain—

CNS—Rarely, reversible hyperactivity, agitation, nervousness, insomnia, confusion, hypertonia, dizziness, hallucinations, and somnolence have been reported.

Transitory abnormalities in clinical laboratory test results have been reported. Although they were of uncertain etiology, they are listed below to serve as alerting information for the physician.

Hepatic—Slight elevations of AST (SGOT), ALT (SGPT), or alkaline phosphatase values (1 in 40).

Hematopoietic—As has also been reported with other β-lactam antibiotics, transient lymphocytosis, leukopenia, and, rarely, hemolytic anemia and reversible neutropenia of possible clinical significance.

There have been rare reports of increased prothrombin time with or without clinical bleeding in patients receiving Ceclor and Coumadin concomitantly.

Renal—Slight elevations in BUN or serum creatinine (less than 1 in 500) or abnormal urinalysis (less than 1 in 200).

OVERDOSAGE

Signs and Symptoms—The toxic symptoms following an overdose of cefaclor may include nausea, vomiting, epigastric distress, and diarrhea. The severity of the epigastric distress and the diarrhea are dose related. If other symptoms are present, it is probable that they are secondary to an underlying disease state, an allergic reaction, or the effects of other intoxication.

Treatment—To obtain up-to-date information about the treatment of overdose, a good resource is your certified Regional Poison Control Center. Telephone numbers of certified poison control centers are listed in the *Physicians' Desk Reference (PDR)*. In managing overdosage, consider the possibility of multiple drug overdoses, interaction among drugs, and unusual drug kinetics in your patient.

Unless 5 times the normal dose of cefaclor has been ingested, gastrointestinal decontamination will not be necessary.

Protect the patient's airway and support ventilation and perfusion. Meticulously monitor and maintain, within acceptable limits, the patient's vital signs, blood gases, serum electrolytes, etc. Absorption of drugs from the gastrointestinal tract may be decreased by giving activated charcoal, which, in many cases, is more effective than emesis or lavage; consider charcoal instead of or in addition to gastric emptying. Repeated doses of charcoal over time may hasten elimination of some drugs that have been absorbed. Safeguard the patient's airway when employing gastric emptying or charcoal.

Forced diuresis, peritoneal dialysis, hemodialysis, or charcoal hemoperfusion have not been established as beneficial for an overdose of cefaclor.

DOSAGE AND ADMINISTRATION

Ceclor is administered orally.

Adults—The usual adult dosage is 250 mg every 8 hours. For more severe infections (such as pneumonia) or those caused by less susceptible organisms, doses may be doubled.

Children—The usual recommended daily dosage for children is 20 mg/kg/day in divided doses every 8 hours. In more serious infections, otitis media, and infections caused by less susceptible organisms, 40 mg/kg/day are recommended, with a maximum dosage of 1 g/day.

	Ceclor Suspension	
	20 mg/kg/day	
Child's Weight	125 mg/5 mL	250 mg/5 mL
9 kg	½ tsp t.i.d.	
18 kg	1 tsp t.i.d.	½ tsp t.i.d.
	40 mg/kg/day	
9 kg	1 tsp t.i.d.	½ tsp t.i.d.
18 kg		1 tsp t.i.d.

B.I.D. Treatment Option—For the treatment of otitis media and pharyngitis, the total daily dosage may be divided and administered every 12 hours.

Continued on next page

*** Identi-Code® symbol. This product information was prepared in June 1996. Current information on these and other products of Eli Lilly and Company may be obtained by direct inquiry to Lilly Research Laboratories, Lilly Corporate Center, Indianapolis, Indiana 46285, 800-545-5979.**

Consult 1997 supplements and future editions for revisions

Lilly—Cont.

Ceclor Suspension
20 mg/kg/day
(Pharyngitis)

Child's Weight	187 mg/5 mL	375 mg/5 mL
9 kg	½ tsp b.i.d.	
18 kg	1 tsp b.i.d.	½ tsp b.i.d.
	40 mg/kg/day (Otitis Media)	
9 kg	1 tsp b.i.d.	½ tsp b.i.d.
18 kg		1 tsp b.i.d.

Ceclor may be administered in the presence of impaired renal function. Under such a condition, the dosage usually is unchanged (*see* Precautions).

In the treatment of β-hemolytic streptococcal infections, a therapeutic dosage of Ceclor should be administered for at least 10 days.

HOW SUPPLIED

Pulvules:

250 mg, purple and white (No. 3061)—(RxPak* of 15) NDC 0002-3061-15; (100s) NDC 0002-3061-02; (ID†100) NDC 0002-3061-33

500 mg, purple and gray (No. 3062)—(RxPak of 15) NDC 0002-3062-15; (100s) NDC 0002-3062-02; (ID100) NDC 0002-3062-33

For Oral Suspension:

125 mg/5 mL, strawberry flavor (M-5057‡)—(75-mL size) NDC 0002-5057-18; (150-mL size) NDC 0002-5057-68

187 mg/5 mL, strawberry flavor (M-5130‡)—(50-mL size) NDC 0002-5130-87; (100-mL size) NDC 0002-5130-48

250 mg/5 mL, strawberry flavor (M-5058‡)—(75-mL size) NDC 0002-5058-18; (150-mL size) NDC 0002-5058-68

375 mg/5 mL, strawberry flavor (M-5132‡)—(50-mL size) NDC 0002-5132-87; (100-mL size) NDC 0002-5132-48

* All RxPaks (prescription packages, Lilly) have safety closures.

† Identi-Dose® (unit dose medication, Lilly).

‡ After mixing, store in a refrigerator. Shake well before using. Keep tightly closed. The mixture may be kept for 14 days without significant loss of potency. Discard unused portion after 14 days.

Store at controlled room temperature, 59° to 86°F (15° to 30°C).

* Bauer AW, Kirby, WMM, Sherris JC, and Turck M: Antibiotic susceptibility testing by a standardized single disk method. *Am J Clin Pathol* 1966;45:493. Standardized disk susceptibility test. *Federal Register* 1974;39:19182-19184.

[010996]

CAUTION-Federal (USA) law prohibits dispensing without prescription.

Literature revised January 9, 1996

Shown in Product Identification Guide, page 322

CEFACLOR, *see* Ceclor® (Cefaclor, USP). ℞

CEFAMANDOLE NAFATE, *see* Mandol® (Cefamandole Nafate, USP). ℞

CEFAZOLIN SODIUM, *see* Kefzol® (Cefazolin Sodium, USP). ℞

CEFTAZIDIME, *see* Tazidime® (Ceftazidime, USP). ℞

CEFUROXIME SODIUM, *see* Kefurox® (Cefuroxime Sodium, USP). ℞

CRYSTODIGIN® ℞

[*krĭs-tō-dĭj´ĭn*]

(digitoxin)

Tablets, USP

DESCRIPTION

Crystodigin® (Digitoxin Tablets, USP, Lilly) is a crystalline-pure single cardiac glycoside obtained from *Digitalis purpurea* and is identical in pharmacologic action with whole-leaf digitalis.

Digitoxin is the most slowly excreted of all digitalis compounds (excretion time is 14 to 21 days). It is most useful in patients with impaired renal function, since excretion and metabolism are independent of renal function.

Crystodigin is noted for its uniform potency, complete absorption, and lack of gastrointestinal irritation. It permits accurate dosage adjustments to produce maximum therapeutic effect smoothly and dependably.

Crystodigin, for oral administration, is available in tablets containing 0.05 mg (0.07 μmol) or 0.1 mg (0.13 μmol) crystalline digitoxin. The tablets also contain cornstarch, lactose, magnesium stearate, and povidone. The 0.05-mg tablet also contains FD&C Yellow No. 6, and the 0.1-mg tablet also contains FD&C Red No. 40.

Digitoxin is a cardiotonic glycoside. The chemical name is card-20 (22)-enolide, 3- [(*O* -2,6-dideoxy-β-D-*ribo*-hexopyranosyl-(1→4) -*O* - 2, 6-dideoxy-β- D - *ribo* -hexopyranosyl- (1→4) - 2,6- dideoxy- β -D- *ribo*-hexopyranosyl)oxy]-14-hydroxy, (3β,-5β) -. The empirical formula of digitoxin is $C_{41}H_{64}O_{13}$, and the structural formula is as follows:

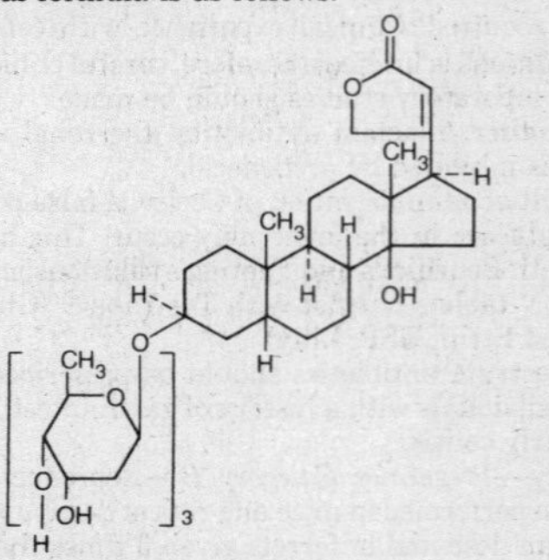

CLINICAL PHARMACOLOGY

The cellular basis for the inotropic effects of digitalis is probably enhancement of excitation-contraction coupling, that process by which chemical energy is converted into mechanical energy when triggered by membrane depolarization. Most evidence relates this process to the entry of calcium ions into the cell during depolarization of the membrane and/or to the release of calcium from intracellular binding sites on the sarcoplasmic reticulum. The free calcium ion mediates the interaction of actin and myosin, resulting in contraction.

The amount of glycoside absorbed depends largely on its polarity, which is a function of the net electronic charge on the molecule. The more nonpolar or lipid-soluble, the better is the absorption, because of the greater permeability of lipid membrane of the intestinal mucosa for lipid-soluble substances. The nonpolar, lipophilic digitoxin is completely absorbed. Other glycosides are not as well absorbed.

Nonpolar digitoxin is over 90% bound to tissue proteins. The firm binding of digitoxin to protein is responsible for its long half-life (7 to 9 days).

Digitoxin differs from other commonly used glycosides not only in its firm binding to protein but also because it is metabolized in the liver, with the only active metabolite being digoxin, which represents only a small fraction of the total metabolites. All other metabolites are inert and are probably excreted as such in the urine. The portion of digitoxin that is not metabolized is excreted in the bile to the intestines and recycled to the liver until it is completely metabolized. The portion of digitoxin that is bound to protein is in equilibrium with free digitoxin in the serum. Thus, as more and more of the free digitoxin is metabolized after a single dose, there is proportionately less bound digitoxin.

INDICATIONS AND USAGE

Crystodigin is indicated in the treatment of heart failure, atrial flutter, atrial fibrillation, and supraventricular tachycardia.

CONTRAINDICATIONS

If the indications are carefully observed, there are few contraindications to digitalis therapy except toxic response or idiosyncrasy to digitalis, ventricular tachycardia, beriberi, heart disease, and some instances of the hypersensitive carotid sinus syndrome.

Patients already taking digitalis preparations must not be given the rapid digitalizing dose of Crystodigin or parenteral calcium.

WARNINGS

Many of the arrhythmias for which digitalis is advised are identical with those reflecting digitalis intoxication. When the possibility of digitalis intoxication cannot be excluded, cardiac glycosides should be withheld temporarily if the clinical situation permits.

The patient with congestive heart failure may complain of nausea and vomiting. Since these symptoms may also be associated with digitalis intoxication, a clinical determination of their cause must be attempted before further administration of the drug.

Cases of idiopathic hypertrophic subaortic stenosis must be managed with extreme care. Unless cardiac failure is severe, it is doubtful whether digitalis should be employed.

NOTE: Digitalis glycosides are an important cause of accidental poisoning in children.

PRECAUTIONS

General —When the risk of digitalis intoxication is great, the use of a short-acting, rapidly eliminated glycoside, such as digoxin, is advisable. Although intoxication cannot always be prevented by the selection of one glycoside over another, certain glycosides may be preferred in patients who have fixed disabilities (eg, liver impairment, drug intolerance). However, digitoxin can be used in patients with impaired renal function.

Special care must be exercised in elderly patients receiving digitalis, because their body mass tends to be small and renal clearance is likely to be reduced. Frequent electrocardiographic monitoring is important in these patients. In addition, digitalis must be used cautiously in the presence of active heart disease, such as acute myocardial infarction or acute myocarditis. In patients with acute or unstable chronic atrial fibrillation, digitalis may not normalize the ventricular rate even when the serum concentration exceeds the usual therapeutic level. Although these patients may be less sensitive to the toxic effects of digitalis than are patients with normal sinus rhythm, dosage should not be increased to potentially toxic levels.

Hypokalemia predisposes to digitalis toxicity, and even a moderate decrease in the concentration of serum potassium can precipitate serious arrhythmias.

Impaired liver function may necessitate reduction in dosage of any digitalis preparation, including digitoxin.

Sensitive radioimmunoassay techniques have been developed for measuring serum levels of digitoxin, and these procedures can be instituted in almost any hospital. Serum levels must, however, be evaluated in conjunction with clinical history and the results of the electrocardiogram and other laboratory tests. A therapeutic serum level for one patient may be excessive or inadequate for another patient.

Drug Interactions —The synthesis of microsomal enzymes that metabolize digitoxin in the liver is subject to stimulation by a number of drugs, such as antihistamines, anticonvulsants, barbiturates, oral hypoglycemic agents, and others.

When digitoxin is the glycoside used for digitalis maintenance, drugs that are liver-microsomal enzyme inducers should not be used at the same time. Phenobarbital, phenylbutazone, and diphenylhydantoin will increase the rate of metabolism of digitoxin. In patients receiving 60 mg of phenobarbital 3 times a day for 12 weeks, the steady-state concentration of digitoxin in plasma fell approximately 50% when the drugs were administered concurrently and returned to previous levels when phenobarbital was discontinued.

When drugs that increase the rate of metabolism of digitoxin in the liver are discontinued, toxicity may occur.

Hypokalemia is most frequently encountered in patients receiving concomitant diuretic therapy, because the most widely used and most effective diuretics (ie, thiazides and furosemide) increase the urinary loss of potassium. Prescribing a potassium-sparing agent (spironolactone or triamterene) together with the potassium-wasting diuretic is a reliable means for maintaining the serum potassium level. Alternatively, potassium chloride supplements may be prescribed.

Mineralocorticoids (eg, prednisone) and, rarely, certain antibiotics (eg, amphotericin B) may also cause increased excretion of potassium.

Usage in Pregnancy —Pregnancy Category C —Animal reproduction studies have not been conducted with Crystodigin. It is also not known whether this drug can cause fetal harm when administered to a pregnant woman or can affect reproduction capacity. Crystodigin should be given to a pregnant woman only if clearly needed.

Labor and Delivery —No information is available concerning the use of Crystodigin in labor and delivery.

Nursing Mothers —It is not known whether this drug is excreted in human breast milk. Because many drugs are excreted in human breast milk, caution should be exercised when Crystodigin is administered to a nursing woman.

ADVERSE REACTIONS

Anorexia, nausea, and vomiting have been reported. These effects are central in origin, but following large oral doses, there is also a local emetic action. Abdominal discomfort or pain and diarrhea may also occur.

OVERDOSAGE

Signs and Symptoms —Symptoms may include alterations in mental status, nausea, vomiting, bradycardia, visual disturbances, heart block, and all known cardiac arrhythmias. Hyperkalemia may be present following acute overdose, whereas hypokalemia is associated with chronic overdose. Peak toxic effects following acute overdose may be delayed up to 12 hours.

Older patients, particularly those with coronary insufficiency, are more susceptible to dysrhythmias. Ventricular fibrillation is the most common cause of death from digitalis poisoning. There is insufficient information to accurately determine the minimum toxic or lethal dose in humans. Death from ventricular fibrillation was reported 24 hours after admission in a patient with a plasma concentration of 124 ng/mL shortly before death.

Treatment —To obtain up-to-date information about the treatment of overdose, a good resource is your certified Regional Poison Control Center. Telephone numbers of certified poison control centers are listed in the *Physicians' Desk Reference (PDR)*. In managing overdosage, consider the possi-

bility of multiple drug overdoses, interaction among drugs, and unusual drug kinetics in your patient.

Continuous ECG monitoring is necessary. For any suspected digitoxin-induced dysrhythmia, discontinue the drug. Monitor potassium and digitoxin concentrations. Severe hyperkalemia may require administration of sodium bicarbonate, glucose, and regular insulin.

Protect the patient's airway and support ventilation and perfusion. Meticulously monitor and maintain, within acceptable limits, the patient's vital signs, blood gases, serum electrolytes, etc. Absorption of drugs from the gastrointestinal tract may be decreased by giving activated charcoal, which, in many cases, is more effective than emesis or lavage; consider charcoal instead of or in addition to gastric emptying. Repeated doses of charcoal over time may hasten elimination of some drugs that have been absorbed. Safeguard the patient's airway when employing gastric emptying or charcoal.

Atropine or a pacemaker may be used for bradycardia and heart block. Phenytoin (15 mg/kg), at a rate not to exceed 50 mg/min, may be useful for treating ventricular dysrhythmias and to improve atrioventricular conduction. Lidocaine may also be used, but impaired AV conduction may require a pacemaker. Consider use of digitalis-specific Fab fragments.

Forced diuresis, peritoneal dialysis, hemodialysis, or charcoal hemoperfusion have not been established as beneficial for an overdose of Crystodigin.

DOSAGE AND ADMINISTRATION

Adults: *Slow Digitalization* —0.2 mg twice daily for a period of 4 days, followed by maintenance dosage.
Rapid Digitalization —Preferably 0.6 mg initially, followed by 0.4 mg and then 0.2 mg at intervals of 4 to 6 hours.
Maintenance Dosage —Ranges from 0.05 to 0.3 mg daily, the most common dose being 0.15 mg daily.

HOW SUPPLIED

Tablets (scored):
0.05 mg. orange (No. 1736)—(100s) NDC 0002-1075-02
0.1 mg, pink (No. 1703)—(100s) NDC 0002-1060-02
Protect from light. Store at controlled room temperature, 59° to 86°F (15° to 30°C).
CAUTION-Federal (USA) law prohibits dispensing without prescription.
Text revised June 5, 1990
Literature revised November 27, 1995   [112795]

CYCLOSERINE, *see* Seromycin® (Cycloserine, USP).

DARVOCET–N® 50
[där'vō-sĕt ĕn]
and
DARVOCET–N® 100
(propoxyphene napsylate
and acetaminophen tablets)
USP

© IV

DARVON–N®
[där'vŏn ĕn]
(propoxyphene napsylate)
USP

DESCRIPTION

Darvon-N® (Propoxyphene Napsylate, USP, Lilly) is an odorless, white crystalline powder with a bitter taste. It is very slightly soluble in water and soluble in methanol, ethanol, chloroform, and acetone. Chemically, it is $(\alpha S,1R)$-α-[2-(Dimethylamino) -1 -methylethyl]- α -phenylphenethyl propionate compound with 2-naphthalenesulfonic acid (1:1) monohydrate, which can be represented by the accompanying structural formula. Its molecular weight is 565.72.

Propoxyphene napsylate

Propoxyphene napsylate differs from propoxyphene hydrochloride in that it allows more stable liquid dosage forms and tablet formulations. Because of differences in molecular weight, a dose of 100 mg (176.8 μmol) of propoxyphene napsylate is required to supply an amount of propoxyphene equivalent to that present in 65 mg (172.9 μmol) of propoxyphene hydrochloride.

Each tablet of Darvocet-N 50 contains 50 mg (88.4 μmol) propoxyphene napsylate and 325 mg (2,150 μmol) acetaminophen.

Each tablet of Darvocet-N 100 contains 100 mg (176.8 μmol) propopoxyphene napsylate and 650 mg (4,300 μmol) acetaminophen.

Each tablet also contains amberlite, cellulose, F D & C Yellow No. 6, magnesium stearate, stearic acid, titanium dioxide, and other inactive ingredients.

CLINICAL PHARMACOLOGY

Propoxyphene is a centrally acting narcotic analgesic agent. Equimolar doses of propoxyphene hydrochloride or napsylate provide similar plasma concentrations. Following administration of 65, 130, or 195 mg of propoxyphene hydrochloride, the bioavailability of propoxyphene is equivalent to that of 100, 200, or 300 mg respectively of propoxyphene napsylate. Peak plasma concentrations of propoxyphene are reached in 2 to 2 $^1/_2$ hours. After a 100-mg oral dose of propoxyphene napsylate, peak plasma levels of 0.05 to 0.1 μg/mL are achieved. As shown in Figure 1, the napsylate salt tends to be absorbed more slowly than the hydrochloride. At or near therapeutic doses, this absorption difference is small when compared with that among subjects and among doses.

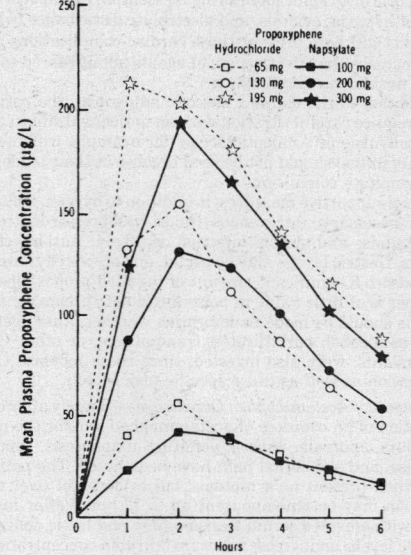

Figure 1. Mean plasma concentrations of propoxyphene in 8 human subjects following oral administration of 65 and 130 mg of the hydrochloride salt and 100 and 200 mg of the napsylate salt and in 7 given 195 mg of the hydrochloride and 300 mg of the napsylate salt.

Because of this several hundredfold difference in solubility, the absorption rate of very large doses of the napsylate salt is significantly lower than that of equimolar doses of the hydrochloride.

Repeated doses of propoxyphene at 6-hour intervals lead to increasing plasma concentrations, with a plateau after the ninth dose at 48 hours.

Propoxyphene is metabolized in the liver to yield norpropoxyphene. Propoxyphene has a half-life of 6 to 12 hours, whereas that of norpropoxyphene is 30 to 36 hours.

Norpropoxyphene has substantially less central-nervous-system-depressant effect than propoxyphene but a greater local anesthetic effect, which is similar to that of amitriptyline and antiarrhythmic agents, such as lidocaine and quinidine.

In animal studies in which propoxyphene and norpropoxyphene were continuously infused in large amounts, intracardiac conduction time (PR and QRS intervals) was prolonged. Any intracardiac conduction delay attributable to high concentrations of norpropoxyphene may be of relatively long duration.

ACTIONS

Propoxyphene is a mild narcotic analgesic structurally related to methadone. The potency of propoxyphene napsylate is from two-thirds to equal that of codeine.

Darvocet-N 50 and Darvocet-N 100 provide the analgesic activity of propoxyphene napsylate and the antipyretic-analgesic activity of acetaminophen.

The combination of propoxyphene and acetaminophen produces greater analgesia than that produced by either propoxyphene or acetaminophen administered alone.

INDICATION

Those products are indicated for the relief of mild to moderate pain, either when pain is present alone or when it is accompanied by fever.

CONTRAINDICATIONS

Hypersensitivity to propoxyphene or acetaminophen

WARNINGS

- **Do not prescribe propoxyphene for patients who are suicidal or addiction-prone.**
- **Prescribe propoxyphene with caution for patients taking tranquilizers or antidepressant drugs and patients who use alcohol in excess.**
- **Tell your patients not to exceed the recommended dose and to limit their intake of alcohol.**

Propoxyphene products in excessive doses, either alone or in combination with other CNS depressants, including alcohol, are a major cause of drug-related deaths. Fatalities within the first hour of overdosage are not uncommon. In a survey of deaths due to overdosage conducted in 1975, in approximately 20% of the fatal cases, death occurred within the first hour (5% occurred within 15 minutes). Propoxyphene should not be taken in doses higher than those recommended by the physician. The judicious prescribing of propoxyphene is essential to the safe use of this drug. With patients who are depressed or suicidal, consideration should be given to the use of non-narcotic analgesics. Patients should be cautioned about the concomitant use of propoxyphene products and alcohol because of potentially serious CNS-additive effects of these agents. Because of its added depressant effects, propoxyphene should be prescribed with caution for those patients whose medical condition requires the concomitant administration of sedatives, tranquilizers, muscle relaxants, antidepressants, or other CNS-depressant drugs. Patients should be advised of the additive depressant effects of these combinations.

Many of the propoxyphene-related deaths have occurred in patients with previous histories of emotional disturbances or suicidal ideation or attempts as well as histories of misuse of tranquilizers, alcohol, and other CNS-active drugs. Some deaths have occurred as a consequence of the accidental ingestion of excessive quantities of propoxyphene alone or in combination with other drugs. Patients taking propoxyphene should be warned not to exceed the dosage recommended by the physician.

Drug Dependence —Propoxyphene, when taken in higher-than-recommended doses over long periods of time, can produce drug dependence characterized by psychic dependence and, less frequently, physical dependence and tolerance. Propoxyphene will only partially suppress the withdrawal syndrome in individuals physically dependent on morphine or other narcotics. The abuse liability of propoxyphene is qualitatively similar to that of codeine although quantitatively less, and propoxyphene should be prescribed with the same degree of caution appropriate to the use of codeine.

Usage in Ambulatory Patients —Propoxyphene may impair the mental and/or physical abilities required for the performance of potentially hazardous tasks, such as driving a car or operating machinery. The patient should be cautioned accordingly.

PRECAUTIONS

General —Propoxyphene should be administered with caution to patients with hepatic or renal impairment since higher serum concentrations or delayed elimination may occur.

Drug Interactions —The CNS-depressant effect of propoxyphene is additive with that of other CNS depressants, including alcohol.

As is the case with many medicinal agents, propoxyphene may slow the metabolism of a concomitantly administered drug. Should this occur, the higher serum concentrations of that drug may result in increased phamacologic or adverse effects of that drug. Such occurrences have been reported when propoxyphene was administered to patients on antidepressants, anticonvulsants, or warfarin-like drugs. Severe neurologic signs, including coma, have occurred with concurrent use of carbamazepine.

Usage in Pregnancy —Safe use in pregnancy has not been established relative to possible adverse effects on fetal development. Instances of withdrawal symptoms in the neonate have been reported following usage during pregnancy. Therefore, propoxyphene should not be used in pregnant women unless, in the judgment of the physician, the potential benefits outweigh the possible hazards.

Continued on next page

• **Identi-Code® symbol. This product information was prepared in June 1996. Current information on these and other products of Eli Lilly and Company may be obtained by direct inquiry to Lilly Research Laboratories, Lilly Corporate Center, Indianapolis, Indiana 46285, 800-545-5979.**

Lilly—Cont.

Usage in Nursing Mothers—Low levels of propoxyphene have been detected in human milk. In postpartum studies involving nursing mothers who were given propoxyphene, no adverse effects were noted in infants receiving mother's milk.
Usage in Children—Propoxyphene is not recommended for use in children, because documented clinical experience has been insufficient to establish safety and a suitable dosage regimen in the pediatric age group.
Usage in the Elderly—The rate of propoxyphene metabolism may be reduced in some patients. Increased dosing interval should be considered.
A Patient Information Sheet is available for these products. See text following "How Supplied" section below.

ADVERSE REACTIONS

In a survey conducted in hospitalized patients, less than 1% of patients taking propoxyphene hydrochloride at recommended doses experienced side effects. The most frequently reported were dizziness, sedation, nausea, and vomiting. Some of these adverse reactions may be alleviated if the patient lies down.
Other adverse reactions include constipation, abdominal pain, skin rashes, lightheadedness, headache, weakness, euphoria, dysphoria, hallucinations, and minor visual disturbances.
Liver dysfunction has been reported in association with both active components of Darvocet-N 50 and Darvocet-N 100. Propoxyphene therapy has been associated with abnormal liver function tests and, more rarely, with instances of reversible jaundice (including cholestatic jaundice). Hepatic necrosis may result from acute overdose of acetaminophen (*see* Management of Overdosage). In chronic ethanol abusers, this has been reported rarely with short-term use of acetaminophen doses of 2.5 to 10 g/day. Fatalities have occurred.
Renal papillary necrosis may result from chronic acetaminophen use, particularly when the dosage is greater than recommended and when combined with aspirin.
Subacute painful myopathy has occurred following chronic propoxyphene overdosage.

DOSAGE AND ADMINISTRATION

These products are given orally. The usual dosage is 100 mg propoxyphene napsylate and 650 mg acetaminophen every 4 hours as needed for pain. The maximum recommended dose of propoxyphene napsylate is 600 mg/day.
Consideration should be given to a reduced total daily dosage in patients with hepatic or renal impairment.

MANAGEMENT OF OVERDOSAGE

In all cases of suspected overdosage, call your regional Poison Control Center to obtain the most up-to-date information about the treatment of overdose. This recommendation is made because, in general, information regarding the treatment of overdosage may change more rapidly than do package inserts.
Initial consideration should be given to the management of the CNS effects of propoxyphene overdosage. Resuscitative measures should be initiated promptly.
Symptoms of Propoxyphene Overdosage—The manifestations of acute overdosage with propoxyphene are those of narcotic overdosage. The patient is usually somnolent but may be stuporous or comatose and convulsing. Respiratory depression is characteristic. The ventilatory rate and/or tidal volume is decreased, which results in cyanosis and hypoxia. Pupils, initially pinpoint, may become dilated as hypoxia increases. Cheyne-Stokes respiration and apnea may occur. Blood pressure and heart rate are usually normal initially, but blood pressure falls and cardiac performance deteriorates, which ultimately results in pulmonary edema and circulatory collapse, unless the respiratory depression is corrected and adequate ventilation is restored promptly. Cardiac arrhythmias and conduction delay may be present. A combined respiratory-metabolic acidosis occurs owing to retained CO_2 (hypercapnia) and to lactic acid formed during anaerobic glycolysis. Acidosis may be severe if large amounts of salicylates have also been ingested. Death may occur.
Treatment of Propoxyphene Overdosage—Attention should be directed first to establishing a patent airway and to restoring ventilation. Mechanically assisted ventilation, with or without oxygen, may be required, and positive pressure respiration may be desirable if pulmonary edema is present. The narcotic antagonist naloxone will markedly reduce the degree of respiratory depression, and 0.4 to 2 mg should be administered promptly, preferably intravenously. If the desired degree of counteraction with improvement in respiratory functions is not obtained, naloxone should be repeated at 2- to 3-minute intervals. The duration of action of the antagonist may be brief. If no response is observed after 10 mg of naloxone have been administered, the diagnosis of propoxyphene toxicity should be questioned. Naloxone may also be administered by continuous intravenous infusion.
Treatment of Propoxyphene Overdosage in Children—The usual initial dose of naloxone in children is 0.01 mg/kg body weight given intravenously. If this dose does not result in the desired degree of clinical improvement, a subsequent increased dose of 0.1 mg/kg body weight may be administered. If an IV route of administration is not available, naloxone may be administered IM or subcutaneously in divided doses. If necessary, naloxone can be diluted with Sterile Water for Injection.
Blood gases, pH, and electrolytes should be monitored in order that acidosis and any electrolyte disturbance present may be corrected promptly. Acidosis, hypoxia, and generalized CNS depression predispose to the development of cardiac arrhythmias. Ventricular fibrillation or cardiac arrest may occur and necessitate the full complement of cardiopulmonary resuscitation (CPR) measures. Respiratory acidosis rapidly subsides as ventilation is restored and hypercapnia eliminated, but lactic acidosis may require intravenous bicarbonate for prompt correction.
Electrocardiographic monitoring is essential. Prompt correction of hypoxia, acidosis, and electrolyte disturbance (when present) will help prevent these cardiac complications and will increase the effectiveness of agents administered to restore normal cardiac function.
In addition to the use of a narcotic antagonist, the patient may require careful titration with an anticonvulsant to control convulsions. Analeptic drugs (for example, caffeine or amphetamine) should not be used because of their tendency to precipitate convulsions.
General supportive measures, in addition to oxygen, include, when necessary, intravenous fluids, vasopressor-inotropic compounds, and, when infection is likely, anti-infective agents. Gastric lavage may be useful, and activated charcoal can adsorb a significant amount of ingested propoxyphene. Dialysis is of little value in poisoning due to propoxyphene. Efforts should be made to determine whether other agents, such as alcohol, barbiturates, tranquilizers, or other CNS depressants, were also ingested, since these increase CNS depression as well as cause specific toxic effects.
Symptoms of Acetaminophen Overdosage—Shortly after oral ingestion of an overdose of acetaminophen and for the next 24 hours, anorexia, nausea, vomiting, diaphoresis, general malaise, and abdominal pain have been noted. The patient may then present no symptoms, but evidence of liver dysfunction may become apparent up to 72 hours after ingestion, with elevated serum transaminase and lactic dehydrogenase levels, an increase in serum bilirubin concentrations, and a prolonged prothrombin time. Death from hepatic failure may result 3 to 7 days after overdosage.
Acute renal failure may accompany the hepatic dysfunction and has been noted in patients who do not exhibit signs of fulminant hepatic failure. Typically, renal impairment is more apparent 6 to 9 days after ingestion of the overdose.
Treatment of Acetaminophen Overdosage—Acetaminophen in massive overdosage may cause hepatic toxicity in some patients. *In all cases of suspected overdose, immediately call your regional poison center or the Rocky Mountain Poison Center's toll-free number* (800-525-6115) for assistance in diagnosis and for directions in the use of N-acetylcysteine as an antidote.
In adults, hepatic toxicity has rarely been reported with acute overdoses of less than 10 g and fatalities with less than 15 g. Importantly, young children seem to be more resistant than adults to the hepatotoxic effect of an acetaminophen overdose. Despite this, the measures outlined below should be initiated in any adult or child suspected of having ingested an acetaminophen overdose.
Because clinical and laboratory evidence of hepatic toxicity may not be apparent until 48 to 72 hours postingestion, liver function studies should be obtained initially and repeated at 24-hour intervals.
Consider emptying the stomach promptly by lavage or by induction of emesis with syrup of ipecac. Patients' estimates of the quantity of a drug ingested are notoriously unreliable. Therefore, if an acetaminophen overdose is suspected, a serum acetaminophen assay should be obtained as early as possible, but no sooner than 4 hours following ingestion. The antidote, N-acetylcysteine, should be administered as early as possible, and within 16 hours of the overdose ingestion for optimal results. Following recovery, there are no residual, structural, or functional hepatic abnormalities.

ANIMAL TOXICOLOGY

The acute lethal doses of the hydrochloride and napsylate salts of propoxyphene were determined in 4 species. The results shown in Figure 2 indicate that, on a molar basis, the napsylate salt is less toxic than the hydrochloride. This may be due to the relative insolubility and retarded absorption of propoxyphene napsylate.

Figure 2. Acute oral toxicity of propoxyphene

Species	Propoxyphene Hydrochloride	Propoxyphene Napsylate
	LD_{50} (mg/kg) ± SE / LD_{50} (mmol/kg)	LD_{50} (mg/kg) ± SE / LD_{50} (mmol/kg)
Mouse	282 ± 39	915 ± 163
	0.75	1.62
Rat	230 ± 44	647 ± 95
	0.61	1.14
Rabbit	*ca.* 82	>183
	0.22	>0.32
Dog	*ca.* 100	>183
	0.27	>0.32

Some indication of the relative insolubility and retarded absorption of propoxyphene napsylate was obtained by measuring plasma propoxyphene levels in 2 groups of 4 dogs following oral administration of equimolar doses of the 2 salts. As shown in Figure 3, the peak plasma concentration observed with propoxyphene hydrochloride was much higher than that obtained after administration of the napsylate salt.

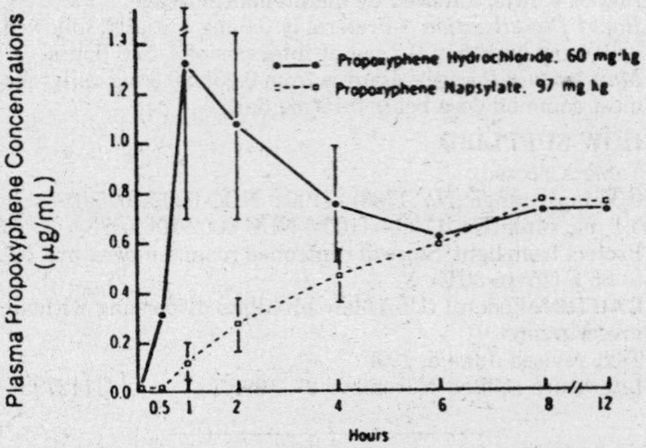

Figure 3. Plasma propoxyphene concentrations in dogs following large doses of the hydrochloride and napsylate salts.

Although none of the animals in this experiment died, 3 of the 4 dogs given propoxyphene hydrochloride exhibited convulsive seizures during the time interval corresponding to the peak plasma levels. The 4 animals receiving the napsylate salt were mildly ataxic but not acutely ill.

HOW SUPPLIED

Darvocet-N® Tablets (No. 1890) are available in:
The 50 mg tablets are dark orange, capsule shaped, film coated, and imprinted with the script "Lilly" and "Darvocet-N 50" on one side of the tablet, using edible black ink. They are available as follows:

Bottles of 100 (RxPak*)	NDC 0002-0351-02 (TA1890)

Darvocet-N® Tablets (No. 1893) are available in:
The 100 mg tablets are dark orange, capsule shaped, film coated, and imprinted with the script "Lilly" on one side and "Darvocet-N 100" on the other side of the tablet, using edible black ink. They are available as follows:

Bottles of 100 (RxPak*)	NDC 0002-0363-02 (TA1893)
Bottles of 500	NDC 0002-0363-03 (TA1893)
ID† 100	NDC 0002-0363-33 (TA1893)
ID† 500	NDC 0002-0363-43 (TA1893)
RN‡ 500	NDC 0002-0363-46 (TA1893)

* All RxPaks (prescription packages, Lilly) have safety closures.
† Identi-Dose® (unit dose medication, Lilly).
‡ Reverse-numbered package.
Store at controlled room temperature, 59° to 86°F (15° to 30°C).

[031496]

The following information, including description of dosage forms and the maximum daily dosage of each, is available to patients receiving Darvon products.

Patient Information Sheet
YOUR PRESCRIPTION FOR A DARVON® (PROPOXYPHENE) PRODUCT ©
Summary

Products containing Darvon are used to relieve pain.
LIMIT YOUR INTAKE OF ALCOHOL WHILE TAKING THIS DRUG. Make sure your doctor knows if you are taking tranquilizers, sleep aids, antidepressants, antihistamines, or any other drugs that make you sleepy. Combining propoxyphene with alcohol or these drugs in excessive doses is dangerous.

Use care while driving a car or using machines until you see how the drug affects you because propoxyphene can make you sleepy. Do not take more of the drug than your doctor prescribed. Dependence has occurred when patients have taken propoxyphene for a long period of time at doses greater than recommended.

The rest of this leaflet gives you more information about propoxyphene. Please read it and keep it for future use.

Uses of Darvon

Products containing Darvon are used for the relief of mild to moderate pain. Products that contain Darvon plus aspirin or acetaminophen are prescribed for the relief of pain or pain associated with fever.

Before Taking Darvon

Make sure your doctor knows if you have ever had an allergic reaction to propoxyphene, aspirin, or acetaminophen. Some forms of propoxyphene products contain aspirin to help relieve the pain. Your doctor should be advised if you have a history of ulcers or if your are taking an anticoagulant ("blood thinner"). The aspirin may irritate the stomach lining and may cause bleeding, particularly if an ulcer is present. Also, bleeding may occur if you are taking an anticoagulant. In a small group of people, aspirin may cause an asthma attack. If you are one of these people, be sure your drug does not contain aspirin.

The effect of propoxyphene in children under 12 has not been studied. Therefore, use of the drug in this age group is not recommended.

Also, due to the possible association between aspirin and Reye Syndrome, those propoxyphene products containing aspirin should not be given to children, including teenagers, with chicken pox or flu unless prescribed by a physician. The following propoxyphene product contains aspirin:

Darvon® Compound-65 (Propoxyphene Hydrochloride, Aspirin, and Caffeine, USP, Lilly)

How to Take Darvon

Follow your doctor's directions exactly. Do not increase the amount you take without your doctor's approval. If you miss a dose of the drug, do not take twice as much the next time.

Pregnancy

Do not take propoxyphene during pregnancy unless your doctor knows you are pregnant and specifically recommends its use. Cases of temporary dependence in the newborn have occurred when the mother has taken propoxyphene consistently in the weeks before delivery. As a general principle, no drug should be taken during pregnancy unless it is clearly necessary.

General Cautions

Heavy use of alcohol with propoxyphene is hazardous and may lead to overdosage symptoms (*see* "Overdose" below). THEREFORE, LIMIT YOUR INTAKE OF ALCOHOL WHILE TAKING PROPOXYPHENE.

Combinations of excessive doses of propoxyphene, alcohol, and tranquilizers are dangerous. Make sure your doctor knows if you are taking tranquilizers, sleep aids, antidepressant drugs, antihistamines, or any other drugs that make you sleepy. The use of these drugs with propoxyphene increases their sedative effects and may lead to overdosage symptoms, including death (*see* "Overdose" below).

Propoxyphene may cause drowsiness or impair your mental and/or physical abilities; therefore, use caution when driving a vehicle or operating dangerous machinery. DO NOT perform any hazardous task until you have seen your response to this drug.

Propoxyphene may increase the concentration in the body of medications, such as anticoagulants ("blood thinners"), antidepressants, or drugs used for epilepsy. The result may be excessive or adverse effects of these medications. Make sure your doctor knows if you are taking any of these medications.

Dependence

You can become dependent on propoxyphene if you take it in higher than recommended doses over a long period of time. Dependence is a feeling of need for the drug and a feeling that you cannot perform normally without it.

Overdose

An overdose of Darvon, alone or in combination with other drugs, including alcohol, may cause weakness, difficulty in breathing, confusion, anxiety, and more severe drowsiness and dizziness. Extreme overdosage may lead to unconsciousness and death.

If the propoxyphene product contains acetaminophen, the overdosage symptoms include nausea, vomiting, lack of appetite, and abdominal pain. Liver damage may occur even after symptoms disappear. Death can occur days later.

When the propoxyphene product contains aspirin, symptoms of taking to much of the drug are headache, dizziness, ringing in the ears, difficulty in hearing, dim vision, confusion, drowsiness, sweating, thirst, rapid breathing, nausea, vomiting, and, occasionally, diarrhea.

In any suspected overdosage situation, contact your doctor or nearest hospital emergency room. GET EMERGENCY HELP IMMEDIATELY.

KEEP THIS DRUG AND ALL DRUGS OUT OF THE REACH OF CHILDREN.

Possible Side Effects

When propoxyphene is taken as directed, side effects are infrequent. Among those reported are drowsiness, dizziness, nausea, and vomiting. If these effects occur, it may help if you lie down and rest.

Less frequently reported side effects are constipation, abdominal pain, skin rashes, lightheadedness, headache, weakness, hallucinations, minor visual disturbances, and feelings of elation or discomfort.

If side effects occur and concern you, contact your doctor.

Other Information

The safe and effective use of propoxyphene depends on your taking it exactly as directed. This drug has been prescribed specifically for you and your present condition. Do not give this drug to others who may have similar symptoms. Do not use it for any other reason.

If you would like more information about propoxyphene, ask your doctor or pharmacist. They have a more technical leaflet (professional labeling) you may read.

Selected Darvon Products

Maximum Daily Dosage		
6	Dark Orange, Capsule Shaped, Film Coated Tablets Imprinted with Script "Lilly" on the one side and "Darvocet-N 100" on the other, using edible black ink	DARVOCET-N® 100 Ⓒ Propoxyphene Napsylate and Acetaminophen Tablets
6	Parabolic-Shaped Capsules Imprinted with Script "Lilly" and "3111" on the opaque gray cap and "Darvon Comp 65" on the opaque red body, using edible black ink	DARVON® COMPOUND-65 Ⓒ Propoxyphene Hydrochloride, Aspirin, and Caffeine Pulvules®
6	Parabolic-Shaped Capsules Imprinted with Script "Lilly" and "H03" on the opaque pink cap and "Darvon" on the opaque pink body, using edible black ink	DARVON® Ⓒ Propoxyphene Hydrochloride Pulvules, 65 mg

Literature revised March 14, 1996

Shown in Product Identification Guide, page 322

DARVON® Ⓒ

[*där'von*]

(propoxyphene hydrochloride)
Capsules, USP

DARVON® COMPOUND-65

(propoxyphene hydrochloride, aspirin, and caffeine)

[*där'vŏn kŏm'pound*]

DESCRIPTION

Darvon® (Propoxyphene Hydrochloride, USP, Lilly) is an odorless, white crystalline powder with a bitter taste. It is freely soluble in water. Chemically, it is (2*S*, 3*R*)-(+)-4-(Dimethylamino)-3-methyl- 1,2-diphenyl-2-butanol propionate (ester) hydrochloride, which can be represented by the accompanying structural formula. Its molecular weight is 375.94.

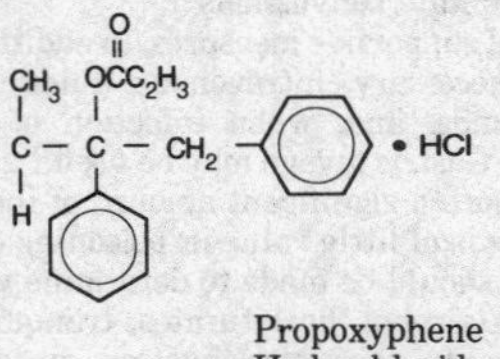

Propoxyphene Hydrochloride

Each Pulvule® Darvon contains 65 mg (172.9 μmol) propoxyphene hydrochloride, 389 mg (2,159 μmol) aspirin, and 32.4 mg (166.8 μmol) caffeine.

It also contains F D & C Red No. 3, F D & C Yellow No. 6, gelatin, glutamic acid hydrochloride, iron oxide, kaolin, silicone, titanium dioxide, and other inactive ingredients.

CLINICAL PHARMACOLOGY

Propoxyphene is a centrally acting narcotic analgesic agent. Equimolar doses of propoxyphene hydrochloride or napsylate provide similar plasma concentrations. Following administration of 65, 130, or 195 mg of propoxyphene hydrochloride, the bioavailability of propoxyphene is equivalent to that of 100, 200, or 300 mg respectively of propoxyphene napsylate. Peak plasma concentrations of propoxyphene are reached in 2 to 2 1/2 hours. After a 65-mg oral dose of propoxyphene hydrochloride, peak plasma levels of 0.05 to 0.1 μg/mL are achieved.

Repeated doses of propoxyphene at 6-hour intervals lead to increasing plasma concentrations, with a plateau after the ninth dose at 48 hours.

Propoxyphene is metabolized in the liver to yield norpropoxyphene. Propoxyphene has a half-life of 6 to 12 hours, whereas that of norpropoxyphene is 30 to 36 hours.

Norpropoxyphene has substantially less central-nervous-system-depressant effect than propoxyphene but a greater local anesthetic effect, which is similar to that of amitriptyline and antiarrhythmic agents, such as lidocaine and quinidine.

In animal studies in which propoxyphene and norpropoxyphene were continuously infused in large amounts, intracardiac conduction time (PR and QRS intervals) was prolonged. Any intracardiac conduction delay attributable to high concentrations of norpropoxyphene may be of relatively long duration.

ACTIONS

Propoxyphene is a mild narcotic analgesic structurally related to methadone. The potency of propoxyphene hydrochloride is from two-thirds to equal that of codeine.

The combination of propoxyphene with a mixture of aspirin and caffeine produces greater analgesia than that produced by either propoxyphene or aspirin and caffeine administered alone.

INDICATION

This product is indicated for the relief of mild to moderate pain, either when pain is present alone or when it is accompanied by fever.

CONTRAINDICATION

Hypersensitivity to propoxyphene, aspirin, or caffeine.

WARNINGS

- **Do not prescribe propoxyphene for patients who are suicidal or addiction-prone.**
- **Prescribe propoxyphene with caution for patients taking tranquilizers or antidepressant drugs and patients who use alcohol in excess.**
- **Tell your patients not to exceed the recommended dose and to limit their intake of alcohol.**

Propoxyphene products in excessive doses, either alone or in combination with other CNS depressants, including alcohol, are a major cause of drug-related deaths. Fatalities within the first hour of overdosage are not uncommon. In a survey of deaths due to overdosage conducted in 1975, in approximately 20% of the fatal cases, death occurred within the first hour (5% occurred within 15 minutes). Propoxyphene should not be taken in doses higher than those recommended by the physician. The judicious prescribing of propoxyphene is essential to the safe use of this drug. With patients who are depressed or suicidal, consideration should be given to the use of non-narcotic analgesics. Patients should be cautioned about the concomitant use of propoxyphene products and alcohol because of potentially serious CNS-additive effects of these agents. Because of its added depressant effects, propoxyphene should be prescribed with caution for those patients whose medical condition requires the concomitant administration of sedatives, tranquilizers, muscle relaxants, antidepressants, or other CNS-depressant drugs. Patients should be advised of the additive depressant effects of these combinations.

Many of the propoxyphene-related deaths have occurred in patients with previous histories of emotional disturbances or suicidal ideation or attempts as well as histories of misuse of tranquilizers, alcohol, and other CNS-active drugs. Some deaths have occurred as a consequence of the accidental ingestion of excessive quantities of propoxyphene alone or in combination with other drugs. Patients taking propoxyphene should be warned not to exceed the dosage recommended by the physician.

Drug Dependence—Propoxyphene, when taken in higher-than-recommended doses over long periods of time, can produce drug dependence characterized by psychic dependence and, less frequently, physical dependence and tolerance. Propoxyphene will only partially suppress the withdrawal syndrome in individuals physically dependent on morphine

Continued on next page

• Identi-Code® symbol. This product information was prepared in June 1996. Current information on these and other products of Eli Lilly and Company may be obtained by direct inquiry to Lilly Research Laboratories, Lilly Corporate Center, Indianapolis, Indiana 46285, 800-545-5979.

Lilly—Cont.

or other narcotics. The abuse liability of propoxyphene is qualitatively similar to that of codeine although quantitatively less, and propoxyphene should be prescribed with the same degree of caution appropriate to the use of codeine.

Usage in Ambulatory Patients —Propoxyphene may impair the mental and/or physical abilities required for the performance of potentially hazardous tasks, such as driving a car or operating machinery. The patient should be cautioned accordingly.

Warning —Reye Syndrome is a rare but serious disease which can follow flu or chicken pox in children and teenagers. While the cause of Reye Syndrome is unknown, some reports claim aspirin (or salicylates) may increase the risk of developing this disease.

PRECAUTIONS

General —Salicylates should be used with extreme caution in the presence of peptic ulcer or coagulation abnormalities. Propoxyphene should be administered with caution to patients with hepatic or renal impairment since higher serum concentrations or delayed elimination may occur.

Drug Interactions —The CNS-depressant effect of propoxyphene is additive with that of other CNS depressants, including alcohol.

Salicylates may enhance the effect of anticoagulants and inhibit the uricosuric effect of uricosuric agents.

As is the case with medicinal agents, propoxyphene may slow the metabolism of a concomitantly administered drug. Should this occur, the higher serum concentrations of that drug may result in increased pharmacologic or adverse effects of that drug. Such occurrences have been reported when propoxyphene was administered to patients on antidepressants, anticonvulsants, or warfarin-like drugs. Severe neurologic signs, including coma, have occurred with concurrent use of carbamazepine.

Usage in Pregnancy —Safe use in pregnancy has not been established relative to possible adverse effects on fetal development. Instances of withdrawal symptoms in the neonate have been reported following usage during pregnancy. Therefore, propoxyphene should not be used in pregnant women unless, in the judgment of the physician, the potential benefits outweigh the possible hazards. Aspirin does not appear to have teratogenic effects. However, prolonged pregnancy and labor with increased bleeding before and after delivery, decreased birth weight, and increased rate of stillbirth were reported with high blood salicylate levels. Because of possible adverse effects on the neonate and the potential for increased maternal blood loss, aspirin should be avoided during the last 3 months of pregnancy.

Usage in Nursing Mothers —Low levels of propoxyphene have been detected in human milk. In postpartum studies involving nursing mothers who were given propoxyphene, no adverse effects were noted in infants receiving mother's milk.

Usage in Children —Propoxyphene is not recommended for use in children, because documented clinical experience has been insufficient to establish safety and a suitable dosage regimen in the pediatric age group.

Usage in the Elderly —The rate of propoxyphene metabolism may be reduced in some patients. Increased dosing interval should be considered.

A Patient Information Sheet is available for this product. See text following "How Supplied" section below.

ADVERSE REACTIONS

In a survey conducted in hospitalized patients, less than 1% of patients taking propoxyphene hydrochloride at recommended doses experienced side effects. The most frequently reported were dizziness, sedation, nausea, and vomiting. Some of these adverse reactions may be alleviated if the patient lies down.

Other adverse reactions include constipation, abdominal pain, skin rashes, lightheadedness, headache, weakness, euphoria, dysphoria, hallucinations, and minor visual disturbances.

Propoxyphene therapy has been associated with abnormal liver function tests and, more rarely, with instances of reversible jaundice (including cholestatic jaundice).

Renal papillary necrosis may result from chronic aspirin use, particularly when the dosage is greater than recommended and when combined with acetaminophen.

Subacute painful myopathy has occurred following chronic propoxyphene overdosage.

DOSAGE AND ADMINISTRATION

This product is given orally. The usual dosage is 65 mg propoxyphene hydrochloride, 389 mg aspirin, and 32.4 mg caffeine every 4 hours as needed for pain.

The maximum recommended dose of propoxyphene hydrochloride is 390 mg/day.

Consideration should be given to a reduced total daily dosage in patients with hepatic or renal impairment.

MANAGEMENT OF OVERDOSAGE

In all cases of suspected overdosage, call your regional Poison Control Center to obtain the most up-to-date information about the treatment of overdose. This recommendation is made because, in general, information regarding the treatment of overdosage may change more rapidly than do package inserts.

Initial consideration should be given to the management of the CNS effects of propoxyphene overdosage. Resuscitative measures should be initiated promptly.

Symptoms of Propoxyphene Overdosage —The manifestations of acute overdosage with propoxyphene are those of narcotic overdosage. The patient is usually somnolent but may be stuporous or comatose and convulsing. Respiratory depression is characteristic. The ventilatory rate and/or tidal volume is decreased, which results in cyanosis and hypoxia. Pupils, initially pinpoint, may become dilated as hypoxia increases. Cheyne-Stokes respiration and apnea may occur. Blood pressure and heart rate are usually normal initially, but blood pressure falls and cardiac performance deteriorates, which ultimately results in pulmonary edema and circulatory collapse, unless the respiratory depression is corrected and adequate ventilation is restored promptly. Cardiac arrhythmias and conduction delay may be present. A combined respiratory-metabolic acidosis occurs owing to retained CO_2 (hypercapnia) and to lactic acid formed during anaerobic glycolysis. Acidosis may be severe if large amounts of salicylates have also been ingested. Death may occur.

Treatment of Propoxyphene Overdosage —Attention should be directed first to establishing a patent airway and to restoring ventilation. Mechanically assisted ventilation, with or without oxygen, may be required, and positive pressure respiration may be desirable if pulmonary edema is present. The narcotic antagonist naloxone will markedly reduce the degree of respiratory depression, and 0.4 to 2 mg should be administered promptly, preferably intravenously. If the desired degree of counteraction with improvement in respiratory functions is not obtained, naloxone should be repeated at 2- to 3-minute intervals. The duration of action of the antagonist may be brief. If no response is observed after 10 mg of naloxone have been administered, the diagnosis of propoxyphene toxicity should be questioned. Naloxone may also be administered by continuous intravenous infusion.

Treatment of Propoxyphene Overdosage in Children —The usual initial dose of naloxone in children is 0.01 mg/kg body weight given intravenously. If this dose does not result in the desired degree of clinical improvement, a subsequent increased dose of 0.1 mg/kg body weight may be administered. If an IV route of administration is not available, naloxone may be administered IM or subcutaneously in divided doses. If necessary, naloxone can be diluted with Sterile Water for Injection.

Blood gases, pH, and electrolytes should be monitored in order that acidosis and any electrolyte disturbance present may be corrected promptly. Acidosis, hypoxia, and generalized CNS depression predispose to the development of cardiac arrhythmias. Ventricular fibrillation or cardiac arrest may occur and necessitate the full complement of cardiopulmonary resuscitation (CPR) measures. Respiratory acidosis rapidly subsides as ventilation is restored and hypercapnia eliminated, but lactic acidosis may require intravenous bicarbonate for prompt correction.

Electrocardiographic monitoring is essential. Prompt correction of hypoxia, acidosis, and electrolyte disturbance (when present) will help prevent these cardiac complications and will increase the effectiveness of agents administered to restore normal cardiac function.

In addition to the use of a narcotic antagonist, the patient may require careful titration with an anticonvulsant to control convulsions. Analeptic drugs (for example, caffeine or amphetamine) should not be used because of their tendency to precipitate convulsions.

General supportive measures, in addition to oxygen, include, when necessary, intravenous fluids, vasopressor-inotropic compounds, and, when infection is likely, anti-infective agents. Gastric lavage may be useful and activated charcoal can adsorb a significant amount of ingested propoxyphene. Dialysis is of little value in poisoning due to propoxyphene. Efforts should be made to determine whether other agents, such as alcohol, barbiturates, tranquilizers, or other CNS depressants, were also ingested, since these increase CNS depression as well as cause specific toxic effects.

Symptoms of Salicylate Overdosage —Such symptoms include central nausea and vomiting, tinnitus and deafness, vertigo and headaches, mental dullness and confusion, diaphoresis, rapid pulse, and increased respiration and respiratory alkalosis.

Treatment of Salicylate Overdosage —When Darvon Compound-65 has been ingested, the clinical picture may be complicated by salicylism.

The treatment of acute salicylate intoxication includes minimizing drug absorption, promoting elimination through the kidneys, and correcting metabolic derangements affecting body temperature, hydration, acid-base balance, and electrolyte balance. The technique to be employed for eliminating salicylate from the bloodstream depends on the degree of drug intoxication.

If the patient is seen within 4 hours of ingestion, the stomach should be emptied by inducing vomiting or by gastric lavage as soon as possible.

The nomogram of Done is a useful prognostic guide in which the expected severity of salicylate intoxication is based on serum salicylate levels and the time interval between ingestion and taking the blood sample.

Exchange transfusion is most feasible for a small infant. Intermittent peritoneal dialysis is useful for cases of moderate severity in adults. Intravenous fluids alkalinized by the addition of sodium bicarbonate or potassium citrate are helpful. Hemodialysis with the artificial kidney is the most effective means of removing salicylate and is indicated for the very severe cases of salicylate intoxication.

HOW SUPPLIED

Darvon® Compound-65 Pulvules® (No. 369) are available in:

The 65 mg parabolic-shaped capsules are imprinted with the script "Lilly" and "3111" on the opaque gray cap and "Darvon Comp 65" on the opaque red body, using edible black ink. They are available as follows:

Bottles of 100 (RxPak*) NDC 0002-3111-02 (PU0369)
Bottles of 500 NDC 0002-3111-03 (PU0369)

* All RxPaks (prescription packages, Lilly) have safety closures.

Store at controlled room temperature, 59° to 86°F (15° to 30°C).

CAUTION—Federal (USA) law prohibits dispensing without prescription.

The following information, including description of dosage forms and the maximum daily dosage of each, is available to patients receiving Darvon products.

Patient Information Sheet
**YOUR PRESCRIPTION FOR A DARVON®
(PROPOXYPHENE) PRODUCT**

Summary: Products containing Darvon are used to relieve pain.

LIMIT YOUR INTAKE OF ALCOHOL WHILE TAKING THIS DRUG. Make sure your doctor knows if you are taking tranquilizers, sleep aids, antidepressants, antihistamines, or any other drugs that make you sleepy. Combining propoxyphene with alcohol or these drugs in excessive doses is dangerous.

Use care while driving a car or using machines until you see how the drug affects you because propoxyphene can make you sleepy. Do not take more of the drug than your doctor prescribed. Dependence has occurred when patients have taken propoxyphene for a long period of time at doses greater than recommended.

The rest of this leaflet gives you more information about propoxyphene. Please read it and keep it for future use.

Uses of Darvon: Products containing Darvon are used for the relief of mild to moderate pain. Products that contain Darvon plus aspirin or acetaminophen are prescribed for the relief of pain or pain associated with fever.

Before Taking Darvon: Make sure your doctor knows if you have ever had an allergic reaction to propoxyphene, aspirin, or acetaminophen. Some forms of propoxyphene products contain aspirin to help relieve the pain. Your doctor should be advised if you have a history of ulcers or if you are taking an anticoagulant ("blood thinner"). The aspirin may irritate the stomach lining and may cause bleeding, particularly if an ulcer is present. Also, bleeding may occur if you are taking an anticoagulant. In a small group of people, aspirin may cause an asthma attack. If you are one of these people, be sure your drug does not contain aspirin.

The effect of propoxyphene in children under 12 has not been studied. Therefore, use of the drug in this age group is not recommended.

Also, due to the possible association between aspirin and Reye Syndrome, those propoxyphene products containing aspirin should not be given to children, including teenagers, with chicken pox or flu unless prescribed by a physician. The following propoxyphene product contains aspirin:

Darvon® Compound-65 (Propoxyphene Hydrochloride, Aspirin, and Caffeine, USP, Lilly)

How to Take Darvon: Follow your doctor's directions exactly. Do not increase the amount you take without your doctor's approval. If you miss a dose of the drug, do not take twice as much the next time.

Pregnancy: Do not take propoxyphene during pregnancy unless your doctor knows you are pregnant and specifically recommends its use. Cases of temporary dependence in the newborn have occurred when the mother has taken propoxyphene consistently in the weeks before delivery. **IT IS ESPECIALLY IMPORTANT NOT TO USE DARVON COMPOUND-65 DURING THE LAST 3 MONTHS OF PREGNANCY UNLESS SPECIFICALLY DIRECTED TO DO SO BY A DOCTOR BECAUSE ASPIRIN MAY CAUSE PROBLEMS IN THE UNBORN CHILD OR COMPLICATIONS DURING DELIVERY.**

As a general principle, no drug should be taken during pregnancy unless it is clearly necessary.

General Cautions: Heavy use of alcohol with propoxyphene is hazardous and may lead to overdose symptoms (*see* "Overdose" below). THEREFORE, LIMIT YOUR INTAKE OF ALCOHOL WHILE TAKING PROPOXYPHENE.

Combinations of excessive doses of propoxyphene, alcohol, and tranquilizers are dangerous. Make sure your doctor knows if you are taking tranquilizers, sleep aids, antidepressant drugs, antihistamines, or any other drugs that make you sleepy. The use of these drugs with propoxyphene increases their sedative effects and may lead to overdosage symptoms, including death (*see* "Overdose" below).

Propoxyphene may cause drowsiness or impair your mental and/or physical abilities; therefore, use caution when driving a vehicle or operating dangerous machinery. DO NOT perform any hazardous task until you have seen your response to this drug.

Propoxyphene may increase the concentration in the body of medications, such as anticoagulants ("blood thinners"), antidepressants, or drugs used for epilepsy. The result may be excessive or adverse effects of these medications. Make sure your doctor knows if you are taking any of these medications.

Dependence: You can become dependent on propoxyphene if you take it in higher than recommended doses over a long period of time. Dependence is a feeling of need for the drug and a feeling that you cannot perform normally without it.

Overdose: An overdose of Darvon, alone or in combination with other drugs, including alcohol, may cause weakness, difficulty in breathing, confusion, anxiety, and more severe drowsiness and dizziness. Extreme overdosage may lead to unconsciousness and death.

If the propoxyphene product contains acetaminophen, the overdosage symptoms include nausea, vomiting, lack of appetite, and abdominal pain. Liver damage may occur.

When the propoxyphene product contains aspirin, symptoms of taking too much of the drug are headache, dizziness, ringing in the ears, difficulty in hearing, dim vision, confusion, drowsiness, sweating, thirst, rapid breathing, nausea, vomiting, and, occasionally, diarrhea.

In any suspected overdosage situation, contact your doctor or nearest hospital emergency room. GET EMERGENCY HELP IMMEDIATELY.

KEEP THIS DRUG AND ALL DRUGS OUT OF THE REACH OF CHILDREN.

Possible Side Effects: When propoxyphene is taken as directed, side effects are infrequent. Among those reported are drowsiness, dizziness, nausea, and vomiting. If these effects occur, it may help if you lie down and rest.

Less frequently reported side effects are constipation, abdominal pain, skin rashes, lightheadedness, headache, weakness, hallucinations, minor visual disturbances, and feelings of elation or discomfort.

If side effects occur and concern you, contact your doctor.

Other Information: The safe and effective use of propoxyphene depends on your taking it exactly as directed. This drug has been prescribed specifically for you and your present condition. Do not give this drug to others who may have similar symptoms. Do not use it for any other reason.

If you would like more information about propoxyphene, ask your doctor or pharmacist. They have a more technical leaflet (professional labeling) you may read.

Selected Darvon Products

Maximum Daily Dosage		
6	Dark Orange, Capsule Shaped, Film Coated Tablets Imprinted with Script "Lilly" on the one side and "Darvocet-N 100" on the other, using edible black ink	DARVOCET-N® 100 ℂ Propoxyphene Napsylate and Acetaminophen Tablets
6	Parabolic-Shaped Capsules Imprinted with Script "Lilly" and "3111" on the opaque gray cap and "Darvon Comp 65" on the opaque red body, using edible black ink	DARVON® COMPOUND-65 ℂ Propoxyphene Hydrochloride, Aspirin, and Caffeine Pulvules®
6	Parabolic-Shaped Capsules Imprinted with Script "Lilly" and "H03" on the opaque pink cap and "Darvon" on the opaque pink body, using edible black ink	DARVON® ℂ Propoxyphene Hydrochloride Pulvules, 65 mg

Literature revised March 14, 1996

Prescription Vial Sticker

Tell your doctor if you are taking tranquilizers, antidepressant drugs, or sleep aids. LIMIT alcohol use with Darvon-N® (propoxyphene napsylate) and Darvon® (propoxyphene hydrochloride) products.

[031496]

DIETHYLSTILBESTROL ℞

[*dī-eth ′ĭl-stĭl-bĕs ′trōl*]
USP

1. USE OF ESTROGENS HAS BEEN REPORTED TO INCREASE THE RISK OF ENDOMETRIAL CARCINOMA

Three independent case-control studies have reported an increased risk of endometrial cancer in postmenopausal women exposed to exogenous estrogens for more than 1 year. This risk was independent of other known risk factors for endometrial cancer. These studies are further supported by the finding that, since 1969, the incidence rate of endometrial cancer has increased sharply in 8 different areas of the United States which have population-based cancer reporting systems.

The 3 case-control studies reported that the risk of endometrial cancer in estrogen users was about 4.5 to 13.9 times greater than in nonusers. The risk appears to depend on both the duration of treatment and the dose of estrogen. In view of these findings, the lowest dose that will control symptoms should be utilized when estrogens are used for the treatment of menopausal symptoms, and medication should be discontinued as soon as possible. When prolonged treatment is medically indicated, a reassessment should be made on at least a semiannual basis to determine the need for continued therapy. Although the evidence must be considered preliminary, one study suggests that cyclic administration of low doses of estrogen may carry less risk than does continuous administration; it therefore appears prudent to utilize such a regimen.

Close clinical surveillance of all women taking estrogens is important. In all cases of undiagnosed persistent or recurring abnormal vaginal bleeding, adequate diagnostic measures should be undertaken to rule out malignancy.

At present, there is no evidence that "natural" estrogens are more or less hazardous than "synthetic" estrogens at equivalent estrogenic doses.

2. ESTROGENS SHOULD NOT BE USED DURING PREGNANCY

The use of female sex hormones, both estrogens and progestagens, during early pregnancy may affect the offspring. It has been reported that females exposed *in utero* to diethylstilbestrol, a nonsteroidal estrogen, may have an increased risk of developing later in life a rare form of vaginal or cervical cancer. This risk has been estimated to be 0.14 to 1.4 per 1,000 exposures. Furthermore, from 30% to 90% of such exposed women have been found to have vaginal adenosis and epithelial changes of the vagina and cervix. Although these changes are histologically benign, it is not known whether they are precursors of malignancy. Even though similar data are not available with the use of other estrogens, it cannot be presumed that they would not induce similar changes.

Several reports suggest that there is an association between intrauterine exposure to female sex hormones and congenital anomalies, including congenital heart defects and limb-reduction defects. One case-control study estimated a 4.7-fold increased risk of limb-reduction defects in infants exposed *in utero* to sex hormones (oral contraceptives, hormone withdrawal tests for pregnancy, or attempted treatment for threatened abortion). Some of these exposures were very short and involved only a few days of treatment. The data suggest that the risk of limb-reduction defects in exposed fetuses is somewhat less than 1 per 1,000.

In the past, female sex hormones have been used during pregnancy in an attempt to treat threatened or habitual abortion; however, their efficacy was never conclusively proved or disproved.

If diethylstilbestrol is administered during pregnancy, or if the patient becomes pregnant while taking this drug, she should be apprised of the potential risks to the fetus and of the advisability of pregnancy continuation.

THIS DRUG PRODUCT SHOULD NOT BE USED AS A POSTCOITAL CONTRACEPTIVE

DESCRIPTION

Diethylstilbestrol is a crystalline synthetic estrogenic substance capable of producing all the pharmacologic and therapeutic responses attributed to natural estrogens. Diethylstilbestrol may be administered orally (in the form of Enseals® [enteric-release tablets, Lilly] and tablets). Chemically, diethylstilbestrol is α,α'-diethyl-4,4′-stilbenediol. The structural formula is as follows:

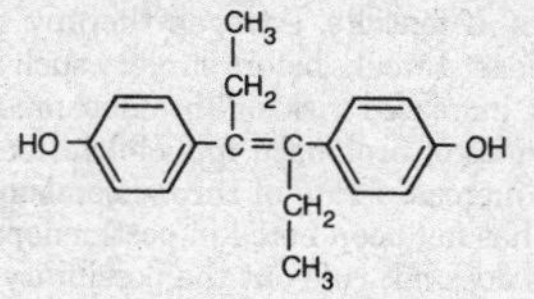

The Enseals contain corn starch, FD&C Blue No. 2, FD&C Red No. 3, FD&C Yellow No. 6, lactose, magnesium stearate, sucrose, talc, titanium dioxide, and other inactive ingredients.

The tablets contain corn starch, lactose, magnesium stearate, and talc.

INDICATIONS AND USAGE

Diethylstilbestrol is indicated in the treatment of:

1. Breast cancer (for palliation only) in appropriately selected women and men with metastatic disease
2. Prostatic carcinoma—palliative therapy of advanced disease

DIETHYLSTILBESTROL SHOULD NOT BE USED FOR ANY PURPOSE DURING PREGNANCY. ITS USE MAY CAUSE SEVERE HARM TO THE FETUS (SEE BOXED WARNING).

CONTRAINDICATIONS

Estrogens should not be used in women (or men) with any of the following conditions:

1. Known or suspected cancer of the breast, except in appropriately selected patients being treated for metastatic disease
2. Known or suspected estrogen-dependent neoplasia
3. Known or suspected pregnancy (*see* boxed Warning)
4. Undiagnosed abnormal genital bleeding
5. Active thrombophlebitis or thromboembolic disorders
6. A past history of thrombophlebitis, thrombosis, or thromboembolic disorders associated with previous use of estrogen (except when used in treatment of breast or prostatic malignancy).

WARNINGS

1. *Induction of malignant neoplasms.* In certain animal species, long-term continuous administration of natural and synthetic estrogens increases the frequency of carcinomas of the breast, cervix, vagina, kidney, and liver. There are now reports that prolonged use of estrogens increases the risk of carcinoma of the endometrium in humans. (*See* boxed Warning.)

At the present time, there is no satisfactory evidence that administration of estrogens to postmenopausal women increases the risk of cancer of the breast. This possibility, however, has been raised by a recent long-term follow-up of one physician's practice. Because of the animal data, there is a need for caution in prescribing estrogens for women with a family history of breast cancer or for women who have breast nodules, fibrocystic disease, or abnormal mammograms.

2. *Gallbladder disease.* A recent study reported a 2 to 3-fold increase in the risk of gallbladder disease occurring in women receiving postmenopausal estrogen therapy, similar to the 2-fold increased risk previously noted in women using oral contraceptives. In the case of oral contraceptives, this increased risk appeared after 2 years of use.

3. *Effects similar to those caused by estrogen-progestagen oral contraceptives.* There are several serious adverse effects associated with the use of oral contraceptives; however, most of these adverse effects have not as yet been documented as consequences of postmenopausal estrogen therapy. This may reflect the comparatively low doses of estrogen used in postmenopausal women. It would be expected that these adverse effects are more likely to occur following administration of the larger doses of estrogen used for treating prostatic or breast cancer. It has, in fact, been shown that there is an increased risk of thrombosis with the administration of estrogens for prostatic cancer in men and for postpartum breast engorgement in women.

a. *Thromboembolic disease.* It is now well established that women taking oral contraceptives run an increased risk of various thromboembolic and thrombotic vascular diseases, such as thrombophlebitis, pulmonary embolism, stroke, and myocardial infarction. Cases of retinal thrombosis, mesenteric thrombosis, and optic neuritis have been reported in users of oral contraceptives. There is evidence that

Continued on next page

• Identi-Code® symbol. This product information was prepared in June 1996. Current information on these and other products of Eli Lilly and Company may be obtained by direct inquiry to Lilly Research Laboratories, Lilly Corporate Center, Indianapolis, Indiana 46285, 800-545-5979.

Lilly—Cont.

the risk of several of these adverse reactions is related to the dose of the drug. An increased risk of postsurgical thromboembolic complications has also been reported in users of oral contraceptives. If feasible, estrogen therapy should be discontinued at least 4 weeks before surgery such as that associated with an increased risk of thromboembolism, or that requiring periods of prolonged immobilization.

Although an increased rate of thromboembolic and thrombotic disease has not been noted in postmenopausal users of estrogen, this does not rule out the possibility that such an increase may be present or that it exists in subgroups of women who have underlying risk factors or who are receiving relatively large doses of estrogens. Therefore, estrogens should not be used in persons with active thrombophlebitis or thromboembolic disorders, nor should they be used (except in treatment of malignancy) in persons with a history of such disorders associated with estrogen therapy. Estrogens should be administered cautiously to patients with cerebral vascular or coronary artery disease and only when such therapy is clearly needed.

In a large prospective clinical trial in men, large doses of estrogen (5 mg of conjugated estrogens per day), comparable to those used to treat cancer of the prostate and breast, have been shown to increase the risk of nonfatal myocardial infarction, pulmonary embolism, and thrombophlebitis. When such large doses of estrogen are used, any of the thromboembolic and thrombotic adverse effects associated with the use of oral contraceptives should be considered a clear risk.

b. *Hepatic adenoma.* Benign hepatic adenomas appear to be associated with the use of oral contraceptives. Although these adenomas are benign and rare, they may rupture and may cause death by intra-abdominal hemorrhage. Such lesions have not yet been reported in association with the administration of other estrogen or progestagen preparations, but they should be considered when abdominal pain and tenderness, abdominal mass, or hypovolemic shock occurs in persons receiving estrogen therapy. Hepatocellular carcinoma has also been reported in women taking estrogen-containing oral contraceptives. The relationship of this malignancy to these drugs is not known at this time.

c. *Elevated blood pressure.* Increased blood pressure is not uncommon in women taking oral contraceptives. There is now one report that this may occur with use of estrogens in the menopause, and blood pressure should be monitored during estrogen therapy, especially if high doses are used.

d. *Glucose tolerance.* A decrease in glucose tolerance has been observed in a significant percentage of patients on estrogen-containing oral contraceptives. For this reason, diabetic patients should be carefully observed while receiving estrogen.

4. *Hypercalcemia.* Administration of estrogens may lead to severe hypercalcemia in patients with breast cancer and bone metastases. If this occurs, the drug should be stopped and appropriate measures taken to reduce the serum calcium level.

PRECAUTIONS

General—1. A complete medical and family history should be taken prior to initiation of any estrogen therapy. In the pretreatment and periodic physical examinations, special consideration should be given to blood pressure, breasts, abdomen, and pelvic organs, and a Papanicolaou smear should be performed. As a general rule, estrogen should not be prescribed for over a year without another physical examination.

2. Fluid retention—Because estrogens may cause some degree of fluid retention, conditions which might be influenced by this factor, such as epilepsy, migraine, and cardiac or renal dysfunction, require careful observation.

3. Certain patients may develop undesirable manifestations of excessive estrogenic stimulation, such as abnormal or excessive uterine bleeding, mastodynia, etc.

4. Oral contraceptives appear to be associated with an increased incidence of mental depression. Although it is not clear whether this is due to the estrogenic or progestogenic component of the contraceptive agent, patients with a history of depression should be carefully observed.

5. Preexisting uterine leiomyomata may increase in size with administration of estrogens.

6. The pathologist should be advised of estrogen therapy when relevant specimens are submitted.

7. Patients with a past history of jaundice during pregnancy run an increased risk of recurrence of jaundice while receiving estrogen-containing oral contraceptive therapy. If jaundice develops in any patient receiving estrogen, the medication should be discontinued while the cause is investigated.

8. Estrogens may be poorly metabolized in patients with impaired liver function, and they should therefore be administered with caution in such patients.

9. Because estrogens influence the metabolism of calcium and phosphorus, they should be used with caution in patients with metabolic bone diseases associated with hypercalcemia or in patients with renal insufficiency.

10. Because of the effects of estrogens on epiphyseal closure, they should be used judiciously in young patients in whom bone growth is not complete.

11. Certain endocrine and liver function tests may be affected by estrogen-containing oral contraceptives. The following similar changes may be expected with larger doses of estrogen:

a. Increased sulfobromophthalein retention.

b. Increased prothrombin and factors VII, VIII, IX, and X; decreased antithrombin 3; increased norepinephrine-induced platelet aggregability.

c. Increased thyroid-binding globulin (TBG) leading to increased circulating total thyroid hormone, as measured by PBI, T_4 by column, or T_4 by radioimmunoassay. Free T_3 resin uptake is decreased, reflecting the elevated TBG; free T_4 concentration is unaltered.

d. Impaired glucose tolerance.

e. Decreased pregnanediol excretion.

f. Reduced response to metyrapone test.

g. Reduced serum folate concentration.

h. Increased serum triglyceride and phospholipid concentration.

Information for the Patient—See text of Patient Package Insert included below.

Pregnancy Category X—See Contraindications and boxed Warning.

Nursing Mothers—As a general principle, the administration of any drug to nursing mothers should be done only when clearly necessary since many drugs are excreted in human milk.

ADVERSE REACTIONS

(*See* Warnings regarding induction of neoplasia, adverse effects on the fetus, increased incidence of gallbladder disease, and adverse effects similar to those of oral contraceptives, including thromboembolism.) The following additional adverse reactions have been reported with estrogenic therapy, including oral contraceptives:

1. *Genitourinary system*
   Breakthrough bleeding, spotting, change in menstrual flow
   Dysmenorrhea
   Premenstrual-like syndrome
   Amenorrhea during and after treatment
   Increase in size of uterine fibromyomata
   Vaginal candidiasis
   Change in cervical eversion and in degree of cervical secretion
   Cystitis-like syndrome
2. *Breasts*
   Tenderness, enlargement, secretion
3. *Gastrointestinal*
   Nausea, vomiting
   Abdominal cramps, bloating
   Cholestatic jaundice
4. *Skin*
   Chloasma or melasma, which may persist when drug is discontinued
   Erythema multiforme
   Erythema nodosum
   Hemorrhagic eruption
   Loss of scalp hair
   Hirsutism
5. *Eyes*
   Steepening of corneal curvature
   Intolerance to contact lenses
6. *CNS*
   Headache, migraine, dizziness
   Mental depression
   Chorea
7. *Miscellaneous*
   Increase or decrease in weight
   Reduced carbohydrate tolerance
   Aggravation of porphyria
   Edema
   Changes in libido

OVERDOSAGE

Signs and Symptoms—Symptoms of acute overdose include anorexia, nausea, vomiting, abdominal cramps, and diarrhea. Withdrawal vaginal bleeding may follow large doses. Chronic toxicity may include salt and water retention, edema, headache, vertigo, leg cramps, gynecomastia, chloasma, and porphyria cutanea tarda. Polydipsia, polyuria, fatigue, and an abnormal glucose tolerance may occur in some patients with preclinical diabetes mellitus.

No information is available on the following: LD_{50}, concentration of diethylstilbestrol in biologic fluids associated with toxicity and/or death, the amount of drug in a single dose usually associated with symptoms of overdosage, or the amount of diethylstilbestrol in a single dose likely to be life threatening.

Treatment—Chronic diethylstilbestrol toxicity should be treated by discontinuing all estrogenic medications and providing supportive care for any symptoms that may be present.

To obtain up-to-date information about the treatment of overdose, a good resource is your certified Regional Poison Control Center. Telephone numbers of certified poison control centers are listed in the *Physicians' Desk Reference (PDR)*. In managing overdosage, consider the possibility of multiple drug overdoses, interaction among drugs, and unusual drug kinetics in your patient.

In treating acute overdose, protect the patient's airway and support ventilation and perfusion. Meticulously monitor and maintain, within acceptable limits, the patient's vital signs, blood gases, serum electrolytes, etc. Absorption of drugs from the gastrointestinal tract may be decreased by giving activated charcoal, which, in many cases, is more effective than emesis or lavage; consider charcoal instead of or in addition to gastric emptying. Repeated doses of charcoal over time may hasten elimination of some drugs that have been absorbed. Safeguard the patient's airway when employing gastric emptying or charcoal.

Forced diuresis, peritoneal dialysis, hemodialysis, or charcoal hemoperfusion have not been established as beneficial for an acute overdose of diethylstilbestrol.

DOSAGE AND ADMINISTRATION

Given chronically:
Inoperable progressing prostatic cancer
1 to 3 mg daily initially, increased in advanced cases; the dosage may later be reduced to an average of 1 mg daily.
Inoperable progressing breast cancer in appropriately selected men and postmenopausal women (see Indications)
15 mg daily.

Patients with an intact uterus should be closely monitored for signs of endometrial cancer, and appropriate diagnostic measures should be taken to rule out malignancy in the event of persistent or recurring abnormal vaginal bleeding.

HOW SUPPLIED

Diethylstilbestrol, USP, is supplied in the following forms:
Enseals:
1 mg (No. 49)—(100s) NDC 0002-0122-02; (1,000s) NDC 0002-0122-04
5 mg (No. 85)—(100s) NDC 0002-0133-02
Tablets:
1 mg (No. 1649)—(100s) NDC 0002-1052-02; (1,000s) NDC 0002-1052-04
5 mg (No. 1685)—(100s) NDC 0002-1054-02   [040894]
CAUTION—Federal (USA) law prohibits dispensing without prescription.

REFERENCES

1. Ziel HK, Finkle WD: Increased risk of endometrial carcinoma among users of conjugated estrogens. *N Engl J Med* 1975;293:1167–1170.
2. Smith DC, Prentic R, Thompson DJ, et al: Association of exogenous estrogen and endometrial carcinoma. *N Engl J Med* 1975;293:1164–1167.
3. Mack TM, Pike MC, Henderson BE, et al: Estrogens and endometrial cancer in a retirement community. *N Engl J Med* 1976;294:1262–1267.
4. Weiss NS, Szekely DR, Austin DF: Increasing incidence of endometrial cancer in the United States. *N Engl J Med* 1976;294:1259–1262.
5. Herbst AL, Ulfelder H, Poskanzer DC: Adenocarcinoma of vagina. *N Engl J Med* 1971;284:878–881.
6. Greenwald P, Barlow J, Nasca P, et al: Vaginal cancer after maternal treatment with synthetic estrogens. *N Engl J Med* 1971;285:390–392.
7. Herbst AL, Cole P, Colton T, et al: Age-incidence and risk of diethylstilbestrol-related clear cell adenocarcinoma of the vagina and cervix. *Am J Obstet Gynecol* 1977;128:43.
8. Herbst A, Kurman R, Scully R: Vaginal and cervical abnormalities after exposure to stilbestrol in utero. *Obstet Gynecol* 1972;40:287–298.
9. Herbst A, Robboy S, Macdonald G, et al: The effects of local progesterone on stilbestrol-associated vaginal adenosis. *Am J Obstet Gynecol* 1974;118:607–615.
10. Herbst A, Poskanzer D, Robboy S, et al: Prenatal exposure to stilbestrol, a prospective comparison of exposed female offspring with unexposed controls. *N Engl J Med* 1975;292:334–339.
11. Stafl A, Mattingly R, Foley D, et al: Clinical diagnosis of vaginal adenosis. *Obstet Gynecol* 1974;43:118–128.
12. Sherman AI, Goldrath M, Berlin A, et al: Cervical-vaginal adenosis after *in utero* exposure to synthetic estrogens. *Obstet Gynecol* 1974;44:531–545.
13. Gal I, Kirman B, Stern J: Hormonal pregnancy tests and congenital malformation. *Nature* 1967;216:83.
14. Levy EP, Cohen A, Fraser FC: Hormone treatment during pregnancy and congenital heart defects. *Lancet* 1973;1:611.
15. Nora J, Nora A: Birth defects and oral contraceptives. *Lancet* 1973;1:941–942.
16. Janerich DT, Piper JM, Glebatis DM: Oral contraceptives and congenital limb-reduction defects. *N Engl J Med* 1974;291:697–700.

17. Estrogens for oral or parenteral use. *Federal Register* 1975;40:8242.
18. Boston Collaborative Drug Surveillance Program: Surgically confirmed gall bladder disease, venous thromboembolism and breast tumors in relation to post-menopausal estrogen therapy. *N Engl J Med* 1974;290:15–19.
19. Hoover R, Gray LA Sr, Cole P, et al: Menopausal estrogens and breast cancer. *N Engl J Med* 1976;295:401–405.
20. Boston Collaborative Drug Surveillance Program: Oral contraceptives and venous thromboembolic disease, surgically confirmed gall bladder disease, and breast tumors. *Lancet* 1973;1:1399–1404.
21. Daniel D, Campbell GH, Turnbull AO: Puerperal thromboembolism and suppression of lactation. *Lancet* 1967;2:287–289.
22. The Veterans Administration Cooperative Urological Research Group: Carcinoma of the prostate: Treatment comparisons. *J Urol* 1967;98:516–522.
23. Baller JC: Thromboembolism and oestrogen therapy. *Lancet* 1967;2:560.
24. Blackard C, Doe R, Mellinger G, et al: Incidence of cardiovascular disease and death in patients receiving diethylstilbestrol for carcinoma of the prostate. *Cancer* 1970;26:249–256.
25. Royal College of General Practitioners: Oral contraception and thromboembolic disease. *J R Coll Gen Pract* 1967;13:267–279.
26. Inman WHW, Vessey MP: Investigation of deaths from pulmonary, coronary, and cerebral thrombosis and embolism in women of childbearing age. *Br Med J* 1968;2:193–199.
27. Vessey MP, Doll R: Investigation of relation between use of oral contraceptives and thromboembolic disease, a further report. *Br Med J* 1969;2:651–657.
28. Sartwell PE, Masi AT, Arthes FG, et al: Thromboembolism and oral contraceptives: An epidemiological case control study. *Am J Epidemiol* 1969;90:365–380.
29. Collaborative Group for the Study of Stroke in Young Women: Oral contraception and increased risk of cerebral ischemia or thrombosis. *N Engl J Med* 1973;288:871–873.
30. Collaborative Group for the Study of Stroke in Young Women: Oral contraceptives and stroke in young women: Associated risk factors. *JAMA* 1975;231:718–722.
31. Mann JI, Inman WHW: Oral contraceptives and death from myocardial infarction. *Br Med J* 1975;2:245–248.
32. Mann JI, Vessey MP, Thorogood M, et al: Myocardial infarction in young women with special reference to oral contraceptive practice. *Br Med J* 1975;2:241–245.
33. Inman WHW, Vessey MP, Westerholm B, et al: Thromboembolic disease and the steroidal content of oral contraceptives. *Br Med J* 1970;2:203–209.
34. Stolley PD, Tonascia JA, Tockman MS, et al: Thrombosis with low-estrogen oral contraceptives. *Am J Epidemiol* 1975;102:197–208.
35. Vessey MP, Doll R, Fairbairn AS, et al: Post-operative thromboembolism and the use of the oral contraceptives. *Br Med J* 1970;3:123–126.
36. Greene GR, Sartwell PE: Oral contraceptive use in patients with thromboembolism following surgery, trauma or infection. *Am J Public Health* 1972;62:680–685.
37. Rosenberg L, Armstrong MB, Jick H: Myocardial infarction and estrogen therapy in postmenopausal women. *N Engl J Med* 1976;294:1256–1259.
38. Coronary Drug Project Research Group: The coronary drug project: Initial findings leading to modification of its research protocol. *JAMA* 1970;214:1303–1313.
39. Baum J, Holtz F, Bookstein JJ, et al: Possible association between benign hepatomas and oral contraceptives. *Lancet* 1973;2:926–928.
40. Mays ET, Christopherson WM, Mahr MM, et al: Hepatic changes in young women ingesting contraceptive steroids, hepatic hemorrhage and primary hepatic tumors. *JAMA* 1976;235:730–732.
41. Edmondson HA, Henderson B, Benton B: Liver cell adenomas associated with the use of oral contraceptives. *N Engl J Med* 1976;294:470–472.
42. Pfeffer RI, Van Den Noore S: Estrogen use and stroke risk in postmenopausal women. *Am J Epidemiol* 1976;103:545–546.

INFORMATION FOR THE PATIENT
DIETHYLSTILBESTROL, USP
FACTS THAT YOU SHOULD KNOW ABOUT ESTROGENS

Estrogens are female hormones produced by the ovaries. The ovaries produce several different kinds of estrogens. In addition, scientists have been able to develop a variety of synthetic estrogens. As far as we know, all these estrogens have similar properties and, therefore, have much the same usefulness and side effects and involve the same risks. This leaflet is intended to help you understand what estrogens are given for, the possible risks involved in their use, and how to use them as safely as possible.

This leaflet contains the most important information about estrogens. If you want to know more, you may ask your doctor or pharmacist to let you read the package insert prepared for the doctor.

USE OF ESTROGEN

Estrogens are prescribed by physicians for a number of purposes, and they may be given:
1. To prevent certain uncomfortable symptoms of estrogen deficiency during a period of adjustment when a woman's ovaries no longer produce estrogen. (All women normally stop producing estrogens, generally between the ages of 45 and 55; this is called the menopause.)
2. To prevent symptoms of estrogen deficiency when a woman's ovaries have been removed surgically before the natural menopause.
3. To prevent pregnancy. (Estrogens are given along with a progestagen, another female hormone; these combinations are called oral contraceptives or birth control pills. Patient information is available to women taking oral contraceptives, and these will not be discussed in this leaflet.)
4. To treat certain cancers in women and men.
NOTE: PREGNANT WOMEN SHOULD NOT TAKE ESTROGENS.

THE USE OF ESTROGENS DURING THE MENOPAUSE

All women eventually experience a decrease in estrogen production during the natural course of life. This usually occurs between the ages of 45 and 55, but it may occur earlier or later. Sometimes, the ovaries may have to be removed by an operation before the natural menopause occurs, thus producing a "surgical menopause."

When the amount of estrogen in the body begins to decrease, many women may develop some of the following typical symptoms: feelings of warmth in the face, neck, and chest, or sudden intense episodes of heat and sweating throughout the body (called "hot flashes" or "hot flushes"). Sometimes these symptoms are quite uncomfortable. A few women may eventually develop changes in the vagina (called "atrophic vaginitis") which cause discomfort, especially during and after intercourse.

Estrogens can be prescribed to treat these symptoms of the menopause. Probably more than half of all women undergoing the menopause have only mild symptoms or none at all and thus do not need estrogens. Some women may require estrogen for only a few months while their bodies adjust to lower estrogen levels, whereas other women will need them for 6 months or longer. In an attempt to avoid overstimulation of the uterus (womb), estrogens are usually given on a cyclic basis each month, that is, 3 weeks of medication followed by 1 week with no medication.

Women sometimes experience nervous symptoms or depression during the menopause. There is no evidence that estrogens are effective for treating such symptoms, and they should not be used for this purpose; however, other treatment may be needed.

You may have heard that taking estrogens for a long period of time (years) after the menopause will keep your skin soft and supple and will keep you feeling young. Unfortunately, there is no evidence that this is true; on the other hand, there may be a significant risk involved in the use of such long-term treatment.

THE DANGER OF ESTROGENS

1. *Endometrial carcinoma.* There may be an increased risk of *endometrial carcinoma*, a form of cancer of the uterus, if estrogens are used for more than a year after the menopause. The chance of this cancer occurring may be approximately 5 to 10 times greater in women taking estrogen than in those women taking no estrogens. To put this another way, a woman who does not take estrogens after the menopause has 1 chance in 1,000 each year of having cancer of the uterus, whereas a woman who takes estrogens has 5 to 10 chances in 1,000 each year. For this reason, *it is important that estrogens be taken only when needed.*

It appears that the longer estrogens are taken, the greater the risk of this cancer; this risk seems to increase when larger doses are taken. For this reason, *it is important to take the lowest dose of estrogen that will control symptoms and to take it only as long as it is needed.* If estrogens are needed for longer periods of time, your doctor will want to reevaluate your need for estrogen at least every 6 months.

Women using estrogens should report to their doctors any irregular vaginal bleeding; such bleeding may be of no importance, but it can also be an early warning of cancer of the uterus. If you have vaginal bleeding, you should *not* use estrogens until your doctor has made a diagnosis and has verified that there is no cancer of the uterus.

If your uterus has been completely removed (total hysterectomy), there is no danger of endometrial carcinoma occurring.

2. *Other possible cancers.* When given to animals for a long period of time, estrogens have caused development of other tumors, such as tumors of the breast, cervix, vagina, or liver.

At present, there is no evidence that there is an increased risk that such tumors will occur in women taking estrogens during the menopause, but there is no way to be sure that there is no risk. One study raises the possibility that the use of estrogens during the menopause may increase the risk that cancer of the breast will develop many years later. This is another reason why estrogens should be used only when clearly needed. While you are taking estrogens, it is important for you to get to your doctor at least once a year for a physical examination. Your doctor may also want to make more frequent examinations of your breasts if members of your family have had breast cancer or if you have breast nodules (lumps) or abnormal mammograms (breast-x-rays).

3. *Gallbladder disease.* Women who use estrogens after the menopause are more likely to develop gallbladder disease than are women who do not use estrogens. Birth control pills have a similar effect.

4. *Abnormal blood clots.* Oral contraceptives increase the risk of blood clots developing in various parts of the body. In rare cases, this can result in a stroke (if the clot is in the brain), a heart attack (a clot in a blood vessel of the heart), or a pulmonary embolus (a clot which forms in the legs or pelvis and then breaks off and travels to the lungs). Any of these can be fatal.

At this time, the use of estrogens during the menopause is not known to cause such blood clots, but this has not been fully studied and could still prove to involve such a risk. If you have blood clots in the legs or lungs or had a heart attack while you were taking estrogens or birth control pills, you should not take estrogens (unless they are being prescribed by your doctor for treating cancer of the breast or prostate). If you have had a stroke or heart attack or if you have angina pectoris, estrogens should be taken with great caution and only if clearly needed (for example, if you have severe symptoms of the menopause).

SPECIAL WARNING ABOUT PREGNANCY

You should not take estrogens if you are pregnant, because, although the possibility remains small, there may be a greater than usual risk that the developing child may be born with a birth defect. In a female child, there may be an increased risk that cancer of the vagina or cervix will develop later in life (in the teens or 20's). If estrogens have been taken during pregnancy, see your doctor.

OTHER EFFECTS OF ESTROGENS

In addition to the serious known risks described above, estrogens have the following side effects and involve the following potential risks:

1. *Nausea and vomiting.* The most common side effect of estrogen therapy is nausea. Vomiting occurs less frequently.
2. *Effects on the breasts.* Estrogens may cause tenderness or enlargement of the breasts and may cause the breasts to secrete a liquid. These effects are not dangerous.
3. *Effects on the uterus.* Estrogens may cause enlargement of benign fibroid tumors of the uterus.

Some women will have menstrual bleeding when they stop taking estrogens; however, if bleeding occurs on days when you are still taking estrogens, you should report this to your doctor.

4. *Effects on the liver.* On very rare occasions, a few women taking oral contraceptives develop a tumor of the liver which can rupture and bleed into the abdomen. So far, these tumors have not been reported in women taking estrogens during the menopause, but any swelling or unusual pain or tenderness in the abdomen should be reported to your doctor immediately.

Women with a past history of jaundice (yellowing of the skin and the white parts of the eyes) may have jaundice again when estrogens are administered. If this occurs, stop taking the estrogen and see your doctor.

5. *Other effects.* Estrogens may cause excess fluid to be retained in the body. This may worsen some conditions, such as epilepsy, migraine, heart disease, or kidney disease.

SUMMARY

Estrogens have important uses, but there also may be risks involved in their use. Together with your doctor, you must decide whether the risks are acceptable to you in view of the benefits of estrogen therapy. Except when your doctor has prescribed estrogens for treatment of special cases of cancer of the breast or prostate, you should not use estrogens if you have cancer of the breast or uterus, if you are pregnant, if you have undiagnosed abnormal vaginal bleeding or clotting in the legs or lungs, or if you have previously had a stroke, heart attack, angina, or clotting in the legs or lungs.

You can use estrogens as safely as possible by understanding that your doctor will want you to have regular physical ex-

Continued on next page

• **Identi-Code® symbol. This product information was prepared in June 1996. Current information on these and other products of Eli Lilly and Company may be obtained by direct inquiry to Lilly Research Laboratories, Lilly Corporate Center, Indianapolis, Indiana 46285, 800-545-5979.**

Lilly—Cont.

aminations while you are taking estrogens, and that he/she will use the smallest dose possible and will try to discontinue the drug as soon as possible. Be alert for signs of trouble, including:
1. Abnormal bleeding from the vagina.
2. Pains in the calves or chest, sudden shortness of breath, or coughing up blood (indicating possible clots in the legs, heart, or lungs).
3. Severe headache, faintness, dizziness, or changes in vision (indicating possible development of clots in the brain or eye).
4. Lumps in the breast. (You should ask your doctor to show you how you can examine your own breast.)
5. Jaundice (yellowing of the skin).
6. Mental depression.
On the basis of his or her assessment of your medical needs, your doctor has prescribed this drug for you. Do not give the drug to anyone else.

HOW SUPPLIED
Diethylstilbestrol is available for oral administration (Enseals® [enteric-release tablets, Lilly] or tablets).

INFORMATION FOR THE PATIENT DIETHYLSTILBESTROL, USP

FACTS THAT YOU SHOULD KNOW ABOUT ESTROGENS
Estrogens are female hormones produced by the ovaries. The ovaries produce several different kinds of estrogens. In addition, scientists have been able to develop a variety of synthetic estrogens. As far as we know, all these estrogens have similar properties and, therefore, have much the same usefulness and side effects and involve the same risks. This leaflet is intended to help you understand what estrogens are given for, the possible risks involved in their use, and how to use them as safely as possible.
This leaflet contains the most important information about estrogens. If you want to know more, you may ask your doctor or pharmacist to let you read the package insert prepared for the doctor.

USES OF ESTROGEN
Estrogens are prescribed by physicians for a number of purposes, and they may be given:
1. To prevent certain uncomfortable symptoms of estrogen deficiency during a period of adjustment when a woman's ovaries no longer produce estrogen. (All women normally stop producing estrogens, generally between the ages of 45 and 55; this is called the menopause.)
2. To prevent symptoms of estrogen deficiency when a woman's ovaries have been removed surgically before the natural menopause.
3. To prevent pregnancy. (Estrogens are given along with a progestagen, another female hormone; these combinations are called oral contraceptives or birth control pills. Patient information is available to women taking oral contraceptives, and these will not be discussed in this leaflet.)
4. To treat certain cancers in women and men.
NOTE: PREGNANT WOMEN SHOULD NOT TAKE ESTROGENS.

THE USE OF ESTROGENS DURING THE MENOPAUSE
All women eventually experience a decrease in estrogen production during the natural course of life. This usually occurs between the ages of 45 and 55, but it may occur earlier or later. Sometimes, the ovaries may have to be removed by an operation before the natural menopause occurs, thus producing a "surgical menopause."
When the amount of estrogen in the body begins to decrease, many women may develop some of the following typical symptoms: feelings of warmth in the face, neck, and chest, or sudden intense episodes of heat and sweating throughout the body (called "hot flashes" or "hot flushes"). Sometimes these symptoms are quite uncomfortable. A few women may eventually develop changes in the vagina (called "atrophic vaginitis") which cause discomfort, especially during and after intercourse.
Estrogens can be prescribed to treat these symptoms of the menopause.
Probably more than half of all women undergoing the menopause have only mild symptoms or none at all and thus do not need estrogens. Some women may require estrogens for only a few months while their bodies adjust to lower estrogen levels, whereas other women will need them for 6 months or longer. In an attempt to avoid overstimulation of the uterus (womb), estrogens are usually given on a cyclic basis each month, that is, 3 weeks of medication followed by 1 week with no medication.
Women sometimes experience nervous symptoms or depression during the menopause. There is no evidence that estrogens are effective for treating such symptoms, and they should not be used for this purpose; however, other treatment may be needed.
You may have heard that taking estrogens for a long period of time (years) after the menopause will keep your skin soft and supple and will keep you feeling young. Unfortunately, there is no evidence that this is true; on the other hand, there may be a significant risk involved in the use of such long-term treatment.

THE DANGER OF ESTROGENS
1. *Endometrial carcinoma.* There may be an increased risk of *endometrial carcinoma,* a form of cancer of the uterus, if estrogens are used for more than a year after the menopause. The chance of this cancer occurring may be approximately 5 to 10 times greater in women taking estrogen than in those women taking no estrogens. To put this another way, a woman who does not take estrogens after the menopause has 1 chance in 1,000 each year of having cancer of the uterus, whereas a woman who takes estrogens has 5 to 10 chances in 1,000 each year. For this reason, *it is important that estrogens be taken only when needed.*
It appears that the longer estrogens are taken, the greater the risk of this cancer; this risk seems to increase when larger doses are taken. For this reason, *it is important to take the lowest dose of estrogen that will control symptoms and to take it only as long as it is needed.* if estrogens are needed for longer periods of time, your doctor will want to reevaluate your need for estrogen at least every 6 months.
Women using estrogens should report to their doctors any irregular vaginal bleeding; such bleeding may be of no importance, but it can also be an early warning of cancer of the uterus. If you have vaginal bleeding, you should *not* use estrogens until your doctor has made a diagnosis and has verified that there is no cancer of the uterus.
If your uterus has been completely removed (total hysterectomy), there is no danger of endometrial carcinoma occurring.
2. *Other possible cancers.* When given to animals for a long period of time, estrogens have caused development of other tumors, such as tumors of the breast, cervix, vagina, or liver. At present, there is no evidence that there is an increased risk that such tumors will occur in women taking estrogens during the menopause, but there is no way to be sure that there is no risk. One study raises the possibility that the use of estrogens during the menopause may increase the risk that cancer of the breast will develop many years later. This is another reason why estrogens should be used only when clearly needed. While you are taking estrogens, it is important for you to go to your doctor at least once a year for a physical examination. Your doctor may also want to make more frequent examinations of your breasts if members of your family have had breast cancer or if you have breast nodules (lumps) or abnormal mammograms (breast-x-rays).
3. *Gallbladder disease.* Women who use estrogens after the menopause are more likely to develop gallbladder disease than are women who do not use estrogens. Birth control pills have a similar effect.
4. *Abnormal blood clots.* Oral contraceptives increase the risk of blood clots developing in various parts of the body. In rare cases, this can result in a stroke (if the clot is in the brain), a heart attack (a clot in a blood vessel of the heart), or a pulmonary embolus (a clot which forms in the legs or pelvis and then breaks off and travels to the lungs). Any of these can be fatal.
At this time, the use of estrogens during the menopause is not known to cause such blood clots, but this has not been fully studied and could still prove to involve such a risk. If you have blood clots in the legs or lungs or had a heart attack while you were taking estrogens or birth control pills, you should not take estrogens (unless they are being prescribed by your doctor for treating cancer of the breast or prostate). If you have had a stroke or heart attack or if you have angina pectoris, estrogens should be taken with great caution and only if clearly needed (for example, if you have severe symptoms of the menopause).

SPECIAL WARNING ABOUT PREGNANCY
You should not take estrogens if you are pregnant, because, although the possibility remains small, there may be a greater than usual risk that the developing child may be born with a birth defect. In a female child, there may be an increased risk that cancer of the vagina or cervix will develop later in life (in the teens or 20's). If estrogens have been taken during pregnancy, see your doctor.

OTHER EFFECTS OF ESTROGENS
In addition to the serious known risks described above, estrogens have the following side effects and involve the following potential risks:
1. *Nausea and vomiting.* The most common side effect of estrogen therapy is nausea. Vomiting occurs less frequently.
2. *Effects on the breasts.* Estrogens may cause tenderness or enlargement of the breasts and may cause the breasts to secrete a liquid. These effects are not dangerous.
3. *Effects on the uterus.* Estrogens may cause enlargement of benign fibroid tumors of the uterus.
Some women will have menstrual bleeding when they stop taking estrogens; however, if bleeding occurs on days when you are still taking estrogens, you should report this to your doctor.
4. *Effects on the liver.* On very rare occasions, a few women taking oral contraceptives develop a tumor of the liver which can rupture and bleed into the abdomen. So far, these tumors have not been reported in women taking estrogens during the menopause, but any swelling or unusual pain or tenderness in the abdomen should be reported to your doctor immediately.
Women with a past history of jaundice (yellowing of the skin and the white parts of the eyes) may have jaundice again when estrogens are administered. If this occurs, stop taking the estrogen and see your doctor.
5. *Other effects.* Estrogens may cause excess fluid to be retained in the body. This may worsen some conditions, such as epilepsy, migraine, heart disease, or kidney disease.

SUMMARY
Estrogens have important uses, but there also may be risks involved in their use. Together with your doctor, you must decide whether the risks are acceptable to you in view of the benefits of estrogen therapy. Except when your doctor has prescribed estrogens for treatment of special cases of cancer of the breast or prostate, you should not use estrogens if you have cancer of the breast or uterus, if you are pregnant, if you have undiagnosed abnormal vaginal bleeding or clotting in the legs or lungs, or if you have previously had a stroke, heart attack, angina, or clotting in the legs or lungs.
You can use estrogens as safely as possible by understanding that your doctor will want you to have regular physical examinations while you are taking estrogens, and that he/she will use the smallest dose possible and will try to discontinue the drug as soon as possible. Be alert for signs of trouble, including:
1. Abnormal bleeding from the vagina.
2. Pains in the calves or chest, sudden shortness of breath, or coughing up blood (indicating possible clots in the legs, heart, or lungs).
3. Severe headache, faintness, dizziness, or changes in vision (indicating possible development of clots in the brain or eye).
4. Lumps in the breast. (You should ask your doctor to show you how you can examine your own breast.)
5. Jaundice (yellowing of the skin).
6. Mental depression.
On the basis of his or her assessment of your medical needs, your doctor has prescribed this drug for you. Do not give the drug to anyone else.
Literature revised April 8, 1994

DOBUTREX® SOLUTION ℞
[*dō'bū-trĕks*]
(dobutamine hydrochloride)
Injection

DESCRIPTION
Dobutrex® Solution (Dobutamine Hydrochloride Injection) is 1,2-benzenediol, 4-[2-[[3-(4-hydroxyphenyl)-1-methylpropyl]amino]ethyl]-, hydrochloride, (±)-. It is a synthetic catecholamine.

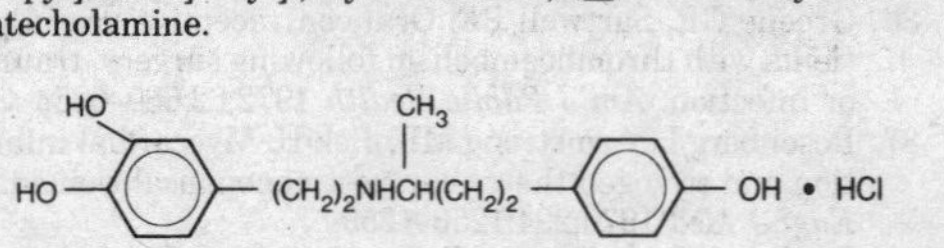
HO
CH3
HO
(CH2)2NHCH(CH2)2
OH • HCl

Molecular Formula: $C_{18}H_{23}NO_3 \cdot HCl$
Molecular Weight: 337.85

The clinical formulation is supplied in a sterile form for intravenous use only. Each mL contains 12.5 mg (41.5 μmol) dobutamine, 0.24 mg sodium bisulfite (added during manufacture), and water for injection, q.s. Hydrochloric acid and/or sodium hydroxide may have been added during manufacture to adjust the pH.

CLINICAL PHARMACOLOGY
Dobutrex Solution is a direct-acting inotropic agent whose primary activity results from stimulation of the β receptors of the heart while producing comparatively mild chronotropic, hypertensive, arrhythmogenic, and vasodilative effects. It does not cause the release of endogenous norepinephrine, as does dopamine. In animal studies, dobutamine hydrochloride produces less increase in heart rate and less decrease in peripheral vascular resistance for a given inotropic effect than does isoproterenol.
In patients with depressed cardiac function, both dobutamine hydrochloride and isoproterenol increase the cardiac output to a similar degree. In the case of dobutamine hydrochloride, this increase is usually not accompanied by marked increases in heart rate (although tachycardia is occasionally observed), and the cardiac stroke volume is usually increased. In contrast, isoproterenol increases the cardiac index primarily by increasing the heart rate while stroke volume changes little or declines.

Facilitation of atrioventricular conduction has been observed in human electrophysiologic studies and in patients with atrial fibrillation.

Systemic vascular resistance is usually decreased with administration of dobutamine hydrochloride. Occasionally, minimum vasoconstriction has been observed.

Most clinical experience with dobutamine hydrochloride is short-term—not more than several hours in duration. In the limited number of patients who were studied for 24, 48, and 72 hours, a persistent increase in cardiac output occurred in some, whereas output returned toward baseline values in others.

The onset of action of Dobutrex Solution is within 1 to 2 minutes; however, as much as 10 minutes may be required to obtain the peak effect of a particular infusion rate.

The plasma half-life of dobutamine hydrochloride in humans is 2 minutes. The principal routes of metabolism are methylation of the catechol and conjugation. In human urine, the major excretion products are the conjugates of dobutamine and 3-O-methyl dobutamine. The 3-O-methyl derivative of dobutamine is inactive.

Alteration of synaptic concentrations of catecholamines with either reserpine or tricyclic antidepressants does not alter the actions of dobutamine in animals, which indicates that the actions of dobutamine are not dependent on presynaptic mechanisms.

INDICATIONS AND USAGE

Dobutrex Solution is indicated when parenteral therapy is necessary for inotropic support in the short-term treatment of adults with cardiac decompensation due to depressed contractility resulting either from organic heart disease or from cardiac surgical procedures.

In patients who have atrial fibrillation with rapid ventricular response, a digitalis preparation should be used prior to institution of therapy with Dobutrex Solution.

CONTRAINDICATIONS

Dobutrex Solution is contraindicated in patients with idiopathic hypertrophic subaortic stenosis and in patients who have shown previous manifestations of hypersensitivity to Dobutrex Solution.

WARNINGS

1. *Increase in Heart Rate or Blood Pressure*—Dobutrex Solution may cause a marked increase in heart rate or blood pressure, especially systolic pressure. Approximately 10% of patients in clinical studies have had rate increases of 30 beats/minute or more, and about 7.5% have had a 50 mm Hg or greater increase in systolic pressure. Usually, reduction of dosage promptly reverses these effects. Because dobutamine hydrochloride facilitates atrioventricular conduction, patients with atrial fibrillation are at risk of developing rapid ventricular response. Patients with preexisting hypertension appear to face an increased risk of developing an exaggerated pressor response.

2. *Ectopic Activity*—Dobutrex Solution may precipitate or exacerbate ventricular ectopic activity, but it rarely has caused ventricular tachycardia.

3. *Hypersensitivity*—Reactions suggestive of hypersensitivity associated with administration of Dobutrex Solution, including skin rash, fever, eosinophilia, and bronchospasm, have been reported occasionally.

4. Dobutrex Solution contains sodium bisulfite, a sulfite that may cause allergic-type reactions, including anaphylactic symptoms and life-threatening or less severe asthmatic episodes, in certain susceptible people. The overall prevalence of sulfite sensitivity in the general population is unknown and probably low. Sulfite sensitivity is seen more frequently in asthmatic than in nonasthmatic people.

PRECAUTIONS

***General*—1. During the administration of Dobutrex Solution, as with any adrenergic agent, ECG and blood pressure should be continuously monitored. In addition, pulmonary wedge pressure and cardiac output should be monitored whenever possible to aid in the safe and effective infusion of Dobutrex Solution.**

2. Hypovolemia should be corrected with suitable volume expanders before treatment with Dobutrex Solution is instituted.

3. No improvement may be observed in the presence of marked mechanical obstruction, such as severe valvular aortic stenosis.

Usage Following Acute Myocardial Infarction—Clinical experience with Dobutrex Solution following myocardial infarction has been insufficient to establish the safety of the drug for this use. There is concern that any agent that increases contractile force and heart rate may increase the size of an infarction by intensifying ischemia, but it is not known whether dobutamine hydrochloride does so.

Laboratory Tests—Dobutamine, like other β_2-agonists, can produce a mild reduction in serum potassium concentration, rarely to hypokalemic levels. Accordingly, consideration should be given to monitoring serum potassium.

Drug Interactions—Animal studies indicate that dobutamine may be ineffective if the patient has recently received a

Dobutrex Solution Infusion Rate (mL/kg/min) for Concentrations of 250, 500, and 1,000 μg/mL

Drug Delivery Rate (μg/kg/min)	Infusion Delivery Rate: 250 μg/mL* (mL/kg/min)	500 μg/mL† (mL/kg/min)	1,000 μg/mL‡ (mL/kg/min)
2.5	0.01	0.005	0.0025
5	0.02	0.01	0.005
7.5	0.03	0.015	0.0075
10	0.04	0.02	0.01
12.5	0.05	0.025	0.0125
15	0.06	0.03	0.015

*250 μg/mL of diluent
†500 μg/mL or 250 mg/500 mL of diluent
‡1,000 μg/mL or 250 mg/250 mL of diluent

β-blocking drug. In such a case, the peripheral vascular resistance may increase.

Preliminary studies indicate that the concomitant use of dobutamine and nitroprusside results in a higher cardiac output and, usually, a lower pulmonary wedge pressure than when either drug is used alone.

There was no evidence of drug interactions in clinical studies in which Dobutrex Solution was administered concurrently with other drugs, including digitalis preparations, furosemide, spironolactone, lidocaine, glyceryl trinitrate, isosorbide dinitrate, morphine, atropine, heparin, protamine, potassium chloride, folic acid, and acetaminophen.

Carcinogenesis, Mutagenesis, Impairment of Fertility—Studies to evaluate the carcinogenic or mutagenic potential of Dobutrex Solution, or its potential to affect fertility, have not been conducted.

Pregnancy—Teratogenic Effects—Pregnancy Category-B—Reproduction studies performed in rats at doses up to the normal human dose (10 μg/kg/min for 24 h, total daily dose of 14.4 mg/kg) and in rabbits at doses up to twice the normal human dose, have revealed no evidence of harm to the fetus due to Dobutrex Solution. There are, however, no adequate and well-controlled studies in pregnant women. Because animal reproduction studies are not always predictive of human response, this drug should be used during pregnancy only if clearly needed.

Labor and Delivery—The effect of Dobutrex Solution on labor and delivery is unknown.

Nursing Mothers—It is not known whether this drug is excreted in human milk. Because many drugs are excreted in human milk, caution should be exercised when Dobutrex Solution is administered to a nursing woman. If a mother requires Dobutrex Solution treatment, breast-feeding should be discontinued for the duration of the treatment.

Pediatric Use—The safety and effectiveness of Dobutrex Solution for use in children have not been studied.

ADVERSE REACTIONS

Increased Heart Rate, Blood Pressure, and Ventricular Ectopic Activity—A 10- to 20-mm increase in systolic blood pressure and an increase in heart rate of 5 to 15 beats/minute have been noted in most patients (*see* Warnings regarding exaggerated chronotropic and pressor effects). Approximately 5% of patients have had increased premature ventricular beats during infusions. These effects are dose related.

Hypotension—Precipitous decreases in blood pressure have occasionally been described in association with Dobutrex Solution therapy. Decreasing the dose or discontinuing the infusion typically results in rapid return of blood pressure to baseline values. In rare cases, however, intervention may be required and reversibility may not be immediate.

Reactions at Sites of Intravenous Infusion—Phlebitis has occasionally been reported. Local inflammatory changes have been described following inadvertent infiltration. Isolated cases of cutaneous necrosis (destruction of skin tissue) have been reported.

Miscellaneous Uncommon Effects—The following adverse effects have been reported in 1% to 3% of patients: nausea, headache, anginal pain, nonspecific chest pain, palpitations, and shortness of breath.

Isolated cases of thrombocytopenia have been reported.

Administration of Dobutrex Solution, like other catecholamines, can produce a mild reduction in serum potassium concentration, rarely to hypokalemic levels (*see* Precautions).

Longer-Term Safety—Infusions of up to 72 hours have revealed no adverse effects other than those seen with shorter infusions.

OVERDOSAGE

Overdoses of Dobutrex Solution have been reported rarely. The following is provided to serve as a guide if such an overdose is encountered.

Signs and Symptoms—Toxicity from Dobutrex Solution is usually due to excessive cardiac β-receptor stimulation. The duration of action of Dobutrex Solution is generally short ($T_{1/2}$ = 2 minutes) because it is rapidly metabolized by catechol-O-methyltransferase. The symptoms of toxicity may include anorexia, nausea, vomiting, tremor, anxiety, palpitations, headache, shortness of breath, and anginal and nonspecific chest pain. The positive inotropic and chronotropic effects of Dobutrex Solution on the myocardium may cause hypertension, tachyarrhythmias, myocardial ischemia, and ventricular fibrillation. Hypotension may result from vasodilation.

Treatment—To obtain up-to-date information about the treatment of overdose, a good resource is your certified Regional Poison Control Center. Telephone numbers of certified poison control centers are listed in the *Physicians' Desk Reference (PDR)*. In managing overdosage, consider the possibility of multiple drug overdoses, interaction among drugs, and unusual drug kinetics in your patient.

The initial actions to be taken in a Dobutrex Solution overdose are discontinuing administration, establishing an airway, and ensuring oxygenation and ventilation. Resuscitative measures should be initiated promptly. Severe ventricular tachyarrhythmias may be successfully treated with propranolol or lidocaine. Hypertension usually responds to a reduction in dose or discontinuation of therapy.

Protect the patient's airway and support ventilation and perfusion. If needed, meticulously monitor and maintain, within acceptable limits, the patient's vital signs, blood gases, serum electrolytes, etc.

If the product is ingested, unpredictable absorption may occur from the mouth and the gastrointestinal tract.

Absorption of drugs from the gastrointestinal tract may be decreased by giving activated charcoal, which, in many cases, is more effective than emesis or lavage; consider charcoal instead of or in addition to gastric emptying. Repeated doses of charcoal over time may hasten elimination of some drugs that have been absorbed. Safeguard the patient's airway when employing gastric emptying or charcoal.

Forced diuresis, peritoneal dialysis, hemodialysis, or charcoal hemoperfusion have not been established as beneficial for an overdose of Dobutrex Solution.

DOSAGE AND ADMINISTRATION

Note—Do not add Dobutrex Solution to 5% Sodium Bicarbonate Injection or to any other strongly alkaline solution. Because of potential physicial incompatibilities, it is recommended that Dobutrex Solution not be mixed with other drugs in the same solution. Dobutrex Solution should not be used in conjunction with other agents or diluents containing both sodium bisulfite and ethanol.

Reconstitution and Stability—At the time of administration, Dobutrex Solution must be further diluted in an IV container to at least a 50-mL solution using one of the following intravenous solutions as a diluent: 5% Dextrose Injection, 5% Dextrose and 0.45% Sodium Chloride Injection, 5% Dextrose and 0.9% Sodium Chloride Injection, 10% Dextrose Injection, Isolyte® M with 5% Dextrose Injection, Lactated Ringer's Injection, 5% Dextrose in Lactated Ringer's Injection, Normosol®-M in D5-W, 20% Osmitrol® in Water for Injection, 0.9% Sodium Chloride Injection, or Sodium Lactate Injection. Intravenous solutions should be used within 24 hours.

Recommended Dosage—The rate of infusion needed to increase cardiac output usually ranged from 2.5 to 15 μg/kg/min (see Table 1). On rare occasions, infusion rates up to 40 μg/kg/min have been required to obtain the desired effect.

[See table above.]

Rates of infusion in mL/h for Dobutrex Solution concentrations of 500 μg/mL, 1,000 μg/mL, and 2,000 μg/mL are given in Table 2.

[See table on top of next column.]

Continued on next page

• Identi-Code® symbol. This product information was prepared in June 1996. Current information on these and other products of Eli Lilly and Company may be obtained by direct inquiry to Lilly Research Laboratories, Lilly Corporate Center, Indianapolis, Indiana 46285, 800-545-5979.

Lilly—Cont.

Table 2
Dobutrex Solution Infusion Rate (mL/h) for 500 μg/mL concentration

Drug Delivery Rate (μg/kg/min)	Patient Body Weight (kg) 30	40	50	60	70	80	90	100	110
2.5	9	12	15	18	21	24	27	30	33
5	18	24	30	36	42	48	54	60	66
7.5	27	36	45	54	63	72	81	90	99
10	36	48	60	72	84	96	108	120	132
12.5	45	60	75	90	105	120	135	150	165
15	54	72	90	108	126	144	162	180	198

Dobutrex Solution Infusion Rate (mL/h) for 1,000 μg/mL concentration

Drug Delivery Rate (μg/kg/min)	Patient Body Weight (kg) 30	40	50	60	70	80	90	100	110
2.5	4.5	6	7.5	9	10.5	12	13.5	15	16.5
5	9	12	15	18	21	24	27	30	33
7.5	13.5	18	22.5	27	31.5	36	40.5	45	49.5
10	18	24	30	36	42	48	54	60	66
12.5	22.5	30	37.5	45	52.5	60	67.5	75	82.5
15	27	36	45	54	63	72	81	90	99

Dobutrex Solution Infusion Rate (mL/h) for 2,000 μg/mL concentration

Drug Delivery Rate (μg/kg/min)	Patient Body Weight (kg) 30	40	50	60	70	80	90	100	110
2.5	2	3	4	4.5	5	6	7	7.5	8
5	4.5	6	7.5	9	10.5	12	13.5	15	16.5
7.5	7	9	11	13.5	16	18	20	22.5	25
10	9	12	15	18	21	24	27	30	33
12.5	11	15	19	22.5	26	30	34	37.5	41
15	13.5	18	22.5	27	31.5	36	40.5	45	49.5

The rate of administration and the duration of therapy should be adjusted according to the patient's response as determined by heart rate, presence of ectopic activity, blood pressure, urine flow, and, whenever possible, measurement of central venous or pulmonary wedge pressure and cardiac output.
Concentrations up to 5,000 μg/mL have been administered to humans (250 mg/50 mL). The final volume administered should be determined by the fluid requirements of the patient.
Intravenous drug products should be inspected visually and should not be used if particulate matter or discoloration is present.

HOW SUPPLIED

Vials:
250 mg,* 20-mL size (No. 7175)—(1s) NDC 0002-7175-01; (Traypak† of 10) NDC 0002-7175-10

* Equivalent to dobutamine hydrochloride.
† Traypak™(multivial carton, Lilly)
Store at controlled room temperature, 59° to 86°F (15° to 30°C).
CAUTION—Federal (USA) law prohibits dispensing without prescription.
Literature revised September 19, 1995 [091995]

FLUOXETINE HYDROCHLORIDE, ℞
see Prozac® (Fluoxetine Hydrochloride).

GEMZAR® ℞
(GEMCITABINE HCl)
FOR INJECTION

DESCRIPTION

Gemzar® (gemcitabine HCl) is a nucleoside analogue that exhibits antitumor activity. Gemcitabine HCl is 2′-deoxy-2′,2′- difluorocytidine monohydrochloride (β-isomer).
The structural formula is as follows:
[See chemical structure at top of next column.]
The empirical formula for gemcitabine HCl is $C_9H_{11}F_2N_3O_4$·HCl. It has a molecular weight of 299.66.
Gemcitabine HCl is a white to off-white solid. It is soluble in water, slightly soluble in methanol, and practically insoluble in ethanol and polar organic solvents.

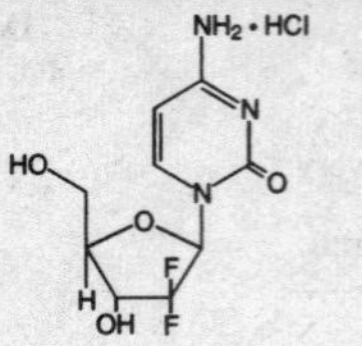

The clinical formulation is supplied in a sterile form for intravenous use only. Vials of Gemzar contain either 200 mg or 1 g of gemcitabine HCl (expressed as free base) formulated with mannitol (200 mg or 1 g, respectively) and sodium acetate (12.5 mg or 62.5 mg, respectively) as a sterile lyophilized powder. Hydrochloric acid and/or sodium hydroxide may have been added for pH adjustment.

CLINICAL PHARMACOLOGY

Gemcitabine exhibits cell phase specificity, primarily killing cells undergoing DNA synthesis (S-phase) and also blocking the progression of cells through the G1/S-phase boundary. Gemcitabine is metabolized intracellularly by nucleoside kinases to the active diphosphate (dFdCDP) and triphosphate (dFdCTP) nucleosides. The cytotoxic effect of gemcitabine is attributed to a combination of two actions of the diphosphate and the triphosphate nucleosides, which leads to inhibition of DNA synthesis. First, gemcitabine diphosphate inhibits ribonucleotide reductase, which is responsible for catalyzing the reactions that generate the deoxynucleoside triphosphates for DNA synthesis. Inhibition of this enzyme by the diphosphate nucleoside causes a reduction in the concentrations of deoxynucleotides, including dCTP. Second, gemcitabine triphosphate competes with dCTP for incorporation into DNA. The reduction in the intracellular concentration of dCTP (by the action of the diphosphate) enhances the incorporation of gemcitabine triphosphate into DNA (self-potentiation). After the gemcitabine nucleotide is incorporated into DNA, only one additional nucleotide is added to the growing DNA strands. After this addition, there is inhibition of further DNA synthesis. DNA polymerase epsilon is unable to remove the gemcitabine nucleotide and repair the growing DNA strands (masked chain termination). In CEM T lymphoblastoid cells, gemcitabine induces internucleosomal DNA fragmentation, one of the characteristics of programmed cell death.
Human Pharmacokinetics—Gemcitabine disposition was studied in five patients who received a single 1000 mg/m²/30 minute infusion of radiolabeled drug. Within one (1) week, 92% to 98% of the dose was recovered, almost entirely in the urine. Gemcitabine (< 10%) and the inactive uracil metabolite, 2′-deoxy-2′, 2′-difluorouridine (dFdU), accounted for 99% of the excreted dose. The metabolite dFdU is also found in plasma. Gemcitabine plasma protein binding is negligible.
The pharmacokinetics of gemcitabine were examined in 353 patients, about 2/3 men, with various solid tumors. Pharmacokinetic parameters were derived using data from patients treated for varying durations of therapy given weekly with periodic rest weeks and using both short infusions (< 70 minutes) and long infusions (70 to 285 minutes). The total Gemzar dose varied from 500 to 3600 mg/m².
Gemcitabine pharmacokinetics are linear and are described by a 2-compartment model. Population pharmacokinetic analyses of combined single and multiple dose studies showed that the volume of distribution of gemcitabine was significantly influenced by duration of infusion and gender. Clearance was affected by age and gender. Differences in either clearance or volume of distribution based on patient characteristics or the duration of infusion result in changes in half-life and plasma concentrations. Table 1 shows plasma clearance and half-life of gemcitabine following short infusions for typical patients by age and gender.

Table 1
Gemcitabine Clearance and Half-Life for the "Typical" Patient

Age	Clearance Men (L/hr/m²)	Clearance Women (L/hr/m²)	Half-Life[a] Men (min)	Half-Life[a] Women (min)
29	92.2	69.4	42	49
45	75.7	57.0	48	57
65	55.1	41.5	61	73
79	40.7	30.7	79	94

[a]Half-life for patients receiving a short infusion (< 70 min)

Gemcitabine half-life for short infusions ranged from 32 to 94 minutes, and the value for long infusions varied from 245 to 638 minutes, depending on age and gender, reflecting a greatly increased volume of distribution with longer infusions. The lower clearance in women and the elderly results in higher concentrations of gemcitabine for any given dose.
The volume of distribution was increased with infusion length. Volume of distribution of gemcitabine was 50 L/m² following infusions lasting < 70 minutes, indicating that gemcitabine, after short infusions, is not extensively distributed into tissues. For long infusions, the volume of distribution rose to 370 L/m², reflecting slow equilibration of gemcitabine within the tissue compartment.
The maximum plasma concentrations of dFdU (inactive metabolite) were achieved up to 30 minutes after discontinuation of the infusions and the metabolite is excreted in urine without undergoing further biotransformation. The metabolite did not accumulate with weekly dosing, but its elimination is dependent on renal excretion, and could accumulate with decreased renal function.
The effects of significant renal or hepatic insufficiency on the disposition of gemcitabine have not been assessed.
The active metabolite, gemcitabine triphosphate, can be extracted from peripheral blood mononuclear cells. The half-life of the terminal phase for gemcitabine triphosphate from mononuclear cells ranges from 1.7 to 19.4 hours.

CLINICAL STUDIES

Data from two clinical trials evaluated the use of Gemzar in patients with locally advanced or metastatic pancreatic cancer. The first trial compared Gemzar to 5-Fluorouracil (5-FU) in patients who had received no prior chemotherapy. A second trial studied the use of Gemzar in pancreatic cancer patients previously treated with 5-FU or a 5-FU-containing regimen. In both studies, the first cycle of Gemzar was administered intravenously at a dose of 1000 mg/m² over 30 minutes once weekly for up to 7 weeks (or until toxicity necessitated holding a dose) followed by a week of rest from treatment with Gemzar. Subsequent cycles consisted of injections once weekly for 3 consecutive weeks out of every 4 weeks.
The primary efficacy parameter in these studies was "clinical benefit response", which is a measure of clinical improvement based on analgesic consumption, pain intensity, performance status, and weight change. Definitions for improvement in these variables were formulated prospectively during the design of the two trials. A patient was considered a clinical benefit responder if either:
i) the patient showed a ≥ 50% reduction in pain intensity (Memorial Pain Assessment Card) or analgesic consumption, or a twenty point or greater improvement in performance status (Karnofsky Performance Scale) for a period of at least four consecutive weeks, without showing any sustained worsening in any of the other parameters. Sustained worsening was defined as four consecutive weeks with either any increase in pain intensity or analgesic consumption or a 20 point decrease in performance status occurring during the first 12 weeks of therapy.

OR:

ii) the patient was stable on all of the aforementioned parameters, and showed a marked, sustained weight gain (≥ 7% increase maintained for ≥ 4 weeks) not due to fluid accumulation.

The first study was a multicenter (17 sites in US and Canada), prospective, single-blinded, two-arm, randomized comparison of Gemzar and 5-FU in patients with locally advanced or metastatic pancreatic cancer who had received no prior treatment with chemotherapy. 5-FU was administered intravenously at a weekly dose of 600 mg/m² for 30 minutes. The results from this randomized trial are shown in Table 2. Patients treated with Gemzar had statistically significant increases in clinical benefit response, survival, and time to progressive disease compared to 5-FU. The Kaplan-Meier curve for survival is shown in Figure 1. No confirmed objective tumor responses were observed with either treatment.
[See Table 2 at top of next page.]

Figure 1
Kaplan-Meier Survival Curve

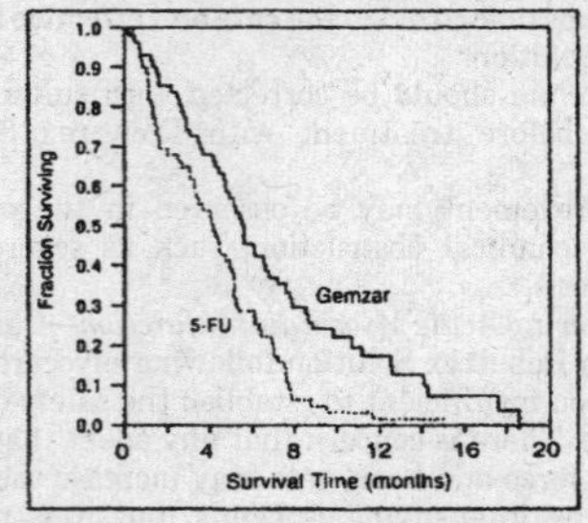

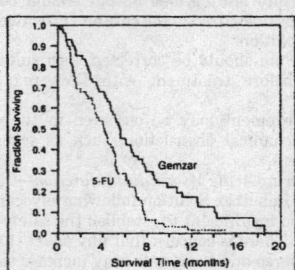

Clinical benefit response was achieved by 14 patients treated with Gemzar and 3 patients treated with 5-FU. One patient on the Gemzar arm showed improvement in all three primary parameters (pain intensity, analgesic consumption, and performance status). Eleven patients on the Gemzar arm and two patients on the 5-FU arm showed improvement in

Table 2
Gemzar Versus 5-FU in Pancreatic Cancer

	Gemzar	5-FU	
Number of Patients	63	63	
Male	34	34	
Female	29	29	
Median Age	62 years	61 years	
Range	37 to 79	36 to 77	
Stage IV Disease	71.4%	76.2%	
Baseline KPS[a] ≤70	69.8%	68.3%	
Clinical benefit response	22.2%	4.8%	p = 0.004
	(N[c] = 14)	(N = 3)	
Survival			p = 0.0009
Median	5.7 months	4.2 months	
6-month probability[b]	(N = 30) 46%	(N = 19) 29%	
9-month probability[b]	(N = 14) 24%	(N = 4) 5%	
1-year probability[b]	(N = 9) 18%	(N = 2) 2%	
Range	0.2 to 18.6 months	0.4 to 15.1+ months	
95% C.I. of the median	4.7 to 6.9 months	3.1 to 5.1 months	
Time to Progressive Disease		p = 0.0013	
Median	2.1 months	0.9 months	
Range	0.1+ to 9.4 months	0.1 to 12.0+ months	
95% C.I. of the median	1.9 to 3.4 months	0.9 to 1.1 months	

a Karnofsky Performance Status
b Kaplan-Meier estimates
c N = number of patients
+No progression at last visit; remains alive.
The p-value for clinical benefit response was calculated using the 2-sided test for difference in binomial proportions. All other p-values were calculated using the Log Rank test for difference in overall time to an event.

Table 3
Selected WHO-Graded Adverse Events in Patients Receiving Gemzar

	All Patients[a]			Pancreatic Cancer Patients[b]			Discontinuations(%)[c]
	All Grades	Grade 3	Grade 4	All Grades	Grade 3	Grade 4	All Patients
Laboratory[d]							
Hematologic							
Anemia	68	7	1	73	8	2	<1
Leukopenia	62	9	<1	64	8	1	<1
Neutropenia	63	19	6	61	17	7	—
Thrombocytopenia	24	4	1	36	7	<1	<1
Hepatic							<1
ALT	68	8	2	72	10	1	
AST	67	6	2	78	12	5	
Alkaline Phosphatase	55	7	2	77	16	4	
Bilirubin	13	2	<1	26	6	2	
Renal							<1
Proteinuria	45	<1	0	32	<1	0	
Hematuria	35	<1	0	23	0	0	
BUN	16	0	0	15	0	0	
Creatinine	8	<1	0	6	0	0	
Nonlaboratory[e]							
Nausea and Vomiting	69	13	1	71	10	2	<1
Pain	48	9	<1	42	6	<1	<1
Fever	41	2	0	38	2	0	<1
Rash	30	<1	0	28	<1	0	<1
Dyspnea	23	3	<1	10	0	<1	<1
Constipation	23	1	<1	31	3	<1	0
Diarrhea	19	1	0	30	3	0	0
Hemorrhage	17	<1	<1	4	2	<1	<1
Infection	16	1	<1	10	2	<1	<1
Alopecia	15	<1	0	16	0	0	0
Stomatitis	11	<1	0	10	<1	0	<1
Somnolence	11	<1	<1	11	2	<1	<1
Paresthesias	10	<1	0	10	<1	0	0

Grade based on criteria from the World Health Organization (WHO)
[a]N = 699–974; all patients with data
[b]N = 161–241; all pancreatic cancer patients with data
[c]N = 979
[d]Regardless of causality
[e]Table includes nonlaboratory data with incidence for all patients ≥ 10%. For approximately 60% of the patients, nonlaboratory events were graded only if assessed to be possibly drug related.

analgesic consumption and/or pain intensity with stable performance status. Two patients on the Gemzar arm showed improvement in analgesic consumption or pain intensity with improvement in performance status. One patient on the 5-FU arm was stable with regard to pain intensity and analgesic consumption, with improvement in performance status. No patient on either arm achieved a clinical benefit response based on weight gain.

The second trial was a multicenter (17 US and Canadian centers), open-label study of Gemzar in 63 patients with advanced pancreatic cancer previously treated with 5-FU or a 5-FU-containing regimen. The study showed a clinical bene-

fit response rate of 27% and median survival of 3.9 months. When Gemzar was administered more frequently than once weekly or with infusions longer than 60 minutes, increased toxicity was observed. Results of a Phase 1 study of Gemzar to assess the maximum tolerated dose (MTD) on a daily × 5 schedule showed that patients developed significant hypotension and severe flu-like symptoms that were intolerable at doses above 10 mg/m^2. The incidence and severity of these events were dose-related. Other Phase 1 studies using a twice-weekly schedule reached MTDs of only 65 mg/m^2 (30-minute infusion) and 150 mg/m^2 (5-minute bolus). The dose-limiting toxicities were thrombocytopenia and flu-like symptoms, particularly asthenia. In a Phase 1 study to assess the maximum tolerated infusion time, clinically significant toxicity, defined as myelosuppression, was seen with weekly doses of 300 mg/m^2 at or above a 270-minute infusion time. The half-life of gemcitabine is influenced by the length of the infusion (see Clinical Pharmacology) and the toxicity appears to be increased if Gemzar is administered more frequently than once weekly or with infusions longer than 60 minutes (see Warnings).

In a single trial where Gemzar at a dose of 1000 mg/m^2 was administered for up to six (6) consecutive weeks concurrently with therapeutic thoracic radiation to patients with NSCLC, significant toxicity in the form of severe, and potentially life-threatening, esophagitis and pneumonitis was observed, particularly in patients receiving large volumes of radiotherapy. The optimum regimen for safe administration of Gemzar with therapeutic doses of radiation has not yet been determined (see Precautions).

INDICATIONS AND USAGE

Therapeutic Indication—Gemzar is indicated as first-line treatment for patients with locally advanced (nonresectable Stage II or Stage III) or metastatic (Stage IV) adenocarcinoma of the pancreas. Gemzar is indicated for patients previously treated with 5-FU.

CONTRAINDICATION

Gemzar is contraindicated in those patients with a known hypersensitivity to the drug (see Adverse Reactions—Allergic).

WARNINGS

Caution—Prolongation of the infusion time beyond 60 minutes and more frequent than weekly dosing have been shown to increase toxicity (see Clinical Studies).

Gemzar can suppress bone marrow function as manifested by leukopenia, thrombocytopenia, and anemia (see Adverse Reactions), and myelosuppression is usually the dose-limiting toxicity. Patients should be monitored for myelosuppression during therapy. See Dosage and Administration for recommended dose adjustments.

Hemolytic-Uremic Syndrome (HUS) has been reported rarely with the use of Gemzar. (see Adverse Reactions—Renal)

Pregnancy—Pregnancy Category D. Gemzar can cause fetal harm when administered to a pregnant woman. Gemcitabine is embryotoxic causing fetal malformations (cleft palate, incomplete ossification) at doses of 1.5 mg/kg/day in mice (about $^1/_{200}$ the recommended human dose on a mg/m^2 basis). Gemcitabine is fetotoxic causing fetal malformations (fused pulmonary artery, absence of gall bladder) at doses of 0.1 mg/kg/day in rabbits (about $^1/_{600}$ the recommended human dose on a mg/m^2 basis). Embryotoxicity was characterized by decreased fetal viability, reduced live litter sizes, and developmental delays. There are no studies of Gemzar in pregnant women. If Gemzar is used during pregnancy, or if the patient becomes pregnant while taking Gemzar, the patient should be apprised of the potential hazard to the fetus.

PRECAUTIONS

General—Patients receiving therapy with Gemzar should be monitored closely by a physician experienced in the use of cancer chemotherapeutic agents. Most adverse events are reversible and do not need to result in discontinuation, although doses may need to be withheld or reduced. There was a greater tendency in women, especially older women, not to proceed to the next cycle.

Laboratory Tests—Patients receiving Gemzar should be monitored prior to each dose with a complete blood count (CBC), including differential and platelet count. Suspension or modification of therapy should be considered when marrow suppression is detected (see Dosage and Administration).

Laboratory evaluation of renal and hepatic function should be performed prior to initiation of therapy and periodically thereafter.

Carcinogenesis, Mutagenesis, Impairment of Fertility—Long-term animal studies to evaluate the carcinogenic potential of

Continued on next page

Lilly—Cont.

Gemzar have not been conducted. Gemcitabine induced forward mutations *in vitro* in a mouse lymphoma (L5178Y) assay and was clastogenic in an *in vivo* mouse micronucleus assay. Gemcitabine was negative when tested using the Ames, *in vivo* sister chromatid exchange, and *in vitro* chromosomal aberration assays, and did not cause unscheduled DNA synthesis *in vitro*. Gemcitabine I.P. doses of 0.5 mg/kg/day (about $^1/_{700}$ the human dose on a mg/m^2 basis) in male mice had an effect on fertility with moderate to severe hypospermatogenesis, decreased fertility, and decreased implantations. In female mice, fertility was not affected but, maternal toxicities were observed at 1.5 mg/kg/day I.V. (about $^1/_{200}$ the human dose on a mg/m^2 basis) and fetotoxicity or embryopethality was observed at 0.25 mg/kg/day I.V. (about $^1/_{1300}$ the human dose on a mg/m^2 basis).

Pregnancy—Category D. *See* Warnings.

Nursing Mothers—It is not known whether Gemzar or its metabolites are excreted in human milk. Because many drugs are excreted in human milk and because of the potential for serious adverse reactions from Gemzar in nursing infants, the mother should be warned and a decision should be made whether to discontinue nursing or to discontinue the drug, taking into account the importance of the drug to the mother and the potential risk to the infant.

Elderly Patients—Gemzar clearance is affected by age (*see* Clinical Pharmacology). There is no evidence, however, that unusual dose adjustment (ie, other than those already recommended in the Dosage and Administration section) are necessary in patients over 65, and, in general adverse reaction rates were similar in patients above and below 65. Grade 3/4 thrombocytopenia was more common in the elderly.

Gender—Gemzar clearance is affected by gender (*see* Clinical Pharmacology). There is no evidence, however, that unusual dose adjustments (ie, other than those already recommended in the Dosage and Administration section) are necessary in women. In general, adverse reaction rates were similar in men and women but women, especially older women were more likely not to proceed to a subsequent cycle and to experience grade 3/4 neutropenia and thrombocytopenia.

Pediatric Patients—Gemzar has not been studied in pediatric patients. Safety and effectiveness in pediatric patients have not been established.

Patients with Renal or Hepatic Impairment—Gemzar should be used with caution in patients with preexisting renal impairment or hepatic insufficiency. Gemzar has not been studied in patients with significant renal or hepatic impairment.

Drug Interactions—No confirmed interactions have been reported with the use of Gemzar. No specific drug interaction studies have been conducted.

Combination Therapy—Safe and effective regimens for the administration of Gemzar with therapeutic doses of radiation have not yet been determined (*See* Clinical Studies).

ADVERSE REACTIONS

Myelosuppression is the principal dose-limiting factor with Gemzar therapy. Dosage adjustments for hematologic toxicity are frequently needed and are described in the Dosage and Administration section.

Data in Table 3 are based on 22 clinical studies (N = 979) of Gemzar administered as a single agent, using starting doses in the range of 800 to 1250 mg/m^2 administered weekly as a 30-minute infusion for treatment of a wide variety of malignancies. Data are also shown for the subset of patients with pancreatic cancer treated in 5 clinical studies. The frequency of all grades and severe (WHO Grade 3 or 4) adverse events were generally similar for the overall safety database and the subset of patients with pancreatic cancer. Adverse reactions reported in the overall database resulted in discontinuation of Gemzar therapy in about 10% of patients. In the comparative trial, the discontinuation rate for adverse reactions was 14.3% for the gemcitabine arm and 4.8% for the 5-FU arm.

All WHO-graded laboratory events are listed in Table 3, regardless of causality. Nonlaboratory adverse events listed in Table 3 or discussed below were those reported, regardless of causality, for at least 10% of all patients, except the categories of Extravasation. Allergic, and Cardiovascular and certain specific events under the Renal, Pulmonary, and Infection categories. Table 4 presents the data from the comparative trial of Gemzar and 5-FU for the same adverse events as Table 3, regardless of incidence.

[See Table 3 on preceding page.]

[See Table 4 above.]

Hematologic—Myelosuppression is the dose-limiting toxicity with Gemzar, but <1% of patients discontinued therapy for either anemia, leukopenia, or thrombocytopenia. Red blood cell transfusions were required by 19% of patients. The incidence of sepsis was less than 1%. Petechiae or mild blood loss (hemorrhage), from any cause, were reported in 16% of patients; less than 1% of patients required platelet transfusions. Patients should be monitored for myelosuppression during Gemzar therapy and dosage modified or suspended

according to the degree of hematologic toxicity (*see* Dosage and Administration).

Gastrointestinal—Nausea and vomiting were commonly reported (69%) but were usually mild to moderate. Severe nausea and vomiting (WHO Grade 3/4) occurred in <15% of patients. Diarrhea was reported by 19% of patients, and stomatitis by 11% of patients.

Hepatic—Gemzar was associated with transient elevations of serum transaminases in approximately two-thirds of patients, but there was no evidence of increasing hepatic toxicity with either longer duration of exposure to Gemzar or with greater total cumulative dose.

Renal—Mild proteinuria and hematuria were commonly reported. Clinical findings consistent with the hemolytic uremic syndrome (HUS) were reported in 6 of 2429 patients (0.25%) receiving Gemzar in clinical trials. Four patients developed HUS on Gemzar therapy, two immediately post-therapy. Renal failure may not be reversible even with discontinuation of therapy, and dialysis may be required.

Fever—The overall incidence of fever was 41%. This is in contrast to the incidence of infection (16%) and indicates that Gemzar may cause fever in the absence of clinical infection. Fever was frequently associated with other flu-like symptoms and was usually mild and clinically manageable.

Rash—Rash was reported in 30% of patients. The rash was typically a macular or finely granular maculopapular pruritic eruption of mild to moderate severity involving the trunk and extremities. Pruritus was reported for 13% of patients.

Pulmonary—Dyspnea was reported in 23% of patients, severe dyspnea in 3%. Dyspnea may be due to underlying disease such as lung cancer (40% of study population) or pulmonary manifestations of other malignancies. Dyspnea was occasionally accompanied by bronchospasm (<2% of patients.) Rare reports of parenchymal lung toxicity consistent with drug induced pneumonitis have been associated with the use of Gemzar.

Edema—Edema (13%), peripheral edema (20%), and generalized edema (<1%) were reported. Less than 1% of patients discontinued due to edema.

Flu-like Symptoms—"Flu syndrome" was reported for 19% of patients. Individual symptoms of fewer, asthenia, anorexia, headache, cough, chills, and myalgia were commonly reported. Fever and asthenia were also reported frequently

as isolated symptoms. Insomia, rhinitis, sweating, and malaise were reported infrequently. Less than 1% of patients discontinued due to flu-like symptoms.

Infection—Infections were reported for 16% of patients. Sepsis was rarely reported (<1%).

Alopecia—Hair loss, usually minimal, was reported by 15% of patients.

Neurotoxicity—There was a 10% incidence of mild paresthesias and a <1% rate of severe paresthesias.

Extravasation—Injection-site related events were reported for 4% of patients. There were no reports of injection site necrosis. Gemzar is not a vesicant.

Allergic—Bronchospasm was reported for less than 2% of patients. Anaphylactoid reaction has been reported rarely. Gemzar should not be administered to patients with a known hypersensitivity to this drug (*see* Contraindication).

Cardiovascular—Two percent of patients discontinued therapy with Gemzar due to cardiovascular events such as myocardial infarction, cerebrovascular accident, arrhythmia, and hypertension. Many of these patients had a prior history of cardiovascular disease.

OVERDOSAGE

There is no known antidote for overdoses of Gemzar. Myelosuppression, paresthesias and severe rash were the principal toxicities seen when a single dose as high as 5700 mg/m^2 was administered by IV infusion over 30 minutes every 2 weeks to several patients in a Phase 1 study. In the event of suspected overdose, the patient should be monitored with appropriate blood counts and should receive supportive therapy, as necessary.

DOSAGE AND ADMINISTRATION

Gemzar is for intravenous use only.

Adults—Gemzar should be administered by intravenous infusion at a dose of 1000 mg/m^2 over 30 minutes once weekly for up to 7 weeks (or until toxicity necessitates reducing or holding a dose), followed by a week of rest from treatment. Subsequent cycles should consist of infusions once weekly for 3 consecutive weeks out of every 4 weeks. Dosage adjustment is based upon the degree of hematologic toxicity experienced by the patient (*see* Warnings). Clearance in women and the elderly is reduced and women were somewhat less able to progress to subsequent cycles (*see* Human Pharmacokinetics and Precautions).

Gemzar® (Gemcitabine HCl)

Table 4
Selected WHO-Graded Adverse Events from Comparative Trial of Gemzar and 5-FU
WHO Grades (% incidence)

	Gemzar[a]			5-FU[b]		
	All Grades	Grade 3	Grade 4	All Grades	Grade 3	Grade 4
Laboratory[c]						
Hematologic						
Anemia	65	7	3	45	0	0
Leukopenia	71	10	0	15	2	0
Neutropenia	62	19	7	18	2	3
Thrombocytopenia	47	10	0	15	2	0
Hepatic						
ALT	72	8	2	38	0	0
AST	72	10	2	52	2	0
Alkaline Phosphatase	71	16	0	64	10	3
Bilirubin	16	2	2	25	6	3
Renal						
Proteinuria	10	0	0	2	0	0
Hematuria	13	0	0	0	0	0
BUN	8	0	0	10	0	0
Creatinine	2	0	0	0	0	0
Nonlaboratory[d]						
Nausea and Vomiting	64	10	3	58	5	0
Pain	10	2	0	7	0	0
Fever	30	0	0	16	0	0
Rash	24	0	0	13	0	0
Dyspnea	6	0	0	3	0	0
Constipation	10	3	0	11	2	0
Diarrhea	24	2	0	31	5	0
Hemorrhage	0	0	0	2	0	0
Infection	8	0	0	3	2	0
Alopecia	18	0	0	16	0	0
Stomatitis	14	0	0	15	0	0
Somnolence	5	2	0	7	2	0
Paresthesias	2	0	0	2	0	0

Grade based on criteria from the World Health Organization (WHO)
[a] N = 58–63; all Gemzar patients with data
[b] N = 61–63; all 5-FU patients with data
[c] Regardless of causality
[d] Nonlaboratory events were graded only if assessed to be possibly drug-related.

Patients receiving Gemzar should be monitored prior to each dose with a complete blood count (CBC), including differential and platelet count. If marrow suppression is detected, therapy should be modified or suspended according to the guidelines in Table 5.

Table 5
Dosage Reduction Guidelines

Absolute granulocyte count ($\times 10^6$/L)		Platelet count ($\times 10^6$/L)	% of full dose
$\geq$ 1,000	and	$\geq$ 100,000	100
500–999	or	50,000–99,000	75
< 500	or	< 50,000	hold

Laboratory evaluation of renal and hepatic function, including transaminases and serum creatinine, should be performed prior to initiation of therapy and periodically thereafter. Gemzar should be administered with caution in patients with evidence of significant renal or hepatic impairment.

Patients who complete an entire 7 week initial cycle of Gemzar therapy or a subsequent 3 week cycle at a dose of 1000 mg/m^2 may have the dose for subsequent cycles increased by 25% (to 1250 mg/m^2), provided that the absolute granulocyte count (AGC) and platelet nadirs exceed 1500 $\times$ 10^6/L and 100,000 $\times$ 10^6/L, respectively, and if nonhematologic toxicity has not been greater than WHO Grade 1. If patients tolerate the subsequent course of Gemzar at a dose of 1250 mg/m^2, the dose for the next cycle can be increased to 1500 mg/m^2, provided again that the AGC and platelet nadirs exceed 1500 $\times$ 10^6/L and 100,000 $\times$ 10^6/L, respectively, and again, if nonhematologic toxicity has not been greater than WHO Grade 1.

Gemzar may be administered on an outpatient basis.

Instructions for Use/Handling—The recommended diluent for reconstitution of Gemzar is 0.9% Sodium Chloride Injection without preservatives. Due to solubility considerations, the maximum concentration for Gemzar upon reconstitution is 40 mg/mL. Reconstitution at concentrations greater than 40 mg/mL may result in incomplete dissolution, and should be avoided.

To reconstitute, add 5 mL of 0.9% Sodium Chloride Injection to the 200 mg vial or 25 mL of 0.9% Sodium Chloride Injection to the 1 g vial. Shake to dissolve. These dilutions each yield a gemcitabine concentration of 40 mg/mL. The appropriate amount of drug may be administered as prepared or further diluted with 0.9% Sodium Chloride Injection to concentrations as low as 0.1 mg/ml.

Reconstituted Gemzar is a clear, colorless to light straw-colored solution. After reconstitution with 0.9% Sodium Chloride Injection, the pH of the resulting solution lies in the range of 2.7 to 3.3. The solution should be inspected visually for particulate matter and discoloration, prior to administration, whenever solution or container permit. If particulate matter or discoloration is found, do not administer.

When prepared as directed, Gemzar solutions are stable for 24 hours at controlled room temperature 20° to 25°C (68° to 77°F) [*See* USP]. Discard unused portion. Solutions of reconstituted Gemzar should not be refrigerated, as crystallization may occur.

The compatibility of Gemzar with other drugs has not been studied. No incompatibilities have been observed with infusion bottles or polyvinyl chloride bags and administration sets.

Unopened vials of Gemzar are stable until the expiration date indicated on the package when stored at controlled room temperature 20° to 25°C (68° to 77°F) [*See* USP].

Caution should be exercised in handling and preparing Gemzar solutions. The use of gloves is recommended. If Gemzar solution contacts the skin or mucosa, immediately wash the skin thoroughly with soap and water or rinse the mucosa with copious amounts of water. Although acute dermal irritation has not been observed in animal studies, two of three rabbits exhibited drug-related systemic toxicities (death, hypoactivity, nasal discharge, shallow breathing) due to dermal absorption.

Procedures for proper handling and disposal of anti-cancer drugs should be considered. Several guidelines on this subject have been published.[1–7] There is no general agreement that all of the procedures recommended in the guidelines are necessary or appropriate.

HOW SUPPLIED

Vials:

200 mg white, lyophilized powder in a 10-mL size sterile single use vial (No. 7501) NDC 0002-7501-01

1 g white, lyophilized powder in a 50-mL size sterile single use vial (No. 7502) NDC 0002-7502-01

Store at controlled room temperature (20° to 25°C) (68° to 77°F). The USP has defined controlled room temperature as "A temperature maintained thermostatically that encompasses the usual and customary working environment of 20° to 25°C (68° to 77°F); that results in a mean kinetic temperature calculated to be not more than 25°C; and that allows for excursions between 15° and 30°C (59° and 86°F) that are experienced in pharmacies, hospitals, and warehouses."

CAUTION—Federal (USA) law prohibits dispensing without prescription.

REFERENCES

1. Recommendations for the safe handling of parenteral antineoplastic drugs. NIH publication No. 83-2621. US Government Printing Office, Washington, DC 20402.
2. Council on Scientific Affairs: Guidelines for handling parenteral antineoplastics. *JAMA* 1985;253:1590.
3. National Study Commission on Cytotoxic Exposure—Recommendations for handling cytotoxic agents, 1987. Available from Louis P Jeffrey, ScD, Director of Pharmacy Services, Rhode Island Hospital, 593 Eddy Street, Providence, Rhode Island 02902.
4. Clinical Oncological Society of Australia: Guidelines and recommendations for safe handling of antineoplastic agents. *Med J Aust* 1983;1:426.
5. Jones RB, et al. Safe handling of chemotherapeutic agents: A report from the Mount Sinai Medical Center. *CA* 1983;33(Sept/Oct):258.
6. American Society of Hospital Pharmacists: Technical assistance bulletin on handling cytotoxic drugs in hospitals. *AM J Hosp Pharm* 1990;47:1033.
7. Yodaiken RE, Bennet D, OSHA work-practice guidelines for personnel dealing with cytotoxic (antineoplastic) drugs. *Am J Hosp Pharm* 1988;43:1193-1204.

Literature issued May 16, 1996 [051696]

GLUCAGON FOR INJECTION ℞
[glōō ′ka-gŏn]
USP

DESCRIPTION

Glucagon, manufactured by Eli Lilly and Company, is extracted from beef and pork pancreas.

Chemically unrelated to insulin, glucagon is a single-chain polypeptide containing 29 amino acid residues and having a molecular weight of 3,483.

The empirical formula is $C_{153}H_{225}N_{43}O_{49}S$. The structure of glucagon is shown below.

His-Ser-Gln-Gly-Thr-Phe-Thr-Ser-Asp-Tyr-Ser-Lys-Tyr-Leu-Asp-Ser-
1 2 3 4 5 6 7 8 9 10 11 12 13 14 15 16

Arg-Arg-Ala-Gln-Asp-Phe-Val-Gln-Trp-Leu-Met-Asn-Thr
17 18 19 20 21 22 23 24 25 26 27 28 29

Crystalline glucagon is a white powder containing less than 0.05% zinc. It is relatively insoluble in water but is soluble at a pH of less than 3 or more than 9.5. Glucagon is stable in lyophilized form at room temperatures.

Glucagon for Injection contains glucagon as the hydrochloride. The 1-mg vials contain 1 mg (1 unit) of glucagon and 49 mg of lactose. One USP unit of glucagon is equivalent to 1 International Unit of glucagon and also to about 1 mg of glucagon.[1] The diluent contains glycerin, 1.6%, with 0.2% phenol as a preservative. Sodium hydroxide and/or hydrochloric acid may have been added during manufacture to adjust the pH.

CLINICAL PHARMACOLOGY

Glucagon causes an increase in blood glucose concentration and is used in the treatment of hypoglycemia. It is effective in small doses, and no evidence of toxicity has been reported with its use. Glucagon acts only on liver glycogen, converting it to glucose.

Parenteral administration of glucagon produces relaxation of the smooth muscle of the stomach, duodenum, small bowel, and colon.

The half-life of glucagon in plasma is approximately 3 to 6 minutes, which is similar to that of insulin.

INDICATIONS AND USAGE

For the treatment of hypoglycemia:

Glucagon is useful in counteracting severe hypoglycemic reactions.

The patient with type I diabetes does not have as great a response in blood glucose levels as does the stable type II diabetes patient. Therefore, supplementary carbohydrate should be given as soon as possible, especially to the child or adolescent patient.

For use as a diagnostic aid:

Glucagon is indicated as a diagnostic aid in the radiologic examination of the stomach, duodenum, small bowel, and colon when a hypotonic state would be advantageous.

Glucagon is as effective for this examination as are the anticholinergic drugs, but it has fewer side effects. When glucagon is administered concomitantly with an anticholinergic agent, the response is not significantly greater than when either drug is used alone. However, the addition of the anticholinergic agent results in increased side effects.

CONTRAINDICATIONS

Glucagon is contraindicated in patients with known hypersensitivity to it or in patients with pheochromocytoma.

WARNINGS

Glucagon should be administered cautiously to patients with a history suggestive of insulinoma and/or pheochromocytoma. In patients with insulinoma, intravenous administration of glucagon will produce an initial increase in blood glucose; however, because of glucagon's insulin-releasing effect, it may cause the insulinoma to release its insulin and subsequently cause hypoglycemia. A patient developing symptoms of hypoglycemia after a dose of glucagon should be given glucose orally, intravenously, or by gavage, whichever is more appropriate.

Exogenous glucagon also stimulates the release of catecholamines. In the presence of pheochromocytoma, glucagon can cause the tumor to release catecholamines, which results in a sudden and marked increase in blood pressure. If a patient suddenly develops a marked increase in blood pressure, 5 to 10 mg of phentolamine mesylate may be administered intravenously in an attempt to control the blood pressure.

Generalized allergic reactions, including urticaria, respiratory distress, and hypotension, have been reported in patients who received glucagon by injection.

PRECAUTIONS

General —Glucagon is helpful in hypoglycemia only if liver glycogen is available. Because glucagon is of little or no help in states of starvation, adrenal insufficiency, or chronic hypoglycemia, glucose should be considered for the treatment of hypoglycemia.

Laboratory Tests —Blood glucose determinations may be obtained to follow the patient in hypoglycemic shock until he or she is asymptomatic.

Carcinogenesis, Mutagenesis, Impairment of Fertility— Because glucagon is usually given in a single dose and has a very short half-life (3 to 6 minutes), no studies have been done regarding carcinogenesis.

Reproduction studies have been performed in rats at doses up to 2 mg/kg b.i.d. (up 120 times the human dose) and have revealed no evidence of impaired fertility.

Usage in Pregnancy —Pregnancy Category B —Reproduction studies have been performed in rats at doses up to 2 mg/kg b.i.d. (up to 120 times the human dose), and have revealed no evidence of harm to the fetus due to glucagon. There are, however, no adequate and well-controlled studies in pregnant women. Because animal reproduction studies are not always predictive of human response, this drug should be used during pregnancy only if clearly needed.

Nursing Mothers —It is not known whether this drug is excreted in human milk. Because many drugs are excreted in human milk, caution should be exercised when glucagon is administered to a nursing woman. If the drug is excreted in human milk during its short half-life, it will be handled like any other polypeptide, ie, it will be hydrolyzed and absorbed. Glucagon is not active when taken orally because it is destroyed in the gastrointestinal tract before it can be absorbed.

ADVERSE REACTIONS

Glucagon is relatively free of adverse reactions except for occasional nausea and vomiting, which may also occur with hypoglycemia. Generalized allergic reactions have been reported (*see* Warnings).

OVERDOSAGE

Signs and Symptoms —No cases of human overdosage of glucagon have been reported. Glucagon is generally well tolerated. If overdosage occurred, it would not be expected to cause consequential toxicity but would be expected to be associated with nausea, vomiting, gastric hypotonicity, and diarrhea.

Intravenous administration of glucagon has been shown to have a positive inotropic and chronotropic effect. A transient increment in both blood pressure and pulse rate may occur following the administration of glucagon. Patients taking β-blockers might be expected to have a greater increment in both pulse and blood pressure. This increase will be transient because of glucagon's short half-life. The increase in blood pressure and pulse rate may require therapy in patients with pheochromocytoma or coronary artery disease.

When glucagon was given in large doses to cardiac patients, investigators reported a positive inotropic effect. These investigators administered glucagon in doses of 0.5 to 16 mg/hour by continuous infusion for periods of 5 to 166 hours. Total doses ranged from 25 to 996 mg, and a 21-month child received approximately 8.25 mg in 165 hours. Side effects

Continued on next page

• Identi-Code® symbol. This product information was prepared in June 1996. Current information on these and other products of Eli Lilly and Company may be obtained by direct inquiry to Lilly Research Laboratories, Lilly Corporate Center, Indianapolis, Indiana 46285, 800-545-5979.

Lilly—Cont.

included nausea, vomiting, and decreasing serum potassium concentration. Serum potassium concentration could be maintained within normal limits with supplemental potassium.

The intravenous median lethal dose for glucagon in mice is approximately 300 mg/kg.

Because glucagon is a polypeptide, it would be rapidly destroyed in the gastrointestinal tract if it were to be accidentally ingested.

Treatment —To obtain up-to-date information about the treatment of overdose, a good resource is your certified Regional Poison Control Center. Telephone numbers of certified poison control centers are listed in the *Physicians' Desk Reference (PDR)*. In managing overdosage, consider the possibility of multiple drug overdoses, interaction among drugs, and unusual drug kinetics in your patient.

In view of the extremely short half-life of glucagon and its prompt destruction and excretion, the treatment of overdosage is symptomatic, primarily for nausea, vomiting, and possible hypokalemia.

If the patient develops a dramatic increase in blood pressure, 5 mg to 10 mg of phentolamine has been shown to be effective in lowering blood pressure for the short time that control would be needed.

Forced diuresis, peritoneal dialysis, hemodialysis, or charcoal hemoperfusion have not been established as beneficial for an overdose of glucagon; it is extremely unlikely that one of these procedures would ever be indicated.

DOSAGE AND ADMINISTRATION

For the treatment of hypoglycemia:
The diluent is provided for use only in the preparation of glucagon for *intermittent* parenteral injection and for no other use.

If glucagon is to be given at doses higher than 2 mg, it should be reconstituted with Sterile Water for Injection instead of the supplied diluting solution and used immediately.

Directions for Use of Glucagon —1. Dissolve the lyophilized glucagon in the accompanying diluent.

2. Glucagon should not be used at concentrations greater than 1 mg (1 unit/mL).

3. Glucagon solutions should not be used unless they are clear and of a water-like consistency.

4. For adults and for children weighing more than 20 kg, give 1 mg (1 unit) by subcutaneous, intramuscular, or intravenous injection.

5. For children weighing less than 20 kg, give 0.5 mg (0.5 unit) or a dose equivalent to 20–30 µg/kg.[2,3,4,5,6]

6. The patient will usually awaken within 15 minutes. If the response is delayed, there is no contraindication to the administration of 1 or 2 additional doses of glucagon; however, in view of the deleterious effects of cerebral hypoglycemia and depending on the duration and depth of coma, the use of parenteral glucose *must* be considered by the physician.

7. Intravenous glucose *must* be given if the patient fails to respond to glucagon.

8. When the patient responds, give supplemental carbohydrate to restore the liver glycogen and prevent secondary hypoglycemia.

Instructions to the Family —Instructions describing the method of using this preparation are included in the literature that accompanies the patient's package. It is advisable for the patient and family members to become familiar with the technique of preparing Glucagon for Injection before an emergency arises. Patients are instructed to use 1 mg (1 unit) for adults and, if recommended by a doctor, $^1/_2$ the adult dose (0.5 mg) [0.5 unit]) for children weighing less than 44 lb (20 kg).

General Management of Hypoglycemia —The following are helpful measures in the prevention of hypoglycemic reactions due to insulin:

1. Reasonable uniformity from day to day with regard to diet, insulin, and exercise.

2. Careful adjustment of the insulin program so that the type (or types) of insulin, dose, and time (or times) of administration are suited to the individual patient.

3. Frequent testing of the blood or urine so that a change in insulin requirements can be foreseen.

4. Routine carrying of sugar, candy, or other readily absorbable carbohydrate by the patient so that it may be taken at the first warning of an oncoming reaction.

If the patient is unaware of the symptoms of hypoglycemia, he/she may lapse into insulin shock; therefore, the physician should instruct the patient in this regard when feasible.

It is important that the patient be aroused as quickly as possible, because prolonged hypoglycemic reactions may result in cortical damage. Glucagon or intravenous glucose will awaken the patient sufficiently so that oral carbohydrates may be taken.

CAUTION—Although the patient may use glucagon for the treatment of hypoglycemia during an emergency, the physician must still be notified when hypoglycemic reactions occur so that the treatment regimen may be adjusted if necessary.

For use as a diagnostic aid:
Dissolve the lyophilized glucagon in the accompanying diluting solution.

Glucagon should not be used at concentrations greater than 1 mg (1 unit/mL).

The following doses may be administered for relaxation of the stomach, duodenum, and small bowel, depending on the time of onset of action and the duration of effect required for the examination. Since the stomach is less sensitive to the effect of glucagon, 0.5 mg (0.5 units) IV or 2 mg (2 units) IM are recommended.

[See table below.]

For examination of the colon, it is recommended that a 2-mg (2 units) dose be administered intramuscularly approximately 10 minutes prior to initiation of the procedure. Relaxation of the colon and reduction of discomfort to the patient will allow the radiologist to perform a more satisfactory examination.

Stability and Storage:

Before Reconstitution—Vials of Glucagon as well as the Diluting Solution for Glucagon for Injection, USP, may be stored at controlled room temperature, 59° to 86°F (15° to 30°C).

After Reconstitution—Glucagon for Injection should be used immediately. **Discard any unused portion.**

HOW SUPPLIED

Vials:

1 mg (1 unit)—(No. 666), with 1-mL vial of diluting solution (No. 667) (1s) NDC 0002-1450-01

Glucagon Emergency Kit (M-8030):

1 mg (1 unit)—(No. 7286), with 1-mL vial of diluting solution (Hyporet* No. 7287) (1s) NDC 0002-8030-01

REFERENCES

1. *Drug Information for the Health Care Professional.* 11th ed. Rockville, Maryland: The United States Pharmacopeial Convention, Inc; 1991; IA: 1380.
2. Gibbs et al: Use of Glucagon to terminate insulin reactions in diabetic children. *Nebr Med J* 1958;43:56–57.
3. Cornblath M, et al: Studies of carbohydrate metabolism in the newborn: Effect of glucagon on concentration of sugar in capillary blood of newborn infant. *Pediatrics* 1958;21:885–892.
4. Carson MJ, Koch R, Clinical studies with glucagon in children. *J Pediatr* 1955;47:167–170.
5. Shipp JC, et al; Treatment of insulin hypoglycemia in diabetic campers. *Diabetes* 1964;13:645–648.
6. Amos J, Wranne L: Hypoglycemia in childhood diabetes II: Effect of subcutaneous or intramuscular injection of different doses of glucagon. *Acta Pediatr Scand* 1988;77:548–553.

*Hyporet® (disposable syringe, Lilly)

CAUTION—Federal (USA) law prohibits dispensing without prescription.
Literature revised December 18, 1995   [121895]

Dose	Route of Administration	Time of Onset of Action	Approximate Duration of Effect
0.25–0.5 mg	IV	1 minute	9–17 minutes
1 mg	IM	8–10 minutes	12–27 minutes
2 mg*	IV	1 minute	22–25 minutes
2 mg*	IM	4–7 minutes	21–32 minutes

*Administration of 2-mg (2 units) doses produces a higher incidence of nausea and vomiting than do lower doses.

HEPARIN SODIUM   ℞

[hĕp'ă-rŭn sō'dē-ŭm]
Injection, USP
WARNING—This is a potent drug, and serious consequences may result if used without constant medical supervision.

DESCRIPTION

Heparin is a heterogenous group of straight-chain anionic mucopolysaccharides, called glycosaminoglycans, having anticoagulant properties. Although others may be present, the main sugars in heparin are: (1) α-L-iduronic acid 2-sulfate, (2) 2-deoxy-2-sulfamino-α-glucose 6-sulfate, (3) β-D-glucuronic acid, (4) 2-acetamido-2-deoxy-α-D-glucose, and (5) α-L-iduronic acid. These sugars are present in decreasing amounts, usually in the order (2) > (1) > (4) > (3) > (5), and are joined by glycosidic linkages, forming polymers of varying sizes. Heparin is strongly acidic because of its covalently linked sulfate and carboxylic acid groups. In heparin sodium, the acidic protons of the sulfate units are partially replaced by sodium ions.

Structure of Heparin Sodium (representative subunits):

Heparin Sodium Injection, USP, is a sterile solution of heparin sodium derived from porcine intestinal mucosa, which is standardized for anticoagulant activity. It is to be administered by intravenous or deep subcutaneous routes. The potency is determined by a biological assay using a USP reference standard based on units of heparin activity per milligram.

Each mL of Vial No. 520 contains 10,000 USP heparin units (derived from porcine intestinal mucosa) and sodium chloride, 0.1%.

During manufacture, 1% benzyl alcohol is added as a preservative to each vial of heparin sodium. Sodium hydroxide and/or hydrochloric acid may be added during manufacture to adjust the pH.

CLINICAL PHARMACOLOGY

Heparin inhibits reactions that lead to the clotting of blood and the formation of fibrin clots both in vitro and in vivo. Heparin acts at multiple sites in the normal coagulation system. Small amounts of heparin in combination with antithrombin III (heparin cofactor) can inhibit thrombosis by inactivating activated Factor X and inhibiting the conversion of prothrombin to thrombin. Once active thrombosis has developed, larger amounts of heparin can inhibit further coagulation by inactivating thrombin and preventing the conversion of fibrinogen to fibrin. Heparin also prevents the formation of a stable fibrin clot by inhibiting the activation of the fibrin stabilizing factor.

Bleeding time is usually unaffected by heparin. Clotting time is prolonged by full therapeutic doses of heparin; in most cases, it is not measurably affected by low doses.

Peak plasma levels of heparin are achieved 2 to 4 hours following subcutaneous administration, although there are considerable individual variations. Log linear plots of heparin plasma concentrations with time for a wide range of dose levels are linear, which suggests the absence of zero order processes. The liver and the reticuloendothelial system are the sites of biotransformation. The biphasic elimination curve, a rapidly declining α phase ($t_{1/2} = 10'$) and, after the age of 40, a slower β phase indicate uptake in organs. The absence of a relationship between anticoagulant half-life and concentration half-life may reflect factors such as protein binding of heparin.

Heparin does not have fibrinolytic activity; therefore, it will not lyse existing clots.

INDICATIONS AND USAGE

Heparin sodium is indicated for:

Anticoagulant therapy in prophylaxis and treatment of venous thrombosis and its extension.

Prevention (in a low-dose regimen) of postoperative deep venous thrombosis and pulmonary embolism in patients undergoing major abdominothoracic surgery or who, for other reasons, are at risk of developing thromboembolic disease (*see* Dosage and Administration)

Prophylaxis and treatment of pulmonary embolism

Atrial fibrillation with embolization

Diagnosis and treatment of acute and chronic consumption coagulopathies (eg, disseminated intravascular coagulation)

Prevention of clotting in arterial and heart surgery
Prophylaxis and treatment of peripheral arterial embolism
As an anticoagulant in blood transfusions, extracorporeal circulation, and dialysis procedures and in blood samples for laboratory purposes

CONTRAINDICATIONS

Heparin sodium should not be used in patients with severe thrombocytopenia or patients for whom suitable blood coagulation tests (eg, tests for whole-blood clotting time and partial thromboplastin time) cannot be performed at appropriate intervals. (This restriction refers to full-dose administration of heparin; it is usually unnecessary to monitor coagulation parameters in patients receiving low-dose heparin). In addition, heparin sodium should not be administered to patients in an uncontrollable active bleeding state (see Warnings), except when this condition is the result of disseminated intravascular coagulation.

WARNINGS

Heparin is not intended for intramuscular use.
Hypersensitivity—Patients with documented hypersensitivity to heparin should be given the drug only in clearly life-threatening situations.
Hemorrhage—Hemorrhage can occur at virtually any site in patients receiving heparin. An unexplained fall in hematocrit, a fall in blood pressure, or any other unexplained symptom warrants consideration of a hemorrhagic event.
Heparin sodium should be used with extreme caution in disease states in which there is increased danger of hemorrhage. Some of the conditions in which this danger exists are as follows:
Cardiovascular—Subacute bacterial endocarditis. Severe hypertension.
Surgical—During and immediately following (a) a spinal tap or spinal anesthesia or (b) major surgery, especially involving the brain, spinal cord, or eye.
Hematologic—Conditions associated with increased bleeding tendencies, such as hemophilia, thrombocytopenia, and some vascular purpuras.
Gastrointestinal—Ulcerative lesions and continuous tube drainage of the stomach or small intestine.
Other—Menstruation and liver disease with impaired hemostasis.
Coagulation Testing—When heparin sodium is administered in therapeutic amounts, its dosage should be regulated by frequent blood coagulation tests. If the coagulation test result is unduly prolonged or if hemorrhage occurs, heparin sodium should be discontinued promptly (see Overdosage).
Thrombocytopenia—Thrombocytopenia occurs in patients receiving heparin with a reported incidence of 0% to 30%. Mild thrombocytopenia (count greater than 100,000/mm^3) may remain stable or reverse, even if heparin is continued. However, thrombocytopenia of any degree should be monitored closely. If the count falls below 100,000/mm^3 or if recurrent thrombosis develops (see Precautions, *White-Clot Syndrome*), the heparin product should be discontinued. If continued heparin therapy is essential, utilize heparin from a different organ source and reinstitute therapy with caution.
Miscellaneous—This product contains benzyl alcohol as a preservative. Benzyl alcohol has been reported to be associated with a fatal "gasping syndrome" in premature infants.

PRECAUTIONS

General—White-Clot Syndrome—It has been reported that patients taking heparin may develop new thrombus formation in association with thrombocytopenia. This development is the result of the irreversible aggregation of platelets induced by heparin, ie, the so-called "white-clot syndrome." The process may lead to severe thromboembolic complications such as skin necrosis, gangrene of the extremities that may lead to amputation, myocardial infarction, pulmonary embolism, stroke, and possibly death. Therefore, heparin administration should be promptly discontinued if a patient develops new thrombosis in association with thrombocytopenia.
Heparin Resistance—Increased resistance to heparin is frequently encountered in cases involving fever, thrombosis, thrombophlebitis, infections with thrombosing tendencies, myocardial infarction, and cancer. Increased resistance can also occur in postsurgical patients.
Increased Risk in Older Women—A higher incidence of bleeding has been reported in women over 60 years of age.
Laboratory Tests—Periodic platelet counts, hematocrit determinations, and tests for occult blood in the stool are recommended during the entire course of heparin therapy, regardless of the route of administration (see Dosage and Administration).
Drug Interactions—Oral anticoagulants: Heparin sodium may prolong the one-stage prothrombin time. Therefore, if a valid prothrombin time is to be obtained when heparin sodium is given with dicumarol or warfarin sodium, a period of at least 5 hours after the last intravenous dose or 24 hours after the last subcutaneous dose should elapse before blood is drawn.

Platelet inhibitors: Drugs such as acetylsalicylic acid, dextran, phenylbutazone, ibuprofen, indomethacin, dipyridamole, hydroxychloroquine, and others that interfere with platelet-aggregation reactions (the main hemostatic defense of heparinized patients) may induce bleeding and should be used with caution in patients receiving heparin sodium.
Other interactions: Digitalis, tetracyclines, nicotine, or antihistamines may partially counteract the anticoagulant action of heparin sodium.
Intravenous nitroglycerin administered to heparinized patients may result in a decrease of the partial thromboplastin time with subsequent rebound effect upon discontinuation of nitroglycerin. Careful monitoring of partial thromboplastin time and adjustment of heparin dosage are recommended during coadministration of heparin and intravenous nitroglycerin.
When clinical circumstances require reversal heparinization, consult the labeling of Protamine Sulfate Injection, USP.
Drug/Laboratory Test Interactions—Hyperaminotransferasemia. Significant elevations of aminotransferase (SGOT and SGPT) levels have occurred in a high percentage of patients (and healthy subjects) who have received heparin. Since aminotransferase determinations are important in the differential diagnosis of myocardial infarction, liver disease, and pulmonary emboli, increases that might be caused by drugs (eg, heparin) should be interpreted with caution.
Carcinogenesis, Mutagenesis, Impairment of Fertility—No long-term studies in animals have been performed to evaluate the carcinogenic potential of heparin. Also, no reproduction studies in animals have been performed concerning mutagenesis or impairment of fertility.
Pregnancy—Teratogenic Effects: Pregnancy Category C—Animal reproduction studies have not been conducted with heparin sodium. It is also not known whether heparin sodium can cause fetal harm when administered to a pregnant woman or can affect reproduction capacity. Heparin sodium should be given to a pregnant woman only if clearly needed.
Nonteratogenic Effects: Heparin does not cross the placental barrier.
Nursing Mothers—Heparin is not excreted in human milk.
Pediatric Use—See Dosage and Administration.

ADVERSE REACTIONS

Hemorrhage—Hemorrhage is the chief complication that may result from heparin therapy (see Warnings). An overly prolonged clotting time or minor bleeding during therapy can usually be controlled by withdrawing the drug (see Overdosage). *Gastrointestinal or urinary tract bleeding during anticoagulant therapy may indicate the presence of an underlying occult lesion.* Bleeding can occur at any site, but certain specific hemorrhagic complications may be difficult to detect:

Adrenal hemorrhage, with resultant acute adrenal insufficiency, has occurred during anticoagulant therapy. Therefore, such treatment should be discontinued in patients who develop signs and symptoms of acute adrenal hemorrhage and insufficiency. Initiation of corrective therapy should not be delayed for laboratory confirmation of the diagnosis, since any delay in an acute situation may result in the patient's death.

Ovarian (corpus luteum) hemorrhage developed in a number of women of reproductive age receiving short- or long-term anticoagulant therapy. If unrecognized, this complication may be fatal.

Retroperitoneal hemorrhage has occurred.

Local Irritation—Local irritation, erythema, mild pain, hematoma, or ulceration may follow deep subcutaneous (intrafat) injection of heparin sodium. These complications are much more common after intramuscular use; therefore, such use is not recommended.
Hypersensitivity—Generalized hypersensitivity reactions have been reported, with chills, fever, and urticaria as the most common manifestations; asthma, rhinitis, lacrimation, headache, nausea and vomiting, and anaphylactoid reactions (including shock) have occurred more rarely. Itching and burning, especially on the plantar site of the feet, may occur.
The occurrence of thrombocytopenia has been reported in patients receiving heparin, with an incidence of 0% to 30%. Although often mild and of no obvious clinical significance, such thrombocytopenia can be accompanied by severe thromboembolic complications, such as skin necrosis, gangrene of the extremities that may lead to amputation, myocardial infarction, pulmonary embolism, stroke, and possibly death (see Warnings *and* Precautions).
Certain episodes of painful, ischemic, and cyanosed limbs have, in the past, been attributed to allergic vasospastic reactions. Whether these are, in fact, identical to the thrombocytopenia-associated complications remains to be determined.
Miscellaneous—Osteoporosis following long-term administration of high doses of heparin, cutaneous necrosis after systemic administration, suppression of aldosterone synthesis, delayed transient alopecia, priapism, and rebound hyper-

lipemia occurring after discontinuation of heparin sodium have also been reported.
Significant elevations of aminotransferase (SGOT and SGPT) levels have occurred in a high percentage of patients (and healthy subjects) who have received heparin.

OVERDOSAGE

Signs and Symptoms—Overdose of heparin may follow parenteral administration, but oral heparin has little systemic effect. Bleeding is the chief sign of heparin overdosage. Excessive heparin effect also increases whole-blood clotting time and activated partial thromboplastin time (APTT). The half-life of heparin ranges from 0.5 to 2.5 hours and may vary widely in cases involving an overdose.
The intravenous median lethal dose in mice is 1,500 mg/kg.
Treatment—To obtain up-to-date information about the treatment of overdose, a good resource is your certified Regional Poison Control Center. Telephone numbers of certified poison control centers are listed in the *Physicians' Desk Reference (PDR)*. In managing overdosage, consider the possibility of multiple drug overdoses, interaction among drugs, and unusual drug kinetics in your patient.
Minor bleeding occurring during therapy with heparin can often be treated by reducing the dose or increasing the dosing interval.
For major bleeding episodes, heparin may be neutralized by protamine; 1 mg of protamine will neutralize approximately 115 units of heparin of porcine intestinal mucosal origin. Protamine dosage may be guided by determining the amount of time by which clotting is shortened in vitro or by the results of other hematologic tests. Note that protamine may cause anaphylactoid reactions that may be life threatening. (See the protamine label for additional information.) The administration of whole blood or fresh frozen plasma should be considered for patients with significant blood losses. Vitamin K will not reverse the activity of heparin.

DOSAGE AND ADMINISTRATION

Parenteral drug products should be inspected visually for particulate matter and discoloration prior to administration if solution and container permit. Slight discoloration does not alter potency.
When heparin is added to an infusion solution for continuous intravenous administration, the container should be inverted at least 6 times to ensure adequate mixing and prevent pooling of the heparin in the solution.
Heparin sodium is not effective by oral administration and should be given by intermittent intravenous injection, intravenous infusion, or deep subcutaneous (intrafat, ie, above the iliac crest or abdominal fat layer) injection. *The intramuscular route of administration should be avoided because of frequent occurrence of hematoma at the injection site.*
The dosage of heparin sodium should be adjusted according to the patient's coagulation test results. When heparin is given by continuous intravenous infusion, the coagulation time should be determined approximately every 4 hours in the early stages of treatment. When the drug is administered intermittently by intravenous injection, coagulation tests should be performed before each injection during the early stages of treatment and at appropriate intervals thereafter. Dosage is considered adequate when the APTT is 1.5 to 2 times normal or when the whole-blood clotting time is elevated approximately 2.5 to 3 times the control value. After deep subcutaneous (intrafat) injections, tests for adequacy of dosage are best performed on samples drawn 4 to 6 hours after the injections.
Periodic platelet counts, hematocrit determinations, and tests for occult blood in the stool are recommended during the entire course of heparin therapy, regardless of the route of administration.
Converting to Oral Anticoagulant—When an oral anticoagulant of the coumarin (or similar) type is to be administered in patients already receiving heparin sodium, baseline and subsequent tests of prothrombin activity must be determined at times during which heparin activity is too low to affect the prothrombin time. Such a time usually occurs about 5 hours after the last IV bolus and 24 hours after the last subcutaneous dose. If heparin is continuously infused by IV, prothrombin time can usually be measured at any time.
In converting from heparin to an oral anticoagulant, the oral anticoagulant should be given in the usual initial amount; thereafter, prothrombin time should be determined at the usual intervals. To ensure continuous anticoagulation, it is advisable to continue full heparin therapy for several days after the prothrombin time has reached the limit of the therapeutic range. Heparin therapy may then be discontinued without tapering.

Continued on next page

• **Identi-Code® symbol. This product information was prepared in June 1996. Current information on these and other products of Eli Lilly and Company may be obtained by direct inquiry to Lilly Research Laboratories, Lilly Corporate Center, Indianapolis, Indiana 46285, 800-545-5979.**

Lilly—Cont.

Method of Administration	Frequency	Recommended Dose*
Deep Subcutaneous (Intrafat) Injection (A different site should be used for each injection to prevent the development of massive hematoma)	Initial dose	5,000 units by IV injection, followed by 10,000–20,000 units of a concentrated solution, subcutaneously
	Every 8 hours or	8,000–10,000 units of a concentrated solution
	Every 12 hours	15,000–20,000 units of a concentrated solution
Intermittent Intravenous Injection	Initial dose	10,000 units, either undiluted or in 50–100 mL of 0.9% Sodium Chloride Injection, USP
	Every 4 to 6 hours	5,000–10,000 units, either undiluted or in 50–100 mL of 0.9% Sodium Chloride Injection, USP
Continuous Intravenous Infusion	Initial dose	5,000 units by IV injection
	Continuous Infusion	20,000–40,000 units/24 hours in 1,000 mL of 0.9% Sodium-Chloride Injection, USP (or in any compatible solution) for infusion

*Based on 150-lb (68-kg) patient.

Therapeutic Anticoagulant Effect With Full-Dose Heparin —Although dosage must be adjusted for the individual patient according to the results of appropriate laboratory tests, the following dosage schedule may be used as a guideline: [See table above.]

Pediatric Use —Follow recommendations of appropriate pediatric reference texts. In general, the following dosage schedule may be used as a guideline:
Initial Dose: 50 units/kg (IV, drip)
Maintenance Dose: 100 units/kg (IV, drip) every 4 hours, or 20,000 units/m^2/24 hours, infused continuously

Surgery of the Heart and Blood Vessels —Patients undergoing total body perfusion for open heart surgery should receive an initial dose of not less than 150 units of heparin sodium per kg of body weight. Frequently, a dose of 300 units/kg is used for procedures estimated to last less than 60 minutes; a dose of 400 units/kg is often used for those procedures likely to last longer than 60 minutes.

Low-Dose Prophylaxis of Postoperative Thromboembolism —A number of well-controlled clinical trials have demonstrated that low-dose heparin prophylaxis, given prior to and after surgery, will reduce the incidences of postoperative deep-vein thrombosis in the legs (as measured by the I-125 fibrinogen technique and venography) and of clinical pulmonary embolism. The most widely used dosage is 5,000 units given 2 hours before surgery and 5,000 units given every 8 to 12 hours thereafter for 7 days or until the patient is fully ambulatory, whichever is longer. The heparin is given by deep subcutaneous (intrafat, ie, above the iliac crest or abdominal fat layer, arm, or thigh) injection with a fine (25- to 26-gauge) needle to minimize tissue trauma. A concentrated solution of heparin sodium is recommended. Such prophylaxis should be reserved for patients over the age of 40 who are undergoing major surgery. Patients with bleeding disorders and those having brain or spinal-cord surgery, spinal anesthesia, eye surgery, or potentially sanguineous operations should be excluded from this treatment, as should patients receiving oral anticoagulants or platelet-active drugs (*see* Warnings). The value of such prophylaxis in hip surgery has not been established. The possibility of increased bleeding during surgery or postoperatively should be borne in mind. If such bleeding occurs, discontinuance of heparin and neutralization with protamine sulfate are advisable. If clinical evidence of thromboembolism develops despite low-dose prophylaxis, full therapeutic doses of anticoagulants should be given unless contraindicated. Prior to initiating heparinization, the physician should rule out the probability of bleeding disorders by taking a thorough history and performing the appropriate laboratory tests. Appropriate coagulation tests should be repeated just prior to surgery. Coagulation test values should be normal or only slightly elevated at these times.

Extracorporeal Dialysis —Follow equipment manufacturers' operating directions carefully.

Blood Transfusion —The addition of 400 to 600 USP units to each 100 mL of whole blood for transfusion is usually employed to prevent coagulation. Usually, 7,500 USP units of heparin sodium are mixed with 100 mL of 0.9% Sodium Chloride Injection, USP (or 75,000 USP units/1,000 mL of 0.9% Sodium Chloride Injection, USP); 6 to 8 mL of this sterile solution is then added to each 100 mL of whole blood used.

Laboratory Samples —70 to 150 units of heparin sodium are usually added per 10- to 20-mL sample of whole blood to prevent coagulation of the sample. Leukocyte counts should be performed on heparinized blood within 2 hours after the addition of the heparin. Heparinized blood should not be used for isoagglutinin, complement, or erythrocyte fragility tests or for taking platelet counts.

Clearing Intermittent Infusion (Heparin Lock) Sets —To prevent clot formation in a heparin lock set following its proper insertion, dilute heparin solution (*see* USP monograph for Heparin Lock Flush Solution, USP) should be injected via the injection hub in a quantity sufficient to fill the entire set to the needle tip. This solution should be replaced each time the heparin lock is used. Aspirate before administering any solution via the lock in order to confirm the patency and location of the needle or catheter tip. If the drug to be administered is incompatible with heparin, the entire heparin lock set should be flushed with sterile water or normal saline before and after the medication is administered; following the second cleansing flush, the dilute heparin solution may be reinstilled in the set. The set manufacturer's instructions should be consulted for specifics concerning the heparin lock set being used at a given time.

NOTE: Since repeated injections of small doses of heparin can alter tests for activated partial thromboplastin time (APTT), a baseline value for APTT should be obtained prior to insertion of a heparin lock set.

HOW SUPPLIED

Multiple-Dose Vials:
10,000 USP heparin units/mL, 5 mL (No. 520)—(1s) NDC 0002-7217-01

Protect from light. Store at controlled room temperature, 59° to 86°F (15° to 30°C).

CAUTION—Federal (USA) law prohibits dispensing without prescription.

Text revised April 2, 1992
Literature revised February 23, 1995 [022395]

HUMALOG® ℞
INSULIN LISPRO INJECTION
(rDNA ORIGIN)

DESCRIPTION

Humalog® (insulin lispro, rDNA origin) is a human insulin analog that is a rapid-acting, parenteral blood glucose-lowering agent. Chemically, it is Lys(B28), Pro(B29) human insulin analog, created when the amino acids at positions 28 and 29 on the insulin B-chain are reversed. Humalog is synthesized in a special non-pathogenic laboratory strain of *Escherichia coli* bacteria that has been genetically altered by the addition of the gene for insulin lispro.

Humalog has the following primary structure:

Figure 1

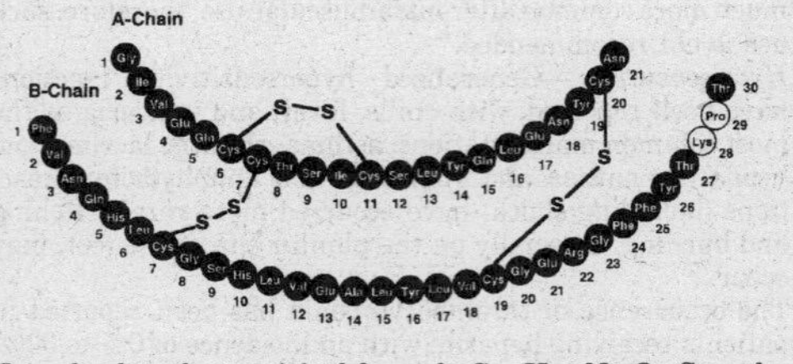

Humalog has the empirical formula $C_{257}H_{383}N_{65}O_{77}S_6$ and a molecular weight of 5808, both identical to that of human insulin.

The vials and cartridges contain a sterile solution of Humalog for use as an injection. Humalog injection consists of zinc-insulin lispro crystals dissolved in a clear aqueous fluid.

Each milliliter of Humalog injection contains insulin lispro 100 Units, 16 mg glycerin, 1.88 mg dibasic sodium phosphate, 3.15 mg *m*-cresol, zinc oxide content adjusted to provide 0.0197 mg zinc ion, trace amounts of phenol, and water for injection. Insulin lispro has a pH of 7.0-7.8. Hydrochloric acid 10% and/or sodium hydroxide 10% may be added to adjust pH.

CLINICAL PHARMACOLOGY

Antidiabetic Activity—The primary activity of insulin, including Humalog, is the regulation of glucose metabolism. In addition, all insulins have several anabolic and anti-catabolic actions on many tissues in the body. In muscle and other tissues (except the brain), insulin causes rapid transport of glucose and amino acids intracellularly, promotes anabolism, and inhibits protein catabolism. In the liver, insulin promotes the uptake and storage of glucose in the form of glycogen, inhibits gluconeogenesis, and promotes the conversion of excess glucose into fat.

Humalog has been shown to be equipotent to human insulin on a molar basis. One unit of Humalog has the same glucose-lowering effect as one unit of human regular insulin, but its effect is more rapid and of shorter duration. The glucose-lowering activity of Humalog and human regular insulin is comparable when administered to normal volunteers by the intravenous route.

Pharmacokinetics—

Absorption and Bioavailability—Humalog is as bioavailable as human regular insulin, with absolute bioavailability ranging between 55%–77% with doses between 0.1–0.2 U/kg, inclusive. Studies in normal volunteers and patients with type I (insulin-dependent) diabetes demonstrated that Humalog is absorbed faster than human regular insulin (U100) (Figure 2).

In normal volunteers given subcutaneous doses of Humalog ranging from 0.1–0.4 U/kg, peak serum levels were seen 30–90 minutes after dosing. When normal volunteers received equivalent doses of human regular insulin, peak insulin doses occurred between 50–120 minutes after dosing. Similar results were seen in patients with type I diabetes. The pharmacokinetic profiles of Humalog and human regular insulin are comparable to one another when administered to normal volunteers by the intravenous route. Humalog was absorbed at a consistently faster rate than human regular insulin in healthy male volunteers given 0.2 U/kg human regular insulin or Humalog at abdominal, deltoid, or femoral sites, the three sites often used by patients with diabetes. After abdominal administration of Humalog, serum drug levels are higher and the duration of action is slightly shorter than after deltoid or thigh administration (*see* DOSAGE AND ADMINISTRATION section). Humalog has less intra- and inter-patient variability compared to human regular insulin.

Figure 2
Serum Humalog and Insulin levels after subcutaneous injection of human regular insulin or Humalog (0.2 U/kg) immediately before a high carbohydrate meal in 10 patients with Type I diabetes.*

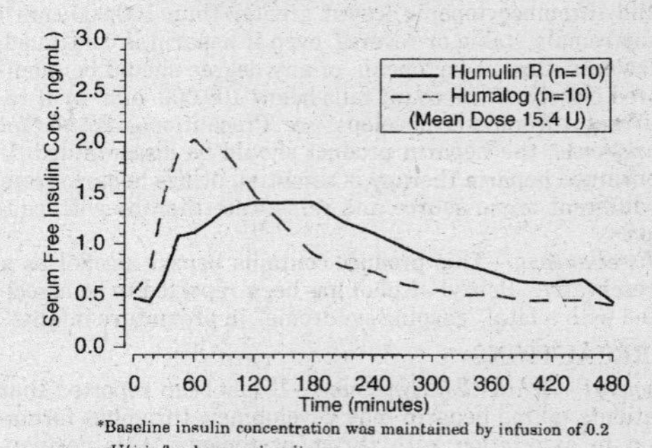

*Baseline insulin concentration was maintained by infusion of 0.2 mU/min/kg human insulin.

Distribution—The volume of distribution for Humalog is identical to that of human regular insulin, with a range of 0.26–0.36 L/kg.

Metabolism—Human metabolism studies have not been conducted. However, animal studies indicate that the metabolism of Humalog is identical to that of human regular insulin.

Elimination—When Humalog is given subcutaneously, its $t_{1/2}$ is shorter than that of human regular insulin (1 vs 1.5 hours, respectively). When given intravenously, Humalog and human regular insulin show identical dose- dependent elimination, with a $t_{1/2}$ of 26 and 52 minutes at 0.1 U/kg and 0.2 U/kg, respectively.

Pharmacodynamics—Studies in normal volunteers and patients with diabetes demonstrated that Humalog has a more rapid onset of glucose-lowering activity, an earlier peak for glucose lowering, and a shorter duration of glucose-lowering activity than human regular insulin (Figure 3). The earlier onset of activity of Humalog is directly related to its more rapid rate of absorption. The time course of action of insulin and insulin analogs such as Humalog may vary considerably in different individuals or within the same individual. The parameters of Humalog activity (time of onset, peak time, and duration) as designated in Figure 3 should be considered only as general guidelines. The rate of insulin absorption and consequently the onset of activity is known to be affected by the site of injection, exercise, and other variables (*see*

PRECAUTIONS, Absorption and Bioavailability sub-section).

Figure 3

Blood glucose levels after subcutaneous injection of human regular insulin or Humalog (0.2 U/kg) immediately before a high carbohydrate meal in 10 patients with Type I diabetes.*

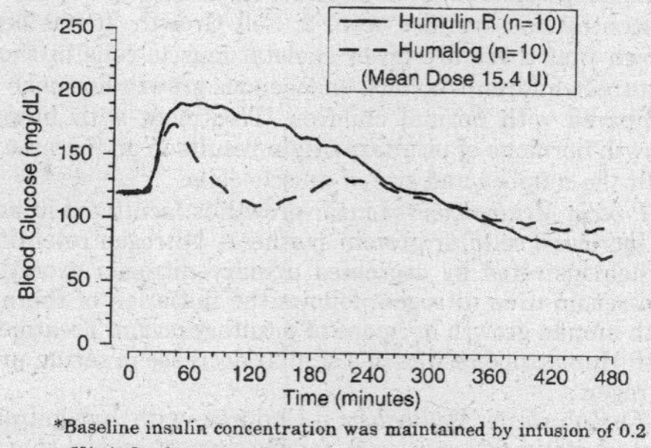

*Baseline insulin concentration was maintained by infusion of 0.2 mU/min/kg human insulin.

In open-label, crossover studies of 1008 patients with type I diabetes and 722 patients with type II (non-insulin-dependent) diabetes, Humalog reduced postprandial glucose compared with human regular insulin (*see* Table). The clinical significance of improvement in postprandial hyperglycemia has not been established.

Comparison of Means of Glycemic Parameters at the End of Combined Treatment Periods. All Randomized Patients in Cross-over Studies (3 months for each treatment)

Type I, N=1008 Glycemic Parameter, (mmol/L)†	Humalog[a]	Humulin® R[a*]	p-value
Premeal Blood Glucose	11.64 ± 5.09	11.34 ± 4.96	.274
1-Hour Postprandial	12.91 ± 5.43	13.89 ± 5.37	<.001
2-Hour Postprandial	11.16 ± 5.30	12.87 ± 5.77	<.001
HbA1c (%)	8.24 ± 1.49	8.17 ± 1.46	.089

Type II, N=722 Glycemic Parameter, (mmol/L)†	Humalog[a]	Humulin R[a]	p-value
Premeal Blood Glucose	10.67 ± 3.77	10.17 ± 3.67	.002
1-Hour Postprandial	13.23 ± 4.43	13.89 ± 4.18	<.001
2-Hour Postprandial	12.08 ± 4.62	13.14 ± 4.48	<.001
HbA1c (%)	8.18 ± 1.30	8.18 ± 1.38	.924

[a] Mean ± Standard Deviation
*Humulin® (Regular insulin human injection, USP, [recombinant DNA origin])
†mg/dL = mmol/L × 18.0

In 12-month parallel studies of type I and type II patients, hemoglobin A_{1c} did not differ between patients treated with human regular insulin and those treated with Humalog. While the overall rate of hypoglycemia did not differ between patients with type I and type II diabetes treated with Humalog compared with human regular insulin, patients with type I diabetes treated with Humalog had fewer hypoglycemic episodes between midnight and 6 a.m. The lower rate of hypoglycemia in the Humalog-treated group may have been related to higher nocturnal blood glucose levels, as reflected by a small increase in mean fasting blood glucose levels.

Special Populations—

Age and Gender—Information on the effect of age and gender on the pharmacokinetics of Humalog is unavailable. However, in large clinical trials, subgroup analysis based on age and gender did not indicate any difference in postprandial glucose parameters between Humalog and human regular insulin.

Smoking—The effect of smoking on the pharmacokinetics and glucodynamics of Humalog has not been studied.

Pregnancy—The effect of pregnancy on the pharmacokinetics and glucodynamics of Humalog has not been studied.

Obesity—The effect of obesity and/or subcutaneous fat thickness on the pharmacokinetics and glucodynamics of Humalog has not been studied. In large clinical trials, which included patients with Body-Mass-Index up to and including 35 kg/m², no consistent differences were seen between Humalog and Humulin R with respect to postprandial glucose parameters.

Renal Impairment—Some studies with human insulin have shown increased circulating levels of insulin in patients with renal failure. Information on the effect of renal impairment on the pharmacokinetics of Humalog is limited. Careful glucose monitoring and dose adjustments of insulin, including Humalog, may be necessary in patients with renal dysfunction.

Hepatic Impairment—Some studies with human insulin have shown increased circulating levels of insulin in patients with hepatic failure. Careful glucose monitoring and dose adjustments of insulin, including Humalog, may be necessary in patients with hepatic dysfunction.

INDICATIONS AND USAGE

Humalog is an insulin analog that is indicated in the treatment of patients with diabetes mellitus for the control of hyperglycemia. Humalog has a more rapid onset and a shorter duration of action than human regular insulin. Therefore, Humalog should be used in regimens including a longer-acting insulin.

CONTRAINDICATIONS

Humalog is contraindicated during episodes of hypoglycemia and in patients sensitive to Humalog or one of its excipients.

WARNINGS

This human insulin analog differs from human regular insulin by its rapid onset of action as well as a shorter duration of activity. When used as a mealtime insulin, the dose of Humalog should be given within 15 minutes before the meal. Because of the short duration of action of Humalog, patients with type I diabetes also require a longer-acting insulin to maintain glucose control.

Hypoglycemia is the most common adverse effect of insulins, including Humalog. As with all insulins, the timing of hypoglycemia may differ among various insulin formulations. Glucose monitoring is recommended for all patients with diabetes[1].

Any change of insulin should be made cautiously and only under medical supervision. Changes in insulin strength, manufacturer, type (e.g., regular, NPH, analog), species (animal, human), or method of manufacture (rDNA versus animal-source insulin) may result in the need for a change in dosage.

PRECAUTIONS

General—Hypoglycemia and hypokalemia are among the potential clinical adverse effects associated with the use of all insulins. Because of differences in the action of Humalog and other insulins, care should be taken in patients in whom such potential side effects might be clinically relevant (e.g., patients who are fasting, have autonomic neuropathy, or are using potassium-lowering drugs). Lipodystrophy and hypersensitivity are among other potential clinical adverse effects associated with the use of all insulins.

As with all insulin preparations, the time course of Humalog action may vary in different individuals or at different times in the same individual and is dependent on site of injection, blood supply, temperature, and physical activity.

Adjustment of dosage of any insulin may be necessary if patients change their physical activity or their usual meal plan. Insulin requirements may be altered during illness, emotional disturbances, or other stress.

Hypoglycemia—As with all insulin preparations, hypoglycemic reactions may be associated with the administration of Humalog. Rapid changes in serum glucose levels may induce symptoms of hypoglycemia in persons with diabetes, regardless of the glucose value. Early warning symptoms of hypoglycemia may be different or less pronounced under certain conditions, such as long duration of diabetes, diabetic nerve disease, use of medications such as beta-blockers, or intensified diabetes control.

Renal Impairment—Although there are no specific data in patients with diabetes, Humalog requirements may be reduced in the presence of renal impairment, similar to observations found with other insulins.

Hepatic Impairment—Although studies have not been performed in diabetes patients with hepatic disease, Humalog requirements may be reduced in the presence of impaired hepatic function, similar to observations found with other insulins.

Allergy—Local Allergy—As with any insulin therapy, patients may experience redness, swelling, or itching at the site of injection. These minor reactions usually resolve in a few days to a few weeks. In some instances, these reactions may be related to factors other than insulin, such as irritants in a skin cleansing agent or poor injection technique.

Systemic Allergy—Less common, but potentially more serious, is generalized allergy to insulin, which may cause rash (including pruritus) over the whole body, shortness of breath, wheezing, reduction in blood pressure, rapid pulse, or sweating. Severe cases of generalized allergy, including anaphylactic reaction, may be life threatening. In controlled clinical trials, pruritus (with or without rash) was seen in 17 patients receiving Humulin R (N=2969) and 30 patients receiving Humalog (N=2944) (p=.053). Localized reactions and generalized myalgias have been reported with the use of cresol as an injectable excipient.

Antibody Production—In large clinical trials, antibodies that cross react with human insulin and insulin lispro were observed in both Humulin R- and Humalog-treatment groups. As expected, the largest increase in the antibody levels during the 12-month clinical trials was observed with patients new to insulin therapy.

Information for Patients—Patients should be informed of the potential risks and advantages of Humalog and alternative therapies. Patients should also be informed about the importance of proper insulin storage, injection technique, timing of dosage, adherence to meal planning, regular physical activity, regular blood glucose monitoring, periodic glycosylated hemoglobin testing, recognition and management of hypo- and hyperglycemia, and periodic assessment for diabetes complications.

Patients should be advised to inform their physician if they are pregnant or intend to become pregnant.

Refer patients to the Information for the Patient circular for information on proper injection technique, timing of Humalog dosing (≤15 minutes before a meal), storing and mixing insulin, and common adverse effects.

Laboratory Tests—As with all insulins, the therapeutic response to Humalog should be monitored by periodic blood glucose tests. Periodic measurement of glycosylated hemoglobin is recommended for the monitoring of long-term glycemic control.

Drug Interactions—(*see* CLINICAL PHARMACOLOGY) Insulin requirements may be increased by medications with hyperglycemic activity such as corticosteroids, isoniazid, certain lipid-lowering drugs (e.g., niacin), estrogens, oral contraceptives, phenothiazines, and thyroid replacement therapy.

Insulin requirements may be decreased in the presence of drugs with hypoglycemic activity, such as oral hypoglycemic agents, salicylates, sulfa antibiotics, and certain antidepressants (monoamine oxidase inhibitors), certain angiotensin-converting-enzyme inhibitors, beta-adrenergic blockers, inhibitors of pancreatic function (e.g., octreotide), and alcohol. Beta-adrenergic blockers may mask the symptoms of hypoglycemia in some patients.

Mixing of Insulins—Care should be taken when mixing all insulins as a change in peak action may occur. The American Diabetes Association warns in its Position Statement on Insulin Administration, "On mixing, physiochemical changes in the mixture may occur (either immediately or over time). As a result, the physiological response to the insulin mixture may differ from that of the injection of the insulins separately."[1] A decrease in the absorption rate, but not total bioavailability, was seen when Humalog was mixed with Humulin N. This decrease in absorption rate was not seen when Humalog was mixed with Humulin U (Figure 4). When Humalog is mixed with either Humulin U or Humulin N, the mixture should be given within 15 minutes before a meal.

Figure 4

Effect of Mixing Humalog and Longer-acting Insulins*

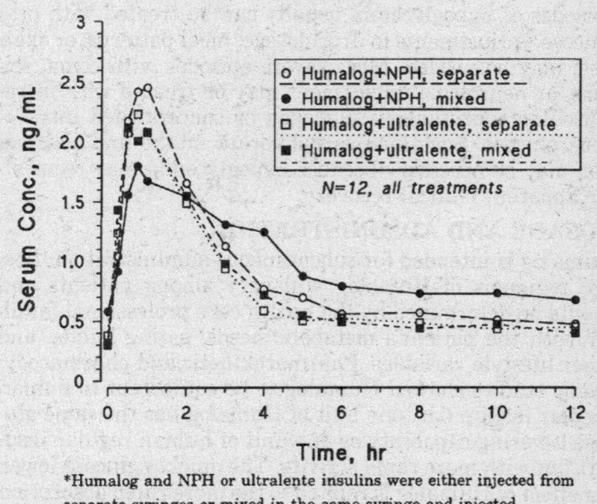

*Humalog and NPH or ultralente insulins were either injected from separate syringes or mixed in the same syringe and injected together.

The effects of mixing Humalog with insulins of animal source or insulin preparations produced by other manufacturers have not been studied (*see* WARNINGS).

If Humalog is mixed with a longer-acting insulin, Humalog should be drawn into the syringe first to prevent clouding of

Continued on next page

• Identi-Code® symbol. This product information was prepared in June 1996. Current information on these and other products of Eli Lilly and Company may be obtained by direct inquiry to Lilly Research Laboratories, Lilly Corporate Center, Indianapolis, Indiana 46285, 800-545-5979.

Lilly—Cont.

the Humalog by the longer-acting insulin. Injection should be made immediately after mixing. Mixtures should not be administered intravenously.

Carcinogenesis, Mutagenesis, Impairment of Fertility—Long-term studies in animals have not been performed to evaluate the carcinogenic potential of Humalog. Humalog was not mutagenic in a battery of *in vitro* and *in vivo* genetic toxicity assays (bacterial mutation tests, unscheduled DNA synthesis, mouse lymphoma assay, chromosomal aberration tests, and a micronucleus test). There is no evidence from animal studies of Humalog-induced impairment of fertility.

Pregnancy—Teratogenic Effects—Pregnancy Category B—Reproduction studies have been performed in pregnant rats and rabbits at parenteral doses up to 4 and 0.3 times, respectively, the average human dose (40 units/day) based on body surface area. The results have revealed no evidence of impaired fertility or harm to the fetus due to Humalog. There are, however, no adequate and well-controlled studies in pregnant women. Because animal reproduction studies are not always predictive of human response, this drug should be used during pregnancy only if clearly needed.

Although there are no clinical studies of the use of Humalog in pregnancy, published studies with human insulins suggest that optimizing overall glycemic control, including postprandial control, before conception and during pregnancy improves fetal outcome. Although the fetal complications of maternal hyperglycemia have been well documented, fetal toxicity also has been reported with maternal hypoglycemia. Insulin requirements usually fall during the first trimester and increase during the second and third trimesters. Careful monitoring of the patient is required throughout pregnancy. During the perinatal period, careful monitoring of infants born to mothers with diabetes is warranted.

Nursing Mothers—It is unknown whether Humalog is excreted in significant amounts in human milk. Many drugs, including human insulin, are excreted in human milk. For this reason, caution should be exercised when Humalog is administered to a nursing woman. Patients with diabetes who are lactating may require adjustments in Humalog dose, meal plan, or both.

Pediatric Use—Safety and effectiveness in patients less than 12 years of age have not been established.

ADVERSE REACTIONS

Clinical studies comparing Humalog with human regular insulin did not demonstrate a difference in frequency of adverse events between the two treatments.

Adverse events commonly associated with human insulin therapy include the following:

Body as a Whole—allergic reactions (*see* PRECAUTIONS)
Skin and Appendages—injection site reaction, lipodystrophy, pruritus, rash
Other—hypoglycemia (see WARNINGS *and* PRECAUTIONS)

OVERDOSAGE

Hypoglycemia may occur as a result of an excess of insulin relative to food intake, energy expenditure, or both. Mild episodes of hypoglycemia usually can be treated with oral glucose. Adjustments in drug dosage, meal patterns, or exercise, may be needed. More severe episodes with coma, seizure, or neurologic impairment may be treated with intramuscular/subcutaneous glucagon or concentrated intravenous glucose. Sustained carbohydrate intake and observation may be necessary because hypoglycemia may recur after apparent clinical recovery.

DOSAGE AND ADMINISTRATION

Humalog is intended for subcutaneous administration. Dosage regimens of Humalog will vary among patients and should be determined by the health care professional familiar with the patient's metabolic needs, eating habits, and other lifestyle variables. Pharmacokinetic and pharmacodynamic studies showed Humalog to be equipotent to human regular insulin (i.e., one unit of Humalog has the same glucose-lowering capability as one unit of human regular insulin), but with more rapid activity. The quicker glucose-lowering effect of Humalog is related to the more rapid absorption rate from subcutaneous tissue. An adjustment of dose or schedule of basal insulin may be needed when a patient changes from other insulins to Humalog, particularly to prevent pre-meal hyperglycemia.

When used as a meal-time insulin, Humalog should be given within 15 minutes before a meal. Human regular insulin is best given 30–60 minutes before a meal. To achieve optimal glucose control, the amount of longer-acting insulin being given may need to be adjusted when using Humalog.

The rate of insulin absorption and consequently the onset of activity is known to be affected by the site of injection, exercise, and other variables. Humalog was absorbed at a consistently faster rate than human regular insulin in healthy male volunteers given 0.2 U/kg human regular insulin or Humalog at abdominal, deltoid, or femoral sites, the three sites often used by patients with diabetes. When not mixed in

the same syringe with other insulins, Humalog maintains its rapid onset of action and has less variability in its onset of action among injection sites compared with human regular insulin (*see* PRECAUTIONS). After abdominal administration, Humalog concentrations are higher than those following deltoid or thigh injections. Also, the duration of action of Humalog is slightly shorter following abdominal injection, compared with deltoid and femoral injections. As with all insulin preparations, the time course of action of Humalog may vary considerably in different individuals or within the same individual. Patients must be educated to use proper injection techniques.

Parenteral drug products should be inspected visually prior to administration whenever the solution and the container permit. If the solution is cloudy, contains particulate matter, is thickened, or is discolored, the contents must not be injected. Humalog should not be used after its expiration date.

Storage—Humalog should be stored in a refrigerator (2° to 8°C [36° to 46°F]), but not in the freezer. If refrigeration is impossible, the vial or cartridge of Humalog in use can be unrefrigerated for up to 28 days, as long as it is kept as cool as possible (not greater than 86°F [30°C]) and away from direct heat and light. Unrefrigerated vials and cartridges must be used within this time period or be discarded. Do not use Humalog if it has been frozen.

HOW SUPPLIED

Humalog (insulin lispro injection) is available in the following package sizes:
100 units per mL (U 100)
    10 mL vials   NDC 0002-7510-01 (VL-7510)
  5– 1.5 mL cartridges* NDC 0002-7515-59 (VL-7515)

*Cartridges are for use only in B-D®† PEN and B-D PEN ULTRA
CAUTION—Federal (USA) law prohibits dispensing without prescription.

REFERENCES
1. American Diabetes Association: Clinical Practice Recommendations 1996, Insulin Administration. *Diabetes Care,* 1996; 19(Supp 1):31-34.

†B-D is a trademark of Becton Dickinson and Company
Literature issued June 14, 1996
ELI LILLY AND COMPANY Indianapolis, IN 46285, USA
PA 6660 AMP

                                           [061496]

HUMATROPE®   ℞
[hū'ma-trōp]
(somatropin (rDNA origin) for injection)

DESCRIPTION

Humatrope® (Somatropin, rDNA Origin, for Injection) is a polypeptide hormone of recombinant DNA origin. Humatrope has 191 amino acid residues and a molecular weight of about 22,125 daltons. The amino acid sequence of the product is identical to that of human growth hormone of pituitary origin. Humatrope is synthesized in a strain of *Escherichia coli* that has been modified by the addition of the gene for human growth hormone.

Humatrope is a sterile, white, lyophilized powder intended for subcutaneous or intramuscular administration after reconstitution. Each vial of Humatrope contains 5 mg somatropin (15 IU* or 225 nanomoles); 25 mg mannitol; 5 mg glycine; and 1.13 mg dibasic sodium phosphate. Phosphoric acid and/or sodium hydroxide may have been added at the time of manufacture to adjust the pH. This product is oxygen sensitive. Each vial is supplied in a combination package with an accompanying 5-mL vial of diluting solution. The diluent contains water for injection with 0.3% *m* -cresol as a preservative and 1.7% glycerin added at the time of manufacture. Humatrope is a highly purified preparation. The 1.7% glycerin content makes the reconstituted product nearly isotonic at a concentration of 2 mg of Humatrope/mL diluent. Reconstituted solutions have a pH of approximately 7.5.

CLINICAL PHARMACOLOGY

Linear Growth—Humatrope stimulates linear growth in children who lack adequate normal endogenous growth hormone. In vitro, preclinical, and clinical testing have demonstrated that Humatrope is therapeutically equivalent to human growth hormone of pituitary origin and achieves equivalent pharmacokinetic profiles in normal adults. Treatment of growth-hormone-deficient children with Humatrope produces increased growth rate and IGF-1 (Insulin-like Growth Factor/Somatomedin-C) concentrations similar to those seen after therapy with human growth hormone of pituitary origin.

In addition, the following actions have been demonstrated for Humatrope and/or human growth hormone of pituitary origin.

A. *Tissue Growth* —1. Skeletal Growth: Humatrope stimulates skeletal growth in patients with growth hormone defi-

ciency. The measurable increase in body length after administration of either Humatrope or human growth hormone of pituitary origin results from an effect on the growth plates of long bones. Concentrations of IGF-1, which may play a role in skeletal growth, are low in the serum of growth-hormone-deficient children but increase during treatment with Humatrope. Elevations in mean serum alkaline phosphatase concentrations are also seen. 2. Cell Growth: It has been shown that there are fewer skeletal muscle cells in short-statured children who lack endogenous growth hormone as compared with normal children. Treatment with human growth hormone of pituitary origin results in an increase in both the number and size of muscle cells.

B. *Protein Metabolism* —Linear growth is facilitated in part by increased cellular protein synthesis. Nitrogen retention, as demonstrated by decreased urinary nitrogen excretion and serum urea nitrogen, follows the initiation of therapy with human growth hormone of pituitary origin. Treatment with Humatrope results in a similar decrease in serum urea nitrogen.

C. *Carbohydrate Metabolism* —Children with hypopituitarism sometimes experience fasting hypoglycemia that is improved by treatment with Humatrope. Large doses of human growth hormone may impair glucose tolerance.

D. *Lipid Metabolism* —In growth-hormone-deficient patients, administration of human growth hormone of pituitary origin has resulted in lipid mobilization, reduction in body fat stores, and increased plasma fatty acids.

E. *Mineral Metabolism* —Retention of sodium, potassium, and phosphorus is induced by human growth hormone of pituitary origin. Serum concentrations of inorganic phosphate increased in patients with growth hormone deficiency after therapy with Humatrope or human growth hormone of pituitary origin. Serum calcium is not significantly altered in patients treated with either human growth hormone of pituitary origin or Humatrope.

INDICATION AND USAGE

Humatrope® (Somatropin, rDNA Origin, for Injection) is indicated only for the long-term treatment of children who have growth failure due to an inadequate secretion of normal endogenous growth hormone.

CONTRAINDICATIONS

Humatrope should not be used in subjects with closed epiphyses.

Humatrope should not be used when there is any evidence of activity of a tumor. Intracranial lesions must be inactive and antitumor therapy complete prior to the institution of therapy. Humatrope should be discontinued if there is evidence of tumor growth.

Humatrope should not be reconstituted with the supplied Diluent for Humatrope by patients with a known sensitivity to either *m*-cresol or glycerin.

WARNING

If sensitivity to the diluent should occur, the vials may be reconstituted with Sterile Water for Injection, USP. When Humatrope is reconstituted in this manner, (1) use only 1 reconstituted dose per vial, (2) refrigerate the solution (36° to 46°F [2° to 8°C]) if it is not used immediately after reconstitution, (3) use the reconstituted dose within 24 hours, and (4) discard the unused portion.

PRECAUTIONS

Therapy with Humatrope should be directed by physicians who are experienced in the diagnosis and management of patients with growth hormone deficiency.

Patients with growth hormone deficiency secondary to an intracranial lesion should be examined frequently for progression or recurrence of the underlying disease process. Patients should be monitored carefully for any malignant transformation of skin lesions.

Because human growth hormone may induce a state of insulin resistance, patients should be observed for evidence of glucose intolerance.

Excessive glucocorticoid therapy will inhibit the growth promoting effect of human growth hormone. Patients with coexisting ACTH deficiency should have their glucocorticoid replacement dose carefully adjusted to avoid an inhibitory effect on growth.

Hypothyroidism may develop during treatment with human growth hormone, and inadequate treatment of hypothyroidism may prevent optimal response to human growth hormone. Therefore, patients should have periodic thyroid function tests and be treated with thyroid hormone when indicated.

Patients with endocrine disorders, including growth hormone deficiency, may develop slipped capital epiphyses more frequently. Any child with the onset of a limp during growth hormone therapy should be evaluated.

Intracranial hypertension (IH) with papilledema, visual changes, headache, nausea and/or vomiting has been reported in a small number of patients treated with growth hormone products. Symptoms usually occurred within the first eight (8) weeks of the initiation of growth hormone therapy. In all reported cases, IH-associated signs and symptoms

resolved after termination of therapy or a reduction of the growth hormone dose. Funduscopic examination of patients is recommended at the initiation and periodically during the course of growth hormone therapy.

Growth hormone has not been shown to increase the incidence of scoliosis. Progression of scoliosis can occur in children who experience rapid growth. Because growth hormone increases growth rate, patients with a history of scoliosis who are treated with growth hormone should be monitored for progression of scoliosis.

Carcinogenesis, Mutagenesis, Impairment of Fertility—Long-term animal studies for carcinogenicity and impairment of fertility with this human growth hormone (Humatrope) have not been performed. There has been no evidence to date of Humatrope-induced mutagenicity.

Pregnancy—Pregnancy Category C—Animal reproduction studies have not been conducted with Humatrope. It is not known whether Humatrope can cause fetal harm when administered to a pregnant woman or can affect reproduction capacity. Humatrope should be given to a pregnant woman only if clearly needed.

Nursing Mothers—There have been no studies conducted with Humatrope in nursing mothers. It is not known whether this drug is excreted in human milk. Because many drugs are excreted in human milk, caution should be exercised when Humatrope is administered to a nursing woman.

Information for Patients—Patients being treated with growth hormone and/or their parents should be informed of the potential benefits and risks associated with treatment. If home use is determined to be desirable by the physician, instructions on appropriate use should be given, including a review of the contents of the patient information insert. This information is intended to aid in the safe and effective administration of the medication. It is not a disclosure of all possible adverse or intended effects.

If home use is prescribed, a puncture resistant container for the disposal of used syringes and needles should be recommended to the patient. Patients and/or parents should be thoroughly instructed in the importance of proper needle disposal and cautioned against any reuse of needles and syringes (*see* Information for the Patient insert).

ADVERSE REACTIONS

Approximately 2% of 481 naive and previously treated clinical trial patients treated with Humatrope have developed antibodies to growth hormone, as demonstrated by a binding capacity determination threshold ≥0.02 μg/mL. Nevertheless, even these patients experienced increases in linear growth and other salutary effects of Humatrope and did not experience any unusual adverse events. Although growth-limiting antibodies have been observed with other growth hormone preparations (including products of pituitary origin), antibodies in patients treated with Humatrope have not limited growth. The long-term implications of antibody development are uncertain at this time.

Of the 232 naive and previously treated clinical trial patients receiving Humatrope for 6 months or more, 4.7% had serum binding of radiolabeled growth hormone in excess of twice the binding observed in control sera when the serum samples were assayed at a tenfold dilution. Among these patients were 160 naive patients, of whom 6.9% had positive serum binding. In comparison, 74.5% of 106 naive patients treated for 6 months or more with somatrem (produced by Lilly) in a similar clinical trial had serum binding of radiolabeled growth hormone of at least twice the binding observed in control sera.

In addition to an evaluation of compliance with the treatment program and of thyroid status, testing for antibodies to human growth hormone should be carried out in any patient who fails to respond to therapy.

In clinical studies in which high doses of Humatrope were administered to healthy adult volunteers, the following events occurred infrequently: headache, localized muscle pain, weakness, mild hyperglycemia, and glucosuria. In studies with growth-hormone-deficient children, injection site pain was reported infrequently. A mild and transient edema, which appeared in 2.5% of patients, was observed early during the course of treatment.

Leukemia has been reported in a small number of children who have been treated with growth hormone, including growth hormone of pituitary origin as well as of recombinant DNA origin (somatrem and somatropin). The relationship, if any, between leukemia and growth hormone therapy is uncertain.

Other adverse drug events that have been reported in growth hormone-treated patients include the following:
1) Metabolic: Infrequent, mild and transient peripheral or generalized edema. 2) Musculoskeletal: Rare carpal tunnel syndrome. 3) Skin: Rare increased growth of pre-existing nevi. Patients should be monitored carefully for malignant transformation. 4) Endocrine: Rare gynecomastia. Rare pancreatitis.

OVERDOSAGE

Acute overdosage could lead initially to hypoglycemia and subsequently to hyperglycemia. Long-term overdosage could result in signs and symptoms of gigantism/acromegaly consistent with the known effects of excess human growth hormone. (See recommended and maximal dosage instructions given below.)

DOSAGE AND ADMINISTRATION

The recommended weekly dosage is 0.18 mg/kg (0.54 IU/kg) of body weight. It should be divided into equal doses given either on 3 alternate days or 6 times per week. The maximal replacement dosage is 0.1 mg/kg (0.30 IU/kg) administered 3 times a week. The route of administration should be by subcutaneous or intramuscular injection. The dosage and administration schedule for Humatrope should be individualized for each patient.

Each 5-mg vial of Humatrope should be reconstituted with 1.5 to 5 mL of Diluent for Humatrope. The diluent should be injected into the vial of Humatrope by aiming the stream of liquid against the glass wall. Following reconstitution, the vial should be swirled with a GENTLE rotary motion until the contents are completely dissolved. DO NOT SHAKE. The resulting solution should be clear, without particulate matter. If the solution is cloudy or contains particulate matter, the contents MUST NOT be injected.

Before and after injection, the septum of the vial should be wiped with rubbing alcohol or an alcoholic antiseptic solution to prevent contamination of the contents by repeated needle insertions. Sterile disposable syringes and/or needles should be used for administration of Humatrope. The volume of the syringe should be small enough so that the prescribed dose can be withdrawn from the vial with reasonable accuracy.

STABILITY AND STORAGE

Before Reconstitution—Vials of Humatrope as well as the Diluent for Humatrope are stable when refrigerated (36° to 46°F [2° to 8°C]). Avoid freezing Diluent for Humatrope. Expiration dates are stated on the labels.

After Reconstitution—Vials of Humatrope are stable for up to 14 days when reconstituted with Diluent for Humatrope and stored in a refrigerator at 36° to 46°F (2° to 8°C). Avoid freezing the reconstituted vial of Humatrope.

HOW SUPPLIED

Vials:
5 mg (No. 7335)—(6s) NDC 0002-7335-16, and 5-mL vials of Diluent for Humatrope (No. 7336)
CAUTION—Federal (USA) law prohibits dispensing without prescription.
Literature revised May 21, 1996 [052196]

*The units per vial of Humatrope have changed from approximately 13 IU to 15 IU. This does not represent a change in product purity or the quantity (mg) of somatropin per vial. The change in units is a result of harmonizing the defined specific activity of the current reference standard with the international WHO (World Health Organization) reference standard. The specific activity of the International Standard for somatropin is defined as 3 International Units per mg of protein (previously designated as approximately 2.67 IU/mg). Humatrope is now labeled based on a specific activity of 3 IU/mg. This change in reference standard activity does not affect the recommended weekly dosage of 0.18 mg of somatropin per kg of body weight. However, due to the reference standard change the weekly units administered will be measured as 0.54 IU/kg of body weight (previously approximately 0.48 IU/kg of body weight).

HUMULIN® 50/50® OTC

[*hū 'mū-lin*]
(50% Human Insulin Isophane Suspension and 50% Human Insulin Injection [Recombinant DNA Origin])

INFORMATION FOR THE PATIENT

WARNINGS

THIS LILLY HUMAN INSULIN PRODUCT DIFFERS FROM ANIMAL-SOURCE INSULINS BECAUSE IT IS STRUCTURALLY IDENTICAL TO THE INSULIN PRODUCED BY YOUR BODY'S PANCREAS AND BECAUSE OF ITS UNIQUE MANUFACTURING PROCESS.

ANY CHANGE OF INSULIN SHOULD BE MADE CAUTIOUSLY AND ONLY UNDER MEDICAL SUPERVISION. CHANGES IN PURITY, STRENGTH, BRAND (MANUFACTURER), TYPE (REGULAR, NPH, LENTE®, ETC), SPECIES (BEEF, PORK, BEEF-PORK, HUMAN), AND/OR METHOD OF MANUFACTURE (RECOMBINANT DNA VERSUS ANIMAL-SOURCE INSULIN) MAY RESULT IN THE NEED FOR A CHANGE IN DOSAGE.

SOME PATIENTS TAKING HUMULIN® (HUMAN INSULIN, RECOMBINANT DNA ORIGIN, LILLY) MAY REQUIRE A CHANGE IN DOSAGE FROM THAT USED WITH ANIMAL-SOURCE INSULINS. IF AN ADJUSTMENT IS NEEDED, IT MAY OCCUR WITH THE FIRST DOSE OR DURING THE FIRST SEVERAL WEEKS OR MONTHS.

DIABETES

Insulin is a hormone produced by the pancreas, a large gland that lies near the stomach. This hormone is necessary for the body's correct use of food, especially sugar. Diabetes occurs when the pancreas does not make enough insulin to meet your body's needs.

To control your diabetes, your doctor has prescribed injections of insulin to keep your blood glucose at a nearly normal level. Proper control of your diabetes requires close and constant cooperation with your doctor. In spite of diabetes, you can lead an active, healthy, and useful life if you eat a balanced diet daily, exercise regularly, and take your insulin injections as prescribed.

You have been instructed to test your blood and/or your urine regularly for glucose. If your blood tests consistently show above- or below-normal glucose levels or your urine tests consistently show the presence of glucose, your diabetes is not properly controlled and you must let your doctor know.

Always keep an extra supply of insulin as well as a spare syringe and needle on hand. Always wear diabetic identification so that appropriate treatment can be given if complications occur away from home.

50/50 HUMAN INSULIN

Description

Humulin is synthesized in a non-disease-producing special laboratory strain of *Escherichia coli* bacteria that has been genetically altered by the addition of the gene for human insulin production. Humulin 50/50 is a mixture of 50% Human Insulin Isophane Suspension and 50% Human Insulin Injection. It is an intermediate-acting insulin combined with the more rapid onset of action of regular insulin. The duration of activity may last up to 24 hours following injection. The time course of action of any insulin may vary considerably in different individuals or at different times in the same individual. As with all insulin preparations, the duration of action of Humulin 50/50 is dependent on dose, site of injection, blood supply, temperature, and physical activity. Humulin 50/50 is a sterile suspension and is for subcutaneous injection only. It should not be used intravenously or intramuscularly. The concentration of Humulin 50/50 is 100 units/mL (U-100).

Identification

Human insulin manufactured by Eli Lilly and Company has the trademark Humulin and is available in 6 formulations—Regular (**R**), NPH (**N**), Lente (**L**), Ultralente® (**U**), 50% Human Insulin Isophane Suspension [NPH]/50% Human Insulin Injection [buffered regular] (**50/50**) and 70% Human Insulin Isophane Suspension [NPH]/30% Human Insulin Injection [buffered regular] (**70/30**). Your doctor has prescribed the type of insulin that he/she believes is best for you. **DO NOT USE ANY OTHER INSULIN EXCEPT ON HIS/HER ADVICE AND DIRECTION.**

Always check the carton and the bottle label for the name and letter designation of the insulin you receive from your pharmacy to make sure it is the same as that your doctor has prescribed. Humulin 50/50 can be identified as follows:

Always examine the appearance of your bottle of insulin before withdrawing each dose. A bottle of Humulin 50/50 must be carefully shaken or rotated before each injection so that the contents are uniformly mixed. Humulin 50/50 should look uniformly cloudy or milky after mixing. Do not use it if the insulin substance (the white material) remains at the bottom of the bottle after mixing. Do not use a bottle of Humulin 50/50 if there are clumps in the insulin after mixing (*Figure 1*). Do not use a bottle of Humulin 50/50 if solid white particles stick to the bottom or wall of the bottle, giving it a frosted appearance (*Figure 2*). Always check the appearance of your bottle of insulin before using, and if you note anything unusual in the appearance of your insulin or notice your insulin requirements changing markedly, consult your doctor.

Storage

Insulin should be stored in a refrigerator but not in the freezer. If refrigeration is not possible, the bottle of insulin that you are currently using can be kept unrefrigerated as long as it is kept as cool as possible (below 86°F [30°C]) and away from heat and light. Do not use insulin if it has been frozen. Do not use a bottle of insulin after the expiration date stamped on the label.

INJECTION PROCEDURES

Correct Syringe

Doses of insulin are measured in **units.** U-100 insulin contains 100 units/mL (1 mL = 1 cc). With Humulin 50/50, it is important to use a syringe that is marked for U-100 insulin preparations. Failure to use the proper syringe can lead to a

Continued on next page

• Identi-Code® symbol. This product information was prepared in June 1996. Current information on these and other products of Eli Lilly and Company may be obtained by direct inquiry to Lilly Research Laboratories, Lilly Corporate Center, Indianapolis, Indiana 46285, 800-545-5979.

Lilly—Cont.

mistake in dosage, causing serious problems for you, such as a blood glucose level that is too low or too high.

Syringe Use

To help avoid contamination and possible infection, follow these instructions exactly.

Disposable syringes and needles should be used only once and then discarded. **NEEDLES AND SYRINGES MUST NOT BE SHARED.**

Reusable syringes and needles must be sterilized before each injection. **Follow the package directions supplied with your syringe.** Described below are 2 methods of sterilizing.

Boiling

1. Put syringe, plunger, and needle in strainer, place in saucepan, and cover with water. Boil for 5 minutes.
2. Remove articles from water. When they have cooled, insert plunger into barrel, and fasten needle to syringe with a slight twist.
3. Push plunger in and out several times until water is completely removed.

Isopropyl Alcohol

If the syringe, plunger, and needle cannot be boiled, as when you are traveling, they may be sterilized by immersion for at least 5 minutes in Isopropyl Alcohol, 91%. Do not use bathing, rubbing, or medicated alcohol for this sterilization. If the syringe is sterilized with alcohol, it must be absolutely dry before use.

Preparing the Dose

1. Wash your hands.
2. Carefully shake or rotate the insulin bottle several times to completely mix the insulin.
3. Inspect the insulin. Humulin 50/50 should look uniformly cloudy or milky. Do not use it if you notice anything unusual in the appearance.
4. If using a new bottle, flip off the plastic protective cap, but **do not** remove the stopper. When using a new bottle, wipe the top of the bottle with an alcohol swab.
5. Draw air into the syringe equal to your insulin dose. Put the needle through rubber top of the insulin bottle and inject the air into the bottle.
6. Turn the bottle and syringe upside down. Hold the bottle and syringe firmly in 1 hand and shake gently.
7. Making sure the tip of the needle is in the insulin, withdraw the correct dose of insulin into the syringe.
8. Before removing the needle from the bottle, check your syringe for air bubbles which reduce the amount of insulin in it. If bubbles are present, hold the syringe straight up and tap its side until the bubbles float to the top. Push them out with the plunger and withdraw the correct dose.
9. Remove the needle from the bottle and lay the syringe down so that the needle does not touch anything.

Injection

Cleanse the skin with alcohol where the injection is to be made. Stabilize the skin by spreading it or pinching up a large area. Insert the needle as instructed by your doctor. Push the plunger in as far as it will go. Pull the needle out and apply gentle pressure over the injection site for several seconds. **Do not rub the area.** To avoid tissue damage, give the next injection at a site at least ½" from the previous site.

DOSAGE

Your doctor has told you which insulin to use, how much, and when and how often to inject it. Because each patient's case of diabetes is different, this schedule has been individualized for you.

Your usual insulin dose may be affected by changes in your food, activity, or work schedule. Carefully follow your doctor's instructions to allow for these changes. Other things that may affect your insulin dose are:

Illness

Illness, especially with nausea and vomiting, may cause your insulin requirements to change. Even if you are not eating, you will still require insulin. You and your doctor should establish a sick day plan for you to use in case of illness. When you are sick, test your blood/urine frequently and call your doctor as instructed.

Pregnancy

Good control of diabetes is especially important for you and your unborn baby. Pregnancy may make managing your diabetes more difficult. If you are planning to have a baby, are pregnant, or are nursing a baby, consult your doctor.

Medication

Insulin requirements may be increased if you are taking other drugs with hyperglycemic activity, such as oral contraceptives, corticosteroids, or thyroid replacement therapy. Insulin requirements may be reduced in the presence of drugs with hypoglycemic activity, such as oral hypoglycemics, salicylates (for example, aspirin), sulfa antibiotics, and certain antidepressants. Always discuss any medications you are taking with your doctor.

Exercise

Exercise may lower your body's need for insulin during and for some time after the activity. Exercise may also speed up the effect of an insulin dose, especially if the exercise involves the area of injection site (for example, the leg should not be used for injection just prior to running). Discuss with your doctor how you should adjust your regimen to accommodate exercise.

Travel

Persons traveling across more than 2 time zones should consult their doctor concerning adjustments in their insulin schedule.

COMMON PROBLEMS OF DIABETES

Hypoglycemia (Insulin Reaction)

Hypoglycemia (too little glucose in the blood) is one of the most frequent adverse events experienced by insulin users. It can be brought about by:

1. Taking too much insulin
2. Missing or delaying meals
3. Exercising or working more than usual
4. An infection or illness (especially with diarrhea or vomiting)
5. A change in the body's need for insulin
6. Diseases of the adrenal, pituitary, or thyroid gland, or progression of kidney or liver disease
7. Interactions with other drugs that lower blood glucose, such as oral hypoglycemics, salicylates (for example, aspirin), sulfa antibiotics, and certain antidepressants
8. Consumption of alcoholic beverages

Symptoms of mild to moderate hypoglycemia may occur suddenly and can include:

- sweating
- dizziness
- palpitation
- tremor
- hunger
- restlessness
- tingling in the hands, feet, lips, or tongue
- lightheadedness
- inability to concentrate
- headache
- drowsiness
- sleep disturbances
- anxiety
- blurred vision
- slurred speech
- depressive mood
- irritability
- abnormal behavior
- unsteady movement
- personality changes

Signs of severe hypoglycemia can include:

- disorientation
- unconsciousness
- seizures
- death

Therefore, it is important that assistance be obtained immediately.

Early warning symptoms of hypoglycemia may be different or less pronounced under certain conditions, such as long duration of diabetes, diabetic nerve disease, medications such as beta-blockers, change in insulin preparations, or intensified control (3 or more insulin injections per day) of diabetes.

A few patients who have experienced hypoglycemic reactions after transfer from animal-source insulin to human insulin have reported that the early warning symptoms of hypoglycemia were less pronounced or different from those experienced with their previous insulin.

Without recognition of early warning symptoms, you may not be able to take steps to avoid more serious hypoglycemia. Be alert for all of the various types of symptoms that may indicate hypoglycemia. Patients who experience hypoglycemia without early warning symptoms should monitor their blood glucose frequently, especially prior to activities such as driving. If the blood glucose is below your normal fasting glucose, you should consider eating or drinking sugar-containing foods to treat your hypoglycemia.

Mild to moderate hypoglycemia may be treated by eating foods or drinks that contain sugar. Patients should always carry a quick source of sugar, such as candy mints or glucose tablets. More severe hypoglycemia may require the assistance of another person. Patients who are unable to take sugar orally or who are unconscious require an injection of glucagon or should be treated with intravenous administration of glucose at a medical facility.

You should learn to recognize your own symptoms of hypoglycemia. If you are uncertain about these symptoms, you should monitor your blood glucose frequently to help you learn to recognize the symptoms that you experience with hypoglycemia.

If you have frequent episodes of hypoglycemia or experience difficulty in recognizing the symptoms, you should consult your doctor to discuss possible changes in therapy, meal plans, and/or exercise programs to help you avoid hypoglycemia.

Hyperglycemia and Diabetic Acidosis

Hyperglycemia (too much glucose in the blood) may develop if your body has too little insulin. Hyperglycemia can be brought about by:

1. Omitting your insulin or taking less than the doctor has prescribed
2. Eating significantly more than your meal plan suggests
3. Developing a fever, infection, or other significant stressful situation.

In patients with insulin-dependent diabetes, prolonged hyperglycemia can result in diabetic acidosis. The first symptoms of diabetic acidosis usually come on gradually, over a period of hours or days, and include a drowsy feeling, flushed face, thirst, loss of appetite, and fruity odor on the breath. With acidosis, urine tests show large amounts of glucose and acetone. Heavy breathing and a rapid pulse are more severe symptoms. If uncorrected, prolonged hyperglycemia or diabetic acidosis can lead to nausea, vomiting, dehydration, loss of consciousness or death. Therefore, it is important that you obtain medical assistance immediately.

Lipodystrophy

Rarely, administration of insulin subcutaneously can result in lipoatrophy (depression in the skin) or lipohypertrophy (enlargement or thickening of tissue). If you notice either of these conditions, consult your doctor. A change in your injection technique may help alleviate the problem.

Allergy to Insulin

Local Allergy—Patients occasionally experience redness, swelling, and itching at the site of injection of insulin. This condition, called local allergy, usually clears up in a few days to a few weeks. In some instances, this condition may be related to factors other than insulin, such as irritants in the skin cleansing agent or poor injection technique. If you have local reactions, contact your doctor.

Systemic Allergy—Less common, but potentially more serious, is generalized allergy to insulin, which may cause rash over the whole body, shortness of breath, wheezing, reduction in blood pressure, fast pulse, or sweating. Severe cases of generalized allergy may be life threatening. If you think you are having a generalized allergic reaction to insulin, notify a doctor immediately.

ADDITIONAL INFORMATION

Additional information about diabetes may be obtained from your diabetes educator.

DIABETES FORECAST is a national magazine designed especially for patients with diabetes and their families and is available by subscription from the American Diabetes Association, National Service Center, 1660 Duke Street, Alexandria, Virginia 22314.

Another publication, **DIABETES COUNTDOWN**, is available from the Juvenile Diabetes Foundation, 432 Park Avenue South, New York, New York 10016-8013.

Literature revised July 12, 1994

HUMULIN® 70/30 OTC

[*hū'mū-lĭn*]

(70% Human Insulin Isophane Suspension and 30% Human Insulin Injection [Recombinant DNA origin])

INFORMATION FOR THE PATIENT

WARNINGS

THIS LILLY HUMAN INSULIN PRODUCT DIFFERS FROM ANIMAL-SOURCE INSULINS BECAUSE IT IS STRUCTURALLY IDENTICAL TO THE INSULIN PRODUCED BY YOUR BODY'S PANCREAS AND BECAUSE OF ITS UNIQUE MANUFACTURING PROCESS.

ANY CHANGE OF INSULIN SHOULD BE MADE CAUTIOUSLY AND ONLY UNDER MEDICAL SUPERVISION. CHANGES IN PURITY, STRENGTH, BRAND (MANUFACTURER), TYPE (REGULAR, NPH, LENTE®, ETC), SPECIES (BEEF, PORK, BEEF-PORK, HUMAN), AND/OR METHOD OF MANUFACTURE (RECOMBINANT DNA VERSUS ANIMAL-SOURCE INSULIN) MAY RESULT IN THE NEED FOR A CHANGE IN DOSAGE.

SOME PATIENTS TAKING HUMULIN® (HUMAN INSULIN, RECOMBINANT DNA ORIGIN, LILLY) MAY REQUIRE A CHANGE IN DOSAGE FROM THAT USED WITH ANIMAL-SOURCE INSULINS. IF AN ADJUSTMENT IS NEEDED, IT MAY OCCUR WITH THE FIRST DOSE OR DURING THE FIRST SEVERAL WEEKS OR MONTHS.

DIABETES

Insulin is a hormone produced by the pancreas, a large gland that lies near the stomach. This hormone is necessary for the body's correct use of food, especially sugar. Diabetes occurs when the pancreas does not make enough insulin to meet your body's needs.

To control your diabetes, your doctor has prescribed injections of insulin to keep your blood glucose at a nearly normal level. Proper control of your diabetes requires close and constant cooperation with your doctor. In spite of diabetes, you can lead an active, healthy, and useful life if you eat a balanced diet daily, exercise regularly, and take your insulin injections as prescribed.

You have been instructed to test your blood and/or your urine regularly for glucose. If your blood tests consistently show above- or below-normal glucose levels or your urine tests consistently show the presence of glucose, your diabetes is not properly controlled and you must let your doctor know. Always keep an extra supply of insulin as well as a spare syringe and needle on hand. Always wear diabetic identification so that appropriate treatment can be given if complications occur away from home.

70/30 HUMAN INSULIN

Description

Humulin is synthesized in a non-disease-producing special laboratory strain of *Escherichia coli* bacteria that has been genetically altered by the addition of the gene for human insulin production. Humulin 70/30 is a mixture of 70% Human Insulin Isophane Suspension and 30% Human Insulin Injection. It is an intermediate-acting insulin combined with the more rapid onset of action of regular insulin. The duration of activity may last up to 24 hours following injection. The time course of action of any insulin may vary considerably in different individuals or at different times in the same individual. As with all insulin preparations, the duration of action of Humulin 70/30 is dependent on dose, site of injection, blood supply, temperature, and physical activity. Humulin 70/30 is a sterile suspension and is for subcutaneous injection only. It should not be used intravenously or intramuscularly. The concentration of Humulin 70/30 is 100 units/mL (U-100).

Identification

Human insulin manufactured by Eli Lilly and Company has the trademark Humulin and is available in 6 formulations—Regular (**R**), NPH (**N**), Lente (**L**), Ultralente® (**U**), 50% Human Insulin Isophane Suspension [NPH]/50% Human Insulin Injection [buffered regular] (**50/50**), and 70% Human Insulin Isophane Suspension [NPH]/30% Human Insulin Injection [buffered regular] (**70/30**). Your doctor has prescribed the type of insulin that he/she believes is best for you. **DO NOT USE ANY OTHER INSULIN EXCEPT ON HIS/HER ADVICE AND DIRECTION.**

Always check the carton and the bottle label for the name and letter designation of the insulin you receive from your pharmacy to make sure it is the same as that your doctor has prescribed. Humulin 70/30 can be identified as follows:

Always examine the appearance of your bottle of insulin before withdrawing each dose. A bottle of Humulin 70/30 must be carefully shaken or rotated before each injection so that the contents are uniformly mixed. Humulin 70/30 should look uniformly cloudy or milky after mixing. Do not use it if the insulin substance (the white material) remains at the bottom of the bottle after mixing. Do not use a bottle of Humulin 70/30 if there are clumps in the insulin after mixing (Figure 1). Do not use a bottle of Humulin 70/30 if solid white particles stick to the bottom or wall of the bottle, giving it a frosted appearance (Figure 2). Always check the appearance of your bottle of insulin before using, and if you note anything unusual in the appearance of your insulin or notice your insulin requirements changing markedly, consult your doctor.

Storage

Insulin should be stored in a refrigerator but not in the freezer. If refrigeration is not possible, the bottle of insulin that you are currently using can be kept unrefrigerated as long as it is kept as cool as possible (below 86°F [30°C]) and away from heat and light. Do not use insulin if it has been frozen. Do not use a bottle of insulin after the expiration date stamped on the label.

INJECTION PROCEDURES

Correct Syringe

Doses of insulin are measured in **units**. U-100 insulin contains 100 units/mL (1 mL=1 cc). With Humulin 70/30, it is important to use a syringe that is marked for U-100 insulin preparations. Failure to use the proper syringe can lead to a mistake in dosage, causing serious problems for you, such as a blood glucose level that is too low or too high.

Syringe Use

To help avoid contamination and possible infection, follow these instructions exactly.

Disposable syringes and needles should be used only once and then discarded. **NEEDLES AND SYRINGES MUST NOT BE SHARED.**

Reusable syringes and needles must be sterilized before each injection. **Follow the package directions supplied with your syringe.** Described below are 2 methods of sterilizing.

Boiling

1. Put syringe, plunger, and needle in strainer, place in saucepan, and cover with water. Boil for 5 minutes.
2. Remove articles from water. When they have cooled, insert plunger into barrel, and fasten needle to syringe with a slight twist.
3. Push plunger in and out several times until water is completely removed.

Isopropyl Alcohol

If the syringe, plunger, and needle cannot be boiled, as when you are traveling, they may be sterilized by immersion for at least 5 minutes in Isopropyl Alcohol, 91%. Do not use bathing, rubbing, or medicated alcohol for this sterilization. If the syringe is sterilized with alcohol, it must be absolutely dry before use.

Preparing the Dose

1. Wash your hands.
2. Carefully shake or rotate the insulin bottle several times to completely mix the insulin.
3. Inspect the insulin. Humulin 70/30 should look uniformly cloudy or milky. Do not use it if you notice anything unusual in the appearance.
4. If using a new bottle, flip off the plastic protective cap, but **do not** remove the stopper. When using a new bottle, wipe the top of the bottle with an alcohol swab.
5. Draw air into the syringe equal to your insulin dose. Put the needle through rubber top of the insulin bottle and inject the air into the bottle.
6. Turn the bottle and syringe upside down. Hold the bottle and syringe firmly in 1 hand and shake gently.
7. Making sure the tip of the needle is in the insulin, withdraw the correct dose of insulin into the syringe.
8. Before removing the needle from the bottle, check your syringe for air bubbles which reduce the amount of insulin in it. If bubbles are present, hold the syringe straight up and tap its side until the bubbles float to the top. Push them out with the plunger and withdraw the correct dose.
9. Remove the needle from the bottle and lay the syringe down so that the needle does not touch anything.

Injection

Cleanse the skin with alcohol where the injection is to be made. Stabilize the skin by spreading it or pinching up a large area. Insert the needle as instructed by your doctor. Push the plunger in as far as it will go. Pull the needle out and apply gentle pressure over the injection site for several seconds. **Do not rub the area.** To avoid tissue damage, give the next injection at a site at least ½" from the previous site.

DOSAGE

Your doctor has told you which insulin to use, how much, and when and how often to inject it. Because each patient's case of diabetes is different, this schedule has been individualized for you.

Your usual insulin dose may be affected by changes in your food, activity, or work schedule. Carefully follow your doctor's instructions to allow for these changes. Other things that may affect your insulin dose are:

Illness

Illness, especially with nausea and vomiting, may cause your insulin requirements to change. Even if you are not eating, you will still require insulin. You and your doctor should establish a sick day plan for you to use in case of illness. When you are sick, test your blood/urine frequently and call your doctor as instructed.

Pregnancy

Good control of diabetes is especially important for you and your unborn baby. Pregnancy may make managing your diabetes more difficult. If you are planning to have a baby, are pregnant, or are nursing a baby, consult your doctor.

Medication

Insulin requirements may be increased if you are taking other drugs with hyperglycemic activity, such as oral contraceptives, corticosteroids, or thyroid replacement therapy. Insulin requirements may be reduced in the presence of drugs with hypoglycemic activity, such as oral hypoglycemics, salicylates (for example, aspirin), sulfa antibiotics, and certain antidepressants. Always discuss any medications you are taking with your doctor.

Exercise

Exercise may lower your body's need for insulin during and for some time after the activity. Exercise may also speed up the effect of an insulin dose, especially if the exercise involves the area of injection site (for example, the leg should not be used for injection just prior to running). Discuss with your doctor how you should adjust your regimen to accommodate exercise.

Travel

Persons traveling across more than 2 time zones should consult their doctor concerning adjustments in their insulin schedule.

COMMON PROBLEMS OF DIABETES

Hypoglycemia (Insulin Reaction)

Hypoglycemia (too little glucose in the blood) is one of the most frequent adverse events experienced by insulin users. It can be brought about by:

1. Taking too much insulin
2. Missing or delaying meals
3. Exercising or working more than usual
4. An infection or illness (especially with diarrhea or vomiting)
5. A change in the body's need for insulin
6. Diseases of the adrenal, pituitary, or thyroid gland, or progression of kidney or liver disease
7. Interactions with other drugs that lower blood glucose, such as oral hypoglycemics, salicylates (for example, aspirin), sulfa antibiotics, and certain antidepressants

8. Consumption of alcoholic beverages

Symptoms of mild to moderate hypoglycemia may occur suddenly and can include:

- sweating
- dizziness
- palpitation
- tremor
- hunger
- restlessness
- tingling in the hands, feet, lips, or tongue
- lightheadedness
- inability to concentrate
- headache
- drowsiness
- sleep disturbances
- anxiety
- blurred vision
- slurred speech
- depressive mood
- irritability
- abnormal behavior
- unsteady movement
- personality changes

Signs of severe hypoglycemia can include:

- disorientation
- unconsciousness
- seizures
- death

Therefore, it is important that assistance be obtained immediately.

Early warning symptoms of hypoglycemia may be different or less pronounced under certain conditions, such as long duration of diabetes, diabetic nerve disease, medications such as beta-blockers, change in insulin preparations, or intensified control (3 or more insulin injections per day) of diabetes.

A few patients who have experienced hypoglycemic reactions after transfer from animal-source insulin to human insulin have reported that the early warning symptoms of hypoglycemia were less pronounced or different from those experienced with their previous insulin.

Without recognition of early warning symptoms, you may not be able to take steps to avoid more serious hypoglycemia. Be alert for all of the various types of symptoms that may indicate hypoglycemia. Patients who experience hypoglycemia without early warning symptoms should monitor their blood glucose frequently, especially prior to activities such as driving. If the blood glucose is below your normal fasting glucose, you should consider eating or drinking sugar-containing foods to treat your hypoglycemia.

Mild to moderate hypoglycemia may be treated by eating foods or drinks that contain sugar. Patients should always carry a quick source of sugar, such as candy mints or glucose tablets. More severe hypoglycemia may require the assistance of another person. Patients who are unable to take sugar orally or who are unconscious require an injection of glucagon or should be treated with intravenous administration of glucose at a medical facility.

You should learn to recognize your own symptoms of hypoglycemia. If you are uncertain about these symptoms, you should monitor your blood glucose frequently to help you learn to recognize the symptoms that you experience with hypoglycemia.

If you have frequent episodes of hypoglycemia or experience difficulty in recognizing the symptoms, you should consult your doctor to discuss possible changes in therapy, meal plans, and/or exercise programs to help you avoid hypoglycemia.

Hyperglycemia and Diabetic Acidosis

Hyperglycemia (too much glucose in the blood) may develop if your body has too little insulin. Hyperglycemia can be brought about by:

1. Omitting your insulin or taking less than the doctor has prescribed
2. Eating significantly more than your meal plan suggests
3. Developing a fever, infection, or other significant stressful situation.

In patients with insulin-dependent diabetes, prolonged hyperglycemia can result in diabetic acidosis. The first symptoms of diabetic acidosis usually come on gradually, over a period of hours or days, and include a drowsy feeling, flushed face, thirst, loss of appetite, and fruity odor on the breath. With acidosis, urine tests show large amounts of glucose and acetone. Heavy breathing and a rapid pulse are more severe symptoms. If uncorrected, prolonged hyperglycemia or diabetic acidosis can lead to nausea, vomiting, dehydration, loss

Continued on next page

• Identi-Code® symbol. **This product information was prepared in June 1996. Current information on these and other products of Eli Lilly and Company may be obtained by direct inquiry to Lilly Research Laboratories, Lilly Corporate Center, Indianapolis, Indiana 46285, 800-545-5979.**

Lilly—Cont.

of consciousness or death. Therefore, it is important that you obtain medical assistance immediately.

Lipodystrophy

Rarely, administration of insulin subcutaneously can result in lipoatrophy (depression in the skin) or lipohypertrophy (enlargement or thickening of tissue). If you notice either of these conditions, consult your doctor. A change in your injection technique may help alleviate the problem.

Allergy to Insulin

Local Allergy—Patients occasionally experience redness, swelling, and itching at the site of injection of insulin. This condition, called local allergy, usually clears up in a few days to a few weeks. In some instances, this condition may be related to factors other than insulin, such as irritants in the skin cleansing agent or poor injection technique. If you have local reactions, contact your doctor.

Systemic Allergy—Less common, but potentially more serious, is generalized allergy to insulin, which may cause rash over the whole body, shortness of breath, wheezing, reduction in blood pressure, fast pulse, or sweating. Severe cases of generalized allergy may be life threatening. If you think you are having a generalized allergic reaction to insulin, notify a doctor immediately.

ADDITIONAL INFORMATION

Additional information about diabetes may be obtained from your diabetes educator.

DIABETES FORECAST is a national magazine designed especially for patients with diabetes and their families and is available by subscription from the American Diabetes Association, National Service Center, 1660 Duke Street, Alexandria, Virginia 22314.

Another publication, **DIABETES COUNTDOWN**, is available from the Juvenile Diabetes Foundation, 432 Park Avenue South, New York, New York 10016-8013.

Text revised July 12, 1994
Literature revised June 26, 1995   [062695]

HUMULIN® L   OTC
[hū'mŭ-lĭn ĕl]
Lente®
(human insulin [recombinant DNA origin]
zinc suspension)

INFORMATION FOR THE PATIENT
WARNINGS

THIS LILLY HUMAN INSULIN PRODUCT DIFFERS FROM ANIMAL-SOURCE INSULINS BECAUSE IT IS STRUCTURALLY IDENTICAL TO THE INSULIN PRODUCED BY YOUR BODY'S PANCREAS AND BECAUSE OF ITS UNIQUE MANUFACTURING PROCESS.

ANY CHANGE OF INSULIN SHOULD BE MADE CAUTIOUSLY AND ONLY UNDER MEDICAL SUPERVISION. CHANGES IN PURITY, STRENGTH, BRAND (MANUFACTURER), TYPE (REGULAR, NPH, LENTE®, ETC), SPECIES (BEEF, PORK, BEEF-PORK, HUMAN), AND/OR METHOD OF MANUFACTURE (RECOMBINANT DNA VERSUS ANIMAL-SOURCE INSULIN) MAY RESULT IN THE NEED FOR A CHANGE IN DOSAGE.

SOME PATIENTS TAKING HUMULIN® (HUMAN INSULIN, RECOMBINANT DNA ORIGIN, LILLY) MAY REQUIRE A CHANGE IN DOSAGE FROM THAT USED WITH ANIMAL-SOURCE INSULINS. IF AN ADJUSTMENT IS NEEDED, IT MAY OCCUR WITH THE FIRST DOSE OR DURING THE FIRST SEVERAL WEEKS OR MONTHS.

DIABETES

Insulin is a hormone produced by the pancreas, a large gland that lies near the stomach. This hormone is necessary for the body's correct use of food, especially sugar. Diabetes occurs when the pancreas does not make enough insulin to meet your body's needs.

To control your diabetes, your doctor has prescribed injections of insulin to keep your blood glucose at a nearly normal level. Proper control of your diabetes requires close and constant cooperation with your doctor. In spite of diabetes, you can lead an active, healthy, and useful life if you eat a balanced diet daily, exercise regularly, and take your insulin injections as prescribed.

You have been instructed to test your blood and/or your urine regularly for glucose. If your blood tests consistently show above- or below-normal glucose levels or your urine tests consistently show the presence of glucose, your diabetes is not properly controlled and you must let your doctor know. Always keep an extra supply of insulin as well as a spare syringe and needle on hand. Always wear diabetic identification so that appropriate treatment can be given if complications occur away from home.

LENTE HUMAN INSULIN

Description

Humulin is synthesized in a special non-disease-producing laboratory strain of *Escherichia coli* bacteria that has been genetically altered by the addition of the gene for human insulin production. Humulin L is an amorphous and crystalline suspension of human insulin with zinc providing an intermediate-acting insulin with a slower onset and a longer duration of activity (up to 24 hours) than regular insulin. The time course of action of any insulin may vary considerably in different individuals or at different times in the same individual. As with all insulin preparations, the duration of action of Humulin L is dependent on dose, site of injection, blood supply, temperature, and physical activity. Humulin L is a sterile suspension and is for subcutaneous injection only. It should not be used intravenously or intramuscularly. The concentration of Humulin L is 100 units/mL (U-100).

Identification

Human insulin manufactured by Eli Lilly and Company has the trademark Humulin and is available in 6 formulations—Regular (**R**), NPH (**N**), Lente (**L**), Ultralente® (**U**), 50% Human Insulin Isophane Suspension [NPH]/50% Human Insulin Injection [buffered regular] (**50/50**), and 70% Human Insulin Isophane Suspension [NPH]/30% Human Insulin Injection [buffered regular] (**70/30**). Your doctor has prescribed the type of insulin that he/she believes is best for you. **DO NOT USE ANY OTHER INSULIN EXCEPT ON HIS/HER ADVICE AND DIRECTION.**

Always check the carton and the bottle label for the name and letter designation of the insulin you receive from your pharmacy to make sure it is the same as that your doctor has prescribed. Humulin L can be identified as follows: [See Figure below.]

Always examine the appearance of your bottle of insulin before withdrawing each dose. A bottle of Humulin L must be carefully shaken or rotated before each injection so that the contents are uniformly mixed. Humulin L should look uniformly cloudy or milky after mixing. Do not use it if the insulin substance (the white material) remains at the bottom of the bottle after mixing (Figure 1). Do not use a bottle of Humulin L if there are clumps in the insulin after mixing (Figure 2). Always check the appearance of your bottle of insulin before using, and if you note anything unusual in the appearance of your insulin or notice your insulin requirements changing markedly, consult your doctor.

Storage

Insulin should be stored in a refrigerator but not in the freezer. If refrigeration is not possible, the bottle of insulin that you are currently using can be kept unrefrigerated as long as it is kept as cool as possible (below 86°F [30°C]) and away from heat and light. Do not use insulin if it has been frozen. Do not use a bottle of insulin after the expiration date stamped on the label.

INJECTION PROCEDURES

Correct Syringe

Doses of insulin are measured in **units**. U-100 insulin contains 100 units/mL (1 mL=1 cc). With Humulin L, it is important to use a syringe that is marked for U-100 insulin preparations. Failure to use the proper syringe can lead to a mistake in dosage, causing serious problems for you, such as a blood glucose level that is too low or too high.

Syringe Use

To help avoid contamination and possible infection, follow these instructions exactly. Disposable syringes and needles should be used only once and then discarded. **NEEDLES AND SYRINGES MUST NOT BE SHARED.** Reusable syringes and needles must be sterilized before each injection. **Follow the package directions supplied with your syringe.** Described below are 2 methods of sterilizing.

Boiling

1. Put syringe, plunger, and needle in strainer, place in saucepan, and cover with water. Boil for 5 minutes.
2. Remove articles from water. When they have cooled, insert plunger into barrel, and fasten needle to syringe with a slight twist.
3. Push plunger in and out several times until water is completely removed.

Isopropyl Alcohol

If the syringe, plunger, and needle cannot be boiled, as when you are traveling, they may be sterilized by immersion for at least 5 minutes in Isopropyl Alcohol, 91%. Do not use bathing, rubbing, or medicated alcohol for this sterilization. If the syringe is sterilized with alcohol, it must be absolutely dry before use.

Preparing the Dose

1. Wash your hands.
2. Carefully shake or rotate the insulin bottle several times to completely mix the insulin.
3. Inspect the insulin. Humulin L should look uniformly cloudy or milky. Do not use it if you notice anything unusual in the appearance.
4. If using a new bottle, flip off the plastic protective cap, but **do not** remove the stopper. When using a new bottle, wipe the top of the bottle witth an alcohol swab.
5. If you are mixing insulins, refer to the instructions for mixing that follow.
6. Draw air into the syringe equal to your insulin dose. Put the needle through rubber top of the insulin bottle and inject the air into the bottle.
7. Turn the bottle and syringe upside down. Hold the bottle and syringe firmly in 1 hand and shake gently.
8. Making sure the tip of the needle is in the insulin, withdraw the correct dose of insulin into the syringe.
9. Before removing the needle from the bottle, check your syringe for air bubbles which reduce the amount of insulin in it. If bubbles are present, hold the syringe straight up and tap its side until the bubbles float to the top. Push them out with the plunger and withdraw the correct dose.
10. Remove the needle from the bottle and lay the syringe down so that the needle does not touch anything.

Mixing Humulin L with Regular or Ultralente Human Insulin

1. Lente human insulin should be mixed with regular or Ultralente human insulin only on the advice of your doctor.
2. Draw air into your syringe equal to the amount of Humulin L you are taking. Insert the needle into the Humulin L bottle and inject the air. Withdraw the needle.
3. Now inject air into your regular or Ultralente human insulin bottle in the same manner, but **do not** withdraw the needle.
4. Turn the bottle and syringe upside down.
5. Making sure the tip of the needle is in the insulin, withdraw the correct dose of regular or Ultralente insulin into the syringe.
6. Before removing the needle from the bottle, check your syringe for air bubbles which reduce the amount of insulin in it. If bubbles are present, hold the syringe straight up and tap its side until the bubbles float to the top. Push them out with the plunger and withdraw the correct dose.
7. Remove the needle from the bottle of regular or Ultralente insulin and insert it into the bottle of Humulin L. Turn the bottle and syringe upside down. Hold the bottle and syringe firmly in 1 hand and shake gently. Making sure the tip of the needle is in the insulin, withdraw your dose of Humulin L.
8. Remove the needle and lay the syringe down so that the needle does not touch anything.

Follow your doctor's instructions on whether to mix your insulins ahead of time or just before giving your injection. It is important to be consistent in your method.

Syringes from different manufacturers may vary in the amount of space between the bottom line and the needle. Because of this, do not change:

- the sequence of mixing, or
- the model and brand of syringe or needle that the doctor has prescribed.

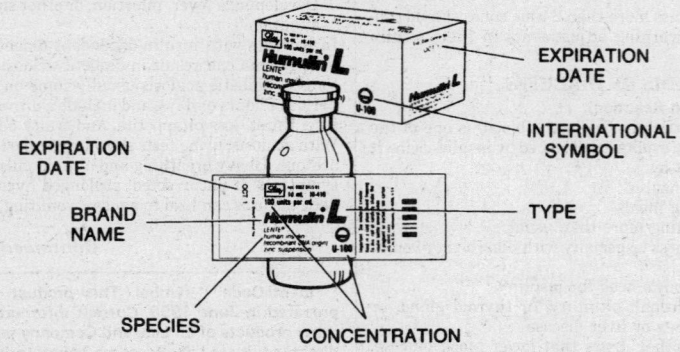

EXPIRATION DATE

INTERNATIONAL SYMBOL

TYPE

EXPIRATION DATE

BRAND NAME

SPECIES

CONCENTRATION

Injection

Cleanse the skin with alcohol where the injection is to be made. Stabilize the skin by spreading it or pinching up a large area. Insert the needle as instructed by your doctor. Push the plunger in as far as it will go. Pull the needle out and apply gentle pressure over the injection site for several seconds. **Do not rub the area.** To avoid tissue damage, give the next injection at a site at least $1/2$" from the previous site.

DOSAGE

Your doctor has told you which insulin to use, how much, and when and how often to inject it. Because each patient's case of diabetes is different, this schedule has been individualized for you.

Your usual insulin dose may be affected by changes in your food, activity, or work schedule. Carefully follow your doctor's instructions to allow for these changes. Other things that may affect your insulin dose are:

Illness

Illness, especially with nausea and vomiting, may cause your insulin requirements to change. Even if you are not eating, you will still require insulin. You and your doctor should establish a sick day plan for you to use in case of illness. When you are sick, test your blood/urine frequently and call your doctor as instructed.

Pregnancy

Good control of diabetes is especially important for you and your unborn baby. Pregnancy may make managing your diabetes more difficult. If you are planning to have a baby, are pregnant, or are nursing a baby, consult your doctor.

Medication

Insulin requirements may be increased if you are taking other drugs with hyperglycemic activity, such as oral contraceptives, corticosteroids, or thyroid replacement therapy. Insulin requirements may be reduced in the presence of drugs with hypoglycemic activity, such as oral hypoglycemics, salicylates (for example, aspirin), sulfa antibiotics, and certain antidepressants. Always discuss any medications you are taking with your doctor.

Exercise

Exercise may lower your body's need for insulin during and for some time after the activity. Exercise may also speed up the effect of an insulin dose, especially if the exercise involves the area of injection site (for example, the leg should not be used for injection just prior to running). Discuss with your doctor how you should adjust your regimen to accommodate exercise.

Travel

Persons traveling across more than 2 time zones should consult their doctor concerning adjustments in their insulin schedule.

COMMON PROBLEMS OF DIABETES

Hypoglycemia (Insulin Reaction)

Hypoglycemia (too little glucose in the blood) is one of the most frequent adverse events experienced by insulin users. It can be brought about by:

1. Taking too much insulin
2. Missing or delaying meals
3. Exercising or working more than usual
4. An infection or illness (especially with diarrhea or vomiting)
5. A change in the body's need for insulin
6. Diseases of the adrenal, pituitary, or thyroid gland, or progression of kidney or liver disease
7. Interactions with other drugs that lower blood glucose, such as oral hypoglycemics, salicylates (for example, aspirin), sulfa antibiotics, and certain antidepressants
8. Consumption of alcoholic beverages

Symptoms of mild to moderate hypoglycemia may occur suddenly and can include:

- sweating
- dizziness
- palpitation
- tremor
- hunger
- restlessness
- tingling in the hands, feet, lips, or tongue
- lightheadedness
- inability to concentrate
- headache
- drowsiness
- sleep disturbances
- anxiety
- blurred vision
- slurred speech
- depressive mood
- irritability
- abnormal behavior
- unsteady movement
- personality changes

Signs of severe hypoglycemia can include:
- disorientation
- unconsciousness

- seizures
- death

Therefore, it is important that assistance be obtained immediately.

Early warning symptoms of hypoglycemia may be different or less pronounced under certain conditions, such as long duration of diabetes, diabetic nerve disease, medications such as beta-blockers, change in insulin preparations, or intensified control (3 or more insulin injections per day) of diabetes.

A few patients who experienced hypoglycemic reactions after transfer from animal-source insulin to human insulin have reported that the early warning symptoms of hypoglycemia were less pronounced or different from those experienced with their previous insulin.

Without recognition of early warning symptoms, you may not be able to take steps to avoid more serious hypoglycemia. Be alert for all of the various types of symptoms that may indicate hypoglycemia. Patients who experience hypoglycemia without early warning symptoms should monitor their blood glucose frequently, especially prior to activities such as driving. If the blood glucose is below your normal fasting glucose, you should consider eating or drinking sugar-containing foods to treat your hypoglycemia.

Mild to moderate hypoglycemia may be treated by eating foods or drinks that contain sugar. Patients should always carry a quick source of sugar, such as candy mints or glucose tablets. More severe hypoglycemia may require the assistance of another person. Patients who are unable to take sugar orally or who are unconscious require an injection of glucagon or should be treated with intravenous administration of glucose at a medical facility.

You should learn to recognize your own symptoms of hypoglycemia. If you are uncertain about these symptoms, you should monitor your blood glucose frequently to help you learn to recognize the symptoms that you experience with hypoglycemia.

If you have frequent episodes of hypoglycemia or experience difficulty in recognizing the symptoms, you should consult your doctor to discuss possible changes in therapy, meal plans, and/or exercise programs to help you avoid hypoglycemia.

Hyperglycemia and Diabetic Acidosis

Hyperglycemia (too much glucose in the blood) may develop if your body has too little insulin. Hyperglycemia can be brought about by:

1. Omitting your insulin or taking less than the doctor has prescribed
2. Eating significantly more than your meal plan suggests
3. Developing a fever, infection, or other significant stressful situation

In patients with insulin-dependent diabetes, prolonged hyperglycemia can result in diabetic acidosis. The first symptoms of diabetic acidosis usually come on gradually, over a period of hours or days, and include a drowsy feeling, flushed face, thirst, loss of appetite, and fruity odor on the breath. With acidosis, urine tests show large amounts of glucose and acetone. Heavy breathing and a rapid pulse are more severe symptoms. If uncorrected, prolonged hyperglycemia or diabetic acidosis can lead to nausea, vomiting, dehydration, loss of consciousness or death. Therefore, it is important that you obtain medical assistance immediately.

Lipodystrophy

Rarely, administration of insulin subcutaneously can result in lipoatrophy (depression in the skin) or lipohypertrophy (enlargement or thickening of tissue). If you notice either of these conditions, consult your doctor. A change in your injection technique may help alleviate the problem.

Allergy to Insulin

Local Allergy—Patients occasionally experience redness, swelling, and itching at the site of injection of insulin. This condition, called local allergy, usually clears up in a few days to a few weeks. In some instances, this condition may be related to factors other than insulin, such as irritants in the skin cleansing agent or poor injection technique. If you have local reactions, contact your doctor.

Systemic Allergy—Less common, but potentially more serious, is generalized allergy to insulin, which may cause rash over the whole body, shortness of breath, wheezing, reduction in blood pressure, fast pulse, or sweating. Severe cases of generalized allergy may be life threatening. If you think you are having a generalized allergic reaction to insulin, notify a doctor immediately.

ADDITIONAL INFORMATION

Additional information about diabetes may be obtained from your diabetes educator.

DIABETES FORECAST is a national magazine designed especially for patients with diabetes and their families and is available by subscription from the American Diabetes Association, National Service Center, 1660 Duke Street, Alexandria, Virginia 22314.

Another publication, **DIABETES COUNTDOWN**, is available from the Juvenile Diabetes Foundation, 432 Park Avenue South, New York, New York 10016–8013.

Literature revised July 12, 1994   [071294]

HUMULIN® N   OTC
[hū'mū-lĭn ĕn]
NPH
(human insulin [recombinant DNA origin] isophane suspension)

INFORMATION FOR THE PATIENT
WARNINGS
THIS LILLY HUMAN INSULIN PRODUCT DIFFERS FROM ANIMAL-SOURCE INSULINS BECAUSE IT IS STRUCTURALLY IDENTICAL TO THE INSULIN PRODUCED BY YOUR BODY'S PANCREAS AND BECAUSE OF ITS UNIQUE MANUFACTURING PROCESS.
ANY CHANGE OF INSULIN SHOULD BE MADE CAUTIOUSLY AND ONLY UNDER MEDICAL SUPERVISION. CHANGES IN PURITY, STRENGTH, BRAND (MANUFACTURER), TYPE (REGULAR, NPH, LENTE®, ETC), SPECIES (BEEF, PORK, BEEF-PORK, HUMAN), AND/OR METHOD OF MANUFACTURE (RECOMBINANT DNA VERSUS ANIMAL-SOURCE INSULIN) MAY RESULT IN THE NEED FOR A CHANGE IN DOSAGE.
SOME PATIENTS TAKING HUMULIN® (HUMAN INSULIN, RECOMBINANT DNA ORIGIN, LILLY) MAY REQUIRE A CHANGE IN DOSAGE FROM THAT USED WITH ANIMAL-SOURCE INSULINS. IF AN ADJUSTMENT IS NEEDED, IT MAY OCCUR WITH THE FIRST DOSE OR DURING THE FIRST SEVERAL WEEKS OR MONTHS.

DIABETES

Insulin is a hormone produced by the pancreas, a large gland that lies near the stomach. This hormone is necessary for the body's correct use of food, especially sugar. Diabetes occurs when the pancreas does not make enough insulin to meet your body's needs.

To control your diabetes, your doctor has prescribed injections of insulin to keep your blood glucose at a nearly normal level. Proper control of your diabetes requires close and constant cooperation with your doctor. In spite of diabetes, you can lead an active, healthy, and useful life if you eat a balanced diet daily, exercise regularly, and take your insulin injections as prescribed.

You have been instructed to test your blood and/or your urine regularly for glucose. If your blood tests consistently show above- or below-normal glucose levels or your urine tests consistently show the presence of glucose, your diabetes is not properly controlled and you must let your doctor know. Always keep an extra supply of insulin as well as a spare syringe and needle on hand. Always wear diabetic identification so that appropriate treatment can be given if complications occur away from home.

NPH HUMAN INSULIN
Description
Humulin is synthesized in a special non-disease-producing laboratory strain of *Escherichia coli* bacteria that has been genetically altered by the addition of the gene for human insulin production. Humulin N is a crystalline suspension of human insulin with protamine and zinc providing an intermediate-acting insulin with a slower onset of action and a longer duration of activity (up to 24 hours) than that of regular insulin. The time course of action of any insulin may vary considerably in different individuals or at different times in the same individual. As with all insulin preparations, the duration of action of Humulin N is dependent on dose, site of injection, blood supply, temperature, and physical activity. Humulin N is a sterile suspension and is for subcutaneous injection only. It should not be used intravenously or intramuscularly. The concentration of Humulin N is 100 units/mL (U-100).

Identification
Human insulin manufactured by Eli Lilly and Company has the trademark Humulin and is available in 6 formulations—Regular (**R**), NPH (**N**), Lente (**L**), Ultralente® (**U**), 50% Human Insulin Isophane Suspension [NPH]/50% Human Insulin Injection [buffered regular] (**50/50**), and 70% Human Insulin Isophane Suspension [NPH]/30% Human Insulin Injection [buffered regular] (**70/30**). Your doctor has prescribed the type of insulin that he/she believes is best for you. **DO NOT USE ANY OTHER INSULIN EXCEPT ON HIS/HER ADVICE AND DIRECTION.**
Always check the carton and the bottle label for the name and letter designation of the insulin you receive from your pharmacy to make sure it is the same as that your doctor has prescribed. Humulin N can be identified as follows:
Always examine the appearance of your bottle of insulin before withdrawing each dose. A bottle of Humulin N must be carefully shaken or rotated before each injection so that

Continued on next page

• **Identi-Code® symbol. This product information was prepared in June 1996. Current information on these and other products of Eli Lilly and Company may be obtained by direct inquiry to Lilly Research Laboratories, Lilly Corporate Center, Indianapolis, Indiana 46285, 800-545-5979.**

Lilly—Cont.

the contents are uniformly mixed. Humulin N should look uniformly cloudy or milky after mixing. Do not use it if the insulin substance (the white material) remains at the bottom of the bottle after mixing. Do not use a bottle of Humulin N if there are clumps in the insulin after mixing (Figure 1). Do not use a bottle of Humulin N if solid white particles stick to the bottom or wall of the bottle, giving it a frosted appearance (Figure 2). Always check the appearance of your bottle of insulin before using, and if you note anything unusual in the appearance of your insulin or notice your insulin requirements changing markedly, consult your doctor.

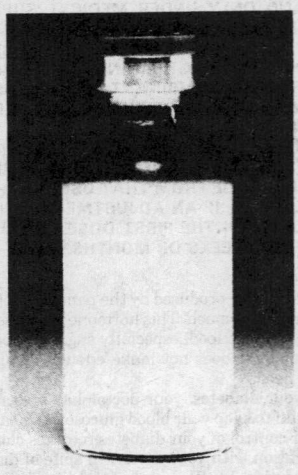

Fig. 1.—Do not use if there are clumps in the insulin after mixing.

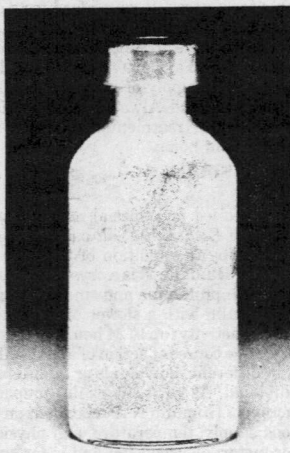

Fig. 2.—Do not use if particles on the bottom or wall give the bottle a frosted appearance.

Storage
Insulin should be stored in a refrigerator but not in the freezer. If refrigeration is not possible, the bottle of insulin that you are currently using can be kept unrefrigerated as long as it is kept as cool as possible (below 86°F [30°C]) and away from heat and light. Do not use insulin if it has been frozen. Do not use a bottle of insulin after the expiration date stamped on the label.

INJECTION PROCEDURES
Correct Syringe
Doses of insulin are measured in units. U-100 insulin contains 100 units/mL (1 mL = 1 cc). With Humulin N, it is important to use a syringe that is marked for U-100 insulin preparations. Failure to use the proper syringe can lead to a mistake in dosage, causing serious problems for you, such as a blood glucose level that is too low or too high.

Syringe Use
To help avoid contamination and possible infection, follow these instructions exactly.
Disposable syringes and needles should be used only once and then discarded. **NEEDLES AND SYRINGES MUST NOT BE SHARED.**
Reusable syringes and needles must be sterilized before each injection. **Follow the package directions supplied with your syringe.** Described below are 2 methods of sterilizing.

Boiling
1. Put syringe, plunger, and needle in strainer, place in saucepan, and cover with water. Boil for 5 minutes.
2. Remove articles from water. When they have cooled, insert plunger into barrel, and fasten needle to syringe with a slight twist.
3. Push plunger in and out several times until water is completely removed.

Isopropyl Alcohol
If the syringe, plunger, and needle cannot be boiled, as when you are traveling, they may be sterilized by immersion for at least 5 minutes in Isopropyl Alcohol, 91%. Do not use bathing, rubbing, or medicated alcohol for this sterilization. If the syringe is sterilized with alcohol, it must be absolutely dry before use.

Preparing the Dose
1. Wash your hands.
2. Carefully shake or rotate the insulin bottle several times to completely mix the insulin.
3. Inspect the insulin. Humulin N should look uniformly cloudy or milky. Do not use it if you notice anything unusual in the appearance.
4. If using a new bottle, flip off the plastic protective cap, but **do not** remove the stopper. When using a new bottle, wipe the top of the bottle with an alcohol swab.
5. If you are mixing insulins, refer to the instructions for mixing that follow.
6. Draw air into the syringe equal to your insulin dose. Put the needle through rubber top of the insulin bottle and inject the air into the bottle.
7. Turn the bottle and syringe upside down. Hold the bottle and syringe firmly in 1 hand and shake gently.
8. Making sure the tip of the needle is in the insulin, withdraw the correct dose of insulin into the syringe.
9. Before removing the needle from the bottle, check your syringe for air bubbles which reduce the amount of insulin in it. If bubbles are present, hold the syringe straight up and tap its side until the bubbles float to the top. Push them out with the plunger and withdraw the correct dose.
10. Remove the needle from the bottle and lay the syringe down so that the needle does not touch anything.

Mixing Humulin N and Regular Human Insulin
1. NPH human insulin should be mixed only with regular human insulin.
2. Draw air into your syringe equal to the amount of Humulin N you are taking. Insert the needle into the Humulin N bottle and inject the air. Withdraw the needle.
3. Now inject air into your regular human insulin bottle in the same manner, but **do not** withdraw the needle.
4. Turn the bottle and syringe upside down.
5. Making sure the tip of the needle is in the insulin, withdraw the correct dose of regular insulin into the syringe.
6. Before removing the needle from the bottle, check your syringe for air bubbles which reduce the amount of insulin in it. If bubbles are present, hold the syringe straight up and tap its side until the bubbles float to the top. Push them out with the plunger and withdraw the correct dose.
7. Remove the needle from the bottle of regular insulin and insert it into the bottle of Humulin N. Turn the bottle and syringe upside down. Hold the bottle and syringe firmly in 1 hand and shake gently. Making sure the tip of the needle is in the insulin, withdraw your dose of Humulin N.
8. Remove the needle and lay the syringe down so that the needle does not touch anything.

Follow your doctor's instructions on whether to mix your insulins ahead of time or just before giving your injection. It is important to be consistent in your method.
Syringes from different manufacturers may vary in the amount of space between the bottom line and the needle. Because of this, do not change:
- the sequence of mixing, or
- the model and brand of syringe or needle that the doctor has prescribed.

Injection
Cleanse the skin with alcohol where the injection is to be made. Stabilize the skin by spreading it or pinching up a large area. Insert the needle as instructed by your doctor. Push the plunger in as far as it will go. Pull the needle out and apply gentle pressure over the injection site for several seconds. **Do not rub the area.** To avoid tissue damage, give the next injection at a site at least 1/2″ from the previous site.

DOSAGE
Your doctor has told you which insulin to use, how much, and when and how often to inject it. Because each patient's case of diabetes is different, this schedule has been individualized for you.
Your usual insulin dose may be affected by changes in your food, activity, or work schedule. Carefully follow your doctor's instructions to allow for these changes. Other things that may affect your insulin dose are:

Illness
Illness, especially with nausea and vomiting, may cause your insulin requirements to change. Even if you are not eating, you will still require insulin. You and your doctor should establish a sick day plan for you to use in case of illness.

When you are sick, test your blood/urine frequently and call your doctor as instructed.

Pregnancy
Good control of diabetes is especially important for you and your unborn baby. Pregnancy may make managing your diabetes more difficult. If you are planning to have a baby, are pregnant, or are nursing a baby, consult your doctor.

Medication
Insulin requirements may be increased if you are taking other drugs with hyperglycemic activity, such as oral contraceptives, corticosteroids, or thyroid replacement therapy. Insulin requirements may be reduced in the presence of drugs with hypoglycemic activity, such as oral hypoglycemics, salicylates (for example, aspirin), sulfa antibiotics, and certain antidepressants. Always discuss any medications you are taking with your doctor.

Exercise
Exercise may lower your body's need for insulin during and for some time after the activity. Exercise may also speed up the effect of an insulin dose, especially if the exercise involves the area of injection site (for example, the leg should not be used for injection just prior to running). Discuss with your doctor how you should adjust your regimen to accomodate exercise.

Travel
Persons traveling across more than 2 time zones should consult their doctor concerning adjustments in their insulin schedule.

COMMON PROBLEMS OF DIABETES
Hypoglycemia (Insulin Reaction)
Hypoglycemia (too little glucose in the blood) is one of the most frequent adverse events experienced by insulin users. It can be brought about by:
1. Taking too much insulin
2. Missing or delaying meals
3. Exercising or working more than usual
4. An infection or illness (especially with diarrhea or vomiting)
5. A change in the body's need for insulin
6. Diseases of the adrenal, pituitary, or thyroid gland, or progression of kidney or liver disease
7. Interactions with other drugs that lower blood glucose, such as oral hypoglycemics, salicylates (for example, aspirin), sulfa antibiotics, and certain antidepressants
8. Consumption of alcoholic beverages

Symptoms of mild to moderate hypoglycemia may occur suddenly and can include:
- sweating
- dizziness
- palpitation
- tremor
- hunger
- restlessness
- tingling in the hands, feet, lips, or tongue
- lightheadedness
- inability to concentrate
- headache
- drowsiness
- sleep disturbances
- anxiety
- blurred vision
- slurred speech
- depressive mood
- irritability
- abnormal behavior
- unsteady movement
- personality changes

Signs of severe hypoglycemia can include:
- disorientation
- unconsciousness
- seizures
- death

Therefore, it is important that assistance be obtained immediately.
Early warning symptoms of hypoglycemia may be different or less pronounced under certain conditions, such as long duration of diabetes, diabetic nerve disease, medications such as beta-blockers, change in insulin preparations, or intensified control (3 or more insulin injections per day) of diabetes.
A few patients who have experienced hypoglycemic reactions after transfer from animal-source insulin to human insulin have reported that the early warning symptoms of hypoglycemia were less pronounced or different from those experienced with their previous insulin.
Without recognition of early warning symptoms, you may not be able to take steps to avoid more serious hypoglycemia. Be alert for all of the various types of symptoms that may indicate hypoglycemia. Patients who experience hypoglycemia without early warning symptoms should monitor their blood glucose frequently, especially prior to activities such as driving. If the blood glucose is below your normal fasting glucose, you should consider eating or drinking sugar-containing foods to treat your hypoglycemia.

Mild to moderate hypoglycemia may be treated by eating foods or drinks that contain sugar. Patients should always carry a quick source of sugar, such as candy mints or glucose tablets. More severe hypoglycemia may require the assistance of another person. Patients who are unable to take sugar orally or who are unconscious require an injection of glucagon or should be treated with intravenous administration of glucose at a medical facility.

You should learn to recognize your own symptoms of hypoglycemia. If you are uncertain about these symptoms, you should monitor your blood glucose frequently to help you learn to recognize the symptoms that you experience with hypoglycemia.

If you have frequent episodes of hypoglycemia or experience difficulty in recognizing the symptoms, you should consult your doctor to discuss possible changes in therapy, meal plans, and/or exercise programs to help you avoid hypoglycemia.

Hyperglycemia and Diabetic Acidosis

Hyperglycemia (too much glucose in the blood) may develop if your body has too little insulin. Hyperglycemia can be brought about by:

1. Omitting your insulin or taking less than the doctor has prescribed
2. Eating significantly more than your meal plan suggests
3. Developing a fever, infection, or other significant stressful situation

In patients with insulin-dependent diabetes, prolonged hyperglycemia can result in diabetic acidosis. The first symptoms of diabetic acidosis usually come on gradually, over a period of hours or days, and include a drowsy feeling, flushed face, thirst, loss of appetite, and fruity odor on the breath. With acidosis, urine tests show large amounts of glucose and acetone. Heavy breathing and a rapid pulse are more severe symptoms. If uncorrected, prolonged hyperglycemia or diabetic acidosis can lead to nausea, vomiting, dehydration, loss of consciousness or death. Therefore, it is important that you obtain medical assistance immediately.

Lipodystrophy

Rarely, administration of insulin subcutaneously can result in lipoatrophy (depression in the skin) or lipohypertrophy (enlargement or thickening of tissue). if you notice either of these conditions, consult your doctor. A change in your injection technique may help alleviate the problem.

Allergy to Insulin

Local Allergy—Patients occasionally experience redness, swelling, and itching at the site of injection of insulin. This condition, called local allergy, usually clears up in a few days to a few weeks. In some instances, this condition may be related to factors other than insulin, such as irritants in the skin cleansing agent or poor injection technique. If you have local reactions, contact your doctor.

Systemic Allergy—Less common, but potentially more serious, is generalized allergy to insulin, which may cause rash over the whole body, shortness of breath, wheezing, reduction in blood pressure, fast pulse, or sweating. Severe cases of generalized allergy may be life threatening. If you think you are having a generalized allergic reaction to insulin, notify a doctor immediately.

ADDITIONAL INFORMATION

Additional information about diabetes may be obtained from your diabetes educator.

DIABETES FORECAST is a national magazine designed especially for patients with diabetes and their families and is available by subscription from the American Diabetes Association, National Service Center, 1660 Duke Street, Alexandria, Virginia 22314.

Another publication, **DIABETES COUNTDOWN**, is available from the Juvenile Diabetes Foundation, 432 Park Avenue South, New York, New York 10016–8013.

Literature revised October 5, 1994 [100594]

HUMULIN® R **OTC**

[*hū´mū-lĭn är*]

Regular

(insulin human injection, USP [recombinant DNA origin])

INFORMATION FOR THE PATIENT

WARNINGS

THIS LILLY HUMAN INSULIN PRODUCT DIFFERS FROM ANIMAL-SOURCE INSULINS BECAUSE IT IS STRUCTURALLY IDENTICAL TO THE INSULIN PRODUCED BY YOUR BODY'S PANCREAS AND BECAUSE OF ITS UNIQUE MANUFACTURING PROCESS.

ANY CHANGE OF INSULIN SHOULD BE MADE CAUTIOUSLY AND ONLY UNDER MEDICAL SUPERVISION. CHANGES IN PURITY, STRENGTH, BRAND (MANUFACTURER), TYPE (REGULAR, NPH, LENTE®, ETC), SPECIES (BEEF, PORK, BEEF-PORK, HUMAN), AND/OR METHOD OF MANUFACTURE (RECOMBINANT DNA VERSUS ANIMAL-SOURCE INSULIN) MAY RESULT IN THE NEED FOR A CHANGE IN DOSAGE.

SOME PATIENTS TAKING HUMULIN® (HUMAN INSULIN, RECOMBINANT DNA ORIGIN, LILLY) MAY REQUIRE A CHANGE IN DOSAGE FROM THAT USED WITH ANIMAL-SOURCE INSULINS. IF AN ADJUSTMENT IS NEEDED, IT MAY OCCUR WITH THE FIRST DOSE OR DURING THE FIRST SEVERAL WEEKS OR MONTHS.

DIABETES

Insulin is a hormone produced by the pancreas, a large gland that lies near the stomach. The hormone is necessary for the body's correct use of food, especially sugar. Diabetes occurs when the pancreas does not make enough insulin to meet your body's needs.

To control your diabetes, your doctor has prescribed injections of insulin to keep your blood glucose at a nearly normal level. Proper control of your diabetes requires close and constant cooperation with your doctor. In spite of diabetes, you can lead an active, healthy, and useful life if you eat a balanced diet daily, exercise regularly, and take your insulin injections as prescribed.

You have been instructed to test your blood and/or your urine regularly for glucose. If your blood tests consistently show above- or below-normal glucose levels or your urine tests consistently show the presence of glucose, your diabetes is not properly controlled and you must let your doctor know.

Always keep an extra supply of insulin as well as a spare syringe and needle on hand. Always wear diabetic identification so that appropriate treatment can be given if complications occur away from home.

REGULAR HUMAN INSULIN

Description

Humulin is synthesized in a special non-disease-producing laboratory strain of *Escherichia coli* bacteria that has been genetically altered by the addition of the gene for human insulin production. Humulin R consists of zinc-insulin crystals dissolved in a clear fluid. Humulin R has had nothing added to change the speed or length of its action. It takes effect rapidly and has a relatively short duration of activity (4 to 12 hours) as compared with other insulins. The time course of action of any insulin may vary considerably in different individuals or at different times in the same individual. As with all insulin preparations, the duration of action of Humulin R is dependent on dose, site of injection, blood supply, temperature, and physical activity. Humulin R is a sterile solution and is for subcutaneous injection. It should not be used intramuscularly. The concentration of Humulin R is 100 units/mL (U-100).

Identification

Human insulin manufactured by Eli Lilly and Company has the trademark Humulin and is available in 6 formulations—Regular (**R**), NPH (**N**), Lente (**L**), Ultralente® (**U**), 50% Human Insulin Isophane Suspension [NPH]/50% Human Insulin Injection [buffered regular] (**50/50**), and 70% Human Insulin Isophane Suspension [NPH]/30% Human Insulin Injection [buffered regular] (**70/30**). Your doctor has prescribed the type of insulin that he/she believes is best for you. **DO NOT USE ANY OTHER INSULIN EXCEPT ON HIS/HER ADVICE AND DIRECTION.**

Always check the carton and the bottle label for the name and letter designation of the insulin you receive from your pharmacy to make sure it is the same as that your doctor has prescribed. Humulin R can be identified as follows:

Always examine the appearance of your bottle of insulin before withdrawing each dose. Humulin R is a clear and colorless liquid with a water-like appearance and consistency. Do not use if it appears cloudy, thickened, or slightly colored or if solid particles are visible. Always check the appearance of your bottle of insulin before using, and if you note anything unusual in the appearance of your insulin or notice your insulin requirements changing markedly, consult your doctor.

Storage

Insulin should be stored in a refrigerator but not in the freezer. If refrigeration is not possible, the bottle of insulin that you are currently using can be kept unrefrigerated as long as it is kept as cool as possible (below 86°F [30°C]) and away from heat and light. Do not use insulin if it has been frozen. Do not use a bottle of insulin after the expiration date stamped on the label.

INJECTION PROCEDURES

Correct Syringe

Doses of insulin are measured in **units**. U-100 insulin contains 100 units/mL (1 mL = 1 cc). With Humulin R, it is important to use a syringe that is marked for U-100 insulin preparations. Failure to use the proper syringe can lead to a mistake in dosage, causing serious problems for you, such as a blood glucose level that is too low or too high.

Syringe Use

To help avoid contamination and possible infection, follow these instructions exactly.

Disposable syringes and needles should be used only once and then discarded. **NEEDLES AND SYRINGES MUST NOT BE SHARED.**

Reusable syringes and needles must be sterilized before each injection.

Follow the package directions supplied with your syringe.

Described below are 2 methods of sterilizing.

Boiling

1. Put syringe, plunger, and needle in strainer, place in saucepan, and cover with water. Boil for 5 minutes.
2. Remove articles from water. When they have cooled, insert plunger into barrel, and fasten needle to syringe with a slight twist.
3. Push plunger in and out several times until water is completely removed.

Isopropyl Alcohol

If the syringe, plunger, and needle cannot be boiled, as when you are traveling, they may be sterilized by immersion for at least 5 minutes in Isopropyl Alcohol, 91%. Do not use bathing, rubbing, or medicated alcohol for this sterilization. If the syringe is sterilized with alcohol, it must be absolutely dry before use.

Preparing the Dose

1. Wash your hands.
2. Inspect the insulin. Humulin R should look clear and colorless. Do not use Humulin R if it appears cloudy, thickened, or slightly colored or if solid particles are visible.
3. If using a new bottle, flip off the plastic protective cap, but **do not** remove the stopper. When using a new bottle, wipe the top of the bottle with an alcohol swab.
4. If you are mixing insulins, refer to instructions for mixing that follow.
5. Draw air into the syringe equal to your insulin dose. Put the needle through rubber top of insulin bottle and inject the air into the bottle.
6. Turn the bottle and syringe upside down. Hold the bottle and syringe firmly in 1 hand.
7. Making sure the tip of the needle is in the insulin, withdraw the correct dose of insulin into the syringe.
8. Before removing the needle from the bottle, check your syringe for air bubbles which reduce the amount of insulin in it. If bubbles are present, hold the syringe straight up and tap its side until the bubbles float to the top. Push them out with the plunger and withdraw the correct dose.
9. Remove the needle from the bottle and lay the syringe down so that the needle dose not touch anything.

Mixing Humulin R with Longer-acting Human Insulins

1. Regular human insulin should be mixed with longer-acting human insulins only on the advice of your doctor.
2. Draw air into your syringe equal to the amount of longer-acting insulin you are taking. Insert the needle into the longer-acting insulin bottle and inject the air. Withdraw the needle.
3. Now inject air into your regular human insulin bottle in the same manner, but **do not** withdraw the needle.
4. Turn the bottle and syringe upside down.
5. Making sure the tip of the needle is in the insulin, withdraw the correct dose of regular insulin into the syringe.
6. Before removing the needle from the bottle, check your syringe for air bubbles which reduce the amount of insulin in it. If bubbles are present, hold the syringe straight up and tap its side until the bubbles float to the top. Push them out with the plunger and withdraw the correct dose.
7. Remove the needle from the bottle of regular insulin and insert it into the bottle of the longer-acting insulin. Turn the bottle and syringe upside down. Hold the bottle and syringe firmly in 1 hand and shake gently. Making sure the tip of the needle is in the insulin, withdraw your dose of longer-acting insulin.
8. Remove the needle and lay the syringe down so that the needle does not touch anything.

Follow your doctor's instructions on whether to mix your insulins ahead of time or just before giving your injection. It is important to be consistent in your method.

Syringes from different manufacturers may vary in the amount of space between the bottom line and the needle. Because of this, do not change:

- the sequence of mixing, or
- the model and brand of syringe or needle that the doctor has prescribed.

Injection

Cleanse the skin with alcohol where the injection is to be made. Stabilize the skin by spreading it or pinching up a large area. Insert the needle as instructed by your doctor. Push the plunger in as far as it will go. Pull the needle out and apply gentle pressure over the injection site for several seconds. **Do not rub area.** To avoid tissue damage, give the next injection at a site at least ½″ from the previous site.

DOSAGE

Your doctor has told you which insulin to use, how much, and when and how often to inject it. Because each patient's

Continued on next page

*** Identi-Code® symbol. This product information was prepared in June 1996. Current information on these and other products of Eli Lilly and Company may be obtained by direct inquiry to Lilly Research Laboratories, Lilly Corporate Center, Indianapolis, Indiana 46285, 800-545-5979.**

Lilly—Cont.

case of diabetes is different, this schedule has been individualized for you.
Your usual insulin dose may be affected by changes in your food, activity, or work schedule. Carefully follow your doctor's instructions to allow for these changes. Other things may affect your insulin dose are:

Illness
Illness, especially with nausea and vomiting, may cause your insulin requirements to change. Even if you are not eating, you will still require insulin. You and your doctor should establish a sick day plan for you to use in case of illness. When you are sick, test your blood/urine frequently and call your doctor as instructed.

Pregnancy
Good control of diabetes is especially important for you and your unborn baby. Pregnancy may make managing your diabetes more difficult. If you are planning to have a baby, are pregnant, or are nursing a baby, consult your doctor.

Medication
Insulin requirements may be increased if you are taking other drugs with hyperglycemic activity, such as oral contraceptives, corticosteroids, or thyroid replacement therapy. Insulin requirements may be reduced in the presence of drugs with hypoglycemic activity, such as oral hypoglycemics, salicylates (for example, aspirin), sulfa antibiotics, and certain antidepressants. Always discuss any medications you are taking with your doctor.

Exercise
Exercise may lower your body's need for insulin during and for some time after the activity. Exercise may also speed up the effect of an insulin dose, especially if the exercise involves the area of injection site (for example, the leg should not be used for injection just prior to running). Discuss with your doctor how you should adjust your regimen to accommodate exercise.

Travel
Persons traveling across more than 2 time zones should consult their doctor concerning adjustments in their insulin schedule.

COMMON PROBLEMS OF DIABETES

Hypoglycemia (Insulin Reaction)
Hypoglycemia (too little glucose in the blood) is one of the most frequent adverse events experienced by insulin users. It can be brought about by:

1. Taking too much insulin
2. Missing or delaying meals
3. Exercising or working more than usual
4. An infection or illness (especially with diarrhea or vomiting)
5. A change in the body's need for insulin
6. Diseases of the adrenal, pituitary, or thyroid gland, or progression of kidney or liver disease
7. Interactions with other drugs that lower blood glucose, such as oral hypoglycemics, salicylates (for example, aspirin), sulfa antibiotics, and certain antidepressants
8. Consumption of alcoholic beverages

Symptoms of mild to moderate hypoglycemia may occur suddenly and can include:

- sweating
- dizziness
- palpitation
- tremor
- hunger
- restlessness
- tingling in the hands, feet, lips, or tongue
- lightheadedness
- inability to concentrate
- headache
- drowsiness
- sleep disturbances
- anxiety
- blurred vision
- slurred speech
- depressive mood
- irritability
- abnormal behavior
- unsteady movement
- personality changes

Signs of severe hypoglycemia can include:

- disorientation
- unconsciousness
- seizures
- death

Therefore, it is important that assistance be obtained immediately.
Early warning symptoms of hypoglycemia may be different or less pronounced under certain conditions, such as long duration of diabetes, diabetic nerve disease, medications such as beta-blockers, change in insulin preparations, or intensified control (3 or more insulin injections per day) of diabetes.

A few patients who have experienced hypoglycemic reactions after transfer from animal-source insulin to human insulin have reported that the early warning symptoms of hypoglycemia were less pronounced or different from those experienced with their previous insulin.
Without recognition of early warning symptoms, you may not be able to take steps to avoid more serious hypoglycemia. Be alert for all of the various types of symptoms that may indicate hypoglycemia. Patients who experience hypoglycemia without early warning symptoms should monitor their blood glucose frequently, especially prior to activities such as driving. If the blood glucose is below your normal fasting glucose, you should consider eating or drinking sugar-containing foods to treat your hypoglycemia.
Mild to moderate hypoglycemia may be treated by eating foods or drinks that contain sugar. Patients should always carry a quick source of sugar, such as candy mints or glucose tablets. More severe hypoglycemia may require the assistance of another person. Patients who are unable to take sugar orally or who are unconscious require an injection of glucagon or should be treated with intravenous administration of glucose at a medical facility.
You should learn to recognize your own symptoms of hypoglycemia. If you are uncertain about these symptoms, you should monitor your blood glucose frequently to help you learn to recognize the symptoms that you experience with hypoglycemia.
If you have frequent episodes of hypoglycemia or experience difficulty in recognizing the symptoms, you should consult your doctor to discuss possible changes in therapy, meal plans, and/or exercise programs to help you avoid hypoglycemia.

Hyperglycemia and Diabetic Acidosis
Hyperglycemia (too much glucose in the blood) may develop if your body has too little insulin. Hyperglycemia can be brought about by:

1. Omitting your insulin or taking less than the doctor has prescribed
2. Eating significantly more than your meal plan suggests
3. Developing a fever, infection, or other significant stressful situation

In patients with insulin-dependent diabetes, prolonged hyperglycemia can result in diabetic acidosis. The first symptoms of diabetic acidosis usually come on gradually, over a period of hours or days, and include a drowsy feeling, flushed face, thirst, loss of appetite, and fruity odor on the breath. With acidosis, urine tests show large amounts of glucose and acetone. Heavy breathing and a rapid pulse are more severe symptoms. If uncorrected, prolonged hyperglycemia or diabetic acidosis can lead to nausea, vomiting, dehydration, loss of consciousness or death. Therefore, it is important that you obtain medical assistance immediately.

Lipodystrophy
Rarely, administration of insulin subcutaneously can result in lipoatrophy (depression in the skin) or lipohypertrophy (enlargement or thickening of tissue). If you notice either of these conditions, consult your doctor. A change in your injection technique may help alleviate the problem.

Allergy to Insulin
Local Allergy—Patients occasionally experience redness, swelling, and itching at the site of injection of insulin. This condition, called local allergy, usually clears up in a few days to a few weeks. In some instances, this condition may be related to factors other than insulin, such as irritants in the skin cleansing agent or poor injection technique. If you have local reactions, contact your doctor.
Systemic Allergy—Less common, but potentially more serious, is generalized allergy insulin, which may cause rash over the whole body, shortness of breath, wheezing, reduction in blood pressure, fast pulse, or sweating. Severe cases of generalized allergy may be life threatening. If you think you are having a generalized allergic reaction to insulin, notify a doctor immediately.

ADDITIONAL INFORMATION

Additional information about diabetes may be obtained from your diabetes educator.
DIABETES FORECAST is a national magazine designed especially for patients with diabetes and their families and is available by subscription from the American Diabetes Association, National Service Center, 1660 Duke Street, Alexandria, Virginia 22314.
Another publication, **DIABETES COUNTDOWN**, is available from the Juvenile Diabetes Foundation, 432 Park Avenue South, New York, New York 10016-8013.
Literature revised July 12, 1994 [071294]

HUMULIN® U — OTC

[*hū'mŭ-lĭn ū*]
Ultralente®
(human Insulin [recombinant DNA origin] extended zinc suspension)

INFORMATION FOR THE PATIENT

WARNINGS

THIS LILLY HUMAN INSULIN PRODUCT DIFFERS FROM ANIMAL-SOURCE INSULINS BECAUSE IT IS STRUCTURALLY IDENTICAL TO THE INSULIN PRODUCED BY YOUR BODY'S PANCREAS AND BECAUSE OF ITS UNIQUE MANUFACTURING PROCESS.
ANY CHANGE OF INSULIN SHOULD BE MADE CAUTIOUSLY AND ONLY UNDER MEDICAL SUPERVISION. CHANGES IN PURITY, STRENGTH, BRAND (MANUFACTURER), TYPE (REGULAR, NPH, LENTE®, ETC), SPECIES (BEEF, PORK, BEEF-PORK, HUMAN), AND/OR METHOD OF MANUFACTURE (RECOMBINANT DNA VERSUS ANIMAL-SOURCE INSULIN) MAY RESULT IN THE NEED FOR A CHANGE IN DOSAGE.
SOME PATIENTS TAKING HUMULIN® (HUMAN INSULIN, RECOMBINANT DNA ORIGIN, LILLY) MAY REQUIRE A CHANGE IN DOSAGE FROM THAT USED WITH ANIMAL-SOURCE INSULINS. IF AN ADJUSTMENT IS NEEDED, IT MAY OCCUR WITH THE FIRST DOSE OR DURING THE FIRST SEVERAL WEEKS OR MONTHS.

DIABETES
Insulin is a hormone produced by the pancreas, a large gland that lies near the stomach. This hormone is necessary for the body's correct use of food, especially sugar. Diabetes occurs when the pancreas does not make enough insulin to meet your body's needs.
To control your diabetes, your doctor has prescribed injections of insulin to keep your blood glucose at a nearly normal level. Proper control of your diabetes requires close and constant cooperation with your doctor. In spite of diabetes, you can lead an active, healthy, and useful life if you eat a balanced diet daily, exercise regularly, and take your insulin injections as prescribed.
You have been instructed to test your blood and/or your urine regularly for glucose. If your blood tests consistently show above- or below-normal glucose levels or your urine tests consistently show the presence of glucose, your diabetes is not properly controlled and you must let your doctor know. Always keep an extra supply of insulin as well as a spare syringe and needle on hand. Always wear diabetic identification so that appropriate treatment can be given if complications occur away from home.

ULTRALENTE HUMAN INSULIN

Description
Humulin is synthesized in a special non-disease-producing laboratory strain of *Escherichia coli* bacteria that has been genetically altered by the addition of the gene for human insulin production. Humulin U is a crystalline suspension of human insulin with zinc providing a slower onset and a longer and less intense duration of activity (up to 28 hours) than regular insulin or the intermediate-acting insulins (NPH and Lente). The time course of action of any insulin may vary considerably in different individuals or at different times in the same individual. As with all insulin preparations, the duration of action of Humulin U is dependent on dose, site of injection, blood supply, temperature, and physical activity. Humulin U is a sterile suspension and is for subcutaneous injection only. It should not be used intravenously or intramuscularly. The concentration of Humulin U is 100 units/mL (U-100).

Identification
Human insulin manufactured by Eli Lilly and Company has the trademark Humulin and is available in 6 formulations—Regular (**R**), NPH (**N**), Lente (**L**), Ultralente (**U**), 50% Human Insulin Isophane Suspension [NPH]/50% Human Insulin Injection [buffered regular] (**50/50**), and 70% Human Insulin Isophane Suspension [NPH]/30% Human Insulin Injection [buffered regular] (**70/30**). Your doctor has prescribed the type of insulin that he/she believes is best for you. **DO NOT USE ANY OTHER INSULIN EXCEPT ON HIS/HER ADVICE AND DIRECTION.**
Always check the carton and the bottle label for the name and letter designation of the insulin you receive from your pharmacy to make sure it is the same as that your doctor has prescribed. Humulin U can be identified as follows:
Always examine the appearance of your bottle of insulin before withdrawing each dose. A bottle of Humulin U must be carefully shaken or rotated before each injection so that the contents are uniformly mixed. Humulin U should look uniformly cloudy or milky after mixing. Do not use it if the insulin substance (the white material) remains at the bottom of the bottle after mixing (Figure 1). Do not use a bottle of Humulin U if there are clumps in the insulin after mixing (Figure 2). Always check the appearance of your bottle of insulin before using, and if you note anything unusual in the appearance of your insulin or notice your insulin requirements changing markedly, consult your doctor.

Storage

Insulin should be stored in a refrigerator but not in the freezer. If refrigeration is not possible, the bottle of insulin that you are currently using can be kept unrefrigerated as long as it is kept as cool as possible (below 86°F [30°C]) and away from heat and light. Do not use insulin if it has been frozen. Do not use a bottle of insulin after the expiration date stamped on the label.

INJECTION PROCEDURES

Correct Syringe

Doses of insulin are measured in **units**. U-100 insulin contains 100 units/mL (1 mL = 1 cc). With Humulin U, it is important to use a syringe that is marked for U-100 insulin preparations. Failure to use the proper syringe can lead to a mistake in dosage, causing serious problems for you, such as a blood glucose level that is too low or too high.

Syringe Use

To help avoid contamination and possible infection, follow these instructions exactly.

Disposable syringes and needles should be used only once and then discarded. **NEEDLES AND SYRINGES MUST NOT BE SHARED.**

Reusable syringes and needles must be sterilized before each injection.

Follow the package directions supplied with your syringe. Described below are 2 methods of sterilizing.

Boiling

1. Put syringe, plunger, and needle in strainer, place in saucepan, and cover with water. Boil for 5 minutes.
2. Remove articles from water. When they have cooled, insert plunger into barrel, and fasten needle to syringe with a slight twist.
3. Push plunger in and out several times until water is completely removed.

Isopropyl Alcohol

If the syringe, plunger, and needle cannot be boiled, as when you are traveling, they may be sterilized by immersion for at least 5 minutes in Isopropyl Alcohol, 91%. Do not use bathing, rubbing, or medicated alcohol for this sterilization. If the syringe is sterilized with alcohol, it must be absolutely dry before use.

Preparing the Dose

1. Wash your hands.
2. Carefully shake or rotate the insulin bottle several times to completely mix the insulin.
3. Inspect the insulin. Humulin U should look uniformly cloudy or milky. Do not use if you notice anything unusual in the appearance.
4. If using a new bottle, flip off the plastic protective cap, but **do not** remove the stopper. When using a new bottle, wipe the top of the bottle with an alcohol swab.
5. If you are mixing insulins, refer to the instructions for mixing that follow.
6. Draw air into the syringe equal to your insulin dose. Put the needle through rubber top of the insulin bottle and inject the air into the bottle.
7. Turn the bottle and syringe upside down. Hold the bottle and syringe firmly in 1 hand and shake gently.
8. Making sure the tip of the needle is in the insulin, withdraw the correct dose of insulin into the syringe.
9. Before removing the needle from the bottle, check your syringe for air bubbles which reduce the amount of insulin in it. If bubbles are present, hold the syringe straight up and tap its side until the bubbles float to the top. Push them out with the plunger and withdraw the correct dose.
10. Remove the needle from the bottle and lay the syringe down so that the needle does not touch anything.

Mixing Humulin U with Regular or Lente Human Insulin

1. Ultralente human insulin should be mixed with regular or Lente human insulin only on the advice of your doctor.
2. Draw air into your syringe equal to the amount of Humulin U you are taking. Insert the needle into the Humulin U bottle and inject the air. Withdraw the needle.
3. Now inject air into your regular or Lente human insulin bottle in the same manner, but **do not** withdraw the needle.
4. Turn the bottle and syringe upside down.
5. Making sure the tip of the needle is in the insulin, withdraw the correct dose of regular or Lente insulin into the syringe.
6. Before removing the needle from the bottle, check your syringe for air bubbles which reduce the amount of insulin in it. If bubbles are present, hold the syringe straight up and tap its side until the bubbles float to the top. Push them out with the plunger and withdraw the correct dose.
7. Remove the needle from the bottle of regular or Lente insulin and insert it into the bottle of Humulin U. Turn the bottle and syringe upside down. Hold the bottle and syringe firmly in 1 hand and shake gently. Making sure the tip of the needle is in the insulin, withdraw your dose of Humulin U.
8. Remove the needle and lay the syringe down so that the needle does not touch anything.

Follow your doctor's instructions on whether to mix your insulins ahead of time or just before giving your injection. It is important to be consistent in your method.

Syringes from different manufacturers may vary in the amount of space between the bottom line and the needle. Because of this, do not change:
- the sequence of mixing, or
- the model and brand of syringe or needle that the doctor has prescribed.

Injection

Cleanse the skin with alcohol where the injection is to be made. Stabilize the skin by spreading it or pinching up a large area. Insert the needle as instructed by your doctor. Push the plunger in as far as it will go. Pull the needle out and apply gentle pressure over the injection site for several seconds. **Do not rub the area.** To avoid tissue damage, give the next injection at a site at least $1/2$″ from the previous site.

DOSAGE

Your doctor has told you which insulin to use, how much, and when and how often to inject it. Because each patient's case of diabetes is different, this schedule has been individualized for you.

Your usual insulin dose may be affected by changes in your food, activity, or work schedule. Carefully follow your doctor's instructions to allow for these changes. Other things that may affect your insulin dose are:

Illness

Illness, especially with nausea and vomiting, may cause your insulin requirements to change. Even if you are not eating, you will still require insulin. You and your doctor should establish a sick day plan for you to use in case of illness. When you are sick, test your blood/urine frequently and call your doctor as instructed.

Pregnancy

Good control of diabetes is especially important for you and your unborn baby. Pregnancy may make managing your diabetes more difficult. If you are planning to have a baby, are pregnant, or are nursing a baby, consult your doctor.

Medication

Insulin requirements may be increased if you are taking other drugs with hyperglycemic activity, such as oral contraceptives, corticosteroids, or thyroid replacement therapy. Insulin requirements may be reduced in the presence of drugs with hypoglycemic activity, such as oral hypoglycemics, salicylates (for example, aspirin), sulfa antibiotics, and certain antidepressants. Always discuss any medications you are taking with your doctor.

Exercise

Exercise may lower your body's need for insulin during and for some time after the activity. Exercise may also speed up the effect of an insulin dose, especially if the exercise involves the area of injection site (for example, the leg should not be used for injection just prior to running). Discuss with your doctor how you should adjust your regimen to accommodate exercise.

Travel

Persons traveling across more than 2 time zones should consult their doctor concerning adjustments in their insulin schedule.

COMMON PROBLEMS OF DIABETES

Hypoglycemia (Insulin Reaction)

Hypoglycemia (too little glucose in the blood) is one of the most frequent adverse events experienced by insulin users. It can be brought about by:
1. Taking too much insulin
2. Missing or delaying meals
3. Exercising or working more than usual
4. An infection or illness (especially with diarrhea or vomiting)
5. A change in the body's need for insulin
6. Diseases of the adrenal, pituitary, or thyroid gland, or progression of kidney or liver disease
7. Interactions with other drugs that lower blood glucose, such as oral hypoglycemics, salicylates (for example, aspirin) sulfa antibiotics, and certain antidepressants
8. Consumption of alcoholic beverages

Symptoms of mild to moderate hypoglycemia may occur suddenly and can include:
- sweating
- dizziness
- palpitation
- tremor
- hunger
- restlessness
- tingling in the hands, feet, lips, or tongue
- lightheadedness
- inability to concentrate
- headache
- drowsiness
- sleep disturbances
- anxiety
- blurred vision
- slurred speech
- depressive mood
- irritability
- abnormal behavior
- unsteady movement
- personality changes

Signs of severe hypoglycemia can include:
- disorientation
- unconsciousness
- seizures
- death

Therefore, it is important that assistance be obtained immediately.

Early warning symptoms of hypoglycemia may be different or less pronounced under certain conditions, such as long duration of diabetes, diabetic nerve disease, medications such as beta-blockers, change in insulin preparations, or intensified control (3 or more insulin injections per day) of diabetes.

A few patients who have experienced hypoglycemic reactions after transfer from animal-source insulin to human insulin have reported that the early warning symptoms of hypoglycemia were less pronounced or different from those experienced with their previous insulin.

Without recognition of early warning symptoms, you may not be able to take steps to avoid more serious hypoglycemia. Be alert for all of the various types of symptoms that may indicate hypoglycemia. Patients who experience hypoglycemia without early warning symptoms should monitor their blood glucose frequently, especially prior to activities such as driving. If the blood glucose is below your normal fasting glucose, you should consider eating or drinking sugar-containing foods to treat your hypoglycemia.

Mild to moderate hypoglycemia may be treated by eating foods or drinks that contain sugar. Patients should always carry a quick source of sugar, such as candy mints or glucose tablets. More severe hypoglycemia may require the assistance of another person. Patients who are unable to take sugar orally or who are unconscious require an injection of glucagon or should be treated with intravenous administration of glucose at a medical facility.

You should learn to recognize your own symptoms of hypoglycemia. If you are uncertain about these symptoms, you should monitor your blood glucose frequently to help you learn to recognize the symptoms that you experience with hypoglycemia.

If you have frequent episodes of hypoglycemia or experience difficulty in recognizing the symptoms, you should consult your doctor to discuss possible changes in therapy, meal plans, and/or exercise programs to help you avoid hypoglycemia.

Hyperglycemia and Diabetic Acidosis

Hyperglycemia (too much glucose in the blood) may develop if your body has too little insulin. Hyperglycemia can be brought about by:
1. Omitting your insulin or taking less than the doctor has prescribed
2. Eating significantly more than your meal plan suggests
3. Developing a fever, infection, or other significant stressful situation

In patients with insulin-dependent diabetes, prolonged hyperglycemia can result in diabetic acidosis. The first symptoms of diabetic acidosis usually come on gradually, over a period of hours or days, and include a drowsy feeling, flushed face, thirst, loss of appetite, and fruity odor on the breath. With acidosis, urine tests show large amounts of glucose and acetone. Heavy breathing and a rapid pulse are more severe symptoms. If uncorrected, prolonged hyperglycemia or diabetic acidosis can lead to nausea, vomiting, dehydration, loss of consciousness or death. Therefore, it is important that you obtain medical assistance immediately.

Lipodystrophy

Rarely, administration of insulin subcutaneously can result in lipoatrophy (depression in the skin) or lipohypertrophy (enlargement or thickening of tissue). If you notice either of these conditions, consult your doctor. A change in your injection technique may help alleviate the problem.

Allergy to Insulin

Local Allergy—Patients occasionally experience redness, swelling, and itching at the site of injection of insulin. This condition, called local allergy, usually clears up in a few days to a few weeks. In some instances, this condition may be related to factors other than insulin, such as irritants in the skin cleansing agent or poor injection technique. If you have local reactions, contact your doctor.

Systemic Allergy—Less common, but potentially more serious, is generalized allergy to insulin, which may cause rash over the whole body, shortness of breath, wheezing, reduc-

Continued on next page

• Identi-Code® symbol. This product information was prepared in June 1996. Current information on these and other products of Eli Lilly and Company may be obtained by direct inquiry to Lilly Research Laboratories, Lilly Corporate Center, Indianapolis, Indiana 46285, 800-545-5979.

Lilly—Cont.

tion in blood pressure, fast pulse, or sweating. Severe cases of generalized allergy may be life threatening. If you think you are having a generalized allergic reaction to insulin, notify a doctor immediately.

ADDITIONAL INFORMATION

Additional information about diabetes may be obtained from your diabetes educator.

DIABETES FORECAST is a national magazine designed especially for patients with diabetes and their families and is available by subscription from the American Diabetes Association, National Service Center, 1660 Duke Street, Alexandria, Virginia 22314.

Another publication, **DIABETES COUNTDOWN**, is available from the Juvenile Diabetes Foundation, 432 Park Avenue South, New York, New York 10016-8013.

Literature revised July 12, 1994 [071294]

KEFTAB® ℞

[*kĕf'tăb*]

(cephalexin hydrochloride)

DESCRIPTION

Keftab® (Cephalexin Hydrochloride) is a semisynthetic cephalosporin antibiotic intended for oral administration. Chemically, it is designated 7-(D-2-amino-2phenylacetamido)-3-methyl-3-cephem-4-carboxylic acid hydrochloride monohydrate, and the chemical formula is $C_{16}H_{17}N_3O_4S \cdot HCl \cdot H_2O$. The molecular weight is 401.86, and it has the following structural formula:

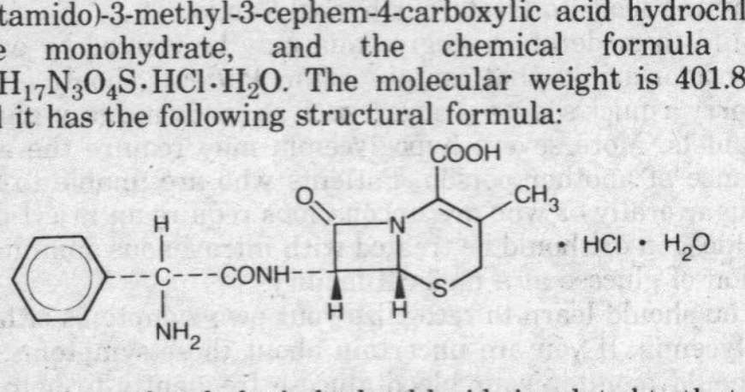

The nucleus of cephalexin hydrochloride is related to that of other cephalosporin antibiotics. The compound is the hydrochloride salt of cephalexin. The isoelectric point of cephalexin in water is approximately 4.5 to 5.

Cephalexin hydrochloride is in crystalline form and is a monohydrate. It is a white crystalline solid having a bitter taste. Solubility in water is high at room temperature; greater than 10 mg/mL may be dissolved readily.

The cephalosporins differ from penicillins in the structure of the bicyclic ring system. Cephalexin has a *D*-phenylglycyl group as substituent at the 7-amino position and an unsubstituted methyl group at the 3-position.

Each tablet contains cephalexin hydrochloride equivalent to 500 mg (1,439 μmol) cephalexin. The tablets also contain D & C Yellow No. 10, F D & C Blue No. 1, F D & C Red No. 40, magnesium stearate, silicon dioxide, stearic acid, sucrose, titanium dioxide, and other inactive ingredients.

CLINICAL PHARMACOLOGY

Human Pharmacology—Keftab is acid stable and may be given without regard to meals. It is rapidly absorbed after oral administration. Following doses of 250 mg and 500 mg, average peak serum levels of approximately 9 and 18 μg/mL respectively were obtained at 1 hour and declined to 1.6 and 3.4 μg/mL respectively at 3 hours. Measurable levels were present 6 hours after administration. Cephalexin is excreted in the urine by glomerular filtration and tubular secretion. Studies showed that approximately 70% of the drug was excreted unchanged in the urine within 12 hours. During the first 6 hours, average urine concentrations following the 250-mg and 500-mg doses were approximately 200 μg/mL (range, 54 to 663) and 500 μg/mL (range, 137 to 1,306) respectively. The average serum half-life is 1.1 hours.

Microbiology—In vitro tests demonstrate that the cephalosporins are bactericidal because of their inhibition of cell-wall synthesis. Keftab is active against the following organisms in vitro:

- β-hemolytic streptococci
- *Staphylococcus aureus,* including penicillinase-producing strains
- *Streptococcus pneumoniae*
- *Escherichia coli*
- *Proteus mirabilis*
- *Klebsiella* sp
- *Haemophilus influenzae*
- *Moraxella (Branhamella) catarrhalis*

Note—Most strains of enterococci (*Enterococcus faecalis* [formerly *Streptococcus faecalis*]) and a few strains of staphylococci are resistant to Keftab. When tested by in vitro methods, staphylococci exhibit cross-resistance between Keftab and methicillin-type antibiotics. Keftab is not active against most strains of *Enterobacter* spp, *Morganella morganii* (formerly *Proteus morganii*), *Serratia* spp, and *Proteus vulgaris*. It has no activity against *Pseudomonas* or *Acinetobacter* spp.

Disk Susceptibility Tests—Quantitative methods that require measurement of zone diameters give the most precise estimates of antibiotic susceptibility. One such procedure[1] has been recommended for use with cephalosporin class (cephalothin) disks for testing susceptibility to cephalexin. The currently accepted zone diameter interpretation for the cephalothin disks[1] are appropriate for determining susceptibility to cephalexin. Interpretations correlate zone diameters of the disk test with MIC values for cephalexin. With this procedure, a report from the laboratory of "resistant" indicates a zone diameter of 14 mm or less and suggests that the infecting organism is not likely to respond to therapy. A report of "susceptibility" indicates a zone diameter of 18 mm or greater. A report of "intermediate susceptibility" indicates zone diameters between 15 and 17 mm and suggests that the organism would be susceptible if the infection is confined to the urine, in which high antibiotic levels can be obtained, or if high dosage is used in other types of infection. Standardized procedures require use of control organisms.[1] The 30-μg cephalothin disk should give zone diameters between 18 and 23 mm and 25 and 37 mm for the reference strains *E. coli* ATCC 25922 and *S. aureus* ATCC 25923 respectively.

[1] 21 CFR 460.1, *Federal Register* 1987; 838–842.

INDICATIONS AND USAGE

Keftab is indicated for the treatment of the following infections when caused by susceptible strains of the designated microorganisms:

Respiratory tract infections caused by *S. pneumoniae* and group A β-hemolytic streptococci (Penicillin is the usual drug of choice in the treatment and prevention of streptococcal infections, including the prophylaxis of rheumatic fever. Keftab is generally effective in the eradication of streptococci from the nasopharynx; however, substantial data establishing the efficacy of Keftab in the subsequent prevention of rheumatic fever are not available at present.)

Skin and skin structure infections caused by *S. aureus* and/or β-hemolytic streptococci.

Bone infections caused by *S. aureus* and/or *P. mirabilis*.

Genitourinary tract infections, including acute prostatitis, caused by *E. coli, P. mirabilis,* and *Klebsiella* spp.

Note—Culture and susceptibility tests should be initiated prior to and during therapy. Renal function studies should be performed when indicated.

CONTRAINDICATION

Keftab is contraindicated in patients with known allergy to the cephalosporin group of antibiotics.

WARNINGS

BEFORE CEPHALEXIN THERAPY IS INSTITUTED, CAREFUL INQUIRY SHOULD BE MADE CONCERNING PREVIOUS HYPERSENSITIVITY REACTIONS TO CEPHALOSPORINS AND PENICILLIN. CEPHALOSPORIN C DERIVATIVES SHOULD BE GIVEN CAUTIOUSLY TO PENICILLIN-SENSITIVE PATIENTS.

SERIOUS ACUTE HYPERSENSITIVITY REACTIONS MAY REQUIRE EPINEPHRINE AND OTHER EMERGENCY MEASURES.

There is some clinical and laboratory evidence of partial cross-allergenicity of the penicillins and the cephalosporins. Patients have been reported to have had severe reactions (including anaphylaxis) to both drugs.

Any patient who has demonstrated some form of allergy, particularly to drugs, should receive antibiotics cautiously. No exception should be made with regard to Keftab.

Pseudomembranous colitis has been reported with virtually all broad-spectrum antibiotics (including macrolides, semisynthetic penicillins, and cephalosporins); therefore, it is important to consider its diagnosis in patients who develop diarrhea in association with the use of antibiotics. Such colitis may range in severity from mild to life threatening.

Treatment with broad-spectrum antibiotics alters the normal flora of the colon and may permit overgrowth of clostridia. Studies indicate that a toxin produced by *Clostridium difficile* is a primary cause of antibiotic-associated colitis.

Mild cases of pseudomembranous colitis usually respond to drug discontinuance alone. In moderate to severe cases, management should include sigmoidoscopy, appropriate bacteriologic studies, and fluid, electrolyte, and protein supplementation. When the colitis does not improve after the drug has been discontinued or when it is severe, treatment with an oral antibacterial drug effective against *C. difficile* is recommended. Other causes of colitis should be ruled out.

PRECAUTIONS

General—Patients should be followed carefully so that any side effects or unusual manifestations of drug idiosyncrasy may be detected. If an allergic reaction to Keftab occurs, the drug should be discontinued and the patient treated with the usual agents (eg, epinephrine or other pressor amines, antihistamines, or corticosteroids).

Prolonged use of Keftab may result in the overgrowth of nonsusceptible organisms. Careful observation of the patient is essential. If superinfection occurs during therapy, appropriate measures should be taken.

Positive direct Coombs' tests have been reported during treatment with the cephalosporin antibiotics. In hematologic studies or in transfusion cross-matching procedures when antiglobulin tests are performed on the minor side or in Coombs' testing of newborns whose mothers have received cephalosporin antibiotics before parturition, it should be recognized that a positive Coombs' test may be due to the drug.

Keftab should be administered with caution in the presence of markedly impaired renal function. Under such conditions, careful clinical observation and laboratory studies should be made because safe dosage may be lower than that usually recommended.

As a result of administration of Keftab, a false-positive reaction for glucose in the urine may occur. This has been observed with Benedict's and Fehling's solutions and also with Clinitest® tablets but not with Tes-Tape® (Glucose Enzymatic Test Strip, USP).

Broad-spectrum antibiotics should be prescribed with caution in individuals with a history of gastrointestinal disease, particularly colitis.

Pregnancy—Pregnancy Category B—Reproduction studies have been performed on rats in doses of 250 or 500 mg/kg/day and have revealed no evidence of impaired fertility or harm to the fetus due to cephalexin. There are, however, no adequate and well-controlled studies in pregnant women. Because animal reproduction studies are not always predictive of human response, this drug should be used during pregnancy only if clearly needed.

Nursing Mothers—The excretion of cephalexin in the milk increased up to 4 hours after a 500-mg dose; the drug reached a maximum level of 4 μg/mL, then decreased gradually, and had disappeared 8 hours after administration. A decision should be considered to discontinue nursing temporarily during therapy with Keftab.

Pediatric Use—Safety and effectiveness in children have not been established.

ADVERSE REACTIONS

Gastrointestinal—Symptoms of pseudomembranous colitis may appear either during or after antibiotic treatment. Nausea and vomiting have been reported rarely. The most frequent side effect has been diarrhea. It was very rarely severe enough to warrant cessation of therapy. Abdominal pain, gastritis, and dyspepsia have also occurred. As with some penicillins and some other cephalosporins, transient hepatitis and cholestatic jaundice have been reported rarely.

Hypersensitivity—Allergic reactions in the form of rash, urticaria, angioedema, and, rarely, erythema multiforme, Stevens-Johnson syndrome, or toxic epidermal necrolysis have been observed. These reactions usually subsided upon discontinuation of the drug. In some of these reactions, supportive therapy may be necessary. Anaphylaxis has also been reported.

Other reactions have included genital and anal pruritus, genital moniliasis, vaginitis and vaginal discharge, dizziness, fatigue, headache, agitation, confusion, hallucinations, arthralgia, arthritis, and joint disorder. Reversible interstitial nephritis has been reported rarely. Eosinophilia, neutropenia, thrombocytopenia, slight elevations in aspartate aminotransferase (AST, SGOT) and alanine aminotransferase (ALT, SGPT), and elevated creatinine and BUN have been reported.

In addition to the adverse reactions listed above that have been observed in patients treated with Keftab, the following adverse reactions and altered laboratory tests have been reported for cephalosporin class antibiotics:

Adverse Reactions—Allergic reactions, including fever, colitis, renal dysfunction, toxic nephropathy, and hepatic dysfunction, including cholestasis.

Several cephalosporins have been implicated in triggering seizures, particularly in patients with renal impairment when the dosage was not reduced (*see* Indications and Usage *and* Precautions, General). If seizures associated with drug therapy should occur, the drug should be discontinued. Anticonvulsant therapy can be given if clinically indicated.

Altered Laboratory Tests—Increased prothrombin time, increased alkaline phosphatase, and leukopenia.

OVERDOSAGE

Signs and Symptoms—Symptoms of oral overdose may include nausea, vomiting, epigastric distress, diarrhea, and hematuria. If other symptoms are present, it is probably secondary to an underlying disease state, an allergic reaction, or toxicity due to ingestion of a second medication.

Treatment—To obtain up-to-date information about the treatment of overdose, a good resource is your certified Regional Poison Control Center. Telephone numbers of certified poison control centers are listed in the *Physicians' Desk Reference (PDR)*. In managing overdosage, consider the possibility of multiple drug overdoses, interaction among drugs, and unusual drug kinetics in your patient.

Unless 5 to 10 times the normal dose of cephalexin has been ingested, gastrointestinal decontamination should not be necessary.

Protect the patient's airway and support ventilation and perfusion. Meticulously monitor and maintain, within acceptable limits, the patient's vital signs, blood gases, serum electrolytes, etc. Absorption of drugs from the gastrointestinal tract may be decreased by giving activated charcoal, which, in many cases, is more effective than emesis or lavage; consider charcoal instead of or in addition to gastric emptying. Repeated doses of charcoal over time may hasten elimination of some drugs that have been absorbed. Safeguard the patient's airway when employing gastric emptying or charcoal.

Forced diuresis, peritoneal dialysis, hemodialysis, or charcoal hemoperfusion have not been established as beneficial for an overdose of cephalexin; however, it would be extremely unlikely that one of these procedures would be indicated.

The oral median lethal dose of cephalexin in rats is 5,000 mg/kg.

DOSAGE AND ADMINISTRATION

Keftab is administered orally.

The adult dosage ranges from 1 to 4 g daily in divided doses. For the following infections, a dosage of 500 mg may be administered every 12 hours: streptococcal pharyngitis, skin and skin structure infections, and uncomplicated cystitis. Cystitis therapy should be continued for 7 to 14 days. For other infections, the usual dose is 250 mg every 6 hours. For more severe infections or those caused by less susceptible organisms, larger doses may be needed. If daily doses of Keftab greater than 4 g are required, parenteral cephalosporins, in appropriate doses, should be considered.

HOW SUPPLIED

Tablets (elliptical-shaped):
500 mg* (dark-green) (No. 4143)—(100s) NDC 0777-4143-02
Store at controlled room temperature, 59° to 86°F (15° to 30°C).

---

* Equivalent to cephalexin.

[050796]

Shown in Product Identification Guide, page 322

LENTE® ILETIN® I   OTC

[*lĕn-ta ī-lĕ-tĭn*]
(Insulin Zinc Suspension, USP, beef-pork)

INFORMATION FOR THE PATIENT

WARNINGS

ANY CHANGE OF INSULIN SHOULD BE MADE CAUTIOUSLY AND ONLY UNDER MEDICAL SUPERVISION. CHANGES IN PURITY, STRENGTH, BRAND (MANUFACTURER), TYPE (REGULAR, NPH, LENTE®, ETC), SPECIES (BEEF, PORK, BEEF-PORK, HUMAN), AND/OR METHOD OF MANUFACTURE (RECOMBINANT DNA VERSUS ANIMAL-SOURCE INSULIN) MAY RESULT IN THE NEED FOR A CHANGE IN DOSAGE. IF AN ADJUSTMENT IS NEEDED, IT MAY OCCUR WITH THE FIRST DOSE OR DURING THE FIRST SEVERAL WEEKS OR MONTHS.

DIABETES

Insulin is a hormone produced by the pancreas, a large gland that lies near the stomach. This hormone is necessary for the body's correct use of food, especially sugar. Diabetes occurs when the pancreas does not make enough insulin to meet your body's needs.

To control your diabetes, your doctor has prescribed injections of insulin to keep your blood glucose at a nearly normal level. Proper control of your diabetes requires close and constant cooperation with your doctor. In spite of diabetes, you can lead an active, healthy, and useful life if you eat a balanced diet daily, exercise regularly, and take your insulin injections as prescribed.

You have been instructed to test your blood and/or your urine regularly for glucose. If your blood tests consistently show above- or below-normal glucose levels or your urine tests consistently show the presence of glucose, your diabetes is not properly controlled and you must let your doctor know. Always keep an extra supply of insulin as well as a spare syringe and needle on hand. Always wear diabetic identification so that appropriate treatment can be given if complications occur away from home.

LENTE BEEF-PORK INSULIN

Description

Lente beef-pork insulin is obtained from beef and pork pancreas.

Lente® Iletin® I (insulin, Lilly) is an amorphous and crystalline suspension of insulin with zinc providing an intermediate-acting insulin with a slower onset and a longer duration of activity (slightly more than 24 hours) than regular insulin. The time course of action of any insulin may vary considerably in different individuals or at different times in the same individual. As with all insulin preparations, the

duration of action of Lente Iletin I is dependent on dose, site of injection, blood supply, temperature, and physical activity. Lente Iletin I is a sterile suspension and is for subcutaneous injection only. It should not be used intravenously or intramuscularly. The concentration of Lente Iletin I is 100 units/mL (U-100).

Identification

This insulin, manufactured by Eli Lilly and Company, has the trademark Iletin I and is available in various types—Regular, NPH, and Lente. Your doctor has prescribed the type of insulin that he/she believes is best for you. DO NOT USE ANY OTHER INSULIN EXCEPT ON HIS/HER ADVICE AND DIRECTION.

Always check the carton and the bottle label for the name and letter designation of the insulin you receive from your pharmacy to make sure it is the same as that your doctor has prescribed.

Always examine the appearance of your bottle of insulin before withdrawing each dose. A bottle of Lente Iletin I must be carefully shaken or rotated before each injection so that the contents are uniformly mixed. Lente Iletin I should look uniformly cloudy or milky after mixing. Do not use it if the insulin substance (the white material) remains at the bottom of the bottle after mixing. Do not use a bottle of Lente Iletin I if there are clumps in the insulin after mixing. Always check the appearance of your bottle of insulin before using, and if you note anything unusual in the appearance of your insulin or notice your insulin requirements changing markedly, consult your doctor.

Storage

Insulin should be stored in a refrigerator but not in the freezer. If refrigeration is not possible, the bottle of insulin that you are currently using can be kept unrefrigerated as long as it is kept as cool as possible (below 86°F [30°C]) and away from heat and light. Do not use insulin if it has been frozen. Do not use a bottle of insulin after the expiration date stamped on the label.

INJECTION PROCEDURES

Correct Syringe

Doses of insulin are measured in **units**. U-100 insulin contains 100 units/mL (1 mL = 1 cc). With Lente Iletin I, it is important to use a syringe that is marked for U-100 insulin preparations. Failure to use the proper syringe can lead to a mistake in dosage, causing serious problems for you, such as a blood glucose level that is too low or too high.

Syringe Use

To help avoid contamination and possible infection, follow these instructions exactly.

Disposable syringes and needles should be used only once and then discarded. NEEDLES AND SYRINGES MUST NOT BE SHARED.

Reusable syringes and needles must be sterilized before each injection. **Follow the package directions supplied with your syringe.** Described below are 2 methods of sterilizing.

Boiling

1. Put syringe, plunger, and needle in strainer, place in saucepan, and cover with water. Boil for 5 minutes.
2. Remove articles from water. When they have cooled, insert plunger into barrel, and fasten needle to syringe with a slight twist.
3. Push plunger in and out several times until water is completely removed.

Isopropyl Alcohol

If the syringe, plunger, and needle cannot be boiled, as when you are traveling, they may be sterilized by immersion for at least 5 minutes in Isopropyl Alcohol, 91%. Do not use bathing, rubbing, or medicated alcohol for this sterilization. If the syringe is sterilized with alcohol, it must be absolutely dry before use.

Preparing the Dose

1. Wash your hands.
2. Carefully shake or rotate the insulin bottle several times to completely mix the insulin.
3. Inspect the insulin. Lente Iletin I should look uniformly cloudy or milky. Do not use it if you notice anything unusual in the appearance.
4. If using a new bottle, flip off the plastic protective cap, but **do not** remove the stopper. When using a new bottle, wipe the top of the bottle with an alcohol swab.
5. If you are mixing insulins, refer to the Warnings below.
6. Draw air into the syringe equal to your insulin dose. Put the needle through rubber top of the insulin bottle and inject the air into the bottle.
7. Turn the bottle and syringe upside down. Hold the bottle and syringe firmly in 1 hand and shake gently.
8. Making sure the tip of the needle is in the insulin, withdraw the correct dose of insulin into the syringe.
9. Before removing the needle from the bottle, check your syringe for air bubbles which reduce the amount of insulin in it. If bubbles are present, hold the syringe straight up and tap its side until the bubbles float to the top. Push them out with the plunger and withdraw the correct dose.
10. Remove the needle from the bottle and lay the syringe down so that the needle does not touch anything.

WARNINGS—SEE ADDITIONAL WARNINGS ABOVE

Patients who have been directed by their doctors to mix 2 types of insulin should be aware that insulin hypodermic syringes of different manufacturers may vary in the amount of space between the bottom line and the needle.

Because of this, do not change:
1. The order of mixing that the doctor has prescribed or
2. The model and brand of syringe or needle without first consulting your doctor.

The mixing should be done immediately prior to injection. Failure to heed this warning could result in a dosage error.

Injection

Cleanse the skin with alcohol where the injection is to be made. Stabilize the skin by spreading it or pinching up a large area. Insert the needle as instructed by your doctor. Push the plunger in as far as it will go. Pull the needle out and apply gentle pressure over the injection site for several seconds. Do not rub the area. To avoid tissue damage, give the next injection at a site at least $1/2''$ from the previous site.

DOSAGE

Your doctor has told you which insulin to use, how much, and when and how often to inject it. Because each patient's case of diabetes is different, this schedule has been individualized for you.

Your usual insulin dose may be affected by changes in your food, activity, or work schedule. Carefully follow your doctor's instructions to allow for these changes. Other things that may affect your insulin dose are:

Illness

Illness, especially with nausea and vomiting, may cause your insulin requirements to change. Even if you are not eating, you will still require insulin. You and your doctor should establish a sick day plan for you to use in case of illness. When you are sick, test your blood/urine frequently and call your doctor as instructed.

Pregnancy

Good control of diabetes is especially important for you and your unborn baby. Pregnancy may make managing your diabetes more difficult. If you are planning to have a baby, are pregnant, or are nursing a baby, consult your doctor.

Medication

Insulin requirements may be increased if you are taking other drugs with hyperglycemic activity, such as oral contraceptives, corticosteroids, or thyroid replacement therapy. Insulin requirements may be reduced in the presence of drugs with hypoglycemic activity, such as oral hypoglycemics, salicylates (for example, aspirin), sulfa antibiotics, and certain antidepressants. Always discuss any medications you are taking with your doctor.

Exercise

Exercise may lower your body's need for insulin during and for some time after the activity. Exercise may also speed up the effect of an insulin dose, especially if the exercise involves the area of injection site (for example, the leg should not be used for injection just prior to running). Discuss with your doctor how you should adjust your regimen to accommodate exercise.

Travel

Persons traveling across more than 2 time zones should consult their doctor concerning adjustments in their insulin schedule.

COMMON PROBLEMS OF DIABETES

Hypoglycemia (Insulin Reaction)

Hypoglycemia (too little glucose in the blood) is one of the most frequent adverse events experienced by insulin users. It can be brought about by:
1. Taking too much insulin
2. Missing or delaying meals
3. Exercising or working more than usual
4. An infection or illness (especially with diarrhea or vomiting)
5. A change in the body's need for insulin
6. Diseases of the adrenal, pituitary, or thyroid gland, or progression of kidney or liver disease
7. Interactions with other drugs that lower blood glucose, such as oral hypoglycemia, salicylates (for example, aspirin), sulfa antibiotics, and certain antidepressants
8. Consumption of alcoholic beverages

Symptoms of mild to moderate hypoglycemia may occur suddenly and can include:
- sweating
- dizziness
- palpitation
- tremor
- hunger

Continued on next page

• Identi-Code® symbol. This product information was prepared in June 1996. Current information on these and other products of Eli Lilly and Company may be obtained by direct inquiry to Lilly Research Laboratories, Lilly Corporate Center, Indianapolis, Indiana 46285, 800-545-5979.

Lilly—Cont.

- restlessness
- tingling in the hands, feet, lips, or tongue
- lightheadedness
- inability to concentrate
- headache
- drowsiness
- sleep disturbances
- anxiety
- blurred vision
- slurred speech
- depressive mood
- irritability
- abnormal behavior
- unsteady movement
- personality changes

Signs of severe hypoglycemia can include:

- disorientation
- unconsciousness
- seizures
- death

Therefore, it is important that assistance be obtained immediately.

Early warning symptoms of hypoglycemia may be different or less pronounced under certain conditions, such as long duration of diabetes, diabetic nerve disease, medications such as beta-blockers, change in insulin preparations, or intensified control (3 or more insulin injections per day) of diabetes.

Without recognition of early warning symptoms, you may not be able to take steps to avoid more serious hypoglycemia. Be alert for all of the various types of symptoms that may indicate hypoglycemia. Patients who experience hypoglycemia without early warning symptoms should monitor their blood glucose frequently, especially prior to activities such as driving. If the blood glucose is below your normal fasting glucose, you should consider eating or drinking sugar-containing foods to treat your hypoglycemia.

Mild to moderate hypoglycemia may be treated by eating foods or taking drinks that contain sugar. Patients should always carry a quick source of sugar, such as candy mints or glucose tablets. More severe hypoglycemia may require the assistance of another person. Patients who are unable to take sugar orally or who are unconscious require an injection of glucagon or should be treated with intravenous administration of glucose at a medical facility.

You should learn to recognize your own symptoms of hypoglycemia. If you are uncertain about these symptoms, you should monitor your blood glucose frequently to help you learn to recognize the symptoms that you experience with hypoglycemia.

If you have frequent episodes of hypoglycemia or experience difficulty in recognizing the symptoms, you should consult your doctor to discuss possible changes in therapy, meal plans, and/or exercise programs to help you avoid hypoglycemia.

Hyperglycemia and Diabetic Acidosis

Hyperglycemia (too much glucose in the blood) may develop if your body has too little insulin. Hyperglycemia can be brought about by:

1. Omitting your insulin or taking less than the doctor has prescribed
2. Eating significantly more than your meal plan suggests
3. Developing a fever or infection

In patients with insulin-dependent diabetes, prolonged hyperglycemia can result in diabetic acidosis. The first symptoms of diabetic acidosis usually come on gradually, over a period of hours or days, and include a drowsy feeling, flushed face, thirst, loss of appetite, and fruity odor on the breath. With acidosis, urine tests show large amounts of glucose and acetone. Heavy breathing and a rapid pulse are more severe symptoms. If uncorrected, prolonged hyperglycemia or diabetic acidosis can result in loss of consciousness or death. Therefore, it is important that you obtain medical assistance immediately.

Lipodystrophy

Rarely, administration of insulin subcutaneously can result in lipoatrophy (depression in the skin) or lipohypertrophy (enlargement or thickening of tissue). If you notice either of these conditions, consult your doctor. A change in your injection technique may help alleviate the problem.

Allergy to Insulin

Local Allergy—Patients occasionally experience redness, swelling, and itching at the site of injection of insulin. This condition, called local allergy, usually clears up in a few days to a few weeks. In some instances, this condition may be related to factors other than insulin, such as irritants in the skin cleansing agent or poor injection technique. If you have local reactions, contact your doctor.

Systemic Allergy—Less common, but potentially more serious, is generalized allergy to insulin, which may cause rash over the whole body, shortness of breath, wheezing, reduction in blood pressure, fast pulse, or sweating. Severe cases of generalized allergy may be life threatening. If you think you are having a generalized allergic reaction to insulin, notify a doctor immediately.

ADDITIONAL INFORMATION

Additional information about diabetes may be obtained from your diabetes educator.

DIABETES FORECAST is a national magazine designed especially for patients with diabetes and their families and is available by subscription from the American Diabetes Association, National Service Center, 1660 Duke Street, Alexandria, Virginia 22314.

Another publication, **DIABETES COUNTDOWN**, is available from the Juvenile Diabetes Foundation, 432 Park Avenue South, New York, New York 10016-8013.

Literature revised October 28, 1992

[102892]

NPH ILETIN® I — OTC

[ĕn'pē-āch ī'lĕ-tĭn]

(Isophane Insulin Suspension, USP, beef-pork)

INFORMATION FOR THE PATIENT

WARNINGS

ANY CHANGE OF INSULIN SHOULD BE MADE CAUTIOUSLY AND ONLY UNDER MEDICAL SUPERVISION. CHANGES IN PURITY, STRENGTH, BRAND (MANUFACTURER), TYPE (REGULAR, NPH, LENTE®, ETC), SPECIES (BEEF, PORK, BEEF-PORK, HUMAN), AND/OR METHOD OF MANUFACTURE (RECOMBINANT DNA VERSUS ANIMAL-SOURCE INSULIN) MAY RESULT IN THE NEED FOR A CHANGE IN DOSAGE. IF AN ADJUSTMENT IS NEEDED, IT MAY OCCUR WITH THE FIRST DOSE OR DURING THE FIRST SEVERAL WEEKS OR MONTHS.

DIABETES

Insulin is a hormone produced by the pancreas, a large gland that lies near the stomach. This hormone is necessary for the body's correct use of food, especially sugar. Diabetes occurs when the pancreas does not make enough insulin to meet your body's needs.

To control your diabetes, your doctor has prescribed injections of insulin to keep your blood glucose at a nearly normal level. Proper control of your diabetes requires close and constant cooperation with your doctor. In spite of diabetes, you can lead an active, healthy, and useful life if you eat a balanced diet daily, exercise regularly, and take your insulin injections as prescribed.

You have been instructed to test your blood and/or your urine regularly for glucose. If your blood tests consistently show above- or below-normal glucose levels or your urine tests consistently show the presence of glucose, your diabetes is not properly controlled and you must let your doctor know.

Always keep an extra supply of insulin as well as a spare syringe and needle on hand. Always wear diabetic identification so that appropriate treatment can be given if complications occur away from home.

NPH BEEF-PORK INSULIN

Description

NPH beef-pork insulin is obtained from beef and pork pancreas.

NPH Iletin® I (insulin, Lilly) is a crystalline suspension of insulin with protamine and zinc providing an intermediate-acting insulin with a slower onset of action and a longer duration of activity (slightly more than 24 hours) than that of regular insulin. The time course of action of any insulin may vary considerably in different individuals or at different times in the same individual. As with all insulin preparations, the duration of action of NPH Iletin I is dependent on dose, site of injection, blood supply, temperature, and physical activity. NPH Iletin I is a sterile suspension and is for subcutaneous injection only. It should not be used intravenously or intramuscularly. The concentration of NPH Iletin I is 100 units/mL (U-100).

Identification

This insulin, manufactured by Eli Lilly and Company, has the trademark Iletin I and is available in various types—Regular, NPH, and Lente. Your doctor has prescribed the type of insulin that he/she believes is best for you. **DO NOT USE ANY OTHER INSULIN EXCEPT ON HIS/HER ADVICE AND DIRECTION.**

Always check the carton and the bottle label for the name and letter designation of the insulin you receive from your pharmacy to make sure it is the same as that your doctor has prescribed.

Always examine the appearance of your bottle of insulin before withdrawing each dose. A bottle of NPH Iletin I must be carefully shaken or rotated before each injection so that the contents are uniformly mixed. NPH Iletin I should look uniformly cloudy or milky after mixing. Do not use it if the insulin substance (the white material) remains at the bottom of the bottle after mixing. Do not use a bottle of NPH Iletin I if there are clumps in the insulin after mixing. Always check the appearance of your bottle of insulin before using, and if you note anything unusual in the appearance of your insulin or notice your insulin requirements changing markedly, consult your doctor.

Storage

Insulin should be stored in a refrigerator but not in the freezer. If refrigeration is not possible, the bottle of insulin that you are currently using can be kept unrefrigerated as long as it is kept as cool as possible (below 86°F [30°C]) and away from heat and light. Do not use insulin if it has been frozen. Do not use a bottle of insulin after the expiration date stamped on the label.

INJECTION PROCEDURES

Correct Syringe

Doses of insulin are measured in **units.** U-100 insulin contains 100 units/mL (1 mL = 1 cc). With NPH Iletin I, it is important to use a syringe that is marked for U-100 insulin preparations. Failure to use the proper syringe can lead to a mistake in dosage, causing serious problems for you, such as a blood glucose level that is too low or too high.

Syringe Use

To help avoid contamination and possible infection, follow these instructions exactly.

Disposable syringes and needles should be used only once and then discarded. **NEEDLES AND SYRINGES MUST NOT BE SHARED.**

Reusable syringes and needles must be sterilized before each injection. **Follow the package directions supplied with your syringe.** Described below are 2 methods of sterilizing.

Boiling

1. Put syringe, plunger, and needle in strainer, place in saucepan, and cover with water. Boil for 5 minutes.
2. Remove articles from water. When they have cooled, insert plunger into barrel, and fasten needle to syringe with a slight twist.
3. Push plunger in and out several times until water is completely removed.

Isopropyl Alcohol

If the syringe, plunger, and needle cannot be boiled, as when you are traveling, they may be sterilized by immersion for at least 5 minutes in Isopropyl Alcohol, 91%. Do not use bathing, rubbing, or medicated alcohol for this sterilization. If the syringe is sterilized with alcohol, it must be absolutely dry before use.

Preparing the Dose

1. Wash your hands.
2. Carefully shake or rotate the insulin bottle several times to completely mix the insulin.
3. Inspect the insulin. NPH Iletin I should look uniformly cloudy or milky. Do not use it if you notice anything unusual in the appearance.
4. If using a new bottle, flip off the plastic protective cap, but **do not** remove the stopper. When using a new bottle, wipe the top of the bottle with an alcohol swab.
5. If you are mixing insulins, refer to the Warnings below.
6. Draw air into the syringe equal to your insulin dose. Put the needle through rubber top of the insulin bottle and inject the air into the bottle.
7. Turn the bottle and syringe upside down. Hold the bottle and syringe firmly in 1 hand and shake gently.
8. Making sure the tip of the needle is in the insulin, withdraw the correct dose of insulin into the syringe.
9. Before removing the needle from the bottle, check your syringe for air bubbles which reduce the amount of insulin in it. If bubbles are present, hold the syringe straight up and tap its side until the bubbles float to the top. Push them out with the plunger and withdraw the correct dose.
10. Remove the needle from the bottle and lay the syringe down so that the needle does not touch anything.

WARNINGS—SEE ADDITIONAL WARNINGS ABOVE

Patients who have been directed by their doctors to mix 2 types of insulin should be aware that insulin hypodermic syringes of different manufacturers may vary in the amount of space between the bottom line and the needle.

Because of this, do not change:

1. The order of mixing that the doctor has prescribed or
2. The model and brand of syringe or needle without first consulting your doctor.

The mixing should be done immediately prior to injection. Failure to heed this warning could result in a dosage error.

Injection

Cleanse the skin with alcohol where the injection is to be made. Stabilize the skin by spreading it or pinching up a large area. Insert the needle as instructed by your doctor. Push the plunger in as far as it will go. Pull the needle out and apply gentle pressure over the injection site for several seconds. **Do not rub the area.** To avoid tissue damage, give the next injection at a site at least ½" from the previous site.

DOSAGE

Your doctor has told you which insulin to use, how much, and when and how often to inject it. Because each patient's

case of diabetes is different, this schedule has been individualized for you.

Your usual insulin dose may be affected by changes in your food, activity, or work schedule. Carefully follow your doctor's instructions to allow for these changes. Other things that may affect your insulin dose are:

Illness

Illness, especially with nausea and vomiting, may cause your insulin requirements to change. Even if you are not eating, you will still require insulin. You and your doctor should establish a sick day plan for you to use in case of illness. When you are sick, test your blood/urine frequently and call your doctor as instructed.

Pregnancy

Good control of diabetes is especially important for you and your unborn baby. Pregnancy may make managing your diabetes more difficult. If you are planning to have a baby, are pregnant, or are nursing a baby, consult your doctor.

Medication

Insulin requirements may be increased if you are taking other drugs with hyperglycemic activity, such as oral contraceptives, corticosteriods, or thyroid replacement therapy. Insulin requirements may be reduced in the presence of drugs with hypoglycemic activity, such as oral hypoglycemics, salicylates (for example, aspirin), sulfa antibiotics, and certain antidepressants. Always discuss any medications you are taking with your doctor.

Exercise

Exercise may lower your body's need for insulin during and for some time after the activity. Exercise may also speed up the effect of an insulin dose, especially if the exercise involves the area of injection site (for example, the leg should not be used for injection just prior to running). Discuss with your doctor how you should adjust your regimen to accommodate exercise.

Travel

Persons traveling across more than 2 times zones should consult their doctor concerning adjustments is their insulin schedule.

COMMON PROBLEMS OF DIABETES

Hypoglycemia (Insulin Reaction)

Hypoglycemia (too little glucose in the blood) is one of the most frequent adverse events experienced by insulin users. It can be brought about by:

1. Taking too much insulin
2. Missing or delaying meals
3. Exercising or working more than usual
4. An infection or illness (especially with diarrhea or vomiting)
5. A change in the body's need for insulin
6. Diseases of the adrenal, pituitary, or thyroid gland, or progression of kidney of liver disease
7. Interactions with other drugs that lower blood glucose, such as oral hypoglycemics, salicylates (for example, aspirin), sulfa antibiotics, and certain antidepressants
8. Consumption of alcoholic beverages

Symptoms of mild to moderate hypoglycemia may occur suddenly and can include:

- sweating
- dizziness
- palpitation
- tremor
- hunger
- restlessness
- tingling in the hands, feet, lips, or tongue
- lightheadedness
- inability to concentrate
- headache
- drowsiness
- sleep disturbances
- anxiety
- blurred vision
- slurred speech
- depressive mood
- irritability
- abnormal behavior
- unsteady movement
- personality changes

Signs of severe hypoglycemia can include:

- disorientation
- unconsciousness
- seizures
- death

Therefore, it is important that assistance be obtained immediately.

Early warning symptoms of hypoglycemia may be different or less pronounced under certain conditions, such as long duration of diabetes, diabetic nerve disease, medications such as beta-blockers, change in insulin preparations, or intensified control (3 or more insulin injections per day) of diabetes.

Without recognition of early warning symptoms, you may not be able to take steps to avoid more serious hypoglycemia. Be alert for all of the various types of symptoms that may indicate hypoglycemia. Patients who experience hypoglycemia without early warning symptoms should monitor their blood glucose frequently, especially prior to activities such as driving. If the blood glucose is below your normal fasting glucose, you should consider eating or drinking sugar-containing foods to treat your hypoglycemia.

Mild to moderate hypoglycemia may be treated by eating foods or taking drinks that contain sugar. Patients should always carry a quick source of sugar, such as candy mints or glucose tablets. More severe hypoglycemia may require assistance of another person. Patients who are unable to take sugar orally or who are unconscious require an injection of glucagon or should be treated with intravenous administration of glucose at a medical facility.

You should learn to recognize your own symptoms of hypoglycemia. If you are uncertain about these symptoms, you should monitor your blood glucose frequently to help you learn to recognize the symptoms that you experience with hypoglycemia.

If you have frequent episodes of hypoglycemia or experience difficulty in recognizing the symptoms, you should consult your doctor to discuss possible changes in therapy, meal plans, and/or exercise programs to help you avoid hypoglycemia.

Hyperglycemia and Diabetic Acidosis

Hyperglycemia (too much glucose in the blood) may develop if your body has too little insulin. Hyperglycemia can be brought about by:

1. Omitting your insulin or taking less than the doctor has prescribed
2. Eating significantly more than your meal plan suggests
3. Developing a fever or infection

In patients with insulin-dependent diabetes, prolonged hyperglycemia can result in diabetic acidosis. The first symptoms of diabetic acidosis usually come on gradually, over a period of hours or days, and include a drowsy feeling, flushed face, thirst, loss of appetite, and fruity odor on the breath. With acidosis, urine tests show large amounts of glucose and acetone. Heavy breathing and a rapid pulse are more severe symptoms. If uncorrected, prolonged hyperglycemia or diabetic acidosis can result in loss of consciousness or death. Therefore, it is important that you obtain medical assistance immediately.

Lipodystrophy

Rarely, administration of insulin subcutaneously can result in lipoatrophy (depression in the skin) or lipohypertrophy (enlargement or thickening of tissue). If you notice either of these conditions, consult your doctor. A change in your injection technique may help alleviate the problem.

Allergy to Insulin

Local Allergy—Patients occasionally experience redness, swelling, and itching at the site of injection of insulin. This condition, called local allergy, usually clears up in a few days to a few weeks. In some instances, this condition may be related to factors other than insulin, such as irritants in the skin cleansing agent or poor injection technique. If you have local reactions, contact your doctor.

Systemic Allergy—Less common, but potentially more serious, is generalized allergy to insulin, which may cause rash over the whole body, shortness of breath, wheezing, reduction in blood pressure, fast pulse, or sweating. Severe cases of generalized allergy may be life threatening. If you think you are having a generalized allergic reaction to insulin, notify a doctor immediately.

ADDITIONAL INFORMATION

Additional information about diabetes may be obtained from your diabetes educator.

DIABETES FORECAST is a national magazine designed especially for patients with diabetes and their families and is available by subscription from the American Diabetes Association, National Service Center, 1660 Duke Street, Alexandria, Virginia 22314.

Another publication, **DIABETES COUNTDOWN**, is available from the Juvenile Diabetes Foundation, 432 Park Avenue South, New York, New York 10016-8013.

Literature revised October 28, 1992

[102892]

ILETIN® (INSULIN)— OTC

[*ī'lĕ-tĭn*]

REGULAR AND MODIFIED INSULIN PRODUCTS

REGULAR ILETIN® I OTC

[*rĕg'ū-lĕr ī'lĕ-tĭn*]

(Insulin Injection, USP, beef-pork)

INFORMATION FOR THE PATIENT

WARNINGS

ANY CHANGE OF INSULIN SHOULD BE MADE CAUTIOUSLY AND ONLY UNDER MEDICAL SUPERVISION. CHANGES IN PURITY, STRENGTH, BRAND (MANUFACTURER), TYPE (REGULAR, NPH, LENTE®, ETC), SPECIES (BEEF, PORK, BEEF-PORK, HUMAN), AND/OR METHOD OF MANUFACTURE (RECOMBINANT DNA VERSUS ANIMAL-SOURCE INSULIN) MAY RESULT IN THE NEED FOR A CHANGE IN DOSAGE. IF AN ADJUSTMENT IS NEEDED, IT MAY OCCUR WITH THE FIRST DOSE OR DURING THE FIRST SEVERAL WEEKS OR MONTHS.

DIABETES

Insulin is a hormone produced by the pancreas, a large gland that lies near the stomach. This hormone is necessary for the body's correct use of food, especially sugar. Diabetes occurs when the pancreas does not make enough insulin to meet your body's needs.

To control your diabetes, your doctor has prescribed injections of insulin to keep your blood glucose at a nearly normal level. Proper control of your diabetes requires close and constant cooperation with your doctor. In spite of diabetes, you can lead an active, healthy, and useful life if you eat a balanced diet daily, exercise regularly, and take your insulin injections as prescribed.

You have been instructed to test your blood and/or your urine regularly for glucose. If your blood tests consistently show above- or below-normal glucose levels or your urine tests consistently show the presence of glucose, your diabetes is not properly controlled and you must let your doctor know. Always keep an extra supply of insulin as well as a spare syringe and needle on hand. Always wear diabetic identification so that appropriate treatment can be given if complications occur away from home.

REGULAR BEEF-PORK INSULIN

Description

Regular beef-pork insulin is obtained from beef and pork pancreas.

Regular Iletin® I (insulin, Lilly) consists of zinc-insulin crystals dissolved in a clear fluid. Regular Iletin I has had nothing added to change the speed or length of its action. It takes effect rapidly and has a relatively short duration of activity (4 to 12 hours) as compared with other insulins. The time course of action of any insulin may vary considerably in different individuals or at different times in the same individual. As with all insulin preparations, the duration of action of Regular Iletin I is dependent on dose, site of injection, blood supply, temperature, and physical activity. Regular Iletin I is a sterile solution and is for subcutaneous injection. It should not be used intramuscularly. The concentration of Regular Iletin I is 100 units/mL (U-100).

Identification

This insulin, manufactured by Eli Lilly and Company, has the trademark Iletin I and is available in various types—Regular, NPH, and Lente. Your doctor has prescribed the type of insulin that he/she believes is best for you. **DO NOT USE ANY OTHER INSULIN EXCEPT ON HIS/HER ADVICE AND DIRECTION.**

Always check the carton and the bottle label for the name and letter designation of the insulin you receive from your pharmacy to make sure it is the same as that your doctor has prescribed.

Always examine the appearance of your bottle of insulin before withdrawing each dose. Regular Iletin I is a clear and colorless liquid with a water-like appearance and consistency. Do not use if it appears cloudy, thickened, or slightly colored or if solid particles are visible. Always check the appearance of your bottle of insulin before using, and if you note anything unusual in the appearance of your insulin or notice your insulin requirements changing markedly, consult your doctor.

Storage

Insulin should be stored in a refrigerator but not in the freezer. If refrigeration is not possible, the bottle of insulin that you are currently using can be kept unrefrigerated as long as it is kept as cool as possible (below 86°F [30°C]) and away from heat and light. Do not use insulin if it has been frozen. Do not use a bottle of insulin after the expiration date stamped on the label.

INJECTION PROCEDURES

Correct Syringe

Doses of insulin are measured in **units**. U-100 insulin contains 100 units/mL (1 mL = 1 cc). With Regular Iletin I, it is important to use a syringe that is marked for U-100 insulin preparations. Failure to use the proper syringe can lead to a mistake in dosage, causing serious problems for you, such as a blood glucose level that is too low or too high.

Syringe Use

To help avoid contamination and possible infection, follow these instructions exactly.

Continued on next page

*** Identi-Code® symbol. This product information was prepared in June 1996. Current information on these and other products of Eli Lilly and Company may be obtained by direct inquiry to Lilly Research Laboratories, Lilly Corporate Center, Indianapolis, Indiana 46285, 800-545-5979.**

Lilly—Cont.

Disposable syringes and needles should be used only once and then discarded. **NEEDLES AND SYRINGES MUST NOT BE SHARED.**

Reusable syringes and needles must be sterilized before each injection. **Follow the package directions supplied with your syringe.** Described below are 2 methods of sterilizing.

Boiling

1. Put syringe, plunger, and needle in strainer, place in saucepan, and cover with water. Boil for 5 minutes.
2. Remove articles from water. When they have cooled, insert plunger into barrel, and fasten needle to syringe with a slight twist.
3. Push plunger in and out several times until water is completely removed.

Isopropyl Alcohol

If the syringe, plunger, and needle cannot be boiled, as when you are traveling, they may be sterilized by immersion for at least 5 minutes in Isopropyl Alcohol, 91%. Do not use bathing, rubbing, or medicated alcohol for this sterilization. If the syringe is sterilized with alcohol, it must be absolutely dry before use.

Preparing the Dose

1. Wash your hands.
2. Inspect the insulin. Regular Iletin I should look clear and colorless. Do not use Regular Iletin I if it appears cloudy, thickened, or slightly colored or if solid particles are visible.
3. If using a new bottle, flip off the plastic protective cap, but **do not** remove the stopper. When using a new bottle, wipe the top of the bottle with an alcohol swab.
4. If you are mixing insulins, refer to the Warnings below.
5. Draw air into the syringe equal to your insulin dose. Put the needle through rubber top of the insulin bottle and inject the air into the bottle.
6. Turn the bottle and syringe upside down. Hold the bottle and syringe firmly in 1 hand.
7. Making sure the tip of the needle is in the insulin, withdraw the correct dose of insulin into the syringe.
8. Before removing the needle from the bottle, check your syringe for air bubbles which reduce the amount of insulin in it. If bubbles are present, hold the syringe straight up and tap its side until the bubbles float to the top. Push them out with the plunger and withdraw the correct dose.
9. Remove the needle from the bottle and lay the syringe down so that the needle does not touch anything.

WARNINGS—SEE ADDITIONAL WARNINGS ABOVE

Patients who have been directed by their doctors to mix 2 types of insulin should be aware that insulin hypodermic syringes of different manufacturers may vary in the amount of space between the bottom line and the needle.

Because of this, do not change:

1. The order of mixing that the doctor has prescribed or
2. The model and brand of syringe or needle without first consulting your doctor.

The mixing should be done immediately prior to injection. Failure to heed this warning could result in a dosage error.

Injection

Cleanse the skin with alcohol where the injection is to be made. Stabilize the skin by spreading it or pinching up a large area. Insert the needle as instructed by your doctor. Push the plunger in as far as it will go. Pull the needle out and apply gentle pressure over the injection site for several seconds. **Do not rub the area.** To avoid tissue damage, give the next injection at a site at least $^1/_2$" from the previous site.

DOSAGE

Your doctor has told you which insulin to use, how much, and when and how often to inject it. Because each patient's case of diabetes is different, this schedule has been individualized for you.

Your usual insulin dose may be affected by changes in your food, activity, or work schedule. Carefully follow your doctor's instructions to allow for these changes. Other things that may affect your insulin dose are:

Illness

Illness, especially with nausea and vomiting, may cause your insulin requirements to change. Even if you are not eating, you will still require insulin. You and your doctor should establish a sick day plan for you to use in case of illness. When you are sick, test your blood/urine frequently and call your doctor as instructed.

Pregnancy

Good control of diabetes is especially important for you and your unborn baby. Pregnancy may make managing your diabetes more difficult. If you are planning to have a baby, are pregnant, or are nursing a baby, consult your doctor.

Medication

Insulin requirements may be increased if you are taking other drugs with hyperglycemic activity, such as oral contraceptives, corticosteroids, or thyroid replacement therapy. Insulin requirements may be reduced in the presence of drugs with hypoglycemic activity, such as oral hypoglyce-mics, salicylates (for example, aspirin), sulfa antibiotics, and certain antidepressants. Always discuss any medications you are taking with your doctor.

Exercise

Exercise may lower your body's need for insulin during and for some time after the activity. Exercise may also speed up the effect of an insulin dose, especially if the exercise involves the area of injection site (for example, the leg should not be used for injection just prior to running). Discuss with your doctor how you should adjust your regimen to accommodate exercise.

Travel

Persons traveling across more than 2 time zones should consult their doctor concerning adjustments in their insulin schedule.

COMMON PROBLEMS OF DIABETES

Hypoglycemia (Insulin Reaction)

Hypoglycemia (too little glucose in the blood) is one of the most frequent adverse events experienced by insulin users. It can be brought about by:

1. Taking too much insulin
2. Missing or delaying meals
3. Exercising or working more than usual
4. An infection or illness (especially with diarrhea or vomiting)
5. A change in the body's need for insulin
6. Diseases of the adrenal, pituitary, or thyroid gland, or progression of kidney or liver disease
7. Interactions with other drugs that lower blood glucose, such as oral hypoglycemics, salicylates (for example, aspirin), sulfa antibiotics, and certain antidepressants
8. Consumption of alcoholic beverages

Symptoms of mild to moderate hypoglycemia may occur suddenly and can include:

- sweating
- dizziness
- palpitation
- tremor
- hunger
- restlessness
- tingling in the hands, feet, lips, or tongue
- lightheadedness
- inability to concentrate
- headache
- drowsiness
- sleep disturbances
- anxiety
- blurred vision
- slurred speech
- depressive mood
- irritability
- abnormal behavior
- unsteady movement
- personality changes

Signs of severe hypoglycemia can include:

- disorientation
- unconsciousness
- seizures
- death

Therefore, it is important that assistance be obtained immediately.

Early warning symptoms of hypoglycemia may be different or less pronounced under certain conditions, such as long duration of diabetes, diabetic nerve disease, medications such as beta-blockers, change in insulin preparations, or intensified control (3 or more insulin injections per day) of diabetes.

Without recognition of early warning symptoms, you may not be able to take steps to avoid more serious hypoglycemia. Be alert for all of the various types of symptoms that may indicate hypoglycemia. Patients who experience hypoglycemia without early warning symptoms should monitor their blood glucose frequently, especially prior to activities such as driving. If the blood glucose is below your normal fasting glucose, you should consider eating or drinking sugar-containing foods to treat your hypoglycemia.

Mild to moderate hypoglycemia may be treated by taking foods or drinks that contain sugar. Patients should always carry a quick source of sugar, such as candy mints or glucose tablets. More severe hypoglycemia may require the assistance of another person. Patients who are unable to take sugar orally or who are unconscious require an injection of glucagon or should be treated with intravenous administration of glucose at a medical facility.

You should learn to recognize your own symptoms of hypoglycemia. If you are uncertain about these symptoms, you should monitor your blood glucose frequently to help you learn to recognize the symptoms that you experience with hypoglycemia.

If you have frequent episodes of hypoglycemia or experience difficulty in recognizing the symptoms, you should consult your doctor to discuss possible changes in therapy, meal plans, and/or exercise programs to help you avoid hypoglycemia.

Hyperglycemia and Diabetic Acidosis

Hyperglycemia (too much glucose in the blood) may develop if your body has too little insulin. Hyperglycemia can be brought about by:

1. Omitting your insulin or taking less than the doctor has prescribed
2. Eating significantly more than your meal plan suggests
3. Developing a fever or infection

In patients with insulin-dependent diabetes, prolonged hyperglycemia can result in diabetic acidosis. The first symptoms of diabetic acidosis usually come on gradually, over a period of hours or days, and include a drowsy feeling, flushed face, thirst, loss of appetite, and fruity odor on the breath. With acidosis, urine tests show large amounts of glucose and acetone. Heavy breathing and a rapid pulse are more severe symptoms. If uncorrected, prolonged hyperglycemia or diabetic acidosis can result in loss of consciousness or death. Therefore, it is important that you obtain medical assistance immediately.

Lipodystrophy

Rarely, administration of insulin subcutaneously can result in lipoatrophy (depression in the skin) or lipohypertrophy (enlargement or thickening of tissue). If you notice either of these conditions, consult your doctor. A change in your injection technique may help alleviate the problem.

Allergy to Insulin

Local Allergy—Patients occasionally experience redness, swelling, and itching at the site of injection of insulin. This condition, called local allergy, usually clears up in a few days to a few weeks. In some instances, this condition may be related to factors other than insulin, such as irritants in the skin cleansing agent or poor injection technique. If you have local reactions, contact your doctor.

Systemic Allergy—Less common, but potentially more serious, is generalized allergy to insulin, which may cause rash over the whole body, shortness of breath, wheezing, reduction in blood pressure, fast pulse, or sweating. Severe cases of generalized allergy may be life threatening. If you think you are having a generalized allergic reaction to insulin, notify a doctor immediately.

ADDITIONAL INFORMATION

Additional information about diabetes may be obtained from your diabetes educator.

DIABETES FORECAST is a national magazine designed especially for patients with diabetes and their families and is available by subscription from the American Diabetes Association, National Service Center, 1660 Duke Street, Alexandria, Virginia 22314.

Another publication, **DIABETES COUNTDOWN,** is available from the Juvenile Diabetes Foundation, 432 Park Avenue South, New York, New York 10016-8013.

[102892]

LENTE® ILETIN® II (PORK)   OTC
[lĕn-tā ī'lĕ-tĭn]
(Insulin Zinc Suspension, USP, purified pork)

INFORMATION FOR THE PATIENT

WARNINGS

ANY CHANGE OF INSULIN SHOULD BE MADE CAUTIOUSLY AND ONLY UNDER MEDICAL SUPERVISION. CHANGES IN PURITY, STRENGTH, BRAND (MANUFACTURER), TYPE (REGULAR, NPH, LENTE®), SPECIES (BEEF, PORK, BEEF-PORK, HUMAN), AND/OR METHOD OF MANUFACTURE (RECOMBINANT DNA VERSUS ANIMAL-SOURCE INSULIN) MAY RESULT IN THE NEED FOR A CHANGE IN DOSAGE. IF AN ADJUSTMENT IS NEEDED, IT MAY OCCUR WITH THE FIRST DOSE OR DURING THE FIRST SEVERAL WEEKS OR MONTHS.

DIABETES

Insulin is a hormone produced by the pancreas, a large gland that lies near the stomach. This hormone is necessary for the body's correct use of food, especially sugar. Diabetes occurs when the pancreas does not make enough insulin to meet your body's needs.

To control your diabetes, your doctor has prescribed injections of insulin to keep your blood glucose at a nearly normal level. Proper control of your diabetes requires close and constant cooperation with your doctor. In spite of diabetes, you can lead an active, healthy, and useful life if you eat a balanced diet daily, exercise regularly, and take your insulin injections as prescribed.

You have been instructed to test your blood and/or your urine regularly for glucose. If your blood tests consistently show above- or below-normal glucose levels or your urine tests consistently show the presence of glucose, your diabetes is not properly controlled and you must let your doctor know. Always keep an extra supply of insulin as well as a spare syringe and needle on hand. Always wear diabetic identification so that appropriate treatment can be given if complications occur away from home.

LENTE PORK INSULIN

Description

Lente pork insulin is obtained from pork pancreas.

Lente® Iletin® II (purified insulin, Lilly) is an amorphous and crystalline suspension of a human insulin with zinc providing an intermediate-acting insulin with a slower onset and a longer duration of activity (slightly more than 24 hours) than regular insulin. The time course of action of any insulin may vary considerably in different individuals or at different times in the same individual. As with all insulin preparations, the duration of action of Lente Iletin II is dependent on dose, site of injection, blood supply, temperature, and physical activity. Lente Iletin II is a sterile suspension and is for subcutaneous injection only. It should not be used intravenously or intramuscularly. The concentration of Lente Iletin II is 100 units/mL (U-100).

Identification

This insulin, manufactured by Eli Lilly and Company, has the trademark Iletin II and is available in various types—Regular, NPH, and Lente. Your doctor has prescribed the type of insulin that he/she believes is best for you. **DO NOT USE ANY OTHER INSULIN EXCEPT ON HIS/HER ADVICE AND DIRECTION.**

Always check the carton and the bottle label for the name and letter designation of the insulin you receive from your pharmacy to make sure it is the same as that your doctor has prescribed.

Always examine the appearance of your bottle of insulin before withdrawing each dose. A bottle of Lente Iletin II must be carefully shaken or rotated before each injection so that the contents are uniformly mixed. Lente Iletin II should look uniformly cloudy or milky after mixing. Do not use it if the insulin substance (the white material) remains at the bottom of the bottle after mixing. Do not use a bottle of Lente Iletin II if there are clumps in the insulin after mixing. Always check the appearance of your bottle of insulin before using, and if you note anything unusual in the appearance of your insulin or notice your insulin requirements changing markedly, consult your doctor.

Storage

Insulin should be stored in a refrigerator but not in the freezer. If refrigeration is not possible, the bottle of insulin that you are currently using can be kept unrefrigerated as long as it is kept as cool as possible (below 86°F [30°C]) and away from heat and light. Do not use insulin if it has been frozen. Do not use a bottle of insulin after the expiration date stamped on the label.

INJECTION PROCEDURES

Correct Syringe

Doses of insulin are measured in **units.** U-100 insulin contains 100 units/mL (1 mL = 1 cc). With Lente Iletin II, it is important to use a syringe that is marked for U-100 insulin preparations. Failure to use the proper syringe can lead to a mistake in dosage, causing serious problems for you, such as a blood glucose level that is too low or too high.

Syringe Use

To help avoid contamination and possible infection, follow these instructions exactly.

Disposable syringes and needles should be used only once and then discarded. **NEEDLES AND SYRINGES MUST NOT BE SHARED.**

Reusable syringes and needles must be sterilized before each injection.

Follow the package directions supplied with your syringe.

Described below are 2 methods of sterilizing.

Boiling

1. Put syringe, plunger, and needle in strainer, place in saucepan, and cover with water. Boil for 5 minutes.
2. Remove articles from water. When they have cooled, insert plunger into barrel, and fasten needle to syringe with a slight twist.
3. Push plunger in and out several times until water is completely removed.

Isopropyl Alcohol

If the syringe, plunger, and needle cannot be boiled, as when you are traveling, they may be sterilized by immersion for at least 5 minutes in Isopropyl Alcohol, 91%. Do not use bathing, rubbing, or medicated alcohol for this sterilization. If the syringe is sterilized with alcohol, it must be absolutely dry before use.

Preparing the Dose

1. Wash your hands.
2. Carefully shake or rotate the insulin bottle several times to completely mix the insulin.
3. Inspect the insulin. Lente Iletin II should look uniformly cloudy or milky. Do not use it if you notice anything unusual in the appearance.
4. If using a new bottle, flip off the plastic protective cap, but **do not** remove the stopper. When using a new bottle, wipe the top of the bottle with an alcohol swab.
5. If you are mixing insulins, refer to the Warnings below.
6. Draw air into the syringe equal to your insulin dose. Put the needle through rubber top of the insulin bottle and inject the air into the bottle.
7. Turn the bottle and syringe upside down. Hold the bottle and syringe firmly in 1 hand and shake gently.
8. Making sure the tip of the needle is in the insulin, withdraw the correct dose of insulin into the syringe.
9. Before removing the needle from the bottle, check your syringe for air bubbles which reduce the amount of insulin in it. If bubbles are present, hold the syringe straight up and tap its side until the bubbles float to the top. Push them out with the plunger and withdraw the correct dose.
10. Remove the needle from the bottle and lay the syringe down so that the needle does not touch anything.

WARNINGS—SEE ADDITIONAL WARNINGS ABOVE

Patients who have been directed by their doctors to mix 2 types of insulin should be aware that insulin hypodermic syringes of different manufacturers may vary in the amount of space between the bottom line and the needle.

Because of this, do not change:

1. The order of mixing that the doctor has prescribed or
2. The model and brand of syringe or needle without first consulting your doctor.

The mixing should be done immediately prior to injection. Failure to heed this warning could result in a dosage error.

Injection

Cleanse the skin with alcohol where the injection is to be made. Stabilize the skin by spreading it or pinching up a large area. Insert the needle as instructed by your doctor. Push the plunger in as far as it will go. Pull the needle out and apply gentle pressure over the injection site for several seconds. **Do not rub the area.** To avoid tissue damage, give the next injection at a side at least 1/2" from the previous site.

DOSAGE

Your doctor has told you which insulin to use, how much, and when and how often to inject it. Because each patient's case of diabetes is different, this schedule has been individualized for you.

Your usual insulin dose may be affected by changes in your food, activity, or work schedule. Carefully follow your doctor's instructions to allow for these changes. Other things that may affect your insulin dose are:

Illness

Illness, especially with nausea and vomiting, may cause your insulin requirements to change. Even if you are not eating, your will still require insulin. You and your doctor should establish a sick day plan for you to use in case of illness. When you are sick, test your blood/urine frequently and call your doctor as instructed.

Pregnancy

Good control of diabetes is especially important for you and your unborn baby. Pregnancy may make managing your diabetes more difficult. If you are planning to have a baby, are pregnant, or are nursing a baby, consult your doctor.

Medication

Insulin requirements may be increased if you are taking other drugs with hyperglycemic activity, such as oral contraceptives, corticosteroids, or thyroid replacement therapy. Insulin requirements may be reduced in the presence of drugs with hypoglycemic activity, such as oral hypoglycemics, salicylates (for example, aspirin), sulfa antibiotics, and certain antidepressants. Always discuss any medications you are taking with your doctor.

Exercise

Exercise may lower your body's need for insulin during and for some time after the activity. Exercise may also speed up the effect of an insulin dose, especially if the exercise involves the area of injection site (for example, the leg should not be used for injection just prior to running). Discuss with your doctor how you should adjust your regimen to accommodate exercise.

Travel

Persons traveling across more than 2 time zones should consult their doctor concerning adjustments in their insulin schedule.

COMMON PROBLEMS OF DIABETES

Hypoglycemia (Insulin Reaction)

Hypoglycemia (too little glucose in the blood) is one of the most frequent adverse events experienced by insulin users. It can be brought about by:

1. Taking too much insulin
2. Missing or delaying meals
3. Exercising or working more than usual
4. An infection or illness (especially with diarrhea or vomiting)
5. A change in the body's need for insulin
6. Diseases of the adrenal, pituitary, or thyroid gland, or progression of kidney or liver disease
7. Interactions with other drugs that lower blood glucose, such as oral hypoglycemics, salicylates (for example, aspirin), sulfa antibiotics, and certain antidepressants
8. Consumption of alcoholic beverages

Symptoms of mild to moderate hypoglycemia may occur suddenly and can include:

- sweating
- dizziness
- palpitation
- tremor
- hunger
- restlessness
- tingling in the hands, feet, lips, or tongue
- lightheadedness
- inability to concentrate
- headache
- drowsiness
- sleep disturbances
- anxiety
- blurred vision
- slurred speech
- depressive mood
- irritability
- abnormal behavior
- unsteady movement
- personality changes

Signs of severe hypoglycemia can include:

- disorientation
- unconsciousness
- seizures
- death

Therefore, it is important that assistance be obtained immediately.

Early warning symptoms of hypoglycemia may be different or less pronounced under certain conditions, such as long duration of diabetes, diabetic nerve disease, medications such as beta-blockers, change in insulin preparations, or intensified control (3 or more insulin injections per day) of diabetes.

Without recognition of early warning symptoms, you may not be able to take steps to avoid more serious hypoglycemia. Be alert for all of the various types of symptoms that may indicate hypoglycemia. Patients who experience hypoglycemia without early warning symptoms should monitor their blood glucose frequently, especially prior to activities such as driving. If the blood glucose is below your normal fasting glucose, you should consider eating or drinking sugar-containing foods to treat your hypoglycemia.

Mild to moderate hypoglycemia may be treated by eating foods or taking drinks that contain sugar. Patients should always carry a quick source of sugar, such as candy mints or glucose tablets. More severe hypoglycemia may require the assistance of another person. Patients who are unable to take sugar orally or who are unconscious require an injection of glucagon or should be treated with intravenous administration of glucose at a medical facility.

You should learn to recognize your own symptoms of hypoglycemia. If you are uncertain about these symptoms, you should monitor your blood glucose frequently to help you learn to recognize the symptoms that you experience with hypoglycemia.

If you have frequent episodes of hypoglycemia or experience difficulty in recognizing the symptoms, you should consult your doctor to discuss possible changes in therapy, meal plans, and/or exercise progams to help you avoid hypoglycemia.

Hyperglycemia and Diabetic Acidosis

Hyperglycemia (too little glucose in the blood) may develop if your body has too little insulin. Hyperglycemia can be brought about by:

1. Omitting your insulin or taking less than the doctor has prescribed
2. Eating significantly more than your meal plan suggests
3. Developing a fever or infection

In patients with insulin-dependent diabetes, prolonged hyperglycemia can result in diabetic acidosis. The first symptoms of diabetic acidosis usually come on gradually, over a period of hours or days, and include a drowsy feeling, flushed face, thirst, loss of appetite, and fruity odor on the breath. With acidosis, urine tests show large amounts of glucose and acetone. Heavy breathing and a rapid pulse are more severe symptoms. If uncorrected, prolonged hyperglycemia or diabetic acidosis can result in loss of consciousness or death. Therefore, it is important that you obtain medical assistance immediately.

Lipodystrophy

Rarely, administration of insulin subcutaneously can result in lipoatrophy (depression in the skin) or lipohypertrophy (enlargement or thickening of tissue). If you notice either of these conditions, consult your doctor. A change in your injection technique may help alleviate the problem.

Continued on next page

• Identi-Code® symbol. This product information was prepared in June 1996. Current information on these and other products of Eli Lilly and Company may be obtained by direct inquiry to Lilly Research Laboratories, Lilly Corporate Center, Indianapolis, Indiana 46285, 800-545-5979.

Lilly—Cont.

Allergy to Insulin

Local Allergy—Patients occasionally experience redness, swelling, and itching at the site of injection of insulin. This condition, called local allergy, usually clears up in a few days to a few weeks. In some instances, this condition may be related to factors other than insulin, such as irritants in the skin cleansing agent or poor injection technique. If you have local reactions, contact your doctor.

Systemic Allergy—Less common, but potentially more serious, is generalized allergy to insulin, which may cause rash over the whole body, shortness of breath, wheezing, reduction in blood pressure, fast pulse, or sweating. Severe cases of generalized allergy may be life threatening. If you think you are having a generalized allergic reaction to insulin, notify a doctor immediately.

ADDITIONAL INFORMATION

Additional information about diabetes may be obtained from your diabetes educator.

DIABETES FORECAST is a national magazine designed especially for patients with diabetes and their families and is available by subscription from the American Diabetes Association, National Service Center, 1660 Duke Street, Alexandria, Virginia 22314.

Another publication, **DIABETES COUNTDOWN**, is available from the Juvenile Diabetes Foundation, 432 Park Avenue South, New York, New York 10016–8013.

Literature revised May 23, 1995

[052395]

NPH ILETIN® II (PORK) OTC

[*ĕn 'pē-āch ī'lĕ-tĭn*]

(Isophane Insulin Suspension, USP, purified pork)

INFORMATION FOR THE PATIENT

WARNINGS

ANY CHANGE OF INSULIN SHOULD BE MADE CAUTIOUSLY AND ONLY UNDER MEDICAL SUPERVISION. CHANGES IN PURITY, STRENGTH, BRAND (MANUFACTURER), TYPE (REGULAR, NPH, LENTE®), SPECIES (BEEF, PORK, BEEF-PORK, HUMAN), AND/OR METHOD OF MANUFACTURE (RECOMBINANT DNA VERSUS ANIMAL-SOURCE INSULIN) MAY RESULT IN THE NEED FOR A CHANGE IN DOSAGE. IF AN ADJUSTMENT IS NEEDED, IT MAY OCCUR WITH THE FIRST DOSE OR DURING THE FIRST SEVERAL WEEKS OR MONTHS.

DIABETES

Insulin is a hormone produced by the pancreas, a large gland that lies near the stomach. This hormone is necessary for the body's correct use of food, especially sugar. Diabetes occurs when the pancreas does not make enough insulin to meet your body's needs.

To control your diabetes, your doctor has prescribed injections of insulin to keep your blood glucose at a nearly normal level. Proper control of your diabetes requires close and constant cooperation with your doctor. In spite of diabetes, you can lead an active, healthy, and useful life if you eat a balanced diet daily, exercise regularly, and take your insulin injections as prescribed.

You have been instructed to test your blood and/or urine regularly for glucose. If your blood tests consistently show above- or below-normal glucose levels or your urine tests consistently show the presence of glucose, your diabetes is not properly controlled and you must let your doctor know.

Always keep an extra supply of insulin as well as a spare syringe and needle on hand. Always wear diabetic identification so that appropriate treatment can be given if complications occur away from home.

NPH PORK INSULIN

Description

NPH pork insulin is obtained from pork pancreas.

NPH Iletin® II (purified insulin, Lilly) is a crystalline suspension of insulin with protamine and zinc providing an intermediate-acting insulin with a slower onset of action and a longer duration of activity (slightly more than 24 hours) than that of regular insulin. The time course of action of any insulin may vary considerably in different individuals or at different times in the same individual. As with all insulin preparations, the duration of action of NPH Iletin II is dependent on dose, site of injection, blood supply, temperature, and physical activity. NPH Iletin II is a sterile suspension and is for subcutaneous injection only. It should not be used intravenously or intramuscularly. The concentration of NPH Iletin II is 100 units/mL (U-100).

Identification

This insulin, manufactured by Eli Lilly and Company, has the trademark Iletin II and is available in various types—Regular, NPH, and Lente. Your doctor has prescribed the type of insulin that he/she believes is best for you. **DO NOT USE ANY OTHER INSULIN EXCEPT ON HIS/HER ADVICE AND DIRECTION.**

Always check the carton and the bottle label for the name and letter designation of the insulin you receive from your pharmacy to make sure it is the same as that your doctor has prescribed.

Always examine the appearance of your bottle of insulin before withdrawing each dose. A bottle of NPH Iletin II must be carefully shaken or rotated before each injection so that the contents are uniformly mixed. NPH Iletin II should look uniformly cloudy or milky after mixing. Do not use it if the insulin substance (the white material) remains at the bottom of the bottle after mixing. Do not use a bottle of NPH Iletin II if there are clumps in the insulin after mixing. Always check the appearance of your bottle of insulin before using, and if you note anything unusual in the appearance of your insulin or notice your insulin requirements changing markedly, consult your doctor.

Storage

Insulin should be stored in a refrigerator but not in the freezer. If refrigeration is not possible, the bottle of insulin that you are currently using can be kept unrefrigerated as long as it is kept as cool as possible (below 86°F [30°C]) and away from heat and light. Do not use insulin if it has been frozen. Do not use a bottle of insulin after the expiration date stamped on the label.

INJECTION PROCEDURES

Correct Syringe

Doses of insulin are measured in **units**. U-100 insulin contains 100 units/mL (1 mL = 1 cc). With NPH Iletin II, it is important to use a syringe that is marked for U-100 insulin preparations. Failure to use the proper syringe can lead to a mistake in dosage, causing serious problems for you, such as a blood glucose level that is too low or too high.

Syringe Use

To help avoid contamination and possible infection, follow these instructions exactly.

Disposable syringes and needles should be used only once and then discarded. **NEEDLES AND SYRINGES MUST NOT BE SHARED.**

Reusable syringes and needles must be sterilized before each injection.

Follow the package directions supplied with your syringe.

Described below are 2 methods of sterilizing.

Boiling

1. Put syringe, plunger, and needle in strainer, place in saucepan, and cover with water. Boil for 5 minutes.
2. Remove articles from water. When they have cooled, insert plunger into barrel, and fasten needle to syringe with a slight twist.
3. Push plunger in and out several times until water is completely removed.

Isopropyl Alcohol

If the syringe, plunger, and needle cannot be boiled, as when you are traveling, they may be sterilized by immersion for at least 5 minutes in Isopropyl Alcohol, 91%. Do not use bathing, rubbing, or medicated alcohol for this sterilization. If the syringe is sterilized with alcohol, it must be absolutely dry before use.

Preparing the Dose

1. Wash your hands.
2. Carefully shake or rotate the insulin bottle several times to completely mix the insulin.
3. Inspect the insulin. NPH Iletin II should look uniformly cloudy or milky. Do not use it if you notice anything unusual in the appearance.
4. If using a new bottle, flip off the plastic protective cap, but **do not** remove the stopper. When using a new bottle, wipe the top of the bottle with an alcohol swab.
5. If you are mixing insulins, refer to the Warnings below.
6. Draw air into the syringe equal to your insulin dose. Put the needle through rubber top of the insulin bottle and inject the air into the bottle.
7. Turn the bottle and syringe upside down. Hold the bottle and syringe firmly in 1 hand and shake gently.
8. Making sure the tip of the needle is in the insulin, withdraw the correct dose of insulin into the syringe.
9. Before removing the needle from the bottle, check your syringe for air bubbles which reduce the amount of insulin in it. If bubbles are present, hold the syringe straight up and tap its side until the bubbles float to the top. Push them out with the plunger and withdraw the correct dose.
10. Remove the needle from the bottle and lay the syringe down so that the needle does not touch anything.

WARNINGS—SEE ADDITIONAL WARNINGS ABOVE

Patients who have been directed by their doctors to mix 2 types of insulin should be aware that insulin hypodermic syringes of different manufacturers may vary in the amount of space between the bottom line and the needle.

Because of this, do not change:

1. The order of mixing that the doctor has prescribed or
2. The model and brand of syringe or needle without first consulting your doctor.

The mixing should be done immediately prior to injection. Failure to heed this warning could result in a dosage error.

Injection

Cleanse the skin with alcohol where the injection is to be made. Stabilize the skin by spreading it or pinching up a large area. Insert the needle as instructed by your doctor. Push the plunger in as far as it will go. Pull the needle out and apply gentle pressure over the injection site for several seconds. **Do not rub the area.** To avoid tissue damage, give the next tissue damage, give the next injection at a site at least $^1/_2$" from the previous site.

DOSAGE

Your doctor has told you which insulin to use, how much, and when and how often to inject it. Because each patient's case of diabetes is different, this schedule has been individualized for you.

Your usual insulin dose may be affected by changes in your food, activity, or work schedule. Carefully follow your doctor's instructions to allow for these changes. Other things that may affect your insulin dose are:

Illness

Illness, especially with nausea and vomiting, may cause your insulin requirements to change. Even if you are not eating, you will still require insulin. You and your doctor should establish a sick day plan for you to use in case of illness. When you are sick, test your blood/urine frequently and call your doctor as instructed.

Pregnancy

Good control of diabetes is especially important for you and your unborn baby. Pregnancy may make managing your diabetes more difficult. If you are planning to have a baby, are pregnant, or are nursing a baby, consult your doctor.

Medication

Insulin requirements may be increased if you are taking other drugs with hyperglycemic activity, such as oral contraceptives, corticosteroids, or thyroid replacement therapy. Insulin requirements may be reduced in the presence of drugs with hypoglycemic activity, such as oral hypoglycemics, salicylates (for example, aspirin), sulfa antibiotics, and certain antidepressants. Always discuss any medications you are taking with your doctor.

Exercise

Exercise may lower your body's need for insulin during and for some time after the activity. Exercise may also speed up the effect of an insulin dose, especially if the exercise involves the area of injection site (for example, the leg should not be used for injection prior to running). Discuss with your doctor how you should adjust your regimen to accommodate exercise.

Travel

Persons traveling across more than 2 times zones should consult their doctor concerning adjustments in their insulin schedule.

COMMON PROBLEMS OF DIABETES

Hypoglycemia (Insulin Reaction)

Hypoglycemia (too little glucose in the blood) is one of the most frequent adverse events experienced by insulin users. It can be brought about by:

1. Taking too much insulin
2. Missing or delaying meals
3. Exercising or working more than usual
4. An infection or illness (especially with diarrhea or vomiting)
5. A change in the body's need for insulin
6. Diseases of the adrenal, pituitary, or thyroid gland, or progression of kidney or liver disease
7. Interactions with other drugs that lower blood glucose, such as oral hypoglycemics, salicylates (for example, aspirin), sulfa antibiotics, and certain antidepressants
8. Consumption of alcoholic beverages

Symptoms of mild to moderate hypoglycemia may occur suddenly and can include:

- sweating
- dizziness
- palpitation
- tremor
- hunger
- restlessness
- tingling in the hands, feet, lips, or tongue
- lightheadedness
- inability to concentrate
- headache
- drowsiness
- sleep disturbances
- anxiety
- blurred vision
- slurred speech
- depressive mood
- irritability
- abnormal behavior
- unsteady movement
- personality changes

Signs of severe hypoglycemia can include:

- disorientation
- unconsciousness

- seizures
- death

Therefore, it is important that assistance be obtained immediately

Early warning symptoms of hypoglycemia may be different or less pronounced under certain conditions, such as long duration of diabetes, diabetic nerve disease, medications such as beta-blockers, change in insulin preparations, or intensified control (3 or more insulin injections per day) of diabetes.

Without recognition of early warning symptoms, you may not be able to take steps to avoid more serious hypoglycemia. Be alert for all of the various types of symptoms that may indicate hypoglycemia. Patients who experience hypoglycemia without early warning symptoms should monitor their blood glucose frequently, especially prior to activities such as driving. If the blood glucose is below your normal fasting glucose, you should consider eating or drinking sugar-containing foods to treat your hypoglycemia.

Mild to moderate hypoglycemia may be treated by eating foods or taking drinks that contain sugar. Patients should always carry a quick source of sugar, such as candy mints or glucose tablets. More severe hypoglycemia may require the assistance of another person. Patients who are unable to take sugar orally or who are unconscious require an injection of glucagon or should be treated with intravenous administration of glucose at a medical facility.

You should learn to recognize your own symptoms of hypoglycemia. If you are uncertain about these symptoms, you should monitor your blood glucose frequently to help you learn to recognize the symptoms that you experience with hypoglycemia.

If you have frequent episodes of hypoglycemia or experience difficulty in recognizing the symptoms, you should consult your doctor to discuss possible changes in therapy, meal plans, and/or exercise programs to help you avoid hypoglycemia.

Hyperglycemia and Diabetic Acidosis

Hyperglycemia (too much glucose in the blood) may develop if your body has too little insulin. Hyperglycemia can be brought about by:

1. Omitting your insulin or taking less than the doctor has prescribed
2. Eating significantly more than your meal plan suggests
3. Developing a fever or infection

In patients with insulin-dependent diabetes, prolonged hyperglycemia can result in diabetic acidosis. The first symptoms of diabetic acidosis usually come on gradually, over a period of hours or days, and include a drowsy feeling, flushed face, thirst, loss of appetite, and fruity odor on the breath. With acidosis, urine tests show large amounts of glucose and acetone. Heavy breathing and a rapid pulse are more severe symptoms. If uncorrected, prolonged hyperglycemia or diabetic acidosis can result in loss of consciousness or death. Therefore, it is important that you obtain medical assistance immediately.

Lipodystrophy

Rarely, administration of insulin subcutaneously can result in lipoatrophy (depression in the skin) or lipohypertrophy (enlargement or thickening of tissue). If you notice either of these conditions, consult your doctor. A change in your injection technique may help alleviate the problem.

Allergy to Insulin

Local Allergy—Patients occasionally experience redness, swelling, and itching at the site of injection of insulin. This condition, called local allergy, usually clears up in a few days to a few weeks. In some instances, this condition may be related to factors other than insulin, such as irritants in the skin cleansing agent or poor injection technique. If you have local reactions, contact your doctor.

Systemic Allergy—Less common, but potentially more serious, is generalized allergy to insulin, which may cause rash over the whole body, shortness of breath, wheezing, reduction in blood pressure, fast pulse, or sweating. Severe cases of generalized allergy may be life threatening. If you think you are having a generalized allergic reaction to insulin, notify a doctor immediately.

ADDITIONAL INFORMATION

Additional information about diabetes may be obtained from your diabetes educator.

DIABETES FORECAST is a national magazine designed especially for patients with diabetes and their families and is available by subscription from the American Diabetes Association, National Service Center, 1660 Duke Street, Alexandria, Virginia 22314.

Another publication, **DIABETES COUNTDOWN**, is available from the Juvenile Diabetes Foundation, 432 Park Avenue South, New York, New York 10016–8013.

Literature revised October 28, 1992

[102892]

REGULAR ILETIN® II (PORK)　　　OTC
[rĕg-ū-lĕr ī′lĕ-tĭn]
(Insulin Injection, USP, purified pork)

INFORMATION FOR THE PATIENT
WARNINGS
ANY CHANGE OF INSULIN SHOULD BE MADE CAUTIOUSLY AND ONLY UNDER MEDICAL SUPERVISION. CHANGES IN PURITY, STRENGTH, BRAND (MANUFACTURER), TYPE (REGULAR, NPH, LENTE®), SPECIES (BEEF, PORK, BEEF-PORK, HUMAN), AND/OR METHOD OF MANUFACTURE (RECOMBINANT DNA VERSUS ANIMAL-SOURCE INSULIN) MAY RESULT IN THE NEED FOR A CHANGE IN DOSAGE. IF AN ADJUSTMENT IS NEEDED, IT MAY OCCUR WITH THE FIRST DOSE OR DURING THE FIRST SEVERAL WEEKS OR MONTHS.

DIABETES

Insulin is a hormone produced by the pancreas, a large gland that lies near the stomach. This hormone is necessary for the body's correct use of food, especially sugar. Diabetes occurs when the pancreas does not make enough insulin to meet your body's needs.

To control your diabetes, your doctor has prescribed injections of insulin to keep your blood glucose at a nearly normal level. Proper control of your diabetes requires close and constant cooperation with your doctor. In spite of diabetes, you can lead an active, healthy, and useful life if you eat a balanced diet daily, exercise regularly, and take your insulin injections as prescribed.

You have been instructed to test your blood and/or your urine regularly for glucose. If your blood tests consistently show above- or below-normal glucose levels or your urine tests consistently show the presence of glucose, your diabetes is not properly controlled and you must let your doctor know. Always keep an extra supply of insulin as well as a spare syringe and needle on hand. Always wear diabetic identification so that appropriate treatment can be given if complications occur away from home.

REGULAR PORK INSULIN
Description
Regular pork insulin is obtained from pork pancreas. Regular Iletin® II (purified insulin, Lilly) consists of zinc-insulin crystals dissolved in a clear fluid. Regular Iletin II has had nothing added to change the speed or length of its action. It takes effect rapidly and has a relatively short duration of activity (4 to 12 hours) as compared with other insulins. The time course of action of any insulin may vary considerably in different individuals or at different times in the same individual. As with all insulin preparations, the duration of action of Regular Iletin II is dependent on dose, site of injection, blood supply, temperature, and physical activity. Regular Iletin II is a sterile solution and is for subcutaneous injection. It should not be used intramuscularly. The concentration of Regular Iletin II is 100 units/mL (U-100).

Identification
This insulin, manufactured by Eli Lilly and Company, has the trademark Iletin II and is available in various types—Regular, NPH, and Lente. Your doctor has prescribed the type of insulin that he/she believes is best for you. DO NOT USE ANY OTHER INSULIN EXCEPT ON HIS/HER ADVICE AND DIRECTION.

Always check the carton and the bottle label for the name and letter designation of the insulin you receive from your pharmacy to make sure it is the same as that your doctor has prescribed.

Always examine the appearance of your bottle of insulin before withdrawing each dose. Regular Iletin II is a clear and colorless liquid with a water-like appearance and consistency. Do not use if it appears cloudy, thickened, or slightly colored or if solid particles are visible. Always check the appearance of your bottle of insulin before using, and if you note anything unusual in the appearance of your insulin or notice your insulin requirements changing markedly, consult your doctor.

Storage
Insulin should be stored in a refrigerator but not in the freezer. If refrigeration is not possible, the bottle of insulin that you are currently using can be kept unrefrigerated as long as it is kept as cool as possible (below 86°F [30°C]) and away from heat and light. Do not use insulin if it has been frozen. Do not use a bottle of insulin after the expiration date stamped on the label.

INJECTION PROCEDURES
Correct Syringe
Doses of insulin are measured in **units**. U-100 insulin contains 100 units/mL (1 mL=1 cc). With Regular Iletin II, it is important to use a syringe that is marked for U-100 insulin preparations. Failure to use the proper syringe can lead to a mistake in dosage, causing serious problems for you, such as a blood glucose level that is too low or too high.
Syringe Use
To help avoid contamination and possible infection, follow these instructions exactly.

Disposable syringes and needles should be used only once and then discarded. **NEEDLES AND SYRINGES MUST NOT BE SHARED.**

Reusable syringes and needles must be sterilized before each injection. **Follow the package directions supplied with your syringe.** Described below are 2 methods of sterilizing.
Boiling
1. Put syringe, plunger, and needle in strainer, place in saucepan, and cover with water. Boil for 5 minutes.
2. Remove articles from water. When they have cooled, insert plunger into barrel, and fasten needle to syringe with a slight twist.
3. Push plunger in and out several times until water is completely removed.
Isopropyl Alcohol
If the syringe, plunger, and needle cannot be boiled, as when you are traveling, they may be sterilized by immersion for at least 5 minutes in Isopropyl Alcohol, 91%. Do not use bathing, rubbing, or medicated alcohol for this sterilization. If the syringe is sterilized with alcohol, it must be absolutely dry before use.
Preparing the Dose
1. Wash your hands.
2. Inspect the insulin. Regular Iletin II should look clear and colorless. Do not use Regular Iletin II if it appears cloudy, thickened, or slightly colored or if solid particles are visible.
3. If using a new bottle, flip off the plastic protective cap, but **do not remove the stopper.** When using a new bottle, wipe the top of the bottle with an alcohol swab.
4. If you are mixing insulins, refer to the Warnings below.
5. Draw air into the syringe equal to your insulin dose. Put the needle through rubber top of the insulin bottle and inject the air into the bottle.
6. Turn the bottle and syringe upside down. Hold the bottle and syringe firmly in 1 hand.
7. Making sure the tip of the needle is in the insulin, withdraw the correct dose of insulin into the syringe.
8. Before removing the needle from the bottle, check your syringe for air bubbles which reduce the amount of insulin in it. If bubbles are present, hold the syringe straight up and tap its side until the bubbles float to the top. Push them out with the plunger and withdraw the correct dose.
9. Remove the needle from the bottle and lay the syringe down so that the needle does not touch anything.

WARNINGS—SEE ADDITIONAL WARNINGS ABOVE
Patients who have been directed by their doctors to mix 2 types of insulin should be aware that insulin hypodermic syringes of different manufacturers may vary in the amount of space between the bottom line and the needle.
Because of this, do not change:
1. The order of mixing that the doctor has prescribed or
2. The model and brand of syringe or needle without first consulting your doctor.
The mixing should be done immediately prior to injection. Failure to heed this warning could result in a dosage error.
Injection
Cleanse the skin with alcohol where the injection is to be made. Stabilize the skin by spreading it or pinching up a large area. Insert the needle as instructed by your doctor. Push the plunger in as far as it will go. Pull the needle out and apply gentle pressure over the injection site for several seconds. Do not rub the area. To avoid tissue damage, give the next injection at a site at least ¹/₂″ from the previous site.
DOSAGE
Your doctor has told you which insulin to use, how much, and when and how often to inject it. Because each patient's case of diabetes is different, this schedule has been individualized for you.

Your usual insulin dose may be affected by changes in your food, activity, or work schedule. Carefully follow your doctor's instructions to allow for these changes. Other things that may affect your insulin dose are:
Illness
Illness, especially with nausea and vomiting, may cause your insulin requirements to change. Even if you are not eating, you will still require insulin. You and your doctor should establish a sick day plan for you to use in case of illness. When you are sick, test your blood/urine frequently and call your doctor as instructed.
Pregnancy
Good control of diabetes is especially important for you and your unborn baby. Pregnancy may make managing your diabetes more difficult. If you are planning to have a baby, are pregnant, or are nursing a baby, consult your doctor.

Continued on next page

• Identi-Code® symbol. This product information was prepared in June 1996. Current information on these and other products of Eli Lilly and Company may be obtained by direct inquiry to Lilly Research Laboratories, Lilly Corporate Center, Indianapolis, Indiana 46285, 800-545-5979.

Lilly—Cont.

Medication

Insulin requirements may be increased if you are taking other drugs with hyperglycemic activity, such as oral contraceptives, corticosteroids, or thyroid replacement therapy. Insulin requirements may be reduced in the presence of drugs with hypoglycemic activity, such as oral hypoglycemics, salicylates (for example, aspirin), sulfa antibiotics, and certain antidepressants. Always discuss any medications you are taking with your doctor.

Exercise

Exercise may lower your body's need for insulin during and for some time after the activity. Exercise may also speed up the effect of an insulin dose, especially if the exercise involves the area of injection site (for example, the leg should not be used for injection just prior to running). Discuss with your doctor how you should adjust your regimen to accommodate exercise.

Travel

Persons traveling across more than 2 time zones should consult their doctor concerning adjustments in their insulin schedule.

COMMON PROBLEMS OF DIABETES

Hypoglycemia (Insulin Reaction)

Hypoglycemia (too little glucose in the blood) is one of the most frequent adverse events experienced by insulin users. It can be brought about by:

1. Taking too much insulin
2. Missing or delaying meals
3. Exercising or working more than usual
4. An infection or illness (especially with diarrhea or vomiting)
5. A change in the body's need for insulin
6. Diseases of the adrenal, pituitary, or thyroid gland, or progression of kidney or liver disease
7. Interactions with other drugs that lower blood glucose, such as oral hypoglycemics, salicylates (for example, aspirin), sulfa antibiotics, and certain antidepressants
8. Consumption of alcoholic beverages

Symptoms of mild to moderate hypoglycemia may occur suddenly and can include:

- sweating
- dizziness
- palpitation
- tremor
- hunger
- restlessness
- tingling in the hands, feet, lips, or tongue
- lightheadedness
- inability to concentrate
- headache
- sleep disturbances
- anxiety
- blurred vision
- slurred speech
- depressive mood
- irritability
- abnormal behavior
- unsteady movement
- personality changes

Signs of severe hypoglycemia can include:

- disorientation
- unconsciousness
- seizures
- death

Therefore, it is important that assistance be obtained immediately.

Early warning symptoms of hypoglycemia may be different or less pronounced under certain conditions, such as long duration of diabetes, diabetic nerve disease, medications such as beta-blockers, change in insulin preparations, or intensified control (3 or more insulin injections per day) of diabetes.

Without recognition of early warning symptoms, you may not be able to take steps to avoid more serious hypoglycemia. Be alert for all of the various types of symptoms that may indicate hypoglycemia. Patients who experience hypoglycemia without early warning symptoms should monitor their blood glucose frequently, especially prior to activities such as driving. If the blood glucose is below your normal fasting glucose, you should consider eating or drinking sugar-containing foods to treat your hypoglycemia.

Mild to moderate hypoglycemia may be treated by taking foods or drinks that contain sugar. Patients should always carry a quick source of sugar, such as candy mints or glucose tablets. More severe hypoglycemia may require the assistance of another person. Patients who are unable to take sugar orally or who are unconscious require an injection of glucagon or should be treated with intravenous administration of glucose at a medical facility.

You should learn to recognize your own symptoms of hypoglycemia. If you are uncertain about these symptoms, you should monitor your blood glucose frequently to help you learn to recognize the symptoms that you experience with hypoglycemia.

If you have frequent episodes of hypoglycemia or experience difficulty in recognizing the symptoms, you should consult your doctor to discuss possible changes in therapy, meal plans, and/or exercise programs to help you avoid hypoglycemia.

Hyperglycemia and Diabetic Acidosis

Hyperglycemia (too much glucose in the blood) may develop if your body has too little insulin. Hyperglycemia can be brought about by:

1. Omitting your insulin or taking less than the doctor has prescribed
2. Eating significantly more than your meal plan suggests
3. Developing a fever or infection

In patients with insulin-dependent diabetes, prolonged hyperglycemia can result in diabetic acidosis. The first symptoms of diabetic acidosis usually come on gradually, over a period of hours or days, and include a drowsy feeling, flushed face, thirst, loss of appetite, and fruity odor on the breath. With acidosis, urine tests show large amounts of glucose and acetone. Heavy breathing and a rapid pulse are more severe symptoms. If uncorrected, prolonged hyperglycemia or diabetic acidosis can result in loss of consciousness or death. Therefore, it is important that you obtain medical assistance immediately.

Lipodystrophy

Rarely, administration of insulin subcutaneously can result in lipoatrophy (depression in the skin) or lipohypertrophy (enlargement or thickening of tissue). If you notice either of these conditions, consult your doctor. A change in your injection technique may help alleviate the problem.

Allergy to Insulin

Local Allergy—Patients occasionally experience redness, swelling, and itching at the site of injection of insulin. This condition, called local allergy, usually clears up in a few days to a few weeks. In some instances, this condition may be related to factors other than insulin, such as irritants in the skin cleansing agent or poor injection technique. If you have local reactions, contact your doctor.

Systemic Allergy—Less common, but potentially serious, is generalized allergy to insulin, which may cause rash over the whole body, shortness of breath, wheezing, reduction in blood pressure, fast pulse, or sweating. Severe cases of generalized allergy may be life threatening. If you think you are having a generalized allergic reaction to insulin, notify a doctor immediately.

ADDITIONAL INFORMATION

Additional information about diabetes may be obtained from your diabetes educator.

DIABETES FORECAST is a national magazine designed especially for patients with diabetes and their families and is available by subscription from the American Diabetes Association, National Service Center, 1660 Duke Street, Alexandria, Virginia 22314.

Another publication, **DIABETES COUNTDOWN**, is available from the Juvenile Diabetes Foundation, 432 Park Avenue South, New York, New York 10016–8013.

Literature revised October 28, 1992

[102892]

REGULAR (CONCENTRATED) ILETIN® II, U-500 ℞

[rĕg-ū-lĕr ī'lĕ-tĭn]

(Insulin Injection, USP, purified pork)

WARNINGS

ANY CHANGE OF INSULIN SHOULD BE MADE CAUTIOUSLY AND ONLY UNDER MEDICAL SUPERVISION. CHANGES IN PURITY, STRENGTH (U-100), BRAND (MANUFACTURER), TYPE (LENTE®, NPH, REGULAR, ETC.), AND/OR SPECIES SOURCE (BEEF, PORK, BEEF-PORK, OR HUMAN) MAY RESULT IN THE NEED FOR A CHANGE IN DOSAGE. SEE BELOW.

IT IS NOT POSSIBLE TO IDENTIFY WHICH PATIENTS WILL REQUIRE A REDUCTION IN DOSE TO AVOID HYPOGLYCEMIA WHEN USING THIS INSULIN. HOWEVER, IT IS KNOWN THAT A SMALL NUMBER OF PATIENTS MAY REQUIRE A SIGNIFICANT CHANGE.

ADJUSTMENT MAY BE NEEDED WITH THE FIRST DOSE OR OCCUR OVER A PERIOD OF SEVERAL WEEKS. BE AWARE OF THE POSSIBILITY OF SYMPTOMS OF EITHER HYPOGLYCEMIA OR HYPERGLYCEMIA.

This insulin is prepared from pork pancreas only. The dose of pork insulin for patients with insulin resistance due to antibodies to beef insulin may be only a fraction of that of beef insulin.

This insulin preparation contains 500 units of insulin in each milliliter. Extreme caution must be observed in the measurement of dosage because inadvertent overdose may result in irreversible insulin shock. Serious consequences may result if it is used other than under constant medical supervision.

DESCRIPTION

This Lilly pork insulin product differs from previous pork insulin preparations because it has undergone additional steps of chromatographic purification.

Regular (Concentrated) Iletin® II, U-500, is an aqueous solution made from the antidiabetic principle of pork pancreas as stated on the label. Each milliliter contains 500 units of regular (unmodified) insulin and approximately 1.6% glycerin (w/v), with approximately 0.25% m-cresol (w/v) as a preservative. Sodium hydroxide and hydrochloric acid are added during manufacture to adjust the pH. All preparations of Iletin® II are made from zinc-insulin crystals.

CLINICAL PHARMACOLOGY

Adequate insulin dosage permits the diabetic patient to utilize carbohydrates and fats in a comparatively satisfactory manner. Regardless of concentration, the action of insulin is basically the same: to enable carbohydrate metabolism to occur and thus to prevent the production of ketone bodies by the liver. Although, under usual circumstances, diabetes can be controlled with doses in the vicinity of 40 to 60 units or less, an occasional patient develops such resistance or becomes so unresponsive to the effect of insulin that daily doses of several hundred, or even several thousand, units are required. Patients who require doses in excess of 300 to 500 units daily usually have impaired receptor function.

Occasionally, a cause of the insulin resistance can be found (such as hemochromatosis, cirrhosis of the liver, some complicating disease of the endocrine glands other than the pancreas, allergy, or infection), but in other cases, no cause of the high insulin requirement can be determined.

Iletin II, U-500, is unmodified by any agent that might prolong its action; however, clinical experience has shown that it frequently has a time action similar to a repository insulin preparation and that a single dose may show activity over a 24-hour period. This effect has been credited to the high concentration of the preparation.

INDICATIONS AND USAGE

Iletin® II, U-500, is especially useful for the treatment of diabetic patients with marked insulin resistance (daily requirements more than 200 units), since a large dose may be administered subcutaneously in a reasonable volume.

CONTRAINDICATIONS

Patients with a history of systemic allergic reactions to pork or mixed beef/pork insulin should not receive the insulin formulation unless they have been successfully desensitized.

PRECAUTIONS

General—Every patient exhibiting insulin resistance who requires Iletin® II, U-500, for control of diabetes should be under close observation until dosage is established. The response will vary among patients. Some can be controlled with a single dose daily; others may require 2 or 3 injections per day. Most patients will show a "tolerance" to insulin, so that minor variations in dosage can occur without the development of untoward symptoms of insulin shock.

Insulin resistance is frequently self-limited; after several weeks or months during which high dosage is required, responsiveness to the pharmacologic effect of insulin may be regained and dosage can be reduced.

Patients with immunologic insulin resistance to beef insulin (this diagnosis is usually confirmed by the finding of increased serum antibody titers) may require an immediate dosage reduction of 20 to 50% when treated with pork insulin.

Information for Patients—Patients should be instructed regarding their dosage and should be reminded that this formulation requires the administration of a smaller volume of solution than is the case with less concentrated formulations.

Laboratory Tests—Blood and urine glucose, glycohemoglobin, and urine ketones should be monitored frequently.

Drug Interactions—The concurrent use of oral hypoglycemic agents with Iletin II, U-500, is not recommended since there are no data to support such use.

Pregnancy—Teratogenic Effects—No reproduction studies have been conducted in animals, and there are no adequate and well-controlled studies in pregnant women. It would be anticipated that the benefits of this insulin preparation would outweigh any risk to the developing fetus.

Nonteratogenic Effects—Insulin does not cross the placenta as does glucose.

Labor and Delivery—Careful monitoring of the patient is required, since the insulin requirement may decrease following delivery.

Nursing Mothers—It is not known whether insulin is excreted in significant amounts in human milk. Because many drugs are excreted in human milk, caution should be exercised when Iletin II, U-500, insulin injection is administered to a nursing woman.

Pediatric Use—There are no special precautions relating to the use of this insulin formulation in the pediatric age group.

ADVERSE REACTIONS

As with other insulin preparations, hypoglycemic reactions may be associated with the administration of Iletin® II, U-500. However, deep secondary hypoglycemic reactions may develop 18 to 24 hours after the original injection of Iletin II, U-500. Consequently, patients should be carefully observed, and prompt treatment of such reactions should be initiated with glucagon injections and/or with glucose by intravenous injection or gavage.

ALLERGIC REACTIONS

Erythema, swelling, or pruritus may occur at injection sites. Such localized allergic manifestations usually resolve within a few days to a few weeks.

Less common, but potentially more serious, is systemic allergy to insulin, manifested by generalized urticaria, dyspnea, and wheezing, which may progress to anaphylaxis. If a severe allergic reaction occurs, the drug should be discontinued and the patient treated with the usual agents (eg, epinephrine, antihistamines, or corticosteroids). Patients who have experienced severe systemic allergic reactions to insulin (eg, generalized urticaria, angioedema, anaphylaxis) should be skin-tested with each new preparation to be used before starting therapy with that preparation. Desensitization procedures may permit resumption of insulin administration.

DOSAGE AND ADMINISTRATION

Iletin® II, U-500, can be administered by both the subcutaneous and the intramuscular routes. It is inadvisable to inject Iletin II, U-500, intravenously because of the possible development of allergic or anaphylactoid reactions.

It is recommended that a tuberculin type of syringe be utilized for the measurement of dosage. Variations in dosage are frequently possible in the insulin-resistant patient, since the individual is unresponsive to the pharmacologic effect of the insulin. Nevertheless, accuracy of measurement is to be encouraged because of the potential danger of the preparation.

HOW SUPPLIED

Insulin should be kept in a cold place, preferably in a refrigerator, but must not be frozen.

Do not inject insulin that is not water-clear. Discoloration, turbidity, or unusual viscosity indicates deterioration or contamination.

Use of a package of insulin should not be started after the expiration date stamped on it.

Vials, U-500, 500 units/mL, 20 mL (No. CP-2500) (1's), NDC 0002-8500-01

CAUTION—Federal (USA) law prohibits dispensing without prescription.

[091394]

KEFUROX® ℞

[*kĕf 'yū-rōeks*]

(sterile cefuroxime sodium)

USP

DESCRIPTION

Kefurox® (Sterile Cefuroxime Sodium, USP) is a semisynthetic, broad-spectrum cephalosporin antibiotic for parenteral administration. Chemically, it is sodium (6R,7R)-7-[2-(2-furyl) glyoxylamido]-3-(hydroxymethyl)-8-oxo-5-thia-1-azabicyclo [4.2.0] oct-2-ene-2-carboxylate, 7^2-(Z)-(*O*-methyloxime), carbamate (ester). The chemical formula is $C_{16}H_{15}N_4NaO_8S$, and the molecular weight is 446.37. Kefurox contains approximately 54.2 mg (2.4 mEq) of sodium per gram of cefuroxime activity. Solutions of Kefurox range from light yellow to amber, depending on the concentration and diluent used. The pH of freshly reconstituted solutions usually ranges from 4.5 to 8.5. This product is oxygen sensitive. The structure is:

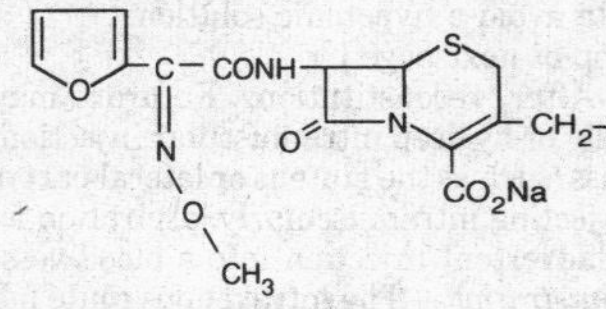

CLINICAL PHARMACOLOGY

After intramuscular injection of a 750-mg dose of cefuroxime to normal volunteers, the mean peak serum concentration was 27 μg/mL. The peak occurred at approximately 45 minutes (range 15 to 60 minutes). Following intravenous doses of 750 mg and 1.5 g, serum concentrations were approximately 50 μg/mL and 100 μg/mL respectively at 15 minutes.

Therapeutic serum concentrations of approximately 2 μg/mL or more were maintained for 5.3 hours and 8 hours or more respectively. There was no evidence of accumulation of cefuroxime in the serum following intravenous administration of 1.5-g doses every 8 hours to normal volunteers. The serum half-life after either intramuscular or intravenous injections is approximately 80 minutes.

Approximately 89% of a dose of cefuroxime is excreted by the kidneys over an 8-hour period, resulting in high urinary concentrations.

Following the intramuscular administration of a 750-mg single dose, urinary concentrations averaged 1,300 μg/mL during the first 8 hours. Intravenous doses of 750 mg and 1.5 g produced urinary levels averaging 1,150 μg/mL and 2,500 μg/mL respectively during the first 8-hour period.

The concomitant oral administration of probenecid with cefuroxime slows tubular secretion, decreases renal clearance by approximately 40%, increases the peak serum level by approximately 30%, and increases the serum half-life by approximately 30%. Kefurox is detectable in therapeutic concentrations in pleural fluid, joint fluid, bile, sputum, bone, cerebrospinal fluid (in patients with meningitis), and aqueous humor.

Cefuroxime is approximately 50% bound to serum protein.

Microbiology—Cefuroxime has in vitro activity against a wide range of gram-positive and gram-negative organisms, and it is highly stable in the presence of β-lactamases of certain gram-negative bacteria. The bactericidal action of cefuroxime results from inhibition of cell-wall synthesis.

Cefuroxime is usually active against the following organisms in vitro.

Gram-Negative—Haemophilus influenzae (including ampicillin-resistant strains), *Haemophilus parainfluenzae, Neisseria gonorrhoeae* (including penicillinase- and non-penicillinase-producing strains), *Neisseria meningitidis, Escherichia coli, Klebsiella* spp (including *Klebsiella pneumoniae), Enterobacter* spp, *Citrobacter* spp, *Salmonella* spp, *Shigella* spp, *Proteus mirabilis, Proteus inconstans* (formerly *Providencia inconstans), Providencia rettgeri* (formerly *Proteus rettgeri), Morganella morganii* (formerly *Proteus morganii).*

Some strains of *M. morganii, Enterobacter cloacae,* and *Citrobacter* spp have been shown by in vitro tests to be resistant to cefuroxime and other cephalosporins.

Gram-Positive—Staphylococcus aureus (including penicillinase- and non-penicillinase-producing strains), *Staphylococcus epidermidis,* and certain strains of streptococci, eg, *Streptococcus pyogenes* and *Streptococcus pneumoniae.*

Certain strains of enterococci, eg, *Enterococcus faecalis* (formerly *Streptococcus faecalis*), are resistant.

Anaerobic Organisms—Gram-positive and gram-negative cocci (including *Peptococcus* and *Peptostreptococcus* spp), gram-positive bacilli (including *Clostridium* spp), gram-negative bacilli (including *Bacteroides* and *Fusobacterium* spp). Most strains of *Bacteroides fragilis* are resistant.

Pseudomonas and *Campylobacter* spp, *Acinetobacter calcoaceticus* (formerly *Mima* and *Herellea* spp), and most strains of *Serratia* spp and *Proteus vulgaris* are resistant to cephalosporins. Methicillin-resistant staphylococci, *Clostridium difficile,* and *Listeria monocytogenes* are resistant to cefuroxime.

Susceptibility Tests—Diffusion Techniques—Quantitative methods that require measurement of zone diameters give the most precise estimates of antibiotic susceptibility. One such procedure[1] has been recommended for use with disks to test susceptibility to cefuroxime. Interpretation involves correlation of the diameters obtained in the disk test with minimal inhibitory concentration (MIC) values for cefuroxime.

Reports from the laboratory giving results of the standardized single-disk susceptibility test[1] using a 30-μg cefuroxime disk should be interpreted according to the following criteria:

1. National Committee for Clinical Laboratory Standards: Performance standards for antimicrobial disk susceptibility test,—5th ed. Approved Standard NCCLS Document M2-A5, Vol 13, No 24, NCCLS, Villanova, PA, 1993.

Susceptible organisms produce zone diameters of ≥ 18 mm, indicating that the tested organism is likely to respond to therapy.

Organisms that produce zones of 15 to 17 mm are expected to be susceptible if high dosage is used or if the infection is confined to tissues and fluids (eg, urine), in which high antibiotic levels are attained.

Resistant organisms produce zones ≤ 14 mm, indicating that other therapy should be selected.

For gram-positive isolates, the test may be performed with either the cephalosporin-class disk (30 μg cephalothin) or the cefuroxime disk (30 μg cefuroxime), and a zone ≥ 18 mm indicates a cefuroxime-susceptible organism.

Gram-negative organisms should be tested with the cefuroxime disk (using the above criteria) because cefuroxime has been shown by in vitro tests to have activity against certain strains of *Enterobacteriaceae* found to be resistant when tested with the cephalosporin-class disk. When using the cephalothin disk, gram-negative organisms with zone diameters < 18 mm do not necessarily indicate either intermediate susceptibility or resistance to cefuroxime.

The cefuroxime disk should not be used for testing susceptibility to other cephalosporins.

Standardized procedures require the use of laboratory control organisms. The 30-μg cefuroxime disk should give zone diameters from 27 to 35 mm for *S. aureus* ATCC 25923. For *E. coli* ATCC 25922, the zone diameters should range from 20 to 26 mm.

Dilution Techniques—A bacterial isolate may be considered susceptible if the MIC value for cefuroxime is ≤ 16 μg/mL. Organisms are considered resistant if the MIC is > 32 μg/mL.

As with standard diffusion methods, dilution procedures require the use of laboratory control organisms. Standard cefuroxime powder should give MIC values that range from 0.5 μg/mL to 2 μg/mL for *S. aureus* ATCC 25923. For *E. coli* ATCC 25922, MIC should range from 2 μg/mL to 8 μg/mL.

INDICATIONS AND USAGE

Kefurox is indicated for the treatment of infections caused by susceptible strains of the designated microorganisms in the diseases listed below:

Lower respiratory infections, including pneumonia caused by *S. pneumoniae, H. influenzae* (including ampicillin-resistant strains), *Klebsiella* spp, *S. aureus* (penicillinase- and non-penicillinase-producing), *S. pyogenes,* and *E. coli.*

Urinary tract infections caused by *E. coli* and *Klebsiella* spp.

Skin and skin structure infections caused by *S. aureus* (penicillinase- and non-penicillinase-producing), *S. pyogenes, E. coli, Klebsiella* spp, and *Enterobacter* spp.

Septicemia caused by *S. aureus* (penicillinase- and non-penicillinase-producing), *S. pneumoniae, E. coli, H. influenzae* (including ampicillin-resistant strains), and *Klebsiella* spp.

Meningitis caused by *S. pneumoniae, H. influenzae* (including ampicillin-resistant strains), *N. meningitidis,* and *S. aureus* (penicillinase- and non-penicillinase-producing). (*See* Adverse Reactions regarding further information on the use of Kefurox in childhood meningitis.)

Gonorrhea—Uncomplicated and disseminated gonococcal infections due to *N. gonorrhoeae* (penicillinase- and non-penicillinase-producing strains) in both males and females.

Bone and joint infections—Caused by *S. aureus* (including penicillinase- and non-penicillinase-producing strains).

Clinical microbiological studies in skin and skin structure infections frequently reveal the growth of susceptible strains of both aerobic and anaerobic organisms. Kefurox has been used successfully in these mixed infections in which several organisms have been isolated. Appropriate cultures and susceptibility studies should be performed to determine the susceptibility of the causative organisms to Kefurox.

Therapy may be started while awaiting the results of these studies; however, once these results become available, the antibiotic treatment should be adjusted accordingly. In certain cases of confirmed or suspected gram-positive or gram-negative sepsis or in patients with other serious infections in which the causative organism has not been identified, Kefurox may be used concomitantly with an aminoglycoside (*see* Precautions *and* Dosage and Administration). If warranted by the severity of the infection and the patient's condition, the recommended doses of both antibiotics may be given.

Prevention: The preoperative prophylactic administration of Kefurox may prevent the growth of susceptible disease-causing bacteria and, thereby, may reduce the incidence of certain postoperative infections in patients undergoing surgical procedures (eg, vaginal hysterectomy) that are classified as clean-contaminated or potentially contaminated procedures. Effective prophylactic use of antibiotics in surgery depends on the time of administration. Kefurox should usually be given ½ to 1 hour before the operation to allow sufficient time to achieve effective antibiotic concentrations in the wound tissues during the procedure. The dose should be repeated intraoperatively if the surgical procedure is lengthy. Prophylactic administration is usually not required after the surgical procedure ends and should be stopped within 24 hours. In the majority of surgical procedures, continuing prophylactic administration of any antibiotic does not reduce the incidence of subsequent infections but will increase the possibility of adverse reactions and the development of bacterial resistance. The perioperative use of Kefurox has also been effective during open heart surgery for surgical patients in whom infections at the operative site would present a serious risk. For these patients, it is recommended that therapy with Kefurox be continued for at least 48 hours after the surgical procedure ends. If an infection is present, specimens for culture should be obtained for the identification of the causative organism and appropriate antimicrobial therapy should be instituted.

Continued on next page

• Identi-Code® symbol. This product information was prepared in June 1996. Current information on these and other products of Eli Lilly and Company may be obtained by direct inquiry to Lilly Research Laboratories, Lilly Corporate Center, Indianapolis, Indiana 46285, 800-545-5979.

Lilly—Cont.

CONTRAINDICATION

Kefurox is contraindicated in patients with known allergy to the cephalosporin group of antibiotics.

WARNINGS

BEFORE THERAPY WITH KEFUROX IS INSTITUTED, CAREFUL INQUIRY SHOULD BE MADE TO DETERMINE WHETHER THE PATIENT HAS HAD PREVIOUS HYPERSENSITIVITY REACTIONS TO CEPHALOSPORINS, PENICILLINS, OR OTHER DRUGS. THIS PRODUCT SHOULD BE GIVEN CAUTIOUSLY TO PENICILLIN-SENSITIVE PATIENTS. ANTIBIOTICS SHOULD BE ADMINISTERED WITH CAUTION TO ANY PATIENT WHO HAS DEMONSTRATED SOME FORM OF ALLERGY, PARTICULARLY TO DRUGS. IF AN ALLERGIC REACTION TO KEFUROX OCCURS, DISCONTINUE THE DRUG. SERIOUS ACUTE HYPERSENSITIVITY REACTIONS MAY REQUIRE EPINEPHRINE AND OTHER EMERGENCY MEASURES.

Pseudomembranous colitis has been reported with the use of cephalosporins (and other broad-spectrum antibiotics); therefore, it is important to consider its diagnosis in patients who develop diarrhea in association with antibiotic use.

Treatment with broad-spectrum antibiotics alters normal flora of the colon and may permit overgrowth of clostridia. Studies indicate a toxin produced by *C. difficile* is one primary cause of antibiotic-associated colitis. Cholestyramine and colestipol resins have been shown to bind the toxin in vitro.

Mild cases of colitis may respond to drug discontinuance alone. Moderate to severe cases should be managed with fluid, electrolyte, and protein supplementation as indicated.

When the colitis is not relieved by drug discontinuance or when it is severe, oral vancomycin is the treatment of choice for antibiotic-associated pseudomembranous colitis produced by *C. difficile*. Other causes of colitis should also be considered.

PRECAUTIONS

Although Kefurox rarely produces alterations in kidney function, evaluation of renal status during therapy is recommended, especially in seriously ill patients receiving the maximum doses. Cephalosporins should be given with caution to patients receiving concurrent treatment with potent diuretics as these regimens are suspected of adversely affecting renal function.

The total daily dose of Kefurox should be reduced in patients with transient or persistent renal insufficiency (*see* Dosage and Administration) because high and prolonged serum antibiotic concentrations can occur in such individuals from usual doses.

As with other antibiotics, prolonged use of Kefurox may result in overgrowth of nonsusceptible organisms. Careful observation of the patient is essential. If superinfection does occur during therapy, appropriate measures should be taken.

Broad-spectrum antibiotics should be prescribed with caution in individuals with a history of gastrointestinal disease, particularly colitis.

Nephrotoxicity has been reported following concomitant administration of aminoglycoside antibiotics and cephalosporins.

Interference with Laboratory Tests—A false-positive reaction for glucose in the urine may occur with copper reduction tests (Benedict's or Fehling's solution or with Clinitest® tablets), but not with enzyme-based tests for glycosuria (eg, Tes-Tape®). A false-negative reaction may occur in the ferricyanide test for blood glucose.

Cefuroxime does not interfere with the assay of serum and urine creatinine by the the alkaline picrate method.

Carcinogenesis, Mutagenesis, and Impairment of Fertility—Although no long-term studies in animals have been performed to evaluate carcinogenic potential, no mutagenic potential of cefuroxime was found in standard laboratory tests.

Reproductive studies revealed no impairment of fertility in animals.

Usage in Pregnancy—Pregnancy Category B—Reproduction studies have been performed in mice and rabbits at doses up to 60 times the human dose and have revealed no evidence of impaired fertility or harm to the fetus due to cefuroxime. There are, however, no adequate well-controlled studies in pregnant women. Because animal reproduction studies are not always predictive of human response, this drug should be used during pregnancy only if clearly needed.

Nursing Mothers—Since Kefurox is excreted in human milk, caution should be exercised when Kefurox is administered to a nursing woman.

Pediatric Use—Safety and effectiveness in children below the age of 3 months have not been established. Accumulation of other members of the cephalosporin class in newborn infants (with resulting prolongation of drug half-life) has been reported.

ADVERSE REACTIONS

Kefurox is generally well tolerated. The most common adverse effects have been local reactions following intravenous administration. Other adverse reactions have been encountered only rarely.

Local Reactions—Thrombophlebitis has occurred with intravenous administration in 1 in 60 patients.

Gastrointestinal—Gastrointestinal symptoms occurred in 1 in 150 patients and included diarrhea (1 in 220 patients) and nausea (1 in 440 patients). Symptoms of pseudomembranous colitis can appear during or after antibiotic treatment. Vomiting has been reported.

Hypersensitivity Reactions—Hypersensitivity reactions have been reported in less than 1% of the patients treated with Kefurox and include rash (1 in 125). Pruritus and urticaria and positive Coombs' test each occurred in less than 1 in 250 patients, and, as with other cephalosporins, cases of anaphylaxis have occurred rarely. Erythema multiforme and Stevens-Johnson syndrome have occurred.

Blood—A decrease in hemoglobin and hematocrit has been observed in 1 in 10 patients and transient eosinophilia in 1 in 14 patients. Less common reactions seen were transient neutropenia (less than 1 in 100 patients) and leukopenia (1 in 750 patients). A similar pattern and incidence were seen with other cephalosporins used in controlled studies. Hemolysis, aplastic anemia, agranulocytosis, pancytopenia, prolonged prothrombin time, and thrombocytopenia have been reported.

Hepatic—Transient rise in AST and ALT (1 in 25 patients), alkaline phosphatase (1 in 50 patients), LDH (1 in 75 patients), and bilirubin (1 in 500 patients) levels has been noted.

Kidney—Elevations in serum creatinine and/or blood urea nitrogen and a decreased creatinine clearance have been observed, but their relationship to cefuroxime is unknown.

Other—Delayed sterilization of cerebrospinal fluid has been reported in occasional children treated with cefuroxime for bacterial meningitis. Moderate to severe hearing impairment has occurred as a complication of meningitis in occasional children treated with cefuroxime for bacterial meningitis. Fever has been reported.

OVERDOSAGE

Signs and Symptoms—Experience with overdose of cefuroxime sodium in humans is limited. The administration of inappropriately large doses of parenteral cephalosporins may cause seizures, particularly in patients with renal failure in whom accumulation is likely to occur.

The oral median lethal dose in the adult mouse was >10 g/kg, representing 83 times the routine maximum adult dose. In animals, doses up to 5 g/kg produced no tissue toxicity. With chronic doses greater than 5 g/kg, tubular necrosis was seen in animals.

Treatment—To obtain up-to-date information about the treatment of overdose, a good resource is your certified Regional Poison Control Center. Telephone numbers of certified poison control centers are listed in the *Physicians' Desk Reference (PDR)*. In managing overdosage, consider the possibility of multiple drug overdoses, interaction among drugs, and unusual drug kinetics in your patient.

Protect the patient's airway and support ventilation and perfusion. Meticulously monitor and maintain, within acceptable limits, the patient's vital signs, blood gases, serum electrolytes, etc. If the patient develops convulsions, the drug should be promptly discontinued; anticonvulsant therapy may be administered if clinically indicated. The use of hemodialysis in the treatment of cefuroxime overdose has not been established.

DOSAGE AND ADMINISTRATION

Adults—The usual adult dosage range for Kefurox is 750 mg to 1.5 g every 8 hours, usually for 5 to 10 days. In uncomplicated urinary tract infections, skin and skin structure infections, disseminated gonococcal infections, and uncomplicated pneumonia, a 750-mg dose every 8 hours is recommended. In severe or complicated infections, a 1.5-g dose every 8 hours is recommended.

In bone and joint infections, a dosage of 1.5 g every 8 hours is recommended. In clinical trials, surgical intervention was performed, when indicated, as an adjunct to therapy with Kefurox. A course of oral antibiotic therapy was administered when appropriate following the completion of parenteral administration of Kefurox.

In life-threatening infections or infections due to less susceptible organisms, 1.5 g every 6 hours may be required. In bacterial meningitis, the dose should not exceed 3.0 g every 8 hours. The recommended dose for uncomplicated gonococcal infection is 1.5 g intramuscularly given as a single dose at two different sites together with 1.0 g of oral probenecid. For preventive use for clean-contaminated or potentially contaminated surgical procedures, a 1.5-g dose administered intravenously just prior to surgery (approximately ½ to 1 hour before the initial incision) is recommended. Thereafter, give 750 mg intravenously or intramuscularly every 8 hours when the procedure is prolonged.

For preventive use during open heart surgery, a 1.5-g dose administered intravenously at the induction of anesthesia and every 12 hours thereafter for a total of 6.0 g is recommended.

Impaired Renal Function—When renal function is impaired, a reduced dosage must be employed. Dosage should be determined by the degree of renal impairment and the susceptibility of the causative organism (see Table 1).

TABLE 1: Dosage of Kefurox in Adults With Reduced Renal Function

Creatinine Clearance (mL/min)	Dose	Frequency
>20	750 mg–1.5 g	Every 8 hours
10–20	750 mg	Every 12 hours
<10	750 mg	Every 24 hours*

*Since Kefurox is dialyzable, patients on hemodialysis should be given a further dose at the end of the dialysis.

When only serum creatinine is available, the following formula (based on sex, weight, and age of the patient) may be used to convert this value into creatinine clearance. The serum creatinine should represent a steady state of renal function.

$$\text{Males:} \quad \frac{\text{Weight (kg)} \times (140 - \text{age})}{72 \times \text{serum creatinine (mg/100 mL)}}$$

$$\text{Females:} \quad 0.9 \times \text{above value}$$

Note: As with antibiotic therapy in general, administration of Kefurox should be continued for a minimum of 48 to 72 hours after the patient becomes asymptomatic or after evidence of bacterial eradication has been obtained; a minimum of 10 days of treatment is recommended in infections caused by *S. pyogenes* in order to guard against the risk of rheumatic fever or glomerulonephritis; frequent bacteriologic and clinical appraisal is necessary during therapy of chronic urinary tract infection and may be required for several months after therapy has been completed; persistent infections may require treatment for several weeks; and doses smaller than those indicated above should not be used. In staphylococcal and other infections involving a collection of pus, surgical drainage should be carried out when indicated.

Infants and Children Above 3 Months of Age—Administration of 50 to 100 mg/kg/day in equally divided doses, every 6 to 8 hours, has been successful for most infections susceptible to cefuroxime. The higher dose of 100 mg/kg/day (not to exceed the maximum adult dose) should be used for the more severe or serious infections.

In cases of bacterial meningitis, larger doses of Kefurox are recommended, initially 200 to 240 mg/kg/day intravenously in divided doses every 6 to 8 hours.

In children with renal insufficiency, the frequency of dosage should be modified to be consistent with the recommendations for adults.

Preparation of Solution and Suspension—The directions for preparing Kefurox for both intravenous and intramuscular use are summarized in Table 2.

For Intramuscular Use—Each 750-mg/10 mL vial of Kefurox should be reconstituted with 3.6 mL of Sterile Water for Injection. Shake gently to disperse and withdraw 3.6 mL of the resulting suspension for injection.

For Intravenous Use—Each 750-mg/10 mL vial should be reconstituted with 9.0 mL of Sterile Water for Injection. Withdraw 8.0 mL of the resulting solution for injection.

Each 1.5-g/20 mL vial should be reconstituted with 14.0 mL of Sterile Water for Injection and the solution completely withdrawn for injection.

For infusion, each 750-mg or 1.5-g dose should be reconstituted with 50 to 100 mL of Sterile Water for Injection, 5% Dextrose Injection, 0.9% Sodium Chloride Injection, or any of the solutions listed under the Intravenous portion of the Compatibility and Stability section. If Sterile Water for Injection is used as the diluent, reconstitute with approximately 20 mL/g to avoid a hypotonic solution.

[See table 2 at top of next page.]

Administration—After reconstitution, Kefurox may be given intravenously or by deep intramuscular injection into a large muscle mass (such as the gluteus or lateral part of the thigh). Prior to injecting intramuscularly, aspiration is necessary to avoid inadvertent injection into a blood vessel.

Intravenous Administration—The intravenous route may be preferable for patients with bacterial septicemia or other severe or life-threatening infections or for patients who may be poor risks because of decreased resistance, particularly if shock is present or impending.

For Direct Intermittent Intravenous Administration—Slowly inject the solution into a vein over a period of 3 to 5 minutes or give it through the tubing system by which the patient is also receiving other intravenous solutions.

For Intermittent Intravenous Infusion with a Y-Type Administration Set—Dosing can be accomplished through the tubing system by which the patient may be receiving other intravenous solutions. However, during infusion of the solution containing Kefurox, it is advisable to temporarily dis-

TABLE 2
Preparation of Solution and Suspension
(Glass Vials, ADD-Vantage®, and Faspak)

Strength	Amount of Diluent to Be Added (mL)		Volume to Be Withdrawn (mL)	Approximate Concentration (mg/mL)
750 mg/10 mL vial	3.6	(IM)	3.6*	220
750 mg/10 mL vial	9	(IV)	8	100
1.5 g/20 mL vial	14	(IV)	Total	100
750 mg/100 mL bottle	50	(IV)	—	15
750 mg/100 mL bottle	100	(IV)	—	7.5
1.5 g/100 mL bottle	50	(IV)	—	30
1.5 g/100 mL bottle	100	(IV)	—	15
750 mg/Faspak	50	(IV)	—	15
750 mg/Faspak	100	(IV)	—	7.5
1.5 g/Faspak	50	(IV)	—	30
1.5 g/Faspak	100	(IV)	—	15
750 mg/ADD-Vantage†	50	(IV)	—	15
750 mg/ADD-Vantage†	100	(IV)	—	7.5
1.5 g/ADD-Vantage†	50	(IV)	—	30
1.5 g/ADD-Vantage†	100	(IV)	—	15

* KEFUROX is a suspension at IM concentrations.
† Instructions for use of the ADD-Vantage Vials are enclosed in the package.

continue administration of any other solutions at the same site.

For Continuous Intravenous Infusion —A solution of Kefurox may be added to an intravenous bottle containing 1 of the following fluids:

0.9% Sodium Chloride Injection, 5% Dextrose Injection, 10% Dextrose Injection, 5% Dextrose and 0.9% Sodium Chloride Injection, 5% Dextrose and 0.45% Sodium Chloride Injection, and M/6 Sodium Lactate Injection

Solutions of Kefurox, like those of most β-lactam antibiotics, should not be added to solutions of aminoglycoside antibiotics because of potential interaction. However, if concurrent therapy with Kefurox and an aminoglycoside is indicated, each of these antibiotics can be administered separately to the same patient.

Compatibility and Stability —Intramuscular—When reconstituted as directed with Sterile Water for Injection, suspensions of Kefurox for intramuscular injection maintain satisfactory potency for 24 hours at room temperature and for 48 hours under refrigeration (5°C).

After the periods mentioned above, any unused suspensions should be discarded.

Intravenous—When the 750-mg and 1.5-g vials are reconstituted as directed with Sterile Water for Injection, the solutions of Kefurox for intravenous administration maintain satisfactory potency for 24 hours at room temperature and for 48 hours under refrigeration (5°C). More dilute solutions, such as 750 mg or 1.5 g reconstituted with 50 to 100 mL of Sterile Water for Injection, 5% Dextrose Injection, or 0.9% Sodium Chloride Injection, maintain satisfactory potency for 24 hours at room temperature and for 7 days under refrigeration.

These solutions may be further diluted to concentrations of between 1 mg/mL and 30 mg/mL in the following solutions and will lose not more than 10% activity for 24 hours at room temperature or for at least 7 days under refrigeration: 0.9% Sodium Chloride Injection, M/6 Sodium Lactate Injection, Ringer's Injection USP, Lactated Ringer's Injection USP, 5% Dextrose and 0.9% Sodium Chloride Injection, 5% Dextrose Injection, 5% Dextrose and 0.45% Sodium Chloride Injection, 5% Dextrose and 0.225% Sodium Chloride Injection, 10% Dextrose Injection, or 10% Invert Sugar in Water for Injection.

Unused solutions should be discarded after the time periods mentioned above.

Kefurox has also been found compatible for 24 hours at room temperature when admixed in intravenous infusion with the following: Heparin (10 and 50 units/mL) in 0.9% Sodium Chloride Injection, or Potassium Chloride (10 and 40 mEq/L) in 0.9% Sodium Chloride Injection.

Note: Prior to administration, parenteral drug products should be inspected visually for particulate matter and discoloration whenever solution and container permit.

As with other cephalosporins, however, cefuroxime powder as well as solutions and suspensions tend to darken depending on storage conditions without adversely affecting product potency.

Protect from light. Prior to reconstitution, store at controlled room temperature, 59° to 86°F (15° to 30°C).

HOW SUPPLIED
Vials:
750 mg,* 10-mL size (No. 7271)—(Traypak† of 25) NDC 0002-7271-25
1.5 g,* 20-mL size (No. 7272)—(Traypak of 10) NDC 0002-7272-10
750 mg,* 100-mL size (No. 7273)—(Traypak of 10) NDC 0002-7273-10

1.5 g,* 100-mL size (No. 7274)—(Traypak of 10) NDC 0002-7274-10
Faspak‡:
750 mg (No. 7276)—(24s) NDC 0002-7276-24
1.5 g (No. 7277)—(24s) NDC 0002-7277-24
ADD-Vantage§ Vials:
750 mg,* (No. 7278)—(Traypak of 25) NDC 0002-7278-25
1.5 g,* (No. 7279)—(Traypak of 10) NDC 0002-7279-10
The above ADD-Vantage Vials are to be used with Abbott Laboratories' ADD-Vantage Antibiotic Diluent Container. Instructions for use of the ADD-Vantage Vials are enclosed in the package.
Also available:
Pharmacy Bulk Package;
7.5 g,* 100-mL size (No. 7275)—(Traypak of 6) NDC 0002-7275-16

* Equivalent to cefuroxime.
† Traypak™ (multivial carton, Lilly)
‡ Faspak® (flexible plastic bag, Lilly)
§ ADD-Vantage® (vials and diluent containers, Abbott).
CAUTION—Federal (USA) law prohibits dispensing without prescription.

[081095]

KEFZOL®   ℞
[kĕf'zōl]
(Cefazolin Sodium)
Sterile, USP

DESCRIPTION
Kefzol® (Sterile Cefazolin Sodium, USP) is a sterile, semisynthetic cephalosporin for intramuscular or intravenous administration. It is 5-Thia-1-azabicyclo[4.2.0]oct-2-ene-2-carboxylic acid, 3-[[(5-methyl-1,3,4-thiadiazol-2-yl)thio]methyl]-8-oxo-7-[[(1H-tetrazol-1-yl) acetyl]amino]-, monosodium salt (6R-trans). The sodium content is 48.3 mg/g of cefazolin sodium. In addition to cefazolin sodium, the Faspak® and the ADD-Vantage® System vial also contain 0.04% polysorbate 80.
The molecular formula is $C_{14}H_{13}N_8NaO_4S_3$. The molecular weight is 476.5. The structural formula is as follows:

The pH of the reconstituted solution is between 4.5 and 6.

CLINICAL PHARMACOLOGY
Human Pharmacology —Table 1 demonstrates the blood levels and duration of cefazolin following intramuscular administration.

TABLE 1. SERUM CONCENTRATIONS AFTER INTRAMUSCULAR ADMINISTRATION

	Serum Concentrations (µg/mL)					
Dose	1/2 h	1 h	2 h	4 h	6 h	8 h
250 mg	15.5	17	13	5.1	2.5	
500 mg	36.2	36.8	37.9	15.5	6.3	3
1 g*	60.1	63.8	54.3	29.3	13.2	7.1

*Average of 2 studies

Clinical pharmacology studies in patients hospitalized with infections indicate that cefazolin produces mean peak serum levels approximately equivalent to those seen in normal volunteers.

In a study (using normal volunteers) of constant intravenous infusion with dosages of 3.5 mg/kg for 1 hour (approximately 250 mg) and 1.5 mg/kg the next 2 hours (approximately 100 mg), cefazolin produced a steady serum level at the 3rd hour of approximately 28 µg/mL. Table 2 shows the average serum concentrations after IV injection of a single 1-g dose; average half-life was 1.4 hours.

TABLE 2. SERUM CONCENTRATIONS AFTER 1-G INTRAVENOUS DOSE

Serum Concentrations (µg/mL)					
5 min	15 min	30 min	1 h	2 h	4 h
188.4	135.8	106.8	73.7	45.6	16.5

Controlled studies on adult normal volunteers receiving 1 g 4 times a day for 10 days, monitoring CBC, AST (SGOT), ALT (SGPT), bilirubin, alkaline phosphatase, BUN, creatinine, and urinalysis, indicated no clinically significant changes attributed to cefazolin.

Cefazolin is excreted unchanged in the urine, primarily by glomerular filtration and, to a lesser degree, by tubular secretion. Following intramuscular injection of 500 mg, 56% to 89% of the administered dose is recovered within 6 hours and 80% to nearly 100% in 24 hours. Cefazolin achieves peak urine concentrations greater than 1,000 µg/mL and 4,000 µg/mL respectively following 500-mg and 1-g intramuscular doses.

In patients undergoing peritoneal dialysis (2 L/h), mean serum levels of cefazolin were approximately 10 and 30 µg/mL after 24 hours' instillation of a dialyzing solution containing 50 µg/mL and 150 µg/mL respectively. Mean peak levels were 29 µg/mL (range 13 to 44 µg/mL) with 50 µg/mL (3 patients) and 72 µg/mL (range 26 to 142 µg/mL) with 150 µg/ mL (6 patients). Intraperitoneal administration of cefazolin is usually well tolerated.

When cefazolin is administered to patients with unobstructed biliary tracts, high concentrations well over serum levels occur in the gallbladder tissue and bile. In the presence of obstruction, however, concentration of the antibiotic is considerably lower in bile than in serum.

Cefazolin readily crosses an inflamed synovial membrane, and the concentration of the antibiotic achieved in the joint space is comparable to levels measured in the serum.

Cefazolin readily crosses the placental barrier into the cord blood and amniotic fluid. It is present in very low concentrations in the milk of nursing mothers.

Microbiology —In vitro tests demonstrate that the bactericidal action of cephalosporins results from inhibition of cellwall synthesis. Kefzol® (Sterile Cefazolin Sodium, USP) is active against the following organisms in vitro and in clinical infections.

Staphylococcus aureus (including penicillinase-producing strains)
Staphylococcus epidermidis
Methicillin-resistant staphylococci are uniformly resistant to cefazolin.
Group A β-hemolytic streptococci and other strains of streptococci (many strains of enterococci are resistant)
Streptococcus pneumoniae
Escherichia coli
Proteus mirabilis
Klebsiella sp.
Enterobacter aerogenes
Haemophilus influenzae
Most strains of indole-positive *Proteus* (*Proteus vulgaris*), *Enterobacter cloacae, Morganella morganii,* and *Providencia rettgeri* are resistant. *Serratia, Pseudomonas,* and *Acinetobacter calcoaceticus* (formerly *Mima* and *Herellea* sp.) are almost uniformly resistant to cefazolin.

Disk Susceptibility Tests —Quantitative methods that require measurement of zone diameters give the most precise estimates of antibiotic susceptibility. One such procedure* has been recommended for use with disks for testing susceptibility to cefazolin. With this procedure, a report from the laboratory of "susceptible" indicates that the infecting organism is likely to respond to therapy. A report of "resistant" indicates that the infecting organism is not likely to respond to therapy. A report of "moderately susceptible"

Continued on next page

Lilly—Cont.

suggests that the organism would be susceptible if high dosage is used or if the infection were confined to tissues and fluids (eg, urine) in which high antibiotic levels are attained.

* National Committee for Clinical Laboratory Standards (NCCLS), 1984. Performance Standards for Antimicrobial Disk Susceptibility Tests, Approved Standard, M2-A3, NCCLS, Villanova, PA 19085.

For gram-positive isolates, a zone of 18 mm is indicative of a cefazolin-susceptible organism when tested with either the cephalosporin-class disk (30 μg cephalothin) or the cefazolin disk (30 μg cefazolin).

Gram-negative organisms should be tested with the cefazolin disk (using the above criteria) because cefazolin has been shown by in vitro tests to have activity against certain strains of *Enterobacteriaceae* found to be resistant when tested with the cephalothin disk. When using the cephalothin disk, gram-negative organisms with zone diameters ≥ 18 mm may be considered susceptible to cefazolin; however, organisms with zone diameters less than 18 mm are not necessarily resistant or moderately susceptible to cefazolin.

The cefazolin disk should not be used for testing susceptibility to other cephalosporins.

Dilution Techniques —A bacterial isolate should be considered susceptible if the minimal inhibitory concentration (MIC) for cefazolin is ≤ 16 μg/mL. Organisms are considered resistant if the MIC is ≥ 64 μg/mL.

INDICATIONS AND USAGE

Kefzol is indicated in the treatment of the following serious infections due to susceptible organisms:

Respiratory tract infections due to *S. pneumoniae, Klebsiella* sp., *H. influenzae, S. aureus* (including penicillinase-producing strains), and group A β-hemolytic streptococci

Injectable penicillin G benzathine is considered to be the drug of choice in the treatment and prevention of streptococcal infections, including the prophylaxis of rheumatic fever. Kefzol is effective in the eradication of streptococci from the nasopharynx; however, data establishing the efficacy of Kefzol in the subsequent prevention of rheumatic fever are not available at present.

Genitourinary tract infections due to *E. coli, P. mirabilis, Klebsiella* sp., and some strains of *Enterobacter* and enterococci

Skin and skin structure infections due to *S. aureus* (including penicillinase-producing strains) and group A β-hemolytic streptococci and other strains of streptococci

Biliary tract infections due to *E. coli*, various strains of streptococci, *P. mirabilis, Klebsiella* sp., and *S. aureus*

Bone and joint infections due to *S. aureus*

Septicemia due to *S. pneumoniae, S. aureus* (penicillin-susceptible and penicillin-resistant), *P. mirabilis, E. coli,* and *Klebsiella* sp.

Endocarditis due to *S. aureus* (penicillin-susceptible and penicillin-resistant) and group A β-hemolytic streptococci

Appropriate culture and susceptibility studies should be performed to determine susceptibility of the causative organism to Kefzol.

Perioperative prophylaxis —The prophylactic administration of Kefzol preoperatively, intraoperatively, and postoperatively may reduce the incidence of certain postoperative infections in patients undergoing surgical procedures that are classified as contaminated or potentially contaminated (eg, vaginal hysterectomy or cholecystectomy in high-risk patients such as those over 70 years of age who have acute cholecystitis, obstructive jaundice, or common-bile-duct stones).

The perioperative use of Kefzol also may be effective in surgical patients in whom infection at the operative site would present a serious risk (eg, during open-heart surgery and prosthetic arthroplasty).

The prophylactic administration of Kefzol should usually be discontinued within a 24-hour period after the surgical procedure. For surgery in which the occurrence of infection may be particularly devastating (eg, open-heart surgery and prosthetic arthroplasty), the prophylactic administration of Kefzol may be continued for 3 to 5 days following the completion of surgery. If there are signs of infection, specimens for culture should be obtained for the identification of the causative organism so that appropriate therapy may be instituted (*see* Dosage and Administration).

CONTRAINDICATION

Kefzol is contraindicated in patients with known allergy to the cephalosporin group of antibiotics.

WARNINGS

BEFORE CEFAZOLIN THERAPY IS INSTITUTED, CAREFUL INQUIRY SHOULD BE MADE CONCERNING PREVIOUS HYPERSENSITIVITY REACTIONS TO CEPHALOSPORINS AND PENICILLIN. CEPHALOSPORIN C DERIVATIVES SHOULD BE GIVEN CAUTIOUSLY TO PENICILLIN-SENSITIVE PATIENTS.

SERIOUS ACUTE HYPERSENSITIVITY REACTIONS MAY REQUIRE EPINEPHRINE AND OTHER EMERGENCY MEASURES.

There is some clinical and laboratory evidence of partial cross-allergenicity of the penicillins and the cephalosporins. Patients have been reported to have had severe reactions (including anaphylaxis) to both drugs.

Antibiotics, including Kefzol, should be administered cautiously to any patient who has demonstrated some form of allergy, particularly to drugs.

Pseudomembranous colitis has been reported with nearly all antibacterial agents, including cefazolin, and may range in severity from mild to life-threatening. Therefore, it is important to consider this diagnosis in patients who present with diarrhea subsequent to the administration of antibacterial agents.

Treatment with antibacterial agents alters the normal flora of the colon and may permit overgrowth of clostridia. Studies indicate that a toxin produced by *Clostridium difficile* is one primary cause of "antibiotic-associated colitis." After the diagnosis of pseudomembranous colitis has been established, therapeutic measures should be initiated. Mild cases of pseudomembranous colitis usually respond to drug discontinuation alone. In moderate to severe cases, consideration should be given to management with fluids and electrolytes, protein supplementation, and treatment with an antibacterial drug clinically effective against *C. difficile* colitis.

Usage in Infants —Safety for use in prematures and infants under 1 month of age has not been established.

PRECAUTIONS

General —If an allergic reaction to Kefzol occurs, the drug should be discontinued and the patient treated with the usual agents (eg, epinephrine or other pressor amines, antihistamines, or corticosteroids).

Prolonged use of Kefzol may result in the overgrowth of nonsusceptible organisms. Careful clinical observation of the patient is essential. If superinfection occurs during therapy, appropriate measures should be taken.

When Kefzol is administered to patients with low urinary output because of impaired renal function, lower daily dosage is required (*see* Dosage and Administration).

The intrathecal administration of Kefzol is not an approved route of administration for this antibiotic; in fact, there have been reports of severe central nervous system (CNS) toxicity including seizures when cefazolin was administered in this manner.

Drug Interactions —Used concurrently, probenecid may decrease renal tubular secretion of cephalosporins, resulting in increased and more prolonged cephalosporin blood levels.

Drug/Laboratory Test Interactions —A false-positive reaction for glucose in the urine may occur with Benedict's solution, Fehling's solution, or Clinitest® tablets but not with enzyme-based tests, such as Clinistix® and Tes-Tape® (Glucose Enzymatic Test Strip, USP, Lilly).

Positive direct and indirect antiglobulin (Coombs') tests have occurred; these may also occur in neonates whose mothers received cephalosporins before delivery.

Broad-spectrum antibiotics should be prescribed with caution in individuals with a history of gastrointestinal disease, particularly colitis.

Carcinogenesis, Mutagenesis, Impairment of Fertility —Mutagenicity studies and long-term studies in animals to determine the carcinogenic potential of cefazolin have not been performed. Studies performed in rats have revealed no evidence of impaired fertility.

Pregnancy: Teratogenic Effects: Pregnancy Category B —Reproduction studies have been performed in rats given doses of 500 mg or 1 g of cefazolin/kg and have revealed no harm to the fetus due to Kefzol. There are, however, no adequate and well-controlled studies in pregnant women. Because animal reproduction studies are not always predictive of human response, this drug should be used during pregnancy only if clearly needed.

Labor and Delivery —When cefazolin has been administered prior to cesarean section, drug levels in cord blood have been measured to be approximately one fourth to one third of maternal drug levels. The drug appears to have no adverse effect on the fetus.

Nursing Mothers —Cefazolin is present in very low concentrations in the milk of nursing mothers. Caution should be exercised when cefazolin is administered to a nursing woman.

ADVERSE REACTIONS

The following reactions have been reported:

Hypersensitivity —Drug fever, skin rash, vulvar pruritus, eosinophilia, and anaphylaxis have occurred.

Blood —Neutropenia, leukopenia, thrombocythemia, and positive direct and indirect Coombs' tests have occurred.

Renal —Transient rise in BUN levels has been observed without clinical evidence of renal impairment. Interstitial nephritis and other renal disorders have been reported rarely. Most patients experiencing these reactions have been seriously ill and were receiving multiple drug therapies. The role of Kefzol in the development of nephropathies has not been determined.

Hepatic —Transient rise in AST, ALT, and alkaline phosphatase levels has been observed rarely. As with some penicillins and some other cephalosporins, transient hepatitis and cholestatic jaundice have been reported rarely.

Gastrointestinal —Symptoms of pseudomembranous colitis may appear either during or after antibiotic treatment. Nausea and vomiting have been reported rarely. Anorexia, diarrhea, and oral candidiasis (oral thrush) have been reported.

Other —Pain on intramuscular injection, sometimes with induration, has occurred infrequently. Phlebitis at the site of injection has been noted. Other reactions have included genital and anal pruritus, genital moniliasis, and vaginitis.

OVERDOSAGE

Signs and Symptoms—Toxic signs and symptoms following an overdose of cefazolin may include pain, inflammation, and phlebitis at the injection site.

The administration of inappropriately large doses of parenteral cephalosporins may cause dizziness, paresthesias, and headaches. Seizures may occur following overdosage with some cephalosporins, particularly in patients with renal impairment in whom accumulation is likely to occur.

Laboratory abnormalities that may occur after an overdose include elevations in creatinine, BUN, liver enzymes and bilirubin, a positive Coombs' test, thrombocytosis, thrombocytopenia, eosinophilia, leukopenia, and prolongation of the prothrombin time.

Treatment—To obtain up-to-date information about the treatment of overdose, a good resource is your certified Regional Poison Control Center. Telephone numbers of certified poison control centers are listed in the *Physicians' Desk Reference (PDR).* In managing overdosage, consider the possibility of multiple drug overdoses, interaction among drugs, and unusual drug kinetics in your patient.

If seizures occur, the drug should be discontinued promptly; anticonvulsant therapy may be administered if clinically indicated. Protect the patient's airway and support ventilation and perfusion. Meticulously monitor and maintain, within acceptable limits, the patient's vital signs, blood gases, serum electrolytes, etc.

In cases of severe overdosage, especially in a patient with renal failure, combined hemodialysis and hemoperfusion may be considered if response to more conservative therapy fails. However, no data supporting such therapy are available.

DOSAGE AND ADMINISTRATION

Kefzol may be administered intramuscularly or intravenously after reconstitution. However, the Faspak containers and the ADD-Vantage vials are for intravenous use only. Total daily dosages are the same for either route of administration.

The intrathecal administration of Kefzol is not an approved route of administration for this antibiotic; in fact, there have been reports of severe CNS toxicity including seizures when cefazolin was administered in this manner.

Intravenous Administration —Kefzol may be administered by intravenous injection or by continuous or intermittent infusion.

Intermittent intravenous infusion: Kefzol can be administered along with primary intravenous fluid management programs in a volume control set or in a separate, secondary IV bottle. Reconstituted 1 g of Kefzol may be diluted in 50 to 100 mL of 1 of the following intravenous solutions: 0.9% Sodium Chloride Injection, 5% or 10% Dextrose Injection, 5% Dextrose in Lactated Ringer's Injection, 5% Dextrose and 0.9% Sodium Chloride Injection (also may be used with 5% Dextrose and 0.45% or 0.2% Sodium Chloride Injection), Lactated Ringer's Injection, 5% or 10% Invert Sugar in Sterile Water for Injection, Ringer's Injection, Normosol®-M in D5-W, Ionosol® B with Dextrose 5%, or Plasma-Lyte® with 5% Dextrose.

ADD-Vantage Vials of Kefzol are to be reconstituted *only* with 0.9% Sodium Chloride Injection or 5% Dextrose Injection in the 50-mL or 100-mL Flexible Diluent Containers.

Intravenous injection (Administer solution directly into vein or though tubing): Dilute the reconstituted 1 g of Kefzol in a minimum of 10 mL of Sterile Water for Injection. Inject solution slowly over 3 to 5 minutes. Do not inject in less than 3 minutes. (NOTE: ADD-VANTAGE VIALS ARE NOT TO BE USED IN THIS MANNER.)

Dosage —The usual adult dosages are given in Table 3.

TABLE 3. USUAL ADULT DOSAGE

Type of Infection	Dose	Frequency
Pneumococcal pneumonia	500 mg	q12h
Mild infections caused by susceptible gram-positive cocci	250 to 500 mg	q8h

Acute uncomplicated urinary tract infections	1 g	q12h
Moderate to severe infections	500 mg to 1 g	q6 to 8h
Severe, life-threatening infections (eg, endocarditis and septicemia)*	1 g to 1.5 g	q6h

*In rare instances, doses up to 12 g of cefazolin per day have been used.

Dosage Adjustment for Patients With Reduced Renal Function—Kefzol may be used in patients with reduced renal function with the following dosage adjustments: Patients with a creatinine clearance of ≥ 55 mL/min or a serum creatinine of ≤ 1.5 mg % can be given full doses. Patients with creatinine clearance rates of 35 to 54 mL/min or serum creatinine of 1.6 to 3.0 mg % can also be given full doses, but dosage should be restricted to at least 8-hour intervals. Patients with creatinine clearance rates of 11 to 34 mL/min or serum creatinine of 3.1 to 4.5 mg % should be given one half the usual dose every 12 hours. Patients with creatinine clearance rates of ≤ 10 mL/min or serum creatinine of ≥ 4.6 mg % should be given one half the usual dose every 18 to 24 hours. All reduced dosage recommendations apply after an initial loading dose appropriate to the severity of the infection. For information about peritoneal dialysis, see *Human Pharmacology*.

Perioperative Prophylactic Use—To prevent postoperative infection in contaminated or potentially contaminated surgery, the recommended doses are as follows:

a. 1 g IV or IM administered one half to 1 hour prior to the start of surgery.
b. For lengthy operative procedures (eg, 2 hours or longer), 0.5 to 1 g IV or IM during surgery (administration modified according to the duration of the operative procedure).
c. 0.5 to 1 g IV or IM every 6 to 8 hours for 24 hours postoperatively.

It is important that (1) the preoperative dose be given just prior (one half to 1 hour) to the start of surgery so that adequate antibiotic levels are present in the serum and tissues at the time of the initial surgical incision and (2) if exposure to infectious organisms is likely, Kefzol be administered at appropriate intervals during surgery in order that sufficient levels of the antibiotic be present when needed.

In surgery in which infection may be particularly devastating (eg, open-heart surgery and prosthetic arthroplasty), the prophylactic administration of Kefzol may be continued for 3 to 5 days following the completion of surgery.

In children, a total daily dosage of 25 to 50 mg/kg (approximately 10 to 20 mg/lb) of body weight, divided into 3 or 4 equal doses, is effective for most mild to moderately severe infections (Table 4). Total daily dosage may be increased to 100 mg/kg (45 mg/lb) of body weight for severe infections.

TABLE 4. PEDIATRIC DOSAGE GUIDE

Weight		25 mg/kg/Day Divided into 3 Doses		25 mg/kg/Day Divided into 4 Doses	
lb	kg	Approximate Single Dose (mg q8h)	Vol (mL) Needed with Dilution of 125 mg/mL	Approximate Single Dose (mg q6h)	Vol (mL) Needed with Dilution of 125 mg/mL
10	4.5	40 mg	0.35 mL	30 mg	0.25 mL
20	9	75 mg	0.6 mL	55 mg	0.45 mL
30	13.6	115 mg	0.9 mL	85 mg	0.7 mL
40	18.1	150 mg	1.2 mL	115 mg	0.9 mL
50	22.7	190 mg	1.5 mL	140 mg	1.1 mL

Weight		50 mg/kg/Day Divided into 3 Doses		50 mg/kg/Day Divided into 4 Doses	
lb	kg	Approximate Single Dose (mg q8h)	Vol (mL) Needed with Dilution of 225 mg/mL	Approximate Single Dose (mg q6h)	Vol (mL) Needed with Dilution of 225 mg/mL
10	4.5	75 mg	0.35 mL	55 mg	0.25 mL
20	9	150 mg	0.7 mL	110 mg	0.5 mL
30	13.6	225 mg	1 mL	170 mg	0.75 mL
40	18.1	300 mg	1.35 mL	225 mg	1 mL
50	22.7	375 mg	1.7 mL	285 mg	1.25 mL

In children with mild to moderate renal impairment (creatinine clearance of 70 to 40 mL/min), 60% of the normal daily dosage given in divided doses every 12 hours should be sufficient. In children with moderate impairment (creatinine clearance of 40 to 20 mL/min), 25% of the normal daily dosage given in divided doses every 12 hours should be sufficient. In children with severe impairment (creatinine clearance of 20 to 5 mL/min), 10% of the normal daily dosage given every 24 hours should be adequate. All dosage recommendations apply after an initial loading dose is administered.

Since safety for use in premature infants and in infants under 1 month of age has not been established, the use of Kefzol in these patients is not recommended.

STABILITY

In those situations in which the drug and diluent have been mixed, but not immediately administered to the patient, the admixture may be stored under the following conditions:

Faspak Containers—Reconstituted Kefzol diluted in Sterile Water for Injection, 5% Dextrose Injection, or 0.9% Sodium Chloride Injection, is stable for 24 hours at room temperature and for 10 days if stored under refrigeration, 2° to 8°C (36° to 46°F).

Solutions of Kefzol in Sterile Water for Injection, 5% Dextrose Injection, or 0.9% Sodium Chloride Injection that are frozen immediately after reconstitution in the original vials or Faspak containers are stable for as long as 12 weeks if stored at −20°C. Once thawed, these solutions are stable for 24 hours at room temperature or for 10 days if stored under refrigeration, 2° to 8°C (36° to 46° F). If the product is warmed, care should be taken to avoid heating it after the thawing is complete. Once thawed, the solution should not be refrozen.

Secondary Diluents—Solutions of Kefzol for infusion in 10% Dextrose Injection, 5% Dextrose in Lactated Ringer's Injection, 5% Dextrose and 0.9% Sodium Chloride Injection (also may be used with 5% Dextrose and 0.45% or 0.2% Sodium Chloride Injection), Lactated Ringer's Injection, 5% or 10% Invert Sugar in Sterile Water for Injection, Ringer's Injection, Normosol®-M in D5-W, Ionosol®-B with Dextrose 5%, or Plasma-Lyte with 5% Dextrose should be used within 24 hours after dilution if stored at room temperature or within 96 hours if stored under refrigeration, 2° to 8° C (36° to 46° F). (DO NOT FREEZE KEFZOL DILUTED WITH THE ABOVE DILUENTS.)

ADD-Vantage Vials—*Only* 0.9% Sodium Chloride Injection and 5% Dextrose Injection in the 50-mL or 100-mL Flexible Diluent Containers are approved for reconstituting ADD-Vantage Kefzol. Ordinarily, ADD-Vantage vials should be reconstituted only when it is certain that the patient is ready to receive the drug. However, reconstituted Kefzol diluted in 5% Dextrose Injection and 0.9% Sodium Chloride Injection is stable for 24 hours at room temperature. (DO NOT REFRIGERATE OR FREEZE KEFZOL IN ADD-VANTAGE VIALS.)

Prior to administration, parenteral drug products should be inspected visually for particulate matter and discoloration whenever solution and container permit.

HOW SUPPLIED

Faspak*:
1 g,† (No. 7202)‡—(Faspak of 96) NDC 0002-7202-74
ADD-Vantage§ Vials:
500 mg,† (No. 7265)—(Traypak‖ of 25) NDC 0002-7265-25
1 g,† (No. 7266)—(Traypak of 25) NDC 0002-7266-25

The above ADD-Vantage Vials are to be used *only* with Abbott Laboratories' 50-mL or 100-mL Flexible Diluent Containers containing 0.9% Sodium Chloride Injection or 5% Dextrose Injection.

Instructions for use of the ADD-Vantage Vials are enclosed in the package.

Also available:
Vials:
500 mg,† 10-mL size (No. 767)—(Traypak of 25) NDC 0002-1497-25
1 gram,† 10-mL size (No. 768)—(Traypak of 25) NDC 0002-1498-25
1 gram,† 100-mL size (No. 7011)‡—(Traypak of 10) NDC 0002-7011-10
Pharmacy Bulk Package:
10 g,† 100-mL size (No. 7014)—(Traypak of 6) NDC 0002-7014-16

* Faspak® (flexible plastic bag, Lilly).
† Equivalent to cefazolin.
‡ For IV use.
‖ Traypak™ (multivial carton, Lilly).
§ ADD-Vantage® (vials and diluent containers, Abbott).

[102093]

LENTE® ILETIN® I AND II   OTC
(insulin zinc suspension, Lilly) See under Iletin® (insulin)

LORABID™   ℞
[lŏr 'ă-bĭd]
(Loracarbef, USP)

DESCRIPTION

LORABID™ (loracarbef, USP) is a synthetic β-lactam antibiotic of the carbacephem class for oral administration. Chemically, carbacephems differ from cephalosporin-class antibiotics in the dihydrothiazine ring where a methylene group has been substituted for a sulfur atom.

The chemical name for loracarbef is (6R, 7S)-7-[(R)-2-amino-2-phenylacetamido]-3-chloro-8-oxo-1-azabicyclo[4.2.0] oct-2-ene-2-carboxylic acid, monohydrate. It is a white to off-white solid with a molecular weight of 367.8. The empirical formula is $C_{16}H_{16}ClN_3O_4 \cdot H_2O$. The structural formula is:

Lorabid Pulvules® (loracarbef capsules, USP) and Lorabid for Oral Suspension (loracarbef for oral suspension, USP) are intended for oral administration only.

Each Pulvule contains loracarbef equivalent to 200 mg (0.57 mmol) or 400 mg (1.14 mmol) anhydrous loracarbef activity. They also contain cornstarch, dimethicone, F D & C Blue No. 2, gelatin, iron oxides, magnesium stearate, titanium dioxide, and other inactive ingredients.

After reconstitution, each 5 mL of Lorabid for Oral Suspension contains loracarbef equivalent to 100 mg (0.286 mmol) or 200 mg (0.57 mmol) anhydrous loracarbef activity. The suspensions also contain cellulose, F D & C Red No. 40, flavors, methylparaben, propylparaben, simethicone emulsion, sodium carboxymethylcellulose, sucrose, and xanthan gum.

CLINICAL PHARMACOLOGY

Loracarbef, after oral administration, was approximately 90% absorbed from the gastrointestinal tract. When capsules were taken with food, peak plasma concentrations were 50% to 60% of those achieved when the drug was administered to fasting subjects and occurred from 30 to 60 minutes later. Total absorption, as measured by urinary recovery and area under the plasma concentration versus time curve (AUC), was unchanged. The effect of food on the rate and extent of absorption of the suspension formulation has not been studied to date.

The pharmacokinetics of loracarbef were linear over the recommended dosage range of 200 to 400 mg, with no accumulation of the drug noted when it was given twice daily. Average peak plasma concentrations after administration of 200-mg or 400-mg single doses of loracarbef as capsules to fasting subjects were approximately 8 and 14 μg/mL, respectively, and were obtained within 1.2 hours after dosing. The average peak plasma concentration in adults following a 400-mg single dose of suspension was 17 μg/mL and was obtained within 0.8 hour after dosing (*see* Table).

Dosage (mg)	Mean Plasma Loracarbef Concentrations (μg/mL)	
	Peak Cmax	Time to Peak Tmax
Capsule (single dose)		
200 mg	8	1.2 h
400 mg	14	1.2 h
Suspension (single dose)		
400 mg (adult)	17	0.8 h
7.5 mg/kg (pediatric)	13	0.8 h
15 mg/kg (pediatric)	19	0.8 h

Following administration of 7.5 and 15 mg/kg single doses of oral suspension to children, average peak plasma concentrations were 13 and 19 μg/mL, respectively, and were obtained within 40 to 60 minutes.

This increased rate of absorption (suspension > capsule) should be taken into consideration if the oral suspension is to be substituted for the capsule, and capsules should not be

Continued on next page

---

* Identi-Code® symbol. This product information was prepared in June 1996. Current information on these and other products of Eli Lilly and Company may be obtained by direct inquiry to Lilly Research Laboratories, Lilly Corporate Center, Indianapolis, Indiana 46285, 800-545-5979.

Lilly—Cont.

substituted for the oral suspension in the treatment of otitis media (*see* **DOSAGE AND ADMINISTRATION**).

The elimination half-life was an average of 1.0 h in patients with normal renal function. Concomitant administration of probenecid decreased the rate of urinary excretion and increased the half-life to 1.5 hours.

In subjects with moderate impairment of renal function (creatinine clearance 10 to 50 mL/min/1.73 m^2), following a single 400-mg dose, the plasma half-life was prolonged to approximately 5.6 hours. In subjects with severe renal impairment (creatinine clearance <10 mL/min/1.73 m^2), the half-life was increased to approximately 32 hours. During hemodialysis the half-life was approximately 4 hours. In patients with severe renal impairment, the C_{max} increased from 15.4 μg/mL to 23 μg/mL (*see* **PRECAUTIONS** *and* **DOSAGE AND ADMINISTRATION**).

In single-dose studies, plasma half-life and AUC were not significantly altered in healthy elderly subjects with normal renal function.

There is no evidence of metabolism of loracarbef in humans. Approximately 25% of circulating loracarbef is bound to plasma proteins.

Middle-ear fluid concentrations of loracarbef were approximately 48% of the plasma concentration 2 hours after drug administration in children. The peak concentration of loracarbef in blister fluid was approximately half that obtained in plasma. Adequate data on CSF levels of loracarbef are not available.

Microbiology—Loracarbef exerts its bactericidal action by binding to essential target proteins of the bacterial cell wall, leading to inhibition of cell-wall synthesis. It is stable in the presence of some bacterial β-lactamases. Loracarbef has been shown to be active against most strains of the following organisms both *in vitro* and in clinical infections (*see* **INDICATIONS AND USAGE**):

Gram-positive aerobes:
- *Staphylococcus aureus* (including penicillinase-producing strains)
  - NOTE: Loracarbef (like most β-lactam antimicrobials) is inactive against methicillin-resistant staphylococci.
- *Staphylococcus saprophyticus*
- *Streptococcus pneumoniae*
- *Streptococcus pyogenes*

Gram-negative aerobes:
- *Escherichia coli*
- *Haemophilus influenzae* (including β-lactamase-producing strains)
- *Moraxella (Branhamella) catarrhalis* (including β-lactamase-producing strains)

The following *in vitro* data are available: however, their clinical significance is unknown.

Loracarbef exhibits *in vitro* minimum inhibitory concentrations (MIC) of 8 μg/mL or less against most strains of the following organisms; however, the safety and efficacy of loracarbef in treating clinical infections due to these organisms have not been established in adequate and well-controlled trials.

Gram-positive aerobes:
- *Staphylococcus epidermidis*
- *Streptococcus agalactiae* (group B streptococci)
- *Streptococcus bovis*
- Streptococci, groups C, F, and G
- viridans group streptococci

Gram-negative aerobes:
- *Citrobacter diversus*
- *Haemophilus parainfluenzae*
- *Klebsiella pneumoniae*
- *Neisseria gonorrhoeae* (including penicillinase-producing strains)
- *Pasteurella multocida*
- *Proteus mirabilis*
- *Salmonella* species
- *Shigella* species
- *Yersinia enterocolitica*

NOTE: Loracarbef is inactive against most strains of *Acinetobacter, Enterobacter, Morganella morganii, Proteus vulgaris, Providencia, Pseudomonas,* and *Serratia.*

Anaerobic organisms:
- *Clostridium perfringens*
- *Fusobacterium necrophorum*
- *Peptococcus niger*
- *Peptostreptococcus intermedius*
- *Propionibacterium acnes*

Susceptibility Testing

Diffusion Techniques—Quantitative methods that require measurement of zone diameters give the most precise estimate of the susceptibility of bacteria to antimicrobial agents. One such standardized method[1] has been recommended for use with the 30-μg loracarbef disk. Interpretation involves the correlation of the diameter obtained in the disk test with MIC for loracarbef.

Reports from the laboratory giving results of the standard single-disk susceptibility test with a 30-μg loracarbef disk should be interpreted according to the following criteria:

Zone Diameter (mm)	Interpretation
≥ 18	(S) Susceptible
15–17	(MS) Moderately Susceptible
≤ 14	(R) Resistant

A report of "susceptible" implies that the pathogen is likely to be inhibited by generally achievable blood concentrations. A report of "moderately susceptible" indicates that inhibitory concentrations of the antibiotic may be achieved if high dosage is used or if the infection is confined to tissues and fluids (e.g., urine) in which high antibiotic concentrations are attained. A report of "resistant" indicates that achievable concentrations of the antibiotic are unlikely to be inhibitory and other therapy should be selected.

Standardized procedures require the use of laboratory control organisms. The 30-μg loracarbef disk should give the following zone diameters with the NCCLS approved procedure:

Organism	Zone Diameter (mm)
E. coli ATCC 25922	23–29
S. aureus ATCC 25923	23–31

Dilution Techniques—Use a standardized dilution method[2] (broth, agar, or microdilution) or equivalent with loracarbef powder. The MIC values obtained should be interpreted according to the following criteria:

MIC (μg/mL)	Interpretation
≤8	(S) Susceptible
16	(MS) Moderately Susceptible
≥32	(R) Resistant

As with standard diffusion methods, dilution procedures require the use of laboratory control organisms. Standard loracarbef powder should give the following MIC values with the NCCLS approved procedure:

Organism	MIC Range (μg/mL)
E. coli ATCC 25922	0.5–2
S. aureus ATCC 29213	0.5–2

INDICATIONS AND USAGE

Lorabid is indicated in the treatment of patients with mild to moderate infections caused by susceptible strains of the designated microorganisms in the conditions listed below. (As recommended dosages, durations of therapy, and applicable patient populations vary among these infections, please see **DOSAGE AND ADMINISTRATION** for specific recommendations.)

Lower Respiratory Tract

Secondary Bacterial Infection of Acute Bronchitis caused by *S. pneumoniae, H. influenzae* (including β-lactamase-producing strains), or *M. catarrhalis* (including β-lactamase-producing strains).

Acute Bacterial Exacerbations of Chronic Bronchitis caused by *S. pneumoniae, H. influenzae* (including β-lactamase-producing strains), or *M. catarrhalis* (including β-lactamase-producing strains).

Pneumonia caused by *S. pneumoniae or H. influenzae* (non-β-lactamase-producing strains only). Data are insufficient at this time to establish efficacy in patients with pneumonia caused by β-lactamase-producing strains of *H. influenzae.*

Upper Respiratory Tract

Otitis Media† caused by *S. pneumoniae, H. influenzae* (including β-lactamase-producing strains), *M. catarrhalis* (including β-lactamase-producing strains), or *S. pyogenes.*

Acute Maxillary Sinusitis† caused by *S. pneumoniae, H. influenzae* (non-β-lactamase-producing strains only), or *M. catarrhalis* (including β-lactamase-producing strains). Data are insufficient at this time to establish efficacy in patients with acute maxillary sinusitis caused by β-lactamase-producing strains of *H. influenzae.*

†NOTE: In a patient population with significant numbers of β-lactamase-producing organisms, loracarbef's clinical cure and bacteriological eradication rates were somewhat less than those observed with a product containing a β-lactamase inhibitor. Lorabid's decreased potential for toxicity compared to products containing β-lactamase inhibitors along with the susceptibility patterns of the common microbes in a given geographic area should be taken into account when considering the use of an antimicrobial (*see* **CLINICAL STUDIES** section).

Pharyngitis and Tonsillitis caused by *S. pyogenes.* (The usual drug of choice in the treatment and prevention of streptococcal infections, including the prophylaxis of rheumatic fever, is penicillin administered by the intramuscular route. Lorabid is generally effective in the eradication of *S. pyogenes* from the nasopharynx; however, data establishing the efficacy of Lorabid in the subsequent prevention of rheumatic fever are not available at present.)

Skin and Skin Structure

Uncomplicated Skin and Skin Structure Infections caused by *S. aureus* (including penicillinase-producing strains) or *S. pyogenes.* Abscesses should be surgically drained as clinically indicated.

Urinary Tract

Uncomplicated Urinary Tract Infections (cystitis) caused by *E. coli* or *S. saprophyticus**.

NOTE: In considering the use of Lorabid in the treatment of cystitis, Lorabid's lower bacterial eradication rates and lower potential for toxicity should be weighed against the increased eradication rates and increased potential for toxicity demonstrated by some other classes of approved agents (*see* **CLINICAL STUDIES** section).

Uncomplicated Pyelonephritis caused by *E. coli.*

* Although treatment of infections due to this organism in this organ system demonstrated a clinically acceptable overall outcome, efficacy was studied in fewer than 10 infections.

Culture and susceptibility testing should be performed when appropriate to determine the causative organism and its susceptibility to loracarbef. Therapy may be started while awaiting the results of these studies. Once these results become available, antimicrobial therapy should be adjusted accordingly.

CONTRAINDICATION

Lorabid is contraindicated in patients with known allergy to loracarbef or cephalosporin-class antibiotics.

WARNINGS

BEFORE THERAPY WITH LORABID IS INSTITUTED, CAREFUL INQUIRY SHOULD BE MADE TO DETERMINE WHETHER THE PATIENT HAS HAD PREVIOUS HYPERSENSITIVITY REACTIONS TO LORACARBEF, CEPHALOSPORINS, PENICILLINS, OR OTHER DRUGS. IF THIS PRODUCT IS TO BE GIVEN TO PENICILLIN-SENSITIVE PATIENTS, CAUTION SHOULD BE EXERCISED BECAUSE CROSS-HYPERSENSITIVITY AMONG β-LACTAM ANTIBIOTICS HAS BEEN CLEARLY DOCUMENTED AND MAY OCCUR IN UP TO 10% OF PATIENTS WITH A HISTORY OF PENICILLIN ALLERGY. IF AN ALLERGIC REACTION TO LORABID OCCURS, DISCONTINUE THE DRUG. SERIOUS ACUTE HYPERSENSITIVITY REACTIONS MAY REQUIRE THE USE OF EPINEPHRINE AND OTHER EMERGENCY MEASURES, INCLUDING OXYGEN, INTRAVENOUS FLUIDS, INTRAVENOUS ANTIHISTAMINES, CORTICOSTEROIDS, PRESSOR AMINES, AND AIRWAY MANAGEMENT, AS CLINICALLY INDICATED.

Pseudomembranous colitis has been reported with nearly all antibacterial agents and may range from mild to life-threatening. Therefore, it is important to consider this diagnosis in patients who present with diarrhea subsequent to the administration of antibacterial agents.

Treatment with broad-spectrum antibiotics alters the normal flora of the colon and may permit overgrowth of clostridia. Studies indicate that a toxin produced by *Clostridium difficile* is a primary cause of "antibiotic-associated colitis."

After the diagnosis of pseudomembranous colitis has been established, therapeutic measures should be initiated. Mild cases of pseudomembranous colitis usually respond to discontinuation of drug alone. In moderate to severe cases, consideration should be given to management with fluids and electrolytes, protein supplementation, and treatment with an antibacterial drug effective against *C. difficile* -associated colitis.

PRECAUTIONS

General—In patients with known or suspected renal impairment (*see* **DOSAGE AND ADMINISTRATION**), careful clinical observation and appropriate laboratory studies should be performed prior to and during therapy. The total daily dose of loracarbef should be reduced in these patients because high and/or prolonged plasma antibiotic concentrations can occur in such individuals administered the usual doses. Loracarbef, like cephalosporins, should be given with caution to patients receiving concurrent treatment with potent diuretics because these diuretics are suspected of adversely affecting renal function.

As with other broad-spectrum antimicrobials, prolonged use of loracarbef may result in the overgrowth of nonsusceptible organisms. Careful observation of the patient is essential. If superinfection occurs during therapy, appropriate measures should be taken.

Loracarbef, as with other broad-spectrum antimicrobials, should be prescribed with caution in individuals with a history of colitis.

Information for Patients—Lorabid should be taken either at least 1 hour prior to eating or at least 2 hours after eating a meal.

Drug Interactions—

Probenecid: As with other β-lactam antibiotics, renal excretion of loracarbef is inhibited by probenecid and resulted in an approximate 80% increase in the AUC for loracarbef (*see* **CLINICAL PHARMACOLOGY**).

Carcinogenesis, Mutagenesis, Impairment of Fertility—Although lifetime studies in animals have not been performed to evaluate carcinogenic potential, no mutagenic potential was found for loracarbef in standard tests of genotoxicity, which included bacterial mutation tests and *in vitro* and *in*

PEDIATRIC DOSAGE CHART
DAILY DOSE 15 mg/kg/day

Weight		100 mg/5 mL Suspension		200 mg/5 mL Suspension	
		Dose given twice daily		Dose given twice daily	
lb	kg	mL	tsp	mL	tsp
15	7	2.6	0.5	—	—
29	13	4.9	1.0	2.5	0.5
44	20	7.5	1.5	3.8	0.75
57	26	9.8	2.0	4.9	1.0

PEDIATRIC DOSAGE CHART
DAILY DOSE 30 mg/kg/day

Weight		100 mg/5 mL Suspension		200 mg/5 mL Suspension	
		Dose given twice daily		Dose given twice daily	
lb	kg	mL	tsp	mL	tsp
15	7	5.2	1.0	2.6	0.5
29	13	9.8	2.0	4.9	1.0
44	20	—	—	7.5	1.5
57	26	—	—	9.8	2.0

vivo mammalian systems. In rats, fertility and reproductive performance were not affected by loracarbef at doses up to 33 times the maximum human exposure in mg/kg (10 times the exposure based on mg/m^2).

Usage in Pregnancy—Pregnancy Category B—Reproduction studies have been performed in mice, rats, and rabbits at doses up to 33 times the maximum human exposure in mg/kg (4, 10, and 4 times the exposure, respectively, based on mg/m^2) and have revealed no evidence of impaired fertility or harm to the fetus due to loracarbef. There are, however, no adequate and well-controlled studies in pregnant women. Because animal reproduction studies are not always predictive of human response, this drug should be used during pregnancy only if clearly needed.

Labor and Delivery—Lorabid has not been studied for use during labor and delivery. Treatment should be given only if clearly needed.

Nursing Mothers—It is not known whether this drug is excreted in human milk. Because many drugs are excreted in human milk, caution should be exercised when Lorabid is administered to a nursing woman.

Pediatric Use—Efficacy and safety in infants less than 6 months of age have not been established.

Geriatric Use—Healthy geriatric volunteers (≥ 65 years old) with normal renal function who received a single 400-mg dose of loracarbef had no significant differences in AUC or clearance when compared to healthy adult volunteers 20 to 40 years of age. In clinical studies, when geriatric patients received the usual recommended adult doses, clinical efficacy and safety were comparable to results in nongeriatric adult patients. Because significant numbers of elderly patients have decreased renal function, evaluation of renal function in this population is recommended (see **DOSAGE AND ADMINISTRATION**).

ADVERSE REACTIONS

The nature of adverse reactions to loracarbef are similar to those observed with orally administered β-lactam antimicrobials. The majority of adverse reactions observed in clinical trials were of a mild and transient nature; 1.5% of patients discontinued therapy because of drug-related adverse reactions. No one reaction requiring discontinuation accounted for > 0.03% of the total patient population; however, of those reactions resulting in discontinuation, gastrointestinal events (diarrhea and abdominal pain) and skin rashes predominated.

All Patients

The following adverse events, irrespective of relationship to drug, have been reported following the use of Lorabid in clinical trials. Incidence rates (combined for all dosing regimens and dosage forms) were less than 1% for the total patient population, except as otherwise noted:

Gastrointestinal: The most commonly observed adverse reactions were related to the gastrointestinal system. The incidence of gastrointestinal adverse reactions increased in patients treated with higher doses. Individual event rates included diarrhea, 4.1%; nausea, 1.9%; vomiting, 1.4%; abdominal pain, 1.4%; and anorexia.

Hypersensitivity: Hypersensitivity reactions including, skin rashes (1.2%), urticaria, pruritus, and erythema multiforme.

Central Nervous System: Headache (2.9%), somnolence, nervousness, insomnia, and dizziness.

Hemic and Lymphatic Systems: Transient thrombocytopenia, leukopenia, and eosinophilia.

Hepatic: Transient elevations in AST (SGOT), ALT (SGPT), and alkaline phosphatase.

Renal: Transient elevations in BUN and creatinine.

Cardiovascular System: Vasodilatation.

Genitourinary: Vaginitis (1.3%), vaginal moniliasis (1.1%). As with other β-lactam antibiotics, the following potentially severe adverse experiences have been reported rarely with loracarbef in worldwide post-marketing surveillance: anaphylaxis, hepatic dysfunction including cholestasis, prolongation of the prothrombin time with clinical bleeding in patients taking anticoagulants, and Stevens-Johnson syndrome.

Pediatric Patients

The incidences of several adverse events, irrespective of relationship to drug, following treatment with Lorabid were significantly different in the pediatric population and the adult population as follows:

Event	Pediatric	Adult
Diarrhea	5.8%	3.6%
Headache	0.9%	3.2%
Rhinitis	6.3%	1.6%
Nausea	0.0%	2.5%
Rash	2.9%	0.7%
Vomiting	3.3%	0.5%
Somnolence	2.1%	0.4%
Anorexia	2.3%	0.3%

β-Lactam Antimicrobial Class Labeling:

The following adverse reactions and altered laboratory test results have been reported in patients treated with β-lactam antibiotics:

Adverse Reactions—Allergic reactions, aplastic anemia, hemolytic anemia, hemorrhage, agranulocytosis, toxic epidermal necrolysis, renal dysfunction, and toxic nephropathy. As with other β-lactam antibiotics, serum sickness-like reactions have been reported rarely with loracarbef.

Several β-lactam antibiotics have been implicated in triggering seizures, particularly in patients with renal impairment when the dosage was not reduced. If seizures associated with drug therapy should occur, the drug should be discontinued. Anticonvulsant therapy can be given if clinically indicated.

Altered Laboratory Tests—Increased prothrombin time, positive direct Coombs' test, elevated LDH, pancytopenia, and neutropenia.

OVERDOSAGE

Signs and Symptoms—The toxic symptoms following an overdose of β-lactams may include nausea, vomiting, epigastric distress, and diarrhea.

Loracarbef is eliminated primarily by the kidneys. Forced diuresis, peritoneal dialysis, hemodialysis, or hemoperfusion have not been established as beneficial for an overdose of loracarbef. Hemodialysis has been shown to be effective in hastening the elimination of loracarbef from plasma in patients with chronic renal failure.

DOSAGE AND ADMINISTRATION

Lorabid is administered orally either at least 1 hour prior to eating or at least 2 hours after eating. The recommended dosages, durations of treatment, and applicable patient populations are described in the following chart:

Population/Infection	Dosage (mg)	Duration (days)
ADULTS (13 years and older)		
Lower Respiratory Tract		
Secondary Bacterial Infection of Acute Bronchitis	200–400 q12h	7
Acute Bacterial Exacerbation of Chronic Bronchitis	400 q12h	7
Pneumonia	400 q12h	14
Upper Respiratory Tract		
Pharyngitis/Tonsillitis	200 q12h	10*
Sinusitis	400 q12h	10
(See **CLINICAL STUDIES** and **INDICATIONS AND USAGE** for further information.)		
Skin and Skin Structure		
Uncomplicated Skin and Skin Structure Infections	200 q12h	7
Urinary Tract		
Uncomplicated cystitis	200 q24h	7
(See **CLINICAL STUDIES** and **INDICATIONS AND USAGE** for further information.)		
Uncomplicated pyelonephritis	400 q12h	14
INFANTS AND CHILDREN (6 months to 12 years)		
Upper Respiratory Tract		
Acute Otitis Media**	30 mg/kg/day in divided doses q12h	10
(See **CLINICAL STUDIES** and **INDICATIONS AND USAGE** for further information.)		
Pharyngitis/Tonsillitis	15 mg/kg/day in divided doses q12h	10*
Skin and Skin Structure		
Impetigo	15 mg/kg/day in divided doses q12h	7

*In the treatment of infections due to *S. pyogenes*, Lorabid should be administered for at least 10 days.

Otitis media should be treated with the suspension. Clinical studies of otitis media were conducted with the suspension formulation only. The suspension is more rapidly absorbed than the capsules, resulting in higher peak plasma concentrations when administered at the same dose. Therefore, the capsule should not be substituted for the suspension in the treatment of otitis media (*see* **CLINICAL PHARMACOLOGY).

[See first table above.]

[See second table above.]

Renal Impairment: Lorabid may be administered to patients with impaired renal function. The usual dose and schedule may be employed in patients with creatinine clearance levels of 50 mL/min or greater. Patients with creatinine clearance between 10 and 49 mL/min may be given half of the recommended dose at the usual dosage interval, or the normal recommended dose at twice the usual dosage interval. Patients with creatinine clearance levels less than 10 mL/min may be treated with the recommended dose given every 3 to 5 days; patients on hemodialysis should receive another dose following dialysis.

When only the serum creatinine is available, the following formula (based on sex, weight, and age of the patient) may be used to convert this value into creatinine clearance (CL_{cr}, mL/min). The equation assumes the patient's renal function is stable.

$$Males = \frac{(weight\ in\ kg) \times (140 - age)}{(72) \times serum\ creatinine\ (mg/100\ mL)}$$

Females = (0.85) × (above value)

Reconstitution Directions for Oral Suspension

Bottle Size	Reconstitution Directions
100 mL	Add 60 mL of water in 2 portions to the dry mixture in the bottle. Shake well after each addition.
50 mL	Add 30 mL of water in 2 portions to the dry mixture in the bottle. Shake well after each addition.

After mixing, the suspension may be kept at room temperature, 59° to 86°F (15° to 30°C), for 14 days without significant loss of potency. Keep tightly closed. Discard unused portion after 14 days.

HOW SUPPLIED

Pulvules:

200 mg, (blue and gray) (No. 3170) (Identi-Code* 3170) (30s) NDC 0002-3170-30

400 mg, (blue and pink) (No. 3171) (Identi-Code 3171) (30s) NDC 0002-3171-30

Keep tightly closed. Store at controlled room temperature, 59° to 86°F (15° to 30°C). Protect from heat.

For Oral Suspension (strawberry bubble gum flavor):

100 mg/5 mL, (M-5135) (50-mL size) NDC 0002-5135-87; (100-mL size) NDC 0002-5135-48

200 mg/5 mL, (M-5136) (50-mL size) NDC 0002-5136-87; (100-mL size) NDC 0002-5136-48

*Identi-Code® (formula identification code, Lilly).

Continued on next page

Lilly—Cont.

Clinical Studies:

Acute Otitis Media

<u>Study 1</u> In a controlled clinical study of acute otitis media performed in the United States where significant rates of β-lactamase-producing organisms were found, loracarbef was compared to an oral antimicrobial agent that contained a specific β-lactamase inhibitor. In this study, using very strict evaluability criteria and microbiologic and clinical response criteria at the 10- to 16-day post therapy follow-up, the following presumptive bacterial eradication/clinical cure outcomes (ie, clinical success) and safety results were obtained:

US Acute Otitis Media Study
Loracarbef vs β-lactamase inhibitor-containing control drug

Efficacy:

Pathogen	% of Cases With Pathogens (n=204)	Outcome
S. pneumoniae	42.6%	Loracarbef equivalent to control
H. influenzae	30.4%	Loracarbef success rate 9% less than control
M. catarrhalis	20.6%	Loracarbef success rate 19% less than control
S. pyogenes	6.4%	Loracarbef equivalent to control
Overall	100.0%	Loracarbef success rate 12% less than control

Safety: The incidences of the following adverse events were clinically and statistically significantly higher in the control arm versus the loracarbef arm.

Event	Loracarbef	Control
Diarrhea	15%	26%
Rash*	8%	15%

*The majority of these involved the diaper area in young children.

<u>Study 2</u> In a controlled clinical study of acute otitis media performed in Europe, loracarbef was compared to amoxicillin. As expected in a European population, this study population had a lower incidence of β-lactamase-producing organisms than usually seen in US trials. In this study, using very strict evaluability criteria and microbiologic and clinical response criteria at the 10- to 16-day post therapy follow-up, the following presumptive bacterial eradication/clinical cure outcomes (ie, clinical success) were obtained:

European Acute Otitis Media Study
Loracarbef vs Amoxicillin

Efficacy:

Pathogen	% of Cases With Pathogens (n=291)	Outcome
S. pneumoniae	51.5%	Loracarbef equivalent to amoxicillin
H. influenzae	29.2%	Loracarbef success rate 14% greater than amoxicillin
M. catarrhalis	15.8%	Loracarbef success rate 31% greater than amoxicillin
S. pyogenes	3.4%	Loracarbef equivalent to amoxicillin
Overall	100.0%	Loracarbef equivalent to amoxicillin

Acute Maxillary Sinusitis

In a controlled clinical study of acute maxillary sinusitis performed in Europe, loracarbef was compared to doxycycline. In this study, there were 210 sinus-puncture evaluable patients. As expected in a European population, this study population had a lower incidence of β-lactamase-producing organisms than usually seen in US trials. In this study, using very strict evaluability criteria and microbiologic and clinical response criteria at the 1- to 2-week post therapy follow-up, the following presumptive bacterial eradication/clinical cure outcomes (ie, clinical success) were obtained:

European Acute Maxillary Sinusitis Study
Loracarbef vs Doxycycline

Efficacy:

Pathogen	% of Cases With Pathogens (n=210)	Outcome
S. pneumoniae	47.6%	Loracarbef equivalent to doxycycline
H. influenzae	41.4%	Loracarbef equivalent to doxycycline
M. catarrhalis	11.0%	Loracarbef equivalent to doxycycline
Overall	100.0%	Loracarbef equivalent to doxycycline

CYSTITIS

<u>Study 1</u> In a controlled clinical study of cystitis performed in the United States, loracarbef was compared to cefaclor. In this study, using very strict evaluability criteria and microbiologic and clinical response criteria at the 5- to 9-day post therapy follow-up, the following bacterial eradication rates were obtained:

U.S. Uncomplicated Cystitis Study
Loracarbef vs Cefaclor

Efficacy:

Pathogen	% of Cases With Pathogens (n=186)	Outcome
E. coli	77.4%	Loracarbef eradication rate 4% greater than cefaclor (loracarbef eradication rate 80%)
Other major Enterobacteriaceae	12.5%	Loracarbef equivalent to cefaclor (loracarbef eradication rate 61%)
S. saprophyticus	3.8%	Loracarbef equivalent to cefaclor

<u>Study 2</u> In a second controlled clinical study of cystitis, performed in Europe, loracarbef was compared to an oral quinolone. In this study, using very strict evaluability criteria and microbiologic and clinical response criteria at the 5- to 9-day post therapy follow-up, the following bacterial eradication rates were obtained:

European Uncomplicated Cystitis Study
Loracarbef vs Quinolone

Efficacy:

Pathogen	% of Cases With Pathogens (n=189)	Outcome
E. coli	82.0%	Loracarbef eradication rate 7% less than quinolone (loracarbef eradication rate 81%)
Other major Enterobacteriaceae	10.1%	Loracarbef eradication rate 32% less than quinolone (loracarbef eradication rate 50%)

REFERENCES

1. National Committee for Clinical Laboratory Standards, M2-A4 performance standards for antimicrobial disk susceptibility tests, ed 4, Villanova, PA, April, 1990.
2. National Committee for Clinical Laboratory Standards, M7-A2 methods for dilution antimicrobial susceptibility tests for bacteria that grow aerobically, ed 2, Villanova, PA, April, 1990.

[040996]

Shown in Product Identification Guide, page 322

MANDOL® ℞

[măn′dŏl]
(Cefamandole Nafate for Injection, USP)

DESCRIPTION

Mandol® (Cefamandole Nafate for Injection, USP) is a semisynthetic broad-spectrum cephalosporin antibiotic for parenteral administration. It is 5-thia-1-azabicyclo[4.2.0]oct-2-ene-2-carboxylic acid, 7-[[(formyloxy)phenylacetyl]amino]-3-[[(1-methyl-1H-tetrazol-5-yl)thio]methyl]-8-oxo-, monosodium salt, [6R-[6α,7β(R *)]]. Cefamandole has the empirical formula $C_{19}H_{17}N_6NaO_6S_2$ representing a molecular weight of 512.49. Mandol also contains 63 mg sodium carbonate/g of cefamandole activity. The total sodium content is approximately 77 mg (3.3 mEq sodium ion) per g of cefamandole activity. After addition of diluent, cefamandole nafate rapidly hydrolyzes to cefamandole, and both compounds have microbiologic activity in vivo. Solutions of Mandol range from light-yellow to amber, depending on concentration and diluent used. The pH of freshly reconstituted solutions usually ranges from 6.0 to 8.5. The structural formula is as follows:

CLINICAL PHARMACOLOGY

After intramuscular administration of a 500-mg dose of cefamandole to normal volunteers, the mean peak serum concentration was 13 μg/mL. After a 1-g dose, the mean peak concentration was 25 μg/mL. These peaks occurred at 30 to 120 minutes. Following intravenous doses of 1, 2, and 3 g, serum concentrations were 139, 240, and 533 μg/mL respectively at

10 minutes. These concentrations declined to 0.8, 2.2, and 2.9 μg/mL at 4 hours. Intravenous administration of 4-g doses every 6 hours produced no evidence of accumulation in the serum. The half-life after an intravenous dose is 32 minutes; after intramuscular administration, the half-life is 60 minutes.

Sixty-five percent to 85% of cefamandole is excreted by the kidneys over an 8-hour period, resulting in high urinary concentrations. Following intramuscular doses of 500 mg and 1 g, urinary concentrations averaged 254 and 1,357 μg/mL respectively. Intravenous doses of 1 and 2 g produced urinary levels averaging 750 and 1,380 μg/mL respectively. Probenecid slows tubular excretion and doubles the peak serum level and the duration of measurable serum concentrations.

The antibiotic reaches therapeutic levels in pleural and joint fluids and in bile and bone.

Microbiology—The bactericidal action of cefamandole results from inhibition of cell-wall synthesis. Cephalosporins have in vitro activity against a wide range of gram-positive and gram-negative organisms. Cefamandole is usually active against the following organisms in vitro and in clinical infections:

Gram-positive
  Staphylococcus aureus, including penicillinase- and non-penicillinase-producing strains
  Staphylococcus epidermidis
  β-hemolytic and other streptococci (Most strains of enterococci, eg, *Enterococcus faecalis* [formerly *Streptococcus faecalis*], are resistant.)
  Streptococcus pneumoniae
Gram-negative
  Escherichia coli
  Klebsiella sp
  Enterobacter sp (Initially susceptible organisms occasionally may become resistant during therapy.)
  Haemophilus influenzae
  Proteus mirabilis
  Providencia rettgeri (formerly *Proteus rettgeri*)
  Morganella morganii (formerly *Proteus morganii*)
  Proteus vulgaris (Some strains of *P. vulgaris* have been shown by in vitro tests to be resistant to cefamandole and other cephalosporins.)
Anaerobic organisms
  Gram-positive and gram-negative cocci (including *Peptococcus* and *Peptostreptococcus* sp)
  Gram-positive bacilli (including *Clostridium* sp)
  Gram-negative bacilli (including *Bacteroides* and *Fusobacterium* sp). Most strains of *Bacteroides fragilis* are resistant.

Pseudomonas, Acinetobacter calcoaceticus (formerly *Mima* and *Herellea* sp), and most *Serratia* strains are resistant to cefamandole and certain other cephalosporins. Cefamandole is resistant to degradation by β-lactamases from certain members of the *Enterobacteriaceae*.

Susceptibility Tests—Quantitative methods that require measurement of zone diameters give the most precise estimates of antibiotic susceptibility. One such procedure[1] has been recommended for use with disks to test susceptibility to cefamandole. Interpretation involves correlation of the diameters obtained in the disk test with minimal inhibitory concentration (MIC) values for cefamandole.

Reports from the laboratory giving results of the standardized single-disk susceptibility test[1] using a 30-μg cefamandole disk should be interpreted according to the following criteria:

Susceptible organisms produce zones of 18 mm or greater, indicating that the tested organism is likely to respond to therapy.

Organisms of intermediate susceptibility produce zones of 15 to 17 mm, indicating that the tested organism would be susceptible if high dosage is used or if the infection is confined to tissues and fluids (eg, urine) in which high antibiotic levels are attained.

Resistant organisms produce zones of 14 mm or less, indicating that other therapy should be selected.

For gram-positive isolates, the test may be performed with either the cephalosporin-class disk (30 μg cephalothin) or the cefamandole disk (30 μg cefamandole), and a zone of 18 mm is indicative of a cefamandole-susceptible organism.

Gram-negative organisms should be tested with the cefamandole disk (using the above criteria), since cefamandole has been shown by in vitro tests to have activity against certain strains of *Enterobacteriaceae* found resistant when tested with the cephalosporin-class disk. Gram-negative organisms having zones of less than 18 mm around the cephalothin disk are not necessarily of intermediate susceptibility or resistant to cefamandole.

The cefamandole disk should not be used for testing susceptibility to other cephalosporins.

A bacterial isolate may be considered susceptible if the MIC value for cefamandole[2] is not more than 16 μg/mL. Organisms are considered resistant if the MIC is greater than 32 μg/mL.

INDICATIONS AND USAGE

Mandol is indicated for the treatment of serious infections caused by susceptible strains of the designated microorganisms in the diseases listed below:

Lower respiratory infections, including pneumonia, caused by *S. pneumoniae*, *H. influenzae*, *Klebsiella* sp, *S. aureus* (penicillinase- and non-penicillinase-producing), β-hemolytic streptococci, and *P. mirabilis*

Urinary tract infections caused by *E. coli*, *Proteus* sp (both indole-negative and indole-positive), *Enterobacter* sp, *Klebsiella* sp, group D streptococci (*Note:* Most enterococci, eg, *E. faecalis*, are resistant), and *S. epidermidis*

Peritonitis caused by *E. coli* and *Enterobacter* sp.

Septicemia caused by *E. coli*, *S. aureus* (penicillinase- and non-penicillinase-producing), *S. pneumoniae*, *S. pyogenes* (group A β-hemolytic streptococci), *H. influenzae*, and *Klebsiella* sp

Skin and skin structure infections caused by *S. aureus* (penicillinase- and non-penicillinase-producing), *S. pyogenes* (group A β-hemolytic streptococci), *H. influenzae*, *E. coli*, *Enterobacter* sp, and *P. mirabilis*

Bone and joint infections caused by *S. aureus* (penicillinase- and non-penicillinase-producing)

Clinical microbiologic studies in nongonococcal pelvic inflammatory disease in females, lower respiratory infections, and skin infections frequently reveal the growth of susceptible strains of both aerobic and anaerobic organisms. Mandol has been used successfully in those infections in which several organisms have been isolated. Most strains of *B. fragilis* are resistant in vitro; however, infections caused by susceptible strains have been treated successfully.

Specimens for bacteriologic cultures should be obtained in order to isolate and identify causative organisms and to determine their susceptibilities to cefamandole. Therapy may be instituted before results of susceptibility studies are known; however, once these results become available, the antibiotic treatment should be adjusted accordingly.

In certain cases of confirmed or suspected gram-positive or gram-negative sepsis or in patients with other serious infections in which the causative organism has not been identified, Mandol may be used concomitantly with an aminoglycoside (*see* Precautions). The recommended doses of both antibiotics may be given, depending on the severity of the infection and the patient's condition. The renal function of the patient should be carefully monitored, especially if higher dosages of the antibiotics are to be administered.

Antibiotic therapy of β-hemolytic streptococcal infections should continue for at least 10 days.

Preventive Therapy —The administration of Mandol preoperatively, intraoperatively, and postoperatively may reduce the incidence of certain postoperative infections in patients undergoing surgical procedures that are classified as contaminated or potentially contaminated (eg, gastrointestinal surgery, cesarean section, vaginal hysterectomy, or cholecystectomy in high-risk patients such as those with acute cholecystitis, obstructive jaundice, or common-bile-duct stones).

In major surgery in which the risk of postoperative infection is low but serious (cardiovascular surgery, neurosurgery, or prosthetic arthroplasty), Mandol may be effective in preventing such infections.

If signs of infection occur, specimens for culture should be obtained for identification of the causative organism so that appropriate antibiotic therapy may be instituted.

CONTRAINDICATION

Mandol is contraindicated in patients with known allergy to the cephalosporin group of antibiotics.

WARNINGS

BEFORE THERAPY WITH MANDOL IS INSTITUTED, CAREFUL INQUIRY SHOULD BE MADE TO DETERMINE WHETHER THE PATIENT HAS HAD PREVIOUS HYPERSENSITIVITY REACTIONS TO CEPHALOSPORINS, PENICILLINS, OR OTHER DRUGS. THIS PRODUCT SHOULD BE GIVEN CAUTIOUSLY TO PENICILLIN-SENSITIVE PATIENTS. ANTIBIOTICS SHOULD BE ADMINISTERED WITH CAUTION TO ANY PATIENT WHO HAS DEMONSTRATED SOME FORM OF ALLERGY, PARTICULARLY TO DRUGS. SERIOUS ACUTE HYPERSENSITIVITY REACTIONS MAY REQUIRE EPINEPHRINE AND OTHER EMERGENCY MEASURES.

In newborn infants, accumulation of other cephalosporin-class antibiotics (with resulting prolongation of drug half-life) has been reported.

Pseudomembranous colitis has been reported with virtually all broad-spectrum antibiotics (including macrolides, semisynthetic penicillins, and cephalosporins); therefore, it is important to consider its diagnosis in patients who develop diarrhea in association with the use of antibiotics. Such colitis may range in severity from mild to life threatening.

Treatment with broad-spectrum antibiotics alters the normal flora of the colon and may permit overgrowth of clostridia. Studies indicate that a toxin produced by *Clostridium difficile* is a primary cause of antibiotic-associated colitis. Mild cases of pseudomembranous colitis usually respond to drug discontinuance alone. In moderate to severe cases, management should include sigmoidoscopy, appropriate bacteriologic studies, and fluid, electrolyte, and protein supplementation. When the colitis does not improve after the drug has been discontinued, or when it is severe, oral vancomycin is the drug of choice for antibiotic-associated pseudomembranous colitis produced by *C. difficile*. Other causes of colitis should be ruled out.

PRECAUTIONS

General —Although Mandol rarely produces alteration in kidney function, evaluation of renal status is recommended, especially in seriously ill patients receiving maximum doses. Prolonged use of Mandol may result in the overgrowth of nonsusceptible organisms. Careful observation of the patient is essential. If superinfection occurs during therapy, appropriate measures should be taken.

Nephrotoxicity has been reported following concomitant administration of aminoglycoside antibiotics and cephalosporins.

A false-positive reaction for glucose in the urine may occur with Benedict's or Fehling's solution or with Clinitest® tablets but not with Tes-Tape® (Glucose Enzymatic Test Strip, USP). There may be a false-positive test for proteinuria with acid and denaturization-precipitation tests.

As with other broad-spectrum antibiotics, hypoprothrombinemia, with or without bleeding, has been reported rarely, but it has been promptly reversed by administration of vitamin K. Such episodes usually have occurred in elderly, debilitated, or otherwise compromised patients with deficient stores of vitamin K. Treatment of such individuals with antibiotics possessing significant gram-negative and/or anaerobic activity is thought to alter the number and/or type of intestinal bacterial flora, with consequent reduction in synthesis of vitamin K. Prophylactic administration of vitamin K may be indicated in such patients, especially when intestinal sterilization and surgical procedures are performed.

In a few patients receiving Mandol, nausea, vomiting, and vasomotor instability with hypotension and peripheral vasodilatation occurred following the ingestion of ethanol.

Cefamandole inhibits the enzyme acetaldehyde dehydrogenase in laboratory animals. This causes accumulation of acetaldehyde when ethanol is administered concomitantly. Broad-spectrum antibiotics should be prescribed with caution in individuals with a history of gastrointestinal disease, particularly colitis.

Carcinogenesis, Mutagenesis, Impairment of Fertility —Certain β-lactam antibiotics containing the N-methylthiotetrazole side chain have been reported to cause delayed maturity of the testicular germinal epithelium when given to neonatal rats during initial spermatogenic development (6 to 36 days of age). In animals that were treated from 6 to 36 days of age with 1,000 mg/kg/day of cefamandole (approximately 5 times the maximum clinical dose), the delayed maturity was pronounced and was associated with decreased testicular weights and a reduced number of germinal cells in the leading waves of spermatogenic development. The effect was slight in rats given 50 or 100 mg/kg/day. Some animals that were given 1,000 mg/kg/day during days 6 to 36 were infertile after becoming sexually mature. No adverse effects have been observed in rats exposed in utero, in neonatal rats (4 days of age or younger) treated prior to the initiation of spermatogenesis, or in older rats (more than 36 days of age) after exposure for up to 6 months. The significance to humans of these findings in rats is unknown because of differences in the time of initiation of spermatogenesis, rate of spermatogenic development, and duration of puberty.

Usage in Pregnancy —Pregnancy Category B —Reproduction studies have been performed in rats given doses of 500 or 1,000 mg/kg/day and have revealed no evidence of impaired fertility or harm to the fetus due to Mandol. There are, however, no adequate and well-controlled studies in pregnant women. Because animal reproduction studies are not always predictive of human response, this drug should be used during pregnancy only if clearly needed.

Nursing Mothers —Caution should be exercised when Mandol is administered to a nursing woman.

Usage in Infancy —Mandol has been effectively used in this age group, but all laboratory parameters have not been extensively studied in infants between 1 and 6 months of age; safety of this product has not been established in prematures and infants under 1 month of age. Therefore, if Mandol is administered to infants, the physician should determine whether the potential benefits outweigh the possible risks involved.

ADVERSE REACTIONS

Gastrointestinal —Symptoms of pseudomembranous colitis may appear either during or after antibiotic treatment. Nausea and vomiting have been reported rarely. As with some penicillins and some other cephalosporins, transient hepatitis and cholestatic jaundice have been reported rarely.

Hypersensitivity —Anaphylaxis, maculopapular rash, urticaria, eosinophilia, and drug fever have been reported. These reactions are more likely to occur in patients with a history of allergy, particularly to penicillin.

Blood —Thrombocytopenia has been reported rarely. Neutropenia has been reported, especially in long courses of treatment. Some individuals have developed positive direct Coombs' tests during treatment with the cephalosporin antibiotics.

Liver —Transient rise in SGOT, SGPT, and alkaline phosphatase levels has been noted.

Kidney —Decreased creatinine clearance has been reported in patients with prior renal impairment. As with some other cephalosporins, transitory elevations of BUN have occasionally been observed with Mandol; their frequency increases in patients over 50 years of age. In some of these cases, there was also a mild increase in serum creatinine.

Local Reactions —Pain on intramuscular injection is infrequent. Thrombophlebitis occurs rarely.

OVERDOSAGE

The administration of inappropriately large doses of parenteral cephalosporins may cause seizures, particularly in patients with renal impairment. Dosage reduction is necessary when renal function is impaired (*see* Dosage and Administration). If seizures occur, the drug should be promptly discontinued; anticonvulsant therapy may be administered if clinically indicated. Hemodialysis may be considered in cases of overwhelming overdosage.

DOSAGE AND ADMINISTRATION

Dosage—Adults: The usual dosage range for cefamandole is 500 mg to 1 g every 4 to 8 hours.

In infections of skin structures and in uncomplicated pneumonia, a dosage of 500 mg every 6 hours is adequate.

In uncomplicated urinary tract infections, a dosage of 500 mg every 8 hours is sufficient. In more serious urinary tract infections, a dosage of 1 g every 8 hours may be needed.

In severe infections, 1-g doses may be given at 4 to 6-hour intervals.

In life-threatening infections or infections due to less susceptible organisms, doses up to 2 g every 4 hours (ie, 12 g/day) may be needed.

Infants and Children: Administration of 50 to 100 mg/kg/day in equally divided doses every 4 to 8 hours has been effective for most infections susceptible to Mandol® (Cefamandole Nafate, USP). This may be increased to a total daily dose of 150 mg/kg (not to exceed the maximum adult dose) for severe infections. (*See* recommendations regarding this age group in Warnings *and* Precautions.)

Note: As with antibiotic therapy in general, administration of Mandol should be continued for a minimum of 48 to 72 hours after the patient becomes asymptomatic or after evidence of bacterial eradication has been obtained; a minimum of 10 days of treatment is recommended in infections caused by group A β-hemolytic streptococci in order to guard against the risk of rheumatic fever or glomerulonephritis; frequent bacteriologic and clinical appraisal is necessary during therapy of chronic urinary tract infection and may be required for several months after therapy has been completed; persistent infections may require treatment for several weeks; and doses smaller than those indicated above should not be used.

For perioperative use of Mandol, the following dosages are recommended:

Adults —1 or 2 g intravenously or intramuscularly ½ to 1 hour prior to the surgical incision followed by 1 or 2 g every 6 hours for 24 to 48 hours.

Children (3 months of age and older) —50 to 100 mg/kg/day in equally divided doses by the routes and schedule designated above.

Note: In patients undergoing prosthetic arthroplasty, administration is recommended for as long as 72 hours.

In patients undergoing cesarean section, the initial dose may be administered just prior to surgery or immediately after the cord has been clamped.

Impaired Renal Function —When renal function is impaired, a reduced dosage must be employed and the serum levels closely monitored. After an initial dose of 1 to 2 g (depending on the severity of infection), a maintenance dosage schedule should be followed (see chart). Continued dosage should be determined by degree of renal impairment, severity of infection, and susceptibility of the causative organism. [See table at top of next page.]

When only serum creatinine is available, the following formula (based on sex, weight, and age of the patient) may be used to convert this value into creatinine clearance. The serum creatinine should represent a steady state of renal function.

Continued on next page

* Identi-Code® symbol. This product information was prepared in June 1996. Current information on these and other products of Eli Lilly and Company may be obtained by direct inquiry to Lilly Research Laboratories, Lilly Corporate Center, Indianapolis, Indiana 46285, 800-545-5979.

Lilly—Cont.

MAINTENANCE DOSAGE GUIDE FOR PATIENTS WITH RENAL IMPAIRMENT

Creatinine Clearance (mL/min/1.73 m²)	Renal Function	Life-Threatening Infections— Maximum Dosage	Less Severe Infections
>80	Normal	2 g q4h	1–2 g q6h
80–50	Mild Impairment	1.5 g q4h OR 2 g q6h	0.75–1.5 g q6h
50–25	Moderate Impairment	1.5 g q6h OR 2 g q8h	0.75–1.5 g q8h
25–10	Severe Impairment	1 g q6h OR 1.25 g q8h	0.5–1 g q8h
10–2	Marked Impairment	0.67 g q8h OR 1 g q12h	0.5–0.75 g q12h
<2	None	0.5 g q8h OR 0.75 g q12h	0.25–0.5 g q12h

Males: $\dfrac{\text{Weight (kg)} \times (140 - \text{age})}{72 \times \text{serum creatinine}}$

Females: 0.9 × above value

Modes of Administration —Mandol may be given intravenously or by deep intramuscular injection into a large muscle mass (such as the gluteus or lateral part of the thigh) to minimize pain.

Intramuscular Administration —Each g of Mandol should be diluted with 3 mL of 1 of the following diluents: Sterile Water for Injection, Bacteriostatic Water for Injection, 0.9% Sodium Chloride Injection, or Bacteriostatic Sodium Chloride Injection. Shake well until dissolved.

Intravenous Administration —The intravenous route may be preferable for patients with bacterial septicemia, localized parenchymal abscesses (such as intra-abdominal abscess), peritonitis, or other severe or life-threatening infections when they may be poor risks because of lowered resistance. In those with normal renal function, the intravenous dosage for such infections is 3 to 12 g of Mandol daily. In conditions such as bacterial septicemia, 6 to 12 g/day may be given initially by the intravenous route for several days, and dosage may then be gradually reduced according to clinical response and laboratory findings.

If combination therapy with Mandol and an aminoglycoside is indicated, each of these antibiotics should be administered in different sites. *Do not mix an aminoglycoside with Mandol in the same intravenous fluid container.*

A SOLUTION OF 1 G OF MANDOL IN 22 ML OF STERILE WATER FOR INJECTION IS ISOTONIC.

The choice of saline, dextrose, or electrolyte solution and the volume to be employed are dictated by fluid and electrolyte management.

For direct intermittent intravenous administration, each g of cefamandole should be reconstituted with 10 mL of Sterile Water for Injection, 5% Dextrose Injection, or 0.9% Sodium Chloride Injection. Slowly inject the solution into the vein over a period of 3 to 5 minutes, or give it through the tubing of an administration set while the patient is also receiving one of the following intravenous fluids: 0.9% Sodium Chloride Injection; 5% Dextrose Injection; 10% Dextrose Injection; 5% Dextrose and 0.9% Sodium Chloride Injection; 5% Dextrose and 0.45% Sodium Chloride Injection; 5% Dextrose and 0.2% Sodium Chloride Injection; or Sodium Lactate Injection (M/6).

Intermittent intravenous infusion with a Y-type administration set or volume control set can also be accomplished while any of the above-mentioned intravenous fluids are being infused. However, during infusion of the solution containing Mandol, it is desirable to discontinue the other solution. When this technique is employed, careful attention should be paid to the volume of the solution containing Mandol so that the calculated dose will be infused. When a Y-tube hookup is used, 100 mL of the appropriate diluent should be added to the 1- or 2-g piggyback (100-mL) vial. If Sterile Water for Injection is used as the diluent, reconstitute with approximately 20 mL/g to avoid a hypotonic solution.

For continuous intravenous infusion, each g of cefamandole should be diluted with 10 mL of Sterile Water for Injection. An appropriate quantity of the resulting solution may be added to an IV bottle containing 1 of the following fluids: 0.9% Sodium Chloride Injection; 5% Dextrose Injection; 10% Dextrose Injection; 5% Dextrose and 0.9% Sodium Chloride Injection; 5% Dextrose and 0.45% Sodium Chloride

Injection; 5% Dextrose and 0.2% Sodium Chloride Injection; or Sodium Lactate Injection (M/6).

STABILITY

Reconstituted Mandol is stable for 24 hours at room temperature (25°C) and for 96 hours if stored under refrigeration (5°C). *During storage at room temperature, carbon dioxide develops inside the vial after reconstitution. This pressure may be dissipated prior to withdrawal of the vial contents, or it may be used to aid withdrawal if the vial is inverted over the syringe needle and the contents are allowed to flow into the syringe.* Solutions of Mandol in Sterile Water for Injection, 5% Dextrose Injection, or 0.9% Sodium Chloride Injection that are frozen immediately after reconstitution in Faspak containers and the conventional vials in which the drugs are supplied are stable for 6 months when stored at −20°C. **If the product is warmed (to a maximum of 37°C), care should be taken to avoid heating it after the thawing is complete. Once thawed, the solution should not be refrozen.**

HOW SUPPLIED

Vials (Dry Powder):

1 g.* 10-mL size (No. 7061)—(Traypak of 25) NDC 0002-7061-25

1 g,* 100-mL size (No. 7068)—(Traypak of 10) NDC 0002-7068-10

2 g,* 20-mL size (No. 7064)—(Traypak of 10) NDC 0002-7064-10

2 g,* 100-mL size (No. 7069)—(Traypak of 10) NDC 0002-7069-10

Faspak‡:

1 g* (No. 7208)—(Faspak of 96) NDC 0002-7208-74

ADD-Vantage§ Vials:

1 g* (No. 7268)—(Traypak of 25) NDC 0002-7268-25

2 g* (No. 7269)—(Traypak of 10) NDC 0002-7269-10

The above ADD-Vantage Vials are to be used only with Abbott Laboratories' ADD-Vantage Diluent Containers. Instructions for use of the ADD-Vantage Vials are enclosed in the package.

Also Available:

Pharmacy Bulk Package:

10 g,* 100-mL size (No. 7072)—(Traypak of 6) NDC 0002-7072-16

---

* Equivalent to cefamandole activity.

†Traypak™ (multivial carton, Lilly).

‡Faspak® (flexible plastic bag, Lilly).

§ADD-Vantage® (vials and diluent containers, Abbott).

[062895]

---

1. Bauer AW, Kirby WMM, et al: Antibiotic susceptibility testing by a standardized single disk method. *Am J Clin Pathol* 1966;45:493. Standardized disk susceptibility test. *Federal Register* 1974;39:19182–19184. National Committee for Clinical Laboratory Standards. Approved Standard: M2-A3 Performance standards for antimicrobial disk susceptibility tests—Fourth Edition, December, 1988.

2. Determined by the ICS agar-dilution method (Ericsson HM, Sherris JC: *Acta Pathol Microbiol Scand* 1971;[suppl 217]: B), or any other method that has been shown to give equivalent results.

NEBCIN® ℞

[*nĕb 'sĭn*]

(Tobramycin Sulfate Injection, USP)

WARNINGS

Patients treated with Nebcin® (Tobramycin Sulfate Injection, USP) and other aminoglycosides should be under close clinical observation, because these drugs have an inherent potential for causing ototoxicity and nephrotoxicity.

Neurotoxicity, manifested as both auditory and vestibular ototoxicity, can occur. The auditory changes are irreversible, are usually bilateral, and may be partial or total. Eighth-nerve impairment and nephrotoxicity may develop, primarily in patients having preexisting renal damage and in those with normal renal function to whom aminoglycosides are administered for longer periods or in higher doses than those recommended. Other manifestations of neurotoxicity may include numbness, skin tingling, muscle twitching, and convulsions. The risk of aminoglycoside-induced hearing loss increases with the degree of exposure to either high peak or high trough serum concentrations. Patients who develop cochlear damage may not have symptoms during therapy to warn them of eighth-nerve toxicity, and partial or total irreversible bilateral deafness may continue to develop after the drug has been discontinued.

Rarely, nephrotoxicity may not become apparent until the first few days after cessation of therapy. Aminoglycoside-induced nephrotoxicity usually is reversible. Renal and eighth-nerve function should be closely monitored in patients with known or suspected renal impairment and also in those whose renal function is initially normal but who develop signs of renal dysfunction during therapy. Peak and trough serum concentrations of aminoglycosides should be monitored periodically during therapy to assure adequate levels and to avoid potentially toxic levels. Prolonged serum concentrations above 12 μg/mL should be avoided. Rising trough levels (above 2 μg/mL) may indicate tissue accumulation. Such accumulation, excessive peak concentrations, advanced age, and cumulative dose may contribute to ototoxicity and nephrotoxicity (see Precautions). Urine should be examined for decreased specific gravity and increased excretion of protein, cells, and casts. Blood urea nitrogen, serum creatinine, and creatinine clearance should be measured periodically. When feasible, it is recommended that serial audiograms be obtained in patients old enough to be tested, particularly high-risk patients. Evidence of impairment of renal, vestibular, or auditory function requires discontinuation of the drug or dosage adjustment.

Nebcin should be used with caution in premature and neonatal infants because of their renal immaturity and the resulting prolongation of serum half-life of the drug. Concurrent and sequential use of other neurotoxic and/or nephrotoxic antibiotics, particularly other aminoglycosides (eg, amikacin, streptomycin, neomycin, kanamycin, gentamicin, and paromomycin), cephaloridine, viomycin, polymyxin B, colistin, cisplatin, and vancomycin, should be avoided. Other factors that may increase patient risk are advanced age and dehydration.

Aminoglycosides should not be given concurrently with potent diuretics, such as ethacrynic acid and furosemide. Some diuretics themselves cause ototoxicity, and intravenously administered diuretics enhance aminoglycoside toxicity by altering antibiotic concentrations in serum and tissue.

Aminoglycosides can cause fetal harm when administered to a pregnant woman (see Precautions).

DESCRIPTION

Tobramycin sulfate, a water-soluble antibiotic of the aminoglycoside group, is derived from the actinomycete *Streptomyces tenebrarius*. Nebcin, Injection, is a clear and colorless sterile aqueous solution for parenteral administration.

Tobramycin sulfate is O-3-amino-3-deoxy-α-D-glucopyranosyl-(1→4)-O-[2,6-diamino-2,3,6-trideoxy-α-D-*ribo*-hexopyranosyl-(1→6)]-2-deoxy-L-streptamine, sulfate (2:5)(salt) and has the chemical formula $(C_{18}H_{37}N_5O_9)_2 \cdot 5H_2SO_4$. The molecular weight is 1,425.39. The structural formula for tobramycin is as follows:

[See chemical structure at top of next column.]

Each mL also contains phenol as a preservative (5 mg, multiple-dose vials; 1.25 mg, ADD-Vantage® vials), sodium bisulfite (3.2 mg, multiple-dose vials; 1.6 mg, ADD-Vantage vials), 0.1 mg edetate disodium, and water for injection, qs. Sulfuric acid and/or sodium hydroxide may have been added to adjust the pH.

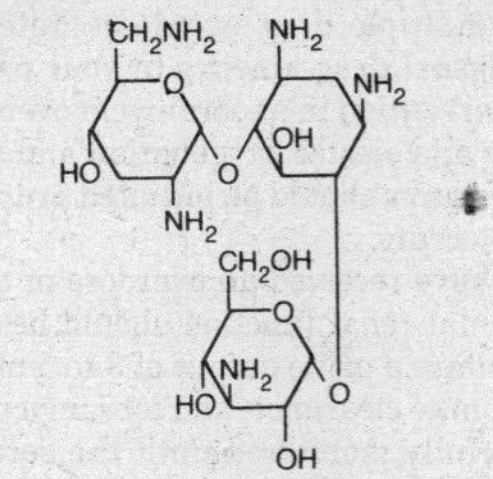

CLINICAL PHARMACOLOGY

Tobramycin is rapidly absorbed following intramuscular administration. Peak serum concentrations of tobramycin occur between 30 and 90 minutes after intramuscular administration. Following an intramuscular dose of 1 mg/kg of body weight, maximum serum concentrations reach about 4 μg/mL, and measurable levels persist for as long as 8 hours. Therapeutic serum levels are generally considered to range from 4 to 6 μg/mL. When Nebcin is administered by intravenous infusion over a 1-hour period, the serum concentrations are similar to those obtained by intramuscular administration. Nebcin is poorly absorbed from the gastrointestinal tract.

In patients with normal renal function, except neonates, Nebcin administered every 8 hours does not accumulate in the serum. However, in those patients with reduced renal function and in neonates, the serum concentration of the antibiotic is usually higher and can be measured for longer periods of time than in normal adults. Dosage for such patients must, therefore, be adjusted accordingly (*see* Dosage and Administration).

Following parenteral administration, little, if any, metabolic transformation occurs, and tobramycin is eliminated almost exclusively by glomerular filtration. Renal clearance is similar to that of endogenous creatinine. Ultrafiltration studies demonstrate that practically no serum protein binding occurs. In patients with normal renal function, up to 84% of the dose is recoverable from the urine in 8 hours and up to 93% in 24 hours.

Peak urine concentrations ranging from 75 to 100 μg/mL have been observed following the intramuscular injection of a single dose of 1 mg/kg. After several days of treatment, the amount of tobramycin excreted in the urine approaches the daily dose administered. When renal function is impaired, excretion of Nebcin is slowed, and accumulation of the drug may cause toxic blood levels.

The serum half-life in normal individuals is 2 hours. An inverse relationship exists between serum half-life and creatinine clearance, and the dosage schedule should be adjusted according to the degree of renal impairment (*see* Dosage and Administration). In patients undergoing dialysis, 25% to 70% of the administered dose may be removed, depending on the duration and type of dialysis.

Tobramycin can be detected in tissues and body fluids after parenteral administration. Concentrations in bile and stools ordinarily have been low, which suggests minimum biliary excretion. Tobramycin has appeared in low concentration in the cerebrospinal fluid following parenteral administration, and concentrations are dependent on dose, rate of penetration, and degree of meningeal inflammation. It has also been found in sputum, peritoneal fluid, synovial fluid, and abscess fluids, and it crosses the placental membranes. Concentrations in the renal cortex are several times higher than the usual serum levels.

Probenecid does not affect the renal tubular transport of tobramycin.

Microbiology – Tobramycin acts by inhibiting synthesis of protein in bacterial cells. In vitro tests demonstrate that tobramycin is bactericidal.

Tobramycin has been shown to be active against most strains of the following organisms both in vitro and in clinical infections as described in the Indications and Usage section:

Aerobic Gram-positive microorganisms

Staphylococcus aureus

Aerobic Gram-negative microorganisms

Citrobacter species
Enterobacter species
Escherichia coli
Klebsiella species
Morganella morganii
Pseudomonas aeruginosa
Proteus mirabilis
Proteus vulgaris
Providencia species
Serratia species

Aminoglycosides have a low order of activity against most gram-positive organisms, including *Streptococcus pyogenes, Streptococcus pneumoniae,* and enterococci.

Although most strains of enterococci demonstrate in vitro resistance, some strains in this group are susceptible. In vitro studies have shown that an aminoglycoside combined with an antibiotic that interferes with cell-wall synthesis affects some enterococcal strains synergistically. The combination of penicillin G and tobramycin results in a synergistic bactericidal effect in vitro against certain strains of *Enterococcus faecalis* . However, this combination is not synergistic against other closely related organisms, eg, *Enterococcus faecium.* Speciation of enterococci alone cannot be used to predict susceptibility. Susceptibility testing and tests for antibiotic synergism are emphasized.

Cross resistance between aminoglycosides may occur.

Susceptibility Tests —

Diffusion techniques: Quantitative methods that require measurement of zone diameters give the most precise estimates of susceptibility of bacteria to antimicrobial agents. One such procedure is the National Committee for Clinical Laboratory Standards (NCCLS)-approved procedure.[1] This method has been recommended for use with disks to test susceptibility to tobramycin. Interpretation involves correlation of the diameters obtained in the disk test with minimum inhibitory concentrations (MIC) for tobramycin.

Reports from the laboratory giving results of the standard single-disk susceptibility test with a 10-μg tobramycin disk should be interpreted according to the following criteria:

Zone Diameter (mm)	Interpretation
≥15	(S) Susceptible
13–14	(I) Intermediate
≤12	(R) Resistant

A report of "Susceptible" indicates that the pathogen is likely to be inhibited by generally achievable blood levels. A report of "Intermediate" suggests that the organism would be susceptible if high dosage is used or if the infection is confined to tissues and fluids in which high antimicrobial levels are obtained. A report of "Resistant" indicates that achievable concentrations are unlikely to be inhibitory and other therapy should be selected.

Standardized procedures require the use of laboratory control organisms. The 10-μg tobramycin disk should give the following zone diameters:

Organism	Zone Diameter (mm)
E. coli ATCC 25922	18–26
P. aeruginosa ATCC 27853	19–25
S. aureus ATCC 25923	19–29

Dilution techniques: Broth and agar dilution methods, such as those recommended by the NCCLS,[2] may be used to determine MICs of tobramycin. MIC test results should be interpreted according to the following criteria:

MIC (μg/mL)	Interpretation
≤4	(S) Susceptible
8	(I) Intermediate
≥16	(R) Resistant

As with standard diffusion methods, dilution procedures require the use of laboratory control organisms. Tobramycin laboratory reagent should give the following MIC values:

Organism	MIC Range (μg/mL)
E. faecalis ATCC 29212	8.0–32.0
E. coli ATCC 25922	0.25–1
P. aeruginosa ATCC 27853	0.12–2
S. aureus ATCC 29213	0.12–1

INDICATIONS AND USAGE

Nebcin is indicated for the treatment of serious bacterial infections caused by susceptible strains of the designated microorganisms in the diseases listed below:

Septicemia in the pediatric patient and adult caused by *P. aeruginosa, E. coli,* and *Klebsiella* spp

Lower respiratory tract infections caused by *P. aeruginosa, Klebsiella* spp, *Enterobacter* spp, *Serratia* spp, *E. coli,* and *S. aureus* (penicillinase- and non-penicillinase-producing strains)

Serious central-nervous-system infections (meningitis) caused by susceptible organisms

Intra-abdominal infections, including peritonitis, caused by *E. coli, Klebsiella* spp, and *Enterobacter* spp

Skin, bone, and skin structure infections caused by *P. aeruginosa, Proteus* spp, *E. coli, Klebsiella* spp, *Enterobacter* spp, and *S. aureus*

Complicated and recurrent urinary tract infections caused by *P. aeruginosa, Proteus* spp (indole-positive and indole-negative), *E. coli, Klebsiella* spp, *Enterobacter* spp, *Serratia* spp, *S. aureus, Providencia* spp, and *Citrobacter* spp

Aminoglycosides, including Nebcin, are not indicated in uncomplicated initial episodes of urinary tract infections unless the causative organisms are not susceptible to antibiotics having less potential toxicity. Nebcin may be considered in serious staphylococcal infections when penicillin or other potentially less toxic drugs are contraindicated and when bacterial susceptibility testing and clinical judgment indicate its use.

Bacterial cultures should be obtained prior to and during treatment to isolate and identify etiologic organisms and to test their susceptibility to tobramycin. If susceptibility tests show that the causative organisms are resistant to tobramycin, other appropriate therapy should be instituted. In patients in whom a serious life-threatening gram-negative infection is suspected, including those in whom concurrent therapy with a penicillin or cephalosporin and an aminoglycoside may be indicated, treatment with Nebcin may be initiated before the results of susceptibility studies are obtained. The decision to continue therapy with Nebcin should be based on the results of susceptibility studies, the severity of the infection, and the important additional concepts discussed in the WARNINGS box above.

CONTRAINDICATIONS

A hypersensitivity to any aminoglycoside is a contraindication to the use of tobramycin. A history of hypersensitivity or serious toxic reactions to aminoglycosides may also contraindicate the use of any other aminoglycoside because of the known cross-sensitivity of patients to drugs in this class.

WARNINGS

See WARNINGS box above.

Nebcin contains sodium bisulfite, a sulfite that may cause allergic-type reactions, including anaphylactic symptoms and life-threatening or less severe asthmatic episodes, in certain susceptible people. The overall prevalence of sulfite sensitivity in the general population is unknown and probably low. Sulfite sensitivity is seen more frequently in asthmatic than in nonasthmatic people.

PRECAUTIONS

Serum and urine specimens for examination should be collected during therapy, as recommended in the WARNINGS box. Serum calcium, magnesium, and sodium should be monitored.

Peak and trough serum levels should be measured periodically during therapy. Prolonged concentrations above 12 μg/mL should be avoided. Rising trough levels (above 2 μg/mL) may indicate tissue accumulation. Such accumulation, advanced age, and cumulative dosage may contribute to ototoxicity and nephrotoxicity. It is particularly important to monitor serum levels closely in patients with known renal impairment.

A useful guideline would be to perform serum level assays after 2 or 3 doses, so that the dosage could be adjusted if necessary, and at 3- to 4-day intervals during therapy. In the event of changing renal function, more frequent serum levels should be obtained and the dosage or dosage interval adjusted according to the guidelines provided in the Dosage and Administration section.

In order to measure the peak level, a serum sample should be drawn about 30 minutes following intravenous infusion or 1 hour after an intramuscular injection. Trough levels are measured by obtaining serum samples at 8 hours or just prior to the next dose of Nebcin. These suggested time intervals are intended only as guidelines and may vary according to institutional practices. It is important, however, that there be consistency within the individual patient program unless computerized pharmacokinetic dosing programs are available in the institution. These serum-level assays may be especially useful for monitoring the treatment of severely ill patients with changing renal function or of those infected with less susceptible organisms or those receiving maximum dosage.

Neuromuscular blockade and respiratory paralysis have been reported in cats receiving very high doses of tobramycin (40 mg/kg). The possibility of prolonged or secondary apnea should be considered if tobramycin is administered to anesthetized patients who are also receiving neuromuscular blocking agents, such as succinylcholine, tubocurarine, or decamethonium, or to patients receiving massive transfusions of citrated blood. If neuromuscular blockade occurs, it may be reversed by the administration of calcium salts.

Cross-allergenicity among aminoglycosides has been demonstrated.

In patients with extensive burns, altered pharmacokinetics may result in reduced serum concentrations of aminoglycosides. In such patients treated with Nebcin, measurement of serum concentration is especially important as a basis for determination of appropriate dosage.

Elderly patients may have reduced renal function that may not be evident in the results of routine screening tests, such as BUN or serum creatinine. A creatinine clearance determination may be more useful. Monitoring of renal function during treatment with aminoglycosides is particularly important in such patients.

An increased incidence of nephrotoxicity has been reported following concomitant administration of aminoglycoside antibiotics and cephalosporins.

Aminoglycosides should be used with caution in patients with muscular disorders, such as myasthenia gravis or parkinsonism, since these drugs may aggravate muscle weak-

Continued on next page

• Identi-Code® symbol. This product information was prepared in June 1996. Current information on these and other products of Eli Lilly and Company may be obtained by direct inquiry to Lilly Research Laboratories, Lilly Corporate Center, Indianapolis, Indiana 46285, 800-545-5979.

Lilly—Cont.

ness because of their potential curare-like effect on neuromuscular function.
Aminoglycosides may be absorbed in significant quantities from body surfaces after local irrigation or application and may cause neurotoxicity and nephrotoxicity.
Aminoglycosides have not been approved for intraocular and/or subconjunctival use. Physicians are advised that macular necrosis has been reported following administration of aminoglycosides, including tobramycin, by these routes.
See WARNINGS box regarding concurrent use of potent diuretics and concurrent and sequential use of other neurotoxic or nephrotoxic drugs.
The inactivation of tobramycin and other aminoglycosides by β-lactam-type antibiotics (penicillins or cephalosporins) has been demonstrated in vitro and in patients with severe renal impairment. Such inactivation has not been found in patients with normal renal function who have been given the drugs by separate routes of administration.
Therapy with tobramycin may result in overgrowth of nonsusceptible organisms. If overgrowth of nonsusceptible organisms occurs, appropriate therapy should be initiated.
Pregnancy Category D—Aminoglycosides can cause fetal harm when administered to a pregnant woman. Aminoglycoside antibiotics cross the placenta, and there have been several reports of total irreversible bilateral congenital deafness in children whose mothers received streptomycin during pregnancy. Serious side effects to mother, fetus, or newborn have not been reported in the treatment of pregnant women with other aminoglycosides. If tobramycin is used during pregnancy or if the patient becomes pregnant while taking tobramycin, she should be apprised of the potential hazard to the fetus.
Pediatric Use —*See* Indications and Usage *and* Dosage and Administration.

ADVERSE REACTIONS

Neurotoxicity—Adverse effects on both the vestibular and auditory branches of the eighth nerve have been noted, especially in patients receiving high doses or prolonged therapy, in those given previous courses of therapy with an ototoxin, and in cases of dehydration. Symptoms include dizziness, vertigo, tinnitus, roaring in the ears, and hearing loss. Hearing loss is usually irreversible and is manifested initially by diminution of high-tone acuity. Tobramycin and gentamicin sulfates closely parallel each other in regard to ototoxic potential.
Nephrotoxicity—Renal function changes, as shown by rising BUN, NPN, and serum creatinine and by oliguria, cylindruria, and increased proteinuria, have been reported, especially in patients with a history of renal impairment who are treated for longer periods or with higher doses than those recommended. Adverse renal effects can occur in patients with initially normal renal function.
Clinical studies and studies in experimental animals have been conducted to compare the nephrotoxic potential of tobramycin and gentamicin. In some of the clinical studies and in the animal studies, tobramycin caused nephrotoxicity significantly less frequently than gentamicin. In some other clinical studies, no significant difference in the incidence of nephrotoxicity between tobramycin and gentamicin was found.
Other reported adverse reactions possibly related to Nebcin include anemia, granulocytopenia, and thrombocytopenia; and fever, rash, exfoliative dermatitis, itching, urticaria, nausea, vomiting, diarrhea, headache, lethargy, pain at the injection site, mental confusion, and disorientation. Laboratory abnormalities possibly related to Nebcin include increased serum transaminases (AST, ALT); increased serum LDH and bilirubin; decreased serum calcium, magnesium, sodium, and potassium; and leukopenia, leukocytosis, and eosinophilia.

OVERDOSAGE

Signs and Symptoms—The severity of the signs and symptoms following a tobramycin overdose are dependent on the dose administered, the patient's renal function, state of hydration, and age and whether or not other medications with similar toxicities are being administered concurrently. Toxicity may occur in patients treated more than 10 days, in adults given more than 5 mg/kg/day, in children given more than 7.5 mg/kg/day, or in patients with reduced renal function where dose has not been appropriately adjusted.
Nephrotoxicity following the parenteral administration of an aminoglycoside is most closely related to the area under the curve of the serum concentration versus time graph. Nephrotoxicity is more likely if trough blood concentrations fail to fall below 2 μg/mL and is also proportional to the average blood concentration. Patients who are elderly, have abnormal renal function, are receiving other nephrotoxic drugs, or are volume depleted are at greater risk for developing acute tubular necrosis. Auditory and vestibular toxicities have been associated with aminoglycoside overdose. These toxicities occur in patients treated longer than 10 days, in patients with abnormal renal function, in dehydrated patients, or in patients receiving medications with additive auditory toxicities. These patients may not have signs or symptoms or may experience dizziness, tinnitus, vertigo, and a loss of high-tone acuity as ototoxicity progresses. Ototoxicity signs and symptoms may not begin to occur until long after the drug has been discontinued.
Neuromuscular blockade or respiratory paralysis may occur following administration of aminoglycosides. Neuromuscular blockade, respiratory failure, and prolonged respiratory paralysis may occur more commonly in patients with myasthenia gravis or Parkinson's disease. Prolonged respiratory paralysis may also occur in patients receiving decamethonium, tubocurarine, or succinylcholine. If neuromuscular blockade occurs, it may be reversed by the administration of calcium salts but mechanical assistance may be necessary.
If tobramycin were ingested, toxicity would be less likely because aminoglycosides are poorly absorbed from an intact gastrointestinal tract.
Treatment—In all cases of suspected overdosage, call your Regional Poison Control Center to obtain the most up-to-date information about the treatment of overdose. This recommendation is made because, in general, information regarding the treatment of overdose may change more rapidly than the package insert. In managing overdosage, consider the possibility of multiple drug overdoses, interaction among drugs, and unusual drug kinetics in your patient.
The initial intervention in a tobramycin overdose is to establish an airway and ensure oxygenation and ventilation. Resuscitative measures should be initiated promptly if respiratory paralysis occurs.
Patients who have received an overdose of tobramycin and who have normal renal function should be adequately hydrated to maintain a urine output of 3 to 5 mL/kg/hr. Fluid balance, creatinine clearance, and tobramycin plasma levels should be carefully monitored until the serum tobramycin level falls below 2 μg/mL.
Patients in whom the elimination half-life is greater than 2 hours or whose renal function is abnormal may require more aggressive therapy. In such patients, hemodialysis may be beneficial.

DOSAGE AND ADMINISTRATION

Nebcin may be given intramuscularly or intravenously. ADD-Vantage vials are not for intramuscular administration. Recommended dosages are the same for both routes. The patient's pretreatment body weight should be obtained for calculation of correct dosage. It is desirable to measure both peak and trough serum concentrations (*see* WARNINGS box *and* Precautions).
Administration for Patients With Normal Renal Function —Adults With Serious Infections: 3 mg/kg/day in 3 equal doses every 8 hours (*see* Table 1).
Adults With Life-Threatening Infections: Up to 5 mg/kg/day may be administered in 3 or 4 equal doses (*see* Table 1). The dosage should be reduced to 3 mg/kg/day as soon as clinically indicated. To prevent increased toxicity due to excessive blood levels, dosage should not exceed 5 mg/kg/day unless serum levels are monitored (*see* WARNINGS box *and* Precautions).
[See table 1 below.]
Pediatric Patients: 6 to 7.5 mg/kg/day in 3 or 4 equally divided doses (2 to 2.5 mg/kg every 8 hours or 1.5 to 1.89 mg/kg every 6 hours).
Premature or Full-Term Neonates 1 Week of Age or Less: Up to 4 mg/kg/day may be administered in 2 equal doses every 12 hours.
It is desirable to limit treatment to a short term. The usual duration of treatment is 7 to 10 days. A longer course of therapy may be necessary in difficult and complicated infections. In such cases, monitoring of renal, auditory, and vestibular functions is advised, because neurotoxicity is more likely to occur when treatment is extended longer than 10 days.
Administration for Patients With Impaired Renal Function —Whenever possible, serum tobramycin concentrations should be monitored during therapy.
Following a loading dose of 1 mg/kg, subsequent dosage in these patients must be adjusted, either with reduced doses administered at 8-hour intervals or with normal doses given at prolonged intervals. Both of these methods are suggested as guides to be used when serum levels of tobramycin cannot be measured directly. They are based on either the creatinine clearance level or the serum creatinine level of the patient because these values correlate with the half-life of tobramycin. The dosage schedule derived from either method should be used in conjunction with careful clinical and laboratory observations of the patient and should be modified as necessary. Neither method should be used when dialysis is being performed.
Reduced dosage at 8-hour intervals: When the creatinine clearance rate is 70 mL or less per minute or when the serum creatinine value is known, the amount of the reduced dose can be determined by multiplying the normal dose from Table 1 by the percent of normal dose from the accompanying nomogram.
[See Figure at top of next column.]
An alternate rough guide for determining reduced dosage at 8-hour intervals (for patients whose steady-state serum creatinine values are known) is to divide the normally recommended dose by the patient's serum creatinine.
Normal dosage at prolonged intervals: If the creatinine clearance rate is not available and the patient's condition is stable, a dosage frequency *in hours* for the dosage given in Table 1 can be determined by multiplying the patient's serum creatinine by 6.
Dosage in Obese Patients—The appropriate dose may be calculated by using the patient's estimated lean body weight plus 40% of the excess as the basic weight on which to figure mg/kg.
Intramuscular Administration—Nebcin may be administered by withdrawing the appropriate dose directly from a vial or by using a prefilled Hyporet®. ADD-Vantage vials are not for intramuscular administration.
Intravenous Administration—For intravenous administration, the usual volume of diluent (0.9% Sodium Chloride Injection or 5% Dextrose Injection) is 50 to 100 mL for adult doses. For pediatric patients, the volume of diluent should be proportionately less than that for adults. The diluted solution usually should be infused over a period of 20 to 60 minutes. Infusion periods of less than 20 minutes are not recom-

TABLE 1. DOSAGE SCHEDULE GUIDE FOR ADULTS WITH NORMAL RENAL FUNCTION
(Dosage at 8-Hour Intervals)

For Patient Weighing kg	lb	Usual Dose for Serious Infections 1 mg/kg q8h (Total, 3 mg/kg/day) mg/dose q8h	mL/dose*	Maximum Dose for Life-Threatening Infections (Reduce as soon as possible) 1.66 mg/kg q8h (Total, 5 mg/kg/day) mg/dose q8h	mL/dose*
120	264	120 mg	3 mL	200 mg	5 mL
115	253	115 mg	2.9 mL	191 mg	4.75 mL
110	242	110 mg	2.75 mL	183 mg	4.5 mL
105	231	105 mg	2.6 mL	175 mg	4.4 mL
100	220	100 mg	2.5 mL	166 mg	4.2 mL
95	209	95 mg	2.4 mL	158 mg	4 mL
90	198	90 mg	2.25 mL	150 mg	3.75 mL
85	187	85 mg	2.1 mL	141 mg	3.5 mL
80	176	80 mg	2 mL	133 mg	3.3 mL
75	165	75 mg	1.9 mL	125 mg	3.1 mL
70	154	70 mg	1.75 mL	116 mg	2.9 mL
65	143	65 mg	1.6 mL	108 mg	2.7 mL
60	132	60 mg	1.5 mL	100 mg	2.5 mL
55	121	55 mg	1.4 mL	91 mg	2.25 mL
50	110	50 mg	1.25 mL	83 mg	2.1 mL
45	99	45 mg	1.1 mL	75 mg	1.9 mL
40	88	40 mg	1 mL	66 mg	1.6 mL

*Applicable to all product forms except Nebcin, Pediatric, Injection (*see* How Supplied).

REDUCED DOSAGE NOMOGRAM*
Creatinine Clearance (mL/min/1.73 m²)

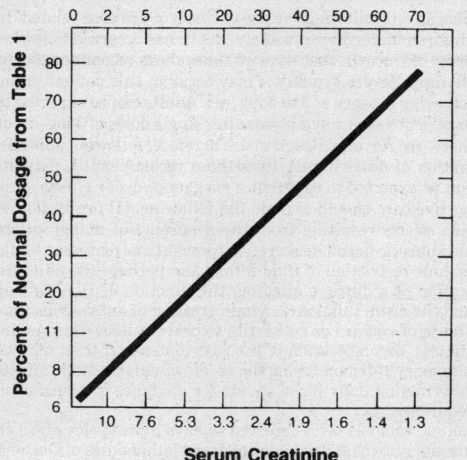

**Serum Creatinine
(mg/100 mL)**

***Scales have been adjusted to
facilitate dosage calculations.***

mended, because peak serum levels may exceed 12 μg/mL (*see* WARNINGS box).

Use of ADD-Vantage Nebcin Vials—ADD-Vantage Nebcin vials are not intended for multiple use and should not be used with a syringe in the conventional way. These products are intended for use only with Abbott ADD-Vantage diluent containers and in those instances in which the physician's order specified 60-mg or 80-mg doses. Use within 24 hours after activation.

Nebcin should not be physically premixed with other drugs but should be administered separately according to the recommended dose and route.

Prior to administration, parenteral drug products should be inspected visually for particulate matter and discoloration whenever solution and container permit.

HOW SUPPLIED

Multiple-Dose Vials:

80 mg*/2 mL, 2 mL (No. 781)—(1s) NDC 0002-1499-01; (Traypak† of 25) NDC 0002-1499-25

Pediatric, 20 mg*/2 mL, 2 mL (No. 782)—(1s) NDC 0002-0501-01

40 mg*/mL, 1.2 g/30 mL (No. 7090)—(Traypak of 6) NDC 0002-7090-16

Hyporets®,‡ each scored with a 10-mg (0.25-mL) fractional dose scale:

60 mg*/1.5 mL, 1.5 mL (No. 55)—(24s) NDC 0002-0509-24
80 mg*/2 mL, 2 mL (No. 42)—(24s) NDC 0002-0503-24

ADD-Vantage§ Vials:

60 mg*/6 mL, 6 mL (No. 7293)—(Traypak of 25) NDC 0002-7293-25

80 mg*/8 mL, 8 mL (No. 7294)—(Traypak of 25) NDC 0002-7294-25

The above ADD-Vantage vials are to be used only with Abbott Laboratories' diluent containers.

Instructions for the use of ADD-Vantage vials are enclosed in the package.

Also Available:

Pharmacy Bulk Vial:

1.2 g* (Dry Powder) (40-mL size) (No. 7040)—(Traypak of 6) NDC 0002-7040-16

Store at controlled room temperature 59° to 86°F (15° to 30°C).

* Equivalent to tobramycin.
† Traypak™ (multivial carton, Lilly).
‡ Hyporet® (disposable syringe, Lilly).
§ ADD-Vantage® (vials and diluent containers, Abbott).

REFERENCES

1. National Committee for Clinical Laboratory Standards, Performance standards for antimicrobial disk susceptibility tests—4th ed. Approved Standard NCCLS Document M2-A5, Vol 13, No 24, NCCLS, Villanova, PA 1993.
2. National Committee for Clinical Laboratory Standards, Methods for dilution antimicrobial susceptibility tests for bacteria that grow aerobically—3rd ed. Approved Standard NCCLS Document M7-A3, Vol 13, No 25, NCCLS, Villanova, PA, 1993.

[040596]

NPH ILETIN® I AND II   OTC
(isophane insulin suspension, Lilly) See Under Iletin®
(insulin)

ONCOVIN®   ℞
[ŏn'kō-vĭn]
**(Vincristine Sulfate Injection, USP)
Solution**

> ### WARNINGS
> *Caution—This preparation should be administered by individuals experienced in the administration of Oncovin. It is extremely important that the intravenous needle or catheter be properly positioned before any vincristine is injected. Leakage into surrounding tissue during intravenous administration of Oncovin may cause considerable irritation. If extravasation occurs, the injection should be discontinued immediately, and any remaining portion of the dose should then be introduced into another vein. Local injection of hyaluronidase and the application of moderate heat to the area of leakage help disperse the drug and are thought to minimize discomfort and the possibility of cellulitis.*
> *FATAL IF GIVEN INTRATHECALLY. FOR INTRAVENOUS USE ONLY. See Warnings section for the treatment of patients given intrathecal Oncovin.*

DESCRIPTION
Oncovin® (Vincristine Sulfate, USP) is vincaleukoblastine, 22-oxo-, sulfate (1:1) (salt). It is the salt of an alkaloid obtained from a common flowering herb, the periwinkle plant (*Vinca rosea* Linn). Originally known as leurocristine, it has also been referred to as LCR and VCR. The empirical formula for vincristine sulfate is $C_{46}H_{56}N_4O_{10} \cdot H_2SO_4$. It has a molecular weight of 923.04. The structural formula is as follows:

$$\cdot H_2SO_4$$

Vincristine sulfate is a white to off-white powder. It is soluble in methanol, freely soluble in water, but only slightly soluble in 95% ethanol.

Each mL contains vincristine sulfate, 1 mg (1.08 μmol); mannitol, 100 mg; methylparaben, 1.3 mg; propylparaben, 0.2 mg; and water for injection, qs. Acetic acid and sodium acetate have been added for pH control. The pH of Oncovin Solution ranges from 3.5 to 5.5. This product is a sterile solution for cancer/oncolytic use.

CLINICAL PHARMACOLOGY
The mechanisms of action of Oncovin remain under investigation.[1] The mechanism of action of Oncovin has been related to the inhibition of microtubule formation in the mitotic spindle, resulting in an arrest of dividing cells at the metaphase stage.

Central-nervous-system leukemia has been reported in patients undergoing otherwise successful therapy with Oncovin. This suggests that Oncovin does not penetrate well into the cerebrospinal fluid.

Pharmacokinetic studies in patients with cancer have shown a triphasic serum decay pattern following rapid intravenous injection. The initial, middle, and terminal half-lives are 5 minutes, 2.3 hours, and 85 hours respectively; however, the range of the terminal half-life in humans is from 19 to 155 hours. The liver is the major excretory organ in humans and animals. The metabolism of vinca alkaloids has been shown to be mediated by hepatic cytochrome P450 isoenzymes in the CYP 3A subfamily. This metabolic pathway may be impaired in patients with hepatic dysfunction or who are taking concomitant potent inhibitors of these isoenzymes (*see* Precautions).[2–3] About 80% of an injected dose of Oncovin appears in the feces and 10% to 20% can be found in the urine. Within 15 to 30 minutes after injection, over 90% of the drug is distributed from the blood into tissue, where it remains tightly, but not irreversibly, bound.[2]

Current principles of cancer chemotherapy involve the simultaneous use of several agents. Generally, each agent used has a unique toxicity and mechanism of action so that therapeutic enhancement occurs without additive toxicity. It is rarely possible to achieve equally good results with single-agent methods of treatment. Thus, Oncovin is often chosen as part of polychemotherapy because of lack of significant bone-marrow suppression (at recommended doses) and of unique clinical toxicity (neuropathy). *See* Dosage and Administration for possible increased toxicity when used in combination therapy.

INDICATIONS AND USAGE
Oncovin is indicated in acute leukemia.

Oncovin has also been shown to be useful in combination with other oncolytic agents in Hodgkin's disease[5], non-Hodgkin's malignant lymphomas[6–8] (lymphocytic, mixed-cell, histiocytic, undifferentiated, nodular, and diffuse types), rhabdomyosarcoma,[9] neuroblastoma,[10] and Wilms' tumor.[11]

CONTRAINDICATIONS
Patients with the demyelinating form of Charcot-Marie-Tooth syndrome should not be given Oncovin. Careful attention should be given to those conditions listed under Warnings *and* Precautions.

WARNINGS

> *This preparation is for intravenous use only. It should be administered by individuals experienced in the administration of Oncovin. The intrathecal administration of Oncovin usually results in death. Syringes containing this product should be labeled, using the auxiliary sticker provided, to state "FATAL IF GIVEN INTRATHECALLY. FOR INTRAVENOUS USE ONLY."*
> Extemporaneously prepared syringes containing this product must be packaged in an overwrap which is labeled "DO NOT REMOVE COVERING UNTIL MOMENT OF INJECTION. FATAL IF GIVEN INTRATHECALLY. FOR INTRAVENOUS USE ONLY."
> Treatment of patients following intrathecal administration of Oncovin has included immediate removal of spinal fluid and flushing with Lactated Ringer's, as well as other solutions and has not prevented ascending paralysis and death. In one case, progressive paralysis in an adult was arrested by the following treatment **initiated immediately after the intrathecal injection:**
> 1. As much spinal fluid was removed as could be safely done through lumbar access.
> 2. The subarachnoid space was flushed with Lactated Ringer's solution infused continuously through a catheter in a cerebral lateral ventricle at the rate of 150 mL/h. The fluid was removed through a lumbar access.
> 3. As soon as fresh frozen plasma became available, the fresh frozen plasma, 25 mL, diluted in 1 L of Lactated Ringer's solution was infused through the cerebral ventricular catheter at the rate of 75 mL/h with removal through the lumbar access. The rate of infusion was adjusted to maintain a protein level in the spinal fluid of 150 mg/dL.
> 4. Glutamic acid, 10 g, was given intravenously over 24 hours followed by 500 mg 3 times daily by mouth for 1 month or until neurological dysfunction stabilized. The role of glutamic acid in this treatment is not certain and may not be essential.

Pregnancy Category D—Oncovin can cause fetal harm when administered to a pregnant woman. When pregnant mice and hamsters were given doses of Oncovin that caused the resorption of 23% to 85% of fetuses, fetal malformations were produced in those that survived. Five monkeys were given single doses of Oncovin between days 27 and 34 of their pregnancies; 3 of the fetuses were normal at term, and 2 viable fetuses had grossly evident malformations at term.[12] In several animal species, Oncovin can induce teratogenesis as well as embryo death at doses that are nontoxic to the pregnant animal. There are no adequate and well-controlled studies in pregnant women. If this drug is used during pregnancy or if the patient becomes pregnant while receiving this drug, she should be apprised of the potential hazard to the fetus. Women of childbearing potential should be advised to avoid becoming pregnant.

PRECAUTIONS
General—Acute uric acid nephropathy, which may occur after the administration of oncolytic agents, has also been

Continued on next page

• **Identi-Code® symbol. This product information was prepared in June 1996. Current information on these and other products of Eli Lilly and Company may be obtained by direct inquiry to Lilly Research Laboratories, Lilly Corporate Center, Indianapolis, Indiana 46285, 800-545-5979.**

Lilly—Cont.

reported with Oncovin. In the presence of leukopenia or a complicating infection, administration of the next dose of Oncovin warrants careful consideration.

If central-nervous-system leukemia is diagnosed, additional agents may be required, because Oncovin does not appear to cross the blood-brain barrier in adequate amounts.

Particular attention should be given to dosage and neurologic side effects if Oncovin is administered to patients with preexisting neuromuscular disease and when other drugs with neurotoxic potential are also being used.

Acute shortness of breath and severe bronchospasm have been reported following the administration of vinca alkaloids. These reactions have been encountered most frequently when the vinca alkaloid was used in combination with mitomycin-C and may require aggressive treatment, particularly when there is preexisting pulmonary dysfunction. The onset of these reactions may occur minutes to several hours after the vinca alkaloid is injected and may occur up to 2 weeks following the dose of mitomycin. Progressive dyspnea requiring chronic therapy may occur. Oncovin should not be readministered.

Care must be taken to avoid contamination of the eye with concentrations of Oncovin used clinically. If accidental contamination occurs, severe irritation (or, if the drug was delivered under pressure, even corneal ulceration) may result. The eye should be washed immediately and thoroughly.

Laboratory Tests—Because dose-limiting clinical toxicity is manifested as neurotoxicity, clinical evaluation (eg, history, physical examination) is necessary to detect the need for dosage modification. Following administration of Oncovin, some individuals may have a fall in the white-blood-cell count or platelet count, particularly when previous therapy or the disease itself has reduced bone-marrow function. Therefore, a complete blood count should be done before administration of each dose. Acute elevation of serum uric acid may also occur during induction of remission in acute leukemia; thus, such levels should be determined frequently during the first 3 to 4 weeks of treatment or appropriate measures taken to prevent uric acid nephropathy. The laboratory performing these tests should be consulted for its range of normal values.

Drug Interaction—The simultaneous oral or intravenous administration of phenytoin and antineoplastic chemotherapy combinations that included vincristine sulfate has been reported to reduce blood levels of the anticonvulsant and to increase seizure activity.[13] Dosage adjustment should be based on serial blood level monitoring. The contribution of vincristine sulfate to this interaction is not certain. The interaction may result from reduced absorption of phenytoin and an increase in the rate of its metabolism and elimination.

Caution should be exercised in patients concurrently taking drugs known to inhibit drug metabolism by hepatic cytochrome P450 isoenzymes in the CYP 3A subfamily, or in patients with hepatic dysfunction. Concurrent administration of vincristine sulfate with itraconazole (a known inhibitor of the metabolic pathway) has been reported to cause an earlier onset and/or an increased severity of neuromuscular side effects (see Adverse Reactions). This interaction is presumed to be related to inhibition of the metabolism of vincristine.

Carcinogenesis, Mutagenesis, Impairment of Fertility—Neither in vivo nor in vitro laboratory tests have conclusively demonstrated the mutagenicity of this product.[12] Fertility following treatment with Oncovin alone for malignant disease has not been studied in humans. Clinical reports of both male and female patients who received multiple-agent chemotherapy that included Oncovin indicate that azoospermia and amenorrhea can occur in postpubertal patients. Recovery occurred many months after completion of chemotherapy in some but not all patients. When the same treatment is administered to prepubertal patients, permanent azoospermia and amenorrhea are much less likely.[14-20]

Patients who received chemotherapy with Oncovin in combination with anticancer drugs known to be carcinogenic have developed second malignancies. The contributing role of Oncovin in this development has not been determined. No evidence of carcinogenicity was found following intraperitoneal administration of Oncovin in rats and mice, although this study was limited.[12]

Usage in Pregnancy—*Pregnancy Category D*—See Warnings.

Nursing Mothers—It is not known whether this drug is excreted in human milk. Because many drugs are excreted in human milk and because of the potential for serious adverse reactions due to Oncovin in nursing infants, a decision should be made either to discontinue nursing or the drug, taking into account the importance of the drug to the mother.

ADVERSE REACTIONS

Prior to the use of this drug, patients and/or their parents/ guardian should be advised of the possibility of untoward symptoms.

In general, adverse reactions are reversible and are related to dosage. The most common adverse reaction is hair loss; the most troublesome adverse reactions are neuromuscular in origin.

When single, weekly doses of the drug are employed, the adverse reactions of leukopenia, neuritic pain, and constipation occur but are usually of short duration (ie, less than 7 days). When the dosage is reduced, these reactions may lessen or disappear. The severity of such reactions seems to increase when the calculated amount of drug is given in divided doses. Other adverse reactions, such as hair loss, sensory loss, paresthesia, difficulty in walking, slapping gait, loss of deep-tendon reflexes, and muscle wasting, may persist for at least as long as therapy is continued. Generalized sensorimotor dysfunction may become progressively more severe with continued treatment. Although most such symptoms usually disappear by about the sixth week after discontinuance of treatment, some neuromuscular difficulties may persist for prolonged periods in some patients. Regrowth of hair may occur while maintenance therapy continues.

The following adverse reactions have been reported:

Hypersensitivity—Rare cases of allergic-type reactions, such as anaphylaxis, rash, and edema, that are temporally related to vincristine therapy have been reported in patients receiving vincristine as a part of multidrug chemotherapy regimens.

Gastrointestinal—Constipation, abdominal cramps, weight loss, nausea, vomiting, oral ulceration, diarrhea, paralytic ileus, intestinal necrosis and/or perforation, and anorexia have occurred. Constipation may take the form of upper-colon impaction, and, on physical examination, the rectum may be empty. Colicky abdominal pain coupled with an empty rectum may mislead the physician. A flat film of the abdomen is useful in demonstrating this condition. All cases have responded to high enemas and laxatives. A routine prophylactic regimen against constipation is recommended for all patients receiving Oncovin.

Paralytic ileus (which mimics the "surgical abdomen") may occur, particularly in young children. The ileus will reverse itself with temporary discontinuance of Oncovin and with symptomatic care.

Genitourinary—Polyuria, dysuria, and urinary retention due to bladder atony have occurred. Other drugs known to cause urinary retention (particularly in the elderly) should, if possible, be discontinued for the first few days following administration of Oncovin.

Cardiovascular—Hypertension and hypotension have occurred. Chemotherapy combinations that have included vincristine sulfate, when given to patients previously treated with mediastinal radiation, have been associated with coronary artery disease and myocardial infarction. Causality has not been established.

Neurologic—Frequently, there is a sequence to the development of neuromuscular side effects. Initially, only sensory impairment and paresthesia may be encountered. With continued treatment, neuritic pain and, later, motor difficulties may occur. There have been no reports of any agent that can reverse the neuromuscular manifestations that may accompany therapy with Oncovin.

Loss of deep-tendon reflexes, foot drop, ataxia, and paralysis have been reported with continued administration. Cranial nerve manifestations, including isolated paresis and/or paralysis of muscles controlled by cranial motor nerves, may occur in the absence of motor impairment elsewhere; extraocular and laryngeal muscles are those most commonly involved. Jaw pain, pharyngeal pain, parotid gland pain, bone pain, back pain, limb pain, and myalgias have been reported; pain in these areas may be severe. Convulsions, frequently with hypertension, have been reported in a few patients receiving Oncovin. Several instances of convulsions followed by coma have been reported in children. Transient cortical blindness and optic atrophy with blindness have been reported. Treatment with vinca alkaloids has resulted rarely in both vestibular and auditory damage to the eighth cranial nerve. Manifestations include partial or total deafness which may be temporary or permanent, and difficulties with balance including dizziness, nystagmus, and vertigo. Particular caution is warranted when Onconvin is used in combination with other agents known to be ototoxic such as the platinum-containing oncolytics.

Pulmonary—See Precautions.

Endocrine—Rare occurrences of a syndrome attributable to inappropriate antidiuretic hormone secretion have been observed in patients treated with Oncovin. This syndrome is characterized by high urinary sodium excretion in the presence of hyponatremia; renal or adrenal disease, hypotension, dehydration, azotemia, and clinical edema are absent. With fluid deprivation, improvement occurs in the hyponatremia and in the renal loss of sodium.

Hematologic—Oncovin does not appear to have any constant or significant effect on platelets or red blood cells. Serious bone-marrow depression is usually not a major dose-limiting event. However, anemia, leukopenia, and thrombocytopenia have been reported. Thrombocytopenia, if present when therapy with Oncovin is begun, may actually improve before the appearance of marrow remission.

Skin—Alopecia and rash have been reported.

Other—Fever and headache have occurred.

OVERDOSAGE

Side effects following the use of Oncovin are dose related. In children under 13 years of age, death has occurred following doses of Oncovin that were 10 times those recommended for therapy. Severe symptoms may occur in this patient group following dosages of 3 to 4 mg/m². Adults can be expected to experience severe symptoms after single doses of 3 mg/m² or more (see Adverse Reactions). Therefore, following administration of doses higher than those recommended, patients can be expected to experience exaggerated side effects. Supportive care should include the following: (1) prevention of side effects resulting from the syndrome of inappropriate antidiuretic hormone secretion (preventive treatment would include restriction of fluid intake and perhaps the administration of a diuretic affecting the function of Henle's loop and the distal tubule); (2) administration of anticonvulsants; (3) use of enemas or cathartics to prevent ileus (in some instances, decompression of the gastrointestinal tract may be necessary); (4) monitoring the cardiovascular system; and (5) determining daily blood counts for guidance in transfusion requirements.

Folinic acid has been observed to have a protective effect in normal mice that were administered lethal doses of Oncovin (*Cancer Res* 1963; 23:1390). Isolated case reports suggest that folinic acid may be helpful in treating humans who have received an overdose of Oncovin. It is suggested that 100 mg of folinic acid be administered intravenously every 3 hours for 24 hours and then every 6 hours for at least 48 hours. Theoretically (based on pharmacokinetic data), tissue levels of Oncovin can be expected to remain significantly elevated for at least 72 hours. Treatment with folinic acid does not eliminate the need for the above-mentioned supportive measures.

Most of an intravenous dose of Oncovin is excreted into the bile after rapid tissue binding (see Clinical Pharmacology). Because only very small amounts of the drug appear in dialysate, hemodialysis is not likely to be helpful in cases of overdosage. An increase in the severity of side effects may be experienced by patients with liver disease that is severe enough to decrease biliary excretion.

Enhanced fecal excretion of parenterally administered vincristine has been demonstrated in dogs pretreated with cholestyramine. There are no published clinical data on the use of cholestyramine as an antidote in humans.

There are no published clinical data on the consequences of oral ingestion of vincristine. Should oral ingestion occur, the stomach should be evacuated. Evacuation should be followed by oral administration of activated charcoal and a cathartic.

DOSAGE AND ADMINISTRATION

This preparation is for intravenous use only (see Warnings). Neurotoxicity appears to be dose related. Extreme care must be used in calculating and administering the dose of Oncovin since overdosage may have a very serious or fatal outcome.

Special Dispensing Information—WHEN DISPENSING VINCRISTINE IN OTHER THAN THE ORIGINAL CONTAINER, IT IS IMPERATIVE THAT IT BE PACKAGED IN THE PROVIDED OVERWRAP WHICH BEARS THE FOLLOWING STATEMENT: "DO NOT REMOVE COVERING UNTIL MOMENT OF INJECTION. FATAL IF GIVEN INTRATHECALLY. FOR INTRAVENOUS USE ONLY". (see Warnings) A syringe containing a specific dose must be labeled, using the auxiliary sticker provided, to state: "FATAL IF GIVEN INTRATHECALLY. FOR INTRAVENOUS USE ONLY."

The concentration of vincristine contained in all vials and Hyporets® of Oncovin is 1 mg/mL. Do not add extra fluid to the vial prior to removal of the dose. Withdraw the solution of Oncovin into an accurate dry syringe, measuring the dose carefully. Do not add extra fluid to the vial in an attempt to empty it completely.

Caution—*It is extremely important that the intravenous needle or catheter be properly positioned before any vincristine is injected. Leakage into surrounding tissue during intravenous administration of Oncovin may cause considerable irritation. If extravasation occurs, the injection should be discontinued immediately, and any remaining portion of the dose should then be introduced into another vein. Local injection of hyaluronidase and the application of moderate heat to the area of leakage will help disperse the drug and may minimize discomfort and the possibility of cellulitis.*

Oncovin must be administered via an intact, free-flowing intravenous needle or catheter. Care should be taken that there is no leakage or swelling occurring during administration (see boxed Warnings).

The solution may be injected either directly into a vein or into the tubing of a running intravenous infusion (see Drug Interactions below). Injection of Oncovin should be accomplished within 1 minute.

The drug is administered intravenously *at weekly intervals.* The usual dose of Oncovin for children is 2 mg/m². For children weighing 10 kg or less, the starting dose should be 0.05 mg/kg, administered once a week. The usual dose of Oncovin

for adults is 1.4 mg/m². A 50% reduction in the dose of Oncovin is recommended for patients having a direct serum bilirubin value above 3 mg/100 mL.[21]

Oncovin should not be given to patients while they are receiving radiation therapy through ports that include the liver. When Oncovin is used in combination with L-asparaginase, Oncovin should be given 12 to 24 hours before administration of the enzyme in order to minimize toxicity; administering L-asparaginase before Oncovin may reduce hepatic clearance of Oncovin.

Drug Interactions —Oncovin should not be diluted in solutions that raise or lower the pH outside the range of 3.5 to 5.5. It should not be mixed with anything other than normal saline or glucose in water.

Whenever solution and container permit, parenteral drug products should be inspected visually for particulate matter and discoloration prior to administration.

Procedures for proper handling and disposal of anticancer drugs should be considered. Several guidelines on this subject have been published.[22-27] There is no general agreement that all of the procedures recommended in the guidelines are necessary or appropriate.

HOW SUPPLIED

Multiple-Dose Vials:
1 mg/1 mL, 1 mL (No. 7194)—(1s) NDC 0002-7194-01
2 mg/2 mL, 2 mL (No. 7195)—(1s) NDC 0002-7195-01
5 mg/5 mL, 5 mL (No. 7196)—(1s) NDC 0002-7196-01
Hyporets,* each marked with a 0.1-mg (0.1-mL) fractional dose scale:
1 mg/1 mL, 1 mL (No. 7198)—(3s) NDC 0002-7198-09
2 mg/2 mL, 2 mL (No. 7199)—(3s) NDC 0002-7199-09
*Hyporet® (disposable syringe, Lilly)

This product should be refrigerated.

CAUTION—Federal (USA) law prohibits dispensing without prescription.

Reference titles are available in the manufacturer's full prescribing information.

Literature revised September 26, 1995
Eli Lilly and Company, Indianapolis, IN 46285, USA
PA 0100 AMP [092695]

PAPAVERINE HYDROCHLORIDE ℞

[pă-păv 'ŭr-ēn hī 'drō-klōr-īd]
Injection, USP

This product is to be used by or under the direction of a physician.

Each ampoule or vial contains a sufficient amount to permit withdrawal and administration of the volume specified on the label.

DESCRIPTION

Papaverine hydrochloride is the hydrochloride of an alkaloid obtained from opium or prepared synthetically. It belongs to the benzylisoquinoline group of alkaloids. It does not contain a phenanthrene group as do morphine and codeine.

Papaverine hydrochloride is 6,7-dimethoxy-1-veratrylisoquinoline hydrochloride and contains, on the dried basis, not less than 98.5% of $C_{20}H_{21}NO_4 \cdot HCl$. The molecular weight is 375.85. The structural formula is as shown:

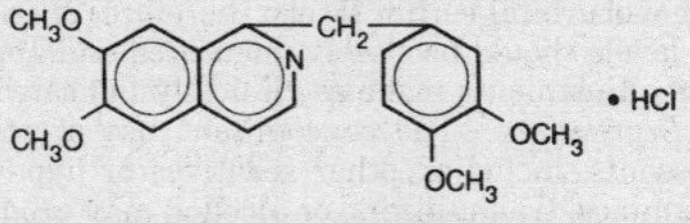

Papaverine hydrochloride occurs as white crystals or white crystalline powder. One g dissolves in about 30 mL of water and in 120 mL of alcohol. It is soluble in chloroform and practically insoluble in ether.

Papaverine Hydrochloride Injection is a clear, colorless to pale-yellow solution.

Papaverine hydrochloride, for parenteral administration, is a smooth-muscle relaxant that is available in ampoules or vials containing 30 mg/mL (88.4 µmol/L) of papaverine base. Each ampoule or vial also contains edetate disodium, 0.005%. Sodium hydroxide may have been added during manufacture to adjust the pH.

CLINICAL PHARMACOLOGY

The most characteristic effect of papaverine is relaxation of the tonus of all smooth muscle, especially when it has been spasmodically contracted. Papaverine hydrochloride apparently acts directly on the muscle itself. This relaxation is noted in the *vascular system* and *bronchial musculature* and in the *gastrointestinal, biliary,* and *urinary tracts.*

The main actions of papaverine are exerted on cardiac and smooth muscle. Papaverine relaxes various smooth muscles, especially those of larger arteries; this relaxation may be prominent if spasm exists. The antispasmodic effect is a direct one and unrelated to muscle innervation, and the muscle still responds to drugs and other stimuli causing contraction. Papaverine has minimal actions on the central nervous system, although very large doses tend to produce some sedation and sleepiness in some patients. In certain circumstances, mild respiratory stimulation can be observed, but this is therapeutically inconsequential. Papaverine stimulates respiration by acting on carotid and aortic body chemoreceptors.

Papaverine relaxes the smooth musculature of the larger blood vessels, including the coronary, cerebral, peripheral, and pulmonary arteries. This action is particularly evident when such vessels are in spasm, induced reflexly or by drugs, and it provides the basis for the clinical use of papaverine in peripheral or pulmonary arterial embolism.

Experimentally in dogs, the alkaloid has been shown to cause fairly marked and long-lasting coronary vasodilatation and an increase in coronary blood flow. However, it also appears to have a direct inotropic effect and, when increased mechanical activity coincides with decreased systemic pressure, increases in coronary blood flow may not be sufficient to prevent brief periods of hypoxic myocardial depression.

Papaverine is effective by all routes of administration. A considerable fraction of the drug localizes in fat depots and in the liver, with the remainder being distributed throughout the body. It is metabolized in the liver. About 90% of the drug is bound to plasma protein. Although estimates of its biologic half-life vary widely, reasonably constant plasma levels can be maintained with oral administration at 6-hour intervals. The drug is excreted in the urine in an inactive form.

INDICATIONS AND USAGE

Papaverine is recommended in various conditions accompanied by spasm of smooth muscle, such as *vascular spasm* associated with acute myocardial infarction (coronary occlusion), angina pectoris, peripheral and pulmonary embolism, peripheral vascular disease in which there is a vasospastic element, or certain cerebral angiospastic states; and *visceral spasm,* as in ureteral, biliary, or gastrointestinal colic.

CONTRAINDICATIONS

Intravenous injection of papaverine is contraindicated in the presence of complete atrioventricular heart block. When conduction is depressed, the drug may produce transient ectopic rhythms of ventricular origin, either premature beats or paroxysmal tachycardia.

Papaverine hydrochloride is not indicated for the treatment of impotence by intracorporeal injection. The intracorporeal injection of papaverine hydrochloride has been reported to have resulted in persistent priapism requiring medical and surgical intervention.

PRECAUTIONS

General —Papaverine Hydrochloride Injection, USP, should not be added to Lactated Ringer's Injection, because precipitation would result.

Papaverine hydrochloride should be used with caution in patients with glaucoma. The medication should be discontinued if hepatic hypersensitivity with gastrointestinal symptoms, jaundice, or eosinophilia becomes evident or if liver function test values become altered.

Usage in Pregnancy —Pregnancy Category C —No teratogenic effects were observed in rats when papaverine hydrochloride was administered subcutaneously as a single agent. It is not known whether papaverine can cause fetal harm when administered to a pregnant woman or can affect reproduction capacity. Papaverine hydrochloride should be given to a pregnant woman only if clearly needed.

Nursing Mothers —It is not known whether this drug is excreted in human milk. Because many drugs are excreted in human milk, caution should be exercised when papaverine hydrochloride is administered to a nursing woman.

Usage in Children —Safety and effectiveness in children have not been established.

ADVERSE REACTIONS

The following side effects have been reported: general discomfort, nausea, abdominal discomfort, anorexia, constipation or diarrhea, skin rash, malaise, vertigo, headache, intensive flushing of the face, perspiration, increase in the depth of respiration, increase in heart rate, a slight rise in blood pressure, and excessive sedation.

Hepatitis, probably related to an immune mechanism, has been reported infrequently. Rarely, this has progressed to cirrhosis.

DRUG ABUSE AND DEPENDENCE

Drug dependence resulting from the abuse of many of the selective depressants, including papaverine hydrochloride, has been reported.

OVERDOSAGE

Signs and Symptoms —The symptoms of toxicity from papaverine hydrochloride often result from vasomotor instability and include nausea, vomiting, weakness, central nervous system depression, nystagmus, diplopia, diaphoresis, flushing, dizziness, and sinus tachycardia. In large overdoses, papaverine is a potent inhibitor of cellular respiration and a weak calcium antagonist. Following an oral overdose of 15 g, metabolic acidosis with hyperventilation, hyperglycemia, and hypokalemia have been reported. No information on toxic serum concentrations is available.

Following intravenous overdosing in animals, seizures, tachyarrhythmias, and ventricular fibrillation have been reported. The oral median lethal dose in rats is 360 mg/kg.

Treatment —To obtain up-to-date information about the treatment of overdose, a good resource is your certified Regional Poison Control Center. Telephone numbers of certified poison control centers are listed in the *Physicians' Desk Reference (PDR).* In managing overdosage, consider the possibility of multiple drug overdoses, interaction among drugs, and unusual drug kinetics in your patient.

Protect the patient's airway and support ventilation and perfusion. Meticulously monitor vital signs, blood gases, blood chemistry values, and other variables.

If convulsions occur, consider diazepam, phenytoin, or phenobarbital. If the seizures are refractory, general anesthesia with thiopental or halothane and paralysis with a neuromuscular blocking agent may be necessary.

For hypotension, consider intravenous fluids, elevation of the legs, and an inotropic vasopressor, such as dopamine or levarteranol. Theoretically, calcium gluconate may be helpful in treating some of the toxic cardiovascular effects of papaverine; monitor the ECG and plasma calcium concentrations.

Forced diuresis, peritoneal dialysis, hemodialysis, or charcoal hemoperfusion have not been established as beneficial for an overdose of papaverine hydrochloride.

DOSAGE AND ADMINISTRATION

Papaverine hydrochloride may be administered intravenously or intramuscularly. The intravenous route is recommended when an immediate effect is desired, but the drug *must* be injected *slowly* over the course of 1 or 2 minutes to avoid uncomfortable or alarming side effects.

Parenteral administration of papaverine hydrochloride in doses of 1 to 4 mL is repeated every 3 hours as indicated. In the treatment of cardiac extrasystoles, 2 doses may be given 10 minutes apart.

HOW SUPPLIED

Multiple-Dose Vials:
30 mg/mL, 10 mL, with 0.5% chlorobutanol (chloroform derivative) (No. 423)—(1s) NDC 0002-1676-01; (25s) NDC 0002-1676-25
Ampoules:
60 mg in 2 mL (No. 396)—(12s) NDC 0002-1664-12; (100s) NDC 0002-1664-02

CAUTION-Federal (USA) law prohibits dispensing without prescription.

[100290]

PHENOBARBITAL Ⓒ IV

[fē 'nō-băr 'bĭ-tăl]
Elixir & Tablets, USP

WARNING: MAY BE HABIT-FORMING

DESCRIPTION

The barbiturates are nonselective central nervous system (CNS) depressants that are primarily used as sedative-hypnotics. In subhypnotic doses, they are also used as anticonvulsants. The barbiturates and their sodium salts are subject to control under the Federal Controlled Substances Act.

Phenobarbital is a barbituric acid derivative and occurs as white, odorless, small crystals or crystalline powder that is very slightly soluble in water; soluble in alcohol, in ether, and in solutions of fixed alkali hydroxides and carbonates; sparingly soluble in chloroform. Phenobarbital is 5-ethyl-5-phenylbarbituric acid and has the empirical formula $C_{12}H_{12}N_2O_3$. Its molecular weight is 232.24. It has the following structural formula:

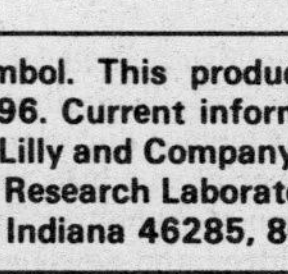

Phenobarbital is a substituted pyrimidine derivative in which the basic structure is barbituric acid, a substance that has no CNS activity. CNS activity is obtained by substituting alkyl, alkenyl, or aryl groups on the pyrimidine ring.

Continued on next page

*** Identi-Code® symbol. This product information was prepared in June 1996. Current information on these and other products of Eli Lilly and Company may be obtained by direct inquiry to Lilly Research Laboratories, Lilly Corporate Center, Indianapolis, Indiana 46285, 800-545-5979.**

Lilly—Cont.

Each 5 mL of the elixir contains 20 mg (0.086 mmol) phenobarbital. The elixir also contains FD & C Red No. 40, flavors, glycerin, sucrose, water, and alcohol, 14%.

The tablets contain 15 mg (0.064 mmol), 30 mg (0.129 mmol), 60 mg (0.258 mmol), or 100 mg (0.431 mmol) phenobarbital. The tablets also contain cornstarch, lactose, magnesium stearate, and talc.

CLINICAL PHARMACOLOGY

Barbiturates are capable of producing all levels of CNS mood alteration, from excitation to mild sedation, hypnosis, and deep coma. Overdosage can produce death. In high enough therapeutic doses, barbiturates induce anesthesia.

Barbiturates depress the sensory cortex, decrease motor activity, alter cerebellar function, and produce drowsiness, sedation, and hypnosis.

Barbiturate-induced sleep differs from physiologic sleep. Sleep laboratory studies have demonstrated that barbiturates reduce the amount of time spent in the rapid eye movement (REM) phase of sleep or the dreaming stage. Also, Stages III and IV sleep are decreased. Following abrupt cessation of barbiturates used regularly, patients may experience markedly increased dreaming, nightmares, and/or insomnia. Therefore, withdrawal of a single therapeutic dose over 5 or 6 days has been recommended to lessen the REM rebound and disturbed sleep that contribute to the drug withdrawal syndrome (for example, the dose should be decreased from 3 to 2 doses/day for 1 week).

In studies, secobarbital sodium and pentobarbital sodium have been found to lose most of their effectiveness for both inducing and maintaining sleep by the end of 2 weeks of continued drug administration even with the use of multiple doses. As with secobarbital sodium and pentobarbital sodium, other barbiturates (including amobarbital) might be expected to lose their effectiveness for inducing and maintaining sleep after about 2 weeks. The short-, intermediate-, and to a lesser degree, long-acting barbiturates have been widely prescribed for treating insomnia. Although the clinical literature abounds with claims that the short-acting barbiturates are superior for producing sleep whereas the intermediate-acting compounds are more effective in maintaining sleep, controlled studies have failed to demonstrate these differential effects. Therefore, as sleep medications, the barbiturates are of limited value beyond short-term use.

Barbiturates have little analgesic action at subanesthetic doses. Rather, in subanesthetic doses, these drugs may increase the reaction to painful stimuli. All barbiturates exhibit anticonvulsant activity in anesthetic doses. However, of the drugs in this class, only phenobarbital, mephobarbital, and metharbital are effective as oral anticonvulsants in subhypnotic doses.

Barbiturates are respiratory depressants, and the degree of respiratory depression is dependent upon the dose. With hypnotic doses, respiratory depression produced by barbiturates is similar to that which occurs during physiologic sleep and is accompanied by a slight decrease in blood pressure and heart rate.

Studies in laboratory animals have shown that barbiturates cause reduction in the tone and contractility of the uterus, ureters, and urinary bladder. However, concentrations of the drugs required to produce this effect in humans are not reached with sedative-hypnotic doses.

Barbiturates do not impair normal hepatic function but have been shown to induce liver microsomal enzymes, thus increasing and/or altering the metabolism of barbiturates and other drugs (*see* Drug Interactions *under* Precautions).

Pharmacokinetics—Barbiturates are absorbed in varying degrees following oral or parenteral administration. The salts are more rapidly absorbed than are the acids. The rate of absorption is increased if the sodium salt is ingested as a dilute solution or taken on an empty stomach.

Duration of action, which is related to the rate at which the barbiturates are redistributed throughout the body, varies among persons and in the same person from time to time.

Phenobarbital is classified as a long-acting barbiturate when taken orally. Its onset of action is 1 hour or longer, and its duration of action ranges from 10 to 12 hours.

Barbiturates are weak acids that are absorbed and rapidly distributed to all tissues and fluids, with high concentrations in the brain, liver, and kidneys. Lipid solubility of the barbiturates is the dominant factor in their distribution within the body. The more lipid soluble the barbiturate, the more rapidly it penetrates all tissues of the body. Barbiturates are bound to plasma and tissue proteins to a varying degree with the degree of binding increasing directly as a function of lipid solubility.

Phenobarbital has the lowest lipid solubility, lowest plasma binding, lowest brain protein binding, the longest delay in onset activity, and the longest duration of action. The plasma half-life for phenobarbital in adults ranges between 53 and 118 hours with a mean of 79 hours. The plasma half-life for phenobarbital in children and newborns (less than 48 hours old) ranges between 60 to 180 hours with a mean of 110 hours.

Barbiturates are metabolized primarily by the hepatic microsomal enzyme system, and the metabolic products are excreted in the urine and, less commonly, in the feces. Approximately 25% to 50% of a dose of phenobarbital is eliminated unchanged in the urine. The excretion of unmetabolized barbiturate is one feature that distinguishes the long-acting category from those belonging to other categories, which are almost entirely metabolized. The inactive metabolities of the barbiturates are excreted as conjugates of glucuronic acid.

INDICATIONS AND USAGE

A. Sedative
B. Anticonvulsant—For the treatment of generalized and partial seizures.

CONTRAINDICATIONS

Phenobarbital is contraindicated in patients who are hypersensitive to barbiturates, in patients with a history of manifest or latent porphyria, and in patients with marked impairment of liver function or respiratory disease in which dyspnea or obstruction is evident.

WARNINGS

1. *Habit Forming*—Phenobarbital may be habit forming. Tolerance and psychological and physical dependence may occur with continued use (*see* Drug Abuse and Dependence *and* Pharmacokinetics *under* Clinical Pharmacology). Patients who have psychologic dependence on barbiturates may increase the dosage or decrease the dosage interval without consulting a physician and may subsequently develop a physical dependence on barbiturates. In order to minimize the possibility of overdosage or the development of dependence, the prescribing and dispensing of sedative-hypnotic barbiturates should be limited to the amount required for the interval until the next appointment. Abrupt cessation after prolonged use in a person who is dependent on the drug may result in withdrawal symptoms, including delirium, convulsions, and possibly death. Barbiturates should be withdrawn gradually from any patient known to be taking excessive doses over long periods of time (*see* Drug Abuse and Dependence).

2. *Acute or Chronic Pain*—Caution should be exercised when barbiturates are administered to patients with acute or chronic pain, because paradoxical excitement could be induced or important symptoms could be masked. However, the use of barbiturates as sedatives in the postoperative surgical period and as adjuncts to cancer chemotherapy is well established.

3. *Usage in Pregnancy*—Barbiturates can cause fetal damage when administered to a pregnant woman. Retrospective, case-controlled studies have suggested a connection between the maternal consumption of barbiturates and a higher than expected incidence of fetal abnormalities. Barbiturates readily cross the placental barrier and are distributed throughout fetal tissues; the highest concentrations are found in the placenta, fetal liver, and brain. Fetal blood levels approach maternal blood levels following parenteral administration.

Withdrawal symptoms occur in infants born to women who receive barbiturates throughout the last trimester of pregnancy (*see* Drug Abuse and Dependence).

If phenobarbital is used during pregnancy or if the patient becomes pregnant while taking this drug, the patient should be apprised of the potential hazard to the fetus.

4. *Usage in Children*—Phenobarbital has been reported to be associated with cognitive deficits in children taking it for complicated febrile seizures.

5. *Synergistic Effects*—The concomitant use of alcohol or other CNS depressants may produce additive CNS depressant effects.

PRECAUTIONS

General—Barbiturates may be habit forming. Tolerance and psychological and physical dependence may occur with continued use (*see* Drug Abuse and Dependence).

Barbiturates should be administered with caution, if at all, to patients who are mentally depressed, have suicidal tendencies, or have a history of drug abuse.

Elderly or debilitated patients may react to barbiturates with marked excitement, depression, or confusion. In some persons, especially children, barbiturates repeatedly produce excitement rather than depression.

In patients with hepatic damage, barbiturates should be administered with caution and initially in reduced doses. Barbiturates should not be administered to patients showing the premonitory signs of hepatic coma.

The systemic effects of exogenous and endogenous corticosteroids may be diminished by phenobarbital. Thus, this product should be administered with caution to patients with borderline hypoadrenal function, regardless of whether it is of pituitary or of primary adrenal origin.

Information for Patients—The following information and instructions should be given to patients receiving barbiturates.

1. The use of barbiturates carries with it an associated risk of psychological and/or physical dependence. The patient should be warned against increasing the dose of the drug without consulting a physician.
2. Barbiturates may impair the mental and/or physical abilities required for the performance of potentially hazardous tasks, such as driving a car or operating machinery. The patient should be cautioned accordingly.
3. Alcohol should not be consumed while taking barbiturates. The concurrent use of the barbiturates with other CNS depressants (eg, alcohol, narcotics, tranquilizers, and antihistamines) may result in additional CNS-depressant effects.

Laboratory Tests—Prolonged therapy with barbiturates should be accompanied by periodic laboratory evaluation of organ systems, including hematopoietic, renal, and hepatic systems (*see* General *under* Precautions *and* Adverse Reactions).

Drug Interactions—Most reports of clinically significant drug interactions occurring with the barbiturates have involved phenobarbital. However, the application of these data to other barbiturates appears valid and warrants serial blood level determinations of the relevant drugs when there are multiple therapies.

1. *Anticoagulants*—Phenobarbital lowers the plasma levels of dicumarol and causes a decrease in anticoagulant activity as measured by the prothrombin time. Barbiturates can induce hepatic microsomal enzymes resulting in increased metabolism and decreased anticoagulant response of oral anticoagulants (eg, warfarin, acenocoumarol, dicumarol, and phenprocoumon). Patients stabilized on anticoagulant therapy may require dosage adjustments if barbiturates are added to or withdrawn from their dosage regimen.
2. *Corticosteroids*—Barbiturates appear to enhance the metabolism of exogenous corticosteroids, probably through the induction of hepatic microsomal enzymes. Patients stabilized on corticosteroid therapy may require dosage adjustments if barbiturates are added to or withdrawn from their dosage regimen.
3. *Griseofulvin*—Phenobarbital appears to interfere with the absorption of orally administered griseofulvin, thus decreasing its blood level. The effect of the resultant decreased blood levels of griseofulvin on therapeutic response has not been established. However, it would be preferable to avoid concomitant administration of these drugs.
4. *Doxycycline*—Phenobarbital has been shown to shorten the half-life of doxycycline for as long as 2 weeks after barbiturate therapy is discontinued. This mechanism is probably through the induction of hepatic microsomal enzymes that metabolize the antibiotic. If phenobarbital and doxycycline are administered concurrently, the clinical response to doxycycline should be monitored closely.
5. *Phenytoin, Sodium Valproate, Valproic Acid*—The effect of barbiturates on the metabolism of phenytoin appears to be variable. Some investigators report an accelerating effect, whereas others report no effect. Because the effect of barbiturates on the metabolism of phenytoin is not predictable, phenytoin and barbiturate blood levels should be monitored more frequently if these drugs are given concurrently. Sodium valproate and valproic acid increase the phenobarbital serum levels; therefore, phenobarbital blood levels should be closely monitored and appropriate dosage adjustments made as clinically indicated.
6. *CNS Depressants*—The concomitant use of other CNS depressants, including other sedatives or hypnotics, antihistamines, tranquilizers, or alcohol, may produce additive depressant effects.
7. *Monoamine Oxidase Inhibitors (MAOIs)*—MAOIs prolong the effects of barbiturates, probably because metabolism of the barbiturate is inhibited.
8. *Estradiol, Estrone, Progesterone, and Other Steroidal Hormones*—Pretreatment with or concurrent administration of phenobarbital may decrease the effect of estradiol by increasing its metabolism. There have been reports of patients treated with antiepileptic drugs (eg, phenobarbital) who become pregnant while taking oral contraceptives. An alternate contraceptive method might be suggested to women taking phenobarbital.

Carcinogenesis—1. *Animal Data.* Phenobarbital sodium is carcinogenic in mice and rats after lifetime administration. In mice, it produced benign and malignant liver cell tumors. In rats, benign liver cell tumors were observed very late in life.

2. *Human Data*—In a 29-year epidemiologic study of 9,136 patients who were treated on an anticonvulsant protocol that included phenobarbital, results indicated a higher than normal incidence of hepatic carcinoma. Previously, some of these patients had been treated with thorotrast, a drug which is known to produce hepatic carcinomas. Thus, this study did not provide sufficient evidence that phenobarbital sodium is carcinogenic in humans.

A retrospective study of 84 children with brain tumors matched to 73 normal controls and 78 cancer controls (malignant disease other than brain tumors) suggested an associa-

tion between exposure to barbiturates prenatally and an increased incidence of brain tumors.

Usage in Pregnancy —1. Teratogenic Effects. Pregnancy Category D —See Usage in Pregnancy *under* Warnings.

2. *Nonteratogenic Effects* —Reports of infants suffering from long-term barbiturate exposure in utero included the acute withdrawal syndrome of seizures and hyperirritability from birth to a delayed onset of up to 14 days (*see* Drug Abuse and Dependence).

Labor and Delivery —Hypnotic doses of barbiturates do not appear to impair uterine activity significantly during labor. Full anesthetic doses of barbiturates decrease the force and frequency of uterine contractions. Administration of sedative-hypnotic barbiturates to the mother during labor may result in respiratory depression in the newborn. Premature infants are particularly susceptible to the depressant effects of barbiturates. If barbiturates are used during labor and delivery, resuscitation equipment should be available.

Data are not available to evaluate the effect of barbiturates when forceps delivery or other intervention is necessary or to determine the effect of barbiturates on the later growth, development, and functional maturation of the child.

Nursing Mothers —Caution should be exercised when phenobarbital is administered to a nursing woman, because small amounts of barbiturates are excreted in the milk.

ADVERSE REACTIONS

The following adverse reactions have been reported:

CNS Depression —Residual sedation or "hangover," drowsiness, lethargy, and vertigo. Emotional disturbances and phobias may be accentuated. In some persons, barbiturates such as phenobarbital repeatedly produce excitement rather than depression, and the patient may appear to be inebriated. Irritability and hyperactivity can occur in children. Like other nonanalgesic hypnotic drugs, barbiturates such as phenobarbital, when given in the presence of pain, may cause restlessness, excitement, and even delirium. Rarely, the use of barbiturates results in localized or diffuse myalgic, neuralgic, or arthritic pain, especially in psychoneurotic patients with insomnia. The pain may appear in paroxysms, is most intense in the early morning hours, and is most frequently located in the region of the neck, shoulder girdle, and upper limbs. Symptoms may last for days after the drug is discontinued.

Respiratory/Circulatory —Respiratory depression, apnea, circulatory collapse.

Allergic —Acquired hypersensitivity to barbiturates consists chiefly in allergic reactions that occur especially in persons who tend to have asthma, urticaria, angioedema, and similar conditions. Hypersensitivity reactions in this category include localized swelling, particularly of the eyelids, cheeks, or lips, and erythematous dermatitis. Rarely, exfoliative dermatitis (eg, Stevens-Johnson syndrome and toxic epidermal necrolysis) may be caused by phenobarbital and can prove fatal. The skin eruption may be associated with fever, delirium, and marked degenerative changes in the liver and other parenchymatous organs. In a few cases, megaloblastic anemia has been associated with the chronic use of phenobarbital.

Other —Nausea and vomiting; headache, osteomalacia.

The following adverse reactions and their incidence were compiled from surveillance of thousands of hospitalized patients who received barbiturates. Because such patients may be less aware of the milder adverse effects of barbiturates, the incidence of these reactions may be somewhat higher in fully ambulatory patients.

More than 1 in 100 Patients

The most common adverse reaction, estimated to occur at a rate of 1 to 3 patients per 100, is:

Nervous System: Somnolence

Less than 1 in 100 Patients

Adverse reactions estimated to occur at a rate of less than 1 in 100 patients are listed below, grouped by organ system and by decreasing order of occurrence:

Nervous System: Agitation, confusion, hyperkinesia, ataxia, CNS depression, nightmares, nervousness, psychiatric disturbance, hallucinations, insomnia, anxiety, dizziness, abnormality in thinking

Respiratory System: Hypoventilation, apnea

Cardiovascular System: Bradycardia, hypotension, syncope

Digestive System: Nausea, vomiting, constipation

Other Reported Reactions: Headache, injection site reactions, hypersensitivity reactions (angioedema, skin rashes, exfoliative dermatitis), fever, liver damage, megaloblastic anemia following chronic phenobarbital use

DRUG ABUSE AND DEPENDENCE

Controlled Substance —Phenobarbital is a Schedule IV drug.

Dependence —Barbiturates may be habit forming. Tolerance, psychological dependence, and physical dependence may occur, especially following prolonged use of high doses of barbiturates. Daily administration in excess of 400 mg of pentobarbital or secobarbital for approximately 90 days is likely to produce some degreee of physical dependence. A dosage of 600 to 800 mg taken for at least 35 days is sufficient to produce withdrawal seizures. The average daily dose for the barbiturate addict is usually about 1.5 g. As tolerance to barbiturates develops, the amount needed to maintain the same level of intoxication increases; tolerance to a fatal dosage, however, does not increase more than twofold. As this occurs, the margin between intoxicating dosage and fatal dosage becomes smaller.

Symptoms of acute intoxication with barbiturates include unsteady gait, slurred speech, and sustained nystagmus. Mental signs of chronic intoxication include confusion, poor judgment, irritability, insomnia, and somatic complaints.

Symptoms of barbiturate dependence are similar to those of chronic alcoholism. If an individual appears to be intoxicated with alcohol to a degree that is radically disproportionate to the amount of alcohol in his or her blood, the use of barbiturates should be suspected. The lethal dose of a barbiturate is far less if alcohol is also ingested.

The symptoms of barbiturate withdrawal can be severe and may cause death. Minor withdrawal symptoms may appear 8 to 12 hours after the last dose of a barbiturate. These symptoms usually appear in the following order: anxiety, muscle twitching, tremor of hands and fingers, progressive weakness, dizziness, distortion in visual perception, nausea, vomiting, insomnia, and orthostatic hypotension. Major withdrawal symptoms (convulsions and delirium) may occur within 16 hours and last up to 5 days after abrupt cessation of barbiturates. The intensity of withdrawal symptoms gradually declines over a period of approximately 15 days. Individuals susceptible to barbiturate abuse and dependence include alcoholics and opiate abusers as well as other sedative-hypnotic and amphetamine abusers.

Drug dependence on barbiturates arises from repeated administration of a barbiturate or agent with barbiturate-like effect on a continuous basis, generally in amounts exceeding therapeutic dose levels. The characteristics of drug dependence on barbiturates include: (a) a strong desire or need to continue taking the drug; (b) a tendency to increase the dose; (c) a psychic dependence on the effects of the drug related to subjective and individual appreciation of those effects; and (d) a physical dependence on the effects of the drug, requiring its presence for maintenance of homeostasis and resulting in a definite, characteristic, and self-limited abstinence syndrome when the drug is withdrawn.

Treatment of barbiturate dependence consists of cautious and gradual withdrawal of the drug. Barbiturate-dependent patients can be withdrawn by using a number of different withdrawal regimens. In all cases, withdrawal requires an extended period of time. One method involves substituting a 30-mg dose of phenobarbital for each 100- to 200-mg dose of barbiturate that the patient has been taking. The total daily amount of phenobarbital is then administered in 3 or 4 divided doses, not to exceed 600 mg daily. If signs of withdrawal occur on the first day of treatment, a loading dose of 100 to 200 mg of phenobarbital may be administered IM in addition to the oral dose. After stabilization on phenobarbital, the total daily dose is decreased by 30 mg/day as long as withdrawal is proceeding smoothly. A modification of this regimen involves initiating treatment at the patient's regular dosage level and decreasing the daily dosage by 10% if tolerated by the patient.

Infants who are physically dependent on barbiturates may be given phenobarbital, 3 to 10 mg/kg/day. After withdrawal symptoms (hyperactivity, disturbed sleep, tremors, and hyperreflexia) are relieved, the dosage of phenobarbital should be gradually decreased and completely withdrawn over a 2-week period.

OVERDOSAGE

Signs and Symptoms —The onset of symptoms following a toxic oral exposure to phenobarbital may not occur until several hours following ingestion. The toxic dose of barbiturates varies considerably. In general, an oral dose of 1 g of most barbiturates produces serious poisoning in an adult. Death commonly occurs after 2 to 10 g of ingested barbiturate. The sedated, therapeutic blood levels of phenobarbital range between 5 to 40 μg/mL; the usual lethal blood level ranges from 100 to 200 μg/mL. Barbiturate intoxication may be confused with alcoholism, bromide intoxication, and various neurologic disorders. Potential tolerance must be considered when evaluating significance of dose and plasma concentration.

The manifestations of a long-acting barbiturate in overdose include nystagmus, ataxia, CNS depression, respiratory depression, hypothermia, and hypotension. Other findings may include absent or depressed reflexes and erythematous or hemorrhagic blisters (primarily at pressure points). Following massive exposure to phenobarbital, pulmonary edema, circulatory collapse with loss of peripheral vascular tone, cardiac arrest, and death may occur.

In extreme overdose, all electrical activity in the brain may cease, in which case a "flat" EEG normally equated with clinical death should not be accepted. This effect is fully reversible unless hypoxic damage occurs.

Consideration should be given to the possibility of barbiturate intoxication even in situations that appear to involve trauma.

Complications such as pneumonia, pulmonary edema, cardiac arrhythmias, congestive heart failure, and renal failure may occur. Uremia may increase CNS sensitivity to barbiturates if renal function is impaired. Differential diagnosis should include hypoglycemia, head trauma, cerebrovascular accidents, convulsive states, and diabetic coma.

Treatment —To obtain up-to-date information about the treatment of overdose, a good resource is your certified Regional Poison Control Center. Telephone numbers of certified poison control centers are listed in the *Physicians' Desk Reference (PDR)*. In managing overdosage, consider the possibility of multiple drug overdoses, interaction among drugs, and unusual drug kinetics in your patient.

Protect the patient's airway and support ventilation and perfusion. Meticulously monitor and maintain, within acceptable limits, the patient's vital signs, blood gases, serum electrolytes, etc. Absorption of drugs from the gastrointestinal tract may be decreased by giving activated charcoal, which, in many cases, is more effective than emesis or lavage; consider charcoal instead of or in addition to gastric emptying. Repeated doses of charcoal over time may hasten elimination of some drugs that have been absorbed. Safeguard the patient's airway when employing gastric emptying or charcoal.

Alkalinization of urine hastens phenobarbital excretion, but dialysis and hemoperfusion are more effective and cause less troublesome alterations in electrolyte equilibrium. If the patient has chronically abused sedatives, withdrawal reactions may be manifest following acute overdose.

DOSAGE AND ADMINISTRATION

The dose of phenobarbital must be individualized with full knowledge of its particular characteristics. Factors of consideration are the patient's age, weight, and condition.

Sedation:

For sedation, the drug may be administered in single does of 30 to 120 mg repeated at intervals: frequency will be determined by the patient's response. It is generally considered that no more than 400 mg of phenobarbital should be administered during a 24-hour period.

Adults:

Daytime Sedation: 30 to 120 mg daily in 2 to 3 divided doses
Oral Hypnotic: 100 to 200 mg.

Anticonvulsant Use —Clinical laboratory reference values should be used to determine the therapeutic anticonvulsant level of phenobarbital in the serum. To achieve the blood levels considered therapeutic in children, higher per-kilogram dosages are generally necessary for phenobarbital and most other anticonvulsants. In children and infants, phenobarbital at a loading dose of 15 to 20 mg/kg produces blood levels of about 20 μg/mL shortly after administration.

Phenobarbital has been used in the treatment and prophylaxis of febrile seizures. However, it has not been established that prevention of febrile seizures influences the subsequent development of epilepsy.

Adults: 60 to 200 mg/day.
Children: 3 to 6 mg/kg/day.

Special Patient Population —Dosage should be reduced in the elderly or debilitated because these patients may be more sensitive to barbiturates. Dosage should be reduced for patients with impaired renal function or hepatic disease.

HOW SUPPLIED

Elixir:
0.4 g/100 mL (No. 227)*—(16 fl oz) NDC 0002-2438-05
Tablets:
15 mg (No. 1544)—(100s) NDC 0002-1031-02; (1000s) NDC 0002-1031-04
30 mg (No. 1545)—(100s) NDC 0002-1032-02; (1000s) NDC 0002-1032-04
60 mg (No. 1574)—(100s) NDC 0002-1037-02; (1000s) NDC 0002-1037-04
100 mg (No. 1546)—(100s) NDC 0002-1033-02

*Contains alcohol, 14%.

Keep tightly closed. Store at controlled room temperature, 59° to 86°F (15° to 30°C).

CAUTION-Federal (USA) law prohibits dispensing without prescription.

[103091]

Continued on next page

• Identi-Code® symbol. This product information was prepared in June 1996. Current information on these and other products of Eli Lilly and Company may be obtained by direct inquiry to Lilly Research Laboratories, Lilly Corporate Center, Indianapolis, Indiana 46285, 800-545-5979.

Lilly—Cont.

PROTAMINE SULFATE ℞

[prō'ta-mēn sŭl'fāt]
Injection, USP

DESCRIPTION
Protamines are simple proteins of low molecular weight that are rich in arginine and strongly basic. They occur in the sperm of salmon and certain other species of fish.
Protamine sulfate occurs as fine white or off-white amorphous or crystalline powder. It is sparingly soluble in water. The pH is between 6 and 7. The cationic hydrogenated protamine at a pH of 6.8 to 7.1 reacts with anionic heparin at a pH of 5.0 to 7.5 to form an inactive complex.
Protamine Sulfate Injection, USP, is a sterile, isotonic solution of protamine sulfate. It acts as a heparin antagonist. It is also a weak anticoagulant.
Each 25-mL vial contains protamine sulfate equivalent to 250 mg of activity. Product also contains 0.9% Sodium Chloride Reagent in Water for Injection, USP. Sodium phosphate and/or sulfuric acid may have been added during manufacture to adjust the pH. Contains no preservative.
Protamine sulfate is administered intravenously.

CLINICAL PHARMACOLOGY
When administered alone, protamine has an anticoagulant effect. However, when it is given in the presence of heparin (which is strongly acidic), a stable salt is formed and the anticoagulant activity of both drugs is lost.
Protamine sulfate has a rapid onset of action. Neutralization of heparin occurs within 5 minutes after intravenous administration of an appropriate dose of protamine sulfate. Although the metabolic fate of the heparin-protamine complex has not been elucidated, it has been postulated that protamine sulfate in the heparin-protamine complex may be partially metabolized or may be attacked by fibrinolysin, thus freeing heparin.

INDICATIONS AND USAGE
Protamine sulfate is indicated in the treatment of heparin overdosage.

CONTRAINDICATION
Protamine sulfate is contraindicated in patients who have shown previous intolerance to the drug.

WARNINGS
Hyperheparinemia or bleeding has been reported in experimental animals and in some patients 30 minutes to 18 hours after cardiac surgery (under cardiopulmonary bypass) in spite of complete neutralization of heparin by adequate doses of protamine sulfate at the end of the operation. It is important to keep the patient under close observation after cardiac surgery. Additional doses of protamine sulfate should be administered if indicated by coagulation studies, such as the heparin titration test with protamine and the determination of plasma thrombin time.
Too-rapid administration of protamine sulfate can cause severe hypotensive and anaphylactoid reactions (*see* Dosage and Administration). Facilities to treat shock should be available.

PRECAUTIONS
***General*—Because of the anticoagulant effect of protamine, it is unwise to give more than 50 mg over a short period unless a larger dose is clearly needed.**
Patients with a history of allergy to fish may develop hypersensitivity reactions to protamine, although to date no relationship has been established between allergic reactions to protamine and fish allergy.
Previous exposure to protamine can induce a humoral immune response and predispose susceptible individuals to the development of untoward reactions from the subsequent use of this drug. Patients exposed to protamine through the use of protamine-containing insulin or during heparin neutralization may experience life-threatening reactions and fatal anaphylaxis upon receiving large doses of protamine intravenously. Severe reactions to intravenous protamine can occur in the absence of local or systemic allergic reactions to subcutaneous injection of protamine-containing insulin.
Reports of the presence of antiprotamine antibodies in the sera of infertile or vasectomized men suggest that some of these individuals may react to use of protamine sulfate.
Fatal anaphylaxis has been reported in one patient with no prior history of allergies.
Drug Interactions —Protamine sulfate has been shown to be incompatible with certain antibiotics, including several of the cephalosporins and penicillins (*see* Dosage and Administration).
Carcinogenesis, Mutagenesis, Impairment of Fertility—Studies have not been performed to determine potential for carcinogenicity, mutagenicity, or impairment of fertility.
Pregnancy—Pregnancy Category C—Animal reproduction studies have not been conducted with protamine sulfate. It is also not known whether protamine sulfate can cause fetal harm when administered to a pregnant woman or can affect reproduction capacity. Protamine sulfate should be given to a pregnant woman only if clearly needed.
Nursing Mothers—It is not known whether this drug is excreted in human milk. Because many drugs are excreted in human milk, caution should be exercised when protamine sulfate is administered to a nursing woman.
Pediatric Use—Safety and effectiveness in children have not been established.

ADVERSE REACTIONS
The intravenous administration of protamine sulfate may cause a sudden fall in blood pressure and bradycardia. Other reactions include transitory flushing and feeling of warmth, dyspnea, nausea, vomiting, and lassitude. Back pain has been reported in conscious patients undergoing such procedures as cardiac catheterization.
Severe adverse reactions have been reported including: (1) Anaphylaxis that resulted in severe respiratory distress, circulatory collapse, and capillary leak (*see* Precautions). Fatal anaphylaxis has been reported in one patient with no prior history of allergies; (2) Anaphylactoid reactions with circulatory collapse, capillary leak, and noncardiogenic pulmonary edema; acute pulmonary hypertension.
Complement activation by the heparin-protamine complexes, release of lysosomal enzymes from neutrophils, and prostaglandin and thromboxane generation have been associated with the development of anaphylactoid reactions.
Severe and potentially irreversible circulatory collapse associated with myocardial failure and reduced cardiac output can also occur. The mechanism(s) of this reaction and the role played by concurrent factors are unclear.
High-protein, noncardiogenic pulmonary edema associated with the use of protamine has been reported in patients on cardiopulmonary bypass who are undergoing cardiovascular surgery. The etiologic role of protamine in the pathogenesis of this condition is uncertain, and multiple factors have been present in most cases. The condition has been reported in association with administration of certain blood products, other drugs, cardiopulmonary bypass alone, and other etiologic factors. It is difficult to treat, and it can be life threatening. Because fatal anaphylactic and anaphylactoid reactions have been reported after the administration of protamine sulfate, the drug should be given only when resuscitation techniques and treatment of anaphylactic and anaphylactoid shock are readily available.

OVERDOSAGE
Signs and Symptoms—Overdose of protamine sulfate may cause bleeding. Protamine has a weak anticoagulant effect due to an interaction with platelets and with many proteins including fibrinogen. This effect should be distinguished from the rebound anticoagulation that may occur 30 minutes to 18 hours following the reversal of heparin with protamine.
Rapid administration of protamine is more likely to result in bradycardia, dyspnea, a sensation of warmth, flushing, and severe hypotension. Hypertension has also occurred.
The median lethal intravenous dose of protamine sulfate is 50 mg/kg in mice. Serum concentrations of protamine sulfate are not clinically useful. Information is not available on the amount of drug in a single dose that is associated with overdosage or is likely to be life threatening.
Treatment—To obtain up-to-date information about the treatment of overdose, a good resource is your certified Regional Poison Control Center. Telephone numbers of certified poison control centers are listed in the *Physicians' Desk Reference (PDR)*. In managing overdosage, consider the possibility of multiple drug overdoses, interaction among drugs, and unusual drug kinetics in your patient.
Replace blood loss with blood transfusions or fresh frozen plasma.
If the patient is hypotensive, consider fluids, epinephrine, dobutamine, or dopamine.

DOSAGE AND ADMINISTRATION
Each mg of protamine sulfate neutralizes approximately 90 USP units of heparin activity derived from lung tissue or about 115 USP units of heparin activity derived from intestinal mucosa.
Protamine Sulfate Injection should be given by very slow intravenous injection over a 10-minute period in doses not to exceed 50 mg (*see* Warnings).
Protamine sulfate is intended for injection without further dilution; however, if further dilution is desired, D5-W or normal saline may be used. Diluted solutions should not be stored since they contain no preservative.
Protamine sulfate should not be mixed with other drugs without knowledge of their compatibility, because protamine sulfate has been shown to be incompatible with certain antibiotics, including several of the cephalosporins and penicillins.
Because heparin disappears rapidly from the circulation, the dose of protamine sulfate required also decreases rapidly with the time elapsed following intravenous injection of heparin. For example, if the protamine sulfate is administered 30 minutes after the heparin, one half the usual dose may be sufficient.
The dosage of protamine sulfate should be guided by blood coagulation studies (*see* Warnings).
Parenteral drug products should be inspected visually for particulate matter and discoloration prior to administration whenever solution and container permit.

HOW SUPPLIED
Vials:
25 mL (No. 735)—(1s) NDC 0002-1462-01
Vials should be stored in the refrigerator between 2° and 8°C (35.6° and 46.4°F).
CAUTION—The total dose of protamine sulfate contained in Vials No. 735 is 250 mg of activity in 25 mL.
The large-size vials (No. 735) are designed for antiheparin treatment only when large doses of heparin have been given during surgery and are to be neutralized by large doses of protamine sulfate after surgical procedures.

[101994]

REGULAR ILETIN® I AND II OTC

(insulin injection, Lilly) See under Iletin® (insulin)

REOPRO™ ℞

(abciximab)
For intravenous administration

DESCRIPTION
Abciximab, ReoPro™, is the Fab fragment of the chimeric human-murine monoclonal antibody 7E3. Abciximab binds to the glycoprotein IIb/IIIa (GPIIb/IIIa) receptor of human platelets and inhibits platelet aggregation.
The chimeric 7E3 antibody is produced by continuous perfusion in mammalian cell culture. The 47,615 dalton Fab fragment is purified from cell culture supernatant by a series of steps involving specific viral inactivation and removal procedures, digestion with papain and column chromatography.
ReoPro™ is a clear, colorless, sterile, non-pyrogenic solution for intravenous (IV) use. Each single-use vial contains 2 mg/mL of Abciximab in a buffered solution (pH 7.2) of 0.01 M sodium phosphate, 0.15 M sodium chloride and 0.001% polysorbate 80 in Water for Injection. No preservatives are added.

CLINICAL PHARMACOLOGY
General: Abciximab binds to the intact GPIIb/IIIa receptor, which is a member of the integrin family of adhesion receptors and the major platelet surface receptor involved in platelet aggregation. Abciximab inhibits platelet aggregation by preventing the binding of fibrinogen, von Willebrand factor, and other adhesive molecules to GPIIb/IIIa receptor sites on activated platelets. The mechanism of action is thought to involve steric hindrance and/or conformational effects to block access of large molecules to the receptor rather than interacting directly with the RGD (arginine-glycine-aspartic acid) binding site of GPIIb/IIIa.
Pre-clinical experience: Maximal inhibition of platelet aggregation was observed *in vivo* when $\geq 80\%$ of GPIIb/IIIa receptors were blocked by Abciximab. In non-human primates, Abciximab bolus doses of 0.25 mg/kg generally achieved a blockade of at least 80% of platelet receptors and fully inhibited platelet aggregation. Inhibition of platelet function was temporary following a bolus dose, but receptor blockade could be sustained at $\geq 80\%$ by continuous intravenous infusion. The inhibitory effects of Abciximab were substantially diminished by the transfusion of platelets in monkeys. The antithrombotic efficacy of prototype antibodies (murine 7E3 Fab and $F(ab')_2$) and Abciximab was evaluated in dog, monkey and baboon models of coronary, carotid, and femoral artery thrombosis. Doses of the murine version of 7E3 or Abciximab sufficient to produce high-grade ($\geq 80\%$) GPIIb/IIIa receptor blockade prevented acute thrombosis and yielded lower rates of thrombosis compared with aspirin and/or heparin.
Pharmacokinetics: Following intravenous bolus administration, free plasma concentrations of Abciximab decrease rapidly with an initial half-life of less than 10 minutes and a second phase half-life of about 30 minutes, probably related to rapid binding to the platelet GPIIb/IIIa receptors. Platelet function generally recovers over the course of 48 hours,[1,2] although Abciximab remains in the circulation for up to 10 days in a platelet-bound state. Intravenous administration of a 0.25 mg/kg bolus dose of Abciximab followed by continuous infusion of 10 μg/min produces approximately constant free plasma concentrations throughout the infusion. At the termination of the infusion period, free plasma concentrations fall rapidly for approximately 6 hours then decline at a slower rate.
Pharmacodynamics: Intravenous administration in humans of single bolus doses of Abciximab from 0.15 mg/kg to

0.30 mg/kg produced rapid dose-dependent inhibition of platelet function as measured by *ex vivo* platelet aggregation in response to adenosine diphosphate (ADP) or by prolongation of bleeding time. At the two highest doses (0.25 and 0.30 mg/kg) at 2 hours post injection, over 80% of the GPIIb/IIIa receptors were blocked and platelet aggregation in response to 20 μM ADP was almost abolished. The median bleeding time increased to over 30 minutes at both doses compared with a baseline value of approximately 5 minutes.

Intravenous administration in humans of a single bolus dose of 0.25 mg/kg followed by a continuous infusion of 10 μg/min for periods of 12 to 96 hours produced sustained high-grade GPIIb/IIIa receptor blockade (≥80%) and inhibition of platelet function (*ex vivo* platelet aggregation in response to 5 μM or 20 μM ADP less than 20% of baseline and bleeding time greater than 30 minutes) for the duration of the infusion in most patients. Results in patients who received the 0.25 mg/kg bolus followed by a 5 μg/min infusion for 24 hours showed a similar initial receptor blockade and inhibition of platelet aggregation, but the response was not maintained throughout the infusion period.

Low levels of GPIIb/IIIa receptor blockade are present for up to 10 days following cessation of the infusion. Bleeding time returned to ≤12 minutes within 12 hours following the end of infusion in 15 of 20 patients (75%), and within 24 hours in 18 of 20 patients (90%). *Ex vivo* platelet aggregation in response to 5 μM ADP returned to ≥50% of baseline within 24 hours following the end of infusion in 11 of 32 patients (34%) and within 48 hours in 23 of 32 patients (72%). In response to 20 μM ADP, *ex vivo* platelet aggregation returned to ≥50% of baseline within 24 hours in 20 of 32 patients (62%) and within 48 hours in 28 of 32 patients (88%).

Clinical safety and efficacy experience: The Evaluation of c7E3 to Prevent Ischemic Complications (EPIC) trial was a multicenter, double-blind, placebo-controlled trial of Abciximab in patients undergoing percutaneous transluminal coronary angioplasty or atherectomy (PTCA)[3]. In the EPIC trial, 2099 patients between 26 and 83 years of age who were at high risk for abrupt closure of the treated coronary vessel were randomly allocated to one of three treatments: 1) an Abciximab bolus (0.25 mg/kg) followed by an Abciximab infusion (10 μg/min) for twelve hours (bolus plus infusion group); 2) an Abciximab bolus (0.25 mg/kg) followed by a placebo infusion (bolus group), or; 3) a placebo bolus followed by a placebo infusion (placebo group). Patients at high risk during or following PTCA were defined as those with unstable angina or a non-Q-wave myocardial infarction (n=489), those with an acute Q-wave myocardial infarction within twelve hours of symptom onset (n=66), and those who were at high risk because of coronary morphology and/or clinical characteristics as defined in INDICATIONS AND USAGE (n=1544). Treatment with study agent in each of the three arms was initiated 10–60 minutes before the onset of PTCA. All patients initially received an intravenous heparin bolus (10,000 to 12,000 units) and boluses of up to 3,000 units thereafter to a maximum of 20,000 units during PTCA. Heparin infusion was continued for twelve hours to maintain a therapeutic elevation of activated partial thromboplastin time (APTT, 1.5–2.5 times normal). Unless contraindicated, aspirin (325 mg) was administered orally two hours prior to the planned procedure and then once daily.

The primary endpoint was the occurrence of any of the following events within 30 days of PTCA: death, myocardial infarction (MI), or the need for urgent intervention for recurrent ischemia (i.e. urgent PTCA, urgent coronary artery bypass graft (CABG) surgery, a coronary stent, or an intra-aortic balloon pump). The 30-day (Kaplan-Meier) primary endpoint event rates for each treatment group by intention-to-treat analysis of all randomized patients are shown in Table 1. The 4.5% lower incidence of the primary endpoint in the bolus plus infusion treatment group, compared with the placebo group, was statistically significant, whereas the 1.3% lower incidence in the bolus treatment group was not. A lower incidence of the primary endpoint was observed in the bolus plus infusion treatment arm for all three high-risk subgroups: patients with unstable angina, patients presenting within twelve hours of the onset of symptoms of an acute myocardial infarction, and patients with other high-risk clinical and/or morphologic characteristics as defined in the INDICATIONS AND USAGE section. The treatment effect was largest in the first two subgroups and smallest in the third subgroup.

[See table above.]

TABLE 1
PRIMARY OUTCOME EVENTS

Event	Placebo (n=696)	Bolus (n=695)	Bolus + Infusion (n=708)
	Number of Patients (%)		
Primary Endpoint[a]	89 (12.8)	79 (11.5)	59 (8.3)
p-value vs. placebo		0.428	0.008
Components of Primary Endpoint[b]			
Death	12 (1.7)	9 (1.3)	12 (1.7)
Acute myocardial infarctions in surviving patients	55 (7.9)	40 (5.8)	31 (4.4)
Urgent interventions in surviving patients without an acute myocardial infarction	22 (3.2)	30 (4.4)	16 (2.2)

[a]Patients who experienced more than one event in the first 30 days are counted only once.
[b]Patients are counted only once under the most serious component (death > acute MI > urgent intervention).

Mortality was uncommon and similar rates were observed in all arms. The rate of acute myocardial infarctions was significantly lower in the groups treated with Abciximab. While 80% of myocardial infarctions in the study were non-Q-wave infarctions, patients in the bolus plus infusion arm experienced a lower incidence of both Q-wave and non-Q-wave infarctions. Urgent intervention rates were lower in the groups treated with Abciximab, mostly because of lower rates of emergency PTCA and, to a lesser extent, emergency CABG surgery. The primary endpoint events in the bolus plus infusion treatment group were reduced mostly in the first 48 hours and this benefit was sustained through 30 days and six months.[3,4] At the 6 months follow-up visit this event rate remained lower in the bolus plus infusion arm (12.3%) than in the placebo arm (17.6%).

INDICATIONS AND USAGE

Abciximab is indicated as an adjunct to percutaneous transluminal coronary angioplasty or atherectomy (PTCA) for the prevention of acute cardiac ischemic complications in patients at high risk for abrupt closure of the treated coronary vessel.

Patients at high risk for abrupt closure include those undergoing PTCA with at least one of the following conditions:

- Unstable angina or a non-Q-wave myocardial infarction
- An acute Q-wave myocardial infarction within 12 hours of the onset of symptoms
- Other high-risk clinical and/or morphologic characteristics (as adapted from the classification of the ACC/AHA) (see footnote):

—two type B lesions in the artery to be dilated,
—one type B lesion in the artery to be dilated in a woman of at least 65 years of age,
—one type B lesion in the artery to be dilated in a patient with diabetes mellitus,
—one type C lesion in the artery to be dilated, or
—angioplasty of an infarct-related lesion within seven days of myocardial infarction.

Abciximab is intended for use with aspirin and heparin and has been studied only in that setting, as described in CLINICAL PHARMACOLOGY.

CONTRAINDICATIONS

Because Abciximab increases the risks of bleeding, it is contraindicated in the following clinical situations:

- **Active internal bleeding**
- **Recent (within six weeks) gastrointestinal (GI) or genitourinary bleeding of clinical significance**
- **History of cerebrovascular accident (CVA) within 2 years, or CVA with a significant residual neurological deficit**
- **Bleeding diathesis**
- **Administration of oral anticoagulants within seven days unless prothrombin time is ≤1.2 times control**
- **Thrombocytopenia (<100,000 cells/μL)**
- **Recent (within six weeks) major surgery or trauma**
- **Intracranial neoplasm, arteriovenous malformation, or aneurysm**
- **Severe uncontrolled hypertension**
- **Presumed or documented history of vasculitis**
- **Use of intravenous dextran before PTCA, or intent to use it during PTCA**

Abciximab is also contraindicated in patients with known hypersensitivity to any component of this product or to murine proteins.

WARNINGS

ADMINISTRATION OF ABCIXIMAB IS ASSOCIATED WITH AN INCREASED FREQUENCY OF MAJOR BLEEDING COMPLICATIONS INCLUDING RETROPERITONEAL BLEEDING, SPONTANEOUS GASTROINTESTINAL AND GENITOURINARY BLEEDING, AND BLEEDING AT THE ARTERIAL ACCESS SITE. THIS RISK IS FURTHER INCREASED IN PATIENTS WHO WEIGH LESS THAN 75 KG. APPROPRIATE MANAGEMENT OF THERAPY AND COMPLICATIONS (as described in PRECAUTIONS: Bleeding Precautions) IS POSSIBLE ONLY WHEN ADEQUATE DIAGNOSIS AND TREATMENT FACILITIES AND QUALIFIED PHYSICIANS ARE READILY AVAILABLE.

Increased Risk of Bleeding: (see ADVERSE REACTIONS)
The most common complication encountered during Abciximab therapy is bleeding. The types of bleeding associated with Abciximab therapy fall into two broad categories:

- Bleeding observed at the arterial access site for cardiac catheterization.
- Internal bleeding, involving the gastrointestinal tract, genitourinary tract, or retroperitoneal sites.

In the following conditions, clinical data suggest that the risks of major bleeds due to Abciximab therapy may be increased and should be weighed against the anticipated benefits:

- Patients who weigh less than 75 kg
- Patients >65 years old
- Patients with a history of prior GI disease
- Patients receiving thrombolytics

The following conditions are also associated with an increased risk of bleeding in the angioplasty setting which may be additive to that of Abciximab:

- PTCA within 12 hours of the onset of symptoms for acute myocardial infarction
- Prolonged PTCA (lasting more than 70 minutes)
- Failed PTCA

Heparin anticoagulation may contribute to the risk of bleeding. See PRECAUTIONS: Bleeding Precautions—Laboratory monitoring.

Should serious bleeding occur that is not controllable with pressure, the infusion of Abciximab and any concomitant heparin should be stopped (see also PRECAUTIONS: Restoration of Platelet Function).

PRECAUTIONS

Readministration: There are no data concerning readministration of Abciximab. Administration of Abciximab may result in human anti-chimeric antibody (HACA) formation (see ADVERSE REACTIONS) that can cause allergic or hypersensitivity reactions (including anaphylaxis), thrombocytopenia or diminished benefit upon readministration of Abciximab.

Use of Thrombolytics, Anticoagulants and Other Antiplatelet Agents
In the EPIC trial, Abciximab was used concomitantly with heparin and aspirin (see CLINICAL PHARMACOLOGY). Because Abciximab inhibits platelet aggregation, caution should be employed when it is used with other drugs that affect hemostasis, including thrombolytics, oral anticoagulants, non-steroidal anti-inflammatory drugs, dipyridamole, and ticlopidine.

In the EPIC trial, there was limited experience with the administration of Abciximab with low molecular weight dextran. Low molecular weight dextran was usually given for the deployment of a coronary stent, for which oral anticoagulants were also given. In the 11 patients who received low molecular weight dextran with Abciximab, 5 had major bleeding events and 4 had minor bleeding events. None of the 5 placebo patients treated with low molecular weight dextran had a major or minor bleeding event (See CONTRAINDICATIONS).

There are limited data on the use of Abciximab in patients receiving thrombolytic agents. Because of concern about synergistic effects on bleeding, systemic thrombolytic therapy should be used judiciously.

Bleeding Precautions: Therapy with Abciximab requires careful attention to all potential bleeding sites (including catheter insertion sites, arterial and venous puncture sites, cutdown sites, needle puncture sites, and gastrointestinal, genitourinary, and retroperitoneal sites).

Femoral artery access site: Abciximab is associated with an increase in bleeding rate particularly at the site of arterial access for femoral sheath placement. Care should be taken when attempting vascular access that only the anterior wall of the femoral artery is punctured, avoiding a Seldinger (through and through) technique for obtaining sheath access. Femoral vein sheath placement should be avoided unless needed. While the vascular sheath is in place, patients should be maintained on complete bed rest with the head of

Continued on next page

• Identi-Code® symbol. This product information was prepared in June 1996. Current information on these and other products of Eli Lilly and Company may be obtained by direct inquiry to Lilly Research Laboratories, Lilly Corporate Center, Indianapolis, Indiana 46285, 800-545-5979.

Lilly—Cont.

the bed ≤30° and the affected limb restrained in a straight position. Heparin should be discontinued at least 4 hours prior to arterial sheath removal. Following sheath removal, pressure should be applied to the femoral artery for at least 30 minutes using either manual compression or a mechanical device for hemostasis. A pressure dressing should be applied following hemostasis. The patient should be maintained on bed rest for 6 to 8 hours following sheath removal or discontinuation of Abciximab, whichever is later.

The sheath insertion site and distal pulses of affected leg(s) should be frequently checked while the femoral artery sheath is in place and for 6 hours after femoral artery sheath removal. Any hematoma should be measured and monitored for enlargement.

General nursing care: Arterial and venous punctures, intramuscular injections, and use of urinary catheters, nasotracheal intubation, nasogastric tubes and automatic blood pressure cuffs should be minimized. When obtaining intravenous access, non-compressible sites (e.g., subclavian or jugular veins) should be avoided. Saline or heparin locks should be considered for blood drawing. Vascular puncture sites should be documented and monitored. Gentle care should be provided when removing dressings.

Laboratory monitoring: Before infusion of Abciximab, platelet count, prothrombin time and APTT should be measured to identify pre-existing hemostatic abnormalities. During and following Abciximab treatment, platelet counts and extent of heparin anticoagulation, as assessed by activated clotting time or APTT, should be monitored closely.

Thrombocytopenia Platelet counts should be monitored prior to treatment, 2 to 4 hours following the bolus dose of Abciximab and at 24 hours or prior to discharge, whichever is first. If a patient experiences an acute platelet decrease (e.g., a platelet decrease to less than 100,000 cells/μL or a decrease of at least 25% from pre-treatment value), additional platelet counts should be determined. These platelet counts should be drawn in separate tubes containing ethylenediaminetetraacetic acid (EDTA), citrate or heparin to exclude pseudothrombocytopenia due to in vitro anticoagulant interaction. If true thrombocytopenia is verified, Abciximab should be immediately discontinued and the condition appropriately monitored and treated. For patients with thrombocytopenia in the EPIC trial, a daily platelet count was obtained until it returned to normal. If a patient's platelet count dropped to 60,000 cells/μL, heparin and aspirin were discontinued. If a patient's platelet count dropped below 50,000 cells/μL, platelets were transfused.

Restoration of Platelet Function: In the event of serious uncontrolled bleeding or the need for surgery (especially major procedures within 48–72 hours of treatment with Abciximab), an Ivy bleeding time should be determined. Preliminary evidence suggests that platelet function may be restored, at least in part, with platelet transfusions.

Allergic Reactions: Anaphylaxis may occur at any time during administration. If it does, administration of Abciximab should be immediately stopped and standard appropriate resuscitative measures should be initiated.

Drug Interactions: Although drug interactions with Abciximab have not been studied systematically, Abciximab has been administered to patients with ischemic heart disease treated concomitantly with a broad range of medications used in the treatment of angina, myocardial infarction and hypertension. These medications have included heparin, warfarin, beta-adrenergic receptor blockers, calcium channel antagonists, angiotensin converting enzyme inhibitors, intravenous and oral nitrates, and aspirin. Heparin, other anticoagulants, thrombolytics, and antiplatelet agents may be associated with an increase in bleeding. Patients with HACA titers may have allergic or hypersensitivity reactions when treated with other diagnostic or therapeutic monoclonal antibodies.

Pregnancy Category C: Animal reproduction studies have not been conducted with Abciximab. It is also not known whether Abciximab can cause fetal harm when administered to a pregnant woman or can affect reproduction capacity. Abciximab should be given to a pregnant woman only if clearly needed.

Pediatric Use: Safety and effectiveness in children have not been studied.

Carcinogenesis, Mutagenesis and Impairment of Fertility: In vitro and in vivo mutagenicity studies have not demonstrated any mutagenic effect. Long-term studies in animals have not been performed to evaluate the carcinogenic potential or effects on fertility in male or female animals.

Nursing Mothers: It is not known whether this drug is excreted in human milk or absorbed systemically after ingestion. Because many drugs are excreted in human milk, caution should be exercised when Abciximab is administered to a nursing woman.

ADVERSE REACTIONS

Bleeding: The most common complication of Abciximab therapy is bleeding. In the EPIC trial, Abciximab treatment

TABLE 2
BLEEDING EVENTS AND TRANSFUSIONS

	Placebo (n=696)	Bolus (n=695)	Bolus + Infusion (n=708)
	Number of Patients (%)		
Major bleeding[a]	46 (6.6)	77 (11.1)	99 (14.0)
p-value vs. placebo		0.003	<0.001
Minor bleeding[a]	68 (9.8)	107 (15.4)	120 (16.9)
p-value vs. placebo		0.002	<0.001
Bleeding requiring transfusions[b]	52 (7.5)	97 (14.0)	119 (16.8)
p-value vs. placebo		<0.002	<0.001

[a] For major and minor bleeding, patients are counted only once according to the most severe classification. Numbers include bleeding events associated with CABG surgery.
[b] Includes transfusions of any type: packed red blood cells, whole blood, platelets, fresh frozen plasma, and cryoprecipitate.

TABLE 3
BLEEDING LOCATIONS IN PATIENTS WITH MAJOR BLEEDING EVENTS[a]

	Placebo	Bolus	Bolus + Infusion
Patients with major bleeding not associated with CABG	23	60	75
Intracranial	2	1	3[b]
Spontaneous gross hematuria	1	4	4
Other genitourinary	2	5	8
Spontaneous hematemesis	0	5	11
Other gastrointestinal	1	11	11
Retroperitoneal	2	2	12
Femoral artery access site	16	43	50
Other access site	1	1	4
Oral	1	4	4
Other[c]	1	9	11
Decrease in Hct/Hgb only	3	7	11

[a] Indicates the number of patients with major bleeding not associated with CABG surgery; patients may be included for more than one bleeding site.
[b] Includes one patient randomized but not treated.
[c] Includes hemoptysis, pulmonary bleeding, epistaxis, ocular bleeding, otic bleeding and bleeding associated with procedures and surgery other than CABG surgery.

was associated with statistically significant increases in both major and minor bleeding events and in bleeding requiring transfusions (see Table 2). Bleeding was classified as major or minor by the criteria of the Thrombolysis in Myocardial Infarction study group[5]. Major bleeding events were defined as either an intracranial hemorrhage or a decrease in hemoglobin greater than 5 g/dL. Minor bleeding events included spontaneous gross hematuria, spontaneous hematemesis, observed blood loss with a hemoglobin decrease of more than 3 g/dL, or a decrease in hemoglobin of at least 4 g/dL without an identified bleeding site. In patients who received transfusions, the number of units of blood lost was estimated through an adaption of the method of Landefeld et al.[6]

[See Table 2 above.]

Major bleeding events occurred most commonly in patients treated with the bolus plus infusion regimen. Ten patients who had major bleeding events died; 5 were in the bolus plus infusion treatment group (one of these 5 patients was randomized, but not treated with Abciximab), 3 were in the bolus treatment group, and 2 were in the placebo treatment group. Of the patients with major bleeding who died, 2 patients (1 patient in the bolus plus infusion treatment group and 1 patient in the placebo treatment group) had deaths attributable to bleeding; both had a hemorrhagic stroke.

Major bleeding events not associated with CABG surgery occurred in 23 (3.3%) patients in the placebo group, 60 (8.6%) patients in the bolus group and 75 (10.6%) patients in the bolus plus infusion group; the sites of bleeding in these patients are listed in Table 3. The incidence of intracranial hemorrhage was similar in all three groups. Approximately 70% of Abciximab-treated patients with major bleeding had bleeding at the arterial access site in the groin. Abciximab-treated patients also had a higher incidence of major bleeding events from gastrointestinal, genitourinary, retroperitoneal, and other sites.

Excess spontaneous major organ bleeding occurred primarily in patients weighing 75 kg or less who received Abciximab.

Although data are limited, Abciximab treatment was not associated with excess major bleeding in patients who underwent CABG surgery. The incidence of CABG surgery-related major blood loss was similar in all 3 groups (3–5%). Some patients with prolonged bleeding times received platelet transfusions to correct the bleeding time prior to surgery.

[See Table 3 above.]

Thrombocytopenia: In the EPIC study, patients treated with Abciximab were more likely than patients treated with

placebo to experience decreases in platelet counts and to require platelet transfusions (see Table 4).

[See table at top of next page.]

Human Anti-chimeric Antibody Development: HACA may appear in response to the administration of Abciximab. In the EPIC trial, positive responses occurred in 6.5% (40/617) of the patients in the bolus plus infusion group versus 0% (0/605) of patients treated with placebo. There was no excess of hypersensitivity or allergic reactions related to Abciximab treatment compared with placebo treatment. See also PRECAUTIONS: Allergic Reactions.

Other Adverse Reactions: Table 5 shows adverse events other than bleeding and thrombocytopenia from the EPIC trial which occurred in patients in the bolus plus infusion arm at an incidence of more than 0.5% higher than in those treated with placebo. Hypotension was often related to bleeding complications associated with Abciximab therapy.

[See Table 5 on top of next page.]

The following additional adverse events from the EPIC trial were reported by investigators for patients treated with a bolus plus infusion of Abciximab at incidences which were less than 0.5% higher than for patients in the placebo arm: *Cardiovascular System*—atrial fibrillation/flutter (3.5%), vascular disorder (1.8%), pulmonary edema (1.5%), complete AV block (1.3%), supraventricular tachycardia (1.0%), weak pulse (1.0%), palpitation (0.7%), intermittent claudication (0.4%), pericardial effusion (0.4%), limb embolism (0.3%), pulmonary embolism (0.3%), ventricular arrhythmia (0.3%); *Gastrointestinal System*—diarrhea (0.9%), constipation (0.3%), ileus (0.3%); *Hemic and Lymphatic System*—hemolytic anemia (0.3%), petechiae (0.3%); *Nervous System*—abnormal thinking (2.1%), dizziness (1.8%), coma (0.4%), brain ischemia (0.3%), insomnia (0.3%); *Musculoskeletal System*—myopathy (0.4%), cellulitis (0.3%), myalgia (0.3%); *Urogenital System*—urinary tract infection (1.9%), urinary retention (0.4%), abnormal renal function (0.3%); *Miscellaneous*—dysphonia (0.3%), pruritus (0.3%).

OVERDOSAGE

There has been no experience of overdosage in human clinical trials. It is recommended that infusion be discontinued after 12 hours to avoid effects of prolonged platelet receptor blockade.

DOSAGE AND ADMINISTRATION

Abciximab is intended for use in patients undergoing PTCA. The safety and efficacy of Abciximab have only been investigated with concomitant administration of heparin and aspirin as described in CLINICAL PHARMACOLOGY.

TABLE 4
THROMBOCYTOPENIA AND PLATELET TRANSFUSIONS[a]

	Placebo (n=696)	Bolus + Infusion (n=708)
	Number of Patients (%)	
Patients with decrease of platelets to <50,000 cells/μL[a]	5 (0.7)	11 (1.6)
Patients with decrease of platelets to <100,000 cells/μL[a]	24 (3.4)	37 (5.2)
Patients who received platelet transfusions[b]	18 (2.6)	39 (5.5)

[a] Patients with a platelet count of <50,000 cells/μL are also included in the category of patients with a platelet count of <100,000 cells/μL.
[b] Includes patients receiving platelet transfusions for thrombocytopenia or any other reason.

TABLE 5
ADVERSE EVENTS AMONG TREATED PATIENTS IN THE EPIC TRIAL

Event	Placebo (n=681)	Bolus + Infusion (n=678)
	Number of Patients (%)	
Cardiovascular System		
Hypotension	82 (12.0)	143 (21.1)
Bradycardia	20 (2.9)	35 (5.2)
Gastrointestinal System		
Nausea	109 (16.0)	125 (18.4)
Vomiting	61 (9.0)	77 (11.4)
Hemic and Lymphatic System		
Anemia	3 (0.4)	8 (1.2)
Leukocytosis	1 (0.1)	7 (1.0)
Nervous System		
Hypesthesia[a]	2 (0.3)	7 (1.0)
Confusion	0 (0.0)	4 (0.6)
Respiratory System		
Pleural Effusion/Pleurisy	2 (0.2)	9 (1.3)
Pneumonia	3 (0.4)	7 (1.0)
Miscellaneous		
Pain[a]	8 (2.6)	23 (3.4)
Peripheral Edema	3 (0.4)	11 (1.6)
Abnormal Vision	1 (0.1)	3 (0.7)

[a] Involving primarily the extremities

In patients with failed PTCAs, the continuous infusion of Abciximab should be stopped because there is no evidence for Abciximab efficacy in that setting.

In the event of serious bleeding that cannot be controlled by compression, Abciximab and heparin should be discontinued immediately (see PRECAUTIONS: Restoration of Platelet Function).

Adults: The recommended dosage of Abciximab is an intravenous bolus of 0.25 mg/kg administered 10–60 minutes before the start of PTCA, followed by a continuous intravenous infusion of 10 μg/min for twelve (12) hours.

Instructions for Administration
1. Parenteral drug products should be inspected visually for particulate matter prior to administration. Preparations of Abciximab containing visibly opaque particles should NOT be used.
2. Hypersensitivity reactions should be anticipated whenever protein solutions such as Abciximab are administered. Epinephrine, dopamine, theophylline, antihistamines and corticosteroids should be available for immediate use. If symptoms of an allergic reaction or anaphylaxis appear, the infusion should be stopped and appropriate treatment given.
3. As with all parenteral drug products, aseptic procedures should be used during the administration of Abciximab.
4. Withdraw the necessary amount of Abciximab (2 mg/mL) for bolus injection through a sterile, non-pyrogenic, low protein-binding 0.2 or 0.22 μm filter (Millipore SLGVO25LS or equivalent) into a syringe. The bolus should be administered 10–60 minutes before the procedure.
5. Withdraw 4.5 mL of Abciximab for the continuous infusion through a sterile, non-pyrogenic, low protein-binding 0.2 or 0.22 μm filter (Millipore SLGVO25LS or equivalent) into a syringe. Inject into 250 mL of sterile 0.9% saline or 5% dextrose and infuse at a rate of 17 mL/hour (10 μg/min) for 12 hours via a continuous infusion pump equipped with an in-line sterile, non-pyrogenic, low protein-binding 0.2 or 0.22 μm filter (Abbott #4524 or equivalent). Discard the unused portion at the end of the 12-hour infusion.
6. Abciximab should be administered in a separate intravenous line; no other medication should be added to the infusion solutions.
7. No incompatibilities have been observed with glass bottles or polyvinyl chloride bags and administration sets.

HOW SUPPLIED
Abciximab (ReoPro™) 2 mg/mL is supplied in 5 mL vials containing 10 mg (NDC 0002-7140-01).

Vials should be stored at 2 to 8°C (36 to 46°F). Do not freeze. Do not shake. Do not use beyond the expiration date. Discard any unused portion left in the vial.

REFERENCES
1. Tcheng J, Ellis SG, George BS. Pharmacodynamics of chimeric glycoprotein IIB/IIIa integrin antiplatelet antibody Fab 7E3 in high risk coronary angioplasty. *Circulation* 1994;**90**:757–764.
2. Simoons ML, de Boer MJ, van der Brand MJBM, et al. Randomized trial of a GPIIb/IIIa platelet receptor blocker in refractory unstable angina. *Circulation* 1994;**89**:596–603.
3. EPIC Investigators. Use of a monoclonal antibody directed against the platelet glycoprotein IIb/IIIa receptor in a high-risk coronary angioplasty. *N Engl J Med* 1994;**330**:956–961.
4. Topol EJ, Califf RM, Weisman HF, et al. Randomised trial of coronary intervention with antibody against platelet IIb/IIIa integrin for reduction of clinical restenosis: results at six months. *The Lancet* 1994;**343**:881–886.
5. Rao AK, Pratt C, Berke A, et al. Thrombolysis in Myocardial Infarction (TIMI) Trial—Phase I: Hemorrhagic manifestations and changes in plasma fibrinogen and the fibrinolytic system in patients treated with recombinant tissue plasminogen activator and streptokinase. *J Am Coll Cardiol* 1988;**11**:1–11.
6. Landefeld CS, Cook EF, Flatley M, et al. Identification and preliminary validation of predictors of major bleeding in hospitalized patients starting anticoagulant therapy. *Am J Med* 1987;**82**:703–713.
7. Ryan TJ, Faxon DP, Gunnar RM, et al. Guidelines for percutaneous transluminal coronary angioplasty: A report of the American College of Cardiology/American Heart Association task force on assessment of diagnostic and therapeutic cardiovascular procedures (Subcommittee on Percutaneous Transluminal Coronary Angioplasty). *J Am Coll Cardiol* 1988;**12**:529–545.

FOOTNOTE
Ryan et al., 1988[7]
Classification of coronary lesions according to ACC/AHA criteria is summarized as follows:

Type A Lesions (high success, >85%; low risk)
- Discrete (<10 mm length)
- Concentric
- Readily accessible
- Nonangulated segment, <45°
- Smooth contour
- Little or no calcification
- Less than totally occlusive
- Not ostial in location
- No major branch involvement
- Absence of thrombus

Type B Lesions (moderate success, 60 to 85%; moderate risk)
- Tubular (10 to 20 mm length)
- Eccentric
- Moderate tortuosity of proximal segment
- Moderately angulated segment >45°, <90°
- Irregular contour
- Moderate to heavy calcification
- Total occlusions <3 months old
- Ostial in location
- Bifurcation lesions requiring double guide wires
- Some thrombus present

Type C Lesions (low success, <60%; high risk)
- Diffuse (>2 cm length)
- Excessive tortuosity of proximal segment
- Extremely angulated segments >90°
- Total occlusion >3 months old
- Inability to protect major side branches
- Degenerated vein grafts with friable lesions

Manufactured by:
Centocor B.V.
Leiden, The Netherlands
U.S. License Number: 1178

Distributed by:
Eli Lilly and Company
Indianapolis, IN 46285 [REV.00]
Shown in Product Identification Guide, page 322

SECONAL® SODIUM
[sĕk'ō-năl sō'dē-ŭm]
(secobarbital sodium)
Capsules, USP
WARNING: MAY BE HABIT-FORMING

DESCRIPTION
The barbiturates are nonselective central nervous system (CNS) depressants that are primarily used as sedative-hypnotics. In subhypnotic doses, they are also used as anticonvulsants. The barbiturates and their sodium salts are subject to control under the Federal Controlled Substances Act. Seconal® Sodium (Secobarbital Sodium Capsules, USP) is a barbituric acid derivative and occurs as a white, odorless, bitter powder that is very soluble in water, soluble in alcohol, and practically insoluble in ether. Chemically, the drug is sodium 5-allyl-5-(1-methylbutyl)barbiturate, with the empirical formula $C_{12}H_{17}N_2NaO_3$. Its molecular weight is 260.27. The structural formula is as follows:

$$CH_2=CHCH_2$$
$$CH_3CH_2CH_2CH$$
$$CH_3$$

Each Pulvule® contains 100 mg (0.38 mmol) of secobarbital sodium. It also contains cornstarch, D & C Yellow No. 10, F D & C Red No. 3, gelatin, magnesium stearate, silicone, and other inactive ingredients.

CLINICAL PHARMACOLOGY
Barbiturates are capable of producing all levels of CNS mood alteration, from excitation to mild sedation, hypnosis, and deep coma. Overdosage can produce death. In high enough therapeutic doses, barbiturates induce anesthesia. Barbiturates depress the sensory cortex, decrease motor activity, alter cerebellar function, and produce drowsiness, sedation, and hypnosis.

Barbiturate-induced sleep differs from physiologic sleep. Sleep laboratory studies have demonstrated that barbiturates reduce the amount of time spent in the rapid eye movement (REM) phase, or dreaming stage of sleep. Also, Stages III and IV sleep are decreased. Following abrupt cessation of regularly used barbiturates, patients may experience markedly increased dreaming, nightmares, and/or insomnia. Therefore, withdrawal of a single therapeutic dose over 5 or 6 days has been recommended to lessen the REM rebound and disturbed sleep that contribute to drug withdrawal syndrome (for example, decreasing the dose from 3 to 2 doses a day for 1 week).

In studies, secobarbital sodium and pentobarbital sodium have been found to lose most of their effectiveness for both

Continued on next page

* Identi-Code® symbol. This product information was prepared in June 1996. Current information on these and other products of Eli Lilly and Company may be obtained by direct inquiry to Lilly Research Laboratories, Lilly Corporate Center, Indianapolis, Indiana 46285, 800-545-5979.

Lilly—Cont.

inducing and maintaining sleep by the end of 2 weeks of continued drug administration, even with the use of multiple doses. As with secobarbital sodium and pentobarbital sodium, other barbiturates (including amobarbital) might be expected to lose their effectiveness for inducing and maintaining sleep after about 2 weeks. The short-, intermediate-, and to a lesser degree, long-acting barbiturates have been widely prescribed for treating insomnia. Although the clinical literature abounds with claims that the short-acting barbiturates are superior for producing sleep whereas the intermediate-acting compounds are more effective in maintaining sleep, controlled studies have failed to demonstrate these differential effects. Therefore, as sleep medications, the barbiturates are of limited value beyond short-term use.

Barbiturates have little analgesic action at subanesthetic doses. Rather, in subanesthetic doses, these drugs may increase the reaction to painful stimuli. All barbiturates exhibit anticonvulsant activity in anesthetic doses. However, of the drugs in this class, only phenobarbital, mephobarbital, and metharbital are effective as oral anticonvulsants in subhypnotic doses.

Barbiturates are respiratory depressants, and the degree of depression is dependent on the dose. With hypnotic doses, respiratory depression is similar to that which occurs during physiologic sleep accompanied by a slight decrease in blood pressure and heart rate.

Studies in laboratory animals have shown that barbiturates cause reduction in the tone and contractility of the uterus, ureters, and urinary bladder. However, concentrations of the drugs required to produce this effect in humans are not reached with sedative-hypnotic doses.

Barbiturates do not impair normal hepatic function, but have been shown to induce liver microsomal enzymes, thus increasing and/or altering the metabolism of barbiturates and other drugs (*see* Drug Interactions *under* Precautions).

Pharmacokinetics—Barbiturates are absorbed in varying degrees following oral or parenteral administration. The salts are more rapidly absorbed than are the acids. The rate of absorption is increased if the sodium salt is ingested as a dilute solution or taken on an empty stomach.

Duration of action, which is related to the rate at which the barbiturates are redistributed throughout the body, varies among persons and in the same person from time to time.

Seconal Sodium is classified as a short-acting barbiturate when taken orally. Its onset of action is 10 to 15 minutes and its duration of action ranges from 3 to 4 hours.

Barbiturates are weak acids that are absorbed and rapidly distributed to all tissues and fluids, with high concentrations in the brain, liver, and kidneys. Lipid solubility of the barbiturates is the dominant factor in their distribution within the body. The more lipid soluble the barbiturate, the more rapidly it penetrates all tissues of the body. Barbiturates are bound to plasma and tissue proteins to a varying degree, with the degree of binding increasing directly as a function of lipid solubility.

Phenobarbital has the lowest lipid solubility, lowest plasma binding, lowest brain protein binding, the longest delay in onset of activity, and the longest duration of action. At the opposite extreme is secobarbital, which has the highest lipid solubility, highest plasma protein binding, highest brain protein binding, the shortest delay in onset of activity, and the shortest duration of action. The plasma half-life for secobarbital sodium in adults ranges between 15 to 40 hours, with a mean of 28 hours. No data are available for children and newborns.

Barbiturates are metabolized primarily by the hepatic microsomal enzyme system, and the metabolic products are excreted in the urine and, less commonly, in the feces. The excretion of unmetabolized barbiturate is 1 feature that distinguishes the long-acting category from those belonging to other categories, which are almost entirely metabolized. The inactive metabolites of the barbiturates are excreted as conjugates of glucuronic acid.

INDICATIONS AND USAGE

A. Hypnotic, for the short-term treatment of insomnia, since it appears to lose its effectiveness for sleep induction and sleep maintenance after 2 weeks (*see* Clinical Pharmacology).

B. Preanesthetic

CONTRAINDICATIONS

Seconal Sodium is contraindicated in patients who are hypersensitive to barbiturates. It is also contraindicated in patients with a history of manifest or latent porphyria, marked impairment of liver function, or respiratory disease in which dyspnea or obstruction is evident.

WARNINGS

1. *Habit-Forming*—Seconal Sodium may be habit-forming. Tolerance and psychological and physical dependence may occur with continued use (*see* Drug Abuse and Dependence *and* Pharmacokinetics *under* Clinical Pharmacology). Patients who have psychological dependence on barbiturates may increase the dosage or decrease the dosage interval without consulting a physician and subsequently may develop a physical dependence on barbiturates. To minimize the possibility of overdosage or development of dependence, the prescribing and dispensing of sedative-hypnotic barbiturates should be limited to the amount required for the interval until the next appointment. The abrupt cessation after prolonged use in a person who is dependent on the drug may result in withdrawal symptoms, including delirium, convulsions, and possibly death. Barbiturates should be withdrawn gradually from any patient known to be taking excessive doses over long periods of time (*see* Drug Abuse and Dependence).

2. *Acute or Chronic Pain*—Caution should be exercised when barbiturates are administered to patients with acute or chronic pain, because paradoxical excitement could be induced or important symptoms could be masked.

3. *Usage in Pregnancy*—Barbiturates can cause fetal harm when administered to a pregnant woman. Retrospective, case-controlled studies have suggested that there may be a connection between the maternal consumption of barbiturates and a higher than expected incidence of fetal abnormalities. Barbiturates readily cross the placental barrier and are distributed throughout fetal tissues; the highest concentrations are found in the placenta, fetal liver, and brain. Fetal blood levels approach maternal blood levels following parenteral administration.

Withdrawal symptoms occur in infants born to women who receive barbiturates throughout the last trimester of pregnancy (*see* Drug Abuse and Dependence). If Seconal Sodium is used during pregnancy or if the patient becomes pregnant while taking this drug, the patient should be apprised of the potential hazard to the fetus.

4. *Synergistic Effects*—The concomitant use of alcohol or other CNS depressants may produce additive CNS-depressant effects.

PRECAUTIONS

General—Barbiturates may be habit-forming. Tolerance and psychological and physical dependence may occur with continuing use (*see* Drug Abuse and Dependence). Barbiturates should be administered with caution, if at all, to patients who are mentally depressed, have suicidal tendencies, or have a history of drug abuse.

Elderly or debilitated patients may react to barbiturates with marked excitement, depression, or confusion. In some persons, especially children, barbiturates repeatedly produce excitement rather than depression.

In patients with hepatic damage, barbiturates should be administered with caution and initially in reduced doses. Barbiturates should not be administered to patients showing the premonitory signs of hepatic coma.

Information for Patients—The following information should be given to patients receiving Seconal Sodium:

1. The use of Seconal Sodium carries with it an associated risk of psychological and/or physical dependence. The patient should be warned against increasing the dose of the drug without consulting a physician.
2. Seconal Sodium may impair the mental and/or physical abilities required for the performance of potentially hazardous tasks, such as driving a car or operating machinery. The patient should be cautioned accordingly.
3. Alcohol should not be consumed while taking Seconal Sodium. The concurrent use of Seconal Sodium with other CNS depressants (eg, alcohol, narcotics, tranquilizers, and antihistamines) may result in additional CNS-depressant effects.

Laboratory Tests—Prolonged therapy with barbiturates should be accompanied by periodic laboratory evaluation of organic systems, including hematopoietic, renal, and hepatic systems (*see* General *under* Precautions *and* Adverse Reactions).

Drug Interactions—Most reports of clinically significant drug interactions occurring with the barbiturates have involved phenobarbital. However, the application of these data to other barbiturates appears valid and warrants serial blood level determinations of the relevant drugs when there are multiple therapies.

1. *Anticoagulants*—Phenobarbital lowers the plasma levels of dicumarol and causes a decrease in anticoagulant activity as measured by the prothrombin time. Barbiturates can induce hepatic microsomal enzymes, resulting in increased metabolism and decreased anticoagulant response of oral anticoagulants (eg, warfarin, acenocoumarol, dicumarol, and phenprocoumon). Patients stabilized on anticoagulant therapy may require dosage adjustments if barbiturates are added to or withdrawn from their dosage regimen.
2. *Corticosteroids*—Barbiturates appear to enhance the metabolism of exogenous corticosteroids, probably through the induction of hepatic microsomal enzymes. Patients stabilized on corticosteroid therapy may require dosage adjustments if barbiturates are added to or withdrawn from their dosage regimen.
3. *Griseofulvin*—Phenobarbital appears to interfere with the absorption of orally administered griseofulvin, thus decreasing its blood level. The effect of the resultant decreased blood levels of griseofulvin on therapeutic response has not been established. However, it would be preferable to avoid concomitant administration of these drugs.
4. *Doxycycline*—Phenobarbital has been shown to shorten the half-life of doxycycline for as long as 2 weeks after barbiturate therapy is discontinued.
   This mechanism is probably through the induction of hepatic microsomal enzymes that metabolize the antibiotic. If barbiturates and doxycycline are administered concurrently, the clinical response to doxycycline should be monitored closely.
5. *Phenytoin, Sodium Valproate, Valproic Acid*—The effect of barbiturates on the metabolism of phenytoin appears to be variable. Some investigators report an accelerating effect, whereas others report no effect. Because the effect of barbiturates on the metabolism of phenytoin is not predictable, phenytoin and barbiturate blood levels should be monitored more frequently if these drugs are given concurrently. Sodium valproate and valproic acid increase secobarbital sodium serum levels; therefore, secobarbital sodium blood levels should be monitored closely and appropriate dosage adjustment made as clinically indicated.
6. *CNS Depressants*—The concomitant use of other CNS depressants, including other sedatives or hypnotics, antihistamines, tranquilizers, or alcohol, may produce additive depressant effects.
7. *Monoamine Oxidase Inhibitors (MAOIs)*—MAOIs prolong the effects of barbiturates, probably because metabolism of the barbiturate is inhibited.
8. *Estradiol, Estrone, Progesterone, and Other Steroidal Hormones*—Pretreatment with or concurrent administration of phenobarbital may decrease the effect of estradiol by increasing its metabolism. There have been reports of patients treated with antiepileptic drugs (eg, phenobarbital) who become pregnant while taking oral contraceptives. An alternate contraceptive method might be suggested to women taking barbiturates.

Carcinogenesis—1. *Animal Data.* Phenobarbital sodium is carcinogenic in mice and rats after lifetime administration. In mice, it produced benign and malignant liver cell tumors. In rats, benign liver cell tumors were observed very late in life.

2. *Human Data*—In a 29-year epidemiologic study of 9,136 patients who were treated on an anticonvulsant protocol that included phenobarbital, results indicated a higher than normal incidence of hepatic carcinoma. Previously, some of these patients had been treated with thorotrast, a drug that is known to produce hepatic carcinomas. Thus, this study did not provide sufficient evidence that phenobarbital sodium is carcinogenic in humans.
   A retrospective study of 84 children with brain tumors matched to 73 normal controls and 78 cancer controls (malignant disease other than brain tumors) suggested an association between exposure to barbiturates prenatally and an increased incidence of brain tumors.

Usage in Pregnancy—1. *Teratogenic Effects. Pregnancy Category D. See* Usage in Pregnancy *under* Warnings.

2. *Nonteratogenic Effects.* Reports of infants suffering from long-term barbiturate exposure in utero included the acute withdrawal syndrome of seizures and hyperirritability from birth to a delayed onset of up to 14 days (*see* Drug Abuse and Dependence).

Labor and Delivery—Hypnotic doses of barbiturates do not appear to impair uterine activity significantly during labor. Full anesthetic doses of barbiturates decrease the force and frequency of uterine contractions. Administration of sedative-hypnotic barbiturates to the mother during labor may result in respiratory depression in the newborn. Premature infants are particularly susceptible to the depressant effects of barbiturates. If barbiturates are used during labor and delivery, resuscitation equipment should be available.

Data are not available to evaluate the effect of barbiturates when forceps delivery or other intervention is necessary or to determine the effect of barbiturates on the later growth, development, and functional maturity of the child.

Nursing Mothers—Caution should be exercised when Seconal Sodium is administered to a nursing woman, because small amounts of barbiturates are excreted in the milk.

ADVERSE REACTIONS

The following adverse reactions and their incidences were compiled from surveillance of thousands of hospitalized patients who received barbiturates. Because such patients may be less aware of some of the milder adverse effects of barbiturates, the incidence of these reactions may be somewhat higher in fully ambulatory patients.

More than 1 in 100 Patients

The most common adverse reaction estimated to occur at a rate of 1 to 3 patients per 100 is the following:

Nervous System: Somnolence

Less than 1 in 100 Patients

Adverse reactions estimated to occur at a rate of less than 1 in 100 patients are listed below, grouped by organ system and by decreasing order of occurrence:

Nervous System: Agitation, confusion, hyperkinesia, ataxia, CNS depression, nightmares, nervousness, psychiatric disturbance, hallucinations, insomnia, anxiety, dizziness, abnormality in thinking

Respiratory System: Hypoventilation, apnea

Cardiovascular System: Bradycardia, hypotension, syncope

Digestive System: Nausea, vomiting, constipation

Other Reported Reactions: Headache, injection site reactions, hypersensitivity reactions (angioedema, skin rashes, exfoliative dermatitis), fever, liver damage, megaloblastic anemia following chronic phenobarbital use

DRUG ABUSE AND DEPENDENCE

Controlled Substance —Seconal Sodium Capsules are a Schedule II drug.

Dependence —Barbiturates may be habit-forming; tolerance, psychological dependence, and physical dependence may occur, especially following prolonged use of high doses of barbiturates. Daily administration in excess of 400 mg of secobarbital for approximately 90 days is likely to produce some degree of physical dependence. A dosage of 600 to 800 mg for at least 35 days is sufficient to produce withdrawal seizures. The average daily dose for the barbiturate addict is usually about 1.5 g. As tolerance to barbiturates develops, the amount needed to maintain the same level of intoxication increases; tolerance to a fatal dosage, however, does not increase more than twofold. As this occurs, the margin between intoxicating dosage and fatal dosage becomes smaller. Symptoms of acute intoxication with barbiturates include unsteady gait, slurred speech, and sustained nystagmus. Mental signs of chronic intoxication include confusion, poor judgment, irritability, insomnia, and somatic complaints. Symptoms of barbiturate dependence are similar to those of chronic alcoholism. If an individual appears to be intoxicated with alcohol to a degree that is radically disproportionate to the amount of alcohol in his or her blood, the use of barbiturates should be suspected. The lethal dose of a barbiturate is far less if alcohol is also ingested.

The symptoms of barbiturate withdrawal can be severe and may cause death. Minor withdrawal symptoms may appear 8 to 12 hours after the last dose of a barbiturate. These symptoms usually appear in the following order: anxiety, muscle twitching, tremor of hands and fingers, progressive weakness, dizziness, distortion in visual perception, nausea, vomiting, insomnia, and orthostatic hypotension. Major withdrawal symptoms (convulsions and delirium) may occur within 16 hours and last up to 5 days after abrupt cessation of barbiturates. Intensity of withdrawal symptoms gradually declines over a period of approximately 15 days. Individuals susceptible to barbiturate abuse and dependence include alcoholics and opiate abusers, as well as other sedative-hypnotic and amphetamine abusers.

Drug dependence on barbiturates arises from repeated administration on a continuous basis, generally in amounts exceeding therapeutic dose levels. The characteristics of drug dependence on barbiturates include the following: (a) a strong desire or need to continue taking the drug; (b) a tendency to increase the dose; (c) a psychic dependence on the effects of the drug related to subjective and individual appreciation of those effects; and (d) a physical dependence on the effects of the drug, requiring its presence for maintenance of homeostasis and resulting in a definite, characteristic, and self-limited abstinence syndrome when the drug is withdrawn.

Treatment of barbiturate dependence consists of cautious and gradual withdrawal of the drug. Barbiturate-dependent patients can be withdrawn by using a number of withdrawal regimens. In all cases, withdrawal takes an extended period. One method involves substituting a 30-mg dose of phenobarbital for each 100- to 200-mg dose of barbiturate that the patient has been taking. The total daily amount of phenobarbital is then administered in 3 or 4 divided doses, not to exceed 600 mg daily. Should signs of withdrawal occur on the first day of treatment, a loading dose of 100 to 200 mg of phenobarbital may be administered IM in addition to the oral dose. After stabilization on phenobarbital, the total daily dose is decreased by 30 mg a day as long as withdrawal is proceeding smoothly. A modification of this regimen involves initiating treatment at the patient's regular dosage level and decreasing the daily dosage by 10% as tolerated by the patient. Infants that are physically dependent on barbiturates may be given phenobarbital, 3 to 10 mg/kg/day. After withdrawal symptoms (hyperactivity, disturbed sleep, tremors, and hyperreflexia) are relieved, the dosage of phenobarbital should be gradually decreased and completely withdrawn over a 2-week period.

OVERDOSAGE

The toxic dose of barbiturates varies considerably. In general, an oral dose of 1 g of most barbiturates produces serious poisoning in an adult. Death commonly occurs after 2 to 10 g of ingested barbiturate. The sedated, therapeutic blood levels of secobarbital range between 0.5 to 5 μg/mL; the usual lethal blood level ranges from 15 to 40 μg/mL. Barbiturate intoxication may be confused with alcoholism, bromide intoxication, and various neurologic disorders. Potential toler-

ance must be considered when evaluating significance of dose and plasma concentration.

Signs and Symptoms —Symptoms of oral overdose may occur within 15 minutes and begin with central nervous system depression, underventilation, hypotension, and hypothermia, which may progress to pulmonary edema and death. Hemorrhagic blisters may develop, especially at pressure points.

In extreme overdose, all electrical activity in the brain may cease, in which case a "flat" EEG normally equated with clinical death cannot be accepted as indicative of brain death. This effect is fully reversible unless hypoxic damage occurs. Consideration should be given to the possibility of barbiturate intoxication even in situations that appear to involve trauma.

Complications such as pneumonia, pulmonary edema, cardiac arrhythmias, congestive heart failure, and renal failure may occur. Uremia may increase CNS sensitivity to barbiturates if renal function is impaired. Differential diagnosis should include hypoglycemia, head trauma, cerebrovascular accidents, convulsive states, and diabetic coma.

Treatment —To obtain up-to-date information about the treatment of overdose, a good resource is your certified Regional Poison Control Center. Telephone numbers of certified poison control centers are listed in the *Physicians' Desk Reference (PDR).* In managing overdosage, consider the possibility of multiple drug overdoses, interaction among drugs, and unusual drug kinetics in your patient.

Protect the patient's airway and support ventilation and perfusion. Meticulously monitor and maintain, within acceptable limits, the patient's vital signs, blood gases, serum electrolytes, etc. Absorption of drugs from the gastrointestinal tract may be decreased by giving activated charcoal, which, in many cases, is more effective than emesis or lavage; consider charcoal instead of or in addition to gastric emptying. Repeated doses of charcoal over time may hasten elimination of some drugs that have been absorbed. Safeguard the patient's airway when employing gastric emptying or charcoal.

Diuresis and peritoneal dialysis are of little value; hemodialysis and hemoperfusion enhance drug clearance and should be considered in serious poisoning. If the patient has chronically abused sedatives, withdrawal reactions may be manifest following acute overdose.

DOSAGE AND ADMINISTRATION

Dosages of barbiturates must be individualized with full knowledge of their particular characteristics. Factors of consideration are the patient's age, weight, and condition.

Adults —As a hypnotic, 100 mg at bedtime. Preoperatively, 200 to 300 mg 1 to 2 hours before surgery.

Children —Preoperatively, 2 to 6 mg/kg, with a maximum dosage of 100 mg.

Special patient population —Dosage should be reduced in the elderly or debilitated because these patients may be more sensitive to barbiturates. Dosage should be reduced for patients with impaired renal function or hepatic disease.

HOW SUPPLIED

Pulvules Seconal Sodium (capsules) (orange):
100 mg (No. 240) (Identi-Code* F40)—(100s) NDC 0002-0640-02; (ID† 100) NDC 0002-0640-33
Store at controlled room temperature, 15° to 30°C (59° to 86°F). Dispense in a tight container.

*Identi-Code® (formula identification code, Lilly)
†Identi-Dose (unit dose medication, Lilly)

[072895]

TAZIDIME®   ℞

[tă΄zĭ-dēm]
(ceftazidime)
for injection
USP

DESCRIPTION

Tazidime® (Ceftazidime, USP) is a semisynthetic, broad-spectrum β-lactam antibiotic for parenteral administration. It is the pentahydrate of pyridinium, 1-[[7-[[(2-amino-4-thiazolyl)](1-carboxy-1-methylethoxy) imino]acetyl]amino]-2-carboxy -8- oxo-5-thia -1-azabicyclo[4.2.0]oct-2-en-3-yl]methyl]-, hydroxide, inner salt, [6R-[6α,7β(Z)]]. It has the following structural formula:

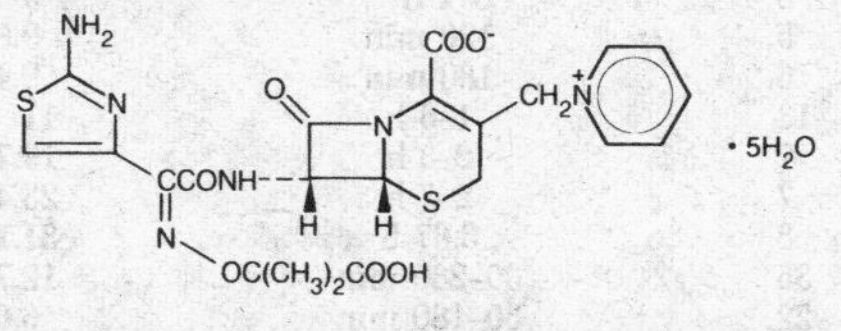

Tazidime is a sterile, dry powder. Tazidime contains 118 mg (18.5 mmol) sodium carbonate/g of ceftazidime activity. The total sodium content of the mixture is approximately 54 mg

(2.3 mEq)/g of ceftazidime activity. Tazidime in sterile crystalline form is supplied in vials equivalent to 500 mg, 1 g, 2 g, or 6 g of anhydrous ceftazidime. Solutions of Tazidime range in color from light yellow to amber, depending on the diluent and volume used. The pH of freshly reconstituted solutions usually ranges from 5.0 to 8.0.

CLINICAL PHARMACOLOGY

After intravenous administration of a 500-mg or a 1-g dose of ceftazidime over 5 minutes to normal adult male volunteers, mean peak serum concentrations were 45 mcg/mL and 90 mcg/mL respectively. Following intravenous infusion of 500-mg, 1-g, and 2-g doses of ceftazidime over 20 to 30 minutes to normal adult male volunteers, mean peak serum concentrations of 42, 69, and 170 mcg/mL respectively were achieved. The average serum concentrations following intravenous infusion of 500-mg, 1-g, and 2-g doses to these volunteers over an 8-hour period are given in Table 1.

Table 1. Ceftazidime Concentrations in Serum

Ceftazidime Dosage (IV)	Serum Concentrations (mcg/mL)				
	$^1/_2$ h	1 h	2 h	4 h	8 h
500 mg	42	25	12	6	2
1 g	60	39	23	11	3
2 g	129	75	42	13	5

The absorption and elimination of ceftazidime were directly proportional to the size of the dose. Following intravenous administration, the half-life was approximately 1.9 hours. Less than 10% of ceftazidime was protein bound. The degree of protein binding was independent of concentration. Following multiple intravenous doses of 1 g and 2 g every 8 hours for 10 days, there was no evidence of accumulation of ceftazidime in the serum in individuals with normal renal function.

Following intramuscular administration of 500-mg and 1-g doses of ceftazidime to normal adult volunteers, the mean peak serum concentrations at approximately 1 hour were 17 mcg/mL and 39 mcg/mL respectively. Serum concentrations remained above 4 mcg/mL for 6 and 8 hours after the intramuscular administration of 500-mg and 1-g doses respectively. The half-life of ceftazidime in these volunteers was approximately 2 hours.

The presence of hepatic dysfunction had no effect on the pharmacokinetics of ceftazidime in individuals who received 2 g intravenously every 8 hours for 5 days. Therefore, a dosage adjustment from the normal recommended dosage is not required for patients with hepatic dysfunction, provided renal function is not impaired.

Approximately 80% to 90% of an intramuscular or intravenous dose of ceftazidime is excreted unchanged by the kidneys over a 24-hour period. After the intravenous administration of a single 500-mg or 1-g dose, approximately 50% of the dose appeared in the urine in the first 2 hours. An additional 20% was excreted 2 to 4 hours after administration, and approximately another 12% of the dose appeared in the urine 4 to 8 hours later. The elimination of ceftazidime by the kidneys resulted in high urinary concentrations. The mean renal clearance of ceftazidime was approximately 100 mL/min. The calculated plasma clearance of approximately 115 mL/min indicated almost complete elimination of ceftazidime by the renal route. The administration of probenecid prior to administration of ceftazidime had no effect on the elimination kinetics of ceftazidime. This suggested that ceftazidime is eliminated by glomerular filtration and is not actively secreted by renal tubular mechanisms.

Since ceftazidime is eliminated almost solely by the kidneys, its serum half-life is significantly prolonged in patients with impaired renal function. Consequently, dosage for such patients must be adjusted (*see* Dosage and Administration).

Therapeutic concentrations of ceftazidime are achieved in tissues and body fluids as listed in Table 2.
[See table at bottom of next page.]

Microbiology —*In vitro* tests demonstrate that ceftazidime is bactericidal, exerting its effect by inhibition of enzymes responsible for cell-wall synthesis. Ceftazidime has *in vitro* activity against a wide range of gram-negative organisms, including strains resistant to gentamicin and other aminoglycosides. In addition, ceftazidime has been shown to be active against gram-positive organisms. It is highly stable to most clinically important β-lactamases, plasmid or chromosomal, that are produced by gram-negative or gram-positive

Continued on next page

Lilly—Cont.

organisms and consequently is active against many strains resistant to ampicillin and other cephalosporins.

Ceftazidime has been shown to be active against the following organisms both *in vitro* and in clinical infections (*see* Indications and Usage):

Aerobes, Gram-Negative
Citrobacter spp (including *Citrobacter freundii* and *Citrobacter diversus*)
Enterobacter spp (including *Enterobacter cloacae* and *Enterobacter aerogenes*)
Escherichia coli
Haemophilus influenzae, including ampicillin-resistant strains
Klebsiella spp (including *Klebsiella pneumoniae*)
Neisseria meningitidis
Proteus mirabilis
Proteus vulgaris
Pseudomonas spp (including *Pseudomonas aeruginosa)*
Serratia spp

Aerobes, Gram-Positive
Staphylococcus aureus, including penicillinase- and non-penicillinase-producing strains
Streptococcus agalactiae (group B streptococci)
Streptococcus pneumoniae
Streptococcus pyogenes (group A β-hemolytic streptococci)

Anaerobes
Bacteroides spp (NOTE: Many strains of *Bacteroides fragilis* are resistant.)

Although clinical efficacy has not been established, ceftazidime has also been shown to demonstrate *in vitro* activity against the following microorganisms:

Acinetobacter spp
Clostridium spp (not including *Clostridium difficile*)
Haemophilus parainfluenzae
Morganella morganii (formerly *Proteus morganii*)
Neisseria gonorrhoeae
Peptococcus spp
Peptostreptococcus spp
Providencia spp (including *Providencia rettgeri,* formerly *Proteus rettgeri*)
Salmonella spp
Shigella spp
Staphylococcus epidermidis
Yersinia enterocolitica

Ceftazidime and the aminoglycosides have been shown to be synergistic *in vitro* against *P. aeruginosa* and the *Enterobacteriaceae.* Ceftazidime and carbenicillin have also been shown to be synergistic *in vitro* against *P. aeruginosa.*

Ceftazidime is not active *in vitro* against methicillin-resistant staphylococci; *Enterococcus faecalis* (formerly *Streptococcus faecalis*) and many other enterococci; *Listeria monocytogenes; Campylobacter* spp; or *C. difficile.*

Disk Susceptibility Tests —Diffusion Techniques: Quantitative methods that require measurement of zone diameters give an estimate of antibiotic susceptibility. One such procedure[1-3] has been recommended for use with disks to test susceptibility to ceftazidime.

Reports from the laboratory giving results of the standard single-disk susceptibility test using a 30-mcg ceftazidime disk should be interpreted according to the following criteria:

Susceptible organisms produce zones of 18 mm or greater, indicating that the tested organism is likely to respond to therapy.

Organisms that produce zones of 15 mm to 17 mm are expected to be susceptible if high dosage is used or if the infection is confined to tissues and fluids (eg, urine) in which high antibiotic levels are attained.

Resistant organisms produce zones of 14 mm or less, indicating that other therapy should be selected.

Organisms should be tested with the ceftazidime disk because ceftazidime has been shown by *in vitro* tests to have activity against certain strains found to be resistant when tested with other β-lactam disks.

Standardized procedures require the use of laboratory control organisms. The 30-µg ceftazidime disk should give zone diameters between 25 mm and 32 mm for *E. coli* ATCC 25922, between 22 mm and 29 mm for *P. aeruginosa* ATCC 27853, and between 16 mm and 20 mm for *S. aureus* ATCC 25923.

Dilution Techniques—In other susceptibility testing procedures (eg, the ICS agar dilution or its equivalent) a bacterial isolate may be considered susceptible if the (minimum inhibitory concentration) MIC value for ceftazidime is not > 16 mcg/mL. Organisms are considered resistant if the (minimum inhibitory concentration) MIC is ≥ 64 mcg/mL. Organisms having an MIC value < 64 mcg/mL but > 16 mcg/mL are expected to be susceptible if high dosage is used or if the infection is confined to tissues and fluids (eg, urine) in which high antibiotic levels are attained.

As with standard diffusion methods, dilution procedures require the use of laboratory control organisms. Standard ceftazidime powder should give MIC values of 4 mcg/mL to 16 mcg/mL for *S. aureus* ATCC 29213, 0.125 mcg/mL to 0.5 mcg/mL for *E. coli* ATCC 25922, and 0.5 mcg/mL to 2 mcg/mL for *P. aeruginosa* ATCC 27853.

INDICATIONS AND USAGE

Tazidime is indicated for the treatment of infections caused by susceptible strains of the designated organisms in the diseases listed below:

*Lower respiratory tract infections,*including pneumonia, caused by *P. aeruginosa* and other *Pseudomonas* spp., *H. influenzae* (including ampicillin-resistant strains), *Klebsiella* spp., *Enterobacter* spp., *P. mirabilis, E. coli, Serratia* spp., *Citrobacter* spp., *S. pneumoniae,* and *S. aureus* (methicillin-susceptible strains)

Skin and skin structure infections caused by *P. aeruginosa, Klebsiella* spp., *E. coli, Proteus* spp. (including *P. mirabilis* and indole-positive *Proteus), Enterobacter* spp., *Serratia* spp., *S. aureus* (methicillin-susceptible strains), and *S. pyogenes* (group A β-hemolytic streptococci)

Urinary tract infections, both complicated and uncomplicated, caused by *P. aeruginosa, Enterobacter* spp., *Proteus* spp. (including *P. mirabilis* and indole-positive *Proteus), Klebsiella* spp., and *E. coli*

Bacterial septicemia caused by *P. aeruginosa, Klebsiella* spp., *H. influenzae, E. coli, Serratia* spp., *S. pneumoniae,* and *S. aureus* (methicillin-susceptible strains)

Bone and joint infections caused by *P. aeruginosa; Klebsiella* spp., *Enterobacter* spp., and *S. aureus* (methicillin-susceptible strains)

Gynecologic infections, including endometritis, pelvic cellulitis, and other infections of the female genital tract caused by *E. coli*

Intra-abdominal infections, including peritonitis, caused by *E. coli, Klebsiella* spp., and *S. aureus* (methicillin-susceptible strains) and polymicrobial infections caused by aerobic and anaerobic organisms and *Bacteroides* spp. (Many strains of *B. fragilis* are resistant.)

Central nervous system infections, including meningitis, caused by *H. influenzae* and *N. meningitidis.* Tazidime has also been used successfully in a limited number of cases of meningitis due to *P. aeruginosa* and *S. pneumoniae*

Specimens for bacteriologic cultures should be obtained prior to therapy in order to isolate and identify causative organisms and to determine their susceptibilities to ceftazidime. Therapy may be instituted before results of susceptibility studies are known; however, once these results become available, the antibiotic treatment should be adjusted accordingly.

Tazidime may be used alone in cases of confirmed or suspected sepsis. Tazidime has been used successfully as empiric therapy in clinical trial cases involving concomitant therapies with other antibiotics.

Tazidime may also be used concomitantly with other antibiotics, such as aminoglycosides, vancomycin, and clindamycin, in severe and life-threatening infections and in the immunocompromised patient. When such concomitant treatment is appropriate, prescribing information in the labeling for the other antibiotics should be followed. The dose depends on the severity of the infection and the patient's condition.

CONTRAINDICATION

Tazidime is contraindicated in patients who have shown hypersensitivity to ceftazidime or the cephalosporin group of antibiotics.

WARNINGS

BEFORE THERAPY WITH TAZIDIME IS INSTITUTED, CAREFUL INQUIRY SHOULD BE MADE TO DETERMINE WHETHER THE PATIENT HAS HAD PREVIOUS HYPERSENSITIVITY REACTIONS TO CEFTAZIDIME, CEPHALOSPORINS, PENICILLINS, OR OTHER DRUGS. IF THIS PRODUCT IS TO BE GIVEN TO PENICILLIN-SENSITIVE PATIENTS, CAUTION SHOULD BE EXERCISED BECAUSE CROSS-HYPERSENSITIVITY AMONG β-LACTAM ANTIBIOTICS HAS BEEN CLEARLY DOCUMENTED AND MAY OCCUR IN UP TO 10% OF PATIENTS WITH A HISTORY OF PENICILLIN ALLERGY. IF AN ALLERGIC REACTION TO TAZIDIME OCCURS, DISCONTINUE THE DRUG. SERIOUS ACUTE HYPERSENSITIVITY REACTIONS MAY REQUIRE TREATMENT WITH EPINEPHRINE AND OTHER EMERGENCY MEASURES, INCLUDING OXYGEN, IV FLUIDS, IV ANTIHISTAMINES, CORTICOSTEROIDS, PRESSOR AMINES, AND AIRWAY MANAGEMENT, AS CLINICALLY INDICATED.

Pseudomembranous colitis has been reported with nearly all antibacterial agents, including ceftazidime, and may range from mild to life threatening. Therefore, it is important to consider this diagnosis in patients who present with diarrhea subsequent to the administration of antibacterial agents.

Treatment with antibacterial agents alters the normal flora of the colon and may permit overgrowth of clostridia. Studies indicate that a toxin produced by *C. difficile* is a primary cause of "antibiotic-associated colitis".

After the diagnosis of pseudomembranous colitis has been established, therapeutic measures should be initiated. Mild cases of pseudomembranous colitis usually respond to drug discontinuation alone. In moderate to severe cases, consideration should be given to management with fluids and electrolytes, protein supplementation, and treatment with an antibacterial drug effective against *C. difficile.*

Elevated levels of ceftazidime in patients with renal insufficiency can lead to seizures, encephalopathy, asterixis, and neuromuscular excitability (*see* Precautions).

PRECAUTIONS

*General —*Tazidime has not been shown to be nephrotoxic; however, because high and prolonged serum antibiotic concentrations can occur from usual doses in patients with transient or persistent reduction of urinary output because of renal insufficiency, the total daily dosage should be reduced when ceftazidime is administered to such patients (*see* Dosage and Administration). Elevated levels of ceftazidime in these patients can lead to seizures, encephalopathy, asterixis, and neuromuscular excitability. Continued dosage should be determined by degree of renal impairment, severity of infection, and susceptibility of the causative organisms.

As with other antibiotics, prolonged use of Tazidime may result in the overgrowth of nonsusceptible organisms. Repeated evaluation of the patient's condition is essential. If superinfection occurs during therapy, appropriate measures should be taken.

Cephalosporins may be associated with a fall in prothrombin activity. Those at risk include patients with renal and hepatic impairment or poor nutritional state, as well as patients receiving a protracted course of antimicrobial therapy. Prothrombin time should be monitored in patients at risk and exogenous vitamin K administered as indicated.

Tazidime should be prescribed with caution in individuals with a history of gastrointestinal disease, particularly colitis.

Drug Interactions —Nephrotoxicity has been reported following the concomitant administration of cephalosporins with aminoglycoside antibiotics or potent diuretics, such as furosemide. Renal function should be carefully monitored because of the potential nephrotoxicity and ototoxicity of aminoglycoside antibiotics, especially if higher dosages of the aminoglycosides are to be administered or if therapy is

Table 2: Ceftazidime Concentration in Tissues and Body Fluids

Tissue or Fluid	Dose/ Route	No. of Patients	Time of Sample Post-Dose	Average Tissue or Fluid Level (mcg/mL)
Urine	500 mg IM	6	0–2 h	2,100
	2 g IV	6	0–2 h	12,000
Bile	2 g IV	3	90 min	36.4
Synovial fluid	2 g IV	13	2 h	25.6
Peritoneal fluid	2 g IV	8	2 h	48.6
Sputum	1 g IV	8	1 h	9
Cerebrospinal fluid	2 g q8h IV	5	120 min	9.8
(inflamed meninges)	2 g q8h IV	6	180 min	9.4
Aqueous humor	2 g IV	13	1–3 h	11
Blister fluid	1 g IV	7	2–3 h	19.7
Lymphatic fluid	1 g IV	7	2–3 h	23.4
Bone	2 g IV	8	0.67 h	31.1
Heart muscle	2 g IV	35	30–280 min	12.7
Skin	2 g IV	22	30–180 min	6.6
Skeletal muscle	2 g IV	35	30–280 min	9.4
Myometrium	2 g IV	31	1–2 h	18.7

prolonged. Nephrotoxicity and ototoxicity were not noted when Tazidime was given alone in clinical trials.

Chloramphenicol has been shown to be antagonistic to beta-lactam antibiotics, including ceftazidime, based on *in vitro* studies and time kill curves with enteric gram-negative bacilli. Due to the possibility of antagonism *in vivo*, particularly when bactericidal activity is desired, this drug combination should be avoided.

Drug/Laboratory Test Interactions—The administration of ceftazidime may result in a false-positive reaction for glucose in the urine when using Clinitest®, Benedict's solution, or Fehling's solution. It is recommended that glucose tests based on enzymatic glucose oxidase reactions (such as Clinistix®) be used.

Carcinogenesis, Mutagenesis, Impairment of Fertility—Long-term studies in animals have not been performed to evaluate carcinogenic potential. However, a mouse micronucleus test and an Ames test were both negative for mutagenic effects.

Usage in Pregnancy—*Pregnancy Category B*—Reproduction studies have been performed in mice and rats at doses up to 40 times the human dose and have revealed no evidence of impaired fertility or harm to the fetus due to Tazidime. There are, however, no adequate and well-controlled studies in pregnant women. Because animal reproduction studies are not always predictive of human response, this drug should be used during pregnancy only if clearly needed.

Nursing Mothers—Ceftazidime is excreted in human milk in low concentrations. Caution should be exercised when Tazidime is administered to a nursing woman.

Pediatric Use—(see Dosage and Administration.)

ADVERSE REACTIONS

Tazidime is generally well tolerated. The incidence of adverse reactions associated with the administration of Tazidime was low in clinical trials. The most common were local reactions following intravenous injection and allergic and gastrointestinal reactions. Other adverse reactions were encountered infrequently. No disulfiram-like reactions were reported.

The following adverse effects during clinical trials were considered to be either related to ceftazidime therapy or of uncertain etiology:

Local effects, reported in < 2% of patients, were phlebitis and inflammation at the site of injection (1 in 69 patients).

Hypersensitivity reactions, reported in 2% of patients, were pruritus, rash and fever. Immediate reactions generally manifested by rash and/or pruritus, occurred in 1 in 285 patients. Angioedema and anaphylaxis (bronchospasm and/or hypotension) have been reported very rarely.

Gastrointestinal symptoms, reported in <2% of patients, were diarrhea (1 in 78), nausea (1 in 156), vomiting (1 in 500), and abdominal pain (1 in 416). The onset of pseudomembranous colitis symptoms may occur during or after treatment (*see* Warnings).

Central Nervous System Reactions (<1%) included headache, dizziness, and paresthesia. Seizures have been reported with several cephalosporins, including ceftazidime. In addition, encephalopathy, asterixis, and neuromuscular excitability have been reported in renally impaired patients treated with unadjusted dosage regimens of ceftazidime (*see* Precautions, General).

Less frequent adverse events (<1%) were candidiasis (including oral thrush) and vaginitis.

Laboratory test changes noted during clinical trials with Tazidime were transient and included eosinophilia (1 in 13), positive Coombs' test without hemolysis (1 in 23), thrombocytosis (1 in 45), and slight elevations in 1 or more of the hepatic enzymes: AST (SGOT) (1 in 16), ALT (SGPT) (1 in 15), LDH (1 in 18), GGT (1 in 19), and alkaline phosphatase (1 in 23). As with some other cephalosporins, transient elevations of blood urea, blood urea nitrogen, and/or serum creatinine were observed occasionally. Transient leukopenia, neutropenia, agranulocytosis, thrombocytopenia, and lymphocytosis were seen very rarely.

In addition to the adverse reactions listed above that have been observed with ceftazidime, the following adverse reactions and altered laboratory tests have been reported for cephalosporin-class antibiotics:

Adverse Reactions—Urticaria, Stevens-Johnson syndrome, erythema multiforme, toxic epidermal necrolysis, colitis, renal dysfunction, toxic nephropathy, hepatic dysfunction including cholestasis, aplastic anemia, hemolytic anemia, and hemorrhage.

Altered Laboratory Tests—Prolonged prothrombin time, false-positive test for urinary glucose, elevated bilirubin, and pancytopenia.

Hematologic—Rare cases of hemolytic anemia have been reported.

OVERDOSAGE

Ceftazidime overdosage has occurred in patients with renal failure. Reactions have included seizure activity, encephalopathy, asterixis, and neuromuscular excitability. Patients who receive an acute overdosage should be carefully observed and given supportive treatment. In the presence of

renal insufficiency, hemodialysis or peritoneal dialysis may aid in the removal of ceftazidime from the body.

DOSAGE AND ADMINISTRATION

Dosage—The usual adult dosage is 1 g administered intravenously or intramuscularly every 8 or 12 hours. The dosage and route of administration should be determined by the susceptibility of the causative organisms, the severity of infection, and the condition and renal function of the patient. The guidelines for dosage of Tazidime are listed in Table 3. The following dosage schedule is recommended:

[See table above.]

Impaired Hepatic Function—No adjustment in dosage is required for patients with hepatic dysfunction.

Impaired Renal Function—Ceftazidime is excreted by the kidneys almost exclusively by glomerular filtration. Therefore, in patients with impaired renal function (GFR <50 mL/min), it is recommended that the dose of Tazidime be reduced to compensate for its slower excretion. In patients with suspected renal insufficiency, an initial loading dose of 1 g of Tazidime may be given. An estimate of GFR should be made to determine the appropriate maintenance dose. The recommended dosage is presented in Table 4.

Table 4. Recommended Maintenance Dosage of Tazidime in Patients With Renal Insufficiency

NOTE: IF THE DOSE RECOMMENDED IN TABLE 3 IS LOWER THAN THAT RECOMMENDED FOR PATIENTS WITH RENAL INSUFFICIENCY AS OUTLINED IN TABLE 4, THE LOWER DOSE SHOULD BE USED.

Creatinine Clearance (mL/min)	Recommended Dose of Tazidime	Frequency
50–31	1 g	q12h
30–16	1 g	q24h
15–6	500 mg	q24h
<5	500 mg	q48h

When only serum creatinine is available, the following formula (Cockcroft's equation)[4] may be used to estimate creatinine clearance. The serum creatinine should represent a steady state of renal function:

$$\text{Males:} \quad \frac{\text{Creatinine Clearance}}{(\text{mL/min})} = \frac{\text{Weight (kg)} \times (140 - \text{age})}{72 \times \text{serum creatinine} \ (\text{mg/dL})}$$

Females: 0.85 × above value

In patients with severe infections who would normally receive 6 g of Tazidime daily were it not for renal insufficiency, the dose given in the above table may be increased by 50% or the dosing frequency increased appropriately. Continued dosage should be determined by therapeutic monitoring, severity of the infection, and susceptibility of the causative organism.

In children, as in adults, the creatinine clearance should be adjusted for body surface area or lean body mass, and the dosing frequency should be reduced in cases of renal insufficiency.

In patients undergoing hemodialysis, a loading dose of 1 g of Tazidime is recommended, followed by 1 g after each hemodialysis period.

Tazidime can also be used in patients undergoing intraperitoneal dialysis (IPD) and continuous ambulatory peritoneal dialysis (CAPD). In such patients, a loading dose of 1 g of Tazidime may be given, followed by 500 mg every 24 hours. In addition to intravenous use, Tazidime can be incorporated in dialysis fluid at a concentration of 250 mg/2 L of dialysis fluid.

NOTE: Tazidime should generally be continued for 2 days after the signs and symptoms of infection have disappeared; however, in complicated infections, longer therapy may be required.

Administration—Tazidime may be given intravenously or by deep intramuscular injection into a large muscle mass (such as the upper outer quadrant of the gluteus maximus or lateral part of the thigh).

Intramuscular Administration—For intramuscular administration, Tazidime should be reconstituted with 1 of the following diluents: Sterile Water for Injection, Bacteriostatic Water for Injection, or 0.5% or 1.0% Lidocaine Hydrochloride Injection. Refer to Table 5.

Intravenous Administration—The IV route is preferable for patients with bacterial septicemia, bacterial meningitis, peritonitis, or other severe or life-threatening infections. It is also preferable for patients who may be poor risks because of lowered resistance resulting from such debilitating conditions as malnutrition, trauma, surgery, diabetes, heart failure, or malignancy, particularly if shock is present or impending.

Direct Intermittent Intravenous Administration—For direct intermittent intravenous administration, reconstitute Tazidime with Sterile Water for Injection (see Table 5). Slowly inject the solution directly into the vein over a period of 3 to 5 minutes or give through the tubing of an administration set while the patient is also receiving 1 of the compatible intravenous fluids (*see* Compatibility and Stability).

Intravenous Infusion—For intravenous infusion, reconstitute the 1-g or 2-g piggyback (100-mL) vial with 100 mL Sterile Water for Injection or 1 of the compatible intravenous fluids listed in the Compatibility and Stability section. Alternatively, reconstitute the 500-mg, 1-g, or 2-g vial, and add an appropriate quantity of the resulting solution to an IV container with 1 of the compatible intravenous fluids.

Intermittent Intravenous Infusion with a Y-type Administration Set—Intermittent intravenous infusion with a Y-type administration set can be accomplished with compatible solutions. However, during infusion of a solution containing ceftazidime, it is desirable to discontinue the other solution. ADD-Vantage® vials are to be used only with Abbott ADD-Vantage diluent bags according to the printed tray card instructions included in each Traypak of vials of Tazidime Reconstitution.

[See table 5 at bottom of next page.]

Continued on next page

Table 3: Recommended Dosage Schedule for Ceftazidime

	Dose	Frequency
Adults		
Usual recommended dose	**1 g IV or IM**	**q8 or 12h**
Uncomplicated urinary tract infections	250 mg IV or IM	q12h
Bone and joint infections	2 g IV	q12h
Complicated urinary tract infections	500 mg IV or IM	q8 or 12h
Uncomplicated pneumonia; mild skin and skin structure infections	500 mg–1 g IV or IM	q8h
Serious gynecologic and intra-abdominal infections	2 g IV	q8h
Meningitis	2 g IV	q8h
Very severe life-threatening infections, especially in immunocompromised patients	2 g IV	q8h
Pseudomonal lung infections in patients with cystic fibrosis with normal renal function*	30–50 mg/kg IV to a maximum of 6 g/day	q8h
Neonates (0 to 4 weeks)	30 mg/kg IV	q12h
Infants and Children (1 month to 12 years of age)	30–50 mg/kg IV to a maximum of 6 g/day†	q8h

* Although clinical improvement has been shown, bacteriologic cures cannot be expected in patients with chronic respiratory disease and cystic fibrosis.

† The higher dose should be reserved for immunocompromised children or children with cystic fibrosis or meningitis.

• **Identi-Code® symbol. This product information was prepared in June 1996. Current information on these and other products of Eli Lilly and Company may be obtained by direct inquiry to Lilly Research Laboratories, Lilly Corporate Center, Indianapolis, Indiana 46285, 800-545-5979.**

Lilly—Cont.

All vials of Tazidime as supplied are under reduced pressure. When Tazidime is dissolved, carbon dioxide is released and a positive pressure develops. For ease of use, please follow the recommended techniques of reconstitution described below. Solutions of Tazidime, like those of most β-lactam antibiotics, should not be added to solutions of aminoglycoside antibiotics because of potential interaction. However, if concurrent therapy with Tazidime and an aminoglycoside is indicated, each of these antibiotics should be administered in different sites.

Instructions for Reconstitution:
For 500-mg IM/IV, 1-g IM/IV, and 2-g IV vials
1. Insert the syringe needle through the vial closure and inject the recommended volume of diluent. The vacuum may assist entry of the diluent. Remove the syringe needle.
2. Shake to dissolve; a clear solution will be obtained in 1 to 2 minutes.
3. Invert the vial. Ensuring that the syringe plunger is fully depressed, insert the needle through the vial closure and withdraw the total volume of solution into the syringe (the pressure in the vial may aid withdrawal). Ensure that the needle remains within the solution and does not enter the headspace. The withdrawn solution may contain some bubbles of carbon dioxide.
Note: As with the administration of all parenteral products, accumulated gases should be expressed from the syringe immediately before injection of Tazidime.
For 1-g and 2-g piggyback vials
1. Insert the syringe needle through the vial closure and inject 10 mL of diluent. The vacuum may assist entry of the diluent. Remove the syringe needle.
2. Shake to dissolve; a clear solution will be obtained in 1 to 2 minutes.
3. Insert a gas relief needle through the vial closure to relieve the internal pressure. With the gas relief needle in position, add the remaining 90 mL of diluent. Remove the gas relief needle and syringe needle; shake the vial and set up for infusion in the normal way.
Note: To preserve product sterility, it is important that a gas relief needle is *not* inserted through the vial closure before the product has dissolved.

COMPATIBILITY AND STABILITY

Intramuscular—Vials of Tazidime, when reconstituted as directed with Sterile Water for Injection, Bacteriostatic Water for Injection, or 0.5% or 1% Lidocaine Hydrochloride Injection, maintain satisfactory potency for 24 hours at room temperature or for 7 days under refrigeration. Solutions in Sterile Water for Injection that are frozen immediately after reconstitution in the original container are stable for 3 months when stored at −20°C. Once thawed, solutions should not be refrozen. Thawed solutions may be stored for up to 8 hours at room temperature or for 4 days in a refrigerator.
Intravenous—Vials of Tazidime, when reconstituted as directed with Sterile Water for Injection, maintain satisfactory potency for 24 hours at room temperature or for 7 days under refrigeration. Solutions in Sterile Water for Injection in the original container or in 0.9% Sodium Chloride Injection or 5% Dextrose Injection in PVC small-volume containers that are frozen immediately after reconstitution are stable for 3 months when stored at −20°C. When it is necessary to warm a large volume of the frozen product (to a maximum of 40°C), care should be taken to avoid heating it after thawing is complete. Once thawed, solutions should not be refrozen. Thawed solutions may be stored for up to 24 hours at room temperature or for 4 days in a refrigerator.
Tazidime is compatible with the more commonly used intravenous infusion fluids. Solutions at concentrations from 1 mg/mL to 40 mg/mL in the following infusion fluids may be

stored for up to 24 hours at room temperature or for 7 days if refrigerated: 0.9% Sodium Chloride Injection; M/6 Sodium Lactate Injection; Ringer's Injection, USP; Lactated Ringer's Injection, USP; 5% Dextrose Injection; 5% Dextrose and 0.225% Sodium Chloride Injection; 5% Dextrose and 0.45% Sodium Chloride Injection; 5% Dextrose and 0.9% Sodium Chloride Injection; 10% Dextrose Injection; 10% Invert Sugar in Water for Injection; and Normosol®-M in 5% Dextrose Injection.
When diluted with Abbott's ADD-Vantage diluents, 0.9% Sodium Chloride Injection and 5% Dextrose Injection, ADD-Vantage Tazidime may be stored for up to 24 hours at room temperature.
Joined vials that have not been activated may be used within a 14-day period; this period corresponds to that for use of Abbott ADD-Vantage containers following removal of the outer packaging (overwrap).
Freezing solutions of Tazidime in the ADD-Vantage system is not recommended.
Tazidime is less stable in Sodium Bicarbonate Injection than in other intravenous fluids. Sodium Bicarbonate Injection is not recommended as a diluent. Solutions of Tazidime in 5% Dextrose or 0.9% Sodium Chloride Injection are stable for at least 6 hours at room temperature in plastic tubing, drip chambers, and volume control devices of common intravenous infusion sets.
At a concentration of 4 mg/mL, Tazidime has been found to be compatible for 24 hours at room temperature or for 7 days under refrigeration in 0.9% Sodium Chloride Injection or 5% Dextrose Injection when admixed with cefuroxime sodium, 3 mg/mL; heparin, 10 units/mL or 50 units/mL; or potassium chloride, 10 mEq/L or 40 mEq/L.
Vancomycin solution exhibits a physical incompatibility when mixed with a number of drugs, including ceftazidime. The likelihood of precipitation with ceftazidime is dependent on the concentrations of vancomycin and ceftazidime present. It is, therefore, recommended that when both drugs are to be administered by intermittent intravenous infusion, they be given separately, flushing the intravenous lines (with one of the compatible intravenous fluids) between the administration of these 2 agents.
Note: Parenteral drug products should be inspected visually for particulate matter whenever solution and container permit.
Tazidime powder and solutions will darken under certain storage conditions. However, product potency is not adversely affected if proper storage conditions and periods are observed.

HOW SUPPLIED

Vials (Dry Powder):
  500 mg,* 10-mL size (No. 7230)—(Traypak† of 25) NDC 0002-7230-25
  1 g,* 20-mL size (No. 7231)—(Traypak of 25) NDC 0002-7231-25
  1 g,* 100-mL size (No. 7238)—(Traypak of 10) NDC 0002-7238-10
  2 g,* 50-mL size (No. 7234)—(Traypak of 10) NDC 0002-7234-10
  2 g,* 100-mL size (No. 7239)—(Traypak of 10) NDC 0002-7239-10

Faspak‡:
  1 g* (No. 7245)—(Faspak of 24) NDC 0002-7245-24
  2 g* (No. 7246)—(Faspak of 24) NDC 0002-7246-24

ADD-Vantage§ Vials:
  1 g* (No. 7290)—(Traypak of 25) NDC 0002-7290-25
  2 g* (No. 7291)—(Traypak of 10) NDC 0002-7291-10
The above ADD-Vantage Vials are to be used only with Abbott Laboratories' ADD-Vantage Diluent Containers.
Instructions for the use of ADD-Vantage Vials are enclosed in the package.

Also available:
Pharmacy Bulk Package:
  6 g,* 100-mL size (No. 7241)—(Traypak of 6) NDC 0002-7241-16

*Equivalent to ceftazidime activity.
†Traypak™(multivial carton, Lilly).
‡Faspak® (flexible plastic bag, Lilly).
§ADD-Vantage® (vials and diluent containers, Abbott).

REFERENCES

1. Bauer AW, Kirby WMM, Sherris J C, et al: Antibiotic susceptibility testing by a standardized single disk method. *Am J Clin Pathol* 1966; 45:483.
2. *Performance standards for antimicrobial disk susceptibility tests,* ed 4, Tentative Standard: M2-T4. NCCLS, Villanova, PA, 1988.
3. Standardized disk susceptibility test. *Federal Register* 1974; 39 (May 30):19182–19184.
4. Cockcroft DW, Gault MH: Prediction of creatinine clearance from serum creatinine. *Nephron* 1978; 16:31–41.

[042296]

TOBRAMYCIN SULFATE ℞

See Nebcin® (Tobramycin Sulfate Injection, USP).

VANCOCIN® HCl ℞

[văn 'kō-sĭn ăch 'sē-ĕl]
(Sterile Vancomycin Hydrochloride, USP)
IntraVenous

DESCRIPTION

Vancocin® HCl (Sterile Vancomycin Hydrochloride, USP), IntraVenous, is a chromatographically purified, tricyclic glycopeptide antibiotic derived from *Amycolatopsis orientalis* (formerly *Nocardia orientalis*) and has the chemical formula $C_{66}H_{75}Cl_2N_9O_{24}$·HCl. The molecular weight is 1,486; 500 mg of the base is equivalent to 0.34 mmol.
Vancomycin hydrochloride has the following structure:

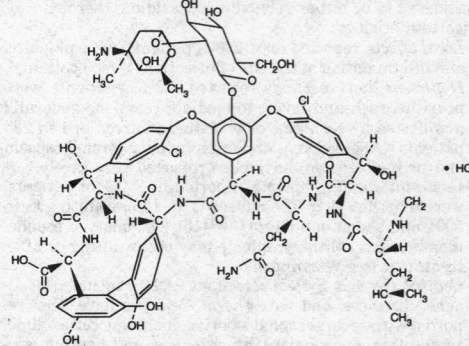

The vials contain sterile vancomycin hydrochloride equivalent to either 500 mg or 1 g vancomycin activity. Vancomycin hydrochloride is an off-white lyophilized plug. When reconstituted in water, it forms a clear solution with a pH range of 2.5 to 4.5. This product is oxygen sensitive.

CLINICAL PHARMACOLOGY

Vancomycin is poorly absorbed after oral administration; it is given intravenously for therapy of systemic infections. Intramuscular injection is painful.
In subjects with normal kidney function, multiple intravenous dosing of 1 g of vancomycin (15 mg/kg) infused over 60 minutes produces mean plasma concentrations of approximately 63 μg/mL immediately after the completion of infusion, mean plasma concentrations of approximately 23 μg/mL 2 hours after infusion, and mean plasma concentrations of approximately 8 μg/mL 11 hours after the end of the infusion. Multiple dosing of 500 mg infused over 30 minutes produces mean plasma concentrations of about 49 μg/mL at the completion of infusion, mean plasma concentrations of about 19 μg/mL 2 hours after infusion, and mean plasma concentrations of about 10 μg/mL 6 hours after infusion. The plasma concentrations during multiple dosing are similar to those after a single dose.
The mean elimination half-life of vancomycin from plasma is 4 to 6 hours in subjects with normal renal function. In the first 24 hours, about 75% of an administered dose of vancomycin is excreted in urine by glomerular filtration. Mean plasma clearance is about 0.058 L/kg/h, and mean renal clearance is about 0.048 L/kg/h. Renal dysfunction slows excretion of vancomycin. In anephric patients, the average half-life of elimination is 7.5 days. The distribution coefficient is from 0.3 to 0.43 L/kg. There is no apparent metabolism of the drug. About 60% of an intraperitoneal dose of vancomycin administered during peritoneal dialysis is absorbed systemically in 6 hours. Serum concentrations of about 10 μg/mL are achieved by intraperitoneal injection of

Table 5: Preparation of Solutions

	Amount of Diluent to Be Added (mL)	Approximate Available Volume (mL)	Approximate Ceftazidime Concentration (mg/mL)
Intramuscular			
500 mg, Vial No. 7230	1.5	1.8	280
1 g, Vial No. 7231	3.0	3.6	280
Intravenous			
500 mg, Vial No. 7230	5	5.3	100
1 g, Vial No. 7231	10	10.6	100
2 g, Vial No. 7234	10	11.2	180
Piggyback (100 mL)			
1 g, Vial No. 7238	100*	100	10
2 g, Vial No. 7239	100*	100	20

*Note: Addition should be in 2 stages (*see* Instructions for Reconstitution *below*).

30 mg/kg of vancomycin. Although vancomycin is not effectively removed by either hemodialysis or peritoneal dialysis, there have been reports of increased vancomycin clearance with hemoperfusion and hemofiltration.

Total systemic and renal clearance of vancomycin may be reduced in the elderly.

Vancomycin is approximately 55% serum protein bound as measured by ultrafiltration at vancomycin serum concentrations of 10 to 100 μg/mL. After IV administration of Vancocin HCl, inhibitory concentrations are present in pleural, pericardial, ascitic, and synovial fluids; in urine; in peritoneal dialysis fluid; and in atrial appendage tissue. Vancocin HCl does not readily diffuse across normal meninges into the spinal fluid; but, when the meninges are inflamed, penetration into the spinal fluid occurs.

Microbiology—The bactericidal action of vancomycin results primarily from inhibition of cell-wall biosynthesis. In addition, vancomycin alters bacterial-cell-membrane permeability and RNA synthesis. There is no cross-resistance between vancomycin and other antibiotics. Vancomycin is active against staphylococci, including *Staphylococcus aureus* and *Staphylococcus epidermidis* (including heterogeneous methicillin-resistant strains); streptococci, including *Streptococcus pyogenes*, *Streptococcus pneumoniae* (including penicillin-resistant strains), *Streptococcus agalactiae*, the viridans group, *Streptococcus bovis*, and enterococci (eg, *Enterococcus faecalis* [formerly *Streptococcus faecalis*]); *Clostridium difficile* (eg, toxigenic strains implicated in pseudomembranous enterocolitis); and diphtheroids. Other organisms that are susceptible to vancomycin in vitro include *Listeria monocytogenes*, *Lactobacillus* species, *Actinomyces* species, *Clostridium* species, and *Bacillus* species.

Vancomycin is not active in vitro against gram-negative bacilli, mycobacteria, or fungi.

Synergy—The combination of vancomycin and an aminoglycoside acts synergistically in vitro against many strains of *S. aureus*, nonenterococcal group D streptococci, enterococci, and *Streptococcus* species (viridans group).

Disk Susceptibility Tests—The standardized disk method described by the National Committee for Clinical Laboratory Standards has been recommended to test susceptibility to vancomycin. Results of standard susceptibility tests with a 30-μg vancomycin hydrochloride disk should be interpreted according to the following criteria: Susceptible organisms produce zones greater than or equal to 12 mm, indicating that the test organism is likely to respond to therapy. Organisms that produce zones of 10 or 11 mm are considered to be of intermediate susceptibility. Organisms in this category are likely to respond if the infection is confined to tissues or fluids in which high antibiotic concentrations are attained. Resistant organisms produce zones of 9 mm or less, indicating that other therapy should be selected.

Using a standardized dilution method, a bacterial isolate may be considered susceptible if the MIC value for vancomycin is 4 μg/mL or less. Organisms are considered resistant to vancomycin if the MIC is greater than or equal to 16 μg/mL. Organisms having an MIC value of less than 16 μg/mL but greater than 4 μg/mL are considered to be of intermediate susceptibility.[1-3]

Standardized procedures require the use of laboratory control organisms. The 30-μg vancomycin disk should give zone diameters between 15 and 19 mm for *S. aureus* ATCC 25923. As with the standard diffusion methods, dilution procedures require the use of laboratory control organisms. Standard vancomycin powder should give MIC values in the range of 0.5 μg/mL to 2.0 μg/mL for *S. aureus* ATCC 29213. For *E. faecalis* ATCC 29212, the MIC range should be 1.0 to 4.0 μg/mL.

INDICATIONS AND USAGE

Vancocin HCl is indicated for the treatment of serious or severe infections caused by susceptible strains of methicillin-resistant (beta-lactam-resistant) staphylococci. It is indicated for penicillin-allergic patients, for patients who cannot receive or who have failed to respond to other drugs, including the penicillins or cephalosporins, and for infections caused by vancomycin-susceptible organisms that are resistant to other antimicrobial drugs. Vancocin HCl is indicated for initial therapy when methicillin-resistant staphylococci are suspected, but after susceptibility data are available, therapy should be adjusted accordingly.

Vancocin HCl is effective in the treatment of staphylococcal endocarditis. Its effectiveness has been documented in other infections due to staphylococci, including septicemia, bone infections, lower respiratory tract infections, and skin and skin structure infections. When staphylococcal infections are localized and purulent, antibiotics are used as adjuncts to appropriate surgical measures.

Vancocin HCl has been reported to be effective alone or in combination with an aminoglycoside for endocarditis caused by *Streptococcus viridans* or *S. bovis*. For endocarditis caused by enterococci (eg, *E. faecalis*), Vancocin HCl has been reported to be effective only in combination with an aminoglycoside.

Vancocin HCl has been reported to be effective for the treatment of diphtheroid endocarditis. Vancocin HCl has been used successfully in combination with either rifampin, an aminoglycoside, or both in early-onset prosthetic valve endocarditis caused by *S. epidermidis* or diphtheroids.

Specimens for bacteriologic cultures should be obtained in order to isolate and identify causative organisms and to determine their susceptibilities to Vancocin HCl.

The parenteral form of Vancocin HCl may be administered orally for treatment of antibiotic-associated pseudomembranous colitis caused by *C. difficile* and for staphylococcal enterocolitis. Parenteral administration of Vancocin HCl alone is of unproven benefit for these indications. **Vancocin HCl is not effective by the oral route for other types of infection.**

Although no controlled clinical efficacy studies have been conducted, intravenous vancomycin has been suggested by the American Heart Association and the American Dental Association as prophylaxis against bacterial endocarditis in penicillin-allergic patients who have congenital heart disease or rheumatic or other acquired valvular heart disease when these patients undergo dental procedures or surgical procedures of the upper respiratory tract.

Note: When selecting antibiotics for the prevention of bacterial endocarditis, the physician or dentist should read the full joint statement of the American Heart Association and the American Dental Association.[4]

CONTRAINDICATION

Vancocin HCl is contraindicated in patients with known hypersensitivity to this antibiotic.

WARNINGS

Rapid bolus administration (eg, over several minutes) may be associated with exaggerated hypotension, and, rarely, cardiac arrest.

Vancocin HCl should be administered in a dilute solution over a period of not less than 60 minutes to avoid rapid-infusion-related reactions. Stopping the infusion usually results in prompt cessation of these reactions.

Ototoxicity has occurred in patients receiving Vancocin HCl. It may be transient or permanent. It has been reported mostly in patients who have been given excessive doses, who have an underlying hearing loss, or who are receiving concomitant therapy with another ototoxic agent, such as an aminoglycoside. Vancomycin should be used with caution in patients with renal insufficiency because the risk of toxicity is appreciably increased by high, prolonged blood concentrations.

Dosage of Vancocin HCl must be adjusted for patients with renal dysfunction (*see* Precautions *and* Dosage and Administration).

Pseudomembranous colitis has been reported with nearly all antibacterial agents, including vancomycin, and may range in severity from mild to life-threatening. Therefore, it is important to consider this diagnosis in patients who present with diarrhea subsequent to the administration of antibacterial agents.

Treatment with antibacterial agents alters the normal flora of the colon and may permit overgrowth of clostridia. Studies indicate that a toxin produced by *Clostridium difficile* is a primary cause of "antibiotic-associated colitis." After the diagnosis of pseudomembranous colitis has been established, therapeutic measures should be initiated. Mild cases of pseudomembranous colitis usually respond to drug discontinuation alone. In moderate to severe cases, consideration should be given to management with fluids and electrolytes, protein supplementation, and treatment with an antibacterial drug clinically effective against *C. difficile* colitis.

PRECAUTIONS

General—Clinically significant serum concentrations have been reported in some patients who have taken multiple oral doses of vancomycin for active *C. difficile*-induced pseudomembranous colitis.

Prolonged use of Vancocin HCl may result in the overgrowth of nonsusceptible organisms. Careful observation of the patient is essential. If superinfection occurs during therapy, appropriate measures should be taken.

In order to minimize the risk of nephrotoxicity when treating patients with underlying renal dysfunction or patients receiving concomitant therapy with an aminoglycoside, serial monitoring of renal function should be performed and particular care should be taken in following appropriate dosing schedules (*see* Dosage and Administration).

Serial tests of auditory function may be helpful in order to minimize the risk of ototoxicity.

Reversible neutropenia has been reported in patients receiving Vancocin HCl (*see* Adverse Reactions). Patients who will undergo prolonged therapy with Vancocin HCl or those who are receiving concomitant drugs that may cause neutropenia should have periodic monitoring of the leukocyte count.

Vancocin HCl is irritating to tissue and must be given by a secure intravenous route of administration. Pain, tenderness, and necrosis occur with intramuscular injection of Vancocin HCl or with inadvertent extravasation. Thrombophlebitis may occur, the frequency and severity of which can be minimized by administering the drug slowly as a dilute solution (2.5 to 5 g/L) and by rotating the sites of infusion.

There have been reports that the frequency of infusion-related events (including hypotension, flushing, erythema, urticaria, and pruritus) increases with the concomitant administration of anesthetic agents. Infusion-related events may be minimized by the administration of Vancocin HCl as a 60-minute infusion prior to anesthetic induction.

The safety and efficacy of vancomycin administration by the intrathecal (intralumbar or intraventricular) routes have not been assessed.

Reports have revealed that administration of sterile vancomycin HCl by the intraperitoneal route during continuous ambulatory peritoneal dialysis (CAPD) has resulted in a syndrome of chemical peritonitis. To date, this syndrome has ranged from a cloudy dialysate alone to a cloudy dialysate accompanied by variable degrees of abdominal pain and fever. This syndrome appears to be short-lived after discontinuation of intraperitoneal vancomycin.

Drug Interactions—Concomitant administration of vancomycin and anesthetic agents has been associated with erythema and histamine-like flushing (*see* Usage in Pediatrics *under* Precautions) and anaphylactoid reactions (*see* Adverse Reactions).

Concurrent and/or sequential systemic or topical use of other potentially neurotoxic and/or nephrotoxic drugs, such as amphotericin B, aminoglycosides, bacitracin, polymyxin B, colistin, viomycin, or cisplatin, when indicated, requires careful monitoring.

Usage in Pregnancy—Pregnancy Category C—Animal reproduction studies have not been conducted with Vancocin HCl. It is not known whether Vancocin HCl can affect reproduction capacity. In a controlled clinical study, the potential ototoxic and nephrotoxic effects of Vancocin HCl on infants were evaluated when the drug was administered to pregnant women for serious staphylococcal infections complicating intravenous drug abuse. Vancocin HCl was found in cord blood. No sensorineural hearing loss or nephrotoxicity attributable to Vancocin HCl was noted. One infant whose mother received Vancocin HCl in the third trimester experienced conductive hearing loss that was not attributed to the administration of Vancocin HCl. Because the number of patients treated in this study was limited and Vancocin HCl was administered only in the second and third trimesters, it is not known whether Vancocin HCl causes fetal harm. Vancocin HCl should be given to a pregnant woman only if clearly needed.

Nursing Mothers—Vancocin HCl is excreted in human milk. Caution should be exercised when Vancocin HCl is administered to a nursing woman. Because of the potential for adverse events, a decision should be made whether to discontinue nursing or to discontinue the drug, taking into account the importance of the drug to the mother.

Usage in Pediatrics—In premature neonates and young infants, it may be appropriate to confirm desired vancomycin serum concentrations. Concomitant administration of vancomycin and anesthetic agents has been associated with erythema and histamine-like flushing in children (*see* Adverse Reactions).

Geriatrics—The natural decrement of glomerular filtration with increasing age may lead to elevated vancomycin serum concentrations if dosage is not adjusted. Vancomycin dosage schedules should be adjusted in elderly patients (*see* Dosage and Administration).

ADVERSE REACTIONS

Infusion-Related Events—During or soon after rapid infusion of Vancocin HCl, patients may develop anaphylactoid reactions, including hypotension, wheezing, dyspnea, urticaria, or pruritus. Rapid infusion may also cause flushing of the upper body ("red neck") or pain and muscle spasm of the chest and back. These reactions usually resolve within 20 minutes but may persist for several hours. In animal studies, hypotension and bradycardia occurred in animals given large doses of vancomycin at high concentrations and rates. Such events are infrequent if Vancocin HCl is given by a slow infusion over 60 minutes. In studies of normal volunteers, infusion-related events did not occur when Vancocin HCl was administered at a rate of 10 mg/min or less.

Nephrotoxicity—Rarely, renal failure, principally manifested by increased serum creatinine or BUN concentrations, especially in patients given large doses of Vancocin HCl, has been reported. Rare cases of interstitial nephritis have been reported. Most of these have occurred in patients who were given aminoglycosides concomitantly or who had preexisting kidney dysfunction. When Vancocin HCl was discontinued, azotemia resolved in most patients.

Continued on next page

* **Identi-Code® symbol. This product information was prepared in June 1996. Current information on these and other products of Eli Lilly and Company may be obtained by direct inquiry to Lilly Research Laboratories, Lilly Corporate Center, Indianapolis, Indiana 46285, 800-545-5979.**

Lilly—Cont.

Gastrointestinal—Onset of pseudomembranous colitis symptoms may occur during or after antibiotic treatment (*see* Warnings).
Ototoxicity—A few dozen cases of hearing loss associated with Vancocin HCl have been reported. Most of these patients had kidney dysfunction or a preexisting hearing loss or were receiving concomitant treatment with an ototoxic drug. Vertigo, dizziness, and tinnitus have been reported rarely.
Hematopoietic—Reversible neutropenia, usually starting 1 week or more after onset of therapy with Vancocin HCl or after a total dosage of more than 25 g, has been reported for several dozen patients. Neutropenia appears to be promptly reversible when Vancocin HCl is discontinued. Thrombocytopenia has rarely been reported.
Although a causal relationship has not been established, reversible agranulocytosis (granulocytes $< 500/mm^3$) has been reported rarely.
Phlebitis—Inflammation at the injection site has been reported.
Miscellaneous—Infrequently, patients have been reported to have had anaphylaxis, drug fever, nausea, chills, eosinophilia, rashes (including exfoliative dermatitis), Stevens-Johnson syndrome, toxic epidermal necrolysis, and rare cases of vasculitis in association with administration of Vancocin HCl.
Chemical peritonitis has been reported following intraperitoneal administration of vancomycin (*see* Precautions).

OVERDOSAGE

Supportive care is advised, with maintenance of glomerular filtration. Vancomycin is poorly removed by dialysis. Hemofiltration and hemoperfusion with polysulfone resin have been reported to result in increased vancomycin clearance.
The median lethal intravenous dose is 319 mg/kg in rats and 400 mg/kg in mice.
To obtain up-to-date information about the treatment of overdose, a good resource is your certified Regional Poison Control Center. Telephone numbers of certified poison control centers are listed in the *Physicians' Desk Reference (PDR)*. In managing overdosage, consider the possibility of multiple drug overdoses, interaction among drugs, and unusual drug kinetics in your patient.

DOSAGE AND ADMINISTRATION

Infusion-related events are related to both concentration and rate of administration of vancomycin. Concentrations of no more than 5 mg/mL and rates of no more than 10 mg/min are recommended in adults (see also age-specific recommendations). In selected patients in need of fluid restriction, a concentration up to 10 mg/mL may be used; use of such higher concentrations may increase the risk of infusion-related events. Infusion-related events may occur, however, at any rate or concentration.
Patients With Normal Renal Function
Adults—The usual daily intravenous dose is 2 g divided either as 500 mg every 6 hours or 1 g every 12 hours. Each dose should be administered at no more than 10 mg/min or over a period of at least 60 minutes, whichever is longer. Other patient factors, such as age or obesity, may call for modification of the usual intravenous daily dose.
Children—The usual intravenous dosage of Vancocin HCl is 10 mg/kg per dose given every 6 hours. Each dose should be administered over a period of at least 60 minutes.
Infants and Neonates—In neonates and young infants, the total daily intravenous dosage may be lower. In both neonates and infants, an initial dose of 15 mg/kg is suggested, followed by 10 mg/kg every 12 hours for neonates in the 1st week of life and every 8 hours thereafter up to the age of 1 month. Each dose should be administered over 60 minutes. Close monitoring of serum concentrations of vancomycin may be warranted in these patients.
Patients With Impaired Renal Function and Elderly Patients
Dosage adjustment must be made in patients with impaired renal function. In premature infants and the elderly, greater dosage reductions than expected may be necessary because of decreased renal function. Measurement of vancomycin serum concentrations can be helpful in optimizing therapy, especially in seriously ill patients with changing renal function. Vancomycin serum concentrations can be determined by use of microbiologic assay, radioimmunoassay, fluorescence polarization immunoassay, fluorescence immunoassay, or high-pressure liquid chromatography.
If creatinine clearance can be measured or estimated accurately, the dosage for most patients with renal impairment can be calculated using the following table. The dosage of Vancocin HCl per day in mg is about 15 times the glomerular filtration rate in mL/min:

DOSAGE TABLE FOR VANCOMYCIN IN PATIENTS WITH IMPAIRED RENAL FUNCTION
(Adapted from Moellering et al[5])

Creatinine Clearance mL/min	Vancomycin Dose mg/24 h
100	1,545
90	1,390
80	1,235
70	1,080
60	925
50	770
40	620
30	465
20	310
10	155

The initial dose should be no less than 15 mg/kg, even in patients with mild to moderate renal insufficiency.

The table is not valid for functionally anephric patients. For such patients, an initial dose of 15 mg/kg of body weight should be given to achieve prompt therapeutic serum concentrations. The dose required to maintain stable concentrations is 1.9 mg/kg/24 h. In patients with marked renal impairment, it may be more convenient to give maintenance doses of 250 to 1,000 mg once every several days rather than administering the drug on a daily basis. In anuria, a dose of 1,000 mg every 7 to 10 days has been recommended.
When only the serum creatinine concentration is known, the following formula (based on sex, weight, and age of the patient) may be used to calculate creatinine clearance. Calculated creatinine clearances (mL/min) are only estimates. The creatinine clearance should be measured promptly.

Men: $\dfrac{\text{Weight (kg)} \times (140 - \text{age in years})}{72 \times \text{serum creatinine concentration (mg/dL)}}$

Women: $0.85 \times$ above value

The serum creatinine must represent a steady state of renal function. Otherwise, the estimated value for creatinine clearance is not valid. Such a calculated clearance is an overestimate of actual clearance in patients with conditions: (1) characterized by decreasing renal function, such as shock, severe heart failure, or oliguria; (2) in which a normal relationship between muscle mass and total body weight is not present, such as obese patients or those with liver disease, edema, or ascites; and (3) accompanied by debilitation, malnutrition, or inactivity.
The safety and efficacy of vancomycin administration by the intrathecal (intralumbar or intraventricular) routes have not been assessed.
Intermittent infusion is the recommended method of administration.

PREPARATION AND STABILITY

At the time of use, reconstitute by adding either 10 mL of Sterile Water for Injection to the 500-mg vial or 20 mL of Sterile Water for Injection to the 1-g vial of dry, sterile vancomycin powder. Vials reconstituted in this manner will give a solution of 50 mg/mL. FURTHER DILUTION IS REQUIRED.
After reconstitution, the vials may be stored in a refrigerator for 14 days without significant loss of potency. Reconstituted solutions containing 500 mg of vancomycin must be diluted with at least 100 mL of diluent. Reconstituted solutions containing 1 g of vancomycin must be diluted with at least 200 mL of diluent. The desired dose, diluted in this manner, should be administered by intermittent intravenous infusion over a period of at least 60 minutes.
Compatibility With Intravenous Fluids—Solutions that are diluted with 5% Dextrose Injection or 0.9% Sodium Chloride Injection may be stored in a refrigerator for 14 days without significant loss of potency. Solutions that are diluted with the following infusion fluids may be stored in a refrigerator for 96 hours:

- 5% Dextrose Injection and 0.9% Sodium Chloride Injection, USP
- Lactated Ringer's Injection, USP
- Lactated Ringer's and 5% Dextrose Injection
- Normosol®-M and 5% Dextrose
- Isolyte® E
- Acetated Ringer's Injection

Vancomycin solution has a low pH and may cause chemical or physical instability when it is mixed with other compounds.
Prior to administration, parenteral drug products should be inspected visually for particulate matter and discoloration whenever solution or container permits.
For Oral Administration—Oral Vancocin HCl is used in treating antibiotic-associated pseudomembranous colitis caused by *C. difficile* and for staphylococcal enterocolitis. Vancocin HCl is not effective by the oral route for other types of infections. The usual adult total daily dosage is 500 mg to 2 g given in 3 or 4 divided doses for 7 to 10 days. The total daily dosage in children is 40 mg/kg of body weight in 3 or 4 divided doses for 7 to 10 days. The total daily dosage should not exceed 2 g. The appropriate dose may be diluted in 1 oz of water and given to the patient to drink. Common flavoring syrups may be added to the solution to improve the taste for oral administration. The diluted solution may be administered via a nasogastric tube.

HOW SUPPLIED

Vancocin HCl Vials are available in:
500 mg,* 10-mL size
NDC 0002-1444-01 (No. 657)—1s
NDC 0002-1444-10 (No. 657)—Traypak† of 10
NDC 0002-1444-25 (No. 657)—Traypack of 25
1 g,* 20-mL size
NDC 0002-7321-10 (No. 7321)—Traypak of 10
NDC 0002-7321-25 (No. 7321)—Traypak of 25
Also available:
Vancocin HCl ADD-Vantage‡ Vials are available in:
500 mg,* 15-mL size
NDC 0002-7297-10 (No. 7297)—Traypak of 10
1 g,* 15-mL size
NDC 0002-7298-10 (No. 7298)—Traypak of 10
Vancocin HCl Pharmacy Bulk Package is available in:
10 g,* 100-mL size
NDC 0002-7355-01 (No. 7355)—1s
Prior to reconstitution, the vials may be stored at room temperature, 59° to 86°F (15° to 30°C).

*Equivalent to vancomycin.
†Traypak™ (multivial carton, Lilly).
‡ADD-Vantage® (vials and diluent containers, Abbott).

ANIMAL PHARMACOLOGY

In animal studies, hypotension and bradycardia occurred in dogs receiving an intravenous infusion of vancomycin hydrochloride, 25 mg/kg, at a concentration of 25 mg/mL and an infusion rate of 13.3 mL/min.

REFERENCES

1. National Committee for Clinical Laboratory Standards, 1984. Performance standards for antimicrobial disk susceptibility tests, MZ-A3, NCCLS, Villanova, PA 19805.
2. National Committee for Clinical Laboratory Standards, 1983. Methods for dilution antimicrobial susceptibility tests for bacteria that grow aerobically, M7-T, NCCLS, Villanova, PA 19805.
3. National Committee for Clinical Laboratory Standards, 1984. Reference agar dilution procedure for antimicrobial susceptibility testing of anaerobic bacteria, M11-A, NCCLS, Villanova, PA 19805.
4. Shulman ST, Amren DP, Bisno AL, et al: Prevention of bacterial endocarditis. *Circulation* 1984, 70:1123A.
5. Moellering RC, Krogstad DJ, Greenblatt DJ: Vancomycin therapy in patients with impaired renal function: A nomogram for dosage. *Ann Intern Med* 1981; 94:343.

[103195]

VANCOCIN® HCl ℞

[*văn´kō-sĭn ăch´sē-ĕl*]
(vancomycin hydrochloride)
For Oral Solution, USP

Pulvules®
Capsules, USP

This preparation for the treatment of colitis is for oral use only and is not systemically absorbed. Vancocin HCl must be given orally for treatment of staphylococcal enterocolitis and antibiotic-associated pseudomembranous colitis caused by *Clostridium difficile*. Orally administered Vancocin HCl is *not* effective for other types of infection.
Parenteral administration of Vancocin HCl is not effective for treatment of staphylococcal enterocolitis and antibiotic-associated pseudomembranous colitis caused by *C. difficile*. If parenteral vancomycin therapy is desired, use Vancocin® HCl (Sterile Vancomycin Hydrochloride, USP), IntraVenous, and consult package insert accompanying that preparation.

DESCRIPTION

Vancocin® HCl for Oral Solution (Vancomycin Hydrochloride for Oral Solution, USP), contain chromatographically purified vancomycin hydrochloride, a tricyclic glycopeptide antibiotic derived from *Amycolatopsis orientalis* (formerly *Nocardia orientalis*), which has the chemical formula $C_{66}H_{75}Cl_2N_9O_{24} \cdot HCl$. The molecular weight of vancomycin hydrochloride is 1,486; 500 mg of the base is equivalent to 0.34 mmol.
Vancocin HCl for Oral Solution contains vancomycin hydrochloride equivalent to 10 g (6.7 mmol) or 1 g (0.67 mmol) vancomycin. Calcium disodium edetate, equivalent to 0.2 mg edetate per gram of vancomycin, is added at the time of manufacture. The 10-g bottle may contain up to 40 mg of ethanol per gram of vancomycin.
Vancomycin hydrochloride has the following structure:
[See chemical structure at top of next column.]

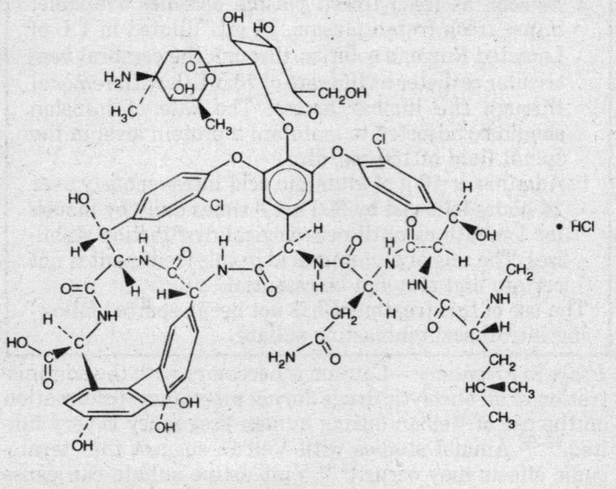

CLINICAL PHARMACOLOGY

Vancomycin is poorly absorbed after oral administration. During multiple dosing of 250 mg every 8 hours for 7 doses, fecal concentrations of vancomycin in volunteers exceeded 100 mg/kg in the majority of samples. No blood concentrations were detected and urinary recovery did not exceed 0.76%. In anephric patients with no inflammatory bowel disease, blood concentrations of vancomycin were barely measurable (0.66 μg/mL) in 2 of 5 subjects who received 2 g of Vancocin HCl for Oral Solution daily for 16 days. No measurable blood concentrations were attained in the other 3 patients. With doses of 2 g daily, very high concentrations of drug can be found in the feces (> 3,100 mg/kg) and very low concentrations (< 1 μg/mL) can be found in the serum of patients with normal renal function who have pseudomembranous colitis. Orally administered vancomycin does not usually enter the systemic circulation even when inflammatory lesions are present. After multiple-dose oral administration of vancomycin, measurable serum concentrations may infrequently occur in patients with active *C. difficile*-induced pseudomembranous colitis, and, in the presence of renal impairment, the possibility of accumulation exists.

Microbiology—The bactericidal action of vancomycin results primarily from inhibition of cell-wall biosynthesis. In addition, vancomycin alters bacterial-cell-membrane permeability and RNA synthesis. There is no cross-resistance between vancomycin and other antibiotics. Vancomycin is active against *C. difficile* (eg, toxigenic strains implicated in pseudomembranous enterocolitis). It is also active against staphylococci, including *Staphylococcus aureus*.

For further information, see prescribing information for Vancocin HCl, IntraVenous.

Vancomycin is not active in vitro against gram-negative bacilli, mycobacteria, or fungi.

Disk Susceptibility Tests—The standardized disk and/or dilution methods described by the National Committee for Clinical Laboratory Standards have been recommended to test susceptibility to vancomycin.

INDICATIONS AND USAGE

Vancocin HCl for Oral Solution is administered orally for treatment of staphylococcal enterocolitis and antiobiotic-associated pseudomembranous colitis caused by *C. difficile*. Parenteral administration of Vancocin HCl is not effective for the above indications; therefore, Vancocin HCl must be given orally for these indications. **Orally administered Vancocin HCl is not effective for other types of infection.**

CONTRAINDICATION

Vancocin HCl is contraindicated in patients with known hypersensitivity to this antibiotic.

PRECAUTIONS

Clinically significant serum concentrations have been reported in some patients who have taken multiple oral doses of vancomycin for active *C. difficile*-induced pseudomembranous colitis; therefore, monitoring of serum concentrations may be appropriate.

Some patients with inflammatory disorders of the intestinal mucosa may have significant systemic absorption of vancomycin and, therefore, may be at risk for the development of adverse reactions associated with the parenteral administration of vancomycin (See package insert accompanying the intravenous preparation.) The risk is greater if renal impairment is present. It should be noted that the total systemic and renal clearances of vancomycin are reduced in the elderly.

Ototoxicity has occurred in patients receiving Vancocin HCl. It may be transient or permanent. It has been reported mostly in patients who have been given excessive intravenous doses, who have an underlying hearing loss, or who are receiving concomitant therapy with another ototoxic agent, such as an aminoglycoside. Serial tests of auditory function may be helpful in order to minimize the risk of ototoxicity.

When patients with underlying renal dysfunction or those receiving concomitant therapy with an aminoglycoside are being treated, serial monitoring of renal function should be performed.

Usage in Pregnancy—Pregnancy Category C—Animal reproduction studies have not been conducted with Vancocin HCl. It is not known whether Vancocin HCl can affect reproduction capacity. In a controlled clinical study, the potential ototoxic and nephrotoxic effects of Vancocin HCl on infants were evaluated when the drug was administered to pregnant women for serious staphylococcal infections complicating intravenous drug abuse. Vancocin HCl was found in cord blood. No sensorineural hearing loss or nephrotoxicity attributable to Vancocin HCl was noted. One infant whose mother received Vancocin HCl in the third trimester experienced conductive hearing loss that was not attributed to the administration of Vancocin HCl. Because the number of patients treated in this study was limited and Vancocin HCl was administered only in the second and third trimesters, it is not known whether Vancocin HCl causes fetal harm. Vancocin HCl should be given to a pregnant woman only if clearly needed.

Nursing Mothers—Vancocin HCl is excreted in human milk based on information obtained with the intravenous administration of Vancocin HCl. Blood concentrations achieved with oral administration are very low (*see* Clinical Pharmacology). Caution should be exercised when Vancocin HCl is administered to a nursing woman. Because of the potential for adverse events, a decision should be made whether to discontinue nursing or discontinue the drug, taking into account the importance of the drug to the mother.

ADVERSE REACTIONS

Nephrotoxicity—Rarely, renal failure, principally manifested by increased serum creatinine or BUN concentrations, especially in patients given large doses of intravenously administered Vancocin HCl has been reported. Rare cases of interstitial nephritis have been reported. Most of these have occurred in patients who were given aminoglycosides concomitantly or who had preexisting kidney dysfunction. When Vancocin HCl was discontinued, azotemia resolved in most patients.

Ototoxicity—A few dozen cases of hearing loss associated with intravenously administered Vancocin HCl have been reported. Most of these patients had kidney dysfunction or a preexisting hearing loss or were receiving concomitant treatment with an ototoxic drug. Vertigo, dizziness, and tinnitus have been reported rarely.

Hematopoietic—Reversible neutropenia, usually starting 1 week or more after onset of intravenous therapy with Vancocin HCl or after a total dosage of more than 25 g, has been reported for several dozen patients. Neutropenia appears to be promptly reversible when Vancocin HCl is discontinued. Thrombocytopenia has rarely been reported.

Miscellaneous—Infrequently, patients have been reported to have had anaphylaxis, drug fever, chills, nausea, eosinophilia, and rashes (including exfoliative dermatitis), Stevens-Johnson syndrome, toxic epidermal necrolysis, and rare cases of vasculitis in association with the administration of Vancocin HCl.

A condition has been reported that is similar to the IV-induced syndrome with symptoms consistent with anaphylactoid reactions, including hypotension, wheezing, dyspnea, urticaria, pruritus, flushing of the upper body ("Red Man Syndrome"), pain and muscle spasm of the chest and back. These reactions usually resolve within 20 minutes but may persist for several hours.

OVERDOSAGE

Supportive care is advised, with maintenance of glomerular filtration. Vancomycin is poorly removed by dialysis. Hemofiltration and hemoperfusion with polysulfone resin have been reported to result in increased vancomycin clearance.

Treatment—To obtain up-to-date information about the treatment of overdose, a good resource is your certified Regional Poison Control Center. Telephone numbers of certified poison control centers are listed in the *Physicians' Desk Reference (PDR)*. In managing overdosage, consider the possibility of multiple drug overdoses, interaction among drugs, and unusual drug kinetics in your patient.

DOSAGE AND ADMINISTRATION

Adults—Oral Vancocin HCl is used in treating antibiotic-associated pseudomembranous colitis caused by *C. difficile* and staphylococcal enterocolitis. Vancocin HCl is not effective by the oral route for other types of infections. The usual adult total daily dosage is 500 mg to 2 g administered orally in 3 or 4 divided doses for 7 to 10 days.

Children—The usual daily dosage is 40 mg/kg in 3 or 4 divided doses for 7 to 10 days. The total daily dosage should not exceed 2 g.

PREPARATION AND STABILITY

The contents of the 10-g bottle may be mixed with distilled or deionized water (115 mL) for oral administration. When mixed with 115 mL of water, each 6 mL provides approximately 500 mg of vancomycin. The contents of the 1-g bottle may be mixed with distilled or deionized water (20 mL). When reconstituted with 20 mL, each 5 mL contains approximately 250 mg of vancomycin. Mix thoroughly to dissolve. These mixtures may be kept for 2 weeks in a refrigerator without significant loss of potency.

The appropriate oral solution dose may be diluted in 1 oz of water and given to the patient to drink. Common flavoring syrups may be added to the solution to improve the taste for oral administration. The diluted material may be administered via nasogastric tube.

HOW SUPPLIED

Vancocin HCl For Oral Solution is available in:

10 g* (in a screw-cap bottle) (No. M-206)—(1s) NDC 0002-2372-37

1 g* (in a screw-cap bottle) (No. M-5105)—(Traypak† of 6) NDC 0002-5105-16

Prior to reconstitution, store at controlled room temperature, 59° to 86°F (15° to 30°C).

Also available:

Vancocin HCl Pulvules®:

Vancocin HCl, 125 mg,* are opaque blue and opaque brown with "Lilly 3125" imprinted on the cap and "Vancocin HCl 125 mg" on the body. They are available in:

NDC 0002-3125-42 (No. 3125)—ID‡20

Vancocin HCl, 250 mg,* are opaque blue and opaque lavender with "Lilly 3126" imprinted on the cap and "Vancocin HCl 250 mg" on the body. They are available in:

NDC 0002-3126-42 (No. 3126)—ID20

*Equivalent to vancomycin.
†Traypak™ (multivial carton, Lilly).
‡Identi-Dose® (unit dose medication, Lilly).

[030596]

VANCOMYCIN HYDROCHLORIDE ℞

See Vancocin® HCl (Vancomycin Hydrochloride, USP).

VELBAN® ℞

[*vĕl' băn*]
(vinblastine sulfate)
Sterile, USP

WARNINGS

Caution—This preparation should be administered by individuals experienced in the administration of Velban. It is extremely important that the needle be properly positioned in the vein before this product is injected. If leakage into surrounding tissue should occur during intravenous administration of Velban, it may cause considerable irritation. The injection should be discontinued immediately, and any remaining portion of the dose should then be introduced into another vein. Local injection of hyaluronidase and the application of moderate heat to the area of leakage help disperse the drug and are thought to minimize discomfort and the possibility of cellulitis.

FATAL IF GIVEN INTRATHECALLY. FOR INTRAVENOUS USE ONLY. *See Warnings section for the treatment of patients given intrathecal Velban.*

DESCRIPTION

Velban® (Sterile Vinblastine Sulfate, USP) is vincaleukoblastine sulfate (1:1) (salt). It is the salt of an alkaloid extracted from *Vinca rosea* Linn,[1–3] a common flowering herb known as the periwinkle (more properly known as *Catharanthus roseus* G. Don). Previously, the generic name was vincaleukoblastine, abbreviated VLB. It is a stathmokinetic oncolytic agent. When treated in vitro with this preparation, growing cells are arrested in metaphase.

Chemical and physical evidence[4,5] indicate that Velban has the empirical formula $C_{46}H_{58}N_4O_9 \cdot H_2SO_4$ and that it is a dimeric alkaloid containing both indole and dihydroindole moieties. It has a molecular weight of 909.06. The structural formula is as follows:

[See chemical structure at top of next column.]

Vinblastine sulfate is a white to off-white powder. It is freely soluble in water, soluble in methanol, and slightly soluble in ethanol. It is insoluble in benzene, ether, and naphtha.

The clinical formulation is supplied in a sterile form for intravenous use only. Vials of Velban contain 10 mg (0.011 mmol) of vinblastine sulfate, in the form of a white, amorphous, solid lyophilized plug, without excipients. After

Continued on next page

* **Identi-Code® symbol. This product information was prepared in June 1996. Current information on these and other products of Eli Lilly and Company may be obtained by direct inquiry to Lilly Research Laboratories, Lilly Corporate Center, Indianapolis, Indiana 46285, 800-545-5979.**

Lilly—Cont.

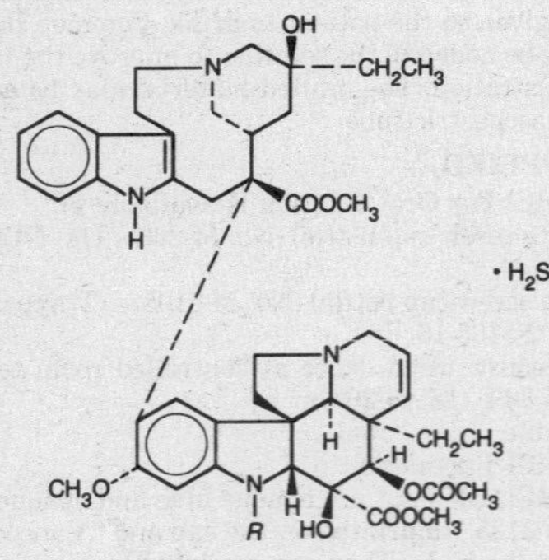

(R is CH_3)

reconstitution with sodium chloride solution, the pH of the resulting solution lies in the range of 3.5 to 5.

CLINICAL PHARMACOLOGY

Experimental data indicate that the action of Velban is different from that of other recognized antineoplastic agents.[8–13] Tissue-culture studies suggest an interference with metabolic pathways of amino acids leading from glutamic acid to the citric acid cycle and to urea.[8–14] In vivo experiments tend to confirm the in vitro results.[13–16] A number of studies in vitro and in vivo have demonstrated that Velban produces a stathmokinetic effect and various atypical mitotic figures.[9,15,17–25] The therapeutic responses, however, are not fully explained by the cytologic changes, since these changes are sometimes observed clinically and experimentally in the absence of any oncolytic effects.

Reversal of the antitumor effect of Velban by glutamic acid or tryptophan has been observed. In addition, glutamic acid and aspartic acid have protected mice from lethal doses of Velban.[13] Aspartic acid was relatively ineffective in reversing the antitumor effect.

Other studies indicate that Velban has an effect on cell-energy production required for mitosis[25] and interferes with nucleic acid synthesis.[26–29] The mechanism of action of Velban has been related to the inhibition of microtubule formation in the mitotic spindle, resulting in an arrest of dividing cells at the metaphase stage.

Pharmacokinetic studies in patients with cancer have shown a triphasic serum decay pattern following rapid intravenous injection. The initial, middle, and terminal half-lives are 3.7 minutes, 1.6 hours, and 24.8 hours respectively. The volume of the central compartment is 70% of body weight, probably reflecting very rapid tissue binding to formed elements of the blood. Extensive reversible tissue binding occurs. Low body stores are present at 48 and 72 hours after injection.[30] Since the major route of excretion may be through the biliary system, toxicity from this drug may be increased when there is hepatic excretory insufficiency. The metabolism of vinca alkaloids has been shown to be mediated by hepatic cytochrome P450 isoenzymes in the CYP 3A subfamily. This metabolic pathway may be impaired in patients with hepatic dysfunction or who are taking concomitant potent inhibitors of these isoenzymes. (*See* Precautions).[31–32] Following injection of titrated vinblastine in the human cancer patient, 10% of the radioactivity was found in the feces and 14% in the urine; the remaining activity was not accounted for.[33] Similar studies in dogs demonstrated that, over 9 days, 30% to 36% of radioactivity was found in the bile and 12% to 17% in the urine. A similar study in the rat demonstrated that the highest concentrations of radioactivity were found in the lung, liver, spleen, and kidney 2 hours after injection.[35,36]

Hematologic Effects—Clinically, leukopenia is an expected effect of Velban, and the level of the leukocyte count is an important guide to therapy with this drug. In general, the larger the dose employed, the more profound and longer lasting the leukopenia will be. The fact that the white-blood-cell count returns to normal levels after drug-induced leukopenia is an indication that the white-cell-producing mechanism is not permanently depressed. Usually, the white count has completely returned to normal after the virtual disappearance of white cells from the peripheral blood.

Following therapy with Velban, the nadir in white-blood-cell count may be expected to occur 5 to 10 days after the last day of drug administration. Recovery of the white blood count is fairly rapid thereafter and is usually complete within another 7 to 14 days. With the smaller doses employed for maintenance therapy, leukopenia may not be a problem.

Although the thrombocyte count ordinarily is not significantly lowered by therapy with Velban, patients whose bone marrow has been recently impaired by prior therapy with radiation or with other oncolytic drugs may show thrombocytopenia (less than 200,000 platelets/mm^3). When other chemotherapy or radiation has not been employed previously, thrombocyte reduction below the level of 200,000/mm^3 is rarely encountered, even when Velban may be causing significant leukopenia. Rapid recovery from thrombocytopenia within a few days is the rule.

The effect of Velban upon the red-cell count and hemoglobin is usually insignificant when other therapy does not complicate the picture. It should be remembered, however, that patients with malignant disease may exhibit anemia even in the absence of any therapy.

INDICATIONS AND USAGE

Vinblastine sulfate is indicated in the palliative treatment of the following:

I. Frequently Responsive Malignancies—
- Generalized Hodgkin's disease (Stages III and IV, Ann Arbor modification of Rye staging system)[37–41]
- Lymphocytic lymphoma (nodular and diffuse, poorly and well differentiated)[42,43]
- Histiocytic lymphoma[42,43]
- Mycosis fungoides (advanced stages)[44]
- Advanced carcinoma of the testis
- Kaposi's sarcoma[45,46]
- Letterer-Siwe disease (histiocytosis X)[47]

II. Less Frequently Responsive Malignancies—
- Choriocarcinoma resistant to other chemotherapeutic agents[48,49]
- Carcinoma of the breast, unresponsive to appropriate endocrine surgery and hormonal therapy[50,53]

Current principles of chemotherapy for many types of cancer include the concurrent administration of several antineoplastic agents. For enhanced therapeutic effect without additive toxicity, agents with different dose-limiting clinical toxicities and different mechanisms of action are generally selected. Therefore, although Velban is effective as a single agent in the aforementioned indications, it is usually administered in combination with other antineoplastic drugs.[53–56] Such combination therapy produces a greater percentage of response than does a single-agent regimen. These principles have been applied, for example, in the chemotherapy of Hodgkin's disease.[50,54–58]

Hodgkin's Disease—Velban has been shown to be one of the most effective single agents for the treatment of Hodgkin's disease.[50,57–59] Advanced Hodgkin's disease has also been successfully treated with several multiple-drug regimens that included Velban.[60–66] Patients who had relapses after treatment with the MOPP program—mechlorethamine hydrochloride (nitrogen mustard), vincristine sulfate (Oncovin [Vincristine Sulfate Injection]), prednisone, and procarbazine—have likewise responded to combination-drug therapy that included Velban.[54,55,67–69] A protocol using cyclophosphamide in place of nitrogen mustard and Velban instead of Oncovin is an alternative therapy for previously untreated patients with advanced Hodgkin's disease.[50,57,58,70]

Advanced testicular germinal-cell cancers (embryonal carcinoma, teratocarcinoma, and choriocarcinoma) are sensitive to Velban alone,[71] but better clinical results are achieved when Velban is administered concomitantly with other antineoplastic agents.[72–77] The effect of bleomycin is significantly enhanced if Velban is administered 6 to 8 hours prior to the administration of bleomycin; this schedule permits more cells to be arrested during metaphase, the stage of the cell cycle in which bleomycin is active.[76,77]

CONTRAINDICATIONS

Velban is contraindicated in patients who have significant granulocytopenia unless this is a result of the disease being treated. It should not be used in the presence of bacterial infections. Such infections must be brought under control prior to the initiation of therapy with Velban.

WARNINGS

This product is for intravenous use only. It should be administered by individuals experienced in the administration of Velban. The intrathecal administration of Velban has resulted in death. Syringes containing this product should be labeled "WARNING—FOR IV USE ONLY."

Extemporaneously prepared syringes containing this product must be packaged in an overwrap that is labeled "DO NOT REMOVE COVERING UNTIL MOMENT OF INJECTION. FATAL IF GIVEN INTRATHECALLY. FOR INTRAVENOUS USE ONLY."

The following treatment successfully arrested progressive paralysis in a single patient mistakenly given the related vinca alkaloid, vincristine sulfate, intrathecally. If Velban is mistakenly administered intrathecally, this treatment is recommended and should be initiated immediately after the intrathecal injection.

1. Remove as much spinal fluid as can be safely done through the lumbar access.
2. Insert a catheter in a lateral cerebral ventricle for the purpose of flushing the subarachnoid space from above with removal through a lumbar access.
3. Initiate flushing through the cerebral catheter with lactated Ringer's solution infused at the rate of 150 mL/h.
4. As soon as fresh frozen plasma becomes available, infuse fresh frozen plasma, 25 mL, diluted in 1 L of Lactated Ringer's solution through the cerebral ventricular catheter at the rate of 75 mL/h with removal through the lumbar access. The rate of infusion should be adjusted to maintain a protein level in the spinal fluid of 150 mg/dL.
5. Administer 10 g of glutamic acid intravenously over 24 hours followed by 500 mg 3 times daily by mouth for 1 month or until neurological dysfunction stabilizes. The role of glutamic acid in this treatment is not certain and may not be essential.

The use of this treatment has not been reported following intrathecal vinblastine sulfate.

Usage in Pregnancy—Caution is necessary with the administration of all oncolytic drugs during pregnancy. Information on the use of Velban during human pregnancy is very limited.[78–82] Animal studies with Velban suggest that teratogenic effects may occur.[83,84] Vinblastine sulfate can cause fetal harm when administered to a pregnant woman. Laboratory animals given this drug early in pregnancy suffer resorption of the conceptus: surviving fetuses demonstrate gross deformities.[85] There are no adequate and well-controlled studies in pregnant women. If this drug is used during pregnancy, or if the patient becomes pregnant while receiving this drug, she should be apprised of the potential hazard to the fetus. Women of childbearing potential should be advised to avoid becoming pregnant.

Aspermia has been reported in man. Animal studies show metaphase arrest and degenerative changes in germ cells.[22,86]

Leukopenia (granulocytopenia) may reach dangerously low levels following administration of the higher recommended doses. It is therefore important to follow the dosage technique recommended under the Dosage and Administration section. Stomatitis and neurologic toxicity, although not common or permanent, can be disabling.

PRECAUTIONS

General—Toxicity may be enhanced in the presence of hepatic insufficiency.

If leukopenia with less than 2,000 white blood cells/mm^3 occurs following a dose of Velban, the patient should be watched carefully for evidence of infection until the white-blood-cell count has returned to a safe level.

When cachexia or ulcerated areas of the skin surface are present, there may be a more profound leukopenic response to the drug; therefore, its use should be avoided in older persons suffering from either of these conditions.

In patients with malignant-cell infiltration of the bone marrow, the leukocyte and platelet counts have sometimes fallen precipitously after moderate doses of Velban. Further use of the drug in such patients is inadvisable.

Acute shortness of breath and severe bronchospasm have been reported following the administration of vinca alkaloids. These reactions have been encountered most frequently when the vinca alkaloid was used in combination with mitomycin-C and may require aggressive treatment, particularly when there is pre-existing pulmonary dysfunction. The onset may be within minutes or several hours after the vinca is injected and may occur up to 2 weeks following a dose of mitomycin. Progressive dyspnea requiring chronic therapy may occur. Velban should not be readministered.

The use of small amounts of Velban daily for long periods is not advised, even though the resulting total weekly dosage may be similar to that recommended. Little or no added therapeutic effect has been demonstrated when such regimens have been used.[87] *Strict adherence to the recommended dosage schedule is very important.* When amounts equal to several times the recommended weekly dosage were given in 7 daily installments for long periods, convulsions, severe and permanent central-nervous-system damage, and even death occurred.[87]

Care must be taken to avoid contamination of the eye with concentrations of Velban used clinically. If accidental contamination occurs, severe irritation (or, if the drug was delivered under pressure, even corneal ulceration) may result. The eye should be washed with water immediately and thoroughly.

It is not necessary to use preservative-containing solvents if unused portions of the remaining solutions are discarded immediately. Unused preservative-containing solutions should be refrigerated for future use.

Information for Patients—The patient should be warned to report immediately the appearance of sore throat, fever, chills, or sore mouth. Advice should be given to avoid constipation, and the patient should be made aware that alopecia may occur and that jaw pain and pain in the organs containing tumor tissue may occur. The latter is thought possibly to result from swelling of tumor tissue during its response to treatment. Scalp hair will regrow to its pretreatment extent even with continued treatment with Velban. Nausea and vomiting, although not common, may occur. Any other serious medical event should be reported to the physician.

Laboratory Tests—Since dose-limiting clinical toxicity is the result of depression of the white-blood-cell count, it is imper-

ative that this count be obtained just before the planned dose of Velban. Following administration of Velban, a fall in the white-blood-cell count may occur. The nadir of this fall is observed from 5 to 10 days following a dose. Recovery to pretreatment levels is usually observed from 7 to 14 days after treatment. These effects will be exaggerated when preexisting bone marrow damage is present and also with the higher recommended doses (*see* Dosage and Administration). The presence of this drug or its metabolites in blood or body tissues is not known to interfere with clinical laboratory tests.

Drug Interactions—Solutions should be made with normal saline (with or without preservative) and should not be combined in the same container with any other chemical. Unused portions of the remaining solutions that do not contain preservatives should be discarded immediately.

The simultaneous oral or intravenous administration of phenytoin and antineoplastic chemotherapy combinations that included vinblastine sulfate has been reported to have reduced blood levels of the anticonvulsant and to have increased seizure activity.[88] Dosage adjustment should be based on serial blood level monitoring. The contribution of vinblastine sulfate to this interaction is not certain. The interaction may result from either reduced absorption of phenytoin or an increase in the rate of its metabolism and elimination.

Caution should be exercised in patients concurrently taking drugs known to inhibit drug metabolism by hepatic cytochrome P450 isoenzymes in the CYP 3A subfamily, or in patients with hepatic dysfunction. Concurrent administration of vinblastine sulfate with an inhibitor of this metabolic pathway may cause an earlier onset and/or an increased severity of side effects (*see* Adverse Reactions).

Carcinogenesis, Mutagenesis, Impairment of Fertility—Aspermia has been reported in man. Animal studies suggest that teratogenic effects may occur. *See* Warnings regarding impaired fertility. Animal studies have shown metaphase arrest and degenerative changes in germ cells.[22] Amenorrhea has occurred in some patients treated with the combination consisting of an alkylating agent, procarbazine, prednisone, and Velban. Its occurrence was related to the total dose of these 4 agents used. Recovery of menses was frequent.[89–92] The same combination of drugs given to male patients produced azoospermia; if spermatogenesis did return, it was not likely to do so with less than 2 years of unmaintained remission.[93–95]

Mutagenicity—Tests in *Salmonella typhimurium* and with the dominant lethal assay in mice failed to demonstrate mutagenicity. Sperm abnormalities have been noted in mice. Velban has produced an increase in micronuclei formation in bone marrow cells of mice; however, since Velban inhibits mitotic spindle formation, it cannot be concluded that this is evidence of mutagenicity.[96] Additional studies in mice demonstrated no reduction in fertility of males. Chromosomal translocations did occur in male mice. First-generation male offspring of these mice were not heterozygous translocation carriers.[96,97]

In vitro tests using hamster lung cells in culture have produced chromosomal changes, including chromatid breaks and exchanges, whereas tests using another type of hamster cell failed to demonstrate mutation.[96] Breaks and aberrations were not observed on chromosome analysis of marrow cells from patients being treated with this drug.[98]

It is not clear from the literature how this drug affects synthesis of DNA and RNA. Some believe that there is no interference.[99] Others believe that vinblastine interferes with nucleic acid metabolism but may not do so by direct effect but possibly as the result of biochemical disturbance in some other part of the molecular organization of the cell.[100] No inhibition of RNA synthesis occurred in rat hepatoma cells exposed in culture to noncytotoxic levels of vinblastine.[101] Conflicting results have been noted by others[102–110] regarding interference with DNA synthesis.

Carcinogenesis—There is no currently available evidence to indicate that Velban itself has been carcinogenic in humans[96] since the inception of its clinical use in the late 1950s. Patients treated for Hodgkin's disease have developed leukemia following radiation therapy and administration of Velban in combination with other chemotherapy including agents known to intercalate with DNA. It is not known to what extent Velban may have contributed to the appearance of leukemia. Available data in rats and mice have failed to demonstrate clearly evidence of carcinogenesis when the animals were treated with the maximum tolerated dose and with one half that dose for 6 months. This testing system demonstrated that other agents were clearly carcinogenic, whereas Velban was in the group of drugs causing slightly increased or the same tumor incidence as controls in one study and 1.5 to twofold increase in tumor incidence over controls in another study.[96,111]

Usage in Pregnancy—*Pregnancy Category D* (*see* Warnings). Velban should be given to a pregnant woman only if clearly needed. Animal studies suggest that teratogenic effects may occur.[83,84]

Pediatric Usage[112,113]—The dosage schedule for children is indicated under Dosage and Administration.

Nursing Mothers—It is not known whether this drug is excreted in human milk. Because many drugs are excreted in human milk and because of the potential for serious adverse reactions from Velban in nursing infants, a decision should be made whether to discontinue nursing or the drug, taking into account the importance of the drug to the mother.

ADVERSE REACTIONS

Prior to the use of the drug, patients should be advised of the possibility of untoward symptoms.

In general, the incidence of adverse reactions attending the use of Velban appears to be related to the size of the dose employed. With the exception of epilation, leukopenia, and neurologic side effects, adverse reactions generally have not persisted for longer than 24 hours. Neurologic side effects are not common; but when they do occur, they often last for more than 24 hours. Leukopenia, the most common adverse reaction, is usually the dose-limiting factor.

The following are manifestations that have been reported as adverse reactions, in decreasing order of frequency. The most common adverse reactions are underlined:

Hematologic—Leukopenia (granulocytopenia), anemia, thrombocytopenia (myelosuppression).

Dermatologic—Alopecia is common. A single case of light sensitivity associated with this product has been reported.

Gastrointestinal—Constipation, anorexia, nausea, vomiting, abdominal pain, ileus, vesiculation of the mouth, pharyngitis, diarrhea, hemorrhagic enterocolitis, bleeding from an old peptic ulcer, rectal bleeding.

Neurologic—Numbness of digits (paresthesias), loss of deep tendon reflexes, peripheral neuritis, mental depression, headache, convulsions.

Treatment with vinca alkaloids has resulted rarely in both vestibular and auditory damage to the eighth cranial nerve. Manifestations include partial or total deafness which may be temporary or permanent, and difficulties with balance including dizziness, nystagmus, and vertigo. Particular caution is warranted when vinblastine sulfate is used in combination with other agents known to be ototoxic such as the platinum-containing oncolytics.

Cardiovascular—Hypertension. Cases of unexpected myocardial infarction and cerebrovascular accidents have occurred in patients undergoing combination chemotherapy with vinblastine, bleomycin, and cisplatin. Raynaud's phenomenon has also been reported with this combination.

Pulmonary—*See* Precautions.

Miscellaneous—Malaise, bone pain, weakness, pain in tumor-containing tissue, dizziness, jaw pain, skin vesiculation, hypertension, Raynaud's phenomenon when patients are being treated with Velban in combination with bleomycin and cis-platinum for testicular cancer. The syndrome of inappropriate secretion of antidiuretic hormone has occurred with higher than recommended doses.

Nausea and vomiting usually may be controlled with ease by antiemetic agents. When epilation develops, it frequently is not total; and, in some cases, hair regrows while maintenance therapy continues.

Extravasation during intravenous injection may lead to cellulitis and phlebitis. If the amount of extravasation is great, sloughing may occur.

OVERDOSAGE

Signs and Symptoms—Side effects following the use of Velban are dose related. Therefore, following administration of more than the recommended dose, patients can be expected to experience these effects in an exaggerated fashion. (*See* Clinical Pharmacology, Contraindications, Warnings, Precautions, and Adverse Reactions.) There is no specific antidote. In addition, neurotoxicity similar to that with Oncovin may be observed. Since the major route of excretion may be through the biliary system, toxicity from this drug may be increased when there is hepatic insufficiency.

Treatment—To obtain up-to-date information about the treatment of overdose, a good resource is your certified Regional Poison Control Center. Telephone numbers of certified poison control centers are listed in the *Physicians' Desk Reference (PDR).* In managing overdosage, consider the possibility of multiple drug overdoses, interaction among drugs, and unusual drug kinetics in your patient. Overdoses of Velban have been reported rarely. The following is provided to serve as a guide should such an overdose be encountered.

Supportive care should include the following: (1) prevention of side effects that result from the syndrome of inappropriate secretion of antidiuretic hormone (this would include restriction of the volume of daily fluid intake to that of the urine output plus insensible loss and perhaps the administration of a diuretic affecting the function of the loop of Henle and the distal tubule); (2) administration of an anticonvulsant; (3) prevention of ileus; (4) monitoring the cardiovascular system; and (5) determining daily blood counts for guidance in transfusion requirements and assessing the risk of infection. The major effect of excessive doses of Velban will be myelosuppression, which may be life threatening. There is no information regarding the effectiveness of dialysis nor of cholestyramine for the treatment of overdosage.

Velban in the dry state is irregularly and unpredictably absorbed from the gastrointestinal tract following oral administration. Absorption of the solution has not been studied. If vinblastine is swallowed, activated charcoal in a water slurry may be given by mouth along with a cathartic. The use of cholestyramine in this situation has not been reported.

Symptoms of overdose will appear when greater-than-recommended doses are given. Any dose of Velban that results in elimination of platelets and neutrophils from blood and marrow and their precursors from marrow should be considered life threatening. The exact dose that will do this in all patients is unknown. Overdoses occurring during prolonged, consecutive-day infusions may be more toxic than the same total dose given by rapid intravenous injection. The intravenous median lethal dose in mice is 10 mg/kg body weight; in rats, it is 2.9 mg/kg.[114] The oral median lethal dose in rats is 7 mg/kg.[86]

Protect the patient's airway and support ventilation and perfusion. Meticulously monitor and maintain, within acceptable limits, the patient's vital signs, blood gases, serum electrolytes, etc. Absorption of drugs from the gastrointestinal tract may be decreased by giving activated charcoal, which, in many cases, is more effective than emesis or lavage; consider charcoal instead of or in addition to gastric emptying if the drug has been swallowed. Repeated doses of charcoal over time may hasten elimination of some drugs that have been absorbed. Safeguard the patient's airway when employing gastric emptying or charcoal.

DOSAGE AND ADMINISTRATION

***Caution*—It is extremely important that the needle be properly positioned in the vein before this product is injected.**

If leakage into surrounding tissue should occur during intravenous administration of Velban, it may cause considerable irritation. The injection should be discontinued immediately, and any remaining portion of the dose should then be introduced into another vein. Local injection of hyaluronidase and the application of moderate heat to the area of leakage help disperse the drug and are thought to minimize discomfort and the possibility of cellulitis.

There are variations in the depth of the leukopenic response that follows therapy with Velban. For this reason, it is recommended that the drug be given no more frequently than *once every 7 days.* It is wise to initiate therapy for adults by administering a single intravenous dose of 3.7 mg/m^2 of body surface area (bsa); the initial dose for children should be 2.5 mg/m^2. Thereafter, white-blood-cell counts should be made to determine the patient's sensitivity to Velban. A reduction of 50% in the dose of Velban is recommended for patients having a direct serum bilirubin value above 3 mg/100 mL. Since metabolism and excretion are primarily hepatic, no modification is recommended for patients with impaired renal function.

A simplified and conservative incremental approach to dosage *at weekly intervals* may be outlined as follows:

	Adults	Children
First dose	3.7 mg/m^2 bsa	2.5 mg/m^2 bsa
Second dose	5.5 mg/m^2 bsa	3.75 mg/m^2 bsa
Third dose	7.4 mg/m^2 bsa	5.0 mg/m^2 bsa
Fourth dose	9.25 mg/m^2 bsa	6.25 mg/m^2 bsa
Fifth dose	11.1 mg/m^2 bsa	7.5 mg/m^2 bsa

The above-mentioned increases may be used until a maximum dose (not exceeding 18.5 mg/m^2 bsa for adults and 12.5 mg/m^2 bsa for children) is reached. The dose should not be increased after that dose which reduces the white-cell count to approximately 3,000 $cells/mm^3$. In some adults, 3.7 mg/m^2 bsa may produce this leukopenia; other adults may require more than 11.1 mg/m^2 bsa; and, very rarely, as much as 18.5 mg/m^2 bsa may be necessary. For most adult patients, however, the weekly dosage will prove to be 5.5 to 7.4 mg/m^2 bsa.

When the dose of Velban which will produce the above degree of leukopenia has been established, a dose of *1 increment smaller* than this should be administered at weekly intervals for maintenance. Thus, the patient is receiving the maximum dose that does not cause leukopenia. *It should be emphasized that, even though 7 days have elapsed, the next dose of Velban should not be given until the white-cell count has returned to at least 4,000/mm^3.* In some cases, oncolytic activity may be encountered before leukopenic effect. When this occurs, there is no need to increase the size of subsequent doses (*see* Precautions).

Continued on next page

• Identi-Code® symbol. This product information was prepared in June 1996. Current information on these and other products of Eli Lilly and Company may be obtained by direct inquiry to Lilly Research Laboratories, Lilly Corporate Center, Indianapolis, Indiana 46285, 800-545-5979.

Lilly—Cont.

The duration of maintenance therapy varies according to the disease being treated and the combination of antineoplastic agents being used. There are differences of opinion regarding the duration of maintenance therapy with the same protocol for a particular disease; for example, various durations have been used with the MOPP program in treating Hodgkin's disease.[55,56,115] Prolonged chemotherapy for maintaining remissions involves several risks, among which are life-threatening infectious diseases, sterility,[113] and possibly the appearance of other cancers through suppression of immune surveillance.[55,116]

In some disorders, survival following complete remission may not be as prolonged as that achieved with shorter periods of maintenance therapy.[37,63] On the other hand, failure to provide maintenance therapy in some patients may lead to unnecessary relapse; complete remissions in patients with testicular cancer, unless maintained for at least 2 years, often result in early relapse.

To prepare a solution containing 1 mg of Velban/mL, add 10 mL of Bacteriostatic Sodium Chloride Injection (preserved with benzyl alcohol) or 10 mL of Sodium Chloride Injection (unpreserved) to the 10 mg of Velban in the sterile vial. Do not use other solutions. The drug dissolves instantly to give a clear solution.

Parenteral drug products should be inspected visually for particulate matter and discoloration prior to administration, whenever solution and container permit.

Unused portions of the remaining solutions made with normal saline that do not contain preservatives should be discarded immediately. Unused preservative-containing solutions made with normal saline may be stored in a refrigerator for future use for a maximum of 28 days.

The dose of Velban (calculated to provide the desired amount) may be injected either into the tubing of a running intravenous infusion or directly into a vein. The latter procedure is readily adaptable to outpatient therapy. In either case, the injection may be completed in about 1 minute. If care is taken to insure that the needle is securely within the vein and that no solution containing Velban is spilled extravascularly, cellulitis and/or phlebitis will not occur. To minimize further the possibility of extravascular spillage, it is suggested that the syringe and needle be rinsed with venous blood before withdrawal of the needle. The dose should not be diluted in large volumes of diluent (ie, 100 to 250 mL) or given intravenously for prolonged periods (ranging from 30 to 60 minutes or more), since this frequently results in irritation of the vein and increases the chance of extravasation.

Because of the enhanced possibility of thrombosis, it is considered inadvisable to inject a solution of Velban into an extremity in which the circulation is impaired or potentially impaired by such conditions as compressing or invading neoplasm, phlebitis, or varicosity.

Procedures for proper handling and disposal of anticancer drugs should be considered. Several guidelines on this subject have been published.[117-122] There is no general agreement that all of the procedures recommended in the guidelines are necessary or appropriate.

Special Dispensing Information —When dispensing Velban in other than the original container, eg, a syringe containing a specific dose, it is imperative that it be packaged in an overwrap bearing the statement: "DO NOT REMOVE COVERING UNTIL MOMENT OF INJECTION. FATAL IF GIVEN INTRATHECALLY. FOR INTRAVENOUS USE ONLY" (*see* Warnings).

HOW SUPPLIED

Vials, 10 mg, 10-mL size (No. 687)—(1s) NDC 0002-1452-01.

The vials should be stored in a refrigerator (2° to 8°C, or 36° to 46°F) to assure extended stability.

Reference titles are available in the manufacturer's full prescribing information.
Literature revised March 6, 1995
ELI LILLY AND COMPANY · Indianapolis, IN 46285, USA
PA 2560 AMP

[030695]

ZINC-INSULIN CRYSTALS   OTC
See under Iletin® (insulin).

Diabetes Patient Education Materials
Managing Your Diabetes Patient Education System
- Comprehensive book on self-care & basic facts
- Topical brochures (eg, insulin and travel)

- Meal planning, gestational diabetes, injecting-insulin 5 part video series
- Self-monitoring records
- Meal plans
- Spanish and English versions

Professional Education Materials and Services
CE programs
Speaker programs
Professional slide series
Diabetes patient management software
For information on these and other educational materials, see your Lilly sales representative.

The Liposome Company, Inc.
ONE RESEARCH WAY
PRINCETON, NJ 08540-6619

Direct Inquiries to:
Customer Service
(800) 335-5476
FAX: (800) 236-4507

For Medical Information Contact:
Gary Horwith, M.D.
Director Clinical Research
(609) 452-7060 or
(800) 547-7243
FAX: (609) 452-8512

ABELCET®   ℞
['ā-bəl- "set]
(Amphotericin B Lipid Complex Injection)

DESCRIPTION

ABELCET® is a sterile, pyrogen-free suspension for intravenous infusion. ABELCET® consists of amphotericin B complexed with two phospholipids in a 1:1 drug-to-lipid molar ratio. The two phospholipids, L-α-dimyristoylphosphatidylcholine (DMPC) and L-α-dimyristoylphosphatidylglycerol (DMPG), are present in a 7:3 molar ratio. ABELCET® is yellow and opaque in appearance, with a pH of 5.5–7.

NOTE: Liposomal encapsulation or incorporation in a lipid complex can substantially affect a drug's functional properties relative to those of the unencapsulated or nonlipid-associated drug. In addition, different liposomal or lipid-complexed products with a common active ingredient may vary from one another in the chemical composition and physical form of the lipid component. Such differences may affect functional properties of these drug products.

Amphotericin B is a polyene, antifungal antibiotic produced from a strain of *Streptomyces nodosus*. Amphotericin B is designated chemically as [1R-(1R*, 3S*, 5R*, 6R*, 9R*, 11R*, 15S*, 16R*, 17R*, 18S*, 19E, 21E, 23E, 25E, 27E, 29E, 31E, 33R*, 35S*, 36R*, 37S*)]-33-[(3-Amino-3, 6-dideoxy-β-D-mannopyranosyl) oxy]-1,3,5,6,9,11,17,37-octahydroxy-15,16,18-trimethyl-13-oxo-14,39-dioxabicyclo[33.3.1]nonatriaconta-19,21,23,25,27,29,31-heptaene-36-carboxylic acid.

It has a molecular weight of 924.09 and a molecular formula of $C_{47}H_{73}NO_{17}$. The structural formula is:

ABELCET® is provided as a sterile, opaque suspension in 20 mL glass, single-use vials. Each vial of ABELCET® contains 100 mg of amphotericin B (see DOSAGE AND ADMINISTRATION), and each mL of ABELCET® contains:

Amphotericin B USP	5 mg
L-α-dimyristoylphosphatidylcholine (DMPC)	3.4 mg
L-α-dimyristoylphosphatidylglycerol (DMPG)	1.5 mg
Sodium Chloride USP	9 mg
Water for Injection USP, q.s. 1 mL	

MICROBIOLOGY

Mechanism of Action
The active component of ABELCET®, amphotericin B, acts by binding to sterols in the cell membrane of susceptible fungi, with a resultant change in the permeability of the membrane. Mammalian cell membranes also contain sterols, and damage to human cells is believed to occur through the same mechanism of action.

Activity *in vitro* and *in vivo*
ABELCET® shows *in vitro* activity against *Aspergillus* sp. (n=3) and *Candida* sp. (n=10), with MICs generally <1 μg/mL. Depending upon the species and strain of *Aspergillus* and *Candida* tested, significant *in vitro* differences in susceptibility to amphotericin B have been reported (MICs ranging from 0.1 to >10μg/mL). However, standardized techniques for susceptibility testing for antifungal agents have not been established, and results of susceptibility studies do not necessarily correlate with clinical outcome.
ABELCET® is active in animal models against *Aspergillus fumigatus, Candida albicans, C. guillermondii, C. stellatoideae*, and *C, tropicalis*, in which end-points were prolonged survival of infected animals and clearance of microorganisms from target organ(s).

Drug Resistance
Mutants with decreased susceptibility to amphotericin B have been isolated from several fungal species after serial passage in culture media containing the drug, and from some patients receiving prolonged therapy. However, the clinical relevance of drug resistance to clinical outcome has not been established.

CLINICAL PHARMACOLOGY

Pharmacokinetics
The assay used to measure amphotericin B in the blood after the administration of ABELCET® does not distinguish amphotericin B that is complexed with the phospholipids of ABELCET® from amphotericin B that is uncomplexed. The pharmacokinetics of amphotericin B after the administration of ABELCET® are nonlinear. Volume of distribution and clearance from blood increase with increasing dose of ABELCET®, resulting in less than proportional increases in blood concentrations of amphotericin B over a dose range of 0.6–5 mg/kg/day. The pharmacokinetics of amphotericin B in whole blood after the administration of ABELCET® and amphotericin B desoxycholate are:
[See table below.]

The large volume of distribution and high clearance value from the blood of amphotericin B after the administration of ABELCET® probably reflect uptake by tissues. The long terminal elimination half-life probably reflects a slow redistribution from tissues. Although amphotericin B is excreted slowly, there is little accumulation in the blood after repeated dosing. AUC of amphotericin B increased approximately 34% from day 1 after the administration of ABELCET® 5 mg/kg/day for 7 days. The effect of gender or ethnicity on the pharmacokinetics of ABELCET® has not been studied.

Pharmacokinetic Parameters of Amphotericin B in Whole Blood
in Patients Administered Multiple Doses of ABELCET® or Amphotericin B Desoxycholate

Pharmacokinetic Parameter	ABELCET® 5mg/kg/day for 5–7 days Mean ±SD	Amphotericin B 0.6 mg/kg/day for 42 days[a] Mean ±SD
Peak Concentration (μg/mL)	1.7 ± 0.8 (n=10)[b]	1.1 ± 0.2 (n=5)
Concentration at End of Dosing Interval (μg/mL)	0.6 ± 0.3 (n=10)[b]	0.4 ± 0.2 (n=5)
Area Under Blood Concentration-Time Curve (AUC_{0-24h}) (μg*h/mL)	14 ± 7 (n=14)[b,c]	17.1 ± 5 (n=5)
Clearance (mL/h/kg)	436 ± 188.5 (n=14)[b,c]	38 ± 15 (n=5)
Apparent Volume of Distribution (Vd_{area}) (L/kg)	131 ± 57.7 (n=8)[c]	5 ± 2.8 (n=5)
Terminal Elimination Half-Life (h)	173.4 ± 78 (n=8)[c]	91.1 ± 40.9 (n=5)
Amount Excreted in Urine Over 24 h After Last Dose (% of dose)[d]	0.9 ± 0.4 (n=8)[c]	9.6 ± 2.5 (n=8)

[a] Data from patients with mucocutaneous leishmaniasis. Infusion rate was 0.25 mg/kg/h.
[b] Data from studies in patients with cytologically proven cancer being treated with chemotherapy or neutropenic patients with presumed or proven fungal infection. Infusion rate was 2.5 mg/kg/h.
[c] Data from patients with mucocutaneous leishmaniasis. Infusion rate was 4 mg/kg/h.
[d] Percentage of dose excreted in 24 hours after last dose.

Tissue concentrations of amphotericin B have been obtained at autopsy from one heart transplant patient who received three doses of ABELCET® at 5.3 mg/kg/day:

Organ	Amphotericin B Tissue Concentration (µg/g)
Spleen	290.0
Lung	222.0
Liver	196.0
Lymph Node	7.6
Kidney	6.9
Heart	5.0
Brain	1.6

This pattern of distribution is consistent with that observed in preclinical studies in dogs in which greatest concentrations of amphotericin B after ABELCET® administration were observed in the liver, spleen, and lung; however, the relationship of tissue concentrations of amphotericin B to its biological activity when administered as ABELCET® is unknown.

Metabolism: The metabolic pathways of ABELCET® are not known. The effect of hepatic impairment on the disposition of ABELCET® is not known.

Renal Impairment: The effect of renal impairment on the disposition of ABELCET® is not known. The effect of dialysis on the elimination of ABELCET® has not been studied; however, amphotericin B is not removed by hemodialysis when administered as amphotericin B desoxycholate.

CLINICAL STUDIES

Aspergillosis: Data were pooled from two emergency-use studies and one small, prospective, single-arm study in which ABELCET® was provided for the treatment of patients with aspergillosis. Most patients enrolled in these studies were judged by the physicians to be clinically refractory to conventional amphotericin B treatment (n=101) or to have developed nephrotoxicity while receiving conventional amphotericin B therapy (n=47). Smaller numbers of patients were entered because they had acute toxicity that contraindicated further conventional amphotericin B therapy (n=13), had preexisting renal insufficiency from other causes that contraindicated conventional amphotericin B therapy (n=11), or were refractory to itraconazole (n=6). Patients were defined by their individual physician as being refractory to or "failing" conventional amphotericin B therapy based on overall clinical judgment after receiving a minimum total dose of 500 mg of amphotericin B. Nephrotoxicity was defined as a serum creatinine that had increased to > 2.5 mg/dL in adults or a creatinine clearance of < 25 mL/min while receiving conventional amphotericin B therapy.

Demographic Characteristics: Patients with Definite or Probable Aspergillosis

Parameter	N = 178
Age (y)	
Median	39
Range	1-82
Gender (M/F)	120/58
Race	
Caucasian	137 (77%)
African-American	18 (10%)
Hispanic	15 (8%)
Asian	4 (2%)
Other	4 (2%)
Baseline Neutrophils (PMN/mm³)	
Median	3,719
<500/mm³	45 (25%)
Underlying Disease, n (%)	
Leukemia	77 (43%)
Lymphoma	14 (8%)
AIDS	11 (6%)
Solid Organ Cancer	11 (6%)
Other[a]	65 (37%)
Site of Infection	
Pulmonary	116 (65%)
Sinus	27 (15%)
CNS	6 (3%)
Other[b]	29 (16%)
Prior Dose of Amphotericin B for Patients Who Were Refractory to Amphotericin B (N=101)	
<7.5 mg/kg	10 (10%)
7.5–15 mg/kg	30 (30%)
>15 mg/kg	59 (58%)
Unknown	2 (2%)

[a] Myelodysplasia (10), transplant (9), congenital immunodeficiency (6), end-stage disease (5), diabetes mellitus (3), cardiovascular disease (3), intravenous drug users (2), cystic fibrosis (1), liver cirrhosis (1), sarcoidosis (1), and unknown (24).
[b] Skin (7), pleural fluid (4), ear (3), spine (3), heart value (2), orbit (2), kidneys (1), lip/face (1), liver (1), penis (1), perianal abscess (1), prostate/urine (1), retroperitoneal abscess (1), and tonsil (1).

Response Rate for Evaluable Patients (n = 111)

Patients Group (n)	Complete Response	Partial Response	Total Responders
Amphotericin B refractory/failure (65)	17%	11%	28%
Nephrotoxicity (37)[a]	22%	30%	51%
Others (9)[b]	22%	44%	67%
Combined	19%	20%	39%

[a] Including 30 patients with nephrotoxicity due to amphotericin B, 7 due to preexisting renal disease.
[b] Including acute toxicity to conventional amphotericin B therapy.

A retrospective response analysis was conducted based on the definitions previously developed by the Mycoses Study Group.[ref1] A "complete response" was defined as resolution of all attributable symptoms, signs, and radiographic and/or bronchoscopic abnormalities present at enrollment; a "partial response" was defined as major improvement of the above-mentioned parameters. The total number of responders was the sum of the number of "complete" and "partial" responses.

Of the 178 patients, 111 were considered evaluable for response. Sixty-seven were excluded on the basis of unconfirmed diagnosis, confounding factors, failure of other drugs, or receiving ≤ 4 doses of ABELCET®. All 178 patients were included in the safety analysis.
[See table above.]

There is no direct comparable control group for the patients described in the above table to be certain how similar patients would have responded had conventional amphotericin B therapy been continued. A retrospective historical control study of patients treated from January 1990 to December 1993 at four medical centers (University of Pittsburgh, H. Lee Moffitt Cancer Center and Research Institute, M.D. Anderson Cancer Center, Fred Hutchinson Cancer Research Center) who developed aspergillosis infection and were treated with conventional amphotericin B as first-line treatment was analyzed using the Mycoses Study Group classification of diagnosis and response. In 60 evaluable patients who had survived at least longer than 4 days after the diagnosis, the response rate was 23%. It should be cautioned that the results are not directly comparable to those of the ABELCET® group.

Renal Function: Patients with aspergillosis who initiated treatment with ABELCET® when serum creatinine was above 2.5 mg/dL experienced a decline in serum creatinine during treatment. Serum creatinine levels were also lower during treatment with ABELCET® when compared to the serum creatinine levels of patients treated with conventional amphotericin B in the historical control group cited above (see figure), although meaningful statistical testing of the differences between these two groups is precluded since these data were obtained from two separate studies.

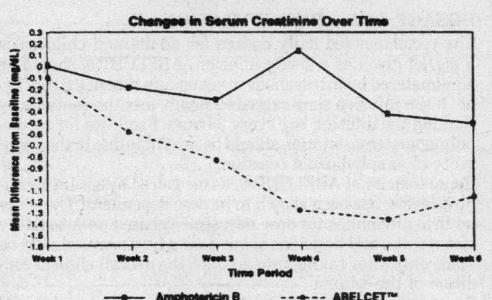

In a randomized study of ABELCET® for the treatment of invasive candidiasis, it was demonstrated in patients with normal baseline renal function that the incidence of nephrotoxicity was significantly less for ABELCET® at a dose of 5 mg/kg/day than for conventional amphotericin B at a dose of 0.7 mg/kg/day.

Despite generally less nephrotoxicity of ABELCET® observed at a dose of 5 mg/kg/day compared with conventional amphotericin B therapy at a dose range of 0.6–1 mg/kg/day, dose-limiting renal toxicity may still be observed with ABELCET®. Renal toxicity of doses greater than 5 mg/kg/day of ABELCET® has not been formally studied.

INDICATIONS AND USAGE

ABELCET® is indicated for the treatment of aspergillosis in patients who are refractory to or intolerant of conventional amphotericin B therapy. This indication is based on results obtained primarily from emergency-use studies of ABELCET® for the treatment of aspergillosis (see CLINICAL STUDIES).

CONTRAINDICATIONS

ABELCET® is contraindicated in patients who have shown hypersensitivity to amphotericin B or any other component in the formulation.

WARNINGS

Anaphylaxis has been reported with amphotericin B desoxycholate and other amphotericin B-containing drugs. One case of anaphylaxis has been reported with ABELCET®. Facilities for cardiopulmonary resuscitation should be available during administration due to the possibility of anaphylactoid reaction. If severe respiratory distress occurs, the infusion should be immediately discontinued. The patient should not receive further infusions of ABELCET®.

PRECAUTIONS

General: As with any amphotericin B-containing product, during the initial dosing of ABELCET®, the drug should be administered intravenously under close clinical observation by medically trained personnel.

Acute reactions including fever and chills may occur 1 to 2 hours after starting an intravenous infusion of ABELCET®. These reactions are usually more common with the first few doses of ABELCET® and generally diminish with subsequent doses. Infusion has been rarely associated with hypotension, bronchospasm, arrhythmias, and shock.

Laboratory Tests: Serum creatinine should be monitored frequently during ABELCET® therapy (see ADVERSE REACTIONS). It is also advisable to regularly monitor liver function, serum electrolytes (particularly magnesium and potassium), and complete blood counts.

Drug Interactions: No formal clinical studies of drug interactions have been conducted with ABELCET®. However, when administered concomitantly, the following drugs are known to interact with amphotericin B; therefore, the following drugs may interact with ABELCET®.

Antineoplastic agents: Concurrent use of antineoplastic agents and amphotericin B may enhance the potential for renal toxicity, bronchospasm, and hypotension. Antineoplastic agents should be given concomitantly with ABELCET® with great caution.

Corticosteroids and corticotropin (ACTH): Concurrent use of corticosteroids and corticotropin (ACTH) with amphotericin B may potentiate hypokalemia which could predispose the patient to cardiac dysfunction. If used concomitantly with ABELCET®, serum electrolytes and cardiac function should be closely monitored.

Cyclosporin A: Data from a prospective study of prophylactic ABELCET® in 22 patients undergoing bone marrow transplantation suggested that concurrent initiation of cyclosporin A and ABELCET® within several days of bone marrow ablation may be associated with increased nephrotoxicity.

Digitalis glycosides: Concurrent use of amphotericin B may induce hypokalemia and may potentiate digitalis toxicity. When administered concomitantly with ABELCET®, serum potassium levels should be closely monitored.

Flucytosine: Concurrent use of flucytosine with amphotericin B-containing preparations may increase the toxicity of flucytosine by possibly increasing its cellular uptake and/or impairing its renal excretion. Flucytosine should be given concomitantly with ABELCET® with caution.

Imidazoles (e.g., ketoconazole, miconazole, clotrimazole, fluconazole, etc.): Antagonism between amphotericin B and imidazole derivatives such as miconazole and ketoconazole, which inhibit ergosterol synthesis, has been reported in both *in vitro* and *in vivo* animal studies. The clinical significance of these findings has not been determined.

Leukocyte transfusions: Acute pulmonary toxicity has been reported in patients receiving intravenous amphotericin B and leukocyte transfusions. Leukocyte transfusions and ABELCET® should not be given concurrently.

Other nephrotoxic medications: Concurrent use of amphotericin B and agents such as aminoglycosides, cyclosporine, and pentamidine may enhance the potential for drug-induced renal toxicity. Aminoglycosides, cyclosporine, and pentamidine should be used concomitantly with ABELCET® only with great caution. Intensive monitoring of renal function is recommended in patients requiring any combination of nephrotoxic medications.

Continued on next page

Liposome Company, Inc.—Cont.

Skeletal muscle relaxants: Amphotericin B-induced hypokalemia may enhance the curariform effect of skeletal muscle relaxants (e.g., tubocurarine) due to hypokalemia. When administered concomitantly with ABELCET®, serum potassium levels should be closely monitored.

Zidovudine: Increased myelotoxicity and nephrotoxicity were observed in dogs when either ABELCET® (at doses 0.16 or 0.5 times the recommended human dose) or amphotericin B desoxycholate (at 0.5 times the recommended human dose) were administered concomitantly with zidovudine for 30 days. If zidovudine is used concomitantly with ABELCET®, renal and hematologic function should be closely monitored.

Carcinogenesis, Mutagenesis, and Impairment of Fertility: No long-term studies in animals have been performed to evaluate the carcinogenic potential of ABELCET®. The following *in vitro* (with and without metabolic activation) and *in vivo* studies to assess ABELCET® for mutagenic potential were conducted: bacterial reverse mutation assay, mouse lymphoma forward mutation assay, chromosomal aberration assay in CHO cells, and *in vivo* mouse micronucleus assay. ABELCET® was found to be without mutagenic effects in all assay systems. Studies demonstrated that ABELCET® had no impact on fertility in male and female rats at doses up to 0.32 times the recommended human dose (based on body surface area considerations).

Pregnancy: Teratogenic Effects. Pregnancy Category B: Reproductive studies in rats and rabbits at doses of ABELCET® up to 0.64 times the human dose revealed no harm to the fetus. There are no reports of pregnant women having been treated with ABELCET®. Because animal reproductive studies are not always predictive of human response, and adequate and well-controlled studies have not been conducted in pregnant women, ABELCET® should be used during pregnancy only after taking into account the importance of the drug to the mother.

Pediatric Use: A small number of children, age 16 years and under, with aspergillosis (n=40), have been treated with ABELCET®. No serious, unexpected adverse events have been reported.

Nursing Mothers: It is not known whether ABELCET® is excreted in human milk. Because many drugs are excreted in human milk, and because of the potential for serious adverse reactions in nursing infants from ABELCET®, taking into account the importance of the drug to the mother, a decision should be made whether to discontinue nursing or to discontinue the drug.

ADVERSE REACTIONS

The total safety data base is composed of 813 patients treated with ABELCET®, of whom 667 were treated with 5 mg/kg/day. Of these 667 patients, 194 patients were treated in four comparative studies, 418 patients were treated in emergency-use studies, and 55 patients were treated in open-label, non-comparative studies. Most had underlying hematologic neoplasms, and many were receiving multiple concomitant medications. In the emergency-use studies, the median duration of therapy was 22 days for ABELCET®-treated patients. Nine percent of ABELCET® patients discontinued treatment due to adverse events, regardless of presumed relationship to drug. In general, the adverse events most commonly reported with ABELCET® were transient chills and fever during infusion of the drug. Shown below are all reported adverse events that occurred with an incidence of ≥3% in the emergency-use studies and the corresponding incidence for patients with documented or suspected aspergillosis.

Adverse Event	All Fungal Infections n=418 %	Aspergillosis n=218 %
Body as a Whole		
Chills	16	15
Fever	12	15
Multiple Organ Failure	10	9
Sepsis	7	9
Headache	4	7
Infection	4	6
Pain	4	4
Abdominal Pain	3	5
Cardiovascular System		
Hypotension	7	6
Cardiac Arrest	5	5
Digestive System		
Nausea	8	6
Vomiting	6	6
Diarrhea	5	10
Gastrointestinal Hemorrhage	3	3
Hemic and Lymphatic System		
Thrombocytopenia	5	4
Leukopenia	4	4
Anemia	4	4
Metabolic and Nutritional Disorders		
Increased Serum Creatinine	11	12
Bilirubinemia	4	5
Hypokalemia	4	6
Acidosis	3	3
Respiratory System		
Respiratory Failure	9	10
Dyspnea	5	8
Respiratory Disorder	4	3
Pneumonia	3	5
Skin and Appendages		
Rash	3	5
Urogenital System		
Kidney Failure	5	4

The following adverse events have also been reported with ABELCET®:

Body as a whole: malaise, weight loss, injection site reaction including inflammation

Allergic: bronchospasm, wheezing, asthma, anaphylactoid and other allergic reactions

Cardiopulmonary: cardiac failure, pulmonary edema, shock, myocardial infarct, hemoptysis, arrhythmias including ventricular fibrillation, hypertension, tachypnea, thrombophlebitis, pulmonary embolus, cardiomyopathy

Dermatological: maculopapular rash, pruritus, exfoliative dermatitis, erythema multiforme

Gastrointestinal: acute liver failure, hepatitis, jaundice, melena, anorexia, dyspepsia, cramping, epigastric pain, veno-occlusive liver disease

Hematologic: coagulation defects, blood dyscrasias including eosinophilia, leukocytosis

Musculoskeletal: myasthenia, generalized pain, including bone, muscle, and joint pains

Neurologic: convulsions, tinnitus, visual impairment, hearing loss, peripheral neuropathy, transient vertigo, diplopia, encephalopathy, extrapyramidal syndrome and other neurologic symptoms

Urogenital: acute renal failure, oliguria, decreased renal function, anuria, renal tubular acidosis, impotence

Altered Laboratory Findings:

Serum electrolyte abnormalities: hypomagnesemia, hyperkalemia, hypocalcemia

Liver function test abnormalities: increased AST, ALT, alkaline phosphatase

Renal function test abnormalities: increased BUN

Other test abnormalities: acidosis, hyperamylasemia, hypoglycemia, hyperglycemia

OVERDOSAGE

Amphotericin B desoxycholate overdose has been reported to result in cardio-respiratory arrest. Ten patients have been reported who have received one or more doses of ABELCET® between 7–13 mg/kg. None of these patients had a serious acute reaction to ABELCET®. If an overdose is suspected, discontinue therapy, monitor the patient's clinical status, and administer supportive therapy as required. ABELCET® is not hemodialyzable.

DOSAGE AND ADMINISTRATION

The recommended daily dosage for adults and children is 5 mg/kg given as a single infusion. ABELCET® should be administered by intravenous infusion at a rate of 2.5 mg/kg/hr. If the infusion time exceeds 2 hours, mix the contents by shaking the infusion bag every 2 hours. Facilities for cardiopulmonary resuscitation should be available due to the possibility of anaphylactoid reaction.

Renal toxicity of ABELCET®, as measured by serum creatinine levels, has been shown to be dose dependent. There are no firm guidelines for dose adjustment based on laboratory test results, and decisions about dose adjustments should be made only after taking into account the overall clinical condition of the patient.

Preparation of Admixture for Infusion: Shake the vial gently until there is no evidence of any yellow sediment at the bottom. Withdraw the appropriate dose of ABELCET® from the required number of vials into one or more sterile 20 mL syringes using an 18-gauge needle. Remove the needle from each syringe filled with ABELCET® and replace with the 5-micron filter needle supplied with each vial. Each filter needle may be used to filter the contents of up to four vials. Insert the filter needle of the syringe into an IV bag containing 5% Dextrose Injection USP, and empty the contents of the syringe into the bag. The infusion concentration should be 1 mg/mL. For pediatric patients and patients with cardiovascular disease the drug may be diluted with 5% Dextrose Injection to a final infusion concentration of 2 mg/mL. Do not use the admixture after dilution with 5% Dextrose Injection if there is any evidence of foreign matter. Vials are for single use. Unused material should be discarded. Aseptic technique must be strictly observed throughout handling of ABELCET® since no bacteriostatic agent or preservative is present.

DO NOT DILUTE WITH SALINE SOLUTIONS OR MIX WITH OTHER DRUGS OR ELECTROLYTES as the compatibility of ABELCET® with these materials has not been established. An existing intravenous line should be flushed with 5% Dextrose Injection before infusion of ABELCET®, or a separate infusion line should be used. *Do not use an in-line filter.*

The diluted ready-for-use admixture is stable for up to 24 hours at either 2° to 8°C (36° to 46°F) or at room temperature.

HOW SUPPLIED

Each vial contains 100 mg of ABELCET® in 20 mL of suspension. Single-use vials along with single-use filter needles are individually packaged. NDC 61799-101-41.

STORAGE

Prior to admixture, ABELCET® should be stored at 2° to 8°C (36° to 46°F) and protected from exposure to light. Do not freeze. ABELCET® should be retained in the carton until time of use.

The admixed ABELCET® and 5% Dextrose Injection may be stored for up to 24 hours at either 2° to 8°C (36° to 46°F) or at room temperature. Do not freeze. Any unused material should be discarded.

U.S. Patent No. 4,973,465

The Liposome Company, Inc.   8/96
Princeton, NJ, USA   1-101-41-US-C

REFERENCE

1. Denning DW, Lee JY, Hostetler JS, et al. NIAID Mycoses Study Group multicenter trial of oral itraconazole therapy for invasive aspergillosis. *Am J Med.* 97:135–144, 1994.
   Shown in Product Identification Guide, page 322

Lotus Biochemical Corporation
P.O. BOX 3586
RADFORD, VA 24143

Direct Inquiries to:
Mike Taylor
(800) 455-5525
FAX: (800) 962-2200

For Medical Information Contact:
In Emergencies:
Lawrence P. Olon
(423) 989-9190
FAX: (423) 989-3532

ADAPIN®   ℞
[ad'uh-pin'']
(doxepin HCl)

DESCRIPTION

Adapin (doxepin HCl) is one of a class of psychotherapeutic agents known as dibenzoxepin tricyclic compounds. The molecular formula of the compound is $C_{19}H_{21}NO$. HCl having a molecular weight of 316. It is a white crystalline solid readily soluble in water, lower alcohols and chloroform.

Its structural formula is:

Chemically, doxepin hydrochloride is a dibenzoxepin derivative and is the first of a family of tricyclic psychotherapeutic agents. Specifically, it is an isomeric mixture of 1-Propanamine, 3-Dibenz[b,e] oxepin-11(6*H*) ylidene-*N,N*-dimethyl-hydrochloride.

All capsule strengths for oral administration contain doxepin base as the hydrochloride and the following inactive ingredients: Gelatin, Magnesium Stearate, Microcrystalline Cellulose, Pregelatinized Starch, Silicon Dioxide, Sodium Lauryl Sulfate, and Titanium Dioxide. In addition the 10 mg capsule contains Blue 1 and Red 28; the 25 mg capsule contains Red 28 and Yellow 10; the 50 mg capsule contains Blue 1, Red 28, Red 33 and Yellow 10; the 75 mg capsule contains Blue 1, Red 28, Red 40 and Yellow 10; the 100 mg capsule contains Blue 1, Red 28 and Yellow 10; and the 150 mg capsule contains Blue 1, Red 28 and Yellow 10.

CLINICAL PHARMACOLOGY

The mechanism of action of doxepin hydrochloride is not definitely known. It is not a central nervous system stimulant nor a monoamine oxidase inhibitor. The current hypothesis is that the clinical effects are due, at least in part, to influences on the adrenergic activity at the synapses so that deactivation of norepinephrine by reuptake into the nerve terminals is prevented. Animal studies suggest that doxepin HCl does not appreciably antagonize the antihypertensive action of guanethidine. In animals studies anticholinergic, antiserotonin antihistamine effects on smooth muscle have been demonstrated. At higher than usual clinical doses nor-

epinephrine response was potentiated in animals. The effect was not demonstrated in humans.

At clinical dosages up to 150 mg per day, **Adapin** can be given to man concomitantly with guanethidine and related compounds without blocking the antihypertensive effect. At dosages above 150 mg per day blocking of the antihypertensive effect of these compounds has been reported.

Adapin is virtually devoid of euphoria as a side effect. Characteristic of this type of compound, **Adapin** has not been demonstrated to produce the physical tolerance or psychological dependence associated with addictive compounds.

INDICATIONS AND USAGE

Adapin is recommended for the treatment of:
1. Psychoneurotic patients with depression and/or anxiety.
2. Depression and/or anxiety associated with alcoholism (not to be taken concomitantly with alcohol).
3. Depression and/or anxiety associated with organic disease (the possibility of drug interaction should be considered if the patient is receiving other drugs concomitantly).
4. Psychotic depressive disorders associated with anxiety including involutional depression and manic-depressive disorders.

The target symptoms of psychoneurosis that respond particularly well to **Adapin** include anxiety, tension, depression, somatic symptoms and concerns, sleep disturbances, guilt, lack of energy, fear, apprehension and worry.

Clinical experience has shown that doxepin HCl is safe and well-tolerated even in the elderly patient. Owing to lack of clinical experience in the pediatric population, **Adapin** is not recommended for use in children under 12 years of age.

CONTRAINDICATIONS

Adapin is contraindicated in patients who have shown hypersensitivity to the drug. Possibility of cross sensitivity with other dibenzoxepines should be kept in mind.

Adapin is contraindicated in patients with glaucoma or a tendency to urinary retention. The disorders should be ruled out particularly in older patients.

WARNINGS

The once-a-day dosage regimen of **Adapin** in patients with intercurrent illness or patients taking other medications should be carefully adjusted. This is especially important in patients receiving other medication with anticholinergic effects.

Usage in Geriatrics: The use of **Adapin** on a once-a-day dosage regimen in geriatric patients should be adjusted carefully based on the patient's condition.

Usage in Pregnancy: Reproduction studies have been performed in rats, rabbits, monkeys and dogs and there was no evidence of harm to the animal fetus. The relevance to humans is not known. Since there is no experience in pregnant women who have received this drug, safety in pregnancy has not been established. There has been a report of apnea and drowsiness occurring in a nursing infant whose mother was taking doxepin HCl.

Usage in Children: The use of **Adapin** in children under 12 years of age is not recommended, because safe conditions for its use have not been established.

DRUG INTERACTIONS

MAO Inhibitors: Serious side effects and even death have been reported following the concomitant use of certain drugs with MAO inhibitors, Therefore, MAO inhibitors should be discontinued at least two weeks prior to the cautious initiation of therapy with **Adapin**. The exact length of time may vary and is dependent upon the particular MAO inhibitor being used, the length of time it has been administered, and the dosage involved.

Cimetidine: Cimetidine has been reported to produce clinically significant fluctuations in steady-state serum concentrations of various tricyclic antidepressants. Serious anticholinergic symptoms (i.e., severe dry mouth, urinary retention and blurred vision) have been associated with elevations in the serum levels of tricyclic antidepressant when cimetidine therapy is initiated. Additonally, higher than expected tricyclic antidepressant levels have been observed when they are begun in patients already taking cimetidine. In patients who have been reported to be well controlled on tricyclic antidepressant receiving concurrent cimetidine therapy, discontinuation of cimetidine has been reported to decrease established steady-state serum tricyclic antidepressant levels and compromise their therapeutic effects.

Usage with Alcohol: It should be borne in mind that alcohol ingestion may increase the danger inherent in any intentional or unintentional **Adapin** overdose. This is especially important in patients who may use alcohol excessively.

PRECAUTIONS

Since drowsiness may occur with the use of this drug patients should be warned of the possibility and cautioned against driving a car or operating hazardous machinery while taking the drug. Patients should also be cautioned that their response to alcohol may be potentiated.

Since suicide is an inherent risk in any depressed patient and may remain so until significant improvement has oc-

curred, patients should be closely supervised during the early course of therapy. Prescriptions should be written for the smallest feasible amount.

Should increased symptoms of psychosis or shift to manic symptomatology occur, it may be necessary to reduce dosage or add a major tranquilizer to the dosage regimen.

Drugs Metabolized by P45011D6: A subset (3% to 10%) of the population has reduced activity of certain drug metabolizing enzymes such as the cytochrome P450 isozyme P45011D6. Such individuals are referred to as "poor metabolizers"of drugs such as debrisoquin, dextromethorphan, and the tricyclic antidepressants. These individuals may have higher than expected plasma concentrations of tricyclic antidepressants when given usual doses. In addition, certain drugs that are metabolized by this isozyme, including many antidepressants (tricyclic antidepressants, selective serotonin reuptake inhibitors, and others), may inhibit the acitivity of this isozyme, and thus may make normal metabolizers resemble poor metabolizers with regard to concomitant therapy with other drugs metabolized by this enzyme system, leading to drug interactions.

Concomitant use of tricyclic antidepressants with other drugs metabolized by cytochrome P45011D6 may require lower doses than usually prescribed for either the tricyclic antidepressants or the other drug.

Therefore, coadministration of tricyclic antidepressants with other drugs that are metabolized by this isoenzyme, including other antidepressants, phenothiazines, carbamazepine, and Type 1C antiarrhythmics (e.g., propafenone, flecainide and encainide), or that inhibits this enzyme (e.g., quinidine), should be approached with caution.

ADVERSE REACTIONS

NOTE: Some of the adverse reactions noted below have not been specifically reported with **Adapin**. However, due to the close pharmacological similarities among the tricyclics, the reactions should be considered when prescribing **Adapin**.

Anticholinergic Effects: Dry mouth, blurred vision, constipation and urinary retention have been reported. If they do not subside with continued therapy or become severe, it may be necessary to reduce the dosage.

Central Nervous System Effects: Drowsiness is the most commonly noticed side effect. This tends to disappear as therapy is continued. Other infrequently reported CNS side effects are confusion, disorientation, hallucinations, numbness, paresthesias, ataxia, extrapyramidal symptoms and seizures.

Cardiovascular Effects: Cardiovascular effects including hypotension and tachycardia have been reported occasionally.

Allergic: Skin rash, edema, photosensitization, and pruritus have occasionally occurred.

Hematologic: Eosinophilia has been reported in a few patients. There have been occasional reports of bone marrow depression manifesting as agranulocytosis, leukopenia, thrombocytopenia, and purpura.

Gastrointestinal: Nausea, vomiting, indigestion, taste disturbances, diarrhea, anorexia, and aphthous stomatitis have been reported. (See anticholinergic effects.)

Endocrine: Raised or lowered libido, testicular swelling, gynecomastia in males, enlargement of breasts and galactorrhea in the female, raising or lowering of blood sugar levels and syndrome of inappropriate antidiuretic hormone secretion have been reported with tricyclic administration.

Other: Dizziness, tinnitus, weight gain, sweating, chills, fatigue, weakness, flushing, jaundice, alopecia, and headache have been occasionally observed as adverse effects.

Withdrawal Symptoms: The possibility of development of withdrawal symptoms upon abrupt cessation of treatment after prolonged **Adapin** should be borne in mind. These are not indicative of addiction and gradual withdrawal of medication should not cause these symptoms.

OVERDOSAGE

A. Signs and symptoms
1. Mild: Drowsiness, stupor, blurred vision, excessive dryness of mouth.
2. Severe: Respiratory depression, hypotension, coma, convulsions, cardiac arrhythmias and tachycardias.
Also: urinary retention (bladder atony), decreased gastrointestinal motility (paralytic ileus), hyperthemia (or hypothermia), hypertension, dilated pupils, hyperactive reflexes.

B. Management and Treatment
1. Mild: Observation and supportive therapy is all that is usually necessary.
2. Severe: Medical management of severe doxepin hydrochloride overdosage consists of aggressive supportive therapy. If the patient is conscious, gastric lavage, with appropriate precautions to prevent pulmonary aspiration, should be performed even though **Adapin** is rapidly absorbed. The use of activated charcoal has been recommended, as has been continuous gastric lavage with saline for 24 hours or more. An adequate airway should be established in comatose patients and assisted ventilation used if necessary. EKG monitoring may be required for

several days, since relapse after apparent recovery has been reported. Arrhythmias should be treated with appropriate antiarrhythmic agents. It has been reported that many of the cardiovascular and CNS symptoms of tricyclic antidepressant poisoning in adults may be reversed by the slow intravenous administration of 1 mg to 3 mg of physostigmine salicylate. Because physostigmine is rapidly metabolized, the dosage should be repeated as required. Convulsions may respond to standard anticonvulsant therapy, however, barbiturates may potentiate any respiratory depression. Dialysis and forced diuresis generally are not of value in the management of overdosage due to high tissue and protein binding of doxepin hydrochloride.

DOSAGE AND ADMINISTRATION

For most patients with illness of mild to moderate severity, a starting daily dose of 75 mg is recommended. Dosage may subsequently be increased or decreased at appropriate intervals and according to individual response. The usual optimum dose range is 75 mg per day to 150 mg per day.

In more severely ill patients higher doses may be required with subsequent gradual increase to 300 mg per day if necessary. Additional therapeutic effect is rarely to be obtained by exceeding a dose of 300 mg per day.

In patients with very mild symptomatology or emotional symptoms accompanying organic disease, lower doses may suffice. Some of these patients have been controlled on doses as low as 25–50 mg per day.

The total daily dosage of **Adapin** may be given on a divided or once-a-day dosage schedule. If the once-a-day schedule is employed the maximum recommended dose is 150 mg per day. This dose may be given at bedtime. **The 150 mg capsule strength is intended for maintenance therapy only and is not recommended for initiation of treatment.**

Antianxiety effect is apparent before the antidepressant effect. Optimal antidepressant effect may not be evident for two to three weeks.

HOW SUPPLIED

Adapin (doxepin hydrochloride capsules, USP) is available containing doxepin hydrochloride, USP equivalent to 10 mg, 25 mg, 50 mg, 75 mg, 100 mg, or 150 mg of doxepin base.

10 mg – Hard shell, opaque, robin egg blue capsules imprinted in black ink with 10 on the body and Adapin on the cap, are supplied as:
NDC# 59417-356-71–Bottle of 100

25 mg – Hard shell, opaque, off-white cap and a yellow body imprinted in black ink with 25 on the body and Adapin on the cap, are supplied as:
NDC# 59417-357-71–Bottle of 100

50 mg – Hard shell, opaque, lavender cap and a cranberry body imprinted in white ink with 50 on the body and Adapin on the cap, are supplied as:
NDC# 59417-358-71–Bottle of 100

75 mg – Hard shell, opaque, plum cap and a pink body imprinted in white ink with 75 on the body and Adapin on the cap, are supplied as:
NDC# 59417-361-71–Bottle of 100

100 mg – Hard shell, opaque, kelly green cap and a white body imprinted in black ink with 100 on the body and Adapin on the cap, are supplied as:
NDC# 59417-359-71–Bottle of 100

150 mg – Hard shell, opaque, gray cap and orange body imprinted in black ink with 150 on the body and Adapin on the cap, are supplied as:
NDC# 59417-370-65–Bottle of 50

Store at controlled room temperature 15–30°C (59–86°F). Protect from light.

Dispense in a tight, light-resistant container using a child-resistant closure.

Manufactured for:
LOTUS BIOCHEMICAL CORPORATION
Radford, VA 24143 USA
Manufactured by:
Lederle Arzneimittel, Cyanamid GmbH
82515 Wolfratshausen, Germany
Adapin is a registered trademark of Lotus Biochemical Corporation.
© 1993, Lotus Biochemical Corporation   REV. 8/93

ERGOMAR® Sublingual Tablets, 2 mg   ℞
[er′go-mar″]
(ergotamine tartrate tablets, USP)

DESCRIPTION

Each sublingual tablet of ERGOMAR contains 2 mg ergotamine tartrate, USP.

Inactive Ingredients: Corn starch, D & C Yellow No. 10, FD & C Blue No. 1, lactose monohydrate NF, magnesium stearate, peppermint oil, saccharin sodium.

Continued on next page

Lotus Biochemical—Cont.

Pharmacological Category: Vasoconstrictor, uterine stimulant, alpha adrenoreceptor antagonist.
Therapeutic Class: Anti-migraine.
Chemical Name: Ergotaman-3′,6′, 18-trione, 12′-hydroxy-2′-methyl-5′-(phenyl-methyl)-,(5′α)-,[R-(R*,R*)]-2, 3-dihydroxy-butanedioate(2:1)(tartrate).
Structural Formula:

CLINICAL PHARMACOLOGY

The pharmacological properties of ergotamine are extremely complex; some of its actions are unrelated to each other, and even mutually antagonistic. The drug has partial agonist and/or antagonist activity against tryptaminergic, dopaminergic and alpha adrenergic receptors depending upon their site, and it is a highly active uterine stimulant. It causes constriction of peripheral and cranial blood vessels and produces depression of central vasomotor centers. The pain of a migraine attack is believed to be due to greatly increased amplitude of pulsations in the cranial arteries, especially the meningeal branches of the external carotid artery. Ergotamine reduces extracranial blood flow, causes a decline in the amplitude of pulsation in the cranial arteries, and decreases hyperperfusion of the territory of the basilar artery. It does not reduce cerebral hemispheric blood flow. Long term usage has established the fact that ergotamine tartrate is effective in controlling up to 70% of acute migraine attacks, so that it is now considered specific for the treatment of this headache syndrome. Ergotamine produces constriction of both arteries and veins. In doses used in the treatment of vascular headaches, ergotamine usually produces only small increases in blood pressure but it does increase peripheral resistance and decrease blood flow in various organs. Small doses of the drug increase the force and frequency of uterine contraction; larger doses increase the resting tone of the uterus also. The gravid uterus is particularly sensitive to these effects of ergotamine. Although specific teratogenic effects attributable to ergotamine have not been found, the fetus suffers if ergotamine is given to the mother. Retarded fetal growth and an increase in intrauterine death and resorption have been seen in animals. These are thought to result from ergotamine induced increases in uterine motility and vasoconstriction in the placental vascular bed.
The bioavailability of sublingually administered ergotamine has not been determined.
Ergotamine is metabolized by the liver by largely undefined pathways, and 90% of the metabolites are excreted in the bile. The unmetabolized drug is erratically secreted in the saliva, and only traces of unmetabolized drug appear in the urine and feces. Ergotamine is secreted into breast milk. The elimination half-life of ergotamine from plasma is about 2 hours, but the drug may be stored in some tissues, which would account for its long lasting therapeutic and toxic actions.

INDICATIONS AND USAGE

ERGOMAR is indicated as therapy to abort or prevent vascular headache, e.g., migraine, migraine variants, or so called "histaminic cephalalgia."

CONTRAINDICATIONS

ERGOMAR is contraindicated in peripheral vascular disease (thromboangitis obliterans, luetic arteritis, severe arteriosclerosis, thrombophlebitis, Raynaud's disease), coronary heart disease, hypertension, impaired hepatic or renal function, severe pruritis, and sepsis. It is also contraindicated in patients who are hypersensitive to any of its components. ERGOMAR may cause fetal harm when administered to a pregnant woman by virtue of its powerful uterine stimulant actions. ERGOMAR is contraindicated in women who are, or may become, pregnant.

PRECAUTIONS

General: Although signs and symptoms of ergotism rarely develop even after long term intermittent use of ergotamine, care should be exercised to remain within the limits of recommended dosage.
Drug Interactions: The effects of ERGOMAR may be potentiated by triacetyloleandomycin which inhibits the metabolism of ergotamine. The pressor effects of ERGOMAR and other vasoconstrictor drugs can combine to cause dangerous hypertension.
Carcinogenesis: No studies have been performed to investigate ERGOMAR for carcinogenic effects.

Pregnancy: Pregnancy Category X—See CONTRAINDICATIONS section.
Nursing Mothers: Ergotamine is secreted into human milk. It can reach the breast-fed infant by this route and exert pharmacologic effects in it. Caution should be exercised when ERGOMAR is administered to a nursing woman. Excessive dosing or prolonged administration of ergotamine may inhibit lactation.

ADVERSE REACTIONS

Nausea and vomiting occur in up to 10% of patients after ingestion of therapeutic doses of ergotamine. Weakness of the legs and pain in limb muscles are also frequent complaints. Numbness and tingling of the fingers and toes, precordial pain, transient changes in heart rate and localized edema and itching may also occur, particularly in patients who are sensitive to the drug.

DRUG ABUSE AND DEPENDENCE

Patients who take ergotamine for extended periods of time may become dependent upon it and require progressively increasing doses for relief of vascular headaches, and for prevention of dysphoric effects which follow withdrawal of the drug.

OVERDOSAGE

Overdosage with ergotamine causes nausea, vomiting, weakness of the legs, pain in limb muscles, numbness and tingling of the fingers and toes, precordial pain, tachycardia or bradycardia, hypertension or hypotension and localized edema and itching together with signs and symptoms of ischemia due to vasoconstriction of peripheral arteries and arterioles. The feet and hands become cold, pale and numb. Muscle pain occurs while walking and later at rest also. Gangrene may ensue. Confusion, depression, drowsiness and convulsions are occasional signs of ergotamine toxicity. Overdosage is particularly likely to occur in patients with sepsis or impaired renal or hepatic function. Patients with peripheral vascular disease are specially at risk of developing peripheral ischemia following treatment with ergotamine. Some cases of ergotamine poisoning have been reported in patients who have taken less than 5 mg of the drug. Usually, however, toxicity is seen in doses of ergotamine tartrate in excess of about 15 mg in 24 hours or 40 mg in a few days.
Treatment of ergotamine overdosage consists of the withdrawal of the drug followed by symptomatic measures including attempts to maintain an adequate circulation in the affected parts. Anticoagulant drugs, low molecular weight dextran and potent vasodilator drugs may all be beneficial. Intravenous infusion of sodium nitroprusside has also been reported to be successful. Vasodilators must be used with special care in the presence of hypotension.
Nausea and vomiting may be relieved by atropine or antiemetic compounds of the phenothiazine group. Ergotamine is dialyzable.

DOSAGE AND ADMINISTRATION

All efforts should be made to initiate therapy as soon as possible after the first symptoms of the attack are noted, since success is proportional to rapidity of treatment, and lower dosages will be effective. At the first sign of an attack or to relieve symptoms after onset of an attack one 2 mg tablet is placed under the tongue. Another tablet should be taken at half-hour intervals thereafter, if necessary, but dosage must not exceed three tablets in any 24 hour period. Dosage should be limited to not more than five tablets (10mg) in any one week.

HOW SUPPLIED

20 tablets (green) each containing 2 mg ergotamine tartrate, supplied in foil strips in a plastic child resistant container. Each tablet is debossed with the following product identification code: LB 2. Protect from light and heat. Keep out of the reach of children.
NDC 59417-120-20 Containers of 20.
Caution: Federal law prohibits dispensing without prescription.
Manufactured for:
LOTUS BIOCHEMICAL CORPORATION
Radford, VA 24143, USA
By: Central Pharmaceuticals, Inc.
    Seymour, IN 47274 USA
©Lotus Biochemical Corporation   REV. 10/95
All Rights Reserved

For information on over-the-counter drugs,
consult PDR For Nonprescription Drugs

Lunsco, Inc.
ROUTE 2, BOX 62
PULASKI, VA 24301

Direct Inquiries to:
(703) 980-4358

For Medical Information Contact:
In Emergencies:
(703) 980-4358

DYTUSS   OTC

COMPOSITION
Ea. Teaspoonful (5mL) contains:
Diphenhydramine HCl 12.5 mg.
Alcohol 5%.

SUPPLIED
Pint.

FETRIN   ℞

COMPOSITION
Each sustained-release capsule contains: Ferrous Fumarate (Equivalent to 66 mg. Elemental Iron) 200 mg., Ascorbic Acid 60 mg., Cyanocobalamin 5 mcg with Intrinsic Factor.

SUPPLIED
Bottles of 100.

PACAPS   ℞

COMPOSITION
Each capsule represents: Butalbital 50 mg., Caffeine 40 mg., Acetaminophen 325 mg.

SUPPLIED
Bottles of 100.

PROTID   ℞

COMPOSITION
Each tablet represents: Acetaminophen 500 mg., Chlorpheniramine Maleate 8 mg., Phenylephrine HCl 40 mg.

SUPPLIED
Bottles of 100.

MDR Fitness Corp.
MEDICAL DOCTORS RESEARCH
14101 NW 4th STREET
SUNRISE, FL 33325

Direct Inquiries to:
(800) MDR-TABS

MDR FITNESS TABS FOR MEN   OTC
MDR FITNESS TABS FOR WOMEN

DESCRIPTION
MDR Fitness Tabs are formulated by Medical Doctors Research based on a two tablet per day system to allow enhanced absorption of nutrients. The A.M. and P.M. dosage allows more absorption of the water soluble vitamins (B-complex and C) which are not readily stored by the body. The AM tablet provides more micronutrients required for energy producing reactions when physical activity is greater. The MDR formulas are free of dyes, yeast, preservatives, fillers, soy, wheat gluten, lactose and other sugars.

INDICATIONS AND USAGE
MDR Fitness Tabs are designed for the maintenance of good health and nutrition for men and women, those 11 years of age or older, and whenever a multi-vitamin, mineral supplement is indicated to help provide nutrients missing from the diet or replace nutrient loss from oral contraceptives, and antacids, excessive alcohol, smoking, physical or emotional stress, exercise, weight loss diets, or illness. Daily use of MDR Fitness Tabs may also play a protective role for good health by assuring adequate intake of essential nutrients,

including antioxidant nutrients shown in recent research to help support the body's natural defenses.
Directions: After the first meal of the day, take one "AM" Fitness Tab. After lunch or dinner, take one "PM" Fitness Tab. Swallow Fitness Tab with a full glass of water.

PRECAUTIONS

Not recommended for persons with severe kidney disease or those undergoing renal dialysis, unless under a physician's supervision. Diabetics may need to adjust insulin dosage and should be monitored. Not recommended for Parkinson patients on levodopa therapy, due to the presence of vitamin B-6 which may decrease levodopa's efficacy. Pregnant and lactating women may need additional supplementation.
Note: MDR Fitness also provides a Stress Defense supplement to be taken with MDR Fitness Tabs when higher dosages are indicated.
Also available: Nite-Cal Calcium, Children's Chewable, Arthritis, and Fibromyalgia Nutritional Support.

For Samples, Product or Order Information Call
1-800-MDR-TABS ext. 5583 or fax (305) 845-9505
or write: Medical Doctors' Research
14101 NW 4th Street
SUNRISE, FL 33325

MGI Pharma, Inc.
SUITE 300 E, OPUS CENTER
9900 BREN ROAD EAST
MINNETONKA, MN 55343-9667

For Medical Information Contact:
Generally:
Medical Affairs
(800) 562-5580
FAX: (612) 935-0468

In Emergencies:
Medical Affairs
(800) 562-5580
FAX: (612) 935-0468

DIDRONEL® I.V. INFUSION ℞
(etidronate disodium)
DILUTE BEFORE USE

DESCRIPTION

Didronel I.V. Infusion is a clear, colorless, sterile solution of etidronate disodium, the disodium salt of (1-hydroxyethylidene) diphosphonic acid. Each 6-ml ampule contains a 5% solution of 300 mg etidronate disodium in water for injection for slow intravenous infusion.
Etidronate disodium is a white powder, highly soluble in water, with a molecular weight of 250 and the following structural formula:

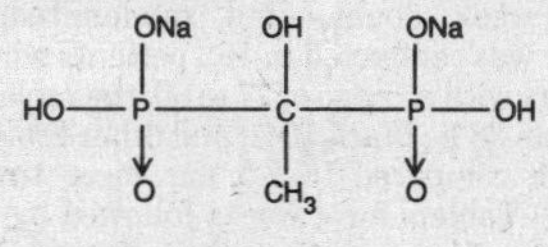

CLINICAL PHARMACOLOGY

Didronel acts primarily on bone. Its major pharmacologic action is the reduction of normal and abnormal bone resorption. Secondarily, it reduces bone formation since formation is coupled to resorption. This reduces bone turnover, but the reduction of bone turnover, *per se*, is not the important action in the reduction of hypercalcemia.
Didronel's reduction of abnormal bone resorption is responsible for its therapeutic benefit in hypercalcemia. The antiresorptive action of Didronel has been demonstrated under a variety of conditions, although the exact mechanism(s) is not fully understood. It may be related to the drug's inhibition of hydroxyapatite crystal dissolution and/or its action on bone resorbing cells. The number of osteoclasts in active bone turnover sites is substantially reduced after Didronel therapy is administered. Didronel also can inhibit the formation and growth of hydroxyapatite crystals and their amorphous precursors at concentrations in excess of those required to inhibit crystal dissolution.
Etidronate disodium is not metabolized. A large fraction of the infused dose is excreted rapidly and unchanged in the urine. The mean residence time in the exchangeable pool is approximately 8.7 ± 1.0 hours. The mean volume of distribution at steady-state in normal humans is 1370 ± 203 ml/kg while the plasma half-life ($t\frac{1}{2}$) is 6.0 ± 0.7 hours. In these same subjects, nonrenal clearance from the exchangeable pool amounts to 30–50% of the infused dose. This nonrenal clearance is considered to be due to uptake of the drug by bone; subsequently the drug is slowly eliminated through bone turnover. The half-life of the dose on bone is in excess of 90 days.
Hyperphosphatemia, which is often observed in association with oral Didronel medication at doses of 10–20 mg/kg/day, occurs less frequently, in association with intravenous medication of patients with hypercalcemia of malignancy.
Hyperphosphatemia is apparently due to increased tubular reabsorption of phosphate by the kidney. No adverse effects have been associated with Didronel-related hyperphosphatemia and its occurrence is not a contraindication to therapy. Serum phosphate elevations usually return to normal 2–4 weeks after medication is discontinued.
The responsiveness of animal tumors susceptible to four commonly employed classes or subclasses of chemotherapeutic agents, antitumor antibiotics (doxorubicin), a classic alkylating agent (cyclophosphamide), a nitrosourea (carmustine), and a pyrimidine antagonist (5-fluorouracil), were not adversely altered by the concurrent administration of intravenous Didronel.
Hypercalcemia of Malignancy: Hypercalcemia of malignancy is usually related to increased bone resorption associated with the presence of neoplastic tissue. It occurs in 8 to 20% of patients with malignant disease. Whereas hypercalcemia is more often seen in patients with demonstrable osteolytic, osteoblastic, or mixed metastatic tumors in bone, discrete skeletal lesions cannot be demonstrated in at least 30% of patients.
Patients with certain types of neoplasms, such as carcinoma of the breast, bronchogenic carcinoma, renal cell carcinoma, cancers of the head and neck, lymphomas, and multiple myeloma, are especially prone to developing hypercalcemia.
As hypercalcemia of malignancy evolves, the renal tubules develop a diminished capacity to concentrate urine. The resultant polyuria and nocturia decrease the extracellular fluid volume. This decrease may be aggravated by vomiting and reduced fluid intake. Thus, the ability of the kidney to eliminate excess calcium is compromised. Renal impairment can eventually cause nitrogen retention, acidosis, renal failure, and further decrease in excretion of calcium. Didronel I.V. Infusion, by inhibiting excessive bone resorption, interrupts this process. Salt loading and use of "high ceiling" or "loop" diuretics may be used to promote calcium excretion, because the rate of renal calcium excretion is directly related to the rate of sodium excretion.
The physiologic derangements induced by excessive serum calcium are due to increased levels of ionized calcium. The pathophysiologic effects of excessive serum calcium are heightened by reductions in serum albumin which normally binds a fraction (about 40%) of the total serum calcium. In patients with hypercalcemia of malignancy, serum albumin is often reduced and this tends to mask the magnitude of the increase in the level of ionized calcium. By reducing the flow of calcium from resorbing bone, Didronel I.V. Infusion effectively reduces total and ionized serum calcium.
In the principal clinical study of Didronel for hypercalcemia of malignancy, patients with elevated calcium levels (10.1–17.4 mg/dl) were treated simultaneously with daily administrations of intravenous Didronel over a 3-day period and up to 3000 ml of saline and 80 mg of loop diuretic. The response to treatment for these patients was compared with that from patients treated with saline and loop diuretics alone. In terms of total serum calcium changes, 88% of patients treated with Didronel I.V. Infusion as described, had reductions of serum calcium of 1 mg/dl or more. Total serum calcium returned to normal in 63% of patients within 7 days compared to 33% of patients treated with hydration alone.
Reductions in urinary calcium excretion, which accompany reductions in excessive bone resorption, became apparent after 24 hours. This was accompanied or followed by maximum decreases in serum calcium which were observed, most frequently, 72 hours after the first infusion.
The physiologically important component of serum calcium is the ionized portion. In most institutions, this cannot be measured directly. It is important to recognize that factors influencing the ratio of free and bound calcium such as serum proteins, particularly albumin, may complicate the interpretation of total serum calcium measurements. If indicated, a corrected serum calcium value should be calculated using an established algorithm.
When the total serum calcium values are adjusted for serum albumin levels, there was a return to normocalcemia in 24% of Didronel-treated patients and in 7% of patients treated with saline infusion. Eighty-seven percent of patients receiving Didronel and 67% of patients on saline had albumin-adjusted serum calcium levels returned to normal or reduced by at least 1 mg/dl.
In the above mentioned study, a second course of Didronel I.V. Infusion was tried in a small number of patients who had a recurrence of hypercalcemia following an initial response to a 3-day infusion of the drug. All patients who received a second 3-day course of Didronel I.V. Infusion showed a decrease of total serum calcium of at least 1 mg/dl. Normalization of total serum calcium occurred in 11 out of 14 patients.
Didronel I.V. Infusion does not appear to alter renal tubular reabsorption of calcium, and does not affect hypercalcemia in patients with hyperparathyroidism where increased calcium reabsorption may be a factor in the hypercalcemia.
Limited clinical study results suggest that continuation of Didronel therapy with oral tablets may maintain clinically acceptable serum calcium levels and prolong normocalcemia.

INDICATIONS AND USAGE

Didronel I.V. Infusion, together with achievement and maintenance of adequate hydration, is indicated for the treatment of hypercalcemia of malignancy inadequately managed by dietary modification and/or oral hydration.
In the treatment of hypercalcemia of malignancy, it is important to initiate rehydration with saline together with "high ceiling" or "loop" diuretics if indicated to restore urine output. This also is intended to increase the renal excretion of calcium and initiate a reduction in serum calcium. Since increased bone resorption is usually the underlying cause of an increased flux of calcium into the vascular compartment, concurrent therapy with Didronel I.V. Infusion is recommended as soon as there is a restoration of urine output. Since Didronel is excreted by the kidney, it is important to know that renal function is adequate to handle not only the increased fluid load but also the excretion of the drug itself. (See WARNINGS.)
Didronel I.V. Infusion is also indicated for the treatment of hypercalcemia of malignancy which persists after adequate hydration has been restored. Patients with and without metastases and with a variety of tumors have been responsive to treatment with Didronel I.V. Infusion. Adequate hydration of patients should be maintained, but in aged patients and in those with cardiac failure, care must be taken to avoid overhydration.

CONTRAINDICATIONS

In patients with Class Dc and higher renal functional impairment (serum creatinine greater than 5.0 mg/dl) Didronel I.V. Infusion should be withheld.

WARNINGS

Occasional mild to moderate abnormalities in renal function (elevated BUN and/or serum creatinine) have been observed when Didronel I.V. Infusion was given as directed to patients with hypercalcemia of malignancy. These changes were reversible or remained stable, without worsening, after completion of the course of Didronel I.V. Infusion. In some patients with pre-existing renal impairment or in those who had received potentially nephrotoxic drugs, further depression of renal function was sometimes seen. This suggests that Didronel I.V. Infusion may produce or aggravate the depression of renal function in approximately 8 of 203 treatment courses when used to treat hypercalcemia of malignancy. Therefore, it is recommended that appropriate monitoring of renal function with serum creatinine and/or BUN be carried out with Didronel I.V. Infusion treatment.
The effects of Didronel I.V. Infusion administration on renal function in patients with serum creatinine greater than 2.5 mg/dl (Class Cc and higher, Classification of Renal Functional Impairment, Council on the Kidney in Cardiovascular Disease, American Heart Association, Ann. Int. Med. 75:251–52, 1971) has not been systematically examined in controlled trials.
Since Didronel is excreted by the kidney, it is important to know that renal function is adequate to handle not only the increased fluid load but also the excretion of the drug itself. Since these capacities are impaired in patients with underlying renal disease and since experience with Didronel I.V. Infusion in patients with serum creatinine >2.5 mg/dl is limited, the use of Didronel I.V. Infusion in such patients should occur only after a careful assessment of renal status or potential risks and potential benefits. (See WARNINGS.)
Reduction of the dose of Didronel I.V. Infusion, if used at all, may be advisable in Class Cc renal functional impairment (serum creatinine 2.5 to 4.9 mg/dl); and, Didronel I.V. Infusion be used only if the potential benefit of hypercalcemia correction will substantially exceed the potential for worsening of renal function. In patients with Class Dc and higher renal functional impairment (serum creatinine greater than 5.0 mg/dl) Didronel I.V. Infusion should be withheld.

PRECAUTIONS

General: Hypercalcemia may cause or exacerbate impaired renal function. In clinical trials, while elevations of serum creatinine or blood urea nitrogen were seen in patients with hypercalcemia of malignancy prior to treatment with Didronel I.V. Infusion, these measurements improved in some patients or remained unchanged in most patients. Nevertheless, elevations in serum creatinine during treatment with Didronel I.V. Infusion have been observed in approximately 10% of patients.
Rare cases of acute renal failure have been reported in association with the use of Didronel I.V. Infusion (See also WARNINGS). Concomitant use of non-steroidal anti-inflam-

Continued on next page

MGI Pharma—Cont.

matory drugs and diuretics in these patients may have contributed to the renal failure.
In animal preclinical studies, administration of Didronel I.V. Infusion in amounts or at rates in excess of those recommended produced transient hypocalcemia or induced proximal renal tubular damage.
In the principal clinical trial of Didronel I.V. Infusion, 33 of 185 patients (18%) treated one or more times with Didronel I.V. Infusion had serum calcium values below the lower limits of normal. When adjusted for levels of reduced serum albumin, less than 1% of the 185 patients are estimated to have hypocalcemic ionized serum calcium levels. No adverse effects have been traced to hypocalcemia.
The hypercalcemia of hyperparathyroidism is refractory to Didronel I.V. Infusion. It is possible for this disease to coexist in patients with malignancy.
Carcinogenesis, Mutagenesis, Impairment of Fertility: Long-term studies in rats indicate that Didronel is not carcinogenic.
Pregnancy: Teratogenic Effects: Pregnancy Category C. Animal reproduction studies have not been conducted with Didronel I.V. Infusion. It is also not known whether Didronel I.V. Infusion can cause fetal harm when administered to a pregnant woman or can affect reproduction capacity. Didronel I.V. Infusion should be given to a pregnant woman only if clearly needed.
Nursing Mothers: It is not known whether this drug is excreted in human milk. Because many drugs are excreted in human milk, caution should be exercised when Didronel I.V. Infusion is administered to a nursing woman.
Pediatric Use: Safety and effectiveness in children have not been established.

ADVERSE REACTIONS

Hypercalcemia of malignancy is frequently associated with abnormal elevations of serum creatinine and BUN. One-third of the patients participating in multiclinic trials had such elevations before receiving Didronel I.V. Infusion. In these trials, the elevations of BUN or serum creatinine improved in some patients, or remained unchanged in most patients; however, in approximately 10% of patients, occasional mild to moderate abnormalities in renal function (increases of > 0.5 mg/dl serum creatinine) were observed during or immediately after treatment. The possibility that Didronel I.V. Infusion contributed to these changes cannot be excluded (see WARNINGS).
Of patients who participated in the controlled hypercalcemia trials, 10 of 221 (5%) treatment courses reported a metallic or altered taste, or loss of taste, which usually disappeared within hours, during and/or shortly after Didronel I.V. Infusion. A few patients with Paget's Disease of bone have reported allergic skin rashes in association with oral Didronel medication.

OVERDOSAGE

Rapid intravenous administration of Didronel at doses above 27 mg/kg has produced ECG changes and bleeding problems in animals. These abnormalities are probably related to marked and/or rapid decreases in ionized calcium levels in blood and tissue fluids. They are thought to be due to chelation of calcium by massive amounts of diphosphonate. These abnormalities have been shown to be reversible in animal studies by the administration of ionizable calcium salts.
Similar problems are not expected to occur in humans treated with Didronel I.V. Infusion used as recommended (see DOSAGE AND ADMINISTRATION). Moreover, signs and symptoms of hypocalcemia such as paresthesias and carpopedal spasms have not been reported. The chelation effects of the diphosphonate, should they occur in man, should be reversible with the intravenous administration of calcium gluconate.
Administration of intravenous etidronate disodium at doses and possibly at rates in excess of those recommended has been reported to be associated with renal insufficiency.

DOSAGE AND ADMINISTRATION

Didronel I.V. Infusion: The recommended dose of Didronel I.V. Infusion is 7.5 mg/kg body weight/day for three successive days. **This daily dose must be diluted in at least 250 ml of sterile normal saline.** Stability studies show that diluted solution stored at controlled room temperature (59°F to 86°F or 15°C to 30°C) shows no loss of drug for a 48-hour period.
THE DILUTED DOSE OF DIDRONEL I.V. INFUSION SHOULD BE ADMINISTERED INTRAVENOUSLY OVER A PERIOD OF AT LEAST 2 HOURS. Didronel I.V. Infusion may be added to volumes of sterile normal saline greater than 250 ml when this is convenient.
REGARDLESS OF THE VOLUME OF SOLUTION IN WHICH DIDRONEL I.V. INFUSION IS DILUTED, SLOW INFUSION IS IMPORTANT TO SAFETY. The minimum infusion time of two hours at the recommended dose, or smaller doses, should be observed. The usual course of treatment is one infusion of 7.5 mg/kg body weight/day on each of 3 consecutive days but some patients have been treated for up to 7 days. When patients are treated for more than 3 days, there may be an increased possibility of producing hypocalcemia.
Retreatment with Didronel I.V. Infusion may be appropriate if hypercalcemia recurs. There should be at least a seven-day interval between courses of treatment with Didronel I.V. Infusion. The dose and manner of retreatment is the same as that for initial treatment. Retreatment for more than three days has not been adequately studied. The safety and efficacy of more than two courses of therapy with Didronel I.V. Infusion have not been studied. In the presence of renal impairment, reduction of the dose may be advisable.
Parenteral drug products should be inspected visually for particulate matter and discoloration prior to administration whenever solution and container permit.
Didronel Oral Tablets: Didronel (etidronate disodium) tablets may be started on the day following the last dose of Didronel I.V. Infusion. The recommended oral dose of Didronel for patients who have had hypercalcemia is 20 mg/kg body weight/day for 30 days. If serum calcium levels remain normal or at clinically acceptable levels, treatment may be extended. Treatment for more than 90 days has not been adequately studied and is not recommended. Please consult the package insert pertaining to oral Didronel tablets for additional prescribing information.

HOW SUPPLIED

Didronel I.V. Infusion is supplied in 6 ml ampules as a 5% solution containing 300 mg etidronate disodium.
NDC 58063-457-01 carton of 6 ampules.
Avoid excessive heat (over 104°F or 40°c) for undiluted product.
Address medical inquires to **MGI PHARMA**, Medical Department, Suite 300E, Opus Center, 9900 Bren Road East, Minnetonka, MN 55343-9667.
CAUTION: Federal law prohibits dispensing without prescription.
Didronel® is a registered trademark of Procter & Gamble Pharmaceuticals, Inc.
Manufactured by
Taylor Pharmacal Company
Decatur, Illinois 62525
for **MGI PHARMA, INC.**
Minnetonka, Minnesota 55343-9667
JULY 1994

Shown in Product Identification Guide, page 322

SALAGEN® TABLETS ℞

[*sal 'ə gən*]
(pilocarpine hydrochloride)

DESCRIPTION

SALAGEN® Tablets contain pilocarpine hydrochloride, a cholinergic agonist for oral use. Pilocarpine hydrochloride is a hygroscopic, odorless, bitter tasting white crystal or powder which is soluble in water and alcohol and virtually insoluble in most non-polar solvents. Pilocarpine hydrochloride, with a chemical name of 2(3H)-Furanone, 3-ethyldihydro-4-[(1-methyl-1H-imidazol-5-yl)methyl] -monohydrochloride, (3S-cis), has a molecular weight of 244.72.

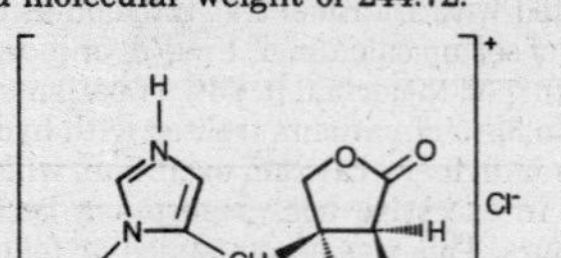

Each SALAGEN® Tablet for oral administration contains 5 mg of pilocarpine hydrochloride. Inactive ingredients in the tablet, the tablet's film coating, polishing, and branding are: carnauba wax, hydroxypropyl methylcellulose, iron oxide, microcrystalline cellulose, stearic acid, titanium dioxide and other ingredients.

CLINICAL PHARMACOLOGY

Pharmacodynamics: Pilocarpine is a cholinergic parasympathomimetic agent exerting a broad spectrum of pharmacologic effects with predominant muscarinic action. Pilocarpine, in appropriate dosage, can increase secretion by the exocrine glands. The sweat, salivary, lacrimal, gastric, pancreatic, and intestinal glands and the mucous cells of the respiratory tract may be stimulated. When applied topically to the eye as a single dose it causes miosis, spasm of accommodation, and may cause a transitory rise in intraocular pressure followed by a more persistent fall. Dose-related smooth muscle stimulation of the intestinal tract may cause increased tone, increased motility, spasm, and tenesmus. Bronchial smooth muscle tone may increase. The tone and motility of urinary tract, gallbladder, and biliary duct smooth muscle may be enhanced. Pilocarpine may have paradoxical effects on the cardiovascular system. The expected effect of a muscarinic agonist is vasodepression, but administration of pilocarpine may produce hypertension after a brief episode of hypotension. Bradycardia and tachycardia have both been reported with use of pilocarpine.
In a study in 12 healthy male volunteers there was a dose-related increase in unstimulated salivary flow following single 5 and 10 mg oral doses of SALAGEN® Tablets. The stimulatory effect was time-related with an onset at 20 minutes and peak at 1 hour with a duration of 3 to 5 hours. (See Pharmacokinetics section.)
In a 12 week randomized, double-blind, placebo-controlled study in 207 patients (placebo, N=65; 5 mg, N=73; 10 mg, N=69), increases from baseline (means 0.072 and 0.112 mL/min, ranges −0.690 to 0.728 and −0.380 to 1.689) of whole saliva flow for the 5 mg (63%) and 10 mg (90%) tablet, respectively, were seen 1 hour after the first dose of SALAGEN® Tablets. Increases in unstimulated parotid flow were seen following the first dose (means 0.025 and 0.046 mL/min, ranges 0 to 0.414 and −0.070 to 1.002 mL/min for the 5 and 10 mg dose, respectively). In this study, no correlation existed between the amount of increase in salivary flow and the degree of symptomatic relief. (See Clinical Studies section for details.)
Pharmacokinetics: In a multiple-dose pharmacokinetic study in male volunteers following 2 days of 5 or 10 mg of oral pilocarpine hydrochloride tablets given at 8 a.m., noontime, and 6 p.m., the mean elimination half-life was 0.76 hours for the 5 mg dose and 1.35 hours for the 10 mg dose. T_{max} values were 1.25 hours and 0.85 hours. C_{max} values were 15 ng/mL and 41 ng/mL. The AUC trapezoidal values were 33 h(ng/mL) and 108 h(ng/mL), respectively, for the 5 and 10 mg doses following the last 6 hour dose.
Pharmacokinetics in elderly male volunteers (n=11) were comparable to those in younger men. In five healthy elderly female volunteers, the mean C_{max} and AUC were approximately twice that of elderly males and young normal male volunteers.
When taken with a high fat meal by 12 healthy male volunteers, there was a decrease in the rate of absorption of pilocarpine from SALAGEN® Tablets. Mean $T_{max's}$ were 1.47 and 0.87 hours, and mean $C_{max's}$ were 51.8 and 59.2 ng/mL for fed and fasted, respectively.
Limited information is available about the metabolism and elimination of pilocarpine in humans. Inactivation of pilocarpine is thought to occur at neuronal synapses and probably in plasma. Pilocarpine and its minimally active or inactive degradation products, including pilocarpic acid, are excreted in the urine.
Clinical Studies: A 12 week randomized, double-blind, placebo-controlled study in 207 patients (142 men, 65 women) was conducted in patients whose mean age was 58.5 years with a range of 19 to 77; the racial distribution was Caucasian 95%, Black 4%, and other 1%. In this population, a statistically significant improvement in mouth dryness occurred in the 5 and 10 mg SALAGEN® Tablet treated patients compared to placebo treated patients. The 5 and 10 mg treated patients could not be distinguished. (See Pharmacodynamics section for flow study details.)
Another 12 week, double-blind, randomized, placebo-controlled study was conducted in 162 patients whose mean age was 57.8 years with a range of 27 to 80; the racial distribution was Caucasian 88%, Black 10%, and other 2%. The effects of placebo were compared to 2.5 mg three times a day of SALAGEN® Tablets for 4 weeks followed by titration to 5 mg three times a day and 10 mg three times a day. Lowering of the dose was necessary because of adverse events in 3 of 67 patients treated with 5 mg of SALAGEN® Tablets and in 7 of 66 patients treated with 10 mg of SALAGEN® Tablets. After 4 weeks of treatment, 2.5 mg of SALAGEN® Tablets three times a day was comparable to placebo in relieving dryness. In patients treated with 5 mg and 10 mg of SALAGEN® Tablets, the greatest improvement in dryness was noted in patients with no measurable salivary flow at baseline.
In both studies, some patients noted improvement in the global assessment of their xerostomia, speaking without liquids, and a reduced need for supplemental oral comfort agents.
In the two placebo-controlled clinical trials, the most common adverse events related to drug, and increasing in rate as dose increases, were sweating, nausea, rhinitis, chills, flushing, urinary frequency, dizziness, and asthenia. The most common adverse experience causing withdrawal from treatment was sweating (5 mg= <1%; 10 mg=12%).

INDICATIONS AND USAGE

SALAGEN® Tablets are indicated for the treatment of symptoms of xerostomia from salivary gland hypofunction caused by radiotherapy for cancer of the head and neck.

CONTRAINDICATIONS

SALAGEN® Tablets are contraindicated in patients with uncontrolled asthma, known hypersensitivity to pilocarpine, and when miosis is undesirable, e.g., in acute iritis and in narrow-angle (angle closure) glaucoma.

WARNINGS

Cardiovascular Disease: Patients with significant cardiovascular disease may be unable to compensate for transient changes in hemodynamics or rhythm induced by pilocarpine. Pulmonary edema has been reported as a complication of pilocarpine toxicity from high ocular doses given for acute angle-closure glaucoma. Pilocarpine should be administered with caution in and under close medical supervision of patients with cardiovascular disease.

Ocular: Careful examination of the fundus should be carried out prior to initiating therapy with pilocarpine. An association of ocular pilocarpine use and retinal detachment in patients with preexisting retinal disease has been reported. The systemic blood level that is associated with this finding is not known.

Ocular formulations of pilocarpine have been reported to cause visual blurring which may result in decreased visual acuity, especially at night and in patients with central lens changes, and to cause impairment of depth perception. Caution should be advised while driving at night or performing hazardous activities in reduced lighting.

Pulmonary Disease: Pilocarpine has been reported to increase airway resistance, bronchial smooth muscle tone, and bronchial secretions. Pilocarpine hydrochloride should be administered with caution to and under close medical supervision in patients with controlled asthma, chronic bronchitis, or chronic obstructive pulmonary disease.

PRECAUTIONS

General: Pilocarpine toxicity is characterized by an exaggeration of its parasympathomimetic effects. These may include: headache, visual disturbance, lacrimation, sweating, respiratory distress, gastrointestinal spasm, nausea, vomiting, diarrhea, atrioventricular block, tachycardia, bradycardia, hypotension, hypertension, shock, mental confusion, cardiac arrhythmia, and tremors.

The dose-related cardiovascular pharmacologic effects of pilocarpine include hypotension, hypertension, bradycardia, and tachycardia.

Pilocarpine should be administered with caution to patients with known or suspected cholelithiasis or biliary tract disease. Contractions of the gallbladder or biliary smooth muscle could precipitate complications including cholecystitis, cholangitis, and biliary obstruction.

Pilocarpine may increase ureteral smooth muscle tone and could theoretically precipitate renal colic (or "ureteral reflux"), particularly in patients with nephrolithiasis.

Cholinergic agonists may have dose-related central nervous system effects. This should be considered when treating patients with underlying cognitive or psychiatric disturbances.

Renal Insufficiency: The pharmacokinetics of orally administered pilocarpine in patients with renal and hepatic disease is not known.

Information for Patients: Patients should be informed that pilocarpine may cause visual disturbances, especially at night, that could impair their ability to drive safely.

If a patient sweats excessively while taking pilocarpine hydrochloride and cannot drink enough liquid, the patient should consult a physician. Dehydration may develop.

Drug Interactions: Pilocarpine should be administered with caution to patients taking beta adrenergic antagonists because of the possibility of conduction disturbances. Drugs with parasympathomimetic effects administered concurrently with pilocarpine would be expected to result in additive pharmacologic effects. Pilocarpine might antagonize the anticholinergic effects of drugs used concomitantly. These effects should be considered when anticholinergic properties may be contributing to the therapeutic effect of concomitant medication (e.g., atropine, inhaled ipratropium).

Carcinogenesis, Mutagenesis, Impairment of Fertility: No definitive long term animal studies have evaluated the carcinogenic potential of pilocarpine hydrochloride.

No evidence that pilocarpine hydrochloride has the potential to cause genetic toxicity was obtained in a series of studies that included: 1) bacterial assays (Salmonella and E. coli) for reverse gene mutations; 2) an *in vitro* chromosome aberration assay in a Chinese hamster ovary cell line; 3) an *in vivo* chromosome aberration assay (micronucleus test) in mice; and 4) a primary DNA damage assay (unscheduled DNA synthesis) in rat hepatocyte primary cultures. In a published report, male rats who received pilocarpine at a dosage of 39 mg/kg/day (approximately 11 times the maximum recommended dose for a 60 kg human based upon body surface area [mg/m^2] estimates) exhibited morphologic evidence of reduced spermatogenesis. The possibility that pilocarpine may impair male fertility in humans cannot be excluded. The effects of pilocarpine on male and female fertility in humans have not been systematically studied.

Pregnancy Category C: Pilocarpine hydrochloride was associated with a reduction in the mean fetal body weight and an increase in the incidence of skeletal variations when given to pregnant rats at a dosage of 90 mg/kg/day (approximately 26 times the maximum recommended dose for a 60 kg human based upon body surface area [mg/m^2] estimates). These effects may have been secondary to maternal toxicity.

There are no adequate and well-controlled studies in pregnant women. SALAGEN® Tablets should be used during pregnancy only if the potential benefit justifies the potential risk to the fetus.

Nursing Mothers: It is not known whether this drug is excreted in human milk. Because many drugs are excreted in human milk and because of the potential for serious adverse reactions in nursing infants from SALAGEN® Tablets, a decision should be made whether to discontinue nursing or to discontinue the drug, taking into account the importance of the drug to the mother.

Pediatrics: Safety and effectiveness of this drug in children have not been established.

Geriatric Use: In the placebo-controlled clinical trials (see Clinical Studies section) the mean age of patients was approximately 58 years (range 19 to 80). Of these patients, 97/369 (61/217 receiving pilocarpine) were over the age of 65 years. In the healthy volunteer studies, 15/150 subjects were over the age of 65 years. In both study populations, the adverse events reported by those over 65 years and those 65 years and younger were comparable. Of the 15 elderly volunteers (5 women, 10 men), the 5 women had higher $C_{max's}$ and AUC's than the men. (See Pharmacokinetics section.)

ADVERSE REACTIONS

In controlled studies, 217 patients received pilocarpine, of whom 68% were men and 32% were women. Race distribution was 91% Caucasian, 8% Black, and 1% of other origin. Mean age was approximately 58 years. The majority of patients were between 50 and 64 years (51%), 33% were 65 years and older and 16% were younger than 50 years of age. The most frequent adverse experiences associated with SALAGEN® Tablets were a consequence of the expected pharmacologic effects of pilocarpine.

Adverse Event	Placebo t.i.d. n=152	5mg t.i.d. n=141	10mg t.i.d. n=121
Sweating	9%	29%	68%
Nausea	4	6	15
Rhinitis	7	5	14
Chills	<1	3	14
Flushing	3	8	13
Urinary Frequency	7	9	12
Dizziness	4	5	12
Asthenia	3	6	12

In addition, the following adverse events (≥1% incidence) were reported at doses of 5 and 10 mg in the controlled clinical trials:

Adverse Event	Placebo t.i.d. n=152	Pilocarpine HCl t.i.d. n=212
Headache	8%	11%
Dyspepsia	5	7
Lacrimation	8	6
Diarrhea	5	6
Edema	4	5
Abdominal Pain	4	4
Amblyopia	2	4
Vomiting	1	4
Pharyngitis	8	3
Hypertension	1	3
Conjunctivitis	4	2
Tachycardia	1	2
Epistaxis	1	2
Tremor	0	2
Dysphagia	<1	2
Voice Alteration	0	2
Rash	4	1
Taste Perversion	2	1
Sinusitis	2	1
Abnormal Vision	1	1
Myalgias	1	1
Pruritis	<1	1

The following events were reported rarely in treated patients (<1%). Causal relation is unknown.
Body as a whole: body odor, hypothermia, mucous membrane abnormality
Cardiovascular: bradycardia, ECG abnormality, palpitations, syncope
Digestive: anorexia, increased appetite, esophagitis, gastrointestinal disorder, tongue disorder
Hematologic: leukopenia, lymphadenopathy
Nervous: anxiety, confusion, depression, abnormal dreams, hyperkinesia, hypesthesia, nervousness, paresthesias, speech disorder, twitching

Respiratory: increased sputum, stridor, yawning
Skin: seborrhea
Special senses: deafness, eye pain, glaucoma
Urogenital: dysuria, metrorrhagia, urinary impairment
In long-term treatment were two patients with underlying cardiovascular disease of whom one experienced a myocardial infarct and another an episode of syncope. The association with drug is uncertain.
The following adverse experiences have been reported rarely with ocular pilocarpine: malignant glaucoma, macular hole, shock, middle ear disturbance, A-V block, depression, delusion, eyelid twitching, visual hallucination, confusion, agitation, dermatitis, ciliary congestion, and iris cysts.

MANAGEMENT OF OVERDOSE

Pilocarpine fatal overdosage resulting from poisoning has been reported in the scientific literature at doses presumed to be greater than 100 mg in two hospitalized patients. 100 mg of pilocarpine is considered potentially fatal. Overdosage should be treated with atropine titration (0.5 mg to 1.0 mg given subcutaneously or intravenously) and supportive measures to maintain respiration and circulation. Epinephrine (0.3 mg to 1.0 mg, subcutaneously or intramuscularly) may also be of value in the presence of severe cardiovascular depression or bronchoconstriction. It is not known if pilocarpine is dialyzable.

DOSAGE AND ADMINISTRATION

The recommended oral dose of SALAGEN® Tablets for the initiation of treatment is 5 mg three times a day. Titration up to 10 mg three times a day may be considered for patients who have not responded adequately and who can tolerate lower doses. The incidence of the most common adverse events increases with dose. The lowest dose that is tolerated and effective should be used for maintenance.

HOW SUPPLIED

SALAGEN® Tablets, 5 mg, are white, film coated, round tablets, coded MGI 705. Each tablet contains 5 mg pilocarpine hydrochloride. They are supplied as follows:
NDC 58063-705-10 bottles of 100
Store at Controlled Room Temperature 15°–30°C (59°–86°F).
Manufactured by:
Boehringer Ingelheim Pharmaceuticals, Inc., Ridgefield, CT 06877
For: MGI PHARMA, INC., Minnetonka, MN 55343–9667
© 1994 MGI PHARMA, INC.   March 1994
Salagen® is a registered trademark of MGI PHARMA, INC.
Shown in Product Identification Guide, page 322

3M Pharmaceuticals
3M CENTER 275-3W-01
P.O. BOX 33275
ST. PAUL, MN 55133-3275

Commercial Customers:
Orders, Returns, Accounting
(800) 447-4537

Trade and Government:
(800) 328-6523

For Medical Matters Contact:
Medical Services Department
3M Pharmaceuticals
3M Center, Bldg. 275-3E-09
PO Box 33275
St. Paul MN, 55133-3275
(800) 328-0255
In Emergencies:
(612) 736-4930 (all hours)

[See table at top of next page.]

ALU-TAB™ Tablets   OTC
(aluminum hydroxide)
and
ALU-CAP™ Capsules
(aluminum hydroxide)

For indications, actions, warnings, dosage, and precautions see container label or call 800-328-0255 for a copy.

HOW SUPPLIED

Bottles of 250 green film-coated Alu-Tab tablets (NDC **0089-0107-25**). Bottles of 100 red and green Alu-Cap capsules (NDC **0089-0105-10**).

Continued on next page

3M—Cont.

The following 3M Pharmaceutical products are available in Military depots:

Military Depot Items	National Stock Number
Norflex™ Tablets 100's	6505-00-138-8462
Norgesic™ Forte Tablets 500's	6505-01-029-9116
Tambocor™ 100 mg Tablets 100's	6505-01-240-5767

CALCIUM DISODIUM VERSENATE ℞
(edetate calcium disodium injection, USP)
STERILE
Injection

> **WARNINGS**
> Calcium Disodium Versenate is capable of producing toxic effects which can be fatal. Lead encephalopathy is relatively rare in adults, but occurs more often in children in whom it may be incipient and thus overlooked. The mortality rate in these children has been high. Patients with lead encephalopathy and cerebral edema may experience a lethal increase in intracranial pressure following intravenous infusion; the intramuscular route is preferred for these patients and for young children. In cases where the intravenous route is necessary, avoid rapid infusion. The dosage schedule should be followed and at no time should the recommended daily dose be exceeded.

DESCRIPTION

Calcium Disodium Versenate (edetate calcium disodium injection, USP) is a sterile, injectable, chelating agent in concentrated solution for intravenous infusion or intramuscular injection. Each 5 ml ampul contains 1000 mg of edetate calcium disodium [equivalent to 200 mg/ml] in water for injection. Chemically, this product is called [[N,N′,-1,2-ethanediylbis[N-(carboxymentyl)-glycinato]](4-)-N,N′,O, $O',O^N,O^{N'}$]-,disodium, hydrate, (OC-6-21)-Calciate(2-).

Structural Formula:

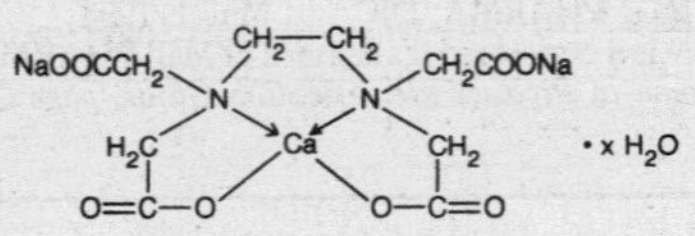

$C_{10}H_{10}CaN_2Na_2O_8 \cdot xH_2O$
Molecular weight 374.27 (anhydrous)

CLINICAL PHARMACOLOGY

The pharmacologic effects of edetate calcium disodium are due to the formation of chelates with divalent and trivalent metals. A stable chelate will form with any metal that has the ability to displace calcium from the molecule, a feature shared by lead, zinc, cadmium, manganese, iron and mercury. The amounts of manganese and iron mobilized are not significant. Copper[1] is not mobilized and mercury is unavailable for chelation because it is too tightly bound to body ligands or it is stored in inaccessible body compartments. The excretion of calcium by the body is not increased following intravenous administration of edetate calcium disodium, but the excretion of zinc is considerably increased.[1]

Edetate calcium disodium is poorly absorbed from the gastrointestinal tract. In blood, all the drug is found in the plasma. Edetate calcium disodium does not appear to penetrate cells; it is distributed primarily in the extracellular fluid with only about 5% of the plasma concentration found in spinal fluid.

The half life of edetate calcium disodium is 20 to 60 minutes. It is excreted primarily by the kidney, with about 50% excreted in one hour and over 95% within 24 hours.[2] Almost none of the compound is metabolized.

The primary source of lead chelated by Calcium Disodium Versenate is from bone; subsequently, soft-tissue lead is redistributed to bone when chelation is stopped.[3,4] There is also some reduction in kidney lead levels following chelation therapy.

It has been shown in animals that following a single dose of Calcium Disodium Versenate urinary lead output increases, blood lead concentration decreasees, but brain lead is significantly increased due to internal redistribution of lead.[5] (See WARNINGS.) These data are in agreement with the recent results of others in experimental animals showing that after a five day course of treatment there is no net reduction in brain lead.[6]

INDICATIONS AND USAGE

Edetate calcium disodium is indicated for the reduction of blood levels and depot stores of lead in lead poisoning (acute and chronic) and lead encephalopathy, in both children and adults.

Chelation therapy should not replace effective measures to eliminate or reduce further exposure to lead.

CONTRAINDICATIONS

Edetate calcium disodium should not be given during periods of anuria, nor to patients with active renal disease or hepatitis.

WARNINGS

See boxed warning.

PRECAUTIONS

General Precautions: Edetate calcium disodium may produce the same renal damage as lead poisoning, such as proteinuria and microscopic hematuria. Treatment-induced nephrotoxicity is dose-dependent and may be reduced by assuring adequate diuresis before therapy begins. Urine flow must be monitored throughout therapy which must be stopped if anuria or severe olyguria develop. The proximal tubule hydropic degeneration usually recovers upon cessation of therapy. Edetate calcium disodium must be used in reduced doses in patients with pre-existing mild renal disease.

Patients should be monitored for cardiac rhythm irregularities and other ECG changes during intravenous therapy.

Information for patients: Patients should be instructed to immediately inform their physician if urine output stops for a period of 12 hours.

Laboratory Tests: Urinarlysis and urine sediment, renal and hepatic function and serum electrolyte levels should be checked before each course of therapy and then be monitored daily during therapy in severe cases, and in less serious cases after the second and fifth day of therapy. Therapy must be discontinued at the first sign of renal toxicity. The presence of large renal epithelial cells or increasing number of red blood cells in urinary sediment or greater proteinuria call for immediate stopping of edetate calcium disodium administration. Alkaline phosphatase values are frequently depressed (possibly due to decreased serum zinc levels), but return to normal within 48 hours after cessation of therapy. Elevated erythrocyte protoporphyrin levels (> 35 mcg/dl of whole blood) indicate the need to perform a venous blood lead determination. If the whole blood lead concentration is between 25–55 mcg/dl a mobilization test can be considered.[7,8] (See Diagnostic Test.) An elevation of urinary coproporphyrin (adults: > 250 mcg/day; children under 80 lbs: > 75 mcg/day) and elevation of urinary delta aminolevulinic acid (ALA) (adults: > 4 mg/day; children: > 3 mg/m²/day) are associated with blood lead levels > 40 mcg/dl. Urinary coproporphyrin may be falsely negative in terminal patients and in severely iron-depleted children who are not regenerating heme.[9] In growing children long bone x-rays showing lead lines and abdominal x-rays showing radio-opaque material in the abdomen may be of help in estimating the level of exposure to lead.

Drug Interactions: There is no known drug interference with standard clinical laboratory tests. Steroids enhance the renal toxicity of edetate calcium disodium in animals.[7] Edetate calcium disodium interferes with the action of zinc insulin preparations by chelating the zinc.[7]

Carcinogenesis, Mutagenesis, Impairment of Fertility: Long term animal studies have not been conducted with edetate calcium disodium to evaluate its carcinogenic potential, mutagenic potential or its effect on fertility.

Pregnancy: Category B: One reproduction study was performed in rats at doses up to 13 times the human dose and revealed no evidence of impaired fertility or harm to the fetus due to Caclium Disodium Versenate.[10] Another reproduction study performed in rats at doses up to about 25 to 40 times the human dose revealed evidence of fetal malformations due to Calcium Disodium Versenate, which were prevented by simultaneous supplementation of dietary zinc.[11] There are, however, no adequate and well-controlled studies in pregnant women. Because animal reproduction studies are not always predictive of human response, this drug should be used during pregnancy only if clearly needed.

Labor and Delivery: Calcium Disodium Versenate has no recognized use during labor and delivery, and its effects during these processes are unknown.

Nursing Mothers: It is not known whether this durg is excreted in human milk. Because many drugs are excreted in human milk, caution should be exercised when Calcium Disodium Versenate is administered to a nursing woman.

Pediatric Use: Since lead poisoning occurs in children and adults but is frequently more severe in children, Calcium Disodium Versenate is used in patients of all ages.

ADVERSE REACTIONS

The following adverse effects have been associated with the use of edetate calcium disodium:

Body as a Whole: pain at intramuscular injection site, fever, chills, malaise, fatigue, myalgia, arthralgia.
Cardiovascular: hypotension, cardiac rhythm irregularities.
Renal: acute necrosis of proximal tubules (which may result in fatal nephrosis), infrequent changes in distal tubules and glomeruli.
Urinary: glycosuria, proteinuria, microscopic hematuria and large epithelial cells in urinary sediment.
Nervous System: tremors, headache, numbness, tingling.
Gastrointestinal: cheilosis, nausea, vomiting, anorexia, excessive thirst.
Hepatic: mild increases in SGOT and SGPT are common, and return to normal within 48 hours after cessation of therapy.
Immunogenic: histamine-like reactions (sneezing, nasal congestion, lacrimation), rash.
Hematopoietic: transient bone marrow depression, anemia.
Metabolic: zinc deficiency, hypercalcemia.

OVERDOSAGE

Symptoms: Inadvertent administration of 5 times the recommended dose, infused intravenously over a 24 hour period, to an asymptomatic 16 month old patient with a blood lead content of 56 mcg/dl did not cause any ill effects. Edetate calcium disodium can aggravate the symptoms of severe lead poisoning, therefore, most toxic effects (cerebral edema, renal tubular necrosis) appear to be associated with lead poisoning. Because of cerebral edema, a therapeutic dose may be lethal to an adult or a child with lead encephalopathy. Higher dosage of edetate calcium disodium may produce a more severe zinc deficiency.

Treatment: Cerebral edema should be treated with repeated doses of mannitol. Steroids enhance the renal toxicity of edetate calcium disodium in animals and, therefore, are no longer recommended.[7] Zinc levels must be monitored. Good urinary output must be maintained because diuresis will enhance drug elimination. It is not known if edetate calcium disodium is dialyzable.

DOSAGE AND ADMINISTRATION

When a source for the lead intoxication has been identified, the patient should be removed from the source, if possible.

The recommended dose of Calcium Disodium Versenate for asymptomatic adults and children whose blood lead level is < 70 mcg/dl but > 20 mcg/dl (World Health Organization recommended upper allowable level) is 1000 mg/m²/day whether given intravenously or intramuscularly. (See Surface Area Nomogram.)

[See table at top of next page.]

For adults with lead nephropathy, the following dosage regimen has been suggested: 500 mg/m² every 24 hours for 5 days for patients with serum creatinine levels of 2–3 mg/dl, every 48 hours for 3 doses for patients with creatinine levels of 3–4 mg/dl, and once weekly for patients with creatinine levels above 4 mg/dl. These regimens may be repeated at one month intervals.[12]

Calcium Disodium Versenate, used alone, may aggravate symptoms in patients with very high blood lead levels. When the blood lead level is > 70 mcg/dl or clinical symptoms consistent with lead poisoning are present, it is recommended that Calcium Disodium Versenate be used in conjunction with BAL (dimercaprol). Please consult published protocols and specialized references for dosage recommendations of combination therapy.[14–18]

Therapy of lead poisoning in adults and children with Calcium Disodium Versenate is continued over a period of five days. Therapy is then interrupted for 2 to 4 days to allow redistribution of the lead and to prevent severe depletion of zinc and other essential metals. Two courses of treatment are usually employed; however, it depends on severity of the lead toxicity and the patient's tolerance of the drug.

Calcium Disodium Versenate is equally effective whether administered intravenously or intramuscularly. The intramuscular route is used for all patients with overt lead encephalopathy and this route is recommended for young children.

Acutely ill individuals may be dehydrated from vomiting. Since edetate calcium disodium is excreted almost exclusively in the urine, it is very important to establish urine flow with intravenous fluid administration before the first dose of the chelating agent is given; however, excessive fluid must be avoided in patients with encephalopathy. Once

SURFACE AREA NOMOGRAM

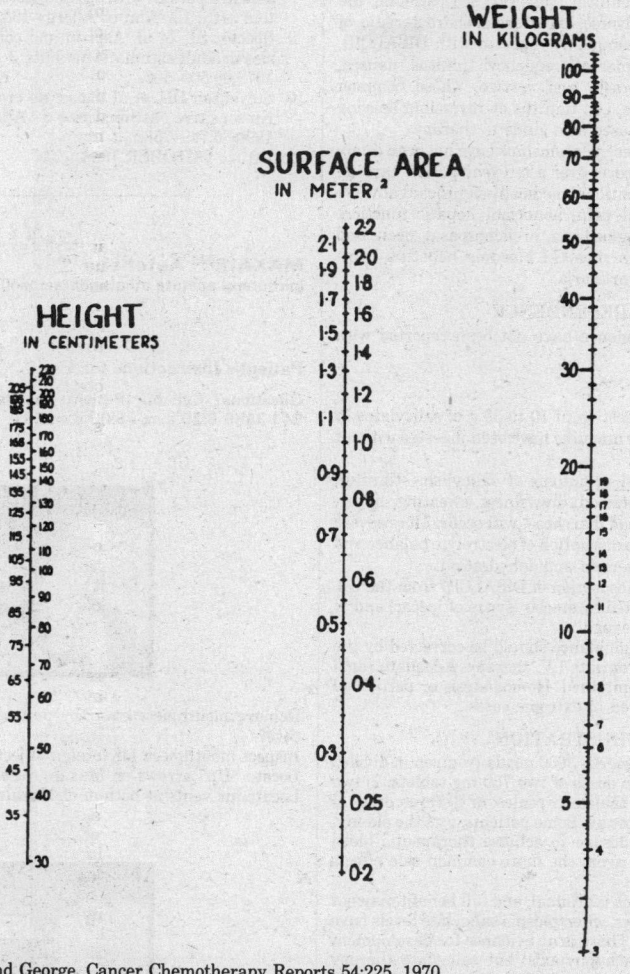

Drawn from Gehan and George, Cancer Chemotherapy Reports 54:225, 1970

urine flow is established, further intravenous fluid is restricted to basal water and electrolyte requirements. Administration of Calcium Disodium Versenate should be stopped whenever there is cessation of urine flow in order to avoid unduly high tissue levels of the drug. Edetate calcium disodium must be used in reduced doses in patients with pre-existing mild renal disease.

Intravenous Administration: Add the total daily dose of Calcium Disodium Versenate (1000 mg/m²/day) to 250–500 ml of 5% dextrose or 0.9% sodium chloride injection. The total daily dose should be infused over a period of 8–12 hours. Calcium Disodium Versenate injection is incompatible with 10% dextrose, 10% invert sugar in 0.9% sodium chloride, lactate Ringer's, Ringer's, one-sixth molar sodium lactate injections, and with injectable amphotericin B and hydralazine hydrochloride.

Intramuscular Administration: The total daily dosage (1000 mg/m²/day) should be divided into equal doses spaced 8–12 hours apart. Lidocaine or procaine should be added to the Calcium Disodium Versenate injection to minimize pain at the injection site. The final lidocaine or procaine concentration of 5 mg/ml (0.5%) can be obtained as follows: 0.25 ml of 10% lidocaine solution per 5 ml (entire content of ampul) concentrated Calcium Disodium Versenate; 1 ml of 1% lidocaine or procaine solution per ml of concentrated Calcium Disodium Versenate. When used alone, regardless of method of administration, Calcium Disodium Versenate should not be given at doses larger than those recommended.

Diagnostic Test: Several methods have been described for lead mobilization tests using edetate calcium disodium to assess body stores.[7,9,12,13,18]
These procedures have advantages and disadvantages that should be reviewed in current references. Edetate calcium disodium mobilization test should not be performed in symptomatic patients and in patients with blood lead levels above 55 mcg/dl for whom appropriate therapy is indicated.
Parenteral drug should be inspected visually for particulate matter and discoloration prior to administration, whenever solution and container permit.

HOW SUPPLIED

Calcium Disodium Versenate injection, 5 ml ampuls containing 200 mg of edetate calcium disodium per ml (1 g per ampul), in boxes containing 6 ampuls (NDC 0089-0510-06).

Store at controlled room temperature 15–30C degrees (59–86F degrees).

CAUTION

Federal law prohibits dispensing without prescription.

REFERENCES

1. Thomas DJ, Chisolm JJ. Lead, zinc and copper decorporation during calcium disodium ethylenediamine tetraacetate treatment of lead-poisoned children. J Pharmacol Exp Therapeu 1986; 239:829-835.
2. The Pharmacological Basis of Therapeutics, 7th edition, Goodman and Gilman, editors. Macmillan Publishing Company, New York, 1985, pp. 1619–1622.
3. Hammond PB, Aronson AL, Olson WC. The mechanism of mobilization of lead by ethylenediaminetetraacetate. J Pharmacol Exp Therapeu 1967; 157:196-206.
4. Van deVyver FL, D'Haese PC, Visser WJ, et al. Bone lead in dialysis patients. Kidney Intl 1988; 33:601-607.
5. Cory-Slecta DA, Weiss B, Cox C. Mobilization and redistribution of lead over the course of calcium disodium ethylenediamine tetraacetate chelation therapy. J Pharmacol Exp Therapeu 1987; 243:804-813.
6. Chisolm JJ. Mobilization of lead by calcium disodium edetate. Am J Dis Child 1987; 141:1256-1257.
7. Drug Evaluations, 6th Edition, American Medical Association, Saunders, Philadelphia, 1986, pp. 1637–1639.
8. Centers for Disease Control: Preventing lead poisoning in young children. Atlanta, GA, Department of Health and Human Services, 1985 Jan.
9. Finberg L, Rajagopal V. Diagnosis and treatment of lead poisoning in children. J Family Med 1985 April: 3–12.
10. Schardein JL, Sakowski R, Petrere J, et al. Teratogenesis studies with EDTA and its salts in rats. Toxicol Appl Pharmacol 1981; 61:423-428.
11. Swenerton H, Hurley LS. Teratogenic effects of a chelating agent and their prevention by zinc. Science 1971; 173:62-64.
12. American Hospital Formulary Service, Drug Information, 1988, pp. 1695–1698.
13. Markowitz ME, Rosen JF. Assessment of lead stores in children: Validation of an 8-hour CaNa₂EDTA (Calcium Disodium Versenate) provocative test. J Pediatrics 1984; 104:337-341.
14. Piomelli S, Rosen JF, Chisolm JJ, et al. Management of childhood lead poisoning. J Pediatrics 1984; 105:523-532.
15. Sachs HK, Blanksma LA, Murray EF, et al. Ambulatory treatment of lead poisoning: Report of 1,155 cases. Pediatrics 1970; 46:389.
16. Chisolm JJ. The use of chelating agents in the treatment of acute and chronic lead intoxication in childhood. J Pediatrics 1968; 73:1.
17. Coffin R, Phillips JL, Staples WI, et al. Treatment of lead encephalopathy in children. J Pediatrics 1966; 69: 198-206.
18. Chisolm JJ. Increased lead absorption and acute lead poisoning. Current Pediatric Therapy 12, Gillis and Kagan, editors, WB Saunders, Philadelphia, 1986, pp. 667–671.

Manufactured for
3M Pharmaceuticals
Northridge, CA 91324
By Sanofi Winthrop Pharmaceuticals
McPherson, Kansas 67460
C-161-14   SEPTEMBER 1992

DISALCID™   ℞
(salsalate)
Tablets and Capsules

DESCRIPTION

DISALCID (salsalate) is a nonsteroidal anti-inflammatory agent for oral administration. Chemically, salsalate (salicylsalicylic acid or 2-hydroxybenzoic acid, 2-carboxyphenyl ester) is a dimer of salicylic acid; its structural formula is shown below.
Chemical Structure:

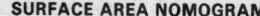

salsalate

Each DISALCID capsule contains 500 mg salsalate and also contains colloidal silicon dioxide, gelatin, magnesium stearate, pregelatinized starch, corn starch, titanium dioxide, FD&C blue #1, and D&C yellow #10.
Each DISALCID tablet contains 500 or 750 mg salsalate and also contains croscarmellose sodium, hydroxypropyl methylcellulose, magnesium stearate, microcrystalline cellulose, polyethylene glycol, polysorbate 80, propylene glycol, talc, titanium dioxide, FD&C blue #1, and D&C yellow #10. (See HOW SUPPLIED.)

CLINICAL PHARMACOLOGY

DISALCID is insoluble in acid gastric fluids (< 0.1 mg/ml at pH 1.0), but readily soluble in the small intestine where it is partially hydrolyzed to two molecules of salicylic acid. A significant portion of the parent compound is absorbed unchanged and undergoes rapid esterase hydrolysis in the body; its half-life is about one hour. About 13% is excreted through the kidneys as a glucuronide conjugate of the parent compound, the remainder as salicylic acid and its metabolites. Thus, the amount of salicylic acid available from DISALCID is about 15% less than from aspirin, when the two drugs are administered on a salicylic acid molar equivalent basis (3.6 g salsalate/5 g aspirin). Salicylic acid biotransformation is saturated at anti-inflammatory doses of DISALCID. Such capacity-limited biotransformation results in an increase in the half-life of salicylic acid from 3.5 to 16 or more hours. Thus, dosing with DISALCID twice a day will satisfactorily maintain blood levels within the desired therapeutic range (10 to 30 mg/100 ml) throughout the 12-hour intervals. Therapeutic blood levels continue for up to 16 hours after the last dose. The parent compound does not show capacity-limited biotransformation, nor does it accumulate in the plasma on multiple dosing. Food slows the absorption of all salicylates including DISALCID.
The mode of anti-inflammatory action of DISALCID and other nonsteroidal anti-inflammatory drugs is not fully defined. Although salicylic acid (the primary metabolite of DISALCID) is a weak inhibitor of prostaglandin synthesis in vitro, DISALCID appears to selectively inhibit prostaglandin synthesis **in vivo**,[1] providing anti-inflammatory activity equivalent to aspirin[2] and indomethacin.[3] Unlike aspirin, DISALCID does not inhibit platelet aggregation.[4]
The usefulness of salicylic acid, the active **in vivo** product of DISALCID, in the treatment of arthritic disorders has been established.[5,6] In contrast to aspirin, DISALCID causes no greater fecal gastrointestinal blood loss than placebo.[7]

Continued on next page

3M—Cont.

INDICATIONS AND USAGE
DISALCID is indicated for relief of the signs and symptoms of rheumatoid arthritis, osteoarthritis and related rheumatic disorders.

CONTRAINDICATIONS
DISALCID is contraindicated in patients hypersensitive to salsalate.

WARNINGS
Reye's Syndrome may develop in individuals who have chicken pox, influenza, or flu symptoms. Some studies suggest a possible association between the development of Reye's Syndrome and the use of medicines containing salicylate or apirin. DISALCID contains a salicylate and therefore is not recommended for use in patients with chicken pox, influenza, or flu symptoms.

PRECAUTIONS
General Precautions: Patients on treatment with DISALCID should be warned not to take other salicylates so as to avoid potentially toxic concentrations. Great care should be exercised when DISALCID is prescribed in the presence of chronic renal insufficiency or peptic ulcer disease. Protein binding of salicylic acid can be influenced by nutritional status, competitive binding of other drugs, and fluctuations in serum proteins caused by disease (rheumatoid arthritis, etc.).

Although cross reactivity, including bronchospasm, has been reported occasionally with non-acetylated salicylates, including salsalate, in aspirin-sensitive patients,[8,9] salsalate is less likely than aspirin to induce asthma in such patients.[10]

Laboratory Tests: Plasma salicylic acid concentrations should be periodically monitored during long-term treatment with DISALCID to aid maintenance of therapeutically effective levels: 10 to 30 mg/100 ml. Toxic manifestations are not usually seen until plasma concentrations exceed 30 mg/100 ml (see OVERDOSAGE). Urinary pH should also be regularly monitored: sudden acidification, as from pH 6.5 to 5.5, can double the plasma level, resulting in toxicity.

Drug Interactions: Salicylates antagonize the uricosuric action of drugs used to treat gout. ASPIRIN AND OTHER SALICYLATE DRUGS WILL BE ADDITIVE TO DISALCID AND MAY INCREASE PLASMA CONCENTRATIONS OF SALICYLIC ACID TO TOXIC LEVELS. Drugs and foods that raise urine pH will increase renal clearance and urinary excretion of salicylic acid, thus lowering plasma levels; acidifying drugs or foods will decrease urinary excretion and increase plasma levels. Salicylates given concomitantly with anticoagulant drugs may predispose to systemic bleeding. Salicylates may enhance the hypoglycemic effect of oral anti-diabetic drugs of the sulfonylurea class. Salicylate competes with a number of drugs for protein binding sites, notably penicillin, thiopental, thyroxine, triiodothyronine, phenytoin, sulfinpyrazone, naproxen, warfarin, methotrexate, and possibly corticosteroids.

Drug/Laboratory Test Interactions: Salicylate competes with thyroid hormone for binding to plasma proteins, which may be reflected in a depressed plasma T_4 value in some patients; thyroid function and basal metabolism are unaffected.

Carcinogenesis: No long-term animal studies have been performed with DISALCID to evaluate its carcinogenic potential.

Use in Pregnancy: Pregnancy Category C: Salsalate and salicylic acid have been shown to be teratogenic and embryocidal in rats when given in doses 4 to 5 times the usual human dose. These effects were not observed at doses twice as great as the usual human dose. There are no adequate and well-controlled studies in pregnant women. DISALCID should be used during pregnancy only if the potential benefit justifies the potential risk to the fetus.

Labor and Delivery: There exist no adequate and well-controlled studies in pregnant women. Although adverse effects on mother or infant have not been reported with DISALCID use during labor, caution is advised when anti-inflammatory dosage is involved. However, other salicylates have been associated with prolonged gestation and labor, maternal and neonatal bleeding sequelae, potentiation of narcotic and barbiturate effects (respiratory or cardiac arrest in the mother), delivery problems and stillbirth.

Nursing Mothers: It is not known whether salsalate per se is excreted in human milk; salicylic acid, the primary metabolite of DISALCID, has been shown to appear in human milk in concentrations approximating the maternal blood level. Thus, the infant of a mother on DISALCID therapy might ingest in mother's milk 30 to 80% as much salicylate per kg body weight as the mother is taking. Accordingly, caution should be exercised when DISALCID is administered to a nursing woman.

Pediatric Use: Safety and effectiveness of DISALCID use in children have not been established. (See WARNINGS section.)

ADVERSE REACTIONS
In two well-controlled clinical trials (n=280 patients), the following reversible adverse experiences characteristic of salicylates were most commonly reported with DISALCID, listed in descending order of frequency: tinnitus, nausea, hearing impairment, rash, and vertigo. These common symptoms of salicylates, i.e., tinnitus or reversible hearing impairment, are often used as a guide to therapy.

Although cause-and-effect relationships have not been established, spontaneous reports over a ten-year period have included the following additional medically significant adverse experiences: abdominal pain, abnormal hepatic function, anaphylactic shock, angioedema, bronchospasm, decreased creatinine clearance, diarrhea, G.I. bleeding, hepatitis, hypotension, nephritis and urticaria.

DRUG ABUSE AND DEPENDENCE
Drug abuse and dependence have not been reported with DISALCID.

OVERDOSAGE
Death has followed ingestion of 10 to 30 g of salicylates in adults, but much larger amounts have been ingested without fatal outcome.

Symptoms: The usual symptoms of salicylism—tinnitus, vertigo, headache, confusion, drowsiness, sweating, hyperventilation, vomiting and diarrhea—will occur. More severe intoxication will lead to disruption of electrolyte balance and blood pH, and hyperthermia and dehydration.

Treatment: Further absorption of DISALCID from the G.I. tract should be prevented by emesis (syrup of ipecac) and, if necessary, by gastric lavage.

Fluid and electrolyte imbalance should be corrected by the administration of appropriate I.V. therapy. Adequate renal function should be maintained. Hemodialysis or peritoneal dialysis may be required in extreme cases.

DOSAGE AND ADMINISTRATION
Adults: The usual dosage is 3000 mg daily, given in divided doses as follows: 1) two doses of two 750 mg tablets; 2) two doses of three 500 mg tablets/capsules; or 3) three doses of two 500 mg tablets/capsules. Some patients, e.g., the elderly, may require a lower dosage to achieve therapeutic blood concentrations and to avoid the more common side effects such as auditory.

Alleviation of symptoms is gradual, and full benefit may not be evident for 3 to 4 days, when plasma salicylate levels have achieved steady state. There is no evidence for development of tissue tolerance (tachyphylaxis) but salicylate therapy may induce increased activity of metabolizing liver enzymes, causing a greater rate of salicyluric acid production and excretion, with a resultant increase in dosage requirement for maintenance of therapeutic serum salicylate levels.

Children: Dosage recommendations and indications for DISALCID use in children have not been established.

HOW SUPPLIED
Each DISALCID 500 mg aqua/white capsule printed with Disalcid/3M is available in:
Bottles of 100 (NDC #0089-0148-10)
Each DISALCID 500 mg aqua, film coated, round, bisected tablet embossed with DISALCID on one side and 3M on the other side is available in:
Bottles of 100 (NDC #0089-0149-10)
Bottles of 500 (NDC #0089-0149-50)
Each DISALCID 750 mg aqua, film coated, capsule shaped, bisected tablet embossed with DISALCID 750 on one side and 3M on the other side is available in:
Bottles of 100 (NDC #0089-0151-10)
Bottles of 500 (NDC #0089-0151-50)
Store at controlled room temperature 15°-30°C (59°-86°F).
CAUTION: Federal law prohibits dispensing without prescription.

REFERENCES
1. Morris HG, et al. Effects of salsalate (non-acetylated salicylate) and aspirin on serum prostaglandins in humans. Thera Drug Mon 1985;7:435–438.
2. April PA, et al. Does the acetyl group of aspirin contribute to the anti-inflammatory efficacy of salicylic acid in the treatment of rheumatoid arthritis? Sem Arth & Rheum 1990;19:(4)2:20–28.
3. Deodhar SD, et al. A short term comparative trial of salsalate and indomethacin in rheumatoid arthritis. Curr Med Res Opin 1977;5:185–188.
4. Estes D, Kaplan K. Lack of platelet effect with the aspirin analog, salsalate. Arth & Rheum 1980;23:1303–1307.
5. Dick C, et al. Effect of anti-inflammatory drug therapy on clearance of ^{133}Xe from knee joints of patients with rheumatoid arthritis. Br Med J 1969;3:278–280.
6. Dick WC, et al. Indices of inflammatory activity. Ann of Rheum Dis 1970;29:643–648.
7. Cohen A, Fecal blood loss and plasma salicylate study of salicylsalicylic acid and aspirin. J Clin Pharmacol 1979;19:242–247.
8. Chudwin DS, et al. Sensitivity to non-acetylated salicylates in a patient with asthma, nasal polyps, and rheumatoid arthritis. Ann of Allergy 1986;57:133–134.
9. Spector SL, et al. Aspirin and concomitant idiosyncrasies in adult asthmatic patients. J Allergy Clin Immunol 1979;64:500–506.
10. Stevenson DD, et al. Salsalate cross sensitivity in aspirin-sensitive asthmatics. J Allergy Clin Immunol 1990;86:749–758.

622500   OCTOBER 1993

MAXAIR™ Autohaler™   ℞
(pirbuterol acetate inhalation aerosol)

Patient's Instructions for Use

Questions? Call our Patient Assistance Line at 1-(800)-841-3885 8:30 a.m.—5:00 p.m. EST.

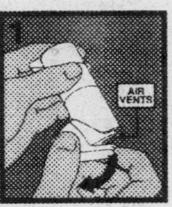

Remove mouthpiece cover by pulling down lip on **back** of cover.
Inspect mouthpiece for foreign objects.
Locate "Up" arrows on Maxair Autohaler.
Locate air vents at bottom of Maxair Autohaler.

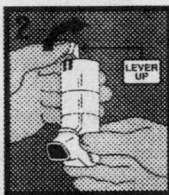

Hold Maxair Autohaler **upright** as shown in figure 2. The arrows should point up.
Maxair Autohaler must be held upright while raising lever.
Raise lever so that it stays up. It will "snap" into place.
Do not lower lever until step 6.

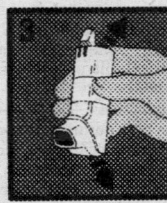

Hold Maxair Autohaler around the middle as shown in figure 3.
Shake Maxair Autohaler gently several times.

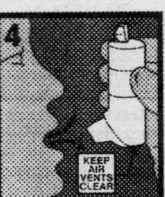

Continue to hold Maxair Autohaler **upright** as shown in figure 4.
Do not block air vents at bottom of Maxair Autohaler.
Exhale normally before use.

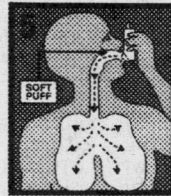

Seal your lips tightly around mouthpiece as shown in figure 5.

Inhale deeply through mouthpiece with **steady, moderate force**. You will hear a "click" and feel a **soft** puff when your inhaling triggers the release of medicine.

Do not stop when you hear and feel the puff. Continue to take a **full, deep breath.**

Take Maxair Autohaler away from your mouth when done inhaling.

Hold your breath for 10 seconds, then exhale slowly.

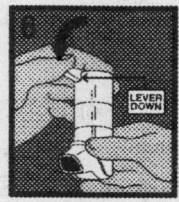

Continue to hold Maxair Autohaler upright while lowering the lever as shown in figure 6. Lower lever after each puff.

If your physician has prescribed additional puffs, wait one minute then repeat steps 2 through 6.

Following use, make sure lever is down and replace mouthpiece cover.

IMPORTANT NOTE:

Use Maxair Autohaler according to the instructions given to you by your physician, who will advise you on the number of puffs to take. If you have previously been using a "press-and-breathe" inhaler, you should take the same number of puffs through your Maxair Autohaler as you did through the "press-and-breathe" inhaler.

General Information

Your Maxair Autohaler is a new type of inhaler designed to be very easy to use. Maxair Autohaler automatically releases a puff of medicine when you inhale.

What will I feel when I use Maxair Autohaler?

Maxair Autohaler provides a **soft spray** of medicine. It is designed to automatically deliver a precisely measured dose of your medicine with each puff, so you can be assured of a consistent dose of medicine.

When medicine is delivered, you will hear a "click" and feel a **soft** puff.

How will I know when there's no more medicine in Maxair Autohaler?

The Maxair Autohaler you receive from the pharmacy contains 400 puffs (the Maxair Autohaler sample contains 80 puffs and says "SAMPLE" on the back; the Maxair Autohaler hospital unit also contains 80 puffs and says "Hospital Pack" on the back). You can estimate how many days it will last by dividing 80 or 400 (total puffs in a unit) by the number of puffs you normally use in a day. The chart below can help you calculate about how long your 400 puff Maxair Autohaler will last. Acutal usage may vary depending on how many puffs you use each day. A total daily dose of 12 puffs should not be exceeded. Discard your Maxair Autohaler when there is no more medicine remaining.

Average Number of Puffs Per Day	Approximate Days of Therapy Available
2 puffs/day	200 days
4 puffs/day	100 days
6 puffs/day	65 days
8 pufffs/day	50 days

How to clean and care for Maxair Autohaler.

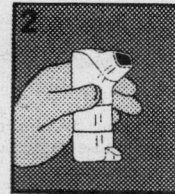

Remove mouthpiece cover by pulling down lip on **back** of cover.

[See figure at top of next column.]

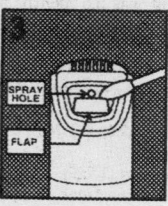

Turn Maxair Autohaler upside down.
Wipe mouthpiece with a clean dry cloth.

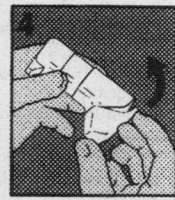

Gently tap back of Maxair Autohaler so flap comes down and spray hole can be seen. With white flap down as shown in the picture, clean the surface of the flap with a dry cotton swab.

Remove mouthpiece cover. When you are not using Maxair Autohaler, make sure lever is down and mouthpiece cover is in place.

Repeat cleaning instructions weekly or as often as required.

Important Information:

Caution: Contents of canister under pressure. Do not puncture. Do not use near heat or open flame. Exposure to temperatures above 120°F may cause bursting. Store between 15° and 30° C (59° to 86° F). Avoid spraying in eyes.

Caution: Federal law prohibits dispensing without a prescription.

Use Maxair Autohaler only as prescribed by your physician.

Handle with care.

DO NOT USE WITH OTHER CANISTERS OR MOUTH-PIECES.

For information on the drug, refer to your doctor or pharmacist.

Keep out of reach of children.

Note: The indented statement below is required by the Federal Government's Clean Air Act for all products containing or manufactured with chlorofluorocarbons (CFC's).

> This product contains trichloromonofluoromethane and dichlorodifluoromethane, substances which harm the environment by destroying ozone in the upper atmosphere.

Your physician has determined that this product is likely to help your personal health. USE THIS PRODUCT AS DIRECTED, UNLESS INSTRUCTED TO DO OTHERWISE BY YOUR PHYSICIAN. If you have any questions about alternatives, consult with your physician.

MAXAIR™ AUTOHALER™   ℞
(pirbuterol acetate inhalation aerosol)
Bronchodilator Aerosol
For Inhalation Only

DESCRIPTION

The active component of MAXAIR AUTOHALER (pirbuterol acetate) is (R,S) a^6-{[(1,1-dimethylethyl)amino]methyl}-3-hydroxy-2,6-pyridine-dimethanol monoacetate salt, a beta-2 adrenergic bronchodilator, having the following chemical structure:

[See chemical structure at top of next column.]

Pirbuterol acetate is a white, crystalline racemic mixture of two optically active isomers. It is a powder, freely soluble in

water, with a molecular weight of 300.3 and empirical formula of $C_{12}H_{20}N_2O_3 \cdot C_2H_4O_2$.

MAXAIR AUTOHALER is a metered dose aerosol unit for oral inhalation. It provides a fine particle suspension of pirbuterol acetate in the propellant mixture of trichloromonofluoromethane and dichlorodifluoromethane, with sorbitan trioleate. Each actuation delivers from the mouthpiece pirbuterol acetate equivalent to 0.2 mg of pirbuterol with the majority of particles less than 5 microns in diameter. The unit is breath-actuated such that the medication is delivered automatically during inspiration without the need for the patient to coordinate actuation with inspiration.

CLINICAL PHARMACOLOGY

In vitro studies and *in vivo* pharmacologic studies have demonstrated that MAXAIR has a preferential effect on beta-2 adrenergic receptors compared with isoproterenol. While it is recognized that beta-2 adrenergic receptors are the predominant receptors in bronchial smooth muscle, recent data indicate that there is a population of beta-2 receptors in the human heart, existing in a concentration between 10–50%. The precise function of these, however, is not yet established (see WARNINGS section).

The pharmacologic effects of beta adrenergic agonist drugs, including pirbuterol, are at least in part attributable to stimulation through beta adrenergic receptors of intracellular adenyl cyclase, the enzyme which catalyzes the conversion of adenosine triphosphate (ATP) to cyclic-3',5'-adenosine monophosphate (c-AMP). Increased c-AMP levels are associated with relaxation of bronchial smooth muscle and inhibition of release of mediators of immediate hypersensitivity from cells, especially from mast cells.

Bronchodilator activity of MAXAIR was manifested clinically by an improvement in various pulmonary function parameters (FEV_1, MMF, PEFR, airway resistance [RAW] and conductance [GA/V_{tg}]).

In controlled double-blind single dose clinical trials, the onset of improvement in pulmonary function occurred within 5 minutes in most patients as determined by forced expiratory volume in one second (FEV_1). FEV_1 and MMF measurements also showed that maximum improvement in pulmonary function generally occurred 30–60 minutes following one (1) or two (2) inhalations of pirbuterol (0.2–0.4 mg). The duration of action of MAXAIR is maintained for 5 hours (the time at which the last observations were made) in a substantial number of patients, based on a 15% or greater increase in FEV_1. In controlled repetitive dose studies of 12 weeks' duration, 74% of 156 patients on pirbuterol and 62% of 141 patients on metaproterenol showed a clinically significant improvement based on a 15% or greater increase in FEV_1 on at least half of the days. Onset and duration were equivalent to that seen in single dose studies. Continued effectiveness was demonstrated over the 12-week period in the majority (94%) of responding patients; however, chronic dosing was associated with the development of tachyphylaxis (tolerance) to the bronchodilator effect in some patients in both treatment groups.

A placebo-controlled double-blind single dose study (24 patients per treatment group), utilizing continuous Holter monitoring for 5 hours after drug administration, showed no significant difference in ectopic activity between the placebo control group and MAXAIR at the recommended dose (0.2–0.4 mg), and twice the recommended dose (0.8 mg). As with other inhaled beta adrenergic agonists, supraventricular and ventricular ectopic beats have been seen with MAXAIR (see WARNINGS).

Recent studies in laboratory animals (minipigs, rodents, and dogs) recorded the occurrence of cardiac arrhythmias and sudden death (with histologic evidence of myocardial necrosis) when beta agonists and methylxanthines were administered concurrently. The significance of these findings when applied to humans is currently unknown.

Two randomized, double-blind, cross-over studies in a total of 97 patients, have compared the clinical effects of either one inhalation or two inhalations of the pirbuterol formulations in the Autohaler actuator and the conventional inhaler and demonstrated no significant difference between the formulations for the means of peak changes in FEV_1, time to peak FEV_1, onset, duration, or area under the FEV_1 curve.

Pharmacokinetics

As expected by extrapolation from oral data, systemic blood levels of pirbuterol are below the limit of assay sensitivity (2–5 ng/ml) following inhalation of doses up to 0.8 mg (twice the maximum recommended dose). A mean of 51% of the dose is recovered in urine as pirbuterol plus its sulfate conjugate following administration by aerosol. Pirbuterol is not metabolized by catechol-O-methyltransferase.

Continued on next page

3M—Cont.

The percent of administered dose recovered as pirbuterol plus its sulfate conjugate does not change significantly over the dose range of 0.4 mg to 0.8 mg and is not significantly different from that after oral administration of pirbuterol. The plasma half-life measured after oral administration is about two hours.

INDICATIONS AND USAGE

MAXAIR AUTOHALER is indicated for the prevention and reversal of bronchospasm in patients with reversible bronchospasm including asthma. It may be used with or without concurrent theophylline and/or steroid therapy.

CONTRAINDICATIONS

MAXAIR is contraindicated in patients with a history of hypersensitivity to any of its ingredients.

WARNINGS

As with other beta adrenergic aerosols, MAXAIR should not be used in excess. Controlled clinical studies and other clinical experience have shown that MAXAIR like other inhaled beta adrenergic agonists can produce a significant cardiovascular effect in some patients, as measured by pulse rate, blood pressure, symptoms, and/or ECG changes. As with other beta adrenergic aerosols, the potential for paradoxical bronchospasm (which can be life threatening) should be kept in mind. If it occurs, the preparation should be discontinued immediately and alternative therapy instituted.

Fatalities have been reported in association with excessive use of inhaled sympathomimetic drugs.

The contents of MAXAIR AUTOHALER are under pressure. Do not puncture. Do not use or store near heat or open flame. Exposure to temperature above 120°F may cause bursting. Never throw container into fire or incinerator. Keep out of reach of children.

PRECAUTIONS

General

Since pirbuterol is a sympathomimetic amine, it should be used with caution in patients with cardiovascular disorders, including ischemic heart disease, hypertension, or cardiac arrhythmias, in patients with hyperthyroidism or diabetes mellitus, and in patients who are unusually responsive to sympathomimetic amines or who have convulsive disorders. Significant changes in systolic and diastolic blood pressure could be expected to occur in some patients after use of any beta adrenergic aerosol bronchodilator.

Information for Patients

MAXAIR effects may last up to five hours or longer. It should not be used more often than recommended and the patient should not increase the number of inhalations or frequency of use without first asking the physician. If symptoms of asthma get worse, adverse reactions occur, or the patient does not respond to the usual dose, the patient should be instructed to contact the physician immediately. The patient should be advised to see the Illustrated Patient's Instructions for Use.

The Autohaler actuator should not be used with any other inhalation aerosol canister. In addition, canisters for use with MAXAIR AUTOHALER should not be utilized with any other actuator.

Drug Interactions

Other beta adrenergic aerosol bronchodilators should not be used concomitantly with MAXAIR because they may have additive effects. Beta adrenergic agonists should be administered with caution to patients being treated with monoamine oxidase inhibitors or tricyclic antidepressants, since the action of beta adrenergic agonists on the vascular system may be potentiated.

Carcinogenesis, Mutagenesis and Impairment of Fertility

Pirbuterol hydrochloride administered in the diet to rats for 24 months and to mice for 18 months was free of carcinogenic activity at doses corresponding to 200 times the maximum human inhalation dose. In addition, the intragastric intubation of the drug at doses corresponding to 6250 times the maximum recommended human daily inhalation dose resulted in no increase in tumors in a 12-month rat study. Studies with pirbuterol revealed no evidence of mutagenesis. Reproduction studies in rats revealed no evidence of impaired fertility.

Teratogenic Effects—Pregnancy Category C

Reproduction studies have been performed in rats and rabbits by the inhalation route at doses up to 12 times (rat) and 16 times (rabbit) the maximum human inhalation dose and have revealed no significant findings. Animal reproduction studies in rats at *oral doses* up to 300 mg/kg and in rabbits at oral doses up to 100 mg/kg have shown no adverse effect on reproductive behavior, fertility, litter size, peri- and postnatal viability or fetal development. In rabbits at the highest dose level given, 300 mg/kg, abortions and fetal mortality were observed. There are no adequate and well controlled studies in pregnant women and MAXAIR should be used during pregnancy only if the potential benefit justifies the potential risk to the fetus.

Nursing Mothers

It is not known whether MAXAIR is excreted in human milk. Therefore, MAXAIR should be used during nursing only if the potential benefit justifies the possible risk to the newborn.

Pediatric Use

MAXAIR AUTOHALER is not recommended for patients under the age of 12 years because of insufficient clinical data to establish safety and effectiveness.

ADVERSE REACTIONS

The following rates of adverse reactions to pirbuterol are based on single and multiple dose clinical trials involving 761 patients, 400 of whom received multiple doses (mean duration of treatment was 2.5 months and maximum was 19 months).

The following were the adverse reactions reported more frequently than 1 in 100 patients:

CNS: nervousness (6.9%), tremor (6.0%), headache (2.0%), dizziness (1.2%).

Cardiovascular: palpitations (1.7%), tachycardia (1.2%).

Respiratory: cough (1.2%).

Gastrointestinal: nausea (1.7%).

The following adverse reactions occurred less frequently than 1 in 100 patients and there may be a causal relationship with pirbuterol:

CNS: depression, anxiety, confusion, insomnia, weakness, hyperkinesia, syncope.

Cardiovascular: hypotension, skipped beats, chest pain.

Gastrointestinal: dry mouth, glossitis, abdominal pain/cramps, anorexia, diarrhea, stomatitis, nausea and vomiting.

Ear, Nose and Throat: smell/taste changes, sore throat.

Dermatological: rash, pruritus.

Other: numbness in extremities, alopecia, bruising, fatigue, edema, weight gain, flushing.

Other adverse reactions were reported with a frequency of less than 1 in 100 patients but a causal relationship between pirbuterol and the reaction could not be determined: migraine, productive cough, wheezing, and dermatitis.

The following rates of adverse reactions during three-month controlled clinical trials involving 310 patients are noted. The table does not include mild reactions.

PERCENT OF PATIENTS WITH MODERATE TO SEVERE ADVERSE REACTIONS

Reaction	Pirbuterol N=157	Metaproterenol N=153
Central Nervous System		
tremors	1.3%	3.3%
nervousness	4.5%	2.6%
headache	1.3%	2.0%
weakness	.0%	1.3%
drowsiness	.0%	0.7%
dizziness	0.6%	.0%
Cardiovascular		
palpitations	1.3%	1.3%
tachycardia	1.3%	2.0%
Respiratory		
chest pain/tightness	1.3%	.0%
cough	.0%	0.7%
Gastrointestinal		
nausea	1.3%	2.0%
diarrhea	1.3%	0.7%
dry mouth	1.3%	1.3%
vomiting	.0%	0.7%
Dermatological		
skin reaction	.0%	0.7%
rash	.0%	1.3%
Other		
bruising	0.6%	.0%
smell/taste change	0.6%	.0%
backache	.0%	0.7%
fatigue	.0%	0.7%
hoarseness	.0%	0.7%
nasal congestion	.0%	0.7%

OVERDOSAGE

The expected symptoms with overdosage are those of excessive beta-stimulation and/or any of the symptoms listed under adverse reactions, e.g., angina, hypertension or hypotension, arrhythmias, nervousness, headache, tremor, dry mouth, palpitation, nausea, dizziness, fatigue, malaise, and insomnia.

Treatment consists of discontinuation of pirbuterol together with appropriate symptomatic therapy.

The oral acute lethal dose in male and female rats and mice was greater than 2000 mg base/kg. The aerosol acute lethal dose was not determined.

DOSAGE AND ADMINISTRATION

The usual dose for adults and children 12 years and older is two inhalations (0.4 mg) repeated every 4–6 hours. One inhalation (0.2 mg) repeated every 4–6 hours may be sufficient for some patients.

A total daily dose of 12 inhalations should not be exceeded.

If a previously effective dosage regimen fails to provide the usual relief, medical advice should be sought immediately as this is often a sign of seriously worsening asthma which would require reassessment of therapy.

HOW SUPPLIED

MAXAIR AUTOHALER is supplied in a pressurized aluminum canister with a light blue plastic breath-activated actuator. DO NOT USE WITH OTHER CANISTERS OR MOUTHPIECES. Each actuation delivers pirbuterol acetate equivalent to 0.2 mg of pirbuterol from the mouthpiece.

Canister with breath-activated Autohaler actuator. Net content weight 14 g, a minimum of 400 inhalations (NDC **0089-0815-21**) and net content weight 2.8 g, a minimum of 80 inhalations (Hospital Pack: NDC **0089-0817-10**, Sample Pack: NDC **0089-0815-08**).

Note: The indented statement below is required by the Federal goverment's Clean Air Act for all products containing or manufactured with chlorofluorocarbons (CFC's).

> **WARNING:** Contains trichloromonofluoromethane and dichlorodifluoromethane, substances which harm public health and environment by destroying ozone in the upper atmosphere.

A notice similar to the above WARNING has been placed in the "Patient's Instructions for Use" of this product pursuant to EPA regulations.

CAUTION

Federal law prohibits dispensing without prescription.

Store between 15° and 30°C (59° to 86°F).

3M

609902 JUNE 1995

Shown in Product Identification Guide, page 322

MAXAIR™ Inhaler ℞

(pirbuterol acetate inhalation aerosol)
Bronchodilator Aerosol
For Inhalation Only

DESCRIPTION

The active component of MAXAIR Inhaler is (R,S)α[6]-{[(1,1-dimethylethyl)amino]methyl}-3-hydroxy-2,6-pyridinedimethanol monoacetate salt, a beta-2 adrenergic bronchodilator, having the following chemical structure:

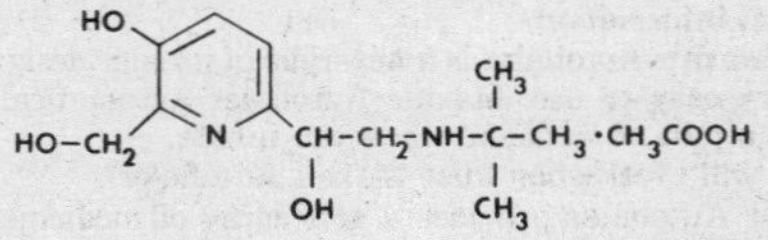

Pirbuterol acetate is a white, crystalline racemic mixture of two optically active isomers. It is a powder, freely soluble in water, with a molecular weight of 300.3 and empirical formula of $C_{12}H_{20}N_2O_3 \cdot C_2H_4O_2$.

MAXAIR Inhaler is a metered dose aerosol unit for oral inhalation. It provides a fine-particle suspension of pirbuterol acetate in the propellant mixture of trichloromonofluoromethane and dichlorodifluoromethane, with sorbitan trioleate. Each actuation delivers from the mouthpiece pirbuterol acetate equivalent to 0.2 mg of pirbuterol with the majority of particles less than 5 microns in diameter. Each canister provides at least 300 inhalations.

CLINICAL PHARMACOLOGY

In vitro studies and *in vivo* pharmacologic studies have demonstrated that MAXAIR has a preferential effect on beta-2 adrenergic receptors compared with isoproterenol. While it is recognized that beta-2 adrenergic receptors are the predominant receptors in bronchial smooth mucle, recent data indicate that there is a population of beta-2 receptors in the human heart, existing in a concentration between 10–50%. The precise function of these, however, is not yet established (see WARNINGS section).

The pharmacologic effects of beta adrenergic agonist drugs, including pirbuterol are at least in part attributable to stimulation through beta adrenergic receptors of intracellular adenyl cyclase, the enzyme which catalyzes the conversion of adenosine triphosphate (ATP) to cyclic-3′,5′-adenosine monophosphate (c-AMP). Increased c-AMP levels are associated with relaxation of bronchial smooth muscle and inhibition of release of mediators of immediate hypersensitivity from cells, especially from mast cells.

Bronchodilator activity of MAXAIR was manifested clinically by an improvement in various pulmonary function parameters (FEV_1, MMF, PEFR, airway resistance [RAW] and conductance [GA/V_{tg}]).

In controlled double-blind single dose clinical trials, the onset of improvement in pulmonary function occurred within 5 minutes in most patients as determined by forced expiratory volume in one second (FEV_1). FEV_1 and MMF measurements also showed that maximum improvement in pulmonary function generally occurred 30–60 minutes follow-

ing one (1) or two (2) inhalations of pirbuterol (0.2–0.4 mg). The duration of action of MAXAIR is maintained for 5 hours (the time at which the last observations were made) in a substantial number of patients, based on a 15% or greater increase in FEV₁. In controlled repetitive dose studies of 12 weeks duration, 74% of 156 patients on pirbuterol and 62% of 141 patients on metaproterenol showed a clinically significant improvement based on a 15% or greater increase in FEV₁ on at least half of the days. Onset and duration were equivalent to that seen in single dose studies. Continued effectiveness was demonstrated over the 12-week period in the majority (94%) of responding patients; however, chronic dosing was associated with the development of tachyphylaxis (tolerance) to the bronchodilator effect in some patients in both treatment groups.

A placebo-controlled double-blind single dose study (24 patients per treatment group), utilizing continuous Holter monitoring for 5 hours after drug administration, showed no significant difference in ectopic activity between the placebo control group and MAXAIR at the recommended dose (0.2–0.4 mg), and twice the recommended dose (0.8 mg). As with other inhaled beta adrenergic agonists, supraventricular and ventricular ectopic beats have been seen with MAXAIR (see WARNINGS).

Recent studies in laboratory animals (minipigs, rodents, and dogs) recorded the occurrence of cardiac arrhythmias and sudden death (with histologic evidence of myocardial necrosis) when beta agonists and methylxanthines were administered concurrently. The significance of these findings when applied to humans is currently unknown.

Pharmacokinetics
As expected by extrapolation from oral data, systemic blood levels of pirbuterol are below the limit of assay sensitivity (2–5 ng/ml) following inhalation of doses up to 0.8 mg (twice the maximum recommended dose). A mean of 51% of the dose is recovered in urine as pirbuterol plus its sulfate conjugate following administration by aerosol. Pirbuterol is not metabolized by catechol-O-methyltransferase. The percent of administered dose recovered as pirbuterol plus its sulfate conjugate does not change significantly over the dose range of 0.4 mg to 0.8 mg and is not significantly different from that after oral administration of pirbuterol. The plasma half-life measured after oral administration is about two hours.

INDICATIONS AND USAGE
MAXAIR Inhaler is indicated for the prevention and reversal of bronchospasm in patients with reversible bronchospasm including asthma. It may be used with or without concurrent theophylline and/or steroid therapy.

CONTRAINDICATIONS
MAXAIR is contraindicated in patients with a history of hypersensitivity to any of its ingredients.

WARNINGS
As with other beta adrenergic aerosols, MAXAIR should not be used in excess. Controlled clinical studies and other clinical experience have shown that MAXAIR like other inhaled beta adrenergic agonists can produce a significant cardiovascular effect in some patients, as measured by pulse rate, blood pressure, symptoms, and/or ECG changes. As with other beta adrenergic aerosols, the potential for paradoxical bronchospasm (which can be life threatening) should be kept in mind. If it occurs, the preparation should be discontinued immediately and alternative therapy instituted.
Fatalities have been reported in association with excessive use of inhaled sympathomimetic drugs.
The contents of MAXAIR Inhaler are under pressure. Do not puncture. Do not use or store near heat or open flame. Exposure to temperature above 120°F may cause bursting. Never throw container into fire or incinerator. Keep out of reach of children.

PRECAUTIONS
General
Since pirbuterol is a sympathomimetic amine, it should be used with caution in patients with cardiovascular disorders, including ischemic heart disease, hypertension, or cardiac arrhythmias, in patients with hyperthyroidism or diabetes mellitus, and in patients who are unusually responsive to sympathomimetic amines or who have convulsive disorders. Significant changes in systolic and diastolic blood pressure could be expected to occur in some patients after use of any beta adrenergic aerosol bronchodilator.
Information for Patients
MAXAIR effects may last up to five hours or longer. It should not be used more often than recommended and the patient should not increase the number of inhalations or frequency of use without first asking the physician. If symptoms of asthma get worse, adverse reactions occur, or the patient does not respond to the usual dose, the patient should be instructed to contact the physician immediately. The patient should be advised to see the Illustrated Directions for Use.
Drug Interactions
Other beta adrenergic aerosol bronchodilators should not be used concomitantly with MAXAIR because they may have

additive effects. Beta adrenergic agonists should be administered with caution to patients being treated with monoamine oxidase inhibitors or tricyclic antidepressants, since the action of beta adrenergic agonists on the vascular system may be potentiated.
Carcinogenesis, Mutagenesis and Impairment of Fertility
Pirbuterol hydrochloride administered in the diet to rats for 24 months and to mice for 18 months was free of carcinogenic activity at doses corresponding to 200 times the maximum human inhalation dose. In addition, the intragastric intubation of the drug at doses corresponding to 6250 times the maximum recommended human daily inhalation dose resulted in no increase in tumors in a 12-month rat study. Studies with pirbuterol revealed no evidence of mutagenesis. Reproduction studies in rats revealed no evidence of impaired fertility.
Teratogenic Effects—Pregnancy Category C
Reproduction studies have been performed in rats and rabbits by the inhalation route at doses up to 12 times (rat) and 16 times (rabbit) the maximum human inhalation dose and have revealed no significant findings. Animal reproduction studies in rats at *oral doses* up to 300 mg/kg and in rabbits at oral doses up to 100 mg/kg have shown no adverse effect on reproductive behavior, fertility, litter size, peri- and postnatal viability or fetal development. In rabbits at the highest dose level given, 300 mg/kg, abortions and fetal mortality were observed. There are no adequate and well controlled studies in pregnant women and MAXAIR should be used during pregnancy only if the potential benefit justifies the potential risk to the fetus.
Nursing Mothers
It is not known whether MAXAIR is excreted in human milk. Therefore, MAXAIR should be used during nursing only if the potential benefit justifies the possible risk to the newborn.
Pediatric Use
MAXAIR Inhaler is not recommended for patients under the age of 12 years because of insufficient clinical data to establish safety and effectiveness.

ADVERSE REACTIONS
The following rates of adverse reactions to pirbuterol are based on single and multiple dose clinical trials involving 761 patients, 400 of whom received multiple doses (mean duration of treatment was 2.5 months and maximum was 19 months).
The following were the adverse reactions reported more frequently than 1 in 100 patients:
CNS: nervousness (6.9%), tremor (6.0%), headache (2.0%), dizziness (1.2%).
Cardiovascular: palpitations (1.7%), tachycardia (1.2%).
Respiratory: cough (1.2%).
Gastrointestinal: nausea (1.7%).
The following adverse reactions occurred less frequently than 1 in 100 patients and there may be a causal relationship with pirbuterol:
CNS: depression, anxiety, confusion, insomnia, weakness, hyperkinesia, syncope.
Cardiovascular: hypotension, skipped beats, chest pain.
Gastrointestinal: dry mouth, glossitis, abdominal pain/cramps, anorexia, diarrhea, stomatitis, nausea and vomiting.
Ear, Nose and Throat: smell/taste changes, sore throat.
Dermatological: rash, pruritus.
Other: numbness in extremities, alopecia, bruising, fatigue, edema, weight gain, flushing.
Other adverse reactions were reported with a frequency of less than 1 in 100 patients but a causal relationship between pirbuterol and the reaction could not be determined: migraine, productive cough, wheezing, and dermatitis.
The following rates of adverse reactions during three-month controlled clinical trials involving 310 patients are noted. The table does not include mild reactions.

PERCENT OF PATIENTS WITH MODERATE TO SEVERE ADVERSE REACTIONS

Reaction	Pirbuterol N=157	Metaproterenol N=153
Central Nervous System		
tremors	1.3%	3.3%
nervousness	4.5%	2.6%
headache	1.3%	2.0%
weakness	.0%	1.3%
drowsiness	.0%	0.7%
dizziness	0.6%	.0%
Cardiovascular		
palpitations	1.3%	1.3%
tachycardia	1.3%	2.0%
Respiratory		
chest pain/tightness	1.3%	.0%
cough	.0%	0.7%
Gastrointestinal		
nausea	1.3%	2.0%
diarrhea	1.3%	0.7%
dry mouth	1.3%	1.3%
vomiting	.0%	0.7%
Dermatological		
skin reaction	.0%	0.7%
rash	.0%	1.3%
Other		
bruising	0.6%	.0%
smell/taste change	0.6%	.0%
backache	.0%	0.7%
fatigue	.0%	0.7%
hoarseness	.0%	0.7%
nasal congestion	.0%	0.7%

OVERDOSAGE
The expected symptoms with overdosage are those of excessive beta-stimulation and/or any of the symptoms listed under adverse reactions, e.g., angina, hypertension or hypotension, arrhythmias, nervousness, headache, tremor, dry mouth, palpitation, nausea, dizziness, fatigue, malaise, and insomnia.
Treatment consists of discontinuation of pirbuterol together with appropriate symptomatic therapy.
The oral acute lethal dose in male and female rats and mice was greater than 2000 mg base/kg. The aerosol acute lethal dose was not determined.

DOSAGE AND ADMINISTRATION
The usual dose for adults and children 12 years and older is two inhalations (0.4 mg) repeated every 4–6 hours. One inhalation (0.2 mg) repeated every 4–6 hours may be sufficient for some patients.
A total daily dose of 12 inhalations should not be exceeded.
If a previously effective dosage regimen fails to provide the usual relief, medical advice should be sought immediately as this is often a sign of seriously worsening asthma which would require reassessment of therapy.

HOW SUPPLIED
MAXAIR Inhaler is supplied in a pressurized aluminum canister with a light-blue plastic actuator and attached white mouthpiece. Each actuation delivers pirbuterol acetate equivalent to 0.2 mg of pirbuterol from the mouthpiece. Net content weight 25.6 g, a minimum of 300 actuations (NDC **0089-0790-21**).
Note: The indented statement below is required by the Federal government's Clean Air Act for all products containing or manufactured with chlorofluorocarbons (CFC's).
> **WARNING:** Contains trichloromonofluoromethane and dichlorodifluoromethane, substances which harm public health and environment by destroying ozone in the upper atmosphere.
A notice similar to the above WARNING has been placed in the "Patient's Instructions for Use" of this product pursuant to EPA regulations.

CAUTION
Federal law prohibits dispensing without prescription.
Store between 15° and 30°C (59° to 86°F).

610000   JUNE 1995

Shown in Product Identification Guide, page 322

MEDIHALER–ISO™   ℞
(isoproterenol sulfate)
Inhalation Aerosol

For full prescribing information see leaflet accompanying product or call 800-328-0255 for a copy.

HOW SUPPLIED
MEDIHALER-ISO (isoproterenol sulfate) is an aerosol device which delivers 0.08 mg isoproterenol sulfate through the oral adapter with each depression of the valve.
15-ml and oral adapter containing 21.0 gm, a minimum of 300 actuations (NDC **0089-0785-21**).
15 ml refill vial only, containing 21.0 gm, a minimum of 300 actuations (NDC **0089-0785-11**)

MINITRAN™   ℞
(nitroglycerin)
Transdermal Delivery System

For full prescribing information see leaflet accompanying product or call 800-328-0255 for a copy.

HOW SUPPLIED
[See table at top of next page.]

Continued on next page

3M—Cont.

MINITRAN System

Rated Release In Vivo	System Size	Total Nitroglycerin in System	NDC Number (30 per carton)
0.1 mg/hr	3.3 cm^2	9 mg	NDC-0089-0301-02
0.2 mg/hr	6.7 cm^2	18 mg	NDC-0089-0302-02*
0.4 mg/hr	13.3 cm^2	36 mg	NDC-0089-0303-02*
0.6 mg/hr	20.0 cm^2	54 mg	NDC-0089-0304-02

*MINITRAN Transdermal Delivery System, 0.2 mg/hr, 0.4 mg/hr, is also available in cartons of 90 patches bearing NDC-0089-0302-09 and NDC-0089-0303-09 respectively.

NORFLEX™ ℞
(orphenadrine citrate)
Tablets and Injection

PRODUCT OVERVIEW

KEY FACTS
Norflex extended-release tablets provide 12 hours relief from the pain of muscle spasm. Also available in injectable form, IV or IM, also given every 12 hours.

MAJOR USES
Norflex is indicated as an adjunct to rest, physical therapy, and other measures for the relief of discomfort associated with painful musculoskeletal disorders.

SAFETY INFORMATION
Contraindicated in patients with glaucoma, pyloric or duodenal obstruction, stenosing peptic ulcers, prostatic hypertrophy or obstruction of the bladder neck, cardiospasm (megaesophagus) and myasthenia gravis. Contraindicated in patients who have a previous sensitivity to the drug.

PRESCRIBING INFORMATION

NORFLEX™ ℞
(orphenadrine citrate)
Tablets and Injection

DESCRIPTION
Orphenadrine citrate is the citrate salt of orphenadrine (2-dimethylaminoethyl 2-methylbenzhydryl ether citrate). It occurs as a white, crystalline powder having a bitter taste. It is practically odorless; sparingly soluble in water, slightly soluble in alcohol.

Each Norflex Tablet contains 100 mg orphenadrine citrate. Norflex Tablets also contain: calcium stearate, ethylcellulose, and lactose. Norflex Injection contains 60 mg of orphenadrine citrate in aqueous solution in each ampul. Norflex Injection also contains: sodium bisulfite NF, 2.0 mg; sodium chloride USP, 5.8 mg; sodium hydroxide, to adjust pH; and water for injection USP, q.s. to 2 mL.

ACTIONS
The mode of therapeutic action has not been clearly identified, but may be related to its analgesic properties. Orphenadrine citrate also possesses anticholinergic actions.

INDICATIONS
Orphenadrine citrate is indicated as an adjunct to rest, physical therapy, and other measures for the relief of discomfort associated with acute painful musculoskeletal conditions. The mode of action of the drug has not been clearly identified, but may be related to its analgesic properties. Orphenadrine citrate does not directly relax tense skeletal muscles in man.

CONTRAINDICATIONS
Contraindicated in patients with glaucoma, pyloric or duodenal obstruction, stenosing peptic ulcers, prostatic hypertrophy or obstruction of the bladder neck, cardio-spasm (megaesophagus) and myasthenia gravis. Contraindicated in patients who have demonstrated a previous hypersensitivity to the drug.

WARNINGS
Some patients may experience transient episodes of light-headedness, dizziness or syncope. Norflex may impair the ability of the patient to engage in potentially hazardous activities such as operating machinery or driving a motor vehicle; ambulatory patients should therefore be cautioned accordingly.
Norflex Injection contains sodium bisulfite, a sulfite that may cause allergic-type reactions including anaphylactic symptoms and life-threatening or less severe asthmatic episodes in certain susceptible people. The overall prevalence of sulfite sensitivity in the general population is unknown and probably low. Sulfite sensitivity is seen more frequently in asthmatic than nonasthmatic people.

PREGNANCY
Pregnancy Category C. Animal reproduction studies have not been conducted with Norflex. It is also not known whether Norflex can cause fetal harm when administered to a pregnant woman or can affect reproduction capacity. Norflex should be given to a pregnant woman only if clearly needed.

USAGE IN CHILDREN
Safety and effectiveness in children have not been established; therefore, this drug is not recommended for use in the pediatric age group.

PRECAUTIONS
Confusion, anxiety and tremors have been reported in a few patients receiving propoxyphene and orphenadrine concomitantly. As these symptoms may be simply due to an additive effect, reduction of dosage and/or discontinuation of one or both agents is recommended in such cases.
Orphenadrine citrate should be used with caution in patients with tachycardia, cardiac decompensation, coronary insufficiency, cardiac arrhythmias.
Safety of continuous long-term therapy with orphenadrine has not been established. Therefore, if orphenadrine is prescribed for prolonged use, periodic monitoring of blood, urine and liver function values is recommended.

ADVERSE REACTIONS
Adverse reactions of orphenadrine are mainly due to the mild anticholinergic action of orphenadrine, and are usually associated with higher dosage. Dryness of the mouth is usually the first adverse effect to appear. When the daily dose is increased, possible adverse effects include: tachycardia, palpitation, urinary hesitancy or retention, blurred vision, dilatation of pupils, increased ocular tension, weakness, nausea, vomiting, headache, dizziness, constipation, drowsiness, hypersensitivity reactions, pruritus, hallucinations, agitation, tremor, gastric irritation, and rarely urticaria and other dermatoses. Infrequently, an elderly patient may experience some degree of mental confusion. These adverse reactions can usually be eliminated by reduction in dosage. Very rare cases of aplastic anemia associated with the use of orphenadrine tablets have been reported. No causal relationship has been established.
Rare instances of anaphylactic reaction have been reported associated with the intramuscular injection of Norflex Injection.

DOSAGE AND ADMINISTRATION
TABLETS: Adults—Two tablets per day; one in the morning and one in the evening.
INJECTION: Adults—One 2 mL ampul (60 mg) intravenously or intramuscularly; may be repeated every 12 hours. Relief may be maintained by 1 Norflex tablet twice daily.

HOW SUPPLIED
TABLETS: Each round, white tablet imprinted with "3M" on one side and "221" on the other. Bottles of 100 (NDC 0089-0221-10) and 500 (NDC 0089-0221-50). Each tablet contains 100 mg of orphenadrine citrate.
INJECTION: Boxes of 6 (NDC 0089-0540-06) 2 mL ampuls, each ampul containing 60 mg of orphenadrine citrate in aqueous solution.

A.H.F.S. Category 12:08

Store at controlled room temperature, 15°–30°C (59°–86°F).

CAUTION
Federal law prohibits dispensing without prescription.
NRF-16   SEPTEMBER 1993
Shown in Product Identification Guide, page 322

NORGESIC™ ℞
and
NORGESIC™ FORTE ℞
Tablets

ACTIONS
Orphenadrine citrate is a centrally acting (brain stem) compound which in animals selectively blocks facilitatory functions of the reticular formation. Orphenadrine does not produce myoneural block, nor does it affect crossed extensor reflexes. Orphenadrine prevents nicotine-induced convulsions but not those produced by strychnine.
Chronic administration of Norgesic to dogs and rats has revealed no drug-related toxicity. No blood or urine changes were observed, nor were there any macroscopic or microscopic pathological changes detected. Extensive experience with combinations containing aspirin and caffeine has established them as safe agents. The addition of orphenadrine citrate does not alter the toxicity of aspirin and caffeine. The mode of therapeutic action of orphenadrine has not been clearly identified, but may be related to its analgesic proper-

ties. Orphenadrine citrate also possesses anticholinergic actions.

INDICATIONS
1. Symptomatic relief of mild to moderate pain of acute musculoskeletal disorders.
2. The orphenadrine component is indicated as an adjunct to rest, physical therapy, and other measures for the relief of discomfort associated with acute painful musculoskeletal conditions.
The mode of action of orphenadrine has not been clearly identified, but may be related to its analgesic properties. Norgesic and Norgesic Forte do not directly relax tense skeletal muscles in man.

CONTRAINDICATIONS
Because of the mild anticholinergic effect of orphenadrine, Norgesic or Norgesic Forte should not be used in patients with glaucoma, pyloric or duodenal obstruction, achalasia, prostatic hypertrophy or obstructions at the bladder neck. Norgesic or Norgesic Forte is also contraindicated in patients with myasthenia gravis and in patients known to be sensitive to aspirin or caffeine.
The drug is contraindicated in patients who have demonstrated a previous hypersensitivity to the drug.

WARNINGS
Reye Syndrome may develop in individuals who have chicken pox, influenza, or flu symptoms. Some studies suggest possible association between the development of Reye Syndrome and the use of medicines containing salicylate or aspirin. Norgesic and Norgesic Forte contain aspirin and therefore are not recommended for use in patients with chicken pox, influenza, or flu symptoms.
Norgesic Forte may impair the ability of the patient to engage in potentially hazardous activities such as operating machinery or driving a motor vehicle; ambulatory patients should therefore be cautioned accordingly.
Aspirin should be used with extreme caution in the presence of peptic ulcers and coagulation abnormalities.

USAGE IN PREGNANCY
Since safety of the use of this preparation in pregnancy, during lactation, or in the childbearing age has not been established, use of the drug in such patients requires that the potential benefits of the drug be weighed against its possible hazard to the mother and child.

USAGE IN CHILDREN
The safe and effective use of this drug in children has not been established. Usage of this drug in children under 12 years of age is not recommended.

PRECAUTIONS
Confusion, anxiety and tremors have been reported in a few patients receiving propoxyphene and orphenadrine concomitantly. As these symptoms may be simply due to an additive effect, reduction of dosage and/or discontinuation of one or both agents is recommended in such cases.
Safety of continuous long term therapy with Norgesic Forte has not been established; therefore, if Norgesic Forte is prescribed for prolonged use, periodic monitoring of blood, urine and liver function values is recommended.

ADVERSE REACTIONS
Side effects of Norgesic or Norgesic Forte are those seen with aspirin and caffeine or those usually associated with mild anticholinergic agents. These may include tachycardia, palpitation, urinary hesitancy or retention, dry mouth, blurred vision, dilatation of the pupil, increased intraocular tension, weakness, nausea, vomiting, headache, dizziness, constipation, drowsiness, and rarely, urticaria and other dermatoses. Infrequently, an elderly patient may experience some degree of confusion. Mild central excitation and occasional hallucinations may be observed. These mild side effects can usually be eliminated by reduction in dosage. One case of aplastic anemia associated with the use of Norgesic has been reported. No causal relationship has been established. Rare G.I. hemorrhage due to aspirin content may be associated with the administration of Norgesic or Norgesic Forte. Some patients may experience transient episodes of light-headedness, dizziness or syncope.

DOSAGE AND ADMINISTRATION
Norgesic: Adults 1 to 2 tablets 3 to 4 times daily.
Norgesic Forte: Adults ½ to 1 tablet 3 to 4 times daily.

HOW SUPPLIED
Norgesic tablets can be identified by their three layers colored light green, white and yellow. Each round tablet is embossed "NORGESIC" on one side and "3M" on the other and contains orphenadrine citrate (2-dimethylaminoethyl 2-methylbenzhydryl ether citrate) 25 mg, aspirin 385 mg, and caffeine 30 mg.
Norgesic Forte tablets are exactly twice the strength of Norgesic. They are identified by their scored capsule shape and by their three layers colored light green, white and yellow. Each capsule shaped tablet is embossed "NORGESIC FORTE" on one side and "3M" on the other and contains

orphenadrine citrate 50 mg, aspirin 770 mg, and caffeine 60 mg.
Norgesic and Norgesic Forte also contain: lactose, polyethylene glycol, povidone, starch, sucrose, zinc stearate, D&C yellow #10, and FD&C blue #1.
Norgesic: Bottles of 100 tablets (NDC **0089-0231-10**) and Bottles of 500 tablets (NDC **0089-0231-50**).
Norgesic Forte: Bottles of 100 tablets (NDC **0089-0233-10**) and bottles of 500 tablets (NDC **0089-0233-50**).
Store below 30°C (86°F).

CAUTION

Federal law prohibits dispensing without prescription.
NG-15 OCTOBER 1993
Shown in Product Identification Guide, page 322

TAMBOCOR™ ℞

[tăm-ba-kōr]
(flecainide acetate)
Tablets

DESCRIPTION

TAMBOCOR™ (flecainide acetate) is an antiarrhythmic drug available in tablets of 50, 100 or 150 mg for oral administration.
Flecainide acetate is benzamide, N-(2-piperidinylmethyl)-2,5-bis(2,2,2-trifluoroethoxy)-, monoacetate. The structural formula is given below.

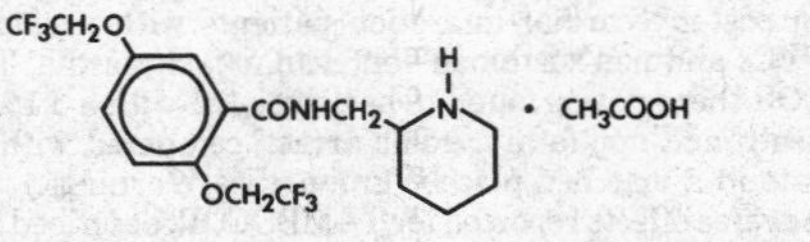

Flecainide acetate is a white crystalline substance with a pK_a of 9.3. It has an aqueous solubility of 48.4 mg/mL at 37°C.
TAMBOCOR tablets also contain: croscarmellose sodium, hydrogenated vegetable oil, magnesium stearate, microcrystalline cellulose and starch.

CLINICAL PHARMACOLOGY

TAMBOCOR has local anesthetic activity and belongs to the membrane stabilizing (Class 1) group of antiarrhythmic agents; it has electrophysiologic effects characteristic of the IC class of antiarrhythmics.
Electrophysiology. In man, TAMBOCOR produces a dose-related decrease in intracardiac conduction in all parts of the heart with the greatest effect on the His-Purkinje system (H-V conduction). Effects upon atrioventricular (AV) nodal conduction time and intra-atrial conduction times, although present, are less pronounced than those on ventricular conduction velocity. Significant effects on refractory periods were observed only in the ventricle. Sinus node recovery times (corrected) following pacing and spontaneous cycle lengths are somewhat increased. This latter effect may become significant in patients with sinus node dysfunction. (See Warnings.)
TAMBOCOR causes a dose-related and plasma-level related decrease in single and multiple PVCs and can suppress recurrence of ventricular tachycardia. In limited studies of patients with a history of ventricular tachycardia, TAMBOCOR has been successful 30–40% of the time in fully suppressing the inducibility of arrhythmias by programmed electrical stimulation. Based on PVC suppression, it appears that plasma levels of 0.2 to 1.0 μg/mL may be needed to obtain the maximal therapeutic effect. It is more difficult to assess the dose needed to suppress serious arrhythmias, but trough plasma levels in patients successfully treated for recurrent ventricular tachycardia were between 0.2 and 1.0 μg/mL. Plasma levels above 0.7–1.0 μg/mL are associated with a higher rate of cardiac adverse experiences such as conduction defects or bradycardia. The relation of plasma levels to proarrhythmic events is not established, but dose reduction in clinical trials of patients with ventricular tachycardia appears to have led to a reduced frequency and severity of such events.
Hemodynamics. TAMBOCOR does not usually alter heart rate, although bradycardia and tachycardia have been reported occasionally.
In animals and isolated myocardium, a negative inotropic effect of flecainide has been demonstrated. Decreases in ejection fraction, consistent with a negative inotropic effect, have been observed after single administration of 200 to 250 mg of the drug in man; both increases and decreases in ejection fraction have been encountered during multidose therapy in patients at usual therapeutic doses. (See Warnings.)
Metabolism in Humans. Following oral administration, the absorption of TAMBOCOR is nearly complete. Peak plasma levels are attained at about three hours in most individuals (range, 1 to 6 hours). Flecainide does not undergo any consequential presystemic biotransformation (first-pass effect). Food or antacid do not affect absorption.
The apparent plasma half-life averages about 20 hours and is quite variable (range, 12 to 27 hours) after multiple oral doses in patients with premature ventricular contractions (PVCs). With multiple dosing, plasma levels increase because of its long half-life with steady-state levels approached in 3 to 5 days; once at steady-state, no additional (or unexpected) accumulation of drug in plasma occurs during chronic therapy. Over the usual therapeutic range, data suggest that plasma levels in an individual are approximately proportional to dose, deviating upwards from linearity only slightly (about 10 to 15% per 100 mg on average).
In healthy subjects, about 30% of a single oral dose (range, 10 to 50%) is excreted in urine as unchanged drug. The two major urinary metabolites are meta-O-dealkylated flecainide (active, but about one-fifth as potent) and the meta-O-dealkylated lactam of flecainide (non-active metabolite). These two metabolites (primarily conjugated) account for most of the remaining portion of the dose. Several minor metabolites (3% of the dose or less) are also found in urine; only 5% of an oral dose is excreted in feces. In patients, free (unconjugated) plasma levels of the two major metabolites are very low (less than 0.05 μg/mL).
When urinary pH is very alkaline (8 or higher), as may occur in rare conditions (e.g., renal tubular acidosis, strict vegetarian diet), flecainide elimination from plasma is much slower.
The elimination of flecainide from the body depends on renal function (i.e., 10 to 50% appears in urine as unchanged drug). With increasing renal impairment, the extent of unchanged drug excretion in urine is reduced and the plasma half-life of flecainide is prolonged. Since flecainide is also extensively metabolized, there is no simple relationship between creatinine clearance and the rate of flecainide elimination from plasma. (See Dosage and Administration.)
In patients with NYHA class III congestive heart failure (CFH), the rate of flecainide elimination from plasma (mean half-life, 19 hours) is moderately slower than for healthy subjects (mean half-life, 14 hours), but similar to the rate for patients with PVCs without CHF. The extent of excretion of unchanged drug in urine is also similar. (See Dosage and Administration.)
From age 20 to 80, plasma levels are only slightly higher with advancing age; flecainide elimination from plasma is somewhat slower in elderly subjects than in younger subjects. Patients up to age 80+ have been safely treated with usual dosages.
The extent of flecainide binding to human plasma proteins is about 40% and is independent of plasma drug level over the range of 0.015 to about 3.4 μg/mL. Thus, clinically significant drug interactions based on protein binding effects would not be expected.
Hemodialysis removes only about 1% of an oral dose as unchanged flecainide.
Small increases in plasma digoxin levels are seen during coadministration of TAMBOCOR with digoxin. Small increases in both flecainide and propranolol plasma levels are seen during coadministration of these two drugs. (See Precautions, Drug Interactions.)
Clinical Trials. In two randomized, crossover, placebo-controlled clinical trials of 16 weeks double-blind duration, 79% of patients with paroxysmal supraventricular tachycardia (PSVT) receiving flecainide were attack free, whereas 15% of patients receiving placebo remained attack free. The median time-before-recurrence of PSVT in patients receiving placebo was 11 to 12 days, whereas over 85% of patients receiving flecainide had no recurrence at 60 days.
In two randomized, crossover, placebo-controlled clinical trials of 16 weeks double-blind duration, 31% of patients with paroxysmal atrial fibrillation/flutter (PAF) receiving flecainide were attack free, whereas 8% receiving placebo remained attack free. The median time-before-recurrence of PAF in patients receiving placebo was about 2 to 3 days, whereas for those receiving flecainide the median time-before recurrence was 15 days.

INDICATIONS AND USAGE

In patients without structural heart disease, TAMBOCOR is indicated for the prevention of
—paroxysmal supraventricular tachycardias (PSVT), including atrioventricular nodal reentrant tachycardia, atrioventricular reentrant tachycardia and other supraventricular tachycardias of unspecified mechanism associated with disabling symptoms
—paroxysmal atrial fibrillation/flutter (PAF) associated with disabling symptoms
TAMBOCOR is also indicated for the prevention of
—documented ventricular arrhythmias, such as sustained ventricular tachycardia (sustained VT), that in the judgment of the physician, are life-threatening.
Use of TAMBOCOR for the treatment of sustained VT, like other antiarrhythmics, should be initiated in the hospital. The use of TAMBOCOR is not recommended in patients with less severe ventricular arrhythmias even if the patients are symptomatic.
Because of the proarrhythmic effects of TAMBOCOR, its use should be reserved for patients in whom, in the opinion of the physician, the benefits of treatment outweigh the risks.
TAMBOCOR should not be used in patients with recent myocardial infarction. (See Boxed Warnings.)
Use of TAMBOCOR in chronic atrial fibrillation has not been adequately studied and is not recommended. (See Boxed Warnings.)
As is the case for other antiarrhythmic agents, there is no evidence from controlled trials that the use of TAMBOCOR favorably affects survival or the incidence of sudden death.

CONTRAINDICATIONS

TAMBOCOR is contraindicated in patients with pre-existing second- or third-degree AV block, or with right bundle branch block when associated with a left hemiblock (bifascicular block), unless a pacemaker is present to sustain the cardiac rhythm should complete heart block occur. TAMBOCOR is also contraindicated in the presence of cardiogenic shock or known hypersensitivity to the drug.

WARNINGS

Mortality. TAMBOCOR was included in the National Heart Lung and Blood Institute's Cardiac Arrhythmia Suppression Trial (CAST), a long-term, multicenter, randomized, double-blind study in patients with asymptomatic non-life-threatening ventricular arrhythmias who had a myocardial infarction more than six days, but less than two years previously. An excessive mortality or non-fatal cardiac arrest rate was seen in patients treated with TAMBOCOR compared with that seen in a carefully matched placebo-treated group. This rate was 16/315 (5.1%) for TAMBOCOR and 7/309 (2.3%) for its matched placebo. The average duration of treatment with TAMBOCOR in this study was 10 months.
Ventricular Pro-arrhythmic Effects in Patients with Atrial Fibrillation/Flutter. A review of the world literature revealed reports of 568 patients treated with oral TAMBOCOR for paroxysmal atrial fibrillation/flutter (PAF). Ventricular tachycardia was experienced in 0.4% (2/568) of these patients. Of 19 patients in the literature with chronic atrial fibrillation (CAF), 10.5% (2) experienced VT or VF. FLECAINIDE IS NOT RECOMMENDED FOR USE IN PATIENTS WITH CHRONIC ATRIAL FIBRILLATION. Case reports of ventricular proarrhythmic effects in patients treated with TAMBOCOR for atrial fibrillation/flutter have included increased PVCs, VT, ventricular fibrillation (VF), and death.
As with other Class I agents, patients treated with TAMBOCOR for atrial flutter have been reported with 1:1 atrioventricular conduction due to slowing the atrial rate. A paradoxical increase in the ventricular rate also may occur in patients with atrial fibrillation who receive TAMBOCOR. Concomitant negative chronotropic therapy such as digoxin or beta-blockers may lower the risk of this complication.

The applicability of the CAST results to other populations (e.g., those without recent infarction) is uncertain, but at present it is prudent to consider the risks of Class IC agents, coupled with the lack of any evidence of improved survival, generally unacceptable in patients whose ventricular arrhythmias are not life-threatening, even if the patients are experiencing unpleasant, but not life-threatening, symptoms or signs.
PROARRHYTHMIC EFFECTS
TAMBOCOR, like other antiarrhythmic agents, can cause new or worsened supraventricular or ventricular arrhythmias. Ventricular proarrhythmic effects range from an increase in frequency of PVCs to the development of more severe ventricular tachycardia, e.g., tachycardia that is more sustained or more resistant to conversion to sinus rhythm, with potentially fatal consequences. In studies of ventricular arrhythmia patients treated with TAMBOCOR, three-fourths of proarrhythmic events were new or worsened ventricular tachyarrhythmias, the remainder being increased frequency of PVCs or new supraventricular arrhythmias. In patients treated with flecainide for sustained ventricular tachycardia, 80% (51/64) of proarrhythmic events occurred within 14 days of the onset of therapy. In studies of 225 patients with supraventricular arrhythmia (108 with paroxysmal supraventricular tachycardia and 117 with paroxysmal atrial fibrillation), there were 9 (4%) proarrhythmic events, 8 of them in patients with paroxysmal atrial fibrillation. Of the 9, 7 (including the one in a PSVT patient) were exacerbations of supraventricular arrhythmias (longer duration, more rapid rate, harder to reverse) while 2 were ventricular arrhythmias, including one fatal case of VT/VF and one wide complex VT (the patient showed inducible VT, however, after withdrawal of flecainide), both in patients with paroxysmal atrial fibrillation and known coronary artery disease.
It is uncertain if TAMBOCOR's risk of proarrhythmia is exaggerated in patients with chronic atrial fibrillation (CAF), high ventricular rate, and/or exercise. Wide complex tachy-

Continued on next page

3M—Cont.

cardia and ventricular fibrillation have been reported in two of 12 CAF patients undergoing maximal exercise tolerance testing.

In patients with complex ventricular arrhythmias, it is often difficult to distinguish a spontaneous variation in the patient's underlying rhythm disorder from drug-induced worsening, so that the following occurrence rates must be considered approximations. Their frequency appears to be related to dose and to the underlying cardiac disease.

Among patients treated for sustained VT (who frequently also had CHF, a low ejection fraction, a history of myocardial infarction and/or an episode of cardiac arrest), the incidence of proarrhythmic events was 13% when dosage was initiated at 200 mg/day with slow upward titration, and did not exceed 300 mg/day in most patients. In early studies in patients with sustained VT utilizing a higher initial dose (400 mg/day) the incidence of proarrhythmic events was 26%; moreover, in about 10% of the patients treated proarrhythmic events resulted in death, despite prompt medical attention. With lower initial doses, the incidence of proarrhythmic events resulting in death decreased to 0.5% of these patients. Accordingly, it is extremely important to follow the recommended dosage schedule. (See Dosage and Administration.)

The relatively high frequency of proarrhythmic events in patients with sustained VT and serious underlying heart disease, and the need for careful titration and monitoring, requires that therapy of patients with sustained VT be started in the hospital. (See Dosage and Administration.)

HEART FAILURE

TAMBOCOR has a negative inotropic effect and may cause or worsen CHF, particularly in patients with cardiomyopathy, preexisting severe heart failure (NYHA functional class III or IV) or low ejection fractions (less than 30%). In patients with supraventricular arrhythmias new or worsened CHF developed in 0.4% (1/225) of patients. In patients with sustained ventricular tachycardia during a mean duration of 7.9 months of TAMBOCOR therapy, 6.3% (20/317) developed new CHF. In patients with sustained ventricular tachycardia and a history of CHF, during a mean duration of 5.4 months of TAMBOCOR therapy, 25.7% (78/304) developed worsened CHF. Exacerbation of preexisting CHF occurred more commonly in studies which included patients with class III or IV failure than in studies which excluded such patients. TAMBOCOR should be used cautiously in patients who are known to have a history of CHF or myocardial dysfunction. The initial dosage in such patients should be no more than 100 mg bid (see Dosage and Administration) and patients should be monitored carefully. Close attention must be given to maintenance of cardiac function, including optimization of digitalis, diuretic, or other therapy. In cases where CHF has developed or worsened during treatment with TAMBOCOR, the time of onset has ranged from a few hours to several months after starting therapy. Some patients who develop evidence of reduced myocardial function while on TAMBOCOR can continue on TAMBOCOR with adjustment of digitalis or diuretics, others may require dosage reduction or discontinuation of TAMBOCOR. When feasible, it is recommended that plasma flecainide levels be monitored. Attempts should be made to keep trough plasma levels below 0.7 to 1.0 μg/mL.

Effects on Cardiac Conduction. TAMBOCOR slows cardiac conduction in most patients to produce dose-related increases in PR, QRS, and QT intervals.

PR interval increases on average about 25% (0.04 seconds) and as much as 118% in some patients. Approximately one-third of patients may develop new first-degree AV heart block (PR interval $\geq$ 0.20 seconds). The QRS complex increases on average about 25% (0.02 seconds) and as much as 150% in some patients. Many patients develop QRS complexes with a duration of 0.12 seconds or more. In one study, 4% of patients developed new bundle branch block while on TAMBOCOR. The degree of lengthening of PR and QRS intervals does not predict either efficacy or the development of cardiac adverse effects. In clinical trials, it was unusual for PR intervals to increase to 0.30 seconds or more, or for QRS intervals to increase to 0.18 seconds or more. Thus, caution should be used when such intervals occur, and dose reductions may be considered. The QT interval widens about 8%, but most of this widening (about 60% to 90%) is due to widening of the QRS duration. The JT interval (QT minus QRS) only widens about 4% on the average. Significant JT prolongation occurs in less than 2% of patients. There have been rare cases of Torsade de Pointes-type arrhythmia associated with TAMBOCOR therapy.

Clinically significant conduction changes have been observed at these rates: sinus node dysfunction such as sinus pause, sinus arrest and symptomatic bradycardia (1.2%), second-degree AV block (0.5%) and third-degree AV block (0.4%). An attempt should be made to manage the patient on the lowest effective dose in an effort to minimize these effects. (See Dosage and Administration.) If second- or third-degree AV block, or right bundle branch block associated with a left hemiblock occur, TAMBOCOR therapy should be discontinued unless a temporary or implanted ventricular pacemaker is in place to ensure an adequate ventricular rate.

Sick Sinus Syndrome (Bradycardia-Tachycardia Syndrome). TAMBOCOR should be used only with extreme caution in patients with sick sinus syndrome because it may cause sinus bradycardia, sinus pause, or sinus arrest.

Effects on Pacemaker Thresholds. TAMBOCOR is known to increase endocardial pacing thresholds and may suppress ventricular escape rhythms. These effects are reversible if flecainide is discontinued. It should be used with caution in patients with permanent pacemakers or temporary pacing electrodes and should not be administered to patients with existing poor thresholds or nonprogrammable pacemakers unless suitable pacing rescue is available.

The pacing threshold in patients with pacemakers should be determined prior to instituting therapy with TAMBOCOR, again after one week of administration and at regular intervals thereafter. Generally threshold changes are within the range of multiprogrammable pacemakers and, when these occur, a doubling of either voltage or pulse width is usually sufficient to regain capture.

Electrolyte Disturbances. Hypokalemia or hyperkalemia may alter the effects of Class I antiarrhythmic drugs. Preexisting hypokalemia or hyperkalemia should be corrected before administration of TAMBOCOR.

PRECAUTIONS

Drug Interactions. TAMBOCOR has been administered to patients receiving **digitalis** preparations or **beta-adrenergic blocking agents** without adverse effects. During administration of multiple oral doses of TAMBOCOR to healthy subjects stabilized on a maintenance dose of **digoxin**, a 13%–19% increase in plasma **digoxin** levels occurred at six hours postdose.

In a study involving healthy subjects receiving TAMBOCOR and **propranolol** concurrently, plasma flecainide levels were increased about 20% and **propranolol** levels were increased about 30% compared to control values. In this formal interaction study, TAMBOCOR and **propranolol** were each found to have negative inotropic effects; when the drugs were administered together, the effects were additive. The effects of concomitant administration of TAMBOCOR and **propranolol** on the PR interval were less than additive. In TAMBOCOR clinical trials, patients who were receiving **beta blockers** concurrently did not experience an increased incidence of side effects. Nevertheless, the possibility of additive negative inotropic effects of **beta blockers** and flecainide should be recognized.

Flecainide is not extensively bound to plasma proteins. In vitro studies with several drugs which may be administered concomitantly showed that the extent of flecainide binding to human plasma proteins is either unchanged or only slightly less. Consequently, interactions with other drugs which are highly protein bound (e.g., **anticoagulants**) would not be expected. TAMBOCOR has been used in a large number of patients receiving **diuretics** without apparent interaction. Limited data in patients receiving known enzyme inducers (**phenytoin, phenobarbital, carbamazepine**) indicate only a 30% increase in the rate of flecainide elimination. In healthy subjects receiving **cimetidine** (1 gm daily) for one week, plasma flecainide levels increased by about 30% and half-life increased by about 10%.

When **amiodarone** is added to flecainide therapy, plasma flecainide levels may increase two-fold or more in some patients, if flecainide dosage is not reduced. (See Dosage and Administration.)

There has been little experience with the coadministration of TAMBOCOR and either **disopyramide** or **verapamil**. Because both of these drugs have negative inotropic properties and the effects of coadministration with TAMBOCOR are unknown, neither **disopyramide** nor **verapamil** should be administered concurrently with TAMBOCOR unless, in the judgment of the physician, the benefits of this combination outweigh the risks. There has been too little experience with the coadministration of TAMBOCOR with **nifedipine** or **diltiazem** to recommend concomitant use.

Carcinogenesis, Mutagenesis, Impairment of Fertility. Long-term studies with flecainide in rats and mice at doses up to 60 mg/kg/day have not revealed any compound-related carcinogenic effects. Mutagenicity studies (Ames test, mouse lymphoma and in vivo cytogenetics) did not reveal any mutagenic effects. A rat reproduction study at doses up to 50 mg/kg/day (seven times the usual human dose) did not reveal any adverse effect on male or female fertility.

Pregnancy. Pregnancy Category C. Flecainide has been shown to have teratogenic effects (club paws, sternebrae and vertebrae abnormalities, pale hearts with contracted ventricular septum) and an embryotoxic effect (increased resorptions) in one breed of rabbit (New Zealand White) when given doses of 30 and 35 mg/kg/day, but not in another breed of rabbit (Dutch Belted) when given doses up to 30 mg/kg/day. No teratogenic effects were observed in rats and mice given doses up to 50 and 80 mg/kg/day, respectively; however, delayed sternebral and vertebral ossification was observed at the high dose in rats. Because there are no adequate and well-controlled studies in pregnant women, TAMBOCOR should be used during pregnancy only if the potential benefit justifies the potential risk to the fetus.

Labor and Delivery. It is not known whether the use of TAMBOCOR during labor or delivery has immediate or delayed adverse effects on the mother or fetus, affects the duration of labor or delivery, or increases the possibility of forceps delivery or other obstetrical intervention.

Nursing Mothers. Results from a multiple dose study conducted in mothers soon after delivery indicates that flecainide is excreted in human breast milk in concentrations as high as 4 times (with average levels about 2.5 times) corresponsing plasma levels; assuming a maternal plasma level at the top of the therapeutic range (1 μg/mL), the calculated daily dose to a nursing infant (assuming about 700 mL breast milk over 24 hours) would be less than 3 mg.

Pediatric Use. The safety and effectiveness of TAMBOCOR in children less than 18 years of age have not been established.

Hepatic Impairment. Since flecainide elimination from plasma can be markedly slower in patients with significant hepatic impairment, TAMBOCOR should not be used in such patients unless the potential benefits clearly outweigh the risks. If used, frequent and early plasma level monitoring is required to guide dosage (see Plasma Level Monitoring); dosage increases should be made very cautiously when plasma levels have plateaued (after more than four days).

ADVERSE REACTIONS

In post-myocardial infarction patients with asymptomatic PVCs and non-sustained ventricular tachycardia, TAMBOCOR therapy was found to be associated with a 5.1% rate of death and non-fatal cardiac arrest, compared with a 2.3% rate in a matched placebo group. (See Warnings.)

Adverse effects reported for TAMBOCOR, described in detail in the Warnings section, were new or worsened arrhythmias which occurred in 1% of 108 patients with PSVT and in 7% of 117 patients with PAF; and new or exacerbated ventricular arrhythmias which occurred in 7% of 1330 patients with PVCs, non-sustained or sustained VT. In patients treated with flecainide for sustained VT, 80% (51/64) of proarrhythmic events occurred within 14 days of the onset of therapy. 198 patients with sustained VT experienced a 13% incidence of new or exacerbated ventricular arrhythmias when dosage was initiated at 200 mg/day with slow upward titration, and did not exceed 300 mg/day in most patients. In some patients, TAMBOCOR treatment has been associated with episodes of unresuscitatable VT or ventricular fibrillation (cardiac arrest). (See Warnings.) New or worsened CHF occurred in 6.3% of 1046 patients with PVCs, non-sustained or sustained VT. Of 297 patients with sustained VT, 9.1% experienced new or worsened CHF. New or worsened CHF was reported in 0.4% of 225 patients with supraventricular arrhythmias. There have also been instances of second- (0.5%) or third-degree (0.4%) AV block. Patients have developed sinus bradycardia, sinus pause, or sinus arrest, about 1.2% altogether (see Warnings). The frequency of most of these serious adverse events probably increases with higher trough plasma levels, especially when these trough levels exceed 1.0 μg/mL.

There have been rare reports of isolated elevations of serum alkaline phosphatase and isolated elevations of serum transaminase levels. These elevations have been asymptomatic and no cause and effect relationship with TAMBOCOR has been established. In foreign postmarketing surveillance studies, there have been rare reports of hepatic dysfunction including reports of cholestasis and hepatic failure, and extremely rare reports of blood dyscrasias. Although no cause and effect relationship has been established, it is advisable to discontinue TAMBOCOR in patients who develop unexplained jaundice or signs of hepatic dysfunction or blood dyscrasias in order to eliminate TAMBOCOR as the possible causative agent.

Incidence figures for other adverse effects in patients with ventricular arrhythmias are based on a multicenter efficacy study, utilizing starting doses of 200 mg/day with gradual upward titration to 400 mg/day. Patients were treated for an average of 4.7 months, with some receiving up to 22 months of therapy. In this trial, 5.4% of patients discontinued due to non-cardiac adverse effects.

[See table at top of next page.]

The following additional adverse experiences, possibly related to TAMBOCOR therapy and occurring in 1% to less than 3% of patients, have been reported in acute and chronic studies: *Body as a Whole*—malaise, fever; *Cardiovascular*—tachycardia, sinus pause or arrest; *Gastrointestinal*—vomiting, diarrhea, dyspepsia, anorexia; *Skin*—rash; *Visual*—diplopia; *Nervous System*—hypoesthesia, paresthesia, paresis, ataxia, flushing, increased sweating, vertigo, syncope, somnolence, tinnitus; *Psychiatric*—anxiety, insomnia, depression.

The following additional adverse experiences, possibly related to TAMBOCOR, have been reported in less than 1% of patients: *Body as a Whole*—swollen lips, tongue and mouth;

Table 1
Most Common Non-Cardiac Adverse Effects in Ventricular Arrhythmia Patients Treated with
TAMBOCOR in the Multicenter Study

Adverse Effect	Incidence in All 429 Patients at Any Dose	Incidence By Dose During Upward Titration 200 mg/Day (N=426)	300 mg/Day (N=293)	400 mg/Day (N=100)
Dizziness*	18.9%	11.0%	10.6%	13.0%
Visual Disturbances†	15.9%	5.4%	12.3%	18.0%
Dyspnea	10.3%	5.2%	7.5%	4.0%
Headache	9.6%	4.5%	6.1%	9.0%
Nausea	8.9%	4.9%	4.8%	6.0%
Fatigue	7.7%	4.5%	4.4%	3.0%
Palpitation	6.1%	3.5%	2.4%	7.0%
Chest Pain	5.4%	3.1%	3.8%	1.0%
Asthenia	4.9%	2.6%	2.0%	4.0%
Tremor	4.7%	2.4%	3.4%	2.0%
Constipation	4.4%	2.8%	2.1%	1.0%
Edema	3.5%	1.9%	1.4%	2.0%
Abdominal pain	3.3%	1.9%	2.4%	1.0%

* Dizziness includes reports of dizziness, lightheadedness, faintness, unsteadiness, near syncope, etc.
† Visual disturbance includes reports of blurred vision, difficulty in focusing, spots before eyes, etc.

arthralgia, bronchospasm, myalgia; *Cardiovascular*—angina pectoris, second-degree and third-degree AV block, bradycardia, hypertension, hypotension; *Gastrointestinal*—flatulence; *Urinary System*—polyuria, urinary retention; *Hematologic*—leukopenia, granulocytopenia, thrombocytopenia; *Skin*—urticaria, exfoliative dermatitis, pruritus, alopecia; *Visual*—eye pain or irritation, photophobia, nystagmus; *Nervous System*—twitching, weakness, change in taste, dry mouth, convulsions, impotence, speech disorder, stupor, neuropathy; *Respiratory*—pneumonitis/pulmonary infiltration possibly due to chronic flecainide treatment. *Psychiatric*—amnesia, confusion, decreased libido, depersonalization, euphoria, morbid dreams, apathy.

For patients with supraventricular arrhythmias, the most commonly reported noncardiac adverse experiences remain consistent with those known for patients treated with TAMBOCOR for ventricular arrhythmias. Dizziness is possibly more frequent in PAF patients.

OVERDOSAGE

No specific antidote has been identified for the treatment of TAMBOCOR overdosage. Overdoses ranging up to 8000 mg have been survived, with peak plasma flecainide concentrations as high as 5.3 µg/mL. Untoward effects in these cases included nausea and vomiting, convulsions, hypotension, bradycardia, syncope, extreme widening of the QRS complex, widening of the QT interval, widening of the PR interval, ventricular tachycardia, AV nodal block, asystole, bundle branch block, cardiac failure, and cardiac arrest. The spectrum of events observed in fatal cases was much the same as that seen in the non-fatal cases. Death has resulted following ingestion of as little as 1000 mg; concomitant overdose of other drugs and/or alcohol in many instances undoubtedly contributed to the fatal outcome. Treatment of overdosage should be supportive and may include the following: removal of unabsorbed drug from the gastrointestinal tract, administration of inotropic agents or cardiac stimulants such as dopamine, dobutamine or isoproterenol; mechanically assisted respiration; circulatory assists such as intra-aortic balloon pumping; and transvenous pacing in the event of conduction block. Because of the long plasma half-life of flecainide (12 to 27 hours in patients receiving usual doses), and the possibility of markedly non-linear elimination kinetics at very high doses, these supportive treatments may need to be continued for extended periods of time. Hemodialysis is not an effective means of removing flecainide from the body. Since flecainide elimination is much slower when urine is very alkaline (pH 8 or higher), theoretically, acidification of urine to promote drug excretion may be beneficial in overdose cases with very alkaline urine. There is no evidence that acidification from normal urinary pH increases excretion.

DOSAGE AND ADMINISTRATION

For patients with sustained VT, no matter what their cardiac status, TAMBOCOR, like other antiarrhythmics, should be initiated in-hospital with rhythm monitoring.

Flecainide has a long half-life (12 to 27 hours in patients). Steady-state plasma levels, in patients with normal renal and hepatic function, may not be achieved until the patient has received 3 to 5 days of therapy at a given dose. Therefore, **increases in dosage should be made no more frequently than once every four days,** since during the first 2 to 3 days of therapy the optimal effect of a given dose may not be achieved. For patients with PSVT and patients with PAF the recommended starting dose is 50 mg every 12 hours. TAMBOCOR doses may be increased in increments of 50 mg bid every four days until efficacy is achieved. For PAF patients, a substantial increase in efficacy without a substantial increase in discontinuations for adverse experiences may be achieved by increasing the TAMBOCOR dose from 50 mg to 100 mg bid. The maximum recommended dose for patients with paroxysmal supraventricular arrhythmias is 300 mg/day.

For sustained VT the recommended starting dose is 100 mg every 12 hours. This dose may be increased in increments of 50 mg bid every four days until efficacy is achieved. Most patients with sustained VT do not require more than 150 mg every 12 hours (300 mg/day), and the maximum dose recommended is 400 mg/day.

In patients with sustained VT, use of higher initial doses and more rapid dosage adjustments have resulted in an increased incidence of proarrhythmic events and CHF, particularly during the first few days of dosing (see Warnings). Therefore, a loading dose is not recommended.

Intravenous lidocaine has been used occasionally with TAMBOCOR while awaiting the therapeutic effect of TAMBOCOR. No adverse drug interactions were apparent. However, no formal studies have been performed to demonstrate the usefulness of this regimen.

An occasional patient not adequately controlled by (or intolerant to) a dose given at 12-hour intervals may be dosed at eight-hour intervals.

Once adequate control of the arrhythmia has been achieved, it may be possible in some patients to reduce the dose as necessary to minimize side effects or effects on conduction. In such patients, efficacy at the lower dose should be evaluated. TAMBOCOR should be used cautiously in patients with a history of CHF or myocardial dysfunction (see Warnings).

In patients with severe renal impairment (creatinine clearance of 35 mL/min/1.73 square meters or less), the initial dosage should be 100 mg once daily (or 50 mg bid); when used in such patients, frequent plasma level monitoring is required to guide dosage adjustments (see Plasma Level Monitoring). In patients with less severe renal disease, the initial dosage should be 100 mg every 12 hours; plasma level monitoring may also be useful in these patients during dosage adjustment. In both groups of patients, dosage increases should be made very cautiously when plasma levels have plateaued (after more than four days), observing the patient closely for signs of adverse cardiac effects or other toxicity. It should be borne in mind that in these patients it may take longer than four days before a new steady-state plasma level is reached following a dosage change.

Based on theoretical considerations, rather than experimental data, the following suggestion is made: when transferring patients from another antiarrhythmic drug to TAMBOCOR allow at least two to four plasma half-lives to elapse for the drug being discontinued before starting TAMBOCOR at the usual dosage. In patients where withdrawal of a previous antiarrhythmic agent is likely to produce life-threatening arrhythmias, the physician should consider hospitalizing the patient.

When flecainide is given in the presence of amiodarone, reduce the usual flecainide dose by 50% and monitor the patient closely for adverse effects. Plasma level monitoring is strongly recommended to guide dosage with such combination therapy (see below).

Plasma Level Monitoring. The large majority of patients successfully treated with TAMBOCOR were found to have trough plasma levels between 0.2 and 1.0 µg/mL. The probability of adverse experiences, especially cardiac, may increase with higher trough plasma levels, especially when these exceed 1.0 µg/mL. Periodic monitoring of trough plasma levels may be useful in patient management. Plasma level monitoring is required in patients with severe renal failure or severe hepatic disease, since elimination of flecainide from plasma may be markedly slower. Monitoring of plasma levels is strongly recommended in patients on concurrent amiodarone therapy and may also be helpful in patients with CHF and in patients with moderate renal disease.

HOW SUPPLIED

All tablets are embossed with 3M on one side and TR 50, TR 100 or TR 150 on the other side.

Tambocor, 50 mg per white, round tablet, is available in
Bottles of 100—NDC #0089-0305-10.

Tambocor, 100 mg per white, round, scored tablet, is available in
Bottles of 100—NDC #0089-0307-10.

Tambocor, 150 mg per white, oval, scored tablet, is available in
Bottles of 100—NDC #0089-0314-10.

Store at controlled room temperature 15°–30°C (59°–86°F) in a tight, light-resistant container.

CAUTION: Federal law prohibits dispensing without prescription.

TR-13   MARCH 1994

Manufactured by
3M Pharmaceuticals
Northridge, CA 91324

Shown in Product Identification Guide, page 322

THEOLAIR™
(theophylline tablets USP)
TABLETS   ℞

THEOLAIR™
(theophylline oral solution)
LIQUID   ℞

For full prescribing information see leaflet accompanying product or call 800-328-0255 for a copy.

HOW SUPPLIED

THEOLAIR™ Tablets:
125 mg tablets—Each round, white, scored tablet imprinted with "3M" on one side and "342" on the other. Bottles of 100 (NDC 0089-0342-10).
250 mg tablets—Each capsule-shaped, white, scored tablet imprinted with "3M" on one side and "THEOLAIR 250" on the other. Bottles of 100 (NDC 0089-0344-10).

THEOLAIR™ Liquid:
1 pint bottles of clear, colorless solution. Each tablespoonful (15 ml) contains theophylline equivalent to 80 mg of theophylline anhydrous (NDC 0089-0960-16).

THEOLAIR™-SR
(anhydrous theophylline, sustained-release)
TABLETS   ℞

For full prescribing information see leaflet accompanying product or call 800-328-0255 for a copy.

HOW SUPPLIED

THEOLAIR-SR Tablets:
200 mg sustained-release tablets—Each round, white, scored tablet imprinted with "3M" on one side and "SR 200" on the other. Bottles of 100 (NDC 0089-0341-10) and 1000 (NDC 0089-0341-80).
250 mg sustained-release tablets—Each round, white, scored tablet imprinted with "3M" on one side and "SR 250" on the other. Bottles of 100 (NDC 0089-0345-10) and 250 (NDC 0089-0345-25).
300 mg sustained-release tablets—Each oval, white, scored tablet imprinted with "3M" on one side and "SR 300" on the other. Bottles of 100 (NDC 0089-0343-10) and 1000 (NDC 0089-0343-80).
500 mg sustained-release tablets—Each capsule-shaped, white, scored tablet imprinted with "3M" on one side and "SR 500" on the other. Bottles of 100 (NDC 0089-0347-10).

UREX™
(methenamine hippurate)   ℞

For full prescribing information see leaflet accompanying product or call 800-328-0255 for a copy.

HOW SUPPLIED

UREX Tablets are capsule-shaped, scored, white imprinted "3M" on one side, and "UREX" on the other. Each tablet contains methenamine hippurate 1 g.
Bottles of 100 tablets (NDC **0089-0371-10**).

Marlyn Health Care
14851 N. SCOTTSDALE RD.
SCOTTSDALE, AZ 85254

Direct Inquiries to:
Kelly Easton
14851 North Scottsdale Road
Scottsdale, AZ 85254
(800) 4-MARLYN
In AZ: (602) 991-0200

HEP–FORTE®   OTC
[hep-for'tay]

DESCRIPTION
Hep Forte is a comprehensive formulation of protein, B factors and other nutritional factors which can be important as a dietary supplement for maintenance and support of normal hepatic function.

COMPOSITION
Each capsule contains:

Vitamin A (Palmitate)	1,200 I.U.
Vitamin E (d-Alpha Tocopherol)	10 I.U.
Vitamin C (Ascorbic Acid)	10 mg.
Folic Acid	0.06 mg.
Vitamin B1 (Thiamine Mononitrate)	1 mg.
Vitamin B2 (Riboflavin)	1 mg.
Niacinamide	10 mg.
Vitamin B6 (Pyridoxine HCl)	0.5 mg.
Vitamin B12 (Cobalamin)	1 mcg.
Biotin	3.3 mcg.
Pantothenic Acid	2 mg.
Choline Bitartrate	21 mg.
Zinc (Zinc Sulfate)	2 mg.
Desiccated Liver	194.4 mg.
Liver Concentrate	64.8 mg.
Liver Fraction Number 2	64.8 mg.
Yeast (Dried)	64.8 mg.
dl-Methionine	10 mg.
Inositol	10 mg.

INDICATIONS
Hep Forte is a balanced formulation of vitamins, minerals, lipotropic factors, and vitamin-protein supplements. It is of value as a nutritional supplement for persons who are receiving professional treatment for alcoholism, hepatic dysfunction due to hepatotoxic drugs and liver poisons, male and female infertility due to hormonal imbalance caused by hepatic dysfunction, and for nutritional supplementation after treatment.

CONTRAINDICATIONS
There are no known contraindications to Hep Forte.

DOSAGE
Three to six capsules daily.

HOW SUPPLIED
Bottles of 100, 300 or 500 capsules.
Literature Available.

MARLYN FORMULA 50®   OTC

PRODUCT OVERVIEW

KEY FACTS
MARLYN FORMULA 50 is a dietary supplement providing a combination of amino acids and B6 in a gelatin capsule which provides protein "building blocks" important to growth and development of all protein containing tissue including nails, hair, and skin.

MAJOR USES
Dermatologists recommend Formula 50 for splitting, peeling nails. Since splitting and peeling nails are often associated with nail fungus, Formula 50 may be recommended in conjunction with drug therapy for nail fungus in order to provide protein necessary to growth and development of nails. OB-Gyn's recommend it for help in controlling excessive hair fall-out after child birth.

SAFETY INFORMATION
There are no known contraindications or adverse reactions.

PRESCRIBING INFORMATION

MARLYN FORMULA 50®
COMPOSITION
Each capsule contains:

Amino Acids	0.3 Gm*
Vitamin B6 (pyridoxine HCl)	1.0 mg.

*Approximate analysis of the amino acids: indispensable amino acids (lysine, tryptophan, phenylalanine, methionine, threonine, leucine, isoleucine, valine), 35.30%; semi-dispensable amino acids (arginine, histidine, tyrosine, cystine, glycine), 19.18%; dispensable amino acids (glutamic acid, alanine, aspartic acid, serine, proline), 45.56%.
Amino acids: Protein "building blocks" important to growth and development of all protein containing tissue including nails, hair, and skin.

DOSAGE AND ADMINISTRATION
The recommended daily dose is 6 capsules daily.

SUPPLY
Bottles of 100, 250 and 500 capsules.

PRO–HEPATONE   OTC

PRODUCT OVERVIEW

KEY FACTS
PRO-HEPATONE is an all-inclusive formulation of vitamins, hematinic factors, amino acids, lipotropic factors, and other nutritional supplements to help overcome dietary deficiencies of these nutrients.

MAJOR USES
PRO-HEPATONE is specially designed to be of help as a nutritional adjuvant for persons under professional care for the avoidance of liver problems that may result from improper diet or excesses of alcohol or drugs, and to be of assistance in some types of occasional impotence.

SAFETY INFORMATION
There are no known contraindications or adverse reactions.

PRESCRIBING INFORMATION

PRO–HEPATONE
EACH TWO CAPSULES SUPPLY:

Choline Bitartrate	100	mg
Methionine	100	mg
Inositol	100	mg
Lecithin	100	mg
Liver Concentrate	64.8	mg
Desiccated Liver	64.8	mg
Unsaturated Fatty Acid	640	mg
Vitamin E (Alpha Tocopheryl)	20	I.U.
Vitamin C (Ascorbic Acid)	20	mg
Vitamin B1 (Thiamine)	5	mg
Vitamin B2 (Riboflavin)	5	mg
Niacinamide (Vitamin P)	20	mg
Vitamin B6 (Pyridoxine HCl)	5	mg
L-Cysteine HCl	10	mg
Gluthathione	5	mg
Desoxycholic Acid	25	mg
Thiotic Acid	5	mg
d-Calcium Pantothenate	20	mg
Vitamin B12 (Cyancobalamin)	64.8	mcg
L-Arginine	5	mg
L-Glutamine	10	mg
L-Aspartic Acid	10	mg
L-Ornithine	5	mg
Ferrous Fumarate	648	mcg
Glycine	100	mg
Fructose	100	mg

DOSAGE AND ADMINISTRATION
The recommended daily dose is 2–3 capsules daily.

SUPPLY
Bottles of 150 capsules

IDENTIFICATION PROBLEM?
Turn to the **Product Identification** Guide,
where you'll find more than
1600 products pictured in actual
size and full color.

Mayrand Pharmaceuticals
(See Merz Pharmaceuticals)

McNeil Consumer Products Company
Division of McNeil-PPC, Inc.
FORT WASHINGTON, PA 19034

Direct Inquiries to:
Consumer Affairs Department
Fort Washington, PA 19034
(215) 233-7000

Children's MOTRIN®   OTC
Ibuprofen Oral Suspension

DESCRIPTION
Children's MOTRIN® Ibuprofen Oral Suspension is an alcohol-free, berry-flavored liquid specially developed for children. Each 5 mL (teaspoon) contains ibuprofen 100 mg.

INDICATIONS
Children's MOTRIN® Ibuprofen Oral Suspension is indicated for temporary relief of fever, and minor aches and pains due to colds, flu, sore throat, headaches and toothaches. One dose lasts 6–8 hours.

DIRECTIONS
Shake well before using. A calibrated dosage cup is provided for accurate dosing of *Children's MOTRIN® Suspension*. If possible, use weight to dose; otherwise use age. 2–3 years (24–35 lbs): 1 tsp, 4–5 years (36–47 lbs): 1.5 tsp, 6–8 years (48–59 lbs): 2 tsp, 9–10 years (60–71 lbs): 2.5 tsp, 11 years (72–95 lbs): 3 tsp. Administer to children under 2 years only on advice of a physician. Repeat dose every 6–8 hours, if needed. Do not use more than 4 times a day.

WARNINGS
ASPIRIN SENSITIVE CHILDREN:
- **This product contains no aspirin, but may cause a severe reaction in people allergic to aspirin.**
- **Do not use this product if your child has had an allergic reaction to aspirin such as asthma, swelling, shock or hives.**

CALL YOUR DOCTOR IF:
- Your child is under a doctor's care for any serious condition or is taking any other drug.
- Your child has problems or serious side effects from taking fever reducers or pain relievers.
- Your child does not get any relief within first day (24 hours) of treatment, or pain or fever gets worse.
- Redness or swelling is present in the painful area.
- Sore throat is severe, lasts for more than 2 days or occurs with fever, headache, rash, nausea or vomiting.
- Any new symptoms appear.

DO NOT USE:
- With any other product that contains ibuprofen, or other pain reliever/fever reducers, unless directed by a doctor.
- For more than **3 days** for fever or pain unless directed by a doctor.
- For stomach pain unless directed by a doctor.
- If your child is dehydrated (significant fluid loss) due to continued vomiting, diarrhea or lack of fluid intake.
- If plastic bottle wrap imprinted with "Safety Seal", or foil inner seal on bottle opening imprinted with "Safety Seal" is broken.

IMPORTANT:
- **Keep this and all drugs out of the reach of children. In case of accidental overdose, seek professional assistance or contact a poison control center immediately.**
- If stomach upset occurs while taking this product, give with food or milk. If stomach upset gets worse or lasts, call your doctor.

INACTIVE INGREDIENTS
Citric acid, corn starch, artificial flavors, glycerin, polysorbate 80, purified water, sodium benzoate, sucrose, xanthan gum, FD&C Red #40, D&C Yellow #10.

HOW SUPPLIED
Orange colored liquid in tamper-resistant bottles of 2 and 4 fl. oz.
Shown in Product Identification Guide, page 322

CHILDREN'S TYLENOL® OTC
acetaminophen
Chewable Tablets, Elixir, Suspension Liquid and Suspension Drops

DESCRIPTION
INFANTS' TYLENOL® Grape Suspension Drops are stable, alcohol-free, grape-flavored and purple in color. ***INFANTS' TYLENOL® Cherry Suspension Drops*** are stable, alcohol-free, cherry-flavored and red in color. Each 0.8 ml (one calibrated dropperful) contains 80 mg acetaminophen. ***CHILDREN'S TYLENOL® Elixir*** is stable and alcohol-free, cherry-flavored, and red in color. ***CHILDREN'S TYLENOL® Suspension Liquid*** is alcohol-free, cherry-flavored, and red in color, or bubble gum flavored, and pink in color or grape flavored and purple in color. Each 5 ml contains 160 mg acetaminophen. Each ***CHILDREN'S TYLENOL® Chewable Tablet*** contains 80 mg acetaminophen in a grape, bubble gum, or fruit burst flavor.

ACTIONS
Acetaminophen is a clinically proven analgesic/antipyretic. Acetaminophen produces analgesia by elevation of the pain threshold and antipyresis through action on the hypothalamic heat regulating center. Acetaminophen is equal to aspirin in analgesic and antipyretic effectiveness and it is unlikely to produce many of the side effects associated with aspirin and aspirin containing products.

INDICATIONS
CHILDREN'S TYLENOL® Chewable Tablets, Elixir, Suspension Liquid and ***Suspension Drops*** are designed for treatment of infants and children with conditions requiring temporary relief of fever and discomfort due to colds and "flu," and of simple pain and discomfort due to teething, immunizations and tonsillectomy.

PRECAUTIONS
If a rare sensitivity reaction occurs, the drug should be stopped.

USUAL DOSAGE
All dosages may be repeated every 4 hours, but not more than 5 times daily. Administer to children under 2 years only on the advice of a physician. ***CHILDREN'S TYLENOL Chewable Tablets:*** 2–3 years: two tablets, 4–5 years: three tablets, 6–8 years: four tablets, 9–10 years: five tablets, 11–12 years: six tablets.
CHILDREN'S TYLENOL® Elixir and ***Suspension Liquid:*** (special cup for measuring dosage is provided) 4–11 months: one-half teaspoon, 12–23 months: three-quarters teaspoon, 2–3 years: one teaspoon, 4–5 years: one and one-half teaspoons, 6–8 years: 2 teaspoons, 9–10 years: two and one-half teaspoons, 11–12 years: three teaspoons.
INFANTS' TYLENOL® Suspension Drops: 0–3 months: 0.4 ml, 4–11 months: 0.8 ml, 12–23 months: 1.2 ml, 2–3 years: 1.6 ml, 4–5 years: 2.4 ml.

WARNINGS
Do not take for pain more than 5 days or for fever for more than 3 days unless directed by a physician. If pain or fever persists or gets worse, if new symptoms occur, or if redness or swelling is present, consult a physician because these could be signs of a serious condition. Keep this and all drugs out of the reach of children. In case of accidental overdose, contact a physician or poison control center immediately. Prompt medical attention is critical even if you do not notice any signs or symptoms. Do not use with other products containing acetaminophen.
NOTE: In addition to the above:
INFANTS' TYLENOL® Suspension Drops—Do not use if printed carton overwrap or printed plastic bottle wrap is broken or missing or if carton is opened.
CHILDREN'S TYLENOL® Elixir and Suspension Liquid—Do not use if printed carton overwrap is broken or missing or if carton is opened. Do not use if printed plastic bottle wrap or printed foil inner seal is broken. Not a USP elixir.
CHILDREN'S TYLENOL® Chewables—Do not use if carton is opened or if printed plastic bottle wrap or printed foil inner seal is broken. Phenylketonurics: grape contains phenylalanine 3 mg per tablet, bubble gum contains 6 mg per tablet, fruit burst contains 4.5 mg per tablet.

OVERDOSAGE INFORMATION
Acetaminophen in massive overdosage may cause hepatic toxicity in some patients. In adults and adolescents, hepatic toxicity has rarely been reported following ingestion of acute overdoses of less than 10 grams. Fatalities are infrequent (less than 3–4% of untreated cases) and have rarely been reported with overdoses of less than 15 grams. In children, an acute overdosage of less than 150 mg/kg has not been associated with hepatic toxicity.
Early symptoms following a potentially hepatotoxic overdose may include: nausea, vomiting, diaphoresis and general malaise. Clinical and laboratory evidence of hepatic toxicity may not be apparent until 48 to 72 hours postingestion.
In adults and adolescents, regardless of the quantity of acetaminophen reported to have been ingested, administer acetylcysteine immediately if 24 hours or less have elapsed from the reported time of ingestion. For full prescribing information, refer to the acetylcysteine package insert. Do not await results of assays for acetaminophen level before initiating treatment with acetylcysteine. The following additional procedures are recommended: The stomach should be emptied promptly by lavage or by induction of emesis with syrup of ipecac. A serum acetaminophen assay should be obtained as early as possible, but no sooner than four hours following ingestion. Liver function studies should be obtained initially and repeated at 24-hour intervals.
Serious toxicity or fatalities are extremely infrequent in children, possibly due to differences in the way they metabolize acetaminophen. In children, the maximum potential amount ingested can be more easily estimated. If more than 150 mg/kg or an unknown amount was ingested, obtain an acetaminophen plasma level. The acetaminophen plasma level should be obtained as soon as possible, but no sooner than 4 hours following the ingestion. Induce emesis using syrup of ipecac. If the plasma level is obtained and falls above the broken line on the acetaminophen overdose nomogram, the acetylcysteine therapy should be initiated and continued for a full course of therapy. If acetaminophen plasma assay capability is not available, and the estimated acetaminophen ingestion exceeds 150 mg/kg, acetylcysteine therapy should be initiated and continued for a full course of therapy.
For additional emergency information, call your regional poison center or call the Rocky Mountain Poison Center toll free, (1-800-525-6115).

INACTIVE INGREDIENTS
CHILDREN'S TYLENOL® Fruit Burst Flavored Chewable Tablets: Aspartame, Cellulose (Microcrystalline), Citric Acid, Corn Starch, Flavors, Magnesium Stearate, Mannitol, Red #7. May contain Ethylcellulose or Cellulose Acetate and Povidone.
CHILDREN'S TYLENOL® Grape Flavored Chewable Tablets: Aspartame, Cellulose, Cellulose Acetate, Citric Acid, Cornstarch, Flavors, Magnesium Stearate, Mannitol, Povidone. Blue #1, Red #7, and Red #30.
CHILDREN'S TYLENOL® Bubble Gum Flavored Chewable Tablets: Aspartame, Cellulose, Flavors, Magnesium Stearate, Maltodextrin, Mannitol, and Red #7. May contain Ethylcellulose or Cellulose Acetate and Povidone.
CHILDREN'S TYLENOL® Elixir: Benzoic Acid, Citric Acid, Flavors, Glycerin, Polyethylene Glycol, Propylene Glycol, Sodium Benzoate, Sorbitol, Sucrose, Purified Water, Red #40, Red #33.
CHILDREN'S TYLENOL® Suspension Liquid: Butylparaben, Cellulose, Citric Acid, Corn Syrup, Flavors, Glycerin, Propylene Glycol, Purified Water, Sodium Benzoate, Sorbitol, Xanthan Gum, FD&C Red #40. In addition to the above ingredients bubble gum flavored suspension contains D&C Red #33, and grape flavored suspension contains D&C Blue #1.
INFANTS' TYLENOL® Cherry Suspension Drops: Butylparaben, Cellulose, Citric Acid, Corn Syrup, Flavors, Glycerin, Propylene Glycol, Purified Water, Sodium Benzoate, Sorbitol, Xanthan Gum, D&C Red #40.
INFANTS' TYLENOL® Grape Suspension Drops: Butylparaben, Cellulose, Citric Acid, Corn Syrup, Flavors, Glycerin, Propylene Glycol, Purified Water, Sodium Benzoate, Sorbitol, Xanthan Gum, D&C Red #33, and FD&C Blue #1.

HOW SUPPLIED
Chewable Tablets (pink colored fruit, purple colored grape, pink colored bubble gum, scored, imprinted "TYLENOL")—Bottles of 30 and also 60's (fruit burst). **Elixir** (cherry colored red)—bottles of 2 and 4 fl. oz. **Suspension liquid** (cherry colored red)—bottles of 2 and 4 fl. oz. (bubble gum flavored colored pink and grape flavored colored purple)—bottle of 4 fl. oz. **Suspension drops** (grape colored purple)—bottles of ½ oz (15 ml) (cherry colored red)—bottles of ½ oz and 1 oz, each with calibrated plastic dropper.
All packages listed above have child-resistant safety caps.
Shown in Product Identification Guide, page 322

CHILDREN'S TYLENOL® COLD OTC
Multi Symptom Chewable Tablets and Liquid

DESCRIPTION
Each ***CHILDREN'S TYLENOL® COLD Multi Symptom Chewable Grape-Flavored Tablet*** contains acetaminophen 80 mg, chlorpheniramine maleate 0.5 mg and pseudoephedrine hydrochloride 7.5 mg. ***CHILDREN'S TYLENOL® COLD Multi Symptom Liquid*** is grape flavored and contains no alcohol. Each teaspoon (5 ml) contains acetaminophen 160 mg, chlorpheniramine maleate 1 mg, and pseudoephedrine hydrochloride 15 mg.

ACTIONS
CHILDREN'S TYLENOL® COLD Multi Symptom Chewable Tablets and Liquid combine the analgesic-antipyretic acetaminophen with the decongestant pseudoephedrine hydrochloride and the antihistamine chlorpheniramine maleate to help relieve nasal congestion, dry runny noses and prevent sneezing as well as to relieve the fever, aches, pains and general discomfort associated with colds and upper respiratory infections.
Acetaminophen is equal to aspirin in analgesic and antipyretic effectiveness and it is unlikely to produce the side effects often associated with aspirin or aspirin-containing products.

INDICATIONS
Provides fast, effective temporary relief of nasal congestion, runny nose, sore throat, sneezing, minor aches and pains, headaches and fever due to the common cold, hay fever or other upper respiratory allergies.

PRECAUTIONS
If a rare sensitivity reaction occurs, the drug should be stopped.

USUAL DOSAGE
All doses may be repeated every 4–6 hours, not to exceed 4 doses in 24 hours.
Administer to children under 6 years only on the advice of a physician. ***CHILDREN'S TYLENOL® COLD Chewable Tablets:*** 2–5 years—2 tablets: 6–11 years—4 tablets.
CHILDREN'S TYLENOL® COLD Liquid Formula: 2–5 years—1 teaspoonful; 6–11 years—2 teaspoonsful. Measuring cup is provided and marked for accurate dosing.

WARNING
KEEP THIS AND ALL MEDICATION OUT OF THE REACH OF CHILDREN. IN CASE OF ACCIDENTAL OVERDOSAGE, CONTACT A PHYSICIAN OR POISON CONTROL CENTER IMMEDIATELY. PROMPT MEDICAL ATTENTION IS CRITICAL EVEN IF YOU DO NOT NOTICE ANY SIGNS OR SYMPTOMS. DO NOT USE WITH OTHER PRODUCTS CONTAINING ACETAMINOPHEN. DO NOT EXCEED RECOMMENDED DOSAGE. Do not take for pain for more than 5 days or for fever for more than 3 days unless directed by a doctor. If pain or fever persists or get worse, if new symptoms occur, or if redness or swelling is present, consult a doctor because these could be signs of a serious condition. If sore throat is severe, persists for more than 2 days, is accompanied or followed by fever, headache, rash, nausea, or vomiting, consult a doctor promptly. If nervousness, dizziness, or sleeplessness, occur discontinue use and consult a doctor. May cause excitability especially in children. Do not give this product to children who have a breathing problem such as chronic bronchitis, or who have glaucoma, heart disease, high blood pressure, thyroid disease, or diabetes without first consulting the child's physician. May cause drowsiness. Sedatives and tranquilizers may increase the drowsiness effect. Do not give this product to children who are taking sedatives or tranquilizers, without first consulting the child's doctor.
NOTE: In addition to the above:
CHILDREN'S TYLENOL® COLD CHEWABLES—DO NOT USE IF CARTON IS OPENED, OR IF PRINTED NECK WRAP OR PRINTED FOIL INNER SEAL IS BROKEN. PHENYLKETONURICS: CONTAINS PHENYLALANINE 6 MG PER TABLET.
CHILDREN'S TYLENOL® COLD LIQUID—DO NOT USE IF CARTON IS OPENED, OR IF PRINTED PLASTIC BOTTLE WRAP OR PRINTED FOIL INNER SEAL IS BROKEN.

DRUG INTERACTION PRECAUTION
Do not give this product to a child who is taking a prescription monamine omidase inhibitor (MAOI) (certain drugs for depression, psychiatric or emotional conditions), or for 2 weeks after stopping the MAOI drug. If you are uncertain whether your child's prescription drug contains an MAOI, consult a health professional before giving this product.

OVERDOSAGE
Acetaminophen in massive overdosage may cause hepatic toxicity in some patients. In adults and adolescents, hepatic toxicity has rarely been reported following ingestion of acute overdosage of less than 10 grams. Fatalities are infrequent (less than 3–4% of untreated cases) and have rarely been reported with overdoses of less than 15 grams. In children, an acute overdosage of less than 150 mg/kg has not been associated with hepatic toxicity.
Early symptoms following a potentially hepatotoxic overdose may include: nausea, vomiting, diaphoresis and general malaise. Clinical and laboratory evidence of hepatic toxicity may not be apparent until 48 to 72 hours postingestion.
In adults and adolescents, regardless of the quantity of acetaminophen reported to have been ingested, administer acetylcysteine immediately if 24 hours or less have elapsed from the reported time of ingestion. For full prescribing informa-

Continued on next page

McNeil Consumer—Cont.

tion, refer to the acetylcysteine package insert. Do not await the results of assays for acetaminophen level before initiating treatment with acetylcysteine. The following additional procedures are recommended: The stomach should be emptied promptly by lavage or by induction of emesis with syrup of ipecac. A plasma acetaminophen assay should be obtained as early as possible, but no sooner than four hours following ingestion. Liver function studies should be obtained initially and repeated at 24-hour intervals.

Serious toxicity or fatalities are extremely infrequent in children, possibly due to differences in the way they metabolize acetaminophen. In children, the maximum potential amount ingested can be more easily estimated. If more than 150 mg/kg or an unknown amount was ingested, obtain an plasma acetaminophen level. The acetaminophen plasma level should be obtained as soon as possible, but no sooner than 4 hours following the ingestion. Induce emesis using syrup of ipecac. If the plasma level is obtained and falls above the broken line on the acetaminophen overdose nomogram, the acetylcysteine therapy should be initiated and continued for a full course of therapy. If acetaminophen plasma assay capability is not available, and the estimated acetaminophen ingestion exceeds 150 mg/kg, acetylcysteine therapy should be initiated and continued for a full course of therapy.

For additional emergency information, call your regional poison center or call the Rocky Mountain Poison Center toll-free, (1-800-525-6115).

Chlorpheniramine toxicity should be treated as you would an antihistamine/anticholinergic overdose and is likely to be present within a few hours after acute ingestion.

Symptoms from pseudoephedrine overdose consist most often of mild anxiety, tachycardia and/or mild hypertension. Symptoms usually appear within 4 to 8 hours of ingestion and are transient, usually requiring no treatment.

INACTIVE INGREDIENTS

Chewable Tablets: Aspartame, Basic Polymuthacrylate, cellulose acetate, citric acid, flavors, hydroxypropyl methylcellulose, magnesium stearate, mannitol, microcrystalline cellulose, Blue #1, Red #7.

Liquid: Benzoic acid, citric acid, flavors, glycerin, malic acid, polyethylene glycol, propylene glycol, sodium benzoate, sorbitol, sucrose, purified water, Blue #1 and Red #40.

HOW SUPPLIED

Chewable Tablets (colored purple, scored, imprinted "Tylenol Cold" on one side and "TC" on opposite side—bottles of 24. **Liquid Formula**—bottles (colored purple) of 4 fl. oz.

Shown in Product Identification Guide, page 322

CHILDREN'S TYLENOL®   OTC
COLD Multi Symptom
PLUS COUGH
Chewable Tablets and Liquid

DESCRIPTION

Each *CHILDREN'S TYLENOL® COLD Multi Symptom Plus Cough Chewable Cherry-Flavored Tablet* contains:
acetaminophen 80 mg
chlorpheniramine maleate 0.5 mg
dextromethorphan hydrobromide 2.5 mg
pseudoephedrine hydrochloride 7.5 mg

CHILDREN'S TYLENOL® COLD Multi Symptom Plus Cough Liquid is cherry flavored and contains no alcohol. Each teaspoon (5 ml) contains acetaminophen 160 mg, chlorpheniramine maleate 1 mg, dextromethorphan hydrobromide 5 mg and pseudoephedrine hydrochloride 15 mg.

ACTIONS

CHILDREN'S TYLENOL® COLD Multi Symptom Plus Cough Chewable Tablets and *Liquid* combines the analgesic-antipyretic acetaminophen with the decongestant pseudoephedrine hydrochloride, the cough suppressant dextromethorphan hydrobromide, and the antihistamine chlorpheniramine maleate to help relieve coughs, nasal congestion, and sore throat, dry runny noses, and prevent sneezing as well as to relieve the fever, aches, pains and general discomfort associated with colds and upper respiratory infections.

Acetaminophen is equal to aspirin in analgesic and antipyretic effectiveness and it is unlikely to produce the side effects often associated with aspirin or aspirin-containing products.

INDICATIONS

For temporary relief of coughs, nasal congestion, runny nose, sore throat, sneezing, minor aches and pains, headaches and fever due to the common cold, hay fever or other upper respiratory allergies.

PRECAUTION

If a rare sensitivity reaction occurs, the drug should be stopped.

DIRECTIONS

All doses may be repeated every 4–6 hours, not to exceed 4 doses in 24 hours.

Administer to children under 6 years only on the advice of a physician.

CHILDREN'S TYLENOL® COLD Plus Cough Chewable Tablets: 2–5 years—2 tablets, 6–11 years—4 tablets.

CHILDREN'S TYLENOL® COLD Plus Cough Liquid Formula: 2–5 years—1 teaspoonful, 6–11 years—2 teaspoonfuls. Measuring cup is provided and marked for accurate dosing.

WARNING

KEEP THIS AND ALL MEDICATION OUT OF THE REACH OF CHILDREN. IN CASE OF ACCIDENTAL OVERDOSE, CONTACT A DOCTOR OR POISON CONTROL CENTER IMMEDIATELY. PROMPT MEDICAL ATTENTION IS CRITICAL EVEN IF YOU DO NOT NOTICE ANY SIGNS OR SYMPTOMS. DO NOT USE WITH OTHER PRODUCTS CONTAINING ACETAMINOPHEN. DO NOT EXCEED RECOMMENDED DOSAGE. Do not take for pain for more than 5 days or for fever for more than 3 days unless directed by a doctor. If pain or fever persists for gets worse, if new symptoms occur, or if redness or swelling is present, consult a doctor because these could be signs of a serious condition. If sore throat is severe, persists for more than 2 days, is accompanied or followed by fever, headache, rash, nausea or vomiting, consult a doctor promptly. If nervousness, dizziness, or sleeplessness occur, discontinue use and consult a doctor. May cause excitability especially in children. Do not give this product to children who have a breathing problem such as chronic bronchitis, or who have glaucoma, heart disease, high blood pressure, thyroid disease, or diabetes, without first consulting the child's doctor. May cause drowsiness. Sedatives and tranquilizers may increase the drowsiness effect. Do not give this product to children who are taking sedatives or tranquilizers, without first consulting the child's doctor. A persistent cough may be a sign of a serious condition. If cough persists for more than 1 week, tends to recur, or is accompanied by fever, rash or persistent headache, consult a doctor. Do not give this product for persistent or chronic cough such as occurs with asthma or if cough is accompanied by excessive phlegm (mucus) unless directed by a doctor. **NOTE:** In addition to the above:

Chewable Tablets—DO NOT USE IF CARTON IS OPENED, OR IF PRINTED NECK WRAP OR PRINTED FOIL INNER SEAL IS BROKEN. **PHENYLKETONURICS: CONTAINS PHENYLALANINE 4 MG PER TABLET.**

Liquid—DO NOT USE IF CARTON IS OPENED, OR IF PRINTED PLASTIC BOTTLE WRAP OR PRINTED FOIL INNER SEAL IS BROKEN.

DRUG INTERACTION PRECAUTION

Do not give this product to a child who is taking a prescription monoamine oxidase inhibitor (MAOI) (certain drugs for depression, psychiatric or emotional conditions), or for 2 weeks after stopping the MAOI drug. If you are uncertain whether your child's prescription drug contains an MAOI, consult a health professional before giving this product.

OVERDOSAGE INFORMATION

Acetaminophen in massive overdosage may cause hepatic toxicity in some patients. In adults and adolescents, hepatic toxicity has rarely been reported following ingestion of acute overdoses of less than 10 grams. Fatalities are infrequent (less than 3–4% of untreated cases) and have rarely been reported with overdoses of less than 15 grams. In children, an acute overdosage of less than 150 mg/kg has not been associated with hepatic toxicity.

Early symptoms following a potentially hepatotoxic overdose may include: nausea, vomiting, diaphoresis and general malaise. Clinical and laboratory evidence of hepatic toxicity may not be apparent until 48 to 72 hours postingestion.

In adults and adolescents, regardless of the quantity of acetaminophen reported to have been ingested, administer acetylcysteine immediately if 24 hours or less have elapsed from the reported time of ingestion. For full prescribing information, refer to the acetylcysteine package insert. Do not await the results of assays for plasma acetaminophen level before initiating treatment with acetylcysteine. The following additional procedures are recommended: The stomach should be emptied promptly by lavage or by induction of emesis with syrup of ipecac. A plasma acetaminophen assay should be obtained as early as possible, but no sooner than four hours following ingestion. If plasma level falls above the lower treatment line on the acetaminophen overdose nomogram, acetylcysteine therapy should be continued. Liver function studies should be obtained initially and repeated at 24-hour intervals.

Serious toxicity or fatalities are extremely infrequent in children, possibly due to differences in the way they metabolize acetaminophen. In children, the maximum potential amount ingested can be more easily estimated. If more than 150 mg/kg or an unknown amount was ingested, obtain an plasma acetaminophen level. The plasma acetaminophen level should be obtained as soon as possible, but no sooner than 4 hours following the ingestion. If plasma level falls

above the lower treatment line on the acetaminophen overdose nomogram, the acetylcysteine therapy should be initiated and continued for a full course of therapy. If plasma acetaminophen assay capability is not available, and the estimated acetaminophen ingestion exceeds 150 mg/kg, acetylcysteine therapy should be initiated and continued for a full course of therapy.

For additional emergency information, call your regional poison center or call the Rocky Mountain Poison Center toll-free, (1-800-525-6115).

Chlorpheniramine toxicity should be treated as you would an antihistamine/anticholinergic overdose and is likely to be present within a few hours after acute ingestion.

Symptoms from pseudoephedrine overdose consist most often of mild anxiety, tachycardia and/or mild hypertension. Symptoms usually appear within 4 to 8 hours of ingestion and are transient, usually requiring no treatment.

Acute dextromethorphan overdose usually does not result in serious signs and symptoms unless massive amounts have been ingested. Signs and symptoms of a substantial overdose may include nausea and vomiting, visual disturbances, CNS disturbances, and urinary retention.

INACTIVE INGREDIENTS

Chewable Tablets: Aspartame, Basic Polymethacrylate, Cellulose Acetate, Colloidal Silicon Dioxide, Flavors, Hydroxypropyl Methylcellulose, Mannitol, Microcrystalline Cellulose, Stearic Acid and Red #7.

Liquid: Citric Acid, Corn Syrup, Flavors, Polyethylene Glycol, Propylene Glycol, Sodium Benzoate, Sodium Carboxymethylcellulose, Sorbitol, Purified Water, Red #33 and Red #40.

HOW SUPPLIED

Chewable Tablets (colored pink, imprinted "TYLENOL C/C" on one side and "TC/C" on the opposite side)—bottles of 24.

Liquid Formula—(red colored) bottles of 4 fl. oz.

Shown in Product Identification Guide, page 323

Children's   OTC
TYLENOL® FLU Suspension Liquid

DESCRIPTION

CHILDREN'S TYLENOL® FLU Suspension Liquid is bubblegum flavored and contains no alcohol or aspirin. Each teaspoon (5 mL) contains acetaminophen 160 mg, pseudoephedrine HCl 15 mg, dextromethorphan HBr 7.5 mg, and chlorpheniramine maleate 1 mg.

ACTIONS

CHILDREN'S TYLENOL® FLU Suspension Liquid combines the analgesic-antipyretic acetaminophen with the decongestant pseudoephedrine hydrochloride, the cough suppressant dextromethorphan hydrobromide and the antihistamine chlorpheniramine maleate to help relieve coughs, nasal congestion, and sore throat, dry runny noses, and prevent sneezing as well as to relieve the fever, aches, pains, and general discomfort associated with colds and upper respiratory infections.

Acetaminophen is equal to aspirin in analgesic and antipyretic effectiveness and it is unlikely to produce the side effects often associated with aspirin or aspirin-containing products.

INDICATIONS

Provides fast, effective, temporary relief of fever, minor aches and pains, headaches, sore throat, nasal congestion, runny nose and coughs due to a cold or "flu".

DOSAGE INSTRUCTIONS

Shake well before using. An Accudose™ measuring cup is provided for accurate dosing of *CHILDREN'S TYLENOL® FLU Suspension Liquid.* 6–11 years (48–95 lbs): 2 tsp. Administer to children under 6 years only on advice of a physician. All doses may be repeated every 6–8 hours. Not to exceed 4 doses in 24 hours.

WARNING

DO NOT USE IF PRINTED CARTON OVERWRAP IS BROKEN OR MISSING OR IF CARTON IS OPENED. DO NOT USE IF PRINTED PLASTIC "SAFETY SEAL" OR PRINTED FOIL INNER SEAL IS BROKEN. KEEP THIS AND ALL DRUGS OUT OF THE REACH OF CHILDREN. IN CASE OF ACCIDENTAL OVERDOSE, CONTACT DOCTOR OR POISON CONTROL CENTER IMMEDIATELY. PROMPT MEDICAL ATTENTION IS CRITICAL FOR ADULTS AS WELL AS CHILDREN EVEN IF YOU DO NOT NOTICE ANY SIGNS OR SYMPTOMS. DO NOT USE WITH OTHER PRODUCTS CONTAINING ACETAMINOPHEN. DO NOT EXCEED RECOMMENDED DOSAGE. Do not take for pain for more than 5 days or for fever for more than 3 days unless directed by a doctor. If pain of fever persists, or gets worse, if new symptoms occur, or if redness or swelling is present, consult a doctor because these could be signs of a serious condition. If sore throat is severe, persists for more than 2 days, is accom-

panied or followed by fever, headache, rash, nausea or vomiting, consult a doctor promptly. A persistent cough may be a sign of a serious condition. If cough persists for more than 1 week, tends to recur or is accompanied by fever, rash, or persistent headache, consult a doctor. Do not give this product for persistent or chronic cough such as occurs with asthma, or if cough is accompanied by excessive phlegm (mucus) unless directed by a doctor. If nervousness, dizziness or sleeplessness occur, discontinue use and consult a doctor. May cause excitability especially in children. Do not give this product to children who have a breathing problem such as chronic bronchitis, or who have glaucoma, heart disease, high blood pressure, thyroid disease or diabetes without first consulting the child's doctor. May cause drowsiness; sedatives and tranquilizers may increase the drowsiness effect. Do not give this product to children who are taking sedatives or tranquilizers without first consulting the child's doctor.

DRUG INTERACTION PRECAUTION

Do not give this product to a child who is taking a prescription monoamine oxidase inhibitor (MAOI) (certain drugs for depression, psychiatric or emotional conditions, or Parkinson's disease), or for 2 weeks after stopping the MAOI drug. If you are uncertain whether your child's prescription drug contains an MAOI, consult a health professional before giving this product.

OVERDOSAGE INFORMATION

Acetaminophen in massive overdosage may cause hepatic toxicity in some patients. In adults and adolescents, hepatic toxicity has rarely been reported following ingestion of acute overdoses of less than 10 grams. Fatalities are infrequent (less than 3–4% of untreated cases) and have rarely been reported with overdoses of less than 15 grams. In children, an acute overdosage of less than 150 mg/kg has not been associated with hepatic toxicity.

Early symptoms following a potentially hepatotoxic overdose may include: nausea, vomiting, diaphoresis and general malaise. Clinical and laboratory evidence of hepatic toxicity may not be apparent until 48 to 72 hours postingestion.

In adults and adolescents, regardless of the quantity of acetaminophen reported to have been ingested, administer acetylcysteine immediately if 24 hours or less have elapsed from the reported time of ingestion. For full prescribing information, refer to the acetylcysteine package insert. Do not await the results of assays for plasma acetaminophen level before initiating treatment wit acetylcysteine. The following additional procedures are recommended: the stomach should be emptied promptly by lavage or by induction of emesis with syrup of ipecac. A plasma acetaminophen assay should be obtained as early as possible, but no sooner than four hours following ingestion. If plasma level falls above the lower treatment line on the acetaminophen overdose nomogram, acetylcysteine therapy should be continued. Liver function studies should be obtained initially and repeated at 24–hour intervals.

Serious toxicity or fatalities are extremely infrequent in children, possibly due to differences in the way they metabolize acetaminophen. In children, the maximum potential amount ingested can be more easily estimated. If more than 150 mg/kg or an unknown amount was ingested, obtain an plasma acetaminophen level. The plasma acetaminophen level should be obtained as soon as possible, but no sooner than 4 hours following the ingestion. If plasma level falls above the lower treatment line on the acetaminophen overdose nomogram, the acetylcysteine therapy should be initiated and continued for a full course of therapy. If plasma acetaminophen assay capability is not available, and the estimated acetaminophen ingestion exceeds 150 mg/kg, acetylcysteine therapy should be initiated and continued for a full course of therapy.

For additional emergency information, call your regional poison center or call the Rocky Mountain Poison Center toll-free (1-800-525-6115).

Chlorpheniramine toxicity should be treated as you would an antihistamine anticholinergic overdose and is likely to be present within a few hours after acute ingestion.

Symptoms from pseudoephedrine overdose consist most often of mild anxiety, tachycardia, and/or mild hypertension. Symptoms usually appear within 4 to 8 hours of ingestion and are transient, usually requiring no treatment.

Acute dextromethorphan overdose usually does not result in serious signs and symptoms unless massive amounts have been ingested. Signs and symptoms of a substantial overdose may include nausea and vomiting, visual disturbances, CNS disturbances, and urinary retention.

INACTIVE INGREDIENTS

Butylparaben, Cellulose, Citric Acid, Corn Syrup, Flavors, Glycerin, Propylene Glycol, Purified Water, Sodium Benzoate, Sodium Carboxymethylcellulose, Sorbitol, Xanthan Gum, D&C Red #33 and FD&C Red #40.

HOW SUPPLIED

Pink colored liquid in child resistant bottles 4 fl. oz.

Shown in Product Identification Guide, page 323

IMODIUM® A–D   OTC
(loperamide hydrochloride)

DESCRIPTION

Each 5 ml (teaspoon) of *IMODIUM® A-D* liquid contains loperamide hydrochloride 1 mg. *IMODIUM A-D* liquid is stable, cherry-mint flavored, and clear in color.

Each caplet of *IMODIUM® AD* contains 2 mg of loperamide and is scored and colored green.

ACTIONS

IMODIUM® A-D contains a clinically proven antidiarrheal medication. Loperamide HCl acts by slowing intestinal motility and by affecting water and electrolyte movement through the bowel.

INDICATION

IMODIUM® A-D is indicated for the control and symptomatic relief of acute nonspecific diarrhea, including travelers' diarrhea.

USUAL DOSAGE

Adults: Take four teaspoonfuls or two caplets after first loose bowel movement. If needed, take two teaspoonfuls or one caplet after each subsequent loose bowel movement. Do not exceed eight teaspoonfuls or four caplets in any 24 hour period, unless directed by a physician.

9–11 years old (60–95 lbs.): Two teaspoonfuls or one caplet after first loose bowel movement, followed by one teaspoonful or one-half caplet after each subsequent loose bowel movement. Do not exceed six teaspoonfuls or three caplets a day.

6–8 years old (48–59 lbs.): Two teaspoonfuls or one caplet after first loose bowel movement, followed by one teaspoonful or one-half caplet after each subsequent loose bowel movement. Do not exceed four teaspoonfuls or two caplets a day.

Professional Dosage Schedule for children two-five years old (24–47 lbs): One teaspoon after first loose bowel movement, followed by one after each subsequent loose bowel movement. Do not exceed three teaspoonfuls a day.

WARNINGS

KEEP THIS AND ALL DRUGS OUT OF THE REACH OF CHILDREN. Do not use for more than two days unless directed by a physician. DO NOT USE IF DIARRHEA IS ACCOMPANIED BY HIGH FEVER (GREATER THAN 101°F), OR IF BLOOD OR MUCUS IS PRESENT IN THE STOOL, OR IF YOU HAVE HAD A RASH OR OTHER ALLERGIC REACTION TO LOPERAMIDE HCl. If you are taking antibiotics or have a history of liver disease, consult a physician before using this product. As with any drug, if you are pregnant or nursing a baby, seek the advice of a health professional before using this product. In case of accidental overdose, seek professional assistance or contact a poison control center immediately.

OVERDOSAGE

Overdosage of loperamide HCl in man may result in constipation, CNS depression and nausea. A slurry of activated charcoal administered promptly after ingestion of loperamide hydrochloride can reduce the amount of drug which is absorbed. If vomiting occurs spontaneously upon ingestion, a slurry of 100 grams of activated charcoal should be administered orally as soon as fluids can be retained. If vomiting has not occurred, and CNS depression is evident, gastric lavage should be performed followed by administration of 100 gms of the activated charcoal slurry through the gastric tube. In the event of overdosage, patients should be monitored for signs of CNS depression for at least 24 hours. Children may be more sensitive to central nervous system effects than adults. If CNS depression is observed, naloxone may be administered. If responsive to naloxone, vital signs must be monitored carefully for recurrence of symptoms of drug overdose for at least 24 hours after the last dose of naloxone.

INACTIVE INGREDIENTS

Liquid: Benzoic acid, citric acid, flavors, glycerin, propylene glycol, purified water, sodium benzoate, sorbitol sucrose, contains 0.5% alcohol.

Caplets: Dibasic calcium phosphate, magnesium stearate, microcrystalline cellulose, colloidal silicon dioxide, FD&C Blue #1 and D&C Yellow #10.

HOW SUPPLIED

Cherry-mint flavored liquid (clear) 2 fl. oz., and 4 fl. oz. tamper resistant bottles with child resistant safety caps and special dosage cups.

Green Scored caplets in 6's and 12's 18's and 24's blister packaging which is tamper resistant and child resistant.

Shown in Product Identification Guide, page 322

INFANTS' TYLENOL® COLD   OTC
Decongestant & Fever Reducer Drops

DESCRIPTION

INFANTS' TYLENOL® COLD Decongestant & Fever Reducer Drops are alcohol-free, bubble gum flavored and red in color. Each 0.8 ml (dropperful) contains acetaminophen 80 mg and pseudoephedrine HCl 7.5 mg.

ACTIONS

Acetaminophen is a clinically proven analgesic/antipyretic. Acetaminophen produces analgesia by elevation of the pain threshold and antipyresis through action on the hypothalamic heat regulating center. Acetaminophen is equal to aspirin in analgesic and antipyretic effectiveness and it is unlikely to produce many of the side effects associated with aspirin and aspirin containing products. Pseudoephedrine hydrochloride is a sympathomimetic amine which provides temporary relief of nasal congestion.

INDICATIONS

INFANTS' TYLENOL® COLD Decongestant & Fever Reducer Drops are indicated for the temporary relief of nasal congestion, minor aches and pains, headaches and fever due to the common cold, hay fever or other upper respiratory allergies.

PRECAUTIONS

If a rare sensitivity reaction occurs, the drug should be stopped.

USUAL DOSAGE

All dosages may be repeated every 4–6 hours, but not more than 4 times daily. Administer to children under 2 years only on the advice of a physician. 0–3 months: 0.4 ml, 4–11 months: 0.8 ml, 12–23 months: 1.2 ml, 2–3 years: 1.6 ml, 4–5 years: 2.4 ml.

WARNINGS

Do not use if printed carton overwrap or printed plastic bottle wrap is broken or missing or if carton is opened. Keep this and all medication out of the reach of children. In case of accidental overdose, contact a doctor or poison control center immediately. Prompt medical attention is critical even if you do not notice any signs or symptoms. Do not exceed recommended dosage. Do not take for pain for more than 5 days or for fever for more than 3 days unless directed by a doctor. If pain or fever persists or gets worse, if new symptoms occur, or if redness or swelling is present, consult a doctor because these could be signs of a serious condition. If nervousness, dizziness or sleeplessness occur, discontinue use and consult a doctor. Do not give this product to a child who has heart disease, high blood pressure, thyroid disease, or diabetes unless directed by a doctor. Do not use with other products containing acetaminophen.

DRUG INTERACTION PRECAUTION

Do not give this product to a child who is taking a prescription monoamine oxidase inhibitor (MAOI) (certain drugs for depression, psychiatric or emotional conditions), or for 2 weeks after stopping the MAOI drug. If you are uncertain whether your child's prescription drug contains an MAOI, consult a health professional before giving this product.

OVERDOSAGE INFORMATION

Acetaminophen in massive overdosage may cause hepatic toxicity in some patients. In adults and adolescents, hepatic toxicity has rarely been reported following ingestion of acute overdoses of less than 10 grams. Fatalities are infrequent (less than 3–4% of untreated cases) and have rarely been reported with overdoses of less than 15 grams. In children, an acute overdosage of less than 150 mg/kg has not been associated with hepatic toxicity.

Early symptoms following a potentially hepatotoxic overdose may include: nausea, vomiting, diaphoresis and general malaise. Clinical and laboratory evidence of hepatic toxicity may not be apparent until 48 to 72 hours postingestion. In adults and adolescents, regardless of the quantity of acetaminophen reported to have been ingested, administer acetylcysteine immediately if 24 hours or less have elapsed from the reported time of ingestion. For full prescribing information, refer to the acetylcysteine package insert. Do not await results of assays for plasma acetaminophen level before initiating treatment with acetylcysteine. The following additional procedures are recommended. The stomach should be emptied promptly by lavage or by induction of emesis with syrup of ipecac. A plasma acetaminophen assay should be obtained as early as possible, but no sooner than four hours following ingestion. If plasma level falls above the lower treatment line on the acetaminophen overdose nomogram, acetylcysteine therapy should be continued. Liver function studies should be obtained initially and repeated at 24-hour intervals.

Serious toxicity or fatalities are extremely infrequent in children, possibly due to differences in the way they metabolize acetaminophen. In children, the maximum potential

Continued on next page

McNeil Consumer—Cont.

amount ingested can be more easily estimated. If more than 150 mg/kg or an unknown amount was ingested, obtain a plasma acetaminophen level. The plasma acetaminophen level should be obtained as soon as possible, but no sooner than 4 hours following the ingestion. If plasma level falls above the lower treatment line on the acetaminophen overdose nomogram, the acetylcysteine therapy should be initiated and continued for a full course of therapy. If plasma acetaminophen assay capability is not available, and the estimated acetaminophen ingestion exceeds 150 mg/kg, acetylcysteine therapy should be initiated and continued for a full course of therapy.
For additional emergency information, call your regional poison center or call the Rocky Mountain Poison Center toll-free, (1-800-525-6115).
Symptoms from pseudoephedrine overdose consist most often of mild anxiety, tachycardia and/or mild hypertension. Symptoms usually appear within 4 to 8 hours of ingestion and are transient, usually requiring no treatment.

INACTIVE INGREDIENTS
Citric acid, corn syrup, flavors, polyethylene glycol, propylene glycol, purified water, sodium benzoate, saccharin, FD&C red #40.

HOW SUPPLIED
Drops (colored red)—bottles of $^1/_2$ fl. oz.
Shown in Product Identification Guide, page 322

JUNIOR STRENGTH TYLENOL® OTC
acetaminophen
Coated Caplets and Chewable Tablets

DESCRIPTION
Each ***JUNIOR STRENGTH TYLENOL® Coated Caplet or Chewable Tablet*** contains 160 mg acetaminophen in a small, coated, capsule shaped tablet or grape or fruit burst flavored chewable tablet.

ACTIONS
Acetaminophen is a clinically proven analgesic/antipyretic. Acetaminophen produces analgesia by elevation of the pain threshold and antipyresis through action on the hypothalamic heat-regulating center. Acetaminophen is equal to aspirin in analgesic and antipyretic effectiveness and it is unlikely to produce many of the side effects associated with aspirin and aspirin-containing products.

INDICATIONS
JUNIOR STRENGTH TYLENOL® Caplets are designed for easy swallowability in older children and young adults. Both ***JUNIOR STRENGTH TYLENOL® Caplets and JUNIOR STRENGTH TYLENOL® Chewable Tablets*** provide fast, effective temporary relief of fever and discomfort due to colds and "flu," and pain and discomfort due to simple headaches, minor muscle aches, sprains and overexertion.

PRECAUTIONS
If a rare sensitivity reaction occurs, the drug should be stopped.

USUAL DOSAGE
Caplets should be taken with liquid. Chewable tablets should be well chewed. All dosages may be repeated every 4 hours, but not more than 5 times daily. For ages: 6–8 years: two caplets or tablets, 9–10 years: two and one-half caplets or tablets, 11 years: three caplets or tablets, 12 years: four caplets or tablets.

WARNING
Do not use if carton is opened or if a blister unit is broken. Do not take for pain for more than 5 days or for fever for more than 3 days unless directed by a physician. If pain or fever persists or gets worse, if new symptoms occur, or if redness or swelling is present, consult a physician because these could be signs of a serious condition. Keep this and all drugs out of reach of children. In case of accidental overdose, contact a physican or poison control center immediately. Prompt medical attention is critical even if you do not notice any signs or symptoms. Do not use with other products containing acetaminophen. As with any drug, if you are pregnant or nursing a baby, seek the advice of a health professional before using this product. In addition the caplet package states: Not for children who have difficulty swallowing tablets. In addition the Grape Chewable Tablet package states: Phenylketonurics: contains phenylalanine 6 mg per tablet, and the Fruit Burst Chewable Tablet package states: Phenylketonurics: contains phenylalanine 9 mg per tablet.

OVERDOSAGE
Acetaminophen in massive overdosage may cause hepatic toxicity in some patients. In adults and adolescents, hepatic toxicity has rarely been reported following ingestion of acute overdosage of less than 10 grams. Fatalities are infrequent (less than 3–4% of untreated cases) and have rarely been reported with overdoses of less than 15 grams. In children, an acute overdosage of less than 150 mg/kg has not been associated with hepatic toxicity.
Early symptoms following a potentially hepatotoxic overdose may include: nausea, vomiting, diaphoresis and general malaise. Clinical and laboratory evidence of hepatic toxicity may not be apparent until 48 to 72 hours postingestion.
In adults and adolescents, regardless of the quantity of acetaminophen reported to have been ingested, administer acetylcysteine immediately if 24 hours or less have elapsed from the reported time of ingestion. For full prescribing information, refer to the acetylcysteine package insert. Do not await the results of assays for acetaminophen level before initiating treatment with acetylcysteine. The following additional procedures are recommended: The stomach should be emptied promptly by lavage or by induction of emesis with syrup of ipecac. A serum acetaminophen assay should be obtained as early as possible, but no sooner than four hours following ingestion. Liver function studies should be obtained initially and repeated at 24-hour intervals.
Serious toxicity or fatalities are extremely infrequent in children, possibly due to differences in the way they metabolize acetaminophen. In children, the maximum potential amount ingested can be more easily estimated. If more than 150 mg/kg or an unknown amount was ingested, obtain an acetaminophen plasma level. The acetaminophen plasma level should be obtained as soon as possible, but no sooner than 4 hours following the ingestion. Induce emesis using syrup of ipecac. If the plasma level is obtained and falls above the broken line on the acetaminophen overdose nomogram, the acetylcysteine therapy should be initiated and continued for a full course of therapy. If acetaminophen plasma assay capability is not available, and the estimated acetaminophen ingestion exceeds 150 mg/kg, acetylcysteine therapy should be initiated and continued for a full course of therapy.
For additional emergency information, call your regional poison center or call the Rocky Mountain Poison Center toll-free, (1-800-525-6115).

INACTIVE INGREDIENTS
Junior Strength Caplets: Cellulose, Cornstarch, Ethylcellulose, Magnesium Stearate, Sodium Lauryl Sulfate, Sodium Starch Glycolate.
Junior Strength Fruit Burst Chewable Tablets: Aspartame, Cellulose, Citric acid, Cornstarch, Flavors, Magnesium Stearate, Mannitol, Red #7. May contain Ethylcellulose or Cellulose Acetate and Povidone.
Junior Strength Grape Flavored Chewable Tablets: Aspartame, Cellulose, Cellulose Acetate, Citric Acid, Cornstarch, Flavors, Magnesium Stearate, Mannitol, Povidone, Blue #1, Red #7 and Red #30.

HOW SUPPLIED
Coated Caplets, (colored white, coated, scored, imprinted "TYLENOL 160") Package of 30.
Chewable Tablets (colored purple or pink, imprinted "TYLENOL 160") Package of 24. All packages are safety sealed and use child resistant blister packaging.
Shown in Product Identification Guide, page 323

LACTAID® Drops OTC
(lactase enzyme)

PRODUCT OVERVIEW

KEY FACTS
LACTAID® is the original dairy digestive supplement that makes milk more digestible. ***LACTAID®*** lactase enzyme hydrolyzes lactose into two digestible simple sugars: glucose and galactose. ***LACTAID® Drops*** are added to milk for *in vitro* hydrolysis of lactose.

MAJOR USES
Lactose intolerance, suspected from gastrointestinal discomfort (ie, gas, bloating, cramps, and diarrhea) after drinking milk.

PRESCRIBING INFORMATION

DESCRIPTION
LACTAID® Drops contain sufficient lactase enzyme (derived from *Kluyveromyces lactis*) to hydrolyze lactose in milk.

ACTION
LACTAID® Drops are a liquid form of the natural lactase enzyme that makes milk more digestible. The lactase enzyme hydrolyzes the lactose sugar (a double sugar) into its simple sugar components, glucose and galactose.

INDICATIONS
Lactose intolerance, suspected from gastrointestinal discomfort (ie, gas, bloating, cramps, and diarrhea) after drinking milk.

USUAL DOSAGE
LACTAID® Drops are a liquid form of the natural lactase enzyme that makes milk more digestible. To use, add ***LACTAID® Drops*** to a quart of milk, shake gently and refrigerate for 24 hours. We recommend starting with 5–7 drops per quart of milk but because sensitivity to lactose can vary, you may have to adjust the number of drops you use. If you are still experiencing discomfort after consuming milk with 5–7 ***LACTAID® Drops*** per quart, you may want to add 10 drops per quart or even 15 drops per quart. 15 drops per quart should remove nearly all of the lactose in the milk. Lactaid can be used with any kind of milk: whole, 1%, 2%, non-fat, skim, powdered and chocolate milk.

WARNING
If you experience any symptoms which are unusual or seem unrelated to the condition for which you took this product, consult a doctor before taking any more of it. Do not use if carton is opened or if printed plastic bodywrap is broken.

INACTIVE INGREDIENTS
Glycerin, Water

HOW SUPPLIED
LACTAID® Drops are available in .22 fl. oz. (7 mL), (30 quart supply). Store at or below room temperature (below 77°F). Refrigerate after opening.
Lactaid Drops are certified kosher from the Orthodox Union.
Also available: 70% lactose reduced Lactaid Milk and 100% lactose-free Lactaid Milk.

LACTAID® Original Strength Caplets OTC
(lactase enzyme)

LACTAID® Extra Strength Caplets
(lactase enzyme)

PRODUCT OVERVIEW

KEY FACTS
LACTAID® is the original lactase dietary supplement that makes milk and dairy foods more digestible. ***LACTAID®*** lactase enzyme hydrolyzes lactose into two digestible simple sugars: glucose and galactose. ***LACTAID® Caplets*** are taken orally for *in vivo* hydrolysis of lactose.

MAJOR USES
Lactose intolerance, suspected from gastrointestinal discomfort (ie, gas, bloating, cramps, and diarrhea) after drinking milk or ingesting other dairy foods such as cheese and ice cream.

PRESCRIBING INFORMATION

DESCRIPTION
Each ***LACTAID® Original Strength Caplet*** contains 3000 FCC (Food Chemical Codex) units of lactase enzyme (derived from *Aspergillus oryzae*).
Each ***LACTAID® Extra Strength Caplet*** contains 4500 FCC units of lactase enzyme (derived from *Aspergillus oryzae*).

ACTION
LACTAID® Caplets work to naturally replenish lactase enzyme that aids in dairy food digestion. Lactase enzyme hydrolyzes lactose sugar (a double sugar) into its simple sugar components, glucose and galactose.

INDICATIONS
Lactose intolerance, suspected from gastrointestinal discomfort (ie, gas, bloating, flatulence, cramps, and diarrhea) after drinking milk or ingesting other dairy foods such as cheese and ice cream.

USUAL DOSAGE
These convenient, portable caplets are easy to swallow or chew and can be used with milk or any dairy food. Original Strength: swallow or chew 3 caplets with the first bite of dairy food. Take no more than 6 caplets at a time. Extra Strength: swallow or chew 2 caplets with first bite of dairy food. Take no more than 4 caplets at a time. Don't be discouraged if at first Lactaid does not work to your satisfaction. Because the degree of enzyme deficiency naturally varies from person to person and from food to food, you may have to adjust the number of caplets up or down to find your own level of comfort. Since Lactaid Caplets work only on the food as you eat it, use them every time you enjoy dairy foods.

WARNING
If you experience any symptoms which are unusual or seem unrelated to the condition for which you took this product, consult a doctor before taking any more of it. Do not use if carton is opened or if printed plastic neckwrap is broken.

INGREDIENTS
Mannitol, Cellulose, Lactase Enzyme, Dextrose, and Sodium Citrate Magnesium Stearate.

HOW SUPPLIED
LACTAID® Original Strength Caplets are available in bottles of 60, and 120 counts. ***LACTAID® Extra Strength Caplets*** are available in bottles of 24, and 50 counts. Store at or below room temperature (below 77°F) but do not refrigerate. Keep away from heat.

LACTAID® Caplets are certified kosher from the Orthodox Union.
Also available: 70% lactose reduced Lactaid Milk and 100% lactose-free Lactaid Milk.

MOTRIN® Ibuprofen Suspension ℞
100 mg/5 mL

MOTRIN® Ibuprofen Oral Drops ℞
40 mg/mL

MOTRIN® Ibuprofen Chewable Tablets ℞
50 mg and 100 mg

MOTRIN® Ibuprofen Caplets ℞
100 mg

DESCRIPTION

The active ingredient in MOTRIN is ibuprofen, which is a member of the propionic acid group of nonsteroidal anti-inflammatory drugs (NSAIDs). Ibuprofen is a racemic mixture of [+]S- and [−]R-enantiomers. It is a white to off-white crystalline powder, with a melting point of 74° to 77°C. It is practically insoluble in water (<0.1 mg/mL), but readily soluble in organic solvents such as ethanol and acetone. Ibuprofen has a pKa of 4.43±0.03 and an n-octanol/water partition coefficient of 11.7 at pH 7.4. The chemical name for ibuprofen is (±)-2-(p-isobutylphenyl) propionic acid. The molecular weight of ibuprofen is 206.28. Its molecular formula is $C_{13}H_{18}O_2$ and it has the following structural formula:

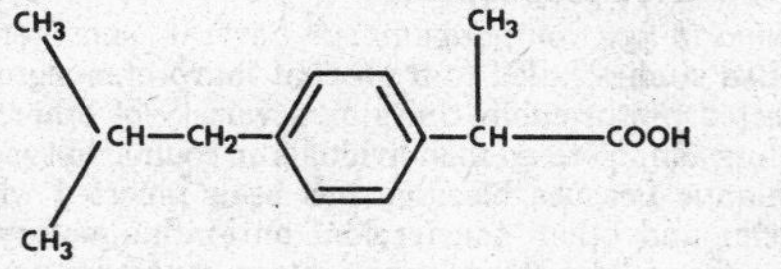

MOTRIN Suspension is a sucrose-sweetened, orange-colored, berry-flavored liquid suspension containing 100 mg of ibuprofen in 5 mL (20 mg/mL). Inactive ingredients include citric acid, glycerin, polysorbate 80, pregelatinized starch, purified water, sodium benzoate, sucrose, xanthan gum, D&C Yellow #10 and FD&C Red #40, and artificial flavors.
MOTRIN Oral Drops (intended for pediatric use only) is a sucrose-sweetened, pink-colored, berry-flavored liquid suspension containing 40 mg of ibuprofen per mL. Inactive ingredients include citric acid, glycerin, polysorbate 80, pregelatinized starch, purified water, sodium benzoate, sorbitol, sucrose, xanthan gum, FD&C Red #40, and artificial flavors.
MOTRIN Chewable Tablets are aspartame-sweetened, citrus-tasting, orange-colored tablets, that contain 50 mg or 100 mg of ibuprofen per tablet. Inactive ingredients include aspartame, citric acid, hydroxyethyl cellulose, hydroxypropyl methylcellulose, magnesium stearate, mannitol, microcrystalline cellulose, povidone, sodium lauryl sulfate, sodium starch glycolate, FD&C Yellow #6, and artificial flavors.
MOTRIN Caplets are unsweetened, white-colored, unflavored, film-coated, capsule-shaped tablets, containing 100 mg of ibuprofen per tablet. Inactive ingredients include carnauba wax, colloidal silicone dioxide, cornstarch, hydroxypropyl methylcellulose, microcrystalline cellulose, polydextrose, polyethylene glycol, pregelatinized starch, propylene glycol, sodium starch glycolate, titanium dioxide, triacetin, D&C Yellow #10, and FD&C Yellow #6.

CLINICAL PHARMACOLOGY

Pharmacodynamics—Ibuprofen is a nonsteroidal anti-inflammatory drug (NSAID) that possesses anti-inflammatory, analgesic and antipyretic activity. Its mode of action, like that of other NSAIDs, is not completely understood, but may be related to prostaglandin synthetase inhibition. After absorption of the racemic ibuprofen, the [−]R-enantiomer undergoes interconversion to the [+]S-form. The biological activities of ibuprofen are associated with the [+]S-enantiomer.
In clinical studies in adult patients with rheumatoid arthritis and osteoarthritis, ibuprofen has been shown to be comparable to aspirin in controlling pain and inflammation, though causing fewer of the mild gastrointestinal side effects (see ADVERSE REACTIONS). MOTRIN may be well tolerated in some patients who have had gastrointestinal side effects with aspirin, but these patients, when treated with MOTRIN, should be carefully followed for signs and symptoms of gastrointestinal ulceration and bleeding. Although it is not definitely known whether ibuprofen causes less peptic ulceration than aspirin, in one study involving 885 adult patients with rheumatoid arthritis treated for up to one year (438 patients on ibuprofen and 447 patients on aspirin), there were no reports of gastric ulceration with ibuprofen whereas frank ulceration was reported in 13 patients in the aspirin group (statistically significant $p<.001$).
Gastroscopic studies at varying doses of ibuprofen showed an increased tendency toward endoscopic lesions at higher doses. However, at clinically comparable doses (2,400 mg of ibuprofen vs. 3,600 mg of aspirin), endoscopic lesions were approximately half that seen with aspirin. Studies using ^{51}Cr-tagged red cells indicate that fecal blood loss associated with ibuprofen in doses up to 2400 mg daily did not exceed the range of normal, and was significantly less than that seen in aspirin-treated patients. The clinical significance of these findings is unknown.

Table 1
Pharmacokinetic Parameters of Ibuprofen Formulations
[Mean Values (% coefficient of variation)]

Dose	200mg (=2.8 mg/kg) in Adults				10 mg/kg in Febrile Children	
Formulation	**Suspension**	**Drops**	**Caplet**	**Chewable Tablet**	**Suspension**	**Chewable Tablet**
Number of Patients	24	24	25	24	18	18
AUCinf (μg·h/mL)	64 (27%)	74 (19%)	60 (19%)	66 (22%)	155 (24%)	176 (25%)
Cmax μg/mL)	19 (22%)	24 (21%)	20 (18%)	15 (24%)	55 (23%)	43 (39%)
Tmax (h)	0.79 (69%)	1.0 (60%)	1.04 (50%)	2.0 (56%)	0.97 (57%)	1.43 (69%)
Cl/F (mL/h/kg)	45.6 (22%)	43.4 (18%)	45.0 (19%)	42.8 (18%)	68.6 (22%)	60.9 (27%)

Legend: AUCinf = Area-under-the-curve to infinity
Tmax = Time-to-peak plasma concentration
Cmax = Peak plasma concentration
Cl/F = Clearance divided by fraction at drug absorbed

Pharmacokinetics—As noted in the DESCRIPTION section, ibuprofen is a racemic mixture of [−]R-and [+]S-isomers. *In vivo* and *in vitro* studies indicate that the [+]S-isomer is responsible for clinial activity. The [−]R-form, while thought to be pharmacologically inactive, is slowly and incompletely (~60%) interconverted into the active [+]S species in adults. The degree of interconversion in children is unknown, but is thought to be similar. The [−]R-isomer serves as a circulating reservoir to maintain levels of active drug. Ibuprofen is well absorbed orally, with less than 1% being excreted in the urine unchanged. It has a biphasic elimination time curve with a plasma half-life of approximately 2 hours. Studies in febrile children have established the dose-proportionality of 5 and 10 mg/kg doses of ibuprofen. Studies in adults have established the dose-proportionality of ibuprofen as a single oral dose from 50 to 600 mg for total drug and up to 1200 mg for free drug.
Absorption—*in vivo* studies indicate that ibuprofen is well absorbed orally from the suspension, drops, caplet and chewable tablet formulations, with peak plasma levels usually occurring within 1 to 2 hours. The pharmacokinetic differences between the products in adults (see Table 1) are due to differences in the rate of absorption of ibuprofen from the various dosage forms. The observed differences in the table between adults and children, in terms of AUC and C_{max}, are due to both differences in dose per body weight and age-or fever-related change in volume of distribution (Vd/F). All of the formulations are equally bioavailable in terms of peak plasma levels (C_{max}) and extent of absorption (AUC), however, the time-to-peak (T_{max}) is different between the products. Clinically, this has been shown to have no effect on either onset or peak fever reduction in children.
[See table 1 above.]
Antacid—A bioavailability study in adults has shown that there was no interference with the absorption of ibuprofen when given in conjunction with an antacid containing both aluminum hydroxide and magnesium hydroxide.
Food Effects—Absorption is most rapid when MOTRIN is given under fasting conditions. Administration of MOTRIN Suspension, MOTRIN Oral Drops, MOTRIN Chewable Tablets and MOTRIN Caplets with food affects the rate but not the extent of absorption. When taken with food, T_{max} is delayed by approximately 30 to 60 minutes, and peak levels are reduced by approximately 30 to 50%.
Distribution—Ibuprofen, like most other drugs of its class, is highly protein bound (>99% bound at 20 μg/mL). Protein binding is saturable and at concentrations >20 μg/mL binding is non-linear. Based on oral dosing data there is an age-or fever-related change in volume of distribution for ibuprofen. Febrile children <11 years old have a volume of approximately 0.2 L/kg while adults have a volume of approximately 0.12 L/kg. The clinical significance of these findings is unknown.
Metabolism—Following oral administration, the majority of the dose was recovered in the urine within 24 hours as the hydroxy-(25%) and carboxypropyl-(37%) phenylpropionic acid metabolites. The percentages of free and conjugated ibuprofen found in the urine were approximately 1% and 14%, respectively. The remainder of the drug was found in the stool as both metabolites and unabsorbed drug.
Elimination—Ibuprofen is rapidly metabolized and eliminated in the urine. The excretion of ibuprofen is virtually complete 24 hours after the last dose. It has a biphasic plasma elimination time curve with a half-life of approximately 2.0 hours. There is no difference in the observed terminal elimination rate or half-life between children and adults, however, there is an age-or fever-related change in total clearance. This suggests that the observed change in clearance is due to changes in the volume of distribution of ibuprofen (see Table 1 for Cl/F values).
Clinical Studies—Controlled clinical trials comparing doses of 5 and 10 mg/kg ibuprofen suspension and 10-15 mg/kg of acetaminophen elixir have been conducted in children 6 months to 12 years of age with fever primarily do to viral illnesses. In these studies there were no differences between treatment in fever reduction for the first hour and maximum fever reduction occurred between 2 and 4 hours. Response after 1 hour was dependent on both the level of temperature elevation as well as the treatment. In children with baseline temperatures at or below 102.5°F both ibuprofen doses and acetaminophen were equally effective in their maximum effect. In children with temperatures above 102.5°F, the ibuprofen 10 mg/kg dose was more effective. By 6 hours, children treated with ibuprofen 5mg/kg tended to have recurrence in fever, whereas children treated with ibuprofen 10 mg/kg still had significant fever reduction at 8 hours. In control groups treated with 10 mg/kg acetaminophen, fever reduction resembled that seen in children treated with 5 mg/kg of ibuprofen, with the exception that temperature elevation tended to return 1-2 hours earlier.
A comparison of MOTRIN Chewable Tablets and MOTRIN Suspension in febrile children showed similar antipyretic effects of the two formulations, lasting between 6 and 8 hours. No clinical studies of fever reduction in children have been performed with MOTRIN Caplets or MOTRIN Oral Drops.
Controlled single-dose clinical analgesia trials comparing doses of 5 and 10 mg/kg ibuprofen suspension with acetaminophen suspension 12.5 mg/kg and placebo, have been conducted in children 5 to 12 years of age, with sore throat pain due to an infectious agent, or ear pain due to acute otitis media. Onset of pain relief provided by ibuprofen was similar to that of acetaminophen, occurring within the first hour, usually around the half-hour mark. All active treatments showed significant pain relief verus placebo, and the 10 mg/kg dose of ibuprofen had a duration of analgesic effect of 6 to 8 hours. Ibuprofen 10 mg/kg provided more overall pain relief than the 5 mg/kg dose.
Controlled studies have demonstrated that ibuprofen is a more effective analgesic than propoxyphene for the relief of episiotomy pain, pain following dental extraction procedures, and for the relief of the symptoms of primary dysmenorrhea.
In patients with primary dysmenorrhea, ibuprofen has been shown to reduce elevated levels of prostaglandin activity in the menstrual fluid and to reduce resting and active intrauterine pressure, as well as the frequency of uterine contractions. The probable mechanism of action is to inhibit prostaglandin synthesis rather than simply to provide analgesia.
In clinical studies in adult patients with rheumatoid arthritis, ibuprofen has been shown to be comparable to indomethacin in controlling the signs and symptoms of disease activity, with a lower incidence of milder gastrointestinal and CNS side effects than indomethacin.
MOTRIN may be used in combination with gold salts and/or corticosteroids.

Continued on next page

McNeil Consumer—Cont.

INDICATIONS AND USAGE

In Children

MOTRIN is indicated:

- For the reduction of fever in patients aged 6 months and older.
- For relief of mild to moderate pain in patients aged 6 months and older.
- For relief of signs and symptoms of juvenille arthritis.

In Adults

MOTRIN is indicated:

- For relief of mild to moderate pain.
- For treatment of primary dysmenorrhea.
- For relief of the signs and symptoms of rheumatoid arthritis and osteoarthritis.

Since there have been no controlled trials to demonstrate whether there is any beneficial effect or harmful interaction with the use of ibuprofen in conjuction with aspirin, the combination cannot be recommended (see PRECAUTIONS—Drug Interactions).

CONTRAINDICATIONS

MOTRIN should not be used in patients with previously demonstrated hypersensitivity to ibuprofen, or in individuals with a history of allergic manifestations to aspirin or other NSAIDs. Severe anaphylactic-like reactions to ibuprofen have been reported in such patients, some with fatal outcome.

WARNINGS

Risk of GI Ulceration, Bleeding and Perforation with NSAID Therapy. Serious gastrointestinal toxicity such as bleeding, ulceration, and perforation, can occur at any time, with or without warning symptoms, in patients treated chronically with NSAID therapy. Although minor upper gastrointestinal problems, such as dyspepsia, are common, usually developing early in therapy, physicians should remain alert for ulceration and bleeding in patients treated chronically with NSAIDs even in the absence of previous GI tract symptoms. In patients observed in clinical trials of several months to two years duration, symptomatic upper GI ulcers, gross bleeding or perforation appear to occur in approximately 1% of patients treated for 3–6 months, and in about 2–4% of patients treated for one year. Physicians should inform patients about the signs and/or symptoms of serious GI toxicity and what steps to take if they occur.

Studies to date have not identified any subset of patients not at risk of developing peptic ulceration and bleeding. Except for a prior history of serious GI events and other risk factors known to be associated with peptic ulcer disease, such as alcoholism, smoking, etc., no risk factors (e.g., age, sex) have been associated with increased risk. Elderly or debilitated patients seem to tolerate ulceration or bleeding less well than other individuals and most spontaneous reports of fatal GI events are in this population. Studies to date are inconclusive concerning the relative risk of various NSAIDs in causing such reactions. High doses of any NSAID probably carry a greater risk of these reactions, although controlled clinical trials showing this do not exist in most cases. In considering the use of relatively large doses (within the recommended dosage range), sufficient benefit should be anticipated to offset the potential increased risk of GI toxicity.

Anaphylactoid Reactions: Anaphylactoid reactions may occur even in patients without prior exposure to ibuprofen. Extreme caution should be exercised when giving MOTRIN to patients with bronchospastic reactivity (e.g., asthma), nasal polyps, or those with a history of angiodema. Emergency help should be sought in case such anaphylactoid reaction occurs.

Advanced Renal Disease: In cases with advanced kidney disease, treatment with MOTRIN should not be initiated; if MOTRIN is used in such cases, close monitoring of the patient's kidney functions is advisable (see PRECAUTIONS—Renal Effects).

PRECAUTIONS

Renal Effects: Caution should be used when initiating treatment with MOTRIN in patients with considerable dehydration. It is advisable to rehydrate patients first and then start therapy with MOTRIN. Caution is also recommended in patients with pre-existing kidney disease (see WARNINGS—Advanced Renal Disease).

As with other NSAIDs, long-term administration of ibuprofen to animals has resulted in renal papillary necrosis and other abnormal renal pathology. In humans, there have been reports of acute interstitial nephritis with hematuria, proteinuria, and occasionally nephrotic syndrome.

A second form of renal toxicity has been seen in patients with prerenal conditions leading to a reduction in renal blood flow or blood volume, where the renal prostaglandins have a supportive role in the maintenance of renal perfusion. In these patients, administration of an NSAID may cause a dose-dependent reduction in prostaglandin formation and may precipitate overt renal decompensation. Patients at greatest risk of this reaction are those with impaired renal function, heart failure, liver dysfunction, those taking diuretics and the elderly. Discontinuation of NSAID therapy is typically followed by recovery to the pre-treatment state.

Those patients at high risk, who chronically take ibuprofen, should have renal function monitored if they have signs or symptoms which may be consistent with mild azotemia, such as malaise, fatigue, loss of appetite, etc. Occasional patients may develop some elevation of serum creatinine and BUN levels without signs or symptoms.

Since ibuprofen is eliminated primarily by the kidneys, patients with significantly impaired renal function should be closely monitored and a reduction in dosage should be anticipated to avoid drug accumulation. Prospective studies on the safety of ibuprofen in patients with chronic renal failure have not been conducted.

Fluid Retention: Fluid retention and edema have been reported in association with ibuprofen, therefore, the drug should be used with caution in patients with a history of cardiac decompensation or hypertension.

Hematologic Effects: MOTRIN can inhibit platelet aggregation but, unlike aspirin, its effect on platelet function is reversible, quantitatively less, and of shorter duration. Because this prolonged bleeding effect may be exaggerated in patients with underlying hemostatic defects, MOTRIN should be used with caution in persons with intrinsic coagulation defects and those on anticoagulant therapy.

Hepatic Effects: As with other nonsteroidal anti-inflammatory drugs, borderline elevations of one or more liver laboratory tests may occur in up to 15% of patients. These abnormalities may progress, may remain essentially unchanged, or may be transient with continued therapy. The ALT (SGPT) test is probably the most sensitive indicator of liver dysfunction. Meaningful (3 times the upper limit of normal) elevations of ALT and AST (SGOT) occurred in controlled clinical trials in less than 1% of patients. A patient with symptoms and/or signs suggesting liver dysfunction, or in whom an abnormal liver test has occurred, should be evaluated for evidence of the development of more severe hepatic reactions while on therapy with MOTRIN. Severe hepatic reactions, including jaundice and cases of fatal hepatitis, have been reported with ibuprofen as with other nonsteroidal anti-inflammatory drugs. Although such reactions are rare, if abnormal liver tests persist or worsen, if clinical signs and symptoms consistent with liver disease develop, or if systemic manifestations occur (e.g., eosinophilia, rash, etc.), treatment with MOTRIN should be discontinued.

Aseptic Meningitis: Aseptic meningitis, with fever and coma, has been observed on rare occasions in patients on ibuprofen therapy. Although it is probably more likely to occur in patients with systemic lupus erythematosus and related connective tissue diseases, it has been reported in patients who do not have an underlying chronic disease. If signs or symptoms of meningitis develop in a patient receiving MOTRIN, the possibility of its being related to ibuprofen should be considered.

Other Precautions—The pharmacological activity of MOTRIN may induce fever reduction and inflammation, thus diminishing their utility as diagnostic signs in detecting underlying conditions.

In order to avoid exacerbation of manifestations of adrenal insufficiency, patients who have been on prolonged corticosteroid therapy should have their therapy tapered slowly rather than discontinued abruptly when ibuprofen is added to the treatment program.

Blurred and/or diminished vision, scotomata, and/or changes in color vision have been reported. If a patient develops such complaints while receiving MOTRIN Chewable Tablets, the drug should be discontinued and the patient should have an ophthalmologic examination which includes central visual fields and color vision testing.

Phenylketonurics: MOTRIN Chewable Tables 50 mg contain phenylalanine 3 mg per tablet, and the 100 mg tablets contain phenylalanine 6 mg per tablet.

Diabetics: MOTRIN Suspension and MOTRIN Oral Drops contains 0.3 g sucrose and 1.6 calories per mL, or 1.5 g sucrose and 8 calories per teaspoon, which should be taken into consideration when treating diabetic patients with this product.

Information for Patients—MOTRIN, like other drugs of its class, is not free of side effects. The side effects of these drugs can cause discomfort and, rarely, there are more serious side effects, such as gastrointestinal bleeding, which may result in hospitalization and even fatal outcomes.

NSAIDs are often essential agents in the management of arthritis, pain and fever, but they also may be commonly employed for conditions which are less serious.

Physicians may wish to discuss with their patients the potential risks (see WARNINGS, PRECAUTIONS, and ADVERSE REACTIONS) and likely benefits of NSAID treatment, particularly when the drugs are used for less serious conditions where treatment without NSAIDs may represent an acceptable alternative to both the patient and physician.

Patients on MOTRIN should report to their physicians signs or symptoms of gastrointestinal ulceration or bleeding, blurred vision or other eye symptoms, skin rash, weight gain, or edema.

Because serious GI tract ulceration and bleeding can occur without warning symptoms, physicians should follow chronically treated patients for the signs and symptoms of ulceration and bleeding and should inform them of the importance of this follow-up (see WARNINGS).

Patients should also be instructed to seek medical emergency help in case of an occurrence of an anaphylactoid reaction (see WARNINGS).

LABORATORY TESTS

Hemoglobin Levels: In cross-study comparisons, in adults, with doses ranging from 1200 mg to 3200 mg daily for several weeks, a slight dose-response decrease in hemoglobin/hematocrit was noted. This has been observed with other nonsteroidal anit-inflammatory drugs; the mechanism is unknown. However, even with daily doses of 3200 mg, the total decrease in hemoglobin usually does not exceed 1 g/dL; if there are no signs of bleeding, it is probably not clinically important.

In two postmarketing clinical studies with ibuprofen, the incidence of a decreased hemoglobin level was greater than previously reported. Decrease in hemoglobin of 1 g/dL or more was observed in 17.1% of 193 patients on 1600 mg ibuprofen daily (osteoarthritis), and 22.8% of 189 patients taking 2400mg of ibuprofen daily (rheumatoid arthritis). Positive stool occult blood tests and elevated serum creatinine levels were also observed in these studies.

DRUG INTERACTIONS

Coumarin-type anticoagulants: Several short-term controlled studies failed to show that iburprofen significantly affected prothrombin times or a variety of other clotting factors administered to individuals on coumarin-type anticoagulants. Because bleeding has been reported when ibuprofen and other nonsteroidal anti-inflammatory agents have been administered to patients on coumarin-type anticoagulants, the physician should be cautious when administering MOTRIN to patients on anticoagulants.

Aspirin: Animal studies show that aspirin given with NSAIDs, including ibuprofen, yields a net decrease in anti-inflammatory activity with lowered blood levels of the non-aspirin drug. Single-dose bioavailability studies in normal volunteers have failed to show an effect of aspirin on ibuprofen blood levels. Correlative clinical studies have not been done.

Methotrexate: Ibuprofen, as well as other NSAIDs, has been reported to competitively inhibit methotrexate accumulation in rabbit kidney slices. This may indicate that ibuprofen could enhance the toxicity of methotrexate. Caution should be used, therefore, if MOTRIN is administered concomitantly with methotrexate.

H-2 Antagonists: In studies with human volunteers, coadministration of cimetidine or ranitidine with ibuprofen had no substantive effect on ibuprofen serum concentrations.

ACE-inhibitors: Reports suggest that NSAIDs, including ibuprofen, may diminish the antihypertensive effect of ACE-inhibitors. This interaction should be given consideration in patients taking MOTRIN concomitantly with ACE-inhibitors.

Furosemide: Clinical studies, as well as random observations, have shown that ibuprofen can reduce the natriuretic effect of furosemide and thiazides in some patients. This response has been attributed to inhibition of renal prostaglandin synthesis. During concomitant therapy with MOTRIN, the patient should be observed closely for signs of renal failure (see PRECAUTIONS, Renal Effects), as well as to assure diuretic efficacy.

Lithium: Ibuprofen produced an elevation of plasma lithium levels and a reduction in renal lithium clearance in a study of eleven normal volunteers. The mean minimum lithium concentration increased 15% and the renal clearance of lithium was decreased by 19% during this period of concomitant drug administration. This effect has been attributed to inhibition of renal prostaglandin synthesis by ibuprofen. Thus, when MOTRIN and lithium are administered concurrently, subjects should be observed carefully for signs of lithium toxicity. (Read circulars for lithium preparation before use of such concurrent therapy.)

Teratogenic Effects—Pregnancy Category B: Reproductive studies conducted in rats and rabbits at doses somewhat less than the maximal clinical dose did not demonstrate evidence of developmental abnormalities. However, animal reproduction studies are not always predictive of human response. As there are no adequate and well-controlled studies in pregnant women, this drug should be used during pregnancy only if clearly needed. Because of the known effects of nonsteroidal anti-inflammatory drugs on the fetal cardiovascular system (closure of ductus arteriosus), use during late pregnancy should be avoided. Administration of MOTRIN is not recommended during pregnancy.

Labor and Delivery: As with other drugs known to inhibit prostaglandin synthesis, an increased incidence of dystocia and delayed parturition occurred in rats. Administration of MOTRIN is not recommended during labor and delivery.

Nursing Mothers: In limited studies, an assay capable of detecting 1 μg/mL did not demonstrate ibuprofen in the milk of lactating mothers. Because of the limited nature of these studies, however, and the possible adverse effects of prostaglandin inhibiting drugs on neonates, MOTRIN is not recommended for use in nursing mothers.

Pediatric Use: Safety and efficacy of MOTRIN in children below the age of 6 months has not been established (see CLINICAL PHARMACOLOGY-Clinical Studies). There is no evidence of age-dependent kinetics in patients 2 to 11 years old (see CLINICAL PHARMACOLOGY-Pharmacokinetics). Dosing of MOTRIN in children 6 months or older should be guided by their body weight (see DOSAGE AND ADMINISTRATION).

ADVERSE REACTIONS

The most frequent type of adverse reaction occurring with ibuprofen is gastrointestinal. In controlled clinical trials, the percentage of adult patients reporting one or more gastrointestinal complaints ranged from 4% to 16%.

In controlled studies in adults, when ibuprofen was compared to aspirin and indomethacin in equally effective doses, the overall incidence of gastrointestinal complaints was about half that seen in either the aspirin- or indomethacin-treated patients.

Adverse reactions observed during controlled clinical trials in adults at an incidence greater than 1% are listed in the chart. Those reactions listed under the heading "Incidence Greater than 1% (but less than 3%) Probable Causal Relationship," encompass observations in approximately 3,000 patients. More than 500 of these patients were treated for periods of at least 54 weeks.

Still other reactions, occurring less frequently than 1 in 100, were reported in controlled clinical trials and from marketing experience. These reactions have been divided into two categories: "Incidence less than 1%—Probable Causal Relationships," lists reactions with Ibuprofen therapy for which the probability of a causal relationship exists; this category was completed over time with postmarketing serious adverse reactions. "Incidence less than 1% —Causal Relationship Unknown," lists reactions with ibuprofen therapy for which a causal relationship has not been established, but are presented as alerting information for physicians.

INCIDENCE OF 1% OR GREATER

Probable Causal Relationship

*Incidence between 3 and 9%=ADR marked with**
Incidence between 1 and <3%=unmarked ADR

Cardiovascular system: Edema, fluid retention (generally responds promptly to drug discontinuation) (See PRECAUTIONS).

Digestive system: Nausea*, epigastric pain*, heartburn*, diarrhea, abdominal distress, nausea and vomiting, indigestion, constipation, abdominal cramps or pain, fullness of GI tract (bloating and flatulence).

Nervous system: Dizziness*, headache, nervousness.

Skin and appendages: Rash* (including maculopapular type), pruritus

Specal senses: Tinnitus.

INCIDENCE LESS THAN 1%

Probable Causal Relationship: The following adverse reactions were reported in clincial trials at an incidence of less than 1%, or were reported from postmarketing or foreign experience. The probability exists between the drug and these adverse reactions.

Body as a whole: Anaphylaxis and anaphylactoid reactions (see WARNINGS).

Cardiovascular system: Cerebrovascular accident, hypotension, congestive heart failure in patients with marginal cardiac function, elevated blood pressure, palpitations.

Digestive system: Gastric or duodenal ulcer with bleeding and/or perforation, gastrointestinal hemorrhage, pancreatitis, melena, gastritis, duodenitis, esophagitis, hematemesis, hepatorenal syndrome, liver necrosis, liver failure, hepatitis, jaundice, abnormal liver tests.

Hematologic system: Neutropenia, agranulocytosis, aplastic anemia, hemolytic anemia (sometimes Coombs positive), thrombocytopenia with or without purpura, eosinophilia, decrease in hemoglobin and hematocrit (see PRECAUTIONS), pancytopenia.

Nervous system: Depression, insomia, confusion, emotional liability, somnolence, convulsions, aseptic meningitis with fever and coma (see PRECAUTIONS).

Respiratory: Bronchospasm, dyspnea, apnea.

Skin and appendages: Vesiculobullous eruptions, urticaria, erythema multiforme, Stevens-Johnson syndrome, alopecia, exfoliative dermatitis, Lyell's syndrome (toxic epidermal necrolysis), photosensitivity reactions.

Special senses: Hearing loss, amblyopia (blurred and/or diminished vision, scotomata and/or changes in color vision) (see PRECAUTIONS—Other Precautions).

Urogenital system: Acute renal failure in patients with pre-existing significantly impaired renal function (see PRECAUTIONS), renal papillary necrosis, tubular necrosis, glomerulitis, decreased creatinine clearance, polyuria, azotemia, cystitis, hematuria.

Miscellaneous: Dry eyes and mouth, gingival ulcer, rhinitis.

INCIDENCE LESS THAN 1%

Causal Relationship Unknown: The following adverse reactions occurred at an incidence of less than 1% in clinical trials, or were suggested by marketing experience under circumstances where a causal relationship could not be definitely established. They are listed as alerting information for the physician.

Allergic: Serum sickness, lupus erythematosus syndrome, Henoch-Schönlein vasculitis, angioedema.

Cardivascular system: Arrhythmias (sinus tachycardia, sinus bradycardia).

Hematologic system: Bleeding episodes (e.g., epistaxis, menorrhagia).

Metabolic/endocrine: Gynecomastia, hypoglycemic reaction, acidosis.

Nervous system: Paresthesias, hallucinations, dream abnormalities, pseudo-tumor cerebri.

Special senses: Conjunctivitis, diplopia, optic neuritis, cataracts.

OVERDOSAGE

The *toxicity of ibuprofen overdose* is dependent upon the amount of drug ingested and the time elapsed since ingestion, though individual response may vary, which makes it necessary to evaluate each case individually. Although uncommon, serious toxicity and death have been reported in the medical literature with ibuprofen overdosage. The most frequently reported symptoms of ibuprofen overdose include abdominal pain, nausea, vomiting, lethargy and drowsiness. Other central nervous system symptoms include headache, tinnitus, CNS depression and seizures. Metabolic acidosis, coma, acute renal failure and apnea (primarily in very young children) may rarely occur. Cardiovascular toxicity, including hypotension, bradycardia, tachycardia and atrial fibrillation, also have been reported.

The *treatment of acute ibuprofen overdose* is primarily supportive. Management hypotension acidosis and gastrointestinal bleeding may be necessary. In cases of acute overdose, the stomach should be emptied through ipecac-induced emesis or lavage. Emesis is most effective if initiated within 30 mintues of ingestion. Orally administered activated charcoal may help in reducing the absorption and reabsorption of ibuprofen.

In children, the estimated amount of ibuprofen ingested per body weight may be helpful to predict the potential for development of toxicity although each case must be evaluated. Ingestion of less than 100 mg/kg is unlikely to produce toxicity. Children ingesting 100 to 200 mg/kg may be managed with induced emesis and a minimal observation time of four hours. Children ingesting 200 to 400 mg/kg of ibuprofen should have immediate gastric emptying and at least four hours observation in a health care facility. Children ingesting greater than 400 mg/kg require immediate medical referral, careful observation and appropriate supportive therapy. Ipecac-induced emesis is not recommended in overdoses greater than 400 mg/kg because of the risk for convulsions and the potential for aspiration of gastric contents.

In adult patients the history of the dose reportedly ingested does not appear to be predictive of toxicity. The need for referral and follow-up must be judged by the circumstances at the time of the overdose ingestion. Symptomatic adults should be admitted to a health care facility for observation.

DOSAGE AND ADMINISTRATION

CHILDREN

Fever reduction: For reduction of fever in children, 6 months to 12 years of age, the dosage should be adjusted on the basis of the initial temperature level (see CLINICAL PHARMACOLOGY). The recommended dose is 5 mg/kg if the baseline temperature is less than 102.5°F, or 10 mg/kg if the baseline temperature is 102.5°F or greater. The duration of fever reduction is generally 6 to 8 hours. The recommended maximum daily dose is 40 mg/kg.

Analgesia: For relief of mild to moderate pain in children, 6 months to 12 years of age, the recommended dosage is 10 mg/kg, every 6 to 8 hours. The recommended maximum daily dose is 40 mg/kg. Doses should be given so as not to disturb the child's sleep pattern. Taking fluids after chewing MOTRIN Chewable Tablets may help to promote absorption of the drug (see CLINICAL PHARMACOLOGY—Pharmacokinetics, and "Individualization of Dosage" in this section).

Juvenile Arthritis: The recommended dose is 30 to 40 mg/kg/day divided into three to four doses (see Individualization of Dosage). Patients with milder disease may be adequately treated with 20 mg/kg/day.

ADULTS

Analgesia: 400 mg every 4 to 6 hours as necessary for the relief of mild to moderate pain in adults. In controlled analgesic clincial trials, doses of MOTRIN greater than 400 mg were no more effective than the 400 mg dose.

Primary Dysmenorrhea: For the treatment of primary dysmenorrhea, beginning with the earliest onset of such pain, MOTRIN should be given in a dose of 400 mg every 4 hours, as necessary, for the relief of pain.

Rheumatoid arthritis and osteoarthritis, including flare-ups of chronic disease: Suggested dosage: 1200-3200 mg daily (300 mg q.i.d or 400 mg, 600 mg or 800 mg t.i.d. or q.i.d). Individual patients may show a better response to 3200 mg daily, as compared with 2400 mg, although in well-controlled clinical trials patients on 3200 mg did not show a better mean response in terms of efficacy. Therefore, when treating patients with 3200 mg/day, the physician should observe sufficient increased clincial benefits to offset potential increased risk.

Individualization of Dosage The dose of MOTRIN should be tailored to each patient, and may be lowered or raised from the suggested doses depending on the severity of symptoms either at time of initiating drug therapy or as the patient responds or fails to respond.

One fever study showed that, after the initial dose of MOTRIN, subsequent doses may be lowered and still provide adequate fever control.

In a situation when low fever would require the MOTRIN 5 mg/kg dose in a child with pain, the dose that will effectively treat the predominant symptom should be chosen.

In chronic conditions, a therapeutic response to MOTRIN therapy is sometimes seen in a few days to a week, but most often is observed by two weeks. After a satisfactory response has been achieved, the patient's dose should be reviewed and adjusted as required.

In patients with juvenile arthritis, doses above 50 mg/kg/day are not recommended because they have not been studied and doses exceeding the upper recommended dose of 40 mg/kg/day may increase the risk of causing serious adverse events. The therapeutic response may require from a few days to several weeks to be achieved. Once a clincial effect is obtained, the dosage should be lowered to the smallest dose of MOTRIN needed to maintain adequate control of symptoms.

In general, patients with rheumatoid arthritis seem to require higher doses than do patients with osteoarthritis. The smallest dose of MOTRIN that yields acceptable control should be employed.

HOW SUPPLIED

MOTRIN® (ibuprofen) Suspension 100 mg/5 mL
Orange-colored, berry-flavored suspension
–Bottles of 120 mL—NDC 0045-0448-04
–Bottles of 480 mL—NDC 0045-0448-16
Shake well before using. Store at controlled room temperature [15° to 30°C (59° to 86°F)]

MOTRIN® (ibuprofen) Oral Drops, 40mg/mL
(intended for pediatric use only)
Pink-colored, berry flavored suspension
–Bottles of 15 ml—NDC 0045-0446-15
Shake well before using. Store at controlled room temperature [15° to 30°C (59° to 86°F)].

MOTRIN® (ibuprofen) Chewable Tablets, 50 mg
Round, orange-colored, citrus-tasting, scored tablet, debossed "MOTRIN 50"
–Bottles of 100 Chewable Tablets—NDC 0045-0361-10
Store at controlled room temperature [15° to 30°C (59° to 86°F)]

MOTRIN® (ibuprofen) Chewable Tablets, 100 mg
Round, orange-colored, citrus-tasting, scored tablet, debossed "MOTRIN 100"
–Bottles of 100 Chewable Tablets—NDC 0045-0431-10
Store at controlled room temperature [15° to 30°C (59° to 86°F)]

MOTRIN® (ibuprofen) Caplets, 100 mg
White-colored, scored capsule-shaped tablet, imprinted "M 100"
–Bottles of 100 Caplets—NDC 0045-0445-10
Store at controlled room temperature [15° to 30°C (59° to 86°F)]

Caution: Federal Law prohibits dispensing without prescription.

McNEIL CONSUMER PRODUCTS CO.
DIVISION OF McNEIL-PPC, INC.
FORT WASHINGTON, PA 19034-USA
DECEMBER 1994

Shown in Product Identification Guide, page 322

NICOTROL® NS ℞

(nicotine nasal spray)
10 mg/mL

DESCRIPTION

Nicotrol® NS (nicotine nasal spray) is an aqueous solution of nicotine intended for administration as a metered spray to the nasal mucosa.

Nicotine is a tertiary amine composed of pyridine and a pyrrolidine ring. It is a colorless to pale yellow, freely water-soluble, strongly alkaline, oily, volatile, hygroscopic liquid obtained from the tobacco plant. Nicotine has a characteristic pungent odor and turns brown on exposure to air or light.

Continued on next page

McNeil Consumer—Cont.

Of its two stereoisomers, S(-)nicotine is the more active. It is the prevalent form in tobacco, and is the form in NICOTROL NS. The free alkaloid is absorbed rapidly through skin, mucous membranes, and the respiratory tract.
Chemical Name: S-3-(1-methyl-2-pyrrolidinyl) pyridine
Molecular Formula $C_{10}H_{14}N_2$
Molecular Weight: 162.23
Ionization Constants: $pKa_1 = 7\ 84$, $pKa_2 = 3\ 04$ at 15°C
Octanol Water Partition Coefficient: 15:1 at pH 7

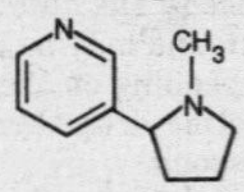

Each 10 ml spray bottle contains 100 mg nicotine (10 mg/mL) in an inactive vehicle containing disodium phosphate, sodium dihydrogen phosphate, citric acid, methylparaben, propylparaben, edetate disodium, sodium chloride, polysorbate 80, aroma and water. The solution is isotonic with a pH of 7. It contains no chlorofluorocarbons.
After priming the delivery system for NICOTROL NS, each actuation of the unit delivers a metered dose spray containing approximately 0.5 mg of nicotine. The size of the droplets produced by the unit is in excess of 8 microns. One NICOTROL NS unit delivers approximately 200 applications.

CLINICAL PHARMACOLOGY

Pharmacologic Action
Nicotine, the chief alkaloid in tobacco products, binds stereoselectively to nicotinic-cholinergic receptors at the autonomic ganglia, in the adrenal medulla, at neuromuscular junctions, and in the brain. Two types of central nervous system effects are believed to be the basis of nicotine's positively reinforcing properties. A stimulating effect is exerted mainly in the cortex via the locus ceruleus and a reward effect is exerted in the limbic system. At low doses, the stimulant effects predominate while at high doses the reward effects predominate. Intermittent intravenous administration of nicotine activates neurohormonal pathways, releasing acetylcholine, norepinephrine, dopamine, serotonin, vasopressin, beta-endorphin, growth hormone, and ACTH.

Pharmacodynamics
The cardiovascular effects of nicotine include peripheral vasoconstriction, tachycardia and elevated blood pressure. Acute and chronic tolerance to nicotine develops from smoking tobacco or ingesting nicotine preparations. Acute tolerance (a reduction in response for a given dose) develops rapidly (less than 1 hour), but not at the same rate for different physiologic effects (skin temperature, heart rate, subjective effects). Withdrawal symptoms such as cigarette craving can be reduced in most individuals by plasma nicotine levels lower than those from smoking.
Withdrawal from nicotine in addicted individuals can be characterized by craving, nervousness, restlessness, irritability, mood lability, anxiety, drowsiness, sleep disturbances, impaired concentration, increased appetite, minor somatic complaints (headache, myalgia, constipation, fatigue), and weight gain. Nicotine toxicity is characterized by nausea, abdominal pain, vomiting, diarrhea, diaphoresis, flushing, dizziness, disturbed hearing and vision, confusion, weakness, palpitations, altered respiration and hypotension.
Both smoking and nicotine can increase circulating cortisol and catecholamines, and tolerance does not develop to the catecholamine-releasing effects of nicotine. Changes in the response to a concomitantly administered adrenergic agonist or antagonist should be watched for when nicotine intake is altered during NICOTROL NS therapy and/or smoking cessation (See **PRECAUTIONS, Drug Interactions**).

PHARMACOKINETICS

Each actuation of NICOTROL NS delivers a metered 50 microliter spray containing approximately 0.5 mg of nicotine. One dose is considered 1 mg of nicotine (2 sprays, one in each nostril).

Absorption
Following administration of 2 sprays of NICOTROL NS approximately 53% ±16% (Mean ±SD) enters the systemic circulation. No significant difference in rate or extent of absorption could be seen due to the deposition of nicotine on different parts of the nasal mucosa. Plasma concentrations of nicotine obtained from 1 dose (1 mg nicotine) of NICOTROL NS rise rapidly, reaching maximum venous concentrations of 2–12 ng/mL in 4–15 minutes. The apparent absorption half-life of nicotine is approximately 3 minutes. There is wide variation among subjects in their plasma nicotine concentrations from the spray. As a result, after a 1 mg dose of spray approximately 20% of the subjects reached peak nicotine concentrations similar to those seen after smoking one cigarette (7–17 ng/mL) (See **DRUG ABUSE AND DEPENDENCE** Section). Figure 1 below plots the mean and 5th and 95th percentile nicotine concentrations after a 1 mg single dose of the nasal spray (n=30).

Figure 1: Mean and Range of the 95th and 5th Percentile Nicotine Concentrations After a 1 mg Dose of NICOTROL NS (n=30)

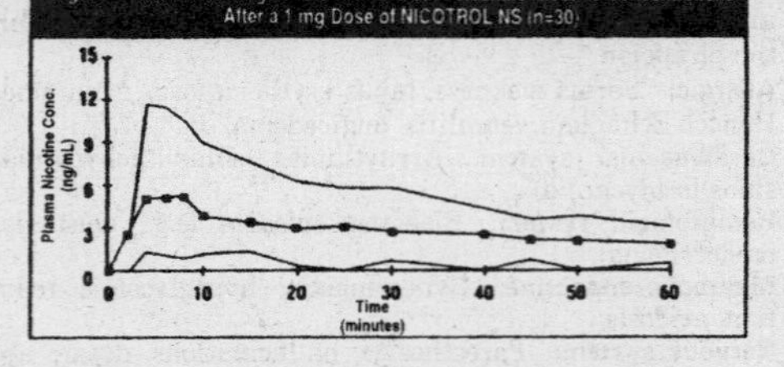

Table 1: Trough Plasma Nicotine Concentrations after 11 Hours of Dosing With 1 mg, 2 mg and 3 mg of NICOTROL NS per hour (n=16)

Dose	Mean (ng/mL) ± SD	(Range)
1 mg every 60 minutes (1 mg/hr)	6 ± 3	(1 7–12)
1 mg every 30 minutes (2 mg/hr)	14 ± 6	(1 5–24)
1 mg every 20 minutes (3 mg/hr)	18 ± 10	(1 2–35)

The data from Table 1 is derived from a three-way cross-over study of repeated applications of NICOTROL NS in sixteen smokers (8 male, 8 female) ranging in age from 18 to 48 years. There is a slight deviation from dose-concentration proportionality from one dose to three doses of NICOTROL NS per hour as shown in Figure 2.

Figure 2: Mean 95th and 5th Percentile Trough Nicotine Plasma Concentrations in Subjects Taking NICOTROL NS for 12 Hours (n=16)

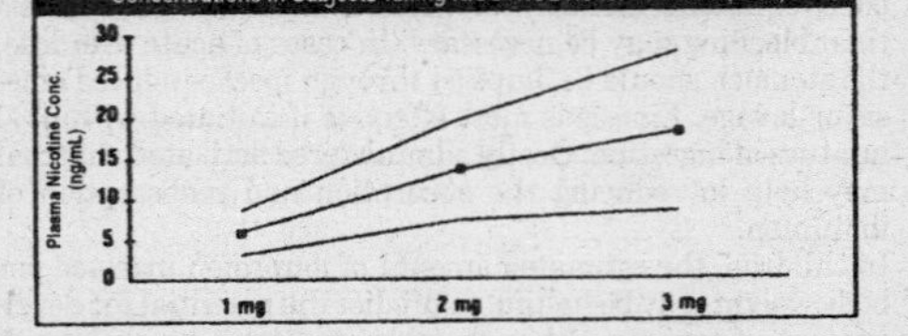

Sixteen smokers (7 males and 9 females) ranging in age from 22 to 44 years were dosed with 1 mg of NICOTROL NS every hour for 10 hours. The pharmacokinetic parameters that were obtained are presented in Table 2.

Table 2 Nicotine Pharmacokinetic Parameters at Steady-State for 1 mg hour of NICOTROL NS Administered Hourly for Ten Hours (Mean ± SD and Range) (n=16)

Parameter	1 mg (2 sprays)	(Range)
Cavg (ng/mL)	8 ± 3	(2 5–12)
Cmax (ng/mL)	9 ± 3	(3 1–14)
Tmax (minutes)	13 ± 5	(10–20)

Cavg: average plasma nicotine concentration for the dosing interval of 10–11 hours
Cmax: maximum measured plasma concentration after last dose administration
Tmax: time of maximum plasma concentration after last dose administration

Distribution
The volume of distribution following IV administration of nicotine is approximately 2 to 3 L/kg. Plasma protein binding of nicotine is <5%. Therefore, changes in nicotine binding from use of concomitant drugs or alterations of plasma proteins by disease status would not be expected to have significant effects on nicotine kinetics.

Metabolsim
More than 20 metabolites of nicotine have been identified, all of which are less active than the parent compound. The primary urinary metabolites are cotinine (15% of the dose) and trans-3-hydroxycotinine (45% of the dose). Cotinine has a half-life of 15 to 20 hours and concentrations that exceed nicotine by 10-fold. The major site for the metabolism of nicotine is the liver. The kidney and lung are also sites of nicotine metabolism.

Elimination
About 10% of the nicotine absorbed is excreted unchanged in the urine. This may be increased to up to 30% with high urine flow rates and urinary acidification below pH 5. The average plasma clearance is about 1.2 L/min in a healthy adult smoker. The apparent elimination half-life of nicotine from NICOTROL NS is 1 to 2 hours.

Pharmacokinetic Model
The data were well described by a two-compartment model with first-order input.
Based on individual fits (N=18) the following parameters were derived after the administration of a 1 mg dose. Absorption rate constant (Ka) $=14.4 \pm 7.3\ hr^{-1}$ (Mean ±SD). elimination rate constant (Ka) $=0.60 \pm 0.53\ hr^{-1}$. Distribution rate constants (K_{12}) $=4.84 \pm 2.57\ hr^{-1}$. (K_{21}) $=4.35 \pm 2.30\ hr^{-1}$. Volume of distribution over fraction absorbed (V/F) $=2.73 \pm 0.82$ L/kg in 8 female and 10 male adults weighing 76 ±15 kg.

Gender Differences
Intersubject variability (50% coefficient of variation) among the pharmacokinetic parameters (AUC C_{max} and Clearance/kg) were observed for both genders. There were no differences between females or males in the kinetics of NICOTROL NS.

Drug/Drug Interactions
The extent of absorption is slightly reduced (approximately 10%) in patients with the common cold/rhinitis. In patients with rhinitis the peak plasma concentration is reduced by approximately 20% (concentrations are lower by 1.5 ng/mL on average) and the time to peak concentration prolonged by approximately 30% (delayed by 7 minutes on average). The use of a nasal vasoconstrictor such as xylometazoline in patients with rhinitis will further prolong the time to peak by approximately 40% (delayed by 15 minutes on average), but the peak plasma concentration remains on average the same as those with rhinitis.

CLINICAL TRIALS

The efficacy of NICOTROL NS therapy as an aid to smoking cessation was demonstrated in three single-center, placebo-controlled, double-blind trials with a total of 730 patients. One of the trials used NICOTROL NS with individual counseling while the other two used group support. Patients with severe or symptomatic cardiovascular disease, hypertension, asthma, diabetes or severe allergy were not included in the studies. The amount of NICOTROL NS used was left to the discretion of each patient, with a minimum dose of 8 mg/day and a maximum dose of 40 mg/day.
In all three studies, the recommended duration of treatment was 3 months; however in two of these trials, 241 patients were permitted to continue to use the product for up to 1 year, if they wished. Among the 64 patients abstinent from cigarettes at the end of a year, 23 (36%) were still using the spray, and probable dependence on the spray was seen in several patients. (See **DRUG ABUSE AND DEPENDENCE**).
Quitting was defined as *total abstinence* from smoking for at least 4 weeks. The "quit rates" are the percentage of all persons initially enrolled who continuously abstained after week 2 or 4.
In all three studies, NICOTROL NS was more effective than placebo at 6 weeks, 3 months, 6 months, and 1 year. The two studies where NICOTROL NS could be used for more than 6 months did not have a better outcome at 1 year than the study in which NICOTROL NS was discontinued at 6 months.
[See table 3 below.]

Table 3 Quit Rates by Treatment (N=730 smokers in 3 Studies)

Group	Size (n)	At 6 Weeks	At 3 Months	At 6 Months	At 1 Year
NICOTROL NS	369	49–58%	41–45%	31–35%	23–27%
Placebo	361	21–32%	17–20%	12–15%	10–15%

Patients treated with NICOTROL NS had more relief of the urge to smoke and withdrawal symptoms compared with placebo-treated patients.
NICOTROL NS allows the patient to vary the dose of nicotine on a short-term basis. As with other variable dose smoking cessation products, NICOTROL NS may be useful in the management of highly dependent smokers.

INDICATIONS AND USAGE

NICOTROL NS is indicated as an aid to smoking cessation for the relief of nicotine withdrawal symptoms. NICOTROL NS therapy should be used as a part of a comprehensive behavioral smoking cessation program.
The safety and efficacy of the continued use of NICOTROL NS for periods longer than 6 months have not been adequately studied and such use is not recommended.

CONTRAINDICATIONS

Use of NICOTROL NS therapy is contraindicated in patients with known hypersensitivity or allergy to nicotine or to any component of the product.

WARNINGS

Nicotine from any source can be toxic and addictive. Smoking causes lung disease, cancer, and heart disease and may adversely affect pregnant women or the fetus. For any smoker, with or without concomitant disease or pregnancy, the risk of nicotine replacement in a smoking cessation program should be weighed against the hazard of continued smoking, and the likelihood of achieving cessation of smoking without nicotine replacement.

Pregnancy, Warning
Tobacco smoke, which has been shown to be harmful to the fetus, contains nicotine, hydrogen cyanide, and carbon monoxide. Nicotine has been shown in animal studies to cause fetal harm. It is therefore presumed that NICOTROL NS can cause fetal harm when administered to a pregnant woman.

The effect of nicotine delivery by NICOTROL NS has not been examined in pregnancy (See **PRECAUTIONS**). **Therefore, pregnant smokers should be encouraged to attempt cessation using educational and behavioral interventions before using pharmacological approaches.** If NICOTROL NS is used during pregnancy, or if the patient becomes pregnant while using it, the patient should be apprised of the potential hazard to the fetus.

Safety Note Concerning Children

The amounts of nicotine that are tolerated by adult smokers can produce symptoms of poisoning and could prove fatal if NICOTROL NS is used or ingested by children or pets. A full bottle of NICOTROL NS contains 100 mg of nicotine, some of which will still be in the bottle when it is discarded. Therefore, patients should be cautioned to keep both used and unused containers of NICOTROL NS out of the reach of children and pets.

PRECAUTIONS

General

The patient should be urged to stop smoking completely when initiating NICOTROL NS therapy (See **DOSAGE AND ADMINISTRATION**). Patients should be informed that if they continue to smoke while using the product, they may experience adverse effects due to peak nicotine levels higher than those experienced from smoking alone. If there is a clinically significant increase in cardiovascular or other effects attributable to nicotine, the treatment should be discontinued (See **WARNINGS**). Physicians should anticipate that concomitant medications may need dosage adjustment (See **Drug Interactions**).

Sustained use (beyond 6 months) of NICOTROL NS by patients who stop smoking is not recommended and should be discouraged (See **DRUG ABUSE AND DEPENDENCE**).

Use of NICOTROL NS is not recommended in patients with known chronic nasal disorders (e.g. allergy, rhinitis, nasal polyps and sinusitis) since such use has not been adequately studied.

Asthma, Bronchospasm and Reactive Airway Disease

Exacerbation of bronchospasm in patients with pre-existing asthma has been reported. Use of NICOTROL NS in patients with severe reactive airway disease is not recommended.

Effect of NICOTROL NS on the Nasal Mucosa

Topical application of either nicotine or tobacco products is irritating to the nasal mucosa and physicians should consider both the risks and benefits to the patient before initiating or continuing NICOTROL NS therapy.

The effect of NICOTROL NS on the nasal mucosa was studied in 39 cigarette smokers who used NICOTROL NS for 1 month. When compared to baseline, random biopsies taken after four weeks of treatment revealed 1 patient with persistence of pre-existing dysplasia and 1 patient with a newly found dysplasia. In both, dysplasia was not seen after a recovery period of eight weeks.

Forty-two patients who used NICOTROL NS for more than 6 months underwent follow-up ear, nose and throat examinations 1 to 3 months after discontinuing the use of the spray. Many reported local irritant effects of the spray during spray use, but none showed persistent mucosal injury that the examining physician could attribute to use of the product. The clinical significance of these findings is not known, but extended use of the product beyond six months is not recommended.

Cardiovascular or Peripheral Vascular Diseases

The risks of nicotine replacement in patients with cardiovascular and peripheral vascular diseases should be weighed against the benefits of including nicotine replacement in a smoking cessation program for them. Specifically, patients with coronary heart disease (history of myocardial infarction and/or angina pectoris), serious cardiac arrhythmias, or vasospastic diseases (Buerger's disease, Prinzmetal's variant angina and Raynaud's phenomena) should be evaluated carefully before nicotine replacement is prescribed.

Tachycardia occurring in association with nicotine replacement therapy has been reported. No serious cardiovascular events were reported in clinical studies with NICOTROL NS, but if symptoms occur, its use should be discontinued.

NICOTROL NS generally should not be used in patients during the immediate post-myocardial infarction period, nor in patients with serious arrhythmias, or with severe or worsening angina.

Renal or Hepatic Insufficiency

The pharmacokinetics of nicotine have not been studied in the elderly or in patients with renal or hepatic impairment. However, given that nicotine is extensively metabolized and that its total system clearance is dependent on liver blood flow, some influence of hepatic impairment on drug kinetics (reduced clearance) should be anticipated. Only severe renal impairment would be expected to affect the clearance of nicotine or its metabolites from the circulation (See **PHARMACOKINETICS**).

Endocrine Diseases

NICOTROL NS therapy should be used with caution in patients with hyperthyroidism, pheochromocytoma or insulin-dependent diabetes, since nicotine causes the release of catecholamines by the adrenal medula.

Peptic Ulcer Disease

Nicotine delays healing in peptic ulcer disease, therefore, NICOTROL NS therapy should be used with caution in patients with active peptic ulcers and only when the benefits of including nicotine replacement in a smoking cessation program outweigh the risks.

Accelerated Hypertension

Nicotine therapy constitutes a risk factor for development of malignant hypertension in patients with accelerated hypertension; therefore, NICOTROL NS therapy should be used with caution in these patients and only when the benefits of including nicotine replacement in a smoking cessation program outweigh the risks.

Information to Patient

A patient instruction sheet is included in the package of NICOTROL NS dispensed to the patient. Patients should be encouraged to read the instruction sheet carefully and to ask their physician and pharmacist about the proper use of the product (See **DOSAGE AND ADMINISTRATION**).

It should be explained to patients that they are likely to experience nasal irritation, which may become less bothersome with continued use.

Patients must be advised to keep both used and unused containers out of the reach of children and pets.

Drug Interactions

The extent of absorption and peak plasma concentration is slightly reduced in patients with the common cold/rhinitis. In addition, the time to peak concentration is prolonged. the use of a nasal vasoconstrictor such as xylometazoline in patients with rhinitis will further prolong the time to peak (See **PHARMACOKINETICS**). Smoking cessation, with or without nicotine replacement, may alter the pharmacokinetics of certain concomitant medications.

May Require A Decrease in Dose at Cessation of Smoking	Possible Mechanism
Acetaminophen caffeine, imipramine, oxazepam, pentazocine, propranolol, or other beta-blockers, theophylline	Deinduction of hepatic enzymes on smoking cessation
Insulin	Increase of subcutaneous insulin absorption with smoking cessation
Adrenergic antagonists (e.g. prazosin labetalol)	Decrease in circulating catecholamines with smoking cessation
May Require an Increase in Dose at Cessation of Smoking	**Possible Mechanism**
Adrenergic agonists (e.g. isoproterenol, phenylephrine)	Decrease in circulating catecholamines with smoking cessation

Carcinogenesis, Mutagenesis, Impairment of Fertility

Nicotine itself does not appear to be a carcinogen in laboratory animals. However, nicotine and its metabolites increased the incidence of tumors in the cheek pouches of hamsters and forestomach of F344 rats, respectively, when given in combination with tumor-initiators. One study, which could not be replicated, suggested that cotinine, the primary metabolite of nicotine, may cause lymphoreticular sarcoma in the large intestine of rats.

Neither nicotine nor cotinine were mutagenic in the Ames salmonella test. Nicotine was shown to be genotoxic in a test system using Chinese hamster ovary cells. In rats and rabbits, implantation can be delayed or inhibited by a reduction in DNA synthesis that appears to be caused by nicotine. Studies have shown a decrease in litter size in rats treated with nicotine during gestation.

PREGNANCY

Pregnancy Category D (See **WARNINGS** sections).

The harmful effects of cigarette smoking on maternal and fetal health are clearly established. These include low birth weight, an increased risk of spontaneous abortion, and increased perinatal mortality. The specific effects of NICOTROL NS on fetal development are unknown. Therefore pregnant smokers should be encouraged to attempt cessation using educational and behavioral interventions before using pharmacological approaches.

Spontaneous abortion during nicotine replacement therapy has been reported; as with smoking, nicotine as a contributing factor cannot be excluded.

NICOTROL NS should be used during pregnancy only if the likelihood of smoking cessation justifies the potential risk of using it by the pregnant patient, who might continue to smoke.

Teratogenicity

Animal Studies Nicotine was shown to produce skeletal abnormalities in the offspring of mice when toxic doses were given to the dams (25 mg/kg IP or SC).

Human Studies Nicotine teratogenicity has not been studied in humans except as a component of cigarette smoke (each cigarette smoked delivers about 1 mg of nicotine). It has not been possible to conclude whether cigarette smoking is teratogenic to humans.

Other Effects

Animal Studies A nicotine bolus (up to 2 mg/kg) to pregnant rhesus monkeys caused acidosis, hypercarbia, and hypotension (fetal and maternal concentrations were about 20 times those achieved after smoking one cigarette in 5 minutes). Fetal breathing movements were reduced in the fetal lamb after intravenous injection of 0.25 mg/kg nicotine to the ewe (equivalent to smoking 1 cigarette every 20 seconds for 5 minutes). Uterine blood flow was reduced about 30% after infusion of 0.1 μg/kg/min nicotine to pregnant rhesus monkeys (equivalent to smoking about six cigarettes every minute for 20 minutes)

Human Experience Cigarette smoking during pregnancy is associated with an increased risk of spontaneous abortion, low birth weight infants and perinatal mortality. Nicotine and carbon monoxide are considered the most likely mediators of these outcomes. The effects of cigarette smoking on fetal cardiovascular parameters have been studied near term. Cigarettes increased fetal aortic blood flow and heart rate and decreased uterine blood flow and fetal breathing movements. NICOTROL NS has not been studied in pregnant women.

Labor and Delivery

NICOTROL NS is not recommended for use during labor and delivery. The effect of nicotine on a mother or the fetus during labor is unknown.

Use in Nursing Mothers

Caution should be exercised when NICOTROL NS is administered to nursing mothers. The safety of NICOTROL NS therapy in nursing infants has not been examined. Nicotine passes freely into breast milk; the milk to plasma ratio averages 2.9. Nicotine is absorbed orally. An infant has the ability to clear nicotine by hepatic first-pass clearance; however, the efficiency of removal is probably lowest at birth. Nicotine concentrations in milk can be expected to be lower with NICOTROL NS when used as recommended than with cigarette smoking, as maternal plasma nicotine concentrations are generally reduced with nicotine replacement. The risk of exposure of the infant to nicotine from NICOTROL NS therapy should be weighed against the risks associated with the infant's exposure to nicotine from continued smoking by the mother (passive smoke exposure and contamination of breast milk with other components of tobacco smoke) and from NICOTROL NS alone, or in combination with continued smoking.

Pediatric Use

NICOTROL NS therapy is not recommended for use in the pediatric population because its safety and effectiveness in children and adolescents who smoke have not been evaluated.

Geriatric Use

Forty-one patients over the age of 60 participated in clinical trials of NICOTROL NS. The spray appeared to be as effective in this age group as in younger smokers. Because medical conditions that are precautions to nicotine use are more common in the elderly, physicians should use care in prescribing this product to these patients.

ADVERSE REACTIONS

Assessment of adverse events in the 730 patients who participated in controlled clinical trials is complicated by the occurrence of signs and symptoms of nicotine withdrawal in some patients and nicotine excess in others. The incidence of adverse events is confounded by the many minor complaints that smokers commonly have, by continued smoking by many patients and the local irritation from both active drug and the pepper placebo. No serious adverse events were reported during the trials.

Common Smoker's Complaints

Common complaints experienced by the smokers in the study (users of both active and placebo spray) include, chest tightness, dyspepsia, paraesthesia (tingling) in limbs, constipation, and stomatitis.

Tobacco Withdrawal Symptoms

Symptoms of tobacco withdrawal were frequent in users of both active and placebo sprays. Common withdrawal symptoms seen in over 5% of patients included: anxiety, irritability, restlessness, cravings, dizziness, impaired concentration, weight increase, emotional lability, somnolence and fatigue, increased sweating, and insomnia. Less frequently seen probable withdrawal symptoms (under 5%) included: confusion, depression, apathy, tremor, increased appetite, incoordination and increased dreaming.

Continued on next page

McNeil Consumer—Cont.

Anxiety, irritability, restlessness and tobacco cravings occurred about equally in both groups, while other symptoms tended to be slightly more common on placebo spray.

Effects of the Spray

NICOTROL NS and the pepper-containing placebo were both associated with irritant side effects on the nasopharyngeal and ocular tissues. During the first 2 days of treatment, nasal irritation was reported by nearly all (94%) of the patients, the majority of whom rated it as either moderate or severe. Both the frequency and severity of nasal irritation declined with continued use of NICOTROL NS but was still experienced by most (81%) of the patients after 3 weeks of treatment, with most patients rating it as moderate or mild. Other common side-effects for both active and placebo groups were runny nose, throat irritation, watering eyes, sneezing, and cough.

The following local events were reported somewhat more commonly for active than for placebo spray: nasal congestion, subjective comments related to the taste or use of the dosage form, sinus irritation, transient epistaxis, eye irritation, transient changes in sense of smell, pharyngitis, paraethesias of the nose, mouth or head, numbness of the nose, or mouth, burning of the nose or eyes, earache, facial flushing, transient changes in sense of taste, hoarseness, nasal ulcer or blister.

Effects of Nicotine

Feelings of dependence on the spray were reported by more patients on active spray than placebo. Drug-like effects such as calming were also more frequent on active spray. (See **DRUG ABUSE AND DEPENDENCE**)

Other Adverse Effects

Adverse events which could not be classified and listed above and which were reported by > 1% of patients on active spray are listed in the following table

Adverse Events Not Attributable to Intercurrent Illness

Adverse Event	Active	Placebo
HEADACHE	18%	15%
BACK PAIN	6%	4%
DYSPNEA	5%	6%
NAUSEA	5%	5%
ARTHRALGIA	5%	1%
MENSTRUAL DISORDER	4%	4%
PALPITATION	4%	4%
FLATULENCE	4%	3%
TOOTH DISORDER	4%	1%
GUM PROBLEMS	4%	1%
MYALGIA	3%	4%
ABDOMINAL PAIN	3%	3%
CONFUSION	3%	3%
ACNE	3%	1%
DYSMENORRHEA	3%	0%
PRURITUS	2%	3%

Adverse events reported with a frequency of < 1% among active spray users are listed below:

Body as a Whole: edema peripheral, pain, numbness, allergy
Gastrointestinal: dry mouth, hiccup, diarrhea
Hematologic: purpura
Neurological: aphasia, amnesia, migraine, numbness
Respiratory: bronchitis, bronchospasm, sputum increased
Skin and appendages: rash, purpura
Special Senses: vision abnormal

DRUG ABUSE AND DEPENDENCE

NICOTROL NS has a dependence potential intermediate between other nicotine-based therapies and cigarettes. This is the result of differences between cigarettes, NICOTROL NS, nicotine gum and nicotine patches in pharmacokinetic and dosing characteristics commonly associated with abuse and dependence. NICOTROL NS is distinct from other nicotine-based smoking cessation therapies in its greater speed of onset, greater capacity for self-titration of dose, and frequent and rapid fluctuations in plasma nicotine concentration.

Dependence on nicotine nasal spray occurred in the clinical trials. Feelings of dependency on the spray were reported by 32% of active spray users and 13% of placebo spray users. Such dependence may represent transference of tobacco-related nicotine dependence to NICOTROL NS.

Fifteen to 20% of patients used the active spray for longer periods than recommended (6 months to 1 year) and 5% used the spray at a higher dose than recommended. Some of these patients experienced anxiety about stopping the spray and some reported craving for the spray rather than for cigarettes.

OVERDOSAGE

The oral LD_{50} for nicotine is > 5 mg/kg in dogs and > 24 mg/kg in rodents. Deaths is due to respiratory paralysis. The oral minimum acute lethal dose for nicotine in adult humans is reported to be 40 to 60 mg (< 1 mg/kg). A full bottle of NICOTROL NS contains 100 mg of nicotine.

NICOTROL NS would be expected to be irritating if sprayed in the eyes, mouth or ears. Eye exposure should be treated with copious irrigation with water for 20 minutes. Large oral nicotine ingestions cause vomiting, and the consequences of an overdose will vary; should this occur, patients should contact their physician immediately. For additional emergency information, call your regional poison center or call the National Capital Poison Center toll-free (1-800-498-8666).

Signs and Symptoms of Nicotine Toxicity

Signs and symptoms of an overdose of NICOTROL NS would be expected to be the same as those of acute nicotine poisoning including: pallor, cold sweat, nausea, salivation, vomiting, abdominal pain, diarrhea, headache, dizziness, disturbed hearing and vision, tremor, mental confusion, and weakness. Prostration, hypotension, and respiratory failure may ensue with large overdoses. Lethal doses produce convulsions quickly and death follows as a result of peripheral or central respiratory paralysis or, less frequently, cardiac failure.

Overdose from Ingestion

If emesis has not occurred, it should be induced in conscious patients with a suitable emetic followed by an appropriate dose of activated charcoal. In unconscious patients with a secure airway, instill activated charcoal via a nasogastric tube. A saline cathartic or sorbitol may be added to the first dose of activated charcoal.

Management of Nicotine Poisoning

Other supportive measures include diazepam or barbiturates for seizures, atropine for excessive bronchial secretions or diarrhea, respiratory support for respiratory failure, and vigorous fluid support for hypotension and cardiovascular collapse.

DOSAGE AND ADMINISTRATION

It is important that patients understand the instructions for use of NICOTROL NS, and have their questions answered. They should clearly understand the directions for using NICOTROL NS and safely disposing of the used container. They should be instructed to stop smoking completely when they begin using the product.

Patients should be instructed not to sniff, swallow or inhale through the nose as the spray is being administered. They should also be advised to administer the spray with the head tilted back slightly.

The dose of NICOTROL NS, should be **individualized** on the basis of each patient's nicotine dependence and the occurrence of symptoms of nicotine excess (See Individualization of Dosage).

Each actuation of NICOTROL NS delivers a metered 50 microliter spray containing 0.5 mg of nicotine. One dose is 1 mg of nicotine (2 sprays, one in each nostril).

Patients should be started with 1 or 2 doses per hour, which may be increased up to a maximum recommended dose of 40 mg (80 sprays, somewhat less than $^1/_2$ bottle) per day). For best results, patients should be encouraged to use at least the recommended minimum of 8 doses per day, as less is unlikely to be effective. In clinicals trials, the patients who successfully quit smoking used the product heavily when nicotine withdrawal was at its peak, sometimes up to the recommended maximum of 40 doses per day (in heavier smokers). Dosing recommendations are summarized in Table 4.

[See table below.]

No tapering strategy has been shown to be optimal in clinical studies. Many patients simply stopped using the spray at their last clinic visit.

Recommended strategies for discontinuation of use include suggesting that patients: use only $^1/_2$ a dose (1 spray) at a time, use the spray less frequently, keep a tally of daily usage, try to meet a steadily reducing usage target, skip a dose by not medicating every hour, or set a planned "quit date" for stopping use of the spray.

Individualization of Dosage

The success or failure of smoking cessation is influenced by the quality, intensity and frequency of supportive care. Patients are more likely to quit smoking if they are seen frequently and participate in formal smoking cessation programs.

The goal of NICOTROL NS therapy is complete abstinence. If a patient is unable to stop smoking by the fourth week of therapy, treatment should probably be discontinued.

Patients who fail to quit on any attempt may benefit from interventions to improve their chances for success on subsequent attempts. Patients who were unsuccessful should be counseled and should then probably be given a "therapy holiday" before the next attempt. A new quit attempt should be encouraged when conditions are more favorable.

Based on the clinical trials, a reasonable approach to assisting patients in their attempt to quit smoking is to begin initial treatment, using the recommended dosage (See **DOSAGE AND ADMINISTRATION**). Regular use of the spray during the first week of treatment may help patients adapt to the irritant effects of the spray. Dosage can then be adjusted in those subjects with signs or symptoms of nicotine withdrawal or excess. Patients who are successfully abstinent on NICOTROL NS should be treated at the selected dosage for up to 8 weeks, following which use of the spray should be discontinued over the next 4 to 6 weeks. Some patients may not require gradual reduction of dosage and may abruptly stop treatment successfully. Treatment with NICOTROL NS for longer periods has not been shown to improve outcome, and the safety of use for periods longer than 6 months has not been established.

The symptoms of nicotine withdrawal overlap those of nicotine excess (See **Pharmacodynamics and ADVERSE REACTIONS** sections). Since patients using NICOTROL NS may also smoke intermittently, it is sometimes difficult to determine if patients are experiencing nicotine withdrawal or nicotine excess. Controlled clinical trials of nicotine products suggest that palpitations, nausea and sweating are more often symptoms of nicotine excess, whereas anxiety, nervousness and irritability are more often symptoms of nicotine withdrawal

SAFETY AND HANDLING

As with all medicines, especially ones in liquid form, care should be taken in handling NICOTROL NS during periods of opening and closing the container (See **WARNINGS and Safety Note Concerning Children**). If it is dropped it may break. If this occurs, the spill should be cleaned up immediately with an absorbent cloth/paper towel. Care should be taken to avoid contact of the solution with the skin. Broken glass should be picked up carefully, using a broom. The area of the spill should be washed several times. Absorbent material may be disposed of as any other household waste. Should even a small amount of NICOTROL NS come in contact with the skin, lips, mouth, eyes or ears, the affected area(s) should be immediately rinsed with water only.

Disposal

Used bottles of NICOTROL NS should be disposed of with their child-resistant caps in place. Used bottles should be disposed of in such a way as to prevent access by children or pets. See patient information for further information on handling and disposal.

HOW SUPPLIED

NDC 0045-0899-01

Nicotrol®NS (nicotine nasal spray) 10 mg/mL, is supplied in individual 10 mL bottles.

Each unit consists of a glass container, mounted with a metered spray pump

A patient information leaflet is enclosed with the package

Store at room temperature not to exceed 30°C/86°F.

CAUTION: Federal law prohibits dispensing without prescription.

Shown in Product Identification Section, page 322

Table 4

Maximum Recommended Duration of Treatment	Recommended Doses per Hour	Maximum Doses per Hour	Maximum Doses per Day
3 months	1–2*	5	40

* One dose = 2 sprays (one in each nostril). One dose delivers 1 mg of nicotine to the nasal mucosa.

NICOTROL® — OTC
NICOTINE TRANSDERMAL SYSTEM

DESCRIPTION

NICOTROL® (nicotine transdermal system) is a multilayered, rectangular, thin film laminated unit containing nicotine as the active ingredient. ***NICOTROL®*** Patch provides systemic delivery of 15 mg of nicotine over 16 hours.

ACTIONS

NICOTROL® (nicotine transdermal system) Patch helps smokers quit by reducing nicotine withdrawal symptoms. Many ***NICOTROL®*** Patch users will be able to stop smoking for a few days but often will start smoking again. Most smokers have to try to quit several times before they completely stop.

Your own chances of quitting smoking depend on how much you want to quit, how strongly you are addicted to nicotine and how closely you follow a quitting program like the PATHWAYS TO CHANGE® Program that comes with the ***NICOTROL®*** Patch.

If you find you cannot stop or if you start smoking again after using ***NICOTROL®*** Patch, please talk to a health care professional who can help you find a program that may work better for you. Remember that breaking this addiction doesn't happen overnight.

Because the *NICOTROL®* Patch provides some nicotine, the *NICOTROL®* Patch will help you stop smoking by reducing nicotine withdrawal symptoms such as nicotine cravings, nervousness and irritability.

INDICATIONS

NICOTROL® Patch is indicated as a stop smoking aid to reduce withdrawal symptoms, including nicotine craving, associated with quitting smoking.

DIRECTIONS

* Stop smoking completely when you begin using the *NICOTROL®* Patch.
* Refer to enclosed patient information leaflet before using this product.
* Use one *NICOTROL®* Patch every day for six weeks. Remove backing from the patch and immediately press onto clean dry hairless skin. Hold for ten seconds. Wash hands.
* The *NICOTROL®* Patch should be worn during awake hours and removed prior to sleep.

FOR BEST RESULTS IN QUITTING SMOKING

1. Firmly commit to quitting smoking.
2. Use enclosed support materials.
3. Use the *NICOTROL®* Patches for six weeks.
4. Stop using *NICOTROL®* Patches at the end of week six. If you still feel the need for *NICOTROL®* Patches talk to your doctor.

WARNINGS

* Keep this and all medication out of reach of children and pets. Even used patches have enough nicotine to poison children and pets. Be sure to fold sticky ends together and throw away out of reach of children and pets. In case of accidental overdose, seek professional assistance or contact a poison control center immediately.
* Nicotine can increase your baby's heart rate. First try to stop smoking without the nicotine patch. As with any drug, if you are pregnant or nursing a baby, seek the advice of a health professional before using this product.
* Do not smoke even when you are not wearing the patch. The nicotine in your skin will still be entering your bloodstream for several hours after you take the patch off.
* If you forget to remove the patch at bedtime you may have vivid dreams or other sleep disruptions.

Do Not Use if You:
* Continue to smoke, chew tobacco, use snuff, or use a nicotine gum or other nicotine containing products.

Ask Your Doctor Before Use if You:
* Are under 18 years of age
* Have heart disease, recent heart attack or irregular heartbeat. Nicotine can increase your heart rate.
* Have high blood pressure not controlled with medication. Nicotine can increase blood pressure.
* Take prescription medicine for depression or asthma. Your prescription dose may need to be adjusted.
* Are allergic to adhesive tape or have skin problems, because you are more likely to get rashes.

Stop Use and See Your Doctor if You Have:
* Skin redness caused by the patch that does not go away after four days, or if your skin swells or you get a rash.
* Irregular heartbeat or palpitations.
* Symptoms of nicotine overdose such as nausea, vomiting, dizziness, weakness and rapid heartbeat.

INACTIVE INGREDIENTS

Polyisobutylenes, polybutene non-woven polyester, pigmented aluminized and clear polyesters.

HOW SUPPLIED

Starter Kit-7 patches, Refill Kit-7 and 14 patches. DO NOT USE IF POUCH IS DAMAGED OR OPEN. Do not Store above 86°F (30°C)
* **Not for sale to those under 18 years of age**
* **Proof of age required.**

---

* Not for sale in vending machines or from any source where proof of age cannot be verified.

Shown in Product Identification Guide, page 322

PEDIACARE® Cough-Cold Liquid   OTC
and Chewable Tablets
PEDIACARE® NightRest
Cough-Cold Liquid
PEDIACARE® Infants' Drops
Decongestant
PEDIACARE® Infants' Drops
Decongestant Plus Cough

DESCRIPTION

Each 5 ml of *PEDIACARE® Cough-Cold Liquid* contains pseudoephedrine hydrochloride 15 mg, chlorpheniramine maleate 1 mg and dextromethorphan hydrobromide 5 mg. Each *PEDIACARE® Cough-Cold Chewable Tablet* contains pseudoephedrine hydrochloride 15 mg, chlorpheniramine maleate 1 mg and dextromethorphan hydrobromide 5 mg. Each 0.8 ml oral dropper of *PEDIACARE® Infants' Drops Decongestant* contains pseudoephedrine hydrochloride 7.5 mg. Each 0.8 oral dropper of *PEDIACARE® Infants' Drops Decongestant Plus Cough* contains pseudoephedrine hydrochloride 7.5 mg and dextromethorphan hydrobromide 2.5 mg. *PEDIACARE® NightRest Cough-Cold Liquid* contains pseudoephedrine hydrochloride 15 mg, chlorpheniramine maleate 1 mg and dextromethorphan hydrobromide 7.5 mg per 5 ml. *PEDIACARE® Cough-Cold Liquid* and *NightRest Cough-Cold Liquid* are stable, cherry flavored and red in color. *PEDIACARE® Infants' Drops* are fruit flavored alcohol free and red in color. *PEDIACARE® Infants' Drops Decongestant Plus Cough* are cherry flavored, alcohol free and clear, non-staining in color. *PEDIACARE® Cough-Cold Chewable Tablets* are fruit flavored and pink in color.

ACTIONS

PEDIACARE Products are available in four different formulas, allowing you to select the ideal product to temporarily relieve the patient's symptoms. *PEDIACARE® Cough-Cold Liquid* and *Chewable Tablets* contain an antihistamine, chlorpheniramine maleate, a nasal decongestant, pseudoephedrine HCl and a cough suppressant, dextromethorphan hydrobromide, to provide temporary relief of nasal congestion, runny nose, sneezing and coughing due to the common cold, hay fever or other upper respiratory allergies. *PEDIACARE® NightRest Cough-Cold Liquid* contains a decongestant, pseudoephedrine hydrochloride, an antihistamine, chlorpheniramine maleate, and a cough suppressant, dextromethorphan hydrobromide, to provide temporary relief of coughs, nasal congestion, runny nose and sneezing due to the common cold hayfever or other upper respiratory allergies. *PEDIACARE® NightRest* may be used day or night to relieve cough and cold symptoms. *PEDIACARE® Infants' Drops Decongestant* contain a decongestant, pseudoephedrine hydrochloride, to provide temporary relief of nasal congestion due to the common cold, hay fever or other upper respiratory allergies. *PEDIACARE® Infants' Drops Decongestant Plus Cough* contain a decongestant, pseudoephedrine hydrochloride, and a cough suppressant, dextromethorphan hydrobromide to provide temporary relief of nasal congestion and coughing due to common cold, hay fever or other upper respiratory allergies.

PROFESSIONAL DOSAGE

A calibrated dosage cup is provided for accurate dosing of the *PEDIACARE* Liquid formulas. A calibrated oral dropper is provided for accurate dosing of *PEDIACARE® Infants' Drops*. All doses of *PEDIACARE® Cough-Cold Liquid* and *Chewable Tablets*, as well as *PEDIACARE® Infants' Drops* may be repeated every 4–6 hours, not to exceed 4 doses in 24

---

hours. *PEDIACARE® NightRest Liquid* may be repeated every 6–8 hrs, not to exceed 4 doses in 24 hours. [See table below.]

WARNINGS

DO NOT USE IF CARTON IS OPENED, OR IF PRINTED PLASTIC BOTTLE WRAP OR FOIL INNER SEAL IS BROKEN. KEEP THIS AND ALL MEDICATION OUT OF THE REACH OF CHILDREN. IN CASE OF ACCIDENTAL OVERDOSAGE, CONTACT A PHYSICIAN OR POISON CONTROL CENTER IMMEDIATELY.

The following information appears on the appropriate package labels:
PEDIACARE® Cough-Cold Chewable Tablets:
PHENYLKETONURICS: CONTAINS PHENYLALANINE 6MG PER TABLET.
PEDIACARE® Cough-Cold Liquid and Chewable Tablets, Night Rest Cough-Cold Liquid: Do not exceed recommended dosage. If nervousness, dizziness or sleeplessness occur, discontinue use and consult a doctor. If symptoms do not improve within 7 days or are accompanied by fever, consult a doctor. A persistent cough may be a sign of a serious condition. If cough persists for more than one week, tends to recur or is accompanied by fever, rash, or persistent headache, consult a doctor. Do not give this product for persistent or chronic cough such as occurs with asthma or if cough is accompanied by excessive phlegm (mucus) unless directed by a doctor. May cause excitability especially in children. May cause drowsiness. Sedatives and tranquilizers may increase the drowsiness effect. Do not give this product to children who are taking sedatives or tranquilizers without first consulting the child's doctor. Do not give this product to children who have a breathing problem such as chronic bronchitis, or who have glaucoma, heart disease, high blood pressure, thyroid disease or diabetes, without first consulting the child's doctor.

PEDIACARE® Infants' Drops Decongestant: Do not exceed the recommended dosage. If nervousness, dizziness or sleeplessness occur discontinue use and consult a doctor. If symptoms do not improve within 7 days or are accompanied by fever, consult a physician. Do not give this product to a child who has heart disease, high blood pressure, thyroid disease or diabetes unless directed by a doctor. Take by mouth only. Not for nasal use.

PEDIACARE® Infants' Drops Decongestant Plus Cough: Do not exceed recommended dosage. If nervousness, dizziness, or sleeplessness occur, discontinue use and consult a doctor. If symptoms do not improve within 7 days or are accompanied by fever, consult a doctor. A persistent cough may be a sign of a serious condition. If cough persists for more than one week, tends to recur or is accompanied by fever, rash, or persistent headache, consult a doctor. Do not give this product for persistent or chronic cough such as occurs with asthma or if cough is accompanied by excessive phlegm (mucus) unless directed by a doctor. Do not give this product to a child who has heart disease, high blood pressure, thyroid disease or diabetes unless directed by a doctor. Take by mouth only. Not for nasal use.

DRUG INTERACTION PRECAUTION

Do not give this product to a child who is taking a prescription monoamine oxidase inhibitor (MAOI) (certain drugs for depression, psychiatric or emotional conditions), or for 2 weeks after stopping the MAOI drug. If you are uncertain whether your child's prescription drug contains an MAOI, consult a health professional before giving this product.

INACTIVE INGREDIENTS

PEDIACARE® Cough-Cold Liquid: Citric acid, corn syrup, flavors, glycerin, propylene glycol, sodium benzoate, sodium carboxymethylcellulose, sorbitol, purified water and Red #40.
PEDIACARE® NightRest Cough-Cold Liquid: Citric acid, corn syrup, flavors, glycerin, propylene glycol, sodium benzo-

---

Age Group	0–3 mos	4–11 mos	12–23 mos	2–3 yrs	4–5 yrs	6–8 yrs	9–10 yrs	11 yrs	Dosage
Weight (lbs)	6–11 lb	12–17 lb	18–23 lb	24–35 lb	36–47 lb	48–59 lb	60–71 lb	72–95 lb	
PEDIACARE® Infants' Drops Decongestant*	½ dropper (0.4 ml)	1 dropper (0.8 ml)	1½ droppers (1.2 ml)	2 droppers (1.6 ml)					q4–6h
PEDIACARE® Infants' Drops Decongestant Plus Cough*	½ dropper (0.4 ml)	1 dropper (0.8 ml)	1½ droppers (1.2 ml)	2 droppers (1.6 ml)					q4–6h
PEDIACARE® Cough-Cold Liquid** and Chewable Tablets**				1 tsp / 1 tab	1½ tsp / 1½ tabs	2 tsp / 2 tabs	2½ tsp / 2½ tabs	3 tsp / 3 tabs	q4–6h
PEDIACARE® NightRest Liquid**				1 tsp	1½ tsp	2 tsp	2½ tsp	3 tsp	q6–8h

* Administer to children under 2 years only on the advice of a physician.
** Administer to children under 6 years only on the advice of a physician.

Continued on next page

Consult 1997 supplements and future editions for revisions

McNeil Consumer—Cont.

ate, sodium carboxymethylcellulose, sorbitol, purified water and Red #40.
PEDIACARE® Cough-Cold Chewable Tablets: Aspartame, cellulose, citric acid, flavors, magnesium stearate, magnesium trisilicate, mannitol, corn starch and Red #7.
PEDIACARE® Infants' Drops Decongestant: Benzoic acid, citric acid, flavors, glycerin, polyethylene glycol, propylene glycol, purified water, sodium benzoate, sorbitol, sucrose and Red #40.
PEDIACARE® Infants's Drops Decongestant Plus Cough- :Citric acid, flavors, glycerin, purified water, sodium benzoate, and sorbitol.

OVERDOSAGE

Acute dextromethorphan overdose usually does not result in serious signs and symptoms unless massive amounts have been ingested. Signs and symptoms of a substantial overdose may include nausea and vomiting, visual disturbances, CNS disturbances, and urinary retention. Symptoms from pseudoephedrine overdose consist most often of mild anxiety, tachycardia and/or mild hypertension. Symptoms usually appear within 4 to 8 hours of ingestion and are transient, usually requiring no treatment. Chlorpheniramine toxicity should be treated as you would an antihistamine/anticholinergic overdose and is likely to be present within a few hours after acute ingestion. Symptoms from pseudoephedrine overdose consist often of mild anxiety, tachycardia and/or mild hypertension. Symptoms usually appear within 4 to 8 hours of ingestion and are transient, usually requiring no treatment.

HOW SUPPLIED

PEDIACARE® Cough-Cold Liquid and NightRest Cough-Cold Liquid (colored red)—bottles of 4 fl. oz. (120 ml) with child-resistant safety cap and calibrated dosage cup. ***PEDIACARE Cough-Cold Chewable Tablets*** (pink, scored)—blister packs of 16. ***PEDIACARE® Infants' Drops Decongestant***(colored red) and ***PEDIACARE® Infants' Drops Decongestant Plus Cough*** (clear)—bottles of ½ fl. oz (15 ml) with calibrated dropper.

Shown in Product Identification Guide, page 322

Maximum Strength SINE-AID® — OTC
Sinus Medication Gelcaps, Caplets and Tablets

DESCRIPTION

Each ***Maximum Strength SINE-AID® Gelcap, Caplet*** or ***Tablet*** contains acetaminophen 500 mg and pseudoephedrine hydrochloride 30 mg.

ACTIONS

Maximum Strength SINE-AID® Gelcaps, Caplets and ***Tablets*** contain a clinically proven analgesic-antipyretic and a decongestant. Maximum allowable non-prescription levels of acetaminophen and pseudoephedrine provide temporary relief of sinus congestion and pain. Acetaminophen is equal to aspirin in analgesic and antipyretic effectiveness and it is unlikely to produce many of the side effects associated with aspirin and aspirin-containing products. Acetaminophen produces analgesia by elevation of the pain threshold and antipyresis through action on the hypothalamic heat-regulating center. Pseudoephedrine hydrochloride is a sympathomimetic amine that promotes sinus cavity drainage by reducing nasopharyngeal mucosal congestion.

INDICATIONS

Maximum Strength SINE-AID® Gelcaps, Caplets and ***Tablets*** provide effective symptomatic relief from sinus headache pain and congestion. SINE-AID® is particularly well-suited in patients with aspirin allergy, hemostatic disturbances (including anticoagulant therapy), and bleeding diatheses (e.g. hemophilia) and upper gastrointestinal disease (e.g. ulcer, gastritis, hiatus hernia).

PRECAUTIONS

If a rare sensitivity occurs, the drug should be discontinued. Although pseudoephedrine is virtually without pressor effect in normotensive patients, it should be used with caution in hypertensives.

DIRECTIONS

Adults & children 12 years of age and older: Two gelcaps, caplets or tablets every four to six hours. Do not exceed eight gelcaps, caplets or tablets in any 24 hour period. Not for use in children under 12 years of age.

WARNINGS

Do not use if carton is open or if blister unit is broken.
Do not take for pain for more than 7 days or for fever for more than 3 days unless directed by a doctor. If pain or fever persists, or gets worse, if new symptoms occur, or if redness or swelling is present, consult a doctor because these could be signs of a serious condition. **Do not exceed recommended dosage.** If nervousness, dizziness or sleeplessness occur, discontinue use and consult a doctor. Do not take this product if you have heart disease, high blood pressure, thyroid disease, diabetes or difficulty in urination due to enlargement of the prostate gland unless directed by a doctor.
As with any drug, if you are pregnant or nursing a baby, seek the advice of a health professional before using this product. Keep this and all drugs out of the reach of children. In case of accidental overdose, contact a doctor or poison control center immediately. Prompt medical attention is critical for adults as well as for children even if you do not notice any signs or symptoms. Do not use with other products containing acetaminophen.

ALCOHOL WARNING

For this and all other pain relievers, including aspirin, ibuprofen, ketoprofen and naproxen sodium, if you generally consume 3 or more alcohol-containing drinks per day, you should consult your physician for advice on when and how you should take pain relievers.

DRUG INTERACTION PRECAUTION

Do not use this product if you are now taking a prescription monoamine oxidase inhibitor (MAOI) (certain drugs for depression, psychiatric or emotional conditions, or Parkinson's disease), or for 2 weeks after stopping the MAOI drug. If you are uncertain whether your prescription drug contains an MAOI, consult a health professional before taking this product.

OVERDOSAGE INFORMATION

Acetaminophen in massive overdosage may cause hepatic toxicity in some patients. In adults and adolescents, hepatic toxicity has rarely been reported following ingestion of acute overdoses of less than 10 grams. Fatalities are infrequent (less than 3–4% of untreated cases) and have rarely been reported with overdoses of less than 15 grams. In children, an acute overdosage of less than 150 mg/kg has not been associated with hepatic toxicity.
Early symptoms following a potentially hepatotoxic overdose may include: nausea, vomiting, diaphoresis and general malaise. Clinical and laboratory evidence of hepatic toxicity may not be apparent until 48 to 72 hours postingestion.
In adults and adolescents, regardless of the quantity of acetaminophen reported to have been ingested, administer acetylcysteine immediately if 24 hours or less have elapsed from the reported time of ingestion. For full prescribing information, refer to the acetylcysteine package insert. Do not await results of assays for plasma acetaminophen level before initiating treatment with acetylcysteine. The following additional procedures are recommended: The stomach should be emptied promptly by lavage or by induction of emesis with syrup of ipecac. A plasma acetaminophen assay should be obtained as early as possible, but no sooner than four hours following ingestion. If plasma level falls above the lower treatment line on the acetaminophen overdose nomogram, acetylcysteine therapy should be continued. Liver function studies should be obtained initially and repeated at 24-hour intervals.
Serious toxicity or fatalities are extremely infrequent in children, possibly due to differences in the way they metabolize acetaminophen. In children, the maximum potential amount ingested can be more easily estimated. If more than 150 mg/kg or an unknown amount was ingested, obtain a plasma acetaminophen level. The plasma acetaminophen level should be obtained as soon as possible, but no sooner than 4 hours following the ingestion. If plasma level falls above the lower treatment line on the acetaminophen overdose nomogram, the acetylcysteine therapy should be initiated and continued for a full course of therapy. If plasma acetaminophen assay capability is not available, and the estimated acetaminophen ingestion exceeds 150 mg/kg, acetylcysteine therapy should be initiated and continued for a full course of therapy.
For additional emergency information, call your regional poison center or call the Rocky Mountain Poison Center toll-free, (1-800-525-6115).
Symptoms from pseudoephedrine overdose consist most often of mild anxiety, tachycardia and/or mild hypertension. Symptoms usually appear within 4 to 8 hours of ingestion and are transient, usually requiring no treatment.

ALCOHOL INFORMATION

Chronic heavy alcohol abusers may be at increased risk of liver toxicity from excessive acetaminophen use, although reports of this event are rare. Reports almost invariably involve cases of severe chronic alcoholics and the dosages of acetaminophen most often exceed recommended doses and often involve substantial overdose. Professionals should alert their patients who regularly consume large amounts of alcohol not to exceed recommended doses of acetaminophen.

INACTIVE INGREDIENTS

Gelcaps: Benzyl Alcohol, Butylparaben, Castor Oil, Cellulose, Corn Starch, Edetate Calcium Disodium, Gelatin, Hydroxypropyl Methylcellulose, Iron Oxide Black, Magnesium Stearate, Methylparaben, Propylparaben, Sodium Lauryl Sulfate, Sodium Propionate, Sodium Starch Glycolate, Titanium Dioxide, FD&C Red #40.
Caplets: Cellulose, Corn Starch, Hydroxypropyl Methylcellulose, Magnesium Stearate, Polyethylene Glycol, Sodium Starch Glycolate, Titanium Dioxide, Blue #1 and Red #40.
Tablets: Cellulose, Corn Starch, Magnesium Stearate and Sodium Starch Glycolate.

HOW SUPPLIED

Gelcaps (colored red and white imprinted "SINE-AID")—blister package of 20 and tamper resistant bottle of 40.
Caplets (colored white imprinted "Maximum SINE-AID")—blister package of 24 and tamper resistant bottle of 50.
Tablets (colored white embossed "SINE-AID")—blister package of 24 and tamper resistant bottle of 50.

Shown in Product Identification Guide, page 323

Extra Strength TYLENOL® acetaminophen — OTC
Gelcaps, Geltabs, Caplets, Tablets

Extra Strength TYLENOL® acetaminophen
Adult Liquid Pain Reliever

Regular Strength TYLENOL® acetaminophen
Caplets and Tablets

TYLENOL® Extended Relief acetaminophen extended release
Caplets

Product information for all dosage forms of Adult TYLENOL acetaminophen have been combined under this heading.

DESCRIPTION

Each ***Extra Strength TYLENOL® Gelcap, Geltab, Caplet, or Tablet*** contains acetaminophen 500 mg.
Each 15 ml (½ fl oz or one tablespoonful) of ***Extra Strength TYLENOL® acetaminophen Adult Liquid Pain Reliever*** contains 500 mg acetaminophen (alcohol 7%).
Each ***Regular Strength TYLENOL® Caplet or Tablet*** contains acetaminophen 325 mg.
Each ***TYLENOL® Extended Relief Caplet*** contains acetaminophen 650 mg.

ACTIONS

Acetaminophen is a clinically proven analgesic and antipyretic. Acetaminophen produces analgesia by elevation of the pain threshold and antipyresis through action on the hypothalamic heat-regulating center. Acetaminophen is equal to aspirin in analgesic and antipyretic effectiveness and it is unlikely to produce many of the side effects associated with aspirin and aspirin-containing products.
Tylenol Extended Relief uses a unique, patented bilayer caplet. The first layer dissolves quickly to provide prompt relief while the second layer is time released to provide up to 8 hours of relief.

INDICATIONS

For the temporary relief of minor aches and pains associated with the common cold, headache, toothache, muscular aches, back ache, for the minor pain of arthritis, for the pain of menstrual cramps and for the reduction of fever.

DIRECTIONS

Extra Strength TYLENOL® Gelcaps, Geltabs, Caplets, or Tablets: Adults and Children 12 years of Age and Older: Take two gelcaps, geltabs, caplets, or tablets every 4 to 6 hours. Not to exceed 8 gelcaps, geltabs, caplets, or tablets in any 24-hour period. Not for use in children under 12 years of age.
Extra Strength TYLENOL® Adult Liquid Pain Reliever: Adults and Children 12 years of Age and Older: Fill measuring cup once to 2-tablespoon line (1,000 mg) which is equivalent to two 500 mg Extra Strength TYLENOL® Gelcaps, Geltabs, Caplets or Tablets. Take every 4–6 hours. No more than 4 doses in any 24-hour period, or as directed by a doctor. Not for use in children under 12 years of age.
Regular Strength TYLENOL® Caplets or Tablets: Adults and Children 12 years of Age and Older: Take two caplets or tablets every 4 to 6 hours. No more than a total of 12 caplets or tablets in any 24-hour period, or as directed by a doctor. Children (6–11): ½ to 1 caplet or tablet every 4 to 6 hours, not to exceed 5 doses in 24 hours. Consult a physician for use by children under 6 years of age.
TYLENOL® Extended Relief Caplets: Adults and Children 12 years of Age and Older: Take two caplets every 8 hours, not to exceed 6 caplets in any 24-hour period. TAKE TWO CAPLETS WITH WATER, SWALLOW EACH CAPLET WHOLE. DO NOT CRUSH, CHEW, OR DISSOLVE THE CAPLET. Not for use in children under 12 years of age.

PRECAUTIONS

If a rare sensitivity reaction occurs, the drug should be discontinued.

WARNINGS

Do not use if carton is opened or printed red neck wrap or printed full inner seal is broken. Do not take for pain for more than 10 days or for fever for more than 3 days unless directed by a physician. If pain or fever persists, or gets worse, if new symptoms occur, or if redness or swelling is present, consult a physician because these could be signs of a serious condition. As with any drug, if you are pregnant or nursing a baby, seek the advice of a health professional before using this product. Keep this and all drugs out of the reach of children. In case of accidental overdose, contact a physician or poison control center immediately. Prompt medical attention is critical for adults as well as for children even if you do not notice any signs or symptoms. Do not use with other products containing acetaminophen.

ALCOHOL WARNING

For this and all other pain relievers, including aspirin, ibuprofen, ketoprofen and naproxen sodium, if you generally consume three or more alcohol-containing drinks per day, you should consult your physician for advice on when and how you should take pain relievers.

OVERDOSAGE INFORMATION

Acetaminophen in massive overdosage may cause hepatic toxicity in some patients. In adults and adolescents, hepatic toxicity has rarely been reported following ingestion of acute overdoses of less than 10 grams. Fatalities are infrequent (less than 3–4% of untreated cases) and have rarely been reported with overdoses of less than 15 grams. In children, an acute overdosage of less than 150 mg/kg has not been associated with hepatic toxicity.

Early symptoms following a potentially hepatotoxic overdose may include: nausea, vomiting, diaphoresis and general malaise. Clinical and laboratory evidence of hepatic toxicity may not be apparent until 48 to 72 hours postingestion. In adults and adolescents, regardless of the quantity of acetaminophen reported to have been ingested, administer acetylcysteine immediately if 24 hours or less have elapsed from the reported time of ingestion. For full prescribing information, refer to the acetylcysteine package insert. Do not await results of assays for plasma acetaminophen level before initiating treatment with acetylcysteine. The following additional procedures are recommended: The stomach should be emptied promptly by lavage or by induction of emesis with syrup of ipecac. A plasma acetaminophen assay should be obtained as early as possible, but no sooner than four hours following ingestion. If an acetaminophen extended release product is involved, it may be appropriate to obtain an additional plasma acetaminophen level 4–6 hours following the initial plasma acetaminophen level. If either plasma level falls above the lower treatment line on the acetaminophen overdose nomogram, acetylcysteine therapy should be continued. Liver function studies should be obtained initially and repeated at 24-hour intervals.

Serious toxicity or fatalities are extremely infrequent in children, possibly due to differences in the way they metabolize acetaminophen. In children, the maximum potential amount ingested can be more easily estimated. If more than 150 mg/kg or an unknown amount was ingested, obtain a plasma acetaminophen level. The plasma level should be obtained as soon as possible, but no sooner than 4 hours following the ingestion. If an acetaminophen *extended release* product is involved, it may be appropriate to obtain an additional plasma acetaminophen level 4–6 hours following the initial plasma acetaminophen level. If either plasma level falls above the lower treatment line on the acetaminophen overdose nomogram, the acetylcysteine therapy should be initiated and continued for a full course of therapy. If plasma acetaminophen assay capability is not available, and the estimated acetaminophen ingestion exceeds 150 mg/kg, acetylcysteine therapy should be initiated and continued for a full course of therapy.

For additional emergency information, call your regional poison center or call the Rocky Mountain Poison Center toll-free, (1-800-525-6115).

ALCOHOL INFORMATION

Chronic heavy alcohol abusers may be at increased risk of liver toxicity from excessive acetaminophen use, although reports of this event are rare. Reports almost invariably involve cases of severe chronic alcoholics and the dosages of acetaminophen most often exceed recommended doses and often involve substantial overdose. Professionals should alert their patients who regularly consume large amounts of alcohol not to exceed recommended doses of acetaminophen.

INACTIVE INGREDIENTS

Extra Strength TYLENOL®: **Tablets:** Magnesium Stearate, Cellulose, Sodium Starch Glycolate and Starch. **Caplets:** Cellulose, Cornstarch, Hydroxypropyl Methylcellulose, Magnesium Stearate, Polyethylene Glycol, Sodium Starch Glycolate, and Red #40. **Gelcaps:** Benzyl Alcohol, Butylparaben, Castor Oil, Cellulose, Edetate Calcium Disodium, Gelatin, Hydroxypropyl Methylcellulose, Magnesium Stearate, Methylparaben, Propylparaben, Sodium Lauryl Sulfate, Sodium Propionate, Sodium Starch Glycolate, Starch, Tita-

nium Dioxide, Blue #1 and #2, Red #40, and Yellow #10. **Geltabs:** Benzyl Alcohol, Butylparaben, Castor Oil, Cellulose, Corn Starch, Edetate Calcium Disodium, Gelatin, Hydroxypropyl Methylcellulose, Magnesium Stearate, Methylparaben, Propylparaben, Sodium Lauryl Sulfate, Sodium Propionate, Sodium Starch Glycolate, Titanium Dioxide, Blue #1 and #2, Red #40, and Yellow #10. **Extra Strength TYLENOL® Adult Liquid Pain Reliever:** Alcohol (7%), Citric Acid, Flavors, Glycerin, Polyethylene Glycol, Purified Water, Sodium Benzoate, Sorbitol, Sucrose, Yellow #6 (Sunset Yellow), Yellow #10 and Blue #1.
Regular Strength TYLENOL®: **Tablets:** Magnesium Stearate, Cellulose, Sodium Starch Glycolate and Starch. **Caplets:** Cellulose, Hydroxypropyl Methylcellulose, Magnesium Stearate, Polyethylene Glycol, Sodium Starch Glycolate, Starch and Red #40.
TYLENOL® Extended Relief Caplets: Corn Starch, Hydroxyethyl Cellulose, Hydroxypropyl Methylcellulose, Magnesium Stearate, Microcrystalline Cellulose, Povidone, Powdered Cellulose, Pregelatinized Starch, Sodium Starch Glycolate, Titanium Dioxide, Triacetin.

HOW SUPPLIED

Extra Strength TYLENOL®: **Tablets** (colored white, imprinted "TYLENOL" and "500")—vials of 10, and tamper-resistant bottles of 30, 60, 100, and 200. **Caplets** (colored white, imprinted "TYLENOL 500 mg")—vials of 10, 10 blister packs, and tamper-resistant bottles of 24, 50, 100, 175, and 250 and FastCap package of 72. **Gelcaps** (colored yellow and red, imprinted "Tylenol 500") vials of 10 and tamper-resistant bottles of 24, 50, 100, and 225 and FastCap package of 72. **Geltabs** (colored yellow and red, imprinted "Tylenol 500") tamper-resistant bottles of 24, 50, and 100.
Extra Strength TYLENOL® Adult Liquid Pain Reliever: Mint-flavored liquid (colored green) 8 fl. oz. tamper-resistant bottle with child resistant safety cap and special dosage cup.
Regular Strength TYLENOL®: **Tablets** (colored white, scored, imprinted "TYLENOL" and "325")—tamper-resistant bottles of 24, 50, 100 and 200. **Caplets** (colored white, "TYLENOL 325")—tamper-resistant bottles of 24, 50, 100.
TYLENOL® Extended Relief Caplets: (colored white, engraved "TYLENOL ER") tamper-resistant bottles of 24, 50, and 100's.

Shown in Product Identification Guide, page 322

TYLENOL® SEVERE ALLERGY OTC
Medication Caplets

Maximum Strength
TYLENOL® ALLERGY SINUS NIGHTTIME
Caplets

Maximum Strength
TYLENOL® ALLERGY SINUS
Caplets and Gelcaps

Product information for all dosage forms of TYLENOL ALLERGY have been combined under this heading.

DESCRIPTION

Each **TYLENOL® SEVERE ALLERGY Caplet** contains acetaminophen 500 mg, and diphenhydramine Hydrochloride 12.5 mg.
Each **Maximum Strength TYLENOL® ALLERGY SINUS NightTime Caplet** contains acetaminophen 500 mg, pseudoephedrine hydrochloride 30 mg, and diphenhydramine hydrochloride 25 mg.
Each **Maximum Strength TYLENOL® ALLERGY SINUS Caplets** or **Gelcap** contains acetaminophen 500 mg, chlorpheniramine maleate 2 mg, and pseudoephedrine hydrochloride 30 mg.

ACTIONS

TYLENOL® SEVERE ALLERGY Caplets contain a clinically proven analgesic-antipyretic and antihistamine. Acetaminophen produces analgesia by elevation of the pain threshold and antipyresis through action on the hypothalamic heat-regulating center. Acetaminophen is equal to aspirin in analgesic and antipyretic effectiveness, and it is unlikely to produce many of the side effects associated with aspirin and aspirin-containing products.
Diphenhydramine is an antihistamine which helps provide temporary relief of itchy, watery eyes, runny nose, sneezing, itching of the nose or throat due to hay fever or other respiratory allergies.
Maximum Strength TYLENOL® ALLERGY SINUS Night-Time contains, in addition to the above ingredients, a decongestant, pseudoephedrine. Pseudoephedrine is a sympathomimetic amine which provides temporary relief of nasal and sinus congestion.
Maximum Strength TYLENOL® ALLERGY SINUS Caplets or **Gelcaps** contains acetaminophen, pseudoephedrine and the antihistamine, chlorpheniramine. Chlorpheniramine is an antihistamine which helps provide temporary relief of runny nose, sneezing and watery and itchy eyes.

INDICATIONS

TYLENOL® SEVERE ALLERGY provides effective temporary relief of itchy, watery eyes, runny nose, sneezing sore or scratchy throat and itching of the nose or throat due to hay fever or other upper respiratory allergies.
TYLENOL® ALLERGY SINUS NightTime and **TYLENOL® ALLERGY SINUS** provide effective temporary relief of runny nose, sneezing, itching of the nose or throat, and itchy, watery eyes due to hay fever or other upper respiratory allergies, nasal and sinus congestion, and sinus pain and headaches.

PRECAUTIONS

TYLENOL® SEVERE ALLERGY: If a rare sensitivity reaction occurs, the drug should be stopped.
TYLENOL® ALLERGY SINUS NightTime and **TYLENOL® ALLERGY SINUS:** If a rare sensitivity reaction occurs, the drug should be stopped. Although pseudoephedrine is virtually without pressor effect in normotensive patients, it should be used with caution in hypertensives.

DIRECTIONS

TYLENOL® SEVERE ALLERGY: Adults and children 12 years of age and older: Two caplets every four to six hours. Do not exceed 8 caplets in any 24 hour period. Not for use in children under 12 years of age.
TYLENOL® ALLERGY SINUS NightTime: Adults and children 12 years of age and older: Two caplets at bedtime. Not for use in children under 12 years of age.
TYLENOL® ALLERGY SINUS: Adults and children 12 years of age and older. Two caplets, gelcaps or geltabs every six hours. Do not exceed 8 caplets, gelcaps, or geltabs in any 24 hour period. Not for use in children under 12 years of age.

WARNINGS

TYLENOL® SEVERE ALLERGY: Do not use if carton is open or if a blister unit is broken. Do not take for pain for more than 10 days or for fever for more than 3 days unless directed by a doctor. If pain or fever persists, or gets worse, if new symptoms occur, or if redness or swelling is present, consult a doctor because these could be signs of a serious condition. If sore throat is severe, persists for more than 2 days, is accompanied or followed by fever, headache, rash, nausea or vomiting, consult a doctor promptly. May cause excitability especially in children. Do not take this product, unless directed by a doctor, if you have a breathing problem such as emphysema or chronic bronchitis, or if you have glaucoma or difficulty in urination due to enlargement of the prostate gland. May cause marked drowsiness: alcohol, sedatives and tranquilizers may increase the drowsiness effect.
Avoid alcoholic beverages while taking this product. Do not take this product if you are taking sedatives or tranquilizers without first consulting your doctor. Use caution while driving a motor vehicle or operating machinery. As with any drug, if you are pregnant or nursing a baby, seek the advice of a health professional before using this product. Keep this and all drugs out of the reach of children. In case of accidental overdose, contact a doctor or poison control center immediately. Prompt medical attention is critical for adults as well as for children even if you do not notice any signs or symptoms. Do not use with other products containing acetaminophen.
TYLENOL® ALLERGY SINUS NightTime and **TYLENOL® ALLERGY SINUS:** Do not use if carton is open or if a blister unit is broken. Do not take for pain for more than 7 days or for fever for more than 3 days unless directed by a doctor. If pain or fever persists, or gets worse, if new symptoms occur, or if redness or swelling is present, consult a doctor because these could be signs of a serious condition. Do not exceed recommended dosage. If nervousness, dizziness or sleeplessness occur, discontinue use and consult a doctor.
May cause excitability, especially in children. Do not take this product unless directed by a doctor, if you have a breathing problem such as emphysema or chronic bronchitis, or if you have glaucoma or difficulty in urination due to enlargement of the prostate gland. Do not take this product if you have heart disease, high blood pressure, thyroid disease or diabetes unless directed by a doctor. May cause marked drowsiness: alcohol, sedatives and tranquilizers may increase the drowsiness effect. Avoid alcoholic beverages while taking this product. Do not take this product if you are taking sedatives or tranquilizers without first consulting your doctor.
Use caution when driving a motor vehicle or operating machinery. As with any drug, if you are pregnant or nursing a baby, seek the advice of a health professional before using this product. Keep this and all drugs out of the reach of children. In case of accidental overdose, contact a doctor or poison control center immediately. Prompt medical attention is critical for adults as well as for children even if you do not notice any signs or symptons. Do not use with other products containing acetaminophen.

Continued on next page

McNeil Consumer—Cont.

ALCOHOL WARNING
For this and all other pain relievers, including aspirin, ibuprofen, ketoprofen and naproxen sodium. if you generally consume 3 or more alcohol-containing drinks per day, you should consult your physician for advice on when and how you should take pain relievers.

DRUG INTERACTION PRECAUTION
TYLENOL® ALLERGY SINUS NightTime and TYLENOL® ALLERGY SINUS: Do not use this product if you are now taking a prescription monoamine oxidase inhibitor (MAOI) (certain drugs for depression, psychiatric or emotional condition, or Parkinson's disease), or for 2 weeks after stopping the MAOI drug. If you are uncertain whether your prescription drug contains an MAOI, consult a health care professional before taking this product.

OVERDOSAGE INFORMATION
Acetaminophen in massive overdosage may cause hepatic toxicity in some patients. In adults and adolescents, hepatic toxicity has rarely been reported following ingestion of acute overdoses of less than 10 grams. Fatalities are infrequent (less than 3–4% of untreated cases) and have rarely been reported with overdoses of less than 15 grams. In children, an acute overdosage of less than 150 mg/kg has not been associated with hepatic toxicity.
Early symptoms following a potentailly hepatotoxic overdose may include: nausea, vomiting, diaphoresis and general malaise. Clinical and laboratory evidence of hepatic toxicity may not be apparent until 48 to 72 hours postingestion. In adults and adolescents, regardless of the quantity of acetaminophen reported to have been ingested, administer acetylcysteine immediately if 24 hours or less have elapsed from the reported time of ingestion. For full prescribing information, refer to the acetylcysteine package insert. Do not await results of assays for plasma acetaminophen level before initiating treatment with acetylcysteine. The following additional procedures are recommended: The stomach should be emptied promptly by lavage or by induction of emesis with syrup of ipecac. A plasma acetaminophen assay should be obtained as early as possible, but no sooner than four hours following ingestion. If plasma level falls above the lower treatment line on the acetaminophen oiverdose nomogram, acetylcysteine therapy should be continued. Liver function studies should be obtained initially and repeated at 24-hour intervals.
Serious toxicity or fatalities are extremely infrequent in children, possibly due to differences in the way they metabolize acetaminophen. In children, the maximum potential amount ingested can be more easily estimated. If more than 150 mg/kg or an unknown amount was ingested, obtain a plasma acetaminophen level. The plasma acetaminophen level should be obtained as soon as possible, but no sooner than 4 hours following the ingestion. If plasma level falls above the lower treatment line on the acetaminophen overdose nomogram, the acetylcysteine therapy should be initiated and continued for a full course of therapy. If plasma acetaminiophen assay capability is not available, and the estimated acetaminophen ingestion exceeds 150 mg/kg, acetylcysteine therapy should be initiated and continued for a full course of therapy.
For additional emergency information, call your regional poison center or call the Rocky Mountain Poison Center toll-free (1–800–525–6115).
Symptoms for pseudoephedrine overdose consist most often of mild anxiety, tachycardia and/or hypertension. Symptoms usually appear within 4 to 8 hours of ingestion and are transient, usually requiring no treatment.
Diphenhydramine and chlorpheniramine toxicity should be treated as ou would an antihistamine/anticholinergic overdose and is likely to be present within a few hours after acute ingestion.

ALCOHOL INFORMATION
Chronic heavy alcohol abusers may be at increased risk of liver toxicity from excessive acetaminophen use, although reports of this event are rare. Reports almost invariably involve cases of severe chronic alcoholics and the dosages of acetaminophen most often exceed recommended doses and often involve substantial overdose. Professionals should alert their patients who regularly consume large amounts of alcohol not to exceed recommended doses of acetaminophen.

INACTIVE INGREDIENTS
TYLENOL® SEVERE ALLERGY Caplets: Cellulose, Corn Starch, Hydroxypropyl, Cellulose, Hydroxypropyl Methylcellulose, Iron Oxide Black, Magnesium Stearate, Polyethylene Glycol, Sodium Citrate, Sodium Starch Glycolate, Titanium Dioxide, Yellow #6 and Yellow #10.
TYLENOL® ALLERGY SINUS NightTime Caplets: Cellulose, Corn Starch, Hydroxypropyl Methylcellulose, Iron Oxide Black, Magnesium Stearate, Polyethylene Glycol, Polysorbate 80, Sodium Citrate, Sodium Starch Glycolate, Titanium Dioxide, Blue #1, and Yellow #10.
TYLENOL® ALLERGY SINUS: **Caplets:** Carnauba Wax, Cellulose, Cornstarch, Hydroxypropyl Cellulose, Hydroxypropyl Methylcellulose, Iron Oxide Black, Magnesium Stearate, Polyethylene Glycol, Sodium Starch Glycolate, Titanium Dioxide, Blue #1, Yellow #6, and Yellow #10. Gelcaps: Benzyl Alcohol, Butylparaben, Castor Oil Cellulose, Cornstarch, Edetate Calcium Disodium, Gelatin, Hydroxypropyl Methylcellulose, Magnesium Stearate, Methylparaben, propylparaben, Sodium Lauryl Sulfate, Sodium Propionate, Sodium Starch Glycolate, Titanium Dioxide, Blue #1 and #2 and Yellow #10.

HOW SUPPLIED
TYLENOL® SEVERE ALLERGY: **Caplets** (dark yellow, imprinted "TYLENOL Severe Allergy") blister packs of 12 and 24.
TYLENOL® ALLERGY SINUS NightTime: **Caplets** (light blue, imprinted "TYLENOL A/S NightTime") child-resistant blister packs of 24.
TYLENOL® ALLERGY SINUS: **Caplets:** (dark yellow, imprinted "TYLENOL Allergy Sinus") Blister packs of 24 and 48.
Gelcaps and Geltabs: (dark green and dark yellow, imprinted "TYLENOL A/S") Blister packs of 24 and 48.
Shown in Product Identification Guide, page 323

TYLENOL® COLD Medication **OTC**
No Drowsiness Formula
Caplets and Gelcaps

Multi-Symptom Formula
TYLENOL® COLD Medication
Tablets and Caplets

TYLENOL® COLD Multi-Symptom
Hot Medication Liquid Packets

Product information for all dosage forms of TYLENOL COLD have been combined under this heading.

DESCRIPTION
Each ***TYLENOL® COLD Medication No Drowsiness Formula Caplet and Gelcap*** contains acetaminophen 325 mg, pseudoephedrine hydrochloride 30 mg, and dextromethorphan hydrobromide 15 mg.
Each ***Multi-Symptom Formula TYLENOL® COLD Tablet or Caplet*** contains acetaminophen 325 mg, chlorpheniramine maleate 2 mg, pseudoephedrine hydrochloride 30 mg, and dextromethorphan hydrobromide 15 mg.
Each packet of ***TYLENOL® COLD Multi-Symptom Hot Medication*** contains acetaminophen 650 mg, chlorpheniramine maleate 4 mg, pseudoephedrine hydrochloride 60 mg, and dextromethorphan hydrobromide 30 mg.

ACTIONS
TYLENOL® COLD Medication No Drowsiness Formula contains a clinically proven analgesic-antipyretic, decongestant and cough suppressant. Acetaminophen produces analgesia by elevation of the pain threshold and antipyresis through action on the hypothalamic heat-regulating center. Acetaminophen is equal to aspirin in analgesic and antipyretic effectiveness and it is unlikely to produce many of the side effects associated with aspirin and aspirin-containing products. Pseudoephedrine is a sympathomimetic amine which provides temporary relief of nasal congestion. Dextromethorphan is a cough suppressant which provides temporary relief of coughs due to minor throat irritations that may occur with the common cold.
Multi-Symptom Formula TYLENOL® COLD Medication and ***TYLENOL® COLD Multi-Symptom Hot Medication*** contain, in addition to the above ingredients, an antihistamine. Chlorpheniramine is an antihistamine which helps provide temporary relief of runny nose, sneezing and watery and itchy eyes.

INDICATIONS
TYLENOL® COLD Medication No Drowsiness Formula provides effective temporary relief of nasal congestion, coughing, and body aches, pains, headache, sore throat and fever due to a cold or "flu."
Multi-Symptom Formula TYLENOL® COLD Medication and ***TYLENOL® COLD Multi-Symptom Hot Medication*** provide effective temporary relief of runny nose, sneezing, watery and itchy eyes, nasal congestion, coughing and body aches, pains, headache, sore throat and fever due to a cold or "flu."

DIRECTIONS
TYLENOL® COLD No Drowsiness Formula and Multi-Symptom Formula TYLENOL® COLD Medication: Adults (12 years and older): Two every 6 hours, not to exceed 8 in 24 hours. Children (6–11 years): One every 6 hours, not to exceed 4 in 24 hours. Not for use in children under 6 years of age.
TYLENOL® COLD Multi-Symptom Hot Medication: Adults (12 years and older): dissolve one packet in 6 oz. cup of hot water. Sip while hot. Sweeten to taste, if desired. May repeat every 6 hours, not to exceed 4 doses in 24 hours. Not for use in children under 12 years of age.

PRECAUTIONS
TYLENOL® COLD Medication No Drowsiness Formula, Multi-Symptom Formula TYLENOL® COLD Medication and ***TYLENOL® COLD Multi-Symptom Hot Medication:*** If a rare sensitivity reaction occurs, the drug should be stopped. Although pseudoephedrine is virtually without pressor effect in normotensive patients, it should be used with caution in hypertensives.
TYLENOL® COLD Medication No Drowsiness Formula: Do not take this product for more than 7 days or for fever for more than 3 days unless directed by a doctor. If pain or fever persists, or gets worse, if new symptoms occur, or if redness or swelling is present, consult a doctor because these could be signs of a serious condition. If sore throat is severe, persists for more than 2 days, is accompanied or followed by fever, headache, rash, nausea or vomiting, consult a doctor promptly. A persistent cough may be a sign of a serious condition. If cough persists for more than 1 week, tends to recur or is accompanied by fever, rash or persistent headache, consult a doctor. Do not take this product for persistent or chronic cough such as occurs with smoking, asthma, emphysema or if cough is accompanied by excessive phlegm (mucus) unless directed by a doctor. Do not exceed recommended dosage because at higher doses, nervousness, dizziness or sleeplessness may occur. Do not take this product if you have heart disease, high blood pressure, thyroid disease, diabetes or difficulty in urination due to enlargement of the prostate gland unless directed by a doctor. Do not use with other products containing acetaminophen.
DO NOT USE IF CARTON IS OPENED OR IF A BLISTER UNIT IS BROKEN. **KEEP THIS AND ALL MEDICATION OUT OF THE REACH OF CHILDREN. AS WITH ANY DRUG, IF YOU ARE PREGNANT OR NURSING A BABY, SEEK THE ADVICE OF A HEALTH PROFESSIONAL BEFORE USING THIS PRODUCT. IN CASE OF ACCIDENTAL OVERDOSE, CONTACT A DOCTOR OR POISON CONTROL CENTER IMMEDIATELY. PROMPT MEDICAL ATTENTION IS CRITICAL FOR ADULTS AS WELL AS FOR CHILDREN EVEN IF YOU DO NOT NOTICE ANY SIGNS OR SYMPTOMS.**
Multi-Symptom Formula TYLENOL® COLD Medication: Do not take this product for more than 7 days or for fever for more than 3 days unless directed by a doctor. If symptoms do not improve or are accompanied by fever, consult a doctor. If sore throat is severe, persists for more than 2 days, is accompanied or followed by fever, headache, rash, nausea or vomiting, consult a doctor promptly. A persistent cough may be a sign of a serious condition. If cough persists for more than 1 week, tends to recur or is accompanied by fever, rash or persistent headache, consult a doctor. Do not take this product for persistent or chronic cough such as occurs with smoking, asthma, emphysema or if cough is accompanied by excessive phlegm (mucus) unless directed by a doctor. Do not exceed recommended dosage because at higher doses, nervousness, dizziness or sleeplessness may occur. May cause excitability in children. Do not take this product unless directed by a doctor, if you have a breathing problem such as emphysema or chronic bronchitis, or if you have glaucoma or difficulty in urination due to enlargement of the prostate gland. Do not take this product if you have heart disease, high blood pressure, thyroid disease or diabetes unless directed by a doctor. May cause drowsiness; alcohol, sedatives and tranquilizers may increase the drowsiness effect. Avoid alcoholic beverages while taking this product. Do not take this product if you are taking sedatives or tranquilizers without first consulting your doctor. Use caution when driving a motor vehicle or operating machinery. Do not use with other products containing acetaminophen.
DO NOT USE IF CARTON IS OPENED OR IF A BLISTER UNIT IS BROKEN. **KEEP THIS AND ALL MEDICATION OUT OF THE REACH OF CHILDREN. AS WITH ANY DRUG, IF YOU ARE PREGNANT OR NURSING A BABY, SEEK THE ADVICE OF A HEALTH PROFESSIONAL BEFORE USING THIS PRODUCT. IN CASE OF ACCIDENTAL OVERDOSE, CONTACT A DOCTOR OR POISON CONTROL CENTER IMMEDIATELY. PROMPT MEDICAL ATTENTION IS CRITICAL FOR ADULTS AS WELL AS FOR CHILDREN EVEN IF YOU DO NOT NOTICE ANY SIGNS OR SYMPTOMS.**

WARNING
TYLENOL® COLD Multi-Symptom Hot Medication: Do not take this product for more than 7 days or for fever for more than 3 days unless directed by a doctor. If symptoms do not improve or are accompanied by fever, consult a doctor. If sore throat is severe, persists for more than 2 days, is accompanied or followed by fever, headache, rash, nausea or vomiting, consult a doctor promptly. A persistent cough may be a sign of a serious condition. If cough persists for more than 1 week, tends to recur or is accompanied by fever, rash or persistent headache, consult a doctor. Do not take this product for persistent or chronic cough such as occurs with smoking, asthma, emphysema or if cough is accompanied by excessive phlegm (mucus) unless directed by a doctor. Do not exceed recommended dosage because at higher doses, nervousness,

dizziness or sleeplessness may occur. May cause excitability especially in children. Do not take this product, unless directed by a doctor, if you have a breathing problem such as emphysema or chronic bronchitis, or if you have glaucoma or difficulty in urination due to enlargement of the prostate gland. Do not take this product if you have heart disease, high blood pressure, thyroid disease or diabetes unless directed by a doctor. May cause drowsiness; alcohol, sedatives and tranquilizers may increase the drowsiness effect. Avoid alcoholic beverages while taking this product. Do not take this product if you are taking sedatives or tranquilizers without first consulting your doctor. Use caution when driving a motor vehicle or operating machinery. Do not use with other products containing acetaminophen.

DO NOT USE IF PRINTED CARTON OVERWRAP IS BROKEN OR MISSING OR IF FOIL PACKET IS TORN OR BROKEN. **KEEP THIS AND ALL MEDICATION OUT OF THE REACH OF CHILDREN. AS WITH ANY DRUG, IF YOU ARE PREGNANT OR NURSING A BABY, SEEK THE ADVICE OF A HEALTH PROFESSIONAL BEFORE USING THIS PRODUCT. IN CASE OF ACCIDENTAL OVERDOSE, CONTACT A DOCTOR OR POISON CONTROL CENTER IMMEDIATELY. PROMPT MEDICAL ATTENTION IS CRITICAL FOR ADULTS AS WELL AS FOR CHILDREN EVEN IF YOU DO NOT NOTICE ANY SIGNS OR SYMPTOMS.**

PHENYLKETONURICS: CONTAINS PHENYLALANINE 11 MG PER PACKET.

ALCOHOL WARNING

For this and all other pain relievers, including aspirin, ibuprofen, ketoprofen and naproxen sodium, if you generally consume 3 or more alcohol-containing drinks per day, you should consult your physician for advice on when and how you should take pain relievers.

DRUG INTERACTION PRECAUTION

TYLENOL® COLD Medication No Drowsiness Formula, Multi-Symptom Formula TYLENOL® COLD Medication and ***TYLENOL® COLD Multi-Symptom Hot Medication:*** Do not take this product if you are presently taking a prescription drug for high blood pressure or you are now taking a prescription monoamine oxidase inhibitor (MAOI) (certain drugs for depression, psychiatric or emotional conditions, or Parkinson's disease), or for 2 weeks after stopping the MAOI drug. If you are uncertain whether your prescription drug contains an MAOI, consult a health professional before taking this product.

OVERDOSAGE INFORMATION

TYLENOL® COLD Medication No Drowsiness Formula, Multi-Symptom Formula TYLENOL® COLD Medication and ***TYLENOL® COLD Multi-Symptom Hot Medication:*** Acetaminophen in massive overdosage may cause hepatic toxicity in some patients. In adults and adolescents, hepatic toxicity has rarely been reported following ingestion of acute overdoses of less than 10 grams. Fatalities are infrequent (less than 3–4% of untreated cases) and have rarely been reported with overdoses of less than 15 grams. In children, an acute overdosage of less than 150 mg/kg has not been associated with hepatic toxicity.

Early symptoms following a potentially hepatotoxic overdose may include: nausea, vomiting, diaphoresis and general malaise. Clinical and laboratory evidence of hepatic toxicity may not be apparent until 48 to 72 hours postingestion. In adults and adolescents, regardless of the quantity of acetaminophen reported to have been ingested, administer acetylcysteine immediately if 24 hours or less have elapsed from the reported time of ingestion. For full prescribing information, refer to the acetylcysteine package insert. Do not await results of assays for plasma acetaminophen level before initiating treatment with acetylcysteine. The following additional procedures are recommended. The stomach should be emptied promptly by lavage or by induction of emesis with syrup of ipecac. A plasma acetaminophen assay should be obtained as early as possible, but no sooner than four hours following ingestion. If plasma level falls above the lower treatment line on the acetaminophen overdose nomogram, acetylcysteine therapy should be continued. Liver function studies should be obtained initially and repeated at 24-hour intervals.

Serious toxicity or fatalities are extremely infrequent in children, possibly due to differences in the way they metabolize acetaminophen. In children, the maximum potential amount ingested can be more easily estimated. If more than 150 mg/kg or an unknown amount was ingested, obtain a plasma acetaminophen level. The plasma acetaminophen level should be obtained as soon as possible, but no sooner than 4 hours following the ingestion. If plasma level falls above the lower treatment line on the acetaminophen overdose nomogram, the acetylcysteine therapy should be initiated and continued for a full course of therapy. If plasma acetaminophen assay capability is not available, and the estimated acetaminophen ingestion exceeds 150 mg/kg, acetylcysteine therapy should be initiated and continued for a full course of therapy.

For additional emergency information, call your regional poison center or call the Rocky Mountain Poison Center toll-free, (1-800-525-6115).

Symptoms from pseudoephedrine overdose consist most often of mild anxiety, tachycardia and/or mild hypertension. Symptoms usually appear within 4 to 8 hours of ingestion and are transient, usually requiring no treatment.

Acute dextromethorphan overdose usually does not result in serious signs and symptoms unless massive amounts have been ingested. Signs and symptoms of a substantial overdose may include nausea and vomiting, visual disturbances, CNS disturbances, and urinary retention.

Chlorpheniramine toxicity should be treated as you would an antihistamine/anticholinergic overdose and is likely to be present within a few hours after acute ingestion.

ALCOHOL INFORMATION

TYLENOL® COLD Medication No Drowsiness Formula, Multi-symptom Formula TYLENOL® COLD Medication and ***TYLENOL® COLD Multi-Symptom Hot Medication:*** Chronic heavy alcohol abusers may be at increased risk of liver toxicity from excessive acetaminophen use, although reports of this event are rare. Reports almost invariably involve cases of severe chronic alcoholics and the dosages of acetaminophen most often exceed recommended doses and often involve substantial overdose. Professionals should alert their patients who regularly consume large amounts of alcohol not to exceed recommended doses of acetaminophen.

INACTIVE INGREDIENTS

TYLENOL® COLD No Drowsiness Formula: Caplets: cellulose, corn starch, glyceryl triacetate, hydroxypropyl methylcellulose, iron oxide black, magnesium stearate, sodium starch glycolate, titanium dioxide, Blue #1 and Yellow #10. Gelcap: benzyl alcohol, butylparaben, castor oil, cellulose, corn starch, edetate calcium disodium, gelatin, hydroxypropyl methylcellulose, magnesium stearate, methylparaben, propylparaben, sodium propionate, sodium lauryl sulfate, sodium starch glycolate, titanium dioxide, Red #40 and Yellow #10.

Multi-Symptom Formula TYLENOL® COLD Medication: Tablets: cellulose, cornstarch, magnesium stearate, Sodium Starch Glycolate Yellow #6 and Yellow #10. **Caplets:** cellulose, cornstarch, glyceryl triacetate, hydroxypropyl methylcellulose, iron oxide black, magnesium stearate, sodium starch glycolate, titanium dioxide, Blue #1 and Yellow #6 and #10.

TYLENOL® COLD Multi-Symptom Hot Medication: Aspartame, citric acid, corn starch, sodium citrate, sucrose, Red #40 and Yellow #10.

HOW SUPPLIED

TYLENOL® COLD No Drowsiness Formula: Caplets (colored white, imprinted "TYLENOL COLD") blister packs of 24. Gelcaps (colored red and tan, imprinted "TYLENOL COLD") blister packs of 24.

Multi-Symptom Formula TYLENOL® COLD Medication: Tablets (colored yellow, imprinted "TYLENOL Cold") blister packs of 24. **Caplets** (light yellow, imprinted "TYLENOL Cold") blister packs of 24.

TYLENOL® COLD Multi-Symptom Hot Medication: Packets of powder (yellow colored) in cartons of 6 tamper-resistant foil packets.

Shown in Product Identification Guide, page 323

MULTI-SYMPTOM TYLENOL® COLD SEVERE CONGESTION — OTC

DESCRIPTION

EACH CAPLET contains acetaminophen 325 mg, pseudoephedrine HCl 30 mg, guaifenesin 200 mg and dextromethorphan HBr 15 mg.

ACTIONS

Multi-Symptom ***TYLENOL® COLD SEVERE CONGESTION Caplets*** contains a clinically proven analgesic-antipyretic, decongestant, expectorant and cough suppressant. Acetaminophen produces analgesia by elevation of the pain threshold and antipyresis through action on the hypothalamic heat-regulating center. Acetaminophen is equal to aspirin in analgesic and antipyretic effectiveness and is unlikely to produce many of the side effects associated with aspirin and aspirin-containing products. Pseudoephedrine is a sympathomimetic amine which provides temporary relief of nasal congestion. Guaifenesin is an expectorant which helps loosen phlegm (mucus) and thin bronchial secretions to make coughs more productive. Dextromethorphan is a cough suppressant which provides temporary relief of coughs due to minor throat irritations that may occur with the common cold.

INDICATIONS

Multi-Symptom ***TYLENOL® COLD SEVERE CONGESTION Caplets*** provide temporary relief without drowsiness of nasal congestion, chest congestion, coughing, sore throat, headaches, body aches and fever.

DOSAGE

Adults and Children 12 years of Age and older: Take two caplets every 6–8 hours, not to exceed 8 caplets in any 24 hour period.

Children 6 to 11 years of age: One caplet every 6–8 hours not to exceed 4 caplets in any 24 hour period. Not for use in children under 6 years of age.

PRECAUTIONS

If a rare sensitivity reaction occurs, the drug should be discontinued. Although pseudoephedrine is virtually without pressor effect in normotensive patients, it should be used with caution in hypertensives.

WARNINGS

DO NOT USE IF CARTON IS OPENED OR IF A BLISTER UNIT IS BROKEN. Do not take for pain for more than 7 days or for fever for more than 3 days unless directed by a doctor. If pain or fever persists, or gets worse, if new symptoms occur, or if redness or swelling is present, consult a doctor because these could be signs of a serious condition. If sore throat is severe, persists for more than 2 days, is accompanied or followed by fever, headache, rash, nausea or vomiting, consult a doctor promptly. A persistent cough may be a sign of a serious condition. If cough persists for more than 1 week, tends to recur or is accompanied by fever, rash or persistent headache, consult a doctor. Do not take this product for persistent or chronic cough such as occurs with smoking, asthma, emphysema or if cough is accompanied by excessive phlegm (mucus) unless directed by a doctor. **Do not exceed recommended dosage.** If nervousness, dizziness, or sleeplessness occur, discontinue use and consult a doctor. Do not take this product if you have heart disease, high blood pressure, thyroid disease, diabetes or difficulty in urination due to enlargement of the prostate gland unless directed by a doctor. As with any drug, if you are pregnant or nursing a baby, seek the advice of a health professional before using this product. Keep this and all drugs out of the reach of children., In case of accidental overdose, contact a doctor or poison control center immediately. Prompt medical attention is critical for adults as well as for children even if you do not notice any signs of symptoms. Do not use with other products containing acetaminophen.

ALCOHOL WARNING

For this and all other pain relievers, including aspirin, ibuprofen, ketoprofen and naproxen sodium, if you generally consume 3 or more alcohol-containing drinks per day you should consult your physician for advice on when and how you should take pain relievers.

OVERDOSAGE INFORMATION

Acetaminophen in massive overdosage may cause hepatic toxicity in some patients. In adults and adolescents, hepatic toxicity has rarely been reported following ingestion of acute overdoses of less than 10 grams. Fatalities are infrequent (less than 3–4% of untreated cases) and have rarely been reported with overdoses of less than 15 grams. In children, an acute overdosage of less than 150 mg/kg has not been associated with hepatic toxicity.

Early symptoms following a potentially hepatotoxic overdose may include: nausea, vomiting, diaphoresis and general malaise. Clinical and laboratory evidence of hepatic toxicity may not be apparent until 48 to 72 hours postingestion. In adults and adolescents, regardless of the quantity of acetaminophen reported to have been ingested, administer acetylcysteine immediately if 24 hours or less have elapsed from the reported time of ingestion. For full prescribing information, refer to the acetylcysteine package insert. Do not await results of assays for plasma acetaminophen level before initiating treatment with acetylcysteine. The following additional procedures are recommended. The stomach should be emptied promptly by lavage or by inducing of emesis with syrup of ipecac. A plasma acetaminophen assay should be obtained as early as possible, but no sooner than four hours following ingestion. If plasma level falls above the lower treatment line on the acetaminophen overdose nomogram, acetylcysteine therapy should be continued. Liver function studies should be obtained initially and repeated at 24-hour intervals.

Serious toxicity or fatalities are extremely infrequent in children, possibly due to differences in the way they metabolize acetaminophen. In children, the maximum potential amount ingested can be more easily estimated. If more than 150 mg/kg or an unknown amount was ingested, obtain a plasma acetaminophen level. The plasma acetaminophen level should be obtained as soon as possible, but no sooner than 4 hours following the ingestion. If plasma level falls above the lower treatment line on the acetaminophen overdose nomogram, the acetylcysteine therapy should be initiated and continued for a full course of therapy. If plasma acetaminophen assay capability is not available, and the

Continued on next page

McNeil Consumer—Cont.

estimated acetaminophen ingestion exceeds 150 mg/kg, acetlcysteine therapy should be initiated and continued for a full course of therapy.
For additional emergency information, call your regional poison center or call the Rocky Mountain Poison Center toll-free, (1-800-525-6115).
Symptoms from pseudoephedrine overdose consist most often of mild anxiety, tachycardia and/or mild hypertension. Symptoms usually appear within 4 to 8 hours of ingestion and are transient, usually requiring no treatment.
Acute dextromethorphan overdose usually does not result in serious signs and symptoms unless massive amounts have been ingested. Signs and symptoms of a substantial overdose may include nausea and vomiting, visual disturbance, CNS disturbances, and urinary retention.
Chlorpheniramine toxicity should be treated as you would an antihistamine/anticholinergic overdose and is likely to be present within a few hours after acute ingestion. Guaifenesin should be treated as a non-toxic ingestion.

ALCOHOL INFORMATION

Chronic heavy alcohol abusers may be at increased risk of liver toxicity from excessive acetaminophen use, although reports of this event are rare. Reports almost invariably involve cases of severe chronic alcoholics and the dosages of acetaminophen most often exceed recommended doses and often involve substantial overdose. Professionals should alert their patients who regularly consume large amounts of alcohol not to exceed recommended doses of acetaminophen.

DRUG INTERACTION PRECAUTION

Do not use this product if you are now taking a prescription monoamine oxidase inhibitor (MAOI) (certain drugs for depression, psychiatric or emotional conditions, or Parkinson's disease), or for 2 weeks after stoppping the MAOI drug. If you are uncertain whether your prescription drug contains an MAOI, consult a health professional before taking this product.

INACTIVE INGREDIENTS

Carnauba Wax, Cellulose, Colloidal Silicon Dioxide, Corn Starch, Hydroxypropyl Methylcellulose, Iron Oxide, Povidone, Pregelatinized Starch, Propylene Glycol, Sodium Starch Glycolate, Stearic Acid, Titanium Dioxide, Triacetin, Blue #1, Yellow #6 and Yellow #10.

HOW SUPPLIED

Caplets (colored buttery-tan, with green imprinted "TYLENOL COLD SC") in blister packs of 12 and 24.
©McN-PPC, Inc. '96 8702830
Shown in Product Identification Guide, page 323

Multi-Symptom TYLENOL® COUGH Medication — OTC

Multi-Symptom TYLENOL® COUGH Medication with Decongestant

Product information for all dosage forms of TYLENOL COUGH have been combined under this heading.

DESCRIPTION

Each 15 ml (3 tsp.) adult dose of ***Multi-Symptom TYLENOL® COUGH Medication*** contains dextromethorphan HBr 30 mg, and acetaminophen 650 mg.
Each 15 ml (3 tsp.) adult dose of ***Multi-Symptom TYLENOL® COUGH Medication with Decongestant*** contains dextromethorphan HBr 30 mg, acetaminophen 650 mg, and pseudoephedrine HCl 60 mg.

ACTIONS

Multi-Symptom TYLENOL® COUGH Medication contains a clinically proven cough suppressant, and an analgesic-antipyretic. Acetaminophen produces analgesia by elevation of the pain threshold and antipyresis through action on the hypothalamic heat-regulating center. Dextromethorphan is a cough suppressant which provides temporary relief of coughs due to minor throat irritations that may occur with the common cold.
Multi-Symptom TYLENOL® COUGH Medication with Decongestant contains, in addition to the above ingredients, a sympathomimetic amine, pseudoephedrine HCl, which provides temporary relief of nasal congestion.

INDICATIONS

Multi-Symptom TYLENOL® COUGH Medication provides effective, temporary relief of coughing, and the aches, pains and sore throat that may accompany a cough due to a cold.
Multi-Symptom TYLENOL® COUGH Medication with Decongestant provides effective, temporary relief of coughing, nasal congestion and the aches, pains and sore throat that may accompany a cough due to a cold.

DIRECTIONS

Multi-Symptom TYLENOL® COUGH Medication and Multi-Symptom TYLENOL® COUGH Medication with Decongestant: Adults (12 years and older): 1 tablespoon or 3 teaspoons every 6–8 hours, not to exceed 4 doses in 24 hours. Children: (ages 6–11) $1^1/_2$ teaspoons every 6–8 hours, not to exceed 4 doses in 24 hours. Not for use in children under 6 years of age.

PRECAUTIONS

Multi-Symptom TYLENOL® COUGH Medication: If a rare sensitivity reaction occurs, the drug should be discontinued.
Multi-Symptom TYLENOL® COUGH Medication with Decongestant: If a rare sensitivity reaction occurs, the drug should be discontinued. Although pseudoephedrine is virtually without pressor effect in normotensive patients, it should be used with caution in hypertensives.

WARNING

Multi-Symptom TYLENOL® COUGH Medication: Do not take this product for more than 10 days or for fever for more than 3 days unless directed by a physician. Severe or recurrent pain or high or continued fever may be indicative of serious illness. Under these conditions, consult a doctor. A persistent cough may be a sign of a serious condition. If cough persists for more than 1 week, tends to recur or is accompanied by fever, rash or persistent headache, consult a doctor. Do not take this product for persistent or chronic cough such as occurs with smoking, asthma, emphysema, or if cough is accompanied by excessive phlegm (mucus) unless directed by a doctor. If sore throat is severe, persists for more than 2 days, is accompanied or followed by fever, headache, rash, nausea or vomiting, consult a doctor promptly. Do not use with other products containing acetaminophen.
DO NOT USE IF PRINTED PLASTIC BOTTLE WRAP OR PRINTED FOIL INNER SEAL IS BROKEN. **As with any drug, if you are pregnant or nursing a baby, seek the advice of a health professional before using this product. Keep this and all medication out of the reach of children. In case of accidental overdosage, contact a doctor or poison control center immediately. Prompt medical attention is critical for adults as well as children even if you do not notice any signs or symptoms.**
Multi-Symptom TYLENOL® COUGH Medication with Decongestant: Do not take this product for more than 7 days or for fever for more than 3 days unless directed by a doctor. If symptoms do not improve or are accompanied by fever, consult a doctor. A persistent cough may be a sign of a serious condition. If cough persists for more than 1 week, tends to recur or is accompanied by fever, rash or persistent headache, consult a doctor. Do not take this product for persistent or chronic cough such as occurs with smoking, asthma, emphysema, or if cough is accompanied by excessive phlegm (mucus) unless directed by a doctor. Do not exceed the recommended dosage because at higher doses nervousness, dizziness or sleeplessness may occur. Do not take this product if you have heart disease, high blood pressure, thyroid disease, diabetes or difficulty in urination due to enlargement of the prostate gland unless directed by a doctor. If sore throat is severe, persists for more than 2 days, is accompanied or followed by fever, headache, rash, nausea or vomiting, consult a doctor promptly. Do not use with other products containing acetaminophen.
DO NOT USE IF PRINTED PLASTIC BOTTLE WRAP OR PRINTED FOIL INNER SEAL IS BROKEN. **As with any drug, if you are pregnant or nursing a baby, seek the advice of a health professional before using this product. Keep this and all medication out of the reach of children. In case of accidental overdosage, contact a doctor or poison control center immediately. Prompt medical attention is critical for adults as well as children even if you do not notice any signs or symptoms.**

ALCOHOL WARNING

Multi-Symptom TYLENOL® COUGH Medication and Multi-Symptom TYLENOL® COUGH Medication with Decongestant: For this and all other pain relievers, including aspirin, ibuprofen, ketoprofen and naproxen sodium; if you generally consume 3 or more alcohol-containing drinks per day, you should consult your physician for advice on when and how you should take pain relievers.

DRUG INTERACTION PRECAUTION

Multi-Symptom TYLENOL® COUGH Medication: Do not use this product if you are presently taking a prescription monoamine oxidase inhibitor (MAOI) (certain drugs for depression, psychiatric or emotional conditions, or Parkinson's Disease), or for 2 weeks after stopping the MAOI drug. If you are uncertain whether your prescription drug contains an MAOI, consult a health professional before taking this product.
Multi-Symptom TYLENOL® COUGH Medication with Decongestant: Do not use this product if you are presently taking a prescription drug for high blood pressure or you are now taking a prescription monoamine oxidase inhibitor (MAOI) (certain drugs for depression or psychiatric or emotional conditions, or Parkinson's Disease), or for 2 weeks after stopping the MAOI drug. If you are uncertain whether your prescription drug contains an MAOI, consult a health professional before taking this product.

OVERDOSAGE INFORMATION

Multi-Symptom TYLENOL® COUGH Medication and Multi-Symptom TYLENOL® COUGH Medication with Decongestant: Acetaminophen in massive overdosage may cause hepatic toxicity in some patients. In adults and adolescents, hepatic toxicity has rarely been reported following ingestion of acute overdoses of less than 10 grams. Fatalities are infrequent (less than 3–4% of untreated cases) and have rarely been reported with overdoses of less than 15 grams. In children, an acute overdosage of less than 150 mg/kg has not been associated with hepatic toxicity.
Early symptoms following a potentially hepatotoxic overdose may include: nausea, vomiting, diaphoresis and general malaise. Clinical and laboratory evidence of hepatic toxicity may not be apparent until 48 to 72 hours postingestion. In adults and adolescents, regardless of the quantity of acetaminophen reported to have been ingested, administer acetylcysteine immediately if 24 hours or less have elapsed from the reported time of ingestion. For full prescribing information, refer to the acetylcysteine package insert. Do not await results of assays for plasma acetaminophen level before initiating treatment with acetylcysteine. The following additional procedures are recommended. The stomach should be emptied promptly by lavage or by induction of emesis with syrup of ipecac. A plasma acetaminophen assay should be obtained as early as possible, but no sooner than four hours following ingestion. If plasma level falls above the lower treatment line on the acetaminophen overdose nomogram, acetylcysteine therapy should be continued. Liver function studies should be obtained initially and repeated at 24-hour intervals.
Serious toxicity or fatalities are extremely infrequent in children, possibly due to differences in the way they metabolize acetaminophen. In children, the maximum potential amount ingested can be more easily estimated. If more than 150 mg/kg or an unknown amount was ingested, obtain a plasma acetaminophen level. The plasma acetaminophen level should be obtained as soon as possible, but no sooner than 4 hours following the ingestion. If the plasma level falls above the lower treatment line on the acetaminophen overdose nomogram, the acetylcysteine therapy should be initiated and continued for a full course of therapy. If plasma acetaminophen assay capability is not available, and the estimated acetaminophen ingestion exceeds 150 mg/kg, acetycysteine therapy should be initiated and continued for a full course of therapy.
For additional emergency information, call your regional poison center or call the Rocky Mountain Poison Center toll-free (1-800-525-6115).
Acute dextromethorphan overdose usually does not result in serious signs and symptoms unless massive amounts have been ingested. Signs and symptoms of a substantial overdose may include nausea and vomiting, visual disturbances, CNS disturbances, and urinary retention.
Symptoms from pseudoephedrine overdose consist most often of mild anxiety, tachycardia and/or mild hypertension. Symptoms usually appear within 4 to 8 hours of ingestion and are transient, usually requiring no treatment.

ALCOHOL INFORMATION

Multi-Symptom TYLENOL® COUGH Medication and Multi-Symptom TYLENOL® COUGH Medication with Decongestant: Chronic heavy alcohol abusers may be at increased risk of liver toxicity from excessive acetaminophen use, although reports of this event are rare. Reports almost invariably involve cases of severe chronic alcoholics and the dosages of acetaminophen most often exceed recommended doses and often involve substantial overdose. Professionals should alert their patients who regularly consume large amounts of alcohol not to exceed recommended doses of acetaminophen.

INACTIVE INGREDIENTS

Multi-Symptom TYLENOL® COUGH Medication: Alcohol (5%), citric acid, flavors, high fructose corn syrup, polyethylene glycol, propylene glycol, purified water, sodium benzoate, sodium carboxymethylcellulose, sodium saccharin, sorbitol, Red #40.
Multi-Symptom TYLENOL® COUGH Medication with Decongestant: Alcohol (5%), citric acid, flavors, high fructose corn syrup. polyethylene glycol, propylene glycol, purified water, sodium benzoate, sodium carboxymethylcellulose, sodium saccharin, sorbitol, Blue #1, and Red #40.

HOW SUPPLIED

Multi-Symptom TYLENOL® COUGH Medication is available in a 4 oz. bottle with child resistant safety cap and tamper resistant packaging.
Multi-Symptom TYLENOL® COUGH Medication with Decongestant is available in a 4 oz. bottle with child resistant safety cap, and tamper resistant packaging.
Shown in Product Identification Guide, page 323

Maximum Strength   OTC
TYLENOL® FLU Medication
No Drowsiness Formula Gelcaps

Maximum Strength
TYLENOL® FLU NightTime
Medication Gelcaps

Maximum Strength
TYLENOL® FLU NightTime
Hot Medication Packets

Product information for all dosage forms of TYLENOL FLU have been combined under this heading.

DESCRIPTION

Each *Maximum Strength TYLENOL® FLU Medication No Drowsiness Formula Gelcap* contains acetaminophen 500 mg, pseudoephedrine hydrochloride 30 mg, and dextromethorphan hydrobromide 15 mg.

Each *Maximum Strength TYLENOL® FLU NightTime Medication Gelcap* contains acetaminophen 500 mg, pseudoephedrine hydrochloride 30 mg, and diphenhydramine hydrochloride 25 mg.

Each packet of *Maximum Strength TYLENOL FLU NightTime Hot Medication* contains acetaminophen 1000 mg, pseudoephedrine hydrochloride 60 mg and diphenhydramine hydrochloride 50 mg.

ACTIONS

Maximum Strength TYLENOL® FLU Medication No Drowsiness Formula contains a clinically proven analgesic-antipyretic, decongestant and cough suppressant. Acetaminophen produces analgesia by elevation of the pain threshold and antipyresis through action on the hypothalamic heat-regulating center. Acetaminophen is equal to aspirin in analgesic and antipyretic effectiveness and it is unlikely to produce many of the side effects associated with aspirin and aspirin-containing products. Pseudoephedrine hydrochloride is a sympathomimetic amine which provides temporary relief of nasal congestion. Dextromethorphan is a cough suppressant which provides temporary relief of coughs due to minor throat irritations that may occur with the common cold. *Maximum Strength TYLENOL® FLU NightTime Medication* and *Maximum Strength TYLENOL® FLU NightTime Hot Medication* contains the same clinically proven analgesic-antipyretic and decongestant as Maximum Strength TYLENOL FLU Medication No Drowsiness Formula along with an antihistamine. Diphenhydramine is an antihistamine which helps provide temporary relief of runny nose and sneezing.

INDICATIONS

Maximum Strength TYLENOL® FLU Medication No Drowsiness Formula provides effective temporary relief of body aches, headaches, fever, sore throat, coughing and nasal congestion due to a cold or "flu."

Maximum Strength TYLENOL® FLU NightTime Medication and *Maximum Strength TYLENOL® FLU NightTime Hot Medication* provides effective temporary relief of body aches, headaches, fever, sore throat, nasal congestion, and runny nose/sneezing due to a cold or "flu" so you can rest.

DIRECTIONS

Maximum Strength TYLENOL® FLU Medication No Drowsiness Formula: Adults (12 years and older): Two gelcaps every 6 hours, not to exceed 8 gelcaps in 24 hours. Not for use in children under 12 years of age.

Maximum Strength TYLENOL® FLU NightTime Medication: Adults (12 years and older): Two gelcaps at bedtime. May repeat every 6 hours, not to exceed 8 gelcaps in 24 hours. Not for use in children under 12 years of age.

Maximum Strength TYLENOL® FLU NightTime Hot Medication: Adults (12 years and older): Dissolve one packet in 6 oz. cup of hot water. Sip while hot. Sweeten to taste, if desired. May repeat every 6 hours, not to exceed 4 doses in 24 hours. Not for use in children under 12 years of age.

PRECAUTIONS

Maximum Strength TYLENOL® FLU Medication No Drowsiness Formula, Maximum Strength TYLENOL® FLU NightTime Medication, and Maximum Strength TYLENOL® FLU NightTime Hot Medication: If a rare sensitivity reaction occurs, the drug should be stopped. Although pseudoephedrine is virtually without pressor effect in normotensive patients, it should be used with caution in hypertensives.

WARNINGS

Maximum Strength TYLENOL® FLU Medication No Drowsiness Formula: Do not take this product for more than 7 days or for fever for more than 3 days unless directed by a doctor. If symptoms do not improve or are accompanied by fever, consult a doctor. A persistent cough may be a sign of a serious condition. If cough persists for more than 1 week, tends to recur or is accompanied by fever, rash or persistent headache, consult a doctor. Do not take this product for persistent or chronic cough such as occurs with smoking, asthma, emphysema or if cough is accompanied by excessive phlegm (mucus) unless directed by a doctor. If sore throat is

severe, persists for more than 2 days, is accompanied or followed by fever, headache, rash, nausea or vomiting, consult a doctor promptly. Do not exceed recommended dosage because at higher doses, nervousness, dizziness or sleeplessness may occur. Do not take this product if you have heart disease, high blood pressure, thyroid disease, diabetes, or difficulty in urination due to enlargement of the prostate gland unless directed by a doctor. Do not use with other products containing acetaminophen.

DO NOT USE IF CARTON IS OPENED OR IF A BLISTER UNIT IS BROKEN. KEEP THIS AND ALL MEDICATION OUT OF THE REACH OF CHILDREN. AS WITH ANY DRUG, IF YOU ARE PREGNANT OR NURSING A BABY, SEEK THE ADVICE OF A HEALTH PROFESSIONAL BEFORE USING THIS PRODUCT. IN CASE OF ACCIDENTAL OVERDOSE, CONTACT A DOCTOR OR POISON CONTROL CENTER IMMEDIATELY. PROMPT MEDICAL ATTENTION IS CRITICAL FOR ADULTS AS WELL AS CHILDREN EVEN IF YOU DO NOT NOTICE ANY SIGNS OR SYMPTOMS.

Maximum Strength TYLENOL® FLU NightTime Medication Gelcaps: Do not exceed the recommended dosage, because at higher doses, nervousness, dizziness or sleeplessness may occur. Do not take this product for more than 7 days or for fever for more than 3 days unless directed by a doctor. If symptoms do not improve or are accompanied by fever, consult a doctor. If sore throat is severe, persists for more than 2 days, is accompanied by fever, headache, rash nausea or vomiting, consult a doctor promptly. May cause excitability, especially in children. Do not take this product, unless directed by a doctor, if you have a breathing problem such as emphysema or chronic bronchitis, or if you have glaucoma or difficulty in urination due to enlargement of the prostate gland. Do not take this product if you have heart disease, high blood pressure, thyroid disease, or diabetes unless directed by a doctor. May cause marked drowsiness: alcohol, sedatives and tranquilizers may increase the drowsiness effect. Avoid alcoholic beverages while taking this product. Do not take this product if you are taking sedatives or tranquilizers without first consulting your doctor. Use caution when driving a motor vehicle or operating machinery. Do not use with other products containing acetaminophen.

DO NOT USE IF CARTON IS OPENED OR IF A BLISTER UNIT IS BROKEN. KEEP THIS AND ALL MEDICATION OUT OF THE REACH OF CHILDREN. AS WITH ANY DRUG, IF YOU ARE PREGNANT OR NURSING A BABY, SEEK THE ADVICE OF A HEALTH PROFESSIONAL BEFORE USING THIS PRODUCT. IN CASE OF ACCIDENTAL OVERDOSE, CONTACT A DOCTOR OR POISON CONTROL CENTER IMMEDIATELY. PROMPT MEDICAL ATTENTION IS CRITICAL FOR ADULTS AS WELL AS CHILDREN EVEN IF YOU DO NOT NOTICE ANY SIGNS OR SYMPTOMS.

Maximum Strength TYLENOL® FLU NightTime Hot Medication: Do not exceed the recommended dosage, because at higher doses, nervousness, dizziness or sleeplessness may occur. Do not take this product for more than 7 days or for fever for more than 3 days unless directed by a doctor. If symptoms do not improve or are accompanied by fever, consult a doctor. If sore throat is severe, persists for more than 2 days, is accompanied or followed by fever, headache, rash, nausea or vomiting, consult a doctor promptly. May cause excitability especially in children. Do not take this product, unless directed by a doctor, if you have a breathing problem such as emphysema or chronic bronchitis, or if you have glaucoma or difficulty in urination due to enlargement of the prostate gland. Do not take this product if you have heart disease, high blood pressure, thyroid disease or diabetes unless directed by a doctor. May cause marked drowsiness: alcohol, sedatives and tranquilizers may increase the drowsiness effect. Avoid alcoholic beverages while taking this product. Do not take this product if you are taking sedatives or tranquilizers without first consulting your doctor. Use caution when driving a motor vehicle or operating machinery. Do not use with other products containing acetaminophen.

DO NOT USE IF PRINTED CARTON OVERWRAP IS BROKEN OR MISSING OR IF CARTON IS OPENED OR FOIL PACKET IS TORN OR BROKEN. KEEP THIS AND ALL MEDICATION OUT OF THE REACH OF CHILDREN. AS WITH ANY DRUG, IF YOU ARE PREGNANT OR NURSING A BABY, SEEK THE ADVICE OF A HEALTH PROFESSIONAL BEFORE USING THIS PRODUCT. IN CASE OF ACCIDENTAL OVERDOSE, CONTACT A DOCTOR OR POISON CONTROL CENTER IMMEDIATELY. PROMPT MEDICAL ATTENTION IS CRITICAL FOR ADULTS AS WELL AS CHILDREN EVEN IF YOU DO NOT NOTICE ANY SIGNS OR SYMPTOMS.

PHENYLKETONURICS: CONTAINS PHENYLALANINE 67 MG PER PACKET.

ALCOHOL WARNING

Maximum Strength TYLENOL® FLU Medication No Drowsiness Formula, Maximum Strength TYLENOL® FLU NightTime Medication, and Maximum Strength TYLENOL® FLU NightTime Hot Medication: For this and all other pain relievers, including aspirin, ibuprofen, ketoprofen and naproxen sodium, if you generally consume 3 or more alcohol-

containing drinks per day, you should consult your physician for advice on when and how you should take pain relievers.

DRUG INTERACTION PRECAUTION

Maximum Strength TYLENOL® FLU Medication No Drowsiness Formula, Maximum Strength TYLENOL® FLU NightTime Medication, and Maximum Strength TYLENOL® FLU NightTime Hot Medication: Do not take this product if you are presently taking a prescription drug for high blood pressure or you are now taking a prescription monoamine oxidase inhibitor (MAOI) (certain drugs for depression, psychiatric or emotional conditions, or Parkinson's disease), or for 2 weeks after stopping the MAOI drug. If you are uncertain whether your prescription drug contains an MAOI, consult a health professional before taking this product.

OVERDOSAGE INFORMATION

Maximum Strength TYLENOL® FLU Medication No Drowsiness Formula, Maximum Strength TYLENOL® FLU NightTime Medication, and Maximum Strength TYLENOL® FLU NightTime Hot Medication: Acetaminophen in massive overdosage may cause hepatic toxicity in some patients. In adults and adolescents, hepatic toxicity has rarely been reported following ingestion of acute overdoses of less than 10 grams. Fatalities are infrequent (less than 3–4% of untreated cases) and have rarely been reported with overdosage of less than 15 grams. In children, an acute overdosage of less than 150 mg/kg has not been associated with hepatic toxicity.

Early symptoms following a potentially hepatotoxic overdose may include: nausea, vomiting, diaphoresis and general malaise. Clinical and laboratory evidence of hepatic toxicity may not be apparent until 48 to 72 hours postingestion. In adults and adolescents, regardless of the quantity of acetaminophen reported to have been ingested, administer acetylcysteine immediately if 24 hours or less have elapsed from the reported time of ingestion. For full prescribing information, refer to the acetylcysteine package insert. Do not await results of assays for plasma acetaminophen level before initiating treatment with acetylcysteine. The following additional procedures are recommended: The stomach should be emptied promptly by lavage or by induction of emesis with syrup of ipecac. A plasma acetaminophen assay should be obtained as early as possible, but not sooner than four hours following ingestion. If plasma level falls above the lower treatment line on the acetaminophen overdose nomogram, acetylcysteine therapy should be continued. Liver function studies should be obtained initially and repeated at 24-hour intervals.

Serious toxicity or fatalities are extremely infrequent in children, possibly due to differences in the way they metabolize acetaminophen. In children, the maximum potential amount ingested can be more easily estimated. If more than 150 mg/kg or an unknown amount was ingested, obtain an plasma acetaminophen level. The plasma acetaminophen level should be obtained as soon as possible, but no sooner than 4 hours following the ingestion. If plasma level falls above the lower treatment line on the acetaminophen overdose nomogram, the acetylcysteine therapy should be initiated and continued for a full course of therapy. If plasma acetaminophen assay capability is not available, and the estimated acetaminophen ingestion exceeds 150 mg/kg, acetylcysteine therapy should be initiated and continued for a full course of therapy.

For additional emergency information, call your regional poison center or call the Rocky Mountain Poison Center toll-free, (1-800-525-6115).

Symptoms from pseudoephedrine overdose consist most often of mild anxiety, tachycardia and/or mild hypertension. Symptoms usually appear within 4 to 8 hours of ingestion and are transient, usually requiring no treatment.

Acute dextromethorphan overdose usually does not result in serious signs and symptoms unless massive amounts have been ingested. Signs and symptoms of a substantial overdose may include nausea and vomiting, visual disturbances, CNS disturbances, and urinary retention.

Diphenhydramine toxicity should be treated as you would an antihistamine/anticholinergic overdose and is likely to be present within a few hours after acute ingestion.

ALCOHOL INFORMATION

Maximum Strength TYLENOL® FLU Medication No Drowsiness Formula, Maximum Strength TYLENOL® FLU NightTime Medication, and Maximum Strength TYLENOL® FLU NightTime Hot Medication: Chronic heavy alcohol abusers may be at increased risk of liver toxicity from excessive acetaminophen use, although reports of this event are rare. Reports almost invariably involve cases of severe chronic alcoholics and the dosages of acetaminophen most often exceed recommended doses and often involve substantial overdose. Professionals should alert their patients who regularly consume large amounts of alcohol not to exceed recommended doses of acetaminophen.

Continued on next page

Consult 1997 supplements and future editions for revisions

McNeil Consumer—Cont.

INACTIVE INGREDIENTS

Maximum Strength TYLENOL® FLU Medication No Drowsiness Formula: Benzyl alcohol, butylparaben, castor oil, cellulose, corn starch edetate calcium disodium, gelatin, hydroxypropyl methylcellulose, iron oxide black, magnesium stearate, methylparaben, propylparaben, sodium lauryl sulfate, sodium propionate, sodium starch glycolate, titanium dioxide, Red #40 and Blue #1.

Maximum Strength TYLENOL® FLU NightTime Medication: Benzyl alcohol, butylparaben, castor oil, cellulose, corn starch, edetate calcium disodium, gelatin, hydroxypropyl methylcellulose, iron oxide black, magnesium stearate, methylparaben, propylparaben, sodium citrate, sodium laurel sulfate, sodium propionate, sodium starch glycolate, titanium dioxide, Red #28 and Blue #1.

Maximum Strength TYLENOL® FLU Hot Medication Packets: Ascorbic acid (vitamin C), aspartame, citric acid, flavors, sodium citrate, sucrose, Yellow #10, Blue #1, Red #40, and Yellow #6. May also contain: silicon dioxide.

HOW SUPPLIED

Maximum Strength TYLENOL® FLU Medication No Drowsiness Formula: **Gelcaps** (colored burgundy and white, imprinted "TYLENOL FLU") in blister packs of 10 and 20.

Maximum Strength TYLENOL® FLU NightTime Medication: **Gelcaps** (colored blue and white, imprinted "TYLENOL FLU NT") in blister packs of 10 and 20.

Maximum Strength TYLENOL® FLU Hot Medication Packets: **Packets of powder** (yellow colored) in cartons of 6 tamper-resistant foil packets.

Shown in Product Identification Guide, page 323

Extra Strength **OTC**

TYLENOL® PM

Pain Reliever/Sleep Aid Caplets, Geltabs and Gelcaps

DESCRIPTION

Each ***Extra Strength TYLENOL® PM Caplet, Geltab*** or ***Gelcap*** contains acetaminophen 500 mg and diphenhydramine HCl 25 mg.

ACTIONS

Extra Strength TYLENOL® PM Caplets, Geltabs and ***Gelcaps*** contain a clinically proven analgesic-antipyretic and an antihistamine. Maximum allowable non-prescription levels of acetaminophen and diphenhydramine provide temporary relief of occasional headaches and minor aches and pains accompanying sleeplessness. Acetaminophen is equal to aspirin in analgesic and antipyretic effectiveness and it is unlikely to produce many of the side effects associated with aspirin containing products. Acetaminophen produces analgesia by elevation of the pain threshold. Diphenhydramine HCl is an antihistamine with sedative properties.

INDICATIONS

Extra Strength TYLENOL® PM Caplets, Geltabs and ***Gelcaps*** provide temporary relief of occasional headaches and minor aches and pains with accompanying sleeplessness.

PRECAUTIONS

If a rare sensitivity reaction occurs, the drug should be discontinued.

DIRECTIONS

Adults and Children 12 years of Age and Older: Two caplets, geltabs or gelcaps at bedtime or as directed by physician. Do not exceed recommended dosage. Not for use in children under 12 years of age.

WARNINGS

Do not use if carton is opened or printed neck wrap or printed foil inner seal is broken. Do not give to children under 12 years of age. If sleeplessness persists continuously for more than 2 weeks, consult your doctor. Insomnia may be a symptom of serious underlying medical illness. Do not take for pain for more than 10 days or for fever for more than 3 days unless directed by a doctor. If pain or fever persists, or gets worse, if new symptoms occur, or if redness or swelling is present, consult a doctor because these could be signs of a serious condition. Do not take this product, unless directed by a doctor, if you have a breathing problem such as emphysema or chronic bronchitis, or if you have glaucoma or difficulty in urination due to enlargement of the prostate gland. Avoid alcoholic beverages while taking this product. Do not take this product if your are taking sedatives or tranquilizers without first consulting your doctor.

As with any drug, if you are pregnant or nursing a baby, seek the advice of a health professional before using this product. Keep this and all drugs out of the reach of children. In case of accidental overdose, contact a doctor or poison control center immediately. Prompt medical attention is critical for adults as well as for children even if you do not notice any signs or symptoms. Do not use with other products containing acetaminophen.

ALCOHOL WARNING

For this and all other pain relievers, including aspirin, ibuprofen, ketoprofen and naproxen sodium, if you generally consume 3 or more alcohol-containing drinks per day, you should consult your physician for advice on when and how you should take pain relievers.

CAUTION

This product will cause drowsiness. Do not drive a motor vehicle or operate machinery after use.

OVERDOSAGE INFORMATION

Acetaminophen in massive overdosage may cause hepatic toxicity in some patients. In adults and adolescents, hepatic toxicity has rarely been reported following ingestion of acute overdoses of less than 10 grams. Fatalities are infrequent (less than 3–4% of untreated cases) and have rarely been reported with overdoses of less than 15 grams. In children, an acute overdosage of less than 150 mg/kg has not been associated with hepatic toxicity.

Early symptoms following a potentially hepatotoxic overdose may include: nausea, vomiting, diaphoresis and general malaise. Clinical and laboratory evidence of hepatic toxicity may not be apparent until 48 to 72 hours postingestion.

In adults and adolescents, regardless of the quantity of acetaminophen reported to have been ingested, administer acetylcysteine immediately if 24 hours or less have elapsed from the reported time of ingestion. For full prescribing information, refer to the acetylcysteine package insert. Do not await results of assays for plasma acetaminophen level before initiating treatment with acetylcysteine. The following additional procedures are recommended. The stomach should be emptied promptly by lavage or by induction of emesis with syrup of ipecac. A plasma acetaminophen assay should be obtained as early as possible, but no sooner than four hours following ingestion. If plasma level falls above the lower treatment line on the acetaminophen overdose nomogram, acetylcysteine therapy should be continued. Liver function studies should be obtained initially and repeated at 24-hour intervals.

Serious toxicity or fatalities are extremely infrequent in children, possibly due to differences in the way they metabolize acetaminophen. In children, the maximum potential amount ingested can be more easily estimated. If more than 150 mg/kg or an unknown amount was ingested, obtain a plasma acetaminophen level. The plasma acetaminophen level should be obtained as soon as possible, but no sooner than 4 hours following the ingestion. If the plasma level falls above the lower treatment line on the acetaminophen overdose nomogram, the acetylcysteine therapy should be initiated and continued for a full course of therapy. If plasma acetaminophen assay capability is not available, and the estimated acetaminophen ingestion exceeds 150 mg/kg, acetylcysteine therapy should be initiated and continued for a full course of therapy.

For additional emergency information, call your regional poison center or call the Rocky Mountain Poison Center toll-free, (1-800-525-6115).

Diphenhydramine toxicity should be treated as you would an antihistamine/anticholinergic overdose and is likely to be present within a few hours after acute ingestion.

ALCOHOL INFORMATION

Chronic heavy alcohol abusers may be at increased risk of liver toxicity from excessive acetaminophen use, although reports of this event are rare. Reports almost invariably involve cases of severe chronic alcoholics and the dosages of acetaminophen most often exceed recommended doses and often involve substantial overdose. Professionals should alert their patients who regularly consume large amounts of alcohol not to exceed recommended doses of acetaminophen.

INACTIVE INGREDIENTS

Caplets: Cellulose, Cornstarch, Hydroxypropyl Methylcellulose, Magnesium Stearate or Stearic Acid and Colloidal Silicon Dioxide, Polyethylene Glycol, Polysorbate 80, Sodium Citrate, Sodium Starch Glycolate, Titanium Dioxide, Blue #1 and Blue #2.

Geltabs/Gelcaps: Benzyl Alcohol, Butylparaben, Castor Oil, Cellulose, Cornstarch, Edetate Calcium Disodium, Gelatin, Hydroxypropyl Methylcellulose, Magnesium Stearate, Propylparaben, Sodium Lauryl Sulfate, Sodium Citrate, Sodium Propionate, Sodium Starch Glycolate, Titanium Dioxide, Blue #1 and Red #28.

HOW SUPPLIED

Caplets (colored light blue imprinted "Tylenol PM") tamper-resistant bottles of 24, 50, 100, and 150.

Geltabs/Gelcaps (colored blue and white imprinted "TYLENOL PM") tamper-resistant bottles of 24 and 50.

Shown in Product Identification Guide, page 323

Maximum Strength **OTC**

TYLENOL® SINUS

Geltabs, Gelcaps, Caplets and Tablets

DESCRIPTION

Each ***Maximum Strength TYLENOL® SINUS Geltab, Gelcap, Caplet or Tablet*** contains acetaminophen 500 mg and pseudoephedrine hydrochloride 30 mg.

ACTIONS

Maximum Strength TYLENOL® SINUS contains a clinically proven analgesic-antipyretic and a decongestant. Maximum allowable non-prescription levels of acetaminophen and pseudoephedrine provide temporary relief of sinus headache and congestion. Acetaminophen is equal to aspirin in analgesic and antipyretic effectiveness and it is unlikely to produce many of the side effects associated with aspirin and aspirin-containing products.

Acetaminophen produces analgesia by elevation of the pain threshold and antipyresis through action on the hypothalamic heat-regulating center. Pseudoephedrine hydrochloride is a sympathomimetic amine which promotes sinus cavity drainage by reducing nasopharyngeal mucosal congestion.

INDICATIONS

Maximum Strength TYLENOL® SINUS provides for the temporary relief of nasal and sinus congestion and sinus pain and headaches. ***Maximum Strength TYLENOL® SINUS*** is particularly well-suited in patients with aspirin allergy, hemostatic disturbances (including anticoagulant therapy), and bleeding diatheses (e.g., hemophilia) and upper gastrointestinal disease (e.g., ulcer, gastritis, hiatus hernia).

PRECAUTIONS

If a rare sensitivity occurs, the drug should be discontinued. Although pseudoephedrine is virtually without pressor effect in normotensive patients, it should be used with caution in hypertensives.

DIRECTIONS

Adults and Children 12 years of Age and Older: Two Tablets, Caplets, Gelcaps, or Geltabs every 4–6 hours. Do not exceed eight Tablets, Caplets, Gelcaps, or Geltabs in any 24-hour period. Not for use in children under 12 years of age.

WARNINGS

Do not use if carton is opened or if blister unit is broken. Do not take for pain for more than 7 days or for fever for more than 3 days unless directed by a doctor. If pain or fever persists. or get worse, if new symptoms occur, or if redness or swelling is present, consult a doctor because these could be signs of a serious condition. **Do not exceed recommended dosage.** If nervousness, dizziness or sleeplessness occur, discontinue use and consult a doctor. Do not take this product if you have heart disease, high blood pressure, thyroid disease, diabetes, or difficulty in urination due to enlargement of the prostate gland unless directed by a doctor.

As with any drug, if you are pregnant or nursing a baby, seek the advice of a health professional before using this product. Keep this and all drugs out of the reach of children. In case of accidental overdose, contact a doctor or poison control center immediately. Prompt medical attention is critical for adults as well as for children even if you do not notice any signs or symptoms. Do not use with other products containing acetaminophen.

ALCOHOL WARNING

For this and all other pain relievers, including aspirin, ibuprofen, ketoprofen and naproxen sodium, if you generally consume 3 or more alcohol-containing drinks per day, you should consult your physician for advice on when and how you should take pain relievers.

DRUG INTERACTION PRECAUTION

Do not use this product if you are now taking a prescription monoamine oxidase inhibitor (MAOI) (certain drugs for depression, psychiatric or emotional conditions, or Parkinson's disease), or for 2 weeks after stopping the MAOI drug. If you are uncertain whether your prescription drug contains an MAOI, consult a health professional before taking this product.

OVERDOSAGE INFORMATION

Acetaminophen in massive overdosage may cause hepatic toxicity in some patients. In adults and adolescents, hepatic toxicity has rarely been reported following ingestion of acute overdoses of less than 10 grams. Fatalities are infrequent (less than 3–4% of untreated cases) and have rarely been reported with overdoses of less than 15 grams. In children, an acute overdosage of less than 150 mg/kg has not been associated with hepatic toxicity.

Early symptoms following a potentially hepatotoxic overdose may include: nausea, vomiting, diaphoresis and general malaise. Clinical and laboratory evidence of hepatic toxicity may not be apparent until 48 to 72 hours postingestion.

In adults and adolescents, regardless of the quantity of acetaminophen reported to have been ingested, administer acetylcysteine immediately if 24 hours or less have elapsed from

the reported time of ingestion. For full prescribing information, refer to the acetylcysteine package insert. Do not await results of assays for plasma acetaminophen level before initiating treatment with acetylcysteine. The following additional procedures are recommended. The stomach should be emptied promptly by lavage or by induction of emesis with syrup of ipecac. A plasma acetaminophen assay should be obtained as early as possible, but no sooner than four hours following ingestion. If plasma level falls above the lower treatment line on the acetaminophen overdose nomogram, acetylcysteine therapy should be continued. Liver function studies should be obtained initially and repeated at 24-hour intervals.

Serious toxicity or fatalities are extremely infrequent in children, possibly due to differences in the way they metabolize acetaminophen. In children, the maximum potential amount ingested can be more easily estimated. If more than 150 mg/kg or an unknown amount was ingested, obtain a plasma acetaminophen level. The plasma acetaminophen level should be obtained as soon as possible, but no sooner than 4 hours following the ingestion. If plasma level falls above the lower treatment line on the acetaminophen overdose nomogram, the acetylcysteine therapy should be initiated and continued for a full course of therapy. If plasma acetaminophen assay capability is not available, and the estimated acetaminophen ingestion exceeds 150 mg/kg, acetylcysteine therapy should be initiated and continued for a full course of therapy.

For additional emergency information, call your regional poison center or call the Rocky Mountain Poison Center toll-free (1-800-525-6115).

Symptoms from pseudoephedrine overdose consist most often of mild anxiety, tachycardia and/or mild hypertension. Symptoms usually appear within 4 to 8 hours after ingestion and are transient, usually requiring no treatment.

ALCOHOL INFORMATION

Chronic heavy alcohol abusers may be at increased risk of liver toxicity from excessive acetaminophen use, although reports of this event are rare. Reports almost invariably involve cases of severe chronic alcoholics and the dosages of acetaminophen most often exceed recommended doses and often involve substantial overdose. Professionals should alert their patients who regularly consume large amounts of alcohol not to exceed recommended doses of acetaminophen.

INACTIVE INGREDIENTS

Caplets: Carnauba Wax, Cellulose, Corn Starch, Hydroxypropyl Methylcellulose, Magnesium Stearate, Polyethylene Glycol, Polysorbate 80, Sodium Starch Glycolate, Titanium Dioxide, Blue #1, Red #40, Yellow #10.
Tablets: Cellulose, Corn Starch, Magnesium Stearate, Sodium Starch Glycolate,. Blue #1, Yellow #6, and Yellow #10.
Gelcaps: Benzyl Alcohol, Butylparaben, Castor Oil, Cellulose, Corn Starch, Edetate Calcium Disodium, Gelatin, Hydroxypropyl Methylcellulose, Iron Oxide Black, Magnesium Stearate, Methylparaben, Propylparaben, Sodium Lauryl Sulfate, Sodium Propionate, Sodium Starch Glycolate, Titanium Dioxide, Blue #1 and Yellow #10.
Geltabs: Benzyl Alcohol, Butylparaben, Castor Oil, Cellulose, Corn Starch, Edetate Calcium Disodium, Gelatin, Hydroxypropyl Methylcellulose, Iron Oxide Black, Magnesium Stearate, Methylparaben, Propylparaben, Sodium Lauryl Sulfate, Sodium Propionate, Sodium Starch Glycolate, Titanium Dioxide, D&C Yellow #10, FD&C Blue #1

HOW SUPPLIED

Tablets: (colored light green, imprinted "Maximum Strength TYLENOL SINUS")—in blister packs of 24.
Caplets: (light green coating, printed "TYLENOL SINUS" in dark green) in blister packs of 24 and 48.
Gelcaps: (colored green and white), printed "TYLENOL SINUS" in blister packs of 24 and 48.
Geltabs: (colored green and white), printed "TYLENOL SINUS" in blister packs of 24 and 48.

Shown in Product Identification Guide, page 323

McNeil Pharmaceutical
RARITAN, NJ 08869-0602

For Medical Information Contact:
Medical Information Department
(800) 542-5365

FLOXIN® TABLETS ℞
[ofloxacin tablets]

DESCRIPTION

FLOXIN® (ofloxacin tablets) Tablets is a synthetic broad-spectrum antimicrobial agent for oral administration. Chemically, ofloxacin, a fluorinated carboxyquinolone, is the racemate, (±)-9-fluoro-2,3-dihydro-3-methyl-10-(4-methyl-1-piperazinyl) -7-oxo-7H-pyrido[1,2,3-de]-1,4-benzoxazine-6-carboxylic acid. The chemical structure is:

Its empirical formula is $C_{18}H_{20}FN_3O_4$, and its molecular weight is 361.4. Ofloxacin is an off-white to pale yellow crystalline powder. The molecule exists as a zwitterion at the pH conditions in the small intestine. The relative solubility characteristics of ofloxacin at room temperature, as defined by USP nomenclature, indicate that ofloxacin is considered to be *soluble* in aqueous solutions with pH between 2 and 5. It is *sparingly* to *slightly soluble* in aqueous solutions with pH 7 and *freely soluble* in aqueous solutions with pH above 9. Ofloxacin has the potential to form stable coordination compounds with many metal ions. This *in vitro* chelation potential has the following formation order: $Fe^{+3} > Al^{+3} > Cu^{+2} > Ni^{+2} > Pb^{+2} > Zn^{+2} > Mg^{+2} > Ca^{+2} > Ba^{+2}$.

FLOXIN Tablets contain the following inactive ingredients: anhydrous lactose, corn starch, hydroxypropyl cellulose, hydroxypropyl methylcellulose, magnesium stearate, polyethylene glycol, polysorbate 80, sodium starch glycolate, titanium dioxide and may also contain synthetic yellow iron oxide.

CLINICAL PHARMACOLOGY

Following oral administration, the bioavailability of ofloxacin in the tablet formulation is approximately 98%. Maximum serum concentrations are achieved one to two hours after an oral dose. Absorption of ofloxacin after single or multiple doses of 200 to 400 mg is predictable, and the amount of drug absorbed increases proportionally with the dose.

Ofloxacin has biphasic elimination. Following multiple oral doses at steady-state administration, the half-lives are approximately 4–5 hours and 20–25 hours. However, the longer half-life represents less than 5% of the total AUC. Accumulation at steady-state can be estimated using a half-life of 9 hours. The total clearance and volume of distribution are approximately similar after single or multiple doses. Elimination is mainly by renal excretion. The following are mean peak serum concentrations in healthy 70–80 kg male volunteers after single oral doses of 200, 300, or 400 mg of ofloxacin or after multiple oral doses of 400 mg.

Oral Dose	Serum Concentration 2 hours after admin. (µg/mL)	Area Under the Curve (AUC$_{(0-\infty)}$) (µg·h/mL)
200 mg single dose	1.5	14.1
300 mg single dose	2.4	21.2
400 mg single dose	2.9	31.4
400 mg steady state	4.6	61.0

Steady-state concentrations were attained after four oral doses and the area under the curve (AUC) was approximately 40% higher than the AUC after single doses. Therefore, after multiple-dose administration of 200 mg and 300 mg doses, peak serum levels of 2.2 µg/mL and 3.6 µg/mL, respectively, are predicted at steady-state.

In vitro, approximately 32% of the drug in plasma is protein bound.

The single dose and steady-state plasma profiles of ofloxacin injection were comparable in extent of exposure (AUC) to those of ofloxacin tablets when the injectable and tablet formulations of ofloxacin were administered in equal doses (mg/mg) to the same group of subjects. The mean steady state AUC$_{(0-12)}$ attained after the intravenous administration of 400 mg over 60 min was 43.5 µg·h/mL; the mean steady state AUC$_{(0-12)}$ attained after the oral administration of 400 mg was 41.2 µg·h/mL (two one-sided t-test, 90% confidence interval was 103–109). (See following chart.)

[See graph below.]

Between 0 and 6 h following the administration of a single 200 mg oral dose of ofloxacin to 12 healthy volunteers, the average urine ofloxacin concentration was approximately 220 µg/mL. Between 12 and 24 hours after administration, the average urine ofloxacin level was approximately 34 µg/mL.

Following oral administration of recommended therapeutic doses, ofloxacin has been detected in blister fluid, cervix, lung tissue, ovary, prostatic fluid, prostatic tissue, skin, and sputum. The mean concentration of ofloxacin in each of these various body fluids and tissues after one or more doses was 0.8 to 1.5 times the concurrent plasma level. Inadequate data are presently available on the distribution or levels of ofloxacin in the cerebrospinal fluid or brain tissue.

Ofloxacin has a pyridobenzoxazine ring that appears to decrease the extent of parent compound metabolism. Between 65% and 80% of an administered oral dose of ofloxacin is excreted unchanged via the kidneys within 48 hours of dosing. Studies indicate that less than 5% of an administered dose is recovered in the urine as the desmethyl or N-oxide metabolites. Four to eight percent of an ofloxacin dose is excreted in the feces. This indicates a small degree of biliary excretion of ofloxacin.

The effect that food has on the absorption of ofloxacin tablets has not been studied.

Following the administration of oral doses of ofloxacin to healthy elderly volunteers (64–74 years of age) with normal renal function, the apparent half-life of ofloxacin was 7 to 8 hours, as compared to approximately 6 hours in younger adults. Drug absorption, however, appears to be unaffected by age.

Clearance of ofloxacin is reduced in patients with impaired renal function (creatinine clearance rate ≤50 mL/min), and dosage adjustment is necessary. (See *PRECAUTIONS: General and DOSAGE AND ADMINISTRATION*.)

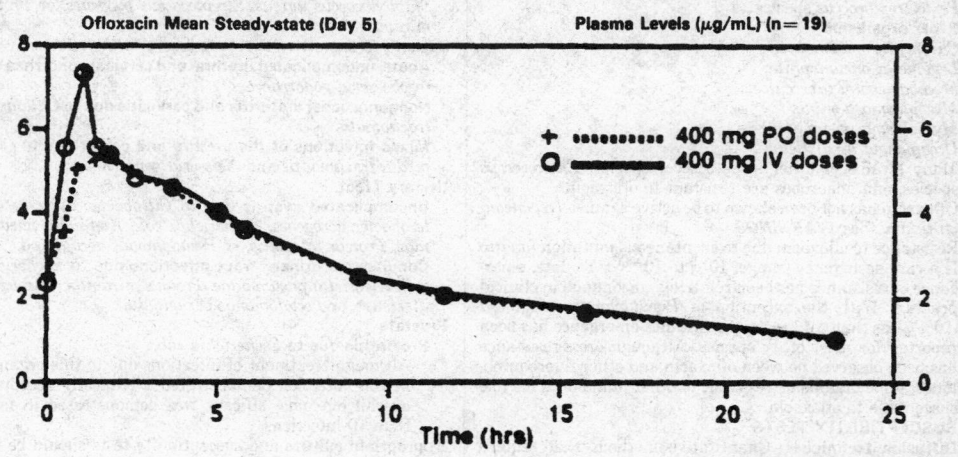

Ofloxacin Mean Steady-state (Day 5) Plasma Levels (µg/mL) (n = 19)

+ ·········· 400 mg PO doses
O ———— 400 mg IV doses

Time (hrs)

Continued on next page

Information on McNeil Pharmaceutical Products is based on labeling in effect in August 1996.

Consult 1997 supplements and future editions for revisions

McNeil—Cont.

MICROBIOLOGY

Ofloxacin has in vitro activity against a broad-spectrum of gram-positive and gram-negative aerobic and anaerobic bacteria. Ofloxacin is often bactericidal at concentrations equal to or slightly greater than inhibitory concentrations. Ofloxacin is thought to exert a bactericidal effect on susceptible microorganisms by inhibiting DNA gyrase, an essential enzyme that is a critical catalyst in the duplication, transcription, and repair of bacterial DNA.

Ofloxacin has been shown to be active against most strains of the following organisms both in vitro and in specific clinical infections; (See INDICATIONS AND USAGE.)

Chlamydia trachomatis
Citrobacter diversus
Enterobacter aerogenes
Escherichia coli
Haemophilus influenzae
Klebsiella pneumoniae
Neisseria gonorrhoeae
Proteus mirabilis
Pseudomonas aeruginosa
Staphylococcus aureus
Streptococcus pneumoniae
Streptococcus pyogenes

The following in vitro data are available; however, their clinical significance is unknown.

Ofloxacin exhibits in vitro minimum inhibitory concentrations of 2 µg/mL or less against most strains of the following organisms; however, the safety and effectiveness of ofloxacin in treating clinical infections due to these organisms have not been established in adequate and well-controlled trials:

Gram-positive aerobes
Enterococcus faecalis
Staphylococcus epidermidis (including methicillin-resistant strains)
Staphylococcus saprophyticus
Streptococcus agalactiae (Group B)
Gram-negative aerobes
Acinetobacter calcoaceticus
Aeromonas hydrophila
Bordetella parapertussis
Bordetella pertussis
Campylobacter jejuni
Citrobacter freundii
Enterobacter cloacae
Haemophilus ducreyi
Klebsiella oxytoca
Moraxella (Branhamella) catarrhalis
Morganella morganii
Neisseria meningitidis
Plesiomonas shigelloides
Proteus vulgaris
Providencia rettgeri
Providencia stuartii
Pseudomonas fluorescens
Serratia marcescens
Anaerobes
Bacteroides fragilis
Bacteroides intermedius
Clostridium perfringens
Clostridium welchii
Eikenella corrodens
Gardnerella vaginalis
Peptococcus niger
Peptostreptococcus species
Other organisms
Chlamydia pneumoniae
Legionella pneumophila
Mycobacterium tuberculosis
Mycoplasma hominis
Mycoplasma pneumoniae
Ureaplasma urealyticum

Many strains of other streptococcal species, Enterococcus species, and anaerobes are resistant to ofloxacin.

Ofloxacin has not been shown to be active against Treponema pallidum. (See WARNINGS.)

Resistance to ofloxacin due to spontaneous mutation in vitro is a rare occurrence (range: 10^{-9} to 10^{-11}). To date, emergence of resistance has been relatively uncommon in clinical practice. With the exception of Pseudomonas aeruginosa (10%), less than a 4% rate of resistance emergence has been reported for most other species. Although cross-resistance has been observed between ofloxacin and other fluoroquinolones, some organisms resistant to other quinolones may be susceptible to ofloxacin.

SUSCEPTIBILITY TESTS

Diffusion techniques: Quantitative methods that require measurement of zone diameters give the most precise estimate of the susceptibility of bacteria to antimicrobial agents. One such standardized procedure[1] that has been recommended for use with disks to test the susceptibility of organisms to ofloxacin uses the 5-µg ofloxacin disk. Interpretation involves correlation of the diameter obtained in the disk test with the minimum inhibitory concentration (MIC) for ofloxacin.

Reports from the laboratory giving results of the standard single-disk susceptibility test with a 5-µg ofloxacin disk should be interpreted according to the following criteria:

Zone diameter (mm)	Interpretation
≥ 16	Susceptible
13–15	Intermediate
≤ 12	Resistant

A report of "Susceptible" indicates that the pathogen is likely to be inhibited by generally achievable drug concentrations. A report of "Intermediate" indicates that the result should be considered equivocal, and, if the organism is not fully susceptible to alternative, clinically feasible drugs, the test should be repeated. This category provides a buffer zone that prevents small uncontrolled technical factors from causing major discrepancies in interpretation. A report of "Resistant" indicates that achievable drug concentrations are unlikely to be inhibitory, and other therapy should be selected.

Standardized susceptibility test procedures require the use of laboratory control organisms. The 5-µg ofloxacin disk should give the following zone diameters:

Organism	Zone diameter (mm)
E. coli ATCC 25922	29–33
P. aeruginosa ATCC 27853	17–21
S. aureus ATCC 25923	24–28

Dilution techniques: Use a standardized dilution method[2] (broth, agar, or microdilution) or equivalent with ofloxacin powder. The MIC values obtained should be interpreted according to the following criteria:

MIC (µg/mL)	Interpretation
≤ 2	(S) Susceptible
4	(I) Intermediate
≥ 8	(R) Resistant

As with standard diffusion methods, dilution procedures require the use of laboratory control organisms. Standard ofloxacin powder should give the following MIC values:

Organism	MIC range (µg/mL)
E. coli ATCC 25922	0.015–0.120
E. faecalis ATCC 29212	1.000–4.000
P. aeruginosa ATCC 27853	1.000–8.000
S. aureus ATCC 25923	0.120–1.000

INDICATIONS AND USAGE

FLOXIN (ofloxacin tablets) Tablets are indicated for the treatment of adults with mild to moderate infections caused by susceptible strains of the designated microorganisms in the infections listed below.

Lower Respiratory Tract
  Acute bacterial exacerbations of chronic bronchitis due to Haemophilus influenzae or Streptococcus pneumoniae.
  Community-acquired Pneumonia due to Haemophilus influenzae or Streptococcus pneumoniae.
Skin and Skin Structures
  Uncomplicated skin and skin structure infections due to Staphylococcus aureus, Streptococcus pyogenes, or Proteus mirabilis*.
Sexually Transmitted Diseases (See WARNINGS.)
  Acute, uncomplicated urethral and cervical gonorrhea due to Neisseria gonorrhoeae.
  Nongonococcal urethritis and cervicitis due to Chlamydia trachomatis.
  Mixed infections of the urethra and cervix due to Chlamydia trachomatis and Neisseria gonorrhoeae.
Urinary Tract
  Uncomplicated cystitis due to Citrobacter diversus, Enterobacter aerogenes, Escherichia coli, Klebsiella pneumoniae, Proteus mirabilis, or Pseudomonas aeruginosa.
  Complicated urinary tract infections due to Escherichia coli, Klebsiella pneumoniae, Proteus mirabilis, Citrobacter diversus*, or Pseudomonas aeruginosa.*
Prostate
  Prostatitis due to Escherichia coli.

* = Although treatment of infections due to this organism in this infection demonstrated a clinically acceptable overall outcome, efficacy was demonstrated in fewer than 10 infections.

Appropriate culture and susceptibility tests should be performed before treatment in order to isolate and identify organisms causing the infection and to determine their susceptibility to ofloxacin. Therapy with ofloxacin may be initiated before results of these tests are known; once results become available, appropriate therapy should be continued.

As with other drugs in this class, some strains of Pseudomonas aeruginosa may develop resistance fairly rapidly during treatment with ofloxacin. Culture and susceptibility testing performed periodically during therapy will provide information not only on the therapeutic effect of the antimicrobial agent but also on the possible emergence of bacterial resistance.

If anaerobic organisms are suspected of contributing to the infection, appropriate therapy for anaerobic pathogens should be administered.

CONTRAINDICATIONS

Ofloxacin is contraindicated in persons with a history of hypersensitivity to ofloxacin or members of the quinolone group of antimicrobial agents.

WARNINGS

THE SAFETY AND EFFICACY OF OFLOXACIN IN CHILDREN, ADOLESCENTS (UNDER THE AGE OF 18 YEARS), PREGNANT WOMEN, AND LACTATING WOMEN HAVE NOT BEEN ESTABLISHED. (SEE PEDIATRIC USE, USE IN PREGNANCY, AND NURSING MOTHERS SUBSECTIONS IN THE PRECAUTIONS SECTION.)

In the immature rat, the oral administration of ofloxacin at 5 to 16 times the recommended maximum human dose based on mg/kg or 1–3 times based on mg/m² increased the incidence and severity of osteochondrosis. The lesions did not regress after 13 weeks of drug withdrawal. Other quinolones also produce similar erosions in the weight-bearing joints and other signs of arthropathy in immature animals of various species. (See ANIMAL PHARMACOLOGY.)

Ofloxacin has not been shown to be effective in the treatment of syphilis. Antimicrobial agents used in high doses for short periods of time to treat gonorrhea may mask or delay the symptoms of incubating syphilis. All patients with gonorrhea should have a serologic test for syphilis at the time of diagnosis. Patients treated with ofloxacin should have a follow-up serologic test for syphilis after three months.

Serious and occasionally fatal hypersensitivity (anaphylactic/anaphylactoid) reactions have been reported in patients receiving therapy with quinolones, including ofloxacin. These reactions often occur following the first dose. Some reactions were accompanied by cardiovascular collapse, hypotension/shock, seizure, loss of consciousness, tingling, angioedema (including tongue, laryngeal, throat or facial edema/swelling, etc.), airway obstruction (including bronchospasm, shortness of breath and acute respiratory distress), dyspnea, urticaria/hives, itching, and other serious skin reactions. A few patients had a history of hypersensitivity reactions. The drug should be discontinued immediately at the first appearance of a skin rash or any other sign of hypersensitivity. Serious acute hypersensitivity reactions may require treatment with epinephrine and other resuscitative measures, including oxygen, intravenous fluids, antihistamines, corticosteroids, pressor amines, and airway management, as clinically indicated. (See PRECAUTIONS and ADVERSE REACTIONS.)

Serious and sometimes fatal events of uncertain etiology have been reported in patients receiving therapy with quinolones including, extremely rarely, ofloxacin. These events may be severe and generally occur following the administration of multiple doses. Clinical manifestations may include one or more of the following: fever, rash or severe dermatologic reactions (e.g., toxic epidermal necrolysis, Stevens-Johnson Syndrome, etc.); vasculitis, arthralgia, myalgia, serum sickness; allergic pneumonitis; interstitial nephritis, acute renal insufficiency/failure; hepatitis, jaundice, acute hepatic necrosis/failure; anemia including hemolytic and aplastic, thrombocytopenia, including thrombotic thrombocytopenic purpura, leukopenia, agranulocytosis, pancytopenia, and/or other hematologic abnormalities. The drug should be discontinued immediately at the first appearance of a skin rash or any other sign of hypersensitivity and supportive measures instituted. (See PRECAUTIONS: Information for Patients and ADVERSE REACTIONS.)

Convulsions, increased intracranial pressure, and toxic psychosis have been reported in patients receiving quinolones, including ofloxacin. Quinolones, including ofloxacin, may also cause central nervous system stimulation which may lead to: tremors, restlessness/agitation, nervousness/anxiety, lightheadedness, confusion, hallucinations, paranoia and depression, nightmares, insomnia, and rarely suicidal thoughts or acts. These reactions may occur following the first dose. If these reactions occur in patients receiving ofloxacin, the drug should be discontinued and appropriate measures instituted. As with all quinolones, ofloxacin should be used with caution in patients with a known or suspected CNS disorder that may predispose to seizures or lower the seizure threshold (e.g., severe cerebral arteriosclerosis, epilepsy, etc.) or in the presence of other risk factors that may predispose to seizures or lower the seizure threshold (e.g., certain drug therapy, renal dysfunction, etc.). (See PRECAUTIONS: General, Drug Interactions and ADVERSE REACTIONS.)

Pseudomembranous colitis has been reported with nearly all antibacterial agents, including ofloxacin, and may range in severity from mild to life-threatening. Therefore, it is impor-

tant to consider this diagnosis in patients who present with diarrhea subsequent to the administration of any antibacterial agents.

Treatment with antibacterial agents alters the normal flora of the colon and may permit overgrowth of clostridia. Studies indicate a toxin produced by *Clostridium difficile* is one primary cause of "antibiotic-associated colitis".

After the diagnosis of pseudomembranous colitis has been established, therapeutic measures should be initiated. Mild cases of pseudomembranous colitis usually respond to drug discontinuation alone. In moderate to severe cases, consideration should be given to management with fluids and electrolytes, protein supplementation, and treatment with an antibacterial drug clinically effective against *C. difficile* colitis. (See ***ADVERSE REACTIONS.***)

PRECAUTIONS

General:

Adequate hydration of patients receiving ofloxacin should be maintained to prevent the formation of a highly concentrated urine.

Administer ofloxacin with caution in the presence of renal or hepatic insufficiency/impairment. In patients with known or suspected renal or hepatic insufficiency/impairment, careful clinical observation and appropriate laboratory studies should be performed prior to and during therapy since elimination of ofloxacin may be reduced. In patients with impaired renal function (creatinine clearance ≤ 50 mg/mL), alteration of the dosage regimen is necessary. (See ***CLINICAL PHARMACOLOGY*** and ***DOSAGE AND ADMINISTRATION.***)

Moderate to severe phototoxicity reactions have been observed in patients exposed to direct sunlight while receiving some drugs in this class, including ofloxacin. Excessive sunlight should be avoided. Therapy should be discontinued if phototoxicity (e.g., a skin eruption, etc.) occurs.

As with all quinolones, ofloxacin should be used with caution in any patient with a known or suspected CNS disorder that may predispose to seizures or lower the seizure threshold (e.g., severe cerebral arteriosclerosis, epilepsy, etc.) or in the presence of other risk factors that may predispose to seizures or lower the seizure threshold (e.g., certain drug therapy, renal dysfunction, etc.). (See ***WARNINGS*** and ***Drug Interactions.***)

As with other quinolones, disturbances of blood glucose, including symptomatic hyper- and hypoglycemia, have been reported, usually in diabetic patients receiving concomitant treatment with an oral hypoglycemic agent (e.g., glyburide/glibenclamide, etc.) or with insulin. In these patients careful monitoring of blood glucose is recommended. If a hypoglycemic reaction occurs in a patient being treated with ofloxacin, discontinue ofloxacin immediately and consult a physician. (See ***Drug Interactions*** and ***ADVERSE REACTIONS.***)

As with any potent drug, periodic assessment of organ system functions, including renal, hepatic, and hematopoietic, is advisable during prolonged therapy. (See ***WARNINGS*** and ***ADVERSE REACTIONS.***)

Information for Patients:

Patients should be advised:

—to drink fluids liberally.

—that mineral supplements, vitamins with iron or minerals, calcium-, aluminum- or magnesium-based antacids or sucralfate should not be taken within the two-hour period before or within the two-hour period after taking ofloxacin. (See ***Drug Interactions.***)

—that ofloxacin should not be taken with food.

—that ofloxacin may cause neurologic adverse effects (e.g., dizziness, lightheadedness, etc.) and that patients should know how they react to ofloxacin before they operate an automobile or machinery or engage in activities requiring mental alertness and coordination. (See ***WARNINGS*** and ***ADVERSE REACTIONS.***)

—that ofloxacin may be associated with hypersensitivity reactions, even following the first dose, to discontinue the drug at the first sign of a skin rash, hives or other skin reactions, a rapid heartbeat, difficulty in swallowing or breathing, any swelling suggesting angioedema (e.g., swelling of the lips, tongue, face; tightness of the throat, hoarseness, etc.), or any other symptom of an allergic reaction. (See ***WARNINGS*** and ***ADVERSE REACTIONS.***)

—to avoid excessive sunlight or artificial ultraviolet light while receiving ofloxacin and to discontinue therapy if phototoxicity (e.g., skin eruption, etc.) occurs.

—that if they are diabetic and are being treated with insulin or an oral hypoglycemic drug, to discontinue ofloxacin immediately if a hypoglycemic reaction occurs and consult a physician. (See ***PRECAUTIONS:*** **General** and ***Drug Interactions.***)

Drug Interactions:

Antacids, Sucralfate, Metal Cations, Multi-Vitamins: Quinolones form chelates with alkaline earth and transition metal cations. Administration of quinolones with antacids containing calcium, magnesium, or aluminum, with sucralfate, with divalent or trivalent cations such as iron, or with multivitamins containing zinc may substantially interfere with the absorption of quinolones resulting in systemic levels considerably lower than desired. These agents should not be taken within the two-hour period before or within the two-hour period after ofloxacin administration. (See ***DOSAGE AND ADMINISTRATION.***)

Caffeine: Interactions between ofloxacin and caffeine have not been detected.

Cimetidine: Cimetidine has demonstrated interference with the elimination of some quinolones. This interference has resulted in significant increases in half-life and AUC of some quinolones. The potential for interaction between ofloxacin and cimetidine has not been studied.

Cyclosporine: Elevated serum levels of cyclosporine have been reported with concomitant use of cyclosporine with some other quinolones. The potential for interaction between ofloxacin and cyclosporine has not been studied.

Drugs metabolized by Cytochrome P450 enzymes: Most quinolone antimicrobial drugs inhibit cytochrome P450 enzyme activity. This may result in a prolonged half-life for some drugs that are also metabolized by this system (e.g., cyclosporine, theophylline/methylxanthines, warfarin, etc.) when co-administered with quinolones. The extent of this inhibition varies among different quinolones. (See other ***Drug Interactions.***)

Non-steroidal anti-inflammatory drugs: The concomitant administration of a non-steroidal anti-inflammatory drug, with a quinolone, including ofloxacin, may increase the risk of CNS stimulation and convulsive seizures. (See ***WARNINGS*** and ***PRECAUTIONS:*** **General.**)

Probenecid: The concomitant use of probenecid with certain other quinolones has been reported to affect renal tubular secretion. The effect of probenecid on the elimination of ofloxacin has not been studied.

Theophylline: Although concurrent administration of some quinolones with theophylline may result in impaired elimination of theophylline, the extent of such impairment varies among different quinolones. Steady-state theophylline levels may increase when ofloxacin and theophylline are administered concurrently. In a pharmacokinetic study involving 15 healthy male subjects, steady-state peak theophylline concentration increased by an average of approximately 9%, and the AUC increased by an average of approximately 13% when oral ofloxacin and theophylline were administered concurrently. In clinical trials with intravenous ofloxacin, theophylline concentrations were determined in 41 patients who were treated with both drugs. In 38 patients, no apparent elevation in the serum theophylline was discernible. Marginal increases above the theophylline therapeutic range were reported in three patients; clinical toxicity was, however, not reported in these three patients. Generally, patients receiving theophylline in clinical trials of the intravenous formulation of ofloxacin reported nausea more frequently than those patients not receiving theophylline. As with some other quinolones, concomitant administration of ofloxacin may prolong the half-life of theophylline, elevate serum theophylline levels, and may increase the risk of theophylline-related adverse reactions. Theophylline levels should be closely monitored and theophylline dosage adjustments made, if appropriate, when ofloxacin is co-administered.

Warfarin: Some quinolones have been reported to enhance the effects of the oral anticoagulant warfarin or its derivatives. Therefore, if a quinolone antimicrobial is administered concomitantly with warfarin or its derivatives, the prothrombin time or other suitable coagulation test should be closely monitored.

Antidiabetic agents (e.g., insulin, glyburide/glibenclamide, etc.): Since disturbances of blood glucose, including hyperglycemia and hypoglycemia, have been reported in patients treated concurrently with quinolones and an antidiabetic agent, careful monitoring of blood glucose is recommended when these agents are used concomitantly. (See ***PRECAUTIONS: General and Information for Patients.***)

Carcinogenesis, Mutagenesis, Impairment of Fertility:

Long-term studies to determine the carcinogenic potential of ofloxacin have not been conducted.

Ofloxacin was not mutagenic in the Ames bacterial test, *in vitro* and *in vivo* cytogenetic assay, sister chromatid exchange (Chinese Hamster and Human Cell Lines), unscheduled DNA Repair (UDS) using human fibroblasts, dominant lethal assays, or mouse micronucleus assay. Ofloxacin was positive in the UDS test using rat hepatocytes and Mouse Lymphoma Assay.

Pregnancy: Teratogenic Effects. Pregnancy Category C.

Ofloxacin has not been shown to have any teratogenic effects at oral doses as high as 810 mg/kg/day (11 times the recommended maximum human dose based on mg/m^2 or 50 times based on mg/kg) and 160 mg/kg/day (4 times the recommended maximum human dose based on mg/m^2 or 10 times based on mg/kg) when administered to pregnant rats and rabbits, respectively. Additional studies in rats with oral doses up to 360 mg/kg/day (5 times the recommended maximum human dose based on mg/m^2 or 23 times based on mg/kg) demonstrated no adverse effect on late fetal development, labor, delivery, lactation, neonatal viability, or growth of the newborn. Doses equivalent to 50 and 10 times the recommended maximum human dose of ofloxacin (based on mg/kg) were fetotoxic (i.e., decreased fetal body weight and increased fetal mortality) in rats and rabbits, respectively. Minor skeletal variations were reported in rats receiving doses of 810 mg/kg/day, which is more than 10 times higher than the recommended maximum human dose based on mg/m^2.

There are, however, no adequate and well-controlled studies in pregnant women. Ofloxacin should be used during pregnancy only if the potential benefit justifies the potential risk to the fetus. (See ***WARNINGS.***)

Nursing Mothers:

In lactating females, a single oral 200-mg dose of ofloxacin resulted in concentrations of ofloxacin in milk that were similar to those found in plasma. Because of the potential for serious adverse reactions from ofloxacin in nursing infants, a decision should be made whether to discontinue nursing or to discontinue the drug, taking into account the importance of the drug to the mother. (See ***WARNINGS*** and ***ADVERSE REACTIONS.***)

Pediatric Use:

Safety and effectiveness in children and adolescents below the age of 18 years have not been established. Ofloxacin causes arthropathy (arthrosis) and osteochondrosis in juvenile animals of several species. (See ***WARNINGS.***)

ADVERSE REACTIONS

The following is a compilation of the data for ofloxacin based on clinical experience with both the oral and intravenous formulations. The incidence of drug-related adverse reactions in patients during Phase 2 and 3 clinical trials was 11%. Among patients receiving multiple-dose therapy, 4% discontinued ofloxacin due to adverse experiences.

In clinical trials, the following events were considered likely to be drug-related in patients receiving multiple doses of ofloxacin:

nausea 3%, insomnia 3%, headache 1%, dizziness 1%, diarrhea 1%, vomiting 1%, rash 1%, pruritus 1%, external genital pruritus in women 1%, vaginitis 1%, dysgeusia 1%.

In clinical trials, the most frequently reported adverse events, regardless of relationship to drug, were:

nausea 10%, headache 9%, insomnia 7%, external genital pruritus in women 6%, dizziness 5%, vaginitis 5%, diarrhea 4%, vomiting 4%.

In clinical trials, the following events, regardless of relationship to drug, occurred in 1 to 3% of patients:

Abdominal pain and cramps, chest pain, decreased appetite, dry mouth, dysgeusia, fatigue, flatulence, gastrointestinal distress, nervousness, pharyngitis, pruritus, fever, rash, sleep disorders, somnolence, trunk pain, vaginal discharge, visual disturbances, and constipation.

Additional events, occurring in clinical trials at a rate of less than 1%, regardless of relationship to drug, were:

Body as a whole: asthenia, chills, malaise, extremity pain, pain, epistaxis

Cardiovascular System: cardiac arrest, edema, hypertension, hypotension, palpitations, vasodilation

Gastroinestinal System: dyspepsia

Genital/Reproductive System: burning, irritation, pain and rash of the female genitalia; dysmenorrhea; menorrhagia; metrorrhagia

Musculoskeletal System: arthralgia, myalgia

Nervous System: seizures, anxiety, cognitive change, depression, dream abnormality, euphoria, hallucinations, paresthesia, syncope, vertigo, tremor, confusion

Nutritional/Metabolic: thirst, weight loss

Respiratory System: respiratory arrest, cough, rhinorrhea

Skin/Hypersenstivity: angioedema, diaphoresis, urticaria, vasculitis

Special Senses: decreased hearing acuity, tinnitus, photophobia

Urinary System: dysuria, urinary frequency, urinary retention

The following laboratory abnormalities appeared in $\geq 1.0\%$ of patients receiving multiple doses of ofloxacin. It is not known whether these abnormalities were caused by the drug or the underlying conditions being treated.

Hematopoietic: anemia, leukopenia, leukocytosis, neutropenia, neutrophilia, increased band forms, lymphocytopenia, eosinophilia, lymphocytosis, thrombocytopenia, thrombocytosis, elevated ESR

Hepatic: elevated: alkaline phosphatase, AST (SGOT), ALT (SGPT)

Serum chemistry: hyperglycemia, hypoglycemia, elevated creatinine, elevated BUN

Urinary: glucosuria, proteinuria, alkalinuria, hyposthenuria, hematuria, pyuria

Continued on next page

Information on McNeil Pharmaceutical Products is based on labeling in effect in August 1996.

McNeil—Cont.

Post-Marketing Adverse Events:
Additional adverse events, regardless of relationship to drug, reported from worldwide marketing experience with quinolones, including ofloxacin:

Clinical:
Cardiovascular System: cerebral thrombosis, pulmonary edema, tachycardia, hypotension/shock, syncope
Endocrine/Metabolic: hyper- or hypoglycemia, especially in diabetic patients on insulin or oral hypoglycemic agents (See **PRECAUTIONS: General** and **Drug Interactions**.)
Gastrointestinal System: hepatic dysfunction including: hepatic necrosis, jaundice (cholestatic or hepatocellular), hepatitis; intestinal perforation; pseudomembranous colitis, GI hemorrhage; hiccough, painful oral mucosa, pyrosis (See **WARNINGS**.)
Genital/Reproductive System: vaginal candidiasis
Hematopoietic: anemia, including hemolytic and aplastic; hemorrhage, pancytopenia, agranulocytosis, leukopenia, reversible bone marrow depression, thrombocytopenia, thrombotic thrombocytopenic purpura, petechiae, ecchymosis/bruising (See **WARNINGS**.)
Musculoskeletal: tendinitis/rupture: weakness
Nervous System: nightmares; suicidal thoughts or acts, disorientation, psychotic reactions, paranoia; phobia, agitation, restlessness, aggressiveness/hostility, manic reaction, emotional lability; peripheral neuropathy, ataxia, incoordination; possible exacerbation of: myasthenia gravis and extrapyramidal disorders; dysphasia, lightheadedness (See **WARNINGS** and **PRECAUTIONS**.)
Respiratory System: dyspnea, bronchospasm, allergic pneumonitis, stridor (See **WARNINGS**.)
Skin/Hypersensitivity: anaphylactic (-toid) reactions/shock; purpura, serum sickness, erythema multiforme/Stevens-Johnson Syndrome, erythema nodosum, exfoliative dermatitis, hyperpigmentation, toxic epidermal necrolysis, conjunctivitis, photosensitivity, vesiculobullous eruption (See **WARNINGS** and **PRECAUTIONS**.)
Special Senses: diplopia, nystagmus, blurred vision, disturbances of: taste, smell, hearing and equilibrium, usually reversible following discontinuation
Urinary System: anuria, polyuria, renal calculi, renal failure, interstitial nephritis, hematuria (See **WARNINGS** and **PRECAUTIONS**.)

Laboratory:
Hematopoietic: prolongation of prothrombin time
Serum chemistry: acidosis, elevation of: serum triglycerides, serum cholesterol, serum potassium, liver function tests including: GGTP, LDH, bilirubin
Urinary: albuminuria, candiduria
In clinical trials using multiple-dose therapy, opthalmologic abnormalities, including cataracts and multiple punctate lenticular opacities, have been noted in patients undergoing treatment with other quinolones. The relationship of the drugs to these events is not presently established.
CRYSTALLURIA and CYLINDRURIA HAVE BEEN REPORTED with other quinolones.

OVERDOSAGE

Information on overdosage with ofloxacin is limited. One incident of accidental overdosage has been reported. In this case, an adult female received 3 grams of ofloxacin intravenously over 45 minutes. A blood sample obtained 15 minutes after the completion of the infusion revealed an ofloxacin level of 39.3 μg/mL. In 7 h, the level had fallen to 16.2 μg/mL, and by 24 h to 2.7 μg/mL. During the infusion, the patient developed drowsiness, nausea, dizziness, hot and cold flushes, subjective facial swelling and numbness, slurring of speech, and mild to moderate disorientation. All complaints except the dizziness subsided within 1 h after discontinuation of the infusion. The dizziness, most bothersome while standing, resolved in approximately 9 h. Laboratory testing reportedly revealed no clinically significant changes in routine parameters in this patient.
In the event of an acute overdose, the stomach should be emptied. The patient should be observed and appropriate hydration maintained. Ofloxacin is not efficiently removed by hemodialysis or peritoneal dialysis.

DOSAGE AND ADMINISTRATION

The usual dose of FLOXIN (ofloxacin tablets) Tablets are 200 mg to 400 mg orally every 12 h as described in the following dosing chart. These recommendations apply to patients with normal renal function (i.e., creatinine clearance > 50 mL/min). For patients with altered renal function (i.e., creatinine clearance ≤ 50 mL/min), see the **Patients with Impaired Renal Function** subsection.

Patients with Normal Renal Function:
[See first table above.]
Antacids containing calcium, magnesium, or aluminum; sucralfate; divalent or trivalent cations such as iron; or mul-

Infection	Description*	Unit Dose	Frequency	Duration	Daily Dose
Lower Respiratory Tract	Exacerbation of Chronic Bronchitis	400 mg	q12h	10 days	800 mg
	Comm. Acquired Pneumonia	400 mg	q12h	10 days	800 mg
Skin and Skin Structures	Uncomplicated infections	400 mg	q12h	10 days	800 mg
Sexually Transmitted Diseases	Acute, uncomplicated gonorrhea	400 mg	single dose	1 day	400 mg
	Cervicitis/urethritis due to C. trachomatis	300 mg	q12h	7 days	600 mg
	Cervicitis/urethritis due to C. trachomatis and N. gonorrhoeae	300 mg	q12h	7 days	600 mg
Urinary Tract	Cystitis due to E. coli or K. pneumoniae	200 mg	q12h	3 days	400 mg
	Cystitis due to other approved pathogens	200 mg	q12h	7 days	400 mg
	Complicated UTI's	200 mg	q12h	10 days	400 mg
Prostate	Prostatitis due to E. coli	300 mg	q12h	6 weeks	600 mg

*   DUE TO THE DESIGNATED PATHOGENS (See **INDICATIONS AND USAGE**.)

Creatinine Clearance	Maintenance Dose	Frequency
10–50 mL/min	the usual recommended unit dose	q24h
<10 mL/min	1/2 the usual recommended unit dose	q24h

tivitamins containing zinc should not be taken within the two-hour period before, or within the two-hour period after ofloxacin administrations. (See **PRECAUTIONS**.)
Patients with Impaired Renal Function:
Dosage should be adjusted for patients with a creatinine clearance ≤ 50 mL/min.
After a normal initial dose, dosage should be adjusted as follows:
[See second table above.]
When only the serum creatinine is known, the following formula may be used to estimate creatinine clearance.

Men: Creatinine

$$\text{clearance (mL/min)} = \frac{\text{Weight (kg)} \times (140 - \text{age})}{72 \times \text{serum creatinine}} \quad \text{(mg/dL)}$$

Women: 0.85 × the value calculated for men.
The serum creatinine should represent a steady-state of renal function.
Patients with Cirrhosis:
The excretion of ofloxacin may be reduced in patients with severe liver function disorders (e.g., cirrhosis with or without ascites). A maximum dose of 400 mg of ofloxacin per day should therefore not be exceeded.

HOW SUPPLIED

FLOXIN (ofloxacin tablets) Tablets are supplied as 200 mg light yellow, 300 mg white, and 400 mg pale gold film-coated tablets. Each tablet is distinguished by 'FLOXIN' and the appropriate strength. FLOXIN Tablets are packaged in bottles of 50 tablets (200 mg and 300 mg), 100 tablets (400 mg), and in unit-dose blister strips of 100 tablets in the following configurations:
200 mg tablets—bottles of 50 (NDC 0062-1540-02)
200 mg tablets—unit-dose/100 tablets (NDC 0062-1540-05)
300 mg tablets—bottles of 50 (NDC 0062-1541-02)
300 mg tablets—unit-dose/100 tablets (NDC 0062-1541-05)
400 mg tablets—bottles of 100 (NDC 0062-1542-01)
400 mg tablets—unit-dose/100 tablets (NDC 0062-1542-05)
FLOXIN Tablets should be stored in well-closed containers. Store below 86°F (30°C).
Also Available:
Ofloxacin is also available for intravenous administration in the following configurations:
FLOXIN (ofloxacin injection) I.V. IN SINGLE-USE VIALS (10 mL and 20 mL) containing a concentrated solution with the equivalent of 400 mg of ofloxacin.
FLOXIN (ofloxacin injection) I.V. PRE-MIXED IN BOTTLES (100 mL) containing a dilute solution with the equivalent of 400 mg of ofloxacin in 5% Dextrose (D5W).
FLOXIN (ofloxacin injection) I.V. PRE-MIXED IN FLEXIBLE CONTAINERS (50 mL and 100 mL) containing a dilute solution with the equivalent of 200 mg or 400 mg of ofloxacin, respectively, in 5% Dextrose (D5W).

ANIMAL PHARMACOLOGY

Ofloxacin, as well as other drugs of the quinolone class, has been shown to cause arthropathies (arthrosis) in immature dogs and rats. In addition, these drugs are associated with an increased incidence of osteochondrosis in rats as compared to the incidence observed in vehicle-treated rats. (See **WARNINGS**.) There is no evidence of arthropathies in fully mature dogs at intravenous doses up to 3 times the recommended maximum human dose (on a mg/m² basis or 5 times based on mg/kg basis), for a one-week exposure period.
Long-term, high-dose systemic use of other quinolones in experimental animals has caused lenticular opacities; however, this finding was not observed in any animal studies with ofloxacin.
Reduced serum globulin and protein levels were observed in animals treated with other quinolones. In one ofloxacin study, minor decreases in serum globulin and protein levels were noted in female cynomolgus monkeys dosed orally with 40 mg/kg ofloxacin for one year. These changes, however, were considered to be within normal limits for monkeys. Crystalluria and ocular toxicity were not observed in any animals treated with ofloxacin.
Caution: Federal (U.S.A.) law prohibits dispensing without prescription.
FLOXIN® is a trademark of Ortho Pharmaceutical Corporation.
U.S. Patent No. 4,382,892

REFERENCES

1. National Committee for Clinical Laboratory Standards, Performance Standards for Antimicrobial Disk Susceptibility Tests—Fourth Edition. Approved Standard NCCLS Document M2-A4, Vol. 10, No. 7, NCCLS, Villanova, PA, 1990.
2. National Committee for Clinical Laboratory Standards, Methods for Dilution Antimicrobial Susceptibility Tests for Bacteria that Grow Aerobically—Second Edition. Approved Standard NCCLS Document M7-A2, Vol. 10, No. 8, NCCLS, Villanova, PA, 1990.

Ortho Pharmaceutical Corporation
Raritan, NJ USA 08869

McNeil Pharmaceutical
Spring House, PA USA 19477
© OPC 1987
Revised June 1994
632-10-270-1
Shown in Product Identification Guide, page 323

FLOXIN®I.V.
(ofloxacin injection)
FOR INTRAVENOUS INFUSION

℞

DESCRIPTION

FLOXIN® (ofloxacin injection) I.V. is a synthetic, broad-spectrum antimicrobial agent for intravenous administra-

tion. Chemically, ofloxacin, a fluorinated carboxyquinolone, is the racemate, $(\pm)$-9-fluoro-2,3-dihydro-3-methyl-10-(4-methyl-1-piperazinyl)-7-oxo -7H-pyrido [1,2,3-de]-1,4-benzoxazine-6-carboxylic acid. The chemical structure is:

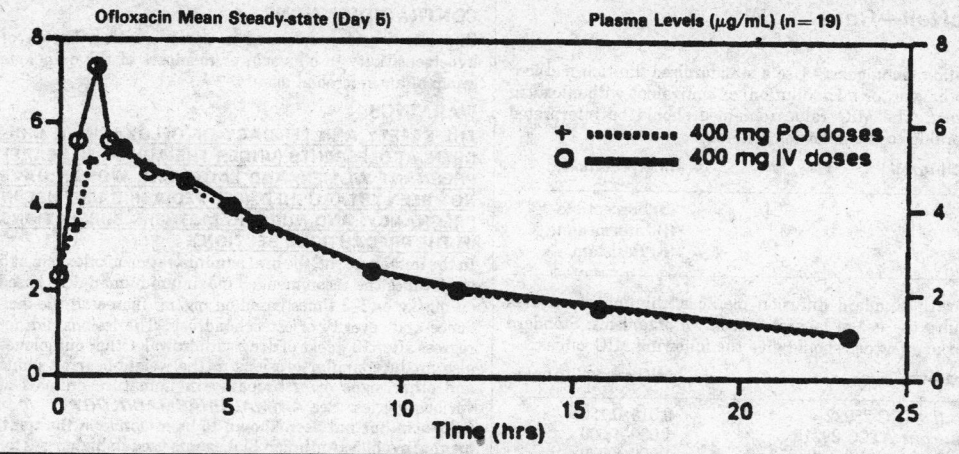

Its empirical formula is $C_{18}H_{20}FN_3O_4$, and its molecular weight is 361.4. Ofloxacin is an off-white to pale yellow crystalline powder. The relative solubility characteristics of ofloxacin at room temperature, as defined by USP nomenclature, indicate that ofloxacin is considered to be *soluble* in aqueous solutions with pH between 2 and 5. It is *sparingly* to *slightly soluble* in aqueous solutions with pH 7 and *freely soluble* in aqueous solutions with pH above 9. Ofloxacin has the potential to form stable coordination compounds with many metal ions. This *in vitro* chelation potential has the following formation order: $Fe^{+3} > Al^{+3} > Cu^{+2} > Ni^{+2} > Pb^{+2} > Zn^{+2} > Mg^{+2} > Ca^{+2} > Ba^{+2}$.

FLOXIN I.V. IN SINGLE-USE VIALS is a sterile, preservative-free aqueous solution of ofloxacin with pH ranging from 3.5 to 5.5. FLOXIN I.V. IN PRE-MIXED BOTTLES and IN PRE-MIXED FLEXIBLE CONTAINERS are sterile, preservative-free aqueous solutions of ofloxacin with pH ranging from 3.8 to 5.8. The color of FLOXIN I.V. may range from light yellow to amber. This does not adversely affect product potency. FLOXIN I.V. IN SINGLE-USE VIALS contains ofloxacin in Water for Injection. FLOXIN I.V. IN PRE-MIXED BOTTLES and IN PRE-MIXED FLEXIBLE CONTAINERS are dilute, non-pyrogenic, nearly isotonic pre-mixed solutions that contain ofloxacin in 5% Dextrose (D_5W). Hydrochloric acid and sodium hydroxide may have been added to adjust the pH.

The flexible container is fabricated from a specially formulated non-plasticized, thermoplastic copolyester (CR3). The amount of water that can permeate from the container into the overwrap is insufficient to affect the solution significantly. Solutions in contact with the flexible container can leach out certain of the container's chemical components in very small amounts within the expiration period. The suitability of the container material has been confirmed by tests in animals according to USP biological tests for plastic containers.

CLINICAL PHARMACOLOGY

Following a single 60-minute intravenous infusion of 200 mg or 400 mg of ofloxacin to normal volunteers, the mean maximum plasma concentrations attained were 2.7 and 4.0 $\mu g/mL$, respectively; the concentrations at 12 hours (h) after dosing were 0.3 and 0.7 $\mu g/mL$, respectively.

Steady-state concentrations were attained after four doses, and the area under the curve (AUC) was approximately 40% higher than the AUC after a single dose. The mean peak and trough plasma steady-state levels attained following intravenous administration of 200 mg of ofloxacin q 12 h for seven days were 2.9 and 0.5 $\mu g/mL$, respectively. Following intravenous doses of 400 mg of ofloxacin q 12 h, the mean peak and trough plasma steady-state levels ranged, in two different studies, from 5.5 to 7.2 $\mu g/mL$ and 1.2 to 1.9 $\mu g/mL$, respectively.

Following 7 days of intravenous administration, the elimination half-life of ofloxacin was 6 h (range 5 to 10 h). The total clearance and the volume of distribution were approximately 15 L/h and 120 L, respectively.

Elimination of ofloxacin is primarily by renal excretion. Approximately 65% of a dose is excreted renally within 48 h. Studies indicate that <5% of an administered dose is recovered in the urine as the desmethyl or N-oxide metabolites. Four to eight percent of an ofloxacin dose is excreted in the feces. This indicates a small degree of biliary excretion of ofloxacin.

In vitro, approximately 32% of the drug in plasma is protein bound.

The single dose and steady-state plasma profiles of ofloxacin injection were comparable in extent of exposure (AUC) to those of ofloxacin tablets when the injectable and tablet formulations of ofloxacin were administered in equal doses (mg/mg). The mean $AUC_{(0-12)}$ attained after the intravenous administration of 400 mg over 60 min was 43.5 $\mu g \cdot h/mL$; the mean $AUC_{(0-12)}$ attained after the oral administration of 400 mg was 41.2 $\mu g \cdot h/mL$ (two one-sided t-test, 90% confidence interval was 103–109). [See following chart.]

[See graph above.]

Between 0 and 6 h following the administration of a single 200 mg oral dose of ofloxacin to 12 healthy volunteers, the average urine ofloxacin concentration was approximately 220 $\mu g/mL$. Between 12 and 24 h after administration, the average urine ofloxacin level was approximately 34 $\mu g/mL$. Following oral administration of recommended therapeutic doses, ofloxacin has been detected in blister fluid, cervix, lung tissue, ovary, prostatic fluid, prostatic tissue, skin, and

sputum. The mean concentration of ofloxacin in each of these various body fluids and tissues after one or more doses was 0.8 to 1.5 times the concurrent plasma level. Inadequate data are presently available on the distribution or levels of ofloxacin in the cerebrospinal fluid or brain tissue.

Following the administration of oral doses of ofloxacin to healthy elderly volunteers (64–74 years of age) with normal renal function, the apparent half-life of ofloxacin was 7 to 8 h, as compared to approximately 6 h in younger adults. Clearance of ofloxacin is reduced in patients with impaired renal function (creatinine clearance ≤ 50 mL/min), and dosage adjustment is necessary. (See *PRECAUTIONS: General* and *DOSAGE AND ADMINISTRATION*.)

MICROBIOLOGY

Ofloxacin has *in vitro* activity against a broad-spectrum of gram-positive and gram-negative aerobic and anaerobic bacteria. Ofloxacin is often bactericidal at concentrations equal to or slightly greater than inhibitory concentrations. Ofloxacin is thought to exert a bactericidal effect on susceptible microorganisms by inhibiting DNA gyrase, an essential enzyme that is a critical catalyst in the duplication, transcription, and repair of bacterial DNA.

Ofloxacin has been shown to be active against most strains of the following organisms both *in vitro* and in specific clinical infections: (See *INDICATIONS AND USAGE*.)

Chlamydia trachomatis
Citrobacter diversus
Enterobacter aerogenes
Escherichia coli
Haemophilus influenzae
Klebsiella pneumoniae
Neisseria gonorrhoeae
Proteus mirabilis
Pseudomonas aeruginosa
Staphylococcus aureus
Streptococcus pneumoniae
Streptococcus pyogenes

The following *in vitro* data are available; **however, their clinical significance is unknown.**

Ofloxacin exhibits *in vitro* minimum inhibitory concentrations of 2 $\mu g/mL$ or less against most strains of the following organisms; however, the safety and effectiveness of ofloxacin in treating clinical infections due to these organisms have not been established in adequate and well-controlled trials:

Gram-positive aerobes
Enterococcus faecalis
Staphylococcus epidermidis (including methicillin-resistant strains)
Staphylococcus saprophyticus
Streptococcus agalactiae (Group B)
Gram-negative aerobes
Acinetobacter calcoaceticus
Aeromonas hydrophila
Bordetella parapertussis
Bordetella pertussis
Campylobacter jejuni
Citrobacter freundii
Enterobacter cloacae
Haemophilus ducreyi
Klebsiella oxytoca
Moraxella (Branhamella) catarrhalis
Morganella morganii
Neisseria meningitidis
Plesiomonas shigelloides
Proteus vulgaris
Providencia rettgeri
Providencia stuartii
Pseudomonas fluorescens
Serratia marcescens
Anaerobes
Bacteroides fragilis
Bacteroides intermedius

Clostridium perfringens
Clostridium welchii
Eikenella corrodens
Gardnerella vaginalis
Peptococcus niger
Peptostreptococcus species
Other organisms
Chlamydia pneumoniae
Legionella pneumophila
Mycobacterium tuberculosis
Mycoplasma hominis
Mycoplasma pneumoniae
Ureaplasma urealyticum

Many strains of other streptococcal species, *Enterococcus* species, and anaerobes are resistant to ofloxacin.

Ofloxacin has not been shown to be active against *Treponema pallidum*. (See *WARNINGS*.)

Resistance to ofloxacin due to spontaneous mutation *in vitro* is a rare occurrence (range: 10^{-9} to 10^{-11}). To date, emergence of resistance has been relatively uncommon in clinical practice. With the exception of *Pseudomonas aeruginosa* (10%), less than a 4% rate of resistance emergence has been reported for most other species. Although cross-resistance has been observed between ofloxacin and other fluoroquinolones, some organisms resistant to other quinolones may be susceptible to ofloxacin.

SUSCEPTIBILITY TESTS

Diffusion techniques: Quantitative methods that require measurement of zone diameters give the most precise estimate of the susceptibility of bacteria to antimicrobial agents. One such standardized procedure[1] that has been recommended for use with disks to test the susceptibility of organisms to ofloxacin uses the 5-μg ofloxacin disk. Interpretation involves correlation of the diameter obtained in the disk test with the minimum inhibitory concentration (MIC) for ofloxacin.

Reports from the laboratory giving results of the standard single-disk susceptibility test with a 5-μg ofloxacin disk should be interpreted according to the following criteria:

Zone diameter (mm)	Interpretation
≥ 16	Susceptible
13–15	Intermediate
≤ 12	Resistant

A report of "Susceptible" indicates that the pathogen is likely to be inhibited by generally achievable drug concentrations. A report of "Intermediate" indicates that the result should be considered equivocal, and, if the organism is not fully susceptible to alternative, clinically feasible drugs, the test should be repeated. This category provides a buffer zone that prevents small uncontrolled technical factors from causing major discrepancies in interpretation. A report of "Resistant" indicates that achievable drug concentrations are unlikely to be inhibitory, and other therapy should be selected.

Standardized susceptibility test procedures require the use of laboratory control organisms. The 5-μg ofloxacin disk should give the following zone diameters:

Organism	Zone diameter (mm)
E. coli ATCC 25922	29–33
P. aeruginosa ATCC 27853	17–21
S. aureus ATCC 25923	24–28

Continued on next page

Information on McNeil Pharmaceutical Products is based on labeling in effect in August 1996.

McNeil—Cont.

Dilution techniques: Use a standardized dilution method[2] (broth, agar, or microdilution) or equivalent with ofloxacin powder. The MIC values obtained should be interpreted according to the following criteria:

MIC (µg/mL)	Interpretation
≤2	(S) Susceptible
4	(I) Intermediate
≥8	(R) Resistant

As with standard diffusion methods, dilution procedures require the use of laboratory control organisms. Standard ofloxacin powder should give the following MIC values:

Organism	MIC range (µg/mL)
E. coli ATCC 25922	0.015–0.120
E. faecalis ATCC 29212	1.000–4.000
P. aeruginosa ATCC 27853	1.000–8.000
S. aureus ATCC 25923	0.120–1.000

INDICATIONS AND USAGE

FLOXIN (ofloxacin injection) I.V. is indicated for the treatment of adults with mild to moderate infections caused by susceptible strains of the designated microorganisms in the infections listed below—when intravenous administration offers a route of administration advantageous to the patient, (*i.e.,* patient cannot tolerate an oral dosage form, etc.).

The safety and effectiveness of the intravenous formulation in treating patients with severe infections have not been established.

NOTE: IN THE ABSENCE OF VOMITING OR OTHER FACTORS INTERFERING WITH THE ABSORPTION OF ORALLY ADMINISTERED DRUG, PATIENTS RECEIVE ESSENTIALLY THE SAME SYSTEMIC ANTIMICROBIAL THERAPY AFTER EQUIVALENT DOSES OF OFLOXACIN ADMINISTERED BY EITHER THE ORAL OR THE INTRAVENOUS ROUTE. THEREFORE, THE INTRAVENOUS FORMULATION DOES NOT PROVIDE A HIGHER DEGREE OF EFFICACY OR MORE POTENT ANTIMICROBIAL ACTIVITY THAN AN EQUIVALENT DOSE OF THE ORAL FORMULATION OF OFLOXACIN.

Lower Respiratory Tract

Acute bacterial exacerbation of chronic bronchitis due to *Haemophilus influenzae* or *Streptococcus pneumoniae.*

Community-acquired Pneumonia due to *Haemophilus influenzae* or *Streptococcus pneumoniae.*

Skin and Skin Structures

Uncomplicated skin and skin structure infections due to *Staphylococcus aureus, Streptococcus pyogenes,* or *Proteus mirabilis.**

Sexually Transmitted Diseases (See ***WARNINGS.***)

Acute, uncomplicated urethral and cervical gonorrhea due to *Neisseria gonorrhoeae.*

Nongonococcal urethritis and cervicitis due to *Chlamydia trachomatis.*

Mixed infections of the urethra and cervix due to *Chlamydia trachomatis* and *Neisseria gonorrhoeae.*

Urinary Tract

Uncomplicated cystitis due to *Citrobacter diversus, Enterobacter aerogenes, Escherichia coli, Klebsiella pneumoniae, Proteus mirabilis,* or *Pseudomonas aeruginosa.*

Complicated urinary tract infections due to *Escherichia coli, Klebsiella pneumoniae, Proteus mirabilis, Citrobacter diversus**, or *Pseudomonas aeruginosa**.

Prostate

Prostatitis due to *Escherichia coli.*

*= Although treatment of infections due to this organism in this infection demonstrated a clinically acceptable overall outcome, efficacy was demonstrated in fewer than 10 infections.

Appropriate culture and susceptibility tests should be performed before treatment in order to isolate and identify organisms causing the infection and to determine their susceptibility to ofloxacin. Therapy with ofloxacin may be initiated before results of these tests are known; once results become available, appropriate therapy should be continued.
As with other drugs in this class, some strains of *Pseudomonas aeruginosa* may develop resistance fairly rapidly during treatment with ofloxacin. Culture and susceptibility testing performed periodically during therapy will provide information not only on the therapeutic effect of the antimicrobial agent but also on the possible emergence of bacterial resistance.
If anaerobic organisms are suspected of contributing to the infection, appropriate therapy for anaerobic pathogens should be administered.

CONTRAINDICATIONS

Ofloxacin is contraindicated in persons with a history of hypersensitivity to ofloxacin or members of the quinolone group of antimicrobial agents.

WARNINGS

THE SAFETY AND EFFICACY OF OFLOXACIN IN CHILDREN, ADOLESCENTS (UNDER THE AGE OF 18 YEARS), PREGNANT WOMEN, AND LACTATING WOMEN HAVE NOT BEEN ESTABLISHED. (SEE PEDIATRIC USE, USE IN PREGNANCY, AND NURSING MOTHERS SUBSECTIONS IN THE PRECAUTIONS SECTION.)

In the immature rat, the oral administration of ofloxacin at 5 to 16 times the recommended maximum human dose based on mg/kg or 1–3 times based on mg/m^2 increased the incidence and severity of osteochondrosis. The lesions did not regress after 13 weeks of drug withdrawal. Other quinolones also produce similar erosions in the weight-bearing joints and other signs of arthropathy in immature animals of various species. (See ***ANIMAL PHARMACOLOGY.***)

Ofloxacin has not been shown to be effective in the treatment of syphilis. Antimicrobial agents used in high doses for short periods of time to treat gonorrhea may mask or delay the symptoms of incubating syphilis. All patients with gonorrhea should have a serologic test for syphilis at the time of diagnosis. Patients treated with ofloxacin should have a follow-up serologic test for syphilis after three months.

Serious and occasionally fatal hypersensitivity (anaphylactic/anaphylactoid) reactions, have been reported in patients receiving therapy with quinolones, including ofloxacin. These reactions often occur following the first dose. Some reactions were accompanied by cardiovascular collapse, hypotension/shock, seizure, loss of consciousness, tingling, angioedema (including tongue, laryngeal, throat or facial edema/swelling, etc.), airway obstruction (including bronchospasm, shortness of breath and acute respiratory distress), dyspnea, urticaria/hives, itching, and other serious skin reactions. A few patients had a history of hypersensitivity reactions. The drug should be discontinued immediately at the first appearance of a skin rash or any other sign of hypersensitivity. Serious acute hypersensitivity reactions may require treatment with epinephrine and other resuscitative measures, including oxygen, intravenous fluids, antihistamines, corticosteroids, pressor amines, and airway management, as clinically indicated. (See ***PRECAUTIONS*** and ***ADVERSE REACTIONS.***)

Serious and sometimes fatal events of uncertain etiology have been reported in patients receiving therapy with quinolones including, extremely rarely, ofloxacin. These events may be severe and generally occur following the administration of multiple doses. Clinical manifestations may include one or more of the following: fever, rash or severe dermatologic reactions (e.g., toxic epidermal necrolysis, Stevens-Johnson Syndrome, etc.); vasculitis, arthralgia, myalgia, serum sickness; allergic pneumonitis; interstitial nephritis, acute renal insufficiency/failure; hepatitis, jaundice, acute hepatic necrosis/failure; anemia including hemolytic and aplastic, thrombocytopenia, including thrombotic thrombocytopenic purpura, leukopenia, agranulocytosis, pancytopenia, and/or other hematologic abnormalities. The drug should be discontinued immediately at the first appearance of a skin rash or any other sign of hypersensitivity and supportive measures instituted. (See ***PRECAUTIONS: Information for Patients*** and ***ADVERSE REACTIONS.***)

Convulsions, increased intracranial pressure, and toxic psychosis have been reported in patients receiving quinolones, including ofloxacin. Quinolones, including ofloxacin, may also cause central nervous system stimulation which may lead to: tremors, restlessness/agitation, nervousness/anxiety, lightheadedness, confusion, hallucinations, paranoia and depression, nightmares, insomnia, and rarely suicidal thoughts or acts. These reactions may occur following the first dose. If these reactions occur in patients receiving ofloxacin, the drug should be discontinued and appropriate measures instituted. As with all quinolones, ofloxacin should be used with caution in patients with a known or suspected CNS disorder that may predispose to seizures or lower the seizure threshold (e.g., severe cerebral arteriosclerosis, epilepsy, etc.) or in the presence of other risk factors that may predispose to seizures or lower the seizure threshold (e.g., certain drug therapy, renal dysfunction, etc.). (See ***PRECAUTIONS: General, Drug Interactions*** and ***ADVERSE REACTIONS.***)

Pseudomembranous colitis has been reported with nearly all antibacterial agents, including ofloxacin, and may range in severity from mild to life-threatening. Therefore, it is important to consider this diagnosis in patients who present with diarrhea subsequent to the administration of any antibacterial agent.

Treatment with antibacterial agents alters the normal flora of the colon and may permit overgrowth of clostridia. Studies indicate a toxin produced by *Clostridium difficile* is one primary cause of "antibiotic-associated colitis".

After the diagnosis of pseudomembranous colitis has been established, therapeutic measures should be initiated. Mild cases of pseudomembranous colitis usually respond to drug discontinuation alone. In moderate to severe cases, consideration should be given to management with fluids and electrolytes, protein supplementation, and treatment with an oral antibacterial drug clinically effective against *C. difficile* colitis. (See ***ADVERSE REACTIONS.***)

PRECAUTIONS

General:

Because a rapid or bolus intravenous injection may result in hypotension, **OFLOXACIN INJECTION SHOULD ONLY BE ADMINISTERED BY SLOW INTRAVENOUS INFUSION OVER A PERIOD OF 60 MINUTES.** (See ***DOSAGE AND ADMINISTRATION.***)

Adequate hydration of patients receiving ofloxacin should be maintained to prevent the formation of a highly concentrated urine.

Administer ofloxacin with caution in the presence of renal or hepatic insufficiency/impairment. In patients with known or suspected renal or hepatic insufficiency/impairment, careful clinical observation and appropriate laboratory studies should be performed prior to and during therapy since elimination of ofloxacin may be reduced. In patients with impaired renal function (creatinine clearance ≤ 50 mg/mL), alteration of the dosage regimen is necessary. (See ***CLINICAL PHARMACOLOGY*** and ***DOSAGE AND ADMINISTRATION.***)

Moderate to severe phototoxicity reactions have been observed in patients exposed to direct sunlight while receiving some drugs in this class, including ofloxacin. Excessive sunlight should be avoided. Therapy should be discontinued if phototoxicity (e.g., a skin eruption, etc.) occurs.

As with all quinolones, ofloxacin should be used with caution in any patient with a known or suspected CNS disorder that may predispose to seizures or lower the seizure threshold (e.g., severe cerebral arteriosclerosis, epilepsy, etc.) or in the presence of other risk factors that may predispose to seizures or lower the seizure threshold (e.g., certain drug therapy, renal dysfunction, etc.). (See ***WARNINGS*** and ***Drug Interactions.***)

As with other quinolones, disturbances of blood glucose, including symptomatic hyper- and hypoglycemia, have been reported, usually in diabetic patients receiving concomitant treatment with an oral hypoglycemic agent (e.g., glyburide/glibenclamide, etc.) or with insulin. In these patients careful monitoring of blood glucose is recommended. If a hypoglycemic reaction occurs in a patient being treated with ofloxacin, discontinue ofloxacin immediately and consult a physician. (See ***Drug Interactions*** and ***ADVERSE REACTIONS.***)

As with any potent drug, periodic assessment of organ system functions, including renal, hepatic, and hematopoietic, is advisable during prolonged therapy. (See ***WARNINGS*** and ***ADVERSE REACTIONS.***)

Information for Patients:

Patients should be advised:

—to drink fluids liberally if able to take fluids by the oral route.

—that ofloxacin may cause neurologic adverse effects (e.g., dizziness, lightheadedness, etc.) and that patients should know how they react to ofloxacin before they operate an automobile or machinery or engage in activities requiring mental alertness and coordination. (See ***WARNINGS*** and ***ADVERSE REACTIONS.***)

—that ofloxacin may be associated with hypersensitivity reactions, even following the first dose, to discontinue the drug at the first sign of a skin rash, hives or other skin reactions, a rapid heartbeat, difficulty in swallowing or breathing, any swelling suggesting angioedema (e.g., swelling of the lips, tongue, face; tightness of the throat, hoarseness, etc.), or any other symptom of an allergic reaction. (See ***WARNINGS*** and ***ADVERSE REACTIONS.***)

—to avoid excessive sunlight or artificial ultraviolet light while receiving ofloxacin and to discontinue therapy if phototoxicity (e.g., skin eruption, etc.) occurs.

—that if they are diabetic and are being treated with insulin or an oral hypoglycemic agent, to discontinue ofloxacin immediately if a hypoglycemic reaction occurs and consult a physician. (See ***PRECAUTIONS: General*** and ***Drug Interactions.***)

Drug Interactions:

Antacids, Sucralfate, Metal Cations, Multi-Vitamins: There are no data concerning an interaction of **intravenous** quinolones with **oral** antacids, sucralfate, multi-vitamins, or metal cations. However, no quinolone should be co-administered with any solution containing multivalent cations, e.g., magnesium, through the same intravenous line. (See ***DOSAGE AND ADMINISTRATION.***)

Caffeine: Interactions between ofloxacin and caffeine have not been detected.

Cimetidine: Cimetidine has demonstrated interference with the elimination of some quinolones. This interference has resulted in significant increases in half-life and AUC of some quinolones. The potential for interaction between ofloxacin and cimetidine has not been studied.

Cyclosporine: Elevated serum levels of cyclosporine have been reported with concomitant use of cyclosporine with

some other quinolones. The potential for interaction between ofloxacin and cyclosporine has not been studied.
Drugs metabolized by Cytochrome P450 enzymes: Most quinolone antimicrobial drugs inhibit cytochrome P450 enzyme activity. This may result in a proloned half-life for some drugs that are also metabolized by this system (e.g., cyclosporine, theophylline/methylxanthines, warfarin, etc.) when co-administered with quinolones. The extent of this inhibition varies among different quinolones. (See other ***Drug Interactions.***)
Non-steroidal anti-inflammatory drugs: The concomitant administration of a non-steroidal anti-inflammatory drug, with a quinolone, including ofloxacin, may increase the risk of CNS stimulation and convulsive seizures. (See ***WARNINGS*** and ***PRECAUTIONS: General.***)
Probenecid: The concomitant use of probenecid with certain other quinolones has been reported to affect renal tubular secretion. The effect of probenecid on the elimination of ofloxacin has not been studied.
Theophylline: Although concurrent administration of some quinolones with theophylline may result in impaired elimination of theophylline, the extent of such impairment varies among different quinolones. Steady-state theophylline levels may increase when ofloxacin and theophylline are administered concurrently. In a pharmacokinetic study involving 15 healthy male subjects, steady-state peak theophylline concentration increased by an average of approximately 9%, and the AUC increased by an average of approximately 13% when oral ofloxacin and theophylline were administered concurrently. In clinical trials with intravenous ofloxacin, theophylline concentrations were determined in 41 patients who were treated with both drugs. In 38 patients, no apparent elevation in the serum theophylline was discernible. Marginal increases above the theophylline therapeutic range were reported in three patients; clinical toxicity was, however, not reported in these three patients. Generally, patients receiving theophylline in clinical trials of the intravenous formulation of ofloxacin reported nausea more frequently than those patients not receiving theophylline. As with some other quinolones, concomitant administration of ofloxacin may prolong the half-life of theophylline, elevate serum theophylline levels, and may increase the risk of theophylline-related adverse reactions. Theophylline levels should be closely monitored and theophylline dosage adjustments made, if appropriate, when ofloxacin is co-administered.
Warfarin: Some quinolones have been reported to enhance the effects of the oral anticoagulant warfarin or its derivatives. Therefore, if a quinolone antimicrobial is administered concomitantly with warfarin or its derivatives, the prothrombin time or other suitable coagulation test should be closely monitored.
Antidiabetic Agents (e.g., insulin, glyburide/glibenclamide, etc.): Since disturbances of blood glucose, including hyperglycemia and hypoglycemia, have been reported in patients treated concurrently with quinolones and an antidiabetic agent, careful monitoring of blood glucose is recommended when these agents are used concomitantly. (See ***PRECAUTIONS: General and Information for Patients.***)

Carcinogenesis, Mutagenesis, Impairment of Fertility:
Long-term studies to determine the carcinogenic potential of ofloxacin have not been conducted.
Ofloxacin was not mutagenic in the Ames bacterial test, *in vitro* and *in vivo* cytogenetic assay, sister chromatid exchange (Chinese Hamster and Human Cell Lines), unscheduled DNA Repair (UDS) using human fibroblasts, dominant lethal assays, or mouse micronucleus assay. Ofloxacin was positive in the UDS test using rat hepatocytes and Mouse Lymphoma Assay.

Pregnancy: Teratogenic Effects. Pregnancy Category C.
Ofloxacin has not been shown to have any teratogenic effects at oral doses as high as 810 mg/kg/day (11 times the recommended maximum human dose based on mg/m^2 or 50 times based on mg/kg) and 160 mg/kg/day (4 times the recommended maximum human dose based on mg/m^2 or 10 times based on mg/kg) when administered to pregnant rats and rabbits, respectively. Additional studies in rats with oral doses up to 360 mg/kg/day (5 times the recommended maximum human dose based on mg/m^2 or 23 times based on mg/kg) demonstrated no adverse effect on late fetal development, labor, delivery, lactation, neonatal viability, or growth of the newborn. Doses equivalent to 50 and 10 times the recommended maximum human dose of ofloxacin (based on mg/kg) were fetotoxic (i.e., decreased fetal body weight and increased fetal mortality) in rats and rabbits, respectively. Minor skeletal variations were reported in rats receiving doses of 810 mg/kg/day, which is more than 10 times higher than the recommended maximum human dose based on mg/m^2.
There are, however, no adequate and well-controlled studies in pregnant women. Ofloxacin should be used during pregnancy only if the potential benefit justifies the potential risk to the fetus. (See ***WARNINGS.***)

Nursing Mothers:
In lactating females, a single oral 200-mg dose of ofloxacin resulted in concentrations of ofloxacin in milk that were similar to those found in plasma. Because of the potential for serious adverse reactions from ofloxacin in nursing infants, a decision should be made whether to discontinue nursing or to discontinue the drug, taking into account the importance of the drug to the mother. (See ***WARNINGS*** and ***ADVERSE REACTIONS.***)

Pediatric Use:
Safety and effectiveness in children and adolescents below the age of 18 years have not been established. Ofloxacin causes arthropathy (arthrosis) and osteochondrosis in juvenile animals of several species. (See ***WARNINGS.***)

ADVERSE REACTIONS

The following is a compilation of the data for ofloxacin based on clinical experience with both the oral and intravenous formulations. The incidence of drug-related adverse reactions in patients during Phase 2 and 3 clinical trials was 11%. Among patients receiving multiple-dose therapy, 4% discontinued ofloxacin due to adverse experiences.
In clinical trials, the following events were considered likely to be drug-related in patients receiving multiple doses of ofloxacin:
nausea 3%, insomnia 3%, headache 1%, dizziness 1%, diarrhea 1%, vomiting 1%, rash 1%, pruritus 1%, external genital pruritus in women 1%, vaginitis 1%, dysgeusia 1%.
Local injection site reactions (phlebitis, swelling, erythema) were reported in approximately 2% of patients treated with the 3.63 mg/mL final infusion concentration of intravenous ofloxacin used in the clnical safety trials. The final infusion concentration of intravenous ofloxacin in the commercially available intravenous preparations is 4.0 mg/mL. To date, individuals administered the 4.0 mg/mL concentration of the intravenous ofloxacin have demonstrated clinically acceptable rates of local injection site reactions. Due to the small difference in concentration, significant differences in local site reactions are unexpected with the 4.0 mg/mL concentration.
In clinical trials, the most frequently reported adverse events, regardless of relationship to drug, were:
nausea 10%, headache 9%, insomnia 7%, external genital pruritus in women 6%, dizziness 5%, vaginitis 5%, diarrhea 4%, vomiting 4%.
In clinical trials, the following events, regardless of relationship to drug occurred in 1 to 3% of patients:
Abdominal pain and cramps, chest pain, decreased appetite, dry mouth, dysgeusia, fatigue, flatulence, gastrointestinal distress, nervousness, pharyngitis, pruritus, fever, rash, sleep disorders, somnolence, trunk pain, vaginal discharge, visual disturbances, and constipation.
Additional events, occurring in clinical trials at a rate of less than 1%, regardless of relationship to drug, were:
Body as a whole: asthenia, chills, malaise, extremity pain, pain, epistaxis
Cardiovascular System: cardiac arrest, edema, hypertension, hypotension, palpitations, vasodilation
Gastrointestinal System: dyspepsia
Genital/Reproductive System: burning, irritation, pain and rash of the female genitalia; dysmenorrhea; menorrhagia; metrorrhagia
Musculoskeletal System: arthralgia, myalgia
Nervous System: seizures, anxiety, cognitive change, depression, dream abnormality, euphoria, hallucinations, paresthesia, syncope, vertigo, tremor, confusion
Nutritional/Metabolic: thirst, weight loss
Respiratory System: respiratory arrest, cough, rhinorrhea
Skin/Hypersensitivity: angioedema, diaphoresis, urticaria, vasculitis
Special Senses: decreased hearing acuity, tinnitus, photophobia
Urinary System: dysuria, urinary frequency, urinary retention
The following laboratory abnormalities appeared in $\geq 1.0\%$ of patients receiving multiple doses of ofloxacin. It is not known whether these abnormalities were caused by the drug or the underlying conditions being treated.
Hematopoietic: anemia, leukopenia, leukocytosis, neutropenia, neutrophilia, increased band forms, lymphocytopenia, eosinophilia, lymphocytosis, thrombocytopenia, thrombocytosis, elevated ESR
Hepatic: elevated: alkaline phosphatase, AST (SGOT), ALT (SGPT)
Serum chemistry: hyperglycemia, hypoglycemia, elevated creatinine, elevated BUN
Urinary: glucosuria, proteinuria, alkalinuria, hyposthenuria, hematuria, pyuria

Post-Marketing Adverse Events:
Additional adverse events, regardless of relationship to drug, reported from worldwide marketing experience with quinolones, including ofloxacin:
<u>Clinical:</u>
Cardiovascular System: cerebral thrombosis, pulmonary edema, tachycardia, hypotension/shock, syncope
Endocrine/Metabolic: hyper- or hypoglycemia, especially in diabetic patients on insulin or oral hypoglycemic agents (See ***PRECAUTIONS: General*** and ***Drug Interactions.***)
Gastrointestinal System: hepatic dysfunction including: hepatic necrosis, jaundice (cholestatic or hepatocellular), hepatitis; intestinal perforation; pseudomembranous colitis, GI hemmorrhage; hiccough, painful oral mucosa, pyrosis (See ***WARNINGS.***)
Genitourinary System: vaginal candidiasis
Hematopoietic: anemia, including hemolytic and aplastic; hemorrhage, pancytopenia, agranulocytosis, leukopenia, reversible bone marrow depression, thrombocytopenia, thrombotic thrombocytopenic purpura, petechiae, ecchymosis/bruising (See ***WARNINGS.***)
Musculoskeletal: tendinitis/rupture: weakness
Nervous System: nightmares; suicidal thoughts or acts, disorientation, psychotic reactions, paranoia; phobia, agitation, restlessness, aggressiveness/hostility, manic reaction, emotional lability; peripheral neuropathy, ataxia, incoordination; possible exacerbation of: myasthenia gravis and extrapyramidal disorders; dysphasia, lightheadedness (See ***WARNINGS*** and ***PRECAUTIONS.***)
Respiratory System: dyspnea, bronchospasm, allergic pneumonitis, stridor (See ***WARNINGS.***)
Skin/Hypersensitivity: anaphylactic (-toid) reactions/shock; purpura, serum sickness, erythema multiforme/Stevens-Johnson syndrome, erythema nodosum, exfoliative dermatitis, hyperpigmentation, toxic epidermal necrolysis, conjunctivitis, photosensitivity, vesiculobullous eruption (See ***WARNINGS*** and ***PRECAUTIONS.***)
Special Senses: diplopia, nystagmus, blurred vision, disturbances of: taste, smell, hearing and equilibrium, usually reversible following discontinuation
Urinary System: anuria, polyuria, renal calculi, renal failure, interstitial nephritis, hematuria (See ***WARNINGS*** and ***PRECAUTIONS.***)
<u>Laboratory:</u>
Hematopoietic: prolongation of prothrombin time
Serum chemistry: acidosis, elevation of: serum triglycerides, serum cholesterol, serum potassium, liver function tests including: GGTP, LDH, bilirubin.
Urinary: albuminuria, candiduria
In clinical trials using multiple-dose therapy, ophthalmologic abnormalities, including cataracts and multiple punctate lenticular opacities, have been noted in patients undergoing treatment with other quinolones. The relationship of the drugs to these events is not presently established.
CRYSTALLURIA and CYLINDRURIA HAVE BEEN REPORTED with other quinolones.

OVERDOSAGE

Information on overdosage with ofloxacin is limited. One incident of accidental overdosage has been reported. In this case, an adult female received 3 grams of ofloxacin intravenously over 45 minutes. A blood sample obtained 15 minutes after the completion of the infusion revealed an ofloxacin level of 39.3 μg/mL. In 7 h, the level had fallen to 16.2 μg/mL, and by 24 h to 2.7 μg/mL. During the infusion, the patient developed drowsiness, nausea, dizziness, hot and cold flushes, subjective facial swelling and numbness, slurring of speech, and mild to moderate disorientation. All complaints except the dizziness subsided within 1 h after discontinuation of the infusion. The dizziness, most bothersome while standing, resolved in approximately 9 h. Laboratory testing reportedly revealed no clinically significant changes in routine parameters in this patient.
In the event of acute overdose, the patient should be observed and appropriate hydration maintained. Ofloxacin is not efficiently removed by hemodialysis or peritoneal dialysis.

DOSAGE AND ADMINISTRATION

FLOXIN I.V. should only be administered by **intravenous** infusion. It is not for intramuscular, intrathecal, intraperitoneal, or subcutaneous administration.

CAUTION: RAPID OR BOLUS INTRAVENOUS INFUSION MUST BE AVOIDED. Ofloxacin injection should be infused intravenously slowly over a period of not less than 60 minutes. (See ***PRECAUTIONS.***)

Single-use vials require dilution prior to administration. (See ***PREPARATION FOR ADMINISTRATION.***)
The usual dose of FLOXIN (ofloxacin injection) I.V. is 200 mg to 400 mg administered by slow infusion over 60 minutes every 12 h as described in the following dosing chart. These recommendations apply to patients with mild to moderate infection and normal renal function (i.e., creatinine clearance > 50 mL/min). For patients with altered renal function (i.e., creatinine clearance ≤ 50 mL/min), see the ***Patients with Impaired Renal Function*** subsection.

Continued on next page

Information on McNeil Pharmaceutical Products is based on labeling in effect in August 1996.

Consult 1997 supplements and future editions for revisions

McNeil—Cont.

Patients with Normal Renal Function:
[See first table at right.]

Patients with Impaired Renal Function:
Dosage should be adjusted for patients with a creatinine clearance ≤50 mL/min.

After a normal initial dose, dosage should be adjusted as follows:
[See second table at right.]

When only the serum creatinine is known, the following formula may be used to estimate creatinine clearance.

Men: Creatinine clearance (mL/min) =

$$\frac{\text{Weight (kg)} \times (140\text{-age})}{72 \times \text{serum creatinine (mg/dL)}}$$

Women: 0.85 × the value calculated for men.

The serum creatinine should represent a steady-state of renal function.

Patients with Cirrhosis:
The excretion of ofloxacin may be reduced in patients with severe liver function disorders (e.g., cirrhosis with or without ascites). A maximum dose of 400 mg of ofloxacin per day should therefore not be exceeded.

PREPARATION OF OFLOXACIN INJECTION FOR ADMINISTRATION

FLOXIN I.V. IN SINGLE-USE VIALS:
FLOXIN I.V. is supplied in single-use vials containing a concentrated ofloxacin solution with the equivalent of 400 mg of ofloxacin in Water for Injection. The 10 mL vials contain 40 mg of ofloxacin/mL, and the 20 mL vials contain 20 mg of ofloxacin/mL. **THESE FLOXIN I.V. SINGLE-USE VIALS MUST BE FURTHER DILUTED WITH AN APPROPRIATE SOLUTION PRIOR TO INTRAVENOUS ADMINISTRATION. (See *COMPATIBLE INTRAVENOUS SOLUTIONS*.)** The concentration of the resulting diluted solution should be 4 mg/mL prior to administration.

This parenteral drug product should be inspected visually for discoloration and particulate matter prior to administration.

Since no preservative or bacteriostatic agent is present in this product, aseptic technique must be used in preparation of the final parenteral solution. Since the vials are for single-use only, any unused portion should be discarded.

Since only limited data are available on the compatibility of ofloxacin intravenous injection with other intravenous substances, **additives or other medications should not be added to FLOXIN I.V. in single-use vials or infused simultaneously through the same intravenous line.** If the same intravenous line is used for sequential infusion of several different drugs, the line should be flushed before and after infusion of FLOXIN I.V. with an infusion solution compatible with FLOXIN I.V. and with any other drug(s) administered via this common line.

Prepare the desired dosage of ofloxacin according to the following chart: [See third table at right.]

For example, to prepare a 200-mg dose using the 10 mL vial (40 mg/mL), withdraw 5 mL and dilute with a compatible intravenous solution to a total volume of 50 mL.

Compatible Intravenous Solutions:
Any of the following intravenous solutions may be used to prepare a 4 mg/mL ofloxacin solution with the approximate pH values: [See fourth table at right.]

FLOXIN I.V. PRE-MIXED IN SINGLE-USE BOTTLES:
FLOXIN I.V. is also supplied in 100 mL bottles containing a pre-mixed, ready-to-use ofloxacin solution in D₅W for single-use. **NO FURTHER DILUTION OF THIS PREPARATION IS NECESSARY. Each 100 mL pre-mixed bottle already contains a dilute solution with the equivalent of 400 mg of ofloxacin (4 mg/mL) in 5% Dextrose (D₅W).**

This parenteral drug product should be inspected visually for discoloration and particulate matter prior to administration.

Since no preservative or bacteriostatic agent is present in this product, aseptic technique must be used in preparation of the final parenteral solution. **Since the pre-mixed bottles are for single-use only, any unused portion should be discarded.**

Since only limited data are available on the compatibility of ofloxacin intravenous injection with other intravenous substances, **additives or other medications should not be added to FLOXIN I.V. in pre-mixed single-use bottles or infused simultaneously through the same intravenous line.** If the same intravenous line is used for sequential infusion of several different drugs, the line should be flushed before and after infusion of FLOXIN I.V. with an infusion solution compatible with FLOXIN I.V. and with any other drug(s) administered via this common line.

FLOXIN I.V. PRE-MIXED IN SINGLE-USE FLEXIBLE CONTAINERS:
FLOXIN I.V. is also supplied in 50 mL and 100 mL flexible containers containing a pre-mixed, ready-to-use ofloxacin solution in D₅W for single-use. **NO FURTHER DILUTION OF**

Infection	Description*	Unit Dose	Frequency	Duration	Daily Dose
Lower Respiratory Tract	Exacerbation of Chronic Bronchitis	400 mg	q12h	10 days	800 mg
	Com. Acq. Pneumonia	400 mg	q12h	10 days	800 mg
Skin and Skin Structures	Uncomplicated infections	400 mg	q12h	10 days	800 mg
Sexually Transmitted Diseases	Acute, uncomplicated gonorrhea	400 mg	single dose	1 day	400 mg
	Cervicitis/urethritis due to *C. trachomatis*	300 mg	q12h	7 days	600 mg
	Cervicitis/urethritis due to *C. trachomatis* and *N. gonorrhoeae*	300 mg	q12h	7 days	600 mg
Urinary Tract	Cystitis due to *E. coli* or *K. pneumoniae*	200 mg	q12h	3 days	400 mg
	Cystitis due to other approved pathogens	200 mg	q12h	7 days	400 mg
	Complicated UTI's	200 mg	q12h	10 days	400 mg
Prostate	Prostatitis due to *E. coli*	300 mg	q12h	6 weeks **	600 mg

* DUE TO THE DESIGNATED PATHOGENS (See *INDICATIONS AND USAGE*.)
** BECAUSE THERE ARE NO SAFETY DATA PRESENTLY AVAILABLE TO SUPPORT THE USE OF THE INTRAVENOUS FORMULATION OF OFLOXACIN FOR MORE THAN 10 DAYS, THERAPY AFTER 10 DAYS SHOULD BE SWITCHED TO THE ORAL TABLET FORMULATION OR OTHER APPROPRIATE THERAPY.

Creatinine Clearance	Maintenance Dose	Frequency
10–50 mL/min	the usual recommended unit dose	q24h
<10 mL/min	¹/₂ the usual recommended unit dose	q24h

Desired Dosage Strength	From 10 mL Vial, Withdraw Volume	From 20 mL Vial, Withdraw Volume	Volume of Diluent	Infusion Time
200 mg	5 mL	10 mL	qs 50 mL	60 min
300 mg	7.5 mL	15 mL	qs 75 mL	60 min
400 mg	10 mL	20 mL	qs 100 mL	60 min

Intravenous Fluids	pH of 4 mg/mL FLOXIN I.V. Solution
0.9% Sodium Chloride Injection, USP	4.69
5% Dextrose Injection, USP	4.57
5% Dextrose/0.9% NaCl Injection	4.56
5% Dextrose in Lactated Ringers	4.94
5% Sodium Bicarbonate Injection	7.95
Plasma/Lyte® 56/5% Dextrose Injection	5.02
5% Dextrose, 0.45% Sodium Chloride, and 0.15% Potassium Chloride Injection	4.64
Sodium Lactate Injection (M/6)	5.64
Water for Injection	4.66

THIS PREPARATION IS NECESSARY. Each 50 mL pre-mixed flexible container already contains a dilute solution with the equivalent of 200 mg of ofloxacin (4 mg/mL) in 5% Dextrose (D₅W). Each 100 mL pre-mixed flexible container already contains a dilute solution with the equivalent of 400 mg of ofloxacin (4 mg/mL) in 5% Dextrose (D₅W).

This parenteral drug product should be inspected visually for discoloration and particulate matter prior to administration.

Since no preservative or bacteriostatic agent is present in this product, aseptic technique must be used in preparation of the final parenteral solution. **Since the pre-mixed flexible containers are for single-use only, any unused portion should be discarded.**

Since only limited data are available on the compatibility of ofloxacin intravenous injection with other intravenous substances, **additives or other medications should not be added to FLOXIN I.V. in flexible containers or infused simultaneously through the same intravenous line.** If the same intravenous line is used for sequential infusion of several different drugs, the line should be flushed before and after infusion of FLOXIN I.V. with an infusion solution compatible with FLOXIN I.V. and with any other drug(s) administered via this common line.

Instructions for the Use of FLOXIN I.V. PRE-MIXED IN FLEXIBLE CONTAINERS:
To open:
1. Tear outer wrap at the notch and remove solution container.

2. Check the container for minute leaks by squeezing the inner bag firmly. If leaks are found, or if the seal is not intact, discard the solution, as the sterility may be compromised.
3. Do not use if the solution is cloudy or a precipitate is present.
4. Use sterile equipment.
5. **WARNING: Do not use flexible containers in series connections.** Such use could result in air embolism due to residual air being drawn from the primary container before administration of the fluid from the secondary container is complete.

Preparation for administration:
1. Close flow control clamp of administration set.
2. Remove cover from port at bottom of container.
3. Insert piercing pin of administration set into port with a twisting motion until the pin is firmly seated.
   NOTE: See full directions on administration set carton.
4. Suspend container from hanger.
5. Squeeze and release drip chamber to establish proper fluid level in chamber during infusion of FLOXIN I.V. IN PRE-MIXED FLEXIBLE CONTAINERS.
6. Open flow control clamp to expel air from set. Close clamp.
7. Regulate rate of administration with flow control clamp.

Stability of FLOXIN I.V. as Supplied:
When stored under recommended conditions, FLOXIN I.V., as supplied in 10 mL and 20 mL vials, 100 mL bottles, and 50 mL and 100 mL flexible containers, is stable through the expiration date printed on the label.

Stability of FLOXIN I.V. Following Dilution:
FLOXIN I.V., when diluted in a compatible intravenous fluid to a concentration between 0.4 mg/mL and 4 mg/mL, is stable for 72 h when stored at or below 75°F or 24°C and for 14 days when stored under refrigeration at 41°F or 5°C in glass bottles or plastic intravenous containers. Solutions that are diluted in a compatible intravenous solution and frozen in glass bottles or plastic intravenous containers are stable for 6 months when stored at −4°F or −20°C. Once thawed, the solution is stable for up to 14 days, if refrigerated at 36°F to 46°F (2°C to 8°C). **THAW FROZEN SOLUTIONS AT ROOM TEMPERATURE (77°F OR 25°C) OR IN A REFRIGERATOR (46°F OR 8°C). DO NOT FORCE THAW BY MICROWAVE IRRADIATION OR WATER BATH IMMERSION. DO NOT RE-FREEZE AFTER INITIAL THAWING.**

HOW SUPPLIED

SINGLE-USE VIALS:
FLOXIN (ofloxacin injection) I.V. is supplied in single-use vials. Each vial contains a concentrated solution with the equivalent of 400 mg of ofloxacin.

40 mg/mL, 10 mL vials (NDC 0062-1550-01)
20 mg/mL, 20 mL vials (NDC 0062-1551-01)

FLOXIN I.V. SINGLE-USE VIALS are manufactured for Ortho Pharmaceutical Corporation and McNeil Pharmaceutical by Schering-Plough Products, Inc., Manati, PR 00674.

PRE-MIXED IN BOTTLES:
FLOXIN (ofloxacin injection) I.V. PRE-MIXED IN BOTTLES is supplied in 100 mL, single-use, pre-mixed bottles. Each bottle contains a dilute solution with the equivalent of 400 mg of ofloxacin in 5% Dextrose (D_5W).

4 mg/mL, 100 mL bottle (NDC 0062-1552-01)

FLOXIN I.V. PRE-MIXED IN BOTTLES is manufactured for Ortho Pharmaceutical Corporation and McNeil Pharmaceutical by Schering-Plough Products, Inc., Manati, PR 00674.

PRE-MIXED IN FLEXIBLE CONTAINERS:
FLOXIN (ofloxacin injection) I.V. PRE-MIXED IN FLEXIBLE CONTAINERS is supplied as a single-use, pre-mixed solution in 50 mL and 100 mL flexible containers. Each contains a dilute solution with the equivalent of 200 mg or 400 mg of ofloxacin, respectively, in 5% Dextrose (D_5W).

4 mg/mL (200 mg), 50 mL flexible container (NDC 0062-1553-01)
4 mg/mL (400 mg), 100 mL flexible container (NDC 0062-1552-02)

FLOXIN I.V. PRE-MIXED IN FLEXIBLE CONTAINERS is manufactured for Ortho Pharmaceutical Corporation and McNeil Pharmaceutical by Abbott Laboratories, North Chicago, IL 60064.
FLOXIN (ofloxacin injection) I.V. IN SINGLE-USE VIALS and PRE-MIXED IN BOTTLES should be stored at controlled room temperature 59°F to 86°F (15°C to 30°C) and protected from light. FLOXIN I.V. PRE-MIXED IN FLEXIBLE CONTAINERS should be stored at or below 77°F or 25°C; however, brief exposure up to 104°F or 40°C does not adversely affect the product. Avoid excessive heat and protect from freezing and light.

Also Available:
TABLETS
Ofloxacin is also available as FLOXIN TABLETS (ofloxacin tablets) 200, 300 and 400 mg.

ANIMAL PHARMACOLOGY:
Ofloxacin, as well as other drugs of the quinolone class, has been shown to cause arthropathies (arthrosis) in immature dogs and rats. In addition, these drugs are associated with an increased incidence of osteochondrosis in rats as compared to the incidence observed in vehicle-treated rats. (See ***WARNINGS.***) There is no evidence of arthropathies in fully mature dogs at intravenous doses up to 3 times the recommended maximum human dose (on a mg/m^2 basis or 5 times based on a mg/kg basis) for a one-week exposure period.
Long-term, high-dose systemic use of other quinolones in experimental animals has caused lenticular opacities; however, this finding was not observed in any animal studies with ofloxacin.
Reduced serum globulin and protein levels were observed in animals treated with other quinolones. In one ofloxacin study, minor decreases in serum globulin and protein levels were noted in female cynomolgus monkeys dosed orally with 40 mg/kg ofloxacin daily for one year. These changes, however, were considered to be within normal limits for monkeys.
Crystalluria and ocular toxicity were not observed in any animals treated with ofloxacin.
Caution: Federal (U.S.A.) law prohibits dispensing without prescription.
FLOXIN® is a trademark of Ortho Pharmaceutical Corporation.
U.S. Patent No. 4,382,892

REFERENCES

1. National Committee for Clinical Laboratory Standards, Performance Standards for Antimicrobial Disk Susceptibility Tests—Fourth Edition. Approved Standard NCCLS Document M2-A4, Vol. 10, No. 7, NCCLS, Villanova, PA, 1990.
2. National Committee for Clinical Laboratory Standards, Methods for Dilution Antimicrobial Susceptibility Tests for Bacteria that Grows Aerobically—Second Edition. Approved Standard NCCLS Document M7-A2, Vol. 10, No. 8, NCCLS, Villanova, PA, 1990.

Ortho Pharmaceutical Corporation
Raritan, NJ USA 08869, and

McNeil Pharmaceutical
Spring House, PA USA 19477
Revised April 1994
©OPC 1991 635-10-290-4

Shown in Product Identification Guide, page 323

HALDOL® ℞
brand of
haloperidol
[hal'dawl]
Tablets/Concentrate/Injection
(For Immediate Release)

DESCRIPTION

Haloperidol is the first of the butyrophenone series of major tranquilizers. The chemical designation is 4-[4-(p-chlorophenyl)-4-hydroxy-piperidino]-4′-fluorobutyrophenone and it has the following structural formula:
[See chemical structure at top of next column.]
HALDOL haloperidol dosage forms include: tablets ($^1/_2$, 1, 2, 5, 10 and 20 mg); a concentrate with 2 mg per mL haloperidol (as the lactate); and a sterile parenteral form for intramuscular injection. The injection provides 5 mg haloperidol (as the lactate) with 1.8 mg methylparaben and 0.2 mg propylparaben per mL, and lactic acid for pH adjustment between 3.0–3.6.

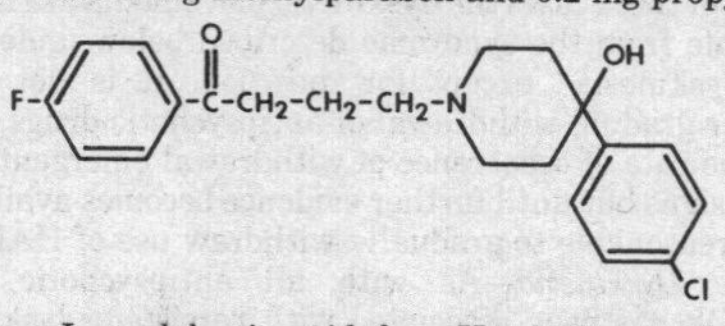

Inactive ingredients: tablets—calcium phosphate, calcium stearate, corn starch, and flavor—1mg contains D&C Yellow No. 10 and FD&C Red No. 40; 2mg contains D&C Red No. 33 and FD&C Blue No. 2; 5mg contains FD&C Blue No. 1, D&C Yellow No. 10 and D&C Red No. 30; 10 mg contains FD&C Blue No. 1, D&C Yellow No. 10 and D&C Red No. 30; and 20 mg contains FD&C Red No. 40; concentrate - lactic acid and methylparaben.

ACTIONS

The precise mechanism of action has not been clearly established.

INDICATIONS

HALDOL haloperidol is indicated for use in the management of manifestations of psychotic disorders.
HALDOL is indicated for the control of tics and vocal utterances of Tourette's Disorder in children and adults.
HALDOL is effective for the treatment of severe behavior problems in children of combative, explosive hyperexcitability (which cannot be accounted for by immediate provocation). HALDOL is also effective in the short-term treatment of hyperactive children who show excessive motor activity with accompanying conduct disorders consisting of some or all of the following symptoms: impulsivity, difficulty sustaining attention, aggressivity, mood lability and poor frustration tolerance. HALDOL should be reserved for these two groups of children only after failure to respond to psychotherapy or medications other than antipsychotics.

CONTRAINDICATIONS

HALDOL haloperidol is contraindicated in severe toxic central nervous system depression or comatose states from any cause and in individuals who are hypersensitive to this drug or have Parkinson's disease.

WARNINGS

Tardive Dyskinesia
A syndrome consisting of potentially irreversible, involuntary, dyskinetic movements may develop in patients treated with antipsychotic drugs. Although the prevalence of the syndrome appears to be highest among the elderly, especially elderly women, it is impossible to rely upon prevalence estimates to predict, at the inception of antipsychotic treatment, which patients are likely to develop the syndrome. Whether antipsychotic drug products differ in their potential to cause tardive dyskinesia is unknown.
Both the risk of developing tardive dyskinesia and the likelihood that it will become irreversible are believed to increase as the duration of treatment and the total cumulative dose of antipsychotic drugs administered to the patient increase. However, the syndrome can develop, although much less commonly, after relatively brief treatment periods at low doses.
There is no known treatment for established cases of tardive dyskinesia, although the syndrome may remit, partially or completely, if antipsychotic treatment is withdrawn. Antipsychotic treatment, itself, however, may suppress (or partially suppress) the signs and symptoms of the syndrome and thereby may possibly mask the underlying process. The effect that symptomatic suppression has upon the long-term course of the syndrome is unknown.
Given these considerations, antipsychotic drugs should be prescribed in a manner that is most likely to minimize the occurrence of tardive dyskinesia. Chronic antipsychotic treatment should generally be reserved for patients who suffer from a chronic illness that, 1) is known to respond to antipsychotic drugs, and 2) for whom alternative, equally effective, but potentially less harmful treatments are not available or appropriate. In patients who do require chronic treatment, the smallest dose and the shortest duration of treatment producing a satisfactory clinical response should be sought. The need for continued treatment should be reassessed periodically.
If signs and symptoms of tardive dyskinesia appear in a patient on antipsychotics, drug discontinuation should be considered. However, some patients may require treatment despite the presence of the syndrome.
(For further information about the description of tardive dyskinesia and its clinical detection, please refer to ADVERSE REACTIONS.)

Neuroleptic Malignant Syndrome (NMS)
A potentially fatal symptom complex sometimes referred to as Neuroleptic Malignant Syndrome (NMS) has been reported in association with antipsychotic drugs. Clinical manifestations of NMS are hyperpyrexia, muscle rigidity, altered mental status (including catatonic signs) and evidence of autonomic instability (irregular pulse or blood pressure, tachycardia, diaphoresis, and cardiac dysrhythmias). Additional signs may include elevated creatine phosphokinase, myoglobinuria (rhabdomyolysis) and acute renal failure.
The diagnostic evaluation of patients with this syndrome is complicated. In arriving at a diagnosis, it is important to identify cases where the clinical presentation includes both serious medical illness (e.g., pneumonia, systemic infection, etc.) and untreated or inadequately treated extrapyramidal signs and symptoms (EPS). Other important considerations in the differential diagnosis include central anticholinergic toxicity, heat stroke, drug fever and primary central nervous system (CNS) pathology.
The management of NMS should include 1) immediate discontinuation of antipsychotic drugs and other drugs not essential to concurrent therapy, 2) intensive symptomatic treatment and medical monitoring, and 3) treatment of any concomitant serious medical problems for which specific treatments are available. There is no general agreement about specific pharmacological treatment regimens for uncomplicated NMS.
If a patient requires antipsychotic drug treatment after recovery from NMS, the potential reintroduction of drug therapy should be carefully considered. The patient should be carefully monitored, since recurrences of NMS have been reported.
Hyperpyrexia and heat stroke, not associated with the above symptom complex, have also been reported with HALDOL.

Usage in Pregnancy
Rodents given 2 to 20 times the usual maximum human dose of haloperidol by oral or parenteral routes showed an increase in incidence of resorption, reduced fertility, delayed delivery and pup mortality. No teratogenic effect has been reported in rats, rabbits or dogs at dosages within this range, but cleft palate has been observed in mice given 15 times the usual maximum human dose. Cleft palate in mice appears to be a non-specific response to stress or nutritional imbalance as well as to a variety of drugs, and there is no evidence to relate this phenomenon to predictable human risk for most of these agents.
There are no well controlled studies with HALDOL haloperidol in pregnant women. There are reports, however, of cases of limb malformations observed following maternal use of HALDOL along with other drugs which have suspected teratogenic potential during the first trimester of pregnancy. Causal relationships were not established in these cases. Since such experience does not exclude the possibility of fetal damage due to HALDOL, this drug should be used during pregnancy or in women likely to become pregnant only if the benefit clearly justifies a potential risk to the fetus. Infants should not be nursed during drug treatment.

Combined Use of HALDOL and Lithium
An encephalopathic syndrome (characterized by weakness, lethargy, fever, tremulousness and confusion, extrapyramidal symptoms, leukocytosis, elevated serum enzymes, BUN, and FBS) followed by irreversible brain damage has occurred

Continued on next page

Information on McNeil Pharmaceutical Products is based on labeling in effect in August 1996.

McNeil—Cont.

in a few patients treated with lithium plus HALDOL. A causal relationship between these events and the concomitant administration of lithium and HALDOL has not been established; however, patients receiving such combined therapy should be monitored closely for early evidence of neurological toxicity and treatment discontinued promptly if such signs appear.

General

A number of cases of bronchopneumonia, some fatal, have followed the use of antipsychotic drugs, including HALDOL. It has been postulated that lethargy and decreased sensation of thirst due to central inhibition may lead to dehydration, hemoconcentration and reduced pulmonary ventilation. Therefore, if the above signs and symptoms appear, especially in the elderly, the physician should institute remedial therapy promptly.

Although not reported with HALDOL, decreased serum cholesterol and/or cutaneous and ocular changes have been reported in patients receiving chemically-related drugs.

HALDOL may impair the mental and/or physical abilities required for the performance of hazardous tasks such as operating machinery or driving a motor vehicle. The ambulatory patient should be warned accordingly.

The use of alcohol with this drug should be avoided due to possible additive effects and hypotension.

PRECAUTIONS

HALDOL haloperidol should be administered cautiously to patients:

—with severe cardiovascular disorders, because of the possibility of transient hypotension and/or precipitation of anginal pain. Should hypotension occur and a vasopressor be required, epinephrine should not be used since HALDOL may block its vasopressor activity and paradoxical further lowering of the blood pressure may occur. Instead, metaraminol, phenylephrine or norepinephrine should be used.

—receiving anticonvulsant medications, with a history of seizures, or with EEG abnormalities, because HALDOL may lower the convulsive threshold. If indicated, adequate anticonvulsant therapy should be concomitantly maintained.

—with known allergies, or with a history of allergic reactions to drugs.

—receiving anticoagulants, since an isolated instance of interference occurred with the effects of one anticoagulant (phenindione).

If concomitant antiparkinson medication is required, it may have to be continued after HALDOL is discontinued because of the difference in excretion rates. If both are discontinued simultaneously, extrapyramidal symptoms may occur. The physician should keep in mind the possible increase in intraocular pressure when anticholinergic drugs, including antiparkinson agents, are administered concomitantly with HALDOL.

As with other antipsychotic agents, it should be noted that HALDOL may be capable of potentiating CNS depressants such as anesthetics, opiates, and alcohol.

When HALDOL is used to control mania in cyclic disorders, there may be a rapid mood swing to depression.

Severe neurotoxicity (rigidity, inability to walk or talk) may occur in patients with thyrotoxicosis who are also receiving antipsychotic medication, including HALDOL.

No mutagenic potential of haloperidol was found in the Ames Salmonella microsomal activation assay. Negative or inconsistent positive findings have been obtained in *in vitro* and *in vivo* studies of effects of haloperidol on chromosome structure and number. The available cytogenetic evidence is considered too inconsistent to be conclusive at this time.

Carcinogenicity studies using oral haloperidol were conducted in Wistar rats (dosed at up to 5 mg/kg daily for 24 months) and in Albino Swiss mice (dosed at up to 5 mg/kg daily for 18 months). In the rat study survival was less than optimal in all dose groups, reducing the number of rats at risk for developing tumors. However, although a relatively greater number of rats survived to the end of the study in high dose male and female groups, these animals did not have a greater incidence of tumors than control animals. Therefore, although not optimal, this study does suggest the absence of a haloperidol related increase in the incidence of neoplasia in rats at doses up to 20 times the usual daily human dose for chronic or resistant patients.

In female mice at 5 and 20 times the highest initial daily dose for chronic or resistant patients, there was a statistically significant increase in mammary gland neoplasia and total tumor incidence; at 20 times the same daily dose there was a statistically significant increase in pituitary gland neoplasia. In male mice, no statistically significant differences in incidences of total tumors or specific tumor types were noted.

Antipsychotic drugs elevate prolactin levels; the elevation persists during chronic administration. Tissue culture experiments indicate that approximately one-third of human breast cancers are prolactin dependent *in vitro*, a factor of potential importance if the prescription of these drugs is contemplated in a patient with a previously detected breast cancer. Although disturbances such as galactorrhea, amenorrhea, gynecomastia, and impotence have been reported, the clinical significance of elevated serum prolactin levels is unknown for most patients. An increase in mammary neoplasms has been found in rodents after chronic administration of antipsychotic drugs. Neither clinical studies nor epidemiologic studies conducted to date, however, have shown an association between chronic administration of these drugs and mammary tumorigenesis; the available evidence is considered too limited to be conclusive at this time.

ADVERSE REACTIONS

CNS Effects:

Extrapyramidal Symptoms (EPS)—EPS during the administration of HALDOL (haloperidol) have been reported frequently, often during the first few days of treatment. EPS can be categorized generally as Parkinson-like symptoms, akathisia, or dystonia (including opisthotonos and oculogyric crisis). While all can occur at relatively low doses, they occur more frequently and with greater severity at higher doses. The symptoms may be controlled with dose reductions or administration of antiparkinson drugs such as benztropine mesylate USP or trihexyphenidyl hydrochloride USP. It should be noted that persistent EPS have been reported; the drug may have to be discontinued in such cases.

Withdrawal Emergent Neurological Signs—Generally, patients receiving short term therapy experience no problems with abrupt discontinuation of antipsychotic drugs. However, some patients on maintenance treatment experience transient dyskinetic signs after abrupt withdrawal. In certain of these cases the dyskinetic movements are indistinguishable from the syndrome described below under "Tardive Dyskinesia" except for duration. It is not known whether gradual withdrawal of antipsychotic drugs will reduce the rate of occurrence of withdrawal emergent neurological signs but until further evidence becomes available, it seems reasonable to gradually withdraw use of HALDOL.

Tardive Dyskinesia—As with all antipsychotic agents HALDOL has been associated with persistent dyskinesias. Tardive dyskinesia, a syndrome consisting of potentially irreversible, involuntary, dyskinetic movements, may appear in some patients on long-term therapy or may occur after drug therapy has been discontinued. The risk appears to be greater in elderly patients on high-dose therapy, especially females. The symptoms are persistent and in some patients appear irreversible. The syndrome is characterized by rhythmical involuntary movements of tongue, face, mouth or jaw (e.g., protrusion of tongue, puffing of cheeks, puckering of mouth, chewing movements). Sometimes these may be accompanied by involuntary movements of extremities and the trunk.

There is no known effective treatment for tardive dyskinesia; antiparkinson agents usually do not alleviate the symptoms of this syndrome. It is suggested that all antipsychotic agents be discontinued if these symptoms appear. Should it be necessary to reinstitute treatment, or increase the dosage of the agent, or switch to a different antipsychotic agent, this syndrome may be masked.

It has been reported that fine vermicular movement of the tongue may be an early sign of tardive dyskinesia and if the medication is stopped at that time the full syndrome may not develop.

Tardive Dystonia—Tardive dystonia, not associated with the above syndrome, has also been reported. Tardive dystonia is characterized by delayed onset of choreic or dystonic movements, is often persistent, and has the potential of becoming irreversible.

Other CNS Effects—Insomnia, restlessness, anxiety, euphoria, agitation, drowsiness, depression, lethargy, headache, confusion, vertigo, grand mal seizures, exacerbation of psychotic symptoms including hallucinations, and catatonic-like behavioral states which may be responsive to drug withdrawal and/or treatment with anticholinergic drugs.

Body as a Whole: Neuroleptic malignant syndrome (NMS), hyperpyrexia and heat stroke have been reported with HALDOL. (See WARNINGS for further information concerning NMS.)

Cardiovascular Effects: Tachycardia, hypotension, hypertension and ECG changes including prolongation of the Q-T interval and ECG pattern changes compatible with the polymorphous configuration of torsades de pointes.

Hematologic Effects: Reports have appeared citing the occurrence of mild and usually transient leukopenia and leukocytosis, minimal decreases in red blood cell counts, anemia, or a tendency toward lymphomonocytosis. Agranulocytosis has rarely been reported to have occurred with the use of HALDOL, and then only in association with other medication.

Liver Effects: Impaired liver function and/or jaundice have been reported.

Dermatologic Reactions: Maculopapular and acneiform skin reactions and isolated cases of photosensitivity and loss of hair.

Endocrine Disorders: Lactation, breast engorgement, mastalgia, menstrual irregularities, gynecomastia, impotence, increased libido, hyperglycemia, hypoglycemia and hyponatremia.

Gastrointestinal Effects: Anorexia, constipation, diarrhea, hypersalivation, dyspepsia, nausea and vomiting.

Autonomic Reactions: Dry mouth, blurred vision, urinary retention, diaphoresis and priapism.

Respiratory Effects: Laryngospasm, bronchospasm and increased depth of respiration.

Special Senses: Cataracts, retinopathy and visual disturbances.

Other: Cases of sudden and unexpected death have been reported in association with the administration of HALDOL. The nature of the evidence makes it impossible to determine definitively what role, if any, HALDOL played in the outcome of the reported cases. The possibility that HALDOL caused death cannot, of course, be excluded, but it is to be kept in mind that sudden and unexpected death may occur in psychotic patients when they go untreated or when they are treated with other antipsychotic drugs.

Postmarketing Events: Hyperammonemia has been reported in a $5^1/_2$ year old child with citrullinemia, an inherited disorder of ammonia excretion, following treatment with HALDOL.

OVERDOSAGE

Manifestations

In general, the symptoms of overdosage would be an exaggeration of known pharmacologic effects and adverse reactions, the most prominent of which would be: 1) severe extrapyramidal reactions, 2) hypotension, or 3) sedation. The patient would appear comatose with respiratory depression and hypotension which could be severe enough to produce a shock-like state. The extrapyramidal reaction would be manifest by muscular weakness or rigidity and a generalized or localized tremor as demonstrated by the akinetic or agitans types respectively. With accidental overdosage, hypertension rather than hypotension occurred in a two-year old child. The risk of ECG changes associated with torsades de pointes should be considered. (For further information regarding torsades de pointes, please refer to ADVERSE REACTIONS.)

Treatment

Gastric lavage or induction of emesis should be carried out immediately followed by administration of activated charcoal. Since there is no specific antidote, treatment is primarily supportive. A patent airway must be established by use of an oropharyngeal airway or endotracheal tube or, in prolonged cases of coma, by tracheostomy. Respiratory depression may be counteracted by artificial respiration and mechanical respirators. Hypotension and circulatory collapse may be counteracted by use of intravenous fluids, plasma, or concentrated albumin, and vasopressor agents such as metaraminol, phenylephrine and norepinephrine. Epinephrine should not be used. In case of severe extrapyramidal reactions, antiparkinson medication should be administered. ECG and vital signs should be monitored especially for signs of Q-T prolongation or dysrhythmias and monitoring should continue until the ECG is normal. Severe arrhythmias should be treated with appropriate anti-arrhythmic measures.

DOSAGE AND ADMINISTRATION

There is considerable variation from patient to patient in the amount of medication required for treatment. As with all antipsychotic drugs, dosage should be individualized according to the needs and response of each patient. Dosage adjustments, either upward or downward, should be carried out as rapidly as practicable to achieve optimum therapeutic control.

To determine the initial dosage, consideration should be given to the patient's age, severity of illness, previous response to other antipsychotic drugs, and any concomitant medication or disease state. Children, debilitated or geriatric patients, as well as those with a history of adverse reactions to antipsychotic drugs, may require less HALDOL haloperidol. The optimal response in such patients is usually obtained with more gradual dosage adjustments and at lower dosage levels, as recommended below.

Clinical experience suggests the following recommendations:

Oral Administration

Initial Dosage Range

Adults

Moderate Symptomatology	0.5 mg to 2.0 mg b.i.d. or t.i.d.
Severe Symptomatology	3.0 mg to 5.0 mg b.i.d. or t.i.d.

To achieve prompt control, higher doses may be required in some cases.

Geriatric or Debilitated Patients	0.5 mg to 2.0 mg b.i.d. or t.i.d.
Chronic or Resistant Patients	3.0 mg to 5.0 mg b.i.d. or t.i.d.

Patients who remain severely disturbed or inadequately controlled may require dosage adjustment. Daily dosages up to 100 mg may be necessary in some cases to achieve an optimal response. Infrequently, HALDOL has been used in doses above 100 mg for severely resistant patients; however, the limited clinical usage has not demonstrated the safety of prolonged administration of such doses.

Children
The following recommendations apply to children between the ages of 3 and 12 years (weight range 15 to 40 kg). HALDOL is not intended for children under 3 years old. Therapy should begin at the lowest dose possible (0.5 mg per day). If required, the dose should be increased by an increment of 0.5 mg at 5 to 7 day intervals until the desired therapeutic effect is obtained. (See chart below).
The total dose may be divided, to be given b.i.d. or t.i.d.

Psychotic Disorders	0.05 mg/kg/day to 0.15 mg/kg/day
Non-Psychotic Behavior Disorders and Tourette's Disorder	0.05 mg/kg/day to 0.075 mg/kg/day

Severely disturbed psychotic children may require higher doses. In severely disturbed, non-psychotic children or in hyperactive children with accompanying conduct disorders, who have failed to respond to psychotherapy or medications other than antipsychotics, it should be noted that since these behaviors may be short-lived, short-term administration of HALDOL may suffice. There is no evidence establishing a maximum effective dosage. There is little evidence that behavior improvement is further enhanced in dosages beyond 6 mg per day.

Maintenance Dosage
Upon achieving a satisfactory therapeutic response, dosage should then be gradually reduced to the lowest effective maintenance level.

Intramuscular Administration
Adults
Parenteral medication, administered intramuscularly in doses of 2 to 5 mg, is utilized for prompt control of the acutely agitated patient with moderately severe to very severe symptoms. Depending on the response of the patient, subsequent doses may be given, administered as often as every hour, although 4 to 8 hour intervals may be satisfactory.
Controlled trials to establish the safety and effectiveness of intramuscular administration in children have not been conducted.
Parenteral drug products should be inspected visually for particulate matter and discoloration prior to administration, whenever solution and container permit.

Switchover Procedure
The oral form should supplant the injectable as soon as practicable. In the absence of bioavailability studies establishing bioequivalence between these two dosage forms the following guidelines for dosage are suggested. For an initial approximation of the total daily dose required, the parenteral dose administered in the preceding 24 hours may be used. Since this dose is only an initial estimate, it is recommended that careful monitoring of clinical signs and symptoms, including clinical efficacy, sedation, and adverse effects, be carried out periodically for the first several days following the initiation of switchover. In this way, dosage adjustments, either upward or downward, can be quickly accomplished. Depending on the patient's clinical status, the first oral dose should be given within 12–24 hours following the last parenteral dose.

HOW SUPPLIED
HALDOL® brand of haloperidol Tablets with a cut-out "H" design, Scored, Imprinted "McNeil" and "HALDOL" with the mg strength of the tablet:

		Bottles Containing 100
1/2 mg, white	NDC 0045-0240-60	x
1 mg, yellow	NDC 0045-0241-60	x
2 mg, pink	NDC 0045-0242-60	x
5 mg, green	NDC 0045-0245-60	x
10 mg, aqua	NDC 0045-0246-60	x
20 mg, salmon	NDC 0045-0248-60	x

HALDOL® brand of haloperidol Concentrate 2 mg per mL (as the lactate) Colorless, Odorless, and Tasteless Solution—NDC 0045-0250-15, bottles of 15 mL and NDC 0045-0250-04, bottles of 120 mL.
HALDOL® brand of haloperidol Injection (For Immediate Release) 5 mg per mL (as the lactate)—NDC 0045-0255-01, units of 10 × 1 mL ampuls and NDC 0045-0255-49, 10 mL multiple-dose vial.
Store HALDOL® haloperidol Tablets at controlled room temperature (15°-30°C, 59°-86°F). Protect from light.
Store HALDOL® haloperidol Concentrate at controlled room temperature (15°-30°C, 59°-86°F). Protect from light. Do not freeze.
Store HALDOL® haloperidol Injection at controlled room temperature (15°-30°C, 59°-86°F). Protect from light. Do not freeze.
Dispense the HALDOL haloperidol tablets and concentrate in a tight, light-resistent container as defined in the official compendium.

McNEIL PHARMACEUTICAL
Spring House, PA 19477

643-94-066-2 Revised 7/6/95
Shown in Product Identification Guide, page 323

HALDOL® Decanoate 50 ℞
HALDOL® Decanoate 100 ℞
[hal'dawl dek"ah-nō'ōt]
(haloperidol) Decanoate Injection
NSN 6505-01-241-8602—1 mL Ampul
NSN 6505-01-293-5628—5 mL MDV

PRODUCT OVERVIEW

KEY FACTS
HALDOL Decanoate 50 and HALDOL Decanoate 100 are the long-acting injectable forms of HALDOL. The basic effects of HALDOL Decanoate 50 and HALDOL Decanoate 100 are those of HALDOL, with the exception of duration of action. HALDOL Decanoate 50 and HALDOL Decanoate 100 reach peak plasma concentration about six days after administration, with an apparent half-life of about three weeks. The recommended interval between doses is four weeks.

MAJOR USES
HALDOL Decanoate 50 and HALDOL Decanoate 100 are intended for use in the management of patients requiring prolonged parenteral antipsychotic therapy.

SAFETY INFORMATION
See complete safety information provided below.

PRESCRIBING INFORMATION

HALDOL® Decanoate 50 ℞
HALDOL® Decanoate 100 ℞
[hal'dawl dek"ah-nō'āt]
(haloperidol) Decanoate Injection

DESCRIPTION
Haloperidol decanoate is the decanoate ester of the butyrophenone, HALDOL haloperidol. It has a markedly extended duration of effect. It is available in sesame oil in sterile form for intramuscular (IM) injection. The structural formula of haloperidol decanoate, 4-(4-chlorophenyl)-1-[4-(4-fluorophenyl)-4-oxobutyl]-4 piperidinyl decanoate, is:

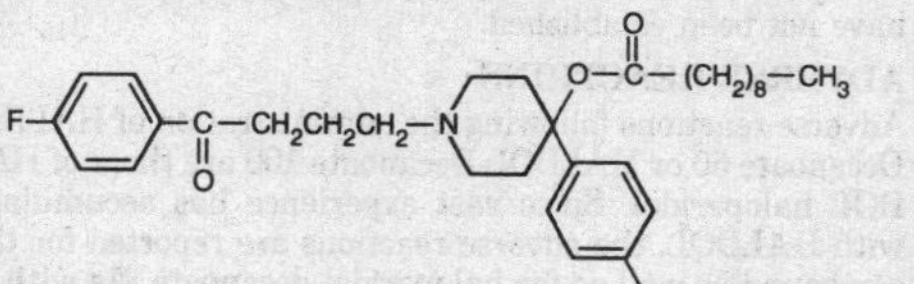

Haloperidol decanoate is almost insoluble in water (0.01 mg/mL), but is soluble in most organic solvents.
Each mL of HALDOL Decanoate 50 for IM injection contains 50 mg haloperidol (present as haloperidol decanoate 70.52 mg) in a sesame oil vehicle, with 1.2% (w/v) benzyl alcohol as a preservative.
Each mL of HALDOL Decanoate 100 for IM injection contains 100 mg haloperidol (present as haloperidol decanoate 141.04 mg) in a sesame oil vehicle, with 1.2% (w/v) benzyl alcohol as a preservative.

CLINICAL PHARMACOLOGY
HALDOL Decanoate 50 and HALDOL Decanoate 100 are the long-acting forms of HALDOL haloperidol. The basic effects of haloperidol decanoate are no different from those of HALDOL with the exception of duration of action. Haloperidol blocks the effects of dopamine and increases its turnover rate; however, the precise mechanism of action is unknown.
Administration of haloperidol decanoate in sesame oil results in slow and sustained release of haloperidol. The plasma concentrations of haloperidol gradually rise, reaching a peak at about 6 days after the injection, and falling thereafter, with an apparent half-life of about 3 weeks. Steady state plasma concentrations are achieved after the third or fourth dose. The relationship between dose of haloperidol decanoate and plasma haloperidol concentration is roughly linear for doses below 450 mg. It should be noted, however, that the pharmacokinetics of haloperidol decanoate following intramuscular injections can be quite variable between subjects.

INDICATIONS AND USAGE
HALDOL Decanoate 50 and HALDOL Decanoate 100 are long-acting parenteral antipsychotic drugs intended for use in the management of patients requiring prolonged parenteral antipsychotic therapy (e.g., patients with chronic schizophrenia).

CONTRAINDICATIONS
Since the pharmacologic and clinical actions of HALDOL Decanoate 50 and HALDOL Decanoate 100 are attributed to HALDOL haloperidol as the active medication, Contraindications, Warnings, and additional information are those of HALDOL, modified only to reflect the prolonged action.
HALDOL is contraindicated in severe toxic central nervous system depression or comatose states from any cause and in individuals who are hypersensitive to this drug or have Parkinson's disease.

WARNINGS
Tardive Dyskinesia
A syndrome consisting of potentially irreversible, involuntary, dyskinetic movements may develop in patients treated with antipsychotic drugs. Although the prevalence of the syndrome appears to be highest among the elderly, especially elderly women, it is impossible to rely upon prevalence estimates to predict, at the inception of antipsychotic treatment, which patients are likely to develop the syndrome. Whether antipsychotic drug products differ in their potential to cause tardive dyskinesia is unknown.
Both the risk of developing tardive dyskinesia and the likelihood that it will become irreversible are believed to increase as the duration of treatment and the total cumulative dose of antipsychotic drugs administered to the patient increase. However, the syndrome can develop, although much less commonly, after relatively brief treatment periods at low doses.
There is no known treatment for established cases of tardive dyskinesia, although the syndrome may remit, partially or completely, if antipsychotic treatment is withdrawn. Antipsychotic treatment, itself, however, may suppress (or partially suppress) the signs and symptoms of the syndrome and thereby may possibly mask the underlying process. The effect that symptomatic suppression has upon the long-term course of the syndrome is unknown.
Given these considerations, antipsychotic drugs should be prescribed in a manner that is most likely to minimize the occurrence of tardive dyskinesia. Chronic antipsychotic treatment should generally be reserved for patients who suffer from a chronic illness that 1) is known to respond to antipsychotic drugs, and 2) for whom alternative, equally effective, but potentially less harmful treatments are **not** available or appropriate. In patients who do require chronic treatment, the smallest dose and the shortest duration of treatment producing a satisfactory clinical response should be sought. The need for continued treatment should be reassessed periodically.
If signs and symptoms of tardive dyskinesia appear in a patient on antipsychotics, drug discontinuation should be considered. However, some patients may require treatment despite the presence of the syndrome. (For further information about the description of tardive dyskinesia and its clinical detection, please refer to ADVERSE REACTIONS.)

Neuroleptic Malignant Syndrome (NMS)
A potentially fatal symptom complex sometimes referred to as Neuroleptic Malignant Syndrome (NMS) has been reported in association with antipsychotic drugs. Clinical manifestations of NMS are hyperpyrexia, muscle rigidity, altered mental status (including catatonic signs) and evidence of autonomic instability (irregular pulse or blood pressure, tachycardia, diaphoresis, and cardiac dysrhythmias). Additional signs may include elevated creatine phosphokinase, myoglobinuria (rhabdomyolysis) and acute renal failure.
The diagnostic evaluation of patients with this syndrome is complicated. In arriving at a diagnosis, it is important to identify cases where the clinical presentation includes both serious medical illness (e.g., pneumonia, systemic infection, etc.) and untreated or inadequately treated extrapyramidal signs and symptoms (EPS). Other important considerations in the differential diagnosis include central anticholinergic toxicity, heat stroke, drug fever and primary central nervous system (CNS) pathology.
The management of NMS should include 1) immediate discontinuation of antipsychotic drugs and other drugs not essential to concurrent therapy, 2) intensive symptomatic

Continued on next page

Information on McNeil Pharmaceutical Products is based on labeling in effect in August 1996.

McNeil—Cont.

treatment and medical monitoring, and 3) treatment of any concomitant serious medical problems for which specific treatments are available. There is no general agreement about specific pharmacological treatment regimens for uncomplicated NMS.

If a patient requires antipsychotic drug treatment after recovery from NMS, the potential reintroduction of drug therapy should be carefully considered. The patient should be carefully monitored, since recurrences of NMS have been reported.

Hyperpyrexia and heat stroke, not associated with the above symptom complex, have also been reported with HALDOL.

General

A number of cases of bronchopneumonia, some fatal, have followed the use of antipsychotic drugs, including HALDOL (haloperidol). It has been postulated that lethargy and decreased sensation of thirst due to central inhibition may lead to dehydration, hemoconcentration and reduced pulmonary ventilation. Therefore, if the above signs and symptoms appear, especially in the elderly, the physician should institute remedial therapy promptly.

Although not reported with HALDOL, decreased serum cholesterol and/or cutaneous and ocular changes have been reported in patients receiving chemically-related drugs.

PRECAUTIONS

HALDOL Decanoate 50 and HALDOL Decanoate 100 should be administered cautiously to patients:

—with severe cardiovascular disorders, because of the possibility of transient hypotension and/or precipitation of anginal pain. Should hypotension occur and a vasopressor be required, epinephrine should not be used since HALDOL haloperidol may block its vasopressor activity, and paradoxical further lowering of the blood pressure may occur. Instead, metaraminol, phenylephrine or norepinephrine should be used.

—receiving anticonvulsant medications, with a history of seizures, or with EEG abnormalities, because HALDOL may lower the convulsive threshold. If indicated, adequate anticonvulsant therapy should be concomitantly maintained.

—with known allergies, or with a history of allergic reactions to drugs.

—receiving anticoagulants, since an isolated instance of interference occurred with the effects of one anticoagulant (phenindione).

If concomitant antiparkinson medication is required, it may have to be continued after HALDOL Decanoate 50 or HALDOL Decanoate 100 is discontinued because of the prolonged action of haloperidol decanoate. If both drugs are discontinued simultaneously, extrapyramidal symptoms may occur. The physician should keep in mind the possible increase in intraocular pressure when anticholinergic drugs, including antiparkinson agents, are administered concomitantly with haloperidol decanoate.

In patients with thyrotoxicosis who are also receiving antipsychotic medication, including haloperidol decanoate, severe neurotoxicity (rigidity, inability to walk or talk) may occur.

When HALDOL is used to control mania in bipolar disorders, there may be a rapid mood swing to depression.

Information for Patients

Haloperidol decanoate may impair the mental and/or physical abilities required for the performance of hazardous tasks such as operating machinery or driving a motor vehicle. The ambulatory patient should be warned accordingly.

The use of alcohol with this drug should be avoided due to possible additive effects and hypotension.

Drug Interactions

An encephalopathic syndrome (characterized by weakness, lethargy, fever, tremulousness and confusion, extrapyramidal symptoms, leukocytosis, elevated serum enzymes, BUN, and FBS) followed by irreversible brain damage has occurred in a few patients treated with lithium plus HALDOL. A causal relationship between these events and the concomitant administration of lithium and HALDOL has not been established; however, patients receiving such combined therapy should be monitored closely for early evidence of neurological toxicity and treatment discontinued promptly if such signs appear.

As with other antipsychotic agents, it should be noted that HALDOL may be capable of potentiating CNS depressants such as anesthetics, opiates, and alcohol.

Carcinogenesis, Mutagenesis, and Impairment of Fertility

No mutagenic potential of haloperidol decanoate was found in the Ames Salmonella microsomal activation assay. Negative or inconsistent positive findings have been obtained in *in vitro* and *in vivo* studies of effects of short-acting haloperidol on chromosome structure and number. The available cytogenetic evidence is considered too inconsistent to be conclusive at this time.

Carcinogenicity studies using oral haloperidol were conducted in Wistar rats (dosed at up to 5 mg/kg daily for 24 months) and in Albino Swiss mice (dosed at up to 5 mg/kg daily for 18 months). In the rat study survival was less than optimal in all dose groups, reducing the number of rats at risk for developing tumors. However, although a relatively greater number of rats survived to the end of the study in high dose male and female groups, these animals did not have a greater incidence of tumors than control animals. Therefore, although not optimal, this study does suggest the absence of a haloperidol related increase in the incidence of neoplasia in rats at doses up to 20 times the usual daily human dose for chronic or resistant patients.

In female mice at 5 and 20 times the highest initial daily dose for chronic or resistant patients, there was a statistically significant increase in mammary gland neoplasia and total tumor incidence; at 20 times the same daily dose there was a statistically significant increase in pituitary gland neoplasia. In male mice, no statistically significant differences in incidences of total tumors or specific tumor types were noted.

Antipsychotic drugs elevate prolactin levels; the elevation persists during chronic administration. Tissue culture experiments indicate that approximately one-third of human breast cancers are prolactin dependent *in vitro*, a factor of potential importance if the prescription of these drugs is contemplated in a patient with a previously detected breast cancer. Although disturbances such as galactorrhea, amenorrhea, gynecomastia, and impotence have been reported, the clinical significance of elevated serum prolactin levels is unknown for most patients.

An increase in mammary neoplasms has been found in rodents after chronic administration of antipsychotic drugs. Neither clinical studies nor epidemiologic studies conducted to date, however, have shown an association between chronic administration of these drugs and mammary tumorigenesis; the available evidence is considered too limited to be conclusive at this time.

Usage in Pregnancy

Pregnancy Category C. Rodents given up to 3 times the usual maximum human dose of haloperidol decanoate showed an increase in incidence of resorption, fetal mortality, and pup mortality. No fetal abnormalities were observed.

Cleft palate has been observed in mice given oral haloperidol at 15 times the usual maximum human dose. Cleft palate in mice appears to be a non-specific response to stress or nutritional imbalance as well as to a variety of drugs, and there is no evidence to relate this phenomenon to predictable human risk for most of these agents.

There are no adequate and well-controlled studies in pregnant women. There are reports, however, of cases of limb malformations observed following maternal use of HALDOL along with other drugs which have suspected teratogenic potential during the first trimester of pregnancy. Causal relationships were not established with these cases. Since such experience does not exclude the possibility of fetal damage due to HALDOL, haloperidol decanoate should be used during pregnancy or in women likely to become pregnant only if the benefit clearly justifies a potential risk to the fetus.

Nursing Mothers

Since haloperidol is excreted in human breast milk, infants should not be nursed during drug treatment with haloperidol decanoate.

Pediatric Use

Safety and effectiveness of haloperidol decanoate in children have not been established.

ADVERSE REACTIONS

Adverse reactions following the administration of HALDOL Decanoate 50 or HALDOL Decanoate 100 are those of HALDOL haloperidol. Since vast experience has accumulated with HALDOL, the adverse reactions are reported for that compound as well as for haloperidol decanoate. As with all injectable medications, local tissue reactions have been reported with haloperidol decanoate.

CNS Effects:

Extrapyramidal Symptoms (EPS)—EPS during the administration of HALDOL (haloperidol) have been reported frequently, often during the first few days of treatment. EPS can be categorized generally as Parkinson-like symptoms, akathisia, or dystonia (including opisthotonos and oculogyric crisis). While all can occur at relatively low doses, they occur more frequently and with greater severity at higher doses. The symptoms may be controlled with dose reductions or administration of antiparkinson drugs such as benztropine mesylate USP or trihexyphenidyl hydrochloride USP. It should be noted that persistent EPS have been reported; the drug may have to be discontinued in such cases.

Withdrawal Emergent Neurological Signs—Generally, patients receiving short term therapy experience no problems with abrupt discontinuation of antipsychotic drugs. However, some patients on maintenance treatment experience transient dyskinetic signs after abrupt withdrawal. In certain of these cases the dyskinetic movements are indistinguishable from the syndrome described below under "Tardive Dyskinesia" except for duration. Although the long acting properties of haloperidol decanoate provide gradual withdrawal, it is not known whether gradual withdrawal of antipsychotic drugs will reduce the rate of occurrence of withdrawal emergent neurological signs.

Tardive Dyskinesia—As with all antipsychotic agents HALDOL has been associated with persistent dyskinesias. Tardive dyskinesia, a syndrome consisting of potentially irreversible, involuntary, dyskinetic movements, may appear in some patients on long-term therapy with haloperidol decanoate or may occur after drug therapy has been discontinued. The risk appears to be greater in elderly patients on high-dose therapy, especially females. The symptoms are persistent and in some patients appear irreversible. The syndrome is characterized by rhythmical involuntary movements of tongue, face, mouth, or jaw (e.g., protrusion of tongue, puffing of cheeks, puckering of mouth, chewing movements). Sometimes these may be accompanied by involuntary movements of extremities and the trunk.

There is no known effective treatment for tardive dyskinesia; antiparkinson agents usually do not alleviate the symptoms of this syndrome. It is suggested that all antipsychotic agents be discontinued if these symptoms appear. Should it be necessary to reinstitute treatment, or increase the dosage of the agent, or switch to a different antipsychotic agent, this syndrome may be masked.

It has been reported that fine vermicular movement of the tongue may be an early sign of tardive dyskinesia and if the medication is stopped at that time the full syndrome may not develop.

Tardive Dystonia—Tardive dystonia, not associated with the above syndrome, has also been reported. Tardive dystonia is characterized by delayed onset of choreic or dystonic movements, is often persistent, and has the potential of becoming irreversible.

Other CNS effects—Insomnia, restlessness, anxiety, euphoria, agitation, drowsiness, depression, lethargy, headache, confusion, vertigo, grand mal seizures, exacerbation of psychotic symptoms including hallucinations, and catatonic-like behavioral states which may be responsive to drug withdrawal and/or treatment with anticholinergic drugs.

Body as a Whole: Neuroleptic malignant syndrome (NMS), hyperpyrexia and heat stroke have been reported with HALDOL. (See WARNINGS for further information concerning NMS.)

Cardiovascular Effects: Tachycardia, hypotension, hypertension and ECG changes including prolongation of the Q-T interval and ECG pattern changes compatible with the polymorphous configuration of torsades de pointes.

Hematologic Effects: Reports have appeared citing the occurrence of mild and usually transient leukopenia and leukocytosis, minimal decreases in red blood cell counts, anemia, or a tendency toward lymphomonocytosis. Agranulocytosis has rarely been reported to have occurred with the use of HALDOL, and then only in association with other medication.

Liver Effects: Impaired liver function and/or jaundice have been reported.

Dermatologic Reactions: Maculopapular and acneiform skin reactions and isolated cases of photosensitivity and loss of hair.

Endocrine Disorders: Lactation, breast engorgement, mastalgia, menstrual irregularities, gynecomastia, impotence, increased libido, hyperglycemia, hypoglycemia and hyponatremia.

Gastrointestinal Effects: Anorexia, constipation, diarrhea, hypersalivation, dyspepsia, nausea and vomiting.

Autonomic Reactions: Dry mouth, blurred vision, urinary retention, diaphoresis and priapism.

Respiratory Effects: Laryngospasm, bronchospasm and increased depth of respiration.

Special Senses: Cataracts, retinopathy and visual disturbances.

Other: Cases of sudden and unexpected death have been reported in association with the administration of HALDOL. The nature of the evidence makes it impossible to determine definitively what role, if any, HALDOL played in the outcome of the reported cases. The possibility that HALDOL caused death cannot, of course, be excluded, but it is to be kept in mind that sudden and unexpected death may occur in psychotic patients when they go untreated or when they are treated with other antipsychotic drugs.

Postmarketing Events: Hyperammonemia has been reported in a $5^1/_2$ year old child with citrullinemia, an inherited disorder of ammonia excretion, following treatment with HALDOL.

OVERDOSAGE

While overdosage is less likely to occur with a parenteral than with an oral medication, information pertaining to HALDOL haloperidol is presented, modified only to reflect the extended duration of action of haloperidol decanoate.

Manifestations—In general, the symptoms of overdosage would be an exaggeration of known pharmacologic effects and adverse reactions, the most prominent of which would be: 1) severe extrapyramidal reactions, 2) hypotension, or 3) sedation. The patient would appear comatose with respiratory depression and hypotension which could be severe enough to produce a shock-like state. The extrapyramidal

reactions would be manifested by muscular weakness or rigidity and a generalized or localized tremor, as demonstrated by the akinetic or agitans types, respectively. With accidental overdosage, hypertension rather than hypotension occurred in a two-year old child. The risk of ECG changes associated with torsades de pointes should be considered. (For further information regarding torsades de pointes, please refer to ADVERSE REACTIONS.)

Treatment—Since there is no specific antidote, treatment is primarily supportive. A patent airway must be established by use of an oropharyngeal airway or endotracheal tube or, in prolonged cases of coma, by tracheostomy. Respiratory depression may be counteracted by artificial respiration and mechanical respirators. Hypotension and circulatory collapse may be counteracted by use of intravenous fluids, plasma, or concentrated albumin, and vasopressor agents such as metaraminol, phenylephrine and norepinephrine. Epinephrine should not be used. In case of severe extrapyramidal reactions, antiparkinson medication should be administered, and should be continued for several weeks, and then withdrawn gradually as extrapyramidal symptoms may emerge. ECG and vital signs should be monitored especially for signs of Q-T prolongation or dysrhythmias and monitoring should continue until the ECG is normal. Severe arrhythmias should be treated with appropriate anti-arrhythmic measures.

DOSAGE AND ADMINISTRATION

HALDOL Decanoate 50 and HALDOL Decanoate 100 should be administered by deep intramuscular injection. A 21 gauge needle is recommended. The maximum volume per injection site should not exceed 3 mL. DO NOT ADMINISTER INTRAVENOUSLY.

Parenteral drug products should be inspected visually for particulate matter and discoloration prior to administration, whenever solution and container permit.

HALDOL Decanoate 50 and HALDOL Decanoate 100 are intended for use in chronic psychotic patients who require prolonged parenteral antipsychotic therapy. These patients should be previously stabilized on antipsychotic medication before considering a conversion to haloperidol decanoate. Furthermore, it is recommended that patients being considered for haloperidol decanoate therapy have been treated with, and tolerate well, short-acting HALDOL haloperidol in order to reduce the possibility of an unexpected adverse sensitivity to haloperidol. Close clinical supervision is required during the initial period of dose adjustment in order to minimize the risk of overdosage or reappearance of psychotic symptoms before the next injection. During dose adjustment or episodes of exacerbation of psychotic symptoms, haloperidol decanoate therapy can be supplemented with short-acting forms of haloperidol.

The dose of HALDOL Decanoate 50 or HALDOL Decanoate 100 should be expressed in terms of its haloperidol content. The starting dose of haloperidol decanoate should be based on the patient's age, clinical history, physical condition, and response to previous antipsychotic therapy. The preferred approach to determining the minimum effective dose is to begin with lower initial doses and to adjust the dose upward as needed. For patients previously maintained on low doses of antipsychotics (e.g. up to the equivalent of 10 mg/day oral haloperidol), it is recommended that the initial dose of haloperidol decanoate be 10–15 times the previous daily dose in oral haloperidol equivalents; limited clinical experience suggests that lower initial doses may be adequate.

Initial Therapy

Conversion from oral haloperidol to haloperidol decanoate can be achieved by using an initial dose of haloperidol decanoate that is 10 to 20 times the previous daily dose in oral haloperidol equivalents.

In patients who are elderly, debilitated, or stable on low doses of oral haloperidol (e.g. up to the equivalent of 10 mg/ day oral haloperidol), a range of 10 to 15 times the previous daily dose in oral haloperidol equivalents is appropriate for initial conversion.

In patients previously maintained on higher doses of antipsychotics for whom a low dose approach risks recurrence of psychiatric decompensation and in patients whose long term use of haloperidol has resulted in a tolerance to the drug, 20 times the previous daily dose in oral haloperidol equivalents should be considered for initial conversion, with downward titration on succeeding injections.

The initial dose of haloperidol decanoate should not exceed 100 mg regardless of previous antipsychotic dose requirements. If, therefore, conversion requires more than 100 mg of haloperidol decanoate as an initial dose, that dose should be administered in two injections, i.e. a maximum of 100 mg initially followed by the balance in 3 to 7 days.

Maintenance Therapy

The maintenance dosage of haloperidol decanoate must be individualized with titration upward or downward based on therapeutic response. The usual maintenance range is 10 to 15 times the previous daily dose in oral haloperidol equivalents dependent on the clinical response of the patient.

HALDOL DECANOATE DOSING RECOMMENDATIONS

PATIENTS	MONTHLY 1ST MONTH	MAINTENANCE
Stabilized on low daily oral doses (up to 10 mg/day)	10–15x Daily Oral Dose	10–15x Previous Daily Oral Dose
Elderly or Debilitated		
High dose	20x Daily Oral Dose	10–15x Previous Daily Oral Dose
Risk of relapse		
Tolerant to oral HALDOL		

Close clinical supervision is required during initiation and stabilization of haloperidol decanoate therapy.

Haloperidol decanoate is usually administered monthly or every 4 weeks. However, variation in patient response may dictate a need for adjustment of the dosing interval as well as the dose (See CLINICAL PHARMACOLOGY).

Clinical experience with haloperidol decanoate at doses greater than 450 mg per month has been limited.

HOW SUPPLIED

HALDOL® (haloperidol) Decanoate 50 for IM injection, 50 mg haloperidol as 70.5 mg per mL haloperidol decanoate—NDC 0045-0253, 10 × 1 mL ampuls, 3 × 1 mL ampuls and 5 mL multiple dose vials.

HALDOL®(haloperidol) Decanoate 100 for IM injection, 100 mg haloperidol as 141.04 mg per mL haloperidol decanoate—NDC 0045-0254, 5 × 1 mL ampuls and 5 mL multiple dose vials.

Store at controlled room temperature (15°–30°C, 59°–86°F). Do not refrigerate or freeze.

Protect from light.

McNeil Pharmaceutical, McNEILAB, INC., Spring House, PA 19477

643-94-253-1   Revised 10/13/92

Shown in Product Identification Guide, page 323

PANCREASE®   ℞

[pan'kre-ace]
(pancrelipase) Capsules
Enteric Coated Microspheres
NSN 6505-01-095-4174—100's
NSN 6505-01-077-2880—250's

DESCRIPTION

PANCREASE pancrelipase capsules are a white, dye-free, orally administered capsule containing enteric coated microspheres of porcine pancreatic enzyme concentrate, predominately steapsin (pancreatic lipase), amylase and protease. Each capsule contains:

Lipase	4,500 U.S.P. Units
Amylase	20,000 U.S.P. Units
Protease	25,000 U.S.P. Units

Inactive ingredients include cellulose acetate phthalate, diethyl phthalate, gelatin, povidone, sodium starch glycollate, corn starch, sugar, talc and titanium dioxide.

CLINICAL PHARMACOLOGY

PANCREASE pancrelipase capsules resist gastric inactivation and deliver predictable, high levels of biologically active enzymes into the duodenum. The enzymes catalyze the hydrolysis of fats into glycerol and fatty acids, protein into proteoses and derived substances, and starch into dextrins and sugars. PANCREASE capsules are effective in controlling steatorrhea and its consequences at low daily dosage levels.

INDICATIONS AND USAGE

PANCREASE pancrelipase capsules are indicated for patients with exocrine pancreatic enzyme deficiency as in but not limited to:
- cystic fibrosis
- chronic pancreatitis
- post-pancreatectomy
- post-gastrointestinal bypass surgery (e.g. Billroth II gastroenterostomy)
- ductal obstruction from neoplasm (e.g. of the pancreas or common bile duct).

CONTRAINDICATIONS

PANCREASE pancrelipase capsules are contraindicated in patients known to be hypersensitive to pork protein.

WARNINGS

Should hypersensitivity occur, discontinue medication and treat symptomatically.

PRECAUTIONS

TO PROTECT ENTERIC COATING, MICROSPHERES SHOULD NOT BE CRUSHED OR CHEWED. Where swallowing of capsules is difficult, they may be opened and the microspheres shaken onto a small quantity of a soft food (e.g. applesauce, gelatin, etc.), which does not require chewing, and swallowed immediately. Contact of the microspheres with foods having a pH greater than 5.5 can dissolve the protective enteric shell.

Pregnancy Category C. Diethyl phthalate, an enteric coating component of PANCREASE pancrelipase capsules has been shown with high intraperitoneal dosing to be tetratogenic in rats. However, when this coating was administered orally to rats up to 100 times the human dose, no teratogenic or embryocidal effects were observed. There were no adequate and well-controlled studies in pregnant women. PANCREASE capsules should be used in pregnancy only if the potential benefit justifies the potential risk to the fetus.

Cases of fibrotic stricture in the ascending colon have been reported in cystic fibrosis patients with the use of enzyme supplements in high doses (approximately 6,500–50,000 USP lipase units/kg/meal). If symptoms suggestive of gastrointestinal obstruction occur, the possibility of bowel strictures should be considered.

Any change in pancreatic enzyme replacement therapy (e.g., dose or brand of medication) should be made cautiously and only under medical supervision.

ADVERSE REACTIONS

The most frequently reported adverse reactions to PANCREASE pancrelipase capsules are gastrointestinal in nature. Less frequently, allergic-type reactions have also been observed. Extremely high doses of exogenous pancreatic enzymes have been associated with hyperuricosuria and hyperuricemia.

DOSAGE AND ADMINISTRATION

Usual dosage: One or two capsules during each meal and one capsule with snacks. Occasionally a third capsule with meals may be required depending upon individual requirements for control of steatorrhea. Dose increases, if required, should be made slowly, with careful monitoring of response and symptomatology.

It is important to ensure adequate hydration of patients at all times while dosing PANCREASE.

HOW SUPPLIED

PANCREASE® pancrelipase capsules (white, dye-free, imprinted "McNeil" and "Pancrease") in bottles of:
100 ....NDC 0045-0095-60
250 ....NDC 0045-0095-69
Keep bottle tightly closed. Store below 25°C (77°F) in a dry place. Do not refrigerate.

643-10-106-2   Revised 6/16/94

Shown in Product Identification Guide, page 323

PANCREASE® MT   ℞

[pan'kre-ace MT]
(pancrelipase) Capsules
Enteric Coated Microtablets
    PANCREASE MT 4 (100's)
NSN 6505-01-287-2188
    PANCREASE MT 10 (100's)
NSN 6505-01-287-2187
    PANCREASE MT 16 (100's)
NSN 6505-01-289-2005
    PANCREASE MT 20 (100's)
Pending

PRODUCT OVERVIEW

KEY FACTS

Microtablet formulation allows for higher enzyme concentrations and smaller capsule size than the original PANCREASE capsules—more enzymatic activity per gram of protein. Enteric coating protects against gastric deactivation and allows delivery of predictable, high levels of biologically active enzymes into the duodenum. Available in four convenient capsule strengths for increased dosage flexibility.

MAJOR USES

PANCREASE MT capsules are indicated for patients with exocrine pancreatic enzyme deficiency.

SAFETY INFORMATION

See complete safety information provided below.

PRESCRIBING INFORMATION

PANCREASE® MT   ℞

[pan'kre-ace MT]
(pancrelipase) Capsules
Enteric Coated Microtablets

DESCRIPTION

PANCREASE MT pancrelipase capsules are orally administered capsules containing enteric coated microtablets of por-

Continued on next page

Information on McNeil Pharmaceutical Products is based on labeling in effect in August 1996.

McNeil—Cont.

cine pancreatic enzyme concentrate, predominately steapsin (pancreatic lipase), amylase and protease.

Each PANCREASE MT 4 capsule contains:
Lipase	4,000 U.S.P. Units
Amylase	12,000 U.S.P. Units
Protease	12,000 U.S.P. Units

Each PANCREASE MT 10 capsule contains:
Lipase	10,000 U.S.P. Units
Amylase	30,000 U.S.P. Units
Protease	30,000 U.S.P. Units

Each PANCREASE MT 16 capsule contains:
Lipase	16,000 U.S.P. Units
Amylase	48,000 U.S.P. Units
Protease	48,000 U.S.P. Units

Each PANCREASE MT 20 capsule contains:
Lipase	20,000 U.S.P. Units
Amylase	56,000 U.S.P. Units
Protease	44,000 U.S.P. Units

Inactive ingredients: cellulose, crospovidone, gelatin, iron oxide, magnesium stearate, methacrylic acid copolymer, polydimethylsiloxane, sodium lauryl sulfate, silicon dioxide, talc, titanium dioxide, triethyl citrate, wax and other trace ingredients.

CLINICAL PHARMACOLOGY

PANCREASE MT pancrelipase capsules resist gastric inactivation and deliver predictable, high levels of biologically active enzymes into the duodenum. The enzymes catalyze the hydrolysis of fats into glycerol and fatty acids, protein into proteoses and derived substances, and starch into dextrins and sugars. PANCREASE MT capsules are effective in controlling steatorrhea and its consequences.

INDICATIONS AND USAGE

PANCREASE MT pancrelipase capsules are indicated for patients with exocrine pancreatic enzyme deficiency such as:
- cystic fibrosis
- chronic pancreatitis
- post-pancreatectomy
- post-gastrointestinal bypass surgery (e.g. Billroth II gastroenterostomy)
- ductal obstruction from neoplasm (e.g. of the pancreas or common bile duct).

CONTRAINDICATIONS

PANCREASE MT pancrelipase capsules are contraindicated in patients known to be hypersensitive to pork protein.
PANCREASE MT capsules are contraindicated in patients with acute pancreatitis or with acute exacerbations of chronic pancreatic diseases.

WARNINGS

Should hypersensitivity occur, discontinue medication and treat symptomatically.

PRECAUTIONS

General
TO PROTECT ENTERIC COATING, MICROTABLETS SHOULD NOT BE CRUSHED OR CHEWED. Where swallowing of capsules is difficult, they may be opened and the microtablets shaken onto a small quantity of a soft food (e.g. applesauce, gelatin, etc.), which does not require chewing, and swallowed immediately. Contact of the microtablets with foods having a pH greater than 6.0 can dissolve the protective enteric shell.
Pregnancy Category C. Animal reproduction studies have not been conducted with PANCREASE MT pancrelipase capsules. It is also not known whether PANCREASE MT can cause fetal harm when administered to a pregnant woman or can affect reproduction capacity. PANCREASE MT should be given to a pregnant woman only if clearly needed.
Cases of fibrotic stricture in the ascending colon have been reported in cystic fibrosis patients with the use of enzyme supplements in high doses (approximately 6,500–50,000 USP lipase units/kg/meal). If symptoms suggestive of gastrointestinal obstruction occur, the possibility of bowel strictures should be considered.
Any change in pancreatic enzyme replacement therapy (e.g., dose or brand of medication) should be made cautiously and only under medical supervision.

ADVERSE REACTIONS

The most frequently reported adverse reactions to pancrelipase-containing products are gastrointestinal in nature. Less frequently, allergic-type reactions have also been observed. Extremely high doses of exogenous pancreatic enzymes have been associated with hyperuricosuria and hyperuricemia when the preparations given were pancrelipase in powdered or capsule form, or pancreatin in tablet form.

DOSAGE AND ADMINISTRATION

Dosage should be adjusted according to the severity of the exocrine pancreatic enzyme deficiency. The number of capsules or capsule strength given with meals and/or snacks should be estimated by assessing which dose minimizes steatorrhea and maintains good nutritional status. Dose in-

creases, if required, should be made slowly, with careful monitoring of response and symptomatology.
It is important to ensure adequate hydration of patients at all times while dosing PANCREASE MT.
In some patients with pancreatic enzyme deficiency, satisfactory responses have been achieved with dosages (expressed in U.S.P. units of lipase) similar to the ones stated below. However, dosages should be adjusted according to the response of the patient.
Children 7 to 12 years: 4,000 to 12,000 units (more if necessary) with each meal and with snacks.
Children 1 to 6 years: 4,000 to 8,000 units with each meal and 4,000 units with snacks.
Children under 1 year: Dosage for children under 6 months of age has not been established. Children 6 months to 1 year have responded to 2,000 units of lipase per meal.
The assessment of the end points in children is aided by charting growth curves.
Adults: 4,000 to 20,000 units (more if necessary) with each meal and with snacks.

HOW SUPPLIED

PANCREASE® MT 4 pancrelipase capsules (yellow and clear, printed "McNEIL" and "Pancrease MT 4") in bottles of 100—NDC 0045-0341-60.
PANCREASE® MT 10 pancrelipase capsules (pink and clear, printed "McNEIL" and "Pancrease MT 10") in bottles of 100—NDC 0045-0342-60.
PANCREASE® MT 16 pancrelipase capsules (salmon and clear, printed "McNEIL" and "Pancrease MT 16") in bottles of 100—NDC 0045-0343-60.
Pancrease® MT 20 pancrelipase capsules (white opaque with yellow bands, printed "McNEIL" and "PANCREASE MT 20") in bottles of 100 NDC 0045-0346-60.
Keep bottle tightly closed. Store below 25°C (77°F) in a dry place. Do not refrigerate.
Dispense in tight container as defined in the official compendium.
Microtablets manufactured by Nordmark Pharmaceutical, Uetersen, Germany.

McNEIL PHARMACEUTICAL
McNEILAB, INC.
SPRING HOUSE, PA 19477
643–10–104–2

Revised 6/16/94
Shown in Product Identification Guide, page 323

PARAFON FORTE® DSC ℞
[par'a-fahn for'ta]
(chlorzoxazone) Caplets 500 mg
NSN 6505-01-264-4453—100's
NSN 6505-01-288-0524—100's (10x10)

DESCRIPTION

Each caplet (capsule shaped tablet) contains:
Chlorzoxazone* .... 500 mg
Inactive ingredients: FD&C Blue No. 1, microcrystalline cellulose, docusate sodium, lactose (hydrous), magnesium stearate, sodium benzoate, sodium starch glycolate, pregelatinized corn starch, D&C Yellow No. 10.

* 5-chlorobenzoxazolinone

ACTIONS

Chlorzoxazone is a centrally-acting agent for painful musculoskeletal conditions. Data available from animal experiments as well as human study indicate that chlorzoxazone acts primarily at the level of the spinal cord and subcortical areas of the brain where it inhibits multisynaptic reflex arcs involved in producing and maintaining skeletal muscle spasm of varied etiology. The clinical result is a reduction of the skeletal muscle spasm with relief of pain and increased mobility of the involved muscles. Blood levels of chlorzoxazone can be detected in people during the first 30 minutes and peak levels may be reached, in the majority of the subjects, in about 1 to 2 hours after oral administration of chlorzoxazone. Chlorzoxazone is rapidly metabolized and is excreted in the urine, primarily in a conjugated form as the glucuronide. Less than one percent of a dose of chlorzoxazone is excreted unchanged in the urine in 24 hours.

INDICATIONS

PARAFON FORTE DSC chlorzoxazone is indicated as an adjunct to rest, physical therapy, and other measures for the relief of discomfort associated with acute, painful musculoskeletal conditions. The mode of action of this drug has not been clearly identified, but may be related to its sedative properties. Chlorzoxazone does not directly relax tense skeletal muscles in man.

CONTRAINDICATIONS

PARAFON FORTE DSC chlorzoxazone is contraindicated in patients with known intolerance to the drug.

WARNINGS

Serious (including fatal) hepatocellular toxicity has been reported rarely in patients receiving chlorzoxazone. The mechanism is unknown but appears to be idiosyncratic and unpredictable. Factors predisposing patients to this rare event are not known. Patients should be instructed to report early signs and/or symptoms of hepatotoxicity such as fever, rash, anorexia, nausea, vomiting, fatigue, right upper quandrant pain, dark urine, or jaundice. Chlorzoxazone should be discontinued immediately and a physician consulted if any of these signs or symptoms develop. Chlorzoxazone use should also be discontinued if a patient develops abnormal liver enzymes (eg. AST, ALT, alkaline phosphatase and bilirubin).
The concomitant use of alcohol or other central nervous system depressants may have an additive effect.
Usage in Pregnancy: The safe use of PARAFON FORTE DSC chlorzoxazone has not been established with respect to the possible adverse effects upon fetal development. Therefore, it should be used in women of childbearing potential only when, in the judgment of the physician, the potential benefits outweigh the possible risks.

PRECAUTIONS

PARAFON FORTE DSC chlorzoxazone should be used with caution in patients with known allergies or with a history of allergic reactions to drugs. If a sensitivity reaction occurs such as urticaria, redness, or itching of the skin, the drug should be stopped.
If any signs or symptoms suggestive of liver dysfunction are observed, the drug should be discontinued.

ADVERSE REACTIONS

Chlorzoxazone containing products are usually well tolerated. It is possible in rare instances that chlorzoxazone may have been associated with gastrointestinal bleeding. Drowsiness, dizziness, light-headedness, malaise, or overstimulation may be noted by an occasional patient. Rarely, allergic-type skin rashes, petechiae, or ecchymoses may develop during treatment. Angioneurotic edema or anaphylactic reactions are extremely rare. There is no evidence that the drug will cause renal damage. Rarely, a patient may note discoloration of the urine resulting from a phenolic metabolite of chlorzoxazone. This finding is of no known clinical significance.

DOSAGE AND ADMINISTRATION

Usual Adult Dosage: One caplet three or four times daily. If adequate reponse is not obtained with this dose, it may be increased to 1$^{1}/_{2}$ caplets (750 mg) three or four times daily. As improvement occurs dosage can usually be reduced.

OVERDOSAGE

Symptoms: Initially, gastrointestinal disturbances such as nausea, vomiting, or diarrhea together with drowsiness, dizziness, lightheadedness or headache may occur. Early in the course there may be malaise or sluggishness followed by marked loss of muscle tone, making voluntary movement impossible. The deep tendon reflexes may be decreased or absent. The sensorium remains intact, and there is no peripheral loss of sensation. Respiratory depression may occur with rapid, irregular respiration and intercostal and substernal retraction. The blood pressure is lowered, but shock has not been observed.
Treatment: Gastric lavage or induction of emesis should be carried out, followed by administration of activated charcoal. Thereafter, treatment is entirely supportive. If respirations are depressed, oxygen and artificial respiration should be employed and a patent airway assured by use of an oropharyngeal airway or endotracheal tube. Hypotension may be counteracted by use of dextran, plasma, concentrated albumin or a vasopressor agent such as norepinephrine. Cholinergic drugs or analeptic drugs are of no value and should not be used.

HOW SUPPLIED

PARAFON FORTE® DSC (chlorzoxazone) 500 mg caplets, (capsule shaped tablet, colored light green, imprinted "PARAFON FORTE DSC" and "McNEIL", scored).
NDC 0045-0325, bottles of 100, 500 and unit dose 100's.
Dispense in a tight container as defined in the official compendium.
Store at controlled room temperature (15°–30°C, 59°–86°F).
643-10-098-2

McNeil Pharmaceutical, McNEILAB, Inc.
Spring House, PA 19477
Shown in Product Identification Guide, page 323

TOLECTIN® 200 (tolmetin sodium) ℞
[*to-lek 'tin*]
200 mg Tablets
TOLECTIN® DS (tolmetin sodium) ℞
400 mg Capsules
TOLECTIN® 600 (tolmetin sodium) ℞
600 mg Tablets
For Oral Administration

PRODUCT OVERVIEW

KEY FACTS

TOLECTIN is rapidly and almost completely absorbed with peak plasma levels being reached within 30–60 minutes. A therapeutic response to TOLECTIN can be expected in a few days to a week. TOLECTIN displays a biphasic elimination from the plasma consisting of a rapid phase with a half-life of one to 2 hours followed by a slower phase with a half-life of about 5 hours. Essentially all of the dose is recovered in the urine in 24 hours.

MAJOR USES

TOLECTIN is indicated for the relief of signs and symptoms of rheumatoid arthritis, osteoarthritis and juvenile rheumatoid arthritis.

SAFETY INFORMATION

See complete safety information provided below.

PRESCRIBING INFORMATION

TOLECTIN® 200 (tolmetin sodium) ℞
[*to-lek 'tin*]
200 mg Tablets
NSN 6505-01-038-7460—100's
TOLECTIN® DS (tolmetin sodium) ℞
400 mg Capsules
NSN 6505-01-091-9624—100's
NSN 6505-01-039-4469—U/D 100's
TOLECTIN® 600 (tolmetin sodium) ℞
600 mg Tablets
NSN 6505-01-322-8539—100's
For Oral Administration

DESCRIPTION

TOLECTIN 200 (tolmetin sodium) tablets for oral administration contain tolmetin sodium as the dihydrate in an amount equivalent to 200 mg of tolmetin (scored for 100 mg). Each tablet contains 18 mg (0.784 mEq) of sodium and the following inactive ingredients: cellulose, magnesium stearate, silicon dioxide, corn starch and talc.

TOLECTIN DS (tolmetin sodium) capsules for oral administration contain tolmetin sodium as the dihydrate in an amount equivalent to 400 mg of tolmetin. Each capsule contains 36 mg (1.568 mEq) of sodium and the following inactive ingredients: gelatin, magnesium stearate, corn starch, talc, FD&C Red No. 3, FD&C Yellow No. 6 and titanium dioxide.

TOLECTIN 600 (tolmetin sodium) tablets for oral administration contain tolmetin sodium as the dihydrate in an amount equivalent to 600 mg of tolmetin. Each tablet contains 54 mg (2.35 mEq) of sodium and the following inactive ingredients: cellulose, silicon dioxide, crospovidone, hydroxypropyl methyl cellulose, magnesium stearate, polyethylene glycol, corn starch, titanium dioxide, FD&C Yellow No. 6 and D&C Yellow No. 10.

The pKa of tolmetin is 3.5 and tolmetin sodium is freely soluble in water.

Tolmetin sodium is a nonsteroidal anti-inflammatory agent. The structural formula is:

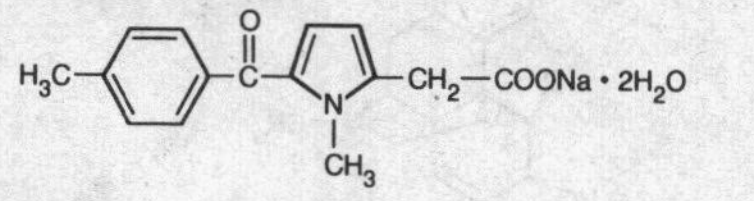

Sodium 1-methyl-5-(4-methylbenzoyl)-1*H*-pyrrole-2-acetate dihydrate.

CLINICAL PHARMACOLOGY

Studies in animals have shown TOLECTIN (tolmetin sodium) to possess anti-inflammatory, analgesic and antipyretic activity. In the rat, TOLECTIN prevents the development of experimentally induced polyarthritis and also decreases established inflammation.

The mode of action of TOLECTIN is not known. However, studies in laboratory animals and man have demonstrated that the anti-inflammatory action of TOLECTIN is *not* due to pituitary-adrenal stimulation. TOLECTIN inhibits prostaglandin synthetase *in vitro* and lowers the plasma level of prostaglandin E in man. This reduction in prostaglandin synthesis may be responsible for the anti-inflammatory action. TOLECTIN does not appear to alter the course of the underlying disease in man.

In patients with rheumatoid arthritis and in normal volunteers, tolmetin sodium is rapidly and almost completely absorbed with peak plasma levels being reached within 30–60 minutes after an oral therapeutic dose. In controlled studies, the time to reach peak tolmetin plasma concentration is approximately 20 minutes longer following administration of a 600 mg tablet, compared to an equivalent dose given as 200 mg tablets. The clinical meaningfulness of this finding, if any, is unknown. Tolmetin displays a biphasic elimination from the plasma consisting of a rapid phase with a half-life of one to 2 hours followed by a slower phase with a half-life of about 5 hours. Peak plasma levels of approximately 40 μg/mL are obtained with a 400 mg oral dose. Essentially all of the administered dose is recovered in the urine in 24 hours either as an inactive oxidative metabolite or as conjugates of tolmetin. An 18-day multiple dose study demonstrated no accumulation of tolmetin when compared with a single dose.

In two fecal blood loss studies of 4 to 6 days duration involving 15 subjects each, TOLECTIN did not induce an increase in blood loss over that observed during a 4-day drug-free control period. In the same studies, aspirin produced a greater blood loss than occurred during the drug-free control period, and a greater blood loss than occurred during the TOLECTIN treatment period. In one of the two studies, indomethacin produced a greater fecal blood loss than occurred during the drug free control period; in the second study, indomethacin did not induce a significant increase in blood loss.

TOLECTIN is effectve in treating both the acute flares and in the long term management of the symptoms of rheumatoid arthritis, osteoarthritis and juvenile rheumatoid arthritis.

In patients with either rheumatoid arthritis or osteaoarthritis, TOLECTIN is as effective as aspirin and indomethacin in controlling disease activity, but the frequency of the milder gastrointestinal adverse effects and tinnitus was less than in aspirin-treated patients, and the incidence of central nervous system adverse effects was less than in indomethacin-treated patients.

In patients with juvenile rheumatoid arthritis, TOLECTIN is as effective as aspirin in controlling disease activity, with a similar incidence of adverse reactions. Mean SGOT values, initially elevated in patients on previous aspirin therapy, remained elevated in the aspirin group and decreased in the TOLECTIN group.

TOLECTIN has produced additional therapeutic benefit when added to a regimen of gold salts and, to a lesser extent, with corticosteroids. TOLECTIN should not be used in conjunction with salicylates since greater benefit from the combination is not likely, but the potential for adverse reactions is increased.

INDICATIONS AND USAGE

TOLECTIN (tolmetin sodium) is indicated for the relief of signs and symptoms of rheumatoid arthritis and osteoarthritis. TOLECTIN is indicated in the treatment of acute flares and the long-term management of the chronic disease.

TOLECTIN is also indicated for treatment of juvenile rheumatoid arthritis. The safety and effectiveness of TOLECTIN have not been established in children under 2 years of age (see PRECAUTIONS—Pediatric Use and DOSAGE AND ADMINISTRATION).

CONTRAINDICATIONS

Anaphylactoid reactions have been reported with TOLECTIN as with other nonsteroidal anti-inflammatory drugs. Because of the possibility of cross-sensitivity to other nonsteroidal anti-inflammatory drugs, particularly zomepirac sodium, anaphylactoid reactions may be more likely to occur in patients who have exhibited allergic reactions to these compounds. For this reason, TOLECTIN should not be given to patients in whom aspirin and other nonsteroidal anti-inflammatory drugs induce symptoms of asthma, rhinitis, urticaria and other symptoms of allergic or anaphylactoid reactions. Patients experiencing anaphylactoid reactions on TOLECTIN should be treated with conventional therapy, such as epinephrine, antihistamines and/or steroids.

WARNINGS

Risk of GI Ulceration, Bleeding and Perforation with NSAID Therapy:

Serious gastrointestinal toxicity such as bleeding, ulceration, and perforation, can occur at any time, with or without symptoms, in patients treated chronically with NSAID (Nonsteroidal Anti-Inflammatory Drug) therapy. Although minor upper gastrointestinal problems, such as dyspepsia, are common, usually developng early in therapy, physicians should remain alert for ulceration and bleeding in patients treated chronically with NSAID's even in the absence of previous GI tract symptoms. In patients observed in clinical trials of several months to two years duration, symptomatic upper GI ulcers, gross bleeding or perforation appear to occur in approximately 1% of patients treated for 3–6 months, and in about 2–4% of patients treated for one year. Physicians should inform patients about the signs and/or symptoms of serious GI toxicity and what steps to take if they occur.

Studies to date have not identified any subset of patients not at risk of developing peptic ulceration and bleeding. Except for a prior history of serious GI events and other risk factors known to be associated with peptic ulcer disease, such as alcoholism, smoking, etc., no risk factor (e.g., age, sex) have been associated with increased risk. Elderly or debilitated patients seem to tolerate ulceration or bleeding less well than other individuals and most spontaneous reports of fatal GI events are in this population. Studies to date are inconclusive concerning the relative risk of various NSAID's in causing such reactions. High doses of any NSAID probably carry a greater risk of these reactions, although controlled clinical trials showing this do not exist in most cases. In considering the use of relatively large doses (within the recommended dosage range), sufficient benefit should be anticipated to offset the potential increased risk of GI toxicity.

PRECAUTIONS

General

Because of ocular changes observed in animals and reports of adverse eye findings with nonsteroidal anti-inflammatory agents, it is recommended that patients who develop visual disturbances during treatment with TOLECTIN have ophthalmologic evaluations.

As with other nonsteroidal anti-inflammatory drugs, long-term administration of tolmetin to animals has resulted in renal papillary necrosis and other abnormal renal pathology. In humans, there have been reports of acute interstitial nephritis with hematuria, proteinuria, and occasionally nephrotic syndrome.

A second form of renal toxicity has been seen in patients with prerenal conditions leading to a reduction in renal blood flow or blood volume, where the renal prostaglandins have a supportive role in the maintenance of renal perfusion. In these patients administration of an NSAID may cause a dose dependent reduction in prostaglandin formation and may precipitate overt renal decompensation. Patients at greatest risk of this reaction are those with heart failure, liver dysfunction, those taking diuretics, and the elderly. Discontinuation of NSAID therapy is typically followed by recovery to the pretreatment state.

Since TOLECTIN and its metabolites are eliminated primarily by the kidneys, patients with impaired renal function should be closely monitored, and it should be anticipated that they will require lower doses.

TOLECTIN prolongs bleeding time. Patients who may be adversely affected by prolongation of bleeding time should be carefully observed when TOLECTIN is administered.

In patients receiving concomitant TOLECTIN-steroid therapy, any reduction in steroid dosage should be gradual to avoid the possible complications of sudden steroid withdrawal.

Peripheral edema has been reported in some patients receiving TOLECTIN therapy. Therefore, as with other nonsteroidal anti-inflammatory drugs, TOLECTIN should be used with caution in patients with compromised cardiac function, hypertension, or other conditions predisposing to fluid retention.

The antipyretic and anti-inflammatory activities of the drug may reduce fever and inflammation, thus diminishing their utility as diagnostic signs in detecting complications of presumed non-infectious, non-inflammatory painful conditions.

As with other nonsteroidal anti-inflammatory drugs, borderline elevations of one or more liver tests may occur in up to 15% of patients. These abnormalities may progress, may remain essentially unchanged, or may be transient with continued therapy. The SGPT (ALT) test is probably the most sensitive indicator of liver dysfunction. Meaningful (3 times the upper limit of normal) elevations of SGPT or SGOT (AST) occurred in controlled clinical trials in less than 1% of patients. A patient with symptoms and/or signs suggesting liver dysfunction, or in whom an abnormal liver test has occurred, should be evaluated for evidence of the development of more severe hepatic reaction while on therapy with TOLECTIN. Severe hepatic reactions, including jaundice and fatal hepatitis, have been reported with TOLECTIN as with other nonsteroidal anti-inflammatory drugs. Although such reactions are rare, if abnormal liver tests persist or worsen, if clinical signs and symptoms consistent with liver disease develop, or if systemic manifestations occur (e.g. eosinophilia, rash, etc.), TOLECTIN should be discontinued.

Carcinogenesis, Mutagenesis, Impairment of Fertility

Tolmetin sodium did not possess any carcinogenic liability in the following long-term studies: a 24-month study in rats at doses as high as 75 mg/kg/day, and an 18-month study in mice at doses as high as 50 mg/kg/day.

No mutagenic potential of tolmetin sodium was found in the Ames Salmonella-Microsomal Activation Test.

Reproductive studies revealed no impairment of fertility in animals. Effects on parturition have been shown, however, as with other prostaglandin inhibitors. This information is detailed in the Pregnancy section below.

Continued on next page

Information on McNeil Pharmaceutical Products is based on labeling in effect in August 1996.

Consult 1997 supplements and future editions for revisions

McNeil—Cont.

Pregnancy
Pregnancy Category C. Reproduction studies in rats and rabbits at doses up to 50 mg/kg (1.5 times the maximum clinical dose based on a body weight of 60 kg) revealed no evidence of teratogenesis or impaired fertility due to TOLECTIN. However, TOLECTIN is an inhibitor of prostaglandin synthetase. Drugs in this class have known effects on the fetal cardiovascular system which may cause constriction of the ductus arteriosus *in utero* during the third trimester of pregnancy, which may result in persistent pulmonary hypertension of the newborn.
There are no adequate and well-controlled studies in pregnant women. TOLECTIN should be used during pregnancy only if the potential benefit justifies the potential risk to the fetus.

Non-Teratogenic Effects
Prostaglandin inhibitors have also been shown to increase the incidence of dystocia and delayed parturition in animals.

Nursing Mothers
TOLECTIN has been shown to be secreted in human milk. Because of the possible adverse effects of prostaglandin inhibiting drugs on neonates, use in nursing mothers should be avoided.

Pediatric Use
The safety and effectiveness of TOLECTIN in children under 2 years of age have not been established.

Drug Interactions
The *in vitro* binding of warfarin to human plasma proteins is unaffected by tolmetin, and tolmetin does not alter the prothrombin time of normal volunteers. However, increased prothrombin time and bleeding have been reported in patients on concomitant TOLECTIN and warfarin therapy. Therefore, caution should be exercised when administering TOLECTIN to patients on anticoagulants.
In adult diabetic patients under treatment with either sulfonylureas or insulin there is no change in the clinical effects of either TOLECTIN or the hypoglycemic agents.
Caution should be used if TOLECTIN is administered concomitantly with methotrexate. TOLECTIN and other nonsteroidal anti-inflammatory drugs have been reported to reduce the tubular secretion of methotrexate in an animal model, possibly enhancing the toxicity of methotrexate.

Laboratory Tests
Because serious GI tract ulceration and bleeding can occur without warning symptoms, physicians should follow chronically treated patients for the signs and symptoms of ulceration and bleeding and should inform them of the importance of this follow-up (see WARNINGS—Risk of GI Ulceration, Bleeding and Perforation with NSAID Therapy).

Drug/Laboratory Test Interaction
The metabolites of tolmetin sodium in urine have been found to give positive tests for proteinuria using tests which rely on acid precipitation as their endpoint (e.g. sulfosalicylic acid). No interference is seen in the tests for proteinuria using dye-impregnated commercially available reagent strips (e.g., Albustix®, Uristix®, etc.).

Drug-Food Interaction
In a controlled single dose study, administration of TOLECTIN with milk had no effect on peak plasma tolmetin concentrations, but decreased total tolmetin bioavailability by 16%. When TOLECTIN was taken immediately after a meal, peak plasma tolmetin concentrations were reduced by 50% while total bioavailability was again decreased by 16%.

Information for Patients
TOLECTIN, like other drugs of its class, is not free of side effects. The side effects of these drugs can cause discomfort and, rarely, there are more serious side effects, such as gastrointestinal bleeding, which may result in hospitalization and even fatal outcomes.
NSAID's (Nonsteroidal Anti-Inflammatory Drugs) are often essential agents in the management of arthritis, but they also may be commonly employed for conditions which are less serious.
Physicians may wish to discuss with their patients the potential risks (see WARNINGS, PRECAUTIONS, and ADVERSE REACTIONS sections) and likely benefits of NSAID treatment, particularly when the drugs are used for less serious conditions where treatment without NSAID's may represent an acceptable alternative to both the patient and physician.

ADVERSE REACTIONS
The adverse reactions which have been observed in clinical trials encompass observations in about 4370 patients treated with TOLECTIN (tolmetin sodium), over 800 of whom have undergone at least one year of therapy. These adverse reactions, reported below by body system, are among those typical of nonsteroidal anti-inflammatory drugs and, as expected, gastrointestinal complaints were most frequent. In clinical trials with TOLECTIN, about 10% of patients dropped out because of adverse reactions, mostly gastrointestinal in nature.

Incidence Greater Than 1%
The following adverse reactions which occurred more frequently than 1 in 100 were reported in controlled clinical trials.
Gastrointestinal: Nausea (11%), dyspepsia,* gastrointestinal distress,* abdominal pain,* diarrhea,* flatulence,* vomiting,* constipation, gastritis, and peptic ulcer. Forty percent of the ulcer patients had a prior history of peptic ulcer disease and/or were receiving concomitant anti-inflammatory drugs including corticosteroids, which are known to produce peptic ulceration.
Body as a Whole: Headache,* asthenia,* chest pain
Cardiovascular: Elevated blood pressure,* edema*
Central Nervous System: Dizziness,* drowsiness, depression
Metabolic/Nutritional: Weight gain,* weight loss*
Dermatologic: Skin irritation
Special Senses: Tinnitus, visual disturbance
Hematologic: Small and transient decreases in hemoglobin and hematocrit not associated with gastrointestinal bleeding have occurred. These are similar to changes reported with other nonsteroidal anti-inflammatory drugs.
Urogenital: Elevated BUN, urinary tract infection

*Reactions occurring in 3% to 9% of patients treated with TOLECTIN. Reactions occurring in fewer than 3% of the patients are unmarked.

Incidence Less Than 1%
(Causal Relationship Probable)
The following adverse reactions were reported less frequently than 1 in 100 in controlled clinical trials or were reported since marketing. The probability exists that there is a causal relationship between TOLECTIN and these adverse reactions.
Gastrointestinal: Gastrointestinal bleeding with or without evidence of peptic ulcer, perforation, glossitis, stomatitis, hepatitis, liver function abnormalities
Body as a Whole: Anaphylactoid reactions, fever, lymphadenopathy, serum sickness
Hematologic: Hemolytic anemia, thrombocytopenia, granulocytopenia, agranulocytosis
Cardiovascular: Congestive heart failure in patients with marginal cardiac function
Dermatologic: Urticaria, purpura, erythema multiforme, toxic epidermal necrolysis
Urogenital: Hematuria, proteinuria, dysuria, renal failure

Incidence Less Than 1%
(Causal Relationship Unknown)
Other adverse reactions were reported less frequently than 1 in 100 in controlled clinical trials or were reported since marketing, but a causal relationship between TOLECTIN and the reaction could not be determined. These rarely reported reactions are being listed as alerting information for the physician since the possibility of a causal relationship cannot be excluded.
Body as Whole: Epistaxis
Special Senses: Optic neuropathy, retinal and macular changes

MANAGEMENT OF OVERDOSAGE
In the event of overdosage, the stomach should be emptied by inducing vomiting or by gastric lavage followed by the administration of activated charcoal.

DOSAGE AND ADMINISTRATION
In adults with rheumatoid arthritis or osteoarthritis, the recommended starting dose is 400 mg three times daily (1200 mg daily), preferably including a dose on arising and a dose at bedtime. To achieve optimal therapeutic effect the dose should be adjusted according to the patient's response after one to two weeks. Control is usually achieved at doses of 600–1800 mg daily in divided doses (generally t.i.d.). Doses larger than 1800 mg/kg have not been studied and are not recommended.
The recommended starting dose for children (2 years and older) is 20 mg/kg/day in divided doses (t.i.d. or q.i.d.). When control has been achieved, the usual dose ranges from 15 to 30 mg/kg/day. Doses higher than 30 mg/kg/day have not been studied and, therefore, are not recommended.
A therapeutic response to TOLECTIN (tolmetin sodium) can be expected in a few days to a week. Progressive improvement can be anticipated during succeeding weeks of therapy. If gastrointestinal symptoms occur, TOLECTIN can be administered with antacids other than sodium bicarbonate. TOLECTIN bioavailability and pharmacokinetics are not significantly affected by acute or chronic administration of magnesium and aluminum hydroxides; however, bioavailability is affected by food or milk (see PRECAUTIONS—Drug-Food Interaction).

HOW SUPPLIED
TOLECTIN® 200 (tolmetin sodium) tablets 200 mg (white, scored, imprinted "TOLECTIN," "200" and "McNEIL"), NDC 0045-0412, bottles of 100.
TOLECTIN® DS (tolmetin sodium) capsules 400 mg (colored orange opaque, with contrasting parallel bands, imprinted "TOLECTIN DS" and "McNEIL"), NDC 0045-0414, bottles of 100, 500 and unit dose of 100's.
TOLECTIN® 600 (tolmetin sodium) tablets 600 mg (colored orange, film coated, imprinted "TOLECTIN 600" and "McNEIL"), NDC 0045-0416, bottles of 100 and 500.
Dispense in tight, light-resistant container as defined in the official compendium.
Store at controlled room temperature (15°-30°C, 59°-86°F). Protect from light.
McNeil Pharmaceutical, McNEILAB, Inc.
Spring House, PA 19477

643-10-089-1

Shown in Product Identification Guide, page 323 and page 324

TYLENOL® with Codeine ℞
[*ti 'len-awl co 'dēn*]
(acetaminophen and codeine phosphate tablets and oral solution USP)
Tablets CIII and Elixir CV
No. 3-NSN 6505-00-400-2054—100's
No. 3-NSN 6505-00-147-8347—500's
No. 3-NSN 6505-01-086-2993—U/D 500's
No. 3-NSN 6505-00-372-3032—1000's
Elixir-NSN 6505-01-035-1963—Pints

DESCRIPTION
Each tablet contains:

No. 2 Codeine Phosphate*	15 mg
Acetaminophen	300 mg
No. 3 Codeine Phosphate*	30 mg
Acetaminophen	300 mg
No. 4 Codeine Phosphate*	60 mg
Acetaminophen	300 mg

Each 5 mL of elixir contains:

Codeine Phosphate*	12 mg
Acetaminophen	120 mg
Alcohol	7%

**Warning* —May be habit forming.
Inactive ingredients: tablets—powdered cellulose, magnesium stearate, sodium metabisulfite†, pregelatinized starch, starch (corn); elixir—alcohol, citric acid, propylene glycol, sodium benzoate, saccharin sodium, sucrose, natural and artificial flavors, FD&C Yellow No.6.
Acetaminophen, 4'-hydroxyacetanilide, is a non-opiate, non-salicylate analgesic and antipyretic which occurs as a white, odorless, crystalline powder, possessing a slightly bitter taste. Its structure is as follows:

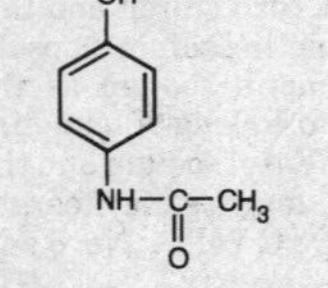

C_8H_9NO M.W. 151.16

Codeine is an alkaloid, obtained from opium or prepared from morphine by methylation. Codeine phosphate occurs as fine, white, needle-shaped crystals, or white, crystalline powder. It is affected by light. Its chemical name is: 7,8-didehydro- 4,5α-epoxy-3-methoxy-17- methylmorphinan-6α-ol phosphate (1:1) (salt) hemihydrate. Its structure is as follows:

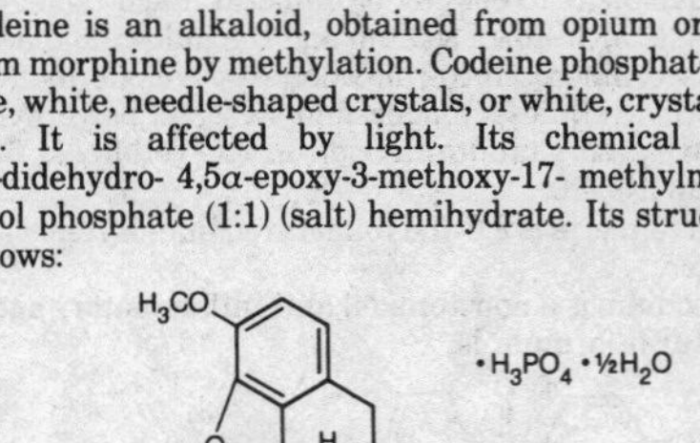

$C_{18}H_{21}NO_3 \cdot H_3PO_4 \cdot {}^1/_2H_2O$ M.W. 406.37

†See WARNINGS

CLINICAL PHARMACOLOGY
TYLENOL with Codeine (acetaminophen and codeine phosphate tablets and oral solution USP) combine the analgesic effects of a centrally acting analgesic, codeine, with a peripherally acting analgesic, acetaminophen. Both ingredients are well absorbed orally. The plasma elimination half-life ranges from 1 to 4 hours for acetaminophen, and from 2.5 to 3 hours for codeine.
Codeine retains at least one-half of its analgesic activity when administered orally. A reduced first-pass metabolism of codeine by the liver accounts for the greater oral efficacy of codeine when compared to most other morphine-like narcotics. Following absorption, codeine is metabolized by the liver and metabolic products are excreted in the urine. Approximately 10 percent of the administered codeine is demethylated to morphine, which may account for its analgesic activity.
Acetaminophen is distributed throughout most fluids of the body, and is metabolized primarily in the liver. Little un-

changed drug is excreted in the urine, but most metabolic products appear in the urine within 24 hours.

INDICATIONS AND USAGE

TYLENOL with Codeine tablets (acetaminophen and codeine phosphate tablets) are indicated for the relief of mild to moderately severe pain.

TYLENOL with Codeine elixir (acetaminophen and codeine phosphate oral solution USP) is indicated for the relief of mild to moderate pain.

CONTRAINDICATIONS

TYLENOL with Codeine tablets or elixir (acetaminophen and codeine phosphate tablets and oral solution USP) should not be administered to patients who have previously exhibited hypersensitivity to any component.

WARNINGS

TYLENOL with Codeine tablets (acetaminophen and codeine phosphate tablets) contain sodium metabisulfite, a sulfite that may cause allergic-type reactions including anaphylactic symptoms and life-threatening or less severe asthmatic episodes in certain susceptible people. The overall prevalence of sulfite sensitivity in the general population is unknown and probably low. Sulfite sensitivity is seen more frequently in asthmatic than in nonasthmatic people.

PRECAUTIONS

General

Head Injury and Increased Intracranial Pressure: The respiratory depressant effects of narcotics and their capacity to elevate cerebrospinal fluid pressure may be markedly exaggerated in the presence of head injury, other intracranial lesions or a pre-existing increase in intracranial pressure. Furthermore, narcotics produce adverse reactions which may obscure the clinical course of patients with head injuries.

Acute Abdominal Conditions: The administration of this product or other narcotics may obscure the diagnosis or clinical course of patients with acute abdominal conditions.

Special Risk Patients: This drug should be given with caution to certain patients such as the elderly or debilitated, and those with severe impairment of hepatic or renal function, hypothyroidism, Addison's disease, and prostatic hypertrophy or urethral stricture.

Information for Patients

Codeine may impair the mental and/or physical abilities required for the performance of potentially hazardous tasks such as driving a car or operating machinery. The patient using this drug should be cautioned accordingly.

The patient should understand the single-dose and 24 hour dose limits, and the time interval between doses.

Drug Interactions

Patients receiving other narcotic analgesics, antipsychotics, antianxiety agents, or other CNS depressants (including alcohol) concomitantly with this drug may exhibit an additive CNS depression. When such combined therapy is contemplated, the dose of one or both agents should be reduced. The concurrent use of anticholinergics with codeine may produce paralytic ileus.

Carcinogenesis, Mutagenesis, Impairment of Fertility

No long-term studies in animals have been performed with acetaminophen or codeine to determine carcinogenic potential or effects on fertility.

Acetaminophen and codeine have been found to have no mutagenic potential using the Ames Salmonella-Microsomal Activation test, the Basc test on Drosophila germ cells, and the Micronucleus test on mouse bone marrow.

Pregnancy

Teratogenic Effects: Pregnancy Category C.

Codeine: A study in rats and rabbits reported no teratogenic effect of codeine administered during the period of organogenesis in doses ranging from 5 to 120 mg/kg. In the rat, doses at the 120 mg/kg level, in the toxic range for the adult animal, were associated with an increase in embryo resorption at the time of implantation. In another study a single 100 mg/kg dose of codeine administered to pregnant mice reportedly resulted in delayed ossification in the offspring.

There are no studies in humans, and the significance of these findings to humans, if any, is not known.

TYLENOL with Codeine (acetaminophen and codeine phosphate tablets and oral solution USP) should be used during pregnancy only if the potential benefit justifies the potential risk to the fetus.

Nonteratogenic Effects:

Dependence has been reported in newborns whose mothers took opiates regularly during pregnancy. Withdrawal signs include irritability, excessive crying, tremors, hyperreflexia, fever, vomiting, and diarrhea. These signs usually appear during the first few days of life.

Labor and Delivery

Narcotic analgesics cross the placental barrier. The closer to delivery and the larger the dose used, the greater the possibility of respiratory depression in the newborn. Narcotic analgesics should be avoided during labor if delivery of a premature infant is anticipated. If the mother has received narcotic analgesics during labor, newborn infants should be observed closely for signs of respiratory depression. Resuscitation may be required (see OVERDOSAGE). The effect of codeine, if any, on the later growth, development, and functional maturation of the child is unknown.

Nursing Mothers

Some studies, but not others, have reported detectable amounts of codeine in breast milk. The levels are probably not clinically significant after usual therapeutic dosage. The possibility of clinically important amounts being excreted in breast milk in individuals abusing codeine should be considered.

Pediatric Use

Safe dosage of TYLENOL with Codeine elixir (acetaminophen and codeine phosphate oral solution USP) has not been established in children below the age of three years.

ADVERSE REACTIONS

The most frequently observed adverse reactions include lightheadedness, dizziness, sedation, shortness of breath, nausea and vomiting. These effects seem to be more prominent in ambulatory than in non-ambulatory patients, and some of these adverse reactions may be alleviated if the patient lies down. Other adverse reactions include allergic reactions, euphoria, dysphoria, constipation, abdominal pain and pruritus.

At higher doses, codeine has most of the disadvantages of morphine including respiratory depression.

DRUG ABUSE AND DEPENDENCE

TYLENOL with Codeine tablets (acetaminophen and codeine phosphate tablets) are a Schedule III controlled substance.

TYLENOL with Codeine elixir (acetaminophen and codeine phosphate oral solution USP) is a Schedule V controlled substance.

Codeine can produce drug dependence of the morphine type and, therefore, has the potential for being abused. Psychic dependence, physical dependence and tolerance may develop upon repeated administration of this drug, and it should be prescribed and administered with the same degree of caution appropriate to the use of other oral narcotic-containing medications.

OVERDOSAGE

Acetaminophen

Signs and Symptoms: In acute acetaminophen overdosage, dose-dependent, potentially fatal hepatic necrosis is the most serious adverse effect. Renal tubular necrosis, hypoglycemic coma and thrombocytopenia may also occur.

In adults, hepatic toxicity has rarely been reported with acute overdoses of less than 10 grams and fatalities with less than 15 grams. Importantly, young children seem to be more resistant than adults to the hepatotoxic effect of an acetaminophen overdose. Despite this, the measures outlined below should be initiated in any adult or child suspected of having ingested an acetaminophen overdose.

Early symptoms following a potentially hepatotoxic overdose may include: nausea, vomiting, diaphoresis and general malaise. Clinical and laboratory evidence of hepatic toxicity may not be apparent until 48 to 72 hours post-ingestion.

Treatment: The stomach should be emptied promptly by lavage or by induction of emesis with syrup of ipecac. Patients' estimates of the quantity of a drug ingested are notoriously unreliable. Therefore, if an acetaminophen overdose is suspected, a serum acetaminophen assay should be obtained as early as possible, but no sooner than four hours following ingestion. Liver function studies should be obtained initially and repeated at 24-hour intervals.

The antidote, N-acetylcysteine, should be administered as early as possible, preferably within 16 hours of the overdose ingestion for optimal results, but in any case, within 24 hours. Following recovery, there are no residual, structural or functional hepatic abnormalities.

Codeine

Signs and Symptoms: Serious overdose with codeine is characterized by respiratory depression (a decrease in respiratory rate and/or tidal volume, Cheyne-Stokes respiration, cyanosis), extreme somnolence progressing to stupor or coma, skeletal muscle flaccidity, cold and clammy skin, and sometimes bradycardia and hypotension. In severe overdosage, apnea, circulatory collapse, cardiac arrest and death may occur.

Treatment: Primary attention should be given to the reestablishment of adequate respiratory exchange through provision of a patent airway and the institution of assisted or controlled ventilation. The narcotic antagonist naloxone is a specific antidote against respiratory depression which may result from overdosage or unusual sensitivity to narcotics, including codeine. Therefore, an appropriate dose of naloxone hydrochloride (see package insert) should be administered, preferably by the intravenous route, and simultaneously with efforts at respiratory resuscitation. Since the duration of action of codeine may exceed that of the antagonist, the patient should be kept under continued surveillance and repeated doses of the antagonist should be administered as needed to maintain adequate respiration.

An antagonist should not be administered in the absence of clinically significant respiratory or cardiovascular depression. Oxygen, intravenous fluids, vasopressors and other supportive measures should be employed as indicated.

Gastric emptying may be useful in removing unabsorbed drug.

DOSAGE AND ADMINISTRATION

Dosage should be adjusted according to severity of pain and response of the patient.

It should be kept in mind, however, that tolerance to codeine can develop with continued use and that the incidence of untoward effects is dose related. Adult doses of codeine higher than 60 mg fail to give commensurate relief of pain but merely prolong analgesia and are associated with an appreciably increased incidence of undesirable side effects. Equivalently high doses in children would have similar effects.

The usual adult dosage for tablets is:

	Single Doses (Range)	Maximum 24 Hour Dose
Codeine Phosphate	15mg–60mg	360mg
Acetaminophen	300mg–1000mg	4000mg

Doses may be repeated up to every 4 hours.

The prescriber must determine the number of tablets per dose, and the maximum number of tablets per 24 hours, based upon the above dosage guidance. This information should be conveyed in the prescription.

For children, the dose of codeine phosphate is 0.5 mg/kg.

TYLENOL with Codeine elixir (acetaminophen and codeine phosphate oral solution USP) contains 120 mg of acetaminophen and 12 mg of codeine phosphate/5 mL and is given orally.

The usual doses are:

Children: *(7 to 12 years):* 10 mL (2 teaspoonfuls) 3 or 4 times daily.
(3 to 6 years): 5 mL (1 teaspoonful) 3 or 4 times daily.
(under 3 years): safe dosage has not been established.

Adults: 15 mL (1 tablespoonful) every 4 hours as needed.

HOW SUPPLIED

TYLENOL with Codeine tablets (acetaminophen and codeine phosphate tablets): (round, white, imprinted "McNEIL," "TYLENOL CODEINE" and either "2," "3," "4"): No.2 – NDC 0045-0511-60 bottles of 100, NDC 0045-0511-72 unit dose (20 × 25); No. 3 – NDC 0045-0513-60 bottles of 100, NDC 0045-0513-70 bottles of 500, NDC 0045-0513-80 bottles of 1000, NDC 0045-0513-72 unit dose (20 × 25); No. 4 — NDC 0045-0515-60 bottles of 100, NDC 0045-0515-70 bottles of 500, NDC 0045-515-72 unit dose (20 × 25).

TYLENOL with Codeine elixir (acetaminophen and codeine phosphate oral solution USP) contains 120 mg acetaminophen and 12 mg codeine phosphate/5 mL (colored amber, cherry flavored) — NDC 0045-0508-16, bottles of 1 pint.

Store TYLENOL with Codeine tablets at controlled room temperature (15–30°C, 59–86°F).

Store TYLENOL with Codeine elixir at controlled room temperature (15–30°C, 59–86°F). Protect from light. Do not refrigerate. Do not freeze.

Dispense in tight, light-resistant container as defined in the official compendium.

McNeil Pharmaceutical, McNEILAB, INC., Spring House, PA 19477

633-10-057-1

Shown in Product Identification Guide, page 324

TYLOX® Capsules ⒸII ℞

[*ti 'lox*]

(oxycodone and acetaminophen capsules USP)

NSN 6505-01-210-4450-100's

NSN 6505-01-211-6803-Unit Dose (100's)

DESCRIPTION

Each capsule of TYLOX (oxycodone and acetaminophen capsules USP) contains:

Oxycodone Hydrochloride USP .... 5 mg*
Warning—May be habit forming.
Acetaminophen USP .... 500 mg

Inactive ingredients: docusate sodium, gelatin, magnesium stearate, sodium benzoate, sodium metabisulfite†, corn starch, FD&C Blue No. 1, FD&C Red No. 3, FD&C Red No. 40, and titanium dioxide.

Continued on next page

Information on McNeil Pharmaceutical Products is based on labeling in effect in August 1996.

McNeil—Cont.

Acetaminophen occurs as a white, odorless crystalline powder, possessing a slightly bitter taste.
The oxycodone component is 14-hydroxydihydrocodeinone, a white, odorless crystalline powder having a saline, bitter taste. It is derived from the opium alkaloid thebaine, and may be represented by the following structural formula:

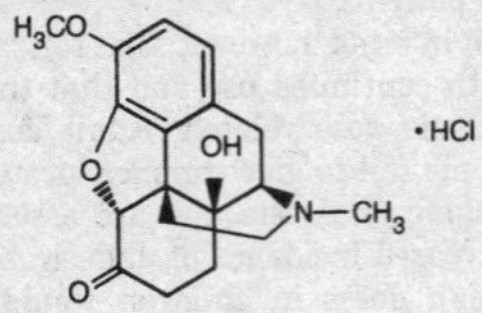

*5 mg oxycodone hydrochloride is equivalent to 4.4815 mg oxycodone
†See WARNINGS

CLINICAL PHARMACOLOGY

The principal ingredient, oxycodone, is a semisynthetic narcotic analgesic with multiple actions qualitatively similar to those of morphine; the most prominent of these involve the central nervous system and organs composed of smooth muscle. The principal actions of therapeutic value of the oxycodone in TYLOX (oxycodone and acetaminophen capsules) are analgesia and sedation.
Oxycodone is similar to codeine and methadone in that it retains at least one-half of its analgesic activity when administered orally.
Acetaminophen is a non-opiate, non-salicylate analgesic and antipyretic.

INDICATIONS AND USAGE

TYLOX (oxycodone and acetaminophen capsules) are indicated for the relief of moderate to moderately severe pain.

CONTRAINDICATIONS

TYLOX (oxycodone and acetaminophen capsules) should not be administered to patients who are hypersensitive to any component.

WARNINGS

Contains sodium metabisulfite, a sulfite that may cause allergic-type reactions including anaphylactic symptoms and life-threatening or less severe asthmatic episodes in certain susceptible people. The overall prevalence of sulfite sensitivity in the general population is unknown and probably low. Sulfite sensitivity is seen more frequently in asthmatic than in nonasthmatic people.

Drug Dependence

Oxycodone can produce drug dependence of the morphine type and, therefore, has the potential for being abused. Psychic dependence, physical dependence and tolerance may develop upon repeated administration of TYLOX (oxycodone and acetaminophen capsules), and it should be prescribed and administered with the same degree of caution appropriate to the use of other oral narcotic-containing medications. Like other narcotic-containing medications, TYLOX is subject to the Federal Control Substances Act (Schedule II).

PRECAUTIONS

General

Head Injury and Increased Intracranial Pressure: The respiratory depressant effects of narcotics and their capacity to elevate cerebrospinal fluid pressure may be markedly exaggerated in the presence of head injury, other intracranial lesions or a pre-existing increase in intracranial pressure. Furthermore, narcotics produce adverse reactions which may obscure the clinical course of patients with head injuries.
Acute Abdominal Conditions: The administration of TYLOX (oxycodone and acetaminophen capsules) or other narcotics may obscure the diagnosis or clinical course in patients with acute abdominal conditions.
Special Risk Patients: TYLOX should be given with caution to certain patients such as the elderly or debilitated, and those with severe impairment of hepatic or renal function, hypothyroidism, Addison's disease, and prostatic hypertrophy or urethral stricture.

Information for Patients

Oxycodone may impair the mental and/or physical abilities required for the performance of potentially hazardous tasks such as driving a car or operating machinery. The patient using TYLOX should be cautioned accordingly.

Drug Interactions

Patients receiving other narcotic analgesics, general anesthetics, phenothiazines, other tranquilizers, sedative-hypnotics or other CNS depressants (including alcohol) concomitantly with TYLOX may exhibit an additive CNS depression. When such combined therapy is contemplated, the dose of one or both agents should be reduced.
The concurrent use of anticholinergics with narcotics may produce paralytic ileus.

Usage in Pregnancy

Pregnancy Category C. Animal reproductive studies have not been conducted with TYLOX. It is also not known whether TYLOX can cause fetal harm when administered to a pregnant woman or can affect reproductive capacity. TYLOX should not be given to a pregnant woman unless in the judgment of the physician, the potential benefits outweigh the possible hazards.
Nonteratogenic Effects: Use of narcotics during pregnancy may produce physical dependence in the neonate.

Labor and Delivery

As with all narcotics, administration of TYLOX to the mother shortly before delivery may result in some degree of respiratory depression in the newborn and the mother, especially if higher doses are used.

Nursing Mothers

It is not known whether the components of TYLOX are excreted in human milk. Because many drugs are excreted in human milk, caution should be exercised when TYLOX is administered to a nursing woman.

Pediatric Use

Safety and effectiveness in children have not been established.

ADVERSE REACTIONS

The most frequently observed adverse reactions include lightheadedness, dizziness, sedation, nausea and vomiting. These effects seem to be more prominent in ambulatory than in non-ambulatory patients, and some of these adverse reactions may be alleviated if the patient lies down.
Other adverse reactions include allergic reactions, euphoria, dysphoria, constipation, skin rash and pruritus. At higher doses, oxycodone has most of the disadvantages of morphine including respiratory depression.

DRUG ABUSE AND DEPENDENCE

TYLOX capsules are a Schedule II controlled substance. Oxycodone can produce drug dependence and has the potential for being abused. (See WARNINGS)

OVERDOSAGE

Acetaminophen

Signs and Symptoms: In acute acetaminophen overdosage, dose-dependent potentially fatal hepatic necrosis is the most serious adverse effect. Renal tubular necrosis, hypoglycemic coma and thrombocytopenia may also occur.
In adults, hepatic toxicity has rarely been reported with acute overdoses of less than 10 grams and fatalities with less than 15 grams. Importantly, young children seem to be more resistant than adults to the hepatotoxic effect of an acetaminophen overdose. Despite this, the measures outlined below should be initiated in any adult or child suspected of having ingested an acetaminophen overdose.
Early symptoms following a potentially hepatotoxic overdose may include: nausea, vomiting, diaphoresis, and general malaise. Clinical and laboratory evidence of hepatic toxicity may not be apparent until 48 to 72 hours post-ingestion.
Treatment: The stomach should be emptied promptly by lavage or by induction of emesis with syrup of ipecac. Patients' estimates of the quantity of a drug ingested are notoriously unreliable. Therefore, if an acetaminophen overdose is suspected, a serum acetaminophen assay should be obtained as early as possible, but no sooner than four hours following ingestion. Liver function studies should be obtained initially and repeated at 24-hour intervals.
The antidote, N-acetylcysteine, should be administered as early as possible, and within 16 hours of the overdose ingestion for optimal results. Following recovery, there are no residual, structural, or functional hepatic abnormalities.

Oxycodone

Signs and symptoms: Serious overdosage with oxycodone is characterized by respiratory depression (a decrease in respiratory rate and/or tidal volume, Cheyne-Stokes respiration, cyanosis), extreme somnolence progressing to stupor or coma, skeletal muscle flaccidity, cold and clammy skin, and sometimes bradycardia and hypotension. In severe overdosage, apnea, circulatory collapse, cardiac arrest, and death may occur.
Treatment: Primary attention should be given to the reestablishment of adequate respiratory exchange through provision of a patent airway and the institution of assisted or controlled ventilation. The narcotic antagonist naloxone hydrochloride is a specific antidote against respiratory depression which may result from overdosage or unusual sensitivity to narcotics, including oxycodone. Therefore, an appropriate dose of naloxone hydrochloride (usual initial adult dose 0.4 mg to 2 mg) should be admininstered preferably by the intravenous route and simultaneously with efforts at respiratory resuscitation (see package insert). Since the duration of action of oxycodone may exceed that of the antagonist, the patient should be kept under continued surveillance and repeated doses of the antagonist should be administered as needed to maintain adequate respiration.
An antagonist should not be administered in the absence of clinically significant respiratory or cardiovascular depression. Oxygen, intravenous fluids, vasopressors and other supportive measures should be employed as indicated.
Gastric emptying may be useful in removing unabsorbed drug.

DOSAGE AND ADMINISTRATION

Dosage should be adjusted according to the severity of the pain and the response of the patient. However, it should be kept in mind that tolerance to oxycodone can develop with continued use and that the incidence of untoward effects is dose related. This product is inappropriate even in high doses for severe or intractable pain.
TYLOX (oxycodone and acetaminophen capsules) are given orally. The usual adult dosage is one TYLOX capsule every 6 hours as needed for pain.

HOW SUPPLIED

TYLOX (oxycodone and acetaminophen capsules USP): (colored red, imprinted "TYLOX" "McNEIL") NDC 0045-0526—bottles of 100 and unit dose 100's.
Dispense in tight, light-resistant container as defined in the official compendium.
Store at controlled room temperature (15°–30° C, 59°–86° F). Protect from moisture.
McNeil Pharmaceutical, McNEILAB, Inc.
Spring House, PA 19477

643-10-561-2

Shown in Product Identification Guide, page 324

ULTRAM® ℞

(tramadol hydrochloride tablets)

DESCRIPTION

ULTRAM® (Tramadol Hydrochloride Tablets) is a centrally acting analgesic. The chemical name for tramadol hydrochloride is (±)*cis*-2-[(dimethylamino)methyl]-1-(3-methoxyphenyl) cyclohexanol hydrochloride. Its structural formula is:

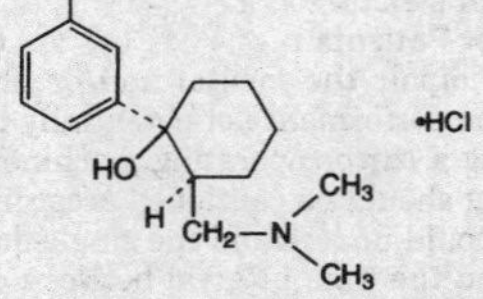

The molecular weight of tramadol hydrochloride is 299.8. Tramadol hydrochloride is a white, bitter, crystalline and odorless powder. It is readily soluble in water and ethanol and has a pKa of 9.41. The water/n-octanol partition coefficient is 1.35 at pH 7. ULTRAM tablets contain 50 mg of tramadol hydrochloride and are white in color. Inactive ingredients in the tablet are corn starch, hydroxypropyl methylcellulose, lactose, magnesium stearate, microcrystalline cellulose, polyethylene glycol, polysorbate 80, sodium starch glycolate, titanium dioxide and wax.

CLINICAL PHARMACOLOGY

Pharmacodynamics

ULTRAM is a centrally acting synthetic analgesic compound. Although its mode of action is not completely understood, from animal tests, at least two complementary mechanisms appear applicable: binding of parent and M1 metabolite to μ-opioid receptors and weak inhibition of reuptake of norepinephrine and serotonin. Opioid activity is due to both low affinity binding of the parent compound and higher affinity binding of the O-demethylated metabolite M1 to μ-opioid receptors. In animal models, M1 is up to 6 times more potent than tramadol in producing analgesia and 200 times more potent in μ-opioid binding. Tramadol-induced analgesia is only partially antagonized by the opiate antagonist naloxone in several animal tests. The relative contribution of both tramadol and M1 to human analgesia is dependent upon the plasma concentrations of each compound (see CLINICAL PHARMACOLOGY, Pharmacokinetics).
Tramadol has been shown to inhibit reuptake of norepinephrine and serotonin *in vitro*, as have some other opioid analgesics. These mechanisms may contribute independently to the overall analgesic profile of ULTRAM. Analgesia in humans begins approximately within one hour after administration and reaches a peak in approximately two to three hours.
Apart from analgesia, ULTRAM administration may produce a constellation of symptoms (including dizziness, somnolence, nausea, constipation, sweating and pruritis) similar to that of an opioid. However, tramadol causes less respiratory depression than morphine at recommended doses (see OVERDOSAGE). In contrast to morphine, tramadol has not been shown to cause histamine release. At therapeutic doses, ULTRAM has no effect on heart rate, left-ventricular function or cardiac index. Orthostatic hypotension has been observed.

Pharmacokinetics

The analgesic activity of ULTRAM is due to both parent drug and the M1 metabolite (see CLINICAL PHARMACOLOGY, Pharmacodynamics). Tramadol is administered as a racemate and both the [−] and [+] forms of both tramadol and M1 are detected in the circulation. Tramadol is well absorbed orally with an absolute bioavailability of 75%. Tramadol has a volume of distribution of approximately 2.7L/kg and is only 20% bound to plasma proteins. Tramadol is extensively metabolized. One metabolite, M1, is pharmacologically active in animal models. The formation of M1 is dependent upon Cytochrome P-450(2D6) and as such is subject to both metabolic induction and inhibition which may affect the therapeutic response (see PRECAUTIONS—Drug Interactions). Tramadol and its metabolites are excreted primarily in the urine with observed plasma half-lives of 6.3 and 7.4 hours for tramadol and M1, respectively. Linear pharmacokinetics have been observed following multiple doses of 50 and 100 mg to steady-state.

Absorption:
Racemic tramadol is rapidly and almost completely absorbed after oral administration. The mean absolute bioavailability of a 100 mg oral dose is approximately 75%. The mean peak plasma concentration of racemic tramadol and M1 occurs at two and three hours, respectively, after administration in healthy adults. In general, both enantiomers of tramadol and M1 follow a parallel time course in the body following single and multiple doses although small differences (~10%) exist in the absolute amount of each enantiomer present.

Steady-state plasma concentrations of both tramadol and M1 are achieved within two days with q.i.d. dosing. There is no evidence of self-induction (see Figure 1 and Table 1 below).

Figure 1: Mean Tramadol and M1 Plasma Concentration Profiles after a Single 100 mg Oral Dose and after Twenty-Nine 100 mg Oral Doses of Tramadol HCl given q.i.d.

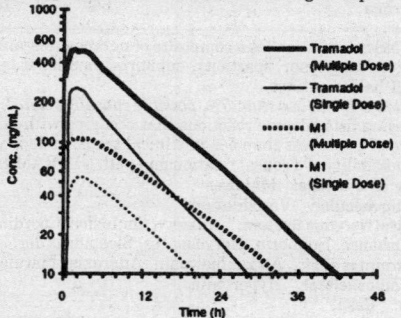

[See table 1 above.]

Food Effects: Oral administration of ULTRAM with food does not significantly affect its rate or extent of absorption, therefore, ULTRAM can be administered without regard to food.

Distribution:
The volume of distribution of tramadol was 2.6 and 2.9 liters/kg in male and female subjects, respectively, following a 100 mg intravenous dose. The binding of tramadol to human plasma proteins is approximately 20% and binding also appears to be independent of concentration up to 10 μg/mL. Saturation of plasma protein binding occurs only at concentrations outside the clinically relevant range. Although not confirmed in humans, tramadol has been shown in rats to cross the blood-brain barrier.

Metabolism:
Tramadol is extensively metabolized after oral administration. Approximately 30% of the dose is excreted in the urine as unchanged drug, whereas 60% of the dose is excreted as metabolites. The remainder is excreted either as unidentified or as unextractable metabolites. The major metabolic pathways appear to be *N*- and *O*-demethylation and glucuronidation or sulfation in the liver. One metabolite (O-desmethyltramadol, denoted M1) is pharmacologically active in animal models. Production of M1 is dependent on the CYP2D6 isoenzyme of cytochrome P-450 and as such is subject to both metabolic induction and inhibition which may affect the therapeutic response (see PRECAUTIONS—Drug Interaction).

Elimination:
The mean terminal plasma elimination half-lives of racemic tramadol and racemic M1 are 6.3 ± 1.4 and 7.4 ± 1.4 hours, respectively. The plasma elimination half-life of racemic tramadol increased from approximately six hours to seven hours upon multiple dosing.

Special Populations
Renal:
Impaired renal function results in a decreased rate and extent of excretion of tramadol and its active metabolite, M1, in patients with creatinine clearances of less than 30 mL/min, adjustment of the dosing regimen is recommended (see DOSAGE AND ADMINISTRATION). The total amount of

Table 1
Mean (%CV) Pharmacokinetic Parameters for Racemic Tramadol and M1 Metabolite

Population/ Dosage Regimen[a]	Parent Drug/ Metabolite	Peak Conc. (ng/mL)	Time to Peak (hrs)	Clearance/F[b] (mL/min/Kg)	$t_{1/2}$ (hrs)
Healthy Adults, 100 mg qid, MD p.o.	Tramadol	592 (30)	2.3 (61)	5.90 (25)	6.7 (15)
	M1	110 (29)	2.4 (46)	c	7.0 (14)
Healthy Adults, 100 mg SD p.o.	Tramadol	308 (25)	1.6 (63)	8.50 (31)	5.6 (20)
	M1	55.0 (36)	3.0 (51)	c	6.7 (16)
Geriatric (> 75 yrs) 50 mg SD p.o.	Tramadol	208 (31)	2.1 (19)	6.89 (25)	7.0 (23)
	M1	d	d	c	d
Hepatic Impaired, 50 mg SD p.o.	Tramadol	217 (11)	1.9 (16)	4.23 (56)	13.3 (11)
	M1	19.4 (12)	9.8 (20)	c	18.5 (15)
Renal Impaired, CL_{cr} 10–30 mL/min 100 mg SD i.v.	Tramadol	c	c	4.23 (54)	10.6 (31)
	M1	c	c	c	11.5 (40)
Renal Impaired, CL_{cr} <5 mL/min 100 mg SD i.v.	Tramadol	c	c	3.73 (17)	11.0 (29)
	M1	c	c	c	16.9 (18)

a SD = Single dose, MD = Multiple dose, p.o. = Oral administration, i.v. = intravenous administration, qid = Four times daily
b F represents the oral bioavailability of tramadol
c Not applicable
d Not measured

tramadol and M1 removed during a 4-hour dialysis period is less than 7% of the administered dose.

Hepatic:
Metabolism of tramadol and M1 is reduced in patients with advanced cirrhosis of the liver, resulting in both a larger area under the concentration time curve for tramadol and longer tramadol and M1 elimination half-lives (13 hrs. for tramadol and 19 hrs. for M1). In cirrhotic patients, adjustment of the dosing regimen is recommended (see DOSAGE AND ADMINISTRATION).

Age:
Healthy elderly subjects aged 65 to 75 years have plasma tramadol concentrations and elimination half-lives comparable to those observed in healthy subjects less than 65 years of age. In subjects over 75 years, maximum serum concentrations are slightly elevated (208 vs. 162 ng/mL) and the elimination half-life is slightly prolonged (7 vs. 6 hours) compared to subjects 65 to 75 years of age. Adjustment of the daily dose is recommended for patients older than 75 years (see DOSAGE AND ADMINISTRATION).

Gender:
The absolute bioavailability of tramadol was 73% in males and 79% in females. The plasma clearance was 6.4 mL/min/kg in males and 5.7 mL/min/kg in females following a 100 mg IV dose of tramadol. Following a single oral dose, and after adjusting for body weight, females had a 12% higher peak tramadol concentration and a 35% higher area under the concentration-time curve compared to males. The clinical significance of this difference is unknown.

Clinical Studies
ULTRAM has been given in single oral doses of 50, 75, 100, 150 and 200 mg to patients with pain following surgical procedures and pain following oral surgery (extraction of impacted molars).

In single-dose models of pain following oral surgery, pain relief was demonstrated in some patients at doses of 50 mg and 75 mg. A dose of 100 mg ULTRAM tended to provide analgesia superior to codeine sulfate 60 mg, but it was not as effective as the combination of aspirin 650 mg with codeine phosphate 60 mg. In single-dose models of pain following surgical procedures, 150 mg provided analgesia generally comparable to the combination of acetaminophen 650 mg with propoxyphene napsylate 100 mg, with a tendency toward later peak effect.

ULTRAM has been studied in three long-term controlled trials involving a total of 820 patients, with 530 patients receiving ULTRAM. Patients with a variety of chronic painful conditions were studied in double-blind trials of one to three months duration. Average daily doses of approximately 250 mg of ULTRAM in divided doses were generally comparable to five doses of acetaminophen 300 mg with codeine phosphate 30 mg (TYLENOL® with Codeine #3) daily, five doses of aspirin 325 mg with codeine phosphate 30 mg daily, or two to three doses of acetaminophen 500 mg with oxycodone hydrochloride 5 mg (TYLOX®) daily.

INDICATIONS AND USAGE
ULTRAM is indicated for the management of moderate to moderately severe pain.

CONTRAINDICATIONS
ULTRAM should not be administered to patients who have previously demonstrated hypersensitivity to tramadol, any other component of this product, or opioids. It is also contraindicated in cases of acute intoxication with alcohol, hypnotics, centrally acting analgesics, opioids or psychotropic drugs.

WARNINGS
Seizure Risk
Seizures have been reported in patients receiving ULTRAM. Post-marketing experience suggests that occurrence of convulsions may be increased with doses of ULTRAM above the recommended range, but seizures have also been reported at doses within the recommended dosing range. Administration of ULTRAM may enhance the seizure risk in patients taking:

- **Tricyclic antidepressants and other tricyclic compounds (e.g., cyclobenzaprine, promethazine, etc.),**
- **Selective serotonin reuptake inhibitors (SSRI antidepressants or anorectics),**
- **MAO inhibitors (see also WARNINGS—Use with MAO inhibitors),**
- **Neuroleptics,**
- **Other drugs that reduce the seizure threshold.**

Risk of convulsions may also increase in patients with epilepsy, those with a history of seizures, or in patients with a recognized risk for seizure (such as head trauma, metabolic disorders, alcohol and drug withdrawal, CNS infections). In ULTRAM overdose, naloxone administration may increase the risk of seizure.

Anaphylactoid Reactions
Serious and rarely fatal anaphylactoid reactions have been reported in patients receiving therapy with ULTRAM. These reactions often occur following the first dose. Other reported reactions include pruritus, hives, bronchospasm, and angioedema. Patients with a history of anaphylactoid reactions to codeine and other opioids may be at increased risk and therefore should not receive ULTRAM (see CONTRAINDICATIONS).

Use in Opioid-dependent Patients
ULTRAM should not be used in opioid-dependent patients. ULTRAM has been shown to reinitiate physical dependence in some patients that have been previously dependent on other opioids. Consequently, in patients with a tendency to opioid abuse or opioid dependence, treatment with ULTRAM is not recommended.

Use with CNS Depressants
ULTRAM should be used with caution and in reduced dosages when administered to patients receiving CNS depres-

Continued on next page

Information on McNeil Pharmaceutical Products is based on labeling in effect in August 1996.

Consult 1997 supplements and future editions for revisions

McNeil—Cont.

sants such as alcohol, opioids, anesthetic agents, phenothiazines, tranquilizers or sedative hypnotics.

Use with MAO Inhibitors

Use ULTRAM with great caution in patients taking monoamine oxidase inhibitors, because animal studies have shown increased deaths with combined administration.

PRECAUTIONS

Respiratory Depression

Administer ULTRAM cautiously in patients at risk for respiratory depression. When large doses of ULTRAM are administered with anesthetic medications or alcohol, respiratory depression may result. Treat such cases as an overdose. If naloxone is to be administered, use cautiously because it may precipitate seizures (see WARNINGS, Seizure Risk and OVERDOSAGE).

Increased Intracranial Pressure or Head Trauma

ULTRAM should be used with caution in patients with increased intracranial pressure or head injury. Pupillary changes (miosis) from tramadol may obscure the existence, extent, or course of intracranial pathology. Clinicians should also maintain a high index of suspicion for adverse drug reaction when evaluating altered mental status in these patients if they are receiving ULTRAM.

Acute Abdominal Conditions

The administration of ULTRAM may complicate the clinical assessment of patients with acute abdominal conditions.

Patients Physically Dependent on Opioids

ULTRAM is not recommended for patients who are dependent on opioids. Patients who have recently taken substantial amounts of opioids may experience withdrawal symptoms. Because of the difficulty in assessing dependence in patients who have previously received substantial amounts of opioid medication, administer ULTRAM cautiously to such patients.

Use in Renal and Hepatic Disease

Impaired renal function results in a decreased rate and extent of excretion of tramadol and its active metabolite, M1. In patients with creatinine clearances of less than 30 mL/min, dosing reduction is recommended (see DOSAGE AND ADMINISTRATION).

Metabolism of tramadol and M1 is reduced in patients with advanced cirrhosis of the liver. In cirrhotic patients, dosing reduction is recommended (see DOSAGE AND ADMINISTRATION).

With the prolonged half-life in these conditions, achievement of steady-state is delayed, so that it may take several days for elevated plasma concentrations to develop.

Information for Patients

- ULTRAM may impair mental or physical abilities required for the performance of potentially hazardous tasks such as driving a car or operating machinery.
- ULTRAM should not be taken with alcohol containing beverages.
- ULTRAM should be used with caution when taking medications such as tranquilizers, hypnotics or other opiate containing analgesics.
- The patient should be instructed to inform the physician if they are pregnant, think they might become pregnant, or are trying to become pregnant (see PRECAUTIONS: Labor and Delivery).
- The patient should understand the single-dose and 24-hour dose limit and the time interval between doses, since exceeding these recommendations can result in respiratory depression and seizures.

Drug Interactions

Tramadol does not appear to induce its own metabolism in humans, since observed maximal plasma concentrations after multiple oral doses are higher than expected based on single-dose data. Tramadol is a mild inducer of selected drug metabolism pathways measured in animals.

Use with Carbamazepine

Concomitant administration of ULTRAM with **carbamazepine** causes a significant increase in tramadol metabolism, presumably through metabolic induction by carbamazepine. Patients receiving chronic carbamazepine doses of up to 800 mg daily may require up to twice the recommended dose of ULTRAM.

Use with Quinidine

Tramadol is metabolized to M1 by the CYP2D6 P-450 isoenzyme. **Quinidine** is a selective inhibitor of that isoenzyme, so that concomitant administration of quinidine and ULTRAM results in increased concentrations of tramadol and reduced concentrations of M1. The clinical consequences of this effect have not been fully investigated, and the effect on quinidine concentrations is unknown.

Use with Cimetidine

Concomitant administration of ULTRAM with **cimetidine** does not result in clinically significant changes in tramadol pharmacokinetics. Therefore, no alteration of the ULTRAM dosage regimen is recommended.

Use with MAO Inhibitors

Interactions with **MAO inhibitors**, due to interference with detoxification mechanisms, have been reported for some centrally acting drugs (see WARNINGS, Use with MAO Inhibitors).

Use with Digoxin and Warfarin

Post-marketing surveillance has revealed rare reports of digoxin toxicity and alteration of warfarin effect, including elevation of prothrombin times.

Carcinogenesis, Mutagenesis, Impairment of Fertility

Tramadol was not mutagenic in the following assays: Ames *Salmonella* microsomal activation test, CHO/HPRT mammalian cell assay, mouse lymphoma assay (in the absence of metabolic activation), dominant lethal mutation tests in mice, chromosome aberration test in Chinese hamsters, and bone marrow micronucleus tests in mice and Chinese hamsters. Weakly mutagenic results occurred in the presence of metabolic activation in the mouse lymphoma assay and micronucleus test in rats. Overall, the weight of evidence from these tests indicates that tramadol does not pose a genotoxic risk to humans.

A slight, but statistically significant, increase in two common murine tumors, pulmonary and hepatic, was observed in a mouse carcinogenicity study, particularly in aged mice (dosing orally up to 30 mg/kg for approximately two years, although the study was not done with the Maximum Tolerated Dose). This finding is not believed to suggest risk in humans. No such finding occurred in a rat carcinogenicity study.

No effects on fertility were observed for tramadol at oral dose levels up to 50 mg/kg in male rats and 75 mg/kg in female rats.

Pregnancy, Teratogenic Effects: *Pregnancy Category C*

There are no adequate and well-controlled studies in pregnant women. ULTRAM should be used during pregnancy only if the potential benefit justifies the potential risk to the fetus.

Tramadol has been shown to be embryotoxic and fetotoxic in mice, rats and rabbits at maternally toxic doses 3 to 15 times the maximum human dose or higher (120 mg/kg in mice, 25 mg/kg or higher in rats and 75 mg/kg or higher in rabbits), but was not teratogenic at these dose levels. No harm to the fetus due to tramadol was seen at doses that were not maternally toxic.

No drug-related teratogenic effects were observed in progeny of mice, rats or rabbits treated with tramadol by various routes (up to 140 mg/kg for mice, 80 mg/kg for rats or 300 mg/kg for rabbits). Embryo and fetal toxicity consisted primarily of decreased fetal weights, skeletal ossification and increased supernumerary ribs at maternally toxic dose levels. Transient delays in developmental or behavioral parameters were also seen in pups from rat dams allowed to deliver. Embryo and fetal lethality were reported only in one rabbit study at 300 mg/kg, a dose that would cause extreme maternal toxicity in the rabbit.

In peri- and post-natal studies in rats, progeny of dams receiving oral (gavage) dose levels of 50 mg/kg or greater had decreased weights, and pup survival was decreased early in lactation at 80 mg/kg (6 to 10 times the maximum human dose). No toxicity was observed for progeny of dams receiving 8, 10, 20, 25, or 40 mg/kg. Maternal toxicity was observed at all dose levels, but effects on progeny were evident only at higher dose levels where maternal toxicity was more severe.

Labor and Delivery

ULTRAM should not be used in pregnant women prior to or during labor unless the potential benefits outweigh the risks. Safe use in pregnancy has not been established. Chronic use during pregnancy may lead to physical dependence and postpartum withdrawal symptoms in the newborn. Tramadol has been shown to cross the placenta. The mean ratio of serum tramadol in the umbilical veins compared to maternal veins was 0.83 for 40 women given tramadol during labor. The effect of ULTRAM, if any, on the later growth, development, and functional maturation of the child is unknown.

Nursing Mothers

ULTRAM is not recommended for obstetrical preoperative medication or for post-delivery analgesia in nursing mothers because its safety in infants and newborns has not been studied. Following a single IV 100 mg dose of tramadol, the cumulative excretion in breast milk within 16 hours postdose was 100 μg of tramadol (0.1% of the maternal dose) and 27 μg of M1.

Pediatric Use

The pediatric use of ULTRAM is not recommended because safety and efficacy in patients under 16 years of age have not been established.

Use in the Elderly

In subjects over the age of 75 years, serum concentrations are slightly elevated and the elimination half-life is slightly prolonged. The aged also can be expected to vary more widely in their ability to tolerate adverse drug effects. Daily doses in excess of 300 mg are not recommended in patients over 75 (see DOSAGE AND ADMINISTRATION).

ADVERSE REACTIONS

ULTRAM was administered to 550 patients during the double-blind or open-label extension periods in U.S. studies of chronic nonmalignant pain. Of these patients, 375 were 65 years old or older. Table 2 reports the cumulative incidence rate of adverse reactions by 7, 30 and 90 days for the most frequent reactions (5% or more by 7 days). The most frequently reported events were in the central nervous system and gastrointestinal system. Although the reactions listed in the table are felt to be probably related to ULTRAM administration, the reported rates also include some events that may have been due to underlying disease or concomitant medication. The overall incidence rates of adverse experiences in these trials were similar for ULTRAM and the active control groups, TYLENOL® with Codeine #3 (acetaminophen 300 mg with codeine phosphate 30 mg), and aspirin 325 mg with codeine phosphate 30 mg.

Table 2
Cumulative Incidence of Adverse Reactions for ULTRAM in Chronic Trials of Nonmalignant Pain (N = 427)

	Up to 7 Days	Up to 30 Days	Up to 90 Days
Dizziness/Vertigo	26%	31%	33%
Nausea	24%	34%	40%
Constipation	24%	38%	46%
Headache	18%	26%	32%
Somnolence	16%	23%	25%
Vomiting	9%	13%	17%
Pruritis	8%	10%	11%
"CNS Stimulation"[1]	7%	11%	14%
Asthenia	6%	11%	12%
Sweating	6%	7%	9%
Dyspepsia	5%	9%	13%
Dry Mouth	5%	9%	10%
Diarrhea	5%	6%	10%

[1] "CNS Stimulation" is a composite of nervousness, anxiety, agitation, tremor, spasticity, euphoria, emotional lability and hallucinations.

Incidence 1% to less than 5%, possibly causally related: the following lists adverse reactions that occurred with an incidence of 1% to less than 5% in clinical trials, and for which the possibility of a causal relationship with ULTRAM exists.

Body as a Whole: Malaise.

Cardiovascular: Vasodilation.

Central Nervous System: Anxiety, Confusion, Coordination disturbance, Euphoria, Nervousness, Sleep disorder.

Gastrointestinal: Abdominal pain, Anorexia, Flatulence.

Musculoskeletal: Hypertonia.

Skin: Rash.

Special Senses: Visual disturbance.

Urogenital: Urinary retention, Urinary frequency, Menopausal symptoms.

Incidence less than 1%, possibly causally related: the following lists adverse reactions that occurred with an incidence of less than 1% in clinical trials and/or reported in post-marketing experience.

Body as a Whole: Allergic reaction, Accidental injury, Weight loss, Anaphylaxis.

Cardiovascular: Syncope, Orthostatic hypotension, Tachycardia.

Central Nervous System: Seizure (see WARNINGS), Paresthesia, Cognitive dysfunction, Hallucinations, Tremor, Amnesia, Difficulty in concentration, Abnormal gait, Depression.

Respiratory: Dyspenia.

Skin: Urticaria, Vesicles, Stevens-Johnson syndrome/Toxic epidermal necrolysis.

Special Senses: Dysgeusia.

Urogenital: Dysuria, Menstrual disorder.

Other adverse experiences, causal relationship unknown: A variety of other adverse events were reported infrequently in patients taking ULTRAM during clinical trials. A causal relationship between ULTRAM and these events has not been determined. However, the most significant events are listed below as alerting information to the physician.

Body as a Whole: Suicidal tendency.

Cardiovascular: Abnormal ECG, Hypertension, Myocardial ischemia, Palpitations.

Central Nervous System: Migraine.

Gastrointestinal: Gastrointestinal bleeding, Hepatitis, Stomatitis.

Laboratory Abnormalities: Creatinine increase, Elevated liver enzymes, Hemoglobin decrease, Proteinuria.

Sensory: Cataracts, Deafness, Tinnitus.

DRUG ABUSE AND DEPENDENCE

ULTRAM has a potential to cause psychic and physical dependence of the morphine-type (μ-opioid). The drug has been associated with craving, drug-seeking behavior and tolerance development. Cases of abuse and dependence on ULTRAM have been reported. ULTRAM should not be used in opioid-dependent patients. ULTRAM can reinitiate physi-

cal dependence in patients that have been previously dependent or chronically using other opioids. In patients with a tendency to drug abuse, a history of drug dependence, or are chronically using opioids, treatment with ULTRAM is not recommended.

DOSAGE AND ADMINISTRATION

For the treatment of painful conditions, ULTRAM 50 mg to 100 mg can be administered as needed for relief every four to six hours, **not to exceed 400 mg per day.** For moderate pain, ULTRAM 50 mg may be adequate as the initial dose, and for more severe pain, ULTRAM 100 mg is usually more effective as the initial dose.

Individualization of Dose

Available data do not suggest that a dosage adjustment is necessary in elderly patients 65 to 75 years of age unless they also have renal or hepatic impairment. For elderly patients **over 75 years old**, not more than 300 mg/day in divided doses as above is recommended. In all patients with **creatinine clearance less than 30 mL/min**, it is recommended that the dosing interval of ULTRAM be increased to 12 hours, with a maximum daily dose of 200 mg. Since only 7% of an administered dose is removed by hemodialysis, **dialysis patients** can receive their regular dose on the day of dialysis. The recommended dose for patients with **cirrhosis** is 50 mg every 12 hours. Patients receiving chronic **carbamazepine** doses up to 800 mg daily may require up to twice the recommended dose of ULTRAM.

OVERDOSAGE

Cases of overdose with tramadol have been reported. Estimates of ingested dose in foreign fatalities have been in the range of 3 to 5 g. A 3 g intentional overdose by a patient in the clinical studies produced emesis and no sequelae. The lowest dose reported to be associated with fatality was possibly between 500 and 1000 mg in a 40 kg woman, but details of the case are not completely known.

Serious potential consequences of overdosage are respiratory depression and seizure. In treating an overdose, primary attention should be given to maintaining adequate ventilation along with general supportive treatment. While naloxone will reverse some, but not all, symptoms caused by overdosage with ULTRAM the risk of seizures is also increased with naloxone administration. In animals convulsions following the administration of toxic doses of tramadol could be suppressed with barbiturates or benzodiazepines but were increased with naloxone. Naloxone administration did not change the lethality of an overdose in mice. Hemodialysis is not expected to be helpful in an overdose because it removes less than 7% of the administered dose in a 4-hour dialysis period.

HOW SUPPLIED

ULTRAM (Tramadol Hydrochloride Tablets) Tablets—50 mg (white, film-coated capsule-shaped tablet) engraved "McNeil" on one side and "659" on the other side.

100's—NDC 0045-0659-60 bottles of 100 tablets
packages of 100 unit doses in blister packs—NDC 0045-0659-10 (10 cards of 10 tablets each).

Dispense in a tight container. Store at controlled room temperature (up to 25°C, 77°F).

Caution: Federal law prohibits dispensing without prescription.

McNEIL PHARMACEUTICAL
Spring House, PA USA 19477,
and

ORTHO PHARMACEUTICAL CORPORATION
Raritan, NJ USA 08869
Revised March 1996   633-10-225-5
Shown in Product Identification Guide, page 324

VASCOR®   ℞
(bepridil hydrochloride)
Tablets
For Oral Administration

DESCRIPTION

VASCOR (bepridil hydrochloride) is a calcium channel blocker that has well characterzied anti-anginal properties and known but poorly characterized type 1 anti-arrhythmic and anti-hypertensive properties. It has inhibitory effects on both the slow calcium and fast sodium inward currents in myocardial and vascular smooth muscle, interferes with calcium binding to calmodulin, and blocks both voltage and receptor operated calcium channels. It is not related chemically to other calcium channel blockers such as diltiazem hydrochloride, nifedipine and verapamil hydrochloride.

Bepridil hydrochloride monohydrate is a white to off-white, crystalline powder with a bitter taste. It is slightly soluble in water, very soluble in ethanol, methanol and chloroform, and freely soluble in acetone. The molecular weight of bepridil hydrochloride monohydrate is 421.02. Its molecular formula is $C_{24}H_{34}N_2O \cdot HCl \cdot H_2O$. The structural formula is:
[See chemical structure at top of next column.]

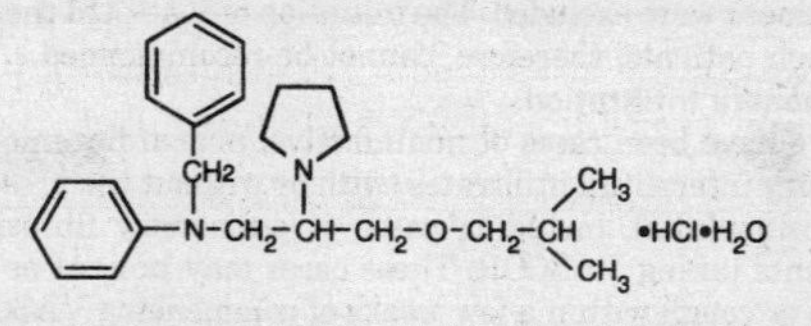

$(\pm)$-β-[(2-Methylpropoxy)methyl]-N-(phenylmethyl)-1-pyrrolidineethanamine monohydrochloride monohydrate

VASCOR is available as film-coated tablets for oral use containing 200, 300, or 400 mg of bepridil hydrochloride monohydrate. Inactive ingredients: hydroxypropyl methylcellulose, lactose, magnesium stearate, microcrystalline cellulose, polyethylene glycol, silicon dioxide, pregelatinized corn starch, corn starch, titanium dioxide, FD&C Blue #1.

CLINICAL PHARMACOLOGY

VASCOR (bepridil hydrochloride) inhibits the transmembrane influx of calcium ions into cardiac and vascular smooth muscle. This has been demonstrated in isolated myocardial and vascular smooth muscle preparations in which both the slope of the calcium dose response curve and the maximum calcium-induced inotropic response were significantly reduced by bepridil hydrochloride. In cardiac myocytes *in vitro*, bepridil hydrochloride was shown to be tightly bound to actin. A negative inotropic effect can be seen in the isolated guinea pig atria.

In *vitro* studies, bepridil hydrochloride has also been demonstrated to inhibit the sodium inward current. Reductions in the maximal upstroke velocity and the amplitude of the action potential, as well as increases in the duration of the normal action potential, have been observed. Additionally, bepridil hydrochloride has been shown to possess local anesthetic activity in isolated myocardial preparations. It effects electrophysiological changes that are observed with several classes of anti-arrhythmic agents.

Clinical Studies

In controlled clinical studies with 200–400 mg of VASCOR, given as a once daily dose, exercise tolerance was improved and angina frequency and daily niitroglycerin use was reduced compared to placebo. Improvement in exercise performance was dose related. In one controlled clinical study, VASCOR was added to propranolol in daily doses of up to 240 mg. The 200–400 mg dose of VASCOR was well tolerated [patients entered were not allowed to be in NYHA Class III or IV heart failure] and there was an added effect of VASCOR on exercise tolerance.

In another controlled clinical study, VASCOR in doses of up to 400 mg/day, significantly improved exercise tolerance compared to diltiazem hydrochloride in patients refractory to diltiazem hydrochloride therapy.

Mechanism of Action: The precise mechanism of action for VASCOR as an anti-anginal agent remains to be fully determined, but is believed to include the following mechanisms: VASCOR regularly reduces heart rate and arterial pressure at rest and at a given level of exercise by dilating peripheral arterioles and reducing total peripheral resistance (afterload) against which the heart works. In exercise tolerance tests in patients with stable angina the heart rate/blood pressure product was reduced with VASCOR for a given work load.

Hemodynamic Effects: VASCOR produces dose dependent slowing of the heart, and reflex tachycardia is not seen. The mean decrease in heart rate in US clinical trials was 3 b.p.m. Orally administered VASCOR also produces modest decreases (less than 5 mm Hg) in systolic and diastolic blood pressure in normotensive patients and somewhat larger decreases in hypertensive patients.

Intravenous administration of VASCOR is associated with a modest reduction in left ventricular contractility (dP/dt), and increased filling pressure, but radionuclide cineangiography studies in angina patients demonstrated improvement in ejection fraction at rest and during exercise following oral VASCOR therapy. Patients with impaired cardiac function [overt heart failure] were not included in these studies.

Electrophysiological Effects: Intravenous administration of VASCOR in man prolongs the effective refractory periods of the atria and ventricles, and the functional refractory period of the AV node. There was a tendency for the AV node effective refractory period and A-H interval to be increased as well. Intravenous and oral administration of VASCOR slow heart rate, prolong the QT and QTc intervals, and alter the morphology of the T-wave (indentation). In clinical trials with angina patients, the mean percent prolongation of the QTc interval was approximately 8%, and of QT about 10%. The prolongation of QT is dose related, varying from about 0.030 sec at doses of 200 mg once a day to 0.055 sec at 400 mg once a day. Upon cessation of therapy, the ECG gradually normalizes. No instances of greater than first-degree heart block have been observed in US controlled and open clinical studies with VASCOR, and first-degree heart block occurred in 0.2% of patients in these studies.

Pulmonary Function: In healthy subjects and asthmatic patients, intravenous VASCOR did not cause bronchocon-

striction. VASCOR has been safely used in asthmatic patients and in patients with chronic obstructive lung disease.

Pharmacokinetics and Metabolism: In studies with healthy volunteers, VASCOR is rapidly and completely absorbed after oral administration. The time to peak bepridil plasma concentration is about 2 to 3 hours. Over a ten day period, approximately 70% of a single dose of VASCOR is excreted in the urine and 22% in the feces, as metabolites of bepridil. Excretion of unmetabolized drug is negligible. In healthy male volunteers, the relationship between dose and steady-state blood levels of bepridil was linear over the range of 200 to 400 mg/day. Elimination of bepridil is biphasic, with a distribution half-life of about 2 hours. The terminal elimination half-life following the cessation of multiple dosing averaged 42 hours (range 26–64 hours). However, during a given dosing interval, decay from the peak concentration occurs relatively rapidly indicating a dosing interval half-life shorter than 24 hours. Following once-daily dosing with therapeutic doses, steady-state was reached in about 8 days in healthy volunteers. The clearance of bepridil decreases after multiple dosing.

Clearance of bepridil in angina patients was lower than that in healthy volunteers, resulting in higher average plasma bepridil concentrations. At steady state, maximum bepridil concentrations averaged 2332 ng/ml (range 1451 to 3609) and mean minimum concentrations were 1174 ng/ml (range 226 to 2639) in angina patients following 300 mg/day doses of VASCOR.

Bepridil is more than 99% bound to plasma proteins. Administration of VASCOR after a meal resulted in a clinically insignificant delay in time to peak concentration, but neither peak bepridil plasma levels nor the extent of absorption was changed.

Bepridil passes through the placental barrier. Bepridil may cause uterine hypotonia.

INDICATIONS AND USAGE

Chronic Stable Angina (Classic Effort-Associated Angina)

VASCOR (bepridil hydrochloride) is indicated for the treatment of chronic stable angina (classic effort-associated angina). Because VASCOR has caused serious ventricular arrhythmias, including torsades de pointes type ventricular tachycardia, and the occurrence of cases of agranulocytosis associated with its use (see **WARNINGS**), it should be reserved for patients who have failed to respond optimally to, or are intolerant of, other anti-anginal medication.

VASCOR may be used alone or in combination with beta blockers and/or nitrates. Controlled clinical studies have shown an added effect when VASCOR is administered to patients already receiving propranolol.

CONTRAINDICATIONS

VASCOR (bepridil hydrochloride) is contraindicated in patients with a known sensitivity to bepridil hydrochloride. VASCOR is contraindicated in (1) patients with a history of serious ventricular arrhythmias (see **WARNINGS**-Induction of New Serious Arrhythmias), (2) patients with sick sinus syndrome or patients with second- or third-degree AV block, except in the presence of a functioning ventricular pacemaker, (3) patients with hypotension (less than 90 mm Hg systolic), (4) patients with uncompensated cardiac insufficiency, (5) patients with congenital QT interval prolongation (see **WARNINGS**), and (6) patients taking other drugs that prolong QT interval (see **PRECAUTIONS**-Drug Interactions).

WARNINGS

Induction of New Serious Arrhythmias

VASCOR (bepridil hydrochloride) has Class 1 anti-arrhythmic properties and, like other such drugs, can induce new arrhythmias, including VT/VF. In addition, because of its ability to prolong the QT interval, VASCOR can cause torsades de pointes type ventricular tachycardia. Because of these properties VASCOR should be reserved for patients in whom other anti-anginal agents do not offer a satisfactory effect.

In US clinical trials, the QT and QTc intervals were commonly prolonged by VASCOR in a dose-related fashion. While the mean prolongation of QTc was 8% and of QT was 10%. Increases of 25% or more were not uncommon, occurring in 5% of the studied population for QTc and 8.7% of the studied population for QT. Increased QT and QTc may be associated with torsades de pointes type VT, which was seen at least briefly, in about 1.0% of patients in US trials; in many cases, however, patients with marked prolongation of QTc were taken off VASCOR therapy. All of the US patients with torsades de pointes had a prolonged QT interval and relatively low

---

Continued on next page

Information on McNeil Pharmaceutical Products is based on labeling in effect in August 1996.

Consult 1997 supplements and future editions for revisions

McNeil—Cont.

serum potassium. French marketing experience has reported over one hundred verified cases of torsades de pointes. While this number, based on total use, represents a rate of only 0.01%, the true rate is undoubtedly much higher, as spontaneous reporting systems all suffer from substantial under reporting.

Torsades de pointes is a polymorphic ventricular tachycardia often but not always associated with a prolonged QT interval, and often drug induced. The relation between the degree of QT prolongation and the development of torsades de pointes is not linear and the likelihood of torsades appears to be increased by hypokalemia, use of potassium wasting diuretics, and the presence of antecedent bradycardia. While the safe upper limit of QT is not defined, it is suggested that the interval not be permitted to exceed 0.52 seconds during treatment. If dose reduction does not eliminate the excessive prolongation, VASCOR should be stopped.

Because most domestic and foreign cases of torsades have developed in patients with hypokalemia, usually related to diuretic use or significant liver disease, if concomitant diuretics are needed, low doses and addition or primary use of a potassium sparing diuretic should be considered and serum potassium should be monitored. VASCOR has been associated with the usual range of pro-arrhythmic effects characteristic of Class 1 antiarrhythmics (increased premature ventricular contraction rates, new sustained VT, and VT/VF that is more resistant to sinus rhythm conversion). Use in patients with severe arrhythmias (who are most susceptible to certain pro-arrhythmic effects) has been limited, so that risk in these patients is not defined.

In the National Heart, Lung and Blood Institute's Cardiac Arrhythmia Suppression Trial (CAST), a long-term, multi-centered, randomized, double-blind study in patients with asymptomatic non-life-threatening ventricular arrhythmias who had myocardial infarctions more than six days but less than two years previously, an excess mortality/non-fatal cardiac arrest rate was seen in patients treated with encainide or flecainide (56/730) compared with that seen in patients assigned to matched placebo-treated groups (22/725). The applicability of these results to other populations (e.g., those without recent myocardial infarction) or to other anti-arrhythmic drugs is uncertain, but at present it is prudent to consider any drug documented to provoke new serious arrhythmias or worsening of pre-existing arrhythmias as having a similar risk and to avoid their use in the post-infarction period.

Agranulocytosis: In US clinical trials of over 800 patients treated with VASCOR for up to five years, two cases of marked leukopenia and neutropenia were reported. Both patients were diabetic and elderly. One died with overwhelming gram-negative sepsis, itself a possible cause of marked leukopenia. The other patient recovered rapidly when VASCOR was stopped.

Congestive Heart Failure: Congestive heart failure has been observed infrequently (about 1%) during US controlled clinical trials, but experience with the use of VASCOR in patients with significantly impaired ventricular function is limited. There is little information on the effect of concomitant administration of VASCOR and digoxin; therefore, caution should be exercised in treating patients with congestive heart failure.

Hepatic Enzyme Elevation: In US clinical studies with VASCOR in about 1000 patients and subjects, clinically significant (at least 2 times the upper limit of normal) transaminase elevations were observed in approximately 1% of the patients. None of these patients became clinically symptomatic or jaundiced and values returned to normal when the drug was stopped.

Hypokalemia: In clinical trials VASCOR has not been reported to reduce serum potassium levels. Because hypokalemia has been associated with ventricular arrhythmias, potassium insufficiency should be corrected before VASCOR therapy is initiated and normal potassium concentrations should be maintained during VASCOR therapy. Serum potassium should be monitored periodically.

PRECAUTIONS

General

Caution should be exercised when using VASCOR (bepridil hydrochloride) in patients with left bundle branch block or sinus bradycardia (less than 50 b.p.m.). Care should also be exercised in patients with serious hepatic or renal disorders because such patients have not been studied and bepridil is highly metabolized, with metabolites excreted primarily in the urine.

Recent Myocardial Infarction

In US clinical trials with VASCOR, patients with myocardial infarctions within three months prior to initiation of drug treatment were excluded. The initiation of VASCOR therapy in such patients, therefore, cannot be recommended.

Pulmonary Infiltration

There have been cases of noninfective, noncardiogenic pulmonary interstitial infiltrates (with or without the presence of eosinophilia), including cases of pulmonary fibrosis in patients taking VASCOR. These cases may present as dyspnea or cough within a few weeks of commencing VASCOR; infiltrates may be seen on chest x-ray.

Although the relationship of pulmonary infiltration to VASCOR is unclear, any patient who develops dyspnea or cough of unspecified etiology should be adequately evaluated. If other causes cannot be identified, discontinuation of VASCOR therapy should be considered.

Information for Patients

Since QT prolongation is not associated with defined symptomatology, patients should be instructed on the importance of maintaining any potassium supplementation or potassium sparing diuretic, and the need for routine electrocardiograms and periodic monitoring of serum potassium.

The following Patient Information is printed on the carton label of each unit of use bottle of 30 tablets:

As with any medication that you take, you should notify your physician of any changes in your overall condition. Be sure to follow your physician's instructions regarding follow-up visits. Please notify any physician who treats you for a medical condition that you are taking VASCOR® (bepridil hydrochloride), as well as any other medications.

Drug Interactions

Nitrates: The concomitant use of VASCOR with long- and short-acting nitrates has been safely tolerated in patients with stable angina pectoris. Sublingual nitroglycerin may be taken if necessary for the control of acute angina attacks during VASCOR therapy.

Beta-blocking Agents: The concomitant use of VASCOR and beta-blocking agents has been well tolerated in patients with stable angina. Available data are not sufficient, however, to predict the effects of concomitant medication on patients with impaired ventricular function or cardiac conduction abnormalities (see **CLINICAL PHARMACOLOGY** and **DOSAGE AND ADMINISTRATION**).

Digoxin: In controlled studies in healthy volunteers, bepridil hydrochloride either had no effect (one study) or was associated with modest increases, about 30% (two studies) in steady-state serum digoxin concentrations. Limited clinical data in angina patients receiving concomitant bepridil hydrochloride and digoxin therapy indicate no discernible changes in serum digoxin levels. Available data are neither sufficient to rule out possible increases in serum digoxin with concomitant treatment in some patients, nor other possible interactions, particularly in patients with cardiac conduction abnormalities (Also see **WARNINGS**-Congestive Heart Failure).

Oral Hypoglycemics: VASCOR has been safely used in diabetic patients without significantly lowering their blood glucose levels or altering their need for insulin or oral hypoglycemic agents.

General Interactions: Certain drugs could increase the likelihood of potentially serious adverse effects with bepridil hydrochloride. In general, these are drugs that have one or more pharmacologic activities similar to bepridil hydrochloride, including anti-arrhythmic agents such as quinidine and procainamide, cardiac glycosides and tricyclic anti-depressants. Anti-arrhythmics and tricyclic anti-depressants could exaggerate the prolongation of the QT interval observed with bepridil hydrochloride. Cardiac glycosides could exaggerate the depression of AV nodal conduction observed with bepridil hydrochloride.

Carcinogenesis, Mutagenesis, Impairment of Fertility

No evidence of carcinogenicity was revealed in one lifetime study in mice at dosages up to 60 times (for a 60 kg subject) the maximum recommended dosage in man. Unilateral follicular adenomas of the thyroid were observed in a study in rats following lifetime administration of high doses of bepridil hydrochloride, i.e., $\geq$ 100 mg/kg/day (20 times the usual recommended dose in man). No mutagenic or other genotoxic potential of bepridil hydrochloride was found in the following standard laboratory tests: the Micronucleus Test for Chromosomal Effects, the Liver Microsome Activated Bacterial Assay for Mutagenicity, the Chinese Hamster Ovary Cell Assay for Mutagenicity, and the Sister Chromatid Exchange Assay. No intrinsic effect on fertility by bepridil hydrochloride was demonstrated in rats.

In monkeys, at 200 mg/kg/day, there was a decrease in testicular weight and spermatogenesis. There were no systematic studies in man related to this point. In rats, at doses up to 300 mg/kg/day, there was no observed alteration of mating behavior nor of reproductive performance.

Usage in Pregnancy

Pregnancy Category C. Reproductive studies (fertility and peri-postnatal) have been conducted in rats. Reduced litter size at birth and decreased pup survival during lactation was observed at maternal dosages 37 times (on a mg/kg basis) the maximum daily recommended therapeutic dosage.

In teratology studies, no effects were observed in rats or rabbits at these same dosages.

There are no well-controlled studies in pregnant women. Use VASCOR in pregnant or nursing women only if the potential benefit justifies the potential risk.

Nursing Mothers

Bepridil is excreted in human milk. Bepridil concentration in human milk is estimated to reach about one third the concentration in serum. Because of the potential for serious adverse reactions in nursing infants from VASCOR a decision should be made whether to discontinue nursing or to discontinue the drug, taking into account the importance of the drug to the mother.

Pediatric Use

The safety and effectiveness of VASCOR in children have not been established.

ADVERSE REACTIONS

Adverse reactions were assessed in placebo and active-drug controlled trials of 4–12 weeks duration and longer-term uncontrolled studies. The most common side effects occurring more frequently than in control groups were upper gastrointestinal complaints (nausea, dyspepsia or GI distress) in about 22%, diarrhea in about 8%, dizziness in about 15%, asthenia in about 10% and nervousness in about 7%. The adverse reactions seen in at least 2% of bepridil patients in controlled trials are shown in the following table.

[See first table on top of next page.]

In one twelve week controlled study, daily doses of 200, 300, and 400 mg were compared to placebo. The following table shows the rates of more common reactions (at least 5% in at least one bepridil group).

[See second table on top of next page.]

Adverse experiences in long-term open studies were generally similar to those seen in controlled trials. Although adverse experiences were frequent (at least one being reported in 71% of patients participating in controlled clinical trials), most were well-tolerated. About 15% of patients however, discontinued bepridil treatment because of adverse experiences. In controlled clinical trials, these were principally gastrointestinal (1.0%), dizziness (1.0%) ventricular arrhythmias (1.0%) and syncope (0.6%). The major reasons for discontinuation, with comparison to control agents, are shown below.

[See third table on top of next page.]

Across all controlled and uncontrolled trials, VASCOR was evaluated in over 800 patients with chronic angina. In addition to the adverse reactions noted above, the following were observed in 0.5 to 2.0% of the VASCOR patients or are rarer, but potentially important events seen in clinical studies or reported in post marketing experience. In most cases it is not possible to determine whether there is a causal relationship to bepridil treatment.

Body as a Whole: Fever, pain, myalgic asthenia, superinfection, flu syndrome.

Cardiovascular/Respiratory: Sinus tachycardia, sinus bradycardia, hypertension, vasodilation, edema, ventricular premature contractions, ventricular tachycardia, prolonged QT interval, rhinitis, cough, pharyngitis.

Gastrointestinal: Flatulence, gastritis, appetite increase, dry mouth, constipation.

Musculoskeletal: Arthritis.

Central Nervous System: Fainting, vertigo, akathisia, drowsiness, insomnia, tremor.

Psychiatric: Depression, anxiousness, adverse behavior effect.

Skin: Rash, sweating, skin irritation.

Special Senses: Blurred vision, tinnitus, taste change.

Urogenital: Loss of libido, impotence.

Abnormal Lab Values: Abnormal liver function test, SGPT increase.

Certain cardiovascular events, such as acute myocardial infarction (about 3% of patients) worsened heart failure (1.9%), worsened angina (4.5%), severe arrhythmia (about 2.4% VT/VF) and sudden death (1.6%) have occurred in patients receiving bepridil, but have not been included as adverse events because they appear to be, and cannot be distinguished from, manifestations of the patient's underlying cardiac disease. Such events as torsades de pointes arrhythmias, prolonged QT/QTc, bradycardia, first degree heart block, which are probably related to bepridil, are included in the tables.

OVERDOSAGE

In the event of overdosage, we recommend close observation in a cardiac care facility for a minimum of 48 hours and use of appropriate supportive measures in addition to gastric lavage. Beta-adrenergic stimulation or parenteral administration of calcium solutions may increase transmembrane calcium ion influx. Clinically significant hypotensive reactions or high-degree AV block should be treated with vasopressor agents or cardiac pacing, respectively. Ventricular tachycardia should be handled by cardioversion and, if persistent, by overdrive pacing.

There has been one experience with overdosage in which a patient inadvertently took a single dose of 1600 mg of

Adverse Experiences by Body System and Treatment in Greater Than 2% of Bepridil Patients in Controlled Trials

Adverse Reaction	Bepridil HCl (N = 529)	Nifedipine (N = 50)	Propranolol (N = 88)	Diltiazem (N = 41)	Placebo (N = 190)
Body as a Whole					
Asthenia	9.83	22.00	22.73	12.20	7.37
Headache	11.34	22.00	13.64	7.32	14.21
Flu Syndrome	2.08	8.00	2.27	—ᵃ	1.05
Cardiovascular/Respiratory					
Palpitations	2.27	6.00	2.27	0.00	1.58
Dyspnea	3.59	4.00	5.68	4.88	2.11
Respiratory Infection	2.84	4.00	3.41	4.88	3.68
Gastrointestinal					
Dyspepsia	6.81	4.00	5.68	4.88	1.58
G.I. Distress	4.35	10.00	6.82	—ᵃ	2.11
Nausea	12.29	14.00	11.36	2.44	3.68
Dry Mouth	3.40	0.00	0.00	2.44	2.63
Anorexia	3.02	0.00	2.27	0.00	1.58
Diarrhea	7.75	2.00	9.09	2.44	2.63
Abdominal Pain	3.02	4.00	1.14	—ᵃ	3.16
Constipation	2.84	6.00	1.14	4.88	2.11
Central Nervous System					
Drowsy	3.78	4.00	4.55	—ᵃ	3.68
Insomnia	2.65	6.00	3.41	—ᵃ	1.05
Dizziness	14.74	30.00	10.23	4.88	9.47
Tremor	4.91	4.00	0.00	—ᵃ	1.05
Tremor of Hand	3.02	4.00	0.00	—ᵃ	0.53
Paresthesia	2.46	2.00	1.14	4.88	3.16
Psychiatric					
Nervous	7.37	16.00	1.14	2.44	3.68

ᵃ No data available.

Adverse Experiences by Body System and Treatment In Greater Than 5% of Bepridil Patients in Controlled Trials

Adverse Reaction	Bepridil HCl 200 mg (N = 43)	Bepridil HCl 300 mg (N = 46)	Bepridil HCl 400 mg (N = 44)	Placebo (N = 44)
Body as a Whole				
Asthenia	13.95	6.52	11.36	2.27
Headache	6.98	8.70	13.64	15.91
Cardiovascular/Respiratory				
Palpitations	0.00	6.52	4.55	0.00
Dyspnea	2.33	8.70	0.00	2.27
Gastrointestinal				
G.I. Distress	6.98	0.00	4.55	4.55
Nausea	6.98	26.09	18.18	2.27
Anorexia	0.00	2.17	6.82	2.27
Diarrhea	0.00	10.87	6.82	0.00
Central Nervous System				
Drowsy	6.98	6.52	0.00	4.55
Dizziness	11.63	15.22	27.27	6.82
Tremor	6.98	0.00	4.55	0.00
Tremor of Hand	9.30	0.00	4.55	0.00
Psychiatric				
Nervous	11.63	8.70	11.36	0.00
Special Senses				
Tinnitus	0.00	6.52	2.27	2.27

Most Common Events Resulting in Discontinuation

Adverse Reaction	Bepridil (N = 515) n (%)	Placebo (N = 288) n (%)	Positive Control (N = 119) n (%)
Dizziness	5 (0.97)	0 (0.0)	2 (1.68)
Gastrointestinal Symptoms	5 (0.97)	0 (0.0)	5 (4.20)
Ventricular Arrhythmia	5 (0.97)	0 (0.0)	0 (0.0)
Syncope	3 (0.58)	0 (0.0)	0 (0.0)

VASCOR (bepridil hydrochloride). The patient was observed for 72 hours in intensive care, but no significant adverse experiences were noted.

DOSAGE AND ADMINISTRATION

Therapy with VASCOR (bepridil hydrochloride) should be individualized according to each patient's response and the physician's clinical judgement. The usual starting dose of VASCOR is 200 mg once daily. After 10 days, dosage may be adjusted upward depending upon the patient's response (e.g., ability to perform activities of daily living, QT interval, heart rate, and frequency and severity of angina). This long interval for dosage adjustment is needed because steady-state blood levels are not achieved until 8 days of therapy. In clinical trials, most patients were maintained at a dose of VASCOR of 300 mg once daily. The maximum daily dose of VASCOR is 400 mg and the established minimum effective dose is 200 mg daily.

The starting dose for elderly patients does not differ from that for young patients. After therapeutic response is demonstrated, however, elderly patients may require more frequent monitoring.

Food does not interfere with the absorption of VASCOR. (see CLINICAL PHARMACOLOGY—Pharmacokinetics and

Metabolism). If nausea is experienced with VASCOR, the drug may be given at meals or at bedtime.

VASCOR has not been studied adequately in patients with impaired hepatic or renal function. It is therefore possible that dosage adjustments may be necessary in these patients.

Concomitant Use with Other Agents

The concomitant use of VASCOR and beta-blocking agents in patients without heart failure is safely tolerated. Physicians wishing to switch patients from beta-blocker therapy to VASCOR therapy may initiate VASCOR before terminating the beta blocker in the usual gradual fashion (see CLINICAL PHARMACOLOGY and PRECAUTIONS).

HOW SUPPLIED

VASCOR® (bepridil hydrochloride) tablets 200 mg (film coated light blue, scored, printed VASCOR and 200), 90 tablets (3 bottles of 30) (NDC 0045-0682-33) and unit dose of 100s (NDC 0045-0682-10) for hospital use.

VASCOR® (bepridil hydrochloride) tablets 300 mg (film coated blue, printed VASCOR and 300), 90 tablets (3 bottles of 30) (NDC 0045-0683-33), and unit dose of 100s (NDC 0045-0683-10) for hospital use.

VASCOR® (bepridil hydrochloride) tablets 400 mg (film coated dark blue, printed VASCOR and 400), 90 tablets (3

bottles of 30) (NDC 0045-0684-33), and unit dose of 100s (NDC 0045-0684-10) for hospital use.

Store at 15°–25° C (59°–77° F). Protect from light.

Co-marketed with:
WALLACE LABORATORIES

633–10–692–2

Manufactured by:
McNEIL PHARMACEUTICAL
MCNEILAB, INC.
SPRING HOUSE, PA 19477-0776
Shown in Product Identification Guide, page 324

EDUCATIONAL MATERIAL

FLOXIN® (ofloxacin tablets/injection)
"AUA Video Library"
"Simple Answers About UTI's" (English and Spanish)
Both are available free to physicians and pharmacists through McNeil representatives or directly from McNeil Pharmaceutical (908) 218-6000.

PANCREASE® (pancrelipase) and **PANCREASE® MT**
"Tree of Life" film and brochure—film available in ¹/₂" videotape.
"The Adventures of Mr. Enzyme" Nutritional Video
Target 100%—Growth and Nutrition brochure—for CF patients and families.
Guide to CF for Patients and Families video and workbook. (English and Spanish)
"Living with CF-Family Guide to Nutrition"
"This is Paul"-book for children with CF
Available free to physicians and pharmacists through McNeil representatives or directly from McNeil Pharmaceutical (908) 218-6000.

PARAFON FORTE® DSC (chlorzoxazone)
"Exercises for Low Back Pain" (English and Spanish)
"Exercises for Cervical Sprain" (English and Spanish)
Both are available free to physicians and pharmacists through McNeil representatives or directly from McNeil Pharmaceutical (908) 218-6000.

TOLECTIN® (tolmetin sodium)
"Six Steps to Control Your Arthritis Symptoms" (English and Spanish)
Available free to physicians and pharmacists through McNeil representatives or directly from McNeil Pharmaceutical (908) 218-6000.

ULTRAM® (tramadol hydrochloride tablets)
"Exercises for Low Back Pain" (English and Spanish)
"Exercises for the Painful Neck and Shoulder (English and Spanish)
Both are available free to physicians and pharmacists through McNeil representatives or directly from McNeil Pharmaceutical (908) 218-6000.

VASCOR® (bepridil hydrochloride) "Patients' Guide" brochure
Available free to physicians and pharmacists through representatives or directly from McNeil Pharmaceutical (908) 218-6000.

Mead Johnson Nutritionals
Mead Johnson & Company
2400 W. LLOYD EXPRESSWAY
EVANSVILLE, INDIANA 47721-0001

Direct Inquiries to:
Medical Services Department
(812) 429-5599

NATALINS® RX   ℞
[nă-tă-lins]
Multivitamin and multimineral supplement with beta-carotene, 1 mg folic acid and 60 mg Iron
Contains no artificial color or flavor from synthetic sources

DESCRIPTION

Natalins Rx tablets provide twelve vitamins and five minerals to supplement the diet during pregnancy or lactation.

Continued on next page

Mead Johnson Nutritionals—Cont.

Each Natalins Rx tablet supplies:
Vitamins
Vitamin A, IU 4,000
Vitamin D, IU 400
Vitamin E, IU 15
Vitamin C (Ascorbic acid), mg 80
Folic acid (Folacin), mg 1
Thiamin (Vitamin B$_1$), mg 1.5
Riboflavin (Vitamin B$_2$), mg 1.6
Niacin, mg 17
Vitamin B$_6$, mg 4
Vitamin B$_{12}$, µg 2.5
Biotin, mg 0.03
Pantothenic acid, mg 7
Minerals
Calcium, mg 200
Iron, mg 60
Magnesium, mg 100
Copper, mg 3
Zinc, mg 25
Active Ingredient
Each tablet contains 1 mg folic acid.
Other Ingredients
Acacia, biotin, calcium carbonate, calcium pantothenate, beta-carotene, cholecalciferol, colloidal silicon dioxide, cupric oxide, cyanocobalamin, ferrous fumarate, hydroxypropyl cellulose, hydroxypropyl methylcellulose, magnesium hydroxide, magnesium stearate, niacinamide, polacrilin potassium, polyethylene glycol, povidone, pyridoxine hydrochloride, riboflavin, sodium ascorbate, thiamine mononitrate, titanium dioxide, dl-alpha-tocopheryl acetate, vitamin A acetate, zinc oxide.

INDICATIONS AND USAGE
Natalins Rx tablets help assure an adequate intake of the vitamins and minerals listed above. Folic acid helps prevent the development of megaloblastic anemia during pregnancy.

CONTRAINDICATIONS
Supplemental vitamins and minerals should not be prescribed for patients with hemochromatosis or Wilson's disease.

WARNING
Keep Natalins Rx tablets out of the reach of children.

PRECAUTIONS
General
Pernicious anemia should be excluded before using this product since folic acid may mask the symptoms of pernicious anemia. The calcium content should be considered before prescribing for patients with kidney stones. Do not exceed the recommended dose.

ADVERSE REACTIONS
No adverse reactions or undesirable side effects have been attributed to the use of Natalins Rx tablets.

DOSAGE AND ADMINISTRATION
One tablet daily, or as prescribed.

HOW SUPPLIED
NDC 0087-0702-01 Bottles of 100
NDC 0087-0702-02 Bottles of 1000

P4757-05/P9735-00

POLY-VI-FLOR® ℞
[pahl-ē-vī'flŏr″]
● 1.0 mg
● 0.5 mg
● 0.25 mg
Multivitamin and fluoride supplement chewable tablets

DESCRIPTION
[See table above.]
Active ingredient for caries prophylaxis: Fluoride as sodium fluoride.
Other ingredients: Ascorbic acid, cholecalciferol, colloidal silicon dioxide, cyanocobalamin, dextrates, FD&C Blue No. 2 (aluminum lake), FD&C Red No. 40 (aluminum lake), FD&C Yellow No. 6 (aluminum lake), folic acid, fruit flavors (artificial), lactose, magnesium stearate, niacinamide, pyridoxine hydrochloride, riboflavin, silica gel, sodium ascorbate, sodium chloride, sucrose, thiamine mononitrate, dl-alpha-tocopheryl acetate, vitamin A acetate. The 1.0 mg tablet does not contain lactose.

| Each tablet supplies: | Poly-Vi-Flor chewable tablets | | | Percentage of U.S. Recommended Daily Allowance | |
	1.0 mg	0.5 mg	0.25 mg	Children Age 2–3 Years	Adults & Children Age 4 Years or More
Vitamin A, IU	2500	2500	2500	100	50
Vitamin D, IU	400	400	400	100	100
Vitamin E, IU	15	15	15	150	50
Vitamin C, mg	60	60	60	150	100
Folic acid, mg	0.3	0.3	0.3	150	75
Thiamine, mg	1.05	1.05	1.05	150	70
Riboflavin, mg	1.2	1.2	1.2	150	70
Niacin, mg	13.5	13.5	13.5	150	68
Vitamin B$_6$, mg	1.05	1.05	1.05	150	53
Vitamin B$_{12}$, µg	4.5	4.5	4.5	150	75
Fluoride, mg	1	0.5	0.25	*	*

* U.S. Recommended Daily Allowance has not been established.

CLINICAL PHARMACOLOGY
It is well established that fluoridation of the water supply (1 ppm fluoride) during the period of tooth development leads to a significant decrease in the incidence of dental caries. Poly-Vi-Flor chewable tablets provide sodium fluoride, and ten essential vitamins in a chewable tablet. Because the tablets are chewable, they provide a *topical* as well as *systemic* source of fluoride.[1,2]
Hydroxyapatite is the principal crystal for all calcified tissue in the human body. The fluoride ion reacts with the *hydroxyapatite* in the tooth as it is formed to produce the more caries-resistant crystal, *fluorapatite*. The reaction may be expressed by the equation:[3]

$$Ca_{10}(PO_4)_6(OH)_2 + 2F^- \rightarrow Ca_{10}(PO_4)_6F_2 + 2OH^-$$
(Hydroxyapatite)   (Fluorapatite)

Three stages of fluoride deposition in tooth enamel can be distinguished:[3]
1. Small amounts (reflecting the low levels of fluoride in tissue fluids) are incorporated into the enamel crystals while they are being formed.
2. After enamel has been laid down, fluoride deposition continues in the surface enamel. Diffusion of fluoride from the surface inward is apparently restricted.
3. After eruption, the surface enamel acquires fluoride from water, food, supplementary fluoride and smaller amounts from saliva.

INDICATIONS AND USAGE
Supplementation of the diet with ten essential vitamins. Supplementation of the diet with the fluoride for caries prophylaxis.
Poly-Vi-Flor 1.0 mg chewable tablets provide fluoride in tablet form for children 3 years and above in areas where the water fluoride level is less than 0.3 ppm.[4]
Poly-Vi-Flor 0.5 mg chewable tablets provide fluoride in tablet form for children 2-3 years of age where the drinking water has a fluoride content of less than 0.3 ppm, and for children 3 years of age and above where the drinking water contains 0.3 through 0.7 ppm of fluoride.[4]
Poly-Vi-Flor 0.25 mg chewable tablets provide fluoride in tablet form for children 2–3 years of age where the drinking water contains 0.3 through 0.7 ppm of fluoride.[4]
Poly-Vi-Flor chewable tablets supply significant amounts of vitamins A, D, E, C, thiamine, riboflavin, niacin, pyridoxine, cyanocobalamin and folic acid to supplement the diet, and to help assure that nutritional deficiencies of these vitamins will not develop. Thus, in a single easy-to-use preparation, children obtain ten essential vitamins and the important mineral, fluoride.
The American Academy of Pediatrics recommends that children up to age 16, in areas where drinking water contains less than optimal levels of fluoride, receive daily fluoride supplementation.
Children using Poly-Vi-Flor chewable tablets regularly should receive semiannual dental examinations. The regular brushing of teeth and attention to good oral hygiene practices are also essential.

WARNINGS
As in the case of all medications, keep out of the reach of children.

PRECAUTIONS
The suggested dose *should not be exceeded*, since dental fluorosis may result from continued ingestion of large amounts of fluoride.
Before prescribing Vi-Flor® products:
1. determine the fluoride content of the drinking water.
2. make sure the child is not receiving significant amounts of fluoride from other medications.
3. periodically check to make sure that the child does not develop significant dental fluorosis.
The Council on Dental Therapeutics of the American Dental Association recommends that no more than 264 mg of sodium fluoride should be dispensed at one time.[5] Therefore, no more than 120 Poly-Vi-Flor 1.0 mg chewable tablets (2.2 mg sodium fluoride per tablet) should be dispensed at one time.

ADVERSE REACTIONS
Allergic rash and other idiosyncrasies have been rarely reported.

DOSAGE AND ADMINISTRATION
One tablet daily or as prescribed.

HOW SUPPLIED
Poly-Vi-Flor 1.0 mg (multivitamin and fluoride supplement) chewable tablets are available in 100- and 1000-tablet bottles.
NDC 0087-0474-02 Bottles of 100
NDC 0087-0474-03 Bottles of 1000
Poly-Vi-Flor 0.5 mg (multivitamin and fluoride supplement) chewable tablets are available in 100 tablet bottles.
NDC 0087-0468-41 Bottles of 100
Poly-Vi-Flor 0.25 mg (multivitamin and fluoride supplement) chewable tablets are available in 100-tablet bottles.
NDC 0087-0487-41 Bottles of 100

LITERATURE AVAILABLE
Yes.

REFERENCES
1. Hennon DK, Stookey GK, Muhler JC. The clinical anti-cariogenic effectiveness of supplementary fluoride-vitamin preparations—Results at the end of three years. *J Dentistry for Children.* January 1966;33:3–12.
2. Hennon DK, Stookey GK, Muhler JC. The clinical anti-cariogenic effectiveness of supplementary fluoride-vitamin preparations—Results at the end of four years. *J Dentistry for Children.* November 1967;34:439–443.
3. Brudevold F, McCann HG. Fluoride and caries control—Mechanism of action. In: Nizel AE, ed. *The Science of Nutrition and Its Application in Clinical Dentistry.* Philadelphia: WB Saunders Co; 1966:331–347.
4. American Academy of Pediatrics Committee on Nutrition: Fluoride supplementation. *Pediatrics.*1986;77:758.
5. Council on Dental Therapeutics, Am Dental Assoc. *Accepted Dental Therapeutics.* 1977, 37th ed, p 294.

POLY-VI-FLOR® ℞
[pahl-ē-vī'flŏr″]
● 0.5 mg
● 0.25 mg
Multivitamin and fluoride supplement drops

DESCRIPTION
[See table at top of next page.]
See INDICATIONS AND USAGE section below for use by infants and children under two years of age.
Active ingredient for caries prophylaxis: Fluoride as sodium fluoride.
Other ingredients: Ascorbic acid, caramel color, cholecalciferol, cyanocobalamin, ferrous sulfate, fruit flavor (artificial), glycerin, niacinamide, polysorbate 80, pyridoxine hydrochloride, riboflavin-5-phosphate sodium, thiamine hydrochloride, d-alpha-tocopheryl acid succinate, vitamin A palmitate, water, and other ingredients.

CLINICAL PHARMACOLOGY
For information on fluoridation see Poly-Vi-Flor chewable tablets.

INDICATIONS AND USAGE
Supplementation of the diet with nine essential vitamins. Supplementation of the diet with fluoride for caries prophylaxis.
The American Academy of Pediatrics recommends that children up to age 16, in areas where drinking water contains

Each 1.0 mL supplies:	Poly-Vi-Flor drops 0.5 mg	0.25 mg	Percentage of U.S. Recommended Daily Allowance Infants	Children Under Age 4 Years
Vitamin A, IU	1500	1500	100	60
Vitamin D, IU	400	400	100	100
Vitamin E, IU	5	5	100	50
Vitamin C, mg	35	35	100	88
Thiamine, mg	0.5	0.5	100	71
Riboflavin, mg	0.6	0.6	100	75
Niacin, mg	8	8	100	89
Vitamin B_6, mg	0.4	0.4	100	57
Vitamin B_{12}, µg	2	2	100	67
Fluoride, mg	0.5	0.25	*	*

* U.S. Recommended Daily Allowance has not been established.

less than optimal levels of fluoride, receive daily fluoride supplementation.
Poly-Vi-Flor 0.5 mg (multivitamin and fluoride supplement) drops provide fluoride in drop form for children ages 2–3 years in areas where the drinking water contains less than 0.3 ppm fluoride; and for children 3 years and above in areas where the drinking water contains 0.3 through 0.7 ppm of fluoride.
Poly-Vi-Flor 0.25 mg (multivitamin and fluoride supplement) drops provide fluoride in drop form for infants and young children from birth to 2 years of age in areas where the drinking water contains less than 0.3 ppm of fluoride and for children ages 2–3 years in areas where the drinking water contains 0.3 through 0.7 ppm of fluoride.
The American Academy of Pediatrics[1] and the American Dental Association[2] currently recommend that infants and children under 2 years of age, in areas where drinking water contains less than 0.3 ppm of fluoride, and children 2-3, in areas where the drinking water contains 0.3 through 0.7 ppm of fluoride, receive 0.25 mg of supplemental fluoride daily which is provided in a full dose (1 mL) of Poly-Vi-Flor® 0.25 mg drops. A half dose (0.5 mL) of Poly-Vi-Flor 0.5 mg drops could also provide a daily fluoride intake of 0.25 mg; however, this dosage reduces vitamin supplementation by half.
Poly-Vi-Flor 0.5 mg drops and 0.25 mg drops supply significant amounts of vitamins A, D, E, C, thiamine, riboflavin, niacin, pyridoxine, and cyanocobalamin to supplement the diet, and to help assure that nutritional deficiencies of these vitamins will not develop. Thus in a single easy-to-use preparation, infants and children obtain nine essential vitamins and fluoride.
A comprehensive 5½ year series of studies of the effectiveness of Tri-Vi-Flor® and Poly-Vi-Flor® products in caries protection has been published.[3-6] Children in this continuing study lived in an area where the water supply contained only 0.05 ppm fluoride. The subjects were divided into two groups, one which used only nonfluoridated Vi-Sol® vitamin products and the other Tri-Vi-Flor and Poly-Vi-Flor vitamin-fluoride products.
The three-year interim report showed 63% fewer carious surfaces in primary teeth and 43% fewer carious surfaces in permanent teeth of the children taking Vi-Flor® vitamin-fluoride products.[3]
After four years the studies continued to support the effectiveness of Tri-Vi-Flor and Poly-Vi-Flor, showing a reduction in carious surfaces of 68% in primary teeth and 46% in permanent teeth.[4]
Results at the end of 5½ years further confirmed the previous findings and indicated that significant reductions in dental caries are apparent with the continued use of Vi-Flor vitamin-fluoride products.[5]

WARNINGS
As in the case of all medications, keep out of the reach of children.

PRECAUTIONS
The suggested dose *should not be exceeded* since dental fluorosis may result from continued ingestion of large amounts of fluoride.
When prescribing Vi-Flor products:
1. determine the fluoride content of the drinking water.
2. make sure the child is not receiving significant amounts of fluoride from other medications.
3. periodically check to make sure that the child does not develop significant dental fluorosis.
Poly-Vi-Flor 0.5 mg drops and 0.25 mg drops should be dispensed in the original plastic container, since contact with glass leads to instability and precipitation. (The amount of sodium fluoride in all Poly-Vi-Flor drops is well below the maximum to be dispensed at one time according to recommendations of the American Dental Association.)

ADVERSE REACTIONS
Allergic rash and other idiosyncrasies have been rarely reported.

DOSAGE AND ADMINISTRATION
1.0 mL daily or as prescribed.
Drops may be dropped directly into mouth with 'Safti-Dropper,' or mixed with cereal, fruit juice or other food.

HOW SUPPLIED
Poly-Vi-Flor 0.5 mg (multivitamin and fluoride supplement) drops are available in bottles of 50 mL.
NDC 0087-0472-02 Bottles of 1⅔ fl oz (50 mL)
FSN 6505-080-0967 (50 mL)
Poly-Vi-Flor 0.25 mg (multivitamin and fluoride supplement) drops are available in bottles of 50 mL.
NDC 0087-0451-41 Bottles of 50 mL.

LITERATURE AVAILABLE
Yes.

REFERENCES
1. American Academy of Pediatrics Committee on Nutrition: Fluoride supplementation. *Pediatrics.* 1986;77:758.
2. American Dental Association. *Accepted Dental Therapeutics.* 38th ed. Chicago: 1979:p 321.
3. Hennon DK, Stookey GK, Muhler JC. The clinical anticariogenic effectiveness of supplementary fluoride-vitamin preparations—Results at the end of three years. *J Dentistry for Children.* January 1966;33:3–12.
4. Hennon DK, Stookey GK, Muhler JC. The clinical anticariogenic effectiveness of supplementary fluoride-vitamin preparations—Results at the end of four years. *J Dentistry for Children.* November 1967;34:439–443.
5. Hennon DK, Stookey GK, Muhler JC. The clinical anticariogenic effectiveness of supplementary fluoride-vitamin preparations—Results at the end of five and a half years. *Phar and Ther In Dent.* 1970;1:1.
6. Hennon DK, Stookey GK, Beiswanger BB. Fluoride-vitamin supplements: Effects on dental caries and fluorosis when used in areas with suboptimum fluoride in the water supply. *J Am Dent Assoc.* 1977;95:965.

TRI-VI-FLOR®   ℞
[trī 'vī-flŏr″]
● 0.5 mg
● 0.25 mg
Vitamins A, D, C and fluoride drops

DESCRIPTION
[See table below.]
See INDICATIONS AND USAGE section below for use by infants and children under two years of age.
Active ingredient for caries prophylaxis: Fluoride as sodium fluoride.
Other ingredients: Ascorbic acid, caramel color, cholecalciferol, fruit flavor (artificial), glycerin, polysorbate 80, sodium hydroxide, vitamin A palmitate, water.

CLINICAL PHARMACOLOGY
For information on fluoridation see Poly-Vi-Flor® chewable tablets.

INDICATIONS AND USAGE
Supplementation of the diet with vitamins A, D and C. Tri-Vi-Flor drops also provide fluoride for caries prophylaxis.
The American Academy of Pediatrics recommends that children up to age 16, in areas where drinking water contains less than optimal levels of fluoride, receive daily fluoride supplementation.
Tri-Vi-Flor 0.5 mg (vitamins A, D, C and fluoride) drops provide fluoride in drop form for children ages 2-3 years in areas where the drinking water contains less than 0.3 ppm fluoride; and for children 3 years and above in areas where the drinking water contains 0.3 through 0.7 ppm of fluoride.
Tri-Vi-Flor 0.25 mg (vitamins A, D, C and fluoride) drops provide fluoride in drop form for infants and young children from birth to 2 years of age in areas where the drinking water contains less than 0.3 ppm of fluoride; and for children ages 2-3 years in areas where the drinking water contains 0.3 through 0.7 ppm of fluoride.
The American Academy of Pediatrics[1] and the American Dental Association[6] currently recommend that infants and children under 2 years of age, in areas where drinking water contains less than 0.3 ppm of fluoride, and children 2-3, in areas where the drinking water contains 0.3 through 0.7 ppm of fluoride, receive 0.25 mg of supplemental fluoride daily which is provided in a full dose (1 mL) of Tri-Vi-Flor® 0.25 mg drops. A half dose (0.5 mL) of Tri-Vi-Flor 0.5 mg drops could also provide a daily fluoride intake of 0.25 mg; however, this dosage reduces vitamin supplementation by half.
A comprehensive 5½ year series of studies of the effectiveness of Tri-Vi-Flor® and Poly-Vi-Flor® products in caries protection has been published.[2-5] Children in this continuing study lived in an area where the water supply contained only 0.05 ppm fluoride. The subjects were divided into two groups, one which used only nonfluoridated Vi-Sol® vitamin products and the other Tri-Vi-Flor and Poly-Vi-Flor vitamin-fluoride products.
The three-year interim report showed 63% fewer carious surfaces in primary teeth and 43% fewer carious surfaces in permanent teeth of the children taking Vi-Flor® vitamin-fluoride products.[2]
After four years the studies continued to support the effectiveness of Tri-Vi-Flor and Poly-Vi-Flor, showing a reduction in carious surfaces of 68% in primary teeth and 46% in permanent teeth.[3]
Results at the end of 5½ years further confirmed the previous findings and indicated that significant reductions in dental caries are apparent with the continued use of Vi-Flor vitamin-fluoride products.[4]

WARNINGS
As in the case of all medications, keep out of the reach of children.

PRECAUTIONS
The suggested dose *should not be exceeded* since dental fluorosis may result from continued ingestion of large amounts of fluoride.
When prescribing Vi-Flor products:
1. determine the fluoride content of the drinking water.
2. make sure the child is not receiving significant amounts of fluoride from other medications.
3. periodically check to make sure that the child does not develop significant dental fluorosis.
Tri-Vi-Flor drops should be dispensed in the original plastic container, since contact with glass leads to instability and precipitation. (The amount of sodium fluoride in all Tri-Vi-Flor drops is well below the maximum to be dispensed at one time acccording to recommendations of the American Dental Association.)

ADVERSE REACTIONS
Allergic rash and other idiosyncrasies have been rarely reported.

DOSAGE AND ADMINISTRATION
1.0 mL daily, or as prescribed.
May be dropped directly into mouth with 'Safti-Dropper,' or mixed with cereal, fruit juice or other food.

HOW SUPPLIED
Tri-Vi-Flor 0.5 mg (vitamins A,D,C, and fluoride) drops are available in bottles of 50 mL.

Each 1.0 mL supplies:	Tri-Vi-Flor Drops 0.5 mg	0.25 mg	Percentage of U.S. Recommended Daily Allowance Infants	Children Under Age 4 Years
Vitamin A, IU	1500	1500	100	60
Vitamin D, IU	400	400	100	100
Vitamin C, mg	35	35	100	88
Fluoride, mg	0.5	0.25	*	*

*U.S. Recommended Daily Allowance has not been established.

Continued on next page

Mead Johnson Nutritionals—Cont.

NDC 0087-0473-02 Bottles of 1⅔ fl oz (50 mL)
Tri-Vi-Flor 0.25 mg (vitamins A, D, C and fluoride) drops are available in bottles of 50 mL.
NDC 0087-0452-41 Bottles of 50 mL.

LITERATURE AVAILABLE

Yes.

REFERENCES

1. American Academy of Pediatrics Committee on Nutrition: Fluoride supplementation. *Pediatrics.* 1986; 77:758.
2. Hennon DK, Stookey GK, Muhler JC. The clinical anticariogenic effectiveness of supplementary fluoride-vitamin preparations—Results at the end of three years. *J Dentistry for Children.* January 1966;33:3–12.
3. Hennon DK, Stookey GK, Muhler JC. The clinical anticariogenic effectiveness of supplementary fluoride-vitamin preparations—Results at the end of four years. *J Dentistry for Children.* November 1967;34:439–443.
4. Hennon DK, Stookey GK, Muhler JC. The clinical anticariogenic effectiveness of supplementary fluoride-vitamin preparations—Results at the end of five and a half years. *Phar and Ther in Dent.* 1970;1:1.
5. Hennon DK, Stookey GK, Beiswanger BB. Fluoride-vitamin supplements: Effects on dental caries and fluorosis when used in areas with suboptimum fluoride in the water supply. *J Am Dent Assoc.* 1977;95:965.
6. American Dental Association. *Accepted Dental Therapeutics.* 38th ed. Chicago: 1979;p 321.

Medeva Pharmaceuticals, Inc.

14801 SOVEREIGN ROAD
FORT WORTH, TEXAS 76155-2645

Direct Inquiries to:
Customer Service Department
P.O. Box 1766
Rochester, NY 14603
(716) 274-5300
(888) 9-MEDEVA
In Emergencies:
(800) 932-1950 (24 hours)

AIRET™ ℞
Albuterol Sulfate Inhalation Solution 0.083%*
(*Potency expressed as albuterol)

PRESCRIBING INFORMATION

DESCRIPTION

Albuterol sulfate inhalation solution is a relatively selective beta$_2$-adrenergic bronchodilator (see **CLINICAL PHARMACOLOGY** section below). Albuterol sulfate, the racemic form of albuterol, has the chemical name α^1-[(*tert*-butylamino)methyl]-4-hydroxy-*m*-xylene-α,α'-diol sulfate (2:1) (salt), and the following chemical structure:

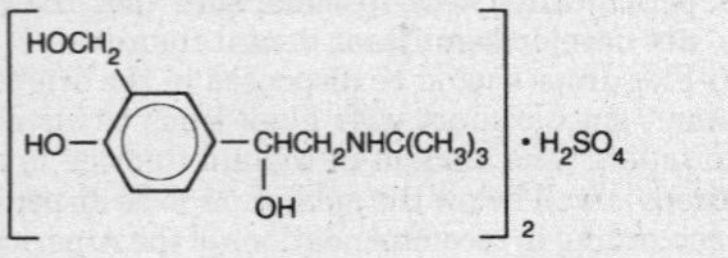

Albuterol sulfate has a molecular weight of 576.7 and the molecular formula $(C_{13}H_{21}NO_3)_2 \cdot H_2SO_4$. Albuterol sulfate is a white or practically white powder, freely soluble in water and slightly soluble in alcohol.
The World Health Organization recommended name for albuterol base is salbutamol.
Albuterol sulfate inhalation solution requires no dilution before administration.
Each mL of albuterol sulfate inhalation solution (0.083%) contains 0.83 mg of albuterol (as 1 mg of albuterol sulfate) in an isotonic, sterile, aqueous solution containing sodium chloride, edetate disodium, sodium citrate, and hydrochloric acid to adjust the pH between 3 and 5. Albuterol sulfate inhalation solution (0.083%) contains no sulfiting agents. It is supplied in 3 mL unit dose vials.
Albuterol sulfate inhalation solution is a clear, colorless to light yellow solution.

CLINICAL PHARMACOLOGY

The prime action of beta-adrenergic drugs is to stimulate adenyl cyclase, the enzyme which catalyzes the formation of cyclic-3′,5′-adenosine monophosphate (cyclic AMP) from adenosine triphosphate (ATP). The cyclic AMP thus formed mediates the cellular responses. *In vitro* studies and *in vivo* pharmacologic studies have demonstrated that albuterol has a preferential effect on beta$_2$-adrenergic receptors compared with isoproterenol. While it is recognized that beta$_2$-adrenergic receptors are the predominant receptors in bronchial smooth muscle, recent data indicate that 10 to 50% of the beta-receptors in the human heart may be beta$_2$-receptors. The precise function of these receptors, however, is not yet established. Albuterol has been shown in most controlled clinical trials to have more effect on the respiratory tract in the form of bronchial smooth muscle relaxation than isoproterenol at comparable doses while producing fewer cardiovascular effects. Controlled clinical studies and other clinical experience have shown that inhaled albuterol, like other beta-adrenergic agonist drugs, can produce a significant cardiovascular effect in some patients, as measured by pulse rate, blood pressure, symptoms, and/or electrocardiographic changes.
Albuterol is longer acting than isoproterenol in most patients by any route of administration because it is not a substrate for the cellular uptake processes for catecholamines nor for catechol-*O*-methyl transferase.
Studies in asthmatic patients have shown that less than 20% of a single albuterol dose was absorbed following the IPPB or nebulizer administration; the remaining amount was recovered from the nebulizer and apparatus and expired air. Most of the absorbed dose was recovered in the urine 24 hours after drug administration. There was a significant dose-related response in FEV_1 (forced expiratory volume in one second) and peak flow rate (PFR). It has been demonstrated that following oral administration of 4 mg albuterol, the elimination half-life was five to six hours.
Animal studies show that albuterol does not pass the blood-brain barrier. Recent studies in laboratory animals (minipigs, rodents, and dogs) recorded the occurrence of cardiac arrhythmias and sudden death (with histologic evidence of myocardial necrosis) when beta-agonists and methylxanthines were administered concurrently. The significance of these findings when applied to humans is currently unknown.
In controlled clinical trials, most patients exhibited an onset of improvement in pulmonary function within 5 minutes as determined by FEV_1. FEV_1 measurements also showed that the maximum average improvement in pulmonary function usually occurred at approximately 1 hour following inhalation of 2.5 mg of albuterol by compressor-nebulizer, and remained close to peak for 2 hours. Clinically significant improvement in pulmonary function (defined as maintenance of a 15% or more increase in FEV_1 over baseline values) continued for 3 to 4 hours in most patients and in some patients continued up to 6 hours.
In repetitive dose studies, continued effectiveness was demonstrated throughout the three-month period of treatment in some patients.

INDICATIONS AND USAGE

Albuterol sulfate inhalation solution is indicated for the relief of bronchospasm in patients with reversible obstructive airway disease and acute attacks of bronchospasm.

CONTRAINDICATIONS

Albuterol sulfate inhalation solution is contraindicated in patients with a history of hypersensitivity to any of its components.

WARNINGS

As with other inhaled beta-adrenergic agonists, albuterol sulfate inhalation solution can produce paradoxical bronchospasm, which can be life threatening. If it occurs, the preparation should be discontinued immediately and alternative therapy instituted.
Fatalities have been reported in association with excessive use of inhaled sympathomimetic drugs and with the home use of nebulizers. It is, therefore, essential that the physician instruct the patient in the need for further evaluation if his/her asthma becomes worse. In individual patients, any beta$_2$-adrenergic agonist, including albuterol solution for inhalation, may have a clinically significant cardiac effect.
Immediate hypersensitivity reactions may occur after administration of albuterol as demonstrated by rare cases of urticaria, angioedema, rash, bronchospasm, and oropharyngeal edema.

PRECAUTIONS

General: Albuterol, as with all sympathomimetic amines, should be used with caution in patients with cardiovascular disorders, especially coronary insufficiency, cardiac arrhythmias and hypertension, in patients with convulsive disorders, hyperthyroidism or diabetes mellitus and in patients who are unusually responsive to sympathomimetic amines.
Large doses of intravenous albuterol have been reported to aggravate pre-existing diabetes mellitus and ketoacidosis. As with other beta-agonists, inhaled and intravenous albuterol may produce a significant hypokalemia in some patients, possibly through intracellular shunting, which has the potential to produce adverse cardiovascular effects. The decrease is usually transient, not requiring supplementation.
Information for Patients: The action of albuterol sulfate inhalation solution may last up to six hours, and therefore it should not be used more frequently than recommended. Do not increase the dose or frequency of medication without medical consultation. If symptoms get worse, medical consultation should be sought promptly. While taking albuterol sulfate inhalation solution, other anti-asthma medicines should not be used unless prescribed.
Drug Interactions: Other sympathomimetic aerosol bronchodilators or epinephrine should not be used concomitantly with albuterol.
Albuterol should be administered with extreme caution to patients being treated with monoamine oxidase inhibitors or tricyclic antidepressants, since the action of albuterol on the vascular system may be potentiated.
Beta-receptor blocking agents and albuterol inhibit the effect of each other.
Carcinogenesis, Mutagenesis, and Impairment of Fertility: Albuterol sulfate, caused a significant dose-related increase in the incidence of benign leiomyomas of the mesovarium in a 2-year study in the rat, at oral doses of 2, 10, and 50 mg/kg, corresponding to 10, 50, and 250 times, respectively, the maximum, nebulization dose for a 50 kg human. In another study, this effect was blocked by the coadministration of propranolol. The relevance of these findings to humans is not known. An 18-month study in mice and a lifetime study in hamsters revealed no evidence of tumorigenicity. Studies with albuterol revealed no evidence of mutagenesis. Reproduction studies in rats revealed no evidence of impaired fertility.
Pregnancy: Teratogenic Effects: Pregnancy Category C: Albuterol has been shown to be teratogenic in mice when given subcutaneously in doses corresponding to the human nebulization dose. There are no adequate and well-controlled studies in pregnant women. Albuterol should be used during pregnancy only if the potential benefit justifies the potential risk to the fetus. A reproduction study in CD-1 mice given albuterol subcutaneously (0.025, 0.25, and 2.5 mg/kg, corresponding to 0.125, 1.25, and 12.5 times, respectively, the maximum nebulization dose for a 50 kg human) showed cleft palate formation in 5 of 111 (4.5%) of fetuses at 0.25 mg/kg and in 10 of 108 (9.3%) of fetuses at 2.5 mg/kg. None were observed at 0.025 mg/kg. Cleft palate also occurred in 22 of 72 (30.5%) fetuses treated with 2.5 mg/kg isoproterenol (positive control). A reproduction study in Stride Dutch rabbits revealed cranioschisis in 7 of 19 (37%) of fetuses at 50 mg/kg, corresponding to 250 times the maximum human nebulization dose.
During worldwide marketing experience, various congenital anomalies, including cleft palate and limb defects, have been rarely reported in the offspring of patients being treated with albuterol. Some of the mothers were taking multiple medications during their pregnancies. No consistent pattern of defects can be discerned, and a relationship between albuterol use and congenital anomalies has not been established.
Labor and Delivery: Oral albuterol has been shown to delay preterm labor in some reports. There are presently no well controlled studies which demonstrate that it will stop preterm labor at term. Therefore, cautious use of albuterol sulfate inhalation solution is required in pregnant patients when given for relief of bronchospasm so as to avoid interference with uterine contractibility.
Nursing Mothers: It is not known whether this drug is excreted in human milk. Because of the potential for tumorigenicity shown for albuterol in some animal studies, a decision should be made whether to discontinue nursing or to discontinue the drug, taking into accord the importance of the drug to the mother.
Pediatric Use: Safety and effectiveness of albuterol solution for inhalation in pediatric patients below the age of 12 years have not been established.

ADVERSE REACTIONS

The results of clinical trials with albuterol sulfate inhalation solution in 135 patients showed the following side effects which were considered probably or possibly drug related:
Central Nervous System: tremors (20%), dizziness (7%), nervousness (4%), headache (3%), insomnia (1%).
Gastrointestinal: nausea (4%), dyspepsia (1%).
Ear, Nose and Throat: pharyngitis (<1%), nasal congestion (1%).
Cardiovascular: tachycardia (1%), hypertension (1%).
Respiratory: bronchospasm (8%), cough (4%), bronchitis (4%), wheezing (1%).
No clinically relevant laboratory abnormalities related to albuterol sulfate inhalation solution administration were determined in these studies.
In comparing the adverse reactions reported for patients treated with albuterol sulfate inhalation solution with those of patients treated with isoproterenol during clinical trials of three months, the following moderate to severe reactions, as judged by the investigators, were reported. This table does not include mild reactions.

Percent Incidence of Moderate to Severe Adverse Reactions

Reaction	Albuterol N=65	Isoproterenol N=65
Central Nervous System		
Tremors	10.7%	13.8%
Headache	3.1%	1.5%
Insomnia	3.1%	1.5%
Cardiovascular		
Hypertension	3.1%	3.1%
Arrhythmias	0%	3%
*Palpitation	0%	22.0%
Respiratory		
**Bronchospasm	15.4%	18%
Cough	3.1%	5%
Bronchitis	1.5%	5%
Wheeze	1.5%	1.5%
Sputum Increase	1.5%	1.5%
Dyspnea	1.5%	1.5%
Gastrointestinal		
Nausea	3.1%	0%
Dyspepsia	1.5%	0%
Systemic		
Malaise	1.5%	0%

*The finding of no arrhythmias and no palpitations after albuterol administration in this clinical study should not be interpreted as indicating that these adverse effects can not occur after the administration of inhaled albuterol.

**In most cases of bronchospasm, this term was generally used to describe exacerbations in the underlying pulmonary disease.

Rare cases of urticaria, angioedema, rash, bronchospasm and oropharyngeal edema have been reported after the use of inhaled albuterol.

OVERDOSAGE

Manifestations of overdosage may include seizures, anginal pain, hypertension, hypokalemia, tachycardia with rates up to 200 beats per minute, and exaggeration of the pharmacological effects listed in **ADVERSE REACTIONS**. The oral LD$_{50}$ in rats and mice was greater than 2,000 mg/kg. The inhalational LD$_{50}$ could not be determined. There is insufficient evidence to determine if dialysis is beneficial for overdosage of albuterol.

DOSAGE AND ADMINISTRATION

The ususal dosage for adults and children 12 years and older is 2.5 mg of albuterol administered 3 or 4 times daily by nebulization. More frequent administration or high doses is not recommended. To administer 2.5 mg of albuterol, use the entire contents of one unit-dose vial (3 mL of 0.083% inhalation solution) by nebulization. The flow rate is regulated to suit the particular nebulizer so that the albuterol sulfate inhalation solution will be delivered over approximately 5 to 15 minutes. (A 2.5 mg dose of albuterol is equivalent to 0.5 mL of a 0.5% solution.)

The use of albuterol sulfate inhalation solution can be continued as medically indicated to control recurring bouts of bronchospasm. During this time most patients gain optimum benefit from regular use of the inhalation solution.

If a previously effective dosage regimen fails to provide the usual relief, medical advice should be sought immediately, as this is often a sign of seriously worsening asthma which would require reassessment of therapy.

HOW SUPPLIED

Unit-dose plastic vial containing AIRET™ Albuterol Sulfate Inhalation Solution 0.083%, 2.5 mg/3mL* (*potency expressed as albuterol.) Equivalent to 0.5 mL albuterol (as the sulfate) 0.5% (2.5 mg albuterol) diluted to 3 mL. Supplied in cartons as listed below.
NDC 53014-075-25
Twenty-five vials per carton.
NDC 53014-075-60
Sixty vials per carton.
Storage: PROTECT FROM LIGHT. RETAIN IN CARTON UNTIL TIME OF USE. Store between 2° and 25°C (36° and 77°F).
CAUTION: Federal law prohibits dispensing without prescription.

Revised: May 1995

AMERICAINE® ANESTHETIC LUBRICANT ℞
[uh-mer'ĭ-kān"]
(benzocaine)
R238C
Rev. 7/96

DESCRIPTION

AMERICAINE Anesthetic Lubricant contains benzocaine 20% with benzethonium chloride 0.1% as a preservative in a water soluble base of polyethylene glycol 300 and 3350.

Benzocaine, a local anesthetic, is chemically ethyl p-aminobenzoate, $C_9H_{11}NO_2$, with a molecular weight of 165.19 and has the following structural formula:

$$NH_2 - \langle \rangle - COOC_2H_5$$

CLINICAL PHARMACOLOGY

Benzocaine reversibly stabilizes the neuronal membrane which decreases its permeability to sodium ions. Depolarization of the neuronal membrane is inhibited thereby blocking the initiation and conduction of nerve impulses.

INDICATIONS AND USAGE

AMERICAINE Anesthetic Lubricant is indicated for general use as a lubricant and topical anesthetic on intratracheal catheters and pharyngeal and nasal airways to obtund the pharyngeal and tracheal reflexes; on nasogastric and endoscopic tubes; urinary catheters; laryngoscopes; proctoscopes; sigmoidoscopes and vaginal specula.

CONTRAINDICATIONS

Known allergy or hypersensitivity to benzocaine.

PRECAUTIONS

General: Medication should be discontinued if sensitivity or irritation occurs.
Carcinogenesis, Mutagenesis, Impairment of Fertility: Long-term studies in animals or humans to evaluate the carcinogenic and mutagenic potential or the effect on fertility have not been conducted.
Pregnancy: Pregnancy Category C. Animal reproduction studies have not been conducted with AMERICAINE Anesthetic Lubricant. It is also not known whether AMERICAINE Anesthetic Lubricant can cause fetal harm when administered to a pregnant woman or can affect reproduction capacity. AMERICAINE Anesthetic Lubricant should be given to a pregnant woman only if clearly needed.
Nursing Mothers: It is not known whether this drug is excreted in human milk. Because many drugs are excreted in human milk, caution should be exercised when AMERICAINE Anesthetic Lubricant is administered to a nursing woman.
Pediatric Use: Do not use in infants under 1 year of age.

ADVERSE REACTIONS

Contact dermatitis and/or hypersensitivity to benzocaine can cause burning, stinging, pruritus, tenderness, erythema, rash, urticaria and edema. Rarely, benzocaine may induce methemoglobinemia causing respiratory distress and cyanosis. Intravenous methylene blue is the specific therapy for this condition.

DOSAGE AND ADMINISTRATION

Apply evenly to exterior of tube or instrument prior to use.

HOW SUPPLIED

AMERICAINE Anesthetic Lubricant (benzocaine) is available in:
NDC 53014-376-16 — 28 g tube
NDC 53014-376-62 — 2.5 g unit dose foil packs, 144 per carton
Store at 15°–25°C (59°–77°F).
CAUTION: Federal law prohibits dispensing without prescription.
MEDEVA PHARMACEUTICALS
Medeva Pharmaceuticals, Inc.
Fort Worth, TX 76155
®Ciba-Geigy Corporation
©1996, Medeva Pharmaceuticals Manufacturing, Inc.

Rev. 7/96
R238C

AMERICAINE® OTIC ℞
[uh-mer'ĭ-kān"]
(benzocaine)
Topical Anesthetic Ear Drops
Rev. 7/96
R239C

DESCRIPTION

AMERICAINE Otic, topical anesthetic ear drops, contains benzocaine 20% (w/w) in a water soluble base of glycerin 1% (w/w) and polyethylene glycol 300 with benzethonium chloride 0.1% as a preservative.
Benzocaine, a local anesthetic, is chemically ethyl p-aminobenzoate, $C_9H_{11}NO_2$, with a molecular weight of 165.19 and has the following structural formula:

$$NH_2 - \langle \rangle - COOC_2H_5$$

CLINICAL PHARMACOLOGY

Benzocaine reversibly stabilizes the neuronal membrane which decreases its permeability to sodium ions. Depolarization of the neuronal membrane is inhibited thereby blocking the initiation and conduction of nerve impulses.

INDICATIONS AND USAGE

AMERICAINE Otic is indicated for relief of pain and pruritus in acute congestive and serous otitis media, acute swimmer's ear, and other forms of otitis externa.

CONTRAINDICATIONS

In the presence of a perforated tympanic membrane or ear discharge.
Known allergy or hypersensitivity to benzocaine.

WARNINGS

Indiscriminate use of anesthetic ear drops may mask symptoms of fulminating infection of the middle ear.

PRECAUTIONS

General: Medication should be discontinued if sensitivity or irritation occurs.
Carcinogenesis, Mutagenesis, Impairment of Fertility: Long-term studies in animals or humans to evaluate the carcinogenic and mutagenic potential or the effect on fertility have not been conducted.
Pregnancy: Pregnancy Category C. Animal reproduction studies have not been conducted with AMERICAINE Otic. It is also not known whether AMERICAINE Otic can cause fetal harm when administered to a pregnant woman or can affect reproduction capacity. AMERICAINE Otic should be given to a pregnant woman only if clearly needed.
Nursing Mothers: It is not known whether this drug is excreted in human milk. Because many drugs are excreted in human milk, caution should be exercised when AMERICAINE Otic is administered to a nursing woman.
Pediatric Use: Do not use in infants under 1 year of age.

ADVERSE REACTIONS

Contact dermatitis and/or hypersensitivity to benzocaine can cause burning, stinging, pruritus, tenderness, erythema, rash, urticaria and edema. Rarely, benzocaine may induce methemoglobinemia causing respiratory distress and cyanosis. Intravenous methylene blue is the specific therapy for this condition.

DOSAGE AND ADMINISTRATION

Instill 4–5 drops of AMERICAINE Otic in the external auditory canal, then insert a cotton pledget into the meatus. Application may be repeated every one to two hours if necessary.

HOW SUPPLIED

AMERICAINE Otic (benzocaine), topical anesthetic ear drops, is available in dropper-top bottles.
NDC 53014-377-51 — 15 mL bottle
Keep bottle tightly closed. Store at 15°–30°C (59°–86°F).
Keep out of the reach of children.
CAUTION: Federal law prohibits dispensing without prescription.
Marketed by:
MEDEVA PHARMACEUTICALS
Medeva Pharmaceuticals, Inc.
Fort Worth, TX 76155
Manufactured by:
Akorn Manufacturing, Inc.
Decatur, IL 62525
® Ciba-Geigy Corporation
© 1996, Medeva Pharmaceuticals Manufacturing, Inc.

Rev. 7/96
R239C

ATROHIST® Pediatric Capsules ℞

DESCRIPTION

Each extended-release capsule contains:
Chlorpheniramine maleate .... 4 mg
Pseudoephedrine hydrochloride .... 60 mg
in a specially prepared base to provide prolonged action. This product contains ingredients of the following therapeutic classes; antihistamine and nasal decongestant.
Inactive Ingredients: dibutyl sebacate, ethylcellulose, fumed silica, hydroxypropyl methylcellulose, methacrylic acid, oleic acid, propylene glycol, sugar spheres NF, and talc NF.

Continued on next page

Information on the Medeva Pharmaceuticals, Inc. products listed on these pages contains the full prescribing information from product circulars in use as of July 1996. For further information, please consult the package insert currently accompanying the product.

Medeva Pharmaceuticals, Inc.—Cont.

CLINICAL PHARMACOLOGY

Chlorpheniramine maleate is an alkylamine type antihistamine. This group of antihistamines is among the most active histamine antagonists and are generally effective in relatively low doses. The drugs are not so prone to produce drowsiness and are among the most suitable agents for day time use; but again, a significant proportion of patients do experience this effect. Pseudoephedrine hydrochloride is a sympathomimetic which acts predominantly on alpha receptors and has little action on beta receptors. It therefore functions as an oral nasal decongestant with minimal CNS stimulation.

INDICATIONS AND USAGE

For the temporary relief of symptoms of the common cold, allergic rhinitis (hay fever) and sinusitis.

CONTRAINDICATIONS

Hypersensitivity to any of the ingredients. Also contraindicated in patients with severe hypertension, severe coronary artery disease, patients on monoamine oxidase inhibitor (MAOI) therapy or for 14 days after stopping MAOI therapy (See **Drug Interactions**), patients with narrow-angle glaucoma, urinary retention, peptic ulcer and during an asthmatic attack.

Should not be used in nursing mothers.

WARNINGS

Considerable caution should be exercised in patients with hypertension, diabetes mellitus, ischemic heart disease, hyperthyroidism, increased intraocular pressure and prostatic hypertrophy. The elderly (60 years or older) are more likely to exhibit adverse reactions.

Antihistamines may cause excitability, especially in pediatric patients. At dosages higher than the recommended dose, nervousness, dizziness or sleeplessness may occur.

PRECAUTIONS

General

Caution should be exercised in patients with high blood pressure, heart disease, diabetes or thyroid disease. The antihistamine in this product may exhibit additive effects with CNS depressants, including alcohol.

Information for Patients: Antihistamine may cause drowsiness and ambulatory patients who operate machinery or motor vehicles should be cautioned accordingly.

Drug Interactions: Do not prescribe this product for use in patients that are now taking a prescription MAOI (certain drugs for depression, psychiatric or emotional conditions, or Parkinson's disease), or for 14 days after stopping the MAOI drug therapy. MAOI and beta adrenergic blockers increase the effects of sympathomimetics. Sympathomimetics may reduce the antihypertensive effects of methyldopa, macamylamine, reserpine and veratrum alkaloids. Concomitant use of antihistamines with alcohol and other CNS depressants may have an additive effect.

Use in Pregnancy: Pregnancy Category C: Animal reproduction studies have not been conducted with Atrohist® Pediatric Capsules. It is also not known whether Atrohist® Pediatric Capsules can cause fetal harm when administered to a pregnant woman or can affect reproduction capacity. Atrohist® Pediatric Capsules should be given to a pregnant woman only if clearly needed.

ADVERSE REACTIONS

Adverse reactions include drowsiness, lassitude, nausea, giddiness, dryness of mouth, blurred vision, cardiac palpitations, flushing, increased irritability or excitement (especially in pediatric patients).

OVERDOSAGE

Acute overdosage with Atrohist® Pediatric Capsules may produce clinical signs of CNS stimulation and variable cardiovascular effects. Pressor amines should be used with great caution in the presence of pseudoephedrine. Patients with signs of stimulation should be treated conservatively.

DOSAGE AND ADMINISTRATION

Adolescents 12 years and older: Two capsules every 12 hours; Children 6 to under 12 years of age: One capsule every 12 hours; Children 2 to under 6 years of age: As determined and directed by physician.

HOW SUPPLIED

NDC 53014-400-10
Bottles of 100 white and yellow Capsules, imprinted "Adams/400"
CAUTION: Federal law prohibits dispensing without prescription.
DISPENSE IN A TIGHT CONTAINER AS DEFINED IN THE USP/NF, WITH A CHILD-RESISTANT CLOSURE.
STORE AT CONTROLLED ROOM TEMPERATURE 15°–30°C (59°–86°F).
August 1995

ATROHIST® Pediatric Suspension   ℞

DESCRIPTION

ATROHIST Pediatric Suspension is an antihistaminic/decongestant combination available for oral administration as **Pediatric Suspension.**
Each 5 mL (teaspoonful) of the Pediatric Suspension contains:
Phenylephrine Tannate .... 5 mg
Chlorpheniramine Tannate .... 2 mg
Pyrilamine Tannate .... 12.5 mg
Other ingredients: Citric acid, D&C Red #28, flavors, glycerin, magnesium aluminum silicate, methylparaben, sodium benzoate, sodium citrate, sodium saccharin, sucrose, xanthan gum.

CLINICAL PHARMACOLOGY

ATROHIST Pediatric Suspension combines the sympathomimetic decongestant effect of phenylephrine with the antihistaminic actions of chlorpheniramine and pyrilamine.

INDICATIONS AND USAGE

ATROHIST Pediatric Suspension is indicated for symptomatic relief of the coryza and nasal congestion associated with the common cold, sinusitis, allergic rhinitis and other upper respiratory tract conditions. Appropriate therapy should be provided for the primary disease.

CONTRAINDICATIONS

ATROHIST Pediatric Suspension is contraindicated for neonates, nursing mothers and patients sensitive to any of the ingredients or related compounds.

WARNINGS

Use with caution in patients with hypertension, cardiovascular disease, hyperthyroidism, diabetes, narrow angle glaucoma or prostatic hypertrophy. Use with caution or avoid use in patients taking monoamine oxidase inhibitors (MAOI). This product contains antihistamines which may cause drowsiness and may have additive central nervous system (CNS) effects with alcohol or other CNS depressants (e.g., hypnotics, sedatives, tranquilizers).

PRECAUTIONS

General: Antihistamines are more likely to cause dizziness, sedation and hypotension in elderly patients. Antihistamines may cause excitation, particularly in pediatric patients, but their combination with sympathomimetics may cause either mild stimulation or mild sedation.

Information for Patients: Caution patients against drinking alcoholic beverages or engaging in potentially hazardous activities requiring alertness, such as driving a car or operating machinery while using this product.

Drug Interactions: Do not prescribe this product for use in patients that are now taking a prescription MAOI (certain drugs for depression, psychiatric or emotional conditions, or Parkinson's disease), or for 14 days after stopping the MAOI drug therapy. MAOI may prolong and intensify the anticholinergic effects of antihistamines and the overall effects of sympathomimetic agents.

Carcinogenesis, Mutagenesis, Impairment of Fertility: No long term animal studies have been performed with ATROHIST.

Pregnancy: Teratogenic Effects: Pregnancy Category C. Animal reproduction studies have not been conducted with ATROHIST Pediatric Suspension. It is also not known whether ATROHIST Pediatric Suspension can cause fetal harm when administered to a pregnant woman or can affect reproduction capacity. ATROHIST Pediatric Suspension should be given to a pregnant woman only if clearly needed.

Nursing Mothers: ATROHIST Pediatric Suspension should not be administered to a nursing mother.

ADVERSE REACTIONS

Adverse effects associated with recommended doses of ATROHIST Pediatric Suspension have been minimal. The most common have been drowsiness, sedation, dryness of mucous membranes, and gastrointestinal effects. Serious side effects with oral antihistamines or sympathomimetics have been rare.

OVERDOSAGE

Signs and Symptoms: May vary from CNS depression to stimulation (restlessness to convulsions). Antihistamine overdosage in pediatric patients may lead to convulsions and death. Antropine-like signs and symptoms may be prominent.

Treatment: Induce vomiting if it has not occurred spontaneously. Precautions must be taken against aspiration especially in pediatric population and comatose patients. If gastric lavage is indicated, isotonic or half-isotonic saline solution is preferred. Stimulants should not be used. If hypotension is a problem, vasopressor agents may be considered.

DOSAGE AND ADMINISTRATION

Administer the recommended dose every 12 hours.
ATROHIST Pediatric Suspension:
Pediatric Patients over six years of age—5 to 10 mL (1 to 2 teaspoonfuls);

Children two to six years of age—2.5 to 5 mL ($^1/_2$ to 1 teaspoonful);
Infants under two years of age—Titrate dose individually.

HOW SUPPLIED

ATROHIST Pediatric Suspension: dark pink with raspberry flavor, in a 4 fl oz unit-of-use container (NDC 53014-026-12) and in pint bottles (NDC 53014-026-47).
Storage:
Store at controlled room temperature, 15°C–25°C (59°F–77°F). Protect from freezing.
264/1095   35260002

ATROHIST® PEDIATRIC SUSPENSION DYE-FREE   ℞

DESCRIPTION

ATROHIST is an antihistamic/decongestant combination available for oral administration as Pediatric Suspension. Each 5 mL (teaspoonful) of the Pediatric Suspension contains:
Phenylephrine Tannate .... 5 mg
Chlorpheniramine Tannate .... 2 mg
Pyrilamine Tannate .... 12.5 mg
Other ingredients: Citric acid, disodium edta, flavors, glycerin, magnesium aluminum silicate, methylparaben, purified water, sodium benzoate, sodium citrate, sodium saccharin, sorbitol, sucrose, xanthan gum.

CLINICAL PHARMACOLOGY

ATROHIST combines the sympathomimetic decongestant effect of phenylephrine with the antihistaminic actions of chlorpheniramine and pyrilamine.

INDICATIONS AND USAGE

ATROHIST is indicated for symptomatic relief of the coryza and nasal congestion associated with the common cold, sinusitis, allergic rhinitis and other upper respiratory tract conditions. Appropriate therapy should be provided for the primary disease.

CONTRAINDICATIONS

ATROHIST is contraindicated for neonates, nursing mothers and patients sensitive to any of the ingredients or related compounds.

WARNINGS

Use with caution in patients with hypertension, cardiovascular disease, hyperthyroidism, diabetes, narrow angle glaucoma or prostatic hypertrophy. Use with caution or avoid use in patients taking monoamine oxidase inhibitors (MAOI). This product contains antihistamines which may cause drowsiness and may have additive central nervous system (CNS) effects with alcohol or other CNS depressants (e.g., hypnotics, sedatives, tranquilizers).

PRECAUTIONS

General: Antihistamines are more likely to cause dizziness, sedation and hypotension in elderly patients. Antihistamines may cause excitation, particularly in pediatric patients, but their combination may cause either mild stimulation or mild sedation.

Information for Patients: Caution patients against drinking alcholic beverages or engaging in potentially hazardous activities requiring alertness, such as driving a car or operating machinery while using this product.

Drug Interactions: Do not prescribe this product for use in patients that are now taking a prescription MAOI (certain drugs for depression, psychiatric or emotional conditions, or Parkinson's disease), or for 14 days after stopping the MAOI drug therapy. MAOI may prolong and intensify the anticholinergic effects of antihistamines and the overall effects of sympathomimetic agents.

Carcinogenesis, Mutagenesis, Impairment of Fertility: No long term animal studies have been performed with ATROHIST.

Pregnancy: Teratoenic Effects: Pregnancy Category C. Animal reproduction studies have not been conducted with ATROHIST. It is also not known whether ATROHIST can cause fetal harm when administered to a pregnant woman or can affect reproduction capacity. ATROHIST should be given to a pregnant woman only if clearly needed.

Nursing Mothers: ATROHIST should not be administered to a nursing mother.

ADVERSE REACTIONS

Adverse effects associated with ATROHIST at recommended doseas have been minimal. The most common have been drowsiness, sedation, dryness of mucous membranes, and gastrointestinal effects. Serious side effects with oral antihistamines or sympathomimetics have been rare.

OVERDOSAGE

Signs and Symptoms: May vary from CNS depression to stimulation (restlessness to convulsions). Antihistamine

overdosage in pediatric patients may lead to convulsions and death. Atropine-like signs and symptoms may be prominent.
Treatment: Induce vomiting if it has not occurred spontaneously. Precautions must be taken against aspiration especially in the pediatric population and comatose patients. If gastric lavage is indicated, isotonic or half-isotonic saline solution is preferred. Stimulants should not be used. If hypotension is a problem, vasopressor agents may be considered.

DOSAGE AND ADMINISTRATION

Administer the recommended dose every 12 hours.
ATROHIST Pediatric Suspension:
Pediatric patients over six years of age–5 to 10 mL (1 to 2 teaspoonfuls);
Pediatric patients two to six yesaards of age–2.5 to 5 mL(1/2 to 1 teaspoonful);
Pediatric patients under two years of age–Titrate dose individually.

HOW SUPPLIED

ATROHIST Pediatric Suspension: Dye Free: Light beige to brown, viscous suspension with raspberry flavor, in a 4 fl oz unit-of-use container (NDC 53014-503-12) and in pint bottles (NDC 53014-503-47).
Storage:
Store at controlled room temperature, 15°C - 25°C (59°F - 77°F). Protect from freezing.
MG #11883
5034/596 35503002

ATROHIST® PLUS Tablets ℞

DESCRIPTION

Each yellow, scored Atrohist PLUS Tablet provides: 25 mg phenylephrine hydrochloride, 50 mg phenylpropanolamine hydrochloride, 8 mg chlorpheniramine maleate, 0.19 mg hyoscyamine sulfate, 0.04 mg atropine sulfate and 0.01 mg scopolamine hydrobromide in a sustained-release formulation.
Atrohist PLUS Tablets are intended for oral administration.
Atrohist PLUS Tablets are a antihistaminic, nasal decongestant and anti-secretory preparation. Inactive ingredients: Dibasic calcium phosphate, ethylcellulose, magnesium stearate, sodium lauryl sulfate, stearic acid, D&C yellow #10 Lake.

INDICATIONS AND USAGE

Atrohist PLUS Tablets provide relief of the symptoms resulting from irritation of sinus, nasal and upper respiratory tract tissues. Phenylephrine and phenylpropanolamine combine to exert a vasoconstrictive and decongestive action while chlorpheniramine maleate decreases the symptoms of watering eyes, post nasal drip and sneezing which may be associated with an allergic-like response. The belladonna alkaloids, hyoscyamine, atropine and scopolamine further augment the anti-secretory activity of Atrohist PLUS Tablets.

CONTRAINDICATIONS

This product is contraindicated in patients with hypersensitivity to antihistamines or sympathomimetics. Atrohist PLUS Tablets are contraindicated in pediatric patients under 12 years of age and in patients with glaucoma, bronchial asthma and women who are pregnant. Concomitant use of monamine oxidase inhibitors (MAOI) is contraindicated. (See **Drug Interactions** section).

WARNINGS

Atrohist PLUS Tablets may cause drowsiness. Patients should be warned of possible additive effects caused by taking antihistamines with alcohol, hypnotics or tranquilizers.

PRECAUTIONS

Atrohist PLUS Tablets contain belladonna alkaloids, and must be administered with care to those patients with urinary bladder neck obstruction. Caution should be exercised when Atrohist PLUS Tablets are given to patients with hypertension, cardiac or peripheral vascular disease or hyperthyroidism. Patients should avoid driving a motor vehicle or operating dangerous machinery. (See **WARNINGS.**)
Drug Interactions: Do not prescribe this product for use in patients that are now taking a prescription MAOI (certain drugs for depression, psychiatric or emotional conditions, or Parkinson's disease), or for 14 days after stopping the MAOI drug therapy.
Use in Pregnancy: Pregnancy Category C: Animal reproduction studies have not been conducted with Atrohist Plus tablets. It is also not known whether Atrohist Plus tablets can cause fetal harm when administered to a pregnant woman or can affect reproduction capacity. Atrohist Plus tablets should be given to a pregnant woman only if clearly needed.

ADVERSE REACTIONS

Hypersensitivity reactions such as rash, urticaria, leukopenia, agranulocytosis, and thrombocytopenia may occur. Large overdoses may cause tachypnea, delirium, fever, stupor, coma and respiratory failure.
Gastrointestinal: nausea, vomiting, diarrhea, constipation, epigastric distress.
Genitourinary System: urinary frequency and dysuria.
Cardiovascular: tightness of the chest, palpitation, tachycardia, hypotension/hypertension.
Central Nervous System: drowsiness, giddiness, faintness, dizziness, headache, incoordination, mydriasis, hyperirritability, nervousness, and insomnia.
Metabolic/Endocrine: lassitude, anorexia.
Miscellaneous: dryness of mucous membranes, xerostomia.
Respiratory: thickening of bronchial secretions.
Special Senses: tinnitus, visual disturbances, blurred vision.

OVERDOSAGE

Since the action of sustained release products may continue for as long as 12 hours, treatment of overdoses directed at reversing the effects of the drug and supporting the patient should be maintained for at least that length of time. In pediatric patients, antihistamine overdosage may produce convulsions and death.

DOSAGE AND ADMINISTRATION

Adults and adolescents over 12 years of age: One tablet every 12 hours not to exceed 2 tablets in 24 hours. Not recommended for use in pediatric patients under 12 years of age. Tablets are to be swallowed whole.

HOW SUPPLIED

Bottles of 100 tablets (NDC 53014-024-10) and 500 tablets (NDC 53014-024-50). Scored, yellow tablets are embossed with "Adams/024". Store at controlled room temperature between 15° C and 30° C (59° F and 86° F). Dispense in tight, light-resistant containers.
CAUTION: Federal law prohibits dispensing without prescription.
June 1996

DECONSAL® II Tablets ℞
(pseudoephedrine hydrochloride & guaifenesin)

DESCRIPTION

DECONSAL® II Tablets: Each scored, dark blue DECONSAL® II Tablet provides 60 mg pseudoephedrine hydrochloride and 600 mg guaifenesin in a sustained-release formulation intended for oral administration. Inactive ingredients: Stearic acid, dibasic calcium phosphate, FD & C Blue #1 Lake, sodium lauryl sulfate, ethyl cellulose, magnesium stearate.
Pseudoephedrine hydrochloride is a nasal decongestant. Chemically, it is [S-(R*,R*)]-α-[1-(methylamino) ethyl] benzenemethanol hydrochloride and has the following structural formula:

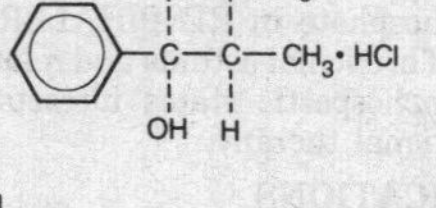

$C_{10}H_{15}NO \cdot HCl$ MW = 201.70

Guaifenesin is an expectorant. Chemically, it is 3-(2-methoxyphenoxy)-1, 2-propanediol and has the following structural formula:

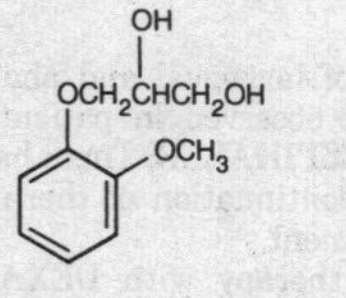

$C_{10}H_{14}O_4$ MW = 198.22

CLINICAL PHARMACOLOGY

Pseudoephedrine hydrochloride is an orally indirect acting sympathomimetic amine and exerts a decongestant action on the nasal mucosa. It does this by vasoconstriction which results in reduction of tissue hyperemia, edema, nasal congestion, and an increase in nasal airway patency. The vasoconstriction action of pseudoephedrine is similar to that of ephedrine. In the usual dose it has minimal vasopressor effects. Pseudoephedrine is rapidly and almost completely absorbed from the gastrointestinal tract. It has a plasma half-life of 6 to 8 hours. Alkaline urine is associated with slower elimination of the drug. The drug is distributed to body tissues and fluids, including the central nervous system (CNS). Approximately 50% to 75% of the administered dose is excreted unchanged in the urine; the remainder is apparently metabolized in the liver to inactive compounds by N-demethylation, parahydroxylation, and oxidative deamination.
Guaifenesin is an expectorant which increases respiratory tract fluid secretions and helps to loosen phlegm and bronchial secretions. By reducing the viscosity of secretions, guaifenesin increases the efficiency of the mucociliary mechanism in removing accumulated secretions from the upper and lower airway. Guaifenesin is readily absorbed from the gastrointestinal tract and is rapidly metabolized and excreted in the urine. Guaifenesin has a plasma half-life of one hour. The major urinary metabolite is β-(2-methoxyphenoxy) lactic acid.

INDICATIONS AND USAGE

DECONSAL® II Tablets are indicated for the temporary relief of nasal congestion and cough associated with respiratory tract infections and related conditions such as sinusitis, pharyngitis, bronchitis, and asthma, when these conditions are complicated by tenacious mucus and/or mucus plugs and congestion. The product is effective in productive as well as non-productive cough, but is of particular value in dry, nonproductive cough which tends to injure the mucous membrane of the air passages.

CONTRAINDICATIONS

This product is contraindicated in patients with hypersensitivity to guaifenesin or with hypersensitivity or idiosyncrasy to sympathomimetic amines which may be manifested by insomnia, dizziness, weakness, tremor or arrhythmias.
Sympathomimetic amines are contraindicated in patients with severe hypertension, severe coronary artery disease, and patients on monoamine oxidase inhibitor (MAOI) therapy and for 14 days after stopping MAOI therapy. (See **Drug Interactions** section).

WARNINGS

Sympathomimetic amines should be used with caution in patients with hypertension, ischemic heart disease, diabetes mellitus, increased intraocular pressure, hyperthyroidism, or prostatic hypertrophy. Sympathomimetics may produce central nervous system stimulation with convulsions or cardiovascular collapse with accompanying hypotension. **Do not exceed recommended dosage.**
Hypertensive crises can occur with concurrent use of pseudoephedrine or phenylephrine and MAOI, and for 14 days after stopping MAOI therapy, indomethacin, or with beta-blockers and methyldopa. If a hypertensive crisis occurs, these drugs should be discontinued immediately and therapy to lower blood pressure should be instituted. Fever should be managed by means of external cooling.

PRECAUTIONS

General: Use with caution in patients with diabetes, hypertension, cardiovascular disease, and intolerance to ephedrine.
Before prescribing medication to suppress or modify cough, it is important to ascertain that the underlying cause of cough is identified, that modification of cough does not increase the risk of clinical or physiologic complications, and that appropriate therapy for the primary disease is instituted.
Information for Patients: Patients should be instructed to check with physician if symptoms do not improve within 5 days or if fever is present.
Pediatric Use: This product is not recommended for use in pediatric patients under 2 years of age.
Use in Elderly: The elderly (60 years and older) are more likely to experience adverse reactions to sympathomimetics. Overdosage of sympathomimetics in this age group may cause hallucinations, convulsions, CNS depression, and death.
Drug Interactions: Do not prescribe this product for use in patients that are now taking a prescription MAOI (certain drugs for depression, psychiatric or emotional conditions, or Parkinson's disease), or for 14 days after stopping the MAOI drug therapy. Beta-adrenergic blockers and MAOI may potentiate the pressor effect of pseudoephedrine. (see **WARNINGS.**) Concurrent use of digitalis glycosides may increase the possibility of cardiac arrhythmias. Sympathomimetics may reduce the hypotensive effects of guanethidine, mecamylamine, methyldopa, reserpine, and veratrum alkaloids. Concurrent use of tricyclic antidepressants may antagonize the effects of pseudoephedrine.
Drug/Laboratory Test Interactions: Guaifenesin may increase renal clearance for urate and thereby lower serum uric acid levels. Guaifenesin may produce an increase in urinary 5-hydroxy-indoleacetic acid and may therefore interfere with the interpretation of this test for the diagnosis of carcinoid syndrome. It may also falsely elevate the VMA test for catechols. Administration of this drug should be discontinued 48 hours prior to the collection of urine specimens for such tests.

Continued on next page

Information on the Medeva Pharmaceuticals, Inc. products listed on these pages contains the full prescribing information from product circulars in use as of July 1996. For further information, please consult the package insert currently accompanying the product.

Medeva Pharmaceuticals, Inc.—Cont.

Carcinogenesis, Mutagenesis, Impairment of Fertility: No data are available on the long-term potential of the components of this product for carcinogenesis, mutagenesis, or impairment of fertility in animals or humans.

Pregnancy: Category C: Animal reproduction studies have not been conducted with DECONSAL® II Tablets. It is also not known whether DECONSAL® II Tablets can cause fetal harm when administered to a pregnant woman or can affect reproduction capacity. DECONSAL® II Tablets should be given to a pregnant woman only if clearly needed.

Nursing Mothers: Pseudoephedrine is excreted in breast milk. Use of this product by nursing mothers is not recommended because of the higher than usual risk for infants from sympathomimetic amines.

ADVERSE REACTIONS

Hyper-reactive individuals may display ephedrine-like reactions such as tachycardia, palpitations, headache, dizziness, or nausea. Sympathomimetics have been associated with certain untoward reactions including fear, anxiety, nervousness, restlessness, tremor, weakness, pallor, respiratory difficulty, dysuria, insomnia, hallucinations, convulsions, CNS depression, arrhythmias, and cardiovascular collapse with hypotension. No serious side effects have been reported with the use of guaifenesin.

OVERDOSAGE

Since DECONSAL® II Tablets contain two pharmacologically different compounds, treatment of overdosage should be based upon the symptomatology of the patient as it relates to the individual ingredients. Treatment of acute overdosage would probably be based upon treating the patient for pseudoephedrine toxicity which may manifest itself as excessive CNS stimulation resulting in excitement, tremor, restlessness, and insomnia. Other effects may include tachycardia, hypertension, pallor, mydriasis, hyperglycemia and urinary retention. Severe overdosage may cause tachypnea or hyperpnea, hallucinations, convulsions or delirium, but in some individuals there may be CNS depression with somnolence, stupor or respiratory depression. Arrhythmias (including ventricular fibrillation) may lead to hypotension and circulatory collapse. Severe hypokalemia can occur, probably due to a compartmental shift rather than a depletion of potassium. No organ damage or significant metabolic derangement is associated with pseudoephedrine overdosage.
Overdosage with guaifenesin is unlikely to produce toxic effects since its toxicity is much lower than that of pseudoephedrine. In severe cases of overdose, it is recommended to monitor the patient in an intensive care setting.
The LD_{50} of pseudoephedrine (single oral dose) has been reported to be 726 mg/kg in the mouse, 2206 mg/kg in the rat and 1177 mg/kg in the rabbit. The toxic and lethal concentrations in human biologic fluids are not known. Urinary excretion increases with acidification and decreases with alkalinization of the urine. There are few published reports of toxicity due to pseudoephedrine and no case of fatal overdosage has been reported. Guaifenesin, when administered by stomach tube to test animals in doses up to 5 grams/kg, produced no signs of toxicity.
Since the action of sustained release products may continue for as long as 12 hours, treatment of overdosage should be directed toward reducing further absorption and supporting the patient for at least that length of time. Gastric emptying (Syrup of Ipecac) and/or lavage is recommended as soon as possible after ingestion, even if the patient has vomited spontaneously. Either isotonic or half-isotonic saline may be used for lavage. Administration of an activated charcoal slurry is beneficial after lavage and/or emesis if less than 4 hours have passed since ingestion. Saline cathartics, such as Milk of Magnesia, are useful for hastening the evacuation of unreleased medication.
Adrenergic receptor blocking agents are antidotes to pseudoephedrine. In practice, the most useful is the beta-blocker propranolol which is indicated when there are signs of cardiac toxicity. Theoretically, pseudoephedrine is dialyzable but procedures have not been clinically established.

DOSAGE AND ADMINISTRATION

Adults and adolescents over 12 years of age: One or two tablets every 12 hours not to exceed 4 tablets in 24 hours. **Children 6 to 12 years:** One tablet every 12 hours not to exceed 2 tablets in 24 hours. **Children 2 to 6 years:** $^{1}/_{2}$ tablet every 12 hours not to exceed 1 tablet in 24 hours.

HOW SUPPLIED

DECONSAL® II Tablets: Bottles of 100 tablets (NDC 53014-017-10) and 500 tablets (NDC 53014-017-50). Scored, dark blue tablets are embossed with "Adams/017". Store at controlled room temperature between 15°C and 30°C (59°F and 86°F). Dispense in tight, light-resistant containers.
CAUTION: Federal law prohibits dispensing without prescription.
August 1995

DEXACORT™ Phosphate ℞
(dexamethasone sodium phosphate) in RESPIHALER® (dispenser)
Aerosol for Oral Inhalation

DESCRIPTION

DEXACORT™ Phosphate (dexamethasone sodium phosphate) in RESPIHALER® (Dispenser) is an aerosol for oral inhalation which contains dexamethasone sodium phosphate, an inorganic ester of dexamethasone, a synthetic adrenocortical steroid with basic glucocorticoid actions and effects.
Each DEXACORT Phosphate in RESPIHALER contains an amount sufficient to deliver at least 170 sprays. The metering valve of the aerosol-mechanism of the RESPIHALER dispenses dexamethasone sodium phosphate equivalent to approximately 0.1 mg of dexamethasone phosphate or approximately 0.084 mg of dexamethasone with each activation. On a regimen of 12 inhalations daily, it has been determined that the patient absorbs approximately 0.4–0.6 mg of dexamethasone. The inactive ingredients are chlorofluorocarbons† included as propellants. Alcohol 2%.
Dexamethasone sodium phosphate, a synthetic adrenocortical steroid, is a white or slightly yellow, crystalline powder. It is freely soluble in water and is exceedingly hygroscopic. It is prepared by a special process to produce particles in the range of 0.5 to 4 microns in size. The molecular weight is 516.41. It is designated chemically as 9-fluoro-11β, 17-dihydroxy-16α-methyl-21-(phosphonooxy) pregna-1, 4-diene-3, 20-dione disodium salt. The empirical formula is: $C_{22}H_{28}FNa_2O_8P$ and the structural formula is:

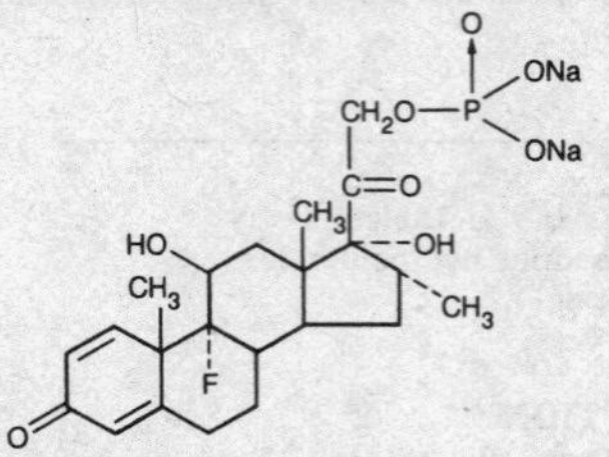

† WARNING: Chlorofluorocarbons (CFCs) are substances which harm public health and environment by destroying ozone in the upper atmosphere.

ACTIONS

Because of the high water solubility of dexamethasone sodium phosphate, the aerosolized particles dissolve readily in the secretions of the bronchial and bronchiolar mucous membrane.

INDICATIONS

DEXACORT Phosphate in RESPIHALER is indicated for the treatment of bronchial asthma and related corticosteroid responsive bronchospastic states intractable to adequate trial of conventional therapy.

CONTRAINDICATIONS

Systemic fungal infections.
Hypersensitivity to any component of this medication.
Persistently positive cultures of the sputum for *Candida albicans.*

WARNINGS

Rare instances of laryngeal and pharyngeal fungal infections have been observed in patients using DEXACORT Phosphate in RESPIHALER. These have usually responded promptly to discontinuation of therapy and institution of antifungal treatment.
In patients on therapy with DEXACORT Phosphate in RESPIHALER subjected to unusual stress, increased dosage of rapidly acting corticosteroids before, during, and after the stressful situation is indicated.
Drug-induced secondary adrenocortical insufficiency may result from too rapid withdrawal of corticosteroids and may be minimized by gradual reduction of dosage. This type of relative insufficiency may persist for months after discontinuation of therapy; therefore, in any situation of stress occurring during that period, hormone therapy should be reinstituted. If the patient is receiving steroids already, dosage may have to be increased. Since mineralocorticoid secretion may be impaired, salt and/or a mineralocorticoid should be administered concurrently.
Dexamethasone may mask some signs of infection, and new infections may appear during its use. There may be decreased resistance and inability to localize infection when corticosteroids are used. Moreover, dexamethasone may affect the nitrobluetetrazolium test for bacterial infection and produce false negative results.
Corticosteroids may activate latent amebiasis. Therefore, it is recommended that latent or active amebiasis be ruled out before initiating corticosteroid therapy in any patient who has spent time in the tropics or any patient with unexplained diarrhea.
Prolonged use of DEXACORT Phosphate in RESPIHALER may produce posterior subcapsular cataracts, glaucoma with possible damage to the optic nerves, and may enhance the establishment of secondary ocular infections due to fungi or viruses.
Usage in pregnancy: Since adequate human reproduction studies have not been done with DEXACORT Phosphate in RESPIHALER, use of this drug in pregnancy or in women of childbearing potential requires that the anticipated benefits be weighed against the possible hazards to the mother and embryo or fetus. Infants born of mothers who have received substantial doses of dexamethasone during pregnancy, should be carefully observed for signs of hypoadrenalism.
Dexamethasone appears in breast milk and could suppress growth, interfere with endogenous corticosteroid production, or cause other unwanted effects. Mothers taking pharmacologic doses of dexamethasone should be advised not to nurse.
Average and large doses of hydrocortisone or cortisone can cause elevation of blood pressure, salt and water retention, and increased excretion of potassium. These effects are less likely to occur with the synthetic derivatives and with DEXACORT Phosphate in RESPIHALER, except when used in large doses. Dietary salt restriction and potassium supplementation may be necessary. All corticosteroids increase calcium excretion.
Administration of live virus vaccines, including smallpox, is contraindicated in individuals receiving immunosuppressive doses of corticosteroids. If inactivated viral or bacterial vaccines are administered to individuals receiving immunosuppressive doses of corticosteroids, the expected serum antibody response may not be obtained.
Patients who are on drugs which suppress the immune system are more susceptible to infections than healthy individuals. Chickenpox and measles, for example, can have a more serious or even fatal course in non-immune children or adults on corticosteroids. In such children or adults who have not had these diseases, particular care should be taken to avoid exposure. The risk of developing a disseminated infection varies among individuals and can be related to the dose, route and duration of corticosteroid administration as well as to the underlying disease. If exposed to chickenpox, prophylaxis with varicella zoster immune globulin (VZIG) may be indicated. If chickenpox develops, treatment with anti-viral agents may be considered. If exposed to measles, prophylaxis with immune globulin (IG) may be indicated. (See the respective package inserts for VZIG and IG for complete prescribing information.)
If DEXACORT Phosphate in RESPIHALER is indicated in patients with latent tuberculosis or tuberculin reactivity, close observation is necessary as reactivation of the disease may occur. During prolonged therapy with DEXACORT Phosphate in RESPIHALER, these patients should receive chemoprophylaxis.
Literature reports suggest an apparent association between use of corticosteroids and left ventricular free wall rupture after a recent myocardial infarction; therefore, therapy with corticosteroids should be used with great caution in these patients.
Keep out of reach of children.

PRECAUTIONS

DEXACORT Phosphate in RESPIHALER is *not* indicated for relief of the occasional mild and isolated attack of asthma which is readily responsive to the immediate, though short-lived, action of epinephrine, isoproterenol, aminophylline, etc. Nor should it be employed for the treatment of severe status asthmaticus where intensive measures are required.
DEXACORT Phosphate in RESPIHALER should be considered only for the following classes of patients: patients not on corticosteroid therapy who have not responded adequately to other treatment; patients already on systemic corticosteroid therapy—in an attempt to reduce or eliminate systemic administration.
Although systemic absorption is low when DEXACORT Phosphate in RESPIHALER is used in the recommended dosage, adrenal suppression may occur. In addition, other systemic effects of steroid administration must be considered as a possibility.
Following prolonged therapy, withdrawal of corticosteroids may result in symptoms of the corticosteroid withdrawal syndrome including fever, myalgia, arthralgia, and malaise. This may occur in patients even without evidence of adrenal insufficiency.
There is an enhanced effect of dexamethasone in patients with hyperthyroidism and in those with cirrhosis.
DEXACORT Phosphate in RESPIHALER should be used cautiously in patients with ocular herpes simplex for fear of corneal perforation.
The lowest possible dose of DEXACORT Phosphate in RESPIHALER should be used to control the condition under treatment, and when reduction in dosage is possible, the reduction must be gradual.
Psychic derangements may appear when dexamethasone is used, ranging from euphoria, insomnia, mood swings, per-

sonality changes, and severe depression, to frank psychotic manifestations. Also, existing emotional instability or psychotic tendencies may be aggravated.

Aspirin should be used cautiously in conjunction with DEXACORT Phosphate in RESPIHALER in hypoprothrombinemia.

DEXACORT Phosphate in RESPIHALER should be used with caution in nonspecific ulcerative colitis, if there is a probability of impending perforation, abscess or other pyogenic infection; also in diverticulitis; fresh intestinal anastomoses; active or latent peptic ulcer; renal insufficiency; hypertension; osteoporosis; and myasthenia gravis. Signs of peritoneal irritation following gastrointestinal perforation in patients receiving large doses of corticosteroids may be minimal or absent. Fat embolism has been reported as a possible complication of hypercortisonism.

Growth and development of infants and children on prolonged therapy with DEXACORT Phosphate in RESPIHALER should be carefully followed.

Dexamethasone may increase or decrease motility and number of spermatozoa in some patients.

Phenytoin, phenobarbital, ephedrine and rifampin may enhance the metabolic clearance of dexamethasone, resulting in decreased blood levels and lessened physiologic activity, thus requiring adjustment in dexamethasone dosage.

The prothrombin time should be checked frequently in patients who are receiving DEXACORT Phosphate in RESPIHALER and coumarin anticoagulants at the same time because of reports that corticosteroids have altered the response to these anticoagulants. Studies have shown that the usual effect produced by adding corticosteroids is inhibition of response to coumarins, although there have been some conflicting reports of potentiation, not substantiated by studies.

When DEXACORT Phosphate in RESPIHALER is used concomitantly with potassium-depleting diuretics, patients should be observed closely for development of hypokalemia.

Since the contents of DEXACORT Phosphate in RESPIHALER are under pressure, the container should not be broken, stored in extreme heat, or incinerated. It should be stored at a temperature below 120°F.

Information for Patients
Susceptible patients who are on immunosuppressant doses of corticosteroids should be warned to avoid exposure to chickenpox or measles. Patients should also be advised that if they are exposed, medical advice should be sought without delay.

ADVERSE REACTIONS

Side effects which may occur in patients treated with DEXACORT Phosphate in RESPIHALER include throat irritation, hoarseness, coughing, and laryngeal and pharyngeal fungal infections.

Patients should be observed for the hormonal effects described below:

Fluid and Electrolyte Disturbances
Sodium retention
Fluid retention
Congestive heart failure in susceptible patients
Potassium loss
Hypokalemic alkalosis
Hypertension

Musculoskeletal
Muscle weakness
Steroid myopathy
Loss of muscle mass
Osteoporosis
Vertebral compression fractures
Aseptic necrosis of femoral and humeral heads
Pathologic fracture of long bones
Tendon rupture

Gastrointestinal
Peptic ulcer with possible subsequent perforation and hemorrhage
Perforation of the small and large bowel, particularly in patients with inflammatory bowel disease
Pancreatitis
Abdominal distention
Ulcerative esophagitis

Dermatologic
Impaired wound healing
Thin fragile skin
Petechiae and ecchymoses
Erythema
Increased sweating
May suppress reactions to skin tests
Other cutaneous reactions, such as allergic dermatitis, urticaria, angioneurotic edema

Neurologic
Convulsions
Increased intracranial pressure with papilledema (pseudotumor cerebri) usually after treatment.
Vertigo
Headache
Psychic disturbances

Endocrine
Menstrual irregularities
Development of cushingoid state
Suppression of growth in children
Secondary adrenocortical and pituitary unresponsiveness, particularly in times of strees, as in trauma, surgery, or illness.
Decreased carbohydrate tolerance
Manifestations of latent diabetics mellitus
Increased requirements for insulin or oral hypoglycemic agents in diabetics
Hirsutism

Ophthalmic
Posterior subcapsular cataracts
Increased intraocular pressure
Glaucoma
Exophthalmos

Metabolic
Negative nitrogen balance due to protein catabolism

Cardiovascular
Myocardial rupture following recent myocardial infarction (see WARNINGS).

Other
Hypersensitivity
Thromboembolism
Weight gain
Increased appetite
Nausea
Malais
Hiccups

OVERDOSAGE

Reports of acute toxicity and/or death following overdosage of glucocorticoids are rare. In the event of overdosage, no specific antidote is available; treatment is supportive and symptomatic.

Significant lethality was observed in female mice at single oral doses of 3630 mg/m^2 (1210 mg/kg) and single intravenous doses of 2382 mg/m^2 (794 mg/kg).

DOSAGE AND ADMINISTRATION

Recommended initial dosage:
Adults—3 inhalations 3 or 4 times per day.
Children—2 inhalations 3 or 4 times per day.

Maximum dosage:
Adults—3 inhalations *per dose;* 12 inhalations *per day.*
Children—2 inhalations *per dose;* 8 inhalations *per day.*

When a favorable response is attained, the dose may be gradually reduced. In patients on systemic corticosteroids, it is recommended that systemic therapy be reduced or eliminated before reduction of RESPIHALER dosage is begun. Gradual reduction of systemic corticosteroid therapy must be emphasized to avoid withdrawal symptoms.

HOW SUPPLIED

DEXACORT Phosphate in RESPIHALER, aerosol for oral inhalation, is supplied as follows: **NDC** 53014-203-13 in a pressurized container, and includes a plastic adapter.

Storage
Store at a temperature below 49°C (120°F).

35203001   2034/794

DEXACORT™ Phosphate   ℞
(dexamethasone sodium phosphate)
in TURBINAIRE® (dispenser)
Aerosol for Intranasal Application

DESCRIPTION

DEXACORT™ Phosphate (dexamethasone sodium phosphate) in TURBINAIRE® (Dispenser) is an aerosol for intranasal application. The inactive ingredients are chlorofluorocarbons† as propellants and alcohol 2%. One cartridge delivers an amount sufficient to ensure delivery of 170 metered sprays, each containing dexamethasone sodium phosphate equivalent to approximately 0.1 mg dexamethasone phosphate or to approximately 0.084 mg dexamethasone. Twelve sprays deliver a theoretical maximum of 1.0 mg dexamethasone.

Dexamethasone sodium phosphate, a synthetic adrenocortical steroid, is a white or slightly yellow, crystalline powder. It is freely soluble in water and is exceedingly hygroscopic. The molecular weight is 516.41. It is designated chemically as 9-fluoro-11β, 17-dihydroxy-16α-methyl-21-(phosphonooxy) pregna-1,4-diene-3, 20-dione disodium salt. The empirical formula is $C_{22}H_{28}FNa_2O_8P$ and the structural formula is: [See chemical structure at top of next column.]

ACTION

Inhibition of inflammatory response to inciting agents of mechanical, chemical or immunological nature.

† WARNING: Chlorofluorocarbons (CFCs) are substances which harm public health and environment by destroying ozone in the upper atmosphere.

INDICATIONS

Allergic or inflammatory nasal conditions, and nasal polyps (excluding polyps originating within the sinuses).

CONTRAINDICATIONS

Systemic fungal infections.
Hypersensitivity to components.
Tuberculous, viral and fungal nasal conditions, ocular herpes simplex.

WARNINGS

In patients on therapy with DEXACORT Phosphate in TURBINAIRE subjected to unusual stress, increased dosage of rapidly acting corticosteroids before, during, and after the stressful situation is indicated.

Drug-induced secondary adrenocortical insufficiency may result from too rapid withdrawal of corticosteroids and may be minimized by gradual reduction of dosage. This type of relative insufficiency may persist for months after discontinuation of therapy; therefore, in any situation of stress occurring during that period, hormone therapy should be reinstituted. If the patient is receiving steroids already, dosage may have to be increased. Since mineralocorticoid secretion may by impaired, salt and/or a mineralocorticoid should be administered concurrently.

Dexamethasone may mask some signs of infection, and new infections may appear during its use. There may be decreased resistance and inability to localize infection when corticosteroids are used. Therefore, patients with bacterial infections should also be given appropriate antibiotic therapy if DEXACORT Phosphate in TURBINAIRE is used. Moreover, dexamethasone may affect the nitrobluetetrazolium test for bacterial infection and produce false negative results.

Corticosteroids may activate latent amebiasis. Therefore, it is recommended that latent or active amebiasis be ruled out before initiating corticosteroid therapy in any patient who has spent time in the tropics or any patient with unexplained diarrhea.

Prolonged use of DEXACORT Phosphate in TURBINAIRE may produce posterior subcapsular cataracts, glaucoma with possible damage to the optic nerves, and may enhance the establishment of secondary ocular infections due to fungi or viruses.

Usage in pregnancy: Since adequate human reproduction studies have not been done with DEXACORT Phosphate in TURBINAIRE, use of this drug in pregnancy or in women of childbearing potential requires that the anticipated benefits be weighed against the possible hazards to the mother and embryo or fetus. Infants born of mothers who have received substantial doses of dexamethasone during pregnancy, should be carefully observed for signs of hypoadrenalism. Dexamethasone appears in breast milk and could suppress growth, interfere with endogenous corticosteroid production, or cause other unwanted effects. Mothers taking pharmacologic doses of dexamethasone should be advised not to nurse. Average and large doses of hydrocortisone or cortisone can cause elevation of blood pressure, salt and water retention, and increased excretion of potassium. These effects are less likely to occur with the synthetic derivatives and with DEXACORT Phosphate in TURBINAIRE, except when used in large doses. Dietary salt restriction and potassium supplementation may be necessary. All corticosteroids increase calcium excretion.

Administration of live virus vaccines, including smallpox, is contraindicated in individuals receiving immunosuppressive doses of corticosteroids. If inactivated viral or bacterial vaccines are administered to individuals receiving immunosuppressive doses of corticosteroids, the expected serum antibody response may not be obtained.

Patients who are on drugs which suppress the immune system are more susceptible to infections than healthy individuals. Chickenpox and measles, for example can have a more serious or even fatal course in non-immune children (see

Continued on next page

Medeva Pharmaceuticals, Inc.—Cont.

PRECAUTIONS regarding use of this product in children) or adults on corticosteroids. In such children or adults who have not had these diseases, particular care should be taken to avoid exposure. The risk of developing a disseminated infection varies among individuals and can be related to the dose, route and duration of corticosteroid administration as well as to the underlying disease. If exposed to chickenpox, prophylaxis with varicella zoster immune globulin (VZIG) may be indicated. If chickenpox develops, treatment with antiviral agents may be considered. If exposed to measles, prophylaxis with immune globulin (IG) may be indicated. (See the respective package inserts for VZIG and IG for complete prescribing information.)

If DEXACORT Phosphate in TURBINAIRE is indicated in patients with latent tuberculosis or tuberculin reactivity, close observation is necessary as reactivation of the disease may occur. During prolonged therapy with DEXACORT Phosphate in TURBINAIRE, these patients should receive chemoprophylaxis.

Literature reports suggest an apparent association between use of corticosteroids and left ventricular free wall rupture after a recent myocardial infarction; therefore, therapy with corticosteroids should be used with great caution in these patients.

Keep out of reach of children.

PRECAUTIONS

During local corticosteroid therapy, the possibility of pharyngeal candidiasis should be kept in mind.

Although systemic absorption is low when DEXACORT Phosphate in TURBINAIRE is used in the recommended dosage, adrenal suppression may occur. In addition, other systemic effects of steroid administration must be considered as a possibility.

Following prolonged therapy, withdrawal of corticosteroids may result in symptoms of the corticosteroid withdrawal syndrome including fever, myalgia, arthralgia, and malaise. This may occur in patients even without evidence of adrenal insufficiency. Replacement of systemic steroid with DEXACORT Phosphate in TURBINAIRE should be gradual and carefully monitored by the physician.

There is an enhanced effect of dexamethasone in patients with hypothyroidism and in those with cirrhosis.

DEXACORT Phosphate in TURBINAIRE should be used cautiously in patients with ocular herpes simplex for fear of corneal perforation.

The lowest possible dose of DEXACORT Phosphate in TURBINAIRE should be used to control the condition under treatment, and when reduction in dosage is possible, the reduction must be gradual. If beneficial effect is not evident within 7 days after initiation of therapy, the patient should be re-evaluated.

Psychic derangements may appear when dexamethasone is used, ranging from euphoria, insomnia, mood swings, personality changes, and severe depression, to frank psychotic manifestations. Also, existing emotional instability or psychotic tendencies may be aggravated.

Aspirin should be used cautiously in conjunction with DEXACORT Phosphate in TURBINAIRE in hypoprothrombinemia.

DEXACORT Phosphate in TURBINAIRE should be used with caution in patients with nonspecific ulcerative colitis, if there is a probability of impending perforation, abscess or other pyogenic infection; also in diverticulitis; fresh intestinal anastomoses; active or latent peptic ulcer; renal insufficiency; hypertension; osteoporosis; and myasthenia gravis.

Signs of peritoneal irritation following gastrointestinal perforation in patients receiving large doses of corticosteroids may be minimal or absent. Fat embolism has been reported as a possible complication of hypercortisonism.

Because clinical studies have not been done, the use of this product in children under the age of 6 years is not recommended. Growth and development of children 6 years of age or older on prolonged therapy with DEXACORT Phosphate in TURBINAIRE should be carefully followed.

Dexamethasone may increase or decrease motility and number of spermatozoa in some patients.

Phenytoin, phenobarbital, ephedrine and rifampin may enhance the metabolic clearance of dexamethasone, resulting in decreased blood levels and lessened physiologic activity, thus requiring adjustment in dexamethasone dosage.

The prothrombin time should be checked frequently in patients who are receiving DEXACORT Phosphate in TURBINAIRE and coumarin anticoagulants at the same time because of reports that corticosteroids have altered the response to these anticoagulants. Studies have shown that the usual effect produced by adding corticosteroids is inhibition of response to coumarins, although there have been some conflicting reports of potentiation, not substantiated by studies.

When DEXACORT Phosphate in TURBINAIRE is used concomitantly with potassium-depleting diuretics, patients should be observed closely for development of hypokelemia.

Since the contents of DEXACORT Phosphate in TURBINAIRE are under pressure, the container should not be broken, stored in extreme heat, or incinerated. It should be stored at a temperature below 120°F.

Information for Patients

Susceptible patients who are on immunuosuppressant doses of corticosteroids should be warned to avoid exposure to chickenpox or measles. Patients should also be advised that if they are exposed, medical advice should be sought without delay.

ADVERSE REACTIONS

Nasal irritation and dryness have been the most common adverse reactions. The following have been reported: headache, lightheadedness, urticaria, nausea, epistaxis, rebound congestion, bronchial asthma, perforation of the nasal septum, and anosmia. Signs of adrenal hypercorticism may occur in some patients, especially with overdosage.

Systemic effects from therapy with DEXACORT Phosphate in TURBINAIRE are less likely to occur than with oral or parenteral corticosteroid therapy because of a lower total dose administered. Nevertheless, patients should be observed for the hormonal effects described below because of absorption of dexamethasone from the nasal mucosa.

Fluid and Electrolyte Disturbances

- Sodium retention
- Fluid retention
- Congestive heart failure in susceptible patients
- Potassium loss
- Hypokalemic alkalosis
- Hypertension

Musculoskeletal

- Muscle weakness
- Steroid myopathy
- Loss of muscle mass
- Osteoporosis
- Vertebral compression fractures
- Aseptic necrosis of femoral and humeral heads
- Pathologic fracture of long bones
- Tendon rupture

Gastrointestinal

- Peptic ulcer with possible subsequent perforation and hemorrhage
- Perforation of the small and large bowel, particularly in patients with inflammatory bowel disease
- Pancreatitis
- Abdominal distention
- Ulcerative esophagitis

Dermatologic

- Impaired wound healing
- Thin fragile skin
- Petechiae and ecchymoses
- Erythema
- Increased sweating
- May suppress reactions to skin tests
- Other cutaneous reactions, such as allergic dermatitis, urticaria, angioneurotic edema

Neurologic

- Convulsions
- Increased intracranial pressure with papilledema (pseudotumor cerebri) usually after treatment.
- Vertigo
- Headache
- Psychic disturbances

Endocrine

- Menstrual irregularities
- Development of cushingoid state
- Suppression of growth in children
- Secondary adrenocortical and pituitary unresponsiveness, particularly in times of stress, as in trauma, surgery, or illness.
- Decreased carbohydrate tolerance
- Manifestations of latent diabetics mellitus
- Increased requirements for insulin or oral hypoglycemic agents in diabetics
- Hirsutism

Ophthalmic

- Posterior subcapsular cataracts
- Increased intraocular pressure
- Glaucoma
- Exophthalmos

Metabolic

- Negative nitrogen balance due to protein catabolism

Cardiovascular

- Myocardial rupture following recent myocardial infarction (see WARNINGS).

Other

- Hypersensitivity
- Thromboembolism
- Weight gain
- Increased appetite
- Nausea
- Malaise
- Hiccups

OVERDOSAGE

Reports of acute toxicity and/or death following overdosage of glucocorticoids are rare. In the event of overdosage, no specific antidote is available; treatment is supportive and symptomatic.

Significant lethality was observed in female mice at single oral doses of 3630 mg/m^2 (1210 mg/kg) and single intravenous doses of 2382 mg/m^2 (794 mg/kg).

DOSAGE AND ADMINISTRATION

DO NOT EXCEED THE RECOMMENDED DOSAGE.

The usual initial dosage of DEXACORT Phosphate in TURBINAIRE is:

Adults—2 sprays in each nostril 2 or 3 times a day.

Children (6 to 12 years of age)—1 or 2 sprays in each nostril 2 times a day depending on age.

See accompanying instructions on the proper use of TURBINAIRE.

When improvement occurs the dosage should be gradually reduced. Some patients will be symptom-free on one spray in each nostril 2 times a day. The maximum daily dosage for adults is 12 sprays, and for children, 8 sprays. Therapy should be discontinued as soon as feasible. It may be reinstituted if recurrence of symptoms occurs.

HOW SUPPLIED

DEXACORT Phosphate in TURBINAIRE, aerosol for intranasal application, is supplied as follows: **NDC** 53014-201-13 in a pressurized container and includes a plastic adapter, 12.6 grams, 170 metered doses.

Storage

Store at a temperature below 49°C (120°F).

35201003 2014/1094

INFLUENZA VIRUS VACCINE ℞
FLUVIRIN™

Purified Surface Antigen Vaccine, Trivalent, Types A and B

1996–1997 FORMULA

DESCRIPTION

Influenza Virus Vaccine, **FLUVIRIN™**, Types A and B (Surface Antigens) is a sterile parenteral for intramuscular use only. The vaccine is a slightly opalescent liquid.

FLUVIRIN™ is prepared from the extraembryonic fluid of embryonated chicken eggs inoculated with a specific type of influenza virus suspension containing neomycin and polymyxin. The fluid containing the virus is harvested and clarified by centrifugation and filtration prior to inactivation with betapropiolactone. The inactivated virus is concentrated and purified by zonal centrifugation. The surface antigens, hemagglutinin and neuraminidase, are obtained from the influenza virus particle by further centrifugation in the presence of Triton® N101, a process which removes most of the internal proteins. The Triton® N101 is removed from the surface antigen preparation and the antigens are suspended in 0.01M phosphate buffered saline. The hemagglutinin content is standardized according to current US Public Health Service requirements. Each 0.5 mL dose contains the recommended ratio of 15μg each of A/Texas/36/91 (H1N1), A/Nanchang/933/95 (H3N2) (A/Wuhan/353/95-like) and B/Harbin/7/94 (B/Beijing/184/93-like) hemagglutinin antigens.

Thimerosal (mercury derivative) 0.01% is added as a preservative. Polymyxin, neomycin, and betapropiolactone cannot be detected in the final product by current assay procedures. This vaccine is manufactured and released by Evan Medical Limited.

CLINICAL PHARMACOLOGY

Influenza A viruses are classified into subtypes on the basis of two surface antigens: hemagglutinin (H) and neuraminidase (N). Three subtypes of hemagglutinin (H1, H2 and H3) and two subtypes of neuraminidase (N1, N2) are recognized among influenza A viruses that have caused widespread human disease. Immunity to these antigens, especially the hemagglutinin, reduces the likelihood of infection and lessens the severity of the disease if infection occurs. Infection with a virus of one subtype confers little or no protection against viruses of other subtypes. Furthermore, over time, antigenic variation (antigenic drift) within a subtype may be so marked that infection or vaccination with one strain may not induce immunity to distantly related strains of the same subtype. Although influenza B viruses have shown more antigenic stability than influenza A viruses, antigenic variation does occur. For these reasons major epidemics of respiratory disease caused by new variants of influenza continue to occur. The antigenic characteristics of circulating strains provide the basis for selecting the virus strains included in each year's vaccine.[1]

Typical influenza illness is characterized by abrupt onset of fever, myalgia, sore throat, and nonproductive cough. Unlike other common respiratory illnesses, influenza can cause

severe malaise lasting several days. More severe illness can result if either primary influenza pneumonia or secondary bacterial pneumonia occurs. During influenza epidemics, high attack rates of acute illness result in both increased numbers of visits to physicians' offices, walk-in clinics, and emergency rooms an increased hospitalizations for management of lower respiratory tract complications.[1]

Elderly persons and persons with underlying health problems are at increased risk of complication from influenza infection. If they become ill with influenza, such members of high risk groups are more likely than the general population to require hospitalization.[1]

During major epidemics, hospitalization rates for persons at high-risk may increase twofold to fivefold, depending on the age group. Previously healthy children and younger adults may also require hospitalization for influenza-related complications, but the relative increase in their hospitalization rates is less for persons who belong to high risk groups.[1]

An increase in mortality further indicates the impact of influenza epidemics. Increased mortality results from not only influenza and pneumonia, but also cardiopulmonary and other chronic diseases that can be exacerbated by influenza infection. It is estimated that >20,000 influenza related deaths occurred during each of ten different U.S. epidemics from 1972–73 to 1990–91, and >40,000 influenza related deaths occurred during each of three of these epidemics. More than 90% of the deaths attributed to pneumonia and influenza occurred among persons ≥ 65 years of age. Because the proportion of elderly persons in the United States population is increasing and because age and its associated chronic diseases are risk factors for severe influenza illness, the number of deaths from influenza can be expected to increase unless control measures are implemented more vigorously. The number of persons <65 years of age at increased risk for influenza-related complications is also increasing. Better survival rates for organ-transplant recipients, the success of neonatal intensive care units, and better management of disease such as cystic fibrosis and acquired immunodeficiency syndrome (AIDS) result in a higher survival rate for younger persons at high risk.[1]

The effectiveness of influenza vaccine in preventing or attenuating illness varies, depending primarily on the age and immunocompetence of the vaccine recipient and the degree of similarity between the virus strains included in the vaccine and those that circulate during the influenza season. When there is a good match between vaccine and circulating viruses, influenza vaccine has been shown to prevent illness in approximately 70% of healthy persons less than 65 years of age. In these circumstances, studies have also indicated that the effectiveness of influenza vaccine in preventing hospitalization for pneumonia and influenza among elderly persons living in settings other than nursing homes or similar chronic-care facilities ranges from 30%–70%.

Among elderly persons residing in nursing homes, influenza vaccine is most effective in preventing severe illness, secondary complications, and death. Studies of this population have indicated that the vaccine can be 50%–60% effective in preventing hospitalization and pneumonia and 80% effective in preventing death, even though efficacy in preventing influenza illness may often be in the range of 30%–40% among the frail elderly. Achieving a high rate of vaccination among nursing home residents may reduce the spread of infection in a facility, thus preventing disease through herd immunity.[1]

Based upon epidemiological studies of circulating influenza virus strains, the Public Health System has recommended that the 1996–1997 vaccine will be trivalent and contain 15μg of hemagglutinin of each strain A/Texas/36/91(H1N1). A/Nanchang/933/95 (H3N2) (A/Wuhan/353/95-like) and B/Harbin/7/94 (B/Beijing/184/93-like) per 0.5 mL dose.[1]

INDICATIONS AND USAGE

FLUVIRIN™ is indicated for immunization of persons 4 years of age and older against influenza viruses containing antigens related to those in the vaccine. The safety and efficacy in children between the ages 6 months through 4 years has not been established for this product. However, the Advisory Committee on Immunization Practices (ACIP) of the US Public Health Service strongly recommends vaccination for any person greater than or equal to 6 months of age, who because of age or underlying medical condition, is at increased risk of complications from influenza.[1] Health care workers and others (including household members) in close contact with persons at high-risk groups should be vaccinated.[1] Guidelines for the use of vaccine among different segments of the population are given below.[1]

Although the current Influenza Virus Vaccine can contain one or more of the antigens administered in previous years, annual vaccination with the current vaccine is necessary because immunity declines in the year following vaccination.[1] **Therefore, a history of immunization in any previous year with a vaccine containing one or more antigens included in the current vaccine does not preclude the need to be reimmunized for the 1996–1997 influenza season.[1]**

Remaining 1995–1996 vaccine should not be used to provide protection for the 1996–1997 influenza season.[1]

TARGET GROUPS FOR SPECIAL IMMUNIZATION PROGRAMS

To maximize protection of high-risk persons, both they and their close contacts should be targeted for organized immunization programs.

Groups at increased risk for influenza-related complications.

1. Persons 65 years of age and older.[1]
2. Residents of nursing homes and other chronic-care facilities housing patients of any age with chronic medical conditions.[1]
3. Adults and children with chronic disorders of the pulmonary or cardiovascular systems, including children with asthma.[1]
4. Adults and children who have required medical follow-up or hospitalization during the preceding year because of chronic metabolic diseases (including diabetes mellitus), renal dysfunction, hemoglobinopathies, or immunosuppression (including immunosuppression caused by medications).[1]
5. Children and teenagers (6 months through 18 years of age) who are receiving long-term aspirin therapy and, therefore, may be at risk of developing Reye syndrome after influenza.[1] Refer to **Indications and Usage** and **Warnings** sections for use of this product in children under the age of 4 years.

Groups that can transmit influenza to persons at high risk.

Persons who are clinically or subclinically infected and who care for or live with members of high risk groups and can transmit influenza virus to them. Some persons at high risk (eg, the elderly, transplant recipients, and persons with acquired immunodeficiency syndrome [AIDS]) can have low antibody responses to influenza vaccine. Efforts to protect these members of high risk groups against influenza may be improved by reducing the likelihood of influenza exposure from their caregivers. Therefore, the following groups should be immunized.[1]

1. Physicians, nurses and other personnel in both hospital and outpatient care settings.[1]
2. Employees of nursing homes and chronic-care facilities who have contact with patients or residents.[1]
3. Providers of home care to persons at high risk (eg, visiting nurses, volunteer workers).[1]
4. Household members (including children) of persons in high risk groups.[1]

IMMUNIZATION OF OTHER GROUPS

General Population.

Physicians should administer influenza vaccine to any person who wishes to reduce the likelihood of becoming ill with influenza. Persons who provide essential community services may be considered for vaccination to minimize disruption of essential activities during influenza outbreaks. Students or other persons in institutional settings (e.g., those who reside in dormitories) should be encouraged to receive vaccine to minimize the disruption of routine activities during epidemics.[1]

Pregnant Women.

Influenza associated excess mortality among pregnant women has not been documented except during the pandemics of 1918–19 and 1957–58.[1] However, because death certificate data often do not indicate whether a woman was pregnant at the time of death, studies are needed to assess influenza-associated risks during pregnancy.[1] Case reports and limited studies suggest that women in the third trimester of pregnancy and early puerperium, including those women without underlying risk factors, might be at increased risk for serious complications following influenza infection.[1] The ACIP states that some of the physiologic changes that occur during pregnancy may increase the risk for such complications; as pregnancy progresses, cardiac output, heart rate, oxygen consumption and stroke volume increase while lung capacity decreases. Immunologic changes during pregnancy may also increase the risk of severe influenza illness. The ACIP also states that health-care workers who provide care for pregnant women should consider administering influenza vaccine to all women who would be in the third trimester of pregnancy or early puerperium during the influenza season.[1] The ACIP has also stated that pregnant women who have medical conditions that increase their risk for complications from influenza should be vaccinated before the influenza season, regardless of the stage of pregnancy. Controlled studies on influenza vaccine have not been conducted to demonstrate safety in pregnant women. **The clinical judgment of the attending physician should prevail at all times in determining whether to administer the vaccine to a pregnant woman (see *PRECAUTIONS*, Use in Pregnancy).**

Persons Infected with Human Immunodeficiency Virus (HIV).

Limited information exists regarding the frequency and severity for influenza illness among HIV-infected persons, but reports suggest that symptoms may be prolonged and the risk of complications increased for some HIV-infected persons. Influenza vaccine has produced protective antibody titers against influenza in vaccinated HIV infected persons who have minimal AIDS-related symptoms and high CD4+ T-lymphocyte cell counts.[1] In patients who have advanced HIV disease and low CD4+ T-lymphocyte cell counts, however, influenza vaccine may not induce protective antibody titers; a second dose of vaccine does not improve the immune response for these persons.[1] Recent studies have examined the effect of influenza vaccination on replication of HIV type 1 (HIV-1). Although some studies have demonstrated a transient (i.e., 2- to 4-week) increase in replication of HIV-1 in the plasma or peripheral blood mononuclear cells of HIV-infected persons after vaccine administration, other studies using similar laboratory techniques have not indicated any substantial increase in replication. Deterioration of CD4+ T-lymphocyte cell counts and progression of clinical HIV disease have not been demonstrated among HIV-infected persons who receive vaccine. Because influenza can result in serious illness and complications and because influenza vaccination may result in protective antibody titers, vaccination will benefit many HIV-infected patients.

Foreign Travelers.

The risk of exposure to influenza during foreign travel varies, depending on season and destination. In the tropics, influenza can occur throughout the year, in the Southern Hemisphere, the most activity occurs from April through September. Because of the short incubation period for influenza, exposure to the virus during travel can result in clinical illness that begins while traveling, an inconvenience or potential danger, especially for those at increased risk for complications. Persons preparing to travel to the tropics at any time of year or the Southern Hemisphere from April through September should review their influenza immunization histories. If not immunized the previous fall/winter, they should consider influenza immunization prior to travel.[1] Persons in the high risk category should be especially encouraged to receive the most current vaccine. Persons at high risk who received the previous seasons vaccine before travel should be revaccinated in the fall or winter with the current vaccine.[1]

TIMING OF IMMUNIZATION

Beginning each September, when vaccine for the upcoming influenza season becomes available, persons at high risk who are seen by health-care providers for routine care or as a result of hospitalization should be offered influenza vaccine. Opportunities to vaccinate persons at high risk for complications of influenza should not be missed.

The optimal time for organized vaccination campaigns for persons at high-risk groups is usually the period between October and mid-November. In the United States, influenza activity generally peaks between late December and early March. High levels of influenza activity infrequently occur in the contiguous 48 states before December. Administering vaccine too far in advance of the influenza season should be avoided in facilities such as nursing homes because antibody levels may begin to decline within a few months of vaccination. Vaccination programs can be undertaken as soon as current vaccine is available if regional influenza activity is expected to begin earlier than December.[1]

Children under 9 years of age who have not been immunized previously should receive two doses of vaccine at least 1 month apart to maximise the likelihood of a satisfactory antibody response to all three vaccine antigens. The second dose should be given before December, if possible. Vaccine should be offered to both children and adults up to and even after influenza virus activity is documented in a community.[1]

CONTRAINDICATIONS

INFLUENZA VIRUS IS PROPAGATED IN EGGS FOR THE PREPARATION OF INFLUENZA VIRUS VACCINE. THUS, THIS VACCINE SHOULD NOT BE ADMINISTERED TO ANYONE WITH A HISTORY OF HYPERSENSITIVITY (ALLERGY) TO CHICKEN EGGS, CHICKEN, CHICKEN FEATHERS OR CHICKEN DANDER.

THE VACCINE IS ALSO CONTRAINDICATED IN INDIVIDUALS HYPERSENSITIVE TO ANY COMPONENT OF THE VACCINE INCLUDING THIMEROSAL (A MERCURY DERIVATIVE) (SEE ADVERSE REACTIONS). EPINEPHRINE INJECTION (1:1000) MUST BE IMMEDIATELY AVAILABLE SHOULD AN ACUTE ANAPHYLACTIC REACTION OCCUR DUE TO ANY COMPONENT OF THE VACCINE.

IMMUNIZATION SHOULD BE DELAYED IN PERSONS WITH AN ACTIVE NEUROLOGICAL DISORDER CHARACTERIZED BY CHANGING NEUROLOGICAL FIND-

Continued on next page

Information on the Medeva Pharmaceuticals, Inc. products listed on these pages contains the full prescribing information from product circulars in use as of July 1996. For further information, please consult the package insert currently accompanying the product.

Medeva Pharmaceuticals, Inc.—Cont.

INGS, BUT SHOULD BE CONSIDERED WHEN THE DISEASE PROCESS HAS BEEN STABILIZED.
THE OCCURRENCE OF ANY NEUROLOGICAL SYMPTOMS OR SIGNS FOLLOWING ADMINISTRATION OF ANY VACCINE IS A CONTRAINDICATION TO FURTHER USE.
THE VACCINE SHOULD NOT BE ADMINISTERED TO PERSONS WITH ACUTE FEBRILE ILLNESSES UNTIL THEIR TEMPORARY SYMPTOMS AND/OR SIGNS HAVE ABATED.
The clinical judgment of the attending physician should prevail at all times.

WARNINGS

The safety and efficacy in children between the ages 6 months through to 4 years has not been established for this product. Influenza Virus Vaccine (Fluvirin™) should not be given to these children unless, in the judgment of the physician, the potential benefits clearly outweigh the risk of administration. In any case, THIS PRODUCT SHOULD NOT BE ADMINISTERED TO CHILDREN YOUNGER THAN 6 MONTHS OF AGE.
THE OCCURRENCE OF A NEUROLOGICAL OR SEVERE HYPERSENSITIVITY REACTION FOLLOWING PREVIOUS IMMUNIZATION WITH INFLUENZA VIRUS VACCINE IS A CONTRAINDICATION TO FURTHER USE OF THIS PRODUCT.
Influenza Virus Vaccine should not be given to individuals with thrombocytopenia or any coagulation disorder that would contraindicate intramuscular injection unless, in the judgment of the physician, the potential benefits clearly outweigh the risk of administration.
Patients with impaired immune responsiveness, whether due to the use of immunosuppressive therapy (including irradiation, corticosteroids, antimetabolites, alkylating agents, and cytotoxic agents), a genetic defect, human immunodeficiency virus (HIV) infection, or other causes, may have a reduced antibody response in active immunization procedures.
Since the likelihood of febrile convulsions from any cause is greater in children between 6 and 35 months, special care should be taken in weighing the relative risks and benefits of immunization in this age group.
As with any vaccine, immunization with Influenza Virus Vaccine may not result in seroconversion of all individuals given the vaccine.
Special care should be taken to prevent injection into a blood vessel.

PRECAUTIONS

General

1. PRIOR TO ADMINISTRATION OF ANY DOSE OF INFLUENZA VIRUS VACCINE, THE PARENT, GUARDIAN, OR ADULT PATIENT SHOULD BE ASKED ABOUT THE RECENT HEALTH STATUS, MEDICAL AND IMMUNIZATION HISTORY OF THE PATIENT TO BE IMMUNIZED IN ORDER TO DETERMINE THE EXISTENCE OF ANY CONTRAINDICATION TO IMMUNIZATION WITH INFLUENZA VIRUS VACCINE (see **CONTRAINDICATIONS, WARNINGS**)
2. BEFORE ADMINISTRATION OF ANY BIOLOGICAL, THE PHYSICIAN SHOULD TAKE ALL PRECAUTIONS KNOWN FOR PREVENTION OF ALLERGIC OR ANY OTHER SIDE REACTIONS. This should include: a review of the patient's history regarding possible sensitivity, the ready availability of epinephrine 1:1000 and other appropriate agents used for control of immediate allergic reactions, and a knowledge of the recent literature pertaining to the use of the biological concerned, including the nature of side effects and adverse reactions that may follow its use.
3. A separate sterile syringe and needle or a sterile disposable unit must be used for each individual patient to prevent transmission of infectious agent from one person to another.

Information for the Patient

PRIOR TO ADMINISTRATION OF THIS VACCINE, HEALTH CARE PERSONNEL SHOULD INFORM THE PARENT, GUARDIAN, OR ADULT PATIENT OF THE BENEFITS AND RISKS OF IMMUNIZATION AGAINST INFLUENZA.

Drug Interactions

Although influenza immunization can inhibit the clearance of warfarin and theophylline, studies have not established any adverse clinical effects attributable to these drugs in patients receiving influenza vaccine.

Use in Pregnancy

Pregnancy Category C.
Animal reproduction studies have not been conducted with Influenza Virus Vaccine (Fluvirin™). Thus it is not known whether Influenza Virus Vaccine (Fluvirin™) can cause fetal harm when administered to a pregnant woman or can affect reproductive capacity. Influenza Virus Vaccine (Fluvirin™) should therefore be given to a pregnant woman ONLY if the clinical judgment of the attending physician considers the established benefits of influenza vaccine justify immunization.
See **INDICATIONS AND USAGE, Pregnant Women. The clinical judgment of the attending physician should prevail at all times in determining whether to administer Influenza Virus Vaccine to a pregnant woman.**

ADVERSE REACTIONS

Because purified surface antigen influenza vaccine contains only noninfectious purified viral proteins, it cannot cause influenza. Respiratory disease after vaccination represents coincidental illness unrelated to influenza vaccination.[1]

Local Symptoms

Slight tenderness, redness or induration at the site of injection lasting for 1 or 2 days may occur in less than one third of recipients.[1]

Systemic Symptoms

Fever, malaise, myalgia, and other systemic symptoms occur infrequently and most often affect persons who have had no exposure to the influenza virus antigens in the vaccine (e.g., young children). These reactions begin 6–12 hours after vaccination and can persist for 1 to 2 days.[1]
Immediate-presumably allergic-reactions (such as hives, angioedema, allergic asthma, or systemic anaphylaxis) occur rarely after influenza vaccination. These reactions probably result from hypersensitivity to some vaccine component - the majority of reactions are most likely related to residual egg protein. Although current influenza vaccines contain only a small quantity of egg protein, this protein may induce immediate hypersensitivity reactions among persons with severe egg allergy. Persons who have developed hives, had swelling of the lips or tongue, or experienced acute respiratory distress or collapse after eating eggs should consult a physician for appropriate evaluation to help determine if vaccine should be administered. Persons with documented immunoglobulin E (IgE)–mediated hypersensitivity to eggs - including those who have had occupational asthma or other allergic responses from exposure to egg protein - may also be at increased risk for reactions from influenza vaccine, and similar consultation should be considered. The ACIP suggest that the protocol for influenza vaccination developed by Murphy and Strunk[2] may be considered for patients who have egg allergies and medical conditions that place them at increased risk for influenza-associated complications.[1]
Unlike the 1976 swine influenza vaccine, subsequent vaccines prepared from other virus strains have not been clearly associated with an increased frequency of Guillain-Barré syndrome (GBS). However, a precise estimate of risk is difficult to determine for a rare condition such as GBS, which has an annual background incidence of only one to two cases per 100,000 adult population. Among persons who received the swine influenza vaccine, the rate of GBS that exceeded the background rate was slightly less than one case per 100,000 vaccinations.[1]
An investigation of GBS cases in 1990–91 indicated no overall increase in frequency of GBS among persons who were administered influenza vaccine; a slight increase in GBS cases among vaccinated persons might have occurred in the age group 18–64 years, but not among persons ≥65 years of age. In contrast to the swine influenza vaccine, the epidemiologic features of the possible association of the 1990–91 vaccine were not as convincing. The rate of GBS cases after vaccination that was passively reported to the Vaccine Adverse Event Reporting System (VAERS) during 1993–94 was estimated to be approximately twice the average rate reported during other recent seasons (i.e., 1990–91, 1991–92, 1992–93, and 1994–95). The data currently available are not sufficient to determine whether this represents an actual risk. However, even if GBS were a true side effect, the very low estimated risk for GBS is less than for severe influenza that could be prevented by vaccination.[1]
Whereas the incidence of GBS in the general population is very low, persons with a history of GBS have a substantially greater likelihood of subsequently developing GBS than persons without such a history. Thus, the likelihood of coincidentally developing GBS after influenza vaccination is expected to be greater among persons with a history of GBS than among persons with no history of this syndrome. Whether influenza vaccination might be causally associated with this risk for recurrence is not known. Although it would seem prudent to avoid a subsequent influenza vaccination in a person known to have developed GBS within 6 weeks of a previous influenza vaccination, for most persons with a history of GBS who are at high risk for severe complications from influenza, the established benefits of influenza vaccination justify yearly immunization.[1]
Other neurological disorders, including encephalopathies not defined as GBS, have been temporarily associated with influenza immunization, but no causal link has been established.[3,4]

DOSAGE AND ADMINISTRATION

For Intramuscular Use Only. Shake well before withdrawing each dose. DO NOT INJECT INTRAVENOUSLY.
Parenteral drug products should be inspected visually for particulate matter and discoloration prior to administration (see **DESCRIPTION**).
Remaining 1995-1996 influenza vaccine should not be used.
Although Influenza Virus Vaccine often contains one or more antigens used in previous years, immunity declines during the year following immunization. Therefore, a history of immunization in any previous year with a vaccine containing one or more antigens included in the current vaccine does NOT preclude the need for reimmunization for the 1996–1997 influenza season in order to provide optimal protection.
See **INDICATIONS AND USAGE** section for information regarding the optimal time of administration of this vaccine.
During the past decade, data on influenza vaccine immunogenicity and side effects have generally been obtained when vaccine has been administered intramuscularly. Because recent influenza vaccines have not been adequately evaluated when administered by other routes, the intramuscular route is recommended. Adults and older children should be immunized in the deltoid muscle; infants and young children in the anterolateral aspect of the thigh.
Before immunization, the skin over the site to be injected should be cleansed with a suitable germicide. After insertion of the needle, aspirate to help avoid inadvertent injection into a blood vessel.

Age Group	Dose	No. of Doses (See below for details)
6 to 35 months*	0.25 mL	1 or 2 Doses
3 years*	0.5 mL	1 or 2 Doses
4 to 8 years	0.5 mL	1 or 2 Doses
9 years and older	0.5 mL	1 Dose

* Refer to **Warnings** section for the use of this product in these age ranges of children.
Two doses administered at least 1 month apart may be required for a satisfactory antibody response among previously unvaccinated children <9 years of age; however, studies of vaccines similar to those being used currently have indicated little or no improvement of antibody responses when a second dose is administered to adults during the same season.[1]
It is recommended that only a purified surface antigen or subvirion vaccine be administered to children under 12 years of age because of lower potential for causing febrile reactions.[1]

Simultaneous Administration with Other Vaccines

The target groups for influenza and pneumococcal immunization overlap considerably. Both vaccines may be given at the same time at different sites without increasing side effects. However, influenza vaccine must be administered each year, whereas pneumococcal vaccine is not. Detailed immunization records should be provided to each patient to record the date when pneumococcal vaccine was administered.[1]
Physicians may prefer not to administer influenza vaccine within 3 days of administration of pertussis containing vaccines. However, the American Academy of Pediatrics now recommends that influenza vaccine may be administered simultaneously (but at a different site and with a different syringe) with other routine vaccinations in children, including pertussis vaccine (DTP or DTaP). Since influenza vaccine in young children can cause fever, DTaP may be preferable in those children 15 months and older who are receiving the fourth (or fifth) dose of pertussis vaccine.[5]

HOW SUPPLIED

NDC 0548-0101-02 5mL vial
NDC 0548-0101-01 5mL pre filled syringe

STORAGE

DO NOT FREEZE. STORE REFRIGERATED, AWAY FROM FREEZER COMPARTMENT, AT 2°C to 8°C (36°F to 46°F).

REFERENCES

1. Prevention and control of influenza. Recommendations of the Immunization Practices Advisory Committee (ACIP). MMWR 1996; 45(RR-5) 1–24.
2. Murphy K R, *et al.:* Safe administration of influenza vaccine in asthmatic children hypersensitive to egg proteins. *J. Pediatr* 1985; 106:931–3.
3. Center for Disease Control: December 1986; Adverse events following immunization: Report No. 2, 1982–1984.
4. Retailliou H, *et al.:* Illness after influenza vaccination reported through a nation-wide surveillance system, 1976–1977. *Am J Epidemiol* 1980; 111:270–278.
5. *American Academy of Pediatrics:* Report of the Committee on Infectious Diseases, ed. 23, 1994, Page 281.

IMPORTANT INFORMATION for Group Immunization Programs: If this vaccine is to be used in an immunization program sponsored by any organization WHERE A TRADITIONAL PHYSICIAN/PATIENT RELATIONSHIP DOES NOT EXIST, each recipient (or legal guardian) must be made aware of the benefits and risks of immunization, and informed consent should be obtained from the recipient (or legal guardian) before immunization. Risks of immunization are summarized in the current labeling. PLEASE CONTACT CDC, or your local State Department of Health to ob-

tain Important Information about influenza and a sample Influenza Consent Form.

Triton® is a registered Trademark of Rohm & Hass Corp.

REV:5-96

GASTROCROM® CAPSULES ℞

[gas ' tro-krōm]

(cromolyn sodium, USP)

Rev. 7/96

R047D

DESCRIPTION

Each gelatin capsule of GASTROCROM (cromolyn sodium, USP) contains 100 mg cromolyn sodium. Cromolyn sodium is a hygroscopic, white powder having little odor. GASTROCROM may leave a slightly bitter aftertaste. It is soluble in water (1 part in 20) and the resulting solution is neutral. It is intended for oral use.

Chemically, cromolyn sodium is the disodium salt of 1,3-bis (2-carboxychromon-5-yloxy)-2-hydroxypropane. The empirical formula is $C_{23}H_{14}Na_2O_{11}$; the molecular weight is 512.34. Its chemical structure is:

Pharmacologic Category: Mast cell stabilizer

Therapeutic Category: Antiallergic

CLINICAL PHARMACOLOGY

In vitro and *in vivo* animal studies have shown that cromolyn sodium inhibits the release of mediators from sensitized mast cells. Cromolyn sodium acts by inhibiting the release of histamine and leukotrienes (SRS-A) from the mast cell. Cromolyn sodium has no intrinsic vasoconstrictor, antihistaminic or anti-inflammatory activity.

Cromolyn sodium is poorly absorbed from the gastrointestinal tract. No more than 1% of an administered dose is absorbed by humans after oral administration, the remainder being excreted in the feces. Very little absorption of cromolyn sodium was seen after oral administration of 500 mg by mouth to each of 12 volunteers. From 0.28 to 0.50% of the administered dose was recovered in the first 24 hours of urinary excretion in 3 subjects. The mean urinary excretion of an administered dose over 24 hours in the remaining 9 subjects was 0.45%.

INDICATIONS AND USAGE

GASTROCROM is indicated in the management of patients with mastocytosis. Use of this product has been associated with improvement in diarrhea, flushing, headaches, vomiting, urticaria, abdominal pain, nausea, and itching in some patients.

CONTRAINDICATIONS

GASTROCROM is contraindicated in those patients who have shown hypersensitivity to cromolyn sodium.

WARNINGS

The recommended dosage should be decreased in patients with decreased renal or hepatic function. Severe anaphylactic reactions may occur rarely in association with cromolyn sodium administration.

PRECAUTIONS

In view of the biliary and renal routes of excretion of GASTROCROM, consideration should be given to decreasing the dosage of the drug in patients with impaired renal or hepatic function.

Carcinogenesis, Mutagenesis, and Impairment of Fertility: Long-term studies in mice (12 months intraperitoneal treatment followed by six months observation), hamsters (12 months intraperitoneal treatment followed by 12 months observation), and rats (18 months subcutaneous treatment) showed no neoplastic effect of cromolyn sodium.

No evidence of chromosomal damage or cytotoxicity was obtained in various mutagenesis studies.

No evidence of impaired fertility was shown in laboratory animal reproduction studies.

Pregnancy: Pregnancy Category B. Reproduction studies with cromolyn sodium administered parenterally to pregnant mice, rats, and rabbits in doses up to 338 times the human clinical dose produced no evidence of fetal malformations. Adverse fetal effects (increased resorption and decreased fetal weight) were noted only at the very high parenteral doses that produced maternal toxicity. There are, however, no adequate and well controlled studies in pregnant women.

Because animal reproduction studies are not always predictive of human response, this drug should be used during pregnancy only if clearly needed.

Drug Interaction During Pregnancy: Cromolyn sodium and isoproterenol were studied following subcutaneous injections in pregnant mice. Cromolyn sodium alone in doses of 60

to 540 mg/kg (38 to 338 times the human dose) did not cause significant increases in resorptions or major malformations. Isoproterenol alone at a dose of 2.7 mg/kg (90 times the human dose) increased both resorptions and malformations. The addition of cromolyn sodium (338 times the human dose) to isoproterenol (90 times the human dose) appears to have increased the incidence of both resorptions and malformations.

Nursing Mothers: It is not known whether this drug is excreted in human milk. Because many drugs are excreted in human milk, caution should be exercised when GASTROCROM is administered to a nursing woman.

Pediatric Use: Animal studies suggest increased risk of toxicity in premature animals when given doses much higher than clinically recommended. In term infants up to six months of age, available clinical data suggest that the dose should not exceed 20 mg/kg/day. The use of this product in pediatric patients less than two years should be reserved for patients with severe disease in which the potential benefits clearly outweigh the risks.

ADVERSE REACTIONS

Most of the adverse events reported in mastocytosis patients have been transient and could represent symptoms of the disease. The most frequently reported adverse events in mastocytosis patients who have received GASTROCROM during clinical studies were headache and diarrhea. Each occurred in 4 of the 87 patients. Pruritus, nausea, and myalgia were each reported in 3 patients and abdominal pain, rash, and irritability in 2 patients each. One report of malaise was also recorded.

A generally similar profile of adverse events has been reported during studies in other clinical conditions. Additional reports which have been received during the course of these studies and spontaneous reports during foreign marketing include: flushing, urticaria/angioedema, arthralgia, dizziness, fatigue, paresthesia, taste perversion, migraine, psychosis, anxiety, depression, insomnia, behavior change, esophagospasm, flatulence, dysphagia, hepatic function test abnormal, edema, dyspnea, polycythemia, neutropenia, dysuria, hallucinations, skin erythema and burning, burning mouth and throat, stiffness and weakness of the legs, and postprandial lightheadedness and lethargy. These events are infrequent, the majority representing only a single report, and in many cases the causal relationship to GASTROCROM is uncertain.

DOSAGE AND ADMINISTRATION

NOT FOR INHALATION. SEE DIRECTIONS FOR USE.

The usual starting dose is as follows:

Adults: Two capsules four times daily one-half hour before meals and at bedtime.

Premature to Term Infants: Not recommended.

Term to 2 years: 20 mg/kg/day in four divided doses. Use of this product in pediatric patients less than 2 years is not recommended and should be attempted only in those patients with severe incapacitating diseases where the benefits clearly outweigh the risks.

Children 2–12 years: One capsule four times daily one-half hour before meals and bedtime.

If satisfactory control of symptoms is not achieved within two to three weeks the dosage may be increased but should not exceed 40 mg/kg/day (30 mg/kg/day for pediatric patients six months to two years).

Patients should be advised that the effect of GASTROCROM therapy is dependent upon its administration at regular intervals, as directed.

Maintenance Dose: Once a therapeutic response has been achieved the dose may be reduced to the minimum required to maintain the patient with a lower degree of symptomatology. To prevent relapses, the dosage should be maintained.

Administration: GASTROCROM should be administered as a solution in water at least $^1/_2$ hour before meals after preparation according to the following directions:

1. Open capsule(s) and pour powder contents of capsule(s) into $^1/_2$ glass of hot water.
2. Stir until completely dissolved (clear solution).
3. Add equal quantity of cold water while stirring.
4. DO NOT MIX WITH FRUIT JUICE, MILK OR FOODS.
5. Drink all of the liquid.

HOW SUPPLIED

GASTROCROM Capsules, each containing 100 mg of cromolyn sodium, are supplied in aluminum cans containing 100 capsules.

Each capsule contains a precisely measured dose. The capsules are intentionally oversized to prevent the powder from spilling when the capsule is opened.

NDC 53014-677-01

Keep tightly closed and out of the reach of children. Store between 15°–30°C (59°–86°F).

CAUTION: Federal law prohibits dispensing without prescription.

MEDEVA PHARMACEUTICALS

Medeva Pharmaceuticals, Inc.

Fort Worth, TX 76155

Made in England

®Fisons plc. 7/96

R047D

© 1996, Medeva Pharmaceuticals Manufacturing, Inc.

GASTROCROM® ℞

[gas 'tro-krōm]

(cromolyn sodium, USP)

Oral Concentrate

For Oral Use Only—Not for Inhalation or Injection

Rev. 7/96

R081B

DESCRIPTION

Each 5 mL ampule of GASTROCROM contains 100 mg cromolyn sodium, USP, in purified water. Cromolyn sodium is a hygroscopic, white powder having little odor. It may leave a slightly bitter aftertaste. GASTROCROM (cromolyn sodium, USP) Oral Concentrate is clear, colorless, and sterile. It is intended for oral use.

Chemically, cromolyn sodium is disodium 5.5′-[(2- hydroxytrimethylene)dioxy]bis[4-oxo-4*H*-1-benzopyran-2- carboxylate]. The empirical formula is $C_{23}H_{14}Na_2O_{11}$: the molecular weight is 512.34. Its chemical structure is:

Pharmacologic Category: Mast cell stabilizer

Therapeutic Category: Antiallergic

CLINICAL PHARMACOLOGY

In vitro and *in vivo* animal studies have shown that cromolyn sodium inhibits the release of mediators from sensitized mast cells. Cromolyn sodium acts by inhibiting the release of histamine and leukotrienes (SRS-A) from the mast cell. Cromolyn sodium has no intrinsic vasoconstrictor, antihistamine, or glucocorticoid activity.

Cromolyn sodium is poorly absorbed from the gastrointestinal tract. No more than 1% of an administered dose is absorbed by humans after oral administration, the remainder being excreted in the feces. Very little absorption of cromolyn sodium was seen after oral administration of 500 mg by mouth to each of 12 volunteers. From 0.28 to 0.50% of the administered dose was recovered in the first 24 hours of urinary excretion in 3 subjects. The mean urinary excretion of an administered dose over 24 hours in the remaining 9 subjects was 0.45%.

CLINICAL STUDIES

Four randomized, controlled clinical trials were conducted with GASTROCROM in patients with either cutaneous or systemic mastocytosis, two of which utilized a placebo-controlled crossover design, one utilized an active-controlled (chlorpheniramine plus cimetidine) crossover design, and one utilized a placebo-controlled parallel group design. Due to the rare nature of this disease, only 36 patients qualified for study entry, of whom 32 were considered evaluable. Consequently, formal statistical analyses were not performed. Clinically significant improvement in gastrointestinal symptoms (diarrhea, abdominal pain) were seen in the majority of patients with some improvement also seen for cutaneous manifestations (urticaria, pruritus, flushing) and cognitive function. The benefit seen with GASTROCROM 200 mg QID was similar to chlorpheniramine (4 mg QID) plus cimetidine (300 mg QID) for both cutaneous and systemic symptoms of mastocytosis.

Clinical improvement occurred within 2–6 weeks of treatment initiation and persisted for 2–3 weeks after treatment withdrawal. GASTROCROM did not affect urinary histamine levels or peripheral eosinophilia, although neither of these variables appeared to correlate with disease severity. Positive clinical benefits were also reported for 37 of 51 patients who received GASTROCROM in United States and foreign humanitarian programs.

Continued on next page

Medeva Pharmaceuticals, Inc.—Cont.

INDICATIONS AND USAGE
GASTROCROM is indicated in the management of patients with mastocytosis. Use of this product has been associated with improvement in diarrhea, flushing, headaches, vomiting, urticaria, abdominal pain, nausea, and itching in some patients.

CONTRAINDICATIONS
GASTROCROM is contraindicated in those patients who have shown hypersensitivity to cromolyn sodium.

WARNINGS
The recommended dosage should be decreased in patients with decreased renal or hepatic function. Severe anaphylactic reactions may occur rarely in association with cromolyn sodium administration.

PRECAUTIONS
In view of the biliary and renal routes of excretion of GASTROCROM, consideration should be given to decreasing the dosage of the drug in patients with impaired renal or hepatic function.
Carcinogenesis, Mutagenesis, and Impairment of Fertility: Long term studies of cromolyn sodium in mice (12 months intraperitoneal administration at doses up to 150 mg/kg three days per week), hamsters, (intraperitoneal administration at doses up to 52.6 mg/kg three days per week for 15 weeks followed by 17.5 mg/kg three days per week for 37 weeks), and rats (18 months subcutaneous administration at doses up to 75 mg/kg six days per week) showed no neoplastic effects. The average daily maximum dose levels administered in these studies were 192.9 mg/m^2 for mice, 47.2 mg/m^2 for hamsters and 385.8 mg/m^2 for rats. These doses correspond to 13%, 3.2%, and 26% of the maximum daily human dose of 1480 mg/m^2.
Cromolyn sodium showed no mutagenic potential in Ames Salmonella/microsome plate assays, mitotic gene conversion in *Saccharomyces cerevisiae* and in an *in vitro* cytogenetic study in human peripheral lymphocytes.
No evidence of impaired fertility was shown in laboratory reproduction studies conducted subcutaneously in rats at the highest doses tested, 175 mg/kg/day (1050 mg/m^2) in males and 100 mg/kg/day (600 mg/m^2) in females. Theses doses are approximately 71% and 41% of the maximum daily human dose, respectively, based on mg/m^2.
Pregnancy: Pregnancy Category B. Reproduction studies with cromolyn sodium administered subcutaneously to pregnant mice and rats at maximum daily dose of 540 mg/kg (1620 mg/m^2) and 164 mg/kg (984 mg/m^2), respectively, and intravenously to rabbits at a maximum daily doses of 485 mg/kg (5820 mg/m^2) produced no evidence of fetal malformations. These doses represent 109%, 66% and 393%, respectively, of the maximum daily human dose on a mg/m^2 basis. Adverse fetal effects (increased resorption and decreased fetal weight) were noted only at very high parenteral doses that produced maternal toxicity. There are, however, no adequate and well controlled studies in pregnant women. Because animal reproduction studies are not always predictive of human response, this drug should be used during pregnancy only if clearly needed.
Drug Interaction During Pregnancy: Cromolyn sodium and isoproterenol were studied following subcutaneous injections in pregnant mice. Cromolyn sodium alone in doses of 60 to 540 mg/kg (38 to 338 times the human dose) did not cause significant increases in resorptions or major malformations. Isoproterenol alone at a dose of 2.7 mg/kg (90 times the human dose) increased both resorptions and malformations. The addition of cromolyn sodium (338 times the human dose) to isoproterenol (90 times the human dose) appears to have increased the incidence of both resorptions and malformations.
Nursing Mothers: It is not known whether this drug is excreted in human milk. Because many drugs are excreted in human milk, caution should be exercised when GASTROCROM is administered to a nursing woman.
Pediatric Use: Animal studies suggest increased risk of toxicity in premature animals when given doses much higher than clinically recommended. In term infants up to six months of age, available clinical data suggest that the dose should not exceed 20 mg/kg/day. The use of this product in pediatric patients less than two years of age should be reserved for patients with severe disease in which the potential benefits clearly outweigh the risks.

ADVERSE REACTIONS
Most of the adverse events reported in mastocytosis patients have been transient and could represent symptoms of the disease. The most frequently reported adverse events in mastocytosis patients who have received GASTROCROM during clinical studies were headache and diarrhea, each of which occurred in 4 of the 87 patients. Pruritus, nausea, and myalgia were each reported in 3 patients and abdominal pain, rash, and irritability in 2 patients each. One report of malaise was also recorded.

Other Adverse Events: Additional adverse events have been reported during studies in other clinical conditions and from worldwide postmarketing experience. In most cases the available information is incomplete and attribution to the drug cannot be determined. The majority of these reports involve the gastrointestinal system and include: diarrhea, nausea, abdominal pain, constipation, dyspepsia, flatulence, glossitis, stomatitis, vomiting, dysphagia, esophagospasm. Other less commonly reported events (the majority representing only a single report) include the following:

Skin:	pruritus, rash, urticaria/angioedema, erythema/burning, photosensitivity
Musculoskeletal:	arthralgia, myalgia, stiffness/weakness of legs
Neurologic:	headache, dizziness, hypoesthesia, paresthesia, migraine, convulsions, flushing
Psychiatric:	psychosis, anxiety, depression, hallucinations, behavior change, insomnia, nervousness
Heart Rate:	tachycardia, premature ventricular contractions (PVCs), palpitations
Respiratory:	pharyngitis, dyspnea
Miscellaneous:	fatigue, edema, unpleasant taste, chest pain, postprandial lightheadedness and lethargy, dysuria, urinary frequency, purpura, hepatic function test abnormal, polycythemia, neutropenia, pancytopenia, tinnitus, lupus erythematosus (LE) syndrome

DOSAGE AND ADMINISTRATION
NOT FOR INHALATION OR INJECTION. SEE DIRECTIONS FOR USE.
The usual starting dose is as follows:
Adults (13 Years and Older): Two ampules four times daily, taken one-half hour before meals and at bedtime.
Children 2–12 Years: One ampule four times daily, taken one-half hour before meals and at bedtime.
Pediatric Patients Under 2 Years: Not recommended.
If satisfactory control of symptoms is not achieved within two to three weeks, the dosage may be increased but should not exceed 40 mg/kg/day.
Patients should be advised that the effect of GASTROCROM therapy is dependent upon its administration at regular intervals, as directed.
Maintenance Dose: Once a therapeutic response has been achieved, the dose may be reduced to the minimum required to maintain the patient with a lower degree of symptomatology. To prevent relapses, the dosage should be maintained.
Administration: GASTROCROM should be administered as a solution at least $^1/_2$ hour before meals and at bedtime after preparation according to the following directions:
1. Break open ampule(s) and squeeze liquid contents of ampule(s) into a glass of water.
2. Stir solution.
3. Drink all of the liquid.

HOW SUPPLIED
GASTROCROM Oral Concentrate is an unpreserved, colorless solution supplied in a low density polyethylene plastic unit dose ampule with 8 ampules per foil pouch. Each 5 mL ampule contains 100 mg cromolyn sodium, USP, in purified water.
NDC 53014-678-70   96 ampules × 5 mL
GASTROCROM Oral Concentrate should be stored between 15°–30°C (59°–86°F) and protected from light. Do not use if it contains a precipitate or becomes discolored. Keep out of the reach of children.
Store ampules in foil pouch until ready for use.
CAUTION: Federal law prohibits dispensing without prescription.
Marketed by:
MEDEVA PHARMACEUTICALS
Medeva Pharmaceuticals, Inc.
Fort Worth, TX 76155

Manufactured by:
Automatic Liquid Packaging, Inc.
Woodstock, IL 60098 USA
®FISONS plc

7/96
R081B
©1996, Medeva Pharmaceuticals Manufacturing, Inc.

HUMIBID® L.A. Tablets
GUAIFENESIN

HUMIBID® Pediatric Capsules
GUAIFENESIN

HUMIBID® DM Tablets
GUAIFENESIN/DEXTROMETHORPHAN HYDROBROMIDE

℞

DESCRIPTION
HUMIBID® L.A. Tablets: Each light green, scored, sustained-release tablet provides 600 mg guaifenesin. Inactive ingredients: Dibasic calcium phosphate, ethylcellulose, FD & C Blue #1 Lake, D & C Yellow #10 Lake, magnesium stearate, sodium lauryl sulfate, stearic acid.
Chemically, guaifenesin is 3-(2-methoxyphenoxy)-1, 2-propanediol and has the following structural formula:

$C_{10}H_{14}O_4$ MW = 198.22

HUMIBID® Pediatric Capsules: Each green and clear capsule provides 300 mg guaifenesin in a sustained-release formulation intended for oral administration. The microencapsulated contents of a capsule may be sprinkled on a small amount of soft food immediately prior to ingestion, making the product ideal for pediatric patients and other patients unable to swallow capsules or tablets. Capsules are oversized to facilitate opening but may also be swallowed whole.
HUMIBID® DM Tablets: Each dark green, scored, sustained-release tablet provides 600 mg guaifenesin and 30 mg dextromethorphan hydrobromide. Inactive ingredients: Dibasic calcium phosphate, stearic acid, FD & C Blue #1 Lake, D & C Yellow #10 Lake, sodium lauryl sulfate, ethylcellulose, magnesium stearate. Chemically, guaifenesin is 3-(2-methoxyphenoxy)-1,2-propanediol and has the following structural formula:

$C_{10}H_{14}O_4$ MW = 198.00

Dextromethorphan hydrobromide is a salt of the methyl ether of the dextrorotatory isomer of levorphanol, a narcotic analgesic. Chemically, it is 3-methoxy-17-methyl-9α, 13α, 14α-morphinan hydrobromide monohydrate and has the following structural formula:

$C_{18}H_{25}NO \cdot HBr \cdot H_2$ MW = 370.33

CLINICAL PHARMACOLOGY
Guaifenesin is an expectorant which increases respiratory tract fluid secretions and helps to loosen phlegm and bronchial secretions. By reducing the viscosity of secretions, guaifenesin increases the efficiency of the mucociliary mechanism in removing accumulated secretions from the upper and lower airway. Guaifenesin is readily absorbed from the gastrointestinal tract and is rapidly metabolized and excreted in the urine. Guaifenesin has a plasma half-life of one hour. The major urinary metabolite is β-(2-methoxyphenoxy) lactic acid.
Dextromethorphan is an antitussive agent which, unlike the isomeric levorphanol, has no analgesic or addictive properties. The drug acts centrally and elevates the threshold for coughing. It is about equal to codeine in depressing the cough reflex. In therapeutic dosage, dextromethorphan does not inhibit ciliary activity. Dextromethorphan is rapidly absorbed from the gastrointestinal tract, metabolized by the liver and excreted primarily in the urine.

INDICATIONS AND USAGE
HUMIBID® L.A. Tablets and **HUMIBID® Pediatric Capsules** are indicated for the temporary relief of coughs associated with respiratory tract infections and related conditions such as sinusitis, pharyngitis and bronchitis, and asthma, when these conditions are complicated by tenacious mucus and/or mucus plugs and congestion.

HUMIBID® DM Tablets are indicated for the temporary relief of coughs associated with upper respiratory tract infections and related conditions such as sinusitis, pharyngitis and bronchitis, particularly when these conditions are complicated by tenacious mucus and/or mucus plugs and congestion.

HUMIBID® L.A. Tablets, HUMIBID® Pediatric Capsules and HUMIBID® DM Tablets are effective in productive as well as non-productive cough, but are of particular value in dry, non-productive cough which tends to injure the mucous membrane of the air passages.

CONTRAINDICATIONS

HUMIBID® L.A. Tablets and HUMIBID® Pediatric Capsules: These products are contraindicated in patients with hypersensitivity to guaifenesin.

HUMIBID® DM Tablets:

This drug is contraindicated in patients with hypersensitivity to guaifenesin or dextromethorphan and in patients receiving monoamine oxidase inhibitor (MAOI) therapy and for 14 days after stopping MAOI therapy. (See **Drug Interactions** section).

PRECAUTIONS

General: Before prescribing medication to suppress or modify cough, it is important that the underlying cause of cough is identified, that modification of cough does not increase the risk of clinical or physiological complications, and that appropriate therapy for the primary disease is instituted.

Dextromethorphan should be used with caution in sedated or debilitated patients, and in patients to be confined to the supine position.

Drug Interactions: HUMIBID® DM Tablets: Do not prescribe this product for use in patients that are now taking a prescription MAOI (certain drugs for depression, psychiatric or emotional conditions, or Parkinson's disease), or for 14 days after stopping the MAOI drug therapy.

Drug/Laboratory Test Interactions: Guaifenesin may increase renal clearance for urate and thereby lower serum uric acid levels. Guaifenesin may produce an increase in urinary 5-hydroxyindoleacetic acid and may therefore interfere with the interpretation of this test for the diagnosis of carcinoid syndrome. It may also falsely elevate the VMA test for catechols. Administration of these products should be discontinued 48 hours prior to the collection of urine specimens for such tests.

Carcinogenesis, Mutagenesis, Impairment of Fertility: No data are available on the long-term potential of guaifenesin or of dextromethorphan for carcinogenesis, mutagenesis, or impairment of fertility in animals or humans.

Pregnancy: Category C: Animal reproduction studies have not been conducted with guaifenesin or with dextromethorphan. It is also not known whether these drugs can cause fetal harm when administered to a pregnant woman or can affect reproduction capacity. Therefore, these products should be given to a pregnant woman only if clearly needed.

Nursing Mothers: It is not known whether guaifenesin or dextromethorphan is excreted in human milk. Because many drugs are excreted in human milk, caution should be exercised when these products are administered to a nursing mother and a decision should be made whether to discontinue nursing or to discontinue the drug, taking into account the importance of the drug to the mother.

ADVERSE REACTIONS

No serious side effects from guaifenesin or dextromethorphan have been reported.

OVERDOSAGE

Overdosage with guaifenesin is unlikely to produce toxic effects since its toxicity is low. Guaifenesin, when administered by stomach tube to test animals in doses up to 5 grams/kg, produced no signs of toxicity. In severe cases of overdosage, treatment should be aimed at reducing further absorption of the drug. Gastric emptying (Syrup of Ipecac) and/or lavage is recommended as soon as possible after ingestion.

Overdosage with dextromethorphan may produce central excitement and mental confusion. Very high doses may produce respiratory depression. One case of toxic psychosis (hyperactivity, marked visual and auditory hallucinations) after ingestion of a single 300 mg dose of dextromethorphan has been reported.

DOSAGE AND ADMINISTRATION

HUMIBID® L.A. Tablets: Adults and adolescents over 12 years of age: One or two tablets every 12 hours not to exceed 4 tablets (2400 mg) in 24 hours. Children 6 to 12 years: One tablet every 12 hours not to exceed 2 tablets (1200 mg) in 24 hours. Children 2 to 6 years: $^1/_2$ tablet every 12 hours not to exceed 1 tablet (600 mg) in 24 hours.

HUMIBID® DM Tablets: Adults and adolescents over 12 years of age: One or two tablets every 12 hours not to exceed 4 tablets in 24 hours. Children 6 to 12 years: One tablet every 12 hours not to exceed 2 tablets in 24 hours. Children 2 to 6 years: $^1/_2$ tablet every 12 hours not to exceed 1 tablet in 24 hours.

HUMIBID® Pediatric Capsules: Adults and adolescents over 12 years of age: Two to four capsules every 12 hours not to exceed 8 capsules in 24 hours. Children 6 to 12 years: Two capsules every 12 hours not to exceed 4 capsules in 24 hours. Children 2 to 6 years: One capsule every 12 hours not to exceed 2 capsules in 24 hours.

HOW SUPPLIED

HUMIBID® L.A. Tablets: Bottles of 100 tablets (NDC 53014-012-10) and 500 tablets (NDC 53014-012-50). Light green, scored tablets are embossed with "Adams/012".

HUMIBID® Pediatric Capsules: Bottles of 100 capsules (NDC 53014-402-10). White beads in a green and clear capsule imprinted with "Adams/402".

HUMIBID® DM Tablets: Bottles of 100 tablets (NDC 53014-030-10) and 500 tablets (NDC 53014-030-50). Dark green, scored tablets are embossed with "Adams/030."

CAUTION: Federal law prohibits dispensing without prescription.

HUMIBID® L.A. Tablets:
August 1995
HUMIBID® DM Tablets:
August 1995
HUMIBID® Pediatric Capsules
August 1995

HYLOREL® Tablets ℞

[hi'lō-rel"]
(guanadrel sulfate tablets, USP)
Rev. 7/96
R253A
814 438 104

DESCRIPTION

HYLOREL Tablets for oral administration contain guanadrel sulfate, an antihypertensive agent belonging to the class of adrenergic neuron blocking drugs. Guanadrel sulfate is (1,4-Dioxaspiro[4.5] dec-2-ylmethyl) guanidine sulfate with a molecular weight of 524.63. The empirical formula is $(C_{10}H_{19}N_3O_2)_2 \cdot H_2SO_4$. It is a white to off-white crystalline powder, which melts with decomposition at about 235°C. It is soluble in water to the extent of 76 mg/mL.

The structural formula is:

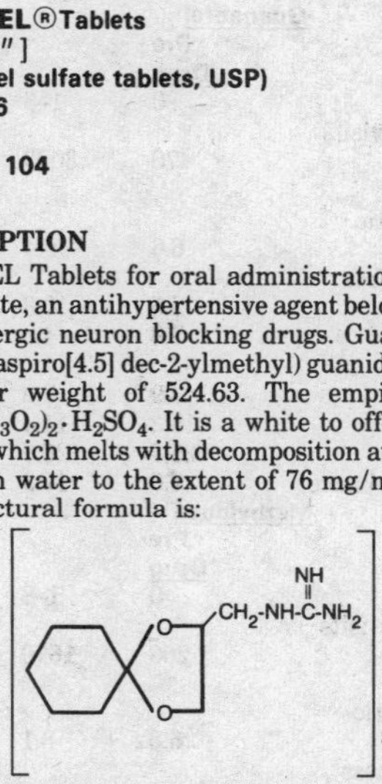

HYLOREL Tablets are available in two strengths: 10 mg and 25 mg. Inactive ingredients: colloidal silicon dioxide, corn starch, lactose monohydrate, magnesium stearate, microcrystalline cellulose and talc. The 10 mg tablet also contains FD&C Yellow No. 6.

CLINICAL PHARMACOLOGY

Guanadrel sulfate is an orally effective antihypertensive agent that lowers both systolic and diastolic arterial blood pressures. Guanadrel sulfate inhibits sympathetic vasoconstriction by inhibiting norepinephrine release from neuronal storage sites in response to stimulation of the nerve and also causes depletion of norepinephrine from the nerve ending. This results in relaxation of vascular smooth muscle which decreases total peripheral resistance, and decreases venous return, both of which reduce the ability to maintain blood pressure in the upright position. The result is a hypotensive effect that is greater in the standing than in the supine position by about 10 mmHg systolic and 3.5 mmHg diastolic, on the average. Heart rate is also decreased usually by about 5 beats/minute. Fluid retention occurs during treatment with guanadrel, particularly when it is not accompanied by a diuretic. The drug does not inhibit parasympathetic nerve function nor does it enter the central nervous system.

Guanadrel sulfate is rapidly absorbed after oral administration. Plasma concentrations generally peak $1^1/_2$ to 2 hours after ingestion. The half-life is about 10 hours, but individual variability is great. Approximately 85% of the drug is eliminated in the urine. Urinary excretion is approximately 85% complete within 24 hours after administration; about 40% of the dose is excreted as unchanged drug. The disposition of guanadrel sulfate is significantly altered in patients with impaired renal function. A study in such patients has shown that as renal function (measured as creatinine clearance) declines, apparent total blody clearance, renal and apparent nonrenal clearances decrease, and the terminal elimination half-life is prolonged. Dosage adjustments may be necessary, especially in patients with creatinine clearances of less than 60 mL/min (see DOSAGE AND ADMINISTRATION).

Guanadrel sulfate begins to decrease blood pressure within two hours and produces maximal decreases in four to six hours. No significant change in cardiac output accompanies the blood pressure decline in normal individuals.

Because drugs of the adrenergic neuron blocking class are transported into the neuron by the "norepinephrine pump", drugs that compete for the pump may block their effects. Tricyclic antidepressants have been shown to block the norepinephrine-depleting effect of guanadrel sulfate in rats and monkeys, and the blood pressure lowering effect of guanadrel sulfate in monkeys. Similar effects have been seen with guanethidine and inhibition of the antihypertensive effects of guanadrel sulfate by tricyclic antidepressants in humans should be presumed.

Therefore caution is recommended if guanadrel sulfate and a tricyclic antidepressant are used concomitantly. Should patients be on both a tricyclic antidepressant and guanadrel sulfate, caution is advised upon discontinuation of the tricyclic antidepressant, especially if discontinued abruptly, as an enhanced effect of guanadrel sulfate may occur.

Chlorpromazine seems to have a similar effect on guanethidine and may affect guanadrel as well. Indirectly acting adrenergic amines are transported into the neuron by the "norepinephrine pump" and may interfere with uptake or may displace blocking agents. Ephedrine rapidly reverses the effects of guanadrel but other agents have not been studied.

Agents of the guanethidine class cause increased sensitivity to circulating norepinephrine, probably by preventing uptake of norepinephrine by adrenergic neurons, the usual mechanism for terminating norepinephrine effects. Agents of this class are thus dangerous in the presence of excess norepinephrine, e.g., in the presence of a pheochromocytoma.

In controlled clinical studies comparing guanadrel to guanethidine and methyldopa, involving about 2000 patients exposed to guanadrel, patients with initial supine blood pressures averaging 160–170/105–110 mmHg had decreases in blood pressure of 20–25/15–20 mmHg in the standing position. The decreases in supine blood pressure were less than the decreases in standing blood pressure by 6–10/2–7 mmHg in different studies. Guanethidine and guanadrel were very similar in effectiveness while methyldopa had a larger effect on supine systolic pressure. Side effects of guanadrel and guanethidine were generally similar in type (see ADVERSE REACTIONS) while methyldopa had more central nervous system effects (depression, drowsiness) but fewer orthostatic effects and less diarrhea.

INDICATIONS AND USAGE

HYLOREL Tablets are indicated for the treatment of hypertension in patients not responding adequately to a thiazide type diuretic. HYLOREL should be added to a diuretic regimen for optimum blood pressure control.

CONTRAINDICATIONS

HYLOREL Tablets are contraindicated in known or suspected pheochromocytoma.

HYLOREL should not be used concurrently with, or within one week of, monoamine oxidase inhibitors.

HYLOREL should not be used in patients hypersensitive to the drug.

HYLOREL should not be used in patients with frank congestive heart failure.

WARNINGS

a. *Orthostatic Hypotension*

Orthostatic hypotension and its consequences (dizziness and weakness) are frequent in people treated with HYLOREL Tablets. Rarely, fainting upon standing or exercise is seen. Careful instructions to the patient can minimize these symptoms, as can recognition by the physician that the supine blood pressure does not constitute an adequate assessment of the effects of this drug. Patients with known regional vascular disease (cerebral, coronary) are at particular risk from marked orthostatic hypotension and HYLOREL should be avoided in them unless drugs with lesser degrees of orthostatic hypotension are ineffective or unacceptable. In such patients hypotensive episodes should be avoided, even if this requires accepting a poorer degree of blood pressure control.

Instructions to patients: Patients should be advised about the risk of orthostatic hypotension and told to sit or lie down immediately at the onset of dizziness or weakness so that they can prevent loss of consciousness. They should be told that postural hypotension is worst in the morning and upon arising, and may be exaggerated by alcohol, fever, hot weather, prolonged standing, or exercise.

Surgery: To reduce the possibility of vascular collapse during anesthesia, guanadrel should be discontinued 48–72 hours before elective surgery. If emergency surgery is required, the anesthesiologist should be made aware that the patient has been taking HYLOREL and that preanesthetic and anesthetic agents should be administered cautiously in reduced dosage. If vasopressors are needed they must be used

Continued on next page

Information on the Medeva Pharmaceuticals, Inc. products listed on these pages contains the full prescribing information from product circulars in use as of July 1996. For further information, please consult the package insert currently accompanying the product.

Medeva Pharmaceuticals, Inc.—Cont.

cautiously, as guanadrel can enhance the pressor response to such agents and increase their arrhythmogenicity.

b. *Drug Interactions*

As discussed above (CLINICAL PHARMACOLOGY), tricyclic antidepressants and indirect-acting sympathomimetics such as ephedrine or phenylpropanolamine, and possibly phenothiazines, can reverse the effects of neuronal blocking agents. IN VIEW OF THE PRESENCE OF SYMPATHOMIMETIC AMINES IN MANY NON-PRESCRIPTION DRUGS FOR THE TREATMENT OF COLDS, ALLERGY, OR ASTHMA, PATIENTS GIVEN GUANADREL SHOULD BE SPECIFICALLY WARNED NOT TO USE SUCH PREPARATIONS WITHOUT THEIR PHYSICIAN'S ADVICE.

Guanadrel enhances the activity of direct-acting sympathomimetics, like norepinephrine, by blocking neuronal uptake. Drugs that affect the adrenergic response by the same or other mechanisms would be expected to potentiate the effects of guanadrel, causing excessive postural hypotension and bradycardia. These include alpha- or beta-adrenergic blocking agents and reserpine. There is no clinical experience with the combination of HYLOREL with alpha-adrenergic blocking agents or reserpine.

When HYLOREL was added to the treatment regimen in hypertensive patients inadequately controlled with a diuretic and propranolol, no significant adverse effects, including bradycardia, were reported in the 26 patients treated concomitantly with the three drugs.

The use of HYLOREL with vasodilators has not been adequately studied and is not generally recommended because concomitant use may increase the potential for symptomatic orthostatic hypotension.

c. *Asthmatic patients*

Special care is needed in patients with bronchial asthma, as their condition may be aggravated by catecholamine depletion and sympathomimetic amines may interfere with the hypotensive effect of guanadrel.

PRECAUTIONS

General: Salt and water retention may occur with the use of HYLOREL Tablets. In clinical studies major problems did not arise because of concomitant diuretic use. Patients with heart failure have not been studied on HYLOREL, but guanadrel could interfere with the adrenergic mechanisms that maintain compensation.

In patients with a history of peptic ulcer, which could be aggravated by a relative increase in parasympathetic tone, HYLOREL should be used cautiously.

In patients with compromised renal function, decreases in renal and nonrenal clearances and an increase in the elimination half-life of guanadrel sulfate have been found. This could possibly lead to an increased incidence of side effects if standard doses are used in these patients. Titration of dose based on the blood pressure response is necessary because of marked interpatient variability (see DOSAGE AND ADMINISTRATION).

A transient increase in blood pressure has been observed in some patients.

Information for patients
See WARNINGS section.
Drug Interactions
See WARNINGS section.
Carcinogenesis, mutagenesis, impairment of fertility: No evidence of carcinogenic potential appeared in a 2-year mouse study of guanadrel sulfate. In a 2-year rat study, an increased number of benign testicular interstitial cell tumors was observed at dosages of 100 mg/kg/day and 400 mg/kg/day. These are common spontaneous tumors in aged rats and their significance to therapy with HYLOREL in man is unknown. Salmonella testing (Ames test) showed no evidence of mutagenic activity.

A reproduction study was performed in male and female rats at dosages of 0, 10, 30 and 100 mg/kg/day. Suppressed libido and reduced fertility were noted at 100 mg/kg/day (12 times the maximum human dose in a 50 kg subject) and libido was suppressed to a lesser extent at 30 mg/kg/day.

Pregnancy Category B
Teratology studies performed in rats and rabbits at doses up to 12 times the maximum recommended human dose (in a 50 kg subject) revealed no significant harm to the fetus due to guanadrel sulfate. There are, however, no adequate and well-controlled studies in pregnant women. Because animal reproduction studies are not always predictive, HYLOREL should be used in pregnant women only when the potential benefit outweighs the potential risk to mother and infant.

Nursing mothers: Whether guanadrel sulfate is excreted in human milk is not known, but because many drugs are excreted in human milk and because of the potential for serious adverse reactions in nursing infants from guanadrel, a decision should be made whether to discontinue nursing or discontinue the drug, taking into account the importance of the drug to the mother.

Pediatric Use: Safety and effectiveness in pediatric patients have not been established.

ADVERSE REACTIONS

The adverse reaction data for guanadrel is derived principally from comparative long-term (6 months to 3 years) studies with methyldopa and guanethidine in which side effects were assessed through use of periodic questionnaires, a method that tends to give high adverse reaction rates. In the tables that follow, some of the adverse effects reported may not be drug-related, but in the absence of a placebo-treated group, these cannot be readily distinguished. Comparative results with two well-known drugs, methyldopa and guanethidine should aid in interpretation of these adverse reaction rates.

The following table displays the frequency of side effects which are believed to be related to sympathetic blocking agents: orthostatic faintness, increased bowel movements and ejaculation disturbances for peripherally acting drugs such as guanadrel and drowsiness for centrally acting drugs such as methyldopa. The frequencies observed were generally higher during the first 8 weeks of therapy. Week 0 frequencies, which were recorded just prior to administration of the antihypertensive drugs while the patients were receiving diuretics, serve as a reference point. Frequency while on therapy is shown for the first 8 weeks and for weeks 9 to 52.

FREQUENCY OF SIDE EFFECTS
Percent of Clinic Visits in
Which Side Effect was Reported

Guanadrel

	Pre Drug		
Week	0	1–8	9–52
Number of clinic visits analyzed	470	3003	4260
Side Effect			
Morning orthostatic faintness	6.6	9.4	6.8
Orthostatic faintness during the day	7.5	10.8	8.5
Other faintness	7.8	4.8	4.5
Increased bowel movements	4.9	7.9	6.1
Drowsiness	15.3	14.4	8.7
Fatigue	25.7	26.6	23.7
Ejaculation disturbance	7.0	17.5	12.0

Methyldopa

	Pre Drug		
Week	0	1–8	9–52
Number of clinic visits analyzed	266	1610	2216
Side Effect			
Morning orthostatic faintness	6.8	8.1	7.4
Orthostatic faintness during the day	7.5	8.0	7.8
Other faintness	6.2	3.7	3.8
Increased bowel movements	4.9	5.9	3.8
Drowsiness	13.2	21.2	18.6
Fatigue	32.9	22.6	27.6
Ejaculation disturbance	10.3	13.4	11.5

Guanethidine

	Pre Drug		
Week	0	1–8	9–52
Number of clinic visits analyzed	215	1421	2009
Side Effect			
Morning orthostatic faintness	4.6	10.7	7.9
Orthostatic faintness during the day	5.6	8.9	6.3
Other faintness	5.9	2.7	2.0
Increased bowel movements	3.7	7.9	9.4
Drowsiness	10.2	10.3	6.4
Fatigue	21.4	20.5	17.5
Ejaculation disturbance	6.9	16.6	18.2

The frequency of side effects over time may be reduced by the discontinuation of drugs in patients who experience intolerable side effects. Reasons for discontinuation of therapy with guanadrel are shown in the following table.

PERCENT OF PATIENTS WHO DISCONTINUED

	Guana-drel	Methyl-dopa	Guane-thidine
Orthostatic faintness	0.6	0.7	6.0*
Syncope	0.4	0.3	2.0
Other faintness	1.2	0.0	0.0
Increased bowel movements	0.8	0.7	1.4
Drowsiness	0.0	1.9*	0.0
Fatigue	0.2	2.6*	0.0
Ejaculation disturbances	0.4	0.0	0.0

* significantly greater than HYLOREL, p < 0.003

The following paragraph shows the incidence of reactions often associated with adrenergic neuron blockers as the percent of patients who reported the event at least once over the treatment periods of 6 months to 3 years. For such long-term studies these incidence rates of side effects, which are found often in untreated patients, tend to be high and accumulate with time. The incidence rates for two well-known comparison drugs, methyldopa and guanethidine should aid in interpreting the high rates. It can be seen that the serious consequences of the orthostatic effect of guanadrel, such as syncope, were very uncommon.

1544 guanadrel, 743 methyldopa and 330 guanethidine patients were evaluated in comparison studies. The observed incidence rates of major drug related side effects for guanadrel, methyldopa and guanethidine, respectively, are as follows: orthostatic faintness: 49%, 41%, 48%; other faintness: 47%, 46%, 45%; increased bowel movements: 31%, 28%, 36%; ejaculation disturbances: 18%, 21%, 22%; impotence: 5.1%, 12.2%, 7.2%; syncope: 0.4%, 0.3%, 2%; urine retention: 0.2%, 0%, 0%.

Apart from these adverse effects, many others were reported. Relationship to therapy is less clear, although some (such as peripheral edema with all three drugs, depression with methyldopa) are in part drug related. All adverse effects reported in at least 1% of guanadrel patients are listed in the following table:

Drug No. pts. treated Event	Guanadrel 1544 %	Methyl-dopa 743 %	Guanethi-dine 330 %
Cardiovascular-Respiratory			
Chest Pain	27.9	37.4	27.3
Coughing	26.9	36.2	21.5
Palpitations	29.5	35.0	24.5
Shortness of breath at rest	18.3	22.3	17.0
Shortness of breath on exertion	45.9	53.2	48.8
Central Nervous System-Special Senses			
Confusion	14.8	22.6	10.9
Depression	1.9	3.9	1.8
Drowsiness	44.6	64.1	28.5
Headache	58.1	69.0	49.7
Paresthesias	25.1	35.1	16.4
Psychological problems	3.8	4.8	3.9
Sleep disorders	2.1	2.3	2.7
Visual disturbances	29.2	35.3	26.1
Gastrointestinal			
Abdominal distress or pain	1.7	1.9	1.5
Anorexia	18.7	23.0	17.6
Constipation	21.0	29.1	20.3
Dry mouth, dry throat	1.7	4.0	0.6
Gas pain	32.0	39.7	29.4
Glossitis	8.4	10.8	4.8
Indigestion	23.7	30.8	18.5
Nausea and/or vomiting	3.9	4.8	3.6
Genitourinary			
Hematuria	2.3	4.2	2.1
Nocturia	48.4	52.4	41.5
Peripheral edema	28.6	37.4	22.7
Urinary urgency or frequency	33.6	39.8	27.6
Miscellaneous			
Excessive weight gain	44.3	53.7	42.4
Excessive weight loss	42.2	51.1	41.5
Fatigue	63.6	76.2	57.0
Musculoskeletal			
Aching limbs	42.9	51.7	33.9
Backache or neckache	1.5	1.1	1.8
Joint pain or inflammation	1.7	2.0	2.4
Leg cramps during the day	21.1	26.0	20.0
Leg cramps during the night	25.6	32.6	21.2

OVERDOSAGE

Overdosage usually produces marked dizziness and blurred vision related to postural hypotension and may progress to syncope on standing. The patient should lie down until these symptoms subside.

If excessive hypotension occurs and persists despite conservative treatment, intensive therapy may be needed to support vital functions. A vasoconstrictor such as phenylephrine will ameliorate the effect of HYLOREL Tablets, but great care must be used because patients may be hypersensitive to such agents.

DOSAGE AND ADMINISTRATION

As with other sympathetic suppressant drugs, the dose response to HYLOREL Tablets varies widely and must be adjusted for each patient until the therapeutic goal is achieved. With long-term therapy, some tolerance may occur and the dosage may have to be increased.

Because HYLOREL has a substantial orthostatic effect, monitoring both supine and standing pressures is essential, especially while dosage is being adjusted.

HYLOREL should be administered in divided doses. The usual starting dosage for treating hypertension is 10 mg per day, which can be given as 5 mg b.i.d. by breaking the 10 mg tablet. The dosage should be adjusted weekly or monthly until blood pressure is controlled. Most patients will require daily dosage in the range of 20 to 75 mg usually in twice daily doses. For larger doses 3 or 4 times daily dosing may be needed. A dosage of more than 400 mg/day is rarely required.

Dosage should be adjusted for patients with impaired renal function (see CLINICAL PHARMACOLOGY and PRECAUTIONS). As a general guideline, it is recommended that initial therapy with HYLOREL in patients with creatinine clearances of 30 to 60 mL/min be reduced to 5 mg every 24 hours. In patients with creatinine clearances less than 30 mL/min, the dosing interval should be increased to 48 hours. The time to achieve steady state will be increased. Dosage increases should be made cautiously at intervals not less than 7 days in patients with moderate renal insufficiency and not less than 14 days in patients with severe renal insufficiency. These recommendations are based upon human pharmacokinetic data and not clinical experience.

HOW SUPPLIED

HYLOREL Tablets are available as follows:

10 mg, scored elliptical tablets (light orange)
Bottles of 100—NDC 53014-787-71

25 mg, scored elliptical tablets (white)
Bottles of 100—NDC 53014-788-71

Store at controlled room temperature 15°–30° C (59°–86°F).
Keep out of the reach of children.

CAUTION: Federal law prohibits dispensing without prescription.

Marketed by:
MEDEVA PHARMACEUTICALS
Medeva Pharmaceuticals, Inc.
Forth Worth, TX 76155
Manufactured by: Rev. 7/96
The Upjohn Company R253A
Kalamazoo, MI 49001, USA 814 438 104
® Fisons Intelmark Holdings, Inc.
691015

IONAMIN® Capsules ℞
[*i "on 'uh-min*]
(phentermine resin)
R195C
Rev. 7/96

DESCRIPTION

IONAMIN '15' and IONAMIN '30' contain 15 mg and 30 mg respectively of phentermine as the cationic exchange resin complex. Phentermine is α, α-dimethyl phenethylamine (phenyl-tertiary-butylamine).

Inactive Ingredients: D&C Yellow No. 10, dibasic calcium phosphate, FD&C Yellow No. 6, gelatin, iron oxides (15 mg capsules only), lactose, magnesium stearate, titanium dioxide.

ACTIONS

IONAMIN is a sympathomimetic amine with pharmacologic activity similar to the prototype drug of this class used in obesity, amphetamine (d- and *dl*-amphetamine). Actions include central nervous system stimulation and elevation of blood pressure. Tachyphylaxis and tolerance have been demonstrated with all drugs of this class in which these phenomena have been looked for.

Drugs of this class used in obesity are commonly known as "anorectics" or "anorexigenics." It has not been established, however, that the action of such drugs in treating obesity is primarily one of appetite suppression. Other central nervous system actions, or metabolic effects may be involved.

Adult obese subjects instructed in dietary management and treated with "anorectic" drugs, lose more weight on the average than those treated with placebo and diet, as determined in relatively short-term clinical trials.

The magnitude of increased weight loss of drug-treated patients over placebo-treated patients is only a fraction of a pound a week. The rate of weight loss is greatest in the first weeks of therapy for both drug and placebo subjects and tends to decrease in succeeding weeks. The possible origins of the increased weight loss due to the various drug effects are not established. The amount of weight loss associated with the use of an "anorectic" drug varies from trial to trial, and the increased weight loss appears to be related in part to variables other than the drugs prescribed, such as the physician-investigator, the population treated, and the diet prescribed. Studies do not permit conclusions as to the relative importance of the drug and non-drug factors on weight loss.

The natural history of obesity is measured in years, whereas the studies cited are restricted to a few weeks' or months' duration; thus, the total impact of drug-induced weight loss over that of diet alone must be considered clinically limited.

The bioavailability of IONAMIN has been studied in humans in which blood levels of phentermine were measured by a gas chromatography method. Blood levels obtained with the 15 mg and 30 mg resin complex formulations indicated slower absorption with a reduced but prolonged peak concentration and without a significant difference in prolongation of blood levels when compared with the same doses of phentermine hydrochloride. The clinical significance of these differences is not known. In clinical trials establishing the efficacy of IONAMIN, a single daily dose produced an effect comparable to that produced by other regimens of "anorectic" drug therapy.

INDICATION

IONAMIN is indicated in the management of exogenous obesity as a short-term (a few weeks) adjunct in a regimen of weight reduction based on caloric restriction. The limited usefulness of agents of this class (see ACTIONS) should be measured against possible risk factors inherent in their use such as those described below.

CONTRAINDICATIONS

Advanced arteriosclerosis, symptomatic cardiovascular disease, moderate to severe hypertension, hyperthyroidism, known hypersensitivity, or idiosyncrasy to the sympathomimetic amines, glaucoma.

Agitated states.

Patients with a history of drug abuse.

During or within 14 days following the administration of monoamine oxidase inhibitors (hypertensive crises may result).

WARNINGS

If tolerance to the "anorectic" effect develops, the recommended dose should not be exceeded in an attempt to increase the effect: rather, the drug should be discontinued.

IONAMIN may impair the ability of the patient to engage in potentially hazardous activities such as operating machinery or driving a motor vehicle; the patient should therefore be cautioned accordingly.

When using CNS active agents, consideration must always be given to the possibility of adverse interactions with alcohol.

Drug Dependence: IONAMIN is related chemically and pharmacologically to amphetamine (d- and *dl*-amphetamine) and other stimulant drugs that have been extensively abused. The possibility of abuse of IONAMIN should be kept in mind when evaluating the desirability of including a drug as part of a weight reduction program. Abuse of amphetamine (d- and *dl*-amphetamine) and related drugs may be associated with intense psychological dependence and severe social dysfunction. There are reports of patients who have increased the dosage of some of these drugs to many times that recommended. Abrupt cessation following prolonged high dosage administration results in extreme fatigue and mental depression; changes are also noted on the sleep EEG. Manifestations of chronic intoxication with anorectic drugs include severe dermatoses, marked insomnia, irritability, hyperactivity, and personality changes. The most severe manifestation of chronic intoxications is psychosis, often clinically indistinguishable from schizophrenia.

Usage in Pregnancy: Safe use in pregnancy has not been established. Use of IONAMIN by women who are or may become pregnant requires that the potential benefit be weighed against the possible hazard to mother and infant.

Usage in Pediatric Patients: IONAMIN is not recommended for use in pediatric patients under 12 years of age.

PRECAUTIONS

Caution is to be exercised in prescribing IONAMIN (phentermine resin) for patients with even mild hypertension. Insulin requirements in diabetes mellitus may be altered in association with the use of IONAMIN and the concomitant dietary regimen.

IONAMIN may decrease the hypotensive effect of adrenergic neuron blocking drugs.

The least amount feasible should be prescribed or dispensed at one time in order to minimize the possibility of overdosage.

ADVERSE REACTIONS

Cardiovascular: Palpitation, tachycardia, elevation of blood pressure.

Central Nervous System: Overstimulation, restlessness, dizziness, insomnia, euphoria, dysphoria, tremor, headache; rarely psychotic episodes at recommended doses with some drugs in this class.

Gastrointestinal: Dryness of the mouth, unpleasant taste, diarrhea, constipation, other gastrointestinal disturbances.

Allergic: Urticaria.

Endocrine: Impotence, changes in libido.

DOSAGE AND ADMINISTRATION

One capsule daily, before breakfast or 10–14 hours before retiring. For individuals exhibiting greater drug responsiveness, IONAMIN '15' will usually suffice. IONAMIN '30' is recommended for less responsive patients. IONAMIN is not recommended for use in pediatric patients under 12 years of age.

IONAMIN capsules should be swallowed whole.

OVERDOSAGE

Manifestations of acute overdosage may include restlessness, tremor, hyperreflexia, rapid respiration, confusion, assaultiveness, hallucinations, panic states.

Fatigue and depression usually follow the central stimulation.

Cardiovascular effects include arrhythmias, hypertension, or hypotension and circulatory collapse. Gastrointestinal symptoms include nausea, vomiting, diarrhea, and abdominal cramps. Overdosage of pharmacologically similar compounds has resulted in fatal poisoning, usually terminating in convulsions and coma.

Management of acute IONAMIN intoxication is largely symptomatic and includes lavage and sedation with a barbiturate. Experience with hemodialysis or peritoneal dialysis is inadequate to permit recommendation in this regard. Intravenous phentolamine (Regitine) has been suggested on pharmacologic grounds for possible acute, severe hypertension, if this complicates overdosage.

HOW SUPPLIED

IONAMIN Capsules (phentermine resin) are available in two strengths:

15 mg, yellow/grey capsules, imprinted with "IONAMIN 15."

NDC 53014-903-71 Bottle of 100's
NDC 53014-903-84 Bottle of 400's

30 mg, yellow/yellow capsules, imprinted with "IONAMIN 30."

NDC 53014-904-71 Bottle of 100's
NDC 53014-904-84 Bottle of 400's

Dispense in a tight container. Store at room temperature.
Keep out of the reach of children.

CAUTION: Federal law prohibits dispensing without prescription.

MEDEVA PHARMACEUTICALS
Medeva Pharmaceuticals, Inc.
Fort Worth, TX 76155
®Fisons BV

Rev. 7/96
R195C

K–NORM® Capsules ℞
[*kā' nórm*]
(potassium chloride
extended-release capsules, USP)
R216D
Rev. 7/96

DESCRIPTION

K-NORM Capsules (potassium chloride extended-release capsules, USP) are a solid oral dosage form of potassium chloride containing 10 mEq (750 mg) of potassium chloride [equivalent to 10 mEq (390 mg) of potassium and 10 mEq (360 mg) of chloride] in a microencapsulated capsule. This formulation is intended to slow the release of potassium so that the likelihood of a high localized concentration of potassium chloride within the gastrointestinal tract is reduced.

K-NORM Capsules are an electrolyte replenisher. The chemical name is potassium chloride, and the structural formula is KCl. Potassium chloride, USP occurs as a white, granular powder or as colorless crystals. It is odorless and has a saline taste. Its solutions are neutral to litmus. It is freely soluble in water and insoluble in alcohol.

Inactive Ingredients: Calcium stearate, gelatin, pharmaceutical glaze, povidone, sugar spheres, talc.

Continued on next page

Information on the Medeva Pharmaceuticals, Inc. products listed on these pages contains the full prescribing information from product circulars in use as of July 1996. For further information, please consult the package insert currently accompanying the product.

Medeva Pharmaceuticals, Inc.—Cont.

CLINICAL PHARMACOLOGY

The potassium ion is the principal intracellular cation of most body tissues. Potassium ions participate in a number of essential physiological processes, including the maintenance of intracellular tonicity, the transmission of nerve impulses, the contraction of cardiac, skeletal and smooth muscle and the maintenance of normal renal function.

The intracellular concentration of potassium is approximately 150 to 160 mEq per liter. The normal adult plasma concentration is 3.5 to 5 mEq per liter. An active ion transport system maintains this gradient across the plasma membrane.

Potassium is a normal dietary constituent and under steady state conditions the amount of potassium absorbed from the gastrointestinal tract is equal to the amount excreted in the urine. The usual dietary intake of potassium is 50 to 100 mEq per day.

Potassium depletion will occur whenever the rate of potassium loss through renal excretion and/or loss from the gastrointestinal tract exceeds the rate of potassium intake. Such depletion usually develops as a consequence of therapy with diuretics, primary or secondary hyperaldosteronism, diabetic ketoacidosis, or inadequate replacement of potassium in patients on prolonged parenteral nutrition. Depletion can develop rapidly with severe diarrhea, especially if associated with vomiting. Potassium depletion due to these causes is usually accompanied by a concomitant loss of chloride and is manifested by hypokalemia and metabolic alkalosis. Potassium depletion may produce weakness, fatigue, disturbances of cardiac rhythm (primarily ectopic beats), prominent U-waves in the electrocardiogram, and, in advanced cases, flaccid paralysis and/or impaired ability to concentrate urine.

If potassium depletion associated with metabolic alkalosis cannot be managed by correcting the fundamental cause of the deficiency, e.g., where the patient requires long term diuretic therapy, supplemental potassium in the form of high potassium food or potassium chloride may be able to restore normal potassium levels.

In rare circumstances (e.g., patients with renal tubular acidosis) potassium depletion may be associated with metabolic acidosis and hyperchloremia. In such patients potassium replacement should be accomplished with potassium salts other than the chloride, such as potassium bicarbonate, potassium citrate, potassium acetate, or potassium gluconate.

INDICATIONS AND USAGE

BECAUSE OF REPORTS OF INTESTINAL AND GASTRIC ULCERATION AND BLEEDING WITH EXTENDED-RELEASE POTASSIUM CHLORIDE PREPARATIONS, THESE DRUGS SHOULD BE RESERVED FOR THOSE PATIENTS WHO CANNOT TOLERATE OR REFUSE TO TAKE LIQUIDS OR EFFERVESCENT POTASSIUM PREPARATIONS OR FOR PATIENTS IN WHOM THERE IS A PROBLEM OF COMPLIANCE WITH THESE PREPARATIONS.

1. For the treatment of patients with hypokalemia, with or without metabolic alkalosis; in digitalis intoxication; and in patients with hypokalemic familial periodic paralysis. If hypokalemia is the result of diuretic therapy, consideration should be given to the use of a lower dose of diuretic therapy, which may be sufficient without leading to hypokalemia.
2. For the prevention of hypokalemia in patients who would be at particular risk if hypokalemia were to develop, e.g., digitalized patients or patients with significant cardiac arrhythmias.

The use of potassium salts in patients receiving diuretics for uncomplicated essential hypertension is often unnecessary when such patients have a normal dietary pattern and when low doses of the diuretic are used. Serum potassium levels should be checked periodically, however, and if hypokalemia occurs, dietary supplementation with potassium-containing foods may be adequate to control milder cases. In more severe cases, and if dose adjustment of the diuretic is ineffective or unwarranted, supplementation with potassium salts may be indicated.

CONTRAINDICATIONS

Potassium supplements are contraindicated in patients with hyperkalemia, since a further increase in serum potassium concentration in such patients can produce cardiac arrest. Hyperkalemia may complicate any of the following conditions: chronic renal failure, systemic acidosis such as diabetic acidosis, acute dehydration, heat cramps, extensive tissue breakdown as in severe burns, adrenal insufficiency, or the administration of a potassium-sparing diuretic (e.g., spironolactone, triamterene, amiloride) (see OVERDOSAGE).

Extended-release formulations of potassium chloride have produced esophageal ulceration in certain cardiac patients with esophageal compression due to an enlarged left atrium.

Potassium supplementation, when indicated in such patients, should be given as a liquid preparation.

All solid oral dosage forms of potassium chloride are contraindicated in any patient in whom there is structural, pathological (e.g., diabetic gastroparesis) or pharmacologic (use of anticholinergic agents or other agents with anticholinergic properties at sufficient doses to exert anticholinergic effects) cause for arrest or delay in capsule passage through the gastrointestinal tract; an oral liquid preparation should be used when indicated in these patients.

WARNINGS

Hyperkalemia: (see OVERDOSAGE) In patients with impaired mechanisms for excreting potassium, the administration of potassium salts can produce hyperkalemia and cardiac arrest. This occurs most commonly in patients given potassium by the intravenous route but may also occur in patients given potassium orally. Potentially fatal hyperkalemia can develop rapidly and be asymptomatic. The use of potassium salts in patients with chronic renal disease, or any other condition which impairs potassium excretion, requires particularly careful monitoring of the serum potassium concentration and appropriate dosage adjustment.

Interaction with Potassium-Sparing Diuretics: Hypokalemia should not be treated by the concomitant administration of potassium salts and a potassium-sparing diuretic (e.g., spironolactone, triamterene or amiloride) since the simultaneous administration of these agents can produce severe hyperkalemia.

Interaction with Angiotensin Converting Enzyme Inhibitors: Angiotensin converting enzyme (ACE) inhibitors (e.g., captopril, enalapril) will produce some potassium retention by inhibiting aldosterone production. Potassium supplements should be given to patients receiving ACE inhibitors only with close monitoring.

Gastrointestinal Lesions: Solid oral dosage forms of potassium chloride can produce ulcerative and/or stenotic lesions of the gastrointestinal tract and deaths. Based on spontaneous adverse reaction reports, enteric coated preparations of potassium chloride are associated with an increased frequency of small bowel lesions (40–50 per 100,000 patient years) compared to extended-release wax matrix formulations (less than one per 100,000 patient years). Because of the lack of extensive marketing experience with microencapsulated products, a comparison between such products and wax matrix or enteric coated products is not available. K-NORM Capsules are microencapsulated capsules formulated to provide a controlled rate of release of potassium chloride and thus to minimize the possibility of a high local concentration of potassium near the gastrointestinal wall. Prospective trials have been conducted in normal human volunteers in which the upper gastrointestinal tract was evaluated by endoscopic inspection before and after one week of solid oral potassium chloride therapy. The ability of this model to predict events occurring in usual clinical practice is unknown. Trials which approximated usual clinical practice did not reveal any clear differences between the wax matrix and microencapsulated dosage forms. In contrast, there was a higher incidence of gastric and duodenal lesions in subjects receiving a high dose of a wax matrix extended-release formulation under conditions which did not resemble usual or recommended clinical practice (i.e., 96 mEq per day in divided doses of potassium chloride administered to fasted patients, in the presence of an anticholinergic drug to delay gastric emptying).

The upper gastrointestinal lesions observed by endoscopy were asymptomatic and were not accompanied by evidence of bleeding (hemoccult testing). The relevance of these findings to the usual conditions (i.e., non-fasting, no anticholinergic agent, smaller doses) under which extended-release potassium chloride products are used is uncertain; epidemiologic studies have not identified an elevated risk, compared to microencapsulated products, for upper gastrointestinal lesions in patients receiving wax matrix formulations. K-NORM Capsules (potassium chloride extended-release capsules, USP) should be discontinued immediately and the possibility of ulceration, obstruction or perforation considered if severe vomiting, abdominal pain, distention, or gastrointestinal bleeding occurs.

Metabolic Acidosis: Hypokalemia in patients with metabolic acidosis should be treated with an alkalinizing potassium salt such as potassium bicarbonate, potassium citrate, potassium acetate, or potassium gluconate.

PRECAUTIONS

General: The diagnosis of potassium depletion is ordinarily made by demonstrating hypokalemia in a patient with a clinical history suggesting some cause for potassium depletion. In interpreting the serum potassium level, the physician should bear in mind that acute alkalosis per se can produce hypokalemia in the absence of a deficit in total body potassium while acute acidosis per se can increase the serum potassium concentration into the normal range even in the presence of a reduced total body potassium. Regular serum potassium determinations are recommended. The treatment of potassium depletion, particularly in the presence of cardiac disease, renal disease, or acidosis requires careful attention to acid-base balance and appropriate monitoring of serum electrolytes, the electrocardiogram, and the clinical status of the patient. Potassium should generally not be given in the immediate postoperative period until urine flow is established.

Information for Patients: Physicians should consider reminding the patient of the following:

To take each dose with meals and with a full glass of water or other liquid.

To take this medicine following the frequency and amount prescribed by the physician. This is especially important if the patient is also taking diuretics and/or digitalis preparations.

To check with the physician if there is trouble swallowing capsules or if the capsules seem to stick in the throat.

To check with the physician at once if tarry stools or other evidence of gastrointestinal bleeding is noticed.

Laboratory Tests: When blood is drawn for analysis of plasma potassium it is important to recognize that artifactual elevations can occur after improper venipuncture technique or as a result of in vitro hemolysis of the sample.

Drug Interactions: Potassium-sparing diuretic, angiotensin converting enzyme inhibitors: see WARNINGS.

Carcinogenesis, Mutagenesis, Impairment of Fertility: Carcinogenity, mutagenicity and fertility studies in animals have not been performed. Potassium is a normal dietary constituent.

Pregnancy: Teratogenic Effects—Pregnancy Category C. Animal reproduction studies have not been conducted with K-NORM Capsules. It is unlikely that potassium supplementation that does not lead to hyperkalemia would have an adverse effect on the fetus or would affect reproductive capacity.

Nursing Mothers: The normal potassium ion content of human milk is about 13 mEq per liter. Since oral potassium becomes part of the potassium pool, so long as body potassium is not excessive, the contribution of potassium chloride supplementation should have little or no effect on the level in human milk.

Pediatric Use: Safety and effectiveness in pediatric patients have not been established.

ADVERSE REACTIONS

One of the most severe adverse effects is hyperkalemia (see CONTRAINDICATIONS, WARNINGS, and OVERDOSAGE). There also have been reports of upper and lower gastrointestinal conditions including obstruction, bleeding, ulceration, and perforation (see CONTRAINDICATIONS and WARNINGS).

The most common adverse reactions to the oral potassium salts are nausea, vomiting, flatulence, abdominal pain/discomfort, and diarrhea. These symptoms are due to irritation of the gastrointestinal tract and are best managed by diluting the preparation further, taking the dose with meals, or reducing the amount taken at one time.

Skin rash has been reported rarely.

OVERDOSAGE

The administration of oral potassium salts to persons with normal excretory mechanisms for potassium rarely causes serious hyperkalemia. However, if excretory mechanisms are impaired, or if potassium is administered too rapidly intravenously, potentially fatal hyperkalemia can result (see CONTRAINDICATIONS and WARNINGS). It is important to recognize that hyperkalemia is usually asymptomatic and may be manifested only by an increased serum potassium concentration (6.5–8.0 mEq/L) and characteristic electrocardiographic changes (peaking of T-waves, loss of P-wave, depression of S-T segment, prolongation of the QT interval), and widening and slurring of the QRS complex. Late manifestations include muscle paralysis and cardiovascular collapse from cardiac arrest. (9–12 mEq/L).

Treatment measures for hyperkalemia include the following:

1. Elimination of foods and medications containing potassium and of any agents with potassium-sparing properties;
2. Intravenous administration of 300 to 500 mL/hr of 10% dextrose solution containing 10–20 units of crystalline insulin per 1,000 mL;
3. Correction of acidosis, if present, with intravenous sodium bicarbonate;
4. Use of exchange resins, hemodialysis, or peritoneal dialysis.

In treating hyperkalemia, it should be recalled that in patients who have been stabilized on digitalis, too rapid a lowering of the serum potassium concentration can produce digitalis toxicity.

DOSAGE AND ADMINISTRATION

The usual dietary potassium intake by the average adult is 50 to 100 mEq per day. Potassium depletion sufficient to cause hypokalemia usually requires the loss of 200 or more mEq of potassium from the total body store.

Dosage must be adjusted to the individual needs of each patient. The dose for the prevention of hypokalemia is typically in the range of 20 mEq per day. Doses of 40–100 mEq per day

or more are used for the treatment of potassium depletion. Dosage should be divided if more than 20 mEq per day is given such that no more than 20 mEq is given in a single dose.

K-NORM Capsules provide 10 mEq of potassium chloride.

K-NORM Capsules should be taken with meals and with a glass of water or other liquid. This product should not be taken on an empty stomach because of its potential for gastric irritation (see WARNINGS). Those patients having difficulty swallowing the capsules may be advised to sprinkle the contents onto a spoonful of soft food to facilitate ingestion.

HOW SUPPLIED

K-NORM Capsules are clear/clear hard gelatin capsules, containing 10 mEq (750 mg) of potassium chloride [equivalent to 10 mEq (390 mg) of potassium and 10 mEq (360 mg) of chloride]. Each capsule is imprinted with "K-NORM" on one side and "10" on the other side.

NDC 53014-010-71 Bottle of 100's
NDC 53014-010-85 Bottle of 500's

Store at controlled room temperature 15°-30°C (59°-86°F).

CAUTION: Federal law prohibits dispensing without prescription.

Marketed by:
MEDEVA PHARMACEUTICALS
Medeva Pharmaceuticals, Inc.
Fort Worth, TX 76155
Manufactured by:
KV Pharmaceutical Company
St. Louis, MO 63144
® Fisons BV

Rev. 7/96
R216D

MYKROX® TABLETS ℞

[*mī'krahks*]
(metolazone tablets, USP)
R156G
Rev. 7/96

DO NOT INTERCHANGE

MYKROX TABLETS ARE A RAPIDLY AVAILABLE FORMULATION OF METOLAZONE FOR ORAL ADMINISTRATION. MYKROX TABLETS AND OTHER FORMULATIONS OF METOLAZONE THAT SHARE ITS MORE RAPID AND COMPLETE BIOAVAILABILITY ARE NOT THERAPEUTICALLY EQUIVALENT TO ZAROXOLYN® TABLETS AND OTHER FORMULATIONS OF METOLAZONE THAT SHARE ITS SLOW AND INCOMPLETE BIOAVAILABILITY. FORMULATIONS BIOEQUIVALENT TO MYKROX AND FORMULATIONS BIOEQUIVALENT TO ZAROXOLYN SHOULD NOT BE INTERCHANGED FOR ONE ANOTHER.

DESCRIPTION

MYKROX Tablets (metolazone tablets, USP) for oral administration contain $^1/_2$ mg of metolazone, USP, a diuretic/saluretic/antihypertensive drug of the quinazoline class.

Metolazone has the molecular formula $C_{16}H_{16}ClN_3O_3S$, the chemical name 7-chloro-1,2,3,4-tetrahydro-2-methyl-3-(2-methylphenyl)-4-oxo-6-quinazolinesulfonamide, and a molecular weight of 365.83. The structural formula is:

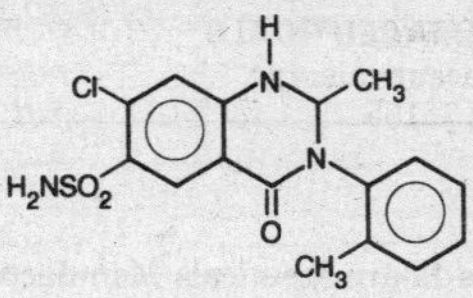

Metolazone is only sparingly soluble in water, but more soluble in plasma, blood, alkali and organic solvents.

Inactive Ingredients: Dibasic calcium phosphate, magnesium stearate, microcrystalline cellulose, pregelatinized starch, sodium starch glycolate.

CLINICAL PHARMACOLOGY

MYKROX (metolazone) is a quinazoline diuretic, with properties generally similar to the thiazide diuretics. The actions of MYKROX result from interference with the renal tubular mechanism of electrolyte reabsorption. MYKROX acts primarily to inhibit sodium reabsorption at the cortical diluting site and to a lesser extent in the proximal convoluted tubule. Sodium and chloride ions are excreted in approximately equivalent amounts. The increased delivery of sodium to the distal tubular exchange site results in increased potassium excretion. MYKROX does not inhibit carbonic anhydrase. A proximal action of metolazone has been shown in humans by increased excretion of phosphate and magnesium ions and by a markedly increased fractional excretion of sodium in patients with severely compromised glomerular filtration. This action has been demonstrated in animals by micropuncture studies.

The antihypertensive mechanism of action of metolazone is not fully understood but is presumed to be related to its saluretic and diuretic properties.

In two double-blind, controlled clinical trials of MYKROX Tablets, the maximum effect on mean blood pressure was achieved within 2 weeks of treatment and showed some evidence of an increased response at 1 mg compared to $^1/_2$ mg. There was no indication of an increased response with 2 mg. After six weeks of treatment, the mean fall in serum potassium was 0.42 mEq/L at $^1/_2$ mg, 0.66 mEq/L at 1 mg and 0.7 mEq/L at 2 mg. Serum uric acid increased by 1.1 to 1.4 mg/dL at increasing doses. There were small falls in serum sodium and chloride and a 1.3–2.1 mg/dL increase in BUN at increasing doses.

The rate and extent of absorption of metolazone from MYKROX Tablets were equivalent to those from an oral solution of metolazone. Peak blood levels are obtained within 2 to 4 hours of oral administration with an elimination half-life of approximately 14 hours. MYKROX Tablets have been shown to produce blood levels that are dose proportional between $^1/_2$–2 mg. Steady state blood levels are usually reached in 4–5 days.

In contrast, other formulations of metolazone produce peak blood concentrations approximately 8 hours following oral administration; absorption continues for an additional 12 hours.

INDICATIONS AND USAGE

MYKROX Tablets are indicated for the treatment of hypertension, alone or in combination with other antihypertensive drugs of a different class.

MYKROX TABLETS HAVE NOT BEEN EVALUATED FOR THE TREATMENT OF CONGESTIVE HEART FAILURE OR FLUID RETENTION DUE TO RENAL OR HEPATIC DISEASE AND THE CORRECT DOSAGE FOR THESE CONDITIONS AND OTHER EDEMA STATES HAS NOT BEEN ESTABLISHED.

SINCE A SAFE AND EFFECTIVE DIURETIC DOSE HAS NOT BEEN ESTABLISHED, MYKROX TABLETS SHOULD NOT BE USED WHEN DIURESIS IS DESIRED.

Usage in Pregnancy

The routine use of diuretics in an otherwise healthy woman is inappropriate and exposes mother and fetus to unnecessary hazard. Diuretics do not prevent development of toxemia of pregnancy, and there is no evidence that they are useful in the treatment of developed toxemia (see PRECAUTIONS).

Edema during pregnancy may arise from pathologic causes or from the physiologic and mechanical consequences of pregnancy. MYKROX is not indicated for the treatment of edema in pregnancy. Dependent edema in pregnancy resulting from restriction of venous return by the expanded uterus is properly treated through elevation of the lower extremities and use of support hose; use of diuretics to lower intravascular volume in this case is illogical and unnecessary. There is hypervolemia during normal pregnancy which is harmful to neither the fetus nor the mother (in the absence of cardiovascular disease), but which is associated with edema, including generalized edema, in the majority of pregnant women. If this edema produces discomfort, increased recumbency will often provide relief. In rare instances, this edema may cause extreme discomfort which is not relieved by rest. In these cases, a short course of diuretics may be appropriate.

CONTRAINDICATIONS

Anuria, hepatic coma or precoma, known allergy or hypersensitivity to metolazone.

WARNINGS

Rapid Onset Hyponatremia

Rarely, the rapid onset of severe hyponatremia and/or hypokalemia has been reported following initial doses of thiazide and non-thiazide diuretics. When symptoms consistent with severe electrolyte imbalance appear rapidly, drug should be discontinued and supportive measures should be initiated immediately. Parenteral electrolytes may be required. Appropriateness of therapy with this class of drugs should be carefully reevaluated.

Hypokalemia

Hypokalemia may occur, with consequent weakness, cramps, and cardiac dysrhythmias. Serum potassium should be determined at regular intervals, and dose reduction, potassium supplementation or addition of a potassium sparing diuretic instituted whenever indicated. Hypokalemia is a particular hazard in patients who are digitalized or who have or have had a ventricular arrhythmia; dangerous or fatal arrhythmias may be precipitated. Hypokalemia is dose related.

In controlled clinical trials, 1.5% of patients taking $^1/_2$ mg and 3.1% of patients taking 1 mg of MYKROX daily developed clinical hypokalemia (defined as hypokalemia accompanied by signs or symptoms); 21% of the patients taking $^1/_2$ mg and 30% of the patients taking 1 mg of MYKROX daily developed hypokalemia (defined as a serum potassium concentration below 3.5 mEq/L); in another controlled clinical trial in which the patients started therapy with a serum potassium level greater than 4.0 mEq/L, 8% of patients taking $^1/_2$ mg of MYKROX daily developed hypokalemia (defined as a serum potassium concentration below 3.5 mEq/L).

Concomitant Therapy

Lithium

In general, diuretics should not be given concomitantly with lithium because they reduce its renal clearance and add a high risk of lithium toxicity. Read prescribing information for lithium preparations before use of such concomitant therapy.

Furosemide: Unusually large or prolonged losses of fluids and electrolytes may result when metolazone is administered concomitantly to patients receiving furosemide (see PRECAUTIONS, DRUG INTERACTIONS).

Other Antihypertensive Drugs: When MYKROX Tablets are used with other antihypertensive drugs, particular care must be taken to avoid excessive reduction of blood pressure, especially during initial therapy.

Cross-Allergy

Cross-allergy, while not reported to date, theoretically may occur when MYKROX Tablets are given to patients known to be allergic to sulfonamide-derived drugs, thiazides, or quinethazone.

Sensitivity Reactions

Sensitivity reactions (e.g., angioedema, bronchospasm) may occur with or without a history of allergy or bronchial asthma and may occur with the first dose of MYKROX.

PRECAUTIONS

DO NOT INTERCHANGE

MYKROX TABLETS ARE A RAPIDLY AVAILABLE FORMULATION OF METOLAZONE FOR ORAL ADMINISTRATION. MYKROX TABLETS AND OTHER FORMULATIONS OF METOLAZONE THAT SHARE ITS MORE RAPID AND COMPLETE BIOAVAILABILITY ARE NOT THERAPEUTICALLY EQUIVALENT TO ZAROXOLYN TABLETS AND OTHER FORMULATIONS OF METOLAZONE THAT SHARE ITS SLOW AND INCOMPLETE BIOAVAILABILITY. FORMULATIONS BIOEQUIVALENT TO MYKROX AND FORMULATIONS BIOEQUIVALENT TO ZAROXOLYN SHOULD NOT BE INTERCHANGED FOR ONE ANOTHER.

GENERAL:

Fluid and Electrolytes

All patients receiving therapy with MYKROX Tablets should have serum electrolyte measurements done at appropriate intervals and be observed for clinical signs of fluid and/or electrolyte imbalance: namely, hyponatremia, hypochloremic alkalosis, and hypokalemia. In patients with severe edema accompanying cardiac failure or renal disease, a low-salt syndrome may be produced, especially with hot weather and a low-salt diet. Serum and urine electrolyte determinations are particularly important when the patient has protracted vomiting, severe diarrhea, or is receiving parenteral fluids. Warning signs of imbalance are: dryness of mouth, thirst, weakness, lethargy, drowsiness, restlessness, muscle pains or cramps, muscle fatigue, hypotension, oliguria, tachycardia, and gastrointestinal disturbances such as nausea and vomiting. Hyponatremia may occur at any time during long term therapy and, on rare occasions, may be life threatening.

The risk of hypokalemia is increased when larger doses are used, when diuresis is rapid, when severe liver disease is present, when corticosteroids are given concomitantly, when oral intake is inadequate or when excess potassium is being lost extrarenally, such as with vomiting or diarrhea.

Thiazide-like diuretics have been shown to increase the urinary excretion of magnesium; this may result in hypomagnesemia.

Glucose Tolerance

Metolazone may raise blood glucose concentrations possibly causing hyperglycemia and glycosuria in patients with diabetes or latent diabetes.

Hyperuricemia

MYKROX regularly causes an increase in serum uric acid and can occasionally precipitate gouty attacks even in patients without a prior history of them.

Azotemia

Azotemia, presumably prerenal azotemia, may be precipitated during the administration of MYKROX Tablets. If azotemia and oliguria worsen during treatment of patients with severe renal disease, MYKROX Tablets should be discontinued.

Renal Impairment

Use caution when administering MYKROX Tablets to patients with severely impaired renal function. As most of the drug is excreted by the renal route, accumulation may occur.

Continued on next page

Information on the Medeva Pharmaceuticals, Inc. products listed on these pages contains the full prescribing information from product circulars in use as of July 1996. For further information, please consult the package insert currently accompanying the product.

Medeva Pharmaceuticals, Inc.—Cont.

Orthostatic Hypotension
Orthostatic hypotension may occur; this may be potentiated by alcohol, barbiturates, narcotics, or concurrent therapy with other antihypertensive drugs. In controlled clinical trials, 1.4% of patients treated with MYKROX Tablets ($^1/_2$ mg) had orthostatic hypotension; this effect was not reported in the placebo group.

Hypercalcemia
Hypercalcemia may infrequently occur with metolazone, especially in patients taking high doses of vitamin D or with high bone turnover states, and may signify hidden hyperparathyroidism. Metolazone should be discontinued before tests for parathyroid function are performed.

Systemic Lupus Erythematosus
Thiazide diuretics have exacerbated or activated systemic lupus erythematosus and this possibility should be considered with MYKROX Tablets.

INFORMATION FOR PATIENTS: Patients should be informed of possible adverse effects, advised to take the medication as directed and promptly report any possible adverse reactions to the treating physician.

DRUG INTERACTIONS:

Diuretics
Furosemide and probably other loop diuretics given concomitantly with metolazone can cause unusually large or prolonged losses of fluid and electrolytes (see WARNINGS).

Other Antihypertensives
When MYKROX Tablets are used with other antihypertensive drugs, care must be taken, especially during initial therapy. Dosage adjustments of other antihypertensives may be necessary.

Alcohol, Barbiturates, and Narcotics
The hypotensive effects of these drugs may be potentiated by the volume contraction that may be associated with metolazone therapy.

Digitalis Glycosides
Diuretic-induced hypokalemia can increase the sensitivity of the myocardium to digitalis. Serious arrhythmias can result.

Corticosteroids or ACTH
May increase the risk of hypokalemia and increase salt and water retention.

Lithium
Serum lithium levels may increase (see WARNINGS).

Curariform Drugs
Diuretic-induced hypokalemia may enhance neuromuscular blocking effects of curariform drugs (such as tubocurarine)—the most serious effect would be respiratory depression which could proceed to apnea. Accordingly, it may be advisable to discontinue MYKROX Tablets three days before elective surgery.

Salicylates and Other Non-Steroidal Anti-Inflammatory Drugs
May decrease the antihypertensive effects of MYKROX Tablets.

Sympathomimetics
Metolazone may decrease arterial responsiveness to norepinephrine, but this diminution is not sufficient to preclude effectiveness of the pressor agent for therapeutic use.

Insulin and Oral Antidiabetic Agents
See Glucose Tolerance under PRECAUTIONS, GENERAL.

Methenamine
Efficacy may be decreased due to urinary alkalizing effect of metolazone.

Anticoagulants
Metolazone, as well as other thiazide-like diuretics, may affect the hypoprothrombinemic response to anticoagulants; dosage adjustments may be necessary.

DRUG/LABORATORY TEST INTERACTIONS: None reported.

CARCINOGENESIS, MUTAGENESIS, IMPAIRMENT OF FERTILITY: Mice and rats administered metolazone 5 days/week for up to 18 and 24 months, respectively, at daily doses of 2, 10 and 50 mg/kg, exhibited no evidence of a tumorigenic effect of the drug. The small number of animals examined histologically and poor survival in the mice limit the conclusions that can be reached from these studies.
Metolazone was not mutagenic *in vitro* in the Ames Test using Salmonella typhimurium strains TA-97, TA-98, TA-100, TA-102 and TA-1535.
Reproductive performance has been evaluated in mice and rats. There is no evidence that metolazone possesses the potential for altering reproductive capacity in mice. In a rat study, in which males were treated orally with metolazone at doses of 2, 10 and 50 mg/kg for 127 days prior to mating with untreated females, an increased number of resorption sites was observed in dams mated with males from the 50 mg/kg group. In addition, the birth weight of offspring was decreased and the pregnancy rate was reduced in dams mated with males from the 10 and 50 mg/kg groups.

PREGNANCY
Teratogenic Effects—Pregnancy Category B.
Reproduction studies performed in mice, rabbits and rats treated during the appropriate periods of gestation at doses up to 50 mg/kg/day have revealed no evidence of harm to the fetus due to metolazone. There are, however, no adequate and well-controlled studies in pregnant women. Because animal reproduction studies are not always predictive of human response, MYKROX Tablets should be used during pregnancy only if clearly needed. Metolazone crosses the placental barrier and appears in cord blood.
Non-Teratogenic Effects
The use of MYKROX Tablets in pregnant women requires that the anticipated benefit be weighed against possible hazards to the fetus. These hazards include fetal or neonatal jaundice, thrombocytopenia, and possibly other adverse reactions which have occurred in the adult. It is not known what effect the use of the drug during pregnancy has on the later growth, development and functional maturation of the child. No such effects have been reported with metolazone.
LABOR AND DELIVERY: Based on clinical studies in which women received metolazone in late pregnancy until the time of delivery, there is no evidence that the drug has any adverse effects on the normal course of labor or delivery.
NURSING MOTHERS: Metolazone appears in breast milk. Because of the potential for serious adverse reactions in nursing infants from metolazone, a decision should be made whether to discontinue nursing or to discontinue the drug, taking into account the importance of the drug to the mother.
PEDIATRIC USE: Safety and effectiveness of MYKROX Tablets in pediatric patients have not been established, and such use is not recommended.

ADVERSE REACTIONS

Adverse experience information is available from more than 14 years of accumulated marketing experience with other formulations of metolazone for which reliable quantitative information is lacking and from controlled clinical trials with MYKROX from which incidences can be calculated.
In controlled clinical trials with MYKROX, adverse experiences resulted in discontinuation of therapy in 6.7–6.8% of patients given $^1/_2$ to 1 mg of MYKROX.
Adverse experiences occurring in controlled clinical trials with MYKROX with an incidence of > 2%, whether or not considered drug-related, are summarized in the following table.

Incidence of Adverse Experiences Volunteered or Elicited (by Patient in Percent)*

	MYKROX n=226†
Dizziness (lightheadedness)	10.2
Headaches	9.3
Muscle Cramps	5.8
Fatigue (malaise, lethargy, lassitude)	4.4
Joint Pain, swelling	3.1
Chest Pain (precordial discomfort)	2.7

* Percent of patients reporting an adverse experience one or more times.

† All doses combined ($^1/_2$, 1 and 2 mg).

Some of the adverse effects reported in association with MYKROX also occur frequently in untreated hypertensive patients, such as headache and dizziness, which occurred in 14.8 and 7.4% of patients in a smaller parallel placebo group. The following adverse effects were reported in less than 2% of the MYKROX treated patients.
Cardiovascular: Cold extremities, edema, orthostatic hypotension, palpitations.
Central and Peripheral Nervous System: Anxiety, depression, dry mouth, impotence, nervousness, neuropathy, weakness, "weird" feeling.
Dermatological: Pruritus, rash, skin dryness.
Eyes, Ears, Nose, Throat: Cough, epistaxis, eye itching, sinus congestion, sore throat, tinnitus.
Gastrointestinal: Abdominal discomfort (pain, bloating), bitter taste, constipation, diarrhea, nausea, vomiting.
Genitourinary: Nocturia.
Musculoskeletal: Back pain.
Other Adverse Experiences:
Adverse experiences reported with other marketed metolazone formulations and most thiazide diuretics, for which quantitative data are not available, are listed in decreasing order of severity within body systems. Several are single or rare occurrences.
Cardiovascular: excessive volume depletion, hemoconcentration, venous thrombosis.
Central and Peripheral Nervous System: syncope, paresthesias, drowsiness, restlessness (sometimes resulting in insomnia).
Dermatologic/Hypersensitivity: necrotizing angiitis (cutaneous vasculitis), purpura, dermatitis, photosensitivity, urticaria.
Gastrointestinal: hepatitis, intrahepatic cholestatic jaundice, pancreatitis, anorexia.

Hematologic: aplastic (hypoplastic) anemia, agranulocytosis, leukopenia.
Metabolic: hypokalemia (see WARNINGS, Hypokalemia), hyponatremia, hyperuricemia, hypochloremia, hypochloremic alkalosis, hyperglycemia, glycosuria, increase in serum urea nitrogen (BUN) or creatinine, hypophosphatemia, hypomagnesemia, hypercalcemia.
Musculoskeletal: acute gouty attacks.
Other: transient blurred vision, chills.
In addition, rare adverse experiences reported in association with similar anti-hypertensive-diuretics but not reported to date for metolazone include: sialadenitis, xanthopsia, respiratory distress (including pneumonitis), thrombocytopenia, and anaphylactic reactions. These experiences could occur with clinical use of metolazone.

OVERDOSAGE

Intentional overdosage has been reported rarely with metolazone and similar diuretic drugs.
Signs and Symptoms
Orthostatic hypotension, dizziness, drowsiness, syncope, electrolyte abnormalities, hemoconcentration and hemodynamic changes due to plasma volume depletion may occur. In some instances depressed respiration may be observed. At high doses, lethargy of varying degree may progress to coma within a few hours. The mechanism of CNS depression with thiazide overdosage is unknown. Also, GI irritation and hypermotility may occur. Temporary elevation of BUN has been reported, especially in patients with impairment of renal function. Serum electrolyte changes and cardiovascular and renal function should be closely monitored.
Treatment
There is no specific antidote available but immediate evacuation of stomach contents is advised. Dialysis is not likely to be effective. Care should be taken when evacuating the gastric contents to prevent aspiration, especially in the stuporous or comatose patient. Supportive measures should be initiated as required to maintain hydration, electrolyte balance, respiration and cardiovascular and renal function.

DOSAGE AND ADMINISTRATION

Therapy should be individualized according to patient response.
For initial treatment of mild to moderate hypertension, the recommended dose is one MYKROX Tablet ($^1/_2$ mg) once daily, usually in the morning. If patients are inadequately controlled with one $^1/_2$ mg tablet, the dose can be increased to two MYKROX Tablets (1 mg) once a day. An increase in hypokalemia may occur. Doses larger than 1 mg do not give increased effectiveness.
The same dose titration is necessary if MYKROX Tablets are to be substituted for other dosage forms of metolazone in the treatment of hypertension.
If blood pressure is not adequately controlled with two MYKROX Tablets alone, the dose should not be increased; rather, another antihypertensive agent with a different mechanism of action should be added to therapy with MYKROX Tablets.

HOW SUPPLIED

MYKROX Tablets (metolazone tablets, USP), $^1/_2$ mg are white, flat-faced, round tablets, debossed "MYKROX" on one side, and "$^1/_2$" on reverse side.
NDC 53014-847-71   Bottle of 100's
Store at room temperature. Dispense in a tight, light-resistant container. Keep out of the reach of children.
CAUTION: Federal law prohibits dispensing without prescription.
MEDEVA PHARMACEUTICALS
Medeva Pharmaceuticals, Inc.
Fort Worth, TX 76155
®Fisons BV

Rev. 7/96
R156G

© 1996, Medeva Pharmaceuticals Manufacturing, Inc.

PEDIAPRED®   ℞

[pēd´ē-uh-pred]
(prednisolone sodium phosphate, USP)
ORAL SOLUTION
R024H
Rev. 7/96

DESCRIPTION

PEDIAPRED (prednisolone sodium phosphate, USP) Oral Solution is a dye free, colorless to light straw colored, raspberry flavored solution. Each 5 mL (teaspoonful) of PEDIAPRED contains 6.7 mg prednisolone sodium phosphate (5 mg prednisolone base) in a palatable, aqueous vehicle.
Inactive Ingredients: Dibasic sodium phosphate, edetate disodium, methylparaben, purified water, sodium biphosphate, sorbitol, natural and artificial raspberry flavor.
Prednisolone sodium phosphate occurs as white or slightly yellow, friable granules or powder. It is freely soluble in water; soluble in methanol; slightly soluble in alcohol and in chloroform; and very slightly soluble in acetone and in diox-

ane. The chemical name of prednisolone sodium phosphate is pregna -1,4- diene-3,20-dione, 11,17-dihydroxy -21- (phosphonooxy)-, disodium salt, (11β)-. The empirical formula is $C_{21}H_{27}Na_2O_8P$; the molecular weight is 484.39. Its chemical structure is:

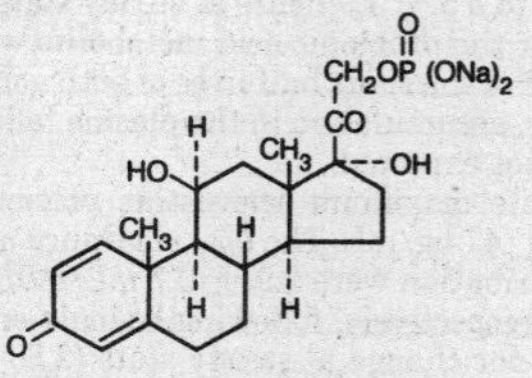

Pharmacological Category: Glucocorticoid

CLINICAL PHARMACOLOGY

Prednisolone is a synthetic adrenocortical steroid drug with predominantly glucocorticoid properties. Some of these properties reproduce the physiological actions of endogenous glucocorticosteroids, but others do not necessarily reflect any of the adrenal hormones' normal functions; they are seen only after administration of large therapeutic doses of the drug. The pharmacological effects of prednisolone which are due to its glucocorticoid properties include: promotion of gluconeogenesis; increased deposition of glycogen in the liver; inhibition of the utilization of glucose; anti-insulin activity; increased catabolism of protein; increased lipolysis; stimulation of fat synthesis and storage; increased glomerular filtration rate and resulting increase in urinary excretion of urate (creatinine excretion remains unchanged); and increased calcium excretion.

Depressed production of eosinophils and lymphocytes occurs, but erythropoiesis and production of polymorphonuclear leukocytes are stimulated. Anti-inflammatory processes (edema, fibrin deposition, capillary dilatation, migration of leukocytes and phagocytosis) and the later stages of wound healing (capillary proliferation, deposition of collagen, cicatrization) are inhibited. Prednisolone can stimulate secretion of various components of gastric juice. Stimulation of the production of corticotropin may lead to suppression of endogenous corticosteroids. Prednisolone has slight mineralocorticoid activity, whereby entry of sodium into cells and loss of intracellular potassium is stimulated. This is particularly evident in the kidney, where rapid ion exchange leads to sodium retention and hypertension.

Prednisolone is rapidly and well absorbed from the gastrointestinal tract following oral administration. PEDIAPRED Oral Liquid produces a 20% higher peak plasma level of prednisolone which occurs approximately 15 minutes earlier than the peak seen with tablet formulations. Prednisolone is 70–90% protein-bound in the plasma and it is eliminated from the plasma with a half-life of 2 to 4 hours. It is metabolized mainly in the liver and excreted in the urine as sulfate and glucuronide conjugates.

INDICATIONS AND USAGE

PEDIAPRED Oral Solution is indicated in the following conditions:

1. Endocrine Disorders
Primary or secondary adrenocortical insufficiency (hydrocortisone or cortisone is the first choice; synthetic analogs may be used in conjunction with mineralocorticoids where applicable; in infancy mineralocorticoid supplementation is of particular importance); congenital adrenal hyperplasia; hypercalcemia associated with cancer; nonsuppurative thyroiditis.

2. Rheumatic Disorders
As adjunctive therapy for short term administration (to tide the patient over an acute episode or exacerbation) in: psoriatic arthritis; rheumatoid arthritis, including juvenile rheumatoid arthritis (selected cases may require low dose maintenance therapy); ankylosing spondylitis; acute and subacute bursitis; acute nonspecific tenosynovitis; acute gouty arthritis; post-traumatic osteoarthritis; synovitis of osteoarthritis; epicondylitis.

3. Collagen Diseases
During an exacerbation or as maintenance therapy in selected cases of: systemic lupus erythematosus; systemic dermatomyositis (polymyositis); acute rheumatic carditis.

4. Dermatologic Diseases
Pemphigus; bullous dermatitis herpetiformis; severe erythema multiforme (Stevens-Johnson syndrome); exfoliative dermatitis; mycosis fungoides; severe psoriasis; severe seborrheic dermatitis.

5. Allergic States
Control of severe or incapacitating allergic conditions intractable to adequate trials of conventional treatment in: seasonal or perennial allergic rhinitis; bronchial asthma; contact dermatitis; atopic dermatitis; serum sickness; drug hypersensitivity reactions.

6. Ophthalmic Diseases
Severe acute and chronic allergic and inflammatory processes involving the eye and its adnexa such as: allergic conjunctivitis; keratitis; allergic corneal marginal ulcers; herpes zoster ophthalmicus; iritis and iridocyclitis; chorioretinitis; anterior segment inflammation; diffuse posterior uveitis and choroiditis; optic neuritis; sympathetic ophthalmia.

7. Respiratory Diseases
Symptomatic sarcoidosis; Loeffler's syndrome not manageable by other means; berylliosis; fulminating or disseminated pulmonary tuberculosis when used concurrently with appropriate antituberculous chemotherapy; aspiration pneumonitis.

8. Hematologic Disorders
Idiopathic thrombocytopenic purpura in adults; secondary thrombocytopenia in adults; acquired (autoimmune) hemolytic anemia; erythroblastopenia (RBC anemia); congenital (erythroid) hypoplastic anemia.

9. Neoplastic Diseases
For palliative management of: leukemias and lymphomas in adults; acute leukemia of childhood.

10. Edematous States
To induce a diuresis or remission of proteinuria in the nephrotic syndrome, without uremia, of the idiopathic type or that due to lupus erythematosus.

11. Gastrointestinal Diseases
To tide the patient over a critical period of the disease in: ulcerative colitis; regional enteritis.

12. Nervous System
Acute exacerbations of multiple sclerosis.

13. Miscellaneous
Tuberculous meningitis with subarachnoid block or impending block when used concurrently with appropriate antituberculous chemotherapy; trichinosis with neurologic or myocardial involvement.

CONTRAINDICATIONS

Systemic fungal infections.

WARNINGS

In patients on corticosteroid therapy subjected to unusual stress, increased dosage of rapidly acting corticosteroids before, during and after the stressful situation is indicated.

Corticosteroids may mask some signs of infection, and new infections may appear during their use. There may be decreased resistance and inability to localize infection when corticosteroids are used.

Prolonged use of corticosteroids may produce posterior subcapsular cataracts, glaucoma with possible damage to the optic nerves, and may enhance the establishment of secondary ocular infections due to fungi or viruses.

Average and large doses of hydrocortisone or cortisone can cause elevation of blood pressure, salt and water retention, and increased excretion of potassium. These effects are less likely to occur with the synthetic derivatives except when used in large doses. Dietary salt restriction and potassium supplementation may be necessary. All corticosteroids increase calcium excretion. **While on corticosteroid therapy patients should not be vaccinated against smallpox. Other immunization procedures should not be undertaken in patients who are on corticosteroids, especially on high doses, because of possible hazards of neurological complications and a lack of antibody response.**

The use of prednisolone in active tuberculosis should be restricted to those cases of fulminating or disseminated tuberculosis in which the corticosteroid is used for the management of the disease in conjunction with an appropriate antituberculous regimen.

If corticosteroids are indicated in patients with latent tuberculosis or tuberculin reactivity, close observation is necessary as reactivation of the disease may occur. During prolonged corticosteroid therapy these patients should receive chemoprophylaxis.

Persons who are on drugs which suppress the immune system are more susceptible to infections than healthy individuals. Chicken pox and measles, for example, can have a more serious or even fatal course in non-immune children or adults on corticosteroids. In such children or adults who have not had these diseases, particular care should be taken to avoid exposure. How the dose, route and duration of corticosteroid administration affects the risk of developing a disseminated infection is not known. The contribution of the underlying disease and/or prior corticosteroid treatment to the risk is also not known. If exposed to chicken pox, prophylaxis with varicella zoster immune globulin (VZIG) may be indicated. If exposed to measles, prophylaxis with pooled intramuscular immunoglobulin (IG) may be indicated. (See the respective package inserts for complete VZIG and IG prescribing information). If chicken pox develops, treatment with antiviral agents may be considered.

Similarly, corticosteroids should be used with great care in patients with known or suspected Strongyloides (threadworm) infestation. In such patients, corticosteroid-induced immunosuppression may lead to Strongyloides hyperinfection and dissemination with widespread larval migration, often accompanied by severe enterocolitis and potentially fatal gram-negative septicemia.

PRECAUTIONS

General: Drug-induced secondary adrenocortical insufficiency may be minimized by gradual reduction of dosage. This type of relative insufficiency may persist for months after discontinuation of therapy; therefore, in any situation of stress occurring during that period, hormone therapy should be reinstituted. Since mineralocorticoid secretion may be impaired, salt and/or a mineralocorticoid should be administered concurrently.

There is an enhanced effect of corticosteroids in patients with hypothyroidism and in those with cirrhosis.

Corticosteroids should be used cautiously in patients with ocular herpes simplex because of possible corneal perforation.

The lowest possible dose of corticosteroid should be used to control the condition under treatment, and when reduction in dosage is possible, the reduction should be gradual.

Psychic derangements may appear when corticosteroids are used, ranging from euphoria, insomnia, mood swings, personality changes, and severe depression, to frank psychotic manifestations. Also, existing emotional instability or psychotic tendencies may be aggravated by corticosteroids.

Aspirin should be used cautiously in conjunction with corticosteroids in hypoprothrombinemia.

Steroids should be used with caution in nonspecific ulcerative colitis, if there is a probability of impending perforation, abscess or other pyogenic infection; diverticulitis; fresh intestinal anastomoses; active or latent peptic ulcer; renal insufficiency; hypertension; osteoporosis; and myasthenia gravis.

Growth and development of infants and children on prolonged corticosteroid therapy should be carefully observed.

Although controlled clinical trials have shown corticosteroids to be effective in speeding the resolution of acute exacerbations of multiple sclerosis, they do not show that they affect the ultimate outcome or natural history of the disease. The studies do show that relatively high doses of corticosteroids are necessary to demonstrate a significant effect. (See DOSAGE AND ADMINISTRATION.)

Since complications of treatment with glucocorticoids are dependent on the size of the dose and the duration of treatment, a risk/benefit decision must be made in each individual case as to dose and duration of treatment and as to whether daily or intermittent therapy should be used.

Information for Patients: Patients should be warned not to discontinue the use of PEDIAPRED abruptly or without medical supervision, to advise any medical attendants that they are taking PEDIAPRED and to seek medical advice at once should they develop fever or other signs of infection.

Persons who are on immunosuppressant doses of corticosteroids should be warned to avoid exposure to chicken pox or measles. Patients should also be advised that if they are exposed, medical advice should be sought without delay.

Drug Interactions: Drugs such as barbiturates which induce hepatic microsomal drug metabolizing enzyme activity may enhance metabolism of prednisolone and require that the dosage of PEDIAPRED be increased.

Pregnancy: Pregnancy Category C—Prednisolone has been shown to be teratogenic in many species when given in doses equivalent to the human dose. There are no adequate and well controlled studies in pregnant women. PEDIAPRED should be used during pregnancy only if the potential benefit justifies the potential risk to the fetus. Animal studies in which prednisolone has been given to pregnant mice, rats and rabbits have yielded an increased incidence of cleft palate in the offspring.

Nursing Mothers: Prednisolone is excreted in breast milk, but only to a small (less than 1% of the administered dose) and probably clinically insignificant extent. Caution should be exercised when PEDIAPRED is administered to a nursing woman.

ADVERSE REACTIONS

Fluid and Electrolyte Disturbances
Sodium retention; fluid retention; congestive heart failure in susceptible patients; potassium loss; hypokalemic alkalosis; hypertension.

Musculoskeletal
Muscle weakness; steroid myopathy; loss of muscle mass; osteoporosis; vertebral compression fractures; aseptic necrosis of femoral and humeral heads; pathologic fracture of long bones.

Gastrointestinal
Peptic ulcer with possible perforation and hemorrhage; pancreatitis; abdominal distention; ulcerative esophagitis.

Continued on next page

Information on the Medeva Pharmaceuticals, Inc. products listed on these pages contains the full prescribing information from product circulars in use as of July 1996. For further information, please consult the package insert currently accompanying the product.

Medeva Pharmaceuticals, Inc.—Cont.

Dermatologic
Impaired wound healing; thin fragile skin; petechiae and ecchymoses; facial erythema; increased sweating; may suppress reactions to skin tests.

Metabolic
Negative nitrogen balance due to protein catabolism.

Neurological
Convulsions; increased intracranial pressure with papilledema (pseudotumor cerebri) usually after treatment; vertigo; headache.

Endocrine
Menstrual irregularities; development of cushingoid state; secondary adrenocortical and pituitary unresponsiveness, particularly in times of stress, as in trauma, surgery or illness; suppression of growth in children; decreased carbohydrate tolerance; manifestations of latent diabetes mellitus; increased requirements for insulin or oral hypoglycemic agents in diabetes.

Ophthalmic
Posterior subcapsular cataracts; increased intraocular pressure; glaucoma; exophthalmos.

OVERDOSAGE

The effects of accidental ingestion of large quantities of prednisolone over a very short period of time have not been reported, but prolonged use of the drug can produce mental symptoms, moon face, abnormal fat deposits, fluid retention, excessive appetite, weight gain, hypertrichosis, acne, striae, ecchymosis, increased sweating, pigmentation, dry scaly skin, thinning scalp hair, increased blood pressure, tachycardia, thrombophlebitis, decreased resistance to infection, negative nitrogen balance with delayed bone and wound healing, headache, weakness, menstrual disorders, accentuated menopausal symptoms, neuropathy, fractures, osteoporosis, peptic ulcer, decreased glucose tolerance, hypokalemia, and adrenal insufficiency. Hepatomegaly and abdominal distention have been observed in children.

Treatment of acute overdosage is by immediate gastric lavage or emesis. For chronic overdosage in the face of severe disease requiring continuous steroid therapy the dosage of prednisolone may be reduced only temporarily, or alternate day treatment may be introduced.

DOSAGE AND ADMINISTRATION

The initial dosage of PEDIAPRED may vary from 5 mL to 60 mL (5 to 60 mg prednisolone base) per day depending on the specific disease entity being treated. In situations of less severity lower doses will generally suffice while in selected patients higher initial doses may be required. The initial dosage should be maintained or adjusted until a satisfactory response is noted. If after a reasonable period of time there is a lack of satisfactory clinical response, PEDIAPRED should be discontinued and the patient transferred to other appropriate therapy. IT SHOULD BE EMPHASIZED THAT DOSAGE REQUIREMENTS ARE VARIABLE AND MUST BE INDIVIDUALIZED ON THE BASIS OF THE DISEASE UNDER TREATMENT AND THE RESPONSE OF THE PATIENT. After a favorable response is noted, the proper maintenance dosage should be determined by decreasing the initial drug dosage in small decrements at appropriate time intervals until the lowest dosage which will maintain an adequate clinical response is reached. It should be kept in mind that constant monitoring is needed in regard to drug dosage. Included in the situations which may make dosage adjustments necessary are changes in clinical status secondary to remissions or exacerbations in the disease process, the patient's individual drug responsiveness, and the effect of patient exposure to stressful situations not directly related to the disease entity under treatment; in this latter situation it may be necessary to increase the dosage of PEDIAPRED for a period of time consistent with the patient's condition. If after long term therapy the drug is to be stopped, it is recommended that it be withdrawn gradually rather than abruptly.

In the treatment of acute exacerbations of multiple sclerosis daily doses of 200 mg of prednisolone for a week followed by 80 mg every other day or 4 to 8 mg dexamethasone every other day for one month have been shown to be effective.

For the purpose of comparison, the following is the equivalent milligram dosage of the various glucocorticoids: cortisone, 25; hydrocortisone, 20; prednisolone, 5; prednisone, 5; methylprednisolone, 4; triamcinolone, 4; paramethasone, 2; betamethasone, 0.75; dexamethasone, 0.75. These dose relationships apply only to oral or intravenous administration of these compounds. When these substances or their derivatives are injected intramuscularly or into joint spaces, their relative properties may be greatly altered.

HOW SUPPLIED

PEDIAPRED (prednisolone sodium phosphate, USP) Oral Solution is a colorless to light straw colored solution containing 6.7 mg prednisolone sodium phosphate (5 mg prednisolone base) per 5 mL (teaspoonful).

NDC 53014-250-01   120 mL bottle

Store at 4°–25°C (39°–77°F). May be refrigerated. Keep tightly closed and out of the reach of children.

CAUTION: Federal law prohibits dispensing without prescription.

MEDEVA PHARMACEUTICALS
Medeva Pharmaceuticals, Inc.
Fort Worth, TX 76155   7/96
® Fisons Corp.   R024H
© 1996, Medeva Pharmaceuticals Manufacturing, Inc.

SEMPREX™-D Capsules ℞
(acrivastine and pseudoephedrine hydrochloride)

CAUTION: Federal law prohibits dispensing without prescription.

DESCRIPTION

SEMPREX-D Capsules (acrivastine and pseudoephedrine HCl) are a fixed combination product formulated for oral administration. Acrivastine is an antihistamine and pseudoephedrine is a decongestant. Each capsule contains 8 mg acrivastine and 60 mg pseudoephedrine HCl and the inactive ingredients: lactose, magnesium stearate and sodium starch glycolate. The green and white capsule shell consists of gelatin, D&C Yellow No. 10, FD&C Green No. 3, and titanium dioxide. The yellow band around the capsule consists of gelatin and D&C Yellow No. 10. The capsules may contain one or more parabens and are printed with edible black and white inks.

The chemical name of acrivastine is (E,E)-3-[6-[1-(4-methylphenyl) -3- (1-pyrrolidinyl)-1-propenyl]-2-pyridinyl] -2-propenoic acid; the molecular formula is $C_{22}H_{24}N_2O_2$. As an analog of triprolidine hydrochloride, acrivastine is classified as an alkylamine antihistamine. Acrivastine is an odorless, white to pale cream crystalline powder that is soluble in chloroform and alcohol and slightly soluble in water.

The chemical name of pseudoephedrine hydrochloride is $[S\text{-}(R^*,R^*)]$ -α- [1-(methylamino)ethyl] benzenemethanol hydrochloride; the molecular formula is $C_{10}H_{15}NO\cdot HCl$. Pseudoephedrine is one of the naturally occurring dextrorotatory diastereoisomers of ephedrine and is classified as an indirect sympathomimetic amine. Pseudoephedrine hydrochloride occurs as odorless, fine white to off-white crystals or powder; the drug is soluble in water, alcohol and chloroform.

Structural formulae for the active ingredients of SEMPREX-D Capsules are as follows:

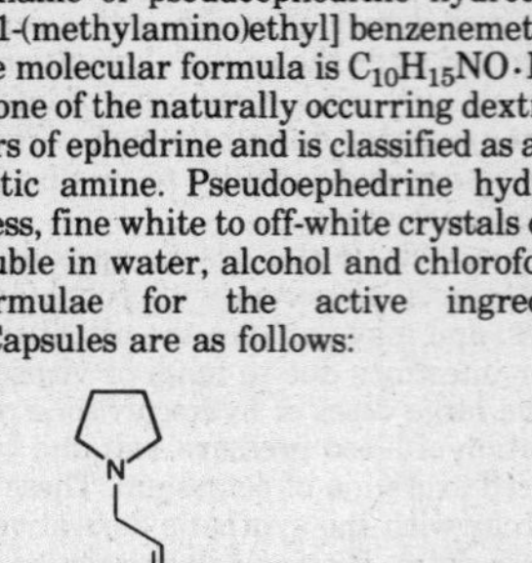

(a) Acrivastine
(Molecular Weight = 348.44)

(b) Pseudoephedrine hydrochloride
(Molecular Weight = 201.70)

CLINICAL PHARMACOLOGY

Acrivastine, a structural analog of triprolidine hydrochloride, exhibits H_1-antihistaminic activity in isolated tissues, animals, and humans, and has sedative effects in humans (see PRECAUTIONS). The propionic acid derivative of acrivastine is a metabolite in several animal species (as well as in man) and also exhibits H_1-antihistaminic activity.

Pseudoephedrine hydrochloride is an indirect sympathomimetic agent; that is, it releases norepinephrine from adrenergic nerves.

In vitro tests and in vivo studies in animals of acrivastine and pseudoephedrine in combination failed to demonstrate evidence of any beneficial or deleterious pharmacologic interaction between the two agents.

Pharmacokinetics and Metabolism

Acrivastine was absorbed rapidly from the combination capsule following oral administration and was as bioavailable as a solution of acrivastine. After administration of SEMPREX-D Capsules, maximum plasma acrivastine concentrations were achieved at 1.14 ± 0.23 hour. A mass balance study in 7 healthy volunteers showed that acrivastine is primarily eliminated by the kidneys. Over a 72-hour collection period, about 84% of the administered total radioactivity was recovered in urine and about 13% in feces, for a combined recovery of about 97%. Further, 67% of the administered radioactive dose was recovered in urine as the

unchanged drug, 11% as the propionic acid metabolite, and 6% as other unknown metabolites.

Acrivastine exhibits linear kinetics over dosages ranging from 2 to 32 mg t.i.d. The mean $\pm$SD terminal half-life for acrivastine was 1.9 ± 0.3 hours following single oral doses and increased to 3.5 ± 1.9 hours at steady state. The terminal half-life for the propionic acid metabolite was 3.8 ± 1.4 hours. Because of the short half-lives of both acrivastine and its metabolites, accumulation in the plasma following multiple dosing is not expected.

The steady-state maximum acrivastine plasma concentration was 227 ± 47 ng/mL. The oral clearance and apparent volume of distribution were 2.9 ± 0.7 mL/min/kg and 0.46 ± 0.05 L/kg, respectively, following a single oral dose; oral clearance did not change at steady state (2.86 ± 0.75 mL/min/kg). The apparent volume of distribution increased to 0.82 ± 0.6 L/kg to parallel the increase in the elimination half-life of the drug.

Acrivastine binding to human plasma proteins was $50 \pm 2.0\%$ and was concentration-independent over the range of 5 to 1000 ng/mL. The main binding protein was serum albumin although the drug was slightly bound to α1-acid glycoprotein. No displacement interaction was observed between acrivastine and either phenytoin or theophylline. The binding of acrivastine was not affected by the presence of pseudoephedrine.

Pseudoephedrine hydrochloride was also rapidly absorbed from the combination capsule, and the capsule was as bioavailable as a solution of pseudoephedrine. Steady state maximum plasma concentration for pseudoephedrine was 498 ± 129 ng/mL. The terminal half-life, oral clearance and apparent volume of distribution were 6.2 ± 1.8 hour, 5.9 ± 1.7 mL/min/kg, and 3.0 ± 0.4 L/kg, respectively. Elimination of pseudoephedrine is primarily through the renal route as 55 to 75% of an administered dose appears unchanged in the urine. Pseudoephedrine elimination, however, is highly dependent upon urine pH; the plasma half-life decreased to about 4 hours at pH 5 and increased to 13 hours at pH 8. Pseudoephedrine did not bind to human plasma proteins over the concentration range of 50 to 2000 ng/mL.

Acrivastine and pseudoephedrine do not influence the pharmacokinetics of the other drug when administered concomitantly.

Special Populations

A single dose pharmacokinetic study showed that the elimination half-lives of acrivastine, the propionic acid metabolite of acrivastine, and pseudoephedrine were prolonged in patients with chronic renal insufficiency. Compared to normal volunteers, the elimination half-life of acrivastine was about 50% increased in patients with mild renal insufficiency (creatinine clearance = 26 to 48 mL/min) and was increased by about 130% in patients with moderate (creatinine clearance = 12 to 17 mL/min) or severe (creatinine clearance 6 to 10 mL/min) renal insufficiency. Oral clearance of acrivastine was diminished by the same magnitude as the half-life was prolonged in each of the three renally impaired groups. The elimination half-life of the propionic acid metabolite of acrivastine was about 140% increased in patients with mild renal insufficiency and about 5 times increased in patients with moderate or severe renal insufficiency.

Compared to normal volunteers, the elimination half-life of pseudoephedrine was about 3 times increased in patients with mild renal insufficiency, about 7 times increased in patients with moderate renal insufficiency, and about 10 times increased in patients with severe renal insufficiency. Oral clearance of pseudoephedrine was diminished by about the same magnitude as the half-life was prolonged in each of the three renally impaired groups (see PRECAUTIONS, Use in Patients with Diminished Renal Function).

The total body load removed by dialysis is approximately 20%, 27% and 38% for acrivastine, the propionic acid metabolite of acrivastine, and pseudoephedrine, respectively, and, therefore, a supplemental dose after a dialysis session is not required.

Based on a multiple dose cross study comparison, the apparent volume of distribution for acrivastine was 44% lower in elderly (n=36, 65–75 yr) than in young volunteers (n=16, 19–33 yr). This difference could be attributed to the decrease in total body water that occurs with aging. Despite this difference, no appreciable differences in plasma acrivastine concentrations were seen in the elderly compared to the young, and no appreciable accumulation of acrivastine occurred in plasma at steady-state. The elimination half-life for pseudoephedrine was 18% longer in elderly (7.9 hours) than in younger subjects (6.7 hours), presumably due to the decline in average renal function that occurs with aging. Despite this difference, clearance of pseudoephedrine was not appreciably different in elderly and younger subjects. Elderly patients should therefore be given the same dosage as younger patients. SEMPREX-D Capsules are not recommended, however, in patients with renal impairment (see PRECAUTIONS, Use in Patients with Diminished Renal Function).

The effect of age and sex on the pharmacokinetic parameters of acrivastine and pseudoephedrine was determined in 93 healthy volunteers who participated in various studies. All

of the 93 volunteers were Caucasian (81 males and 12 females); 57 were between the ages of 18 and 38 years and 36 were between the ages of 65 and 75 years. There were no age- or sex-related differences in the pharmacokinetic parameters of either acrivastine or pseudoephedrine.

The effect of race on acrivastine and pseudoephedrine pharmacokinetics was examined by screening data obtained from 1035 patients, age 12 to 71 years, who participated in the 8 safety and efficacy studies. No race-related differences were observed in the pharmacokinetics of either acrivastine or pseudoephedrine.

Clinical Studies

In healthy volunteers, histamine-induced wheal and flare areas were significantly reduced relative to placebo at 30 minutes after administration of a single dose of acrivastine 8 mg. Maximum reductions of wheal and flare occurred by 1 to 2 hours and significant reductions relative to placebo persisted for up to 6 hours after a single oral dose of acrivastine 8 mg. No additional reductions of wheal and flare were observed following single doses of acrivastine up to 24 mg. The exact correlation between responses on skin testing and clinical efficacy is not established.

Five randomized, placebo- and/or active-controlled trials compared SEMPREX-D with its acrivastine and pseudoephedrine components for the symptomatic relief of seasonal allergic rhinitis. In these studies, 696 patients received four daily doses of acrivastine 8 mg plus pseudoephedrine hydrochloride 60 mg (i.e., SEMPREX-D Capsules or bioequivalent formulations administered concurrently) or the same doses of the components for 14 days. The combination reduced the intensity of sneezing, rhinorrhea, pruritus, and lacrimation more than pseudoephedrine and reduced the intensity of nasal congestion more than acrivastine, demonstrating a contribution of each of the components. The onset of antihistaminic and nasal decongestant actions occurred within one or two hours after the first dose of SEMPREX-D Capsules. Somnolence occurred in about 12% of patients given SEMPREX-D compared with about 6% on placebo.

INDICATIONS AND USAGE

SEMPREX-D Capsules are indicated for relief of symptoms associated with seasonal allergic rhinitis such as sneezing, rhinorrhea, pruritus, lacrimation, and nasal congestion. SEMPREX-D Capsules should be administered when both the antihistaminic activity of acrivastine and the nasal decongestant activity of pseudoephedrine are desired (see CLINICAL PHARMACOLOGY). The efficacy of SEMPREX-D Capsules beyond 14 days of continuous treatment in patients with seasonal allergic rhinitis has not been adequately investigated in clinical trials.

SEMPREX-D Capsules have not been adequately studied for effectiveness in relieving the symptoms of the common cold.

CONTRAINDICATIONS

SEMPREX-D Capsules are contraindicated in patients with a known sensitivity to acrivastine, other alkylamine antihistamines (e.g., triprolidine), pseudoephedrine, other sympathomimetic amines (e.g., phenylpropanolamine), or to any other components of the formulation. SEMPREX-D Capsules are contraindicated in patients with severe hypertension or severe coronary artery disease. SEMPREX-D Capsules are contraindicated in patients taking monoamine oxidase (MAO) inhibitors and for two weeks after stopping use of an MAO inhibitor (see Drug Interactions).

WARNINGS

SEMPREX-D Capsules should be used with caution in patients with hypertension, diabetes mellitus, ischemic heart disease, increased intraocular pressure, hyperthyroidism, prostatic hypertrophy, stenosing peptic ulcer, or pyloroduodenal obstruction. Overdose of sympathomimetic amines may produce CNS stimulation with convulsions or cardiovascular collapse with accompanying hypotension. The elderly are more likely to have adverse reactions to sympathomimetic amines.

PRECAUTIONS

General: Acrivastine is sedating in some patients. In controlled clinical trials, somnolence (i.e., drowsiness, sedation, sleepiness) was more common with SEMPREX-D Capsules (by an average of 6%) than with placebo (see ADVERSE EXPERIENCES).

Patients should be advised to assess their individual responses to SEMPREX-D Capsules before engaging in any activity requiring mental alertness, such as driving a motor vehicle or operating machinery. Concurrent use of SEMPREX-D Capsules with alcohol or other CNS depressants may cause additional reductions in alertness and impairment of CNS performance and should be avoided (see Drug Interactions).

Use in Patients with Diminished Renal Function: Acrivastine and pseudoephedrine are excreted primarily through the kidney. Both compounds therefore accumulate in patients with impaired renal function. Due to the differential effects of renal failure on the serum half-life and clearance of acrivastine and pseudoephedrine, use of SEMPREX-D Capsules, a fixed combination product, in patients with renal impairment (creatinine clearance ≤ 48 mL/min) is not recommended (see OVERDOSAGE and CLINICAL PHARMACOLOGY).

ADVERSE EVENTS REPORTED IN CLINICAL TRIALS* (PERCENT OF PATIENTS REPORTING)†

	Controlled Studies			
	Placebo (N=1767)	Acrivastine (N=1935)	Pseudoephedrine (N=887)	Acrivastine plus Pseudoephedrine (N=1650)
CNS				
Somnolence‡	6	12	8	12
Headache	18	19	19	19
Dizziness	2	3	3	3
Nervousness‡	1	2	4	3
Insomnia	1	1	6	4
MISCELLANEOUS				
Nausea	2	3	3	2
Dry Mouth‡	2	3	5	7
Asthenia	2	3	2	2
Dyspepsia	1	1	2	2
Pharyngitis	2	1	1	3
Cough Increase	1	2	1	2
Dysmenorrhea	1	2	3	2

* Includes all events regardless of causal relationship to treatment.
† Includes all adverse events with a reported frequency of > 1% for the acrivastine plus pseudoephedrine treatment group.
‡ SEMPREX-D demonstrates a statistically higher frequency of events than placebo. p ≤0.05.

Information to Patients: Patients taking SEMPREX-D Capsules should receive the following information. SEMPREX-D Capsules are prescribed to reduce symptoms associated with seasonal allergic rhinitis. Patients should be instructed to take SEMPREX-D Capsules only as prescribed and not to exceed the prescribed dose. Patients should be advised against the concurrent use of SEMPREX-D with over-the-counter antihistamines and decongestants. Patients who are or may become pregnant should be told that this product should be used in pregnancy or during lactation only if the potential benefit justifies the potential risks to the fetus or nursing infant. Due to the risk of hypertensive crisis, patients should be instructed not to take SEMPREX-D Capsules if they are presently taking a monoamine oxidase inhibitor or for two weeks after stopping use of a MAO inhibitor. Patients should be advised to assess their individual responses to SEMPREX-D Capsules before engaging in any activity requiring mental alertness, such as driving a car or operating machinery. Patients should be advised that the concurrent use of SEMPREX-D Capsules with alcohol and other CNS depressants may lead to additional reductions in alertness and impairment of CNS performance and should be avoided.

Use in the Elderly (Approximately 60 Years or Older): Elderly patients who participated in clinical trials did not differ in effectiveness or adverse effects from younger patients. Antihistamines, however, as a pharmaceutical class, are more likely to cause dizziness, sedation, bladder-neck obstruction, and hypotension in elderly patients. The elderly are also more likely to have adverse reactions to sympathomimetics such as pseudoephedrine (see CLINICAL PHARMACOLOGY and WARNINGS).

Drug Interactions: MAO inhibitors and beta-adrenergic agonists increase the effects of sympathomimetic amines. Concomitant use of sympathomimetic amines with MAO inhibitors can result in a hypertensive crisis (see CONTRAINDICATIONS). Because MAO inhibitors are long-acting, SEMPREX-D Capsules should not be taken with a MAO inhibitor or for two weeks after stopping use of a MAO inhibitor.

Because of their pseudoephedrine content, SEMPREX-D Capsules may reduce the antihypertensive effects of drugs that interfere with sympathetic activity. Care should be taken in the administration of SEMPREX-D Capsules concomitantly with other sympathomimetic amines because the combined effects of the cardiovascular system may be harmful to the patient.

Concomitant administration of SEMPREX-D Capsules with alcohol and other CNS depressants may result in additional reduction in alertness and impairment of CNS performance and should be avoided.

No formal drug interaction studies between SEMPREX-D Capsules and other possibly co-administered drugs have been performed.

Carcinogenesis, Mutagenesis, and Impairment of Fertility: Carcinogenicity studies with the combination of acrivastine and pseudoephedrine have not been performed. Oral doses of acrivastine alone at levels up to 40 mg/kg/day (236 mg/m^2/day or 10 times the recommended human daily dose) for 20 to 22 months in rats and up to 250 mg/kg/day (750 mg/m^2/day or 32 times the recommended human daily dose) for 20 to 24 months in mice revealed no evidence of carcinogenic potential. No evidence of mutagenicity (with or without metabolic activation) was observed in the Ames Salmonella mutagenicity assay or in the L5178Y/tk$^{+/-}$ mouse lymphoma assay. In an in vitro cytogenetic study performed in cultured human lymphocytes, acrivastine induced structural chromosomal abnormalities in the absence of metabolic activation, but not in its presence. In an in vivo cytogenetic study in rats given single oral doses of acrivastine up to 1000 mg/kg (5900 mg/m^2 or 249 times the recommended human daily dose) there were no structural chromosomal alterations.

Reproduction-fertility studies in rats given acrivastine alone at levels up to 200 mg/kg/day (1180 mg/m^2/day or 50 times the recommended human daily dose) had no effect on male or female fertility. Similarly, no effect on fertility was seen in male rats given acrivastine 20 mg/kg/day and pseudoephedrine 100 mg/kg/day (118 and 590 mg/m^2/day or 5 and 3 times the recommended human daily doses, respectively) or in female rats given acrivastine 4 mg/kg/day and pseudoephedrine 20 mg/kg/day (23.6 and 118 mg/m^2/day or 1 and 0.7 times the recommended human daily doses, respectively).

Pregnancy: Pregnancy Category B:

Teratogenic Effects: No evidence of teratogenicity was seen in rats and rabbits given acrivastine 1000 and 400 mg/kg/day, respectively (5900 and 4720 mg/m^2/day or 249 and 200 times the recommended human daily dose). No evidence of teratogenicity was seen in rats given a combination of acrivastine 30 mg/kg/day and pseudoephedrine 150 mg/kg/day (177 and 885 mg/m^2/day or 8 and 5 times the recommended human daily dose, respectively). Similarly, no evidence of teratogenicity was observed in rabbits given acrivastine 20 mg/kg/day and pseudoephedrine 100 mg/kg/day (236 and 1180 mg/m^2/day or 10 and 7 times the recommended human daily dose, respectively). There are, however, no adequate and well-controlled studies in pregnant women. Because animal teratology studies are not always predictive of human responses, SEMPREX-D Capsules should be used during pregnancy only if the potential benefit justifies the potential risks to the fetus.

Nonteratogenic Effects: In a perinatal-postnatal study in rats, acrivastine given alone at levels up to 500 mg/kg/day (2950 mg/m^2/day or 124 times the recommended human daily dose) was associated with maternal and neonatal mortality at the maximum dose level. Neonatal survival was decreased in rats given a combination of acrivastine 20 mg/kg/day and pseudoephedrine 100 mg/kg/day (118 and 590 mg/m^2/day or 5 and 3 times the human dose respectively).

Nursing Mothers: It is not known whether acrivastine is excreted in human milk; pseudoephedrine is excreted in human milk. SEMPREX-D Capsules should only be used in nursing mothers when the potential benefit justifies the potential risks to the nursing infant.

Pediatric Use: Safety and effectiveness of SEMPREX-D Capsules in children under the age of 12 years have not been established.

ADVERSE EXPERIENCES

Information on the incidence of adverse events in clinical investigations conducted in the U.S. was obtained from 33 controlled and 15 uncontrolled clinical studies in which 2499 patients received acrivastine and 2631 patients received acrivastine plus pseudoephedrine hydrochloride for treatment periods ranging from one day to one year. The majority of patients in clinical trials were exposed to acrivastine or acrivastine plus pseudoephedrine for less than 90 days. Acrivastine dosages ranged from 3 to 96 mg/day; 1336 patients received dosages equal to or greater than acrivastine

Continued on next page

Information on the Medeva Pharmaceuticals, Inc. products listed on these pages contains the full prescribing information from product circulars in use as of July 1996. For further information, please consult the package insert currently accompanying the product.

Medeva Pharmaceuticals, Inc.—Cont.

24 mg/day. Acrivastine plus pseudoephedrine hydrochloride dosages ranged from acrivastine 8 to 48 mg/day plus pseudoephedrine hydrochloride 60 to 240 mg/day. A total of 2335 patients received three or four daily doses of acrivastine 8 mg plus pseudoephedrine hydrochloride 60 mg.

In controlled clinical trials, only 12 spontaneously elicited adverse events were reported with frequencies greater than 1% in the acrivastine plus pseudoephedrine hydrochloride treatment group (see table).

[See table on top of preceding page.]

The nature and overall frequencies of adverse events from international clinical trials (35 studies involving approximately 1600 patients) were similar to the results obtained in the U.S. studies.

Post-marketing clinical experience reports with acrivastine and acrivastine plus pseudoephedrine have included rare serious hypersensitivity reactions manifested by anaphylaxis, angioedema, bronchospasm, and erythema multiforme. No deaths associated with use of acrivastine or acrivastine plus pseudoephedrine have been reported.

Pseudoephedrine may cause ephedrine-like reactions such tachycardia, palpitations, headache, dizziness, or nausea (see WARNINGS and OVERDOSAGE).

OVERDOSAGE

There have been no reports of overdosage with SEMPREX-D Capsules. In the clinical trial program and in international post-marketing experience, there have been two reported overdoses with acrivastine. Doses were 72 mg and 322 mg. Both patients recovered without sequelae. Adverse events included trembling, loss of consciousness and possible convulsions in the first patient and somnolence in the second.

Since acrivastine and pseudoephedrine have pharmacologically different actions, it is difficult to predict how an individual will respond to overdosage with SEMPREX-D Capsules. However, acute overdosage with SEMPREX-D Capsules may produce clinical signs of either CNS stimulation or depression. Overdosage of sympathomimetics has been associated with the following events: fear, anxiety, tenseness, restlessness, tremor, weakness, pallor, respiratory difficulty, dysuria, insomnia, hallucinations, convulsions, CNS depression, arrhythmias, and cardiovascular collapse with hypotension. Treatment for overdosage with SEMPREX-D Capsules should follow general symptomatic and supportive principles.

In a placebo-controlled, double-bind clinical trial in 18 healthy male subjects, single doses of acrivastine up to 400 mg (50 times the recommended antihistaminic dose) produced only a weak vagolytic effect, manifested as an increase in heart rate, and did not cause cardiac repolarization delays (i.e., increased QTc). Daily doses of acrivastine up to 2400 mg (75 times the recommended antihistamine dose) in an uncontrolled study in 38 cancer patients produced a 15 beats per minute increase in mean heart rate and occasional episodes of nausea and vomiting. The effects of acrivastine plus pseudoephedrine at single or multiple doses higher than the recommended daily dose of SEMPREX-D Capsules (i.e., 32 mg acrivastine plus 240 mg pseudoephedrine) on heart rate and cardiac repolarization have been investigated in clinical trials.

The mean LD_{50} (single, oral dose) of acrivastine is greater than 4000 mg/kg (23600 mg/m^2 or 1000 times the recommended human daily dose) in rats and greater than 1200 mg/kg (3600 mg/m^2 or 153 times the recommended human daily dose) in mice. The mean LD_{50} (single, oral dose) of pseudoephedrine hydrochloride is 2206 mg/kg (13015 mg/m^2 or 73 times the recommended human daily dose) in rats 726 mg/kg (2178 mg/m^2 or 12 times the recommended human daily dose) in mice. The toxic and lethal concentrations of acrivastine and pseudoephedrine in human biologic fluids are not known. Based upon pharmacokinetic screening data from clinical trials, the maximum plasma acrivastine concentration after dosing with acrivastine 8 mg was 393 ng/mL and the maximum plasma pseudoephedrine concentration after dosing with pseudoephedrine hydrochloride 60 mg was 1308 ng/mL.

DOSAGE AND ADMINISTRATION

The recommended dosage for adults and children 12 years and older is one capsule administered orally, every 4 to 6 hours four times a day.

HOW SUPPLIED

SEMPREX-D Capsules (dark green opaque cap and white opaque body with a yellow band) contain acrivastine 8 mg and pseudoephedrine hydrochloride 60 mg. The cap is printed with "Wellcome" and the unicorn logo in white ink, and the body is printed with "SEMPREX-D" in black ink.

Bottles of 100 (NDC 0081-0280-55).

The capsules should be stored at 15° to 25°C (59° to 77°F) in a dry place and protected from light.

U.S. Patent Nos. 4501893 and 4650807.

BURROUGHS WELLCOME CO.
Research Triangle Park, NC 27709
April 1994 466027

SYN™-Rx Tablets ℞
14 Day Treatment Regimen

DESCRIPTION

Each SYN-Rx 14 Day Treatment Regimen pack of 56 tablets consists of two different drug treatment phases as follows: an **A.M. Treatment Phase** comprised of 28 dark blue scored controlled-release tablets, each containing 60 mg pseudoephedrine HCl and 600 mg guaifenesin, embossed with "Adams/017"; and a **P.M. Treatment Phase** comprised of 28 light green scored controlled-release tablets, each containing 600 mg guaifenesin, embossed with "Adams/012".

SYN-Rx 14 Day Treatment Regimen contains ingredients of two therapeutic classes: nasal decongestant and expectorant. Pseudoephedrine hydrochloride is a nasal decongestant. Chemically, it is [S-(R*,R*)]-α-[1-(methylamino)ethyl] benzenemethanol hydrochloride and has the following structural formula:

Molecular weight = 207.70; chemical formula = $C_{10}H_{15}NO \cdot HCl$

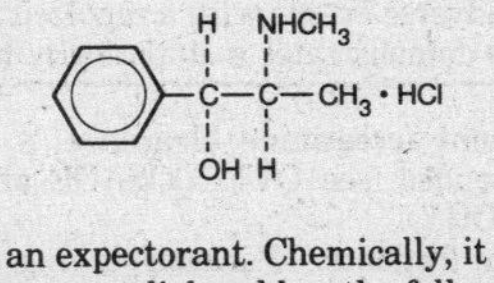

Guaifenesin is an expectorant. Chemically, it is 3-(2-methoxyphenoxy)-1, 2-propanediol and has the following structural formula:

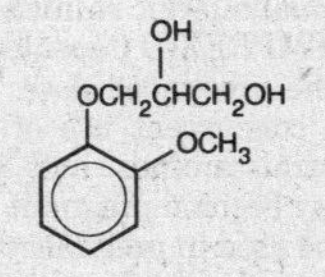

Molecular weight = 198.22; chemical formula = $C_{10}H_{14}O_4$

Inactive Ingredients: Each dark blue A.M. tablet and light green P.M. tablet contains stearic acid, dibasic calcium phosphate, sodium lauryl sulfate, ethylcellulose, magnesium stearate, FD&C Blue #1 Lake; each light green P.M. tablet also contains D & C Yellow #10 Lake.

CLINICAL PHARMACOLOGY

Pseudoephedrine hydrochloride is an orally indirect acting sympathomimetic amine and exerts a decongestant action on the nasal mucosa. It does this by vasoconstriction which results in reduction of tissue hyperemia, edema, nasal congestion, and an increase in nasal airway patency. In the usual dose it has minimal vasopressor effects. Pseudoephedrine is rapidly and almost completely absorbed from the gastrointestinal tract. It has a plasma half-life of 6 to 8 hours. Alkaline urine is associated with slower elimination of the drug. The drug is distributed to body tissues and fluids, including the central nervous system (CNS). Approximately 50% to 75% of the administered dose is excreted unchanged in the urine; the remainder is apparently metabolized in the liver to inactive compounds by N-demethylation, parahydroxylation and oxidative deamination.

Guaifenesin is an expectorant which increases respiratory tract fluid secretions and helps to loosen phlegm, bronchial and nasal secretions. By reducing the viscosity of secretions, guaifenesin increases the efficiency of the mucociliary mechanism in removing accumulated secretions from the upper and lower airway. Guaifenesin is readily absorbed from the gastrointestinal tract and is rapidly metabolized and excreted in the urine. Guaifenesin has a plasma half-life of one hour. The major urinary metabolite is β-(2-methoxyphenoxy) lactic acid.

INDICATIONS AND USAGE

SYN-Rx 14 Day Treatment Regimen is indicated for the temporary relief of nasal congestion associated with respiratory tract infections and related conditions such as sinusitis, bronchitis, and asthma, when these conditions are complicated by tenacious mucus, and/or mucus plugs and congestion. In the treatment of bacterial sinusitis this treatment regimen may be used concomitantly with appropriate antibiotic therapy.

CONTRAINDICATIONS

This product is contraindicated in patients with hypersensitivity to guaifenesin and pseudoephedrine HCl, or with hypersensitivity or idiosyncrasy to sympathomimetic amines which may be manifested by insomnia, dizziness, weakness, tremor or arrhythmias.

Sympathomimetic amines are contraindicated in patients with severe hypertension, severe coronary artery disease and patients on monoamine oxidase inhibitor (MAOI) therapy and for 14 days after stopping MAOI therapy. (see **Drug Interactions** section).

WARNINGS

Sympathomimetic amines should be used in caution in patients with hypertension, ischemic heart disease, diabetes mellitus, increased intraocular pressure, hyperthyroidism, or prostatic hypertrophy. Sympathomimetics may produce central nervous system stimulation with convulsions or cardiovascular collapse with accompanying hypotension. **Do not exceed recommended dosage.**

Hypertensive crises can occur with concurrent use of pseudoephedrine or phenylephrine and monoamine oxidase inhibitors (MAOI), and for 14 days after stopping the MAOI drug therapy, indomethacin, or with beta-blockers and methyldopa. If a hypertensive crisis occurs, these drugs should be discontinued immediately and therapy to lower blood pressure should be instituted. Fever should be managed by means of external cooling.

PRECAUTIONS

General: Use with caution in patients with diabetes, hypertension, cardiovascular disease and intolerance to ephedrine.

Failure of symptoms to completely resolve should alert the patient and physician that further diagnostic studies are indicated.

Pediatric Use: This product is not recommended for use in pediatric patients under 12 years of age.

Use in Elderly: The elderly (60 years and older) are more likely to experience adverse reactions to sympathomimetics. Overdosage of sympathomimetics in this age group may cause hallucinations, convulsions, CNS depression, and death.

Drug Interactions: Do not prescribe this product for use in patients that are now taking a monoamine oxidate inhibitor (MAOI) drug (certain drugs for depression, psychiatric or emotional conditions; or Parkinson's disease) or for 14 days after stopping the MAOI drug therapy. Beta-adrenergic blockers and inhibitors (MAOI) may potentiate the pressor effect of pseudoephedrine. Concurrent use of digitalis glycosides may increase the possibility of cardiac arrhythmias. Sympathomimetics may reduce the hypotensive effects of guanethidine, mecamylamine, methyldopa, reserpine and veratrum alkaloids. Concurrent use of tricylic antidepressants may antagonize the effects of pseudoephedrine.

Drug/Laboratory Test Interactions: Guaifenesin may increase renal clearance for urate and thereby lower serum uric acid levels. Guaifenesin may produce an increase in urinary 5-hydroxy-indoleacetic acid and may therefore interfere with the interpretation of this test for the diagnosis of carcinoid syndrome. It may also falsely elevate the VMA test for catechols. Administration of this drug should be discontinued 48 hours prior to the collection of urine specimens for such tests.

Carcinogenesis, Mutagenesis, Impairment of Fertility: No data are available on the long-term potential of the components of this product for carcinogenesis, mutagenesis, or impairment of fertility in animals or humans.

Pregnancy Category C: Animal reproduction studies have not been conducted with Syn™-Rx Tablets. It is also not known whether Syn-Rx Tablets can cause fetal harm when administered to a pregnant woman or can affect reproduction capacity. Syn-Rx Tablets should be given to a pregnant woman only if clearly needed.

Nursing Mothers: Pseudoephedrine is excreted in breast milk. Use of this product by nursing mothers is not recommended because of the higher than usual risk for pediatric patients from sympathomimetic amines.

ADVERSE REACTIONS

Some individuals may display sympathomimetic amine effects such as tachycardia, palpitations, headache, dizziness or nausea. Sympathomimetics have been associated with certain untoward reactions including fear, anxiety, nervousness, restlessness, tremor, weakness, pallor, respiratory difficulty, dysuria, insomnia, hallucinations, convulsions, CNS depression, arrhythmias, and cardiovascular collapse with hypotension. No serious side effects have been reported with the use of guaifenesin.

OVERDOSAGE

Since Syn-Rx 14 Day Treatment Regimen contains two pharmacologically different compounds, treatment of overdosage should be based upon the symptomatology of the patient as it relates to the individual ingredients. Treatment of acute overdosage would probably be based upon treating the patient for pseudoephedrine toxicity which may manifest itself as excessive CNS stimulation resulting in excitement, tremor, restlessness, and insomnia. Other effects may include tachycardia, hypertension, pallor, mydriasis, hyperglycemia and urinary retention. Severe overdosage may cause tachypnea or hyperpnea, hallucinations, convulsions or delirium, but in some individuals there may be CNS depression with somnolence, stupor or respiratory depression. Arrhythmias (including ventricular fibrillation) may lead to

hypotension and circulatory collapse. Severe hypokalemia can occur, probably due to a compartmental shift rather than a depletion of potassium. No organ damage or significant metabolic derangement is associated with pseudoephedrine overdosage. Overdosage with guaifenesin is unlikely to produce toxic effects since its toxicity is much lower than that of pseudoephedrine. In severe cases of overdosage, it is recommended to monitor the patient in an intensive care setting.

The LD_{50} of pseudoephedrine (single oral dose) has been reported to be 726 mg/kg in the mouse, 2206 mg/kg in the rat and 1177 mg/kg in the rabbit. The toxic and lethal concentrations in human biologic fluids are not known. Urinary excretion increases with acidification and decreases with alkalinization of the urine. There are few published reports of toxicity due to pseudoephedrine and no case of fatal overdosage has been reported. Guaifenesin, when administered by stomach tube to test animals in doses up to 5 grams/kg, produced no signs of toxicity.

Since the action of sustained release products may continue for as long as 12 hours, treatment of overdosage should be directed toward reducing further absorption and supporting the patient for at least that length of time. Gastric emptying (Syrup of Ipecac) and/or lavage is recommended as soon as possible after ingestion, even if the patient has vomited spontaneously. Either isotonic or half-isotonic saline may be used for lavage. Administration of an activated charcoal slurry is beneficial after lavage and/or emesis if less than 4 hours have passed since ingestion. Saline cathartics, such as Milk of Magnesia, are useful for hastening the evacuation of unreleased medication.

Adrenergic receptor blocking agents are antidotes to pseudoephedrine. In practice, the most useful is the beta-blocker propranolol which is indicated when there are signs of cardiac toxicity. Theoretically, pseudoepnedrine is dialyzable but procedures have not been clinically established.

DOSAGE AND ADMINISTRATION

Adults and adolescents over 12 years of age: 1 or 2 dark blue A.M. tablet(s) in the morning and 1 or 2 light green P.M. tablet(s) 12 hours later. Repeat A.M. and P.M. dosing cycle every 12 hours for 14 days.

Tablets should not be crushed or chewed prior to swallowing.

HOW SUPPLIED

NDC 53014-308-14 SYN-Rx 14 Day Treatment Regimen, is available as a shelf-pak consisting of three 14 Day Treatment Regiment packs. Each 14 Day Treatment Regimen contains 56 controlled-release tablets as follows:

NDC 53014-017, 28 dark blue elongated and scored A.M. tablets embossed with "Adams/017", each containing 60 mg pseudoephedrine HCl and 600 mg guaifenesin.

NDC 53014-012, 28 light green elongated and scored P.M. tablets embossed with "Adams/012", each containing 600 mg guaifenesin.

Store at controlled room temperature between 15°C and 30°C (59°F–86°F).

Dispense as a complete 14 day pack.

Caution: Federal law prohibits dispensing without prescription.

February 1996

SYN™-Rx DM Tablets ℞
14 Day Treatment Regimen

DESCRIPTION

Each SYN-Rx DM 14 Day Treatment Regimen pack of 56 tablets consists of two different drug treatment phases as follows: an **A.M. Treatment Phase** comprised of 28 light blue scored controlled-release tablets, each containing 60 mg psuedoephedrine HCl and 600 mg guaifenesin, embossed with "Adams/310"; and a **P.M. Treatment Phase** comprised of 28 yellow scored controlled-release tablets, each containing 30 mg dextromethorphan hydrobromide and 600 mg guaifenesin, embossed with "Adams/309".

Syn-Rx DM 14 Day Treatment Regimen contains ingredients of three therapeutic classes: nasal decongestant, antitussive, and expectorant.

Pseudoephedrine hydrochloride is a nasal decongestant. Chemically, it is [S-(R*,R*)]-α-[1-(methylamino)ethyl] benzenemethanol hydrochloride and has the following structural formula:

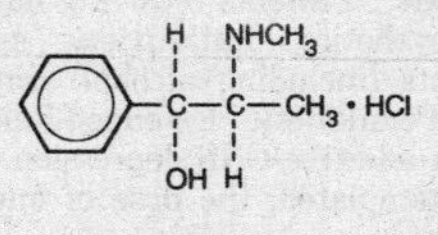

Molecular weight = 201.70;
chemical formula = $C_{10}H_{15}NO \cdot HCl$

Dextromethorphan hydrobromide is a salt of the methyl ether of the dextrorotatory isomer of levorphanol, a narcotic analgesic. Chemically, it is 3-methoxy-17-methyl-9α, 13α, 14α - morphinan hydrobromide monohydrate and has the following structural formula:

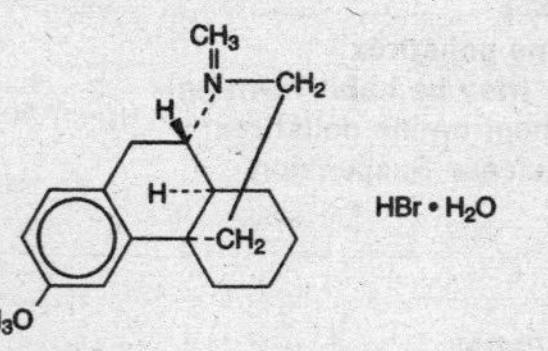

$C_{18}H_{25}NO \cdot HBr \cdot H_2O$ MW = 370.33

Guaifenesin is an expectorant. Chemically, it is 3-(2-methoxyphenoxy)-1, 2-propanediol and has the following structural formula:

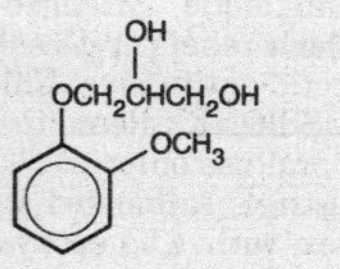

Molecular weight = 198.22; chemical formula = $C_{10}H_{14}O_4$

Inactive Ingredients: Each light blue A.M. tablet and yellow P.M. tablet contains stearic acid, dibasic calcium phosphate, sodium lauryl sulfate, ethylcellulose, magnesium stearate. Each light blue A.M. tablet also contains FD&C Blue #1 Aluminum Lake. Each yellow P.M. tablet also contains D & C Yellow #10 Lake.

CLINICAL PHARMACOLOGY

Pseudoephedrine hydrochloride is an orally indirect acting sympathomimetic amine and exerts a decongestant action on the nasal mucosa. It does this by vasoconstriction which results in reduction of tissue hyperemia, edema, nasal congestion, and an increase in nasal airway patency. In the usual dose it has minimal vasopressor effects. Pseudoephedrine is rapidly and almost completely absorbed from the gastrointestinal tract. It has a plasma half-life of 6 to 8 hours. Alkaline urine is associated with slower elimination of the drug. The drug is distributed to body tissues and fluids, including the central nervous system (CNS). Approximately 50% to 75% of the administered dose is excreted unchanged in the urine; the remainder is apparently metabolized in the liver to inactive compounds by N-demethylation, parahydroxylation and oxidative deamination.

Dextromethorphan is an antitussive agent which, unlike the isomeric levorphanol, has no analgesic or addictive properties. The drug acts centrally and elevates the threshold for coughing. It is about equal to codeine in depressing the cough reflex. In therapeutic dosage, dextromethorphan does not inhibit ciliary activity. Dextromethorphan is rapidly absorbed from the gastrointestinal tract, metabolized by the liver and excreted primarily in the urine.

Guaifenesin is an expectorant which increases respiratory tract fluid secretions and helps to loosen phlegm, bronchial and nasal secretions. By reducing the viscosity of secretions, guaifenesin increases the efficiency of the mucociliary mechanism in removing accumulated secretions from the upper and lower airway. Guaifenesin is readily absorbed from the gastrointestinal tract and is rapidly metabolized and excreted in the urine. Guaifenesin has a plasma half-life of one hour. The major urinary metabolite is β-(2-methoxyphenoxy) lactic acid.

INDICATIONS AND USAGE

SYN-Rx DM 14 Day Treatment Regimen is indicated for the temporary relief of nasal congestion and cough associated with respiratory tract infections and related conditions such as sinusitis, bronchitis, and asthma, when these conditions are complicated by tenacious mucus, and/or mucus plugs and congestion. In the treatment of bacterial sinusitis this treatment regimen may be used concomitantly with appropriate antibiotic therapy. The product is effective in productive as well as nonproductive cough, but is of particular value in dry, nonproductive cough which tends to injure the mucous membrane of the air passages.

CONTRAINDICATIONS

This product is contraindicated in patients with hypersensitivity to guaifenesin, dextromethorphan HBr, or psuedoephedrine HCl, or with hypersensitivity or idiosyncrasy to sympathomimetic amines which may be manifested by insomnia, dizziness, weakness, tremor or arrhythmias.

Sympathomimetic amines are contraindicated in patients with severe hypertension and severe coronary artery disease.

The product is contraindicated in patients on monoamine oxidase inhibitor (MAOI) therapy and for 14 days after stopping MAOI therapy. (see **Drug Interaction** section).

WARNINGS

Sympathomimetic amines should be used with caution in patients with hypertension, ischemic heart disease, diabetes mellitus, increased intraocular pressure, hyperthyroidism, or prostatic hypertrophy. Sympathomimetics may produce central nervous system stimulation with convulsions or cardiovascular collapse with accompanying hypotension. **Do not exceed recommended dosage.**

Do not prescribe this product for use in patients that are now taking a prescription MAOI (certain drugs for depression, psychiatric or emotional conditions, or Parkinson's disease), or for 14 days after stopping the MAOI drug therapy.

Hypertensive crises can occur with concurrent use of pseudoephedrine and monoamine oxidase inhibitors (MAOI), and for 14 days after stopping the MAOI drug therapy, indomethacine, or with beta-blockers and methyldopa. If a hypertensive crisis occurs, these drugs should be discontinued immediately and therapy to lower blood pressure should be instituted. Fever should be managed by means of external cooling.

PRECAUTIONS

General: Use with caution in patients with diabetes, hypertenson, cardiovascular disease and intolerance to ephedrine. Before prescribing medication to suppress or modify cough, it is important that the underlying cause of cough is identified, that modification of cough does not increase the risk of clinical or physiological complications, and that appropriate therapy for the primary disease is instituted.

Dextromethorphan should be used with caution in sedated or debilitated patients, and in patients confined to the supine position.

Failure of symptoms to completely resolve should alert the patient and physician that further diagnostic studies are indicated.

Pediatric Use: This product is not recommended for use in pediatric patients under 12 years of age.

Use in Elderly: The elderly (60 years and older) are more likely to experience adverse reactions to sympathomimetics. Overdosage of sympathomimetics in this age group may cause hallucinations, convulsions, CNS depression and death.

Drug Interactions: Do not prescribe this product for use in patients that are now taking a monoamine oxidase inhibitor (MAOI) drug (certain drugs for depression, psychiatric or emotional conditions, or Parkinson's disease) or for 14 days after stopping the MAOI drug therapy. Beta-adrenergic blockers and inhibitors (MAOI) may potentiate the pressor effect of pseudoephedrine. Concurrent use of digitalis glycosides may increase the possibility of cardiac arrhythmias. Sympathomimetics may reduce the hypotensive effects of guanethidine, mecamylamine, methyldopa, reserpine and veratrum alkaloids. Concurrent use of tricyclic antidepressants may antagonize the effects of pseudoephedrine.

Drug/Laboratory Test Interactions: Guaifenesin may increase renal clearance for urate and thereby lower serum uric acid levels. Guaifenesin may produce and increase in urinary 5-hydroxyindoleacetic acid and may therefore interfere with the interpretation of this test for the diagnosis of carcinoid syndrome. It may also falsely elevate the VMA test for catechols. Administration of this drug should be discontinued 48 hours prior to the collection of urine specimens for such tests.

Carcinogenesis, Mutagenesis, Impairment of Fertility: No data are available on the long-term potential of the components of this product for carcinogenesis, mutagenesis, or impairment of fertility in animals or humans.

Pregnancy Category C: Animal reproduction studies have not been conducted with Syn-Rx DM Tablets. It is also not known whether Syn-Rx DM Tablets can cause fetal harm when administered to a pregnant woman or can affect reproduction capacity. Syn-Rx DM Tablets should be given to pregnant woman only if clearly needed.

Nursing Mothers: Pseudoephedrine is excreted in breast milk. Use of this product by nursing mothers is not recommended because of the higher than usual risk for pediatric patients from sympathomimetic amines.

ADVERSE REACTIONS

Some individuals may display sympathomimetic amine effects such as tachycardia, palpitations, headache, dizziness or nausea. Sympathomimetics have been associated with certain untoward reactions including fear, anxiety, nervousness, restlessness, tremor, weakness, pallor, respiratory difficulty, dysuria, insomnia, hallucinations, convulsions, CNS depression, arrhythmias, and cardiovascular collapse with hypotension. No serious side effects have been reported with the use of guaifenesin or dextromethorphan HBr.

Continued on next page

Information on the Medeva Pharmaceuticals, Inc. products listed on these pages contains the full prescribing information from product circulars in use as of July 1996. For further information, please consult the package insert currently accompanying the product.

Medeva Pharmaceuticals, Inc.—Cont.

OVERDOSAGE

Since SYN-Rx DM 14 Day Treatment Regimen contains three pharmacologically different compounds, treatment of overdosage should be based upon the symptomatology of the patient as it relates to the individual ingredients. Treatment of acute overdosage would probably be based upon treating the patient for pseudoephedrine toxicity which may manifest itself as excessive CNS stimulation resulting in excitement, tremor, restlessness, and insomnia. Other effects may include tachycardia, hypertension, pallor, mydriasis, hyperglycemia and urinary retention. Severe overdosage may cause tachypnea or hypernea, hallucinations, convulsions, or delirium, but in some individuals there may be CNS depression with somnolence, stupor or respiratory depression. Arrhythmias (including ventricular fibrillation) may lead to hypotension and circulatory collapse. Severe hypokalemia can occur, probably due to a compartmental shift rather than a depletion of potassium. No organ damage or significant metabolic derangement is associated with pseudoephedrine overdosage. Overdosage with guaifenesin is unlikely to produce toxic effects since its toxicity is much lower than that of pseudoephedrine. In severe cases of overdosage, it is recommended to monitor the patient in an intensive care setting.

The LD_{50} of pseudoephedrine (single oral dose) has been reported to be 726 mg/kg in the mouse, 2206 mg/kg in the rat and 1177 mg/kg in the rabbit. The toxic and lethal concentrations in human biologic fluids are not known. Urinary excretion increases with acidification and decreases with alkalinization of the urine. There are few published reports of toxicity due to pseudoephedrine and no case of fatal overdosage has been reported. Guaifenesin, when administered by stomach tube to test animals in doses up to 5 grams/kg, produced no signs of toxicity.

Overdosage with dextromethorphan may produce central excitement and mental confusion. Very high doses may produce respiratory depression. One case of toxic psychosis (hyperactivity, marked visual and auditory hallucinations) after ingestion of a single 300 mg dose of dextromethorphan has been reported.

Since the action of sustained release products may continue for as long as 12 hours, treatment of overdosage should be directed toward reducing further absorption and supporting the patient for at least that length of time. Gastric emptying (Syrup of Ipecac) and/or lavage is recommended as soon as possible after ingestion, even if the patient has vomited spontaneously. Either isotonic or half-isotonic saline may be used for lavage. Administration of an activated charcoal slurry is beneficial after lavage and/or emesis if less than 4 hours have passed since ingestion. Saline cathartics, such as Milk of Magnesia, are useful for hastening the evacuation of unreleased medication.

Adrenergic receptor blocking agents are antidotes to pseudoephedrine. In practice, the most useful is the beta-blocker propranolol which is indicated when there are signs of cardiac toxicity. Theoretically, pseudoephedrine is dialyzable but procedures have not been clinically established.

DOSAGE AND ADMINISTRATION

Adults and adolescents over 12 years of age: 1 or 2 light blue A.M. tablets in the morning and 1 or 2 yellow P.M. tablets 12 hours later. Repeat A.M. and P.M. dosing cycle every 12 hours for 14 days. **Do not crush or chew tablets prior to swallowing.**

HOW SUPPLIED

NDC 53014-311-14 SYN-Rx DM 14 Day Treatment Regimen, containing 56 controlled-release tablets as follows:
NDC 53014-310, 28 light blue elongated and scored A.M. tablets embossed with "Adams/310", each containing 60 mg pseudoephedrine HCl and 600 mg guaifenesin;
NDC 53014-309, 28 yellow elongated and scored P.M. tablets embossed with "Adams/309", each containing 30 mg dextromethorphan HBr and 600 mg guaifenesin.

Store at controlled room temperature between 15°C and 30°C (59°F–86°F).

Dispense as a complete 14 day pack.

Caution: Federal law prohibits dispensing without prescription.
January 1996

TUSSIONEX® ℞
Pennkinetic®
[tus'e-uh-nex]
(hydrocodone polistirex
[Warning: May be habit forming]
and chlorpheniramine polistirex)
Extended-Release Suspension
R 240G
Rev. 7/96

DESCRIPTION

Each teaspoonful (5 mL) of TUSSIONEX Pennkinetic Extended-Release Suspension contains hydrocodone polistirex equivalent to 10 mg of hydrocodone bitartrate (Warning: May be habit-forming) and chlorpheniramine polistirex equivalent to 8 mg of chlorpheniramine maleate. TUSSIONEX Pennkinetic Extended-Release Suspension provides up to 12-hour relief per dose. Hydrocodone is a centrally-acting narcotic antitussive. Chlorpheniramine is an antihistamine. TUSSIONEX Pennkinetic Extended-Release Suspension is for oral use only.
Hydrocodone Polistirex: sulfonated styrene-divinylbenzene copolymer complex with 4,5α-epoxy-3-methoxy-17-methylmorphinan-6-one.

Chlorpheniramine Polistirex: sulfonated styrene-divinylbenzene copolymer complex with 2-[p-chloro-α-[2-(dimethylamino)ethyl]-benzyl]pyridine.

Inactive Ingredients: Ascorbic acid, D&C Yellow No. 10, ethylcellulose, FD&C Yellow No. 6, flavor, high fructose corn syrup, methylparaben, polyethylene glycol 3350, polysorbate 80, pregelatinized starch, propylene glycol, propylparaben, purified water, sucrose, vegetable oil, xanthan gum.

CLINICAL PHARMACOLOGY

Hydrocodone is a semisynthetic narcotic antitussive and analgesic with multiple actions qualitatively similar to those of codeine. The precise mechanism of action of hydrocodone and other opiates is not known; however, hydrocodone is believed to act directly on the cough center. In excessive doses, hydrocodone, like other opium derivatives, will depress respiration. The effects of hydrocodone in therapeutic doses on the cardiovascular system are insignificant. Hydrocodone can produce miosis, euphoria, physical and psychological dependence.

Chlorpheniramine is an antihistamine drug (H_1 receptor antagonist) that also possesses anticholinergic and sedative activity. It prevents released histamine from dilating capillaries and causing edema of the respiratory mucosa.

Hydrocodone release from TUSSIONEX Pennkinetic Extended-Release Suspension is controlled by the Pennkinetic System, an extended-release drug delivery system which combines an ion-exchange polymer matrix with a diffusion rate-limiting permeable coating. Chlorpheniramine release is prolonged by use of an ion-exchange polymer system.

Following multiple dosing with TUSSIONEX Pennkinetic Extended-Release Suspension, hydrocodone mean (S.D.) peak plasma concentrations of 22.8 (5.9) ng/mL occurred at 3.4 hours. Chlorpheniramine mean (S.D.) peak plasma concentrations of 58.4 (14.7) ng/mL occurred at 6.3 hours following multiple dosing. Peak plasma levels obtained with an immediate-release syrup occurred at approximately 1.5 hours for hydrocodone and 2.8 hours for chlorpheniramine. The plasma half-lives of hydrocodone and chlorpheniramine have been reported to be approximately 4 and 16 hours, respectively.

INDICATIONS AND USAGE

TUSSIONEX Pennkinetic Extended-Release Suspension is indicated for relief of cough and upper respiratory symptoms associated with allergy or a cold.

CONTRAINDICATIONS

Known allergy or sensitivity to hydrocodone or chlorpheniramine.

WARNINGS

Respiratory Depression: As with all narcotics, TUSSIONEX Pennkinetic Extended-Release Suspension produces dose-related respiratory depression by directly acting on brain stem respiratory centers. Hydrocodone affects the center that controls respiratory rhythm, and may produce irregular and periodic breathing. Caution should be exercised when TUSSIONEX Pennkinetic Extended-Release Suspension is used postoperatively and in patients with pulmonary disease or whenever ventilatory function is depressed. If respiratory depression occurs, it may be antagonized by the use of naloxone hydrochloride and other supportive measures when indicated (see OVERDOSAGE).
Head Injury and Increased Intracranial Pressure: The respiratory depressant effects of narcotics and their capacity to elevate cerebrospinal fluid pressure may be markedly exaggerated in the presence of head injury, other intracranial lesions or a pre-existing increase in intracranial pressure. Furthermore, narcotics produce adverse reactions which may obscure the clinical course of patients with head injuries.
Acute Abdominal Conditions: The administration of narcotics may obscure the diagnosis or clinical course of patients with acute abdominal conditions.
Obstructive Bowel Disease: Chronic use of narcotics may result in obstructive bowel disease especially in patients with underlying intestinal motility disorder.
Pediatric Use: In pediatric patients, as well as adults, the respiratory center is sensitive to the depressant action of narcotic cough suppressants in a dose-dependent manner. Benefit to risk ratio should be carefully considered especially in pediatric patients with respiratory embarrassment (e.g., croup) (see PRECAUTIONS).

PRECAUTIONS

General
Caution is advised when prescribing this drug to patients with narrow-angle glaucoma, asthma or prostatic hypertrophy.
Special Risk Patients: As with any narcotic agent, TUSSIONEX Pennkinetic Extended-Release Suspension should be used with caution in elderly or debilitated patients and those with severe impairment of hepatic or renal function, hypothyroidism, Addison's disease, prostatic hypertrophy or urethral stricture. The usual precautions should be observed and the possibility of respiratory depression should be kept in mind.
Information for Patients: As with all narcotics, TUSSIONEX Pennkinetic Extended-Release Suspension may produce marked drowsiness and impair the mental and/or physical abilities required for the performance of potentially hazardous tasks such as driving a car or operating machinery; patients should be cautioned accordingly. TUSSIONEX Pennkinetic Extended-Release Suspension must not be diluted with fluids or mixed with other drugs as this may alter the resin-binding and change the absorption rate, possibly increasing the toxicity.
Keep out of the reach of children.
Cough Reflex: Hydrocodone suppresses the cough reflex; as with all narcotics, caution should be exercised when TUSSIONEX Pennkinetic Extended-Release Suspension is used postoperatively, and in patients with pulmonary disease.
Drug Interactions: Patients receiving narcotics, antihistaminics, antipsychotics, antianxiety agents or other CNS depressants (including alcohol) concomitantly with TUSSIONEX Pennkinetic Extended-Release Suspension may exhibit an additive CNS depression. When combined therapy is contemplated, the dose of one or both agents should be reduced.
The use of MAO inhibitors or tricyclic antidepressants with hydrocodone preparations may increase the effect of either the antidepressant or hydrocodone.
The concurrent use of other anticholinergics with hydrocodone may produce paralytic ileus.

Carcinogenesis, Mutagenesis, Impairment of Fertility: Carcinogenicity, mutagenicity and reproductive studies have not been conducted with TUSSIONEX Pennkinetic Extended-Release Suspension.

Pregnancy: Teratogenic Effects—Pregnancy Category C. Hydrocodone has been shown to be teratogenic in hamsters when given in doses 700 times the human dose. There are no adequate and well-controlled studies in pregnant women. TUSSIONEX Pennkinetic Extended-Release Suspension should be used during pregnancy only if the potential benefit justifies the potential risk to the fetus.

Nonteratogenic Effects: Babies born to mothers who have been taking opioids regularly prior to delivery will be physically dependent. The withdrawal signs include irritability and excessive crying, tremors, hyperactive reflexes, increased respiratory rate, increased stools, sneezing, yawning, vomiting and fever. The intensity of the syndrome does not always correlate with the duration of maternal opioid use or dose.

Labor and Delivery: As with all narcotics, administration of TUSSIONEX Pennkinetic Extended-Release Suspension to the mother shortly before delivery may result in some degree of respiratory depression in the newborn, especially if higher doses are used.

Nursing Mothers: It is not known whether this drug is excreted in human milk. Because many drugs are excreted in human milk and because of the potential for serious adverse reactions in nursing infants from TUSSIONEX Pennkinetic Extended-Release Suspension, a decision should be made whether to discontinue nursing or to discontinue the drug, taking into account the importance of the drug to the mother.

Pediatric Use: Safety and effectiveness of TUSSIONEX Pennkinetic Extended-Release Suspension in pediatric patients under six years have not been established.

ADVERSE REACTIONS

Central Nervous System: Sedation, drowsiness, mental clouding, lethargy, impairment of mental and physical performance, anxiety, fear, dysphoria, euphoria, dizziness, psychic dependence, mood changes.

Dermatologic System: Rash, pruritus.

Gastrointestinal System: Nausea and vomiting may occur; they are more frequent in ambulatory than in recumbent patients. Prolonged administration of TUSSIONEX Pennkinetic Extended-Release Suspension may produce constipation.

Genitourinary System: Ureteral spasm, spasm of vesicle sphincters and urinary retention have been reported with opiates.

Respiratory Depression: TUSSIONEX Pennkinetic Extended-Release Suspension may produce dose-related respiratory depression by acting directly on brain stem respiratory centers (see OVERDOSAGE).

Respiratory System: Dryness of the pharynx, occasional tightness of the chest.

DRUG ABUSE AND DEPENDENCE

TUSSIONEX Pennkinetic Extended-Release Suspension is a Schedule III narcotic. Psychic dependence, physical dependence and tolerance may develop upon repeated administration of narcotics; therefore, TUSSIONEX Pennkinetic Extended-Release Suspension should be prescribed and administered with caution. However, psychic dependence is unlikely to develop when TUSSIONEX Pennkinetic Extended-Release Suspension is used for a short time for the treatment of cough. Physical dependence, the condition in which continued administration of the drug is required to prevent the appearance of a withdrawal syndrome, assumes clinically significant proportions only after several weeks of continued oral narcotic use, although some mild degree of physical dependence may develop after a few days of narcotic therapy.

OVERDOSAGE

Signs and Symptoms: Serious overdosage with hydrocodone is characterized by respiratory depression (a decrease in respiratory rate and/or tidal volume, Cheyne-Stokes respiration, cyanosis), extreme somnolence progressing to stupor or coma, skeletal muscle flaccidity, cold and clammy skin, and sometimes bradycardia and hypotension. Although miosis is characteristic of narcotic overdose, mydriasis may occur in terminal narcosis or severe hypoxia. In severe overdosage apnea, circulatory collapse, cardiac arrest and death may occur. The manifestations of chlorpheniramine overdosage may vary from central nervous system depression to stimulation.

Treatment: Primary attention should be given to the reestablishment of adequate respiratory exchange through provision of a patent airway and the institution of assisted or controlled ventilation. The narcotic antagonist naloxone hydrochloride is a specific antidote for respiratory depression which may result from overdosage or unusual sensitivity to narcotics including hydrocodone. Therefore, an appropriate dose of naloxone hydrochloride should be administered, preferably by the intravenous route, simultaneously with efforts at respiratory resuscitation. Since the duration of action of hydrocodone in this formulation may exceed that

of the antagonist, the patient should be kept under continued surveillance and repeated doses of the antagonist should be administered as needed to maintain adequate respiration. For further information, see full prescribing information for naloxone hydrochloride. An antagonist should not be administered in the absence of clinically significant respiratory depression. Oxygen, intravenous fluids, vasopressors and other supportive measures should be employed as indicated. Gastric emptying may be useful in removing unabsorbed drug.

DOSAGE AND ADMINISTRATION

Shake well before using.

Adults: 1 teaspoonful (5 mL) every 12 hours; do not exceed 2 teaspoonfuls in 24 hours.

Children 6–12: $1/2$ teaspoonful every 12 hours; **do not exceed 1 teaspoonful in 24 hours.**

Not recommended for pediatric patients under 6 years of age (see PRECAUTIONS).

HOW SUPPLIED

TUSSIONEX Pennkinetic (hydrocodone polistirex and chlorpheniramine polistirex) Extended-Release Suspension is a gold-colored suspension.

| NDC 53014-548-67 | 473 mL bottle |
| NDC 53014-548-91 | 900 mL bottle |

Shake well. Dispense in a well-closed container. Store at 59°–86°F (15°–30°C).

CAUTION: Federal law prohibits dispensing without prescription.

MEDEVA PHARMACEUTICALS
Medeva Pharmaceuticals, Inc.
Fort Worth, TX 76155
® Fisons BV
© 1996, Medeva Pharmaceuticals Manufacturing, Inc.
Rev. 7/96
R 240G

ZAROXOLYN® TABLETS ℞
[zar″ ox ′ uh-lin]
(metolazone tablets, USP)
R 241F
Rev. 7/96

DO NOT INTERCHANGE

DO NOT INTERCHANGE ZAROXOLYN TABLETS AND OTHER FORMULATIONS OF METOLAZONE THAT SHARE ITS SLOW AND INCOMPLETE BIOAVAILABILITY AND ARE NOT THERAPEUTICALLY EQUIVALENT AT THE SAME DOSES TO MYKROX® TABLETS, A MORE RAPIDLY AVAILABLE AND COMPLETELY BIOAVAILABLE METOLAZONE PRODUCT. FORMULATIONS BIOEQUIVALENT TO ZAROXOLYN AND FORMULATIONS BIOEQUIVALENT TO MYKROX SHOULD NOT BE INTERCHANGED FOR ONE ANOTHER.

DESCRIPTION

ZAROXOLYN Tablets (metolazone tablets, USP) for oral administration contain $2^{1}/_{2}$, 5 or 10 mg of metolazone, USP, a diuretic/saluretic/antihypertensive drug of the quinazoline class.

Metolazone has the molecular formula $C_{16}H_{16}ClN_3O_3S$, the chemical name 7-chloro-1,2,3,4-tetrahydro-2-methyl-3-(2-methylphenyl)-4-oxo-6-quinazolinesulfonamide and a molecular weight of 365.83. The structural formula is:

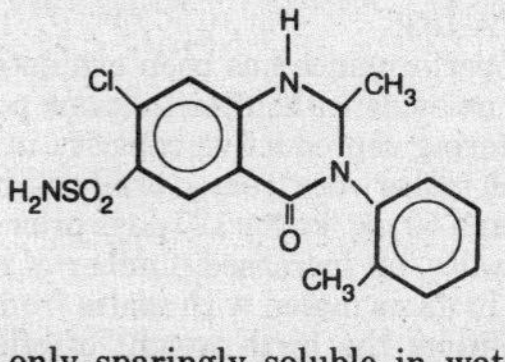

Metolazone is only sparingly soluble in water, but more soluble in plasma, blood, alkali and organic solvents.

Inactive Ingredients: magnesium stearate, microcrystalline cellulose and dye: $2^{1}/_{2}$ mg-D&C Red No. 33; 5 mg-FD&C Blue No. 2; 10 mg-D&C Yellow No. 10 and FD&C Yellow No. 6.

CLINICAL PHARMACOLOGY

ZAROXOLYN (metolazone) is a quinazoline diuretic, with properties generally similar to the thiazide diuretics. The actions of ZAROXOLYN result from interference with the renal tubular mechanism of electrolyte reabsorption. ZAROXOLYN acts primarily to inhibit sodium reabsorption at the cortical diluting site and to a lesser extent in the proximal convoluted tubule. Sodium and chloride ions are excreted in approximately equivalent amounts. The increased delivery of sodium to the distal tubular exchange site results in increased potassium excretion. ZAROXOLYN does not inhibit carbonic anhydrase. A proximal action of metolazone has been shown in humans by increased excretion of phosphate and magnesium ions and by a markedly increased fractional excretion of sodium in patients with severely com-

promised glomerular filtration. This action has been demonstrated in animals by micropuncture studies.

When ZAROXOLYN Tablets are given, diuresis and saluresis usually begin within one hour and may persist for 24 hours or more. For most patients, the duration of effect can be varied by adjusting the daily dose. High doses may prolong the effect. A single daily dose is recommended. When a desired therapeutic effect has been obtained, it may be possible to reduce dosage to a lower maintenance level.

The diuretic potency of ZAROXOLYN at maximum therapeutic dosage is approximately equal to thiazide diuretics. However, unlike thiazides, ZAROXOLYN may produce diuresis in patients with glomerular filtration rates below 20 mL/min.

ZAROXOLYN and furosemide administered concurrently have produced marked diuresis in some patients where edema or ascites was refractory to treatment with maximum recommended doses of these or other diuretics administered alone. The mechanism of this interaction is unknown (see WARNINGS and PRECAUTIONS, DRUG INTERACTIONS).

Maximum blood levels of metolazone are found approximately eight hours after dosing. A small fraction of metolazone is metabolized. Most of the drug is excreted in the unconverted form in the urine.

INDICATIONS AND USAGE

ZAROXOLYN is indicated for the treatment of salt and water retention including:

—edema accompanying congestive heart failure;

—edema accompanying renal diseases, including the nephrotic syndrome and states of diminished renal function.

ZAROXOLYN is also indicated for the treatment of hypertension, alone or in combination with other antihypertensive drugs of a different class. MYKROX Tablets, a more rapidly available form of metolazone, are intended for the treatment of new patients with mild to moderate hypertension. A dose titration is necessary if MYKROX Tablets are to be substituted for ZAROXOLYN in the treatment of hypertension. See package circular for MYKROX Tablets (Medeva).

Usage in Pregnancy

The routine use of diuretics in an otherwise healthy woman is inappropriate and exposes mother and fetus to unnecessary hazard. Diuretics do not prevent development of toxemia of pregnancy, and there is no evidence that they are useful in the treatment of developed toxemia. Edema during pregnancy may arise from pathologic causes or from the physiologic and mechanical consequences of pregnancy. ZAROXOLYN is indicated in pregnancy when edema is due to pathologic causes, just as it is in the absence of pregnancy (see PRECAUTIONS). Dependent edema in pregnancy resulting from restriction of venous return by the expanded uterus is properly treated through elevation of the lower extremities and use of support hose; use of diuretics to lower intravascular volume in this case is illogical and unnecessary. There is hypervolemia during normal pregnancy which is harmful to neither the fetus nor the mother (in the absence of cardiovascular disease), but which is associated with edema, including generalized edema, in the majority of pregnant women. If this edema produces discomfort, increased recumbency will often provide relief. In rare instances, this edema may cause extreme discomfort which is not relieved by rest. In these cases, a short course of diuretics may be appropriate.

CONTRAINDICATIONS

Anuria, hepatic coma or precoma, known allergy or hypersensitivity to metolazone.

WARNINGS

Rapid Onset Hyponatremia

Rarely, the rapid onset of severe hyponatremia and/or hypokalemia has been reported following initial doses of thiazide and non-thiazide diuretics. When symptoms consistent with severe electrolyte imbalance appear rapidly, drug should be discontinued and supportive measures should be initiated immediately. Parenteral electrolytes may be required. Appropriateness of therapy with this class of drugs should be carefully reevaluated.

Hypokalemia

Hypokalemia may occur with consequent weakness, cramps, and cardiac dysrhythmias. Serum potassium should be determined at regular intervals, and dose reduction, potassium supplementation or addition of a potassium-sparing diuretic instituted whenever indicated. Hypokalemia is a particular hazard in patients who are digitalized or who have or have had a ventricular arrhythmia; dangerous or fatal arrhythmias may be precipitated. Hypokalemia is dose related.

Continued on next page

Medeva Pharmaceuticals, Inc.—Cont.

Concomitant Therapy
Lithium
In general, diuretics should not be given concomitantly with lithium because they reduce its renal clearance and add a high risk of lithium toxicity. Read prescribing information for lithium preparations before use of such concomitant therapy.

Furosemide: Unusually large or prolonged losses of fluids and electrolytes may result when ZAROXOLYN is administered concomitantly to patients receiving furosemide (see PRECAUTIONS, DRUG INTERACTIONS).

Other Antihypertensive Drugs: When ZAROXOLYN is used with other antihypertensive drugs, particular care must be taken to avoid excessive reduction of blood pressure, especially during initial therapy.

Cross-Allergy
Cross-allergy, while not reported to date, theoretically may occur when ZAROXOLYN is given to patients known to be allergic to sulfonamide-derived drugs, thiazides, or quinethazone.

Sensitivity Reactions: Sensitivity reactions (e.g., angioedema, bronchospasm) may occur with or without a history of allergy or bronchial asthma and may occur with the first dose of ZAROXOLYN.

PRECAUTIONS

DO NOT INTERCHANGE
DO NOT INTERCHANGE ZAROXOLYN TABLETS AND OTHER FORMULATIONS OF METOLAZONE THAT SHARE ITS SLOW AND INCOMPLETE BIOAVAILABILITY AND ARE NOT THERAPEUTICALLY EQUIVALENT AT THE SAME DOSES TO MYKROX TABLETS, A MORE RAPIDLY AVAILABLE AND COMPLETELY BIOAVAILABLE METOLAZONE PRODUCT. FORMULATIONS BIOEQUIVALENT TO ZAROXOLYN AND FORMULATIONS BIOEQUIVALENT TO MYKROX SHOULD NOT BE INTERCHANGED FOR ONE ANOTHER.

GENERAL:
Fluid and Electrolytes
All patients receiving therapy with ZAROXOLYN Tablets should have serum electrolyte measurements done at appropriate intervals and be observed for clinical signs of fluid and/or electrolyte imbalance: namely, hyponatremia, hypochloremic alkalosis, and hypokalemia. In patients with severe edema accompanying cardiac failure or renal disease, a low-salt syndrome may be produced, especially with hot weather and a low-salt diet. Serum and urine electrolyte determinations are particularly important when the patient has protracted vomiting, severe diarrhea, or is receiving parenteral fluids. Warning signs of imbalance are: dryness of mouth, thirst, weakness, lethargy, drowsiness, restlessness, muscle pains or cramps, muscle fatigue, hypotension, oliguria, tachycardia, and gastrointestinal disturbances such as nausea and vomiting. Hyponatremia may occur at any time during long term therapy and, on rare occasions, may be life threatening.

The risk of hypokalemia is increased when larger doses are used, when diuresis is rapid, when severe liver disease is present, when corticosteroids are given concomitantly, when oral intake is inadequate or when excess potassium is being lost extrarenally, such as with vomiting or diarrhea. Thiazide-like diuretics have been shown to increase the urinary excretion of magnesium; this may result in hypomagnesemia.

Glucose Tolerance
Metolazone may raise blood glucose concentrations possibly causing hyperglycemia and glycosuria in patients with diabetes or latent diabetes.

Hyperuricemia
ZAROXOLYN regularly causes an increase in serum uric acid and can occasionally precipitate gouty attacks even in patients without a prior history of them.

Azotemia
Azotemia, presumably prerenal azotemia, may be precipitated during the administration of ZAROXOLYN. If azotemia and oliguria worsen during treatment of patients with severe renal disease, ZAROXOLYN should be discontinued.

Renal Impairment
Use caution when administering ZAROXOLYN Tablets to patients with severely impaired renal function. As most of the drug is excreted by the renal route, accumulation may occur.

Orthostatic Hypotension
Orthostatic hypotension may occur; this may be potentiated by alcohol, barbiturates, narcotics, or concurrent therapy with other antihypertensive drugs.

Hypercalcemia
Hypercalcemia may infrequently occur with metolazone, especially in patients taking high doses of vitamin D or with high bone turnover states, and may signify hidden hyperparathyroidism. Metolazone should be discontinued before tests for parathyroid function are performed.

Systemic Lupus Erythematosus
Thiazide diuretics have exacerbated or activated systemic lupus erythematosus and this possibility should be considered with ZAROXOLYN Tablets.

INFORMATION FOR PATIENTS: Patients should be informed of possible adverse effects, advised to take the medication as directed and promptly report any possible adverse reactions to the treating physician.

DRUG INTERACTIONS:
Diuretics
Furosemide and probably other loop diuretics given concomitantly with metolazone can cause unusually large or prolonged losses of fluid and electrolytes (see WARNINGS).

Other Antihypertensives
When ZAROXOLYN Tablets are used with other antihypertensive drugs, care must be taken, especially during initial therapy. Dosage adjustments of other antihypertensives may be necessary.

Alcohol, Barbiturates, and Narcotics
The hypotensive effects of these drugs may be potentiated by the volume contraction that may be associated with metolazone therapy.

Digitalis Glycosides
Diuretic-induced hypokalemia can increase the sensitivity of the myocardium to digitalis. Serious arrhythmias can result.

Corticosteroids or ACTH
May increase the risk of hypokalemia and increase salt and water retention.

Lithium
Serum lithium levels may increase (see WARNINGS).

Curariform Drugs
Diuretic-induced hypokalemia may enhance neuromuscular blocking effects of curariform drugs (such as tubocurarine) — the most serious effect would be respiratory depression which could proceed to apnea. Accordingly, it may be advisable to discontinue ZAROXOLYN Tablets three days before elective surgery.

Salicylates and Other Non-Steroidal Anti-Inflammatory Drugs
May decrease the antihypertensive effects of ZAROXOLYN Tablets.

Sympathomimetics
Metolazone may decrease arterial responsiveness to norepinephrine, but this diminution is not sufficient to preclude effectiveness of the pressor agent for therapeutic use.

Insulin and Oral Antidiabetic Agents
See Glucose Tolerance under PRECAUTIONS, GENERAL.

Methenamine
Efficacy may be decreased due to urinary alkalizing effect of metolazone.

Anticoagulants: Metolazone, as well as other thiazide-like diuretics, may affect the hypoprothrombinemic response to anticoagulants; dosage adjustments may be necessary.

DRUG/LABORATORY TEST INTERACTIONS: None reported.

CARCINOGENESIS, MUTAGENESIS, IMPAIRMENT OF FERTILITY: Mice and rats administered metolazone 5 days/week for up to 18 and 24 months, respectively, at daily doses of 2, 10 and 50 mg/kg, exhibited no evidence of a tumorigenic effect of the drug. The small number of animals examined histologically and poor survival in the mice limit the conclusions that can be reached from these studies. Metolazone was not mutagenic *in vitro* in the Ames Test using Salmonella typhimurium strains TA-97, TA-98, TA-100, TA-102 and TA-1535.

Reproductive performance has been evaluated in mice and rats. There is no evidence that metolazone possesses the potential for altering reproductive capacity in mice. In a rat study, in which males were treated orally with metolazone at doses of 2, 10 and 50 mg/kg for 127 days prior to mating with untreated females, an increased number of resorption sites was observed in dams mated with males from the 50 mg/kg group. In addition, the birth weight of offspring was decreased and the pregnancy rate was reduced in dams mated with males from the 10 and 50 mg/kg groups.

PREGNANCY:
Teratogenic Effects—Pregnancy Category B.
Reproduction studies performed in mice, rabbits and rats treated during the appropriate period of gestation at doses up to 50 mg/kg/day have revealed no evidence of harm to the fetus due to metolazone. There are, however, no adequate and well-controlled studies in pregnant women. Because animal reproduction studies are not always predictive of human response, ZAROXOLYN Tablets should be used during pregnancy only if clearly needed. Metolazone crosses the placental barrier and appears in cord blood.

Non-Teratogenic Effects
The use of ZAROXOLYN Tablets in pregnant women requires that the anticipated benefit be weighed against possible hazards to the fetus. These hazards include fetal or neonatal jaundice, thrombocytopenia, and possibly other adverse reactions which have occurred in the adult. It is not known what effect the use of the drug during pregnancy has on the later growth, development and functional maturation

of the child. No such effects have been reported with metolazone.

LABOR AND DELIVERY: Based on clinical studies in which women received metolazone in late pregnancy until the time of delivery, there is no evidence that the drug has any adverse effects on the normal course of labor or delivery.

NURSING MOTHERS: Metolazone appears in breast milk. Because of the potential for serious adverse reactions in nursing infants from metolazone, a decision should be made whether to discontinue nursing or to discontinue the drug, taking into account the importance of the drug to the mother.

PEDIATRIC USE: Safety and effectiveness in pediatric patients have not been established and such use is not recommended.

ADVERSE REACTIONS
ZAROXOLYN is usually well tolerated, and most reported adverse reactions have been mild and transient. Many ZAROXOLYN related adverse reactions represent extensions of its expected pharmacologic activity and can be attributed to either its antihypertensive action or its renal/metabolic actions. The following adverse reactions have been reported. Several are single or comparably rare occurrences. Adverse reactions are listed in decreasing order of severity within body systems.

Cardiovascular: Chest pain/discomfort, orthostatic hypotension, excessive volume depletion, hemoconcentration, venous thrombosis, palpitations.

Central and Peripheral Nervous System: Syncope, neuropathy, vertigo, paresthesias, psychotic depression, impotence, dizziness/light-headedness, drowsiness, fatigue, weakness, restlessness (sometimes resulting in insomnia), headache.

Dermatologic/Hypersensitivity: Necrotizing angiitis (cutaneous vasculitis), purpura, dermatitis (photosensitivity), urticaria and skin rashes.

Gastrointestinal: Hepatitis, intrahepatic cholestatic jaundice, pancreatitis, vomiting, nausea, epigastric distress, diarrhea, constipation, anorexia, abdominal bloating.

Hematologic: Aplastic/hypoplastic anemia, agranulocytosis, leukopenia.

Metabolic: Hypokalemia, hyponatremia, hyperuricemia, hypochloremia, hypochloremic alkalosis, hyperglycemia, glycosuria, increase in serum urea nitrogen (BUN) or creatinine, hypophosphatemia, hypomagnesemia, hypercalcemia.

Musculoskeletal: Joint pain, acute gouty attacks, muscle cramps or spasm.

Other: Transient blurred vision, chills.

In addition, adverse reactions reported with similar antihypertensive-diuretics, but which have not been reported to date for ZAROXOLYN include: bitter taste, dry mouth, sialadenitis, xanthopsia, respiratory distress (including pneumonitis), thrombocytopenia and anaphylactic reactions. These reactions should be considered as possible occurrences with clinical usage of ZAROXOLYN.

Whenever adverse reactions are moderate or severe, ZAROXOLYN dosage should be reduced or therapy withdrawn.

OVERDOSAGE
Intentional overdosage has been reported rarely with metolazone and similar diuretic drugs.

Signs and Symptoms
Orthostatic hypotension, dizziness, drowsiness, syncope, electrolyte abnormalities, hemoconcentration and hemodynamic changes due to plasma volume depletion may occur. In some instances depressed respiration may be observed. At high doses, lethargy of varying degree may progress to coma within a few hours. The mechanism of CNS depression with thiazide overdosage is unknown. Also, GI irritation and hypermotility may occur. Temporary elevation of BUN has been reported, especially in patients with impairment of renal function. Serum electrolyte changes and cardiovascular and renal function should be closely monitored.

Treatment
There is no specific antidote available but immediate evacuation of stomach contents is advised. Dialysis is not likely to be effective. Care should be taken when evacuating the gastric contents to prevent aspiration, especially in the stuporous or comatose patient. Supportive measures should be initiated as required to maintain hydration, electrolyte balance, respiration, and cardiovascular and renal function.

DOSAGE AND ADMINISTRATION
Effective dosage of ZAROXOLYN should be individualized according to indication and patient response. A single daily dose is recommended. Therapy with ZAROXOLYN should be titrated to gain an initial therapeutic response and to determine the minimal dose possible to maintain the desired therapeutic response.

Usual Single Daily Dosage Schedules
Suitable initial dosages will usually fall in the ranges given.
Edema of cardiac failure:
 ZAROXOLYN 5 to 20 mg once daily.
Edema of renal disease:
 ZAROXOLYN 5 to 20 mg once daily.

Mild to moderate essential hypertension:
ZAROXOLYN $2^1/_2$ to 5 mg once daily.

New patients—MYKROX Tablets (metolazone tablets, USP) (see MYKROX package circular). If considered desirable to switch patients currently on ZAROXOLYN to MYKROX, the dose should be determined by titration starting at one tablet ($^1/_2$ mg) once daily and increasing to two tablets (1 mg) once daily if needed.

Treatment of Edematous States

The time interval required for the initial dosage to produce an effect may vary. Diuresis and saluresis usually begin within one hour and persist for 24 hours or longer. When a desired therapeutic effect has been obtained, it may be advisable to reduce the dose if possible. The daily dose depends on the severity of the patient's condition, sodium intake and responsiveness. A decision to change the daily dose should be based on the results of thorough clinical and laboratory evaluations. If antihypertensive drugs or diuretics are given concurrently with ZAROXOLYN, more careful dosage adjustment may be necessary. For patients who tend to experience paroxysmal nocturnal dyspnea, it may be advisable to employ a larger dose to ensure prolongation of diuresis and saluresis for a full 24-hour period.

Treatment of Hypertension

The time interval required for the initial dosage regimen to show effect may vary from three or four days to three to six weeks in the treatment of elevated blood pressure. Doses should be adjusted at appropriate intervals to achieve maximum therapeutic effect.

HOW SUPPLIED

ZAROXOLYN TABLETS (metolazone tablets, USP) are shallow biconvex, round tablets, and are available in three strengths: $2^1/_2$ mg, pink, debossed "ZAROXOLYN" on one side, and "$2^1/_2$" on reverse side.

NDC 53014-975-71	Bottle of 100's
NDC 53014-975-90	Bottle of 1000's
NDC 53014-975-72	Carton of 100's, unit dose

5 mg. blue, debossed "ZAROXOLYN" on one side, and "5" on reverse side.

NDC 53014-850-71	Bottle of 100's
NDC 53014-850-90	Bottle of 1000's
NDC 53014-850-72	Carton of 100's, unit dose

10 mg, yellow, debossed "ZAROXOLYN" on one side, and "10" on reverse side.

NDC 53014-835-71	Bottle of 100's
NDC 53014-835-90	Bottle of 1000's
NDC 53014-835-72	Carton of 100's, unit dose

Store at room temperature. Dispense in a tight, light-resistant container. Keep out of the reach of children.

CAUTION: Federal law prohibits dispensing without prescription.

MEDEVA PHARMACEUTICALS

Medeva Pharmaceuticals, Inc.
Fort Worth, TX 76155
® Fisons BV
© 1996, Medeva Pharmaceuticals Manufacturing, Inc.

Rev. 7/96
R 241F

EDUCATIONAL MATERIAL

For educational information, please write to Medeva Pharmaceuticals, Inc., PO Box 1766, Rochester, NY 14603.

Medicis Dermatologics, Inc.
4343 EAST CAMELBACK RD
PHOENIX, AZ 85018

For Medical Information Contact:
Generally:
Medical Affairs Department
(602) 808-8800
FAX: (602) 808-0822

In Emergencies:
(602) 808-8800

BENZASHAVE® 5%
Benzoyl Peroxide, USP 5%
Medicated Shave Cream

℞

BENZASHAVE® 10%
Benzoyl Peroxide, USP 10%
Medicated Shave Cream

℞

DESCRIPTION

BENZASHAVE 5% and BENZASHAVE 10% Benzoyl Peroxide, USP (5% and 10%) are topical shave cream preparations for use in the treatment of pseudofolliculitis (*p. barbae;* ingrown hairs, razor bumps) and acne vulgaris associated with shaving. Benzoyl peroxide is an oxidizing agent which possesses antibacterial properties and is classified as a keratolytic agent. Benzoyl peroxide ($C_{14}H_{10}O_4$) is represented by the following chemical structure:

INGREDIENTS

BENZASHAVE 5% & 10% contain: ACTIVES: Benzoyl Peroxide, USP, 5% or 10%; INACTIVES: Stearic Acid, Mineral Oil, Triethanolamine, Diisopropyl Dimerate, PEG-15 Cocamine, Carbomer 940, Aloe Vera, Purified Water; PRESERVATIVES: Diazolidinyl Urea, Methylparaben and Propylparaben.

CLINICAL PHARMACOLOGY

The mechanism of action of benzoyl peroxide has not been determined but may be related to its antibacterial activity against *Propionibacterium acnes* and its ability to cause drying and peeling. Benzoyl peroxide reduces the concentration of free fatty acids in the sebum. Little is known about the percutaneous penetration, metabolism and excretion of benzoyl peroxide, although it is likely that benzoic acid is a major metabolite. There is no evidence of systemic toxicity caused by benzoyl peroxide in humans.

INDICATIONS AND USAGE

These products are indicated for the topical treatment of acne vulgaris.

CONTRAINDICATIONS

These products are contraindicated in patients with a history of hypersensitivity to any of the components of the preparations.

PRECAUTIONS

General: For external use only. Not for ophthalmic use. If severe irritation develops, discontinue use and institute appropriate therapy. After the reaction clears, treatment may often be resumed with less frequent application. This preparation should not be used in or near the eyes or on mucous membranes.

Information for Patients: Avoid contact with eyes, eyelids, lips and mucous membranes. If accidental contact occurs, rinse with water. May bleach hair and colored fabrics. If excessive irritation develops, discontinue use and consult your physician.

Carcinogensis, Mutagenesis, Impairment of Fertility: Data from several studies using mice known to be highly susceptible to cancer suggest that benzoyl peroxide acts as a tumor promotor. The clinical significance of these findings to humans is unknown.

Pregnancy: Pregnancy Category C: Animal reproduction studies have not been conducted with benzoyl peroxide. It is also *not* known whether benzoyl peroxide can cause fetal harm when administered to a pregnant woman or can affect reproduction capacity. Benzoyl peroxide should be used by a pregnant woman only if clearly needed. There are no data available on the effect of benzoyl peroxide on the growth, development and functional maturation of the unborn child.

Nursing Mothers: It is not known whether this drug is excreted in human milk. Because many drugs are excreted in human milk, caution should be exercised when benzoyl peroxide is administered to a nursing woman.

Pediatric Use: Safety and effectiveness in children have not been established.

ADVERSE REACTIONS

Allergic contact dermatitis has been reported with topical benzoyl peroxide therapy.

DOSAGE AND ADMINISTRATION

Wet area to be shaved. Apply a small amount of BENZASHAVE with fingertips. Gently rub over entire area and shave.

HOW SUPPLIED

BENZASHAVE® Benzoyl Peroxide, USP (5%), 4 oz (113.4g) tube, NDC 99207-530-04.
BENZASHAVE® Benzoyl Peroxide, USP (10%), 4 oz (113.4g) tube, NDC 99207-540-04.

Keep out of reach of children.
Store at Controlled Room Temperature 15°–30°C (59°–86°F).
For external use only. Not for ophthalmic use.
Lot number and expiration date on package.

CAUTION

Federal law prohibits dispensing without prescription.
Manufactured specially for:
Medicis® Dermatologics, Inc.
The Dermatology Company™
Phoenix, AZ 85018
by: Zenith Goldline Dermatologicals, Inc.
Syosset, NY 11791

DYNACIN®
[dī 'nă-cən]
(MINOCYCLINE
HCl CAPSULES, USP)

℞

DESCRIPTION

Minocycline hydrochloride, a semisynthetic derivative of tetracycline, is [4S-(4α, 4aα, 5aα, 12aα)]-4,7-bis(dimethylamino) -1,4,4a,5,5a,6,11,12a -octahydro -3,10,12,12a -tetrahydroxy-1,11-dioxo-2-naphthacenecarboxamide monohydrochloride. The structural formula is represented below:

$C_{23}H_{27}N_3O_7 \cdot HCl$ M.W. 493.94

Each minocycline hydrochloride capsule for oral administration contains the equivalent of 50 mg or 100 mg of minocycline. In addition each capsule contains the following inactive ingredients: D&C Yellow No. 10, D&C Red No. 28, gelatin, magnesium stearate, starch (corn) and titanium dioxide.

Minocycline Hydrochloride Capsules, USP 100 mg also contain black iron oxide.

CLINICAL PHARMACOLOGY

Following oral administration of minocycline hydrochloride capsules, absorption from the gastrointestinal tract is rapid. Maximum serum concentrations following a single dose of minocycline hydrochloride to normal fasting adult volunteers were attained in 1 to 4 hours. The serum half-life in normal volunteers ranges from approximately 11 hours to 22 hours.

When minocycline hydrochloride capsules were given concomitantly with a meal which included dairy products, the extent of absorption of minocycline hydrochloride capsules was not noticably influenced. The peak plasma concentrations were slightly decreased and delayed by one hour when administered with food, compared to dosing under fasting conditions.

In previous studies with other minocycline dosage forms, the minocycline serum half-life ranged from 11 to 16 hours in 7 patients with hepatic dysfunction, and from 18 to 69 hours in 5 patients with renal dysfunction. The urinary and fecal recovery of minocycline when administered to 12 normal volunteers is one-half to one-third that of other tetracyclines.

Microbiology: The tetracyclines are primarily bacteriostatic and are thought to exert their antimicrobial effect by the inhibition of protein synthesis. The tetracyclines, including minocycline, have similar antimicrobial spectra of activity against a wide range of gram-positive and gram-negative organisms. Cross-resistance of these organisms to tetracyclines is common.

While *in vitro* studies have demonstrated the susceptibility of most strains of the following microorganisms, clinical efficacy for infections other than those included in the **INDICATIONS AND USAGE** section has not been documented.

Gram-Negative Bacteria
Bartonella bacilliformis
Brucella species
Campylobacter fetus
Francisella tularensis
Haemophilus ducreyi
Haemophilus influenzae
Listeria monocytogenes
Neisseria gonorrhoeae
Vibrio cholerae
Yersinia pestis

Because many strains of the following groups of gram-negative microorganisms have been shown to be resistant to tetracyclines, culture and susceptibility tests are especially recommended:

Continued on next page

Medicis—Cont.

Acinetobacter species
Bacteroides species
Enterobacter aerogenes
Escherichia coli
Klebsiella species
Shigella species

Gram-Positive Bacteria

Because many strains of the following groups of gram-positive microorganisms have been shown to be resistant to tetracyclines, culture and susceptibility testing are especially recommended. Up to 44 percent of *Streptococcus pyogenes* strains have been found to be resistant to tetracycline drugs. Therefore, tetracyclines should not be used for streptococcal disease unless the organism has been demonstrated to be susceptible.

Alpha-hemolytic streptococci (viridans group)
Streptococcus pneumoniae
Streptococcus pyogenes

Other Microorganisms

Actinomyces species
Bacillus anthracis
Balantidium coli
Borrelia recurrentis
Chlamydia psittaci
Chlamydia trachomatis
Clostridium species
Entamoeba species
Fusobacterium fusiforme
Propionibacterium acnes
Treponema pallidum
Treponema pertenue
Ureaplasma urealyticum

Susceptibility Tests: *Diffusion Techniques:* The use of antibiotic disk susceptibility test methods which measure zone diameter give an accurate estimation of susceptibility of microorganisms to minocycline. One such standard procedure[1] has been recommended for use with disks for testing antimicrobials. Either the 30 mcg tetracycline-class disk or the 30 mcg minocycline disk should be used for the determination of the susceptibility of microorganisms to minocycline.

With this type of procedure a report of "susceptible" from the laboratory indicates that the infecting organism is likely to respond to therapy. A report of "intermediate susceptibility" suggests that the organism would be susceptible if a high dosage is used or if the infection is confined to tissues and fluids (e.g., urine) in which high antibiotic levels are attained. A report of "resistant" indicates that the infecting organism is not likely to respond to therapy. With either the tetracycline-class disk or the minocycline disk, zone sizes of 19 mm or greater indicate susceptibility, zone sizes of 14 mm or less indicate resistance, and zone sizes of 15 to 18 mm indicate intermediate susceptibility.

Standardized procedures require the use of laboratory control organisms. The 30 mcg tetracycline disk should give zone diameters between 19 and 28 mm for *Staphylococcus aureus* ATCC 25923 and between 18 and 25 mm for *Escherichia coli* ATCC 25922. The 30 mcg minocycline disk should give zone diameters between 25 and 30 mm for *S aureus* ATCC 25923 and between 19 and 25 mm for *E coli* ATCC 25922.

Dilution Techniques: When using the NCCLS agar dilution or broth dilution (including microdilution) method[2] or equivalent, a bacterial isolate may be considered susceptible if the MIC (minimal inhibitory concentration) of minocycline is 4 mcg/mL or less. Organisms are considered resistant if the MIC is 16 mcg/mL or greater. Organisms with an MIC value of less than 16 mcg/mL but greater than 4 mcg/mL are expected to be susceptible if a high dosage is used or if the infection is confined to tissues and fluids (e.g., urine) in which high antibiotic levels are attained.

As with standard diffusion methods, dilution procedures require the use of laboratory control organisms. Standard tetracycline or minocycline powder should give MIC values of 0.25 mcg/mL to 1.0 mcg/mL for *S aureus* ATCC 25923, and 1.0 mcg/mL to 4.0 mcg/mL for *E coli* ATCC 25922.

INDICATIONS AND USAGE

Minocycline Hydrochloride Capsules are indicated in the treatment of the following infections due to susceptible strains of the designated microorganisms:

Rocky Mountain spotted fever, typhus fever and the typhus group, Q fever, rickettsialpox and tick fevers caused by Rickettsiae

Respiratory tract infections caused by *Mycoplasma pneumoniae*

Lymphogranuloma venereum caused by *Chlamydia trachomatis*

Psittacosis (Ornithosis) due to *Chlamydia psittaci*

Trachoma caused by *Chlamydia trachomatis*, although the infectious agent is not always eliminated, as judged by immunofluorescence

Inclusion conjunctivitis caused by *Chlamydia trachomatis*

Nongonococcal urethritis in adults caused by *Ureaplasma urealyticum* or *Chlamydia trachomatis*

Relapsing fever due to *Borrelia recurrentis*

Chancroid caused by *Haemophilus ducreyi*

Plague due to *Yersinia pestis*

Tularemia due to *Francisella tularensis*

Cholera caused by *Vibrio cholerae*

Campylobacter fetus infections caused by *Campylobacter fetus*

Brucellosis due to *Brucella* species (in conjunction with streptomycin)

Bartonellosis due to *Bartonella bacilliformis*

Granuloma inguinale caused by *Calymmatobacterium granulomatis*

Minocycline is indicated for treatment of infections caused by the following gram-negative microorganisms, when bacteriologic testing indicates appropriate susceptibility to the drug:

Escherichia coli
Enterobacter aerogenes
Shigella species
Acinetobacter species

Respiratory tract infections caused by *Haemophilus influenzae*

Respiratory tract and urinary tract infections caused by *Klebsiella* species

Minocycline hydrochloride capsules are indicated for the treatment of infections caused by the following gram-positive microorganisms when bacteriologic testing indicates appropriate susceptibility to the drug:

Upper respiratory tract infections caused by *Streptococcus pneumoniae*

Skin and skin structure infections caused by *Staphylococcus aureus*. (Note: Minocycline is not the drug of choice in the treatment of any type of staphylococcal infection.)

Uncomplicated urethritis in men due to *Neisseria gonorrhoeae* and for the treatment of other gonococcal infections when penicillin is contraindicated .

When penicillin is contraindicated, minocycline is an alternative drug in the treatment of the following infections:

Infections in women caused by *Neisseria gonorrhoeae*

Syphilis caused by *Treponema pallidum*

Yaws caused by *Treponema pertenue*

Listeriosis due to *Listeria monocytogenes*

Anthrax due to *Bacillus anthracis*

Vincent's infection caused by *Fusobacterium fusiforme*

Actinomycosis caused by *Actinomyces israelii*

Infections caused by *Clostridium* species

In *acute intestinal amebiasis,* minocycline may be a useful adjunct to amebicides.

In severe acne, minocycline may be useful adjunctive therapy.

Oral minocycline is indicated in the treatment of asymptomatic carriers of *Neisseria meningitidis* to eliminate meningococci from the nasopharynx. In order to preserve the usefulness of minocycline in the treatment of asymptomatic meningococcal carrier, diagnostic laboratory procedures, including serotyping and susceptibility testing, should be performed to establish the carrier state and the correct treatment. It is recommended that the prophylactic use of minocycline be reserved for situations in which the risk of meningococcal meningitis is high.

Oral minocycline is not indicated for the treatment of meningococcal infection.

Although no controlled clinical efficacy studies have been conducted, limited clinical data show that oral minocycline hydrochloride has been used successfully in the treatment of infections caused by *Mycobacterium marinum.*

CONTRAINDICATIONS

This drug is contraindicated in persons who have shown hypersensitivity to any of the tetracyclines.

WARNINGS

MINOCYCLINE, LIKE OTHER TETRACYCLINE-CLASS ANTIBIOTICS, CAN CAUSE FETAL HARM WHEN ADMINISTERED TO A PREGNANT WOMAN. IF ANY TETRACYCLINE IS USED DURING PREGNANCY OR IF THE PATIENT BECOMES PREGNANT WHILE TAKING THESE DRUGS, THE PATIENT SHOULD BE APPRISED OF THE POTENTIAL HAZARD TO THE FETUS. THE USE OF DRUGS OF THE TETRACYCLINE CLASS DURING TOOTH DEVELOPMENT (LAST HALF OF PREGNANCY, INFANCY, AND CHILDHOOD TO THE AGE OF 8 YEARS) MAY CAUSE PERMANENT DISCOLORATION OF THE TEETH (YELLOW-GRAY-BROWN).

This adverse reaction is more common during long-term use of the drug but has been observed following repeated short-term courses. Enamel hypoplasia has also been reported. TETRACYCLINE DRUGS, THEREFORE, SHOULD NOT BE USED DURING TOOTH DEVELOPMENT UNLESS OTHER DRUGS ARE NOT LIKELY TO BE EFFECTIVE OR ARE CONTRAINDICATED.

All tetracyclines form a stable calcium complex in any bone-forming tissue. A decrease in fibula growth rate has been

observed in young animals (rats and rabbits) given oral tetracycline in doses of 25 mg/kg every six hours. This reaction was shown to be reversible when the drug was discontinued. Results of animal studies indicate that tetracyclines cross the placenta, are found in fetal tissues, and can have toxic effects on the developing fetus (often related to retardation of skeletal development). Evidence of embryotoxicity has been noted in animals treated early in pregnancy.

The anti-anabolic action of the tetracyclines may cause an increase in BUN. While this is not a problem in those with normal renal function, in patients with significantly impaired function, higher serum levels of tetracycline may lead to azotemia, hyperphosphatemia, and acidosis. If renal impairment exists, even usual oral or parenteral doses may lead to excessive systemic accumulations of the drug and possible liver toxicity. Under such conditions, lower than usual total doses are indicated, and if therapy is prolonged, serum level determinations of the drug may be advisable.

Photosensitivity manifested by an exaggerated sunburn reaction has been observed in some individuals taking tetracyclines. This has been reported rarely with minocycline. Central nervous system side effects including lightheadedness, dizziness, or vertigo have been reported with minocycline therapy.

Patients who experience these symptoms should be cautioned about driving vehicles or using hazardous machinery while on minocycline therapy. These symptoms may disappear during therapy and usually disappear rapidly when the drug is discontinued.

PRECAUTIONS

General: As with other antibiotic preparations, use of this drug may result in overgrowth of nonsusceptible organisms, including fungi. If superinfection occurs, the antibiotic should be discontinued and appropriate therapy instituted.

Pseudotumor cerebri (benign intracranial hypertension) in adults has been associated with the use of tetracyclines. The usual clinical manifestations are headache and blurred vision. Bulging fontanels have been associated with the use of tetracyclines in infants. While both of these conditions and related symptoms usually resolve after discontinuation of tetracycline, the possibility for permanent sequelae exists. Incision and drainage or other surgical procedures should be performed in conjunction with antibiotic therapy when indicated.

Information for Patients: Photosensitivity manifested by an exaggerated sunburn reaction has been observed in some individuals taking tetracyclines. Patients apt to be exposed to direct sunlight or ultraviolet light should be advised that this reaction can occur with tetracycline drugs, and treatment should be discontinued at the first evidence of skin erythema. This reaction has been reported rarely with use of minocycline.

Patients who experience central nervous system symptoms (see **WARNINGS**) should be cautioned about driving vehicles or using hazardous machinery while on minocycline therapy.

Concurrent use of tetracycline may render oral contraceptives less effective (see **Drug Interactions**).

Laboratory Tests: In venereal disease when coexistent syphilis is suspected, a dark-field examination should be done before treatment is started and the blood serology repeated monthly for at least four months.

In long-term therapy, periodic laboratory evaluations of organ systems, including hematopoietic, renal, and hepatic studies should be performed.

Drug Interactions: Because tetracyclines have been shown to depress plasma prothrombin activity, patients who are on anticoagulant therapy may require downward adjustment of their anticoagulant dosage.

Since bacteriostatic drugs may interfere with the bactericidal action of penicillin, it is advisable to avoid giving tetracycline-class drugs in conjunction with penicillin.

Absorption of tetracyclines is impaired by antacids containing aluminum, calcium or magnesium, and iron-containing preparations. The concurrent use of tetracycline and methoxyflurane has been reported to result in fatal renal toxicity.

Concurrent use of tetracyclines may render oral contraceptives less effective.

Drug/Laboratory Test Interactions: False elevations of urinary catecholamine levels may occur due to interference with the fluorescence test.

Carcinogenesis, Mutagenesis, Impairment of Fertility: Dietary administration of minocycline in long-term tumorigenicity studies in rats resulted in evidence of thyroid tumor production. Minocycline has also been found to produce thyroid hyperplasia in rats and dogs. In addition, there has been evidence of oncogenic activity in rats in studies with a related antibiotic, oxytetracycline (i.e., adrenal and pituitary tumors). Likewise, although mutagenicity studies of minocycline have not been conducted, positive results in *in vitro* mammalian cell assays (i.e., mouse lymphoma and Chinese hamster lung cells) have been reported for related antibiotics (tetracycline hydrochloride and oxytetracycline). Segment I

(fertility and general reproduction) studies have provided evidence that minocycline impairs fertility in male rats.

Teratogenic Effects: *Pregnancy:* Pregnancy Category D (See **WARNINGS**.)

Labor and Delivery: The effect of tetracyclines on labor and delivery is unknown.

Nursing Mothers: Tetracyclines are excreted in human milk. Because of the potential for serious adverse reactions in nursing infants from the tetracyclines, a decision should be made whether to discontinue nursing or discontinue the drug, taking into account the importance of the drug to the mother (See **WARNINGS**).

Pediatric Use: (See **WARNINGS**).

ADVERSE REACTIONS

Due to oral minocycline's virtually complete absorption, side effects to the lower bowel, particularly diarrhea, have been infrequent. The following adverse reactions have been observed in patients receiving tetracyclines.

Gastrointestinal: Anorexia, nausea, vomiting, diarrhea, glossitis, dysphagia, enterocolitis, pancreatitis, and inflammatory lesions (with monilial overgrowth) in the anogenital region, increases in liver enzymes. Rarely, hepatitis and liver failure have been reported. Rare instances of esophagitis and esophageal ulcerations have been reported in patients taking the tetracycline-class anitibiotics in capsule and tablet form. Most of these patients took the medication immediately before going to bed (see **DOSAGE AND ADMINISTRATION**).

Skin: Maculopapular and erythematous rashes. Exfoliative dermatitis has been reported but is uncommon. Fixed drug eruptions, including balanitis, have been rarely reported. Erythema multiforme and rarely Stevens-Johnson syndrome have been reported. Photosensitivity is discussed above (see **WARNINGS**). Pigmentation of the skin and mucous membranes has been reported.

Renal toxicity: Elevations in BUN have been reported and are apparently dose related (See **WARNINGS**).

Hypersensitivity reactions: Urticaria, angioneurotic edema, anaphylaxis, anaphylactoid purpura, pericarditis, exacerbation of systemic lupus erythematosus and rarely pulmonary infiltrates with eosinophilia have been reported. A transient, lupus-like syndrome has also been reported.

Blood: Hemolytic anemia, thrombocytopenia, neutropenia, and eosinophilia have been reported.

Central Nervous System: Bulging fontanels in infants and benign intracranial hypertension (Pseudotumor cerebri) in adults (see **PRECAUTIONS-General**) have been reported. Headache has also been reported.

Other: When given over prolonged periods, tetracyclines have been reported to produce brown-black microscopic discoloration of the thyroid glands. Very rare cases of abnormal thyroid function have been reported. Decreased hearing has been rarely reported in patients on minocycline hydrochloride.

Tooth discoloration in children less than 8 years of age (see **WARNINGS**) and also, rarely, in adults have been reported.

OVERDOSAGE

In case of overdosage, discontinue medication, treat symptomatically and institute supportive measures.

DOSAGE AND ADMINISTRATION

THE USUAL DOSAGE AND FREQUENCY OF ADMINISTRATION OF MINOCYCLINE DIFFERS FROM THAT OF THE OTHER TETRACYCLINES. EXCEEDING THE RECOMMENDED DOSAGE MAY RESULT IN AN INCREASED INCIDENCE OF SIDE EFFECTS.

Minocycline hydrochloride capsules may be taken with or without food. (See **CLINICAL PHARMACOLOGY**.)

Adults: The usual dosage of minocycline hydrochloride is 200 mg initially followed by 100 mg every 12 hours. Alternatively, if more frequent doses are preferrred, two or four 50 mg capsules may be given initially followed by one 50 mg capsule four times daily.

For children above 8 years of age: The usual dosage of minocycline hydrochloride is 4 mg/kg initially followed by 2 mg/kg every 12 hours.

Uncomplicated gonococcal infections other than urethritis and anorectal infections in men: 200 mg initially, followed by 100 mg every 12 hours for a minimum of four days, with post-therapy cultures within 2 to 3 days.

In the treatment of uncomplicated gonococcal urethritis in men, 100 mg every 12 hours for five days is recommended. For the treatment of syphilis, the usual dosage of minocycline should be administered over a period of 10 to 15 days. Close follow-up, including laboratory tests, is recommended.

In the treatment of meningococcal carrier state, the recommended dosage is 100 mg every 12 hours for five days.

Mycobacterium marinum infections: Although optimal doses have not been established, 100 mg every 12 hours for 6 to 8 weeks have been used successfully in a limited number of cases.

Uncomplicated nongonococcal urethral infection in adults caused by *Chlamydia trachomatis* or *Ureaplasma urealyticum:* 100 mg orally, every 12 hours for at least seven days.

Ingestion of adequate amounts of fluids along with capsule forms of drugs in the tetracycline-class is recommended to reduce the risk of esophageal irritation and ulceration.

In patients with renal impairment (see **WARNINGS**), the total dosage should be decreased by either reducing the recommended individual doses and/or extending the time intervals between doses.

HOW SUPPLIED

DYNACIN® (Minocycline Hydrochloride Capsules, USP) equivalent to 50 mg minocycline are opaque yellow capsules supplied in bottles of 100 and 500.

DYNACIN® (Minocycline Hydrochloride Capsules, USP) equivalent to 100 mg minocycline are opaque dark gray and opaque yellow capsules supplied in bottles of 50 and 500.

Dispense in tight, light-resistant container with child-resistant closure.

Store at controlled room temperature, 15°–30°C (59°–86°F).

Protect from light, moisture and excessive heat.

CAUTION

Federal law prohibits dispensing without prescription.

ANIMAL PHARMACOLOGY AND TOXICOLOGY: Minocycline hydrochloride has been observed to cause a dark discoloration of the thyroid in experimental animals (rats, minipigs, dogs and monkeys). In the rat, chronic treatment with minocycline hydrochloride has resulted in goiter accompanied by elevated radioactive iodine uptake, and evidence of thyroid tumor production. Minocycline hydrochloride has also been found to produce thyroid hyperplasia in rats and dogs.

REFERENCES

1. National Committee for Clinical Laboratory Standards, Approved Standard: *Performance Standards for Antimicrobial Disk Susceptibility Tests,* 3rd Edition, Vol. 4(16):M2-A3, Villanova, PA, December 1984.
2. National Committee for Clinical Laboratory Standards, Approved Standard: *Methods for Dilution Antimicrobial Susceptibility Tests for Bacteria that Grow Aerobically,* 2nd Edition, Vol. 5(22):M7-A, Villanova, PA, December 1985.

Manufactured specially for:

MEDICIS DERMATOLOGICS, INC.
Phoenix, AZ 85018
by
DANBURY PHARMACAL INC.
Danbury, CT 06810

MG6432

THERAMYCIN™ Z ℞
ERYTHROMYCIN
2% SOLUTION

DESCRIPTION

THERAMYCIN Z (Erythromycin 2% Solution) is an antibiotic produced from a strain of *Streptomyces erythraeus.* It is basic and readily forms salts with acids. The active ingredient is represented by the following structure:

CONTENTS

Each mL of THERAMYCIN Z (Erythromycin 2% Solution) Contains: ACTIVE: Erythromycin, USP, 20mg in a clear solution vehicle of; INACTIVES: SD Alcohol 40B 81% (by weight) equivalent to Absolute Alcohol 86% (by volume), Propylene Glycol, Lauramide DEA, Hydroxypropyl Cellulose, Fragrance and Zinc Acetate.

CLINICAL PHARMACOLOGY

Although the mechanism by which Erythromycin 2% Solution acts in reducing inflammatory lesions of acne vulgaris is unknown, it is presumably due to its antibiotic action.

INDICATIONS AND USAGE

Erythromycin 2% Solution is indicated for the topical control of acne vulgaris.

CONTRAINDICATIONS

Erythromycin 2% Solution is contraindicated in persons who have shown hypersensitivity to erythromycin or any of the other listed ingredients.

WARNING

The safe use of Erythromycin 2% Solution during pregnancy or lactation has *not* been established.

PRECAUTIONS

General—The use of antibiotic agents may be associated with the overgrowth of antibiotic-resistant organisms. If this occurs, administration of this drug should be discontinued and appropriate measures taken.

Information for Patients—Erythromycin 2% Solution is for external use only and should be kept away from the eyes, nose, mouth and other mucous membranes. Concomitant topical acne therapy should be used with caution because a cumulative irritant effect may occur, especially with the use of peeling, desquamating, or abrasive agents.

Carcinogenesis, Mutagenesis, Impairment of Fertility—Long-term animal studies to evaluate carcinogenic potential, mutagenicity, or the effect on fertility of erythromycin have *not* been performed.

Pregnancy—Pregnancy Category C. Animal reproduction studies have *not* been conducted with erythromycin. It is also *not* known whether erythromycin can cause fetal harm when administered to a pregnant woman or can affect reproduction capacity. Erythromycin should be given to a pregnant woman only if clearly needed.

Nursing Mothers—Erythromycin is excreted in breast milk. Caution should be exercised when erythromycin is administered to a nursing mother.

ADVERSE REACTIONS

Adverse conditions reported include dryness, pruritus, desquamation, erythema, oiliness, and burning sensation. Irritation of the eyes has also been reported. A case of generalized urticarial reaction, possibly related to the drug, which required the use of systemic steroid therapy has been reported.

DOSAGE AND ADMINISTRATION

THERAMYCIN Z (Erythromycin 2% Solution) should be applied (ball type applicator should be rubbed) twice a day, once in the morning and once in the evening, to areas usually affected by acne. These areas should be washed with warm water and soap and patted dry before applying the THERAMYCIN Z. Acne lesions on the face, neck, shoulder, chest, and back may be treated in this manner. Shake well before using and close tightly after each use.

HOW SUPPLIED

THERAMYCIN Z (Erythromycin 2% Solution), 2 fl oz (59.14 mL) in a 60 mL plastic bottle with applicator attached—NDC 99207-550-02.

STORAGE

THERAMYCIN Z (Erythromycin 2% Solution) should be stored at Controlled Room Temperature 15°–30° C (59°–86°F). Preserve in a light-resistant container.

INSTRUCTIONS FOR INSTALLING APPLICATOR

1. Remove and discard temporary shipping cap.
2. Push applicator firmly into bottle using white cap as holder.
3. Screw cap down to seat applicator.

WARNINGS: Contains Alcohol—Do not use near open flame.

For external use only. Not for ophthalmic use.

Keep out of reach of children.

CAUTION: Federal law prohibits dispensing without prescription.

Manufactured specially for:
Medicis® Dermatologics, Inc.
The Dermatology Company™
Phoenix, AZ 85018
by: Zenith Goldline Dermatologicals, Inc.
Syosset; NY 11791

TRIAZ™ ℞

DESCRIPTION

TRIAZ 6%, TRIAZ 10% Gels and TRIAZ Cleanser are topical, gel-based, benzoyl peroxide containing preparations for use in the treatment of acne vulgaris. Benzoyl peroxide is an oxidizing agent that possesses antibacterial properties and is classified as a keratolytic. Benzoyl peroxide ($C_{14}H_{10}O_4$) is represented by the following chemical structure:

TRIAZ 6% and TRIAZ 10% Gels contain, respectively, benzoyl peroxide 6% and 10% as the active ingredient in a gel-based formulation consisting of: Water, C12-15 Alkyl Benzoate, Glycerin, Cetyl Stearyl Alcohol, Glycolic Acid, Polyacrylamide (and) C13-14 Isoparaffin (and) Laureth-7, PEG-100 Stearate, Stearth S-2, Sodium Hydroxide, Stearth S-20, Dimethicone, Zinc Lactate, Disodium EDTA.

Continued on next page

Medicis—Cont.

TRIAZ Cleanser contains benzoyl peroxide 10% as the active ingredient in a vehicle consisting of: Glycerin, Petrolatum, C12-15 Alkyl Benzoate, Sodium Cocoyl Isethionate, Water, Special Petrolatum Fraction, Sodium C14-16 Olefin Sulfonate, Zinc Lactate, Carbomer, Potassium Polymetaphosphate, Titanium Dioxide, Glycolic Acid, Sodium Hydroxide, Lavender Extract, Menthol.

CLINICAL PHARMACOLOGY

The mechanism of action of benzoyl peroxide is not totally understood but its antibacterial activity against *Propionibacterium acnes* is thought to be a major mode of action. In addition, patients treated with benzoyl peroxide show a reduction in lipids and free fatty acids and mild desquamation (drying and peeling activity) with simultaneous reduction in comedones and acne lesions.

Little is known about the percutaneous penetration, metabolism, and excretion of benzoyl peroxide, although it has been shown that benzoyl peroxide absorbed by the skin is metabolized to benzoic acid and then excreted as benzoate in the urine. There is no evidence of systemic toxicity caused by benzoyl peroxide in humans.

INDICATIONS AND USAGE

TRIAZ 6% and TRIAZ 10% Gels and TRIAZ Cleanser are indicated for the topical treatment of acne vulgaris.

CONTRAINDICATIONS

These preparations are contraindicated in patients with a history of hypersensitivity to any of their components.

WARNINGS

When using this product, avoid unnecessary sun exposure and use a sunscreen.

PRECAUTIONS

General: For external use only. If severe irritation develops, discontinue use and institute appropriate therapy. After reaction clears, treatment may often be resumed with less frequent application. These preparations should not be used in or near the eyes or on mucous membranes.

Information for patients: Avoid contact with eyes, eyelids, lips and mucous membranes. If accidental contact occurs, rinse with water. Contact with any colored material (including hair and fabric) may result in bleaching or discoloration. If excessive irritation develops, discontinue use and consult your physician.

Carcinogenesis, Mutagenesis, Impairment of Fertility: Data from several studies employing a strain of mice that are highly susceptible to developing cancer suggest that benzoyl peroxide acts as a tumor promoter. The clinical significance of these findings to humans is unknown. Benzoyl peroxide has not been found to be mutagenic (Ames Test) and there are no published data indicating it impairs fertility.

Pregnancy: Teratogenic Effects: *Pregnancy Category C:* Animal reproduction studies have not been conducted with benzoyl peroxide. It is not known whether benzoyl peroxide can cause fetal harm when administered to a pregnant woman or can affect reproduction capacity. Benzoyl peroxide should be used by a pregnant woman only if clearly needed. There are no available data on the effect of benzoyl peroxide on the later growth, development and functional maturation of the unborn child.

Nursing Mothers: It is not known whether this drug is excreted in human milk. Because many drugs are excreted in human milk, caution should be exercised when benzoyl peroxide is administered to a nursing woman.

Pediatric Use: Safety and effectiveness in children have not been established.

ADVERSE REACTIONS

Allergic contact dermatitis and dryness have been reported with topical benzoyl peroxide therapy.

OVERDOSAGE

If excessive scaling, erythema or edema occurs, the use of this preparation should be discontinued. To hasten resolution of the adverse effects, cool compresses may be used. After symptoms and signs subside, a reduced dosage schedule may be cautiously tried if the reaction is judged to be due to excessive use and not allergenicity.

DOSAGE AND ADMINISTRATION

TRIAZ Gels: Apply once or twice daily to cover affected areas, or as directed by your dermatologist. Use after washing with a mild cleanser, such as TRIAZ Cleanser, and water.

TRIAZ Cleanser: Wash affected areas once or twice daily, or as directed by your dermatologist. Avoid contact with eyes or mucous membranes. Wet skin and liberally apply to areas to be cleansed; massage gently into skin for 10–20 seconds working to a full lather; rinse thoroughly and pat dry. If drying occurs, it may be controlled by rinsing cleanser off sooner or using less often.

HOW SUPPLIED

TRIAZ 6% Gel—1.5 oz. (42.5g) tube, NDC 99207-051-01.
TRIAZ 10% Gel—1.5 oz. (42.5g) tube, NDC 99207-210-01.
TRIAZ Cleanser—3 oz. (85.1 g) tube, NDC 99207-106-02.

Caution: Federal law prohibits dispensing without prescription. Store at controlled room temperature (59°–86°F).

Manufactured specially for:
Medicis® Dermatologics, Inc. 10/95
The Dermatology Company™
Phoenix, AZ 85018
by: PACO Pharmaceutical Services, Inc.
Lakewood, NJ 08701

MedImmune, Inc.
35 WEST WATKINS MILL ROAD
GAITHERSBURG, MD 20878

Direct Inquiries to:
Professional Services:
(800) 949-3789
Customer Services:
(301) 527-4300

For Medical Information Contact:
In Emergencies:
(301) 527-4300

CYTOMEGALOVIRUS ℞
IMMUNE GLOBULIN INTRAVENOUS (HUMAN)
CYTOGAM® Liquid Formulation Solvent Detergent Treated

DESCRIPTION

CytoGam®, Cytomegalovirus Immune Globulin Intravenous (Human) (CMV-IGIV), is an immunoglobulin G (IgG) containing a standardized amount of antibody to Cytomegalovirus (CMV). CMV-IGIV is formulated in final vial as a sterile liquid. The globulin is stabilized with 5% sucrose and 1% Albumin (Human). CytoGam® contains no preservative. The purified immunoglobulin is derived from pooled adult human plasma selected for high titers of antibody for Cytomegalovirus (CMV).[1] Source material for fractionation may be obtained from another U.S. licensed manufacturer. Pooled plasma was fractionated by ethanol precipitation of the proteins according to Cohn Methods 6 and 9, modified to yield a product suitable for intravenous administration. A widely utilized solvent-detergent viral inactivation process is also.[2] Certain manufacturing operations may be performed by other firms. Each milliliter contains: 50 ± 10 mg of immunoglobulin, primarily IgG, and trace amounts of IgA and IgM; 50 mg of sucrose; 10 mg of Albumin (Human). The sodium content is 20–30 mEq per liter; i.e. 0.4–0.6 mEq per 20 ml or 1.0–1.5 mEq per 50 ml. The solution should appear colorless and translucent.

CLINICAL PHARMACOLOGY

CytoGam® contains IgG antibodies representative of the large number of normal persons who contributed to the plasma pools from which the product was derived. The globulin contains a relatively high concentration of antibodies directed against Cytomegalovirus (CMV). In the case of persons who may be exposed to CMV, CytoGam® can raise the relevant antibodies to levels sufficient to attenuate or reduce the incidence of serious CMV disease.

In two separate clinical trials, CytoGam® was shown to provide effective prophylaxis in renal-transplant recipients at risk for primary CMV disease. In the first randomized trial,[3] the incidence of virologically confirmed CMV-associated syndromes was reduced from 60% in controls ($n=35$) to 21% in recipients of CMV immune globulin ($n=24$) ($P<0.01$); marked leukopenia was reduced from 37% in controls to 4% in globulin recipients ($P<0.01$); and fungal or parasite superinfections were not seen in globulin recipients but occurred in 20% of controls. ($P=0.05$). Serious CMV disease was reduced from 46% to 13%. There was a concomitant but not statistically significant reduction in the incidence of CMV pneumonia (17% of controls is as compared with 4% of globulin recipients). There was no effect on rates of viral isolation or seroconversion although the rate of viremia was less in CytoGam® recipients. In a subsequent nonrandomized trial in renal transplant recipients ($n=36$),[4] the incidence of virologically confirmed CMV-associated syndrome was reduced to 36% in the globulin recipients. The rates of CMV-associated pneumonia, CMV-associated hepatitis, and concomitant fungal and parasitic superinfection were similar to those in the first trial.

INDICATIONS AND USAGE

Cytomegalovirus Immune Globulin Intravenous (Human) is indicated for the attenuation of primary (1°) Cytomegalovirus disease associated with kidney transplantation. Specifically, the product is indicated for kidney transplant recipients who are seronegative for CMV and who receive a kidney from a CMV seropositive donor. In a population of seronegative recipients of seropositive kidneys approximately 75% of the untreated recipients would be expected to develop CMV disease.[1,5] Clinical studies have shown a 50% reduction in 1° CMV disease in renal transplant patients given Cytomegalovirus Immune Globulin Intravenous (Human).[3,4,6]

CONTRAINDICATIONS

CytoGam® should not be used in individuals with a history of a prior severe reaction associated with the administration of this or other human immunoglobulin preparations. Persons with selective immunoglobulin A deficiency have the potential for developing antibodies to immunoglobulin A and could have anaphylactic reactions to subsequent administration of blood products that contain immunoglobulin A, including CytoGam®.

WARNINGS

During administration, the patient's vital signs should be monitored continuously and careful observation made for any symptoms throughout the infusion. Epinephrine should be available for the treatment of an acute anaphylactic reaction (see PRECAUTIONS section).

PRECAUTIONS

Although systemic allergic reactions are rare (see ADVERSE REACTIONS section), epinephrine and diphenhydramine should be available for treatment of acute allergic symptoms. If hypertension or anaphylaxis occur, the administration of the immunoglobulin should be discontinued immediately and an antidote should be given as noted above.

An aseptic meningitis syndrome (AMS) has been reported to occur infrequently in association with immune Globulin Intravenous (Human) (IGIV) treatment (7–10). The syndrome usually begins with several hours to two days following IGIV treatment. It is characterized by symptoms and signs including severe headache, nuchal rigidity, drowsiness, fever, photophobia, painful eye movements, and nausea and vomiting. Cerebrospinal fluid studies are frequently positive with pleocytosis up to several thousand cells per cu.mm., predominantly from the granulocytic series, and elevated protein levels up to several hundred mg/dl. Patients exhibiting such symptoms and signs should receive a thorough neurological examination, including CSF studies, to rule out other causes of meningitis. AMS may occur more frequently in association with high dose (2 g/kg) IGIV treatment. Discontinuation of IGIV treatment. Discontinuation of IGIV treatment has resulted in remission of AMS within several days without sequelae.

CMV-IGIV is made from human plasma and, like other plasma products, carries the possibility for transmission of blood-borne vial agents. The risk of transmission of recognized blood-borne viruses is considered to be low because of the viral inactivation and removal properties in the Cohn-Oncley cold ethanol precipitation procedure used for purification of immune globulin products (11–13). Until 1993, cold ethanol manufactured immune globulins licensed in the United States had not been documented to transmit any viral agent. However, during a brief period in late 1993 to early 1994, intravenous immune globulin made by one U.S. manufacturer was associated with transmission of Hepatitis C virus (14). To further guard against possible transmission of blood-borne viruses, including Hepatitis C, CMV-IGIV is treated with a solvent detergent viral inactivation procedure (2) known to inactivate a wide spectrum of lipid enveloped viruses, including HIV-1, HIV-2, Hepatitis B, and Hepatitis C (15). However, because new blood-borne viruses may yet emerge, some of which may not be inactivated by the manufacturing process or by solvent detergent treatment, CMV-IGIV, like any other blood product, should be given only if a benefit is expected.

CytoGam® does not contain a preservative. The vial should be entered only once for administration purposes and the infusion should begin within 6 hours. The infusion schedule should be adhered to closely (see INFUSION section). Do not use if the solution is turbid.

Drug Interaction: Antibodies present in immune globulin preparations may interfere with the immune response to live virus vaccines such as measles, mumps, and rubella; therefore, vaccination with live virus vaccines should be deferred until approximately three months after administration of CytoGam®. If such vaccinations were given shortly after CytoGam®, a revaccination may be necessary. Admixture of CytoGam® with other drugs have not been evaluated. It is recommended that CytoGam® be administered separately from other drugs or medications which the patient may be receiving (see ADMINISTRATION section).

Pregnancy Category C: Animal reproduction studies have not been conducted with Cytomegalovirus Immune Globulin Intravenous (Human). It is also not known whether Cytomegalovirus Immune Globulin Intravenous (Human) can cause fetal harm when administered to a pregnant woman or can affect reproduction capacity. Cytomegalovirus Immune Globulin Intravenous (Human) should be given to a pregnant woman only if clearly needed.

ADVERSE REACTIONS

Minor reactions such as flushing, chills, muscle cramps, back pain, fever, nausea, arthralgia, and wheezing were the most

frequent adverse reactions observed during the clinical trials of CytoGam®. The incidence of these reactions during the clinical trials was less than 5.0% of all infusions and were most often related to infusion rates. A potential side reaction might be hypotension but this has not been observed in over 200 infusions. If a patient develops a minor side effect, slow the rate immediately or temporarily interrupt the infusion. Severe reactions such as angloneurotic edema and anaphylactic shock, although not observed during clinical trials, are a possibility. Clinical anaphylaxis may occur even when the patient is not known to be sensitized to immune globulin products. A reaction may be related to the rate of infusion; therefore, carefully adhere to the infusion rates as outlined under "DOSAGE AND ADMINISTRATION." If anaphylaxis or drop in blood pressure occurs, *discontinue infusion* and use antidote such as diphenhydramine and adrenalin.

OVERDOSAGE

Although little data are available, clinical experience with other immunoglobulin preparations suggests that the major manifestations would be those related to volume overload.

DOSAGE AND ADMINISTRATION

The maximum recommended total dosage per infusion is 150 mg/kg, administered according to the following schedule:

Within:	72 hours of transplant:	150 mg/kg
	2 weeks post transplant:	100 mg/kg
	4 weeks post transplant:	100 mg/kg
	6 weeks post transplant:	100 mg/kg
	8 weeks post transplant:	100 mg/kg
	12 weeks post transplant:	50 mg/kg
	16 weeks post transplant:	50 mg/kg

Preparation for Administration. Remove the tab portion of the vial cap and clean the rubber stopper with 70% alcohol or equivalent. DO NOT SHAKE VIAL; AVOID FOAMING. Parenteral drug products should be inspected visually for particulate matter and discoloration prior to administration whenever solution and container permit. Infuse the solution only if it is colorless, free of particulate matter and not turbid.

Infusion. Infusion should begin within 6 hours after entering the vial and should be complete within 12 hours of entering the vial. Vital signs should be taken preinfusion, midway and post-infusion as well as before any rate increase. CytoGam® should be administered through an intravenous line using a constant infusion pump (i.e., IVAC pump or equivalent). Pre-dilution of CytoGam® before infusion is not recommended. CytoGam® should be administered through a separate intravenous line. If this is not possible, CytoGam® may be "piggybacked" into a pre-existing line if that line contains either Sodium Chloride, Injection, USP, or one of the following dextrose solutions (with or without NaCl added): 2.5% dextrose in water, 5% dextrose in water, 10% dextrose in water, 20% dextrose in water. If a preexisting line must be used, the CytoGam® should not be diluted more than 1:2 with any of the above-named solutions. Admixtures of CytoGam® with any other solutions have not been evaluated. While filters are not necessary, and in-line filter may be used for the infusion of CytoGam®.

Initial Dose. Administer Intravenously at 15 mg per kg body weight per hour. If no adverse reactions occur after 30 minutes, the rate may be increased to 30 mg/kg/hr; If no adverse reactions occur after a subsequent 30 minutes, then the Infusion may be increased to 60 mg/kg/hr (volume not to exceed 75 ml/hour). DO NOT EXCEED THIS RATE OF ADMINISTRATION. The patient should be monitored closely during and after each rate change.

Subsequent Doses. Administer at 15 mg/kg/hr for 15 minutes. If no adverse reactions occur, increase to 30 mg/kg/hr for 15 minutes and then increase to a maximum rate of 60 mg/kg/hr (volume not to exceed 75 ml/hour). DO NOT EXCEED THIS RATE OF ADMINISTRATION. The patient should be monitored closely during each rate change.

Potential adverse reactions are: flushing, chills, muscle cramps, back pain, fever, nausea, vomiting, wheezing, drop in blood pressure. Minor adverse reactions have been infusion rate related-if the patient develops a minor side effect (i.e., nausea, back pain, flushing), slow the rate or temporarily interrupt the infusion. If anaphylaxis or drop in blood pressure occurs, discontinue infusion and use antidote such as diphenhydramine and adrenalin.

To prevent the transmission of hepatitis viruses or other infectious agents from one person to another, sterile disposable syringes and needles should be used. The syringes and needles should not be reused.

HOW SUPPLIED

CytoGam®, Cytomegalovirus Immune Globulin Intravenous (Human), is supplied in two single-dose vial forms:

NDC No.	Total Quantity of Immunoglobulin	Volume	Concentration
60574-3102-1	1000 mg ± 200 mg	20 ml	50 ± 10 mg/ml
60574-3101-1	2500 mg ± 500 mg	50 ml	50 ± 10 mg/ml

STORAGE

CytoGam® should be stored between 2°C and 8°C (35.6°F and 46.4°F), and used within 6 hours after entering the vial.

REFERENCES

1. Snydman, D.R., McIver, J., Leszczynski, J., Cho, S.I., Werner, B.G., Berardi, V.P., LoGerfo, F., HeinzeLacey, B., Grady, G.F. A Pilot Trial of a Novel Cytomegalovirus Immune Globulin in Renal Transplant Recipients. Transplantation 38(5):553–557, 1984.
2. Horowitz, B., Wiebe, M.E., Lippin, A. et al. Inactivation of Viruses in Labile Blood Derivatives. Transfusion; 25:516–522, 1985.
3. Snydman, D.R., Werner, B.G., and Heinze-Lacey, B.H., et al. Use of Cytomegalovirus Immune Globulin to Prevent Cytomegalovirus Disease in Renal Transplant Recipients. NEJM 317:1049–1054, 1987.
4. Snydman, D.R., Werner, B.G., and Tilney, N.L., et al. A Final Analysis of Primary Cytomegalovirus Disease Prevention in Renal Transplant Recipient with a Cytomegalovirus Immune Globulin:Comparison of Randomized and Open-Label Trials. Transplant. Proceed. 23(1):1357–1360, 1991.
5. Ho, M., Suwansirikul, S., Dowling, J.N., et al. The Transplant Kidney as a Source of Cytomegalovirus Infection. NEJM 293 (2):1109–1112, 1975.
6. Werner, B.G., Snydman, D.R., Freeman, R., et al. Cytomegalovirus Immune Globulin for the Prevention of Primary CMV Disease in Renal Transplant Patients: Analysis of Usage Under Treatment IND Status. Transplant. Proceed. 25(1):1441–1443, 1993.
7. Sekul E, Culper E. Dalaks M. Aseptic meningitis associated with high-dose intravenous immunoglobulin therapy: Frequency and risk factors. Ann Int Med; 123:259–262, 1994.
8. Kato E, Shindo S, Eto Y, Hashimoto N, Yamamoto M, Sakata Y, Hiyoshi Y, Administration of immune globulin associated with aseptic meningitis. JAMA; 3269–3270, 1988.
9. Casteels Van Daele M, Wijndaele L, Hunnick K, Gillis P. Intravenous immunoglobulin and acute aseptic meningitis. N Engl J Med; 323(9):614–615, 1990.
10. Scribner C, Kapit R, Philips E, Rickels N. Aseptic meningitis and intravenous immunoglobulin therapy. Ann Intern Med; 121:305–306, 1994.
11. Bossell, et al. Safety of therapeutic immune globulin preparations with respect to transmission of human T-lymphotropic virus type III/lymphodenopathy-associated virus infection MMWR vol. 35 (14):231–233, April 11, 1986.
12. Wells MA, Wittek AE, Epstein JS, et al. Inactivation and partition of human T-cell lymphotropic virus, type III, during ethanol fractionation of plasma. Transfusion 26:210–213, 1986.
13. McIver, J. Grady, G. Immunoglobulin preparations. In:-Churchill WH and Kurtz SR, (ed): Transfusion Medicine. Boston: Blackwell; 1988.
14. Schneider L, Geha R. Outbreak of Hepatitis C associated with intravenous immunoglobulin administration-United States, October 1993–June 1994. MMWR vol. 43 (28):505–509, July 22, 1994.
15. Edwards CA, Piet MP J, China S. Horowitz B. Tri(n Butyl) phosphate detergent treatment of licensed therapeutic and experimental blood derivatives. Vox Sang 52:53–59, 1987.

For additional information concerning Cytomegalovirus Immune Globulin Intravenous (Human) contact:

Professional Services
Medimmune, Inc.
35 West Watkins Mill Road
Gaithersburg, MD 20878, USA
1-800-949-3789

Manufactured by:
MASSACHUSETTS PUBLIC HEALTH
BIOLOGICAL LABORATORIES
Boston, Massachusetts 02130, USA
U.S. Govt. License No. 64

Selling Agent:
MedImmune, Inc.
35 West Watkins Mill Road
Gaithersburg, MD 20878, USA

3AA1201
Product Information as of August, 1995 Ed.002
2754

RESPIRATORY SYNCYTIAL VIRUS IMMUNE GLOBULIN INTRAVENOUS (HUMAN), (RSV-IGIV) ℞

RespiGam™ Liquid Formulation
Solvent Detergent Treated

DESCRIPTION

RespiGam™, Respiratory Syncytial Virus Immune Globulin Intravenous (Human) (RSV-IGIV) is a sterile liquid immunoglobulin G containing neutralizing antibody to Respiratory Syncytial Virus (RSV). Each lot of RespiGam™ meets the minimum potency specifications when compared to the validated Reference Standard. The globulin is stabilized with 5% sucrose and 1% Albumin (Human). RespiGam™ contains no preservative. The immunoglobulin is purified from pooled adult human plasma selected for high titers of neutralizing antibody against RSV using a proprietary patented screening assay (1). Source material for fractionation may be obtained from another U.S.-licensed manufacturer. Pooled plasma is fractionated by ethanol precipitation of the proteins according to Cohn Method 6 and Oncley Method 9, with additional steps to yield a product suitable for intravenous administration. A widely utilized solvent-detergent viral inactivation process is used to decrease the possibility of transmission of bloodborne pathogens (2). Certain manufacturing operations may be performed by other firms. Each milliliter contains 50 ± 10 mg immunoglobulin, primarily IgG, and trace amounts of IgA and IgM; 50 mg sucrose; and 10 mg Albumin (Human). The sodium content is 20–30 mEq per liter, i.e., 1.0–1.5 mEq per 50 ml. The solution should appear colorless and translucent.

CLINICAL PHARMACOLOGY

RespiGam™ contains IgG antibodies representative of the large number of normal healthy persons who contributed to the plasma pools from which the product was derived. The immune globulin contains a high concentration of neutralizing and protective antibodies directed against RSV (3). In vitro tests demonstrated that RespiGam™ neutralized each of 62 different RSV clinical isolates of both subgroup A (n=39) and subgroup B (n=23). In the PREVENT study monthly doses of 750 mg/kg of RespiGam™ attained trough geometric mean serum RSV neutralization antibody titers of 1:297 ± 38 (SE) one month after the first infusion, 1:477 ± 85 one month after the second infusion, 1:490 ± 61 one month after the third infusion and 1:429 ± 23 one month after the fourth infusion. The mean half-life of serum RSV neutralizing antibodies after RespiGam™ infusion is 22–28 days (4).

INDICATIONS AND USAGE

RespiGam™ is indicated for the prevention of serious lower respiratory tract infection caused by RSV in children under 24 months of age with bronchopulmonary dysplasia (BPD) or a history of premature birth (≤35 weeks gestation). RespiGam™ has been demonstrated to be safe and effective in reducing the incidence and duration of RSV hospitalization and the severity of RSV illness in these high risk infants.

CLINICAL STUDIES

In randomized, controlled studies of RSV disease prophylaxis, monthly doses of 750 mg/kg of RespiGam™ were effective in reducing the incidence of RSV hospitalization in high-risk children. Children with BPD may be at high risk for serious RSV disease up to 60 months of age (5). Children born prematurely may be at high risk for serious RSV disease during the first year of life (6). Summarized below are the results of the pivotal trial and three additional studies supportive of the safety and efficacy of RespiGam™.

Prevent Trial:

The pivotal trial known as the PREVENT trial was a 54 center, randomized, placebo-controlled, double-blind study of the safety and effectiveness of RespiGam™ in the prophylaxis of RSV disease in infants and children with BPD ≤24 months of age or premature birth (≤35 weeks gestation) ≤6 months of age at study entry. The age of premature infants at the end of the study ranged from 4.8 to 11.4 months. In this trial, 510 patients were randomized to receive monthly infusions in November through April of either 750 mg/kg (15 ml/kg) RespiGam™ or 15 ml/kg 1% Albumin (Human) serum as a control. The efficacy analyses of this study were conducted on an "intent-to-treat" basis that included all randomized patients. The prospectively defined endpoints for the study are shown in Table 1. RespiGam™ reduced the incidence of RSV hospitalization by 41%, (p=0.047) total days of RSV hospitalization by 53%, (p=0.045) total RSV hospital days with increased supplemental oxygen requirement by 60%, (p=0.007) and total RSV hospital days with a moderate or severe lower respiratory tract infection by 54% (p=0.049). A trend in reduction in total intensive care unit (ICU) days (44%) was observed although it was not statistically significant (p=0.407).

Continued on next page

MedImmune, Inc.—Cont.

Two additional endpoints were evaluated. The incidence of any hospitalization due to respiratory illness was compared between placebo control and children receiving RespiGam™. The incidence in placebo controls was 69/260 (26.5%) versus 41/250 (16.4%) in the RespiGam™ recipients. This represents a 38% reduction (p=0.005) in the incidence of respiratory hospitalization for RespiGam™ recipients. The total days of hospitalization for respiratory illness per 100 randomized children were compared between placebo controls and RespiGam™ recipients. There were 317 days per 100 control children and 170 days per 100 RespiGam™ children. This represents a 46% reduction (p=0.005) in the total days of hospitalization for respiratory illness per 100 randomized children for RespiGam™ recipients.

[See Table 1 below.]

PREVENT was not designed nor powered to detect treatment differences among subsets of participants. Reductions in RSV hospitalization ranging from 17% to 58% were observed in RespiGam™ treated subgroups defined by gender, categorical age (< or > 6 months at entry) and diagnosis. The largest reductions were seen in children >6 months of age, all of whom had BPD. The smallest observed reduction was seen among children age <6 months. This subgroup also had a low incidence of RSV hospitalization which limited the ability to quantify the magnitude of the treatment effect. Consequently, the effectiveness of RespiGam™ in the subgroup of premature infants without BPD could not be definitively established in this study. Analyses using weight as a categorical variable revealed that children with entry weight below the median (4.3 kg) had a 49% observed reduction in the incidence of RSV hospitalization.

RespiGam™ has not been investigated for its effect in the prevention of RSV related apnea or RSV related apnea-hypothermia-sepsis syndrome.

NIAID Trial:

The NIAID study was supportive, multi-center, randomized, non-placebo controlled, single-blind study of the safety and effectiveness of RespiGam™ in the prophylaxis of RSV disease in 274 infants and children at high risk of RSV disease due to chronic pulmonary disease (principally BPD), congenital heart disease (CHD), or premature birth (≤35 weeks gestation) (7,8,9). Compared to control children (n=90), children randomized to receive 750 mg/kg RespiGam™, Respiratory Syncytial Virus Immune Globulin Intravenous (Human) (RSV-IGIV) (n=92) showed a 57% (p=0.029) reduction in the incidence of RSV hospitalization, a 59% (p=0.030) reduction in total days of RSV hospitalization per 100 children, a 97% (p=0.049) reduction in RSV ICU days per 100 children and 100% reduction in mechanical ventilation per 100 children.

Cardiac Trial:

The CARDIAC trial was a supportive multi-center, randomized non-placebo controlled, single-blind study conducted to further assess the safety and efficacy of RespiGam™ in 429 children with congenital heart disease (CHD) of less than 48 months of age at enrollment. The mean age of children at entry was 9 months and ranged from 0 to 47 months. Although trends toward RespiGam™ efficacy were observed, the data were not statistically significant. The efficacy and safety of RespiGam™ has not been established in children with CHD (see WARNING SECTION).

Open Label Trial:

A third supportive clinical trial was conducted to determine the safety and pharmacokinetics of monthly 750 mg/kg doses of RespiGam™ in 68 children with BPD or prematurity. This multi-center study was open-label in design. During the study, seven children (10.3%) were hospitalized for RSV. RSV hospital days were 54 per 100 children (mean = 5.3 days, n=7) and RSV ICU days were 15 per 100 children (mean = 10 days, n=1).

RespiGam™ has not been demonstrated to be effective for the treatment of RSV infection.

CONTRAINDICATIONS

RespiGam™ should not be used in patients with a history of a severe prior reaction associated with the administration of RespiGam™ or other human immunoglobulin preparations. Patients with selective IgA deficiency have the potential for developing antibodies to IgA and could have anaphylactic or allergic reactions to subsequent administration of blood products that contain IgA, including RespiGam™.

WARNINGS

Infants with underlying pulmonary disease may be sensitive to extra fluid volume. Infusion of RespiGam™, particularly in children with BPD, may precipitate symptoms of fluid overload. Overall, 8.4% of participants (1% premature and 13% BPD) received new or extra diuretics during the period 24 hours before through 48 hours after at least one of their infusions in the PREVENT trial. The reason for this use was not recorded (e.g. prophylaxis, treatment, or part of routine care during a clinical visit). RespiGam™-related fluid overload was reported in 3 patients (1.2%) and RespiGam™-related respiratory distress was reported in 4 patients (1.6%); all had underlying BPD. With the exception of one child with respiratory distress (part of an acute allergic reaction) for whom RespiGam™ was discontinued, these children were managed with diuretics and/or modification of the infusion rate and went on to receive subsequent infusions. Complications related to fluid volume were recorded as a reason for incomplete or prolonged infusion in 2.0% of children receiving RespiGam™ (2.5% BPD and 1.1% premature) and in 1.5% of children receiving placebo in the PREVENT trial. Children with clinically apparent fluid overload should not be infused with RespiGam™.

RespiGam™ should be administered cautiously (see DOSAGE AND ADMINISTRATION). During administration, a patient's vital signs should be monitored frequently, and a patient should be observed for increases in heart rate, respiratory rate, retractions, and rales. **A loop diuretic such as furosemide or bumetanide should be available for management of fluid overload.**

Severe reactions, such as anaphylaxis or angioneurotic edema, have been reported in association with intravenous immunoglobulins even in patients not known to be sensitive to human immunoglobulins or blood products. Serious allergic reaction was noted in 2 patients in the PREVENT trial. These reactions were manifest as an acute episode of cyanosis, mottling and fever in one patient and respiratory distress in the other. The rate of allergic reaction appears to be low and consistent with rates observed for other Immune Globulin Intravenous (Human) [IGIV] products. **If hypotension, anaphylaxis, or severe allergic reaction occurs, discontinue infusion and administer epinephrine (1:1000), as required.**

The safety and efficacy of RespiGam™ in children with CHD has not been established. Although equivalent proportions of children in the RespiGam™ and control groups in the CARDIAC trial had adverse events, a larger number of RespiGam™ recipients had severe or life-threatening adverse events. These events were most frequently observed in infants with CHD with right to left shunts who underwent cardiac surgery.

PRECAUTIONS

Except for hypersensitivity reactions, adverse reactions to IGIVs may be related to the rate of administration. Careful adherence to the infusion rate outlined under DOSAGE AND ADMINISTRATION is therefore important. Loop diuretics should be available for the management of patients who are at risk for fluid overload. Although systemic allergic reactions are rare (see ADVERSE REACTIONS), epinephrine and diphenhydramine should be available for treatment of acute allergic symptoms.

Rare occurrences of aseptic meningitis syndrome (AMS) have been reported in association with Immune Globulin Intravenous (Human) (IGIV) treamtent (10, 11, 12, 13). AMS usually begins within several hours to two days following IGIV treatment and is characterized by symptoms and signs including severe headache, drowsiness, fever, photophobia, painful eye movements, muscle rigidity, and nausea and vomiting. Cerebrospinal fluid studies generally demonstrate pleocytosis, predominantly granulocytic, and elevated protein levels. Patients exhibiting such symptoms and signs should be thoroughly evaluated to rule out other causes of meningitis. AMS may occur more frequently in association with high dose (2 g/kg) IGIV treatment. Discontinuation of IGIV treatment has resulted in remission of AMS within several days without sequelae.

RespiGam™ is made from human plasma and, like other plasma products, carries the possibility for transmission of bloodborne pathogenic agents. The risk of transmission of recognized blood-borne viruses is considered to be low because of screening of plasma donors, an added viral inactivation step and removal properties in the Cohn-Oncley cold ethanol precipitation procedure used for purification of immune globulin products (14, 15, 16). Until 1993, cold ethanol manufactured immune globulins licensed in the United States had not been documented to transmit any viral agent. However, during a brief period in late 1993 to early 1994, intravenous immune globulin made by one U.S. manufacturer was associated with transmission of Hepatitis C virus (17). To further guard against possible transmission of blood-borne viruses, RespiGam™ is treated with a solvent-detergent viral inactivation procedure (2) known to inactivate a wide spectrum of lipid enveloped viruses, including HIV-1, HIV-2, Hepatitis B Virus and Hepatitis C Virus (18). However, because new blood-borne agents may yet emerge, some of which may not be inactivated or eliminated by the manufacturing process or by solvent-detergent treatment, RespiGam™, like any other blood product, should be given only if a benefit is expected.

RespiGam™ does not contain a preservative. The single-use vial should be entered only once for administration purposes and the infusion should begin within 6 hours. The infusion schedule should be adhered to closely (see DOSAGE AND ADMINISTRATION). Do not use if the solution is turbid.

Drug Interactions:

Antibodies present in immune globulin preparations may interfere with the immune response to live virus vaccines, such as mumps, rubella, and particularly measles. If such vaccines are given during or within 10 months after RespiGam™ infusion, reimmunization is recommended, if appropriate (19). Studies have suggested that responses to non-live childhood vaccines (e.g. DPT) are not substantially influenced by IGIVs administration (20). Limited information available from infants who received RespiGam™ concurrently with one or more doses of their primary immunization series indicates that antibody responses to diphtheria, tetanus pertussis and H. Influenza b may be lower in RespiGam™ recipients than in controls. It is not known whether antibody responses to trivalent oral polio vaccine might be affected by concurrent RespiGam™. Physicians may wish to consider giving a booster dose of these vaccines three or four months after the last dose of RespiGam™ in order to ensure immunity to DPT (diphtheria, pertussis, tetanus), DaPT (Diphtheria, acellular pertussis, tetanus), Hib (hemophilus influenza b) and OPV (oral poliovirus). The effect of human immunoglobulin on immunization with eIPV (enhanced, inactivated poliovirus vaccine) has not been evaluated.

Admixtures of RespiGam™ with other drugs have not been studied; however, it is recommended that RespiGam™ be administered separately from other drugs or medications that the patient may be receiving (see DOSAGE AND ADMINISTRATION).

Pregnancy Category C:

Animal reproduction studies have not been conducted with RespiGam™, Respiratory Syncytial Virus Immune Globulin Intravenous (Human) (RSV-IGIV). It is also not known whether RespiGam™ can cause fetal harm when administered to a pregnant woman or could affect reproduction capacity. RespiGam™ should be given to a pregnant woman only if clearly indicated.

ADVERSE REACTIONS

RespiGam™ is generally well tolerated. In the PREVENT trial of RespiGam™ in children with BPD or prematurity, there was no difference in the proportion of children in the RespiGam™ and placebo groups who reported adverse events.

Table 2 illustrates adverse events which the investigator judged potentially related to study drug (RespiGam™ or Placebo) and which were reported at an incidence of 1% or greater in the RespiGam™ group in the PREVENT trial. The number of children reporting one or more of these adverse events were evenly distributed between the two treatment groups (35 of 260 in placebo, and 43 of 250 in RespiGam™ patients, p=0.269). In addition, the distribution of severity of adverse events was not significantly different between the two groups (p=0.216). Respiratory distress occurred in 2% (6 of 250) of children receiving RespiGam™. Patients in the RespiGam™ group reported a slightly higher incidence of fever compared to the placebo group.

Table 1—Summary of PREVENT Trial Results

Clinical Endpoint	Control N=260	RespiGam™ (RSV-IGIV) (750 mg/kg) N=250	% Reduction
Incidence of RSV Hospitalization	35 (13.5%)	20 (8.0%)	41%
RSV Hospital Days/100 Children	129	60	53%
RSV Hospital Days with Increased Supplemental O_2/100 Children	85	34	60%
RSV Hospital Days with Moderate to Severe LRI*/100 Children	106	49	54%
RSV ICU Days/100 Children	50	28	44%
Days of RSV Mechanical Ventilation/100 Children	20	18	10%

*Lower Respiratory Tract Infection/Illness

Table 2
Potentially Drug Related* Adverse Events Reported at an Incidence of 1% in the RespiGam™ (RSV-IGIV) Group in the PREVENT Clinical Study of RespiGam™

	Placebo		RespiGam™	
Number in study	n=260		n=250	
Number of children with any	n	%	n	%
drug related adverse event	35	13	43	15
Number of children with drug related [1]:				
fever/pyrexia	6	2%	15	6%
respiratory distress	1	<1%	6	2%
vomiting/emesis	3	1%	5	2%
wheezing	4	2%	4	2%
diarrhea	1	<1%	3	1%
rales	0	0%	3	1%
fluid overload	0	0%	3	1%
tachycardia/increased pulse rate	0	0%	3	1%
rash	5	2%	3	1%
hypertension	0	0%	2	1%
hypoxia/hypoxemia	2	1%	2	1%
tachypnea	1	<1%	2	1%
gastroenteritis	1	<1%	2	1%
injection site inflammation	2	1%	2	1%
overdose effect	1	<1%	2	1%

* = events possibly, probably, or definitely related to study drug.
[1] a child may be represented in more than one category.

The incidence of serious adverse events potentially related to study drug was equivalent for both treatment groups with 2% of children in the placebo group and 2% of children in the RespiGam™ group reporting such events (p=0.538). The rate of serious adverse events is similar to the rate reported for other IGIVs.

Infrequent adverse reactions were reported (rate of less than one percent) in the PREVENT trial as potentially related to the use of RespiGam™ including: edema, pallor, hypotension, heart murmur, gagging, cyanosis, sleepiness, cough, rhinorrhea, eczema, skin cold and clammy, and conjunctival hemorrhage. Adverse events occurring only in the placebo group are not listed.

Reactions similar to those reported with other IGIVs may occur with RespiGam™. These include: dizziness, flushing, blood pressure changes, anxiety, palpitations, chest tightness, dyspnea, abdominal cramps, pruritus, myalgia or arthralgia (see WARNINGS). Such reactions are often related to the rate of infusion. Immediate allergic, anaphylactic, or hypersensitivity reactions may be observed (see CONTRAINDICATIONS). Rarely, aseptic meningitis syndrome (AMS) has been reported in association with IGIV treatment, particularly at high dosage (2 g/kg) (10–13) (see PRECAUTIONS). In the PREVENT trial, 3 children developed aseptic meningitis of unknown etiology; one had a presumptive diagnosis of enteroviral infection, another child had an unconfirmed diagnosis of Herpes simplex meningitis which improved in association with acyclovir treatment and a third child developed fever, vomiting and malaise associated with 21 cells/mm^3 in cerebrospinal fluid. Also, one child was initially reported to have hepatitis but was subsequently diagnosed with hemosiderosis judged unrelated to RespiGam™.

Other Safety Experience:
In the single-blind, controlled NIAID trial in children with BPD, CHD or prematurity, adverse reactions were reported in 3% of all RespiGam™ infusions. Five of 160 children were considered to have had mild fluid overload associated with infusion. The remaining adverse reactions consisted of mild decreases in oxygen saturation (n=8) and fever (n=5).

In the Open-label study in children with BPD or prematurity (n=68) infusion-associated adverse reactions were noted in 14 of 294 (4.8%) infusions. Six adverse events were considered related to infusion, including 4 mild and 2 moderate events.

In the CARDIAC study, children with CHD with right to left shunts appeared to have an increased frequency of cardiac surgery and had a greater frequency of severe and life-threatening adverse events associated with cardiac surgery (see WARNINGS).

OVERDOSAGE

Although few data are available, clinical experience with other immune globulin preparations suggests that the major manifestations would be those related to fluid volume overload.

DOSAGE AND ADMINISTRATION

The maximum recommended total dosage per monthly infusion is 750 mg/kg, administered according to the following schedule:

Time After Start of Infusion	Rate of Infusion (ml/kg of Body Mass per Hour)
0–15 minutes	1.5 ml/kg/hr
15–30 minutes	3.0 ml/kg/hr
30 minutes to end of infusion	6.0 ml/kg/hr

Administer RespiGam™ intravenously at 1.5 ml/kg/hr for 15 minutes. If the clinical condition does not contraindicate a higher rate, increase the rate to 3.0 ml/kg/hr for 15 minutes and finally increase to a maximum rate of 6.0 ml/kg/hr. DO NOT EXCEED THIS RATE OF ADMINISTRATION. Monitor the patient closely during and after each rate change. In especially ill children with BPD, slower rates of infusion may be indicated.

A physician may want to consider factors such as other clinical illness, how well the child has grown and the risk of exposure from siblings or daycare when determining whether to use RespiGam™, Respiratory Syncytial Virus Immune Globulin Intravenous (Human) (RSV-IGIV). The first dose should be administered prior to commencement of the RSV season and subsequent doses should be administered monthly throughout the RSV season in order to maintain protection. In the Northern Hemisphere the RSV season typically commences in November and runs through April. Children should be infused from early November through April, unless RSV activity begins earlier or persists later in a community. It is recommended that RespiGam™ be administered separately from other drugs or medications that the patient may be receiving. It is recommended that children infected with RSV continue to receive monthly doses of RespiGam™ for the duration of the RSV season.

Preparation for Administration:
Remove the tab portion of the vial cap and clean the rubber stopper with 70% alcohol or equivalent. RespiGam™, like all parenteral drug products, should be inspected for particulate matter and discoloration prior to administration. Infuse the solution only if it is colorless and not turbid. DO NOT SHAKE VIAL; AVOID FOAMING.

Infusion:
Infusion should begin within 6 hours and should be completed within 12 hours after the single-use vial is entered. The patient's vital signs and cardiopulmonary status should be assessed prior to infusion, before each rate increase, and thereafter at 30-minute intervals until 30 minutes following completion of the infusion. RespiGam™ should be administered through an intravenous line using a constant infusion pump (i.e. IVAC pump or equivalent). Predilution of RespiGam™ before infusion is not recommended. If possible, RespiGam™ should be administered through a separate intravenous line, although it may be "piggy-backed" into a pre-existing line if that line contains one of the following dextrose solutions (with or without sodium chloride): 2.5%, 5%, 10%, or 20% dextrose in water. If a pre-existing line must be used, the RespiGam™ should not be diluted more than 1:2 with any other of the above-named solutions. Admixtures of RespiGam™ with any other solutions have not been evaluated. While filters are not necessary, an in-line filter with a pore size larger than 15 micrometers may be used for the infusion of RespiGam™.

To prevent the transmission of hepatitis viruses or infectious agents from one person to another, sterile disposable syringes and needles should be used. Do not reuse syringes and needles.

HOW SUPPLIED

RespiGam™, Respiratory Syncytial Virus Immune Globulin Intravenous (Human) is supplied in a single-use vial containing:

NDC no.	Total Quantity of Immunoglobulin	Volume	Concentration
60574-2101-1	2500 mg ± 500 mg	50 ml	50 mg ± 10 mg/ml

STORAGE

RespiGam™ should be stored between 2° C and 8° C (35.6° F and 46.4° F). Do not freeze.

REFERENCES

1. Siber GR, Leszczynski J, Pena-Cruz V, et al. Protective Activity of a Human Respiratory Syncytial Virus Immune Globulin Prepared from Donors Screened by Microneutralization Assay. *J. Infect. Dis*; 165:456-463, 1992.
2. Horowitz B, Wiebe ME, Lippin A, et al. Inactivation of Viruses in Labile Blood Derivatives. *Transfusion*; 25:516-522, 1985.
3. Siber GR, Leombruno D, Leszczynski J, et al. Comparison of Antibody Concentrations and Protective Activity of Respiratory Syncytial Virus (RSV) Immune Globulin and Conventional Immune Globulin. *J. Infect. Dis*; 169:1368-1373, 1994.
4. Groothuis JR, Simoes EAF, Lehr MV, et al. Safety and Bioequivalency of Three Formulations of Respiratory Syncytial Virus-enriched Immunoglobulin. *Antimicrob. Agents Chemother*, 39:668-671, 1995.
5. Groothuis JR, Gutierrez M, Lauer B, Respiratory Syncytial Virus Infection in Children with Bronchopulmonary Dysplasia. *Pediatrics*; 82:199-203, 1988.
6. Green, Brayer, Schenkman and Wald, *Ped. Inf. Dis. J*;. 8:601-605, 1989.
7. Groothuis JR, Simoes EAF, Hemming VG, et al. Prophylactic Administration of Respiratory Syncytial Virus (RSV) Immune Globulin in High Risk Infants and Young Children. *N. Engl. J. Med*; 329:1524-30, 1993.
8. Ellenberg SS, Epstein JS, Fratantoni JC, et al. A Trial of RSV Immune Globulin in Infants and Young Children; The FDA's View. *N. Engl. J. Med*; 331:203-204, 1994.
9. Groothuis JR, Hemming VR, Siber GR, et al. Reply to ibid. *N. Engl. J. Med.* 331:204-205, 1994.
10. Sekul E, Culper E, Dalaks M. Aseptic Meningitis Associated with High-dose Intravenous Immunoglobulin Therapy: Frequency and Risk Factors. *Ann Int. Med*; 123:259-262, 1994.
11. Kato E, Shindo S, Eto Y, et al. Administration of Immune Globulin Associated with Aseptic Meningitis. *JAMA*; 3269-3270, 1988.
12. Casteels Van Daele M, Wijndaele L, Hunnick K, et al. Intravenous Immunoglobulin and Acute Aseptic Meningitis. *N. Eng. J. Med*,; 323:614-615, 1990.
13. Scribner C, Kapit R, Phillips E, et al. Aseptic Meningitis and Intravenous Immunoglobulin Therapy. *Ann. Int. Med*; 121:305-306, 1994.
14. Bossell J, Safety of Therapeutic Immune Globulin Preparations with Respect to Transmission of Human T-lymphotropic Virus Type III/Lymphadenopathy-Associated Virus Infection. *MMWR*; 35:231-233, 1986.
15. Wells MA, Wittek AE, Epstein JS, et al. Inactivation and Partition of Human T-cell Lymphotrophic Virus, Type III, During Ethanol Fractionation of Plasma. *Transfusion*; 26:210-213, 1986.
16. Mclver J, Grady G. Immunoglobulin Preparations. In: Churchill WH and Kurtz S R, (ed): *Transfusion Medicine.* Boston: Blackwell; 1988.
17. Schneider L, Geha R. Outbreak of Hepatitis C Associated with Intravenous Immunoglobulin Administration—United States October 1993-June 1994. *MMWR*; 43:505-509, 1994.
18. Edwards CA, Piet MPJ, Chin S, et al. Tri(n Butyl) Phosphate Detergent Treatment of Licensed Therapeutic and Experimental Blood Derivatives. *Vox Sang*; 52:53-59, 1987.
19. Siber GR, Werner BG, Halsey NA, et al. Interference of Immune Globulin with Measles and Rubella Immunization. *J. Pediatrics*; 122:204-211, 1993.
20. General Recommendations on Immunization. Recommendations of the Advisory Committee on Immunization Practices. *MMWR*; 43:1-38, 1994.

For additional information concerning RespiGam™ (Respiratory Syncytial Virus Immune Globulin Intravenous [Human]) (RSV-IGIV), contact:
Professional Services
MedImmune, Inc.
35 West Watkins Mill Road
Gaithersburg, MD 20878, USA
Product Information as of January, 1996
1-800-949-3789
Manufactured by:
MASSACHUSETTS PUBLIC HEALTH BIOLOGIC LABORATORIES
Boston, Massachusetts 02130, USA
U.S. Govt. License No. 64
Selling Agent: **MedImmune, Inc.**
Gaithersburg, MD 20878
Product information as of January, 1996

Medisan Pharmaceuticals Inc.
400 LANIDEX PLAZA
PARSIPPANY, NJ 07054

Direct Inquiries to:
Jane Flynn
800-763-3472 (TELEPHONE)
201-515-9799 (FAX)

HYSKON® Hysteroscopy Fluid ℞
32% (w/v) dextran 70 in dextrose

DESCRIPTION

HYSKON® Hysteroscopy Fluid is a clear, viscid, sterile, non-pyrogenic solution of dextran 70 (32% w/v) in dextrose (10% w/v). Dextran 70 is that fraction of dextran, a branched polysaccharide composed of glucose units, having a weight average molecular weight of 70,000. The fluid is electrolyte-free and non-conductive. At room temperature HYSKON® Hysteroscopy Fluid has a viscosity of 220 cS.

Continued on next page

Medisan Pharmaceuticals—Cont.

HYSKON® has a tendency to crystallize when subjected to temperature variations or when stored for long periods. If flakes of dextran are present, heat at 100–110° C until complete dissolution is achieved.

INDICATIONS AND USAGE

HYSKON® Hysteroscopy Fluid is indicated for use with the hysteroscope as an aid in distending the uterine cavity and in irrigating and visualizing its surfaces.

CONTRAINDICATIONS

HYSKON® Hysteroscopy Fluid should not be instilled in patients known to be hypersensitive to dextran. All other contraindications are those related to the hysteroscopic procedure itself, such as pregnancy, endometrial carcinoma, etc.

WARNINGS

It is possible that during hysteroscopy dextran may leak into the peritoneal cavity, the precise amount depending on the volume of HYSKON® instilled and the instillation pressure. Slow absorption from the peritoneal cavity (peak blood levels are reached in 3–4 days) (1) may result in systemic effects varying from simple plasma volume expansion or a transient prolongation of the bleeding time, to severe, fatal anaphylactic reactions. It is also reported that dextran may enter the pleural cavity through a pathway that has yet to be defined (2). When HYSKON® is employed during diagnostic hysteroscopy dextran absorption also may occur, but adverse effects are rare. In hysteroscopic surgery greater volumes of HYSKON® are instilled over a longer period of time and the exposed blood vessels of the freshly traumatized endometrium allow the dextran direct access to the systemic circulation. Elevated blood levels of dextran have been observed within 30 minutes of a hysteroscopic procedure (3). For each 100 mL of HYSKON® absorbed into the systemic circulation, the intravascular volume is expanded by up to 800 mL. Therefore, patients should be observed for signs of circulatory overload, including pulmonary edema.

Because of the potential for rapid absorption of dextran, there is the potential for these patients to rapidly develop adverse systemic effects, in particular pulmonary edema (3). Patients are considered at increased risk of developing pulmonary edema if:

1. They undergo a surgical procedure lasting more than 45 minutes when HYSKON® is being used to distend the uterus.
2. Greater than 250 ml of HYSKON® remain in the body.
3. Large areas of endometrium are traumatized during surgery.
4. The volume of intravascular fluids being administered concurrently is beyond maintenance needs.

ADVERSE REACTIONS

The following adverse reactions, although rare, have been reported for HYSKON®: fatal anaphylactic reaction, generalized itching, macular rash, urticaria, nasal congestion, flushing, hypotension, dyspnea, tightness of chest, cyanosis, wheezing, coughing, peripheral edema, pulmonary edema, pleural effusion, ascites, nausea, vomiting, fever, joint pains, oliguria, convulsions and increased clotting time. In one large series, the incidence of pulmonary edema was 2/1793 or 0.11%. When greater than 500 mL were instilled, the incidence was 2/138 or 1.4% (4).

DOSAGE AND ADMINISTRATION

The amount of HYSKON® Hysteroscopy Fluid required depends on a numberr of factors, including the type and length of the procedure and whether manipulation or surgery is performed. When using a 30 to 60 mL syringe and catheter tube, HYSKON® should be introduced into the uterine cavity through the cannula of the hysteroscope until the uterus is sufficiently distended to permit adequate visualization. The intrauterine pressure needed to distend the uterus when using this method ranges between 50 and 100 mm Hg. If a pump or other mechanical device is used to instill HYSKON® the pressure should be monitored using a pressure manometer and the apparatus set so that a maximum intrauterine pressure of 150 mm Hg is not exceeded. Should the uterus fail to distend or if adequate distension cannot be maintained without the use of excessive pressure the procedure should be terminated and the cause determined. During the hysteroscopic examination, HYSKON® should be instilled at a rate which is not greater than that necessary to maintain suitable distension and visualization if blood or debris is present. To avoid the possibility of uterine rupture and to reduce the risk of injecting HYSKON® through the tubes and into the tissues of the uterus and parametria, the flow should not exceed the minimum needed for adequate distension and uterine irrigation to achieve good visualization.

CARE SHOULD BE TAKEN TO MEASURE THE AMOUNT OF HYSKON® INSTILLED AND THE AMOUNT RECOVERED EVERY 15 MINUTES IN ORDER TO DETERMINE THE VOLUME OF HYSKON® REMAINING IN THE BODY. CAREFUL MONITORING IS ESSENTIAL IN ORDER TO PREVENT EXCESSIVE INTRAVASATION AND SUBSEQUENT INTRAVASCULAR VOLUME EXPANSION. CAUTION REGARDING INTRAVASCULAR VOLUME EXPANSION SHOULD BE EXERCISED WHENEVER THE VOLUME OF HYSKON® REMAINING IN THE BODY EXCEEDS 250 ML AND/OR WITH PROCEDURES LASTING MORE THAN 45 MINUTES, OR WITH THE APPEARANCE OF TYPICAL CLINICAL SIGNS THAT MIGHT INDICATE INTRAVASCULAR VOLUME EXPANSION.

These signs might include, but are not limited to: tachycardia, tachypnea, blood pressure elevation, hypoxia, lung rales and cardiac gallops (see WARNINGS). For high risk procedures as defined above, the laboratory monitoring of intravascular volume expansion may be helpful. Compared with a pre-operative value, the lowering of the hematocrit during or immediately after the procedure, could indicate that a significant intravascular volume expansion has occurred.

OVERDOSAGE

If a circulatory fluid overload with pulmonary edema occurs associated with HYSKON® administration, intravenous diuretic administration along with other therapies may be indicated. If the fluid overload is not responsive, e.g., in connection with impaired renal function, other measures including phlebotomy or plasmapheresis, may be considered.

HOW SUPPLIED

HYSKON® Hysteroscopy Fluid (32% w/v dextran 70 in 10% w/v dextrose) is available as a sterile, non-pyrogenic solution in 100 mL bottles packed 12 to a carton (NDC 61563-0231-61).

Store at 20–25°C (68–77°F). Protect from cold.

CAUTION

Federal law restricts this device to sale by or on the order of a physician.

REFERENCES

1. Cleary R.E., Howard T., diZerega G.S.: Plasma dextran levels after abdominal instillation of 32% dextran 70: Evidence for prolonged intraperitoneal retention. Am J Obstet Gynecol 152:78–79, 1985.
2. Adoni A., Adatto-Levy R., Mogle P., Palti Z.: Post-operative pleural effusion caused by dextran. Int J Gyn Obs 18:243–244, 1980.
3. Baggish M.S., Davauluri C., Rodriguez F., Camporesi E.: Vascular uptake of HYSKON® (Dextran 70) during operative and diagnostic hysteroscopy. J Gynecol Surg 8:211–217, 1992.
4. Ruiz J., Neuwirth R.: The incidence of complications associated with the use of HYSKON® during hysteroscopy: Experience in 1793 consecutive patients. J Gynecol Surg 8:219–224, 1992.

(Rev. June, 1995)

Manufactured by:
Pharmacia Inc.
Clayton, NC 27520 USA
For:
Medisan Pharmaceuticals Inc.
Parsippany, NJ 07054 USA

PROMIT® ℞

[prō'mit]
(dextran 1)

15% Dextran 1 in 0.6% Sodium Chloride Injection. 20 ml.

RHEOMACRODEX® ℞

[re"o-mak'ro-dex]
(Plasma Volume Expander)

10% Dextran 40 in 5% Dextrose Injection. 500 ml.
10% Dextran 40 in 0.9% Sodium Chloride Injection. 500 ml.

For EMERGENCY telephone numbers, consult the **Manufacturers Index**.

Medtronic, Inc.
Neurological Division
800 53rd AVENUE NE
MINNEAPOLIS, MN 55421

Direct Inquiries to:
(800) 328-0810
(612) 572-5000

LIORESAL® INTRATHECAL ℞

[lye-oar' eh-sal]
(baclofen injection)

DESCRIPTION

LIORESAL INTRATHECAL (baclofen injection) is a muscle relaxant and antispastic. Its chemical name is 4-amino-3-(4-chlorophenyl) butanoic acid, and its structural formula is:

Baclofen is a white to off-white, odorless or practically odorless crystalline powder, with a molecular weight of 213.66. It is slightly soluble in water, very slightly soluble in methanol, and insoluble in chloroform.

LIORESAL INTRATHECAL is a sterile, pyrogen-free, isotonic solution free of antioxidants, preservatives or other potentially neurotoxic additives indicated only for intrathecal administration. The drug is stable in solution at 37° C and compatible with CSF. Each milliliter of LIORESAL INTRATHECAL contains baclofen U.S.P. 500 mcg or 2000 mcg and sodium chloride 9 mg in Water for Injection; pH range is 5.0–7.0. Each ampule is intended for SINGLE USE ONLY. Discard any unused portion. DO NOT AUTOCLAVE.

CLINICAL PHARMACOLOGY

The precise mechanism of action of baclofen as a muscle relaxant and antispasticity agent is not fully understood. Baclofen inhibits both monosynaptic and polysynaptic reflexes at the spinal level, possibly by decreasing excitatory neurotransmitter release from primary afferent terminals, although actions at supraspinal sites may also occur and contribute to its clinical effect. Baclofen is a structural analog of the inhibitory neurotransmitter gamma-aminobutyric acid (GABA), and may exert its effects by stimulation of the GABAB receptor subtype.

LIORESAL INTRATHECAL when introduced directly into the intrathecal space permits effective CSF concentrations to be achieved with resultant plasma concentrations 100 times less than those occurring with oral administration.

In people, as well as in animals, baclofen has been shown to have general CNS depressant properties as indicated by the production of sedation with tolerance, somnolence, ataxia, and respiratory and cardiovascular depression.

Pharmacodynamics of LIORESAL INTRATHECAL:

Intrathecal Bolus:

Adult Patients: The onset of action is generally one-half hour to one hour after an intrathecal bolus. Peak spasmolytic effect is seen at approximately four hours after dosing and effects may last four to eight hours. Onset, peak response, and duration of action may vary with individual patients depending on the dose and severity of symptoms.

Pediatric Patients: The onset, peak response and duration of action is similar to those seen in adult patients.

Continuous Infusion:

LIORESAL INTRATHECAL'S antispastic action is first seen at 6 to 8 hours after initiation of continuous infusion. Maximum activity is observed in 24 to 48 hours.

Continuous Infusion: No additional information is available for pediatric patients.

Pharmacokinetics of LIORESAL INTRATHECAL:

The pharmacokinetics of CSF clearance of LIORESAL INTRATHECAL calculated from intrathecal bolus or continuous infusion studies approximates CSF turnover, suggesting elimination is by bulk flow removal of CSF.

Intrathecal Bolus: After a bolus lumbar injection of 50 or 100 mcg LIORESAL INTRATHECAL in seven patients, the average CSF elimination half-life was 1.51 hours over the first four hours and the average CSF clearance was approximately 30 ml/hour.

Continuous Infusion: The mean CSF clearance for LIORESAL INTRATHECAL (baclofen injection) was approximately 30 ml/hour in a study involving ten patients on continuous intrathecal infusion.

Concurrent plasma concentrations of baclofen during intrathecal administration are expected to be low (0–5 ng/ml).

Limited pharmacokinetic data suggest that a lumbar-cisternal concentration gradient of about 4:1 is established along the neuroaxis during baclofen infusion. This is based upon simultaneous CSF sampling via cisternal and lumbar tap in 5 patients receiving continuous baclofen infusion at the lumbar level at doses associated with therapeutic efficacy; the interpatient variability was great. The gradient was not altered by position.

Six pediatric patients (age 8–18 years) receiving continuous intrathecal baclofen infusion at doses of 77–400 mcg/day had plasma baclofen levels near or below 10 ng/ml.

INDICATIONS

LIORESAL INTRATHECAL is indicated for use in the management of severe spasticity. Patients should first respond to a screening dose of intrathecal baclofen prior to consideration for long term infusion via an implantable pump. For spasticity of spinal cord origin, chronic infusion of LIORESAL INTRATHECAL via an implantable pump should be reserved for patients unresponsive to oral baclofen therapy, or those who experience intolerable CNS side effects at effective doses.

Patients with spasticity due to traumatic brain injury should wait at least one year after the injury before consideration of long term intrathecal baclofen therapy. LIORESAL INTRATHECAL (baclofen injection) is intended for use by the intrathecal route in single bolus test doses (via spinal catheter or lumbar puncture) and, for chronic use, only in implantable pumps approved by the FDA specifically for the administration of LIORESAL INTRATHECAL into the intrathecal space.

Spasticity of Spinal Cord Origin: Evidence supporting the efficacy of LIORESAL INTRATHECAL was obtained in randomized, controlled investigations that compared the effects of either a single intrathecal dose or a three day intrathecal infusion of LIORESAL INTRATHECAL to placebo in patients with severe spasticity and spasms due to either spinal cord trauma or multiple sclerosis. LIORESAL INTRATHECAL was superior to placebo on both principal outcome measures employed: change from baseline in the Ashworth rating of spasticity and the frequency of spasms.

Spasticity of Cerebral Origin: The efficacy of LIORESAL INTRATHECAL was investigated in three controlled clinical trials; two enrolled patients with cerebral palsy and one enrolled patient with spasticity due to previous brain injury. The first study, a randomized controlled cross-over trial of 51 patients with cerebral palsy, provided strong, statistically significant results; LIORESAL INTRATHECAL was superior to placebo in reducing spasticity as measured by the Ashworth Scale. A second cross-over study was conducted in 11 patients with spasticity arising from brain injury. Despite the small sample size, the study yielded a nearly significant test statistic (p=0.066) and provided directionally favorable results. The last study, however, did not provide data that could be reliably analyzed.

LIORESAL INTRATHECAL therapy may be considered an alternative to destructive neurosurgical procedures. Prior to implantation of a device for chronic intrathecal infusion of LIORESAL INTRATHECAL, patients must show a response to LIORESAL INTRATHECAL in a screening trial (see Dosage and Administration).

CONTRAINDICATIONS

Hypersensitivity to baclofen. LIORESAL INTRATHECAL is not recommended for intravenous, intramuscular, subcutaneous or epidural administration.

WARNINGS

LIORESAL INTRATHECAL is for use in single bolus intrathecal injections (via a catheter placed in the lumbar intrathecal space or injection by lumbar puncture) and in implantable pumps approved by the FDA specifically for the intrathecal administration of baclofen. Because of the possibility of potentially life-threatening CNS depression, cardiovascular collapse, and/or respiratory failure, physicians must be adequately trained and educated in chronic intrathecal infusion therapy.

The pump system should not be implanted until the patient's response to bolus LIORESAL INTRATHECAL injection is adequately evaluated. Evaluation (consisting of a screening procedure: see Dosage and Administration) requires that LIORESAL INTRATHECAL be administered into the intrathecal space via a catheter or lumbar puncture. Because of the risks associated with the screening procedure and the adjustment of dosage following pump implantation, these phases must be conducted in a medically supervised and adequately equipped environment following the instructions outlined in the Dosage and Administration section.

Resuscitative equipment should be available.

Following surgical implantation of the pump, particularly during the initial phases of pump use, the patient should be monitored closely until it is certain that the patient's response to the infusion is acceptable and reasonably stable. On each occasion that the dosing rate of the pump and/or the concentration of LIORESAL INTRATHECAL (baclofen injection) in the reservoir is adjusted, close medical monitoring is required until it is certain that the patient's response to the infusion is acceptable and reasonably stable.

It is mandatory that the patient, all patient care givers, and the physicians responsible for the patient receive adequate information regarding the risks of this mode of treatment. All medical personnel and care givers should be instructed in 1) the signs and symptoms of overdose, 2) procedures to be followed in the event of overdose and 3) proper home care of the pump and insertion site.

Overdose: Signs of overdose may appear suddenly or insidiously. Acute massive overdose may present as coma. Less sudden and/or less severe forms of overdose may present with signs of drowsiness, lightheadedness, dizziness, somnolence, respiratory depression, seizures, rostral progression of hypotonia and loss of consciousness progressing to coma. Should overdose appear likely, the patient should be taken immediately to a hospital for assessment and emptying of the pump reservoir. In cases reported to date, overdose has generally been related to pump malfunction or dosing error. (See Drug Overdose Symptoms and Treatment.)

Extreme caution must be used when filling an FDA approved implantable pump. Such pumps should only be refilled through the reservoir refill septum. However, some pumps are also equipped with a catheter access port that allows direct access to the intrathecal catheter. Direct injection into this catheter access port may cause a life-threatening overdose.

Hallucinations have occurred after abrupt withdrawal of LIORESAL INTRATHECAL.

Seizures have been reported during overdose and with withdrawal from LIORESAL INTRATHECAL as well as in patients maintained on therapeutic doses of LIORESAL INTRATHECAL.

Fatalities:

Spasticity of Spinal Cord Origin: There were 16 deaths reported among the 576 U.S. patients treated with LIORESAL INTRATHECAL (baclofen injection) in pre- and post-marketing studies evaluated as of December 1992. Because these patients were treated under uncontrolled clinical settings, it is impossible to determine definitively what role, if any, LIORESAL INTRATHECAL played in their deaths.

As a group, the patients who died were relatively young (mean age was 47 with a range from 25 to 63), but the majority suffered from severe spasticity of many years duration, were nonambulatory, had various medical complications such as pneumonia, urinary tract infections, and decubiti, and/or had received multiple concomitant medications. A case-by-case review of the clinical course of the 16 patients who died failed to reveal any unique signs, symptoms, or laboratory results that would suggest that treatment with LIORESAL INTRATHECAL caused their deaths. Two patients, however, did suffer sudden and unexpected death within 2 weeks of pump implantation and one patient died unexpectedly after screening.

One patient, a 44 year-old male with MS, died in hospital on the second day following pump implantation. An autopsy demonstrated severe fibrosis of the coronary conduction system. A second patient, a 52 year-old woman with MS and a history of an inferior wall myocardial infarction, was found dead in bed 12 days after pump implantation, 2 hours after having had documented normal vital signs. An autopsy revealed pulmonary congestion and bilateral pleural effusions. It is impossible to determine whether LIORESAL INTRATHECAL contributed to these deaths. The third patient underwent three baclofen screening trials. His medical history included SCI, aspiration pneumonia, septic shock, disseminated intravascular coagulopathy, severe metabolic acidosis, hepatic toxicity, and status epilepticus. Twelve days after screening (he was not implanted), he again experienced status epilepticus with subsequent significant neurological deterioration. Based upon prior instruction, extraordinary resuscitative measures were not pursued and the patient died.

Spasticity of Cerebral Origin: There were three deaths occurring among the 211 patients treated with LIORESAL INTRATHECAL in pre-marketing studies as of March 1996. These deaths were not attributed to the therapy.

PRECAUTIONS

Children should be of sufficient body mass to accommodate the implantable pump for chronic infusion. Please consult pump manufacturer's manual for specific recommendations. The safe use of LIORESAL INTRATHECAL in children under age 4 has not been established.

Screening

Patients should be infection-free prior to the screening trial with LIORESAL INTRATHECAL (baclofen injection) because the presence of a systemic infection may interfere with an assessment of the patient's response to bolus LIORESAL INTRATHECAL.

Pump Implantation

Patients should be infection-free prior to pump implantation because the presence of infection may increase the risk of surgical complications. Moreover, a systemic infection may complicate dosing.

Pump Dose Adjustment and Titration

In most patients, it will be necessary to increase the dose gradually over time to maintain effectiveness; a sudden requirement for substantial dose escalation typically indicates a catheter complication (i.e., catheter kink or dislodgement). Reservoir refilling must be performed by fully trained and qualified personnel following the directions provided by the pump manufacturer. Refill intervals should be carefully calculated to prevent depletion of the reservoir, as this would result in the return of severe spasticity and possibly symptoms of withdrawal.

Strict aseptic technique in filling is required to avoid bacterial contamination and serious infection. A period of observation appropriate to the clinical situation should follow each refill or manipulation of the drug reservoir.

Extreme caution must be used when filling an FDA approved implantable pump equipped with an injection port that allows direct access to the intrathecal catheter. Direct injection into the catheter through the catheter access port may cause a life-threatening overdose.

Additional considerations pertaining to dosage adjustment: It may be important to titrate the dose to maintain some degree of muscle tone and allow occasional spasms to: 1) help support circulatory function, 2) possibly prevent the formation of deep vein thrombosis, 3) optimize activities of daily living and ease of care.

Except in overdose related emergencies, the dose of LIORESAL INTRATHECAL should ordinarily be reduced slowly if the drug is discontinued for any reason.

An attempt should be made to discontinue concomitant oral antispasticity medication to avoid possible overdose or adverse drug interactions, either prior to screening or following implant and initiation of chronic LIORESAL INTRATHECAL infusion. Reduction and discontinuation of oral antispasmotics should be done slowly and with careful monitoring by the physician. Abrupt reduction or discontinuation of concomitant antispastics should be avoided.

Drowsiness: Drowsiness has been reported in patients on LIORESAL INTRATHECAL. Patients should be cautioned regarding the operation of automobiles or other dangerous machinery, and activities made hazardous by decreased alertness. Patients should also be cautioned that the central nervous system depressant effects of LIORESAL INTRATHECAL (baclofen injection) may be additive to those of alcohol and other CNS depressants.

Precautions in special patient populations: Careful dose titration of LIORESAL INTRATHECAL is needed when spasticity is necessary to sustain upright posture and balance in locomotion or whenever spasticity is used to obtain optimal function and care.

Patients suffering from psychotic disorders, schizophrenia, or confusional states should be treated cautiously with LIORESAL INTRATHECAL and kept under careful surveillance, because exacerbations of these conditions have been observed with oral administration.

LIORESAL INTRATHECAL should be used with caution in patients with a history of autonomic dysreflexia. The presence of nociceptive stimuli or abrupt withdrawal of LIORESAL INTRATHECAL (baclofen injection) may cause an autonomic dysreflexic episode.

Because LIORESAL is primarily excreted unchanged by the kidneys, it should be given with caution in patients with impaired renal function and it may be necessary to reduce the dosage.

LABORATORY TESTS

No specific laboratory tests are deemed essential for the management of patients on LIORESAL INTRATHECAL.

DRUG INTERACTIONS

There is inadequate systematic experience with the use of LIORESAL INTRATHECAL in combination with other medications to predict specific drug-drug interactions. Interactions attributed to the combined use of LIORESAL INTRATHECAL and epidural morphine include hypotension and dyspnea.

CARCINOGENESIS, MUTAGENESIS, AND IMPAIRMENT OF FERTILITY

No increase in tumors was seen in rats receiving LIORESAL (baclofen USP) orally for two years at approximately 30–60 times on a mg/kg basis, or 10–20 times on a mg/m^2 basis, the maximum oral dose recommended for human use. Mutagenicity assays with LIORESAL have not been performed.

PREGNANCY CATEGORY C

LIORESAL (baclofen USP) given orally has been shown to increase the incidence of omphaloceles (ventral hernias) in fetuses of rats given approximately 13 times on a mg/kg basis, or 3 times on a mg/m^2 basis, the maximum oral dose recommended for human use; this dose also caused reductions in food intake and weight gain in the dams.

This abnormality was not seen in mice or rabbits. There are no adequate and well-controlled studies in pregnant women. LIORESAL should be used during pregnancy only if the potential benefit justifies the potential risk to the fetus.

Continued on next page

Medtronic Neurological—Cont.

NURSING MOTHERS

In mothers treated with oral LIORESAL (baclofen USP) in therapeutic doses, the active substance passes into the breast milk. It is not known whether detectable levels of drug are present in breast milk of nursing mothers receiving LIORESAL INTRATHECAL. As a general rule, nursing should be undertaken while a patient is receiving LIORESAL INTRATHECAL only if the potential benefit justifies the potential risks to the infant.

PEDIATRIC USE

Children should be of sufficient body mass to accommodate the implantable pump for chronic infusion. Please consult pump manufacturer's manual for specific recommendations. The safe use of LIORESAL INTRATHECAL in children under age 4 has not been established.

Considerations based on experience with oral LIORESAL (baclofen USP)

A dose-related increase in incidence of ovarian cysts was observed in female rats treated chronically with oral LIORESAL. Ovarian cysts have been found by palpation in about 4% of the multiple sclerosis patients who were treated with oral LIORESAL for up to one year. In most cases these cysts disappeared spontaneously while patients continued to receive the drug. Ovarian cysts are estimated to occur spontaneously in approximately 1% to 5% of the normal female population.

ADVERSE DRUG EVENTS

Spasticity of Spinal Cord Origin:

Commonly Observed in Patients with Spasticity of Spinal Origin—In pre- and post-marketing clinical trials, the most commonly observed adverse events associated with use of LIORESAL INTRATHECAL (baclofen injection) which were not seen at an equivalent incidence among placebo-treated patients were: somnolence, dizziness, nausea, hypotension, headache, convulsions and hypotonia.

Associated with Discontinuation of Treatment—8/474 patients with spasticity of spinal cord origin receiving long term infusion of LIORESAL INTRATHECAL in pre- and post-marketing clinical studies in the U.S. discontinued treatment due to adverse events. These include: pump pocket infections (3), meningitis (2), wound dehiscence (1), gynecological fibroids (1), and pump overpressurization (1) with unknown, if any, sequela. Eleven patients who developed coma secondary to overdose had their treatment temporarily suspended, but all were subsequently re-started and were not, therefore, considered to be true discontinuations.

Fatalities—See Warnings.

Spasticity of Spinal Cord Origin:

Incidence in Controlled Trials—Experience with LIORESAL INTRATHECAL (baclofen injection) obtained in parallel, placebo-controlled, randomized studies provides only a limited basis for estimating the incidence of adverse events because the studies were of very brief duration (up to three days of infusion) and involved only a total of 63 patients. The following events occurred among the 31 patients receiving LIORESAL INTRATHECAL (baclofen injection) in two randomized, placebo-controlled trials: hypotension (2), dizziness (2), headache (2), dyspnea (1). No adverse events were reported among the 32 patients receiving placebo in these studies.

Events Observed during the Pre- and Post-marketing Evaluation of LIORESAL INTRATHECAL—Adverse events associated with the use of LIORESAL INTRATHECAL reflect experience gained with 576 patients followed prospectively in the United States. They received LIORESAL INTRATHECAL for periods of one day (screening) (N=576) to over eight years (maintenance) (N=10). The usual screening bolus dose administered prior to pump implantation in these studies was typically 50 mcg. The maintenance dose ranged from 12 mcg to 2003 mcg per day. Because of the open, uncontrolled nature of the experience, a causal linkage between events observed and the administration of LIORESAL INTRATHECAL cannot be reliably assessed in many cases and many of the adverse events reported are known to occur in association with the underlying conditions being treated. Nonetheless, many of the more commonly reported reactions—hypotonia, somnolence, dizziness, paresthesia, nausea/vomiting and headache—appear clearly drug-related.

Adverse experiences reported during all U.S. studies (both controlled and uncontrolled) are shown in the following table. Eight of 474 patients who received chronic infusion via implanted pumps had adverse experiences which led to a discontinuation of long term treatment in the pre- and post-marketing studies.

[See table below.]

In addition to the more common (1% or more) adverse events reported in the prospectively followed 576 domestic patients in pre- and post-marketing studies, experience from an additional 194 patients exposed to LIORESAL INTRATHECAL (baclofen injection) from foreign studies has been reported. The following adverse events, not described in the table, and arranged in decreasing order of frequency, and classified by body system, were reported:

Nervous System: Abnormal gait, thinking abnormal, tremor, amnesia, twitching, vasodilitation, cerebrovascular accident, nystagmus, personality disorder, psychotic depression, cerebral ischemia, emotional lability, euphoria, hypertonia, ileus, drug dependence, incoordination, paranoid reaction and ptosis.

Digestive System: Flatulence, dysphagia, dyspepsia and gastroenteritis.

Cardiovascular: Postural hypotension, bradycardia, palpitations, syncope, arrhythmia ventricular, deep thrombophlebitis, pallor and tachycardia.

Respiratory: Respiratory disorder, aspiration pneumonia, hyperventilation, pulmonary embolus and rhinitis.

Urogenital: Hematuria and kidney failure.

Skin and Appendages: Alopecia and sweating.

Metabolic and Nutritional Disorders: Weight loss, albuminuria, dehydration and hyperglycemia.

Special Senses: Abnormal vision, abnormality of accomodation, photophobia, taste loss and tinnitus.

Body as a Whole: Suicide, lack of drug effect, abdominal pain, hypothermia, neck rigidity, chest pain, chills, face edema, flu syndrome and overdose.

Hemic and Lymphatic System: Anemia.

Spasticity of Cerebral Origin:

Commonly Observed—In pre-marketing clinical trials, the most commonly observed adverse events associated with use of LIORESAL INTRATHECAL (baclofen injection) which were not seen at an equivalent incidence among placebo-treated patients included: agitation, constipation, somnolence, leukocytosis, chills, urinary retention and hypotonia.

Associated with Discontinuation of Treatment—Nine of 211 patients receiving LIORESAL INTRATHECAL in pre-marketing clinical studies in the U.S. discontinued long term infusion due to adverse events associated with intrathecal therapy.

The nine adverse events leading to discontinuation were: infection (3), CSF leaks (2), meningitis (2), drainage (1), and unmanageable trunk control (1).

Fatalities—Three deaths, none of which were attributed to LIORESAL INTRATHECAL, were reported in patients in clinical trials involving patients with spasticity of cerebral origin. See *Warnings* on other deaths reported in spinal spasticity patients.

Incidence in Controlled Trials—Experience with LIORESAL INTRATHECAL (baclofen injection) obtained in parallel, placebo-controlled, randomized studies provides only a limited basis for estimating the incidence of adverse events because the studies involved a total of 62 patients exposed to a single 50 mcg intrathecal bolus. The following events occurred among the 62 patients receiving LIORESAL INTRATHECAL in two randomized, placebo-controlled trials involving cerebral palsy and head injury patients, respectively: agitation, constipation, somnolence, leukocytosis, nausea, vomiting, nystagmus, chills, urinary retention, and hypotonia.

Events Observed during the Pre-marketing Evaluation of LIORESAL INTRATHECAL—Adverse events associated with the use of LIORESAL INTRATHECAL reflect experience gained with a total of 211 U.S. patients with spasticity of cerebral origin, of whom 112 were pediatric patients (under age 16 at enrollment). They received LIORESAL INTRATHECAL for periods of one day (screening) (N=211) to 84 months (maintenance) (N=1). The usual screening bolus dose administered prior to pump implantation in these studies was 50–75 mcg. The maintenance dose ranged from 22 mcg to 1400 mcg per day. Doses used in this patient population for long term infusion are generally lower than those required for patients with spasticity of spinal cord origin. Because of the open, uncontrolled nature of the experience, a causal linkage between events observed and the administration of LIORESAL INTRATHECAL cannot be reliably assessed in many cases. Nonetheless, many of the more commonly reported reactions—somnolence, dizziness, headache, nausea, hypotension, hypotonia and coma—appear clearly drug-related.

The most frequent (≥1%) adverse events reported during all clinical trials are shown in the following table. Nine patients discontinued long term treatment due to adverse events.

[See table at top of next page.]

The more common (1% or more) adverse events reported in the prospectively followed 211 patients exposed to LIORESAL INTRATHECAL (baclofen injection) have been reported. In the total cohort, the following adverse events, not described in the table, and arranged in decreasing order of frequency, and classified by body system, were reported:

INCIDENCE OF MOST FREQUENT (≥ 1%) ADVERSE EVENTS IN PATIENTS WITH SPASTICITY OF SPINAL ORIGIN IN PROSPECTIVELY MONITORED CLINICAL TRIALS

	Percent of Patients Reporting Events		
Adverse Event	N = 576 Screening[a] Percent	N = 474 Titration[b] Percent	N = 430 Maintenance[c] Percent
Hypotonia	5.4	13.5	25.3
Somnolence	5.7	5.9	20.9
Dizziness	1.7	1.9	7.9
Paresthesia	2.4	2.1	6.7
Nausea and Vomiting	1.6	2.3	5.6
Headache	1.6	2.5	5.1
Constipation	0.2	1.5	5.1
Convulsion	0.5	1.3	4.7
Urinary Retention	0.7	1.7	1.9
Dry Mouth	0.2	0.4	3.3
Accidental Injury	0.0	0.2	3.5
Asthenia	0.7	1.3	1.4
Confusion	0.5	0.6	2.3
Death	0.2	0.4	3.0
Pain	0.0	0.6	3.0
Speech Disorder	0.0	0.2	3.5
Hypotension	1.0	0.2	1.9
Ambylopia	0.5	0.2	2.3
Diarrhea	0.0	0.8	2.3
Hypoventilation	0.2	0.8	2.1
Coma	0.0	1.5	0.9
Impotence	0.2	0.4	1.6
Peripheral Edema	0.0	0.0	2.3
Urinary Incontinence	0.0	0.8	1.4
Insomnia	0.0	0.4	1.6
Anxiety	0.2	0.4	0.9
Depression	0.0	0.0	1.6
Dyspnea	0.3	0.0	1.2
Fever	0.5	0.2	0.7
Pneumonia	0.2	0.2	1.2
Urinary Frequency	0.0	0.6	0.9
Urticaria	0.2	0.2	1.2
Anorexia	0.0	0.4	0.9
Diplopia	0.0	0.4	0.9
Dysautonomia	0.2	0.2	0.9
Hallucinations	0.3	0.4	0.5
Hypertension	0.2	0.2	0.5

[a] Following administration of test bolus
[b] Two month period following implant
[c] Beyond two months following implant
N=total number of patients entering each period
%=% of patients evaluated

Nervous System: Akathisia, ataxia, confusion, depression, opisthotonos, amnesia, anxiety, hallucinations, hysteria, insomnia, nystagmus, personality disorder, reflexes decreased, and vasodilitation.

Digestive System: Dysphagia, fecal incontinence, gastrointestinal hemorrhage and tongue disorder.

Cardiovascular: Bradycardia.

Respiratory: Apnea, dyspnea and hyperventilation.

Urogenital: Abnormal ejaculation, kidney calculus, oliguria and vaginitis.

Skin and Appendages: Rash, sweating, alopecia, contact dermatitis and skin ulcer.

Special Senses: Abnormality of accomodation.

Body as a Whole: Death, fever, abdominal pain, carcinoma, malaise and hypothermia.

Hemic and Lymphatic System: Leukocytosis and petechial rash.

DRUG OVERDOSE

Special attention must be given to recognizing the signs and symptoms of overdosage, especially during the initial screening and dose-titration phase of treatment, but also during reintroduction of LIORESAL INTRATHECAL after a period of interruption in therapy.

Symptoms of LIORESAL INTRATHECAL Overdose: Drowsiness, lightheadedness, dizziness, somnolence, respiratory depression, seizures, rostral progression of hypotonia and loss of consciousness progressing to coma of up to 72 hrs. duration. In most cases reported, coma was reversible without sequelae after drug was discontinued.

Symptoms of LIORESAL INTRATHECAL overdose were reported in a sensitive adult patient after receiving a 25 mcg intrathecal bolus.

Treatment Suggestions for Overdose:

There is no specific antidote for treating overdoses of LIORESAL INTRATHECAL (baclofen injection); however, the following steps should ordinarily be undertaken:

1) Residual LIORESAL INTRATHECAL solution should be removed from the pump as soon as possible.

2) Patients with respiratory depression should be intubated if necessary, until the drug is eliminated.

Anecdotal reports suggest that intravenous physostigmine may reverse central side effects, notably drowsiness and respiratory depression. Caution in administering physostigmine is advised, however, because its use has been associated with the induction of seizures, bradycardia, and cardiac conduction disturbances.

Physostigmine Doses for Adult Patients: A total dose of 1–2 mg physostigmine may be tried intravenously over 5–10 minutes. Patients should be monitored closely during this time. Repeat doses of 1 mg may be administered at 30–60 minute intervals in an attempt to maintain adequate respiration and alertness if the patient shows a positive response.

Physostigmine Doses for Pediatric Patients: Administer 0.02 mg/kg physostigmine intravenously, do not give more than 0.5 mg per minute. The dosage may be repeated at 5 to 10 minute intervals until a therapeutic effect is obtained or a maximum dose of 2 mg is attained.

Physostigmine may not be effective in reversing large overdoses and patients may need to be maintained with respiratory support.

If lumbar puncture is not contraindicated, consideration should be given to withdrawing 30–40 ml of CSF to reduce CSF baclofen concentration.

DOSAGE AND ADMINISTRATION

Refer to the manufacturer's manual for the implantable pump approved for intrathecal infusion for specific instructions and precautions for programming the pump and/or refilling the reservoir.

Screening Phase: Prior to pump implantation and initiation of chronic infusion of LIORESAL INTRATHECAL (baclofen injection), patients must demonstrate a positive clinical response to a LIORESAL INTRATHECAL bolus dose administered intrathecally in a screening trial. The screening trial employs LIORESAL INTRATHECAL which must be diluted to a concentration of 50 mcg per ml. The screening procedure is as follows. An initial bolus containing 50 micrograms in a volume of 1 milliliter is administered into the intrathecal space by barbotage over a period of not less than one minute. The patient is observed over the ensuing 4 to 8 hours. A positive response consists of a significant decrease in muscle tone and/or frequency and/or severity of spasms. If the initial response is less than desired, a second bolus injection may be administered 24 hours after the first. The second screening bolus dose consists of 75 micrograms in 1.5 milliliters. Again, the patient should be observed for an interval of 4 to 8 hours. If the response is still inadequate, a final bolus screening dose of 100 micrograms in 2 milliliters may be administered 24 hours later.

Pediatric Patients: The starting screening dose for pediatric patients is the same as in adult patients, i.e., 50 mcg. However, for very small patients, a screening dose of 25 mcg may be tried first.

INCIDENCE OF MOST FREQUENT (≥ 1%) ADVERSE EVENTS IN PATIENTS WITH SPASTICITY OF CEREBRAL ORIGIN IN PROSPECTIVELY MONITORED CLINICAL TRIALS

Adverse Event	Percent of Patients Reporting Events		
	N = 211 Screening[a] Percent	N = 153 Titration[b] Percent	N = 150 Maintenance[c] Percent
Hypotonia	2.4	14.4	34.7
Somnolence	7.6	10.5	18.7
Headache	6.6	7.8	10.7
Nausea and Vomiting	6.6	10.5	4.0
Vomiting	6.2	8.5	4.0
Urinary Retention	0.9	6.5	8.0
Convulsion	0.9	3.3	10.0
Dizziness	2.4	2.6	8.0
Nausea	1.4	3.3	7.3
Hypoventilation	1.4	1.3	4.0
Hypertonia	0.0	0.7	6.0
Paresthesia	1.9	0.7	3.3
Hypotension	1.9	0.7	2.0
Increased Salivation	0.0	2.6	2.7
Back Pain	0.9	0.7	2.0
Constipation	0.5	1.3	2.0
Pain	0.0	0.0	4.0
Pruritus	0.0	0.0	4.0
Diarrhea	0.5	0.7	2.0
Peripheral Edema	0.0	0.0	3.3
Thinking Abnormal	0.5	1.3	0.7
Agitation	0.5	0.0	1.3
Asthenia	0.0	0.0	2.0
Chills	0.5	0.0	1.3
Coma	0.5	0.0	1.3
Dry Mouth	0.5	0.0	1.3
Pneumonia	0.0	0.0	2.0
Speech Disorder	0.5	0.7	0.7
Tremor	0.5	0.0	1.3
Urinary Incontinence	0.0	0.0	2.0
Urination Impaired	0.0	0.0	2.0

[a] Following administration of test bolus
[b] Two month period following implant
[c] Beyond two months following implant
N=Total number of patients entering each period. 211 patients received drug; (1 of 212) received placebo only.

Patients who do not respond to a 100 mcg intrathecal bolus should not be considered candidates for an implanted pump for chronic infusion.

Post-Implant Dose Titration Period: To determine the initial total daily dose of LIORESAL INTRATHECAL following implant, the screening dose that gave a positive effect should be doubled and administered over a 24-hour period, unless the efficacy of the bolus dose was maintained for more than 8 hours, in which case the starting daily dose should be the screening dose delivered over a 24-hour period. No dose increases should be given in the first 24 hours (i.e., until the steady state is achieved).

Adult Patients with Spasticity of Spinal Cord Origin: After the first 24 hours, for adult patients, the daily dosage should be increased slowly by 10–30% increments and only once every 24 hours, until the desired clinical effect is achieved.

Adult Patients with Spasticity of Cerebral Origin: After the first 24 hours, the daily dose should be increased slowly by 5–15% only once every 24 hours, until the desired clinical effect is achieved.

Pediatric Patients: After the first 24 hours, the daily dose should be increased slowly by 5–15% only once every 24 hours, until the desired clinical effect is achieved.

If there is not a substantive clinical response to increases in the daily dose, check for proper pump function and catheter patency.

Patients must be monitored closely in a fully equipped and staffed environment during the screening phase and dose-titration period immediately following implant. Resuscitative equipment should be immediately available for use in case of life-threatening or intolerable side effects.

Maintenance Therapy:

Spasticity of Spinal Cord Origin Patients: The clinical goal is to maintain muscle tone as close to normal as possible, and to minimize the frequency and severity of spasms to the extent possible, without inducing intolerable side effects. Very often, the maintenance dose needs to be adjusted during the first few months of therapy while patients adjust to changes in life style due to the alleviation of spasticity. During periodic refills of the pump, the daily dose may be increased by 10–40%, but no more than 40%, to maintain adequate symptom control. The daily dose may be reduced by 10–20% if patients experience side effects. Most patients require gradual increases in dose over time to maintain optimal response during chronic therapy. A sudden large requirement for dose escalation suggests a catheter complication (i.e., catheter kink or dislodgement).

Maintenance dosage for long term continuous infusion of LIORESAL INTRATHECAL (baclofen injection) has ranged from 12 mcg/day to 2,003 mcg/day, with most patients adequately maintained on 300 micrograms to 800 micrograms per day. There is limited experience with daily doses greater than 1000 mcg/day. Determination of the optimal LIORESAL INTRATHECAL dose requires individual titration. The lowest dose with an optimal response should be used.

Spasticity of Cerebral Origin Patients: The clinical goal is to maintain muscle tone as close to normal as possible and to minimize the frequency and severity of spasms to the extent possible, without inducing intolerable side effects, or to titrate the dose to the desired degree of muscle tone for optimal functions. Very often the maintenance dose needs to be adjusted during the first few months of therapy while patients adjust to changes in life style due to the alleviation of spasticity. During periodic refills of the pump, the daily dose may be increased by 5–20%, but no more than 20%, to maintain adequate symptom control. The daily dose may be reduced by 10–20% if patients experience side effects. Many patients require gradual increases in dose over time to maintain optimal response during chronic therapy. A sudden large requirement for dose escalation suggests a catheter complication (i.e., catheter kink or dislodgement).

Maintenance dosage for long term continuous infusion of LIORESAL INTRATHECAL (baclofen injection) has ranged from 22 mcg/day to 1400 mcg/day, with most patients adequately maintained on 90 micrograms to 703 micrograms per day. In clinical trials, only 3 of 150 patients required daily doses greater than 1000 mcg/day.

Pediatric Patients: Use same dosing recommendations for patients with spasticity of cerebral origin. Pediatric patients under 12 years seemed to require a lower daily dose in clinical trials. Average daily dose for patients under 12 years was 274 mcg/day, with a range of 24 to 1199 mcg/day. Dosage requirement for pediatric patients over 12 years does not seem to be different from that of adult patients. Determination of the optimal LIORESAL INTRATHECAL dose requires individual titration. The lowest dose with an optimal response should be used.

Potential need for dose adjustments in chronic use: During long term treatment, approximately 5% (28/627) of patients become refractory to increasing doses. There is not sufficient experience to make firm recommendations for tolerance treatment; however, this "tolerance" has been treated on occasion, in hospital, by a "drug holiday" consisting of the gradual reduction of LIORESAL INTRATHECAL over a to 4 week period and switching to alternative methods

Continued on next page

Medtronic Neurological—Cont.

of spasticity management. After the "drug holiday," LIORESAL INTRATHECAL may be restarted at the initial continuous infusion dose.

Stability
Parenteral drug products should be inspected for particulate matter and discoloration prior to administration, whenever solution and container permit.

Delivery Specifications
The specific concentration that should be used depends upon the total daily dose required as well as the delivery rate of the pump. LIORESAL INTRATHECAL may require dilution when used with certain implantable pumps. Please consult manufacturer's manual for specific recommendations.

Dilution Instruction:
Screening
Both strengths of LIORESAL INTRATHECAL (10 mg/5 ml and 10 mg/20 ml) must be diluted to a 50 mcg/ml concentration for bolus injection into the subarachnoid space.
Maintenance
For patients who require concentrations other than 500 mcg/ml or 2000 mcg/ml, LIORESAL INTRATHECAL **must be diluted.**
LIORESAL INTRATHECAL **must be diluted** with sterile preservative free Sodium Chloride for Injection, U.S.P.

Delivery Regimen:
LIORESAL INTRATHECAL is most often administered in a continuous infusion mode immediately following implant. For those patients implanted with programmable pumps who have achieved relatively satisfactory control on continuous infusion, further benefit may be attained using more complex schedules of LIORESAL INTRATHECAL delivery. For example, patients who have increased spasms at night may require a 20% increase in their hourly infusion rate. Changes in flow rate should be programmed to start two hours before the time of desired clinical effect.

HOW SUPPLIED

LIORESAL INTRATHECAL (baclofen injection) is available in single use ampules packaged in a Refill Kit for intrathecal administration.
Model 8561 LIORESAL INTRATHECAL Refill Kit contains one ampule of 10 mg/20 ml (500 mcg/ml) (NDC 58281-0560-01).
Model 8562 LIORESAL INTRATHECAL Refill Kit contains two ampules of 10 mg/5 ml (2000 mcg/ml) (NDC 58281-0561-02).
Model 8564 LIORESAL INTRATHECAL Refill Kit contains four ampules of 10 mg/5 ml (2000 mcg/ml) (NDC 58281-0561-04).

STORAGE
Does not require refrigeration.
Do not store above 86°F (30°C).
Do not freeze.
Do not heat sterilize.
Manufactured by CIBA-GEIGY Ltd., Basle, Switzerland, for Medtronic, Inc., Minneapolis, Minnesota 55421 USA.
PN 187012-003
Revised June 1996
Medtronic
Medtronic, Inc.
Neurological Division
800 53rd Avenue N.E.
Minneapolis, MN 55421
Telephone: (612) 572-5000
Toll-free: 1-800-328-0810
Visit Medtronic at:
http://www.medtronic.com

IDENTIFICATION PROBLEM?
Turn to the **Product Identification** Guide,
where you'll find more than
1600 products pictured in actual
size and full color.

Merck & Co., Inc.
WEST POINT, PA 19486

For Medical Information Contact:
Generally:
Product and service information:
Call the Merck National Service Center, 8:00 AM to 7:00 PM (ET), Monday through Friday:
(800) NSC-MERCK
(800) 672-6372
FAX: (800) MERCK-68
FAX: (800) 637-2568
Adverse Drug Experiences:
Call the Merck National Service Center, 8:00 AM to 7:00 PM (ET), Monday through Friday:
(800) NSC-MERCK
(800) 672-6372
In Emergencies:
24-hour emergency information for healthcare professionals:
(800) NSC-MERCK
(800) 672-6372
Sales and Ordering:
For product orders and direct account inquiries only, call the Order Management Center,
8:00 AM to 7:00 PM (ET), Monday through Friday:
(800) MERCK RX
(800) 637-2579

ALDOCLOR® Tablets   ℞
(Methyldopa-Chlorothiazide), U.S.P.

WARNING
This fixed combination drug is not indicated for initial therapy of hypertension. Hypertension requires therapy titrated to the individual patient. If the fixed combination represents the dosage so determined, its use may be more convenient in patient management. The treatment of hypertension is not static, but must be re-evaluated as conditions in each patient warrant.

DESCRIPTION

ALDOCLOR* (Methyldopa-Chlorothiazide) combines two antihypertensives: methyldopa and chlorothiazide.
Methyldopa
Methyldopa is an antihypertensive and is the *L*-isomer of alpha-methyldopa. It is levo-3-(3,4-dihydroxyphenyl)-2-methylalanine. Its empirical formula is $C_{10}H_{13}NO_4$, with a molecular weight of 211.22, and its structural formula is:

Methyldopa is a white to yellowish white, odorless fine powder, and is soluble in water.
Chlorothiazide
Chlorothiazide is a diuretic and antihypertensive. It is 6-chloro-2*H*-1, 2, 4-benzothiadiazine-7-sulfonamide 1, 1-dioxide. Its empirical formula is $C_7H_6ClN_3O_4S_2$ and its structural formula is:

It is a white, or practically white crystalline powder with a molecular weight of 295.72, which is very slightly soluble in water, but readily soluble in dilute aqueous sodium hydroxide. It is soluble in urine to the extent of about 150 mg per 100 mL at pH 7.
ALDOCLOR is supplied as tablets in two strengths for oral use:
ALDOCLOR 150, contains 250 mg of methyldopa and 150 mg of chlorothiazide.
ALDOCLOR 250, contains 250 mg of methyldopa and 250 mg of chlorothiazide.
Each tablet contains the following inactive ingredients: calcium disodium edetate, cellulose, citric acid, D&C Yellow 10, ethylcellulose, FD&C Yellow 6, gelatin, glycerin, guar gum, hydroxypropyl methylcellulose, magnesium stearate, starch, talc, and titanium dioxide. ALDOCLOR 150 also con-

tains iron oxides. ALDOCLOR 250 also contains FD&C Blue 2.

*Registered trademark of MERCK & CO., INC.

CLINICAL PHARMACOLOGY

Methyldopa
Methyldopa is an aromatic-amino-acid decarboxylase inhibitor in animals and in man. Although the mechanism of action has yet to be conclusively demonstrated, the antihypertensive effect of methyldopa probably is due to its metabolism to alpha-methylnorepinephrine, which then lowers arterial pressure by stimulation of central inhibitory alpha-adrenergic receptors, false neurotransmission, and/or reduction of plasma renin activity. Methyldopa has been shown to cause a net reduction in the tissue concentration of serotonin, dopamine, norepinephrine, and epinephrine.
Only methyldopa, the *L*-isomer of alpha-methyldopa, has the ability to inhibit dopa decarboxylase and to deplete animal tissues of norepinephrine. In man, the antihypertensive activity appears to be due solely to the *L*-isomer. About twice the dose of the racemate (*DL*-alpha-methyldopa) is required for equal antihypertensive effect.
Methyldopa has no direct effect on cardiac function and usually does not reduce glomerular filtration rate, renal blood flow, or filtration fraction. Cardiac output usually is maintained without cardiac acceleration. In some patients the heart rate is slowed.
Normal or elevated plasma renin activity may decrease in the course of methyldopa therapy.
Methyldopa reduces both supine and standing blood pressure. It usually produces highly effective lowering of the supine pressure with infrequent symptomatic postural hypotension. Exercise hypotension and diurnal blood pressure variations rarely occur.
Chlorothiazide
The mechanism of the antihypertensive effect of thiazides is unknown. Chlorothiazide does not usually affect normal blood pressure.
Chlorothiazide affects the distal renal tubular mechanism of electrolyte reabsorption. At maximal therapeutic dosage all thiazides are approximately equal in their diuretic efficacy. Chlorothiazide increases excretion of sodium and chloride in approximately equivalent amounts. Natriuresis may be accompanied by some loss of potassium and bicarbonate. After oral use diuresis begins within 2 hours, peaks in about 4 hours and lasts about 6 to 12 hours.
Pharmacokinetics and Metabolism
Methyldopa
The maximum decrease in blood pressure occurs four to six hours after oral dosage. After withdrawal, blood pressure usually returns to pretreatment levels within 24–48 hours. Methyldopa is extensively metabolized. The known urinary metabolites are: α-methyldopa mono-0-sulfate; 3-0 methyl-α-methyldopa; 3,4,-dihydroxyphenylacetone; α-methyldopamine; 3-0-methyl-α-methyldopamine and their conjugates. Approximately 70 percent of the drug which is absorbed is excreted in the urine as methyldopa and its mono-0-sulfate conjugate. The renal clearance is about 130 mL/min in normal subjects and is diminished in renal insufficiency. The plasma half-life of methyldopa is 105 minutes. After oral doses, excretion is essentially complete in 36 hours.
Methyldopa crosses the placental barrier, appears in cord blood, and appears in breast milk.
Chlorothiazide
Chlorothiazide is not metabolized but is eliminated rapidly by the kidney. The plasma half-life is 45–120 minutes. After oral doses, 20–24 percent of the dose is excreted unchanged in the urine. Chlorothiazide crosses the placental but not the blood-brain barrier and is excreted in breast milk.

INDICATION AND USAGE

Hypertension (see box warning).

CONTRAINDICATIONS

ALDOCLOR is contraindicated in patients:
—with active hepatic disease, such as acute hepatitis and active cirrhosis
—with liver disorders previously associated with methyldopa therapy (see WARNINGS)
—with anuria
—with hypersensitivity to methyldopa, or to chlorothiazide or other sulfonamide-derived drugs
—on therapy with monoamine oxidase (MAO) inhibitors.

WARNINGS

Methyldopa
It is important to recognize that a positive Coombs test, hemolytic anemia, and liver disorders may occur with methyldopa therapy. The rare occurrences of hemolytic anemia or liver disorders could lead to potentially fatal complications

unless properly recognized and managed. Read this section carefully to understand these reactions.

With prolonged methyldopa therapy, 10 to 20 percent of patients develop a positive direct Coombs test which usually occurs between 6 and 12 months of methyldopa therapy. Lowest incidence is at daily dosage of 1 g or less. This on rare occasions may be associated with hemolytic anemia, which could lead to potentially fatal complications. One cannot predict which patients with a positive direct Coombs test may develop hemolytic anemia.

Prior existence or development of a positive direct Coombs test is not in itself a contraindication to use of methyldopa. If a positive Coombs test develops during methyldopa therapy, the physician should determine whether hemolytic anemia exists and whether the positive Coombs test may be a problem. For example, in addition to a positive direct Coombs test there is less often a positive indirect Coombs test which may interfere with cross matching of blood.

Before treatment is started, it is desirable to do a blood count (hematocrit, hemoglobin, or red cell count) for a baseline or to establish whether there is anemia. Periodic blood counts should be done during therapy to detect hemolytic anemia. It may be useful to do a direct Coombs test before therapy and at 6 and 12 months after the start of therapy.

If Coombs-positive hemolytic anemia occurs, the cause may be methyldopa and the drug should be discontinued. Usually the anemia remits promptly. If not, corticosteroids may be given and other causes of anemia should be considered. If the hemolytic anemia is related to methyldopa, the drug should not be reinstituted.

When methyldopa causes Coombs positivity alone or with hemolytic anemia, the red cell is usually coated with gamma globulin of the IgG (gamma G) class only. The positive Coombs test may not revert to normal until weeks to months after methyldopa is stopped.

Should the need for transfusion arise in a patient receiving methyldopa, both a direct and an indirect Coombs test should be performed. In the absence of hemolytic anemia, usually only the direct Coombs test will be positive. A positive direct Coombs test alone will not interfere with typing or cross matching. If the indirect Coombs test is also positive, problems may arise in the major cross match and the assistance of a hematologist or transfusion expert will be needed.

Occasionally, fever has occurred within the first three weeks of methyldopa therapy, associated in some cases with eosinophilia or abnormalities in one or more liver function tests, such as serum alkaline phosphatase, serum transaminases (SGOT, SGPT), bilirubin, and prothrombin time. Jaundice, with or without fever, may occur with onset usually within the first two to three months of therapy. In some patients the findings are consistent with those of cholestasis. In others the findings are consistent with hepatitis and hepatocellular injury.

Rarely, fatal hepatic necrosis has been reported after use of methyldopa. These hepatic changes may represent hypersensitivity reactions. Periodic determination of hepatic function should be done particularly during the first 6 to 12 weeks of therapy or whenever an unexplained fever occurs. If fever, abnormalities in liver function tests, or jaundice appear, stop therapy with methyldopa. If caused by methyldopa, the temperature and abnormalities in liver function characteristically have reverted to normal when the drug was discontinued. Methyldopa should not be reinstituted in such patients.

Rarely, a reversible reduction of the white blood cell count with a primary effect on the granulocytes has been seen. The granulocyte count returned promptly to normal on discontinuance of the drug. Rare cases of granulocytopenia have been reported. In each instance, upon stopping the drug, the white cell count returned to normal. Reversible thrombocytopenia has occurred rarely.

Chlorothiazide

Use with caution in severe renal disease. In patients with renal disease, thiazides may precipitate azotemia. Cumulative effects of the drug may develop in patients with impaired renal function.

Thiazides should be used with caution in patients with impaired hepatic function or progressive liver disease, since minor alterations of fluid and electrolyte balance may precipitate hepatic coma.

Thiazides may add to or potentiate the action of other antihypertensive drugs.

Sensitivity reactions may occur in patients with or without a history of allergy or bronchial asthma.

The possibility of exacerbation or activation of systemic lupus erythematosus has been reported.

Lithium generally should not be given with diuretics (see PRECAUTIONS, *Drug Interactions*).

PRECAUTIONS

General

Methyldopa

Methyldopa should be used with caution in patients with a history of previous liver disease or dysfunction (see WARNINGS).

Some patients taking methyldopa experience clinical edema or weight gain which may be controlled by use of a diuretic. Methyldopa should not be continued if edema progresses or signs of heart failure appear.

Hypertension has recurred occasionally after dialysis in patients given methyldopa because the drug is removed by this procedure.

Rarely, involuntary choreoathetotic movements have been observed during therapy with methyldopa in patients with severe bilateral cerebrovascular disease. Should these movements occur, stop therapy.

Chlorothiazide

All patients receiving diuretic therapy should be observed for evidence of fluid or electrolyte imbalance: namely, hyponatremia, hypochloremic alkalosis, and hypokalemia. Serum and urine electrolyte determinations are particularly important when the patient is vomiting excessively or receiving parenteral fluids. Warning signs or symptoms of fluid and electrolyte imbalance, irrespective of cause include dryness of mouth, thirst, weakness, lethargy, drowsiness, restlessness, confusion, seizures, muscle pains or cramps, muscular fatigue, hypotension, oliguria, tachycardia, and gastrointestinal disturbances such as nausea and vomiting.

Hypokalemia may develop, especially after prolonged therapy or when severe cirrhosis is present (see CONTRAINDICATIONS and WARNINGS).

Interference with adequate oral electrolyte intake will also contribute to hypokalemia. Hypokalemia may cause cardiac arrhythmia and may also sensitize or exaggerate the response of the heart to the toxic effects of digitalis (e.g., increased ventricular irritability). Hypokalemia may be avoided or treated by use of potassium sparing diuretics or potassium supplements such as foods with a high potassium content.

Although any chloride deficit is generally mild and usually does not require specific treatment except under extraordinary circumstances (as in liver disease or renal disease), chloride replacement may be required in the treatment of metabolic alkalosis.

Dilutional hyponatremia may occur in edematous patients in hot weather; appropriate therapy is water restriction, rather than administration of salt, except in rare instances when the hyponatremia is life threatening. In actual salt depletion, appropriate replacement is the therapy of choice.

Hyperuricemia may occur or acute gout may be precipitated in certain patients receiving thiazides.

In diabetic patients dosage adjustments of insulin or oral hypoglycemic agents may be required. Hyperglycemia may occur with thiazide diuretics. Thus latent diabetes mellitus may become manifest during thiazide therapy.

The antihypertensive effects of the drug may be enhanced in the postsympathectomy patient.

If progressive renal impairment becomes evident, consider withholding or discontinuing diuretic therapy.

Thiazides have been shown to increase the urinary excretion of magnesium; this may result in hypomagnesemia.

Thiazides may decrease urinary calcium excretion. Thiazides may cause intermittent and slight elevation of serum calcium in the absence of known disorders of calcium metabolism. Marked hypercalcemia may be evidence of hidden hyperparathyroidism. Thiazides should be discontinued before carrying out tests for parathyroid function.

Increases in cholesterol and triglyceride levels may be associated with thiazide diuretic therapy.

Laboratory Tests

Methyldopa

Blood count, Coombs test and liver function tests are recommended before initiating therapy and at periodic intervals (see WARNINGS).

Chlorothiazide

Periodic determination of serum electrolytes to detect possible electrolyte imbalance should be done at appropriate intervals.

Drug Interactions

Methyldopa

When methyldopa is used with other antihypertensive drugs, potentiation of antihypertensive effect may occur. Patients should be followed carefully to detect side reactions or unusual manifestations of drug idiosyncrasy.

Patients may require reduced doses of anesthetics when on methyldopa. If hypotension does occur during anesthesia, it usually can be controlled by vasopressors. The adrenergic receptors remain sensitive during treatment with methyldopa.

Monoamine oxidase (MAO) inhibitors: See CONTRAINDICATIONS.

Chlorothiazide

When given concurrently the following drugs may interact with thiazide diuretics.

Alcohol, barbiturates, or narcotics—potentiation of orthostatic hypotension may occur.

Antidiabetic drugs (oral agents and insulin)—dosage adjustment of the antidiabetic drug may be required.

Other antihypertensive drugs—additive effect or potentiation.

Cholestyramine and colestipol resins—Both cholestyramine and colestipol resins have the potential of binding thiazide diuretics and reducing diuretic absorption from the gastrointestinal tract.

Corticosteroids, ACTH—intensified electrolyte depletion, particularly hypokalemia.

Pressor amines (e.g., norepinephrine)—possible decreased response to pressor amines but not sufficient to preclude their use.

Skeletal muscle relaxants, nondepolarizing (e.g., tubocurarine)—possible increased responsiveness to the muscle relaxant.

Lithium—generally should not be given with diuretics. Diuretic agents reduce the renal clearance of lithium and add a high risk of lithium toxicity. Refer to the package insert for lithium preparations before use of such preparations with ALDOCLOR.

Non-steroidal Anti-inflammatory Drugs—In some patients, the administration of a non-steroidal anti-inflammatory agent can reduce the diuretic, natriuretic, and antihypertensive effects of loop, potassium-sparing and thiazide diuretics. Therefore, when ALDOCLOR and non-steroidal anti-inflammatory agents are used concomitantly, the patient should be observed closely to determine if the desired effect of the diuretic is obtained.

Drug/Laboratory Test Interactions

Methyldopa

Methyldopa may interfere with measurement of: urinary uric acid by the phosphotungstate method, serum creatinine by the alkaline picrate method, and SGOT by colorimetric methods. Interference with spectrophotometric methods for SGOT analysis has not been reported.

Since methyldopa causes fluorescence in urine samples at the same wave lengths as catecholamines, falsely high levels of urinary catecholamines may be reported. This will interfere with the diagnosis of pheochromocytoma. It is important to recognize this phenomenon before a patient with a possible pheochromocytoma is subjected to surgery. Methyldopa does not interfere with measurement of VMA (vanillylmandelic acid), a test for pheochromocytoma, by those methods which convert VMA to vanillin. Methyldopa is not recommended for the treatment of patients with pheochromocytoma. Rarely, when urine is exposed to air after voiding, it may darken because of breakdown of methyldopa or its metabolites.

Chlorothiazide

Thiazides should be discontinued before carrying out tests for parathyroid function (see PRECAUTIONS, *General*).

Carcinogenesis, Mutagenesis, Impairment of Fertility

Studies to evaluate the carcinogenic or mutagenic potential of the methyldopa-chlorothiazide combination, or the effects of this combination on fertility have not been performed.

Methyldopa

No evidence of a tumorigenic effect was seen when methyldopa was given for two years to mice at doses up to 1800 mg/kg/day or to rats at doses up to 240 mg/kg/day (30 and 4 times the maximum recommended human dose in mice and rats, respectively, when compared on the basis of body weight; 2.5 and 0.6 times the maximum recommended human dose in mice and rats, respectively, when compared on the basis of body surface area; calculations assume a patient weight of 50 kg).

Methyldopa was not mutagenic in the Ames Test and did not increase chromosomal aberration or sister chromatid exchanges in Chinese hamster ovary cells. These *in vitro* studies were carried out both with and without exogenous metabolic activation.

Fertility was unaffected when methyldopa was given to male and female rats at 100 mg/kg/day (1.7 times the maximum daily human dose when compared on the basis of body weight; 0.2 times the maximum daily human dose when compared on the basis of body surface area). Methyldopa decreased sperm count, sperm motility, the number of late spermatids and the male fertility index when given to male rats of 200 and 400 mg/kg/day (3.3 and 6 times the maximum daily human dose when compared on the basis of body weight; 0.5 and 1 times the maximum daily human dose when compared on the basis of body surface area).

Continued on next page

Information on the Merck & Co., Inc. products listed on these pages is the full prescribing information from product circulars in use September 30, 1996.

Merck & Co.—Cont.

Chlorothiazide
Carcinogenicity studies have not been done with chlorothiazide.
Chlorothiazide was not mutagenic *in vitro* in the Ames microbial mutagen test (using a maximum concentration of 5 mg/plate and *Salmonella typhimurium* strains TA98 and TA100) and was not mutagenic and did not induce miotic nondis junction to diploid-strains of *Aspergillus nidulans*.
Chlorothiazide had no adverse effects on fertility in female rats at doses up to 60/mg/kg/day and no adverse effects on fertility in male rats at doses up to 40 mg/kg/day. These doses are 1.5 and 1.0 times* the recommended maximum human dose, respectively, when compared on a body weight basis.

---

*Calculations based on a human body weight of 50 kg.

Pregnancy

Use of diuretics during normal pregnancy is inappropriate and exposes mother and fetus to unnecessary hazard. Diuretics do not prevent development of toxemia of pregnancy and there is no satisfactory evidence that they are useful in treatment of toxemia.
Teratogenic Effects—Pregnancy Category C: Reproduction studies in the rat, at doses up to 40 mg/kg/day (3–4 times the maximum recommended human dose), did not impair fertility or cause abnormalities of the fetus due to ALDOCLOR. There are no adequate and well-controlled studies with ALDOCLOR in pregnant women. Because animal reproduction studies are not always predictive of human response, this drug should be used during pregnancy only if clearly needed.
Chlorothiazide: Thiazides cross the placental barrier and appear in cord blood.
Although reproduction studies performed with chlorothiazide doses of 50 mg/kg/day in rabbits, 60 mg/kg/day in rats and 500 mg/kg/day in mice revealed no external abnormalities or impairment of neonatal growth and survival due to chlorothiazide, such studies did not include complete visceral and skeletal examinations.
Methyldopa: Reproduction studies performed with methyldopa at oral doses up to 1000 mg/kg in mice, 200 mg/kg in rabbits, and 100 mg/kg in rats revealed no evidence of harm to the fetus. These doses are 16.6 times, 3.3 times and 1.7 times, respectively, the maximum daily human dose when compared on the basis of body weight: 1.4 times, 1.1 times and 0.2 times, respectively, when compared on the basis of body surface area: calculations assume a patient weight of 50 kg. There are, however, no adequate and well-controlled studies in pregnant women in the first trimester of pregnancy. Because animal reproduction studies are not always predictive of human response, methyldopa should be used during pregnancy only if clearly needed.
Published reports of the use of methyldopa during all trimesters indicate that if this drug is used during pregnancy the possibility of fetal harm appears remote. In five studies, three of which were controlled, involving 332 pregnant hypertensive women, treatment with methyldopa was associated with an improved fetal outcome. The majority of these women were in the third trimester when methyldopa therapy was begun.
In one study, women who had begun methyldopa treatment between weeks 16 and 20 of pregnancy gave birth to infants whose average head circumference was reduced by a small amount (34.2 ± 1.7 cm vs. 34.6 ± 1.3 cm [mean ± 1 S.D.]). Long-term follow up of 195 (97.5%) of the children born to methyldopa-treated pregnant women (including those who began treatment between weeks 16 and 20) failed to uncover any significant adverse effect on the children. At four years of age, the developmental delay commonly seen in children born to hypertensive mothers was less evident in those whose mothers were treated with methyldopa during pregnancy than those whose mothers were untreated. The children of the treated group scored consistently higher than the children of the untreated group on five major indices of intellectual and motor development. At age seven and one-half developmental scores and intelligence indices showed no significant differences in children of treated or untreated hypertensive women.
Nonteratogenic Effects: These may include fetal or neonatal jaundice, thrombocytopenia, and possibly other adverse reactions which have occurred in the adult.
Nursing Mothers
Methyldopa and thiazides appear in breast milk. Therefore, because of the potential for serious adverse reactions in nursing infants from chlorothiazide, a decision should be made whether to discontinue nursing or to discontinue the drug, taking into account the importance of the drug to the mother.
Pediatric Use
Safety and effectiveness of ALDOCLOR in children has not been established.

ADVERSE REACTIONS

The following adverse reactions have been reported and, within each category, are listed in order of decreasing severity.
Methyldopa
Sedation, usually transient, may occur during the initial period of therapy or whenever the dose is increased. Headache, asthenia, or weakness may be noted as early and transient symptoms. However, significant adverse effects due to methyldopa have been infrequent and this agent usually is well tolerated.
Cardiovascular: Aggravation of angina pectoris, congestive heart failure, prolonged carotid sinus hypersensitivity, orthostatic hypotension (decrease daily dosage), edema or weight gain, bradycardia.
Digestive: Pancreatitis, colitis, vomiting, diarrhea, sialadenitis, sore or "black" tongue, nausea, constipation, distension, flatus, dryness of mouth.
Endocrine: Hyperprolactinemia.
Hematologic: Bone marrow depression, leukopenia, granulocytopenia, thrombocytopenia, hemolytic anemia; positive tests for antinuclear antibody, LE cells, and rheumatoid factor, positive Coombs test.
Hepatic: Liver disorders including hepatitis, jaundice, abnormal liver function tests (see WARNINGS).
Hypersensitivity: Myocarditis, pericarditis, vasculitis, lupus-like syndrome, drug-related fever.
Nervous System/Psychiatric: Parkinsonism, Bell's palsy, decreased mental acuity, involuntary choreoathetotic movements, symptoms of cerebrovascular insufficiency, psychic disturbances including nightmares and reversible mild psychoses or depression, headache, sedation, asthenia or weakness, dizziness, lightheadedness, paresthesias.
Metabolic: Rise in BUN.
Musculoskeletal: Arthralgia, with or without joint swelling; myalgia.
Respiratory: Nasal stuffiness.
Skin: Toxic epidermal necrolysis, rash.
Urogenital: Amenorrhea, breast enlargement, gynecomastia, lactation, impotence, decreased libido.
Chlorothiazide
Body as a Whole: Weakness.
Cardiovascular: Hypotension including orthostatic hypotension (may be aggravated by alcohol, barbiturates, narcotics or antihypertensive drugs).
Digestive: Pancreatitis, jaundice (intrahepatic cholestatic jaundice), diarrhea, vomiting, sialadenitis, cramping, constipation, gastric irritation, nausea, anorexia.
Hematologic: Aplastic anemia, agranulocytosis, leukopenia, hemolytic anemia, thrombocytopenia.
Hypersensitivity: Anaphylactic reactions, necrotizing angiitis (vasculitis and cutaneous vasculitis), respiratory distress including pneumonitis and pulmonary edema, photosensitivity, fever, urticaria, rash, purpura.
Metabolic: Electrolyte imbalance (see PRECAUTIONS), hyperglycemia, glycosuria, hyperuricemia.
Musculoskeletal: Muscle spasm.
Nervous System/Psychiatric: Vertigo, paresthesias, dizziness, headache, restlessness.
Renal: Renal failure, renal dysfunction, interstitial nephritis. (See WARNINGS.)
Skin: Erythema multiforme including Stevens-Johnson syndrome, exfoliative dermatitis including toxic epidermal necrolysis, alopecia.
Special Senses: Transient blurred vision, xanthopsia.
Urogenital: Impotence.

OVERDOSAGE

Acute overdosage may produce acute hypotension with other responses attributable to brain and gastrointestinal malfunction (excessive sedation, weakness, bradycardia, dizziness, lightheadedness, constipation, distention, flatus, diarrhea, nausea, vomiting).
In the event of overdosage, symptomatic and supportive measures should be employed. When ingestion is recent, gastric lavage or emesis may reduce absorption. Otherwise, management includes special attention to cardiac rate and output, blood volume, electrolyte imbalance, paralytic ileus, urinary function and cerebral activity.
Sympathomimetic drugs [e.g., levarterenol, epinephrine, ARAMINE* (Metaraminol Bitartrate)] may be indicated. Methyldopa is dialyzable. The degree to which chlorothiazide is removed by hemodialysis has not been established.
The oral LD_{50} of methyldopa is greater than 1.5 g/kg in both the mouse and the rat. The oral LD_{50} of chlorothiazide is 8.5 g/kg, greater than 10 g/kg, and greater than 1 g/kg in the mouse, rat, and dog respectively.

---

*Registered trademark of MERCK & CO., INC.

DOSAGE AND ADMINISTRATION

DOSAGE MUST BE INDIVIDUALIZED, AS DETERMINED BY TITRATION OF THE INDIVIDUAL COMPONENTS (see box warning). Once the patient has been successfully titrated, ALDOCLOR may be substituted if the previously determined titrated doses are the same as in the combination. The usual starting dosage is one tablet of ALDOCLOR 150 or one tablet of ALDOCLOR 250 two or three times a day.
When administered individually, the usual daily dosage of chlorothiazide is 0.5 g to 1.0 g in single or divided doses and that of methyldopa is 500 mg to 2 g. To minimize the sedation associated with methyldopa, start dosage increases in the evening.
Occasionally tolerance to methyldopa may occur, usually between the second and third month of therapy. Additional separate doses of methyldopa or replacement of ALDOCLOR with single entity agents is necessary until the new effective dose ratio is re-established by titration. The maximum recommended daily dose of methyldopa is 3 g. When ALDOCLOR 150 is used to provide 1 g of methyldopa, 0.6 g of chlorothiazide is delivered. When ALDOCLOR 250 is used to provide 1 g of methyldopa, 1 g of chlorothiazide is delivered. It is prudent, if greater than 1 g of methyldopa per day is required, to provide the additional methyldopa as methyldopa alone.
If ALDOCLOR does not adequately control blood pressure, additional doses of other agents may be given. When ALDOCLOR is given with antihypertensives other than thiazides, the initial dosage of methyldopa should be limited to 500 mg daily in divided doses and the dose of these other agents may need to be adjusted to effect a smooth transition.
Since both components of ALDOCLOR have a relatively short duration of action, withdrawal is followed by return of hypertension usually within 48 hours. This is not complicated by an overshoot of blood pressure.
Since methyldopa is largely excreted by the kidney, patients with impaired renal function may respond to smaller doses. Syncope in older patients may be related to an increased sensitivity and advanced arteriosclerotic vascular disease. This may be avoided by lower doses.

HOW SUPPLIED

No. 3318—Tablets ALDOCLOR 150 are beige, oval, film coated tablets coded MSD 612. Each tablet contains 250 mg of methyldopa and 150 mg of chlorothiazide. They are supplied as follows:
NDC 0006-0612-68 bottles of 100.
Shown in Product Identification Guide, page 324
No. 3319—Tablets ALDOCLOR 250 are green, oval, film coated tablets coded MSD 634. Each tablet contains 250 mg of methyldopa and 250 mg of chlorothiazide. They are supplied as follows:
NDC 0006-0634-68 bottles of 100.
Shown in Product Identification Guide, page 324
Storage
Keep container tightly closed. Protect from moisture, light, and freezing, −20°C (−4°F) and store at room temperature, 15–30°C (59–86°F).
7899643 Issued October 1994

ALDOMET® Tablets ℞
(Methyldopa), U.S.P.
ALDOMET® Oral Suspension ℞
(Methyldopa), U.S.P.

DESCRIPTION

ALDOMET* (Methyldopa) is an antihypertensive drug.
Methyldopa, the *L*-isomer of alpha-methyldopa is levo-3-(3,4-dihydroxyphenyl)-2-methylalanine. Its empirical formula is $C_{10}H_{13}NO_4$, with a molecular weight of 211.22, and its structural formula is:

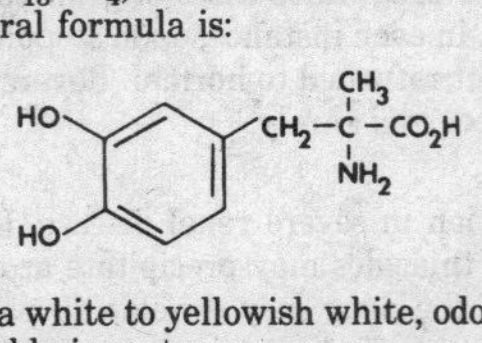

Methyldopa is a white to yellowish white, odorless fine powder, and is soluble in water.
ALDOMET is supplied as tablets, for oral use, in three strengths: 125 mg, 250 mg, or 500 mg of methyldopa per tablet. Inactive ingredients in the tablets are: calcium disodium edetate, cellulose, citric acid, colloidal silicon dioxide, D&C Yellow 10, ethylcellulose, guar gum, hydroxypropyl methylcellulose, iron oxide, magnesium stearate, propylene glycol, talc, and titanium dioxide.
Oral Suspension ALDOMET is supplied as a white to off-white preparation; each 5 mL contains 250 mg of methyldopa and alcohol 1 percent, with benzoic acid 0.1 percent and sodium bisulfite 0.2 percent added as preservatives. Inactive ingredients in the oral suspension are: artificial and natural

flavors, cellulose, citric acid, confectioner's sugar, disodium edetate, glycerin, polysorbate, purified water, and sodium carboxymethylcellulose.

*Registered trademark of MERCK & CO., INC.

CLINICAL PHARMACOLOGY

ALDOMET is an aromatic-amino-acid decarboxylase inhibitor in animals and in man. Although the mechanism of action has yet to be conclusively demonstrated, the antihypertensive effect of methyldopa probably is due to its metabolism to alpha-methylnorepinephrine, which then lowers arterial pressure by stimulation of central inhibitory alpha-adrenergic receptors, false neurotransmission, and/or reduction of plasma renin activity. Methyldopa has been shown to cause a net reduction in the tissue concentration of serotonin, dopamine, norepinephrine, and epinephrine.

Only methyldopa, the *L*-isomer of alpha-methyldopa, has the ability to inhibit dopa decarboxylase and to deplete animal tissues of norepinephrine. In man the antihypertensive activity appears to be due solely to the *L*-isomer. About twice the dose of the racemate (*DL*-alpha-methyldopa) is required for equal antihypertensive effect.

Methyldopa has no direct effect on cardiac function and usually does not reduce glomerular filtration rate, renal blood flow, or filtration fraction. Cardiac output usually is maintained without cardiac acceleration. In some patients the heart rate is slowed.

Normal or elevated plasma renin activity may decrease in the course of methyldopa therapy.

ALDOMET reduces both supine and standing blood pressure. Methyldopa usually produces highly effective lowering of the supine pressure with infrequent symptomatic postural hypotension. Exercise hypotension and diurnal blood pressure variations rarely occur.

Pharmacokinetics and Metabolism

The maximum decrease in blood pressure occurs four to six hours after oral dosage. Once an effective dosage level is attained, a smooth blood pressure response occurs in most patients in 12 to 24 hours. After withdrawal, blood pressure usually returns to pretreatment levels within 24–48 hours.

Methyldopa is extensively metabolized. The known urinary metabolites are: α-methyldopa mono-0-sulfate; 3-0-methyl-α-methyldopa; 3,4-dihydroxyphenylacetone; α-methyldopamine; 3-0-methyl-α-methyldopamine and their conjugates.

Approximately 70% of the drug which is absorbed is excreted in the urine as methyldopa and its mono-0-sulfate conjugate. The renal clearance is about 130 mL/min in normal subjects and is diminished in renal insufficiency. The plasma half-life of methyldopa is 105 minutes. After oral doses, excretion is essentially complete in 36 hours.

Methyldopa crosses the placental barrier, appears in cord blood, and appears in breast milk.

INDICATION AND USAGE

Hypertension.

CONTRAINDICATIONS

ALDOMET is contraindicated in patients:

—with active hepatic disease, such as acute hepatitis and active cirrhosis

—with liver disorders previously associated with methyldopa therapy (see WARNINGS)

—with hypersensitivity to any component of these products, including sulfites contained in Oral Suspension ALDOMET (see WARNINGS). (Tablets ALDOMET do not contain sulfites.)

—on therapy with monoamine oxidase (MAO) inhibitors.

WARNINGS

It is important to recognize that a positive Coombs test, hemolytic anemia, and liver disorders may occur with methyldopa therapy. The rare occurrences of hemolytic anemia or liver disorders could lead to potentially fatal complications unless properly recognized and managed. Read this section carefully to understand these reactions.

With prolonged methyldopa therapy, 10 to 20 percent of patients develop a positive direct Coombs test which usually occurs between 6 and 12 months of methyldopa therapy. Lowest incidence is at daily dosage of 1 g or less. This on rare occasions may be associated with hemolytic anemia, which could lead to potentially fatal complications. One cannot predict which patients with a positive direct Coombs test may develop hemolytic anemia.

Prior existence or development of a positive direct Coombs test is not in itself a contraindication to use of methyldopa. If a positive Coombs test develops during methyldopa therapy, the physician should determine whether hemolytic anemia exists and whether the positive Coombs test may be a problem. For example, in addition to a positive direct Coombs test there is less often a positive indirect Coombs test which may interfere with cross matching of blood.

Before treatment is started, it is desirable to do a blood count (hematocrit, hemoglobin, or red cell count) for a baseline or to establish whether there is anemia. Periodic blood counts should be done during therapy to detect hemolytic anemia. It may be useful to do a direct Coombs test before therapy and at 6 and 12 months after the start of therapy.

If Coombs-positive hemolytic anemia occurs, the cause may be methyldopa and the drug should be discontinued. Usually the anemia remits promptly. If not, corticosteroids may be given and other causes of anemia should be considered. If the hemolytic anemia is related to methyldopa, the drug should not be reinstituted.

When methyldopa causes Coombs positivity alone or with hemolytic anemia, the red cell is usually coated with gamma globulin of the IgG (gamma G) class only. The positive Coombs test may not revert to normal until weeks to months after methyldopa is stopped.

Should the need for transfusion arise in a patient receiving methyldopa, both a direct and an indirect Coombs test should be performed. In the absence of hemolytic anemia, usually only the direct Coombs test will be positive. A positive direct Coombs test alone will not interfere with typing or cross matching. If the indirect Coombs test is also positive, problems may arise in the major cross match and the assistance of a hematologist or transfusion expert will be needed.

Occasionally, fever has occurred within the first 3 weeks of methyldopa therapy, associated in some cases with eosinophilia or abnormalities in one or more liver function tests, such as serum alkaline phosphatase, serum transaminases (SGOT, SGPT), bilirubin, and prothrombin time. Jaundice, with or without fever, may occur with onset usually within the first 2 to 3 months of therapy. In some patients the findings are consistent with those of cholestasis. In others the findings are consistent with hepatitis and hepatocellular injury.

Rarely, fatal hepatic necrosis has been reported after use of methyldopa. These hepatic changes may represent hypersensitivity reactions. Periodic determinations of hepatic function should be done particularly during the first 6 to 12 weeks of therapy or whenever an unexplained fever occurs. If fever, abnormalities in liver function tests, or jaundice appear, stop therapy with methyldopa. If caused by methyldopa, the temperature and abnormalities in liver function characteristically have reverted to normal when the drug was discontinued. Methyldopa should not be reinstituted in such patients.

Rarely, a reversible reduction of the white blood cell count with a primary effect on the granulocytes has been seen. The granulocyte count returned promptly to normal on discontinuance of the drug. Rare cases of granulocytopenia have been reported. In each instance, upon stopping the drug, the white cell count returned to normal. Reversible thrombocytopenia has occurred rarely.

Oral Suspension ALDOMET (but not Tablets ALDOMET) contains sodium bisulfite, a sulfite that may cause allergic-type reactions including anaphylactic symptoms and life-threatening or less severe asthmatic episodes in certain susceptible people. The overall prevalence of sulfite sensitivity in the general population is unknown and probably low. Sulfite sensitivity is seen more frequently in asthmatic than in nonasthmatic people.

PRECAUTIONS

General

Methyldopa should be used with caution in patients with a history of previous liver disease or dysfunction (see WARNINGS).

Some patients taking methyldopa experience clinical edema or weight gain which may be controlled by use of a diuretic. Methyldopa should not be continued if edema progresses or signs of heart failure appear.

Hypertension has recurred occasionally after dialysis in patients given methyldopa because the drug is removed by this procedure.

Rarely involuntary choreoathetotic movements have been observed during therapy with methyldopa in patients with severe bilateral cerebrovascular disease. Should these movements occur, stop therapy.

Laboratory Tests

Blood count, Coombs test, and liver function tests are recommended before initiating therapy and at periodic intervals (see WARNINGS).

Drug Interactions

When methyldopa is used with other antihypertensive drugs, potentiation of antihypertensive effect may occur. Patients should be followed carefully to detect side reactions or unusual manifestations of drug idiosyncrasy.

Patients may require reduced doses of anesthetics when on methyldopa. If hypotension does occur during anesthesia, it usually can be controlled by vasopressors. The adrenergic receptors remain sensitive during treatment with methyldopa.

When methyldopa and lithium are given concomitantly the patient should be carefully monitored for symptoms of lithium toxicity. Read the circular for lithium preparations.

Monoamine oxidase (MAO) inhibitors: see CONTRAINDICATIONS.

Drug/Laboratory Test Interactions

Methyldopa may interfere with measurement of: urinary uric acid by the phosphotungstate method, serum creatinine by the alkaline picrate method, and SGOT by colorimetric methods. Interference with spectrophotometric methods for SGOT analysis has not been reported.

Since methyldopa causes fluorescence in urine samples at the same wave lengths as catecholamines, falsely high levels of urinary catecholamines may be reported. This will interfere with the diagnosis of pheochromocytoma. It is important to recognize this phenomenon before a patient with a possible pheochromocytoma is subjected to surgery. Methyldopa does not interfere with measurement of VMA (vanillylmandelic acid), a test for pheochromocytoma, by those methods which convert VMA to vanillin. Methyldopa is not recommended for the treatment of patients with pheochromocytoma. Rarely, when urine is exposed to air after voiding, it may darken because of breakdown of methyldopa or its metabolites.

Carcinogenesis, Mutagenesis, Impairment of Fertility

No evidence of a tumorigenic effect was seen when methyldopa was given for two years to mice at doses up to 1800 mg/kg/day or to rats at doses up to 240 mg/kg/day (30 and 4 times the maximum recommended human dose in mice and rats, respectively, when compared on the basis of body weight; 2.5 and 0.6 times the maximum recommended human dose in mice and rats, respectively, when compared on the basis of body surface area; calculations assume a patient weight of 50 kg).

Methyldopa was not mutagenic in the Ames Test and did not increase chromosomal aberration or sister chromatid exchanges in Chinese hamster ovary cells. These *in vitro* studies were carried out both with and without exogenous metabolic activation.

Fertility was unaffected when methyldopa was given to male and female rats at 100 mg/kg/day (1.7 times the maximum daily human dose when compared on the basis of body weight; 0.2 times the maximum daily human dose when compared on the basis of body surface area). Methyldopa decreased sperm count, sperm motility, the number of late spermatids and the male fertility index when given to male rats at 200 and 400 mg/kg/day (3.3 and 6.7 times the maximum daily human dose when compared on the basis of body weight; 0.5 and 1 times the maximum daily human dose when compared on the basis of body surface area).

Pregnancy

Pregnancy Category B. Reproduction studies performed with methyldopa at oral doses up to 1000 mg/kg in mice, 200 mg/kg in rabbits and 100 mg/kg in rats revealed no evidence of harm to the fetus. These doses are 16.6 times, 3.3 times and 1.7 times, respectively, the maximum daily human dose when compared on the basis of body weight; 1.4 times, 1.1 times and 0.2 times, respectively, when compared on the basis of body surface area; calculations assume a patient weight of 50 kg. There are, however, no adequate and well-controlled studies in pregnant women in the first trimester of pregnancy. Because animal reproduction studies are not always predictive of human response, ALDOMET should be used during pregnancy only if clearly needed.

Published reports of the use of methyldopa during all trimesters indicate that if this drug is used during pregnancy the possibility of fetal harm appears remote. In five studies, three of which were controlled, involving 332 pregnant hypertensive women, treatment with ALDOMET was associated with an improved fetal outcome. The majority of these women were in the third trimester when methyldopa therapy was begun.

In one study, women who had begun methyldopa treatment between weeks 16 and 20 of pregnancy gave birth to infants whose average head circumference was reduced by a small amount (34.2 $\pm$ 1.7 cm vs. 34.6 $\pm$ 1.3 cm [mean $\pm$ 1 S.D.]). Long-term follow up of 195 (97.5%) of the children born to methyldopa-treated pregnant women (including those who began treatment between weeks 16 and 20) failed to uncover any significant adverse effect on the children. At four years of age, the developmental delay commonly seen in children born to hypertensive mothers was less evident in those whose mothers were treated with methyldopa during pregnancy than those whose mothers were untreated. The children of the treated group scored consistently higher than the children of the untreated group on five major indices of intellectual and motor development. At age seven and one-half

Continued on next page

Information on the Merck & Co., Inc. products listed on these pages is the full prescribing information from product circulars in use September 30, 1996.

Merck & Co.—Cont.

developmental scores and intelligence indices showed no significant differences in children of treated or untreated hypertensive women.

Nursing Mothers

Methyldopa appears in breast milk. Therefore, caution should be exercised when methyldopa is given to a nursing woman.

ADVERSE REACTIONS

Sedation, usually transient, may occur during the initial period of therapy or whenever the dose is increased. Headache, asthenia, or weakness may be noted as early and transient symptoms. However, significant adverse effects due to ALDOMET have been infrequent and this agent usually is well tolerated.

The following adverse reactions have been reported and, within each category, are listed in order of decreasing severity.

Cardiovascular: Aggravation of angina pectoris, congestive heart failure, prolonged carotid sinus hypersensitivity, orthostatic hypotension (decrease daily dosage), edema or weight gain, bradycardia.

Digestive: Pancreatitis, colitis, vomiting, diarrhea, sialadenitis, sore or "black" tongue, nausea, constipation, distension, flatus, dryness of mouth.

Endocrine: Hyperprolactinemia.

Hematologic: Bone marrow depression, leukopenia, granulocytopenia, thrombocytopenia, hemolytic anemia; positive tests for antinuclear antibody, LE cells, and rheumatoid factor, positive Coombs test.

Hepatic: Liver disorders including hepatitis, jaundice, abnormal liver function tests (see WARNINGS).

Hypersensitivity: Myocarditis, pericarditis, vasculitis, lupus-like syndrome, drug-related fever.

Nervous System/Psychiatric: Parkinsonism, Bell's palsy, decreased mental acuity, involuntary choreoathetotic movements, symptoms of cerebrovascular insufficiency, psychic disturbances including nightmares and reversible mild psychoses or depression, headache, sedation, asthenia or weakness, dizziness, lightheadedness, paresthesias.

Metabolic: Rise in BUN.

Musculoskeletal: Arthralgia, with or without joint swelling; myalgia.

Respiratory: Nasal stuffiness.

Skin: Toxic epidermal necrolysis, rash.

Urogenital: Amenorrhea, breast enlargement, gynecomastia, lactation, impotence, decreased libido.

OVERDOSAGE

Acute overdosage may produce acute hypotension with other responses attributable to brain and gastrointestinal malfunction (excessive sedation, weakness, bradycardia, dizziness, lightheadedness, constipation, distention, flatus, diarrhea, nausea, vomiting).

In the event of overdosage, symptomatic and supportive measures should be employed. When ingestion is recent, gastric lavage or emesis may reduce absorption. When ingestion has been earlier, infusions may be helpful to promote urinary excretion. Otherwise, management includes special attention to cardiac rate and output, blood volume, electrolyte balance, paralytic ileus, urinary function and cerebral activity.

Sympathomimetic drugs [e.g., levarterenol, epinephrine, ARAMINE* (Metaraminol Bitartrate)] may be indicated. Methyldopa is dialyzable.

The oral LD_{50} of methyldopa is greater than 1.5 g/kg in both the mouse and the rat.

*Registered trademark of MERCK & CO., INC.

DOSAGE AND ADMINISTRATION

ADULTS

Initiation of Therapy

The usual starting dosage of ALDOMET is 250 mg two or three times a day in the first 48 hours. The daily dosage then may be increased or decreased, preferably at intervals of not less than two days, until an adequate response is achieved. To minimize the sedation, start dosage increases in the evening. By adjustment of dosage, morning hypotension may be prevented without sacrificing control of afternoon blood pressure.

When methyldopa is given to patients on other antihypertensives, the dose of these agents may need to be adjusted to effect a smooth transition. When ALDOMET is given with antihypertensives other than thiazides, the initial dosage of ALDOMET should be limited to 500 mg daily in divided doses; when ALDOMET is added to a thiazide, the dosage of thiazide need not be changed.

Maintenance Therapy

The usual daily dosage of ALDOMET is 500 mg to 2 g in two to four doses. Although occasional patients have responded to higher doses, the maximum recommended daily dosage is 3 g. Once an effective dosage range is attained, a smooth blood pressure response occurs in most patients in 12 to 24 hours. Since methyldopa has a relatively short duration of action, withdrawal is followed by return of hypertension usually within 48 hours. This is not complicated by an overshoot of blood pressure.

Occasionally tolerance may occur, usually between the second and third month of therapy. Adding a diuretic or increasing the dosage of methyldopa frequently will restore effective control of blood pressure. A thiazide may be added at any time during methyldopa therapy and is recommended if therapy has not been started with a thiazide or if effective control of blood pressure cannot be maintained on 2 g of methyldopa daily.

Methyldopa is largely excreted by the kidney and patients with impaired renal function may respond to smaller doses. Syncope in older patients may be related to an increased sensitivity and advanced arteriosclerotic vascular disease. This may be avoided by lower doses.

CHILDREN

Initial dosage is based on 10 mg/kg of body weight daily in two to four doses. The daily dosage then is increased or decreased until an adequate response is achieved. The maximum dosage is 65 mg/kg or 3 g daily, whichever is less.

HOW SUPPLIED

No. 3341—Tablets ALDOMET, 125 mg, are yellow, film coated, round tablets, coded MSD 135. They are supplied as follows:

NDC 0006-0135-68 bottles of 100.

Shown in Product Identification Guide, page 324

No. 3290—Tablets ALDOMET, 250 mg, are yellow, film coated, round tablets, coded MSD 401. They are supplied as follows:

NDC 0006-0401-68 bottles of 100
(6505-00-890-1856, 250 mg 100's)
NDC 0006-0401-28 unit dose packages of 100
(6505-00-149-0090, 250 mg individually sealed 100's)
NDC 0006-0401-78 unit of use bottles of 100
NDC 0006-0401-82 bottles of 1000
(6505-00-931-6646, 250 mg 1000's).

Shown in Product Identification Guide, page 324

No. 3292—Tablets ALDOMET, 500 mg, are yellow, film coated, round tablets, coded MSD 516. They are supplied as follows:

NDC 0006-0516-68 bottles of 100
NDC 0006-0516-28 unit dose packages of 100
(6505-01-046-3616, 500 mg individually sealed 100's)
NDC 0006-0516-78 unit of use bottles of 100
NDC 0006-0516-74 bottles of 500
(6505-01-199-8339, 500 mg 500's).

Shown in Product Identification Guide, page 324

No. 3382—Oral Suspension ALDOMET, 250 mg per 5 mL, is an off-white, creamy suspension with a citric orange-pineapple flavor. It is supplied as follows:

NDC 0006-3382-74 bottles of 473 mL.

Storage

Store Oral Suspension ALDOMET below 26°C (78°F) in a tight, light-resistant container. Protect from freezing.

7843429 Issued March 1994

COPYRIGHT © MERCK & CO., INC., 1985
All rights reserved

ALDOMET® Ester HCl Injection (Methyldopate HCl), U.S.P. ℞

DESCRIPTION

Injection ALDOMET* Ester Hydrochloride (Methyldopate HCl) is an antihypertensive agent for intravenous use. Methyldopate hydrochloride [levo-3-(3,4-dihydroxyphenyl)-2-methylalanine, ethyl ester hydrochloride]is the ethyl ester of methyldopa, supplied as the hydrochloride salt with a molecular weight of 275.73. Methyldopate hydrochloride is more soluble and stable in solution than methyldopa and is the preferred form for intravenous use.

The empirical formula for methyldopate hydrochloride is $C_{12}H_{17}NO_4 \cdot HCl$ and its structural formula is:

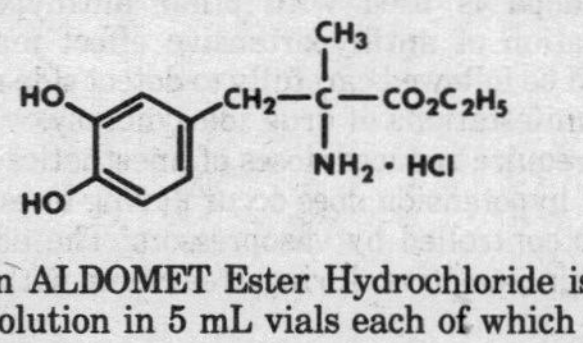
CH3
HO
CH2—C—CO2C2H5
NH2 · HCl
HO

Injection ALDOMET Ester Hydrochloride is supplied as a sterile solution in 5 mL vials each of which contains:

Methyldopate hydrochloride	250.0 mg
Inactive ingredients:	
Citric acid anhydrous	25.0 mg
Disodium edetate	2.5 mg
Monothioglycerol	10.0 mg
Sodium hydroxide to adjust pH	
Water for Injection, q.s. to 5 mL	

Methylparaben 7.5 mg, propylparaben 1 mg, and sodium bisulfite 16 mg added as preservatives.

*Registered trademark of MERCK & CO., INC.

CLINICAL PHARMACOLOGY

ALDOMET (Methyldopa), an antihypertensive, is an aromatic-amino-acid decarboxylase inhibitor in animals and in man. Although the mechanism of action has yet to be conclusively demonstrated, the antihypertensive effect of methyldopa probably is due to its metabolism to alpha-methyl-norepinephrine, which then lowers arterial pressure by stimulation of central inhibitory alpha-adrenergic receptors, false neurotransmission, and/or reduction of plasma renin activity. Methyldopa has been shown to cause a net reduction in the tissue concentration of serotonin, dopamine, norepinephrine, and epinephrine.

Only methyldopa, the *L*-isomer of alpha-methyldopa, has the ability to inhibit dopa decarboxylase and to deplete animal tissues of norepinephrine. In man the antihypertensive activity appears to be due solely to the *L*-isomer. About twice the dose of the racemate (*DL*-alpha-methyldopa) is required for equal antihypertensive effect.

Methyldopa has no direct effect on cardiac function and usually does not reduce glomerular filtration rate, renal blood flow, or filtration fraction. Cardiac output usually is maintained without cardiac acceleration. In some patients the heart rate is slowed.

Normal or elevated plasma renin activity may decrease in the course of methyldopa therapy.

Methyldopa reduces both supine and standing blood pressure. It usually produces highly effective lowering of the supine pressure with infrequent symptomatic postural hypotension. Exercise hypotension and diurnal blood pressure variations rarely occur.

Pharmacokinetics and Metabolism

Methyldopate hydrochloride is the ethyl ester of methyldopa hydrochloride and possesses the same pharmacologic attributes.

Methyldopa is extensively metabolized. The known urinary metabolites are: α-methyldopa mono-0-sulfate; 3-0-methyl-α-methyldopa; 3,4-dihydroxyphenylacetone; α-methyldopamine; 3-0-methyl-α-methyldopamine and their conjugates.

Following intravenous administration of methyldopate hydrochloride a decrease in blood pressure may occur in four to six hours and last 10 to 16 hours.

Approximately 49 percent of the dose of methyldopate hydrochloride is excreted in the urine as methyldopa and its mono-0-sulfate. The renal clearance of methyldopa following methyldopate hydrochloride is about 156 mL/min in normal subjects and is diminished in renal insufficiency. Following methyldopate hydrochloride injection the plasma half-life of methyldopa is 90–127 mins. Approximately 17 percent of a dose of methyldopate hydrochloride given to normal subjects appears in plasma as free methyldopa.

Methyldopa crosses the placental barrier, appears in cord blood, and appears in breast milk.

INDICATION AND USAGE

Hypertension, when parenteral medication is indicated.

The treatment of hypertensive crises may be initiated with Injection ALDOMET Ester Hydrochloride.

CONTRAINDICATIONS

Injection ALDOMET Ester Hydrochloride is contraindicated in patients:

—with active hepatic disease, such as acute hepatitis and active cirrhosis

—with liver disorders previously associated with methyldopa therapy (see WARNINGS)

—with hypersensitivity to any component of this product, including sulfites (see WARNINGS)

—on therapy with monoamine oxidase (MAO) inhibitors.

WARNINGS

It is important to recognize that a positive Coombs test, hemolytic anemia, and liver disorders may occur with methyldopa therapy. The rare occurrences of hemolytic anemia or liver disorders could lead to potentially fatal complications unless properly recognized and managed. Read this section carefully to understand these reactions.

With prolonged methyldopa therapy, 10 to 20 percent of patients develop a positive direct Coombs test which usually

occurs between 6 and 12 months of methyldopa therapy. Lowest incidence is at daily dosage of 1 g or less. This on rare occasions may be associated with hemolytic anemia, which could lead to potentially fatal complications. One cannot predict which patients with a positive direct Coombs test may develop hemolytic anemia.

Prior existence or development of a positive direct Coombs test is not in itself a contraindication to use of methyldopa. If a positive Coombs test develops during methyldopa therapy, the physician should determine whether hemolytic anemia exists and whether the positive Coombs test may be a problem. For example, in addition to a positive direct Coombs test there is less often a positive indirect Coombs test which may interfere with cross matching of blood.

Before treatment is started, it is desirable to do a blood count (hematocrit, hemoglobin, or red cell count) for a baseline or to establish whether there is anemia. Periodic blood counts should be done during therapy to detect hemolytic anemia. It may be useful to do a direct Coombs test before therapy and at 6 and 12 months after the start of therapy.

If Coombs-positive hemolytic anemia occurs, the cause may be methyldopa and the drug should be discontinued. Usually the anemia remits promptly. If not, corticosteroids may be given and other causes of anemia should be considered. If the hemolytic anemia is related to methyldopa, the drug should not be reinstituted.

When methyldopa causes Coombs positivity alone or with hemolytic anemia, the red cell is usually coated with gamma globulin of the IgG (gamma G) class only. The positive Coombs test may not revert to normal until weeks to months after methyldopa is stopped.

Should the need for transfusion arise in a patient receiving methyldopa, both a direct and an indirect Coombs test should be performed. In the absence of hemolytic anemia, usually only the direct Coombs test will be positive. A positive direct Coombs test alone will not interfere with typing or cross matching. If the indirect Coombs test is also positive, problems may arise in the major cross match and the assistance of a hematologist or transfusion expert will be needed.

Occasionally, fever has occurred within the first three weeks of methyldopa therapy, associated in some cases with eosinophilia or abnormalities in one or more liver function tests, such as serum alkaline phosphatase, serum transaminases (SGOT, SGPT), bilirubin and prothrombin time. Jaundice, with or without fever, may occur with onset usually within the first two to three months of therapy. In some patients the findings are consistent with those of cholestasis. In others the findings are consistent with hepatitis and hepatocellular injury.

Rarely fatal hepatic necrosis has been reported after use of methyldopa. These hepatic changes may represent hypersensitivity reactions. Periodic determination of hepatic function should be done particularly during the first 6 to 12 weeks of therapy or whenever an unexplained fever occurs. If fever, abnormalities in liver function tests, or jaundice appear, stop therapy with methyldopa. If caused by methyldopa, the temperature and abnormalities in liver function characteristically have reverted to normal when the drug was discontinued. Methyldopa should not be reinstituted in such patients.

Rarely, a reversible reduction of the white blood cell count with a primary effect on the granulocytes has been seen. The granulocyte count returned promptly to normal on discontinuance of the drug. Rare cases of granulocytopenia have been reported. In each instance, upon stopping the drug, the white cell count returned to normal. Reversible thrombocytopenia has occurred rarely.

Injection ALDOMET Ester Hydrochloride contains sodium bisulfite, a sulfite that may cause allergic-type reactions including anaphylactic symptoms and life-threatening or less severe asthmatic episodes in certain susceptible people. The overall prevalence of sulfite sensitivity in the general population is unknown and probably low. Sulfite sensitivity is seen more frequently in asthmatic than in nonasthmatic people.

PRECAUTIONS

General

Methyldopa should be used with caution in patients with a history of previous liver disease or dysfunction (see WARNINGS).

Some patients taking methyldopa experience clinical edema or weight gain which may be controlled by use of a diuretic. Methyldopa should not be continued if edema progresses or signs of heart failure appear.

A paradoxical pressor response has been reported with intravenous administration of ALDOMET Ester Hydrochloride.

Hypertension has recurred occasionally after dialysis in patients given methyldopa because the drug is removed by this procedure.

Rarely involuntary choreoathetotic movements have been observed during therapy with methyldopa in patients with severe bilateral cerebrovascular disease. Should these movements occur, stop therapy.

Laboratory Tests

Blood count, Coombs test, and liver function tests are recommended before initiating therapy and at periodic intervals (see WARNINGS).

Drug Interactions

When methyldopa is used with other antihypertensive drugs, potentiation of antihypertensive effect may occur. Patients should be followed carefully to detect side reactions or unusual manifestations of drug idiosyncrasy.

Patients may require reduced doses of anesthetics when on methyldopa. If hypotension does occur during anesthesia, it usually can be controlled by vasopressors. The adrenergic receptors remain sensitive during treatment with methyldopa.

When methyldopa and lithium are given concomitantly the patient should be carefully monitored for symptoms of lithium toxicity. Read the circular for lithium preparations.

Monoamine oxidase (MAO) inhibitors: See CONTRAINDICATIONS.

Drug/Laboratory Test Interactions

Methyldopa may interfere with measurement of: urinary uric acid by the phosphotungstate method, serum creatinine by the alkaline picrate method, and SGOT by colorimetric methods. Interference with spectrophotometric methods for SGOT analysis has not been reported.

Since methyldopa causes fluorescence in urine samples at the same wave lengths as catecholamines, falsely high levels of urinary catecholamines may be reported. This will interfere with the diagnosis of pheochromocytoma. It is important to recognize this phenomenon before a patient with a possible pheochromocytoma is subjected to surgery. Methyldopa does not interfere with measurement of VMA (vanillylmandelic acid), a test for pheochromocytoma, by those methods which convert VMA to vanillin. Methyldopa is not recommended for the treatment of patients with pheochromocytoma. Rarely, when urine is exposed to air after voiding, it may darken because of breakdown of methyldopa or its metabolites.

Carcinogenesis, Mutagenesis, Impairment of Fertility

No evidence of a tumorigenic effect was seen when methyldopa was given for two years to mice at doses up to 1800 mg/kg/day or to rats at doses up to 240 mg/kg/day (30 and 4 times the maximum recommended human dose in mice and rats, respectively, when compared on the basis of body weight; 2.5 and 0.6 times the maximum recommended human dose in mice and rats, respectively, when compared on the basis of body surface area; calculations assume a patient weight of 50 kg).

Methyldopa was not mutagenic in the Ames Test and did not increase chromosomal aberration or sister chromatid exchanges in Chinese hamster ovary cells. These *in vitro* studies were carried out both with and without exogenous metabolic activation.

Fertility was unaffected when methyldopa was given to male and female rats at 100 mg/kg/day (1.7 times the maximum daily human dose when compared on the basis of body weight; 0.2 times the maximum daily human dose when compared on the basis of body surface area). Methyldopa decreased sperm count, sperm motility, the number of late spermatids and the male fertility index when given to male rats at 200 and 400 mg/kg/day (3.3 and 6.7 times the maximum daily human dose when compared on the basis of body weight; 0.5 and 1 times the maximum daily human dose when compared on the basis of body surface area).

Long-term studies in animals have not been performed to evaluate the carcinogenic potential of methyldopate hydrochloride; nor have evaluations of this ester's mutagenic potential or potential to affect fertility been carried out.

Pregnancy

Pregnancy Category C. Animal reproduction studies have not been conducted with ALDOMET Ester Hydrochloride. It is also not known whether ALDOMET Ester Hydrochloride can affect reproduction capacity or can cause fetal harm when given to a pregnant woman. ALDOMET Ester Hydrochloride should be given to a pregnant woman only if clearly needed.

Nursing Mothers

Methyldopa appears in breast milk. Therefore, caution should be exercised when methyldopa is given to a nursing woman.

ADVERSE REACTIONS

Sedation, usually transient, may occur during the initial period of therapy or whenever the dose is increased. Headache, asthenia, or weakness may be noted as early and transient symptoms. However, significant adverse effects due to methyldopa have been infrequent and this agent usually is well tolerated.

The following adverse reactions have been reported and, within each category, are listed in order of decreasing severity.

Cardiovascular: Aggravation of angina pectoris, congestive heart failure, prolonged carotid sinus hypersensitivity, paradoxical pressor response with intravenous use, orthostatic hypotension (decrease daily dosage), edema or weight gain, bradycardia.

Digestive: Pancreatitis, colitis, vomiting, diarrhea, sialadenitis, sore or "black" tongue, nausea, constipation, distension, flatus, dryness of mouth.

Endrocrine: Hyperprolactinemia.

Hematologic: Bone marrow depression, leukopenia, granulocytopenia, thrombocytopenia, hemolytic anemia; positive tests for antinuclear antibody, LE cells, and rheumatoid factor, positive Coombs tests.

Hepatic: Liver disorders including hepatitis, jaundice, abnormal liver function tests (see WARNINGS).

Hypersensitivity: Myocarditis, pericarditis, vasculitis, lupus-like syndrome, drug-related fever.

Nervous System/Psychiatric: Parkinsonism, Bell's palsy, decreased mental acuity, involuntary choreoathetotic movements, symptoms of cerebrovascular insufficiency, psychic disturbances including nightmares and reversible mild psychoses or depression, headache, sedation, asthenia or weakness, dizziness, lightheadedness, paresthesias.

Metabolic: Rise in BUN.

Musculoskeletal: Arthralgia, with or without joint swelling; myalgia.

Respiratory: Nasal stuffiness.

Skin: Toxic epidermal necrolysis, rash.

Urogenital: Amenorrhea, breast enlargement, gynecomastia, lactation, impotence, decreased libido.

OVERDOSAGE

Acute overdosage may produce acute hypotension with other responses attributable to brain and gastrointestinal malfunction (excessive sedation, weakness, bradycardia, dizziness, lightheadedness, constipation, distention, flatus, diarrhea, nausea, vomiting).

In the event of overdosage, symptomatic and supportive measures should be employed. Management includes special attention to cardiac rate and output, blood volume, electrolyte balance, paralytic ileus, urinary function and cerebral activity.

Sympathomimetic drugs [e.g. levarterenol, epinephrine, ARAMINE* (Metaraminol Bitartrate)] may be indicated.

The acute intravenous LD_{50} of ALDOMET Ester Hydrochloride in the mouse is 321 mg/kg.

*Registered trademark of MERCK & CO., INC.

DOSAGE AND ADMINISTRATION

Injection ALDOMET Ester Hydrochloride, when given intravenously in effective doses, causes a decline in blood pressure that may begin in four to six hours and last 10 to 16 hours after injection.

Add the desired dose of Injection ALDOMET Ester Hydrochloride to 100 mL of 5 percent Dextrose Injection USP. Alternatively the desired dose may be given in 5% dextrose in water in a concentration of 100 mg/10 mL. Give this intravenous infusion slowly over a period of 30 to 60 minutes.

The vial containing Injection ALDOMET Ester Hydrochloride should be inspected visually for particulate matter and discoloration before use whenever solution and container permit.

ADULTS

The usual adult dosage intravenously is 250 to 500 mg at six hour intervals as required. The maximum recommended intravenous dose is 1 g every six hours.

When control has been obtained, oral therapy with Tablets ALDOMET (Methyldopa) may be substituted for intravenous therapy, starting with the same dosage schedule used for the parenteral route. The effectiveness and anticipated responses are described in the circular for Tablets ALDOMET (Methyldopa).

Since methyldopa has a relatively short duration of action, withdrawal is followed by return of hypertension usually within 48 hours. This is not complicated by an overshoot of blood pressure.

Occasionally tolerance may occur, usually between the second and third month of therapy. Adding a diuretic or increasing the dosage of methyldopa frequently will restore effective control of blood pressure. A thiazide may be added at any time during methyldopa therapy and is recommended if therapy has not been started with a thiazide or if effective control of blood pressure cannot be maintained on 2 g of methyldopa daily.

Methyldopa is largely excreted by the kidney and patients with impaired renal function may respond to smaller doses. Syncope in older patients may be related to an increased

Continued on next page

Information on the Merck & Co., Inc. products listed on these pages is the full prescribing information from product circulars in use September 30, 1996.

Merck & Co.—Cont.

sensitivity and advanced arteriosclerotic vascular disease. This may be avoided by lower doses.

CHILDREN

The recommended daily dosage is 20 to 40 mg/kg of body weight in divided doses every six hours. The maximum dosage is 65 mg/kg or 3 g daily, whichever is less. When the blood pressure is under control, continue with oral therapy using Tablets ALDOMET (Methyldopa) in the same dosage as for the parenteral route.

HOW SUPPLIED

No. 3293—Injection ALDOMET Ester Hydrochloride, 250 mg per 5 mL, is a clear, colorless solution and is supplied as follows:

NDC 0006-3293-05 in 5 mL vials
(6505-01-096-2735, 5 mL vial).

Storage

Store below 30°C (86°F).
Protect from freezing.

7900437 Issued March 1994

COPYRIGHT © MERCK & CO., INC., 1989
All rights reserved

ALDORIL® Tablets ℞
(Methyldopa-Hydrochlorothiazide), U.S.P.

> **WARNING**
>
> This fixed combination drug is not indicated for initial therapy of hypertension. Hypertension requires therapy titrated to the individual patient. If the fixed combination represents the dosage so determined, its use may be more convenient in patient management. The treatment of hypertension is not static, but must be re-evaluated as conditions in each patient warrant.

DESCRIPTION

ALDORIL* (Methyldopa-Hydrochlorothiazide) combines two antihypertensives: methyldopa and hydrochlorothiazide.

Methyldopa

Methyldopa is an antihypertensive and is the *L*-isomer of alphamethyldopa. It is levo-3-(3,4-dihydroxyphenyl)-2-methylalanine. Its empirical formula is $C_{10}H_{13}NO_4$, with a molecular weight of 211.22, and its structural formula is:

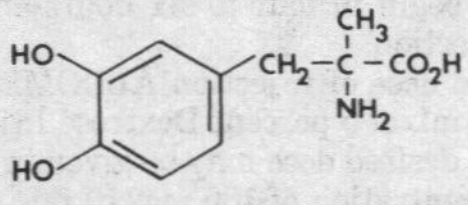

Methyldopa is a white to yellowish white, odorless fine powder, and is soluble in water.

Hydrochlorothiazide

Hydrochlorothiazide is a diuretic and antihypertensive. It is the 3,4-dihydro derivative of chlorothiazide. Its chemical name is 6-chloro-3,4-dihydro-2*H*-1,2,4-benzothiadiazine-7-sulfonamide 1,1-dioxide. Its empirical formula is $C_7H_8ClN_3O_4S_2$ and its structural formula is:

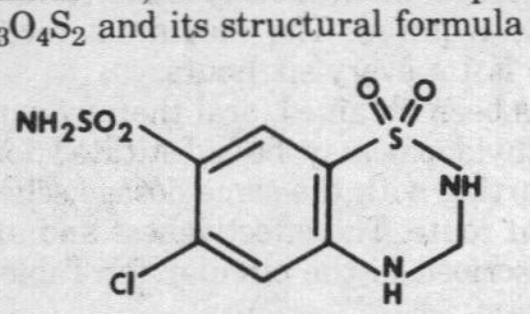

Hydrochlorothiazide is a white, or practically white, crystalline powder with a molecular weight of 297.72, which is slightly soluble in water, but freely soluble in sodium hydroxide solution.

ALDORIL is supplied as tablets in four strengths for oral use:

ALDORIL 15, contains 250 mg of methyldopa and 15 mg of hydrochlorothiazide.

ALDORIL 25, contains 250 mg of methyldopa and 25 mg of hydrochlorothiazide.

ALDORIL D30, contains 500 mg of methyldopa and 30 mg of hydrochlorothiazide.

ALDORIL D50, contains 500 mg of methyldopa and 50 mg of hydrochlorothiazide.

Each tablet contains the following inactive ingredients: calcium disodium edetate, calcium phosphate, cellulose, citric acid, colloidal silicon dioxide, ethylcellulose, guar gum, hydroxypropyl methylcellulose, magnesium stearate, propylene glycol, talc, and titanium dioxide. ALDORIL 15 and ALDORIL D30 also contain iron oxide.

---

*Registered trademark of MERCK & CO., INC.

CLINICAL PHARMACOLOGY

Methyldopa

Methyldopa is an aromatic-amino-acid decarboxylase inhibitor in animals and in man. Although the mechanism of action has yet to be conclusively demonstrated, the antihypertensive effect of methyldopa probably is due to its metabolism to alpha-methylnorepinephrine, which then lowers arterial pressure by stimulation of central inhibitory alpha-adrenergic receptors, false neurotransmission, and/or reduction of plasma renin activity. Methyldopa has been shown to cause a net reduction in the tissue concentration of serotonin, dopamine, norepinephrine, and epinephrine.

Only methyldopa, the *L*-isomer of alpha-methyldopa, has the ability to inhibit dopa decarboxylase and to deplete animal tissues of norepinephrine. In man, the antihypertensive activity appears to be due solely to the *L*-isomer. About twice the dose of the racemate (*DL*-alpha-methyldopa) is required for equal antihypertensive effect.

Methyldopa has no direct effect on cardiac function and usually does not reduce glomerular filtration rate, renal blood flow, or filtration fraction. Cardiac output usually is maintained without cardiac acceleration. In some patients the heart rate is slowed.

Normal or elevated plasma renin activity may decrease in the course of methyldopa therapy.

Methyldopa reduces both supine and standing blood pressure. It usually produces highly effective lowering of the supine pressure with infrequent symptomatic postural hypotension. Exercise hypotension and diurnal blood pressure variations rarely occur.

Hydrochlorothiazide

The mechanism of the antihypertensive effect of thiazides is unknown. Hydrochlorothiazide does not usually affect normal blood pressure.

Hydrochlorothiazide affects the distal renal tubular mechanism of electrolyte reabsorption. At maximal therapeutic dosage all thiazides are approximately equal in their diuretic efficacy.

Hydrochlorothiazide increases excretion of sodium and chloride in approximately equivalent amounts. Natriuresis may be accompanied by some loss of potassium and bicarbonate.

After oral use diuresis begins within 2 hours, peaks in about 4 hours and lasts about 6 to 12 hours.

Pharmacokinetics and Metabolism

Methyldopa

The maximum decrease in blood pressure occurs four to six hours after oral dosage. Once an effective dosage level is attained, a smooth blood pressure response occurs in most patients in 12 to 24 hours. After withdrawal, blood pressure usually returns to pretreatment levels within 24–48 hours.

Methyldopa is extensively metabolized. The known urinary metabolites are: α-methyldopa mono-0-sulfate; 3-0-methyl-α-methyldopa; 3,4-dihydroxyphenylacetone; α-methyldopamine; 3-0-methyl-α-methyldopamine and their conjugates.

Approximately 70 percent of the drug which is absorbed is excreted in the urine as methyldopa and its mono-0-sulfate conjugate. The renal clearance is about 130 mL/min in normal subjects and is diminished in renal insufficiency. The plasma half-life of methyldopa is 105 minutes. After oral doses, excretion is essentially complete in 36 hours.

Methyldopa crosses the placental barrier, appears in cord blood, and appears in breast milk.

Hydrochlorothiazide

Hydrochlorothiazide is not metabolized but is eliminated rapidly by the kidney. When plasma levels have been followed for at least 24 hours, the plasma half-life has been observed to vary between 5.6 and 14.8 hours. At least 61 percent of the oral dose is eliminated unchanged within 24 hours. Hydrochlorothiazide crosses the placental but not the blood-brain barrier and is excreted in breast milk.

INDICATION AND USAGE

Hypertension (see box warning).

CONTRAINDICATIONS

ALDORIL is contraindicated in patients:

—with active hepatic disease, such as acute hepatitis and active cirrhosis
—with liver disorders previously associated with methyldopa therapy (see WARNINGS)
—with anuria
—with hypersensitivity to methyldopa, or to hydrochlorothiazide or other sulfonamide-derived drugs
—on therapy with monoamine oxidase (MAO) inhibitors.

WARNINGS

Methyldopa

It is important to recognize that a positive Coombs test, hemolytic anemia, and liver disorders may occur with methyldopa therapy. The rare occurrences of hemolytic anemia or liver disorders could lead to potentially fatal complications unless properly recognized and managed. Read this section carefully to understand these reactions.

With prolonged methyldopa therapy, 10 to 20 percent of patients develop a positive direct Coombs test which usually occurs between 6 and 12 months of methyldopa therapy. Lowest incidence is at daily dosage of 1 g or less. This on rare occasions may be associated with hemolytic anemia, which could lead to potentially fatal complications. One cannot predict which patients with a positive direct Coombs test may develop hemolytic anemia.

Prior existence or development of a positive direct Coombs test is not in itself a contraindication to use of methyldopa. If a positive Coombs test develops during methyldopa therapy, the physician should determine whether hemolytic anemia exists and whether the positive Coombs test may be a problem. For example, in addition to a positive direct Coombs test there is less often a positive indirect Coombs test which may interfere with cross matching of blood.

Before treatment is started it is desirable to do a blood count (hematocrit, hemoglobin, or red cell count) for a baseline or to establish whether there is anemia. Periodic blood counts should be done during therapy to detect hemolytic anemia. It may be useful to do a direct Coombs test before therapy and at 6 and 12 months after the start of therapy.

If Coombs-positive hemolytic anemia occurs, the cause may be methyldopa and the drug should be discontinued. Usually the anemia remits promptly. If not, corticosteroids may be given and other causes of anemia should be considered. If the hemolytic anemia is related to methyldopa, the drug should not be reinstituted.

When methyldopa causes Coombs positivity alone or with hemolytic anemia, the red cell is usually coated with gamma globulin of the IgG (gamma G) class only. The positive Coombs test may not revert to normal until weeks to months after methyldopa is stopped.

Should the need for transfusion arise in a patient receiving methyldopa, both a direct and an indirect Coombs test should be performed. In the absence of hemolytic anemia, usually only the direct Coombs test will be positive. A positive direct Coombs test alone will not interfere with typing or cross matching. If the indirect Coombs test is also positive, problems may arise in the major cross match and the assistance of a hematologist or transfusion expert will be needed.

Occasionally, fever has occurred within the first three weeks of methyldopa therapy, associated in some cases with eosinophilia or abnormalities in one or more liver function tests, such as serum alkaline phosphatase, serum transaminases (SGOT, SGPT), bilirubin, and prothrombin time. Jaundice, with or without fever, may occur with onset usually within the first two to three months of therapy. In some patients the findings are consistent with those of cholestasis. In others the findings are consistent with hepatitis and hepatocellular injury.

Rarely fatal hepatic necrosis has been reported after use of methyldopa. These hepatic changes may represent hypersensitivity reactions. Periodic determination of hepatic function should be done particularly during the first 6 to 12 weeks of therapy or whenever an unexplained fever occurs. If fever, abnormalities in liver function tests, or jaundice appear, stop therapy with methyldopa. If caused by methyldopa, the temperature and abnormalities in liver function characteristically have reverted to normal when the drug was discontinued. Methyldopa should not be reinstituted in such patients.

Rarely, a reversible reduction of the white blood cell count with a primary effect on the granulocytes has been seen. The granulocyte count returned promptly to normal on discontinuance of the drug. Rare cases of granulocytopenia have been reported. In each instance, upon stopping the drug, the white cell count returned to normal. Reversible thrombocytopenia has occurred rarely.

Hydrochlorothiazide

Use with caution in severe renal disease. In patients with renal disease, thiazides may precipitate azotemia. Cumulative effects of the drug may develop in patients with impaired renal function.

Thiazides should be used with caution in patients with impaired hepatic function or progressive liver disease, since minor alterations of fluid and electrolyte balance may precipitate hepatic coma.

Thiazides may add to or potentiate the action of other antihypertensive drugs.

Sensitivity reactions may occur in patients with or without a history of allergy or bronchial asthma.

The possibility of exacerbation or activation of systemic lupus erythematosus has been reported.

Lithium generally should not be given with diuretics (see PRECAUTIONS, *Drug Interactions*).

PRECAUTIONS

General
Methyldopa
Methyldopa should be used with caution in patients with a history of previous liver disease or dysfunction (see WARNINGS).
Some patients taking methyldopa experience clinical edema or weight gain which may be controlled by use of a diuretic. Methyldopa should not be continued if edema progresses or signs of heart failure appear.
Hypertension has recurred occasionally after dialysis in patients given methyldopa because the drug is removed by this procedure.
Rarely involuntary choreoathetotic movements have been observed during therapy with methyldopa in patients with severe bilateral cerebrovascular disease. Should these movements occur, stop therapy.
Hydrochlorothiazide
All patients receiving diuretic therapy should be observed for evidence of fluid or electrolyte imbalance: namely; hyponatremia, hypochloremic alkalosis, and hypokalemia. Serum and urine electrolyte determinations are particularly important when the patient is vomiting excessively or receiving parenteral fluids. Warning signs or symptoms of fluid and electrolyte imbalance, irrespective of cause, include dryness of mouth, thirst, weakness, lethargy, drowsiness, restlessness, confusion, seizures, muscle pains or cramps, muscular fatigue, hypotension, oliguria, tachycardia, and gastrointestinal disturbances such as nausea and vomiting.
Hypokalemia may develop especially after prolonged therapy or when severe cirrhosis is present (see CONTRAINDICATIONS and WARNINGS).
Interference with adequate oral electrolyte intake will also contribute to hypokalemia. Hypokalemia may cause cardiac arrhythmia and may also sensitize or exaggerate the response of the heart to the toxic effects of digitalis (e.g., increased ventricular irritability). Hypokalemia may be avoided or treated by use of potassium sparing diuretics or potassium supplements such as foods with a high potassium content.
Although any chloride deficit is generally mild and usually does not require specific treatment except under extraordinary circumstances (as in liver disease or renal disease), chloride replacement may be required in the treatment of metabolic alkalosis.
Dilutional hyponatremia may occur in edematous patients in hot weather; appropriate therapy is water restriction, rather than administration of salt, except in rare instances when the hyponatremia is life threatening. In actual salt depletion, appropriate replacement is the therapy of choice.
Hyperuricemia may occur or acute gout may be precipitated in certain patients receiving thiazides.
In diabetic patients dosage adjustment of insulin or oral hypoglycemic agents may be required. Hyperglycemia may occur with thiazide diuretics. Thus latent diabetes mellitus may become manifest during thiazide therapy.
The antihypertensive effects of the drug may be enhanced in the postsympathectomy patient.
If progressive renal impairment becomes evident, consider withholding or discontinuing diuretic therapy.
Thiazides have been shown to increase the urinary excretion of magnesium; this may result in hypomagnesemia.
Thiazides may decrease urinary calcium excretion. Thiazides may cause intermittent and slight elevation of serum calcium in the absence of known disorders of calcium metabolism. Marked hypercalcemia may be evidence of hidden hyperparathyroidism. Thiazides should be discontinued before carrying out tests for parathyroid function.
Increases in cholesterol and triglyceride levels may be associated with thiazide diuretic therapy.
Laboratory Tests
Methyldopa
Blood count, Coombs test and liver function test, are recommended before initiating therapy and at periodic intervals (see WARNINGS).
Hydrochlorothiazide
Periodic determination of serum electrolytes to detect possible electrolyte imbalance should be done at appropriate intervals.
Drug Interactions
Methyldopa
When methyldopa is used with other antihypertensive drugs, potentiation of antihypertensive effect may occur. Patients should be followed carefully to detect side reactions or unusual manifestations of drug idiosyncrasy.
Patients may require reduced doses of anesthetics when on methyldopa. If hypotension does occur during anesthesia, it usually can be controlled by vasopressors. The adrenergic receptors remain sensitive during treatment with methyldopa.
Monoamine oxidase (MAO) inhibitors: see CONTRAINDICATIONS.
Hydrochlorothiazide
When given concurrently the following drugs may interact with thiazide diuretics.
Alcohol, barbiturates, or narcotics—potentiation of orthostatic hypotension may occur.
Antidiabetic drugs (oral agents and insulin)—dosage adjustment of the antidiabetic drug may be required.
Other antihypertensive drugs—additive effect or potentiation.
Cholestyramine and colestipol resins—Absorption of hydrochlorothiazide is impaired in the presence of anionic exchange resins. Single doses of either cholestyramine or colestipol resins bind the hydrochlorothiazide and reduce its absorption from the gastrointestinal tract by up to 85 and 43 percent, respectively.
Corticosteroids, ACTH—intensified electrolyte depletion, particularly hypokalemia.
Pressor amines (e.g., norepinephrine)—possible decreased response to pressor amines but not sufficient to preclude their use.
Skeletal muscle relaxants, nondepolarizing (e.g., tubocurarine)—possible increased responsiveness to the muscle relaxant.
Lithium—generally should not be given with diuretics. Diuretic agents reduce the renal clearance of lithium and add a high risk of lithium toxicity. Refer to the package insert for lithium preparations before use of such preparations with ALDORIL.
Non-steroidal Anti-inflammatory Drugs—In some patients, the administration of a non-steroidal anti-inflammatory agent can reduce the diuretic, natriuretic, and antihypertensive effects of loop, potassium-sparing and thiazide diuretics. Therefore, when ALDORIL and non-steroidal anti-inflammatory agents are used concomitantly, the patient should be observed closely to determine if the desired effect of the diuretic is obtained.
Drug/Laboratory Test Interactions
Methyldopa
Methyldopa may interfere with measurement of: urinary uric acid by the phosphotungstate method, serum creatinine by the alkaline picrate method, and SGOT by colorimetric methods. Interference with spectrophotometric methods for SGOT analysis has not been reported.
Since methyldopa causes fluorescence in urine samples at the same wave lengths as catecholamines, falsely high levels of urinary catecholamines may be reported. This will interfere with the diagnosis of pheochromocytoma. It is important to recognize this phenomenon before a patient with a possible pheochromocytoma is subjected to surgery. Methyldopa does not interfere with measurement of VMA (vanillylmandelic acid), a test for pheochromocytoma, by those methods which convert VMA to vanillin. Methyldopa is not recommended for the treatment of patients with pheochromocytoma. Rarely, when urine is exposed to air after voiding, it may darken because of breakdown of methyldopa or its metabolites.
Hydrochlorothiazide
Thiazides should be discontinued before carrying out tests for parathyroid function (see PRECAUTIONS, *General*).
Carcinogenesis, Mutagenesis,
Impairment of Fertility
Long-term studies in animals have not been performed to evaluate the effects upon fertility, mutagenic or carcinogenic potential of the combination.
Methyldopa
No evidence of a tumorigenic effect was seen when methyldopa was given for two years to mice at doses up to 1800 mg/kg/day or to rats at doses up to 240 mg/kg/day (30 and 4 times the maximum recommended human dose in mice and rats, respectively, when compared on the basis of body weight; 2.5 and 0.6 times the maximum recommended human dose in mice and rats, respectively, when compared on the basis of body surface area; calculations assume a patient weight of 50 kg).
Methyldopa was not mutagenic in the Ames Test and did not increase chromosomal aberration or sister chromatid exchanges in Chinese hamster ovary cells. These *in vitro* studies were carried out both with and without exogenous metabolic activation.
Fertility was unaffected when methyldopa was given to male and female rats at 100 mg/kg/day (1.7 times the maximum daily human dose when compared on the basis of body weight; 0.2 times the maximum daily human dose when compared on the basis of body surface area). Methyldopa decreased sperm count, sperm motility, the number of late spermatids and the male fertility index when given to male rats at 200 and 400 mg/kg/day (3.3 and 6.7 times the maximum daily human dose when compared on the basis of body weight; 0.5 and 1 times the maximum daily human dose when compared on the basis of body surface area).
Hydrochlorothiazide
Two-year feeding studies in mice and rats conducted under the auspices of the National Toxicology Program (NTP) uncovered no evidence of a carcinogenic potential of hydrochlorothiazide in female mice (at doses of up to approximately 600 mg/kg/day) or in male and female rats (at doses of up to approximately 100 mg/kg/day). The NTP, however, found equivocal evidence for hepatocarcinogenicity in male mice.
Hydrochlorothiazide was not genotoxic *in vitro* in the Ames mutagenicity assay of *Salmonella typhimurium* strains TA 98, TA 100, TA 1535, TA 1537, and TA 1538 and in the Chinese Hamster Ovary (CHO) test for chromosomal aberrations, or *in vivo* in assays using mouse germinal cell chromosomes, Chinese hamster bone marrow chromosomes, and the *Drosophila* sex-linked recessive lethal trait gene. Positive test results were obtained only in the *in vitro* CHO Sister Chromatid Exchange (clastogenicity) and in the Mouse Lymphoma Cell (mutagenicity) assays, using concentrations of hydrochlorothiazide from 43 to 1300 μg/mL, and in the *Aspergillus nidulans* non-disjunction assay at an unspecified concentration.
Hydrochlorothiazide had no adverse effects on the fertility of mice and rats of either sex in studies wherein these species were exposed, via their diet, to doses of up to 100 and 4 mg/kg, respectively, prior to conception and throughout gestation.
Pregnancy
Use of diuretics during normal pregnancy is inappropriate and exposes mother and fetus to unnecessary hazard. Diuretics do not prevent development of toxemia of pregnancy and there is no satisfactory evidence that they are useful in the treatment of toxemia.
Teratogenic Effects—Pregnancy Category C: Animal reproduction studies have not been conducted with ALDORIL. It is also not known whether ALDORIL can affect reproduction capacity or can cause fetal harm when given to a pregnant woman. ALDORIL should be given to a pregnant woman only if clearly needed.
Hydrochlorothiazide: Studies in which hydrochlorothiazide was orally administered to pregnant mice and rats during their respective periods of major organogenesis at doses up to 3000 and 1000 mg hydrochlorothiazide/kg, respectively, provided no evidence of harm to the fetus. There are, however, no adequate and well-controlled studies in pregnant women.
Methyldopa: Reproduction studies performed with methyldopa at oral doses up to 1000 mg/kg in mice, 200 mg/kg in rabbits and 100 mg/kg in rats revealed no evidence of harm to the fetus. These doses are 16.6 times, 3.3 times and 1.7 times, respectively, the maximum daily human dose when compared on the basis of body weight; 1.4 times, 1.1 times and 0.2 times, respectively, when compared on the basis of body surface area; calculations assume a patient weight of 50 kg. There are, however, no adequate and well-controlled studies in pregnant women in the first trimester of pregnancy. Because animal reproduction studies are not always predictive of human response, methyldopa should be used during pregnancy only if clearly needed.
Published reports of the use of methyldopa during all trimesters indicate that if this drug is used during pregnancy the possibility of fetal harm appears remote. In five studies, three of which were controlled, involving 332 pregnant hypertensive women, treatment with methyldopa was associated with an improved fetal outcome. The majority of these women were in the third trimester when methyldopa therapy was begun.
In one study, women who had begun methyldopa treatment between weeks 16 and 20 of pregnancy gave birth to infants whose average head circumference was reduced by a small amount (34.2 ± 1.7 cm vs. 34.6 ± 1.3 cm [mean ± 1 S.D.]). Long term follow-up of 195 (97.5%) of the children born to methyldopa-treated pregnant women (including those who began treatment between weeks 16 and 20) failed to uncover any significant adverse effect on the children. At four years of age, the developmental delay commonly seen in children born to hypertensive mothers was less evident in those whose mothers were treated with methyldopa during pregnancy than those whose mothers were untreated. The children of the treated group scored consistently higher than the children of the untreated group on five major indices of intellectual and motor development. At age 7 and one-half developmental scores and intelligence indices showed no significant differences in children of treated or untreated hypertensive women.
Nonteratogenic Effects: Thiazides cross the placental barrier and appear in cord blood. There is a risk of fetal or neonatal jaundice, thrombocytopenia, and possibly other adverse reactions that have occurred in adults.
Nursing Mothers
Methyldopa and thiazides appear in breast milk. Therefore, because of the potential for serious adverse reactions in nursing infants from hydrochlorothiazide, a decision should be made whether to discontinue nursing or to discontinue the

Continued on next page

Information on the Merck & Co., Inc. products listed on these pages is the full prescribing information from product circulars in use September 30, 1996.

Merck & Co.—Cont.

drug, taking into account the importance of the drug to the mother.

Pediatric Use
Safety and effectiveness of ALDORIL in children have not been established.

ADVERSE REACTIONS

The following adverse reactions have been reported and, within each category, are listed in order of decreasing severity.

Methyldopa
Sedation, usually transient, may occur during the initial period of therapy or whenever the dose is increased. Headache, asthenia, or weakness may be noted as early and transient symptoms. However, significant adverse effects due to methyldopa have been infrequent and this agent usually is well tolerated.

Cardiovascular: Aggravation of angina pectoris, congestive heart failure, prolonged carotid sinus hypersensitivity, orthostatic hypotension (decrease daily dosage), edema or weight gain, bradycardia.

Digestive: Pancreatitis, colitis, vomiting, diarrhea, sialadenitis, sore or "black" tongue, nausea, constipation, distention, flatus, dryness of mouth.

Endocrine: Hyperprolactinemia.

Hematologic: Bone marrow depression, leukopenia, granulocytopenia, thrombocytopenia, hemolytic anemia; positive tests for antinuclear antibody, LE cells, and rheumatoid factor, positive Coombs test.

Hepatic: Liver disorders including hepatitis, jaundice, abnormal liver function tests (see WARNINGS).

Hypersensitivity: Myocarditis, pericarditis, vasculitis, lupus-like syndrome, drug-related fever.

Nervous System/Psychiatric: Parkinsonism, Bell's palsy, decreased mental acuity, involuntary choreoathetotic movements, symptoms of cerebrovascular insufficiency, psychic disturbances including nightmares and reversible mild psychoses or depression, headache, sedation, asthenia or weakness, dizziness, lightheadedness, paresthesias.

Metabolic: Rise in BUN.

Musculoskeletal: Arthralgia, with or without joint swelling; myalgia.

Respiratory: Nasal stuffiness.

Skin: Toxic epidermal necrolysis, rash.

Urogenital: Amenorrhea, breast enlargement, gynecomastia, lactation, impotence, decreased libido.

Hydrochlorothiazide
Body as a Whole: Weakness.

Cardiovascular: Hypotension including orthostatic hypotension (may be aggravated by alcohol, barbiturates, narcotics or antihypertensive drugs).

Digestive: Pancreatitis, jaundice (intrahepatic cholestatic jaundice), diarrhea, vomiting, sialadenitis, cramping, constipation, gastric irritation, nausea, anorexia.

Hematologic: Aplastic anemia, agranulocytosis, leukopenia, hemolytic anemia, thrombocytopenia.

Hypersensitivity: Anaphylactic reactions, necrotizing angiitis (vasculitis and cutaneous vasculitis), respiratory distress including pneumonitis and pulmonary edema, photosensitivity, fever, urticaria, rash, purpura.

Metabolic: Electrolyte imbalance (see PRECAUTIONS), hyperglycemia, glycosuria, hyperuricemia.

Musculoskeletal: Muscle spasm.

Nervous System/Psychiatric: Vertigo, paresthesias, dizziness, headache, restlessness.

Renal: Renal failure, renal dysfunction, interstitial nephritis. (See WARNINGS.)

Skin: Erythema multiforme including Stevens-Johnson syndrome, exfoliative dermatitis including toxic epidermal necrolysis, alopecia.

Special Senses: Transient blurred vision, xanthopsia.

Urogenital: Impotence.

OVERDOSAGE

Acute overdosage may produce acute hypotension with other responses attributable to brain and gastrointestinal malfunction (excessive sedation, weakness, bradycardia, dizziness, lightheadedness, constipation, distention, flatus, diarrhea, nausea, vomiting).

In the event of overdosage, symptomatic and supportive measures should be employed. When ingestion is recent, gastric lavage or emesis may reduce absorption. When ingestion has been earlier, infusions may be helpful to promote urinary excretion. Otherwise, management includes special attention to cardiac rate and output, blood volume, electrolyte balance, paralytic ileus, urinary function and cerebral activity.

Sympathomimetic drugs [e.g., levarterenol, epinephrine, ARAMINE* (Metaraminol Bitartrate)] may be indicated. Methyldopa is dialyzable. The degree to which hydrochloro-

thiazide is removed by hemodialysis has not been established.

The oral LD_{50} of methyldopa is greater than 1.5 g/kg in both the mouse and the rat. The oral LD_{50} of hydrochlorothiazide is greater than 10 g/kg in the mouse and rat.

---

*Registered trademark of MERCK & CO., INC.

DOSAGE AND ADMINISTRATION

DOSAGE MUST BE INDIVIDUALIZED, AS DETERMINED BY TITRATION OF THE INDIVIDUAL COMPONENTS (see box warning). Once the patient has been successfully titrated, ALDORIL may be substituted if the previously determined titrated doses are the same as in the combination. The usual starting dosage is one tablet of ALDORIL 15 two or three times a day or one tablet of ALDORIL 25 two times a day. For those patients requiring higher doses, one tablet of ALDORIL D30 or ALDORIL D50 two times a day may be used.

Patients usually do not require doses of hydrochlorothiazide in excess of 50 mg daily when combined with other antihypertensive agents. The usual daily dosage of methyldopa is 500 mg to 2 g. To minimize the sedation associated with methyldopa, start dosage increases in the evening.

Occasionally tolerance to methyldopa may occur, usually between the second and third month of therapy. Additional separate doses of methyldopa or replacement of ALDORIL with single entity agents is necessary until the new effective dose ratio is re-established by titration. The maximum recommended daily dose of methyldopa is 3 g and of hydrochlorothiazide is 200 mg.

If ALDORIL does not adequately control blood pressure, additional doses of other agents may be given. When ALDORIL is given with antihypertensives other than thiazides, the initial dosage of methyldopa should be limited to 500 mg daily in divided doses and the dose of these other agents may need to be adjusted to effect a smooth transition.

Since both components of ALDORIL have a relatively short duration of action, withdrawal is followed by return of hypertension usually within 48 hours. This is not complicated by an overshoot of blood pressure.

Since methyldopa is largely excreted by the kidney, patients with impaired renal function may respond to smaller doses. Syncope in older patients may be related to an increased sensitivity and advanced arteriosclerotic vascular disease. This may be avoided by lower doses.

HOW SUPPLIED

No. 3294—Tablets ALDORIL 15 are salmon, round, film coated tablets, coded MSD 423. Each tablet contains 250 mg of methyldopa and 15 mg of hydrochlorothiazide. They are supplied as follows:

NDC 0006-0423-68 bottles of 100
NDC 0006-0423-82 bottles of 1000
  Shown in Product Identification Guide, page 324
No. 3295—Tablets ALDORIL 25 are white, round, film coated tablets, coded MSD 456. Each tablet contains 250 mg of methyldopa and 25 mg of hydrochlorothiazide. They are supplied as follows:

NDC 0006-0456-68 bottles of 100
NDC 0006-0456-28 unit dose packages of 100
NDC 0006-0456-82 bottles of 1000
  Shown in Product Identification Guide, page 324
No. 3362—Tablets ALDORIL D30 are salmon, oval, film coated tablets, coded MSD 694. Each tablet contains 500 mg of methyldopa and 30 mg of hydrochlorothiazide. They are supplied as follows:

NDC 0006-0694-68 bottles of 100
  Shown in Product Identification Guide, page 324
No. 3363—Tablets ALDORIL D50 are white, oval, film coated tablets, coded MSD 935. Each tablet contains 500 mg of methyldopa and 50 mg of hydrochlorothiazide. They are supplied as follows:

NDC 0006-0935-68 bottles of 100
  Shown in Product Identification Guide, page 324
Storage
Keep container tightly closed. Protect from light, moisture, freezing, −20°C (−4°F) and store at controlled room temperature, 15–30°C (59–86°F).
    7843550   Issued March 1994
COPYRIGHT © MERCK & CO., INC., 1986
All rights reserved

AMINOHIPPURATE SODIUM "PAH" ℞
Injection, U.S.P.

DESCRIPTION

Aminohippurate sodium* is an agent to measure effective renal plasma flow (ERPF). It is the sodium salt of para-aminohippuric acid, commonly abbreviated "PAH." It is water

soluble, lipid-insoluble, and has a pKa of 3.83. The empirical formula of the anhydrous salt is $C_9H_9N_2NaO_3$ and its structural formula is:

It is provided as a sterile, non-preserved 20 percent aqueous solution for injection, with a pH of 6.7 to 7.6. Each 10 mL contains: Aminohippurate sodium 2 g. Inactive ingredients: Sodium hydroxide to adjust pH, water for injection, q.s.

---

*Formerly referred to as Sodium para-Aminohippurate.

CLINICAL PHARMACOLOGY

PAH is filtered by the glomeruli and is actively secreted by the proximal tubules. At low plasma concentrations (1.0 to 2.0 mg/100 mL), an average of 90 percent of PAH is cleared by the kidneys from the renal blood stream in a single circulation. It is ideally suited for measurement of ERPF since it has a high clearance, is essentially nontoxic at the plasma concentrations reached with recommended doses and its analytical determination is relatively simple and accurate. PAH is also used to measure the functional capacity of the renal tubular secretory mechanism or transport maximum (Tm_{PAH}). This is accomplished by elevating the plasma concentration to levels (40–60 mg/100 mL) sufficient to saturate the maximal capacity of the tubular cells to secrete PAH. Inulin clearance is generally measured during Tm_{PAH} determinations since glomerular filtration rate (GFR) must be known before calculations of secretory Tm measurements can be done (See *Calculations*).

INDICATIONS AND USAGE

Estimation of effective renal plasma flow.
Measurement of the functional capacity of the renal tubular secretory mechanism.

CONTRAINDICATIONS

Hypersensitivity to this product or to its components.

PRECAUTIONS

General
Intravenous solutions must be given with caution to patients with low cardiac reserve, since a rapid increase in plasma volume can precipitate congestive heart failure.
For measurement of ERPF, small doses of PAH are used. However, in research procedures to measure Tm_{PAH}, high plasma levels are required to saturate the capacity of the tubular cells. During these procedures the intravenous administration of PAH solutions should be carried out slowly and with caution. The patient should be continuously observed for any adverse reactions.
Drug Interactions
Renal clearance measurements of PAH cannot be made with any significant accuracy in patients receiving sulfonamides, procaine, or thiazolesulfone. These compounds interfere with chemical color development essential to the analytical procedures.
Probenecid depresses tubular secretion of certain weak acids such as PAH. Therefore, patients receiving probenecid will have erroneously low ERPF and Tm_{PAH} values.
Carcinogenesis, Mutagenesis, Impairment of Fertility
Long-term studies in animals have not been done to evaluate any effects upon fertility or carcinogenic potential of PAH.
Pregnancy
Pregnancy Category C. Animal reproduction studies have not been done with PAH. It is also not known whether PAH can cause fetal harm when given to a pregnant woman or can affect reproduction capacity. PAH should be given to a pregnant woman only if clearly needed.
Nursing Mothers
It is not known whether this drug is excreted in human milk. Because many drugs are excreted in human milk, caution should be exercised when PAH is administered to a nursing woman.
Pediatric Use
Safety and effectiveness in children have not been established.

ADVERSE REACTIONS

Vasomotor disturbances, flushing, tingling, nausea, vomiting, and cramps may occur.
Patients may have a sensation of warmth or the desire to defecate or urinate during or shortly following initiation of infusion.

OVERDOSAGE

The intravenous LD_{50} in female mice is 7.22 g/kg.

DOSAGE AND ADMINISTRATION

For intravenous use only
Clearance measurements using single injection technics are generally inaccurate, particularly in the measurement of ERPF. For this reason, intravenous infusions at fixed rates are used to sustain the plasma PAH concentration at the desired level.

To measure ERPF, the concentration of PAH in the plasma should be maintained at 2 mg per 100 mL, which can be achieved with a priming dose of 6 to 10 mg/kg and an infusion dose of 10 to 24 mg/min.

As a research procedure for the measurement of Tm_{PAH}, the plasma level of PAH must be sufficient to saturate the capacity of the tubular secretory cells. Concentrations of from 40 to 60 mg per 100 mL are usually necessary.

Technical details of these tests may be found in Smith[1]; Wesson[2]; Bauer[3]; Pitts[4]; and Schnurr.[5]

Parenteral drug products should be inspected visually for particulate matter and discoloration prior to use, whenever solution and container permit. NOTE: The normal color range for this product is a colorless to yellow/brown solution. The efficacy is not affected by color changes within this range.

Calculations
Effective Renal Plasma Flow (ERPF)
The clearance of PAH, which is extracted almost completely from the blood during its passage through the renal circulation, constitutes a measure of ERPF. Hence:

$$ERPF = \frac{U_{PAH}V}{P_{PAH}}$$

Where U_{PAH} = concentration of PAH (mg/mL) in the urine
V = rate of urine excretion (mL/min), and
P_{PAH} = plasma concentration of PAH (mg/mL).

Example U_{PAH} = 8.0 mg/mL
V = 1.5 mL/min
P_{PAH} = 0.02 mg/mL

$$ERPF = \frac{8.0 \times 1.5}{0.02} = 600 \text{ mL/min.}$$

Based on PAH clearance studies, the normal values for ERPF are:

men 675 ± 150 mL/min.
women 595 ± 125 mL/min.

Maximum Tubular Secretory
Mechanism (Tm_{PAH})
The quantity of PAH, secreted by the tubules (Tm_{PAH}) is given by the difference between the total rate of excretion ($U_{PAH}V$) and the quantity filtered by the glomeruli ($GFR \times P_{PAH}$). Hence:

$$Tm_{PAH} = U_{PAH}V - (GFR \times P_{PAH} \times 0.83)$$

The factor, 0.83, corrects for that portion of PAH which is bound to plasma protein and hence is unfilterable.

Example U_{PAH} = 9.55 mg/mL
V = 16.68 mL/min
GFR = 120 mL/min
P_{PAH} = 0.60 mg/mL

Then Tm_{PAH} = 9.55 × 16.68 − (120 × 0.60 × 0.83) = 100 mg/min.

Average normal values of Tm_{PAH} are 80–90 mg/min.

The value of the expression $U_{PAH}V$, used in calculations of ERPF and Tm_{PAH}, may be found by determining the amount of PAH in a measured volume of urine excreted within a specific period of time.

These calculations are based on a body surface area of 1.73 m^2. Corrections for variations in surface area are made by multiplying the values obtained for ERPF and Tm_{PAH} by 1.73/A, where A is the subject surface area.

HOW SUPPLIED

No. 95—Aminohippurate Sodium, 20 percent sterile solution for intravenous injection, is supplied as follows:
NDC 0006-3395-11 in 10 mL vials.
Storage
Avoid storage at temperatures below −20℃ (−4°F) and above 40℃ (104°F).

REFERENCES

1. Smith, H. W.: Lectures on the kidney, University Extension Division, University of Kansas, Lawrence, Kansas, 1943.
2. Wesson, L. G., Jr.: "Physiology of the Human Kidney," New York, Grune & Stratton, 1969, pp. 632–655.
3. Bauer, J. D.; Ackermann, P. G.; Toro, G.: "Brays Clinical Laboratory Methods," ed. 7, St. Louis, Mosby, 1968.
4. Pitts, R. F.: "Physiology of the Kidney and Body Fluids," ed. 2, Chicago, Year Book Medical Publishers, 1968.
5. Schnurr, E., Lahme, W., Kuppers, H.: Measurement of renal clearance of inulin and PAH in the steady state without urine collection; Clinical Nephrology, *13* (1): (26–29), 1980.

7470620 Issued March 1994

ANTIVENIN ℞
(Latrodectus mactans), U.S.P.
(Black Widow Spider Antivenin)
Equine Origin

DESCRIPTION

Antivenin (Latrodectus mactans) is a sterile, non-pyrogenic preparation derived by drying a frozen solution of specific venom-neutralizing globulins obtained from the blood serum of healthy horses immunized against venom of black widow spiders (Latrodectus mactans). It is standardized by biological assay on mice, in terms of one dose of antivenin neutralizing the venom in not less than 6000 mouse LD_{50} of Latrodectus mactans. Thimerosal (mercury derivative) 1:10,000 is added as a preservative. When constituted as specified, it is opalescent, ranging in color from light (straw) to very dark (iced tea), and contains not more than 20.0 percent of solids. Each vial contains not less than 6000 Antivenin units. One unit of Antivenin will neutralize one average mouse lethal dose of black widow spider venom when the Antivenin and the venom are injected simultaneously in mice under suitable conditions.

CLINICAL PHARMACOLOGY

The pharmacological mode of action is unknown and metabolic and pharmacokinetic data in humans are unavailable.

INDICATIONS AND USAGE

Antivenin (Latrodectus mactans) is used to treat patients with symptoms due to bites by the black widow spider (Latrodectus mactans). Early use of the Antivenin is emphasized for prompt relief.

Local muscular cramps begin from 15 minutes to several hours after the bite which usually produces a sharp pain similar to that caused by puncture with a needle. The exact sequence of symptoms depends somewhat on the location of the bite. The venom acts on the myoneural junctions or on the nerve endings, causing an ascending motor paralysis or destruction of the peripheral nerve endings. The groups of muscles most frequently affected at first are those of the thigh, shoulder, and back. After a varying length of time, the pain becomes more severe, spreading to the abdomen, and weakness and tremor usually develop. The abdominal muscles assume a boardlike rigidity, but tenderness is slight. Respiration is thoracic. The patient is restless and anxious. Feeble pulse, cold, clammy skin, labored breathing and speech, light stupor, and delirium may occur. Convulsions also may occur, particularly in small children. The temperature may be normal or slightly elevated. Urinary retention, shock, cyanosis, nausea and vomiting, insomnia, and cold sweats also have been reported. The syndrome following the bite of the black widow spider may be confused easily with any medical or surgical condition with acute abdominal symptoms.

The symptoms of black widow spider bite increase in severity for several hours, perhaps a day, and then very slowly become less severe, gradually passing off in the course of two or three days except in fatal cases. Residual symptoms such as general weakness, tingling, nervousness, and transient muscle spasm may persist for weeks or months after recovery from the acute stage.

If possible, the patient should be hospitalized. Other additional measures giving greatest relief are prolonged warm baths and intravenous injection of 10 mL of 10 percent solution of calcium gluconate repeated as necessary to control muscle pain. Morphine also may be required to control pain. Barbiturates may be used for extreme restlessness. However, as the venom is a neurotoxin, it can cause respiratory paralysis. This must be borne in mind when considering use of morphine or a barbiturate. Adrenocorticosteroids have been used with varying degrees of success. Supportive therapy is indicated by the condition of the patient. Local treatment of the site of the bite is of no value. Nothing is gained by applying a tourniquet or by attempting to remove venom from the site of the bite by incision and suction.

In otherwise healthy individuals between the ages of 16 and 60, the use of Antivenin may be deferred and treatment with muscle relaxants may be considered.

WARNINGS

Prior to treatment with any product prepared from horse serum, a careful review of the patient's history should be taken emphasizing prior exposure to horse serum or any allergies. Serious sickness and even death could result from the use of horse serum in a sensitive patient. A skin or conjunctival test should be performed prior to administration of Antivenin.

Skin test: Inject into (not under) the skin not more than 0.02 mL of the test material (1:10 dilution of normal horse serum in physiologic saline). Evaluate result in 10 minutes. A positive reaction is an urticarial wheal surrounded by a zone of erythema. A control test using Sodium Chloride Injection facilitates interpretation of the results.

Conjunctival test: For adults instill into the conjunctival sac one drop of a 1:10 dilution of horse serum and for children one drop of 1:100 dilution. Itching of the eye and reddening of the conjunctiva indicate a positive reaction, usually within 10 minutes.

Patients should be observed for serum sickness for an average of 8 to 12 days following administration of Antivenin. Desensitization should be attempted only when the administration of Antivenin is considered necessary to save life. Epinephrine must be available in case of untoward reaction.

Desensitization: If the history is positive or the results of the sensitivity tests are mildly or questionably positive, Antivenin should be administered as follows to reduce the risk of an immediate severe allergic reaction:

1. In separate sterile vials or syringes prepare 1:10 or 1:100 dilutions of Antivenin in Sodium Chloride for Injection.

2. Allow at least 15 but preferably 30 minutes between injections and only proceed with the next dose if no reactions occurred following the previous dose.

3. Using a tuberculin syringe, inject subcutaneously 0.1, 0.2 and 0.5 mL of the 1:100 dilution at 15 or 30 minute intervals; repeat with the 1:10 dilution, and finally the undiluted Antivenin.

4. If there is a reaction after any of the injections, place a tourniquet proximal to the sites of injection and administer epinephrine, 1:1000 (0.3 to 1.0 mL subcutaneously, 0.05 to 0.1 mL intravenously), proximal to the tourniquet or into another extremity. Wait at least 30 minutes before giving another injection of Antivenin, the amount of which should be the same as the last one not evoking a reaction.

5. If no reaction has occurred after 0.5 mL of undiluted Antivenin has been given, it is probably safe to continue the dose at 15 minute intervals until the entire dose has been injected.

PRECAUTIONS

Carcinogenesis, Mutagenesis, Impairment of Fertility
No long term studies in animals have been performed to evaluate the potential for carcinogenesis, mutagenesis, or impairment of fertility.

Pregnancy
Pregnancy Category C. Animal reproduction studies have not been conducted with Black Widow Spider Antivenin. It is also not known whether Black Widow Spider Antivenin can cause fetal harm when administered to a pregnant woman or can affect reproduction capacity. Black Widow Spider Antivenin should be given to a pregnant woman only if clearly needed.

Nursing Mothers
It is not known whether this drug is excreted in human milk. Because many drugs are excreted in human milk, caution should be exercised when Black Widow Spider Antivenin is administered to a nursing woman.

Pediatric Use
Controlled clinical studies for safety and effectiveness in children have not been conducted; however, there have been virtually no adverse effects reported in those children who have received the product.

ADVERSE REACTIONS

Anaphylaxis and serum sickness have been reported following use of Antivenin.

DOSAGE AND ADMINISTRATION

Using a sterile syringe, remove from the accompanying vial 2.5 mL of Sterile Diluent for Antivenin and inject into the vial of Antivenin. With the needle still in the rubber stopper, shake the vial to dissolve the contents completely.

Continued on next page

Merck & Co.—Cont.

Parenteral drug products should be inspected visually for particulate matter prior to administration, whenever solution and container permit (see DESCRIPTION).

The dose for adults and children is the entire contents of a restored vial (2.5 mL) of Antivenin. It may be given intramuscularly, preferably in the region of the anterolateral thigh so that a tourniquet may be applied in the event of a systemic reaction. Symptoms usually subside in 1 to 3 hours. Although one dose of Antivenin usually is adequate, a second dose may be necessary in some cases.

Antivenin also may be given intravenously in 10 to 50 mL of saline solution over a 15 minute period. It is the preferred route in severe cases, or when the patient is under 12, or in shock. One restored vial usually is enough.

HOW SUPPLIED

No. 4084—Antivenin (Latrodectus mactans) equine origin is a white to grey crystalline powder, each vial containing not less than 6000 Antivenin units. Thimerosal (mercury derivative) 1:10,000 is added as preservative, NDC 0006-4084-00. A 2.5 mL vial of Sterile Diluent for Antivenin is included. Also supplied is a 1 mL vial of normal horse serum (1:10 dilution) for sensitivity testing. Thimerosal (mercury derivative) 1:10,000 is added as preservative.

Storage

Antivenin must be stored and shipped at 2–8°C (36–46°F). When reconstituted as directed, the color of Antivenin ranges from light (straw) to very dark (iced tea), but the color has no effect on potency. *Do not freeze.*

A.H.F.S. Category: 80:04

7972114 Issued March 1995

AquaMEPHYTON® Injection
(Phytonadione), U.S.P.
Aqueous Colloidal Solution of Vitamin K₁

R

> **WARNING—INTRAVENOUS USE**
>
> Severe reactions, including fatalities, have occurred during and immediately after INTRAVENOUS injection of AquaMEPHYTON* (Phytonadione), even when precautions have been taken to dilute the AquaMEPHYTON and to avoid rapid infusion. Typically these severe reactions have resembled hypersensitivity or anaphylaxis, including shock and cardiac and/or respiratory arrest. Some patients have exhibited these severe reactions on receiving AquaMEPHYTON for the first time. Therefore the INTRAVENOUS route should be restricted to those situations where other routes are not feasible and the serious risk involved is considered justified.

*Registered trademark of MERCK & CO., INC.

DESCRIPTION

Phytonadione is a vitamin, which is a clear, yellow to amber, viscous, odorless or nearly odorless liquid. It is insoluble in water, soluble in chloroform and slightly soluble in ethanol. It has a molecular weight of 450.70.

Phytonadione is 2-methyl-3-phytyl-1,4-naphthoquinone. Its empirical formula is $C_{31}H_{46}O_2$ and its structural formula is:

AquaMEPHYTON injection is a yellow, sterile, aqueous colloidal solution of vitamin K₁, with a pH of 5.0 to 7.0, available for injection by the intravenous, intramuscular, and subcutaneous routes. Each milliliter contains:

Phytonadione .... 2 mg or 10 mg
Inactive ingredients:
  Polyoxyethylated fatty acid
    derivative .... 70 mg
  Dextrose .... 37.5 mg
  Water for Injection, q.s. .... 1 mL
Added as preservative:
  Benzyl alcohol 0.9%

CLINICAL PHARMACOLOGY

AquaMEPHYTON aqueous colloidal solution of vitamin K₁ for parenteral injection, possesses the same type and degree of activity as does naturally-occurring vitamin K, which is necessary for the production via the liver of active prothrom-

bin (factor II), proconvertin (factor VII), plasma thromboplastin component (factor IX), and Stuart factor (factor X). The prothrombin test is sensitive to the levels of three of these four factors—II, VII, and X. Vitamin K is an essential cofactor for a microsomal enzyme that catalyzes the post-translational carboxylation of multiple, specific, peptide-bound glutamic acid residues in inactive hepatic precursors of factors II, VII, IX, and X. The resulting gamma-carboxyglutamic acid residues convert the precursors into active coagulation factors that are subsequently secreted by liver cells into the blood.

Phytonadione is readily absorbed following intramuscular administration. After absorption, phytonadione is initially concentrated in the liver, but the concentration declines rapidly. Very little vitamin K accumulates in tissues. Little is known about the metabolic fate of vitamin K. Almost no free unmetabolized vitamin K appears in bile or urine.

In normal animals and humans, phytonadione is virtually devoid of pharmacodynamic activity. However, in animals and humans deficient in vitamin K, the pharmacological action of vitamin K is related to its normal physiological function, that is, to promote the hepatic biosynthesis of vitamin K dependent clotting factors.

The action of the aqueous colloidal solution, when administered intravenously, is generally detectable within an hour or two and hemorrhage is usually controlled within 3 to 6 hours. A normal prothrombin level may often be obtained in 12 to 14 hours.

In the prophylaxis and treatment of hemorrhagic disease of the newborn, phytonadione has demonstrated a greater margin of safety than that of the water-soluble vitamin K analogues.

INDICATIONS AND USAGE

AquaMEPHYTON is indicated in the following coagulation disorders which are due to faulty formation of factors II, VII, IX and X when caused by vitamin K deficiency or interference with vitamin K activity.

AquaMEPHYTON injection is indicated in:
  — anticoagulant-induced prothrombin deficiency caused by coumarin or indanedione derivatives;
  — prophylaxis and therapy of hemorrhagic disease of the newborn;
  — hypoprothrombinemia due to antibacterial therapy;
  — hypoprothrombinemia secondary to factors limiting absorption or synthesis of vitamin K, e.g., obstructive jaundice, biliary fistula, sprue, ulcerative colitis, celiac disease, intestinal resection, cystic fibrosis of the pancreas, and regional enteritis;
  — other drug-induced hypoprothrombinemia where it is definitely shown that the result is due to interference with vitamin K metabolism, e.g., salicylates.

CONTRAINDICATION

Hypersensitivity to any component of this medication.

WARNINGS

Benzyl alcohol as a preservative in Bacteriostatic Sodium Chloride Injection has been associated with toxicity in newborns. Data are unavailable on the toxicity of other preservatives in this age group. There is no evidence to suggest that the small amount of benzyl alcohol contained in AquaMEPHYTON, when used as recommended, is associated with toxicity.

An immediate coagulant effect should not be expected after administration of phytonadione. It takes a minimum of 1 to 2 hours for measurable improvement in the prothrombin time.

AquaMEPHYTON
Summary of Dosage Guidelines
(See circular text for details)

Newborns	Dosage
Hemorrhagic Disease of the Newborn	
Prophylaxis	0.5–1 mg IM within 1 hour of birth
Treatment	1 mg SC or IM (Higher doses may be necessary if the mother has been receiving oral anticoagulants)
Adults	**Initial Dosage**
Anticoagulant-Induced Prothrombin Deficiency (caused by coumarin or indanedione derivatives)	2.5 mg–10 mg or up to 25 mg (rarely 50 mg)
Hypoprothrombinemia due to other causes (Antibiotics; Salicylates or other drugs; Factors limiting absorption or synthesis)	2.5 mg–25 mg or more (rarely up to 50 mg)

Whole blood or component therapy may also be necessary if bleeding is severe.

Phytonadione will not counteract the anticoagulant action of heparin.

When vitamin K₁ is used to correct excessive anticoagulant-induced hypoprothrombinemia, anticoagulant therapy still being indicated, the patient is again faced with the clotting hazards existing prior to starting the anticoagulant therapy. Phytonadione is not a clotting agent, but overzealous therapy with vitamin K₁ may restore conditions which originally permitted thromboembolic phenomena. Dosage should be kept as low as possible, and prothrombin time should be checked regularly as clinical conditions indicate.

Repeated large doses of vitamin K are not warranted in liver disease if the response to initial use of the vitamin is unsatisfactory. Failure to respond to vitamin K may indicate that the condition being treated is inherently unresponsive to vitamin K.

PRECAUTIONS

Drug Interactions

Temporary resistance to prothrombin-depressing anticoagulants may result, especially when larger doses of phytonadione are used. If relatively large doses have been employed, it may be necessary when reinstituting anticoagulant therapy to use somewhat larger doses of the prothrombin-depressing anticoagulant, or to use one which acts on a different principle, such as heparin sodium.

Laboratory Tests

Prothrombin time should be checked regularly as clinical conditions indicate.

Carcinogenesis, Mutagenesis, Impairment of Fertility

Studies of carcinogenicity, mutagenesis or impairment of fertility have not been conducted with AquaMEPHYTON.

Pregnancy

Pregnancy Category C: Animal reproduction studies have not been conducted with AquaMEPHYTON. It is also not known whether AquaMEPHYTON can cause fetal harm when administered to a pregnant woman or can affect reproduction capacity. AquaMEPHYTON should be given to a pregnant woman only if clearly needed.

Nursing Mothers

It is not known whether this drug is excreted in human milk. Because many drugs are excreted in human milk, caution should be exercised when AquaMEPHYTON is administered to a nursing woman.

Pediatric Use

Hemolysis, jaundice, and hyperbilirubinemia in newborns, particularly in premature infants, may be related to the dose of AquaMEPHYTON. Therefore, the recommended dose should not be exceeded (see ADVERSE REACTIONS and DOSAGE AND ADMINISTRATION).

ADVERSE REACTIONS

Deaths have occurred after intravenous administration. (See Box Warning at beginning of circular.)

Transient "flushing sensations" and "peculiar" sensations of taste have been observed, as well as rare instances of dizziness, rapid and weak pulse, profuse sweating, brief hypotension, dyspnea, and cyanosis.

Pain, swelling, and tenderness at the injection site may occur.

The possibility of allergic sensitivity, including an anaphylactoid reaction, should be kept in mind.

Infrequently, usually after repeated injection, erythematous, indurated, pruritic plaques have occurred; rarely, these

have progressed to sclerodermalike lesions that have persisted for long periods. In other cases, these lesions have resembled erythema perstans.

Hyperbilirubinemia has been observed in the newborn following administration of phytonadione. This has occurred rarely and primarily with doses above those recommended. (See PRECAUTIONS, *Pediatric Use.*)

OVERDOSAGE

The intravenous LD_{50} of AquaMEPHYTON in the mouse is 41.5 and 52 mL/kg for the 0.2% and 1% concentrations respectively.

DOSAGE AND ADMINISTRATION

Whenever possible, AquaMEPHYTON should be given by the subcutaneous or intramuscular route. When intravenous administration is considered unavoidable, the drug should be injected very slowly, not exceeding 1 mg per minute. Protect from light at all times.

Parenteral drug products should be inspected visually for particulate matter and discoloration prior to administration, whenever solution and container permit.

Directions for Dilution
AquaMEPHYTON may be diluted with 0.9% Sodium Chloride Injection, 5% Dextrose Injection, or 5% Dextrose and Sodium Chloride Injection. Benzyl alcohol as a preservative has been associated with toxicity in newborns. *Therefore, all of the above diluents should be preservative-free* (see WARNINGS). *Other diluents should not be used.* When dilutions are indicated, administration should be started immediately after mixture with the diluent, and unused portions of the dilution should be discarded, as well as unused contents of the ampul.

Prophylaxis of Hemorrhagic Disease of the Newborn
The American Academy of Pediatrics recommends that vitamin K_1 be given to the newborn. A single intramuscular dose of AquaMEPHYTON 0.5 to 1 mg within one hour of birth is recommended.

Treatment of Hemorrhagic Disease of the Newborn
Empiric administration of vitamin K_1 should not replace proper laboratory evaluation of the coagulation mechanism. A prompt response (shortening of the prothrombin time in 2 to 4 hours) following administration of vitamin K_1 is usually diagnostic of hemorrhagic disease of the newborn, and failure to respond indicates another diagnosis or coagulation disorder.

AquaMEPHYTON 1 mg should be given either subcutaneously or intramuscularly. Higher doses may be necessary if the mother has been receiving oral anticoagulants. [See table on top of preceding page.]

Whole blood or component therapy may be indicated if bleeding is excessive. This therapy, however, does not correct the underlying disorder and AquaMEPHYTON should be given concurrently.

Anticoagulant-Induced Prothrombin Deficiency in Adults
To correct excessively prolonged prothrombin time caused by oral anticoagulant therapy—2.5 to 10 mg or up to 25 mg initially is recommended. In rare instances 50 mg may be required. Frequency and amount of subsequent doses should be determined by prothrombin time response or clinical condition (see WARNINGS). If in 6 to 8 hours after parenteral administration the prothrombin time has not been shortened satisfactorily, the dose should be repeated.

In the event of shock or excessive blood loss, the use of whole blood or component therapy is indicated.

Hypoprothrombinemia Due to Other Causes in Adults
A dosage of 2.5 to 25 mg or more (rarely up to 50 mg) is recommended, the amount and route of administration depending upon the severity of the condition and response obtained.

If possible, discontinuation or reduction of the dosage of drugs interfering with coagulation mechanisms (such as salicylates, antibiotics) is suggested as an alternative to administering concurrent AquaMEPHYTON. The severity of the coagulation disorder should determine whether the immediate administration of AquaMEPHYTON is required in addition to discontinuation or reduction of interfering drugs.

HOW SUPPLIED

Injection AquaMEPHYTON is a yellow, sterile, aqueous colloidal solution and is supplied in the following concentrations:
No. 7780—10 mg of vitamin K_1 per mL
NDC 0006-7780-64 boxes of 6 × 1 mL ampuls
(6505-00-854-2499 10 mg 1 mL 6's)
NDC 0006-7780-66 boxes of 25 × 1 mL ampuls.
No. 7782—10 mg of vitamin K_1 per mL
NDC 0006-7782-30 in 2.5 mL multiple dose vials
NDC 0006-7782-03 in 5 mL multiple dose vials.
No. 7784—1 mg of vitamin K_1 per 0.5 mL
NDC 0006-7784-33 boxes of 25 × 0.5 mL ampuls
(6505-00-180-6372 1 mg 0.5 mL 25's).
7349820   Issued April 1995

ARAMINE® Injection
(Metaraminol Bitartrate), U.S.P.   ℞

DESCRIPTION

Metaraminol bitartrate is a potent sympathomimetic amine that increases both systolic and diastolic blood pressure. Metaraminol bitartrate is $[R\text{-}(R^*,S^*)]\text{-}\alpha\text{-}(1\text{-aminoethyl})\text{-}3\text{-hy}$droxybenzenemethanol $[R\text{-}(R^*,R^*)]\text{-}2,3\text{-dihydroxy}$butanedioate (1:1) (salt), which is levorotatory. Its empirical formula is $C_9H_{13}NO_2 \cdot C_4H_6O_6$ and its structural formula is:

Metaraminol bitartrate is a white, crystalline powder with a molecular weight of 317.29, is freely soluble in water, slightly soluble in alcohol, and practically insoluble in chloroform and in ether.

Injection ARAMINE* (Metaraminol Bitartrate) is a sterile solution. Each mL contains:

Metaraminol bitartrate equivalent to metaraminol	10 mg
Inactive ingredients:	
Sodium chloride	4.4 mg
Water for Injection q.s. ad	1 mL

Methylparaben 0.15%, propylparaben 0.02%, and sodium bisulfite 0.2% added as preservatives.

*Registered trademark of MERCK & CO., INC.

CLINICAL PHARMACOLOGY

The pressor effect of ARAMINE begins in 1 to 2 minutes after intravenous infusion, in about 10 minutes after intramuscular injection, and in 5 to 20 minutes after subcutaneous injection. The effect lasts from about 20 minutes to one hour. ARAMINE has a positive inotropic effect on the heart and a peripheral vasoconstrictor action.

Renal, coronary, and cerebral blood flow are a function of perfusion pressure and regional resistance. In patients with insufficient or failing vasoconstriction, there is additional advantage to the peripheral action of ARAMINE, but in most patients with shock, vasoconstriction is adequate and any further increase is unnecessary. Blood flow to vital organs may decrease with ARAMINE if regional resistance increases excessively.

The pressor effect of ARAMINE is decreased but not reversed by alpha-adrenergic blocking agents. Primary or secondary fall in blood pressure and tachyphylactic response to repeated use are uncommon.

INDICATIONS AND USAGE

ARAMINE is indicated for prevention and treatment of the acute hypotensive state occurring with spinal anesthesia. It is also indicated as adjunctive treatment of hypotension due to hemorrhage, reactions to medications, surgical complications, and shock associated with brain damage due to trauma or tumor.

CONTRAINDICATIONS

Use of ARAMINE with cyclopropane or halothane anesthesia should be avoided, unless clinical circumstances demand such use.

Hypersensitivity to any component of this product, including sulfites (see WARNINGS).

WARNINGS

Use of sympathomimetic amines with monoamine oxidase inhibitors or tricyclic antidepressants may result in potentiation of the pressor effect. (See PRECAUTIONS, *Drug Interactions.*)

ARAMINE contains sodium bisulfite, a sulfite that may cause allergic-type reactions including anaphylactic symptoms and life-threatening or less severe asthmatic episodes in certain susceptible people. The overall prevalence of sulfite sensitivity in the general population is unknown and probably low. Sulfite sensitivity is seen more frequently in asthmatic than in nonasthmatic people.

PRECAUTIONS

General
Caution should be used to avoid excessive blood pressure response. Rapidly induced hypertensive responses have been reported to cause acute pulmonary edema, arrhythmias, cerebral hemorrhage, or cardiac arrest.

Patients with cirrhosis should be treated with caution, with adequate restoration of electrolytes if diuresis ensues. Fatal ventricular arrhythmia was reported in one patient with Laennec's cirrhosis while receiving metaraminol bitartrate. In several instances, ventricular extrasystoles that appeared during infusion of this vasopressor subsided promptly when the rate of infusion was reduced.

With the prolonged action of ARAMINE, a cumulative effect is possible. If there is an excessive vasopressor response there may be a prolonged elevation of blood pressure even after discontinuation of therapy.

When vasopressor amines are used for long periods, the resulting vasoconstriction may prevent adequate expansion of circulating volume and may cause perpetuation of shock. There is evidence that plasma volume may be reduced in all types of shock, and that the measurement of central venous pressure is useful in assessing the adequacy of the circulating blood volume. Therefore, blood or plasma volume expanders should be used when the principal reason for hypotension or shock is decreased circulating volume.

Because of its vasoconstrictor effect ARAMINE should be given with caution in heart or thyroid disease, hypertension, or diabetes. Sympathomimetic amines may provoke a relapse in patients with a history of malaria.

Drug Interactions
ARAMINE should be used with caution in digitalized patients, since the combination of digitalis and sympathomimetic amines may cause ectopic arrhythmias.

Monoamine oxidase inhibitors or tricyclic antidepressants may potentiate the action of sympathomimetic amines. Therefore, when initiating pressor therapy in patients receiving these drugs, the initial dose should be small and given with caution. (See WARNINGS.)

Carcinogenesis, Mutagenesis, Impairment of Fertility
Studies in animals have not been performed to evaluate the mutagenic or carcinogenic potential of ARAMINE or its potential to affect fertility.

Pregnancy
Pregnancy Category C. Animal reproduction studies have not been conducted with ARAMINE. It is not known whether ARAMINE can cause fetal harm when given to a pregnant woman or can affect reproduction capacity. ARAMINE should be given to a pregnant woman only if clearly needed.

Nursing Mothers
It is not known whether this drug is secreted in human milk. Because many drugs are secreted in human milk, caution should be exercised when ARAMINE is given to a nursing woman.

Pediatric Use
Safety and effectiveness in children have not been established.

ADVERSE REACTIONS

Sympathomimetic amines, including ARAMINE, may cause sinus or ventricular tachycardia, or other arrhythmias, especially in patients with myocardial infarction. (See PRECAUTIONS.)

In patients with a history of malaria, these compounds may provoke a relapse.

Abscess formation, tissue necrosis, or sloughing rarely may follow the use of ARAMINE. In choosing the site of injection, it is important to avoid those areas recognized as *not* suitable for use of any pressor agent and to discontinue the infusion immediately if infiltration or thrombosis occurs. Although the physician may be forced by the urgent nature of the patient's condition to choose injection sites that are not recognized as suitable, he should, when possible, use the preferred areas of injection. The larger veins of the antecubital fossa or the thigh are preferred to veins in the dorsum of the hand or ankle veins, particularly in patients with peripheral vascular disease, diabetes mellitus, Buerger's disease, or conditions with coexistent hypercoagulability.

OVERDOSAGE

Overdosage may result in severe hypertension accompanied by headache, constricting sensation in the chest, nausea, vomiting, euphoria, diaphoresis, pulmonary edema, tachycardia, bradycardia, sinus arrhythmia, atrial or ventricular arrhythmias, cerebral hemorrhage, myocardial infarction, cardiac arrest or convulsions.

Continued on next page

Merck & Co.—Cont.

Should an excessive elevation of blood pressure occur, it may be immediately relieved by a sympatholytic agent, e.g. phentolamine. An appropriate antiarrhythmic agent may also be required.

The oral LD_{50} in the rat and mouse is 240 mg/kg and 99 mg/kg, respectively.

DOSAGE AND ADMINISTRATION

ARAMINE may be given intramuscularly, subcutaneously, or intravenously, the route depending on the nature and severity of the indication.

Parenteral drug products should be inspected visually for particulate matter and discoloration prior to use, whenever solution and container permit.

Allow at least 10 minutes to elapse before increasing the dose because the maximum effect is not immediately apparent. When the vasopressor is discontinued, observe the patient carefully as the effect of the drug tapers off, so that therapy can be reinitiated promptly if the blood pressure falls too rapidly. The response to vasopressors may be poor in patients with coexistent shock and acidosis. When indicated, established methods of shock management should be used, such as blood or fluid replacement.

Intramuscular or Subcutaneous Injection (for prevention of hypotension—see INDICATIONS): The recommended dose is 2 to 10 mg (0.2 to 1 mL). As with other agents given subcutaneously, only the preferred sites of injection, as set forth in standard texts, should be used.

Intravenous Infusion (for adjunctive treatment of hypotension—see INDICATIONS): The recommended dose is 15 to 100 mg (1.5 to 10 mL) in 500 mL of Sodium Chloride Injection or 5% Dextrose Injection, adjusting the rate of infusion to maintain the blood pressure at the desired level. Higher concentrations of ARAMINE, 150 to 500 mg per 500 mL of infusion fluid, have been used.

If the patient needs more saline or dextrose solution at a rate of flow that would provide an excessive dose of the vasopressor, the recommended volume of infusion fluid (500 mL) should be increased accordingly. ARAMINE may also be added to *less* than 500 mL of infusion fluid if a smaller volume is desired.

Compatibility Information

In addition to Sodium Chloride Injection and Dextrose Injection 5%, the following infusion solutions were found physically and chemically compatible with Injection ARAMINE when 5 mL of Injection ARAMINE, 10 mg/mL (metaraminol equivalent), was added to 500 mL of infusion solution: Ringer's Injection, Lactated Ringer's Injection, Dextran 6% in Saline†, Normosol®-R pH 7.4†, and Normosol®-M in D5-W†.

When Injection ARAMINE is mixed with an infusion solution, sterile precautions should be observed. Since infusion solutions generally do not contain preservatives, mixtures should be used within 24 hours.

Direct Intravenous Injection: In severe shock, when time is of great importance, this agent should be given by direct intravenous injection. The suggested dose is 0.5 to 5 mg (0.05 to 0.5 mL), followed by an infusion of 15 to 100 mg (1.5 to 10 mL) in 500 mL of infusion fluid as described previously. Vials may be sterilized by autoclaving or by immersion in a sterilizing solution.

†Product of Abbott Laboratories

HOW SUPPLIED

No. 3222X—Injection ARAMINE 1%, containing metaraminol bitartrate equivalent to 10 mg of metaraminol per mL, is a clear, colorless solution and is supplied as follows:
NDC 0006-3222-10 in 10 mL vials
(6505-00-753-9601 10 mL vial).

Storage
Protect from light. Store container in carton until contents have been used.
Avoid storage at temperatures below -20°C (-4°F) and above 40°C (104°F).

7348523   Issued January 1994
COPYRIGHT © MERCK & CO., INC., 1987
All rights reserved

ATTENUVAX®   ℞
(Measles Virus Vaccine Live), U.S.P.
(More Attenuated Enders' Strain)

DESCRIPTION

ATTENUVAX* (Measles Virus Vaccine Live) is a live virus vaccine for immunization against measles (rubeola).

ATTENUVAX is a sterile lyophilized preparation of a more attenuated line of measles virus derived from Enders' attenuated Edmonston strain. The further modification of the virus in ATTENUVAX was achieved in the Merck Institute for Therapeutic Research by multiple passage of Edmonston strain virus in cell cultures of chick embryo at low temperature.

The reconstituted vaccine is for subcutaneous administration. When reconstituted as directed, the dose for injection is 0.5 mL and contains not less than the equivalent of 1,000 $TCID_{50}$ (tissue culture infectious doses) of the U.S. Reference Measles Virus. Each dose also contains approximately 25 mcg of neomycin. The product contains no preservative. Sorbitol and hydrolized gelatin are added as stabilizers.

---

* Registered trademark of MERCK & CO., INC.

CLINICAL PHARMACOLOGY

ATTENUVAX produces a modified measles infection in susceptible persons. Fever and rash may appear. Extensive clinical trials have demonstrated that ATTENUVAX is highly immunogenic and generally well tolerated. A single injection of the vaccine has been shown to induce measles hemagglutination-inhibiting (HI) antibodies in 97 percent or more of susceptible persons. Vaccine-induced antibody levels have been shown to persist for at least 13 years without substantial decline. Continued surveillance will be necessary to determine further duration of antibody persistence.

INDICATIONS AND USAGE

ATTENUVAX is indicated for immunization against measles (rubeola) in persons 15 months of age or older. A second dose of ATTENUVAX is recommended (see *Revaccination*). Infants who are less than 15 months of age may fail to respond to the vaccine due to presence in the circulation of residual measles antibody of maternal origin; the younger the infant, the lower the likelihood of seroconversion. In geographically isolated or other relatively inaccessible populations for whom immunization programs are logistically difficult, and in population groups in which natural measles infection may occur in a significant proportion of infants before 15 months of age, it may be desirable to give the vaccine to infants at an earlier age. Infants vaccinated under these conditions at less than 12 months of age should be revaccinated after reaching 15 months of age. There is some evidence to suggest that infants immunized at less than one year of age may not develop sustained antibody levels when later reimmunized. The advantage of early protection must be weighed against the chance for failure to respond adequately on reimmunization.

According to ACIP recommendations, most persons born in 1956 or earlier are likely to have been infected naturally and generally need not be considered susceptible. All children, adolescents, and adults born after 1956 are considered susceptible and should be vaccinated, if there are no contraindications. This includes persons who may be immune to measles but who lack adequate documentation of immunity as evidenced by: (1) physician-diagnosed measles, (2) laboratory evidence of measles immunity, or (3) adequate immunization with live measles vaccine on or after the first birthday. ATTENUVAX given immediately after exposure to natural measles may provide some protection. If, however, the vaccine is given a few days before exposure, substantial protection may be provided.

Individuals planning travel outside the United States, if not immune, can acquire measles, mumps or rubella and import these diseases to the United States. Therefore, prior to International travel, individuals known to be susceptible to one or more of these diseases can receive either a single antigen vaccine (measles, mumps or rubella), or a combined antigen vaccine as appropriate. However, M-M-R* II (Measles, Mumps, and Rubella Virus Vaccine Live) is preferred for persons likely to be susceptible to mumps and rubella; and if single-antigen measles vaccine is not readily available, travelers should receive M-M-R II (Measles, Mumps, and Rubella Virus Vaccine Live) regardless of their immune status to mumps or rubella.

Revaccination: Children first vaccinated when younger than 12 months of age should be revaccinated at 15 months of age, particularly if vaccine was administered with immune serum globulin or measles immune globulin, a standardized globulin preparation.

The American Academy of Pediatrics (AAP), the Immunization Practices Advisory Committee (ACIP), and some state and local health agencies have recommended guidelines for routine measles revaccination and to help control measles outbreaks.**

Vaccines available for revaccination include monovalent measles vaccine (ATTENUVAX) and polyvalent vaccines containing measles [e.g., M-M-R II (Measles, Mumps, and Rubella Virus Vaccine Live), M-R-VAX* II (Measles and Rubella Virus Vaccine Live)]. If the prevention of sporadic measles outbreaks is the sole objective, revaccination with a

monovalent measles vaccine should be considered (see appropriate product circular). If concern also exists about immune status regarding mumps or rubella, revaccination with appropriate monovalent or polyvalent vaccines should be considered after consulting the appropriate product circulars. Unnecessary doses of a vaccine are best avoided by ensuring that written documentation of vaccination is preserved and a copy given to each vaccinee's parent or guardian.

Despite the risk of reactions (see ADVERSE REACTIONS), persons born since 1956 who have previously been given inactivated vaccine alone or followed by live vaccine within 3 months should be revaccinated with live vaccine to reduce the risk of the severe atypical form of natural measles that may occur.

Use with other Vaccines

Routine administration of DTP (diphtheria, tetanus, pertussis) and/or OPV (oral poliovirus vaccine) concomitantly with measles, mumps and rubella vaccines is not recommended because there are insufficient data relating to the simultaneous administration of these antigens. However, the American Academy of Pediatrics has noted that in some circumstances, particularly when the patient may not return, some practitioners prefer to administer all these antigens on a single day. If done, separate sites and syringes should be used for DTP and ATTENUVAX.

ATTENUVAX should not be given less than one month before or after administration of other virus vaccines.

---

* Registered trademark of MERCK & CO., INC.
** NOTE: A primary difference among these recommendations is the timing of revaccination: the ACIP recommends routine revaccination at entry into kindergarten or first grade, whereas the AAP recommends routine revaccination at entrance to middle school or junior high school. In addition, some public health jurisdictions mandate the age for revaccination. The complete text of applicable guidelines should be consulted.

CONTRAINDICATIONS

Do not give ATTENUVAX to pregnant females; the possible effects of the vaccine on fetal development are unknown at this time. If vaccination of postpubertal females is undertaken, pregnancy should be avoided for three months following vaccination (see PRECAUTIONS, *Pregnancy*).

Anaphylactic or anaphylactoid reactions to neomycin (each dose of reconstituted vaccine contains approximately 25 mcg of neomycin).

History of anaphylactic or anaphylactoid reactions to eggs (see HYPERSENSITIVITY TO EGGS below).

Any febrile respiratory illness or other active febrile infection.

Active untreated tuberculosis.

Patients receiving immunosuppressive therapy. This contraindication does not apply to patients who are receiving corticosteroids as replacement therapy, e.g., for Addison's disease.

Individuals with blood dyscrasias, leukemia, lymphomas of any type, or other malignant neoplasms affecting the bone marrow or lymphatic systems.

Primary and acquired immunodeficiency states, including patients who are immunosuppressed in association with AIDS or other clinical manifestations of infection with human immunodeficiency viruses; cellular immune deficiencies; and hypogammaglobulinemic and dysgammaglobulinemic states.

Individuals with a family history of congenital or hereditary immunodeficiency, until the immune competence of the potential vaccine recipient is demonstrated.

HYPERSENSITIVITY TO EGGS

Live measles vaccine is produced in chick embryo cell culture. Persons with a history of anaphylactic, anaphylactoid or other immediate reactions (e.g., hives, swelling of the mouth and throat, difficulty breathing, hypotension and shock) subsequent to egg ingestion should not be vaccinated. Evidence indicates that persons are not at increased risk if they have egg allergies that are not anaphylactic or anaphylactoid in nature. Such persons should be vaccinated in the usual manner. There is no evidence to indicate that persons with allergies to chickens or feathers are at increased risk of reaction to the vaccine.

PRECAUTIONS

General
Adequate treatment provisions including epinephrine, should be available for immediate use should an anaphylactic or anaphylactoid reaction occur.

Due caution should be employed in administration of measles vaccine to persons with a history of cerebral injury, individual or family histories of convulsions, or of any other condition in which stress due to fever should be avoided. The physician should be alert to the temperature elevation

which may occur following vaccination. (See ADVERSE REACTIONS.)
Children and young adults who are known to be infected with human immunodeficiency viruses but without overt clinical manifestations of immunosuppression may be vaccinated; however, the vaccinees should be monitored closely for vaccine-preventable diseases because immunization may be less effective than for uninfected persons.
Vaccination should be deferred for at least 3 months following blood or plasma transfusions, or administration of human immune serum globulin.
There are no reports of transmission of live attenuated measles virus from vaccinees to susceptible contacts.
It has been reported that attenuated measles virus vaccine, live, may result in a temporary depression of tuberculin skin sensitivity. Therefore, if a tuberculin test is to be done, it should be administered either before or simultaneously with ATTENUVAX.
Children under treatment for tuberculosis have not experienced exacerbation of the disease when immunized with live measles virus vaccine; no studies have been reported to date of the effect of measles virus vaccines on untreated tuberculous children.
As for any vaccine, vaccination with ATTENUVAX may not result in seroconversion in 100% of susceptible persons given the vaccine.

Pregnancy

Pregnancy Category C

Animal reproduction studies have not been conducted with ATTENUVAX. It is also not known whether ATTENUVAX can cause fetal harm when administered to a pregnant woman or can affect reproduction capacity. Therefore, the vaccine should not be administered to pregnant females; furthermore, pregnancy should be avoided for three months following vaccination (see CONTRAINDICATIONS).
Reports have indicated that contracting of natural measles during pregnancy enhances fetal risk. Increased rates of spontaneous abortion, stillbirth, congenital defects and prematurity have been observed subsequent to natural measles during pregnancy. There are no adequate studies of the attenuated (vaccine) strain of measles virus in pregnancy. However, it would be prudent to assume that the vaccine strain of virus is also capable of inducing adverse fetal effects for up to three months following vaccination.
Vaccine administration to postpubertal females entails a potential for inadvertent immunization during pregnancy. Theoretical risks involved should be weighed against the risks that measles poses to the unimmunized adolescent or adult. Advisory committees reviewing this matter have recommended vaccination of postpubertal females who are presumed to be susceptible to measles and not known to be pregnant. If a measles exposure occurs during pregnancy, one should consider the possibility of providing temporary passive immunity through the administration of immune globulin (human).

Nursing Mothers

It is not known whether measles vaccine virus is secreted in human milk. Therefore, because many drugs are excreted in human milk, caution should be exercised when ATTENUVAX is administered to a nursing woman.

ADVERSE REACTIONS

Burning and/or stinging of short duration at the injection site have been reported.
Anaphylaxis and anaphylactoid reactions have been reported.

Occasional

Moderate fever [101–102.9°F (38.3–39.4°C)] may occur during the month after vaccination. Generally, fever, rash, or both appear between the 5th and the 12th days. Cough and rhinitis have also been reported. Rash, when it occurs, is usually minimal, but rarely may be generalized. Erythema multiforme has also been reported rarely.

Less Common

High fever [over 103°F (39.4°C)].
Mild lymphadenopathy has been reported.

Rare

Reactions at injection site. Allergic reactions such as wheal and flare at the injection site or urticaria have been reported.
Diarrhea has been reported after vaccination with measles-containing vaccines.
Children developing fever may, on rare occasions, exhibit febrile convulsions. Afebrile convulsions or seizures have occurred rarely following vaccination with live attenuated measles vaccine. Syncope, particularly at the time of mass vaccination, has been reported.
Thrombocytopenia and purpura have occurred rarely.
Vasculitis has been reported rarely.
Forms of optic neuritis, including retrobulbar neuritis, papillitis, and retinitis may infrequently follow viral infections, and have been reported to occur 1 to 3 weeks following inoculation with some live virus vaccines.
Experience from more than 80 million doses of all live measles vaccines given in the U.S. through 1975 indicates that significant central nervous system reactions such as encephalitis and encephalopathy, occurring within 30 days after vaccination, have been temporally associated with measles vaccine very rarely. In no case has it been shown that reactions were actually caused by vaccine. The Center for Disease Control has pointed out that "a certain number of cases of encephalitis may be expected to occur in a large childhood population in a defined period of time even when no vaccines are administered". However, the data suggest the possibility that some of these cases may have been caused by measles vaccines. The risk of such serious neurological disorders following live measles virus vaccine administration remains far less than that for encephalitis and encephalopathy with natural measles (one per two thousand reported cases).
There have been rare reports of ocular palsies, Guillain-Barré syndrome, or ataxia occurring after immunization with vaccines containing live attenuated measles virus. The ocular palsies have occurred approximately 3–24 days following vaccination. No definite causal relationship has been established between either of these events and vaccination.
There have been reports of subacute sclerosing panencephalitis (SSPE) in children who did not have a history of natural measles but did receive measles vaccine. Some of these cases may have resulted from unrecognized measles in the first year of life or possibly from the measles vaccination. Based on estimated nationwide measles vaccine distribution, the association of SSPE cases to measles vaccination is about one case per million vaccine doses distributed. This is far less than the association with natural measles, 6–22 cases of SSPE per million cases of measles. The results of a retrospective case-controlled study conducted by the Center for Disease Control suggest that the overall effect of measles vaccine has been to protect against SSPE by preventing measles with its inherent higher risk of SSPE.
Local reactions characterized by marked swelling, redness and vesiculation at the injection site of attenuated live virus measles vaccines, and systemic reactions including atypical measles, have occurred in persons who have previously received killed measles vaccine. Rarely, more severe reactions that require hospitalization, including prolonged high fevers, panniculitis, and extensive local reactions, have been reported.

DOSAGE AND ADMINISTRATION

FOR SUBCUTANEOUS ADMINISTRATION

Do not inject intravenously

The dosage of vaccine is the same for all persons. Inject the total volume of the single dose vial (about 0.5 mL) or 0.5 mL of the multiple dose vial of reconstituted vaccine subcutaneously, preferably into the outer aspect of upper arm. *Do not give immune globulin (IG) concurrently with* ATTENUVAX.
During shipment, to insure that there is no loss of potency, the vaccine must be maintained at a temperature of 10°C (50°F) or less.
Before reconstitution, store ATTENUVAX at 2–8°C (36–46°F). *Protect from light.*
CAUTION: A sterile syringe free of preservatives, antiseptics, and detergents should be used for each injection and/or reconstitution of the vaccine because these substances may inactivate the live virus vaccine. A 25 gauge, ⅝" needle is recommended.
To reconstitute, use only the diluent supplied, since it is free of preservatives or other antiviral substances which might inactivate the vaccine.

Single Dose Vial—First withdraw the entire volume of diluent into the syringe to be used for reconstitution. Inject all the diluent in the syringe into the vial of lyophilized vaccine, and agitate to mix thoroughly. Withdraw the entire contents into a syringe and inject the total volume of restored vaccine subcutaneously.
It is important to use a separate sterile syringe and needle for each individual patient to prevent transmission of hepatitis B and other infectious agents from one person to another.

10 Dose Vial (available only to government agencies/institutions)—Withdraw the entire contents (7 mL) of the diluent vial into the sterile syringe to be used for reconstitution, and introduce into the 10 dose vial of lyophilized vaccine. Agitate to ensure thorough mixing. The outer labeling suggests "For Jet Injector or Syringe Use". Use with separate sterile syringes is permitted for containers of 10 doses or less. The vaccine and diluent do not contain preservatives; therefore, the user must recognize the potential contamination hazards and exercise special precautions to protect the sterility and potency of the product. The use of aseptic techniques and proper storage prior to and after restoration of the vaccine and subsequent withdrawal of the individual doses is essential. Use 0.5 mL of the reconstituted vaccine for subcutaneous injection.
It is important to use a separate sterile syringe and needle for each individual patient to prevent transmission of hepatitis B and other infectious agents from one person to another.

50 Dose Vial (available only to government agencies/institutions)—Withdraw the entire contents (30 mL) of diluent vial into the sterile syringe to be used for reconstitution and introduce into the 50 dose vial of lyophilized vaccine. Agitate to ensure thorough mixing. With full aseptic precautions, attach the vial to the sterilized multidose jet injector apparatus. Use 0.5 mL of the reconstituted vaccine for subcutaneous injection.

Each dose of ATTENUVAX contains not less than 1,000 $TCID_{50}$ (tissue culture infectious doses) of measles virus vaccine expressed in terms of the assigned titer of the U.S. Reference Measles Virus.
Parenteral drug products should be inspected visually for particulate matter and discoloration prior to administration. ATTENUVAX, when reconstituted, is clear yellow.

HOW SUPPLIED

No. 4709—ATTENUVAX is supplied as a single-dose vial of lyophilized vaccine, **NDC** 0006-4709-00, and a vial of diluent.
No. 4589X/4309—ATTENUVAX is supplied as follows: (1) a box of 10 single-dose vials of lyophilized vaccine (package A), **NDC** 0006-4589-00; and (2) a box of 10 vials of diluent (package B). To conserve refrigerator space, the diluent may be stored separately at room temperature
(6505-01-038-0794, Ten Pack).

Available only to government agencies/institutions:

No. 4614X—ATTENUVAX is supplied as one 10 dose vial of lyophilized vaccine, **NDC** 0006-4614-00, and one 7 mL vial of diluent.
No. 4591X—ATTENUVAX is supplied as one 50 dose vial of lyophilized vaccine, **NDC** 0006-4591-00, and one 30 mL vial of diluent
(6505-01-222-6467, 50 Dose).

Storage

It is recommended that the vaccine be used as soon as possible after reconstitution. Protect vaccine from light at all times, since such exposure may inactivate the virus. Store reconstituted vaccine in the vaccine vial in a dark place at 2–8°C (36–46°F) and discard if not used within 8 hours.

A.H.F.S. Category: 80:12
7680014 Issued March 1995
COPYRIGHT © MERCK & CO., INC., 1990
All rights reserved

BENEMID® Tablets ℞
(Probenecid), U.S.P.

DESCRIPTION

BENEMID* (Probenecid) is a uricosuric and renal tubular transport blocking agent.
Probenecid is the generic name for 4-[(dipropylamino) sulfonyl] benzoic acid (molecular weight 285.36). It has the following structural formula:

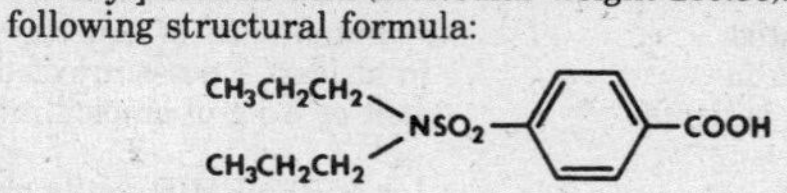

Probenecid is a white or nearly white, fine, crystalline powder. Probenecid is soluble in dilute alkali, in alcohol, in chloroform, and in acetone; it is practically insoluble in water and in dilute acids.
Each tablet contains 0.5 g probenecid and the following inactive ingredients: calcium stearate, D&C Yellow 10, gelatin, hydroxypropyl methylcellulose, iron oxide, magnesium carbonate, polyethylene glycol, starch, talc, and titanium dioxide.

*Registered trademark of MERCK & CO., INC.

ACTIONS

BENEMID is a uricosuric and renal tubular blocking agent. It inhibits the tubular reabsorption of urate, thus increasing the urinary excretion of uric acid and decreasing serum urate levels. Effective uricosuria reduces the miscible urate pool, retards urate deposition, and promotes resorption of urate deposits.
BENEMID inhibits the tubular secretion of penicillin and usually increases penicillin plasma levels by any route the antibiotic is given. A 2-fold to 4-fold elevation has been demonstrated for various penicillins.

Continued on next page

Information on the Merck & Co., Inc. products listed on these pages is the full prescribing information from product circulars in use September 30, 1996.

Merck & Co.—Cont.

BENEMID also has been reported to inhibit the renal transport of many other compounds including aminohippuric acid (PAH), aminosalicylic acid (PAS), indomethacin, sodium iodomethamate and related iodinated organic acids, 17-ketosteroids, pantothenic acid, phenolsulfonphthalein (PSP), sulfonamides, and sulfonylureas. See also DRUG INTERACTIONS.

BENEMID decreases both hepatic and renal excretion of sulfobromophthalein (BSP). The tubular reabsorption of phosphorus is inhibited in hypoparathyroid but not in euparathyroid individuals.

BENEMID does not influence plasma concentrations of salicylates, nor the excretion of streptomycin, chloramphenicol, chlortetracycline, oxytetracycline, or neomycin.

INDICATIONS

For treatment of the hyperuricemia associated with gout and gouty arthritis.

As an adjuvant to therapy with penicillin or with ampicillin, methicillin, oxacillin, cloxacillin, or nafcillin, for elevation and prolongation of plasma levels by whatever route the antibiotic is given.

CONTRAINDICATIONS

Hypersensitivity to this product.
Children under 2 years of age.
Not recommended in persons with known blood dyscrasias or uric acid kidney stones.
Therapy with BENEMID should not be started until an acute gouty attack has subsided.

WARNINGS

Exacerbation of gout following therapy with BENEMID may occur; in such cases colchicine or other appropriate therapy is advisable.

BENEMID increases plasma concentrations of methotrexate in both animals and humans. In animal studies, increased methotrexate toxicity has been reported. If BENEMID is given with methotrexate, the dosage of methotrexate should be reduced and serum levels may need to be monitored.

In patients on BENEMID the use of salicylates in either small or large doses is contraindicated because it antagonizes the uricosuric action of BENEMID. The biphasic action of salicylates in the renal tubules accounts for the so-called "paradoxical effect" of uricosuric agents. In patients on BENEMID who require a mild analgesic agent the use of acetaminophen rather than small doses of salicylates would be preferred.

Rarely, severe allergic reactions and anaphylaxis have been reported with the use of BENEMID. Most of these have been reported to occur within several hours after readministration following prior usage of the drug.

The appearance of hypersensitivity reactions requires cessation of therapy with BENEMID.

Use in Pregnancy: BENEMID crosses the placental barrier and appears in cord blood. The use of any drug in women of childbearing potential requires that the anticipated benefit be weighed against possible hazards.

PRECAUTIONS

General

Hematuria, renal colic, costovertebral pain, and formation of uric acid stones associated with the use of BENEMID in gouty patients may be prevented by alkalization of the urine and a liberal fluid intake (*see* DOSAGE AND ADMINISTRATION). In these cases when alkali is administered, the acid-base balance of the patient should be watched.

Use with caution in patients with a history of peptic ulcer. BENEMID has been used in patients with some renal impairment but dosage requirements may be increased. BENEMID may not be effective in chronic renal insufficiency particularly when the glomerular filtration rate is 30 mL/minute or less. Because of its mechanism of action, BENEMID is not recommended in conjunction with a penicillin in the presence of *known* renal impairment.

A reducing substance may appear in the urine of patients receiving BENEMID. This disappears with discontinuance of therapy. Suspected glycosuria should be confirmed by using a test specific for glucose.

Drug Interactions

When BENEMID is used to elevate plasma concentrations of penicillin or other beta-lactams, or when such drugs are given to patients taking BENEMID therapeutically, high plasma concentrations of the other drug may increase the incidence of adverse reactions associated with that drug. In the case of penicillin or other beta-lactams, psychic disturbances have been reported.

The use of salicylates antagonizes the uricosuric action of BENEMID (*see* WARNINGS). The uricosuric action of BENEMID is also antagonized by pyrazinamide.

BENEMID produces an insignificant increase in free sulfonamide plasma concentrations but a significant increase in total sulfonamide plasma levels. Since BENEMID decreases the renal excretion of conjugated sulfonamides, plasma concentrations of the latter should be determined from time to time when a sulfonamide and BENEMID are coadministered for prolonged periods. BENEMID may prolong or enhance the action of oral sulfonylureas and thereby increase the risk of hypoglycemia.

It has been reported that patients receiving BENEMID require significantly less thiopental for induction of anesthesia. In addition, ketamine and thiopental anesthesia were significantly prolonged in rats receiving probenecid.

The concomitant administration of probenecid increases the

BENEMID® (Probenecid) Penicillin Therapy (Gonorrhea)*

	Recommended Regimens**	Remarks
Uncomplicated gonococcal infection in men and women (urethral, cervical, rectal)	4.8 million units of aqueous procaine penicillin G† I.M., in at least 2 doses injected at different sites at one visit + 1 g of BENEMID (Probenecid) orally just before injections *or* 3.5 g of ampicillin† orally + 1 g of BENEMID orally given simultaneously.	Follow-up: Obtain urethral and other appropriate cultures from men, and cervical, anal, and other appropriate cultures from women, 7 to 14 days after completion of treatment. Treatment of sexual partners: Persons with known recent exposure to gonorrhea should receive same treatment as those known to have gonorrhea. Examination and treatment of male sex partners of persons with gonorrhea are essential because of high prevalence of nonsymptomatic urethral gonococcal infection in such men.
Pharyngeal gonococcal infection in men and women	4.8 million units of aqueous procaine penicillin G† I.M., in at least 2 doses injected at different sites at one visit + 1 g of BENEMID orally just before injections	Pharyngeal gonococcal infections may be more difficult to treat than anogenital gonorrhea. Posttreatment cultures are essential.
Uncomplicated gonorrhea in pregnant patients	4.8 million units of aqueous procaine penicillin G† I.M., in at least 2 doses injected at different sites at one visit *or* 3.5 g of ampicillin† orally + 1 g of BENEMID orally given simultaneously	
Acute gonococcal salpingitis	*Outpatients:* Aqueous procaine penicillin G† or ampicillin† with BENEMID as for gonorrhea in pregnancy, followed by 500 mg of ampicillin 4 times a day for 10 days *Hospitalized patients:* See details in CDC recommendations	Follow-up of patients with acute salpingitis is essential. All patients should receive repeat pelvic examinations and cultures for *Neisseria gonorrhoeae* after treatment. Examination and appropriate treatment of male sex partners are essential because of high prevalence of nonsymptomatic urethral gonorrhea in such men.
Disseminated gonococcal infection (arthritis-dermatitis syndrome)	10 million units of aqueous crystalline penicillin G† I.V. a day for 3 days or till significant clinical improvement occurs. May be followed with 500 mg of ampicillin† 4 times a day orally to complete 7 days of treatment *or* 3.5 g of ampicillin† orally with 1 g of BENEMID, followed by 500 mg of ampicillin† 4 times a day for at least 7 days	
Gonococcal infection in children	For postpubertal children and/or those weighing over 45 kg (100 lb) use the dosage regimens given above for adults Uncomplicated vulvovaginitis and urethritis: aqueous procaine penicillin G† 75,000—100,000 units/kg I.M., with BENEMID 23 mg/kg orally	See CDC recommendations for detailed information about prevention and treatment of neonatal gonococcal infection and gonococcal ophthalmia.

Note: Before treating gonococcal infections in patients with suspected primary or secondary syphilis, perform proper diagnostic procedures including darkfield examinations. If concomitant syphilis is suspected, perform monthly serological tests for at least 4 months.

* Recommended by Venereal Disease Control Advisory Committee, Center for Disease Control, U.S. Department of Health, Education, and Welfare, Public Health Service (Morbidity and Mortality Weekly Report, Vol. 23: 341, 342, 347, 348, Oct. 11, 1974).

** See CDC recommendations for definition of regimens of choice, alternative regimens, treatment of hypersensitive patients, and other aspects of therapy.

† See package circulars of manufacturers for detailed information about contraindications, warnings, precautions, and adverse reactions.

Information will be superseded by supplements and subsequent editions

mean plasma elimination half-life of a number of drugs which can lead to increased plasma concentrations. These include agents such as indomethacin, acetaminophen, naproxen, ketoprofen, meclofenamate, lorazepam, and rifampin. Although the clinical significance of this observation has not been established, a lower dosage of the drug may be required to produce a therapeutic effect, and increases in dosage of the drug in question should be made cautiously and in small increments when probenecid is being co-administered. Although specific instances of toxicity due to this potential interaction have not been observed to date physicians should be alert to this possibility.
Probenecid given concomitantly with sulindac had only a slight effect on plasma sulfide levels, while plasma levels of sulindac and sulfone were increased. Sulindac was shown to produce a modest reduction in the uricosuric action of probenecid, which probably is not significant under most circumstances.
In animals and in humans, BENEMID has been reported to increase plasma concentrations of methotrexate (*see* WARNINGS).
Falsely high readings for theophylline have been reported in an *in vitro* study, using the Schack and Waxler technic, when therapeutic concentrations of theophylline and BENEMID were added to human plasma.

ADVERSE REACTIONS

The following adverse reactions have been observed and within each category are listed in order of decreasing severity.
Central Nervous System: headache, dizziness.
Metabolic: precipitation of acute gouty arthritis.
Gastrointestinal: hepatic necrosis, vomiting, nausea, anorexia, sore gums.
Genitourinary: nephrotic syndrome, uric acid stones with or without hematuria, renal colic, costovertebral pain, urinary frequency.
Hypersensitivity: anaphylaxis, fever, urticaria, pruritus.
Hematologic: aplastic anemia, leukopenia, hemolytic anemia which in some patients could be related to genetic deficiency of glucose -6- phosphate dehydrogenase in red blood cells, anemia.
Integumentary: dermatitis, alopecia, flushing.

DOSAGE AND ADMINISTRATION

Gout
Therapy with BENEMID should not be *started* until an acute gouty attack has subsided. However, if an acute attack is precipitated *during* therapy, BENEMID may be continued without changing the dosage, and full therapeutic dosage of colchicine or other appropriate therapy should be given to control the acute attack.
The recommended adult dosage is 0.25 g (½ tablet of BENEMID) twice a day for one week, followed by 0.5 g (1 tablet) twice a day thereafter.
Some degree of renal impairment may be present in patients with gout. A daily dosage of 1 g may be adequate. However, if necessary, the daily dosage may be increased by 0.5 g increments every 4 weeks within tolerance (and usually not above 2 g per day) if symptoms of gouty arthritis are not controlled or the 24 hour uric acid excretion is not above 700 mg. As noted, BENEMID may not be effective in chronic renal insufficiency particularly when the glomerular filtration rate is 30 mL/minute or less.
Gastric intolerance may be indicative of overdosage, and may be corrected by decreasing the dosage.
As uric acid tends to crystallize out of an acid urine, a liberal fluid intake is recommended, as well as sufficient sodium bicarbonate (3 to 7.5 g daily) or potassium citrate (7.5 g daily) to maintain an alkaline urine (*see* PRECAUTIONS).
Alkalization of the urine is recommended until the serum urate level returns to normal limits and tophaceous deposits disappear, i.e., during the period when urinary excretion of uric acid is at a high level. Thereafter, alkalization of the urine and the usual restriction of purine-producing foods may be somewhat relaxed.
BENEMID should be continued at the dosage that will maintain normal serum urate levels. When acute attacks have been absent for 6 months or more and serum urate levels remain within normal limits, the daily dosage may be decreased by 0.5 g every 6 months. The maintenance dosage should not be reduced to the point where serum urate levels tend to rise.
BENEMID *and Penicillin Therapy (General)*
Adults:
The recommended dosage is 2 g (4 tablets of BENEMID) daily in divided doses. This dosage should be reduced in older patients in whom renal impairment may be present.
Children 2-14 years of age:
Initial dose: 25 mg/kg body weight (*or* 0.7 g/square meter body surface).
Maintenance dose: 40 mg/kg body weight (*or* 1.2 g/square meter body surface) per day, divided into 4 doses.
For children weighing more than 50 kg (110 lb) the adult dosage is recommended.
BENEMID is contraindicated in children under 2 years of age.
The PSP excretion test may be used to determine the effectiveness of BENEMID in retarding penicillin excretion and maintaining therapeutic levels. The renal clearance of PSP is reduced to about one-fifth the normal rate when dosage of BENEMID is adequate.
Penicillin Therapy (Gonorrhea)
[See table on preceding page.]

HOW SUPPLIED

No. 3337—Tablets BENEMID, 0.5 g, are yellow, capsule shaped, scored, film coated tablets, coded MSD 501. They are supplied as follows:
NDC 0006-0501-68 bottles of 100
(6505-00-527-6885 100's)
NDC 0006-0501-28 unit dose packages of 100
NDC 0006-0501-82 bottles of 1000
(6505-00-181-8387 1000's).

Shown in Product Identification Guide, page 324

7876122 Issued August 1988

BIAVAX®$_{II}$ ℞
(Rubella and Mumps Virus Vaccine Live), U.S.P.

DESCRIPTION

BIAVAX* II (Rubella and Mumps Virus Vaccine Live) is a live virus vaccine for immunization against rubella (German measles) and mumps.
BIAVAX II is a sterile lyophilized preparation of the Wistar RA 27/3 strain of live attenuated rubella virus grown in human diploid cell (WI-38) culture; and the Jeryl Lynn (B level) strain of mumps virus grown in cell cultures of chick embryo. The vaccine viruses are the same as those used in the manufacture of MERUVAX* II (Rubella Virus Vaccine Live) and MUMPSVAX* (Mumps Virus Vaccine Live). The two viruses are mixed before being lyophilized.
The reconstituted vaccine is for subcutaneous administration. When reconstituted as directed, the dose for injection is 0.5 mL and contains not less than the equivalent of 1,000 $TCID_{50}$ of the U.S. Reference Rubella Virus and 20,000 $TCID_{50}$ of the U.S. Reference Mumps Virus. Each dose contains approximately 25 mcg of neomycin. The product contains no preservative. Sorbitol and hydrolized gelatin are added as stabilizers.

*Registered trademark of MERCK & CO., INC.

CLINICAL PHARMACOLOGY

Clinical studies of 73 double seronegative children 12 months to 2 years of age demonstrated that BIAVAX II is highly immunogenic and generally well tolerated. In these studies, a single injection of the vaccine induced rubella hemagglutination-inhibition (HI) antibodies in 100 percent, and mumps neutralizing antibodies in 97 percent of the susceptible children.
The RA 27/3 rubella strain in BIAVAX II elicits higher immediate post-vaccination HI, complement-fixing and neutralizing antibody levels than other strains of rubella vaccine and has been shown to induce a broader profile of circulating antibodies including anti-theta and anti-iota precipitating antibodies. The RA 27/3 rubella strain immunologically simulates natural infection more closely than other rubella vaccine viruses. The increased levels and broader profile of antibodies produced by RA 27/3 strain rubella virus vaccine appear to correlate with greater resistance to subclinical reinfection with the wild virus, and provide greater confidence for lasting immunity.
Vaccine induced antibody levels following administration of BIAVAX II have been shown to persist for at least two years without substantial decline. Antibody levels after immunization with BIAVAX (Rubella and Mumps Virus Vaccine Live), containing the HPV-77 strain of rubella, have persisted for 10.5 years without substantial decline. If the present pattern continues, it will provide a basis for the expectation that immunity following vaccination will be permanent. However, continued surveillance will be required to demonstrate this point.

INDICATIONS AND USAGE

BIAVAX II is indicated for simultaneous immunization against rubella and mumps in persons 12 months of age or older. A booster is not needed.
The vaccine is not recommended for infants younger than 12 months because they may retain maternal rubella and mumps neutralizing antibodies which may interfere with the immune response.
Previously unimmunized children of susceptible pregnant women should receive live attenuated rubella vaccine, because an immunized child will be less likely to acquire natural rubella and introduce the virus into the household.
Individuals planning travel outside the United States, if not immune, can acquire measles, mumps or rubella and import these diseases to the United States. Therefore, prior to International travel, individuals known to be susceptible to one or more of these diseases can receive either a single antigen vaccine (measles, mumps, or rubella), or a combined antigen vaccine as appropriate. However, M-M-R* II (Measles, Mumps, and Rubella Virus Vaccine Live) is preferred for persons likely to be susceptible to mumps and rubella; and if single-antigen measles vaccine is not readily available, travelers should receive M-M-R II (Measles, Mumps, and Rubella Virus Vaccine Live) regardless of their immune status to mumps or rubella.
Non-Pregnant Adolescent and Adult Females
Immunization of susceptible non-pregnant adolescent and adult females of childbearing age with live attenuated rubella virus vaccine is indicated if certain precautions are observed (see below and PRECAUTIONS). Vaccinating susceptible postpubertal females confers individual protection against subsequently acquiring rubella infection during pregnancy, which in turn prevents infection of the fetus and consequent congenital rubella injury.
Women of childbearing age should be advised not to become pregnant for three months after vaccination and should be informed of the reasons for this precaution.**
It is recommended that rubella susceptibility be determined by serologic testing prior to immunization.***
If immune, as evidenced by a specific rubella antibody titer of 1:8 or greater (hemagglutination-inhibition test), vaccination is unnecessary. Congenital malformations do occur in up to seven percent of all live births. Their chance appearance after vaccination could lead to misinterpretation of the cause, particularly if the prior rubella-immune status of vaccinees is unknown.
Postpubertal females should be informed of the frequent occurrence of generally self-limited arthralgia and/or arthritis beginning 2 to 4 weeks after vaccination (see ADVERSE REACTIONS).
Postpartum Women
It has been found convenient in many instances to vaccinate rubella-susceptible women in the immediate postpartum period. (See *Nursing Mothers*).
Revaccination: Children vaccinated when younger than 12 months of age should be revaccinated. Based on available evidence, there is no reason to routinely revaccinate persons who were vaccinated originally when 12 months of age or older. However, persons should be revaccinated if there is evidence to suggest that initial immunization was ineffective.
Use with other Vaccines
Routine administration of DTP (diphtheria, tetanus, pertussis) and/or OPV (oral poliovirus vaccine) concomitantly with measles, mumps and rubella vaccines is not recommended because there are insufficient data relating to the simultaneous administration of these antigens. However, the American Academy of Pediatrics has noted that in some circumstances, particularly when the patient may not return, some practitioners prefer to administer all these antigens on a single day. If done, separate sites and syringes should be used for DTP and BIAVAX II.
BIAVAX II should not be given less than one month before or after administration of other virus vaccines.

* Registered trademark of MERCK & CO., INC.
** NOTE: The Immunization Practices Advisory Committee (ACIP) has recommended "In view of the importance of protecting this age group against rubella, reasonable precautions in a rubella immunization program include asking females if they are pregnant, excluding those who say they are, and explaining the theoretical risks to the others."
*** NOTE: The Immunization Practices Advisory Committee (ACIP) has stated "When practical, and when reliable laboratory services are available, potential vaccinees of childbearing age can have serologic tests to determine susceptibility to rubella. . . . However, routinely performing serologic tests for all females of childbearing age to determine susceptibility so that vaccine is given only to proven susceptibles is expensive and has been ineffective in some areas. Accordingly, the ACIP believes that rubella vaccination of a woman who is not known to be pregnant and has no history of vaccination is justifiable without serologic testing."

Continued on next page

Information on the Merck & Co., Inc. products listed on these pages is the full prescribing information from product circulars in use September 30, 1996.

Merck & Co.—Cont.

CONTRAINDICATIONS

Do not give BIAVAX II to pregnant females; the possible effects of the vaccine on fetal development are unknown at this time. If vaccination of postpubertal females is undertaken, pregnancy should be avoided for three months following vaccination. (See PRECAUTIONS, *Pregnancy*).
Anaphylactic or anaphylactoid reactions to neomycin (each dose of reconstituted vaccine contains approximately 25 mcg of neomycin).
History of anaphylactic or anaphylactoid reactions to eggs (see HYPERSENSITIVITY TO EGGS below).
Any febrile respiratory illness or other active febrile infection.
Active untreated tuberculosis.
Patients receiving immunosuppressive therapy. This contraindication does not apply to patients who are receiving corticosteroids as replacement therapy, e.g., for Addison's disease.
Individuals with blood dyscrasias, leukemia, lymphomas of any type, or other malignant neoplasms affecting the bone marrow or lymphatic systems.
Primary and acquired immunodeficiency states, including patients who are immunosuppressed in association with AIDS or other clinical manifestations of infection with human immunodeficiency viruses; cellular immune deficiencies; and hypogammaglobulinemic and dysgammaglobulinemic states.
Individuals with a family history of congenital or hereditary immunodeficiency, until the immune competence of the potential vaccine recipient is demonstrated.

HYPERSENSITIVITY TO EGGS

Live mumps vaccine is produced in chick embryo cell culture. Persons with a history of anaphylactic, anaphylactoid, or other immediate reactions (e.g., hives, swelling of the mouth and throat, difficulty breathing, hypotension, or shock) subsequent to egg ingestion should not be vaccinated. Evidence indicates that persons are not at increased risk if they have egg allergies that are not anaphylactic or anaphylactoid in nature. Such persons may be vaccinated in the usual manner. There is no evidence to indicate that persons with allergies to chickens or feathers are at increased risk of reaction to the vaccine.

PRECAUTIONS

General
Adequate treatment provisions including epinephrine, should be available for immediate use should an anaphylactic or anaphylactoid reaction occur.
Children and young adults who are known to be infected with human immunodeficiency viruses but without overt clinical manifestations of immunosuppression may be vaccinated; however, the vaccinees should be monitored closely for vaccine-preventable diseases because immunization may be less effective than for uninfected persons.
Vaccination should be deferred for at least 3 months following blood or plasma transfusions, or administration of human immune serum globulin.
Excretion of small amounts of the live attenuated rubella virus from the nose and throat has occurred in the majority of susceptible individuals 7–28 days after vaccination. There is no confirmed evidence to indicate that such virus is transmitted to susceptible persons who are in contact with the vaccinated individuals. Consequently, transmission through close personal contact, while accepted as a theoretical possibility, is not regarded as a significant risk. However, transmission of the rubella vaccine virus to infants via breast milk has been documented (see *Nursing Mothers*).
There are no reports of transmission of live attenuated mumps virus from vaccinees to susceptible contacts.
It has been reported that live attenuated rubella and mumps virus vaccines given individually may result in a temporary depression of tuberculin skin sensitivity. Therefore, if a tuberculin test is to be done, it should be administered either before or simultaneously with BIAVAX II.
As for any vaccine, vaccination with BIAVAX II may not result in seroconversion in 100% of susceptible persons given the vaccine.
Pregnancy
Pregnancy Category C
Animal reproduction studies have not been conducted with BIAVAX II. It is also not known whether BIAVAX II can cause fetal harm when administered to a pregnant woman or can affect reproduction capacity. Therefore, the vaccine should not be administered to pregnant females; furthermore, pregnancy should be avoided for three months following vaccination (see CONTRAINDICATIONS).
In counseling women who are inadvertently vaccinated when pregnant or who become pregnant within 3 months of vaccination, the physician should be aware of the following: (1) In a 10 year survey involving over 700 pregnant women who received rubella vaccine within 3 months before or after conception, (of whom 189 received the Wistar RA 27/3 strain) none of the newborns had abnormalities compatible with congenital rubella syndrome; and (2) although mumps virus is capable of infecting the placenta and fetus, there is no good evidence that it causes congenital malformations in humans. Mumps vaccine virus also has been shown to infect the placenta, but the virus has not been isolated from the fetal tissues from susceptible women who were vaccinated and underwent elective abortions.
Nursing Mothers
It is not known whether mumps vaccine virus is secreted in human milk. Recent studies have shown that lactating postpartum women immunized with live attenuated rubella vaccine may secrete the virus in breast milk and transmit it to breast-fed infants. In the infants with serological evidence of rubella infection, none exhibited severe disease; however, one exhibited mild clinical illness typical of acquired rubella. Caution should be exercised when BIAVAX II is administered to a nursing woman.

ADVERSE REACTIONS

Burning and/or stinging of short duration at the injection site have been reported.
The adverse clinical reactions associated with the use of BIAVAX II are those expected to follow administration of the monovalent vaccines given separately. These may include malaise, sore throat, cough, rhinitis, headache, dizziness, fever, rash, nausea, vomiting or diarrhea; mild local reactions such as erythema, induration, tenderness and regional lymphadenopathy; parotitis, orchitis, nerve deafness, thrombocytopenia and purpura; allergic reactions such as wheal and flare at the injection site or urticaria; polyneuritis; and arthralgia and/or arthritis (usually transient and rarely chronic).
Anaphylaxis and anaphylactoid reactions have been reported.
Vasculitis has been reported rarely.
Moderate fever [101–102.9°F (38.3–39.4°C)] occurs occasionally, and high fever [above 103°F (39.4°C)] occurs less commonly. On rare occasions, children developing fever may exhibit febrile convulsions. Syncope, particularly at the time of mass vaccination, has been reported. Rash occurs infrequently and is usually minimal, but rarely may be generalized. Erythema multiforme has also been reported rarely.
Forms of optic neuritis, including retrobulbar neuritis and papillitis may infrequently follow viral infections, and have been reported to occur 1 to 3 weeks following inoculation with some live virus vaccines.
Isolated reports of polyneuropathy including Guillain-Barré syndrome have been reported after immunization with rubella-containing vaccines.
Clinical experience with live attenuated rubella and mumps virus vaccines given individually indicates that encephalitis and other nervous system reactions have occurred very rarely. These might occur also with BIAVAX II.
Arthralgia and/or arthritis (usually transient and rarely chronic), and polyneuritis are features of natural rubella and vary in frequency and severity with age and sex, being greatest in adult females and least in prepubertal children. This type of involvement as well as myalgia and paresthesia have also been reported following administration of MERUVAX II (Rubella Virus Vaccine Live).
Chronic arthritis has been associated with natural rubella infection and has been related to persistent virus and/or viral antigen isolated from body tissues. Only rarely have vaccine recipients developed chronic joint symptoms.
Following vaccination in children, reactions in joints are uncommon and generally of brief duration. In women, incidence rates for arthritis and arthralgia are generally higher than those seen in children (children: 0–3%; women: 12–20%), and the reactions tend to be more marked and of longer duration. Symptoms may persist for a matter of months or on rare occasions for years. In adolescent girls, the reactions appear to be intermediate in incidence between those seen in children and in adult women. Even in older women (35–45 years), these reactions are generally well tolerated and rarely interfere with normal activities.

DOSAGE AND ADMINISTRATION

FOR SUBCUTANEOUS ADMINISTRATION
Do not inject intravenously.
The dosage of vaccine is the same for all persons. Inject the total volume (about 0.5 mL) of reconstituted vaccine subcutaneously, preferably into the outer aspect of upper arm. *Do not give immune globulin (IG) concurrently with* BIAVAX II.
During shipment, to insure that there is no loss of potency, the vaccine must be maintained at a temperature of 10°C (50°F) or less.
Before reconstitution, store BIAVAX II at 2–8°C (36–46°F).
Protect from light.
CAUTION: A sterile syringe free of preservatives, antiseptics, and detergents should be used for each injection of the vaccine because these substances may inactivate the live virus vaccine. A 25 gauge, ⅝″ needle is recommended.
To reconstitute, use only the diluent supplied, since it is free of preservatives or other antiviral substances which might inactivate the vaccine. First withdraw the entire volume of diluent into the syringe to be used for reconstitution. Inject all the diluent in the syringe into the vial of lyophilized vaccine, and agitate to mix thoroughly. Withdraw the entire contents into a syringe and inject the total volume of restored vaccine subcutaneously.
It is important to use a separate sterile syringe and needle for each individual patient to prevent transmission of hepatitis B virus and other infectious agents from one person to another.
Each dose of BIAVAX II contains not less than the equivalent of 1,000 $TCID_{50}$ of the U.S. Reference Rubella Virus and 20,000 $TCID_{50}$ of the U.S. Reference Mumps Virus.
Parenteral drug products should be inspected visually for particulate matter and discoloration prior to administration. BIAVAX II, when reconstituted, is clear yellow.

HOW SUPPLIED

No. 4746—BIAVAX II is supplied as a single-dose vial of lyophilized vaccine, **NDC** 0006-4746-00, and a vial of diluent.
No. 4669/4309—BIAVAX II is supplied as follows: (1) a box of 10 single-dose vials of lyophilized vaccine (package A), **NDC** 0006-4669-00; and (2) a box of 10 vials of diluent (package B). To conserve refrigerator space, the diluent may be stored separately at room temperature.
Storage
It is recommended that the vaccine be used as soon as possible after reconstitution. Protect the vaccine from light at all times, since such exposure may inactivate the virus. Store reconstituted vaccine in the vaccine vial in a dark place at 2–8°C (36–46°F) and discard if not used within eight hours.

A.H.F.S. Category: 80:12
7680116 Issued March 1995

COPYRIGHT © MERCK & CO., INC., 1990
All rights reserved

BLOCADREN® Tablets ℞
(Timolol Maleate), U.S.P.

DESCRIPTION

BLOCADREN* (Timolol Maleate) is a non-selective beta-adrenergic receptor blocking agent. The chemical name for timolol maleate is (*S*)-1-[(1,1-dimethylethyl)amino] -3-[[4-(4-morpholinyl)-1,2,5-thiadiazol-3-yl]oxy]-2-propanol (*Z*)-2-butenedioate (1:1) salt. It possesses an asymmetric carbon atom in its structure and is provided as the levo isomer. Its empirical formula is $C_{13}H_{24}N_4O_3S \cdot C_4H_4O_4$ and its structural formula is:

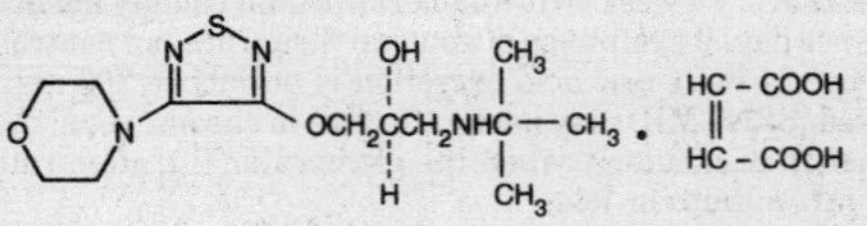

Timolol maleate has a molecular weight of 432.50. It is a white, odorless, crystalline powder which is soluble in water, methanol, and alcohol.
BLOCADREN is supplied as tablets in three strengths containing 5 mg, 10 mg or 20 mg timolol maleate for oral administration. Inactive ingredients are cellulose, FD&C Blue 2, magnesium stearate, and starch.

*Registered trademark of MERCK & CO., INC.

CLINICAL PHARMACOLOGY

BLOCADREN is a $beta_1$ and $beta_2$ (non-selective) adrenergic receptor blocking agent that does not have significant intrinsic sympathomimetic, direct myocardial depressant, or local anesthetic activity.
Pharmacodynamics
Clinical pharmacology studies have confirmed the beta-adrenergic blocking activity as shown by (1) changes in resting heart rate and response of heart rate to changes in posture; (2) inhibition of isoproterenol-induced tachycardia; (3) alteration of the response to the Valsalva maneuver and amyl nitrite administration; and (4) reduction of heart rate and blood pressure changes on exercise.
BLOCADREN decreases the positive chronotropic, positive inotropic, bronchodilator, and vasodilator responses caused by beta-adrenergic receptor agonists. The magnitude of this decreased response is proportional to the existing sympathe-

tic tone and the concentration of BLOCADREN at receptor sites.
In normal volunteers, the reduction in heart rate response to a standard exercise was dose dependent over the test range of 0.5 to 20 mg, with a peak reduction at 2 hours of approximately 30% at higher doses.
Beta-adrenergic receptor blockade reduces cardiac output in both healthy subjects and patients with heart disease. In patients with severe impairment of myocardial function beta-adrenergic receptor blockade may inhibit the stimulatory effect of the sympathetic nervous system necessary to maintain adequate cardiac function.
Beta-adrenergic receptor blockade in the bronchi and bronchioles results in increased airway resistance from unopposed parasympathetic activity. Such an effect in patients with asthma or other bronchospastic conditions is potentially dangerous.
Clinical studies indicate that BLOCADREN at a dosage of 20–60 mg/day reduces blood pressure without causing postural hypotension in most patients with essential hypertension. Administration of BLOCADREN to patients with hypertension results initially in a decrease in cardiac output, little immediate change in blood pressure, and an increase in calculated peripheral resistance. With continued administration of BLOCADREN, blood pressure decreases within a few days, cardiac output usually remains reduced, and peripheral resistance falls toward pretreatment levels. Plasma volume may decrease or remain unchanged during therapy with BLOCADREN. In the majority of patients with hypertension BLOCADREN also decreases plasma renin activity. Dosage adjustment to achieve optimal antihypertensive effect may require a few weeks. When therapy with BLOCADREN is discontinued, the blood pressure tends to return to pretreatment levels gradually. In most patients the antihypertensive activity of BLOCADREN is maintained with long-term therapy and is well tolerated.
The mechanism of the antihypertensive effects of beta-adrenergic receptor blocking agents is not established at this time. Possible mechanisms of action include reduction in cardiac output, reduction in plasma renin activity, and a central nervous system sympatholytic action.
A Norwegian multi-center, double-blind study compared the effects of timolol maleate with placebo in 1,884 patients who had survived the acute phase of a myocardial infarction. Patients with systolic blood pressure below 100 mm Hg, sick sinus syndrome and contraindications to beta blockers, including uncontrolled heart failure, second or third degree AV block and bradycardia (<50 beats per minute), were excluded from the multi-center trial. Therapy with BLOCADREN, begun 7 to 28 days following infarction, was shown to reduce overall mortality; this was primarily attributable to a reduction in cardiovascular mortality. BLOCADREN significantly reduced the incidence of sudden deaths (deaths occurring without symptoms or within 24 hours of the onset of symptoms), including those occurring within one hour, and particularly instantaneous deaths (those occurring without preceding symptoms). The protective effect of BLOCADREN was consistent regardless of age, sex or site of infarction. The effect was clearest in patients with a first infarction who were considered at a high risk of dying, defined as those with one or more of the following characteristics during the acute phase: transient left ventricular failure, cardiomegaly, newly appearing atrial fibrillation or flutter, systolic hypotension, or SGOT (ASAT) levels greater than four times the upper limit of normal. Therapy with BLOCADREN also reduced the incidence of non-fatal reinfarction. The mechanism of the protective effect of BLOCADREN is unknown.
BLOCADREN was studied for the prophylactic treatment of migraine headache in placebo-controlled clinical trials involving 400 patients, mostly women between the ages of 18 and 66 years. Common migraine was the most frequent diagnosis. All patients had at least two headaches per month at baseline. Approximately 50 percent of patients who received BLOCADREN had a reduction in the frequency of migraine headache of at least 50 percent, compared to a similar decrease in frequency in 30 percent of patients receiving placebo. The most common cardiovascular adverse effect was bradycardia (5%).
Pharmacokinetics and Metabolism
BLOCADREN is rapidly and nearly completely absorbed (about 90%) following oral ingestion. Detectable plasma levels of timolol occur within one-half hour and peak plasma levels occur in about one to two hours. The drug half-life in plasma is approximately 4 hours and this is essentially unchanged in patients with moderate renal insufficiency. Timolol is partially metabolized by the liver and timolol and its metabolites are excreted by the kidney. Timolol is not extensively bound to plasma proteins; i.e., <10% by equilibrium dialysis and approximately 60% by ultrafiltration. An *in vitro* hemodialysis study, using ^{14}C timolol added to human plasma or whole blood, showed that timolol was readily dialyzed from these fluids; however, a study of patients with renal failure showed that timolol did not dialyze readily. Plasma levels following oral administration are about half those following intravenous administration indicating approximately 50% first pass metabolism. The level of beta sympathetic activity varies widely among individuals, and no simple correlation exists between the dose or plasma level of timolol maleate and its therapeutic activity. Therefore, objective clinical measurements such as reduction of heart rate and/or blood pressure should be used as guides in determining the optimal dosage for each patient.

INDICATIONS AND USAGE

Hypertension
BLOCADREN is indicated for the treatment of hypertension. It may be used alone or in combination with other antihypertensive agents, especially thiazide-type diuretics.
Myocardial Infarction
BLOCADREN is indicated in patients who have survived the acute phase of a myocardial infarction, and are clinically stable, to reduce cardiovascular mortality and the risk of reinfarction.
Migraine
BLOCADREN is indicated for the prophylaxis of migraine headache.

CONTRAINDICATIONS

BLOCADREN is contraindicated in patients with bronchial asthma or with a history of bronchial asthma, or severe chronic obstructive pulmonary disease (see WARNINGS); sinus bradycardia; second and third degree atrioventricular block; overt cardiac failure (see WARNINGS); cardiogenic shock; hypersensitivity to this product.

WARNINGS

Cardiac Failure
Sympathetic stimulation may be essential for support of the circulation in individuals with diminished myocardial contractility, and its inhibition by beta-adrenergic receptor blockade may precipitate more severe failure. Although beta blockers should be avoided in overt congestive heart failure, they can be used, if necessary, with caution in patients with a history of failure who are well-compensated, usually with digitalis and diuretics. Both digitalis and timolol maleate slow AV conduction. If cardiac failure persists, therapy with BLOCADREN should be withdrawn.
In Patients Without a History of Cardiac Failure continued depression of the myocardium with beta-blocking agents over a period of time can, in some cases, lead to cardiac failure. At the first sign or symptom of cardiac failure, patients receiving BLOCADREN should be digitalized and/or be given a diuretic, and the response observed closely. If cardiac failure continues, despite adequate digitalization and diuretic therapy, BLOCADREN should be withdrawn.

Exacerbation of Ischemic Heart Disease Following Abrupt Withdrawal—Hypersensitivity to catecholamines has been observed in patients withdrawn from beta blocker therapy; exacerbation of angina and, in some cases, myocardial infarction have occurred after *abrupt* discontinuation of such therapy. When discontinuing chronically administered timolol maleate, particularly in patients with ischemic heart disease, the dosage should be gradually reduced over a period of one to two weeks and the patient should be carefully monitored. If angina markedly worsens or acute coronary insufficiency develops, timolol maleate administration should be reinstituted promptly, at least temporarily, and other measures appropriate for the management of unstable angina should be taken. Patients should be warned against interruption or discontinuation of therapy without the physician's advice. Because coronary artery disease is common and may be unrecognized, it may be prudent not to discontinue timolol maleate therapy abruptly even in patients treated only for hypertension.

Obstructive Pulmonary Disease
PATIENTS WITH CHRONIC OBSTRUCTIVE PULMONARY DISEASE (e.g., CHRONIC BRONCHITIS, EMPHYSEMA) OF MILD OR MODERATE SEVERITY, BRONCHOSPASTIC DISEASE OR A HISTORY OF BRONCHOSPASTIC DISEASE (OTHER THAN BRONCHIAL ASTHMA OR A HISTORY OF BRONCHIAL ASTHMA, IN WHICH 'BLOCADREN' IS CONTRAINDICATED, see CONTRAINDICATIONS), SHOULD IN GENERAL NOT RECEIVE BETA BLOCKERS, INCLUDING 'BLOCADREN'. However, if BLOCADREN is necessary in such patients, then the drug should be administered with caution since it may block bronchodilation produced by endogenous and exogenous catecholamine stimulation of $beta_2$ receptors.
Major Surgery
The necessity or desirability of withdrawal of beta-blocking therapy prior to major surgery is controversial. Beta-adrenergic receptor blockade impairs the ability of the heart to respond to beta-adrenergically mediated reflex stimuli. This may augment the risk of general anesthesia in surgical procedures. Some patients receiving beta-adrenergic receptor blocking agents have been subject to protracted severe hypotension during anesthesia. Difficulty in restarting and maintaining the heartbeat has also been reported. For these reasons, in patients undergoing elective surgery, some authorities recommend gradual withdrawal of beta-adrenergic receptor blocking agents.
If necessary during surgery, the effects of beta-adrenergic blocking agents may be reversed by sufficient doses of such agonists as isoproterenol, dopamine, dobutamine or levarterenol (see OVERDOSAGE).
Diabetes Mellitus
BLOCADREN should be administered with caution in patients subject to spontaneous hypoglycemia or to diabetic patients (especially those with labile diabetes) who are receiving insulin or oral hypoglycemic agents. Beta-adrenergic receptor blocking agents may mask the signs and symptoms of acute hypoglycemia.
Thyrotoxicosis
Beta-adrenergic blockade may mask certain clinical signs (e.g., tachycardia) of hyperthyroidism. Patients suspected of developing thyrotoxicosis should be managed carefully to avoid abrupt withdrawal of beta blockade which might precipitate a thyroid storm.

PRECAUTIONS

General
Impaired Hepatic or Renal Function: Since BLOCADREN is partially metabolized in the liver and excreted mainly by the kidneys, dosage reductions may be necessary when hepatic and/or renal insufficiency is present.
Dosing in the Presence of Marked Renal Failure: Although the pharmacokinetics of BLOCADREN are not greatly altered by renal impairment, marked hypotensive responses have been seen in patients with marked renal impairment undergoing dialysis after 20 mg doses. Dosing in such patients should therefore be especially cautious.
Muscle Weakness: Beta-adrenergic blockade has been reported to potentiate muscle weakness consistent with certain myasthenic symptoms (e.g., diplopia, ptosis, and generalized weakness). Timolol has been reported rarely to increase muscle weakness in some patients with myasthenia gravis or myasthenic symptoms.
Cerebrovascular Insufficiency: Because of potential effects of beta-adrenergic blocking agents relative to blood pressure and pulse, these agents should be used with caution in patients with cerebrovascular insufficiency. If signs or symptoms suggesting reduced cerebral blood flow are observed, consideration should be given to discontinuing these agents.
Drug Interactions
Close observation of the patient is recommended when BLOCADREN is administered to patients receiving catecholamine-depleting drugs such as reserpine, because of possible additive effects and the production of hypotension and/or marked bradycardia, which may produce vertigo, syncope, or postural hypotension.
Blunting of the antihypertensive effect of beta-adrenoceptor blocking agents by non-steroidal anti-inflammatory drugs has been reported. When using these agents concomitantly, patients should be observed carefully to confirm that the desired therapeutic effect has been obtained.
Literature reports suggest that oral calcium antagonists may be used in combination with beta-adrenergic blocking agents when heart function is normal, but should be avoided in patients with impaired cardiac function. Hypotension, AV conduction disturbances, and left ventricular failure have been reported in some patients receiving beta-adrenergic blocking agents when an oral calcium antagonist was added to the treatment regimen. Hypotension was more likely to occur if the calcium antagonist were a dihydropyridine derivative, e.g. nifedipine, while left ventricular failure and AV conduction disturbances were more likely to occur with either verapamil or diltiazem.
Intravenous calcium antagonists should be used with caution in patients receiving beta-adrenergic blocking agents.
The concomitant use of beta-adrenergic blocking agents with digitalis and either diltiazem or verapamil may have additive effects in prolonging AV conduction time.
Risk from Anaphylactic Reaction: While taking beta-blockers, patients with a history of atopy or a history of severe anaphylactic reaction to a variety of allergens may be more reactive to repeated accidental, diagnostic, or therapeutic challenge with such allergens. Such patients may be unresponsive to the usual doses of epinephrine used to treat anaphylactic reactions.

Continued on next page

Information on the Merck & Co., Inc. products listed on these pages is the full prescribing information from product circulars in use September 30, 1996.

Merck & Co.—Cont.

Carcinogenesis, Mutagenesis, Impairment of Fertility
In a two-year study of timolol maleate in rats, there was a statistically significant increase in the incidence of adrenal pheochromocytomas in male rats administered 300 mg/kg/day (250 times* the maximum recommended human dose). Similar differences were not observed in rats administered doses equivalent to approximately 20 or 80 times* the maximum recommended human dose.

In a lifetime study in mice, there were statistically significant increases in the incidence of benign and malignant pulmonary tumors, benign uterine polyps and mammary adenocarcinoma in female mice at 500 mg/kg/day (approximately 400 times* the maximum recommended human dose), but not at 5 or 50 mg/kg/day. In a subsequent study in female mice, in which post-mortem examinations were limited to uterus and lungs, a statistically significant increase in the incidence of pulmonary tumors was again observed at 500 mg/kg/day.

The increased occurrence of mammary adenocarcinoma was associated with elevations in serum prolactin that occurred in female mice administered timolol at 500 mg/kg/day, but not at doses of 5 or 50 mg/kg/day. An increased incidence of mammary adenocarcinomas in rodents has been associated with administration of several other therapeutic agents which elevate serum prolactin, but no correlation between serum prolactin levels and mammary tumors has been established in man. Furthermore, in adult human female subjects who received oral dosages of up to 60 mg of timolol maleate, the maximum recommended human oral dosage, there were no clinically meaningful changes in serum prolactin.

Timolol maleate was devoid of mutagenic potential when evaluated *in vivo* (mouse) in the micronucleus test and cytogenetic assay (doses up to 800 mg/kg) and *in vitro* in a neoplastic cell transformation assay (up to 100 μg/mL). In Ames tests the highest concentrations of timolol employed, 5000 or 10,000 μg/plate, were associated with statistically significant elevations of revertants observed with tester strain TA100 (in seven replicate assays), but not in three additional strains. In the assays with tester strain TA100, no consistent dose response relationship was observed, nor did the ratio of test to control revertants reach 2. A ratio of 2 is usually considered the criterion for a positive Ames test. Reproduction and fertility studies in rats showed no adverse effect on male or female fertility at doses up to 125 times* the maximum recommended human dose.

---

* Based on patient weight of 50 kg
Pregnancy
Pregnancy Category C. Teratogenicity studies with timolol in mice, rats and rabbits at doses up to 50 mg/kg/day (approximately 40 times* the maximum recommended daily human dose) showed no evidence of fetal malformations. Although delayed fetal ossification was observed at this dose in rats, there were no adverse effects on postnatal development of offspring. Doses of 1000 mg/kg/day (approximately 830 times* the maximum recommended daily human dose) were maternotoxic in mice and resulted in an increased number of fetal resorptions. Increased fetal resorptions were also seen in rabbits at doses of approximately 40 times* the maximum recommended daily human dose, in this case without apparent maternotoxicity. There are no adequate and well-controlled studies in pregnant women. BLOCADREN should be used during pregnancy only if the potential benefit justifies the potential risk to the fetus.

---

* Based on patient weight of 50 kg
Nursing Mothers
Timolol maleate has been detected in human milk. Because of the potential for serious adverse reactions from timolol in nursing infants, a decision should be made whether to discontinue nursing or to discontinue the drug, taking into account the importance of the drug to the mother.
Pediatric Use
Safety and effectiveness in pediatric patients have not been established.

ADVERSE REACTIONS

BLOCADREN is usually well tolerated in properly selected patients. Most adverse effects have been mild and transient. In a multicenter (12-week) clinical trial comparing timolol maleate and placebo in hypertensive patients, the following adverse reactions were reported spontaneously and considered to be causally related to timolol maleate:

	Timolol Maleate (n = 176) %	Placebo (n = 168) %
BODY AS A WHOLE		
fatigue/tiredness	3.4	0.6
headache	1.7	1.8
chest pain	0.6	0
asthenia	0.6	0
CARDIOVASCULAR		
bradycardia	9.1	0
arrhythmia	1.1	0.6
syncope	0.6	0
edema	0.6	1.2
DIGESTIVE		
dyspepsia	0.6	0.6
nausea	0.6	0
SKIN		
pruritus	1.1	0
NERVOUS SYSTEM		
dizziness	2.3	1.2
vertigo	0.6	0
paresthesia	0.6	0
PSYCHIATRIC		
decreased libido	0.6	0
RESPIRATORY		
dyspnea	1.7	0.6
bronchial spasm	0.6	0
rales	0.6	0
SPECIAL SENSES		
eye irritation	1.1	0.6
tinnitus	0.6	0

These data are representative of the incidence of adverse effects that may be observed in properly selected patients treated with BLOCADREN, i.e., excluding patients with bronchospastic disease, congestive heart failure or other contraindications to beta blocker therapy.

In patients with migraine the incidence of bradycardia was 5 percent.

In a coronary artery disease population studied in the Norwegian multi-center trial (see CLINICAL PHARMACOLOGY), the frequency of the principal adverse reactions and the frequency with which these resulted in discontinuation of therapy in the timolol and placebo groups were:
[See table below.]

The following additional adverse effects have been reported in clinical experience with the drug: *Body as a Whole:* extremity pain, decreased exercise tolerance, weight loss, fever; *Cardiovascular:* cardiac arrest, cardiac failure, cerebrovascular accident, worsening of angina pectoris, worsening of arterial insufficiency, Raynaud's phenomenon, palpitations, vasodilatation; *Digestive:* gastrointestinal pain, hepatomegaly, vomiting, diarrhea, dyspepsia; *Hematologic:* nonthrombocytopenic purpura; *Endocrine:* hyperglycemia, hypoglycemia; *Skin:* rash, skin irritation, increased pigmentation, sweating, alopecia; *Musculoskeletal:* arthralgia; *Nervous System:* local weakness, increase in signs and symptoms of myasthenia gravis; *Psychiatric:* depression, nightmares, somnolence, insomnia, nervousness, diminished concentration, hallucinations; *Respiratory:* cough; *Special Senses:* visual disturbances, diplopia, ptosis, dry eyes; *Urogenital:* impotence, urination difficulties.

There have been reports of retroperitoneal fibrosis in patients receiving timolol maleate and in patients receiving other beta-adrenergic blocking agents. A causal relationship between this condition and therapy with beta-adrenergic blocking agents has not been established.

Potential Adverse Effects: In addition, a variety of adverse effects not observed in clinical trials with BLOCADREN, but reported with other beta-adrenergic blocking agents, should be considered potential adverse effects of BLOCADREN: *Nervous System:* Reversible mental depression progressing to catatonia; an acute reversible syndrome characterized by disorientation for time and place, short-term memory loss, emotional lability, slightly clouded sensorium, and decreased performance on neuropsychometrics; *Cardiovascular:* Intensification of AV block (see CONTRAINDICATIONS); *Digestive:* Mesenteric arterial thrombosis, ischemic colitis; *Hematologic:* Agranulocytosis, thrombocytopenic purpura; *Allergic:* Erythematous rash, fever combined with aching and sore throat, laryngospasm with respiratory distress; *Miscellaneous:* Peyronie's disease.

There have been reports of a syndrome comprising psoriasiform skin rash, conjunctivitis sicca, otitis, and sclerosing serositis attributed to the beta-adrenergic receptor blocking agent, practolol. This syndrome has not been reported with BLOCADREN.

Clinical Laboratory Test Findings: Clinically important changes in standard laboratory parameters were rarely associated with the administration of BLOCADREN. Slight increases in blood urea nitrogen, serum potassium, uric acid, and triglycerides, and slight decreases in hemoglobin, hematocrit and HDL cholesterol occurred, but were not progressive or associated with clinical manifestations. Increases in liver function tests have been reported.

OVERDOSAGE

Overdosage has been reported with Tablets BLOCADREN. A 30-year-old female ingested 650 mg of BLOCADREN (maximum recommended daily dose—60 mg) and experienced second and third degree heart block. She recovered without treatment but approximately two months later developed irregular heartbeat, hypertension, dizziness, tinnitus, faintness, increased pulse rate and borderline first degree heart block.

The oral LD_{50} of the drug is 1190 and 900 mg/kg in female mice and female rats, respectively.

An *in vitro* hemodialysis study, using ^{14}C timolol added to human plasma or whole blood, showed that timolol was readily dialyzed from these fluids; however, a study of patients with renal failure showed that timolol did not dialyze readily.

The most common signs and symptoms to be expected with overdosage with a beta-adrenergic receptor blocking agent are symptomatic bradycardia, hypotension, bronchospasm, and acute cardiac failure. Therapy with BLOCADREN should be discontinued and the patient observed closely. The following additional therapeutic measures should be considered:

(1) *Gastric lavage*

(2) *Symptomatic bradycardia:* Use atropine sulfate intravenously in a dosage of 0.25 mg to 2 mg to induce vagal blockade. If bradycardia persists, intravenous isoproterenol hydrochloride should be administered cautiously. In refractory cases the use of a transvenous cardiac pacemaker may be considered.

(3) *Hypotension:* Use sympathomimetic pressor drug therapy, such as dopamine, dobutamine or levarterenol. In refractory cases the use of glucagon hydrochloride has been reported to be useful.

(4) *Bronchospasm:* Use isoproterenol hydrochloride. Additional therapy with aminophylline may be considered.

(5) *Acute cardiac failure:* Conventional therapy with digitalis, diuretics, and oxygen should be instituted immediately. In refractory cases the use of intravenous aminophylline is suggested. This may be followed if necessary by glucagon hydrochloride which has been reported to be useful.

(6) *Heart block (second or third degree):* Use isoproterenol hydrochloride or a transvenous cardiac pacemaker.

DOSAGE AND ADMINISTRATION

Hypertension
The usual initial dosage of BLOCADREN is 10 mg twice a day, whether used alone or added to diuretic therapy. Dosage may be increased or decreased depending on heart rate and blood pressure response. The usual total maintenance dosage is 20–40 mg per day. Increases in dosage to a maximum of 60 mg per day divided into two doses may be necessary.

BLOCADREN	Adverse Reaction†		Withdrawal‡	
	Timolol (n = 945) %	Placebo (n = 939) %	Timolol (n = 945) %	Placebo (n = 939) %
Asthenia or Fatigue	5	1	<1	<1
Heart Rate <40 beats/minute	5	<1	4	<1
Cardiac Failure—Nonfatal	8	7	3	2
Hypotension	3	2	3	1
Pulmonary Edema—Nonfatal	2	<1	<1	<1
Claudication	3	3	1	<1
AV Block 2nd or 3rd degree	<1	<1	<1	<1
Sinoatrial Block	<1	<1	<1	<1
Cold Hands and Feet	8	<1	<1	0
Nausea or Digestive Disorders	8	6	1	<1
Dizziness	6	4	1	0
Bronchial Obstruction	2	<1	1	<1

† When an adverse reaction recurred in a patient, it is listed only once.
‡ Only principal reason for withdrawal in each patient is listed.
These adverse reactions can also occur in patients treated for hypertension.

There should be an interval of at least seven days between increases in dosages.

BLOCADREN may be used with a thiazide diuretic or with other antihypertensive agents. Patients should be observed carefully during initiation of such concomitant therapy.

Myocardial Infarction

The recommended dosage for long-term prophylactic use in patients who have survived the acute phase of a myocardial infarction is 10 mg given twice daily (see CLINICAL PHARMACOLOGY).

Migraine

The usual initial dosage of BLOCADREN is 10 mg twice a day. During maintenance therapy the 20 mg daily dosage may be administered as a single dose. Total daily dosage may be increased to a maximum of 30 mg, given in divided doses, or decreased to 10 mg once per day, depending on clinical response and tolerability. If a satisfactory response is not obtained after 6-8 weeks use of the maximum daily dosage, therapy with BLOCADREN should be discontinued.

HOW SUPPLIED

No. 3343—Tablets BLOCADREN, 5 mg, are light blue, round, compressed tablets, with code MSD 59 on one side and BLOCADREN on the other. They are supplied as follows:
  NDC 0006-0059-68 bottles of 100.
    Shown in Product Identification Guide, page 324
No. 3344—Tablets BLOCADREN, 10 mg, are light blue, round, scored, compressed tablets, with code MSD 136 on one side and BLOCADREN on the other. They are supplied as follows:
  NDC 0006-0136-68 bottles of 100
  (6505-01-132-0651, 10 mg 100's)
  NDC 0006-0136-28 unit dose packages of 100.
    Shown in Product Identification Guide, page 324
No. 3371—Tablets BLOCADREN, 20 mg, are light blue, capsule shaped, scored, compressed tablets, with code MSD 437 on one side and BLOCADREN on the other. They are supplied as follows:
  NDC 0006-0437-68 bottles of 100
  (6505-01-132-0652, 20 mg 100's).
    Shown in Product Identification Guide, page 324
Storage
Store at controlled room temperature. 15–30°C (59–86°F). Keep container tightly closed. Protect from light.
        7901230   Issued May 1995
COPYRIGHT © MERCK & CO., INC., 1985
All rights reserved

CHIBROXIN®   ℞
(Norfloxacin)
Sterile Ophthalmic Solution

DESCRIPTION

CHIBROXIN* (Norfloxacin) Ophthalmic Solution is a synthetic broad-spectrum antibacterial agent supplied as a sterile isotonic solution for topical ophthalmic use. Norfloxacin, a fluoroquinolone, is 1-ethyl-6-fluoro-1,4-dihydro-4-oxo-7-(1-piperazinyl)-3-quinoline-carboxylic acid. Its empirical formula is $C_{16}H_{18}FN_3O_3$ and the structural formula is:

Norfloxacin is a white to pale yellow crystalline powder with a molecular weight of 319.34 and a melting point of about 221°C. It is freely soluble in glacial acetic acid and very slightly soluble in ethanol, methanol and water.
CHIBROXIN Ophthalmic Solution 0.3% is supplied as a sterile isotonic solution. Each mL contains 3 mg norfloxacin. Inactive ingredients: disodium edetate, sodium acetate, sodium chloride, hydrochloric acid (to adjust pH) and water for injection, Benzalkonium chloride 0.0025% is added as preservative. The pH of CHIBROXIN is approximately 5.2 and the osmolarity is approximately 285 mOsmol/liter.
Norfloxacin, a fluoroquinolone, differs from quinolones by having a fluorine atom at the 6 position and a piperazine moiety at the 7 position.

*Registered trademark of MERCK & CO., INC.

CLINICAL PHARMACOLOGY

Microbiology
Norfloxacin has *in vitro* activity against a broad spectrum of gram-positive and gram-negative aerobic bacteria. The fluorine atom at the 6 position provides increased potency against gram-negative organisms and the piperazine moiety at the 7 position is responsible for anti-pseudomonal activity.

Norfloxacin inhibits bacterial deoxyribonucleic acid synthesis and is bactericidal. At the molecular level three specific events are attributed to CHIBROXIN in *E. coli* cells:
1) inhibition of the ATP-dependent DNA supercoiling reaction catalyzed by DNA gyrase;
2) inhibition of the relaxation of supercoiled DNA;
3) promotion of double-stranded DNA breakage.
There is generally no cross-resistance between norfloxacin and other classes of antibacterial agents. Therefore, norfloxacin generally demonstrates activity against indicated organisms resistant to some other antimicrobial agents. When such cross-resistance does occur, it is probably due to decreased entry of the drugs into the bacterial cells. Antagonism has been demonstrated *in vitro* between norfloxacin and nitrofurantoin.
Norfloxacin has been shown to be active against most strains of the following organisms both *in vitro* and clinically in ophthalmic infections (see INDICATIONS AND USAGE):
Gram-positive bacteria including:
  Staphylococcus aureus
  Staphylococcus epidermidis
  Staphylococcus warnerii
  Streptococcus pneumoniae
Gram-negative bacteria including:
  Acinetobacter calcoaceticus
  Aeromonas hydrophila
  Haemophilus influenzae
  Proteus mirabilis
  Pseudomonas aeruginosa
  Serratia marcescens
Norfloxacin has been shown to be active *in vitro* against most strains of the following organisms; however, *the clinical significance of these data in ophthalmic infections is unknown.*
Gram-positive bacteria:
  Bacillus cereus
  Enterococcus faecalis (formerly *Streptococcus faecalis*)
  Staphylococcus saprophyticus
Gram-negative bacteria:
  Citrobacter diversus
  Citrobacter freundii
  Edwardsiella tarda
  Enterobacter aerogenes
  Enterobacter cloacae
  Escherichia coli
  Hafnia alvei
  Haemophilus aegyptius (Koch-Weeks bacillus)
  Klebsiella oxytoca
  Klebsiella pneumoniae
  Klebsiella rhinoscleromatis
  Morganella morganii
  Neisseria gonorrhoeae
  Proteus vulgaris
  Providencia alcalifaciens
  Providencia rettgeri
  Providencia stuartii
  Salmonella typhi
  Vibrio cholerae
  Vibrio parahemolyticus
  Yersinia enterocolitica
Other:
  Ureaplasma urealyticum
Norfloxacin is not active against obligate anaerobes.
Clinical Studies
Clinical studies were conducted comparing CHIBROXIN Ophthalmic Solution (n=152) with ophthalmic solutions of tobramycin, gentamicin, and chloramphenicol (n=158) in patients with conjunctivitis and positive bacterial cultures. After seven days of therapy with CHIBROXIN Ophthalmic Solution, 72 percent of patients were clinically cured. Of those cured, 85 percent had all their pathogens eradicated. Eradication was also achieved in 62 percent (23/37) of patients whose clinical outcome was not completely cured by day seven. These results were similar among all treatment groups.
Another clinical study compared CHIBROXIN Ophthalmic Solution with placebo in patients with conjunctivitis and positive bacterial cultures. Placebo in this study was the liquid vehicle for CHIBROXIN Ophthalmic Solution and the preservative. After five days of therapy, 64 percent (36/56) of patients on CHIBROXIN Ophthalmic Solution were clinically cured compared to 50 percent (23/46) of patients receiving placebo. Of those cured, 78 percent had all their pathogens eradicated. Eradication was also achieved in 50 percent (10/20) of patients whose clinical outcome was not completely cured. The response to CHIBROXIN Ophthalmic Solution was statistically significantly better than the response to placebo.

INDICATIONS AND USAGE

CHIBROXIN Ophthalmic Solution is indicated for the treatment of conjunctivitis when caused by susceptible strains of the following bacteria:

  Acinetobacter calcoaceticus *
  Aeromonas hydrophila *
  Haemophilus influenzae
  Proteus mirabilis *
  Pseudomonas aeruginosa *
  Serratia marcescens *
  Staphylococcus aureus
  Staphylococcus epidermidis
  Staphylococcus warnerii *
  Streptococcus pneumoniae
Appropriate monitoring of bacterial response to topical antibiotic therapy should accompany the use of CHIBROXIN Ophthalmic Solution.

---

* Efficacy for this organism was studied in fewer than 10 infections.

CONTRAINDICATIONS

CHIBROXIN Ophthalmic Solution is contraindicated in patients with a history of hypersensitivity to norfloxacin, or the other members of the quinolone group of antibacterial agents or any other component of this medication.

WARNINGS

NOT FOR INJECTION INTO THE EYE.
Serious and occasionally fatal hypersensitivity (anaphylactoid or anaphylactic) reactions, some following the first dose, have been reported in patients receiving systemic quinolone therapy. Some reactions were accompanied by cardiovascular collapse, loss of consciousness, tingling, pharyngeal or facial edema, dyspnea, urticaria, and itching. Only a few patients had a history of hypersensitivity reactions. Serious anaphylactoid or anaphylactic reactions require immediate emergency treatment with epinephrine. Oxygen, intravenous steroids and airway management, including intubation, should be administered as indicated.

PRECAUTIONS

General
As with other antibiotic preparations, prolonged use may result in overgrowth of nonsusceptible organisms, including fungi. If superinfection occurs, appropriate measures should be initiated. Whenever clinical judgment dictates, the patient should be examined with the aid of magnification, such as slit lamp biomicroscopy and, where appropriate, fluorescein staining.
Information For Patients
Patients should be instructed to avoid allowing the tip of the dispensing container to contact the eye or surrounding structures.
Patients should be advised that norfloxacin may be associated with hypersensitivity reactions, even following a single dose, and to discontinue the drug at the first sign of a skin rash or other allergic reaction.
Patients being treated for bacterial conjunctivitis generally should not wear contact lenses. However, if the physician considers the use of contact lenses appropriate, patients should be instructed to wait at least 15 minutes after instilling CHIBROXIN Ophthalmic Solution before inserting their lenses because the preservative in CHIBROXIN Ophthalmic Solution, benzalkonium chloride, may be absorbed by contact lenses.
Drug Interactions
Specific drug interaction studies have not been conducted with norfloxacin ophthalmic solution. However, the systemic administration of some quinolones has been shown to elevate plasma concentrations of theophylline, interfere with the metabolism of caffeine, and enhance the effects of the oral anticoagulant warfarin and its derivatives. Elevated serum levels of cyclosporine have been reported with concomitant use of cyclosporine with norfloxacin. Therefore, cyclosporine serum levels should be monitored and appropriate cyclosporine dosage adjustments made when these drugs are used concomitantly.
Carcinogenesis, Mutagenesis, Impairment of Fertility
No increase in neoplastic changes was observed with norfloxacin as compared to controls in a study in rats, lasting up to 96 weeks at doses eight to nine times the usual human oral dose*.
Norfloxacin was tested for mutagenic activity in a number of *in vivo* and *in vitro* tests. Norfloxacin had no mutagenic effect in the dominant lethal test in mice and did not cause chromosomal aberrations in hamsters or rats at doses 30 to 60 times the usual oral dose*. Norfloxacin had no mutagenic activity *in vitro* in the Ames microbial mutagen test, Chinese

---

Continued on next page

Merck & Co.—Cont.

hamster fibroblasts and V-79 mammalian cell assay. Although norfloxacin was weakly positive in the Rec-assay for DNA repair, all other mutagenic assays were negative including a more sensitive test (V-79).
Norfloxacin did not adversely affect the fertility of male and female mice at oral doses up to 33 times the usual human oral dose*.
Pregnancy
Pregnancy Category C: Norfloxacin has been shown to produce embryonic loss in monkeys when given in doses 10 times the maximum human oral dose* (400 mg b.i.d.), with peak plasma levels that are two to three times those obtained in humans. There has been no evidence of a teratogenic effect in any of the animal species tested (rat, rabbit, mouse, monkey) at 6 to 50 times the human oral dose. There are no adequate and well-controlled studies in pregnant women. CHIBROXIN Ophthalmic Solution should be used during pregnancy only if the potential benefit justifies the potential risk to the fetus.
Nursing Mothers
It is not known whether norfloxacin is excreted in human milk following ocular administration. Because many drugs are excreted in human milk, and because of the potential for serious adverse reactions in nursing infants from norfloxacin, a decision should be made to discontinue nursing or to discontinue the drug, taking into account the importance of the drug to the mother (see ANIMAL PHARMACOLOGY).
Pediatric Use
Safety and effectiveness in infants below the age of one year have not been established.
Although quinolones including norfloxacin have been shown to cause arthropathy in immature animals after oral administration, topical ocular administration of other quinolones to immature animals has not shown any arthropathy and there is no evidence that the ophthalmic dosage form of those quinolones has any effects on the weight-bearing joints.

* All factors are based on a standard patient weight of 50 kg. The usual oral dose of norfloxacin is 800 mg daily. One drop of CHIBROXIN Ophthalmic Solution 0.3% contains about 1/6,666 of this dose (0.12 mg).

ADVERSE REACTIONS

In clinical trials, the most frequently reported drug-related adverse reaction was local burning or discomfort. Other drug-related adverse reactions were conjunctival hyperemia, chemosis, photophobia and a bitter taste following instillation.

DOSAGE AND ADMINISTRATION

The recommended dose in adults and pediatric patients (one year and older) is one or two drops of CHIBROXIN Ophthalmic Solution applied topically to the affected eye(s) four times daily for up to seven days. Depending on the severity of the infection, the dosage for the first day of therapy may be one or two drops every two hours during the waking hours.

HOW SUPPLIED

CHIBROXIN Ophthalmic Solution is a clear, colorless to light yellow solution.
No. 3526—CHIBROXIN Ophthalmic Solution 0.3% is supplied in a white, opaque, plastic OCUMETER* ophthalmic dispenser with a controlled drop tip as follows:
NDC 0006-3526-03, 5 mL.
Storage
Store CHIBROXIN Ophthalmic Solution at room temperature, 15°-30°C (59°-86°F). Protect from light.

*Registered trademark of MERCK & CO., INC.

ANIMAL PHARMACOLOGY

The oral administration of single doses of norfloxacin, six times the recommended human oral dose**, caused lameness in immature dogs. Histologic examination of the weight-bearing joints of these dogs revealed permanent lesions of the cartilage. Related drugs also produced erosions of the cartilage in weight-bearing joints and other signs of arthropathy in immature animals of various species.

** All factors are based on a standard patient weight of 50 kg. The usual oral dose of norfloxacin is 800 mg daily. One drop of CHIBROXIN Ophthalmic Solution 0.3% contains about 1/6,666 of this dose (0.12 mg).

ADDITIONAL CAUTIONARY INFORMATION

Norfloxacin is available as an oral dosage form in addition to the ophthalmic dosage form. The following adverse effects, while they have not been reported with the ophthalmic dosage form, have been reported with the oral dosage form. However, it should be noted that the usual dosage of oral norfloxacin (800 mg/day) contains 6,666 times the amount in one drop of CHIBROXIN Ophthalmic Solution 0.3% (0.12 mg).
Convulsions have been reported in patients receiving oral norfloxacin. Convulsions, increased intracranial pressure, and toxic psychoses have been reported with other drugs in this class. Orally administered quinolones may also cause central nervous system (CNS) stimulation which may lead to tremors, restlessness, lightheadedness, confusion and hallucinations. If these reactions occur in patients receiving norfloxacin, the drug should be discontinued and appropriate measures instituted.
The effects of norfloxacin on brain function or on the electrical activity of the brain have not been tested. Therefore, as with all quinolones, norfloxacin should be used with caution in patients with known or suspected CNS disorders, such as severe cerebral arteriosclerosis, epilepsy, and other factors which predispose to seizures.
The following adverse effects have been reported with Tablets NOROXIN* (Norfloxacin). *Hypersensitivity Reactions:* Hypersensitivity reactions including anaphylactoid reactions, angioedema, dyspnea, vasculitis, urticaria, arthritis, arthralgia, myalgia; *Gastrointestinal:* Pseudomembranous colitis, hepatitis, jaundice, including cholestatic jaundice, pancreatitis; *Hematologic:* Neutropenia, leukopenia, thrombocytopenia; *Nervous System/Psychiatric:* CNS effects characterized as generalized seizures and myoclonus; neurological changes such as ataxia, diplopia and possible exacerbation of myasthenia gravis; psychic disturbances including psychotic reactions and confusion, depression; *Renal:* Interstitial nephritis, renal failure; *Skin:* Toxic epidermal necrolysis, Stevens-Johnson syndrome and erythema multiforme, exfoliative dermatitis, rash, photosensitivity; *Special Senses:* Transient hearing loss.
Abnormal laboratory values observed with oral norfloxacin included elevation of ALT (SGPT) and AST (SGOT), alkaline phosphatase, BUN, serum creatinine, and LDH.
Please consult the package circular for Tablets NOROXIN (Norfloxacin) for additional information concerning these and other adverse effects and other cautionary information.

* Registered trademark of MERCK & CO., INC.
DC 7679104 Issued June 1993

CLINORIL® Tablets (Sulindac), U.S.P. ℞

DESCRIPTION

Sulindac is a non-steroidal, anti-inflammatory indene derivative designated chemically as (Z)-5-fluoro-2-methyl-1-[[*p*-(methylsulfinyl) phenyl]methylene]-1*H*-indene-3-acetic acid. It is not a salicylate, pyrazolone or propionic acid derivative. Its empirical formula is $C_{20}H_{17}FO_3S$, with a molecular weight of 356.42. Sulindac, a yellow crystalline compound, is a weak organic acid practically insoluble in water below pH 4.5, but very soluble as the sodium salt or in buffers of pH 6 or higher.
CLINORIL* (Sulindac) is available in 150 and 200 mg tablets for oral administration. Each tablet contains the following inactive ingredients: cellulose, magnesium stearate, starch.
Following absorption, sulindac undergoes two major biotransformations—reversible reduction to the sulfide metabolite, and irreversible oxidation to the sulfone metabolite. Available evidence indicates that the biological activity resides with the sulfide metabolite.
The structural formulas of sulindac and its metabolites are: [See chemical structures at top of next column.]

* Registered trademark of MERCK & CO., INC.

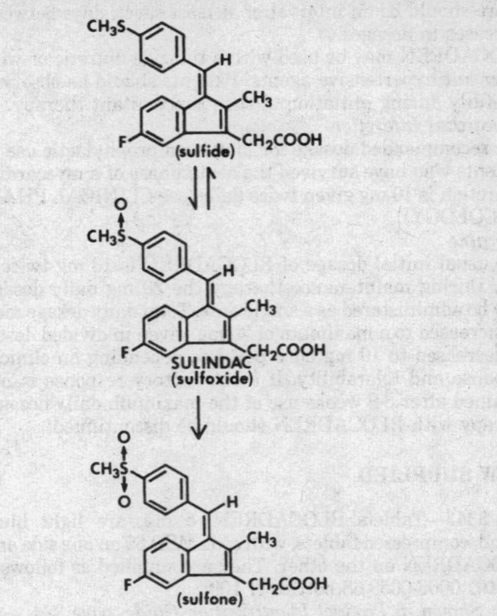

CLINICAL PHARMACOLOGY

CLINORIL is a non-steroidal anti-inflammatory drug, also possessing analgesic and antipyretic activities. Its mode of action, like that of other non-steroidal, anti-inflammatory agents, is not known; however, its therapeutic action is not due to pituitary-adrenal stimulation. Inhibition of prostaglandin synthesis by the sulfide metabolite may be involved in the anti-inflammatory action of CLINORIL.
Sulindac is approximately 90% absorbed in man after oral administration. The peak plasma concentrations of the biologically active sulfide metabolite are achieved in about two hours when sulindac is administered in the fasting state, and in about three to four hours when sulindac is administered with food. The mean half-life of sulindac is 7.8 hours while the mean half-life of the sulfide metabolite is 16.4 hours. Sustained plasma levels of the sulfide metabolite are consistent with a prolonged anti-inflammatory action which is the rationale for a twice per day dosage schedule.
Sulindac and its sulfone metabolite undergo extensive enterohepatic circulation relative to the sulfide metabolite in animals. Studies in man have also demonstrated that recirculation of the parent drug, sulindac, and its sulfone metabolite, is more extensive than that of the active sulfide metabolite. The active sulfide metabolite accounts for less than six percent of the total intestinal exposure to sulindac and its metabolites.
The primary route of excretion in man is via the urine as both sulindac and its sulfone metabolite (free and glucuronide conjugates). Approximately 50% of the administered dose is excreted in the urine, with the conjugated sulfone metabolite accounting for the major portion. Less than 1% of the administered dose of sulindac appears in the urine as the sulfide metabolite. Approximately 25% is found in the feces, primarily as the sulfone and sulfide metabolites.
The bioavailability of sulindac, as assessed by urinary excretion, was not changed by concomitant administration of an antacid containing magnesium hydroxide 200 mg and aluminum hydroxide 225 mg per 5 mL.
Because CLINORIL is excreted in the urine primarily as biologically inactive forms, it may possibly affect renal function to a lesser extent than other non-steroidal anti-inflammatory drugs, however, renal adverse experiences have been reported with CLINORIL (see ADVERSE REACTIONS). In a study of patients with chronic glomerular disease treated with therapeutic doses of CLINORIL, no effect was demonstrated on renal blood flow, glomerular filtration rate, or urinary excretion of prostaglandin E_2 and the primary metabolite of prostacyclin, 6-keto-$PGF_1\alpha$. However, in other studies in healthy volunteers and patients with liver disease, CLINORIL was found to blunt the renal responses to intravenous furosemide, i.e., the diuresis, natriuresis, increments in plasma renin activity and urinary excretion of prostaglandins. These observations may represent a differentiation of the effects of CLINORIL on renal functions based on differences in pathogenesis of the renal prostaglandin dependence associated with differing dose-response relationships of different NSAIDs to the various renal functions influenced by prostaglandins. These observations need further clarification and in the interim, sulindac should be used with caution in patients whose renal function may be impaired (see PRECAUTIONS).
In healthy men, the average fecal blood loss, measured over a two-week period during administration of 400 mg per day of CLINORIL, was similar to that for placebo, and was statistically significantly less than that resulting from 4800 mg per day of aspirin.
In controlled clinical studies CLINORIL was evaluated in the following five conditions:
1. *Osteoarthritis*
In patients with osteoarthritis of the hip and knee, the anti-inflammatory and analgesic activity of CLINORIL was demonstrated by clinical measurements that included: assessments by both patient and investigator of overall response; decrease in disease activity as assessed by both patient and investigator; improvement in ARA Functional Class; relief of night pain; improvement in overall evaluation of pain, including pain on weight bearing and pain on active and passive motion; improvement in joint mobility, range of motion, and functional activities; decreased swelling and tenderness; and decreased duration of stiffness following prolonged inactivity.
In clinical studies in which dosages were adjusted according to patient needs, CLINORIL 200 to 400 mg daily was shown to be comparable in effectiveness to aspirin 2400 to 4800 mg

daily. CLINORIL was generally well tolerated, and patients on it had a lower overall incidence of total adverse effects, of milder gastrointestinal reactions, and of tinnitus than did patients on aspirin. (See ADVERSE REACTIONS.)

2. *Rheumatoid Arthritis*

In patients with rheumatoid arthritis, the anti-inflammatory and analgesic activity of CLINORIL was demonstrated by clinical measurements that included: assessments by both patient and investigator of overall response; decrease in disease activity as assessed by both patient and investigator; reduction in overall joint pain; reduction in duration and severity of morning stiffness; reduction in day and night pain; decrease in time required to walk 50 feet; decrease in general pain as measured on a visual analog scale; improvement in the Ritchie articular index; decrease in proximal interphalangeal joint size; improvement in ARA Functional Class; increase in grip strength; reduction in painful joint count and score; reduction in swollen joint count and score; and increased flexion and extension of the wrist.

In clinical studies in which dosages were adjusted according to patient needs, CLINORIL 300 to 400 mg daily was shown to be comparable in effectiveness to aspirin 3600 to 4800 mg daily. CLINORIL was generally well tolerated, and patients on it had a lower overall incidence of total adverse effects, of milder gastrointestinal reactions, and of tinnitus than did patients on aspirin. (See ADVERSE REACTIONS.)

In patients with rheumatoid arthritis, CLINORIL may be used in combination with gold salts at usual dosage levels. In clinical studies, CLINORIL added to the regimen of gold salts usually resulted in additional symptomatic relief but did not alter the course of the underlying disease.

3. *Ankylosing spondylitis*

In patients with ankylosing spondylitis, the anti-inflammatory and analgesic activity of CLINORIL was demonstrated by clinical measurements that included: assessments by both patient and investigator of overall response; decrease in disease activity as assessed by both patient and investigator; improvement in ARA Functional Class; improvement in patient and investigator evaluation of spinal pain, tenderness and/or spasm; reduction in the duration of morning stiffness; increase in the time to onset of fatigue; relief of night pain; increase in chest expansion; and increase in spinal mobility evaluated by fingers-to-floor distance, occiput to wall distance, the Schober Test, and the Wright Modification of the Schober Test. In a clinical study in which dosages were adjusted according to patient need, CLINORIL 200 to 400 mg daily was as effective as indomethacin 75 to 150 mg daily. In a second study, CLINORIL 300 to 400 mg daily was comparable in effectiveness to phenylbutazone 400 to 600 mg daily. CLINORIL was better tolerated than phenylbutazone. (See ADVERSE REACTIONS.)

4. *Acute painful shoulder (Acute subacromial bursitis/ supraspinatus tendinitis)*

In patients with acute painful shoulder (acute subacromial bursitis/supraspinatus tendinitis), the anti-inflammatory and analgesic activity of CLINORIL was demonstrated by clinical measurements that included: assessments by both patient and investigator of overall response; relief of night pain, spontaneous pain, and pain on active motion; decrease in local tenderness; and improvement in range of motion measured by abduction, and internal and external rotation. In clinical studies in acute painful shoulder, CLINORIL 300 to 400 mg daily and oxyphenbutazone 400 to 600 mg daily were shown to be equally effective and well tolerated.

5. *Acute gouty arthritis*

In patients with acute gouty arthritis, the anti-inflammatory and analgesic activity of CLINORIL was demonstrated by clinical measurements that included: assessments by both the patient and investigator of overall response; relief of weight-bearing pain; relief of pain at rest and on active and passive motion; decrease in tenderness; reduction in warmth and swelling; increase in range of motion; and improvement in ability to function. In clinical studies, CLINORIL at 400 mg daily and phenylbutazone at 600 mg daily were shown to be equally effective. In these short-term studies in which reduction of dosage was permitted according to response, both drugs were equally well tolerated.

INDICATIONS AND USAGE

CLINORIL is indicated for acute or long-term use in the relief of signs and symptoms of the following:
1. Osteoarthritis
2. Rheumatoid arthritis*
3. Ankylosing spondylitis
4. Acute painful shoulder (Acute subacromial bursitis/ supraspinatus tendinitis)
5. Acute gouty arthritis

---

*The safety and effectiveness of CLINORIL have not been established in rheumatoid arthritis patients who are designated in the American Rheumatism Association classification as Functional Class IV (incapacitated, largely or wholly bedridden, or confined to wheelchair; little or no self-care).

CONTRAINDICATIONS

CLINORIL should not be used in:
Patients who are hypersensitive to this product.
Patients in whom acute asthmatic attacks, urticaria, or rhinitis are precipitated by aspirin or other non-steroidal anti-inflammatory agents.

WARNINGS

Gastrointestinal Effects

Peptic ulceration and gastrointestinal bleeding have been reported in patients receiving CLINORIL. Fatalities have occurred. Gastrointestinal bleeding is associated with higher morbidity and mortality in patients acutely ill with other conditions, the elderly and patients with hemorrhagic disorders. In patients with active gastrointestinal bleeding or an active peptic ulcer, an appropriate ulcer regimen should be instituted, and the physician must weigh the benefits of therapy with CLINORIL against possible hazards, and carefully monitor the patient's progress. When CLINORIL is given to patients with a history of either upper or lower gastrointestinal tract disease, it should be given under close supervision and only after consulting the ADVERSE REACTIONS section.

Risk of GI Ulcerations, Bleeding and Perforation with NSAID Therapy

Serious gastrointestinal toxicity such as bleeding, ulceration, and perforation, can occur at any time, with or without warning symptoms, in patients treated chronically with NSAID therapy. Although minor upper gastrointestinal problems, such as dyspepsia, are common, usually developing early in therapy, physicians should remain alert for ulceration and bleeding in patients treated chronically with NSAIDs even in the absence of previous GI tract symptoms. In patients observed in clinical trials of several months to two years duration, symptomatic upper GI ulcers, gross bleeding or perforation appear to occur in approximately 1% of patients treated for 3-6 months, and in about 2-4% of patients treated for one year. Physicians should inform patients about the signs and/or symptoms of serious GI toxicity and what steps to take if they occur.

Studies to date have not identified any subset of patients not at risk of developing peptic ulceration and bleeding. Except for a prior history of serious GI events and other risk factors known to be associated with peptic ulcer disease, such as alcoholism, smoking, etc., no risk factors (e.g., age, sex) have been associated with increased risk. Elderly or debilitated patients seem to tolerate ulceration or bleeding less well than other individuals and most spontaneous reports of fatal GI events are in this population. Studies to date are inconclusive concerning the relative risk of various NSAIDs in causing such reactions. High doses of any NSAID probably carry a greater risk of these reactions, although controlled clinical trials showing this do not exist in most cases. In considering the use of relatively large doses (within the recommended dosage range), sufficient benefit should be anticipated to offset the potential increased risk of GI toxicity.

Hypersensitivity

Rarely, fever and other evidence of hypersensitivity (see ADVERSE REACTIONS) including abnormalities in one or more liver function tests and severe skin reactions have occurred during therapy with CLINORIL. Fatalities have occurred in these patients. Hepatitis, jaundice, or both, with or without fever, may occur usually within the first one to three months of therapy. Determinations of liver function should be considered whenever a patient on therapy with CLINORIL develops unexplained fever, rash or other dermatologic reactions or constitutional symptoms. If unexplained fever or other evidence of hypersensitivity occurs, therapy with CLINORIL should be discontinued. The elevated temperature and abnormalities in liver function caused by CLINORIL characteristically have reverted to normal after discontinuation of therapy. Administration of CLINORIL should not be reinstituted in such patients.

Hepatic Effects

In addition to hypersensitivity reactions involving the liver, in some patients the findings are consistent with those of cholestatic hepatitis. As with other non-steroidal anti-inflammatory drugs, borderline elevations of one or more liver tests without any other signs and symptoms may occur in up to 15% of patients. These abnormalities may progress, may remain essentially unchanged, or may be transient with continued therapy. The SGPT (ALT) test is probably the most sensitive indicator of liver dysfunction. Meaningful (3 times the upper limit of normal) elevations of SGPT or SGOT (AST) occurred in controlled clinical trials in less than 1% of patients. A patient with symptoms and/or signs suggesting liver dysfunction, or in whom an abnormal liver test has occurred, should be evaluated for evidence of the development of more severe hepatic reaction while on therapy with CLINORIL. Although such reactions as described above are rare, if abnormal liver tests persist or worsen, if clinical signs and symptoms consistent with liver disease develop, or if

systemic manifestations occur (e.g. eosinophilia, rash, etc.), CLINORIL should be discontinued.

In clinical trials with CLINORIL, the use of doses of 600 mg/ day has been associated with an increased incidence of mild liver test abnormalities (see DOSAGE AND ADMINISTRATION for maximum dosage recommendation).

PRECAUTIONS

General

Non-steroidal anti-inflammatory drugs, including CLINORIL, may mask the usual signs and symptoms of infection. Therefore, the physician must be continually on the alert for this and should use the drug with extra care in the presence of existing infection.

Although CLINORIL has less effect on platelet function and bleeding time than aspirin, it is an inhibitor of platelet function; therefore, patients who may be adversely affected should be carefully observed when CLINORIL is administered.

Pancreatitis has been reported in patients receiving CLINORIL (see ADVERSE REACTIONS). Should pancreatitis be suspected, the drug should be discontinued and not restarted, supportive medical therapy instituted, and the patient monitored closely with appropriate laboratory studies (e.g., serum and urine amylase, amylase/creatinine clearance ratio, electrolytes, serum calcium, glucose, lipase, etc.). A search for other causes of pancreatitis as well as those conditions which mimic pancreatitis should be conducted.

Because of reports of adverse eye findings with non-steroidal anti-inflammatory agents, it is recommended that patients who develop eye complaints during treatment with CLINORIL have ophthalmologic studies.

In patients with poor liver function, delayed, elevated and prolonged circulating levels of the sulfide and sulfone metabolites may occur. Such patients should be monitored closely; a reduction of daily dosage may be required.

Edema has been observed in some patients taking CLINORIL. Therefore, as with other non-steroidal anti-inflammatory drugs, CLINORIL should be used with caution in patients with compromised cardiac function, hypertension, or other conditions predisposing to fluid retention.

CLINORIL may allow a reduction in dosage or the elimination of chronic corticosteroid therapy in some patients with rheumatoid arthritis. However, it is generally necessary to reduce corticosteroids gradually over several months in order to avoid an exacerbation of disease or signs and symptoms of adrenal insufficiency. Abrupt withdrawal of chronic corticosteroid treatment is generally not recommended even when patients have had a serious complication of chronic corticosteroid therapy.

Renal Effects

As with other non-steroidal anti-inflammatory drugs, long term administration of sulindac to animals has resulted in renal papillary necrosis and other abnormal renal pathology. In humans, there have been reports of acute interstitial nephritis with hematuria, proteinuria, and occasionally nephrotic syndrome.

A second form of renal toxicity has been seen in patients with prerenal and renal conditions leading to a reduction in renal blood flow or blood volume, where the renal prostaglandins have a supportive role in the maintenance of renal perfusion. In these patients administration of an NSAID may cause a dose dependent reduction in prostaglandin formation and may precipitate overt renal decompensation. CLINORIL may affect renal function less than other NSAIDs in patients with chronic glomerular renal disease (see CLINICAL PHARMACOLOGY). Until these observations are better understood and clarified, however, and because renal adverse experiences have been reported with CLINORIL (see ADVERSE REACTIONS), caution should be exercised when administering the drug to patients with conditions associated with increased risk of the effects of non-steroidal anti-inflammatory drugs on renal function, such as those with renal or hepatic dysfunction, diabetes mellitus, advanced age, extracellular volume depletion from any cause, congestive heart failure, septicemia, pyelonephritis, or concomitant use of any nephrotoxic drug. Discontinuation of NSAID therapy is typically followed by recovery to the pretreatment state.

Since CLINORIL is eliminated primarily by the kidneys, patients with significantly impaired renal function should be closely monitored; a lower daily dosage should be anticipated to avoid excessive drug accumulation.

Sulindac metabolites have been reported rarely as the major or a minor component in renal stones in association with other calculus components. CLINORIL should be used with

Continued on next page

Information on the Merck & Co., Inc. products listed on these pages is the full prescribing information from product circulars in use September 30, 1996.

Merck & Co.—Cont.

caution in patients with a history of renal lithiasis, and they should be kept well hydrated while receiving CLINORIL.

Information for Patients

CLINORIL, like other drugs of its class, is not free of side effects. The side effects of these drugs can cause discomfort and, rarely, there are more serious side effects such as gastrointestinal bleeding, which may result in hospitalization and even fatal outcomes.

NSAIDs (Non-steroidal Anti-inflammatory Drugs) are often essential agents in the management of arthritis, but they also may be commonly employed for conditions which are less serious.

Physicians may wish to discuss with their patients the potential risks (see WARNINGS, PRECAUTIONS and ADVERSE REACTIONS) and likely benefits of NSAID treatment, particularly when the drugs are used for less serious conditions where treatment without NSAIDs may represent an acceptable alternative to both the patient and physician.

Laboratory Tests

Because serious GI tract ulceration and bleeding can occur without warning symptoms, physicians should follow chronically treated patients for the signs and symptoms of ulceration and bleeding and should inform them of the importance of this follow-up (see WARNINGS, *Risk of GI Ulcerations, Bleeding and Perforation with NSAID Therapy).*

Use in Pregnancy

CLINORIL is not recommended for use in pregnant women, since safety for use has not been established. The known effects of drugs of this class on the human fetus during the third trimester of pregnancy include: constriction of the ductus arteriosus prenatally, tricuspid incompetence, and pulmonary hypertension; non-closure of the ductus arteriosus postnatally which may be resistant to medical management; myocardial degenerative changes, platelet dysfunction with resultant bleeding, intracranial bleeding, renal dysfunction or failure, renal injury/dysgenesis which may result in prolonged or permanent renal failure, oligohydramnios, gastrointestinal bleeding or perforation, and increased risk of necrotizing enterocolitis.

In reproduction studies in the rat, a decrease in average fetal weight and an increase in numbers of dead pups were observed on the first day of the postpartum period at dosage levels of 20 and 40 mg/kg/day (2½ and 5 times the usual maximum daily dose in humans), although there was no adverse effect on the survival and growth during the remainder of the postpartum period. CLINORIL prolongs the duration of gestation in rats, as do other compounds of this class which also may cause dystocia and delayed parturition in pregnant animals. Visceral and skeletal malformations observed in low incidence among rabbits in some teratology studies did not occur at the same dosage levels in repeat studies, nor at a higher dosage level in the same species.

Nursing Mothers

Nursing should not be undertaken while a patient is on CLINORIL. It is not known whether sulindac is secreted in human milk; however, it is secreted in the milk of lactating rats.

Use in Children

Safety and effectiveness in children have not been established.

Drug Interactions

DMSO should not be used with sulindac. Concomitant administration has been reported to reduce the plasma levels of the active sulfide metabolite and potentially reduce efficacy. In addition, this combination has been reported to cause peripheral neuropathy.

Although sulindac and its sulfide metabolite are highly bound to protein, studies, in which CLINORIL was given at a dose of 400 mg daily, have shown no clinically significant interaction with oral anticoagulants or oral hypoglycemic agents. However, patients should be monitored carefully until it is certain that no change in their anticoagulant or hypoglycemic dosage is required. Special attention should be paid to patients taking higher doses than those recommended and to patients with renal impairment or other metabolic defects that might increase sulindac blood levels.

The concomitant administration of aspirin with sulindac significantly depressed the plasma levels of the active sulfide metabolite. A double-blind study compared the safety and efficacy of CLINORIL 300 or 400 mg daily given alone or with aspirin 2.4 g/day for the treatment of osteoarthritis. The addition of aspirin did not alter the types of clinical or laboratory adverse experiences for CLINORIL; however, the combination showed an increase in the incidence of gastrointestinal adverse experiences. Since the addition of aspirin did not have a favorable effect on the therapeutic response to CLINORIL, the combination is not recommended.

The concomitant use of CLINORIL with other NSAIDs is not recommended due to the increased possibility of gastrointestinal toxicity, with little or no increase in efficacy.

Caution should be used if CLINORIL is administered concomitantly with methotrexate. Nonsteroidal anti-inflammatory drugs have been reported to decrease the tubular secretion of methotrexate and to potentiate its toxicity.

Administration of non-steroidal anti-inflammatory drugs concomitantly with cyclosporine has been associated with an increase in cyclosporine-induced toxicity, possibly due to decreased synthesis of renal prostacyclin. NSAIDs should be used with caution in patients taking cyclosporine, and renal function should be carefully monitored.

The concomitant administration of CLINORIL and diflunisal in normal volunteers resulted in lowering of the plasma levels of the active sulindac sulfide metabolite by approximately one-third.

Probenecid given concomitantly with sulindac had only a slight effect on plasma sulfide levels, while plasma levels of sulindac and sulfone were increased. Sulindac was shown to produce a modest reduction in the uricosuric action of probenecid, which probably is not significant under most circumstances.

Neither propoxyphene hydrochloride nor acetaminophen had any effect on the plasma levels of sulindac or its sulfide metabolite.

ADVERSE REACTIONS

The following adverse reactions were reported in clinical trials or have been reported since the drug was marketed. The probability exists of a causal relationship between CLINORIL and these adverse reactions. The adverse reactions which have been observed in clinical trials encompass observations in 1,865 patients, including 232 observed for at least 48 weeks.

Incidence Greater Than 1%

Gastrointestinal

The most frequent types of adverse reactions occurring with CLINORIL are gastrointestinal; these include gastrointestinal pain (10%), dyspepsia*, nausea* with or without vomiting, diarrhea*, constipation*, flatulence, anorexia and gastrointestinal cramps.

Dermatologic

Rash*, pruritus.

Central Nervous System

Dizziness*, headache*, nervousness.

Special Senses

Tinnitus.

Miscellaneous

Edema (see PRECAUTIONS).

*Incidence between 3% and 9%. Those reactions occurring in 1% to 3% of patients are not marked with an asterisk.

Incidence Less Than 1 in 100

Gastrointestinal

Gastritis, gastroenteritis or colitis. Peptic ulcer and gastrointestinal bleeding have been reported. GI perforation and intestinal strictures (diaphragms) have been reported rarely.

Liver function abnormalities; jaundice, sometimes with fever; cholestasis; hepatitis; hepatic failure.

There have been rare reports of sulindac metabolites in common bile duct "sludge" and in biliary calculi in patients with symptoms of cholecystitis who underwent a cholecystectomy.

Pancreatitis (see PRECAUTIONS).

Ageusia; glossitis.

Dermatologic

Stomatitis, sore or dry mucous membranes, alopecia, photosensitivity.

Erythema multiforme, toxic epidermal necrolysis, Stevens-Johnson syndrome, and exfoliative dermatitis have been reported.

Cardiovascular

Congestive heart failure, especially in patients with marginal cardiac function; palpitation; hypertension.

Hematologic

Thrombocytopenia; ecchymosis; purpura; leukopenia; agranulocytosis; neutropenia; bone marrow depression, including aplastic anemia; hemolytic anemia; increased prothrombin time in patients on oral anticoagulants (see PRECAUTIONS).

Genitourinary

Urine discoloration; dysuria; vaginal bleeding; hematuria; proteinuria; crystalluria; renal impairment, including renal failure; interstitial nephritis; nephrotic syndrome.

Renal calculi containing sulindac metabolites have been observed rarely.

Metabolic

Hyperkalemia.

Musculoskeletal

Muscle weakness.

Psychiatric

Depression; psychic disturbances including acute psychosis.

Nervous System

Vertigo; insomnia; somnolence; paresthesia; convulsions; syncope; aseptic meningitis.

Special Senses

Blurred vision; visual disturbances; decreased hearing; metallic or bitter taste.

Respiratory

Epistaxis.

Hypersensitivity Reactions

Anaphylaxis; angioneurotic edema; bronchial spasm; dyspnea.

Hypersensitivity vasculitis.

A potentially fatal apparent hypersensitivity syndrome has been reported. This syndrome may include constitutional symptoms (fever, chills, diaphoresis, flushing), cutaneous findings (rash or other dermatologic reactions—see above), conjunctivitis, involvement of major organs (changes in liver function including hepatic failure, jaundice, pancreatitis, pneumonitis with or without pleural effusion, leukopenia, leukocytosis, eosinophilia, disseminated intravascular coagulation, anemia, renal impairment, including renal failure), and other less specific findings (adenitis, arthralgia, arthritis, myalgia, fatigue, malaise, hypotension, chest pain, tachycardia).

Causal Relationship Unknown

A rare occurrence of fulminant necrotizing fasciitis, particularly in association with Group A β-hemolytic streptococcus, has been described in persons treated with non-steroidal anti-inflammatory agents, sometimes with fatal outcome (see also PRECAUTIONS, *General).*

Other reactions have been reported in clinical trials or since the drug was marketed, but occurred under circumstances where a causal relationship could not be established. However, in these rarely reported events, that possibility cannot be excluded. Therefore, these observations are listed to serve as alerting information to physicians.

Cardiovascular

Arrhythmia.

Metabolic

Hyperglycemia.

Nervous System

Neuritis.

Special Senses

Disturbances of the retina and its vasculature.

Miscellaneous

Gynecomastia.

MANAGEMENT OF OVERDOSAGE

Cases of overdosage have been reported and rarely, deaths have occurred. The following signs and symptoms may be observed following overdosage: stupor, coma, diminished urine output and hypotension.

In the event of overdosage, the stomach should be emptied by inducing vomiting or by gastric lavage, and the patient carefully observed and given symptomatic and supportive treatment.

Animal studies show that absorption is decreased by the prompt administration of activated charcoal and excretion is enhanced by alkalinization of the urine.

DOSAGE AND ADMINISTRATION

CLINORIL should be administered orally twice a day with food. The maximum dosage is 400 mg per day. Dosages above 400 mg per day are not recommended.

In osteoarthritis, rheumatoid arthritis, and ankylosing spondylitis, the recommended starting dosage is 150 mg twice a day. The dosage may be lowered or raised depending on the response.

A prompt response (within one week) can be expected in about one-half of patients with osteoarthritis, ankylosing spondylitis, and rheumatoid arthritis. Others may require longer to respond.

In acute painful shoulder (acute subacromial bursitis/supraspinatus tendinitis) and acute gouty arthritis, the recommended dosage is 200 mg twice a day. After a satisfactory response has been achieved, the dosage may be reduced according to the response. In acute painful shoulder, therapy for 7–14 days is usually adequate. In acute gouty arthritis, therapy for 7 days is usually adequate.

HOW SUPPLIED

No. 3360—Tablets CLINORIL 150 mg are yellow, hexagon-shaped, compressed tablets, coded MSD 941 on one side and CLINORIL on the other. They are supplied as follows:

NDC 0006-0941-68 in bottles of 100
(6505-01-071-5559 100's)

Shown in Product Identification Guide, page 324

No. 3353—Tablets CLINORIL 200 mg are yellow, hexagon-shaped, scored, compressed tablets, coded MSD 942 on one side and CLINORIL on the other. They are supplied as follows:

NDC 0006-0942-68 in bottles of 100
(6505-01-072-3426 100's)

Shown in Product Identification Guide, page 324

7858634 Issued August 1995

COGENTIN® Tablets ℞
(Benztropine Mesylate), U.S.P.
COGENTIN® Injection ℞
(Benztropine Mesylate), U.S.P.

DESCRIPTION

Benztropine mesylate is a synthetic compound containing structural features found in atropine and diphenhydramine. It is designated chemically as 8-azabicyclo[3.2.1] octane, 3-(diphenylmethoxy)-,*endo*, methanesulfonate. Its empirical formula is $C_{21}H_{25}NO \cdot CH_4O_3S$, and its structural formula is:

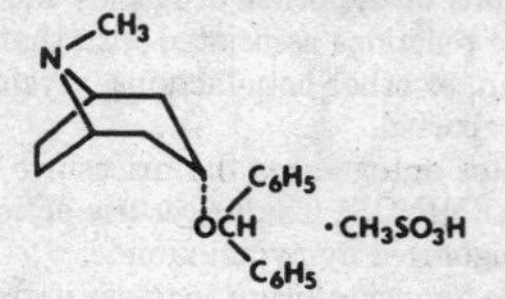

Benztropine mesylate is a crystalline white powder, very soluble in water, and has a molecular weight of 403.54.
COGENTIN* (Benztropine Mesylate) is supplied as tablets in three strengths (0.5 mg, 1 mg, and 2 mg per tablet), and as a sterile injection for intravenous and intramuscular use.
Tablets COGENTIN contain 0.5, 1 or 2 mg of benztropine mesylate. Each tablet contains the following inactive ingredients: calcium phosphate, cellulose, lactose, magnesium stearate and starch.
Each milliliter of the injection contains:

Benztropine mesylate	1 mg
Sodium chloride	9 mg
Water for Injection q.s.	1 mL

*Registered trademark of MERCK & CO., INC.

ACTIONS

COGENTIN possesses both anticholinergic and antihistaminic effects, although only the former have been established as therapeutically significant in the management of parkinsonism.
In the isolated guinea pig ileum, the anticholinergic activity of this drug is about equal to that of atropine; however, when administered orally to unanesthetized cats, it is only about half as active as atropine.
In laboratory animals, its antihistaminic activity and duration of action approach those of pyrilamine maleate.

INDICATIONS

For use as an adjunct in the therapy of all forms of parkinsonism.
Useful also in the control of extrapyramidal disorders (except tardive dyskinesia—see PRECAUTIONS) due to neuroleptic drugs (e.g., phenothiazines).

CONTRAINDICATIONS

Hypersensitivity to COGENTIN tablets or to any component of COGENTIN injection.
Because of its atropine-like side effects, this drug is contraindicated in children under three years of age, and should be used with caution in older children.

WARNINGS

Safe use in pregnancy has not been established.
COGENTIN may impair mental and/or physical abilities required for performance of hazardous tasks, such as operating machinery or driving a motor vehicle.
When COGENTIN is given concomitantly with phenothiazines, haloperidol, or other drugs with anticholinergic or antidopaminergic activity, patients should be advised to report gastrointestinal complaints, fever or heat intolerance promptly. Paralytic ileus, hyperthermia and heat stroke, all of which have sometimes been fatal, have occurred in patients taking anticholinergic-type antiparkinsonism drugs, including COGENTIN, in combination with phenothiazines and/or tricyclic antidepressants.
Since COGENTIN contains structural features of atropine, it may produce anhidrosis. For this reason, it should be administered with caution during hot weather, especially when given concomitantly with other atropine-like drugs to the chronically ill, the alcoholic, those who have central nervous system disease, and those who do manual labor in a hot environment. Anhidrosis may occur more readily when some disturbance of sweating already exists. If there is evidence of anhidrosis, the possibility of hyperthermia should be considered. Dosage should be decreased at the discretion of the physician so that the ability to maintain body heat equilibrium by perspiration is not impaired. Severe anhidrosis and fatal hyperthermia have occurred.

PRECAUTIONS

General
Since COGENTIN has cumulative action, continued supervision is advisable. Patients with a tendency to tachycardia and patients with prostatic hypertrophy should be observed closely during treatment.
Dysuria may occur, but rarely becomes a problem. Urinary retention has been reported with COGENTIN.
The drug may cause complaints of weakness and inability to move particular muscle groups, especially in large doses. For example, if the neck has been rigid and suddenly relaxes, it may feel weak, causing some concern. In this event, dosage adjustment is required.
Mental confusion and excitement may occur with large doses, or in susceptible patients. Visual hallucinations have been reported occasionally. Furthermore, in the treatment of extrapyramidal disorders due to neuroleptic drugs (e.g., phenothiazines), in patients with mental disorders, occasionally there may be intensification of mental symptoms. In such cases, antiparkinsonian drugs can precipitate a toxic psychosis. Patients with mental disorders should be kept under careful observation, especially at the beginning of treatment or if dosage is increased.
Tardive dyskinesia may appear in some patients on long-term therapy with phenothiazines and related agents, or may occur after therapy with these drugs has been discontinued. Antiparkinsonism agents do not alleviate the symptoms of tardive dyskinesia, and in some instances may aggravate them. COGENTIN is not recommended for use in patients with tardive dyskinesia.
The physician should be aware of the possible occurrence of glaucoma. Although the drug does not appear to have any adverse effect on simple glaucoma, it probably should not be used in angle-closure glaucoma.
Drug Interactions
Antipsychotic drugs such as phenothiazines or haloperidol; tricyclic antidepressants (see WARNINGS).

ADVERSE REACTIONS

The adverse reactions below, most of which are anticholinergic in nature, have been reported and within each category are listed in order of decreasing severity.
Cardiovascular
Tachycardia.
Digestive
Paralytic ileus, constipation, vomiting, nausea, dry mouth.
If dry mouth is so severe that there is difficulty in swallowing or speaking, or loss of appetite and weight, reduce dosage, or discontinue the drug temporarily.
Slight reduction in dosage may control nausea and still give sufficient relief of symptoms. Vomiting may be controlled by temporary discontinuation, followed by resumption at a lower dosage.
Nervous System
Toxic psychosis, including confusion, disorientation, memory impairment, visual hallucinations; exacerbation of pre-existing psychotic symptoms; nervousness; depression; listlessness; numbness of fingers.
Special Senses
Blurred vision, dilated pupils.
Urogenital
Urinary retention, dysuria.
Metabolic/Immune or Skin
Occasionally, an allergic reaction, e.g., skin rash, develops. If this can not be controlled by dosage reduction, the medication should be discontinued.
Other
Heat stroke, hyperthermia, fever.

DOSAGE AND ADMINISTRATION

COGENTIN tablets should be used when patients are able to take oral medication.
The injection is especially useful for psychotic patients with acute dystonic reactions or other reactions that make oral medication difficult or impossible. It is recommended also when a more rapid response is desired than can be obtained with the tablets.
Since there is no significant difference in onset of effect after intravenous or intramuscular injection, usually there is no need to use the intravenous route. The drug is quickly effective after either route, with improvement sometimes noticeable a few minutes after injection. In emergency situations, when the condition of the patient is alarming, 1 to 2 mL of the injection normally will provide quick relief. If the parkinsonian effect begins to return, the dose can be repeated.
Because of cumulative action, therapy should be initiated with a low dose which is increased gradually at five or six-day intervals to the smallest amount necessary for optimal relief. Increases should be made in increments of 0.5 mg, to a maximum of 6 mg, or until optimal results are obtained without excessive adverse reactions.
Postencephalitic and
Idiopathic Parkinsonism—
The usual daily dose is 1 to 2 mg, with a range of 0.5 to 6 mg orally or parenterally.
As with any agent used in parkinsonism, dosage must be individualized according to age and weight, and the type of parkinsonism being treated. Generally, older patients and thin patients cannot tolerate large doses. Most patients with postencephalitic parkinsonism need fairly large doses and tolerate them well. Patients with a poor mental outlook are usually poor candidates for therapy.
In idiopathic parkinsonism, therapy may be initiated with a single daily dose of 0.5 to 1 mg at bedtime. In some patients, this will be adequate; in others 4 to 6 mg a day may be required.
In postencephalitic parkinsonism, therapy may be initiated in most patients with 2 mg a day in one or more doses. In highly sensitive patients, therapy may be initiated with 0.5 mg at bedtime, and increased as necessary.
Some patients experience greatest relief by taking the entire dose at bedtime; others react more favorably to divided doses, two to four times a day. Frequently, one dose a day is sufficient, and divided doses may be unnecessary or undesirable.
The long duration of action of this drug makes it particularly suitable for bedtime medication when its effects may last throughout the night, enabling patients to turn in bed during the night more easily, and to rise in the morning.
When COGENTIN is started, do not terminate therapy with other antiparkinsonian agents abruptly. If the other agents are to be reduced or discontinued, it must be done gradually. Many patients obtain greatest relief with combination therapy.
COGENTIN may be used concomitantly with SINEMET* (Carbidopa-Levodopa), or with levodopa, in which case periodic dosage adjustment may be required in order to maintain optimum response.
Drug-Induced Extrapyramidal Disorders—In treating extrapyramidal disorders due to neuroleptic drugs (e.g., phenothiazines), the recommended dosage is 1 to 4 mg once or twice a day orally or parenterally. Dosage must be individualized according to the need of the patient. Some patients require more than recommended; others do not need as much.
In acute dystonic reactions, 1 to 2 mL of the injection usually relieves the condition quickly. After that, the tablets, 1 to 2 mg twice a day, usually prevent recurrence.
When extrapyramidal disorders develop soon after initiation of treatment with neuroleptic drugs (e.g., phenothiazines), they are likely to be transient. One to 2 mg of COGENTIN tablets two or three times a day usually provides relief within one or two days. After one or two weeks, the drug should be withdrawn to determine the continued need for it. If such disorders recur, COGENTIN can be reinstituted.
Certain drug-induced extrapyramidal disorders that develop slowly may not respond to COGENTIN.

*Registered trademark of MERCK & CO., INC.

OVERDOSAGE

Manifestations—May be any of those seen in atropine poisoning or antihistamine overdosage: CNS depression, preceded or followed by stimulation; confusion; nervousness; listlessness; intensification of mental symptoms or toxic psychosis in patients with mental illness being treated with neuroleptic drugs (e.g., phenothiazines); hallucinations (especially visual); dizziness; muscle weakness; ataxia; dry mouth; mydriasis; blurred vision; palpitations; tachycardia; elevated blood pressure; nausea; vomiting; dysuria; numbness of fingers; dysphagia; allergic reactions, e.g., skin rash; headache; hot, dry, flushed skin; delirium; coma; shock; convulsions; respiratory arrest; anhidrosis; hyperthermia; glaucoma; constipation.
Treatment—Physostigmine salicylate, 1 to 2 mg, SC or IV, reportedly will reverse symptoms of anticholinergic intoxication.* A second injection may be given after 2 hours if required. Otherwise treatment is symptomatic and supportive. Induce emesis or perform gastric lavage (contraindicated in precomatose, convulsive, or psychotic states). Maintain respiration. A short-acting barbiturate may be used for CNS excitement, but with caution to avoid subsequent depression; supportive care for depression (avoid convulsant stimulants such as picrotoxin, pentylenetetrazol, or bemegride); artificial respiration for severe respiratory depression; a local

Continued on next page

Information on the Merck & Co., Inc. products listed on these pages is the full prescribing information from product circulars in use September 30, 1996.

Merck & Co.—Cont.

miotic for mydriasis and cycloplegia; ice bags or other cold applications and alcohol sponges for hyperpyrexia, a vasopressor and fluids for circulatory collapse. Darken room for photophobia.

*Duvoisin, R.C.; Katz, R.J.; Amer. Med. Ass. *206*:1963–1965, Nov. 25, 1968.

HOW SUPPLIED

No. 3297—Tablets COGENTIN, 0.5 mg, are white, round, scored, compressed tablets, coded MSD 21 on one side and COGENTIN on the other. They are supplied as follows:
NDC 0006-0021-68 in bottles of 100.
Shown in Product Identification Guide, page 324
No. 3334—Tablets COGENTIN, 1 mg, are white, oval shaped, scored, compressed tablets, coded MSD 635 on one side and COGENTIN on the other. They are supplied as follows:
NDC 0006-0635-68 in bottles of 100
NDC 0006-0635-28 unit dose packages of 100.
Shown in Product Identification Guide, page 324
No. 3172—Tablets COGENTIN, 2 mg, are white, round, scored, compressed tablets, coded MSD 60 on one side and COGENTIN on the other. They are supplied as follows:
NDC 0006-0060-68 in bottles of 100
(6505-01-230-8726, 2 mg 100's)
NDC 0006-0060-28 unit dose packages of 100
NDC 0006-0060-82 in bottles of 1000.
Shown in Product Identification Guide, page 324
No. 3275—Injection COGENTIN, 1 mg per mL, is a clear, colorless solution and is supplied as follows:
NDC 0006-3275-16 in boxes of 6×2 mL ampuls.
7924120 Issued November 1991

ColBENEMID® Tablets (Probenecid-Colchicine), U.S.P. ℞

DESCRIPTION

ColBENEMID* (Probenecid-Colchicine) contains probenecid, which is a uricosuric agent, and colchicine, which has antigout activity, the mechanism of which is unknown.
Probenecid is the generic name for 4-[(dipropylamino) sulfonyl] benzoic acid (molecular weight 285.36). It has the following structural formula:

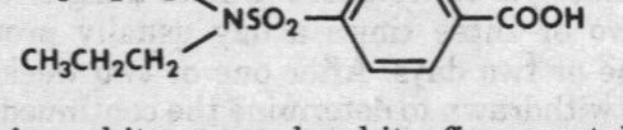

Probenecid is a white or nearly white, fine, crystalline powder. It is soluble in dilute alkali, in alcohol, in chloroform, and in acetone; it is practically insoluble in water and in dilute acids.
Colchicine is an alkaloid obtained from various species of Colchicum. The chemical name for colchicine is (*S*)-*N*-(5,6,7,9-tetrahydro-1,2,3,10-tetramethoxy-9-oxobenzo [*a*] heptalen-7-yl) acetamide (molecular weight 399.43). It has the following structural formula:

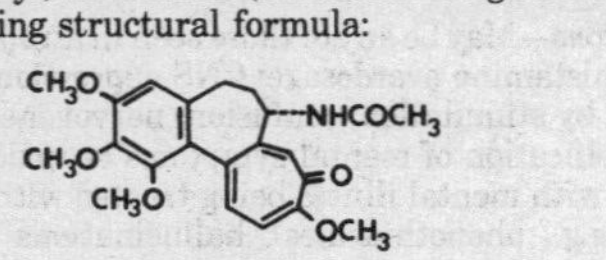

Colchicine consists of pale yellow scales or powder; it darkens on exposure to light. Colchicine is soluble in water, freely soluble in alcohol and in chloroform, and slightly soluble in ether.
Each tablet contains 0.5 g probenecid and 0.5 mg colchicine and the following inactive ingredients: calcium stearate, gelatin, magnesium carbonate, starch.

*Registered trademark of MERCK & CO., INC.

ACTIONS

Probenecid is a uricosuric and renal tubular blocking agent. It inhibits the tubular reabsorption of urate, thus increasing the urinary excretion of uric acid and decreasing serum urate levels. Effective uricosuria reduces the miscible urate pool, retards urate deposition, and promotes resorption of urate deposits.
Probenecid inhibits the tubular secretion of penicillin and usually increases penicillin plasma levels by any route the antibiotic is given. A 2-fold to 4-fold elevation has been demonstrated for various penicillins.
Probenecid also has been reported to inhibit the renal transport of many other compounds including aminohippuric acid (PAH), aminosalicylic acid (PAS), indomethacin, sodium iodomethamate and related iodinated organic acids, 17-ketosteroids, pantothenic acid, phenolsulfonphthalein (PSP), sulfonamides, and sulfonylureas. See also DRUG INTERACTIONS.
Probenecid decreases both hepatic and renal excretion of sulfobromophthalein (BSP). The tubular reabsorption of phosphorus is inhibited in hypoparathyroid but not in euparathyroid individuals.
Probenecid does not influence plasma concentrations of salicylates, nor the excretion of streptomycin, chloramphenicol, chlortetracycline, oxytetracycline, or neomycin.
The mode of action of colchicine in gout is unknown. It is not an analgesic, though it relieves pain in acute attacks of gout. It is not a uricosuric agent and will not prevent progression of gout to chronic gouty arthritis. It does have a prophylactic, suppressive effect that helps to reduce the incidence of acute attacks and to relieve the residual pain and mild discomfort that patients with gout occasionally feel.
In man and certain other animals, colchicine can produce a temporary leukopenia that is followed by leukocytosis.
Colchicine has other pharmacologic actions in animals: It alters neuromuscular function, intensifies gastrointestinal activity by neurogenic stimulation, increases sensitivity to central depressants, heightens response to sympathomimetic compounds, depresses the respiratory center, constricts blood vessels, causes hypertension by central vasomotor stimulation, and lowers body temperature.

INDICATIONS

For the treatment of chronic gouty arthritis when complicated by frequent, recurrent acute attacks of gout.

CONTRAINDICATIONS

Hypersensitivity to this product or to probenecid or colchicine.
Children under 2 years of age.
Not recommended in persons with known blood dyscrasias or uric acid kidney stones.
Therapy with ColBENEMID should not be started until an acute gouty attack has subsided.
Pregnancy: Probenecid crosses the placental barrier and appears in cord blood. Colchicine can arrest cell division in animals and plants. In certain species of animal under certain conditions, colchicine has produced teratogenic effects. The possibility of such effects in humans also has been reported. Because of the colchicine component, ColBENEMID is contraindicated in pregnant patients. The use of any drug in women of childbearing potential requires that the anticipated benefit be weighed against possible hazards.

WARNINGS

Exacerbation of gout following therapy with ColBENEMID may occur; in such cases additional colchicine or other appropriate therapy is advisable.
Probenecid increases plasma concentrations of methotrexate in both animals and humans. In animal studies, increased methotrexate toxicity has been reported. If ColBENEMID is given with methotrexate, the dosage of methotrexate should be reduced and serum levels may need to be monitored.
In patients on ColBENEMID the use of salicylates in either small or large doses is contraindicated because it antagonizes the uricosuric action of probenecid. The biphasic action of salicylates in the renal tubules accounts for the so-called "paradoxical effect" of uricosuric agents. In patients on ColBENEMID who require a mild analgesic agent the use of acetaminophen rather than small doses of salicylates would be preferred.
Rarely, severe allergic reactions and anaphylaxis have been reported with the use of ColBENEMID. Most of these have been reported to occur within several hours after readministration following prior usage of the drug.
The appearance of hypersensitivity reactions requires cessation of therapy with ColBENEMID.
Colchicine has been reported to adversely affect spermatogenesis in animals. Reversible azoospermia has been reported in one patient.

PRECAUTIONS

General
Hematuria, renal colic, costovertebral pain, and formation of uric acid stones associated with the use of ColBENEMID in gouty patients may be prevented by alkalization of the urine and a liberal fluid intake (*see* DOSAGE AND ADMINISTRATION). In these cases when alkali is administered, the acid-base balance of the patient should be watched.
Use with caution in patients with a history of peptic ulcer.
ColBENEMID has been used in patients with some renal impairment but dosage requirements may be increased. ColBENEMID may not be effective in chronic renal insufficiency particularly when the glomerular filtration rate is 30 mL/minute or less.
A reducing substance may appear in the urine of patients receiving probenecid. This disappears with discontinuance of therapy. Suspected glycosuria should be confirmed by using a test specific for glucose.
Adequate animal studies have not been conducted to determine the carcinogenicity potential of probenecid or this drug combination. Since colchicine is an established mutagen, its ability to act as a carcinogen must be suspected and administration of ColBENEMID should involve a weighing of the benefit-vs-risk when long-term administration is contemplated.
Drug Interactions
When probenecid is used to elevate plasma concentrations of penicillin, or other beta-lactams, or when such drugs are given to patients taking probenecid therapeutically, high plasma concentrations of the other drug may increase the incidence of adverse reactions associated with that drug. In the case of penicillin, or other beta-lactams, psychic disturbances have been reported.
The use of salicylates antagonizes the uricosuric action of probenecid (*see* WARNINGS). The uricosuric action of probenecid is also antagonized by pyrazinamide.
Probenecid produces an insignificant increase in free sulfonamide plasma concentrations but a significant increase in total sulfonamide plasma levels. Since probenecid decreases the renal excretion of conjugated sulfonamides, plasma concentrations of the latter should be determined from time to time when a sulfonamide and ColBENEMID are coadministered for prolonged periods. Probenecid may prolong or enhance the action of oral sulfonylureas and thereby increase the risk of hypoglycemia.
It has been reported that patients receiving probenecid require significantly less thiopental for induction of anesthesia. In addition, ketamine and thiopental anesthesia were significantly prolonged in rats receiving probenecid.
The concomitant administration of probenecid increases the mean plasma elimination half-life of a number of drugs which can lead to increased plasma concentrations. These include agents such as indomethacin, acetaminophen, naproxen, ketoprofen, meclofenamate, lorazepam, and rifampin. Although the clinical significance of this observation has not been established, a lower dosage of the drug may be required to produce a therapeutic effect, and increases in dosage of the drug in question should be made cautiously and in small increments when probenecid is being co-administrated. Although specific instances of toxicity due to this potential interaction have not been observed to date, physicians should be alert to this possibility.
Probenecid given concomitantly with sulindac had only a slight effect on plasma sulfide levels, while plasma levels of sulindac and sulfone were increased. Sulindac was shown to produce a modest reduction in the uricosuric action of probenecid, which probably is not significant under most circumstances.
In animals and in humans, probenecid has been reported to increase plasma concentrations of methotrexate (*see* WARNINGS).
Falsely high readings for theophylline have been reported in an *in vitro* study, using the Schack and Waxler technic, when therapeutic concentrations of theophylline and probenecid were added to human plasma.

ADVERSE REACTIONS

The following adverse reactions have been observed and within each category are listed in order of decreasing severity.
Probenecid
Central Nervous System: headache, dizziness.
Metabolic: precipitation of acute gouty arthritis.
Gastrointestinal: hepatic necrosis, vomiting, nausea, anorexia, sore gums.
Genitourinary: nephrotic syndrome, uric acid stones with or without hematuria, renal colic, costovertebral pain, urinary frequency.
Hypersensitivity: anaphylaxis, fever, urticaria, pruritus.
Hematologic: aplastic anemia, leukopenia, hemolytic anemia which in some patients could be related to genetic deficiency of glucose -6- phosphate dehydrogenase in red blood cells, anemia.
Integumentary: dermatitis, alopecia, flushing.
Colchicine
Side effects due to colchicine appear to be a function of dosage. The possibility of increased colchicine toxicity in the presence of hepatic dysfunction should be considered. The appearance of any of the following symptoms may require reduction of dosage or discontinuance of the drug.
Central Nervous System: peripheral neuritis.
Musculoskeletal: muscular weakness.
Gastrointestinal: nausea, vomiting, abdominal pain, or diarrhea may be particularly troublesome in the presence of peptic ulcer or spastic colon.

Hypersensitivity: urticaria.
Hematologic: aplastic anemia, agranulocytosis.
Integumentary: dermatitis, purpura, alopecia.
At toxic doses, colchicine may cause severe diarrhea, generalized vascular damage, and renal damage with hematuria and oliguria.

DOSAGE AND ADMINISTRATION

Therapy with ColBENEMID should not be *started* until an acute gouty attack has subsided. However, if an acute attack is precipitated *during* therapy, ColBENEMID may be continued without changing the dosage, and additional colchicine or other appropriate therapy should be given to control the acute attack.

The recommended adult dosage is 1 tablet of ColBENEMID daily for one week, followed by 1 tablet twice a day thereafter.

Some degree of renal impairment may be present in patients with gout. A daily dosage of 2 tablets may be adequate. However, if necessary, the daily dosage may be increased by 1 tablet every four weeks within tolerance (and usually not above 4 tablets per day) if symptoms of gouty arthritis are not controlled or the 24 hour uric acid excretion is not above 700 mg. As noted, probenecid may not be effective in chronic renal insufficiency particularly when the glomerular filtration rate is 30 mL/minute or less.

Gastric intolerance may be indicative of overdosage, and may be corrected by decreasing the dosage.

As uric acid tends to crystallize out of an acid urine, a liberal fluid intake is recommended, as well as sufficient sodium bicarbonate (3 to 7.5 g daily) or potassium citrate (7.5 g daily) to maintain an alkaline urine (*see* PRECAUTIONS).

Alkalization of the urine is recommended until the serum urate level returns to normal limits and tophaceous deposits disappear, i.e., during the period when urinary excretion of uric acid is at a high level. Thereafter, alkalization of the urine and the usual restriction of purine-producing foods may be somewhat relaxed.

ColBENEMID (or probenecid) should be continued at the dosage that will maintain normal serum urate levels. When acute attacks have been absent for six months or more and serum urate levels remain within normal limits, the daily dosage of ColBENEMID may be decreased by 1 tablet every six months. The maintenance dosage should not be reduced to the point where serum urate levels tend to rise.

HOW SUPPLIED

No. 3283—Tablets ColBENEMID are white to off-white, capsule-shaped, scored tablets, coded MSD 614. Each tablet contains 0.5 g of probenecid and 0.5 mg of colchicine. They are supplied as follows:
NDC 0006-0614-68 bottles of 100.
Shown in Product Identification Guide, page 324
Storage
Protect from light.
      7876427 Issued May 1989

CORTONE® Acetate Sterile Suspension   ℞
(Cortisone Acetate), U.S.P.

For intramuscular injection only
NOT FOR INTRAVENOUS USE

DESCRIPTION

Cortisone acetate, a synthetic adrenocortical steroid, is a white or practically white, odorless, crystalline powder. It is stable in air. It is insoluble in water. The molecular weight is 402.49. It is designated chemically as 21-(acetyloxy)-17-hydroxypregn-4-ene-3,11,20-trione. The empirical formula is $C_{23}H_{30}O_6$ and the structural formula is:

CORTONE* Acetate (Cortisone Acetate) sterile suspension is a sterile suspension containing 50 mg per milliliter of cortisone acetate in an aqueous medium (pH 5.0 to 7.0). Inactive ingredients per mL: sodium chloride, 9 mg; polysorbate 80, 4 mg; sodium carboxymethylcellulose, 5 mg; Water for Injection q.s. 1 mL. Benzyl alcohol, 9 mg, added as preservative.
No attempt should be made to alter CORTONE Acetate ster-

ile suspension. Diluting it or mixing it with other substances may affect the state of suspension or change the rate of absorption and reduce its effectiveness.

---

*Registered trademark of MERCK & CO., INC.

ACTIONS

CORTONE Acetate sterile suspension has a slow onset but long duration of action when compared with more soluble preparations. When daily corticosteroid therapy is required and oral therapy is not feasible, the required daily dosage may be given in a single intramuscular injection of this preparation.

Naturally occurring glucocorticoids (hydrocortisone and cortisone), which also have salt-retaining properties, are used as replacement therapy in adrenocortical deficiency states. They are also used for their potent anti-inflammatory effects in disorders of many organ systems.

Glucocorticoids cause profound and varied metabolic effects. In addition, they modify the body's immune responses to diverse stimuli.

INDICATIONS

When oral therapy is not feasible:
1. *Endocrine disorders*
Primary or secondary adrenocortical insufficiency (hydrocortisone or cortisone is the drug of choice; synthetic analogs may be used in conjunction with mineralocorticoids where applicable; in infancy, mineralocorticoid supplementation is of particular importance)
Acute adrenocortical insufficiency (hydrocortisone or cortisone is the drug of choice; mineralocorticoid supplementation may be necessary, particularly when synthetic analogs are used)
Preoperatively, and in the event of serious trauma or illness, in patients with known adrenal insufficiency or when adrenocortical reserve is doubtful
Shock unresponsive to conventional therapy if adrenocortical insufficiency exists or is suspected
    Congenital adrenal hyperplasia
    Nonsuppurative thyroiditis
    Hypercalcemia associated with cancer
2. *Rheumatic disorders*
As adjunctive therapy for short-term administration (to tide the patient over an acute episode or exacerbation) in:
    Post-traumatic osteoarthritis
    Synovitis of osteoarthritis
    Rheumatoid arthritis, including juvenile rheumatoid arthritis (selected cases may require low-dose maintenance therapy)
    Acute and subacute bursitis
    Epicondylitis
    Acute nonspecific tenosynovitis
    Acute gouty arthritis
    Psoriatic arthritis
    Ankylosing spondylitis
3. *Collagen diseases*
During an exacerbation or as maintenance therapy in selected cases of:
    Systemic lupus erythematosus
    Acute rheumatic carditis
    Systemic dermatomyositis (polymyositis)
4. *Dermatologic diseases*
    Pemphigus
    Severe erythema multiforme (Stevens-Johnson syndrome)
    Exfoliative dermatitis
    Bullous dermatitis herpetiformis
    Severe seborrheic dermatitis
    Severe psoriasis
    Mycosis fungoides
5. *Allergic states*
Control of severe or incapacitating allergic conditions intractable to adequate trials of conventional treatment in:
    Bronchial asthma
    Contact dermatitis
    Atopic dermatitis
    Serum sickness
    Seasonal or perennial allergic rhinitis
    Drug hypersensitivity reactions
    Urticarial transfusion reactions
    Acute noninfectious laryngeal edema (epinephrine is the drug of first choice)
6. *Ophthalmic diseases*
Severe acute and chronic allergic and inflammatory processes involving the eye, such as:
    Herpes zoster ophthalmicus
    Iritis, iridocyclitis
    Chorioretinitis
    Diffuse posterior uveitis and choroiditis
    Optic neuritis
    Sympathetic ophthalmia
    Anterior segment inflammation
    Allergic conjunctivitis

    Keratitis
    Allergic corneal marginal ulcers
7. *Gastrointestinal diseases*
To tide the patient over a critical period of the disease in:
    Ulcerative colitis (Systemic therapy)
    Regional enteritis (Systemic therapy)
8. *Respiratory diseases*
    Symptomatic sarcoidosis
    Berylliosis
    Fulminating or disseminated pulmonary tuberculosis when used concurrently with appropriate antituberculous chemotherapy
    Loeffler's syndrome not manageable by other means
    Aspiration pneumonitis
9. *Hematologic disorders*
    Acquired (autoimmune) hemolytic anemia
    Erythroblastopenia (RBC anemia)
    Congenital (erythroid) hypoplastic anemia
10. *Neoplastic diseases*
    For palliative management of:
    Leukemias and lymphomas in adults
    Acute leukemia of childhood
11. *Edematous states*
    To induce diuresis or remission of proteinuria in the nephrotic syndrome, without uremia, of the idiopathic type, or that due to lupus erythematosus
12. *Miscellaneous*
    Tuberculous meningitis with subarachnoid block or impending block when used concurrently with appropriate antituberculous chemotherapy
    Trichinosis with neurologic or myocardial involvement.

CONTRAINDICATIONS

Systemic fungal infections
Hypersensitivity to any component of this product

WARNINGS

Because rare instances of anaphylactoid reactions have occurred in patients receiving parenteral corticosteroid therapy, appropriate precautionary measures should be taken prior to administration, especially when the patient has a history of allergy to any drug. Anaphylactoid and hypersensitivity reactions have been reported for Sterile Suspension CORTONE Acetate (see ADVERSE REACTIONS).

In patients on corticosteroid therapy subjected to any unusual stress, increased dosage of rapidly acting corticosteroids before, during, and after the stressful situation is indicated.

Drug-induced secondary adrenocortical insufficiency may result from too rapid withdrawal of corticosteroids and may be minimized by gradual reduction of dosage. This type of relative insufficiency may persist for months after discontinuation of therapy; therefore, in any situation of stress occurring during that period, hormone therapy should be reinstituted. If the patient is receiving steroids already, dosage may have to be increased. Since mineralocorticoid secretion may be impaired, salt and/or a mineralocorticoid should be administered concurrently.

Corticosteroids may mask some signs of infection, and new infections may appear during their use. There may be decreased resistance and inability to localize infection when corticosteroids are used. Moreover, corticosteroids may affect the nitroblue-tetrazolium test for bacterial infection and produce false negative results.

In cerebral malaria, a double-blind trial has shown that the use of corticosteroids is associated with prolongation of coma and a higher incidence of pneumonia and gastrointestinal bleeding.

Corticosteroids may activate latent amebiasis. Therefore, it is recommended that latent or active amebiasis be ruled out before initiating corticosteroid therapy in any patient who has spent time in the tropics or any patient with unexplained diarrhea.

Prolonged use of corticosteroids may produce posterior subcapsular cataracts, glaucoma with possible damage to the optic nerves, and may enhance the establishment of secondary ocular infections due to fungi or viruses.

Usage in pregnancy. Since adequate human reproduction studies have not been done with corticosteroids, use of these drugs in pregnancy or in women of childbearing potential requires that the anticipated benefits be weighed against the possible hazards to the mother and embryo or fetus. Infants born of mothers who have received substantial doses of corticosteroids during pregnancy should be carefully observed for signs of hypoadrenalism.

Corticosteroids appear in breast milk and could suppress growth, interfere with endogenous corticosteroid production,

Continued on next page

Merck & Co.—Cont.

or cause other unwanted effects. Mothers taking pharmacologic doses of corticosteroids should be advised not to nurse.
Average and large doses of cortisone or hydrocortisone can cause elevation of blood pressure, salt and water retention, and increased excretion of potassium. These effects are less likely to occur with the synthetic derivatives except when used in large doses. Dietary salt restriction and potassium supplementation may be necessary. All corticosteroids increase calcium excretion.

Administration of live virus vaccines, including smallpox, is contraindicated in individuals receiving immunosuppressive doses of corticosteroids. If inactivated viral or bacterial vaccines are administered to individuals receiving immunosuppressive doses of corticosteroids, the expected serum antibody response may not be obtained.

Patients who are on drugs which suppress the immune system are more susceptible to infections than healthy individuals. Chickenpox and measles, for example, can have a more serious or even fatal course in non-immune children or adults on corticosteroids. In such children or adults who have not had these diseases, particular care should be taken to avoid exposure. The risk of developing a disseminated infection varies among individuals and can be related to the dose, route and duration of corticosteroid administration as well as to the underlying disease. If exposed to chickenpox, prophylaxis with varicella zoster immune globulin (VZIG) may be indicated. If chickenpox develops, treatment with antiviral agents may be considered. If exposed to measles, prophylaxis with immune globulin (IG) may be indicated. (See the respective package inserts for VZIG and IG for complete prescribing information.)

Similarly, corticosteroids should be used with great care in patients with known or suspected Strongyloides (threadworm) infestation. In such patients, corticosteroid-induced immunosuppression may lead to Strongyloides hyperinfection and dissemination with widespread larval migration, often accompanied by severe enterocolitis and potentially fatal gram-negative septicemia.

The use of CORTONE Acetate sterile suspension in active tuberculosis should be restricted to those cases of fulminating or disseminated tuberculosis in which the corticosteroid is used for the management of the disease in conjunction with an appropriate antituberculous regimen.

If corticosteroids are indicated in patients with latent tuberculosis or tuberculin reactivity, close observation is necessary as reactivation of the disease may occur. During prolonged corticosteroid therapy, these patients should receive chemoprophylaxis.

Literature reports suggest an apparent association between use of corticosteroids and left ventricular free wall rupture after a recent myocardial infarction; therefore, therapy with corticosteroids should be used with great caution in these patients.

PRECAUTIONS

CORTONE Acetate sterile suspension, like many other steroid formulations, is sensitive to heat. Therefore, it should not be autoclaved when it is desirable to sterilize the exterior of the vial.

Following prolonged therapy, withdrawal of corticosteroids may result in symptoms of the corticosteroid withdrawal syndrome including fever, myalgia, arthralgia, and malaise. This may occur in patients even without evidence of adrenal insufficiency.

There is an enhanced effect of corticosteroids in patients with hypothyroidism and in those with cirrhosis.

Corticosteroids should be used cautiously in patients with ocular herpes simplex for fear of corneal perforation.

The lowest possible dose of corticosteroid should be used to control the condition under treatment, and when reduction in dosage is possible, the reduction must be gradual.

Psychic derangements may appear when corticosteroids are used, ranging from euphoria, insomnia, mood swings, personality changes, and severe depression to frank psychotic manifestations. Also, existing emotional instability or psychotic tendencies may be aggravated by corticosteroids.

Aspirin should be used cautiously in conjunction with corticosteroids in hypoprothrombinemia.

Steroids should be used with caution in nonspecific ulcerative colitis, if there is a probability of impending perforation, abscess, or other pyogenic infection, also in diverticulitis, fresh intestinal anastomoses, active or latent peptic ulcer, renal insufficiency, hypertension, osteoporosis, and myasthenia gravis. Signs of peritoneal irritation following gastrointestinal perforation in patients receiving large doses of corticosteroids may be minimal or absent. Fat embolism has been reported as a possible complication of hypercortisonism.

When large doses are given, some authorities advise that antacids be administered between meals to help to prevent peptic ulcer.

Growth and development of infants and children on prolonged corticosteroid therapy should be carefully followed.

Steroids may increase or decrease motility and number of spermatozoa in some patients.

Phenytoin, phenobarbital, ephedrine, and rifampin may enhance the metabolic clearance of corticosteroids, resulting in decreased blood levels and lessened physiologic activity, thus requiring adjustment in corticosteroid dosage.

The prothrombin time should be checked frequently in patients who are receiving corticosteroids and coumarin anticoagulants at the same time because of reports that corticosteroids have altered the response to these anticoagulants. Studies have shown that the usual effect produced by adding corticosteroids is inhibition of response to coumarins, although there have been some conflicting reports of potentiation not substantiated by studies.

When corticosteroids are administered concomitantly with potassium-depleting diuretics, patients should be observed closely for development of hypokalemia.

Injection of a steroid into an infected site is to be avoided.

Information for Patients

Susceptible patients who are on immunosuppressant doses of corticosteroids should be warned to avoid exposure to chickenpox or measles. Patients should also be advised that if they are exposed, medical advice should be sought without delay.

ADVERSE REACTIONS

Fluid and electrolyte disturbances
 Sodium retention
 Fluid retention
 Congestive heart failure in susceptible patients
 Potassium loss
 Hypokalemic alkalosis
 Hypertension
Musculoskeletal
 Muscle weakness
 Steroid myopathy
 Loss of muscle mass
 Osteoporosis
 Vertebral compression fractures
 Aseptic necrosis of femoral and humeral heads
 Pathologic fracture of long bones
 Tendon rupture
Gastrointestinal
 Peptic ulcer with possible subsequent perforation and hemorrhage
 Perforation of the small and large bowel, particularly in patients with inflammatory bowel disease
 Pancreatitis
 Abdominal distention
 Ulcerative esophagitis
Dermatologic
 Impaired wound healing
 Thin fragile skin
 Petechiae and ecchymoses
 Erythema
 Increased sweating
 May suppress reactions to skin tests
 Other cutaneous reactions, such as allergic dermatitis, urticaria, angioneurotic edema
Neurologic
 Convulsions
 Increased intracranial pressure with papilledema (pseudo-tumor cerebri) usually after treatment
 Vertigo
 Headache
 Psychic disturbances
Endocrine
 Menstrual irregularities
 Development of cushingoid state
 Suppression of growth in children
 Secondary adrenocortical and pituitary unresponsiveness, particularly in times of stress, as in trauma, surgery, or illness
 Decreased carbohydrate tolerance
 Manifestations of latent diabetes mellitus
 Increased requirements for insulin or oral hypoglycemic agents in diabetics
 Hirsutism
Ophthalmic
 Posterior subcapsular cataracts
 Increased intraocular pressure
 Glaucoma
 Exophthalmos
Metabolic
 Negative nitrogen balance due to protein catabolism
Cardiovascular
 Myocardial rupture following recent myocardial infarction (see WARNINGS).
Other
 Anaphylactoid or hypersensitivity reactions
 Thromboembolism
 Weight gain
 Increased appetite
 Nausea
 Malaise

The following *additional* adverse reactions are related to parenteral corticosteroid therapy:
 Rare instances of blindness associated with intralesional therapy around the face and head
 Hyperpigmentation or hypopigmentation
 Subcutaneous and cutaneous atrophy
 Sterile abscess

OVERDOSAGE

Reports of acute toxicity and/or death following overdosage of glucocorticoids are rare. In the event of overdosage, no specific antidote is available; treatment is supportive and symptomatic.

The intraperitoneal LD_{50} of cortisone acetate in female mice was 1405 mg/kg.

DOSAGE AND ADMINISTRATION

For intramuscular injection only
NOT FOR INTRAVENOUS USE
DOSAGE REQUIREMENTS ARE VARIABLE AND MUST BE INDIVIDUALIZED ON THE BASIS OF THE DISEASE AND THE RESPONSE OF THE PATIENT.

The initial dosage varies from 20 to 300 mg a day depending on the disease being treated. In less severe diseases doses lower than 20 mg may suffice, while in severe diseases doses higher than 300 mg may be required. The initial dosage should be maintained or adjusted until the patient's response is satisfactory. If a satisfactory clinical response does not occur after a reasonable period of time, discontinue CORTONE Acetate sterile suspension and transfer the patient to other therapy.

After a favorable initial response, the proper maintenance dosage should be determined by decreasing the initial dosage in small amounts to the lowest dosage that maintains an adequate clinical response.

Patients should be observed closely for signs that might require dosage adjustment, including changes in clinical status resulting from remissions or exacerbations of the disease, individual drug responsiveness, and the effect of stress (e.g., surgery, infection, trauma). During stress it may be necessary to increase dosage temporarily.

If the drug is to be stopped after more than a few days of treatment, it usually should be withdrawn gradually.

HOW SUPPLIED

No. 7069—Sterile Suspension CORTONE Acetate is a white, mobile suspension, each mL containing 50 mg cortisone acetate, and is supplied as follows:
NDC 0006-7069-10 in 10 mL vials.
Storage
Sensitive to heat. Do not autoclave.
Protect from freezing.
 7411917   Issued October 1995

CORTONE® Acetate Tablets   ℞
(Cortisone Acetate), U.S.P.

DESCRIPTION

Glucocorticoids are adrenocortical steroids, both naturally occurring and synthetic, which are readily absorbed from the gastrointestinal tract.

Cortisone acetate is a white or practically white, odorless, crystalline powder. It is stable in air. It is insoluble in water. The molecular weight is 402.49. It is designated chemically as 21-(acetyloxy)-17-hydroxypregn-4-ene-3,11,20-trione. The empirical formula is $C_{23}H_{30}O_6$ and the structural formula is:

CORTONE* Acetate (Cortisone Acetate) tablets contain 25 mg of cortisone acetate in each tablet.
Inactive ingredients are lactose, magnesium stearate, and starch.

*Registered trademark of MERCK & CO., INC.

ACTIONS

Naturally occurring glucocorticoids (hydrocortisone and cortisone), which also have salt-retaining properties, are

used as replacement therapy in adrenocortical deficiency states. They are also used for their potent anti-inflammatory effects in disorders of many organ systems.

Glucocorticoids cause profound and varied metabolic effects. In addition, they modify the body's immune responses to diverse stimuli.

INDICATIONS

1. *Endocrine Disorders*
Primary or secondary adrenocortical insufficiency (hydrocortisone or cortisone is the first choice; synthetic analogs may be used in conjunction with mineralocorticoids where applicable; in infancy mineralocorticoid supplementation is of particular importance).
    Congenital adrenal hyperplasia
    Nonsuppurative thyroiditis
    Hypercalcemia associated with cancer

2. *Rheumatic Disorders*
As adjunctive therapy for short-term administration (to tide the patient over an acute episode or exacerbation) in:
    Psoriatic arthritis
    Rheumatoid arthritis, including juvenile rheumatoid arthritis (selected cases may require low-dose maintenance therapy)
    Ankylosing spondylitis
    Acute and subacute bursitis
    Acute nonspecific tenosynovitis
    Acute gouty arthritis
    Post-traumatic osteoarthritis
    Synovitis of osteoarthritis
    Epicondylitis

3. *Collagen Diseases*
During an exacerbation or as maintenance therapy in selected cases of—
    Systemic lupus erythematosus
    Acute rheumatic carditis
    Systemic dermatomyositis (polymyositis)

4. *Dermatologic Diseases*
    Pemphigus
    Bullous dermatitis herpetiformis
    Severe erythema multiforme (Stevens-Johnson syndrome)
    Exfoliative dermatitis
    Mycosis fungoides
    Severe psoriasis
    Severe seborrheic dermatitis

5. *Allergic States*
Control of severe or incapacitating allergic conditions intractable to adequate trials of conventional treatment:
    Seasonal or perennial allergic rhinitis
    Bronchial asthma
    Contact dermatitis
    Atopic dermatitis
    Serum sickness
    Drug hypersensitivity reactions

6. *Ophthalmic Diseases*
Severe acute and chronic allergic and inflammatory processes involving the eye and its adnexa, such as—
    Allergic conjunctivitis
    Keratitis
    Allergic corneal marginal ulcers
    Herpes zoster ophthalmicus
    Iritis and iridocyclitis
    Chorioretinitis
    Anterior segment inflammation
    Diffuse posterior uveitis and choroiditis
    Optic neuritis
    Sympathetic ophthalmia

7. *Respiratory Diseases*
    Symptomatic sarcoidosis
    Loeffler's syndrome not manageable by other means
    Berylliosis
    Fulminating or disseminated pulmonary tuberculosis when used concurrently with appropriate antituberculous chemotherapy
    Aspiration pneumonitis

8. *Hematologic Disorders*
    Idiopathic thrombocytopenic purpura in adults
    Secondary thrombocytopenia in adults
    Acquired (autoimmune) hemolytic anemia
    Erythroblastopenia (RBC anemia)
    Congenital (erythroid) hypoplastic anemia

9. *Neoplastic Diseases*
For palliative management of:
    Leukemias and lymphomas in adults
    Acute leukemia of childhood

10. *Edematous States*
To induce a diuresis or remission of proteinuria in the nephrotic syndrome, without uremia, of the idiopathic type or that due to lupus erythematosus

11. *Gastrointestinal Diseases*
To tide the patient over a critical period of the disease in:
    Ulcerative colitis
    Regional enteritis

12. *Miscellaneous*
Tuberculous meningitis with subarachnoid block or impending block when used concurrently with appropriate antituberculous chemotherapy
Trichinosis with neurologic or myocardial involvement

CONTRAINDICATIONS

Systemic fungal infections
Hypersensitivity to this product

WARNINGS

In patients on corticosteroid therapy subjected to unusual stress, increased dosage of rapidly acting corticosteroids before, during, and after the stressful situation is indicated.

Drug-induced secondary adrenocortical insufficiency may result from too rapid withdrawal of corticosteroids and may be minimized by gradual reduction of dosage. This type of relative insufficiency may persist for months after discontinuation of therapy; therefore, in any situation of stress occurring during that period, hormone therapy should be reinstituted. If the patient is receiving steroids already, dosage may have to be increased. Since mineralocorticoid secretion may be impaired, salt and/or a mineralocorticoid should be administered concurrently.

Corticosteroids may mask some signs of infection, and new infections may appear during their use. There may be decreased resistance and inability to localize infection when corticosteroids are used. Moreover, corticosteroids may affect the nitroblue-tetrazolium test for bacterial infection and produce false negative results.

In cerebral malaria, a double-blind trial has shown that the use of corticosteroids is associated with prolongation of coma and a higher incidence of pneumonia and gastrointestinal bleeding.

Corticosteroids may activate latent amebiasis. Therefore, it is recommended that latent or active amebiasis be ruled out before initiating corticosteroid therapy in any patient who has spent time in the tropics or any patient with unexplained diarrhea.

Prolonged use of corticosteroids may produce posterior subcapsular cataracts, glaucoma with possible damage to the optic nerves, and may enhance the establishment of secondary ocular infections due to fungi or viruses.

Usage in pregnancy: Since adequate human reproduction studies have not been done with corticosteroids, use of these drugs in pregnancy or in women of childbearing potential requires that the anticipated benefits be weighed against the possible hazards to the mother and embryo or fetus. Infants born of mothers who have received substantial doses of corticosteroids during pregnancy should be carefully observed for signs of hypoadrenalism.

Corticosteroids appear in breast milk and could suppress growth, interefere with endogenous corticosteroid production, or cause other unwanted effects. Mothers taking pharmacologic doses of corticosteroids should be advised not to nurse.

Average and large doses of hydrocortisone or cortisone can cause elevation of blood pressure, salt and water retention, and increased excretion of potassium. These effects are less likely to occur with the synthetic derivatives except when used in large doses. Dietary salt restriction and potassium supplementation may be necessary. All corticosteroids increase calcium excretion.

Administration of live virus vaccines, including smallpox, is contraindicated in individuals receiving immunosuppressive doses of corticosteroids. If inactivated viral or bacterial vaccines are administered to individuals receiving immunosuppressive doses of corticosteroids, the expected serum antibody response may not be obtained. However, immunization procedures may be undertaken in patients who are receiving corticosteroids as replacement therapy, e.g., for Addison's disease.

Patients who are on drugs which suppress the immune system are more susceptible to infections than healthy individuals. Chickenpox and measles, for example, can have a more serious or even fatal course in non-immune children or adults on corticosteroids. In such children or adults who have not had these diseases, particular care should be taken to avoid exposure. The risk of developing a disseminated infection varies among individuals and can be related to the dose, route and duration of corticosteroid administration as well as to the underlying disease. If exposed to chickenpox, prophylaxis with varicella zoster immune globulin (VZIG) may be indicated. If chickenpox develops, treatment with antiviral agents may be considered. If exposed to measles, prophylaxis with immune globulin (IG) may be indicated. (See the respective package inserts for VZIG and IG for complete prescribing information.)

Similarly, corticosteroids should be used with great care in patients with known or suspected Strongyloides (threadworm) infestation. In such patients, corticosteroid-induced immunosuppression may lead to Strongyloides hyperinfection and dissemination with widespread larval migration, often accompanied by severe enterocolitis and potentially fatal gram-negative septicemia.

The use of CORTONE Acetate tablets in active tuberculosis should be restricted to those cases of fulminating or disseminated tuberculosis in which the corticosteroid is used for the management of the disease in conjunction with an appropriate antituberculous regimen.

If corticosteroids are indicated in patients with latent tuberculosis or tuberculin reactivity, close observation is necessary as reactivation of the disease may occur. During prolonged corticosteroid therapy, these patients should receive chemoprophylaxis.

Literature reports suggest an apparent association between use of corticosteroids and left ventricular free wall rupture after a recent myocardial infarction; therefore, therapy with corticosteroids should be used with great caution in these patients.

PRECAUTIONS

Following prolonged therapy, withdrawal of corticosteroids may result in symptoms of the corticosteroid withdrawal syndrome including fever, myalgia, arthralgia, and malaise. This may occur in patients even without evidence of adrenal insufficiency.

There is an enhanced effect of corticosteroids in patients with hypothyroidism and in those with cirrhosis.

Corticosteroids should be used cautiously in patients with ocular herpes simplex because of possible corneal perforation.

The lowest possible dose of corticosteroid should be used to control the condition under treatment, and when reduction in dosage is possible, the reduction should be gradual.

Psychic derangements may appear when corticosteroids are used, ranging from euphoria, insomnia, mood swings, personality changes, and severe depression, to frank psychotic manifestations. Also, existing emotional instability or psychotic tendencies may be aggravated by corticosteroids.

Aspirin should be used cautiously in conjunction with corticosteroids in hypoprothrombinemia.

Steroids should be used with caution in nonspecific ulcerative colitis, if there is a probability of impending perforation, abscess, or other pyogenic infection, diverticulitis, fresh intestinal anastomoses, active or latent peptic ulcer, renal insufficiency, hypertension, osteoporosis, and myasthenia gravis. Signs of peritoneal irritation following gastrointestinal perforation in patients receiving large doses of corticosteroids may be minimal or absent. Fat embolism has been reported as a possible complication of hypercortisonism.

When large doses are given, some authorities advise that corticosteroids be taken with meals and antacids taken between meals to help to prevent peptic ulcer.

Growth and development of infants and children on prolonged corticosteroid therapy should be carefully observed.

Steroids may increase or decrease motility and number of spermatozoa in some patients.

Phenytoin, phenobarbital, ephedrine, and rifampin may enhance the metabolic clearance of corticosteroids, resulting in decreased blood levels and lessened physiologic activity, thus requiring adjustment in corticosteroid dosage.

The prothrombin time should be checked frequently in patients who are receiving corticosteroids and coumarin anticoagulants at the same time because of reports that corticosteroids have altered the response to these anticoagulants. Studies have shown that the usual effect produced by adding corticosteroids is inhibition of response to coumarins, although there have been some conflicting reports of potentiation not substantiated by studies.

When corticosteroids are administered concomitantly with potassium-depleting diuretics, patients should be observed closely for development of hypokalemia.

Information for Patients
Susceptible patients who are on immunosuppressant doses of corticosteroids should be warned to avoid exposure to chickenpox or measles. Patients should also be advised that if they are exposed, medical advice should be sought without delay.

ADVERSE REACTIONS

Fluid and Electrolyte Disturbances
    Sodium retention
    Fluid retention
    Congestive heart failure in susceptible patients
    Potassium loss
    Hypokalemic alkalosis
    Hypertension

Continued on next page

Information on the Merck & Co., Inc. products listed on these pages is the full prescribing information from product circulars in use September 30, 1996.

Consult 1997 supplements and future editions for revisions

Merck & Co.—Cont.

Musculoskeletal
  Muscle weakness
  Steroid myopathy
  Loss of muscle mass
  Osteoporosis
  Vertebral compression fractures
  Aseptic necrosis of femoral and humeral heads
  Pathologic fracture of long bones
  Tendon rupture
Gastrointestinal
  Peptic ulcer with possible perforation and hemorrhage
  Perforation of the small and large bowel, particularly in patients with inflammatory bowel disease
  Pancreatitis
  Abdominal distention
  Ulcerative esophagitis
Dermatologic
  Impaired wound healing
  Thin fragile skin
  Petechiae and ecchymoses
  Erythema
  Increased sweating
  May suppress reactions to skin tests
  Other cutaneous reactions, such as allergic dermatitis, urticaria, angioneurotic edema
Neurologic
  Convulsions
  Increased intracranial pressure with papilledema (pseudotumor cerebri), usually after treatment
  Vertigo
  Headache
  Psychic disturbances
Endocrine
  Menstrual irregularities
  Development of cushingoid state
  Suppression of growth in children
  Secondary adrenocortical and pituitary unresponsiveness, particularly in times of stress, as in trauma, surgery, or illness
  Decreased carbohydrate tolerance
  Manifestations of latent diabetes mellitus
  Increased requirements for insulin or oral hypoglycemic agents in diabetics
  Hirsutism
Ophthalmic
  Posterior subcapsular cataracts
  Increased intraocular pressure
  Glaucoma
  Exophthalmos
Metabolic
  Negative nitrogen balance due to protein catabolism
Cardiovascular
  Myocardial rupture following recent myocardial infarction (see WARNINGS).
Other
  Hypersensitivity
  Thromboembolism
  Weight gain
  Increased appetite
  Nausea
  Malaise

OVERDOSAGE

Reports of acute toxicity and/or death following overdosage of glucocorticoids are rare. In the event of overdosage, no specific antidote is available; treatment is supportive and symptomatic.
The intraperitoneal LD_{50} of cortisone acetate in female mice was 1405 mg/kg.

DOSAGE AND ADMINISTRATION

For oral administration
DOSAGE REQUIREMENTS ARE VARIABLE AND MUST BE INDIVIDUALIZED ON THE BASIS OF THE DISEASE AND THE RESPONSE OF THE PATIENT.
The initial dosage varies from 25 to 300 mg a day depending on the disease being treated. In less severe diseases doses lower than 25 mg may suffice, while in severe diseases doses higher than 300 mg may be required. The initial dosage should be maintained or adjusted until the patient's response is satisfactory. If satisfactory clinical response does not occur after a reasonable period of time, discontinue CORTONE Acetate tablets and transfer the patient to other therapy.
After a favorable initial response, the proper maintenance dosage should be determined by decreasing the initial dosage in small amounts to the lowest dosage that maintains an adequate clinical response.
Patients should be observed closely for signs that might require dosage adjustment, including changes in clinical status resulting from remissions or exacerbations of the disease,

individual drug responsiveness, and the effect of stress (e.g., surgery, infection, trauma). During stress it may be necessary to increase dosage temporarily.
If the drug is to be stopped after more than a few days of treatment, it usually should be withdrawn gradually.

HOW SUPPLIED

No. 7063—Tablets Cortone Acetate, 25 mg each, are white, round, scored, compressed tablets, coded MSD 219 on one side and CORTONE on the other. They are supplied as follows:
NDC 0006-0219-68 in bottles of 100.
  Shown in Product Identification Guide, page 324
  7930631   Issued October 1995

COSMEGEN® for Injection
(Dactinomycin for Injection), U.S.P.
(Actinomycin D)

℞

> ### WARNING
> Dactinomycin is extremely corrosive to soft tissue. If extravasation occurs during intravenous use, severe damage to soft tissues will occur. In at least one instance, this has led to contracture of the arms.
>
> ### DOSAGE
> The dosage of COSMEGEN* (Dactinomycin for Injection) is calculated in micrograms (mcg). The usual adult dosage is 500 micrograms (0.5 mg) daily intravenously for a maximum of five days. The dosage for adults or children should not exceed 15 mcg/kg or 400–600 mcg/square meter of body surface daily intravenously for five days. Calculation of the dosage for obese or edematous patients should be on the basis of surface area in an effort to relate dosage to lean body mass.

*Registered trademark of MERCK & CO., INC.

DESCRIPTION

Dactinomycin is one of the actinomycins, a group of antibiotics produced by various species of *Streptomyces*. Dactinomycin is the principal component of the mixture of actinomycins produced by *Streptomyces parvullus*. Unlike other species of *Streptomyces*, this organism yields an essentially pure substance that contains only traces of similar compounds differing in the amino acid content of the peptide side chains. The empirical formula is $C_{62}H_{86}N_{12}O_{16}$ and the structural formula is:

COSMEGEN is a sterile, yellow lyophilized powder for injection by the intravenous route or by regional perfusion after reconstitution. Each vial contains 0.5 mg (500 mcg) of dactinomycin and 20.0 mg of mannitol.

CLINICAL PHARMACOLOGY

Action
Generally, the actinomycins exert an inhibitory effect on gram-positive and gram-negative bacteria and on some fungi. However, the toxic properties of the actinomycins (including dactinomycin) in relation to antibacterial activity are such as to preclude their use as antibiotics in the treatment of infectious diseases.
Because the actinomycins are cytotoxic, they have an antineoplastic effect which has been demonstrated in experimental animals with various types of tumor implant. This cytotoxic action is the basis for their use in the palliative treatment of certain types of cancer.
Pharmacokinetics and Metabolism
Results of a study in patients with malignant melanoma indicate that dactinomycin (^{3}H actinomycin D) is minimally metabolized, is concentrated in nucleated cells, and does not

penetrate the blood brain barrier. Approximately 30% of the dose was recovered in urine and feces in one week. The terminal plasma half-life for radioactivity was approximately 36 hours.

INDICATIONS AND USAGE

Wilms' Tumor
The neoplasm responding most frequently to COSMEGEN is Wilms' tumor. With low doses of both dactinomycin and radiotherapy, temporary objective improvement may be as good as and may last longer than with higher doses of each given alone. In the National Wilms' Tumor study, combination therapy with dactinomycin and vincristine together with surgery and radiotherapy, was shown to have significantly improved the prognosis of patients in groups II and III. Dactinomycin and vincristine were given for a total of seven cycles, so that maintenance therapy continued for approximately 15 months.
Postoperative radiotherapy in group I patients and optimal combination chemotherapy for those in group IV are unsettled issues. About 70 percent of lung metastases have disappeared with an appropriate combination of radiation, dactinomycin and vincristine.
Rhabdomyosarcoma
Temporary regression of the tumor and beneficial subjective results have occurred with dactinomycin in rhabdomyosarcoma which, like most soft tissue sarcomas, is comparatively radio-resistant.
Several groups have reported successful use of cyclophosphamide, vincristine, dactinomycin and doxorubicin hydrochloride in various combinations. Effective combinations have included vincristine and dactinomycin; vincristine, dactinomycin and cyclophosphamide (VAC therapy) and all four drugs in sequence. At present, the most effective treatment for children with inoperable or metastatic rhabdomyosarcoma has been VAC chemotherapy. Two-thirds of these children were doing well without evidence of disease at a median time of three years after diagnosis.
Carcinoma of Testis and Uterus
The sequential use of dactinomycin and methotrexate, along with meticulous monitoring of human chorionic gonadotropin levels until normal, has resulted in survival in the majority of women with metastatic choriocarcinoma. Sequential therapy is used if there is:
1. Stability in gonadotropin titers following two successive courses of an agent.
2. Rising gonadotropin titers during treatment.
3. Severe toxicity preventing adequate therapy.
In patients with nonmetastatic choriocarcinoma, dactinomycin or methotrexate or both, have been used successfully, with or without surgery.
Dactinomycin has been beneficial as a single agent in the treatment of metastatic nonseminomatour testicular carcinoma when used in cycles of 500 mcg/day for five consecutive days, every 6–8 weeks for periods of four months or longer.
Other Neoplasms
Dactinomycin has been given intravenously or by regional perfusion, either alone or with other antineoplastic compounds or x-ray therapy, in the palliative treatment of Ewing's sarcoma and sarcoma botryoides. For nonmetastatic Ewing's sarcoma, promising results were obtained when dactinomycin (45 mcg/m^2) and cyclophosphamide (1200 mg/m^2) were given sequentially and with radiotherapy, over an 18 month period. Those with metastatic disease remain the subject of continued investigation with a more aggressive chemotherapeutic regimen employed initially.
Temporary objective improvement and relief of pain and discomfort have followed the use of dactinomycin usually in conjunction with radiotherapy for sarcoma botryoides. This palliative effect ranges from transitory inhibition of tumor growth to a considerable but temporary regression in tumor size.
COSMEGEN (Dactinomycin for Injection) and Radiation Therapy
Much evidence suggests that dactinomycin potentiates the effects of x-ray therapy. The converse also appears likely; i.e., dactinomycin may be more effective when radiation therapy also is given.
With combined dactinomycin-radiation therapy, the normal skin, as well as the buccal and pharyngeal mucosa, show early erythema. A smaller than usual x-ray dose when given with dactinomycin causes erythema and vesiculation, which progress more rapidly through the stages of tanning and desquamation. Healing may occur in four to six weeks rather than two to three months. Erythema from previous x-ray therapy may be reactivated by dactinomycin alone, even when irradiation occurred many months earlier, and especially when the interval between the two forms of therapy is brief. This potentiation of radiation effect represents a special problem when the irradiation treatment area includes the mucous membrane. When irradiation is directed toward the nasopharynx, the combination may produce severe oropharyngeal mucositis. *Severe reactions may ensue if high*

doses of both dactinomycin and radiation therapy are used or if the patient is particularly sensitive to such combined therapy.
Because of this potentiating effect, dactinomycin may be tried in radio-sensitive tumors not responding to doses of x-ray therapy that can be tolerated. Objective improvement in tumor size and activity may be observed when lower, better tolerated doses of both types of therapy are employed.
COSMEGEN (Dactinomycin for Injection) and Perfusion Technic
Dactinomycin alone or with other antineoplastic agents has also been given by the isolation-perfusion technic, either as palliative treatment or as an adjunct to resection of a tumor. Some tumors considered resistant to chemotherapy and radiation therapy may respond when the drug is given by the perfusion technic. Neoplasms in which dactinomycin has been tried by this technic include various types of sarcoma, carcinoma, and adenocarcinoma.
In some instances tumors regressed, pain was relieved for variable periods, and surgery made possible. On other occasions, however, the outcome has been less favorable. Nevertheless, in selected cases, the drug by perfusion may provide more effective palliation than when given systemically.
Dactinomycin by the isolation-perfusion technic offers certain advantages, provided leakage of the drug through the general circulation into other areas of the body is minimal. By this technic the drug is in continuous contact with the tumor for the duration of treatment. The dose may be increased well over that used by the systemic route, usually without adding to the danger of toxic effects. If the agent is confined to an isolated part, it should not interfere with the patient's defense mechanism. Systemic absorption of toxic products from neoplastic tissue can be minimized by removing the perfusate when the procedure is finished.

CONTRAINDICATIONS

If dactinomycin is given at or about the time of infection with chicken pox or herpes zoster, a severe generalized disease, which may result in death, may occur.

PRECAUTIONS

General
COSMEGEN should be administered only under the supervision of a physician who is experienced in the use of cancer chemotherapeutic agents.
This drug is highly toxic and both powder and solution must be handled and administered with care. Inhalation of dust or vapors and contact with skin or mucous membranes, especially those of the eyes, must be avoided. Should accidental eye contact occur, copious irrigation with water should be instituted immediately, followed by prompt ophthalmologic consultation. Should accidental skin contact occur, the affected part must be irrigated immediately with copious amounts of water for at least 15 minutes.
As with all antineoplastic agents, dactinomycin is a toxic drug and very careful and frequent observation of the patient for adverse reactions is necessary. These reactions may involve any tissue of the body. The possibility of an anaphylactoid reaction should be borne in mind.
Increased incidence of gastrointestinal toxicity and marrow suppression has been reported when dactinomycin was given with x-ray therapy.
Particular caution is necessary when administering dactinomycin within two months of irradiation for the treatment of right-sided Wilms' tumor, since hepatomegaly and elevated SGOT levels have been noted.
Nausea and vomiting due to dactinomycin make it necessary to give this drug intermittently. It is extremely important to observe the patient daily for toxic side effects when multiple chemotherapy is employed, since a full course of therapy occasionally is not tolerated. If stomatitis, diarrhea, or severe hemopoietic depression appear during therapy, these drugs should be discontinued until the patient has recovered.
Recent reports indicate an increased incidence of second primary tumors following treatment with radiation and anti-neoplastic agents, such as dactinomycin. Multi-modal therapy creates the need for careful, long-term observation of cancer survivors.
Laboratory Tests
Many abnormalities of renal, hepatic, and bone marrow function have been reported in patients with neoplastic disease and receiving dactinomycin. It is advisable to check renal, hepatic, and bone marrow functions frequently.
Drug/Laboratory Test Interactions
It has been reported that dactinomycin may interfere with bioassay procedures for the determination of antibacterial drug levels.
Carcinogenesis, Mutagenesis, Impairment of Fertility
The International Agency on Research on Cancer has judged that dactinomycin is a positive carcinogen in animals. Local sarcomas were produced in mice and rats after repeated subcutaneous or intraperitoneal injection. Mesenchymal tumors occurred in male F344 rats given intraperitoneal injections of 0.05 mg/kg, 2 to 5 times per week for 18 weeks. The first tumor appeared at 23 weeks.
Dactinomycin has been shown to be mutagenic in a number of test systems *in vitro* and *in vivo* including human fibroblasts and leucocytes, and HELA cells. DNA damage and cytogenetic effects have been demonstrated in the mouse and the rat.
Adequate fertility studies have not been reported.
Pregnancy
Pregnancy Category C. COSMEGEN has been shown to cause malformations and embryotoxicity in the rat, rabbit and hamster when given in doses of 50–100 mcg/kg intravenously (3–7 times the maximum recommended human dose). There are no adequate and well-controlled studies in pregnant women. COSMEGEN should be used during pregnancy only if the potential benefit justifies the potential risk to the fetus.
Nursing Mothers
It is not known whether this drug is excreted in human milk. Because many drugs are excreted in human milk and because of the potential for serious adverse reactions in nursing infants from COSMEGEN, a decision should be made whether to discontinue nursing or to discontinue the drug, taking into account the importance of the drug to the mother.
Pediatric Use
The greater frequency of toxic effects of dactinomycin in infants suggest that this drug should be given to infants only over the age of 6 to 12 months.

ADVERSE REACTIONS

Toxic effects (excepting nausea and vomiting) usually do not become apparent until two to four days after a course of therapy is stopped, and may not be maximal before one to two weeks have elapsed. Deaths have been reported. However, adverse reactions are usually reversible on discontinuance of therapy. They include the following:
Miscellaneous: malaise, fatigue, lethargy, fever, myalgia, proctitis, hypocalcemia.
Oral: cheilitis, dysphagia, esophagitis, ulcerative stomatitis, pharyngitis.
Gastrointestinal: anorexia, nausea, vomiting, abdominal pain, diarrhea, gastrointestinal ulceration, liver toxicity including ascites, hepatomegaly, hepatitis, and liver function test abnormalities. Nausea and vomiting, which occur early during the first few hours after administration, may be alleviated by giving antiemetics.
Hematologic: anemia, even to the point of aplastic anemia, agranulocytosis, leukopenia, thrombopenia, pancytopenia, reticulopenia. Platelet and white cell counts should be done *daily* to detect severe hemopoietic depression. If either count markedly decreases, the drug should be withheld to allow marrow recovery. This often takes up to three weeks.
Dermatologic: alopecia, skin eruptions, acne, flare-up of erythema or increased pigmentation of previously irradiated skin.
Soft tissues. Dactinomycin is extremely corrosive. If extravasation occurs during intravenous use, severe damage to soft tissues will occur. In at least one instance, this has led to contracture of the arms.

OVERDOSAGE

The intravenous LD_{50} of COSMEGEN in the rat is 460 mcg/kg.

DOSAGE AND ADMINISTRATION

Toxic reactions due to dactinomycin are frequent and may be severe (see ADVERSE REACTIONS), thus limiting in many instances the amount that may be given. However, the severity of toxicity varies markedly and is only partly dependent on the dose employed. The drug must be given in short courses.
Intravenous Use
The dosage of dactinomycin varies depending on the tolerance of the patient, the size and location of the neoplasm, and the use of other forms of therapy. It may be necessary to decrease the usual dosages suggested below when other chemotherapy or x-ray therapy is used concomitantly or has been used previously.
The dosage for adults or children should not exceed 15 mcg/kg or 400–600 mcg/square meter of body surface daily intravenously for five days. Calculation of the dosage for obese or edematous patients should be on the basis of surface area in an effort to relate dosage to lean body mass.
Adults: The usual adult dosage is 500 mcg (0.5 mg) daily intravenously for a maximum of five days.
Children: In children 15 mcg (0.015 mg) per kilogram of body weight is given intravenously daily for five days. An alternative schedule is a total dosage of 2500 mcg (2.5 mg) per square meter of body surface given intravenously over a one week period.
In both adults and children, a second course may be given after at least three weeks have elapsed, provided all signs of toxicity have disappeared.
Reconstitute COSMEGEN by adding 1.1 ml of **Sterile Water for Injection (without preservative)** using aseptic precautions. The resulting solution of dactinomycin will contain approximately 500 mcg (0.5 mg) per mL.
Parenteral drug products should be inspected visually for particulate matter and discoloration prior to administration, whenever solution and container permit. When reconstituted, COSMEGEN is a clear, gold-colored solution.
Once reconstituted, the solution of dactinomycin can be added to infusion solutions of Dextrose Injection 5 percent or Sodium Chloride Injection either directly or to the tubing of a running intravenous infusion.
Although reconstituted COSMEGEN is chemically stable, the product does not contain a preservative and accidental microbial contamination might result. Any unused portion should be discarded. Use of water containing preservatives (benzyl alcohol or parabens) to reconstitute COSMEGEN for Injection, results in the formation of a precipitate.
Partial removal of dactinomycin from intravenous solutions by cellulose ester membrane filters used in some intravenous in-line filters has been reported.
Since dactinomycin is extremely corrosive to soft tissue, precautions for materials of this nature should be observed.
If the drug is given directly into the vein without the use of an infusion, the "two-needle technic" should be used. Reconstitute and withdraw the calculated dose from the vial with one sterile needle. Use another sterile needle for direct injection into the vein.
Discard any unused portion of the dactinomycin solution.
Isolation-Perfusion Technic
The dosage schedules and the technic itself vary from one investigator to another; the published literature, therefore, should be consulted for details. In general, the following doses are suggested:

50 mcg (0.05 mg) per kilogram of body weight for lower extremity or pelvis.
35 mcg (0.035 mg) per kilogram of body weight for upper extremity.

It may be advisable to use lower doses in obese patients, or when previous chemotherapy or radiation therapy has been employed.
Complications of the perfusion technic are related mainly to the amount of drug that escapes into the systemic circulation and may consist of hemopoietic depression, absorption of toxic products from massive destruction of neoplastic tissue, increased susceptibility to infection, impaired wound healing, and superficial ulceration of the gastric mucosa. Other side effects may include edema of the extremity involved, damage to soft tissues of the perfused area, and (potentially) venous thrombosis.

HOW SUPPLIED

No. 3298—COSMEGEN for Injection is a lyophilized powder. In the dry form the compound is an amorphous yellow powder. The solution is clear and gold-colored. COSMEGEN for Injection is supplied as follows:
NDC 0006-3298-22 in vials containing 0.5 mg (500 micrograms) of dactinomycin and 20.0 mg of mannitol.
(6505-00-902-1222, 0.5 mg)
Storage
Store at controlled room temperature, 15–30°C (59–86°F). Protect from light and humidity.
Special Handling
Due to the drug's toxic and mutagenic properties, appropriate precautions including the use of appropriate safety equipment are recommended for the preparation of COSMEGEN for parenteral administration. The National Institutes of Health presently recommends that the preparation of injectable antineoplastic drugs should be performed in a Class II laminar flow biological safety cabinet and that personnel preparing drugs of this class should wear surgical gloves and a closed front surgical-type gown with knit cuffs.
7496527 Issued March 1995

Continued on next page

Information on the Merck & Co., Inc. products listed on these pages is the full prescribing information from product circulars in use September 30, 1996.

Merck & Co.—Cont.

COZAAR® ℞
(Losartan Potassium Tablets)

USE IN PREGNANCY
When used in pregnancy during the second and third trimesters, drugs that act directly on the renin-angiotensin system can cause injury and even death to the developing fetus. When pregnancy is detected, COZAAR should be discontinued as soon as possible. See WARNINGS: *Fetal/Neonatal Morbidity and Mortality.*

DESCRIPTION

COZAAR* (losartan potassium), the first of a new class of antihypertensives, is an angiotensin II receptor (type AT_1) antagonist.
Losartan potassium, a non-peptide molecule, is chemically described as 2-butyl-4-chloro-1-[*p*-(*o*-1*H*-tetrazol-5-ylphenyl)-benzyl]imidazole-5-methanol monopotassium salt.
Its empirical formula is $C_{22}H_{22}ClKN_6O$, and its structural formula is:

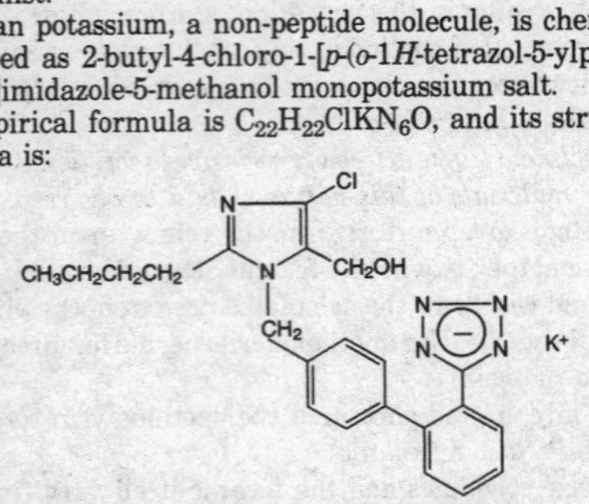

Losartan potassium is a white to off-white free-flowing crystalline powder with a molecular weight of 461.01. It is freely soluble in water, soluble in alcohols, and slightly soluble in common organic solvents, such as acetonitrile and methyl ethyl ketone. Oxidation of the 5-hydroxymethyl group on the imidazole ring results in the active metabolite of losartan.
COZAAR is available for oral administration containing either 25 mg or 50 mg of losartan potassium and the following inactive ingredients: microcrystalline cellulose, lactose hydrous, pregelatinized starch, magnesium stearate, hydroxypropyl cellulose, hydroxypropyl methylcellulose, titanium dioxide, D&C yellow No. 10 aluminum lake and FD&C blue No. 2 aluminum lake.
COZAAR 25 mg and 50 mg contain potassium in the following amounts: 2.12 mg (0.054 mEq) and 4.24 mg (0.108 mEq), respectively.

*Registered trademark of E. I. du Pont de Nemours and Company, Wilmington, Delaware, USA

CLINICAL PHARMACOLOGY

Mechanism of Action
Angiotensin II [formed from angiotensin I in a reaction catalyzed by angiotensin converting enzyme (ACE, kininase II)], is a potent vasoconstrictor, the primary vasoactive hormone of the renin-angiotensin system and an important component in the pathophysiology of hypertension. It also stimulates aldosterone secretion by the adrenal cortex. Losartan and its principal active metabolite block the vasoconstrictor and aldosterone-secreting effects of angiotensin II by selectively blocking the binding of angiotensin II to the AT_1 receptor found in many tissues, (e.g., vascular smooth muscle, adrenal gland). There is also an AT_2 receptor found in many tissues but it is not known to be associated with cardiovascular homeostatis. Both losartan and its principal active metabolite do not exhibit any partial agonist activity at the AT_1 receptor and have much greater affinity (about 1000-fold) for the AT_1 receptor than for the AT_2 receptor. *In vitro* binding studies indicate that losartan is a reversible, competitive inhibitor of the AT_1 receptor. The active metabolite is 10 to 40 times more potent by weight than losartan and appears to be a reversible, non-competitive inhibitor of the AT_1 receptor.
Neither losartan nor its active metabolite inhibits ACE (kininase II, the enzyme that converts angiotensin I to angiotensin II and degrades bradykinin); nor do they bind to or block other hormone receptors or ion channels known to be important in cardiovascular regulation.
Pharmacokinetics
General
Losartan is an orally active agent that undergoes substantial first-pass metabolism by cytochrome P450 enzymes. It is converted, in part, to an active carboxylic acid metabolite that is responsible for most of the angiotensin II receptor antagonism that follows losartan treatment. The terminal half-life of losartan is about 2 hours and of the metabolite is about 6–9 hours. The pharmacokinetics of losartan and its active metabolite are linear with oral losartan doses up to 200 mg and do not change over time. Neither losartan nor its metabolite accumulate in plasma upon repeated once-daily dosing.
Following oral administration, losartan is well absorbed (based on absorption of radiolabeled losartan) and undergoes substantial first-pass metabolism; the systemic bioavailability of losartan is approximately 33%. About 14% of an orally-administered dose of losartan is converted to the active metabolite. Mean peak concentrations of losartan and its active metabolite are reached in 1 hour and in 3–4 hours, respectively. While maximum plasma concentrations of losartan and its active metabolite are approximately equal, the AUC of the metabolite is about 4 times as great as that of losartan. A meal slows absorption of losartan and decreases its C_{max} but has only minor effects on losartan AUC or on the AUC of the metabolite (about 10% decreased).
Both losartan and its active metabolite are highly bound to plasma proteins, primarily albumin, with plasma free fractions of 1.3% and 0.2% respectively. Plasma protein binding is constant over the concentration range achieved with recommended doses. Studies in rats indicate that losartan crosses the blood-brain barrier poorly, if at all.
Losartan metabolites have been identified in human plasma and urine. In addition to the active carboxylic acid metabolite, several inactive metabolites are formed. Following oral and intravenous administration of ^{14}C-labeled losartan potassium, circulating plasma radioactivity is primarily attributed to losartan and its active metabolite. *In vitro* studies indicate that cytochrome P450 2C9 and 3A4 are involved in the biotransformation of losartan to its metabolites. Minimal conversion of losartan to the active metabolite (less than 1% of the dose compared to 14% of the dose in normal subjects) was seen in about one percent of individuals studied.
The volume of distribution of losartan is about 34 liters and of the active metabolite is about 12 liters. Total plasma clearance of losartan and the active metabolite is about 600 mL/min and 50 mL/min, respectively, with renal clearance of about 75 mL/min and 25 mL/min, respectively. When losartan is administered orally, about 4% of the dose is excreted unchanged in the urine and about 6% is excreted in urine as active metabolite. Biliary excretion contributes to the elimination of losartan and its metabolites. Following oral ^{14}C-labeled losartan, about 35% of radioactivity is recovered in the urine and about 60% in the feces. Following an intravenous dose of ^{14}C-labeled losartan, about 45% of radioactivity is recovered in the urine and 50% in the feces.
Special Populations
Pediatric: Losartan pharmacokinetics have not been investigated in patients <18 years of age.
Geriatric and Gender: Losartan pharmacokinetics have been investigated in the elderly (65–75 years) and in both genders. Plasma concentrations of losartan and its active metabolite are similar in elderly and young hypertensives. Plasma concentrations of losartan were about twice as high in female hypertensives as male hypertensives, but concentrations of the active metabolite were similar in males and females. No dosage adjustment is necessary (see DOSAGE AND ADMINISTRATION).
Race: Pharmacokinetic differences due to race have not been studied.
Renal Insufficiency: Plasma concentrations of losartan are not altered in patients with creatinine clearance above 30 mL/min. In patients with lower creatinine clearance, AUCs are about 50% greater and they are doubled in hemodialysis patients. Plasma concentrations of the active metabolite are not significantly altered in patients with renal impairment or in hemodialysis patients. Neither losartan nor its active metabolite can be removed by hemodialysis. No dosage adjustment is necessary for patients with renal impairment unless they are volume-depleted (see WARNINGS, *Hypotension—Volume-Depleted Patients* and DOSAGE AND ADMINISTRATION).
Hepatic Insufficiency: Following oral administration in patients with mild to moderate alcoholic cirrhosis of the liver, plasma concentrations of losartan and its active metabolite were, respectively, 5-times and about 1.7-times those in young male volunteers. Compared to normal subjects the total plasma clearance of losartan in patients with hepatic insufficiency was about 50% lower and the oral bioavailability was about 2-times higher. A lower starting dose is recommended for patients with a history of hepatic impairment (see DOSAGE AND ADMINISTRATION).
Drug Interactions
Losartan, administered for 12 days, did not affect the pharmacokinetics or pharmacodynamics of a single dose of warfarin. Losartan did not affect the pharmacokinetics of oral or intravenous digoxin. Coadministration of losartan and cimetidine led to an increase of about 18% in AUC of losartan but did not affect the pharmacokinetics of its active metabolite. Coadministration of losartan and phenobarbital led to a reduction of about 20% in the AUC of losartan and that of its active metabolite. There is no pharmacokinetic interaction between losartan and hydrochlorothiazide.
Pharmacodynamics and Clinical Effects
Losartan inhibits the pressor effect of angiotensin II (as well as angiotensin I) infusions. A dose of 100 mg inhibits the pressor effect by about 85% at peak with 25–40% inhibition persisting for 24 hours. Removal of the negative feedback of angiotensin II causes a 2–3 fold rise in plasma renin activity and consequent rise in angiotensin II plasma concentration in hypertensive patients. Losartan does not affect the response to bradykinin, whereas ACE inhibitors increase the response to bradykinin. Aldosterone plasma concentrations fall following losartan administration. In spite of the effect of losartan on aldosterone secretion, very little effect on serum potassium was observed.
In a single-dose study in normal volunteers, losartan had no effects on glomerular filtration rate, renal plasma flow or filtration fraction. In multiple dose studies in hypertensive patients, there were no notable effects on systemic or renal prostaglandin concentrations, fasting triglycerides, total cholesterol or HDL-cholesterol or fasting glucose concentrations. There was a small uricosuric effect leading to a minimal decrease in serum uric acid (mean decrease <0.4 mg/dL) during chronic oral administration.
The antihypertensive effects of COZAAR were demonstrated principally in 4 placebo-controlled 6–12 week trials of dosages from 10 to 150 mg per day in patients with baseline diastolic blood pressures of 95–115. The studies allowed comparisons of two doses (50–100 mg/day) as once-daily or twice-daily regimens, comparisons of peak and trough effects, and comparisons of response by gender, age, and race. Three additional studies examined the antihypertensive effects of losartan and hydrochlorothiazide in combination.
The 4 studies of losartan monotherapy included a total of 1075 patients randomized to several doses of losartan and 334 to placebo. The 10 and 25 mg doses produced some effect at peak (6 hours after dosing) but small and inconsistent trough (24 hour) responses. Doses of 50, 100 and 150 mg once daily gave statistically significant systolic/diastolic mean decreases in blood pressure, compared to placebo in the range of 5.5–10.5/3.5–7.5 mmHg, with the 150 mg dose giving no greater effect than 50–100 mg. Twice-daily dosing at 50–100 mg/day gave consistently larger trough responses than once-daily dosing at the same total dose. Peak (6 hour) effects were uniformly, but moderately, larger than trough effects, with the trough-to-peak ratio for systolic and diastolic responses 50–95% and 60–90%, respectively.
Addition of a low dose of hydrochlorothiazide (12.5 mg) to losartan 50 mg once daily resulted in placebo-adjusted blood pressure reduction of 15.5/9.2 mmHg.
Analysis of age, gender, and race subgroups of patients showed that men and women, and patients over and under 65, had generally similar responses. Black patients, however, had notably smaller responses to losartan monotherapy.
The effect of losartan is substantially present within one week but in some studies the maximal effect occurred in 3–6 weeks. In long-term follow-up studies (without placebo control) the effect of losartan appeared to be maintained for up to a year. There is no apparent rebound effect after abrupt withdrawal of losartan. There was essentially no change in average heart rate in losartan-treated patients in controlled trials.
Persistent dry cough (with an incidence of a few percent) has been associated with ACE inhibitor use and in practice can be a cause of discontinuation of ACE inhibitor therapy. Two prospective, parallel-group, double-blind, randomized, controlled trials were conducted to assess the effects of losartan on the incidence of cough in hypertensive patients who had experienced cough while receiving ACE inhibitor therapy. Patients who had typical ACE inhibitor cough when challenged with lisinopril, whose cough disappeared on placebo, were randomized to losartan 50 mg, lisinopril 20 mg, or either placebo (one study, n=97) or 25 mg hydrochlorothiazide (n=135). The double-blind treatment period lasted up to 8 weeks. The incidence of cough is shown below.

Study 1†	HCTZ	Losartan	Lisinopril
Cough	25%	17%	69%
Study 2††	**Placebo**	**Losartan**	**Lisinopril**
Cough	35%	29%	62%

† Demographics = (89% caucasian, 64% female)
†† Demographics = (90% caucasian, 51% female)

These studies demonstrate that the incidence of cough associated with losartan therapy, in a population that all had cough associated with ACE inhibitor therapy, is similar to that associated with hydrochlorothiazide or placebo therapy.

INDICATIONS AND USAGE

COZAAR is indicated for the treatment of hypertension. It may be used alone or in combination with other antihypertensive agents.
In considering the use of monotherapy with COZAAR, it should be noted that in controlled trials COZAAR had an

effect on blood pressure that was notably less in black patients than in non-blacks, a finding similar to the small effect of angiotensin converting enzyme inhibitors in blacks.

CONTRAINDICATIONS

COZAAR is contraindicated in patients who are hypersensitive to any component of this product.

WARNINGS

Fetal/Neonatal Morbidity and Mortality

Drugs that act directly on the renin-angiotensin system can cause fetal and neonatal morbidity and death when administered to pregnant women. Several dozen cases have been reported in the world literature in patients who were taking angiotensin converting enzyme inhibitors. When pregnancy is detected, COZAAR should be discontinued as soon as possible.

The use of drugs that act directly on the renin-angiotensin system during the second and third trimesters of pregnancy has been associated with fetal and neonatal injury, including hypotension, neonatal skull hypoplasia, anuria, reversible or irreversible renal failure, and death. Oligohydramnios has also been reported, presumably resulting from decreased fetal renal function; oligohydramnios in this setting has been associated with fetal limb contractures, craniofacial deformation, and hypoplastic lung development. Prematurity, intrauterine growth retardation, and patent ductus arteriosus have also been reported, although it is not clear whether these occurrences were due to exposure to the drug.

These adverse effects do not appear to have resulted from intrauterine drug exposure that has been limited to the first trimester.

Mothers whose embryos and fetuses are exposed to an angiotensin II receptor antagonist only during the first trimester should be so informed. Nonetheless, when patients become pregnant, physicians should have the patient discontinue the use of COZAAR as soon as possible.

Rarely (probably less often than once in every thousand pregnancies), no alternative to an angiotensin II receptor antagonist will be found. In these rare cases, the mothers should be apprised of the potential hazards to their fetuses, and serial ultrasound examinations should be performed to assess the intraamniotic environment.

If oligohydramnios is observed, COZAAR should be discontinued unless it is considered life-saving for the mother. Contraction stress testing (CST), a non-stress test (NST), or biophysical profiling (BPP) may be appropriate, depending upon the week of pregnancy. Patients and physicians should be aware, however, that oligohydramnios may not appear until after the fetus has sustained irreversible injury.

Infants with histories of *in utero* exposure to an angiotensin II receptor antagonist should be closely observed for hypotension, oliguria, and hyperkalemia. If oliguria occurs, attention should be directed toward support of blood pressure and renal perfusion. Exchange transfusion or dialysis may be required as means of reversing hypotension and/or substituting for disordered renal function.

Losartan potassium has been shown to produce adverse effects in rat fetuses and neonates, including decreased body weight, delayed physical and behavioral development, mortality and renal toxicity. With the exception of neonatal weight gain (which was affected at doses as low as 10 mg/kg/day), doses associated with these effects exceeded 25 mg/kg/day (approximately three times the maximum recommended human dose of 100 mg on a mg/m^2 basis). These findings are attributed to drug exposure in late gestation and during lactation. Significant levels of losartan and its active metabolite were shown to be present in rat fetal plasma during late gestation and in rat milk.

Hypotension—Volume-Depleted Patients

In patients who are intravascularly volume-depleted (e.g., those treated with diuretics), symptomatic hypotension may occur after initiation of therapy with COZAAR. These conditions should be corrected prior to administration of COZAAR, or a lower starting dose should be used (see DOSAGE AND ADMINISTRATION).

PRECAUTIONS

General

Based on pharmacokinetic data which demonstrate significantly increased plasma concentrations of losartan in cirrhotic patients, a lower dose should be considered for patients with impaired liver function (see DOSAGE AND ADMINISTRATION and CLINICAL PHARMACOLOGY, *Pharmacokinetics*).

Hypersensitivity. See ADVERSE REACTIONS, *Post-Marketing Experience.*

Impaired Renal Function

As a consequence of inhibiting the renin-angiotensin-aldosterone system, changes in renal function have been reported in susceptible individuals treated with COZAAR; in some patients, these changes in renal function were reversible upon discontinuation of therapy.

In patients whose renal function may depend on the activity of the renin-angiotensin-aldosterone system (e.g., patients with severe congestive heart failure), treatment with angiotensin converting enzyme inhibitors has been associated with oliguria and/or progressive azotemia and (rarely) with acute renal failure and/or death. Similar outcomes have been reported with COZAAR.

In studies of ACE inhibitors in patients with unilateral or bilateral renal artery stenosis, increases in serum creatinine or BUN have been reported. Similar effects have been reported with COZAAR; in some patients, these effects were reversible upon discontinuation of therapy.

Information for Patients

Pregnancy: Female patients of childbearing age should be told about the consequences of second- and third-trimester exposure to drugs that act on the renin-angiotensin system, and they should also be told that these consequences do not appear to have resulted from intrauterine drug exposure that has been limited to the first trimester. These patients should be asked to report pregnancies to their physicians as soon as possible.

Drug Interactions

No significant drug-drug pharmacokinetic interactions have been found in interaction studies with hydrochlorothiazide, digoxin, warfarin, cimetidine and phenobarbital. (See CLINICAL PHARMACOLOGY, *Drug Interactions.*) Potent inhibitors of cytochrome P450 3A4 and 2C9 have not been studied clinically but *in vitro* studies show significant inhibition of the formation of the active metabolite by inhibitors of P450 3A4 (ketoconazole, troleandomycin, gestodene), or P450 2C9 (sulfaphenazole) and nearly complete inhibition by the combination of sulfaphenazole and ketoconazole. The pharmacodynamic consequences of concomitant use of losartan and these inhibitors have not been examined.

Carcinogenesis, Mutagenesis, Impairment of Fertility

Losartan potassium was not carcinogenic when administered at maximally tolerated dosages to rats and mice for 105 and 92 weeks, respectively. Female rats given the highest dose (270 mg/kg/day) had a slightly higher incidence of pancreatic acinar adenoma. The maximally tolerated dosages (270 mg/kg/day in rats, 200 mg/kg/day in mice) provided systemic exposures for losartan and its pharmacologically active metabolite that were approximately 160- and 90-times (rats) and 30- and 15-times (mice) the exposure of a 50 kg human given 100 mg per day.

Losartan potassium was negative in the microbial mutagenesis and V-79 mammalian cell mutagenesis assays and in the *in vitro* alkaline elution and *in vitro* and *in vivo* chromosomal aberration assays. In addition, the active metabolite showed no evidence of genotoxicity in the microbial mutagenesis, *in vitro* alkaline elution, and *in vitro* chromosomal aberration assays.

Fertility and reproductive performance were not affected in studies with male rats given oral doses of losartan potassium up to approximately 150 mg/kg/day. The administration of toxic dosage levels in females (300/200 mg/kg/day) was associated with a significant ($p < 0.05$) decrease in the number of corpora lutea/female, implants/female, and live fetuses/female at C-section. At 100 mg/kg/day only a decrease in the number of corpora lutea/female was observed. The relationship of these findings to drug-treatment is uncertain since there was no effect at these dosage levels on implants/pregnant female, percent post-implantation loss, or live animals/litter at parturition. In nonpregnant rats dosed at 135 mg/kg/day for 7 days, systemic exposure (AUCs) for losartan and its active metabolite were approximately 66 and 26 times the exposure achieved in man at the maximum recommended human daily dosage (100 mg).

Pregnancy

Pregnancy Categories C (first trimester) and D (second and third trimesters). See WARNINGS, *Fetal/Neonatal Morbidity and Mortality.*

Nursing Mothers

It is not known whether losartan is excreted in human milk, but significant levels of losartan and its active metabolite were shown to be present in rat milk. Because of the potential for adverse effects on the nursing infant, a decision should be made whether to discontinue nursing or discontinue the drug, taking into account the importance of the drug to the mother.

Pediatric Use

Safety and effectiveness in pediatric patients have not been established.

Use in the Elderly

Of the total number of patients receiving COZAAR in controlled clinical studies, 391 patients (19%) were 65 years and over, while 37 patients (2%) were 75 years and over. No overall differences in effectiveness or safety were observed between these patients and younger patients, but greater sensitivity of some older individuals cannot be ruled out.

ADVERSE REACTIONS

COZAAR has been evaluated for safety in more than 3300 patients treated for essential hypertension and 4058 patients/subjects overall. Over 1200 patients were treated for over 6 months and more than 800 for over one year. In general, treatment with COZAAR was well-tolerated. The overall incidence of adverse experiences reported with COZAAR was similar to placebo.

In controlled clinical trials, discontinuation of therapy due to clinical adverse experiences was required in 2.3 percent of patients treated with COZAAR and 3.7 percent of patients given placebo.

The following table of adverse events is based on four 6–12 week placebo controlled trials involving over 1000 patients on various doses (10–150 mg) of losartan and over 300 patients given placebo. All doses of losartan are grouped because none of the adverse events appeared to have a dose-related frequency. The table includes all adverse events, whether or not attributed to the treatment, occurring in at least 1% of patients treated with losartan and that were more frequent on losartan than placebo.

	Losartan (n=1075) Incidence	Placebo (n=334) Incidence
Digestive		
Diarrhea	2.4	2.1
Dyspepsia	1.3	1.2
Musculoskeletal		
Cramp, muscle	1.1	0.3
Myalgia	1.0	0.9
Pain, back	1.8	1.2
Pain, leg	1.0	0.0
Nervous System/Psychiatric		
Dizziness	3.5	2.1
Insomnia	1.4	0.6
Respiratory		
Congestion, nasal	2.0	1.2
Cough	3.4	3.3
Infection, upper respiratory	7.9	6.9
Sinus disorder	1.5	1.2
Sinusitis	1.0	0.3

The following adverse events were also reported at a rate of 1% or greater in patients treated with losartan, but were as, or more frequent, in the placebo group: asthenia/fatigue, edema/swelling, abdominal pain, chest pain, nausea, headache, pharyngitis.

Adverse events occurred at about the same rates in men and women, older and younger patients, and black and non-black patients.

A patient with known hypersensitivity to aspirin and penicillin, when treated with COZAAR, was withdrawn from study due to swelling of the lips and eyelids and facial rash, reported as angioedema, which returned to normal 5 days after therapy was discontinued.

Superficial peeling of palms and hemolysis was reported in one subject.

In addition to the adverse events above, potentially important events that occurred in at least two patients/subjects exposed to losartan or other adverse events that occurred in <1% of patients in clinical studies are listed below. It cannot be determined whether these events were causally related to losartan: *Body as a Whole:* facial edema, fever, orthostatic effects, syncope; *Cardiovascular:* angina pectoris, second degree AV block, CVA, hypotension, myocardial infarction, arrhythmias including atrial fibrillation, palpitation, sinus bradycardia, tachycardia, ventricular tachycardia, ventricular fibrillation; *Digestive:* anorexia, constipation, dental pain, dry mouth, flatulence, gastritis, vomiting; *Hematologic:* anemia; *Metabolic:* gout; *Musculoskeletal:* arm pain, hip pain, joint swelling, knee pain, musculoskeletal pain, shoulder pain, stiffness, arthralgia, arthritis, fibromyalgia, muscle weakness; *Nervous System/ Psychiatric:* anxiety, anxiety disorder, ataxia, confusion, depression, dream abnormality, hypesthesia, decreased libido, memory impairment, migraine, nervousness, paresthesia, peripheral neuropathy, panic disorder, sleep disorder, somnolence, tremor, vertigo; *Respiratory:* dyspnea, bronchitis, pharyngeal discomfort, epistaxis, rhinitis, respiratory congestion; *Skin:* alopecia, dermatitis, dry skin, ecchymosis, erythema, flushing, photosensitivity, pruritus, rash, sweating, urticaria; *Special Senses:* blurred vision, burning/stinging in the eye, conjunctivitis, taste perversion, tinnitus, decrease in visual acuity; *Urogenital:* impotence, nocturia, urinary frequency, urinary tract infection.

Post-Marketing Experience

The following adverse reactions have been reported in post-marketing experience: *Hypersensitivity:* Angioedema (involv-

Continued on next page

Information on the Merck & Co., Inc. products listed on these pages is the full prescribing information from product circulars in use September 30, 1996.

Merck & Co.—Cont.

ing swelling of the face, lips, and/or tongue) has been reported rarely in patients treated with losartan.

Laboratory Test Findings

In controlled clinical trials, clinically important changes in standard laboratory parameters were rarely associated with administration of COZAAR.

Creatinine, Blood Urea Nitrogen: Minor increases in blood urea nitrogen (BUN) or serum creatinine were observed in less than 0.1 percent of patients with essential hypertension treated with COZAAR alone. No patient discontinued taking COZAAR alone due to increased BUN or serum creatinine. (See PRECAUTIONS, *Impaired Renal Function.*)

Hemoglobin and Hematocrit: Small decreases in hemoglobin and hematocrit (mean decreases of approximately 0.11 grams percent and 0.09 volume percent, respectively) occurred frequently in patients treated with COZAAR alone, but were rarely of clinical importance. No patients were discontinued due to anemia.

Liver Function Tests: Occasional elevations of liver enzymes and/or serum bilirubin have occurred. In patients with essential hypertension treated with COZAAR alone, one patient ($<0.1\%$) was discontinued due to these laboratory adverse experiences.

OVERDOSAGE

Significant lethality was observed in mice and rats after oral administration of 1000 mg/kg and 2000 mg/kg, respectively, about 44 and 170 times the maximum recommended human dose on a mg/m^2 basis.

Limited data are available in regard to overdosage in humans. The most likely manifestation of overdosage would be hypotension and tachycardia; bradycardia could occur from parasympathetic (vagal) stimulation. If symptomatic hypotension should occur, supportive treatment should be instituted.

Neither losartan nor its active metabolite can be removed by hemodialysis.

DOSAGE AND ADMINISTRATION

The usual starting dose of COZAAR is 50 mg once daily, with 25 mg used in patients with possible depletion of intravascular volume (e.g., patients treated with diuretics) (see WARNINGS, *Hypotension—Volume-Depleted Patients*) and patients with a history of hepatic impairment (see PRECAUTIONS, *General*). COZAAR can be administered once or twice daily with total daily doses ranging from 25 mg to 100 mg.

If the antihypertensive effect measured at trough using once-a-day dosing is inadequate, a twice-a-day regimen at the same total daily dose or an increase in dose may give a more satisfactory response.

If blood pressure is not controlled by COZAAR alone, a low dose of a diuretic may be added. Hydrochlorothiazide has been shown to have an additive effect (see CLINICAL PHARMACOLOGY, *Pharmacodynamics and Clinical Effects*).

No initial dosage adjustment is necessary for elderly patients or for patients with renal impairment, including patients on dialysis.

COZAAR may be administered with other antihypertensive agents.

COZAAR may be administered with or without food.

HOW SUPPLIED

No. 3612—Tablets COZAAR, 25 mg, are light green, teardrop-shaped, film-coated tablets with code MRK on one side and 951 on the other. They are supplied as follows:

NDC 0006-0951-54 unit of use bottles of 90
(6505-01-414-4064, 25 mg 90's)

NDC 0006-0951-58 unit of use bottles of 100
(6505-01-414-4059, 25 mg 100's)

NDC 0006-0951-28 unit dose packages of 100
(6505-01-414-4063, 25 mg individually sealed 100's).

Shown in Product Identification Guide, page 324

No. 3613—Tablets COZAAR, 50 mg, are green, teardrop-shaped, film-coated tablets with code MRK 952 on one side and COZAAR on the other. They are supplied as follows:

NDC 0006-0952-31 unit of use bottles of 30
(6505-01-414-4062, 50 mg 30's)

NDC 0006-0952-54 unit of use bottles of 90
(6505-01-414-4060, 50 mg 90's)

NDC 0006-0952-58 unit of use bottles of 100
(6505-01-414-4058, 50 mg 100's)

NDC 0006-0952-28 unit dose packages of 100
(6505-01-414-4061, 50 mg individually sealed 100's)

NDC 0006-0952-82 bottles of 1,000.

Shown in Product Identification Guide, page 324

Storage

Store at controlled room temperature, 15–30°C (59–86°F). Keep container tightly closed. Protect from light.

Manufactured for:
MERCK & CO., INC., West Point, PA 19486, USA
by:
Du Pont Pharmaceuticals, Wilmington, DE 19880 USA
7882903 Issued April 1996

CRIXIVAN® Capsules ℞
(indinavir sulfate)

> **WARNING**
> CRIXIVAN is indicated for the treatment of HIV infection in adults when antiretroviral therapy is warranted. This indication is based on analyses of surrogate endpoints in studies of up to 24 weeks in duration. At present, there are no results from controlled clinical trials evaluating the effect of therapy with CRIXIVAN on clinical progression of HIV infection, such as survival or the incidence of opportunistic infections.

DESCRIPTION

CRIXIVAN* (indinavir sulfate) is an inhibitor of the human immunodeficiency virus (HIV) protease. CRIXIVAN Capsules are formulated as a sulfate salt and are available for oral administration in strengths of 200 and 400 mg of indinavir (corresponding to 250 and 500 mg indinavir sulfate, respectively). Each capsule also contains the inactive ingredients anhydrous lactose and magnesium stearate. The capsule shell has the following inactive ingredients and dyes: gelatin, titanium dioxide, silicon dioxide and sodium lauryl sulfate.

The chemical name for indinavir sulfate is [1(1*S*,2*R*),5(*S*)]-2,3,5-trideoxy-*N*-(2,3-dihydro-2-hydroxy-1*H*-inden-1-yl)-5-[2-[[(1,1-dimethylethyl)amino]carbonyl]-4-(3-pyridinylmethyl)-1-piperazinyl]-2-(phenylmethyl)-D-*erythro*-pentonamide sulfate (1:1) salt. Indinavir sulfate has the following structural formula:

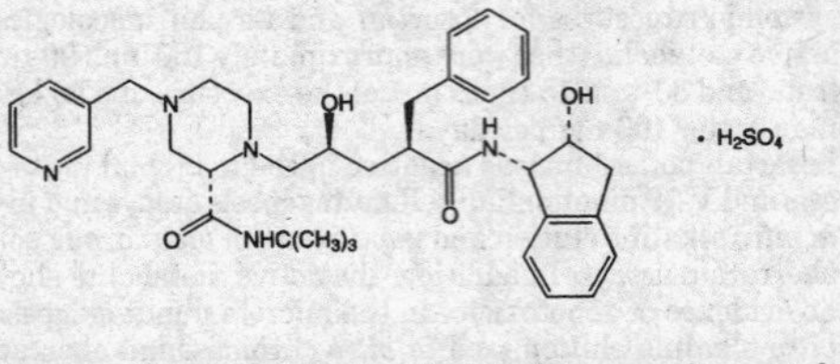

Indinavir sulfate is a white to off-white, hygroscopic, crystalline powder with the molecular formula $C_{36}H_{47}N_5O_4 \cdot H_2SO_4$ and a molecular weight of 711.88. It is very soluble in water and in methanol.

---

*Registered trademark of MERCK & CO., Inc.

CLINICAL PHARMACOLOGY

Mechanism of Action: HIV protease is an enzyme required for the proteolytic cleavage of the viral polyprotein precursors into the individual functional proteins found in infectious HIV. Indinavir binds to the protease active site and inhibits the activity of the enzyme. This inhibition prevents cleavage of the viral polyproteins resulting in the formation of immature non-infectious viral particles.

Antiretroviral Activity In Vitro: The relationship between *in vitro* susceptibility of HIV to indinavir and inhibition of HIV replication in humans has not been established. The *in vitro* activity of indinavir was assessed in cell lines of lymphoblastic and monocytic origin and in peripheral blood lymphocytes. HIV variants used to infect the different cell types include laboratory-adapted variants, primary clinical isolates and clinical isolates resistant to nucleoside analogue and nonnucleoside inhibitors of the HIV reverse transcriptase. The IC_{95} (95% inhibitory concentration) of indinavir in these test systems was in the range of 25 to 100 nM. In drug combination studies with the nucleoside analogues zidovudine and didanosine, as well as with an investigational nonnucleoside (L-697,661), indinavir showed synergistic activity in cell culture.

Drug Resistance: Isolates of HIV with reduced susceptibility to the drug have been recovered from some patients treated with indinavir. Viral resistance was correlated with the accumulation of mutations that resulted in the expression of amino acid substitutions in the viral protease. Eleven amino acid residue positions, at which substitutions are associated with resistance, have been identified. Resistance was mediated by the co-expression of multiple and variable substitutions at these positions. In general, higher levels of resistance were associated with the co-expression of greater numbers of substitutions.

Cross-Resistance to other antiviral agents: Cross-resistance between indinavir and HIV reverse transcriptase inhibitors is unlikely because the enzyme targets involved are different. Cross-resistance was noted between indinavir and the protease inhibitor ritonavir. Varying degrees of cross-resistance have been observed between indinavir and other HIV-protease inhibitors.

Pharmacokinetics

Absorption: Indinavir was rapidly absorbed in the fasted state with a time to peak plasma concentration (T_{max}) of 0.8 $\pm$ 0.3 hours (mean $\pm$ S.D.) (n=11). A greater than dose-proportional increase in indinavir plasma concentrations was observed over the 200–1000 mg dose range. At a dosing regimen of 800 mg every 8 hours, steady-state area under the plasma concentration time curve (AUC) was 30,691 $\pm$ 11,407 nM·hour (n=16), peak plasma concentration (C_{max}) was 12,617 $\pm$ 4037 nM (n=16), and plasma concentration eight hours post dose (trough) was 251 $\pm$ 178 nM (n=16).

Effect of Food on Oral Absorption: Administration of indinavir with a meal high in calories, fat, and protein (784 kcal, 48.6 g fat, 31.3 g protein) resulted in a 77% $\pm$ 8% reduction in AUC and an 84% $\pm$ 7% reduction in C_{max} (n=10). Administration with lighter meals (e.g., a meal of dry toast with jelly, apple juice, and coffee with skim milk and sugar or a meal of corn flakes, skim milk and sugar) resulted in little or no change in AUC, C_{max} or trough concentration.

Distribution: Indinavir was approximately 60% bound to human plasma proteins over a concentration range of 81 nM to 16,300 nM.

Metabolism: Following a 400-mg dose of ^{14}C-indinavir, 83 $\pm$ 1% (n=4) and 19 $\pm$3% (n=6) of the total radioactivity was recovered in feces and urine, respectively; radioactivity due to parent drug in feces and urine was 19.1% and 9.4%, respectively. Seven metabolites have been identified, one glucuronide conjugate and six oxidative metabolites. *In vitro* studies indicate that cytochrome P-450 3A4 (CYP3A4) is the major enzyme responsible for formation of the oxidative metabolites.

Elimination: Less than 20% of indinavir is excreted unchanged in the urine. Mean urinary excretion of unchanged drug was 10.4 $\pm$ 4.9% (n=10) and 12.0 $\pm$ 4.9% (n=10) following a single 700-mg and 1000-mg dose, respectively. Indinavir was rapidly eliminated with a half-life of 1.8 $\pm$ 0.4 hours (n=10). Significant accumulation was not observed after multiple dosing at 800 mg every 8 hours.

Special Populations

Hepatic Insufficiency: Patients with mild to moderate hepatic insufficiency and clinical evidence of cirrhosis had evidence of decreased metabolism of indinavir resulting in approximately 60% higher mean AUC following a single 400-mg dose (n=12). The half-life of indinavir increased to 2.8 $\pm$ 0.5 hours. Indinavir pharmacokinetics have not been studied in patients with severe hepatic insufficiency (see DOSAGE AND ADMINISTRATION, *Hepatic Insufficiency*).

Renal Insufficiency: The pharmacokinetics of indinavir have not been studied in patients with renal insufficiency.

Gender: Pharmacokinetics of indinavir appear to be comparable in men and women based on pharmacokinetic studies including 32 women (15 HIV-positive).

Race: Pharmacokinetics of indinavir appear to be comparable in Caucasians and Blacks based on pharmacokinetic studies including 42 Caucasians (26 HIV-positive) and 16 Blacks (4 HIV-positive).

Drug Interactions (also see PRECAUTIONS, *Drug Interactions)*

Specific drug interaction studies were performed with indinavir and a number of drugs.

Drugs Requiring Dose Modification

Rifabutin: Administration of indinavir (800 mg every 8 hours) with rifabutin (300 mg once daily) for 10 days resulted in a 32% $\pm$ 19% decrease in indinavir AUC and a 204% $\pm$ 142% increase in rifabutin AUC (see DOSAGE AND ADMINISTRATION, *Concomitant Therapy*).

Ketoconazole: Administration of a 400-mg dose of ketoconazole with a 400-mg dose of indinavir resulted in a 68% $\pm$ 48% increase in indinavir AUC (see DOSAGE AND ADMINISTRATION, *Concomitant Therapy*). The effects of administering a 400- or 800-mg dose of ketoconazole with an 800-mg dose of indinavir are not known.

Drugs Not Requiring Dose Modification

Nucleoside analogue antiretroviral agents: Administration of indinavir (1000 mg every 8 hours) with zidovudine (200 mg every 8 hours) for one week resulted in a 13% $\pm$ 48% increase in indinavir AUC and a 17% $\pm$ 23% increase in zidovudine AUC. In another study, administration of indinavir (800 mg every 8 hours) with zidovudine (200 mg every 8 hours) in combination with lamivudine (150 mg twice daily) for one week resulted in no change in indinavir AUC, a 36% increase in zidovudine AUC, and a 6% decrease in lamivudine AUC. Administration of indinavir (800 mg every 8 hours) in combination with stavudine (40 mg every 12 hours) for one week resulted in no change in indinavir AUC and a 25% $\pm$ 26% increase in stavudine AUC.

ORTHO-NOVUM 1/35**: Administration of indinavir (800 mg every 8 hours) with ORTHO-NOVUM 1/35 for one week resulted in a 24% ± 17% increase in ethinyl estradiol AUC and a 26% ± 14% increase in norethindrone AUC.

Cimetidine, Quinidine, Grapefruit Juice: Administration of a single 400-mg dose of indinavir following six days of cimetidine (600 mg every 12 hours) did not affect indinavir AUC. Administration of a single 400-mg dose of indinavir with 8 oz. of grapefruit juice resulted in a decrease in indinavir AUC (26% ± 18%). Administration of a single 400-mg dose of indinavir with 200 mg of quinidine sulfate resulted in a 10% ± 26% increase in indinavir AUC.

Trimethoprim/Sulfamethoxazole, Fluconazole, Isoniazid, Clarithromycin: Administration of indinavir (400 mg every 6 hours) with trimethoprim/sulfamethoxazole (one double strength tablet every 12 hours) for one week resulted in no change in indinavir AUC, a 19% ± 31% increase in trimethoprim AUC, and no change in sulfamethoxazole AUC. Administration of indinavir (1000 mg every 6 hours) with fluconazole (400 mg once daily) for one week resulted in a 19% ± 33% decrease in indinavir AUC and no change in fluconazole AUC. Administration of indinavir (800 mg every 8 hours) with isoniazid (300 mg once daily) for one week resulted in no change in indinavir AUC and a 13% ± 15% increase in isoniazid AUC. Administration of indinavir (800 mg every 8 hours) with clarithromycin (500 mg every 12 hours) for one week resulted in a 29% ± 42% increase in indinavir AUC and a 53% ± 36% increase in clarithromycin AUC.

**Registered trademark of Ortho Pharmaceutical Corporation

INDICATIONS AND USAGE

CRIXIVAN is indicated for the treatment of HIV infection in adults when antiretroviral therapy is warranted. This indication is based on analyses of surrogate endpoints in studies of up to 24 weeks in duration evaluating patients who received CRIXIVAN in combination with other antiretroviral agents or alone. At present, there are no results from controlled trials evaluating the effect of therapy with CRIXIVAN on clinical progression of HIV infection, such as survival or the incidence of opportunistic infection.

Description of Studies

Study 028 is an ongoing multicenter, double-blind, randomized clinical endpoint trial in patients with no prior antiretroviral therapy. The effects of CRIXIVAN on CD4 cell counts and serum viral RNA were evaluated in a cohort of 224 HIV-1 seropositive adults (75% male, 90% Caucasian) over a 24-week period. At baseline, patients were randomized to one of three treatment groups: CRIXIVAN alone, zidovudine alone, and CRIXIVAN plus zidovudine. The median age for these patients was 34 years (range 20–67 years). The mean baseline CD4 cell count over all patients was 145.0 cells/mm³, and the serum viral RNA was 4.40 $\log_{10}$ copies/mL (25,330 copies/mL). Mean changes in CD4 cell counts and $\log_{10}$ serum viral RNA are summarized in Figures 1 and 2, respectively.

Study 028: Figure 1

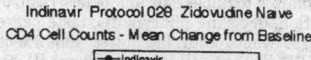
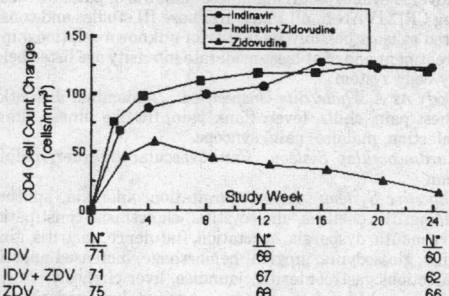

Indinavir Protocol 028 Zidovudine Naive
CD4 Cell Counts - Mean Change from Baseline

	N*	N*	N*
IDV	71	69	60
IDV + ZDV	71	67	62
ZDV	75	69	66

* N = Number with CD4 cell count measurement at weeks 0, 12, 24

[See Figure 2 at top of next column.]

At 24 weeks of therapy, 22 of 59 (37%) of patients receiving indinavir alone, 21 of 58 (36%) of patients receiving indinavir in combination with zidovudine, and 4 of 62 (7%) of patients receiving zidovudine alone had serum viral RNA levels at or below 500 copies/mL, the limit of detection of the assay; the clinical significance of this finding is unknown. Study 033 is an ongoing, multicenter, double-blind, randomized clinical trial in patients without prior antiretroviral therapy. The effects of CRIXIVAN on CD4 cell counts and serum viral RNA were evaluated in 266 HIV-1 seropositive adults (91% male, 85% Caucasian) over a 24-week period. At baseline, patients were randomized to one of three treatment groups: CRIXIVAN alone, zidovudine alone, and CRIXIVAN plus zidovudine. The median age for these patients was 37

Study 028: Figure 2

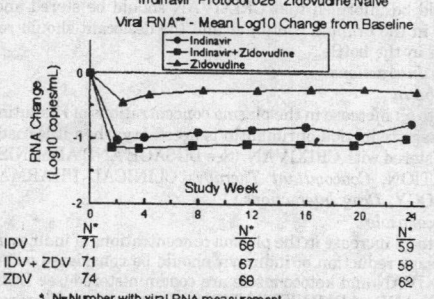

Indinavir Protocol 028 Zidovudine Naive
Viral RNA** - Mean Log10 Change from Baseline

	N*	N*	N*
IDV	71	68	59
IDV + ZDV	71	67	58
ZDV	74	68	62

* N = Number with viral RNA measurement
** The clinical significance of changes in serum viral RNA measurements during treatment with CRIXIVAN has not been established

years (range 22–76 years). The mean baseline CD4 cell count over all patients was 254.4 cells/mm³, and the mean baseline serum viral RNA was 4.28 $\log_{10}$ copies/mL (19,210 copies/mL). Mean changes in CD4 cell counts and $\log_{10}$ serum viral RNA are summarized in Figures 3 and 4, respectively.

Study 033: Figure 3

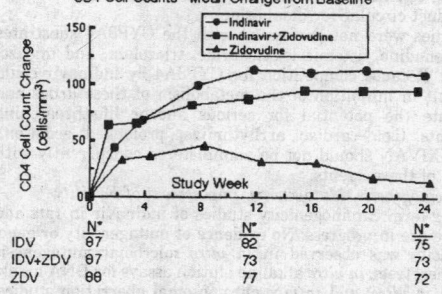

Indinavir Protocol 033 Zidovudine Naive
CD4 Cell Counts - Mean Change from Baseline

	N*	N*	N*
IDV	87	82	75
IDV+ZDV	87	73	73
ZDV	88	77	72

* N = Number with CD4 cell count measurement at weeks 0, 12, 24

Study 033: Figure 4

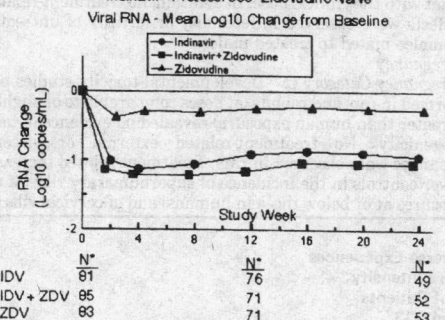

Indinavir Protocol 033 Zidovudine Naive
Viral RNA - Mean Log10 Change from Baseline

	N*	N*	N*
IDV	81	76	49
IDV + ZDV	85	71	52
ZDV	83	71	53

* N=Number with viral RNA measurement

At 24 weeks of therapy, 18 of 49 (37%) of patients receiving indinavir alone, 29 of 52 (56%) of patients receiving indinavir in combination with zidovudine, and 1 of 53 (2%) of patients receiving zidovudine alone had serum viral RNA levels at or below 500 copies/mL, the limit of detection of the assay; the clinical significance of this finding is unknown. Study 035 is an ongoing multicenter, double-blind, randomized clinical trial in HIV-1 seropositive patients with prior zidovudine experience (median time of zidovudine therapy—30.9 months). The effects of CRIXIVAN on CD4 cell counts and serum viral RNA were evaluated in a cohort of 96 patients (85% male), with zidovudine experience, over a 24-week period. At baseline, patients were randomized to one of three treatment groups: CRIXIVAN, zidovudine plus lamivudine or CRIXIVAN plus zidovudine plus lamivudine. The median age for these patients was 39 years (range 18–67 years), with 72% Caucasian. The mean baseline CD4 cell count over all patients was 174.8 cells/mm³, and the mean baseline serum viral RNA was 4.58 $\log_{10}$ copies/mL (38,400 copies/mL). Mean changes in CD4 cell counts and $\log_{10}$ serum viral RNA are summarized in Figures 5 and 6, respectively.

[See Figures at top of next column.]

At 24 weeks of therapy, 7 of 20 (35%) of patients receiving indinavir alone, 20 of 22 (91%) of patients receiving indinavir in combination with zidovudine and lamivudine, and

Study 035: Figure 5

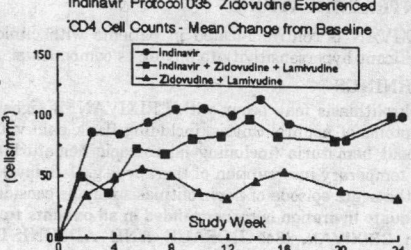

Indinavir Protocol 035 Zidovudine Experienced
CD4 Cell Counts - Mean Change from Baseline

	N*	N*	N*
IDV	31	29	23
IDV+ZDV+L	32	28	25
ZDV+L	33	31	24

* N = Number with CD4 cell count measurement at weeks 0, 12, 24

Study 035: Figure 6

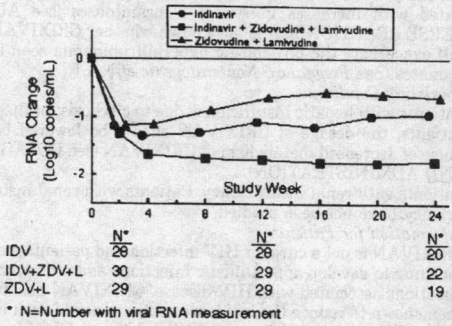

Indinavir Protocol 035 Zidovudine Experienced
Viral RNA - Mean Log10 Change from Baseline

	N*	N*	N*
IDV	28	28	20
IDV+ZDV+L	30	29	22
ZDV+L	29	29	19

* N=Number with viral RNA measurement

0 of 19 (0%) of patients receiving zidovudine plus lamivudine had serum viral RNA levels at or below 500 copies/mL, the limit of detection of the assay; the clinical significance of this finding is unknown.

Additional Studies

In open-label study 020, 78 zidovudine- and didanosine-naive HIV-infected patients were randomized to one of three treatment groups: CRIXIVAN 600 mg every 6 hours, zidovudine plus didanosine, and CRIXIVAN plus zidovudine plus didanosine. At 24 weeks of therapy, all three groups had a significant increase in CD4 cell counts and decrease in serum viral RNA compared to baseline; however, there were no differences in mean CD4 cell count changes between treatment arms. Patients treated with CRIXIVAN plus zidovudine plus didanosine had a greater mean decline in serum viral RNA than those treated with indinavir alone or zidovudine plus didanosine.

Study 021 was a randomized trial in which 70 HIV-seropositive patients received CRIXIVAN at one of three doses (800 mg every 8 hours, 1000 mg every 8 hours and 800 mg every 6 hours). At 24 weeks, changes in CD4 cell counts and serum viral RNA were similar in all three treatment groups.

Genotypic Resistance in Clinical Studies

Study 006 was a dose-ranging study in which patients were initially treated with CRIXIVAN at a dose of < 2.4 g/day followed by 2.4 g/day. Study 019 was a randomized comparison of CRIXIVAN 600 mg every 6 hours, CRIXIVAN plus zidovudine, and zidovudine alone. Table 1 shows the incidence of genotypic resistance at 24 weeks in these studies.

Table 1
Genotypic Resistance at 24 Weeks

Treatment Group	Resistance to IDV n/N*	Resistance to ZVD n/N*
IDV	—	—
< 2.4g/day	31/37 (84%)	—
2.4g/day	9/21 (43%)	1/17 (6%)
IDV/ZDV	4/22 (18%)	1/22 (5%)
ZDV	1/18 (6%)	11/17 (65%)

* N–includes patients with non-amplifiable virus at 24 weeks who had amplifiable virus at week 0.

Continued on next page

Merck & Co.—Cont.

CONTRAINDICATIONS

CRIXIVAN is contraindicated in patients with clinically significant hypersensitivity to any of its components.

WARNINGS

Nephrolithiasis may occur with CRIXIVAN. If signs and symptoms of nephrolithiasis, including flank pain with or without hematuria (including microscopic hematuria), occur, temporary interruption of therapy (e.g., 1–3 days) during the acute episode of nephrolithiasis may be considered. **Adequate hydration is recommended in all patients treated with CRIXIVAN. (See DOSAGE AND ADMINISTRATION,** *Nephrolithiasis.*)

Indinavir should not be administered concurrently with terfenadine, astemizole, cisapride, triazolam, and midazolam because competition for CYP3A4 by indinavir could result in inhibition of the metabolism of these drugs and create the potential for serious and/or life-threatening events (i.e., cardiac arrhythmias, prolonged sedation).

PRECAUTIONS

General
Indirect hyperbilirubinemia has occurred frequently during treatment with CRIXIVAN and has infrequently been associated with increases in serum transaminases (see ADVERSE REACTIONS). It is not known whether CRIXIVAN will exacerbate the physiologic hyperbilirubinemia seen in neonates (See *Pregnancy, Nonteratogenic effects.*)

Coexisting Conditions
Patients with hepatic insufficiency due to cirrhosis: In these patients, the dosage of CRIXIVAN should be lowered because of decreased metabolism of CRIXIVAN (see DOSAGE AND ADMINISTRATION).
Patients with renal insufficiency: Patients with renal insufficiency have not been studied.

Information for Patients
CRIXIVAN is not a cure for HIV infection and patients may continue to develop opportunistic infections and other complications associated with HIV disease. CRIXIVAN has not been shown to reduce the incidence or frequency of such illnesses. The long-term effects of CRIXIVAN are unknown at this time. CRIXIVAN has not been shown to reduce the risk of transmission of HIV to others through sexual contact or blood contamination.
Patients should be advised to remain under the care of a physician when using CRIXIVAN and should not modify or discontinue treatment without first consulting the physician. Therefore, if a dose is missed, patients should take the next dose at the regularly scheduled time and should not double this dose. Therapy with CRIXIVAN should be initiated and maintained at the recommended dosage.
For optimal absorption, CRIXIVAN should be administered without food but with water 1 hour before or 2 hours after a meal. Alternatively, CRIXIVAN may be administered with other liquids such as skim milk, juice, coffee, or tea, or with a light meal, e.g., dry toast with jelly, juice, and coffee with skim milk and sugar; or corn flakes, skim milk and sugar (see CLINICAL PHARMACOLOGY, *Effect of Food on Oral Absorption* and DOSAGE AND ADMINISTRATION). Ingestion

of CRIXIVAN with a meal high in calories, fat, and protein reduces the absorption of indinavir.
CRIXIVAN Capsules are sensitive to moisture. Patients should be informed that CRIXIVAN should be stored and used in the original container and the desiccant should remain in the bottle.

Drug Interactions
Rifabutin
Due to an increase in the plasma concentrations of rifabutin, a dosage reduction of rifabutin is necessary when it is coadministered with CRIXIVAN. (See DOSAGE AND ADMINISTRATION, *Concomitant Therapy*; CLINICAL PHARMACOLOGY, *Drug Interactions.*)
Ketoconazole
Due to an increase in the plasma concentrations of indinavir, a dosage reduction of indinavir should be considered when CRIXIVAN and ketoconazole are coadministered (see DOSAGE AND ADMINISTRATION, *Concomitant Therapy*; CLINICAL PHARMACOLOGY, *Drug Interactions*).
Rifampin
Because rifampin is a potent inducer of P-450 3A4 which could markedly diminish plasma concentrations of indinavir, coadministration of CRIXIVAN and rifampin is not recommended.
Other
If CRIXIVAN and didanosine are administered concomitantly, they should be administered at least one hour apart on an empty stomach; a normal (acidic) gastric pH may be necessary for optimum absorption of indinavir, whereas acid rapidly degrades didanosine which is formulated with buffering agents to increase pH (consult the manufacturer's product circular for didanosine).
Studies were not performed with the CYP3A4 substrates terfenadine, astemizole, cisapride, triazolam, and midazolam. Because competition for CYP3A4 by indinavir could result in inhibition of the metabolism of these drugs and create the potential for serious and/or life-threatening events (i.e., cardiac arrhythmias, prolonged sedation), CRIXIVAN should not be administered concurrently with any of these agents.

Carcinogenesis, Mutagenesis, Impairment of Fertility
Long-term carcinogenicity studies of indinavir in rats and mice are in progress. No evidence of mutagenicity or genotoxicity was observed in *in vitro* microbial mutagenesis (Ames) tests, *in vitro* alkaline elution assays for DNA breakage, *in vitro* and *in vivo* chromosomal aberration studies, and *in vitro* mammalian cell mutagenesis assays. No treatment-related effects on mating, fertility, or embryo survival were seen in female rats and no treatment-related effects on mating performance were seen in male rats at doses providing systemic exposure comparable to or slightly higher than that with the clinical dose. In addition, no treatment-related effects were observed in fecundity or fertility of untreated females mated to treated males.

Pregnancy
Pregnancy Category C: Developmental toxicity studies performed in rats and rabbits (at doses comparable to or slightly greater than human exposure) revealed no evidence of teratogenicity. No treatment-related external or visceral changes were observed in rats. Treatment-related increases over controls in the incidence of supernumerary ribs (at exposures at or below those in humans) and of cervical ribs (at

exposures comparable to or slightly greater than those in humans) were seen in rats. No treatment-related external, visceral, or skeletal changes were observed in rabbits. In both species, no treatment-related effects on embryonic/fetal survival or fetal weights were observed. *In utero* exposure to indinavir was significant in rats. Since fetal exposure was low in the rabbit, a developmental toxicity study in dogs is in progress. There are no adequate and well controlled studies in pregnant women. CRIXIVAN should be used during pregnancy only if the potential benefit justifies the potential risk to the fetus.

Nonteratogenic effects
Hyperbilirubinemia has occurred during treatment with CRIXIVAN (see PRECAUTIONS and ADVERSE REACTIONS). It is unknown whether CRIXIVAN administered to the mother in the perinatal period will exacerbate physiologic hyperbilirubinemia in neonates.

Nursing Mothers
Studies in lactating rats have demonstrated that indinavir is excreted in milk. Although it is not known whether CRIXIVAN is excreted in human milk, there exists the potential for adverse effects from indinavir in nursing infants. Mothers should be instructed to discontinue nursing if they are receiving CRIXIVAN. This is consistent with the recommendation by the U.S. Public Health Service Centers for Disease Control and Prevention that HIV-infected mothers not breast-feed their infants to avoid risking postnatal transmission of HIV.

Pediatric Use
Safety and effectiveness in pediatric patients have not been established.

ADVERSE REACTIONS

Nephrolithiasis, including flank pain with or without hematuria (including microscopic hematuria), has been reported in approximately 4% (79/2205) of patients receiving CRIXIVAN in clinical trials. In general, these events were not associated with renal dysfunction and resolved with hydration and temporary interruption of therapy (e.g., 1–3 days). Following the acute episode, 9.2% (7/76) of patients discontinued therapy. (See WARNINGS and DOSAGE AND ADMINISTRATION, *Nephrolithiasis.*)
Asymptomatic hyperbilirubinemia (total bilirubin ≥ 2.5 mg/dL), reported predominantly as elevated indirect bilirubin, has occurred in approximately 10% of patients treated with CRIXIVAN. In <1% this was associated with elevations in ALT or AST.
Hyperbilirubinemia and nephrolithiasis occurred more frequently at doses exceeding 2.4 g/day compared to doses ≤2.4 g/day.
Drug-related clinical adverse experiences of moderate or severe intensity in ≥ 2% of patients treated with CRIXIVAN alone, CRIXIVAN in combination with zidovudine, or zidovudine alone are presented in Table 2.
[See table below.]
In Phase I and II controlled trials, the following adverse events were reported significantly more frequently by those randomized to CRIXIVAN-containing arms than by those randomized to nucleoside analogues: rash, upper respiratory infection, dry skin, pharyngitis, taste perversion.
Adverse events occurring in less than 2% of patients receiving CRIXIVAN in all Phase II/Phase III studies and considered at least possibly related or of unknown relationship to treatment and of at least moderate intensity are listed below by body system.
Body As A Whole/Site Unspecified: Abdominal distention, chest pain, chills, fever, flank pain, flu-like illness, fungal infection, malaise, pain, syncope.
Cardiovascular System: Cardiovascular disorder, palpitation.
Digestive System: Acid regurgitation, anorexia, aphthous stomatitis, cheilitis, cholecystitis, cholestasis, constipation, dry mouth, dyspepsia, eructation, flatulence, gastritis, gingivitis, glossodynia, gingival hemorrhage, increased appetite, infectious gastroenteritis, jaundice, liver cirrhosis.
Hemic and Lymphatic System: Anemia, lymphadenopathy, spleen disorder.
Metabolic/Nutritional/Immune: Food allergy.
Musculoskeletal System: Arthralgia, back pain, leg pain, myalgia, muscle cramps, muscle weakness, musculoskeletal pain, shoulder pain, stiffness.
Nervous System and Psychiatric: Agitation, anxiety, anxiety disorder, bruxism, decreased mental acuity, depression, dizziness, dream abnormality, dysesthesia, excitement, fasciculation, hypesthesia, nervousness, neuralgia, neurotic disorder, paresthesia, peripheral neuropathy, sleep disorder, somnolence, tremor, vertigo.
Respiratory System: Cough, dyspnea, halitosis, pharyngeal hyperemia, pharyngitis, pneumonia, rales/rhonchi, respiratory failure, sinus disorder, sinusitis, upper respiratory infection.
Skin and Skin Appendage: Body odor, contact dermatitis, dermatitis, dry skin, flushing, folliculitis, herpes simplex,

Table 2
Drug-Related Clinical Adverse Experiences
of Moderate or Severe Intensity
Reported in ≥ 2% of Patients
Studies 028 and 033

Adverse Experience	CRIXIVAN Percent (n=196)	CRIXIVAN plus Zidovudine Percent (n=196)	Zidovudine Percent (n=195)
Body as a Whole			
Abdominal pain	8.7	8.2	5.1
Asthenia/fatigue	3.6	9.2	7.7
Flank pain	2.6	1.0	0
Malaise	0.5	2.0	1.5
Digestive System			
Nausea	11.7	32.1	14.4
Diarrhea	4.6	4.1	2.1
Vomiting	4.1	12.2	4.6
Acid regurgitation	2.0	2.0	0.5
Anorexia	0.5	2.0	3.1
Dry mouth	0.5	0	2.1
Musculoskeletal System			
Back pain	2.0	1.0	1.5
Nervous System/Psychiatric			
Headache	5.6	11.7	5.1
Insomnia	3.1	1.5	0
Dizziness	1.0	3.6	0.5
Somnolence	1.0	1.5	3.6
Special Senses			
Taste perversion	2.6	3.6	2.1

Table 3
Selected Laboratory Abnormalities Reported in
Studies 028 and 033

	CRIXIVAN	CRIXIVAN plus zidovudine	Zidovudine
	Percent (n=196)	Percent (n=196)	Percent (n=195)
Hematology			
Decreased hemoglobin <8.0g/dL	0.5	1.1	0.5
Decreased platelet count <50 THS/mm³	0.5	0.5	0
Decreased neutrophils <0.75 THS/mm³	1.1	1.6	3.8
Blood chemistry			
Increased ALT >500% ULN*	3.1	3.2	2.1
Increased AST >500% ULN	2.1	2.1	1.1
Total serum bilirubin >2.5 mg/dL	7.8	7.4	0.5
Increased serum amylase >200% ULN	1.0	2.1	0.5

*Upper limit of the normal range.

herpes zoster, night sweats, pruritis, seborrhea, skin disorder, skin infection, sweating, urticaria.

Special Senses: Accommodation disorder, blurred vision, eye pain, eye swelling, orbital edema, taste disorder.

Urogenital System: Dysuria, hematuria, hydronephrosis, nocturia, premenstrual syndrome, proteinuria, renal colic, urinary frequency, urinary tract infection, urine abnormality, urine sediment abnormality, urolithiasis.
[See table 3 above.]

OVERDOSAGE

No reports are available with regard to overdosage in humans. It is not known whether CRIXIVAN is dialyzable by peritoneal or hemodialysis. Single oral or intraperitoneal doses of indinavir up to 20 times the related human dose in rats and 10 times the related human dose in mice caused no lethality.

DOSAGE AND ADMINISTRATION

The recommended dosage of CRIXIVAN is 800 mg (**two 400-mg capsules**) orally every 8 hours. The dosage is the same whether CRIXIVAN is used alone or in combination with other antiretroviral agents. The antiretroviral activity of CRIXIVAN **may** be increased when used in combination with approved reverse transcriptase inhibitors (See INDICATIONS AND USAGE, *Description of Studies* and *Genotypic Resistance in Clinical Studies.*)

CRIXIVAN must be taken at intervals of 8 hours. For optimal absorption, CRIXIVAN should be administered without food but with water 1 hour before or 2 hours after a meal. Alternatively, CRIXIVAN may be administered with other liquids such as skim milk, juice, coffee, or tea, or with a light meal, e.g., dry toast with jelly, juice, and coffee with skim milk and sugar; or corn flakes, skim milk and sugar. (See CLINICAL PHARMACOLOGY, *Effect of Food on Oral Absorption.*)

To ensure adequate hydration, it is recommended that the patient drink at least 1.5 liters (approximately 48 ounces) of liquids during the course of 24 hours.

Concomitant Therapy
Dose reduction of rifabutin to half the standard dose is recommended (consult the manufacturer's product circular). Dose reduction of CRIXIVAN to 600 mg every 8 hours should be considered when administering ketoconazole concurrently.
If indinavir and didanosine are administered concomitantly, they should be administered at least one hour apart on an empty stomach (consult the manufacturer's product circular for didanosine).

Hepatic Insufficiency
The dosage of CRIXIVAN should be reduced to 600 mg every 8 hours in patients with mild-to-moderate hepatic insufficiency due to cirrhosis.

Nephrolithiasis
In addition to adequate hydration, medical management in patients who experience nephrolithiasis may include temporary interruption of therapy (e.g., 1–3 days) during the acute episode of nephrolithiasis or discontinuation of therapy.

HOW SUPPLIED

CRIXIVAN Capsules are supplied as follows:
No. 3756—200 mg capsules: white opaque capsules coded "CRIXIVAN™ 200 mg" in blue. Available as:

NDC 0006-0571-42 unit-of-use bottles of 270 (with desiccant).
NDC 0006-0571-43 unit-of-use bottles of 360 (with desiccant).
Shown in Product Identification Guide, page 324

No. 3758—400 mg capsules: white opaque capsules coded "CRIXIVAN™ 400 mg" in green. Available as:
NDC 0006-0573-62 unit-of-use bottles of 180 (with desiccant).
Shown in Product Identification Guide, page 324

Storage
Store in a tightly-closed container at room temperature, 15–30°C (59–86°). Protect from moisture.
CRIXIVAN Capsules are sensitive to moisture. CRIXIVAN should be dispensed and stored in the original container. The desiccant should remain in the original bottle.

7979800   Issued March 1996
Copyright © MERCK & CO., Inc., 1996

CUPRIMINE® Capsules
(Penicillamine), U.S.P.   ℞

> Physicians planning to use penicillamine should thoroughly familiarize themselves with its toxicity, special dosage considerations, and therapeutic benefits. Penicillamine should never be used casually. Each patient should remain constantly under the close supervision of the physician. Patients should be warned to report promptly any symptoms suggesting toxicity.

DESCRIPTION

Penicillamine is a chelating agent used in the treatment of Wilson's disease. It is also used to reduce cystine excretion in cystinuria and to treat patients with severe, active rheumatoid arthritis unresponsive to conventional therapy (see INDICATIONS). It is 3-mercapto-D-valine. It is a white or practically white, crystalline powder, freely soluble in water, slightly soluble in alcohol, and insoluble in ether, acetone, benzene, and carbon tetrachloride. Although its configuration is D, it is levorotatory as usually measured:

$$[\alpha]\!_D^{25°} = -62.5° \pm 2° \ (c = 1, \ 1N \ NaOH),$$

calculated on a dried basis.
The empirical formula is $C_5H_{11}NO_2S$, giving it a molecular weight of 149.21. The structural formula is:

$$(CH_3)_2C\!\!\underset{SH}{\overset{}{|}}\!\!\!-\!\!\underset{NH_2}{\overset{}{|}}\!\!CHCOOH$$

It reacts readily with formaldehyde or acetone to form a thiazolidine-carboxylic acid.
Capsules CUPRIMINE* (Penicillamine) for oral administration contain either 125 mg or 250 mg of penicillamine. Each capsule contains the following inactive ingredients: D & C Yellow 10, gelatin, lactose, magnesium stearate, and titanium dioxide. The 125 mg capsule also contains iron oxide.

---

*Registered trademark of MERCK & CO., INC.

CLINICAL PHARMACOLOGY

Penicillamine is a chelating agent recommended for the removal of excess copper in patients with Wilson's disease. From *in vitro* studies which indicate that one atom of copper combines with two molecules of penicillamine, it would ap-

pear that one gram of penicillamine should be followed by the excretion of about 200 milligrams of copper; however, the actual amount excreted is about one percent of this.
Penicillamine also reduces excess cystine excretion in cystinuria. This is done, at least in part, by disulfide interchange between penicillamine and cystine, resulting in formation of penicillamine-cysteine disulfide, a substance that is much more soluble than cystine and is excreted readily.
Penicillamine interferes with the formation of cross-links between tropocollagen molecules and cleaves them when newly formed.
The mechanism of action of penicillamine in rheumatoid arthritis is unknown although it appears to suppress disease activity. Unlike cytotoxic immunosuppressants, penicillamine markedly lowers IgM rheumatoid factor but produces no significant depression in absolute levels of serum immunoglobulins. Also unlike cytotoxic immunosuppressants which act on both, penicillamine *in vitro* depresses T-cell activity but not B-cell activity.
In vitro, penicillamine dissociates macroglobulins (rheumatoid factor) although the relationship of the activity to its effect in rheumatoid arthritis is not known.
In rheumatoid arthritis, the onset of therapeutic response to CUPRIMINE may not be seen for two or three months. In those patients who respond, however, the first evidence of suppression of symptoms such as pain, tenderness, and swelling is generally apparent within three months. The optimum duration of therapy has not been determined. If remissions occur, they may last from months to years, but usually require continued treatment (see DOSAGE AND ADMINISTRATION).
In all patients receiving penicillamine, it is important that CUPRIMINE be given on an empty stomach, at least one hour before meals or two hours after meals, and at least one hour apart from any other drug, food, or milk. This permits maximum absorption and reduces the likelihood of inactivation by metal binding in the gastrointestinal tract.
Methodology for determining the bioavailability of penicillamine is not available; however, penicillamine is known to be a very soluble substance.

INDICATIONS

CUPRIMINE is indicated in the treatment of Wilson's disease, cystinuria, and in patients with severe, active rheumatoid arthritis who have failed to respond to an adequate trial of conventional therapy. Available evidence suggests that CUPRIMINE is not of value in ankylosing spondylitis.
Wilson's Disease—Wilson's disease (hepatolenticular degeneration) results from the interaction of an inherited defect and an abnormality in copper metabolism. The metabolic defect, which is the consequence of the autosomal inheritance of one abnormal gene from each parent, manifests itself in a greater positive copper balance than normal. As a result, copper is deposited in several organs and appears eventually to produce pathologic effects most prominently seen in the brain, where degeneration is widespread; in the liver, where fatty infiltration, inflammation, and hepatocellular damage progress to postnecrotic cirrhosis; in the kidney, where tubular and glomerular dysfunction results; and in the eye, where characteristic corneal copper deposits are known as Kayser-Fleischer rings.
Two types of patients require treatment for Wilson's disease: (1) the symptomatic, and (2) the asymptomatic in whom it can be assumed the disease will develop in the future if the patient is not treated.
Diagnosis, suspected on the basis of family or individual history, physical examination, or a low serum concentration of ceruloplasmin*, is confirmed by the demonstration of Kayser-Fleischer rings or, particularly in the asymptomatic patient, by the quantitative demonstration in a liver biopsy specimen of a concentration of copper in excess of 250 mcg/g dry weight.
Treatment has two objectives:
  (1) to minimize dietary intake and absorption of copper.
  (2) to promote excretion of copper deposited in tissues.
The first objective is attained by a daily diet that contains no more than one or two milligrams of copper. Such a diet should exclude, most importantly, chocolate, nuts, shellfish, mushrooms, liver, molasses, broccoli, and cereals enriched with copper, and be composed to as great an extent as possible of foods with a low copper content. Distilled or demineralized water should be used if the patient's drinking water contains more than 0.1 mg of copper per liter.
For the second objective, a copper chelating agent is used. In symptomatic patients this treatment usually produces marked neurologic improvement, fading of Kayser-Fleischer rings, and gradual amelioration of hepatic dysfunction and psychic disturbances.

Continued on next page

Information on the Merck & Co., Inc. products listed on these pages is the full prescribing information from product circulars in use September 30, 1996.

Merck & Co.—Cont.

Clinical experience to date suggests that life is prolonged with the above regimen.
Noticeable improvement may not occur for one to three months. Occasionally, neurologic symptoms become worse during initiation of therapy with CUPRIMINE. Despite this, the drug should not be discontinued permanently, although temporary interruption may result in clinical improvement of the neurological symptoms but it carries an increased risk of developing a sensitivity reaction upon resumption of therapy (see WARNINGS).
Treatment of asymptomatic patients has been carried out for over ten years. Symptoms and signs of the disease appear to be prevented indefinitely if daily treatment with CUPRIMINE can be continued.
Cystinuria—Cystinuria is characterized by excessive urinary excretion of the dibasic amino acids, arginine, lysine, ornithine, and cystine, and the mixed disulfide of cysteine and homocysteine. The metabolic defect that leads to cystinuria is inherited as an autosomal, recessive trait. Metabolism of the affected amino acids is influenced by at least two abnormal factors: (1) defective gastrointestinal absorption and (2) renal tubular dysfunction.
Arginine, lysine, ornithine, and cysteine are soluble substances, readily excreted. There is no apparent pathology connected with their excretion in excessive quantities.
Cystine, however, is so slightly soluble at the usual range of urinary pH that it is not excreted readily, and so crystallizes and forms stones in the urinary tract. Stone formation is the only known pathology in cystinuria.
Normal daily output of cystine is 40 to 80 mg. In cystinuria, output is greatly increased and may exceed 1 g/day. At 500 to 600 mg/day, stone formation is almost certain. When it is more than 300 mg/day, treatment is indicated.
Conventional treatment is directed at keeping urinary cystine diluted enough to prevent stone formation, keeping the urine alkaline enough to dissolve as much cystine as possible, and minimizing cystine production by a diet low in methionine (the major dietary precursor of cystine). Patients must drink enough fluid to keep urine specific gravity below 1.010, take enough alkali to keep urinary pH at 7.5 to 8, and maintain a diet low in methionine. This diet is not recommended in growing children and probably is contraindicated in pregnancy because of its low protein content (see PRECAUTIONS).
When these measures are inadequate to control recurrent stone formation, CUPRIMINE may be used as additional therapy. When patients refuse to adhere to conventional treatment, CUPRIMINE may be a useful substitute. It is capable of keeping cystine excretion to near normal values, thereby hindering stone formation and the serious consequences of pyelonephritis and impaired renal function that develop in some patients.
Bartter and colleagues depict the process by which penicillamine interacts with cystine to form penicillamine-cysteine mixed disulfide as:

$$\text{CSSC} + \text{PS}' \rightleftarrows \text{CS}' + \text{CSSP}$$
$$\text{PSSP} + \text{CS}' \rightleftarrows \text{PS}' + \text{CSSP}$$
$$\text{CSSC} + \text{PSSP} \rightleftarrows 2\,\text{CSSP}$$

CSSC = cystine
CS′ = deprotonated cysteine
PSSP = penicillamine
PS′ = deprotonated penicillamine sulfhydryl
CSSP = penicillamine-cysteine mixed disulfide

In this process, it is assumed that the deprotonated form of penicillamine, PS′, is the active factor in bringing about the disulfide interchange.
Rheumatoid Arthritis—Because CUPRIMINE can cause severe adverse reactions, its use in rheumatoid arthritis should be restricted to patients who have severe, active disease and who have failed to respond to an adequate trial of conventional therapy. Even then, benefit-to-risk ratio should be carefully considered. Other measures, such as rest, physiotherapy, salicylates, and corticosteroids should be used, when indicated, in conjunction with CUPRIMINE (see PRECAUTIONS).

* For quantitative test for serum ceruloplasmin see: Morell, A.G.; Windsor, J.; Sternlieb, I.; Scheinberg, I.H.: Measurement of the concentration of ceruloplasmin in serum by determination of its oxidase activity, in "Laboratory Diagnosis of Liver Disease", F.W. Sunderman; F.W. Sunderman, Jr. (eds.), St. Louis, Warren H. Green, Inc., 1968, pp. 193-195.

CONTRAINDICATIONS

Except for the treatment of Wilson's disease or certain cases of cystinuria, use of penicillamine during pregnancy is contraindicated (see WARNINGS).
Although breast milk studies have not been reported in animals or humans, mothers on therapy with penicillamine should not nurse their infants.
Patients with a history of penicillamine-related aplastic anemia or agranulocytosis should not be restarted on penicillamine (see WARNINGS and ADVERSE REACTIONS).
Because of its potential for causing renal damage, penicillamine should not be administered to rheumatoid arthritis patients with a history or other evidence of renal insufficiency.

WARNINGS

The use of penicillamine has been associated with fatalities due to certain diseases such as aplastic anemia, agranulocytosis, thrombocytopenia, Goodpasture's syndrome, and myasthenia gravis.
Because of the potential for serious hematological and renal adverse reactions to occur at any time, routine urinalysis, white and differential blood cell count, hemoglobin determination, and direct platelet count must be done every two weeks for at least the first six months of penicillamine therapy and monthly thereafter. Patients should be instructed to report promptly the development of signs and symptoms of granulocytopenia and/or thrombocytopenia such as fever, sore throat, chills, bruising or bleeding. The above laboratory studies should then be promptly repeated.
Leukopenia and thrombocytopenia have been reported to occur in up to five percent of patients during penicillamine therapy. Leukopenia is of the granulocytic series and may or may not be associated with an increase in eosinophils. A confirmed reduction in WBC below 3500/mm^3 mandates discontinuance of penicillamine therapy. Thrombocytopenia may be on an idiosyncratic basis, with decreased or absent megakaryocytes in the marrow, when it is part of an aplastic anemia. In other cases the thrombocytopenia is presumably on an immune basis since the number of megakaryocytes in the marrow has been reported to be normal or sometimes increased. The development of a platelet count below 100,000/mm^3, even in the absence of clinical bleeding, requires at least temporary cessation of penicillamine therapy. A progressive fall in either platelet count or WBC in three successive determinations, even though values are still within the normal range, likewise requires at least temporary cessation.
Proteinuria and/or hematuria may develop during therapy and may be warning signs of membranous glomerulopathy which can progress to a nephrotic syndrome. Close observation of these patients is essential. In some patients the proteinuria disappears with continued therapy; in others, penicillamine must be discontinued. When a patient develops proteinuria or hematuria the physician must ascertain whether it is a sign of drug-induced glomerulopathy or is unrelated to penicillamine.
Rheumatoid arthritis patients who develop moderate degrees of proteinuria may be continued cautiously on penicillamine therapy, provided that quantitative 24-hour urinary protein determinations are obtained at intervals of one to two weeks. Penicillamine dosage should not be increased under these circumstances. Proteinuria which exceeds 1 g/24 hours, or proteinuria which is progressively increasing, requires either discontinuance of the drug or a reduction in the dosage. In some patients, proteinuria has been reported to clear following reduction in dosage.
In rheumatoid arthritis patients, penicillamine should be discontinued if unexplained gross hematuria or persistent microscopic hematuria develops.
In patients with Wilson's disease or cystinuria the risks of continued penicillamine therapy in patients manifesting potentially serious urinary abnormalities must be weighed against the expected therapeutic benefits.
When penicillamine is used in cystinuria, an annual x-ray for renal stones is advised. Cystine stones form rapidly, sometimes in six months.
Up to one year or more may be required for any urinary abnormalities to disappear after penicillamine has been discontinued.
Because of rare reports of intrahepatic cholestasis and toxic hepatitis, liver function tests are recommended every six months for the duration of therapy.
Goodpasture's syndrome has occurred rarely. The development of abnormal urinary findings associated with hemoptysis and pulmonary infiltrates on x-ray requires immediate cessation of penicillamine.
Obliterative bronchiolitis has been reported rarely. The patient should be cautioned to report immediately pulmonary symptoms such as exertional dyspnea, unexplained cough or wheezing. Pulmonary function studies should be considered at that time.
Myasthenic syndrome sometimes progressing to myasthenia gravis has been reported. Ptosis and diplopia, with weakness of the extraocular muscles, are often early signs of myasthenia. In the majority of cases, symptoms of myasthenia have receded after withdrawal of penicillamine.
Most of the various forms of pemphigus have occurred during treatment with penicillamine. Pemphigus vulgaris and pemphigus foliaceus are reported most frequently, usually as a late complication of therapy. The seborrhea-like characteristics of pemphigus foliaceus may obscure an early diagnosis. When pemphigus is suspected, CUPRIMINE should be discontinued. Treatment has consisted of high doses of corticosteroids alone or, in some cases, concomitantly with an immunosuppressant. Treatment may be required for only a few weeks or months, but may need to be continued for more than a year.
Once instituted for Wilson's disease or cystinuria, treatment with penicillamine should, as a rule, be continued on a daily basis. Interruptions for even a few days have been followed by sensitivity reactions after reinstitution of therapy.
Use in Pregnancy—Penicillamine has been shown to be teratogenic in rats when given in doses 6 times higher than the highest dose recommended for human use. Skeletal defects, cleft palates and fetal toxicity (resorptions) have been reported.
There are no controlled studies on the use of penicillamine in pregnant women. Although normal outcomes have been reported, characteristic congenital cutis laxa and associated birth defects have been reported in infants born of mothers who received therapy with penicillamine during pregnancy. Penicillamine should be used in women of childbearing potential only when the expected benefits outweigh the possible hazards. Women on therapy with penicillamine who are of childbearing potential should be apprised of this risk, advised to report promptly any missed menstrual periods or other indications of possible pregnancy, and followed closely for early recognition of pregnancy.
Wilson's Disease—Reported experience* shows that continued treatment with penicillamine throughout pregnancy protects the mother against relapse of the Wilson's disease, and that discontinuation of penicillamine has deleterious effects on the mother.
If penicillamine is administered during pregnancy to patients with Wilson's disease, it is recommended that the daily dosage be limited to 1 g. If cesarean section is planned, the daily dosage should be limited to 250 mg during the last six weeks of pregnancy and postoperatively until wound healing is complete.
Cystinuria—If possible, penicillamine should not be given during pregnancy to women with cystinuria (see CONTRAINDICATIONS). There are reports of women with cystinuria on therapy with penicillamine who gave birth to infants with generalized connective tissue defects who died following abdominal surgery. If stones continue to form in these patients, the benefits of therapy to the mother must be evaluated against the risk to the fetus.
Rheumatoid Arthritis—Penicillamine should not be administered to rheumatoid arthritis patients who are pregnant (see CONTRAINDICATIONS) and should be discontinued promptly in patients in whom pregnancy is suspected or diagnosed.
There is a report that a woman with rheumatoid arthritis treated with less than one gram a day of penicillamine during pregnancy gave birth (cesarean delivery) to an infant with growth retardation, flattened face with broad nasal bridge, low set ears, short neck with loose skin folds, and unusually lax body skin.

* Scheinberg, I.H., Sternlieb, I.: N. Engl. J. Med. *293*: 1300-1302, Dec. 18, 1975.

PRECAUTIONS

Some patients may experience drug fever, a marked febrile response to penicillamine, usually in the second to third week following initiation of therapy. Drug fever may sometimes be accompanied by a macular cutaneous eruption.
In the case of drug fever in patients with Wilson's disease or cystinuria, penicillamine should be temporarily discontinued until the reaction subsides. Then penicillamine should be reinstituted with a small dose that is gradually increased until the desired dosage is attained. Systemic steroid therapy may be necessary, and is usually helpful, in such patients in whom toxic reactions develop a second or third time.
In the case of drug fever in rheumatoid arthritis patients, because other treatments are available, penicillamine should be discontinued and another therapeutic alternative tried since experience indicates that the febrile reaction will recur in a very high percentage of patients upon readministration of penicillamine.
The skin and mucous membranes should be observed for allergic reactions. Early and late rashes have occurred. Early rash occurs during the first few months of treatment and is more common. It is usually a generalized pruritic, erythematous, maculopapular or morbilliform rash and resembles the allergic rash seen with other drugs. Early rash usually disappears within days after stopping penicillamine and seldom recurs when the drug is restarted at a lower dosage. Pruritus and early rash may often be controlled by the concomitant administration of antihistamines. Less commonly, a late rash may be seen, usually after six months or more of treatment, and requires discontinuation of penicillamine. It is usually on the trunk, is accompanied by intense pruritus, and is usually unresponsive to topical corticoste-

roid therapy. Late rash may take weeks to disappear after penicillamine is stopped and usually recurs if the drug is restarted.

The appearance of a drug eruption accompanied by fever, arthralgia, lymphadenopathy or other allergic manifestations usually requires discontinuation of penicillamine.

Certain patients will develop a positive antinuclear antibody (ANA) test and some of these may show a lupus erythematosus-like syndrome similar to drug-induced lupus associated with other drugs. The lupus erythematosus-like syndrome is not associated with hypocomplementemia and may be present without nephropathy. The development of a positive ANA test does not mandate discontinuance of the drug; however, the physician should be alerted to the possibility that a lupus erythematosus-like syndrome may develop in the future.

Some patients may develop oral ulcerations which in some cases have the appearance of aphthous stomatitis. The stomatitis usually recurs on rechallenge but often clears on a lower dosage. Although rare, cheilosis, glossitis and gingivostomatitis have also been reported. These oral lesions are frequently dose-related and may preclude further increase in penicillamine dosage or require discontinuation of the drug.

Hypogeusia (a blunting or diminution in taste perception) has occurred in some patients. This may last two to three months or more and may develop into a total loss of taste; however, it is usually self-limited despite continued penicillamine treatment. Such taste impairment is rare in patients with Wilson's disease.

Penicillamine should not be used in patients who are receiving concurrently gold therapy, antimalarial or cytotoxic drugs, oxyphenbutazone or phenylbutazone because these drugs are also associated with similar serious hematologic and renal adverse reactions. Patients who have had gold salt therapy discontinued due to a major toxic reaction may be at greater risk of serious adverse reactions with penicillamine but not necessarily of the same type.

Patients who are allergic to penicillin may theoretically have cross-sensitivity to penicillamine. The possibility of reactions from contamination of penicillamine by trace amounts of penicillin has been eliminated now that penicillamine is being produced synthetically rather than as a degradation product of penicillin.

Because of their dietary restrictions, patients with Wilson's disease and cystinuria should be given 25 mg/day of pyridoxine during therapy, since penicillamine increases the requirement for this vitamin. Patients also may receive benefit from a multivitamin preparation, although there is no evidence that deficiency of any vitamin other than pyridoxine is associated with penicillamine. In Wilson's disease, multivitamin preparations must be copper-free.

Rheumatoid arthritis patients whose nutrition is impaired should also be given a daily supplement of pyridoxine. Mineral supplements should not be given, since they may block the response to penicillamine.

Iron deficiency may develop, especially in children and in menstruating women. In Wilson's disease, this may be a result of adding the effects of the low copper diet, which is probably also low in iron, and the penicillamine to the effects of blood loss or growth. In cystinuria, a low methionine diet may contribute to iron deficiency, since it is necessarily low in protein. If necessary, iron may be given in short courses, but a period of two hours should elapse between administration of penicillamine and iron, since orally administered iron has been shown to reduce the effects of penicillamine.

Penicillamine causes an increase in the amount of soluble collagen. In the rat this results in inhibition of normal healing and also a decrease in tensile strength of intact skin. In man this may be the cause of increased skin friability at sites especially subject to pressure or trauma, such as shoulders, elbows, knees, toes, and buttocks. Extravasations of blood may occur and may appear as purpuric areas, with external bleeding if the skin is broken, or as vesicles containing dark blood. Neither type is progressive. There is no apparent association with bleeding elsewhere in the body and no associated coagulation defect has been found. Therapy with penicillamine may be continued in the presence of these lesions. They may not recur if dosage is reduced. Other reported effects probably due to the action of penicillamine on collagen are excessive wrinkling of the skin and development of small, white papules at venipuncture and surgical sites.

The effects of penicillamine on collagen and elastin make it advisable to consider a reduction in dosage to 250 mg/day, when surgery is contemplated. Reinstitution of full therapy should be delayed until wound healing is complete.

Carcinogenesis—Long-term animal carcinogenicity studies have not been done with penicillamine. There is a report that five of ten autoimmune disease-prone NZB hybrid mice developed lymphocytic leukemia after 6 months' intraperitoneal treatment with a dose of 400 mg/kg penicillamine 5 days per week.

Nursing Mothers —See CONTRAINDICATIONS.

Usage in Children —The efficacy of CUPRIMINE in juvenile rheumatoid arthritis has not been established.

ADVERSE REACTIONS

Penicillamine is a drug with a high incidence of untoward reactions, some of which are potentially fatal. Therefore, it is mandatory that patients receiving penicillamine therapy remain under close medical supervision throughout the period of drug administration (see WARNINGS and PRECAUTIONS).

Reported incidences (%) for the most commonly occurring adverse reactions in rheumatoid arthritis patients are noted, based on 17 representative clinical trials reported in the literature (1270 patients).

Allergic—Generalized pruritus, early and late rashes (5%), pemphigus (see WARNINGS), and drug eruptions which may be accompanied by fever, arthralgia, or lymphadenopathy have occurred (see WARNINGS and PRECAUTIONS). Some patients may show a lupus erythematosus-like syndrome similar to drug-induced lupus produced by other pharmacological agents (see PRECAUTIONS).

Urticaria and exfoliative dermatitis have occurred.

Thyroiditis has been reported; hypoglycemia in association with anti-insulin antibodies has been reported. These reactions are extremely rare.

Some patients may develop a migratory polyarthralgia, often with objective synovitis (see DOSAGE AND ADMINISTRATION).

Gastrointestinal—Anorexia, epigastric pain, nausea, vomiting, or occasional diarrhea may occur (17%).

Isolated cases of reactivated peptic ulcer have occurred, as have hepatic dysfunction and pancreatitis. Intrahepatic cholestasis and toxic hepatitis have been reported rarely. There have been a few reports of increased serum alkaline phosphatase, lactic dehydrogenase, and positive cephalin flocculation and thymol turbidity tests.

Some patients may report a blunting, diminution, or total loss of taste perception (12%); or may develop oral ulcerations. Although rare, cheilosis, glossitis, and gingivostomatitis have been reported (see PRECAUTIONS).

Gastrointestinal side effects are usually reversible following cessation of therapy.

Hematological—Penicillamine can cause bone marrow depression (see WARNINGS). Leukopenia (2%) and thrombocytopenia (4%) have occurred. Fatalities have been reported as a result of thrombocytopenia, agranulocytosis, aplastic anemia, and sideroblastic anemia.

Thrombotic thrombocytopenic purpura, hemolytic anemia, red cell aplasia, monocytosis, leukocytosis, eosinophilia, and thrombocytosis have also been reported.

Renal—Patients on penicillamine therapy may develop proteinuria (6%) and/or hematuria which, in some, may progress to the development of the nephrotic syndrome as a result of an immune complex membranous glomerulopathy (see WARNINGS).

Central Nervous System—Tinnitus, optic neuritis and peripheral sensory and motor neuropathies (including polyradiculoneuropathy, i.e., Guillain-Barre syndrome) have been reported. Muscular weakness may or may not occur with the peripheral neuropathies. Visual and psychic disturbances have been reported.

Neuromuscular—Myasthenia gravis (see WARNINGS).

Other—Adverse reactions that have been reported rarely include thrombophlebitis; hyperpyrexia (see PRECAUTIONS); falling hair or alopecia; lichen planus; polymyositis; dermatomyositis; mammary hyperplasia; elastosis perforans serpiginosa; toxic epidermal necrolysis; anetoderma (cutaneous macular atrophy); and Goodpasture's syndrome, a severe and ultimately fatal glomerulonephritis associated with intra-alveolar hemorrhage (see WARNINGS). Fatal renal vasculitis has also been reported. Allergic alveolitis, obliterative bronchiolitis, interstitial pneumonitis and pulmonary fibrosis have been reported in patients with severe rheumatoid arthritis, some of whom were receiving penicillamine. Bronchial asthma also has been reported.

Increased skin friability, excessive wrinkling of skin, and development of small white papules at venipuncture and surgical sites have been reported (see PRECAUTIONS).

The chelating action of the drug may cause increased excretion of other heavy metals such as zinc, mercury and lead.

There have been reports associating penicillamine with leukemia. However, circumstances involved in these reports are such that a cause and effect relationship to the drug has not been established.

DOSAGE AND ADMINISTRATION

In all patients receiving penicillamine, it is important that CUPRIMINE be given on an empty stomach, at least one hour before meals or two hours after meals, and at least one hour apart from any other drug, food, or milk. Because penicillamine increases the requirement for pyridoxine, patients may require a daily supplement of pyridoxine (see PRECAUTIONS).

Wilson's Disease — Optimal dosage can be determined by measurement of urinary copper excretion and the determination of free copper in the serum. The urine must be collected in copper-free glassware, and should be quantitatively analyzed for copper before and soon after initiation of therapy with CUPRIMINE.

Determination of 24-hour urinary copper excretion is of greatest value in the first week of therapy with penicillamine. In the absence of any drug reaction, a dose between 0.75 and 1.5 g that results in an initial 24-hour cupriuresis of over 2 mg should be continued for about three months, by which time the most reliable method of monitoring maintenance treatment is the determination of free copper in the serum. This equals the difference between quantitatively determined total copper and ceruloplasmin-copper. Adequately treated patients will usually have less than 10 mcg free copper/dL of serum. It is seldom necessary to exceed a dosage of 2 g/day. If the patient is intolerant to therapy with CUPRIMINE, alternative treatment is trientine hydrochloride.

In patients who cannot tolerate as much as 1 g/day initially, initiating dosage with 250 mg/day, and increasing gradually to the requisite amount, gives closer control of the effects of the drug and may help to reduce the incidence of adverse reactions.

Cystinuria —It is recommended that CUPRIMINE be used along with conventional therapy. By reducing urinary cystine, it decreases crystalluria and stone formation. In some instances, it has been reported to decrease the size of, and even to dissolve, stones already formed.

The usual dosage of CUPRIMINE in the treatment of cystinuria is 2 g/day for adults, with a range of 1 to 4 g/day. For children, dosage can be based on 30 mg/kg/day. The total daily amount should be divided into four doses. If four equal doses are not feasible, give the larger portion at bedtime. If adverse reactions necessitate a reduction in dosage, it is important to retain the bedtime dose.

Initiating dosage with 250 mg/day, and increasing gradually to the requisite amount, gives closer control of the effects of the drug and may help to reduce the incidence of adverse reactions.

In addition to taking CUPRIMINE, patients should drink copiously. It is especially important to drink about a pint of fluid at bedtime and another pint once during the night when urine is more concentrated and more acid than during the day. The greater the fluid intake, the lower the required dosage of CUPRIMINE.

Dosage must be individualized to an amount that limits cystine excretion to 100–200 mg/day in those with no history of stones, and below 100 mg/day in those who have had stone formation and/or pain. Thus, in determining dosage, the inherent tubular defect, the patient's size, age, and rate of growth, and his diet and water intake all must be taken into consideration.

The standard nitroprusside cyanide test has been reported useful as a qualitative measure of the effective dose*: Add 2 mL of freshly prepared 5 percent sodium cyanide to 5 mL of a 24-hour aliquot of protein-free urine and let stand ten minutes. Add 5 drops of freshly prepared 5 percent sodium nitroprusside and mix. Cystine will turn the mixture magenta. If the result is negative, it can be assumed that cystine excretion is less than 100 mg/g creatinine.

Although penicillamine is rarely excreted unchanged, it also will turn the mixture magenta. If there is any question as to which substance is causing the reaction, a ferric chloride test can be done to eliminate doubt: Add 3 percent ferric chloride dropwise to the urine. Penicillamine will turn the urine an immediate and quickly fading blue. Cystine will not produce any change in appearance.

*Lotz, M., Potts, J.T. and Bartter, F.C.: Brit. Med. J. *2*:521, Aug. 28, 1965 (in Medical Memoranda).

Rheumatoid Arthritis —The principal rule of treatment with CUPRIMINE in rheumatoid arthritis is patience. The onset of therapeutic response is typically delayed. Two or three months may be required before the first evidence of a clinical response is noted (see CLINICAL PHARMACOLOGY).

When treatment with CUPRIMINE has been interrupted because of adverse reactions or other reasons, the drug should be reintroduced cautiously by starting with a lower dosage and increasing slowly.

Initial Therapy—The currently recommended dosage regimen in rheumatoid arthritis begins with a single daily dose of 125 mg or 250 mg which is thereafter increased at one to three month intervals, by 125 mg or 250 mg/day, as patient response and tolerance indicate. If a satisfactory remission of symptoms is achieved, the dose associated with the remission should be continued (see *Maintenance Therapy*). If there is no improvement and there are no signs of potentially serious toxicity after two to three months of treatment with doses of

Continued on next page

Information on the Merck & Co., Inc. products listed on these pages is the full prescribing information from product circulars in use September 30, 1996.

Merck & Co.—Cont.

500–750 mg/day, increases of 250 mg/day at two to three month intervals may be continued until a satisfactory remission occurs (see *Maintenance Therapy*) or signs of toxicity develop (see WARNINGS and PRECAUTIONS). If there is no discernible improvement after three to four months of treatment with 1000 to 1500 mg of penicillamine/day, it may be assumed the patient will not respond and CUPRIMINE should be discontinued.

Maintenance Therapy—The maintenance dosage of CUPRIMINE must be individualized, and may require adjustment during the course of treatment. Many patients respond satisfactorily to a dosage within the 500–750 mg/day range. Some need less.

Changes in maintenance dosage levels may not be reflected clinically or in the erythrocyte sedimentation rate for two to three months after each dosage adjustment.

Some patients will subsequently require an increase in the maintenance dosage to achieve maximal disease suppression. In those patients who do respond, but who evidence incomplete suppression of their disease after the first six to nine months of treatment, the daily dosage of CUPRIMINE may be increased by 125 mg or 250 mg/day at three-month intervals. It is unusual in current practice to employ a dosage in excess of 1 g/day, but up to 1.5 g/day has sometimes been required.

Management of Exacerbations—During the course of treatment some patients may experience an exacerbation of disease activity following an initial good response. These may be self-limited and can subside within twelve weeks. They are usually controlled by the addition of non-steroidal anti-inflammatory drugs, and only if the patient has demonstrated a true "escape" phenomenon (as evidenced by failure of the flare to subside within this time period) should an increase in the maintenance dose ordinarily be considered.

In the rheumatoid patient, migratory polyarthralgia due to penicillamine is extremely difficult to differentiate from an exacerbation of the rheumatoid arthritis. Discontinuance or a substantial reduction in dosage of CUPRIMINE for up to several weeks will usually determine which of these processes is responsible for the arthralgia.

Duration of Therapy—The optimum duration of therapy with CUPRIMINE in rheumatoid arthritis has not been determined. If the patient has been in remission for six months or more, a gradual, stepwise dosage reduction in decrements of 125 mg or 250 mg/day at approximately three month intervals may be attempted.

Concomitant Drug Therapy—CUPRIMINE should not be used in patients who are receiving concomitant gold therapy, antimalarial or cytotoxic drugs, oxyphenbutazone, or phenylbutazone (see PRECAUTIONS). Other measures, such as salicylates, other non-steroidal anti-inflammatory drugs, or systemic corticosteroids, may be continued when penicillamine is initiated. After improvement commences, analgesic and anti-inflammatory drugs may be slowly discontinued as symptoms permit. Steroid withdrawal must be done gradually, and many months of treatment with CUPRIMINE may be required before steroids can be completely eliminated.

Dosage Frequency—Based on clinical experience dosages up to 500 mg/day can be given as a single daily dose. Dosages in excess of 500 mg/day should be administered in divided doses.

HOW SUPPLIED

No. 3299—Capsules CUPRIMINE, 250 mg, are ivory-colored capsules containing a white or nearly white powder, and are coded MSD 602. They are supplied as follows:
NDC 0006-0602-68 in bottles of 100
(6505-01-049-9494, 250 mg 100's).
   Shown in Product Identification Guide, page 324
No. 3350—Capsules CUPRIMINE, 125 mg, are opaque ivory and gray capsules containing a white or nearly white powder, and are coded MSD 672. They are supplied as follows:
NDC 0006-0672-68 in bottles of 100.
   Shown in Product Identification Guide, page 324
Storage
Keep container tightly closed.
     7873239   Issued March 1989
COPYRIGHT © MERCK & CO., INC., 1985, 1989
All rights reserved

DARANIDE® Tablets   ℞
(Dichlorphenamide), U.S.P.

DESCRIPTION

DARANIDE* (Dichlorphenamide) is an oral carbonic anhydrase inhibitor. Dichlorphenamide, a dichlorinated benzenedisulfonamide, is known chemically as 4,5-dichloro-

1,3-benzenedisulfonamide. Its empirical formula is $C_6H_6Cl_2N_2O_4S_2$ and its structural formula is:

Dichlorphenamide is a white or practically white, crystalline compound with a molecular weight of 305.16. It is very slightly soluble in water but soluble in dilute solutions of sodium carbonate and sodium hydroxide. Dilute alkaline solutions of dichlorphenamide are stable at room temperature.

DARANIDE is supplied as tablets, for oral administration, each containing 50 mg dichlorphenamide. Inactive ingredients are D&C Yellow 10, lactose, magnesium stearate, and starch.

---

*Registered trademark of MERCK & CO., INC.

CLINICAL PHARMACOLOGY

Carbonic anhydrase inhibitors reduce intraocular pressure by partially suppressing the secretion of aqueous humor (inflow), although the mechanism by which they do this is not fully understood. Evidence suggests that HCO_3^- ions are produced in the ciliary body by hydration of carbon dioxide under the influence of carbonic anhydrase and diffuse into the posterior chamber with Na^+ ions. The aqueous fluid contains more Na^+ and HCO_3^- ions than does plasma and consequently is hypertonic. Water is attracted to the posterior chamber by osmosis. Systemic administration of a carbonic anhydrase inhibitor has been shown to inactivate carbonic anhydrase in the ciliary body of the rabbit's eye and to reduce the high concentration of HCO_3^- ions in ocular fluids. As is the case with all carbonic anhydrase inhibitors, DARANIDE in high doses causes some decrease in renal blood flow and glomerular filtration rate.

In man, DARANIDE begins to act within an hour and maximal effect is observed in two to four hours. The lowered intraocular tension may be maintained for approximately 6 to 12 hours.

INDICATIONS AND USAGE

For adjunctive treatment of: chronic simple (open-angle) glaucoma, secondary glaucoma, and preoperatively in acute angle-closure glaucoma where delay of surgery is desired in order to lower intraocular pressure.

CONTRAINDICATIONS

DARANIDE is contraindicated in hepatic insufficiency, renal failure, adrenocortical insufficiency, hyperchloremic acidosis, or in conditions in which serum levels of sodium or potassium are depressed. DARANIDE should not be used in patients with severe pulmonary obstruction who are unable to increase their alveolar ventilation since their acidosis may be increased.

DARANIDE is contraindicated in patients who are hypersensitive to this product.

PRECAUTIONS

General
Potassium excretion is increased by DARANIDE and hypokalemia may develop with brisk diuresis, when severe cirrhosis is present, or during concomitant use of steroids or ACTH.

Interference with adequate oral electrolyte intake will also contribute to hypokalemia. Hypokalemia can sensitize or exaggerate the response of the heart to the toxic effects of digitalis (e.g., increased ventricular irritability). Hypokalemia may be avoided or treated by use of potassium supplements such as foods with a high potassium content. DARANIDE should be used with caution in patients with respiratory acidosis.

Drug Interactions
Caution is advised in patients receiving concomitant high-dose aspirin and carbonic anhydrase inhibitors, as anorexia, tachypnea, lethargy and coma have been rarely reported due to a possible drug interaction.

Carcinogenesis, Mutagenesis, Impairment of Fertility
Long-term studies in animals have not been performed to evaluate the effects upon fertility or carcinogenic potential of DARANIDE.

Pregnancy
Pregnancy Category C. Dichlorphenamide has been shown to be teratogenic in the rat (skeletal anomalies) when given in doses 100 times the human dose. There are no adequate and well-controlled studies in pregnant women. DARANIDE

should not be used in women of childbearing age or in pregnancy, especially during the first trimester, unless the potential benefits outweigh the potential risks.
Nursing Mothers
It is not known whether dichlorphenamide is excreted in human milk. Because many drugs are excreted in human milk, caution should be exercised when dichlorphenamide is administered to a nursing woman.
Pediatric Use
Safety and effectiveness in children have not been established.

ADVERSE REACTIONS

Certain side effects characteristic of carbonic anhydrase inhibitors may occur with DARANIDE, particularly with increasing doses. The most common effects include gastrointestinal disturbances (anorexia, nausea, and vomiting), drowsiness and paresthesias.

Included in the listing which follows are some adverse reactions which have not been reported with DARANIDE. However, pharmacological similarities among the carbonic anhydrase inhibitors make it advisable to consider the following reactions when dichlorphenamide is administered. *Central Nervous System/Psychiatric:* ataxia, tremor, tinnitus, headache, weakness, nervousness, globus hystericus, lassitude, depression, confusion, disorientation, dizziness; *Gastrointestinal:* constipation, hepatic insufficiency; *Metabolic:* loss of weight, metabolic acidosis, electrolyte imbalance (hypokalemia, hyperchloremia), hyperuricemia; *Hypersensitivity:* skin eruptions, pruritus, fever; *Hematologic:* leukopenia, agranulocytosis, thrombocytopenia; *Genitourinary:* urinary frequency, renal colic, renal calculi, phosphaturia.

OVERDOSAGE

The oral LD_{50} of DARANIDE is 1710 and 2600 mg/kg in the mouse and rat respectively.

Symptoms of overdosage or toxicity may include drowsiness, anorexia, nausea, vomiting, dizziness, paresthesias, ataxia, tremor and tinnitus.

In the event of overdosage, induce emesis or perform gastric lavage. The electrolyte disturbance most likely to be encountered from overdosage is hyperchloremic acidosis that may respond to bicarbonate administration. Potassium supplementation may be required. The patient should be carefully observed and given supportive treatment.

DOSAGE AND ADMINISTRATION

DARANIDE is usually given in conjunction with topical ocular hypotensive agents. In acute angle-closure glaucoma, it may be used together with miotics and osmotic agents in an attempt to reduce intraocular tension rapidly. If this is not quickly relieved, surgery may be mandatory.

Dosage must be adjusted carefully to meet the requirements of the individual patient. A priming dose of 100 to 200 mg of DARANIDE (2 to 4 tablets) is suggested for adults, followed by 100 mg (2 tablets) every 12 hours until the desired response has been obtained. The recommended maintenance dosage for adults is 25 to 50 mg (½ to 1 tablet) once to three times daily.

HOW SUPPLIED

No. 3256—Tablets DARANIDE, 50 mg each, are yellow, round, scored, compressed tablets, coded MSD 49. They are supplied as follows:
NDC 0006-0049-68 bottles of 100.
       7870318   Issued May 1994
COPYRIGHT © MERCK & CO., INC., 1985
All rights reserved

DECADRON® Elixir   ℞
(Dexamethasone), U.S.P.

DESCRIPTION

Glucocorticoids are adrenocortical steroids, both naturally occurring and synthetic, which are readily absorbed from the gastrointestinal tract.

Dexamethasone, a synthetic adrenocortical steroid, is a white to practically white, odorless, crystalline powder. It is stable in air. It is practically insoluble in water. The molecular weight is 392.47. It is designated chemically as 9-fluoro-11β,17,21-trihydroxy-16α-methylpregna -1, 4- diene-3,20-dione. The empirical formula is $C_{22}H_{29}FO_5$ and the structural formula is:
[See chemical structure at top of next column.]
DECADRON* (Dexamethasone) elixir contains 0.5 mg of dexamethasone in each 5 mL. Benzoic acid, 0.1%, is added as a preservative. It also contains alcohol 5%. Inactive ingredi-

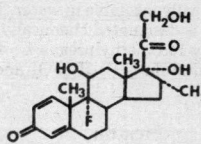

ents are FD&C Red 40, flavors, glycerin, purified water, and sodium saccharin.

*Registered trademark of MERCK & CO., INC.

ACTIONS

Naturally occurring glucocorticoids (hydrocortisone and cortisone), which also have salt-retaining properties, are used as replacement therapy in adrenocortical deficiency states. Their synthetic analogs, including dexamethasone, are primarily used for their potent anti-inflammatory effects in disorders of many organ systems.

Glucocorticoids cause profound and varied metabolic effects. In addition, they modify the body's immune responses to diverse stimuli.

At equipotent anti-inflammatory doses, dexamethasone almost completely lacks the sodium-retaining property of hydrocortisone and closely related derivatives of hydrocortisone.

INDICATIONS

1. *Endocrine Disorders*
   Primary or secondary adrenocortical insufficiency (hydrocortisone or cortisone is the first choice; synthetic analogs may be used in conjunction with mineralocorticoids where applicable; in infancy mineralocorticoid supplementation is of particular importance)
   Congenital adrenal hyperplasia
   Nonsuppurative thyroiditis
   Hypercalcemia associated with cancer
2. *Rheumatic Disorders*
   As adjunctive therapy for short-term administration (to tide the patient over an acute episode or exacerbation) in:
   Psoriatic arthritis
   Rheumatoid arthritis, including juvenile rheumatoid arthritis (selected cases may require low-dose maintenance therapy)
   Ankylosing spondylitis
   Acute and subacute bursitis
   Acute nonspecific tenosynovitis
   Acute gouty arthritis
   Post-traumatic osteoarthritis
   Synovitis of osteoarthritis
   Epicondylitis
3. *Collagen Diseases*
   During an exacerbation or as maintenance therapy in selected cases of—
   Systemic lupus erythematosus
   Acute rheumatic carditis
4. *Dermatologic Diseases*
   Pemphigus
   Bullous dermatitis herpetiformis
   Severe erythema multiforme (Stevens-Johnson syndrome)
   Exfoliative dermatitis
   Mycosis fungoides
   Severe psoriasis
   Severe seborrheic dermatitis
5. *Allergic States*
   Control of severe or incapacitating allergic conditions intractable to adequate trials of conventional treatment:
   Seasonal or perennial allergic rhinitis
   Bronchial asthma
   Contact dermatitis
   Atopic dermatitis
   Serum sickness
   Drug hypersensitivity reactions
6. *Ophthalmic Diseases*
   Severe acute and chronic allergic and inflammatory processes involving the eye and its adnexa, such as—
   Allergic conjunctivitis
   Keratitis
   Allergic corneal marginal ulcers
   Herpes zoster ophthalmicus
   Iritis and iridocyclitis
   Chorioretinitis
   Anterior segment inflammation
   Diffuse posterior uveitis and choroiditis
   Optic neuritis
   Sympathetic ophthalmia
7. *Respiratory Diseases*
   Symptomatic sarcoidosis

   Loeffler's syndrome not manageable by other means
   Berylliosis
   Fulminating or disseminated pulmonary tuberculosis when used concurrently with appropriate antituberculous chemotherapy
   Aspiration pneumonitis
8. *Hematologic Disorders*
   Idiopathic thrombocytopenic purpura in adults
   Secondary thrombocytopenia in adults
   Acquired (autoimmune) hemolytic anemia
   Erythroblastopenia (RBC anemia)
   Congenital (erythroid) hypoplastic anemia
9. *Neoplastic Diseases*
   For palliative management of:
   Leukemias and lymphomas in adults
   Acute leukemia of childhood
10. *Edematous States*
    To induce a diuresis or remission of proteinuria in the nephrotic syndrome, without uremia, of the idiopathic type or that due to lupus erythematosus
11. *Gastrointestinal Diseases*
    To tide the patient over a critical period of the disease in:
    Ulcerative colitis
    Regional enteritis
12. *Miscellaneous*
    Tuberculous meningitis with subarachnoid block or impending block when used concurrently with appropriate antituberculous chemotherapy
    Trichinosis with neurologic or myocardial involvement
13. *Diagnostic testing of adrenocortical hyperfunction.*

CONTRAINDICATIONS

Systemic fungal infections
Hypersensitivity to this product

WARNINGS

In patients on corticosteroid therapy subjected to unusual stress, increased dosage of rapidly acting corticosteroids before, during, and after the stressful situation is indicated.

Drug-induced secondary adrenocortical insufficiency may result from too rapid withdrawal of corticosteroids and may be minimized by gradual reduction of dosage. This type of relative insufficiency may persist for months after discontinuation of therapy; therefore, in any situation of stress occurring during that period, hormone therapy should be reinstituted. If the patient is receiving steroids already, dosage may have to be increased. Since mineralocorticoid secretion may be impaired, salt and/or a mineralocorticoid should be administered concurrently.

Corticosteroids may mask some signs of infection, and new infections may appear during their use. There may be decreased resistance and inability to localize infection when corticosteroids are used. Moreover, corticosteroids may affect the nitroblue-tetrazolium test for bacterial infection and produce false negative results.

In cerebral malaria, a double-blind trial has shown that the use of corticosteroids is associated with prolongation of coma and a higher incidence of pneumonia and gastrointestinal bleeding.

Corticosteroids may activate latent amebiasis. Therefore, it is recommended that latent or active amebiasis be ruled out before initiating corticosteroid therapy in any patient who has spent time in the tropics or any patient with unexplained diarrhea.

Prolonged use of corticosteroids may produce posterior subcapsular cataracts, glaucoma with possible damage to the optic nerves, and may enhance the establishment of secondary ocular infections due to fungi or viruses.

Usage in pregnancy: Since adequate human reproduction studies have not been done with corticosteroids, use of these drugs in pregnancy or in women of childbearing potential requires that the anticipated benefits be weighed against the possible hazards to the mother and embryo or fetus. Infants born of mothers who have received substantial doses of corticosteroids during pregnancy should be carefully observed for signs of hypoadrenalism.

Corticosteroids appear in breast milk and could suppress growth, interfere with endogenous corticosteroid production, or cause other unwanted effects. Mothers taking pharmacologic doses of corticosteroids should be advised not to nurse.

Average and large doses of hydrocortisone or cortisone can cause elevation of blood pressure, salt and water retention, and increased excretion of potassium. These effects are less likely to occur with the synthetic derivatives except when used in large doses. Dietary salt restriction and potassium supplementation may be necessary. All corticosteroids increase calcium excretion.

Administration of live virus vaccines, including smallpox, is contraindicated in individuals receiving immunosuppressive doses of corticosteroids. If inactivated viral or bacterial vaccines are administered to individuals receiving immunosuppressive doses of corticosteroids, the expected serum antibody response may not be obtained. However, immunization

procedures may be undertaken in patients who are receiving corticosteroids as replacement therapy, e.g., for Addison's disease.

Patients who are on drugs which suppress the immune system are more susceptible to infections than healthy individuals. Chickenpox and measles, for example, can have a more serious or even fatal course in non-immune children or adults on corticosteroids. In such children or adults who have not had these diseases, particular care should be taken to avoid exposure. The risk of developing a disseminated infection varies among individuals and can be related to the dose, route and duration of corticosteroid administration as well as to the underlying disease. If exposed to chickenpox, prophylaxis with varicella zoster immune globulin (VZIG) may be indicated. If chickenpox develops, treatment with antiviral agents may be considered. If exposed to measles, prophylaxis with immune globulin (IG) may be indicated. (See the respective package inserts for VZIG and IG for complete prescribing information.)

Similarly, corticosteroids should be used with great care in patients with known or suspected Strongyloides (threadworm) infestation. In such patients, corticosteroid-induced immunosuppression may lead to Strongyloides hyperinfection and dissemination with widespread larval migration, often accompanied by severe enterocolitis and potentially fatal gram-negative septicemia.

The use of DECADRON elixir in active tuberculosis should be restricted to those cases of fulminating or disseminated tuberculosis in which the corticosteroid is used for the management of the disease in conjunction with an appropriate antituberculous regimen.

If corticosteroids are indicated in patients with latent tuberculosis or tuberculin reactivity, close observation is necessary as reactivation of the disease may occur. During prolonged corticosteroid therapy, these patients should receive chemoprophylaxis.

Literature reports suggest an apparent association between use of corticosteroids and left ventricular free wall rupture after a recent myocardial infarction; therefore, therapy with corticosteroids should be used with great caution in these patients.

PRECAUTIONS

Following prolonged therapy, withdrawal of corticosteroids may result in symptoms of the corticosteroid withdrawal syndrome including fever, myalgia, arthralgia, and malaise. This may occur in patients even without evidence of adrenal insufficiency.

There is an enhanced effect of corticosteroids in patients with hypothyroidism and in those with cirrhosis.

Corticosteroids should be used cautiously in patients with ocular herpes simplex because of possible corneal perforation.

The lowest possible dose of corticosteroid should be used to control the condition under treatment, and when reduction in dosage is possible, the reduction should be gradual.

Psychic derangements may appear when corticosteroids are used, ranging from euphoria, insomnia, mood swings, personality changes, and severe depression, to frank psychotic manifestations. Also, existing emotional instability or psychotic tendencies may be aggravated by corticosteroids.

Aspirin should be used cautiously in conjunction with corticosteroids in hypoprothrombinemia.

Steroids should be used with caution in nonspecific ulcerative colitis, if there is a probability of impending perforation, abscess, or other pyogenic infection, diverticulitis, fresh intestinal anastomoses, active or latent peptic ulcer, renal insufficiency, hypertension, osteoporosis, and myasthenia gravis. Signs of peritoneal irritation following gastrointestinal perforation in patients receiving large doses of corticosteroids may be minimal or absent. Fat embolism has been reported as a possible complication of hypercortisonism.

When large doses are given, some authorities advise that corticosteroids be taken with meals and antacids taken between meals to help to prevent peptic ulcer.

Growth and development of infants and children on prolonged corticosteroid therapy should be carefully observed. Steroids may increase or decrease motility and number of spermatozoa in some patients.

Phenytoin, phenobarbital, ephedrine, and rifampin may enhance the metabolic clearance of corticosteroids, resulting in decreased blood levels and lessened physiologic activity, thus requiring adjustment in corticosteroid dosage. These interactions may interfere with dexamethasone suppression tests which should be interpreted with caution during administration of these drugs.

Continued on next page

Information on the Merck & Co., Inc. products listed on these pages is the full prescribing information from product circulars in use September 30, 1996.

Merck & Co.—Cont.

False-negative results in the dexamethasone suppression test (DST) in patients being treated with indomethacin have been reported. Thus, results of the DST should be interpreted with caution in these patients.

The prothrombin time should be checked frequently in patients who are receiving corticosteroids and coumarin anticoagulants at the same time because of reports that corticosteroids have altered the response to these anticoagulants. Studies have shown that the usual effect produced by adding corticosteroids is inhibition of response to coumarins, although there have been some conflicting reports of potentiation not substantiated by studies.

When corticosteroids are administered concomitantly with potassium-depleting diuretics, patients should be observed closely for development of hypokalemia.

Information for Patients

Susceptible patients who are on immunosuppressant doses of corticosteroids should be warned to avoid exposure to chickenpox or measles. Patients should also be advised that if they are exposed, medical advice should be sought without delay.

ADVERSE REACTIONS

Fluid and Electrolyte Disturbances
  Sodium retention
  Fluid retention
  Congestive heart failure in susceptible patients
  Potassium loss
  Hypokalemic alkalosis
  Hypertension
Musculoskeletal
  Muscle weakness
  Steroid myopathy
  Loss of muscle mass
  Osteoporosis
  Vertebral compression fractures
  Aseptic necrosis of femoral and humeral heads
  Pathologic fracture of long bones
  Tendon rupture
Gastrointestinal
  Peptic ulcer with possible perforation and hemorrhage
  Perforation of the small and large bowel, particularly in patients with inflammatory bowel disease
  Pancreatitis
  Abdominal distention
  Ulcerative esophagitis
Dermatologic
  Impaired wound healing
  Thin fragile skin
  Petechiae and ecchymoses
  Erythema
  Increased sweating
  May suppress reactions to skin tests
  Other cutaneous reactions, such as allergic dermatitis, urticaria, angioneurotic edema
Neurologic
  Convulsions
  Increased intracranial pressure with papilledema (pseudotumor cerebri) usually after treatment
  Vertigo
  Headache
  Psychic disturbances
Endocrine
  Menstrual irregularities
  Development of cushingoid state
  Suppression of growth in children
  Secondary adrenocortical and pituitary unresponsiveness, particularly in times of stress, as in trauma, surgery, or illness
  Decreased carbohydrate tolerance
  Manifestations of latent diabetes mellitus
  Increased requirements for insulin or oral hypoglycemic agents in diabetics
  Hirsutism
Ophthalmic
  Posterior subcapsular cataracts
  Increased intraocular pressure
  Glaucoma
  Exophthalmos
Metabolic
  Negative nitrogen balance due to protein catabolism
Cardiovascular
  Myocardial rupture following recent myocardial infarction (see WARNINGS).
Other
  Hypersensitivity
  Thromboembolism
  Weight gain
  Increased appetite
  Nausea
  Malaise
  Hiccups

OVERDOSAGE

Reports of acute toxicity and/or death following overdosage of glucocorticoids are rare. In the event of overdosage, no specific antidote is available; treatment is supportive and symptomatic.

The oral LD$_{50}$ of dexamethasone in female mice was 6.5 g/kg.

DOSAGE AND ADMINISTRATION

For oral administration

DOSAGE REQUIREMENTS ARE VARIABLE AND MUST BE INDIVIDUALIZED ON THE BASIS OF THE DISEASE AND THE RESPONSE OF THE PATIENT.

The initial dosage varies from 0.75 to 9 mg a day depending on the disease being treated. In less severe diseases doses lower than 0.75 mg may suffice, while in severe diseases doses higher than 9 mg may be required. The initial dosage should be maintained or adjusted until the patient's response is satisfactory. If satisfactory clinical response does not occur after a reasonable period of time, discontinue DECADRON elixir and transfer the patient to other therapy. After a favorable initial response, the proper maintenance dosage should be determined by decreasing the initial dosage in small amounts to the lowest dosage that maintains an adequate clinical response.

Patients should be observed closely for signs that might require dosage adjustment, including changes in clinical status resulting from remissions or exacerbations of the disease, individual drug responsiveness, and the effect of stress (e.g., surgery, infection, trauma). During stress it may be necessary to increase dosage temporarily.

If the drug is to be stopped after more than a few days of treatment, it usually should be withdrawn gradually.

The following milligram equivalents facilitate changing to DECADRON from other glucocorticoids:

DECADRON	Methylprednisolone and Triamcinolone	Hydrocortisone	Prednisolone and Prednisone	Cortisone
0.75 mg =	4 mg =	5 mg =	20 mg =	25 mg

Dexamethasone suppression tests
1.   Tests for Cushing's syndrome
     Give 1.0 mg of DECADRON orally at 11:00 p.m. Blood is drawn for plasma cortisol determination at 8:00 a.m. the following morning.
     For greater accuracy, give 0.5 mg of DECADRON orally every 6 hours for 48 hours. Twenty-four hour urine collections are made for determination of 17-hydroxycorticosteroid excretion.
2.   Test to distinguish Cushing's syndrome due to pituitary ACTH excess from Cushing's syndrome due to other causes
     Give 2.0 mg of DECADRON orally every 6 hours for 48 hours. Twenty-four hour urine collections are made for determination of 17-hydroxycorticosteroid excretion.

HOW SUPPLIED

No. 7622—Elixir DECADRON, 0.5 mg dexamethasone per 5 mL, is a clear, red liquid and is supplied as follows:
NDC 0006-7622-55 bottles of 100 mL with calibrated dropper assembly
NDC 0006-7622-66 bottles of 237 mL without dropper assembly
(6505-01-137-8465, 237 mL).
Storage
Keep container tightly closed.
        7412729   Issued October 1995

DECADRON® Tablets   ℞
(Dexamethasone), U.S.P.

DESCRIPTION

Glucocorticoids are adrenocortical steroids, both naturally occurring and synthetic, which are readily absorbed from the gastrointestinal tract.

Dexamethasone, a synthetic adrenocortical steroid, is a white to practically white, odorless, crystalline powder. It is

stable in air. It is practically insoluble in water. The molecular weight is 392.47. It is designated chemically as 9-fluoro-11β, 17, 21-trihydroxy-16α-methylpregna-1, 4-diene-3,20-dione. The empirical formula is $C_{22}H_{29}FO_5$ and the structural formula is:

DECADRON* (Dexamethasone) tablets are supplied in six potencies, 0.25 mg, 0.5 mg, 0.75 mg, 1.5 mg, 4 mg, and 6 mg. Inactive ingredients are calcium phosphate, lactose, magnesium stearate, and starch. Tablets DECADRON 0.25 mg also contain FD&C Yellow 6. Tablets DECADRON 0.5 mg also contain D&C Yellow 10 and FD&C Yellow 6. Tablets DECADRON 0.75 mg also contain FD&C Blue 1. Tablets DECADRON 1.5 mg also contain FD&C Red 40. Tablets DECADRON 6 mg also contain FD&C Blue 1 and iron oxide.

---

*Registered trademark of MERCK & CO., INC.

ACTIONS

Naturally occurring glucocorticoids (hydrocortisone and cortisone), which also have salt-retaining properties, are used as replacement therapy in adrenocortical deficiency states. Their synthetic analogs including dexamethasone are primarily used for their potent anti-inflammatory effects in disorders of many organ systems.

Glucocorticoids cause profound and varied metabolic effects. In addition, they modify the body's immune responses to diverse stimuli.

At equipotent anti-inflammatory doses, dexamethasone almost completely lacks the sodium-retaining property of hydrocortisone and closely related derivatives of hydrocortisone.

INDICATIONS

1. *Endocrine Disorders*
   Primary or secondary adrenocortical insufficiency (hydrocortisone or cortisone is the first choice; synthetic analogs may be used in conjunction with mineralocorticoids where applicable; in infancy mineralocorticoid supplementation is of particular importance)
     Congenital adrenal hyperplasia
     Nonsuppurative thyroiditis
     Hypercalcemia associated with cancer
2. *Rheumatic Disorders*
   As adjunctive therapy for short-term administration (to tide the patient over an acute episode or exacerbation) in:
     Psoriatic arthritis
     Rheumatoid arthritis, including juvenile rheumatoid arthritis (selected cases may require low-dose maintenance therapy)
     Ankylosing spondylitis
     Acute and subacute bursitis
     Acute nonspecific tenosynovitis
     Acute gouty arthritis
     Post-traumatic osteoarthritis
     Synovitis of osteoarthritis
     Epicondylitis
3. *Collagen Diseases*
   During an exacerbation or as maintenance therapy in selected cases of—
     Systemic lupus erythematosus
     Acute rheumatic carditis
4. *Dermatologic Diseases*
     Pemphigus
     Bullous dermatitis herpetiformis
     Severe erythema multiforme (Stevens-Johnson syndrome)
     Exfoliative dermatitis
     Mycosis fungoides
     Severe psoriasis
     Severe seborrheic dermatitis
5. *Allergic States*
   Control of severe or incapacitating allergic conditions intractable to adequate trials of conventional treatment:
     Seasonal or perennial allergic rhinitis
     Bronchial asthma
     Contact dermatitis
     Atopic dermatitis
     Serum sickness
     Drug hypersensitivity reactions
6. *Ophthalmic Diseases*
   Severe acute and chronic allergic and inflammatory processes involving the eye and its adnexa, such as—

Allergic conjunctivitis
Keratitis
Allergic corneal marginal ulcers
Herpes zoster ophthalmicus
Iritis and iridocyclitis
Chorioretinitis
Anterior segment inflammation
Diffuse posterior uveitis and choroiditis
Optic neuritis
Sympathetic ophthalmia
7. *Respiratory Diseases*
Symptomatic sarcoidosis
Loeffler's syndrome not manageable by other means
Berylliosis
Fulminating or disseminated pulmonary tuberculosis when used concurrently with appropriate antituberculous chemotherapy
Aspiration pneumonitis
8. *Hematologic Disorders*
Idiopathic thrombocytopenic purpura in adults
Secondary thrombocytopenia in adults
Acquired (autoimmune) hemolytic anemia
Erythroblastopenia (RBC anemia)
Congenital (erythroid) hypoplastic anemia
9. *Neoplastic Diseases*
For palliative management of:
Leukemias and lymphomas in adults
Acute leukemia of childhood
10. *Edematous States*
To induce a diuresis or remission of proteinuria in the nephrotic syndrome, without uremia, of the idiopathic type or that due to lupus erythematosus
11. *Gastrointestinal Diseases*
To tide the patient over a critical period of the disease in:
Ulcerative colitis
Regional enteritis
12. *Cerebral Edema* associated with primary or metastatic brain tumor, craniotomy, or head injury. Use in cerebral edema is not a substitute for careful neurosurgical evaluation and definitive management such as neurosurgery or other specific therapy.
13. *Miscellaneous*
Tuberculous meningitis with subarachnoid block or impending block when used concurrently with appropriate antituberculous chemotherapy
Trichinosis with neurologic or myocardial involvement
14. *Diagnostic testing of adrenocortical hyperfunction.*

CONTRAINDICATIONS

Systemic fungal infections
Hypersensitivity to this drug

WARNINGS

In patients on corticosteroid therapy subjected to unusual stress, increased dosage of rapidly acting corticosteroids before, during, and after the stressful situation is indicated.
Drug-induced secondary adrenocortical insufficiency may result from too rapid withdrawal of corticosteroids and may be minimized by gradual reduction of dosage. This type of relative insufficiency may persist for months after discontinuation of therapy; therefore, in any situation of stress occurring during that period, hormone therapy should be reinstituted. If the patient is receiving steroids already, dosage may have to be increased. Since mineralocorticoid secretion may be impaired, salt and/or a mineralocorticoid should be administered concurrently.
Corticosteroids may mask some signs of infection, and new infections may appear during their use. There may be decreased resistance and inability to localize infection when corticosteroids are used. Moreover, corticosteroids may affect the nitroblue-tetrazolium test for bacterial infection and produce false negative results.
In cerebral malaria, a double-blind trial has shown that the use of corticosteroids is associated with prolongation of coma and a higher incidence of pneumonia and gastrointestinal bleeding.
Corticosteroids may activate latent amebiasis. Therefore, it is recommended that latent or active amebiasis be ruled out before initiating corticosteroid therapy in any patient who has spent time in the tropics or any patient with unexplained diarrhea.
Prolonged use of corticosteroids may produce posterior subcapsular cataracts, glaucoma with possible damage to the optic nerves, and may enhance the establishment of secondary ocular infections due to fungi or viruses.
Usage in pregnancy: Since adequate human reproduction studies have not been done with corticosteroids, use of these drugs in pregnancy or in women of childbearing potential requires that the anticipated benefits be weighed against the possible hazards to the mother and embryo or fetus. Infants born of mothers who have received substantial doses of corticosteroids during pregnancy should be carefully observed for signs of hypoadrenalism.

Corticosteroids appear in breast milk and could suppress growth, interfere with endogenous corticosteroid production, or cause other unwanted effects. Mothers taking pharmacologic doses of corticosteroids should be advised not to nurse.
Average and large doses of hydrocortisone or cortisone can cause elevation of blood pressure, salt and water retention, and increased excretion of potassium. These effects are less likely to occur with the synthetic derivatives except when used in large doses. Dietary salt restriction and potassium supplementation may be necessary. All corticosteroids increase calcium excretion.
Administration of live virus vaccines, including smallpox, is contraindicated in individuals receiving immunosuppressive doses of corticosteroids. If inactivated viral or bacterial vaccines are administered to individuals receiving immunosuppressive doses of corticosteroid the expected serum antibody response may not be obtained. However, immunization procedures may be undertaken in patients who are receiving corticosteroids as replacement therapy, e.g., for Addison's disease.
Patients who are on drugs which suppress the immune system are more susceptible to infections than healthy individuals. Chickenpox and measles, for example, can have a more serious or even fatal course in non-immune children or adults on corticosteroids. In such children or adults who have not had these diseases, particular care should be taken to avoid exposure. The risk of developing a disseminated infection varies among individuals and can be related to the dose, route and duration of corticosteroid administration as well as to the underlying disease. If exposed to chickenpox, prophylaxis with varicella zoster immune globulin (VZIG) may be indicated. If chickenpox develops, treatment with antiviral agents may be considered. If exposed to measles, prophylaxis with immune globulin (IG) may be indicated. (See the respective package inserts for VZIG and IG for complete prescribing information.)
Similarly, corticosteroids should be used with great care in patients with known or suspected Strongyloides (threadworm) infestation. In such patients, corticosteroid-induced immunosuppression may lead to Strongyloides hyperinfection and dissemination with widespread larval migration, often accompanied by severe enterocolitis and potentially fatal gram-negative septicemia.
The use of DECADRON tablets in active tuberculosis should be restricted to those cases of fulminating or disseminated tuberculosis in which the corticosteroid is used for the management of the disease in conjunction with an appropriate antituberculous regimen.
If corticosteroids are indicated in patients with latent tuberculosis or tuberculin reactivity, close observation is necessary as reactivation of the disease may occur. During prolonged corticosteroid therapy, these patients should receive chemoprophylaxis.
Literature reports suggest an apparent association between use of corticosteroids and left ventricular free wall rupture after a recent myocardial infarction; therefore, therapy with corticosteroids should be used with great caution in these patients.

PRECAUTIONS

Following prolonged therapy, withdrawal of corticosteroids may result in symptoms of the corticosteroid withdrawal syndrome including fever, myalgia, arthralgia, and malaise. This may occur in patients even without evidence of adrenal insufficiency.
There is an enhanced effect of corticosteroids in patients with hypothyroidism and in those with cirrhosis.
Corticosteroids should be used cautiously in patients with ocular herpes simplex because of possible corneal perforation.
The lowest possible dose of corticosteroids should be used to control the condition under treatment, and when reduction in dosage is possible, the reduction should be gradual.
Psychic derangements may appear when corticosteroids are used, ranging from euphoria, insomnia, mood swings, personality changes, and severe depression, to frank psychotic manifestations. Also, existing emotional instability or psychotic tendencies may be aggravated by corticosteroids.
Aspirin should be used cautiously in conjunction with corticosteroids in hypoprothrombinemia.
Steroids should be used with caution in nonspecific ulcerative colitis, if there is a probability of impending perforation, abscess, or other pyogenic infection, diverticulitis, fresh intestinal anastomoses, active or latent peptic ulcer, renal insufficiency, hypertension, osteoporosis, and myasthenia gravis. Signs of peritoneal irritation following gastrointestinal perforation in patients receiving large doses of corticosteroids may be minimal or absent. Fat embolism has been reported as a possible complication of hypercortisonism.
When large doses are given, some authorities advise that corticosteroids be taken with meals and antacids taken between meals to help to prevent peptic ulcer.
Growth and development of infants and children on prolonged corticosteroid therapy should be carefully observed.

Steroids may increase or decrease motility and number of spermatozoa in some patients.
Phenytoin, phenobarbital, ephedrine, and rifampin may enhance the metabolic clearance of corticosteroids, resulting in decreased blood levels and lessened physiologic activity, thus requiring adjustment in corticosteroid dosage. These interactions may interfere with dexamethasone suppression tests which should be interpreted with caution during administration of these drugs.
False-negative results in the dexamethasone suppression test (DST) in patients being treated with indomethacin have been reported. Thus, results of the DST should be interpreted with caution in these patients.
The prothrombin time should be checked frequently in patients who are receiving corticosteroids and coumarin anticoagulants at the same time because of reports that corticosteroids have altered the response to these anticoagulants. Studies have shown that the usual effect produced by adding corticosteroids is inhibition of response to coumarins, although there have been some conflicting reports of potentiation not substantiated by studies.
When corticosteroids are administered concomitantly with potassium-depleting diuretics, patients should be observed closely for development of hypokalemia.
Information for Patients
Susceptible patients who are on immunosuppressant doses of corticosteroids should be warned to avoid exposure to chickenpox or measles. Patients should also be advised that if they are exposed, medical advice should be sought without delay.

ADVERSE REACTIONS

Fluid and Electrolyte Disturbances
Sodium retention
Fluid retention
Congestive heart failure in susceptible patients
Potassium loss
Hypokalemic alkalosis
Hypertension
Musculoskeletal
Muscle weakness
Steroid myopathy
Loss of muscle mass
Osteoporosis
Vertebral compression fractures
Aseptic necrosis of femoral and humeral heads
Pathologic fracture of long bones
Tendon rupture
Gastrointestinal
Peptic ulcer with possible perforation and hemorrhage
Perforation of the small and large bowel, particularly in patients with inflammatory bowel disease
Pancreatitis
Abdominal distention
Ulcerative esophagitis
Dermatologic
Impaired wound healing
Thin fragile skin
Petechiae and ecchymoses
Erythema
Increased sweating
May suppress reactions to skin tests
Other cutaneous reactions, such as allergic dermatitis, urticaria, angioneurotic edema
Neurologic
Convulsions
Increased intracranial pressure with papilledema (pseudotumor cerebri) usually after treatment
Vertigo
Headache
Psychic disturbances
Endocrine
Menstrual irregularities
Development of cushingoid state
Suppression of growth in children
Secondary adrenocortical and pituitary unresponsiveness, particularly in times of stress, as in trauma, surgery, or illness
Decreased carbohydrate tolerance
Manifestations of latent diabetes mellitus
Increased requirements for insulin or oral hypoglycemic agents in diabetics
Hirsutism
Ophthalmic
Posterior subcapsular cataracts
Increased intraocular pressure
Glaucoma
Exophthalmos

Continued on next page

Information on the Merck & Co., Inc. products listed on these pages is the full prescribing information from product circulars in use September 30, 1996.

Merck & Co.—Cont.

Metabolic
Negative nitrogen balance due to protein catabolism
Cardiovascular
Myocardial rupture following recent myocardial infarction (see WARNINGS).
Other
Hypersensitivity
Thromboembolism
Weight gain
Increased appetite
Nausea
Malaise
Hiecups

OVERDOSAGE

Reports of acute toxicity and/or death following overdosage of glucocorticoids are rare. In the event of overdosage, no specific antidote is available; treatment is supportive and symptomatic.
The oral LD_{50} of dexamethasone in female mice was 6.5 g/kg.

DOSAGE AND ADMINISTRATION

For oral administration
DOSAGE REQUIREMENTS ARE VARIABLE AND MUST BE INDIVIDUALIZED ON THE BASIS OF THE DISEASE AND THE RESPONSE OF THE PATIENT.
The initial dosage varies from 0.75 to 9 mg a day depending on the disease being treated. In less severe diseases doses lower than 0.75 mg may suffice, while in severe diseases doses higher than 9 mg may be required. The initial dosage should be maintained or adjusted until the patient's response is satisfactory. If satisfactory clinical response does not occur after a reasonable period of time, discontinue DECADRON tablets and transfer the patient to other therapy.
After a favorable initial response, the proper maintenance dosage should be determined by decreasing the initial dosage in small amounts to the lowest dosage that maintains an adequate clinical response.
Patients should be observed closely for signs that might require dosage adjustment, including changes in clinical status resulting from remissions or exacerbations of the disease, individual drug responsiveness, and the effect of stress (e.g., surgery, infection, trauma). During stress it may be necessary to increase dosage temporarily.
If the drug is to be stopped after more than a few days of treatment, it usually should be withdrawn gradually.
The following milligram equivalents facilitate changing to DECADRON from other glucocorticoids:

DECADRON	Methylprednisolone and Triamcinolone	Prednisolone and Prednisone Hydrocortisone		Cortisone
0.75 mg =	4 mg =	5 mg =	20 mg =	25 mg

In *acute, self-limited allergic disorders or acute exacerbations of chronic allergic disorders,* the following dosage schedule combining parenteral and oral therapy is suggested:
DECADRON* Phosphate (Dexamethasone Sodium Phosphate) injection, 4 mg per mL:
First Day
1 or 2 mL, intramuscularly
DECADRON tablets, 0.75 mg:
Second Day
4 tablets in two divided doses
Third Day
4 tablets in two divided doses
Fourth Day
2 tablets in two divided doses
Fifth Day
1 tablet
Sixth Day
1 tablet
Seventh Day
No treatment
Eighth Day
Follow-up visit
This schedule is designed to ensure adequate therapy during acute episodes, while minimizing the risk of overdosage in chronic cases.

In *cerebral edema,* DECADRON Phosphate (Dexamethasone Sodium Phosphate) injection is generally administered initially in a dosage of 10 mg intravenously followed by 4 mg every six hours intramuscularly until the symptoms of cerebral edema subside. Response is usually noted within 12 to 24 hours and dosage may be reduced after two to four days and gradually discontinued over a period of five to seven days. For palliative management of patients with recurrent or inoperable brain tumors, maintenance therapy with either DECADRON Phosphate (Dexamethasone Sodium Phosphate) injection or DECADRON tablets in a dosage of two mg two or three times daily may be effective.
Dexamethasone suppression tests
1. Tests for Cushing's syndrome
    Give 1.0 mg of DECADRON orally at 11:00 p.m. Blood is drawn for plasma cortisol determination at 8:00 a.m. the following morning.
    For greater accuracy, give 0.5 mg of DECADRON orally every 6 hours for 48 hours. Twenty-four hour urine collections are made for determination of 17-hydroxycorticosteroid excretion.
2. Test to distinguish Cushing's syndrome due to pituitary ACTH excess from Cushing's syndrome due to other causes
    Give 2.0 mg of DECADRON orally every 6 hours for 48 hours. Twenty-four hour urine collections are made for determination of 17-hydroxycorticosteroid excretion.

*Registered trademark of MERCK & CO., INC.

HOW SUPPLIED

Tablets DECADRON are compressed, pentagonal-shaped tablets, colored to distinguish potency. They are scored and coded on one side and embossed with DECADRON on the other. They are available as follows:
No. 7648—6 mg, green in color and coded MSD 147.
NDC 0006-0147-50 bottles of 50.
    Shown in Product Identification Guide, page 324
No. 7645—4 mg, white in color and coded MSD 97.
NDC 0006-0097-50 bottles of 50
    Shown in Product Identification Guide, page 324
No. 7638—1.5 mg, pink in color and coded MSD 95.
NDC 0006-0095-50 bottles of 50.
    Shown in Product Identification Guide, page 324
No. 7601—0.75 mg, bluish-green in color and coded MSD 63.
NDC 0006-0063-12 5-12 PAK* (package of 12)
NDC 0006-0063-68 bottles of 100.
    Shown in Product Identification Guide, page 324
No. 7598—0.5 mg, yellow in color and coded MSD 41.
NDC 0006-0041-68 bottles of 100.
    Shown in Product Identification Guide, page 324
No. 7592—0.25 mg, orange in color and coded MSD 20.
NDC 0006-0020-68 bottles of 100.
    Shown in Product Identification Guide, page 324

*Registered trademark of MERCK & CO., INC.
7921147   Issued October 1995

DECADRON® Phosphate Injection (Dexamethasone Sodium Phosphate), U.S.P.   ℞

DESCRIPTION

Dexamethasone sodium phosphate, a synthetic adrenocortical steroid, is a white or slightly yellow, crystalline powder. It is freely soluble in water and is exceedingly hygroscopic. The molecular weight is 516.41. It is designated chemically as 9-fluoro-11β, 17-dihydroxy-16α-methyl-21-(phosphonooxy)pregna-1, 4-diene-3, 20-dione disodium salt. The empirical formula is $C_{22}H_{28}FNa_2O_8P$ and the structural formula is:

DECADRON* Phosphate (Dexamethasone Sodium Phosphate) injection is a sterile solution (pH 7.0 to 8.5) of dexamethasone sodium phosphate, sealed under nitrogen, and is supplied in two concentrations: 4 mg/mL and 24 mg/mL. The 24 mg/mL concentration offers the advantage of less volume in indications where high doses of corticosteroids by the intravenous route are needed.
Each milliliter of DECADRON Phosphate injection, 4 mg/mL, contains dexamethasone sodium phosphate equivalent to 4 mg dexamethasone phosphate or 3.33 mg dexamethasone. Inactive ingredients per mL: 8 mg creatinine, 10 mg sodium citrate, sodium hydroxide to adjust pH, and Water

for Injection q.s., with 1 mg sodium bisulfite, 1.5 mg methylparaben, and 0.2 mg propylparaben added as preservatives. Each milliliter of DECADRON Phosphate injection, 24 mg/mL, contains dexamethasone sodium phosphate equivalent to 24 mg dexamethasone phosphate or 20 mg dexamethasone. Inactive ingredients per mL: 8 mg creatinine, 10 mg sodium citrate, 0.5 mg disodium edetate, sodium hydroxide to adjust pH, and Water for Injection q.s., with 1 mg sodium bisulfite, 1.5 mg methylparaben, and 0.2 mg propylparaben added as preservatives.

*Registered trademark of MERCK & CO., INC.

ACTIONS

DECADRON Phosphate injection has a rapid onset but short duration of action when compared with less soluble preparations. Because of this, it is suitable for the treatment of acute disorders responsive to adrenocortical steroid therapy.
Naturally occurring glucocorticoids (hydrocortisone and cortisone), which also have salt-retaining properties, are used as replacement therapy in adrenocortical deficiency states. Their synthetic analogs, including dexamethasone, are primarily used for their potent anti-inflammatory effects in disorders of many organ systems.
Glucocorticoids cause profound and varied metabolic effects. In addition, they modify the body's immune responses to diverse stimuli.
At equipotent anti-inflammatory doses, dexamethasone almost completely lacks the sodium-retaining property of hydrocortisone and closely related derivatives of hydrocortisone.

INDICATIONS

A. By intravenous or intramuscular injection when oral therapy is not feasible:
1. *Endocrine disorders*
Primary or secondary adrenocortical insufficiency (hydrocortisone or cortisone is the drug of choice; synthetic analogs may be used in conjunction with mineralocorticoids where applicable; in infancy, mineralocorticoid supplementation is of particular importance)
Acute adrenocortical insufficiency (hydrocortisone or cortisone is the drug of choice; mineralocorticoid supplementation may be necessary, particularly when synthetic analogs are used)
Preoperatively, and in the event of serious trauma or illness, in patients with known adrenal insufficiency or when adrenocortical reserve is doubtful
Shock unresponsive to conventional therapy if adrenocortical insufficiency exists or is suspected
Congenital adrenal hyperplasia
Nonsuppurative thyroiditis
Hypercalcemia associated with cancer
2. *Rheumatic disorders*
As adjunctive therapy for short-term administration (to tide the patient over an acute episode or exacerbation) in:
Post-traumatic osteoarthritis
Synovitis of osteoarthritis
Rheumatoid arthritis, including juvenile rheumatoid arthritis (selected cases may require low-dose maintenance therapy)
Acute and subacute bursitis
Epicondylitis
Acute nonspecific tenosynovitis
Acute gouty arthritis
Psoriatic arthritis
Ankylosing spondylitis
3. *Collagen diseases*
During an exacerbation or as maintenance therapy in selected cases of:
Systemic lupus erythematosus
Acute rheumatic carditis
4. *Dermatologic diseases*
Pemphigus
Severe erythema multiforme (Stevens-Johnson syndrome)
Exfoliative dermatitis
Bullous dermatitis herpetiformis
Severe seborrheic dermatitis
Severe psoriasis
Mycosis fungoides
5. *Allergic states*
Control of severe or incapacitating allergic conditions intractable to adequate trials of conventional treatment in:
Bronchial asthma
Contact dermatitis
Atopic dermatitis
Serum sickness
Seasonal or perennial allergic rhinitis
Drug hypersensitivity reactions
Urticarial transfusion reactions
Acute noninfectious laryngeal edema (epinephrine is the drug of first choice)

6. *Ophthalmic diseases*
Severe acute and chronic allergic and inflammatory processes involving the eye, such as:
Herpes zoster ophthalmicus
Iritis, iridocyclitis
Chorioretinitis
Diffuse posterior uveitis and choroiditis
Optic neuritis
Sympathetic ophthalmia
Anterior segment inflammation
Allergic conjunctivitis
Keratitis
Allergic corneal marginal ulcers
7. *Gastrointestinal diseases*
To tide the patient over a critical period of the disease in:
Ulcerative colitis (Systemic therapy)
Regional enteritis (Systemic therapy)
8. *Respiratory diseases*
Symptomatic sarcoidosis
Berylliosis
Fulminating or disseminated pulmonary tuberculosis when used concurrently with appropriate antituberculous chemotherapy
Loeffler's syndrome not manageable by other means
Aspiration pneumonitis
9. *Hematologic disorders*
Acquired (autoimmune) hemolytic anemia
Idiopathic thrombocytopenic purpura in adults (I.V. only; I.M. administration is contraindicated)
Secondary thrombocytopenia in adults
Erythroblastopenia (RBC anemia)
Congenital (erythroid) hypoplastic anemia
10. *Neoplastic diseases*
For palliative management of:
Leukemias and lymphomas in adults
Acute leukemia of childhood
11. *Edematous states*
To induce diuresis or remission of proteinuria in the nephrotic syndrome, without uremia, of the idiopathic type, or that due to lupus erythematosus
12. *Miscellaneous*
Tuberculous meningitis with subarachnoid block or impending block when used concurrently with appropriate antituberculous chemotherapy
Trichinosis with neurologic or myocardial involvement
13. *Diagnostic testing of adrenocortical hyperfunction*
14. *Cerebral Edema* associated with primary or metastatic brain tumor, craniotomy, or head injury. Use in cerebral edema is not a substitute for careful neurosurgical evaluation and definitive management such as neurosurgery or other specific therapy.
B. By intra-articular or soft tissue injection:
As adjunctive therapy for short-term administration (to tide the patient over an acute episode or exacerbation) in:
Synovitis of osteoarthritis
Rheumatoid arthritis
Acute and subacute bursitis
Acute gouty arthritis
Epicondylitis
Acute nonspecific tenosynovitis
Post-traumatic osteoarthritis.
C. By intralesional injection:
Keloids
Localized hypertrophic, infiltrated, inflammatory lesions of: lichen planus, psoriatic plaques, granuloma annulare, and lichen simplex chronicus (neurodermatitis)
Discoid lupus erythematosus
Necrobiosis lipoidica diabeticorum
Alopecia areata
May also be useful in cystic tumors of an aponeurosis or tendon (ganglia).

CONTRAINDICATIONS

Systemic fungal infections. (See WARNINGS regarding amphotericin B)
Hypersensitivity to any component of this product, including sulfites (see WARNINGS).

WARNINGS

Because rare instances of anaphylactoid reactions have occurred in patients receiving parenteral corticosteroid therapy, appropriate precautionary measures should be taken prior to administration, especially when the patient has a history of allergy to any drug. Anaphylactoid and hypersensitivity reactions have been reported for Injection DECADRON Phosphate (see ADVERSE REACTIONS).
Injection DECADRON Phosphate contains sodium bisulfite, a sulfite that may cause allergic-type reactions including anaphylactic symptoms and life-threatening or less severe asthmatic episodes in certain susceptible people. The overall prevalence of sulfite sensitivity in the general population is unknown and probably low. Sulfite sensitivity is seen more frequently in asthmatic than in nonasthmatic people.
Corticosteroids may exacerbate systemic fungal infections and therefore should not be used in the presence of such infections unless they are needed to control drug reactions due to amphotericin B. Moreover, there have been cases reported in which concomitant use of amphotericin B and hydrocortisone was followed by cardiac enlargement and congestive failure.
In patients on corticosteroid therapy subjected to any unusual stress, increased dosage of rapidly acting corticosteroids before, during, and after the stressful situation is indicated.
Drug-induced secondary adrenocortical insufficiency may result from too rapid withdrawal of corticosteroids and may be minimized by gradual reduction of dosage. This type of relative insufficiency may persist for months after discontinuation of therapy; therefore, in any situation of stress occurring during that period, hormone therapy should be reinstituted. If the patient is receiving steroids already, dosage may have to be increased. Since mineralocorticoid secretion may be impaired, salt and/or a mineralocorticoid should be administered concurrently.
Corticosteroids may mask some signs of infection, and new infections may appear during their use. There may be decreased resistance and inability to localize infection when corticosteroids are used. Moreover, corticosteroids may affect the nitroblue-tetrazolium test for bacterial infection and produce false negative results.
In cerebral malaria, a double-blind trial has shown that the use of corticosteroids is associated with prolongation of coma and a higher incidence of pneumonia and gastrointestinal bleeding.
Corticosteroids may activate latent amebiasis. Therefore, it is recommended that latent or active amebiasis be ruled out before initiating corticosteroid therapy in any patient who has spent time in the tropics or any patient with unexplained diarrhea.
Prolonged use of corticosteroids may produce posterior subcapsular cataracts, glaucoma with possible damage to the optic nerves, and may enhance the establishment of secondary ocular infections due to fungi or viruses.
Usage in pregnancy. Since adequate human reproduction studies have not been done with corticosteroids, use of these drugs in pregnancy or in women of childbearing potential requires that the anticipated benefits be weighed against the possible hazards to the mother and embryo or fetus. Infants born of mothers who have received substantial doses of corticosteroids during pregnancy should be carefully observed for signs of hypoadrenalism.
Corticosteroids appear in breast milk and could suppress growth, interfere with endogenous corticosteroid production, or cause other unwanted effects. Mothers taking pharmacologic doses of corticosteroids should be advised not to nurse.
Average and large doses of cortisone or hydrocortisone can cause elevation of blood pressure, salt and water retention, and increased excretion of potassium. These effects are less likely to occur with the synthetic derivatives except when used in large doses. Dietary salt restriction and potassium supplementation may be necessary. All corticosteroids increase calcium excretion.
Administration of live virus vaccines, including smallpox, is contraindicated in individuals receiving immunosuppressive doses of corticosteroids. If inactivated viral or bacterial vaccines are administered to individuals receiving immunosuppressive doses of corticosteroids, the expected serum antibody response may not be obtained. However, immunization procedures may be undertaken in patients who are receiving corticosteroids as replacement therapy, e.g., for Addison's disease.
Patients who are on drugs which suppress the immune system are more susceptible to infections than healthy individuals. Chickenpox and measles, for example, can have a more serious or even fatal course in non-immune children or adults on corticosteroids. In such children or adults who have not had these diseases, particular care should be taken to avoid exposure. The risk of developing a disseminated infection varies among individuals and can be related to the dose, route and duration of corticosteroid administration as well as to the underlying disease. If exposed to chickenpox, prophylaxis with varicella zoster immune globulin (VZIG) may be indicated. If chickenpox develops, treatment with antiviral agents may be considered. If exposed to measles, prophylaxis with immune globulin (IG) may be indicated. (See the respective package inserts for VZIG and IG for complete prescribing information.)
Similarly, corticosteroids should be used with great care in patients with known or suspected Strongyloides (threadworm) infestation. In such patients, corticosteroid-induced immunosuppression may lead to Strongyloides hyperinfection and dissemination with widespread larval migration, often accompanied by severe enterocolitis and potentially fatal gram-negative septicemia.
The use of DECADRON Phosphate injection in active tuberculosis should be restricted to those cases of fulminating or disseminated tuberculosis in which the corticosteroid is used for the management of the disease in conjunction with an appropriate antituberculous regimen.
If corticosteroids are indicated in patients with latent tuberculosis or tuberculin reactivity, close observation is necessary as reactivation of the disease may occur. During prolonged corticosteroid therapy, these patients should receive chemoprophylaxis.
Literature reports suggest an apparent association between use of corticosteroids and left ventricular free wall rupture after a recent myocardial infarction; therefore, therapy with corticosteroids should be used with great caution in these patients.

PRECAUTIONS

This product, like many other steroid formulations, is sensitive to heat. Therefore, it should not be autoclaved when it is desirable to sterilize the exterior of the vial.
Following prolonged therapy, withdrawal of corticosteroids may result in symptoms of the corticosteroid withdrawal syndrome including fever, myalgia, arthralgia, and malaise. This may occur in patients even without evidence of adrenal insufficiency.
There is an enhanced effect of corticosteroids in patients with hypothyroidism and in those with cirrhosis.
Corticosteroids should be used cautiously in patients with ocular herpes simplex for fear of corneal perforation.
The lowest possible dose of corticosteroid should be used to control the condition under treatment, and when reduction in dosage is possible, the reduction must be gradual.
Psychic derangements may appear when corticosteroids are used, ranging from euphoria, insomnia, mood swings, personality changes, and severe depression to frank psychotic manifestations. Also, existing emotional instability or psychotic tendencies may be aggravated by corticosteroids.
Aspirin should be used cautiously in conjunction with corticosteroids in hypoprothrombinemia.
Steroids should be used with caution in nonspecific ulcerative colitis, if there is a probability of impending perforation, abscess, or other pyogenic infection, also in diverticulitis, fresh intestinal anastomoses, active or latent peptic ulcer, renal insufficiency, hypertension, osteoporosis, and myasthenia gravis. Signs of peritoneal irritation following gastrointestinal perforation in patients receiving large doses of corticosteroids may be minimal or absent. Fat embolism has been reported as a possible complication of hypercortisonism.
When large doses are given, some authorities advise that antacids be administered between meals to help to prevent peptic ulcer.
Growth and development of infants and children on prolonged corticosteroid therapy should be carefully followed.
Steroids may increase or decrease motility and number of spermatozoa in some patients.
Phenytoin, phenobarbital, ephedrine, and rifampin may enhance the metabolic clearance of corticosteroids resulting in decreased blood levels and lessened physiologic activity, thus requiring adjustment in corticosteroid dosage. These interactions may interfere with dexamethasone suppression tests which should be interpreted with caution during administration of these drugs.
False negative results in the dexamethasone suppression test (DST) in patients being treated with indomethacin have been reported. Thus, results of the DST should be interpreted with caution in these patients.
The prothrombin time should be checked frequently in patients who are receiving corticosteroids and coumarin anticoagulants at the same time because of reports that corticosteroids have altered the response to these anticoagulants. Studies have shown that the usual effect produced by adding corticosteroids is inhibition of response to coumarins, although there have been some conflicting reports of potentiation not substantiated by studies.
When corticosteroids are administered concomitantly with potassium-depleting diuretics, patients should be observed closely for development of hypokalemia.
Intra-articular injection of a corticosteroid may produce systemic as well as local effects.
Appropriate examination of any joint fluid present is necessary to exclude a septic process.
A marked increase in pain accompanied by local swelling, further restriction of joint motion, fever, and malaise is suggestive of septic arthritis. If this complication occurs and the diagnosis of sepsis is confirmed, appropriate antimicrobial therapy should be instituted.
Injection of a steroid into an infected site is to be avoided.
Corticosteroids should not be injected into unstable joints.
Patients should be impressed strongly with the importance of not overusing joints in which symptomatic benefit has

Continued on next page

Information on the Merck & Co., Inc. products listed on these pages is the full prescribing information from product circulars in use September 30, 1996.

Merck & Co.—Cont.

been obtained as long as the inflammatory process remains active.

Frequent intra-articular injection may result in damage to joint tissues.

The slower rate of absorption by intramuscular administration should be recognized.

Information for Patients

Susceptible patients who are on immunosuppressant doses of corticosteroids should be warned to avoid exposure to chickenpox or measles. Patients should also be advised that if they are exposed, medical advice should be sought without delay.

ADVERSE REACTIONS

Fluid and electrolyte disturbances
Sodium retention
Fluid retention
Congestive heart failure in susceptible patients
Potassium loss
Hypokalemic alkalosis
Hypertension
Musculoskeletal
Muscle weakness
Steroid myopathy
Loss of muscle mass
Osteoporosis
Vertebral compression fractures
Aseptic necrosis of femoral and humeral heads
Pathologic fracture of long bones
Tendon rupture
Gastrointestinal
Peptic ulcer with possible subsequent perforation and hemorrhage
Perforation of the small and large bowel, particularly in patients with inflammatory bowel disease
Pancreatitis
Abdominal distention
Ulcerative esophagitis
Dermatologic
Impaired wound healing
Thin fragile skin
Petechiae and ecchymoses
Erythema
Increased sweating
May suppress reactions to skin tests
Burning or tingling, especially in the perineal area (after I.V. injection)
Other cutaneous reactions, such as allergic dermatitis, urticaria, angioneurotic edema
Neurologic
Convulsions
Increased intracranial pressure with papilledema (pseudotumor cerebri) usually after treatment
Vertigo
Headache
Psychic disturbances
Endocrine
Menstrual irregularities
Development of cushingoid state
Suppression of growth in children
Secondary adrenocortical and pituitary unresponsiveness, particularly in times of stress, as in trauma, surgery, or illness
Decreased carbohydrate tolerance
Manifestations of latent diabetes mellitus
Increased requirements for insulin or oral hypoglycemic agents in diabetics
Hirsutism
Ophthalmic
Posterior subcapsular cataracts
Increased intraocular pressure
Glaucoma
Exophthalmos
Metabolic
Negative nitrogen balance due to protein catabolism
Cardiovascular
Myocardial rupture following recent myocardial infarction (see WARNINGS).
Other
Anaphylactoid or hypersensitivity reactions
Thromboembolism
Weight gain
Increased appetite
Nausea
Malaise
Hiccups
The following *additional* adverse reactions are related to parenteral corticosteroid therapy:
Rare instances of blindness associated with intralesional therapy around the face and head

Hyperpigmentation or hypopigmentation
Subcutaneous and cutaneous atrophy
Sterile abscess
Postinjection flare (following intra-articular use)
Charcot-like arthropathy

OVERDOSAGE

Reports of acute toxicity and/or death following overdosage of glucocorticoids are rare. In the event of overdosage, no specific antidote is available; treatment is supportive and symptomatic.

Significant lethality was observed in female mice at single oral doses of 3630 mg/m^2 (1210 mg/kg) and single intravenous doses of 2382 mg/m^2 (794 mg/kg).

DOSAGE AND ADMINISTRATION

DECADRON Phosphate injection, 4 mg/mL—*For intravenous, intramuscular, intra-articular, intralesional, and soft tissue injection.*

DECADRON Phosphate injection, 24 mg/mL—*For intravenous injection only.*

DECADRON Phosphate injection can be given directly from the vial, or it can be added to Sodium Chloride Injection or Dextrose Injection and administered by intravenous drip. Solutions used for intravenous administration or further dilution of this product should be preservative-free when used in the neonate, especially the premature infant.

When it is mixed with an infusion solution, sterile precautions should be observed. Since infusion solutions generally do not contain preservatives, mixtures should be used within 24 hours.

DOSAGE REQUIREMENTS ARE VARIABLE AND MUST BE INDIVIDUALIZED ON THE BASIS OF THE DISEASE AND THE RESPONSE OF THE PATIENT.

Intravenous and Intramuscular Injection

The initial dosage of DECADRON Phosphate injection varies from 0.5 to 9 mg a day depending on the disease being treated. In less severe diseases doses lower than 0.5 mg may suffice, while in severe diseases doses higher than 9 mg may be required.

The initial dosage should be maintained or adjusted until the patient's response is satisfactory. If a satisfactory clinical response does not occur after a reasonable period of time, discontinue DECADRON Phosphate injection and transfer the patient to other therapy.

After a favorable initial response, the proper maintenance dosage should be determined by decreasing the initial dosage in small amounts to the lowest dosage that maintains an adequate clinical response.

Patients should be observed closely for signs that might require dosage adjustment, including changes in clinical status resulting from remissions or exacerbations of the disease, individual drug responsiveness, and the effect of stress (e.g., surgery, infection, trauma). During stress it may be necessary to increase dosage temporarily.

If the drug is to be stopped after more than a few days of treatment, it usually should be withdrawn gradually.

When the intravenous route of administration is used, dosage usually should be the same as the oral dosage. In certain overwhelming, acute, life-threatening situations, however, administration in dosages exceeding the usual dosages may be justified and may be in multiples of the oral dosages. The slower rate of absorption by intramuscular administration should be recognized.

Shock

There is a tendency in current medical practice to use high (pharmacologic) doses of corticosteroids for the treatment of unresponsive shock. The following dosages of DECADRON phosphate injection have been suggested by various authors:

Author[*]	*Dosage*
Cavanagh[1]	3 mg/kg of body weight per 24 hours by constant intravenous infusion after an initial intravenous injection of 20 mg
Dietzman[2]	2 to 6 mg/kg of body weight as a single intravenous injection
Frank[3]	40 mg initially followed by repeat intravenous injection every 4 to 6 hours while shock persists
Oaks[4]	40 mg initially followed by repeat intravenous injection every 2 to 6 hours while shock persists
Schumer[5]	1 mg/kg of body weight as a single intravenous injection

Administration of high dose corticosteroid therapy should be continued only until the patient's condition has stabilized and usually not longer than 48 to 72 hours.

Although adverse reactions associated with high dose, short term corticosteroid therapy are uncommon, peptic ulceration may occur.

[*]1. Cavanagh, D.; Singh, K. B.: Endotoxin shock in pregnancy and abortion, in "Corticosteroids in the Treatment of Shock", Schumer, W.; Nyhus, L. M., Editors, Urbana, University of Illinois Press, 1970, pp. 86-96.
2. Dietzman, R. H.; Ersek, R. A.; Bloch, J. M.; Lillehei, R. C.: High-output, low-resistance gram-negative septic shock in man, Angiology 20: 691-700, Dec. 1969.
3. Frank, E.: Clinical observations in shock and management (In: Shields, T. F., ed.: Symposium on current concepts and management of shock), J. Maine Med. Ass. 59: 195-200, Oct. 1968.
4. Oaks, W. W.; Cohen, H. E.: Endotoxin shock in the geriatric patient, Geriat. 22: 120-130, Mar. 1967.
5. Schumer, W.; Nyhus, L. M.: Corticosteroid effect on biochemical parameters of human oligemic shock, Arch. Surg. 100: 405-408, Apr. 1970.

Cerebral Edema

DECADRON Phosphate injection is generally administered initially in a dosage of 10 mg intravenously followed by 4 mg every six hours intramuscularly until the symptoms of cerebral edema subside. Response is usually noted within 12 to 24 hours and dosage may be reduced after two to four days and gradually discontinued over a period of five to seven days. For palliative management of patients with recurrent or inoperable brain tumors, maintenance therapy with two mg two or three times a day may be effective.

Acute Allergic Disorders

In acute, self-limited allergic disorders or acute exacerbations of chronic allergic disorders, the following dosage schedule combining parenteral and oral therapy is suggested:

DECADRON Phosphate injection, 4 mg/mL: *first day,* 1 or 2 mL (4 or 8 mg), intramuscularly.

DECADRON* (Dexamethasone) tablets, 0.75 mg: *second and third days,* 4 tablets in two divided doses each day; *fourth day,* 2 tablets in two divided doses; *fifth and sixth days,* 1 tablet each day; *seventh day,* no treatment; *eighth day,* follow-up visit.

This schedule is designed to ensure adequate therapy during acute episodes, while minimizing the risk of overdosage in chronic cases.

*Registered trademark of MERCK & CO., INC.

Intra-articular, Intralesional, and Soft Tissue Injection

Intra-articular, intralesional, and soft tissue injections are generally employed when the affected joints or areas are limited to one or two sites. Dosage and frequency of injection varies depending on the condition and the site of injection. The usual dose is from 0.2 to 6 mg. The frequency usually ranges from once every three to five days to once every two to three weeks. Frequent intra-articular injection may result in damage to joint tissues.

Some of the usual single doses are:

Site of Injection	Amount of Dexamethasone Phosphate (mg)
Large Joints (e.g., Knee)	2 to 4
Small Joints (e.g., Interphalangeal, Temporomandibular)	0.8 to 1
Bursae	2 to 3
Tendon Sheaths	0.4 to 1
Soft Tissue Infiltration	2 to 6
Ganglia	1 to 2

DECADRON Phosphate injection is particularly recommended for use in conjunction with one of the less soluble, longer-acting steroids for intra-articular and soft tissue injection.

HOW SUPPLIED

No 7628X—Injection DECADRON Phosphate, 4 mg per mL, is a clear, colorless solution, and is available in 1 mL, 5 mL, and 25 mL vials as follows:
NDC 0006-7628-66, boxes of 25 × 1 mL vials
NDC 0006-7628-03, 5 mL vial
(6505-00-963-5355, 5 mL vial)
NDC 0006-7628-25, 25 mL vial.
FOR INTRAVENOUS USE ONLY:
No. 7646—Injection DECADRON Phosphate, 24 mg per mL, is a clear, colorless to light yellow solution and is available in 5 mL and 10 mL vials as follows:

NDC 0006-7646-03, 5 mL vial
NDC 0006-7646-10, 10 mL vial.
Storage
Sensitive to heat. Do not autoclave.
Protect from freezing.
Protect from light. Store container in carton until contents have been used.
7347229 Issued October 1995

DECADRON® Phosphate with XYLOCAINE® ℞
Injection, Sterile
(Dexamethasone Sodium Phosphate-Lidocaine Hydrochloride)

For local injection only

NOT FOR INTRAVENOUS USE

DESCRIPTION

Dexamethasone sodium phosphate is a white or slightly yellow, crystalline powder. It is freely soluble in water and is exceedingly hygroscopic. The molecular weight is 516.41. It is designated chemically as 9-fluoro-11β,17-dihydroxy-16α-methyl-21-(phosphonooxy)pregna-1,4-diene-3,20-dione disodium salt. The empirical formula is $C_{22}H_{28}FNa_2O_8P$ and the structural formula is:

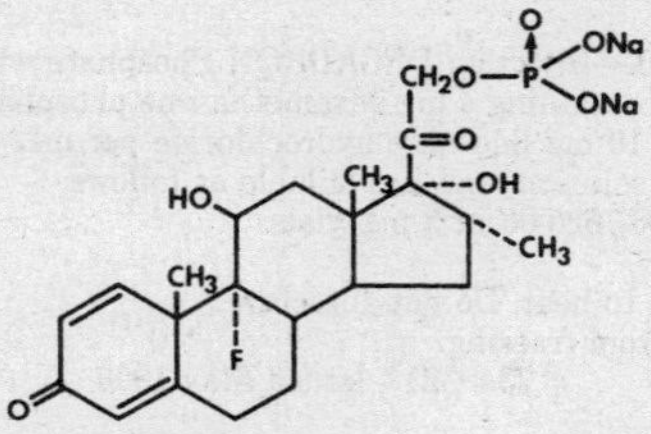

Lidocaine hydrochloride is a white, crystalline powder that is very soluble in water and alcohol, soluble in chloroform, and insoluble in ether. The molecular weight is 288.82. It is designated chemically as 2-(diethylamino)-*N*-(2,6- dimethylphenyl)acetamide, monohydrochloride, monohydrate. The empirical formula is $C_{14}H_{22}N_2O \cdot HCl \cdot H_2O$ and the structural formula is:

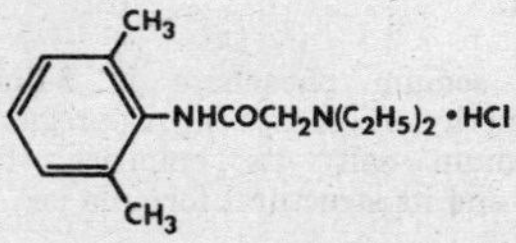

DECADRON* Phosphate with XYLOCAINE** (Dexamethasone Sodium Phosphate-Lidocaine Hydrochloride) injection is provided as a sterile solution (pH 6.5 to 6.9), sealed under nitrogen, for the convenience of physicians who prefer to treat patients with simultaneous administration of a corticosteroid and a local anesthetic.
Each milliliter contains dexamethasone sodium phosphate equivalent to dexamethasone phosphate, 4 mg; and lidocaine hydrochloride, 10 mg. Inactive ingredients per mL: citric acid anhydrous, 10 mg; creatinine, 8 mg; sodium bisulfite, 0.5 mg; disodium edetate, 0.5 mg; sodium hydroxide to adjust pH; and Water for Injection, q.s., 1 mL.
Methylparaben, 1.5 mg, and propylparaben, 0.2 mg, added as preservatives.

*Registered trademark of MERCK & CO., INC.
**Registered trademark of Astra Pharmaceutical Products, Inc.

ACTIONS

DECADRON Phosphate (Dexamethasone Sodium Phosphate) is a synthetic glucocorticoid used primarily for its potent anti-inflammatory effects in disorders of many organ systems. Glucocorticoids cause profound and varied metabolic effects. In addition, they modify the body's immune responses to diverse stimuli.
XYLOCAINE (Lidocaine Hydrochloride) is a local anesthetic with a rapid onset and moderate duration of action.
Local anesthesia appears within a few minutes after injection of DECADRON Phosphate with XYLOCAINE and lasts 45 minutes to one hour. By the time the anesthesia wears off, steroid activity usually has begun. If the anesthesia wears off before full steroid effect appears, there may be some discomfort beginning about an hour after injection and relief of pain may be delayed for a short time.

INDICATIONS

Acute and subacute bursitis
Acute and subacute nonspecific tenosynovitis

CONTRAINDICATIONS

Hypersensitivity to any component of this product, including sulfites (see WARNINGS).
Dexamethasone Sodium Phosphate
Systemic fungal infections
Lidocaine Hydrochloride
Patients with known history of hypersensitivity to local anesthetics of the amide type (e.g., mepivacaine, prilocaine)
Severe shock
Heart block

WARNINGS

Because rare instances of anaphylactoid reactions have occurred in patients receiving parenteral corticosteroid therapy, appropriate precautionary measures should be taken prior to administration, especially when the patient has a history of allergy to any drug. Anaphylactoid and hypersensitivity reactions have been reported for Injection DECADRON Phosphate with XYLOCAINE (see ADVERSE REACTIONS).
Injection DECADRON Phosphate with XYLOCAINE contains sodium bisulfite, a sulfite that may cause allergic-type reactions including anaphylactic symptoms and life-threatening or less severe asthmatic episodes in certain susceptible people. The overall prevalence of sulfite sensitivity in the general population is unknown and probably low. Sulfite sensitivity is seen more frequently in asthmatic than in nonasthmatic people.
Lidocaine Hydrochloride
RESUSCITATIVE EQUIPMENT AND DRUGS SHOULD BE IMMEDIATELY AVAILABLE WHEN ANY LOCAL ANESTHETIC IS USED.
Usage in pregnancy: The safe use of lidocaine hydrochloride has not been established with respect to adverse effects upon fetal development. Careful consideration should be given to this fact before administering this drug to women of childbearing potential, particularly during early pregnancy.
Dexamethasone Sodium Phosphate
In patients on corticosteroid therapy subjected to unusual stress, increased dosage of rapidly acting corticosteroids before, during, and after the stressful situation is indicated.
Drug-induced secondary adrenocortical insufficiency may result from too rapid withdrawal of corticosteroids and may be minimized by gradual reduction of dosage. This type of relative insufficiency may persist for months after discontinuation of therapy: therefore, in any situation of stress occurring during that period, hormone therapy should be reinstituted. If the patient is receiving steroids already, dosage may have to be increased. Since mineralocorticoid secretion may be impaired, salt and/or a mineralocorticoid should be administered concurrently.
Corticosteroids may mask some signs of infection, and new infections may appear during their use. There may be decreased resistance and inability to localize infection when corticosteroids are used. Moreover, corticosteroids may affect the nitroblue-tetrazolium test for bacterial infection and produce false negative results.
Corticosteroids may activate latent amebiasis. Therefore, it is recommended that latent or active amebiasis be ruled out before initiating corticosteroid therapy in any patient who has spent time in the tropics or any patient with unexplained diarrhea.
Prolonged use of corticosteroids may produce posterior subcapsular cataracts, glaucoma with possible damage to the optic nerves, and may enhance the establishment of secondary ocular infections due to fungi or viruses.
Usage in pregnancy: Since adequate human reproduction studies have not been done with corticosteroids, use of these drugs in pregnancy or in women of childbearing potential requires that the anticipated benefits be weighed against the possible hazards to the mother and embryo or fetus. Infants born of mothers who have received substantial doses of corticosteroids during pregnancy should be carefully observed for signs of hypoadrenalism.
Corticosteroids appear in breast milk and could suppress growth, interfere with endogenous corticosteroid production, or cause other unwanted effects. Mothers taking pharmacologic doses of corticosteroids should be advised not to nurse.
Average and large doses of cortisone or hydrocortisone can cause elevation of blood pressure, salt and water retention, and increased excretion of potassium. These effects are less likely to occur with the synthetic derivatives except when used in large doses. Dietary salt restriction and potassium supplementation may be necessary. All corticosteroids increase calcium excretion.
Administration of live virus vaccines, including smallpox, is contraindicated in individuals receiving immunosuppressive doses of corticosteroids. If inactivated viral or bacterial vaccines are administered to individuals receiving immunosuppressive doses of corticosteroids, the expected serum antibody response may not be obtained.
Patients who are on drugs which suppress the immune system are more susceptible to infections than healthy individuals. Chickenpox and measles, for example, can have a more serious or even fatal course in non-immune children or adults on corticosteroids. In such children or adults who have not had these diseases, particular care should be taken to avoid exposure. The risk of developing a disseminated infection varies among individuals and can be related to the dose, route and duration of corticosteroid administration as well as to the underlying disease. If exposed to chickenpox, prophylaxis with varicella zoster immune globulin (VZIG) may be indicated. If chickenpox develops, treatment with antiviral agents may be considered. If exposed to measles, prophylaxis with immune globulin (IG) may be indicated. (See the respective package inserts for VZIG and IG for complete prescribing information.)
Similarly, corticosteroids should be used with great care in patients with known or suspected Strongyloides (threadworm) infestation. In such patients, corticosteroid-induced immunosuppression may lead to Strongyloides hyperinfection and dissemination with widespread larval migration, often accompanied by severe enterocolitis and potentially fatal gram-negative septicemia.
If corticosteroids are indicated in patients with latent tuberculosis or tuberculin reactivity, close observation is necessary as reactivation of the disease may occur. During prolonged corticosteroid therapy, these patients should receive chemoprophylaxis.
Literature reports suggest an apparent association between use of corticosteroids and left ventricular free wall rupture after a recent myocardial infarction; therefore, therapy with corticosteroids should be used with great caution in these patients.

PRECAUTIONS

This product, like many other steroid formulations, is sensitive to heat. Therefore, it should not be autoclaved when it is desirable to sterilize the exterior of the vial.
Therapy with this preparation does not eliminate the need for conventional supportive measures. Although capable of ameliorating symptoms, and even suppressing them completely in some patients, it is not a cure. Neither the hormone nor the anesthetic has any effect on the basic cause of inflammation.
Supportive measures, such as analgesics, pertinent orthopedic procedures, heat or cold, rest, rehabilitation, and physiotherapy must be used as applicable. If physiotherapy is applied immediately following injection, it may cause severe pain.
In some patients, a single injection fully restores mobility. Patients should be strongly impressed with the importance of not overusing the affected part as long as the inflammatory process remains active.
Injection into an infected site is to be avoided.
Dexamethasone Sodium Phosphate
Following prolonged therapy, withdrawal of corticosteroids may result in symptoms of the corticosteroid withdrawal syndrome including fever, myalgia, arthralgia, and malaise. This may occur in patients even without evidence of adrenal insufficiency.
There is an enhanced effect of corticosteroids in patients with hypothyroidism and in those with cirrhosis.
Corticosteroids should be used cautiously in patients with ocular herpes simplex for fear of corneal perforation.
Psychic derangements may appear when corticosteroids are used, ranging from euphoria, insomnia, mood swings, personality changes, and severe depression to frank psychotic manifestations. Also, existing emotional instability or psychotic tendencies may be aggravated by corticosteroids.
Aspirin should be used cautiously in conjunction with corticosteroids in hypoprothrombinemia.
Steroids should be used with caution in non-specific ulcerative colitis, if there is a probability of impending perforation, abscess, or other pyogenic infection, also in diverticulitis, fresh intestinal anastomoses, active or latent peptic ulcer, renal insufficiency, hypertension, osteoporosis, and myasthenia gravis. Signs of peritoneal irritation following gastrointestinal perforation in patients receiving large doses of corticosteroids may be minimal or absent. Fat embolism has been reported as a possible complication of hypercortisonism.
When large doses are given, some authorities advise that antacids be administered between meals to help to prevent peptic ulcer.

Continued on next page

Information on the Merck & Co., Inc. products listed on these pages is the full prescribing information from product circulars in use September 30, 1996.

Consult 1997 supplements and future editions for revisions

Merck & Co.—Cont.

Growth and development of infants and children on prolonged corticosteroid therapy should be carefully followed. Steroids may increase or decrease motility and number of spermatozoa in some patients.

Phenytoin, phenobarbital, ephedrine, and rifampin may enhance the metabolic clearance of corticosteroids, resulting in decreased blood levels and lessened physiologic activity, thus requiring adjustment in corticosteroid dosage.

The prothrombin time should be checked frequently in patients who are receiving corticosteroids and coumarin anticoagulants at the same time because of reports that corticosteroids have altered the response to these anticoagulants. Studies have shown that the usual effect produced by adding corticosteroids is inhibition of response to coumarins, although there have been some conflicting reports of potentiation not substantiated by studies.

When corticosteroids are administered concomitantly with potassium-depleting diuretics, patients should be observed closely for development of hypokalemia.

Lidocaine Hydrochloride
The safety and effectiveness of lidocaine hydrochloride depend on proper dosage, correct technique, adequate precautions, and readiness for emergencies.

Injection of repeated doses may cause significant increases in blood levels with each repeated dose due to slow accumulation of the drug or its metabolites. Tolerance varies with the status of the patient. Debilitated, elderly patients, acutely ill patients, and children should be given reduced doses commensurate with their age and physical status. INJECTIONS SHOULD ALWAYS BE MADE SLOWLY AND WITH FREQUENT ASPIRATIONS. Aspiration is advisable since it reduces the possibility of intravascular injection, thereby keeping the incidence of side effects and anesthetic failures to a minimum. Consult standard textbooks for specific techniques and precautions for various local anesthetic procedures.

Lidocaine hydrochloride should be used with caution in persons with known drug sensitivities. Patients allergic to para-aminobenzoic acid derivatives (procaine, tetracaine, benzocaine, etc.) have not shown cross sensitivity to lidocaine hydrochloride.

Local anesthetics react with certain metals and cause the release of their respective ions which, if injected, may cause severe local irritation. Adequate precaution should be taken to avoid this type of interaction.

Information for Patients
Susceptible patients who are on immunosuppressant doses of corticosteroids should be warned to avoid exposure to chickenpox or measles. Patients should also be advised that if they are exposed, medical advice should be sought without delay.

ADVERSE REACTIONS

Dexamethasone Sodium Phosphate
Fluid and electrolyte disturbances
  Sodium retention
  Fluid retention
  Congestive heart failure in susceptible patients
  Potassium loss
  Hypokalemic alkalosis
  Hypertension
Musculoskeletal
  Muscle weakness
  Steroid myopathy
  Loss of muscle mass
  Osteoporosis
  Vertebral compression fractures
  Aseptic necrosis of femoral and humeral heads
  Pathologic fracture of long bones
  Tendon rupture
Gastrointestinal
  Peptic ulcer with possible subsequent perforation and hemorrhage
  Perforation of the small and large bowel, particularly in patients with inflammatory bowel disease
  Pancreatitis
  Abdominal distention
  Ulcerative esophagitis
Dermatologic
  Impaired wound healing
  Thin fragile skin
  Petechiae and ecchymoses
  Erythema
  Increased sweating
  May suppress reactions to skin tests
  Other cutaneous reactions, such as allergic dermatitis, urticaria, angioneurotic edema
Neurologic
  Convulsions
  Increased intracranial pressure with papilledema (pseudotumor cerebri) usually after treatment
  Vertigo
  Headache
  Psychic disturbances
Endocrine
  Menstrual irregularities
  Development of cushingoid state
  Suppression of growth in children
  Secondary adrenocortical and pituitary unresponsiveness, particularly in times of stress, as in trauma, surgery, or illness
  Decreased carbohydrate tolerance
  Manifestations of latent diabetes mellitus
  Increased requirements for insulin or oral hypoglycemic agents in diabetics
  Hirsutism
Ophthalmic
  Posterior subcapsular cataracts
  Increased intraocular pressure
  Glaucoma
  Exophthalmos
Metabolic
  Negative nitrogen balance due to protein catabolism
Cardiovascular
  Myocardial rupture following recent myocardial infarction (see WARNINGS).
Other
  Anaphylactoid or hypersensitivity reactions
  Thromboembolism
  Weight gain
  Increased appetite
  Nausea
  Malaise
  Hiccups
The following *additional* adverse reactions are related to parenteral corticosteroid therapy:
  Rare instances of blindness associated with intralesional therapy around the face and head
  Hyperpigmentation or hypopigmentation
  Subcutaneous and cutaneous atrophy
  Sterile abscess
  Charcot-like arthropathy
Lidocaine Hydrochloride
Adverse reactions may result from high plasma levels due to excessive dosage, rapid absorption or inadvertent intravascular injection, or may result from a hypersensitivity, idiosyncrasy or diminished tolerance on the part of the patient. Such reactions are systemic in nature and involve the central nervous system and/or the cardiovascular system.

CNS reactions are excitatory and/or depressant, and may be characterized by nervousness, dizziness, blurred vision, and tremors followed by drowsiness, convulsions, unconsciousness, and possibly respiratory arrest. The excitatory reactions may be very brief or may not occur at all, in which case the first manifestations of toxicity may be drowsiness merging into unconsciousness and respiratory arrest.

Cardiovascular reactions are depressant, and may be characterized by hypotension, myocardial depression, bradycardia and possibly cardiac arrest.

Treatment of a patient with toxic manifestations consists of assuring and maintaining a patent airway and supporting ventilation using oxygen and assisted or controlled respiration as required. This usually will be sufficient in the management of most reactions. Should circulatory depression occur, vasopressors, such as ephedrine or metaraminol, and intravenous fluids may be used. Should a convulsion persist despite oxygen therapy, small increments of an ultra-short acting barbiturate (thiopental or thiamylal) or a short acting barbiturate (pentobarbital or secobarbital) may be given intravenously.

Allergic reactions are characterized by cutaneous lesions, urticaria, edema or anaphylactoid reactions. The detection of sensitivity by skin testing is of doubtful value.

DOSAGE AND ADMINISTRATION

For local injection only

NOT FOR INTRAVENOUS USE
DOSAGE AND FREQUENCY OF INJECTION ARE VARIABLE AND MUST BE INDIVIDUALIZED ON THE BASIS OF THE DISEASE AND THE RESPONSE OF THE PATIENT.
Injections should always be made slowly and with frequent aspiration.
The initial dose ranges from 0.1 to 0.75 mL depending on the disease being treated and the size of the area to be injected. Frequency of injection depends on symptomatic response. In some patients, acute conditions are controlled adequately by a single injection. In others, additional injections are required, usually at intervals of four to seven days. If satisfactory clinical response does not occur after a reasonable period of time, discontinue DECADRON Phosphate with XYLOCAINE Injection and transfer the patient to other therapy.

Patients should be observed closely for signs that might require dosage adjustment, including changes in clinical status resulting from remissions or exacerbations of the disease, and individual drug responsiveness.
The usual doses are:

	Acute and Subacute Bursitis	Acute and Subacute Nonspecific Tenosynovitis
Amount of injection (mL)	0.5 to 0.75	0.1 to 0.25
Amount of dexamethasone sodium phosphate (mg)	2 to 3	0.4 to 1
Amount of lidocaine hydrochloride (mg)	5 to 7.5	1 to 2.5

DECADRON Phosphate with XYLOCAINE may be given undiluted directly from the vial, or it may be diluted with Sterile Water for Injection or Sodium Chloride Injection, using up to five parts of diluent to each part of injection. Dilutions should be used within one hour, since there is a possibility of change in pH, and this may adversely affect the stability or activity of the components.

HOW SUPPLIED

No. 7625X—Injection DECADRON Phosphate with XYLOCAINE, containing 4 mg dexamethasone phosphate equivalent and 10 mg lidocaine hydrochloride per mL, is a clear, colorless solution, and is available as follows:
NDC 0006-7625-03 in 5 mL vials.
Storage
Sensitive to heat. Do not autoclave.
Protect from freezing.
  7349321 Issued May 1996

DECADRON® Phosphate ℞
(Dexamethasone Sodium Phosphate), U.S.P.
0.05% Dexamethasone Phosphate Equivalent
Sterile Ophthalmic Ointment

DESCRIPTION

Dexamethasone sodium phosphate is 9-fluoro-11β,17-dihydroxy-16α -methyl-21-(phosphonooxy)pregna-1,4-diene-3,20-dione disodium salt. Its empirical formula is $C_{22}H_{28}FNa_2O_8P$ and its structural formula is:

Glucocorticoids are adrenocortical steroids, both naturally occurring and synthetic. Dexamethasone is a synthetic analog of naturally occurring glucocorticoids (hydrocortisone and cortisone). Dexamethasone sodium phosphate is a water soluble, inorganic ester of dexamethasone. Its molecular weight is 516.41.

Sterile Ophthalmic Ointment DECADRON* Phosphate (Dexamethasone Sodium Phosphate) is a topical steroid ointment containing dexamethasone sodium phosphate equivalent to 0.5 mg (0.05%) dexamethasone phosphate in each gram. Inactive ingredients: white petrolatum and mineral oil.

Dexamethasone sodium phosphate is an inorganic ester of dexamethasone.

*Registered trademark of MERCK & CO., INC.

CLINICAL PHARMACOLOGY

Dexamethasone sodium phosphate suppresses the inflammatory response to a variety of agents and it probably delays or slows healing. No generally accepted explanation of these steroid properties have been advanced.

INDICATIONS AND USAGE

For the treatment of the following conditions:
Steroid responsive inflammatory conditions of the palpebral and bulbar conjunctiva, cornea, and anterior segment of the globe, such as allergic conjunctivitis, acne rosacea, superficial punctate keratitis, herpes zoster keratitis, iritis, cyclitis, selected infective conjunctivitis when the inherent hazard of steroid use is accepted to obtain an advisable diminution in edema and inflammation; corneal injury from chemical or thermal burns, or penetration of foreign bodies.

CONTRAINDICATIONS

Epithelial herpes simplex keratitis (dendritic keratitis).
Acute infectious stages of vaccinia, varicella, and many other viral diseases of the cornea and conjunctiva.
Mycobacterial infection of the eye.
Fungal diseases of ocular structures.
Hypersensitivity to a component of the medication.

WARNINGS

Prolonged use may result in ocular hypertension and/or glaucoma, with damage to the optic nerve, defects in visual acuity and fields of vision, and posterior subcapsular cataract formation. Prolonged use may suppress the host response and thus increase the hazard of secondary ocular infections. In those diseases causing thinning of the cornea or sclera, perforations have been known to occur with the use of topical corticosteroids. In acute purulent conditions of the eye, corticosteroids may mask infection or enhance existing infection. If these products are used for 10 days or longer, intraocular pressure should be routinely monitored even though it may be difficult in children and uncooperative patients.
Employment of corticosteroid medication in the treatment of herpes simplex other than epithelial herpes simplex keratitis, in which it is contraindicated, requires great caution; periodic slit-lamp microscopy is essential.

PRECAUTIONS

General
The possibility of persistent fungal infections of the cornea should be considered after prolonged corticosteroid dosing. There have been reports of bacterial keratitis associated with the use of multiple dose containers of topical ophthalmic products. These containers had been inadvertently contaminated by patients who, in most cases, had a concurrent corneal disease or a disruption of the ocular epithelial surface. (See PRECAUTIONS, *Information for Patients.*)
Information for Patients
Patients should be instructed to avoid allowing the tip of the dispensing container to contact the eye or surrounding structures.
Patients should also be instructed that ocular preparations, if handled improperly, can become contaminated by common bacteria known to cause ocular infections. Serious damage to the eye and subsequent loss of vision may result from using contaminated preparations. (See PRECAUTIONS, *General.*)
Patients should also be advised that if they develop an intercurrent ocular condition (e.g., trauma, ocular surgery or infection), they should immediately seek their physician's advice concerning the continued use of the present multidose container.
Carcinogenesis, Mutagenesis, Impairment of Fertility
Long-term animal studies have not been performed to evaluate the carcinogenic potential or the effect on fertility of Ophthalmic Ointment DECADRON Phosphate.
Pregnancy
Pregnancy Category C. Dexamethasone has been shown to be teratogenic in mice and rabbits following topical ophthalmic application in multiples of the therapeutic dose.
In the mouse, corticosteroids produce fetal resorptions and a specific abnormality, cleft palate. In the rabbit, corticosteroids have produced fetal resorptions and multiple abnormalities involving the head, ears, limbs, palate, etc.
There are no adequate or well-controlled studies in pregnant women. Ophthalmic Ointment DECADRON Phosphate should be used during pregnancy only if the potential benefit to the mother justifies the potential risk to the embryo or fetus. Infants born of mothers who have received substantial doses of corticosteroids during pregnancy should be observed carefully for signs of hypoadrenalism.
Nursing Mothers
Topically applied steroids are absorbed systemically. Therefore, because of the potential for serious adverse reactions in nursing infants from dexamethasone sodium phosphate, a decision should be made whether to discontinue nursing or discontinue the drug, taking into account the importance of the drug to the mother.
Pediatric Use
Safety and effectiveness in children have not been established.

ADVERSE REACTIONS

Glaucoma with optic nerve damage, visual acuity and field defects, posterior subcapsular cataract formation, secondary ocular infection from pathogens including herpes simplex, perforation of the globe.
Rarely, filtering blebs have been reported when topical steroids have been used following cataract surgery.
Rarely, stinging or burning may occur.

DOSAGE AND ADMINISTRATION

The duration of treatment will vary with the type of lesion and may extend from a few days to several weeks, according to therapeutic response. Relapses, more common in chronic active lesions than in self-limited conditions, usually respond to retreatment.
Apply a thin coating of ointment three or four times a day. When a favorable response is observed, reduce the number of daily applications to two, and later to one a day as a maintenance dose if this is sufficient to control symptoms.
Ophthalmic Ointment DECADRON Phosphate is particularly convenient when an eye pad is used. It may also be the preparation of choice for patients in whom therapeutic benefit depends on prolonged contact of the active ingredients with ocular tissues.

HOW SUPPLIED

No. 7615—0.05% Sterile Ophthalmic Ointment DECADRON Phosphate is a clear unctuous ointment and is supplied as follows:
NDC 0006-7615-04 in 3.5 g tubes
(6505-00-961-5508 0.05% 3.5 g).

7612331   Issued October 1993

DECADRON® Phosphate   ℞
(Dexamethasone Sodium Phosphate), U.S.P.
0.1% Dexamethasone Phosphate Equivalent
Sterile Ophthalmic Solution

DESCRIPTION

Dexamethasone sodium phosphate is 9-fluoro-11β,17-dihydroxy-16α-methyl-21-(phosphonooxy)pregna-1,4-diene-3,20-dione disodium salt. Its empirical formula is $C_{22}H_{28}FNa_2O_8P$ and its structural formula is:

Glucocorticoids are adrenocortical steroids, both naturally occurring and synthetic. Dexamethasone is a synthetic analog of naturally occurring glucocorticoids (hydrocortisone and cortisone). Dexamethasone sodium phosphate is a water soluble, inorganic ester of dexamethasone. It is approximately three thousand times more soluble in water at 25°C than hydrocortisone. Its molecular weight is 516.41.
Ophthalmic Solution DECADRON* Phosphate (Dexamethasone Sodium Phosphate) in the 5 mL OCUMETER* ophthalmic dispenser is a topical steroid solution containing dexamethasone sodium phosphate equivalent to 1 mg (0.1%) dexamethasone phosphate in each milliliter of buffered solution. Inactive ingredients: creatinine, sodium citrate, sodium borate, polysorbate 80, disodium edetate, hydrochloric acid to adjust pH, and water for injection. Sodium bisulfite 0.1%, phenylethanol 0.25% and benzalkonium chloride 0.02% added as preservatives.

---

*Registered trademark of MERCK & CO., INC.

CLINICAL PHARMACOLOGY

Dexamethasone sodium phosphate suppresses the inflammatory response to a variety of agents and it probably delays or slows healing. No generally accepted explanation of these steroid properties have been advanced.

INDICATIONS AND USAGE

For the treatment of the following conditions:
Ophthalmic:
Steroid responsive inflammatory conditions of the palpebral and bulbar conjunctiva, cornea, and anterior segment of the globe, such as allergic conjunctivitis, acne rosacea, superficial punctate keratitis, herpes zoster keratitis, iritis, cyclitis, selected infective conjunctivitis when the inherent hazard of steroid use is accepted to obtain an advisable diminution in edema and inflammation; corneal injury from chemical or thermal burns, or penetration of foreign bodies.
Otic:
Steroid responsive inflammatory conditions of the external auditory meatus, such as allergic otitis externa, selected purulent and nonpurulent infective otitis externa when the hazard of steroid use is accepted to obtain an advisable diminution in edema and inflammation.

CONTRAINDICATIONS

Epithelial herpes simplex keratitis (dendritic keratitis).
Acute infectious stages of vaccinia, varicella, and many other viral diseases of the cornea and conjunctiva.
Mycobacterial infection of the eye.
Fungal diseases of ocular or auricular structures.
Hypersensitivity to any component of this product, including sulfites (see WARNINGS).
Perforation of a drum membrane.

WARNINGS

Prolonged use may result in ocular hypertension and/or glaucoma, with damage to the optic nerve, defects in visual acuity and fields of vision, and posterior subcapsular cataract formation. Prolonged use may suppress the host response and thus increase the hazard of secondary ocular infections. In those diseases causing thinning of the cornea or sclera, perforations have been known to occur with the use of topical corticosteroids. In acute purulent conditions of the eye or ear, corticosteroids may mask infection or enhance existing infection. If these products are used for 10 days or longer, intraocular pressure should be routinely monitored even though it may be difficult in children and uncooperative patients.
Employment of corticosteroid medication in the treatment of herpes simplex other than epithelial herpes simplex keratitis, in which it is contraindicated, requires great caution; periodic slit-lamp microscopy is essential.
Ophthalmic Solution DECADRON Phosphate contains sodium bisulfite, a sulfite that may cause allergic-type reactions including anaphylactic symptoms and life-threatening or less severe asthmatic episodes in certain susceptible people. The overall prevalence of sulfite sensitivity in the general population is unknown and probably low. Sulfite sensitivity is seen more frequently in asthmatic than in nonasthmatic people.

PRECAUTIONS

General
The possibility of persistent fungal infections of the cornea should be considered after prolonged corticosteroid dosing. There have been reports of bacterial keratitis associated with the use of multiple dose containers of topical ophthalmic products. These containers had been inadvertently contaminated by patients who, in most cases, had a concurrent corneal disease or a disruption of the ocular epithelial surface. (See PRECAUTIONS, *Information for Patients.*)
Information for Patients
Patients should be instructed to avoid allowing the tip of the dispensing container to contact the eye or surrounding structures.
Patients should also be instructed that ocular solutions, if handled improperly, can become contaminated by common bacteria known to cause ocular infections. Serious damage to the eye and subsequent loss of vision may result from using contaminated solutions. (See PRECAUTIONS, *General.*)
Patients should also be advised that if they develop an intercurrent ocular condition (e.g., trauma, ocular surgery or infection), they should immediately seek their physician's advice concerning the continued use of the present multidose container.
One of the preservatives in Ophthalmic Solution DECADRON Phosphate, benzalkonium chloride, may be absorbed by soft contact lenses. Patients wearing soft contact lenses should be instructed to wait at least 15 minutes after instilling Ophthalmic Solution DECADRON Phosphate before they insert their lenses.
Carcinogenesis, Mutagenesis, Impairment of Fertility
Long-term animal studies have not been performed to evaluate the carcinogenic potential or the effect on fertility of Ophthalmic Solution DECADRON Phosphate.

Continued on next page

Merck & Co.—Cont.

Pregnancy
Pregnancy Category C. Dexamethasone has been shown to be teratogenic in mice and rabbits following topical ophthalmic application in multiples of the therapeutic dose.
In the mouse, corticosteroids produce fetal resorptions and a specific abnormality, cleft palate. In the rabbit, corticosteroids have produced fetal resorptions and multiple abnormalities involving the head, ears, limbs, palate, etc.
There are no adequate or well-controlled studies in pregnant women. Ophthalmic Solution DECADRON Phosphate should be used during pregnancy only if the potential benefit to the mother justifies the potential risk to the embryo or fetus. Infants born of mothers who have received substantial doses of corticosteroids during pregnancy should be observed carefully for signs of hypoadrenalism.
Nursing Mothers
Topically applied steroids are absorbed systemically. Therefore, because of the potential for serious adverse reactions in nursing infants from dexamethasone sodium phosphate, a decision should be made whether to discontinue nursing or discontinue the drug, taking into account the importance of the drug to the mother.
Pediatric Use
Safety and effectiveness in children have not been established.

ADVERSE REACTIONS

Glaucoma with optic nerve damage, visual acuity and field defects, posterior subcapsular cataract formation, secondary ocular infection from pathogens including herpes simplex, perforation of the globe.
Rarely, filtering blebs have been reported when topical steroids have been used following cataract surgery.
Rarely, stinging or burning may occur.

DOSAGE AND ADMINISTRATION

The duration of treatment will vary with the type of lesion and may extend from a few days to several weeks, according to therapeutic response. Relapses, more common in chronic active lesions than in self-limited conditions, usually respond to retreatment.
Eye—Instill one or two drops of solution into the conjunctival sac every hour during the day and every two hours during the night as initial therapy. When a favorable response is observed, reduce dosage to one drop every four hours. Later, further reduction in dosage to one drop three or four times daily may suffice to control symptoms.
Ear—Clean the aural canal thoroughly and sponge dry. Instill the solution directly into the aural canal. A suggested initial dosage is three or four drops two or three times a day. When a favorable response is obtained, reduce dosage gradually and eventually discontinue.
If preferred, the aural canal may be packed with a gauze wick saturated with solution. Keep the wick moist with the preparation and remove from the ear after 12 to 24 hours. Treatment may be repeated as often as necessary at the discretion of the physician.

HOW SUPPLIED

Sterile Ophthalmic Solution DECADRON Phosphate is a clear, colorless to pale yellow solution.
No. 7643—Ophthalmic Solution DECADRON Phosphate is supplied as follows:
NDC 0006-7643-03 in 5 mL white, opaque, plastic OCUMETER ophthalmic dispenser with a controlled drop tip.
(6505-00-007-4536 0.1% 5 mL).
7261521 Issued October 1993

DECADRON® Phosphate Topical Cream ℞
(Dexamethasone Sodium Phosphate), U.S.P.
0.1% Dexamethasone Phosphate Equivalent

DESCRIPTION

DECADRON* Phosphate (Dexamethasone Sodium Phosphate) Topical Cream is a topical steroid preparation.
The topical corticosteroids constitute a class of primarily synthetic steroids used as anti-inflammatory and anti-pruritic agents.
Dexamethasone sodium phosphate is 9-fluoro-11β,17-dihydroxy -16α -methyl -21- (phosphonooxy) pregna-1,4-diene-3,20-dione disodium salt. Its empirical formula is $C_{22}H_{28}FNa_2O_8P$ and its structural formula is:
[See chemical structure at top of next column.]
Dexamethasone sodium phosphate has a molecular weight of 516.41.

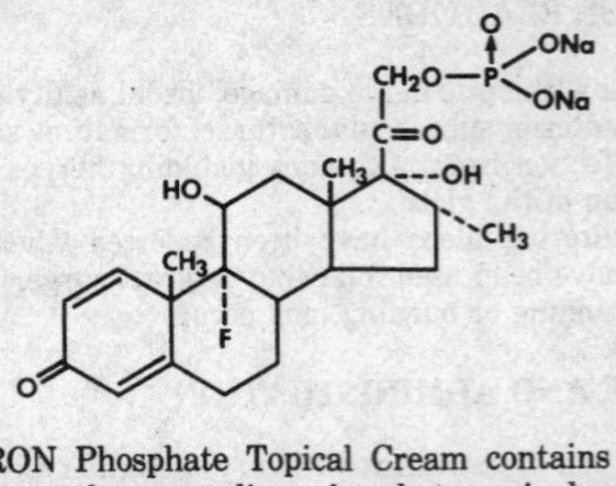

DECADRON Phosphate Topical Cream contains in each gram: dexamethasone sodium phosphate equivalent to 1 mg (0.1%) dexamethasone phosphate in a greaseless bland base. Inactive ingredients: stearyl alcohol, cetyl alcohol, mineral oil, polyoxyl 40 stearate, sorbitol solution, methyl polysilicone emulsion, creatinine, sodium citrate, disodium edetate, sodium hydroxide to adjust pH, and purified water. Methylparaben, 0.15%, and sorbic acid, 0.1% added as preservatives.

*Registered trademark of MERCK & CO., INC.

CLINICAL PHARMACOLOGY

Topical corticosteroids share anti-inflammatory, anti-pruritic and vasoconstrictive actions.
The mechanism of anti-inflammatory activity of the topical corticosteroids is unclear. Various laboratory methods, including vasoconstrictor assays, are used to compare and predict potencies and/or clinical efficacies of the topical corticosteroids. There is some evidence to suggest that a recognizable correlation exists between vasoconstrictor potency and therapeutic efficacy in man.
Pharmacokinetics
The extent of percutaneous absorption of topical corticosteroids is determined by many factors including the vehicle, the integrity of the epidermal barrier, and the use of occlusive dressings.
Topical corticosteroids can be absorbed from normal intact skin. Inflammation and/or other disease processes in the skin increase percutaneous absorption. Occlusive dressings substantially increase the percutaneous absorption of topical corticosteroids. Thus, occlusive dressings may be a valuable therapeutic adjunct for treatment of resistant dermatoses. (See DOSAGE AND ADMINISTRATION)
Once absorbed through the skin, topical corticosteroids are handled through pharmacokinetic pathways similar to systemically administered corticosteroids. Corticosteroids are bound to plasma proteins in varying degrees. Corticosteroids are metabolized primarily in the liver and are then excreted by the kidneys. Some of the topical corticosteroids and their metabolites are also excreted into the bile.

INDICATIONS AND USAGE

DECADRON Phosphate Topical Cream is indicated for relief of the inflammatory and pruritic manifestations of corticosteroid-responsive dermatoses.

CONTRAINDICATIONS

Topical corticosteroids are contraindicated in those patients with a history of hypersensitivity to any of the components of the preparation.

WARNING

Topically applied steroids are absorbed systemically. There may be rare instances in which this absorption results in immunosuppression. Patients who are on drugs which suppress the immune system are more susceptible to infections than healthy individuals. Chickenpox and measles, for example, can have a more serious or even fatal course in non-immune children (see PRECAUTIONS, *Pediatric Use*) or adults on corticosteroids. In such children or adults who have not had these diseases, particular care should be taken to avoid exposure. The risk of developing a disseminated infection varies among individuals and can be related to the dose, route and duration of corticosteroid administration as well as to the underlying disease. If exposed to chickenpox, prophylaxis with varicella zoster immune globulin (VZIG) may be indicated. If chickenpox develops, treatment with antiviral agents may be considered. If exposed to measles, prophylaxis with immune globulin (IG) may be indicated. (See the respective package inserts for VZIG and IG for complete prescribing information.)

PRECAUTIONS

General
Systemic absorption of topical corticosteroids has produced reversible hypothalamic-pituitary-adrenal (HPA) axis suppression, manifestations of Cushing's syndrome, hyperglycemia, and glycosuria in some patients.
Conditions which augment systemic absorption include the application of the more potent corticosteroids, use over large surface areas, prolonged use, and the addition of occlusive dressings.
Therefore, patients receiving a large dose of a potent topical corticosteroid applied to a large surface area or under an occlusive dressing should be evaluated periodically for evidence of HPA axis suppression by using urinary free cortisol and ACTH stimulation tests. If HPA axis suppression is noted, an attempt should be made to withdraw the drug, to reduce the frequency of application, or to substitute a less potent corticosteroid.
Recovery of HPA axis function is generally prompt and complete upon discontinuation of the drug. Infrequently, signs and symptoms of corticosteroid withdrawal may occur, requiring supplemental systemic corticosteroids.
Children may absorb proportionally larger amounts of topical corticosteroids and thus be more susceptible to systemic toxicity (See PRECAUTIONS, *Pediatric Use*).
If irritation develops, topical corticosteroids should be discontinued and appropriate therapy instituted.
In the presence of dermatological infections, the use of an appropriate antifungal or antibacterial agent should be instituted. If a favorable response does not occur promptly, the corticosteroid should be discontinued until the infection has been adequately controlled.
This product is not for ophthalmic use. However, if applied to the eyelids or skin near the eyes, the drug may enter the eyes. In patients with a history of herpes simplex keratitis, ocular exposure to corticosteroids may lead to a recurrence. Prolonged ocular exposure may cause steroid glaucoma.
Generally, occlusive dressings should not be used on weeping or exudative lesions.
If occlusive dressing therapy is used, inspect lesions between dressings for development of infection. If infection develops, the technique should be discontinued and appropriate anti-microbial therapy instituted.
When large areas of the body are covered with an occlusive dressing, thermal homeostasis may be impaired. If elevation of body temperature occurs, use of the occlusive dressing should be discontinued.
Information for the Patient
Patients using topical corticosteroids should receive the following information and instructions:

1. This medication is to be used as directed by the physician. It is for external use only. Avoid contact with the eyes.
2. Patients should be advised not to use this medication for any disorder other than that for which it was prescribed.
3. The treated skin area should not be bandaged or otherwise covered or wrapped so as to be occlusive unless directed by the physician.
4. Patients should report any signs of local adverse reactions, especially under occlusive dressing.
5. Parents of pediatric patients should be advised not to use tight-fitting diapers or plastic pants on a child being treated in the diaper area, as these garments may constitute occlusive dressings.
6. Susceptible patients who are on immunosuppressant doses of corticosteroids should be warned to avoid exposure to chickenpox or measles. Patients should also be advised that if they are exposed, medical advice should be sought without delay.

Laboratory Tests
The following tests may be helpful in evaluating the HPA axis suppression:

- Urinary free cortisol test
- ACTH stimulation test

Carcinogenesis, Mutagenesis, and Impairment of Fertility
Long-term animal studies have not been performed to evaluate the carcinogenic potential or the effect on fertility of topical corticosteroids.
Studies to determine mutagenicity with prednisolone and hydrocortisone have revealed negative results.
Pregnancy
Pregnancy Category C: Corticosteroids are generally teratogenic in laboratory animals when administered systemically at relatively low dosage levels. The more potent corticosteroids have been shown to be teratogenic after dermal application in laboratory animals. There are no adequate and well-controlled studies in pregnant women on teratogenic effects from topically applied corticosteroids. Therefore, topical corticosteroids should be used during pregnancy only if the potential benefit justifies the potential risk to the fetus. Drugs of this class should not be used extensively on pregnant patients, in large amounts, or for prolonged periods of time.
Nursing Mothers
It is not known whether topical administration of corticosteroids could result in sufficient systemic absorption to produce detectable quantities in breast milk. Systemically administered corticosteroids are secreted into breast milk in quantities *not* likely to have a deleterious effect on the infant. Nevertheless, caution should be exercised when topical corticosteroids are administered to a nursing woman.

Pediatric Use

Pediatric patients may demonstrate greater susceptibility to topical corticosteroid-induced HPA axis suppression and Cushing's syndrome than mature patients because of a larger skin surface area to body weight ratio.

Hypothalamic-pituitary-adrenal (HPA) axis suppression, Cushing's syndrome, and intracranial hypertension have been reported in children receiving topical corticosteroids. Manifestations of adrenal suppression in children include linear growth retardation, delayed weight gain, low plasma cortisol levels, and absence of response to ACTH stimulation. Manifestations of intracranial hypertension include bulging fontanelles, headaches, and bilateral papilledema. Administration of topical corticosteroids to children should be limited to the least amount compatible with an effective therapeutic regimen. Chronic corticosteroid therapy may interfere with the growth and development of children.

ADVERSE REACTIONS

The following adverse reactions are reported infrequently with topical corticosteroids, but may occur more frequently with the use of occlusive dressings. These reactions are listed in an approximate decreasing order of occurrence:

Burning
Itching
Irritation
Dryness
Folliculitis
Hypertrichosis
Acneiform eruptions
Hypopigmentation
Perioral dermatitis
Allergic contact dermatitis
Maceration of the skin
Secondary infection
Skin atrophy
Striae
Miliaria

OVERDOSAGE

Topically applied corticosteroids can be absorbed in sufficient amounts to produce systemic effects (See PRECAUTIONS).

DOSAGE AND ADMINISTRATION

Apply to the affected area as a thin film three or four times daily.
Occlusive dressings may be used for the management of psoriasis or recalcitrant conditions.
Before using this preparation in the *ear*, clean the aural canal thoroughly and sponge dry. Confirm that the eardrum is intact. With a cotton-tipped applicator, apply a thin coating of the cream to the affected canal area three or four times a day.

HOW SUPPLIED

No. 7616X — 0.1% Topical Cream DECADRON Phosphate is a white cream, and is supplied as follows:
NDC 0006-7616-12 in 15 g tubes
NDC 0006-7616-24 in 30 g tubes.
　　　DC 7612525　Issued April 1993
Copyright © MERCK & CO., INC., 1983
All rights reserved

DECADRON-LA® Sterile Suspension　　　　℞
(Dexamethasone Acetate), U.S.P.

NOT FOR INTRAVENOUS USE

DESCRIPTION

Dexamethasone acetate, a synthetic adrenocortical steroid, is a white to practically white, odorless powder. It is a practically insoluble ester of dexamethasone. The structural formula is:

Dexamethasone acetate is present in DECADRON-LA* (Dexamethasone Acetate) sterile suspension as the monohydrate, with the empirical formula, $C_{24}H_{31}FO_6 \cdot H_2O$, and molecular weight, 452.52. Dexamethasone acetate is designated chemically as 21-(acetyloxy)-9-fluoro-11β,17-dihydroxy-16α-methylpregna-1,4-diene-3,20-dione.

DECADRON-LA sterile suspension is a sterile white suspension (pH 5.0 to 7.5) that settles on standing, but is easily resuspended by mild shaking.
Each milliliter contains dexamethasone acetate equivalent to 8 mg dexamethasone. Inactive ingredients per mL: 6.67 mg sodium chloride; 5 mg creatinine; 0.5 mg disodium edetate; 5 mg sodium carboxymethylcellulose; 0.75 mg polysorbate 80; sodium hydroxide to adjust pH; and Water for Injection, q.s. 1 mL, with 9 mg benzyl alcohol, and 1 mg sodium bisulfite added as preservatives.

*Registered trademark of MERCK & CO., INC.

ACTIONS

DECADRON-LA sterile suspension is a long-acting, repository adrenocorticosteroid preparation with a prompt onset of action. It is suitable for intramuscular or local injection, but not when an immediate effect of short duration is desired. Naturally occurring glucocorticoids (hydrocortisone and cortisone), which also have salt-retaining properties, are used as replacement therapy in adrenocortical deficiency states. Their synthetic analogs, including dexamethasone, are primarily used for their potent anti-inflammatory effects in disorders of many organ systems.
Glucocorticoids cause profound and varied metabolic effects. In addition, they modify the body's immune responses to diverse stimuli.
At equipotent anti-inflammatory doses, dexamethasone almost completely lacks the sodium-retaining property of hydrocortisone.

INDICATIONS

A.　By intramuscular injection when oral therapy is not feasible:
1.　*Endocrine disorders*
Congenital adrenal hyperplasia
Nonsuppurative thyroiditis
Hypercalcemia associated with cancer
2.　*Rheumatic disorders*
As adjunctive therapy for short-term administration (to tide the patient over an acute episode or exacerbation) in:
Post-traumatic osteoarthritis
Synovitis of osteoarthritis
Rheumatoid arthritis, including juvenile rheumatoid arthritis (selected cases may require low-dose maintenance therapy)
Acute and subacute bursitis
Epicondylitis
Acute nonspecific tenosynovitis
Acute gouty arthritis
Psoriatic arthritis
Ankylosing spondylitis
3.　*Collagen diseases*
During an exacerbation or as maintenance therapy in selected cases of:
Systemic lupus erythematosus
Acute rheumatic carditis
4.　*Dermatologic diseases*
Pemphigus
Severe erythema multiforme (Stevens-Johnson syndrome)
Exfoliative dermatitis
Bullous dermatitis herpetiformis
Severe seborrheic dermatitis
Severe psoriasis
Mycosis fungoides
5.　*Allergic states*
Control of severe or incapacitating allergic conditions intractable to adequate trials of conventional treatment in:
Bronchial asthma
Contact dermatitis
Atopic dermatitis
Serum sickness
Seasonal or perennial allergic rhinitis
Drug hypersensitivity reactions
Urticarial transfusion reactions
6.　*Ophthalmic diseases*
Severe acute and chronic allergic and inflammatory processes involving the eye, such as:
Herpes zoster ophthalmicus
Iritis, Iridocyclitis
Chorioretinitis
Diffuse posterior uveitis and choroiditis
Optic neuritis
Sympathetic ophthalmia
Anterior segment inflammation
Allergic conjunctivitis
Keratitis
Allergic corneal marginal ulcers
7.　*Gastrointestinal diseases*
To tide the patient over a critical period of the disease in:
Ulcerative colitis (Systemic therapy)
Regional enteritis (Systemic therapy)

8.　*Respiratory diseases*
Symptomatic sarcoidosis
Berylliosis
Loeffler's syndrome not manageable by other means
Aspiration pneumonitis
9.　*Hematologic disorders*
Acquired (autoimmune) hemolytic anemia
Secondary thrombocytopenia in adults
Erythroblastopenia (RBC anemia)
Congenital (erythroid) hypoplastic anemia
10.　*Neoplastic diseases*
For palliative management of:
Leukemias and lymphomas in adults
Acute leukemia of childhood
11.　*Edematous states*
To induce diuresis or remission of proteinuria in the nephrotic syndrome, without uremia, of the idiopathic type, or that due to lupus erythematosus
12.　*Miscellaneous*
Trichinosis with neurologic or myocardial involvement.
B.　By intra-articular or soft tissue injection as adjunctive therapy for short-term administration (to tide the patient over an acute episode or exacerbation) in:
Synovitis of osteoarthritis
Rheumatoid arthritis
Acute and subacute bursitis
Acute gouty arthritis
Epicondylitis
Acute nonspecific tenosynovitis
Post-traumatic osteoarthritis.
C.　By intralesional injection in:
Keloids
Localized hypertrophic, infiltrated, inflammatory lesions of: lichen planus, psoriatic plaques, granuloma annulare, and lichen simplex chronicus (neurodermatitis)
Discoid lupus erythematosus
Necrobiosis lipoidica diabeticorum
Alopecia areata
May also be useful in cystic tumors of an aponeurosis or tendon (ganglia).

CONTRAINDICATIONS

Systemic fungal infections
Hypersensitivity to any component of this product, including sulfites (see WARNINGS).

WARNINGS

DO NOT INJECT INTRAVENOUSLY
Because rare instances of anaphylactoid reactions have occurred in patients receiving parenteral corticosteroid therapy, appropriate precautionary measures should be taken prior to administration, especially when the patient has a history of allergy to any drug. Anaphylactoid and hypersensitivity reactions have been reported for Sterile Suspension DECADRON-LA (see ADVERSE REACTIONS).
Sterile Suspension DECADRON-LA contains sodium bisulfite, a sulfite that may cause allergic-type reactions including anaphylactic symptoms and life-threatening or less severe asthmatic episodes in certain susceptible people. The overall prevalence of sulfite sensitivity in the general population is unknown and probably low. Sulfite sensitivity is seen more frequently in asthmatic than in nonasthmatic people.
In patients on corticosteroid therapy subjected to any unusual stress, increased dosage of rapidly acting corticosteroids before, during, and after the stressful situation is indicated.
Drug-induced secondary adrenocortical insufficiency may result from too rapid withdrawal of corticosteroids and may be minimized by gradual reduction of dosage. This type of relative insufficiency may persist for months after discontinuation of therapy; therefore, in any situation of stress occurring during that period, hormone therapy should be reinstituted. If the patient is receiving steroids already, dosage may have to be increased. Since mineralocorticoid secretion may be impaired, salt and/or a mineralocorticoid should be administered concurrently.
Corticosteroids may mask some signs of infection, and new infections may appear during their use. There may be decreased resistance and inability to localize infection when corticosteroids are used. Moreover, corticosteroids may affect the nitroblue-tetrazolium test for bacterial infection and produce false negative results.
In cerebral malaria, a double-blind trial has shown that the use of corticosteroids is associated with prolongation of coma and a higher incidence of pneumonia and gastrointestinal bleeding.

Continued on next page

Information on the Merck & Co., Inc. products listed on these pages is the full prescribing information from product circulars in use September 30, 1996.

Consult 1997 supplements and future editions for revisions

Merck & Co.—Cont.

Corticosteroids may activate latent amebiasis. Therefore, it is recommended that latent or active amebiasis be ruled out before initiating corticosteroid therapy in any patient who has spent time in the tropics or any patient with unexplained diarrhea.

Prolonged use of corticosteroids may produce posterior subcapsular cataracts, glaucoma with possible damage to the optic nerves, and may enhance the establishment of secondary ocular infections due to fungi or viruses.

Usage in pregnancy. Since adequate human reproduction studies have not been done with corticosteroids, use of these drugs in pregnancy or in women of childbearing potential requires that the anticipated benefits be weighed against the possible hazards to the mother and embryo or fetus. Infants born of mothers who have received substantial doses of corticosteroids during pregnancy should be carefully observed for signs of hypoadrenalism.

Corticosteroids appear in breast milk and could suppress growth, interfere with endogenous corticosteroid production, or cause other unwanted effects. Mothers taking pharmacologic doses of corticosteroids should be advised not to nurse.

Average and large doses of cortisone or hydrocortisone can cause elevation of blood pressure, salt and water retention, and increased excretion of potassium. These effects are less likely to occur with the synthetic derivatives except when used in large doses. Dietary salt restriction and potassium supplementation may be necessary. All corticosteroids increase calcium excretion.

Administration of live virus vaccines, including smallpox, is contraindicated in individuals receiving immunosuppressive doses of corticosteroids. If inactivated viral or bacterial vaccines are administered to individuals receiving immunosuppressive doses of corticosteroids, the expected serum antibody response may not be obtained.

Patients who are on drugs which suppress the immune system are more susceptible to infections than healthy individuals. Chickenpox and measles, for example, can have a more serious or even fatal course in non-immune children or adults on corticosteroids. In such children or adults who have not had these diseases, particular care should be taken to avoid exposure. The risk of developing a disseminated infection varies among individuals and can be related to the dose, route and duration of corticosteroid administration as well as to the underlying disease. If exposed to chickenpox, prophylaxis with varicella zoster immune globulin (VZIG) may be indicated. If chickenpox develops, treatment with antiviral agents may be considered. If exposed to measles, prophylaxis with immune globulin (IG) may be indicated. (See the respective package inserts for VZIG and IG for complete prescribing information.)

Similarly, corticosteroids should be used with great care in patients with known or suspected Strongyloides (threadworm) infestation. In such patients, corticosteroid-induced immunosuppression may lead to Strongyloides hyperinfection and dissemination with widespread larval migration, often accompanied by severe enterocolitis and potentially fatal gram-negative septicemia.

If corticosteroids are indicated in patients with latent tuberculosis or tuberculin reactivity, close observation is necessary as reactivation of the disease may occur. During prolonged corticosteroid therapy, these patients should receive chemoprophylaxis.

Repository adrenocorticosteroid preparations may cause atrophy at the site of injection. To minimize the likelihood and/or severity of atrophy, do not inject subcutaneously, avoid injection into the deltoid muscle, and avoid repeated intramuscular injections into the same site if possible.

Dosage in children under 12 has not been established.

Literature reports suggest an apparent association between use of corticosteroids and left ventricular free wall rupture after a recent myocardial infarction; therefore, therapy with corticosteroids should be used with great caution in these patients.

PRECAUTIONS

DECADRON-LA sterile suspension is not recommended as initial therapy in acute, life-threatening situations.

This product, like many other steroid formulations, is sensitive to heat. Therefore, it should not be autoclaved when it is desirable to sterilize the exterior of the vial.

Following prolonged therapy, withdrawal of corticosteroids may result in symptoms of the corticosteroid withdrawal syndrome including fever, myalgia, arthralgia, and malaise. This may occur in patients even without evidence of adrenal insufficiency.

There is an enhanced effect of corticosteroids in patients with hypothyroidism and in those with cirrhosis.

Corticosteroids should be used cautiously in patients with ocular herpes simplex for fear of corneal perforation.

Psychic derangements may appear when corticosteroids are used, ranging from euphoria, insomnia, mood swings, personality changes, and severe depression to frank psychotic manifestations. Also, existing emotional instability or psychotic tendencies may be aggravated by corticosteroids.

Aspirin should be used cautiously in conjunction with corticosteroids in hypoprothrombinemia.

Steroids should be used with caution in nonspecific ulcerative colitis, if there is a probability of impending perforation, abscess, or other pyogenic infection, also in diverticulitis, fresh intestinal anastomoses, active or latent peptic ulcer, renal insufficiency, hypertension, osteoporosis, and myasthenia gravis. Signs of peritoneal irritation following gastrointestinal perforation in patients receiving large doses of corticosteroids may be minimal or absent. Fat embolism has been reported as a possible complication of hypercortisonism.

When large doses are given, some authorities advise that antacids be administered between meals to help to prevent peptic ulcer.

Growth and development of infants and children on prolonged corticosteroid therapy should be carefully followed.

Steroids may increase or decrease motility and number of spermatozoa in some patients.

Phenytoin, phenobarbital, ephedrine, and rifampin may enhance the metabolic clearance of corticosteroids, resulting in decreased blood levels and lessened physiologic activity, thus requiring adjustment in corticosteroid dosage.

The prothrombin time should be checked frequently in patients who are receiving corticosteroids and coumarin anticoagulants at the same time because of reports that corticosteroids have altered the response to these anticoagulants. Studies have shown that the usual effect produced by adding corticosteroids is inhibition of response to coumarins, although there have been some conflicting reports of potentiation not substantiated by studies.

When corticosteroids are administered concomitantly with potassium-depleting diuretics, patients should be observed closely for development of hypokalemia.

Intra-articular injection of a corticosteroid may produce systemic as well as local effects.

Appropriate examination of any joint fluid present is necessary to exclude a septic process.

A marked increase in pain accompanied by local swelling, further restriction of joint motion, fever, and malaise is suggestive of septic arthritis. If this complication occurs and the diagnosis of sepsis is confirmed, appropriate antimicrobial therapy should be instituted.

Injection of a steroid into an infected site is to be avoided. Corticosteroids should not be injected into unstable joints.

Patients should be impressed strongly with the importance of not overusing joints in which symptomatic benefit has been obtained as long as the inflammatory process remains active.

Frequent intra-articular injection may result in damage to joint tissues.

Information for Patients

Susceptible patients who are on immunosuppressant doses of corticosteroids should be warned to avoid exposure to chickenpox or measles. Patients should also be advised that if they are exposed, medical advice should be sought without delay.

ADVERSE REACTIONS

Fluid and electrolyte disturbances
Sodium retention
Fluid retention
Congestive heart failure in susceptible patients
Potassium loss
Hypokalemic alkalosis
Hypertension
Musculoskeletal
Muscle weakness
Steroid myopathy
Loss of muscle mass
Osteoporosis
Vertebral compression fractures
Aseptic necrosis of femoral and humeral heads
Pathologic fracture of long bones
Tendon rupture
Gastrointestinal
Peptic ulcer with possible subsequent perforation and hemorrhage
Perforation of the small and large bowel, particularly in patients with inflammatory bowel disease
Pancreatitis
Abdominal distention
Ulcerative esophagitis
Dermatologic
Impaired wound healing
Thin fragile skin
Petechiae and ecchymoses
Erythema
Increased sweating
May suppress reactions to skin tests

Other cutaneous reactions, such as allergic dermatitis, urticaria, angioneurotic edema
Neurologic
Convulsions
Increased intracranial pressure with papilledema (pseudotumor cerebri) usually after treatment
Vertigo
Headache
Psychic disturbances
Endocrine
Menstrual irregularities
Development of cushingoid state
Suppression of growth in children
Secondary adrenocortical and pituitary unresponsiveness, particularly in times of stress, as in trauma, surgery, or illness
Decreased carbohydrate tolerance
Manifestations of latent diabetes mellitus
Increased requirements for insulin or oral hypoglycemic agents in diabetics
Hirsutism
Ophthalmic
Posterior subcapsular cataracts
Increased intraocular pressure
Glaucoma
Exophthalmos
Metabolic
Negative nitrogen balance due to protein catabolism
Cardiovascular
Myocardial rupture following recent myocardial infarction (see WARNINGS).
Other
Anaphylactoid or hypersensitivity reactions
Thromboembolism
Weight gain
Increased appetite
Nausea
Malaise

The following *additional* adverse reactions are related to parenteral corticosteroid therapy:
Rare instances of blindness associated with intralesional therapy around the face and head
Hyperpigmentation or hypopigmentation
Subcutaneous and cutaneous atrophy
Sterile abscess
Postinjection flare (following intra-articular use)
Charcot-like arthropathy
Scarring
Induration
Inflammation
Paresthesia
Delayed pain or soreness
Muscle twitching, ataxia, hiccups, and nystagmus have been reported in low incidence after injection of DECADRON-LA sterile suspension.

OVERDOSAGE

Reports of acute toxicity and/or death following overdosage of glucocorticoids are rare. In the event of overdosage, no specific antidote is available; treatment is supportive and symptomatic.

The intraperitoneal LD_{50} of dexamethasone acetate in female mice was 424 mg/kg.

DOSAGE AND ADMINISTRATION

For intramuscular, intralesional, intra-articular, and soft tissue injection.

Dosage Requirements Are Variable and Must Be Individualized on the Basis of the Disease and the Response of the Patient.

Dosage in children under 12 has not been established.

Intramuscular Injection
Dosage ranges from 1 to 2 mL, equivalent to 8 to 16 mg of dexamethasone. If further treatment is needed, dosage may be repeated at intervals of 1 to 3 weeks.

Intralesional Injection
The usual dose is 0.1 to 0.2 mL, equivalent to 0.8 to 1.6 mg of dexamethasone, per injection site.

Intra-articular and Soft Tissue Injection
The dose varies, depending on the location and the severity of inflammation. The usual dose is 0.5 to 2 mL, equivalent to 4 to 16 mg of dexamethasone. If further treatment is needed, dosage may be repeated at intervals of 1 to 3 weeks. Frequent intra-articular injection may result in damage to joint tissues.

HOW SUPPLIED

No. 7644—Sterile Suspension DECADRON-LA, 8 mg dexamethasone equivalent per mL, is a sterile white suspension, and is supplied as follows:
NDC 0006-7644-01 in 1 mL vials
NDC 0006-7644-03 in 5 mL vials.

Storage
Sensitive to heat. Do not autoclave.
Protect from freezing.
7498419   Issued October 1995

DECASPRAY® Topical Aerosol ℞
(Dexamethasone), U.S.P.

DESCRIPTION

Topical Aerosol DECASPRAY* (Dexamethasone) is a topical steroid preparation, each 25 g of which contains 10 mg of dexamethasone. The topical corticosteroids constitute a class of primarily synthetic steroids used as anti-inflammatory and anti-pruritic agents.

Dexamethasone is 9-fluoro-11β,17,21-trihydroxy-16α-methylpregna-1, 4-diene-3, 20 dione. Its empirical formula is $C_{22}H_{29}FO_5$ and its structural formula is:

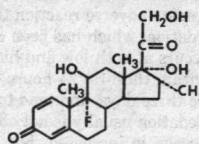

Dexamethasone has a molecular weight of 392.47.
The inactive ingredients are isopropyl myristate, and isobutane. Each second of spray dispenses approximately 0.075 mg of dexamethasone.

---

*Registered trademark of MERCK & CO., INC.

CLINICAL PHARMACOLOGY

Topical corticosteroids share anti-inflammatory, anti-pruritic, and vasoconstrictive actions.
The mechanism of anti-inflammatory activity of the topical corticosteroids is unclear. Various laboratory methods, including vasoconstrictor assays, are used to compare and predict potencies and/or clinical efficacies of the topical corticosteroids. There is some evidence to suggest that a recognizable correlation exists between vasoconstrictor potency and therapeutic efficacy in man.
Pharmacokinetics
The extent of percutaneous absorption of topical corticosteroids is determined by many factors including the vehicle, the integrity of the epidermal barrier, and the use of occlusive dressings.
Topical corticosteroids can be absorbed from normal intact skin. Inflammation and/or other disease processes in the skin increase percutaneous absorption. Occlusive dressings substantially increase the percutaneous absorption of topical corticosteroids. Thus, occlusive dressings may be a valuable therapeutic adjunct for treatment of resistant dermatoses. (See DOSAGE AND ADMINISTRATION.)
Once absorbed through the skin, topical corticosteroids are handled through pharmacokinetic pathways similar to systemically administered corticosteroids. Corticosteroids are bound to plasma proteins in varying degrees. Corticosteroids are metabolized primarily in the liver and are then excreted by the kidneys. Some of the topical corticosteroids and their metabolites are also excreted into the bile.

INDICATIONS AND USAGE

DECASPRAY Topical Aerosol is indicated for relief of the inflammatory and pruritic manifestations of corticosteroid-responsive dermatoses.

CONTRAINDICATIONS

Topical corticosteroids are contraindicated in those patients with a history of hypersensitivity to any of the components of the preparation.

WARNINGS

Avoid spraying in eyes or nose. Contents under pressure. Do not puncture or burn. Keep out of reach of children. Use only as directed. Intentional misuse by deliberately concentrating and inhaling the contents can be harmful or fatal.
Topically applied steroids are absorbed systemically. There may be rare instances in which this absorption results in immunosuppression. Patients who are on drugs which suppress the immune system are more susceptible to infections than healthy individuals. Chickenpox and measles, for example, can have a more serious or even fatal course in non-immune children or adults on corticosteroids. In such children or adults who have not had these diseases, particular care should be taken to avoid exposure. The risk of developing a disseminated infection varies among individuals and can be related to the dose, route and duration of corticosteroid administration as well as to the underlying disease. If exposed to chickenpox, prophylaxis with varicella zoster immune globulin (VZIG) may be indicated. If chickenpox develops, treatment with antiviral agents may be considered. If exposed to measles, prophylaxis with immune globulin (IG) may be indicated. (See the respective package inserts for VZIG and IG for complete prescribing information.)

PRECAUTIONS

General
Systemic absorption of topical corticosteroids has produced reversible hypothalamic-pituitary-adrenal (HPA) axis suppression, manifestations of Cushing's syndrome, hyperglycemia, and glycosuria in some patients.
Conditions which augment systemic absorption include the application of the more potent corticosteroids, use over large surface areas, prolonged use, and the addition of occlusive dressings.
Therefore, patients receiving a large dose of a potent topical corticosteroid applied to a large surface area or under an occlusive dressing should be evaluated periodically for evidence of HPA axis suppression by using urinary free cortisol and ACTH stimulation tests. If HPA axis suppression is noted, an attempt should be made to withdraw the drug, to reduce the frequency of application, or to substitute a less potent corticosteroid.
Recovery of HPA axis function is generally prompt and complete upon discontinuation of the drug. Infrequently, signs and symptoms of corticosteroid withdrawal may occur, requiring supplemental systemic corticosteroids.
Children may absorb proportionally larger amounts of topical corticosteroids and thus be more susceptible to systemic toxicity (See PRECAUTIONS, *Pediatric Use*).
If irritation develops, topical corticosteroids should be discontinued and appropriate therapy instituted.
In the presence of dermatological infections, the use of an appropriate antifungal or antibacterial agent should be instituted. If a favorable response does not occur promptly, the corticosteroid should be discontinued until the infection has been adequately controlled.
The product is not for ophthalmic use. However, if applied to the eyelids or skin near the eyes, the drug may enter the eyes. In patients with a history of herpes simplex keratitis ocular exposure to corticosteroids may lead to a recurrence. Prolonged ocular exposure may cause steroid glaucoma.
A few individuals may be sensitive to one or more of the components of this product. If any reaction indicating sensitivity is observed, discontinue use.
Generally, occlusive dressings should not be used on weeping or exudative lesions.
If occlusive dressing therapy is used, inspect lesions between dressings for development of infection. If infection develops, the technique should be discontinued and appropriate antimicrobial therapy instituted.
When large areas of the body are covered with an occlusive dressing, thermal homeostasis may be impaired. If elevation of body temperature occurs, use of the occlusive dressing should be discontinued.
CAUTION: Flammable. Do not use around open flame or while smoking.
Information for the Patient
Patients using topical corticosteroids should receive the following information and instructions:
1. This medication is to be used as directed by the physician. It is for external use only. Avoid contact with the eyes.
2. Patients should be advised not to use this medication for any disorder other than that for which it was prescribed.
3. The treated skin area should not be bandaged or otherwise covered or wrapped so as to be occlusive unless directed by the physician.
4. Patients should report any signs of local adverse reactions, especially under occlusive dressing.
5. Parents of pediatric patients should be advised not to use tight-fitting diapers or plastic pants on a child being treated in the diaper area, as these garments may constitute occlusive dressings.
6. Susceptible patients who are on immunosuppressant doses of corticosteroids should be warned to avoid exposure to chickenpox or measles. Patients should also be advised that if they are exposed, medical advice should be sought without delay.
Laboratory Tests
The following tests may be helpful in evaluating the HPA axis suppression:
• Urinary free cortisol test
• ACTH stimulation test
Carcinogenesis, Mutagenesis, and Impairment of Fertility
Long-term animal studies have not been performed to evaluate the carcinogenic potential or the effect on fertility of topical corticosteroids.
Studies to determine mutagenicity with prednisolone and hydrocortisone have revealed negative results.
Pregnancy
Pregnancy Category C: Corticosteroids are generally teratogenic in laboratory animals when administered systemically at relatively low dosage levels. The more potent corticosteroids have been shown to be teratogenic after dermal application in laboratory animals. There are no adequate and well-controlled studies in pregnant women on teratogenic effects from topically applied corticosteroids. Therefore, topical corticosteroids should be used during pregnancy only if the potential benefit justifies the potential risk to the fetus. Drugs of this class should not be used extensively on pregnant patients, in large amounts, or for prolonged periods of time.
Nursing Mothers
It is not known whether topical administration of corticosteroids could result in sufficient systemic absorption to produce detectable quantities in breast milk. Systemically administered corticosteroids are secreted into breast milk in quantities *not* likely to have a deleterious effect on the infant. Nevertheless, caution should be exercised when topical corticosteroids are administered to a nursing woman.
Pediatric Use
Pediatric patients may demonstrate greater susceptibility to topical corticosteroid-induced HPA axis suppression and Cushing's syndrome than mature patients because of a larger skin surface area to body weight ratio.
Hypothalamic-pituitary-adrenal (HPA) axis suppression, Cushing's syndrome, and intracranial hypertension have been reported in children receiving topical corticosteroids. Manifestations of adrenal suppression in children include linear growth retardation, delayed weight gain, low plasma cortisol levels, and absence of response to ACTH stimulation. Manifestations of intracranial hypertension include bulging fontanelles, headaches, and bilateral papilledema.
Administration of topical corticosteroids to children should be limited to the least amount compatible with an effective therapeutic regimen. Chronic corticosteroid therapy may interfere with the growth and development of children.

ADVERSE REACTIONS

The following adverse reactions are reported infrequently with topical corticosteroids, but may occur more frequently with the use of occlusive dressings. These reactions are listed in an approximate decreasing order of occurrence:

Burning
Itching
Irritation
Dryness
Folliculitis
Hypertrichosis
Acneiform eruptions
Hypopigmentation
Perioral dermatitis
Allergic contact dermatitis
Maceration of the skin
Secondary infection
Skin atrophy
Striae
Miliaria

OVERDOSAGE

Topically applied corticosteroids can be absorbed in sufficient amounts to produce systemic effects (See PRECAUTIONS).

DOSAGE AND ADMINISTRATION

Patients should be instructed in the correct way to use DECASPRAY. The preparation is readily applied, even on hairy areas. It does not have to be rubbed into the skin.
Optimal effects will be obtained with DECASPRAY when these directions are followed:
1. Keep the affected area clean to reduce the possibility of infection.
2. Shake the container *gently* once or twice each time before using. Hold it about six inches from the area to be treated. Effective medication may be obtained with the container held either upright or inverted, since it is fitted with a special valve that dispenses approximately the same dosage in either position.
3. Spray each four inch square of affected area for one or two seconds three or four times a day, depending on the nature of the condition and the response to therapy.
4. When a favorable response is obtained, reduce dosage gradually and eventually discontinue.
5. Occlusive dressings may be used for the management of psoriasis or recalcitrant conditions.

Continued on next page

Information on the Merck & Co., Inc. products listed on these pages is the full prescribing information from product circulars in use September 30, 1996.

Merck & Co.—Cont.

HOW SUPPLIED

No. 7623X—DECASPRAY is supplied as follows:
NDC 0006-7623-25 in a 25 g pressurized container.
DC 7413319 Issued April 1993

COPYRIGHT © MERCK & CO., INC., 1983
All rights reserved

DEMSER® Capsules ℞
(Metyrosine), U.S.P.

DESCRIPTION

DEMSER* (Metyrosine) is (−)-α-methyl-*L*-tyrosine or (α-MPT). It has the following structural formula:

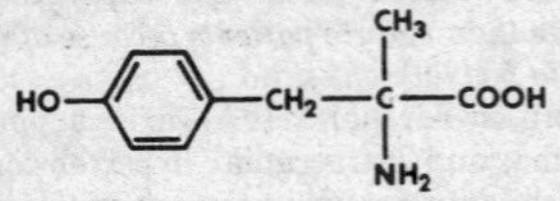

Metyrosine is a white, crystalline compound of molecular weight 195. It is very slightly soluble in water, acetone, and methanol, and insoluble in chloroform and benzene. It is soluble in acidic aqueous solutions. It is also soluble in alkaline aqueous solutions, but is subject to oxidative degradation under these conditions.
DEMSER is supplied as capsules, for oral administration. Each capsule contains 250 mg metyrosine. Inactive ingredients are colloidal silicon dioxide, gelatin, hydroxypropyl cellulose, magnesium stearate, and titanium dioxide. The capsules may also contain any combination of D&C Red 33, D&C Yellow 10, FD&C Blue 1, and FD&C Blue 2.

*Registered trademark of MERCK & CO., INC.

CLINICAL PHARMACOLOGY

DEMSER inhibits tyrosine hydroxylase, which catalyzes the first transformation in catecholamine biosynthesis, i.e., the conversion of tyrosine to dihydroxyphenylalanine (DOPA). Because the first step is also the rate-limiting step, blockade of tyrosine hydroxylase activity results in decreased endogenous levels of catecholamines, usually measured as decreased urinary excretion of catecholamines and their metabolites.
In patients with pheochromocytoma, who produce excessive amounts of norepinephrine and epinephrine, administration of one to four grams of DEMSER per day has reduced catecholamine biosynthesis from about 35 to 80 percent as measured by the total excretion of catecholamines and their metabolites (metanephrine and vanillylmandelic acid). The maximum biochemical effect usually occurs within two to three days, and the urinary concentration of catecholamines and their metabolites usually returns to pretreatment levels within three to four days after DEMSER is discontinued. In some patients the total excretion of catecholamines and catecholamine metabolites may be lowered to normal or near normal levels (less than 10 mg/24 hours). In most patients the duration of treatment has been two to eight weeks, but several patients have received DEMSER for periods of one to 10 years.
Most patients with pheochromocytoma treated with DEMSER experience decreased frequency and severity of hypertensive attacks with their associated headache, nausea, sweating, and tachycardia. In patients who respond, blood pressure decreases progressively during the first two days of therapy with DEMSER; after withdrawal, blood pressure usually increases gradually to pretreatment values within two to three days.
Metyrosine is well absorbed from the gastrointestinal tract. From 53 to 88 percent (mean 69 percent) was recovered in the urine as unchanged drug following maintenance oral doses of 600 to 4000 mg/24 hours in patients with pheochromocytoma or essential hypertension. Less than 1% of the dose was recovered as catechol metabolites. These metabolites are probably not present in sufficient amounts to contribute to the biochemical effects of metyrosine. The quantities excreted, however, are sufficient to interfere with accurate determination of urinary catecholamines determined by routine techniques.
Plasma half-life of metyrosine determined over an 8-hour period after single oral doses was 3.4–3.7 hours in three patients.
For further information, refer to: Sjoerdsma, A.; Engelman, K.; Waldman, T. A.; Cooperman, L. H.; Hammond, W. G.: Pheochromocytoma: Current concepts of diagnosis and treatment, Ann. Intern. Med. *65:* 1302–1326, Dec. 1966.

INDICATIONS AND USAGE

DEMSER is indicated in the treatment of patients with pheochromocytoma for:
1. Preoperative preparation of patients for surgery
2. Management of patients when surgery is contraindicated
3. Chronic treatment of patients with malignant pheochromocytoma.

DEMSER is not recommended for the control of essential hypertension.

CONTRAINDICATIONS

DEMSER is contraindicated in persons known to be hypersensitive to this compound.

WARNINGS

Maintain Fluid Volume During and After Surgery
When DEMSER is used preoperatively, alone or especially in combination with alpha-adrenergic blocking drugs, adequate intravascular volume must be maintained intraoperatively (especially after tumor removal) and postoperatively to avoid hypotension and decreased perfusion of vital organs resulting from vasodilatation and expanded volume capacity. Following tumor removal, large volumes of plasma may be needed to maintain blood pressure and central venous pressure within the normal range.
In addition, life-threatening arrhythmias may occur during anesthesia and surgery, and may require treatment with a beta blocker or lidocaine. During surgery, patients should have continuous monitoring of blood pressure and electrocardiogram.
Intraoperative Effects
While the preoperative use of DEMSER in patients with pheochromocytoma is thought to decrease intraoperative problems with blood pressure control, DEMSER does not eliminate the danger of hypertensive crises or arrhythmias during manipulation of the tumor, and the alpha-adrenergic blocking drug, phentolamine, may be needed.
Interaction with Alcohol
DEMSER may add to the sedative effects of alcohol and other CNS depressants, e.g., hypnotics, sedatives, and tranquilizers. (See PRECAUTIONS, *Information for Patients and Drug Interactions.*)

PRECAUTIONS

General
Metyrosine Crystalluria: **Crystalluria and urolithiasis have been found in dogs treated with DEMSER (Metyrosine) at doses similar to those used in humans, and crystalluria has also been observed in a few patients. To minimize the risk of crystalluria, patients should be urged to maintain water intake sufficient to achieve a daily urine volume of 2000 mL or more, particularly when doses greater than 2 g per day are given. Routine examination of the urine should be carried out. Metyrosine will crystallize as needles or rods. If metyrosine crystalluria occurs, fluid intake should be increased further. If crystalluria persists, the dosage should be reduced or the drug discontinued.**
Relatively Little Data Regarding Long-term Use: The total human experience with the drug is quite limited and few patients have been studied long-term. Chronic animal studies have not been carried out. Therefore, suitable laboratory tests should be carried out periodically in patients requiring prolonged use of DEMSER and caution should be observed in patients with impaired hepatic or renal function.
Information for Patients
When receiving DEMSER, patients should be warned about engaging in activities requiring mental alertness and motor coordination, such as driving a motor vehicle or operating machinery. DEMSER may have additive sedative effects with alcohol and other CNS depressants, e.g., hypnotics, sedatives, and tranquilizers.
Patients should be advised to maintain a liberal fluid intake. (See PRECAUTIONS, *General.*)
Drug Interactions
Caution should be observed in administering DEMSER to patients receiving phenothiazines or haloperidol because the extrapyramidal effects of these drugs can be expected to be potentiated by inhibition of catecholamine synthesis.
Concurrent use of DEMSER with alcohol or other CNS depressants can increase their sedative effects. (See WARNINGS and PRECAUTIONS, *Information for Patients.*)
Laboratory Test Interference
Spurious increases in urinary catecholamines may be observed in patients receiving DEMSER due to the presence of metabolites of the drug.
Carcinogenesis, Mutagenesis, Impairment of Fertility
Long-term carcinogenic studies in animals and studies on mutagenesis and impairment of fertility have not been performed with metyrosine.
Pregnancy
Pregnancy Category C. Animal reproduction studies have not been conducted with DEMSER. It is also not known whether DEMSER can cause fetal harm when administered to a pregnant woman or can affect reproduction capacity. DEMSER should be given to a pregnant woman only if clearly needed.
Nursing Mothers
It is not known whether DEMSER is excreted in human milk. Because many drugs are excreted in human milk, caution should be exercised when DEMSER is administered to a nursing woman.
Pediatric Use
Safety and effectiveness in children under 12 years of age have not been established.

ADVERSE REACTIONS

Central Nervous System
Sedation: The most common adverse reaction to DEMSER is moderate to severe sedation, which has been observed in almost all patients. It occurs at both low and high dosages. Sedative effects begin within the first 24 hours of therapy, are maximal after two to three days, and tend to wane during the next few days. Sedation usually is not obvious after one week unless the dosage is increased, but at dosages greater than 2000 mg/day some degree of sedation or fatigue may persist.
In most patients who experience sedation, temporary changes in sleep pattern occur following withdrawal of the drug. Changes consist of insomnia that may last for two or three days and feelings of increased alertness and ambition. Even patients who do not experience sedation while on DEMSER may report symptoms of psychic stimulation when the drug is discontinued.
Extrapyramidal Signs: Extrapyramidal signs such as drooling, speech difficulty, and tremor have been reported in approximately 10 percent of patients. These occasionally have been accompanied by trismus and frank parkinsonism.
Anxiety and Psychic Disturbances: Anxiety and psychic disturbances such as depression, hallucinations, disorientation, and confusion may occur. These effects seem to be dose-dependent and may disappear with reduction of dosage.
Diarrhea
Diarrhea occurs in about 10 percent of patients and may be severe. Anti-diarrheal agents may be required if continuation of DEMSER is necessary.
Miscellaneous
Infrequently, slight swelling of the breast, galactorrhea, nasal stuffiness, decreased salivation, dry mouth, headache, nausea, vomiting, abdominal pain, and impotence or failure of ejaculation may occur. Crystalluria (see PRECAUTIONS) and transient dysuria and hematuria have been observed in a few patients. Hematologic disorders (including eosinophilia, anemia, thrombocytopenia, and thrombocytosis), increased SGOT levels, peripheral edema, and hypersensitivity reactions such as urticaria and pharyngeal edema have been reported rarely.

OVERDOSAGE

Signs of metyrosine overdosage include those central nervous system effects observed in some patients even at low dosages.
At doses exceeding 2000 mg/day, some degree of sedation or feeling of fatigue may persist. Doses of 2000–4000 mg/day can result in anxiety or agitated depression, neuromuscular effects (including fine tremor of the hands, gross tremor of the trunk, tightening of the jaw with trismus), diarrhea, and decreased salivation with dry mouth.
Reduction of drug dose or cessation of treatment results in the disappearance of these symptoms.
The acute toxicity of metyrosine was 442 mg/kg and 752 mg/kg in the female mouse and rat respectively.

DOSAGE AND ADMINISTRATION

The recommended initial dosage of DEMSER for adults and children 12 years of age and older is 250 mg orally four times daily. This may be increased by 250 mg to 500 mg every day to a maximum of 4.0 g/day in divided doses. When used for preoperative preparation, the optimally effective dosage of DEMSER should be given for at least five to seven days.
Optimally effective dosages of DEMSER usually are between 2.0 and 3.0 g/day, and the dose should be titrated by monitoring clinical symptoms and catecholamine excretion. In patients who are hypertensive, dosage should be titrated to achieve normalization of blood pressure and control of clinical symptoms. In patients who are usually normotensive, dosage should be titrated to the amount that will reduce urinary metanephrines and/or vanillylmandelic acid by 50 percent or more.
If patients are not adequately controlled by the use of DEMSER, an alpha-adrenergic blocking agent (phenoxybenzamine) should be added.

Use of DEMSER in children under 12 years of age has been limited and a dosage schedule for this age group cannot be given.

HOW SUPPLIED

No. 3355—Capsules DEMSER, 250 mg, are opaque, two-toned blue capsules coded MSD 690 on one side and DEMSER on the other. They are supplied as follows:
NDC 0006-0690-68 bottles of 100.
Shown in Product Identification Guide, page 324
7900806 Issued September 1985
COPYRIGHT© MERCK & CO., INC., 1985
All rights reserved

DIUPRES® Tablets ℞
(Reserpine-Chlorothiazide), U.S.P.

<table>
<tr><td>

WARNING

This fixed combination drug is not indicated for initial therapy of hypertension. Hypertension requires therapy titrated to the individual patient. If the fixed combination represents the dosage so determined, its use may be more convenient in patient management. The treatment of hypertension is not static, but must be re-evaluated as conditions in each patient warrant.

</td></tr>
</table>

DESCRIPTION

DIUPRES* (Reserpine-Chlorothiazide) combines two antihypertensives: DIURIL* (Chlorothiazide) and reserpine.
Chlorothiazide
Chlorothiazide is a diuretic and antihypertensive. Its chemical name is 6-chloro-2H-1,2,4-benzothiadiazine-7-sulfonamide 1,1-dioxide. Its empirical formula is $C_7H_6ClN_3O_4S_2$ and its structural formula is:

Chlorothiazide is a white, or practically white, crystalline powder with a molecular weight of 295.73, which is very slightly soluble in water, but readily soluble in dilute aqueous sodium hydroxide. It is soluble in urine to the extent of about 150 mg per 100 mL at pH 7.
Reserpine
The chemical name of reserpine is 11,17α-dimethoxy-18β-[(3, 4, 5-trimethoxybenzoyl)oxy] -3β,20α-yohimban- 16 β-carboxylic acid methylester. It is a crystalline alkaloid derived from Rauwolfia serpentina. Its empirical formula is $C_{33}H_{40}N_2O_9$ and its structural formula is:

Reserpine is a white or pale buff to slightly yellowish, odorless, crystalline powder with a molecular weight of 608.69, is insoluble in water and freely soluble in glacial acetic acid. DIUPRES is supplied as tablets in two strengths for oral use:
DIUPRES-250*, contains 250 mg of chlorothiazide and 0.125 mg of reserpine.
DIUPRES-500*, contains 500 mg of chlorothiazide and 0.125 mg of reserpine.
Each tablet contains the following inactive ingredients: FD&C Red 3, gelatin, lactose, magnesium stearate, starch and talc.

---

*Registered trademark of MERCK & CO., INC.

CLINICAL PHARMACOLOGY

Chlorothiazide
The mechanism of the antihypertensive effect of thiazides is unknown. Chlorothiazide does not usually affect normal blood pressure.
Chlorothiazide affects the distal renal tubular mechanism of electrolyte reabsorption. At maximal therapeutic dosage all thiazides are approximately equal in their diuretic efficacy.

Chlorothiazide increases excretion of sodium and chloride in approximately equivalent amounts. Natriuresis may be accompanied by some loss of potassium and bicarbonate. After oral use diuresis begins within 2 hours, peaks in about 4 hours and lasts about 6 to 12 hours.
Reserpine
Reserpine has antihypertensive, bradycardic, and tranquilizing properties. It lowers arterial blood pressure by depletion of catecholamines. Reserpine is beneficial in relieving anxiety, tension, and headache in the hypertensive patient. It acts at the hypothalamic level of the central nervous system to promote relaxation without hypnosis or analgesia. The sleep pattern shown by the electroencephalogram following barbiturates does not occur with this drug. In laboratory animals spontaneous activity and response to external stimuli are decreased, but confusion or difficulty of movement is not evident.
The bradycardic action of reserpine promotes relaxation and may eliminate sinus tachycardia. It is most pronounced in subjects with sinus tachycardia and usually is not prominent in persons with a normal pulse rate.
Miosis, relaxation of the nictitating membrane, ptosis, hypothermia, and increased gastrointestinal activity are noted in animals given reserpine, sometimes in subclinical doses. None of these effects, except increased gastrointestinal activity, has been found to be clinically significant in man with therapeutic doses.
Pharmacokinetics and Metabolism
Chlorothiazide
Chlorothiazide is not metabolized but is eliminated rapidly by the kidney. The plasma half-life of chlorothiazide is 45-120 minutes. After oral doses, 10-15 percent is excreted unchanged in the urine. Chlorothiazide crosses the placental but not the blood-brain barrier and is excreted in breast milk.
Reserpine
Oral reserpine is rapidly absorbed from the gastrointestinal tract. Methylreserpate and trimethoxybenzoic acid are the primary metabolites which result from the hydrolytic cleavage of reserpine. Maximal blood levels are achieved approximately 2 hours after the oral dosage of ^{3}H-reserpine to six normal volunteers; within 96 hours approximately 8 percent was excreted in urine and 62 percent in feces. Reserpine appears in human breast milk. Reserpine crosses the placental barrier in guinea pigs.

INDICATIONS AND USAGE

Hypertension (see box warning).

CONTRAINDICATIONS

Chlorothiazide is contraindicated in anuria.
DIUPRES is contraindicated in hypersensitivity to chlorothiazide or other sulfonamide-derived drugs or to reserpine.
Electroshock therapy should not be given to patients while on reserpine, as severe and even fatal reactions have been reported with minimal convulsive electroshock dosage. After discontinuing reserpine, allow at least seven days before starting electroshock therapy.
Reserpine is contraindicated in patients:
—with active peptic ulcer
—with ulcerative colitis
—with a history of mental depression, especially suicidal tendencies.
—on therapy with monoamine oxidase (MAO) inhibitors.

WARNINGS

Chlorothiazide
Use with caution in severe renal disease. In patients with renal disease, thiazides may precipitate azotemia. Cumulative effects of the drug may develop in patients with impaired renal function.
Thiazides should be used with caution in patients with impaired hepatic function or progressive liver disease, since minor alterations of fluid and electrolyte balance may precipitate hepatic coma.
Thiazides may add to or potentiate the action of other antihypertensive drugs.
Sensitivity reactions may occur in patients with or without a history of allergy or bronchial asthma.
The possibility of exacerbation or activation of systemic lupus erythematosus has been reported.
Lithium generally should not be given with diuretics (see PRECAUTIONS, *Drug Interactions*).
Reserpine
Reserpine may cause mental depression. Recognition of depression may be difficult because this condition may often be disguised by somatic complaints (masked depression). The drug should be discontinued at first signs of depression such as despondency, early morning insomnia, loss of appetite, impotence or self-deprecation. Drug-induced depression may persist for several months after drug withdrawal and may be severe enough to result in suicide.

The occurrence of mental depression due to reserpine in doses of 0.25 mg daily or less is unusual. In any event, DIUPRES should be discontinued at the first sign of depression.

PRECAUTIONS

General
Chlorothiazide
All patients receiving diuretic therapy should be observed for evidence of fluid or electrolyte imbalance: namely, hyponatremia, hypochloremic alkalosis, and hypokalemia. Serum and urine electrolyte determinations are particularly important when the patient is vomiting excessively or receiving parenteral fluids. Warning signs or symptoms of fluid and electrolyte imbalance, irrespective of cause, include dryness of mouth, thirst, weakness, lethargy, drowsiness, restlessness, confusion, seizures, muscle pains or cramps, muscular fatigue, hypotension, oliguria, tachycardia, and gastrointestinal disturbances such as nausea and vomiting.
Hypokalemia may develop, especially with brisk diuresis, when severe cirrhosis is present or after prolonged therapy. Interference with adequate oral electrolyte intake will contribute to hypokalemia. Hypokalemia may cause cardiac arrhythmia and may also sensitize or exaggerate the response of the heart to the toxic effects of digitalis (e.g., increased ventricular irritability). Hypokalemia may be avoided or treated by use of potassium sparing diuretics or potassium supplements such as foods with a high potassium content.
Although any chloride deficit is generally mild and usually does not require specific treatment except under extraordinary circumstances (as in liver disease or renal disease), chloride replacement may be required in the treatment of metabolic alkalosis.
Dilutional hyponatremia may occur in edematous patients in hot weather. Appropriate therapy is water restriction, rather than administration of salt, except in rare instances when the hyponatremia is life threatening. In actual salt depletion, appropriate replacement is the therapy of choice.
Hyperuricemia may occur or acute gout may be precipitated in certain patients receiving thiazides.
In diabetic patients dosage adjustments of insulin or oral hypoglycemic agents may be required. Hyperglycemia may occur with thiazide diuretics. Thus latent diabetes mellitus may become manifest during thiazide therapy.
The antihypertensive effect of the drug may be enhanced in the postsympathectomy patient.
If progressive renal impairment becomes evident, consider withholding or discontinuing diuretic therapy.
Thiazides have been shown to increase the urinary excretion of magnesium; this may result in hypomagnesemia.
Thiazides may decrease urinary calcium excretion. Thiazides may cause intermittent and slight elevation of serum calcium in the absence of known disorders of calcium metabolism. Marked hypercalcemia may be evidence of hidden hyperparathyroidism. Thiazides should be discontinued before carrying out tests for parathyroid function.
Increases in cholesterol and triglyceride levels may be associated with thiazide diuretic therapy.
Reserpine
Since reserpine may increase gastric secretion and motility, it should be used cautiously in patients with a history of peptic ulcer, ulcerative colitis, or other gastrointestinal disorder. This compound may precipitate biliary colic in patients with gallstones, or bronchial asthma in susceptible persons. Reserpine may cause hypotension including orthostatic hypotension.
Anxiety or depression, as well as psychosis, may develop during reserpine therapy. If depression is present when therapy is begun, it may be aggravated. Mental depression is unusual with reserpine doses of 0.25 mg daily or less. In any case, DIUPRES should be discontinued at the first sign of depression. Extreme caution should be used in treating patients with a history of mental depression, and the possibility of suicide should be kept in mind.
As with most antihypertensive therapy, caution should be exercised when treating hypertensive patients with renal insufficiency, since they adjust poorly to lowered blood pressure.
When two or more antihypertensives are given, the individual dosages may have to be reduced to prevent excessive drop in blood pressure. In hypertensive patients with coronary artery disease, it is important to avoid a precipitous drop in blood pressure.

Continued on next page

Merck & Co.—Cont.

Laboratory Tests
Periodic determination of serum electrolytes to detect possible electrolyte imbalance should be done at appropriate intervals.
Drug Interactions
Chlorothiazide
When given concurrently the following drugs may interact with thiazide diuretics.
Alcohol, barbiturates, or narcotics—potentiation of orthostatic hypotension may occur.
Antidiabetic drugs (oral agents and insulin)—dosage adjustment of the antidiabetic drug may be required.
Other antihypertensive drugs—additive effect or potentiation.
Cholestyramine and colestipol resins—Both cholestyramine and colestipol resins have the potential of binding thiazide diuretics and reducing diuretic absorption from the gastrointestinal tract.
Corticosteroids, ACTH—intensified electrolyte depletion, particularly hypokalemia.
Pressor amines (e.g., norepinephrine)—possible decreased response to pressor amines but not sufficient to preclude their use.
Skeletal muscle relaxants, nondepolarizing (e.g., tubocurarine)—possible increased responsiveness to the muscle relaxant.
Lithium—generally should not be given with diuretics. Diuretic agents reduce the renal clearance of lithium and add a high risk of lithium toxicity. Refer to the package insert for lithium preparations before use of such preparations with DIUPRES.
Non-steroidal Anti-inflammatory Drugs—In some patients, the administration of a non-steroidal anti-inflammatory agent can reduce the diuretic, natriuretic, and antihypertensive effects of loop, potassium-sparing and thiazide diuretics. Therefore, when DIUPRES and non-steroidal anti-inflammatory agents are used concomitantly, the patient should be observed closely to determine if the desired effect of the diuretic is obtained.
Reserpine
In hypertensive patients on reserpine therapy significant hypotension and bradycardia may develop during surgical anesthesia. The anesthesiologist should be aware that reserpine has been taken, since it may be necessary to give vagal blocking agents parenterally to prevent or reverse hypotension and/or bradycardia.
Use reserpine cautiously with digitalis and quinidine; cardiac arrhythmias have occurred with reserpine preparations.
Barbiturates enhance the central nervous system depressant effects of reserpine.
Monoamine oxidase (MAO) inhibitors: see CONTRAINDICATIONS.
Drug/Laboratory Test Interactions
Thiazides should be discontinued before carrying out tests for parathyroid function (see PRECAUTIONS, *General*).
Carcinogenesis, Mutagenesis, Impairment of Fertility
Carcinogenicity and mutagenicity studies have not been conducted with combinations of reserpine/chlorothiazide.
In a two-litter study in the rat at an oral dose of 50.0/0.025 mg/kg, the combination of chlorothiazide/reserpine did not impair fertility or produce abnormalities in the fetus.
Chlorothiazide
Carcinogenicity studies have not been done with chlorothiazide.
Chlorothiazide was not mutagenic *in vitro* in the Ames microbial mutagen test (using a maximum concentration of 5 mg/plate and *Salmonella typhimurium* strains TA 98 and TA 100) and was not mutagenic and did not induce mitotic nondisjunction in diploid-strains of *Aspergillus nidulans*.
Chlorothiazide had no adverse effects on fertility in female rats at doses up to 60 mg/kg/day and no adverse effects on fertility in male rats at doses up to 40 mg/kg/day.
Reserpine
Reserpine at a concentration of 1 to 5000 mcg/plate had no mutagenic activity against four strains of *S. typhimurium in vitro* in the Ames microbial mutagen test with or without metabolic activation. Reserpine did not induce malignant transformation of mouse fibroblasts *in vitro* at concentrations of 0.3 to 10 mcg/mL.
A few chromosomal aberrations were induced by reserpine *in vitro* in cultured mouse mammary carcinoma cells but were considered negative in this study. The drug did not produce chromosomal aberrations in human peripheral leucocyte cultures although an increase in mitotic figures occurred. One study reported chromosomal aberrations and dominant lethal mutations in mice at doses up to 10 mg/kg of reserpine in the form of a pharmaceutical preparation. Another study did not show dominant lethal mutations in mice at IP doses of 0.92 and 4.6 mg/kg of reserpine.
Reserpine did not impair fertility in a two-litter study in the rat at an oral dose of 0.025 mg/kg.

Rodent studies have shown that reserpine is an animal tumorigen, causing an increased incidence of mammary fibroadenomas in female mice, malignant tumors of the seminal vesicle in male mice, and malignant adrenal medullary tumors in male rats. These findings arose in two year studies in which the drug was administered in the feed at concentrations of 5 and 10 ppm—about 100 to 300 times the usual human dose. The breast neoplasms are thought to be related to reserpine's prolactin-elevating effect. Several other prolactin-elevating drugs have also been associated with an increased incidence of mammary neoplasia in rodents.
The extent to which these findings indicate a risk to humans is uncertain. Tissue culture experiments show that about one-third of human breast tumors are prolactin-dependent *in vitro*, a factor of considerable importance if the use of the drug is contemplated in a patient with previously detected breast cancer. The possibility of an increased risk of breast cancer in reserpine users has been studied extensively; however, no firm conclusion has emerged. Although a few epidemiologic studies have suggested a slightly increased risk (less than twofold in all studies except one) in women who have used reserpine, other studies of generally similar design have not confirmed this. Epidemiologic studies conducted using other drugs (neuroleptic agents) that, like reserpine, increase prolactin levels and therefore would be considered rodent mammary carcinogens, have not shown an association between chronic administration of the drug and human mammary tumorigenesis. While long-term clinical observation has not suggested such an association, the available evidence is considered too limited to be conclusive at this time. An association of reserpine intake with pheochromocytoma or tumors of the seminal vesicles has not been explored.
Pregnancy
Use of diuretics during normal pregnancy is inappropriate and exposes mother and fetus to unnecessary hazard. Diuretics do not prevent development of toxemia of pregnancy and there is no satisfactory evidence that they are useful in the treatment of toxemia.
Teratogenic Effects—Pregnancy Category C: There are no adequate and well-controlled studies with DIUPRES or other combinations of reserpine/chlorothiazide in animals or pregnant women. DIUPRES may cause fetal harm when given to a pregnant woman. DIUPRES should be used during pregnancy only if the potential benefit justifies the potential risk to the fetus.
Reserpine: Reproduction studies in rats have shown that reserpine is teratogenic at doses of 1-2 mg/kg (125–250 times the maximum recommended human dose) IM or IP given early in pregnancy. A variety of abnormalities was produced including anophthalmia, absence of the axial skeleton, hydronephrosis, etc. Pregnancy in rabbits was interrupted when doses as low as 0.04 mg/kg (10 times the maximum recommended human dose) were given early or late in pregnancy.
Chlorothiazide: Thiazides cross the placental barrier and appear in cord blood.
Although reproduction studies performed with chlorothiazide doses of 50 mg/kg/day in rabbits, 60 mg/kg/day in rats and 500 mg/kg/day in mice revealed no external abnormalities of the fetus or impairment of growth and survival of the fetus due to chlorothiazide, such studies did not include complete examinations for visceral and skeletal abnormalities.
Nonteratogenic Effects
Reserpine: Reserpine has been demonstrated to cross the placental barrier in guinea pigs with depression of adrenal catecholamine stores in the newborn. There is some evidence that side effects such as nasal congestion, lethargy, depressed Moro reflex, and bradycardia may appear in infants born of reserpine-treated mothers.
Chlorothiazide: Chlorothiazide may cause fetal or neonatal jaundice, thrombocytopenia, and possibly other adverse reactions which have occurred in the adult.
Nursing Mothers
Thiazides and reserpine appear in breast milk. Because of the potential for serious adverse reactions in nursing infants from DIUPRES, a decision should be made whether to discontinue nursing or to discontinue the drug, taking into account the importance of the drug to the mother.
Pediatric Use
Safety and effectiveness of DIUPRES in pediatric patients have not been established.

ADVERSE REACTIONS

The following adverse reactions have been reported and, within each category, are listed in order of decreasing severity.
Chlorothiazide
Body as a Whole: Weakness.
Cardiovascular: Hypotension including orthostatic hypotension (may be aggravated by alcohol, barbiturates, narcotics or antihypertensive drugs).
Digestive: Pancreatitis, jaundice (intrahepatic cholestatic jaundice), diarrhea, vomiting, sialadenitis, cramping, constipation, gastric irritation, nausea, anorexia.

Hematologic: Aplastic anemia, agranulocytosis, leukopenia, hemolytic anemia, thrombocytopenia.
Hypersensitivity: Anaphylactic reactions, necrotizing angiitis (vasculitis and cutaneous vasculitis), respiratory distress including pneumonitis and pulmonary edema, photosensitivity, fever, urticaria, rash, purpura.
Metabolic: Electrolyte imbalance (see PRECAUTIONS), hyperglycemia, glycosuria, hyperuricemia.
Musculoskeletal: Muscle spasm.
Nervous System/Psychiatric: Vertigo, paresthesias, dizziness, headache, restlessness.
Renal: Renal failure, renal dysfunction, interstitial nephritis. (See WARNINGS.)
Skin: Erythema multiforme including Stevens-Johnson syndrome, exfoliative dermatitis including toxic epidermal necrolysis, alopecia.
Special Senses: Transient blurred vision, xanthopsia.
Urogenital: Impotence.
Reserpine
Cardiovascular: Angina pectoris, arrhythmia, premature ventricular contractions, other direct cardiac effects (e.g., fluid retention, congestive heart failure), bradycardia.
Digestive: Vomiting, diarrhea, nausea, hypersecretion and increased motility, anorexia, dryness of mouth, increased salivation.
Hematologic: Thrombocytopenic purpura, excessive bleeding following prostatic surgery.
Hypersensitivity: Pruritis, rash, flushing of skin.
Metabolic: Weight gain.
Musculoskeletal: Muscular aches.
Nervous System/Psychiatric: Mental depression, dull sensorium, syncope, paradoxical anxiety, excessive sedation, nightmares, headache, dizziness, nervousness, parkinsonism (usually reversible with decreased dosage or discontinuance of therapy).
Respiratory: Dyspnea, epistaxis, nasal congestion, enhanced susceptibility to colds.
Special Senses: Optic atrophy, uveitis, deafness, glaucoma, conjunctival injection, blurred vision.
Urogenital: Dysuria, impotence, decreased libido, nonpuerperal lactation.

OVERDOSAGE

Overdosage may lead to excessive sedation, mental depression, severe hypotension, extrapyramidal reactions.
There is no specific antidote. In the event of overdosage, symptomatic and supportive measures should be employed. Emesis should be induced or gastric lavage performed. Correct dehydration, electrolyte imbalance, hepatic coma and hypotension by established procedures. If required, give oxygen or artificial respiration for respiratory impairment. In the event of severe hypotension from the reserpine component, intravenous use of a vasopressor is indicated [e.g., ARAMINE* (Metaraminol Bitartrate), levarterenol, phenylephrine]. Anticholinergics may be needed to relieve gastrointestinal distress from reserpine. Because the effects of the rauwolfia alkaloids are prolonged, the patient should be closely observed for at least 72 hours.
Reserpine is not dialyzable. The degree to which chlorothiazide is removed by hemodialysis has not been established. The oral LD$_{50}$ of chlorothiazide is 8.5 g/kg, greater than 10 g/kg, and greater than 1 g/kg, in the mouse, rat and dog, respectively. The oral LD$_{50}$ of reserpine in the mouse is 390 mg/kg.

DOSAGE AND ADMINISTRATION

The initial dosage of DIUPRES should conform to the dosages of the individual components established during titration (see box warning).
The usual adult dosage of DIUPRES-250* is 1 or 2 tablets once or twice a day; that of DIUPRES-500* is 1 tablet once or twice a day.
Dosage may require adjustment according to the blood pressure response of the patient. For maintenance, dosage should be adjusted to the lowest requirement of the individual patient. Doses higher than 0.25 mg daily of reserpine should be used cautiously, because occurrence of serious mental depression and other side effects may increase considerably (see WARNINGS).

*Registered trademark of MERCK & CO., Inc.

HOW SUPPLIED

No. 3261—Tablets DIUPRES-250 are pink, round, scored, compressed tablets, coded MSD 230 on one side and DIUPRES on the other. Each tablet contains 250 mg of chlorothiazide and 0.125 mg of reserpine. They are supplied as follows:

NDC 0006-0230-68 in bottles of 100
NDC 0006-0230-82 in bottles of 1000.
Shown in Product Identification Guide, page 324
No. 3262—Tablets DIUPRES-500 are pink, round, scored, compressed tablets, coded MSD 405 on one side and DIUPRES on the other. Each tablet contains 500 mg of chlorothiazide and 0.125 mg of reserpine. They are supplied as follows:
NDC 0006-0405-68 in bottles of 100
NDC 0006-0405-82 in bottles of 1000.
Shown in Product Identification Guide, page 324
Storage
Keep container tightly closed. Protect from light, moisture, freezing, -20°C (-4°F) and store at room temperature, 15–30°C (59–86°F).
7900347 Issued March 1995
COPYRIGHT © MERCK & CO., INC., 1986
All rights reserved

DIURIL® Sodium Intravenous (Chlorothiazide Sodium), U.S.P. ℞

DESCRIPTION

Intravenous Sodium DIURIL* (Chlorothiazide Sodium) is a diuretic and antihypertensive. It is 6-chloro-2*H*-1,2,4-benzothiadiazine-7-sulfonamide 1,1-dioxide monosodium salt and its molecular weight is 317.71. Its empirical formula is $C_7H_5ClN_3NaO_4S_2$ and its structural formula is:

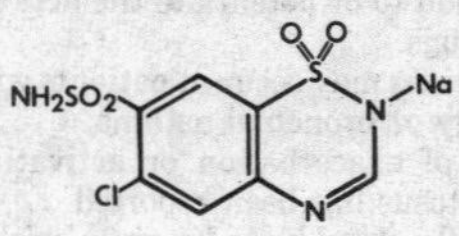

Intravenous Sodium DIURIL is a sterile lyophilized white powder and is supplied in a vial containing:
Chlorothiazide sodium equivalent to chlorothiazide .... 0.5 g
Inactive ingredients:
Mannitol .... 0.25 g
Sodium hydroxide to adjust pH, with 0.4 mg thimerosal (mercury derivative) added as preservative.
DIURIL* (Chlorothiazide) is a diuretic and antihypertensive. It is 6-chloro-2*H*-1,2,4-benzothiadiazine-7-sulfonamide 1,1-dioxide. Its empirical formula is $C_7H_6ClN_3O_4S_2$ and its structural formula is:

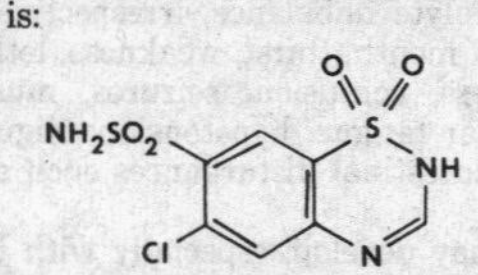

It is a white, or practically white, crystalline powder with a molecular weight of 295.72, which is very slightly soluble in water, but readily soluble in dilute aqueous sodium hydroxide. It is soluble in urine to the extent of about 150 mg per 100 mL at pH 7.

*Registered trademark of MERCK & CO., INC.

CLINICAL PHARMACOLOGY

The mechanism of the antihypertensive effect of thiazides is unknown. DIURIL (Chlorothiazide) does not usually affect normal blood pressure.
DIURIL (Chlorothiazide) affects the distal renal tubular mechanism of electrolyte reabsorption. At maximal therapeutic dosage all thiazides are approximately equal in their diuretic efficacy.
DIURIL (Chlorothiazide) increases excretion of sodium and chloride in approximately equivalent amounts. Natriuresis may be accompanied by some loss of potassium and bicarbonate.
After oral use diuresis begins within 2 hours, peaks in about 4 hours and lasts about 6 to 12 hours. Following intravenous use of Sodium DIURIL, onset of the diuretic action occurs in 15 minutes and the maximal action in 30 minutes.
Pharmacokinetics and Metabolism
DIURIL is not metabolized but is eliminated rapidly by the kidney; 96 percent of an intravenous dose is excreted unchanged in the urine within 23 hours. The plasma half-life of chlorothiazide is 45–120 minutes. Chlorothiazide crosses the placental but not the blood-brain barrier and is excreted in breast milk.

INDICATIONS AND USAGE

Intravenous Sodium DIURIL is indicated as adjunctive therapy in edema associated with congestive heart failure, hepatic cirrhosis, and corticosteroid and estrogen therapy.
Intravenous Sodium DIURIL has also been found useful in edema due to various forms of renal dysfunction such as nephrotic syndrome, acute glomerulonephritis, and chronic renal failure.
Use in Pregnancy. Routine use of diuretics during normal pregnancy is inappropriate and exposes mother and fetus to unnecessary hazard. Diuretics do not prevent development of toxemia of pregnancy and there is no satisfactory evidence that they are useful in the treatment of toxemia.
Edema during pregnancy may arise from pathologic causes or from the physiologic and mechanical consequences of pregnancy. Thiazides are indicated in pregnancy when edema is due to pathologic causes, just as they are in the absence of pregnancy (see PRECAUTIONS, *Pregnancy*).
Dependent edema in pregnancy, resulting from restriction of venous return by the gravid uterus, is properly treated through elevation of the lower extremities and use of support stockings. Use of diuretics to lower intravascular volume in this instance is illogical and unnecessary. During normal pregnancy there is hypervolemia which is not harmful to the fetus or the mother in the absence of cardiovascular disease. However, it may be associated with edema, rarely generalized edema. If such edema causes discomfort, increased recumbency will often provide relief. Rarely this edema may cause extreme discomfort which is not relieved by rest. In these instances, a short course of diuretic therapy may provide relief and be appropriate.

CONTRAINDICATIONS

Anuria.
Hypersensitivity to any component of this product or to other sulfonamide-derived drugs.

WARNINGS

Intravenous use in infants and children has been limited and is not generally recommended.
Use with caution in severe renal disease. In patients with renal disease, thiazides may precipitate azotemia. Cumulative effects of the drug may develop in patients with impaired renal function.
Thiazides should be used with caution in patients with impaired hepatic function or progressive liver disease, since minor alterations of fluid and electrolyte balance may precipitate hepatic coma.
Thiazides may add to or potentiate the action of other antihypertensive drugs.
Sensitivity reactions may occur in patients with or without a history of allergy or bronchial asthma.
The possibility of exacerbation or activation of systemic lupus erythematosus has been reported.
Lithium generally should not be given with diuretics (see PRECAUTIONS, *Drug Interactions*).

PRECAUTIONS

General
All patients receiving diuretic therapy should be observed for evidence of fluid or electrolyte imbalance: namely, hyponatremia, hypochloremic alkalosis, and hypokalemia. Serum and urine electrolyte determinations are particularly important when the patient is vomiting excessively or receiving parenteral fluids. Warning signs or symptoms of fluid and electrolyte imbalance, irrespective of cause, include dryness of mouth, thirst, weakness, lethargy, drowsiness, restlessness, confusion, seizures, muscle pains or cramps, muscular fatigue, hypotension, oliguria, tachycardia, and gastrointestinal disturbances such as nausea and vomiting.
Hypokalemia may develop especially with brisk diuresis, when severe cirrhosis is present or after prolonged therapy. Interference with adequate oral electrolyte intake will also contribute to hypokalemia. Hypokalemia may cause cardiac arrhythmias and may also sensitize or exaggerate the response of the heart to the toxic effects of digitalis (e.g., increased ventricular irritability). Hypokalemia may be avoided or treated by use of potassium sparing diuretics or potassium supplements such as foods with a high potassium content.
Although any chloride deficit is generally mild and usually does not require specific treatment except under extraordinary circumstances (as in liver disease or renal disease), chloride replacement may be required in the treatment of metabolic alkalosis.
Dilutional hyponatremia may occur in edematous patients in hot weather; appropriate therapy is water restriction, rather than administration of salt, except in rare instances when the hyponatremia is life threatening. In actual salt depletion, appropriate replacement is the therapy of choice.
Hyperuricemia may occur or acute gout may be precipitated in certain patients receiving thiazides.
In diabetic patients dosage adjustments of insulin or oral hypoglycemic agents may be required. Hyperglycemia may occur with thiazide diuretics. Thus latent diabetes mellitus may become manifest during thiazide therapy.
The antihypertensive effects of the drug may be enhanced in the postsympathectomy patient.
If progressive renal impairment becomes evident, consider withholding or discontinuing diuretic therapy.
Thiazides have been shown to increase the urinary excretion of magnesium; this may result in hypomagnesemia.
Thiazides may decrease urinary calcium excretion. Thiazides may cause intermittent and slight elevation of serum calcium in the absence of known disorders of calcium metabolism. Marked hypercalcemia may be evidence of hidden hyperparathyroidism. Thiazides should be discontinued before carrying out tests for parathyroid function.
Increases in cholesterol and triglyceride levels may be associated with thiazide diuretic therapy.
Laboratory Tests
Periodic determination of serum electrolytes to detect possible electrolyte imbalance should be done at appropriate intervals.
Drug Interactions
When given concurrently the following drugs may interact with thiazide diuretics.
Alcohol, barbiturates, or narcotics—potentiation of orthostatic hypotension may occur.
Antidiabetic drugs—(oral agents and insulin)—dosage adjustment of the antidiabetic drug may be required.
Other antihypertensive drugs—additive effect or potentiation.
Corticosteroids, ACTH—intensified electrolyte depletion, particularly hypokalemia.
Pressor amines (e.g., norepinephrine)—possible decreased response to pressor amines but not sufficient to preclude their use.
Skeletal muscle relaxants, nondepolarizing (e.g., tubocurarine)—possible increased responsiveness to the muscle relaxant.
Lithium—generally should not be given with diuretics. Diuretic agents reduce the renal clearance of lithium and add a high risk of lithium toxicity. Refer to the package insert for lithium preparations before use of such preparations with Sodium DIURIL.
Non-steroidal Anti-inflammatory Drugs—In some patients, the administration of a non-steroidal anti-inflammatory agent can reduce the diuretic, natriuretic, and antihypertensive effects of loop, potassium-sparing and thiazide diuretics. Therefore, when Sodium DIURIL and non-steroidal anti-inflammatory agents are used concomitantly, the patient should be observed closely to determine if the desired effect of the diuretic is obtained.
Drug/Laboratory Test Interactions
Thiazides should be discontinued before carrying out tests for parathyroid function (see PRECAUTIONS, *General*).
Carcinogenesis, Mutagenesis, Impairment of Fertility
Carcinogenicity studies have not been conducted with chlorothiazide.
Chlorothiazide was not mutagenic *in vitro* in the Ames microbial mutagen test (using a maximum concentration of 5 mg/plate and *Salmonella typhimurium* strains TA98 and TA100) and was not mutagenic and did not induce mitotic nondisjunction in diploid-strains of *Aspergillus nidulans.*
Chlorothiazide had no adverse effects on fertility in female rats at doses up to 60 mg/kg/day and no adverse effects on fertility in male rats at doses up to 40 mg/kg/day. These doses are 1.5 and 1.0 times* the recommended maximum human dose, respectively, when compared on a body weight basis.

*Calculations based on a human body weight of 50 kg
Pregnancy
Teratogenic Effects—Pregnancy Category C: Although reproduction studies performed with chlorothiazide doses of 50 mg/kg/day in rabbits, 60 mg/kg/day in rats and 500 mg/kg/day in mice revealed no external abnormalities of the fetus or impairment of growth and survival of the fetus due to chlorothiazide, such studies did not include complete examinations for visceral and skeletal abnormalities. It is not known whether chlorothiazide can cause fetal harm when administered to a pregnant woman; however, thiazides cross the placental barrier and appear in cord blood. DIURIL should be used during pregnancy only if clearly needed (see INDICATIONS AND USAGE).
Nonteratogenic Effects: Chlorothiazide may cause fetal or neonatal jaundice, thrombocytopenia, and possibly other adverse reactions which have occurred in the adult.
Nursing Mothers
Because of the potential for serious adverse reactions in nursing infants from Intravenous Sodium DIURIL, a deci-

Continued on next page

Information on the Merck & Co., Inc. products listed on these pages is the full prescribing information from product circulars in use September 30, 1996.

Merck & Co.—Cont.

sion should be made whether to discontinue nursing or to discontinue the drug, taking into account the importance of the drug to the mother.

Pediatric Use

Safety and effectiveness of Intravenous Sodium DIURIL in pediatric patients have not been established.

ADVERSE REACTIONS

The following adverse reactions have been reported and, within each category, are listed in order of decreasing severity.

Body as a Whole: Weakness.

Cardiovascular: Hypotension including orthostatic hypotension (may be aggravated by alcohol, barbiturates, narcotics or antihypertensive drugs).

Digestive: Pancreatitis, jaundice (intrahepatic cholestatic jaundice), diarrhea, vomiting, sialadenitis, cramping, constipation, gastric irritation, nausea, anorexia.

Hematologic: Aplastic anemia, agranulocytosis, leukopenia, hemolytic anemia, thrombocytopenia.

Hypersensitivity: Anaphylactic reactions, necrotizing angiitis (vasculitis and cutaneous vasculitis), respiratory distress including pneumonitis and pulmonary edema, photosensitivity, fever, urticaria, rash, purpura.

Metabolic: Electrolyte imbalance (see PRECAUTIONS), hyperglycemia, glycosuria, hyperuricemia.

Musculoskeletal: Muscle spasm.

Nervous System/Psychiatric: Vertigo, paresthesias, dizziness, headache, restlessness.

Skin: Erythema multiforme including Stevens-Johnson syndrome, exfoliative dermatitis including toxic epidermal necrolysis, alopecia.

Special Senses: Transient blurred vision, xanthopsia.

Renal: Renal failure, renal dysfunction, interstitial nephritis (see WARNINGS); hematuria (following intravenous use).

Urogenital: Impotence.

Whenever adverse reactions are moderate or severe, thiazide dosage should be reduced or therapy withdrawn.

OVERDOSAGE

The most common signs and symptoms observed are those caused by electrolyte depletion (hypokalemia, hypochloremia, hyponatremia) and dehydration resulting from excessive diuresis. If digitalis has also been administered, hypokalemia may accentuate cardiac arrhythmias.

In the event of overdosage, symptomatic and supportive measures should be employed. Correct dehydration, electrolyte imbalance, hepatic coma and hypotension by established procedures. If required, give oxygen or artificial respiration for respiratory impairment.

The degree to which chlorothiazide sodium is removed by hemodialysis has not been established.

The intravenous LD_{50} of chlorothiazide in the mouse is 1.1 g/kg.

DOSAGE AND ADMINISTRATION

Intravenous Sodium DIURIL should be reserved for patients unable to take oral medication or for emergency situations.

Therapy should be individualized according to patient response. Use the smallest dosage necessary to achieve the required response.

Intravenous use in infants and children has been limited and is not generally recommended.

When medication can be taken orally, therapy with DIURIL tablets or oral suspension may be substituted for intravenous therapy, using the same dosage schedule as for the parenteral route.

Intravenous Sodium DIURIL may be given slowly by direct intravenous injection or by intravenous infusion.

Add 18 mL of Sterile Water for Injection to the vial to form an isotonic solution for intravenous injection. Never add less than 18 mL. When reconstituted with 18 mL of Sterile Water, the final concentration of Intravenous Sodium DIURIL is 28 mg/mL. Unused solution may be stored at room temperature for 24 hours, after which it must be discarded. Parenteral drug products should be inspected visually for particulate matter and discoloration prior to use whenever solution and container permit. The solution is compatible with dextrose or sodium chloride solutions for intravenous infusion. Avoid simultaneous administration of solutions of chlorothiazide with whole blood or its derivatives.

Extravasation must be rigidly avoided. Do not give subcutaneously or intramuscularly.

The usual adult dosage is 0.5 to 1.0 g once or twice a day. Many patients with edema respond to intermittent therapy, i.e., administration on alternate days or on three to five days each week. With an intermittent schedule, excessive response and the resulting undesirable electrolyte imbalance are less likely to occur.

HOW SUPPLIED

No. 3250—Intravenous Sodium DIURIL is a dry, sterile lyophilized white powder usually in plug form, supplied in vials containing chlorothiazide sodium equivalent to 0.5 g of chlorothiazide.

NDC 0006-3250-32.

Storage

Store lyophilized powder between 2–25°C (36–77°F).

Store reconstituted solution at room temperature, 15–30°C (59–86°F), and discard unused portion after 24 hours.

7413535 Issued June 1995

COPYRIGHT © MERCK & CO., INC., 1986
All rights reserved

DIURIL® Tablets ℞
(Chlorothiazide), U.S.P.
DIURIL® Oral Suspension ℞
(Chlorothiazide), U.S.P.

DESCRIPTION

DIURIL* (Chlorothiazide) is a diuretic and antihypertensive. It is 6-chloro-2*H*-1,2,4-benzothiadiazine-7-sulfonamide 1,1-dioxide. Its empirical formula is $C_7H_6ClN_3O_4S_2$ and its structural formula is:

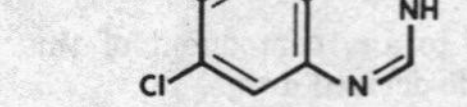

It is a white, or practically white, crystalline powder with a molecular weight of 295.73, which is very slightly soluble in water, but readily soluble in dilute aqueous sodium hydroxide. It is soluble in urine to the extent of about 150 mg per 100 mL at pH 7.

DIURIL is supplied as 250 mg and 500 mg tablets, for oral use. Each tablet contains the following inactive ingredients: gelatin, magnesium stearate, starch and talc. The 250 mg tablet also contains lactose.

Oral Suspension DIURIL contains 250 mg of chlorothiazide per 5 mL, alcohol 0.5 percent, with methylparaben 0.12 percent, propylparaben 0.02 percent, and benzoic acid 0.1 percent added as preservatives. The inactive ingredients are D&C Yellow 10, flavors, glycerin, purified water, sodium saccharin, sucrose and tragacanth.

---

*Registered trademark of MERCK & CO., INC.

CLINICAL PHARMACOLOGY

The mechanism of the antihypertensive effect of thiazides is unknown. DIURIL does not usually affect normal blood pressure.

DIURIL affects the distal renal tubular mechanism of electrolyte reabsorption. At maximal therapeutic dosage all thiazides are approximately equal in their diuretic efficacy. DIURIL increases excretion of sodium and chloride in approximately equivalent amounts. Natriuresis may be accompanied by some loss of potassium and bicarbonate.

After oral use diuresis begins within 2 hours, peaks in about 4 hours and lasts about 6 to 12 hours.

Pharmacokinetics and Metabolism

DIURIL is not metabolized but is eliminated rapidly by the kidney. The plasma half-life of chlorothiazide is 45–120 minutes. After oral doses, 10–15 percent of the dose is excreted unchanged in the urine. Chlorothiazide crosses the placental but not the blood-brain barrier and is excreted in breast milk.

INDICATIONS AND USAGE

DIURIL is indicated as adjunctive therapy in edema associated with congestive heart failure, hepatic cirrhosis, and corticosteroid and estrogen therapy.

DIURIL has also been found useful in edema due to various forms of renal dysfunction such as nephrotic syndrome, acute glomerulonephritis, and chronic renal failure.

DIURIL is indicated in the management of hypertension either as the sole therapeutic agent or to enhance the effectiveness of other antihypertensive drugs in the more severe forms of hypertension.

Use in Pregnancy. Routine use of diuretics during normal pregnancy is inappropriate and exposes mother and fetus to unnecessary hazard. Diuretics do not prevent development of toxemia of pregnancy and there is no satisfactory evidence that they are useful in the treatment of toxemia.

Edema during pregnancy may arise from pathologic causes or from the physiologic and mechanical consequences of pregnancy. Thiazides are indicated in pregnancy when edema is due to pathologic causes, just as they are in the absence of pregnancy (see PRECAUTIONS, *Pregnancy*). Dependent edema in pregnancy, resulting from restriction of venous return by the gravid uterus, is properly treated through elevation of the lower extremities and use of support stockings. Use of diuretics to lower intravascular volume in this instance is illogical and unnecessary. During normal pregnancy there is hypervolemia which is not harmful to the fetus or the mother in the absence of cardiovascular disease. However, it may be associated with edema, rarely generalized edema. If such edema causes discomfort, increased recumbency will often provide relief. Rarely this edema may cause extreme discomfort which is not relieved by rest. In these instances, a short course of diuretic therapy may provide relief and be appropriate.

CONTRAINDICATIONS

Anuria.

Hypersensitivity to this product or to other sulfonamide-derived drugs.

WARNINGS

Use with caution in severe renal disease. In patients with renal disease, thiazides may precipitate azotemia. Cumulative effects of the drug may develop in patients with impaired renal function.

Thiazides should be used with caution in patients with impaired hepatic function or progressive liver disease, since minor alterations of fluid and electrolyte balance may precipitate hepatic coma.

Thiazides may add to or potentiate the action of other antihypertensive drugs.

Sensitivity reactions may occur in patients with or without a history of allergy or bronchial asthma.

The possibility of exacerbation or activation of systemic lupus erythematosus has been reported.

Lithium generally should not be given with diuretics (see PRECAUTIONS, *Drug Interactions*).

PRECAUTIONS

General

All patients receiving diuretic therapy should be observed for evidence of fluid or electrolyte imbalance: namely, hyponatremia, hypochloremic alkalosis, and hypokalemia. Serum and urine electrolyte determinations are particularly important when the patient is vomiting excessively or receiving parenteral fluids. Warning signs or symptoms of fluid and electrolyte imbalance, irrespective of cause, include dryness of mouth, thirst, weakness, lethargy, drowsiness, restlessness, confusion, seizures, muscle pains or cramps, muscular fatigue, hypotension, oliguria, tachycardia, and gastrointestinal disturbances such as nausea and vomiting.

Hypokalemia may develop, especially with brisk diuresis, when severe cirrhosis is present or after prolonged therapy. Interference with adequate oral electrolyte intake will also contribute to hypokalemia. Hypokalemia may cause cardiac arrhythmias and may also sensitize or exaggerate the response of the heart to the toxic effects of digitalis (e.g., increased ventricular irritability). Hypokalemia may be avoided or treated by use of potassium sparing diuretics or potassium supplements such as foods with a high potassium content.

Although any chloride deficit is generally mild and usually does not require specific treatment except under extraordinary circumstances (as in liver disease or renal disease), chloride replacement may be required in the treatment of metabolic alkalosis.

Dilutional hyponatremia may occur in edematous patients in hot weather; appropriate therapy is water restriction, rather than administration of salt, except in rare instances when the hyponatremia is life-threatening. In actual salt depletion, appropriate replacement is the therapy of choice.

Hyperuricemia may occur or acute gout may be precipitated in certain patients receiving thiazides.

In diabetic patients dosage adjustments of insulin or oral hypoglycemic agents may be required. Hyperglycemia may occur with thiazide diuretics. Thus latent diabetes mellitus may become manifest during thiazide therapy.

The antihypertensive effects of the drug may be enhanced in the post-sympathectomy patient.

If progressive renal impairment becomes evident, consider withholding or discontinuing diuretic therapy.

Thiazides have been shown to increase the urinary excretion of magnesium; this may result in hypomagnesemia.

Thiazides may decrease urinary calcium excretion. Thiazides may cause intermittent and slight elevation of serum calcium in the absence of known disorders of calcium metabolism. Marked hypercalcemia may be evidence of hidden hyperparathyroidism. Thiazides should be discontinued before carrying out tests for parathyroid function.

Increases in cholesterol and triglyceride levels may be associated with thiazide diuretic therapy.

Laboratory Tests
Periodic determination of serum electrolytes to detect possible electrolyte imbalance should be done at appropriate intervals.
Drug Interactions
When given concurrently the following drugs may interact with thiazide diuretics.
Alcohol, barbiturates, or narcotics—potentiation of orthostatic hypotension may occur.
Antidiabetic drugs (oral agents and insulin)—dosage adjustment of the antidiabetic drug may be required.
Other antihypertensive drugs—additive effect or potentiation.
Cholestyramine and colestipol resins—Both cholestyramine and colestipol resins have the potential of binding thiazide diuretics and reducing diuretic absorption from the gastrointestinal tract.
Corticosteroids, ACTH—intensified electrolyte depletion, particularly hypokalemia.
Pressor amines (e.g., norepinephrine)—possible decreased response to pressor amines but not sufficient to preclude their use.
Skeletal muscle relaxants, nondepolarizing (e.g., tubocurarine)—possible increased responsiveness to the muscle relaxant.
Lithium—generally should not be given with diuretics. Diuretic agents reduce the renal clearance of lithium and add a high risk of lithium toxicity. Refer to the package insert for lithium preparations before use of such preparations with DIURIL.
Non-steroidal Anti-inflammatory Drugs—In some patients, the administration of a non-steroidal anti-inflammatory agent can reduce the diuretic, natriuretic, and antihypertensive effects of loop, potassium-sparing and thiazide diuretics. Therefore, when DIURIL and non-steroidal anti-inflammatory agents are used concomitantly, the patient should be observed closely to determine if the desired effect of the diuretic is obtained.
Drug/Laboratory Test Interactions
Thiazides should be discontinued before carrying out tests for parathyroid function (see PRECAUTIONS, *General*).
Carcinogenesis, Mutagenesis, Impairment of Fertility
Carcinogenicity studies have not been conducted with chlorothiazide.
Chlorothiazide was not mutagenic *in vitro* in the Ames microbial mutagen test (using a maximum concentration of 5 mg/plate and *Salmonella typhimurium* strains TA98 and TA100) and was not mutagenic and did not induce mitotic nondisjunction in diploid-strains of *Aspergillus nidulans*.
Chlorothiazide had no adverse effects on fertility in female rats at doses up to 60 mg/kg/day and no adverse effects on fertility in male rats at doses up to 40 mg/kg/day. These doses are 1.5 and 1.0 times* the recommended maximum human dose, respectively, when compared on a body weight basis.

*Calculations based on a human body weight of 50 kg

Pregnancy
Teratogenic Effects—Pregnancy Category C: Although reproduction studies performed with chlorothiazide doses of 50 mg/kg/day in rabbits, 60 mg/kg/day in rats and 500 mg/kg/day in mice revealed no external abnormalities of the fetus or impairment of growth and survival of the fetus due to chlorothiazide, such studies did not include complete examinations for visceral and skeletal abnormalities. It is not known whether chlorothiazide can cause fetal harm when administered to a pregnant woman; however, thiazides cross the placental barrier and appear in cord blood. DIURIL should be used during pregnancy only if clearly needed (see INDICATIONS AND USAGE).
Nonteratogenic Effects: Chlorothiazide may cause fetal or neonatal jaundice, thrombocytopenia, and possibly other adverse reactions which have occurred in the adult.
Nursing Mothers
Because of the potential for serious adverse reactions in nursing infants from DIURIL, a decision should be made whether to discontinue nursing or to discontinue the drug, taking into account the importance of the drug to the mother.

ADVERSE REACTIONS

The following adverse reactions have been reported and, within each category, are listed in order of decreasing severity.
Body as a Whole: Weakness.
Cardiovascular: Hypotension including orthostatic hypotension (may be aggravated by alcohol, barbiturates, narcotics or antihypertensive drugs).
Digestive: Pancreatitis, jaundice (intrahepatic cholestatic jaundice), diarrhea, vomiting, sialadenitis, cramping, constipation, gastric irritation, nausea, anorexia.
Hematologic: Aplastic anemia, agranulocytosis, leukopenia, hemolytic anemia, thrombocytopenia.
Hypersensitivity: Anaphylactic reactions, necrotizing angiitis (vasculitis and cutaneous vasculitis), respiratory distress including pneumonitis and pulmonary edema, photosensitivity, fever, urticaria, rash, purpura.
Metabolic: Electrolyte imbalance (see PRECAUTIONS), hyperglycemia, glycosuria, hyperuricemia.
Musculoskeletal: Muscle spasm.
Nervous System/Psychiatric: Vertigo, paresthesias, dizziness, headache, restlessness.
Renal: Renal failure, renal dysfunction, interstitial nephritis. (See WARNINGS.)
Skin: Erythema multiforme including Stevens-Johnson syndrome, exfoliative dermatitis including toxic epidermal necrolysis, alopecia.
Special Senses: Transient blurred vision, xanthopsia.
Urogenital: Impotence.
Whenever adverse reactions are moderate or severe, thiazide dosage should be reduced or therapy withdrawn.

OVERDOSAGE

The most common signs and symptoms observed are those caused by electrolyte depletion (hypokalemia, hypochloremia, hyponatremia) and dehydration resulting from excessive diuresis. If digitalis has also been administered, hypokalemia may accentuate cardiac arrhythmias.
In the event of overdosage, symptomatic and supportive measures should be employed. Emesis should be induced or gastric lavage performed. Correct dehydration, electrolyte imbalance, hepatic coma and hypotension by established procedures. If required, give oxygen or artificial respiration for respiratory impairment.
The degree to which chlorothiazide sodium is removed by hemodialysis has not been established.
The oral LD_{50} of chlorothiazide is 8.5 g/kg, greater than 10 g/kg, and greater than 1 g/kg, in the mouse, rat and dog respectively.

DOSAGE AND ADMINISTRATION

Therapy should be individualized according to patient response. Use the smallest dosage necessary to achieve the required response.

Adults

For Edema
The usual adult dosage is 0.5 to 1.0 g once or twice a day. Many patients with edema respond to intermittent therapy, i.e., administration on alternate days or on three to five days each week. With an intermittent schedule, excessive response and the resulting undesirable electrolyte imbalance are less likely to occur.
For Control of Hypertension
The usual adult starting dosage is 0.5 or 1.0 g a day as a single or divided dose. Dosage is increased or decreased according to blood pressure response. Rarely some patients may require up to 2.0 g a day in divided doses.

Pediatric Patients
For Diuresis and For Control of Hypertension
The usual pediatric dosage is 5 to 10 mg per pound (10 to 20 mg/kg) per day in single or two divided doses, not to exceed 375 mg per day (2.5 to 7.5 mL or ½ to 1½ teaspoonfuls of the oral suspension daily) in infants up to 2 years of age or 1 g per day in pediatric patients 2 to 12 years of age. In infants less than 6 months of age, doses up to 15 mg per pound (30 mg/kg) per day in two divided doses may be required.

HOW SUPPLIED

No. 3244—Tablets DIURIL, 250 mg, are white, round, scored, compressed tablets, coded MSD 214 on one side and DIURIL on the other. They are supplied as follows:
NDC 0006-0214-68 bottles of 100
NDC 0006-0214-82 bottles of 1000.
Shown in Product Identification Guide, page 324
No. 3245—Tablets DIURIL, 500 mg, are white, round, scored, compressed tablets, coded MSD 432 on one side and DIURIL on the other. They are supplied as follows:
NDC 0006-0432-68 bottles of 100
NDC 0006-0432-82 bottles of 1000
NDC 0006-0432-86 bottles of 5000.
Shown in Product Identification Guide, page 324
No. 3239—Oral Suspension DIURIL, 250 mg of chlorothiazide per 5 mL, is a yellow, creamy suspension, and is supplied as follows:
NDC 0006-3239-66 bottles of 237 mL
(6505-01-156-1600, 250 mg/5 mL, 237 mL).
Storage
Tablets DIURIL: Keep container tightly closed. Protect from moisture, freezing, -20°C (-4°F) and store at room temperature, 15–30°C (59–86°F).
Oral Suspension DIURIL: Keep container tightly closed. Protect from freezing, -20°C (-4°F) and store at room temperature, 15–30°C (59–86°F).

7897958 Issued June 1995
COPYRIGHT © MERCK & CO., INC., 1986
All rights reserved

DOLOBID® Tablets ℞
(Diflunisal), U.S.P.

DESCRIPTION

Diflunisal is 2′, 4′-difluoro-4-hydroxy-3-biphenylcarboxylic acid. Its empirical formula is $C_{13}H_8F_2O_3$ and its structural formula is:

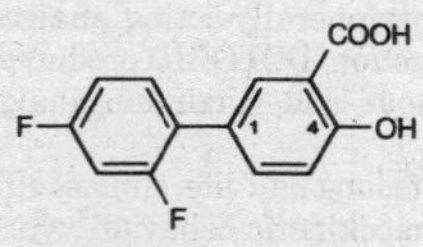

Diflunisal has a molecular weight of 250.20. It is a stable, white, crystalline compound with a melting point of 211–213°C. It is practically insoluble in water at neutral or acidic pH. Because it is an organic acid, it dissolves readily in dilute alkali to give a moderately stable solution at room temperature. It is soluble in most organic solvents including ethanol, methanol, and acetone.
DOLOBID* (Diflunisal) is available in 250 and 500 mg tablets for oral administration. Tablets DOLOBID contain the following inactive ingredients: cellulose, FD&C Yellow 6 hydroxypropyl cellulose, hydroxypropyl methylcellulose, magnesium stearate, starch, talc, and titanium dioxide.

*Registered trademark of MERCK & CO., INC.

CLINICAL PHARMACOLOGY

Action
DOLOBID is a non-steroidal drug with analgesic, anti-inflammatory and antipyretic properties. It is a peripherally-acting non-narcotic analgesic drug. Habituation, tolerance and addiction have not been reported.
Diflunisal is a difluorophenyl derivative of salicylic acid. Chemically, diflunisal differs from aspirin (acetylsalicylic acid) in two respects. The first of these two is the presence of a difluorophenyl substituent at carbon 1. The second difference is the removal of the 0-acetyl group from the carbon 4 position. Diflunisal is not metabolized to salicylic acid, and the fluorine atoms are not displaced from the difluorophenyl ring structure.
The precise mechanism of the analgesic and anti-inflammatory actions of diflunisal is not known. Diflunisal is a prostaglandin synthetase inhibitor. In animals, prostaglandins sensitize afferent nerves and potentiate the action of bradykinin in inducing pain. Since prostaglandins are known to be among the mediators of pain and inflammation, the mode of action of diflunisal may be due to a decrease of prostaglandins in peripheral tissues.
Pharmacokinetics and Metabolism
DOLOBID is rapidly and completely absorbed following oral administration with peak plasma concentrations occurring between 2 to 3 hours. The drug is excreted in the urine as two soluble glucuronide conjugates accounting for about 90% of the administered dose. Little or no diflunisal is excreted in the feces. Diflunisal appears in human milk in concentrations of 2–7% of those in plasma. More than 99% of diflunisal in plasma is bound to proteins.
As is the case with salicylic acid, concentration-dependent pharmacokinetics prevail when DOLOBID is administered; a doubling of dosage produces a greater than doubling of drug accumulation. The effect becomes more apparent with repetitive doses. Following single doses, peak plasma concentrations of 41 ± 11 μg/mL (mean ± S.D.) were observed following 250 mg doses, 87 ± 17 μg/mL were observed following 500 mg and 124 ± 11 μg/mL following single 1000 mg doses. However, following administration of 250 mg b.i.d., a mean peak level of 56 ± 14 μg/mL was observed on day 8, while the mean peak level after 500 mg b.i.d. for 11 days was 190 ± 33 μg/mL. In contrast to salicylic acid which has a plasma half-life of 2½ hours, the plasma half-life of diflunisal is 3 to 4 times longer (8 to 12 hours), because of a difluorophenyl substituent at carbon 1. Because of its long half-life and nonlinear pharmacokinetics, several days are required for diflunisal plasma levels to reach steady state following multiple doses. For this reason, an initial loading dose is necessary to shorten the time to reach steady state levels, and 2 to 3 days of observation are necessary for evalu-

Continued on next page

Information on the Merck & Co., Inc. products listed on these pages is the full prescribing information from product circulars in use September 30, 1996.

Merck & Co.—Cont.

ating changes in treatment regimens if a loading dose is not used.

Studies in baboons to determine passage across the blood-brain barrier have shown that only small quantities of diflunisal, under normal or acidotic conditions are transported into the cerebrospinal fluid (CSF). The ratio of blood/CSF concentrations after intravenous doses of 50 mg/kg or oral doses of 100 mg/kg of diflunisal was 100:1. In contrast, oral doses of 500 mg/kg of aspirin resulted in a blood/CSF ratio of 5:1.

Mild to Moderate Pain

DOLOBID is a peripherally-acting analgesic agent with a long duration of action. DOLOBID produces significant analgesia within 1 hour and maximum analgesia within 2 to 3 hours.

Consistent with its long half-life, clinical effects of DOLOBID mirror its pharmacokinetic behavior, which is the basis for recommending a loading dose when instituting therapy. Patients treated with DOLOBID, on the first dose, tend to have a slower onset of pain relief when compared with drugs achieving comparable peak effects. However, DOLOBID produces longer-lasting responses than the comparative agents.

Comparative single dose clinical studies have established the analgesic efficacy of DOLOBID at various dose levels relative to other analgesics. Analgesic effect measurements were derived from hourly evaluations by patients during eight and twelve-hour postdosing observation periods. The following information may serve as a guide for prescribing DOLOBID.

DOLOBID 500 mg was comparable in analgesic efficacy to aspirin 650 mg, acetaminophen 600 mg or 650 mg, and acetaminophen 650 mg with propoxyphene napsylate 100 mg. Patients treated with DOLOBID had longer lasting responses than the patients treated with the comparative analgesics.

DOLOBID 1000 mg was comparable in analgesic efficacy to acetaminophen 600 mg with codeine 60 mg. Patients treated with DOLOBID had longer lasting responses than the patients who received acetaminophen with codeine.

A loading dose of 1000 mg provides faster onset of pain relief, shorter time to peak analgesic effect, and greater peak analgesic effect than an initial 500 mg dose.

In contrast to the comparative analgesics, a significantly greater proportion of patients treated with DOLOBID did not remedicate and continued to have a good analgesic effect eight to twelve hours after dosing. Seventy-five percent (75%) of patients treated with DOLOBID continued to have a good analgesic response at four hours. When patients having a good analgesic response at four hours were followed, 78% of these patients continued to have a good analgesic response at eight hours and 64% at twelve hours.

Chronic Anti-inflammatory Therapy in Osteoarthritis and Rheumatoid Arthritis

In the controlled, double-blind clinical trials in which DOLOBID (500 mg to 1000 mg a day) was compared with anti-inflammatory doses of aspirin (2–4 grams a day), patients treated with DOLOBID had a significantly lower incidence of tinnitus and of adverse effects involving the gastrointestinal system than patients treated with aspirin. (See also *Effect on Fecal Blood Loss*).

Osteoarthritis

The effectiveness of DOLOBID for the treatment of osteoarthritis was studied in patients with osteoarthritis of the hip and/or knee. The activity of DOLOBID was demonstrated by clinical improvement in the signs and symptoms of disease activity.

In a double-blind multicenter study of 12 weeks' duration in which dosages were adjusted according to patient response, DOLOBID, 500 or 750 mg daily, was shown to be comparable in effectiveness to aspirin, 2000 or 3000 mg daily. In open-label extensions of this study to 24 or 48 weeks, DOLOBID continued to show similar effectiveness and generally was well tolerated.

Rheumatoid Arthritis

In controlled clinical trials, the effectiveness of DOLOBID was established for both acute exacerbations and long-term management of rheumatoid arthritis. The activity of DOLOBID was demonstrated by clinical improvement in the signs and symptoms of disease activity.

In a double-blind multicenter study of 12 weeks' duration in which dosages were adjusted according to patient response, DOLOBID 500 or 750 mg daily was comparable in effectiveness to aspirin 2,600 or 3,900 mg daily. In open-label extensions of this study to 52 weeks, DOLOBID continued to be effective and was generally well tolerated.

DOLOBID 500, 750, or 1000 mg daily was compared with aspirin 2000, 3000, or 4000 mg daily in a multicenter study of 8 weeks' duration in which dosages were adjusted according to patient response. In this study, DOLOBID was comparable in efficacy to aspirin.

In a double-blind multicenter study of 12 weeks' duration in which dosages were adjusted according to patient needs, DOLOBID 500 or 750 mg daily and ibuprofen 1600 or 2400 mg daily were comparable in effectiveness and tolerability.

In a double-blind multicenter study of 12 weeks' duration, DOLOBID 750 mg daily was comparable in efficacy to naproxen 750 mg daily. The incidence of gastrointestinal adverse effects and tinnitus was comparable for both drugs. This study was extended to 48 weeks on an open-label basis. DOLOBID continued to be effective and generally well tolerated.

In patients with rheumatoid arthritis, DOLOBID and gold salts may be used in combination at their usual dosage levels. In clinical studies, DOLOBID added to the regimen of gold salts usually resulted in additional symptomatic relief but did not alter the course of the underlying disease.

Antipyretic Activity

DOLOBID is not recommended for use as an antipyretic agent. In single 250 mg, 500 mg, or 750 mg doses, DOLOBID produced measurable but not clinically useful decreases in temperature in patients with fever; however, the possibility that it may mask fever in some patients, particularly with chronic or high doses, should be considered.

Uricosuric Effect

In normal volunteers, an increase in the renal clearance of uric acid and a decrease in serum uric acid was observed when DOLOBID was administered at 500 mg or 750 mg daily in divided doses. Patients on long-term therapy taking DOLOBID at 500 mg to 1000 mg daily in divided doses showed a prompt and consistent reduction across studies in mean serum uric acid levels, which were lowered as much as 1.4 mg%. It is not known whether DOLOBID interferes with the activity of other uricosuric agents.

Effect on Platelet Function

As an inhibitor of prostaglandin synthetase, DOLOBID has a dose-related effect on platelet function and bleeding time. In normal volunteers, 250 mg b.i.d. for 8 days had no effect on platelet function, and 500 mg b.i.d., the usual recommended dose, had a slight effect. At 1000 mg b.i.d., which exceeds the maximum recommended dosage, however, DOLOBID inhibited platelet function. In contrast to aspirin, these effects of DOLOBID were reversible, because of the absence of the chemically labile and biologically reactive 0-acetyl group at the carbon 4 position. Bleeding time was not altered by a dose of 250 mg b.i.d., and was only slightly increased at 500 mg b.i.d. At 1000 mg b.i.d., a greater increase occurred, but was not statistically significantly different from the change in the placebo group.

Effect on Fecal Blood Loss

When DOLOBID was given to normal volunteers at the usual recommended dose of 500 mg twice daily, fecal blood loss was not significantly different from placebo. Aspirin at 1000 mg four times daily produced the expected increase in fecal blood loss. DOLOBID at 1000 mg twice daily (NOTE: exceeds the recommended dosage) caused a statistically significant increase in fecal blood loss, but this increase was only one-half as large as that associated with aspirin 1300 mg twice daily.

Effect on Blood Glucose

DOLOBID did not affect fasting blood sugar in diabetic patients who were receiving tolbutamide or placebo.

INDICATIONS AND USAGE

DOLOBID is indicated for acute or long-term use for symptomatic treatment of the following:

1. Mild to moderate pain
2. Osteoarthritis
3. Rheumatoid arthritis

CONTRAINDICATIONS

Patients who are hypersensitive to this product.

Patients in whom acute asthmatic attacks, urticaria, or rhinitis are precipitated by aspirin or other non-steroidal anti-inflammatory drugs.

WARNINGS

Peptic ulceration and gastrointestinal bleeding have been reported in patients receiving DOLOBID. Fatalities have occurred rarely. Gastrointestinal bleeding is associated with higher morbidity and mortality in patients acutely ill with other conditions, the elderly and patients with hemorrhagic disorders. In patients with active gastrointestinal bleeding or an active peptic ulcer, the physician must weigh the benefits of therapy with DOLOBID against possible hazards, institute an appropriate ulcer regimen, and carefully monitor the patient's progress. When DOLOBID is given to patients with a history of either upper or lower gastrointestinal tract disease, it should be given only after consulting the ADVERSE REACTIONS section and under close supervision.

Risk of GI Ulcerations, Bleeding and Perforation with NSAID Therapy

Serious gastrointestinal toxicity such as bleeding, ulceration, and perforation, can occur at any time, with or without warning symptoms, in patients treated chronically with NSAID therapy. Although minor upper gastrointestinal problems, such as dyspepsia, are common, usually developing early in therapy, physicians should remain alert for ulceration and bleeding in patients treated chronically with NSAIDs even in the absence of previous GI tract symptoms. In patients observed in clinical trials of several months to two years duration, symptomatic upper GI ulcers, gross bleeding or perforation appear to occur in approximately 1% of patients treated for 3–6 months, and in about 2–4% of patients treated for one year. Physicians should inform patients about the signs and/or symptoms of serious GI toxicity and what steps to take if they occur.

Studies to date have not identified any subset of patients not at risk of developing peptic ulceration and bleeding. Except for a prior history of serious GI events and other risk factors known to be associated with peptic ulcer disease, such as alcoholism, smoking, etc., no risk factors (e.g., age, sex) have been associated with increased risk. Elderly or debilitated patients seem to tolerate ulceration or bleeding less well than other individuals and most spontaneous reports of fatal GI events are in this population. Studies to date are inconclusive concerning the relative risk of various NSAIDs in causing such reactions. High doses of any NSAID probably carry a greater risk of these reactions, although controlled clinical trials showing this do not exist in most cases. In considering the use of relatively large doses (within the recommended dosage range), sufficient benefit should be anticipated to offset the potential increased risk of GI toxicity.

PRECAUTIONS

General

Non-steroidal anti-inflammatory drugs, including DOLOBID, may mask the usual signs and symptoms of infection. Therefore, the physician must be continually on the alert for this and should use the drug with extra care in the presence of existing infection.

Although DOLOBID has less effect on platelet function and bleeding time than aspirin, at higher doses it is an inhibitor of platelet function; therefore, patients who may be adversely affected should be carefully observed when DOLOBID is administered (see CLINICAL PHARMACOLOGY).

Because of reports of adverse eye findings with agents of this class, it is recommended that patients who develop eye complaints during treatment with DOLOBID have ophthalmologic studies.

Peripheral edema has been observed in some patients taking DOLOBID. Therefore, as with other drugs in this class, DOLOBID should be used with caution in patients with compromised cardiac function, hypertension, or other conditions predisposing to fluid retention.

Acetylsalicylic acid has been associated with Reye syndrome. Because diflunisal is a derivative of salicylic acid, the possibility of its association with Reye syndrome cannot be excluded.

Hypersensitivity Syndrome

A potentially life-threatening, apparent hypersensitivity syndrome has been reported. This multisystem syndrome includes constitutional symptoms (fever, chills), and cutaneous findings (see ADVERSE REACTIONS, *Dermatologic*). It may also include involvement of major organs (changes in liver function, jaundice, leukopenia, thrombocytopenia, eosinophilia, disseminated intravascular coagulation, renal impairment, including renal failure), and less specific findings (adenitis, arthralgia, myalgia, arthritis, malaise, anorexia, disorientation). If evidence of hypersensitivity occurs, therapy with DOLOBID should be discontinued.

Renal Effects

As with other non-steroidal anti-inflammatory drugs, long term administration of diflunisal to animals has resulted in renal papillary necrosis and other abnormal renal pathology. In humans, there have been reports of acute interstitial nephritis with hematuria and proteinuria and occasionally nephrotic syndrome.

A second form of renal toxicity has been seen in patients with prerenal and renal conditions leading to a reduction in renal blood flow or blood volume, where the renal prostaglandins have a supportive role in the maintenance of renal perfusion. In these patients administration of an NSAID may cause a dose dependent reduction in prostaglandin formation and may precipitate overt renal decompensation. Patients at greatest risk of this reaction are those with conditions such as renal or hepatic dysfunction, diabetes mellitus, advanced age, extracellular volume depletion from any cause, congestive heart failure, septicemia, pyelonephritis, or concomitant use of any nephrotoxic drug. DOLOBID or other NSAIDs should be given with caution and renal function should be monitored in any patient who may have reduced renal reserve. Discontinuation of NSAID therapy is typically followed by recovery to the pretreatment state.

Since DOLOBID is eliminated primarily by the kidneys, patients with significantly impaired renal function should be closely monitored; a lower daily dosage should be anticipated to avoid excessive drug accumulation.

Information for Patients

DOLOBID, like other drugs of its class, is not free of side effects. The side effects of these drugs can cause discomfort and, rarely, there are more serious side effects such as gastrointestinal bleeding, which may result in hospitalization and even fatal outcomes.

NSAIDs (Non-steroidal Anti-inflammatory Drugs) are often essential agents in the management of arthritis and have a major role in the treatment of pain, but they also may be commonly employed for conditions which are less serious. Physicians may wish to discuss with their patients the potential risks (see WARNINGS, PRECAUTIONS and ADVERSE REACTIONS) and likely benefits of NSAID treatment, particularly when the drugs are used for less serious conditions where treatment without NSAIDs may represent an acceptable alternative to both the patient and physician.

Laboratory Tests

Liver Function Tests: As with other non-steroidal anti-inflammatory drugs, borderline elevations of one or more liver tests may occur in up to 15% of patients. These abnormalities may progress, may remain essentially unchanged, or may be transient with continued therapy. The SGPT (ALT) test is probably the most sensitive indicator of liver dysfunction. Meaningful (3 times the upper limit of normal) elevations of SGPT or SGOT (AST) occurred in controlled clinical trials in less than 1% of patients. A patient with symptoms and/or signs suggesting liver dysfunction, or in whom an abnormal liver test has occurred, should be evaluated for evidence of the development of more severe hepatic reactions while on therapy with DOLOBID. Severe hepatic reactions, including jaundice, have been reported with DOLOBID as well as with other non-steroidal anti-inflammatory drugs. Although such reactions are rare, if abnormal liver tests persist or worsen, if clinical signs and symptoms consistent with liver disease develop, or if systemic manifestations occur (e.g., eosinophilia, rash, etc.), DOLOBID should be discontinued, since liver reactions can be fatal.

Gastrointestinal: Because serious GI tract ulceration and bleeding can occur without warning symptoms, physicians should follow chronically treated patients for the signs and symptoms of ulceration and bleeding and should inform them of the importance of this follow-up (see WARNINGS, *Risk of GI Ulcerations, Bleeding and Perforation with NSAID Therapy*).

Drug Interactions

Oral Anticoagulants: In some normal volunteers, the concomitant administration of DOLOBID and warfarin, acenocoumarol, or phenprocoumon resulted in prolongation of prothrombin time. This may occur because diflunisal competitively displaces coumarins from protein binding sites. Accordingly, when DOLOBID is administered with oral anticoagulants, the prothrombin time should be closely monitored during and for several days after concomitant drug administration. Adjustment of dosage of oral anticoagulants may be required.

Tolbutamide: In diabetic patients receiving DOLOBID and tolbutamide, no significant effects were seen on tolbutamide plasma levels or fasting blood glucose.

Hydrochlorothiazide: In normal volunteers, concomitant administration of DOLOBID and hydrochlorothiazide resulted in significantly increased plasma levels of hydrochlorothiazide. DOLOBID decreased the hyperuricemic effect of hydrochlorothiazide.

Furosemide: In normal volunteers, the concomitant administration of DOLOBID and furosemide had no effect on the diuretic activity of furosemide. DOLOBID decreased the hyperuricemic effect of furosemide.

Antacids: Concomitant administration of antacids may reduce plasma levels of DOLOBID. This effect is small with occasional doses of antacids, but may be clinically significant when antacids are used on a continuous schedule.

Acetaminophen: In normal volunteers, concomitant administration of DOLOBID and acetaminophen resulted in an approximate 50% increase in plasma levels of acetaminophen. Acetaminophen had no effect on plasma levels of DOLOBID. Since acetaminophen in high doses has been associated with hepatotoxicity, concomitant administration of DOLOBID and acetaminophen should be used cautiously, with careful monitoring of patients.

Concomitant administration of DOLOBID and acetaminophen in dogs, but not in rats, at approximately 2 times the recommended maximum human therapeutic dose of each (40-52 mg/kg/day of DOLOBID/acetaminophen), resulted in greater gastrointestinal toxicity than when either drug was administered alone. The clinical significance of these findings has not been established.

Methotrexate: Caution should be used if DOLOBID is administered concomitantly with methotrexate. Non-steroidal anti-inflammatory drugs have been reported to decrease the tubular secretion of methotrexate and to potentiate its toxicity.

Cyclosporine: Administration of non-steroidal anti-inflammatory drugs concomitantly with cyclosporine has been associated with an increase in cyclosporine-induced toxicity, possibly due to decreased synthesis of renal prostacyclin. NSAIDs should be used with caution in patients taking cyclosporine, and renal function should be carefully monitored.

Drug Interactions: Non-steroidal Anti-inflammatory Drugs

The administration of diflunisal to normal volunteers receiving indomethacin decreased the renal clearance and significantly increased the plasma levels of indomethacin. In some patients the combined use of indomethacin and DOLOBID has been associated with fatal gastrointestinal hemorrhage. Therefore, indomethacin and DOLOBID should not be used concomitantly.

The concomitant use of DOLOBID and other NSAIDs is not recommended due to the increased possibility of gastrointestinal toxicity, with little or no increase in efficacy. The following information was obtained from studies in normal volunteers.

Aspirin: In normal volunteers, a small decrease in diflunisal levels was observed when multiple doses of DOLOBID and aspirin were administered concomitantly.

Sulindac: The concomitant administration of DOLOBID and sulindac in normal volunteers resulted in lowering of the plasma levels of the active sulindac sulfide metabolite by approximately one-third.

Naproxen: The concomitant administration of DOLOBID and naproxen in normal volunteers had no effect on the plasma levels of naproxen, but significantly decreased the urinary excretion of naproxen and its glucuronide metabolite. Naproxen had no effect on plasma levels of DOLOBID.

Drug/Laboratory Test Interactions

Serum Salicylate Assays: Caution should be used in interpreting the results of serum salicylate assays when diflunisal is present. Salicylate levels have been found to be falsely elevated with some assay methods.

Carcinogenesis, Mutagenesis, Impairment of Fertility

Diflunisal did not affect the type or incidence of neoplasia in a 105-week study in the rat given doses up to 40 mg/kg/day (equivalent to approximately 1.3 times the maximum recommended human dose), or in long-term carcinogenic studies in mice given diflunisal at doses up to 80 mg/kg/day (equivalent to approximately 2.7 times the maximum recommended human dose). It was concluded that there was no carcinogenic potential for DOLOBID.

Diflunisal passes the placental barrier to a minor degree in the rat. Diflunisal had no mutagenic activity after oral administration in the dominant lethal assay, in the Ames microbial mutagen test or in the V-79 Chinese hamster lung cell assay.

No evidence of impaired fertility was found in reproduction studies in rats at doses up to 50 mg/kg/day.

Pregnancy

Pregnancy Category C. A dose of 60 mg/kg/day of diflunisal (equivalent to two times the maximum human dose) was maternotoxic, embryotoxic, and teratogenic in rabbits. In three of six studies in rabbits, evidence of teratogenicity was observed at doses ranging from 40 to 50 mg/kg/day. Teratology studies in mice, at doses up to 45 mg/kg/day, and in rats at doses up to 100 mg/kg/day, revealed no harm to the fetus due to diflunisal. Aspirin and other salicylates have been shown to be teratogenic in a wide variety of species, including the rat and rabbit, at doses ranging from 50 to 400 mg/kg/day (approximately one to eight times the human dose).

There are no adequate and well controlled studies with diflunisal in pregnant women. DOLOBID should be used during the first two trimesters of pregnancy only if the potential benefit justifies the potential risk to the fetus. The known effects of drugs of this class on the human fetus during the third trimester of pregnancy include: constriction of the ductus arteriosus prenatally, tricuspid incompetence, and pulmonary hypertension; non-closure of the ductus arteriosus postnatally which may be resistant to medical management; myocardial degenerative changes, platelet dysfunction with resultant bleeding, intracranial bleeding, renal dysfunction or failure, renal injury/dysgenesis which may result in prolonged or permanent renal failure, oligohydramnios, gastrointestinal bleeding or perforation, and increased risk of necrotizing enterocolitis. Use during the third trimester of pregnancy is not recommended.

In rats at a dose of one and one-half times the maximum human dose, there was an increase in the average length of gestation. Similar increases in the length of gestation have been observed with aspirin, indomethacin, and phenylbutazone, and may be related to inhibition of prostaglandin synthetase. Drugs of this class may cause dystocia and delayed parturition in pregnant animals.

Nursing Mothers

Diflunisal is excreted in human milk in concentrations of 2–7% of those in plasma. Because of the potential for serious adverse reactions in nursing infants from DOLOBID, a decision should be made whether to discontinue nursing or to discontinue the drug, taking into account the importance of the drug to the mother.

Pediatric Use

The adverse effects observed following diflunisal administration to neonatal animals appear to be species, age, and dose-dependent. At dose levels approximately 3 times the usual human therapeutic dose, both aspirin (200 to 400 mg/kg/day) and diflunisal (80 mg/kg/day) resulted in death, leukocytosis, weight loss, and bilateral cataracts in neonatal (4 to 5-day-old) beagle puppies after 2 to 10 doses. Administration of an 80 mg/kg/day dose of diflunisal to 25-day-old puppies resulted in lower mortality, and did not produce cataracts. In newborn rats, a 400 mg/kg/day dose of aspirin resulted in increased mortality and some cataracts, whereas the effects of diflunisal administration at doses up to 140 mg/kg/day were limited to a decrease in average body weight gain.

Safety and effectiveness in infants and children have not been established, and use of the drug in children below the age of 12 years is not recommended.

ADVERSE REACTIONS

The adverse reactions observed in controlled clinical trials encompass observations in 2,427 patients.

Listed below are the adverse reactions reported in the 1,314 of these patients who received treatment in studies of two weeks or longer. Five hundred thirteen patients were treated for at least 24 weeks, 255 patients were treated for at least 48 weeks, and 46 patients were treated for 96 weeks. In general, the adverse reactions listed below were 2 to 14 times less frequent in the 1,113 patients who received short-term treatment for mild to moderate pain.

Incidence Greater Than 1%

Gastrointestinal

The most frequent types of adverse reactions occurring with DOLOBID are gastrointestinal: these include nausea*, vomiting, dyspepsia*, gastrointestinal pain*, diarrhea*, constipation, and flatulence.

Psychiatric

Somnolence, insomnia.

Central Nervous System

Dizziness.

Special Senses

Tinnitus.

Dermatologic

Rash*.

Miscellaneous

Headache*, fatigue/tiredness.

Incidence Less Than 1 in 100

The following adverse reactions, occurring less frequently than 1 in 100, were reported in clinical trials or since the drug was marketed. The probability exists of a causal relationship between DOLOBID and these adverse reactions.

Dermatologic

Erythema multiforme, exfoliative dermatitis, Stevens-Johnson syndrome, toxic epidermal necrolysis, urticaria, pruritus, sweating, dry mucous membranes, stomatitis, photosensitivity.

Gastrointestinal

Peptic ulcer, gastrointestinal bleeding, anorexia, eructation, gastrointestinal perforation, gastritis.

Liver function abnormalities; jaundice, sometimes with fever; cholestasis; hepatitis.

Hematologic

Thrombocytopenia; agranulocytosis; hemolytic anemia.

Genitourinary

Dysuria; renal impairment, including renal failure; interstitial nephritis; hematuria; proteinuria.

Psychiatric

Nervousness, depression, hallucinations, confusion, disorientation.

Central Nervous System

Vertigo; light-headedness; paresthesias.

Special Senses

Transient visual disturbances including blurred vision.

Hypersensitivity Reactions

Acute anaphylactic reaction with bronchospasm; angioedema; flushing.

Hypersensitivity vasculitis.

Hypersensitivity syndrome (see PRECAUTIONS).

Miscellaneous

Asthenia, edema.

Causal Relationship Unknown

Other reactions have been reported in clinical trials or since the drug was marketed, but occurred under circumstances where a causal relationship could not be established. However, in these rarely reported events, that possibility cannot be excluded. Therefore, these observations are listed to serve as alerting information to physicians.

Continued on next page

Information on the Merck & Co., Inc. products listed on these pages is the full prescribing information from product circulars in use September 30, 1996.

Merck & Co.—Cont.

Respiratory
Dyspnea.
Cardiovascular
Palpitation, syncope.
Musculoskeletal
Muscle cramps.
Genitourinary
Nephrotic syndrome.
Miscellaneous
Chest pain.

A rare occurrence of fulminant necrotizing fasciitis, particularly in association with Group A β-hemolytic streptococcus, has been described in persons treated with non-steroidal anti-inflammatory agents, including diflunisal, sometimes with fatal outcome (see also PRECAUTIONS, *General*).

Potential Adverse Effects
In addition, a variety of adverse effects not observed with DOLOBID in clinical trials or in marketing experience, but reported with other non-steroidal analgesic/anti-inflammatory agents, should be considered potential adverse effects of DOLOBID.

*Incidence between 3% and 9%. Those reactions occurring in 1% to 3% are not marked with an asterisk.

OVERDOSAGE

Cases of overdosage have occurred and deaths have been reported. Most patients recovered without evidence of permanent sequelae. The most common signs and symptoms observed with overdosage were drowsiness, vomiting, nausea, diarrhea, hyperventilation, tachycardia, sweating, tinnitus, disorientation, stupor and coma. Diminished urine output and cardiorespiratory arrest have also been reported. The lowest dosage of DOLOBID at which a death has been reported was 15 grams without the presence of other drugs. In a mixed drug overdose, ingestion of 7.5 grams of DOLOBID resulted in death.

In the event of overdosage, the stomach should be emptied by inducing vomiting or by gastric lavage, and the patient carefully observed and given symptomatic and supportive treatment. Because of the high degree of protein binding, hemodialysis may not be effective.

The oral LD_{50} of the drug is 500 mg/kg and 826 mg/kg in female mice and female rats respectively.

DOSAGE AND ADMINISTRATION

Concentration-dependent pharmacokinetics prevail when DOLOBID is administered; a doubling of dosage produces a greater than doubling of drug accumulation. The effect becomes more apparent with repetitive doses.

For mild to moderate pain, an initial dose of 1000 mg followed by 500 mg every 12 hours is recommended for most patients. Following the initial dose, some patients may require 500 mg every 8 hours.

A lower dosage may be appropriate depending on such factors as pain severity, patient response, weight, or advanced age; for example, 500 mg initially, followed by 250 mg every 8–12 hours.

For osteoarthritis and rheumatoid arthritis, the suggested dosage range is 500 mg to 1000 mg daily in two divided doses. The dosage of DOLOBID may be increased or decreased according to patient response.

Maintenance doses higher than 1500 mg a day are not recommended.

DOLOBID may be administered with water, milk or meals. Tablets should be swallowed whole, not crushed or chewed.

HOW SUPPLIED

Tablets DOLOBID are capsule-shaped, film-coated tablets supplied as follows:
No. 3390—250 mg peach colored, coded DOLOBID on one side and MSD 675 on the other.
NDC 0006-0675-28 unit dose package of 100
(6505-01-203-6282, 250 mg individually sealed 100's)
NDC 0006-0675-61 unit of use bottles of 60
(6505-01-164-0501, 250 mg 60's).
Shown in Product Identification Guide, page 324
No. 3392—500 mg orange colored, coded DOLOBID on one side and MSD 697 on the other.
NDC 0006-0697-28 unit dose package of 100
(6505-01-154-4287, 500 mg individually sealed 100's)
NDC 0006-0697-61 unit of use bottles of 60
(6505-01-144-9724, 500 mg 60's).
Shown in Product Identification Guide, page 324
7928831   Issued August 1995
COPYRIGHT © MERCK & CO., INC., 1988
All rights reserved

EDECRIN® Tablets ℞
(Ethacrynic Acid), U.S.P.
Intravenous
SODIUM EDECRIN® ℞
(Ethacrynate Sodium), U.S.P.

EDECRIN* (Ethacrynic Acid) is a potent diuretic which, if given in excessive amounts, may lead to profound diuresis with water and electrolyte depletion. Therefore, careful medical supervision is required, and dose and dose schedule must be adjusted to the individual patient's needs (see DOSAGE AND ADMINISTRATION).

DESCRIPTION

Ethacrynic acid is an unsaturated ketone derivative of an aryloxyacetic acid. It is designated chemically as [2,3-dichloro-4-(2-methylene-1-oxobutyl)phenoxy] acetic acid, and has a molecular weight of 303.14. Ethacrynic acid is a white, or practically white, crystalline powder, very slightly soluble in water, but soluble in most organic solvents such as alcohols, chloroform, and benzene. Its empirical formula is $C_{13}H_{12}Cl_2O_4$ and its structural formula is:

Ethacrynate sodium, the sodium salt of ethacrynic acid, is soluble in water at 25°C to the extent of about 7 percent. Solutions of the sodium salt are relatively stable at about pH 7 at room temperature for short periods, but as the pH or temperature increases the solutions are less stable. The molecular weight of ethacrynate sodium is 325.12. Its empirical formula is $C_{13}H_{11}Cl_2NaO_4$ and its structural formula is:

EDECRIN is supplied as 25 mg and 50 mg tablets for oral use. Each tablet contains the following inactive ingredients: colloidal silicon dioxide, lactose, magnesium stearate, starch and talc. The 50 mg tablet also contains D&C Yellow 10, FD&C Blue 1 and FD&C Yellow 6. Intravenous SODIUM EDECRIN* (Ethacrynate Sodium) is a sterile freeze-dried powder and is supplied in a vial containing:

Ethacrynate sodium equivalent to ethacrynic acid	50.0 mg
Inactive ingredients:	
Mannitol	62.5 mg
with 0.1 mg thimerosal (mercury derivative) added as preservative.	

*Registered trademark of MERCK & CO., INC.

CLINICAL PHARMACOLOGY

Pharmacokinetics and Metabolism
EDECRIN acts on the ascending limb of the loop of Henle and on the proximal and distal tubules. Urinary output is usually dose dependent and related to the magnitude of fluid accumulation. Water and electrolyte excretion may be increased several times over that observed with thiazide diuretics, since EDECRIN inhibits reabsorption of a much greater proportion of filtered sodium than most other diuretic agents. Therefore, EDECRIN is effective in many patients who have significant degrees of renal insufficiency (see WARNINGS concerning deafness). EDECRIN has little or no effect on glomerular filtration or on renal blood flow, except following pronounced reductions in plasma volume when associated with rapid diuresis.

The electrolyte excretion pattern of ethacrynic acid varies from that of the thiazides and mercurial diuretics. Initial sodium and chloride excretion is usually substantial and chloride loss exceeds that of sodium. With prolonged administration, chloride excretion declines, and potassium and hydrogen ion excretion may increase. EDECRIN is effective whether or not there is clinical acidosis or alkalosis. Although EDECRIN, in carefully controlled studies in animals and experimental subjects, produces a more favorable sodium/potassium excretion ratio than the thiazides, in pa-

tients with increased diuresis excessive amounts of potassium may be excreted.

Onset of action is rapid, usually within 30 minutes after an oral dose of EDECRIN or within 5 minutes after an intravenous injection of SODIUM EDECRIN. After oral use, diuresis peaks in about 2 hours and lasts about 6 to 8 hours.

The sulfhydryl binding propensity of ethacrynic acid differs somewhat from that of the organomercurials. Its mode of action is not by carbonic anhydrase inhibition.

Ethacrynic acid does not cross the blood-brain barrier.

INDICATIONS AND USAGE

EDECRIN is indicated for treatment of edema when an agent with greater diuretic potential than those commonly employed is required.

1. Treatment of the edema associated with congestive heart failure, cirrhosis of the liver, and renal disease, including the nephrotic syndrome.
2. Short-term management of ascites due to malignancy, idiopathic edema, and lymphedema.
3. Short-term management of hospitalized pediatric patients, other than infants, with congenital heart disease or the nephrotic syndrome.
4. Intravenous SODIUM EDECRIN is indicated when a rapid onset of diuresis is desired, e.g., in acute pulmonary edema, or when gastrointestinal absorption is impaired or oral medication is not practicable.

CONTRAINDICATIONS

All diuretics, including ethacrynic acid, are contraindicated in anuria. If increasing electrolyte imbalance, azotemia, and/or oliguria occur during treatment of severe, progressive renal disease, the diuretic should be discontinued.

In a few patients this diuretic has produced severe, watery diarrhea. If this occurs, it should be discontinued and not used again.

Until further experience in infants is accumulated, therapy with oral and parenteral EDECRIN is contraindicated.

Hypersensitivity to any component of this product.

WARNINGS

The effects of EDECRIN on electrolytes are related to its renal pharmacologic activity and are dose dependent. The possibility of profound electrolyte and water loss may be avoided by weighing the patient throughout the treatment period, by careful adjustment of dosage, by initiating treatment with small doses, and by using the drug on an intermittent schedule when possible. When excessive diuresis occurs, the drug should be withdrawn until homeostasis is restored. When excessive electrolyte loss occurs, the dosage should be reduced or the drug temporarily withdrawn.

Initiation of diuretic therapy with EDECRIN in the cirrhotic patient with ascites is best carried out in the hospital. When maintenance therapy has been established, the individual can be satisfactorily followed as an outpatient.

EDECRIN should be given with caution to patients with advanced cirrhosis of the liver, particularly those with a history of previous episodes of electrolyte imbalance or hepatic encephalopathy. Like other diuretics it may precipitate hepatic coma and death.

Too vigorous a diuresis, as evidenced by rapid and excessive weight loss, may induce an acute hypotensive episode. In elderly cardiac patients, rapid contraction of plasma volume and the resultant hemoconcentration should be avoided to prevent the development of thromboembolic episodes, such as cerebral vascular thromboses and pulmonary emboli which may be fatal. Excessive loss of potassium in patients receiving digitalis glycosides may precipitate digitalis toxicity. Care should also be exercised in patients receiving potassium-depleting steroids.

A number of possibly drug-related deaths have occurred in critically ill patients refractory to other diuretics. These generally have fallen into two categories: (1) patients with severe myocardial disease who have been receiving digitalis and presumably developed acute hypokalemia with fatal arrhythmia; (2) patients with severely decompensated hepatic cirrhosis with ascites, with or without accompanying encephalopathy, who were in electrolyte imbalance and died because of intensification of the electrolyte defect.

Deafness, tinnitus, and vertigo with a sense of fullness in the ears have occurred, most frequently in patients with severe impairment of renal function. These symptoms have been associated most often with intravenous administration and with doses in excess of those recommended. The deafness has usually been reversible and of short duration (one to 24 hours). However, in some patients the hearing loss has been permanent. A number of these patients were also receiving drugs known to be ototoxic. EDECRIN may increase the ototoxic potential of other drugs (see PRECAUTIONS, subsection *Drug Interactions*).

Lithium generally should not be given with diuretics (see PRECAUTIONS, subsection *Drug Interactions*).

PRECAUTIONS

General

Weakness, muscle cramps, paresthesias, thirst, anorexia, and signs of hyponatremia, hypokalemia, and/or hypochloremic alkalosis may occur following vigorous or excessive diuresis and these may be accentuated by rigid salt restriction. Rarely tetany has been reported following vigorous diuresis. *During therapy with ethacrynic acid, liberalization of salt intake and supplementary potassium chloride are often necessary.*

When a metabolic alkalosis may be anticipated, e.g., in cirrhosis with ascites, the use of potassium chloride or a potassium-sparing agent before and during therapy with EDECRIN may mitigate or prevent the hypokalemia.

Loop diuretics have been shown to increase the urinary excretion of magnesium; this may result in hypomagnesemia.

The safety and efficacy of ethacrynic acid in hypertension have not been established. However, the dosage of coadministered antihypertensive agents may require adjustment.

Orthostatic hypotension may occur in patients receiving other antihypertensive agents when given ethacrynic acid. EDECRIN has little or no effect on glomerular filtration or on renal blood flow, except following pronounced reductions in plasma volume when associated with rapid diuresis. A transient increase in serum urea nitrogen may occur. Usually, this is readily reversible when the drug is discontinued. As with other diuretics used in the treatment of renal edema, hypoproteinemia may reduce responsiveness to ethacrynic acid and the use of salt-poor albumin should be considered.

A number of drugs, including ethacrynic acid, have been shown to displace warfarin from plasma protein; a reduction in the usual anticoagulant dosage may be required in patients receiving both drugs.

EDECRIN may increase the risk of gastric hemorrhage associated with corticosteroid treatment.

Laboratory Tests

Frequent serum electrolyte, CO_2 and BUN determinations should be performed early in therapy and periodically thereafter during active diuresis. Any electrolyte abnormalities should be corrected or the drug temporarily withdrawn.

Increases in blood glucose and alterations in glucose tolerance tests have been observed in patients receiving EDECRIN.

Drug Interactions

Lithium generally should not be given with diuretics because they reduce its renal clearance and add a high risk of lithium toxicity. Read circulars for lithium preparations before use of such concomitant therapy.

EDECRIN may increase the ototoxic potential of other drugs such as aminoglycoside and some cephalosporin antibiotics. Their concurrent use should be avoided.

A number of drugs, including ethacrynic acid, have been shown to displace warfarin from plasma protein; a reduction in the usual anticoagulant dosage may be required in patients receiving both drugs.

In some patients, the administration of a non-steroidal anti-inflammatory agent can reduce the diuretic, natriuretic, and antihypertensive effects of loop, potassium-sparing and thiazide diuretics. Therefore, when EDECRIN and non-steroidal anti-inflammatory agents are used concomitantly, the patient should be observed closely to determine if the desired effect of the diuretic is obtained.

Carcinogenesis, Mutagenesis, Impairment of Fertility

There was no evidence of a tumorigenic effect in a 79-week oral chronic toxicity study in rats at doses up to 45 times the human dose.

Ethacrynic acid had no effect on fertility in a two-litter study in rats or a two-generation study in mice at 10 times the human dose.

Pregnancy

Pregnancy Category B: Reproduction studies in the mouse and rabbit at doses up to 50 times the human dose showed no evidence of external abnormalities of the fetus due to EDECRIN.

In a two-litter study in the dog and rat, oral doses of 5 or 20 mg/kg/day (2½ or 10 times the human dose), respectively, did not interfere with pregnancy or with growth and development of the pups. Although there was reduction in the mean body weights of the fetuses in a teratogenic study in the rat at a dose level of 100 mg/kg (50 times the human dose), there was no effect on mortality or postnatal development. Functional and morphologic abnormalities were not observed. There are, however, no adequate and well-controlled studies in pregnant women. Since animal reproduction studies are not always predictive of human response, EDECRIN should be used during pregnancy only if clearly needed.

Nursing Mothers

It is not known whether this drug is excreted in human milk. Because many drugs are excreted in human milk and because of the potential for serious adverse reactions in nursing infants from EDECRIN, a decision should be made whether to discontinue nursing or to discontinue the drug,

taking into account the importance of the drug to the mother.

Pediatric Use

For information on oral use in pediatrics, other than infants, see INDICATIONS AND USAGE and DOSAGE AND ADMINISTRATION.

Safety and effectiveness in infants have not been established (see CONTRAINDICATIONS).

Safety and effectiveness of intravenous use in children have not been established (see DOSAGE AND ADMINISTRATION, *Intravenous Use*).

ADVERSE REACTIONS

Gastrointestinal

Anorexia, malaise, abdominal discomfort or pain, dysphagia, nausea, vomiting, and diarrhea have occurred. These are more frequent with large doses or after one to three months of continuous therapy. A few patients have had sudden onset of profuse, watery diarrhea. Discontinue EDECRIN if diarrhea is severe and do not give it again. Gastrointestinal bleeding has occurred in some patients. Rarely, acute pancreatitis has been reported.

Metabolic

Reversible hyperuricemia and acute gout have been reported. Acute symptomatic hypoglycemia with convulsions occurred in two uremic patients who received doses above those recommended. Hyperglycemia has been reported. Rarely, jaundice and abnormal liver function tests have been reported in seriously ill patients receiving multiple drug therapy, including EDECRIN.

Hematologic

Agranulocytosis or severe neutropenia has been reported in a few critically ill patients also receiving agents known to produce this effect. Thrombocytopenia has been reported rarely. Henoch-Schönlein purpura has been reported rarely in patients with rheumatic heart disease receiving multiple drug therapy, including EDECRIN.

Special Senses (See WARNINGS)

Deafness, tinnitus and vertigo with a sense of fullness in the ears, and blurred vision have occurred.

Central Nervous System

Headache, fatigue, apprehension, confusion.

Miscellaneous

Skin rash, fever, chills, hematuria.

SODIUM EDECRIN occasionally has caused local irritation and pain after intravenous use.

OVERDOSAGE

Overdosage may lead to excessive diuresis with electrolyte depletion and dehydration.

In the event of overdosage, symptomatic and supportive measures should be employed. Emesis should be induced or gastric lavage performed. Correct dehydration, electrolyte imbalance, hepatic coma, and hypotension by established procedures. If required, give oxygen or artificial respiration for respiratory impairment.

In the mouse, the oral LD_{50} of ethacrynic acid is 627 mg/kg and the intravenous LD_{50} of ethacrynate sodium is 175 mg/kg.

DOSAGE AND ADMINISTRATION

Dosage must be regulated carefully to prevent a more rapid or substantial loss of fluid or electrolyte than is indicated or necessary. The magnitude of diuresis and natriuresis is largely dependent on the degree of fluid accumulation present in the patient. Similarly, the extent of potassium excretion is determined in large measure by the presence and magnitude of aldosteronism.

Oral Use

EDECRIN is available for oral use as 25 mg and 50 mg tablets.

Dosage: To Initiate Diuresis

In Adults: The smallest dose required to produce gradual weight loss (about 1 to 2 pounds per day) is recommended. Onset of diuresis usually occurs at 50 to 100 mg for adults. After diuresis has been achieved, the minimally effective dose (usually from 50 to 200 mg daily) may be given on a continuous or intermittent dosage schedule. Dosage adjustments are usually in 25 to 50 mg increments to avoid derangement of water and electrolyte excretion.

The patient should be weighed under standard conditions before and during the institution of diuretic therapy with this compound. Small alterations in dose should effectively prevent a massive diuretic response. The following schedule may be helpful in determining the smallest effective dose.

  Day 1—50 mg (single dose) after a meal
  Day 2—50 mg twice daily after meals, if necessary
  Day 3—100 mg in the morning and 50 to 100 mg following
         the afternoon or evening meal, depending upon
         response to the morning dose
A few patients may require initial and maintenance doses as high as 200 mg twice daily. These higher doses, which should

be achieved gradually, are most often required in patients with severe, refractory edema.

In children (excluding infants, see CONTRAINDICATIONS): The initial dose should be 25 mg. Careful stepwise increments in dosage of 25 mg should be made to achieve effective maintenance.

Maintenance Therapy

It is usually possible to reduce the dosage and frequency of administration once dry weight has been achieved.

EDECRIN (Ethacrynic Acid) may be given intermittently after an effective diuresis is obtained with the regimen outlined above. Dosage may be on an alternate daily schedule or more prolonged periods of diuretic therapy may be interspersed with rest periods. Such an intermittent dosage schedule allows time for correction of any electrolyte imbalance and may provide a more efficient diuretic response.

The chloruretic effect of this agent may give rise to retention of bicarbonate and a metabolic alkalosis. This may be corrected by giving chloride (ammonium chloride or arginine chloride). Ammonium chloride should not be given to cirrhotic patients.

EDECRIN has additive effects when used with other diuretics. For example, a patient who is on maintenance dosage of an oral diuretic may require additional intermittent diuretic therapy, such as an organomercurial, for the maintenance of basal weight. The intermittent use of EDECRIN orally may eliminate the need for injections of organomercurials. Small doses of EDECRIN may be added to existing diuretic regimens to maintain basal weight. This drug may potentiate the action of carbonic anhydrase inhibitors, with augmentation of natriuresis and kaliuresis. Therefore, when adding EDECRIN the initial dose and changes of dose should be in 25 mg increments, to avoid electrolyte depletion. Rarely, patients who failed to respond to ethacrynic acid have responded to older established agents.

While many patients do not require supplemental potassium, the use of potassium chloride or potassium-sparing agents, or both, during treatment with EDECRIN is advisable, especially in cirrhotic or nephrotic patients and in patients receiving digitalis.

Salt liberalization usually prevents the development of hyponatremia and hypochloremia. During treatment with EDECRIN, salt may be liberalized to a greater extent than with other diuretics. Cirrhotic patients, however, usually require at least moderate salt restriction concomitant with diuretic therapy.

Intravenous Use

Intravenous SODIUM EDECRIN is for intravenous use when oral intake is impractical or in urgent conditions, such as acute pulmonary edema.

The usual intravenous dose for the average sized adult is 50 mg, or 0.5 to 1.0 mg per kg of body weight. Usually only one dose has been necessary; occasionally a second dose at a new injection site, to avoid possible thrombophlebitis, may be required. A single intravenous dose not exceeding 100 mg has been used in critical situations.

Insufficient pediatric experience precludes recommendation for this age group.

To reconstitute the dry material, add 50 mL of 5 percent Dextrose Injection, or Sodium Chloride Injection to the vial. Occasionally, some 5 percent Dextrose Injection solutions may have a low pH (below 5). The resulting solution with such a diluent may be hazy or opalescent. Intravenous use of such a solution is not recommended. Inspect the vial containing Intravenous SODIUM EDECRIN for particulate matter and discoloration before use.

The solution may be given slowly through the tubing of a running infusion or by direct intravenous injection over a period of several minutes. Do not mix this solution with whole blood or its derivatives. Discard unused reconstituted solution after 24 hours.

SODIUM EDECRIN should not be given subcutaneously or intramuscularly because of local pain and irritation.

HOW SUPPLIED

No. 3321—Tablets EDECRIN, 25 mg, are white, capsule shaped, scored tablets, coded MSD 65. They are supplied as follows:

NDC 0006-0065-68 in bottles of 100.

 Shown in Product Identification Guide, page 324

No. 3322—Tablets EDECRIN, 50 mg, are green, capsule shaped, scored tablets, coded MSD 90. They are supplied as follows:

NDC 0006-0090-68 in bottles of 100.

 Shown in Product Identification Guide, page 324

No. 3330—Intravenous SODIUM EDECRIN is a dry white material either in a plug form or as a powder. It is supplied in

Continued on next page

Information on the Merck & Co., Inc. products listed on these pages is the full prescribing information from product circulars in use September 30, 1996.

Merck & Co.—Cont.

vials containing ethacrynate sodium equivalent to 50 mg of ethacrynic acid, **NDC 0006-3330-50.**

7901425   Issued October 1985
COPYRIGHT © MERCK & CO., INC., 1984
All rights reserved

ELSPAR®
(Asparaginase)

℞

WARNING

IT IS RECOMMENDED THAT ASPARAGINASE BE ADMINISTERED TO PATIENTS ONLY IN A HOSPITAL SETTING UNDER THE SUPERVISION OF A PHYSICIAN WHO IS QUALIFIED BY TRAINING AND EXPERIENCE TO ADMINISTER CANCER CHEMOTHERAPEUTIC AGENTS, BECAUSE OF THE POSSIBILITY OF SEVERE REACTIONS, INCLUDING ANAPHYLAXIS AND SUDDEN DEATH. THE PHYSICIAN MUST BE PREPARED TO TREAT ANAPHYLAXIS AT EACH ADMINISTRATION OF THE DRUG.
IN THE TREATMENT OF EACH PATIENT THE PHYSICIAN MUST WEIGH CAREFULLY THE POSSIBILITY OF ACHIEVING THERAPEUTIC BENEFIT VERSUS THE RISK OF TOXICITY. THE FOLLOWING DATA SHOULD BE THOROUGHLY REVIEWED BEFORE ADMINISTERING THE COMPOUND.

DESCRIPTION

ELSPAR* (Asparaginase) contains the enzyme L-asparagine amidohydrolase, type EC-2, derived from *Escherichia coli*. It is a white crystalline powder that is freely soluble in water and practically insoluble in methanol, acetone and chloroform. Its activity is expressed in terms of International Units (I.U.) according to the recommendation of the International Union of Biochemistry. The specific activity of ELSPAR is at least 225 I.U. per milligram of protein and each vial contains 10,000 I.U. of asparaginase and 80 mg of mannitol, an inactive ingredient, as a sterile, white lyophilized plug or powder for intravenous or intramuscular injection after reconstitution.

*Registered trademark of MERCK & CO., INC.

CLINICAL PHARMACOLOGY

Action
In a significant number of patients with acute leukemia, particularly lymphocytic, the malignant cells are dependent on an exogenous source of asparagine for survival. Normal cells, however, are able to synthesize asparagine and thus are affected less by the rapid depletion produced by treatment with the enzyme asparaginase. This is a unique approach to therapy based on a metabolic defect in asparagine synthesis of some malignant cells. ELSPAR, derived from *Escherichia coli*, is effective in inducing remissions in some patients with acute lymphocytic leukemia.

Asparagine Dependence Test
An asparagine dependence test has been utilized during the investigational studies. In this test leukemic cells obtained from some marrow cultures could be shown to require asparagine in *vitro*, suggesting sensitivity to asparaginase therapy in *vivo*. However, present data indicate that the correlation between asparagine dependence in such tests and the final response to therapy is sufficiently poor that the test is not recommended as a basis for selection of patients for treatment.

Pharmacokinetics and Metabolism
In a study in patients with metastatic cancer and leukemia, initial plasma levels of L-asparaginase following intravenous administration were correlated to dose. Daily administration resulted in a cumulative increase in plasma levels. Plasma half-life varied from 8 to 30 hours; it did not appear to be influenced by dosage, either single or repetitive, and could not be correlated with age, sex, surface area, renal or hepatic function, diagnosis or extent of disease. Apparent volume of distribution was approximately 70–80% of estimated plasma volume. There was some slow movement of asparaginase from vascular to extravascular, extracellular space. L-asparaginase was detected in the lymph. Cerebrospinal fluid levels were less than 1% of concurrent plasma levels. Only trace amounts appeared in the urine.
In a study in which patients with leukemia and metastatic cancer received intramuscular L-asparaginase, peak plasma levels of asparaginase were reached 14 to 24 hours after dosing. Plasma half-life was 39 to 49 hours. No asparaginase was detected in the urine.

INDICATIONS AND USAGE

ELSPAR is indicated in the therapy of patients with acute lymphocytic leukemia. This agent is useful primarily in combination with other chemotherapeutic agents in the induction of remissions of the disease in children. ELSPAR should not be used as the sole induction agent unless combination therapy is deemed inappropriate. ELSPAR is not recommended for maintenance therapy.

CONTRAINDICATIONS

ELSPAR is contraindicated in patients with pancreatitis or a history of pancreatitis. Acute hemorrhagic pancreatitis, in some instances fatal, has been reported following asparaginase administration. Asparaginase is also contraindicated in patients who have had previous anaphylactic reactions to it.

WARNINGS

Allergic reactions to asparaginase are frequent and may occur during the primary course of therapy. They are not completely predictable on the basis of the intradermal skin test. Anaphylaxis and death have occurred even in a hospital setting with experienced observers.
Once a patient has received ELSPAR as part of a treatment regimen, retreatment with this agent at a later time is associated with increased risk of hypersensitivity reactions. In patients found by skin testing to be hypersensitive to asparaginase, and in any patient who has received a previous course of therapy with asparaginase, therapy with this agent should be instituted or reinstituted only after successful desensitization, and then only if in the judgement of the physician the possible benefit is greater than the increased risk. Desensitization itself may be hazardous. (See DOSAGE AND ADMINISTRATION, *Intradermal Skin Test.*)
In view of the unpredictability of the adverse reactions to asparaginase, it is recommended that this product be used in a hospital setting. Asparaginase has an adverse effect on liver function in the majority of patients. Therapy with asparaginase may increase pre-existing liver impairment caused by prior therapy or the underlying disease. Because of this there is a possibility that asparaginase may increase the toxicity of other medications.
The administration of ELSPAR *intravenously concurrently with or immediately before* a course of vincristine and prednisone may be associated with increased toxicity. (See DOSAGE AND ADMINISTRATION, *Recommended Induction Regimens.*)

PRECAUTIONS

General
This drug may be a contact irritant and both powder and solution must be handled and administered with care. Inhalation of dust or vapors and contact with skin or mucous membranes, especially those of the eyes, must be avoided. In case of contact, wash with copious amounts of water for at least 15 minutes.
Asparaginase has been reported to have immunosuppressive activity in animal experiments. Accordingly, the possibility that use of the drug in man may predispose to infection should be considered.
Asparaginase toxicity is reported to be greater in adults than in children.

Laboratory Tests
The fall in circulating lymphoblasts often is quite marked; normal or below normal leukocyte counts are noted frequently within the first several days after initiating therapy. This may be accompanied by a marked rise in serum uric acid. The possible development of uric acid nephropathy should be borne in mind. Appropriate preventive measures should be taken, e.g., allopurinol, increased fluid intake, alkalization of urine. As a guide to the effects of therapy, the patient's peripheral blood count and bone marrow should be monitored frequently.
Frequent serum amylase determinations should be obtained to detect early evidence of pancreatitis. If pancreatitis occurs, therapy should be stopped and not reinstituted.
Blood sugar should be monitored during therapy with ELSPAR because hyperglycemia may occur.

Drug Interactions
Tissue culture and animal studies indicate that ELSPAR can diminish or abolish the effect of methotrexate on malignant cells. This effect on methotrexate activity persists as long as plasma asparagine levels are suppressed. These results would seem to dictate against the clinical use of methotrexate with ELSPAR, or during the period following ELSPAR therapy when plasma asparagine levels are below normal.

Drug/Laboratory Test Interactions
L-asparaginase has been reported to interfere with the interpretation of thyroid function tests by producing a rapid and marked reduction in serum concentrations of thyroxine-binding globulin within two days after the first dose. Serum concentrations of thyroxine-binding globulin returned to

pretreatment values within four weeks of the last dose of L-asparaginase.

Animal Toxicology
A one-month intravenous toxicity study of ELSPAR in dogs at doses of 250, 1000, and 2000 I.U./kg/day revealed reduced serum total protein and albumin with loss of body weight at the highest dose level and anorexia, emesis, and diarrhea at all dosage levels. A similar study in monkeys at doses of 100, 300, and 1000 I.U./kg/day also revealed reduction of serum total protein and albumin and body weight loss at all dosage levels. Bromsulfalein retention and fatty changes in the liver were noted in monkeys that were given 300 and 1000 I.U./kg/day. The rabbit was unusually sensitive to ELSPAR since a single intravenous dose of 1000 I.U./kg caused hypocalcemia associated with necrosis of the parathyroid cells, convulsions, and death in about one third of the animals. Some rabbits that died showed small thymic and lymph node hemorrhages and necrosis of the germinal centers in the lymph nodes and spleen. The intravenous administration of calcium gluconate alleviated or prevented the adverse effects.
Changes in the pancreatic islets (not pancreatitis) ranging from edema to necrosis were observed in the rabbits in the acute intravenous toxicity studies (doses of 12,500 to 50,000 I.U./kg) but not in rabbits that received 1000 I.U./kg. The anatomical changes and the hypocalcemia found in the rabbits were not observed in the subacute intravenous studies in the dogs and monkeys.

Carcinogenesis, Mutagenesis, Impairment of Fertility
The intraperitoneal injection of 2500 I.U./kg/ day for 4 days in newborn Swiss mice resulted in a small increase in pulmonary adenomas; lymphatic leukemia was not increased. L-asparaginase at concentrations of 152-909 I.U./plate was not mutagenic in the Ames microbial mutagen test with or without metabolic activation.
There are no adequate studies on the effects of asparaginase on fertility.

Pregnancy
Pregnancy Category C. In mice and rats ELSPAR has been shown to retard the weight gain of mothers and fetuses when given in doses of more than 1000 I.U./kg (the recommended human dose). Resorptions, gross abnormalities and skeletal abnormalities were observed. The intravenous administration of 50 or 100 I.U./kg (one-twentieth or one-tenth of the human dose) to pregnant rabbits on Day 8 and 9 of gestation resulted in dose dependent embryotoxicity and gross abnormalities. There are no adequate and well-controlled studies in pregnant women. ELSPAR should be used during pregnancy only if the potential benefit justifies the potential risk to the fetus.

Nursing Mothers
It is not known whether this drug is secreted in human milk. Because many drugs are secreted in human milk and because of the potential for serious adverse reactions in nursing infants from ELSPAR, a decision should be made whether to discontinue nursing or to discontinue the drug, taking into account the importance of the drug to the mother.

ADVERSE REACTIONS

Allergic reactions, including skin rashes, urticaria, arthralgia, respiratory distress, and acute anaphylaxis have been reported. (See WARNINGS.) Acute reactions have occurred in the absence of a positive skin test and during continued maintenance of therapeutic serum levels of ELSPAR.
In children with advanced leukemia, a lower incidence of anaphylaxis has been reported with intramuscular administration, although there was a higher incidence of milder hypersensitivity reactions than with intravenous administration.
Fatal hyperthermia has been reported.
Pancreatitis, sometimes fulminant and fatal, has occurred during or following therapy with ELSPAR.
Hyperglycemia with glucosuria and polyuria has been reported in low incidence. Serum and urine acetone usually have been absent or negligible in these patients; this syndrome thus resembles hyperosmolar, nonketotic, hyperglycemia induced by a variety of other agents. This complication usually responds to discontinuance of ELSPAR, judicious use of intravenous fluid, and insulin, but may be fatal on occasion.
In addition to hypofibrinogenemia, depression of various other clotting factors has been reported. Most marked has been a decrease in plasma levels of factors V and VIII with a variable decrease in factors VII and IX. A decrease in circulating platelets has occurred in low incidence which, together with the increased levels of fibrin degradation products in the serum, may indicate development of a consumption coagulopathy. Bleeding has been a problem in only a minority of patients with demonstrable coagulopathy. However, intracranial hemorrhage and fatal bleeding associated with low fibrinogen levels have been reported. Increased fibrinolytic activity, apparently compensatory in nature, also has occurred.

Some patients have shown central nervous system effects consisting of depression, somnolence, fatigue, coma, confusion, agitation, and hallucinations varying from mild to severe. Rarely, a Parkinson-like syndrome has occurred, with tremor and a progressive increase in muscular tone. These side effects usually have reversed spontaneously after treatment was stopped. Therapy with ELSPAR is associated with an increase in blood ammonia during the conversion of asparagine to aspartic acid by the enzyme. No clear correlation exists between the degree of elevation of blood ammonia levels and the appearance of CNS changes. Chills, fever, nausea, vomiting, anorexia, abdominal cramps, weight loss, headache, and irritability may occur and usually are mild.
Azotemia, usually pre-renal, occurs frequently. Acute renal shut down and fatal renal insufficiency have been reported during treatment. Proteinuria has occurred infrequently.
A variety of liver function abnormalities have been reported, including elevations of SGOT, SGPT, alkaline phosphatase, bilirubin (direct and indirect), and depression of serum albumin, cholesterol (total and esters), and plasma fibrinogen. Increases and decreases of total lipids have occurred. Marked hypoalbuminemia associated with peripheral edema has been reported. However, these abnormalities usually are reversible on discontinuance of therapy and some reversal may occur during the course of therapy. Fatty changes in the liver have been documented by biopsy. Malabsorption syndrome has been reported.
Rarely, transient bone marrow depression has been observed, as evidenced by a delay in return of hemoglobin or hematocrit levels to normal in patients undergoing hematologic remission of leukemia. Marked leukopenia has been reported.

OVERDOSAGE

The acute intravenous LD_{50} of ELSPAR for mice was about 500,000 I.U./kg and for rabbits about 22,000 I.U./kg.

DOSAGE AND ADMINISTRATION

As a component of selected multiple agent induction regimens, ELSPAR may be administered by either the intravenous or the intramuscular route. When administered intravenously this enzyme should be given over a period of not less than thirty minutes through the side arm of an already running infusion of Sodium Chloride Injection or Dextrose Injection 5% (D_5W). ELSPAR has little tendency to cause phlebitis when given intravenously. Anaphylactic reactions require the immediate use of epinephrine, oxygen, and intravenous steroids.
When administering ELSPAR intramuscularly, the volume at a single injection site should be limited to 2 ml. If a volume greater than 2 ml is to be administered, two injection sites should be used.
Unfavorable interactions of ELSPAR with some antitumor agents have been demonstrated. It is recommended therefore, that ELSPAR be used in combination regimens only by physicians familiar with the benefits and risks of a given regimen. During the period of its inhibition of protein synthesis and cell replication ELSPAR may interfere with the action of drugs such as methotrexate which require cell replication for their lethal effect. ELSPAR may interfere with the enzymatic detoxification of other drugs, particularly in the liver.
Recommended Induction Regimens:
When using chemotherapeutic agents in combination for the induction of remissions in patients with acute lymphocytic leukemia, regimens are sought which provide maximum chance of success while avoiding excessive cumulative toxicity or negative drug interactions.
One of the following combination regimens incorporating ELSPAR is recommended for acute lymphocytic leukemia in children:
In the regimens below, Day 1 is considered to be the first day of therapy.
Regimen I
Prednisone 40 mg/square meter of body surface area per day orally in three divided doses for 15 days, followed by tapering of the dosage as follows:
20 mg/square meter for 2 days, 10 mg/square meter for 2 days, 5 mg/square meter for 2 days, 2.5 mg/square meter for 2 days and then discontinue.
Vincristine sulfate 2 mg/square meter of body surface area intravenously once weekly on Days 1, 8, and 15 of the treatment period. The maximum single dose should not exceed 2.0 mg.
Asparaginase 1,000 I.U./kg/day intravenously for ten successive days beginning on Day 22 of the treatment period.
Regimen II
Prednisone 40 mg/square meter of body surface area per day orally in three divided doses for 28 days (the total daily dose should be to the nearest 2.5 mg), following which the dosage of prednisone should be discontinued gradually over a 14 day period.
Vincristine sulfate 1.5 mg/square meter of body surface area intravenously weekly for four doses, on Days 1, 8, 15, and 22 of the treatment period. The maximum single dose should not exceed 2.0 mg.
Asparaginase 6,000 I.U./square meter of body surface area intramuscularly on Days 4, 7, 10, 13, 16, 19, 22, 25, and 28 of the treatment period. When a remission is obtained with either of the above regimens, appropriate maintenance therapy must be instituted. ELSPAR should not be used as part of a maintenance regimen. The above regimens do not preclude a need for special therapy directed toward the prevention of central nervous system leukemia.
It should be noted that ELSPAR has been used in combination regimens other than those recommended above. It is important to keep in mind that ELSPAR administered intravenously concurrently with or immediately before a course of vincristine and prednisone may be associated with increased toxicity. Physicians using a given regimen should be thoroughly familiar with its benefits and risks. Clinical data are insufficient for a recommendation concerning the use of combination regimens in adults. Asparaginase toxicity is reported to be greater in adults than in children.
Use of ELSPAR as the sole induction agent should be undertaken only in an unusual situation when a combined regimen is inappropriate because of toxicity or other specific patient-related factors, or in cases refractory to other therapy. When ELSPAR is to be used as the sole induction agent for children or adults the recommended dosage regimen is 200 I.U./kg/ day intravenously for 28 days. When complete remissions were obtained with this regimen, they were of short duration, 1 to 3 months. ELSPAR has been used as the sole induction agent in other regimens. Physicians using a given regimen should be thoroughly familiar with its benefits and risks.
Patients undergoing induction therapy must be carefully monitored and the therapeutic regimen adjusted according to response and toxicity.
Such adjustments should always involve decreasing dosages of one or more agents or discontinuation depending on the degree of toxicity. Patients who have received a course of ELSPAR, if retreated, have an increased risk of hypersensitivity reactions. Therefore, retreatment should be undertaken only when the benefit of such therapy is weighed against the increased risk.
Intradermal Skin Test:
Because of the occurrence of allergic reactions, an intradermal skin test should be performed prior to the initial administration of ELSPAR and when ELSPAR is given after an interval of a week or more has elapsed between doses. The skin test solution may be prepared as follows: Reconstitute the contents of a 10,000 I.U. vial with 5.0 ml of diluent. From this solution (2,000 I.U./ml) withdraw 0.1 ml and inject it into another vial containing 9.9 ml of diluent, yielding a skin test solution of approximately 20.0 I.U./ml. Use 0.1 ml of this solution (about 2.0 I.U.) for the intradermal skin test. The skin test site should be observed for at least one hour for the appearance of a wheal or erythema either of which indicates a positive reaction. An allergic reaction even to the skin test dose in certain sensitized individuals may rarely occur. A negative skin test reaction does not preclude the possibility of the development of an allergic reaction.

Desensitization:
Desensitization should be performed before administering the first dose of ELSPAR on initiation of therapy in positive reactors, and on retreatment of any patient in whom such therapy is deemed necessary after carefully weighing the increased risk of hypersensitivity reactions. Rapid desensitization of the patient may be attempted with progressively increasing amounts of intravenously administered ELSPAR provided adequate precautions are taken to treat an acute allergic reaction should it occur. One reported schedule begins with a total of 1 I.U. given intravenously and doubles the dose every 10 minutes, provided no reaction has occurred, until the accumulated total amount given equals the planned doses for that day.
For convenience the following table is included to calculate the number of doses necessary to reach the patient's total dose for that day:

Injection Number	ELSPAR Dose in I.U.	Accumulated Total Dose
1	1	1
2	2	3
3	4	7
4	8	15
5	16	31
6	32	63
7	64	127
8	128	255
9	256	511
10	512	1023
11	1024	2047
12	2048	4095
13	4096	8191
14	8192	16383
15	16384	32767
16	32768	65535
17	65536	131071
18	131072	262143

For example: A patient weighing 20 kg who is to receive 200 I.U./kg (total dose 4000 I.U.) would receive injections 1 through 12 during desensitization.

DIRECTIONS FOR RECONSTITUTION

Parenteral drug products should be inspected visually for particulate matter and discoloration prior to administration whenever solution and container permit. When reconstituted, ELSPAR should be a clear, colorless solution. If the solution becomes cloudy, discard.
For Intravenous Use
Reconstitute with Sterile Water for Injection or with Sodium Chloride Injection. The volume recommended for reconstitution is 5 ml for the 10,000 unit vials. Ordinary shaking during reconstitution does not inactivate the enzyme. This solution may be used for direct intravenous administration within an eight hour period following restoration. For administration by infusion, solutions should be diluted with the isotonic solutions, Sodium Chloride Injection or Dextrose Injection 5%. These solutions should be infused within eight hours and only if clear.
Occasionally, a very small number of gelatinous fiber-like particles may develop on standing. Filtration through a 5.0 micron filter during administration will remove the particles with no resultant loss in potency. Some loss of potency has been observed with the use of a 0.2 micron filter.
For Intramuscular Use
When ELSPAR is administered intramuscularly according to the schedule cited in the induction regimen, reconstitution is carried out by adding 2 ml Sodium Chloride Injection to the 10,000 unit vial. The resulting solution should be used within eight hours and only if clear.

HOW SUPPLIED

No. 4612 — ELSPAR is a white lyophilized plug or powder supplied as follows:
NDC 0006-4612-00 in a sterile 10 ml vial containing 10,000 I.U. of asparaginase and 80 mg mannitol, an inactive ingredient.
(6505-01-153-9650 10 mL vial)
Personnel preparing ELSPAR should avoid drug contact with skin, mucous membranes, or eyes and avoid inhaling the dust or vapor.
Store at 2–8°C (36–46°F). ELSPAR does not contain a preservative. Unused, reconstituted solution should be stored at 2 to 8°C (36 to 46°F) and discarded after eight hours, or sooner if it becomes cloudy.

A.H.F.S. Category: 44:00
7407111 Issued March 1995

FLEXERIL® Tablets ℞
(Cyclobenzaprine HCl), U.S.P.

DESCRIPTION

Cyclobenzaprine hydrochloride is a white, crystalline tricyclic amine salt with the empirical formula $C_{20}H_{21}N \cdot HCl$ and a molecular weight of 311.9. It has a melting point of 217°C, and a pK_a of 8.47 at 25°C. It is freely soluble in water and alcohol, sparingly soluble in isopropanol, and insoluble in hydrocarbon solvents. If aqueous solutions are made alkaline, the free base separates. Cyclobenzaprine HCl is designated chemically as 3-(5*H*-dibenzo[*a,d*]cyclohepten-5-ylidene)-*N, N*-dimethyl-1-propanamine hydrochloride, and has the following structural formula:

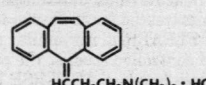

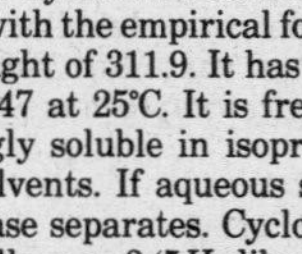
HCCH2CH2N(CH3)2 · HCl

FLEXERIL* (Cyclobenzaprine HCl) is supplied as 10 mg tablets for oral administration.
Tablets FLEXERIL contain the following inactive ingredients: hydroxypropyl cellulose, hydroxypropyl methylcellu-

Continued on next page

Information on the Merck & Co., Inc. products listed on these pages is the full prescribing information from product circulars in use September 30, 1996.

Merck & Co.—Cont.

lose, iron oxide, lactose, magnesium stearate, starch, and titanium dioxide.

---

*Registered trademark of MERCK & CO., INC.

CLINICAL PHARMACOLOGY

Cyclobenzaprine HCl relieves skeletal muscle spasm of local origin without interfering with muscle function. It is ineffective in muscle spasm due to central nervous system disease. Cyclobenzaprine reduced or abolished skeletal muscle hyperactivity in several animal models. Animal studies indicate that cyclobenzaprine does not act at the neuromuscular junction or directly on skeletal muscle. Such studies show that cyclobenzaprine acts primarily within the central nervous system at brain stem as opposed to spinal cord levels, although its action on the latter may contribute to its overall skeletal muscle relaxant activity. Evidence suggests that the net effect of cyclobenzaprine is a reduction of tonic somatic motor activity, influencing both gamma (γ) and alpha (α) motor systems.

Pharmacological studies in animals showed a similarity between the effects of cyclobenzaprine and the structurally related tricyclic antidepressants, including reserpine antagonism, norepinephrine potentiation, potent peripheral and central anticholinergic effects, and sedation. Cyclobenzaprine caused slight to moderate increase in heart rate in animals.

Cyclobenzaprine is well absorbed after oral administration, but there is a large intersubject variation in plasma levels. Cyclobenzaprine is eliminated quite slowly with a half-life as long as one to three days. It is highly bound to plasma proteins, is extensively metabolized primarily to glucuronide-like conjugates, and is excreted primarily via the kidneys. No significant effect on plasma levels or bioavailability of FLEXERIL or aspirin was noted when single or multiple doses of the two drugs were administered concomitantly. Concomitant administration of FLEXERIL and aspirin is usually well tolerated and no unexpected or serious clinical or laboratory adverse effects have been observed. No studies have been performed to indicate whether FLEXERIL enhances the clinical effect of aspirin or other analgesics, or whether analgesics enhance the clinical effect of FLEXERIL in acute musculoskeletal conditions.

Clinical Studies
Controlled clinical studies show that FLEXERIL significantly improves the signs and symptoms of skeletal muscle spasm as compared with placebo. The clinical responses include improvement in muscle spasm as determined by palpation, reduction in local pain and tenderness, increased range of motion, and less restriction in activities of daily living. When daily observations were made, clinical improvement was observed as early as the first day of therapy.

Eight double-blind controlled clinical studies were performed in 642 patients comparing FLEXERIL, diazepam*, and placebo. Muscle spasm, local pain and tenderness, limitation of motion, and restriction in activities of daily living were evaluated. In three of these studies there was a significantly greater improvement with FLEXERIL than with diazepam, while in the other studies the improvement following both treatments was comparable.

Although the frequency and severity of adverse reactions observed in patients treated with FLEXERIL were comparable to those observed in patients treated with diazepam, dry mouth was observed more frequently in patients treated with FLEXERIL and dizziness more frequently in those treated with diazepam. The incidence of drowsiness, the most frequent adverse reaction, was similar with both drugs. Analysis of the data from controlled studies shows that FLEXERIL produces clinical improvement whether or not sedation occurs.

---

*VALIUM® (diazepam, Roche)

Surveillance Program
A post-marketing surveillance program was carried out in 7607 patients with acute musculoskeletal disorders, and included 297 patients treated for 30 days or longer. The overall effectiveness of FLEXERIL was similar to that observed in the double-blind controlled studies; the overall incidence of adverse effects was less (see ADVERSE REACTIONS).

INDICATIONS AND USAGE

FLEXERIL is indicated as an adjunct to rest and physical therapy for relief of muscle spasm associated with acute, painful musculoskeletal conditions.

Improvement is manifested by relief of muscle spasm and its associated signs and symptoms, namely, pain, tenderness, limitation of motion, and restriction in activities of daily living.

FLEXERIL (Cyclobenzaprine HCl) should be used only for short periods (up to two or three weeks) because adequate evidence of effectiveness for more prolonged use is not available and because muscle spasm associated with acute, painful musculoskeletal conditions is generally of short duration and specific therapy for longer periods is seldom warranted.
FLEXERIL has not been found effective in the treatment of spasticity associated with cerebral or spinal cord disease, or in children with cerebral palsy.

CONTRAINDICATIONS

Hypersensitivity to the drug.
Concomitant use of monoamine oxidase inhibitors or within 14 days after their discontinuation.
Acute recovery phase of myocardial infarction, and patients with arrhythmias, heart block or conduction disturbances, or congestive heart failure.
Hyperthyroidism.

WARNINGS

Cyclobenzaprine is closely related to the tricyclic antidepressants, e.g., amitriptyline and imipramine. In short term studies for indications other than muscle spasm associated with acute musculoskeletal conditions, and usually at doses somewhat greater than those recommended for skeletal muscle spasm, some of the more serious central nervous system reactions noted with the tricyclic antidepressants have occurred (see WARNINGS, below, and ADVERSE REACTIONS).
FLEXERIL may interact with monoamine oxidase (MAO) inhibitors. Hyperpyretic crisis, severe convulsions, and deaths have occurred in patients receiving tricyclic antidepressants and MAO inhibitor drugs.
Tricyclic antidepressants have been reported to produce arrhythmias, sinus tachycardia, prolongation of the conduction time leading to myocardial infarction and stroke.
FLEXERIL may enhance the effects of alcohol, barbiturates, and other CNS depressants.

PRECAUTIONS

General
Because of its atropine-like action, FLEXERIL should be used with caution in patients with a history of urinary retention, angle-closure glaucoma, increased intraocular pressure, and in patients taking anticholinergic medication.
Information for Patients
FLEXERIL may impair mental and/or physical abilities required for performance of hazardous tasks, such as operating machinery or driving a motor vehicle.
Drug Interactions
FLEXERIL may enhance the effects of alcohol, barbiturates, and other CNS depressants.
Tricyclic antidepressants may block the antihypertensive action of guanethidine and similarly acting compounds.
Carcinogenesis, Mutagenesis, Impairment of Fertility
In rats treated with FLEXERIL for up to 67 weeks at doses of approximately 5 to 40 times the maximum recommended human dose, pale, sometimes enlarged, livers were noted and there was a dose-related hepatocyte vacuolation with lipidosis. In the higher dose groups this microscopic change was seen after 26 weeks and even earlier in rats which died prior to 26 weeks; at lower doses, the change was not seen until after 26 weeks.
Cyclobenzaprine did not affect the onset, incidence or distribution of neoplasia in an 81-week study in the mouse or in a 105-week study in the rat.
At oral doses of up to 10 times the human dose, cyclobenzaprine did not adversely affect the reproductive performance or fertility of male or female rats. Cyclobenzaprine did not demonstrate mutagenic activity in the male mouse at dose levels of up to 20 times the human dose.
Pregnancy
Pregnancy Category B: Reproduction studies have been performed in rats, mice and rabbits at doses up to 20 times the human dose, and have revealed no evidence of impaired fertility or harm to the fetus due to FLEXERIL. There are, however, no adequate and well-controlled studies in pregnant women. Because animal reproduction studies are not always predictive of human response, this drug should be used during pregnancy only if clearly needed.
Nursing Mothers
It is not known whether this drug is excreted in human milk. Because cyclobenzaprine is closely related to the tricyclic antidepressants, some of which are known to be excreted in human milk, caution should be exercised when FLEXERIL is administered to a nursing woman.
Pediatric Use
Safety and effectiveness of FLEXERIL in children below the age of 15 have not been established.

ADVERSE REACTIONS

The following list of adverse reactions is based on the experience in 473 patients treated with FLEXERIL in controlled clinical studies, 7607 patients in the post-marketing surveillance program, and reports received since the drug was marketed. The overall incidence of adverse reactions among patients in the surveillance program was less than the incidence in the controlled clinical studies.

The adverse reactions reported most frequently with FLEXERIL were drowsiness, dry mouth and dizziness. The incidence of these common adverse reactions was lower in the surveillance program than in the controlled clinical studies:

	Clinical Studies	Surveillance Program
drowsiness	39%	16%
dry mouth	27%	7%
dizziness	11%	3%

Among the less frequent adverse reactions, there was no appreciable difference in incidence in controlled clinical studies or in the surveillance program. Adverse reactions which were reported in 1% to 3% of the patients were: fatigue/tiredness, asthenia, nausea, constipation, dyspepsia, unpleasant taste, blurred vision, headache, nervousness, and confusion.

Incidence Less Than 1 in 100
The following adverse reactions have been reported at an incidence of less than 1 in 100:
Body as a Whole: Syncope; malaise.
Cardiovascular: Tachycardia; arrhythmia; vasodilatation; palpitation; hypotension.
Digestive: Vomiting; anorexia; diarrhea; gastrointestinal pain; gastritis; thirst; flatulence; edema of the tongue; abnormal liver function and rare reports of hepatitis, jaundice and cholestasis.
Hypersensitivity: Anaphylaxis; angioedema; pruritus; facial edema; urticaria; rash.
Musculoskeletal: Local weakness.
Nervous System and Psychiatric: Ataxia; vertigo; dysarthria; tremors; hypertonia; convulsions; muscle twitching; disorientation; insomnia; depressed mood; abnormal sensations; anxiety; agitation; abnormal thinking and dreaming; hallucinations; excitement; paresthesia; diplopia.
Skin: Sweating.
Special Senses: Ageusia; tinnitus.
Urogenital: Urinary frequency and/or retention.
Causal Relationship Unknown
Other reactions, reported rarely for FLEXERIL under circumstances where a causal relationship could not be established or reported for other tricyclic drugs, are listed to serve as alerting information to physicians:
Body as a Whole: Chest pain; edema.
Cardiovascular: Hypertension; myocardial infarction; heart block; stroke.
Digestive: Paralytic ileus; tongue discoloration; stomatitis; parotid swelling.
Endocrine: Inappropriate ADH syndrome.
Hematic and Lymphatic: Purpura; bone marrow depression; leukopenia; eosinophilia; thrombocytopenia.
Metabolic, Nutritional and Immune: Elevation and lowering of blood sugar levels; weight gain or loss.
Musculoskeletal: Myalgia.
Nervous System and Psychiatric: Decreased or increased libido; abnormal gait; delusions; peripheral neuropathy; Bell's palsy; alteration in EEG patterns; extrapyramidal symptoms.
Respiratory: Dyspnea.
Skin: Photosensitization; alopecia.
Urogenital: Impaired urination; dilatation of urinary tract; impotence; testicular swelling; gynecomastia; breast enlargement; galactorrhea.

DRUG ABUSE AND DEPENDENCE

Pharmacologic similarities among the tricyclic drugs require that certain withdrawal symptoms be considered when FLEXERIL is administered, even though they have not been reported to occur with this drug. Abrupt cessation of treatment after prolonged administration may produce nausea, headache, and malaise. These are not indicative of addiction.

OVERDOSAGE

Manifestations: High doses may cause temporary confusion, disturbed concentration, transient visual hallucinations, agitation, hyperactive reflexes, muscle rigidity, vomiting, or hyperpyrexia, in addition to anything listed under ADVERSE REACTIONS. Based on the known pharmacologic actions of the drug, overdosage may cause drowsiness, hypothermia, tachycardia and other cardiac rhythm abnormalities such as bundle branch block, ECG evidence of impaired conduction, and congestive heart failure. Other manifestations may be dilated pupils, convulsions, severe hypotension, stupor, and coma.
The acute oral LD_{50} of FLEXERIL is approximately 338 and 425 mg/kg in mice and rats, respectively.
Treatment: Treatment is symptomatic and supportive. Empty the stomach as quickly as possible by emesis, followed

---

by gastric lavage. After gastric lavage, activated charcoal may be administered. Twenty to 30 g of activated charcoal may be given every four to six hours during the first 24 to 48 hours after ingestion. An ECG should be taken and close monitoring of cardiac function must be instituted if there is any evidence of dysrhythmia. Maintenance of an open airway, adequate fluid intake, and regulation of body temperature are necessary.
The intravenous administration of 1-3 mg of physostigmine salicylate is reported to reverse symptoms of poisoning by atropine and other drugs with anticholinergic activity. Physostigmine may be helpful in the treatment of cyclobenzaprine overdose. Because physostigmine is rapidly metabolized, the dosage of physostigmine should be repeated as required, particularly if life-threatening signs such as arrhythmias, convulsions, and deep coma recur or persist after the initial dosage of physostigmine. Because physostigmine itself may be toxic, it is not recommended for routine use.
Standard medical measures should be used to manage circulatory shock and metabolic acidosis. Cardiac arrhythmias may be treated with neostigmine, pyridostigmine, or propranolol. When signs of cardiac failure occur, the use of a short-acting digitalis preparation should be considered. Close monitoring of cardiac function for not less than five days is advisable.
Anticonvulsants may be given to control seizures.
Dialysis is probably of no value because of low plasma concentrations of the drug.
Since overdosage is often deliberate, patients may attempt suicide by other means during the recovery phase. Deaths by deliberate or accidental overdosage have occurred with this class of drugs.

DOSAGE AND ADMINISTRATION

The usual dosage of FLEXERIL is 10 mg three times a day, with a range of 20 to 40 mg a day in divided doses. Dosage should not exceed 60 mg a day. Use of FLEXERIL for periods longer than two or three weeks is not recommended. (See INDICATIONS AND USAGE.)

HOW SUPPLIED

No. 3358—Tablets FLEXERIL, 10 mg, are butterscotch yellow, D-shaped, film coated tablets, coded MSD 931. They are supplied as follows:
NDC 0006-0931-68 in bottles of 100
(6505-01-062-8010, 10 mg 100's)
NDC 0006-0931-28 unit dose packages of 100.
Shown in Product Identification Guide, page 324
7897213 Issued August 1990
COPYRIGHT © MERCK & CO., INC., 1985
All rights reserved

FOSAMAX® ℞
(ALENDRONATE SODIUM TABLETS)

DESCRIPTION

FOSAMAX* (alendronate sodium) is an aminobisphosphonate that acts as a specific inhibitor of osteoclast-mediated bone resorption. Bisphosphonates are synthetic analogs of pyrophosphate that bind to the hydroxyapatite found in bone.
Alendronate sodium is chemically described as (4-amino-1-hydroxybutylidene) bisphosphonic acid monosodium salt trihydrate.
The empirical formula of alendronate sodium is $C_4H_{12}NNaO_7P_2 \cdot 3H_2O$ and its formula weight is 325.12. The structural formula is:

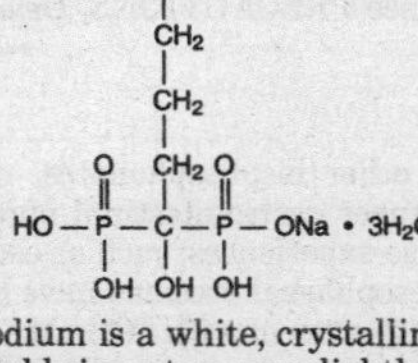

Alendronate sodium is a white, crystalline, nonhygroscopic powder. It is soluble in water, very slightly soluble in alcohol, and practically insoluble in chloroform.
Tablets FOSAMAX for oral administration contain either 13.05 mg or 52.21 mg of alendronate monosodium salt trihydrate, which is the molar equivalent of 10.0 mg and 40.0 mg, respectively, of free acid, and the following inactive ingredients: microcrystalline cellulose, anhydrous lactose, croscarmellose sodium, and magnesium stearate.

*Registered trademark of MERCK & CO., Inc.

CLINICAL PHARMACOLOGY

Mechanism of Action
Animal studies have indicated the following mode of action. At the cellular level, alendronate shows preferential localization to sites of bone resorption, specifically under osteoclasts. The osteoclasts adhere normally to the bone surface but lack the ruffled border that is indicative of active resorption. Alendronate does not interfere with osteoclast recruitment or attachment, but it does inhibit osteoclast activity. Studies in mice on the localization of radioactive [^{3}H]alendronate in bone showed about 10-fold higher uptake on osteoclast surfaces than on osteoblast surfaces. Bones examined 6 and 49 days after [^{3}H]alendronate administration in rats and mice, respectively, showed that normal bone was formed on top of the alendronate, which was incorporated inside the matrix. While incorporated in bone matrix, alendronate is not pharmacologically active. Thus, alendronate must be continuously administered to suppress osteoclasts on newly formed resorption surfaces. Histomorphometry in baboons and rats showed that alendronate treatment reduces bone turnover (i.e., the number of sites at which bone is remodeled). In addition, bone formation exceeds bone resorption at these remodeling sites, leading to progressive gains in bone mass.
Pharmacokinetics
Absorption
Relative to an intravenous (IV) reference dose, the mean oral bioavailability of alendronate in women was 0.7% for doses ranging from 5 to 40 mg when administered after an overnight fast and two hours before a standardized breakfast. Oral bioavailability of the 10 mg tablet in men (0.59%) was similar to that in women (0.78%) when administered after an overnight fast and 2 hours before breakfast.
A study examining the effect of timing of a meal on the bioavailability of alendronate was performed in 49 postmenopausal women. Bioavailability was decreased (by approximately 40%) when 10 mg alendronate was administered either 0.5 or 1 hour before a standardized breakfast, when compared to dosing 2 hours before eating. Bioavailability was negligible whether alendronate was administered with or up to two hours after a standardized breakfast. Concomitant administration of alendronate with coffee or orange juice reduced bioavailability by approximately 60%.
In a trial in elderly patients given 5 mg of alendronate (n = 86) 30 minutes before breakfast, similar bone mineral density changes were noted when compared to pivotal trials, in which one of the treatment arms was 5 mg alendronate administered 60 minutes before breakfast.
Distribution
Preclinical studies (in male rats) show that alendronate transiently distributes to soft tissues following 1 mg/kg IV administration but is then rapidly redistributed to bone or excreted in the urine. The mean steady-state volume of distribution, exclusive of bone, is at least 28 L in humans. Concentrations of drug in plasma following therapeutic oral doses are too low (less than 5 ng/mL) for analytical detection. Protein binding in human plasma is approximately 78%.
Metabolism
There is no evidence that alendronate is metabolized in animals or humans.
Excretion
Following a single IV dose of [^{14}C]alendronate, approximately 50% of the radioactivity was excreted in the urine within 72 hours and little or no radioactivity was recovered in the feces. Following a single 10 mg IV dose, the renal clearance of alendronate was 71 mL/min, and systemic clearance did not exceed 200 mL/min. Plasma concentrations fell by more than 95% within 6 hours following IV administration. The terminal half-life in humans is estimated to exceed 10 years, probably reflecting release of alendronate from the skeleton. Based on the above, it is estimated that after 10 years of oral treatment with FOSAMAX (10 mg daily) the amount of alendronate released daily from the skeleton is approximately 25% of that absorbed from the gastrointestinal tract.
Special Populations
Pediatric: Alendronate pharmacokinetics have not been investigated in patients <18 years of age.
Gender: Bioavailability and the fraction of an IV dose excreted in urine were similar in men and women.
Geriatric: Bioavailability and disposition (urinary excretion) were similar in elderly (≥ 65 years of age) and younger patients. No dosage adjustment is necessary (see DOSAGE AND ADMINISTRATION).
Race: Pharmacokinetic differences due to race have not been studied.
Renal Insufficiency: Preclinical studies show that, in rats with kidney failure, increasing amounts of drug are present in plasma, kidney, spleen, and tibia. In healthy controls, drug that is not deposited in bone is rapidly excreted in the urine. No evidence of saturation of bone uptake was found after 3 weeks dosing with cumulative IV doses of 35 mg/kg in young male rats. Although no clinical information is available, it is likely that, as in animals, elimination of alendronate via the kidney will be reduced in patients with impaired renal function. Therefore, somewhat greater accumulation of alendronate in bone might be expected in patients with impaired renal function.
No dosage adjustment is necessary for patients with mild-to-moderate renal insufficiency (creatinine clearance 35 to 60 mL/min). **FOSAMAX is not recommended for patients with more severe renal insufficiency (creatinine clearance <35 mL/min) due to lack of experience.**
Hepatic Insufficiency: As there is evidence that alendronate is not metabolized or excreted in the bile, no studies were conducted in patients with hepatic insufficiency. No dosage adjustment is necessary.
Drug Interactions (also see PRECAUTIONS, *Drug Interactions*)
Intravenous ranitidine was shown to double the bioavailability of oral alendronate. The clinical significance of this increased bioavailability and whether similar increases will occur in patients given oral H_2-antagonists is unknown; no other specific drug interaction studies were performed.
Products containing calcium and other multivalent cations likely will interfere with absorption of alendronate.

Summary of Pharmacokinetic Parameters in the Normal Population

	Mean	90% Confidence Interval
Absolute bioavailability of 10 mg tablet, taken 2 hours before first meal of the day	0.78% (females)	(0.61, 1.04)
	0.59% (males)	(0.43, 0.81)
Absolute bioavailability of 40 mg tablet, taken 2 hours before first meal of the day	0.60% (females)	(0.46, 0.78)
Renal Clearance (mL/min) (n=6)	71	(64, 78)

Pharmacodynamics
Osteoporosis in postmenopausal women
Osteoporosis is characterized by low bone mass that leads to an increased risk of fracture. The diagnosis can be confirmed by the finding of low bone mass, evidence of fracture on x-ray, a history of osteoporotic fracture, or height loss or kyphosis, indicative of vertebral fracture. Osteoporosis occurs in both males and females but is most common among women following the menopause, when bone turnover increases and the rate of bone resorption exceeds that of bone formation. These changes result in progressive bone loss and lead to osteoporosis in a significant proportion of women over age 50. Fractures, usually of the spine, hip, and wrist, are the common consequences. From age 50 to age 90, the risk of hip fracture in white women increases 50-fold and the risk of vertebral fracture 15- to 30-fold. It is estimated that approximately 40% of 50-year-old women will sustain one or more osteoporosis-related fractures of the spine, hip, or wrist during their remaining lifetimes. Hip fractures, in particular, are associated with substantial morbidity, disability, and mortality.
Alendronate is an aminobisphosphonate that binds to bone hydroxyapatite and specifically inhibits the activity of osteoclasts, the bone-resorbing cells. Alendronate reduces bone resorption with no direct effect on bone formation, although the latter process is ultimately reduced because bone resorption and formation are coupled during bone turnover. Alendronate thus reduces the elevated rate of bone turnover observed in postmenopausal women to approximate more closely that in premenopausal women.
Daily oral doses of alendronate (5, 20, and 40 mg for six weeks) in postmenopausal women produced biochemical changes indicative of dose-dependent inhibition of bone resorption, including decreases in urinary calcium and urinary markers of bone collagen degradation (such as deoxypyridinoline and cross-linked N-telopeptides of type I collagen). These biochemical changes tended to return toward baseline values as early as 3 weeks following the discontinuation of therapy with alendronate and did not differ from placebo after 7 months.
In long-term (two- or three-year) studies, FOSAMAX 10 mg/day reduced urinary excretion of markers of bone resorption, including deoxypyridinoline and cross-linked N-telopeptides

Continued on next page

Information on the Merck & Co., Inc. products listed on these pages is the full prescribing information from product circulars in use September 30, 1996.

Merck & Co.—Cont.

of type I collagen, by approximately 50–60% to reach levels similar to those seen in healthy premenopausal women. The decrease in the rate of bone resorption indicated by these markers was evident as early as one month and at three to six months reached a plateau that was maintained for the entire duration of treatment with FOSAMAX. In addition, the markers of bone formation, serum osteocalcin and alkaline phosphatase, were also reduced by approximately 50% and 25 to 30%, respectively, to a plateau after 6 to 12 months. These data indicate that the rate of bone turnover reached a new steady-state, despite the progressive increase in the total amount of alendronate deposited within bone. As a result of inhibition of bone resorption, asymptomatic reductions in serum calcium and phosphate concentrations were also observed following treatment with FOSAMAX. In the long-term studies, reductions from baseline in serum calcium (approximately 2%) and phosphate (approximately 4 to 6%) were evident the first month after the initiation of FOSAMAX 10 mg, but no further decreases were observed for the three-year duration of the studies. The reduction in serum phosphate may reflect not only the positive bone mineral balance due to FOSAMAX but also a decrease in renal phosphate reabsorption.

Paget's disease of bone

Paget's disease of bone is a chronic, focal skeletal disorder characterized by greatly increased and disorderly bone remodeling. Excessive osteoclastic bone resorption is followed by osteoblastic new bone formation, leading to the replacement of the normal bone architecture by disorganized, enlarged, and weakened bone structure.

Clinical manifestations of Paget's disease range from no symptoms to severe morbidity due to bone pain, bone deformity, pathological fractures, and neurological and other complications. Serum alkaline phosphatase, the most frequently used biochemical index of disease activity, provides an objective measure of disease severity and response to therapy.

FOSAMAX decreases the rate of bone resorption directly, which leads to an indirect decrease in bone formation. In clinical trials, FOSAMAX 40 mg once daily for six months produced highly significant decreases in serum alkaline phosphatase as well as in urinary markers of bone collagen degradation. As a result of the inhibition of bone resorption, FOSAMAX induced generally mild, transient, and asymptomatic decreases in serum calcium and phosphate.

Clinical Studies

Osteoporosis in postmenopausal women

The efficacy of FOSAMAX 10 mg once daily in postmenopausal women, 44 to 84 years of age, with osteoporsorsis (lumbar spine bone mineral density [BMD] of at least 2 standard deviations below the premenopausal mean) was demonstrated in four double-blind, placebo-controlled clinical studies of two or three years' duration. These included two large three-year, multicenter studies of virtually identical design, one performed in the United States (U.S.) and the other in 15 different countries (Multinational), which enrolled 478 and 516 patients, respectively. The following graph shows the mean increases in BMD of the lumbar spine, femoral neck, and trochanter in patients receiving FOSAMAX 10 mg/day relative to placebo-treated patients at three years for each of these studies.

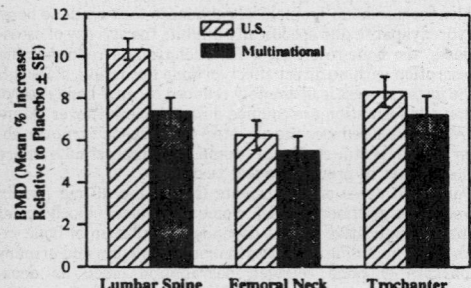

Increase in BMD
FOSAMAX 10 mg/day in Two Studies at Three Years

Highly significant increases in BMD, relative both to baseline and placebo, were seen at each measurement site in each study in patients who received FOSAMAX 10 mg/day. Total body BMD also increased significantly in each study, suggesting that the increases in bone mass of the spine and hip did not occur at the expense of other skeletal sites. Increases in BMD were evident as early as three months and continued throughout the three years of treatment. (See figures below for lumbar spine results.) Thus, FOSAMAX appears to reverse the progression of osteoporosis. FOSAMAX was similarly effective regardless of age, race, baseline rate of bone turnover, and baseline BMD in the range studied (at least 2 standard deviations below the premenopausal mean).

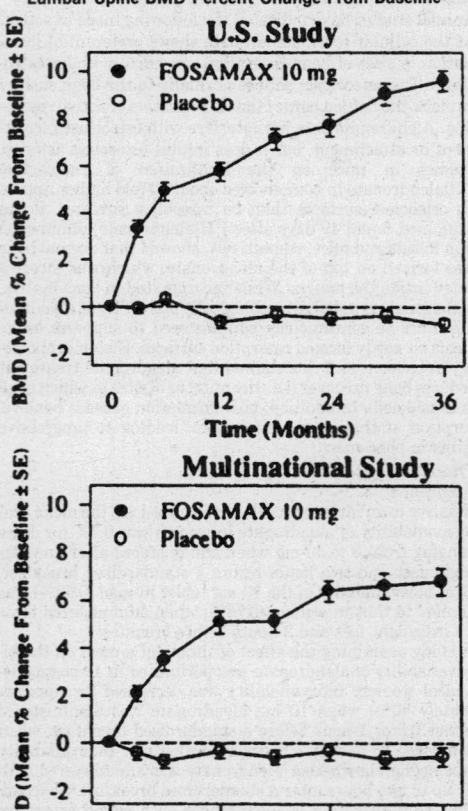

Time Course of Effect of FOSAMAX 10 mg/day
Versus Placebo:
Lumbar Spine BMD Percent Change From Baseline

U.S. Study

Multinational Study

To assess the effects of FOSAMAX on vertebral fracture incidence, the U.S. and Multinational studies were combined in an analysis that compared placebo to the pooled dosage groups of FOSAMAX (5 or 10 mg for three years or 20 mg for two years followed by 5 mg for one year). There was a significant 48% reduction in the proportion of patients treated with FOSAMAX experiencing one or more new vertebral fractures relative to those treated with placebo (3.2% vs. 6.2%). A reduction in the total number of new vertebral fractures (4.2 vs. 11.3 per 100 patients) was also observed. In the pooled analysis, patients who received FOSAMAX had a statistically significant smaller loss in stature than those who received placebo (-3.0 mm vs. -4.6 mm). Furthermore, of patients who sustained any vertebral fracture, those treated with FOSAMAX experienced less height loss (5.9 mm vs. 23.3 mm) due to a reduction in both the number and severity of fractures.

The effects of treatment withdrawal were assessed in a study that included patients treated with FOSAMAX for one or two years. Following discontinuation, neither further increases in bone mass nor accelerated rate of bone loss was noted. These data indicate that continuous daily treatment with FOSAMAX is required to maintain the effect of the drug.

Bone histology in 270 postmenopausal patients with osteoporosis treated with FOSAMAX at doses ranging from 1 to 20 mg/day for one, two, or three years revealed normal mineralization and structure, as well as the expected decrease in bone turnover relative to placebo. These data, together with the normal bone histology and increased bone strength observed in rats and baboons exposed to long-term alendronate treatment, support the conclusion that bone formed during therapy with FOSAMAX is of normal quality.

Paget's disease of bone

The efficacy of FOSAMAX 40 mg once daily for six months was demonstrated in two double-blind clinical studies of male and female patients with moderate to severe Paget's disease (alkaline phosphatase at least twice the upper limit of normal): a placebo-controlled multinational study and a U.S. comparative study with etidronate disodium 400 mg/day. The following figure shows the mean percent changes from baseline in serum alkaline phosphatase for up to six months of randomized treatment.

[See Figure at top of next column.]

At six months the suppression in alkaline phosphatase in patients treated with FOSAMAX was significantly greater than that achieved with etidronate and contrasted with the complete lack of response in placebo-treated patients. Re-

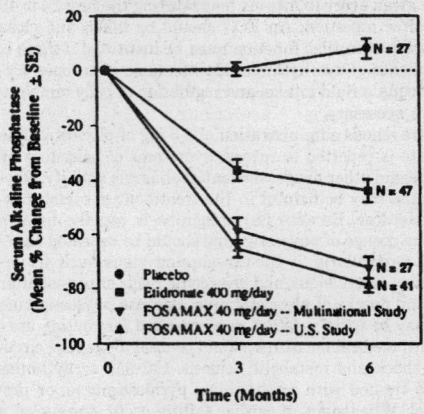

Effect on Serum Alkaline Phosphatase of FOSAMAX 40 mg/day
versus Placebo or Etidronate 400 mg/day

sponse (defined as either normalization of serum alkaline phosphatase or decrease from baseline $\geq 60\%$) occurred in approximately 85% of patients treated with FOSAMAX in the combined studies vs. 30% in the etidronate group and 0% in the placebo group. FOSAMAX was similarly effective irrespective of age, gender, race, prior use of other bisphosphonates, or baseline alkaline phosphatase within the range studied (at least twice the upper limit of normal).

Bone histology was evaluated in 33 patients with Paget's disease treated with FOSAMAX 40 mg/day for 6 months. As in patients treated for osteoporosis (see *Clinical Studies, Osteoporosis in postmenopausal women*), FOSAMAX did not impair mineralization, and the expected decrease in the rate of bone turnover was observed. Normal lamellar bone was produced during the treatment with FOSAMAX, even where preexisting bone was woven and disorganized. Overall, bone histology data support the conclusion that bone formed during the treatment with FOSAMAX is of normal quality.

ANIMAL PHARMACOLOGY

The relative inhibitory activities on bone resorption and mineralization of alendronate and etidronate were compared in the Schenk assay, which is based on histological examination of the epiphyses of growing rats. In this assay, the lowest dose of alendronate that interfered with bone mineralization (leading to osteomalacia) was 6000-fold the antiresponsive dose. The corresponding ratio for etidronate was one to one. These data suggest that alendronate administered in therapeutic doses is highly unlikely to induce osteomalacia.

INDICATIONS AND USAGE

FOSAMAX is indicated for the treatment of:
- Osteoporosis in postmenopausal women
  Osteoporosis may be confirmed by the finding of low bone mass (for example, at least 2 standard deviations below the premenopausal mean) or by the presence or history of osteoporotic fracture. (See CLINICAL PHARMACOLOGY, *Pharmacodynamics*.)
- Paget's disease of bone
  Treatment is indicated in patients with Paget's disease of bone having alkaline phosphatase at least two times the upper limit of normal, or those who are symptomatic, or those at risk for future complications from their disease.

CONTRAINDICATIONS

- Abnormalities of the esophagus which delay esophageal emptying such as stricture or achalasia
- Inability to stand or sit upright for at least 30 minutes
- Hypersensitivity to any component of this product
- Hypocalcemia (see PRECAUTIONS, *General*)

WARNINGS

FOSAMAX, like other bisphosphonates, may cause local irritation of the upper gastrointestinal mucosa.

Esophageal adverse experiences, such as esophagitis, esophageal ulcers and esophageal erosions have been reported in patients receiving treatment with FOSAMAX. In some cases these have been severe and required hospitalization. Physicians should therefore be alert to any signs or symptoms signaling a possible esophageal reaction and patients should be instructed to discontinue FOSAMAX and seek medical attention if they develop dysphagia, odynophagia or retrosternal pain.

The risk of severe esophageal adverse experiences appears to be greater in patients who lie down after taking FOSAMAX and/or who fail to swallow it with a full glass (6–8 oz) of water, and/or who continue to take FOSAMAX after develop-

ing symptoms suggestive of esophageal irritation. Therefore, it is very important that the full dosing instructions are provided to, and understood by, the patient (see DOSAGE AND ADMINISTRATION).

Because of possible irritant effects of FOSAMAX on the upper gastrointestinal mucosa, caution should be used when FOSAMAX is given to patients with active upper gastrointestinal problems, such as dysphagia, esophageal diseases, gastritis, duodenitis, or ulcers.

PRECAUTIONS

General

FOSAMAX is not recommended for patients with renal insufficiency (creatinine clearance <35 mL/min). (See DOSAGE AND ADMINISTRATION.)

Causes of osteoporosis other than estrogen deficiency and aging should be considered.

Hypocalcemia must be corrected before initiating therapy with FOSAMAX (see CONTRAINDICATIONS). Other disturbances of mineral metabolism (such as vitamin D deficiency) should also be effectively treated. Presumably due to the effects of FOSAMAX on increasing bone mineral, small, asymptomatic decreases in serum calcium and phosphate may occur, especially in patients with Paget's disease, in whom the pretreatment rate of bone turnover may be greatly elevated. Adequate calcium and vitamin D intake should be ensured to provide for these enhanced needs.

Information for Patients

Patients should be instructed that the expected benefits of FOSAMAX may only be obtained when each tablet is swallowed with plain water the first thing upon arising for the day at least 30 minutes before the first food, beverage, or medication of the day. Even dosing with orange juice or coffee has been shown to markedly reduce the absorption of FOSAMAX (see CLINICAL PHARMACOLOGY, *Pharmacokinetics, Absorption*).

To facilitate delivery to the stomach and thus reduce the potential for esophageal irritation patients should be instructed to swallow FOSAMAX with a full glass of water (6–8 oz) and not to lie down for at least 30 minutes and until after their first food of the day. Patients should not chew or suck on the tablet. Patients should be specifically instructed not to take FOSAMAX at bedtime or before arising for the day. Patients should be informed that failure to follow these instructions may increase their risk of esophageal problems. Patients should be instructed that if they develop symptoms of esophageal disease (such as difficulty or pain upon swallowing, retrosternal pain or new or worsening heartburn) they should stop taking FOSAMAX and consult their physician.

Patients should be instructed to take supplemental calcium and vitamin D, if daily dietary intake is inadequate. Weight-bearing exercise should be considered along with the modification of certain behavioral factors, such as excessive cigarette smoking, and/or alcohol consumption, if these factors exist.

Physicians should instruct their patients to read the patient package insert before starting therapy with FOSAMAX and to reread it each time the prescription is renewed.

Drug Interactions (also see CLINICAL PHARMACOLOGY, *Pharmacokinetics, Drug Interactions*)

Estrogen

A small number of postmenopausal women in the osteoporosis trials received estrogen (intravaginal, transdermal, or oral) while taking FOSAMAX. No adverse experiences attributable to their concomitant use were identified.

Concomitant use of hormone replacement therapy and FOSAMAX in the treatment of osteoporosis in postmenopausal women is not recommended because of lack of clinical experience.

Calcium Supplements/Antacids

It is likely that calcium supplements, antacids, and some oral medications will interfere with absorption of FOSAMAX. Therefore, patients must wait at least one-half hour after taking FOSAMAX before taking any other drug.

Aspirin

In clinical studies, the incidence of upper gastrointestinal adverse events was increased in patients receiving concomitant therapy with doses of FOSAMAX greater than 10 mg/day and aspirin-containing compounds.

Other

Although specific interaction studies were not performed, FOSAMAX 10 mg/day was used in postmenopausal osteoporosis studies with a wide range of commonly prescribed drugs without evidence of clinical adverse interactions. These included antacids, anticholinergics, aspirin-containing compounds, benzodiazepines, beta-blockers, calcium channel blockers, diuretics, gastric acid secretion inhibitors, glucocorticoids, nonsteroidal anti-inflammatory drugs (NSAIDs), sedative hypnotics, thiazides, thyroid hormones, vasoconstrictors, and vasodilators.

Carcinogenesis, Mutagenesis, Impairment of Fertility

Harderian gland (a retroorbital gland not present in humans) adenomas were increased in high-dose female mice (p=0.003) in a 92-week carcinogenicity study at doses of alendronate of 1, 3, and 10 mg/kg/day (males) or 1, 2, and 5 mg/kg/day (females). These doses are equivalent to 0.5 to 4 times the 10 mg human dose based on surface area, mg/m^2. Parafollicular cell (thyroid) adenomas were increased in high-dose male rats (p=0.003) in a 2-year carcinogenicity study at doses of 1 and 3.75 mg/kg body weight. These doses are equivalent to 1 and 3 times the 10 mg human dose based on surface area.

Alendronate was not genotoxic in the *in vitro* microbial mutagenesis assay with and without metabolic activation, in an *in vitro* mammalian cell mutagenesis assay, in an *in vitro* alkaline elution assay in rat hepatocytes, and in an *in vivo* chromosomal aberration assay in mice. In an *in vitro* chromosomal aberration assay in Chinese hamster ovary cells, however, alendronate was weakly positive at concentrations ≥5 mM in the presence of cytotoxicity.

Alendronate had no effect on fertility (male or female) in rats at oral doses up to 5 mg/kg/day (four times the 10 mg human dose based on surface area).

Pregnancy

Pregnancy Category C:

Reproduction studies in rats showed decreased postimplantation survival at 2 mg/kg/day and decreased body weight gain in normal pups at 1 mg/kg/day. Sites of incomplete fetal ossification were statistically significantly increased in rats beginning at 10 mg/kg/day in vertebral (cervical, thoracic, and lumbar), skull, and sternebral bones. The above doses ranged from 1 times (1 mg/kg) to 9 times (10 mg/kg) the 10 mg human dose based on surface area, mg/m^2. No similar fetal effects were seen when pregnant rabbits were treated at doses up to 35 mg/kg/day (50 times the 10 mg human dose based on surface area, mg/m^2).

Both total and ionized calcium decreased in pregnant rats at 15 mg/kg/day (13 times the 10 mg human dose based on surface area) resulting in delays and failures of delivery. Protracted parturition due to maternal hypocalcemia occurred in rats at doses as low as 0.5 mg/kg/day (0.5 times the recommended human dose) when rats were treated from before mating through gestation. Maternotoxicity (late pregnancy deaths) occurred in the female rats treated with 15 mg/kg/day for varying periods of time ranging from treatment only during pre-mating to treatment only during early, middle, or late gestation; these deaths were lessened but not eliminated by cessation of treatment. Calcium supplementation either in the drinking water or by minipump could not ameliorate the hypocalcemia or prevent maternal and neonatal deaths due to delays in delivery; calcium supplementation IV prevented maternal, but not fetal deaths.

There are no studies in pregnant women. FOSAMAX should be used during pregnancy only if the potential benefit justifies the potential risk to the mother and fetus.

Nursing Mothers

Alendronate was secreted in the milk of rats after an IV dose. It is not known whether alendronate is excreted in human milk. FOSAMAX has not been studied in nursing women and should not be given to them.

Pediatric Use

Safety and effectiveness in pediatric patients have not been established.

Use in the Elderly

Of the patients receiving FOSAMAX in the two large osteoporosis studies and Paget's disease studies (see CLINICAL PHARMACOLOGY, *Clinical Studies*), 45% and 70%, respectively, were 65 years of age or over. No overall differences in efficacy or safety were observed between these patients and younger patients but greater sensitivity of some older individuals cannot be ruled out.

Use in Men

Safety and effectiveness in male osteoporosis have not been established.

ADVERSE REACTIONS

Clinical Studies

In clinical studies adverse experiences associated with FOSAMAX usually were mild, and generally did not require discontinuation of therapy.

Osteoporosis in postmenopausal women

FOSAMAX has been evaluated for safety in clinical studies in more than 1800 postmenopausal patients. In two large, three-year, placebo-controlled, double-blind, multicenter studies (United States and Multinational), discontinuation of therapy due to any clinical adverse experience occurred in 4.1% of 196 patients treated with FOSAMAX 10 mg/day and 6.0% of 397 patients treated with placebo. Adverse experiences reported by the investigators as possibly, probably, or definitely drug related in ≥1% of patients treated with either FOSAMAX 10 mg/day or placebo are presented in the following table.

[See table on top of next column.]

Drug-Related** Adverse Experiences
Reported in ≥1% of Patients

	FOSAMAX 10 mg/day % (n = 196)	Placebo % (n = 397)
Gastrointestinal		
abdominal pain	6.6	4.8
nausea	3.6	4.0
dyspepsia	3.6	3.5
constipation	3.1	1.8
diarrhea	3.1	1.8
flatulence	2.6	0.5
acid regurgitation	2.0	4.3
esophageal ulcer	1.5	0.0
vomiting	1.0	1.5
dysphagia	1.0	0.0
abdominal distention	1.0	0.8
gastritis	0.5	1.3
Musculoskeletal		
musculoskeletal pain	4.1	2.5
muscle cramp	0.0	1.0
Nervous System/Psychiatric		
headache	2.6	1.5
dizziness	0.0	1.0
Special Senses		
taste perversion	0.5	1.0

**Considered possibly, probably, or definitely drug related as assessed by the investigators

Rarely, rash and erythema have occurred.

One patient treated with FOSAMAX (10 mg/day), who had a history of peptic ulcer disease and gastrectomy and who was taking concomitant aspirin developed an anastomotic ulcer with mild hemorrhage, which was considered drug related. Aspirin and FOSAMAX were discontinued and the patient recovered.

The adverse experience profile was similar for the 401 patients treated with either 5 or 20 mg doses of FOSAMAX in the United States and Multinational studies.

Paget's disease of bone

In clinical studies (osteoporosis and Paget's disease), adverse experiences reported in 175 patients taking FOSAMAX 40 mg/day for 3–12 months were similar to those in postmenopausal women treated with FOSAMAX 10 mg/day. However, there was an apparent increased incidence of upper gastrointestinal adverse experiences in patients taking FOSAMAX 40 mg/day (17.7% FOSAMAX vs. 10.2% placebo). One case of esophagitis and two cases of gastritis resulted in discontinuation of treatment.

Additionally, musculoskeletal pain, which has been described in patients with Paget's disease treated with other bisphosphonates, was reported by the investigators as possibly, probably, or definitely drug related in approximately 6% of patients treated with FOSAMAX 40 mg/day versus approximately 1% of patients treated with placebo, but rarely resulted in discontinuation of therapy. Discontinuation of therapy due to any clinical adverse experience occurred in 6.4% of patients with Paget's disease treated with FOSAMAX 40 mg/day and 2.4% of patients treated with placebo.

Laboratory Test Findings

In double-blind, multicenter, controlled studies, asymptomatic, mild, and transient decreases in serum calcium phosphate were observed in approximately 18% and 10%, respectively, of patients taking FOSAMAX versus approximately 12% and 3% of those taking placebo. However, the incidences of decreases in serum calcium to <8.0 mg/dL (2.0 mM) and serum phosphate to ≤2.0 mg/dL (0.65 mM) were similar in both treatment groups.

Post-Marketing Experience

The following adverse reactions have been reported in post-marketing use: esophagitis, esophageal erosions and esophageal ulcers (see WARNINGS and DOSAGE AND ADMINISTRATION).

OVERDOSAGE

Significant lethality after single oral doses was seen in female rats and mice at 552 mg/kg (3256 mg/m^2) and 966 mg/kg (2898 mg/m^2), respectively. In males, these values were slightly higher, 626 and 1280 mg/kg, respectively. There was no lethality in dogs at oral doses up to 200 mg/kg (4000 mg/m^2).

No specific information is available on the treatment of overdosage with FOSAMAX. Hypocalcemia, hypophosphatemia, and upper gastrointestinal adverse events, such as upset stomach, heartburn, esophagitis, gastritis, or ulcer, may result from oral overdosage. Milk or antacids should be given

Continued on next page

Information on the Merck & Co., Inc. products listed on these pages is the full prescribing information from product circulars in use September 30, 1996.

Merck & Co.—Cont.

to bind alendronate. Due to the risk of esophageal irritation, vomiting should not be induced and the patient should remain fully upright.

Dialysis would not be beneficial.

DOSAGE AND ADMINISTRATION

FOSAMAX must be taken *at least* one-half hour before the first food, beverage, or medication of the day with plain water only (see PRECAUTIONS, *Information for Patients*). Other beverages (including mineral water), food, and some medications are likely to reduce the absorption of FOSAMAX (see PRECAUTIONS, *Drug Interactions*). Waiting less than 30 minutes, or taking FOSAMAX with food, beverages (other than plain water) or other medications will lessen the effect of FOSAMAX by decreasing its absorption into the body.

To facilitate delivery to the stomach and thus reduce the potential for esophageal irritation, FOSAMAX should only be swallowed upon arising for the day with a full glass of water (6–8 oz) and patients should not lie down for at least 30 minutes <u>and</u> until after their first food of the day. FOSAMAX should not be taken at bedtime or before arising for the day. Failure to follow these instructions may increase the risk of esophageal adverse experiences (see WARNINGS).

Patients with osteoporosis or Paget's disease should receive supplemental calcium and vitamin D, if dietary intake is inadequate (see PRECAUTIONS, *General*).

No dosage adjustment is necessary for the elderly or for patients with mild-to-moderate renal insufficiency (creatinine clearance 35 to 60 mL/min). FOSAMAX is not recommended for patients with more severe renal insufficiency (creatinine clearance <35 mL/min) due to lack of experience.

Osteoporosis in postmenopausal women
The recommended dosage is 10 mg once a day.
Safety of treatment with FOSAMAX for longer than four years has not been studied; extension studies are ongoing.

Paget's disease of bone
The recommended treatment regimen is 40 mg once a day for six months.

Retreatment of Paget's disease
In clinical studies in which patients were followed every six months, relapses during the 12 months following therapy occurred in 9% (3 out of 32) of patients who responded to treatment with FOSAMAX. Specific retreatment data are not available, although responses to FOSAMAX were similar in patients who had received prior bisphosphonate therapy and those who had not. Retreatment with FOSAMAX may be considered, following a six-month post-treatment evaluation period in patients who have relapsed, based on increases in serum alkaline phosphatase, which should be measured periodically. Retreatment may also be considered in those who failed to normalize their serum alkaline phosphatase.

HOW SUPPLIED

No. 3600—Tablets FOSAMAX, 10 mg, are white, round, uncoated tablets with a bone image and code MRK 936 on one side and a bone image and FOSAMAX on the other. They are supplied as follows:
NDC 0006-0936-31 unit-of-use bottles of 30
(6505-01-424-1106, 10 mg 30's)
NDC 0006-0936-58 unit-of-use bottles of 100
NDC 0006-0936-28 unit dose packages of 100
(6505-01-424-1113, 10 mg 100's)
NDC 0006-0936-82 bottles of 1000.

Shown in Product Identification Guide, page 324

No. 3592—Tablets FOSAMAX, 40 mg, are white, triangular-shaped, uncoated tablets, with code MRK 212 on one side and FOSAMAX on the other. They are supplied as follows:
NDC 0006-0212-31 unit-of-use bottles of 30
(6505-01-424-1111, 40 mg 30's).

Shown in Product Identification Guide, page 324

Storage
Store in a well-closed container at room temperature, 15–30°C (59–86°F).

7957003   Issued April 1996
COPYRIGHT © MERCK & CO., Inc., 1995
All rights reserved.

HEP-B-GAMMAGEE®   ℞
(Hepatitis B Immune Globulin [Human], MSD), U.S.P.

DESCRIPTION

HEP-B-GAMMAGEE* [Hepatitis B Immune Globulin (Human), MSD] is a sterile solution of human immunoglobulin (10–18% protein) intended for intramuscular injection. The high levels of antibody to hepatitis B surface antigen (anti-HBs) found in the product are derived from a small group of well-monitored individuals who were hyperimmunized with hepatitis B vaccine. The potency is adjusted by the addition of IgG obtained from large pools of normal plasma. The pooled plasma is processed by MSD and/or Armour Pharmaceutical Company using Cohn cold ethanol fractionation procedures. The product is dissolved in 0.3 molar glycine and contains thimerosal (mercury derivative) 1:10,000 added as a preservative. The solution has a pH of 6.8 ± 0.4 adjusted with hydrochloric acid or sodium hydroxide. Each vial of HEP-B-GAMMAGEE contains anti-HBs equivalent to or exceeding the potency of anti-HBs in a U.S. reference Hepatitis B Immune Globulin (Office of Biologics Research and Review FDA).

There is no evidence to suggest that the causative virus of AIDS (HIV) has been transmitted by HEP-B-GAMMAGEE prepared by the Cohn cold ethanol process.

---

* Registered trademark of MERCK & CO., INC.

CLINICAL PHARMACOLOGY

Hepatitis B Immune Globulin (Human) provides passive immunization for individuals exposed to the hepatitis B virus (HBV) as evidenced by a reduction in the attack rate of hepatitis B following its use. The administration of the usual recommended dose of HEP-B-GAMMAGEE generally results in a detectable level of circulating antibody to hepatitis B surface antigen (anti-HBs) which persists for approximately 2 months or longer. Peak serum levels of anti-HBs are seen at 3–7 days after intramuscular administration of hepatitis B immunoglobulin. The half-life of this antibody ranges from 17.5–25 days. The possibility of hepatitis B transmission is remote, as it is with other immune globulins prepared by the cold ethanol process.

INDICATIONS AND USAGE

HEP-B-GAMMAGEE is indicated for post-exposure prophylaxis following either parenteral exposure, direct mucous membrane contact, sexual exposure or oral ingestion involving HBsAg-positive materials such as blood, plasma or serum. Such exposures might occur by accidental "needlestick", accidental splash, or a pipetting accident. HEP-B-GAMMAGEE is also indicated for post-exposure prophylaxis in infants born to hepatitis B-positive (HBsAg-positive) mothers.

CONTRAINDICATIONS

Hypersensitivity to any component of the product.

WARNINGS

Persons with isolated immunoglobulin A deficiency have the potential for developing antibodies to immunoglobulin A and could have anaphylactic reactions to subsequent administration of blood products that contain immunoglobulin A. Therefore, as with any immunoglobulin preparation, Hepatitis B Immune Globulin (Human) should be given to such persons only if the expected benefits outweigh the potential risks.

In patients who have severe thrombocytopenia or any coagulation disorder that would contraindicate intramuscular injections, Hepatitis B Immune Globulin (Human) should be given only if the expected benefits outweigh the potential risks.

PRECAUTIONS

General
HEP-B-GAMMAGEE should be given with caution to patients with a history of prior systemic allergic reactions following the administration of human immune globulin preparations. Hypersensitivity reactions to injections of immunoglobulin occur rarely. The incidence of these reactions may be increased in patients receiving large intramuscular doses or in patients receiving repeated injections of immunoglobulin.

HEP-B-GAMMAGEE *must not be administered intravenously* because of the potential for serious reactions. Injections should be made intramuscularly. Care should be taken to draw back on the plunger of the syringe before injection in order to be certain that the needle is not in a blood vessel. Epinephrine should be available for treatment of acute allergic symptoms.

There is no evidence that the causative virus of AIDS (HIV-1) is transmitted by HEP-B-GAMMAGEE which is prepared by the Cohn cold ethanol process.

Some investigational intravenous immunoglobulin products have been linked to transmission of non-A, non-B hepatitis; however, there have been no reports of this in association with HEP-B-GAMMAGEE.

Drug Interactions
Antibodies present in immunoglobulin preparations may interfere with the immune response to live virus vaccines such as measles, mumps, and rubella. Therefore, vaccination with live virus vaccines should be deferred until approximately three months after administration of Hepatitis B Immune Globulin (Human). It may be necessary to revaccinate persons who received Hepatitis B Immune Globulin (Human) shortly after live virus vaccination.

Pregnancy
Pregnancy Category C. Animal reproduction studies have not been conducted with HEP-B-GAMMAGEE. It is also not known whether HEP-B-GAMMAGEE can cause fetal harm when administered to a pregnant woman or can affect reproduction capacity. HEP-B-GAMMAGEE should be given to a pregnant woman only if clearly needed.

Nursing Mothers
It is not known whether this drug is excreted in human milk. Because many drugs are excreted in human milk, caution should be exercised when HEP-B-GAMMAGEE is administered to a nursing woman.

ADVERSE REACTIONS

Local pain and tenderness at the injection site, urticaria and angioedema may occur. Anaphylactic reactions, although rare, have been reported following the injection of human immunoglobulin preparations. Anaphylaxis is more likely to occur if Hepatitis B Immune Globulin (Human) is given intravenously; therefore, Hepatitis B Immune Globulin (Human) must be administered *only* intramuscularly. In highly allergic individuals, repeated injections may lead to anaphylactic shock.

OVERDOSAGE

Although no data are available, clinical experience with other immunoglobulin preparations suggests that the only manifestations would be pain and tenderness at the injection site.

DOSAGE AND ADMINISTRATION

Parenteral drug products should be inspected visually for particulate matter and discoloration prior to administration, whenever solution and container permit. HEP-B-GAMMAGEE is a clear, very slightly amber, moderately viscous liquid.

HEP-B-GAMMAGEE is administered *intramuscularly. It must not be injected intravenously.*

It is important to use a separate sterile syringe and needle for each individual patient to prevent transmission of hepatitis B and other infectious agents from one person to another.

Known or Presumed Exposure to HBsAg
There are no prospective studies directly testing the efficacy of a combination of Hepatitis B Immune Globulin (Human) and hepatitis B vaccine (HEPTAVAX-B† [Hepatitis B Vaccine, MSD] or RECOMBIVAX HB† [Hepatitis B Vaccine (Recombinant), MSD]) in preventing clinical hepatitis B following percutaneous, ocular or mucous membrane exposure to hepatitis B virus. However, since most persons with such exposures (e.g., health-care workers) are candidates for the hepatitis B vaccine and since combined Hepatitis B Immune Globulin (Human) plus vaccine is more efficacious than Hepatitis B Immune Globulin (Human) alone in perinatal exposures, the following guidelines are recommended for persons who have been exposed to hepatitis B virus such as through (1) percutaneous (needlestick), ocular, mucous membrane exposure to blood known or presumed to contain HBsAg, (2) human bites by known or presumed HBsAg carriers, that penetrate the skin, or (3) following intimate sexual contact with known or presumed HBsAg carriers:

Recommendations for adults who have not been previously vaccinated against hepatitis B:
Hepatitis B Immune Globulin (Human) (0.06 mL/kg) should be given intramuscularly as soon as possible after exposure and within 24 hours if possible. Hepatitis B vaccine (see HEPTAVAX-B (Hepatitis B Vaccine, MSD) or RECOMBIVAX HB [Hepatitis B Vaccine (Recombinant), MSD] circular for appropriate dosage recommendations) should be given intramuscularly within 7 days of exposure and second and third doses given one and six months, respectively, after the first dose.

Recommendations for adults who have been previously vaccinated against hepatitis B:
Prior recipients of a recommended course of hepatitis B vaccine should have their anti-HBs titer checked promptly. For those with known adequate antibody (10 MIU/mL anti-HBs, approximately equal to 10 SRU) nothing is required. Those with inadequate or unknown titers should receive a dose of Hepatitis B Immune Globulin (Human) and a dose of hepatitis B vaccine simultaneously at two different sites as soon as possible.

Dosage for Infants Born of HBsAg Positive Mothers:

Infants born to HBsAg positive mothers are at high risk of becoming chronic carriers of hepatitis B virus and of developing the chronic sequelae of hepatitis B virus infection. Well-controlled studies have shown that administration of three 0.5 mL doses of Hepatitis B Immune Globulin (Human) starting at birth is 75% effective in preventing establishment of the chronic carrier state in these infants during the first year of life. Protection can be transient, whereupon the effectiveness of the Hepatitis B Immune Globulin (Human) would decline thereafter. Results from clinical studies indicate that administration of one 0.5 mL dose of Hepatitis B Immune Globulin (Human) at birth and the recommended three doses of HEPTAVAX-B (Hepatitis B Vaccine, MSD) or RECOMBIVAX HB [Hepatitis B Vaccine (Recombinant), MSD] (see Table below), were effective in preventing establishment of the chronic carrier state in infants born to HBsAg and HBeAg positive mothers.

Testing for HBsAg and anti-HBs is recommended at 12–15 months of age. If HBsAg is not detectable, and anti-HBs is present, the child has been protected.

The recommended dosage for infants born to HBsAg positive mothers is as follows:

	Birth	Within 7 days	1 month	6 months
Hepatitis B vaccine**		0.5 mL*	0.5 mL	0.5 mL
Hepatitis B Immune Globulin (Human)	0.5 mL	—	—	—

* The first dose of hepatitis B vaccine may be given at birth at the same time as Hepatitis B Immune Globulin (Human); but should be administered in the opposite anterolateral thigh.

** See DOSAGE AND ADMINISTRATION section of RECOMBIVAX HB [Hepatitis B Vaccine (Recombinant), MSD] circular.

† Registered trademark of MERCK & CO., INC.

HOW SUPPLIED

No. 4692—HEP-B-GAMMAGEE is supplied as follows:
NDC 0006-4692-00 in 5 mL vials.
Store at 2–8°C (36–46°F). Do not freeze. Do not use after expiration date.

A.H.F.S. Category: 80:04
DC 7413911   Issued April 1992
COPYRIGHT © MERCK & CO., INC., 1988
All rights reserved

**HUMORSOL® Sterile Ophthalmic Solution   ℞
(Demecarium Bromide), U.S.P.
For Topical Application into the
Conjunctival Sac Only**

DESCRIPTION

Ophthalmic Solution HUMORSOL* (Demecarium Bromide) is a sterile solution supplied in two dosage strengths: 0.125 percent and 0.25 percent. The inactive ingredients are sodium chloride and water for injection; benzalkonium chloride 1:5000 is added as preservative. Demecarium bromide is a quaternary ammonium compound with a molecular weight of 716.60. Its chemical name is 3,3'-[1,10-decanediylbis [(methylimino)carbonyloxy]] bis [N,N,N-trimethylbenzenaminium] dibromide. Its empirical formula is $C_{32}H_{52}Br_2N_4O_4$ and its structural formula is:

*Registered trademark of MERCK & CO., INC.

CLINICAL PHARMACOLOGY

HUMORSOL is a cholinesterase inhibitor with sustained activity. It acts mainly on true (erythrocyte) cholinesterase. Application of HUMORSOL to the eye produces intense miosis and ciliary muscle contraction due to inhibition of cholinesterase, allowing acetylcholine to accumulate at sites of cholinergic transmission. These effects are accompanied by increased capillary permeability of the ciliary body and iris, increased permeability of the blood-aqueous barrier, and vasodilation. Myopia may be induced or, if present, may be augmented by the increased refractive power of the lens that results from the accommodative effect of the drug. HUMORSOL indirectly produces some of the muscarinic and nicotinic effects of acetylcholine as quantities of the latter accumulate.

INDICATIONS AND USAGE

Open-angle glaucoma (HUMORSOL should be used in glaucoma only when shorter-acting miotics have proved inadequate.)
Conditions obstructing aqueous outflow, such as synechial formation, that are amenable to miotic therapy
Following iridectomy
Accommodative esotropia (accommodative convergent strabismus)

CONTRAINDICATIONS

Hypersensitivity to any component of this product.
Because of the toxicity of cholinesterase inhibitors in general, HUMORSOL is contraindicated in women who are or who may become pregnant. If this drug is used during pregnancy, or if the patient becomes pregnant while taking this drug, the patient should be apprised of the potential hazard to the fetus.
Because miotics may aggravate inflammation, HUMORSOL should not be used in active uveal inflammation and/or glaucoma associated with iridocyclitis.

WARNINGS

In patients receiving cholinesterase inhibitors such as HUMORSOL, succinylcholine should be administered with extreme caution before and during general anesthesia.
Because of possible adverse additive effects, HUMORSOL should be administered only with extreme caution to patients with myasthenia gravis who are receiving systemic anticholinesterase therapy; conversely, extreme caution should be exercised in the use of an anticholinesterase drug for the treatment of myasthenia gravis patients who are already undergoing topical therapy with cholinesterase inhibitors.

PRECAUTIONS

General
Gonioscopy is recommended prior to medication with HUMORSOL.
HUMORSOL should be used with caution in patients with chronic angle-closure (narrow-angle) glaucoma or in patients with narrow angles, because of the possibility of producing pupillary block and increasing angle blockage.
When an intraocular inflammatory process is present, the intensity and persistence of miosis and ciliary muscle contraction that result from anticholinesterase therapy require abstention from, or cautious use of, HUMORSOL.
Systemic effects are infrequent when HUMORSOL is instilled carefully. Compression of the lacrimal duct for several seconds immediately following instillation minimizes drainage into the nasal chamber with its extensive absorption surface. Wash the hands immediately after instillation.
Discontinue HUMORSOL if salivation, urinary incontinence, diarrhea, profuse sweating, muscle weakness, respiratory difficulties, shock, or cardiac irregularities occur.
Persons receiving cholinesterase inhibitors who are exposed to organophosphate-type insecticides and pesticides (gardeners, organophosphate plant or warehouse workers, farmers, residents of communities which are undergoing insecticide spraying or dusting, etc.) should be warned of the added systemic effects possible from absorption through the respiratory tract or skin. Wearing of respiratory masks, frequent washing, and clothing changes may be advisable.
Anticholinesterase drugs should be used with extreme caution, if at all, in patients with marked vagotonia, bronchial asthma, spastic gastrointesinal disturbances, peptic ulcer, pronounced bradycardia and hypotension, recent myocardial infarction, epilepsy, parkinsonism, and other disorders that may respond adversely to vagotonic effects.
After long-term use of HUMORSOL, dilation of blood vessels and resulting greater permeability increase the possibility of hyphema during ophthalmic surgery. Therefore, this drug should be discontinued before surgery.
Despite observance of all precautions and the use of only the recommended dose, there is some evidence that repeated administration may cause depression of the concentration of cholinesterase in the serum and erythrocytes, with resultant systemic effects.
There have been reports of bacterial keratitis associated with the use of multiple dose containers of topical ophthalmic products. These containers had been inadvertently contaminated by patients who, in most cases, had a concurrent corneal disease or a disruption of the ocular epithelial surface. (See PRECAUTIONS, *Information for Patients.*)

Information for Patients
Patients should be instructed to avoid allowing the tip of the dispensing container to contact the eye or surrounding structures.
Patients should also be instructed that ocular solutions, if handled improperly, can become contaminated by common bacteria known to cause ocular infections. Serious damage to the eye and subsequent loss of vision may result from using contaminated solutions. (See PRECAUTIONS, *General*.)
Patients should also be advised that if they develop an intercurrent ocular condition (e.g., trauma, ocular surgery or infection), they should immediately seek their physician's advice concerning the continued use of the present multidose container.
The preservative in HUMORSOL, benzalkonium chloride, may be absorbed by soft contact lenses. Patients wearing soft contact lenses should be instructed to wait at least 15 minutes after instilling HUMORSOL before they insert their lenses.
Drug Interactions
See WARNINGS regarding possible drug interactions of HUMORSOL with succinylcholine or with other anticholinesterase agents.
Carcinogenesis, Mutagenesis, Impairment of Fertility
Long-term studies in animals have not been performed to evaluate the effects of HUMORSOL on fertility or carcinogenic potential.
Pregnancy
Pregnancy Category X: See CONTRAINDICATIONS.
Nursing Mothers
It is not known whether this drug is excreted in human milk. Because of the potential for serious adverse reactions in nursing infants from HUMORSOL, a decision should be made whether to discontinue nursing or to discontinue the drug, taking into account the importance of the drug to the mother.
Pediatric Use
The occurrence of iris cysts is more frequent in children. (See ADVERSE REACTIONS and DOSAGE AND ADMINISTRATION.)
Extreme caution should be exercised in children receiving HUMORSOL who may require general anesthesia (see WARNINGS).
Since HUMORSOL is a potent cholinesterase inhibitor it should be kept out of the reach of children.

ADVERSE REACTIONS

Stinging, burning, lacrimation, lid muscle twitching, conjunctival and ciliary redness, brow ache, headache, and induced myopia with visual blurring may occur.
Activation of latent iritis or uveitis may occur.
As with all miotic therapy, retinal detachment has been reported occasionally.
Iris cysts may form, enlarge, and obscure vision. Occurrence is more frequent in children. The iris cyst usually shrinks upon discontinuance of the miotic. Rarely, the cyst may rupture or break free into the aqueous. Frequent examination for this occurrence is advised.
Lens opacities have been reported in patients on miotic therapy. Routine slit-lamp examinations, including the lens, should accompany prolonged use.
Paradoxical increase in intraocular pressure may follow anticholinesterase instillation. This may be alleviated by pupil-dilating medication.
Prolonged use may cause conjunctival thickening and obstruction of nasolacrimal canals.
Systemic effects, which occur rarely, are suggestive of increased cholinergic activity. Such effects may include nausea, vomiting, abdominal cramps, diarrhea, urinary incontinence, salivation, sweating, difficulty in breathing, bradycardia, or cardiac irregularities. Medical management of systemic effects may be indicated (see TREATMENT OF ADVERSE EFFECTS).

TREATMENT OF ADVERSE EFFECTS

If HUMORSOL is taken systemically by accident, or if systemic effects occur after topical application in the eye or from accidental skin contact, administer atropine sulfate parenterally (intravenously if necessary) in a dose (for adults) of 0.4 to 0.6 mg or more. The recommended dosage of atropine in infants and children up to 12 years of age is 0.01 mg/kg repeated every two hours as needed until the desired effect is obtained, or adverse effects of atropine preclude further usage. The maximum single dose should not exceed 0.4 mg.

Continued on next page

Merck & Co.—Cont.

The use of much larger doses of atropine in treating anticholinesterase intoxication in adults has been reported in the literature. Initially 2 to 6 mg may be given followed by 2 mg every hour or more often, as long as muscarinic effects continue. The greater possibility of atropinization with large doses, particularly in sensitive individuals, should be borne in mind.

Pralidoxime* chloride has been reported to be useful in treating systemic effects due to cholinesterase inhibitors. However, its use is recommended in addition to and not as substitute for atropine.

A short-acting barbiturate is indicated if convulsions occur that are not entirely relieved by atropine. Barbiturate dosage should be carefully adjusted to avoid central respiratory depression. Marked weakness or paralysis of muscles of respiration should be treated promptly by artificial respiration and maintenance of a clear airway.

The oral LD_{50} of HUMORSOL is 2.96 mg/kg in the mouse.

---

*PROTOPAM® Chloride (Pralidoxime Chloride). Ayerst Laboratories

DOSAGE AND ADMINISTRATION

HUMORSOL *is intended solely for topical use in the conjunctival sac.*

As HUMORSOL is an extremely potent drug, the physician should thoroughly familiarize himself with its use and the technic of instillation.

The required dose is applied in the conjunctival sac, with the patient supine, care being taken not to touch the cornea with the tip of the OCUMETER** ophthalmic dispenser. *The patient or person administering the medication should apply continuous gentle pressure on the lacrimal duct with the index finger for several seconds immediately following instillation of the drops. This is to prevent drainage overflow of solution into the nasal and pharyngeal spaces, which might cause systemic absorption. Wash the hands immediately after administration.*

HUMORSOL *should not be used more often than directed. Caution is necessary to avoid overdosage.*

Initial titration and dosage adjustments with HUMORSOL must be individualized to obtain maximal therapeutic effect. The patient must be closely observed during the initial period. If the response is not adequate within the first 24 hours, other measures should be considered.

Keep frequency of use to a minimum in all patients, but especially in children, to reduce the chance of iris cyst development (see ADVERSE REACTIONS).

Glaucoma

For initial therapy with HUMORSOL (0.125 percent or 0.25 percent) place 1 drop (children) or 1 or 2 drops (adults) in the glaucomatous eye. A decrease in intraocular pressure should occur within a few hours. During this period, keep the patient under supervision and make tonometric examinations at least hourly for 3 or 4 hours to be sure that no immediate rise in pressure occurs (see ADVERSE REACTIONS).

Duration of effect varies with the individual. The usual dosage can vary from as much as 1 or 2 drops twice a day to as little as 1 or 2 drops twice a week. The 0.125 percent strength used twice a day usually results in smooth control of the physiologic diurnal variation in intraocular pressure. This is probably the preferred dosage for most wide (open) angle glaucoma patients.

Strabismus

Essentially equal visual acuity of both eyes is a prerequisite to the successful treatment of esotropia with HUMORSOL. For initial evaluation it may be used as a diagnostic aid to determine if an accommodative factor exists. This is especially useful preoperatively in young children and in patients with normal hypermetropic refractive errors. One drop is given daily for 2 weeks, then 1 drop every 2 days for 2 to 3 weeks. If the eyes become straighter, an accommodative factor is demonstrated. This technic may supplement or complement standard testing with atropine and trial with glasses for the accommodative factor.

In esotropia uncomplicated by amblyopia or anisometropia, HUMORSOL may be instilled in both eyes, *not more than 1 drop at a time every day for 2 to 3 weeks,* as too severe a degree of miosis may interfere with vision. Then reduce the dosage to 1 drop every other day for 3 to 4 weeks and reevaluate the patient's status.

HUMORSOL may be continued in a dosage of 1 drop every 2 days to 1 drop twice a week. (The latter dosage may be maintained for several months.) Evaluate the patient's condition every 4 to 12 weeks. If improvement continues, change the schedule to 1 drop once a week and eventually to a trial without medication. However, if after 4 months, control of the condition still requires 1 drop every 2 days, therapy with HUMORSOL should be stopped.

**Registered trademark of MERCK & CO., INC.

HOW SUPPLIED

Sterile Ophthalmic Solution HUMORSOL is a clear, colorless, aqueous solution and is supplied in a 5 mL white, opaque, plastic OCUMETER ophthalmic dispenser with a controlled-drop tip:
No. 3255—0.125 percent solution.
  NDC 0006-3255-03.
No. 3267—0.25 percent solution.
  NDC 0006-3267-03.
Storage
Protect from freezing and excessive heat.
      DC 7414314   Issued May 1993
COPYRIGHT © MERCK & CO., INC., 1987
All rights reserved

HYDELTRASOL® Injection, Sterile   ℞
(Prednisolone Sodium Phosphate), U.S.P.

DESCRIPTION

Prednisolone sodium phosphate, a synthetic adrenocortical steroid, is a white or slightly yellow powder that is slightly hygroscopic and is freely soluble in water. The molecular weight is 484.39. It is designated chemically as $11\beta,17$-dihydroxy-21-(phosphonooxy)pregna-1,4-diene-3,20-dione disodium salt. The empirical formula is $C_{21}H_{27}Na_2O_8P$ and the structural formula is:

HYDELTRASOL* (Prednisolone Sodium Phosphate) injection is a sterile solution (pH 7.0 to 8.0) sealed under nitrogen, for intravenous, intramuscular, intra-articular, intralesional, and soft tissue administration.

Each milliliter contains prednisolone sodium phosphate equivalent to 20 mg prednisolone phosphate. Inactive ingredients per mL: niacinamide, 25 mg; sodium hydroxide to adjust pH; disodium edetate, 0.5 mg; Water for Injection, q.s. 1 mL. Sodium bisulfite, 1 mg, and phenol, 5 mg, added as preservatives.

---

*Registered trademark of MERCK & CO., INC.

ACTIONS

HYDELTRASOL injection has a rapid onset but short duration of action when compared with less soluble preparations. Because of this, it is suitable for the treatment of acute disorders responsive to adrenocortical steroid therapy.

Naturally occurring glucocorticoids (hydrocortisone and cortisone), which also have salt-retaining properties, are used as replacement therapy in adrenocortical deficiency states. Their synthetic analogs, including prednisolone, are primarily used for their potent anti-inflammatory effects in disorders of many organ systems.

Glucocorticoids cause profound and varied metabolic effects. In addition, they modify the body's immune responses to diverse stimuli.

At equipotent anti-inflammatory doses, prednisolone has less tendency to cause salt and water retention than either hydrocortisone or cortisone.

INDICATIONS

A. By intravenous or intramuscular injection when oral therapy is not feasible:
1. *Endocrine disorders*

Primary or secondary adrenocortical insufficiency (hydrocortisone or cortisone is the drug of choice; synthetic analogs may be used in conjunction with mineralocorticoids where applicable; in infancy, mineralocorticoid supplementation is of particular importance)

Acute adrenocortical insufficiency (hydrocortisone or cortisone is the drug of choice; mineralocorticoid supplementation may be necessary, particularly when synthetic analogs are used)

Preoperatively, and in the event of serious trauma or illness, in patients with known adrenal insufficiency or when adrenocortical reserve is doubtful

Congenital adrenal hyperplasia
Nonsuppurative thyroiditis
Hypercalcemia associated with cancer
2. *Rheumatic disorders*

As adjunctive therapy for short-term administration (to tide the patient over an acute episode or exacerbation) in:
Post-traumatic osteoarthritis
Synovitis of osteoarthritis
Rheumatoid arthritis, including juvenile rheumatoid arthritis (selected cases may require low-dose maintenance therapy)
Acute and subacute bursitis
Epicondylitis
Acute nonspecific tenosynovitis
Acute gouty arthritis
Psoriatic arthritis
Ankylosing spondylitis
3. *Collagen diseases*

During an exacerbation or as maintenance therapy in selected cases of:
Systemic lupus erythematosus
Acute rheumatic carditis
Systemic dermatomyositis (polymyositis)
4. *Dermatologic diseases*
Pemphigus
Severe erythema multiforme (Stevens-Johnson syndrome)
Exfoliative dermatitis
Bullous dermatitis herpetiformis
Severe seborrheic dermatitis
Severe psoriasis
Mycosis fungoides
5. *Allergic states*

Control of severe or incapacitating allergic conditions intractable to adequate trials of conventional treatment in:
Bronchial asthma
Contact dermatitis
Atopic dermatitis
Serum sickness
Seasonal or perennial allergic rhinitis
Drug hypersensitivity reactions
Urticarial transfusion reactions
Acute noninfectious laryngeal edema (epinephrine is the drug of first choice)
6. *Ophthalmic diseases*

Severe acute and chronic allergic and inflammatory processes involving the eye, such as:
Herpes zoster ophthalmicus
Iritis, iridocyclitis
Chorioretinitis
Diffuse posterior uveitis and choroiditis
Optic neuritis
Sympathetic ophthalmia
Anterior segment inflammation
Allergic conjunctivitis
Keratitis
Allergic corneal marginal ulcers
7. *Gastrointestinal diseases*

To tide the patient over a critical period of the disease in:
Ulcerative colitis (Systemic therapy)
Regional enteritis (Systemic therapy)
8. *Respiratory diseases*
Symptomatic sarcoidosis
Berylliosis
Fulminating or disseminated pulmonary tuberculosis when used concurrently with appropriate antituberculous chemotherapy
Loeffler's syndrome not manageable by other means
Aspiration pneumonitis
9. *Hematologic disorders*
Acquired (autoimmune) hemolytic anemia
Idiopathic thrombocytopenic purpura in adults (I.V. only; I.M. administration is contraindicated)
Secondary thrombocytopenia in adults
Erythroblastopenia (RBC anemia)
Congenital (erythroid) hypoplastic anemia
10. *Neoplastic diseases*

For palliative management of:
Leukemias and lymphomas in adults
Acute leukemia of childhood
11. *Edematous states*

To induce diuresis or remission of proteinuria in the nephrotic syndrome, without uremia, of the idiopathic type, or that due to lupus erythematosus
12. *Miscellaneous*

Tuberculous meningitis with subarachnoid block or impending block when used concurrently with appropriate antituberculous chemotherapy
Trichinosis with neurologic or myocardial involvement.
B. By intra-articular or soft tissue injection:

As adjunctive therapy for short-term administration (to tide the patient over an acute episode or exacerbation) in:
Synovitis of osteoarthritis
Rheumatoid arthritis
Acute and subacute bursitis
Acute gouty arthritis
Epicondylitis

Acute nonspecific tenosynovitis
Post-traumatic osteoarthritis.
C. By intralesional injection:
Keloids
Localized hypertrophic, infiltrated, inflammatory lesions of: lichen planus, psoriatic plaques, granuloma annulare, and lichen simplex chronicus (neurodermatitis)
Discoid lupus erythematosus
Necrobiosis lipoidica diabeticorum
Alopecia areata
May also be useful in cystic tumors of an aponeurosis or tendon (ganglia).

CONTRAINDICATIONS

Systemic fungal infections (see WARNINGS regarding amphotericin B)
Hypersensitivity to any component of this product, including sulfites (see WARNINGS).

WARNINGS

Because rare instances of anaphylactoid reactions have occurred in patients receiving parenteral corticosteroid therapy, appropriate precautionary measures should be taken prior to administration, especially when the patient has a history of allergy to any drug. Anaphylactoid and hypersensitivity reactions have been reported for Injection HYDELTRASOL (see ADVERSE REACTIONS).
Injection HYDELTRASOL contains sodium bisulfite, a sulfite that may cause allergic-type reactions including anaphylactic symptoms and life-threatening or less severe asthmatic episodes in certain susceptible people. The overall prevalence of sulfite sensitivity in the general population is unknown and probably low. Sulfite sensitivity is seen more frequently in asthmatic than in nonasthmatic people.
Corticosteroids may exacerbate systemic fungal infections and therefore should not be used in the presence of such infections unless they are needed to control drug reactions due to amphotericin B. Moreover, there have been cases reported in which concomitant use of amphotericin B and hydrocortisone was followed by cardiac enlargement and congestive failure.
In patients on corticosteroid therapy subjected to any unusual stress, increased dosage of rapidly acting corticosteroids before, during, and after the stressful situation is indicated.
Drug-induced secondary adrenocortical insufficiency may result from too rapid withdrawal of corticosteroids and may be minimized by gradual reduction of dosage. This type of relative insufficiency may persist for months after discontinuation of therapy; therefore, in any situation of stress occurring during that period, hormone therapy should be reinstituted. If the patient is receiving steroids already, dosage may have to be increased. Since mineralocorticoid secretion may be impaired, salt and/or a mineralocorticoid should be administered concurrently.
Corticosteroids may mask some signs of infection, and new infections may appear during their use. There may be decreased resistance and inability to localize infection when corticosteroids are used. Moreover, corticosteroids may affect the nitroblue-tetrazolium test for bacterial infection and produce false negative results.
In cerebral malaria, a double-blind trial has shown that the use of corticosteroids is associated with prolongation of coma and a higher incidence of pneumonia and gastrointestinal bleeding.
Corticosteroids may activate latent amebiasis. Therefore, it is recommended that latent or active amebiasis be ruled out before initiating corticosteroid therapy in any patient who has spent time in the tropics or any patient with unexplained diarrhea.
Prolonged use of corticosteroids may produce posterior subcapsular cataracts, glaucoma with possible damage to the optic nerves, and may enhance the establishment of secondary ocular infections due to fungi or viruses.
Usage in pregnancy. Since adequate human reproduction studies have not been done with corticosteroids, use of these drugs in pregnancy or in women of childbearing potential requires that the anticipated benefits be weighed against the possible hazards to the mother and embryo or fetus. Infants born of mothers who have received substantial doses of corticosteroids during pregnancy should be carefully observed for signs of hypoadrenalism.
Corticosteroids appear in breast milk and could suppress growth, interfere with endogenous corticosteroid production, or cause other unwanted effects. Mothers taking pharmacologic doses of corticosteroids should be advised not to nurse.
Average and large doses of cortisone or hydrocortisone can cause elevation of blood pressure, salt and water retention, and increased excretion of potassium. These effects are less likely to occur with the synthetic derivatives except when used in large doses. Dietary salt restriction and potassium supplementation may be necessary. All corticosteroids increase calcium excretion.
Administration of live virus vaccines, including smallpox, is contraindicated in individuals receiving immunosuppressive doses of corticosteroids. If inactivated viral or bacterial vaccines are administered to individuals receiving immunosuppressive doses of corticosteroids, the expected serum antibody response may not be obtained. However, immunization procedures may be undertaken in patients who are receiving corticosteroids as replacement therapy, e.g., for Addison's disease.
Patients who are on drugs which suppress the immune system are more susceptible to infections than healthy individuals. Chickenpox and measles, for example, can have a more serious or even fatal course in non-immune children or adults on corticosteroids. In such children or adults who have not had these diseases, particular care should be taken to avoid exposure. The risk of developing a disseminated infection varies among individuals and can be related to the dose, route and duration of corticosteroid administration as well as to the underlying disease. If exposed to chickenpox, prophylaxis with varicella zoster immune globulin (VZIG) may be indicated. If chickenpox develops, treatment with antiviral agents may be considered. If exposed to measles, prophylaxis with immune globulin (IG) may be indicated. (See the respective package inserts for VZIG and IG for complete prescribing information.)
The use of HYDELTRASOL injection in active tuberculosis should be restricted to those cases of fulminating or disseminated tuberculosis in which the corticosteroid is used for the management of the disease in conjunction with appropriate antituberculous regimen.
If corticosteroids are indicated in patients with latent tuberculosis or tuberculin reactivity, close observation is necessary as reactivation of the disease may occur. During prolonged corticosteroid therapy, these patients should receive chemoprophylaxis.
Literature reports suggest an apparent association between use of corticosteroids and left ventricular free wall rupture after a recent myocardial infarction; therefore, therapy with corticosteroids should be used with great caution in these patients.

PRECAUTIONS

This product, like many other steroid formulations, is sensitive to heat. Therefore, it should not be autoclaved when it is desirable to sterilize the exterior of the vial.
Following prolonged therapy, withdrawal of corticosteroids may result in symptoms of the corticosteroid withdrawal syndrome including fever, myalgia, arthralgia, and malaise. This may occur in patients even without evidence of adrenal insufficiency.
There is an enhanced effect of corticosteroids in patients with hypothyroidism and in those with cirrhosis.
Corticosteroids should be used cautiously in patients with ocular herpes simplex for fear of corneal perforation.
The lowest possible dose of corticosteroid should be used to control the condition under treatment, and when reduction in dosage is possible, the reduction must be gradual.
Psychic derangements may appear when corticosteroids are used, ranging from euphoria, insomnia, mood swings, personality changes, and severe depression to frank psychotic manifestations. Also, existing emotional instability or psychotic tendencies may be aggravated by corticosteroids.
Aspirin should be used cautiously in conjunction with corticosteroids in hypoprothrombinemia.
Steroids should be used with caution in nonspecific ulcerative colitis, if there is a probability of impending perforation, abscess, or other pyogenic infection, also in diverticulitis, fresh intestinal anastomoses, active or latent peptic ulcer, renal insufficiency, hypertension, osteoporosis, and myasthenia gravis. Signs of peritoneal irritation following gastrointestinal perforation in patients receiving large doses of corticosteroids may be minimal or absent. Fat embolism has been reported as a possible complication of hypercortisonism.
When large doses are given, some authorities advise that antacids be administered between meals to help to prevent peptic ulcer.
Growth and development of infants and children on prolonged corticosteroid therapy should be carefully followed.
Steroids may increase or decrease motility and number of spermatozoa in some patients.
Phenytoin, phenobarbital, ephedrine, and rifampin may enhance the metabolic clearance of corticosteroids, resulting in decreased blood levels and lessened physiologic activity, thus requiring adjustment in corticosteroid dosage.
The prothrombin time should be checked frequently in patients who are receiving corticosteroids and coumarin anticoagulants at the same time because of reports that corticosteroids have altered the response to these anticoagulants. Studies have shown that the usual effect produced by adding corticosteroids is inhibition of response to coumarins, although there have been some conflicting reports of potentiation not substantiated by studies.
When corticosteroids are administered concomitantly with potassium-depleting diuretics, patients should be observed closely for development of hypokalemia.
Intra-articular injection of a corticosteroid may produce systemic as well as local effects.
Appropriate examination of any joint fluid present is necessary to exclude a septic process.
A marked increase in pain accompanied by local swelling, further restriction of joint motion, fever, and malaise is suggestive of septic arthritis. If this complication occurs and the diagnosis of sepsis is confirmed, appropriate antimicrobial therapy should be instituted.
Injection of a steroid into an infected site is to be avoided.
Corticosteroids should not be injected into unstable joints.
Patients should be impressed strongly with the importance of not overusing joints in which symptomatic benefit has been obtained as long as the inflammatory process remains active.
Frequent intra-articular injection may result in damage to joint tissues.
The slower rate of absorption by intramuscular administration should be recognized.
Information for Patients
Susceptible patients who are on immunosuppressant doses of corticosteroids should be warned to avoid exposure to chickenpox or measles. Patients should also be advised that if they are exposed, medical advice should be sought without delay.

ADVERSE REACTIONS

Fluid and electrolyte disturbances
Sodium retention
Fluid retention
Congestive heart failure in susceptible patients
Potassium loss
Hypokalemic alkalosis
Hypertension
Musculoskeletal
Muscle weakness
Steroid myopathy
Loss of muscle mass
Osteoporosis
Vertebral compression fractures
Aseptic necrosis of femoral and humeral heads
Pathologic fracture of long bones
Tendon rupture
Gastrointestinal
Peptic ulcer with possible subsequent perforation and hemorrhage
Perforation of the small and large bowel, particularly in patients with inflammatory bowel disease
Pancreatitis
Abdominal distention
Ulcerative esophagitis
Dermatologic
Impaired wound healing
Thin fragile skin
Petechiae and ecchymoses
Erythema
Increased sweating
May suppress reactions to skin tests
Burning or tingling, especially in the perineal area (after I.V. injection)
Other cutaneous reactions, such as allergic dermatitis, urticaria, angioneurotic edema
Neurologic
Convulsions
Increased intracranial pressure with papilledema (pseudotumor cerebri) usually after treatment
Vertigo
Headache
Psychic disturbances
Endocrine
Menstrual irregularities
Development of cushingoid state
Suppression of growth in children
Secondary adrenocortical and pituitary unresponsiveness, particularly in times of stress, as in trauma, surgery, or illness
Decreased carbohydrate tolerance
Manifestations of latent diabetes mellitus
Increased requirements for insulin or oral hypoglycemic agents in diabetics
Hirsutism
Ophthalmic
Posterior subcapsular cataracts
Increased intraocular pressure
Glaucoma
Exophthalmos

Continued on next page

Information on the Merck & Co., Inc. products listed on these pages is the full prescribing information from product circulars in use September 30, 1996.

Merck & Co.—Cont.

| | Doses | |
Site of Injection	Amount of Injection (mL)	Amount of Prednisolone Phosphate (mg)
Large Joints (e.g., Knee)	0.5 to 1	10 to 20
Small Joints (e.g., Interphalangeal, Temporomandibular)	0.2 to 0.25	4 to 5
Bursae	0.5 to 0.75	10 to 15
Tendon Sheaths	0.1 to 0.25	2 to 5
Soft Tissue Infiltration	0.5 to 1.5	10 to 30
Ganglia	0.25 to 0.5	5 to 10

Metabolic
Negative nitrogen balance due to protein catabolism
Cardiovascular
Myocardial rupture following recent myocardial infarction (see WARNINGS).
Other
Anaphylactoid or hypersensitivity reactions
Thromboembolism
Weight gain
Increased appetite
Nausea
Malaise
The following *additional* adverse reactions are related to parenteral corticosteroid therapy:
Rare instances of blindness associated with intralesional therapy around the face and head
Hyperpigmentation or hypopigmentation
Subcutaneous and cutaneous atrophy
Sterile abscess
Postinjection flare (following intra-articular use)
Charcot-like arthropathy.

OVERDOSAGE

Reports of acute toxicity and/or death following overdosage of glucocorticoids are rare. In the event of overdosage, no specific antidote is available; treatment is supportive and symptomatic.
The intraperitoneal LD_{50} of prednisolone phosphate disodium in female mice was 1190 mg/kg.

DOSAGE AND ADMINISTRATION

For intravenous, intramuscular, intra-articular, intralesional, and soft tissue injection.
DOSAGE REQUIREMENTS ARE VARIABLE AND MUST BE INDIVIDUALIZED ON THE BASIS OF THE DISEASE AND THE RESPONSE OF THE PATIENT.

Intravenous and Intramuscular Injection
HYDELTRASOL injection can be given directly from the vial, or it can be added to Sodium Chloride Injection or Dextrose Injection and given by intravenous drip.
Benzyl alcohol as a preservative has been associated with toxicity in premature infants. Solutions used for intravenous administration or further dilution of this product should be preservative-free when used in the neonate, especially the premature infant.
When it is mixed with an infusion solution, sterile precautions should be observed. Since infusion solutions generally do not contain preservatives, mixtures should be used within 24 hours.
The initial dosage varies from 4 to 60 mg a day depending on the disease being treated. In less severe diseases doses lower than 4 mg may suffice, while in severe diseases doses higher than 60 mg may be required. Usually the daily parenteral dose of HYDELTRASOL injection is the same as the daily oral dose of prednisolone and the dosage interval is every 4 to 8 hours.
The initial dosage should be maintained or adjusted until the patient's response is satisfactory. If a satisfactory clinical response does not occur after a reasonable period of time, discontinue HYDELTRASOL injection and transfer the patient to other therapy.
After a favorable initial response, the proper maintenance dosage should be determined by decreasing the initial dosage in small amounts to the lowest dosage that maintains an adequate clinical response.
Patients should be observed closely for signs that might require dosage adjustment, including changes in clinical status resulting from remissions or exacerbations of the disease, individual drug responsiveness, and the effect of stress (e.g., surgery, infection, trauma). During stress it may be necessary to increase dosage temporarily.

If the drug is to be stopped after more than a few days of treatment, it usually should be withdrawn gradually.
Intra-articular, Intralesional, and Soft Tissue Injection
Intra-articular, intralesional, and soft tissue injections are generally employed when the affected joints or areas are limited to one or two sites. Dosage and frequency of injection vary depending on the condition being treated and the site of injection. The usual dose is from 2 to 30 mg. The frequency usually ranges from once every three to five days to once every two to three weeks Frequent intra-articular injection may result in damage to joint tissues.
Some of the usual single doses are:
[See table above.]
HYDELTRASOL injection is particularly recommended for use in conjunction with one of the less soluble, longer-acting steroids, such as HYDELTRA-T.B.A.* (Prednisolone Tebutate) suspension or HYDROCORTONE* Acetate (Hydrocortisone Acetate) sterile suspension, available for intra-articular and soft tissue injection.

---

*Registered trademark of MERCK & CO., INC.

HOW SUPPLIED

No. 7577X—Injection HYDELTRASOL, 20 mg prednisolone phosphate equivalent per mL, is a clear, colorless to slightly yellow solution, and is supplied as follows:
NDC 0006-7577-02 in 2 mL vials
NDC 0006-7577-03 in 5 mL vials
(6505-00-890-1496 20 mg/mL 5 mL vial).
Storage
Sensitive to heat. Do not autoclave.
Protect from light. Store container in carton until contents have been used.
7407228   Issued February 1993

HYDELTRA–T.B.A.® Sterile Suspension (Prednisolone Tebutate), U.S.P.

℞

For intra-articular, intralesional, and soft tissue injection only.

NOT FOR INTRAVENOUS USE
DESCRIPTION

Prednisolone tebutate, a synthetic adrenocortical steroid, is a white to slightly yellow powder sparingly soluble in alcohol, freely soluble in chloroform, and very slightly soluble in water. The molecular weight is 476.61 (monohydrate). It is designated chemically as $11\beta,17$-dihydroxy-21-[(3,3-dimethyl-1-oxobutyl)oxy]pregna-1,4-diene-3,20-dione. The empirical formula is $C_{27}H_{38}O_6$ and the structural formula is:

HYDELTRA-T.B.A.* (Prednisolone Tebutate) sterile suspension is a white to slightly yellow suspension (pH 6.0 to 8.0) that settles upon standing. Each mL contains prednisolone tebutate, 20 mg. Inactive ingredients per mL: sodium citrate, 1 mg; polysorbate 80, 1 mg; sorbitol solution, 0.5 mL (equal to

450 mg d-sorbitol); Water for Injection, q.s., 1 mL. Benzyl alcohol, 9 mg, added as preservative.

*Registered trademark of MERCK & CO., INC.

ACTIONS

HYDELTRA-T.B.A. has a slow onset but long duration of action when compared with more soluble preparations. Because of its slight solubility, it is suitable for intra-articular, intralesional, and soft tissue injection where its anti-inflammatory effects are confined mainly to the area in which it has been injected, although it is capable of producing systemic hormonal effects.
Naturally occurring glucocorticoids (hydrocortisone and cortisone), which also have salt-retaining properties, are used as replacement therapy in adrenocortical deficiency states. Their synthetic analogs, including prednisolone, are primarily used for their potent anti-inflammatory effects in disorders of many organ systems.
Glucocorticoids cause profound and varied metabolic effects. In addition, they modify the body's immune responses to diverse stimuli.

INDICATIONS

A. By intra-articular or soft tissue injection:
As adjunctive therapy for short-term administration (to tide the patient over an acute episode or exacerbation) in:
Synovitis of osteoarthritis
Rheumatoid arthritis
Acute and subacute bursitis
Acute gouty arthritis
Epicondylitis
Acute nonspecific tenosynovitis
Post-traumatic osteoarthritis
B. By intralesional injection:
May be useful in cystic tumors of an aponeurosis or tendon (ganglia).

CONTRAINDICATIONS

Systemic fungal infections
Hypersensitivity to any component of this product

WARNINGS

Because rare instances of anaphylactoid reactions have occurred in patients receiving parenteral corticosteroid therapy, appropriate precautionary measures should be taken prior to administration, especially when the patient has a history of allergy to any drug. Anaphylactoid and hypersensitivity reactions have been reported for Sterile Suspension HYDELTRA-T.B.A. (see ADVERSE REACTIONS).
In patients on corticosteroid therapy subjected to any unusual stress, increased dosage of rapidly acting corticosteroids before, during, and after the stressful situation is indicated.
Drug-induced secondary adrenocortical insufficiency may result from too rapid withdrawal of corticosteroids and may be minimized by gradual reduction of dosage. This type of relative insufficiency may persist for months after discontinuation of therapy; therefore, in any situation of stress occurring during that period, hormone therapy should be reinstituted. If the patient is receiving steroids already, dosage may have to be increased. Since mineralocorticoid secretion may be impaired, salt and/or a mineralocorticoid should be administered concurrently.
Corticosteroids may mask some signs of infection, and new infections may appear during their use. There may be decreased resistance and inability to localize infection when corticosteroids are used. Moreover, corticosteroids may affect the nitroblue-tetrazolium test for bacterial infection and produce false negative results.
In cerebral malaria, a double-blind trial has shown that the use of corticosteroids is associated with prolongation of coma and a higher incidence of pneumonia and gastrointestinal bleeding.
Corticosteroids may activate latent amebiasis. Therefore, it is recommended that latent or active amebiasis be ruled out before initiating corticosteroid therapy in any patient who has spent time in the tropics or any patient with unexplained diarrhea.
Prolonged use of corticosteroids may produce posterior subcapsular cataracts, glaucoma with possible damage to the optic nerves, and may enhance the establishment of secondary ocular infections due to fungi or viruses.
Usage in pregnancy. Since adequate human reproduction studies have not been done with corticosteroids, use of these drugs in pregnancy or in women of childbearing potential requires that the anticipated benefits be weighed against the possible hazards to the mother and embryo or fetus. Infants born of mothers who have received substantial doses of corticosteroids during pregnancy should be carefully observed for signs of hypoadrenalism.

Corticosteroids appear in breast milk and could suppress growth, interfere with endogenous corticosteroid production, or cause other unwanted effects. Mothers taking pharmacologic doses of corticosteroids should be advised not to nurse.

Average and large doses of cortisone or hydrocortisone can cause elevation of blood pressure, salt and water retention, and increased excretion of potassium. These effects are less likely to occur with the synthetic derivatives except when used in large doses. Dietary salt restriction and potassium supplementation may be necessary. All corticosteroids increase calcium excretion.

Administration of live virus vaccines, including smallpox, is contraindicated in individuals receiving immunosuppressive doses of corticosteroids. If inactivated viral or bacterial vaccines are administered to individuals receiving immunosuppressive doses of corticosteroids, the expected serum antibody response may not be obtained.

Patients who are on drugs which suppress the immune system are more susceptible to infections than healthy individuals. Chickenpox and measles, for example, can have a more serious or even fatal course in non-immune children or adults on corticosteroids. In such children or adults who have not had these diseases, particular care should be taken to avoid exposure. The risk of developing a disseminated infection varies among individuals and can be related to the dose, route and duration of corticosteroid administration as well as to the underlying disease. If exposed to chickenpox, prophylaxis with varicella zoster immune globulin (VZIG) may be indicated. If chickenpox develops, treatment with antiviral agents may be considered. If exposed to measles, prophylaxis with immune globulin (IG) may be indicated. (See the respective package inserts for VZIG and IG for complete prescribing information.)

Similarly, corticosteroids should be used with great care in patients with known or suspected Strongyloides (threadworm) infestation. In such patients, corticosteroid-induced immunosuppression may lead to Strongyloides hyperinfection and dissemination with widespread larval migration, often accompanied by severe enterocolitis and potentially fatal gram-negative septicemia.

If corticosteroids are indicated in patients with latent tuberculosis or tuberculin reactivity, close observation is necessary as reactivation of the disease may occur. During prolonged corticosteroid therapy, these patients should receive chemoprophylaxis.

Literature reports suggest an apparent association between use of corticosteroids and left ventricular free wall rupture after a recent myocardial infarction; therefore, therapy with corticosteroids should be used with great caution in these patients.

PRECAUTIONS

This product, like many other steroid formulations, is sensitive to heat. Therefore, it should not be autoclaved when it is desirable to sterilize the exterior of the vial.

Following prolonged therapy, withdrawal of corticosteroids may result in symptoms of the corticosteroid withdrawal syndrome including fever, myalgia, arthralgia, and malaise. This may occur in patients even without evidence of adrenal insufficiency.

There is an enhanced effect of corticosteroids in patients with hypothyroidism and in those with cirrhosis.

Corticosteroids should be used cautiously in patients with ocular herpes simplex for fear of corneal perforation.

Psychic derangements may appear when corticosteroids are used, ranging from euphoria, insomnia, mood swings, personality changes, and severe depression to frank psychotic manifestations. Also, existing emotional instability or psychotic tendencies may be aggravated by corticosteroids.

Aspirin should be used cautiously in conjunction with corticosteroids in hypoprothrombinemia.

Steroids should be used with caution in nonspecific ulcerative colitis, if there is a probability of impending perforation, abscess, or other pyogenic infection, also in diverticulitis, fresh intestinal anastomoses, active or latent peptic ulcer, renal insufficiency, hypertension, osteoporosis, and myasthenia gravis. Signs of peritoneal irritation following gastrointestinal perforation in patients receiving large doses of corticosteroids may be minimal or absent. Fat embolism has been reported as a possible complication of hypercortisonism.

When large doses are given, some authorities advise that antacids be administered between meals to help to prevent peptic ulcer.

Growth and development of infants and children on prolonged corticosteroid therapy should be carefully followed.

Steroids may increase or decrease motility and number of spermatozoa in some patients.

Phenytoin, phenobarbital, ephedrine, and rifampin may enhance the metabolic clearance of corticosteroids, resulting in decreased blood levels and lessened physiologic activity, thus requiring adjustment in corticosteroid dosage.

The prothrombin time should be checked frequently in patients who are receiving corticosteroids and coumarin anticoagulants at the same time because of reports that corticosteroids have altered the response to these anticoagulants. Studies have shown that the usual effect produced by adding corticosteroids is inhibition of response to coumarins, although there have been some conflicting reports of potentiation not substantiated by studies.

When corticosteroids are administered concomitantly with potassium-depleting diuretics, patients should be observed closely for development of hypokalemia.

Intra-articular injection of a corticosteroid may produce systemic as well as local effects.

Appropriate examination of any joint fluid present is necessary to exclude a septic process.

A marked increase in pain accompanied by local swelling, further restriction of joint motion, fever, and malaise is suggestive of septic arthritis. If this complication occurs and the diagnosis of sepsis is confirmed, appropriate antimicrobial therapy should be instituted.

Injection of a steroid into an infected site is to be avoided. Corticosteroids should not be injected into unstable joints. Patients should be impressed strongly with the importance of not overusing joints in which symptomatic benefit has been obtained as long as the inflammatory process remains active.

Frequent intra-articular injection may result in damage to joint tissues.

Information for Patients

Susceptible patients who are on immunosuppressant doses of corticosteroids should be warned to avoid exposure to chickenpox or measles. Patients should also be advised that if they are exposed, medical advice should be sought without delay.

ADVERSE REACTIONS

Fluid and electrolyte disturbances
  Sodium retention
  Fluid retention
  Congestive heart failure in susceptible patients
  Potassium loss
  Hypokalemic alkalosis
  Hypertension
Musculoskeletal
  Muscle weakness
  Steroid myopathy
  Loss of muscle mass
  Osteoporosis
  Vertebral compression fractures
  Aseptic necrosis of femoral and humeral heads
  Pathologic fracture of long bones
  Tendon rupture
Gastrointestinal
  Peptic ulcer with possible subsequent perforation and hemorrhage
  Perforation of the small and large bowel, particularly in patients with inflammatory bowel disease
  Pancreatitis
  Abdominal distention
  Ulcerative esophagitis
Dermatologic
  Impaired wound healing
  Thin fragile skin
  Petechiae and ecchymoses
  Erythema
  Increased sweating
  May suppress reactions to skin tests
  Other cutaneous reactions, such as allergic dermatitis, urticaria, angioneurotic edema
Neurologic
  Convulsions
  Increased intracranial pressure with papilledema (pseudotumor cerebri) usually after treatment
  Vertigo
  Headache
  Psychic disturbances
Endocrine
  Menstrual irregularities
  Development of cushingoid state
  Suppression of growth in children
  Secondary adrenocortical and pituitary unresponsiveness, particularly in times of stress, as in trauma, surgery, or illness
  Decreased carbohydrate tolerance
  Manifestations of latent diabetes mellitus
  Increased requirements for insulin or oral hypoglycemic agents in diabetics
  Hirsutism
Ophthalmic
  Posterior subcapsular cataracts
  Increased intraocular pressure
  Glaucoma
  Exophthalmos
Metabolic
  Negative nitrogen balance due to protein catabolism

Cardiovascular
  Myocardial rupture following recent myocardial infarction (see WARNINGS).
Other
  Anaphylactoid or hypersensitivity reactions
  Thromboembolism
  Weight gain
  Increased appetite
  Nausea
  Malaise
  Foreign body granulomatous reactions involving the synovium have been reported with repeated injections of HYDELTRA-T.B.A.

Localized pain and swelling, sometimes distal to the site of injection and persisting for several days, have been reported. The following *additional* adverse reactions are related to injection of corticosteroids:

  Rare instances of blindness associated with intralesional therapy around the face and head
  Hyperpigmentation or hypopigmentation
  Subcutaneous and cutaneous atrophy
  Sterile abscess
  Postinjection flare (following intra-articular use)
  Charcot-like arthropathy

DOSAGE AND ADMINISTRATION

> For intra-articular, intralesional, and soft tissue injection only.

NOT FOR INTRAVENOUS USE

DOSAGE AND FREQUENCY OF INJECTION ARE VARIABLE AND MUST BE INDIVIDUALIZED ON THE BASIS OF THE DISEASE AND THE RESPONSE OF THE PATIENT.

The initial dose varies from 4 to 40 mg depending on the disease being treated and the size of the area to be injected. Frequency of injection depends on symptomatic response, and usually is once every two or three weeks. Severe conditions may require injection once a week. Frequent intra-articular injection may result in damage to joint tissues. If satisfactory clinical response does not occur after a reasonable period of time, discontinue HYDELTRA-T.B.A. sterile suspension and transfer the patient to other therapy.

Patients should be observed closely for signs that might require dosage adjustment, including changes in clinical status resulting from remissions or exacerbations of the disease, and individual drug responsiveness.

For rapid onset of action, a soluble adrenocortical hormone preparation, such as DECADRON* Phosphate (Dexamethasone Sodium Phosphate) injection or HYDELTRASOL* (Prednisolone Sodium Phosphate) injection, may be given with HYDELTRA-T.B.A.

If desired, a local anesthetic may be used, and may be injected before HYDELTRA-T.B.A., or mixed in a syringe with HYDELTRA-T.B.A. and given simultaneously.

If used prior to intra-articular injection of the steroid, inject most of the anesthetic into the soft tissues of the surrounding area and instill a small amount into the joint.

If given together, mixing should be done in the injection syringe by drawing the steroid in *first,* then the anesthetic. In this way, the anesthetic will not be introduced inadvertently into the vial of steroid. *The mixture must be used immediately and any unused portion discarded.*

Some of the usual single doses are:

Large Joints (e.g., Knee)	20 mg (1 mL), occasionally 30 mg (1.5 mL). Doses over 40 mg (2 mL) not recommended.
Small Joints (e.g., Interphalangeal, Temporomandibular)	8 to 10 mg (0.4 to 0.5 mL).
Bursae	20 to 30 mg (1 to 1.5 mL).
Tendon Sheaths	4 to 10 mg (0.2 to 0.5 mL).
Ganglia	10 to 20 mg (0.5 to 1 mL).

*Registered trademark of MERCK & CO., INC.

Continued on next page

Merck & Co.—Cont.

HOW SUPPLIED

No. 7572—Sterile Suspension HYDELTRA-T.B.A., 20 mg per mL, is a white, milky suspension, and is supplied as follows:
NDC 0006-7572-01 in 1 mL vials
(6505-00-225-7499 1 mL vial)
NDC 0006-7572-03 in 5 mL vials
(6505-00-890-1353 5 mL vial).
Storage
Sensitive to heat. Do not autoclave.
Protect from freezing.
Protect from light. Store container in carton until contents have been used.

7498027   Issued October 1995

HYDROCORTONE®   ℞
Acetate Sterile Suspension
(Hydrocortisone Acetate), U.S.P.

For intra-articular, intralesional, and soft tissue injection only.

NOT FOR INTRAVENOUS USE

DESCRIPTION

Hydrocortisone acetate, a synthetic adrenocortical steroid, is a white to practically white, odorless, crystalline powder. It is insoluble in water and slightly soluble in alcohol and chloroform. The molecular weight is 404.50. It is designated chemically as 21-(acetyloxy)-11β,17-dihydroxypregn-4-ene-3,20-dione. The empirical formula is $C_{23}H_{32}O_6$ and the structural formula is:

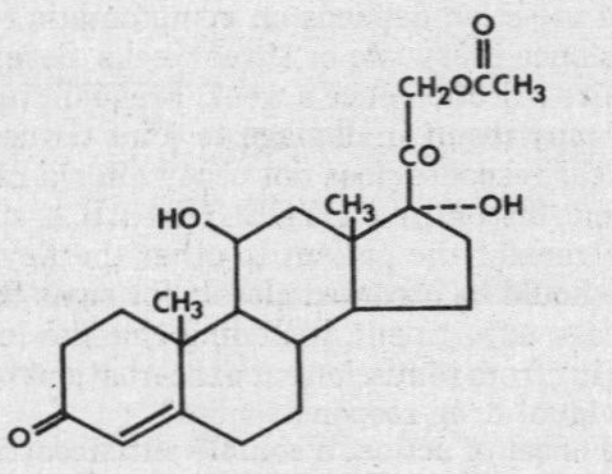

HYDROCORTONE* Acetate (Hydrocortisone Acetate) sterile suspension is a sterile suspension containing 50 mg per milliliter of hydrocortisone acetate in a suitable aqueous medium (pH -5.0 to 7.0). Inactive ingredients per mL: sodium chloride, 9 mg; polysorbate 80, 4 mg; sodium carboxymethylcellulose, 5 mg; and Water for Injection, q.s., 1 mL. Benzyl alcohol, 9 mg, added as preservative.

---

* Registered trademark of MERCK & CO., Inc.

ACTIONS

HYDROCORTONE Acetate sterile suspension has a slow onset but long duration of action when compared with more soluble preparations. Because of its insolubility, it is suitable for intra-articular, intralesional, and soft tissue injection where its anti-inflammatory effects are confined mainly to the area in which it has been injected, although it is capable of producing systemic hormonal effects.
Naturally occurring glucocorticoids (hydrocortisone and cortisone), which also have salt-retaining properties, are used as replacement therapy in adrenocortical deficiency states. They are also used for their potent anti-inflammatory effect in disorders of many organ systems.
Glucocorticoids cause profound and varied metabolic effects. In addition, they modify the body's immune responses to diverse stimuli.

INDICATIONS

A. By intra-articular or soft tissue injection:
As adjunctive therapy for short-term administration (to tide the patient over an acute episode or exacerbation) in:
Synovitis of osteoarthritis
Rheumatoid arthritis
Acute and subacute bursitis
Acute gouty arthritis
Epicondylitis
Acute nonspecific tenosynovitis
Post-traumatic osteoarthritis
B. By intralesional injection:
Keloids

Localized hypertrophic, infiltrated, inflammatory lesions of: lichen planus, psoriatic plaques, granuloma annulare, and lichen simplex chronicus (neurodermatitis)
Discoid lupus erythematosus
Necrobiosis lipoidica diabeticorum
Alopecia areata
May also be useful in cystic tumors of an aponeurosis or tendon (ganglia).

CONTRAINDICATIONS

Systemic fungal infections
Hypersensitivity to any component of this product

WARNINGS

Because rare instances of anaphylactoid reactions have occurred in patients receiving parenteral corticosteroid therapy, appropriate precautionary measures should be taken prior to administration, especially when the patient has a history of allergy to any drug.
In patients on corticosteroid therapy subjected to any unusual stress, increased dosage of rapidly acting corticosteroids before, during, and after the stressful situation is indicated.
Drug-induced secondary adrenocortical insufficiency may result from too rapid withdrawal of corticosteroids and may be minimized by gradual reduction of dosage. This type of relative insufficiency may persist for months after discontinuation of therapy; therefore, in any situation of stress occurring during that period, hormone therapy should be reinstituted. If the patient is receiving steroids already, dosage may have to be increased. Since mineralocorticoid secretion may be impaired, salt and/or a mineralocorticoid should be administered concurrently.
Corticosteroids may mask some signs of infection, and new infections may appear during their use. There may be decreased resistance and inability to localize infection when corticosteroids are used. Moreover, corticosteroids may affect the nitroblue-tetrazolium test for bacterial infection and produce false negative results.
In cerebral malaria, a double-blind trial has shown that the use of corticosteroids is associated with prolongation of coma and a higher incidence of pneumonia and gastrointestinal bleeding.
Corticosteroids may activate latent amebiasis. Therefore, it is recommended that latent or active amebiasis be ruled out before initiating corticosteroid therapy in any patient who has spent time in the tropics or any patient with unexplained diarrhea.
Prolonged use of corticosteroids may produce posterior subcapsular cataracts, glaucoma with possible damage to the optic nerves, and may enhance the establishment of secondary ocular infections due to fungi or viruses.
Usage in pregnancy: Since adequate human reproduction studies have not been done with corticosteroids, use of these drugs in pregnancy or in women of childbearing potential requires that the anticipated benefits be weighed against the possible hazards to the mother and embryo or fetus. Infants born of mothers who have received substantial doses of corticosteroids during pregnancy should be carefully observed for signs of hypoadrenalism.
Corticosteroids appear in breast milk and could suppress growth, interfere with endogenous corticosteroid production, or cause other unwanted effects. Mothers taking pharmacologic doses of corticosteroids should be advised not to nurse.
Average and large doses of cortisone or hydrocortisone can cause elevation of blood pressure, salt and water retention, and increased excretion of potassium. These effects are less likely to occur with the synthetic derivatives except when used in large doses. Dietary salt restriction and potassium supplementation may be necessary. All corticosteroids increase calcium excretion.
Administration of live virus vaccines, including smallpox, is contraindicated in individuals receiving immunosuppressive doses of corticosteroids. If inactivated viral or bacterial vaccines are administered to individuals receiving immunosuppressive doses of corticosteroids, the expected serum antibody response may not be obtained.
Patients who are on drugs which suppress the immune system are more susceptible to infections than healthy individuals. Chickenpox and measles, for example, can have a more serious or even fatal course in non-immune children or adults on corticosteroids. In such children or adults who have not had these diseases, particular care should be taken to avoid exposure. The risk of developing a disseminated infection varies among individuals and can be related to the dose, route and duration of corticosteroid administration as well as to the underlying disease. If exposed to chickenpox, prophylaxis with varicella zoster immune globulin (VZIG) may be indicated. If chickenpox develops, treatment with antiviral agents may be considered. If exposed to measles, prophylaxis with immune globulin (IG) may be indicated. (See the respective package inserts for VZIG and IG for complete prescribing information.)

Similarly, corticosteroids should be used with great care in patients with known or suspected Strongyloides (threadworm) infestation. In such patients, corticosteroid-induced immunosuppression may lead to Strongyloides hyperinfection and dissemination with widespread larval migration, often accompanied by severe enterocolitis and potentially fatal gram-negative septicemia.
If corticosteroids are indicated in patients with latent tuberculosis or tuberculin reactivity, close observation is necessary as reactivation of the disease may occur. During prolonged corticosteroid therapy, these patients should receive chemoprophylaxis.
Literature reports suggest an apparent association between use of corticosteroids and left ventricular free wall rupture after a recent myocardial infarction; therefore, therapy with corticosteroids should be used with great caution in these patients.

PRECAUTIONS

This product, like many other steroid formulations, is sensitive to heat. Therefore, it should not be autoclaved when it is desirable to sterilize the exterior of the vial.
Following prolonged therapy, withdrawal of corticosteroids may result in symptoms of the corticosteroid withdrawal syndrome including fever, myalgia, arthralgia, and malaise. This may occur in patients even without evidence of adrenal insufficiency.
There is an enhanced effect of corticosteroids in patients with hypothyroidism and in those with cirrhosis.
Corticosteroids should be used cautiously in patients with ocular herpes simplex for fear of corneal perforation.
Psychic derangements may appear when corticosteroids are used, ranging from euphoria, insomnia, mood swings, personality changes, and severe depression to frank psychotic manifestations. Also, existing emotional instability or psychotic tendencies may be aggravated by corticosteroids.
Aspirin should be used cautiously in conjunction with corticosteroids in hypoprothrombinemia.
Steroids should be used with caution in nonspecific ulcerative colitis, if there is a probability of impending perforation, abscess, or other pyogenic infection, also in diverticulitis, fresh intestinal anastomoses, active or latent peptic ulcer, renal insufficiency, hypertension, osteoporosis, and myasthenia gravis. Signs of peritoneal irritation following gastrointestinal perforation in patients receiving large doses of corticosteroids may be minimal or absent. Fat embolism has been reported as a possible complication of hypercortisonism.
When large doses are given, some authorities advise that antacids be administered between meals to help to prevent peptic ulcer.
Growth and development of infants and children on prolonged corticosteroid therapy should be carefully followed. Steroids may increase or decrease motility and number of spermatozoa in some patients.
Phenytoin, phenobarbital, ephedrine, and rifampin may enhance the metabolic clearance of corticosteroids resulting in decreased blood levels and lessened physiologic activity, thus requiring adjustment in corticosteroid dosage.
The prothrombin time should be checked frequently in patients who are receiving corticosteroids and coumarin anticoagulants at the same time because of reports that corticosteroids have altered the response to these anticoagulants. Studies have shown that the usual effect produced by adding corticosteroids is inhibition of response to coumarins, although there have been some conflicting reports of potentiation not substantiated by studies.
When corticosteroids are administered concomitantly with potassium-depleting diuretics, patients should be observed closely for development of hypokalemia.
Intra-articular injection of a corticosteroid may produce systemic as well as local effects.
Appropriate examination of any joint fluid present is necessary to exclude a septic process.
A marked increase in pain accompanied by local swelling, further restriction of joint motion, fever, and malaise is suggestive of septic arthritis. If this complication occurs and the diagnosis of sepsis is confirmed, appropriate antimicrobial therapy should be instituted.
Injection of a steroid into an infected site is to be avoided. Corticosteroids should not be injected into unstable joints. Patients should be impressed strongly with the importance of not overusing joints in which symptomatic benefit has been obtained as long as the inflammatory process remains active.
Frequent intra-articular injection may result in damage to joint tissues.
Information for Patients
Susceptible patients who are on immunosuppressant doses of corticosteroids should be warned to avoid exposure to chickenpox or measles. Patients should also be advised that if they are exposed, medical advice should be sought without delay.

Information will be superseded by supplements and subsequent editions

ADVERSE REACTIONS

Fluid and electrolyte disturbances
Sodium retention
Fluid retention
Congestive heart failure in susceptible patients
Potassium loss
Hypokalemic alkalosis
Hypertension

Musculoskeletal
Muscle weakness
Steroid myopathy
Loss of muscle mass
Osteoporosis
Vertebral compression fractures
Aseptic necrosis of femoral and humeral heads
Pathologic fracture of long bones
Tendon rupture

Gastrointestinal
Peptic ulcer with possible subsequent perforation and hemorrhage
Perforation of the small and large bowel, particularly in patients with inflammatory bowel disease
Pancreatitis
Abdominal distention
Ulcerative esophagitis

Dermatologic
Impaired wound healing
Thin fragile skin
Petechiae and ecchymoses
Erythema
Increased sweating
May suppress reactions to skin tests
Other cutaneous reactions, such as allergic dermatitis, urticaria, angioneurotic edema

Neurologic
Convulsions
Increased intracranial pressure with papilledema (pseudotumor cerebri) usually after treatment
Vertigo
Headache
Psychic disturbances

Endocrine
Menstrual irregularities
Development of cushingoid state
Suppression of growth in children
Secondary adrenocortical and pituitary unresponsiveness, particularly in times of stress, as in trauma, surgery, or illness
Decreased carbohydrate tolerance
Manifestations of latent diabetes mellitus
Increased requirements for insulin or oral hypoglycemic agents in diabetics
Hirsutism

Ophthalmic
Posterior subcapsular cataracts
Increased intraocular pressure
Glaucoma
Exophthalmos

Metabolic
Negative nitrogen balance due to protein catabolism

Cardiovascular
Myocardial rupture following recent myocardial infarction (see WARNINGS).

Other
Anaphylactoid or hypersensitivity reactions
Thromboembolism
Weight gain
Increased appetite
Nausea
Malaise

The following *additional* adverse reactions are related to injection of corticosteroids:
Rare instances of blindness associated with intralesional therapy around the face and head
Hyperpigmentation or hypopigmentation
Subcutaneous and cutaneous atrophy
Sterile abscess
Postinjection flare (following intra-articular use)
Charcot-like arthropathy.

OVERDOSAGE

Reports of acute toxicity and/or death following overdosage of glucocorticoids are rare. In the event of overdosage, no specific antidote is available; treatment is supportive and symptomatic.

DOSAGE AND ADMINISTRATION

For intra-articular, intralesional, and soft tissue injection only

NOT FOR INTRAVENOUS USE

DOSAGE AND FREQUENCY OF INJECTION ARE VARIABLE AND MUST BE INDIVIDUALIZED ON THE BASIS OF THE DISEASE AND THE RESPONSE OF THE PATIENT.
The initial dose varies from 5 to 75 mg depending on the disease being treated and the size of the area to be injected. Frequency of injection depends on symptomatic response, and usually is once every two or three weeks. Severe conditions may require injection once a week. Frequent intra-articular injection may result in damage to joint tissues. If satisfactory clinical response does not occur after a reasonable period of time, discontinue HYDROCORTONE Acetate sterile suspension and transfer the patient to other therapy.
Patients should be observed closely for signs that might require dosage adjustment, including changes in clinical status resulting from remissions or exacerbations of the disease, and individual drug responsiveness.
Some of the usual single doses are:

Large Joints (e.g., Knee)	25 mg, occasionally 37.5 mg. Doses over 50 mg not recommended
Small Joints (e.g, Interphalangeal, Temporomandibular)	10 to 25 mg
Bursae	25 to 37.5 mg
Tendon Sheaths	5 to 12.5 mg
Soft Tissue Infiltration	25 to 50 mg, occasionally 75 mg
Ganglia	12.5 to 25 mg

For rapid onset of action, a soluble adrenocortical hormone preparation, such as DECADRON* Phosphate (Dexamethasone Sodium Phosphate) injection or HYDELTRASOL* (Prednisolone Sodium Phosphate) injection, may be given with HYDROCORTONE Acetate sterile suspension.
If desired, a local anesthetic may be used, and may be injected before HYDROCORTONE Acetate sterile suspension or mixed in a syringe with HYDROCORTONE Acetate sterile suspension and given simultaneously.
If used prior to intra-articular injection of the steroid, inject most of the anesthetic into the soft tissues of the surrounding area and instill a small amount into the joint.
If given together, mixing should be done in the injection syringe by drawing the steroid in *first* , then the anesthetic. In this way, the anesthetic will not be introduced inadvertently into the vial of steroid. *The mixture must be used immediately and any unused portion discarded.*

* Registered trademark of MERCK & CO., INC.

HOW SUPPLIED

No. 7519—Sterile suspension HYDROCORTONE Acetate is a white, mobile suspension, containing 50 mg hydrocortisone acetate in each mL, and is supplied as follows:
NDC 0006-7519-03 in 5 mL vials.
Storage
Sensitive to heat. Do not autoclave.
Protect from freezing.
7348728   Issued October 1995

HYDROCORTONE® Phosphate Injection, Sterile ℞
(Hydrocortisone Sodium Phosphate), U.S.P.

DESCRIPTION

Hydrocortisone sodium phosphate, a synthetic adrenocortical steroid, is a white to light yellow, odorless or practically odorless powder. It is freely soluble in water and is exceedingly hygroscopic. The molecular weight is 486.41. It is designated chemically as 11β,17-dihydroxy-21-(phosphonooxy)-pregn-4-ene-3,20-dione disodium salt. The empirical formula is $C_{21}H_{29}Na_2O_8P$ and the structural formula is:
[See chemical structure at top of next column.]
HYDROCORTONE* Phosphate (Hydrocortisone Sodium Phosphate) injection is a sterile solution (pH 7.5 to 8.5), sealed under nitrogen, for intravenous, intramuscular, and subcutaneous administration.
Each milliliter contains hydrocortisone sodium phosphate equivalent to 50 mg hydrocortisone. Inactive ingredients per mL: 8 mg creatinine, 10 mg sodium citrate, sodium hydrox-

ide to adjust pH, and Water for Injection, q.s. 1 mL, with 3.2 mg sodium bisulfite, 1.5 mg methylparaben, and 0.2 mg propylparaben added as preservatives.

* Registered trademark of MERCK & CO., INC.

ACTIONS

HYDROCORTONE Phosphate injection has a rapid onset but short duration of action when compared with less soluble preparations. Because of this, it is suitable for the treatment of acute disorders responsive to adrenocortical steroid therapy.
Naturally occurring glucocorticoids (hydrocortisone and cortisone), which also have salt-retaining properties, are used as replacement therapy in adrenocortical deficiency states. They are also used for their potent anti-inflammatory effects in disorders of many organ systems.
Glucocorticoids cause profound and varied metabolic effects. In addition, they modify the body's immune responses to diverse stimuli.

INDICATIONS

When oral therapy is not feasible:
1. *Endocrine disorders*
   Primary or secondary adrenocortical insufficiency (hydrocortisone or cortisone is the drug of choice; synthetic analogs may be used in conjunction with mineralocorticoids where applicable; in infancy, mineralocorticoid supplementation is of particular importance)
   Acute adrenocortical insufficiency (hydrocortisone or cortisone is the drug of choice; mineralocorticoid supplementation may be necessary, particularly when synthetic analogs are used)
   Preoperatively, and in the event of serious trauma or illness, in patients with known adrenal insufficiency or when adrenocortical reserve is doubtful
   Shock unresponsive to conventional therapy if adrenocortical insufficiency exists or is suspected
   Congenital adrenal hyperplasia
   Nonsuppurative thyroiditis
   Hypercalcemia associated with cancer
2. *Rheumatic disorders*
   As adjunctive therapy for short-term administration (to tide the patient over an acute episode or exacerbation) in:
   Post-traumatic osteoarthritis
   Synovitis of osteoarthritis
   Rheumatoid arthritis, including juvenile rheumatoid arthritis (selected cases may require low-dose maintenance therapy)
   Acute and subacute bursitis
   Epicondylitis
   Acute nonspecific tenosynovitis
   Acute gouty arthritis
   Psoriatic arthritis
   Ankylosing spondylitis
3. *Collagen diseases*
   During an exacerbation or as maintenance therapy in selected cases of:
   Systemic lupus erythematosus
   Acute rheumatic carditis
   Systemic dermatomyositis (polymyositis)
4. *Dermatologic diseases*
   Pemphigus
   Severe erythema multiforme (Stevens-Johnson syndrome)
   Exfoliative dermatitis
   Bullous dermatitis herpetiformis
   Severe seborrheic dermatitis
   Severe psoriasis
   Mycosis fungoides
5. *Allergic states*
   Control of severe or incapacitating allergic conditions intractable to adequate trials of conventional treatment in:

Continued on next page

Merck & Co.—Cont.

Bronchial asthma
Contact dermatitis
Atopic dermatitis
Serum sickness
Seasonal or perennial allergic rhinitis
Drug hypersensitivity reactions
Urticarial transfusion reactions
Acute noninfectious laryngeal edema (epinephrine is the drug of first choice)

6. *Ophthalmic diseases*
Severe acute and chronic allergic and inflammatory processes involving the eye, such as:
Herpes zoster ophthalmicus
Iritis, iridocyclitis
Chorioretinitis
Diffuse posterior uveitis and choroiditis
Optic neuritis
Sympathetic ophthalmia
Anterior segment inflammation
Allergic conjunctivitis
Keratitis
Allergic corneal marginal ulcers

7. *Gastrointestinal diseases*
To tide the patient over a critical period of the disease in:
Ulcerative colitis (Systemic therapy)
Regional enteritis (Systemic therapy)

8. *Respiratory diseases*
Symptomatic sarcoidosis
Berylliosis
Fulminating or disseminated pulmonary tuberculosis when used concurrently with appropriate antituberculous chemotherapy
Loeffler's syndrome not manageable by other means
Aspiration pneumonitis

9. *Hematologic disorders*
Acquired (autoimmune) hemolytic anemia
Idiopathic thrombocytopenic purpura in adults (I.V. only; I.M. administration is contraindicated)
Secondary thrombocytopenia in adults
Erythroblastopenia (RBC anemia)
Congenital (erythroid) hypoplastic anemia

10. *Neoplastic diseases*
For palliative management of:
Leukemias and lymphomas in adults
Acute leukemia of childhood

11. *Edematous states*
To induce diuresis or remission of proteinuria in the nephrotic syndrome, without uremia, of the idiopathic type, or that due to lupus erythematosus

12. *Miscellaneous*
Tuberculous meningitis with subarachnoid block or impending block when used concurrently with appropriate antituberculous chemotherapy
Trichinosis with neurologic or myocardial involvement

CONTRAINDICATIONS

Systemic fungal infections (see WARNINGS regarding amphotericin B)
Hypersensitivity to any component of this product, including sulfites (see WARNINGS).

WARNINGS

Because rare instances of anaphylactoid reactions have occurred in patients receiving parenteral corticosteroid therapy, appropriate precautionary measures should be taken prior to administration, especially when the patient has a history of allergy to any drug. Anaphylactoid and hypersensitivity reactions have been reported for Injection HYDROCORTONE Phosphate (see ADVERSE REACTIONS).

Injection HYDROCORTONE Phosphate contains sodium bisulfite, a sulfite that may cause allergic-type reactions including anaphylactic symptoms and life-threatening or less severe asthmatic episodes in certain susceptible people. The overall prevalence of sulfite sensitivity in the general population is unknown and probably low. Sulfite sensitivity is seen more frequently in asthmatic than in nonasthmatic people.

Corticosteroids may exacerbate systemic fungal infections and therefore should not be used in the presence of such infections unless they are needed to control drug reactions due to amphotericin B. Moreover, there have been cases reported in which concomitant use of amphotericin B and hydrocortisone was followed by cardiac enlargement and congestive failure.

In patients on corticosteroid therapy subjected to any unusual stress, increased dosage of rapidly acting corticosteroids before, during, and after the stressful situation is indicated.

Drug-induced secondary adrenocortical insufficiency may result from too rapid withdrawal of corticosteroids and may be minimized by gradual reduction of dosage. This type of relative insufficiency may persist for months after discontinuation of therapy; therefore, in any situation of stress occurring during that period, hormone therapy should be reinstituted. If the patient is receiving steroids already, dosage may have to be increased. Since mineralocorticoid secretion may be impaired, salt and/or a mineralocorticoid should be administered concurrently.

Corticosteroids may mask some signs of infection, and new infections may appear during their use. There may be decreased resistance and inability to localize infection when corticosteroids are used. Moreover, corticosteroids may affect the nitroblue-tetrazolium test for bacterial infection and produce false negative results.

In cerebral malaria, a double-blind trial has shown that the use of corticosteroids is associated with prolongation of coma and a higher incidence of pneumonia and gastrointestinal bleeding.

Corticosteroids may activate latent amebiasis. Therefore, it is recommended that latent or active amebiasis be ruled out before initiating corticosteroid therapy in any patient who has spent time in the tropics or any patient with unexplained diarrhea.

Prolonged use of corticosteroids may produce posterior subcapsular cataracts, glaucoma with possible damage to the optic nerves, and may enhance the establishment of secondary ocular infections due to fungi or viruses.

Usage in pregnancy. Since adequate human reproduction studies have not been done with corticosteroids, use of these drugs in pregnancy or in women of childbearing potential requires that the anticipated benefits be weighed against the possible hazards to the mother and embryo or fetus. Infants born of mothers who have received substantial doses of corticosteroids during pregnancy should be carefully observed for signs of hypoadrenalism.

Corticosteroids appear in breast milk and could suppress growth, interfere with endogenous corticosteroid production, or cause other unwanted effects. Mothers taking pharmacologic doses of corticosteroids should be advised not to nurse.

Average and large doses of cortisone or hydrocortisone can cause elevation of blood pressure, salt and water retention, and increased excretion of potassium. These effects are less likely to occur with the synthetic derivatives except when used in large doses. Dietary salt restriction and potassium supplementation may be necessary. All corticosteroids increase calcium excretion.

Administration of live virus vaccines, including smallpox, is contraindicated in individuals receiving immunosuppressive doses of corticosteroids. If inactivated viral or bacterial vaccines are administered to individuals receiving immunosuppressive doses of corticosteroids, the expected serum antibody response may not be obtained. However, immunization procedures may be undertaken in patients who are receiving corticosteroids as replacement therapy, e.g., for Addison's disease.

Patients who are on drugs which suppress the immune system are more susceptible to infections than healthy individuals. Chickenpox and measles, for example, can have a more serious or even fatal course in non-immune children or adults on corticosteroids. In such children or adults who have not had these diseases, particular care should be taken to avoid exposure. The risk of developing a disseminated infection varies among individuals and can be related to the dose, route and duration of corticosteroid administration as well as to the underlying disease. If exposed to chickenpox, prophylaxis with varicella zoster immune globulin (VZIG) may be indicated. If chickenpox develops, treatment with antiviral agents may be considered. If exposed to measles, prophylaxis with immune globulin (IG) may be indicated. (See the respective package inserts for VZIG and IG for complete prescribing information.)

Similarly, corticosteroids should be used with great care in patients with known or suspected Strongyloides (threadworm) infestation. In such patients, corticosteroid-induced immunosuppression may lead to Strongyloides hyperinfection and dissemination with widespread larval migration, often accompanied by severe enterocolitis and potentially fatal gram-negative septicemia.

The use of HYDROCORTONE Phosphate injection in active tuberculosis should be restricted to those cases of fulminating or disseminated tuberculosis in which the corticosteroid is used for the management of the disease in conjunction with an appropriate antituberculous regimen.

If corticosteroids are indicated in patients with latent tuberculosis or tuberculin reactivity, close observation is necessary as reactivation of the disease may occur. During prolonged corticosteroid therapy, these patients should receive chemoprophylaxis.

Literature reports suggest an apparent association between use of corticosteroids and left ventricular free wall rupture after a recent myocardial infarction; therefore, therapy with corticosteroids should be used with great caution in these patients.

PRECAUTIONS

This product, like many other steroid formulations, is sensitive to heat. Therefore, it should not be autoclaved when it is desirable to sterilize the exterior of the vial.

Following prolonged therapy, withdrawal of corticosteroids may result in symptoms of the corticosteroid withdrawal syndrome including fever, myalgia, arthralgia, and malaise. This may occur in patients even without evidence of adrenal insufficiency.

There is an enhanced effect of corticosteroids in patients with hypothyroidism and in those with cirrhosis.

Corticosteroids should be used cautiously in patients with ocular herpes simplex for fear of corneal perforation.

The lowest possible dose of corticosteroid should be used to control the condition under treatment, and when reduction in dosage is possible, the reduction must be gradual.

Psychic derangements may appear when corticosteroids are used, ranging from euphoria, insomnia, mood swings, personality changes, and severe depression to frank psychotic manifestations. Also, existing emotional instability or psychotic tendencies may be aggravated by corticosteroids.

Aspirin should be used cautiously in conjunction with corticosteroids in hypoprothrombinemia.

Steroids should be used with caution in nonspecific ulcerative colitis, if there is a probability of impending perforation, abscess, or other pyogenic infection, also in diverticulitis, fresh intestinal anastomoses, active or latent peptic ulcer, renal insufficiency, hypertension, osteoporosis, and myasthenia gravis. Signs of peritoneal irritation following gastrointestinal perforation in patients receiving large doses of corticosteroids may be minimal or absent. Fat embolism has been reported as a possible complication of hypercortisonism.

When large doses are given, some authorities advise that antacids be administered between meals to help to prevent peptic ulcer.

Growth and development of infants and children on prolonged corticosteroid therapy should be carefully followed.

Steroids may increase or decrease motility and number of spermatozoa in some patients.

Phenytoin, phenobarbital, ephedrine, and rifampin may enhance the metabolic clearance of corticosteroids, resulting in decreased blood levels and lessened physiologic activity, thus requiring adjustment in corticosteroid dosage.

The prothrombin time should be checked frequently in patients who are receiving corticosteroids and coumarin anticoagulants at the same time because of reports that corticosteroids have altered the response to these anticoagulants. Studies have shown that the usual effect produced by adding corticosteroids is inhibition of response to coumarins, although there have been some conflicting reports of potentiation not substantiated by studies.

When corticosteroids are administered concomitantly with potassium-depleting diuretics, patients should be observed closely for development of hypokalemia.

Injection of a steroid into an infected site is to be avoided. The slower rate of absorption by intramuscular administration should be recognized.

Information for Patients
Susceptible patients who are on immunosuppressant doses of corticosteroids should be warned to avoid exposure to chickenpox or measles. Patients should also be advised that if they are exposed, medical advice should be sought without delay.

ADVERSE REACTIONS

Fluid and electrolyte disturbances
Sodium retention
Fluid retention
Congestive heart failure in susceptible patients
Potassium loss
Hypokalemic alkalosis
Hypertension

Musculoskeletal
Muscle weakness
Steroid myopathy
Loss of muscle mass
Osteoporosis
Vertebral compression fractures
Aseptic necrosis of femoral and humeral heads
Pathologic fracture of long bones
Tendon rupture

Gastrointestinal
Peptic ulcer with possible subsequent perforation and hemorrhage
Perforation of the small and large bowel, particularly in patients with inflammatory bowel disease
Pancreatitis
Abdominal distention
Ulcerative esophagitis

Dermatologic
Impaired wound healing
Thin fragile skin

Petechiae and ecchymoses
Erythema
Increased sweating
May suppress reactions to skin tests
Burning or tingling, especially in the perineal area (after I.V. injection)
Other cutaneous reactions, such as allergic dermatitis, urticaria, angioneurotic edema

Neurologic
Convulsions
Increased intracranial pressure with papilledema (pseudotumor cerebri) usually after treatment
Vertigo
Headache
Psychic disturbances

Endocrine
Menstrual irregularities
Development of cushingoid state
Suppression of growth in children
Secondary adrenocortical and pituitary unresponsiveness, particularly in times of stress, as in trauma, surgery, or illness
Decreased carbohydrate tolerance
Manifestations of latent diabetes mellitus
Increased requirements for insulin or oral hypoglycemic agents in diabetics
Hirsutism

Ophthalmic
Posterior subcapsular cataracts
Increased intraocular pressure
Glaucoma
Exophthalmos

Metabolic
Negative nitrogen balance due to protein catabolism

Cardiovascular
Myocardial rupture following recent myocardial infarction (see WARNINGS).

Other
Anaphylactoid or hypersensitivity reactions
Thromboembolism
Weight gain
Increased appetite
Nausea
Malaise

The following *additional* adverse reactions are related to parenteral corticosteroid therapy:
Rare instances of blindness associated with intralesional therapy around the face and head
Hyperpigmentation or hypopigmentation
Subcutaneous and cutaneous atrophy
Sterile abscess

OVERDOSAGE

Reports of acute toxicity and/or death following overdosage of glucocorticoids are rare. In the event of overdosage, no specific antidote is available; treatment is supportive and symptomatic.
The intraperitoneal LD_{50} of hydrocortisone in female mice was 1740 mg/kg.

DOSAGE AND ADMINISTRATION

For intravenous, intramuscular, and subcutaneous injection. For single dose use only. Maintenance of sterility cannot be assured when used as a multiple dose vial.
HYDROCORTONE Phosphate injection can be given directly from the vial, or it can be added to Sodium Chloride Injection or Dextrose Injection and administered by intravenous drip.
Benzyl alcohol as a preservative has been associated with toxicity in premature infants. Solutions used for intravenous administration or further dilution of this product should be preservative-free when used in the neonate, especially the premature infant.
When it is mixed with an infusion solution, sterile precautions should be observed. Since infusion solutions generally do not contain preservatives, mixtures should be used within 24 hours.
DOSAGE REQUIREMENTS ARE VARIABLE AND MUST BE INDIVIDUALIZED ON THE BASIS OF THE DISEASE AND THE RESPONSE OF THE PATIENT.
The initial dosage varies from 15 to 240 mg a day depending on the disease being treated. In less severe diseases doses lower than 15 mg may suffice, while in severe diseases doses higher than 240 mg may be required. Usually the parenteral dosage ranges are one-third to one-half the oral dose given every 12 hours. However, in certain overwhelming, acute, life-threatening situations, administration in dosages exceeding the usual dosages may be justified and may be in multiples of the oral dosages.
The initial dosage should be maintained or adjusted until the patient's response is satisfactory. If a satisfactory clinical response does not occur after a reasonable period of time,

discontinue HYDROCORTONE Phosphate injection and transfer the patient to other therapy.
After a favorable initial response, the proper maintenance dosage should be determined by decreasing the initial dosage in small amounts to the lowest dosage that maintains an adequate clinical response.
Patients should be observed closely for signs that might require dosage adjustment, including changes in clinical status resulting from remissions or exacerbations of the disease, individual drug responsiveness, and the effect of stress (e.g., surgery, infection, trauma). During stress it may be necessary to increase dosage temporarily.
If the drug is to be stopped after more than a few days of treatment, it usually should be withdrawn gradually.

HOW SUPPLIED

No. 7633—Injection HYDROCORTONE Phosphate, 50 mg hydrocortisone equivalent per mL, is a clear, light yellow solution, and is supplied as follows:
NDC 0006-7633-04 in 2 mL single dose vials.
Storage
Sensitive to heat. Do not autoclave.
7498328   Issued March 1996

HYDROCORTONE® Tablets
(Hydrocortisone), U.S.P.   ℞

DESCRIPTION

Glucocorticoids are adrenocortical steroids, both naturally occurring and synthetic, which are readily absorbed from the gastrointestinal tract.
Hydrocortisone is a white to practically white, odorless, crystalline powder, very slightly soluble in water. The molecular weight is 362.47. It is designated chemically as 11β,17,21-trihydroxypregn-4-ene-3,20-dione. The empirical formula is $C_{21}H_{30}O_5$ and the structural formula is:

Hydrocortisone is believed to be the principal hormone secreted by the adrenal cortex.
HYDROCORTONE* (Hydrocortisone) tablets contain 10 mg of hydrocortisone in each tablet.
Inactive ingredients are lactose, magnesium stearate, and starch.

* Registered trademark of MERCK & CO., INC.

ACTIONS

Naturally occurring glucocorticoids (hydrocortisone and cortisone), which also have salt-retaining properties, are used as replacement therapy in adrenocortical deficiency states. They are also used for their potent anti-inflammatory effects in disorders of many organ systems.
Glucocorticoids cause profound and varied metabolic effects. In addition, they modify the body's immune responses to diverse stimuli.

INDICATIONS

1. *Endocrine Disorders*
Primary or secondary adrenocortical insufficiency (hydrocortisone or cortisone is the first choice; synthetic analogs may be used in conjunction with mineralocorticoids where applicable; in infancy mineralocorticoid supplementation is of particular importance)
Congenital adrenal hyperplasia
Nonsuppurative thyroiditis
Hypercalcemia associated with cancer
2. *Rheumatic Disorders*
As adjunctive therapy for short-term administration (to tide the patient over an acute episode or exacerbation) in:
Psoriatic arthritis
Rheumatoid arthritis, including juvenile rheumatoid arthritis (selected cases may require low-dose maintenance therapy)
Ankylosing spondylitis
Acute and subacute bursitis
Acute nonspecific tenosynovitis
Acute gouty arthritis
Post-traumatic osteoarthritis

Synovitis of osteoarthritis
Epicondylitis
3. *Collagen Diseases*
During an exacerbation or as maintenance therapy in selected cases of—
Systemic lupus erythematosus
Acute rheumatic carditis
Systemic dermatomyositis (polymyositis)
4. *Dermatologic Diseases*
Pemphigus
Bullous dermatitis herpetiformis
Severe erythema multiforme (Stevens-Johnson syndrome)
Exfoliative dermatitis
Mycosis fungoides
Severe psoriasis
Severe seborrheic dermatitis
5. *Allergic States*
Control of severe or incapacitating allergic conditions intractable to adequate trials of conventional treatment:
Seasonal or perennial allergic rhinitis
Bronchial asthma
Contact dermatitis
Atopic dermatitis
Serum sickness
Drug hypersensitivity reactions
6. *Ophthalmic Diseases*
Severe acute and chronic allergic and inflammatory processes involving the eye and its adnexa, such as—
Allergic conjunctivitis
Keratitis
Allergic corneal marginal ulcers
Herpes zoster ophthalmicus
Iritis and iridocyclitis
Chorioretinitis
Anterior segment inflammation
Diffuse posterior uveitis and choroiditis
Optic neuritis
Sympathetic ophthalmia
7. *Respiratory Diseases*
Symptomatic sarcoidosis
Loeffler's syndrome not manageable by other means
Berylliosis
Fulminating or disseminated pulmonary tuberculosis when used concurrently with appropriate antituberculous chemotherapy
Aspiration pneumonitis
8. *Hematologic Disorders*
Idiopathic thrombocytopenic purpura in adults
Secondary thrombocytopenia in adults
Acquired (autoimmune) hemolytic anemia
Erythroblastopenia (RBC anemia)
Congenital (erythroid) hypoplastic anemia
9. *Neoplastic Diseases*
For palliative management of:
Leukemias and lymphomas in adults
Acute leukemia of childhood
10. *Edematous States*
To induce a diuresis or remission of proteinuria in the nephrotic syndrome, without uremia, of the idiopathic type or that due to lupus erythematosus
11. *Gastrointestinal Diseases*
To tide the patient over a critical period of the disease in:
Ulcerative colitis
Regional enteritis
12. *Miscellaneous*
Tuberculous meningitis with subarachnoid block or impending block when used concurrently with appropriate antituberculous chemotherapy
Trichinosis with neurologic or myocardial involvement

CONTRAINDICATIONS

Systemic fungal infections
Hypersensitivity to this product

WARNINGS

In patients on corticosteroid therapy subjected to unusual stress, increased dosage of rapidly acting corticosteroids before, during, and after the stressful situation is indicated. Drug-induced secondary adrenocortical insufficiency may result from too rapid wthdrawal of corticosteroids and may be minimized by gradual reduction of dosage. This type of relative insufficiency may persist for months after discontinuation of therapy; therefore, in any situation of stress occurring during that period, hormone therapy should be reinstituted. If the patient is receiving steroids already, dosage may have to be increased. Since mineralocorticoid secre-

Continued on next page

Merck & Co.—Cont.

tion may be impaired, salt and/or a mineralocorticoid should be administered concurrently.
Corticosteroids may mask some signs of infection, and new infections may appear during their use. There may be decreased resistance and inability to localize infection when corticosteroids are used. Moreover, corticosteroids may affect the nitroblue-tetrazolium test for bacterial infection and produce false negative results.
In cerebral malaria, a double-blind trial has shown that the use of corticosteroids is associated with prolongation of coma and a higher incidence of pneumonia and gastrointestinal bleeding.
Corticosteroids may activate latent amebiasis. Therefore, it is recommended that latent or active amebiasis be ruled out before initiating corticosteroid therapy in any patient who has spent time in the tropics or any patient with unexplained diarrhea.
Prolonged use of corticosteroids may produce posterior subcapsular cataracts, glaucoma with possible damage to the optic nerves, and may enhance the establishment of secondary ocular infections due to fungi or viruses.
Usage in pregnancy: Since adequate human reproduction studies have not been done with corticosteroids, use of these drugs in pregnancy or in women of childbearing potential requires that the anticipated benefits be weighed against the possible hazards to the mother and embryo or fetus. Infants born of mothers who have received substantial doses of corticosteroids during pregnancy should be carefully observed for signs of hypoadrenalism.
Corticosteroids appear in breast milk and could suppress growth, interfere with endogenous corticosteroid production, or cause other unwanted effects. Mothers taking pharmacologic doses of corticosteroids should be advised not to nurse.
Average and large doses of hydrocortisone or cortisone can cause elevation of blood pressure, salt and water retention, and increased excretion of potassium. These effects are less likely to occur with the synthetic derivatives except when used in large doses. Dietary salt restriction and potassium supplementation may be necessary. All corticosteroids increase calcium excretion.
Administration of live virus vaccines, including smallpox, is contraindicated in individuals receiving immunosuppressive doses of corticosteroids. If inactivated viral or bacterial vaccines are administered to individuals receiving immunosuppressive doses of corticosteroids, the expected serum antibody response may not be obtained. However, immunization procedures may be undertaken in patients who are receiving corticosteroids as replacement therapy, e.g., for Addison's disease.
Patients who are on drugs which suppress the immune system are more susceptible to infections than healthy individuals. Chickenpox and measles, for example, can have a more serious or even fatal course in non-immune children or adults on corticosteroids. In such children or adults who have not had these diseases, particular care should be taken to avoid exposure. The risk of developing a disseminated infection varies among individuals and can be related to the dose, route and duration of corticosteroid administration as well as to the underlying disease. If exposed to chickenpox, prophylaxis with varicella zoster immune globulin (VZIG) may be indicated. If chickenpox develops, treatment with antiviral agents may be considered. If exposed to measles, prophylaxis with immune globulin (IG) may be indicated. (See the respective package inserts for VZIG and IG for complete prescribing information.)
Similarly, corticosteroids should be used with great care in patients with known or suspected Strongyloides (threadworm) infestation. In such patients, corticosteroid-induced immunosuppression may lead to Strongyloides hyperinfection and dissemination with widespread larval migration, often accompanied by severe enterocolitis and potentially fatal gram-negative septicemia.
The use of HYDROCORTONE tablets in active tuberculosis should be restricted to those cases of fulminating or disseminated tuberculosis in which the corticosteroid is used for the management of the disease in conjunction with an appropriate antituberculous regimen.
If corticosteroids are indicated in patients with latent tuberculosis or tuberculin reactivity, close observation is necessary as reactivation of the disease may occur. During prolonged corticosteroid therapy, these patients should receive chemoprophylaxis.
Literature reports suggest an apparent association between use of corticosteroids and left ventricular free wall rupture after a recent myocardial infarction; therefore, therapy with corticosteroids should be used with great caution in these patients.

PRECAUTIONS

Following prolonged therapy, withdrawal of corticosteroids may result in symptoms of the corticosteroid withdrawal syndrome including fever, myalgia, arthralgia, and malaise. This may occur in patients even without evidence of adrenal insufficiency.
There is an enhanced effect of corticosteroids in patients with hypothyroidism and in those with cirrhosis.
Corticosteroids should be used cautiously in patients with ocular herpes simplex because of possible corneal perforation.
The lowest possible dose of corticosteroid should be used to control the condition under treatment, and when reduction in dosage is possible, the reduction should be gradual.
Psychic derangements may appear when corticosteroids are used, ranging from euphoria, insomnia, mood swings, personality changes, and severe depression, to frank psychotic manifestations. Also, existing emotional instability or psychotic tendencies may be aggravated by corticosteroids.
Aspirin should be used cautiously in conjunction with corticosteroids in hypoprothrombinemia.
Steroids should be used with caution in nonspecific ulcerative colitis, if there is a probability of impending perforation, abscess, or other pyogenic infection, diverticulitis, fresh intestinal anastomoses, active or latent peptic ulcer, renal insufficiency, hypertension, osteoporosis, and myasthenia gravis. Signs of peritoneal irritation following gastrointestinal perforation in patients receiving large doses of corticosteroids may be minimal or absent. Fat embolism has been reported as a possible complication of hypercortisonism.
When large doses are given, some authorities advise that corticosteroids be taken with meals and antacids taken between meals to help to prevent peptic ulcer.
Growth and development of infants and children on prolonged corticosteroid therapy should be carefully observed.
Steroids may increase or decrease motility and number of spermatozoa in some patients.
Phenytoin, phenobarbital, ephedrine, and rifampin may enhance the metabolic clearance of corticosteroids, resulting in decreased blood levels and lessened physiologic activity, thus requiring adjustment in corticosteroid dosage.
The prothrombin time should be checked frequently in patients who are receiving corticosteroids and coumarin anticoagulants at the same time because of reports that corticosteroids have altered the response to these anticoagulants. Studies have shown that the usual effect produced by adding corticosteroids is inhibition of response to coumarins, although there have been some conflicting reports of potentiation not substantiated by studies.
When corticosteroids are administered concomitantly with potassium-depleting diuretics, patients should be observed closely for development of hypokalemia.
Information for Patients
Susceptible patients who are on immunosuppressant doses of corticosteroids should be warned to avoid exposure to chickenpox or measles. Patients should also be advised that if they are exposed, medical advice should be sought without delay.

ADVERSE REACTIONS

Fluid and Electrolyte Disturbances
- Sodium retention
- Fluid retention
- Congestive heart failure in susceptible patients
- Potassium loss
- Hypokalemic alkalosis
- Hypertension

Musculoskeletal
- Muscle weakness
- Steroid myopathy
- Loss of muscle mass
- Osteoporosis
- Vertebral compression fractures
- Aseptic necrosis of femoral and humeral heads
- Pathologic fracture of long bones
- Tendon rupture

Gastrointestinal
- Peptic ulcer with possible perforation and hemorrhage
- Perforation of the small and large bowel, particularly in patients with inflammatory bowel disease
- Pancreatitis
- Abdominal distention
- Ulcerative esophagitis

Dermatologic
- Impaired wound healing
- Thin fragile skin
- Petechiae and ecchymoses
- Erythema
- Increased sweating
- May suppress reactions to skin tests
- Other cutaneous reactions, such as allergic dermatitis, urticaria, angioneurotic edema

Neurologic
- Convulsions
- Increased intracranial pressure with papilledema (pseudotumor cerebri) usually after treatment
- Vertigo
- Headache
- Psychic disturbances

Endocrine
- Menstrual irregularities
- Development of cushingoid state
- Suppression of growth in children
- Secondary adrenocortical and pituitary unresponsiveness, particularly in times of stress, as in trauma, surgery, or illness
- Decreased carbohydrate tolerance
- Manifestations of latent diabetes mellitus
- Increased requirements for insulin or oral hypoglycemic agents in diabetics
- Hirsutism

Ophthalmic
- Posterior subcapsular cataracts
- Increased intraocular pressure
- Glaucoma
- Exophthalmos

Metabolic
- Negative nitrogen balance due to protein catabolism

Cardiovascular
- Myocardial rupture following recent myocardial infarction (see WARNINGS).

Other
- Hypersensitivity
- Thromboembolism
- Weight gain
- Increased appetite
- Nausea
- Malaise

OVERDOSAGE

Reports of acute toxicity and/or death following overdosage of glucocorticoids are rare. In the event of overdosage, no specific antidote is available; treatment is supportive and symptomatic.
The intraperitoneal LD_{50} of hydrocortisone in female mice was 1740 mg/kg.

DOSAGE AND ADMINISTRATION

For oral administration
DOSAGE REQUIREMENTS ARE VARIABLE AND MUST BE INDIVIDUALIZED ON THE BASIS OF THE DISEASE AND THE RESPONSE OF THE PATIENT.
The initial dosage varies from 20 to 240 mg a day depending on the disease being treated. In less severe diseases doses lower than 20 mg may suffice, while in severe diseases doses higher than 240 mg may be required. The initial dosage should be maintained or adjusted until the patient's response is satisfactory. If satisfactory clinical response does not occur after a reasonable period of time, discontinue HYDROCORTONE tablets and transfer the patient to other therapy.
After a favorable initial response, the proper maintenance dosage should be determined by decreasing the initial dosage in small amounts to the lowest dosage that maintains an adequate clinical response.
Patients should be observed closely for signs that might require dosage adjustment, including changes in clinical status resulting from remissions or exacerbations of the disease, individual drug responsiveness, and the effect of stress (e.g, surgery, infection, trauma). During stress it may be necessary to increase dosage temporarily.
If the drug is to be stopped after more than a few days of treatment, it usually should be withdrawn gradually.

HOW SUPPLIED

No. 7604—Tablets HYDROCORTONE, 10 mg each, are white, oval shaped compressed tablets, scored on one side, coded MSD 619, and are supplied as follows:
NDC 0006-0619-68 in bottles of 100.

Shown in Product Identification Guide, page 324
7920527 Issued October 1995

HydroDIURIL® Tablets (Hydrochlorothiazide), U.S.P. ℞

DESCRIPTION

HydroDIURIL* (Hydrochlorothiazide) is a diuretic and antihypertensive. It is the 3,4-dihydro derivative of chlorothiazide. Its chemical name is 6-chloro-3,4-dihydro-2*H*-1,2,4-benzothiadiazine-7-sulfonamide 1,1-dioxide. Its empirical formula is $C_7H_8ClN_3O_4S_2$ and its structural formula is:

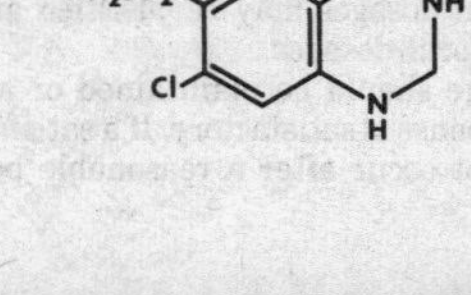

It is a white, or practically white, crystalline powder with a molecular weight of 297.72, which is slightly soluble in water, but freely soluble in sodium hydroxide solution. HydroDIURIL is supplied as 25 mg, 50 mg and 100 mg tablets for oral use. Each tablet contains the following inactive ingredients: calcium phosphate, FD&C Yellow 6, gelatin, lactose, magnesium stearate, starch and talc.

---

*Registered trademark of MERCK & CO., INC.

CLINICAL PHARMACOLOGY

The mechanism of the antihypertensive effect of thiazides is unknown. HydroDIURIL does not usually affect normal blood pressure.
HydroDIURIL affects the distal renal tubular mechanism of electrolyte reabsorption. At maximal therapeutic dosage all thiazides are approximately equal in their diuretic efficacy. HydroDIURIL increases excretion of sodium and chloride in approximately equivalent amounts. Natriuresis may be accompanied by some loss of potassium and bicarbonate.
After oral use diuresis begins within 2 hours, peaks in about 4 hours and lasts about 6 to 12 hours.
Pharmacokinetics and Metabolism
HydroDIURIL is not metabolized but is eliminated rapidly by the kidney. When plasma levels have been followed for at least 24 hours, the plasma half-life has been observed to vary between 5.6 and 14.8 hours. At least 61 percent of the oral dose is eliminated unchanged within 24 hours. Hydrochlorothiazide crosses the placental but not the blood-brain barrier and is excreted in breast milk.

INDICATIONS AND USAGE

HydroDIURIL is indicated as adjunctive therapy in edema associated with congestive heart failure, hepatic cirrhosis, and corticosteroid and estrogen therapy.
HydroDIURIL has also been found useful in edema due to various forms of renal dysfunction such as nephrotic syndrome, acute glomerulonephritis, and chronic renal failure. HydroDIURIL is indicated in the management of hypertension either as the sole therapeutic agent or to enhance the effectiveness of other antihypertensive drugs in the more severe forms of hypertension.
Use in Pregnancy. Routine use of diuretics during normal pregnancy is inappropriate and exposes mother and fetus to unnecessary hazard. Diuretics do not prevent development of toxemia of pregnancy and there is no satisfactory evidence that they are useful in the treatment of toxemia.
Edema during pregnancy may arise from pathologic causes or from the physiologic and mechanical consequences of pregnancy. Thiazides are indicated in pregnancy when edema is due to pathologic causes, just as they are in the absence of pregnancy (see PRECAUTIONS, *Pregnancy*). Dependent edema in pregnancy, resulting from restriction of venous return by the gravid uterus, is properly treated through elevation of the lower extremities and use of support stockings. Use of diuretics to lower intravascular volume in this instance is illogical and unnecessary. During normal pregnancy there is hypervolemia which is not harmful to the fetus or the mother in the absence of cardiovascular disease. However, it may be associated with edema, rarely generalized edema. If such edema causes discomfort, increased recumbency will often provide relief. Rarely this edema may cause extreme discomfort which is not relieved by rest. In these instances, a short course of diuretic therapy may provide relief and be appropriate.

CONTRAINDICATIONS

Anuria.
Hypersensitivity to this product or to other sulfonamide-derived drugs.

WARNINGS

Use with caution in severe renal disease. In patients with renal disease, thiazides may precipitate azotemia. Cumulative effects of the drug may develop in patients with impaired renal function.
Thiazides should be used with caution in patients with impaired hepatic function or progressive liver disease, since minor alterations of fluid and electrolyte balance may precipitate hepatic coma.
Thiazides may add to or potentiate the action of other antihypertensive drugs.
Sensitivity reactions may occur in patients with or without a history of allergy or bronchial asthma.
The possibility of exacerbation or activation of systemic lupus erythematosus has been reported.
Lithium generally should not be given with diuretics (see PRECAUTIONS, *Drug Interactions*).

PRECAUTIONS

General
All patients receiving diuretic therapy should be observed for evidence of fluid or electrolyte imbalance: namely, hyponatremia, hypochloremic alkalosis, and hypokalemia. Serum and urine electrolyte determinations are particularly important when the patient is vomiting excessively or receiving parenteral fluids. Warning signs or symptoms of fluid and electrolyte imbalance, irrespective of cause, include dryness of mouth, thirst, weakness, lethargy, drowsiness, restlessness, confusion, seizures, muscle pains or cramps, muscular fatigue, hypotension, oliguria, tachycardia, and gastrointestinal disturbances such as nausea and vomiting.
Hypokalemia may develop, especially with brisk diuresis, when severe cirrhosis is present or after prolonged therapy. Interference with adequate oral electrolyte intake will also contribute to hypokalemia. Hypokalemia may cause cardiac arrhythmia and may also sensitize or exaggerate the response of the heart to the toxic effects of digitalis (e.g., increased ventricular irritability). Hypokalemia may be avoided or treated by use of potassium sparing diuretics or potassium supplements such as foods with a high potassium content.
Although any chloride deficit is generally mild and usually does not require specific treatment except under extraordinary circumstances (as in liver disease or renal disease), chloride replacement may be required in the treatment of metabolic alkalosis.
Dilutional hyponatremia may occur in edematous patients in hot weather; appropriate therapy is water restriction, rather than administration of salt, except in rare instances when the hyponatremia is life threatening. In actual salt depletion, appropriate replacement is the therapy of choice.
Hyperuricemia may occur or acute gout may be precipitated in certain patients receiving thiazides.
In diabetic patients dosage adjustments of insulin or oral hypoglycemic agents may be required. Hyperglycemia may occur with thiazide diuretics. Thus latent diabetes mellitus may become manifest during thiazide therapy.
The antihypertensive effects of the drug may be enhanced in the post-sympathectomy patient.
If progressive renal impairment becomes evident, consider withholding or discontinuing diuretic therapy.
Thiazides have been shown to increase the urinary excretion of magnesium; this may result in hypomagnesemia.
Thiazides may decrease urinary calcium excretion. Thiazides may cause intermittent and slight elevation of serum calcium in the absence of known disorders of calcium metabolism. Marked hypercalcemia may be evidence of hidden hyperparathyroidism. Thiazides should be discontinued before carrying out tests for parathyroid function.
Increases in cholesterol and triglyceride levels may be associated with thiazide diuretic therapy.
Laboratory Tests
Periodic determination of serum electrolytes to detect possible electrolyte imbalance should be done at appropriate intervals.
Drug Interactions
When given concurrently the following drugs may interact with thiazide diuretics.
Alcohol, barbiturates, or narcotics —potentiation of orthostatic hypotension may occur.
Antidiabetic drugs —(oral agents and insulin)—dosage adjustment of the antidiabetic drug may be required.
Other antihypertensive drugs —additive effect or potentiation.
Cholestyramine and colestipol resins—Absorption of hydrochlorothiazide is impaired in the presence of anionic exchange resins. Single doses of either cholestyramine or colestipol resins bind the hydrochlorothiazide and reduce its absorption from the gastrointestinal tract by up to 85 and 43 percent, respectively.
Corticosteroids, ACTH —intensified electrolyte depletion, particularly hypokalemia.
Pressor amines (e.g., norepinephrine) —possible decreased response to pressor amines but not sufficient to preclude their use.
Skeletal muscle relaxants, nondepolarizing (e.g., tubocurarine) —possible increased responsiveness to the muscle relaxant.
Lithium —generally should not be given with diuretics. Diuretic agents reduce the renal clearance of lithium and add a high risk of lithium toxicity. Refer to the package insert for lithium preparations before use of such preparations with HydroDIURIL.
Non-steroidal Anti-inflammatory Drugs —In some patients, the administration of a non-steroidal anti-inflammatory agent can reduce the diuretic, natriuretic, and antihypertensive effects of loop, potassium-sparing and thiazide diuretics. Therefore, when HydroDIURIL and non-steroidal anti-inflammatory agents are used concomitantly, the patient should be observed closely to determine if the desired effect of the diuretic is obtained.
Drug/Laboratory Test Interactions
Thiazides should be discontinued before carrying out tests for parathyroid function (see PRECAUTIONS, *General*).
Carcinogenesis, Mutagenesis, Impairment of Fertility
Two-year feeding studies in mice and rats conducted under the auspices of the National Toxicology Program (NTP) uncovered no evidence of a carcinogenic potential of hydrochlorothiazide in female mice (at doses of up to approximately 600 mg/kg/day) or in male and female rats (at doses of up to approximately 100 mg/kg/day). The NTP, however, found equivocal evidence for hepatocarcinogenicity in male mice. Hydrochlorothiazide was not genotoxic *in vitro* in the Ames mutagenicity assay of *Salmonella typhimurium* strains TA 98, TA 100, TA 1535, TA 1537, and TA 1538 and in the Chinese Hamster Ovary (CHO) test for chromosomal aberrations, or *in vivo* in assays using mouse germinal cell chromosomes, Chinese hamster bone marrow chromosomes, and the *Drosophila* sex-linked recessive lethal trait gene. Positive test results were obtained only in the *in vitro* CHO Sister Chromatid Exchange (clastogenicity) and in the Mouse Lymphoma Cell (mutagenicity) assays, using concentrations of hydrochlorothiazide from 43 to 1300 μg/mL, and in the *Aspergillus nidulans* non-disjunction assay at an unspecified concentration.
Hydrochlorothiazide had no adverse effects on the fertility of mice and rats of either sex in studies wherein these species were exposed, via their diet, to doses of up to 100 and 4 mg/kg, respectively, prior to conception and throughout gestation.
Pregnancy
Teratogenic Effects—Pregnancy Category B: Studies in which hydrochlorothiazide was orally administered to pregnant mice and rats during their respective periods of major organogenesis at doses up to 3000 and 1000 mg hydrochlorothiazide/kg, respectively, provided no evidence of harm to the fetus.
There are, however, no adequate and well-controlled studies in pregnant women. Because animal reproduction studies are not always predictice of human response, this drug should be used during pregnancy only if clearly needed.
Nonteratogenic Effects: Thiazides cross the placental barrier and appear in cord blood. There is a risk of fetal or neonatal jaundice, thrombocytopenia, and possibly other adverse reactions that have occurred in adults.
Nursing Mothers
Thiazides are excreted in breast milk. Because of the potential for serious adverse reactions in nursing infants, a decision should be made whether to discontinue nursing or to discontinue hydrochlorothiazide, taking into account the importance of the drug to the mother.
Pediatric Use
Safety and effectiveness in children have not been established.

ADVERSE REACTIONS

The following adverse reactions have been reported and, within each category, are listed in order of decreasing severity.
Body as a Whole: Weakness.
Cardiovascular: Hypotension including orthostatic hypotension (may be aggravated by alcohol, barbiturates, narcotics or antihypertensive drugs).
Digestive: Pancreatitis, jaundice (intrahepatic cholestatic jaundice), diarrhea, vomiting, sialadenitis, cramping, constipation, gastric irritation, nausea, anorexia.
Hematologic: Aplastic anemia, agranulocytosis, leukopenia, hemolytic anemia, thrombocytopenia.
Hypersensitivity: Anaphylactic reactions, necrotizing angiitis (vasculitis and cutaneous vasculitis), respiratory distress including pneumonitis and pulmonary edema, photosensitivity, fever, urticaria, rash, purpura.
Metabolic: Electrolyte imbalance (see PRECAUTIONS), hyperglycemia, glycosuria, hyperuricemia.
Musculoskeletal: Muscle spasm.
Nervous System/Psychiatric: Vertigo, paresthesias, dizziness, headache, restlessness.
Renal: Renal failure, renal dysfunction, interstitial nephritis. (See WARNINGS.)
Skin: Erythema multiforme including Stevens-Johnson syndrome, exfoliative dermatitis including toxic epidermal necrolysis, alopecia.
Special Senses: Transient blurred vision, xanthopsia.
Urogenital: Impotence.
Whenever adverse reactions are moderate or severe, thiazide dosage should be reduced or therapy withdrawn.

Continued on next page

Information on the Merck & Co., Inc. products listed on these pages is the full prescribing information from product circulars in use September 30, 1996.

Merck & Co.—Cont.

OVERDOSAGE

The most common signs and symptoms observed are those caused by electrolyte depletion (hypokalemia, hypochloremia, hyponatremia) and dehydration resulting from excessive diuresis. If digitalis has also been administered, hypokalemia may accentuate cardiac arrhythmias.

In the event of overdosage, symptomatic and supportive measures should be employed. Emesis should be induced or gastric lavage performed. Correct dehydration, electrolyte imbalance, hepatic coma and hypotension by established procedures. If required, give oxygen or artificial respiration for respiratory impairment. The degree to which hydrochlorothiazide is removed by hemodialysis has not been established.

The oral LD$_{50}$ of hydrochlorothiazide is greater than 10 g/kg in the mouse and rat.

DOSAGE AND ADMINISTRATION

Therapy should be individualized according to patient response. Use the smallest dosage necessary to achieve the required response.

Adults
For Edema
The usual adult dosage is 25 to 100 mg daily as a single or divided dose. Many patients with edema respond to intermittent therapy, i.e., administration on alternate days or on three to five days each week. With an intermittent schedule, excessive response and the resulting undesirable electrolyte imbalance are less likely to occur.
For Control of Hypertension
The usual initial dose in adults is 25 mg daily given as a single dose. The dose may be increased to 50 mg daily, given as a single or two divided doses. Doses above 50 mg are often associated with marked reductions in serum potassium (see also PRECAUTIONS).
Patients usually do not require doses in excess of 50 mg of hydrochlorothiazide daily when used concomitantly with other antihypertensive agents.

Infants and Children
For Diuresis and For Control of Hypertension
The usual pediatric dosage is 0.5 to 1 mg per pound (1 to 2 mg/kg) per day in single or two divided doses, not to exceed 37.5 mg per day in infants up to 2 years of age or 100 mg per day in children 2 to 12 years of age. In infants less than 6 months of age, doses up to 1.5 mg per pound (3 mg/kg) per day in two divided doses may be required.

HOW SUPPLIED

No. 3263—Tablets HydroDIURIL, 25 mg, are peach-colored, round, scored, compressed tablets, coded MSD 42. They are supplied as follows:
NDC 0006-0042-68 bottles of 100
NDC 0006-0042-82 bottles of 1000.
Shown in Product Identification Guide, page 324
No. 3264—Tablets HydroDIURIL, 50 mg, are peach-colored, round, scored, compressed tablets, coded MSD 105. They are supplied as follows:
NDC 0006-0105-68 bottles of 100
NDC 0006-0105-82 bottles of 1000
NDC 0006-0105-86 bottles of 5000.
Shown in Product Identification Guide, page 324
No. 3340—Tablets HydroDIURIL, 100 mg, are peach-colored, round, scored, compressed tablets, coded MSD 410. They are supplied as follows:
NDC 0006-0410-68 bottles of 100.
Shown in Product Identification Guide, page 324
Storage
Keep container tightly closed. Protect from light, moisture, freezing. −20℃ (−4℉) and store at room temperature, 15–30℃ (59–86℉).
      7897449   Issued February 1994
COPYRIGHT © MERCK & CO., INC., 1986
All rights reserved

HYDROPRES® Tablets   ℞
(Reserpine-Hydrochlorothiazide), U.S.P.

WARNING

This fixed combination drug is not indicated for initial therapy of hypertension. Hypertension requires therapy titrated to the individual patient. If the fixed combination represents the dosage so determined, its use may be more convenient in patient management. The treatment of hypertension is not static, but must be re-evaluated as conditions in each patient warrant.

DESCRIPTION

HYDROPRES* (Reserpine-Hydrochlorothiazide) combines two antihypertensives: HydroDIURIL* (Hydrochlorothiazide) and reserpine.
Hydrochlorothiazide
Hydrochlorothiazide is a diuretic and antihypertensive. It is the 3,4-dihydro derivative of chlorothiazide. Its chemical name is 6-chloro-3,4-dihydro-2H-1,2,4-benzothiadiazine-7-sulfonamide 1,1-dioxide. Its empirical formula is $C_7H_8ClN_3O_4S_2$ and its structural formula is:

Hydrochlorothiazide is a white, or practically white, crystalline powder with a molecular weight of 297.72, which is slightly soluble in water, but freely soluble in sodium hydroxide solution.
Reserpine
The chemical name for reserpine is (11, 17α-dimethoxy -18β-[(3,4,5-trimethoxybenzoyl) oxy]-3β, 20α-yohimban-16β-carboxylic acid methyl ester). It is a crystalline alkaloid derived from Rauwolfia serpentina. Its empirical formula is $C_{33}H_{40}N_2O_9$ and its structural formula is:

Reserpine is a white or pale buff to slightly yellowish, odorless, crystalline powder with a molecular weight of 608.69, is insoluble in water, and freely soluble in glacial acetic acid.
HYDROPRES is supplied as tablets in two strengths for oral use:
HYDROPRES 25, contains 25 mg of hydrochlorothiazide and 0.125 mg of reserpine.
HYDROPRES 50, contains 50 mg of hydrochlorothiazide and 0.125 mg of reserpine.
Each tablet contains the following inactive ingredients: calcium phosphate, D&C Yellow 10, FD&C Blue 1, FD&C Yellow 6, lactose, magnesium stearate, starch and talc.

---

*Registered trademark of MERCK & CO., INC.

CLINICAL PHARMACOLOGY

Hydrochlorothiazide
The mechanism of the antihypertensive effect of thiazides is unknown. Hydrochlorothiazide does not usually affect normal blood pressure.
Hydrochlorothiazide affects the distal renal tubular mechanism of electrolyte reabsorption. At maximal therapeutic dosage all thiazides are approximately equal in their diuretic efficacy.
Hydrochlorothiazide increases excretion of sodium and chloride in approximately equivalent amounts. Natriuresis may be accompanied by some loss of potassium and bicarbonate. After oral use, diuresis begins within 2 hours, peaks in about 4 hours and lasts about 6 to 12 hours.
Reserpine
Reserpine has antihypertensive, bradycardic, and tranquilizing properties. It lowers arterial blood pressure by depletion of catecholamines. Reserpine is beneficial in relieving anxiety, tension, and headache in the hypertensive patient. It acts at the hypothalamic level of the central nervous system to promote relaxation without hypnosis or analgesia. The sleep pattern shown by the electroencephalogram following barbiturates does not occur with this drug. In laboratory animals spontaneous activity and response to external stimuli are decreased, but confusion or difficulty of movement is not evident.
The bradycardic action of reserpine promotes relaxation and may eliminate sinus tachycardia. It is most pronounced in subjects with sinus tachycardia and usually is not prominent in persons with a normal pulse rate.
Miosis, relaxation of the nictitating membrane, ptosis, hypothermia, and increased gastrointestinal activity are noted in animals given reserpine, sometimes in subclinical doses.

None of these effects, except increased gastrointestinal activity, has been found to be clinically significant in man with therapeutic doses.
Pharmacokinetics and Metabolism
Hydrochlorothiazide
Hydrochlorothiazide is not metabolized but is eliminated rapidly by the kidney. When plasma levels have been followed for at least 24 hours, the plasma half-life has been observed to vary between 5.6 and 14.8 hours. At least 61 percent of the oral dose is eliminated unchanged within 24 hours. Hydrochlorothiazide crosses the placental but not the blood-brain barrier and is excreted in breast milk.
Reserpine
Oral reserpine is rapidly absorbed from the gastrointestinal tract. Methylreserpate and trimethoxybenzoic acid are the primary metabolites which result from the hydrolytic cleavage of reserpine. Maximal blood levels were achieved approximately 2 hours after the oral dosage of ^{3}H-reserpine to six normal volunteers; within 96 hours approximately 8 percent was excreted in urine and 62 percent in feces. Reserpine appears in human breast milk. Reserpine crosses the placental barrier in guinea pigs.

INDICATION AND USAGE

Hypertension (see box warning).

CONTRAINDICATIONS

Hydrochlorothiazide is contraindicated in anuria.
HYDROPRES is contraindicated in hypersensitivity to hydrochlorothiazide or other sulfonamide-derived drugs or to reserpine.
Electroshock therapy should not be given to patients while on reserpine, as severe and even fatal reactions have been reported with minimal convulsive electroshock dosage. After discontinuing reserpine, allow at least seven days before starting electroshock therapy.
Reserpine is contraindicated in patients:
—with active peptic ulcer
—with ulcerative colitis
—with active or a history of mental depression, especially suicidal tendencies
—on therapy with monoamine oxidase (MAO) inhibitors.

WARNINGS

Hydrochlorothiazide
Use with caution in severe renal disease. In patients with renal disease, thiazides may precipitate azotemia. Cumulative effects of the drug may develop in patients with impaired renal function.
Thiazides should be used with caution in patients with impaired hepatic function or progressive liver disease, since minor alterations of fluid and electrolyte balance may precipitate hepatic coma.
Thiazides may add to or potentiate the action of other antihypertensive drugs.
Sensitivity reactions may occur in patients with or without a history of allergy or bronchial asthma.
The possibility of exacerbation or activation of systemic lupus erythematosus has been reported.
Lithium generally should not be given with diuretics (see PRECAUTIONS, *Drug Interactions*).
Reserpine
Reserpine may cause mental depression. Recognition of depression may be difficult because this condition may often be disguised by somatic complaints (masked depression). The drug should be discontinued at first signs of depression such as despondency, early morning insomnia, loss of appetite, impotence or self depression. Drug induced depression may persist for several months after drug withdrawal and may be severe enough to result in suicide.
The occurrence of mental depression due to reserpine in doses of 0.25 mg daily or less is unusual. In any event, HYDROPRES should be discontinued at the first sign of depression.

PRECAUTIONS

General
Hydrochlorothiazide
All patients receiving diuretic therapy should be observed for evidence of fluid or electrolyte imbalance: namely, hyponatremia, hypochloremic alkalosis, and hypokalemia. Serum and urine electrolyte determinations are particularly important when the patient is vomiting excessively or receiving parenteral fluids. Warning signs or symptoms of fluid and electrolyte imbalance irrespective of cause, include dryness of mouth, thirst, weakness, lethargy, drowsiness, restlessness, confusion, seizures, muscle pains or cramps, muscular fatigue, hypotension, oliguria, tachycardia, and gastrointestinal disturbances such as nausea and vomiting. Hypokalemia may develop, especially with brisk diuresis, when severe cirrhosis is present or after prolonged therapy.

Interference with adequate oral electrolyte intake will contribute to hypokalemia. Hypokalemia may cause cardiac arrhythmia and may also sensitize or exaggerate the response of the heart to the toxic effects of digitalis (e.g., increased ventricular irritability). Hypokalemia may be avoided or treated by use of potassium sparing diuretic or potassium supplements such as foods with a high potassium content.
Although any chloride deficit is generally mild and usually does not require specific treatment except under extraordinary circumstances (as in liver disease or renal disease), chloride replacement may be required in the treatment of metabolic alkalosis.
Dilutional hyponatremia may occur in edematous patients in hot weather. Appropriate therapy is water restriction, rather than administration of salt, except in rare instances when the hyponatremia is life threatening. In actual salt depletion, appropriate replacement is the therapy of choice.
Hyperuricemia may occur or acute gout may be precipitated in certain patients receiving thiazides.
In diabetic patients dosage adjustment of insulin or oral hypoglycemic agents may be required. Hyperglycemia may occur with thiazide diuretics. Thus latent diabetes mellitus may become manifest during thiazide therapy.
The antihypertensive effect of the drug may be enhanced in the postsympathectomy patient.
If progressive renal impairment becomes evident, consider withholding or discontinuing diuretic therapy.
Thiazides have been shown to increase the urinary excretion of magnesium; this may result in hypomagnesemia.
Thiazides may decrease urinary calcium excretion. Thiazides may cause intermittent and slight elevation of serum calcium in the absence of known disorders of calcium metabolism. Marked hypercalcemia may be evidence of hidden hyperparathyroidism. Thiazides should be discontinued before carrying out tests for parathyroid function.
Increases in cholesterol and triglyceride levels may be associated with thiazide diuretic therapy.

Reserpine

Since reserpine may increase gastric secretion and motility, it should be used cautiously in patients with a history of peptic ulcer, ulcerative colitis, or other gastrointestinal disorder. This compound may precipitate biliary colic in patients with gallstones, or bronchial asthma in susceptible persons.
Reserpine may cause hypotension including orthostatic hypotension.
Anxiety or depression, as well as psychosis, may develop during reserpine therapy. If depression is present when therapy is begun, it may be aggravated. Mental depression is unusual with reserpine doses of 0.25 mg daily or less. In any case, HYDROPRES should be discontinued at the first sign of depression. Extreme caution should be used in treating patients with a history of mental depression, and the possibility of suicide should be kept in mind.
As with most antihypertensive therapy, caution should be exercised when treating hypertensive patients with renal insufficiency, since they adjust poorly to lowered blood pressure.
When two or more antihypertensives are given, the individual dosages may have to be reduced to prevent excessive drop in blood pressure. In hypertensive patients with coronary artery disease, it is important to avoid a precipitous drop in blood pressure.

Laboratory Tests

Periodic determination of serum electrolytes to detect possible electrolyte imbalance should be done at appropriate intervals.

Drug Interactions

Hydrochlorothiazide

When given concurrently the following drugs may interact with thiazide diuretics.
Alcohol, barbiturates, or narcotics—potentiation of orthostatic hypotension may occur.
Antidiabetic drugs (oral agents and insulin)—dosage adjustment of the antidiabetic drug may be required.
Other antihypertensive drugs—additive effect or potentiation.
Cholestyramine and colestipol resins—Absorption of hydrochlorothiazide is impaired in the presence of anionic exchange resins. Single doses of either cholestyramine or colestipol resins bind the hydrochlorothiazide and reduce its absorption from the gastrointestinal tract by up to 85 and 43 percent, respectively.
Corticosteroids, ACTH—intensified electrolyte depletion, particularly hypokalemia.
Pressor amines (e.g., norepinephrine)—possible decreased response to pressor amines but not sufficient to preclude their use.
Skeletal muscle relaxants, nondepolarizing (e.g., tubocurarine)—possible increased responsiveness to the muscle relaxant.
Lithium—generally should not be given with diuretics. Diuretic agents reduce the renal clearance of lithium and add a high risk of lithium toxicity. Refer to the package insert for lithium preparations before use of such preparations with HYDROPRES.
Non-steroidal Anti-inflammatory Drugs—In some patients, the administration of a non-steroidal anti-inflammatory agent can reduce the diuretic, natriuretic, and antihypertensive effects of loop, potassium-sparing and thiazide diuretics. Therefore, when HYDROPRES and non-steroidal anti-inflammatory agents are used concomitantly, the patient should be observed closely to determine if the desired effect of the diuretic is obtained.

Reserpine

In hypertensive patients on reserpine therapy significant hypotension and bradycardia may develop during surgical anesthesia. The anesthesiologist should be aware that reserpine has been taken, since it may be necessary to give vagal blocking agents parenterally to prevent or reverse hypotension and/or bradycardia.
Use reserpine cautiously with digitalis and quinidine; cardiac arrhythmias have occurred with reserpine preparations.
Barbiturates enhance the central nervous system depressant effects of reserpine.
Monoamine oxidase (MAO) inhibitors: See CONTRAINDICATIONS.

Drug/Laboratory Test Interactions

Thiazides should be discontinued before carrying out tests for parathyroid function (see PRECAUTIONS, *General*).

Carcinogenesis, Mutagenesis, Impairment of Fertility

Carcinogenicity and mutagenicity studies have not been conducted with combinations of reserpine/hydrochlorothiazide.
In a two-litter study in the rat at an oral dose of 5.0/0.25 mg/kg, the combination of hydrochlorothiazide/reserpine did not impair fertility or produce abnormalities in the fetus.

Hydrochlorothiazide

Two-year feeding studies in mice and rats conducted under the auspices of the National Toxicology Program (NTP) uncovered no evidence of a carcinogenic potential of hydrochlorothiazide in female mice (at doses of up to approximately 600 mg/kg/day) or in male and female rats (at doses of up to approximately 100 mg/kg/day). The NTP, however, found equivocal evidence for hepatocarcinogenicity in male mice.
Hydrochlorothiazide was not genotoxic *in vitro* in the Ames mutagenicity assay of *Salmonella typhimurium* strains TA 98, TA 100, TA 1535, TA 1537, and TA 1538 and in the Chinese Hamster Ovary (CHO) test for chromosomal aberrations, or *in vivo* in assays using mouse germinal cell chromosomes, Chinese hamster bone marrow chromosomes, and the *Drosophila* sex-linked recessive lethal trait gene. Positive test results were obtained only in the *in vitro* CHO Sister Chromatid Exchange (clastogenicity) and in the Mouse Lymphoma Cell (mutagenicity) assays, using concentrations of hydrochlorothiazide from 43 to 1300 μg/mL, and in the *Aspergillus nidulans* non-disjunction assay at an unspecified concentration.
Hydrochlorothiazide had no adverse effects on the fertility of mice and rats of either sex in studies wherein these species were exposed, via their diet, to doses of up to 100 and 4 mg/kg, respectively, prior to conception and throughout gestation.

Reserpine

Reserpine at a concentration of 1 to 5000 mcg/plate had no mutagenic activity against four strains of *S. typhimurium in vitro* in the Ames microbial mutagen test with or without metabolic activation. Reserpine did not induce malignant transformation of mouse fibroblasts *in vitro* at concentrations of 0.3 to 10 mcg/mL.
A few chromosomal aberrations were induced by reserpine *in vitro* in cultured mouse mammary carcinoma cells but were considered negative in this study. The drug did not produce chromosomal aberrations in human peripheral leucocyte cultures although an increase in mitotic figures occurred. One study reported chromosomal aberrations and dominant lethal mutations in mice at doses up to 10 mg/kg of reserpine in the form of a pharmaceutical preparation. Another study did not show dominant lethal mutations in mice at IP doses of 0.92 and 4.6 mg/kg of reserpine.
Reserpine did not impair fertility in a two-litter study in the rat at an oral dose of 0.025 mg/kg.
Rodent studies have shown that reserpine is an animal tumorigen, causing an increased incidence of mammary fibroadenomas in female mice, malignant tumors of the seminal vesicles in male mice, and malignant adrenal medullary tumors in male rats. These findings arose in 2 year studies in which the drug was administered in the feed at concentrations of 5 and 10 ppm—about 100 to 300 times the usual human dose. The breast neoplasms are thought to be related to reserpine's prolactin-elevating effect. Several other prolactin-elevating drugs have also been associated with an increased incidence of mammary neoplasia in rodents.
The extent to which these findings indicate a risk to humans is uncertain. Tissue culture experiments show that about one-third of human breast tumors are prolactin-dependent *in vitro*, a factor of considerable importance if the use of the drug is contemplated in a patient with previously detected breast cancer. The possibility of an increased risk of breast cancer in reserpine users has been studied extensively; however, no firm conclusion has emerged. Although a few epidemiologic studies have suggested a slightly increased risk (less than twofold in all studies except one) in women who have used reserpine, other studies of generally similar design have not confirmed this. Epidemiologic studies conducted using other drugs (neuroleptic agents) that, like reserpine, increase prolactin levels and therefore would be considered rodent mammary carcinogens, have not shown an association between chronic administration of the drug and human mammary tumorigenesis. While long-term clinical observation has not suggested such an association, the available evidence is considered too limited to be conclusive at this time. An association of reserpine intake with pheochromocytoma or tumors of the seminal vesicles has not been explored.

Pregnancy

Use of diuretics during normal pregnancy is inappropriate and exposes mother and fetus to unnecessary hazard. Diuretics do not prevent development of toxemia of pregnancy and there is no satisfactory evidence that they are useful in the treatment of toxemia.
Teratogenic Effects—Pregnancy Category C: HYDROPRES may cause fetal harm when given to a pregnant woman. There are no adequate and well-controlled studies with HYDROPRES or other combinations of reserpine/hydrochlorothiazide in animals or pregnant women. HYDROPRES should be used during pregnancy only if the potential benefit justifies the potential risk to the fetus.
Reserpine: Reproduction studies in rats have shown that reserpine is teratogenic at doses of 1–2 mg/kg (125 to 250 times the maximum recommended human dose) IM or IP given early in pregnancy. A variety of abnormalities was produced including anophthalmia, absence of the axial skeleton, hydronephrosis, etc. Pregnancy in rabbits was interrupted when doses as low as 0.04 mg/kg (10 times the maximum recommended human dose) were given early or late in pregnancy.
Hydrochlorothiazide: Studies in which hydrochlorothiazide was orally administered to pregnant mice and rats during their respective periods of major organogenesis at doses up to 3000 and 1000 mg hydrochlorothiazide/kg, respectively, provided no evidence of harm to the fetus.

Nonteratogenic Effects

Reserpine: Reserpine has been demonstrated to cross the placental barrier in guinea pigs with depression of adrenal catecholamine stores in the newborn. There is some evidence that side effects such as nasal congestion, lethargy, depressed Moro reflex, and bradycardia may appear in infants born of reserpine-treated mothers.
Hydrochlorothiazide: Thiazides cross the placental barrier and appear in cord blood. There is a risk of fetal or neonatal jaundice, thrombocytopenia, and possibly other adverse reactions that have occurred in adults.

Nursing Mothers

Thiazides and reserpine appear in breast milk. Because of the potential for serious adverse reactions in nursing infants from HYDROPRES, a decision should be made whether to discontinue nursing or to discontinue the drug, taking into account the importance of the drug to the mother.

Pediatric Use

Safety and effectiveness of HYDROPRES in children has not been established.

ADVERSE REACTIONS

The following adverse reactions have been reported and, within each category, are listed in order of decreasing severity.

Hydrochlorothiazide

Body as a Whole: Weakness.
Cardiovascular: Hypotension including orthostatic hypotension (may be aggravated by alcohol, barbiturates, narcotics or antihypertensive drugs).
Digestive: Pancreatitis, jaundice (intrahepatic cholestatic jaundice), diarrhea, vomiting, sialadenitis, cramping, constipation, gastric irritation, nausea, anorexia.
Hematologic: Aplastic anemia, agranulocytosis, leukopenia, hemolytic anemia, thrombocytopenia.
Hypersensitivity: Anaphylactic reactions, necrotizing angiitis (vasculitis and cutaneous vasculitis), respiratory distress including pneumonitis and pulmonary edema, photosensitivity, fever, urticaria, rash, purpura.
Metabolic: Electrolyte imbalance (see PRECAUTIONS), hyperglycemia, glycosuria, hyperuricemia.
Musculoskeletal: Muscle spasm.
Nervous System/Psychiatric: Vertigo, paresthesias, dizziness, headache, restlessness.
Renal: Renal failure, renal dysfunction, interstitial nephritis. (See WARNINGS.)

Continued on next page

Information on the Merck & Co., Inc. products listed on these pages is the full prescribing information from product circulars in use September 30, 1996.

Merck & Co.—Cont.

Skin: Erythema multiforme including Stevens-Johnson syndrome, exfoliative dermatitis including toxic epidermal necrolysis, alopecia.
Special Senses: Transient blurred vision, xanthopsia.
Urogenital: Impotence.
Reserpine
Cardiovascular: Angina pectoris, arrhythmia, premature ventricular contractions, other direct cardiac effects (e.g., fluid retention, congestive heart failure), bradycardia.
Digestive: Vomiting, diarrhea, nausea, hypersecretion and increased motility, anorexia, dryness of mouth, increased salivation.
Hematologic: Thrombocytopenic purpura, excessive bleeding following prostatic surgery.
Hypersensitivity: Pruritus, rash, flushing of skin.
Metabolic: Weight gain.
Musculoskeletal: Muscular aches.
Nervous System/Psychiatric: Mental depression, dull sensorium, syncope, paradoxical anxiety, excessive sedation, nightmares, headache, dizziness, nervousness, parkinsonism (usually reversible with decreased dosage or discontinuance of therapy).
Respiratory: Dyspnea, epistaxis, nasal congestion, enhanced susceptibility to colds.
Special Senses: Optic atrophy, uveitis, deafness, glaucoma, conjunctival injection, blurred vision.
Urogenital: Dysuria, impotence, decreased libido, nonpuerperal lactation.

OVERDOSAGE

Overdosage may lead to excessive sedation, mental depression, severe hypotension, extrapyramidal reactions.
There is no specific antidote. In the event of overdosage, symptomatic and supportive measures should be employed. Emesis should be induced or gastric lavage performed. Correct dehydration, electrolyte imbalance, hepatic coma and hypotension by established procedures. If required, give oxygen or artificial respiration for respiratory impairment. In the event of severe hypotension from the reserpine component, intravenous use of a vasopressor is indicated [e.g., ARAMINE* (Metaraminol Bitartrate), levarterenol, phenylephrine]. Anticholinergics may be needed to relieve gastrointestinal distress from reserpine. Because the effects of the rauwolfia alkaloids are prolonged, the patient should be closely observed for at least 72 hours.
Reserpine is not dialyzable. The degree to which hydrochlorothiazide is removed by hemodialysis has not been established.
The oral LD_{50} of hydrochlorothiazide is greater than 10 g/kg in the mouse and rat. The oral LD_{50} of reserpine in the mouse is 390 mg/kg.

*Registered trademark of MERCK & CO., INC.

DOSAGE AND ADMINISTRATION

The initial dosage of HYDROPRES should conform to the dosages of the individual components established during titration (see box warning).
The usual adult dosage of HYDROPRES 25 is 1 or 2 tablets once a day; that of HYDROPRES 50 is 1 tablet once a day. Patients usually do not require doses in excess of 50 mg of hydrochlorothiazide daily when combined with other antihypertensive agents. Dosage may require adjustment according to the blood pressure response of the patient. For maintenance, dosage should be adjusted to the lowest requirements of the individual patient. Doses higher than 0.25 mg daily of reserpine should be used cautiously, because occurrence of serious mental depression and other side effects may increase considerably (see WARNINGS).

HOW SUPPLIED

No. 3265—Tablets HYDROPRES 25 are green, round, scored, compressed tablets, coded MSD 53. Each tablet contains 25 mg of hydrochlorothiazide and 0.125 mg of reserpine. They are supplied as follows:
NDC 0006-0053-68 in bottles of 100
NDC 0006-0053-82 in bottles of 1000.
Shown in Product Identification Guide, page 324
No. 3266—Tablets HYDROPRES 50 are green, round, scored, compressed tablets, coded MSD 127. Each tablet contains 50 mg of hydrochlorothiazide and 0.125 mg of reserpine. They are supplied as follows:
NDC 0006-0127-68 in bottles of 100
NDC 0006-0127-82 in bottles of 1000.
Shown in Product Identification Guide, page 324
Storage
Keep container tightly closed. Protect from light, moisture, freezing. −20°C (−4°F) and store at room temperature, 15–30°C (59–86°F).

7899046 Issued February 1995

HYZAAR® ℞
(Losartan Potassium-Hydrochlorothiazide Tablets)

USE IN PREGNANCY
When used in pregnancy during the second and third trimesters, drugs that act directly on the renin-angiotensin system can cause injury and even death to the developing fetus. When pregnancy is detected, HYZAAR should be discontinued as soon as possible. See WARNINGS: *Fetal/Neonatal Morbidity and Mortality.*

DESCRIPTION

HYZAAR* (losartan potassium-hydrochlorothiazide), combines an angiotensin II receptor (type AT_1) antagonist and a diuretic, hydrochlorothiazide.
Losartan potassium, a non-peptide molecule, is chemically described as 2-butyl-4-chloro-1-[*p*-(*o*-1*H*-tetrazol-5-ylphenyl)-benzyl]imidazole-5-methanol monopotassium salt. Its empirical formula is $C_{22}H_{22}ClKN_6O$, and its structural formula is:

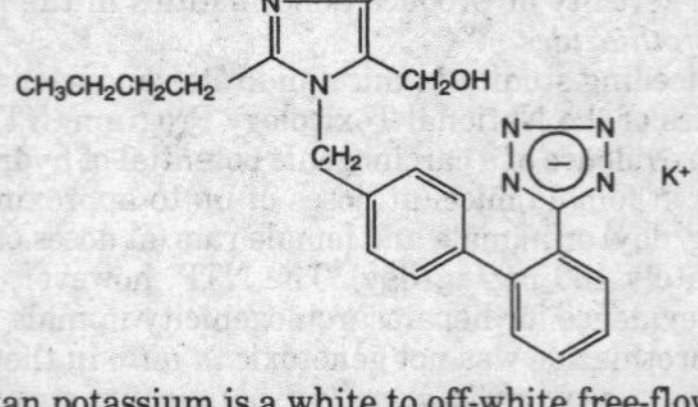

Losartan potassium is a white to off-white free-flowing crystalline powder with a molecular weight of 461.01. It is freely soluble in water, soluble in alcohols, and slightly soluble in common organic solvents, such as acetonitrile and methyl ethyl ketone.
Oxidation of the 5-hydroxymethyl group on the imidazole ring results in the active metabolite of losartan.
Hydrochlorothiazide is 6-chloro-3,4-dihydro-2*H*-1,2,4-benzothiadiazine-7-sulfonamide 1,1-dioxide. Its empirical formula is $C_7H_8ClN_3O_4S_2$ and its structural formula is:

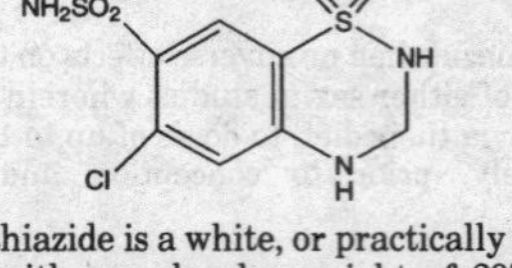

Hydrochlorothiazide is a white, or practically white, crystalline powder with a molecular weight of 297.74, which is slightly soluble in water, but freely soluble in sodium hydroxide solution.
HYZAAR is available for oral administration containing 50 mg of losartan potassium, 12.5 mg of hydrochlorothiazide and the following inactive ingredients: microcrystalline cellulose, lactose hydrous, pregelatinized starch, magnesium stearate, hydroxypropyl cellulose, hydroxypropyl methylcellulose, titanium dioxide and D&C yellow No. 10 aluminum lake.
HYZAAR contains 4.24 mg (0.108 mEq) of potassium.

*Registered trademark of E.I. du Pont de Nemours and Company, Wilmington, Delaware, USA

CLINICAL PHARMACOLOGY

Mechanism of Action
Angiotensin II [formed from angiotensin I in a reaction catalyzed by angiotensin converting enzyme (ACE, kininase II)], is a potent vasoconstrictor, the primary vasoactive hormone of the renin-angiotensin system and an important component in the pathophysiology of hypertension. It also stimulates aldosterone secretion by the adrenal cortex. Losartan and its principal active metabolite block the vasoconstrictor and aldosterone-secreting effects of angiotensin II by selectively blocking the binding of angiotensin II to the AT_1 receptor found in many tissues, (e.g., vascular smooth muscle, adrenal gland). There is also an AT_2 receptor found in many tissues but it is not known to be associated with cardiovascular homeostasis. Both losartan and its principal active metabolite do not exhibit any partial agonist activity at the AT_1 receptor and have much greater affinity (about 1000-fold) for the AT_1 receptor than for the AT_2 receptor. *In vitro* binding studies indicate that losartan is a reversible, competitive inhibitor of the AT_1 receptor. The active metabolite is 10 to 40 times more potent by weight than losartan and appears to be a reversible, non-competitive inhibitor of the AT_1 receptor.
Neither losartan nor its active metabolite inhibits ACE (kininase II, the enzyme that converts angiotensin I to angiotensin II and degrades bradykinin); nor do they bind to or block other hormone receptors or ion channels known to be important in cardiovascular regulation.
Hydrochlorothiazide is a thiazide diuretic. Thiazides affect the renal tubular mechanisms of electrolyte reabsorption, directly increasing excretion of sodium and chloride in approximately equivalent amounts. Indirectly, the diuretic action of hydrochlorothiazide reduces plasma volume, with consequent increases in plasma renin activity, increases in aldosterone secretion, increases in urinary potassium loss, and decreases in serum potassium. The renin-aldosterone link is mediated by angiotensin II, so coadministration of an angiotensin II receptor antagonist tends to reverse the potassium loss associated with these diuretics.
The mechanism of the antihypertensive effect of thiazides is unknown.
Pharmacokinetics
General
Losartan Potassium
Losartan is an orally active agent that undergoes substantial first-pass metabolism by cytochrome P450 enzymes. It is converted, in part, to an active carboxylic acid metabolite that is responsible for most of the angiotensin II receptor antagonism that follows losartan treatment. The terminal half-life of losartan is about 2 hours and of the metabolite is about 6–9 hours. The pharmacokinetics of losartan and its active metabolite are linear with oral losartan doses up to 200 mg and do not change over time. Neither losartan nor its metabolite accumulate in plasma upon repeated once-daily dosing.
Following oral administration, losartan is well absorbed (based on absorption of radiolabeled losartan) and undergoes substantial first-pass metabolism; the systemic bioavailability of losartan is approximately 33%. About 14% of an orally-administered dose of losartan is converted to the active metabolite. Mean peak concentrations of losartan and its active metabolite are reached in 1 hour and in 3–4 hours, respectively. While maximum plasma concentrations of losartan and its active metabolite are approximately equal, the AUC of the metabolite is about 4 times as great as that of losartan. A meal slows absorption of losartan and decreases its C_{max} but has only minor effects on losartan AUC or on the AUC of the metabolite (about 10% decreased).
Both losartan and its active metabolite are highly bound to plasma proteins, primarily albumin, with plasma free fractions of 1.3% and 0.2% respectively. Plasma protein binding is constant over the concentration range achieved with recommended doses. Studies in rats indicate that losartan crosses the blood-brain barrier poorly, if at all.
Losartan metabolites have been identified in human plasma and urine. In addition to the active carboxylic acid metabolite, several inactive metabolites are formed. Following oral and intravenous administration of ^{14}C-labeled losartan potassium, circulating plasma radioactivity is primarily attributed to losartan and its active metabolite. *In vitro* studies indicate that cytochrome P450 2C9 and 3A4 are involved in the biotransformation of losartan to its metabolites. Minimal conversion of losartan to the active metabolite (less than 1% of the dose compared to 14% of the dose in normal subjects) was seen in about one percent of individuals studied.
The volume of distribution of losartan is about 34 liters and of the active metabolite is about 12 liters. Total plasma clearance of losartan and the active metabolite is about 600 mL/min and 50 mL/min, respectively, with renal clearance of about 75 mL/min and 25 mL/min, respectively. When losartan is administered orally, about 4% of the dose is excreted unchanged in the urine and about 6% is excreted in urine as active metabolite. Biliary excretion contributes to the elimination of losartan and its metabolites. Following oral ^{14}C-labeled losartan, about 35% of radioactivity is recovered in the urine and about 60% in the feces. Following an intravenous dose of ^{14}C-labeled losartan, about 45% of radioactivity is recovered in the urine and 50% in the feces.
Special Populations
Pediatric: Losartan pharmacokinetics have not been investigated in patients < 18 years of age.
Geriatric and Gender: Losartan pharmacokinetics have been investigated in the elderly (65–75 years) and in both genders. Plasma concentrations of losartan and its active metabolite are similar in elderly and young hypertensives. Plasma concentrations of losartan were about twice as high in female hypertensives as male hypertensives, but concentrations of the active metabolite were similar in males and females.
Race: Pharmacokinetic differences due to race have not been studied.
Renal Insufficiency: Plasma concentrations of losartan are not altered in patients with creatinine clearance above 30 mL/min. In patients with lower creatinine clearance, AUCs are about 50% greater and are doubled in hemodialysis patients. Plasma concentrations of the active metabolite are not significantly altered in patients with renal impairment

or in hemodialysis patients. Neither losartan nor its active metabolite can be removed by hemodialysis.

Hepatic Insufficiency: Following oral administration in patients with mild to moderate alcoholic cirrhosis of the liver, plasma concentrations of losartan and its active metabolite were, respectively, 5 times and about 1.7 times those in young male volunteers. Compared to normal subjects the total plasma clearance of losartan in patients with hepatic insufficiency was about 50% lower and the oral bioavailability was about 2-times higher. The lower starting dose of losartan recommended for use in patients with hepatic impairment cannot be given using HYZAAR. Its use in such patients as a means of losartan titration is, therefore, not recommended (see DOSAGE AND ADMINISTRATION).

Drug Interactions

Losartan Potassium

Losartan, administered for 12 days, did not affect the pharmacokinetics or pharmacodynamics of a single dose of warfarin. Losartan did not affect the pharmacokinetics of oral or intravenous digoxin. Coadministration of losartan and cimetidine led to an increase of about 18% in AUC of losartan but did not affect the pharmacokinetics of its active metabolite. Coadministration of losartan and phenobarbital led to a reduction of about 20% in the AUC of losartan and that of its active metabolite. There is no pharmacokinetic interaction between losartan and hydrochlorothiazide.

Hydrochlorothiazide

After oral administration of hydrochlorothiazide, diuresis begins within 2 hours, peaks in about 4 hours and lasts about 6 to 12 hours.

Hydrochlorothiazide is not metabolized but is eliminated rapidly by the kidney. When plasma levels have been followed for at least 24 hours, the plasma half-life has been observed to vary between 5.6 and 14.8 hours. At least 61 percent of the oral dose is eliminated unchanged within 24 hours. Hydrochlorothiazide crosses the placental but not the blood-brain barrier and is excreted in breast milk.

Pharmacodynamics and Clinical Effects

Losartan Potassium

Losartan inhibits the pressor effect of angiotensin II (as well as angiotensin I) infusions. A dose of 100 mg inhibits the pressor effect by about 85% at peak with 25–40% inhibition persisting for 24 hours. Removal of the negative feedback of angiotensin II causes a 2–3 fold rise in plasma renin activity and consequent rise in angiotensin II plasma concentration in hypertensive patients. Losartan does not affect the response to bradykinin, whereas ACE inhibitors increase the response to bradykinin. Aldosterone plasma concentrations fall following losartan administration. In spite of the effect of losartan on aldosterone secretion, very little effect on serum potassium was observed.

In a single-dose study in normal volunteers, losartan had no effects on glomerular filtration rate, renal plasma flow or filtration fraction. In multiple dose studies in hypertensive patients, there were no notable effects on systemic or renal prostaglandin concentrations, fasting triglycerides, total cholesterol or HDL-cholesterol or fasting glucose concentrations. There was a small uricosuric effect leading to a minimal decrease in serum uric acid (mean decrease <0.4 mg/dL) during chronic oral administration.

The antihypertensive effects of losartan were demonstrated principally in 4 placebo-controlled 6–12 week trials of dosages from 10 to 150 mg per day in patients with baseline diastolic blood pressures of 95–115. The studies allowed comparisons of two doses (50–100 mg/day) as once-daily or twice-daily regimens, comparisons of peak and trough effects, and comparisons of response by gender, age, and race. Three additional studies examined the antihypertensive effects of losartan and hydrochlorothiazide in combination.

The 4 studies of losartan monotherapy included a total of 1075 patients randomized to several doses of losartan and 334 to placebo. The 10 and 25 mg doses produced some effect at peak (6 hours after dosing) but small and inconsistent trough (24 hour) responses. Doses of 50, 100, and 150 mg once daily gave statistically significant systolic/diastolic mean decreases in blood pressure, compared to placebo in the range of 5.5–10.5/3.5–7.5 mmHg, with the 150 mg dose giving no greater effect than 50–100 mg. Twice-daily dosing at 50–100 mg/day gave consistently larger trough responses than once daily dosing at the same total dose. Peak (6 hour) effects were uniformly, but moderately larger than trough effects, with the trough to peak ratio for systolic and diastolic responses 50–95% and 60–90% respectively.

Analysis of age, gender, and race subgroups of patients showed that men and women, and patients over and under 65, had generally similar responses. Black patients, however, had notably smaller responses to losartan monotherapy.

The effect of losartan is substantially present within one week but in some studies the maximal effect occurred in 3–6 weeks. In long-term follow-up studies (without placebo control) the effect of losartan appeared to be maintained for up to a year. There is no apparent rebound effect after abrupt withdrawal of losartan. There was essentially no change in average heart rate in losartan-treated patients in controlled trials.

Persistent dry cough (with an incidence of a few percent) has been associated with ACE inhibitor use and in practice can be a cause of discontinuation of ACE inhibitor therapy. Two prospective, parallel-group, double-blind, randomized, controlled trials were conducted to assess the effects of losartan on the incidence of cough in hypertensive patients who had experienced cough while receiving ACE inhibitor therapy. Patients who had typical ACE inhibitor cough when challenged with lisinopril, whose cough disappeared on placebo, were randomized to losartan 50 mg, lisinopril 20 mg, or either placebo (one study, n=97) or 25 mg hydrochlorothiazide (n=135). The double-blind treatment period lasted up to 8 weeks. The incidence of cough is shown below.

Study 1†	HCTZ	Losartan	Lisinopril
Cough	25%	17%	69%
Study 2††	**Placebo**	**Losartan**	**Lisinopril**
Cough	35%	29%	62%

† Demographics = (89% caucasian, 64% female)
†† Demographics = (90% caucasian, 51% female)

These studies demonstrate that the incidence of cough associated with losartan therapy, in a population that all had cough associated with ACE inhibitor therapy, is similar to that associated with hydrochlorothiazide or placebo therapy.

Losartan Potassium-Hydrochlorothiazide

The 3 controlled studies of losartan and hydrochlorothiazide included over 1300 patients assessing the antihypertensive efficacy of various doses of losartan (25, 50 and 100 mg) and concomitant hydrochlorothiazide (6.25, 12.5 and 25 mg). A factorial study compared the combination of losartan/hydrochlorothiazide 50/12.5 mg with its components and placebo. The combination of losartan/hydrochlorothiazide 50/12.5 mg resulted in an approximately additive placebo-adjusted systolic/diastolic response (15.5/9.0 mmHg for the combination compared to 8.5/5.0 mmHg for losartan alone and 7.0/3.0 mmHg for hydrochlorothiazide alone). Another study investigated the dose-response relationship of various doses of hydrochlorothiazide (6.25, 12.5 and 25 mg) or placebo on a background of losartan (50 mg) in patients not adequately controlled (SiDBP 93–120 mmHg) on losartan (50 mg) alone. The third study investigated the dose-response relationship of various doses of losartan (25, 50 and 100 mg) or placebo on a background of hydrochlorothiazide (25 mg) in patients not adequately controlled (SiDBP 93–120 mmHg) on hydrochlorothiazide (25 mg) alone. These studies showed an added antihypertensive response at trough (24 hours post-dosing) of hydrochlorothiazide 12.5 or 25 mg added to losartan 50 mg of 5.5/3.5 and 10.0/6.0 mmHg, respectively. Similarly, there was an added antihypertensive response at trough when losartan 50 or 100 mg was added to hydrochlorothiazide 25 mg of 9.0/5.5 and 12.5/6.5 mmHg, respectively. There was no significant effect on heart rate.

There was no difference in response for men and women or in patients over or under 65 years of age.

Black patients had a larger response to hydrochlorothiazide than non-black patients and a smaller response to losartan. The overall response to the combination was similar for black and non-black patients.

INDICATIONS AND USAGE

HYZAAR is indicated for the treatment of hypertension. This fixed dose combination is not indicated for initial therapy (see DOSAGE AND ADMINISTRATION).

CONTRAINDICATIONS

HYZAAR is contraindicated in patients who are hypersensitive to any component of this product.

Because of the hydrochlorothiazide component, this product is contraindicated in patients with anuria or hypersensitivity to other sulfonamide-derived drugs.

WARNINGS

Fetal/Neonatal Morbidity and Mortality

Drugs that act directly on the renin-angiotensin system can cause fetal and neonatal morbidity and death when administered to pregnant women. Several dozen cases have been reported in the world literature in patients who were taking angiotensin converting enzyme inhibitors. When pregnancy is detected, HYZAAR should be discontinued as soon as possible.

The use of drugs that act directly on the renin-angiotensin system during the second and third trimesters of pregnancy has been associated with fetal and neonatal injury, including hypotension, neonatal skull hypoplasia, anuria, reversible or irreversible renal failure, and death. Oligohydramnios has also been reported, presumably resulting from decreased fetal renal function; oligohydramnios in this setting has been associated with fetal limb contractures, craniofacial deformation, and hypoplastic lung development. Prematurity, intrauterine growth retardation, and patent ductus arteriosus have also been reported, although it is not clear whether these occurrences were due to exposure to the drug.

These adverse effects do not appear to have resulted from intrauterine drug exposure that has been limited to the first trimester.

Mothers whose embryos and fetuses are exposed to an angiotensin II receptor antagonist only during the first trimester should be so informed. Nonetheless, when patients become pregnant, physicians should have the patient discontinue the use of HYZAAR as soon as possible.

Rarely (probably less often than once in every thousand pregnancies), no alternative to an angiotensin II receptor antagonist will be found. In these rare cases, the mothers should be apprised of the potential hazards to their fetuses, and serial ultrasound examinations should be performed to assess the intra-amniotic environment.

If oligohydramnios is observed, HYZAAR should be discontinued unless it is considered life-saving for the mother. Contraction stress testing (CST), a non-stress test (NST), or biophysical profiling (BPP) may be appropriate, depending upon the week of pregnancy. Patients and physicians should be aware, however, that oligohydramnios may not appear until after the fetus has sustained irreversible injury.

Infants with histories of *in utero* exposure to an angiotensin II receptor antagonist should be closely observed for hypotension, oliguria, and hyperkalemia. If oliguria occurs, attention should be directed toward support of blood pressure and renal perfusion. Exchange transfusion or dialysis may be required as means of reversing hypotension and/or substituting for disordered renal function.

There was no evidence of teratogenicity in rats or rabbits treated with a maximum losartan potassium dose of 10 mg/kg/day in combination with 2.5 mg/kg/day of hydrochlorothiazide. At these dosages, respective exposures (AUCs) of losartan, its active metabolite, and hydrochlorothiazide in rabbits were approximately 5-, 1.5-, and 1.0-times those achieved in humans with 100 mg losartan in combination with 25 mg hydrochlorothiazide. AUC values for losartan, its active metabolite and hydrochlorothiazide, extrapolated from data obtained with losartan administered to rats at a dose of 50 mg/kg/day in combination with 12.5 mg/kg/day of hydrochlorothiazide, were approximately 6, 2, and 2 times greater than those achieved in humans with 100 mg of losartan in combination with 25 mg of hydrochlorothiazide.

Fetal toxicity in rats, as evidenced by a slight increase in supernumerary ribs, was observed when females were treated prior to and throughout gestation with 10 mg/kg/day losartan in combination with 2.5 mg/kg/day hydrochlorothiazide. As also observed in studies with losartan alone, adverse fetal and neonatal effects, including decreased body weight, renal toxicity, and mortality, occurred when pregnant rats were treated during late gestation and/or lactation with 50 mg/kg/day losartan in combination with 12.5 mg/kg/day hydrochlorothiazide. Respective AUCs for losartan, its active metabolite and hydrochlorothiazide at these dosages in rats were approximately 35, 10 and 10 times greater than those achieved in humans with the administration of 100 mg of losartan in combination with 25 mg hydrochlorothiazide. When hydrochlorothiazide was administered without losartan to pregnant mice and rats during their respective periods of major organogenesis, at doses up to 3000 and 1000 mg/kg/day, respectively, there was no evidence of harm to the fetus.

Thiazides cross the placental barrier and appear in cord blood. There is a risk of fetal or neonatal jaundice, thrombocytopenia, and possibly other adverse reactions that have occurred in adults.

Hypotension—Volume-Depleted Patients

In patients who are intravascularly volume-depleted (e.g., those treated with diuretics), symptomatic hypotension may occur after initiation of therapy with HYZAAR. This condition should be corrected prior to administration of HYZAAR (see DOSAGE AND ADMINISTRATION).

Impaired Hepatic Function

Losartan Potassium-Hydrochlorothiazide

HYZAAR is not recommended for patients with hepatic impairment who require titration with losartan. The lower starting dose of losartan recommended for use in patients with hepatic impairment cannot be given using HYZAAR.

Hydrochlorothiazide

Thiazides should be used with caution in patients with impaired hepatic function or progressive liver disease, since minor alterations of fluid and electrolyte balance may precipitate hepatic coma.

Continued on next page

Information on the Merck & Co., Inc. products listed on these pages is the full prescribing information from product circulars in use September 30, 1996.

Merck & Co.—Cont.

Hypersensitivity Reaction
Hypersensitivity reactions to hydrochlorothiazide may occur in patients with or without a history of allergy or bronchial asthma, but are more likely in patients with such a history.
Systemic Lupus Erythematosus
Thiazide diuretics have been reported to cause exacerbation or activation of systemic lupus erythematosus.
Lithium Interaction
Lithium generally should not be given with thiazides (see PRECAUTIONS, *Drug Interactions, Hydrocholorothiazide, Lithium*).

PRECAUTIONS

General
Losartan Potassium-Hydrochlorothiazide
In double-blind clinical trials of various doses of losartan potassium and hydrochlorothiazide, the incidence of hypertensive patients who developed hypokalemia (serum potassium < 3.5 mEq/L) was 6.7% versus 3.5% for placebo; the incidence of hyperkalemia (serum potassium > 5.7 mEq/L) was 0.4%. No patient discontinued due to increases or decreases in serum potassium. The mean decrease in serum potassium in patients treated with various doses of losartan and hydrochlorothiazide was 0.123 mEq/L. In patients treated with various doses of losartan and hydrochlorothiazide, there was also a dose-related decrease in the hypokalemic response to hydrochlorothiazide as the dose of losartan was increased, as well as a dose-related decrease in serum uric acid with increasing doses of losartan.
Hydrochlorothiazide
Periodic determination of serum electrolytes to detect possible electrolyte imbalance should be performed at appropriate intervals.
All patients receiving thiazide therapy should be observed for clinical signs of fluid or electrolyte imbalance: hyponatremia, hypochloremic alkalosis, and hypokalemia. Serum and urine electrolyte determinations are particularly important when the patient is vomiting excessively or receiving parenteral fluids. Warning signs or symptoms of fluid and electrolyte imbalance, irrespective of cause, include dryness of mouth, thirst, weakness, lethargy, drowsiness, restlessness, confusion, seizures, muscle pains or cramps, muscular fatigue, hypotension, oliguria, tachycardia, and gastrointestinal disturbances such as nausea and vomiting.
Hypokalemia may develop, especially with brisk diuresis, when severe cirrhosis is present, or after prolonged therapy. Interference with adequate oral electrolyte intake will also contribute to hypokalemia. Hypokalemia may cause cardiac arrhythmia and may also sensitize or exaggerate the response of the heart to the toxic effects of digitalis (e.g., increased ventricular irritability).
Although any chloride deficit is generally mild and usually does not require specific treatment except under extraordinary circumstances (as in liver disease or renal disease), chloride replacement may be required in the treatment of metabolic alkalosis.
Dilutional hyponatremia may occur in edematous patients in hot weather; appropriate therapy is water restriction, rather than administration of salt except in rare instances when the hyponatremia is life-threatening. In actual salt depletion, appropriate replacement is the therapy of choice.
Hyperuricemia may occur or frank gout may be precipitated in certain patients receiving thiazide therapy. Because losartan decreases uric acid, losartan in combination with hydrochlorothiazide attenuates the diuretic-induced hyperuricemia.
In diabetic patients dosage adjustments of insulin or oral hypoglycemic agents may be required. Hyperglycemia may occur with thiazide diuretics. Thus latent diabetes mellitus may become manifest during thiazide therapy.
The antihypertensive effects of the drug may be enhanced in the postsympathectomy patient.
If progressive renal impairment becomes evident consider withholding or discontinuing diuretic therapy.
Thiazides have been shown to increase the urinary excretion of magnesium; this may result in hypomagnesemia.
Thiazides may decrease urinary calcium excretion. Thiazides may cause intermittent and slight elevation of serum calcium in the absence of known disorders of calcium metabolism. Marked hypercalcemia may be evidence of hidden hyperparathyroidism. Thiazides should be discontinued before carrying out tests for parathyroid function.
Increases in cholesterol and triglyceride levels may be associated with thiazide diuretic therapy.
Hypersensitivity. See ADVERSE REACTIONS, *Post-Marketing Experience.*
Impaired Renal Function
As a consequence of inhibiting the renin-angiotensin-aldosterone system, changes in renal function have been reported in susceptible individuals treated with losartan; in

some patients, these changes in renal function were reversible upon discontinuation of therapy.
In patients whose renal function may depend on the activity of the renin-angiotensin-aldosterone system (e.g., patients with severe congestive heart failure), treatment with angiotensin converting enzyme inhibitors has been associated with oliguria and/or progressive azotemia and (rarely) with acute renal failure and/or death. Similar outcomes have been reported with losartan.
In studies of ACE inhibitors in patients with unilateral or bilateral renal artery stenosis, increases in serum creatinine or BUN have been reported. Similar effects have been reported with losartan; in some patients, these effects were reversible upon discontinuation of therapy.
Thiazides should be used with caution in severe renal disease. In patients with renal disease, thiazides may precipitate azotemia. Cumulative effects of the drug may develop in patients with impaired renal function.
Information for Patients
Pregnancy: Female patients of childbearing age should be told about the consequences of second- and third-trimester exposure to drugs that act on the renin-angiotensin system, and they should also be told that these consequences do not appear to have resulted from intrauterine drug exposure that has been limited to the first trimester. These patients should be asked to report pregnancies to their physicians as soon as possible.
Symptomatic Hypotension: A patient receiving HYZAAR should be cautioned that lightheadedness can occur, especially during the first days of therapy, and that it should be reported to the prescribing physician. The patients should be told that if syncope occurs, HYZAAR should be discontinued until the physician has been consulted.
All patients should be cautioned that inadequate fluid intake, excessive perspiration, diarrhea, or vomiting can lead to an excessive fall in blood pressure, with the same consequences of lightheadedness and possible syncope.
Potassium Supplements: A patient receiving HYZAAR should be told not to use potassium supplements or salt substitutes containing potassium without consulting the prescribing physician.
Drug Interactions
Losartan Potassium
No significant drug-drug pharmacokinetic interactions have been found in interaction studies with hydrochlorothiazide, digoxin, warfarin, cimetidine and phenobarbital. (See CLINICAL PHARMACOLOGY, *Drug Interactions.*) Potent inhibitors of cytochrome P450 3A4 and 2C9 have not been studied clinically but *in vitro* studies show significant inhibition of the formation of the active metabolite by inhibitors of P450 3A4 (ketoconazole, troleandomycin, gestodene), or P450 2C9 (sulfaphenazole) and nearly complete inhibition by the combination of sulfaphenazole and ketoconazole. The pharmacodynamic consequences of concomitant use of losartan and these inhibitors have not been examined.
Hydrochlorothiazide
When administered concurrently the following drugs may interact with thiazide diuretics:
Alcohol, barbiturates, or narcotics—potentiation of orthostatic hypotension may occur.
Antidiabetic drugs (oral agents and insulin)—dosage adjustment of the antidiabetic drug may be required.
Other antihypertensive drugs—additive effect or potentiation.
Cholestyramine and colestipol resins—Absorption of hydrochlorothiazide is impaired in the presence of anionic exchange resins. Single doses of either cholestyramine or colestipol resins bind the hydrochlorothiazide and reduce its absorption from the gastrointestinal tract by up to 85 and 43 percent, respectively.
Corticosteroids, ACTH—intensified electrolyte depletion, particularly hypokalemia.
Pressor amines (e.g., *norepinephrine*)—possible decreased response to pressor amines but not sufficient to preclude their use.
Skeletal muscle relaxants, nondepolarizing (e.g., *tubocurarine*)—possible increased responsiveness to the muscle relaxant.
Lithium—should not generally be given with diuretics. Diuretic agents reduce the renal clearance of lithium and add a high risk of lithium toxicity. Refer to the package insert for lithium preparations before use of such preparations with HYZAAR.
Non-steroidal Anti-inflammatory Drugs—In some patients, the administration of a non-steroidal anti-inflammatory agent can reduce the diuretic, natriuretic, and antihypertensive effects of loop, potassium-sparing and thiazide diuretics. Therefore, when HYZAAR and non-steroidal anti-inflammatory agents are used concomitantly, the patient should be observed closely to determine if the desired effect of the diuretic is obtained.
Carcinogenesis, Mutagenesis, Impairment of Fertility
Losartan Potassium-Hydrochlorothiazide
No carcinogenicity studies have been conducted with the losartan potassium-hydrochlorothiazide combination.

Losartan potassium-hydrochlorothiazide when tested at a weight ratio of 4:1, was negative in the Ames microbial mutagenesis assay and the V-79 Chinese hamster lung cell mutagenesis assay. In addition, there was no evidence of direct genotoxicity in the *in vitro* alkaline elution assay in rat hepatocytes and *in vitro* chromosomal aberration assay in Chinese hamster ovary cells at noncytotoxic concentrations. Losartan potassium, coadministered with hydrochlorothiazide, had no effect on the fertility or mating behavior of male rats of dosages up to 135 mg/kg/day of losartan and 33.75 mg/kg/day of hydrochlorothiazide. These dosages have been shown to provide respective systemic exposures (AUCs) for losartan, its active metabolite and hydrochlorothiazide that are approximately 60, 60 and 30 times greater than those achieved in humans with 100 mg of losartan potassium in combination with 25 mg of hydrochlorothiazide. In female rats, however, the coadministration of doses as low as 10 mg/kg/day of losartan and 2.5 mg/kg/day of hydrochlorothiazide was associated with slight but statistically significant decreases in fecundity and fertility indices. AUC values for losartan, its active metabolite and hydrochlorothiazide, extrapolated from data obtained with losartan administered to rats at a dose of 50 mg/kg/day in combination with 12.5 mg/kg/day of hydrochlorothiazide, were approximately 6, 2, and 2 times greater than those achieved in humans with 100 mg of losartan in combination with 25 mg of hydrochlorothiazide.
Losartan Potassium
Losartan potassium was not carcinogenic when administered at maximally tolerated dosages to rats and mice for 105 and 92 weeks, respectively. Female rats given the highest dose (270 mg/kg/day) had a slightly higher incidence of pancreatic acinar adenoma. The maximally tolerated dosages (270 mg/kg/day in rats, 200 mg/kg/day in mice) provided systemic exposures for losartan and its pharmacologically active metabolite that were approximately 160 and 90 times (rats) and 30 and 15 times (mice) the exposure of a 50 kg human given 100 mg per day.
Losartan potassium was negative in the microbial mutagenesis and V-79 mammalian cell mutagenesis assays and in the *in vitro* alkaline elution and *in vitro* and *in vivo* chromosomal aberration assays. In addition, the active metabolite showed no evidence of genotoxicity in the microbial mutagenesis, *in vitro* alkaline elution, and *in vitro* chromosomal aberration assays.
Fertility and reproductive performance were not affected in studies with male rats given oral doses of losartan potassium up to approximately 150 mg/kg/day. The administration of toxic dosage levels in females (300/200 mg/kg/day) was associated with a significant (p < 0.05) decrease in the number of corpora lutea/female, implants/female, and live fetuses/female at C-section. At 100 mg/kg/day only a decrease in the number of corpora lutea/female was observed. The relationship of these findings to drug-treatment is uncertain since there was no effect at these dosage levels on implants/pregnant female, percent post-implantation loss, or live animals/litter at parturition. In nonpregnant rats dosed at 135 mg/kg/day for 7 days, systemic exposure (AUCs) for losartan and its active metabolite were approximately 66 and 26 times the exposure achieved in man at the maximum recommended human daily dosage (100 mg).
Hydrochlorothiazide
Two-year feeding studies in mice and rats conducted under the auspices of the National Toxicology Program (NTP) uncovered no evidence of a carcinogenic potential of hydrochlorothiazide in female mice (at doses of up to approximately 600 mg/kg/day) or in male and female rats (at doses of up to approximately 100 mg/kg/day). The NTP, however, found equivocal evidence for hepatocarcinogenicity in male mice. Hydrochlorothiazide was not genotoxic *in vitro* in the Ames mutagenicity assay of *Salmonella typhimurium* strains TA 98, TA 100, TA 1535, TA 1537, and TA 1538 and in the Chinese Hamster Ovary (CHO) test for chromosomal aberrations, or *in vivo* in assays using mouse germinal cell chromosomes, Chinese hamster bone marrow chromosomes, and the *Drosophila* sex-linked recessive lethal trait gene. Positive test results were obtained only in the *in vitro* CHO Sister Chromatid Exchange (clastogenicity) and in the Mouse Lymphoma Cell (mutagenicity) assays, using concentrations of hydrochlorothiazide from 43 to 1300 μg/mL, and in the *Aspergillus nidulans* non-disjunction assay at an unspecified concentration.
Hydrochlorothiazide had no adverse effects on the fertility of mice and rats of either sex in studies wherein these species were exposed, via their diet, to doses of up to 100 and 4 mg/kg, respectively, prior to mating and throughout gestation.
Pregnancy
Pregnancy Categories C (first trimester) and D (second and third trimesters). See WARNINGS, *Fetal/Neonatal Morbidity and Mortality.*
Nursing Mothers
It is not known whether losartan is excreted in human milk, but significant levels of losartan and its active metabolite were shown to be present in rat milk. Thiazides appear in human milk. Because of the potential for adverse effects on the nursing infant, a decision should be made whether to

discontinue nursing or discontinue the drug, taking into account the importance of the drug to the mother.

Pediatric Use

Safety and effectiveness in pediatric patients have not been established.

Use in the Elderly

Of the total number of patients in controlled clinical studies of hypertension with HYZAAR, 107 patients (12.5%) were 65 years and over, while 9 patients (1.0%) were 75 years and over. No overall differences in effectiveness or safety were observed between these patients and younger patients, but greater sensitivity of some older individuals cannot be ruled out.

ADVERSE REACTIONS

Losartan potassium-hydrochlorothiazide has been evaluated for safety in 858 patients treated for essential hypertension. In clinical trials with losartan potassium-hydrochlorothiazide, no adverse experiences peculiar to this combination drug have been observed. Adverse experiences have been limited to those that were reported previously with losartan potassium and/or hydrochlorothiazide. The overall incidence of adverse experiences reported with the combination was comparable to placebo.

In general, treatment with losartan potassium-hydrochlorothiazide was well tolerated. For the most part, adverse experiences have been mild and transient in nature and have not required discontinuation of therapy. In controlled clinical trials, discontinuation of therapy due to clinical adverse experiences was required in only 2.8% and 2.3% of patients treated with the combination and placebo, respectively.

In these double-blind controlled clinical trials, the following adverse experiences reported with HYZAAR occurred in ≥ 1 percent of patients, and more often on drug than placebo, regardless of drug relationship:

	Losartan Potassium-Hydrochlorothiazide (n=858)	Placebo (n=173)
Body as a Whole		
Abdominal pain	1.2	0.6
Edema/swelling	1.3	1.2
Cardiovascular		
Palpitation	1.4	0.0
Musculoskeletal		
Back pain	2.1	0.6
Nervous/Psychiatric		
Dizziness	5.7	2.9
Respiratory		
Cough	2.6	2.3
Sinusitis	1.2	0.6
Upper respiratory infection	6.1	4.6
Skin		
Rash	1.4	0.0

The following adverse events were also reported at a rate of 1% or greater, but were as, or more, common in the placebo group: asthenia/fatigue, diarrhea, nausea, headache, bronchitis, pharyngitis.

Adverse events occurred at about the same rates in men and women, older and younger patients, and black and non-black patients.

A patient with known hypersensitivity to aspirin and penicillin, when treated with losartan potassium, was withdrawn from study due to swelling of the lips and eyelids and facial rash, reported as angioedema, which returned to normal 5 days after therapy was discontinued.

Superficial peeling of palms and hemolysis was reported in one subject treated with losartan potassium.

Losartan Potassium

Other adverse experiences that have been reported with losartan, without regard to causality, are listed below:

Body as a Whole: chest pain, facial edema, fever, orthostatic effects, syncope; *Cardiovascular:* angina pectoris, arrhythmias including atrial fibrillation, sinus bradycardia, tachycardia, ventricular tachycardia and ventricular fibrillation, CVA, hypotension, myocardial infarction, second degree AV block; *Digestive:* anorexia, constipation, dental pain, dry mouth, dyspepsia, flatulence, gastritis, vomiting; *Hematologic:* anemia; *Metabolic:* gout; *Musculoskeletal:* arm pain, arthralgia, arthritis, fibromyalgia, hip pain, joint swelling, knee pain, leg pain, muscle cramps, muscle weakness, musculoskeletal pain, myalgia, shoulder pain, stiffness; *Nervous System/Psychiatric:* anxiety, anxiety disorder, ataxia, confusion, depression, dream abnormality, hypesthesia, insomnia, libido decreased, memory impairment, migraine, nervousness, panic disorder, paresthesia, peripheral neuropathy, sleep disorder, somnolence, tremor, vertigo; *Respiratory:* dyspnea, epistaxis, nasal congestion, pharyngeal discomfort, respiratory congestion, rhinitis, sinus disorder; *Skin:* alopecia, dermatitis, dry skin, ecchymosis, erythema, flushing, photosensitivity, pruritus, sweating, urticaria; *Special Senses:* blurred vision, burning/stinging in the eye, conjunctivitis, decrease in visual acuity, taste perversion, tinnitus; *Urogenital:* impotence, nocturia, urinary frequency, urinary tract infection.

Hydrochlorothiazide

Other adverse experiences that have been reported with hydrochlorothiazide, without regard to causality, are listed below:

Body as a Whole: weakness; *Digestive:* pancreatitis, jaundice (intrahepatic cholestatic jaundice), sialadenitis, cramping, gastric irritation; *Hematologic:* aplastic anemia, agranulocytosis, leukopenia, hemolytic anemia, thrombocytopenia; *Hypersensitivity:* purpura, photosensitivity, urticaria, necrotizing angiitis (vasculitis and cutaneous vasculitis), fever, respiratory distress including pneumonitis and pulmonary edema, anaphylactic reactions; *Metabolic:* hyperglycemia, glycosuria, hyperuricemia; *Musculoskeletal:* muscle spasm; *Nervous System/Psychiatric:* restlessness; *Renal:* renal failure, renal dysfunction, interstitial nephritis; *Skin:* erythema multiforme including Stevens-Johnson syndrome, exfoliative dermatitis including toxic epidermal necrolysis; *Special Senses:* transient blurred vision, xanthopsia.

Post-Marketing Experience

The following adverse reactions have been reported in post-marketing experience: *Hypersensitivity:* Angioedema (involving swelling of the face, lips, and/or tongue) has been reported rarely in patients treated with losartan.

Laboratory Test Findings

In controlled clinical trials, clinically important changes in standard laboratory parameters were rarely associated with administration of HYZAAR.

Creatinine, Blood Urea Nitrogen: Minor increases in blood urea nitrogen (BUN) or serum creatinine were observed in 0.6 and 0.8 percent, respectively, of patients with essential hypertension treated with HYZAAR alone. No patient discontinued taking HYZAAR due to increased BUN. One patient discontinued taking HYZAAR due to a minor increase in serum creatinine.

Hemoglobin and Hematocrit: Small decreases in hemoglobin and hematocrit (mean decreases of approximately 0.14 grams percent and 0.72 volume percent, respectively) occurred frequently in patients treated with HYZAAR alone, but were rarely of clinical importance. No patients were discontinued due to anemia.

Liver Function Tests: Occasional elevations of liver enzymes and/or serum bilirubin have occurred. In patients with essential hypertension treated with HYZAAR alone, no patients were discontinued due to these laboratory adverse experiences.

Serum Electrolytes: See PRECAUTIONS.

OVERDOSAGE

Losartan Potassium

Significant lethality was observed in mice and rats after oral administration of 1000 mg/kg and 2000 mg/kg, respectively, about 44 and 170 times the maximum recommended human dose on a mg/m^2 basis.

Limited data are available in regard to overdosage in humans. The most likely manifestation of overdosage would be hypotension and tachycardia; bradycardia could occur from parasympathetic (vagal) stimulation. If symptomatic hypotension should occur, supportive treatment should be instituted.

Neither losartan nor its active metabolite can be removed by hemodialysis.

Hydrochlorothiazide

The oral LD_{50} of hydrochlorothiazide is greater than 10 g/kg in both mice and rats. The most common signs and symptoms observed are those caused by electrolyte depletion (hypokalemia, hypochloremia, hyponatremia) and dehydration resulting from excessive diuresis. If digitalis has also been administered, hypokalemia may accentuate cardiac arrhythmias. The degree to which hydrochlorothiazide is removed by hemodialysis has not been established.

DOSAGE AND ADMINISTRATION

The usual starting dose of losartan is 50 mg once daily, with 25 mg recommended for patients with intravascular volume depletion (e.g., patients treated with diuretics) (see WARNINGS, *Hypotension—Volume-Depleted Patients*) and patients with a history of hepatic impairment (see WARNINGS, *Impaired Hepatic Function*). Losartan can be administered once or twice daily at total daily doses of 25 to 100 mg. If the antihypertensive effect measured at trough using once-a-day dosing is inadequate, a twice-a-day regimen at the same total daily dose or an increase in dose may give a more satisfactory response.

Hydrochlorothiazide is effective in doses of 12.5 to 100 mg once daily and can be given at doses of 12.5 to 25 mg as HYZAAR.

To minimize dose-independent side effects, it is usually appropriate to begin combination therapy only after a patient has failed to achieve the desired effect with monotherapy.

The side effects (see WARNINGS) of losartan are generally rare and apparently independent of dose; those of hydrochlorothiazide are a mixture of dose-dependent (primarily hypokalemia) and dose-independent phenomena (e.g., pancreatitis), the former much more common than the latter. Therapy with any combination of losartan and hydrochlorothiazide will be associated with both sets of dose-independent side effects.

Replacement Therapy: The combination may be subtituted for the titrated components.

Dose Titration by Clinical Effect: A patient whose blood pressure is not adequately controlled with losartan monotherapy (see above) may be switched to HYZAAR (losartan 50 mg/hydrochlorothiazide 12.5 mg) once daily. If blood pressure remains uncontrolled after about 3 weeks of therapy, the dose may be increased to two tablets once daily.

A patient whose blood pressure is inadequately controlled by 25 mg once daily of hydrochlorothiazide, or is controlled but who experiences hypokalemia with this regimen, may be switched to HYZAAR (losartan 50 mg/hydrochlorothiazide 12.5 mg) once daily, reducing the dose of hydrochlorothiazide without reducing the overall expected antihypertensive response. The clinical response to HYZAAR should be subsequently evaluated and if blood pressure remains uncontrolled after about 3 weeks of therapy, the dose may be increased to two tablets once daily.

The usual dose of HYZAAR is one tablet once daily. More than two tablets once daily is not recommended. The maximal antihypertensive effect is attained about 3 weeks after initiation of therapy.

Use in Patients with Renal Impairment: The usual regimens of therapy with HYZAAR may be followed as long as the patient's creatinine clearance is > 30 mL/min. In patients with more severe renal impairment, loop diuretics are preferred to thiazides, so HYZAAR is not recommended.

Patients with Hepatic Impairment: HYZAAR is not recommended for titration in patients with hepatic impairment (see WARNINGS, *Impaired Hepatic Function*) because the appropriate 25 mg starting dose of losartan cannot be given.

HYZAAR may be administered with other antihypertensive agents.

HYZAAR may be administered with or without food.

HOW SUPPLIED

No. 3502—Tablets HYZAAR, 50-12.5 are yellow, teardrop shaped, film-coated tablets, coded MRK 717 on one side and HYZAAR on the other. Each tablet contains 50 mg of losartan potassium and 12.5 mg of hydrochlorothiazide. They are supplied as follows:

NDC 0006-0717-31 unit of use bottles of 30
NDC 0006-0717-54 unit of use bottles of 90
NDC 0006-0717-58 unit of use bottles of 100
(6505-01-416-4329, 50-12.5 100's).
NDC 0006-0717-28 unit dose packages of 100.

Storage

Store at controlled room temperature, 15–30°C (59–86°F). Keep container tightly closed. Protect from light.

Manufactured for:
MERCK & CO., INC., West Point, PA 19486, USA
by:
Du Pont Pharmaceuticals, Wilmington, DE 19880 USA
7892802 Issued April 1996

COPYRIGHT © MERCK & CO., Inc., 1995
All rights reserved.

Shown in Product Identification Guide, page 324

INDOCIN® Capsules, Oral Suspension and Suppositories (Indomethacin), U.S.P. ℞
INDOCIN® SR Capsules (Indomethacin), U.S.P. ℞

DESCRIPTION

INDOCIN* (Indomethacin) cannot be considered a simple analgesic and should not be used in conditions other than those recommended under INDICATIONS.

INDOCIN is supplied in four dosage forms. Capsules INDOCIN for oral administration contain either 25 mg or 50 mg of indomethacin and the following inactive ingredients: colloidal silicon dioxide, FD & C Blue 1, FD & C Red 3, gelatin, lactose, lecithin, magnesium stearate, and titanium dioxide. Capsules INDOCIN SR for sustained release oral administration contain 75 mg of indomethacin and the following inactive ingredients: cellulose, confectioner's sugar, FD & C Blue 1, FD & C Blue 2, FD & C Red 3, gelatin, hydroxypropyl methylcellulose, magnesium stearate, polyvinyl acetate-

Continued on next page

Information on the Merck & Co., Inc. products listed on these pages is the full prescribing information from product circulars in use September 30, 1996.

Merck & Co.—Cont.

crotonic acid copolymer, starch, and titanium dioxide. Capsules INDOCIN SR conform to the requirements of the USP Drug Release Test 1 for Indomethacin Extended-release Capsules. Suspension INDOCIN for oral use contains 25 mg of indomethacin per 5 mL, alcohol 1%, and sorbic acid 0.1% added as a preservative and the following inactive ingredients: antifoam AF emulsion, flavors, purified water, sodium hydroxide or hydrochloric acid to adjust pH, sorbitol solution, tragacanth. Suppositories INDOCIN for rectal use contain 50 mg of indomethacin and the following inactive ingredients: butylated hydroxyanisole, butylated hydroxytoluene, edetic acid, glycerin, polyethylene glycol 3350, polyethylene glycol 8000 and sodium chloride. Indomethacin is a non-steroidal anti-inflammatory indole derivative designated chemically as 1-(4-chlorobenzoyl)-5-methoxy-2-methyl-1*H*-indole-3-acetic acid. Indomethacin is practically insoluble in water and sparingly soluble in alcohol. It has a pKa of 4.5 and is stable in neutral or slightly acidic media and decomposes in strong alkali. The suspension has a pH of 4.0–5.0. The structural formula is:

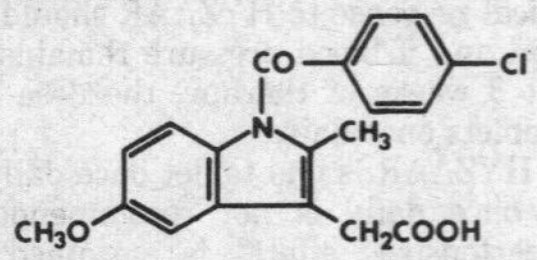

*Registered trademark of MERCK & CO., INC.

CLINICAL PHARMACOLOGY

INDOCIN is a non-steroidal drug with anti-inflammatory, antipyretic and analgesic properties. Its mode of action, like that of other anti-inflammatory drugs, is not known. However, its therapeutic action is not due to pituitary-adrenal stimulation.

INDOCIN is a potent inhibitor of prostaglandin synthesis *in vitro.* Concentrations are reached during therapy which have been demonstrated to have an effect *in vivo* as well. Prostaglandins sensitize afferent nerves and potentiate the action of bradykinin in inducing pain in animal models. Moreover, prostaglandins are known to be among the mediators of inflammation. Since indomethacin is an inhibitor of prostaglandin synthesis, its mode of action may be due to a decrease of prostaglandins in peripheral tissues.

INDOCIN has been shown to be an effective anti-inflammatory agent, appropriate for long-term use in rheumatoid arthritis, ankylosing spondylitis, and osteoarthritis.

INDOCIN affords relief of symptoms; it does not alter the progressive course of the underlying disease.

INDOCIN suppresses inflammation in rheumatoid arthritis as demonstrated by relief of pain, and reduction of fever, swelling and tenderness. Improvement in patients treated with INDOCIN for rheumatoid arthritis has been demonstrated by a reduction in joint swelling, average number of joints involved, and morning stiffness; by increased mobility as demonstrated by a decrease in walking time; and by improved functional capability as demonstrated by an increase in grip strength.

Indomethacin has been reported to diminish basal and CO_2 stimulated cerebral blood flow in healthy volunteers following acute oral and intravenous administration. In one study after one week of treatment with orally administered indomethacin, this effect on basal cerebral blood flow had disappeared. The clinical significance of this effect has not been established.

Capsules INDOCIN have been found effective in relieving the pain, reducing the fever, swelling, redness, and tenderness of acute gouty arthritis. Capsules INDOCIN rather than Capsules INDOCIN SR are recommended for treatment of acute gouty arthritis—see INDICATIONS.

Following single oral doses of Capsules INDOCIN 25 mg or 50 mg, indomethacin is readily absorbed, attaining peak plasma concentrations of about 1 and 2 mcg/mL, respectively, at about 2 hours. Orally administered Capsules INDOCIN are virtually 100% bioavailable, with 90% of the dose absorbed within 4 hours. A single 50 mg dose of Oral Suspension INDOCIN was found to be bioequivalent to a 50 mg INDOCIN capsule when each was administered with food.

Capsules INDOCIN SR 75 mg are designed to release 25 mg of the drug initially and the remaining 50 mg over approximately 12 hours (90% of dose absorbed by 12 hours). When measured over a 24-hour period, the cumulative amount and time-course of indomethacin absorption from a single Capsule INDOCIN SR are comparable to those of 3 doses of 25 mg Capsules INDOCIN given at 4–6 hour intervals.

Plasma concentrations of indomethacin fluctuate less and are more sustained following administration of Capsules INDOCIN SR than following administration of 25 mg Capsules INDOCIN given at 4–6 hour intervals. In multiple-dose comparisons, the mean daily steady-state plasma level of indomethacin attained with daily administration of Capsules INDOCIN SR 75 mg was indistinguishable from that following Capsules INDOCIN 25 mg given at 0, 6 and 12 hours daily. However, there was a significant difference in indomethacin plasma levels between the two dosage regimens especially after 12 hours.

Controlled clinical studies of safety and efficacy in patients with osteoarthritis have shown that one Capsule INDOCIN SR was clinically comparable to one 25 mg Capsule INDOCIN t.i.d.; and in controlled clinical studies in patients with rheumatoid arthritis, one Capsule INDOCIN SR taken in the morning and one in the evening were clinically indistinguishable from one 50 mg Capsule INDOCIN t.i.d.

Indomethacin is eliminated via renal excretion, metabolism, and biliary excretion. Indomethacin undergoes appreciable enterohepatic circulation. The mean half-life of indomethacin is estimated to be about 4.5 hours. With a typical therapeutic regimen of 25 or 50 mg t.i.d., the steady-state plasma concentrations of indomethacin are an average 1.4 times those following the first dose.

The rate of absorption is more rapid from the rectal suppository than from Capsules INDOCIN. Ordinarily, therefore, the total amount absorbed from the suppository would be expected to be at least equivalent to the capsule. In controlled clinical trials, however, the amount of indomethacin absorbed was found to be somewhat less (80–90%) than that absorbed from Capsules INDOCIN. This is probably because some subjects did not retain the material from the suppository for the one hour necessary to assure complete absorption. Since the suppository dissolves rather quickly rather than melting slowly, it is seldom recovered in recognizable form if the patient retains the suppository for more than a few minutes.

Indomethacin exists in the plasma as the parent drug and its desmethyl, desbenzoyl, and desmethyl-desbenzoyl metabolites, all in the unconjugated form. About 60 percent of an oral dosage is recovered in urine as drug and metabolites (26 percent as indomethacin and its glucuronide), and 33 percent is recovered in feces (1.5 percent as indomethacin).

About 99% of indomethacin is bound to protein in plasma over the expected range of therapeutic plasma concentrations. Indomethacin has been found to cross the blood-brain barrier and the placenta.

In a gastroscopic study in 45 healthy subjects, the number of gastric mucosal abnormalities was significantly higher in the group receiving Capsules INDOCIN than in the group taking Suppositories INDOCIN or placebo.

In a double-blind comparative clinical study involving 175 patients with rheumatoid arthritis, however, the incidence of upper gastrointestinal adverse effects with Suppositories or Capsules INDOCIN was comparable. The incidence of lower gastrointestinal adverse effects was greater in the suppository group.

INDICATIONS

Indomethacin has been found effective in active stages of the following:

1. Moderate to severe rheumatoid arthritis including acute flares of chronic disease.
2. Moderate to severe ankylosing spondylitis.
3. Moderate to severe osteoarthritis.
4. Acute painful shoulder (bursitis and/or tendinitis).
5. Acute gouty arthritis.

Capsules INDOCIN SR are recommended for all of the indications for Capsules INDOCIN except acute gouty arthritis.

INDOCIN may enable the reduction of steroid dosage in patients receiving steroids for the more severe forms of rheumatoid arthritis. In such instances the steroid dosage should be reduced slowly and the patients followed very closely for any possible adverse effects.

The use of INDOCIN in conjunction with aspirin or other salicylates is not recommended. Controlled clinical studies have shown that the combined use of INDOCIN and aspirin does not produce any greater therapeutic effect than the use of INDOCIN alone. Furthermore, in one of these clinical studies, the incidence of gastrointestinal side effects was significantly increased with combined therapy (see DRUG INTERACTIONS).

CONTRAINDICATIONS

INDOCIN should not be used in:

Patients who are hypersensitive to this product.

Patients in whom acute asthmatic attacks, urticaria, or rhinitis are precipitated by aspirin or other non-steroidal anti-inflammatory agents.

Suppositories INDOCIN are contraindicated in patients with a history of proctitis or recent rectal bleeding.

WARNINGS

General:

Because of the variability of the potential of INDOCIN to cause adverse reactions in the individual patient, the following are strongly recommended:

1. The lowest possible effective dose for the individual patient should be prescribed. Increased dosage tends to increase adverse effects, particularly in doses over 150–200 mg/day, without corresponding increase in clinical benefits.
2. Careful instructions to, and observations of, the individual patient are essential to the prevention of serious adverse reactions. As advancing years appear to increase the possibility of adverse reactions, INDOCIN should be used with greater care in the aged.
3. Effectiveness of INDOCIN in children has not been established. INDOCIN should not be prescribed for children 14 years of age and younger unless toxicity or lack of efficacy associated with other drugs warrants the risk.

   In experience with more than 900 children reported in the literature or to Merck Sharp and Dohme who were treated with Capsules INDOCIN, side effects in children were comparable to those reported in adults. Experience in children has been confined to the use of Capsules INDOCIN.

   If a decision is made to use indomethacin for children two years of age or older, such patients should be monitored closely and periodic assessment of liver function is recommended. There have been cases of hepatotoxicity reported in children with juvenile rheumatoid arthritis, including fatalities. If indomethacin treatment is instituted, a suggested starting dose is 2 mg/kg/day given in divided doses. Maximum daily dosage should not exceed 4 mg/kg/day or 150–200 mg/day, whichever is less. As symptoms subside, the total daily dosage should be reduced to the lowest level required to control symptoms, or the drug should be discontinued.
4. If Capsules INDOCIN SR are used for initial therapy or during dosage adjustment, observe the patient closely (see DOSAGE AND ADMINISTRATION).

Gastrointestinal Effects:

Single or multiple ulcerations, including perforation and hemorrhage of the esophagus, stomach, duodenum or small and large intestine, have been reported to occur with INDOCIN. Fatalities have been reported in some instances. Rarely, intestinal ulceration has been associated with stenosis and obstruction.

Gastrointestinal bleeding without obvious ulcer formation and perforation of pre-existing sigmoid lesions (diverticulum, carcinoma, etc.) have occurred. Increased abdominal pain in ulcerative colitis patients or the development of ulcerative colitis and regional ileitis have been reported to occur rarely.

Because of the occurrence, and at times severity, of gastrointestinal reactions to INDOCIN, the prescribing physician must be continuously alert for any sign or symptom signaling a possible gastrointestinal reaction. The risks of continuing therapy with INDOCIN in the face of such symptoms must be weighed against the possible benefits to the individual patient.

INDOCIN should not be given to patients with active gastrointestinal lesions or with a history of recurrent gastrointestinal lesions except under circumstances which warrant the very high risk and where patients can be monitored very closely.

The gastrointestinal effects may be reduced by giving Capsules INDOCIN or Capsules INDOCIN SR immediately after meals, with food, or with antacids.

Risk of GI Ulcerations, Bleeding and Perforation with NSAID Therapy

Serious gastrointestinal toxicity such as bleeding, ulceration, and perforation, can occur at any time, with or without warning symptoms, in patients treated chronically with NSAID therapy. Although minor upper gastrointestinal problems, such as dyspepsia, are common, usually developing early in therapy, physicians should remain alert for ulceration and bleeding in patients treated chronically with NSAIDs even in the absence of previous GI tract symptoms. In patients observed in clinical trials of several months to two years duration, symptomatic upper GI ulcers, gross bleeding or perforation appear to occur in approximately 1% of patients treated for 3–6 months, and in about 2–4% of patients treated for one year. Physicians should inform patients about the signs and/or symptoms of serious GI toxicity and what steps to take if they occur.

Studies to date have not identified any subset of patients not at risk of developing peptic ulceration and bleeding. Except for a prior history of serious GI events and other risk factors known to be associated with peptic ulcer disease, such as alcoholism, smoking, etc., no risk factors (e.g., age, sex) have been associated with increased risk. Elderly or debilitated patients seem to tolerate ulceration or bleeding less well than other individuals and most spontaneous reports of fatal GI events are in this population. Studies to date are inconclusive concerning the relative risk of various NSAIDs in causing such reactions. High doses of any NSAID probably carry a greater risk of these reactions, although controlled clinical trials showing this do not exist in most cases. In considering the use of relatively large doses (within the recommended dosage range), sufficient benefit should be anticipated to offset the potential increased risk of GI toxicity.

Renal Effects:

As with other non-steroidal anti-inflammatory drugs, long term administration of indomethacin to animals has resulted in renal papillary necrosis and other abnormal renal pathology. In humans, there have been reports of acute interstitial nephritis with hematuria, proteinuria, and occasionally nephrotic syndrome.

A second form of renal toxicity has been seen in patients with prerenal and renal conditions leading to a reduction in renal blood flow or blood volume, where the renal prostaglandins have a supportive role in the maintenance of renal perfusion. In these patients administration of an NSAID may cause a dose dependent reduction in prostaglandin formation and may precipitate overt renal decompensation. Patients at greatest risk of this reaction are those with conditions such as renal or hepatic dysfunction, diabetes mellitus, advanced age, extracellular volume depletion from any cause, congestive heart failure, septicemia, pyelonephritis, or concomitant use of any nephrotoxic drug. INDOCIN or other NSAIDs should be given with caution and renal function should be monitored in any patient who may have reduced renal reserve. Discontinuation of NSAID therapy is typically followed by recovery to the pretreatment state. Increases in serum potassium concentration, including hyperkalemia, have been reported, even in some patients without renal impairment. In patients with normal renal function, these effects have been attributed to a hyporeninemic-hypoaldosteronism state (see PRECAUTIONS, *Drug Interactions*).

Since INDOCIN is eliminated primarily by the kidneys, patients with significantly impaired renal function should be closely monitored; a lower daily dosage should be anticipated to avoid excessive drug accumulation.

Ocular Effects:

Corneal deposits and retinal disturbances, including those of the macula, have been observed in some patients who had received prolonged therapy with INDOCIN. The prescribing physician should be alert to the possible association between the changes noted and INDOCIN. It is advisable to discontinue therapy if such changes are observed. Blurred vision may be a significant symptom and warrants a thorough ophthalmological examination. Since these changes may be asymptomatic, ophthalmologic examination at periodic intervals is desirable in patients where therapy is prolonged.

Central Nervous System Effects:

INDOCIN may aggravate depression or other psychiatric disturbances, epilepsy, and parkinsonism, and should be used with considerable caution in patients with these conditions. If severe CNS adverse reactions develop, INDOCIN should be discontinued.

INDOCIN may cause drowsiness; therefore, patients should be cautioned about engaging in activities requiring mental alertness and motor coordination, such as driving a car. INDOCIN may also cause headache. Headache which persists despite dosage reduction requires cessation of therapy with INDOCIN.

Use in Pregnancy and the Neonatal Period

INDOCIN is not recommended for use in pregnant women, since safety for use has not been established. The known effects of indomethacin and other drugs of this class on the human fetus during the third trimester of pregnancy include: constriction of the ductus arteriosus prenatally, tricuspid incompetence, and pulmonary hypertension; nonclosure of the ductus arteriosus postnatally which may be resistant to medical management; myocardial degenerative changes, platelet dysfunction with resultant bleeding, intracranial bleeding, renal dysfunction or failure, renal injury/dysgenesis which may result in prolonged or permanent renal failure, oligohydramnios, gastrointestinal bleeding or perforation, and increased risk of necrotizing enterocolitis. Teratogenic studies were conducted in mice and rats at dosages of 0.5, 1.0, 2.0, and 4.0 mg/kg/day. Except for retarded fetal ossification at 4 mg/kg/day considered secondary to the decreased average fetal weights, no increase in fetal malformations was observed as compared with control groups. Other studies reported in the literature using higher doses (5 to 15 mg/kg/day) have described maternal toxicity and death, increased fetal resorptions, and fetal malformations. Comparable studies in rodents using high doses of aspirin have shown similar maternal and fetal effects.

As with other non-steroidal anti-inflammatory agents which inhibit prostaglandin synthesis, indomethacin has been found to delay parturition in rats.

In rats and mice, 4.0 mg/kg/day given during the last three days of gestation caused a decrease in maternal weight gain and some maternal and fetal deaths. An increased incidence of neuronal necrosis in the diencephalon in the live-born fetuses was observed. At 2.0 mg/kg/day, no increase in neuronal necrosis was observed as compared to the control groups. Administration of 0.5 or 4.0 mg/kg/day during the first three days of life did not cause an increase in neuronal necrosis at either dose level.

Use in Nursing Mothers

INDOCIN is excreted in the milk of lactating mothers. INDOCIN is not recommended for use in nursing mothers.

Incidence greater than 1%	Incidence less than 1%	
GASTROINTESTINAL		
nausea* with or without vomiting	anorexia	gastrointestinal bleeding without obvious ulcer formation and perforation of pre-existing sigmoid lesions (diverticulum, carcinoma, etc.)
dyspepsia* (including indigestion, heartburn and epigastric pain)	bloating (includes distention)	
	flatulence	
	peptic ulcer	
	gastroenteritis	
diarrhea	rectal bleeding	
abdominal distress or pain	proctitis	
constipation	single or multiple ulcerations, including perforation and hemorrhage of the esophagus, stomach, duodenum or small and large intestines	development of ulcerative colitis and regional ileitis
		ulcerative stomatitis
		toxic hepatitis and jaundice (some fatal cases have been reported)
	intestinal ulceration associated with stenosis and obstruction	intestinal strictures (diaphragms)
CENTRAL NERVOUS SYSTEM		
headache (11.7%)	anxiety (includes nervousness)	light-headedness
dizziness*		syncope
vertigo	muscle weakness	paresthesia
somnolence	involuntary muscle movements	aggravation of epilepsy and parkinsonism
depression and fatigue (including malaise and listlessness)	insomnia	depersonalization
	muzziness	coma
	psychic disturbances including psychotic episodes	peripheral neuropathy
		convulsions
		dysarthria
	mental confusion	
	drowsiness	
SPECIAL SENSES		
tinnitus	ocular—corneal deposits and retinal disturbances, including those of the macula, have been reported in some patients on prolonged therapy with INDOCIN	blurred vision
		diplopia
		hearing disturbances, deafness

PRECAUTIONS

General

Non-steroidal anti-inflammatory drugs, including INDOCIN, may mask the usual signs and symptoms of infection. Therefore, the physician must be continually on the alert for this and should use the drug with extra care in the presence of existing infection.

Fluid retention and peripheral edema have been observed in some patients taking INDOCIN. Therefore, as with other non-steroidal anti-inflammatory drugs, INDOCIN should be used with caution in patients with cardiac dysfunction, hypertension, or other conditions predisposing to fluid retention.

In a study of patients with severe heart failure and hyponatremia, INDOCIN was associated with significant deterioration of circulatory hemodynamics, presumably due to inhibition of prostaglandin dependent compensatory mechanisms. INDOCIN, like other non-steroidal anti-inflammatory agents, can inhibit platelet aggregation. This effect is of shorter duration than that seen with aspirin and usually disappears within 24 hours after discontinuation of INDOCIN. INDOCIN has been shown to prolong bleeding time (but within the normal range) in normal subjects. Because this effect may be exaggerated in patients with underlying hemostatic defects, INDOCIN should be used with caution in persons with coagulation defects.

As with other non-steroidal anti-inflammatory drugs, borderline elevations of one or more liver tests may occur in up to 15% of patients. These abnormalities may progress, may remain essentially unchanged, or may be transient with continued therapy. The SGPT (ALT) test is probably the most sensitive indicator of liver dysfunction. Meaningful (3 times the upper limit of normal) elevations of SGPT or SGOT (AST) occurred in controlled clinical trials in less than 1% of patients. A patient with symptoms and/or signs suggesting liver dysfunction, or in whom an abnormal liver test has occurred, should be evaluated for evidence of the development of more severe hepatic reaction while on therapy with INDOCIN. Severe hepatic reactions, including jaundice and cases of fatal hepatitis, have been reported with INDOCIN as with other non-steroidal anti-inflammatory drugs. Although such reactions are rare, if abnormal liver tests persist or worsen, if clinical signs and symptoms consistent with liver disease develop, or if systemic manifestations occur (e.g., eosinophilia, rash, etc.), INDOCIN should be discontinued.

Information for Patients

INDOCIN, like other drugs of its class, is not free of side effects. The side effects of these drugs can cause discomfort and, rarely, there are more serious side effects such as gastrointestinal bleeding, which may result in hospitalization and even fatal outcomes.

NSAIDs (Non-steroidal Anti-inflammatory Drugs) are often essential agents in the management of arthritis; but they also may be commonly employed for conditions which are less serious.

Physicians may wish to discuss with their patients the potential risks (see WARNINGS, PRECAUTIONS and ADVERSE REACTIONS) and likely benefits of NSAID treatment, particularly when the drugs are used for less serious conditions where treatment without NSAIDs may represent an acceptable alternative to both the patient and physician.

Laboratory Tests

Because serious GI tract ulceration and bleeding can occur without warning symptoms, physicians should follow chronically treated patients for the signs and symptoms of ulceration and bleeding and should inform them of the importance of this follow-up (see WARNINGS, *Risk of GI Ulcerations, Bleeding and Perforation with NSAID Therapy*).

Carcinogenesis, Mutagenesis, Impairment of Fertility

In an 81-week chronic oral toxicity study in the rat at doses up to 1 mg/kg/day, indomethacin had no tumorigenic effect. Indomethacin produced no neoplastic or hyperplastic changes related to treatment in carcinogenic studies in the rat (dosing period 73–110 weeks) and the mouse (dosing period 62–88 weeks) at doses up to 1.5 mg/kg/day.

Indomethacin did not have any mutagenic effect in *in vitro* bacterial tests (Ames test and *E. coli* with or without metabolic activation) and a series of *in vivo* tests including the host-mediated assay, sex-linked recessive lethals in *Drosophila*, and the micronucleus test in mice.

Indomethacin at dosage levels up to 0.5 mg/kg/day had no effect on fertility in mice in a two generation reproduction study or a two litter reproduction study in rats.

Continued on next page

Information on the Merck & Co., Inc. products listed on these pages is the full prescribing information from product circulars in use September 30, 1996.

Merck & Co.—Cont.

Drug Interactions

In normal volunteers receiving indomethacin, the administration of diflunisal decreased the renal clearance and significantly increased the plasma levels of indomethacin. In some patients, combined use of INDOCIN and diflunisal has been associated with fatal gastrointestinal hemorrhage. Therefore, diflunisal and INDOCIN should not be used concomitantly.

In a study in normal volunteers, it was found that chronic concurrent administration of 3.6 g of aspirin per day decreases indomethacin blood levels approximately 20%.

The concomitant use of INDOCIN with other NSAIDs is not recommended due to the increased possibility of gastrointestinal toxicity, with little or no increase in efficacy.

Clinical studies have shown that INDOCIN does not influence the hypoprothrombinemia produced by anticoagulants. However, when any additional drug, including INDOCIN, is added to the treatment of patients on anticoagulant therapy, the patients should be observed for alterations of the prothrombin time.

When INDOCIN is given to patients receiving probenecid, the plasma levels of indomethacin are likely to be increased. Therefore, a lower total daily dosage of INDOCIN may produce a satisfactory therapeutic effect. When increases in the dose of INDOCIN are made, they should be made carefully and in small increments.

Caution should be used if INDOCIN is administered simultaneously with methotrexate. INDOCIN has been reported to decrease the tubular secretion of methotrexate and to potentiate its toxicity.

Administration of non-steroidal anti-inflammatory drugs concomitantly with cyclosporine has been associated with an increase in cyclosporine-induced toxicity, possibly due to decreased synthesis of renal prostacyclin. NSAIDs should be used with caution in patients taking cyclosporine, and renal function should be monitored.

Capsules INDOCIN 50 mg t.i.d. produced a clinically relevant elevation of plasma lithium and reduction in renal lithium clearance in psychiatric patients and normal subjects with steady state plasma lithium concentrations. This effect has been attributed to inhibition of prostaglandin synthesis. As a consequence, when INDOCIN and lithium are given concomitantly, the patient should be carefully observed for signs of lithium toxicity. (Read circulars for lithium preparations before use of such concomitant therapy.) In addition, the frequency of monitoring serum lithium concentration should be increased at the outset of such combination drug treatment.

INDOCIN given concomitantly with digoxin has been reported to increase the serum concentration and prolong the half-life of digoxin. Therefore, when INDOCIN and digoxin are used concomitantly, serum digoxin levels should be closely monitored.

In some patients, the administration of INDOCIN can reduce the diuretic, natriuretic, and, antihypertensive effects of loop, potassium-sparing, and thiazide diuretics. Therefore, when INDOCIN and diuretics are used concomitantly, the patient should be observed closely to determine if the desired effect of the diuretic is obtained.

INDOCIN reduces basal plasma renin activity (PRA), as well as those elevations of PRA induced by furosemide administration, or salt or volume depletion. These facts should be considered when evaluating plasma renin activity in hypertensive patients.

It has been reported that the addition of triamterene to a maintenance schedule of INDOCIN resulted in reversible acute renal failure in two of four healthy volunteers. INDOCIN and triamterene should not be administered together. INDOCIN and potassium-sparing diuretics each may be associated with increased serum potassium levels. The potential effects of INDOCIN and potassium-sparing diuretics on potassium kinetics and renal function should be considered when these agents are administered concurrently.

Most of the above effects concerning diuretics have been attributed, at least in part, to mechanisms involving inhibition of prostaglandin synthesis by INDOCIN.

Blunting of the antihypertensive effect of beta-adrenoceptor blocking agents by non-steroidal anti-inflammatory drugs including INDOCIN has been reported. Therefore, when using these blocking agents to treat hypertension, patients should be observed carefully in order to confirm that the desired therapeutic effect has been obtained. There are reports that INDOCIN can reduce the antihypertensive effect of captopril in some patients.

False-negative results in the dexamethasone suppression test (DST) in patients being treated with INDOCIN have been reported. Thus, results of the DST should be interpreted with caution in these patients.

Pediatric Use

Effectiveness in children 14 years of age and younger has not been established (see WARNINGS).

Incidence greater than 1%	Incidence less than 1%
CARDIOVASCULAR	
none	hypertension / congestive heart failure
	hypotension / arrhythmia;
	tachycardia / palpitations
	chest pain	
METABOLIC	
none	edema / hyperglycemia
	weight gain / glycosuria
	fluid retention / hyperkalemia
	flushing or sweating	
INTEGUMENTARY	
none	pruritus / exfoliative dermatitis
	rash; urticaria / erythema nodosum
	petechiae or / loss of hair
	ecchymosis / Stevens-Johnson
	/ syndrome
	/ erythema multiforme
	/ toxic epidermal
	/ necrolysis
HEMATOLOGIC	
none	leukopenia / aplastic anemia
	bone marrow / hemolytic anemia
	depression / agranulocytosis
	anemia secondary / thrombocytopenic
	to obvious or / purpura
	occult / disseminated intravascular
	gastrointestinal / coagulation
	bleeding	
HYPERSENSITIVITY	
none	acute anaphylaxis / dyspnea
	acute respiratory / asthma
	distress / purpura
	rapid fall in blood / angiitis
	pressure / pulmonary edema
	resembling a / fever
	shock-like state	
	angioedema	
GENITOURINARY	
none	hematuria / BUN elevation
	vaginal bleeding / renal insufficiency,
	proteinuria / including renal
	nephrotic syndrome / failure
	interstitial nephritis	
MISCELLANEOUS	
none	epistaxis
	breast changes,
	including
	enlargement and
	tenderness, or
	gynecomastia

*Reactions occurring in 3% to 9% of patients treated with INDOCIN. (Those reactions occurring in less than 3% of the patients are unmarked.)

ADVERSE REACTIONS

The adverse reactions for Capsules INDOCIN listed in the following table have been arranged into two groups: (1) incidence greater than 1%; and (2) incidence less than 1%. The incidence for group (1) was obtained from 33 double-blind controlled clinical trials reported in the literature (1,092 patients). The incidence for group (2) was based on reports in clinical trials, in the literature, and on voluntary reports since marketing. The probability of a causal relationship exists between INDOCIN and these adverse reactions, some of which have been reported only rarely.

In controlled clinical trials, the incidence of adverse reactions to Capsules INDOCIN SR and equal 24-hour doses of Capsules INDOCIN were similar.

The adverse reactions reported with Capsules INDOCIN may occur with use of the suppositories. In addition, rectal irritation and tenesmus have been reported in patients who have received the suppositories.

The adverse reactions reported with Capsules INDOCIN may also occur with use of the suspension.

[See table at top of preceding page and above.]

Causal relationship unknown: Other reactions have been reported but occurred under circumstances where a causal relationship could not be established. However, in these rarely reported events, the possibility cannot be excluded. Therefore, these observations are being listed to serve as alerting information to physicians:

Cardiovascular: Thrombophlebitis

Hematologic: Although there have been several reports of leukemia, the supporting information is weak.

Genitourinary: Urinary frequency.

A rare occurrence of fulminant necrotizing fasciitis, particularly in association with Group A β-hemolytic streptococcus, has been described in persons treated with non-steroidal anti-inflammatory agents, including indomethacin, sometimes with fatal outcome (see also PRECAUTIONS, *General*).

OVERDOSAGE

The following symptoms may be observed following overdosage: nausea, vomiting, intense headache, dizziness, mental confusion, disorientation, or lethargy. There have been reports of paresthesias, numbness, and convulsions.

Treatment is symptomatic and supportive. The stomach should be emptied as quickly as possible if the ingestion is recent. If vomiting has not occurred spontaneously, the patient should be induced to vomit with syrup of ipecac. If the patient is unable to vomit, gastric lavage should be performed. Once the stomach has been emptied, 25 or 50 g of activated charcoal may be given. Depending on the condition of the patient, close medical observation and nursing care may be required. The patient should be followed for several days because gastrointestinal ulceration and hemorrhage have been reported as adverse reactions of indomethacin. Use of antacids may be helpful.

The oral LD_{50} of indomethacin in mice and rats (based on 14 day mortality response) was 50 and 12 mg/kg, respectively.

DOSAGE AND ADMINISTRATION

INDOCIN is available as 25 and 50 mg Capsules INDOCIN, 75 mg Capsules INDOCIN SR for oral use, Oral Suspension INDOCIN, containing 25 mg of indomethacin per 5 mL, and 50 mg Suppositories INDOCIN for rectal use. Capsules INDOCIN SR 75 mg once a day can be substituted for Capsules INDOCIN 25 mg t.i.d. However, there will be significant differences between the two dosage regimens in indomethacin blood levels, especially after 12 hours (see CLINICAL PHARMACOLOGY). In addition, Capsules INDOCIN SR 75 mg b.i.d. can be substituted for Capsules INDOCIN 50 mg t.i.d. Capsules INDOCIN SR may be substituted for all the indications for Capsules INDOCIN except acute gouty arthritis. Adverse reactions appear to correlate with the size of the dose of INDOCIN in most patients but not all. Therefore, every effort should be made to determine the smallest effective dosage for the individual patient.

Always give Capsules INDOCIN, Capsules INDOCIN SR, or Oral Suspension INDOCIN with food, immediately after meals, or with antacids to reduce gastric irritation.

Pediatric Use

INDOCIN ordinarily should not be prescribed for children 14 years of age and under (see WARNINGS).

Adult Use

Dosage Recommendations for Active Stages of the Following:

1. Moderate to severe rheumatoid arthritis including acute flares of chronic disease; moderate to severe ankylosing spondylitis; and moderate to severe osteoarthritis.
   Suggested Dosage:
   Capsules INDOCIN 25 mg b.i.d. or t.i.d. If this is well tolerated, increase the daily dosage by 25 or by 50 mg, if required by continuing symptoms, at weekly intervals until a satisfactory response is obtained or until a total daily dose of 150–200 mg is reached. DOSES ABOVE THIS AMOUNT GENERALLY DO NOT INCREASE THE EFFECTIVENESS OF THE DRUG.

In patients who have persistent night pain and/or morning stiffness, the giving of a large portion, up to a maximum of 100 mg, of the total daily dose at bedtime, either orally or by rectal suppositories, may be helpful in affording relief. The total daily dose should not exceed 200 mg. In acute flares of chronic rheumatoid arthritis, it may be necessary to increase the dosage by 25 mg or, if required, by 50 mg daily.

If Capsules INDOCIN SR 75 mg are used for initiating indomethacin treatment, one capsule daily should be the usual starting dose in order to observe patient tolerance since 75 mg per day is the maximum recommended starting dose for indomethacin (see above). If Capsules INDOCIN SR are used to increase the daily dose, patients should be observed for possible signs and symptoms of intolerance since the daily increment will exceed the daily increment recommended for the other dosage forms. For patients who require 150 mg of INDOCIN per day and have demonstrated acceptable tolerance, INDOCIN SR may be prescribed as one capsule twice daily.

If minor adverse effects develop as the dosage is increased, reduce the dosage rapidly to a tolerated dose and OBSERVE THE PATIENT CLOSELY.

If severe adverse reactions occur, STOP THE DRUG. After the acute phase of the disease is under control, an attempt to reduce the daily dose should be made repeatedly until the patient is receiving the smallest effective dose or the drug is discontinued.

Careful instructions to, and observations of, the individual patient are essential to the prevention of serious, irreversible, including fatal, adverse reactions.

As advancing years appear to increase the possibility of adverse reactions, INDOCIN should be used with greater care in the aged.

2. Acute painful shoulder (bursitis and/or tendinitis).
   Initial Dose:
   75–150 mg daily in 3 or 4 divided doses.
   The drug should be discontinued after the signs and symptoms of inflammation have been controlled for several days. The usual course of therapy is 7–14 days.
3. Acute gouty arthritis.
   Suggested Dosage:
   Capsules INDOCIN 50 mg t.i.d. until pain is tolerable. The dose should then be rapidly reduced to complete cessation of the drug. Definite relief of pain has been reported within 2 to 4 hours. Tenderness and heat usually subside in 24 to 36 hours, and swelling gradually disappears in 3 to 5 days.

HOW SUPPLIED

No. 3316—Capsules INDOCIN, 25 mg are opaque blue and white capsules, coded INDOCIN and MSD 25. They are supplied as follows:

NDC 0006-0025-68 bottles of 100
(6505-00-926-2154, 25 mg 100's)

NDC 0006-0025-82 bottles of 1000
(6505-00-931-0680, 25 mg 1000's).

Shown in Product Identification Guide, page 324

No. 3317—Capsules INDOCIN, 50 mg are opaque blue and white capsules, coded INDOCIN and MSD 50. They are supplied as follows:

NDC 0006-0050-68 bottles of 100.

Shown in Product Identification Guide, page 324

No. 3376—Oral Suspension INDOCIN, 25 mg per 5 mL, is an off-white suspension with a pineapple coconut mint flavor. It is supplied as follows:

NDC 0006-3376-66 in bottles of 237 mL.

No. 3370—Capsules INDOCIN SR, 75 mg each, are capsules with an opaque blue cap and clear body containing a mixture of blue and white pellets, coded INDOCIN SR and MSD 693. They are supplied as follows:

NDC 0006-0693-31 unit of use bottles of 30
(6505-01-135-7391, 75 mg 30's)

NDC 0006-0693-61 unit of use bottles of 60
(6505-01-137-4629, 75 mg 60's).

Shown in Product Identification Guide, page 324

No. 3354—Suppositories INDOCIN, 50 mg each, are white, opaque, rectal suppositories and are supplied as follows:

NDC 0006-0150-30, boxes of 30.

Shown in Product Identification Guide, page 324

Storage

Store Oral Suspension INDOCIN below 30°C (86°F). Avoid temperatures above 50°C (122°F). Protect from freezing. Store Suppositories INDOCIN below 30°C (86°F). Avoid transient temperatures above 40°C (104°F).

Suppositories INDOCIN are distributed by:
MERCK SHARP & DOHME, Division of Merck & Co., INC.
West Point, Pa. 19486

Manufactured by:
MERCK SHARP & DOHME
(Italia) S.p.A.
27100—Pavia, Italy

Capsules and Oral Suspension INDOCIN® and Capsules INDOCIN® SR are distributed and manufactured by:
MERCK SHARP & DOHME, Division of Merck & Co., INC.
West Point, Pa. 19486

7873324 Issued August 1995

COPYRIGHT © MERCK & CO., INC., 1988
All rights reserved

INDOCIN® I.V. ℞

(Indomethacin Sodium Trihydrate)

DESCRIPTION

Sterile INDOCIN* I.V. (Indomethacin Sodium Trihydrate) for intravenous administration is lyophilized indomethacin sodium trihydrate. Each vial contains indomethacin sodium trihydrate equivalent to 1 mg indomethacin as a white to yellow lyophilized powder or plug. Variations in the size of the lyophilized plug and the intensity of color have no relationship to the quality or amount of indomethacin present in the vial.

Indomethacin sodium trihydrate is designated chemically as 1-(4-chlorobenzoyl) -5- methoxy-2-methyl-1*H*-indole-3-acetic acid, sodium salt, trihydrate. Its molecular weight is 433.82. Its empirical formula is $C_{19}H_{15}ClNNaO_4 \cdot 3H_2O$ and its structural formula is:

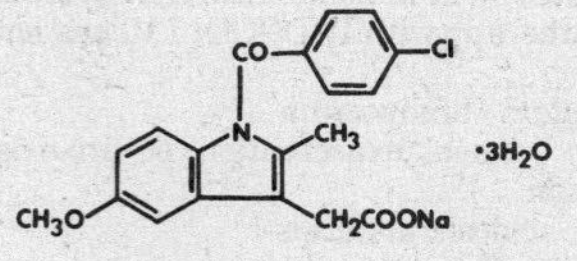

*Registered trademark of MERCK & CO., INC.

CLINICAL PHARMACOLOGY

Although the exact mechanism of action through which indomethacin causes closure of a patent ductus arteriosus is not known, it is believed to be through inhibition of prostaglandin synthesis. Indomethacin has been shown to be a potent inhibitor of prostaglandin synthesis, both *in vitro* and *in vivo*. In human newborns with certain congenital heart malformations, PGE 1 dilates the ductus arteriosus. In fetal and newborn lambs, E type prostaglandins have also been shown to maintain the patency of the ductus, and as in human newborns, indomethacin causes its constriction.

Studies in healthy young animals and in premature infants with patent ductus arteriosus indicated that, after the first dose of intravenous indomethacin, there was a transient reduction in cerebral blood flow velocity and cerebral blood flow. The clinical significance of this effect has not been established.

In double-blind placebo-controlled studies of INDOCIN I.V. in 460 small pre-term infants, weighing 1750 g or less, the infants treated with placebo had a ductus closure rate after 48 hours of 25 to 30 percent, whereas those treated with INDOCIN I.V. had a 75 to 80 percent closure rate. In one of these studies, a multicenter study, involving 405 pre-term infants, later re-opening of the ductus arteriosus occurred in 26 percent of infants treated with INDOCIN I.V., however, 70 percent of these closed subsequently without the need for surgery or additional indomethacin.

Pharmacokinetics and Metabolism

The disposition of indomethacin following intravenous administration (0.2 mg/kg) in pre-term neonates with patent ductus arteriosus has not been extensively evaluated. Even though the plasma half-life of indomethacin was variable among premature infants, it was shown to vary inversely with postnatal age and weight. In one study, of 28 infants who could be evaluated, the plasma half-life in those infants less than 7 days old averaged 20 hours (range: 3–60 hours, n = 18). In infants older than 7 days, the mean plasma half-life of indomethacin was 12 hours (range: 4–38 hours, n = 10). Grouping the infants by weight, mean plasma half-life in those weighing less than 1000 g was 21 hours (range: 9–60 hours, n = 10); in those infants weighing more than 1000 g, the mean plasma half-life was 15 hours (range: 3–52 hours, n = 18).

Following intravenous administration in adults, indomethacin is eliminated via renal excretion, metabolism, and biliary excretion. Indomethacin undergoes appreciable enterohepatic circulation. The mean plasma half-life of indomethacin is 4.5 hours. In the absence of enterohepatic circulation, it is 90 minutes. Indomethacin has been found to cross the blood-brain barrier and the placenta.

In adults, about 99 percent of indomethacin is bound to protein in plasma over the expected range of therapeutic plasma concentrations. The percent bound in neonates has not been studied. In controlled trials in premature infants, however, no evidence of bilirubin displacement has been observed as evidenced by increased incidence of bilirubin encephalopathy (kernicterus).

INDICATIONS AND USAGE

INDOCIN I.V. is indicated to close a hemodynamically significant patent ductus arteriosus in premature infants weighing between 500 and 1750 g when after 48 hours usual medical management (e.g., fluid restriction, diuretics, digitalis, respiratory support, etc.) is ineffective. Clear-cut clinical evidence of a hemodynamically significant patent ductus arteriosus should be present, such as respiratory distress, a continuous murmur, a hyperactive precordium, cardiomegaly and pulmonary plethora on chest x-ray.

CONTRAINDICATIONS

INDOCIN I.V. is contraindicated in: infants with proven or suspected infection that is untreated; infants who are bleeding, especially those with active intracranial hemorrhage or gastrointestinal bleeding; infants with thrombocytopenia; infants with coagulation defects; infants with or who are suspected of having necrotizing enterocolitis; infants with significant impairment of renal function; infants with congenital heart disease in whom patency of the ductus arteriosus is necessary for satisfactory pulmonary or systemic blood flow (e.g., pulmonary atresia, severe tetralogy of Fallot, severe coarctation of the aorta).

WARNINGS

Gastrointestinal Effects:

In the collaborative study, major gastrointestinal bleeding was no more common in those infants receiving indomethacin than in those infants on placebo. However, minor gastrointestinal bleeding (i.e., chemical detection of blood in the stool) was more commonly noted in those infants treated with indomethacin. Severe gastrointestinal effects have been reported in adults with various arthritic disorders treated chronically with oral indomethacin. [For further information, see package circular for Capsules INDOCIN* (Indomethacin)].

Central Nervous System Effects:

Prematurity per se, is associated with an increased incidence of spontaneous intraventricular hemorrhage. Because indomethacin may inhibit platelet aggregation, the potential for intraventricular bleeding may be increased. However, in the large multi-center study of INDOCIN I.V. (see CLINICAL PHARMACOLOGY), the incidence of intraventricular hemorrhage in babies treated with INDOCIN I.V. was not significantly higher than in the control infants.

Renal Effects:

INDOCIN I.V. may cause significant reduction in urine output (50 percent or more) with concomitant elevations of blood urea nitrogen and creatinine, and reductions in glomerular filtration rate and creatinine clearance. These effects in most infants are transient, disappearing with cessation of therapy with INDOCIN I.V. However, because adequate renal function can depend upon renal prostaglandin synthesis, INDOCIN I.V. may precipitate renal insuffi-

Continued on next page

Information on the Merck & Co., Inc. products listed on these pages is the full prescribing information from product circulars in use September 30, 1996.

Merck & Co.—Cont.

ciency, including acute renal failure, especially in infants with other conditions that may adversely affect renal function (e.g., extracellular volume depletion from any cause, congestive heart failure, sepsis, concomitant use of any nephrotoxic drug, hepatic dysfunction). When significant suppression of urine volume occurs after a dose of INDOCIN I.V., no additional dose should be given until the urine output returns to normal levels.

INDOCIN I.V. in pre-term infants may suppress water excretion to a greater extent than sodium excretion. When this occurs, a significant reduction in serum sodium values (i.e., hyponatremia) may result. Infants should have serum electrolyte determinations done during therapy with INDOCIN I.V. Renal function and serum electrolytes should be monitored (see PRECAUTIONS, *Drug Interactions* and DOSAGE AND ADMINISTRATION).

* Registered trademark of MERCK & CO., INC.

PRECAUTIONS

General

INDOCIN (Indomethacin) may mask the usual signs and symptoms of infection. Therefore, the physician must be continually on the alert for this and should use the drug with extra care in the presence of existing controlled infection.

Severe hepatic reactions have been reported in adults treated chronically with oral indomethacin for arthritic disorders. [For further information, see package circular for Capsules INDOCIN (Indomethacin)]. If clinical signs and symptoms consistent with liver disease develop in the neonate, or if systemic manifestations occur, INDOCIN I.V. should be discontinued.

INDOCIN I.V. may inhibit platelet aggregation. In one small study, platelet aggregation was grossly abnormal after indomethacin therapy (given orally to premature infants to close the ductus arteriosus). Platelet aggregation returned to normal by the tenth day. Premature infants should be observed for signs of bleeding.

The drug should be administered carefully to avoid extravascular injection or leakage as the solution may be irritating to tissue.

Drug Interactions

Since renal function may be reduced by INDOCIN I.V., consideration should be given to reduction in dosage of those medications that rely on adequate renal function for their elimination. Because the half-life of digitalis (given frequently to pre-term infants with patent ductus arteriosus and associated cardiac failure) may be prolonged when given concomitantly with indomethacin, the infant should be observed closely; frequent ECGs and serum digitalis levels may be required to prevent or detect digitalis toxicity early. Furthermore, in one study of premature infants treated with INDOCIN I.V. and also receiving either gentamicin or amikacin, both peak and trough levels of these aminoglycosides were significantly elevated.

Therapy with indomethacin may blunt the natriuretic effect of furosemide. This response has been attributed to inhibition of prostaglandin synthesis by non-steroidal anti-inflammatory drugs. In a study of 19 premature infants with patent ductus arteriosus treated with either INDOCIN I.V. alone or a combination of INDOCIN I.V. and furosemide, results showed that infants receiving both INDOCIN I.V. and furosemide had significantly higher urinary output, higher levels of sodium and chloride excretion, and higher glomerular filtration rates than did those infants receiving INDOCIN I.V. alone. In this study, the data suggested that therapy with furosemide helped to maintain renal function in the premature infant when INDOCIN I.V. was added to the treatment of patent ductus arteriosus.

Neonatal Effects

In rats and mice, oral indomethacin 4.0 mg/kg/day given during the last three days of gestation caused a decrease in maternal weight gain and some maternal and fetal deaths. An increased incidence of neuronal necrosis in the diencephalon in the live-born fetuses was observed. At 2.0 mg/kg/day, no increase in neuronal necrosis was observed as compared to the control groups. Administration of 0.5 or 4.0 mg/kg/day during the first three days of life did not cause an increase in neuronal necrosis at either dose level.

Pregnant rats, given 2.0 mg/kg/day and 4.0 mg/kg/day during the last trimester of gestation, delivered offspring whose pulmonary blood vessels were both reduced in number and excessively muscularized. These findings are similar to those observed in the syndrome of persistent pulmonary hypertension of the newborn.

ADVERSE REACTIONS

In a double-blind placebo-controlled trial of 405 premature infants weighing less than or equal to 1750 g with evidence of large ductal shunting, in those infants treated with indomethacin (n = 206), there was a statistically significantly greater incidence of bleeding problems, including gross or microscopic bleeding into the gastrointestinal tract, oozing from the skin after needle stick, pulmonary hemorrhage, and disseminated intravascular coagulopathy. There was no statistically significant difference between treatment groups with reference to intracranial hemorrhage.

The infants treated with indomethacin sodium trihydrate also had a significantly higher incidence of transient oliguria and elevations of serum creatinine (greater than or equal to 1.8 mg/dL) than did the infants treated with placebo.

The incidences of retrolental fibroplasia (grades III and IV) and pneumothorax in infants treated with INDOCIN I.V. were no greater than in placebo controls and were statistically significantly lower than in surgically-treated infants.

The following additional adverse reactions in infants have been reported from the collaborative study, anecdotal case reports, from other studies using rectal, oral, or intravenous indomethacin for treatment of patent ductus arteriosus or in marketed use. The rates are calculated from a database which contains experience of 849 indomethacin-treated infants reported in the medical literature, regardless of the route of administration. One year follow-up is available on 175 infants and shows no long-term sequelae which could be attributed to indomethacin. In controlled clinical studies, only electrolyte imbalance and renal dysfunction (of the reactions listed below) occurred statistically significantly more frequently after INDOCIN I.V. than after placebo. Reactions marked with a single asterick (*) occurred in 3–9 percent of indomethacin-treated infants: those marked with a double asterisk (**) occurred in 3–9 percent of both indomethacin- and placebo-treated infants. Unmarked reactions occurred in less than 3 percent of infants.

Renal: renal dysfunction in 41 percent of infants, including one or more of the following: reduced urinary output; reduced urine sodium, chloride, or potassium urine osmolality, free water clearance, or glomerular filtration, rate; elevated serum creatinine or BUN; uremia.

Cardiovascular: intracranial bleeding**, pulmonary hypertension.

Gastrointestinal: gastrointestinal bleeding*, vomiting, abdominal distention, transient ileus, localized perforation(s) of the small and/or large intestine.

Metabolic: hyponatremia*, elevated serum potassium*, reduction in blood sugar, including hypoglycemia, increased weight gain (fluid retention).

Coagulation: decreased platelet aggregation (see PRECAUTIONS).

The following adverse reactions have also been reported in infants treated with indomethacin, however, a causal relationship to therapy with INDOCIN I.V. has not been established:

Cardiovascular: bradycardia.

Respiratory: apnea, exacerbation of pre-existing pulmonary infection.

Metabolic: acidosis/alkalosis.

Hematologic: disseminated intravascular coagulation.

Gastrointestinal: necrotizing enterocolitis.

Ophthalmic: retrolental fibroplasia.**

A variety of additional adverse experiences have been reported in adults treated with oral indomethacin for moderate to severe rheumatoid arthritis, osteoarthritis, ankylosing spondylitis, acute painful shoulder and acute gouty arthritis (see section ADDITIONAL ADVERSE REACTIONS—ADULTS). Their relevance to the pre-term neonate receiving indomethacin for patent ductus arteriosus is unknown, however, the possibility exists that these experiences may be associated with the use of INDOCIN I.V. in pre-term neonates.

DOSAGE AND ADMINISTRATION

FOR INTRAVENOUS ADMINISTRATION ONLY.

Dosage recommendations for closure of the ductus arteriosus depends on the age of the infant at the time of therapy. A course of therapy is defined as three intravenous doses of INDOCIN I.V. given at 12–24 hour intervals, with careful attention to urinary output. If anuria or marked oliguria (urinary output < 0.6 mL/kg/hr) is evident at the scheduled time of the second or third dose of INDOCIN I.V., no additional doses should be given until laboratory studies indicate that renal function has returned to normal (see WARNINGS, *Renal Effects*).

Dosage according to age is as follows:

AGE at 1st dose	DOSAGE (mg/kg)		
	1st	2nd	3rd
Less than 48 hours	0.2	0.1	0.1
2–7 days	0.2	0.2	0.2
over 7 days	0.2	0.25	0.25

If the ductus arteriosus closes or is significantly reduced in size after an interval of 48 hours or more from completion of the first course of INDOCIN I.V., no further doses are necessary. If the ductus arteriosus re-opens, a second course of 1–3 doses may be given, each dose separated by a 12–24 hour interval as described above.

If the infant remains unresponsive to therapy with INDOCIN I.V. after 2 courses, surgery may be necessary for closure of the ductus arteriosus. If severe adverse reactions occur, STOP THE DRUG.

Directions for Use

Parenteral drug products should be inspected visually for particulate matter and discoloration prior to administration whenever solution and container permit.

The solution should be prepared only with 1 to 2 mL of preservative-free sterile Sodium Chloride Injection, 0.9 percent or preservative-free Sterile Water for Injection. Benzyl alcohol as a preservative has been associated with toxicity in newborns. Therefore, all diluents should be preservative-free. If 1 mL of diluent is used, the concentration of indomethacin in the solution will equal approximately 0.1 mg/0.1 mL; if 2 mL of diluent are used, the concentration of the solution will equal approximately 0.05 mg/0.1 mL. Any unused portion of the solution should be discarded because there is no preservative contained in the vial. A fresh solution should be prepared just prior to each administration. Once reconstituted, the indomethacin solution may be injected intravenously over 5–10 seconds.

Further dilution with intravenous infusion solutions is not recommended. INDOCIN I.V. is not buffered, and reconstitution with solutions at pH values below 6.0 may result in precipitation of the insoluble indomethacin free acid moiety.

HOW SUPPLIED

No. 3406—Sterile INDOCIN I.V. is a lyophilized white to yellow powder or plug supplied as single dose vials containing indomethacin sodium trihydrate, equivalent to 1 mg indomethacin.

NDC 0006-3406-17
(6505-01-209-1192, 3 single dose vials).

Storage

Store below 30°C (86°F). *Protect from light.* Store container in carton until contents have been used.

ADDITIONAL ADVERSE REACTIONS—ADULTS

The following adverse reactions have been reported in adults treated with oral indomethacin for moderate to severe rheumatoid arthritis, osteoarthritis, ankylosing spondylitis, acute painful shoulder and acute gouty arthritis. Complaints not of relevance in the treatment of the premature infant, such as anorexia, psychic disturbances, and blurred vision, are not listed.

Incidence 1% to 3%	Incidence less than 1%	
GASTROINTESTINAL		
diarrhea constipation	bloating (includes distention) flatulence peptic ulcer gastroenteritis rectal bleeding proctitis single or multiple ulcerations, including perforation and hemorrhage of the esophagus, stomach, duodenum or small and large intestines intestinal ulceration associated with stenosis and obstruction	gastrointestinal bleeding without obvious ulcer formation and perforation of pre-existing sigmoid lesions development of ulcerative stomatitis toxic hepatitis and jaundice (some fatal cases have been reported) intestinal strictures (diaphragms)
CENTRAL NERVOUS SYSTEM		
none	involuntary muscle movements	aggravation of epilepsy coma peripheral neuropathy convulsions
SPECIAL SENSES		
none	hearing disturbances, deafness	
CARDIOVASCULAR		
none	hypertension hypotension tachycardia	arrhythmia congestive heart failure thrombophlebitis
METABOLIC		
none	edema weight gain flushing	hyperglycemia glycosuria hyperkalemia

INTEGUMENTARY		
none	rash; urticaria	exfoliative dermatitis
	petechiae or	erythema nodosum
	ecchymosis	loss of hair
		Stevens-Johnson
		syndrome
		erythema multiforme
		toxic epidermal
		necrolysis
HEMATOLOGIC		
none	leukopenia	aplastic anemia
	bone marrow	hemolytic anemia
	depression	agranulocytosis
	anemia secondary to	thrombocytopenic
	obvious or occult	purpura
	gastrointestinal	
	bleeding	
HYPERSENSITIVITY		
none	acute anaphylaxis	dyspnea
	acute respiratory	asthma
	distress	purpura
	rapid fall in blood	angiitis
	pressure resembling	pulmonary edema
	a shock-like state	
GENITOURINARY		
none	hematuria	renal insufficiency,
	vaginal bleeding	including renal
		failure
MISCELLANEOUS		
none	epistaxis	
	breast changes,	
	including en-	
	largement and	
	tenderness, or	
	gynecomastia	

See package circular for Capsules INDOCIN (Indomethacin) for additional information concerning adverse reactions and other cautionary statements.

7414814   Issued August 1995

INVERSINE® Tablets ℞
(Mecamylamine HCl), U.S.P.

DESCRIPTION

INVERSINE* (Mecamylamine HCl) is a potent, oral antihypertensive agent and ganglion blocker, and is a secondary amine. It is $N,2,3,3$-tetramethylbicyclo[2.2.1] heptan-2-amine hydrochloride. Its empirical formula is $C_{11}H_{21}N \cdot HCl$ and its structural formula is:

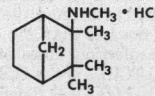

It is a white, odorless, or practically odorless, crystalline powder, is highly stable, soluble in water and has a molecular weight of 203.75.

INVERSINE is supplied as tablets for oral use, each containing 2.5 mg mecamylamine HCl. Inactive ingredients are acacia, calcium phosphate, D&C Yellow 10, FD&C Yellow 6, lactose, magnesium stearate, starch, and talc.

*Registered trademark of MERCK & CO., INC.

CLINICAL PHARMACOLOGY

Mecamylamine reduces blood pressure in both normotensive and hypertensive individuals. It has a gradual onset of action ($^1/_2$ to 2 hours) and a long-lasting effect (usually 6 to 12 hours or more). A small oral dosage often produces a smooth and predictable reduction of blood pressure. Although this antihypertensive effect is predominantly orthostatic, the supine blood pressure is also significantly reduced.

Pharmacokinetics and Metabolism
Mecamylamine is almost completely absorbed from the gastrointestinal tract, resulting in consistent lowering of blood pressure in most patients with hypertensive cardiovascular disease. Mecamylamine is excreted slowly in the urine in the unchanged form. The rate of its renal elimination is influenced markedly by urinary pH. Alkalinization of the urine reduces, and acidification promotes, renal excretion of mecamylamine.
Mecamylamine crosses the blood-brain and placental barriers.

INDICATIONS AND USAGE

For the management of moderately severe to severe essential hypertension and in uncomplicated cases of malignant hypertension.

CONTRAINDICATIONS

INVERSINE should not be used in mild, moderate, labile hypertension and may prove unsuitable in uncooperative patients. It is contraindicated in coronary insufficiency or recent myocardial infarction.
INVERSINE should be given with great discretion, if at all, when renal insufficiency is manifested by a rising or elevated BUN. The drug is contraindicated in uremia. Patients receiving antibiotics and sulfonamides should generally not be treated with ganglion blockers. Other contraindications are glaucoma, organic pyloric stenosis or hypersensitivity to the product.

WARNINGS

Mecamylamine, a secondary amine, readily penetrates into the brain and thus may produce central nervous sytem effects. Tremor, choreiform movements, mental aberrations, and convulsions may occur rarely. These have occurred most often when large doses of INVERSINE were used, especially in patients with cerebral or renal insufficiency.
When ganglion blockers or other potent antihypertensive drugs are discontinued suddenly, hypertensive levels return. In patients with malignant hypertension and others, this may occur abruptly and may cause fatal cerebral vascular accidents or acute congestive heart failure. When INVERSINE is withdrawn, this should be done gradually and other antihypertensive therapy usually must be substituted. On the other hand, the effects of INVERSINE sometimes may last from hours to days after therapy is discontinued.

PRECAUTIONS

General
The patient's condition should be evaluated carefully, particularly as to renal and cardiovascular function. When renal, cerebral, or coronary blood flow is deficient, any additional impairment, which might result from added hypotension, must be avoided. The use of INVERSINE in patients with marked cerebral and coronary arteriosclerosis or after a recent cerebral accident requires caution.
The action of INVERSINE may be potentiated by excessive heat, fever, infection, hemorrhage, pregnancy, anesthesia, surgery, vigorous exercise, other antihypertensive drugs, alcohol, and salt depletion as a result of diminished intake or increased excretion due to diarrhea, vomiting, excessive sweating, or diuretics.
During therapy with INVERSINE, sodium intake should not be restricted but, if necessary, the dosage of the ganglion blocker must be adjusted.
Since urinary retention may occur in patients on ganglion blockers, caution is required in patients with prostatic hypertrophy, bladder neck obstruction, and urethral stricture. Frequent loose bowel movements with abdominal distention and decreased borborygmi may be the first signs of paralytic ileus. If these are present, INVERSINE should be discontinued immediately and remedial steps taken.
Information for Patients
INVERSINE may cause dizziness, lightheadedness, or fainting, especially when rising from a lying or sitting position. This effect may be increased by alcoholic beverages, exercise, or during hot weather. Getting up slowly may help alleviate such a reaction.
Drug Interactions
Patients receiving antibiotics and sulfonamides generally should not be treated with ganglion blockers.
The action of INVERSINE may be potentiated by anesthesia, other antihypertensive drugs and alcohol.
Carcinogenesis, Mutagenesis, Impairment of Fertility
Long-term studies in animals have not been performed to evaluate the effects upon fertility, mutagenic or carcinogenic potential of INVERSINE.
Pregnancy
Pregnancy Category C. Animal reproduction studies have not been conducted with INVERSINE. It is not known whether INVERSINE can cause fetal harm when given to a pregnant woman or can affect reproductive capacity. INVERSINE should be given to a pregnant woman only if clearly needed.
Nursing Mothers
Because of the potential for serious adverse reactions in nursing infants from INVERSINE, a decision should be made whether to discontinue nursing or to discontinue the drug, taking into account the importance of the drug to the mother.

ADVERSE REACTIONS

The following adverse reactions have been reported and within each category are listed in order of decreasing severity.
Gastrointestinal: Ileus, constipation (sometimes preceded by small, frequent liquid stools), vomiting, nausea, anorexia, glossitis and dryness of mouth.

Cardiovascular: Orthostatic dizziness and syncope, postural hypotension.
Nervous System/Psychiatric: Convulsions, choreiform movements, mental aberrations, tremor, and paresthesias (see WARNINGS).
Respiratory: Interstitial pulmonary edema and fibrosis.
Urogenital: Urinary retention, impotence, decreased libido.
Special Senses: Blurred vision, dilated pupils.
Miscellaneous: Weakness, fatigue, sedation.

OVERDOSAGE

Signs of overdosage include: hypotension (which may progress to peripheral vascular collapse), postural hypotension, nausea, vomiting, diarrhea, constipation, paralytic ileus, urinary retention, dizziness, anxiety, dry mouth, mydriasis, blurred vision, or palpitations. A rise in intraocular pressure may occur.
Pressor amines may be used to counteract excessive hypotension. Since patients being treated with ganglion blockers are more than normally reactive to pressor amines, small doses of the latter are recommended to avoid excessive response. The oral LD_{50} of mecamylamine in the mouse is 92 mg/kg.

DOSAGE AND ADMINISTRATION

Therapy is usually started with one 2.5 mg tablet of INVERSINE twice a day. This initial dosage should be modified by increments of one 2.5 mg tablet at intervals of not less than 2 days until the desired blood pressure response occurs (the criterion being a dosage just under that which causes signs of mild postural hypotension).
The average total daily dosage of INVERSINE is 25 mg, usually in three divided doses. However, as little as 2.5 mg daily may be sufficient to control hypertension in some patients. A range of two to four or even more doses may be required in severe cases when smooth control is difficult to obtain. In severe or urgent cases, larger increments at smaller intervals may be needed. Partial tolerance may develop in certain patients, requiring an increase in the daily dosage of INVERSINE.
Administration of INVERSINE after meals may cause a more gradual absorption and smoother control of excessively high blood pressure. The timing of doses in relation to meals should be consistent. Since the blood pressure response to antihypertensive drugs is increased in the early morning, the larger dose should be given at noontime and perhaps in the evening. The morning dose, as a rule, should be relatively small and in some instances may even be omitted.
The *initial regulation of dosage* should be determined by blood pressure readings in the erect position at the time of maximal effect of the drug, as well as by other signs and symptoms of orthostatic hypotension.
The *effective maintenance dosage* should be regulated by blood pressure readings in the erect position and by limitation of dosage to that which causes slight faintness or dizziness in this position. If the patient or a relative can use a sphygmomanometer, instructions may be given to reduce or omit a dose if readings fall below a designated level or if faintness or lightheadedness occurs. However, *no change should be instituted without the knowledge of the physician.* Close supervision and education of the patient, as well as critical adjustment of dosage, are essential to successful therapy.
Other Antihypertensive Agents
When INVERSINE is given with other antihypertensive drugs, the dosage of these other agents, as well as that of INVERSINE, should be reduced to avoid excessive hypotension. However, thiazides should be continued in their usual dosage, while that of INVERSINE is decreased by at least 50 percent.

HOW SUPPLIED

No. 3219—Tablets INVERSINE, 2.5 mg, are yellow, round, scored, compressed tablets, coded MSD 52. They are supplied as follows:
NDC 0006-0052-68 in bottles of 100.
Shown in Product Identification Guide, page 324
7898722   Issued March 1994

Continued on next page

Merck & Co.—Cont.

LACRISERT® Sterile Ophthalmic Insert ℞
(Hydroxypropyl Cellulose), U.S.P.

DESCRIPTION

LACRISERT* (Hydroxypropyl Cellulose) is a sterile, translucent, rod-shaped, water soluble, ophthalmic insert made of hydroxypropyl cellulose, for administration into the inferior cul-de-sac of the eye.

The chemical name for hydroxypropyl cellulose is cellulose, 2-hydroxypropyl ether. It is an ether of cellulose in which hydroxypropyl groups ($-CH_2CHOHCH_3$) are attached to the hydroxyls present in the anhydroglucose rings of cellulose by ether linkages. A representative structure of the monomer is:

$$R=CH_2CHCH_3$$
$$OH$$

The molecular weight is typically 1×10^6.

Hydroxypropyl cellulose is an off-white, odorless, tasteless powder. It is soluble in water below 38°C, and in many polar organic solvents such as ethanol, propylene glycol, dioxane, methanol, isopropyl alcohol (95%), dimethyl sulfoxide, and dimethyl formamide.

Each LACRISERT is 5 mg of hydroxypropyl cellulose. LACRISERT contains no preservatives or other ingredients. It is about 1.27 mm in diameter by about 3.5 mm long. LACRISERT is supplied in packages of 60 units, together with illustrated instructions and a special applicator for removing LACRISERT from the unit dose blister and inserting it into the eye. A spare applicator is included in each package.

*Registered trademark of MERCK & CO., INC.

CLINICAL PHARMACOLOGY

Pharmacodynamics

LACRISERT acts to stabilize and thicken the precorneal tear film and prolong the tear film breakup time which is usually accelerated in patients with dry eye states. LACRISERT also acts to lubricate and protect the eye. LACRISERT usually reduces the signs and symptoms resulting from moderate to severe dry eye syndromes, such as conjunctival hyperemia, corneal and conjunctival staining with rose bengal, exudation, itching, burning, foreign body sensation, smarting, photophobia, dryness and blurred or cloudy vision. Progressive visual deterioration which occurs in some patients may be retarded, halted, or sometimes reversed.

In a multicenter crossover study the 5 mg LACRISERT administered once a day during the waking hours was compared to artificial tears used four or more times daily. There was a prolongation of tear film breakup time and a decrease in foreign body sensation associated with dry eye syndrome in patients during treatment with inserts as compared to artificial tears; these findings were statistically significantly different between the treatment groups. Improvement, as measured by amelioration of symptoms, by slit-lamp examination and by rose bengal staining of the cornea and conjunctiva, was greater in most patients with moderate to severe symptoms during treatment with LACRISERT. Patient comfort was usually better with LACRISERT than with artificial tears solution, and most patients preferred LACRISERT.

In most patients treated with LACRISERT for over one year, improvement was observed as evidenced by amelioration of symptoms generally associated with keratoconjunctivitis sicca such as burning, tearing, foreign body sensation, itching, photophobia and blurred or cloudy vision.

During studies in healthy volunteers, a thickened precorneal tear film was usually observed through the slit-lamp while LACRISERT was present in the conjunctival sac.

Pharmacokinetics and Metabolism

Hydroxypropyl cellulose is a physiologically inert substance. In a study of rats fed hydroxypropyl cellulose or unmodified cellulose at levels up to 5% of their diet, it was found that the two were biologically equivalent in that neither was metabolized.

Studies conducted in rats fed ^{14}C-labeled hydroxypropyl cellulose demonstrated that when orally administered, hydroxypropyl cellulose is not absorbed from the gastrointestinal tract and is quantitatively excreted in the feces.

Dissolution studies in rabbits showed that hydroxypropyl cellulose inserts became softer within 1 hour after they were placed in the conjunctival sac. Most of the inserts dissolved completely in 14 to 18 hours; with a single exception, all had disappeared by 24 hours after insertion. Similar dissolution of the inserts was observed during prolonged administration (up to 54 weeks).

INDICATIONS AND USAGE

LACRISERT is indicated in patients with moderate to severe dry eye syndromes, including keratoconjunctivitis sicca. LACRISERT is indicated especially in patients who remain symptomatic after an adequate trial of therapy with artificial tear solutions.

LACRISERT is also indicated for patients with:
Exposure keratitis
Decreased corneal sensitivity
Recurrent corneal erosions

CONTRAINDICATIONS

LACRISERT is contraindicated in patients who are hypersensitive to hydroxypropyl cellulose.

WARNINGS

Instructions for inserting and removing LACRISERT should be carefully followed.

PRECAUTIONS

General

If improperly placed, LACRISERT may result in corneal abrasion (see DOSAGE AND ADMINISTRATION).

Information for Patients

Patients should be advised to follow the instructions for using LACRISERT which accompany the package.

Because this product may produce transient blurring of vision, patients should be instructed to exercise caution when operating hazardous machinery or driving a motor vehicle.

Drug Interactions

Application of hydroxypropyl cellulose inserts to the eyes of unanesthetized rabbits immediately prior to or two hours before instilling pilocarpine, proparacaine HCl (0.5%), or phenylephrine (5%) did not markedly alter the magnitude and/or duration of the miotic, local corneal anesthetic, or mydriatic activity, respectively, of these agents.

Under various treatment schedules, the anti-inflammatory effect of ocularly instilled dexamethasone (0.1%) in unanesthetized rabbits with primary uveitis was not affected by the presence of hydroxypropyl cellulose inserts.

Carcinogenesis, Mutagenesis, Impairment of Fertility

Feeding of hydroxypropyl cellulose to rats at levels up to 5% of their diet produced no gross or histopathologic changes or other deleterious effects.

ADVERSE REACTIONS

The following adverse reactions have been reported in patients treated with LACRISERT, but were in most instances mild and transient:

Transient blurring of vision (See PRECAUTIONS)
Ocular discomfort or irritation
Matting or stickiness of eyelashes
Photophobia
Hypersensitivity
Edema of the eyelids
Hyperemia

DOSAGE AND ADMINISTRATION

One LACRISERT ophthalmic insert in each eye once daily is usually sufficient to relieve the symptoms associated with moderate to severe dry eye syndromes. Individual patients may require more flexibility in the use of LACRISERT; some patients may require twice daily use for optimal results.

Clinical experience with LACRISERT indicates that in some patients several weeks may be required before satisfactory improvement of symptoms is achieved.

LACRISERT is inserted into the inferior cul-de-sac of the eye beneath the base of the tarsus, not in apposition to the cornea, nor beneath the eyelid at the level of the tarsal plate. If not properly positioned, it will be expelled into the interpalpebral fissure, and may cause symptoms of a foreign body. Illustrated instructions are included in each package. While in the licensed practitioner's office, the patient should read the instructions, then practice insertion and removal of LACRISERT until proficiency is achieved.

NOTE: Occasionally LACRISERT is inadvertently expelled from the eye, especially in patients with shallow conjunctival fornices. The patient should be cautioned against rubbing the eye(s) containing LACRISERT, especially upon awakening, so as not to dislodge or expel the insert. If re-

quired, another LACRISERT ophthalmic insert may be inserted. If experience indicates that transient blurred vision develops in an individual patient, the patient may want to remove LACRISERT a few hours after insertion to avoid this. Another LACRISERT ophthalmic insert may be inserted if needed.

If LACRISERT causes worsening of symptoms, the patient should be instructed to inspect the conjunctival sac to make certain LACRISERT is in the proper location, deep in the inferior cul-de-sac of the eye beneath the base of the tarsus. If these symptoms persist, LACRISERT should be removed and the patient should contact the practitioner.

HOW SUPPLIED

No. 3380—LACRISERT, a sterile, translucent, rod-shaped, water soluble, ophthalmic insert made of hydroxypropyl cellulose, 5 mg, is supplied as follows:

NDC 0006-3380-60 in packages containing 60 unit doses, two reusable applicators and a storage container.
(6505-01-153-4360, 5 mg 60's).

Storage

Store below 30°C (86°F).

7415109   Issued August 1989

COPYRIGHT © MERCK & CO., INC., 1988
All rights reserved

M–M–R®II ℞
(Measles, Mumps, and Rubella Virus Vaccine
Live), U.S.P.

DESCRIPTION

M-M-R* II (Measles, Mumps, and Rubella Virus Vaccine Live) is a live virus vaccine for immunization against measles (rubeola), mumps and rubella (German measles).

M-M-R II is a sterile lyophilized preparation of (1) ATTENUVAX* (Measles Virus Vaccine Live), a more attenuated line of measles virus, derived from Enders' attenuated Edmonston strain and grown in cell cultures of chick embryo; (2) MUMPSVAX* (Mumps Virus Vaccine Live), the Jeryl Lynn (B level) strain of mumps virus grown in cell cultures of chick embryo; and (3) MERUVAX* II (Rubella Virus Vaccine Live), the Wistar RA 27/3 strain of live attenuated rubella virus grown in human diploid cell (WI-38) culture. The vaccine viruses are the same as those used in the manufacture of ATTENUVAX (Measles Virus Vaccine Live), MUMPSVAX (Mumps Virus Vaccine Live) and MERUVAX II (Rubella Virus Vaccine Live). The three viruses are mixed before being lyophilized. The product contains no preservative.

The reconstituted vaccine is for subcutaneous administration. When reconstituted as directed, the dose for injection is 0.5 mL and contains not less than the equivalent of 1,000 $TCID_{50}$ (tissue culture infectious doses) of the U.S. Reference Measles Virus; 20,000 $TCID_{50}$ of the U.S. Reference Mumps Virus; and 1,000 $TCID_{50}$ of the U.S. Reference Rubella Virus. Each dose contains approximately 25 mcg of neomycin. The product contains no preservative. Sorbitol and hydrolyzed gelatin are added as stabilizers.

* Registered trademark of MERCK & CO., INC.

CLINICAL PHARMACOLOGY

Clinical studies of 279 triple seronegative children, 11 months to 7 years of age, demonstrated that M-M-R II is highly immunogenic and generally well tolerated. In these studies, a single injection of the vaccine induced measles hemagglutination-inhibition (HI) antibodies in 95 percent, mumps neutralizing antibodies in 96 percent, and rubella HI antibodies in 99 percent of susceptible persons.

The RA 27/3 rubella strain in M-M-R II elicits higher immediate post-vaccination HI, complement-fixing and neutralizing antibody levels than other strains of rubella vaccine and has been shown to induce a broader profile of circulating antibodies including anti-theta and anti-iota precipitating antibodies. The RA 27/3 rubella strain immunologically simulates natural infection more closely than other rubella vaccine viruses. The increased levels and broader profile of antibodies produced by RA 27/3 strain rubella virus vaccine appear to correlate with greater resistance to subclinical reinfection with the wild virus, and provide greater confidence for lasting immunity.

Vaccine induced antibody levels following administration of M-M-R II have been shown to persist up to 11 years without substantial decline. Continued surveillance will be necessary to determine further duration of antibody persistence.

INDICATIONS AND USAGE

M-M-R II is indicated for simultaneous immunization against measles, mumps, and rubella in persons 15 months of

age or older. A second dose of M-M-R II or monovalent measles vaccine is recommended (see *Revaccination*).

Infants who are less than 15 months of age may fail to respond to the measles component of the vaccine due to presence in the circulation of residual measles antibody of maternal origin, the younger the infant, the lower the likelihood of seroconversion. In geographically isolated or other relatively inaccessible populations for whom immunization programs are logistically difficult, and in population groups in which natural measles infection may occur in a significant proportion of infants before 15 months of age, it may be desirable to give the vaccine to infants at an earlier age. Infants vaccinated under these conditions at less than 12 months of age should be revaccinated after reaching 15 months of age. There is some evidence to suggest that infants immunized at less than one year of age may not develop sustained antibody levels when later reimmunized. The advantage of early protection must be weighed against the chance for failure to respond adequately on reimmunization.

Previously unimmunized children of susceptible pregnant women should receive live attenuated rubella vaccine, because an immunized child will be less likely to acquire natural rubella and introduce the virus into the household.

Individuals planning travel outside the United States, if not immune, can acquire measles, mumps or rubella and import these diseases to the United States. Therefore, prior to International travel, individuals known to be susceptible to one or more of these diseases can receive either a single antigen vaccine (measles, mumps or rubella), or a combined antigen vaccine as appropriate. However, M-M-R II is preferred for persons likely to be susceptible to mumps and rubella; and if single-antigen measles vaccine is not readily available, travelers should receive M-M-R II regardless of their immune status to mumps or rubella.

Non-Pregnant Adolescent and Adult Females
Immunization of susceptible non-pregnant adolescent and adult females of childbearing age with live attenuated rubella virus vaccine is indicated if certain precautions are observed (see below and PRECAUTIONS). Vaccinating susceptible postpubertal females confers individual protection against subsequently acquiring rubella infection during pregnancy, which in turn prevents infection of the fetus and consequent congenital rubella injury.

Women of childbearing age should be advised not to become pregnant for three months after vaccination and should be informed of the reasons for this precaution.*

It is recommended that rubella susceptibility be determined by serologic testing prior to immunization.** If immune, as evidenced by a specific rubella antibody titer of 1:8 or greater (hemagglutination-inhibition test), vaccination is unnecessary. Congenital malformations do occur in up to seven percent of all live births. Their chance appearance after vaccination could lead to misinterpretation of the cause, particularly if the prior rubella-immune status of vaccinees is unknown.

Postpubertal females should be informed of the frequent occurrence of generally self-limited arthralgia and/or arthritis beginning 2 to 4 weeks after vaccination (see ADVERSE REACTIONS).

Postpartum Women
It has been found convenient in many instances to vaccinate rubella-susceptible women in the immediate postpartum period. (See *Nursing Mothers*).

Revaccination: Children first vaccinated when younger than 12 months of age should be revaccinated at 15 months of age.

The American Academy of Pediatrics (AAP), the Immunization Practices Advisory Committee (ACIP), and some state and local health agencies have recommended guidelines for routine measles revaccination and to help control measles outbreaks.†

Vaccines available for revaccination include monovalent measles vaccine [ATTENUVAX (Measles Virus Vaccine Live)] and polyvalent vaccines containing measles [e.g., M-M-R II, M-R-VAX‡ II (Measles and Rubella Virus Vaccine Live)]. If the prevention of sporadic measles outbreaks is the sole objective, revaccination with a monovalent measles vaccine should be considered (see appropriate product circular). If concern also exists about immune status regarding mumps or rubella, revaccination with appropriate monovalent or polyvalent vaccine should be considered after consulting the appropriate product circulars. Unnecessary doses of a vaccine are best avoided by ensuring that written documentation of vaccination is preserved and a copy given to each vaccinee's parent or guardian.

Use with other Vaccines
Routine administration of DTP (diphtheria, tetanus, pertussis) and/or OPV (oral poliovirus vaccine) concomitantly with measles, mumps, and rubella vaccines is not recommended because there are limited data relating to the simultaneous administration of these antigens. M-M-R II should be given one month before or after administration of other vaccines. However, other schedules have been used. For example, the American Academy of Pediatrics has noted that when the patient may not return, some practitioners prefer to administer DTP, OPV, and M-M-R II on a single day. If done, separate sites and syringes should be used for DTP and M-M-R II. The Immunization Practices Advisory Committee (ACIP) recommends routine simultaneous administration of M-M-R II, DTP and OPV or inactivated polio vaccine (IPV) to all children ≥ 15 months who are eligible to receive these vaccines on the basis that there are equivalent antibody responses and no clinically significant increases in the frequency of adverse events when DTP, M-M-R II and OPV or IPV are administered either simultaneously at different sites or separately.†† Administration of M-M-R II at 15 months followed by DTP and OPV (or IPV) at 18 months remains an acceptable alternative, especially for children with caregivers known to be generally compliant with other health-care recommendations.

---

*NOTE: The Immunization Practices Advisory Committee (ACIP) has recommended "In view of the importance of protecting this age group against rubella, reasonable precautions in a rubella immunization program include asking females if they are pregnant, excluding those who say they are, and explaining the theoretical risks to the others."

**NOTE: The Immunization Practices Advisory Committee (ACIP) has stated "When practical, and when reliable laboratory services are available, potential vaccinees of childbearing age can have serologic tests to determine susceptibility to rubella. . . . However, routinely performing serologic tests for all females of childbearing age to determine susceptibility so that vaccine is given only to proven susceptibles is expensive and has been ineffective in some areas. Accordingly, the ACIP believes that rubella vaccination of a woman who is not known to be pregnant and has no history of vaccination is justifiable without serologic testing."

†NOTE: A primary difference among these recommendations is the timing of revaccination: the ACIP recommends routine revaccination at entry into kindergarten or first grade, whereas the AAP recommends routine revaccination at entrance to middle school or junior high school. In addition, some public health jurisdictions mandate the age for revaccination. The complete text of applicable guidelines should be consulted.

††NOTE: The Immunization Practices Advisory Committee (ACIP) recommends administering M-M-R II concomitantly with the fourth dose of DTP and the third dose of OPV to children 15 months of age or older providing that 6 months have elapsed since DTP-3; or, if fewer than three DTPs have been received, at least 6 weeks have elapsed since the last dose of DTP and OPV.

‡Registered trademark of MERCK & CO., INC.

CONTRAINDICATIONS

Do not give M-M-R II to pregnant females; the possible effects of the vaccine on fetal development are unknown at this time. If vaccination of postpubertal females is undertaken, pregnancy should be avoided for three months following vaccination. (See PRECAUTIONS, *Pregnancy*).

Anaphylactic or anaphylactoid reactions to neomycin (each dose of reconstituted vaccine contains approximately 25 mcg of neomycin).

History of anaphylactic or anaphylactoid reactions to eggs (see HYPERSENSITIVITY TO EGGS below).

Any febrile respiratory illness or other active febrile infection.

Active untreated tuberculosis.

Patients receiving immunosuppressive therapy. This contraindication does not apply to patients who are receiving corticosteroids as replacement therapy, e.g., for Addison's disease.

Individuals with blood dyscrasias, leukemia, lymphomas of any type, or other malignant neoplasms affecting the bone marrow or lymphatic systems.

Primary and acquired immunodeficiency states, including patients who are immunosuppressed in association with AIDS or other clinical manifestations of infection with human immunodeficiency viruses; cellular immune deficiencies; and hypogammaglobulinemic and dysgammaglobulinemic states.

Individuals with a family history of congenital or hereditary immunodeficiency, until the immune competence of the potential vaccine recipient is demonstrated.

HYPERSENSITIVITY TO EGGS

Live measles vaccine and live mumps vaccine are produced in chick embryo cell culture. Persons with a history of anaphylactic, anaphylactoid, or other immediate reactions (e.g., hives, swelling of the mouth and throat, difficulty breathing, hypotension, or shock) subsequent to egg ingestion should not be vaccinated. Evidence indicates that persons are not at increased risk if they have egg allergies that are not anaphylactic or anaphylactoid in nature. Such persons may be vaccinated in the usual manner. There is no evidence to indicate that persons with allergies to chickens or feathers are at increased risk of reaction to the vaccine.

PRECAUTIONS

General
Adequate treatment provisions including epinephrine, should be available for immediate use should an anaphylactic or anaphylactoid reaction occur.

Due caution should be employed in administration of M-M-R II to persons with a history of cerebral injury, individual or family histories of convulsions, or any other condition in which stress due to fever should be avoided. The physician should be alert to the temperature elevation which may occur following vaccination. (See ADVERSE REACTIONS).

Children and young adults who are known to be infected with human immunodeficiency viruses but without overt clinical manifestations of immunosuppression may be vaccinated; however, the vaccinees should be monitored closely for vaccine-preventable diseases because immunization may be less effective than for uninfected persons.

Vaccination should be deferred for at least 3 months following blood or plasma transfusions, or administration of human immune serum globulin.

Excretion of small amounts of the live attenuated rubella virus from the nose or throat has occurred in the majority of susceptible individuals 7–28 days after vaccination. There is no confirmed evidence to indicate that such virus is transmitted to susceptible persons who are in contact with the vaccinated individuals. Consequently, transmission through close personal contact, while accepted as a theoretical possibility, is not regarded as a significant risk. However, transmission of the rubella vaccine virus to infants via breast milk has been documented (see *Nursing Mothers*).

There are no reports of transmission of live attenuated measles or mumps viruses from vaccinees to susceptible contacts. It has been reported that live attenuated measles, mumps and rubella virus vaccines given individually may result in a temporary depression of tuberculin skin sensitivity. Therefore, if a tuberculin test is to be done, it should be administered either before or simultaneously with M-M-R II.

Children under treatment for tuberculosis have not experienced exacerbation of the disease when immunized with live measles virus vaccine; no studies have been reported to date of the effect of measles virus vaccines on untreated tuberculous children.

As for any vaccine, vaccination with M-M-R II may not result in seroconversion in 100% of susceptible persons given the vaccine.

Pregnancy
Pregnancy Category C
Animal reproduction studies have not been conducted with M-M-R II. It is also not known whether M-M-R II can cause fetal harm when administered to a pregnant woman or can affect reproduction capacity. Therefore, the vaccine should not be administered to pregnant females; furthermore, pregnancy should be avoided for three months following vaccination (see CONTRAINDICATIONS).

In counseling women who are inadvertently vaccinated when pregnant or who become pregnant within 3 months of vaccination, the physician should be aware of the following: (1) In a 10 year survey involving over 700 pregnant women who received rubella vaccine within 3 months before or after conception (of whom 189 received the Wistar RA 27/3 strain), none of the newborns had abnormalities compatible with congenital rubella syndrome; (2) Although mumps virus is capable of infecting the placenta and fetus, there is no good evidence that it causes congenital malformations in humans. Mumps vaccine virus also has been shown to infect the placenta, but the virus has not been isolated from the fetal tissues from susceptible women who were vaccinated and underwent elective abortions; and (3) Reports have indicated that contracting of natural measles during pregnancy enhances fetal risk. Increased rates of spontaneous abortion, stillbirth, congenital defects and prematurity have been observed subsequent to natural measles during pregnancy. There are no adequate studies of the attenuated (vaccine) strain of measles virus in pregnancy. However, it would be prudent to assume that the vaccine strain of virus is also capable of inducing adverse fetal effects.

Nursing Mothers
It is not known whether measles or mumps vaccine virus is secreted in human milk. Recent studies have shown that lactating postpartum women immunized with live attenuated rubella vaccine may secrete the virus in breast milk and transmit it to breast-fed infants. In the infants with serological evidence of rubella infection, none exhibited severe disease; however, one exhibited mild clinical illness typical of

Continued on next page

Information on the Merck & Co., Inc. products listed on these pages is the full prescribing information from product circulars in use September 30, 1996.

Merck & Co.—Cont.

acquired rubella. Caution should be exercised when M-M-R II is administered to a nursing woman.

ADVERSE REACTIONS

Burning and/or stinging of short duration at the injection site have been reported.

The adverse clinical reactions associated with the use of M-M-R II are those expected to follow administration of the monovalent vaccines given separately. These may include malaise, sore throat, cough, rhinitis, headache, dizziness, fever, rash, nausea, vomiting or diarrhea; mild local reactions such as erythema, induration, tenderness and regional lymphadenopathy; parotitis, orchitis, nerve deafness, thrombocytopenia and purpura; allergic reactions such as wheal and flare at the injection site or urticaria; polyneuritis; and arthralgia and/or arthritis (usually transient and rarely chronic).

Anaphylaxis and anaphylactoid reactions have been reported.

Vasculitis has been reported rarely.

Otitis media and conjunctivitis have been reported.

Moderate fever [101-102.9°F (38.3-39.4°C)] occurs occasionally, and high fever [above 103°F (39.4°C)] occurs less commonly. On rare occasions, children developing fever may exhibit febrile convulsions. Afebrile convulsions or seizures have occurred rarely following vaccination with live attenuated measles vaccine. Syncope, particularly at the time of mass vaccination, has been reported. Rash occurs infrequently and is usually minimal, but rarely may be generalized. Erythema multiforme has also been reported rarely. Forms of optic neuritis, including retrobulbar neuritis, papillitis, and retinitis may infrequently follow viral infections, and have been reported to occur 1 to 3 weeks following inoculation with some live virus vaccines.

Clinical experience with live attenuated measles, mumps and rubella virus vaccines given individually indicates that encephalitis and other nervous system reactions have occurred very rarely. These might occur also with M-M-R II. Experience from more than 80 million doses of all live measles vaccines given in the U.S. through 1975 indicates that significant central nervous system reactions such as encephalitis and encephalopathy, occurring within 30 days after vaccination, have been temporally associated with measles vaccine very rarely. In no case has it been shown that reactions were actually caused by vaccine. The Center for Disease Control has pointed out that "a certain number of cases of encephalitis may be expected to occur in a large childhood population in a defined period of time even when no vaccines are administered". However, the data suggest the possibility that some of these cases may have been caused by measles vaccines. The risk of such serious neurological disorders following live measles virus vaccine administration remains far less than that for encephalitis and encephalopathy with natural measles (one per two thousand reported cases).

There have been rare reports of ocular palsies, Guillain-Barré syndrome, or ataxia occurring after immunization with vaccines containing live attenuated measles virus. The ocular palsies have occurred approximately 3–24 days following vaccination. No definite causal relationship has been established between these events and vaccination. Isolated reports of polyneuropathy including Guillain-Barré syndrome have also been reported after immunization with rubella-containing vaccines.

There have been reports of subacute sclerosing panencephalitis (SSPE) in children who did not have a history of natural measles but did receive measles vaccine. Some of these cases may have resulted from unrecognized measles in the first year of life or possibly from the measles vaccination. Based on estimated nationwide measles vaccine distribution, the association of SSPE cases to measles vaccination is about one case per million vaccine doses distributed. This is far less than the association with natural measles, 6–22 cases of SSPE per million cases of measles. The results of a retrospective case-controlled study conducted by the Center for Disease Control suggest that the overall effect of measles vaccine has been to protect against SSPE by preventing measles with its inherent higher risk of SSPE.

Local reactions characterized by marked swelling, redness and vesiculation at the injection site of attenuated live measles virus vaccines, and systemic reactions including atypical measles, have occurred in persons who received killed measles vaccine previously. M-M-R II was not given under this condition in clinical trials. Rarely, more severe reactions that require hospitalization, including prolonged high fevers and extensive local reactions, have been reported. Panniculitis has been reported rarely following administration of measles vaccine.

Arthralgia and/or arthritis (usually transient and rarely chronic), and polyneuritis are features of natural rubella and vary in frequency and severity with age and sex, being greatest in adult females and least in prepubertal children. This type of involvement as well as myalgia and paresthesia, have also been reported following administration of MERUVAX II (Rubella Virus Vaccine Live).

Chronic arthritis has been associated with natural rubella infection and has been related to persistent virus and/or viral antigen isolated from body tissues. Only rarely have vaccine recipients developed chronic joint symptoms. Following vaccination in children, reactions in joints are uncommon and generally of brief duration. In women, incidence rates for arthritis and arthralgia are generally higher than those seen in children (children: 0–3%; women: 12–20%), and the reactions tend to be more marked and of longer duration. Symptoms may persist for a matter of months or on rare occasions for years. In adolescent girls, the reactions appear to be intermediate in incidence between those seen in children and in adult women. Even in older women (35–45 years), these reactions are generally well tolerated and rarely interfere with normal activities.

DOSAGE AND ADMINISTRATION

FOR SUBCUTANEOUS ADMINISTRATION
Do not inject intravenously.

The dosage of vaccine is the same for all persons. Inject the total volume of the single dose vial (about 0.5 mL) or 0.5 mL of the 10 dose vial of reconstituted vaccine subcutaneously, preferably into the outer aspect of upper arm. *Do not give immune globulin (IG) concurrently with M-M-R II.*

During shipment, to insure that there is no loss of potency, the vaccine must be maintained at a temperature of 10°C (50°F) or less.

Before reconstitution, store M-M-R II at 2–8°C (36–46°F). *Protect from light.*

CAUTION: A sterile syringe free of preservatives, antiseptics, and detergents should be used for each injection and/or reconstitution of the vaccine because these substances may inactivate the live virus vaccine. A 25 gauge, ⅝″ needle is recommended.

To reconstitute, use only the diluent supplied, since it is free of preservatives or other antiviral substances which might inactivate the vaccine.

Single Dose Vial —First withdraw the entire volume of diluent into the syringe to be used for reconstitution. Inject all the diluent in the syringe into the vial of lyophilized vaccine, and agitate to mix thoroughly. Withdraw the entire contents into a syringe and inject the total volume of restored vaccine subcutaneously.

It is important to use a separate sterile syringe and needle for each individual patient to prevent transmission of hepatitis B and other infectious agents from one person to another.

10 Dose Vial (available only to government agencies/institutions)

Withdraw the entire contents (7 mL) of the diluent vial into the sterile syringe to be used for reconstitution, and introduce into the 10 dose vial of lyophilized vaccine. Agitate to ensure thorough mixing. The outer labeling suggests "For Jet Injector or Syringe Use". Use with separate sterile syringes is permitted for containers of 10 doses or less. The vaccine and diluent do not contain preservatives; therefore, the user must recognize the potential contamination hazards and exercise special precautions to protect the sterility and potency of the product. The use of aseptic techniques and proper storage prior to and after restoration of the vaccine and subsequent withdrawal of the individual doses is essential. Use 0.5 mL of the reconstituted vaccine for subcutaneous injection.

It is important to use a separate sterile syringe and needle for each individual patient to prevent transmission of hepatitis B and other infectious agents from one person to another.

Each dose contains not less than the equivalent of 1,000 TCID$_{50}$ of the U.S. Reference Measles Virus, 20,000 TCID$_{50}$ of the U.S. Reference Mumps Virus and 1,000 TCID$_{50}$ of the U.S. Reference Rubella Virus.

Parenteral drug products should be inspected visually for particulate matter and discoloration prior to administration. M-M-R II, when reconstituted, is clear yellow.

HOW SUPPLIED

No. 4749—M-M-R II is supplied as a single-dose vial of lyophilized vaccine, **NDC** 0006-4749-00, and a vial of diluent.

No. 4681/4309—M-M-R II is supplied as follows: (1) a box of 10 single-dose vials of lyophilized vaccine (package A), **NDC** 0006-4681-00; and (2) a box of 10 vials of diluent (package B). To conserve refrigerator space, the diluent may be stored separately at room temperature (6505-00-165-6519, Ten Pack).

Available only to government agencies/institutions

No. 4682X—M-M-R II is supplied as one 10 dose vial of lyophilized vaccine, **NDC** 0006-4682-00, and one 7 mL vial of diluent.

Storage

It is recommended that the vaccine be used as soon as possible after reconstitution. Protect vaccine from light at all times, since such exposure may inactivate the virus. Store reconstituted vaccine in the vaccine vial in a dark place at 2–8°C (36–46°F) and discard if not used within 8 hours.

A.H.F.S. Category: 80:12
7678915   Issued March 1995

M-R-VAX®II   ℞
(Measles and Rubella Virus Vaccine Live), U.S.P.

DESCRIPTION

M-R-VAX* II (Measles and Rubella Virus Vaccine Live), is a live virus vaccine for immunization against measles (rubeola) and rubella (German measles).

M-R-VAX II is a sterile lyophilized preparation of (1) ATTENUVAX* (Measles Virus Vaccine Live), a more attenuated line of measles virus, derived from Enders' attenuated Edmonston strain and grown in cell cultures of chick embryo; and (2) MERUVAX* II (Rubella Virus Vaccine Live), the Wistar RA 27/3 strain of live attenuated rubella virus grown in human diploid cell (WI-38) culture. The vaccine viruses are the same as those used in the manufacture of ATTENUVAX (Measles Virus Vaccine Live) and MERUVAX II (Rubella Virus Vaccine Live). The two viruses are mixed before being lyophilized. The product contains no preservative.

The reconstituted vaccine is for subcutaneous administration. When reconstituted as directed, the dose for injection is 0.5 mL and contains not less than the equivalent of 1,000 TCID$_{50}$ (tissue culture infectious doses) of the U.S. Reference Measles Virus; and 1,000 TCID$_{50}$ of the U.S. Reference Rubella Virus. Each dose contains approximately 25 mcg of neomycin. The product contains no preservative. Sorbitol and hydrolized gelatin are added as stabilizers.

* Registered trademark of MERCK & CO., INC.

CLINICAL PHARMACOLOGY

Clinical studies of 237 double seronegative children, 10 months to 10 years of age, demonstrated that M-R-VAX II is highly immunogenic and generally well tolerated. In these studies, a single injection of the vaccine induced measles hemagglutination-inhibition (HI) antibodies in 95 percent and rubella HI antibodies in 99 percent of susceptible persons.

The RA 27/3 rubella strain in M-R-VAX II elicits higher immediate post-vaccination HI, complement-fixing and neutralizing antibody levels than other strains of rubella vaccine and has been shown to induce a broader profile of circulating antibodies including anti-theta and anti-iota precipitating antibodies. The RA 27/3 rubella strain immunologically simulates natural infection more closely than other rubella vaccine viruses. The increased levels and broader profile of antibodies produced by RA 27/3 strain rubella virus vaccine appear to correlate with greater resistance to subclinical reinfection with the wild virus, and provide greater confidence for lasting immunity.

Vaccine induced antibody levels following administration of M-R-VAX II have been shown to persist up to 11 years without substantial decline. Continued surveillance will be necessary to determine further duration of antibody persistence.

INDICATIONS AND USAGE

M-R-VAX II is indicated for simultaneous immunization against measles and rubella in persons 15 months of age or older. A second dose of M-R-VAX II or monovalent measles vaccine is recommended (see *Revaccination*).

Infants who are less than 15 months of age may fail to respond to the measles component of the vaccine due to presence in the circulation of residual measles antibody of maternal origin; the younger the infant, the lower the likelihood of seroconversion. In geographically isolated or other relatively inaccessible populations for whom immunization programs are logistically difficult, and in population groups in which natural measles infection may occur in a significant proportion of infants before 15 months of age, it may be desirable to give the vaccine to infants at an earlier age. Infants vaccinated under these conditions at less than 12 months of age should be revaccinated after reaching 15 months of age. There is some evidence to suggest that infants immunized at less than one year of age may not develop sustained antibody levels when later reimmunized. The advantage of early protection must be weighed against the chance for failure to respond adequately on reimmunization.

Previously unimmunized children of susceptible pregnant women should receive live attenuated rubella vaccine, be-

cause an immunized child will be less likely to acquire natural rubella and introduce the virus into the household.
Individuals planning travel outside the United States, if not immune, can acquire measles, mumps or rubella and import these diseases to the United States. Therefore, prior to International travel, individuals known to be susceptible to one or more of these diseases can receive either a single antigen vaccine (measles, mumps, or rubella), or a combined antigen vaccine as appropriate. However, M-M-R† II (Measles, Mumps, and Rubella Virus Vaccine Live) is preferred for persons likely to be susceptible to mumps and rubella; and if a single-antigen measles vaccine is not readily available, travelers should receive M-M-R II (Measles, Mumps, and Rubella Virus Vaccine Live) regardless of their immune status to mumps or rubella.

Non-Pregnant Adolescent and Adult Females

Immunization of susceptible non-pregnant adolescent and adult females of childbearing age with live attenuated rubella virus vaccine is indicated if certain precautions are observed (see below and PRECAUTIONS). Vaccinating susceptible postpubertal females confers individual protection against subsequently acquiring rubella infection during pregnancy, which in turn prevents infection of the fetus and consequent congenital rubella injury.
Women of childbearing age should be advised not to become pregnant for three months after vaccination and should be informed of the reason for this precaution.*
It is recommended that rubella susceptibility be determined by serologic testing prior to immunization.** If immune, as evidenced by a specific rubella antibody titer of 1:8 or greater (hemagglutination-inhibition test), vaccination is unnecessary. Congenital malformations do occur in up to seven percent of all live births. Their chance appearance after vaccination could lead to misinterpretation of the cause, particularly if the prior rubella-immune status of vaccinees is unknown.
Postpubertal females should be informed of the frequent occurrence of generally self-limited arthralgia and/or arthritis beginning 2 to 4 weeks after vaccination (see ADVERSE REACTIONS).

Postpartum Women

It has been found convenient in many instances to vaccinate rubella-susceptible women in the immediate postpartum period. (See *Nursing Mothers*).

Revaccination: Children first vaccinated when younger than 12 months of age should be revaccinated at 15 months of age.
The American Academy of Pediatrics (AAP), the Immunization Practices Advisory Committee (ACIP), and some state and local health agencies have recommended guidelines for routine measles revaccination and to help control measles outbreaks.***
Vaccines available for revaccination include monovalent measles vaccine [ATTENUVAX (Measles Virus Vaccine Live)] and polyvalent vaccines containing measles [e.g., M-M-R II (Measles, Mumps, and Rubella Virus Vaccine Live), M-R-VAX II]. If the prevention of sporadic measles outbreaks is the sole objective, revaccination with a monovalent measles vaccine should be considered (see appropriate product circular). If concern also exists about immune status regarding mumps or rubella, revaccination with appropriate monovalent or polyvalent vaccines should be considered after consulting the appropriate product circulars. Unnecessary doses of a vaccine are best avoided by ensuring that written documentation of vaccination is preserved and a copy given to each vaccinee's parent or guardian.

Use with other Vaccines

Routine administration of DTP (diphtheria, tetanus, pertussis) and/or OPV (oral poliovirus vaccine) concomitantly with measles, mumps and rubella vaccines is not recommended because there are insufficient data relating to the simultaneous administration of these antigens. However, the American Academy of Pediatrics has noted that in some circumstances, particularly when the patient may not return, some practitioners prefer to administer all these antigens on a single day. If done, separate sites and syringes should be used for DTP and M-R-VAX II.
M-R-VAX II should not be given less than one month before or after administration of other virus vaccines.

† Registered trademark of MERCK & CO., INC.

* NOTE: The Immunization Practices Advisory Committee (ACIP) has recommended "In view of the importance of protecting this age group against rubella, reasonable precautions in a rubella immunization program include asking females if they are pregnant, excluding those who say they are, and explaining the theoretical risks to the others."

** NOTE: The Immunization Practices Advisory Committee (ACIP) has stated "When practical, and when reliable laboratory services are available, potential vaccinees of childbearing age can have serologic tests to determine susceptibility to rubella. . . . However, routinely performing serologic tests for all females of childbearing age to determine susceptibility so that vaccine is given only to proven susceptibles is expensive and has been ineffective in some areas. Accordingly, the ACIP believes that rubella vaccination of a woman who is not known to be pregnant and has no history of vaccination is justifiable without serologic testing."

*** NOTE: A primary difference among these recommendations is the timing of revaccination: the ACIP recommends routine revaccination at entry into Kindergarten or first grade, whereas the AAP recommends routine revaccination at entrance to middle school or junior high school. In addition, some public health jurisdictions mandate the age for revaccination. The complete text of applicable guidelines should be consulted.

CONTRAINDICATIONS

Do not give M-R-VAX II to pregnant females; the possible effects of the vaccine on fetal development are unknown at this time. If vaccination of postpubertal females is undertaken, pregnancy should be avoided for three months following vaccination. (See PRECAUTIONS, *Pregnancy*).
Anaphylactic or anaphylactoid reactions to neomycin (each dose of reconstituted vaccine contains approximately 25 mcg of neomycin).
History of anaphylactic or anaphylactoid reactions to eggs (see HYPERSENSITIVITY TO EGGS below).
Any febrile respiratory illness or other active febrile infection.
Active untreated tuberculosis.
Patients receiving immunosuppressive therapy. This contraindication does not apply to patients who are receiving corticosteroids as replacement therapy, e.g., for Addison's disease.
Individuals with blood dyscrasias, leukemia, lymphomas of any type, or other malignant neoplasms affecting the bone marrow or lymphatic systems.
Primary and acquired immunodeficiency states, including patients who are immunosuppressed in association with AIDS or other clinical manifestations of infection with human immunodeficiency viruses; cellular immune deficiencies; and hypogammaglobulinemic and dysgammaglobulinemic states.
Individuals with a family history of congenital or hereditary immunodeficiency, until the immune competence of the potential vaccine recipient is demonstrated.

HYPERSENSITIVITY TO EGGS

Live measles vaccine is produced in chick embryo cell culture. Persons with a history of anaphylactic, anaphylactoid, or other immediate reactions (e.g., hives, swelling of the mouth and throat, difficulty breathing, hypotension, or shock) subsequent to egg ingestion should not be vaccinated. Evidence indicates that persons are not at increased risk if they have egg allergies that are not anaphylactic or anaphylactoid in nature. Such persons may be vaccinated in the usual manner. There is no evidence to indicate that persons with allergies to chickens or feathers are at increased risk of reaction to the vaccine.

PRECAUTIONS

General

Adequate treatment provisions including epinephrine, should be available for immediate use should an anaphylactic or anaphylactoid reaction occur.
Due caution should be employed in administration of M-R-VAX II to persons with a history of cerebral injury, individual or family histories of convulsions, or any other condition in which stress due to fever should be avoided. The physician should be alert to the temperature elevation which may occur following vaccination. (See ADVERSE REACTIONS.)
Children and young adults who are known to be infected with human immunodeficiency viruses but without overt clinical manifestations of immunosuppression may be vaccinated; however, the vaccinees should be monitored closely for vaccine-preventable diseases because immunization may be less effective than for uninfected persons.
Vaccination should be deferred for at least 3 months following blood or plasma transfusions, or administration of human immune serum globulin.
Excretion of small amounts of the live attenuated rubella virus from the nose or throat has occurred in the majority of susceptible individuals 7–28 days after vaccination. There is no confirmed evidence to indicate that such virus is transmitted to susceptible persons who are in contact with the vaccinated individuals. Consequently, transmission through close personal contact, while accepted as a theoretical possibility, is not regarded as a significant risk. However, transmission of the rubella vaccine virus to infants via breast milk has been documented (see *Nursing Mothers*).
There are no reports of transmission of live attenuated measles virus from vaccinees to susceptible contacts.
It has been reported that live attenuated measles and rubella virus vaccines given individually may result in a temporary depression of tuberculin skin sensitivity. Therefore, if a tuberculin test is to be done, it should be administered either before or simultaneously with M-R-VAX II.
Children under treatment for tuberculosis have not experienced exacerbation of the disease when immunized with live measles virus vaccine; no studies have been reported to date of the effect of measles virus vaccines on untreated tuberculous children.
As for any vaccine, vaccination with M-R-VAX II may not result in seroconversion in 100% of susceptible persons given the vaccine.

Pregnancy

Pregnancy Category C

Animal reproduction studies have not been conducted with M-R-VAX II. It is also not known whether M-R-VAX II can cause fetal harm when administered to a pregnant woman or can affect reproduction capacity. Therefore, the vaccine should not be administered to pregnant females; futhermore, pregnancy should be avoided for three months following vaccination (see CONTRAINDICATIONS).
In counseling women who are inadvertently vaccinated when pregnant or who become pregnant within 3 months of vaccination, the physician should be aware of the following: (1) In a 10 year survey involving over 700 pregnant women who received rubella vaccine within 3 months before or after conception, (of whom 189 received the Wistar RA 27/3 strain), none of the newborns had abnormalities compatible with congenital rubella syndrome; (2) Reports have indicated that contracting of natural measles during pregnancy enhances fetal risk. Increased rates of spontaneous abortion, stillbirth, congenital defects and prematurity have been observed subsequent to natural measles during pregnancy. There are no adequate studies of the attenuated (vaccine) strain of measles virus in pregnancy. However, it would be prudent to assume that the vaccine strain of virus is also capable of inducing adverse fetal effects.

Nursing Mothers

It is not known whether measles vaccine virus is secreted in human milk. Recent studies have shown that lactating postpartum women immunized with live attenuated rubella vaccine may secrete the virus in breast milk and transmit it to breast-fed infants. In the infants with serological evidence of rubella infection, none exhibited severe disease; however, one exhibited mild clinical illness typical of acquired rubella. Caution should be exercised when M-R-VAX II is administered to a nursing woman.

ADVERSE REACTIONS

Burning and/or stinging of short duration at the injection site have been reported.
The adverse clinical reactions associated with the use of M-R-VAX II are those expected to follow administration of the monovalent vaccines given separately. These may include malaise, sore throat, cough, rhinitis, headache, dizziness, fever, rash, nausea, vomiting or diarrhea; mild local reactions such as erythema, induration, tenderness and regional lymphadenopathy; thrombocytopenia and purpura; allergic reactions such as wheal and flare at the injection site or urticaria; polyneuritis, and arthralgia and/or arthritis (usually transient and rarely chronic).
Anaphylaxis and anaphylactoid reactions have been reported.
Vasculitis has been reported rarely.
Moderate fever [101–102.9°F (38.3–39.4°C)] occurs occasionally, and high fever [above 103°F (39.4°C)] occurs less commonly. On rare occasions, children developing fever may exhibit febrile convulsions. Afebrile convulsions or seizures have occurred rarely following vaccination with live attenuated measles vaccine. Syncope, particularly at the time of mass vaccination, has been reported. Rash occurs infrequently and is usually minimal, but rarely may be generalized. Erythema multiforme has also been reported rarely.
Forms of optic neuritis, including retrobulbar neuritis, papillitis, and retinitis may infrequently follow viral infections, and have been reported to occur 1 to 3 weeks following inoculation with some live virus vaccines.
Clinical experience with live attenuated measles and rubella virus vaccines given individually indicates that encephalitis and other nervous system reactions have occurred very rarely. These might occur also with M-R-VAX II.
Experience from more than 80 million doses of all live measles vaccines given in the U.S. through 1975 indicates that significant central nervous system reactions such as encephalitis and encephalopathy, occurring within 30 days after vaccination, have been temporally associated with measles vaccine very rarely. In no case has it been shown that reactions were actually caused by vaccine. The Center for Disease Control has pointed out that "a certain number of cases

Continued on next page

Information on the Merck & Co., Inc. products listed on these pages is the full prescribing information from product circulars in use September 30, 1996.

Merck & Co.—Cont.

of encephalitis may be expected to occur in a large childhood population in a defined period of time even when no vaccines are administered". However, the data suggest the possibility that some of these cases may have been caused by measles vaccines. The risk of such serious neurological disorders following live measles virus vaccine administration remains far less than that for encephalitis and encephalopathy with natural measles (one per two thousand reported cases).

There have been rare reports of ocular palsies, Guillain-Barré syndrome, or ataxia occurring after immunization with vaccines containing live attenuated measles virus. The ocular palsies have occurred approximately 3–24 days following vaccination. No definite causal relationship has been established between these events and vaccination. Isolated reports of polyneuropathy including Guillain-Barré syndrome have also been reported after immunization with rubella-containing vaccines.

There have been reports of subacute sclerosing panencephalitis (SSPE) in children who did not have a history of natural measles but did receive measles vaccine. Some of these cases may have resulted from unrecognized measles in the first year of life or possibly from the measles vaccination. Based on estimated nationwide measles vaccine distribution, the association of SSPE cases to measles vaccination is about one case per million vaccine doses distributed. This is far less than the association with natural measles, 6–22 cases of SSPE per million cases of measles. The results of a retrospective case-controlled study conducted by the Center for Disease Control suggest that the overall effect of measles vaccine has been to protect against SSPE by preventing measles with its inherent higher risk of SSPE.

Local reactions characterized by marked swelling, redness and vesiculation at the injection site of attenuated live measles virus vaccines, and systemic reactions including atypical measles, have occurred in persons who received killed measles vaccine previously. M-R-VAX II was not given under this condition in clinical trials. Rarely, more severe reactions that require hospitalization, including prolonged high fevers and extensive local reactions, have been reported. Panniculitis has been reported rarely following administration of measles vaccine.

Arthralgia and/or arthritis (usually transient and rarely chronic), and polyneuritis are features of natural rubella and vary in frequency and severity with age and sex, being greatest in adult females and least in prepubertal children. This type of involvement as well as myalgia and paresthesia have also been reported following administration of MERUVAX II (Rubella Virus Vaccine Live).

Chronic arthritis has been associated with natural rubella infection and has been related to persistent virus and/or viral antigen isolated from body tissues. Only rarely have vaccine recipients developed chronic joint symptoms.

Following vaccination in children, reactions in joints are uncommon and generally of brief duration. In women, incidence rates for arthritis and arthralgia are generally higher than those seen in children (children: 0–3%; women: 12–20%), and the reactions tend to be more marked and of longer duration. Symptoms may persist for a matter of months or on rare occasions for years. In adolescent girls, the reactions appear to be intermediate in incidence between those seen in children and in adult women. Even in older women (35–45 years), these reactions are generally well tolerated and rarely interfere with normal activities.

DOSAGE AND ADMINISTRATION

FOR SUBCUTANEOUS ADMINISTRATION
Do not inject intravenously

The dosage of vaccine is the same for all persons. Inject the total volume of the single dose vial (about 0.5 mL) or 0.5 mL of the multiple dose vial of reconstituted vaccine subcutaneously, preferably into the outer aspect of upper arm. *Do not give immune globulin (IG) concurrently with* M-R-VAX II.

During shipment, to insure that there is no loss of potency, the vaccine must be maintained at a temperature of 10°C (50°F) or less.

Before reconstitution, store M-R-VAX II at 2–8°C (36–46°F). *Protect from light.*

CAUTION: A sterile syringe free of preservatives, antiseptics, and detergents should be used for each injection and/or reconstitution of the vaccine because these substances may inactivate the live virus vaccine. A 25 gauge, 5/8" needle is recommended.

To reconstitute, use only the diluent supplied, since it is free of preservatives or other antiviral substances which might inactivate the vaccine.

Single Dose Vial—First withdraw the entire volume of diluent into the syringe to be used for reconstitution. Inject all the diluent in the syringe into the vial of lyophilized vaccine, and agitate to mix thoroughly. Withdraw the entire contents into a syringe and inject the total volume of restored vaccine subcutaneously.

It is important to use a separate sterile syringe and needle for each individual patient to prevent transmission of hepatitis B and other infectious agents from one person to another.

10 Dose Vial (available only to government agencies/institutions)—Withdraw the entire contents (7 mL) of the diluent vial into the sterile syringe to be used for reconstitution, and introduce into the 10 dose vial of lyophilized vaccine. Agitate to ensure thorough mixing. The outer labeling suggests "For Jet Injector or Syringe Use". Use with separate sterile syringes is permitted for containers of 10 doses or less. The vaccine and diluent do not contain preservatives; therefore, the user must recognize the potential contamination hazards and exercise special precautions to protect the sterility and potency of the product. The use of aseptic techniques and proper storage prior to and after restoration of the vaccine and subsequent withdrawal of the individual doses is essential. Use 0.5 mL of the reconstituted vaccine for subcutaneous injection.

It is important to use a separate sterile syringe and needle for each individual patient to prevent transmission of hepatitis B and other infectious agents from one person to another.

50 Dose Vial (available only to government agencies/institutions)—Withdraw the entire contents (30 mL) of diluent vial into the sterile syringe to be used for reconstitution and introduce into the 50 dose vial of lyophilized vaccine. Agitate to ensure thorough mixing. With full aseptic precautions, attach the vial to the sterilized multidose jet injector apparatus. Use 0.5 mL of the reconstituted vaccine for subcutaneous injection.

Each dose contains not less than the equivalent of 1,000 $TCID_{50}$ of the U.S. Reference Measles Virus and 1,000 $TCID_{50}$ of the U.S. Reference Rubella Virus.

Parenteral drug products should be inspected visually for particulate matter and discoloration prior to administration. M-R-VAX II, when reconstituted, is clear yellow.

HOW SUPPLIED

No. 4751—M-R-VAX II is supplied as a single-dose vial of lyophilized vaccine, **NDC** 0006-4751-00, and a vial of diluent.

No. 4677/4309—M-R-VAX II is supplied as follows: (1) a box of 10 single-dose vials of lyophilized vaccine (package A), **NDC** 0006-4677-00; and (2) a box of 10 vials of diluent (package B). To conserve refrigerator space, the diluent may be stored separately at room temperature (6505-01-098-8004, Ten Pack).

Available only to government agencies/institutions:

No. 4678—M-R-VAX II is supplied as one 10 dose vial of lyophilized vaccine, **NDC** 0006-4678-00, and one 7 mL vial of diluent.

No. 4679—M-R-VAX II is supplied as one 50 dose vial of lyophilized vaccine, **NDC** 0006-4679-00, and one 30 mL vial of diluent (6505-01-098-8005, 50 dose).

Storage

It is recommended that the vaccine be used as soon as possible after reconstitution. Protect vaccine from light at all times, since such exposure may inactivate the virus. Store reconstituted vaccine in the vaccine vial in a dark place at 2–8°C (36–46°F) and discard if not used within 8 hours.

A.H.F.S. Category: 80:12
7680217 Issued March 1995

COPYRIGHT © MERCK & CO., INC., 1990
All rights reserved

MEFOXIN® ℞
(Cefoxitin Sodium), U.S.P.

DESCRIPTION

MEFOXIN* (Sterile Cefoxitin Sodium) is a semi-synthetic, broad-spectrum cepha antibiotic sealed under nitrogen for parenteral administration. It is derived from cephamycin C, which is produced by *Streptomyces lactamdurans.* It is the sodium salt of 3-(hydroxymethyl)-7α-methoxy-8-oxo-7-[2-(2-thienyl) acetamido]-5-thia-1-azabicyclo [4.2.0] oct-2-ene-2-carboxylate carbamate (ester). The empirical formula is $C_{16}H_{16}N_3NaO_7S_2$, and the structural formula is:

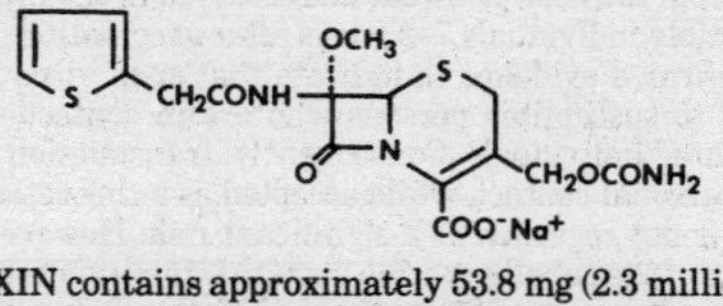

MEFOXIN contains approximately 53.8 mg (2.3 milliequivalents) of sodium per gram of cefoxitin activity. Solutions of MEFOXIN range from colorless to light amber in color. The pH of freshly constituted solutions usually ranges from 4.2 to 7.0.

*Registered trademark of MERCK & CO., INC.

CLINICAL PHARMACOLOGY

Clinical Pharmacology

After intramuscular administration of a 1 gram dose of MEFOXIN to normal volunteers, the mean peak serum concentration was 24 mcg/mL. The peak occurred at 20 to 30 minutes. Following an intravenous dose of 1 gram, serum concentrations were 110 mcg/mL at 5 minutes, declining to less than 1 mcg/mL at 4 hours. The half-life after an intravenous dose is 41 to 59 minutes; after intramuscular administration, the half-life is 64.8 minutes. Approximately 85 percent of cefoxitin is excreted unchanged by the kidneys over a 6-hour period, resulting in high urinary concentrations. Following an intramuscular dose of 1 gram, urinary concentrations greater than 3000 mcg/mL were observed. Probenecid slows tubular excretion and produces higher serum levels and increases the duration of measurable serum concentrations.

Cefoxitin passes into pleural and joint fluids and is detectable in antibacterial concentrations in bile.

Clinical experience has demonstrated that MEFOXIN can be administered to patients who are also receiving carbenicillin, kanamycin, gentamicin, tobramycin, or amikacin (see PRECAUTIONS and ADMINISTRATION).

Microbiology

The bactericidal action of cefoxitin results from inhibition of cell wall synthesis. Cefoxitin has *in vitro* activity against a wide range of gram-positive and gram-negative organisms. The methoxy group in the 7α position provides MEFOXIN with a high degree of stability in the presence of beta-lactamases, both penicillinases and cephalosporinases, of gram-negative bacteria. Cefoxitin is usually active against the following organisms *in vitro* and in clinical infections:

Gram-positive
- *Staphylococcus aureus,* including penicillinase and non-penicillinase producing strains.
- *Staphylococcus epidermidis*
- Beta-hemolytic and other streptococci (most strains of enterococci, e.g., *Streptococcus faecalis,* are resistant)
- *Streptococcus pneumoniae*

Gram-negative
- *Escherichia coli*
- *Klebsiella* species (including *K. pneumoniae*)
- *Hemophilus influenzae*
- *Neisseria gonorrhoeae,* including penicillinase and non-penicillinase producing strains
- *Proteus mirabilis*
- *Morganella morganii*
- *Proteus vulgaris*
- *Providencia* species, including *Providencia rettgeri*

Anaerobic organisms
- *Peptococcus* species
- *Peptostreptococcus* species
- *Clostridium* species
- *Bacteroides* species, including the *B. fragilis* group (includes *B. fragilis, B. distasonis, B. ovatus, B. thetaiotaomicron, B. vulgatus*)

MEFOXIN is inactive *in vitro* against most strains of *Pseudomonas aeruginosa* and enterococci and many strains of *Enterobacter cloacae.*

Methicillin-resistant staphylococci are almost uniformly resistant to MEFOXIN.

Susceptibility Tests

For fast-growing aerobic organisms, quantitative methods that require measurements of zone diameters give the most precise estimates of antibiotic susceptibility. One such procedure* has been recommended for use with discs to test susceptibility to cefoxitin. Interpretation involves correlation of the diameters obtained in the disc test with minimal inhibitory concentration (MIC) values for cefoxitin.

Reports from the laboratory giving results of the standardized single disc susceptibility test* using a 30 mcg cefoxitin disc should be interpreted according to the following criteria: Organisms producing zones of 18 mm or greater are considered susceptible, indicating that the tested organism is likely to respond to therapy.

Organisms of intermediate susceptibility produce zones of 15 to 17 mm, indicating that the tested organism would be susceptible if high dosage is used or if the infection is confined to tissues and fluids (e.g., urine) in which high antibiotic levels are attained.

Resistant organisms produce zones of 14 mm or less, indicating that other therapy should be selected.

The cefoxitin disc should be used for testing cefoxitin susceptibility.

Cefoxitin has been shown by *in vitro* tests to have activity against certain strains of *Enterobacteriaceae* found resistant when tested with the cephalosporin class disc. For this reason, the cefoxitin disc should not be used for testing susceptibility to cephalosporins, and cephalosporin discs should not be used for testing susceptibility to cefoxitin.

Dilution methods, preferably the agar plate dilution procedure, are most accurate for susceptibility testing of obligate anaerobes.

A bacterial isolate may be considered susceptible if the MIC value for cefoxitin† is not more than 16 mcg/mL. Organisms are considered resistant if the MIC is greater than 32 mcg/mL.

* Bauer, A. W.; Kirby, W. M. M.; Sherris, J. C.; Turck, M.: Antibiotic susceptibility testing by a standardized single disc method, Amer. J. Clin. Path. *45* : 493–496, Apr. 1966. Standardized disc susceptibility test, Federal Register *37*: 20527–20529, 1972. National Committee for Clinical Laboratory Standards: Approved Standard: ASM-2, Performance Standards for Antimicrobial Disc Susceptibility Tests, July 1975.
† Determined by the ICS agar dilution method (Ericsson and Sherris, Acta Path. Microbiol. Scand. (B) Suppl. No. 217, 1971) or any other method that has been shown to give equivalent results.

INDICATIONS AND USAGE

Treatment
MEFOXIN is indicated for the treatment of serious infections caused by susceptible strains of the designated microorganisms in the diseases listed below.
(1) **Lower respiratory tract infections,** including pneumonia and lung abscess, caused by *Streptococcus pneumoniae*, other streptococci (excluding enterococci, e.g., *Streptococcus faecalis*), *Staphylococcus aureus* (penicillinase and non-penicillinase producing), *Escherichia coli*, *Klebsiella* species, *Hemophilus influenzae*, and *Bacteroides* species.
(2) **Genitourinary infections.** Urinary tract infections caused by *Escherichia coli*, *Klebsiella* species, *Proteus mirabilis*, indole-positive Proteus (which include the organisms now called *Morganella morganii* and *Proteus vulgaris*), and *Providencia* species (including *Providencia rettgeri*). Uncomplicated gonorrhea due to *Neisseria gonorrhoeae* (penicillinase and non-penicillinase producing).
(3) **Intra-abdominal infections,** including peritonitis and intra-abdominal abscess, caused by *Escherichia coli*, *Klebsiella* species, *Bacteroides* species including the *Bacteroides fragilis* group**, and *Clostridium* species.
(4) **Gynecological infections,** including endometritis, pelvic cellulitis, and pelvic inflammatory disease caused by *Escherichia coli*, *Neisseria gonorrhoeae* (penicillinase and non-penicillinase producing), *Bacteroides* species including the *Bacteroides fragilis* group**, *Clostridium* species, *Peptococcus* species, *Peptostreptococcus* species, and Group B streptococci.
MEFOXIN, like cephalosporins, has no activity against *Chlamydia trachomatis*. Therefore, when MEFOXIN is used in the treatment of patients with pelvic inflammatory disease and *C. trachomatis* is one of the suspected pathogens, appropriate anti-chlamydial coverage should be added.
(5) **Septicemia** caused by *Streptococcus pneumoniae*, *Staphylococcus aureus* (penicillinase and non-penicillinase producing), *Escherichia coli*, *Klebsiella* species, and *Bacteroides* species including the *Bacteroides fragilis* group.**
(6) **Bone and joint infections** caused by *Staphylococcus aureus* (penicillinase and non-penicillinase producing).
(7) **Skin and skin structure infections** caused by *Staphylococcus aureus* (penicillinase and non-penicillinase producing), *Staphylococcus epidermidis*, streptococci (excluding enterococci, e.g., *Streptococcus faecalis*), *Escherichia coli*, *Proteus mirabilis*, *Klebsiella* species, *Bacteroides* species including the *Bacteroides fragilis* group**, *Clostridium* species, *Peptococcus* species, and *Peptostreptococcus* species.
Appropriate culture and susceptibility studies should be performed to determine the susceptibility of the causative organisms to MEFOXIN. Therapy may be started while awaiting the results of these studies.
In randomized comparative studies, MEFOXIN and cephalothin were comparably safe and effective in the management of infections caused by gram-positive cocci and gram-negative rods susceptible to the cephalosporins. MEFOXIN has a high degree of stability in the presence of bacterial beta-lactamases, both penicillinases and cephalosporinases.
Many infections caused by aerobic and anaerobic gram-negative bacteria resistant to some cephalosporins respond to MEFOXIN. Similarly, many infections caused by aerobic and anaerobic bacteria resistant to some penicillin antibiotics (ampicillin, carbenicillin, penicillin G) respond to treatment with MEFOXIN. Many infections caused by mixtures of susceptible aerobic and anaerobic bacteria respond to treatment with MEFOXIN.
Prevention
MEFOXIN is indicated for the prophylaxis of infection in patients undergoing uncontaminated gastrointestinal surgery, vaginal hysterectomy, abdominal hysterectomy, or cesarean section.
Effective prophylactic use depends on the time of administration. MEFOXIN usually should be given one-half to one hour before the operation, which is sufficient time to achieve effective levels in the wound during the procedure. Prophy-

lactic administration should usually be stopped within 24 hours since continuing administration of any antibiotic increases the possibility of adverse reactions but, in the majority of surgical procedures, does not reduce the incidence of subsequent infection.
If there are signs of infection, specimens for culture should be obtained for identification of the causative organism so that appropriate treatment may be instituted.

** *B. fragilis*, *B. distasonis*, *B. ovatus*, *B. thetaiotaomicron*, *B. vulgatus*.

CONTRAINDICATIONS

MEFOXIN is contraindicated in patients who have shown hypersensitivity to cefoxitin and the cephalosporin group of antibiotics.

WARNINGS

BEFORE THERAPY WITH 'MEFOXIN' IS INSTITUTED, CAREFUL INQUIRY SHOULD BE MADE TO DETERMINE WHETHER THE PATIENT HAS HAD PREVIOUS HYPERSENSITIVITY REACTIONS TO CEFOXITIN, CEPHALOSPORINS, PENICILLINS, OR OTHER DRUGS. THIS PRODUCT SHOULD BE GIVEN WITH CAUTION TO PENICILLIN-SENSITIVE PATIENTS. ANTIBIOTICS SHOULD BE ADMINISTERED WITH CAUTION TO ANY PATIENT WHO HAS DEMONSTRATED SOME FORM OF ALLERGY, PARTICULARLY TO DRUGS. IF AN ALLERGIC REACTION TO 'MEFOXIN' OCCURS, DISCONTINUE THE DRUG. SERIOUS HYPERSENSITIVITY REACTIONS MAY REQUIRE EPINEPHRINE AND OTHER EMERGENCY MEASURES.
Pseudomembranous colitis has been reported with virtually all antibiotics (including cephalosporins); therefore, it is important to consider its diagnosis in patients who develop diarrhea in association with antibiotic use. This colitis may range from mild to life threatening in severity.
Treatment with broad-spectrum antibiotics alters normal flora of the colon and may permit overgrowth of clostridia. Studies indicate a toxin produced by *Clostridium difficile* is one primary cause of antibiotic-associated colitis.
Mild cases of pseudomembranous colitis may respond to drug discontinuance alone. In more severe cases, management may include sigmoidoscopy, appropriate bacteriological studies, fluid, electrolyte and protein supplementation, and the use of a drug such as oral vancomycin as indicated. Isolation of the patient may be advisable. Other causes of colitis should also be considered.

PRECAUTIONS

General
The total daily dose should be reduced when MEFOXIN is administered to patients with transient or persistent reduction of urinary output due to renal insufficiency (see DOSAGE), because high and prolonged serum antibiotic concentrations can occur in such individuals from usual doses.
Antibiotics (including cephalosporins) should be prescribed with caution in individuals with a history of gastrointestinal disease, particularly colitis.
As with other antibiotics, prolonged use of MEFOXIN may result in overgrowth of nonsusceptible organisms. Repeated evaluation of the patient's condition is essential. If superinfection occurs during therapy, appropriate measures should be taken.
Drug Interactions
Increased nephrotoxicity has been reported following concomitant administration of cephalosporins and aminoglycoside antibiotics.
Drug/Laboratory Test Interactions
As with cephalothin, high concentrations of cefoxitin (> 100 micrograms/mL) may interfere with measurement of serum and urine creatinine levels by the Jaffé reaction, and produce false increases of modest degree in the levels of creatinine reported. Serum samples from patients treated with cefoxitin should not be analyzed for creatinine if withdrawn within 2 hours of drug administration.
High concentrations of cefoxitin in the urine may interfere with measurement of urinary 17-hydroxy-corticosteroids by the Porter-Silber reaction, and produce false increases of modest degree in the levels reported.
A false-positive reaction for glucose in the urine may occur. This has been observed with CLINITEST* reagent tablets.
Carcinogenesis, Mutagenesis, Impairment of Fertility
Long-term studies in animals have not been performed with cefoxitin to evaluate carcinogenic or mutagenic potential. Studies in rats treated intravenously with 400 mg/kg of cefoxitin (approximately three times the maximum recommended human dose) revealed no effects on fertility or mating ability.
Pregnancy
Pregnancy Category B. Reproduction studies performed in rats and mice at parenteral doses of approximately one to

seven and one-half times the maximum recommended human dose did not reveal teratogenic or fetal toxic effects, although a slight decrease in fetal weight was observed. There are, however, no adequate and well-controlled studies in pregnant women. Because animal reproduction studies are not always predictive of human response, this drug should be used during pregnancy only if clearly needed.
In the rabbit, cefoxitin was associated with a high incidence of abortion and maternal death. This was not considered to be a teratogenic effect but an expected consequence of the rabbit's unusual sensitivity to antibiotic-induced changes in the population of the microflora of the intestine.
Nursing Mothers
MEFOXIN is excreted in human milk in low concentrations. Caution should be exercised when MEFOXIN is administered to a nursing woman.
Pediatric Use
Safety and efficacy in infants from birth to three months of age have not yet been established. In children three months of age and older, higher doses of MEFOXIN have been associated with an increased incidence of eosinophilia and elevated SGOT.

* Registered trademark of Ames Company, Division of Miles Laboratories, Inc.

ADVERSE REACTIONS

MEFOXIN is generally well tolerated. The most common adverse reactions have been local reactions following intravenous or intramuscular injection. Other adverse reactions have been encountered infrequently.
Local Reactions
Thrombophlebitis has occurred with intravenous administration. Pain, induration, and tenderness after intramuscular injections have been reported.
Allergic Reactions
Rash (including exfoliative dermatitis and toxic epidermal necrolysis), pruritus, eosinophilia, fever, dyspnea, and other allergic reactions including anaphylaxis, interstitial nephritis and angioedema have been noted.
Cardiovascular
Hypotension
Gastrointestinal
Diarrhea, including documented pseudomembranous colitis which can appear during or after antibiotic treatment. Nausea and vomiting have been reported rarely.
Neuromuscular
Possible exacerbation of myasthenia gravis
Blood
Eosinophilia, leukopenia, including granulocytopenia, neutropenia, anemia, including hemolytic anemia, thrombocytopenia, and bone marrow depression. A positive direct Coombs test may develop in some individuals, especially those with azotemia.
Liver Function
Transient elevations in SGOT, SGPT, serum LDH, serum alkaline phosphatase; and jaundice have been reported.
Renal Function
Elevations in serum creatinine and/or blood urea nitrogen levels have been observed. As with the cephalosporins, acute renal failure has been reported rarely. The role of MEFOXIN in changes in renal function tests is difficult to assess, since factors predisposing to prerenal azotemia or to impaired renal function usually have been present.

OVERDOSAGE

The acute intravenous LD_{50} in the adult female mouse and rabbit was about 8.0 g/kg and greater than 1.0 g/kg respectively. The acute intraperitoneal LD_{50} in the adult rat was greater than 10.0 g/kg.

DOSAGE

TREATMENT
Adults
The usual adult dosage range is 1 gram to 2 grams every six to eight hours. Dosage and route of administration should be determined by susceptibility of the causative organisms, severity of infection, and the condition of the patient (see Table 1 for dosage guidelines).
If *C. trachomatis* is a suspected pathogen, appropriate anti-chlamydial coverage should be added, because cefoxitin sodium has no activity against this organism.
[See table 1 at bottom of next page.]
MEFOXIN may be used in patients with reduced renal function with the following dosage adjustments:

Continued on next page

Information on the Merck & Co., Inc. products listed on these pages is the full prescribing information from product circulars in use September 30, 1996.

Merck & Co.—Cont.

In adults with renal insufficiency, an initial loading dose of 1 gram to 2 grams may be given. After a loading dose, the recommendations for *maintenance dosage* (Table 2) may be used as a guide.
[See table at right.]

When only the serum creatinine level is available, the following formula (based on sex, weight, and age of the patient) may be used to convert this value into creatinine clearance. The serum creatinine should represent a steady state of renal function.

Males:

$$\text{Males:} \quad \frac{\text{Weight (kg)} \times (140 - \text{age})}{72 \times \text{serum creatinine (mg/100 mL)}}$$

Females: $0.85 \times$ above value

In patients undergoing hemodialysis, the loading dose of 1 to 2 grams should be given after each hemodialysis, and the maintenance dose should be given as indicated in Table 2. Antibiotic therapy for group A beta-hemolytic streptococcal infections should be maintained for at least 10 days to guard against the risk of rheumatic fever or glomerulonephritis. In staphylococcal and other infections involving a collection of pus, surgical drainage should be carried out where indicated. The recommended dosage of MEFOXIN **for uncomplicated gonorrhea** is 2 grams intramuscularly, with 1 gram of BENEMID* (Probenecid) given by mouth at the same time or up to ½ hour before MEFOXIN.

Infants and Children
The recommended dosage in children three months of age and older is 80 to 160 mg/kg of body weight per day divided into four to six equal doses. The higher dosages should be used for more severe or serious infections. The total daily dosage should not exceed 12 grams.
At this time no recommendation is made for children from birth to three months of age (See PRECAUTIONS).
In children with renal insufficiency the dosage and frequency of dosage should be modified consistent with the recommendations for adults (see Table 2).

PREVENTION
For prophylactic use in uncontaminated gastrointestinal surgery, vaginal hysterectomy, or abdominal hysterectomy, the following doses are recommended:
Adults:
2 grams administered intravenously or intramuscularly just prior to surgery (approximately one-half to one hour before the initial incision) followed by 2 grams every 6 hours after the first dose for no more than 24 hours.
Children (3 months and older):
30 to 40 mg/kg doses may be given at the times designated above.
For prophylactic use in vaginal hysterectomy, a single 2.0 gram dose administered intramuscularly one-half to one hour prior to surgery is recommended.
Cesarean section patients:
For patients undergoing cesarean section, either a single 2 gram dose administered intravenously as soon as the umbilical cord is clamped OR a 3-dose regimen consisting of 2 grams given intravenously as soon as the umbilical cord is clamped followed by 2 grams 4 and 8 hours after the initial dose is recommended. (See CLINICAL STUDIES.)

* Registered trademark of MERCK & CO., INC.

PREPARATION OF SOLUTION

Table 3 is provided for convenience in constituting MEFOXIN for both intravenous and intramuscular administration.
[See table 3 at top of next page.]
For intravenous use, 1 gram should be constituted with at least 10 mL of Sterile Water for Injection, and 2 grams, with 10 or 20 mL. The 10 gram bulk package should be constituted with 43 or 93 mL of Sterile Water for Injection or any of the solutions listed under the *Intravenous* portion of the COMPATIBILITY AND STABILITY section. CAUTION: THE 10 GRAM BULK STOCK SOLUTION IS NOT FOR DIRECT INFUSION. One or 2 grams of MEFOXIN for infusion may be constituted with 50 or 100 mL of 0.9 percent Sodium Chloride Injection, 5 percent or 10 percent Dextrose Injection, or any of the solutions listed under the *Intravenous* portion of the COMPATIBILITY AND STABILITY section.
Benzyl alcohol as a preservative has been associated with toxicity in neonates. While toxicity has not been demonstrated in infants greater than three months of age, in whom use of MEFOXIN may be indicated, small infants in this age range may also be at risk for benzyl alcohol toxicity. Therefore, diluent containing benzyl alcohol should not be used when MEFOXIN is constituted for administration to infants.
For ADD-Vantage®† vials, see separate INSTRUCTIONS FOR USE OF MEFOXIN IN ADD-Vantage® VIALS. MEFOXIN in ADD-Vantage® vials should be constituted with ADD-Vantage® diluent containers containing 50 mL or 100 mL of either 0.9 percent Sodium Chloride Injection or 5 percent Dextrose Injection. MEFOXIN in ADD-Vantage® vials is for IV use only.
For intramuscular use, each gram of MEFOXIN may be constituted with 2 mL of Sterile Water for Injection, *or —*
For intramuscular use ONLY: each gram of MEFOXIN may be constituted with 2 mL of 0.5 percent lidocaine hydrochloride solution** (without epinephrine) to minimize the discomfort of intramuscular injection.

†Registered trademark of Abbott Laboratories.
**See package circular of manufacturer for detailed information concerning contraindications, warnings, precautions, and adverse reactions.

ADMINISTRATION

MEFOXIN may be administered intravenously or intramuscularly after constitution.
Parenteral drug products should be inspected visually for particulate matter and discoloration prior to administration whenever solution and container permit.
Intravenous Administration
The intravenous route is preferable for patients with bacteremia, bacterial septicemia, or other severe or life-threatening infections, or for patients who may be poor risks because of lowered resistance resulting from such debilitating conditions as malnutrition, trauma, surgery, diabetes, heart failure, or malignancy, particularly if shock is present or impending.
For intermittent intravenous administration, a solution containing 1 gram or 2 grams in 10 mL of Sterile Water for Injection can be injected over a period of three to five minutes. Using an infusion system, it may also be given over a longer period of time through the tubing system by which the patient may be receiving other intravenous solutions. However, during infusion of the solution containing MEFOXIN, it is advisable to temporarily discontinue administration of any other solutions at the same site.
For the administration of higher doses by continuous intravenous infusion, a solution of MEFOXIN may be added to an intravenous bottle containing 5 percent Dextrose Injection, 0.9 percent Sodium Chloride Injection, 5 percent Dextrose and 0.9 percent Sodium Chloride Injection, or 5 percent Dextrose Injection with 0.02 percent sodium bicarbonate solution. BUTTERFLY† or scalp vein-type needles are preferred for this type of infusion.

Solutions of MEFOXIN, like those of most beta-lactam antibiotics, should not be added to aminoglycoside solutions (e.g., gentamicin sulfate, tobramycin sulfate, amikacin sulfate) because of potential interaction. However, MEFOXIN and aminoglycosides may be administered separately to the same patient.
Intramuscular Administration
As with all intramuscular preparations, MEFOXIN should be injected well within the body of a relatively large muscle such as the upper outer quadrant of the buttock (i.e., gluteus maximus); aspiration is necessary to avoid inadvertent injection into a blood vessel.

† Registered trademark of Abbott Laboratories.

COMPATIBILITY AND STABILITY

Intravenous
MEFOXIN, as supplied in vials or the bulk package and constituted to 1 gram/10 mL with Sterile Water for Injection, Bacteriostatic Water for Injection (see PREPARATION OF SOLUTION), 0.9 percent Sodium Chloride Injection, or 5 percent Dextrose Injection, maintains satisfactory potency for 24 hours at room temperature, for one week under refrigeration (below 5°C), and for at least 30 weeks in the frozen state.
These three primary solutions may be further diluted in 50 to 1000 mL of the following solutions and maintain potency for 24 hours at room temperature and at least 48 hours under refrigeration:
  Sterile Water for Injection‡
  0.9 percent Sodium Chloride Injection
  5 percent or 10 percent Dextrose Injection‡
  5 percent Dextrose and 0.9 percent Sodium Chloride Injection
  5 percent Dextrose Injection with 0.02 percent sodium bicarbonate solution
  5 percent Dextrose Injection with 0.2 percent or 0.45 percent saline solution
  Ringer's Injection
  Lactated Ringer's Injection‡
  5 percent dextrose in Lactated Ringer's Injection‡
  5 percent or 10 percent invert sugar in water
  10 percent invert sugar in saline solution
  5 percent Sodium Bicarbonate Injection
  Neut (sodium bicarbonate)*‡
  M/6 sodium lactate solution
  NORMOSOL-M in D5-W*‡
  IONOSOL B w/Dextrose 5 percent*‡
  POLYONIC M 56 in 5 percent Dextrose**
  Mannitol 5% and 2.5%
  Mannitol 10%‡
  ISOLYTE*** E
  ISOLYTE*** E with 5% dextrose
MEFOXIN, as supplied in infusion bottles and constituted with 50 to 100 mL of 0.9 percent Sodium Chloride Injection, or 5 percent or 10 percent Dextrose Injection, maintains satisfactory potency for 24 hours at room temperature or for 1 week under refrigeration (below 5°C).
MEFOXIN is supplied in single dose ADD-Vantage® vials and should be prepared as directed in the accompanying INSTRUCTIONS FOR USE OF MEFOXIN IN ADD-Vantage® VIALS using ADD-Vantage® diluent containers containing 50 mL or 100 mL of either 0.9 percent Sodium Chloride Injection or 5 percent Dextrose Injection. When prepared with either of these diluents, MEFOXIN maintains satisfactory potency for 24 hours at room temperature.
Limited studies with solutions of MEFOXIN in 0.9 percent Sodium Chloride Injection, Lactated Ringer's Injection, and 5 percent Dextrose Injection in VIAFLEX† intravenous bags show stability for 24 hours at room temperature, 48 hours under refrigeration or 26 weeks in the frozen state and 24 hours at room temperature thereafter. Also, solutions of MEFOXIN in 0.9 percent Sodium Chloride Injection show similar stability in plastic tubing, drip chambers, and volume control devices of common intravenous infusion sets.
After constitution with Sterile Water for Injection and subsequent storage in disposable plastic syringes, MEFOXIN is stable for 24 hours at room temperature and 48 hours under refrigeration.
After the periods mentioned above, any unused solutions or frozen material should be discarded. Do not refreeze.

Table 2—Maintenance Dosage of MEFOXIN in Adults with Reduced Renal Function

Renal Function	Creatinine Clearance (mL/min)	Dose (grams)	Frequency
Mild impairment	50–30	1–2	every 8–12 hours
Moderate impairment	29–10	1–2	every 12–24 hours
Severe impairment	9–5	0.5–1	every 12–24 hours
Essentially no function	<5	0.5–1	every 24–48 hours

Table 1—Guidelines for Dosage of MEFOXIN

Type of Infection	Daily Dosage	Frequency and Route
Uncomplicated forms* of infections such as pneumonia, urinary tract infection, cutaneous infection	3–4 grams	1 gram every 6–8 hours IV or IM
Moderately severe or severe infections	6–8 grams	1 gram every 4 hours *or* 2 grams every 6–8 hours IV
Infections commonly needing antibiotics in higher dosage (e.g., gas gangrene)	12 grams	2 grams every 4 hours *or* 3 grams every 6 hours IV

*Including patients in whom bacteremia is absent or unlikely

Table 3—Preparation of Solution
MEFOXIN

Strength	Amount of Diluent to be Added (mL)*	Approximate Withdrawable Volume (mL)	Approximate Average Concentration (mg/mL)
1 gram Vial	2 (Intramuscular)	2.5	400
2 gram Vial	4 (Intramuscular)	5	400
1 gram Vial	10 (IV)	10.5	95
2 gram Vial	10 or 20 (IV)	11.1 or 21.0	180 or 95
1 gram Infusion Bottle	50 or 100 (IV)	50 or 100	20 or 10
2 gram Infusion Bottle	50 or 100 (IV)	50 or 100	40 or 20
10 gram Bulk	43 or 93 (IV)	49 or 98.5	200 or 100

*Shake to dissolve and let stand until clear.

Intramuscular

MEFOXIN, as constituted with Sterile Water for Injection, Bacteriostatic Water for Injection, or 0.5 percent or 1 percent lidocaine hydrochloride solution (without epinephrine), maintains satisfactory potency for 24 hours at room temperature, for one week under refrigeration (below 5℃), and for at least 30 weeks in the frozen state.

After the periods mentioned above, any unused solutions or frozen material should be discarded. Do not refreeze.

MEFOXIN has also been found compatible when admixed in intravenous infusions with the following:

Heparin 0.1 units/mL at room temperature—8 hours
Heparin 100 units/mL at room temperature—24 hours
M.V.I.†† concentrate at room temperature 24 hours; under refrigeration 48 hours
BEROCCA††† C-500 at room temperature 24 hours; under refrigeration 48 hours
Insulin in Normal Saline at room temperature 24 hours; under refrigeration 48 hours
Insulin in 10% invert sugar at room temperature 24 hours; under refrigeration 48 hours

*   Registered trademark of Abbott Laboratories.
**   Registered trademark of Cutter Laboratories, Inc.
***   Registered trademark of American Hospital Supply Corporation.
‡   In these solutions, MEFOXIN has been found to be stable for a period of one week under refrigeration.
†   Registered trademark of Baxter International, Ltd.
††   Registered trademark of USV Pharmaceutical Corp.
†††   Registered trademark of Roche Laboratories.

HOW SUPPLIED

Sterile MEFOXIN is a dry white to off-white powder supplied in vials and infusion bottles containing cefoxitin sodium as follows:
No. 3356—1 gram cefoxitin equivalent
NDC 0006-3356-45 in trays of 25 vials
(6505-01-119-6005, 1 g 25's).
No. 3368—1 gram cefoxitin equivalent
NDC 0006-3368-71 in trays of 10 infusion bottles
(6505-01-195-0649, 1 g infusion bottle 10's).
No. 3357—2 gram cefoxitin equivalent
NDC 0006-3357-53 in trays of 25 vials
(6505-01-104-6393, 2 g 25's).
No. 3369—2 gram cefoxitin equivalent
NDC 0006-3369-73 in trays of 10 infusion bottles
(6505-01-185-2624, 2 g infusion bottle 10's).
No. 3388—10 gram cefoxitin equivalent
NDC 0006-3388-67 in trays of 6 bulk bottles
(6505-01-263-0730, 10 g 6's).
No. 3548—1 gram cefoxitin equivalent
NDC 0006-3548-45 in trays of 25 ADD-Vantage® vials.
(6505-01-262-9509, 1 g ADD-Vantage® 25's).
No. 3549—2 gram cefoxitin equivalent
NDC 0006-3549-53 in trays of 25 ADD-Vantage® vials.
(6505-01-263-4531, 2 g ADD-Vantage® 25's).

Special storage instructions

MEFOXIN in the dry state should be stored below 30℃. Avoid exposure to temperatures above 50℃. The dry material as well as solutions tend to darken, depending on storage conditions; product potency, however, is not adversely affected.

CLINICAL STUDIES

A prospective, randomized, double-blind, placebo-controlled clinical trial was conducted to determine the efficacy of short-term prophylaxis with MEFOXIN in patients undergoing cesarean section who were at high risk for subsequent endometritis because of ruptured membranes. Patients were randomized to receive either three doses of placebo (n=58), a single dose of MEFOXIN (2 g) followed by two doses of placebo (n=64), or a three-dose regimen of MEFOXIN (each dose consisting of 2 g) (n=60), given intravenously, usually beginning at the time of clamping of the umbilical cord, with the second and third doses given 4 and 8 hours post-operatively. Endometritis occurred in 16/58 (27.6%) patients

given placebo, 5/63 (7.9%) patients given a single dose of MEFOXIN, and 3/58 (5.2%) patients given three doses of MEFOXIN. The differences between the two groups treated with MEFOXIN and placebo with respect to endometritis were statistically significant (p < 0.01) in favor of MEFOXIN. The differences between the one-dose and three-dose regimens of MEFOXIN were not statistically significant.

Two double-blind, randomized studies compared the efficacy of a single 2 gram intravenous dose of MEFOXIN to a single 2 gram dose of cefotetan in the prevention of surgical site-related infection (major morbidity) and non-site-related infections (minor morbidity) in patients following cesarean section. In the first study, 82/98 (83.7%) patients treated with MEFOXIN and 71/95 (74.7%) patients treated with cefotetan experienced no major or minor morbidity. The difference in the outcomes in this study (95% CI: −0.03, +0.21) was not statistically significant. In the second study, 65/75 (86.7%) patients treated with MEFOXIN and 62/76 (81.6%) patients treated with cefotetan experienced no major or minor morbidity. The difference in the outcomes in this study (95% CI: −0.08, +0.18) was not statistically significant.

7882333   Issued February 1995
COPYRIGHT © MERCK & CO., INC. 1985, 1995
All rights reserved

MEFOXIN® Premixed Intravenous Solution   ℞
(Cefoxitin Sodium Injection)

DESCRIPTION

Cefoxitin sodium is a semi-synthetic, broad-spectrum cepha antibiotic for intravenous administration. It is derived from cephamycin C, which is produced by *Streptomyces lactamdurans*. It is the sodium salt of 3-(hydroxymethyl) -7α- methoxy-8-oxo -7- [2- (2-thienyl) acetamido]-5-thia-1-azabicyclo [4.2.0] oct-2-ene-2-carboxylate carbamate (ester). The empirical formula is $C_{16}H_{16}N_3NaO_7S_2$, and the molecular weight is 449.44. The structural formula is:

Cefoxitin sodium contains approximately 53.8 mg (2.3 milliequivalents) of sodium per gram of cefoxitin activity.

Premixed Intravenous Solution MEFOXIN* (Cefoxitin Sodium Injection) is supplied as a sterile, nonpyrogenic, frozen, iso-osmotic solution of cefoxitin sodium. Each 50 mL contains cefoxitin sodium equivalent to either 1 gram or 2 grams cefoxitin. Dextrose hydrous USP has been added to the above dosages to adjust osmolality (approximately 2 grams and 1.1 grams to 1 gram and 2 gram dosages, respectively). The pH is adjusted with sodium bicarbonate and may have been adjusted with hydrochloric acid. The pH is approximately 6.5. After thawing, the solution is intended for intravenous use only. Solutions of MEFOXIN range from colorless to light amber.

The plastic container is fabricated from a specially designed multilayer plastic (PL 2040). Solutions are in contact with the polyethylene layer of this container and can leach out certain chemical components of the plastic in very small amounts within the expiration period. The suitability and safety of the plastic have been confirmed in tests in animals according to the USP biological tests for plastic containers, as well as by tissue culture toxicity studies.

*Registered trademark of MERCK & CO., INC.

CLINICAL PHARMACOLOGY

Clinical Pharmacology

Following an intravenous dose of 1 gram of cefoxitin, serum concentrations were 110 mcg/mL at 5 minutes, declining to

less than 1 mcg/mL at 4 hours. The half-life after an intravenous dose is 41 to 59 minutes. Approximately 85 percent of cefoxitin is excreted unchanged by the kidneys over a 6-hour period, resulting in high urinary concentrations. Probenecid slows tubular excretion and produces higher serum levels and increases the duration of measurable serum concentrations.

Cefoxitin passes into pleural and joint fluids and is detectable in antibacterial concentrations in bile.

Clinical experience has demonstrated that cefoxitin can be administered to patients who are also receiving carbenicillin, kanamycin, gentamicin, tobramycin, or amikacin (see PRECAUTIONS and DOSAGE AND ADMINISTRATION, ADMINISTRATION).

Microbiology

The bactericidal action of cefoxitin results from inhibition of cell wall synthesis. Cefoxitin has *in vitro* activity against a wide range of gram-positive and gram-negative organisms. The methoxy group in the 7α position provides MEFOXIN with a high degree of stability in the presence of beta-lactamases, both penicillinases and cephalosporinases, of gram-negative bacteria. Cefoxitin is usually active against the following organisms *in vitro* and in clinical infections:

Gram-positive

Staphylococcus aureus, including penicillinase and non-penicillinase producing strains
Staphylococcus epidermidis
Beta-hemolytic and other streptococci (most strains of enterococci, e.g., *Streptococcus faecalis,* are resistant)
Streptococcus pneumoniae

Gram-negative

Escherichia coli
Klebsiella species (including *K. pneumoniae*)
Hemophilus influenzae
Neisseria gonorrhoeae, including penicillinase and non-penicillinase producing strains
Proteus mirabilis
Morganella morganii
Proteus vulgaris
Providencia species, including *Providencia rettgeri*

Anaerobic organisms

Peptococcus species
Peptostreptococcus species
Clostridium species
Bacteroides species, including the *B. fragilis* group (includes *B. fragilis, B. distasonis, B. ovatus, B. thetaiotaomicron, B. vulgatus*)

MEFOXIN is inactive *in vitro* against most strains of *Pseudomonas aeruginosa* and enterococci and many strains of *Enterobacter cloacae.*

Methicillin-resistant staphylococci are almost uniformly resistant to MEFOXIN.

Susceptibility Tests

For fast-growing aerobic organisms, quantitative methods that require measurements of zone diameters give the most precise estimates of antibiotic susceptibility. One such procedure* has been recommended for use with discs to test susceptibility to cefoxitin. Interpretation involves correlation of the diameters obtained in the disc test with minimal inhibitory concentration (MIC) values for cefoxitin.

Reports from the laboratory giving results of the standardized single disc susceptibility test* using a 30 mcg cefoxitin disc should be interpreted according to the following criteria:

Organisms producing zones of 18 mm or greater are considered susceptible, indicating that the tested organism is likely to respond to therapy.

Organisms of intermediate susceptibility produce zones of 15 to 17 mm, indicating that the tested organism would be susceptible if high dosage is used or if the infection is confined to tissues and fluids (e.g., urine) in which high antibiotic levels are attained.

Resistant organisms produce zones of 14 mm or less, indicating that other therapy should be selected.

The cefoxitin disc should be used for testing cefoxitin susceptibility.

Cefoxitin has been shown by *in vitro* tests to have activity against certain strains of *Enterobacteriaceae* found resistant when tested with the cephalosporin class disc. For this reason, the cefoxitin disc should not be used for testing susceptibility to cephalosporins, and cephalosporin discs should not be used for testing susceptibility to cefoxitin.

Dilution methods, preferably the agar plate dilution procedure, are most accurate for susceptibility testing of obligate anaerobes.

Continued on next page

Merck & Co.—Cont.

A bacterial isolate may be considered susceptible if the MIC value for cefoxitin** is not more than 16 mcg/mL. Organisms are considered resistant if the MIC is greater than 32 mcg/mL.

---

* Bauer, A. W.; Kirby, W. M. M.; Sherris, J. C.; Turck, M.: Antibiotic susceptibility testing by a standardized single disc method, Amer. J. Clin. Path. 45 : 493–496, Apr. 1966. Standardized disc susceptibility test, Federal Register 37 : 20527–20529, 1972. National Committee for Clinical Laboratory Standards: Approved Standard: M2-A3, Performance Standards for Antimicrobial Disk Susceptibility Tests, 1984.

** Determined by the ICS agar dilution method (Ericsson and Sherris, Acta Path. Microbiol. Scand. [B] Suppl. No. 217, 1971) or any other method that has been shown to give equivalent results.

INDICATIONS AND USAGE

MEFOXIN, supplied as a premixed solution in plastic containers, is intended for intravenous use only. For indications specifically concerning the intramuscular use of cefoxitin (e.g., gonococcal urethritis) or for adverse reactions associated only with intramuscular administration, please refer to the product circular for MEFOXIN (Sterile Cefoxitin Sodium) supplied as dry powder.

Treatment

MEFOXIN is indicated for the treatment of serious infections caused by susceptible strains of the designated microorganisms in the diseases listed below.

(1) **Lower respiratory tract infections,** including pneumonia and lung abscess, caused by *Streptococcus pneumoniae,* other streptococci (excluding enterococci, e.g., *Streptococcus faecalis*), *Staphylococcus aureus* (penicillinase and non-penicillinase producing), *Escherichia coli, Klebsiella* species, *Hemophilus influenzae,* and *Bacteroides* species.

(2) **Genitourinary infections.** Urinary tract infections caused by *Escherichia coli, Klebsiella* species, *Proteus mirabilis,* indole-positive Proteus , (which include *Morganella morganii* and *Proteus vulgaris*), and *Providencia* species (including *Providencia rettgeri*). Uncomplicated gonorrhea due to *Neisseria gonorrhoeae* (penicillinase and non-penicillinase producing).

(3) **Intra-abdominal infections,** including peritonitis and intra-abdominal abscess, caused by *Escherichia coli, Klebsiella* species, *Bacteroides* species including the *Bacteroides fragilis* group***, and *Clostridium* species.

(4) **Gynecological infections,** including endometritis, pelvic cellulitis, and pelvic inflammatory disease caused by *Escherichia coli, Neisseria gonorrhoeae* (penicillinase and non-penicillinase producing), *Bacteroides* species including the *Bacteroides fragilis* group***, *Clostridium* species, *Peptococcus* species, *Peptostreptococcus* species, and Group B streptococci. MEFOXIN, like cephalosporins, has no activity against *Chlamydia trachomatis.* Therefore, when MEFOXIN is used in the treatment of patients with pelvic inflammatory disease and *C. trachomatis* is one of the suspected pathogens, appropriate anti-chlamydial coverage should be added.

(5) **Septicemia** caused by *Streptococcus pneumoniae, Staphylococcus aureus* (penicillinase and non-penicillinase producing), *Escherichia coli, Klebsiella* species, and *Bacteroides* species including the *Bacteroides fragilis* group.***

(6) **Bone and joint infections** caused by *Staphylococcus aureus* (penicillinase and non-penicillinase producing).

(7) **Skin and skin structure infections** caused by *Staphylococcus aureus* (penicillinase and non-penicillinase producing), *Staphylococcus epidermidis,* streptococci (excluding enterococci, e.g., *Streptococcus faecalis*), *Escherichia coli, Proteus mirabilis, Klebsiella* species, *Bacteroides* species including the *Bacteroides fragilis* group***, *Clostridium* species, *Peptococcus* species, and *Peptostreptococcus* species.

Appropriate culture and susceptibility studies should be performed to determine the susceptibility of the causative organisms to MEFOXIN. Therapy may be started while awaiting the results of these studies.

In randomized comparative studies, cefoxitin and cephalothin were comparably safe and effective in the management of infections caused by gram-positive cocci and gram-negative rods susceptible to the cephalosporins. MEFOXIN has a high degree of stability in the presence of bacterial beta-lactamases, both penicillinases and cephalosporinases.

Many infections caused by aerobic and anaerobic gram-negative bacteria resistant to some cephalosporins respond to MEFOXIN. Similarly, many infections caused by aerobic and anaerobic bacteria resistant to some penicillin antibiotics (ampicillin, carbenicillin, penicillin G) respond to treatment with MEFOXIN. Many infections caused by mixtures of susceptible aerobic and anaerobic bacteria respond to treatment with MEFOXIN.

Prevention

MEFOXIN is indicated for the prophylaxis of infection in patients undergoing uncontaminated gastrointestinal surgery, vaginal hysterectomy, abdominal hysterectomy, or cesarean section.

Effective prophylactic use depends on the time of administration. MEFOXIN usually should be given one-half to one hour before the operation, which is sufficient time to achieve effective levels in the wound during the procedure. Prophylactic administration should usually be stopped within 24 hours since continuing administration of any antibiotic increases the possibility of adverse reactions but, in the majority of surgical procedures, does not reduce the incidence of subsequent infection.

If there are signs of infection, specimens for culture should be obtained for identification of the causative organism so that appropriate treatment may be instituted.

*** B. fragilis, B. distasonis, B. ovatus, B. thetaiotaomicron, B. vulgatus.

CONTRAINDICATIONS

MEFOXIN is contraindicated in patients who have shown hypersensitivity to cefoxitin and the cephalosporin group of antibiotics.

WARNINGS

BEFORE THERAPY WITH 'MEFOXIN' IS INSTITUTED, CAREFUL INQUIRY SHOULD BE MADE TO DETERMINE WHETHER THE PATIENT HAS HAD PREVIOUS HYPERSENSITIVITY REACTIONS TO CEFOXITIN, CEPHALOSPORINS, PENICILLINS, OR OTHER DRUGS. THIS PRODUCT SHOULD BE GIVEN WITH CAUTION TO PENICILLIN-SENSITIVE PATIENTS. ANTIBIOTICS SHOULD BE ADMINISTERED WITH CAUTION TO ANY PATIENT WHO HAS DEMONSTRATED SOME FORM OF ALLERGY, PARTICULARLY TO DRUGS. IF AN ALLERGIC REACTION TO 'MEFOXIN' OCCURS, DISCONTINUE THE DRUG. SERIOUS HYPERSENSITIVITY REACTIONS MAY REQUIRE EPINEPHRINE AND OTHER EMERGENCY MEASURES.

Pseudomembranous colitis has been reported with virtually all antibiotics (including cephalosporins); therefore, it is important to consider its diagnosis in patients who develop diarrhea in association with antibiotic use. This colitis may range from mild to life threatening in severity.

Treatment with broad-spectrum antibiotics alters normal flora of the colon and may permit overgrowth of clostridia. Studies indicate a toxin produced by *Clostridium difficile* is one primary cause of antibiotic-associated colitis.

Mild cases of pseudomembranous colitis may respond to drug discontinuance alone. In more severe cases, management may include sigmoidoscopy, appropriate bacteriological studies, fluid, electrolyte and protein supplementation, and the use of a drug such as oral vancomycin as indicated. Isolation of the patient may be advisable. Other causes of colitis should also be considered.

PRECAUTIONS

General

The total daily dose should be reduced when MEFOXIN is administered to patients with transient or persistent reduction of urinary output due to renal insufficiency (see DOSAGE AND ADMINISTRATION, *TREATMENT),* because high and prolonged serum antibiotic concentrations can occur in such individuals from usual doses.

Antibiotics (including cephalosporins) should be prescribed with caution in individuals with a history of gastrointestinal disease, particularly colitis.

As with other antibiotics, prolonged use of MEFOXIN may result in overgrowth of nonsusceptible organisms. Repeated evaluation of the patient's condition is essential. If superinfection occurs during therapy, appropriate measures should be taken.

Do not use unless solution is clear and seal is intact.

Drug Interactions

Increased nephrotoxicity has been reported following concomitant administration of cephalosporins and aminoglycoside antibiotics.

Drug/Laboratory Test Interactions

As with cephalothin, high concentrations of cefoxitin (>100 micrograms/mL) may interfere with measurement of serum and urine creatinine levels by the Jaffé reaction, and produce false increases of modest degree in the levels of creatinine reported. Serum samples from patients treated with cefoxitin should not be analyzed for creatinine if withdrawn within 2 hours of drug administration.

High concentrations of cefoxitin in the urine may interfere with measurement of urinary 17-hydroxy-corticosteroids by the Porter-Silber reaction, and produce false increases of modest degree in the levels reported.

A false-positive reaction for glucose in the urine may occur. This has been observed with CLINITEST* reagent tablets.

---

* Registered trademark of Ames Company, Division of Miles Laboratories, Inc.

Carcinogenesis, Mutagenesis, Impairment of Fertility

Long term studies in animals have not been performed with cefoxitin to evaluate carcinogenic or mutagenic potential. Studies in rats treated intravenously with 400 mg/kg of cefoxitin (approximately three times the maximum recommended human dose) revealed no effects on fertility or mating ability.

Pregnancy

Pregnancy Category B. Reproduction studies performed in rats and mice at parenteral doses of approximately one to seven and one-half times the maximum recommended human dose did not reveal teratogenic or fetal toxic effects, although a slight decrease in fetal weight was observed. There are, however, no adequate and well-controlled studies in pregnant women. Because animal reproduction studies are not always predictive of human response, this drug should be used during pregnancy only if clearly needed. In the rabbit, cefoxitin was associated with a high incidence of abortion and maternal death. This was not considered to be a teratogenic effect but an expected consequence of the rabbit's unusual sensitivity to antibiotic-induced changes in the population of the microflora of the intestine.

Nursing Mothers

Cefoxitin is excreted in human milk in low concentrations. Caution should be exercised when MEFOXIN is administered to a nursing woman.

Pediatric Use

Safety and efficacy in infants from birth to three months of age have not yet been established. In children three months of age and older, higher doses of cefoxitin have been associated with an increased incidence of eosinophilia and elevated SGOT.

The potential for toxic effects in children from chemicals that may leach from the single-dose I.V. preparation in plastic has not been determined.

ADVERSE REACTIONS

Cefoxitin is generally well tolerated. The most common adverse reactions have been local reactions following intravenous injection. Other adverse reactions have been encountered infrequently.

Local Reactions

Thrombophlebitis has occurred with intravenous administration.

Allergic Reactions

Rash (including exfoliative dermatitis and toxic epidermal necrolysis), pruritus, eosinophilia, fever, dyspnea, and other allergic reactions including anaphylaxis, interstitial nephritis and angioedema have been noted.

Cardiovascular

Hypotension

Gastrointestinal

Diarrhea, including documented pseudomembranous colitis which can appear during or after antibiotic treatment. Nausea and vomiting have been reported rarely.

Neuromuscular

Possible exacerbation of myasthenia gravis.

Blood

Eosinophilia, leukopenia including granulocytopenia, neutropenia, anemia, including hemolytic anemia, thrombocytopenia, and bone marrow depression. A positive direct Coombs test may develop in some individuals, especially those with azotemia.

Liver Function

Transient elevations in SGOT, SGPT, serum LDH, and serum alkaline phosphatase; and jaundice have been reported.

Renal Function

Elevations in serum creatinine and/or blood urea nitrogen levels have been observed. As with the cephalosporins, acute renal failure has been reported rarely. The role of MEFOXIN in changes in renal function tests is difficult to assess, since factors predisposing to prerenal azotemia or to impaired renal function usually have been present.

OVERDOSAGE

The acute intravenous LD_{50} in the adult female mouse and rabbit was about 8.0 g/kg and greater than 1.0 g/kg respectively. The acute intraperitoneal LD_{50} in the adult rat was greater than 10.0 g/kg.

DOSAGE AND ADMINISTRATION

NOTE: MEFOXIN® in Galaxy† container is for intravenous infusion only.

TREATMENT

Adults

The usual adult dosage range is 1 gram to 2 grams every six to eight hours. Dosage and route of administration should be determined by susceptibility of the causative organisms, severity of infection, and the condition of the patient (see Table 1 for dosage guidelines).

If *C. trachomatis* is a suspected pathogen, appropriate antichlamydial coverage should be added, because cefoxitin sodium has no activity against this organism.

MEFOXIN may be used in patients with reduced renal function with the following dosage adjustments:

In adults with renal insufficiency, an initial loading dose of 1 gram to 2 grams may be given. After a loading dose, the recommendations for *maintenance dosage* (Table 2) may be used as a guide.

When only the serum creatinine level is available, the following formula (based on sex, weight, and age of the patient) may be used to convert this value into creatinine clearance. The serum creatinine should represent a steady state of renal function.

Males:
$$\frac{\text{Weight (kg)} \times (140 - \text{age})}{72 \times \text{serum creatinine (mg/100 mL)}}$$

Females: $0.85 \times$ male value

In patients undergoing hemodialysis, the loading dose of 1 to 2 grams should be given after each hemodialysis, and the maintenance dose should be given as indicated in Table 2.

Antibiotic therapy for group A beta-hemolytic streptococcal infections should be maintained for at least 10 days to guard against the risk of rheumatic fever or glomerulonephritis. In staphylococcal and other infections involving a collection of pus, surgical drainage should be carried out where indicated.

Infants and Children

The recommended dosage in children three months of age and older is 80 to 160 mg/kg of body weight per day divided into four to six equal doses. The higher dosages should be used for more severe or serious infections. The total daily dosage should not exceed 12 grams.

At this time no recommendation is made for children from birth to three months of age (see PRECAUTIONS).

In children with renal insufficiency the dosage and frequency of dosage should be modified consistent with the recommendations for adults (see Table 2).

PREVENTION

For prophylactic use in uncontaminated gastrointestinal surgery, vaginal hysterectomy, or abdominal hysterectomy, the following doses are recommended:

Adults:

2 grams administered intravenously just prior to surgery (approximately one-half to one hour before the initial incision) followed by 2 grams every 6 hours after the first dose for no more than 24 hours.

Children (3 months and older):

30 to 40 mg/kg doses may be given at the times designated above.

Cesarean section patients:

For patients undergoing cesarean section, either a single 2 gram dose administered intravenously as soon as the umbilical cord is clamped OR a 3-dose regimen consisting of 2 grams given intravenously as soon as the umbilical cord is clamped followed by 2 grams 4 and 8 hours after the initial dose is recommended. (See CLINICAL STUDIES.)

[See table 1 above.]

ADMINISTRATION

This premixed solution is for intravenous use only. Premixed Intravenous Solution MEFOXIN in Galaxy® containers (PL 2040 Plastic) is to be administered either as a continuous or intermittent infusion using sterile equipment. Scalp vein-type needles are preferred for this type of infusion. It is recommended that the intravenous administration apparatus be replaced at least once every 48 hours.

The intravenous route is preferred for patients with bacteremia, bacterial septicemia, or other severe or life-threatening infections, or for patients who may be poor risks because of lowered resistance resulting from such debilitating conditions as malnutrition, trauma, surgery, diabetes, heart failure, or malignancy, particularly if shock is present or impending.

Directions for Use of Galaxy® Containers (PL 2040 Plastic)

Thaw frozen container at room temperature, 25°C (77°F), or under refrigeration, 2–8°C (36–46°F). DO NOT FORCE THAW BY IMMERSION IN WATER BATHS OR BY MICROWAVE IRRADIATION.

After thawing, check for minute leaks by squeezing container firmly. If leaks are detected, discard solution as sterility may be impaired.

The container should be visually inspected for particulate matter and discoloration prior to administration. Components of the solution may precipitate in the frozen state and will dissolve upon reaching room temperature with little or no agitation. Agitate after solution has reached room temperature.

Table 1—Guidelines for Dosage of MEFOXIN

Type of Infection	Daily Dosage	Frequency and Route
Uncomplicated forms* of infections such as pneumonia, urinary tract infection, cutaneous infection	3–4 grams	1 gram every 6–8 hours IV
Moderately severe or severe infections	6–8 grams	1 gram every 4 hours or 2 grams every 6–8 hours IV
Infections commonly needing antibiotics in higher dosage (e.g., gas gangrene)	12 grams	2 grams every 4 hours or 3 grams every 6 hours IV

*Including patients in whom bacteremia is absent or unlikely.

Table 2—Maintenance Dosage of MEFOXIN in Adults with Reduced Renal Function

Renal Function	Creatinine Clearance (mL/min)	Dose (grams)	Frequency
Mild impairment	50–30	1–2	every 8–12 hours
Moderate impairment	29–10	1–2	every 12–24 hours
Severe impairment	9–5	0.5–1	every 12–24 hours
Essentially no function	<5	0.5–1	every 24–48 hours

Do not use if the solution is cloudy or a precipitate has formed. If any seals or outlet ports are not intact, the container should be discarded. Solutions of MEFOXIN tend to darken depending on storage conditions; product potency, however, is not adversely affected.

Additives should not be introduced into this solution.

CAUTION: Do not use plastic containers in series connections. Such use would result in air embolism due to residual air being drawn from the primary container before administration of the fluid from the secondary container is complete.

Preparation for Intravenous Administration:

1. Suspend container from eyelet support.
2. Remove plastic protector from outlet port at bottom of container.
3. Attach administration set. Refer to complete directions accompanying set.

MEFOXIN may be administered through the tubing system by which the patient may be receiving other intravenous solutions. However, during infusion of the solution containing MEFOXIN, it is advisable to temporarily discontinue administration of any other solutions at the same site.

Solutions of MEFOXIN, like those of most beta-lactam antibiotics, should not be added to aminoglycoside solutions (e.g., gentamicin sulfate, tobramycin sulfate, amikacin sulfate) because of potential interaction. However, MEFOXIN and aminoglycosides may be administered separately to the same patient.

†Galaxy® is a registered trademark of Baxter International Inc.

STABILITY

MEFOXIN, supplied as frozen, premixed, iso-osmotic solution in Galaxy® containers (PL 2040 Plastic), maintains satisfactory potency after thawing for 24 hours at a room temperature of 25°C (77°F) or 21 days under refrigeration, 2–8°C (36–46°F). After these periods, any unused solutions should be discarded.

DO NOT REFREEZE.

HOW SUPPLIED

Premixed Intravenous Solution MEFOXIN is supplied in single dose Galaxy® containers (PL 2040 Plastic) containing cefoxitin sodium as follows:

No. 2G3506—1 gram cefoxitin equivalent, iso-osmotic in 50 mL diluent containing approximately 2 grams dextrose hydrous USP
NDC 0006-3545-24 in boxes of 24.

No. 2G3507—2 gram cefoxitin equivalent, iso-osmotic in 50 mL diluent containing approximately 1.1 grams dextrose hydrous USP
NDC 0006-3547-25 in boxes of 24.

Special storage instructions

Store at or below −20°C (−4°F). [See Directions for Use of Galaxy® container (PL 2040 Plastic)].

MEFOXIN is also available in dry powder form in vials and infusion bottles containing sterile cefoxitin sodium equivalent to either 1 gram or 2 grams of cefoxitin, and in vials for pharmacy bulk use containing sterile cefoxitin sodium equivalent to 10 grams of cefoxitin, for constitution and either intravenous or intramuscular administration (see appropriate product circular).

CLINICAL STUDIES

A prospective, randomized, double-blind, placebo-controlled clinical trial was conducted to determine the efficacy of short-term prophylaxis with MEFOXIN in patients undergoing cesarean section who were at high risk for subsequent endometritis because of ruptured membranes. Patients were randomized to receive either three doses of placebo (n = 58), a single dose of MEFOXIN (2 g) followed by two doses of placebo (n = 64), or a three-dose regimen of MEFOXIN (each dose consisting of 2 g) (n = 60), given intravenously, usually beginning at the time of clamping of the umbilical cord, with the second and third doses given 4 and 8 hours post-operatively. Endometritis occurred in 16/58 (27.6%) patients given placebo, 5/63 (7.9%) patients given a single dose of MEFOXIN, and 3/58 (5.2%) patients given three doses of MEFOXIN. The differences between the two groups treated with MEFOXIN and placebo with respect to endometritis were statistically significant (p < 0.01) in favor of MEFOXIN. The differences between the one-dose and three-dose regimens of MEFOXIN were not statistically significant.

Two double-blind, randomized studies compared the efficacy of a single 2 gram intravenous dose of MEFOXIN to a single 2 gram intravenous dose of cefotetan in the prevention of surgical site-related infection (major morbidity) and non-site-related infections (minor morbidity) in patients following cesarean section. In the first study, 82/98 (83.7%) patients treated with MEFOXIN and 71/95 (74.7%) patients treated with cefotetan experienced no major or minor morbidity. The difference in the outcomes in this study (95% CI: −0.03, +0.21) was not statistically significant. In the second study, 65/75 (86.7%) patients treated with MEFOXIN and 62/76 (81.6%) patients treated with cefotetan experienced no major or minor morbidity. The difference in the outcomes in this study (95% CI: −0.08, +0.18) was not statistically significant.

Manufactured for:
MERCK & CO., INC., WEST POINT, PA 19486, USA
By:
BAXTER HEALTHCARE CORPORATION
Deerfield, Illinois 60015, USA
7948517   Issued February 1995
COPYRIGHT © MERCK & CO., INC., 1985, 1995
All rights reserved

MEPHYTON® Tablets
(Phytonadione), U.S.P.
Vitamin K₁
℞

DESCRIPTION

Phytonadione is a vitamin which is a clear, yellow to amber, viscous, and nearly odorless liquid. It is insoluble in water, soluble in chloroform and slightly soluble in ethanol. It has a molecular weight of 450.70.

Phytonadione is 2-methyl-3-phytyl-1, 4-naphthoquinone. Its empirical formula is $C_{31}H_{46}O_2$ and its structural formula is:

Continued on next page

Information on the Merck & Co., Inc. products listed on these pages is the full prescribing information from product circulars in use September 30, 1996.

Consult 1997 supplements and future editions for revisions

Merck & Co.—Cont.

MEPHYTON* (Phytonadione) tablets containing 5 mg of phytonadione are yellow, compressed tablets, scored on one side. Inactive ingredients are acacia, calcium phosphate, colloidal silicon dioxide, lactose, magnesium stearate, starch, and talc.

* Registered trademark of MERCK & CO., INC.

CLINICAL PHARMACOLOGY

MEPHYTON tablets possess the same type and degree of activity as does naturally-occurring vitamin K, which is necessary for the production via the liver of active prothrombin (factor II), proconvertin (factor VII), plasma thromboplastin component (factor IX), and Stuart factor (factor X). The prothrombin test is sensitive to the levels of three of these four factors—II, VII, and X. Vitamin K is an essential cofactor for a microsomal enzyme that catalyzes the post-translational carboxylation of multiple, specific, peptide-bound glutamic acid residues in inactive hepatic precursors of factors II, VII, IX, and X. The resulting gamma-carboxyglutamic acid residues convert the precursors into active coagulation factors that are subsequently secreted by liver cells into the blood. Oral phytonadione is adequately absorbed from the gastrointestinal tract only if bile salts are present. After absorption, phytonadione is initially concentrated in the liver, but the concentration declines rapidly. Very little vitamin K accumulates in tissues. Little is known about the metabolic fate of vitamin K. Almost no free unmetabolized vitamin K appears in bile or urine.

In normal animals and humans, phytonadione is virtually devoid of pharmacodynamic activity. However, in animals and humans deficient in vitamin K, the pharmacological action of vitamin K is related to its normal physiological function; that is, to promote the hepatic biosynthesis of vitamin K-dependent clotting factors.

MEPHYTON tablets generally exert their effect within 6 to 10 hours.

INDICATIONS AND USAGE

MEPHYTON is indicated in the following coagulation disorders which are due to faulty formation of factors II, VII, IX and X when caused by vitamin K deficiency or interference with vitamin K activity.

MEPHYTON tablets are indicated in:

—anticoagulant-induced prothrombin deficiency caused by coumarin or indanedione derivatives;

—hypoprothrombinemia secondary to antibacterial therapy;

—hypoprothrombinemia secondary to administration of salicylates;

—hypoprothrombinemia secondary to obstructive jaundice or biliary fistulas but only if bile salts are administered concurrently, since otherwise the oral vitamin K will not be absorbed.

CONTRAINDICATION

Hypersensitivity to any component of this medication.

WARNINGS

An immediate coagulant effect should not be expected after administration of phytonadione.

Phytonadione will not counteract the anticoagulant action of heparin.

When vitamin K$_1$ is used to correct excessive anticoagulant-induced hypoprothrombinemia, anticoagulant therapy still being indicated, the patient is again faced with the clotting hazards existing prior to starting the anticoagulant therapy. Phytonadione is not a clotting agent, but overzealous therapy with vitamin K$_1$ may restore conditions which originally permitted thromboembolic phenomena. Dosage should be kept as low as possible, and prothrombin time should be checked regularly as clinical conditions indicate.

Repeated large doses of vitamin K are not warranted in liver disease if the response to initial use of the vitamin is unsatisfactory. Failure to respond to vitamin K may indicate a congenital coagulation defect or that the condition being treated is unresponsive to vitamin K.

PRECAUTIONS

General

Temporary resistance to prothrombin-depressing anticoagulants may result, especially when larger doses of phytonadione are used. If relatively large doses have been employed, it may be necessary when reinstituting anticoagulant therapy to use somewhat larger doses of the prothrombin-depressing anticoagulant, or to use one which acts on a different principle, such as heparin sodium.

Laboratory Tests

Prothrombin time should be checked regularly as clinical conditions indicate.

Carcinogenesis, Mutagenesis, Impairment of Fertility

Studies of carcinogenicity or impairment of fertility have not been performed with MEPHYTON. MEPHYTON at concentrations up to 2000 mcg/plate with or without metabolic activation, was negative in the Ames microbial mutagen test.

Pregnancy

Pregnancy Category C: Animal reproduction studies have not been conducted with MEPHYTON. It is also not known whether MEPHYTON can cause fetal harm when administered to a pregnant woman or can affect reproduction capacity. MEPHYTON should be given to a pregnant woman only if clearly needed.

Pediatric Use

Safety and effectiveness in pediatric patients have not been established with MEPHYTON. Hemolysis, jaundice, and hyperbilirubinemia in newborns, particularly in premature infants, have been reported with vitamin K.

Nursing Mothers

It is not known whether this drug is excreted in human milk. Because many drugs are excreted in human milk, caution should be exercised when MEPHYTON is administered to a nursing woman.

ADVERSE REACTIONS

Transient "flushing sensations" and "peculiar" sensations of taste have been observed with parenteral phytonadione, as well as rare instances of dizziness, rapid and weak pulse, profuse sweating, brief hypotension, dyspnea, and cyanosis. Hyperbilirubinemia has been observed in the newborn following administration of parenteral phytonadione. This has occurred rarely and primarily with doses above those recommended.

OVERDOSAGE

The intravenous and oral LD$_{50}$s in the mouse are approximately 1.17 g/kg and greater than 24.18 g/kg, respectively.

DOSAGE AND ADMINISTRATION

MEPHYTON
Summary of Dosage Guidelines
(See circular text for details)

Adults	Initial Dosage
Anticoagulant-Induced Prothrombin Deficiency (caused by coumarin or indanedione derivatives)	2.5 mg–10 mg or up to 25 mg (rarely 50 mg)
Hypoprothrombinemia due to other causes (Antibiotics; Salicylates or other drugs; Factors limiting absorption or synthesis)	2.5 mg–25 mg or more (rarely up to 50 mg)

Anticoagulant-Induced Prothrombin Deficiency in Adults

To correct excessively prolonged prothrombin times caused by oral anticoagulant therapy—2.5 to 10 mg or up to 25 mg initially is recommended. In rare instances 50 mg may be required. Frequency and amount of subsequent doses should be determined by prothrombin time response or clinical condition. (See WARNINGS.) If, in 12 to 48 hours after oral administration, the prothrombin time has not been shortened satisfactorily, the dose should be repeated.

Hypoprothrombinemia Due to Other Causes in Adults

If possible, discontinuation or reduction of the dosage of drugs interfering with coagulation mechanisms (such as salicylates, antibiotics) is suggested as an alternative to administering concurrent MEPHYTON. The severity of the coagulation disorder should determine whether the immediate administration of MEPHYTON is required in addition to discontinuation or reduction of interfering drugs.

A dosage of 2.5 to 25 mg or more (rarely up to 50 mg) is recommended, the amount and route of administration depending upon the severity of the condition and response obtained. The oral route should be avoided when the clinical disorder would prevent proper absorption. Bile salts must be given with the tablets when the endogenous supply of bile to the gastrointestinal tract is deficient.

HOW SUPPLIED

No. 7776—Tablets MEPHYTON, 5 mg vitamin K$_1$, are yellow, round, scored, compressed tablets, coded MSD 43 on one side and MEPHYTON on the other. They are supplied as follows:

NDC 0006-0043-68 bottles of 100
(6505-00-660-0460, 5 mg 100's).

Shown in Product Identification Guide, page 324

Storage:
Protect from light.

7918715   Issued August 1995
COPYRIGHT © MERCK & CO., INC., 1986, 1991
All rights reserved

MERUVAX®II   ℞
(Rubella Virus Vaccine Live), U.S.P.
Wistar RA 27/3 Strain

DESCRIPTION

MERUVAX* II (Rubella Virus Vaccine Live) is a live virus vaccine for immunization against rubella (German measles). MERUVAX II is a sterile lyophilized preparation of the Wistar Institute RA 27/3 strain of live attenuated rubella virus. The virus was adapted to and propagated in human diploid cell (WI-38) culture.

The reconstituted vaccine is for subcutaneous administration. When reconstituted as directed, the dose for injection is 0.5 mL and contains not less than the equivalent of 1,000 TCID$_{50}$ (tissue culture infectious doses) of the U.S. Reference Rubella Virus. Each dose also contains approximately 25 mcg of neomycin. The product contains no preservative. Sorbitol and hydrolyzed gelatin are added as stabilizers.

* Registered trademark of MERCK & CO., INC.

CLINICAL PHARMACOLOGY

MERUVAX II produces a modified, non-communicable rubella infection in susceptible persons.

Extensive clinical trials of rubella virus vaccines, prepared using RA 27/3 strain rubella virus, have been carried out in more than 28,000 human subjects (approximately 11,000 with MERUVAX II) in the U.S.A. and more than 20 additional countries. A single injection of the vaccine has been shown to induce rubella hemagglutination-inhibiting (HI) antibodies in 97% or more of susceptible persons. The RA 27/3 rubella strain elicits higher immediate post-vaccination HI, complement-fixing and neutralizing antibody levels than other strains of rubella vaccine and has been shown to induce a broader profile of circulating antibodies including anti-theta and anti-iota precipitating antibodies. The RA 27/3 rubella strain immunologically simulates natural infection more closely than other rubella vaccine viruses. The increased levels and broader profile of antibodies produced by RA 27/3 strain rubella virus vaccine appear to correlate with greater resistance to subclinical reinfection with the wild virus, and provide greater confidence for lasting immunity.

Vaccine-induced antibody levels have been shown to persist for at least 10 years without substantial decline. If the present pattern continues, it will provide a basis for the expectation that immunity following vaccination will be permanent. However, continued surveillance will be required to demonstrate this point.

INDICATIONS AND USAGE†

1. *Children Between 12 Months of Age and Puberty*
MERUVAX II is indicated for immunization against rubella (German measles) in persons from 12 months of age to puberty. A booster is not needed. It is not recommended for infants younger than 12 months because they may retain maternal rubella neutralizing antibodies that may interfere with the immune response. Children in kindergarten and the first grades of elementary school deserve priority for vaccination because often they are epidemiologically the major source of virus dissemination in the community. A history of rubella illness is usually not reliable enough to exclude children from immunization.

Previously unimmunized children of susceptible pregnant women should receive live attenuated rubella vaccine, because an immunized child will be less likely to acquire natural rubella and introduce the virus into the household.

2. *Adolescent and Adult Males*
Vaccination of adolescent or adult males may be a useful procedure in preventing or controlling outbreaks of rubella in circumscribed population groups (e.g., military bases and schools).

3. *Non-Pregnant Adolescent and Adult Females*
Immunization of susceptible non-pregnant adolescent and adult females of childbearing age with live attenuated ru-

bella virus vaccine is indicated if certain precautions are observed (see below and PRECAUTIONS). Vaccinating susceptible postpubertal females confers individual protection against subsequently acquiring rubella infection during pregnancy, which in turn prevents infection of the fetus and consequent congenital rubella injury.

Women of childbearing age should be advised not to become pregnant for three months after vaccination and should be informed of the reason for this precaution.*

It is recommended that rubella susceptibility be determined by serologic testing prior to immunization.** If immune, as evidenced by a specific rubella antibody titer of 1:8 or greater (hemagglutination-inhibition test), vaccination is unnecessary. Congenital malformations do occur in up to seven percent of all live births. Their chance appearance after vaccination could lead to misinterpretation of the cause, particularly if the prior rubella-immune status of vaccinees is unknown.

Postpubertal females should be informed of the frequent occurrence of generally self-limited arthralgia and/or arthritis beginning 2 to 4 weeks after vaccination (see ADVERSE REACTIONS).

4. *Postpartum Women*

It has been found convenient in many instances to vaccinate rubella-susceptible women in the immediate postpartum period (see *Nursing Mothers*).

5. *International Travelers*

Individuals planning travel outside the United States, if not immune, can acquire measles, mumps or rubella and import these diseases to the United States. Therefore, prior to International travel, individuals known to be susceptible to one or more of these diseases can receive either a single antigen vaccine (measles, mumps or rubella), or a combined antigen vaccine as appropriate. However, M-M-R‡ II (Measles, Mumps, and Rubella Virus Vaccine Live) is preferred for persons likely to be susceptible to mumps and rubella; and if single-antigen measles vaccine is not readily available, travelers should receive M-M-R II (Measles, Mumps, and Rubella Virus Vaccine Live) regardless of their immune status to mumps or rubella.

Revaccination:

Children vaccinated when younger than 12 months of age should be revaccinated. Based on available evidence, there is no reason to routinely revaccinate persons who were vaccinated originally when 12 months of age or older. However, persons should be revaccinated if there is evidence to suggest that initial immunization was ineffective.

Use with Other Vaccines

Routine administration of DTP (diphtheria, tetanus, pertussis) and/or OPV (oral poliovirus vaccine) concomitantly with measles, mumps and rubella vaccines is not recommended because there are insufficient data relating to the simultaneous administration of these antigens. However, the American Academy of Pediatrics has noted that in some circumstances, particularly when the patient may not return, some practitioners prefer to administer all these antigens on a single day. If done, separate sites and syringes should be used for DTP and MERUVAX II.

MERUVAX II should not be given less than one month before or after administration of other virus vaccines.

---

†Based in part on the recommendation for rubella vaccine use of the Immunization Practices Advisory Committee (ACIP), Morbidity and Mortality Weekly Report: *33* (22): 301–310, 315–318, June 8, 1984.

*NOTE: The Immunization Practices Advisory Committee (ACIP) has recommended "In view of the importance of protecting this age group against rubella, reasonable precautions in a rubella immunization program include asking females if they are pregnant, excluding those who say they are, and explaining the theoretical risks to the others."

**NOTE: The Immunization Practices Advisory Committee (ACIP) has stated "When practical, and when reliable laboratory services are available, potential vaccinees of childbearing age can have serologic tests to determine susceptibility to rubella. . . . However, routinely performing serologic tests for all females of childbearing age to determine susceptibility so that vaccine is given only to proven susceptibles is expensive and has been ineffective in some areas. Accordingly, the ACIP believes that rubella vaccination of a woman who is not known to be pregnant and has no history of vaccination is justifiable without serologic testing."

‡Registered trademark of MERCK & CO., INC.

CONTRAINDICATIONS

Do not give MERUVAX II to pregnant females; the possible effects of the vaccine on fetal development are unknown at this time. If vaccination of postpubertal females is undertaken, pregnancy should be avoided for three months following vaccination. (See PRECAUTIONS, *Pregnancy*).

Anaphylactic or anaphylactoid reactions to neomycin (each dose of reconstituted vaccine contains approximately 25 mcg of neomycin).

Any febrile respiratory illness or other active febrile infection.

Active untreated tuberculosis.

Patients receiving immunosuppressive therapy. This contraindication does not apply to patients who are receiving corticosteroids as replacement therapy, e.g., for Addison's disease.

Individuals with blood dyscrasias, leukemia, lymphomas of any type, or other malignant neoplasms affecting the bone marrow or lymphatic systems.

Primary and acquired immunodeficiency states, including patients who are immunosuppressed in association with AIDS or other clinical manifestations of infection with human immunodeficiency viruses; cellular immune deficiencies; and hypogammaglobulinemic and dysgammaglobulinemic states.

Individuals with a family history of congenital or hereditary immunodeficiency, until the immune competence of the potential vaccine recipient is demonstrated.

PRECAUTIONS

General

Adequate treatment provisions including epinephrine, should be available for immediate use should an anaphylactic or anaphylactoid reaction occur.

Excretion of small amounts of the live attenuated rubella virus from the nose or throat has occurred in the majority of susceptible individuals 7–28 days after vaccination. There is no confirmed evidence to indicate that such virus is transmitted to susceptible persons who are in contact with the vaccinated individuals. Consequently, transmission through close personal contact, while accepted as a theoretical possibility, is not regarded as a significant risk. However, transmission of the vaccine virus to infants via breast milk has been documented (see *Nursing Mothers*).

There is no evidence that live rubella virus vaccine given after exposure to natural rubella virus will prevent illness. There is, however, no contraindication to vaccinating children already exposed to natural rubella.

Children and young adults who are known to be infected with human immunodeficiency viruses but without overt clinical manifestations of immunosuppression may be vaccinated; however, the vaccinees should be monitored closely for vaccine-preventable diseases because immunization may be less effective than for uninfected persons.

Vaccination should be deferred for at least three months following blood or plasma transfusions, or administration of human immune serum globulin. However, susceptible postpartum patients who received blood products may receive MERUVAX II prior to discharge provided that a repeat HI titer is drawn 6–8 weeks after vaccination to insure seroconversion. Similarly, although studies with other live rubella virus vaccines suggest that MERUVAX II may be given in the immediate postpartum period to those non-immune women who have received anti-Rho (D) globulin (human) without interfering with vaccine effectiveness, a follow-up post-vaccination HI titer should also be determined.

It has been reported that attenuated rubella virus vaccine, live, may result in a temporary depression of tuberculin skin sensitivity. Therefore, if a tuberculin test is to be done, it should be administered either before or simultaneously with MERUVAX II.

As for any vaccine, vaccination with MERUVAX II may not result in seroconversion in 100% of susceptible persons given the vaccine.

Pregnancy

Pregnancy Category C

Animal reproduction studies have not been conducted with MERUVAX II. It is also not known whether MERUVAX II can cause fetal harm when administered to a pregnant woman or can affect reproduction capacity. There is evidence suggesting transmission of rubella vaccine viruses to products of conception. Therefore, rubella vaccine should not be administered to pregnant females (see CONTRAINDICATIONS).

In counseling women who are inadvertently vaccinated when pregnant or who become pregnant within 3 months of vaccination, the physician should be aware of the following: In a 10 year survey involving over 700 pregnant women who received rubella vaccine within 3 months before or after conception, (of whom 189 received the Wistar RA 27/3 strain) none of the newborns had abnormalities compatible with congenital rubella syndrome.

Nursing Mothers

Recent studies have shown that lactating postpartum women immunized with live attenuated rubella vaccine may secrete the virus in breast milk and transmit it to breast-fed infants. In the infants with serological evidence of rubella infection, none exhibited severe disease; however, one exhibited mild clinical illness typical of acquired rubella. Caution should be exercised when MERUVAX II is administered to a nursing woman.

ADVERSE REACTIONS

Burning and/or stinging of short duration at the injection site have been reported.

Symptoms of the same kind as those seen following natural rubella may occur after vaccination. These include mild regional lymphadenopathy, urticaria, rash, malaise, sore throat, fever, headache, dizziness, nausea, vomiting, diarrhea, polyneuritis, and arthralgia and/or arthritis (usually transient and rarely chronic). Local pain, wheal and flare, induration, and erythema may occur at the site of injection. Reactions are usually mild and transient. Erythema multiforme has also been reported rarely.

Cough and rhinitis have also been reported.

Vasculitis has been reported rarely.

Anaphylaxis and anaphylactoid reactions have been reported.

Moderate fever [101–102.9°F (38.3–39.4°C)] occurs occasionally, and high fever [over 103°F (39.4°C)] occurs less commonly.

Syncope, particularly at the time of mass vaccination, has been reported.

Chronic arthritis has been associated with natural rubella infection and has been related to persistent virus and/or viral antigen isolated from body tissues. Only rarely have vaccine recipients developed chronic joint symptoms.

Following vaccination in children, reactions in joints are uncommon and generally of brief duration. In women, incidence rates for arthritis and arthralgia are generally higher than those seen in children (children: 0–3%; women: 12–20%) and the reactions tend to be more marked and of longer duration. Symptoms may persist for a matter of months or on rare occasions for years. In adolescent girls, the reactions appear to be intermediate in incidence between those seen in children and in adult women. Even in older women (35–45 years), these reactions are generally well tolerated and rarely interfere with normal activities. Myalgia and paresthesia have been reported rarely after administration of MERUVAX II.

Forms of optic neuritis, including retrobulbar neuritis and papillitis may infrequently follow viral infections, and have been reported to occur 1 to 3 weeks following inoculation with some live virus vaccines.

Isolated reports of polyneuropathy including Guillain-Barré syndrome have been reported after immunization with rubella-containing vaccines.

Clinical experience with live rubella vaccines thus far indicates that encephalitis and other nervous system reactions have occurred very rarely in subjects who were given the vaccines, but a cause and effect relationship has not been established.

Thrombocytopenia with or without purpura has been reported.

DOSAGE AND ADMINISTRATION

FOR SUBCUTANEOUS ADMINISTRATION

Do not inject intravenously

The dosage of vaccine is the same for all persons. Inject the total volume of the single dose vial (about 0.5 mL) or 0.5 mL of the multiple dose vial of reconstituted vaccine subcutaneously, preferably into the outer aspect of upper arm. *Do not give immune globulin (IG) concurrently with* MERUVAX II.

To insure that there is no loss of potency during shipment, the vaccine must be maintained at a temperature of 10°C (50°F) or less.

Before reconstitution, store MERUVAX II at 2–8°C (36–46°F). *Protect from light.*

CAUTION: A sterile syringe free of preservatives, antiseptics, and detergents should be used for each injection and/or reconstitution of the vaccine because these substances may inactivate the live virus vaccine. A 25 gauge, $^5/_8$″ needle is recommended.

To reconstitute, use only the diluent supplied, since it is free of preservatives or other antiviral substances which might inactivate the vaccine.

Single Dose Vial—First withdraw the entire volume of diluent into the syringe to be used for reconstitution. Inject all the diluent in the syringe into the vial of lyophilized vaccine, and agitate to mix thoroughly. Withdraw the entire contents into a syringe and inject the total volume of restored vaccine subcutaneously.

It is important to use a separate sterile syringe and needle for each individual patient to prevent transmission of hep-

Continued on next page

Information on the Merck & Co., Inc. products listed on these pages is the full prescribing information from product circulars in use September 30, 1996.

Merck & Co.—Cont.

atitis B and other infectious agents from one person to another.

10 Dose Vial (available only to government agencies/institutions)—Withdraw the entire contents (7 mL) of the diluent vial into the sterile syringe to be used for reconstitution, and introduce into the 10 dose vial of lyophilized vaccine. Agitate to ensure thorough mixing. The outer labeling suggests "For Jet Injector or Syringe Use". Use with separate sterile syringes is permitted for containers of 10 doses or less. The vaccine and diluent do not contain preservatives; therefore, the user must recognize the potential contamination hazards and exercise special precautions to protect the sterility and potency of the product. The use of aseptic techniques and proper storage prior to and after restoration of the vaccine and subsequent withdrawal of the individual doses is essential. Use 0.5 mL of the reconstituted vaccine for subcutaneous injection.

It is important to use a separate sterile syringe and needle for each individual patient to prevent transmission of hepatitis B and other infectious agents from one person to another.

50 Dose Vial (available only to government agencies/institutions)—Withdraw the entire contents (30 mL) of diluent vial into the sterile syringe to be used for reconstitution and introduce into the 50 dose vial of lyophilized vaccine. Agitate to ensure thorough mixing. With full aseptic precautions, attach the vial to the sterilized multidose jet injector apparatus. Use 0.5 mL of the reconstituted vaccine for subcutaneous injection.

Each dose contains not less than the equivalent of 1,000 $TCID_{50}$ of the U.S. Reference Rubella Virus.

Parenteral drug products should be inspected visually for particulate matter and discoloration prior to administration. MERUVAX II, when reconstituted, is clear yellow.

HOW SUPPLIED

No. 4747—MERUVAX II is supplied as a single-dose vial of lyophilized vaccine,
NDC 0006-4747-00, and a vial of diluent.

No. 4673/4309—MERUVAX II is supplied as follows: (1) a box of 10 single-dose vials of lyophilized vaccine (package A), **NDC** 0006-4673-00; and (2) a box of 10 vials of diluent (package B). To conserve refrigerator space, the diluent may be stored separately at room temperature.
(6505-00-145-0180, Ten Pack).

Available only to government agencies/institutions:

No. 4674—MERUVAX II is supplied as one 10 dose vial of lyophilized vaccine,
NDC 0006-4674-00, and one 7 mL vial of diluent.

No. 4675—MERUVAX II is supplied as one 50 dose vial of lyophilized vaccine,
NDC 0006-4675-00, and one 30 mL vial of diluent.
(6505-01-222-6468, 50 Dose).

Storage

It is recommended that the vaccine be used as soon as possible after reconstitution. Protect vaccine from light at all times, since such exposure may inactivate the virus. Store reconstituted vaccine in the vaccine vial in a dark place at 2–8°C (36–46°F) and discard if not used within 8 hours.

A.H.F.S. Category: 80:12
7680317 Issued March 1995

COPYRIGHT © MERCK & CO., INC., 1990
All rights reserved

MEVACOR® Tablets ℞
(Lovastatin), U.S.P.

DESCRIPTION

MEVACOR* (Lovastatin), is a cholesterol lowering agent isolated from a strain of *Aspergillus terreus.* After oral ingestion, lovastatin, which is an inactive lactone, is hydrolyzed to the corresponding β-hydroxyacid form. This is a principal metabolite and an inhibitor of 3-hydroxy-3-methylglutaryl-coenzyme A (HMG-CoA) reductase. This enzyme catalyzes the conversion of HMG-CoA to mevalonate, which is an early and rate limiting step in the biosynthesis of cholesterol.

Lovastatin is [1*S*-[1α(*R* *),3α,7β,8β(2*S* *,4*S* *),8aβ]]-1,2,3,7,8,8a-hexahydro-3,7-dimethyl-8-[2-(tetrahydro-4-hydroxy-6-oxo-2*H*-pyran-2-yl)ethyl]-1-naphthalenyl 2-methylbutanoate. The empirical formula of lovastatin is $C_{24}H_{36}O_5$ and its molecular weight is 404.55. Its structural formula is:

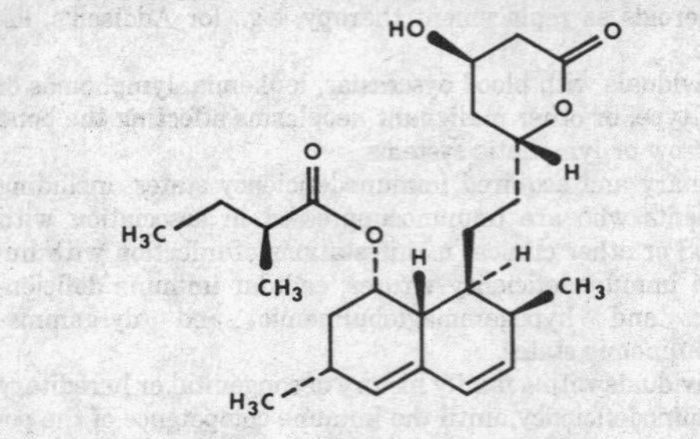

Lovastatin is a white, nonhygroscopic crystalline powder that is insoluble in water and sparingly soluble in ethanol, methanol, and acetonitrile.

Tablets MEVACOR are supplied as 10 mg, 20 mg and 40 mg tablets for oral administration. In addition to the active ingredient lovastatin, each tablet contains the following inactive ingredients: cellulose, lactose, magnesium stearate, and starch. Butylated hydroxyanisole (BHA) is added as a preservative. Tablets MEVACOR 10 mg also contain red ferric oxide and yellow ferric oxide. Tablets MEVACOR 20 mg also contain FD&C Blue 2. Tablets MEVACOR 40 mg also contain D&C Yellow 10 and FD&C Blue 2.

*Registered trademark of MERCK & CO., INC.

CLINICAL PHARMACOLOGY

The involvement of low-density lipoprotein (LDL) cholesterol in atherogenesis has been well-documented in clinical and pathological studies, as well as in many animal experiments. Epidemiological studies have established that high LDL (low-density lipoprotein) cholesterol and low HDL (high-density lipoprotein) cholesterol are both risk factors for coronary heart disease. The Lipid Research Clinics Coronary Primary Prevention Trial (LRC-CPPT), coordinated by the National Institutes of Health (NIH) studied men aged 35–59 with total cholesterol levels 265 mg/dL (6.8 mmol/L) or greater, LDL cholesterol values 175 mg/dL (4.5 mmol/L) or greater and triglyceride levels not more than 300 mg/dL (3.4 mmol/L). This seven-year, double-blind, placebo-controlled study demonstrated that lowering LDL cholesterol with diet and cholestyramine decreased the combined rate of coronary heart disease death plus non-fatal myocardial infarction.

MEVACOR has been shown to reduce both normal and elevated LDL cholesterol concentrations. LDL is formed from VLDL and is catabolized predominantly by the high affinity LDL receptor. The mechanism of the LDL-lowering effect of MEVACOR may involve both reduction of VLDL cholesterol concentration, and induction of the LDL receptor, leading to reduced production and/or increased catabolism of LDL cholesterol. Apolipoprotein B also falls substantially during treatment with MEVACOR. Since each LDL particle contains one molecule of apolipoprotein B, and since little apolipoprotein B is found in other lipoproteins, this strongly suggests that MEVACOR does not merely cause cholesterol to be lost from LDL, but also reduces the concentration of circulating LDL particles. In addition, MEVACOR can produce increases of variable magnitude in HDL cholesterol, and modestly reduces VLDL cholesterol and plasma triglycerides (see Tables I–IV under *Clinical Studies*). The effects of MEVACOR on Lp(a), fibrinogen, and certain other independent biochemical risk markers for coronary heart disease are unknown.

MEVACOR is a specific inhibitor of HMG-CoA reductase, the enzyme which catalyzes the conversion of HMG-CoA to mevalonate. The conversion of HMG-CoA to mevalonate is an early step in the biosynthetic pathway for cholesterol.

Pharmacokinetics

Lovastatin is a lactone which is readily hydrolyzed *in vivo* to the corresponding β-hydroxyacid, a potent inhibitor of HMG-CoA reductase. Inhibition of HMG-CoA reductase is the basis for an assay in pharmacokinetic studies of the β-hydroxyacid metabolites (active inhibitors) and, following base hydrolysis, active plus latent inhibitors (total inhibitors) in plasma following administration of lovastatin.

Following an oral dose of ^{14}C-labeled lovastatin in man, 10% of the dose was excreted in urine and 83% in feces. The latter represents absorbed drug equivalents excreted in bile, as well as any unabsorbed drug. Plasma concentrations of total radioactivity (lovastatin plus ^{14}C-metabolites) peaked at 2 hours and declined rapidly to about 10% of peak by 24 hours postdose. Absorption of lovastatin, estimated relative to an intravenous reference dose, in each of four animal species tested, averaged about 30% of an oral dose. In animal studies, after oral dosing, lovastatin had high selectivity for the liver, where it achieved substantially higher concentrations than in non-target tissues. Lovastatin undergoes extensive first-pass extraction in the liver, its primary site of action, with subsequent excretion of drug equivalents in the bile. As a consequence of extensive hepatic extraction of lovastatin, the availability of drug to the general circulation is low and variable. In a single dose study in four hypercholesterolemic patients, it was estimated that less than 5% of an oral dose of lovastatin reaches the general circulation as active inhibitors. Following administration of lovastatin tablets the coefficient of variation, based on between-subject variability, was approximately 40% for the area under the curve (AUC) of total inhibitory activity in the general circulation.

Both lovastatin and its β-hydroxyacid metabolite are highly bound (>95%) to human plasma proteins. Animal studies demonstrated that lovastatin crosses the blood-brain and placental barriers.

The major active metabolites present in human plasma are the β-hydroxyacid of lovastatin, its 6′-hydroxy derivative, and two additional metabolites. Peak plasma concentrations of both active and total inhibitors were attained within 2 to 4 hours of dose administration. While the recommended therapeutic dose range is 10 to 80 mg/day, linearity of inhibitory activity in the general circulation was established by a single dose study employing lovastatin tablet dosages from 60 to as high as 120 mg. With a once-a-day dosing regimen, plasma concentrations of total inhibitors over a dosing interval achieved a steady state between the second and third days of therapy and were about 1.5 times those following a single dose. When lovastatin was given under fasting conditions, plasma concentrations of total inhibitors were on average about two-thirds those found when lovastatin was administered immediately after a standard test meal.

In a study of patients with severe renal insufficiency (creatinine clearance 10–30 mL/min), the plasma concentrations of total inhibitors after a single dose of lovastatin were approximately two-fold higher than those in healthy volunteers.

Clinical Studies

MEVACOR has been shown to be highly effective in reducing total and LDL cholesterol in heterozygous familial and non-familial forms of primary hypercholesterolemia and in mixed hyperlipidemia. A marked response was seen within 2 weeks, and the maximum therapeutic response occurred within 4–6 weeks. The response was maintained during continuation of therapy. Single daily doses given in the evening were more effective than the same dose given in the morning, perhaps because cholesterol is synthesized mainly at night.

In multicenter, double-blind studies in patients with familial or non-familial hypercholesterolemia, MEVACOR, administered in doses ranging from 10 mg q.p.m. to 40 mg b.i.d., was compared to placebo. MEVACOR consistently and significantly decreased total plasma cholesterol (TOTAL-C), LDL cholesterol (LDL-C), total cholesterol/HDL cholesterol (TOTAL-C/HDL-C) ratio and LDL cholesterol/HDL cholesterol (LDL-C/HDL-C) ratio. In addition, MEVACOR produced increases of variable magnitude in HDL cholesterol (HDL-C), and modestly decreased VLDL cholesterol (VLDL-C) and plasma triglycerides (TRIG.) (see Tables I through IV for dose response results).

The results of a study in patients with primary hypercholesterolemia are presented in Table I.
[See table below.]

MEVACOR was compared to cholestyramine in a randomized open parallel study and to probucol in a double-blind, parallel study. Both studies were performed with patients with hypercholesterolemia who were at high risk of myocardial infarction. Summary results of these two comparative studies are presented in Tables II & III.
[See tables at top of next page.]

MEVACOR was studied in controlled trials in hypercholesterolemic patients with well-controlled non-insulin dependent diabetes mellitus with normal renal function. The effect of MEVACOR on lipids and lipoproteins and the safety profile of MEVACOR were similar to that demonstrated in studies in nondiabetics. MEVACOR had no clinically important effect on glycemic control or on the dose requirement of oral hypoglycemic agents.

TABLE I
MEVACOR vs Placebo
(Mean Percent Change from Baseline After 6 Weeks)

DOSAGE	N	TOTAL-C	LDL-C	HDL-C	LDL-C/ HDL-C	TOTAL-C/ HDL/C	TRIG.
Placebo	33	−2	−1	−1	0	+1	+9
MEVACOR							
10 mg q.p.m.	33	−16	−21	+5	−24	−19	−10
20 mg q.p.m.	33	−19	−27	+6	−30	−23	+9
10 mg b.i.d.	32	−19	−28	+8	−33	−25	−7
40 mg q.p.m.	33	−22	−31	+5	−33	−25	−8
20 mg b.i.d.	36	−24	−32	+2	−32	−24	−6

TABLE II
MEVACOR vs. Cholestyramine
(Percent Change from Baseline After 12 Weeks)

TREATMENT	N	TOTAL-C (mean)	LDL-C (mean)	HDL-C (mean)	LDL-C/ HDL-C (mean)	TOTAL-C/ HDL-C (mean)	VLDL-C (median)	TRIG. (median)
MEVACOR								
20 mg b.i.d.	85	−27	−32	+9	−36	−31	−34	−21
40 mg b.i.d.	88	−34	−42	+8	−44	−37	−31	−27
Cholestyramine								
12 g b.i.d.	88	−17	−23	+8	−27	−21	+2	+11

TABLE III
MEVACOR vs. Probucol
(Percent Change from Baseline After 14 Weeks)

TREATMENT	N	TOTAL-C (mean)	LDL-C (mean)	HDL-C (mean)	LDL-C/ HDL-C (mean)	TOTAL-C/ HDL-C (mean)	VLDL-C (median)	TRIG. (median)
MEVACOR								
40 mg q.p.m.	47	−25	−32	+9	−38	−31	−37	−18
80 mg q.p.m.	49	−30	−37	+11	−42	−36	−27	−17
40 mg b.i.d.	47	−33	−40	+12	−45	−39	−40	−25
Probucol								
500 mg b.i.d.	97	−10	−8	−23	+26	+23	−13	+1

TABLE IV
MEVACOR vs. Placebo
(Percent Change from Baseline—
Average Values Between Weeks 12 and 48)

DOSAGE	N**	TOTAL-C (mean)	LDL-C (mean)	HDL-C (mean)	LDL-C/ HDL-C (mean)	TOTAL-C/ HDL-C (mean)	TRIG. (median)
Placebo	1663	+0.7	+0.4	+2.0	+0.2	+0.6	+4
MEVACOR							
20 mg q.p.m.	1642	−17	−24	+6.6	−27	−21	−10
40 mg q.p.m.	1645	−22	−30	+7.2	−34	−26	−14
20 mg b.i.d.	1646	−24	−34	+8.6	−38	−29	−16
40 mg b.i.d.	1649	−29	−40	+9.5	−44	−34	−19
**Patients enrolled							

Expanded Clinical Evaluation of Lovastatin (EXCEL) Study
MEVACOR was compared to placebo in 8,245 patients with hypercholesterolemia (total cholesterol 240–300 mg/dL [6.2 mmol/L–7.6 mmol/L], LDL cholesterol >160 mg/dL [4.1 mmol/L]) in the randomized, double-blind, parallel, 48-week EXCEL study. All changes in the lipid measurements (Table IV) in MEVACOR treated patients were dose-related and significantly different from placebo (p ≤0.001). These results were sustained throughout the study.
[See Table IV above.]
Atherosclerosis
In the Canadian Coronary Atherosclerosis Intervention Trial (CCAIT), the effect of therapy with lovastatin on coronary atherosclerosis was assessed by coronary angiography in hyperlipidemic patients. In this randomized, double-blind, controlled clinical trial, patients were treated with conventional measures (usually diet and 325 mg of aspirin every other day) and either lovastatin 20–80 mg daily or placebo. Angiograms were evaluated at baseline and at two years by computerized quantitative coronary angiography (QCA). Lovastatin significantly slowed the progression of lesions as measured by the mean change per-patient in minimum lumen diameter (the primary endpoint) and percent diameter stenosis, and decreased the proportions of patients categorized with disease progression (33% vs. 50%) and with new lesions (16% vs. 32%).
In a similarly designed trial, the Monitored Atherosclerosis Regression Study (MARS), patients were treated with diet and either lovastatin 80 mg daily or placebo. No statistically significant difference between lovastatin and placebo was seen for the primary endpoint (mean change per patient in percent diameter stenosis of all lesions), or for most secondary QCA endpoints. Visual assessment by angiographers who formed a consensus opinion of overall angiographic change (Global Change Score) was also a secondary endpoint. By this endpoint, significant slowing of disease was seen, with regression in 23% of patients treated with lovastatin compared to 11% of placebo patients.
In the Familial Atherosclerosis Treatment Study (FATS), either lovastatin or niacin in combination with a bile acid sequestrant for 2.5 years in hyperlipidemic subjects significantly reduced the frequency of progression and increased the frequency of regression of coronary atherosclerotic lesions by QCA compared to diet and, in some cases, low-dose resin.
The effect of lovastatin on the progression of atherosclerosis in the coronary arteries has been corroborated by similar findings in another vasculature. In the Asymptomatic Carotid Artery Progression Study (ACAPS), the effect of therapy with lovastatin on carotid atherosclerosis was assessed by B-mode ultrasonography in hyperlipidemic patients with early carotid lesion and without known coronary heart disease at baseline. In this double-blind, controlled clinical trial, 919 patients were randomized in a 2 x 2 factorial design to placebo, lovastatin 10–40 mg daily and/or warfarin. Ultrasonograms of the carotid walls were used to determine the

change per patient from baseline to three years in mean maximum intimal-medial thickness (IMT) of 12 measured segments. There was a significant regression of carotid lesions in patients receiving lovastatin alone compared to those receiving placebo alone (p=0.001). The predictive value of changes in IMT for stroke has not yet been established. In the lovastatin group there was a significant reduction in the number of patients with major cardiovascular events relative to the placebo group (5 vs. 14) and a significant reduction in all-cause mortality (1 vs. 8).
Eye
There was a high prevalence of baseline lenticular opacities in the patient population included in the early clinical trials with lovastatin. During these trials the appearance of new opacities was noted in both the lovastatin and placebo groups. There was no clinically significant change in visual acuity in the patients who had new opacities reported nor was any patient, including those with opacities noted at baseline, discontinued from therapy because of a decrease in visual acuity.
A three-year, double-blind, placebo-controlled study in hypercholesterolemic patients to assess the effect of lovastatin on the human lens demonstrated that there were no clinically or statistically significant differences between the lovastatin and placebo groups in the incidence, type or progression of lenticular opacities. There are no controlled clinical data assessing the lens available for treatment beyond three years.

INDICATIONS AND USAGE

Therapy with lipid-altering agents should be a component of multiple risk factor intervention in those individuals at significantly increased risk for artherosclerotic vascular disease due to hypercholesterolemia. MEVACOR is indicated as an adjunct to diet for the reduction of elevated total and LDL cholesterol levels in patients with primary hypercholesterolemia (Types IIa and IIb***), when the response to diet restricted in saturated fat and cholesterol and to other nonpharmacological measures alone has been inadequate.
MEVACOR is also indicated to slow the progression of coronary atherosclerosis in patients with coronary heart disease as part of a treatment strategy to lower total and LDL cholesterol to target levels. Most subjects in the angiographic studies were middle-aged men; therefore, it is not clear to what extent these data can be extrapolated to women and the elderly (see CLINICAL PHARMACOLOGY, *Clinical Studies*).
Prior to initiating therapy with lovastatin, secondary causes for hypercholesterolemia (e.g., poorly controlled diabetes mellitus, hypothyroidism, nephrotic syndrome, dysproteinemias, obstructive liver disease, other drug therapy, alcoholism) should be excluded, and a lipid profile performed to measure TOTAL-C, HDL-C, and triglycerides (TG). For patients with TG less than 400 mg/dL (<4.5 mmol/L), LDL-C can be estimated using the following equation:
LDL-C = Total cholesterol − [0.2 × (triglycerides) + HDL-C]

For TG levels > 400 mg/dL (>4.5 mmol/L), this equation is less accurate and LDL-C concentrations should be determined by ultracentrifugation. In hypertriglyceridemic patients, LDL-C may be low or normal despite elevated TOTAL-C. In such cases, MEVACOR is not indicated.
The National Cholesterol Education Program (NCEP) Treatment Guidelines are summarized below:

		LDL-Cholesterol mg/dL (mmol/L)	
Definite Atherosclerotic Disease[†]	Two or More Other Risk Factors[††]	Initiation Level	Goal
NO	NO	≥190 (≥4.9)	<160 (<4.1)
NO	YES	≥160 (≥4.1)	<130 (<3.4)
YES	YES or NO	≥130 (≥3.4)	<100 (≤2.6)

[†] Coronary heart disease or peripheral vascular disease (including symptomatic carotid artery disease).
[††] Other risk factors for coronary heart disease (CHD) include: age (males: ≥45 years; females: ≥55 years of premature menopause without estrogen replacement therapy); family history of premature CHD; current cigarette smoking; hypertension; confirmed HDL-C <35 mg/dL (<0.91 mmol/L); and diabetes mellitus. Subtract one risk factor if HDL-C is ≥60 mg/dL (≥1.6 mmol/L).

Since the goal of treatment is to lower LDL-C, the NCEP recommends that LDL-C levels be used to initiate and assess treatment response. Only if LDL-C levels are not available, should the TOTAL-C be used to monitor therapy.
Although MEVACOR may be useful to reduce elevated LDL cholesterol levels in patients with combined hypercholesterolemia and hypertriglyceridemia where hypercholesterolemia is the major abnormality (Type IIb hyperlipoproteinemia), it has not been studied in conditions where the major abnormality is elevation of chylomicrons, VLDL or IDL (i.e., hyperlipoproteinemia types I, III, IV, or V).***

***Classification of Hyperlipoproteinemias

Type	Lipoproteins elevated	Lipid Elevations major	Lipid Elevations minor
I (rare)	chylomicrons	TG	→C
IIa	LDL	C	—
IIb	LDL, VLDL	C	TG
III (rare)	IDL	C/TG	—
IV	VLDL	TG	→C
V (rare)	chylomicrons, VLDL	TG	→C

C = cholesterol, TG = triglycerides,
LDL = low-density lipoprotein,
VLDL = very low-density lipoprotein,
IDL = intermediate-density lipoprotein.

CONTRAINDICATIONS

Hypersensitivity to any component of this medication.
Active liver disease or unexplained persistent elevations of serum transaminases (see WARNINGS).
Pregnancy and lactation. Atherosclerosis is a chronic process and the discontinuation of lipid-lowering drugs during pregnancy should have little impact on the outcome of long-term therapy of primary hypercholesterolemia. Moreover, cholesterol and other products of the cholesterol biosynthesis pathway are essential components for fetal development, including synthesis of steroids and cell membranes. Because of the ability of inhibitors of HMG-CoA reductase such as MEVACOR to decrease the synthesis of cholesterol and possibly other products of the cholesterol biosynthesis pathway, MEVACOR may cause fetal harm when administered to a pregnant woman. Therefore, lovastatin is contraindicated during pregnancy. **Lovastatin should be administered to women of childbearing age only when such patients are highly unlikely to conceive.** If the patient becomes pregnant while taking this drug, lovastatin should be discontinued and the patient should be apprised of the potential hazard to the fetus.

WARNINGS

Liver Dysfunction
Marked persistent increases (to more than 3 times the upper limit of normal) in serum transaminases occurred in 1.9% of

Continued on next page

Merck & Co.—Cont.

adult patients who received lovastatin for at least one year in early clinical trials (see ADVERSE REACTIONS). When the drug was interrupted or discontinued in these patients, the transaminase levels usually fell slowly to pretreatment levels. The increases usually appeared 3 to 12 months after the start of therapy with lovastatin, and were not associated with jaundice or other clinical signs or symptoms. There was no evidence of hypersensitivity. In the EXCEL study (see CLINICAL PHARMACOLOGY, *Clinical Studies*), the incidence of marked persistent increases in serum transaminases over 48 weeks was 0.1% for placebo, 0.1% at 20 mg/day, 0.9% at 40 mg/day, and 1.5% at 80 mg/day in patients on lovastatin. However, in post-marketing experience with MEVACOR, symptomatic liver disease has been reported rarely at all dosages (see ADVERSE REACTIONS).

It is recommended that liver function tests be performed before the initiation of treatment, at 6 and 12 weeks after initiation of therapy or elevation of dose, and periodically thereafter (e.g., semiannually). Patients who develop increased transaminase levels should be monitored with a second liver function evaluation to confirm the finding and be followed thereafter with frequent liver function tests until the abnormality(ies) return to normal. Should an increase in AST or ALT of three times the upper limit of normal or greater persist, withdrawal of therapy with MEVACOR is recommended.

The drug should be used with caution in patients who consume substantial quantities of alcohol and/or have a past history of liver disease. Active liver disease or unexplained transaminase elevations are contraindications to the use of lovastatin.

As with other lipid-lowering agents, moderate (less than three times the upper limit of normal) elevations of serum transaminases have been reported following therapy with MEVACOR (see ADVERSE REACTIONS). These changes appeared soon after initiation of therapy with MEVACOR, were often transient, were not accompanied by any symptoms and interruption of treatment was not required.

Skeletal Muscle
Rhabdomyolysis has been associated with lovastatin therapy alone, when combined with immunosuppressive therapy including cyclosporine in cardiac transplant patients, and when combined in non-transplant patients with either gemfibrozil or lipid-lowering doses (≥ 1 g/day) of nicotinic acid. Some of the affected patients had pre-existing renal insufficiency, usually as a consequence of long-standing diabetes. Acute renal failure from rhabdomyolysis has been seen more commonly with the lovastatin-gemfibrozil combination, and has also been reported in transplant patients receiving lovastatin plus cyclosporine.

Rhabdomyolysis with renal failure has been reported in a renal transplant patient receiving cyclosporine and lovastatin shortly after a dose increase in the systemic antifungal agent itraconazole. Another transplant patient on cyclosporine and a different HMG-CoA reductase inhibitor experienced muscle weakness accompanied by marked elevation of creatine phosphokinase following the initiation of systemic itraconazole therapy. The HMG-CoA reductase inhibitors and the azole derivative antifungal agents inhibit cholesterol biosynthesis at different points in the biosynthetic pathway. In patients receiving cyclosporine, lovastatin should be temporarily discontinued if systemic azole derivative antifungal therapy is required; patients not taking cyclosporine should be carefully monitored if systemic azole derivative antifungal therapy is required.

Rhabdomyolysis with or without renal impairment has been reported in seriously ill patients receiving erythromycin concomitantly with lovastatin. Therefore, patients receiving concomitant lovastatin and erythromycin should be carefully monitored.

Fulminant rhabdomyolysis has been seen as early as three weeks after initiation of combined therapy with gemfibrozil and lovastatin, but may be seen after several months. For these reasons, it is felt that, in most subjects who have had an unsatisfactory lipid response to either drug alone, the possible benefits of combined therapy with lovastatin and gemfibrozil do not outweigh the risks of severe myopathy, rhabdomyolysis, and acute renal failure. While it is not known whether this interaction occurs with fibrates other than gemfibrozil, myopathy and rhabdomyolysis have occasionally been associated with the use of other fibrates alone, including clofibrate. Therefore, the combined use of lovastatin with other fibrates should generally be avoided.

Physicians contemplating combined therapy with lovastatin and lipid-lowering doses of nicotinic acid or with immunosuppressive drugs should carefully weigh the potential benefits and risks and should carefully monitor patients for any signs and symptoms of muscle pain, tenderness, or weakness, particularly during the initial months of therapy and during any periods of upward dosage titration of either drug.

Periodic CPK determinations may be considered in such situations, but there is no assurance that such monitoring will prevent the occurrence of severe myopathy. The monitoring of lovastatin drug and metabolite levels may be considered in transplant patients who are treated with immunosuppressives and lovastatin.

Lovastatin therapy should be temporarily withheld or discontinued in any patient with an acute, serious condition suggestive of a myopathy or having a risk factor predisposing to the development of renal failure secondary to rhabdomyolysis, including: severe acute infection, hypotension, major surgery, trauma, severe metabolic, endocrine and electrolyte disorders, and uncontrolled seizures.

Myalgia has been associated with lovastatin therapy. Transient, mildly elevated creatine phosphokinase levels are commonly seen in lovastatin-treated patients. However, in early clinical trials, approximately 0.5% of patients developed a myopathy, i.e., myalgia or muscle weakness associated with markedly elevated CPK levels. In the EXCEL study (see CLINICAL PHARMACOLOGY, *Clinical Studies*), five (0.1%) patients taking lovastatin alone (one at 40 mg q.p.m., and four at 40 mg b.i.d.) developed myopathy (muscle symptoms and CPK levels >10 times the upper limit of normal). Myopathy should be considered in any patient with diffuse myalgias, muscle tenderness or weakness, and/or marked elevation of CPK. Patients should be advised to report promptly unexplained muscle pain, tenderness or weakness, particularly if accompanied by malaise or fever. Lovastatin therapy should be discontinued if markedly elevated CPK levels occur or myopathy is diagnosed or suspected.

Most of the patients who have developed myopathy (including rhabdomyolysis) were taking lovastatin concomitantly with immunosuppressive drugs, gemfibrozil, or lipid-lowering doses of nicotinic acid. In initial clinical trials, about 30 percent of patients on concomitant immunosuppressive therapy including cyclosporine developed myopathy. Most of these patients were receiving lovastatin at doses of 40 to 80 mg/day. In reports from 7 subsequent studies, 148 cyclosporine-treated patients (105 cardiac and 43 renal) received concurrent lovastatin doses of 10 to 60 mg/day (the majority receiving 20 mg/day) for mean periods of 3 to 15 months. There was one case of rhabdomyolysis (0.6%) and one case of significant CPK elevation. In earlier studies of patients taking lovastatin in combination with gemfibrozil or niacin, the incidences of myopathy were approximately 5% and 2%, respectively.

In six patients with cardiac transplants taking immunosuppressive therapy including cyclosporine concomitantly with lovastatin 20 mg/day, the average plasma level of active metabolites derived from lovastatin was elevated to approximately four times the expected levels. Because of an apparent relationship between increased plasma levels of active metabolites derived from lovastatin and myopathy, the daily dosage in patients taking immunosuppressants should not exceed 20 mg/day (see DOSAGE AND ADMINISTRATION). Even at this dosage, the benefits and risks of using lovastatin in patients taking immunosuppressants should be carefully considered.

PRECAUTIONS

General
Before instituting therapy with MEVACOR, an attempt should be made to control hypercholesterolemia with appropriate diet, exercise, weight reduction in obese patients, and to treat other underlying medical problems (see INDICATIONS AND USAGE).
Lovastatin may elevate creatine phosphokinase and transaminase levels (see WARNINGS and ADVERSE REACTIONS). This should be considered in the differential diagnosis of chest pain in a patient on therapy with lovastatin.
Homozygous Familial Hypercholesterolemia
MEVACOR is less effective in patients with the rare homozygous familial hypercholesterolemia, possibly because these patients have no functional LDL receptors. MEVACOR appears to be more likely to raise serum transaminases (see ADVERSE REACTIONS) in these homozygous patients.
Information for Patients
Patients should be advised to report promptly unexplained muscle pain, tenderness or weakness, particularly if accompanied by malaise or fever.
Drug Interactions
Immunosuppressive Drugs, Itraconazole, Gemfibrozil, Niacin (Nicotinic Acid), Erythromycin: See WARNINGS, *Skeletal Muscle.*
Coumarin Anticoagulants: In a small clinical trial in which lovastatin was administered to warfarin treated patients, no effect on prothrombin time was detected. However, another HMG-CoA reductase inhibitor has been found to produce a less than two seconds increase in prothrombin time in healthy volunteers receiving low doses of warfarin. Also, bleeding and/or increased prothrombin time have been reported in a few patients taking coumarin anticoagulants concomitantly with lovastatin. It is recommended that in

patients taking anticoagulants, prothrombin time be determined before starting lovastatin and frequently enough during early therapy to insure that no significant alteration of prothrombin time occurs. Once a stable prothrombin time has been documented, prothrombin times can be monitored at the intervals usually recommended for patients on coumarin anticoagulants. If the dose of lovastatin is changed, the same procedure should be repeated. Lovastatin therapy has not been associated with bleeding or with changes in prothrombin time in patients not taking anticoagulants.
Antipyrine: Because lovastatin had no effect on the pharmacokinetics of antipyrine or its metabolites, interactions of other drugs metabolized via the same cytochrome isozymes are not expected.
Propranolol: In normal volunteers, there was no clinically significant pharmacokinetic or pharmacodynamic interaction with concomitant administration of single doses of lovastatin and propranolol.
Digoxin: In patients with hypercholesterolemia, concomitant administration of lovastatin and digoxin resulted in no effect on digoxin plasma concentrations.
Oral Hypoglycemic Agents: In pharmacokinetic studies of MEVACOR in hypercholesterolemic non-insulin dependent diabetic patients, there was no drug interaction with glipizide or with chlorpropamide (see CLINICAL PHARMACOLOGY, *Clinical Studies*).
Other Concomitant Therapy: Although specific interaction studies were not performed, in clinical studies, lovastatin was used concomitantly with beta blockers, calcium channel blockers, diuretics and nonsteroidal anti-inflammatory drugs (NSAIDs) without evidence of clinically significant adverse interactions.
Endocrine Function
HMG-CoA reductase inhibitors interfere with cholesterol synthesis and as such might theoretically blunt adrenal and/or gonadal steroid production. Results of clinical trials with drugs in this class have been inconsistent with regard to drug effects on basal and reserve steroid levels. However, clinical studies have shown that lovastatin does not reduce basal plasma cortisol concentration or impair adrenal reserve, and does not reduce basal plasma testosterone concentration. Another HMG-CoA reductase inhibitor has been shown to reduce the plasma testosterone response to HCG. In the same study, the mean testosterone response to HCG was slightly but not significantly reduced after treatment with lovastatin 40 mg daily for 16 weeks in 21 men. The effects of HMG-CoA reductase inhibitors on male fertility have not been studied in adequate numbers of male patients. The effects, if any, on the pituitary-gonadal axis in premenopausal women are unknown. Patients treated with lovastatin who develop clinical evidence of endocrine dysfunction should be evaluated appropriately. Caution should also be exercised if an HMG-CoA reductase inhibitor or other agent used to lower cholesterol levels is administered to patients also receiving other drugs (e.g., ketoconazole, spironolactone, cimetidine) that may decrease the levels or activity of endogenous steroid hormones.
CNS Toxicity
Lovastatin produced optic nerve degeneration (Wallerian degeneration of retinogeniculate fibers) in clinically normal dogs in a dose-dependent fashion starting at 60 mg/kg/day, a dose that produced mean plasma drug levels about 30 times higher than the mean drug level in humans taking the highest recommended dose (as measured by total enzyme inhibitory activity). Vestibulocochlear Wallerian-like degeneration and retinal ganglion cell chromatolysis were also seen in dogs treated for 14 weeks at 180 mg/kg/day, a dose which resulted in a mean plasma drug level (C_{max}) similar to that seen with the 60 mg/kg/day dose.
CNS vascular lesions, characterized by perivascular hemorrhage and edema, mononuclear cell infiltration of perivascular spaces, perivascular fibrin deposits and necrosis of small vessels, were seen in dogs treated with lovastatin at a dose of 180 mg/kg/day, a dose which produced plasma drug levels (C_{max}) which were about 30 times higher than the mean values in humans taking 80 mg/day.
Similar optic nerve and CNS vascular lesions have been observed with other drugs of this class.
Cataracts were seen in dogs treated for 11 and 28 weeks at 180 mg/kg/day and 1 year at 60 mg/kg/day.
Carcinogenesis, Mutagenesis, Impairment of Fertility
In a 21-month carcinogenic study in mice, there was a statistically significant increase in the incidence of hepatocellular carcinomas and adenomas in both males and females at 500 mg/kg/day. This dose produced a total plasma drug exposure 3 to 4 times that of humans given the highest recommended dose of lovastatin (drug exposure was measured as total HMG-CoA reductase inhibitory activity in extracted plasma). Tumor increases were not seen at 20 and 100 mg/kg/day, doses that produced drug exposures of 0.3 to 2 times that of humans at the 80 mg/day dose. A statistically significant increase in pulmonary adenomas was seen in female mice at approximately 4 times the human drug exposure. (Although mice were given 300 times the human dose [HD] on a mg/kg body weight basis, plasma levels of total inhibi-

tory activity were only 4 times higher in mice than in humans given 80 mg of MEVACOR.)

There was an increase in incidence of papilloma in the non-glandular mucosa of the stomach of mice beginning at exposures of 1 to 2 times that of humans. The glandular mucosa was not affected. The human stomach contains only glandular mucosa.

In a 24-month carcinogenicity study in rats, there was a positive dose response relationship for hepatocellular carcinogenicity in males at drug exposures between 2–7 times that of human exposure at 80 mg/day (doses in rats were 5, 30 and 180 mg/kg/day).

An increased incidence of thyroid neoplasms in rats appears to be a response that has been seen with other HMG-CoA reductase inhibitors.

A chemically similar drug in this class was administered to mice for 72 weeks at 25, 100, and 400 mg/kg body weight, which resulted in mean serum drug levels approximately 3, 15, and 33 times higher than the mean human serum drug concentration (as total inhibitory activity) after a 40 mg oral dose. Liver carcinomas were significantly increased in high dose females and mid- and high dose males, with a maximum incidence of 90 percent in males. The incidence of adenomas of the liver was significantly increased in mid- and high dose females. Drug treatment also significantly increased the incidence of lung adenomas in mid- and high dose males and females. Adenomas of the Harderian gland (a gland of the eye of rodents) were significantly higher in high dose mice than in controls.

No evidence of mutagenicity was observed in a microbial mutagen test using mutant strains of *Salmonella typhimurium* with or without rat or mouse liver metabolic activation. In addition, no evidence of damage to genetic material was noted in an *in vitro* alkaline elution assay using rat or mouse hepatocytes, a V-79 mammalian cell forward mutation study, an *in vitro* chromosome aberration study in CHO cells, or an *in vivo* chromosomal aberration assay in mouse bone marrow.

Drug-related testicular atrophy, decreased spermatogenesis, spermatocytic degeneration and giant cell formation were seen in dogs starting at 20 mg/kg/day. Similar findings were seen with another drug in this class. No drug-related effects on fertility were found in studies with lovastatin in rats. However, in studies with a similar drug in this class, there was decreased fertility in male rats treated for 34 weeks at 25 mg/kg body weight, although this effect was not observed in a subsequent fertility study when this same dose was administered for 11 weeks (the entire cycle of spermatogenesis, including epididymal maturation). In rats treated with this same reductase inhibitor at 180 mg/kg/day, seminiferous tubule degeneration (necrosis and loss of spermatogenic epithelium) was observed. No microscopic changes were observed in the testes from rats of either study. The clinical significance of these findings is unclear.

Pregnancy
Pregnancy Category X
See CONTRAINDICATIONS.

Safety in pregnant women has not been established. Lovastatin has been shown to produce skeletal malformations at plasma levels 40 times the human exposure (for mouse fetus) and 80 times the human exposure (for rat fetus) based on mg/m² surface area (doses were 800 mg/kg/day). No drug-induced changes were seen in either species at multiples of 8 times (rat) or 4 times (mouse) based on surface area. No evidence of malformations was noted in rabbits at exposures up to 3 times the human exposure (dose of 15 mg/kg/day, highest tolerated dose). Rare reports of congenital anomalies have been received following intrauterine exposure to HMG-CoA reductase inhibitors. There has been one report of severe congenital bony deformity, tracheo-esophageal fistula, and anal atresia (VATER association) in a baby born to a woman who took lovastatin with dextroamphetamine sulfate during the first trimester of pregnancy. MEVACOR should be administered to women of child-bearing potential only when such patients are highly unlikely to conceive and have been informed of the potential hazards. If the woman becomes pregnant while taking MEVACOR, it should be discontinued and the patient advised again as to the potential hazards to the fetus.

Nursing Mothers
It is not known whether lovastatin is excreted in human milk. Because a small amount of another drug in this class is excreted in human breast milk and because of the potential for serious adverse reactions in nursing infants, women taking MEVACOR should not nurse their infants (see CONTRAINDICATIONS).

Pediatric Use
Safety and effectiveness in children and adolescents have not been established. Because children and adolescents are not likely to benefit from cholesterol lowering for at least a decade and because experience with this drug is limited (no studies in subjects below the age of 20 years), treatment of children with lovastatin is not recommended at this time.

	MEVACOR (N=613) %	Placebo (N=82) %	Cholestyramine (N=88) %	Probucol (N=97) %
Gastrointestinal				
Constipation	4.9	—	34.1	2.1
Diarrhea	5.5	4.9	8.0	10.3
Dyspepsia	3.9	—	13.6	3.1
Flatus	6.4	2.4	21.6	2.1
Abdominal pain/cramps	5.7	2.4	5.7	5.2
Heartburn	1.6	—	8.0	—
Nausea	4.7	3.7	9.1	6.2
Musculoskeletal				
Muscle cramps	1.1	—	1.1	—
Myalgia	2.4	1.2	—	—
Nervous System/Psychiatric				
Dizziness	2.0	1.2	—	1.0
Headache	9.3	4.9	4.5	8.2
Skin				
Rash/pruritus	5.2	—	4.5	—
Special Senses				
Blurred vision	1.5	—	1.1	3.1
Dysgeusia	0.8	—	1.1	—

	Placebo (N=1663) %	MEVACOR 20 mg q.p.m. (N=1642) %	MEVACOR 40 mg q.p.m. (N=1645) %	MEVACOR 20 mg b.i.d. (N=1646) %	MEVACOR 40 mg b.i.d. (N=1649) %
Body As a Whole					
Asthenia	1.4	1.7	1.4	1.5	1.2
Gastrointestinal					
Abdominal pain	1.6	2.0	2.0	2.2	2.5
Constipation	1.9	2.0	3.2	3.2	3.5
Diarrhea	2.3	2.6	2.4	2.2	2.6
Dyspepsia	1.9	1.3	1.3	1.0	1.6
Flatulence	4.2	3.7	4.3	3.9	4.5
Nausea	2.5	1.9	2.5	2.2	2.2
Musculoskeletal					
Muscle cramps	0.5	0.6	0.8	1.1	1.0
Myalgia	1.7	2.6	1.8	2.2	3.0
Nervous System/Psychiatric					
Dizziness	0.7	0.7	1.2	0.5	0.5
Headache	2.7	2.6	2.8	2.1	3.2
Skin					
Rash	0.7	0.8	1.0	1.2	1.3
Special Senses					
Blurred vision	0.8	1.1	0.9	0.9	1.2

ADVERSE REACTIONS

MEVACOR is generally well tolerated; adverse reactions usually have been mild and transient. Less than 1% of patients were discontinued from controlled clinical studies of up to 14 weeks due to adverse experiences attributable to MEVACOR. About 3% of patients were discontinued from extensions of these studies due to adverse experiences attributable to MEVACOR; about half of these patients were discontinued due to increases in serum transaminases. The median duration of therapy in these extensions was 5.2 years.

In the EXCEL study (see CLINICAL PHARMACOLOGY, *Clinical Studies*), 4.6% of the patients treated up to 48 weeks were discontinued due to clinical or laboratory adverse experiences which were rated by the investigator as possibly, probably or definitely related to therapy with MEVACOR. The value for the placebo group was 2.5%.

Clinical Adverse Experiences
Adverse experiences reported in patients treated with MEVACOR in controlled clinical studies are shown in the table below:
[See first table above.]

Laboratory Tests
Marked persistent increases of serum transaminases have been noted (see WARNINGS).

About 11% of patients had elevations of creatine phosphokinase (CPK) levels of at least twice the normal value on one or more occasions. The corresponding values for the control agents were cholestyramine, 9 percent and probucol, 2 percent. This was attributable to the noncardiac fraction of CPK. Large increases in CPK have sometimes been reported (see WARNINGS, *Skeletal Muscle*).

Expanded Clinical Evaluation of Lovastatin
(EXCEL) Study
Clinical Adverse Experiences
MEVACOR was compared to placebo in 8,245 patients with hypercholesterolemia (total cholesterol 240–300 mg/dL [6.2–7.8 mmol/L]) in the randomized, double-blind, parallel, 48-week EXCEL study. Clinical adverse experiences reported as possibly, probably or definitely drug-related in ≥1% in any treatment group are shown in the table below. For no event was the incidence on drug and placebo statistically different.
[See second table above.]

Other clinical adverse experiences reported as possibly, probably or definitely drug-related in 0.5 to 1.0 percent of patients in any drug-related group are listed below. In all these cases the incidence on drug and placebo was not statistically different. *Body as a Whole:* chest pain; *Gastrointestinal:* acid regurgitation, dry mouth, vomiting; *Musculoskeletal:* leg pain, shoulder pain, arthralgia; *Nervous System/Psychiatric:* insomnia, paresthesia; *Skin:* alopecia, pruritus; *Special Senses:* eye irritation.

Concomitant Therapy
In controlled clinical studies in which lovastatin was administered concomitantly with cholestyramine, no adverse reactions peculiar to this concomitant treatment were observed. The adverse reactions that occurred were limited to those reported previously with lovastatin or cholestyramine. Other lipid-lowering agents were not administered concomitantly with lovastatin during controlled clinical studies. Preliminary data suggests that the addition of either probucol or gemfibrozil to therapy with lovastatin is not associated with greater reduction in LDL cholesterol than that achieved with lovastatin alone. In uncontrolled clinical studies, most of the patients who have developed myopathy were receiving concomitant therapy with immunosuppressive drugs, gemfibrozil or niacin (nicotinic acid) (see WARNINGS, *Skeletal Muscle*).

The following effects have been reported with drugs in this class. Not all the effects listed below have necessarily been associated with lovastatin therapy.
Skeletal: muscle cramps, myalgia, myopathy, rhabdomyolysis, arthralgias.
Neurological: dysfunction of certain cranial nerves (including alteration of taste, impairment of extra-ocular movement, facial paresis), tremor, dizziness, vertigo, memory loss, paresthesia, peripheral neuropathy, peripheral nerve palsy, psychic disturbances, anxiety, insomnia, depression.
Hypersensitivity Reactions: An apparent hypersensitivity syndrome has been reported rarely which has included one or more of the following features: anaphylaxis, angioedema, lupus erythematous-like syndrome, polymyalgia rheumatica, vasculitis, purpura, thrombocytopenia, leukopenia, hemolytic anemia, positive ANA, ESR increase, eosinophilia, arthritis, arthralgia, urticaria, asthenia, photosensitivity, fever, chills, flushing, malaise, dyspnea, toxic epidermal

Continued on next page

Information on the Merck & Co., Inc. products listed on these pages is the full prescribing information from product circulars in use September 30, 1996.

Merck & Co.—Cont.

necrolysis, erythema multiforme, including Stevens-Johnson syndrome.
Gastrointestinal: pancreatitis, hepatitis, including chronic active hepatitis, cholestatic jaundice, fatty change in liver; and rarely, cirrhosis, fulminant hepatic necrosis, and hepatoma; anorexia, vomiting.
Skin: alopecia, pruritus. A variety of skin changes (e.g., nodules, discoloration, dryness of skin/mucous membranes, changes to hair/nails) have been reported.
Reproductive: gynecomastia, loss of libido, erectile dysfunction.
Eye: progression of cataracts (lens opacities), ophthalmoplegia.
Laboratory Abnormalities: elevated transaminases, alkaline phosphatase, γ-glutamyl transpeptidase, and bilirubin; thyroid function abnormalities.

OVERDOSAGE

After oral administration of MEVACOR to mice the median lethal dose observed was >15 g/m^2.
Five healthy human volunteers have received up to 200 mg of lovastatin as a single dose without clinically significant adverse experiences. A few cases of accidental overdosage have been reported; no patients had any specific symptoms, and all patients recovered without sequelae. The maximum dose taken was 5–6 g.
Until further experience is obtained, no specific treatment of overdosage with MEVACOR can be recommended.
The dialyzability of lovastatin and its metabolites in man is not known at present.

DOSAGE AND ADMINISTRATION

The patient should be placed on a standard cholesterol-lowering diet before receiving MEVACOR and should continue on this diet during treatment with MEVACOR (see NCEP Treatment Guidelines for details on dietary therapy). MEVACOR should be given with meals.
The usual recommended starting dose is 20 mg once a day given with the evening meal. The recommended dosing range is 10–80 mg/day in single or two divided doses; the maximum recommended dose is 80 mg/day. Doses should be individualized according to the recommended goal of therapy (see NCEP Guidelines) and the patient's response (see Tables I to IV under CLINICAL PHARMACOLOGY, *Clinical Studies* for dose response results). Patients requiring reductions in LDL cholesterol of 20% or more to achieve their goal (see INDICATIONS AND USAGE) should be started on 20 mg/day of MEVACOR. A starting dose of 10 mg may be considered for patients requiring smaller reductions. Adjustments should be made at intervals of 4 weeks or more.
In patients taking immunosuppressive drugs concomitantly with lovastatin (see WARNINGS, *Skeletal Muscle*), therapy should begin with 10 mg of MEVACOR and should not exceed 20 mg/day.
Cholesterol levels should be monitored periodically and consideration should be given to reducing the dosage of MEVACOR if cholesterol levels fall significantly below the targeted range.
Concomitant Therapy
Preliminary evidence suggests that the cholesterol-lowering effects of lovastatin and the bile acid sequestrant, cholestyramine, are additive.
Dosage in Patients with Renal Insufficiency
In patients with severe renal insufficiency (creatinine clearance <30 mL/min), dosage increases above 20 mg/day should be carefully considered and, if deemed necessary, implemented cautiously (see CLINICAL PHARMACOLOGY and WARNINGS, *Skeletal Muscle*).

HOW SUPPLIED

No. 3560—Tablets MEVACOR 10 mg are peach, octagonal tablets, coded MSD 730 on one side and MEVACOR on the other. They are supplied as follows:
NDC 0006-0730-61 unit of use bottles of 60.
Shown in Product Identification Guide, page 324
No. 3561—Tablets MEVACOR 20 mg are light blue, octagonal tablets, coded MSD 731 on one side and MEVACOR on the other. They are supplied as follows:
NDC 0006-0731-37 unit of use bottles of 30
NDC 0006-0731-61 unit of use bottles of 60
(6505-01-267-2497, 20 mg 60's)
NDC 0006-0731-94 unit of use bottles of 90
NDC 0006-0731-28 unit dose packages of 100
(6505-01-267-7925, 20 mg 100's)
NDC 0006-0731-78 unit of use bottles of 100
NDC 0006-0731-98 unit of use bottles of 180
NDC 0006-0731-82 bottles of 1000
(6505-01-359-1865, 20 mg 1000's)
NDC 0006-0731-87 bottles of 10,000
(6505-01-379-7905, 20 mg 10,000's).
Shown in Product Identification Guide, page 324
No. 3562—Tablets MEVACOR 40 mg are green, octagonal tablets, coded MSD 732 on one side and MEVACOR on the other. They are supplied as follows:
NDC 0006-0732-61 unit of use bottles of 60
(6505-01-310-0615, 40 mg 60's)
NDC 0006-0732-94 unit of use bottles of 90
NDC 0006-0732-82 bottles of 1000
NDC 0006-0732-87 bottles of 10,000
(6505-01-379-7903, 40 mg 10,000's).
Shown in Product Identification Guide, page 324
Storage
Store between 5–30°C (41–86°F). Tablets MEVACOR must be protected from light and stored in a well-closed, light-resistant container.
7825336 Issued February 1996
COPYRIGHT © MERCK & CO., INC., 1987, 1989, 1991
All rights reserved

MIDAMOR® Tablets ℞
(Amiloride HCl), U.S.P.

DESCRIPTION

Amiloride HCl, an antikaliuretic-diuretic agent, is a pyrazine-carbonyl-guanidine that is unrelated chemically to other known antikaliuretic or diuretic agents. It is the salt of a moderately strong base (pKa 8.7). It is designated chemically as 3,5-diamino-6-chloro-*N*-(diaminomethylene) pyrazinecarboxamide monohydrochloride, dihydrate and has a molecular weight of 302.14. Its empirical formula is $C_6H_8ClN_7O \cdot HCl \cdot 2H_2O$ and its structural formula is:

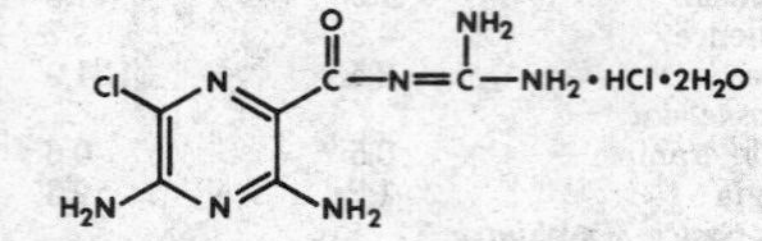

MIDAMOR* (Amiloride HCl) is available for oral use as tablets containing 5 mg of anhydrous amiloride HCl. Each tablet contains the following inactive ingredients: calcium phosphate, D&C Yellow 10, iron oxide, lactose, magnesium stearate and starch.

*Registered trademark of MERCK & CO., INC.

CLINICAL PHARMACOLOGY

MIDAMOR is a potassium-conserving (antikaliuretic) drug that possesses weak (compared with thiazide diuretics) natriuretic, diuretic, and antihypertensive activity. These effects have been partially additive to the effects of thiazide diuretics in some clinical studies. When administered with a thiazide or loop diuretic, MIDAMOR has been shown to decrease the enhanced urinary excretion of magnesium which occurs when a thiazide or loop diuretic is used alone. MIDAMOR has potassium-conserving activity in patients receiving kaliuretic-diuretic agents.
MIDAMOR is not an aldosterone antagonist and its effects are seen even in the absence of aldosterone.
MIDAMOR exerts its potassium sparing effect through the inhibition of sodium reabsorption at the distal convoluted tubule, cortical collecting tubule and collecting duct; this decreases the net negative potential of the tubular lumen and reduces both potassium and hydrogen secretion and their subsequent excretion. This mechanism accounts in large part for the potassium sparing action of amiloride.
MIDAMOR usually begins to act within 2 hours after an oral dose. Its effect on electrolyte excretion reaches a peak between 6 and 10 hours and lasts about 24 hours. Peak plasma levels are obtained in 3 to 4 hours and the plasma half-life varies from 6 to 9 hours. Effects on electrolytes increase with single doses of amiloride HCl up to approximately 15 mg.
Amiloride HCl is not metabolized by the liver but is excreted unchanged by the kidneys. About 50 percent of a 20 mg dose of MIDAMOR is excreted in the urine and 40 percent in the stool within 72 hours. MIDAMOR has little effect on glomerular filtration rate or renal blood flow. Because amiloride HCl is not metabolized by the liver, drug accumulation is not anticipated in patients with hepatic dysfunction, but accumulation can occur if the hepatorenal syndrome develops.

INDICATIONS AND USAGE

MIDAMOR is indicated as adjunctive treatment with thiazide diuretics or other kaliuretic-diuretic agents in congestive heart failure or hypertension to:

a. help restore normal serum potassium levels in patients who develop hypokalemia on the kaliuretic diuretic
b. prevent development of hypokalemia in patients who would be exposed to particular risk if hypokalemia were to develop, e.g., digitalized patients or patients with significant cardiac arrhythmias.

The use of potassium-conserving agents is often unnecessary in patients receiving diuretics for uncomplicated essential hypertension when such patients have a normal diet. MIDAMOR has little additive diuretic or antihypertensive effect when added to a thiazide diuretic.
MIDAMOR should rarely be used alone. It has weak (compared with thiazides) diuretic and antihypertensive effects. Used as single agents, potassium sparing diuretics, including MIDAMOR, result in an increased risk of hyperkalemia (approximately 10% with amiloride). MIDAMOR should be used alone only when persistent hypokalemia has been documented and only with careful titration of the dose and close monitoring of serum electrolytes.

CONTRAINDICATIONS

Hyperkalemia
MIDAMOR should not be used in the presence of elevated serum potassium levels (greater than 5.5 mEq per liter).
Antikaliuretic Therapy or Potassium Supplementation
MIDAMOR should not be given to patients receiving other potassium-conserving agents, such as spironolactone or triamterene. Potassium supplementation in the form of medication, potassium-containing salt substitutes or a potassium-rich diet should not be used with MIDAMOR except in severe and/or refractory cases of hypokalemia. Such concomitant therapy can be associated with rapid increases in serum potassium levels. If potassium supplementation is used, careful monitoring of the serum potassium level is necessary.
Impaired Renal Function
Anuria, acute or chronic renal insufficiency, and evidence of diabetic nephropathy are contraindications to the use of MIDAMOR. Patients with evidence of renal functional impairment (blood urea nitrogen [BUN] levels over 30 mg per 100 mL or serum creatinine levels over 1.5 mg per 100 mL) or diabetes mellitus should not receive the drug without careful, frequent and continuing monitoring of serum electrolytes, creatinine, and BUN levels. Potassium retention associated with the use of an antikaliuretic agent is accentuated in the presence of renal impairment and may result in the rapid development of hyperkalemia.
Hypersensitivity
MIDAMOR is contraindicated in patients who are hypersensitive to this product.

WARNINGS

Hyperkalemia

> Like other potassium-conserving agents, amiloride may cause hyperkalemia (serum potassium levels greater than 5.5 mEq per liter) which, if uncorrected, is potentially fatal. Hyperkalemia occurs commonly (about 10%) when amiloride is used without a kaliuretic diuretic. This incidence is greater in patients with renal impairment, diabetes mellitus (with or without recognized renal insufficiency), and in the elderly. When MIDAMOR is used concomitantly with a thiazide diuretic in patients without these complications, the risk of hyperkalemia is reduced to about 1–2 percent. It is thus essential to monitor serum potassium levels carefully in any patient receiving amiloride, particularly when it is first introduced, at the time of diuretic dosage adjustments, and during any illness that could affect renal function.

The risk of hyperkalemia may be increased when potassium-conserving agents, including MIDAMOR, are administered concomitantly with an angiotensin-converting enzyme inhibitor. (See PRECAUTIONS, *Drug Interactions.*) Warning signs or symptoms of hyperkalemia include paresthesias, muscular weakness, fatigue, flaccid paralysis of the extremities, bradycardia, shock, and ECG abnormalities. Monitoring of the serum potassium level is essential because mild hyperkalemia is not usually associated with an abnormal ECG.
When abnormal, the ECG in hyperkalemia is characterized primarily by tall, peaked T waves or elevations from previous tracings. There may also be lowering of the R wave and increased depth of the S wave, widening and even disappearance of the P wave, progressive widening of the QRS complex, prolongation of the PR interval, and ST depression.
Treatment of hyperkalemia: If hyperkalemia occurs in patients taking MIDAMOR, the drug should be discontinued immediately. If the serum potassium level exceeds 6.5 mEq per liter, active measures should be taken to reduce it. Such measures include the intravenous administration of sodium bicarbonate solution or oral or parenteral glucose with a rapid-acting insulin preparation. If needed, a cation exchange resin such as sodium polystyrene sulfonate may be given orally or by enema. Patients with persistent hyperkalemia may require dialysis.
Diabetes Mellitus
In diabetic patients, hyperkalemia has been reported with the use of all potassium-conserving diuretics, including MIDAMOR, even in patients without evidence of diabetic

nephropathy. Therefore, MIDAMOR should be avoided, if possible, in diabetic patients and, if it is used, serum electrolytes and renal function must be monitored frequently. MIDAMOR should be discontinued at least three days before glucose tolerance testing.

Metabolic or Respiratory Acidosis

Antikaliuretic therapy should be instituted only with caution in severely ill patients in whom respiratory or metabolic acidosis may occur, such as patients with cardiopulmonary disease or poorly controlled diabetes. If MIDAMOR is given to these patients, frequent monitoring of acid-base balance is necessary. Shifts in acid-base balance alter the ratio of extracellular/intracellular potassium, and the development of acidosis may be associated with rapid increases in serum potassium levels.

PRECAUTIONS

General

Electrolyte Imbalance and BUN Increases

Hyponatremia and hypochloremia may occur when MIDAMOR is used with other diuretics and increases in BUN levels have been reported. These increases usually have accompanied vigorous fluid elimination, especially when diuretic therapy was used in seriously ill patients, such as those who had hepatic cirrhosis with ascites and metabolic alkalosis, or those with resistant edema. Therefore, when MIDAMOR is given with other diuretics to such patients, careful monitoring of serum electrolytes and BUN levels is important. In patients with pre-existing severe liver disease, hepatic encephalopathy, manifested by tremors, confusion, and coma, and increased jaundice, have been reported in association with diuretics, including amiloride HCl.

Drug Interactions

When amiloride HCl is administered concomitantly with an angiotensin-converting enzyme inhibitor, the risk of hyperkalemia may be increased. Therefore, if concomitant use of these agents is indicated because of demonstrated hypokalemia, they should be used with caution and with frequent monitoring of serum potassium. (See WARNINGS.)

Lithium generally should not be given with diuretics because they reduce its renal clearance and add a high risk of lithium toxicity. Read circulars for lithium preparations before use of such concomitant therapy.

In some patients, the administration of a non-steroidal anti-inflammatory agent can reduce the diuretic, natriuretic, and antihypertensive effects of loop, potassium-sparing and thiazide diuretics. Therefore, when MIDAMOR and non-steroidal anti-inflammatory agents are used concomitantly, the patient should be observed closely to determine if the desired effect of the diuretic is obtained. Since indomethacin and potassium-sparing diuretics, including MIDAMOR, each may be associated with increased serum potassium levels, the potential effects on potassium kinetics and renal function should be considered when these agents are administered concurrently.

Carcinogenicity, Mutagenicity, Impairment of Fertility

There was no evidence of a tumorigenic effect when amiloride HCl was administered for 92 weeks to mice at doses up to 10 mg/kg/day (25 times the maximum daily human dose). Amiloride HCl has also been administered for 104 weeks to male and female rats at doses up to 6 and 8 mg/kg/day (15 and 20 times the maximum daily dose for humans, respectively) and showed no evidence of carcinogenicity. Amiloride HCl was devoid of mutagenic activity in various strains of *Salmonella typhimurium* with or without a mammalian liver microsomal activation system (Ames test).

Pregnancy

Pregnancy Category B. Teratogenicity studies with amiloride HCl in rabbits and mice given 20 and 25 times the maximum human dose, respectively, revealed no evidence of harm to the fetus, although studies showed that the drug crossed the placenta in modest amounts. Reproduction studies in rats at 20 times the expected maximum daily dose for humans showed no evidence of impaired fertility. At approximately 5 or more times the expected maximum daily dose for humans, some toxicity was seen in adult rats and rabbits and a decrease in rat pup growth and survival occurred. There are, however, no adequate and well-controlled studies in pregnant women. Because animal reproduction studies are not always predictive of human response, this drug should be used during pregnancy only if clearly needed.

Nursing Mothers

Studies in rats have shown that amiloride is excreted in milk in concentrations higher than that found in blood, but it is not known whether MIDAMOR is excreted in human milk. Because many drugs are excreted in human milk and because of the potential for serious adverse reactions in nursing infants from MIDAMOR, a decision should be made whether to discontinue nursing or to discontinue the drug, taking into account the importance of the drug to the mother.

Pediatric Use

Safety and effectiveness in children have not been established.

ADVERSE REACTIONS

MIDAMOR is usually well tolerated and, except for hyperkalemia (serum potassium levels greater than 5.5 mEq per liter—see WARNINGS), significant adverse effects have been reported infrequently. Minor adverse reactions were reported relatively frequently (about 20%) but the relationship of many of the reports to amiloride HCl is uncertain and the overall frequency was similar in hydrochlorothiazide treated groups. Nausea/anorexia, abdominal pain, flatulence, and mild skin rash have been reported and probably are related to amiloride. Other adverse experiences that have been reported with amiloride are generally those known to be associated with diuresis, or with the underlying disease being treated.

The adverse reactions for MIDAMOR listed in the following table have been arranged into two groups: (1) incidence greater than one percent; and (2) incidence one percent or less. The incidence for group (1) was determined from clinical studies conducted in the United States (837 patients treated with MIDAMOR). The adverse effects listed in group (2) include reports from the same clinical studies and voluntary reports since marketing. The probability of a causal relationship exists between MIDAMOR and these adverse reactions, some of which have been reported only rarely.

Incidence > 1%	Incidence ≤ 1%
Body as a Whole	
Headache*	Back pain
Weakness	Chest pain
Fatigability	Neck/shoulder ache
	Pain, extremities
Cardiovascular	
None	Angina pectoris
	Orthostatic hypotension
	Arrhythmia
	Palpitation
Digestive	
Nausea/anorexia*	Jaundice
Diarrhea*	GI bleeding
Vomiting*	Abdominal fullness
Abdominal pain	GI disturbance
Gas pain	Thirst
Appetite changes	Heartburn
Constipation	Flatulence
	Dyspepsia
Metabolic	
Elevated serum potassium levels (> 5.5 mEq per liter)†	None
Skin	
None	Skin rash
	Itching
	Dryness of mouth
	Pruritus
	Alopecia
Musculoskeletal	
Muscle cramps	Joint pain
	Leg ache
Nervous	
Dizziness	Paresthesia
Encephalopathy	Tremors
	Vertigo
Psychiatric	
None	Nervousness
	Mental confusion
	Insomnia
	Decreased libido
	Depression
	Somnolence
Respiratory	
Cough	Shortness of breath
Dyspnea	
Special Senses	
None	Visual disturbances
	Nasal congestion
	Tinnitus
	Increased intraocular pressure
Urogenital	
Impotence	Polyuria
	Dysuria
	Urinary frequency
	Bladder spasms
	Gynecomastia

* Reactions occurring in 3% to 8% of patients treated with MIDAMOR. (Those reactions occurring in less than 3% of the patients are unmarked.)

† See WARNINGS.

Causal Relationship Unknown

Other reactions have been reported but occurred under circumstances where a causal relationship could not be established. However, in these rarely reported events, that possibility cannot be excluded. Therefore, these observations are listed to serve as alerting information to physicians.

Activation of probable pre-existing peptic ulcer
Aplastic anemia
Neutropenia
Abnormal liver function

OVERDOSAGE

No data are available in regard to overdosage in humans. The oral LD_{50} of amiloride hydrochloride (calculated as the base) is 56 mg/kg in mice and 36 to 85 mg/kg in rats, depending on the strain.

It is not known whether the drug is dialyzable.

The most likely signs and symptoms to be expected with overdosage are dehydration and electrolyte imbalance. These can be treated by established procedures. Therapy with MIDAMOR should be discontinued and the patient observed closely. There is no specific antidote. Emesis should be induced or gastric lavage performed. Treatment is symptomatic and supportive. If hyperkalemia occurs, active measures should be taken to reduce the serum potassium levels.

DOSAGE AND ADMINISTRATION

MIDAMOR should be administered with food.

MIDAMOR, one 5 mg tablet daily, should be added to the usual antihypertensive or diuretic dosage of a kaliuretic diuretic. The dosage may be increased to 10 mg per day, if necessary. More than two 5 mg tablets of MIDAMOR daily usually are not needed, and there is little controlled experience with such doses. If persistent hypokalemia is documented with 10 mg, the dose can be increased to 15 mg, then 20 mg, with careful monitoring of electrolytes.

In treating patients with congestive heart failure after an initial diuresis has been achieved, potassium loss may also decrease and the need for MIDAMOR should be reevaluated. Dosage adjustment may be necessary. Maintenance therapy may be on an intermittent basis.

If it is necessary to use MIDAMOR alone (see INDICATIONS), the starting dosage should be one 5 mg tablet daily. This dosage may be increased to 10 mg per day, if necessary. More than two 5 mg tablets usually are not needed, and there is little controlled experience with such doses. If persistent hypokalemia is documented with 10 mg, the dose can be increased to 15 mg, then 20 mg, with careful monitoring of electrolytes.

HOW SUPPLIED

No. 3381—Tablets MIDAMOR, 5 mg, are yellow, diamond-shaped, compressed tablets, coded MSD 92. They are supplied as follows:

NDC 0006-0092-68 bottles of 100
(6505-01-127-8721 5 mg, 100's).

Shown in Product Identification Guide, page 325

Storage

Protect from moisture, freezing and excessive heat.
7905115   Issued April 1992
COPYRIGHT © MERCK & CO., INC., 1985
All rights reserved

MINTEZOL® Chewable Tablets ℞
(Thiabendazole), U.S.P.

MINTEZOL® Suspension ℞
(Thiabendazole), U.S.P.

DESCRIPTION

MINTEZOL* (Thiabendazole) is an anthelmintic provided as 500 mg chewable tablets, and as a suspension, containing 500 mg thiabendazole per 5 mL. The suspension also contains sorbic acid 0.1% added as a preservative. Inactive ingredients in the tablets are acacia, calcium phosphate, flavors, lactose, magnesium stearate, mannitol, methylcellulose, and sodium saccharin. Inactive ingredients in the suspension are an antifoam agent, flavors, polysorbate, purified water, sorbitol solution, and tragacanth.

Thiabendazole is a white to off-white odorless powder with a molecular weight of 201.26, which is practically insoluble in water but readily soluble in dilute acid and alkali. Its chemical name is 2-(4-thiazolyl)-1H-benzimidazole. The empirical formula is $C_{10}H_7N_3S$ and the structural formula is:

Continued on next page

Information on the Merck & Co., Inc. products listed on these pages is the full prescribing information from product circulars in use September 30, 1996.

Merck & Co.—Cont.

*Registered trademark of MERCK & CO., INC.

CLINICAL PHARMACOLOGY

In man, thiabendazole is rapidly absorbed and peak plasma concentration is reached within 1 to 2 hours after the oral administration of a suspension. It is metabolized almost completely to the 5-hydroxy form which appears in the urine as glucuronide or sulfate conjugates. In 48 hours, about 5% of the administered dose is recovered from the feces and about 90% from the urine. Most is excreted in the first 24 hours.

Mechanism of Action

The precise mode of action of thiabendazole on the parasite is unknown, but it may inhibit the helminth-specific enzyme fumarate reductase.

Thiabendazole is vermicidal and/or vermifugal against *Ascaris lumbricoides* ("common roundworm"), *Strongyloides stercoralis* (threadworm), *Necator americanus*, and *Ancylostoma duodenale* (hookworm), *Trichuris trichiura* (whipworm), *Ancylostoma braziliense* (dog and cat hookworm), *Toxocara canis* and *Toxocara cati* (ascarids), and *Enterobius vermicularis* (pinworm).

Its effect on larvae of *Trichinella spiralis* that have migrated to muscle is questionable.

Thiabendazole also suppresses egg and/or larval production and may inhibit the subsequent development of those eggs or larvae which are passed in the feces.

INDICATIONS AND USAGE

MINTEZOL is indicated for the treatment of:
Strongyloidiasis (threadworm)
Cutaneous larva migrans (creeping eruption)
Visceral larva migrans
Trichinosis: Relief of symptoms and fever and a reduction of eosinophilia have followed the use of MINTEZOL during the invasion stage of the disease.

Although not indicated as primary therapy, when enterobiasis (pinworm) occurs with any of the conditions listed above, additional therapy is not required for most patients. MINTEZOL should be used only in the following infestations when more specific therapy is not available or cannot be used or when further therapy with a second agent is desirable: Uncinariasis (hookworm: *Necator americanus* and *Ancylostoma duodenale*); Trichuriasis (whipworm); Ascariasis (large roundworm).

CONTRAINDICATION

Hypersensitivity to this product.

WARNINGS

If hypersensitivity reactions occur, the drug should be discontinued immediately and not be resumed. Erythema multiforme has been associated with thiabendazole therapy; in severe cases (Stevens-Johnson syndrome), fatalities have occurred.

Because CNS side effects may occur quite frequently, activities requiring mental alertness should be avoided.

PRECAUTIONS

General

MINTEZOL is not suitable for the treatment of mixed infections with ascaris because it may cause these worms to migrate.

Ideally, supportive therapy is indicated for anemic, dehydrated or malnourished patients prior to initiation of the anthelmintic therapy.

In the presence of hepatic or renal dysfunction, patients should be carefully monitored.

MINTEZOL should be used only in patients in whom susceptible worm infestation has been diagnosed and should not be used prophylactically.

Information for Patients

Because CNS side effects may occur quite frequently, activities requiring mental alertness should be avoided.

Laboratory Tests

Rarely, a transient rise in cephalin flocculation and SGOT has occurred in patients receiving MINTEZOL.

Drug Interactions

Thiabendazole may compete with other drugs, such as theophylline, for sites of metabolism in the liver, thus elevating the serum levels of such compounds to potentially toxic levels. Therefore, when concomitant use of thiabendazole and xanthine derivatives is anticipated, it may be necessary to monitor blood levels and/or reduce the dosage of such compounds. Such concomitant use should be administered under careful medical supervision.

Carcinogenesis, Mutagenesis, Impairment of Fertility

Thiabendazole has been used in numerous short- and long-term studies in animals at doses up to 15 times the usual human dose and was without carcinogenic effects. It did not adversely affect fertility in the mouse at 2½ times the usual human dose or in the rat at a dose equivalent to the usual human dose. Thiabendazole had no mutagenic activity in *in vitro* microbial mutagen test, the micronucleus test and the host mediated assay *in vivo*.

Pregnancy

Pregnancy Category C: Reproduction and teratogenic studies done in the rabbit at a dose up to 15 times the usual human dose, in the rat at a dose equivalent to the human dose, and in the mouse at a dose up to 2½ times the usual human dose, revealed no evidence of harm to the fetus. In an additional study in the mouse, no defects were observed when thiabendazole was given in an aqueous suspension, at a dose 10 times the usual human dose; however, cleft palate and axial skeletal defects were observed when thiabendazole was suspended in olive oil and given at the same dose. There are no adequate and well controlled studies in pregnant women. MINTEZOL should be used during pregnancy only if the potential benefit justifies the potential risk to the fetus.

Nursing Mothers

It is not known whether this drug is excreted in human milk. Because of the potential for serious adverse reactions in nursing infants from MINTEZOL, a decision should be made whether to discontinue nursing or to discontinue the drug, taking into account the importance of the drug to the mother.

Pediatric Use

The safety and effectiveness of thiabendazole for the treatment of Strongyloidiasis, Ascariasis, Uncinariasis, Trichuriasis and Trichinosis in children weighing less than 30 lbs has been limited.

ADVERSE REACTIONS

Gastrointestinal: anorexia, nausea, vomiting, diarrhea, epigastric distress, jaundice, cholestasis and parenchymal liver damage.

Central Nervous System: dizziness, weariness, drowsiness, giddiness, headache, numbness, hyperirritability, convulsions, collapse, psychic disturbances.

Special Senses: tinnitus, abnormal sensation in eyes, xanthopsia, blurring of vision, drying of mucous membranes (mouth, eyes, etc.).

Cardiovascular: hypotension.

Metabolic: hyperglycemia.

Hematologic: transient leukopenia.

Genitourinary: hematuria, enuresis, malodor of the urine, crystalluria.

Hypersensitivity: pruritus, fever, facial flush, chills, conjunctival injection, angioedema, anaphylaxis, skin rashes (including perianal), erythema multiforme (including Stevens-Johnson syndrome), and lymphadenopathy.

Miscellaneous: appearance of live Ascaris in the mouth and nose.

OVERDOSAGE

Overdosage may be associated with transient disturbances of vision and psychic alterations.

There is no specific antidote in the event of overdosage. Therefore, symptomatic and supportive measures should be employed. Emesis should be induced or gastric lavage performed carefully.

The oral LD_{50} of MINTEZOL is 3.6 g/kg, 3.1 g/kg and 3.8 g/kg in the mouse, rat, and rabbit respectively.

DOSAGE AND ADMINISTRATION

The recommended maximum daily dose of MINTEZOL is 3 grams.

MINTEZOL should be given after meals if possible. Tablets MINTEZOL should be chewed before swallowing. Dietary restriction, complementary medications and cleansing enemas are not needed.

The usual dosage schedule for all conditions is two doses per day. The dosage is determined by the patient's weight. A weight-dose chart follows:

Weight	Each Dose	
	g	mL
30 lb	0.25	2.5
	(½ tablet)	(½ teaspoon)
50 lb	0.5	5.0
	(1 tablet)	(1 teaspoon)
75 lb	0.75	7.5
	(1½ tablets)	(1½ teaspoons)
100 lb	1.0	10.0
	(2 tablets)	(2 teaspoons)
125 lb	1.25	12.5
	(2½ tablets)	(2½ teaspoons)
150 lb	1.5	15.0
& over	(3 tablets)	(3 teaspoons)

The regimen for each indication follows:
[See table at left.]

HOW SUPPLIED

No. 3331 — MINTEZOL Suspension, 500 mg per 5 mL, is white to off-white and is supplied as follows:
NDC 0006-3331-60 in bottles of 120 mL
(6505-00-935-5835, 0.5 g/5 mL, 120 mL).
No. 3332 — MINTEZOL Chewable Tablets, 500 mg, are white to off-white, orange-flavored, round, scored, compressed tablets, coded MSD 907. They are supplied as follows:
NDC 0006-0907-36 in boxes of 36 strip packaged, individually foil-wrapped tablets
(6505-01-226-9909, 500 mg chewable, 36's).
Shown in Product Identification Guide, page 324
7930812 Issued June 1985
COPYRIGHT © MERCK & CO., INC., 1983
All rights reserved

MODURETIC® Tablets ℞
(Amiloride HCl-Hydrochlorothiazide), U.S.P.

DESCRIPTION

MODURETIC* (Amiloride HCl-Hydrochlorothiazide) combines the potassium-conserving action of amiloride HCl with the natriuretic action of hydrochlorothiazide.

Therapeutic Regimens

Indication	Regimen	Comments
*STRONGYLOIDIASIS	2 doses per day for 2 successive days.	A single dose of 20 mg/lb or 50 mg/kg may be employed as an alternative schedule, but a higher incidence of side effects should be expected.
CUTANEOUS LARVA MIGRANS (Creeping Eruption)	2 doses per day for 2 successive days.	If active lesions are still present 2 days after completion of therapy, a second course is recommended.
VISCERAL LARVA MIGRANS	2 doses per day for 7 successive days.	Safety and efficacy data on the seven-day treatment course are limited.
*TRICHINOSIS	2 doses per day for 2–4 successive days according to the response of the patient.	The optimal dosage for the treatment of trichinosis has not been established.
Other Indications		
* Intestinal roundworms (including Ascariasis, Uncinariasis and Trichuriasis)	2 doses per day for 2 successive days.	A single dose of 20 mg/lb or 50 mg/kg may be employed as an alternative schedule, but a higher incidence of side effects should be expected.

* Clinical experience with thiabendazole for treatment of each of these conditions in children weighing less than 30 lbs has been limited.

Amiloride HCl is designated chemically as 3,5-diamino-6- chloro -*N*- (diaminomethylene) pyrazinecarboxamide monohydrochloride, dihydrate and has a molecular weight of 302.14. Its empirical formula is $C_6H_8ClN_7O \cdot HCl \cdot 2H_2O$ and its structural formula is:

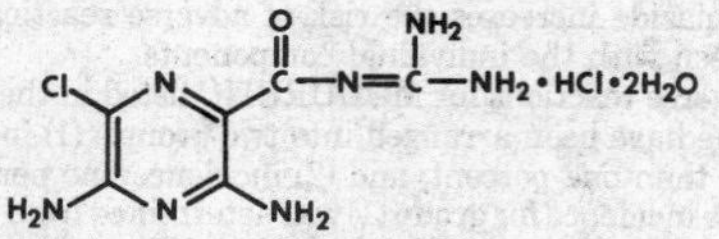

Hydrochlorothiazide is designated chemically as 6-chloro-3,4-dihydro-2*H* -1,2,4-benzothiadiazine-7-sulfonamide 1,1-dioxide. Its empirical formula is $C_7H_8ClN_3O_4S_2$ and its structural formula is:

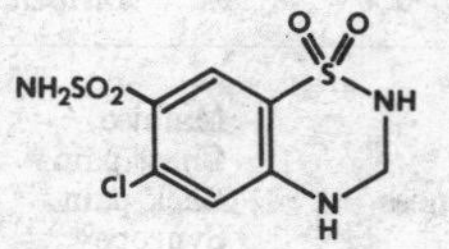

It is a white, or practically white, crystalline powder with a molecular weight of 297.72, which is slightly soluble in water, but freely soluble in sodium hydroxide solution.
MODURETIC is available for oral use as tablets containing 5 mg of anhydrous amiloride HCl and 50 mg of hydrochlorothiazide. Each tablet contains the following inactive ingredients: calcium phosphate, FD&C Yellow 6, guar gum, lactose, magnesium stearate and starch.

---

*Registered trademark of MERCK & CO., INC.

CLINICAL PHARMACOLOGY

MODURETIC provides diuretic and antihypertensive activity (principally due to the hydrochlorothiazide component), while acting through the amiloride component to prevent the excessive potassium loss that may occur in patients receiving a thiazide diuretic. Due to its amiloride component, the urinary excretion of magnesium is less with MODURETIC than with a thiazide or loop diuretic used alone (see PRECAUTIONS). The onset of the diuretic action of MODURETIC is within 1 to 2 hours and this action appears to be sustained for approximately 24 hours.

Amiloride HCl

Amiloride HCl is a potassium-conserving (antikaliuretic) drug that possesses weak (compared with thiazide diuretics) natriuretic, diuretic, and antihypertensive activity. These effects have been partially additive to the effects of thiazide diuretics in some clinical studies. Amiloride HCl has potassium-conserving activity in patients receiving kaliuretic-diuretic agents.
Amiloride HCl is not an aldosterone antagonist and its effects are seen even in the absence of aldosterone.
Amiloride HCl exerts its potassium sparing effect through the inhibition of sodium reabsorption at the distal convoluted tubule, cortical collecting tubule and collecting duct; this decreases the net negative potential of the tubular lumen and reduces both potassium and hydrogen secretion and their subsequent excretion. This mechanism accounts in large part for the potassium sparing action of amiloride.
Amiloride HCl usually begins to act within 2 hours after an oral dose. Its effect on electrolyte excretion reaches a peak between 6 and 10 hours and lasts about 24 hours. Peak plasma levels are obtained in 3 to 4 hours and the plasma half-life varies from 6 to 9 hours. Effects on electrolytes increase with single doses of amiloride HCl up to approximately 15 mg.
Amiloride HCl is not metabolized by the liver but is excreted unchanged by the kidneys. About 50 percent of a 20 mg dose of amiloride HCl is excreted in the urine and 40 percent in the stool within 72 hours. Amiloride HCl has little effect on glomerular filtration rate or renal blood flow. Because amiloride HCl is not metabolized by the liver, drug accumulation is not anticipated in patients with hepatic dysfunction, but accumulation can occur if the hepatorenal syndrome develops.

Hydrochlorothiazide

The mechanism of the antihypertensive effect of thiazides is unknown. Thiazides do not usually affect normal blood pressure.
Hydrochlorothiazide is a diuretic and antihypertensive. It affects the distal renal tubular mechanism of electrolyte reabsorption. Hydrochlorothiazide increases excretion of sodium and chloride in approximately equivalent amounts. Natriuresis may be accompanied by some loss of potassium and bicarbonate.
After oral use diuresis begins within two hours, peaks in about four hours and lasts about 6 to 12 hours.
Hydrochlorothiazide is not metabolized but is eliminated rapidly by the kidney. When plasma levels have been followed for at least 24 hours, the plasma half-life has been observed to vary between 5.6 and 14.8 hours. At least 61 percent of the oral dose is eliminated unchanged within 24 hours. Hydrochlorothiazide crosses the placental but not the blood-brain barrier and is excreted in breast milk.

INDICATIONS AND USAGE

MODURETIC is indicated in those patients with hypertension or with congestive heart failure who develop hypokalemia when thiazides or other kaliuretic diuretics are used alone, or in whom maintenance of normal serum potassium levels is considered to be clinically important, e.g., digitalized patients, or patients with significant cardiac arrhythmias.
The use of potassium-conserving agents is often unnecessary in patients receiving diuretics for uncomplicated essential hypertension when such patients have a normal diet.
MODURETIC may be used alone or as an adjunct to other antihypertensive drugs, such as methyldopa or beta blockers. Since MODURETIC enhances the action of these agents, dosage adjustments may be necessary to avoid an excessive fall in blood pressure and other unwanted side effects.
This fixed combination drug is not indicated for the initial therapy of edema or hypertension except in individuals in whom the development of hypokalemia cannot be risked.

CONTRAINDICATIONS

Hyperkalemia

MODURETIC should not be used in the presence of elevated serum potassium levels (greater than 5.5 mEq per liter).

Antikaliuretic Therapy or Potassium Supplementation

MODURETIC should not be given to patients receiving other potassium-conserving agents, such as spironolactone or triamterene. Potassium supplementation in the form of medication, potassium-containing salt substitutes or a potassium-rich diet should not be used with MODURETIC except in severe and/or refractory cases of hypokalemia. Such concomitant therapy can be associated with rapid increases in serum potassium levels. If potassium supplementation is used, careful monitoring of the serum potassium level is necessary.

Impaired Renal Function

Anuria, acute or chronic renal insufficiency, and evidence of diabetic nephropathy are contraindications to the use of MODURETIC. Patients with evidence of renal functional impairment (blood urea nitrogen [BUN] levels over 30 mg per 100 mL or serum creatinine levels over 1.5 mg per 100 mL) or diabetes mellitus should not receive the drug without careful, frequent and continuing monitoring of serum electrolytes, creatinine, and BUN levels. Potassium retention associated with the use of an antikaliuretic agent is accentuated in the presence of renal impairment and may result in the rapid development of hyperkalemia.

Hypersensitivity

MODURETIC is contraindicated in patients who are hypersensitive to this product, or to other sulfonamide-derived drugs.

WARNINGS

Hyperkalemia

> Like other potassium-conserving diuretic combinations, MODURETIC may cause hyperkalemia (serum potassium levels greater than 5.5 mEq per liter). In patients without renal impairment or diabetes mellitus, the risk of hyperkalemia with MODURETIC is about 1-2 percent. This risk is higher in patients with renal impairment or diabetes mellitus (even without recognized diabetic nephropathy). Since hyperkalemia, if uncorrected, is potentially fatal, it is essential to monitor serum potassium levels carefully in any patient receiving MODURETIC, particularly when it is first introduced, at the time of dosage adjustments, and during any illness that could affect renal function.

The risk of hyperkalemia may be increased when potassium-conserving agents, including MODURETIC, are administered concomitantly with an angiotensin-converting enzyme inhibitor. (See PRECAUTIONS, *Drug Interactions.*) Warning signs or symptoms of hyperkalemia include paresthesias, muscular weakness, fatigue, flaccid paralysis of the extremities, bradycardia, shock, and ECG abnormalities. Monitoring of the serum potassium level is essential because mild hyperkalemia is not usually associated with an abnormal ECG.
When abnormal, the ECG in hyperkalemia is characterized primarily by tall, peaked T waves or elevations from previous tracings. There may also be lowering of the R wave and increased depth of the S wave, widening and even disappearance of the P wave, progressive widening of the QRS complex, prolongation of the PR interval, and ST depression.

Treatment of hyperkalemia: If hyperkalemia occurs in patients taking MODURETIC, the drug should be discontinued immediately. If the serum potassium level exceeds 6.5 mEq per liter, active measures should be taken to reduce it. Such measures include the intravenous administration of sodium bicarbonate solution or oral or parenteral glucose with a rapid-acting insulin preparation. If needed, a cation exchange resin such as sodium polystyrene sulfonate may be given orally or by enema. Patients with persistent hyperkalemia may require dialysis.

Diabetes Mellitus

In diabetic patients, hyperkalemia has been reported with the use of all potassium-conserving diuretics, including amiloride HCl, even in patients without evidence of diabetic nephropathy. Therefore, MODURETIC should be avoided, if possible, in diabetic patients and, if it is used, serum electrolytes and renal function must be monitored frequently.
MODURETIC should be discontinued at least three days before glucose tolerance testing.

Metabolic or Respiratory Acidosis

Antikaliuretic therapy should be instituted only with caution in severely ill patients in whom respiratory or metabolic acidosis may occur, such as patients with cardiopulmonary disease or poorly controlled diabetes. If MODURETIC is given to these patients, frequent monitoring of acid-base balance is necessary. Shifts in acid-base balance alter the ratio of extracellular/intracellular potassium, and the development of acidosis may be associated with rapid increases in serum potassium levels.

PRECAUTIONS

General

Electrolyte Imbalance and BUN Increases

Determination of serum electrolytes to detect possible electrolyte imbalance should be performed at appropriate intervals.
Patients should be observed for clinical signs of fluid or electrolyte imbalance: i.e., hyponatremia, hypochloremic alkalosis, and hypokalemia. Serum and urine electrolyte determinations are particularly important when the patient is vomiting excessively or receiving parenteral fluids. Warning signs or symptoms of fluid and electrolyte imbalance, irrespective of cause, include dryness of mouth, thirst, weakness, lethargy, drowsiness, restlessness, confusion, seizures, muscle pains or cramps, muscular fatigue, hypotension, oliguria, tachycardia, and gastrointestinal disturbances such as nausea and vomiting.
Hyponatremia and hypochloremia may occur during the use of thiazides and other diuretics. Any chloride deficit during thiazide therapy is generally mild and may be lessened by the amiloride HCl component of MODURETIC. Hypochloremia usually does not require specific treatment except under extraordinary circumstances (as in liver disease or renal disease). Dilutional hyponatremia may occur in edematous patients in hot weather; appropriate therapy is water restriction, rather than administration of salt, except in rare instances when the hyponatremia is life-threatening. In actual salt depletion, appropriate replacement is the therapy of choice.
Hypokalemia may develop during thiazide therapy, especially with brisk diuresis, when severe cirrhosis is present, during concomitant use of corticosteroids or ACTH, or after prolonged therapy. However, this usually is prevented by the amiloride HCl component of MODURETIC.
Interference with adequate oral electrolyte intake will also contribute to hypokalemia. Hypokalemia may cause cardiac arrhythmia and may also sensitize or exaggerate the response of the heart to the toxic effects of digitalis (e.g., increased ventricular irritability).
Thiazides have been shown to increase the urinary excretion of magnesium; this may result in hypomagnesemia. Amiloride HCl, a component of MODURETIC, has been shown to decrease the enhanced urinary excretion of magnesium which occurs when a thiazide or loop diuretic is used alone.
Increases in BUN levels have been reported with amiloride HCl and with hydrochlorothiazide. These increases usually have accompanied vigorous fluid elimination, especially when diuretic therapy was used in seriously ill patients, such as those who had hepatic cirrhosis with ascites and metabolic alkalosis, or those with resistant edema. Therefore, when MODURETIC is given to such patients, careful monitoring of serum electrolyte and BUN levels is important. In patients with pre-existing severe liver disease, hepatic encephalopathy, manifested by tremors, confusion, and coma, and increased jaundice, have been reported in association

Continued on next page

Information on the Merck & Co., Inc. products listed on these pages is the full prescribing information from product circulars in use September 30, 1996.

Merck & Co.—Cont.

with diuretic therapy including amiloride HCl and hydrochlorothiazide.

In patients with renal disease, diuretics may precipitate azotemia. Cumulative effects of the components of MODURETIC may develop in patients with impaired renal function. If renal impairment becomes evident, MODURETIC should be discontinued (see CONTRAINDICATIONS and WARNINGS).

Drug Interactions

In some patients, the administration of a non-steroidal anti-inflammatory agent can reduce the diuretic, natriuretic, and antihypertensive effects of loop, potassium-sparing and thiazide diuretics. Therefore, when MODURETIC and non-steroidal anti-inflammatory agents are used concomitantly, the patient should be observed closely to determine if the desired effect of the diuretic is obtained. Since indomethacin and potassium-sparing diuretics, including MODURETIC, each may be associated with increased serum potassium levels, the potential effects on potassium kinetics and renal function should be considered when these agents are administered concurrently.

Amiloride HCl

When amiloride HCl is administered concomitantly with an angiotensin-converting enzyme inhibitor, the risk of hyperkalemia may be increased. Therefore, if concomitant use of these agents in indicated because of demonstrated hypokalemia, they should be used with caution and with frequent monitoring of serum potassium. (See WARNINGS.)

Hydrochlorothiazide

When given concurrently the following drugs may interact with thiazide diuretics.

Alcohol, barbiturates, or narcotics—potentiation of orthostatic hypotension may occur.

Antidiabetic drugs (oral agents and insulin)—dosage adjustment of the antidiabetic drug may be required.

Other antihypertensive drugs—additive effect or potentiation.

Cholestyramine and colestipol resins—Absorption of hydrochlorothiazide is impaired in the presence of anionic exchange resins. Single doses of either cholestyramine or colestipol resins bind the hydrochlorothiazide and reduce its absorption from the gastrointestinal tract by up to 85 and 43 percent, respectively.

Corticosteroids, ACTH—intensified electrolyte depletion, particularly hypokalemia.

Pressor amines (e.g., norepinephrine)—possible decreased response to pressor amines but not sufficient to preclude their use.

Skeletal muscle relaxants, nondepolarizing (e.g., tubocurarine)—possible increased responsiveness to the muscle relaxant.

Lithium—generally should not be given with diuretics. Diuretic agents reduce the renal clearance of lithium and add a high risk of lithium toxicity. Refer to the package insert for lithium preparations before use of such preparations with MODURETIC.

Metabolic and Endocrine Effects

In diabetic patients, insulin requirements may be increased, decreased, or unchanged due to the hydrochlorothiazide component. Diabetes mellitus that has been latent may become manifest during administration of thiazide diuretics.

Because calcium excretion is decreased by thiazides, MODURETIC should be discontinued before carrying out tests for parathyroid function. Pathologic changes in the parathyroid glands, with hypercalcemia and hypophosphatemia have been observed in a few patients on prolonged thiazide therapy; however, the common complications of hyperparathyroidism such as renal lithiasis, bone resorption, and peptic ulceration have not been seen.

Hyperuricemia may occur or acute gout may be precipitated in certain patients receiving thiazide therapy.

Other Precautions

In patients receiving thiazides, sensitivity reactions may occur with or without a history of allergy or bronchial asthma. The possibility of exacerbation or activation of systemic lupus erythematosus has been reported with the use of thiazides.

Increases in cholesterol and triglyceride levels may be associated with thiazide diuretic therapy.

Carcinogenicity, Mutagenicity, Impairment of Fertility

Long-term studies in animals have not been performed to evaluate the effects upon fertility, mutagenicity or carcinogenic potential of MODURETIC.

Amiloride HCl

There was no evidence of a tumorigenic effect when amiloride HCl was administered for 92 weeks to mice at doses up to 10 mg/kg/day (25 times the maximum daily human dose). Amiloride HCl has also been administered for 104 weeks to male and female rats at doses up to 6 and 8 mg/kg/day (15 and 20 times the maximum daily dose for humans, respectively) and showed no evidence of carcinogenicity.

Amiloride HCl was devoid of mutagenic activity in various strains of *Salmonella typhimurium* with or without a mammalian liver microsomal activation system (Ames test).

Hydrochlorothiazide

Two-year feeding studies in mice and rats conducted under the auspices of the National Toxicology Program (NTP) uncovered no evidence of a carcinogenic potential of hydrochlorothiazide in female mice (at doses of up to approximately 600 mg/kg/day) or in male and female rats (at doses of up to approximately 100 mg/kg/day). The NTP, however, found equivocal evidence for hepatocarcinogenicity in male mice.

Hydrochlorothiazide was not genotoxic *in vitro* in the Ames mutagenicity assay of *Salmonella typhimurium* strains TA 98, TA 100, TA 1535, TA 1537, and TA 1538 and in the Chinese Hamster Ovary (CHO) test for chromosomal aberrations, or *in vivo* in assays using mouse germinal cell chromosomes, Chinese hamster bone marrow chromosomes, and the *Drosophila* sex-linked recessive lethal trait gene. Positive test results were obtained only in the *in vitro* CHO Sister Chromatid Exchange (clastogenicity) and in the Mouse Lymphoma Cell (mutagenicity) assays, using concentrations of hydrochlorothiazide from 43 to 1300 μg/mL, and in the *Aspergillus nidulans* non-disjunction assay at an unspecified concentration.

Hydrochlorothiazide had no adverse effects on the fertility of mice and rats of either sex in studies wherein these species were exposed, via their diet, to doses of up to 100 and 4 mg/kg, respectively, prior to conception and throughout gestation.

Pregnancy

Pregnancy Category B. Teratogenicity studies have been performed with combinations of amiloride HCl and hydrochlorothiazide in rabbits and mice at doses up to 25 times the expected maximum daily dose for humans and have revealed no evidence of harm to the fetus. No evidence of impaired fertility in rats was apparent at dosage levels up to 25 times the expected maximum human daily dose. A perinatal and postnatal study in rats showed a reduction in maternal body weight gain during and after gestation at a daily dose of 25 times the expected maximum daily dose for humans. The body weights of alive pups at birth and at weaning were also reduced at this dose level. There are no adequate and well-controlled studies in pregnant women. Because animal reproduction studies are not always predictive of human responses, and because of the data listed below with the individual components, this drug should be used during pregnancy only if clearly needed.

Amiloride HCl

Teratogenicity studies with amiloride HCl in rabbits and mice given 20 and 25 times the maximum human dose, respectively, revealed no evidence of harm to the fetus, although studies showed that the drug crossed the placenta in modest amounts. Reproduction studies in rats at 20 times the expected maximum daily dose for humans showed no evidence of impaired fertility. At approximately 5 or more times the expected maximum daily dose for humans, some toxicity was seen in adult rats and rabbits and a decrease in rat pup growth and survival occurred.

Hydrochlorothiazide

Teratogenic Effects: Studies in which hydrochlorothiazide was orally administered to pregnant mice and rats during their respective periods of major organogenesis at doses up to 3000 and 1000 mg hydrochlorothiazide/kg, respectively, provided no evidence of harm to the fetus. There are, however, no adequate and well-controlled studies in pregnant women.

Nonteratogenic Effects: Thiazides cross the placental barrier and appear in cord blood. There is a risk of fetal or neonatal jaundice, thrombocytopenia, and possibly other adverse reactions that have occurred in adults.

Nursing Mothers

Studies in rats have shown that amiloride is excreted in milk in concentrations higher than that found in blood, but it is not known whether amiloride HCl is excreted in human milk. However, thiazides appear in breast milk. Because of the potential for serious adverse reactions in nursing infants, a decision should be made whether to discontinue nursing or to discontinue the drug, taking into account the importance of the drug to the mother.

Pediatric Use

Safety and effectiveness in children have not been established.

ADVERSE REACTIONS

MODURETIC is usually well tolerated and significant clinical adverse effects have been reported infrequently. The risk of hyperkalemia (serum potassium levels greater than 5.5 mEq per liter) with MODURETIC is about 1–2 percent in patients without renal impairment or diabetes mellitus (see WARNINGS). Minor adverse reactions to amiloride HCl have been reported relatively frequently (about 20%) but the relationship of many of the reports to amiloride HCl is uncertain and the overall frequency was similar in hydrochlorothiazide treated groups. Nausea/anorexia, abdominal pain, flatulence, and mild skin rash have been reported and probably are related to amiloride. Other adverse experiences that have been reported with MODURETIC are generally those known to be associated with diuresis, thiazide therapy, or with the underlying disease being treated. Clinical trials have not demonstrated that combining amiloride and hydrochlorothiazide increases the risk of adverse reactions over those seen with the individual components.

The adverse reactions for MODURETIC listed in the following table have been arranged into two groups: (1) incidence greater than one percent; and (2) incidence one percent or less. The incidence for group (1) was determined from clinical studies conducted in the United States (607 patients treated with MODURETIC). The adverse effects listed in group (2) include reports from the same clinical studies and voluntary reports since marketing. The probability of a causal relationship exists between MODURETIC and these adverse reactions, some of which have been reported only rarely.

Incidence > 1%	*Incidence ≤ 1%*
Body as a Whole	
Headache*	Malaise
Weakness*	Chest pain
Fatigue/tiredness	Back pain
	Syncope
Cardiovascular	
Arrhythmia	Tachycardia
	Digitalis toxicity
	Orthostatic hypotension
	Angina pectoris
Digestive	
Nausea/anorexia*	Constipation
Diarrhea	GI bleeding
Gastrointestinal pain	GI disturbance
	Appetite changes
Abdominal pain	Abdominal fullness
	Hiccups
	Thirst
	Vomiting
	Anorexia
	Flatulence
Metabolic	
Elevated serum	Gout
potassium levels	Dehydration
(>5.5 mEq	Symptomatic
per liter)†	hyponatremia**
Musculoskeletal	
Leg ache	Muscle cramps/spasm
	Joint pain
Nervous	
Dizziness*	Paresthesia/numbness
	Stupor
	Vertigo
Psychiatric	
None	Insomnia
	Nervousness
	Depression
	Sleepiness
	Mental confusion
Respiratory	
Dyspnea	None
Skin	
Rash*	Flushing
Pruritus	Diaphoresis
	Erythema multiforme including Stevens-Johnson syndrome
	Exfoliative dermatitis including toxic epidermal necrolysis
	Alopecia
Special Senses	
None	Bad taste
	Visual disturbance
	Nasal congestion
Urogenital	
None	Impotence
	Nocturia
	Dysuria
	Incontinence
	Renal dysfunction including renal failure
	Gynecomastia

* Reactions occurring in 3% to 8% of patients treated with MODURETIC. (Those reactions occurring in less than 3% of the patients are unmarked.)

† See WARNINGS.

** See PRECAUTIONS.

Other adverse reactions that have been reported with the individual components and within each category are listed in order of decreasing severity:

Amiloride—*Body as a Whole:* Painful extremities, neck/shoulder ache, fatigability; *Cardiovascular:* Palpitation; *Di-*

gestive: Activation of probable pre-existing peptic ulcer, abnormal liver function, jaundice, dyspepsia, heartburn; Hematologic: Aplastic anemia, neutropenia; Integumentary: Alopecia, itching, dry mouth; Nervous System/Psychiatric: Encephalopathy, tremors, decreased libido; Respiratory: Shortness of breath, cough; Special Senses: Increased intraocular pressure, tinnitus; Urogenital: Bladder spasms, polyuria, urinary frequency.

Hydrochlorothiazide—Digestive: Pancreatitis, jaundice (intrahepatic cholestatic jaundice), sialadenitis, cramping, gastric irritation; Hematologic: Aplastic anemia, agranulocytosis, leukopenia, hemolytic anemia, thrombocytopenia; Hypersensitivity: Anaphylactic reactions, necrotizing angiitis (vasculitis, cutaneous vasculitis), respiratory distress including pneumonitis and pulmonary edema, photosensitivity, fever, urticaria, purpura; Metabolic: Electrolyte imbalance (see PRECAUTIONS), hyperglycemia, glycosuria, hyperuricemia; Nervous System/Psychiatric: Restlessness; Special Senses: Transient blurred vision, xanthopsia; Urogenital: Interstitial nephritis (see WARNINGS).

OVERDOSAGE

No data are available in regard to overdosage in humans. The oral LD_{50} of the combination drug is 189 and 422 mg/kg for female mice and female rats, respectively.

It is not known whether the drug is dialyzable.

No specific information is available on the treatment of overdosage with MODURETIC, and no specific antidote is available. Treatment is symptomatic and supportive. Therapy with MODURETIC should be discontinued and the patient observed closely. Suggested measures include induction of emesis and/or gastric lavage.

Amiloride HCl: No data are available in regard to overdosage in humans.

The oral LD_{50} of amiloride HCl (calculated as the base) is 56 mg/kg in mice and 36 to 85 mg/kg in rats, depending on the strain.

The most common signs and symptoms to be expected with overdosage are dehydration and electrolyte imbalance. If hyperkalemia occurs, active measures should be taken to reduce the serum potassium levels.

Hydrochlorothiazide: The oral LD_{50} of hydrochlorothiazide is greater than 10.0 g/kg in both mice and rats.

The most common signs and symptoms observed are those caused by electrolyte depletion (hypokalemia, hypochloremia, hyponatremia) and dehydration resulting from excessive diuresis. If digitalis has also been administered, hypokalemia may accentuate cardiac arrhythmias.

DOSAGE AND ADMINISTRATION

MODURETIC should be administered with food.

The usual starting dosage is 1 tablet a day. The dosage may be increased to 2 tablets a day, if necessary. More than 2 tablets of MODURETIC daily usually are not needed and there is no controlled experience with such doses. The daily dose is usually given as a single dose but may be given in divided doses. Once an initial diuresis has been achieved, dosage adjustment may be necessary. Maintenance therapy may be on an intermittent basis.

HOW SUPPLIED

No. 3385—Tablets MODURETIC are peach-colored, diamond-shaped, scored, compressed tablets, coded MSD 917. Each tablet contains 5 mg of anhydrous amiloride HCl and 50 mg of hydrochlorothiazide. They are supplied as follows: NDC 0006-0917-68 in bottles of 100
(6505-01-139-1498 100's)
NDC 0006-0917-28 unit dose packages of 100.
Shown in Product Identification Guide, page 325
Storage
Keep container tightly closed. Protect from light, moisture, freezing, -20°C (-4°F) and store at room temperature, 15–30 °C (59–86°F).

7887324   Issued May 1993
COPYRIGHT © MERCK & CO., INC., 1988
All rights reserved

MUMPSVAX®   ℞
(Mumps Virus Vaccine Live), U.S.P.
Jeryl Lynn Strain

DESCRIPTION

MUMPSVAX* (Mumps Virus Vaccine Live) is a live virus vaccine for immunization against mumps.
MUMPSVAX is a sterile lyophilized preparation of the Jeryl Lynn (B level) strain of mumps virus. The virus was adapted to and propagated in cell cultures of chick embryo free of avian leukosis virus and other adventitious agents.

The reconstituted vaccine is for subcutaneous administration. When reconstituted as directed, the dose for injection is 0.5 mL and contains not less than the equivalent of 20,000 $TCID_{50}$ (tissue culture infectious doses) of the U.S. Reference Mumps Virus. Each dose contains approximately 25 mcg of neomycin. The product contains no preservative. Sorbitol and hydrolized gelatin are added as stabilizers.

*Registered trademark of MERCK & CO., INC.

CLINICAL PHARMACOLOGY

MUMPSVAX produces a modified, non-communicable mumps infection in susceptible persons. Extensive clinical trials have demonstrated that MUMPSVAX is highly immunogenic and well tolerated. A single injection of the vaccine has been shown to induce mumps neutralizing antibodies in approximately 97 percent of susceptible children and approximately 93 percent of susceptible adults. The pattern of antibody response closely resembles that observed for natural mumps. Although the antibody level is significantly lower than that following natural infection, it is protective and long lasting. Vaccine-induced antibody levels have been shown to persist for at least 15 years with a rate of decline comparable to that seen in natural infection. If the present pattern continues, it will provide a basis for the expectation that immunity following vaccination will be permanent. However, continued surveillance will be required to demonstrate this point.

INDICATIONS AND USAGE

MUMPSVAX is indicated for immunization against mumps in persons 12 months of age or older. Most adults are likely to have been infected naturally and generally may be considered immune, even if they did not have clinically recognizable disease. A booster is not needed. It is not recommended for infants younger than 12 months because they may retain maternal mumps neutralizing antibodies which may interfere with the immune response.

Evidence indicates that the vaccine will not offer protection when given after exposure to natural mumps. Passively acquired antibody can interfere with the response to live, attenuated-virus vaccines. Therefore, administration of mumps virus vaccine should be deferred until approximately three months after passive immunization.

Individuals planning travel outside the United States, if not immune, can acquire measles, mumps or rubella and import these diseases to the United States. Therefore, prior to International travel, individuals known to be susceptible to one or more of these diseases can receive either a single antigen vaccine (measles, mumps or rubella), or a combined antigen vaccine as appropriate. However, M-M-R* II (Measles, Mumps, and Rubella Virus Vaccine Live) is preferred for persons likely to be susceptible to mumps and rubella; and if single-antigen measles vaccine is not readily available, travelers should receive M-M-R II (Measles, Mumps, and Rubella Virus Vaccine Live) regardless of their immune status to mumps or rubella.

Revaccination: Children vaccinated when younger than 12 months of age should be revaccinated. Based on available evidence, there is no reason to routinely revaccinate persons who were vaccinated originally when 12 months of age or older. However, persons should be revaccinated if there is evidence to suggest that initial immunization was ineffective.

Use with other Vaccines
Routine administration of DTP (diphtheria, tetanus, pertussis) and/or OPV (oral poliovirus vaccine) concomitantly with measles, mumps and rubella vaccines is not recommended because there are insufficient data relating to the simultaneous administration of these antigens. However, the American Academy of Pediatrics has noted that in some circumstances, particularly when the patient may not return, some practitioners prefer to administer all these antigens on a single day. If done, separate sites and syringes should be used for DTP and MUMPSVAX.

MUMPSVAX should not be given less than one month before or after administration of other virus vaccines.

*Registered trademark of MERCK & CO., INC.

CONTRAINDICATIONS

Do not give MUMPSVAX to pregnant females; the possible effects of the vaccine on fetal development are unknown at this time. If vaccination of postpubertal females is undertaken, pregnancy should be avoided for three months following vaccination (see PRECAUTIONS, Pregnancy).

Anaphylactic or anaphylactoid reactions to neomycin (each dose of reconstituted vaccine contains approximately 25 mcg of neomycin).

History of anaphylactic or anaphylactoid reactions to eggs (see HYPERSENSITIVITY TO EGGS below).

Any febrile respiratory illness or other active febrile infection.

Active untreated tuberculosis.

Patients receiving immunosuppressive therapy. This contraindication does not apply to patients who are receiving corticosteroids as replacement therapy, e.g., for Addison's disease.

Individuals with blood dyscrasias, leukemia, lymphomas of any type, or other malignant neoplasms affecting the bone marrow or lymphatic systems.

Primary and acquired immunodeficiency states, including patients who are immunosuppressed in association with AIDS or other clinical manifestations of infection with human immunodeficiency viruses; cellular immune deficiencies; and hypogammaglobulinemic and dysgammaglobulinemic states.

Individuals with a family history of congenital or hereditary immunodeficiency, until the immune competence of the potential vaccine recipient is demonstrated.

HYPERSENSITIVITY TO EGGS

Live mumps vaccine is produced in chick embryo cell culture. Persons with a history of anaphylactic, anaphylactoid, or other immediate reactions (e.g., hives, swelling of the mouth and throat, difficulty breathing, hypotension, or shock) subsequent to egg ingestion should be vaccinated only with extreme caution. Evidence indicates that persons are not at increased risk if they have egg allergies that are not anaphylactic or anaphylactoid in nature. Such persons may be vaccinated in the usual manner. There is no evidence to indicate that persons with allergies to chickens or feathers are at increased risk of reaction to the vaccine.

PRECAUTIONS

General
Adequate treatment provisions including epinephrine, should be available for immediate use should an anaphylactic or anaphylactoid reaction occur.

Children and young adults who are known to be infected with human immunodeficiency viruses but without overt clinical manifestations of immunosuppression may be vaccinated; however, the vaccinees should be monitored closely for vaccine-preventable diseases because immunization may be less effective than for uninfected persons.

Vaccination should be deferred for at least 3 months following blood or plasma transfusions, or administration of human immune serum globulin.

There are no reports of transmission of live mumps virus from vaccinees to susceptible contacts.

It has been reported that mumps virus vaccine, live, may result in a temporary depression of tuberculin skin sensitivity. Therefore, if a tuberculin test is to be done, it should be administered either before or simultaneously with MUMPSVAX.

As for any vaccine, vaccination with MUMPSVAX may not result in seroconversion in 100% of susceptible persons given the vaccine.

Pregnancy
Pregnancy Category C
Animal reproduction studies have not been conducted with MUMPSVAX. It is also not known whether MUMPSVAX can cause fetal harm when administered to a pregnant woman or can affect reproduction capacity. Therefore, mumps virus vaccine should not be given to persons known to be pregnant; furthermore, pregnancy should be avoided for three months following vaccination. Although mumps virus is capable of infecting the placenta and fetus, there is no good evidence that it causes congenital malformations in humans. Mumps vaccine virus also has been shown to infect the placenta, but the virus has not been isolated from the fetal tissues from susceptible women who were vaccinated and underwent elective abortions.

Nursing Mothers
It is not known whether mumps vaccine virus is secreted in human milk. Therefore, because many drugs are excreted in human milk, caution should be exercised when MUMPSVAX is administered to a nursing woman.

ADVERSE REACTIONS

Burning and/or stinging of short duration at the injection site have been reported.

Anaphylaxis and anaphylactoid reactions have been reported.

Mild fever occurs occasionally. Fever above 103°F (39.4°C) is uncommon.

Continued on next page

Information on the Merck & Co., Inc. products listed on these pages is the full prescribing information from product circulars in use September 30, 1996.

Consult 1997 supplements and future editions for revisions

Merck & Co.—Cont.

Mild lymphadenopathy has been reported.
Cough and rhinitis have been reported after vaccination with other mumps-containing vaccines.
Diarrhea has been reported after vaccination with mumps-containing vaccines.
Vasculitis has been reported rarely after vaccination with other mumps-containing vaccines.
Parotitis has been reported to occur in very low incidence, and orchitis rarely, in persons who were vaccinated. In most instances investigated, prior exposure to natural mumps was established. In other instances, whether or not this was due to vaccine or to prior natural mumps exposure or to other causes has not been established.
Reports of purpura and allergic reactions such as wheal and flare at the injection site or urticaria have been extremely rare. Erythema multiforme has also been reported rarely.
Forms of optic neuritis, including retrobulbar neuritis and papillitis may infrequently follow viral infections, and have been reported to occur 1 to 3 weeks following inoculation with some live virus vaccines.
Syncope, particularly at the time of mass vaccination, has been reported.
Very rarely encephalitis, febrile seizures, nerve deafness and other nervous system reactions have occurred in vaccinees. A cause-effect relationship has not been established.

DOSAGE AND ADMINISTRATION

FOR SUBCUTANEOUS ADMINISTRATION
Do not inject intravenously
The dosage of vaccine is the same for all persons. Inject the total volume (about 0.5 mL) of reconstituted vaccine subcutaneously, preferably into the outer aspect of upper arm. *Do not give immune serum globulin (ISG) concurrently with* MUMPSVAX.
During shipment, to insure that there is no loss of potency, the vaccine must be maintained at a temperature of 10°C (50°F) or less.
Before reconstitution, store MUMPSVAX at 2–8°C (36–46°F). *Protect from light.*
CAUTION: A sterile syringe free of preservatives, antiseptics, and detergents should be used for each injection and/or reconstitution of the vaccine because these substances may inactivate the live virus vaccine. A 25 gauge, ⅝" needle is recommended.
To reconstitute, use only the diluent supplied, since it is free of preservatives or other antiviral substances which might inactivate the vaccine.

Single Dose Vial—First withdraw the entire volume of diluent into the syringe to be used for reconstitution. Inject all the diluent in the syringe into the vial of lyophilized vaccine, and agitate to mix thoroughly. Withdraw the entire contents into a syringe and inject the total volume of restored vaccine subcutaneously.
It is important to use a separate sterile syringe and needle for each individual patient to prevent transmission of hepatitis B and other infectious agents from one person to another.
10 Dose Vial (available only to government agencies/institutions)—Withdraw the entire contents (7 mL) of the diluent vial into the sterile syringe to be used for reconstitution, and introduce into the 10 dose vial of lyophilized vaccine. Agitate to ensure thorough mixing. The outer labeling suggests "For Jet Injector or Syringe Use". Use with separate sterile syringes is permitted for containers of 10 doses or less. The vaccine and diluent do not contain preservatives; therefore, the user must recognize the potential contamination hazards and exercise special precautions to protect the sterility and potency of the product. The use of aseptic techniques and proper storage prior to and after restoration of the vaccine and subsequent withdrawal of the individual doses is essential. Use 0.5 mL of the reconstituted vaccine for subcutaneous injection.
It is important to use a separate sterile syringe and needle for each individual patient to prevent transmission of hepatitis B and other infectious agents from one person to another.
50 Dose Vial (available only to government agencies/institutions)—Withdraw the entire contents (30 mL) of the diluent vial into the sterile syringe to be used for reconstitution and introduce into the 50 dose vial of lyophilized vaccine. Agitate to ensure thorough mixing. With full aseptic precautions, attach the vial to the sterilized multidose jet injector apparatus. Use 0.5 mL of the reconstituted vaccine for subcutaneous injection.

Each dose of MUMPSVAX contains not less than the equivalent of 20,000 $TCID_{50}$ of the U.S. Reference Mumps Virus.
Parenteral drug products should be inspected visually for particulate matter and discoloration prior to administration. MUMPSVAX, when reconstituted, is clear yellow.

HOW SUPPLIED

No. 4753—MUMPSVAX is supplied as a single-dose vial of lyophilized vaccine, **NDC** 0006-4753-00, and a vial of diluent.
No. 4584X/4309—MUMPSVAX is supplied as follows: (1) a box of 10 single-dose vials of lyophilized vaccine (package A), **NDC** 0006-4584-00; and (2) a box of 10 vials of diluent (package B). To conserve refrigerator space, the diluent may be stored separately at room temperature (6505-01-037-6792, Ten Pack).
Available only to government agencies/institutions:
No. 4664X—MUMPSVAX is supplied as one 10 dose vial of lyophilized vaccine, **NDC** 0006-4664-00, and one 7 mL vial of diluent.
No. 4593X—MUMPSVAX is supplied as one 50 dose vial of lyophilized vaccine, **NDC** 0006-4593-00, and one 30 mL vial of diluent.
Storage
It is recommended that the vaccine be used as soon as possible after reconstitution. Protect vaccine from light at all times, since such exposure may inactivate the virus. Store reconstituted vaccine in the vaccine vial in a dark place at 2–8°C (36–46°F) and discard if not used within 8 hours.

A.H.F.S. Category: 80:12
DC 7680412 Issued March 1995

COPYRIGHT © MERCK & CO., INC., 1990
All rights reserved

MUSTARGEN®, Trituration of (Mechlorethamine HCl for Injection), U.S.P. ℞

DESCRIPTION

MUSTARGEN* (Mechlorethamine HCl), an antineoplastic nitrogen mustard also known as HN2 hydrochloride, is a nitrogen analog of sulfur mustard. It is a light yellow brown, crystalline, hygroscopic powder that is very soluble in water and also soluble in alcohol.
Mechlorethamine hydrochloride is designated chemically as 2-chloro-*N*-(2-chloroethyl)-*N*-methylethanamine hydrochloride. The molecular weight is 192.52 and the melting point is 108–111°C. The empirical formula is $C_5H_{11}Cl_2N \cdot HCl$, and the structural formula is:

$$CH_3N(CH_2CH_2Cl)_2 \cdot HCl$$

Trituration of MUSTARGEN is a sterile, light yellow brown crystalline powder for injection by the intravenous or intracavitary routes after dissolution. Each vial of MUSTARGEN contains 10 mg of mechlorethamine hydrochloride triturated with sodium chloride q.s. 100 mg. When dissolved with 10 mL Sterile Water for Injection or 0.9% Sodium Chloride Injection, the resulting solution has a pH of 3–5 at a concentration of 1 mg mechlorethamine HCl per mL.

*Registered trademark of MERCK & CO., INC.

CLINICAL PHARMACOLOGY

Mechlorethamine, a biologic alkylating agent, has a cytotoxic action which inhibits rapidly proliferating cells.
Pharmacokinetics and Metabolism
In water or body fluids, mechlorethamine undergoes rapid chemical transformation and combines with water or reactive compounds of cells, so that the drug is no longer present in active form a few minutes after administration.

INDICATIONS AND USAGE

Before using MUSTARGEN *see CONTRAINDICATIONS, WARNINGS, PRECAUTIONS, ADVERSE REACTIONS, DOSAGE AND ADMINISTRATION, and HOW SUPPLIED, Special Handling.*
MUSTARGEN, administered intravenously, is indicated for the palliative treatment of Hodgkin's disease (Stages III and IV), lymphosarcoma, chronic myelocytic or chronic lymphocytic leukemia, polycythemia vera, mycosis fungoides, and bronchogenic carcinoma.
MUSTARGEN, administered intrapleurally, intraperitoneally, or intrapericardially, is indicated for the palliative treatment of metastatic carcinoma resulting in effusion.

CONTRAINDICATIONS

The use of MUSTARGEN is contraindicated in the presence of known infectious diseases and in patients who have had previous anaphylactic reactions to MUSTARGEN.

WARNINGS

Extravasation of the drug into subcutaneous tissues results in a painful inflammation. The area usually becomes indurated and sloughing may occur. If leakage of drug is obvious, prompt infiltration of the area with sterile isotonic sodium thiosulfate (⅙ molar) and application of an ice compress for 6 to 12 hours may minimize the local reaction. For a ⅙ molar solution of sodium thiosulfate, use 4.14 g of sodium thiosulfate per 100 mL of Sterile Water for Injection or 2.64 g of anhydrous sodium thiosulfate per 100 mL or dilute 4 mL of Sodium Thiosulfate Injection (10%) with 6 mL of Sterile Water for Injection.

Before using MUSTARGEN, *an accurate histologic diagnosis of the disease, a knowledge of its natural course, and an adequate clinical history are important. The hematologic status of the patient must first be determined. It is essential to understand the hazards and therapeutic effects to be expected. Careful clinical judgment must be exercised in selecting patients. If the indication for its use is not clear, the drug should not be used.*
As nitrogen mustard therapy may contribute to extensive and rapid development of amyloidosis, it should be used only if foci of acute and chronic suppurative inflammation are absent.
Usage in Pregnancy
Mechlorethamine hydrochloride can cause fetal harm when administered to a pregnant woman. MUSTARGEN has been shown to produce fetal malformations in the rat and ferret when given as single subcutaneous injections of 1 mg/kg (2–3 times the maximum recommended human dose). There are no adequate and well controlled studies in pregnant women. If this drug is used during pregnancy, or if the patient becomes pregnant while taking this drug, the patient should be apprised of the potential hazard to the fetus. Women of childbearing potential should be advised to avoid becoming pregnant.

PRECAUTIONS

General
This drug is highly toxic and both powder and solution must be handled and administered with care. Since MUSTARGEN is a powerful vesicant, it is intended primarily for intravenous use, and in most instances is given by this route. Inhalation of dust or vapors and contact with skin or mucous membranes, especially those of the eyes, must be avoided. Rubber gloves should be worn when handling MUSTARGEN. (See DOSAGE AND ADMINISTRATION and HOW SUPPLIED, *Special Handling.*)
Because of the toxicity of MUSTARGEN, and the unpleasant side effects following its use, the potential risk and discomfort from the use of this drug in patients with inoperable neoplasms or in the terminal stage of the disease must be balanced against the limited gain obtainable. These gains will vary with the nature and the status of the disease under treatment. The routine use of MUSTARGEN in all cases of widely disseminated neoplasms is to be discouraged.
The use of MUSTARGEN in patients with leukopenia, thrombocytopenia, and anemia, due to invasion of the bone marrow by tumor carries a greater risk. In such patients a good response to treatment with disappearance of the tumor from the bone marrow may be associated with improvement of bone marrow function. However, in the absence of a good response or in patients who have been previously treated with chemotherapeutic agents, hematopoiesis may be further compromised, and leukopenia, thrombocytopenia and anemia may become more severe and lead to the demise of the patient.
Tumors of bone and nervous tissue have responded poorly to therapy. Results are unpredictable in disseminated and malignant tumors of different types.
Precautions must be observed with the use of MUSTARGEN and x-ray therapy or other chemotherapy in alternating courses. Hematopoietic function is characteristically depressed by either form of therapy, and neither MUSTARGEN following x-ray therapy nor x-ray therapy subsequent to the drug should be given until bone marrow function has recovered. In particular, irradiation of such areas as sternum, ribs, and vertebrae shortly after a course of nitrogen mustard may lead to hematologic complications.
MUSTARGEN has been reported to have immunosuppressive activity. Therefore, it should be borne in mind that use of the drug may predispose the patient to bacterial, viral or fungal infection.
Hyperuricemia may develop during therapy with MUSTARGEN. The problem of urate precipitation should be anticipated, particularly in the treatment of the lymphomas, and adequate methods for control of hyperuricemia should be instituted and careful attention directed toward adequate fluid intake before treatment.
Since drug toxicity, especially sensitivity to bone marrow failure, seems to be more common in chronic lymphatic leukemia than in other conditions, the drug should be given in this condition with great caution, if at all.
Extreme caution must be used in exceeding the average recommended dose. (See OVERDOSAGE.)

Laboratory Tests
Many abnormalities of renal, hepatic, and bone marrow function have been reported in patients with neoplastic disease and receiving mechlorethamine. It is advisable to check renal, hepatic, and bone marrow functions frequently.
Carcinogenesis, Mutagenesis, Impairment of Fertility
Therapy with alkylating agents such as MUSTARGEN may be associated with an increased incidence of a second malignant tumor, especially when such therapy is combined with other antineoplastic agents or radiation therapy.
Young-adult female RF mice were injected intravenously with four doses of 2.4 mg/kg of mechlorethamine (0.1% solution) at 2-week intervals with observations for up to 2 years. An increased incidence of thymic lymphomas and pulmonary adenomas was observed. Painting mechlorethamine on the skin of mice for periods up to 33 weeks resulted in squamous cell tumors in 9 of 33 mice.
Mechlorethamine induced mutations in the Ames test, in *E. coli*, and *Neurospora crassa*. Mechlorethamine caused chromosome aberrations in a variety of plant and mammalian cells. Dominant lethal mutations were produced in ICR/Ha Swiss mice.
Mechlorethamine impaired fertility in the rat at a daily dose of 500 mg/kg intravenously for two weeks.
Pregnancy
Pregnancy Category D. See WARNINGS.
Nursing Mothers
It is not known whether this drug is excreted in human milk. Because many drugs are excreted in human milk and because of the potential for serious adverse reactions in nursing infants from MUSTARGEN, a decision should be made whether to discontinue nursing or to discontinue the drug, taking into account the importance of the drug to the mother.
Pediatric Use
Safety and effectiveness in children have not been established by well-controlled studies. Use of MUSTARGEN in children has been quite limited. MUSTARGEN has been used in Hodgkin's disease, stages III and IV, in combination with other oncolytic agents (MOPP schedule). The MOPP chemotherapy combination includes mechlorethamine, vincristine, procarbazine, and prednisone or prednisolone.

ADVERSE REACTIONS

Clinical use of MUSTARGEN *usually is accompanied by toxic manifestations.*
Local Toxicity
Thrombosis and thrombophlebitis may result from direct contact of the drug with the intima of the injected vein. Avoid high concentration and prolonged contact with the drug, especially in cases of elevated pressure in the antebrachial vein (e.g., in mediastinal tumor compression from severe vena cava syndrome).
Systemic Toxicity
General: Hypersensitivity reactions, including anaphylaxis, have been reported. Nausea, vomiting and depression of formed elements in the circulating blood are dose-limiting side effects and usually occur with the use of full doses of MUSTARGEN. Jaundice, alopecia, vertigo, tinnitus and diminished hearing may occur infrequently. Rarely, hemolytic anemia associated with such diseases as the lymphomas and chronic lymphocytic leukemia may be precipitated by treatment with alkylating agents including MUSTARGEN. Also, various chromosomal abnormalities have been reported in association with nitrogen mustard therapy.
MUSTARGEN is given preferably at night in case sedation for side effects is required. Nausea and vomiting usually occur 1 to 3 hours after use of the drug. Emesis may disappear in the first 8 hours, but nausea may persist for 24 hours. Nausea and vomiting may be so severe as to precipitate vascular accidents in patients with a hemorrhagic tendency. Premedication with antiemetics, in addition to sedatives, may help control severe nausea and vomiting. Anorexia, weakness and diarrhea may also occur.
Hematologic: The usual course of MUSTARGEN (total dose of 0.4 mg/kg either given as a single intravenous dose or divided into two or four daily doses of 0.2 or 0.1 mg/kg respectively) generally produces a lymphocytopenia within 24 hours after the first injection; significant granulocytopenia occurs within 6 to 8 days and lasts for 10 days to 3 weeks. Agranulocytosis appears to be relatively infrequent and recovery from leukopenia in most cases is complete within two weeks of the maximum reduction. Thrombocytopenia is variable but the time course of the appearance and recovery from reduced platelet counts generally parallels the sequence of granulocyte levels. In some cases severe thrombocytopenia may lead to bleeding from the gums and gastrointestinal tract, petechiae, and small subcutaneous hemorrhages; these symptoms appear to be transient and in most cases disappear with return to a normal platelet count. However, a severe and even uncontrollable depression of the hematopoietic system occasionally may follow the usual dose of MUSTARGEN, particularly in patients with widespread disease and debility and in patients previously treated with other antineoplastic agents or x-ray. Persistent pancytopenia has been reported. In rare instances, hemorrhagic complications may be due to hyperheparinemia. Erythrocyte and hemoglobin levels may decline during the first 2 weeks after therapy but rarely significantly. Depression of the hematopoietic system may be found up to 50 days or more after starting therapy.
Integumentary: Occasionally, a maculopapular skin eruption occurs, but this may be idiosyncratic and does not necessarily recur with subsequent courses of the drug. Erythema multiforme has been observed. Herpes zoster, a common complicating infection in patients with lymphomas, may first appear after therapy is instituted and on occasion may be precipitated by treatment. Further treatment should be discontinued during the acute phase of this illness to avoid progression to generalized herpes zoster.
Reproductive: Since the gonads are susceptible to MUSTARGEN, treatment may be followed by delayed catamenia, oligomenorrhea, or temporary or permanent amenorrhea. Impaired spermatogenesis, azoospermia, and total germinal aplasia have been reported in male patients treated with alkylating agents, especially in combination with other drugs. In some instances spermatogenesis may return in patients in remission, but this may occur only several years after intensive chemotherapy has been discontinued. Patients should be warned of the potential risk to their reproductive capacity.

OVERDOSAGE

With total doses exceeding 0.4 mg/kg of body weight for a single course, severe leukopenia, anemia, thrombocytopenia and a hemorrhagic diathesis with subsequent delayed bleeding may develop. Death may follow. The only treatment in instances of excessive dosage appears to be repeated blood product transfusions, antibiotic treatment of complicating infections and general supportive measures.
The intravenous LD_{50} of MUSTARGEN is 2 mg/kg and 1.6 mg/kg in the mouse and rat, respectively.

DOSAGE AND ADMINISTRATION

Intravenous Administration
The dosage of MUSTARGEN varies with the clinical situation, the therapeutic response and the magnitude of hematologic depression. A total dose of 0.4 mg/kg of body weight for each course usually is given either as a single dose or in divided doses of 0.1 to 0.2 mg/kg per day. Dosage should be based on ideal dry body weight. The presence of edema or ascites must be considered so that dosage will be based on actual weight unaugmented by these conditions.
The margin of safety in therapy with MUSTARGEN *is narrow and considerable care must be exercised in the matter of dosage.* Repeated examinations of blood are *mandatory* as a guide to subsequent therapy. (See OVERDOSAGE.)
Within a few minutes after intravenous injection, MUSTARGEN undergoes chemical transformation, combines with reactive compounds, and is no longer present in its active form in the blood stream. Subsequent courses should not be given until the patient has recovered hematologically from the previous course; this is best determined by repeated studies of the peripheral blood elements awaiting their return to normal levels. It is often possible to give repeated courses of MUSTARGEN as early as three weeks after treatment.
Preparation of Solution for Intravenous Administration
This drug is highly toxic and both powder and solution must be handled and administered with care. Since MUSTARGEN is a powerful vesicant, it is intended primarily for intravenous use, and in most instances is given by this route. Inhalation of dust or vapors and contact with skin or mucous membranes, especially those of the eyes, must be avoided. Rubber gloves should be worn when handling MUSTARGEN. Should accidental eye contact occur, copious irrigation with water, normal saline or a balanced salt ophthalmic irrigating solution should be instituted immediately, followed by prompt ophthalmologic consultation. Should accidental skin contact occur, the affected part must be irrigated immediately with copious amounts of water, for at least 15 minutes, followed by 2 percent sodium thiosulfate solution. (See also box warning and *Special Handling.*)
Each vial of MUSTARGEN contains 10 mg of mechlorethamine hydrochloride triturated with sodium chloride q.s. 100 mg. In neutral or alkaline aqueous solution it undergoes rapid chemical transformation and is highly unstable. Although solutions prepared according to instructions are acidic and do not decompose as rapidly, they should be prepared immediately before each injection since they will decompose on standing. When reconstituted, MUSTARGEN is a clear colorless solution. *Do not use if the solution is discolored or if droplets of water are visible within the vial prior to reconstitution.*
Using a sterile 10 mL syringe, inject 10 mL of Sterile Water for Injection or 10 mL Sodium Chloride Injection into a vial of MUSTARGEN. With the needle (syringe attached) still in the rubber stopper, shake the vial several times to dissolve the drug completely. The resultant solution contains 1 mg of mechlorethamine hydrochloride per mL.
Parenteral drug products should be inspected visually for particulate matter and discoloration prior to administration whenever solution and container permit.
Special Handling
Due to the drug's toxic and mutagenic properties, appropriate precautions including the use of appropriate safety equipment are recommended for the preparation of MUSTARGEN for parenteral administration. The National Institutes of Health presently recommends that the preparation of injectable anti-neoplastic drugs should be performed in a Class II laminar flow biological safety cabinet and that personnel preparing drugs of this class should wear surgical gloves and a closed front surgical-type gown with knit cuffs. Several other guidelines for proper handling and disposal of anti-cancer drugs have been published and should be considered. There is no general agreement that all of the procedures recommended in the guidelines are necessary or appropriate.
Accidental contact: Should accidental eye contact occur, copious irrigation with water, normal saline or a balanced salt ophthalmic irrigating solution should be instituted immediately, followed by prompt ophthalmologic consultation. Should accidental skin contact occur, the affected part must be irrigated immediately with copious amounts of water, for at least 15 minutes, followed by 2 percent sodium thiosulfate solution. (See also box warning.)
Technique for Intravenous Administration
Withdraw into the syringe the calculated volume of solution required for a single injection. *Dispose of any remaining solution after neutralization* (see below). Although the drug may be injected directly into any suitable vein, it is injected preferably into the rubber or plastic tubing of a flowing intravenous infusion set. This reduces the possibility of severe local reactions due to extravasation or high concentration of the drug. Injecting the drug into the tubing rather than adding it to the entire volume of the infusion fluid minimizes a chemical reaction between the drug and the solution. The rate of injection apparently is not critical provided it is completed within a few minutes.
Intracavitary Administration
Nitrogen mustard has been used by intracavitary administration with varying success in certain malignant conditions for the control of pleural, peritoneal, and pericardial effusions caused by malignant cells.
The technic and the dose used by any of these routes varies. Therefore, if MUSTARGEN is given by the intracavitary route, the published articles concerning such use should be consulted. *Because of the inherent risks involved, the physician should be experienced in the appropriate injection technics, and be thoroughly aware of the indications, dosages, hazards, and precautions as set forth in the published literature. When using* MUSTARGEN *by the intracavitary route, the general precautions concerning this agent should be borne in mind.*
As a general guide, reference is made especially to the technics of Weisberger et al. Intracavitary use is indicated in the presence of pleural, peritoneal, or pericardial effusion due to metastatic tumors. Local therapy with nitrogen mustard is used only when malignant cells are demonstrated in the effusion. Intracavitary injection is not recommended when the accumulated fluid is chylous in nature, since results are likely to be poor.
Paracentesis is first performed with most of the fluid being removed from the pleural or peritoneal cavity. The intracavitary use of MUSTARGEN may exert at least some of its effect through production of a chemical poudrage. Therefore, the removal of excess fluid allows the drug to more easily contact the peritoneal and pleural linings. For intrapleural or intrapericardial injection nitrogen mustard is introduced directly through the thoracentesis needle. For intraperitoneal injection it is given through a rubber catheter inserted into the trocar used for paracentesis or through a No. 18 gauge needle inserted at another site. This drug should be injected slowly, with frequent aspiration to ensure that a free flow of fluid is present. If fluid cannot be aspirated, pain and necrosis due to injection of solution outside the cavity may occur. Free flow of fluid also is necessary to prevent injection into a loculated pocket and to ensure adequate dissemination of nitrogen mustard.
The usual dose of nitrogen mustard for intracavitary injection is 0.4 mg/kg of body weight, though 0.2 mg/kg (or 10 to 20 mg) has been used by the intrapericardial route. The solution is prepared, as previously described for intravenous injection, by adding 10 mL of Sterile Water for Injection or 10 mL of Sodium Chloride Injection to the vial containing 10 mg of mechlorethamine hydrochloride. (Amounts of diluent

Continued on next page

Information on the Merck & Co., Inc. products listed on these pages is the full prescribing information from product circulars in use September 30, 1996.

Merck & Co.—Cont.

of 50 to 100 mL of normal saline have also been used.) The position of the patient should be changed every 5 to 10 minutes for an hour after injection to obtain more uniform distribution of the drug throughout the serous cavity. The remaining fluid may be removed from the pleural or peritoneal cavity by paracentesis 24 to 36 hours later. The patient should be followed carefully by clinical and x-ray examination to detect reaccumulation of fluid.
Pain occurs rarely with intrapleural use; it is common with intraperitoneal injection and is often associated with nausea, vomiting, and diarrhea of 2 to 3 days duration. Transient cardiac irregularities may occur with intrapericardial injection. Death, possibly accelerated by nitrogen mustard, has been reported following the use of this agent by the intracavitary route. Although absorption of MUSTARGEN when given by the intracavitary route is probably not complete because of its rapid deactivation by body fluids, the systemic effect is unpredictable. The acute side effects such as nausea and vomiting are usually mild. Bone marrow depression is generally milder than when the drug is given intravenously. Care should be taken to avoid use by the intracavitary route when other agents which may suppress bone marrow function are being used systemically.
Neutralization of Equipment and Unused Solution
To clean rubber gloves, tubing, glassware, etc., after giving MUSTARGEN, soak them in an aqueous solution containing equal volumes of sodium thiosulfate (5%) and sodium bicarbonate (5%) for 45 minutes. Excess reagents and reaction products are washed away easily with water. Any unused injection solution should be neutralized by mixing with an equal volume of sodium thiosulfate/sodium bicarbonate solution. Allow the mixture to stand for 45 minutes. Vials that have contained MUSTARGEN should be treated in the same way with thiosulfate/bicarbonate solution before disposal.

HOW SUPPLIED

No. 7753—Trituration of MUSTARGEN is a light yellow brown crystalline powder, each vial containing 10 mg mechlorethamine hydrochloride with sodium chloride q.s. 100 mg, and is supplied as follows:
NDC 0006-7753-31 in treatment sets of 4 vials.
Storage
Store at controlled room temperature 15–30°C (59–86°F). Protect from light and humidity. Solutions of mechlorethamine HCl decompose on standing; therefore, solutions of the drug should be prepared immediately before use.
7417930 Issued September 1994
COPYRIGHT © MERCK & CO., INC., 1985
All rights reserved

MYOCHRYSINE® Injection
(Gold Sodium Thiomalate), U.S.P. ℞

Physicians planning to use MYOCHRYSINE* *(Gold Sodium Thiomalate) should thoroughly familiarize themselves with its toxicity and its benefits. The possibility of toxic reactions should always be explained to the patient before starting therapy. Patients should be warned to report promptly any symptoms suggesting toxicity. Before each injection of* MYOCHRYSINE, *the physician should review the results of laboratory work, and see the patient to determine the presence or absence of adverse reactions since some of these can be severe or even fatal.*

*Registered trademark of MERCK & CO., INC.

DESCRIPTION

MYOCHRYSINE is a sterile aqueous solution of gold sodium thiomalate. It contains 0.5 percent benzyl alcohol added as a preservative. The pH of the product is 5.8–6.5.
Gold sodium thiomalate is a mixture of the mono- and disodium salts of gold thiomalic acid. The structural formula is:

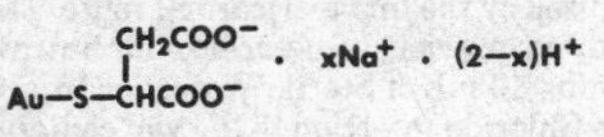
CH2COO⁻ · xNa+ · (2−x)H+
Au—S—CHCOO⁻

mercaptobutanedioic acid, monogold (1+) sodium salt

The molecular weight for $C_4H_3AuNa_2O_4S$ (the disodium salt) is 390.07 and for $C_4H_4AuNaO_4S$ (the monosodium salt) is 368.09.
MYOCHRYSINE is supplied as a solution for intramuscular injection containing 50 mg of gold sodium thiomalate per mL.

CLINICAL PHARMACOLOGY

The mode of action of gold sodium thiomalate is unknown. The predominant action appears to be a suppressive effect on the synovitis of active rheumatoid disease.

INDICATIONS AND USAGE

MYOCHRYSINE is indicated in the treatment of selected cases of active rheumatoid arthritis— both adult and juvenile type. The greatest benefit occurs in the early active stage. In late stages of the illness when cartilage and bone damage have occurred, gold can only check the progression of rheumatoid arthritis and prevent further structural damage to joints. It cannot repair damage caused by previously active disease.
MYOCHRYSINE should be used only as *one part* of a complete program of therapy; alone it is not a complete treatment.

CONTRAINDICATIONS

Hypersensitivity to any component of this product.
Severe toxicity resulting from previous exposure to gold or other heavy metals.
Severe debilitation.
Systemic lupus erythematosus.

WARNINGS

Before treatment is started, the patient's hemoglobin, erythrocyte, white blood cell, differential and platelet counts should be determined, and urinalysis should be done to serve as basic reference. Urine should be analyzed for protein and sediment changes prior to each injection. Complete blood counts including platelet estimation should be made before every second injection throughout treatment. The occurrence of purpura or ecchymoses at any time always requires a platelet count.
Danger signals of possible gold toxicity include: rapid reduction of hemoglobin, leukopenia below 4000 WBC/mm^3, eosinophilia above 5 percent, platelet decrease below 100,000/mm^3, albuminuria, hematuria, pruritus, skin eruption, stomatitis, or persistent diarrhea. No additional injections of MYOCHRYSINE should be given unless further studies show these abnormalities to be caused by conditions other than gold toxicity.

PRECAUTIONS

General
Gold salts should not be used concomitantly with penicillamine.
The safety of coadministration with cytotoxic drugs has not been established.
Caution is indicated in the use of MYOCHRYSINE in patients with the following:
1. a history of blood dyscrasias such as granulocytopenia or anemia caused by drug sensitivity,
2. allergy or hypersensitivity to medications,
3. skin rash,
4. previous kidney or liver disease,
5. marked hypertension,
6. compromised cerebral or cardiovascular circulation.

Diabetes mellitus or congestive heart failure should be under control before gold therapy is instituted.
Carcinogenicity
Renal adenomas have been reported in long-term toxicity studies of rats receiving MYOCHRYSINE at high dose levels (2 mg/kg weekly for 45 weeks, followed by 6 mg/kg daily for 47 weeks), approximately 2 to 42 times the usual human dose. These adenomas are histologically similar to those produced in rats by chronic administration of experimental gold compounds and other heavy metals, such as lead. No reports have been received of renal adenomas in man in association with the use of MYOCHRYSINE.
Pregnancy
Pregnancy Category C.
MYOCHRYSINE has been shown to be teratogenic during the organogenetic period in rats and rabbits when given in doses, respectively, of 140 and 175 times the usual human dose. Hydrocephaly and microphthalmia were the malformations observed in rats when MYOCHRYSINE was administered subcutaneously at a dose of 25 mg/kg/day from day 6 through day 15 of gestation. In rabbits, limb malformations and gastroschisis were the malformations observed when MYOCHRYSINE was administered subcutaneously at doses of 20–45 mg/kg/day from day 6 through day 18 of gestation. There are no adequate and well-controlled studies in pregnant women. MYOCHRYSINE should be used during pregnancy only if the potential benefit to the mother justifies the potential risk to the fetus.
Nursing Mothers
The presence of gold has been demonstrated in the milk of lactating mothers. In addition, gold has been found in the serum and red blood cells of a nursing infant. In view of the above findings and because of the potential for serious adverse reactions in nursing infants from MYOCHRYSINE, a decision should be made whether to discontinue nursing or to discontinue the drug, taking into account the importance of the drug to the mother. The slow excretion and persistence of gold in the mother, even after therapy is discontinued, must also be kept in mind.

ADVERSE REACTIONS

A variety of adverse reactions may develop during the initial phase (weekly injections) of therapy or during maintenance treatment. Adverse reactions are observed most frequently when the cumulative dose of MYOCHRYSINE administered is between 400 and 800 mg. Very uncommonly, complications occur days to months after cessation of treatment.
Cutaneous reactions: Dermatitis is the most common reaction. *Any eruption, especially if pruritic, that develops during treatment with* MYOCHRYSINE *should be considered a reaction to gold until proven otherwise.* Pruritus often exists before dermatitis becomes apparent, and therefore should be considered a warning signal of impending cutaneous reaction. The most serious form of cutaneous reaction is generalized exfoliative dermatitis which may lead to alopecia and shedding of nails. Gold dermatitis may be aggravated by exposure to sunlight or an actinic rash may develop.
Mucous membrane reactions: Stomatitis is the second most common adverse reaction. Shallow ulcers on the buccal membranes, on the borders of the tongue, and on the palate or in the pharynx may occur as the only adverse reaction, or along with dermatitis. Sometimes diffuse glossitis or gingivitis develops. A metallic taste may precede these oral mucous membrane reactions and should be considered a warning signal.
Conjunctivitis is a rare reaction.
Renal reactions: Gold may be toxic to the kidney and produce a nephrotic syndrome or glomerulitis with hematuria. These renal reactions are usually relatively mild and subside completely if recognized early and treatment is discontinued. They may become severe and chronic if treatment is continued after onset of the reaction. Therefore, it is important to perform a *urinalysis before every injection,* and to discontinue treatment promptly if proteinuria or hematuria develops.
Hematologic reactions: Blood dyscrasia due to gold toxicity is rare, but because of the potential serious consequences it must be constantly watched for and recognized early by frequent blood examinations done throughout treatment. Granulocytopenia; thrombocytopenia, with or without purpura; hypoplastic and aplastic anemia; and eosinophilia have all been reported. These hematologic disorders may occur separately or in combinations.
Nitritoid and allergic reactions: Reactions of the "nitritoid type" which may resemble anaphylactoid effects have been reported. Flushing, fainting, dizziness and sweating are most frequently reported. Other symptoms that may occur include: nausea, vomiting, malaise, headache, and weakness. More severe, but less common effects include: anaphylactic shock, syncope, bradycardia, thickening of the tongue, difficulty in swallowing and breathing, and angioneurotic edema. These effects may occur almost immediately after injection or as late as 10 minutes following injection. They may occur at any time during the course of therapy and if observed, treatment with MYOCHRYSINE should be discontinued.
Miscellaneous reactions: Gastrointestinal reactions have been reported, including nausea, vomiting, anorexia, abdominal cramps and diarrhea. Ulcerative enterocolitis, which can be severe or even fatal, has been reported rarely.
There have been rare reports of reactions involving the eye such as iritis, corneal ulcers, and gold deposits in ocular tissues. Peripheral and central nervous system complications have been reported rarely. Peripheral neuropathy, with or without fasciculations, sensorimotor effects (including Guillain-Barré syndrome) and elevated spinal fluid protein have been reported. Central nervous system complications have included confusion, hallucinations and seizures. Usually these signs and symptoms cleared upon discontinuation of gold therapy.
Hepatitis, jaundice, with or without cholestasis, gold bronchitis, pulmonary injury manifested by interstitial pneumonitis and fibrosis, partial or complete hair loss and fever have also been reported.
Sometimes arthralgia occurs for a day or two after an injection of MYOCHRYSINE; this reaction usually subsides after the first few injections.

MANAGEMENT OF ADVERSE REACTIONS

Treatment with MYOCHRYSINE should be discontinued immediately when toxic reactions occur. Minor complications such as localized dermatitis, mild stomatitis, or slight proteinuria generally require no other therapy and resolve spontaneously with suspension of MYOCHRYSINE. Moderately severe skin and mucous membrane reactions often

benefit from topical corticosteroids, oral antihistaminics, and soothing or anesthetic lotions.

If stomatitis or dermatitis becomes severe or more generalized, systemic corticosteroids (generally, prednisone 10 to 40 mg daily in divided doses) may provide symptomatic relief. For serious renal, hematologic, pulmonary, and enterocolitic complications, high doses of systemic corticosteroids (prednisone 40 to 100 mg daily in divided doses) are recommended. The optimum duration of corticosteroid treatment varies with the response of the individual patient. Therapy may be required for many months when adverse effects are unusually severe or progressive.

In patients whose complications do not improve with high-dose corticosteroid treatment, or who develop significant steroid-related adverse reactions, a chelating agent may be given to enhance gold excretion. Dimercaprol (BAL) has been used successfully, but patients must be monitored carefully as numerous untoward reactions may attend its use. Corticosteroids and a chelating agent may be used concomitantly.

MYOCHRYSINE *should not be reinstituted after severe or idiosyncratic reactions.*

MYOCHRYSINE may be readministered following resolution of mild reactions, using a reduced dosage schedule. If an initial test dose of 5 mg MYOCHRYSINE is well-tolerated, progressively larger doses (5 to 10 mg increments) may be given at weekly to monthly intervals until a dose of 25 to 50 mg is reached.

DOSAGE AND ADMINISTRATION

MYOCHRYSINE should be administered only by intramuscular injection, preferably intragluteally. It should be given with the patient lying down. He should remain recumbent for approximately 10 minutes after the injection.

Therapeutic effects from MYOCHRYSINE occur slowly. Early improvement, often limited to a reduction in morning stiffness, may begin after six to eight weeks of treatment, but beneficial effects may not be observed until after months of therapy.

Parenteral drug products should be inspected visually for particulate matter and discoloration prior to administration. Do not use if material has darkened. Color should not exceed pale yellow.

For the adult of average size the following dosage schedule is suggested:

Weekly Injections

1st injection	10 mg
2nd injection	25 mg

3rd and subsequent injections, 25 to 50 mg until there is toxicity or major clinical improvement, or, in the absence of either of these, the cumulative dose of MYOCHRYSINE reaches one gram.

MYOCHRYSINE is continued until the cumulative dose reaches one gram unless toxicity or major clinical improvement occurs. If significant clinical improvement occurs before a cumulative dose of one gram has been administered, the dose may be decreased or the interval between injections increased as with maintenance therapy. Maintenance doses of 25 to 50 mg every other week for two to 20 weeks are recommended. If the clinical course remains stable, injections of 25 to 50 mg may be given every third and subsequently every fourth week indefinitely. Some patients may require maintenance treatment at intervals of one to three weeks. Should the arthritis exacerbate during maintenance therapy, weekly injections may be resumed temporarily until disease activity is suppressed.

Should a patient fail to improve during initial therapy (cumulative dose of one gram), several options are available:

1— the patient may be considered to be unresponsive and MYOCHRYSINE is discontinued
2— the same dose (25 to 50 mg) of MYOCHRYSINE may be continued for approximately ten additional weeks
3— the dose of MYOCHRYSINE may be increased by increments of 10 mg every one to four weeks, not to exceed 100 mg in a single injection.

If significant clinical improvement occurs using option 2 or 3, the maintenance schedule described above should be initiated. If there is no significant improvement or if toxicity occurs, therapy with MYOCHRYSINE should be stopped. The higher the individual dose of MYOCHRYSINE, the greater the risk of gold toxicity. Selection of one of these options for chrysotherapy should be based upon a number of factors, including the physician's experience with gold salt therapy, the course of the patient's condition, the choice of alternative treatments, and the availability of the patient for the close supervision required.

Juvenile Rheumatoid Arthritis

The pediatric dose of MYOCHRYSINE is proportional to the adult dose on a weight basis. After the initial test dose of 10 mg, the recommended dose for children is one mg per kilogram body weight, not to exceed 50 mg for a single injection. Otherwise, the guidelines given above for administration to adults also apply to children.

Concomitant Drug Therapy —Gold salts should not be used concomitantly with penicillamine.

The safety of coadministration with cytotoxic drugs has not been established. Other measures, such as salicylates, other non-steroidal anti-inflammatory drugs, or systemic corticosteroids, may be continued when MYOCHRYSINE is initiated. After improvement commences, analgesic and anti-inflammatory drugs may be discontinued slowly as symptoms permit.

HOW SUPPLIED

Injection MYOCHRYSINE is a light yellow to yellow solution which must be protected from light. It is supplied as follows:

No. 7762—50 mg of gold sodium thiomalate per mL as
NDC 0006-7762-64 in boxes of 6 x 1 mL ampuls
NDC 0006-7762-10 in 10 mL vials
(6505-00-973-8579, 10 mL vial).

Storage
Protect from light.
Store container in carton until contents have been used.

7594528   Issued April 1994
COPYRIGHT © MERCK & CO., INC., 1985

NEODECADRON® ℞
Sterile Ophthalmic Ointment
(Neomycin Sulfate-Dexamethasone
Sodium Phosphate), U.S.P.

DESCRIPTION

Sterile Ophthalmic Ointment NEODECADRON* (Neomycin Sulfate-Dexamethasone Sodium Phosphate) is a topical corticosteroid-antibiotic ointment for ophthalmic use.

Dexamethasone sodium phosphate is 9-fluoro-11β, 17-dihydroxy-16α-methyl-21-(phosphonooxy)pregna-1, 4-diene-3, 20-dione disodium salt. Its empirical formula is $C_{22}H_{28}FNa_2O_8P$ and its structural formula is:

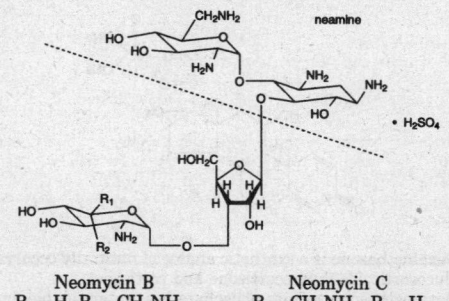

Dexamethasone is a synthetic analog of naturally occurring glucocorticoids (hydrocortisone and cortisone).

Dexamethasone sodium phosphate is a water soluble, inorganic ester of dexamethasone. Its molecular weight is 516.41. Neomycin sulfate, an antibiotic of the aminoglycoside group, is a mixture of the sulfate salts of neomycin, produced by the growth of *Streptomyces fradiae* Waksman (Fam. Streptomycetaceae). Neomycin is a complex typically containing 8–13% neomycin C, less than 0.2% neomycin A, and the rest, neomycin B. The empirical formula for both neomycin B and neomycin C is $C_{23}H_{46}N_6O_{13}$, and the molecular weight for each is 614.65. Neomycin A (also referred to as neamine) has an empirical formula of $C_{12}H_{26}N_4O_6$ and a molecular weight of 322.36. The structural formulae for neomycin sulfate are:

neamine

Neomycin B
R_1=H, R_2=CH_2NH_2

Neomycin C
R_1=CH_2NH_2, R_2=H

$\cdot H_2SO_4$

Ophthalmic Ointment NEODECADRON contains in each gram: dexamethasone sodium phosphate equivalent to 0.5 mg (0.05%) dexamethasone phosphate and neomycin sulfate equivalent to 3.5 mg neomycin base. Inactive ingredients: white petrolatum and mineral oil.

---

*Registered trademark of MERCK & CO., INC.

CLINICAL PHARMACOLOGY

Corticosteroids suppress the inflammatory response to a variety of agents, and they probably delay or slow healing. Since corticosteroids may inhibit the body's defense mechanism against infection, a concomitant antimicrobial drug may be used when this inhibition is considered to be clinically significant in a particular case.

When a decision to administer both a corticosteroid and an antimicrobial is made, the administration of such drugs in combination has the advantage of greater patient compliance and convenience, with the added assurance that the appropriate dosage of both drugs is administered, plus assured compatibility of ingredients when both types of drug are in the same formulation and, particularly, that the correct volume of drug is delivered and retained.

The relative potency of corticosteroids depends on the molecular structure, concentration, and release from the vehicle.

Microbiology

The anti-infective component in Ophthalmic Ointment NEODECADRON is included to provide action against specific organisms susceptible to it. Neomycin sulfate is active *in vitro* against susceptible strains of the following microorganisms: *Staphylococcus aureus, Escherichia coli, Haemophilus influenzae, Klebsiella/Enterobacter* species, and *Neisseria* species. The product does not provide adequate coverage against: *Pseudomonas aeruginosa, Serratia marcescens,* and streptococci, including *Streptococcus pneumoniae.* (See INDICATIONS AND USAGE.)

INDICATIONS AND USAGE

For steroid-responsive inflammatory ocular conditions for which a corticosteroid is indicated and where bacterial infection or a risk of bacterial ocular infection exists.

Ocular steroids are indicated in inflammatory conditions of the palpebral and bulbar conjunctiva, cornea, and anterior segment of the globe where the inherent risk of steroid use in certain infective conjunctivities is accepted to obtain a diminution in edema and inflammation. They are also indicated in chronic anterior uveitis and corneal injury from chemical, radiation, or thermal burns, or penetration of foreign bodies. The use of a combination drug with an anti-infective component is indicated where the risk of infection is high or where there is an expectation that potentially dangerous numbers of bacteria will be present in the eye.

The particular anti-infective drug in this product is active against the following common bacterial eye pathogens:

Staphylococcus aureus
Escherichia coli
Haemophilus influenzae
Klebsiella/Enterobacter species
Neisseria species

The product does not provide adequate coverage against:

Pseudomonas aeruginosa
Serratia marcescens
Streptococci, including *Streptococcus pneumoniae*

CONTRAINDICATIONS

NEODECADRON is contraindicated in most viral diseases of the cornea and conjunctiva including epithelial herpes simplex keratitis (dendritic keratitis), vaccinia varicella, and also in mycobacterial infection of the eye and fungal diseases of ocular structures. NEODECADRON is also contraindicated in individuals with known or suspected hypersensitivity to any of the ingredients of this preparation and to other corticosteroids (see WARNINGS). Hypersensitivity to the antibiotic component occurs at a higher rate than for other components.

WARNINGS

NOT FOR INJECTION INTO THE EYE

Prolonged use of corticosteroids may result in ocular hypertension and/or glaucoma with damage to the optic nerve, defects in visual acuity and fields of vision, and in posterior subcapsular cataract formation.

Prolonged use of corticosteroids may suppress the host response and thus increase the hazard of secondary ocular infections. In those diseases causing thinning of the cornea or sclera, perforations have been known to occur with the use of topical corticosteroids. In acute purulent conditions of the eye, corticosteroids may mask infection or enhance existing infection.

Continued on next page

Merck & Co.—Cont.

If this product is used for 10 days or longer, intraocular pressure should be routinely monitored even though it may be difficult in children and uncooperative patients. Corticosteroids should be used with caution in the presence of ocular hypertension and/or glaucoma. Intraocular pressure should be checked frequently.

The use of corticosteroids after cataract surgery may delay healing and increase the incidence of filtering blebs.

Use of ocular corticosteroids may prolong the course and may exacerbate the severity of many viral infections of the eye (including herpes simplex). Employment of a corticosteroid medication in the treatment of patients with a history of herpes simplex requires great caution; periodic slit lamp microscopy is essential. (See CONTRAINDICATIONS.)

Neomycin sulfate may occasionally cause cutaneous sensitization. If any reaction indicating such sensitivity is observed, discontinue use.

PRECAUTIONS

General
The initial prescription and renewal of the medication order beyond 8 grams should be made by a physician only after examination of the patient with the aid of magnification, such as slit-lamp biomicroscopy and, where appropriate, fluorescein staining. If signs and symptoms fail to improve after two days, the patient should be re-evaluated.

The possibility of fungal infections of the cornea should be considered after prolonged corticosteroid dosing. Fungal cultures should be taken when appropriate.

If this product is used for 10 days or longer, intraocular pressure should be monitored (see WARNINGS).

There have been reports of bacterial keratitis associated with the use of multiple dose containers of topical ophthalmic products. These containers had been inadvertently contaminated by patients who, in most cases, had a concurrent corneal disease or a disruption of the ocular epithelial surface. (See PRECAUTIONS, *Information for Patients*.)

Information for Patients
Patients should be instructed to avoid allowing the tip of the dispensing container to contact the eye, eyelid, fingers, or any other surface. The use of this product by more than one person may spread infection. Keep tightly closed when not in use.

Patients should also be instructed that ocular preparations, if handled improperly, can become contaminated by common bacteria known to cause ocular infections. Serious damage to the eye and subsequent loss of vision may result from using contaminated preparations. (See PRECAUTIONS, *General*.)

If redness, irritation, swelling or pain persists or becomes aggravated, the patient should be advised to consult a physician. Patients should also be advised that if they have ocular surgery or develop an intercurrent ocular condition (e.g., trauma or infection), they should immediately seek their physician's advice.

Keep out of the reach of children.

Carcinogenesis, Mutagenesis, Impairment of Fertility
Long term animal studies have not been performed to evaluate the carcinogenic potential or the effect on fertility of Ophthalmic Ointment NEODECADRON. Treatment of human lymphocytes *in-vitro* with neomycin increased the frequency of chromosome aberrations at the highest concentration (80μg/mL) tested; however, the effects of neomycin on carcinogenesis and mutagenesis in humans are unknown.

Pregnancy
Teratogenic effects
Pregnancy Category C
Corticosteroids have been found to be teratogenic in animal studies. Ocular administration of 0.1% dexamethasone resulted in 15.6% and 32.3% incidence of fetal anomalies in two groups of pregnant rabbits. Fetal growth retardation and increased mortality rates have been observed in rats with chronic dexamethasone therapy. There are no adequate and well-controlled studies in pregnant women. Ophthalmic Ointment NEODECADRON should be used during pregnancy only if the potential benefit justifies the potential risk to the fetus. Infants born of mothers who have received substantial doses of corticosteroids during pregnancy should be observed carefully for signs of hypoadrenalism.

Nursing Mothers
It is not known whether topical administration of corticosteroids could result in sufficient systemic absorption to produce detectable quantities in human milk. Systemically-administered corticosteroids appear in human milk and could suppress growth, interfere with endogenous corticosteroid production, or cause other untoward effects. Because of the potential for serious adverse reactions in nursing infants from Ophthalmic Ointment NEODECADRON, a decision should be made whether to discontinue nursing or to discontinue the drug, taking into account the importance of the drug to the mother.

Pediatric Use
Safety and effectiveness in pediatric patients have not been established.

ADVERSE REACTIONS

Adverse reactions have occurred with corticosteroid/anti-infective combination drugs which can be attributed to the corticosteroid component, the anti-infective component, or the combination. Exact incidence figures are not available since no denominator of treated patients is available.

Reactions occurring most often from the presence of the anti-infective ingredient are allergic sensitizations. The reactions due to the corticosteroid component in decreasing order of frequency are: elevation of intraocular pressure (IOP) with possible development of glaucoma, and infrequent optic nerve damage; posterior subcapsular cataract formation; and delayed wound healing.

Secondary Infection: The development of secondary infection has occurred after use of combinations containing corticosteroids and antimicrobials. Fungal and viral infections of the cornea are particularly prone to develop coincidentally with long-term applications of a corticosteroid. The possibility of fungal invasion must be considered in any persistent corneal ulceration where corticosteroid treatment has been used.

DOSAGE AND ADMINISTRATION

NOT FOR INJECTION INTO THE EYE
The duration of treatment will vary with the type of lesion and may extend from a few days to several weeks, according to therapeutic response.

Apply a thin coating of Ophthalmic Ointment NEODECADRON three or four times a day. When a favorable response is observed, reduce the number of daily applications to two, and later to one a day as maintenance dose if this is sufficient to control symptoms.

Not more than 8 grams should be prescribed initially and the prescription should not be refilled without further evaluation as outlined in PRECAUTIONS above.

HOW SUPPLIED

No. 7617—Sterile Ophthalmic Ointment NEODECADRON is a clear, unctuous ointment, and is supplied as follows:
NDC 0006-7617-04 in 3.5 g tubes
(6505-00-982-0291 0.05% 3.5 g)
Storage
Store at controlled room temperature, 15°–30°C (59°–86°F).
7612628   Issued December 1995
COPYRIGHT © MERCK & CO., Inc., 1985, 1995

NEODECADRON®   ℞
Sterile Ophthalmic Solution
(Neomycin Sulfate-Dexamethasone
Sodium Phosphate), U.S.P.

DESCRIPTION

Ophthalmic Solution NEODECADRON* (Neomycin Sulfate-Dexamethasone Sodium Phosphate) is a topical corticosteroid-antibiotic solution for ophthalmic use.

Dexamethasone sodium phosphate is 9-fluoro-11β, 17-dihydroxy-16α-methyl-21-(phosphonooxy)pregna-1, 4-diene-3, 20-dione disodium salt. Its empirical formula is $C_{22}H_{28}FNa_2O_8P$ and its structural formula is:

Dexamethasone is a synthetic analog of naturally occurring glucocorticoids (hydrocortisone and cortisone).

Dexamethasone sodium phosphate is a water soluble, inorganic ester of dexamethasone. Its molecular weight is 516.41. Neomycin sulfate, an antibiotic of the aminoglucoside group, is a mixture of the sulfate salts of neomycin, produced by the growth of *Streptomyces fradiae* Waksman (Fam. Stretomycetaceae). Neomycin is a complex typically containing 8–13% neomycin C, less than 0.2% neomycin A, and the rest, neomycin B. The empirical formula for both neomycin B and neomycin C is $C_{23}H_{46}N_6O_{13}$, and the molecular weight for each is 614.65. Neomycin A (also referred to as neamine)

has an empirical formula of $C_{12}H_{26}N_4O_6$ and a molecular weight of 322.36. The structural formulae for neomycin sulfate are:

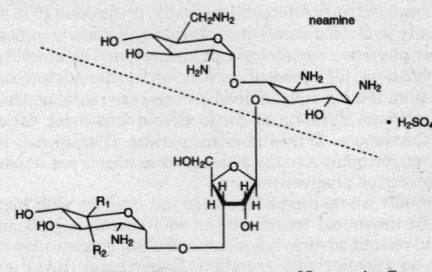

Neomycin B   Neomycin C
$R_1=H$, $R_2=CH_2NH_2$ $R_1=CH_2NH_2$, $R_2=H$

Each milliliter of buffered Ophthalmic Solution NEODECADRON in the OCUMETER* ophthalmic dispenser contains: dexamethasone sodium phosphate equivalent to 1 mg (0.1%) dexamethasone phosphate, and neomycin sulfate equivalent to 3.5 mg neomycin base. Inactive ingredients: creatinine, sodium citrate, sodium borate, polysorbate 80, disodium edetate, hydrochloric acid to adjust pH to 6.6–7.2, and water for injection. Benzalkonium chloride 0.02% and sodium bisulfite 0.1% added as preservatives.

* Registered trademark of MERCK & CO., Inc.

CLINICAL PHARMACOLOGY

Corticosteroids suppress the inflammatory response to a variety of agents, and they probably delay or slow healing. Since corticosteroids may inhibit the body's defense mechanism against infection, a concomitant antimicrobial drug may be used when this inhibition is considered to be clinically significant in a particular case.

When a decision to administer both a corticosteroid and an antimicrobial is made, the administration of such drugs in combination has the advantage of greater patient compliance and convenience, with the added assurance that the appropriate dosage of both drugs is administered, plus assured compatibility of ingredients when both types of drug are in the same formulation and, particularly, that the correct volume of drug is delivered and retained.

The relative potency of corticosteroids depends on the molecular structure, concentration, and release from the vehicle.

Microbiology
The anti-infective component in Ophthalmic Solution NEODECADRON is included to provide action against specific organisms susceptible to it. Neomycin sulfate is active *in vitro* against susceptible strains of the following microorganisms: *Staphylococcus aureus*, *Escherichia coli*, *Haemophilus influenzae*, *Klebsiella/Enterobacter* species, and *Neisseria* species. The product does not provide adequate coverage against: *Pseudomonas aeruginosa*, *Serratia marcescens*, and streptococci, including *Streptococcus pneumoniae*. (See INDICATIONS AND USAGE.)

INDICATIONS AND USAGE

For steroid-responsive inflammatory ocular conditions for which a corticosteroid is indicated and where bacterial infection a risk of bacterial ocular infection exists.

Ocular steroids are indicated in inflammatory conditions of the palpebral and bulbar conjunctiva, cornea, and anterior segment of the globe where the inherent risk of steroid use in certain infective conjunctivities is accepted to obtain a diminution in edema and inflammation. They are also indicated in chronic anterior uveitis and corneal injury from chemical, radiation, or thermal burns, or penetration of foreign bodies.

The use of a combination drug with an anti-infective component is indicated where the risk of infection is high or where there is an expectation that potentially dangerous numbers of bacteria will be present in the eye.

The particular anti-infective drug in this product is active against the following common bacterial eye pathogens:
Staphylococcus aureus
Escherichia coli
Haemophilus influenzae
Klebsiella/Enterobacter species
Neisseria species
The product does not provide adequate coverage against:
Pseudomonas aeruginosa
Serratia marcescens
Streptococci, including *Streptococcus pneumoniae*

CONTRAINDICATIONS

NEODECADRON is contraindicated in most viral diseases of the cornea and conjunctiva including epithelial herpes simplex keratitis (dendritic keratitis), vaccinia, varicella, and also in mycobacterial infection of the eye and fungal diseases

of ocular structures. NEODECADRON is also contraindicated in individuals with known or suspected hypersensitivity to any of the ingredients of this preparation, including sulfites, and to other corticosteroids (see WARNINGS). (Hypersensitivity to the antibiotic component occurs at a higher rate than for other components.)

WARNINGS

NOT FOR INJECTION INTO THE EYE
Prolonged use of corticosteroids may result in ocular hypertension and/or glaucoma with damage to the optic nerve, defects in visual acuity and fields of vision, and in posterior subcapsular cataract formation.

Prolonged use of corticosteroids may suppress the host response and thus increase the hazard of secondary ocular infections. In those diseases causing thinning of the cornea or sclera, perforations have been known to occur with the use of topical corticosteroids. In acute purulent conditions of the eye, corticosteroids may mask infection or enhance existing infection.

If this product is used for 10 days or longer, intraocular pressure should be routinely monitored even though it may be difficult in children and uncooperative patients. Corticosteroids should be used with caution in the presence of ocular hypertension and/or glaucoma. Intraocular pressure should be checked frequently.

The use of corticosteroids after cataract surgery may delay healing and increase the incidence of filtering blebs.

Use of ocular corticosteroids may prolong the course and may exacerbate the severity of many viral infections of the eye (including herpes simplex). Employment of a corticosteroid medication in the treatment of patients with a history of herpes simplex requires great caution; periodic slit lamp microscopy is essential. (See CONTRAINDICATIONS.)

Neomycin sulfate may occasionally cause cutaneous sensitization. If any reaction indicating such sensitivity is observed, discontinue use.

Ophthalmic Solution NEODECADRON contains sodium bisulfite, a sulfite that may cause allergic-type reactions including anaphylactic symptoms and life-threatening or less severe asthmatic episodes in certain susceptible people. The overall prevalence of sulfite sensitivity in the general population is unknown and probably low. Sulfite sensitivity is seen more frequently in asthmatic than in nonasthmatic people.

PRECAUTIONS

General
The initial prescription and renewal of the medication order beyond 20 milliliters should be made by a physician only after examination of the patient with the aid of magnification, such as slit lamp biomicroscopy and, where appropriate, fluorescein staining. If signs and symptoms fail to improve after two days, the patient should be re-evaluated.

The possibility of fungal infections of the cornea should be considered after prolonged corticosteroid dosing. Fungal cultures should be taken when appropriate.

If this product is used for 10 days or longer, intraocular pressure should be monitored (see WARNINGS).

There have been reports of bacterial keratitis associated with the use of multiple dose containers of topical ophthalmic products. These containers had been inadvertently contaminated by patients who, in most cases, had a concurrent corneal disease or a disruption of the ocular epithelial surface. (See PRECAUTIONS, Information for Patients.)

Information for Patients
Patients should be instructed to avoid allowing the tip of the dispensing container to contact the eye, eyelid, fingers, or any other surface. The use of this product by more than one person may spread infection. Keep tightly closed when not in use.

Patients should also be instructed that ocular preparations, if handled improperly, can become contaminated by common bacteria known to cause ocular infections. Serious damage to the eye and subsequent loss of vision may result from using contaminated preparations (see PRECAUTIONS, General).

If redness, irritation, swelling or pain persists or becomes aggravated, the patient should be advised to consult a physician. Patients should also be advised that if they have ocular surgery or develop an intercurrent ocular condition (e.g., trauma or infection), they should immediately seek their physician's advice.

One of the preservatives in Ophthalmic Solution NEODECADRON, benzalkonium chloride, may be absobed by soft contact lenses. Patients wearing soft contact lenses should be instructed to wait at least 15 minutes after instilling Ophthalmic Solution NEODECADRON before they insert their lenses.

Keep out of the reach of children.

Carcinogenesis, Mutagenesis, Impairment of Fertility
Long term animal studies have not been performed to evaluate the carcinogenic potential or the effect on fertility of Ophthalmic Solution NEODECADRON. Treatment of human lymphocytes in-vitro with neomycin increased the frequency of chromosome aberrations at the highest concentration (80 μg/mL) tested; however, the effects of neomycin on carcinogenesis and mutagenesis in humans are unknown.

Pregnancy
Teratogenic effects
Pregnancy Category C.
Corticosteroids have been found to be teratogenic in animal studies. Ocular administration of 0.1% dexamethasone resulted in 15.6% and 32.3% incidence of fetal anomalies in two groups of pregnant rabbits. Fetal growth retardation and increased mortality rates have been observed in rats with chronic dexamethasone therapy. There are no adequate and well-controlled studies in pregnant women. Ophthalmic Solution NEODECADRON should be used during pregnancy only if the potential benefit justifies the potential risk to the fetus. Infants born of mothers who have received substantial doses of corticosteroids during pregnancy should be observed carefully for signs of hypoadrenalism.

Nursing Mothers
It is not known whether topical administration of corticosteroids could result in sufficient systemic absorption to produce detectable quantities in human milk. Systemically-administered corticosteroids appear in human milk and could suppress growth, interfere with endogenous corticosteroid production, or cause other untoward effects. Because of the potential for serious adverse reactions in nursing infants from Ophthalmic Solution NEODECADRON, a decision should be made whether to discontinue nursing or to discontinue the drug, taking into account the importance of the drug to the mother.

Pediatric Use
Safety and effectiveness in pediatric patients have not been established.

ADVERSE REACTIONS

Adverse reactions have occurred with corticosteroid/anti-infective combination drugs which can be attributed to the corticosteroid component, the anti-infective component, the combination, or any other component of the product. Exact incidence figures are not available since no denominator of treated patients is available.

Reactions occurring most often from the presence of the anti-infective ingredient are allergic sensitizations. The reactions due to the corticosteroid component in decreasing order of frequency are: elevation of intraocular pressure (IOP) with possible development of glaucoma, and infrequent optic nerve damage; posterior subcapsular cataract formation; and delayed wound healing.

Secondary Infection:
The development of secondary infection has occurred after use of combinations containing corticosteroids and antimicrobials. Fungal and viral infections of the cornea are particularly prone to develop coincidentally with long-term applications of a corticosteroid. The possibility of fungal invasion must be considered in any persistent corneal ulceration where corticosteroid treatment has been used.

DOSAGE AND ADMINISTRATION

The duration of treatment will vary with the type of lesion and may extend from a few days to several weeks, according to therapeutic response.

Instill one or two drops of Ophthalmic Solution NEODECADRON into the conjunctival sac every hour during the day and every two hours during the night as initial therapy. When a favorable response is observed, reduce dosage to one drop every four hours. Later, further reduction in dosage to one drop three or four times daily may suffice to control symptoms.

Not more than 20 milliliters should be prescribed initially and the prescription should not be refilled without further evaluation as outlined in PRECAUTIONS above.

HOW SUPPLIED

Sterile Ophthalmic Solution NEODECADRON is a clear, colorless to pale yellow solution.

No. 7639—Ophthalmic Solution NEODECADRON is supplied as follows:

NDC 0006-7639-03 in 5 mL white opaque, plastic OCUMETER ophthalmic dispenser with a controlled drop tip. (6505-01-039-4352 0.1% 5 mL).

Storage
Store at controlled room temperature, 15°–30°C (59°–86°F). Protect from light.

7261326   Issued December 1995
COPYRIGHT © MERCK & CO., Inc., 1989, 1995
All rights reserved

NEODECADRON® Topical Cream
(Neomycin Sulfate-Dexamethasone Sodium Phosphate), U.S.P. ℞

DESCRIPTION

NEODECADRON* (Neomycin Sulfate-Dexamethasone Sodium Phosphate) Topical Cream is a topical steroid-antibiotic preparation.

NEODECADRON Topical Cream contains in each gram: dexamethasone sodium phosphate equivalent to 1 mg (0.1%) dexamethasone phosphate, and neomycin sulfate equivalent to 3.5 mg neomycin base, in a greaseless bland base. Inactive ingredients: stearyl alcohol, cetyl alcohol, mineral oil, polyoxyl 40 stearate, sorbitol solution, methyl polysilicone emulsion, creatinine, disodium edetate, sodium citrate, sodium hydroxide to adjust pH, and purified water. Methylparaben 0.15%, sodium bisulfite 0.18%, and sorbic acid 0.1% added as preservatives.

Dexamethasone sodium phosphate is 9-fluoro-11β,17-dihydroxy-16α-methyl-21-(phosphonooxy)pregna-1,4-diene-3,20-dione disodium salt. Its empirical formula is $C_{22}H_{28}FNa_2O_8P$ and its structural formula is:

Dexamethasone sodium phosphate has a molecular weight of 516.41.

Glucocorticoids are adrenocortical steroids, both naturally occurring and synthetic. Dexamethasone is a synthetic analog of naturally occurring glucocorticoids (hydrocortisone and cortisone).

Neomycin sulfate is a mixture of the sulfate salts of neomycin, an antibacterial substance produced by the growth of Streptomyces fradiae Waksman (Fam. Streptomycetaceae). Neomycin is a complex typically containing 8–13% neomycin C, less than 0.2% neomycin A and the rest, neomycin B. The empirical formulas and molecular weights for the three components are: neomycin B, $C_{23}H_{46}N_6O_{13}$, molecular weight 614.65; neomycin C, $C_{23}H_{46}N_6O_{13}$, molecular weight 614.65; neomycin A, (also referred to as neamine), $C_{12}H_{26}N_4O_6$, molecular weight 322.36. The structural formula for neomycin B sulfate is:

Neomycin B

*Registered trademark of MERCK & CO., INC.

CLINICAL PHARMACOLOGY

Topical corticosteroids share anti-inflammatory, anti-pruritic, and vasoconstrictive actions.

The mechanism of anti-inflammatory activity of the topical corticosteroids is unclear. Various laboratory methods, including vasoconstrictor assays, are used to compare and predict potencies and/or clinical efficacies of the topical corticosteroids. There is some evidence to suggest that a recognizable correlation exists between vasoconstrictor potency and therapeutic efficacy in man.

Pharmacokinetics
The extent of percutaneous absorption of topical corticosteroids is determined by many factors including the vehicle, the integrity of the epidermal barrier, and the use of occlusive dressings.

Continued on next page

Merck & Co.—Cont.

Topical corticosteroids can be absorbed from normal intact skin. Inflammation and/or other disease processes in the skin increase percutaneous absorption. Occlusive dressings substantially increase the percutaneous absorption of topical corticosteroids. Thus, occlusive dressings may be a valuable therapeutic adjunct for treatment of resistant dermatoses. (See DOSAGE AND ADMINISTRATION.)
Once absorbed through the skin, topical corticosteroids are handled through pharmacokinetic pathways similar to systemically administered corticosteroids. Corticosteroids are bound to plasma proteins in varying degrees. Corticosteroids are metabolized primarily in the liver and are then excreted by the kidneys. Some of the topical corticosteroids and their metabolites are also excreted into the bile.
The antibiotic component, neomycin, is bactericidal to many gram-positive and gram-negative bacteria.

INDICATIONS AND USAGE

For the treatment of corticosteroid-responsive dermatoses with secondary infection. It has not been demonstrated that this steroid-antibiotic combination provides greater benefit than the steroid component alone after 7 days of treatment (see WARNINGS).

CONTRAINDICATIONS

Hypersensitivity to any component of this product, including sulfites (see WARNINGS).

WARNINGS

Topical Cream NEODECADRON contains sodium bisulfite, a sulfite that may cause allergic-type reactions including anaphylactic symptoms and life-threatening or less severe asthmatic episodes in certain susceptible people. The overall prevalence of sulfite sensitivity in the general population is unknown and probably low. Sulfite sensitivity is seen more frequently in asthmatic than in nonasthmatic people.
Because of the concern of nephrotoxicity and ototoxicity associated with neomycin, this combination product should not be used over a wide area or for extended periods of time.
Topically applied steroids are absorbed systemically. There may be rare instances in which this absorption results in immunosuppression. Patients who are on drugs which suppress the immune system are more susceptible to infections than healthy individuals. Chickenpox and measles, for example, can have a more serious or even fatal course in non-immune children or adults on corticosteroids. In such children or adults who have not had these diseases, particular care should be taken to avoid exposure. The risk of developing a disseminated infection varies among individuals and can be related to the dose, route and duration of corticosteroid administration as well as to the underlying disease. If exposed to chickenpox, prophylaxis with varicella zoster immune globulin (VZIG) may be indicated. If chickenpox develops, treatment with antiviral agents may be considered. If exposed to measles, prophylaxis with immune globulin (IG) may be indicated. (See the respective package inserts for VZIG and IG for complete prescribing information.)

PRECAUTIONS

General
Systemic absorption of topical corticosteroids has produced reversible hypothalamic-pituitary-adrenal (HPA) axis suppression, manifestations of Cushing's syndrome, hyperglycemia, and glycosuria in some patients.
Conditions which augment systemic absorption include the application of the more potent corticosteroids, use over large surface areas, prolonged use, and the addition of occlusive dressings.
Therefore, patients receiving a large dose of a potent topical corticosteroid applied to a large surface area or under an occlusive dressing should be evaluated periodically for evidence of HPA axis suppression by using urinary free cortisol and ACTH stimulation tests. If HPA axis suppression is noted, an attempt should be made to withdraw the drug, to reduce the frequency of application, or to substitute a less potent corticosteroid.
Recovery of HPA axis function is generally prompt and complete upon discontinuation of the drug. Infrequently, signs and symptoms of corticosteroid withdrawal may occur, requiring supplemental systemic corticosteroids.
Children may absorb proportionally larger amounts of topical corticosteroids and thus be more susceptible to systemic toxicity (see PRECAUTIONS, *Pediatric Use*).
Corticosteroids may mask some signs of infection, and new infections may appear during their use. There may be decreased resistance and inability to localize infection when corticosteroids are used. Therefore, patients with bacterial infections should also be given appropriate antibiotic therapy if Topical Cream NEODECADRON is used. Moreover, corticosteroids may affect the nitroblue-tetrazolium test for bacterial infection and produce false-negative results.
Corticosteroid therapy exerts its major immunosuppressive effects by impairing the normal function of the T-lymphocyte population and macrophages. When T-cell and/or macrophage function is impaired, latent disease may be activated or there may be an exacerbation of intercurrent infections due to pathogens, including those caused by Candida, Mycobacterium, Ameba, Toxoplasma, Strongyloides, Pneumocystis, Cryptococcus, Nocardia, etc. Products containing steroids should be used with caution in patients with impaired T-cell function or in patients receiving other immunosuppressive therapy.
In the presence of dermatological infections, the use of an appropriate antifungal or antibacterial agent should be instituted. If a favorable response does not occur promptly, the corticosteroid should be discontinued until the infection has been adequately controlled.
If irritation develops, topical corticosteroids should be discontinued and appropriate therapy instituted.
This product is not for ophthalmic use. However, if applied to the eyelids or skin near the eyes, the drug may enter the eyes. In patients with a history of herpes simplex keratitis, ocular exposure to corticosteroids may lead to a recurrence. Prolonged ocular exposure may cause steroid glaucoma.
A few individuals may be sensitive to one or more of the components of this product. Sensitivity to neomycin may occasionally develop, especially when it is applied to abraded skin. If any reaction indicating sensitivity is observed, discontinue use. There are reports in the current medical literature that indicate an increase in the prevalence of persons sensitive to neomycin.
Generally, occlusive dressings should not be used on weeping or exudative lesions.
If the occlusive dressing technique is employed, caution should be exercised with regard to the use of plastic films which are often inflammable and may pose a suffocation hazard for children.
When large areas of the body are covered with an occlusive dressing, thermal homeostasis may be impaired. If elevation of body temperature occurs, use of the occlusive dressing should be discontinued.

Information for the Patient
Patients using topical corticosteroids should receive the following information and instructions:

1. This medication is to be used as directed by the physician. It is for external use only. Avoid contact with the eyes.
2. Patients should be advised not to use this medication for any disorder other than that for which it was prescribed.
3. The treated skin area should not be bandaged or otherwise covered or wrapped so as to be occlusive unless directed by the physician.
4. Patients should report any signs of local adverse reactions, especially under occlusive dressings.
5. Parents of pediatric patients should be advised not to use tight-fitting diapers or plastic pants on a child being treated in the diaper area, as these garments may constitute occlusive dressings.
6. Susceptible patients who are on immunosuppressant doses of corticosteroids should be warned to avoid exposure to chickenpox or measles. Patients should also be advised that if they are exposed, medical advice should be sought without delay.

Laboratory Tests
The following tests may be helpful in evaluating the HPA axis suppression:

- Urinary free cortisol test
- ACTH stimulation test

Carcinogenesis, Mutagenesis and Impairment of Fertility
Long-term animal studies have not been performed to evaluate the carcinogenic potential or the effect on fertility of Topical Cream NEODECADRON.
Studies to determine mutagenicity with prednisolone and hydrocortisone have revealed negative results.

Pregnancy
Pregnancy Category C: Corticosteroids are generally teratogenic in laboratory animals when administered systemically at relatively low dosage levels. The more potent corticosteroids have been shown to be teratogenic after dermal application in laboratory animals. There are no adequate and well controlled studies in pregnant women on teratogenic effects from topically applied corticosteroids. Therefore, topical corticosteroids should be used during pregnancy only if the potential benefit justifies the potential risk to the fetus. Drugs of this class should not be used extensively on pregnant patients, in large amounts, or for prolonged periods of time.

Nursing Mothers
It is not known whether topical administration of corticosteroids could result in sufficient systemic absorption to produce detectable quantities in breast milk. Systemically administered corticosteroids are secreted into breast milk in quantities *not* likely to have a deleterious effect on the infant. Nevertheless, caution should be exercised when topical corticosteroids are administered to a nursing woman.

Pediatric Use
Pediatric patients may demonstrate greater susceptibility to topical corticosteroid-induced HPA axis suppression and Cushing's syndrome than mature patients bcause of a larger skin surface area to body weight ratio.
Hypothalamic-pituitary-adrenal (HPA) axis suppression, Cushing's syndrome, and intracranial hypertension have been reported in children receiving topical corticosteroids. Manifestations of adrenal suppression in children include linear growth retardation, delayed weight gain, low plasma cortisol levels, and absence of response to ACTH stimulation. Manifestations of intracranial hypertension include bulging fontanelles, headaches, and bilateral papilledema.
Administration of topical corticosteroids to children should be limited to the least amount compatible with an effective therapeutic regimen. Chronic corticosteroid therapy may interfere with the growth and development of children.

ADVERSE REACTIONS

The following adverse reactions are reported infrequently with topical corticosteroids, but may occur more frequently with the use of occlusive dressings. These reactions are listed in an approximate decreasing order of occurrence:

Burning
Itching
Irritation
Dryness
Folliculitis
Hypertrichosis
Acneiform eruptions
Hypopigmentation
Perioral dermatitis
Allergic contact dermatitis
Maceration of the skin
Secondary infection
Skin atrophy
Striae
Miliaria

Prevalence of neomycin hypersensitivity is increasing. Ototoxicity and nephrotoxicity have been reported with prolonged use or use of large amounts of topical neomycin preparations.

OVERDOSAGE

Topically applied corticosteroids can be absorbed in sufficient amounts to produce systemic effects (see PRECAUTIONS).

DOSAGE AND ADMINISTRATION

Apply to the affected area as a thin film three or four times daily.
Before using NEODECADRON Topical Cream in the *ear*, clean the aural canal thoroughly and sponge dry. Confirm that the eardrum is intact. With a cotton-tipped applicator, apply a thin coating of the cream to the affected canal area two or three times a day. When a favorable response is obtained, reduce the number of daily applications to one or two, and eventually discontinue.

HOW SUPPLIED

No. 7607—Topical Cream NEODECADRON is a white cream, and is supplied as follows:
NDC 0006-7607-12 in 15 g tubes
NDC 0006-7607-24 in 30 g tubes
DC 7612428 Issued April 1993

COPYRIGHT © MERCK & CO. INC., 1985
All rights reserved

NOROXIN® Tablets ℞
(Norfloxacin), U.S.P.

This product is manufactured by Merck & Co., Inc. and distributed by Roberts Laboratories, Inc. Please call 1-800-828-2088 for additional product information.

DESCRIPTION

NOROXIN+ (Norfloxacin) is a synthetic, broad-spectrum antibacterial agent for oral administration. Norfloxacin, a fluoroquinolone, is 1-ethyl-6-fluoro-1,4-dihydro-4-oxo-7-(1-piperazinyl)-3-quinolinec arboxylic acid. Its empirical formula is $C_{16}H_{18}FN_3O_3$ and the structural formula is:

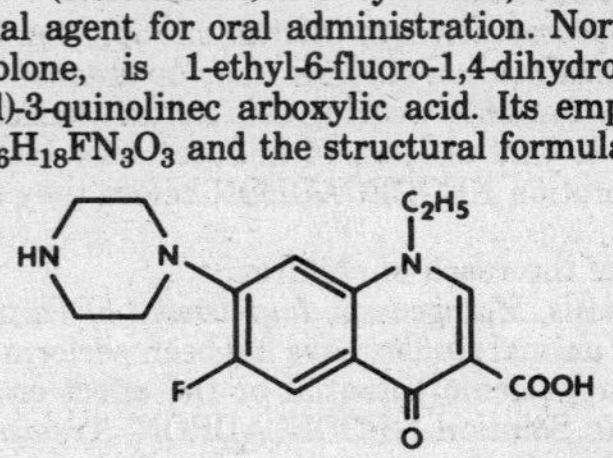

Norfloxacin is a white to pale yellow crystalline powder with a molecular weight of 319.34 and a melting point of about 221°C. It is freely soluble in glacial acetic acid, and very slightly soluble in ethanol, methanol and water.

NOROXIN is available in 400-mg tablets. Each tablet contains the following inactive ingredients: cellulose, croscarmellose sodium, hydroxypropyl cellulose, hydroxypropyl methylcellulose, iron oxide, magnesium stearate, and titanium dioxide.

Norfloxacin, a fluoroquinolone, differs from non-fluorinated quinolones by having a fluorine atom at the 6 position and a piperazine moiety at the 7 position.

---

†Registered trademark of MERCK & CO., INC.

CLINICAL PHARMACOLOGY

In fasting healthy volunteers, at least 30–40% of an oral dose of NOROXIN is absorbed. Absorption is rapid following single doses of 200 mg, 400 mg and 800 mg. At the respective doses, mean peak serum and plasma concentrations of 0.8, 1.5 and 2.4 μg/mL are attained approximately one hour after dosing. The presence of food may decrease absorption. The effective half-life of norfloxacin in serum and plasma is 3–4 hours. Steady-state concentrations of norfloxacin will be attained within two days of dosing.

In healthy elderly volunteers (65–75 years of age with normal renal function for their age), norfloxacin is eliminated more slowly because of their slightly decreased renal function. Drug absorption appears unaffected. However, the effective half-life of norfloxacin in these elderly subjects is 4 hours.

The disposition of norfloxacin in patients with creatinine clearance rates greater than 30 mL/min/1.73m² is similar to that in healthy volunteers. In patients with creatinine clearance rates equal to or less than 30 mL/min/1.73m², the renal elimination of norfloxacin decreases so that the effective serum half-life is 6.5 hours. In these patients, alteration of dosage is necessary (see DOSAGE AND ADMINISTRATION). Drug absorption appears unaffected by decreasing renal function.

Norfloxacin is eliminated through metabolism, biliary excretion, and renal excretion. After a single 400-mg dose of NOROXIN, mean antimicrobial activities equivalent to 278, 773, and 82 μg of norfloxacin/g of feces were obtained at 12, 24, and 48 hours, respectively. Renal excretion occurs by both glomerular filtration and tubular secretion as evidenced by the high rate of renal clearance (approximately 275 mL/min). Within 24 hours of drug administration, 26 to 32% of the administered dose is recovered in the urine as norfloxacin with an additional 5–8% being recovered in the urine as six active metabolites of lesser antimicrobial potency. Only a small percentage (less than 1%) of the dose is recovered thereafter. Fecal recovery accounts for another 30% of the administered dose.

Two to three hours after a single 400-mg dose, urinary concentrations of 200 μg/mL or more are attained in the urine. In healthy volunteers, mean urinary concentrations of norfloxacin remain above 30 μg/mL for at least 12 hours following a 400-mg dose. The urinary pH may affect the solubility of norfloxacin. Norfloxacin is least soluble at urinary pH of 7.5 with greater solubility occurring at pHs above and below this value. The serum protein binding of norfloxacin is between 10 and 15%.

The following are mean concentrations of norfloxacin in various fluids and tissues measured 1 to 4 hours post-dose after two 400-mg doses, unless otherwise indicated:

Renal Parenchyma	7.3 μg/g
Prostate	2.5 μg/g
Seminal Fluid	2.7 μg/mL
Testicle	1.6 μg/g
Uterus/Cervix	3.0 μg/g
Vagina	4.3 μg/g
Fallopian Tube	1.9 μg/g
Bile	6.9 μg/mL (after two 200-mg doses)

Microbiology

Norfloxacin has *in vitro* activity against a broad range of gram-positive and gram-negative aerobic bacteria. The fluorine atom at the 6 position provides increased potency against gram-negative organisms, and the piperazine moiety at the 7 position is responsible for anti-pseudomonal activity.

Norfloxacin inhibits bacterial deoxyribonucleic acid synthesis and is bactericidal. At the molecular level, three specific events are attributed to norfloxacin in *E. coli* cells:

1) inhibition of the ATP-dependent DNA supercoiling reaction catalyzed by DNA gyrase,
2) inhibition of the relaxation of supercoiled DNA,
3) promotion of double-stranded DNA breakage.

Resistance to norfloxacin due to spontaneous mutation *in vitro* is a rare occurrence (range: 10^{-9} to 10^{-12} cells). Resistant organisms have emerged during therapy with norfloxacin in less than 1% of patients treated. Organisms in which development of resistance is greatest are the following:

Pseudomonas aeruginosa
Klebsiella pneumoniae
Acinetobacter species
Enterococcus species

For this reason, when there is a lack of satisfactory clinical response, repeat culture and susceptibility testing should be done. Nalidixic acid-resistant organisms are generally susceptible to norfloxacin *in vitro;* however, these organisms may have higher MICs to norfloxacin than nalidixic acid-susceptible strains. There is generally no cross-resistance between norfloxacin and other classes of antibacterial agents. Therefore, norfloxacin may demonstrate activity against indicated organisms resistant to some other antimicrobial agents including the aminoglycosides, penicillins, cephalosporins, tetracyclines, macrolides, and sulfonamides, including combinations of sulfamethoxazole and trimethoprim. Antagonism has been demonstrated *in vitro* between norfloxacin and nitrofurantoin.

Norfloxacin has been shown to be active against most strains of the following organisms both *in vitro* and in clinical infections (see INDICATIONS AND USAGE):

Gram-positive aerobes:
Enterococcus faecalis
Staphylococcus aureus
Staphylococcus epidermidis
Staphylococcus saprophyticus
Streptococcus agalactiae

Gram-negative aerobes:
Citrobacter freundii
Enterobacter aerogenes
Enterobacter cloacae
Escherichia coli
Klebsiella pneumoniae
Neisseria gonorrhoeae
Proteus mirabilis
Proteus vulgaris
Pseudomonas aeruginosa
Serratia marcescens

Norfloxacin has been shown to be active *in vitro* against most strains of the following organisms; however, the clinical significance of these data is unknown.

Gram-positive aerobes:
Bacillus cereus

Gram-negative aerobes:
Acinetobacter calcoaceticus
Aeromonas species
Alcaligenes species
Campylobacter species
Citrobacter diversus
Edwardsiella tarda
Flavobacterium species
Hafnia alvei
Klebsiella oxytoca
Klebsiella rhinoscleromatis
Morganella morganii
Providencia alcalifaciens
Providencia rettgeri
Providencia stuartii
Salmonella species
Shigella species
Vibrio cholerae
Vibrio parahemolyticus
Yersinia enterocolitica

Other:
Ureaplasma urealyticum

NOROXIN is not generally active against obligate anaerobes.

Norfloxacin has not been shown to be active against *Treponema pallidum.* (See WARNINGS.)

Susceptibility Tests

Diffusion Techniques: Quantitative methods that require measurement of zone diameters give the most precise estimate of the susceptibility of bacteria to antimicrobial agents. One such procedure is the National Committee for Clinical Laboratory Standards (NCCLS) approved procedure (M2-A4–Performance Standards for Antimicrobial Disk Susceptibility Tests 1990). This method has been recommended for use with the 10-μg norfloxacin disk to test susceptibility to norfloxacin. Interpretation involves correlation of the diameters obtained in the disk test with minimum inhibitory concentration (MIC) for norfloxacin. Reports from the laboratory giving results of the standard single-disk susceptibility test with a 10-μg norfloxacin disk should be interpreted according to the following criteria **(these criteria apply to isolates from urinary tract or prostatic infections):**

Zone diameter (mm)	Interpretation
≥17	(S) Susceptible
13–16	(I) Intermediate
≤12	(R) Resistant

A report of "Susceptible" indicates that the pathogen is likely to be inhibited by generally achievable urine/prostatic tissue levels. A report of "Intermediate" indicates that the test results be considered equivocal or indeterminate. A report of "Resistant" indicates that achievable concentrations of the antibiotic are unlikely to be inhibitory and other therapy should be selected.

Standardized procedures require the use of laboratory control organisms. The 10-μg norfloxacin disk should give the following zone diameter:

Organism	Zone diameter (mm)
E. coli ATCC 25922	28–35
P. aeruginosa ATCC 27853	22–29
S. aureus ATCC 25923	17–28

Other quinolone antibacterial disks should not be substituted when performing susceptibility tests for norfloxacin because of spectrum differences with norfloxacin. The 10-μg norfloxacin disk should be used for all *in vitro* testing of isolates using diffusion techniques.

Dilution Techniques: Broth and agar dilution methods, such as those recommended by the NCCLS (M7-A2—Methods for Dilution Antimicrobial Susceptibility Tests for Bacteria that Grow Aerobically 1990), may be used to determine the minimum inhibitory concentration (MIC) of norfloxacin. MIC test results should be interpreted according to the following criteria **(these criteria apply to isolates from urinary tract or prostatic infections):**

MIC (μg/mL)	Interpretation
≤4	(S) Susceptible
8	(I) Intermediate
≥16	(R) Resistant

As with standard diffusion methods, dilution procedures require the use of laboratory control organisms. Standard norfloxacin powder should give the following MIC values:

Organism	MIC range (μg/mL)
E. coli ATCC 25922	0.03–0.12
E. faecalis ATCC 29212	2.0–8.0
P. aeruginosa ATCC 27853	1.0–4.0
S. aureus ATCC 29213	0.05–2.0

INDICATIONS AND USAGE

NOROXIN is indicated for the treatment of adults with the following infections caused by susceptible strains of the designated microorganisms:

Urinary tract infections:

Uncomplicated urinary tract infections (including cystitis) due to *Enterococcus faecalis, Escherichia coli, Klebsiella pneumoniae, Proteus mirabilis, Pseudomonas aeruginosa, Staphylococcus epidermidis, Staphylococcus saprophyticus, Citrobacter freundii*, Enterobacter aerogenes*, Enterobacter cloacae*, Proteus vulgaris*, Staphylococcus aureus**, or *Streptococcus agalactiae**.

Complicated urinary tract infections due to *Enterococcus faecalis, Escherichia coli, Klebsiella pneumoniae, Proteus mirabilis, Pseudomonas aeruginosa*, or *Serratia marcescens**.

Sexually transmitted diseases (See WARNINGS.):

Uncomplicated urethral and cervical gonorrhea due to *Neisseria gonorrhoeae.*

Prostatitis:

Prostatitis due to *Escherichia coli.*

(See DOSAGE AND ADMINISTRATION for appropriate dosing instructions.)

Penicillinase production should have no effect on norfloxacin activity.

Appropriate culture and susceptibility tests should be performed before treatment in order to isolate and identify organisms causing the infection and to determine their susceptibility to norfloxacin. Therapy with norfloxacin may be initiated before results of these tests are known; once results become available, appropriate therapy should be given. Repeat culture and susceptibility testing performed periodically during therapy will provide information not only on the therapeutic effect of the antimicrobial agents but also on the possible emergence of bacterial resistance.

---

* Efficacy for this organism in this organ system was studied in fewer than 10 infections.

CONTRAINDICATIONS

NOROXIN (norfloxacin) is contraindicated in persons with a history of hypersensitivity, tendinitis, or tendon rupture associated with the use of norfloxacin or any member of the quinolone group of antimicrobial agents.

WARNINGS

THE SAFETY AND EFFICACY OF ORAL NORFLOXACIN IN CHILDREN, ADOLESCENTS (UNDER THE AGE OF 18), PREGNANT WOMEN, AND NURSING MOTHERS HAVE NOT BEEN ESTABLISHED. (See PRECAUTIONS—*Pregnancy, Nursing Mothers* and *Pediatric Use.*) The oral administration of single doses of norfloxacin, 6 times** the recommended human clinical dose (on a mg/kg basis), caused lame-

Continued on next page

Information on the Merck & Co., Inc. products listed on these pages is the full prescribing information from product circulars in use September 30, 1996.

Merck & Co.—Cont.

ness in immature dogs. Histologic examination of the weight-bearing joints of these dogs revealed permanent lesions of the cartilage. Other quinolones also produced erosions of the cartilage in weight-bearing joints and other signs of arthropathy in immature animals of various species. (See ANIMAL PHARMACOLOGY.)

Convulsions have been reported in patients receiving norfloxacin. Convulsions, increased intracranial pressure, and toxic psychoses have been reported in patients receiving drugs in this class. Quinolones may also cause central nervous system (CNS) stimulation which may lead to tremors, restlessness, lightheadedness, confusion, and hallucinations. If these reactions occur in patients receiving norfloxacin, the drug should be discontinued and appropriate measures instituted.

The effects of norfloxacin on brain function or on the electrical activity of the brain have not been tested. Therefore, until more information becomes available, norfloxacin, like all other quinolones, should be used with caution in patients with known or suspected CNS disorders, such as severe cerebral arteriosclerosis, epilepsy, and other factors which predispose to seizures. (See ADVERSE REACTIONS.)

Serious and occasionally fatal hypersensitivity (anaphylactoid or anaphylactic) reactions, some following the first dose, have been reported in patients receiving quinolone therapy. Some reactions were accompanied by cardiovascular collapse, loss of consciousness, tingling, pharyngeal or facial edema, dyspnea, urticaria and itching. Only a few patients had a history of hypersensitivity reactions. If an allergic reaction to norfloxacin occurs, discontinue the drug. Serious acute hypersensitivity reactions may require immediate emergency treatment with epinephrine. Oxygen, intravenous fluids, antihistamines, corticosteroids, pressor amines, and airway management, including intubation, should be administered as indicated.

Pseudomembranous colitis has been reported with nearly all antibacterial agents, including norfloxacin, and may range in severity from mild to life-threatening. Therefore, it is important to consider this diagnosis in patients who present with diarrhea subsequent to the administration of antibacterial agents.

Treatment with antibacterial agents alters the normal flora of the colon and may permit overgrowth of clostridia. Studies indicate that a toxin produced by *Clostridium difficile* is one primary cause of "antibiotic-associated colitis."

After the diagnosis of pseudomembranous colitis has been established, therapeutic measures should be initiated. Mild cases of pseudomembranous colitis usually respond to drug discontinuation alone. In moderate to severe cases, consideration should be given to management with fluids and electrolytes, protein supplementation, and treatment with an antibacterial drug clinically effective against *C. difficile* colitis.

Ruptures of the shoulder, hand, and Achilles tendons that required surgical repair or resulted in prolonged disability have been reported with norfloxacin. Norfloxacin should be discontinued if the patient experiences pain, inflammation, or rupture of a tendon. Patients should rest and refrain from exercise until the diagnosis of tendinitis or tendon rupture has been confidently excluded. Tendon rupture can occur at any time during or after therapy with norfloxacin.

Norfloxacin has not been shown to be effective in the treatment of syphilis. Antimicrobial agents used in high doses for short periods of time to treat gonorrhea may mask or delay the symptoms of incubating syphilis. All patients with gonorrhea should have a serologic test for syphilis at the time of diagnosis. Patients treated with norfloxacin should have a follow-up serologic test for syphilis after three months.

**Based on a patient weight of 50 kg.

PRECAUTIONS

General:
Needle-shaped crystals were found in the urine of some volunteers who received either placebo, 800 mg norfloxacin, or 1600 mg norfloxacin (at or twice the recommended daily dose, respectively) while participating in a double-blind, crossover study comparing single doses of norfloxacin with placebo. While crystalluria is not expected to occur under usual conditions with a dosage regimen of 400 mg b.i.d., as a precaution, the daily recommended dosage should not be exceeded and the patient should drink sufficient fluids to ensure a proper state of hydration and adequate urinary output.

Alteration in dosage regimen is necessary for patients with impaired renal function (see DOSAGE AND ADMINISTRATION).

Moderate to severe phototoxicity reactions have been observed in patients who are exposed to excessive sunlight while receiving some members of this drug class. Excessive sunlight should be avoided. Therapy should be discontinued if phototoxicity occurs.

Rarely, hemolytic reactions have been reported in patients with latent or actual defects in glucose-6-phosphate dehydrogenase activity who take quinolone antibacterial agents, including norfloxacin. (See ADVERSE REACTIONS.)

Information for Patients
Patients should be advised:
—to drink fluids liberally.
—that norfloxacin should be taken at least one hour before or at least two hours after a meal or milk ingestion.
—that multivitamins or other products containing iron or zinc, or antacids should not be taken within the two-hour period before or within the two-hour period after taking norfloxacin. (See *Drug Interactions.*)
—that norfloxacin can cause dizziness and lightheadedness and, therefore, patients should know how they react to norfloxacin before they operate an automobile or machinery or engage in activities requiring mental alertness and coordination.
—to discontinue treatment and inform their physician if they experience pain, inflammation, or rupture of a tendon, and to rest and refrain from exercise until the diagnosis of tendinitis or tendon rupture has been confidently excluded.
—that norfloxacin may be associated with hypersensitivity reactions, even following the first dose, and to discontinue the drug at the first sign of a skin rash or other allergic reaction.
—to avoid undue exposure to excessive sunlight while receiving norfloxacin and to discontinue therapy if phototoxicity occurs.
—that some quinolones may increase the effects of theophylline and/or caffeine. (See *Drug Interactions.*)

Laboratory Tests
As with any potent antibacterial agent, periodic assessment of organ system functions, including renal, hepatic, and hematopoietic, is advisable during prolonged therapy.

Drug Interactions
Elevated plasma levels of theophylline have been reported with concomitant quinolone use. There have been reports of theophylline-related side effects in patients on concomitant therapy with norfloxacin and theophylline. Therefore, monitoring of theophylline plasma levels should be considered and dosage of theophylline adjusted as required.

Elevated serum levels of cyclosporine have been reported with concomitant use of cyclosporine with norfloxacin. Therefore cyclosporine serum levels should be monitored and appropriate cyclosporine dosage adjustments made when these drugs are used concomitantly.

Quinolones, including norfloxacin, may enhance the effects of the oral anticoagulant warfarin or its derivatives. When these products are administered concomitantly, prothrombin time or other suitable coagulation tests should be closely monitored.

Diminished urinary excretion of norfloxacin has been reported during the concomitant administration of probenecid and norfloxacin.

The concomitant use of nitrofurantoin is not recommended since nitrofurantoin may antagonize the antibacterial effect of NOROXIN in the urinary tract.

Multivitamins, or other products containing iron or zinc, antacids or sucralfate should not be administered concomitantly with, or within 2 hours of, the administration of norfloxacin, because they may interfere with absorption resulting in lower serum and urine levels of norfloxacin.

Some quinolones have also been shown to interfere with the metabolism of caffeine. This may lead to reduced clearance of caffeine and a prolongation of its plasma half-life.

Carcinogenesis, Mutagenesis, Impairment of Fertility
No increase in neoplastic changes was observed with norfloxacin as compared to controls in a study in rats, lasting up to 96 weeks at doses 8–9 times** the usual human dose (on a mg/kg basis).

Norfloxacin was tested for mutagenic activity in a number of *in vivo* and *in vitro* tests. Norfloxacin had no mutagenic effect in the dominant lethal test in mice and did not cause chromosomal aberrations in hamsters or rats at doses 30–60 times** the usual human dose (on a mg/kg basis). Norfloxacin had no mutagenic activity *in vitro* in the Ames microbial mutagen test, Chinese hamster fibroblasts and V-79 mammalian cell assay. Although norfloxacin was weakly positive in the Rec-assay for DNA repair, all other mutagenic assays were negative including a more sensitive test (V-79).

Norfloxacin did not adversely affect the fertility of male and female mice at oral doses up to 30 times** the usual human dose (on a mg/kg basis).

Pregnancy
Teratogenic Effects. Pregnancy Category C. Norfloxacin has been shown to produce embryonic loss in monkeys when given in doses 10 times** the maximum daily total human dose (on a mg/kg basis). At this dose, peak plasma levels obtained in monkeys were approximately 2 times those obtained in humans. There has been no evidence of a teratogenic effect in any of the animal species tested (rat, rabbit, mouse, monkey) at 6–50 times** the maximum daily human dose (on a mg/kg basis). There are, however, no adequate and well controlled studies in pregnant women. Norfloxacin

should be used during pregnancy only if the potential benefit justifies the potential risk to the fetus.

Nursing Mothers
It is not known whether norfloxacin is excreted in human milk.

When a 200-mg dose of NOROXIN was administered to nursing mothers, norfloxacin was not detected in human milk. However, because the dose studied was low, because other drugs in this class are secreted in human milk, and because of the potential for serious adverse reactions from norfloxacin in nursing infants, a decision should be made to discontinue nursing or to discontinue the drug, taking into account the importance of the drug to the mother.

Pediatric Use
The safety and effectiveness of oral norfloxacin in children and adolescents below the age of 18 years have not been established. Norfloxacin causes arthropathy in juvenile animals of several animal species. (See WARNINGS and ANIMAL PHARMACOLOGY.)

**Based on a patient weight of 50 kg.

ADVERSE REACTIONS

Single-Dose Studies
In clinical trials involving 82 healthy subjects and 228 patients with gonorrhea, treated with a single dose of norfloxacin, 6.5% reported drug-related adverse experiences. However, the following incidence figures were calculated without reference to drug relationship.

The most common adverse experiences (> 1.0%) were: dizziness (2.6%), nausea (2.6%), headache (2.0%), and abdominal cramping (1.6%).

Additional reactions (0.3%–1.0%) were: anorexia, diarrhea, hyperhidrosis, asthenia, anal/rectal pain, constipation, dyspepsia, flatulence, tingling of the fingers, and vomiting.

Laboratory adverse changes considered drug-related were reported in 4.5% of patients/subjects. These laboratory changes were: increased AST (SGOT) (1.6%), decreased WBC (1.3%), decreased platelet count (1.0%), increased urine protein (1.0%), decreased hematocrit and hemoglobin (0.6%), and increased eosinophils (0.6%).

Multiple-Dose Studies
In clinical trials involving 52 healthy subjects and 1980 patients with urinary tract infections or prostatitis, treated with multiple doses of norfloxacin, 3.6% reported drug-related adverse experiences. However, the incidence figures below were calculated without reference to drug relationship.

The most common adverse experiences (> 1.0%) were: nausea (4.2%), headache (2.8%), dizziness (1.7%), and asthenia (1.3%).

Additional reactions (0.3%–1.0%) were: abdominal pain, back pain, constipation, diarrhea, dry mouth, dyspepsia/heartburn, fever, flatulence, hyperhidrosis, loose stools, pruritus, rash, somnolence, and vomiting.

Less frequent reactions (0.1%–0.2%) included: abdominal swelling, allergies, anorexia, anxiety, bitter taste, blurred vision, bursitis, chest pain, chills, depression, dysmenorrhea, edema, erythema, foot or hand swelling, insomnia, mouth ulcer, myocardial infarction, palpitation, pruritus ani, renal colic, sleep disturbances, and urticaria.

Abnormal laboratory values observed in these patients/subjects were: eosinophilia (1.5%), elevation of ALT (SGPT) (1.4%), decreased WBC and/or neutrophil count (1.4%), elevation of AST (SGOT) (1.4%), and increased alkaline phosphatase (1.1%). Those occurring less frequently included increased BUN, increased LDH, increased serum creatinine, decreased hematocrit, and glycosuria.

Post Marketing
The most frequently reported adverse reaction in post-marketing experience is rash.

CNS effects characterized as generalized seizures and myoclonus have been reported with NOROXIN®. A causal relationship to NOROXIN® has not been established (see WARNINGS). Visual disturbances have been reported with drugs in this class.

The following additional adverse reactions have been reported since the drug was marketed:

Hypersensitivity Reactions
Hypersensitivity reactions have been reported including anaphylactoid reactions, angioedema, dyspnea, vasculitis, urticaria, arthritis, arthralgia and myalgia (see WARNINGS).

Skin
Toxic epidermal necrolysis, Stevens-Johnson syndrome and erythema multiforme, exfoliative dermatitis, photosensitivity

Gastrointestinal
Pseudomembranous colitis, hepatitis, jaundice including cholestatic jaundice, pancreatitis (rare), stomatitis. The onset of pseudomembranous colitis symptoms may occur during or after antibacterial treatment. (See WARNINGS.)

Infection	Description	Unit Dose	Frequency	Duration	Daily Dose
Urinary Tract	Uncomplicated UTI's (crystitis) due to *E. coli*, *K. pneumoniae*, or *P. mirabilis*	400 mg	q12h	3 days	800 mg
	Uncomplicated UTI's due to other indicated organisms	400 mg	q12h	7–10 days	800 mg
	Complicated UTI's	400 mg	q12h	10–21 days	800 mg
Sexually Transmitted Diseases	Uncomplicated Gonorrhea	800 mg	single dose	1 day	800 mg
Prostatitis	Acute or Chronic	400 mg	q12h	28 days	800 mg

Renal
Interstitial nephritis, renal failure

Nervous System/Psychiatric
Peripheral neuropathy, Guillain-Barré syndrome, ataxia, paresthesia; psychic disturbances including psychotic reactions and confusion

Musculoskeletal
Tendinitis, tendon rupture, possible exacerbation of myasthenia gravis

Hematologic
Neutropenia, leukopenia, hemolytic anemia, sometimes associated with glucose-6-phosphate dehydrogenase deficiency; thrombocytopenia

Special Senses
Transient hearing loss (rare), tinnitus, diplopia

Other adverse events reported with quinolones include: agranulocytosis, albuminuria, candiduria, crystalluria, cylindruria, dysphagia, elevation of blood glucose, elevation of serum cholesterol, elevation of serum potassium, elevation of serum triglycerides, hematuria, hepatic necrosis, symptomatic hypoglycemia, nystagmus, postural hypotension, prolongation of prothrombin time, and vaginal candidiasis.

OVERDOSAGE

No significant lethality was observed in male and female mice and rats at single oral doses up to 4 g/kg.
In the event of acute overdosage, the stomach should be emptied by inducing vomiting or by gastric lavage, and the patient carefully observed and given symptomatic and supportive treatment. Adequate hydration must be maintained.

DOSAGE AND ADMINISTRATION

Tablets NOROXIN should be taken at least one hour before or at least two hours after a meal or milk ingestion. Tablets NOROXIN should be taken with a glass of water. Patients receiving NOROXIN should be well hydrated (see PRECAUTIONS).

Normal Renal Function
The recommended daily dose of NOROXIN is as described in the following chart:
[See table above.]

Renal Impairment
NOROXIN may be used for the treatment of urinary tract infections in patients with renal insufficiency. In patients with a creatinine clearance rate of 30 mL/min/1.73m² or less, the recommended dosage is one 400-mg tablet once daily for the duration given above. At this dosage, the urinary concentration exceeds the MICs for most urinary pathogens susceptible to norfloxacin, even when the creatinine clearance is less than 10 mL/min/1.73m².
When only the serum creatinine level is available, the following formula (based on sex, weight, and age of the patient) may be used to convert this value into creatinine clearance. The serum creatinine should represent a steady state of renal function.

Males:

$$\frac{\text{(weight in kg)} \times (140 - \text{age})}{(72) \times \text{serum creatinine (mg/100 mL)}}$$

Females: $(0.85) \times$ (above value)

Elderly
Elderly patients being treated for urinary tract infections who have a creatinine clearance of greater than 30 mL/min/1.73m² should receive the dosages recommended under *Normal Renal Function.*
Elderly patients being treated for urinary tract infections who have a creatinine clearance of 30 mL/min/1.73m² or less should receive 400 mg once daily as recommended under *Renal Impairment.*

HOW SUPPLIED

No. 3522—Tablets NOROXIN 400 mg are dark pink, oval shaped, film-coated tablets, coded MSD 705 on one side and NOROXIN on the other. They are supplied as follows:
NDC 54092-097-01 bottles of 100
(6505-01-258-9542 100's)
NDC 54092-097-20 unit of use bottles of 20
NDC 54092-097-52 unit dose packages of 100.
Shown in Product Identification Guide, page 325
Storage
Tablets NOROXIN should be stored in a tightly-closed container. Avoid storage at temperatures above 40°C (104°F).

ANIMAL PHARMACOLOGY

Norfloxacin and related drugs have been shown to cause arthropathy in immature animals of most species tested (see WARNINGS).
Crystalluria has occurred in laboratory animals tested with norfloxacin. In dogs, needle-shaped drug crystals were seen in the urine at doses of 50 mg/kg/day. In rats, crystals were reported following doses of 200 mg/kg/day.
Embryo lethality and slight maternotoxicity (vomiting and anorexia) were observed in cynomolgus monkeys at doses of 150 mg/kg/day or higher.
Ocular toxicity, seen with some related drugs, was not observed in any norfloxacin-treated animals.

7898525   Issued November 1995

PedvaxHIB®   ℞
[Haemophilus b Conjugate Vaccine
(Meningococcal Protein Conjugate)]

DESCRIPTION

PedvaxHIB* [Haemophilus b Conjugate Vaccine (Meningococcal Protein Conjugate)] is a highly purified capsular polysaccharide (polyribosylribitol phosphate or PRP) of *Haemophilus influenzae* type b (Haemophilus b, Ross strain) that is covalently bound to an outer membrane protein complex (OMPC) of the B11 strain of *Neisseria meningitidis* serogroup B. The covalent bonding of the PRP to the OMPC which is necessary for enhanced immunogenicity of the PRP is confirmed by analysis of the conjugate's components by chemical treatment which yields a unique amino acid. This PRP-OMPC conjugate vaccine is a lyophilized preparation containing lactose as a stabilizer.
PedvaxHIB, when reconstituted as directed, is a sterile suspension for intramuscular use formulated to contain: 15 mcg of Haemophilus b PRP, 250 mcg of *Neisseria meningitidis* OMPC, 225 mcg of aluminum as aluminum hydroxide, thimerosal (a mercury derivative) at 1:20,000 as a preservative, and 2.0 mg of lactose, in 0.9% sodium chloride.

* Registered trademark of MERCK & CO., INC.

CLINICAL PHARMACOLOGY

Haemophilus influenzae type b (Haemophilus b) is the most frequent cause of bacterial meningitis and a leading cause of serious, systemic bacterial disease in young children worldwide.
Haemophilus b disease occurs primarily in children under 5 years of age and in the United States prior to the initiation of a vaccine program was estimated to account for nearly 20,000 cases of invasive infections annually, approximately 12,000 of which are meningitis. The mortality rate from Haemophilus b meningitis is about 5%. In addition, up to 35% of survivors develop neurologic sequelae including seizures, deafness, and mental retardation. Other invasive diseases caused by this bacterium include cellulitis, epiglottitis,

sepsis, pneumonia, septic arthritis, osteomyelitis and pericarditis.
It has been estimated that 17% of all cases of Haemophilus b disease occur in infants less than 6 months of age. The peak incidence of Haemophilus b meningitis occurs between 6 to 11 months of age. Forty-seven percent of all cases occur by one year of age with the remaining 53% of cases occurring over the next four years.
Among children under 5 years of age, the risk of invasive Haemophilus b disease is further increased in certain populations including the following:
● Daycare attendees
● Lower socio-economic groups
● Blacks (especially those who lack the Km(1) immunoglobulin allotype)
● Caucasians who lack the G2m(n or 23) immunoglobulin allotype
● Native Americans
● Household contacts of cases
● Individuals with asplenia, sickle cell disease, or antibody deficiency syndromes
An important virulence factor of the Haemophilus b bacterium is its polysaccharide capsule (PRP). Antibody to PRP (anti-PRP) has been shown to correlate with protection against Haemophilus b disease. While the anti-PRP level associated with protection using conjugated vaccines has not yet been determined, the level of anti-PRP associated with protection in studies using bacterial polysaccharide immune globulin or nonconjugated PRP vaccines ranged from ≥ 0.15 to ≥ 1.0 mcg/mL.
Nonconjugated PRP vaccines are capable of stimulating B-lymphocytes to produce antibody without the help of T-lymphocytes (T-independent). The responses to many other antigens are augmented by helper T-lymphocytes (T-dependent). PedvaxHIB is a PRP-conjugate vaccine in which the PRP is covalently bound to the OMPC carrier producing an antigen which is postulated to convert the T-independent antigen (PRP alone) into a T-dependent antigen resulting in both an enhanced antibody response and immunologic memory.
Clinical Evaluation of PedvaxHIB
The protective efficacy, safety, and antibody responses to PedvaxHIB were evaluated in 3,486 Native American (Navajo) infants who completed the primary two-dose regimen in a randomized, double-blind, placebo-controlled study (The Protective Efficacy Study). This population has a much higher incidence of Haemophilus b disease than the United States population as a whole and also has a lower antibody response to Haemophilus b conjugate vaccines, including PedvaxHIB.
Each infant in this study received two doses of either placebo or PedvaxHIB with the first dose administered at a mean of 8 weeks of age and the second administered approximately two months later; DTP and OPV were administered concomitantly. Antibody levels were measured in a subset of each group (Table 1).
[See table at top of next page.]
In this study, 22 cases of invasive Haemophilus b disease occurred in the placebo group (8 cases after the first dose and 14 cases after the second dose) and only 1 case in the vaccine group (none after the first dose and 1 after the second dose). Following the recommended two-dose regimen, the protective efficacy of PedvaxHIB was calculated to be 93% with a 95% confidence interval of 57%–98% (p = 0.001, two-tailed). In the two months between the first and second doses, the difference in number of cases of disease between placebo and vaccine recipients (8 vs 0 cases, respectively) was statistically significant (p = 0.008, two-tailed); however, a primary two-dose regimen is required for infants 2–14 months of age. A subset of 1,368 infants from this study was followed to 15 months of age with no additional cases of invasive Haemophilus b disease occurring after the primary two-dose regimen of PedvaxHIB (see DOSAGE AND ADMINISTRATION, including *Booster Dose*).
Since protective efficacy with PedvaxHIB was demonstrated in such a high risk population, it would be expected to be predictive of efficacy in other populations.
The safety and immunogenicity of PedvaxHIB were evaluated in infants and children in other clinical studies that were conducted in various locations throughout the United States. PedvaxHIB was highly immunogenic in all age groups studied.
Antibody responses from these clinical studies (excluding Native Americans) are shown in Table 2. These data were derived by evaluating the sera in one laboratory using a radioimmunoassay which correlated with both the Finnish National Public Health Institute assay and that recommended by the Center for Biologics Evaluation and Research of the FDA (Table 1, Table 2).

Continued on next page

Information on the Merck & Co., Inc. products listed on these pages is the full prescribing information from product circulars in use September 30, 1996.

Merck & Co.—Cont.

Since the magnitude of initial antibody response is lower among younger infants, a booster dose is required in infants who complete the primary two-dose regimen before 12 months of age (see Table 1 and DOSAGE AND ADMINISTRATION). [See table 2 at right.]

Antibodies to the OMPC of *N. meningitidis* (see DESCRIPTION) have been demonstrated in vaccinee sera but the clinical relevance of these antibodies has not been established. In a multicenter study of immunogenicity and safety in different subpopulations in the United States, antibody responses to PedvaxHIB were evaluated in infants initially vaccinated between the ages of 2 and 3 months (Table 3). [See table at top of next page.]

PedvaxHIB induced antibody levels greater than 1.0 mcg/mL in children who were poor responders to nonconjugated PRP vaccines. In a study involving such a subpopulation 34 children ranging in age from 27 to 61 months who developed invasive Haemophilus b disease despite previous vaccination with nonconjugated PRP vaccines were randomly assigned to 2 groups. One group (n = 14) was immunized with PedvaxHIB and the other group (n = 20) with a nonconjugated PRP vaccine at a mean interval of approximately 12 months after recovery from disease. All 14 children immunized with PedvaxHIB but only 6 of 20 children re-immunized with a nonconjugated PRP vaccine achieved an antibody level of > 1.0 mcg/mL. The 14 children who had not responded to revaccination with the nonconjugated PRP vaccine were then immunized with a single dose of PedvaxHIB; following this vaccination, all achieved antibody levels of > 1.0 mcg/mL. In addition, PedvaxHIB has been studied in children at high risk of Haemophilus b disease because of genetically-related deficiencies [Blacks who were Km(1) allotype negative and Caucasians who were G2m(23) allotype negative] and are considered hyporesponsive to nonconjugated PRP vaccines on this basis. The hyporesponsive children had anti-PRP responses comparable to those of allotype positive children of similar age range when vaccinated with PedvaxHIB. All children achieved anti-PRP levels of > 1.0 mcg/mL.

INDICATIONS AND USAGE

PedvaxHIB is indicated for routine immunization against invasive disease caused by *Haemophilus influenzae* type b in infants and children 2 to 71 months of age.

PedvaxHIB will not protect against disease caused by *Haemophilus influenzae* other than type b or against other microorganisms that cause invasive disease such as meningitis or sepsis.

Revaccination
Infants completing the primary two-dose regimen before 12 months of age should receive a booster dose (see DOSAGE AND ADMINISTRATION).

Use with Other Vaccines
Studies have been conducted in which PedvaxHIB has been administered concomitantly with the primary vaccination series of DTP and OPV, or concomitantly with M-M-R* II (Measles, Mumps, and Rubella Virus Vaccine Live) (using separate sites and syringes) or with a booster dose of OPV plus DTP (using separate sites and syringes for PedvaxHIB and DTP). No impairment of immune response to individual tested vaccine antigens was demonstrated. The type, frequency and severity of adverse experiences observed in these studies with PedvaxHIB were similar to those seen when the other vaccines were given alone.

PedvaxHIB IS NOT RECOMMENDED FOR USE IN INFANTS YOUNGER THAN 2 MONTHS OF AGE.

---

*Registered trademark of MERCK & CO., INC.

CONTRAINDICATIONS

Hypersensitivity to any component of the vaccine or the diluent.

WARNINGS

USE ONLY THE ALUMINUM HYDROXIDE DILUENT SUPPLIED.

If PedvaxHIB is used in persons with malignancies or those receiving immunosuppressive therapy or who are otherwise immunocompromised, the expected immune response may not be obtained.

PRECAUTIONS

General
As for any vaccine, adequate treatment provisions, including epinephrine, should be available for immediate use should an anaphylactoid reaction occur.

As with other vaccines, PedvaxHIB may not induce protective antibody levels immediately following vaccination.

As with any vaccine, vaccination with PedvaxHIB may not result in a protective antibody response in all individuals given the vaccine.

As reported with Haemophilus b Polysaccharide Vaccine and another Haemophilus b Conjugate Vaccine, cases of Haemophilus b disease may occur in the week after vaccination, prior to the onset of the protective effects of the vaccines.

There is insufficient evidence that PedvaxHIB given immediately after exposure to natural *Haemophilus influenzae* type b will prevent illness.

Any acute infection or febrile illness is reason for delaying use of PedvaxHIB except when in the opinion of the physician, withholding the vaccine entails a greater risk.

Laboratory Test Interactions
Sensitive tests (e.g., Latex Agglutination Kits) may detect PRP derived from the vaccine in urine of some vaccinees for at least 30 days following vaccination with PedvaxHIB; in clinical studies with PedvaxHIB, such children demonstrated normal immune response to the vaccine.

Carcinogenesis, Mutagenesis, and Impairment of Fertility
PedvaxHIB has not been evaluated for its carcinogenic or mutagenic potential, or its potential to impair fertility.

Pregnancy
Pregnancy Category C: Animal reproduction studies have not been conducted with PedvaxHIB. It is also not known whether PedvaxHIB can cause fetal harm when administered to a pregnant woman or can affect reproductive capacity. PedvaxHIB is not recommended for use in a pregnant woman.

ADVERSE REACTIONS

In early clinical studies involving the administration of 8,086 doses of PedvaxHIB alone to 5,027 healthy infants and children 2 months to 71 months of age, PedvaxHIB was generally well tolerated. No serious adverse reactions were reported.

During a two-day period following vaccination with PedvaxHIB in a subset of these infants and children, the most frequently reported adverse reactions, excluding those shown in Table 4, in decreasing order of frequency included irritability, sleepiness, respiratory infection/symptoms and ear infection/otitis media. Urticaria was reported in two children. Thrombocytopenia was seen in one child. A cause and effect relationship between these side effects and the vaccination has not been established.

Selected objective observations reported by parents over a 48-hour period in infants and children 2 to 71 months of age

following primary vaccination with PedvaxHIB alone are summarized in Table 4.

In The Protective Efficacy Study (see CLINICAL PHARMACOLOGY), 4,459 healthy Navajo infants 6 to 12 weeks of age received PedvaxHIB or placebo. Most of these infants received DTP/OPV concomitantly. No differences were seen in the type and frequency of serious health problems expected in this Navajo population or in serious adverse experiences reported among those who received PedvaxHIB and those who received placebo, and none was reported to be related to PedvaxHIB. Only one serious reaction (tracheitis) was reported as possibly related to PedvaxHIB and only one (diarrhea) as possibly related to placebo. Seizures occurred infrequently in both groups (9 occurred in vaccine recipients, 8 of whom also received DTP; 8 occurred in placebo recipients, 7 of whom also received DTP) and were not reported to be related to PedvaxHIB. The frequencies of fever and local reactions occurring in a subset of these infants during a 48-hour period following each dose were similar to those seen in early clinical studies (Table 4).

[See table 4 on next page.]

As with any vaccine, there is the possibility that broad use of PedvaxHIB could reveal adverse reactions not observed in clinical trials. The following additional adverse reactions have been reported with use of the marketed vaccine:

Hemic and Lymphatic System
Lymphadenopathy.
Nervous System
Febrile seizures.
Skin
Sterile injection site abscess; pain at the injection site.
Potential Adverse Reactions
The use of Haemophilus b Polysaccharide Vaccines and another Haemophilus b Conjugate Vaccine has been associated with the following additional adverse effects: early onset Haemophilus b disease and Guillain-Barré syndrome. A cause and effect relationship between these side effects and the vaccination was not established.

DOSAGE AND ADMINISTRATION

FOR INTRAMUSCULAR ADMINISTRATION
DO NOT INJECT INTRAVENOUSLY

2 to 14 Months of Age
Infants 2 to 14 months of age should receive a 0.5 mL dose of vaccine ideally beginning at 2 months of age followed by a 0.5 mL dose 2 months later (or as soon as possible thereafter). When the primary two-dose regimen is completed before 12 months of age, a booster dose is required (see below and Table 5).

TABLE 1
Antibody Responses in Navajo Infants

Vaccine	No. of Subjects	Time	% Subjects with > 0.15 mcg/mL	> 1.0 mcg/mL	Anti-PRP GMT (mcg/mL)
PedvaxHIB*	416†	Pre-Vaccination	44	10	0.16
	416	Dose 1	88	52	0.95
	416	Dose 2	91	60	1.43
Placebo*	461†	Pre-Vaccination	44	9	0.16
	461	Dose 1	21	2	0.09
	461	Dose 2	14	1	0.08
PedvaxHIB	27**	Prebooster	70	33	0.51
	27	Postbooster***	100	89	8.39

* Post vaccination values obtained approximately 1–3 months after each dose.
† The Protective Efficacy Study.
** Immunogenicity Trial.
*** Booster given at 12 months of age; post vaccination values obtained 1 month after administration of booster dose.

TABLE 2
Antibody Responses* to PedvaxHIB in Other Clinical Studies

Age (Months)	Time	No. of Subjects	% Subjects Responding with > 0.15 mcg/mL	> 1.0 mcg/mL	Post-Vaccination Anti-PRP GMT (mcg/mL)
2–3	Dose 1**	113	97	81	2.48
	Dose 2***	113	98	88	4.60
4–14	Dose 1**	252	98	75	2.53
	Dose 2***	252	100	92	6.04
15–17	Single Dose***	59	100	83	3.11
18–23	Single Dose***	59	98	97	7.43
24–71	Dose ***	52	98	92	10.55

* Only subjects with prevaccination anti-PRP ≤ 0.15 mcg/mL are included in this table (excluding native Americans).
** Two months post vaccination.
*** One month post vaccination.

TABLE 3
Antibody Responses* After Two Doses of PedvaxHIB Among Infants Initially Vaccinated at 2–3 Months of Age By Racial/Ethnic Group

Racial/Ethnic Groups	No. of Subjects	% With Anti-PRP		GMT (mcg/mL)
		> 0.15 mcg/mL	> 1.0 mcg/mL	
Native American†	44	95	68	2.24
Caucasian	155	99	85	4.00
Hispanic	16	100	94	4.60
Black	18	100	94	8.57

† Apache and Navajo
* One month after the second dose

TABLE 4
Fever or Local Reactions in Subjects 2 to 71 Months of Age Vaccinated with PedvaxHIB Alone Other Clinical Studies

Age (Months)	Reaction	No. of Subjects Evaluated	Dose 1 6 hr	24	48	No. of Subjects Evaluated	Dose 2 6 hr	24	48
				Percentage					
2–14*	Fever > 38.3°C (101°F) Rectal	532	2.4	3.8	1.9	329	3.0	4.3	3.6
	Erythema > 2.5 cm diameter	1026	0.2	1.0	0.4	585	0.9	1.2	0.7
	Swelling/ Induration > 2.5 cm diameter	1026	0.6	1.5	1.6	585	0.9	2.8	3.7
15–71**	Fever > 38.3°C (101°F) Rectal	149	4.0	4.0	6.7				
	Erythema > 2.5 cm diameter	572	0.0	0.3	0.2				
	Swelling/ Induration > 2.5 cm diameter	572	0.9	2.1	1.4				

*Additional complaints reported following vaccination with the first and second dose of PedvaxHIB, respectively, in the indicated number of subjects were: nausea, vomiting and/or diarrhea (101, 41), crying for more than one-half hour (43, 15), rash (16, 17), and unusual high-pitched crying (4, 4).

**Additional complaints reported following vaccination with 1 dose of PedvaxHIB in the indicated number of subjects were: nausea, vomiting and/or diarrhea (44), crying for more than one-half hour (19), rash (12), and unusual high-pitched crying (0).

15 Months of Age and Older
Children 15 months of age and older previously unvaccinated against Haemophilus b disease should receive a single 0.5 mL dose of vaccine.

Booster Dose
In infants completing the primary two-dose regimen before 12 months of age, a booster dose (0.5 mL) should be administered at 12 to 15 months of age but not earlier than 2 months after the second dose.

DATA ARE NOT AVAILABLE REGARDING THE INTERCHANGEABILITY OF OTHER HAEMOPHILUS b CONJUGATE VACCINES AND PedvaxHIB.

Vaccination regimens by age group are outlined in Table 5.

TABLE 5
(see circular text above for details)

Age (Months) at First Dose	Primary	Age (Months) at Booster Dose
2–10	2 doses, 2 mo. apart	12–15
11–14	2 doses, 2 mo. apart	—
15–71	1 dose	—

TO RECONSTITUTE, USE ONLY THE ALUMINUM HYDROXIDE DILUENT SUPPLIED.
First, agitate the diluent vial, then, using sterile technique, withdraw the entire volume of aluminum hydroxide diluent into the syringe to be used for reconstitution. Inject all the aluminum hydroxide diluent in the syringe into the vial of lyophilized vaccine, and agitate to mix thoroughly.

Withdraw the entire contents into the syringe and inject the total volume of reconstituted vaccine (0.5 mL) intramuscularly, preferably into the anterolateral thigh or the outer aspect of the upper arm.

It is recommended that the vaccine be used as soon as possible after reconstitution. Store reconstituted vaccine in the vaccine vial at 2–8°C (36–46°F) and discard if not used with 24 hours. Agitate prior to injection.

Parenteral drug products should be inspected visually for extraneous particulate matter and discoloration prior to administration whenever solution and container permit. Aluminum hydroxide diluent and PedvaxHIB when reconstituted are slightly opaque white suspensions; the flocculated appearance of reconstituted PedvaxHIB does not affect the usability of the vaccine.

Special care should be taken to ensure that the injection does not enter a blood vessel.

It is important to use a separate sterile syringe and needle for each patient to prevent transmission of hepatitis B or other infectious agents from one person to another.

HOW SUPPLIED
No. 4792—PedvaxHIB is supplied as a single-dose vial of lyophilized vaccine, **NDC** 0006-4792-00, and a vial of aluminum hydroxide diluent.

No. 4797—PedvaxHIB is supplied as follows: a box of 5 single-dose vials of lyophilized vaccine, **NDC** 0006-4797-00, and 5 vials of aluminum hydroxide diluent.

Storage
Before reconstitution, store the vial of lyophilized vaccine and the vial of the aluminum hydroxide diluent at 2–8°C (36–46°F).

Store reconstituted vaccine in the vaccine vial at 2–8°C (36–46°F) and discard if not used within 24 hours.
DO NOT FREEZE the aluminum hydroxide diluent or the reconstituted vaccine.
7611809   Issued November 1995
COPYRIGHT © MERCK & CO., INC., 1990
All rights reserved

PEPCID® Tablets ℞
(Famotidine), U.S.P.
PEPCID® ℞
(Famotidine) for Oral Suspension

DESCRIPTION

The active ingredient in PEPCID* (Famotidine), is a histamine H_2-receptor antagonist. Famotidine is N'-(aminosulfonyl) -3- [[[2-[(diaminomethylene)amino] -4- thiazolyl]methyl]thio]propanimidamide. The empirical formula of famotidine is $C_8H_{15}N_7O_2S_3$ and its molecular weight is 337.43. Its structural formula is:

Famotidine is a white to pale yellow crystalline compound that is freely soluble in glacial acetic acid, slightly soluble in methanol, very slightly soluble in water, and practically insoluble in ethanol.

Each tablet for oral administration contains either 20 mg or 40 mg of famotidine and the following inactive ingredients: hydroxypropyl cellulose, hydroxypropyl methylcellulose, iron oxides, magnesium stearate, microcrystalline cellulose, corn starch, talc, titanium dioxide.

Each 5 mL of the oral suspension when prepared as directed contains 40 mg of famotidine and the following inactive ingredients: citric acid, flavors, microcrystalline cellulose and carboxymethylcellulose sodium, sucrose and xanthan gum. Added as preservatives are sodium benzoate 0.1%, sodium methylparaben 0.1%, and sodium propylparaben 0.02%.

*Registered trademark of MERCK & CO., INC.

CLINICAL PHARMACOLOGY

GI Effects
PEPCID is a competitive inhibitor of histamine H_2-receptors. The primary clinically important pharmacologic activity of PEPCID is inhibition of gastric secretion. Both the acid concentration and volume of gastric secretion are suppressed by PEPCID, while changes in pepsin secretion are proportional to volume output.

In normal volunteers and hypersecretors, PEPCID inhibited basal and nocturnal gastric secretion, as well as secretion stimulated by food and pentagastrin. After oral administration, the onset of the antisecretory effect occurred within one hour; the maximum effect was dose-dependent, occurring within one to three hours. Duration of inhibition of secretion by doses of 20 and 40 mg was 10 to 12 hours.

Single evening oral doses of 20 and 40 mg inhibited basal and nocturnal acid secretion in all subjects; mean nocturnal gastric acid secretion was inhibited by 86% and 94%, respectively, for a period of at least 10 hours. The same doses given in the morning suppressed food-stimulated acid secretion in all subjects. The mean suppression was 76% and 84% respectively 3 to 5 hours after administration, and 25% and 30% respectively 8 to 10 hours after administration. In some subjects who received the 20 mg dose, however, the antisecretory effect was dissipated within 6–8 hours. There was no cumulative effect with repeated doses. The nocturnal intragastric pH was raised by evening doses of 20 and 40 mg of PEPCID to mean values of 5.0 and 6.4, respectively. When PEPCID was given after breakfast, the basal daytime interdigestive pH at 3 and 8 hours after 20 or 40 mg of PEPCID was raised to about 5.

PEPCID had little or no effect on fasting or postprandial serum gastrin levels. Gastric emptying and exocrine pancreatic function were not affected by PEPCID.

Other Effects
Systemic effects of PEPCID in the CNS, cardiovascular, respiratory or endocrine systems were not noted in clinical pharmacology studies. Also, no antiandrogenic effects were noted. (See ADVERSE REACTIONS.) Serum hormone levels, including prolactin, cortisol, thyroxine (T_4), and testosterone, were not altered after treatment with PEPCID.

Continued on next page

Merck & Co.—Cont.

Pharmacokinetics
PEPCID is incompletely absorbed. The bioavailability of oral doses is 40–45%. PEPCID Tablets and PEPCID Oral Suspension are bioequivalent. Bioavailability may be slightly increased by food, or slightly decreased by antacids; however, these effects are of no clinical consequence. PEPCID undergoes minimal first-pass metabolism. After oral doses, peak plasma levels occur in 1–3 hours. Plasma levels after multiple doses are similar to those after single doses. Fifteen to 20% of PEPCID in plasma is protein bound. PEPCID has an elimination half-life of 2.5–3.5 hours. PEPCID is eliminated by renal (65–70%) and metabolic (30–35%) routes. Renal clearance is 250–450 mL/min, indicating some tubular excretion. Twenty-five to 30% of an oral dose and 65–70% of an intravenous dose are recovered in the urine as unchanged compound. The only metabolite identified in man is the S-oxide.

There is a close relationship between creatinine clearance values and the elimination half-life of PEPCID. In patients with severe renal insufficiency, i.e., creatinine clearance less than 10 mL/min, the elimination half-life of PEPCID may exceed 20 hours and adjustment of dose or dosing intervals may be necessary (see PRECAUTIONS, DOSAGE AND ADMINISTRATION).

In elderly patients, there are no clinically significant age-related changes in the pharmacokinetics of PEPCID.

Clinical Studies
Duodenal Ulcer
In a U.S. multicenter, double-blind study in outpatients with endoscopically confirmed duodenal ulcer, orally administered PEPCID was compared to placebo. As shown in Table 1, 70% of patients treated with PEPCID 40 mg h.s. were healed by week 4.

Table 1
Outpatients with Endoscopically
Confirmed Healed Duodenal Ulcers

	PEPCID 40 mg h.s. (N=89)	PEPCID 20 mg b.i.d. (N=84)	Placebo h.s. (N=97)
Week 2	*32%	*38%	17%
Week 4	*70%	*67%	31%

* Statistically significantly different than placebo (p < 0.001)
Patients not healed by week 4 were continued in the study. By week 8, 83% of patients treated with PEPCID had healed versus 45% of patients treated with placebo. The incidence of ulcer healing with PEPCID was significantly higher than with placebo at each time point based on proportion of endoscopically confirmed healed ulcers.

In this study, time to relief of daytime and nocturnal pain was significantly shorter for patients receiving PEPCID than for patients receiving placebo; patients receiving PEPCID also took less antacid than the patients receiving placebo.

Long-Term Maintenance
Treatment of Duodenal Ulcers
PEPCID, 20 mg p.o. h.s. was compared to placebo h.s. as maintenance therapy in two double-blind, multicenter studies of patients with endoscopically confirmed healed duodenal ulcers. In the U.S. study the observed ulcer incidence within 12 months in patients treated with placebo was 2.4 times greater than in the patients treated with PEPCID. The 89 patients treated with PEPCID had a cumulative observed ulcer incidence of 23.4% compared to an observed ulcer incidence of 56.6% in the 89 patients receiving placebo (p < 0.01). These results were confirmed in an international study where the cumulative observed ulcer incidence within 12 months in the 307 patients treated with PEPCID was 35.7%, compared to an incidence of 75.5% in the 325 patients treated with placebo (p < 0.01).

Gastric Ulcer
In both a U.S. and an international multicenter, double-blind study in patients with endoscopically confirmed active benign gastric ulcer, orally administered PEPCID, 40 mg h.s., was compared to placebo h.s. Antacids were permitted during the studies, but consumption was not significantly different between the PEPCID and placebo groups. As shown in Table 2, the incidence of ulcer healing (dropouts counted as unhealed) with PEPCID was statistically significantly better than placebo at weeks 6 and 8 in the U.S. study, and at weeks 4, 6 and 8 in the international study, based on the number of ulcers that healed, confirmed by endoscopy.

Table 2
Patients with Endoscopically
Confirmed Healed Gastric Ulcers

	U.S. Study PEPCID 40 mg h.s. (N=74)	U.S. Study Placebo h.s. (N=75)	International Study PEPCID 40 mg h.s. (N=149)	International Study Placebo h.s. (N=145)
Week 4	45%	39%	**47%	31%
Week 6	**66%	44%	**65%	46%
Week 8	*78%	64%	**80%	54%

*,** Statistically significantly better than placebo (p ≤ 0.05, p ≤ 0.01 respectively)

Time to complete relief of daytime and nighttime pain was statistically significantly shorter for patients receiving PEPCID than for patients receiving placebo; however, in neither study was there a statistically significant difference in the proportion of patients whose pain was relieved by the end of the study (week 8).

Gastroesophageal Reflux Disease (GERD)
Orally administered PEPCID was compared to placebo in a U.S. study that enrolled patients with symptoms of GERD and without endoscopic evidence of erosion or ulceration of the esophagus. PEPCID 20 mg b.i.d. was statistically significantly superior to 40 mg h.s. and to placebo in providing a successful symptomatic outcome, defined as moderate or excellent improvement of symptoms (Table 3).

Table 3
% Successful Symptomatic Outcome

	PEPCID 20 mg b.i.d. (N=154)	PEPCID 40 mg h.s. (N=149)	Placebo (N=73)
Week 6	82**	69	62

** p ≤ 0.01) vs Placebo

By two weeks of treatment, symptomatic success was observed in a greater percentage of patients taking PEPCID 20 mg b.i.d. compared to placebo (p ≤ 0.01).
Symptomatic improvement and healing of endoscopically verified erosion and ulceration were studied in two additional trials. Healing was defined as complete resolution of all erosions or ulcerations visible with endoscopy. The U.S. study comparing PEPCID 40 mg p.o. b.i.d. to placebo and PEPCID 20 mg p.o. b.i.d. showed a significantly greater percentage of healing for PEPCID 40 mg b.i.d. at weeks 6 and 12 (Table 4).

Table 4
% Endoscopic Healing—U.S. Study

	PEPCID 40 mg b.i.d. (N=127)	PEPCID 20 mg b.i.d. (N=125)	Placebo (N=66)
Week 6	48**,++	32	18
Week 12	69**,+	54**	29

** p ≤ 0.01 vs Placebo
+ p ≤ 0.05 vs PEPCID 20 mg b.i.d.
++ p ≤ 0.01 vs PEPCID 20 mg b.i.d.

As compared to placebo, patients who received PEPCID had faster relief of daytime and nighttime heartburn and a greater percentage of patients experienced complete relief of nighttime heartburn. These differences were statistically significant.
In the international study, when PEPCID 40 mg p.o. b.i.d. was compared to ranitidine 150 mg p.o. b.i.d., a statistically significantly greater percentage of healing was observed with PEPCID 40 mg b.i.d. at week 12 (Table 5). There was, however, no significant difference among treatments in symptom relief.

Table 5
% Endoscopic Healing—International Study

	PEPCID 40 mg b.i.d. (N=175)	PEPCID 20 mg b.i.d. (N=93)	Ranitidine 150 mg b.i.d. (N=172)
Week 6	48	52	42
Week 12	71*	68	60

* p ≤ 0.05 vs Ranitidine 150 mg b.i.d.

Pathological Hypersecretory Conditions (e.g., Zollinger-Ellison Syndrome, Multiple Endocrine Adenomas)
In studies of patients with pathological hypersecretory conditions such as Zollinger-Ellison Syndrome with or without multiple endocrine adenomas, PEPCID significantly inhibited gastric acid secretion and controlled associated symptoms. Orally administered doses from 20 to 160 mg q 6 h maintained basal acid secretion below 10 mEq/hr; initial doses were titrated to the individual patient need and subsequent adjustments were necessary with time in some patients. PEPCID was well tolerated at these high dose levels for prolonged periods (greater than 12 months) in eight patients, and there were no cases reported of gynecomastia, increased prolactin levels, or impotence which were considered to be due to the drug.

INDICATIONS AND USAGE

PEPCID is indicated in:
1. *Short term treatment of active duodenal ulcer.* Most patients heal within 4 weeks; there is rarely reason to use PEPCID at full dosage for longer than 6 to 8 weeks. Studies have not assessed the safety of famotidine in uncomplicated active duodenal ulcer for periods of more than eight weeks.
2. *Maintenance therapy for duodenal ulcer patients at reduced dosage after healing of an active ulcer.* Controlled studies have not extended beyond one year.
3. *Short term treatment of active benign gastric ulcer.* Most patients heal within 6 weeks. Studies have not assessed

the safety or efficacy of famotidine in uncomplicated active benign gastric ulcer for periods of more than 8 weeks.
4. *Short term treatment of gastroesophageal reflux disease (GERD).* PEPCID is indicated for short term treatment of patients with symptoms of GERD (see CLINICAL PHARMACOLOGY, *Clinical Studies*).
   PEPCID is also indicated for the short term treatment of esophagitis due to GERD including erosive or ulcerative disease diagnosed by endoscopy (see CLINICAL PHARMACOLOGY, *Clinical Studies*).
5. *Treatment of pathological hypersecretory conditions (e.g., Zollinger-Ellison Syndrome, multiple endocrine adenomas).*

CONTRAINDICATIONS

Hypersensitivity to any component of these products.

PRECAUTIONS

General
Symptomatic response to therapy with PEPCID does not preclude the presence of gastric malignancy.
Patients with Severe Renal Insufficiency
Longer intervals between doses or lower doses may need to be used in patients with severe renal insufficiency (creatinine clearance < 10 mL/min) to adjust for the longer elimination half-life of famotidine. (See CLINICAL PHARMACOLOGY and DOSAGE AND ADMINISTRATION.) However, currently, no drug-related toxicity has been found with high plasma concentrations of famotidine.
Information for Patients
The patient should be instructed to shake the oral suspension vigorously for 5–10 seconds prior to each use. Unused constituted oral suspension should be discarded after 30 days.
Drug Interactions
No drug interactions have been identified. Studies with famotidine in man, in animal models, and *in vitro* have shown no significant interference with the disposition of compounds metabolized by the hepatic microsomal enzymes, e.g., cytochrome P450 system. Compounds tested in man include warfarin, theophylline, phenytoin, diazepam, aminopyrine and antipyrine. Indocyanine green as an index of hepatic drug extraction has been tested and no significant effects have been found.
Carcinogenesis, Mutagenesis, Impairment of Fertility
In a 106 week study in rats and a 92 week study in mice given oral doses of up to 2000 mg/kg/day (approximately 2500 times the recommended human dose for active duodenal ulcer), there was no evidence of carcinogenic potential for PEPCID.
Famotidine was negative in the microbial mutagen test (Ames test) using *Salmonella typhimurium* and *Escherichia coli* with or without rat liver enzyme activation at concentrations up to 10,000 mcg/plate. In *in vivo* studies in mice, with a micronucleus test and a chromosomal aberration test, no evidence of a mutagenic effect was observed.
In studies with rats given oral doses of up to 2000 mg/kg/day or intravenous doses of up to 200 mg/kg/day, fertility and reproductive performance were not affected.
Pregnancy
Pregnancy Category B
Reproductive studies have been performed in rats and rabbits at oral doses of up to 2000 and 500 mg/kg/day respectively and in both species at I.V. doses of up to 200 mg/kg/day, and have revealed no significant evidence of impaired fertility or harm to the fetus due to PEPCID. While no direct fetotoxic effects have been observed, sporadic abortions occurring only in mothers displaying marked decreased food intake were seen in some rabbits at oral doses of 200 mg/kg/day (250 times the usual human dose) or higher. There are, however, no adequate or well-controlled studies in pregnant women. Because animal reproductive studies are not always predictive of human response, this drug should be used during pregnancy only if clearly needed.
Nursing Mothers
Studies performed in lactating rats have shown that famotidine is secreted into breast milk. Transient growth depression was observed in young rats suckling from mothers treated with maternotoxic doses of at least 600 times the usual human dose. Famotidine is detectable in human milk. Because of the potential for serious adverse reactions in nursing infants from PEPCID, a decision should be made whether to discontinue nursing or discontinue the drug, taking into account the importance of the drug to the mother.
Pediatric Use
Safety and effectiveness in children have not been established.
Use in Elderly Patients
No dosage adjustment is required based on age (see CLINICAL PHARMACOLOGY, *Pharmacokinetics*). Dosage adjustment in the case of severe renal impairment may be necessary.

ADVERSE REACTIONS

The adverse reactions listed below have been reported during domestic and international clinical trials in approximately 2500 patients. In those controlled clinical trials in which PEPCID Tablets were compared to placebo, the incidence of adverse experiences in the group which received PEPCID Tablets, 40 mg at bedtime, was similar to that in the placebo group.

The following adverse reactions have been reported to occur in more than 1% of patients on therapy with PEPCID in controlled clinical trials, and may be causally related to the drug: headache (4.7%), dizziness (1.3%), constipation (1.2%) and diarrhea (1.7%).

The following other adverse reactions have been reported infrequently in clinical trials or since the drug was marketed. The relationship to therapy with PEPCID has been unclear in many cases. Within each category the adverse reactions are listed in order of decreasing severity:

Body as a Whole: fever, asthenia, fatigue

Cardiovascular: arrhythmia, AV block, palpitation

Gastrointestinal: cholestatic jaundice, liver enzyme abnormalities, vomiting, nausea, abdominal discomfort, anorexia, dry mouth

Hematologic: rare cases of agranulocytosis, pancytopenia, leukopenia, thrombocytopenia

Hypersensitivity: anaphylaxis, angioedema, orbital or facial edema, urticaria, rash, conjunctival injection

Musculoskeletal: musculoskeletal pain including muscle cramps, arthralgia

Nervous System/Psychiatric: grand mal seizure; psychic disturbances, which were reversible in cases for which follow-up was obtained, including hallucinations, confusion, agitation, depression, anxiety, decreased libido; paresthesia; insomnia; somnolence

Respiratory: bronchospasm

Skin: toxic epidermal necrolysis (very rare), alopecia, acne, pruritus, dry skin, flushing

Special Senses: tinnitus, taste disorder

Other: rare cases of impotence and rare cases of gynecomastia have been reported; however, in controlled clinical trials, the incidences were not greater than those seen with placebo.

The adverse reactions reported for PEPCID Tablets may also occur with PEPCID for Oral Suspension.

OVERDOSAGE

There is no experience to date with deliberate overdosage. Oral doses of up to 640 mg/day have been given to patients with pathological hypersecretory conditions with no serious adverse effects. In the event of overdosage, treatment should be symptomatic and supportive. Unabsorbed material should be removed from the gastrointestinal tract, the patient should be monitored, and supportive therapy should be employed.

The oral LD_{50} of famotidine in male and female rats and mice was greater than 3000 mg/kg and the minimum lethal acute oral dose in dogs exceeded 2000 mg/kg. Famotidine did not produce overt effects at high oral doses in mice, rats, cats and dogs, but induced significant anorexia and growth depression in rabbits starting with 200 mg/kg/day orally. The intravenous LD_{50} of famotidine for mice and rats ranged from 254–563 mg/kg and the minimum lethal single I.V. dose in dogs was approximately 300 mg/kg. Signs of acute intoxication in I.V. treated dogs were emesis, restlessness, pallor of mucous membranes or redness of mouth and ears, hypotension, tachycardia and collapse.

DOSAGE AND ADMINISTRATION

Duodenal Ulcer

Acute Therapy: The recommended adult oral dosage for active duodenal ulcer is 40 mg once a day at bedtime. Most patients heal within 4 weeks; there is rarely reason to use PEPCID at full dosage for longer than 6 to 8 weeks. A regimen of 20 mg b.i.d. is also effective.

Maintenance Therapy: The recommended oral dose is 20 mg once a day at bedtime.

Benign Gastric Ulcer

Acute Therapy: The recommended adult oral dosage for active benign gastric ulcer is 40 mg once a day at bedtime.

Gastroesophageal Reflux Disease (GERD)

The recommended oral dosage for treatment of patients with symptoms of GERD is 20 mg b.i.d. for up to 6 weeks. The recommended oral dosage for the treatment of patients with esophagitis including erosions and ulcerations and accompanying symptoms due to GERD is 20 or 40 mg b.i.d. for up to 12 weeks (see CLINICAL PHARMACOLOGY, *Clinical Studies*).

Pathological Hypersecretory Conditions (e.g., Zollinger-Ellison Syndrome, Multiple Endocrine Adenomas)

The dosage of PEPCID in patients with pathological hypersecretory conditions varies with the individual patient. The recommended adult oral starting dose for pathological hypersecretory conditions is 20 mg q 6 h. In some patients, a higher starting dose may be required. Doses should be adjusted to individual patient needs and should continue as long as clinically indicated. Doses up to 160 mg q 6 h have been administered to some patients with severe Zollinger-Ellison Syndrome.

Oral Suspension

PEPCID Oral Suspension may be substituted for PEPCID Tablets in any of the above indications. Each five mL contains 40 mg of famotidine after constitution of the powder with 46 mL of Purified Water as directed.

Directions for Preparing PEPCID Oral Suspension

Prepare suspension at time of dispensing. Slowly add 46 mL of Purified Water. Shake vigorously for 5–10 seconds immediately after adding the water and immediately before use.

Stability of PEPCID Oral Suspension

Unused constituted oral suspension should be discarded after 30 days.

Concomitant Use of Antacids

Antacids may be given concomitantly if needed.

Dosage Adjustment for Patients with Severe Renal Insufficiency

In patients with severe renal insufficiency, i.e., with a creatinine clearance less than 10 mL/min, the elimination half-life of PEPCID may exceed 20 hours, reaching approximately 24 hours in anuric patients. Although no relationship of adverse effects to high plasma levels has been established, to avoid excess accumulation of the drug, the dose of PEPCID may be reduced to 20 mg h.s. or the dosing interval may be prolonged to 36–48 hours as indicated by the patient's clinical response.

HOW SUPPLIED

No. 3535—PEPCID Tablets, 20 mg, are beige colored, U-shaped, film-coated tablets coded MSD 963 on one side and PEPCID on the other. They are supplied as follows:

NDC 0006-0963-31 unit of use bottles of 30
(6505-01-260-0902, 20 mg 30's)
NDC 0006-0963-94 unit of use bottles of 90
NDC 0006-0963-58 unit of use bottles of 100
NDC 0006-0963-28 unit dose package of 100
NDC 0006-0963-82 bottles of 1,000
NDC 0006-0963-87 bottles of 10,000
NDC 0006-0963-72 carton of 25
UNIBLISTER™ cards of 31 tablets each.

Shown in Product Identification Guide, page 325

No. 3536—PEPCID Tablets, 40 mg, are light brownish-orange, U-shaped, film-coated tablets coded MSD 964 on one side and PEPCID on the other. They are supplied as follows:

NDC 0006-0964-31 unit of use bottles of 30
(6505-01-257-3164, 40 mg 30's)
NDC 0006-0964-94 unit of use bottles of 90
NDC 0006-0964-58 unit of use bottles of 100
NDC 0006-0964-28 unit dose package of 100
(6505-01-318-0464, 40 mg individually sealed 100's)
NDC 0006-0964-82 bottles of 1,000
NDC 0006-0964-87 bottles of 10,000
NDC 0006-0964-72 carton of 25
UNIBLISTER™ cards of 31 tablets each.

Shown in Product Identification Guide, page 325

No. 3538—Oral Suspension PEPCID is a white to off-white powder containing 400 mg of famotidine for constitution. When constituted as directed, PEPCID Oral Suspension is a smooth, mobile, off-white, homogeneous suspension with a cherry-banana-mint flavor, containing 40 mg of famotidine per 5 mL.

NDC 0006-3538-92, bottles containing 400 mg famotidine.

Storage

Avoid storage of PEPCID Tablets at temperatures above 40°C (104°F).

Avoid storage of the powder for oral suspension at temperatures above 40°C (104°F). After constitution store the suspension below 30°C (86°F). Do not freeze. Discard unused suspension after 30 days.

7825028 Issued May 1996

COPYRIGHT © MERCK & CO., INC., 1986, 1988, 1991
All rights reserved

PEPCID® Injection Premixed ℞
(Famotidine)

PEPCID® Injection ℞
(Famotidine)

DESCRIPTION

The active ingredient in PEPCID* (Famotidine) Injection Premixed and PEPCID (famotidine) Injection is a histamine H_2-receptor antagonist. Famotidine is *N′*-(aminosulfonyl)-3-[[[2-[(diaminomethylene)amino]-4-thiazolyl]methyl]thio]-propanimidamide. The empirical formula of famotidine is $C_8H_{15}N_7O_2S_3$ and its molecular weight is 337.43. Its structural formula is:

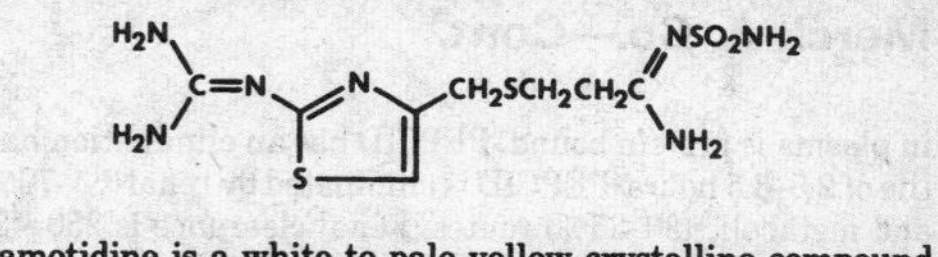

Famotidine is a white to pale yellow crystalline compound that is freely soluble in glacial acetic acid, slightly soluble in methanol, very slightly soluble in water, and practically insoluble in ethanol.

PEPCID Injection Premixed is supplied as a sterile solution, for intravenous use only, in plastic single dose containers. Each 50 mL of the premixed, iso-osmotic intravenous injection contains 20 mg famotidine, USP, and the following inactive ingredients: L-aspartic acid 6.8 mg, sodium chloride, USP, 450 mg, and Water for Injection. The pH ranges from 5.7 to 6.4 and may have been adjusted with additional L-aspartic acid or with sodium hydroxide.

The plastic container is fabricated from a specially designed multi-layer plastic (PL 2501). Solutions are in contact with the polyethylene layer of the container and can leach out certain chemical components of the plastic in very small amounts within the expiration period. The suitability and safety of the plastic have been confirmed in tests in animals according to the USP biological tests for plastic containers, as well as by tissue culture toxicity studies.

PEPCID (famotidine) Injection is supplied as a sterile concentrated solution for intravenous injection. Each mL of the solution contains 10 mg of famotidine and the following inactive ingredients: L-aspartic acid 4 mg, mannitol 20 mg, and Water for Injection q.s. 1 mL. The multidose injection also contains benzyl alcohol 0.9% added as preservative.

---

*Registered trademark of MERCK & CO., INC.

CLINICAL PHARMACOLOGY

GI Effects

PEPCID is a competitive inhibitor of histamine H_2-receptors. The primary clinically important pharmacologic activity of PEPCID is inhibition of gastric secretion. Both the acid concentration and volume of gastric secretion are suppressed by PEPCID, while changes in pepsin secretion are proportional to volume output.

In normal volunteers and hypersecretors, PEPCID inhibited basal and nocturnal gastric secretion, as well as secretion stimulated by food and pentagastrin. After oral administration, the onset of the antisecretory effect occurred within one hour; the maximum effect was dose-dependent, occurring within one to three hours. Duration of inhibition of secretion by doses of 20 and 40 mg was 10 to 12 hours.

After intravenous administration, the maximum effect was achieved within 30 minutes. Single intravenous doses of 10 and 20 mg inhibited nocturnal secretion for a period of 10 to 12 hours. The 20 mg dose was associated with the longest duration of action in most subjects.

Single evening oral doses of 20 and 40 mg inhibited basal and nocturnal acid secretion in all subjects; mean nocturnal gastric acid secretion was inhibited by 86% and 94%, respectively, for a period of at least 10 hours. The same doses given in the morning suppressed food-stimulated acid secretion in all subjects. The mean suppression was 76% and 84% respectively, 3 to 5 hours after administration, and 25% and 30%, respectively, 8 to 10 hours after administration. In some subjects who received the 20 mg dose, however, the antisecretory effect was dissipated within 6–8 hours. There was no cumulative effect with repeated doses. The nocturnal intragastric pH was raised by evening doses of 20 and 40 mg of PEPCID to mean values of 5.0 and 6.4, respectively. When PEPCID was given after breakfast, the basal daytime interdigestive pH at 3 and 8 hours after 20 or 40 mg of PEPCID was raised to about 5.

PEPCID had little or no effect on fasting or postprandial serum gastrin levels. Gastric emptying and exocrine pancreatic function were not affected by PEPCID.

Other Effects

Systemic effects of PEPCID in the CNS, cardiovascular, respiratory or endocrine systems were not noted in clinical pharmacology studies. Also, no antiandrogenic effects were noted. (See ADVERSE REACTIONS.) Serum hormone levels, including prolactin, cortisol, thyroxine (T_4), and testosterone, were not altered after treatment with PEPCID.

Pharmacokinetics

Orally administered PEPCID is incompletely absorbed and its bioavailability is 40–45%. PEPCID undergoes minimal first-pass metabolism. After oral doses, peak plasma levels occur in 1–3 hours. Plasma levels after multiple doses are similar to those after single doses. Fifteen to 20% of PEPCID

Continued on next page

Information on the Merck & Co., Inc. products listed on these pages is the full prescribing information from product circulars in use September 30, 1996.

Merck & Co.—Cont.

in plasma is protein bound. PEPCID has an elimination half-life of 2.5–3.5 hours. PEPCID is eliminated by renal (65–70%) and metabolic (30–35%) routes. Renal clearance is 250–450 mL/min, indicating some tubular excretion. Twenty-five to 30% of an oral dose and 65–70% of an intravenous dose are recovered in the urine as unchanged compound. The only metabolite identified in man is the S-oxide.

There is a close relationship between creatinine clearance values and the elimination half-life of PEPCID. In patients with severe renal insufficiency, i.e., creatinine clearance less than 10 mL/min, the elimination half-life of PEPCID may exceed 20 hours and adjustment of dose or dosing intervals may be necessary (see PRECAUTIONS, DOSAGE AND ADMINISTRATION).

In elderly patients, there are no clinically significant age-related changes in the pharmacokinetics of PEPCID.

Clinical Studies
The majority of clinical study experience involved oral administration of PEPCID Tablets, and is provided herein for reference.

Duodenal Ulcer
In a U.S. multicenter, double-blind study in outpatients with endoscopically confirmed duodenal ulcer, orally administered PEPCID was compared to placebo. As shown in Table 1, 70% of patients treated with PEPCID 40 mg h.s. were healed by week 4.

Table 1
Outpatients with Endoscopically
Confirmed Healed Duodenal Ulcers

	PEPCID 40 mg h.s. (N=89)	PEPCID 20 mg b.i.d. (N=84)	Placebo h.s. (N=97)
Week 2	*32%	*38%	17%
Week 4	*70%	*67%	31%

*Statistically significantly different than placebo (p < 0.001)

Patients not healed by week 4 were continued in the study. By week 8, 83% of patients treated with PEPCID had healed versus 45% of patients treated with placebo. The incidence of ulcer healing with PEPCID was significantly higher than with placebo at each time point based on proportion of endoscopically confirmed healed ulcers.

In this study, time to relief of daytime and nocturnal pain was significantly shorter for patients receiving PEPCID than for patients receiving placebo; patients receiving PEPCID also took less antacid than the patients receiving placebo.

Long-Term Maintenance
Treatment of Duodenal Ulcers
PEPCID, 20 mg p.o. h.s. was compared to placebo h.s. as maintenance therapy in two double-blind, multicenter studies of patients with endoscopically confirmed healed duodenal ulcers. In the U.S. study the observed ulcer incidence within 12 months in patients treated with placebo was 2.4 times greater than in the patients treated with PEPCID. The 89 patients treated with PEPCID had a cumulative observed ulcer incidence of 23.4% compared to an observed ulcer incidence of 56.6% in the 89 patients receiving placebo (p < 0.01). These results were confirmed in an international study where the cumulative observed ulcer incidence within 12 months in the 307 patients treated with PEPCID was 35.7%, compared to an incidence of 75.5% in the 325 patients treated with placebo (p < 0.01).

Gastric Ulcer
In both a U.S. and an international multicenter, double-blind study in patients with endoscopically confirmed active benign gastric ulcer, orally administered PEPCID, 40 mg h.s., was compared to placebo h.s. Antacids were permitted during the studies, but consumption was not significantly different between the PEPCID and placebo groups. As shown in Table 2, the incidence of ulcer healing (dropouts counted as unhealed) with PEPCID was statistically significantly better than placebo at weeks 6 and 8 in the U.S. study, and at weeks 4, 6 and 8 in the international study, based on the number of ulcers that healed, confirmed by endoscopy.

Table 2
Patients with Endoscopically
Confirmed Healed Gastric Ulcers

	U.S. Study		International Study	
	PEPCID 40 mg h.s. (N=74)	Placebo h.s. (N=75)	PEPCID 40 mg h.s. (N=149)	Placebo h.s. (N=145)
Week 4	45%	39%	**47%	31%
Week 6	**66%	44%	**65%	46%
Week 8	*78%	64%	**80%	54%

*,** Statistically significantly better than placebo (p ≤ 0.05, p ≤ 0.01 respectively)

Time to complete relief of daytime and nighttime pain was statistically significantly shorter for patients receiving PEPCID than for patients receiving placebo; however, in neither study was there a statistically significant difference in the proportion of patients whose pain was relieved by the end of the study (week 8).

Gastroesophageal Reflux Disease (GERD)
Orally administered PEPCID was compared to placebo in a U.S. study that enrolled patients with symptoms of GERD and without endoscopic evidence of erosion or ulceration of the esophagus. PEPCID 20 mg b.i.d. was statistically significantly superior to 40 mg h.s. and to placebo in providing a successful symptomatic outcome, defined as moderate or excellent improvement of symptoms (Table 3).

Table 3
% Successful Symptomatic Outcome

	PEPCID 20 mg b.i.d. (N=154)	PEPCID 40 mg h.s. (N=149)	Placebo (N=73)
Week 6	82**	69	62

**p ≤ 0.01 vs Placebo

By two weeks of treatment, symptomatic success was observed in a greater percentage of patients taking PEPCID 20 mg b.i.d. compared to placebo (p ≤ 0.01).

Symptomatic improvement and healing of endoscopically verified erosion and ulceration were studied in two additional trials. Healing was defined as complete resolution of all erosions or ulcerations visible with endoscopy. The U.S. study comparing PEPCID 40 mg p.o. b.i.d. to placebo and PEPCID 20 mg p.o. b.i.d., showed a significantly greater percentage of healing for PEPCID 40 mg b.i.d. at weeks 6 and 12 (Table 4).

Table 4
% Endoscopic Healing—U.S. Study

	PEPCID 40 mg b.i.d. (N=127)	PEPCID 20 mg b.i.d. (N=125)	Placebo (N=66)
Week 6	48**,++	32	18
Week 12	69**,+	54**	29

** p ≤ 0.01 vs Placebo
+ p ≤ 0.05 vs PEPCID 20 mg b.i.d.
++ p ≤ 0.01 vs PEPCID 20 mg b.i.d.

As compared to placebo, patients who received PEPCID had faster relief of daytime and nighttime heartburn and a greater percentage of patients experienced complete relief of nighttime heartburn. These differences were statistically significant.

In the international study, when PEPCID 40 mg p.o. b.i.d. was compared to ranitidine 150 mg p.o. b.i.d., a statistically significantly greater percentage of healing was observed with PEPCID 40 mg b.i.d. at week 12 (Table 5). There was, however, no significant difference among treatments in symptom relief.

Table 5
% Endoscopic Healing—International Study

	PEPCID 40 mg b.i.d. (N=175)	PEPCID 20 mg b.i.d. (N=93)	Ranitidine 150 mg b.i.d. (N=172)
Week 6	48	52	42
Week 12	71*	68	60

*p ≤ 0.05 vs Ranitidine 150 mg b.i.d.

Pathological Hypersecretory Conditions
(e.g., Zollinger-Ellison Syndrome,
Multiple Endocrine Adenomas)
In studies of patients with pathological hypersecretory conditions such as Zollinger-Ellison Syndrome with or without multiple endocrine adenomas, PEPCID significantly inhibited gastric acid secretion and controlled associated symptoms. Orally administered doses from 20 to 160 mg q 6 h maintained basal acid secretion below 10 mEq/hr; initial doses were titrated to the individual patient need and subsequent adjustments were necessary with time in some patients. PEPCID was well tolerated at these high dose levels for prolonged periods (greater than 12 months) in eight patients, and there were no cases reported of gynecomastia, increased prolactin levels, or impotence which were considered to be due to the drug.

INDICATIONS AND USAGE

PEPCID Injection Premixed, supplied as a premixed solution in plastic containers (PL 2501 Plastic), and PEPCID Injection, supplied as a concentrated solution for intravenous injection, are intended for intravenous use only. PEPCID Injection Premixed and PEPCID Injection are indicated in some hospitalized patients with pathological hypersecretory conditions or intractable ulcers, or as an alternative to the oral dosage forms for short term use in patients who are unable to take oral medication for the following conditions:

1. *Short term treatment of active duodenal ulcer.* Most patients heal within 4 weeks; there is rarely reason to use PEPCID at full dosage for longer than 6 to 8 weeks. Studies have not assessed the safety of famotidine in uncomplicated active duodenal ulcer for periods of more than eight weeks.

2. *Maintenance therapy for duodenal ulcer patients at reduced dosage after healing of an active ulcer.* Controlled studies have not extended beyond one year.

3. *Short term treatment of active benign gastric ulcer.* Most patients heal within 6 weeks. Studies have not assessed the safety or efficacy of famotidine in uncomplicated active benign gastric ulcer for periods of more than 8 weeks.

4. *Short term treatment of gastroesophageal reflux disease (GERD).* PEPCID is indicated for short term treatment of patients with symptoms of GERD (see CLINICAL PHARMACOLOGY, *Clinical Studies*).
PEPCID is also indicated for the short term treatment of esophagitis due to GERD including erosive or ulcerative disease diagnosed by endoscopy (see CLINICAL PHARMACOLOGY, *Clinical Studies*).

5. *Treatment of pathological hypersecretory conditions (e.g., Zollinger-Ellison Syndrome, multiple endocrine adenomas).*

CONTRAINDICATIONS

Hypersensitivity to any component of these products.

PRECAUTIONS

General
Symptomatic response to therapy with PEPCID does not preclude the presence of gastric malignancy.
Patients with Severe Renal Insufficiency
Longer intervals between doses or lower doses may need to be used in patients with severe renal insufficiency (creatinine clearance < 10 mL/min) to adjust for the longer elimination half-life of famotidine. (See CLINICAL PHARMACOLOGY, DOSAGE AND ADMINISTRATION.) However, currently, no drug-related toxicity has been found with high plasma concentrations of famotidine.
Drug Interactions
No drug interactions have been identified. Studies with famotidine in man, in animal models, and in vitro have shown no significant interference with the disposition of compounds metabolized by the hepatic microsomal enzymes, e.g., cytochrome P450 system. Compounds tested in man include warfarin, theophylline, phenytoin, diazepam, aminopyrine and antipyrine. Indocyanine green as an index of hepatic drug extraction has been tested and no significant effects have been found.
Carcinogenesis, Mutagenesis,
Impairment of Fertility
In a 106 week study in rats and a 92 week study in mice given oral doses of up to 2000 mg/kg/day (approximately 2500 times the recommended human dose for active duodenal ulcer), there was no evidence of carcinogenic potential for PEPCID.
Famotidine was negative in the microbial mutagen test (Ames test) using *Salmonella typhimurium* and *Escherichia coli* with or without rat liver enzyme activation at concentrations up to 10,000 mcg/plate. In *in vivo* studies in mice, with a micronucleus test and a chromosomal aberration test, no evidence of a mutagenic effect was observed.
In studies with rats given oral doses of up to 2000 mg/kg/day or intravenous doses of up to 200 mg/kg/day fertility and reproductive performance were not affected.
Pregnancy
Pregnancy Category B
Reproductive studies have been performed in rats and rabbits at oral doses of up to 2000 and 500 mg/kg/day, respectively, and in both species at I.V. doses of up to 200 mg/kg/day, and have revealed no significant evidence of impaired fertility or harm to the fetus due to PEPCID. While no direct fetotoxic effects have been observed, sporadic abortions occurring only in mothers displaying marked decreased food intake were seen in some rabbits at oral doses of 200 mg/kg/day (250 times the usual human dose) or higher. There are, however, no adequate or well-controlled studies in pregnant women. Because animal reproductive studies are not always predictive of human response, this drug should be used during pregnancy only if clearly needed.
Nursing Mothers
Studies performed in lactating rats have shown that famotidine is secreted into breast milk. Transient growth depression was observed in young rats suckling from mothers treated with maternotoxic doses of at least 600 times the usual human dose. Famotidine is detectable in human milk. Because of the potential for serious adverse reactions in nursing infants from PEPCID, a decision should be made whether to discontinue nursing or discontinue the drug, taking into account the importance of the drug to the mother.
Pediatric Use
Safety and effectiveness in children have not been established.
Use in Elderly Patients
No dosage adjustment is required based on age (see CLINICAL PHARMACOLOGY, *Pharmacokinetics*). Dosage adjustment in the case of severe renal impairment may be necessary.

ADVERSE REACTIONS

The adverse reactions listed below have been reported during domestic and international clinical trials in approximately 2500 patients. In those controlled clinical trials in which PEPCID Tablets were compared to placebo, the incidence of adverse experiences in the group which received PEPCID Tablets, 40 mg at bedtime, was similar to that in the placebo group.

The following adverse reactions have been reported to occur in more than 1% of patients on therapy with PEPCID in controlled clinical trials, and may be causally related to the drug: headache (4.7%), dizziness (1.3%), constipation (1.2%) and diarrhea (1.7%).

The following other adverse reactions have been reported infrequently in clinical trials or since the drug was marketed. The relationship to therapy with PEPCID has been unclear in many cases. Within each category the adverse reactions are listed in order of decreasing severity:

Body as a Whole: fever, asthenia, fatigue

Cardiovascular: arrhythmia, AV block, palpitation

Gastrointestinal: cholestatic jaundice, liver enzyme abnormalities, vomiting, nausea, abdominal discomfort, anorexia, dry mouth

Hematologic: rare cases of agranulocytosis, pancytopenia, leukopenia, thrombocytopenia

Hypersensitivity: anaphylaxis, angioedema, orbital or facial edema, urticaria, rash, conjunctival injection

Musculoskeletal: musculoskeletal pain including muscle cramps, arthralgia

Nervous System/Psychiatric: grand mal seizure; psychic disturbances, which were reversible in cases for which follow-up was obtained, including hallucinations, confusion, agitation, depression, anxiety, decreased libido; paresthesia; insomnia; somnolence

Respiratory: bronchospasm

Skin: toxic epidermal necrolysis (very rare), alopecia, acne, pruritus, dry skin, flushing

Special Senses: tinnitus, taste disorder

Other: rare cases of impotence and rare cases of gynecomastia have been reported; however, in controlled clinical trials, the incidences were not greater than those seen with placebo.

The adverse reactions reported for PEPCID Tablets may also occur with PEPCID for Oral Suspension, PEPCID Injection Premixed or PEPCID Injection. In addition, transient irritation at the injection site has been observed with PEPCID Injection.

OVERDOSAGE

There is no experience to date with deliberate overdosage. Oral doses of up to 640 mg/day have been given to patients with pathological hypersecretory conditions with no serious adverse effects. In the event of overdosage, treatment should be symptomatic and supportive. Unabsorbed material should be removed from the gastrointestinal tract, the patient should be monitored, and supportive therapy should be employed.

The intravenous LD_{50} of famotidine for mice and rats ranged from 254–563 mg/kg and the minimum lethal single I.V. dose in dogs was approximately 300 mg/kg. Signs of acute intoxication in I.V. treated dogs were emesis, restlessness, pallor of mucous membranes or redness of mouth and ears, hypotension, tachycardia and collapse. The oral LD_{50} of famotidine in male and female rats and mice was greater than 3000 mg/kg and the minimum lethal acute oral dose in dogs exceeded 2000 mg/kg. Famotidine did not produce overt effects at high oral doses in mice, rats, cats and dogs, but induced significant anorexia and growth depression in rabbits starting with 200 mg/kg/day orally.

DOSAGE AND ADMINISTRATION

In some hospitalized patients with pathological hypersecretory conditions or intractable ulcers, or in patients who are unable to take oral medication, PEPCID Injection Premixed or PEPCID Injection may be administered until oral therapy can be instituted.

The recommended dosage for PEPCID Injection Premixed and PEPCID Injection is 20 mg q 12 h.

The doses and regimen for parenteral administration in patients with GERD have not been established.

Dosage Adjustments for Patients with Severe Renal Insufficiency

In patients with severe renal insufficiency, i.e., with a creatinine clearance less than 10 mL/min, the elimination half-life of PEPCID may exceed 20 hours, reaching approximately 24 hours in anuric patients. Although no relationship of adverse effects to high plasma levels has been established, to avoid excess accumulation of the drug, the dose of PEPCID Injection Premixed or PEPCID Injection may be reduced to 20 mg h.s. or the dosing interval may be prolonged to 36–48 hours as indicated by the patient's clinical response.

Pathological Hypersecretory Conditions (e.g., Zollinger-Ellison Syndrome, Multiple Endocrine Adenomas)

The dosage of PEPCID in patients with pathological hypersecretory conditions varies with the individual patient. The recommended adult intravenous dose is 20 mg q 12 h. Doses should be adjusted to individual patient needs and should continue as long as clinically indicated. In some patients, a higher starting dose may be required. Oral doses up to 160 mg q 6 h have been administered to some patients with severe Zollinger-Ellison Syndrome.

PEPCID Injection Premixed

PEPCID Injection Premixed, supplied in Galaxy** containers (PL 2501 Plastic), is a 50 mL iso-osmotic solution premixed with 0.9% sodium chloride for administration as an infusion over a 15–30 minute period. *This premixed solution is for intravenous use only using sterile equipment.*

Directions for Use of Galaxy® Containers

Check the container for minute leaks prior to use by squeezing the bag firmly. If leaks are found, discard solution as sterility may be impaired. Do not add supplementary medication. Do not use unless solution is clear and seal is intact.

CAUTION: Do not use plastic containers in series connections. Such use could result in air embolism due to residual air being drawn from the primary container before administration of the fluid from the secondary container is complete.

Preparation for administration:

1. Suspend container from eyelet support.
2. Remove plastic protector from outlet port at bottom of container.
3. Attach administration set. Refer to complete directions accompanying set.

To prepare PEPCID intravenous solutions, aseptically dilute 2 mL of PEPCID Injection (solution containing 10 mg/mL) with 0.9% Sodium Chloride Injection or other compatible intravenous solution to a total volume of either 5 mL or 10 mL and inject over a period of not less than 2 minutes.

To prepare PEPCID intravenous infusion solutions, aseptically dilute 2 mL of PEPCID Injection with 100 mL of 5% dextrose or other compatible solution, and infuse over a 15–30 minute period.

Concomitant Use of Antacids

Antacids may be given concomitantly if needed.

Stability

Parenteral drug products should be inspected visually for particulate matter and discoloration prior to administration whenever solution and container permit.

PEPCID Injection Premixed

PEPCID Injection Premixed, as supplied premixed in 0.9% sodium chloride in Galaxy® containers (PL 2501 Plastic), is stable through the labeled expiration date when stored under the recommended conditions. (See HOW SUPPLIED, *Storage*).

PEPCID Injection

When added to or diluted with most commonly used intravenous solutions, e.g., Water for Injection, 0.9% Sodium Chloride Injection, 5% and 10% Dextrose Injection, Lactated Ringer's Injection, or Sodium Bicarbonate Injection, 5%, diluted PEPCID Injection is physically and chemically stable (i.e., maintains at least 90% of initial potency) for 7 days at room temperature—see HOW SUPPLIED, *Storage*.

** Galaxy® is a registered trademark of Baxter International Inc.

HOW SUPPLIED

FOR INTRAVENOUS USE ONLY

No. 3537—PEPCID (famotidine) Injection Premixed 20 mg per 50 mL is a clear, non-preserved, sterile solution premixed in a vehicle made iso-osmotic with Sodium Chloride, and is supplied as follows:

NDC 0006-3537-50, 50 mL single dose Galaxy® containers (PL 2501 Plastic).

No. 3539—PEPCID Injection 10 mg per 1 mL, is a non-preserved, clear, colorless solution and is supplied as follows:

NDC 0006-3539-04, 10 × 2 mL single dose vials (6505-01-281-1249, 10 mg per mL, 2 mL 10's).

No. 3541—PEPCID Injection 10 mg per 1 mL, is a clear, colorless solution and is supplied as follows:

NDC 0006-3541-14, 4 mL vials (6505-01-282-1180, 10 mg per mL, 4 mL)

NDC 0006-3541-20, 20 mL vials.

NDC 0006-3541-49, 10 ×20 mL vials.

Storage

Store PEPCID Injection Premixed in Galaxy® containers (PL 2501 Plastic) at room temperature (25°C, 77°F). Exposure of the premixed product to excessive heat should be avoided. Brief exposure to temperatures up to 35°C (95°F) does not adversely affect the product.

Store PEPCID Injection at 2–8°C (36–46°F). If solution freezes, bring to room temperature; allow sufficient time to solubilize all the components.

Although diluted PEPCID Injection has been shown to be physically and chemically stable for 7 days at room temperature, there are no data on the maintenance of sterility after dilution. Therefore, it is recommended that if not used immediately after preparation, diluted solutions of PEPCID Injection should be refrigerated and used within 48 hours (see DOSAGE AND ADMINISTRATION).

PEPCID (famotidine) Injection Premixed is manufactured for:

MERCK & CO., INC., West Point, PA 19486, USA

By:

BAXTER HEALTHCARE CORPORATION

Deerfield, Illinois 60015 USA

PEPCID (famotidine) Injection is manufactured by:

MERCK & CO., INC., West Point, PA 19486, USA

7866204 Issued March 1996

COPYRIGHT © MERCK & CO., INC., 1993, 1995
All rights reserved

PERIACTIN® Tablets ℞
(Cyproheptadine HCl), U.S.P.
PERIACTIN® Syrup ℞
(Cyproheptadine HCl), U.S.P.

DESCRIPTION

PERIACTIN* (Cyproheptadine HCl) is an antihistaminic and antiserotonergic agent.

Cyproheptadine hydrochloride is a white to slightly yellowish, crystalline solid, with a molecular weight of 350.89, which is soluble in water, freely soluble in methanol, sparingly soluble in ethanol, soluble in chloroform, and practically insoluble in ether. It is the sesquihydrate of 4-(5*H*-dibenzo[*a,d*]cyclohepten-5-ylidene)-1-methylpiperidine hydrochloride. The empirical formula of the anhydrous salt is $C_{21}H_{21}N \cdot HCl$ and the structural formula of the anhydrous salt is:

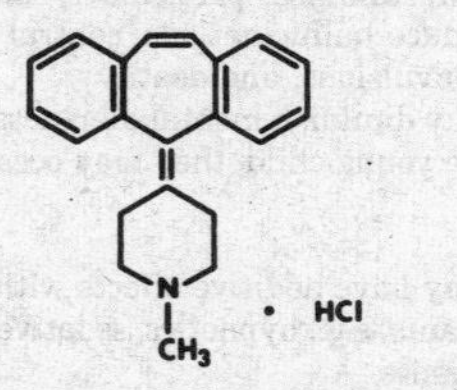

PERIACTIN is available in tablets, containing 4 mg of cyproheptadine hydrochloride, and as a syrup in which 5 mL contains 2 mg of cyproheptadine hydrochloride, with a pH range of 3.5 to 4.5.

The tablets also contain the following inactive ingredients: calcium phosphate, lactose, magnesium stearate, and starch. The syrup contains the following inactive ingredients: alcohol 5%, D & C Yellow 10, artificial flavors, glycerin, purified water, sodium saccharin, and sucrose, with sorbic acid 0.1% added as preservative.

*Registered trademark of MERCK & CO., INC.

CLINICAL PHARMACOLOGY

PERIACTIN is a serotonin and histamine antagonist with anticholinergic and sedative effects. Antiserotonin and antihistamine drugs appear to compete with serotonin and histamine, respectively, for receptor sites.

Pharmacokinetics and Metabolism

After a single 4 mg oral dose of ^{14}C-labelled cyproheptadine HCl in normal subjects, given as tablets or syrup, 2-20% of the radioactivity was excreted in the stools. Only about 34% of the stool radioactivity was unchanged drug, corresponding to less than 5.7% of the dose. At least 40% of the administered radioactivity was excreted in the urine. No significant difference in the mean urinary excretion exists between the tablet and syrup formulations. No detectable amounts of unchanged drug were present in the urine of patients on chronic 12-20 mg daily doses of PERIACTIN Syrup. The principal metabolite found in human urine has been identified as a quaternary ammonium glucuronide conjugate of cyproheptadine. Elimination is diminished in renal insufficiency.

INDICATIONS AND USAGE

Perennial and seasonal allergic rhinitis
Vasomotor rhinitis
Allergic conjunctivitis due to inhalant allergens and foods
Mild, uncomplicated allergic skin manifestations of urticaria and angioedema

Continued on next page

Information on the Merck & Co., Inc. products listed on these pages is the full prescribing information from product circulars in use September 30, 1996.

Merck & Co.—Cont.

Amelioration of allergic reactions to blood or plasma
Cold urticaria
Dermatographism
As therapy for anaphylactic reactions *adjunctive* to epinephrine and other standard measures after the acute manifestations have been controlled.

CONTRAINDICATIONS

Newborn or Premature Infants
This drug should *not* be used in newborn or premature infants.

Nursing Mothers
Because of the higher risk of antihistamines for infants generally and for newborns and prematures in particular, antihistamine therapy is contraindicated in nursing mothers.

Other Conditions
Hypersensitivity to cyproheptadine and other drugs of similar chemical structure:

  Monoamine oxidase inhibitor therapy
    (see DRUG INTERACTIONS)
  Angle-closure glaucoma
  Stenosing peptic ulcer
  Symptomatic prostatic hypertrophy
  Bladder neck obstruction
  Pyloroduodenal obstruction
  Elderly, debilitated patients

WARNINGS

Children
Overdosage of antihistamines, particularly in infants and children, may produce hallucinations, central nervous system depression, convulsions, and death.
Antihistamines may diminish mental alertness; conversely, particularly, in the young child, they may occasionally produce excitation.

CNS Depressants
Antihistamines may have additive effects with alcohol and other CNS depressants, e.g., hypnotics, sedatives, tranquilizers, antianxiety agents.

Activities Requiring Mental Alertness
Patients should be warned about engaging in activities requiring mental alertness and motor coordination, such as driving a car or operating machinery.
Antihistamines are more likely to cause dizziness, sedation, and hypotension in elderly patients.

PRECAUTIONS

General
Cyproheptadine has an atropine-like action and, therefore, should be used with caution in patients with:

  History of bronchial asthma
  Increased intraocular pressure
  Hyperthyroidism
  Cardiovascular disease
  Hypertension

Information for Patients
Antihistamines may diminish mental alertness; conversely, particularly, in the young child, they may occasionally produce excitation.
Patients should be warned about engaging in activities requiring mental alertness and motor coordination, such as driving a car or operating machinery.

Drug Interactions
MAO inhibitors prolong and intensify the anticholinergic effects of antihistamines.
Antihistamines may have additive effects with alcohol and other CNS depressants, e.g., hypnotics, sedatives, tranquilizers, antianxiety agents.

Carcinogenesis, Mutagenesis, Impairment of Fertility
Long-term carcinogenic studies have not been done with cyproheptadine.
Cyproheptadine had no effect on fertility in a two-litter study in rats or a two generation study in mice at about 10 times the human dose.
Cyproheptadine did not produce chromosome damage in human lymphocytes or fibroblasts *in vitro;* high doses $(10^{-4}$ M) were cytotoxic. Cyproheptadine did not have any mutagenic effect in the Ames microbial mutagen test; concentrations of above 500 mcg/plate inhibited bacterial growth.

Pregnancy
Pregnancy Category B: Reproduction studies have been performed in rabbits, mice, and rats at oral or subcutaneous doses up to 32 times the maximum recommended human oral dose and have revealed no evidence of impaired fertility or harm to the fetus due to cyproheptadine. Cyproheptadine has been shown to be fetotoxic in rats when given by intra-

peritoneal injection in doses four times the maximum recommended human oral dose. Two studies in pregnant women, however, have not shown that cyproheptadine increases the risk of abnormalities when administered during the first, second and third trimesters of pregnancy. No teratogenic effects were observed in any of the newborns. Nevertheless, because the studies in humans cannot rule out the possibility of harm, cyproheptadine should be used during pregnancy only if clearly needed.

Nursing Mothers
It is not known whether this drug is excreted in human milk. Because many drugs are excreted in human milk, and because of the potential for serious adverse reactions in nursing infants from PERIACTIN, a decision should be made whether to discontinue nursing or to discontinue the drug, taking into account the importance of the drug to the mother (see CONTRAINDICATIONS).

Pediatric Use
Safety and effectiveness in children below the age of two have not been established. See CONTRAINDICATIONS, *Newborn Premature Infants*, and WARNINGS, *Children*.

ADVERSE REACTIONS

Adverse reactions which have been reported with the use of antihistamines are as follows:
Central Nervous System: Sedation and sleepiness (often transient), dizziness, disturbed coordination, confusion, restlessness, excitation, nervousness, tremor, irritability, insomnia, paresthesias, neuritis, convulsions, euphoria, hallucinations, hysteria, faintness.
Integumentary: Allergic manifestation of rash and edema, excessive perspiration, urticaria, photosensitivity.
Special Senses: Acute labyrinthitis, blurred vision, diplopia, vertigo, tinnitus.
Cardiovascular: Hypotension, palpitation, tachycardia, extrasystoles, anaphylactic shock.
Hematologic: Hemolytic anemia, leukopenia, agranulocytosis, thrombocytopenia.
Digestive System: Dryness of mouth, epigastric distress, anorexia, nausea, vomiting, diarrhea, constipation, jaundice.
Genitourinary: Urinary frequency, difficult urination, urinary retention, early menses.
Respiratory: Dryness of nose and throat, thickening of bronchial secretions, tightness of chest and wheezing, nasal stuffiness.
Miscellaneous: Fatigue, chills, headache, increased appetite/weight gain.

OVERDOSAGE

Antihistamine overdosage reactions may vary from central nervous system depression to stimulation especially in children. Also, atropine-like signs and symptoms (dry mouth; fixed, dilated pupils; flushing, etc.) as well as gastrointestinal symptoms may occur.
If vomiting has not occurred spontaneously the patient should be induced to vomit with syrup of ipecac.
If the patient is unable to vomit, perform gastric lavage followed by activated charcoal. Isotonic or $^1/_2$ isotonic saline is the lavage of choice. Precautions against aspiration must be taken especially in infants and children.
When life threatening CNS signs and symptoms are present, intravenous physostigmine salicylate may be considered. Dosage and frequency of administration are dependent on age, clinical response, and recurrence after response. (See package circulars for physostigmine products.)
Saline cathartics, as milk of magnesia, by osmosis draw water into the bowel and, therefore, are valuable for their action in rapid dilution of bowel content.
Stimulants should *not* be used.
Vasopressors may be used to treat hypotension.
The oral LD_{50} of cyproheptadine is 123 mg/kg, and 295 mg/kg in the mouse and rat, respectively.

DOSAGE AND ADMINISTRATION

DOSAGE SHOULD BE INDIVIDUALIZED ACCORDING TO THE NEEDS AND THE RESPONSE OF THE PATIENT.
Each PERIACTIN tablet contains 4 mg of cyproheptadine hydrochloride. Each 5 mL of PERIACTIN syrup contains 2 mg of cyproheptadine hydrochloride.
Although intended primarily for administration to children, the syrup is also useful for administration to adults who cannot swallow tablets.

Children
The total daily dosage for children may be calculated on the basis of body weight or body area using approximately 0.25 mg/kg/day (0.11 mg/lb/day) or 8 mg per square meter of body surface (8 mg/m^2). In small children for whom the calculation of dosage based upon body size is most important, it may be necessary to use PERIACTIN syrup to permit accurate dosage.

Age 2 to 6 years
The usual dose is 2 mg ($^1/_2$ tablet or 1 teaspoon) two or three times a day, adjusted as necessary to the size and response of the patient. The dose is not to exceed 12 mg a day.
Age 7 to 14 years
The usual dose is 4 mg (1 tablet or 2 teaspoons) two or three times a day, adjusted as necessary to the size and response of the patient. The dose is not to exceed 16 mg a day.
Adults
The total daily dose for adults should not exceed 0.5 mg/kg/day (0.23 mg/lb/day).
The therapeutic range is 4 to 20 mg a day, with the majority of patients requiring 12 to 16 mg a day. An occasional patient may require as much as 32 mg a day for adequate relief. It is suggested that dosage be initiated with 4 mg (1 tablet or 2 teaspoons) three times a day and adjusted according to the size and response of the patient.

HOW SUPPLIED

No. 3276—Tablets PERIACTIN, containing 4 mg of cyproheptadine hydrochloride each, are white, round, scored, compressed tablets, coded MSD 62 on one side and PERIACTIN on the other. They are supplied as follows:
NDC 0006-0062-68 bottles of 100
(6505-00-890-1884 4 mg 100's).
  Shown in Product Identification Guide, page 325
No. 3289X—Syrup PERIACTIN, 2 mg per 5 mL is a clear, yellow, syrupy liquid and is supplied as follows:
NDC 0006-3289-74 bottles of 473 mL.
Storage
Store Tablets PERIACTIN at controlled room temperature, 15–30°C (59–86°F), in a well-closed container.
Store Syrup PERIACTIN at controlled room temperature, 15–30°C (59–86°F), in a container which is kept tightly closed. Because of the risk of breakage, avoid freezing bottle.
    7926420   Issued October 1994
COPYRIGHT © MERCK & CO., INC., 1985
All rights reserved

PNEUMOVAX® 23   ℞
(Pneumococcal Vaccine Polyvalent)

DESCRIPTION

PNEUMOVAX* 23 (Pneumococcal Vaccine Polyvalent), is a sterile, liquid vaccine for intramuscular or subcutaneous injection. It consists of a mixture of highly purified capsular polysaccharides from the 23 most prevalent or invasive pneumococcal types accounting for at least 90% of pneumococcal blood isolates and at least 85% of all pneumococcal isolates from sites which are generally sterile as determined by ongoing surveillance of U.S. data.
PNEUMOVAX 23 is manufactured according to methods developed by the MERCK Research Laboratories. Each 0.5 mL dose of vaccine contains 25 µg of each polysaccharide type dissolved in isotonic saline solution containing 0.25% phenol as preservative.
Type 6B pneumococcal polysaccharide exhibits somewhat greater stability in purified form than does Type 6A. A high degree of cross-reactivity between the two types has been demonstrated in adult volunteers. Therefore, Type 6B has replaced Type 6A, which had been used in the 14-valent vaccine. Although contained in the 14-valent vaccine, Type 25 is not included in PNEUMOVAX 23 because it has recently become a rare isolate in many parts of the world including the United States, Canada and Europe.
[See table on bottom of next page.]

* Registered trademark of MERCK & CO., INC.

CLINICAL PHARMACOLOGY

Pneumococcal infection is a leading cause of death throughout the world and a major cause of pneumonia, meningitis, and otitis media. The emergence of strains of pneumococci with increased resistance to one or more of the common antibiotics and recent isolations of pneumococci with multiple antibiotic resistance emphasize the importance of vaccine prophylaxis against pneumococcal disease. Based on projection from limited observations in the United States, it has been estimated that 400,000 to 500,000 cases of pneumococcal pneumonia may occur annually. The overall case fatality rate ranges from 5–10%. Populations at high risk are the elderly; individuals with immune deficiencies; patients with asplenia or splenic deficiencies, including sickle cell anemia and other severe hemoglobinopathies; alcoholics; and patients with the following diseases: Hodgkin's disease, multiple myeloma and nephrotic syndrome. About 25% of all persons with pneumococcal pneumonia develop bacteremia. Death occurs in about 28% of these bacteremic patients over 50 years of age. Of all patients with pneumococcal bacteremia who died despite treatment with penicillin or tetracy-

cline, as many as 60% died within five days of onset of the illness.
The annual incidence of pneumococcal meningitis is approximately 1.5 to 2.5 per 100,000 population. One-half of the cases occur in children, in whom the fatality rate is about 40%. Children with sickle cell disease have been estimated to have a risk of pneumococcal meningitis nearly 600 times greater than normal children. Other illnesses caused by pneumococci include acute exacerbations of chronic bronchitis, sinusitis, arthritis and conjunctivitis.
Invasive pneumococcal disease causes high morbidity and mortality in spite of effective antimicrobial control by antibiotics. These effects of pneumococcal disease appear due to irreversible physiologic damage caused by the bacteria during the first 5 days following onset of illness, and occur irrespective of antimicrobial therapy. Vaccination offers an effective means of further reducing the mortality and morbidity of this disease.
At present, there are 83 known pneumococcal capsular types. However, the preponderance of pneumococcal diseases is caused by only some capsular types. For example, a 10-year (1952–1962) surveillance at a New York medical center, showed that 56% of all deaths due to pneumococcal pneumonia were caused by 6 capsular types and that approximately 78% of all pneumococcal pneumonias were caused by 12 capsular types. Such unequal distribution of pneumococcal capsular types causing disease has been shown throughout the world. It is on the basis of this information that the pneumococcal vaccine is composed of 23 capsular types, designed to provide coverage of approximately 90% of the most frequently reported types.
It has been established that the purified pneumococcal capsular polysaccharides induce antibody production and that such antibody is effective in preventing pneumococcal disease. Studies in humans have demonstrated the immunogenicity (antibody-stimulating capability) of each of the 23 capsular types when tested in polyvalent vaccines. Adults of all ages responded immunologically to the vaccines. Earlier studies with 12- and 14-valent pneumococcal vaccines in children two years of age and older and in adults showed immunogenic responses. Protective capsular type-specific antibody levels develop by the third week following vaccination.
The protective efficacy of pneumococcal vaccines containing 6 and 12 capsular polysaccharides was investigated in controlled studies of gold miners in South Africa, in whom there is a high attack rate for pneumococcal pneumonia. Capsular type-specific attack rates for pneumococcal pneumonia were observed for the period from 2 weeks through about 1 year after vaccination. The rates for pneumonia caused by the same capsular types represented in the vaccines are given in the table. Protective efficacy was 76% and 92%, respectively, in the two studies for the capsular types represented.
[See table above.]

PNEUMOVAX 23

Number of Capsular Types in Pneumococcal Vaccine	Rate/1000 for Pneumonia Caused by Homologous Capsular Types		Protective Efficacy
	Vaccinated Group	Control Group	
6	9.2	38.3	76%
12	1.8	22.0	92%

In similar studies carried out by Dr. R. Austrian and associates using similar pneumococcal vaccines prepared for the National Institute of Allergy and Infectious Diseases, the reduction in pneumonias caused by the capsular types contained in the vaccines was 79%. Reduction in type-specific pneumococcal bacteremia was 82%. A preliminary report suggests that in patients with sickle cell anemia and/or anatomical or functional asplenia, the vaccine was highly effective in persons over two years of age in preventing severe pneumococcal disease and bacteremia.
The duration of protective effect of PNEUMOVAX 23 is presently unknown, but it has been shown in previous studies with other pneumococcal vaccines that antibody induced by the vaccine may persist for as long as 5 years. Type-specific antibody levels induced by PNEUMOVAX (Pneumococcal Vaccine Polyvalent) (14-valent) have been observed to decline over a 42-month period of observation, but remain significantly above prevaccination levels in almost all recipients who manifest an initial response.

INDICATIONS AND USAGE

PNEUMOVAX 23 is indicated for immunization against pneumococcal disease caused by those pneumococcal types included in the vaccine. Effectiveness of the vaccine in the prevention of pneumococcal pneumonia and pneumococcal bacteremia has been demonstrated in controlled trials.
PNEUMOVAX 23 *will not immunize against capsular types of pneumococcus other than those contained in the vaccine.*
Use in selected individuals over 2 years of age as follows: (1) patients who have anatomical asplenia or who have splenic dysfunction due to sickle cell disease or other causes; (2) persons with chronic illnesses in which there is an increased risk of pneumococcal disease, such as functional impairment of cardiorespiratory, hepatic and renal systems; (3) persons 50 years of age or older; (4) patients with other chronic illnesses who may be at greater risk of developing pneumococcal infection or experiencing more severe pneumococcal illness as a result of alcohol abuse or coexisting diseases including diabetes mellitus, chronic cerebrospinal fluid leakage, or conditions associated with immunosuppression; (5) patients with Hodgkin's disease if immunization can be given at least 10 days prior to treatment. For maximal antibody response immunization should be given at least 14 days prior to the start of treatment with radiation or chemotherapy. Immunization of patients less than 10 days prior to or during treatment is not recommended. (see CONTRAINDICATIONS.)
Use in communities. Persons over 2 years of age as follows: (1) closed groups such as those in residential schools, nursing homes and other institutions. (To decrease the likelihood of acute outbreaks of pneumococcal disease in closed institutional populations where there is increased risk that the disease may be severe, vaccination of the entire closed population should be considered where there are no other contraindications.); (2) groups epidemiologically at risk in the community when there is a generalized outbreak in the population due to a single pneumococcal type included in the vaccine; (3) patients at high risk of influenza complications, particularly pneumonia.
PNEUMOVAX 23 may not be effective in preventing infection resulting from basilar skull fracture or from external communication with cerebrospinal fluid.
Simultaneous administration of pneumococcal polysaccharide vaccine and whole-virus influenza vaccine gives satisfactory antibody response without increasing the occurrence of adverse reactions. Simultaneous administration of the pneumococcal vaccine and split-virus influenza vaccine may also be expected to yield satisfactory results.

Revaccination

Adults

Routine revaccination of adults previously vaccinated with PNEUMOVAX 23 is not recommended except for those at highest risk of pneumococcal infection described in the Immunization Practices Advisory Committee (ACIP) guidelines below. An increased incidence and severity of adverse reactions (generally local reactions) have been reported among healthy adults revaccinated with pneumococcal vaccines at intervals under three years. This was probably due to sustained high antibody levels.
Based on a clinical study, revaccination with PNEUMOVAX 23 is recommended for adults at highest risk of fatal pneumococcal infection who were initially vaccinated with PNEUMOVAX* (Pneumococcal Vaccine Polyvalent) (14-valent) without serious or severe reaction four or more years previously.
The Immunization Practices Advisory Committee (ACIP) has stated that, without more information: persons who received the 14-valent pneumococcal vaccine should not be routinely revaccinated with the 23-valent vaccine, as increased coverage is modest and duration of protection is not well defined. However, revaccination with the 23-valent vaccine should be strongly considered for persons who received the 14-valent vaccine if they are at highest risk of fatal pneumococcal infection (e.g., asplenic patients). Revaccination should also be considered for adults at highest risk who received the 23-valent vaccine ≥ 6 years before and for those shown to have rapid decline in pneumococcal antibody levels (e.g., patients with nephrotic syndrome, renal failure, or transplant recipients).

Children

Children at highest risk of pneumococcal infection (e.g., children with asplenia, sickle cell disease or nephrotic syndrome) may have lower peak antibody levels and/or more rapid antibody decline than do healthy adults. There is evidence that some of these high-risk children (e.g., asplenic children) benefit from revaccination with vaccine containing antigen types 7F, 8, 19F. The Immunization Practices Advisory Committee (ACIP) recommends that revaccination after three to five years should be considered for children at highest risk of pneumococcal infection (e.g., children with asplenia, sickle cell disease or nephrotic syndrome) who would be ten years old or younger at revaccination.

* Registered trademark of MERCK & CO., INC.

CONTRAINDICATIONS

Hypersensitivity to any component of the vaccine. Epinephrine injection (1:1000) must be immediately available should an acute anaphylactoid reaction occur due to any component of the vaccine.
Revaccination with PNEUMOVAX 23 is contraindicated except for those at highest risk of pneumococcal infections (see INDICATIONS AND USAGE, *Revaccination*).
Patients with Hodgkin's disease immunized less than 7 to 10 days prior to immunosuppressive therapy have in some instances been found to have post-immunization antibody levels below their pre-immunization levels. Because of these results, immunization less than 10 days prior to or during treatment is contraindicated.
Patients with Hodgkin's disease who have received extensive chemotherapy and/or nodal irradiation have been shown to have an impaired antibody response to a 12-valent pneumococcal vaccine. Because, in some intensively treated patients, administration of that vaccine depressed pre-existing levels of antibody to some pneumococcal types, PNEUMOVAX 23 is not recommended at this time for patients who have received these forms of therapy for Hodgkin's disease.

WARNINGS

If the vaccine is used in persons receiving immunosuppressive therapy, the expected serum antibody response may not be obtained.
Intradermal administration may cause severe local reactions.

PRECAUTIONS

General

Caution and appropriate care should be exercised in administering PNEUMOVAX 23 to individuals with severely compromised cardiac and/or pulmonary function in whom a systemic reaction would pose a significant risk.
Any febrile respiratory illness or other active infection is reason for delaying use of PNEUMOVAX 23, except when, in the opinion of the physician, withholding the agent entails even greater risk.
In patients who require penicillin (or other antibiotic) prophylaxis against pneumococcal infection, such prophylaxis should not be discontinued after vaccination with PNEUMOVAX 23.

Pregnancy

Pregnancy Category C: Animal reproduction studies have not been conducted with PNEUMOVAX 23. It is also not known whether PNEUMOVAX 23 can cause fetal harm when administered to a pregnant woman or can affect reproduction capacity. PNEUMOVAX 23 should be given to a pregnant woman only if clearly needed.

Nursing Mothers

It is not known whether this drug is excreted in human milk. Because many drugs are excreted in human milk, caution should be exercised when PNEUMOVAX 23 is administered to a nursing woman.

Pediatric Use

Children less than 2 years of age do not respond satisfactorily to the capsular types of PNEUMOVAX 23 that are most often the cause of pneumococcal disease in this age group. Safety and effectiveness in children below the age of 2 years have not been established. Accordingly, PNEUMOVAX 23 is not recommended in this age group.

ADVERSE REACTIONS

Local reactions including local injection site soreness, warmth, erythema and swelling, usually of less than 48 hours duration, occurs commonly; local induration occurs

Continued on next page

23 Pneumococcal Capsular Types Included in PNEUMOVAX 23

Nomenclature	Pneumococcal Types																						
Danish	1	2	3	4	5	6B	7F	8	9N	9V	10A	11A	12F	14	15B	17F	18C	19F	19A	20	22F	23F	33F
U.S.	1	2	3	4	5	26	51	8	9	68	34	43	12	14	54	17	56	19	57	20	22	23	70

Information on the Merck & Co., Inc. products listed on these pages is the full prescribing information from product circulars in use September 30, 1996.

Consult 1997 supplements and future editions for revisions

Merck & Co.—Cont.

less commonly. In a study of PNEUMOVAX 22 (containing 22 capsular types) in 29 adults, 21 (71%) showed local reaction characterized principally by local soreness and/or induration at the injection site within 2 days after vaccination. Rash, urticaria, arthritis, arthralgia, serum sickness, and adenitis have been reported rarely.

Low grade fever (less than 100.9°F) occurs occasionally and is usually confined to the 24-hour period following vaccination. Although rare, fever over 102°F has been reported. Malaise, myalgia, headache, nausea, vomiting and asthenia also have been reported.

Patients with otherwise stabilized idiopathic thrombocytopenic purpura have, on rare occasions, experienced a relapse in their thrombocytopenia, occurring 2 to 14 days after vaccination, and lasting up to 2 weeks.

Reactions of greater severity, duration, or extent are unusual. Neurological disorders such as paresthesias and acute radiculoneuropathy including Guillain-Barré syndrome have been rarely reported in temporal association with administration of pneumococcal vaccine. No cause and effect relationship has been established. Rarely, anaphylactoid reactions have been reported.

DOSAGE AND ADMINISTRATION

Do not inject intravenously. Intradermal administration should be avoided.

Parenteral drug products should be inspected visually for particulate matter and discoloration prior to administration, whenever solution and container permit. PNEUMOVAX 23 is a clear, colorless solution.

Administer a single 0.5 mL dose of PNEUMOVAX 23 subcutaneously or intramuscularly (preferably in the deltoid muscle or lateral mid-thigh), with appropriate precautions to avoid intravascular administration.

Single-Dose and 5-Dose Vials

For Syringe Use Only: Withdraw 0.5 mL from the vial using a sterile needle and syringe free of preservatives, antiseptics and detergents.

It is important to use a separate sterile syringe and needle for each individual patient to prevent transmission of hepatitis B and other infectious agents from one person to another. Store unopened and opened vials at 2–8°C (36–46°F). The vaccine is used directly as supplied. No dilution or reconstitution is necessary. Phenol 0.25% added as preservative. All vaccine must be discarded after the expiration date.

HOW SUPPLIED

No. 4739—PNEUMOVAX 23 contains one 5-dose vial of liquid vaccine, **NDC** 0006-4739-00. For use with syringe only (6505-01-092-0391).

No. 4741—PNEUMOVAX 23 is supplied as follows: **NDC** 0006-4741-00. A box of 5 individual cartons, each containing a single-dose vial of vaccine.

7497411   Issued March 1995
COPYRIGHT © MERCK & CO., INC., 1986
All rights reserved

PRIMAXIN® I.M.   ℞
(Imipenem-Cilastatin Sodium for Suspension)

For Intramuscular Injection Only

DESCRIPTION

Sterile PRIMAXIN† I.M. (Imipenem-Cilastatin Sodium for Suspension) is a formulation of imipenem (a thienamycin antibiotic) and cilastatin sodium (the inhibitor of the renal dipeptidase, dehydropeptidase I). PRIMAXIN I.M. is a potent broad spectrum antibacterial agent for intramuscular administration.

Imipenem (N-formimidoylthienamycin monohydrate) is a crystalline derivative of thienamycin, which is produced by *Streptomyces cattleya*. Its chemical name is [5R-[5α, 6α (R*)]]-6-(1-hydroxyethyl)-3-[[2-[(iminomethyl)amino] ethyl] thio]-7-oxo-1-azabicyclo [3.2.0] hept-2-ene-2-carboxylic acid monohydrate. It is an off-white, nonhygroscopic crystalline compound with a molecular weight of 317.37. It is sparingly soluble in water, and slightly soluble in methanol. Its empirical formula is $C_{12}H_{17}N_3O_4S \cdot H_2O$, and its structural formula is:

Cilastatin sodium is the sodium salt of a derivatized heptenoic acid. Its chemical name is [R-[R*,S*-(Z)]]-7-[(2-

amino-2-carboxyethyl)thio]-2-[[(2,   2-dimethylcyclopropyl) carbonyl]amino]-2-heptenoic acid, monosodium salt. It is an off-white to yellowish-white, hygroscopic, amorphous compound with a molecular weight of 380.43. It is very soluble in water and in methanol. Its empirical formula is $C_{16}H_{25}N_2O_5SNa$, and its structural formula is:

PRIMAXIN I.M. 500 contains 32 mg of sodium (1.4 mEq) and PRIMAXIN I.M. 750 contains 48 mg of sodium (2.1 mEq). Prepared PRIMAXIN I.M. suspensions are white to light tan in color. Variations of color within this range do not affect the potency of the product.

†Registered trademark of MERCK & CO., INC.

CLINICAL PHARMACOLOGY

Following intramuscular administrations of 500 or 750 mg doses of imipenem-cilastatin sodium in a 1:1 ratio with 1% lidocaine, peak plasma levels of imipenem antimicrobial activity occur within 2 hours and average 10 and 12 mcg/mL, respectively. For cilastatin, peak plasma levels average 24 and 33 mcg/mL, respectively, and occur within 1 hour. When compared to intravenous administration of imipenem-cilastatin sodium, imipenem is approximately 75% bioavailable following intramuscular administration while cilastatin is approximately 95% bioavailable. The absorption of imipenem from the IM injection site continues for 6 to 8 hours while that for cilastatin is essentially complete within 4 hours. This prolonged absorption of imipenem following the administration of the intramuscular formulation of imipenem-cilastatin sodium results in an effective plasma half-life of imipenem of approximately 2 to 3 hours and plasma levels of the antibiotic which remain above 2 mcg/mL for at least 6 or 8 hours, following a 500 mg or 750 mg dose, respectively. This plasma profile for imipenem permits IM administration of the intramuscular formulation of imipenem-cilastatin sodium every 12 hours with no accumulation of cilastatin and only slight accumulation of imipenem.

A comparison of plasma levels of imipenem after a single dose of 500 mg or 750 mg of imipenem-cilastatin sodium (intravenous formulation) administered intravenously or of imipenem-cilastatin sodium (intramuscular formulation) diluted with 1% lidocaine and administered intramuscularly is as follows:

PLASMA CONCENTRATIONS OF IMIPENEM
(mcg/mL)

	500 MG		750 MG	
TIME	I.V.	I.M.	I.V.	I.M.
25 min	45.1	6.0	57.0	6.7
1 hr	21.6	9.4	28.1	10.0
2 hr	10.0	9.9	12.0	11.4
4 hr	2.6	5.6	3.4	7.3
6 hr	0.6	2.5	1.1	3.8
12 hr	ND†	0.5	ND†	0.8

† ND: Not Detectable (<0.3 mcg/mL)

Imipenem urine levels remain above 10 mcg/mL for the 12 hour dosing interval following the administration of 500 mg or 750 mg doses of the intramuscular formulation of imipenem-cilastatin sodium. Total urinary excretion of imipenem averages 50% while that for cilastatin averages 75% following either dose of the intramuscular formulation of imipenem-cilastatin sodium.

Imipenem, when administered alone, is metabolized in the kidneys by dehydropeptidase I resulting in relatively low levels in urine. Cilastatin sodium, an inhibitor of this enzyme, effectively prevents renal metabolism of imipenem so that when imipenem and cilastatin sodium are given concomitantly, increased levels of imipenem are achieved in the urine. The binding of imipenem to human serum proteins is approximately 20% and that of cilastatin is approximately 40%.

In a clinical study in which a 500 mg dose of the intramuscular formulation of imipenem-cilastatin sodium was administered to healthy subjects, the average peak level of imipenem in interstitial fluid (skin blister fluid) was approximately 5.0 mcg/mL within 3.5 hours after administration. Imipenem-cilastatin sodium is hemodialyzable. However, usefulness of this procedure in the overdosage setting is questionable (see OVERDOSAGE).

Microbiology

The bactericidal activity of imipenem results from the inhibition of cell wall synthesis. Its greatest affinity is for penicillin-binding proteins (PBPs) 1A, 1B, 2, 4, 5 and 6 of *Escheri-*

chia coli, and 1A, 1B, 2, 4 and 5 of *Pseudomonas aeruginosa*. The lethal effect is related to binding to PBP 2 and PBP 1B.

Imipenem has a high degree of stability in the presence of beta-lactamases, including penicillinases and cephalosporinases produced by gram-negative and gram-positive bacteria. It is a potent inhibitor of beta-lactamases from certain gram-negative bacteria which are inherently resistant to many beta-lactam antibiotics, e.g., *Pseudomonas aeruginosa*, *Serratia* spp. and *Enterobacter* spp.

Imipenem has *in vitro* activity against a wide range of gram-positive and gram-negative organisms. Imipenem is active against most strains of the following microorganisms *in vitro* and in clinical infections treated with the intramuscular formulation of imipenem-cilastatin sodium (see INDICATIONS AND USAGE).

Gram-positive aerobes:
Staphylococcus aureus including penicillinase-producing strains
    (NOTE: Methicillin-resistant staphylococci should be reported as resistant to imipenem.)
Group D streptococcus including *Enterococcus faecalis* (formerly *S. faecalis*)
    (NOTE: Imipenem is inactive *in vitro* against *Enterococcus faecium* [formerly *S. faecium*].)
Streptococcus pneumoniae
Streptococcus pyogenes (Group A streptococcus)
Streptococcus viridans group

Gram-negative aerobes:
Acinetobacter spp., including *A. calcoaceticus*
Citrobacter spp.
Enterobacter cloacae
Escherichia coli
Haemophilus influenzae
Klebsiella pneumoniae
Pseudomonas aeruginosa
    (NOTE: Imipenem is inactive *in vitro* against *Xanthomonas (Pseudomonas) maltophilia* and *P. cepacia*.)

Gram-positive anaerobes:
Peptostreptococcus spp.

Gram-negative anaerobes:
Bacteroides spp., including
    Bacteroides distasonis
    Bacteroides intermedius (formerly *B. melaninogenicus intermedius*)
    Bacteroides fragilis
    Bacteroides thetaiotaomicron
Fusobacterium spp.

Imipenem has been shown to be active *in vitro* against the following microorganisms; however, the clinical significance of these data is unknown.

Gram-positive aerobes:
Listeria monocytogenes
Nocardia spp.
Staphylococcus epidermidis including penicillinase-producing strains.
    (NOTE: Methicillin-resistant staphylococci should be reported as resistant to imipenem.)
Streptococcus agalactiae (Group B streptococcus)
Group C streptococcus
Group G streptococcus

Gram-negative aerobes:
Achromobacter spp.
Aeromonas hydrophila
Alcaligenes spp.
Bordetella bronchiseptica
Campylobacter spp.
Enterobacter spp.
Gardnerella vaginalis
Haemophilus parainfluenzae
Hafnia spp., including *H. alvei*
Klebsiella spp., including *K. oxytoca*
Moraxella spp.
Morganella morganii
Neisseria gonorrhoeae including penicillinase-producing strains
Pasteurella multocida
Plesiomonas shigelloides
Proteus mirabilis
Proteus vulgaris
Providencia rettgeri
Providencia stuartii
Salmonella spp.
Serratia spp., including *S. marcescens* and *S. proteamaculans* (formerly *S. liquefaciens*)
Shigella spp.
Yersinia spp., including *Y. enterocolitica* and *Y. pseudotuberculosis*

Gram-positive anaerobes:
Actinomyces spp.
Clostridium spp., including *C. perfringens*
Eubacterium spp.
Peptococcus niger
Propionibacterium spp., including *P. acnes*

Gram-negative anaerobes:
Bacteroides bivius
Bacteroides disiens

Bacteroides ovatus
Bacteroides vulgatus
Porphyromonas asaccharolytica (formerly *Bacteroides asaccharolyticus*)
Veillonella spp.

In vitro tests show imipenem to act synergistically with aminoglycoside antibiotics against some isolates of *Pseudomonas aeruginosa.*

Susceptibility Tests:
Diffusion techniques:
Quantitative methods that require measurement of zone diameters give the most precise estimate of antibiotic susceptibility. One such standard procedure[1], which has been recommended for use with disks to test susceptibility of organisms to imipenem, uses the 10-mcg imipenem disk. Interpretation involves the correlation of the diameters obtained in the disk test with the minimum inhibitory concentration (MIC) for imipenem.

Reports from the laboratory giving results of the standard single-disk susceptibility test with a 10-mcg imipenem disk should be interpreted according to the following criteria:

Zone Diameter (mm)	Interpretation
≥16	Susceptible
14–15	Moderately Susceptible
≤13	Resistant

A report of "susceptible" indicates that the pathogen is likely to be inhibited by generally achievable blood levels. A report of "moderately susceptible" suggests that the organism would be susceptible if high dosage is used or if the infection is confined to tissues and fluids in which high antibiotic levels are attained. A report of "resistant" indicates that achievable concentrations are unlikely to be inhibitory and other therapy should be selected.

Standardized procedures require the use of laboratory control organisms. The 10-mcg imipenem disk should give the following zone diameters:

Organism	Zone Diameter (mm)
E. coli ATCC 25922	26–32
P. aeruginosa ATCC 27853	20–28

Dilution techniques:
Use a standardized dilution method[2] (broth, agar, microdilution) or equivalent with imipenem powder. The MIC values obtained should be interpreted according to the following criteria:

MIC (mcg/mL)	Interpretation
≤4	Susceptible
8	Moderately Susceptible
≥16	Resistant

As with standard diffusion techniques, dilution methods require the use of laboratory control organisms. Standard imipenem powder should provide the following MIC values:

Organism	MIC (mcg/mL)
E. coli ATCC 25922	0.06–0.25
S. aureus ATCC 29213	0.015–0.06
E. faecalis ATCC 29212	0.5–2.0
P. aeruginosa ATCC 27853	1.0–4.0

For anaerobic bacteria, the MIC of imipenem can be determined by agar or broth dilution (including microdilution) techniques.[3]

INDICATIONS AND USAGE

PRIMAXIN I.M. is indicated for the treatment of serious infections (listed below) of mild to moderate severity for which intramuscular therapy is appropriate. **PRIMAXIN I.M. is not intended for the therapy of severe or life-threatening infections, including bacterial sepsis or endocarditis, or in instances of major physiological impairments such as shock.**

PRIMAXIN I.M. is indicated for the treatment of infections caused by susceptible strains of the designated microorganisms in the conditions listed below:

(1) **Lower respiratory tract infections,** including pneumonia and bronchitis as an exacerbation of COPD, caused by *Streptococcus pneumoniae* and *Haemophilus influenzae.*
(2) **Intra-abdominal infections,** including acute gangrenous or perforated appendicitis and appendicitis with peritonitis, caused by Group D streptococcus including *Enterococcus faecalis*; Streptococcus viridans* group*; *Escherichia coli; Klebsiella pneumoniae*; Pseudomonas aeruginosa*; Bacteroides* species including *B. fragilis, B. distasonis*, B. intermedius** and *B. thetaiotaomicron*; Fusobacterium* species and *Peptostreptococcus** species.
(3) **Skin and skin structure infections,** including abscesses, cellulitis, infected skin ulcers and wound infections caused by *Staphylococcus aureus* including penicillinase-producing strains; *Streptococcus pyogenes**; Group D streptococcus including *Enterococcus faecalis; Acinetobacter* species* including *A. calcoaceticus*; Citrobacter* species*; *Escherichia coli; Enterobacter cloacae; Klebsiella pneumoniae*; Pseudomonas aeruginosa** and *Bacteroides* species* including *B. fragilis*.*
(4) **Gynecologic infections,** including postpartum endomyometritis, caused by Group D streptococcus including *Enterococcus faecalis*; Escherichia coli; Klebsiella pneumoniae*; Bacteroides intermedius**; and *Peptostreptococcus* species*.

As with other beta-lactam antibiotics, some strains of *Pseudomonas aeruginosa* may develop resistance fairly rapidly during treatment with PRIMAXIN I.M. During therapy of *Pseudomonas aeruginosa* infections, periodic susceptibility testing should be done when clinically appropriate.

* Efficacy for this organism in this organ system was studied in fewer than 10 infections.

CONTRAINDICATIONS

PRIMAXIN I.M. is contraindicated in patients who have shown hypersensitivity to any component of this product. Due to the use of lidocaine hydrochloride diluent, this product is contraindicated in patients with a known hypersensitivity to local anesthetics of the amide type and in patients with severe shock or heart block. (Refer to the package circular for lidocaine hydrochloride).

WARNINGS

SERIOUS AND OCCASIONALLY FATAL HYPERSENSITIVITY (anaphylactic) REACTIONS HAVE BEEN REPORTED IN PATIENTS RECEIVING THERAPY WITH BETA-LACTAMS. THESE REACTIONS ARE MORE LIKELY TO OCCUR IN INDIVIDUALS WITH A HISTORY OF SENSITIVITY TO MULTIPLE ALLERGENS. THERE HAVE BEEN REPORTS OF INDIVIDUALS WITH A HISTORY OF PENICILLIN HYPERSENSITIVITY WHO HAVE EXPERIENCED SEVERE REACTIONS WHEN TREATED WITH ANOTHER BETA-LACTAM. BEFORE INITIATING THERAPY WITH PRIMAXIN® I.M., CAREFUL INQUIRY SHOULD BE MADE CONCERNING PREVIOUS HYPERSENSITIVITY REACTIONS TO PENICILLINS, CEPHALOSPORINS, OTHER BETA-LACTAMS, AND OTHER ALLERGENS. IF AN ALLERGIC REACTION OCCURS, PRIMAXIN® SHOULD BE DISCONTINUED. **SERIOUS ANAPHYLACTIC REACTIONS REQUIRE IMMEDIATE EMERGENCY TREATMENT WITH EPINEPHRINE. OXYGEN, INTRAVENOUS STEROIDS, AND AIRWAY MANAGEMENT, INCLUDING INTUBATION, MAY ALSO BE ADMINISTERED AS INDICATED.**

Pseudomembranous colitis has been reported with nearly all antibacterial agents, including PRIMAXIN, and may range in severity from mild to life-threatening. Therefore, it is important to consider this diagnosis in patients who present with diarrhea subsequent to the administration of antibacterial agents.

Treatment with antibacterial agents alters the normal flora of the colon and may permit overgrowth of clostridia. Studies indicate that a toxin produced by *Clostridium difficile* is one primary cause of "antibiotic-associated colitis".

After the diagnosis of pseudomembranous colitis has been established, therapeutic measures should be initiated. Mild cases of pseudomembranous colitis usually respond to drug discontinuation alone. In moderate to severe cases, consideration should be given to management with fluids and electrolytes, protein supplementation and treatment with an antibacterial drug effective against *C. difficile.*

Lidocaine HCl —Refer to the package circular for lidocaine HCl.

PRECAUTIONS

General
CNS adverse experiences such as myoclonic activity, confusional states, or seizures have been reported with PRIMAXIN I.V. (Imipenem-Cilastatin Sodium for Injection). These experiences have occurred most commonly in patients with CNS disorders (e.g., brain lesions or history of seizures) who also have compromised renal function. However, there were reports in which there was no recognized or documented underlying CNS disorder. These adverse CNS effects have not been seen with PRIMAXIN I.M.; however, should they occur during treatment, PRIMAXIN I.M. should be discontinued. Anticonvulsant therapy should be continued in patients with a known seizure disorder.

As with other antibiotics, prolonged use of PRIMAXIN I.M. may result in overgrowth of nonsusceptible organisms. Repeated evaluation of the patient's condition is essential. If superinfection occurs during therapy, appropriate measures should be taken.

Caution should be taken to avoid inadvertent injection into a blood vessel (see DOSAGE AND ADMINISTRATION). For additional precautions, refer to the package circular for lidocaine HCl.

Drug Interactions
Since concomitant administration of PRIMAXIN (Imipenem-Cilastatin Sodium) and probenecid results in only minimal increases in plasma levels of imipenem and plasma half-life, it is not recommended that probenecid be given with PRIMAXIN I.M.

PRIMAXIN I.M. should not be mixed with or physically added to other antibiotics. However, PRIMAXIN I.M. may be administered concomitantly with other antibiotics, such as aminoglycosides.

Carcinogenesis, Mutagenesis, Impairment of Fertility
Long term studies in animals have not been performed to evaluate carcinogenic potential of imipenem-cilastatin. Genetic toxicity studies were performed in a variety of bacterial and mammalian tests *in vivo* and *in vitro.* The tests used were: V79 mammalian cell mutagenesis assay (imipenem-cilastatin sodium alone and imipenem alone), Ames test (cilastatin sodium alone and imipenem alone), unscheduled DNA synthesis assay (imipenem-cilastatin sodium) and *in vivo* mouse cytogenetics test (imipenem-cilastatin sodium). None of these tests showed any evidence of genetic alterations.

Reproductive tests in male and female rats were performed with imipenem-cilastatin sodium at dosage levels up to 11 times† the maximum daily recommended human dose of the intramuscular formulation (on a mg/kg basis). Slight decreases in live fetal body weight were restricted to the highest dosage level. No other adverse effects were observed on fertility, reproductive performance, fetal viability, growth or postnatal development of pups. Similarly, no adverse effects on the fetus or on lactation were observed when imipenem-cilastatin sodium was administered to rats late in gestation.

Pregnancy: Teratogenic Effects
Pregnancy Category C: Teratology studies with cilastatin sodium in rabbits and rats at 10 and 33 times† the maximum recommended daily human dose of the intramuscular formulation (30 mg/kg/day) of PRIMAXIN, respectively, showed no evidence of adverse effects on the fetus. No evidence of teratogenicity was observed in rabbits and rats given imipenem at doses up to 2 and 30 times† the maximum recommended daily human dose of the intramuscular formulation of PRIMAXIN, respectively.

Teratology studies with imipenem-cilastatin sodium at doses up to 11 times† the maximum recommended human dose in pregnant mice and rats during the period of major organogenesis revealed no evidence of teratogenicity.

Imipenem-cilastatin sodium, when administered to pregnant rabbits at dosages above the usual human dose of the intramuscular formulation (1000–1500 mg/day), caused body weight loss, diarrhea, and maternal deaths. When comparable doses of imipenem-cilastatin sodium were given to non-pregnant rabbits, body weight loss, diarrhea, and deaths were also observed. This intolerance is not unlike that seen with other beta-lactam antibiotics in this species and is probably due to alteration of gut flora.

A teratology study in pregnant cynomolgus monkeys given imipenem-cilastatin sodium at doses of 40 mg/kg/day (bolus intravenous injection) or 160 mg/kg/day (subcutaneous injection) resulted in maternal toxicity including emesis, inappetence, body weight loss, diarrhea, abortion and death in some cases. In contrast, no significant toxicity was observed when nonpregnant cynomolgus monkeys were given doses of imipenem-cilastatin sodium up to 180 mg/kg/day (subcutaneous injection). When doses of imipenem-cilastatin sodium (approximately 100 mg/kg/day or approximately 3 times† the maximum daily recommended human dose of the intramuscular formulation) were administered to pregnant cynomolgus monkeys at an intraveous infusion rate which mimics human clinical use, there was minimal maternal intolerance (occasional emesis), no maternal deaths, no evidence of teratogenicity, but an increase in embryonic loss relative to the control groups.

There are, however, no adequate and well-controlled studies in pregnant women. PRIMAXIN I.M. should be used during pregnancy only if the potential benefit justifies the potential risk to the mother and fetus.

Nursing Mothers
It is not known whether imipenem-cilastatin sodium or lidocaine HCl (diluent) is excreted in human milk. Because many drugs are excreted in human milk, caution should be exercised when PRIMAXIN I.M. is administered to a nursing woman.

Pediatric Use
Safety and effectiveness in children below the age of 12 years have not been established.

† Based on patient weight of 50 kg.

ADVERSE REACTIONS

PRIMAXIN I.M.
In 686 patients in multiple dose clinical trials of PRIMAXIN I.M., the following adverse reactions were reported:

Continued on next page

Information on the Merck & Co., Inc. products listed on these pages is the full prescribing information from product circulars in use September 30, 1996.

Merck & Co.—Cont.

Local Adverse Reactions
The most frequent adverse local clinical reaction that was reported as possibly, probably or definitely related to therapy with PRIMAXIN I.M. was pain at the injection site (1.2%).
Systemic Adverse Reactions
The most frequently reported systemic adverse clinical reactions that were reported as possibly, probably or definitely related to PRIMAXIN I.M. were nausea (0.6%), diarrhea (0.6%), vomiting (0.3%) and rash (0.4%).
Adverse Laboratory Changes
Adverse laboratory changes without regard to drug relationship that were reported during clinical trials were:
Hemic: decreased hemoglobin and hematocrit, eosinophilia, increased and decreased WBC, increased and decreased platelets, decreased erythrocytes, and increased prothrombin time.
Hepatic: increased AST, ALT, alkaline phosphatase, and bilirubin.
Renal: increased BUN and creatinine.
Urinalysis: presence of red blood cells, white blood cells, casts, and bacteria in the urine.
Potential ADVERSE EFFECTS:
In addition, a variety of adverse effects, not observed in clinical trials with PRIMAXIN I.M., have been reported with intravenous administration of PRIMAXIN I.V. (Imipenem-Cilastatin Sodium for Injection). Those listed below are to serve as alerting information to physicians.
Systemic Adverse Reactions
The most frequently reported systemic adverse clinical reactions that were reported as possibly, probably or definitely related to PRIMAXIN I.V. (Imipenem-Cilastatin Sodium for Injection) were fever, hypotension, seizures (see PRECAUTIONS), dizziness, pruritus, urticaria, and somnolence.
Additional adverse systemic clinical reactions reported possibly, probably or definitely drug related or reported since the drug was marketed are listed within each body system in order of decreasing severity: *Gastrointestinal:* pseudomembranous colitis (the onset of pseudomembranous colitis symptoms may occur during or after antibiotic treatment, see WARNINGS), hemorrhagic colitis, hepatitis, jaundice, gastroenteritis, abdominal pain, glossitis, tongue papillar hypertrophy, staining of the teeth, heartburn, pharyngeal pain, increased salivation; *Hematologic:* pancytopenia, bone marrow depression, thrombocytopenia, neutropenia, leukopenia, hemolytic anemia; *CNS:* encephalopathy, tremor, confusion, myoclonus, paresthesia, vertigo, headache, psychic disturbances including hallucinations; *Special Senses:* hearing loss, tinnitus, taste perversion; *Respiratory:* chest discomfort, dyspnea, hyperventilation, thoracic spine pain; *Cardiovascular:* palpitations, tachycardia; *Renal:* acute renal failure, oliguria/anuria, polyuria, urine discoloration; *Skin:* toxic epidermal necrolysis, Stevens-Johnson syndrome, erythema multiforme, angioneurotic edema, flushing, cyanosis, hyperhidrosis, skin texture changes, candidiasis, pruritus vulvae; *Body as a whole:* polyarthralgia, asthenia/ weakness.
Adverse Laboratory Changes
Adverse laboratory changes without regard to drug relationship that were reported during clinical trials or reported since the drug was marketed were:
Hepatic: increased LDH; *Hemic:* positive Coombs test, decreased neutrophils, agranulocytosis, increased monocytes, abnormal prothrombin time, increased lymphocytes, increased basophils; *Electrolytes:* decreased serum sodium, increased potassium, increased chloride; *Urinalysis:* presence of urine protein, urine bilirubin, and urine urobilinogen.
Lidocaine HCl —Refer to the package circular for lidocaine HCl.

OVERDOSAGE

The acute intravenous toxicity of imipenem-cilastatin sodium in a ratio of 1:1 was studied in mice at doses of 751 to 1359 mg/kg. Following drug administration, ataxia was rapidly produced and clonic convulsions were noted in about 45 minutes. Deaths occurred within 4–56 minutes at all doses. The acute intravenous toxicity of imipenem-cilastatin sodium was produced within 5–10 minutes in rats at doses of 771 to 1583 mg/kg. In all dosage groups, females had de-

creased activity, bradypnea and ptosis with clonic convulsions preceding death; in males, ptosis was seen at all dose levels while tremors and clonic convulsions were seen at all but the lowest dose (771 mg/kg). In another rat study, female rats showed ataxia, bradypnea and decreased activity in all but the lowest dose (550 mg/kg); deaths were preceded by clonic convulsions. Male rats showed tremors at all doses and clonic convulsions and ptosis were seen at the two highest doses (1130 and 1734 mg/kg). Deaths occurred between 6 and 88 minutes with doses of 771 to 1734 mg/kg.
In the case of overdosage, discontinue PRIMAXIN I.M., treat symptomatically, and institute supportive measures as required. Imipenem-cilastatin sodium is hemodialyzable. However, usefulness of this procedure in the overdosage setting is questionable.

DOSAGE AND ADMINISTRATION

PRIMAXIN I.M. is for intramuscular use only.
The dosage recommendations for PRIMAXIN I.M. represent the quantity of imipenem to be administered. An equivalent amount of cilastatin is also present.
Patients with lower respiratory tract infections, skin and skin structure infections, and gynecologic infections of mild to moderate severity may be treated with 500 mg or 750 mg administered every 12 hours depending on the severity of the infection.
Intra-abdominal infection may be treated with 750 mg every 12 hours. [See table below.]
Total daily IM dosages greater than 1500 mg per day are not recommended.
The dosage for any particular patient should be based on the location of and severity of the infection, the susceptibility of the infecting pathogen(s), and renal function.
The duration of therapy depends upon the type and severity of the infection. Generally, PRIMAXIN I.M. should be continued for at least two days after the signs and symptoms of infection have resolved. Safety and efficacy of treatment beyond fourteen days have not been established.
PRIMAXIN I.M. should be administered by deep intramuscular injection into a large muscle mass (such as the gluteal muscles or lateral part of the thigh) with a 21 gauge 2″ needle. Aspiration is necessary to avoid inadvertent injection into a blood vessel.

ADULTS WITH IMPAIRED RENAL FUNCTION

The safety and efficacy of PRIMAXIN I.M. have not been studied in patients with creatinine clearance of less than 20 mL/ min/1.73m^2. Serum creatinine alone may not be a sufficiently accurate measure of renal function. Creatinine clearance (T_{cc}) may be estimated from the following equation:

$$T_{cc} \text{ (Males)} = \frac{\text{(wt. in kg) } (140 - \text{age})}{(72) \text{ (creatinine in mg/dL)}}$$

$$T_{cc} \text{ (Females)} = 0.85 \times \text{above value}$$

PREPARATION FOR ADMINISTRATION

PRIMAXIN I.M. should be prepared for use with 1.0% lidocaine HCl solution† (without epinephrine). PRIMAXIN I.M. 500 should be prepared with 2 mL and PRIMAXIN I.M. 750 with 3 mL of lidocaine HCl. Agitate to form a suspension then withdraw and inject the entire contents of vial intramuscularly. The suspension of PRIMAXIN I.M. in lidocaine HCl should be used within one hour after preparation. **Note: The IM formulation is not for IV use.**

---

† Refer to the package circular for lidocaine HCl for detailed information concerning CONTRAINDICATIONS, WARNINGS, PRECAUTIONS, and ADVERSE REACTIONS.

COMPATIBILITY AND STABILITY

Before reconsitution:
The dry powder should be stored at a temperature below 30℃ (86°F).
Suspensions for IM Administration
Suspensions of PRIMAXIN I.M. are white to light tan in color. Variations of color within this range do not affect the potency of the product.
The suspension of PRIMAXIN I.M. in lidocaine HCl should be used within one hour after preparation.
PRIMAXIN I.M. should not be mixed with or physically added to other antibiotics. However, PRIMAXIN I.M. may be

administered concomitantly but at separate sites with other antibiotics, such as aminoglycosides.

HOW SUPPLIED

PRIMAXIN I.M. is supplied as a sterile powder mixture in vials for IM administration as follows:
No. 3582—500 mg imipenem equivalent and 500 mg cilastatin equivalent
NDC 0006-3582-75 in trays of 10 vials
(6505-01-337-3131 500 mg, 10's).
No. 3583—750 mg imipenem equivalent and 750 mg cilastatin equivalent
NDC 0006-3583-76 in trays of 10 vials
(6505-01-337-3130 750 mg, 10's).

REFERENCES

1. National Committee for Clinical Laboratory Standards, Performance Standards for Antimicrobial Disk Susceptibility Tests— Fourth Edition. Approved Standard NCCLS Document M2-A4, Vol. 10, No. 7 NCCLS, Villanova, PA, 1990.
2. National Committee for Clinical Laboratory Standards, Methods for Dilution Antimicrobial Susceptibility Tests for Bacteria that Grow Aerobically—Second Edition. Approved Standard NCCLS Document M7-A2, Vol. 10, No. 8 NCCLS, Villanova, PA, 1990.
3. National Committee for Clinical Laboratory Standards, Methods for Antimicrobial Susceptibility Testing of Anaerobic Bacteria—Second Edition. Tentative Standard NCCLS Document M11-T2, Villanova, PA, 1988.
7632906   Issued June 1994

PRIMAXIN® I.V.   ℞
(Imipenem-Cilastatin Sodium for Injection)

For Intravenous Injection Only

DESCRIPTION

PRIMAXIN† I.V. (Imipenem-Cilastatin Sodium for Injection) is a sterile formulation of imipenem (a thienamycin antibiotic) and cilastatin sodium (the inhibitor of the renal dipeptidase, dehydropeptidase I), with sodium bicarbonate added as a buffer. PRIMAXIN I.V. is a potent broad spectrum antibacterial agent for intravenous administration. Imipenem (N-formimidoylthienamycin monohydrate) is a crystalline derivative of thienamycin, which is produced by *Streptomyces cattleya.* Its chemical name is (5R,6S)-3-[[2-(formimidoylamino)ethyl]thio]-6-[(R)-1-hydroxyethyl]-7-oxo-1-azabicyclo[3.2.0]hept-2-ene-2-carboxylic acid monohydrate. It is an off-white, nonhygroscopic crystalline compound with a molecular weight of 317.37. It is sparingly soluble in water, and slightly soluble in methanol. Its empirical formula is $C_{12}H_{17}N_3O_4S \cdot H_2O$, and its structural formula is:

Cilastatin sodium is the sodium salt of a derivatized heptenoic acid. Its chemical name is sodium (Z)-7-[[(R)-2-amino-2-carboxyethyl]thio] -2- [(S) - 2,2- dimethylcyclopropanecarboxamido]-2-heptenoate. It is an off-white to yellowish-white, hygroscopic, amorphous compound with a molecular weight of 380.43. It is very soluble in water and in methanol. Its empirical formula is $C_{16}H_{25}N_2O_5S$ Na, and its structural formula is:

PRIMAXIN I.V. is buffered to provide solutions in the pH range of 6.5 to 7.5. There is no significant change in pH when solutions are prepared and used as directed. (See **COMPATIBILITY AND STABILITY**.) PRIMAXIN I.V. 250 contains 18.8 mg of sodium (0.8 mEq) and PRIMAXIN I.V. 500 contains 37.5 mg of sodium (1.6 mEq). Solutions of PRIMAXIN I.V. range from colorless to yellow. Variations of color within this range do not affect the potency of the product.

---

†Registered trademark of MERCK & CO., INC.

DOSAGE GUIDELINES		
Type†/Location of Infection	Severity	Dosage Regimen
Lower respiratory tract Skin and skin structure Gynecologic	Mild/Moderate	500 or 750 mg q 12 h depending on the severity of infection
Intra-abdominal	Mild/Moderate	750 mg q 12 h

†See INDICATIONS AND USAGE section.

CLINICAL PHARMACOLOGY

Intravenous Administration

Intravenous infusion of PRIMAXIN I.V. over 20 minutes results in peak plasma levels of imipenem antimicrobial activity that range from 14 to 24 µg/mL for the 250 mg dose, from 21 to 58 µg/mL for the 500 mg dose and from 41 to 83 µg/mL for the 1000 mg dose. At these doses, plasma levels of imipenem antimicrobial activity decline to below 1 µg/mL or less in 4 to 6 hours. Peak plasma levels of cilastatin following a 20-minute intravenous infusion of PRIMAXIN I.V., range from 15 to 25 µg/mL for the 250 mg dose, from 31 to 49 µg/mL for the 500 mg dose and from 56 to 88 µg/mL for the 1000 mg dose.

General

The plasma half-life of each component is approximately 1 hour. The binding of imipenem to human serum proteins is approximately 20% and that of cilastatin is approximately 40%. Approximately 70% of the administered imipenem is recovered in the urine within 10 hours after which no further urinary excretion is detectable. Urine concentrations of imipenem in excess of 10 µg/mL can be maintained for up to 8 hours with PRIMAXIN I.V. at the 500 mg dose. Approximately 70% of the cilastatin sodium dose is recovered in the urine within 10 hours of administration of PRIMAXIN I.V. No accumulation of PRIMAXIN I.V. in plasma or urine is observed with regimens administered as frequently as every 6 hours in patients with normal renal function.

Imipenem, when administered alone, is metabolized in the kidneys by dehydropeptidase I resulting in relatively low levels in urine. Cilastatin sodium, an inhibitor of this enzyme, effectively prevents renal metabolism of imipenem so that when imipenem and cilastatin sodium are given concomitantly, fully adequate antibacterial levels of imipenem are achieved in the urine.

After a 1 gram dose of PRIMAXIN I.V., the following average levels of imipenem were measured (usually at 1 hour post-dose except where indicated) in the tissues and fluids listed:

[See table above.]

Imipenem-cilastatin sodium is hemodialyzable. However, usefulness of this procedure in the overdosage setting is questionable. (See **OVERDOSAGE**.)

Microbiology

The bactericidal activity of imipenem results from the inhibition of cell wall synthesis. Its greatest affinity is for penicillin binding proteins (PBPs) 1A, 1B, 2, 4, 5 and 6 of *Escherichia coli*, and 1A, 1B, 2, 4 and 5 of *Pseudomonas aeruginosa*. The lethal effect is related to binding to PBP 2 and PBP 1B. Imipenem has a high degree of stability in the presence of beta-lactamases, both penicillinases and cephalosporinases produced by gram-negative and gram-positive bacteria. It is a potent inhibitor of beta-lactamases from certain gram-negative bacteria which are inherently resistant to most beta-lactam antibiotics, e.g., *Pseudomonas aeruginosa*, *Serratia* spp., and *Enterobacter* spp.

Imipenem has *in vitro* activity against a wide range of gram-positive and gram-negative organisms. Imipenem is active against most strains of the following microorganisms *in vitro* and in clinical infections treated with the intravenous formulation of imipenem-cilastatin sodium. (See **INDICATIONS AND USAGE**.)

Gram-positive aerobes:
Enterococcus faecalis (formerly *S. faecalis*)
 (NOTE: Imipenem is inactive *in vitro* against *Enterococcus faecium* [formerly *S. faecium*].)
Staphylococcus aureus including penicillinase-producing strains
Staphylococcus epidermidis including penicillinase-producing strains
 (NOTE: Methicillin-resistant staphylococci should be reported as resistant to imipenem.)
Streptococcus agalactiae (Group B streptococcus)
Streptococcus pneumoniae
Streptococcus pyogenes
Gram-negative aerobes:
Acinetobacter spp.
Citrobacter spp.
Enterobacter spp.
Escherichia coli
Gardnerella vaginalis
Haemophilus influenzae
Haemophilus parainfluenzae
Klebsiella spp.
Morganella morganii
Proteus vulgaris
Providencia rettgeri
Pseudomonas aeruginosa
 (NOTE: Imipenem is inactive *in vitro* against *Xanthomonas (Pseudomonas) maltophilia* and some strains of *P. cepacia*.)
Serratia spp., including *S. marcescens*
Gram-positive anaerobes:
Bifidobacterium spp.
Clostridium spp.

Tissue or Fluid	n	Imipenem Level µg/mL or µg/g	Range
Vitreous Humor	3	3.4 (3.5 hours post dose)	2.88–3.6
Aqueous Humor	5	2.99 (2 hours post dose)	2.4–3.9
Lung Tissue	8	5.6 (median)	3.5–15.5
Sputum	1	2.1	—
Pleural	1	22.0	
Peritoneal	12	23.9 S.D. ±5.3 (2 hours post dose)	—
Bile	2	5.3 (2.25 hours post dose)	4.6 to 6.0
CSF (uninflamed)	5	1.0 (4 hours post dose)	0.26–2.0
CSF (inflamed)	7	2.6 (2 hours post dose)	0.5–5.5
Fallopian Tubes	1	13.6	—
Endometrium	1	11.1	—
Myometrium	1	5.0	—
Bone	10	2.6	0.4–5.4
Interstitial Fluid	12	16.4	10.0–22.6
Skin	12	4.4	NA
Fascia	12	4.4	NA

Eubacterium spp.
Peptococcus spp.
Peptostreptococcus spp.
Propionibacterium spp.
Gram-negative anaerobes:
Bacteroides spp., including *B. fragilis*
Fusobacterium spp.
The following *in vitro* data are available, **but their clinical significance is unknown.**
Imipenem exhibits *in vitro* minimum inhibitory concentrations (MIC's) of 4 µg/mL or less against most (≥ 90%) strains of the following microorganisms; however, the safety and effectiveness of imipenem in treating clinical infections due to these microorganisms have not been established in adequate and well-controlled clinical trials.
Gram-positive aerobes:
Listeria monocytogenes
Nocardia spp.
Group C streptococcus
Group G streptococcus
Viridans group streptococci
Gram-negative aerobes:
Achromobacter spp.
Aeromonas hydrophila
Alcaligenes spp.
Bordetella bronchiseptica
Campylobacter spp.
Hafnia alvei
Klebsiella oxytoca
Klebsiella pneumoniae
Moraxella spp.
Neisseria gonorrhoeae including penicillinase-producing strains
Pasteurella multocida
Plesiomonas shigelloides
Proteus mirabilis
Providencia stuartii
Salmonella spp.
Serratia proteamaculans (formerly *S. liquefaciens*)
Shigella spp.
Yersinia spp., including *Y. enterocolitica* and *Y. pseudotuberculosis*
Gram-positive anaerobes:
Actinomyces spp.
Clostridium perfringens
Propionibacterium acnes
Gram-negative anaerobes:
Bacteroides spp., including *B. bivius*, *B. disiens*, *B. distasonis*, *B. intermedius* (formerly *B. melaninogenicus intermedius*), *B. ovatus*, *B. thetaiotaomicron*, and *B. vulgatus*
Porphyromonas asaccharolytica (formerly *B. asaccharolyticus*)
Veillonella spp.
In vitro tests show imipenem to act synergistically with aminoglycoside antibiotics against some isolates of *Pseudomonas aeruginosa*.

Susceptibility Tests:
Measurement of MIC or minimum bactericidal concentration (MBC) and achieved antimicrobial compound concentrations may be appropriate to guide therapy in some infections. (See **CLINICAL PHARMACOLOGY** section for further information on drug concentrations achieved in infected body sites and other pharmacokinetic properties of this antimicrobial drug product.)

Diffusion techniques:
Quantitative methods that require measurement of zone diameters provide reproducible estimates of the susceptibility of bacteria to antimicrobial compounds. One such standardized procedure[1] that has been recommended for use with disks to test the susceptibility of microorganisms to imipenem uses the 10-µg imipenem disk. Interpretation involves correlation of the diameter obtained in the disk test with the MIC for imipenem.
Reports from the laboratory providing results of the standard single-disk susceptibility test with a 10-µg imipenem disk should be interpreted according to the following criteria:

Zone Diameter (mm)	Interpretation
≥ 16	Susceptible (S)
14–15	Intermediate (I)
≤ 13	Resistant (R)

A report of "Susceptible" indicates that the pathogen is likely to be inhibited by usually achievable concentrations of the antimicrobial compound in blood. A report of "Intermediate" indicates that the result should be considered equivocal, and, if the microorganism is not fully susceptible to alternative, clinically feasible drugs, the test should be repeated. This category implies possible clinical applicability in body sites where the drug is physiologically concentrated or in situations where high dosage of drug can be used. This category also provides a buffer zone that prevents small uncontrolled technical factors from causing major discrepancies in interpretation. A report of "Resistant" indicates that usually achievable concentrations of the antimicrobial compound in the blood are unlikely to be inhibitory and that other therapy should be selected.

Standardized susceptibility test procedures require the use of laboratory control microorganisms. The 10-µg imipenem disk should provide the following diameters in these laboratory test quality control strains:

Microorganism	Zone Diameter (mm)
E. coli ATCC 25922	26–32
P. aeruginosa ATCC 27853	20–28

Dilution techniques:
Quantitative methods that are used to determine MIC's provide reproducible estimates of the susceptibility of bacteria to antimicrobial compounds. One such procedure uses a standardized dilution method[2] (broth, agar, or microdilution) or equivalent with imipenem powder.
The MIC values obtained should be interpreted according to the following criteria:

MIC (µg/mL)	Interpretation
≤ 4	Susceptible (S)
8	Intermediate (I)
≥ 16	Resistant (R)

Interpretation should be as stated above for results using diffusion techniques.
As with standard diffusion techniques, dilution methods require the use of laboratory control microorganisms. Standard imipenem powder should provide the following MIC values:

Microorganism	MIC (µg/mL)
E. coli ATCC 25922	0.06–0.25
S. aureus ATCC 29213	0.015–0.06
E. faecalis ATCC 29212	0.5–2.0
P. aeruginosa ATCC 27853	1.0–4.0

Anaerobic techniques:
For anaerobic bacteria, the susceptibility to imipenem can be determined by the reference agar dilution method or by alternate standardized test methods.[3]
As with other susceptibility techniques, the use of laboratory control microorganisms is required. Standard imipenem powder should provide the following MIC values:
Reference Agar Dilution Testing:

Microorganism	MIC (µg/mL)
B. fragilis ATCC 25285	0.03–0.12
B. thetaiotaomicron ATCC 29741	0.06–0.25
E. lentum ATCC 43055	0.25–1.0

Continued on next page

Merck & Co.—Cont.

Broth Microdilution Testing:

Microorganism	MIC (µg/mL)
B. thetaiotaomicron ATCC 29741	0.06–0.25
E. lentum ATCC 43055	0.12–0.5

INDICATIONS AND USAGE

PRIMAXIN I.V. is indicated for the treatment of serious infections caused by susceptible strains of the designated microorganisms in the diseases listed below:

(1) **Lower respiratory tract infections.** *Staphylococcus aureus* (penicillinase-producing strains), *Acinetobacter* species, *Enterobacter* species, *Escherichia coli*, *Haemophilus influenzae*, *Haemophilus parainfluenzae**, *Klebsiella* species, *Serratia marcescens*.

(2) **Urinary tract infections** (complicated and uncomplicated). *Enterococcus faecalis*, *Staphylococcus aureus* (penicillinase-producing strains)*, *Enterobacter* species, *Escherichia coli*, *Klebsiella* species, *Morganella morganii**, *Proteus vulgaris**, *Providencia rettgeri**, *Pseudomonas aeruginosa*.

(3) **Intra-abdominal infections.** *Enterococcus faecalis*, *Staphylococcus aureus* (penicillinase-producing strains)*, *Staphylococcus epidermidis*, *Citrobacter* species, *Enterobacter* species, *Escherichia coli*, *Klebsiella* species, *Morganella morganii**, *Proteus* species (indole positive and indole negative), *Pseudomonas aeruginosa*, *Bifidobacterium* species, *Clostridium* species, *Eubacterium* species, *Peptococcus* species, *Peptostreptococcus* species, *Propionibacterium* species*, *Bacteroides* species including *B. fragilis*, *Fusobacterium* species.

(4) **Gynecologic infections.** *Enterococcus faecalis*, *Staphylococcus aureus* (penicillinase-producing strains)*, *Staphylococcus epidermidis*, *Streptococcus agalactiae* (Group B streptococcus), *Enterobacter* species*, *Escherichia coli*, *Gardnerella vaginalis*, *Klebsiella* species*, *Proteus* species (indole positive and indole negative), *Bifidobacterium* species*, *Peptococcus* species*, *Peptostreptococcus* species, *Propionibacterium* species*, *Bacteroides* species including *B. fragilis**.

(5) **Bacterial septicemia.** *Enterococcus faecalis*, *Staphylococcus aureus* (penicillinase-producing strains), *Enterobacter* species, *Escherichia coli*, *Klebsiella* species, *Pseudomonas aeruginosa*, *Serratia* species*, *Bacteroides* species including *B. fragilis**.

(6) **Bone and joint infections.** *Enterococcus faecalis*, *Staphylococcus aureus* (penicillinase-producing strains), *Staphylococcus epidermidis*, *Enterobacter* species, *Pseudomonas aeruginosa*.

(7) **Skin and skin structure infections.** *Enterococcus faecalis*, *Staphylococcus aureus* (penicillinase-producing strains), *Staphylococcus epidermidis*, *Acinetobacter* species, *Citrobacter* species, *Enterobacter* species, *Escherichia coli*, *Klebsiella* species, *Morganella morganii*, *Proteus vulgaris*, *Providencia rettgeri**, *Pseudomonas aeruginosa*, *Serratia* species, *Peptococcus* species, *Peptostreptococcus* species, *Bacteroides* species including *B. fragilis*, *Fusobacterium* species*.

(8) **Endocarditis.** *Staphylococcus aureus* (penicillinase-producing strains).

(9) **Polymicrobic infections.** PRIMAXIN I.V. is indicated for polymicrobic infections including those in which *S. pneumoniae* (pneumonia, septicemia), Group A beta-hemolytic streptococcus (skin and skin structure), or nonpenicillinase-producing *S. aureus* is one of the causative organisms. However, monobacterial infections due to these organisms are usually treated with narrower spectrum antibiotics, such as penicillin G.

PRIMAXIN I.V. is not indicated in patients with meningitis because safety and efficacy have not been established.

Because of its broad spectrum of bactericidal activity against gram-positive and gram-negative aerobic and anaerobic bacteria, PRIMAXIN I.V. is useful for the treatment of mixed infections and as presumptive therapy prior to the identification of the causative organisms.

Although clinical improvement has been observed in patients with cystic fibrosis, chronic pulmonary disease, and lower respiratory tract infections caused by *Pseudomonas aeruginosa*, bacterial eradication may not necessarily be achieved.

As with other beta-lactam antibiotics, some strains of *Pseudomonas aeruginosa* may develop resistance fairly rapidly during treatment with PRIMAXIN I.V. During therapy of *Pseudomonas aeruginosa* infections, periodic susceptibility testing should be done when clinically appropriate.

Infections resistant to other antibiotics, for example, cephalosporins, penicillin, and aminoglycosides, have been shown to respond to treatment with PRIMAXIN I.V.

---

* Efficacy for this organism in this organ system was studied in fewer than 10 infections.

CONTRAINDICATIONS

PRIMAXIN I.V. is contraindicated in patients who have shown hypersensitivity to any component of this product.

WARNINGS

SERIOUS AND OCCASIONALLY FATAL HYPERSENSITIVITY (anaphylactic) REACTIONS HAVE BEEN REPORTED IN PATIENTS RECEIVING THERAPY WITH BETA-LACTAMS. THESE REACTIONS ARE MORE APT TO OCCUR IN PERSONS WITH A HISTORY OF SENSITIVITY TO MULTIPLE ALLERGENS.

THERE HAVE BEEN REPORTS OF PATIENTS WITH A HISTORY OF PENICILLIN HYPERSENSITIVITY WHO HAVE EXPERIENCED SEVERE HYPERSENSITIVITY REACTIONS WHEN TREATED WITH ANOTHER BETA-LACTAM. BEFORE INITIATING THERAPY WITH PRIMAXIN I.V., CAREFUL INQUIRY SHOULD BE MADE CONCERNING PREVIOUS HYPERSENSITIVITY REACTIONS TO PENICILLINS, CEPHALOSPORINS, OTHER BETA-LACTAMS, AND OTHER ALLERGENS. IF AN ALLERGIC REACTION OCCURS, PRIMAXIN SHOULD BE DISCONTINUED.

SERIOUS ANAPHYLACTIC REACTIONS REQUIRE IMMEDIATE EMERGENCY TREATMENT WITH EPINEPHRINE. OXYGEN, INTRAVENOUS STEROIDS, AND AIRWAY MANAGEMENT, INCLUDING INTUBATION, MAY ALSO BE ADMINISTERED AS INDICATED.

Seizures and other CNS adverse experiences, such as confusional states and myoclonic activity, have been reported during treatment with PRIMAXIN I.V. (See **PRECAUTIONS**.)

Pseudomembranous colitis has been reported with nearly all antibacterial agents, including imipenem-cilastatin sodium, and may range in severity from mild to life threatening. Therefore, it is important to consider this diagnosis in patients who present with diarrhea subsequent to the administration of antibacterial agents.

Treatment with antibacterial agents alters the normal flora of the colon and may permit overgrowth of clostridia. Studies indicate that a toxin produced by *Clostridium difficile* is one primary cause of "antibiotic-associated colitis."

After the diagnosis of pseudomembranous colitis has been established, therapeutic measures should be initiated. Mild cases of pseudomembranous colitis usually respond to drug discontinuation alone. In moderate to severe cases, consideration should be given to management with fluids and electrolytes, protein supplementation and treatment with an antibacterial drug clinically effective against *C. difficile* colitis.

PRECAUTIONS

General

CNS adverse experiences such as confusional states, myoclonic activity, and seizures have been reported during treatment with PRIMAXIN I.V., especially when recommended dosages were exceeded. These experiences have occurred most commonly in patients with CNS disorders (e.g., brain lesions or history of seizures) and/or compromised renal function. However, there have been reports of CNS adverse experiences in patients who had no recognized or documented underlying CNS disorder or compromised renal function.

When recommended doses were exceeded, adult patients with creatinine clearances of ≤ 20 mL/min/1.73 m², whether or not undergoing hemodialysis, had a higher risk of seizure activity than those without impairment of renal function. Therefore, close adherence to the dosing guidelines for these patients is recommended. (See **DOSAGE AND ADMINISTRATION**.)

Patients with creatinine clearances of ≤ 5 mL/min/1.73 m² should not receive PRIMAXIN I.V. unless hemodialysis is instituted within 48 hours.

For patients on hemodialysis, PRIMAXIN I.V. is recommended only when the benefit outweighs the potential risk of seizures.

Close adherence to the recommended dosage and dosage schedules is urged, especially in patients with known factors that predispose to convulsive activity. Anticonvulsant therapy should be continued in patients with known seizure disorders. If focal tremors, myoclonus, or seizures occur, patients should be evaluated neurologically, placed on anticonvulsant therapy if not already instituted, and the dosage of PRIMAXIN I.V. re-examined to determine whether it should be decreased or the antibiotic discontinued.

As with other antibiotics, prolonged use of PRIMAXIN I.V. may result in overgrowth of nonsusceptible organisms. Repeated evaluation of the patient's condition is essential. If superinfection occurs during therapy, appropriate measures should be taken.

Laboratory Tests

While PRIMAXIN I.V. possesses the characteristic low toxicity of the beta-lactam group of antibiotics, periodic assess-

ment of organ system functions, including renal, hepatic, and hematopoietic, is advisable during prolonged therapy.

Drug Interactions

Generalized seizures have been reported in patients who received ganciclovir and PRIMAXIN. These drugs should not be used concomitantly unless the potential benefits outweigh the risks.

Since concomitant administration of PRIMAXIN and probenecid results in only minimal increases in plasma levels of imipenem and plasma half-life, it is not recommended that probenecid be given with PRIMAXIN.

PRIMAXIN should not be mixed with or physically added to other antibiotics. However, PRIMAXIN may be administered concomitantly with other antibiotics, such as aminoglycosides.

Carcinogenesis, Mutagenesis, Impairment of Fertility

Long term studies in animals have not been performed to evaluate carcinogenic potential of imipenem-cilastatin. Genetic toxicity studies were performed in a variety of bacterial and mammalian tests in *in vivo* and *in vitro*. The tests used were: V79 mammalian cell mutagenesis assay (imipenem-cilastatin sodium alone and imipenem alone), Ames test (cilastatin sodium alone and imipenem alone), unscheduled DNA synthesis assay (imipenem-cilastatin sodium) and *in vivo* mouse cytogenetics test (imipenem-cilastatin sodium). None of these tests showed any evidence of genetic alterations.

Reproductive tests in male and female rats were performed with imipenem-cilastatin sodium at dosage levels up to 11 times† the usual human dose of the intravenous formulation (on a mg/kg basis). Slight decreases in live fetal body weight were restricted to the highest dosage level. No other adverse effects were observed on fertility, reproductive performance, fetal viability, growth or postnatal development of pups. Similarly, no adverse effects on the fetus or on lactation were observed when imipenem-cilastatin sodium was administered to rats late in gestation.

Pregnancy: Teratogenic Effects

Pregnancy Category C: Teratology studies with cilastatin sodium in rabbits and rats at 6 and 20 times† the maximum recommended human dose of the intravenous formulation of imipenem-cilastatin sodium (50 mg/kg/day†), respectively, showed no evidence of adverse effect on the fetus. No evidence of teratogenicity was observed in rabbits and rats given imipenem at doses up to 1 and 18 times† the maximum recommended daily human dose of the intravenous formulation of imipenem-cilastatin sodium, respectively.

Teratology studies with imipenem-cilastatin sodium at doses up to 11 times† the usual recommended human dose of the intravenous formulation (30 mg/kg/day†) in pregnant mice and rats during the period of major organogenesis revealed no evidence of teratogenicity.

Imipenem-cilastatin sodium, when administered to pregnant rabbits at dosages equivalent to the usual human dose of the intravenous formulation and higher, caused body weight loss, diarrhea, and maternal deaths. When comparable doses of imipenem-cilastatin sodium were given to non-pregnant rabbits, body weight loss, diarrhea, and deaths were also observed. This intolerance is not unlike that seen with other beta-lactam antibiotics in this species and is probably due to alteration of gut flora.

A teratology study in pregnant cynomolgus monkeys given imipenem-cilastatin sodium at doses of 40 mg/kg/day (bolus intravenous injection) or 160 mg/kg/day (subcutaneous injection) resulted in maternal toxicity including emesis, inappetence, body weight loss, diarrhea, abortion and death in some cases. In contrast, no significant toxicity was observed when non-pregnant cynomolgus monkeys were given doses of imipenem-cilastatin sodium up to 180 mg/kg/day (subcutaneous injection). When doses of imipenem-cilastatin sodium (approximately 100 mg/kg/day or approximately 2 times† the maximum recommended daily human dose of the intravenous formulation) were administered to pregnant cynomolgus monkeys at an intravenous infusion rate which mimics human clinical use, there was minimal maternal intolerance (occasional emesis), no maternal deaths, no evidence of teratogenicity, but an increase in embryonic loss relative to control groups.

There are, however, no adequate and well-controlled studies in pregnant women. PRIMAXIN I.V. should be used during pregnancy only if the potential benefit justifies the potential risk to the mother and fetus.

Nursing Mothers

It is not known whether imipenem-cilastatin sodium is excreted in human milk. Because many drugs are excreted in human milk, caution should be exercised when PRIMAXIN I.V. is administered to a nursing woman.

Pediatric Use

Safety and effectiveness in infants and children below 12 years of age have not yet been established.

---

† Based on patient weight of 70 kg.

ADVERSE REACTIONS

PRIMAXIN I.V. is generally well tolerated. Many of the 1,723 patients treated in clinical trials were severely ill and had multiple background diseases and physiological impairments, making it difficult to determine causal relationship of adverse experiences to therapy with PRIMAXIN I.V.

Local Adverse Reactions

Adverse local clinical reactions that were reported as possibly, probably or definitely related to therapy with PRIMAXIN I.V. were:

Phlebitis/thrombophlebitis—3.1%
Pain at the injection site—0.7%
Erythema at the injection site—0.4%
Vein induration—0.2%
Infused vein infection—0.1%

Systemic Adverse Reactions

The most frequently reported systemic adverse clinical reactions that were reported as possibly, probably, or definitely related to PRIMAXIN I.V. were nausea (2.0%), diarrhea (1.8%), vomiting (1.5%), rash (0.9%), fever (0.5%), hypotension (0.4%), seizures (0.4%) (see **PRECAUTIONS**), dizziness (0.3%), pruritus (0.3%), urticaria (0.2%), somnolence (0.2%). Additional adverse systemic clinical reactions reported as possibly, probably or definitely drug related occurring in less than 0.2% of the patients or reported since the drug was marketed are listed within each body system in order of decreasing severity: *Gastrointestinal* —pseudomembranous colitis (the onset of pseudomembranous colitis symptoms may occur during or after antibacterial treatment, see **WARNINGS**), hemorrhagic colitis, hepatitis, jaundice, gastroenteritis, abdominal pain, glossitis, tongue papillar hypertrophy, staining of the teeth, heartburn, pharyngeal pain, increased salivation; *Hematologic* —pancytopenia, bone marrow depression, thrombocytopenia, neutropenia, leukopenia, hemolytic anemia; *CNS* —encephalopathy, tremor, confusion, myoclonus, paresthesia, vertigo, headache, psychic disturbances including hallucinations; *Special Senses* —hearing loss, tinnitus, taste perversion; *Respiratory* —chest discomfort, dyspnea, hyperventilation, thoracic spine pain; *Cardiovascular* —palpitations, tachycardia; *Skin* —Stevens-Johnson syndrome, toxic epidermal necrolysis, erythema multiforme, angioneurotic edema, flushing, cyanosis, hyperhidrosis, skin texture changes, candidiasis, pruritus vulvae; *Body as a whole* —polyarthralgia, asthenia/weakness; *Renal* —acute renal failure, oliguria/anuria, polyuria, urine discoloration. The role of PRIMAXIN I.V. in changes in renal function is difficult to assess, since factors predisposing to pre-renal azotemia or to impaired renal function usually have been present.

Adverse Laboratory Changes

Adverse laboratory changes without regard to drug relationship that were reported during clinical trials or reported since the drug was marketed were:

Hepatic: Increased ALT (SGPT), AST (SGOT), alkaline phosphatase, bilirubin and LDH.
Hemic: Increased eosinophils, positive Coombs test, increased WBC, increased platelets, decreased hemoglobin and hematocrit, agranulocytosis, increased monocytes, abnormal prothrombin time, increased lymphocytes, increased basophils.
Electrolytes: Decreased serum sodium, increased potassium, increased chloride.
Renal: Increased BUN, creatinine.

Urinalysis: Presence of urine protein, urine red blood cells, urine white blood cells, urine casts, urine bilirubin, and urine urobilinogen.

OVERDOSAGE

The acute intravenous toxicity of imipenem-cilastatin sodium in a ratio of 1:1 was studied in mice at doses of 751 to 1359 mg/kg. Following drug administration, ataxia was rapidly produced and clonic convulsions were noted in about 45 minutes. Deaths occurred within 4–56 minutes at all doses. The acute intravenous toxicity of imipenem-cilastatin sodium was produced within 5–10 minutes in rats at doses of 771 to 1583 mg/kg. In all dosage groups, females had decreased activity, bradypnea and ptosis with clonic convulsions preceding death; in males, ptosis was seen at all dose levels while tremors and clonic convulsions were seen at all but the lowest dose (771 mg/kg). In another rat study, female rats showed ataxia, bradypnea and decreased activity in all but the lowest dose (550 mg/kg); deaths were preceded by clonic convulsions. Male rats showed tremors at all doses and clonic convulsions and ptosis were seen at the two highest doses (1130 and 1734 mg/kg). Deaths occurred between 6 and 88 minutes with doses of 771 to 1734 mg/kg.

In the case of overdosage, discontinue PRIMAXIN I.V., treat symptomatically, and institute supportive measures as required. Imipenem-cilastatin sodium is hemodialyzable. However, usefulness of this procedure in the overdosage setting is questionable.

DOSAGE AND ADMINISTRATION

The dosage recommendations for PRIMAXIN I.V. represent the quantity of imipenem to be administered. An equivalent amount of cilastatin is also present in the solution. Each 125 mg, 250 mg or 500 mg dose should be given by intravenous administration over 20 to 30 minutes. Each 750 mg or 1000 mg dose should be infused over 40 to 60 minutes. In patients who develop nausea during the infusion, the rate of infusion may be slowed.

The total daily dosage for PRIMAXIN I.V. should be based on the type or severity of infection and given in equally divided doses based on consideration of degree of susceptibility of the pathogen(s), renal function and body weight. Patients with impaired renal function, as judged by creatinine clearance ≤ 70 mL/min/1.73 m^2, require adjustment of dosage as described in the succeeding section of these guidelines.

Intravenous Dosage Schedule for Adults with Normal Renal Function and Body Weight ≥ 70 kg

Doses cited in Table I are based on a patient with normal renal function and a body weight of 70 kg. These doses should be used for a patient with a creatinine clearance of ≥ 71 mL/min/1.73 m^2 and a body weight of ≥ 70 kg. A reduction in dose must be made for a patient with a creatinine clearance ≤ 70 mL/min/1.73 m^2 and/or a body weight less than 70 kg. (See Tables II and III.)

Dosage regimens in column A of Table I are recommended for infections caused by fully susceptible organisms which represent the majority of pathogenic species. Dosage regimens in column B of Table I are recommended for infections caused by organisms with moderate susceptibility to imipenem, primarily some strains of *P. aeruginosa*.

TABLE I
INTRAVENOUS DOSAGE SCHEDULE FOR ADULTS WITH NORMAL RENAL FUNCTION AND BODY WEIGHT ≥ 70 kg

Type or Severity of Infection	A Fully susceptible organisms including gram-positive and gram-negative aerobes and anaerobes	B Moderately susceptible organisms, primarily some strains of *P. aeruginosa*
Mild	250 mg q6h (TOTAL DAILY DOSE=1.0g)	500 mg q6h (TOTAL DAILY DOSE=2.0g)
Moderate	500 mg q8h (TOTAL DAILY DOSE =1.5g) or 500 mg q6h (TOTAL DAILY DOSE=2.0g)	500 mg q6h (TOTAL DAILY DOSE=2.0g) or 1 g q8h (TOTAL DAILY DOSE=3.0g)
Severe, life threatening only	500 mg q6h (TOTAL DAILY DOSE=2.0g)	1 g q8h (TOTAL DAILY DOSE=3.0g) or 1 g q6h (TOTAL DAILY DOSE=4.0g)
Uncomplicated urinary tract infection	250 mg q6h (TOTAL DAILY DOSE=1.0g)	250 mg q6h (TOTAL DAILY DOSE=1.0g)
Complicated urinary tract infection	500 mg q6h (TOTAL DAILY DOSE=2.0g)	500 mg q6h (TOTAL DAILY DOSE=2.0g)

Due to the high antimicrobial activity of PRIMAXIN I.V., it is recommended that the maximum total daily dosage not exceed 50 mg/kg/day or 4.0 g/day, whichever is lower. There is no evidence that higher doses provide greater efficacy. However, patients over twelve years of age with cystic fibrosis and normal renal function have been treated with PRIMAXIN I.V. at doses up to 90 mg/kg/day in divided doses, not exceeding 4.0 g/day.

Reduced Intravenous Dosage Schedule for Adults with Impaired Renal Function and/or Body Weight <70 kg

Patients with creatinine clearance of ≤ 70 mL/min/1.73 m^2 and/or body weight less than 70 kg require dosage reduction of PRIMAXIN I.V. as indicated in the tables below. Creatinine clearance may be calculated from serum creatinine concentration by the following equation:

$$T_{cc} \text{ (Males)} = \frac{(\text{wt. in kg}) (140 - \text{age})}{(72) (\text{creatinine in mg/dL})}$$

$$T_{cc} \text{ (Females)} = 0.85 \times \text{above value}$$

To determine the dose for adults with impaired renal function and/or reduced body weight:

1. Choose a total daily dose from Table I based on infection characteristics.
2. a) If the total daily dose is 1.0 g, 1.5 g or 2.0 g, use the appropriate subsection of Table II and continue with step 3.
   b) If the total daily dose is 3.0 g or 4.0 g, use the appropriate subsection of Table III and continue with step 3.
3. From Table II or III:
   a) Select the body weight on the far left which is closest to the patient's body weight (kg).
   b) Select the patient's creatinine clearance category.
   c) Where the row and column intersect is the reduced dosage regimen.

[See Table II at left.]

[See Table III on top of next page.]

Patients with creatinine clearances of 6 to 20 mL/min/1.73 m^2 should be treated with PRIMAXIN I.V. 125 mg or 250 mg every 12 hours for most pathogens. There may be an increased risk of seizures when doses of 500 mg every 12 hours are administered to these patients.

Patients with creatinine clearance ≤ 5 mL/min/1.73 m^2 should not receive PRIMAXIN I.V. unless hemodialysis is instituted within 48 hours. There is inadequate information to recommend usage of PRIMAXIN I.V. for patients undergoing peritoneal dialysis.

Continued on next page

Information on the Merck & Co., Inc. products listed on these pages is the full prescribing information from product circulars in use September 30, 1996.

TABLE II
REDUCED INTRAVENOUS DOSAGE OF PRIMAXIN I.V. IN ADULT PATIENTS WITH IMPAIRED RENAL FUNCTION AND/OR BODY WEIGHT <70 kg

and Body Weight (kg) is:	If TOTAL DAILY DOSE from TABLE I is:											
	1.0 g/day				1.5 g/day				2.0 g/day			
	and creatinine clearance (mL/min/1.73m²) is:				and creatinine clearance (mL/min/1.73m²) is:				and creatinine clearance (mL/min/1.73m²) is:			
	≥71	41–70	21–40	6–20	≥71	41–70	21–40	6–20	≥71	41–70	21–40	6–20
	then the reduced dosage regimen (mg) is:				then the reduced dosage regimen (mg) is:				then the reduced dosage regimen (mg) is:			
≥70	250 q6h	250 q8h	250 q12h	250 q12h	500 q8h	250 q6h	250 q8h	250 q12h	500 q6h	500 q8h	250 q6h	250 q12h
60	250 q8h	125 q6h	250 q12h	125 q12h	250 q6h	250 q8h	250 q8h	250 q12h	500 q8h	250 q6h	250 q8h	250 q12h
50	125 q6h	125 q6h	125 q8h	125 q12h	250 q6h	250 q8h	250 q12h	250 q12h	250 q6h	250 q8h	250 q8h	250 q12h
40	125 q6h	125 q6h	125 q8h	125 q12h	250 q6h	125 q6h	125 q8h	125 q12h	250 q6h	250 q8h	250 q8h	250 q12h
30	125 q8h	125 q8h	125 q12h	125 q12h	125 q6h	125 q8h	125 q8h	125 q12h	250 q8h	125 q6h	125 q8h	125 q12h

Merck & Co.—Cont.

TABLE III
REDUCED INTRAVENOUS DOSAGE OF PRIMAXIN I.V. IN ADULT PATIENTS WITH IMPAIRED RENAL FUNCTION AND/OR BODY WEIGHT <70 kg

and Body Weight (kg) is:	If TOTAL DAILY DOSE from TABLE I is:							
	3.0 g/day				4.0 g/day			
	and creatinine clearance (mL/min/1.73m²) is:				and creatinine clearance (mL/min/1.73m²) is:			
	≥71	41–70	21–40	6–20	≥71	41–70	21–40	6–20
	then the reduced dosage regimen (mg) is:				then the reduced dosage regimen (mg) is:			
≥70	1000 q8h	500 q6h	500 q8h	500 q12h	1000 q6h	750 q8h	500 q6h	500 q12h
60	750 q8h	500 q8h	500 q8h	500 q12h	1000 q8h	750 q8h	500 q8h	500 q12h
50	500 q6h	500 q8h	250 q6h	250 q12h	750 q8h	500 q6h	500 q8h	500 q12h
40	500 q8h	250 q6h	250 q8h	250 q12h	500 q8h	500 q8h	250 q6h	250 q12h
30	250 q6h	250 q8h	250 q8h	250 q12h	500 q8h	250 q6h	250 q8h	250 q12h

Hemodialysis

When treating patients with <u>creatinine clearances of ≤5 mL/min/1.73 m² who are undergoing hemodialysis</u>, use the dosage recommendations for patients with creatinine clearances of 6–20 mL/min/1.73 m². (See *Reduced Intravenous Dosage Schedule for Adults with Impaired Renal Function and/or Body Weight < 70 kg.*) Both imipenem and cilastatin are cleared from the circulation during hemodialysis. The patient should receive PRIMAXIN I.V. after hemodialysis and at 12 hour intervals timed from the end of that hemodialysis session. Dialysis patients, especially those with background CNS disease, should be carefully monitored; for patients on hemodialysis, PRIMAXIN I.V. is recommended only when the benefit outweighs the potential risk of seizures. (See **PRECAUTIONS**.)

PREPARATION OF SOLUTION

Infusion Bottles

Contents of the infusion bottles of PRIMAXIN I.V. Powder should be restored with 100 mL of diluent (see list of diluents under **COMPATIBILITY AND STABILITY**) and shaken until a clear solution is obtained.

Vials

Contents of the vials must be suspended and transferred to 100 mL of an appropriate infusion solution.

A suggested procedure is to add approximately 10 mL from the appropriate infusion solution (see list of diluents under **COMPATIBILITY AND STABILITY**) to the vial. Shake well and transfer the resulting suspension to the infusion solution container.

CAUTION: THE SUSPENSION IS NOT FOR DIRECT INFUSION.

Repeat with an additional 10 mL of infusion solution to ensure complete transfer of vial contents to the infusion solution. **The resulting mixture should be agitated until clear.**

ADD-Vantage®† Vials

See separate INSTRUCTIONS FOR USE OF 'PRIMAXIN I.V.' IN ADD-Vantage® VIALS. PRIMAXIN I.V. in ADD-Vantage® vials should be reconstituted with ADD-Vantage® diluent containers containing 100 mL of either 0.9% Sodium Chloride Injection or 100 mL 5% Dextrose Injection.

—————
†Registered trademark of Abbott Laboratories, Inc.

COMPATIBILITY AND STABILITY

Before reconstitution:

The dry powder should be stored at a temperature below 25°C (77°F).

Reconstituted solutions:

Solutions of PRIMAXIN I.V. range from colorless to yellow. Variations of color within this range do not affect the potency of the product.

PRIMAXIN I.V., as supplied in infusion bottles and vials and reconstituted as above with the following diluents, maintains satisfactory potency for four hours at room temperature or for 24 hours under refrigeration (5°C). Solutions of PRIMAXIN I.V. should not be frozen.

0.9% Sodium Chloride Injection
5% or 10% Dextrose Injection
5% Dextrose and 0.9% Sodium Chloride Injection
5% Dextrose Injection with 0.225% or 0.45% saline solution
5% Dextrose Injection with 0.15% potassium chloride solution
Mannitol 5% and 10%

PRIMAXIN I.V. is supplied in single dose ADD-Vantage® vials and should be prepared as directed in the accompany-ing INSTRUCTIONS FOR USE OF 'PRIMAXIN I.V.' IN ADD-Vantage® VIALS using ADD-Vantage® diluent containers containing 100 mL of either 0.9% Sodium Chloride Injection or 5% Dextrose Injection. When prepared with either of these diluents, PRIMAXIN I.V. maintains satisfactory potency for 8 hours at room temperature.

PRIMAXIN I.V. should not be mixed with or physically added to other antibiotics. However, PRIMAXIN I.V. may be administered concomitantly with other antibiotics, such as aminoglycosides.

HOW SUPPLIED

PRIMAXIN I.V. is supplied as a sterile powder mixture in vials and infusion bottles containing imipenem (anhydrous equivalent) and cilastatin sodium as follows:

No. 3514—250 mg imipenem equivalent and 250 mg cilastatin equivalent and 10 mg sodium bicarbonate as a buffer **NDC** 0006-3514-58 in trays of 25 vials (6505-01-332-4793 250 mg, 25's).

No. 3516—500 mg imipenem equivalent and 500 mg cilastatin equivalent and 20 mg sodium bicarbonate as a buffer **NDC** 0006-3516-59 in trays of 25 vials (6505-01-332-4794 500 mg, 25's).

No. 3515—250 mg imipenem equivalent and 250 mg cilastatin equivalent and 10 mg sodium bicarbonate as a buffer **NDC** 0006-3515-74 in trays of 10 infusion bottles (6505-01-246-4126 infusion bottle, 10's).

No. 3517—500 mg imipenem equivalent and 500 mg cilastatin equivalent and 20 mg sodium bicarbonate as a buffer **NDC** 0006-3517-75 in trays of 10 infusion bottles (6505-01-234-0240 infusion bottle, 10's).

No. 3551—250 mg imipenem equivalent and 250 mg cilastatin equivalent and 10 mg sodium bicarbonate as a buffer **NDC** 0006-3551-58 in trays of 25 ADD-Vantage® vials.

No. 3552—500 mg imipenem equivalent and 500 mg cilastatin equivalent and 20 mg sodium bicarbonate as a buffer **NDC** 0006-3552-59 in trays of 25 ADD-Vantage® vials (6505-01-279-9627 500 mg ADD-Vantage®, 25's).

REFERENCES

1. National Committee for Clinical Laboratory Standards, Performance Standards for Antimicrobial Disk Susceptibility Tests—Fifth Edition. Approved Standard NCCLS Document M2-A5, Vol. 13, No. 24 NCCLS, Villanova, PA, 1993.
2. National Committee for Clinical Laboratory Standards, Methods for Dilution Antimicrobial Susceptibility Tests for Bacteria that Grow Aerobically—Third Edition. Approved Standard NCCLS Document M7-A3, Vol. 13, No. 25 NCCLS, Villanova, PA, 1993.
3. National Committee for Clinical Laboratory Standards, Method for Antimicrobial Susceptibility Testing of Anaerobic Bacteria—Third Edition. Approved Standard NCCLS Document M11-A3, Vol. 13, No. 26 NCCLS, Villanova, PA, 1993.

7882121   Issued September 1995

PRINIVIL® Tablets
(Lisinopril)   ℞

DESCRIPTION

PRINIVIL* (Lisinopril), a synthetic peptide derivative, is an oral long-acting angiotensin converting enzyme inhibitor. Lisinopril is chemically described as (S)-1-[N^2-(1-carboxy-3-phenylpropyl)-L-lysyl]-L-proline dihydrate. Its empirical formula is $C_{21}H_{31}N_3O_5 \cdot 2H_2O$ and its structural formula is:

Lisinopril is a white to off-white, crystalline powder, with a molecular weight of 441.52. It is soluble in water and sparingly soluble in methanol and practically insoluble in ethanol.

PRINIVIL is supplied as 2.5 mg, 5 mg, 10 mg, 20 mg and 40 mg tablets for oral administration. In addition to the active ingredient lisinopril, each tablet contains the following inactive ingredients: calcium phosphate, mannitol, magnesium stearate, and starch. The 10 mg, 20 mg and 40 mg tablets also contain iron oxide.

* Registered trademark of MERCK & CO., INC.

CLINICAL PHARMACOLOGY

Mechanism of Action

Lisinopril inhibits angiotensin-converting enzyme (ACE) in human subjects and animals. ACE is a peptidyl dipeptidase that catalyzes the conversion of angiotensin I to the vasoconstrictor substance, angiotensin II. Angiotensin II also stimulates aldosterone secretion by the adrenal cortex. The beneficial effects of lisinopril in hypertension and heart failure appear to result primarily from suppression of the renin-angiotensin-aldosterone system. Inhibition of ACE results in decreased plasma angiotensin II which leads to decreased vasopressor activity and to decreased aldosterone secretion. The latter decrease may result in a small increase of serum potassium. In hypertensive patients with normal renal function treated with PRINIVIL alone for up to 24 weeks, the mean increase in serum potassium was approximately 0.1 mEq/L; however, approximately 15 percent of patients had increases greater than 0.5 mEq/L and approximately six percent had a decrease greater than 0.5 mEq/L. In the same study, patients treated with PRINIVIL and hydrochlorothiazide for up to 24 weeks had a mean decrease in serum potassium of 0.1 mEq/L; approximately 4 percent of patients had increases greater than 0.5 mEq/L and approximately 12 percent had a decrease greater than 0.5 mEq/L. (See PRECAUTIONS.) Removal of angiotensin II negative feedback on renin secretion leads to increased plasma renin activity. ACE is identical to kininase, an enzyme that degrades bradykinin. Whether increased levels of bradykinin, a potent vasodepressor peptide, play a role in the therapeutic effects of PRINIVIL remains to be elucidated.

While the mechanism through which PRINIVIL lowers blood pressure is believed to be primarily suppression of the renin-angiotensin-aldosterone system, PRINIVIL is antihypertensive even in patients with low-renin hypertension. Although PRINIVIL was antihypertensive in all races studied, black hypertensive patients (usually a low-renin hypertensive population) had a smaller average response to monotherapy than non-black patients. Concomitant administration of PRINIVIL and hydrochlorothiazide further reduced blood pressure in black and non-black patients and any racial difference in blood pressure response was no longer evident.

Pharmacokinetics and Metabolism

Following oral administration of PRINIVIL, peak serum concentrations of lisinopril occur within about 7 hours, although there was a trend to a small delay in time taken to reach peak serum concentrations in acute myocardial infarction patients. Declining serum concentrations exhibit a prolonged terminal phase which does not contribute to drug accumulation. This terminal phase probably represents saturable binding to ACE and is not proportional to dose. Lisinopril does not appear to be bound to other serum proteins. Lisinopril does not undergo metabolism and is excreted unchanged entirely in the urine. Based on urinary recovery, the mean extent of absorption of lisinopril is approximately 25 percent, with large intersubject variability (6–60 percent) at all doses tested (5–80 mg). Lisinopril absorption is not influenced by the presence of food in the gastrointestinal tract. The absolute bioavailability of lisinopril is reduced to about 16% in patients with stable NYHA Class II-IV congestive heart failure, and the volume of distribution appears to be slightly smaller than that in normal subjects.

The oral bioavailability of lisinopril in patients with acute myocardial infarction is similar to that in healthy volunteers.

Upon multiple dosing, lisinopril exhibits an effective half-life of accumulation of 12 hours.

Impaired renal function decreases elimination of lisinopril, which is excreted principally through the kidneys, but this decrease becomes clinically important only when the glomerular filtration rate is below 30 mL/min. Above this glomerular filtration rate, the elimination half-life is little changed. With greater impairment, however, peak and trough lisinopril levels increase, time to peak concentration increases and time to attain steady state is prolonged. Older patients, on average, have (approximately doubled) higher blood levels and area under the plasma concentration time curve (AUC) than younger patients. (See DOSAGE AND ADMINISTRATION.) Lisinopril can be removed by hemodialysis.

Studies in rats indicate that lisinopril crosses the blood-brain barrier poorly. Multiple doses of lisinopril in rats do not result in accumulation in any tissues. Milk of lactating rats contains radioactivity following administration of ^{14}C lisinopril. By whole body autoradiography, radioactivity was found in the placenta following administration of labeled drug to pregnant rats, but none was found in the fetuses.

Pharmacodynamics and Clinical Effects

Hypertension: Administration of PRINIVIL to patients with hypertension results in a reduction of supine and standing blood pressure to about the same extent with no compensatory tachycardia. Symptomatic postural hypotension is usually not observed although it can occur and should be anticipated in volume and/or salt-depleted patients. (See WARNINGS.) When given together with thiazide-type diuretics, the blood pressure lowering effects of the two drugs are approximately additive.

In most patients studied, onset of antihypertensive activity was seen at one hour after oral administration of an individual dose of PRINIVIL, with peak reduction of blood pressure achieved by six hours. Although an antihypertensive effect was observed 24 hours after dosing with recommended single daily doses, the effect was more consistent and the mean effect was considerably larger in some studies with doses of 20 mg or more than with lower doses. However, at all doses studied, the mean antihypertensive effect was substantially smaller 24 hours after dosing than it was six hours after dosing.

In some patients achievement of optimal blood pressure reduction may require two to four weeks of therapy.

The antihypertensive effects of PRINIVIL are maintained during long-term therapy. Abrupt withdrawal of PRINIVIL has not been associated with a rapid increase in blood pressure or a significant increase in blood pressure compared to pretreatment levels.

Two dose-response studies utilizing a once daily regimen were conducted in 438 mild to moderate hypertensive patients not on a diuretic. Blood pressure was measured 24 hours after dosing. An antihypertensive effect of PRINIVIL was seen with 5 mg in some patients. However, in both studies blood pressure reduction occurred sooner and was greater in patients treated with 10, 20, or 80 mg of PRINIVIL. In controlled clinical studies, PRINIVIL 20–80 mg has been compared in patients with mild to moderate hypertension to hydrochlorothiazide 12.5–50 mg and with atenolol 50–200 mg; and in patients with moderate to severe hypertension to metoprolol 100–200 mg. It was superior to hydrochlorothiazide in effects on systolic and diastolic blood pressure in a population that was $^{3}/_{4}$ caucasian. PRINIVIL was approximately equivalent to atenolol and metoprolol in effects on diastolic blood pressure and had somewhat greater effects on systolic blood pressure.

PRINIVIL had similar effectiveness and adverse effects in younger and older (> 65 years) patients. It was less effective in blacks than in caucasians.

In hemodynamic studies in patients with essential hypertension, blood pressure reduction was accompanied by a reduction in peripheral arterial resistance with little or no change in cardiac output and in heart rate. In a study in nine hypertensive patients, following administration of PRINIVIL, there was an increase in mean renal blood flow that was not significant. Data from several small studies are inconsistent with respect to the effect of PRINIVIL on glomerular filtration rate in hypertensive patients with normal renal function, but suggest that changes, if any, are not large.

In patients with renovascular hypertension PRINIVIL has been shown to be well tolerated and effective in controlling blood pressure (see PRECAUTIONS).

Heart Failure: During baseline-controlled clinical trials, in patients receiving digitalis and diuretics, single doses of PRINIVIL resulted in decreases in pulmonary capillary wedge pressure, systemic vascular resistance and blood pressure accompanied by an increase in cardiac output and no change in heart rate.

In two placebo controlled, 12-week clinical studies, PRINIVIL as adjunctive therapy to digitalis and diuretics improved the following signs and symptoms due to congestive heart failure: edema, rales, paroxysmal nocturnal dyspnea and jugular venous distention. In one of the studies beneficial response was also noted for: orthopnea, presence of third heart sound and the number of patients classified as NYHA Class III and IV. Exercise tolerance was also improved in this study. The effect of lisinopril on mortality in patients with heart failure has not been evaluated.

Acute Myocardial Infarction: The Gruppo Italiano per lo Studio della Sopravvienza nell'Infarto Miocardico (GISSI-3) study was a multicenter, controlled, randomized, unblinded clinical trial conducted in 19,394 patients with acute myocardial infarction admitted to a coronary care unit. It was designed to examine the effects of short-term (6 week) treatment with lisinopril, nitrates, their combination, or no therapy on short-term (6 week) mortality and on long-term death and markedly impaired cardiac function. Patients presenting within 24 hours of the onset of symptoms who were hemodynamically stable were randomized, in a 2 × 2 factorial design, to six weeks of either

1) PRINIVIL alone (n = 4841),
2) nitrates alone (n = 4869),
3) PRINIVIL plus nitrates (n = 4841), or
4) open control (n = 4843).

All patients received routine therapies, including thrombolytics (72%), aspirin (84%), and a beta-blocker (31%), as appropriate, normally utilized in acute myocardial infarction (MI) patients.

The protocol excluded patients with hypotension (systolic blood pressure ≤100 mmHg), severe heart failure, cardiogenic shock and renal dysfunction (serum creatinine >2 mg/dL and/or proteinuria >500 mg/24 h). Doses of PRINIVIL were adjusted as necessary according to protocol. (See DOSAGE AND ADMINISTRATION.)

Study treatment was withdrawn at six weeks except where clinical conditions indicated continuation of treatment.

The primary outcomes of the trial were the overall mortality at six weeks and a combined endpoint at six months after the myocardial infarction, consisting of the number of patients who died, had late (day 4) clinical congestive heart failure, or had extensive left ventricular damage defined as ejection fraction ≤35%, or an akinetic-dyskinetic [A-D] score ≥45%. Patients receiving PRINIVIL (n = 9646) alone or with nitrates, had an 11 percent lower risk of death (2p [two-tailed] = 0.04) compared to patients receiving no PRINIVIL (n = 9672) (6.4 percent versus 7.2 percent, respectively) at six weeks. Although patients randomized to receive PRINIVIL for up to six weeks also fared numerically better on the combined endpoint at 6 months, the open nature of the assessment of heart failure, substantial loss of follow-up echocardiography, and substantial excess use of lisinopril between 6 weeks and 6 months in the group randomized to 6 weeks of lisinopril, preclude any conclusion about this endpoint.

Patients with acute myocardial infarction, treated with PRINIVIL had a higher (9.0 percent versus 3.7 percent, respectively) incidence of persistent hypotension (systolic blood pressure <90 mmHg for more than 1 hour) and renal dysfunction (2.4 percent versus 1.1 percent) in-hospital and at six weeks (increasing creatinine concentration to over 3 mg/dL or a doubling or more of the baseline serum creatinine concentration). See ADVERSE REACTIONS, *ACUTE MYOCARDIAL INFARCTION.*

INDICATIONS AND USAGE

Hypertension

PRINIVIL is indicated for the treatment of hypertension. It may be used alone as initial therapy or concomitantly with other classes of antihypertensive agents.

Heart Failure

PRINIVIL is indicated as adjunctive therapy in the management of heart failure in patients who are not responding adequately to diuretics and digitalis.

Acute Myocardial Infarction

PRINIVIL is indicated for the treatment of hemodynamically stable patients within 24 hours of acute myocardial infarction, to improve survival. Patients should receive, as appropriate, the standard recommended treatments such as thrombolytics, aspirin and beta-blockers.

In using PRINIVIL, consideration should be given to the fact that another angiotensin converting enzyme inhibitor, captopril, has caused agranulocytosis, particularly in patients with renal impairment or collagen vascular disease, and that available data are insufficient to show that PRINIVIL does not have a similar risk. (See WARNINGS.)

In considering use of PRINIVIL, it should be noted that in controlled clinical trials ACE inhibitors have an effect on blood pressure that is less in black patients than in non-blacks. In addition, it should be noted that black patients receiving ACE inhibitors have been reported to have a higher incidence of angioedema compared to non-blacks.

CONTRAINDICATIONS

PRINIVIL is contraindicated in patients who are hypersensitive to this product and in patients with a history of angioedema related to previous treatment with an angiotensin converting enzyme inhibitor.

WARNINGS

Anaphylactoid and Possibly Related Reactions

Presumably because angiotensin-converting enzyme inhibitors affect the metabolism of eicosanoids and polypeptides, including endogenous bradykinin, patients receiving ACE inhibitors (including PRINIVIL) may be subject to a variety of adverse reactions, some of them serious.

Angioedema: Angioedema of the face, extremities, lips, tongue, glottis and/or larynx has been reported in patients treated with angiotensin converting enzyme inhibitors, including PRINIVIL. This may occur at any time during treatment. In such cases PRINIVIL should be promptly discontinued and appropriate therapy and monitoring should be provided until complete and sustained resolution of signs and symptoms has occurred. In instances where swelling has been confined to the face and lips the condition has generally resolved without treatment, although antihistamines have been useful in relieving symptoms. Angioedema associated with laryngeal edema may be fatal. **Where there is involvement of the tongue, glottis or larynx, likely to cause airway obstruction, appropriate therapy, e.g., subcutaneous epinephrine solution 1:1000 (0.3 mL to 0.5 mL) and/or measures necessary to ensure a patent airway, should be promptly provided.** (See ADVERSE REACTIONS.)

Patients with a history of angioedema unrelated to ACE inhibitor therapy may be at increased risk of angioedema while receiving an ACE inhibitor (see also INDICATIONS AND USAGE and CONTRAINDICATIONS).

Anaphylactoid reactions during desensitization: Two patients undergoing desensitizing treatment with hymenoptera venom while receiving ACE inhibitors sustained life-threatening anaphylactoid reactions. In the same patients, these reactions were avoided when ACE inhibitors were temporarily withheld, but they reappeared upon inadvertent rechallenge.

Anaphylactoid reactions during membrane exposure: Anaphylactoid reactions have been reported in patients dialyzed with high-flux membranes and treated concomitantly with an ACE inhibitor. Anaphylactoid reactions have also been reported in patients undergoing low-density lipoprotein apheresis with dextran sulfate absorption (a procedure dependent upon devices not approved in the United States).

Hypotension

Excessive hypotension is rare in patients with uncomplicated hypertension treated with PRINIVIL alone.

Patients with heart failure given PRINIVIL commonly have some reduction in blood pressure with peak blood pressure reduction occurring 6 to 8 hours post dose, but discontinuation of therapy because of continuing symptomatic hypotension usually is not necessary when dosing instructions are followed; caution should be observed when initiating therapy. (See DOSAGE AND ADMINISTRATION.)

Patients at risk of excessive hypotension, sometimes associated with oliguria and/or progressive azotemia, and rarely with acute renal failure and/or death, include those with the following conditions or characteristics: heart failure with systolic blood pressure below 100 mmHg, hyponatremia, high dose diuretic therapy, recent intensive diuresis or increase in diuretic dose, renal dialysis, or severe volume and/or salt depletion of any etiology. It may be advisable to eliminate the diuretic (except in patients with heart failure), reduce the diuretic dose or increase salt intake cautiously before initiating therapy with PRINIVIL in patients at risk for excessive hypotension who are able to tolerate such adjustments. (See PRECAUTIONS, *Drug Interactions,* and ADVERSE REACTIONS.)

Patients with acute myocardial infarction in the GISSI-3 study had a higher (9.0 versus 3.7 percent) incidence of persistent hypotension (systolic blood pressure <90 mmHg for more than 1 hour) when treated with PRINIVIL. Treatment with PRINIVIL must not be initiated in acute myocardial infarction patients at risk of further serious hemodynamic deterioration after treatment with a vasodilator (e.g., systolic blood pressure of 100 mmHg or lower) or cardiogenic shock.

In patients at risk of excessive hypotension, therapy should be started under very close medical supervision and such patients should be followed closely for the first two weeks of treatment and whenever the dose of PRINIVIL and/or diuretic is increased. Similar considerations may apply to patients with ischemic heart or cerebrovascular disease, or in patients with acute myocardial infarction, in whom an excessive fall in blood pressure could result in a myocardial infarction or cerebrovascular accident.

Continued on next page

Information on the Merck & Co., Inc. products listed on these pages is the full prescribing information from product circulars in use September 30, 1996.

Merck & Co.—Cont.

If excessive hypotension occurs, the patient should be placed in the supine position and, if necessary, receive an intravenous infusion of normal saline. A transient hypotensive response is not a contraindication to further doses of PRINIVIL which usually can be given without difficulty once the blood pressure has stabilized. If symptomatic hypotension develops, a dose reduction or discontinuation of PRINIVIL or concomitant diuretic may be necessary.

Neutropenia/Agranulocytosis
Another angiotensin converting enzyme inhibitor, captopril, has been shown to cause agranulocytosis and bone marrow depression, rarely in uncomplicated patients but more frequently in patients with renal impairment especially if they also have a collagen vascular disease. Available data from clinical trials of PRINIVIL are insufficient to show that PRINIVIL does not cause agranulocytosis at similar rates. Marketing experience has revealed rare cases of neutropenia and bone marrow depression in which a causal relationship to lisinopril cannot be excluded. Periodic monitoring of white blood cell counts in patients with collagen vascular disease and renal disease should be considered.

Hepatic Failure: Rarely, ACE inhibitors have been associated with a syndrome that starts with cholestatic jaundice and progresses to fulminant hepatic necrosis, and (sometimes) death. The mechanism of this syndrome is not understood. Patients receiving ACE inhibitors who develop jaundice or marked elevations of hepatic enzymes should discontinue the ACE inhibitor and receive appropriate medical follow-up.

Fetal/Neonatal Morbidity and Mortality
ACE inhibitors can cause fetal and neonatal morbidity and death when administered to pregnant women. Several dozen cases have been reported in the world literature. When pregnancy is detected, ACE inhibitors should be discontinued as soon as possible.

The use of ACE inhibitors during the second and third trimesters of pregnancy has been associated with fetal and neonatal injury, including hypotension, neonatal skull hypoplasia, anuria, reversible or irreversible renal failure, and death. Oligohydramnios has also been reported, presumably resulting from decreased fetal renal function; oligohydramnios in this setting has been associated with fetal limb contractures, craniofacial deformation, and hypoplastic lung development. Prematurity, intrauterine growth retardation, and patent ductus arteriosus have also been reported, although it is not clear whether these occurrences were due to the ACE-inhibitor exposure.

These adverse effects do not appear to have resulted from intrauterine ACE-inhibitor exposure that has been limited to the first trimester. Mothers whose embryos and fetuses are exposed to ACE inhibitors only during the first trimester should be so informed. Nonetheless, when patients become pregnant, physicians should make every effort to discontinue the use of PRINIVIL as soon as possible.

Rarely (probably less often than once in every thousand pregnancies), no alternative to ACE inhibitors will be found. In these rare cases, the mothers should be apprised of the potential hazards to their fetuses, and serial ultrasound examinations should be performed to assess the intraamniotic environment.

If oligohydramnios is observed, PRINIVIL should be discontinued unless it is considered lifesaving for the mother. Contraction stress testing (CST), a non-stress test (NST), or biophysical profiling (BPP) may be appropriate, depending upon the week of pregnancy. Patients and physicians should be aware, however, that oligohydramnios may not appear until after the fetus has sustained irreversible injury.

Infants with histories of *in utero* exposure to ACE inhibitors should be closely observed for hypotension, oliguria, and hyperkalemia. If oliguria occurs, attention should be directed toward support of blood pressure and renal perfusion. Exchange transfusion or dialysis may be required as means of reversing hypotension and/or substituting for disordered renal function. Lisinopril, which crosses the placenta, has been removed from neonatal circulation by peritoneal dialysis with some clinical benefit, and theoretically may be removed by exchange transfusion, although there is no experience with the latter procedure.

No teratogenic effects of lisinopril were seen in studies of pregnant rats, mice, and rabbits. On a mg/kg basis, the doses used were up to 625 times (in mice), 188 times (in rats), and 0.6 times (in rabbits) the maximum recommended human dose.

PRECAUTIONS

General
Impaired Renal Function: As a consequence of inhibiting the renin-angiotensin-aldosterone system, changes in renal function may be anticipated in susceptible individuals. In patients with severe congestive heart failure whose renal function may depend on the activity of the renin-angioten-

sin-aldosterone system, treatment with angiotensin converting enzyme inhibitors, including PRINIVIL, may be associated with oliguria and/or progressive azotemia and rarely with acute renal failure and/or death.

In hypertensive patients with unilateral or bilateral renal artery stenosis, increases in blood urea nitrogen and serum creatinine may occur. Experience with another angiotensin converting enzyme inhibitor suggests that these increases are usually reversible upon discontinuation of PRINIVIL and/or diuretic therapy. In such patients renal function should be monitored during the first few weeks of therapy. Some patients with hypertension or heart failure with no apparent pre-existing renal vascular disease have developed increases in blood urea nitrogen and serum creatinine, usually minor and transient, especially when PRINIVIL has been given concomitantly with a diuretic. This is more likely to occur in patients with pre-existing renal impairment. Dosage reduction and/or discontinuation of the diuretic and/or PRINIVIL may be required.

Patients with acute myocardial infarction in the GISSI-3 study, treated with PRINIVIL, had a higher (2.4 percent versus 1.1 percent) incidence of renal dysfunction in-hospital and at six weeks (increasing creatinine concentration to over 3 mg/dL or a doubling or more of the baseline serum creatinine concentration). In acute myocardial infarction, treatment with PRINIVIL should be initiated with caution in patients with evidence of renal dysfunction, defined as serum creatinine concentration exceeding 2 mg/dL. If renal dysfunction develops during treatment with PRINIVIL (serum creatinine concentration exceeding 3 mg/dL or a doubling from the pre-treatment value) then the physician should consider withdrawal of PRINIVIL.

Evaluation of patients with hypertension, heart failure, or myocardial infarction should always include assessment of renal function. (See DOSAGE AND ADMINISTRATION.)

Hyperkalemia: In clinical trials hyperkalemia (serum potassium greater than 5.7 mEq/L) occurred in approximately 2.2 percent of hypertensive patients and 4.8 percent of patients with heart failure. In most cases these were isolated values which resolved despite continued therapy. Hyperkalemia was a cause of discontinuation of therapy in approximately 0.1 percent of hypertensive patients, 0.6 percent of patients with heart failure and 0.1 percent of patients with myocardial infarction. Risk factors for the development of hyperkalemia include renal insufficiency, diabetes mellitus, and the concomitant use of potassium-sparing diuretics, potassium supplements and/or potassium-containing salt substitutes, which should be used cautiously, if at all, with PRINIVIL. (See *Drug Interactions*.)

Cough: Presumably due to the inhibition of the degradation of endogenous bradykinin, persistent nonproductive cough has been reported with all ACE inhibitors, always resolving after discontinuation of therapy. ACE inhibitor-induced cough should be considered in the differential diagnosis of cough.

Surgery/Anesthesia: In patients undergoing major surgery or during anesthesia with agents that produce hypotension, PRINIVIL may block angiotensin II formation secondary to compensatory renin release. If hypotension occurs and is considered to be due to this mechanism, it can be corrected by volume expansion.

Information for Patients
Angioedema: Angioedema, including laryngeal edema, may occur at any time during treatment with angiotensin converting enzyme inhibitors, including lisinopril. Patients should be so advised and told to report immediately any signs or symptoms suggesting angioedema (swelling of face, extremities, eyes, lips, tongue, difficulty in swallowing or breathing) and to take no more drug until they have consulted with the prescribing physician.

Symptomatic Hypotension: Patients should be cautioned to report lightheadedness especially during the first few days of therapy. If actual syncope occurs, the patients should be told to discontinue the drug until they have consulted with the prescribing physician.

All patients should be cautioned that excessive perspiration and dehydration may lead to an excessive fall in blood pressure because of reduction in fluid volume. Other causes of volume depletion such as vomiting or diarrhea may also lead to a fall in blood pressure; patients should be advised to consult with their physician.

Hyperkalemia: Patients should be told not to use salt substitutes containing potassium without consulting their physician.

Neutropenia: Patients should be told to report promptly any indication of infection (e.g., sore throat, fever) which may be a sign of neutropenia.

Pregnancy: Female patients of childbearing age should be told about the consequences of second- and third-trimester exposure to ACE inhibitors, and they should also be told that these consequences do not appear to have resulted from intrauterine ACE-inhibitor exposure that has been limited to the first trimester. These patients should be asked to report pregnancies to their physicians as soon as possible.

NOTE: As with many other drugs, certain advice to patients being treated with PRINIVIL is warranted. This infor-

mation is intended to aid in the safe and effective use of this medication. It is not a disclosure of all possible adverse or intended effects.

Drug Interactions
Hypotension—Patients on Diuretic Therapy: Patients on diuretics, and especially those in whom diuretic therapy was recently instituted, may occasionally experience an excessive reduction of blood pressure after initiation of therapy with PRINIVIL. The possibility of hypotensive effects with PRINIVIL can be minimized by either discontinuing the diuretic or increasing the salt intake prior to initiation of treatment with PRINIVIL. If it is necessary to continue the diuretic, initiate therapy with PRINIVIL at a dose of 5 mg daily, and provide close medical supervision after the initial dose until blood pressure has stabilized. (See WARNINGS, and DOSAGE AND ADMINISTRATION.) When a diuretic is added to the therapy of a patient receiving PRINIVIL, an additional antihypertensive effect is usually observed. Studies with ACE inhibitors in combination with diuretics indicate that the dose of the ACE inhibitor can be reduced when it is given with a diuretic. (See DOSAGE AND ADMINISTRATION.)

Indomethacin: In a study in 36 patients with mild to moderate hypertension where the antihypertensive effects of PRINIVIL alone were compared to PRINIVIL given concomitantly with indomethacin, the use of indomethacin was associated with a reduced effect, although the difference between the two regimens was not significant.

Other Agents: PRINIVIL has been used concomitantly with nitrates and/or digoxin without evidence of clinically significant adverse interactions. This included post myocardial infarction patients who were receiving intravenous or transdermal nitroglycerin. No clinically important pharmacokinetic interactions occurred when PRINIVIL was used concomitantly with propranolol or hydrochlorothiazide. The presence of food in the stomach does not alter the bioavailability of PRINIVIL.

Agents Increasing Serum Potassium: PRINIVIL attenuates potassium loss caused by thiazide-type diuretics. Use of PRINIVIL with potassium-sparing diuretics (e.g., spironolactone, triamterene, or amiloride), potassium supplements, or potassium-containing salt substitutes may lead to significant increases in serum potassium. Therefore, if concomitant use of these agents is indicated because of demonstrated hypokalemia, they should be used with caution and with frequent monitoring of serum potassium. Potassium sparing agents should generally not be used in patients with heart failure who are receiving PRINIVIL.

Lithium: Lithium toxicity has been reported in patients receiving lithium concomitantly with drugs which cause elimination of sodium, including ACE inhibitors. Lithium toxicity was usually reversible upon discontinuation of lithium and the ACE inhibitor. It is recommended that serum lithium levels be monitored frequently if PRINIVIL is administered concomitantly with lithium.

Carcinogenesis, Mutagenesis, Impairment of Fertility
There was no evidence of a tumorigenic effect when lisinopril was administered for 105 weeks to male and female rats at doses up to 90 mg/kg/day (about 56 times* the maximum recommended daily human dose) or when lisinopril was administered for 92 weeks to (male and female) mice at doses up to 135 mg/kg/day (about 84 times* the maximum recommended daily human dose).

Lisinopril was not mutagenic in the Ames microbial mutagen test with or without metabolic activation. It was also negative in a forward mutation assay using Chinese hamster lung cells. Lisinopril did not produce single strand DNA breaks in an *in vitro* alkaline elution rat hepatocyte assay. In addition, lisinopril did not produce increases in chromosomal aberrations in an *in vitro* test in Chinese hamster ovary cells or in an *in vivo* study in mouse bone marrow. There were no adverse effects on reproductive performance in male and female rats treated with up to 300 mg/kg/day of lisinopril.

Pregnancy
Pregnancy Categories C (first trimester) *and D* (second and third trimesters). See WARNINGS, *Fetal/Neonatal Morbidity and Mortality.*

Nursing Mothers
Milk of lactating rats contains radioactivity following administration of ^{14}C lisinopril. It is not known whether this drug is secreted in human milk. Because many drugs are secreted in human milk, caution should be exercised when PRINIVIL is given to a nursing mother.

Pediatric Use
Safety and effectiveness in pediatric patients have not been established.

---

*Based on patient weight of 50 kg

ADVERSE REACTIONS

PRINIVIL has been found to be generally well tolerated in controlled clinical trials involving 1969 patients with hyper-

tension or heart failure. For the most part, adverse experiences were mild and transient.

HYPERTENSION

In clinical trials in patients with hypertension treated with PRINIVIL, discontinuation of therapy due to clinical adverse experiences occurred in 5.7 percent of patients. The overall frequency of adverse experiences could not be related to total daily dosage within the recommended therapeutic dosage range.

For adverse experiences occurring in greater than one percent of patients with hypertension treated with PRINIVIL or PRINIVIL plus hydrochlorothiazide in controlled clinical trials and more frequently with PRINIVIL and/or PRINIVIL plus hydrochlorothiazide than placebo, comparative incidence data are listed in the table below:

[See table at right.]

Chest pain and back pain were also seen but were more common on placebo than PRINIVIL.

HEART FAILURE

In patients with heart failure treated with PRINIVIL for up to four years, discontinuation of therapy due to clinical adverse experiences occurred in 11.0 percent of patients. In controlled studies in patients with heart failure, therapy was discontinued in 8.1 percent of patients treated with PRINIVIL for up to 12 weeks, compared to 7.7 percent of patients treated with placebo for 12 weeks.

The following table lists those adverse experiences which occurred in greater than one percent of patients with heart failure treated with PRINIVIL or placebo for up to 12 weeks in controlled clinical trials and more frequently on PRINIVIL than placebo.

	Controlled Trials PRINIVIL (n = 407) Incidence (discontinuation) 12 weeks	Placebo (n = 155) Incidence (discontinuation) 12 weeks
Body As A Whole		
Chest Pain	3.4 (0.2)	1.3 (0.0)
Abdominal Pain	2.2 (0.7)	1.9 (0.0)
Cardiovascular		
Hypotension	4.4 (1.7)	0.6 (0.6)
Digestive		
Diarrhea	3.7 (0.5)	1.9 (0.0)
Nervous/Psychiatric		
Dizziness	11.8 (1.2)	4.5 (1.3)
Headache	4.4 (0.2)	3.9 (0.0)
Respiratory		
Upper Respiratory Infection	1.5 (0.0)	1.3 (0.0)
Skin		
Rash	1.7 (0.5)	0.6 (0.6)

Also observed at > 1% with PRINIVIL but more frequent or as frequent on placebo than PRINIVIL in controlled trials were asthenia, angina pectoris, nausea, dyspnea, cough and pruritus.

Worsening of heart failure, anorexia, increased salivation, muscle cramps, back pain, myalgia, depression, chest sound abnormalities and pulmonary edema were also seen in controlled clinical trials, but were more common on placebo than PRINIVIL.

ACUTE MYOCARDIAL INFARCTION

In the GISSI-3 trial, in patients treated with PRINIVIL for six weeks following acute myocardial infarction, discontinuation of therapy occurred in 17.6 percent of patients. Patients treated with PRINIVIL had a significantly higher incidence of hypotension and renal dysfunction compared with patients not taking PRINIVIL.

In the GISSI-3 trial, hypotension (9.7 percent), renal dysfunction (2.0 percent), cough (0.5 percent), post-infarction angina (0.3 percent), skin rash and generalized edema (0.01 percent), and angioedema (0.01 percent) resulted in withdrawal of treatment. In elderly patients treated with PRINIVIL, discontinuation due to renal dysfunction was 4.2 percent.

Other clinical adverse experiences occurring in 0.3 to 1.0 percent of patients with hypertension or heart failure treated with PRINIVIL in controlled trials and rarer, serious, possibly drug-related events reported in uncontrolled studies or marketing experience are listed below, and within each category, are in order of decreasing severity:

Body as a Whole: Anaphylactoid reactions (see WARNINGS, *Anaphylactoid and Possible Related Reactions*), syncope, orthostatic effects, chest discomfort, pain, pelvic pain, flank pain, edema, facial edema, virus infection, fever, chills, malaise.

Cardiovascular: Cardiac arrest; myocardial infarction or cerebrovascular accident, possibly secondary to excessive hypotension in high risk patients (see WARNINGS, *Hypotension*); pulmonary embolism and infarction, arrhythmias (including ventricular tachycardia, atrial tachycardia, atrial fibrillation, bradycardia and premature ventricular contractions), palpitations, transient ischemic attacks, paroxysmal nocturnal dyspnea, orthostatic hypotension, decreased blood pressure, peripheral edema, vasculitis.

	Percent of Patients in Controlled Studies		
	PRINIVIL (n = 1349) Incidence (discontinuation)	PRINIVIL/ Hydrochlorothiazide (n = 629) Incidence (discontinuation)	Placebo (n =207) Incidence (discontinuation)
Body As A Whole			
Fatigue	2.5 (0.3)	4.0 (0.5)	1.0 (0.0)
Asthenia	1.3 (0.5)	2.1 (0.2)	1.0 (0.0)
Orthostatic Effects	1.2 (0.0)	3.5 (0.2)	1.0 (0.0)
Cardiovascular			
Hypotension	1.2 (0.5)	1.6 (0.5)	0.5 (0.5)
Digestive			
Diarrhea	2.7 (0.2)	2.7 (0.3)	2.4 (0.0)
Nausea	2.0 (0.4)	2.5 (0.2)	2.4 (0.0)
Vomiting	1.1 (0.2)	1.4 (0.1)	0.5 (0.0)
Dyspepsia	0.9 (0.0)	1.9 (0.0)	0.0 (0.0)
Musculoskeletal			
Muscle Cramps	0.5 (0.0)	2.9 (0.8)	0.5 (0.0)
Nervous/Psychiatric			
Headache	5.7 (0.2)	4.5 (0.5)	1.9 (0.0)
Dizziness	5.4 (0.4)	9.2 (1.0)	1.9 (0.0)
Paresthesia	0.8 (0.1)	2.1 (0.2)	0.0 (0.0)
Decreased Libido	0.4 (0.1)	1.3 (0.1)	0.0 (0.0)
Vertigo	0.2 (0.1)	1.1 (0.2)	0.0 (0.0)
Respiratory			
Cough	3.5 (0.7)	4.6 (0.8)	1.0 (0.0)
Upper Respiratory Infection	2.1 (0.1)	2.7 (0.1)	0.0 (0.0)
Common Cold	1.1 (0.1)	1.3 (0.1)	0.0 (0.0)
Nasal Congestion	0.4 (0.1)	1.3 (0.1)	0.0 (0.0)
Influenza	0.3 (0.1)	1.1 (0.1)	0.0 (0.0)
Skin			
Rash	1.3 (0.4)	1.6 (0.2)	0.5 (0.5)
Urogenital			
Impotence	1.0 (0.4)	1.6 (0.5)	0.0 (0.0)

Digestive: Pancreatitis, hepatitis (hepatocellular or cholestatic jaundice) (see WARNINGS, *Hepatic Failure*), vomiting, gastritis, dyspepsia, heartburn, gastrointestinal cramps, constipation, flatulence, dry mouth.

Hematologic: Rare cases of bone marrow depression, neutropenia, and thrombocytopenia.

Endocrine: Diabetes mellitus.

Metabolic: Weight loss, dehydration, fluid overload, gout, weight gain.

Musculoskeletal: Arthritis, arthralgia, neck pain, hip pain, low back pain, joint pain, leg pain, knee pain, shoulder pain, arm pain, lumbago.

Nervous System/Psychiatric: Stroke, ataxia, memory impairment, tremor, peripheral neuropathy (e.g., dysesthesia) spasm, paresthesia, confusion, insomnia, somnolence, hypersomnia, irritability, and nervousness.

Respiratory System: Malignant lung neoplasms, hemoptysis, pulmonary infiltrates, bronchospasm, asthma, pleural effusion, pneumonia, bronchitis, wheezing, orthopnea, painful respiration, epistaxis, laryngitis, sinusitis, pharyngeal pain, pharyngitis, rhinitis, rhinorrhea.

Skin: Urticaria, alopecia, herpes zoster, photosensitivity, skin lesions, skin infections, pemphigus, erythema, flushing, diaphoresis. Other severe skin reactions (including toxic epidermal necrolysis and Stevens-Johnson syndrome) have been reported rarely; causal relationship has not been established.

Special Senses: Visual loss, diplopia, blurred vision, tinnitus, photophobia.

Urogenital System: Acute renal failure, oliguria, anuria, uremia, progressive azotemia, renal dysfunction (see PRECAUTIONS and DOSAGE AND ADMINISTRATION), pyelonephritis, dysuria, urinary tract infection, breast pain.

Miscellaneous: A symptom complex has been reported which may include a positive ANA, an elevated erythrocyte sedimentation rate, arthralgia/arthritis, myalgia, fever, vasculitis, leukocytosis, eosinophilia, photosensitivity, rash, and other dermatological manifestations.

Angioedema: Angioedema has been reported in patients receiving PRINIVIL with an incidence higher in black than in non-black patients. Angioedema associated with laryngeal edema may be fatal. If angioedema of the face, extremities, lips, tongue, glottis and/or larynx occurs, treatment with PRINIVIL should be discontinued and appropriate therapy instituted immediately. (See WARNINGS.)

Hypotension: In hypertensive patients, hypotension occurred in 1.2 percent and syncope in 0.1 percent of patients. Hypotension or syncope was a cause for discontinuation of therapy in 0.5 percent of hypertensive patients. In patients with heart failure, hypotension occurred in 5.3 percent and syncope occurred in 1.8 percent of patients. These adverse experiences were causes for discontinuation of therapy in 1.8 percent of these patients. In patients treated with PRINIVIL for six weeks after acute myocardial infarction, hypotension (systolic blood pressure 100 mmHg) resulted in discontinuation of therapy in 9.7 percent of the patients. (See WARNINGS.)

Fetal/Neonatal Morbidity and Mortality: See WARNINGS, *Fetal/Neonatal Morbidity and Mortality.*

Cough: See PRECAUTIONS, *Cough.*

Clinical Laboratory Test Findings

Serum Electrolytes: Hyperkalemia (see PRECAUTIONS), hyponatremia.

Creatinine, Blood Urea Nitrogen: Minor increases in blood urea nitrogen and serum creatinine, reversible upon discontinuation of therapy, were observed in about 2.0 percent of patients with essential hypertension treated with PRINIVIL alone. Increases were more common in patients receiving concomitant diuretics and in patients with renal artery stenosis. (See PRECAUTIONS.) Reversible minor increases in blood urea nitrogen and serum creatinine were observed in approximately 11.6 percent of patients with heart failure on concomitant diuretic therapy. Frequently, these abnormalities resolved when the dosage of the diuretic was decreased.

Hemoglobin and Hematocrit: Small decreases in hemoglobin and hematocrit (mean decreases of approximately 0.4 g percent and 1.3 vol percent, respectively) occurred frequently in patients treated with PRINIVIL but were rarely of clinical importance in patients without some other cause of anemia. In clinical trials, less than 0.1 percent of patients discontinued therapy due to anemia. Hemolytic anemia has been reported; a causal relationship to lisinopril cannot be excluded.

Liver Function Tests: Rarely, elevations of liver enzymes and/or serum bilirubin have occurred (see WARNINGS, *Hepatic Failure*).

In hypertensive patients, 2.0 percent discontinued therapy due to laboratory adverse experiences, principally elevations in blood urea nitrogen (0.6 percent), serum creatinine (0.5 percent) and serum potassium (0.4 percent). In the heart failure trials, 3.4 percent of patients discontinued therapy due to laboratory adverse experiences, 1.8 percent due to elevations in blood urea nitrogen and/or creatinine and 0.6 percent due to elevations in serum potassium. In the myocardial infarction trial, 2.0 percent of patients receiving PRINIVIL discontinued therapy due to renal dysfunction (increasing creatinine concentration to over 3 mg/dL or a doubling or more of the baseline serum creatinine concentration); less than 1.0 percent of patients discontinued therapy due to other laboratory adverse experiences: 0.1 percent with hyperkalemia and less than 0.1 percent with hepatic enzyme alterations.

OVERDOSAGE

The oral LD$_{50}$ of lisinopril is greater than 20 g/kg in mice and rats. The most likely manifestation of overdosage would

Continued on next page

Information on the Merck & Co., Inc. products listed on these pages is the full prescribing information from product circulars in use September 30, 1996.

Merck & Co.—Cont.

be hypotension, for which the usual treatment would be intravenous infusion of normal saline solution.
Lisinopril can be removed by hemodialysis.

DOSAGE AND ADMINISTRATION

Hypertension
Initial Therapy: In patients with uncomplicated essential hypertension not on diuretic therapy, the recommended initial dose is 10 mg once a day. Dosage should be adjusted according to blood pressure response. The usual dosage range is 20 to 40 mg per day administered in a single daily dose. The antihypertensive effect may diminish toward the end of the dosing interval regardless of the administered dose, but most commonly with a dose of 10 mg daily. This can be evaluated by measuring blood pressure just prior to dosing to determine whether satisfactory control is being maintained for 24 hours. If it is not, an increase in dose should be considered. Doses up to 80 mg have been used but do not appear to give a greater effect. If blood pressure is not controlled with PRINIVIL alone, a low dose of a diuretic may be added. Hydrochlorothiazide 12.5 mg has been shown to provide an additive effect. After the addition of a diuretic, it may be possible to reduce the dose of PRINIVIL.
Diuretic Treated Patients: In hypertensive patients who are currently being treated with a diuretic, symptomatic hypotension may occur occasionally following the initial dose of PRINIVIL. The diuretic should be discontinued, if possible, for two to three days before beginning therapy with PRINIVIL to reduce the likelihood of hypotension. (See WARNINGS.) The dosage of PRINIVIL should be adjusted according to blood pressure response. If the patient's blood pressure is not controlled with PRINIVIL alone, diuretic therapy may be resumed as described above.
If the diuretic cannot be discontinued, an initial dose of 5 mg should be used under medical supervision for at least two hours and until blood pressure has stabilized for at least an additional hour. (See WARNINGS and PRECAUTIONS, *Drug Interactions.*)
Concomitant administration of PRINIVIL with potassium supplements, potassium salt substitutes, or potassium-sparing diuretics may lead to increases of serum potassium (see PRECAUTIONS).
Dosage Adjustment in Renal Impairment: The usual dose of PRINIVIL (10 mg) is recommended for patients with a creatinine clearance > 30 mL/min (serum creatinine of up to approximately 3 mg/dL). For patients with creatinine clearance ≥ 10 mL/min ≤ 30 mL/min (serum creatinine ≥ 3 mg/dL), the first dose is 5 mg once daily. For patients with creatinine clearance < 10 mL/min (usually on hemodialysis) the recommended initial dose is 2.5 mg. The dosage may be titrated upward until blood pressure is controlled or to a maximum of 40 mg daily.

Renal Status	Creatinine-Clearance mL/min	Initial Dose mg/day
Normal Renal Function to Mild Impairment	> 30 mL/min	10 mg
Moderate to Severe Impairment	≥ 10 ≤ 30 mL/min	5 mg
Dialysis Patients*	< 10 mL/min	2.5 mg**

* See PRECAUTIONS, *Hemodialysis Patients.*
** *Dosage or dosing interval should be adjusted depending on the blood pressure response.*

Heart Failure
PRINIVIL is indicated as adjunctive therapy with diuretics and digitalis. The recommended starting dose is 5 mg once a day.
When initiating treatment with lisinopril in patients with heart failure, the initial dose should be administered under medical observation, especially in those patients with low blood pressure (systolic blood pressure below 100 mmHg). The mean peak blood pressure lowering occurs six to eight hours after dosing. Observation should continue until blood pressure is stable. The concomitant diuretic dose should be reduced, if possible, to help minimize hypovolemia which may contribute to hypotension. (See WARNINGS and PRECAUTIONS, *Drug Interactions.*) The appearance of hypotension after the initial dose of PRINIVIL does not preclude subsequent careful dose titration with the drug, following effective management of the hypotension.
The usual effective dosage range is 5 to 20 mg per day administered as a single daily dose.
Dosage Adjustment in Patients with Heart Failure and Renal Impairment or Hyponatremia: In patients with heart failure who have hyponatremia (serum sodium < 130 mEq/L) or moderate to severe renal impairment (creatinine clearance ≤ 30 mL/min or serum creatinine > 3 mg/dL), therapy with PRINIVIL should be initiated at a dose of 2.5 mg once a day under close medical supervision. (See WARNINGS and PRECAUTIONS, *Drug Interactions.*)
Acute Myocardial Infarction
In hemodynamically stable patients within 24 hours of the onset of acute myocardial infarction, the first dose of PRINIVIL is 5 mg given orally, followed by 5 mg after 24 hours, 10 mg after 48 hours and then 10 mg of PRINIVIL once daily. Dosing should continue for six weeks. Patients should receive, as appropriate, the standard recommended treatments such as thrombolytics, aspirin and beta-blockers. Patients with a low systolic blood pressure (≤120 mmHg) when treatment is started or during the first 3 days after the infarct should be given a lower 2.5 mg oral dose of PRINIVIL (see WARNINGS). If hypotension occurs (systolic blood pressure ≤100 mmHg) a daily maintenance dose of 5 mg may be given with temporary reductions to 2.5 mg if needed. If prolonged hypotension occurs (systolic blood pressure <90 mmHg for more than 1 hour) PRINIVIL should be withdrawn. For patients who develop symptoms of heart failure, see DOSAGE AND ADMINISTRATION, *Heart Failure.*
Dosage Adjustment in Patients with Myocardial Infarction with Renal Impairment: In acute myocardial infarction, treatment with PRINIVIL should be initiated with caution in patients with evidence of renal dysfunction, defined as serum creatinine concentration exceeding 2 mg/dL. No evaluation of dosage adjustment in myocardial infarction patients with severe renal impairment has been performed.
Use in Elderly: In general, blood pressure response and adverse experiences were similar in younger and older patients given similar doses of PRINIVIL. Pharmacokinetic studies, however, indicate that maximum blood levels and area under the plasma concentration time curve (AUC) are doubled in older patients so that dosage adjustments should be made with particular caution.

HOW SUPPLIED

No. 3658—Tablets PRINIVIL, 2.5 mg, are white, round flat-faced beveled edged compressed tablets, coded MSD on one side and 15 on the other. They are supplied as follows:
NDC 0006-0015-28 unit dose packages of 100
NDC 0006-0015-31 unit of use bottles of 30
NDC 0006-0015-58 unit of use bottles of 100.
Shown in Product Identification Guide, page 325
No. 3577—Tablets PRINIVIL, 5 mg, are white, shield shaped, scored, compressed tablets, with code MSD 19 on one side and PRINIVIL on the other. They are supplied as follows:
NDC 0006-0019-28 unit dose packages of 100
NDC 0006-0019-58 unit of use bottles of 100
(6505-01-281-2771, 5 mg 100's)
NDC 0006-0019-94 unit of use bottles of 90
NDC 0006-0019-82 bottles of 1,000
NDC 0006-0019-86 bottles of 5,000
(6505-01-367-8874, 5 mg 5,000's)
NDC 0006-0019-87 bottles of 10,000
(6505-01-377-8061, 5 mg 10,000's).
Shown in Product Identification Guide, page 325
No. 3578—Tablets PRINIVIL, 10 mg, are light yellow, shield shaped, compressed tablets, with code MSD 106 on one side and PRINIVIL on the other. They are supplied as follows:
NDC 0006-0106-28 unit dose packages of 100
(6505-01-342-4861, 10 mg individually sealed 100's
NDC 0006-0106-31 unit of use bottles of 30
NDC 0006-0106-58 unit of use bottles of 100
(6505-01-275-0061, 10 mg 100's)
NDC 0006-0106-94 unit of use bottles of 90
NDC 0006-0106-82 bottles of 1,000
NDC 0006-0106-86 bottles of 5,000
(6505-01-368-6604, 10 mg 5,000's)
NDC 0006-0106-87 bottles of 10,000
(6505-01-8064, 10 mg 10,000's).
Shown in Product Identification Guide, page 325
No. 3579—Tablets PRINIVIL, 20 mg, are peach, shield shaped, compressed tablets, with code MSD 207 on one side and PRINIVIL on the other. They are supplied as follows:
NDC 0006-0207-28 unit dose packages of 100
NDC 0006-0207-31 unit of use bottles of 30
NDC 0006-0207-58 unit of use bottles of 100
(6505-01-282-6327, 20 mg 100's)
NDC 0006-0207-94 unit of use bottles of 90
NDC 0006-0207-82 bottles of 1,000
NDC 0006-0207-86 bottles of 5,000
NDC 0006-0207-87 bottles of 10,000
(6505-01-8066, 20 mg 10,000's).
Shown in Product Identification Guide, page 325
No. 3580—Tablets PRINIVIL, 40 mg, are rose red, shield shaped, compressed tablets, with code MSD 237 on one side and PRINIVIL on the other. They are supplied as follows:
NDC 0006-0237-58 unit of use bottles of 100.
Shown in Product Identification Guide, page 325

Storage
Store at room temperature, 15–30°C (59–86°F), and protect from moisture.
Dispense in a tight container, if product package is subdivided.
7825239 Issued November 1995
COPYRIGHT © MERCK & CO., INC., 1988, 1989, 1992, 1993
All rights reserved

PRINZIDE® Tablets ℞
(Lisinopril-Hydrochlorothiazide)

> **USE IN PREGNANCY**
> **When used in pregnancy during the second and third trimesters, ACE inhibitors can cause injury and even death to the developing fetus.** When pregnancy is detected, PRINZIDE should be discontinued as soon as possible. See WARNINGS, *Pregnancy, Lisinopril, Fetal/Neonatal Morbidity and Mortality.*

DESCRIPTION

PRINZIDE* (Lisinopril-Hydrochlorothiazide) combines an angiotensin converting enzyme inhibitor, lisinopril, and a diuretic, hydrochlorothiazide.
Lisinopril, a synthetic peptide derivative, is an oral long-acting angiotensin converting enzyme inhibitor. It is chemically described as (*S*)-1-[N^2-(1-carboxy-3-phenylpropyl)-L-lysyl]-L-proline dihydrate. Its empirical formula is $C_{21}H_{31}N_3O_5 \cdot 2H_2O$ and its structural formula is:

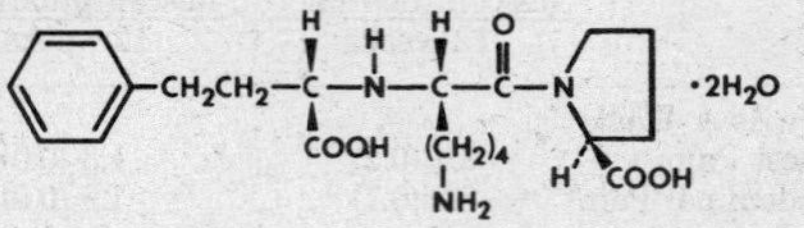

Lisinopril is a white to off-white, crystalline powder, with a molecular weight of 441.52. It is soluble in water, sparingly soluble in methanol, and practically insoluble in ethanol.
Hydrochlorothiazide is 6-chloro-3,4-dihydro-2*H*-1,2,4-benzothiadiazine-7-sulfonamide 1,1-dioxide. Its empirical formula is $C_7H_8ClN_3O_4S_2$ and its structural formula is:

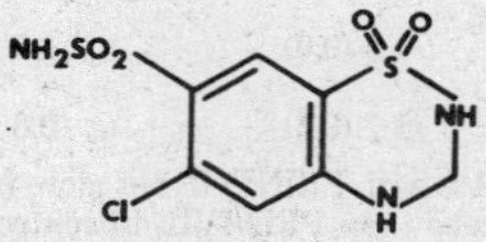

Hydrochlorothiazide is a white, or practically white, crystalline powder with a molecular weight of 297.73, which is slightly soluble in water, but freely soluble in sodium hydroxide solution.
PRINZIDE is available for oral use in three tablet combinations of lisinopril with hydrochlorothiazide: PRINZIDE 10-12.5, containing 10 mg lisinopril and 12.5 mg hydrochlorothiazide. PRINZIDE 20-12.5, containing 20 mg lisinopril and 12.5 mg hydrochlorothiazide and PRINZIDE 20-25, containing 20 mg lisinopril and 25 mg hydrochlorothiazide.
Inactive ingredients are calcium phosphate, magnesium stearate, mannitol, and starch. PRINZIDE 10-12.5 also contains FD&C Blue #2 aluminum lake. PRINZIDE 20-12.5 and PRINZIDE 20-25 also contain iron oxide.

*Registered trademark of MERCK & CO., INC.

CLINICAL PHARMACOLOGY

Lisinopril-Hydrochlorothiazide
As a result of its diuretic effects, hydrochlorothiazide increases plasma renin activity, increases aldosterone secretion, and decreases serum potassium. Administration of lisinopril blocks the renin-angiotensin-aldosterone axis and tends to reverse the potassium loss associated with the diuretic.
In clinical studies, the extent of blood pressure reduction seen with the combination of lisinopril and hydrochlorothiazide was approximately additive. The PRINZIDE 10-12.5 combination worked equally well in black and white patients. The PRINZIDE 20-12.5 and PRINZIDE 20-25 combinations appeared somewhat less effective in black patients, but relatively few black patients were studied. In most patients, the antihypertensive effect of PRINZIDE was sustained for at least 24 hours.
In a randomized, controlled comparison, the main antihypertensive effects of PRINZIDE 20-12.5 and PRINZIDE 20-25 were similar, suggesting that many patients who respond adequately to the latter combination may be controlled with

PRINZIDE 20-12.5. (See DOSAGE AND ADMINISTRATION.)

Concomitant administration of lisinopril and hydrochlorothiazide has little or no effect on the bioavailability of either drug. The combination tablet is bioequivalent to concomitant administration of the separate entities.

Lisinopril
Mechanism of Action

Lisinopril inhibits angiotensin-converting enzyme (ACE) in human subjects and animals. ACE is a peptidyl dipeptidase that catalyzes the conversion of angiotensin I to the vasoconstrictor substance, angiotensin II. Angiotensin II also stimulates aldosterone secretion by the adrenal cortex. Inhibition of ACE results in decreased plasma angiotensin II which leads to decreased vasopressor activity and to decreased aldosterone secretion. The latter decrease may result in a small increase of serum potassium. Removal of angiotensin II negative feedback on renin secretion leads to increased plasma renin activity. In hypertensive patients with normal renal function treated with lisinopril alone for up to 24 weeks, the mean increase in serum potassium was less than 0.1 mEq/L; however, approximately 15 percent of patients had increases greater than 0.5 mEq/L and approximately six percent had a decrease greater than 0.5 mEq/L. In the same study, patients treated with lisinopril plus a thiazide diuretic showed essentially no change in serum potassium. (See PRECAUTIONS.)

ACE is identical to kininase, an enzyme that degrades bradykinin. Whether increased levels of bradykinin, a potent vasodepressor peptide, play a role in the therapeutic effects of lisinopril remains to be elucidated.

While the mechanism through which lisinopril lowers blood pressure is believed to be primarily suppression of the renin-angiotensin-aldosterone system, lisinopril is antihypertensive even in patients with low-renin hypertension. Although lisinopril was antihypertensive in all races studied, black hypertensive patients (usually a low-renin hypertensive population) had a smaller average response to lisinopril monotherapy than non-black patients.

Pharmacokinetics and Metabolism

Following oral administration of lisinopril, peak serum concentrations occur within about 7 hours. Declining serum concentrations exhibit a prolonged terminal phase which does not contribute to drug accumulation. This terminal phase probably represents saturable binding to ACE and is not proportional to dose. Lisinopril does not appear to be bound to other serum proteins.

Lisinopril does not undergo metabolism and is excreted unchanged entirely in the urine. Based on urinary recovery, the mean extent of absorption of lisinopril is approximately 25 percent, with large intersubject variability (6–60 percent) at all doses tested (5–80 mg). Lisinopril absorption is not influenced by the presence of food in the gastrointestinal tract. Upon multiple dosing, lisinopril exhibits an effective half-life of accumulation of 12 hours.

Impaired renal function decreases elimination of lisinopril, which is excreted principally through the kidneys, but this decrease becomes clinically important only when the glomerular filtration rate is below 30 mL/min. Above this glomerular filtration rate, the elimination half-life is little changed. With greater impairment, however, peak and trough lisinopril levels increase, time to peak concentration increases and time to attain steady state is prolonged. Older patients, on average, have (approximately doubled) higher blood levels and area under the plasma concentration time curve (AUC) than younger patients. (See DOSAGE AND ADMINISTRATION.) Lisinopril can be removed by hemodialysis.

Studies in rats indicate that lisinopril crosses the blood-brain barrier poorly. Multiple doses of lisinopril in rats do not result in accumulation in any tissues. However, milk of lactating rats contains radioactivity following administration of ^{14}C lisinopril. By whole body autoradiography, radioactivity was found in the placenta following administration of labeled drug to pregnant rats, but none was found in the fetuses.

Pharmacodynamics

Administration of lisinopril to patients with hypertension results in a reduction of supine and standing blood pressure to about the same extent with no compensatory tachycardia. Symptomatic postural hypotension is usually not observed although it can occur and should be anticipated in volume and/or salt-depleted patients. (See WARNINGS.)

In most patients studied, onset of antihypertensive activity was seen at one hour after oral administration of an individual dose of lisinopril, with peak reduction of blood pressure achieved by six hours.

In some patients achievement of optimal blood pressure reduction may require two to four weeks of therapy.

At recommended single daily doses, antihypertensive effects have been maintained for at least 24 hours after dosing, although the effect at 24 hours was substantially smaller than the effect six hours after dosing.

The antihypertensive effects of lisinopril have continued during long-term therapy. Abrupt withdrawal of lisinopril has not been associated with a rapid increase in blood pressure; nor with a significant overshoot of pretreatment blood pressure.

In hemodynamic studies in patients with essential hypertension, blood pressure reduction was accompanied by a reduction in peripheral arterial resistance with little or no change in cardiac output and in heart rate. In a study in nine hypertensive patients, following administration of lisinopril, there was an increase in mean renal blood flow that was not significant. Data from several small studies are inconsistent with respect to the effect of lisinopril on glomerular filtration rate in hypertensive patients with normal renal function, but suggest that changes, if any, are not large.

In patients with renovascular hypertension lisinopril has been shown to be well tolerated and effective in controlling blood pressure (see PRECAUTIONS).

Hydrochlorothiazide

The mechanism of the antihypertensive effect of thiazides is unknown. Thiazides do not usually affect normal blood pressure.

Hydrochlorothiazide is a diuretic and antihypertensive. It affects the distal renal tubular mechanism of electrolyte reabsorption. Hydrochlorothiazide increases excretion of sodium and chloride in approximately equivalent amounts. Natriuresis may be accompanied by some loss of potassium and bicarbonate.

After oral use diuresis begins within two hours, peaks in about four hours and lasts about 6 to 12 hours.

Hydrochlorothiazide is not metabolized but is eliminated rapidly by the kidney. When plasma levels have been followed for at least 24 hours, the plasma half-life has been observed to vary between 5.6 and 14.8 hours. At least 61 percent of the oral dose is eliminated unchanged within 24 hours. Hydrochlorothiazide crosses the placental but not the blood-brain barrier.

INDICATIONS AND USAGE

PRINZIDE is indicated for the treatment of hypertension. These fixed-dose combinations are not indicated for initial therapy (see DOSAGE AND ADMINISTRATION).

In using PRINZIDE, consideration should be given to the fact that an angiotensin converting enzyme inhibitor, captopril, has caused agranulocytosis, particularly in patients with renal impairment or collagen vascular disease, and that available data are insufficient to show that lisinopril does not have a similar risk. (See WARNINGS.)

In considering use of PRINZIDE, it should be noted that black patients receiving ACE inhibitor monotherapy have been reported to have a higher incidence of angioedema compared to non-blacks. (See WARNINGS, *Angioedema*.)

CONTRAINDICATIONS

PRINZIDE is contraindicated in patients who are hypersensitive to any component of this product and in patients with a history of angioedema related to previous treatment with an angiotensin converting enzyme inhibitor. Because of the hydrochlorothiazide component, this product is contraindicated in patients with anuria or hypersensitivity to other sulfonamide-derived drugs.

WARNINGS

General
Lisinopril
Anaphylactoid and Possibly Related Reactions:
Presumably because angiotensin-converting enzyme inhibitors affect the metabolism of eicosanoids and polypeptides, including endogenous bradykinin, patients receiving ACE inhibitors (including PRINZIDE) may be subject to a variety of adverse reactions, some of them serious.

Angioedema: Angioedema of the face, extremities, lips, tongue, glottis and/or larynx has been reported rarely in patients treated with angiotensin converting enzyme inhibitors, including lisinopril. This may occur at any time during treatment. In such cases PRINZIDE should be promptly discontinued and appropriate therapy and monitoring should be provided until complete and sustained resolution of signs and symptoms has occurred. In instances where swelling has been confined to the face and lips the condition has generally resolved without treatment, although antihistamines have been useful in relieving symptoms. Angioedema associated with laryngeal edema may be fatal. **Where there is involvement of the tongue, glottis or larynx, likely to cause airway obstruction, subcutaneous epinephrine solution 1:1000 (0.3 mL to 0.5 mL) and/or measures necessary to ensure a patent airway, should be promptly provided.** (See ADVERSE REACTIONS.)

Patients with a history of angioedema unrelated to ACE inhibitor therapy may be at increased risk of angioedema while receiving an ACE inhibitor (see also INDICATIONS AND USAGE and CONTRAINDICATIONS).

Anaphylactoid reactions during desensitization: Two patients undergoing desensitizing treatment with hymenoptera venom while receiving ACE inhibitors sustained life-threatening anaphylactoid reactions. In the same patients, these reactions were avoided when ACE inhibitors were temporarily withheld, but they reappeared upon inadvertent rechallenge.

Anaphylactoid reactions during membrane exposure: Anaphylactoid reactions have been reported in patients dialyzed with high-flux membranes and treated concomitantly with an ACE inhibitor. Anaphylactoid reactions have also been reported in patients undergoing low-density lipoprotein apheresis with dextran sulfate absorption (a procedure dependent upon devices not approved in the United States).

Hypotension and Related Effects:
Excessive hypotension was rarely seen in uncomplicated hypertensive patients but is a possible consequence of lisinopril use in salt/volume-depleted persons, such as those treated vigorously with diuretics or patients on dialysis. (See PRECAUTIONS, *Drug Interactions* and ADVERSE REACTIONS.)

Syncope has been reported in 0.8 percent of patients receiving PRINZIDE. In patients with hypertension receiving lisinopril alone, the incidence of syncope was 0.1 percent. The overall incidence of syncope may be reduced by proper titration of the individual components. (See PRECAUTIONS, *Drug Interactions*, ADVERSE REACTIONS and DOSAGE AND ADMINISTRATION.)

In patients with severe congestive heart failure, with or without associated renal insufficiency, excessive hypotension has been observed and may be associated with oliguria and/or progressive azotemia, and rarely with acute renal failure and/or death. Because of the potential fall in blood pressure in these patients, therapy should be started under very close medical supervision. Such patients should be followed closely for the first two weeks of treatment and whenever the dose of lisinopril and/or diuretic is increased. Similar considerations apply to patients with ischemic heart or cerebrovascular disease in whom an excessive fall in blood pressure could result in a myocardial infarction or cerebrovascular accident.

If hypotension occurs, the patient should be placed in supine position and, if necessary, receive an intravenous infusion of normal saline. A transient hypotensive response is not a contraindication to further doses which usually can be given without difficulty once the blood pressure has increased after volume expansion.

Neutropenia/Agranulocytosis:
Another angiotensin converting enzyme inhibitor, captopril, has been shown to cause agranulocytosis and bone marrow depression, rarely in uncomplicated patients but more frequently in patients with renal impairment, especially if they also have a collagen vascular disease. Available data from clinical trials of lisinopril are insufficient to show that lisinopril does not cause agranulocytosis at similar rates. Marketing experience has revealed rare cases of neutropenia and bone marrow depression in which a causal relationship to lisinopril cannot be excluded. Periodic monitoring of white blood cell counts in patients with collagen vascular disease and renal disease should be considered.

Hepatic Failure:
Rarely, ACE inhibitors have been associated with a syndrome that starts with cholestatic jaundice and progresses to fulminant hepatic necrosis, and (sometimes) death. The mechanism of this syndrome is not understood. Patients receiving ACE inhibitors who develop jaundice or marked elevations of hepatic enzymes should discontinue the ACE inhibitor and receive appropriate medical follow-up.

Hydrochlorothiazide
Thiazides should be used with caution in severe renal disease. In patients with renal disease, thiazides may precipitate azotemia. Cumulative effects of the drug may develop in patients with impaired renal function.

Thiazides should be used with caution in patients with impaired hepatic function or progressive liver disease, since minor alterations of fluid and electrolyte balance may precipitate hepatic coma.

Sensitivity reactions may occur in patients with or without a history of allergy or bronchial asthma.

The possibility of exacerbation or activation of systemic lupus erythematosus has been reported.

Lithium generally should not be given with thiazides (see PRECAUTIONS, *Drug Interactions, Lisinopril* and *Hydrochlorothiazide*).

Pregnancy
Lisinopril-Hydrochlorothiazide
Teratogenicity studies were conducted in mice and rats with up to 90 mg/kg/day of lisinopril (56 times the maximum recommended human dose) in combination with 10 mg/kg/day of hydrochlorothiazide (2.5 times the maximum recommended human dose). Maternal or fetotoxic effects were not

Continued on next page

Information on the Merck & Co., Inc. products listed on these pages is the full prescribing information from product circulars in use September 30, 1996.

Merck & Co.—Cont.

seen in mice with the combination. In rats decreased maternal weight gain and decreased fetal weight occurred down to 3/10 mg/kg/day (the lowest dose tested). Associated with the decreased fetal weight was a delay in fetal ossification. The decreased fetal weight and delay in fetal ossification were not seen in saline-supplemented animals given 90/10 mg/kg/day.

When used in pregnancy during the second and third trimesters, ACE inhibitors can cause injury and even death to the developing fetus. When pregnancy is detected, PRINZIDE should be discontinued as soon as possible. (See *Lisinopril, Fetal/Neonatal Morbidity and Mortality*, below.)

Lisinopril

Fetal/Neonatal Morbidity and Mortality: ACE inhibitors can cause fetal and neonatal morbidity and death when administered to pregnant women. Several dozen cases have been reported in the world literature. When pregnancy is detected, ACE inhibitors should be discontinued as soon as possible.

The use of ACE inhibitors during the second and third trimesters of pregnancy has been associated with fetal and neonatal injury, including hypotension, neonatal skull hypoplasia, anuria, reversible or irreversible renal failure, and death. Oligohydramnios has also been reported, presumably resulting from decreased fetal renal function; oligohydramnios in this setting has been associated with fetal limb contractures, craniofacial deformation, and hypoplastic lung development. Prematurity, intrauterine growth retardation, and patent ductus arteriosus have also been reported, although it is not clear whether these occurrences were due to the ACE-inhibitor exposure.

These adverse effects do not appear to have resulted from intrauterine ACE-inhibitor exposure that has been limited to the first trimester. Mothers whose embryos and fetuses are exposed to ACE inhibitors only during the first trimester should be so informed. Nonetheless, when patients become pregnant, physicians should make every effort to discontinue the use of PRINZIDE as soon as possible.

Rarely (probably less often than once in every thousand pregnancies), no alternative to ACE inhibitors will be found. In these rare cases, the mothers should be apprised of the potential hazards to their fetuses, and serial ultrasound examinations should be performed to assess the intraamniotic environment.

If oligohydramnios is observed, PRINZIDE should be discontinued unless it is considered lifesaving for the mother. Contraction stress testing (CST), a non-stress test (NST), or biophysical profiling (BPP) may be appropriate, depending upon the week of pregnancy. Patients and physicians should be aware, however, that oligohydramnios may not appear until after the fetus has sustained irreversible injury.

Infants with histories of *in utero* exposure to ACE inhibitors should be closely observed for hypotension, oliguria, and hyperkalemia. If oliguria occurs, attention should be directed toward support of blood pressure and renal perfusion. Exchange transfusion or dialysis may be required as means of reversing hypotension and/or substituting for disordered renal function. Lisinopril, which crosses the placenta, has been removed from neonatal circulation by peritoneal dialysis with some clinical benefit, and theoretically may be removed by exchange transfusion, although there is no experience with the latter procedure.

No teratogenic effects of lisinopril were seen in studies of pregnant rats, mice, and rabbits. On a mg/kg basis, the doses used were up to 625 times (in mice), 188 times (in rats), 0.6 times (in rabbits) the maximum recommended human dose.

Hydrochlorothiazide

Teratogenic Effects: Reproduction studies in the rabbit, the mouse and the rat at doses up to 100 mg/kg/day (50 times the human dose) showed no evidence of external abnormalities of the fetus due to hydrochlorothiazide. Hydrochlorothiazide given in a two-litter study in rats at doses of 4 - 5.6 mg/kg/day (approximately 1 - 2 times the usual daily human dose) did not impair fertility or produce birth abnormalities in the offspring. Thiazides cross the placental barrier and appear in cord blood.

Nonteratogenic Effects: These may include fetal or neonatal jaundice, thrombocytopenia, and possibly other adverse reactions which have occurred in the adult.

PRECAUTIONS

General

Lisinopril

Impaired Renal Function: As a consequence of inhibiting the renin-angiotensin-aldosterone system, changes in renal function may be anticipated in susceptible individuals. In patients with severe congestive heart failure whose renal function may depend on the activity of the renin-angiotensin-aldosterone system, treatment with angiotensin converting enzyme inhibitors, including lisinopril, may be associated with oliguria and/or progressive azotemia and rarely with acute renal failure and/or death.

In hypertensive patients with unilateral or bilateral renal artery stenosis, increases in blood urea nitrogen and serum creatinine may occur. Experience with another angiotensin converting enzyme inhibitor suggests that these increases are usually reversible upon discontinuation of lisinopril and/ or diuretic therapy. In such patients renal function should be monitored during the first few weeks of therapy. Some hypertensive patients with no apparent pre-existing renal vascular disease have developed increases in blood urea and serum creatinine, usually minor and transient, especially when lisinopril has been given concomitantly with a diuretic. This is more likely to occur in patients with pre-existing renal impairment. Dosage reduction of lisinopril and/or discontinuation of the diuretic may be required.

Evaluation of the hypertensive patient should always include assessment of renal function. (See DOSAGE AND ADMINISTRATION.)

Hyperkalemia: In clinical trials hyperkalemia (serum potassium greater than 5.7 mEq/L) occurred in approximately 1.4 percent of hypertensive patients treated with lisinopril plus hydrochlorothiazide. In most cases these were isolated values which resolved despite continued therapy. Hyperkalemia was not a cause of discontinuation of therapy. Risk factors for the development of hyperkalemia include renal insufficiency, diabetes mellitus, and the concomitant use of potassium-sparing diuretics, potassium supplements and/or potassium-containing salt substitutes, which should be used cautiously if at all with PRINZIDE. (See *Drug Interactions*.)

Cough: Presumably due to the inhibition of the degradation of endogenous bradykinin, persistent nonproductive cough has been reported with all ACE inhibitors, always resolving after discontinuation of therapy. ACE inhibitor-induced cough should be considered in the differential diagnosis of cough.

Surgery/Anesthesia: In patients undergoing major surgery or during anesthesia with agents that produce hypotension, lisinopril may block angiotensin II formation secondary to compensatory renin release. If hypotension occurs and is considered to be due to this mechanism, it can be corrected by volume expansion.

Hydrochlorothiazide

Periodic determination of serum electrolytes to detect possible electrolyte imbalance should be performed at appropriate intervals.

All patients receiving thiazide therapy should be observed for clinical signs of fluid or electrolyte imbalance: namely, hyponatremia, hypochloremic alkalosis, and hypokalemia. Serum and urine electrolyte determinations are particularly important when the patient is vomiting excessively or receiving parenteral fluids. Warning signs or symptoms of fluid and electrolyte imbalance, irrespective of cause, include dryness of mouth, thirst, weakness, lethargy, drowsiness, restlessness, confusion, seizures, muscle pains or cramps, muscular fatigue, hypotension, oliguria, tachycardia, and gastrointestinal disturbances such as nausea and vomiting.

Hypokalemia may develop, especially with brisk diuresis, when severe cirrhosis is present, or after prolonged therapy. Interference with adequate oral electrolyte intake will also contribute to hypokalemia. Hypokalemia may cause cardiac arrhythmia and may also sensitize or exaggerate the response of the heart to the toxic effects of digitalis (e.g., increased ventricular irritability). Because lisinopril reduces the production of aldosterone, concomitant therapy with lisinopril attenuates the diuretic-induced potassium loss (see *Drug Interactions, Agents Increasing Serum Potassium*).

Although any chloride deficit is generally mild and usually does not require specific treatment, except under extraordinary circumstances (as in liver disease or renal disease), chloride replacement may be required in the treatment of metabolic alkalosis.

Dilutional hyponatremia may occur in edematous patients in hot weather; appropriate therapy is water restriction, rather than administration of salt except in rare instances when the hyponatremia is life-threatening. In actual salt depletion, appropriate replacement is the therapy of choice.

Hyperuricemia may occur or frank gout may be precipitated in certain patients receiving thiazide therapy.

In diabetic patients dosage adjustments of insulin or oral hypoglycemic agents may be required. Hyperglycemia may occur with thiazide diuretics. Thus latent diabetes mellitus may become manifest during thiazide therapy.

The antihypertensive effects of the drug may be enhanced in the postsympathectomy patient.

If progressive renal impairment becomes evident consider withholding or discontinuing diuretic therapy.

Thiazides have been shown to increase the urinary excretion of magnesium; this may result in hypomagnesemia.

Thiazides may decrease urinary calcium excretion. Thiazides may cause intermittent and slight elevation of serum calcium in the absence of known disorders of calcium metabolism. Marked hypercalcemia may be evidence of hidden hyperparathyroidism. Thiazides should be discontinued before carrying out tests for parathyroid function.

Increases in cholesterol and triglyceride levels may be associated with thiazide diuretic therapy.

Information for Patients

Angioedema: Angioedema, including laryngeal edema, may occur at any time during treatment with angiotensin converting enzyme inhibitors, including lisinopril. Patients should be so advised and told to report immediately any signs or symptoms suggesting angioedema (swelling of face, extremities, eyes, lips, tongue, difficulty in swallowing or breathing) and to take no more drug until they have consulted with the prescribing physician.

Symptomatic Hypotension: Patients should be cautioned to report lightheadedness especially during the first few days of therapy. If actual syncope occurs, the patients should be told to discontinue the drug until they have consulted with the prescribing physician.

All patients should be cautioned that excessive perspiration and dehydration may lead to an excessive fall in blood pressure because of reduction in fluid volume. Other causes of volume depletion such as vomiting or diarrhea may also lead to a fall in blood pressure; patients should be advised to consult with their physician.

Hyperkalemia: Patients should be told not to use salt substitutes containing potassium without consulting their physician.

Neutropenia: Patients should be told to report promptly any indication of infection (e.g., sore throat, fever) which may be a sign of neutropenia.

Pregnancy: Female patients of childbearing age should be told about the consequences of second- and third-trimester exposure to ACE inhibitors, and they should also be told that these consequences do not appear to have resulted from intrauterine ACE-inhibitor exposure that has been limited to the first trimester. These patients should be asked to report pregnancies to their physicians as soon as possible.

NOTE: As with many other drugs, certain advice to patients being treated with PRINZIDE is warranted. This information is intended to aid in the safe and effective use of this medication. It is not a disclosure of all possible adverse or intended effects.

Drug Interactions

Lisinopril

Hypotension —Patients on Diuretic Therapy: Patients on diuretics, and especially those in whom diuretic therapy was recently instituted, may occasionally experience an excessive reduction of blood pressure after initiation of therapy with lisinopril. The possibility of hypotensive effects with lisinopril can be minimized by either discontinuing the diuretic or increasing the salt intake prior to initiation of treatment with lisinopril. If it is necessary to continue the diuretic, initiate therapy with lisinopril at a dose of 5 mg daily, and provide close medical supervision after the initial dose for at least two hours and until blood pressure has stabilized for at least an additional hour. (See WARNINGS and DOSAGE AND ADMINISTRATION.) When a diuretic is added to the therapy of a patient receiving lisinopril, an additional antihypertensive effect is usually observed. (See DOSAGE AND ADMINISTRATION.)

Indomethacin: In a study in 36 patients with mild to moderate hypertension where the antihypertensive effects of lisinopril alone were compared to lisinopril given concomitantly with indomethacin, the use of indomethacin was associated with a reduced effect, although the difference between the two regimens was not significant.

Other Agents: Lisinopril has been used concomitantly with nitrates and/or digoxin without evidence of clinically significant adverse interactions. No meaningful clinically important pharmacokinetic interactions occurred when lisinopril was used concomitantly with propranolol, digoxin, or hydrochlorothiazide. The presence of food in the stomach does not alter the bioavailability of lisinopril.

Agents Increasing Serum Potassium: Lisinopril attenuates potassium loss caused by thiazide-type diuretics. Use of lisinopril with potassium-sparing diuretics (e.g., spironolactone, triamterene, or amiloride), potassium supplements, or potassium-containing salt substitutes may lead to significant increases in serum potassium. Therefore, if concomitant use of these agents is indicated, because of demonstrated hypokalemia, they should be used with caution and with frequent monitoring of serum potassium.

Lithium: Lithium toxicity has been reported in patients receiving lithium concomitantly with drugs which cause elimination of sodium, including ACE inhibitors. Lithium toxicity was usually reversible upon discontinuation of lithium and the ACE inhibitor. It is recommended that serum lithium levels be monitored frequently if lisinopril is administered concomitantly with lithium.

Hydrochlorothiazide

When administered concurrently the following drugs may interact with thiazide diuretics.

Alcohol, barbiturates, or narcotics —potentiation of orthostatic hypotension may occur.

Antidiabetic drugs (oral agents and insulin)—dosage adjustment of the antidiabetic drug may be required.

Other antihypertensive drugs —additive effect or potentiation.

Cholestyramine and colestipol resins —Absorption of hydrochlorothiazide is impaired in the presence of anionic exchange resins. Single doses of either cholestyramine or colestipol resins bind the hydrochlorothiazide and reduce its absorption from the gastrointestinal tract by up to 85 and 43 percent, respectively.

Corticosteroids, ACTH —intensified electrolyte depletion, particularly hypokalemia.

Pressor amines (e.g., norepinephrine) —possible decreased response to pressor amines but not sufficient to preclude their use.

Skeletal muscle relaxants, nondepolarizing (e.g., tubocurarine) —possible increased responsiveness to the muscle relaxant.

Lithium —should not generally be given with diuretics. Diuretic agents reduce the renal clearance of lithium and add a high risk of lithium toxicity. Refer to the package insert for lithium preparations before use of such preparations with PRINZIDE.

Non-steroidal Anti-inflammatory Drugs —In some patients, the administration of a non-steroidal anti-inflammatory agent can reduce the diuretic, natriuretic, and antihypertensive effects of loop, potassium-sparing and thiazide diuretics. Therefore, when PRINZIDE and non-steroidal anti-inflammatory agents are used concomitantly, the patient should be observed closely to determine if the desired effect of PRINZIDE is obtained.

Carcinogenesis, Mutagenesis, Impairment of Fertility
Lisinopril-Hydrochlorothiazide
Lisinopril in combination with hydrochlorothiazide was not mutagenic in a microbial mutagen test using *Salmonella typhimurium* (Ames test) or *Escherichia coli* with or without metabolic activation or in a forward mutation assay using Chinese hamster lung cells. Lisinopril-hydrochlorothiazide did not produce DNA single strand breaks in an *in vitro* alkaline elution rat hepatocyte assay. In addition, it did not produce increases in chromosomal aberrations in an *in vitro* test in Chinese hamster ovary cells or in an *in vivo* study in mouse bone marrow.
Lisinopril
There was no evidence of a tumorigenic effect when lisinopril was administered for 105 weeks to male and female rats at doses up to 90 mg/kg/day (about 56 times* the maximum recommended daily human dose). Lisinopril has also been administered for 92 weeks to (male and female) mice at doses up to 135 mg/kg/day (about 84 times* the maximum recommended daily human dose) and showed no evidence of carcinogenicity.

Lisinopril was not mutagenic in the Ames microbial mutagen test with or without metabolic activation. It was also negative in a forward mutation assay using Chinese hamster lung cells. Lisinopril did not produce single strand DNA breaks in an *in vitro* alkaline elution rat hepatocyte assay. In addition, lisinopril did not produce increases in chromosomal aberrations in an *in vitro* test in Chinese hamster ovary cells or in an *in vivo* study in mouse bone marrow. There were no adverse effects on reproductive performance in male and female rats treated with up to 300 mg/kg/day of lisinopril.

---
*Based on patient weight of 50 kg

Hydrochlorothiazide
Two-year feeding studies in mice and rats conducted under the auspices of the National Toxicology Program (NTP) uncovered no evidence of a carcinogenic potential of hydrochlorothiazide in female mice (at doses of up to approximately 600 mg/kg/day) or in male and female rats (at doses of up to approximately 100 mg/kg/day). The NTP, however, found equivocal evidence for hepatocarcinogenicity in male mice.

Hydrochlorothiazide was not genotoxic *in vitro* in the Ames mutagenicity assay of *Salmonella typhimurium* strains TA 98, TA 100, TA 1535, TA 1537, and TA 1538 and in the Chinese Hamster Ovary (CHO) test for chromosomal aberrations, or *in vivo* in assays using mouse germinal cell chromosomes, Chinese hamster bone marrow chromosomes, and the *Drosophila* sex-linked recessive lethal trait gene. Positive test results were obtained only in the *in vitro* CHO Sister Chromatid Exchange (clastogenicity) and in the Mouse Lymphoma Cell (mutagenicity) assays, using concentrations of hydrochlorothiazide from 43 to 1300 µg/mL, and in the *Aspergillus nidulans* non-disjunction assay at an unspecified concentration.

Hydrochlorothiazide had no adverse effects on the fertility of mice and rats of either sex in studies wherein these species were exposed, via their diet, to doses of up to 100 and 4 mg/kg, respectively, prior to conception and throughout gestation.
Pregnancy
Pregnancy Categories C (first trimester) and D (second and third trimesters). See WARNINGS, Pregnancy, Lisinopril, Fetal/Neonatal Morbidity and Mortality.
Nursing Mothers
It is not known whether lisinopril is secreted in human milk. However, milk of lactating rats contains radioactivity following administration of ^{14}C lisinopril. In another study, lisino-

pril was present in rat milk at levels similar to plasma levels in the dams. Thiazides do appear in human milk. Because of the potential for serious reactions in nursing infants from hydrochlorothiazide and the unknown effects of lisinopril in infants, a decision should be made whether to discontinue nursing or to discontinue PRINZIDE, taking into account the importance of the drug to the mother.
Pediatric Use
Safety and effectiveness in pediatric patients have not been established.

ADVERSE REACTIONS

PRINZIDE has been evaluated for safety in 930 patients, including 100 patients treated for 50 weeks or more.
In clinical trials with PRINZIDE no adverse experiences peculiar to this combination drug have been observed. Adverse experiences that have occurred have been limited to those that have been previously reported with lisinopril or hydrochlorothiazide.
The most frequent clinical adverse experiences in controlled trials (including open label extensions) with any combination of lisinopril and hydrochlorothiazide were: dizziness (7.5 percent), headache (5.2 percent), cough (3.9 percent), fatigue (3.7 percent) and orthostatic effects (3.2 percent), all of which were more common than in placebo-treated patients. Generally, adverse experiences were mild and transient in nature; but see WARNINGS regarding angioedema and excessive hypotension or syncope. Discontinuation of therapy due to adverse effects was required in 4.4 percent of patients, principally because of dizziness, cough, fatigue and muscle cramps.
Adverse experiences occurring in greater than one percent of patients treated with lisinopril plus hydrochlorothiazide in controlled clinical trials are shown below.
[See table above.]

	Percent of Patients in Controlled Studies	
	Lisinopril-Hydrochlorothiazide (n=930) Incidence (discontinuation)	Placebo (n=207) Incidence
Dizziness	7.5 (0.8)	1.9
Headache	5.2 (0.3)	1.9
Cough	3.9 (0.6)	1.0
Fatigue	3.7 (0.4)	1.0
Orthostatic Effects	3.2 (0.1)	1.0
Diarrhea	2.5 (0.2)	2.4
Nausea	2.2 (0.1)	2.4
Upper Respiratory Infection	2.2 (0.0)	0.0
Muscle Cramps	2.0 (0.4)	0.5
Asthenia	1.8 (0.2)	1.0
Paresthesia	1.5 (0.1)	0.0
Hypotension	1.4 (0.3)	0.5
Vomiting	1.4 (0.1)	0.5
Dyspepsia	1.3 (0.0)	0.0
Rash	1.2 (0.1)	0.5
Impotence	1.2 (0.3)	0.0

Clinical adverse experiences occurring in 0.3 to 1.0 percent of patients in controlled trials included: *Body as a Whole:* Chest pain, abdominal pain, syncope, chest discomfort, fever, trauma, virus infection. *Cardiovascular:* Palpitation, orthostatic hypotension. *Digestive:* Gastrointestinal cramps, dry mouth, constipation, heartburn. *Musculoskeletal:* Back pain, shoulder pain, knee pain, back strain, myalgia, foot pain. *Nervous/Psychiatric:* Decreased libido, vertigo, depression, somnolence. *Respiratory:* Common cold, nasal congestion, influenza, bronchitis, pharyngeal pain, dyspnea, pulmonary congestion, chronic sinusitis, allergic rhinitis, pharyngeal discomfort. *Skin:* Flushing, pruritus, skin inflammation, diaphoresis. *Special Senses:* Blurred vision, tinnitus, otalgia. *Urogenital:* Urinary tract infection.
Angioedema: Angioedema has been reported in patients receiving PRINZIDE, with an incidence higher in black than in non-black patients. Angioedema associated with laryngeal edema may be fatal. If angioedema of the face, extremities, lips, tongue, glottis and/or larynx occurs, treatment with PRINZIDE should be discontinued and appropriate therapy instituted immediately. (See WARNINGS.)
Hypotension: In clinical trials, adverse effects relating to hypotension occurred as follows: hypotension (1.4), orthostatic hypotension (0.5), other orthostatic effects (3.2). In addition syncope occurred in 0.8 percent of patients. (See WARNINGS.)
Cough: See PRECAUTIONS, *Cough.*
Clinical Laboratory Test Findings
Serum Electrolytes: See PRECAUTIONS.
Creatinine, Blood Urea Nitrogen: Minor reversible increases in blood urea nitrogen and serum creatinine were observed in patients with essential hypertension treated with PRINZIDE. More marked increases have also been reported and were more likely to occur in patients with renal artery stenosis. (See PRECAUTIONS.)

Serum Uric Acid, Glucose, Magnesium, Cholesterol, Triglycerides and Calcium: See PRECAUTIONS.
Hemoglobin and Hematocrit: Small decreases in hemoglobin and hematocrit (mean decreases of approximately 0.5 g percent and 1.5 vol percent, respectively) occurred frequently in hypertensive patients treated with PRINZIDE but were rarely of clinical importance unless another cause of anemia coexisted. In clinical trials, 0.4 percent of patients discontinued therapy due to anemia.
Liver Function Tests: Rarely, elevations of liver enzymes and/or serum bilirubin have occurred (see WARNINGS, *Hepatic Failure*).

Other adverse reactions that have been reported with the individual components are listed below:
Lisinopril: In clinical trials adverse reactions which occurred with lisinopril were also seen with PRINZIDE. In addition, and since lisinopril has been marketed, the following adverse reactions have been reported with lisinopril and should be considered potential adverse reactions for PRINZIDE: *Body as a Whole:* Anaphylactoid reactions (see WARNINGS, *Anaphylactoid and Possibly Related Reactions),* malaise, edema, facial edema, pain, pelvic pain, flank pain, chills; *Cardiovascular:* Cardiac arrest, myocardial infarction or cerebrovascular accident, possibly secondary to excessive hypotension in high risk patients (see WARNINGS, *Hypotension),* pulmonary embolism and infarction, worsening of heart failure, arrhythmias (including tachycardia, ventricular tachycardia, atrial tachycardia, atrial fibrillation, bradycardia, and premature ventricular contractions), angina pectoris, transient ischemic attacks, paroxysmal nocturnal dyspnea, decreased blood pressure, peripheral edema, vasculitis; *Digestive:* Pancreatitis, hepatitis (hepatocellular or cholestatic jaundice) (see WARNINGS, *Hepatic Failure*), gastritis, anorexia, flatulence, increased salivation; *Endocrine:* Diabetes mellitus; *Hematologic:* Rare cases of neutropenia, thrombocytopenia, and bone marrow depression have been reported. Hemolytic anemia has been reported; a causal relationship to lisinopril cannot be excluded; *Metabolic:* Gout, weight loss, dehydration, fluid overload, weight gain; *Musculoskeletal:* Arthritis, arthralgia, neck pain, hip pain, joint pain, leg pain, arm pain, lumbago; *Nervous System/Psychiatric:* Ataxia, memory impairment, tremor, insomnia, stroke, nervousness, confusion, peripheral neuropathy (e.g., paresthesia, dysesthesia), spasm, hypersomnia, irritability; *Respiratory:* Malignant lung neoplasms, hemoptysis, pulmonary edema, pulmonary infiltrates, bronchospasm, asthma, pleural effusion, pneumonia, wheezing, orthopnea, painful respiration, epistaxis, laryngitis, sinusitis, pharyngitis, rhinitis, rhinorrhea, chest sound abnormalities; *Skin:* Urticaria, alopecia, herpes zoster, photosensitivity, skin lesions, skin infections, pemphigus, erythema. Other severe skin reactions (including toxic epidermal necrolysis and Stevens-Johnson syndrome) have been reported rarely; causal relationship has not been established; *Speical Senses:* Visual loss, diplopia, photophobia; *Urogenital:* Acute renal failure, oliguria, anuria, uremia, progressive azotemia, renal dysfunction (see PRECAUTIONS and DOSAGE AND ADMINISTRATION), pyelonephritis, dysuria, breast pain.
Miscellaneous: A symptom complex has been reported which may include a positive ANA, an elevated erythrocyte sedimentation rate, arthralgia/arthritis, myalgia, fever, vasculitis, leukocytosis, eosinophilia, photosensitivity, rash, and other dermatological manifestations.

Continued on next page

Information on the Merck & Co., Inc. products listed on these pages is the full prescribing information from product circulars in use September 30, 1996.

Merck & Co.—Cont.

Fetal/Neonatal Morbidity and Mortality: See WARNINGS, *Pregnancy, Lisinopril, Fetal/Neonatal Morbidity and Mortality.*
Hydrochlorothiazide—Body as a Whole: Weakness; *Digestive:* Anorexia, gastric irritation, cramping, jaundice (intrahepatic cholestatic jaundice), pancreatitis, sialadenitis, constipation; *Hematologic:* Leukopenia, agranulocytosis, thrombocytopenia, aplastic anemia, hemolytic anemia; *Musculoskeletal:* Muscle spasm; *Nervous System/Psychiatric:* Restlessness; *Renal:* Renal failure, renal dysfunction, interstitial nephritis (see WARNINGS); *Skin:* Erythema multiforme including Stevens-Johnson syndrome, exfoliative dermatitis including toxic epidermal necrolysis, alopecia; *Special Senses:* Xanthopsia; *Hypersensitivity:* Purpura, photosensitivity, urticaria, necrotizing angiitis (vasculitis and cutaneous vasculitis), respiratory distress including pneumonitis and pulmonary edema, anaphylactic reactions.

OVERDOSAGE

No specific information is available on the treatment of overdosage with PRINZIDE. Treatment is symptomatic and supportive. Therapy with PRINZIDE should be discontinued and the patient observed closely. Suggested measures include induction of emesis and/or gastric lavage, and correction of dehydration, electrolyte imbalance and hypotension by established procedures.
Lisinopril
The oral LD_{50} of lisinopril is greater than 20 g/kg in mice and rats. The most likely manifestation of overdosage would be hypotension, for which the usual treatment would be intravenous infusion of normal saline solution.
Lisinopril can be removed by hemodialysis.
Hydrochlorothiazide
The oral LD_{50} of hydrochlorothiazide is greater than 10.0 g/kg in both mice and rats. The most common signs and symptoms observed are those caused by electrolyte depletion (hypokalemia, hypochloremia, hyponatremia) and dehydration resulting from excessive diuresis. If digitalis has also been administered, hypokalemia may accentuate cardiac arrhythmias.

DOSAGE AND ADMINISTRATION

Lisinopril is an effective treatment of hypertension in once-daily doses of 10–80 mg, while hydrochlorothiazide is effective in doses of 25–100 mg. In clinical trials of lisinopril/hydrochlorothiazide combination therapy using lisinopril doses of 10–80 mg and hydrochlorothiazide doses of 6.25–50 mg, the antihypertensive response rates generally increased with increasing dose of either component.
The side effects (see WARNINGS) of lisinopril are generally rare and apparently independent of dose; those of hydrochlorothiazide are a mixture of dose-dependent phenomena (primarily hypokalemia) and dose-independent phenomena (e.g., pancreatitis), the former much more common than the latter. Therapy with any combination of lisinopril and hydrochlorothiazide will be associated with both sets of dose-independent side effects, but addition of lisinopril in clinical trials blunted the hypokalemia normally seen with diuretics.
To minimize dose-independent side effects, it is usually appropriate to begin combination therapy only after a patient has failed to achieve the desired effect with monotherapy.
Dose Titration Guided by Clinical Effect
A patient whose blood pressure is not adequately controlled with either lisinopril or hydrochlorothiazide monotherapy may be switched to PRINZIDE 10/12.5 or PRINZIDE 20/12.5. Further increases of either or both components could depend on clinical response. The hydrochlorothiazide dose should generally not be increased until 2–3 weeks have elapsed. Patients whose blood pressures are adequately controlled with 25 mg of daily hydrochlorothiazide, but who experience significant potassium loss with this regimen, may achieve similar or greater blood pressure control with less potassium loss if they are switched to PRINZIDE 10/12.5.
Replacement Therapy
The combination may be substituted for the titrated individual components.
Use in Renal Impairment
The usual regimens of therapy with PRINZIDE need not be adjusted as long as the patient's creatinine clearance is >30 mL /min/1.73 m^2 (serum creatinine approximately ≤ 3 mg/dL or 265 μmol/L. In patients with more severe renal impairment, loop diuretics are preferred to thiazides, so PRINZIDE is not recommended (see WARNINGS, *Anaphylactoid reactions during membrane exposure*).
Use in Elderly In general, blood pressure response and adverse experiences were similar in younger and older patients given PRINZIDE. However, in a multiple dose pharmacokinetic study in elderly versus young patients using the lisinopril/hydrochlorothiazide combination, area under the plasma concentration time curve (AUC) increased approximately 120% for lisinopril and approximately 80% for hydrochlorothiazide in older patients. Therefore, dosage adjustments in elderly patients should be made with particular caution.

HOW SUPPLIED

No. 3616—Tablets PRINZIDE 10-12.5 are blue hexagon-shaped tablets, coded MSD 145 on one side and PRINZIDE on the other. Each tablet contains 10 mg of lisinopril and 12.5 mg of hydrochlorothiazide. They are supplied as follows:
NDC 0006-0145-31 unit of use bottles of 30.
NDC 0006-0145-58 unit of use bottles of 100.
Shown in Product Identification Guide, page 325
No. 3594—Tablets PRINZIDE 20-12.5 are yellow, round, fluted-edge tablets, coded MSD 140 on one side and PRINZIDE on the other. Each tablet contains 20 mg of lisinopril and 12.5 mg of hydrochlorothiazide. They are supplied as follows:
NDC 0006-0140-31 unit of use bottles of 30
NDC 0006-0140-58 unit of use bottles of 100.
Shown in Product Identification Guide, page 325
No. 3595—Tablets PRINZIDE 20-25 are peach, round, fluted-edge tablets, coded MSD 142 on one side and PRINZIDE on the other. Each tablet contains 20 mg of lisinopril and 25 mg of hydrochlorothiazide. They are supplied as follows:
NDC 0006-0142-31 unit of use bottles of 30
NDC 0006-0142-58 unit of use bottles of 100.
Shown in Product Identification Guide, page 325
Storage
Store at controlled room temperature. 15–30°C (59–86°F).
Protect from excessive light and humidity.
Dispense in a well-closed container, if product package is subdivided.

7836327 Issued July 1995

PROSCAR® Tablets
(Finasteride) ℞

DESCRIPTION

PROSCAR* (finasteride), a synthetic 4-azasteroid compound, is a specific inhibitor of steroid 5α-reductase, an intracellular enzyme that converts testosterone into the potent androgen 5α-dihydrotestosterone (DHT).
Finasteride is 4-azaandrost-1-ene-17-carboxamide, *N*-(1,1-dimethylethyl)-3-oxo-,(5α, 17β)-. The empirical formula of finasteride is $C_{23}H_{36}N_2O_2$ and its molecular weight is 372.55. Its structural formula is:

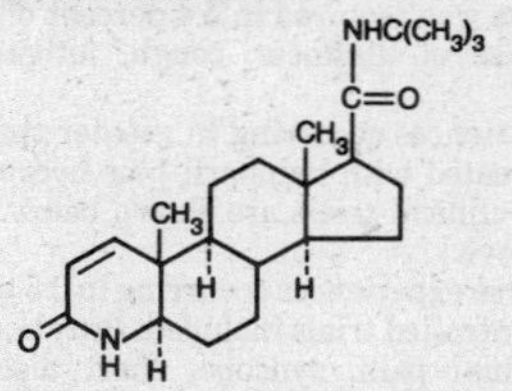

Finasteride is a white crystalline powder with a melting point near 250°C. It is freely soluble in chloroform and in lower alcohol solvents, but is practically insoluble in water.
PROSCAR (finasteride) tablets for oral administration are film-coated tablets that contain 5 mg of finasteride and the following inactive ingredients: docusate sodium, FD&C Blue 2 aluminum lake, hydrous lactose, hydroxypropyl cellulose LF, hydroxypropylmethyl cellulose, magnesium stearate, microcrystalline cellulose, pregelatinized starch, purified water, sodium starch glycolate, talc, titanium dioxide and yellow iron oxide.

* Registered trademark of MERCK & CO., INC.

CLINICAL PHARMACOLOGY

Progressive enlargement of the prostate gland is often associated with urinary symptoms and a decrease in urine flow, although a precise correlation between increased gland size and symptoms has not been demonstrated. Benign prostatic hyperplasia (BPH) produces symptoms in the majority of men over the age of 50 and its prevalence increases with age.
The development of the prostate gland is dependent on the potent androgen, 5α-dihydrotestosterone (DHT). The enzyme 5α-reductase metabolizes testosterone to DHT in the prostate gland, liver and skin. DHT induces androgenic effects by binding to androgen receptors in the cell nuclei of these organs.
Finasteride is a competitive and specific inhibitor of 5α-reductase with which it slowly forms a stable enzyme complex. Turnover from this complex is extremely slow ($t_{1/2}$ ~30 days). This has been demonstrated both *in vivo* and *in vitro*. Finasteride has no affinity for the androgen receptor. In man, the 5α-reduced steroid metabolites in blood and urine are decreased after administration of finasteride.
In man, a single 5-mg oral dose of PROSCAR produces a rapid reduction in serum DHT concentration, with the maximum effect observed 8 hours after the first dose. The suppression of DHT is maintained throughout the 24-hour dosing interval and with continued treatment. Daily dosing of PROSCAR at 5 mg/day for up to 24 months has been shown to reduce the serum DHT concentration by approximately 70%. The median circulating level of testosterone increased by 10% but remained within the physiologic range.
Adult males with genetically inherited 5α-reductase deficiency also have decreased levels of DHT. Except for the associated urogenital defects present at birth, no other clinical abnormalities related to 5α-reductase deficiency have been observed in these individuals. These individuals have a small prostate gland throughout life and do not develop BPH.
In patients with BPH treated with finasteride (1–100 mg/day) for 7–10 days prior to prostatectomy, an approximate 80% lower DHT content was measured in prostatic tissue removed at surgery, compared to placebo; testosterone tissue concentration was increased up to 10 times over pretreatment levels, relative to placebo. Intraprostatic content of prostate-specific antigen (PSA) was also decreased.
In healthy male volunteers treated with PROSCAR for 14 days, discontinuation of therapy resulted in a return of DHT levels to pretreatment levels in approximately 2 weeks. In patients treated for three months, prostate volume returned to close to baseline value after approximately three months of discontinuation of therapy.
In patients with BPH, PROSCAR had no effect on circulating levels of cortisol, estradiol, prolactin, thyroid-stimulating hormone, or thyroxine. Nor did it affect the plasma lipid profile (i.e. total cholesterol, low density lipoproteins, high density lipoproteins and triglycerides) of 56 patients receiving PROSCAR for 12 weeks. The effects of long-term administration of PROSCAR on the plasma lipid profile are unknown. Increases of about 10% were observed in luteinizing hormone (LH), follicle-stimulating hormone (FSH) and testosterone levels in patients receiving PROSCAR, but levels remained within the normal range. In healthy volunteers, treatment with PROSCAR did not alter the response of LH and FSH to gonadotropin-releasing hormone, indicating that the hypothalamic-pituitary-testicular axis was not affected.
Treatment with PROSCAR for 12 weeks to evaluate semen parameters in healthy male volunteers revealed no effects on total sperm per ejaculate, sperm motility or morphology. A 0.5 mL median decrease in ejaculate volume was observed and was reversible upon discontinuation of drug.
Pharmacokinetics
Following an oral dose of ^{14}C-finasteride in man, a mean of 39% (range, 32–46%) of the dose was excreted in the urine in the form of metabolites; 57% (range, 51–64%) was excreted in the feces. The major compound isolated from urine was the monocarboxylic acid metabolite; virtually no unchanged drug was recovered. The t-butyl side chain monohydroxylated metabolite has been isolated from plasma. These metabolites possess no more than 20% of the 5α-reductase inhibitory activity of finasteride.
In a study in 15 healthy male subjects, the mean bioavailability of a 5-mg PROSCAR tablet was 63% (range, 34–108%), based on the ratio of AUC relative to a 5-mg intravenous dose infused over 60 minutes. Maximum finasteride plasma concentration averaged 37 ng/mL (range, 27–49 ng/mL) and was reached 1 to 2 hours postdose. The mean plasma half-life of elimination was 6 hours (range, 3–16 hours). Following the intravenous infusion, mean plasma clearance was 165 mL/min (range, 70–279 mL/min) and mean steady-state volume of distribution was 76 liters (range, 44–96 liters). In a separate study, the bioavailability of finasteride was not affected by food.
Approximately 90% of circulating finasteride is bound to plasma proteins. Finasteride has been found to cross the blood-brain barrier.
There is a slow accumulation phase for finasteride after multiple dosing. After dosing with 5 mg/day of finasteride for 17 days, plasma concentrations of finasteride were 47% and 54% higher than after the first dose in men 45–60 years old (n=12) and ≥ 70 years old (n=12), respectively. Mean trough concentrations after 17 days of dosing were 6.2 ng/mL (range, 2.4–9.8 ng/mL) and 8.1 ng/mL (range, 1.8–19.7 ng/mL), respectively in the two age groups. Although steady state was not reached in this study, mean trough plasma concentration in another study in patients with BPH (mean age, 65 years) receiving 5 mg/day was 9.4 ng/mL (range, 7.1–13.3 ng/mL; n=22) after over a year of dosing.
The elimination rate of finasteride is decreased in the elderly, but no dosage adjustment is necessary. The mean terminal half-life of finasteride in subjects ≥ 70 years of age was approximately 8 hours (range, 6–15 hours) compared to 6 hours (range, 4–12 hours) in subjects 45–60 years of age. As a result, mean AUC (0–24 hr) after 17 days of dosing was 15% higher in subjects ≥ 70 years of age (p=0.02).

FIGURE 1
Prostate Volume

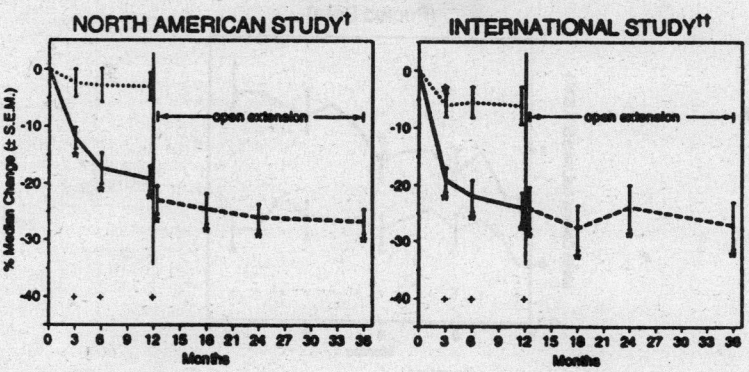

NORTH AMERICAN STUDY†   INTERNATIONAL STUDY††

*   p < 0.05 vs Baseline
+   p < 0.001 vs Placebo

	North America		International	
	Baseline			Baseline
	n	(mL)	n	(mL)
— PROSCAR 5 mg—Patients treated during 12-month controlled Phase III studies	270	52.0	218	45.1
... Placebo—Patients treated during 12-month controlled Phase III studies	281	50.9	222	41.6
-- PROSCAR 5 mg—Patients continued beyond 12 months (open extension)	123	52.5	84	45.9

†   Prostate volume measured by magnetic resonance imaging
††   Prostate volume measured by ultrasound

FIGURE 2
Maximum Urinary Flow Rate†

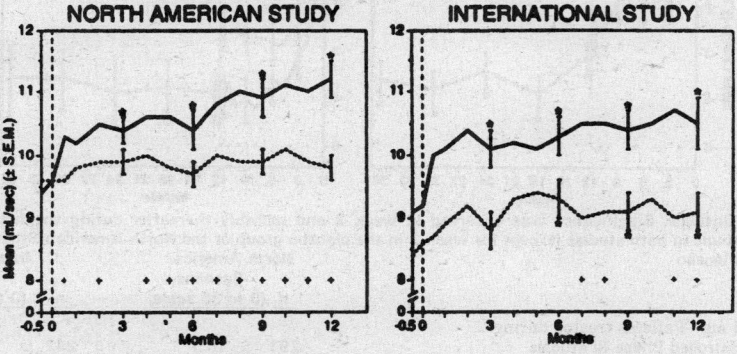

NORTH AMERICAN STUDY   INTERNATIONAL STUDY

*   p < 0.05 vs Baseline
+   p < 0.05 vs Placebo

	North America		International	
	Baseline			Baseline
	n	(mL/sec)	n	(mL/sec)
— PROSCAR 5 mg	270	9.6	182	9.2
... Placebo	281	9.6	186	8.6

†   Maximum urinary flow rates (voided volumes ≥ 150 mL) were measured with a non-invasive urinary flow meter.
NOTE: Area of the graph to the left of time 0 is a two-week placebo run-in period.

No dosage adjustment is necessary in patients with renal insufficiency. In patients with chronic renal impairment, with creatinine clearances ranging from 9.0 to 55 mL/min, area under the curve, maximum plasma concentration, half-life, and protein binding after a single dose of ^{14}C-finasteride were similar to values obtained in healthy volunteers. Urinary excretion of metabolites was decreased in patients with renal impairment. This decrease was associated with an increase in fecal excretion of metabolites. Plasma concentrations of metabolites were significantly higher in patients with renal impairment (based on a 60% increase in total radioactivity AUC). However, finasteride has been well tolerated in BPH patients with normal renal function receiving up to 80 mg/day for 12 weeks where exposure of these patients to metabolites would presumably be much greater.

In 16 subjects receiving PROSCAR 5 mg/day, finasteride concentrations in semen ranged from undetectable (<1 ng/mL) to 21 ng/mL. Based on a 5 mL ejaculate volume, the amount of finasteride in ejaculate was estimated to be less than 1/50 of the dose of finasteride (5 micrograms) that had no effect on circulating DHT levels in adults.

Clinical Studies

Patients with BPH were treated with either PROSCAR 5 mg/day or placebo in North American and international multicenter, double-blind, 12-month studies and their 24-month open extensions for a total of 36 months. Of 543 patients originally randomized to receive PROSCAR 5 mg/day, 297 completed 36 months and were available for analysis. The efficacy parameters were regression of the enlarged prostate, improvement in maximum urinary flow rate, and improvement in total and obstructive symptoms as measured by a decrease in symptom scores.

By week 2, a reduction of serum DHT was noted and was accompanied by regression of the enlarged prostate at the first evaluation at 3 months. These reductions were statistically significant when compared to both baseline and placebo and were maintained through month 36 (Figure 1).

In both studies the groups treated with PROSCAR demonstrated statistically significant improvement compared to baseline in maximum urinary flow rate (Table 1) and total symptom score (Figure 4) within 2 weeks, which was maintained in uncontrolled studies through month 36. Moreover, when compared to placebo, statistically significant increases in maximum urinary flow rates were observed in both studies. In the North American study, these were observed by month 4 and maintained through month 12, and in the international study were observed at months 7, 8, 11, and 12. (See Figures 2 and 3 and Table 1.) Most patients treated with PROSCAR experienced at least a 10% increase in urinary flow rate. (See INDICATIONS AND USAGE.)

[See Figures 1 and 2 above.]

[See table 1 on top of next column.]

TABLE 1
Mean Increase in Maximum Urinary Flow Rate (mL/sec)† from Baseline

	North American Study		International Study	
	PROSCAR 5 mg (n=297)	Placebo (n=300)	PROSCAR 5 mg (n=246)	Placebo (n=255)
Baseline flow rate (mL/sec)	9.6	9.6	9.2	8.6
Week 2	0.5*	−0.2	0.6	0.2
Month 1	0.5	0.2	0.7	0.3
Month 2	0.9*	0.3	1.1	0.6
Month 3	0.8	0.3	0.8	0.2
Month 4	1.0*	0.4	1.0	0.6
Month 5	1.0**	0.2	0.9	0.8
Month 6	0.8*	0.1	1.1	0.7
Month 7	1.2**	0.4	1.3*	0.4
Month 8	1.4***	0.3	1.3*	0.5
Month 9	1.3**	0.3	1.2	0.4
Month 10	1.5***	0.5	1.3	0.7
Month 11	1.4***	0.3	1.5**	0.4
Month 12	1.6***	0.2	1.3*	0.4

†   Maximum urinary flow rates (voided volumes ≥ 150 mL) were measured with a non-invasive urinary flow meter.
*,**,*** p < 0.05, p < 0.01, p < 0.001 vs placebo, respectively
[See Figure 3 on next page.]

Obstructive and total symptom scores were calculated based on patient responses to a validated questionnaire. The obstructive symptoms evaluated were hesitancy, feeling of incomplete bladder emptying, interruption of urinary stream, impairment of size and force of urinary stream and terminal urinary dribbling. The total symptom score also included straining to start urinary flow, dysuria, frequency of clothes wetting and urgency to urinate. The scale used to evaluate symptoms ranged from 0 (absence of all symptoms) to 36 (worst response for all symptoms).

The mean total symptom scores of patients in the North American and international studies decreased from baseline starting at week 2 of treatment with either PROSCAR or placebo. Statistical significance compared to placebo (p < 0.05) was reached starting at month 7 in the international study and at month 10 in the North American study (Figure 4). Similar results were observed with the obstructive symptom scores. Most patients treated with PROSCAR experienced at least a 30% improvement in symptoms. (See INDICATIONS AND USAGE.)

[See Figure 4 on next page.]

Blinded global assessments of overall urinary function and symptoms were performed. Greater improvement in patients treated with PROSCAR as compared to placebo was demonstrated by both the investigator's assessment (N.Am. and Int'l, p ≤ 0.01) and the patient's own assessment (N.Am.) p ≤ 0.01; Int'l, p ≤ 0.1).

In both of these 12-month studies, patients treated with PROSCAR 5 mg had progressively decreasing prostate volumes, increasing maximum urinary flow rates and improvement of symptoms associated with BPH, suggesting an arrest in the disease process. These improvements were maintained through the long-term open extensions for up to 36 months.[1]

In addition, regression of the enlarged prostate gland and a decrease in PSA levels were maintained in approximately 50 patients who were treated with PROSCAR for 48 months.

Additional Clinical Trials

Urodynamic effects of finasteride in the treatment of bladder outlet obstruction due to BPH were assessed by invasive techniques in a 24-week, double-blind, placebo-controlled study of 36 patients with moderate to severe symptoms of urinary obstruction and a maximum flow rate of less than 15 cc/sec. Relief of obstruction, as evidenced by significant improvement in detrusor pressure and increased mean flow rate, was demonstrated in patients treated with 5 mg PROSCAR compared to placebo.[2]

The effect of finasteride on the volume of the peripheral and periurethral zones of the prostate in 20 men with BPH was evaluated by magnetic resonance imaging in a one-year, double-blind, placebo-controlled study. Patients treated with PROSCAR, but not those treated with placebo, experienced a significant decrease [11.5 ± 3.2 cc (SE)] in total gland size,

Continued on next page

Information on the Merck & Co., Inc. products listed on these pages is the full prescribing information from product circulars in use September 30, 1996.

Merck & Co.—Cont.

largely accounted for by a reduction [6.2 ± 3 cc] in the size of the periurethral zone.

[1] Stoner, E.; Members of the Finasteride Study Group: Three-year safety and efficacy data on the use of finasteride in the treatment of benign prostatic hyperplasia, Urology. 43 (3): 284–294, March 1994.

[2] Tammela, T.L.J.; Kontturi, M.J.: Urodynamic effects of finasteride in the treatment of bladder outlet obstruction due to benign prostatic hyperplasia, J. Urology. 149 (2): 342–344, February 1993.

INDICATIONS AND USAGE

PROSCAR is indicated for the treatment of symptomatic benign prostatic hyperplasia (BPH). There is a rapid regression of the enlarged prostate gland in most treated patients. Approximately 60% of patients experience an increase in urinary flow (of greater than 10%) and improvement in symptoms of BPH (of greater than 30%) when treated with PROSCAR. (See CLINICAL PHARMACOLOGY.)

The long-term effects of PROSCAR on the incidence of surgery, acute urinary obstruction or other complications of BPH are yet to be determined.

Although some patients may respond sooner, a minimum of 6 months treatment may be necessary to determine whether an individual will respond to PROSCAR. It is not possible to identify prospectively those patients who will respond.

Prior to initiating therapy with PROSCAR, appropriate evaluation should be performed to identify other conditions, such as infection, prostate cancer, stricture disease, hypotonic bladder or other neurogenic disorders, that might mimic BPH.

CONTRAINDICATIONS

PROSCAR is contraindicated in the following:
Hypersensitivity to any component of this medication.
Pregnancy. Finasteride is contraindicated in women who are or may become pregnant. Because of the ability of 5α-reductase inhibitors to inhibit the conversion of testosterone to DHT, finasteride may cause abnormalities of the external genitalia of a male fetus of a pregnant woman who receives finasteride. If this drug is used during pregnancy, or if pregnancy occurs while taking this drug, the pregnant woman should be apprised of the potential hazard to the male fetus. (See also WARNINGS, *Exposure of Women—Risk to Male Fetus* and PRECAUTIONS, *Information for Patients* and *Pregnancy*.) In female rats, low doses of finasteride administered during pregnancy have produced abnormalities of the external genitalia in male offspring.

WARNINGS

PROSCAR is not indicated for use in pediatric patients (see PRECAUTIONS, *Pediatric Use*) or women (see also CLINICAL PHARMACOLOGY, *Pharmacokinetics*; WARNINGS, *Exposure of Women—Risk to Male Fetus*; PRECAUTIONS, *Information for Patients* and *Pregnancy*: and HOW SUPPLIED).

Exposure of Women—Risk to Male Fetus
It is not known whether the amount of finasteride that could potentially be absorbed by a pregnant woman through either direct contact with crushed PROSCAR tablets or from the semen of a patient taking PROSCAR can adversely affect a developing male fetus (see CLINICAL PHARMACOLOGY, *Pharmacokinetics*; CONTRAINDICATIONS; PRECAUTIONS, *Information for Patients* and *Pregnancy*; and HOW SUPPLIED). Therefore, because of the potential risk to a male fetus, a woman who is pregnant or who may become pregnant should not handle crushed PROSCAR tablets; in addition, when the patient's sexual partner is or may become pregnant, the patient should either avoid exposure of his partner to semen or he should discontinue PROSCAR.

PRECAUTIONS

General
Digital rectal examinations, as well as other evaluations for prostate cancer, should be performed on patients with BPH prior to initiating therapy with PROSCAR and periodically thereafter. Although currently not indicated for this purpose, serum PSA is being increasingly used as one of the components of the screening process to detect prostate cancer.[3] Generally, a baseline PSA > 10 ng/mL (Hybritech) prompts further evaluation and consideration of biopsy; for PSA levels between 4 and 10 ng/mL, further evaluation is generally considered advisable. The physician should be aware that a baseline PSA < 4 ng/mL does not exclude the diagnosis of prostate cancer.

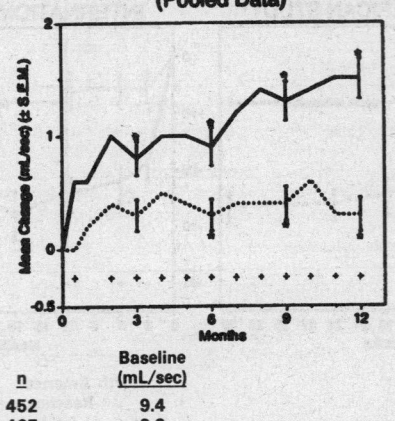

FIGURE 3
Mean Increase in Maximum Urinary Flow Rate (mL/sec)[†]
(Pooled Data)

	n	Baseline (mL/sec)
— PROSCAR 5 mg	452	9.4
... Placebo	467	9.2

* $p < 0.05$ vs Baseline
+ $p < 0.05$ vs Placebo
† Maximum urinary flow rates (voided volumes ≥ 150 mL) were measured with a non-invasive urinary flow meter.

FIGURE 4
Total Symptom Score

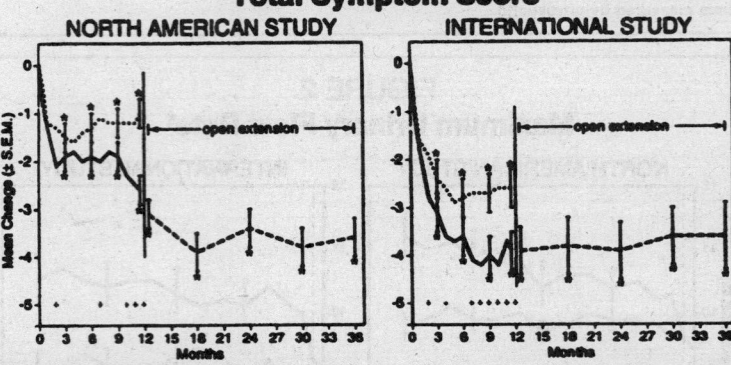

NORTH AMERICAN STUDY   INTERNATIONAL STUDY

* $p < 0.05$ vs Baseline. Significance was observed at week 2 and monthly thereafter during the first year for both treatment groups in both studies (except for week 2 in the placebo group of the North American Study).
+ $p < 0.05$ vs Placebo

	North America		International	
	n	Baseline (0 to 36 scale)	n	Baseline (0 to 36 scale)
— PROSCAR 5 mg—Patients treated during 12-month controlled Phase III studies	291	10.1	242	10.6
... Placebo—Patients treated during 12-month controlled Phase III studies	299	9.8	254	10.2
-- PROSCAR 5 mg—Patients continued beyond 12 months (open extension)	192	9.8	105	9.0

PROSCAR causes a decrease in serum PSA levels in patients with BPH even in the presence of prostate cancer (see *Drug/Laboratory Test Interactions*). This reduction of PSA levels should be considered when evaluating PSA laboratory data and does not suggest a beneficial effect of PROSCAR on prostate cancer. In controlled clinical trials PROSCAR did not appear to alter the rate of prostate cancer detection.

Any sustained increases in PSA levels while on PROSCAR should be carefully evaluated, including consideration of non-compliance to therapy with PROSCAR (see *Drug/Laboratory Test Interactions*).

Since not all patients demonstrate a response to PROSCAR, patients with a large residual urinary volume and/or severely diminished urinary flow should be carefully monitored for obstructive uropathy. These patients may not be candidates for this therapy.

Caution should be used in the administration of PROSCAR in those patients with liver function abnormalities, as finasteride is metabolized extensively in the liver.

[3] Catalona, W.J.; Smith, D.S.; Ratliff, T.I.; Dodds, K.M.; Coplen, M.D.; Yuan, J.J.J.; Petros, J.A.; Andriole, G.L.: Measurement of prostate-specific antigen in serum as a screening test for prostate cancer, N.Eng.J.Med. 324(17): 1156–1161, April 25, 1991.

Information for Patients
Crushed PROSCAR tablets should not be handled by a woman who is pregnant or who may become pregnant because of the potential for absorption of finasteride and the subsequent potential risk to the male fetus. Similarly, when the patient's sexual partner is or may become pregnant, the patient should either avoid exposure of his partner to semen or he should discontinue PROSCAR (see CLINICAL PHARMACOLOGY, *Pharmacokinetics*; CONTRAINDICATIONS; WARNINGS, *Exposure of Women—Risk to Male Fetus*; PRECAUTIONS, *Pregnancy*; and HOW SUPPLIED).

Physicians should inform patients that the volume of ejaculate may be decreased in some patients during treatment with PROSCAR. This decrease does not appear to interfere with normal sexual function. However, impotence and decreased libido may occur in patients treated with PROSCAR (see ADVERSE REACTIONS, *Twelve-Month Controlled Clinical Trials*).

Physicians should instruct their patients to read the patient package insert before starting therapy with PROSCAR and to reread it each time the prescription is renewed so that they are aware of current information for patients regarding PROSCAR.

Drug/Laboratory Test Interactions
Serum PSA concentration is correlated with patient age and prostatic volume, and prostatic volume is correlated with patient age.[4] When PSA laboratory determinations are evaluated, consideration should be given to the fact that PSA levels generally decrease in patients treated with PROSCAR (see PRECAUTIONS, *General*). In most patients, a rapid decrease in PSA is seen within the first months of therapy, after which time PSA levels stabilize to a new baseline. The post-treatment baseline approximates half of the pre-treatment value. This decrease is predictable over the entire range of PSA values, although it may vary in individual patients. Therefore, in typical patients treated with PROSCAR for six months or more, PSA values should be doubled for comparison to normal ranges in untreated men. There is

considerable overlap in PSA levels among men with and without prostate cancer. Therefore, in men with BPH, PSA values within the normal reference range do not rule out prostate cancer, regardless of finasteride treatment.[5,6]

Based on a comparison of PSA levels between men diagnosed with prostate cancer while taking PROSCAR (n=10) and men not diagnosed with prostate cancer while taking PROSCAR, any ability of PSA to distinguish between BPH and cancer was not adversely affected by treatment with PROSCAR.[6]

---

[4] Oesterling, J.E.; Jacobsen, S.J.; Chute, C.G.; Guess, H.A.; Girman, C.J.; Panser, L.A.; Lieber, M.M.; Serum prostate-specific antigen in a community-based population of healthy men, JAMA. 270(7): 860-864, August 18, 1993.
[5] Guess, H.A.; et al.: Effect of finasteride on serum PSA concentration in men with benign prostatic hyperplasia. Urol. Clin. N. Amer. 20(4): 627-636, November 1993.
[6] Guess, H.A.; Heyse, J.F.; Gormley, G.J.: The effect of finasteride on prostate-specific antigen in men with benign prostatic hyperplasia, Prostate. 22(1): 31-37, 1993.

Drug Interactions
Antipyrine: Antipyrine is used as a model for drugs that are metabolized by the same isoenzymatic cytochrome P450 system. In 12 subjects receiving PROSCAR 10 mg/day for 28 days, PROSCAR had no effect on the pharmacokinetic parameters of antipyrine or its metabolites.
Propranolol: In 19 normal volunteers receiving PROSCAR 5 mg/day for 10 days, PROSCAR did not affect the beta-adrenergic blocking activity or plasma concentrations of propranolol enantiomers after a single dose of propranolol.
Digoxin: In 17 normal volunteers receivng PROSCAR 5 mg/day for 10 days, concomitant administration of multiple doses of PROSCAR and a single dose of digoxin resulted in no effect on plasma concentrations of digoxin and its immunoreactive metabolites.
Theophylline: In 12 normal volunteers receiving PROSCAR 5 mg/day for 8 days, PROSCAR significantly increased theophylline clearance by 7% and decreased its half-life by 10% after intravenous administration of aminophylline. These changes were not clinically significant.
Warfarin: In 12 patients chronically treated with warfarin, the prothrombin times and plasma concentrations of warfarin enantiomers were not altered after treatment with PROSCAR 5 mg/day for 14 days.
Other Concomitant Therapy: Although specific interaction studies were not performed, PROSCAR was concomitantly used in clinical studies with α-blockers, angiotensin-converting enzyme (ACE) inhibitors, analgesics, anti-convulsants, beta-adrenergic blocking agents, diuretics, calcium channel blockers, cardiac nitrates, HMG-CoA reductase inhibitors, nonsteroidal anti-inflammatory drugs (NSAIDs), benzodiazepines, H$_2$ antagonists and quinolone anti-infectives without evidence of clinically significant advers interactions.
Carcinogenesis, Mutagenesis, Impairment of Fertility
No evidence of a tumorigenic effect was observed in a 24-month study in Sprague-Dawley rats receiving doses of finasteride up to 160 mg/kg/day in males and 320 mg/kg/day in females. These doses produced respective systemic exposure in rats of 111 and 274 times those observed in man receiving the recommended human dose of 5 mg/day. All exposure calculations were based on calculated AUC(0–24hr) for animals and mean AUC(0–24hr) for man (0.4 μg·hr/mL).
In a 19-month carcinogenicity study in CD-1 mice, a statistically significant (p ≤ 0.05) increase in the incidence of testicular Leydig cell adenomas was observed at a dose of 250 mg/kg/day (228 times the human exposure). In mice at a dose of 25 mg/kg/day (23 times the human exposure, estimated) and in rats at a dose of ≥ 40 mg/kg/day (39 times the human exposure) an increase in the incidence of Leydig cell hyperplasia was observed. A positive correlation between the proliferative changes in the Leydig cells and an increase in serum LH levels (2–3 fold above control) has been demonstrated in both rodent species treated with high doses of finasteride. No drug-related Leydig cell changes were seen in either rats or dogs treated with finasteride for 1 year at doses of 20 mg/kg/day and 45 mg/kg/day (30 and 350 times, respectively, the human exposure) or in mice treated for 19 months at a dose of 2.5 mg/kg/day (2.3 times the human exposure, estimated).
No evidence of mutagenicity was observed in an *in vitro* bacterial mutagenesis assay, a mammalian cell mutagenesis assay, or in an *in vitro* alkaline elution assay. In an *in vitro* chromosome aberration assay, when Chinese hamster ovary cells were treated with high concentrations (450–550 μmol) of finasteride, there was a slight increase in chromosome aberrations. These concentrations correspond to 4000–5000 times the peak plasma levels in man given a total dose of 5 mg. Further, the concentrations (450–550 μmol) used in *in vitro* studies are not achievable in a biological system. In an *in vivo* chromosome aberration assay in mice, no treatment-related increase in chromosome aberration was observed with finasteride at the maximum tolerated dose of 250 mg/kg/day (228 times the human exposure) as determined in the carcinogenicity studies.

In sexually mature male rabbits treated with finasteride at 80 mg/kg/day (543 times the human exposure) for up to 12 weeks, no effect on fertility, sperm count, or ejaculate volume was seen. In sexually mature male rats treated with 80 mg/kg/day of finasteride (61 times the human exposure), there were no significant effects on fertility after 6 or 12 weeks of treatment; however, when treatment was continued for up to 24 or 30 weeks, there was an apparent decrease in fertility, fecundity and an associated significant decrease in the weights of the seminal vesicles and prostate. All these effects were reversible within 6 weeks of discontinuation of treatment. No drug-related effect on testes or on mating performance has been seen in rats or rabbits. This decrease in fertility in finasteride-treated rats is secondary to its effect on accessory sex organs (prostate and seminal vesicles) resulting in failure to form a seminal plug. The seminal plug is essential for normal fertility in rats and is not relevant in man.
Pregnancy
Pregnancy Category X
See CONTRAINDICATIONS.
PROSCAR is not indicated for use in women.
Administration of finasteride to pregnant rats at doses ranging from 100 μg/kg/day to 100 mg/kg/day (1–1000 times the recommended human dose) resulted in dose-dependent development of hypospadias in 3.6 to 100% of male offspring. Pregnant rats produced male offspring with decreased prostatic and seminal vesicular weights, delayed preputial separation and transient nipple development when given finasteride at ≥ 30 μg/kg/day (≥ 3/10 of the recommended human dose) and decreased anogenital distance when given finasteride at ≥ 3 μg/kg/day (≥ 3/100 of the recommended human dose). The critical period during which these effects can be induced in male rats has been defined to be days 16–17 of gestation. The changes described above are expected pharmacological effects of drugs belonging to the class of 5α-reductase inhibitors and are similar to those reported in male infants with a genetic deficiency of 5α-reductase. No abnormalities were observed in female offspring exposed to any dose of finasteride *in utero*.
No developmental abnormalities have been observed in first filial generation (F$_1$) male or female offspring resulting from mating finasteride-treated male rats (80 mg/kg/day; 61 times the human exposure) with untreated females. Administration of finasteride at 3 mg/kg/day (30 times the recommended human dose) during the late gestation and lactation period resulted in slightly decreased fertility in F$_1$ male offspring. No effects were seen in female offspring. No evidence of malformations has been observed in rabbit fetuses exposed to finasteride *in utero* from days 6–18 of gestation at doses up to 100 mg/kg/day (1000 times the recommended human dose). However, effects on male genitalia would not be expected since the rabbits were not exposed during the critical period of genital system development.
Nursing Mothers
PROSCAR is not indicated for use in women.
It is not known whether finasteride is excreted in human milk.
Pediatric Use
PROSCAR is not indicated for use in pediatric patients.
Safety and effectiveness in pediatric patients have not been established.

ADVERSE REACTIONS

PROSCAR is generally well tolerated; adverse reactions usually have been mild and transient.
Twelve-Month Controlled Clinical Trials
In North American and international clinical trials, 543 patients were treated with 5 mg of PROSCAR for 12 months. Seven of these patients (1.3%) were discontinued due to adverse experiences that were considered to be possibly, probably or definitely drug-related; only 1 of these patients (0.2%) discontinued therapy with PROSCAR because of a sexual adverse experience.
The following clinical adverse reactions were reported as possibly, probably or definitely drug-related in ≥ 1% of patients treated for 12 months with 5 mg/day of PROSCAR or placebo, respectively: impotence (3.7%, 1.1%), decreased libido (3.3%, 1.6%), decreased volume of ejaculate (2.8%, 0.9%).
The adverse experience profile for an additional 547 patients treated with 1 mg/day of PROSCAR for 12 months was similar to that observed in patients treated for 12 months with 5 mg/day of PROSCAR.
Long-Term Open Extensions
The adverse experience profile for approximately 1100 patients who were maintained on PROSCAR 5 mg/day for 24 months and 400 patients treated for 36 months was similar to that observed in the controlled studies. In addition, a similar safety profile was observed in 50 patients treated with PROSCAR 5 mg/day for 48 months. There is no evidence of increased adverse experiences with increased duration of treatment with PROSCAR. The annual incidence of drug-related sexual adverse experiences decreased with duration

of treatment. Sexual adverse experiences resolved with continued treatment in over 60% of patients who reported them.
The following additional adverse effects have been reported in post-marketing experience:
—breast tenderness and enlargement
—hypersensitivity reactions, including lip swelling and skin rash

OVERDOSAGE

Patients have received single doses of PROSCAR up to 400 mg and multiple doses of PROSCAR up to 80 mg/day for three months without adverse effects. Until further experience is obtained, no specific treatment for an overdose with PROSCAR can be recommended.
Significant lethality was observed in male and female mice at single oral doses of 1500 mg/m^2 (500 mg/kg) and in female and male rats at single oral doses of 2360 mg/m^2 (400 mg/kg) and 5900 mg/m^2 (1000 mg/kg), respectively.

DOSAGE AND ADMINISTRATION

The recommended dose is 5 mg once a day.
Although early improvement may be seen, at least 6–12 months of therapy with PROSCAR may be necessary in some patients to assess whether a beneficial response has been achieved. Periodic follow-up evaluations should be performed to determine whether a clinical response has occurred.
PROSCAR may be administered with or without meals.
No dosage adjustment is necessary for patients with renal impairment or for the elderly (see CLINICAL PHARMACOLOGY, *Pharmacokinetics*).

HOW SUPPLIED

No. 3094—PROSCAR tablets 5 mg are blue, modified apple-shaped, film-coated tablets, with the code MSD 72 on one side and PROSCAR on the other. They are supplied as follows:
  NDC 0006-0072-31 unit of use bottles of 30
  (6505-01-362-5331, 5 mg 30's)
  NDC 0006-0072-58 unit of use bottles of 100
  (6505-01-362-7422, 5 mg 100's)
  NDC 0006-0072-28 unit dose packages of 100
  (6505-01-362-5332, 5 mg individually sealed 100's).
  Shown in Product Identification Guide, page 325
Storage and Handling
Store at room temperatures below 30°C (86°F). Protect from light and keep container tightly closed.
If the film coating of PROSCAR tablets has been broken (e.g., crushed), the tablets should not be handled by a woman who is pregnant or who may become pregnant because of the potential for absorption of finasteride and the subsequent potential risk to a male fetus (see CLINICAL PHARMACOLOGY, *Pharmacokinetics*; WARNINGS, *Exposure of Women—Risk to Male Fetus*; and PRECAUTIONS, *Information for Patients* and *Pregnancy*).
Distributed by:
MERCK & CO., INC.
West Point, PA 19486, USA
        7819205 Issued April 1996
COPYRIGHT © MERCK & CO., INC., 1992, 1995
All rights reserved.

RECOMBIVAX HB®   ℞
Hepatitis B Vaccine (Recombinant)

DESCRIPTION

RECOMBIVAX HB* Hepatitis B Vaccine (Recombinant) is a non-infectious subunit viral vaccine derived from Hepatitis B surface antigen (HBsAg) produced in yeast cells. A portion of the hepatitis B virus gene, coding for HBsAg, is cloned into yeast, and the vaccine for hepatitis B is produced from cultures of this recombinant yeast strain according to methods developed in the Merck Research Laboratories.
The antigen is harvested and purified from fermentation cultures of a recombinant strain of the yeast *Saccharomyces cerevisiae* containing the gene for the *adw* subtype of HBsAg. The HBsAg protein is released from the yeast cells by cell disruption and purified by a series of physical and chemical methods. The vaccine contains no detectable yeast DNA but may contain not more than 1% yeast protein. The vaccine produced by the Merck method has been shown to be comparable to the plasma-derived vaccine in terms of animal

Continued on next page

Information on the Merck & Co., Inc. products listed on these pages is the full prescribing information from product circulars in use September 30, 1996.

Consult 1997 supplements and future editions for revisions

Merck & Co.—Cont.

potency (mouse, monkey, and chimpanzee) and protective efficacy (chimpanzee and human).

The vaccine against hepatitis B, prepared from recombinant yeast cultures, is free of association with human blood or blood products.

Each lot of hepatitis B vaccine is tested for safety, in mice and guinea pigs, and for sterility.

RECOMBIVAX HB is a sterile suspension for intramuscular injection. However, for persons at risk of hemorrhage following intramuscular injection, the vaccine may be administered subcutaneously. (See DOSAGE AND ADMINISTRATION).

RECOMBIVAX HB Hepatitis B Vaccine, (Recombinant) is supplied in four formulations.

Pediatric Formulation, 5 mcg/mL: each 0.5 mL dose contains 2.5 mcg of hepatitis B surface antigen.

Adolescent/High-Risk Infant, 10 mcg/mL: each 0.5 mL dose contains 5 mcg of hepatitis B surface antigen.

Adult Formulation, 10 mcg/mL: each 1 mL dose contains 10 mcg of hepatitis B surface antigen.

Dialysis Formulation, 40 mcg/mL: each 1 mL dose contains 40 mcg of hepatitis B surface antigen.

Each formulation contains thimerosal (mercury derivative) 1:20,000 added as a preservative and has been treated with formaldehyde prior to adsorption onto aluminum hydroxide. In each formulation, hepatitis B surface antigen is adsorbed onto approximately 0.5 mg of aluminum (provided as aluminum hydroxide) per mL of vaccine. The vaccine is of the *adw* subtype. RECOMBIVAX HB is indicated for vaccination of persons at risk of infection from hepatitis B virus including all known subtypes. RECOMBIVAX HB Dialysis Formulation is indicated for vaccination of adult predialysis and dialysis patients against infection caused by all known subtypes of hepatitis B virus.

---

* Registered trademark of MERCK & CO., INC.

CLINICAL PHARMACOLOGY

Hepatitis B virus is one of at least three hepatitis viruses that cause a systemic infection, with a major pathology in the liver. The others include hepatitis A virus, and non-A, non-B hepatitis viruses.

Hepatitis B virus is an important cause of viral hepatitis. There is no specific treatment for this disease. The incubation period for hepatitis B is relatively long; six weeks to six months may elapse between exposure and the onset of clinical symptoms. The prognosis following infection with hepatitis B virus is variable and dependent on at least three factors: (1) Age—Infants and younger children usually experience milder initial disease than older persons; (2) Dose of virus—The higher the dose, the more likely acute icteric hepatitis B will result; and, (3) Severity of associated underlying disease—underlying malignancy or pre-existing hepatic disease predisposes to increased mortality and morbidity.

Persistence of viral infection (the chronic hepatitis B virus carrier state) occurs in 5–10% of persons following acute hepatitis B, and occurs more frequently after initial anicteric hepatitis B than after initial icteric disease. Consequently, carriers of hepatitis B surface antigen (HBsAg) frequently give no history of having had recognized acute hepatitis. It has been estimated that more than 170 million people in the world today are persistently infected with hepatitis B virus. The Centers for Disease Control and Prevention (CDC) estimates that there are approximately 0.75 to 1 million chronic carriers of hepatitis B virus in the USA. Chronic carriers represent the largest human reservoir of hepatitis B virus.

The serious complications and sequelae of hepatitis B virus infection include massive hepatic necrosis, cirrhosis of the liver, chronic active hepatitis, and hepatocellular carcinoma. Chronic carriers of HBsAg appear to be at increased risk of developing hepatocellular carcinoma. Although a number of etiologic factors are associated with development of hepatocellular carcinoma, the single most important etiologic factor appears to be active infection with the hepatitis B virus.

There is also evidence that several diseases other than hepatitis have been associated with hepatitis B virus infection through an immunologic mechanism involving antigen-antibody complexes. Such diseases include a syndrome with rash, urticaria, and arthralgia resembling serum sickness; periarteritis nodosa; membranous glomerulonephritis; and infantile papular acrodermatitis.

Although the vehicles for transmission of the virus are often blood and blood products, viral antigen has also been found in tears, saliva, breast milk, urine, semen and vaginal secretions. Hepatitis B virus is capable of surviving for days on environmental surfaces exposed to body fluids containing hepatitis B virus. Infection may occur when hepatitis B virus, transmitted by infected body fluids, is implanted via mucous surfaces or percutaneously introduced through accidental or deliberate breaks in the skin.

Transmission of hepatitis B virus infection is often associated with close interpersonal contact with an infected individual and with crowded living conditions. In such circumstances, transmission by inoculation via routes other than overt percutaneous ones may be quite common. Perinatal transmission of hepatitis B infection from infected mother to child, at or shortly after birth, can occur if the mother is a hepatitis B surface antigen (HBsAg) carrier or if the mother has an acute hepatitis B infection in the third trimester. Infection in infancy by the hepatitis B virus usually leads to the chronic carrier state. Among infants born to women whose sera are positive for both the hepatitis B surface antigen and the e antigen, 85–90% are infected and become chronic carriers. Well-controlled studies have shown that administration of three 0.5 mL doses of Hepatitis B Immune Globulin (Human) starting at birth is 75% effective in preventing establishment of the chronic carrier state in these infants during the first year of life. However, the protective effect of Hepatitis B Immune Globulin (Human) is transient. Hepatitis B is endemic throughout the world and is a serious medical problem in population groups at increased risk. Because vaccination limited to high-risk individuals has failed to substantially lower the overall incidence of hepatitis B infection, both the immunization Practices Advisory Committee (ACIP) and the Committee on Infectious Diseases of the American Academy of Pediatrics (AAP) have also endorsed universal infant immunization as part of a comprehensive strategy for the control of hepatitis B infection. These advisory groups further recommend broad-based vaccination of adolescents. The ACIP encourages universal hepatitis B vaccination of adolescents in communities where use of illicit injectable drugs, pregnancy among teenagers, and/or sexually transmitted diseases are common. Similarly, the AAP recommends that universal immunization of all adolescents should be implemented when resources permit with emphasis on those individuals in high-risk settings. (Refer to INDICATIONS AND USAGE.)

Numerous epidemiological studies have shown that persons who develop anti-HBs following active infection with the hepatitis B virus are protected against the disease on reexposure to the virus.

Clinical studies have shown that RECOMBIVAX HB when injected into the deltoid muscle induced protective levels of antibody in 96% of 1213 healthy adults who received the recommended 3-dose regimen. Antibody responses varied with age; a protective level of antibody was induced in 98% of 787 young adults 20–29 years of age, 94% of 249 adults 30–39 years of age and in 89% of 177 adults ≥ 40 years of age. Studies with hepatitis B vaccine derived from plasma have shown that a lower response rate (81%) to vaccine may be obtained if the vaccine is administered as a buttock injection. Seroconversion rates and geometric mean antibody titers were measured 1 to 2 months after the 3rd dose. Multiple clinical studies have defined a protective antibody (anti-HBs) level as 1) 10 or more sample ratio units (SRU) as determined by radioimmunoassay or 2) a positive result as determined by enzyme immunoassay. Note: 10 SRU is comparable to 10 mIU/mL of antibody.

RECOMBIVAX HB is highly immunogenic in younger individuals. In clinical studies, 99% of 94 infants under 1 year of age born of non-carrier mothers, 96% of 48 children 1–10 years of age, and 99% of 112 children and adolescents 11–19 years of age developed a protective level of antibody following the recommended 3-dose regimen of vaccine (see DOSAGE AND ADMINISTRATION).

The protective efficacy of three 5 mcg doses of RECOMBIVAX HB has been demonstrated in neonates born of mothers positive for both HBsAg and HBeAg (a core-associated antigenic complex which correlates with high infectivity). In a clinical study of infants who received one dose of Hepatitis B Immune Globulin at birth followed by the recommended three dose regimen of RECOMBIVAX HB, chronic infection had not occurred in 96% of 130 infants after nine months of follow-up. The estimated efficacy in prevention of chronic hepatitis B infection was 95% as compared to the infection rate in untreated historical controls. Significantly fewer neonates became chronically infected when given one dose of Hepatitis B Immune Globulin at birth followed by the recommended three dose regimen of RECOMBIVAX HB when compared to historical controls who received only a single dose of Hepatitis B Immune Globulin. Testing for HBsAg and anti-HBs is recommended at 12–15 months of age. If HBsAg is not detectable, and anti-HBs is present, the child has been protected.

As demonstrated in the above study, Hepatitis B Immune Globulin, when administered simultaneously with RECOMBIVAX HB at separate body sites, did not interfere with the induction of protective antibodies against hepatitis B virus elicited by the vaccine.

The duration of the protective effect of RECOMBIVAX HB in healthy vaccinees is unknown at present and the need for booster doses is not yet defined. However, long-term follow-up (5 to 9 years) of approximately 3000 high-risk vaccinees (infants of carrier mothers, male homosexuals, Alaskan Natives) who developed an anti-HBs titer of ≥ 10 mIU/mL when given a similar plasma-derived vaccine of intervals of 0, 1, and 6 months showed that no subjects developed clinically apparent hepatitis B infection and that 5 subjects developed antigenemia, even though up to half of the subjects failed to maintain a titer at this level. Persistence of immunologic memory was demonstrated by an anamnestic antibody response to a booster dose of RECOMBIVAX HB in healthy adults given plasma-derived vaccine 5 to 7 years earlier at intervals of 0, 1, and 6 months.

Predialysis and Dialysis Patients

Predialysis and dialysis adult patients respond less well to hepatitis B vaccines than do healthy individuals. In addition, the responses to these vaccines may be lower if the vaccine is administered as a buttock injection. When 40 mcg of Hepatitis B Vaccine (Recombinant) was administered in the deltoid muscle, 89% of 28 participants developed anti-HBs with 86% achieving levels ≥ 10 mIU/mL. However, when the same dosage of this vaccine was administered inappropriately either in the buttock or a combination of buttock and deltoid, 62% of 47 participants developed anti-HBs with 55% achieving levels of ≥ 10 mIU/mL. Revaccination with RECOMBIVAX HB Dialysis Formulation may be considered in predialysis/dialysis patients if the anti-HBs level is less than 10 mIU/mL.

Reports in the literature describe a more virulent form of hepatitis B associated with superinfections or coinfections by delta virus, an imcomplete RNA virus. Delta virus can only infect and cause illness in persons infected with hepatitis B virus since the delta agent requires a coat of HBsAg in order to become infectious. Therefore, persons immune to hepatitis B virus infection should also be immune to delta virus infection.

Interchangeability of Plasma-Derived and Recombinant Hepatitis B Vaccines

Although there have been no clinical studies in which a three-dose vaccine series was initiated with HEPTAVAX-B* (Hepatitis B Vaccine) and completed with RECOMBIVAX HB, or vice versa, extensive *in vitro* and *in vivo* studies have demonstrated that two vaccines are immunologically comparable.

---

* Registered trademark of MERCK & CO., INC.

INDICATIONS AND USAGE

RECOMBIVAX HB is indicated for vaccination against infection caused by all known subtypes of hepatitis B virus. RECOMBIVAX HB Dialysis Formulation is indicated for vaccination of adult predialysis and dialysis patients against infection caused by all known subtypes of hepatitis B virus.

Vaccination with RECOMBIVAX HB is recommended for:

1) Infants including those born to HBsAg positive mothers (high-risk infants).

2) Adolescents (see CLINICAL PHARMACOLOGY).

3) Other persons of all ages in areas of high prevalence or those who are or may be at increased risk of infection with hepatitis B virus, such as:

- *Health Care Personnel*
  Dentists and oral surgeons.
  Physicians and surgeons.
  Nurses.
  Paramedical personnel and custodial staff who may be exposed to the virus via blood or other patient specimens.
  Dental hygienists and dental nurses.
  Laboratory personnel handling blood, blood products, and other patient specimens.
  Dental, medical and nursing students.
- *Selected Patients and Patient Contacts*
  Staff in hemodialysis units and hematology/oncology units.
  Patients requiring frequent and/or large volume blood transfusions or clotting factor concentrates (e.g., persons with hemophilia, thalassemia).
  Clients (residents) and staff of institutions for the mentally handicapped.
  Classroom contacts of deinstitutionalized mentally handicapped persons who have persistent hepatitis B surface antigenemia and who show aggressive behavior.
  Household and other intimate contacts of persons with persistent hepatitis B surface antigenemia.
- *Sub-populations with a known high incidence of the disease,* such as:
  Alaskan Natives.
  Pacific Islanders.
  Refugees from areas where hepatitis B virus infection is endemic.
- *Military Personnel identified as being at increased risk*
- *Morticians and Embalmers*
- *Blood bank and plasma fractionation workers*
- *Persons at Increased Risk of the Disease Due to Their Sexual Practices,* such as:
  Persons who have heterosexual activity with multiple partners.

Persons who repeatedly contract sexually transmitted diseases.

Homosexually active males.

Female prostitutes.

- *Prisoners*
- *Users of illicit injectable drugs*

Neither dosage strength will prevent hepatitis caused by other agents, such as hepatitis A virus, non-A, non-B hepatitis viruses, or other viruses known to infect the liver.

Revaccination

See CLINICAL PHARMACOLOGY

Use with Other Vaccines

Specific data are not yet available for the simultaneous administration of RECOMBIVAX HB with other vaccines. However, the Immunization Practices Advisory Committee states that, in general, simultaneous administration of certain live and inactivated pediatric vaccines has not resulted in impaired antibody responses or increased rates of adverse reactions. Separate sites and syringes should be used for simultaneous administration of injectable vaccines.

CONTRAINDICATIONS

Hypersensitivity to yeast or any component of the vaccine.

WARNINGS

Patients who develop symptoms suggestive of hypersensitivity after an injection should not receive further injections of the vaccine (see CONTRAINDICATIONS).

Because of the long incubation period for hepatitis B, it is possible for unrecognized infection to be present at the time the vaccine is given. The vaccine may not prevent hepatitis B in such patients.

PRECAUTIONS

General

As with any percutaneous vaccine, epinephrine should be available for immediate use should an anaphylactoid reaction occur.

Any serious active infection is reason for delaying use of the vaccine except when in the opinion of the physician, withholding the vaccine entails a greater risk.

Caution and appropriate care should be exercised in administering the vaccine to individuals with severely compromised cardiopulmonary status or to others in whom a febrile or systemic reaction could pose a significant risk.

Pregnancy

Pregnancy Category C: Animal reproduction studies have not been conducted with the vaccine. It is also not known whether the vaccine can cause fetal harm when administered to a pregnant woman or can affect reproduction capacity. The vaccine should be given to a pregnant woman only if clearly needed.

Nursing Mothers

It is not known whether the vaccine is excreted in human milk. Because many drugs are excreted in human milk, cautions should be exercised when the vaccine is administered to a nursing woman.

Pediatric Use

RECOMBIVAX HB has been shown to be usually well-tolerated and highly immunogenic in infants and children of all ages. Newborns also respond well; maternally transferred antibodies do not interfere with the active immune response to the vaccine. See DOSAGE AND ADMINISTRATION for recommended pediatric dosage and for recommended dosage for infants born to HBsAg positive mothers.

The safety and effectiveness of RECOMBIVAX HB Dialysis Formulation in children have not been established.

ADVERSE REACTIONS

RECOMBIVAX HB and RECOMBIVAX HB Dialysis Formulation are generally well-tolerated. No serious adverse reactions attributable to the vaccine have been reported during the course of clinical trials. No adverse experiences were reported during clinical trials which could be related to changes in the titers of antibodies to yeast. As with any vaccine, there is the possibility that broad use of the vaccine could reveal adverse reactions not observed in clinical trials.

In a group of studies, 1636 doses of RECOMBIVAX HB were administered to 653 healthy infants and children (up to 10 years of age) who were monitored for 5 days after each dose. Injection site complaints (including erythema and swelling) and systemic complaints were reported following 8% and 17% of the injections, respectively. The most frequently reported systemic adverse reactions (>1% injections), in decreasing order of frequency, were irritability, tiredness, fever (>101°F oral equivalent), crying, diarrhea, vomiting, diminished appetite, and insomnia.

In a group of studies, 3258 doses of RECOMBIVAX HB were administered to 1252 healthy adults who were monitored for 5 days after each dose. Injection site and systemic complaints were reported following 17% and 15% of the

injections, respectively. The following adverse reactions were reported:

Incidence Equal to or
Greater Than 1% of Injections

LOCAL REACTION (INJECTION SITE)

Injection site reactions consisting principally of soreness, and including pain, tenderness, pruritus, erythema, ecchymosis, swelling, warmth, and nodule formation.

BODY AS A WHOLE

The most frequent systemic complaints include fatigue/weakness; headache; fever (≥ 100°F); and malaise.

DIGESTIVE SYSTEM

Nausea; and diarrhea

RESPIRATORY SYSTEM

Pharyngitis; and upper respiratory infection

Incidence Less than 1% of Injections

BODY AS A WHOLE

Sweating; achiness; sensation of warmth; lightheadedness; chills; and flushing

DIGESTIVE SYSTEM

Vomiting; abdominal pains/cramps; dyspepsia; and diminished appetite

RESPIRATORY SYSTEM

Rhinitis; influenza; and cough

NERVOUS SYSTEM

Vertigo/dizziness; and paresthesia

INTEGUMENTARY SYSTEM

Pruritus; rash (non-specified); angioedema; and urticaria

MUSCULOSKELETAL SYSTEM

Arthralgia including monoarticular; myalgia; back pain, neck pain; shoulder pain; and neck stiffness

HEMIC/LYMPHATIC SYSTEM

Lymphadenopathy

PSYCHIATRIC/BEHAVIORAL

Insomnia/Disturbed sleep

SPECIAL SENSES

Earache

UROGENITAL SYSTEM

Dysuria

CARDIOVASCULAR SYSTEM

Hypotension

Marketed Experience

The following additional adverse reactions have been reported with use of the marketed vaccine. In many instances, the relationship to the vaccine was unclear.

Hypersensitivity

Anaphylaxis and symptoms of immediate hypersensitivity reactions including rash, pruritus, urticaria, edema, angioedema, dyspnea, chest discomfort, bronchial spasm, palpitation, or symptoms consistent with a hypotensive episode have been reported within the first few hours after vaccination. An apparent hypersensitivity syndrome (serum-sickness-like) of delayed onset has been reported days to weeks after vaccination, including: arthralgia/arthritis (usually transient), fever, and dermatologic reactions such as urticaria, erythema multiforme, ecchymoses and erythema nodosum (See WARNINGS and PRECAUTIONS).

Digestive System

Elevation of liver enzymes; constipation.

Nervous System

Guillain-Barré Syndrome; multiple sclerosis; myelitis including transverse myelitis; peripheral neuropathy including Bell's Palsy; radiculopathy; herpes zoster; migraine; muscle weakness; hypesthesia.

Integumentary System

Stevens-Johnson Syndrome; petechiae.

Musculoskeletal System

Arthritis.

Hematologic

Increased erythrocyte sedimentation rate; thrombocytopenia.

Immune System

Lupus-like syndrome.

Psychiatric/Behavioral

Irritability; agitation; somnolence.

Special Senses

Optic neuritis; tinnitus; conjunctivitis; visual disturbances.

Cardiovascular System

Syncope; tachycardia.

The following adverse reaction has been reported with another Heaptitis B Vaccine (Recombinant) but not with RECOMBIVAX HB: keratitis.

DOSAGE AND ADMINISTRATION

Do not inject intravenously or intradermally.

RECOMBIVAX HB [Hepatitis B Vaccine (Recombinant)] DIALYSIS FORMULATION (40 mcg/mL) IS INTENDED ONLY FOR ADULT PREDIALYSIS/DIALYSIS PATIENTS.

RECOMBIVAX HB [Hepatitis B Vaccine (Recombinant)] PEDIATRIC, ADOLESCENT/HIGH-RISK INFANT, and ADULT FORMULATIONS (5 mcg/mL or 10 mcg/mL) ARE NOT INTENDED FOR USE IN PREDIALYSIS/DIALYSIS PATIENTS.

Table 1 summarizes the dose and formulation of RECOMBIVAX HB for specific populations. The vaccination regimen for each population EXCEPT Infants of HBsAg Positive Mothers (see Table 2) consists of 3 doses of vaccine given according to the following schedule:

1st dose: at elected date

2nd dose: 1 month later

3rd dose: 6 months after the first dose

Table 1

Group	Dose*	Formulation	Color Code
Infants born of:			
HBsAg Negative Mothers	2.5 mcg (0.5 mL)	Pediatric	Brown
HBsAg Positive Mothers†	5 mcg (0.5 mL)	Adolescent/ High-Risk Infant	Yellow
1–10 years of age	2.5 mcg (0.5 mL)	Pediatric	Brown
11–19 years of age	5 mcg (0.5 mL)	Adolescent/ High-Risk Infant	Yellow
≥ 20 years of age	10 mcg (1.0 mL)	Adult	Green
Predialysis and Dialysis Patients**	40 mcg/ 1.0 mL	Dialysis	Blue

† See Table 2

* If the suggested formulation is not available, the appropriate dosage can be achieved from another formulation provided that the total volume of vaccine administered does not exceed 1 mL. However, the Dialysis Formulation may be used only for adult predialysis/dialysis patients.

** See also recommendations for revaccination of Predialysis and Dialysis Patients under *Revaccination*, DOSAGE AND ADMINISTRATION.

RECOMBIVAX HB is for intramuscular injection. The *deltoid muscle* is the preferred site for intramuscular injection in adults. Data suggests that injections given in the buttocks frequently are given into fatty tissue instead of into muscle. Such injections have resulted in a lower seroconversion rate than was expected. The *anterolateral thigh* is the recommended site for intramuscular injection in infants and young children.

For persons at risk of hemorrhage following intramuscular injection, RECOMBIVAX HB may be administered subcutaneously. However, when other aluminum-adsorbed vaccines have been administered subcutaneously, an increased incidence of local reactions including subcutaneous nodules has been observed. Therefore, subcutaneous administration should be used only in persons (e.g., hemophiliacs) who are at risk of hemorrhage following intramuscular injections.

The vaccine should be used as supplied; no dilution or reconstitution is necessary. The full recommended dose of the vaccine should be used.

For Vial and Pre-filled Single Dose Syringe: Shake well before use. Thorough agitation at the time of administration is necessary to maintain suspension of the vaccine.

Parenteral drug products should be inspected visually for particulate matter and discoloration prior to administration. After thorough agitation, the vaccine is a slightly opaque, white suspension.

For Vial: Withdraw the recommended dose from the vial using a sterile needle and syringe free of preservatives, antiseptics, and detergents.

It is important to use a separate sterile syringe and needle for each individual patient to prevent transmission of hepatitis and other infectious agents from one person to another. Injection must be accomplished with a needle long enough to ensure intramuscular deposition of the vaccine.

The Immunization Practices Advisory Committee has recommended that "for an intramuscular injection, the needle and syringe should be of sufficient length and bore to reach the muscle mass itself and prevent vaccine from seeping into subcutaneous tissue. For children, a 20- or 22-gauge needle 1 to 1$^1/_4$ inches long is recommended. For small infants, a 25-gauge $^5/_8$-inch-long needle may be adequate. For adults, the suggested needle length is 1$^1/_2$ inches."

Dosage for Infants Born of HBsAg Positive Mothers (High-Risk Infants) or Mothers of Unknown HBsAg Status

The recommended regimen for infants born of HBsAg positive mothers is as follows:

Table 2

	Birth*	Within 7 days	1 month	6 months
RECOMBIVAX HB Adolescent/High-Risk Infant yellow color code		5 mcg** (0.5 mL)	5 mcg (0.5 mL)	5 mcg (0.5 mL)

Continued on next page

Merck & Co.—Cont.

HEPATITIS B IMMUNE GLOBULIN	0.5 mL	—	—	—

* The first 5 mcg/0.5 mL dose of RECOMBIVAX HB is given preferably within the first 12 hours of birth but may be given within the first 7 days.

** The first 5 mcg/0.5 mL dose of RECOMBIVAX HB may be given at birth at the same time as Hepatitis B Immune Globulin, but should be administered in the opposite anterolateral thigh.

Recommendations from the Immunization Practices Advisory Committee for infants born of mothers of unknown HBsAg status are summarized as follows: In the event that a mother's HBsAg status is unknown, vaccination should be initiated as soon as possible with a 5 mcg/0.5 mL dose of vaccine (Adolescent/High-Risk Infant, yellow color code). If within 7 days of delivery the mother is determined to be HBsAg positive, the infant should also be given a dose of Hepatitis B Immune Globulin immediately; the vaccination series should then be completed with 5 mcg/0.5 mL dosages. If the mother's HBsAg antigen test is negative, then complete the vaccination series with 2.5 mcg/0.5 mL dosages (Pediatric Formulation, brown color code).

Revaccination

The duration of the protective effect of RECOMBIVAX HB in healthy vaccinees is unknown at present and the need for booster doses is not yet defined.

A booster dose or revaccination with RECOMBIVAX HB Dialysis Formulation (blue color code) may be considered in predialysis/dialysis patients if the anti-HBs level is less than 10 MIU/mL 1 to 2 months after the 3rd dose.

Known or Presumed Exposure to HBsAg

There are no prospective studies directly testing the efficacy of a combination of Hepatitis B Immune Globulin (Human) and RECOMBIVAX HB in preventing clinical hepatitis B following percutaneous, ocular or mucous membrane exposure to hepatitis B virus. However, since most persons with such exposures (e.g., health-care workers) are candidates for RECOMBIVAX HB and since combined Hepatitis B Immune Globulin (Human) plus vaccine is more efficacious than Hepatitis B Immune Globulin (Human) alone in perinatal exposures, the following guidelines are recommended for persons who have been exposed to hepatitis B virus such as through (1) percutaneous (needlestick), ocular, mucous membrane exposure to blood known or presumed to contain HBsAg, (2) human bites by known or presumed HBsAg carriers, that penetrate the skin, or (3) following intimate sexual contact with known or presumed HBsAg carriers:

Hepatitis B Immune Globulin (Human) (0.06 mL/kg) should be given intramuscularly as soon as possible after exposure and within 24 hours if possible. RECOMBIVAX HB (see dosage recommendation) should be given intramuscularly at a separate site within 7 days of exposure and second and third doses given one and six months, respectively, after the first dose.

HOW SUPPLIED

PEDIATRIC FORMULATION

No. 4799—RECOMBIVAX HB for pediatric use is supplied as 2.5 mcg/0.5 mL of HBsAg in a 0.5 mL single-dose vial, color coded with a brown cap and stripe on the vial labels and cartons, **NDC** 0006-4799-00.

No. 4761—RECOMBIVAX HB for pediatric use is supplied as 2.5 mcg/0.5 mL of HBsAg in a 3 mL multiple-dose vial, color coded with a brown cap and stripe on the vial labels and cartons, **NDC** 0006-4761-00.

No. 4874—RECOMBIVAX HB for pediatric use is supplied as 2.5 mcg/0.5 mL of HBsAg in a 0.5 mL single-dose vial, in a box of 10 single-dose vials, color coded with a brown cap and stripe on the vial labels and cartons, **NDC** 0006-4874-00.

No. 4875—RECOMBIVAX HB for pediatric use is supplied as 2.5 mcg/0.5 mL of HBsAg in a 3 mL multiple-dose vial, in a box of 10 multi-dose vials, color coded with a brown cap and stripe on the vial labels and cartons, **NDC** 0006-4875-00 (6505-01-415-9815 2.5 mcg/0.5 mL, 3 mL).

No. 4851—RECOMBIVAX HB for pediatric use is supplied as 2.5 mcg/0.5 mL of HBsAg in a 0.5 mL pre-filled single-dose syringe, in a box of 5 pre-filled single-dose syringes, color coded with a brown plunger rod and stripe on the syringe labels and cartons, **NDC** 0006-4851-00.

ADOLESCENT/HIGH-RISK INFANT

No. 4769—RECOMBIVAX HB for adolescent use and for infants born of HBsAg+ mothers is supplied as 5 mcg/0.5 mL of HBsAg in a 0.5 mL single-dose vial, color coded with a yellow cap and stripe on the vial labels and cartons, **NDC** 0006-4769-00.

No. 4876—RECOMBIVAX HB for adolescent use and for infants born of HBsAg+ mothers is supplied as 5 mcg/0.5 mL of HBsAg in a 0.5 mL single-dose vial, in a box of 10 single-dose vials, color coded with a yellow cap and stripe on the vial labels and cartons, **NDC** 0006-4876-00 (6505-01-415-9813 5 mcg/0.5 mL, 0.5 mL).

No. 4849—RECOMBIVAX HB for adolescent use and for infants born of HBsAg+ mothers is supplied as 5 mcg/0.5 mL of HBsAg in a 0.5 mL pre-filled single-dose syringe, in a box of 5 pre-filled single-dose syringes, color coded with a yellow plunger rod and stripe on the syringe labels and cartons, **NDC** 0006-4849-00.

ADULT FORMULATION

No. 4775—RECOMBIVAX HB for adult use is supplied as 10 mcg/mL of HBsAg in a 1 mL single-dose vial, color coded with a green cap and stripe on the vial labels and cartons, **NDC** 0006-4775-00.
(6505-01-312-6410 10 mcg/1.0 mL, 1 mL).

No. 4773—RECOMBIVAX HB for adult use is supplied as 10 mcg/mL of HBsAg in a 3 mL multiple-dose vial, color coded with a green cap and stripe on the vial labels and cartons, **NDC** 0006-4773-00
(6505-01-266-3780 10 mcg/mL, 3 mL).

No. 4872—RECOMBIVAX HB for adult use is supplied as 10 mcg/mL of HBsAg in a 1 mL single-dose vial, in a box of 10 single-dose vials, color coded with a green cap and stripe on the vial labels and cartons, **NDC** 0006-4872-00.

No.4873—RECOMBIVAX HB for adult use is supplied as 10 mcg/mL of HBsAg in a 3 mL multiple-dose vial, in a box of 10 multi-dose vials, color coded with a green cap and stripe on the vial labels and cartons, **NDC** 0006-4873-00
(6505-10-415-9816 10 mcg/1.0 mL, 3 mL).

No. 4848—RECOMBIVAX HB for adult use is supplied as 10 mcg/mL of HBsAg in a 1 mL pre-filled single-dose syringe, in a box of 5 pre-filled single-dose syringes, color coded with a green plunger rod and stripe on the syringe labels and cartons, **NDC** 0006-4848-00.

DIALYSIS FORMULATION

No. 4776—RECOMBIVAX HB Dialysis Formulation is supplied as 40 mcg/mL of HBsAg in a 1 mL single-dose vial, color coded with a blue cap and stripe on the vial labels and cartons, **NDC** 0006-4776-00
(6505-01-317-1132 40 mcg/mL, 1 mL).

Storage

Store vials and syringes at 2–8°C (36°–46°F). Storage above or below the recommended temperature may reduce potency.

Do not freeze since freezing destroys potency.

7462214 Issued February 1996

COPYRIGHT © MERCK & CO., INC., 1986, 1989, 1993
All rights reserved

SYPRINE® Capsules ℞
(Trientine Hydrochloride), U.S.P.
(Formerly 'CUPRID®')

DESCRIPTION

Trientine hydrochloride is *N,N'*-bis (2-aminoethyl)-1,2-ethanediamine dihydrochloride. It is a white to pale yellow crystalline hygroscopic powder. It is freely soluble in water, soluble in methanol, slightly soluble in ethanol, and insoluble in chloroform and ether.

The empirical formula is $C_6H_{18}N_4 \cdot 2HCl$ with a molecular weight of 219.2. The structural formula is:

$$NH_2(CH_2)_2NH(CH_2)_2NH(CH_2)_2NH_2 \cdot 2HCl$$

Trientine hydrochloride is a chelating compound for removal of excess copper from the body. SYPRINE* (Trientine Hydrochloride) is available as 250 mg capsules for oral administration. Capsules SYPRINE contain gelatin, iron oxides, stearic acid, and titanium dioxide as inactive ingredients.

*Registered trademark of MERCK & CO., INC.

CLINICAL PHARMACOLOGY

Introduction

Wilson's disease (hepatolenticular degeneration) is an autosomal inherited metabolic defect resulting in an inability to maintain a near-zero balance of copper. Excess copper accumulates possibly because the liver lacks the mechanism to excrete free copper into the bile. Hepatocytes store excess copper but when their capacity is exceeded copper is released into the blood and is taken up into extrahepatic sites. This condition is treated with a low copper diet and the use of chelating agents that bind copper to facilitate its excretion from the body.

Clinical Summary

Forty-one patients (18 male and 23 female) between the ages of 6 and 54 with a diagnosis of Wilson's disease and who were intolerant of d-penicillamine were treated in two separate studies with trientine hydrochloride. The dosage varied from 450 to 2400 mg per day. The average dosage required to achieve an optimal clinical response varied between 1000 mg and 2000 mg per day. The mean duration of trientine hydrochloride therapy was 48.7 months (range 2–164 months). Thirty-four of the 41 patients improved, 4 had no change in clinical global response, 2 were lost to follow-up and one showed deterioration in clinical condition. One of the patients who improved while on therapy with trientine hydrochloride experienced a recurrence of the symptoms of systemic lupus erythematosus which had appeared originally during therapy with penicillamine. Therapy with trientine hydrochloride was discontinued. No other adverse reactions, except iron deficiency, were noted among any of these 41 patients.

One investigator treated 13 patients with trientine hydrochloride following their development of intolerance to d-penicillamine. Retrospectively, he compared these patients to an additional group of 12 patients with Wilson's disease who were both tolerant of and controlled with d-penicillamine therapy, but who failed to continue any copper chelation therapy. The mean age at onset of disease of the latter group was 12 years as compared to 21 years for the former group. The trientine hydrochloride group received d-penicillamine for an average of 4 years as compared to an average of 10 years for the non-treated group.

Various laboratory parameters showed changes in favor of the patients treated with trientine hydrochloride. Free and total serum copper, SGOT, and serum bilirubin all showed mean increases over baseline in the untreated group which were significantly larger than with the patients treated with trientine hydrochloride. In the 13 patients treated with trientine hydrochloride, previous symptoms and signs relating to d-penicillamine intolerance disappeared in 8 patients, improved in 4 patients, and remained unchanged in one patient. The neurological status in the trientine hydrochloride group was unchanged or improved over baseline, whereas in the untreated group, 6 patients remained unchanged and 6 worsened. Kayser-Fleischer rings improved significantly during trientine hydrochloride treatment.

The clinical outcome of the two groups also differed markedly. Of the 13 patients on therapy with trientine hydrochloride (mean duration of therapy 4.1 years; range 1 to 13 years), all were alive at the data cutoff date, and in the non-treated group (mean years with no therapy 2.7 years; range 3 months to 9 years), 9 of the 12 died of hepatic disease.

Chelating Properties

Preclinical Studies

Studies in animals have shown that trientine hydrochloride has cupriuretic activities in both normal and copper-loaded rats. In general, the effects of trientine hydrochloride on urinary copper excretion are similar to those of equimolar doses of penicillamine, although in one study they were significantly smaller.

Human Studies

Renal clearance studies were carried out with penicillamine and trientine hydrochloride on separate occasions in selected patients treated with penicillamine for at least one year. Six-hour excretion rates of copper were determined off treatment and after a single dose of 500 mg of penicillamine or 1.2 g of trientine hydrochloride. The mean urinary excretion rates of copper were as follows:

No. of Patients	Single Dose Treatment	Basal Excretion Rate ($\mu g\ Cu^{++}$/6hr)	Test-dose Excretion Rate ($\mu g\ Cu^{++}$/6hr)
6	Trientine, 1.2 g	19	234
4	Penicillamine, 500 mg	17	320

In patients *not* previously treated with chelating agents, a similar comparison was made:

No. of Patients	Single Dose Treatment	Basal Excretion Rate ($\mu g\ Cu^{++}$/6hr)	Test-dose Excretion Rate ($\mu g\ Cu^{++}$/6hr)
8	Trientine, 1.2 g	71	1326
7	Penicillamine, 500 mg	68	1074

These results demonstrate that SYPRINE is effective as a cupriuretic agent in patients with Wilson's disease although on a molar basis it appears to be less potent or less effective than penicillamine. Evidence from a radio-labelled copper study indicates that the different cupriuretic effect between these two drugs could be due to a difference in selectivity of the drugs for different copper pools within the body.

Pharmacokinetics

Data on the pharmacokinetics of trientine hydrochloride are not available. Dosage adjustment recommendations are based upon clinical use of the drug (see DOSAGE AND ADMINISTRATION).

INDICATIONS AND USAGE

SYPRINE is indicated in the treatment of patients with Wilson's disease who are intolerant of penicillamine. Clinical

experience with SYPRINE is limited and alternate dosing regimens have not been well-characterized; all endpoints in determining an individual patient's dose have not been well defined. SYPRINE and penicillamine cannot be considered interchangeable. SYPRINE should be used when continued treatment with penicillamine is no longer possible because of intolerable or life endangering side effects.
Unlike penicillamine, SYPRINE is not recommended in cystinuria or rheumatoid arthritis. The absence of a sulfhydryl moiety renders it incapable of binding cystine and, therefore, it is of no use in cystinuria. In 15 patients with rheumatoid arthritis, SYPRINE was reported not to be effective in improving any clinical or biochemical parameter after 12 weeks of treatment.
SYPRINE is not indicated for treatment of biliary cirrhosis.

CONTRAINDICATIONS

Hypersensitivity to this product.

WARNINGS

Patient experience with trientine hydrochloride is limited (see CLINICAL PHARMACOLOGY). Patients receiving SYPRINE should remain under regular medical supervision throughout the period of drug administration. Patients (especially women) should be closely monitored for evidence of iron deficiency anemia.

PRECAUTIONS

General
There are no reports of hypersensitivity in patients who have been administered trientine hydrochloride for Wilson's disease. However, there have been reports of asthma, bronchitis and dermatitis occurring after prolonged environmental exposure in workers who use trientine hydrochloride as a hardener of epoxy resins. Patients should be observed closely for signs of possible hypersensitivity.

Information for Patients
Patients should be directed to take SYPRINE on an empty stomach, at least one hour before meals or two hours after meals and at least one hour apart from any other drug, food, or milk. The capsules should be swallowed whole with water and should not be opened or chewed. Because of the potential for contact dermatitis, any site of exposure to the capsule contents should be washed with water promptly. For the first month of treatment, the patient should have his temperature taken nightly, and he should be asked to report any symptom such as fever or skin eruption.

Laboratory Tests
The most reliable index for monitoring treatment is the determination of free copper in the serum, which equals the difference between quantitatively determined total copper and ceruloplasmin-copper. Adequately treated patients will usually have less than 10 mcg free copper/dL of serum.
Therapy may be monitored with a 24 hour urinary copper analysis periodically (i.e., every 6–12 months). Urine must be collected in copper-free glassware. Since a low copper diet should keep copper absorption down to less than one milligram a day, the patient probably will be in the desired state of negative copper balance if 0.5 to 1.0 milligram of copper is present in a 24-hour collection of urine.

Drug Interactions
In general, mineral supplements should not be given since they may block the absorption of SYPRINE. However, iron deficiency may develop, especially in children and menstruating or pregnant women, or as a result of the low copper diet recommended for Wilson's disease. If necessary, iron may be given in short courses, but since iron and SYPRINE each inhibit absorption of the other, two hours should elapse between administration of SYPRINE and iron.
It is important that SYPRINE be taken on an empty stomach, at least one hour before meals or two hours after meals and at least one hour apart from any other drug, food, or milk. This permits maximum absorption and reduces the likelihood of inactivation of the drug by metal binding in the gastrointestinal tract.

Carcinogenesis, Mutagenesis, Impairment of Fertility
Data on carcinogenesis, mutagenesis, and impairment of fertility are not available.

Pregnancy
Pregnancy Category C. Trientine hydrochloride was teratogenic in rats at doses similar to the human dose. The frequencies of both resorptions and fetal abnormalities, including hemorrhage and edema, increased while fetal copper levels decreased when trientine hydrochloride was given in the maternal diets of rats. There are no adequate and well-controlled studies in pregnant women. SYPRINE should be used during pregnancy only if the potential benefit justifies the potential risk to the fetus.

Nursing Mothers
It is not known whether this drug is excreted in human milk. Because many drugs are excreted in human milk, caution should be exercised when SYPRINE is administered to a nursing mother.

Pediatric Use
Controlled studies of the safety and effectiveness of SYPRINE in children have not been conducted. It has been used clinically in children as young as 6 years with no reported adverse experiences.

ADVERSE REACTIONS

Clinical experience with SYPRINE has been limited. The following adverse reactions have been reported in patients with Wilson's disease who were on therapy with trientine hydrochloride: iron deficiency, systemic lupus erythematosus (see CLINICAL PHARMACOLOGY).
SYPRINE is not indicated for treatment of biliary cirrhosis, but in one study of 4 patients treated with trientine hydrochloride for primary biliary cirrhosis, the following adverse reactions were reported: heartburn; epigastric pain and tenderness; thickening, fissuring and flaking of the skin; hypochromic microcytic anemia; acute gastritis; aphthoid ulcers; abdominal pain; melena; anorexia; malaise; cramps; muscle pain; weakness; rhabdomyolysis. A causal relationship of these reactions to drug therapy could not be rejected or established.

OVERDOSAGE

There is a report of an adult woman who ingested 30 grams of trientine hydrochloride without apparent ill effects. No other data on overdosage are available.

DOSAGE AND ADMINISTRATION

Systemic evaluation of dose and/or interval between dose has not been done. However, on limited clinical experience, the recommended initial dose of SYPRINE is 500–750 mg/day for children and 750–1250 mg/day for adults given in divided doses two, three or four times daily. This may be increased to a maximum of 2000 mg/day for adults or 1500 mg/day for children age 12 or under. The daily dose of SYPRINE should be increased only when the clinical response is not adequate or the concentration of free serum copper is persistently above 20 mcg/dL. Optimal long-term maintenance dosage should be determined at 6–12 month intervals (see PRECAUTIONS, *Laboratory Tests*).
It is important that SYPRINE be given on an empty stomach, at least one hour before meals or two hours after meals and at least one hour apart from any other drug, food, or milk. The capsules should be swallowed whole with water and should not be opened or chewed.

HOW SUPPLIED

No. 3408—Capsules SYPRINE, 250 mg, are light brown opaque capsules and are coded MSD 661. They are supplied as follows:
NDC 0006-0661-68 in bottles of 100.
Shown in Product Identification Guide, page 325

Storage
Keep container tightly closed.
Store at 2°–8°C (36°–46°F).
7664601 Issued March 1989
COPYRIGHT © MERCK & CO., INC., 1985, 1989
All rights reserved

TIMOLIDE® Tablets ℞
(Timolol Maleate-Hydrochlorothiazide), U.S.P.

DESCRIPTION

TIMOLIDE* (Timolol Maleate-Hydrochlorothiazide) is for the treatment of hypertension. It combines the antihypertensive activity of two agents: a non-selective beta-adrenergic receptor blocking agent (timolol maleate) and a diuretic (hydrochlorothiazide).
Timolol maleate is (*S*)-1-[(1, 1-dimethylethyl) amino]-3-[[4-(4-morpholinyl)-1, 2, 5-thiadiazol -3- yl] oxy]-2-propanol (*Z*)-2-butenedioate (1:1) salt. Its empirical formula is $C_{13}H_{24}N_4O_3S \cdot C_4H_4O_4$ and its structural formula is:

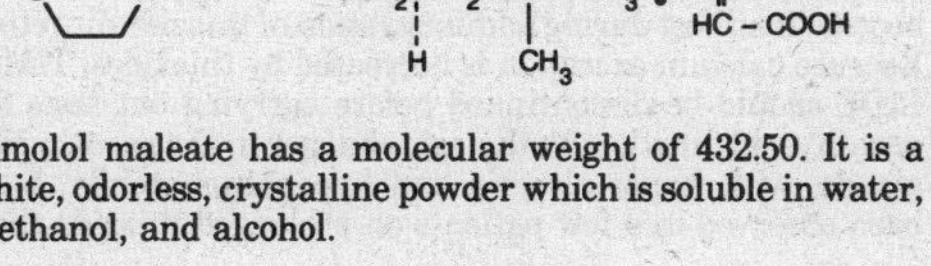

Timolol maleate has a molecular weight of 432.50. It is a white, odorless, crystalline powder which is soluble in water, methanol, and alcohol.
Hydrochlorothiazide is 6-chloro-3,4-dihydro-2*H*-1,2,4-benzothiadiazine-7-sulfonamide 1, 1- dioxide. Its empirical formula is $C_7H_8ClN_3O_4S_2$ and its structural formula is:

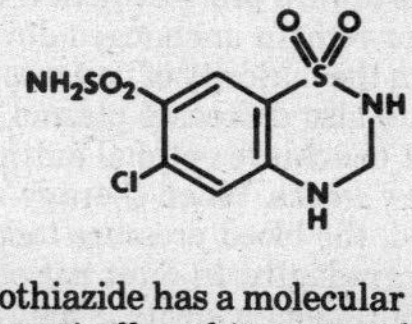

Hydrochlorothiazide has a molecular weight of 297.73. It is a white, or practically white, crystalline powder which is slightly soluble in water, but freely soluble in sodium hydroxide solution.
TIMOLIDE is supplied as tablets containing 10 mg of timolol maleate and 25 mg of hydrochlorothiazide for oral administration. Inactive ingredients are cellulose, FD&C Blue 2, magnesium stearate, and starch.

* Registered trademark of MERCK & CO., INC.

CLINICAL PHARMACOLOGY

TIMOLIDE
Timolol maleate and hydrochlorothiazide have been used singly and concomitantly for the treatment of hypertension. The antihypertensive effects of these agents are additive. The two components of TIMOLIDE have similar dosage schedules, and studies have shown that there is no interference with bioavailability when these agents are given together in the single combination tablet. Therefore, this combination provides a convenient formulation for the concomitant administration of these two entities.
In controlled clinical trials with TIMOLIDE in selected patients with mild to moderate essential hypertension, about 90 percent had a good to excellent response. In patients with more severe hypertension, TIMOLIDE may be administered with other antihypertensives such as ALDOMET* (Methyldopa) or a vasodilator.
Although the mechanisms of action of timolol maleate and hydrochlorothiazide in the treatment of hypertension have not been established, they are thought to be different; for example, hydrochlorothiazide increases plasma renin activity while timolol maleate reduces plasma renin activity.

Timolol Maleate
Timolol maleate is a $beta_1$ and $beta_2$ (non-selective) adrenergic receptor blocking agent that does not have significant intrinsic sympathomimetic, direct myocardial depressant, or local anesthetic activity.

Pharmacodynamics
Clinical pharmacology studies have confirmed the beta-adrenergic blocking activity as shown by (1) changes in resting heart rate and response of heart rate to changes in posture; (2) inhibition of isoproterenol-induced tachycardia; (3) alteration of the response to the Valsalva maneuver and amyl nitrite administration; and (4) reduction of heart rate and blood pressure changes on exercise.
Timolol maleate decreases the positive chronotropic, positive inotropic, bronchodilator, and vasodilator responses caused by beta-adrenergic receptor agonists. The magnitude of this decreased response is proportional to the existing sympathetic tone and the concentration of timolol maleate at receptor sites.
In normal volunteers, the reduction in heart rate response to a standard exercise was dose dependent over the test range of 0.5 to 20 mg, with a peak reduction at 2 hours of approximately 30% at higher doses.
Beta-adrenergic receptor blockade reduces cardiac output in both healthy subjects and patients with heart disease. In patients with severe impairment of myocardial function beta-adrenergic receptor blockade may inhibit the stimulatory effect of the sympathetic nervous system necessary to maintain adequate cardiac function.
Beta-adrenergic receptor blockade in the bronchi and bronchioles results in increased airway resistance from unopposed parasympathetic activity. Such an effect in patients with asthma or other bronchospastic conditions is potentially dangerous.
Clinical studies indicate that timolol maleate at a dosage of 20–60 mg/day reduces blood pressure without causing postural hypotension in most patients with essential hypertension. Administration of timolol maleate to patients with hypertension results initially in a decrease in cardiac output, little immediate change in blood pressure, and an increase in calculated peripheral resistance. With continued administration of timolol maleate blood pressure decreases within a few days, cardiac output usually remains reduced, and pe-

Continued on next page

Information on the Merck & Co., Inc. products listed on these pages is the full prescribing information from product circulars in use September 30, 1996.

Merck & Co.—Cont.

ripheral resistance falls toward pretreatment levels. Plasma volume may decrease or remain unchanged during therapy with timolol maleate. In the majority of patients with hypertension, timolol maleate also decreases plasma renin activity. Dosage adjustment to achieve optimal antihypertensive effect may require a few weeks. When therapy with timolol maleate is discontinued, the blood pressure tends to return to pretreatment levels gradually. In most patients the antihypertensive activity of timolol maleate is maintained with long-term therapy and is well tolerated.

The mechanism of the antihypertensive effects of beta-adrenergic receptor blocking agents is not established at this time. Possible mechanisms of action include reduction in cardiac output, reduction in plasma renin activity, and a central nervous system sympatholytic action.

Pharmacokinetics and Metabolism

Timolol maleate is rapidly and nearly completely absorbed (about 90%) following oral ingestion. Detectable plasma levels of timolol occur within one-half hour and peak plasma levels occur in about one to two hours. The drug half-life in plasma is approximately 4 hours and this is essentially unchanged in patients with moderate renal insufficiency. Timolol is partially metabolized by the liver and timolol and its metabolites are excreted by the kidney. Timolol is not extensively bound to plasma proteins; i.e., < 10% by equilibrium dialysis and approximately 60% by ultrafiltration. An *in vitro* hemodialysis study, using ^{14}C timolol added to human plasma or whole blood, showed that timolol was readily dialyzed from these fluids; however, a study of patients with renal failure showed that timolol did not dialyze readily. Plasma levels following oral administration are about half those following intravenous administration indicating approximately 50% first pass metabolism. The level of beta sympathetic activity varies widely among individuals, and no simple correlation exists between the dose or plasma level of timolol maleate and its therapeutic activity. Therefore, objective clinical measurements such as reduction of heart rate and/or blood pressure should be used as guides in determining the optimal dosage for each patient.

Hydrochlorothiazide

Hydrochlorothiazide is a diuretic and antihypertensive agent. It affects the renal tubular mechanism of electrolyte reabsorption. Hydrochlorothiazide increases excretion of sodium and chloride in approximately equivalent amounts. Natriuresis may be accompanied by some loss of potassium and bicarbonate. The mechanism of the antihypertensive effect of thiazides may be related to the excretion and redistribution of body sodium. Hydrochlorothiazide usually does not cause clinically important changes in normal blood pressure.

---

* Registered trademark of MERCK & CO., INC.

INDICATIONS AND USAGE

TIMOLIDE is indicated for the treatment of hypertension. **This fixed combination drug is not indicated for initial therapy of hypertension. If the fixed combination represents the dose titrated to an individual patient's needs, it may be more convenient than the separate components.**

CONTRAINDICATIONS

TIMOLIDE is contraindicated in patients with bronchial asthma or with a history of bronchial asthma, or severe chronic obstructive pulmonary disease (see WARNINGS); sinus bradycardia; second and third degree atrioventricular block; overt cardiac failure (see WARNINGS); cardiogenic shock; anuria; hypersensitivity to this product or to sulfonamide-derived drugs.

WARNINGS

Cardiac Failure

Sympathetic stimulation may be essential for support of the circulation in individuals with diminished myocardial contractility, and its inhibition by beta-adrenergic receptor blockade may precipitate more severe failure. Although beta blockers should be avoided in overt congestive heart failure, they can be used, if necessary, with caution in patients with a history of failure who are well-compensated, usually with digitalis and diuretics. Both digitalis and timolol maleate slow AV conduction. If cardiac failure persists, therapy with TIMOLIDE should be withdrawn.

In Patients Without a History of Cardiac Failure continued depression of the myocardium with beta-blocking agents over a period of time can, in some cases, lead to cardiac failure. At the first sign or symptom of cardiac failure, patients receiving TIMOLIDE should be digitalized and/or be given additional diuretic therapy. Observe the patient closely. If cardiac failure continues, despite adequate digitalization and diuretic therapy, TIMOLIDE should be withdrawn.

Renal and Hepatic Disease and Electrolyte Disturbances

Since timolol maleate is partially metabolized in the liver and excreted mainly by the kidneys, dosage reductions may be necessary when hepatic and/or renal insufficiency is present.

Although the pharmacokinetics of timolol maleate are not greatly altered by renal impairment, marked hypotensive responses have been seen in patients with marked renal impairment undergoing dialysis after 20 mg doses. Dosing in such patients should therefore be especially cautious.

In patients with renal disease, thiazides may precipitate azotemia, and cumulative effects may develop in the presence of impaired renal function. If progressive renal impairment becomes evident, TIMOLIDE should be discontinued. In patients with impaired hepatic function or progressive liver disease, even minor alterations in fluid and electrolyte balance may precipitate hepatic coma. Hepatic encephalopathy, manifested by tremors, confusion, and coma, has been reported in association with diuretic therapy including hydrochlorothiazide.

Exacerbation of Ischemic Heart Disease Following Abrupt Withdrawal —Hypersensitivity to catecholamines has been observed in patients withdrawn from beta blocker therapy; exacerbation of angina and, in some cases, myocardial infarction have occurred after *abrupt* discontinuation of such therapy. When discontinuing chronically administered timolol maleate, particularly in patients with ischemic heart disease, the dosage should be gradually reduced over a period of one to two weeks and the patient should be carefully monitored. If angina markedly worsens or acute coronary insufficiency develops, timolol maleate administration should be reinstituted promptly, at least temporarily, and other measures appropriate for the management of unstable angina should be taken. Patients should be warned against interruption or discontinuation of therapy without the physician's advice. Because coronary artery disease is common and may be unrecognized, it may be prudent not to discontinue timolol maleate therapy abruptly even in patients treated only for hypertension.

Obstructive Pulmonary Disease

PATIENTS WITH CHRONIC OBSTRUCTIVE PULMONARY DISEASE (e.g., CHRONIC BRONCHITIS, EMPHYSEMA) OF MILD OR MODERATE SEVERITY, BRONCHOSPASTIC DISEASE OR A HISTORY OF BRONCHOSPASTIC DISEASE (OTHER THAN BRONCHIAL ASTHMA OR A HISTORY OF BRONCHIAL ASTHMA, IN WHICH 'TIMOLIDE' IS CONTRAINDICATED, see CONTRAINDICATIONS), SHOULD IN GENERAL NOT RECEIVE BETA BLOCKERS, INCLUDING 'TIMOLIDE'. However, if TIMOLIDE is necessary in such patients, then the drug should be administered with caution since it may block bronchodilation produced by endogenous and exogenous catecholamine stimulation of beta$_2$ receptors.

Major Surgery

The necessity or desirability of withdrawal of beta-blocking therapy prior to major surgery is controversial. Beta-adrenergic receptor blockade impairs the ability of the heart to respond to beta-adrenergically mediated reflex stimuli. This may augment the risk of general anesthesia in surgical procedures. Some patients receiving beta-adrenergic receptor blocking agents have been subject to protracted severe hypotension during anesthesia. Difficulty in restarting and maintaining the heartbeat has also been reported. For these reasons, in patients undergoing elective surgery, some authorities recommend gradual withdrawal of beta-adrenergic receptor blocking agents.

If necessary during surgery, the effects of beta-adrenergic blocking agents may be reversed by sufficient doses of such agonists as isoproterenol, dopamine, dobutamine or levarterenol (see OVERDOSAGE).

Metabolic and Endocrine Effects

Beta-adrenergic blockade may mask certain clinical signs (e.g., tachycardia) of hyperthyroidism. Patients suspected of developing thyrotoxicosis should be managed carefully to avoid abrupt withdrawal of beta blockade which might precipitate a thyroid storm. Thiazides may decrease serum PBI levels without signs of thyroid disturbance.

Beta-adrenergic receptor blocking agents may mask the signs and symptoms of acute hypoglycemia. Therefore, TIMOLIDE should be administered with caution to patients subject to spontaneous hypoglycemia, or to diabetic patients (especially those with labile diabetes) who are receiving insulin or oral hypoglycemic agents. Insulin requirements in diabetic patients may be increased, decreased, or unchanged by thiazides. Diabetes mellitus which has been latent may become manifest during administration of thiazide diuretics. Because calcium excretion is decreased by thiazides, TIMOLIDE should be discontinued before carrying out tests for parathyroid function. Pathologic changes in the parathyroid glands, with hypercalcemia and hypophosphatemia, have been observed in a few patients on prolonged thiazide therapy; however, the common complications of hyperparathyroidism such as renal lithiasis, bone resorption, and peptic ulceration have not been seen.

Hyperuricemia may occur or acute gout may be precipitated in certain patients receiving thiazide therapy.

PRECAUTIONS

General

Electrolyte and Fluid Balance Status: Periodic determination of serum electrolytes to detect possible electrolyte imbalance should be performed at appropriate intervals.

Patients should be observed for clinical signs of fluid or electrolyte imbalance, i.e., hyponatremia, hypochloremic alkalosis, and hypokalemia. Serum and urine electrolyte determinations are particularly important when the patient is vomiting excessively or receiving parenteral fluids. Warning signs or symptoms of fluid and electrolyte imbalance, irrespective of cause, include dryness of the mouth, thirst, weakness, lethargy, drowsiness, restlessness, confusion, seizures, muscle pains or cramps, muscular fatigue, hypotension, oliguria, tachycardia, and gastrointestinal disturbances such as nausea and vomiting.

Hypokalemia may develop, especially with brisk diuresis, when severe cirrhosis is present, or during concomitant use of corticosteroids or ACTH.

Interference with adequate oral electrolyte intake will also contribute to hypokalemia. Hypokalemia may cause cardiac arrhythmia and may also sensitize or exaggerate the response of the heart to the toxic effects of digitalis (e.g., increased ventricular irritability). Hypokalemia may be avoided or treated by use of potassium sparing diuretics or potassium supplements such as foods with a high potassium content.

Any chloride deficit during thiazide therapy is generally mild and usually does not require specific treatment except under extraordinary circumstances (as in liver disease or renal disease). Dilutional hyponatremia may occur in edematous patients in hot weather; appropriate therapy is water restriction rather than administration of salt except in rare instances when the hyponatremia is life threatening. In actual salt depletion, appropriate replacement is the therapy of choice.

Thiazides have been shown to increase urinary excretion of magnesium, which may result in hypomagnesemia.

Effects on Cholesterol and Triglyceride Levels: Increases in cholesterol and triglyceride levels may be associated with thiazide diuretic therapy.

Muscle Weakness: Beta-adrenergic blockade has been reported to potentiate muscle weakness consistent with certain myasthenic symptoms (e.g., diplopia, ptosis, and generalized weakness). Timolol has been reported rarely to increase muscle weakness in some patients with myasthenia gravis or myasthenic symptoms.

Cerebrovascular Insufficiency: Because of potential effects of beta-adrenergic blocking agents relative to blood pressure and pulse, these agents should be used with caution in patients with cerebrovascular insufficiency. If signs or symptoms suggesting reduced cerebral blood flow are observed, consideration should be given to discontinuing these agents.

Drug Interactions

TIMOLIDE may potentiate the action of other antihypertensive agents used concomitantly. Close observation of the patient is recommended when TIMOLIDE is administered to patients receiving catecholamine-depleting drugs such as reserpine, because of possible additive effects and the production of hypotension and/or marked bradycardia, which may produce vertigo, syncope, or postural hypotension.

Blunting of the antihypertensive effect of beta-adrenoceptor blocking agents by non-steroidal anti-inflammatory drugs has been reported. In some patients, the administration of a non-steroidal anti-inflammatory agent can reduce the diuretic, natriuretic, and antihypertensive effects of loop, potassium-sparing and thiazide diuretics. Therefore, when TIMOLIDE and non-steroidal anti-inflammatory agents are used concomitantly, the patient should be observed closely to determine if the desired therapeutic effect has been obtained.

Literature reports suggest that oral calcium antagonists may be used in combination with beta-adrenergic blocking agents when heart function is normal, but should be avoided in patients with impaired cardiac function. Hypotension, AV conduction disturbances, and left ventricular failure have been reported in some patients receiving beta-adrenergic blocking agents when an oral calcium antagonist was added to the treatment regimen. Hypotension was more likely to occur if the calcium antagonist were a dihydropyridine derivative, e.g., nifedipine, while left ventricular failure and AV conduction disturbances were more likely to occur with either verapamil or diltiazem.

Intravenous calcium antagonists should be used with caution in patients receiving beta-adrenergic blocking agents. The concomitant use of beta-adrenergic blocking agents with digitalis and either diltiazem or verapamil may have additive effects in prolonging AV conduction time.

Risk from Anaphylactic Reaction: While taking beta-blockers, patients with a history of atopy or a history of severe anaphylactic reaction to a variety of allergens may be more reactive to repeated accidental, diagnostic, or therapeutic challenge with such allergens. Such patients may be unresponsive to the usual doses of epinephrine used to treat anaphylactic reactions.

In patients receiving thiazides, sensitivity reactions may occur with or without a history of allergy or bronchial asthma. The possible exacerbation or activation of systemic lupus erythematosus has been reported. The antihypertensive effects of thiazides may be enhanced in the post-sympathectomy patient.

Thiazides may decrease arterial responsiveness to norepinephrine. This diminution is not sufficient to preclude the therapeutic effectiveness of norepinephrine. Thiazides may increase the responsiveness to tubocurarine.

Lithium generally should not be given with diuretics because they reduce its renal clearance and add a high risk of lithium toxicity. Read circulars for lithium preparations before use of such preparations with TIMOLIDE.

Absorption of hydrochlorothiazide is impaired in the presence of anionic exchange resins. Single doses of either cholestyramine or colestipol resins bind the hydrochlorothiazide and reduce its absorption from the gastrointestinal tract by up to 85 and 43 percent, respectively.

Carcinogenesis, Mutagenesis, Impairment of Fertility

Carcinogenicity, mutagenicity, and fertility studies have not been conducted in animals with TIMOLIDE.

Timolol maleate: In a two-year study of timolol maleate in rats, there was a statistically significant increase in the incidence of adrenal pheochromocytomas in male rats administered 300 mg/kg/day (250 times* the maximum recommended daily human dose). Similar differences were not observed in rats administered doses equivalent to approximately 20 or 80 times* the maximum recommended daily human dose.

In a lifetime study in mice, there were statistically significant increases in the incidence of benign and malignant pulmonary tumors, benign uterine polyps and mammary adenocarcinoma in female mice at 500 mg/kg/day (approximately 400 times* the maximum recommended daily human dose), but not at 5 or 50 mg/kg/day. In a subsequent study in female mice, in which post-mortem examinations were limited to uterus and lungs, a statistically significant increase in the incidence of pulmonary tumors was again observed at 500 mg/kg/day.

The increased occurrence of mammary adenocarcinoma was associated with elevations of serum prolactin that occurred in female mice administered timolol at 500 mg/kg/day, but not at doses of 5 or 50 mg/kg/day. An increased incidence of mammary adenocarcinomas in rodents has been associated with administration of several other therapeutic agents which elevate serum prolactin, but no correlation between serum prolactin levels and mammary tumors has been established in man. Furthermore, in adult human female subjects who received oral dosages of up to 60 mg of timolol maleate, the maximum recommended daily human oral dosage, there were no clinically meaningful changes in serum prolactin.

Timolol maleate was devoid of mutagenic potential when evaluated *in vivo* (mouse) in the micronucleus test and cytogenetic assay (doses up to 800 mg/kg) and *in vitro* in a neoplastic cell transformation assay (up to 100 μg/mL). In Ames tests the highest concentrations of timolol employed, 5000 or 10,000 μg/plate, were associated with statistically significant elevations of revertants observed with tester strain TA100 (in seven replicate assays), but not in three additional strains. In the assays with tester strain TA100, no consistent dose response relationship was observed, nor did the ratio of test to control revertants reach 2. A ratio of 2 is usually considered the criterion for a positive Ames test.

Reproduction and fertility studies in rats showed no adverse effect on male or female fertility at doses up to 125 times* the maximum recommended daily human dose.

Hydrochlorothiazide: Two-year feeding studies in mice and rats conducted under the auspices of the National Toxicology Program (NTP) uncovered no evidence of a carcinogenic potential of hydrochlorothiazide in female mice (at doses of up to approximately 600 mg/kg/day) or in male and female rats (at doses of up to approximately 100 mg/kg/day). The NTP, however, found equivocal evidence for hepatocarcinogenicity in male mice.

Hydrochlorothiazide was not genotoxic *in vitro* in the Ames mutagenicity assay of *Salmonella typhimurium* strains TA 98, TA 100, TA 1535, TA 1537, and TA 1538 and in the Chinese Hamster Ovary (CHO) test for chromosomal aberrations, or *in vivo* in assays using mouse germinal cell chromosomes, Chinese hamster bone marrow chromosomes, and the *Drosophila* sex-linked recessive lethal trait gene. Positive test results were obtained only in the *in vitro* CHO Sister Chromatid Exchange (clastogenicity) and in the Mouse Lymphoma Cell (mutagenicity) assay, using concentrations of hydrochlorothiazide from 43 to 1300 μg/mL, and in the *Aspergillus nidulans* nondisjunction assay at an unspecified concentration.

Hydrochlorothiazide had no adverse effects on the fertility of mice and rats of either sex in studies wherein these species were exposed, via their diet, to doses of up to 100 and 4 mg/kg, respectively, prior to conception and throughout gestation.

---

*Based on patient weight of 50 kg

Pregnancy

Teratogenic Effects—Pregnancy Category C. Combinations of timolol maleate and hydrochlorothiazide were studied for teratogenic potential in the mouse and rabbit. The timolol maleate/hydrochlorothiazide combinations were administered orally to pregnant mice and pregnant rabbits at dosage levels of 1/2.5, 4/10, or 8/10 mg/kg/day. No teratogenic, embryotoxic, fetotoxic, or maternotoxic effects attributable to treatment were observed in either species. There are no adequate and well-controlled studies in pregnant women with TIMOLIDE. Because of the data listed below with the individual components, TIMOLIDE should be used during pregnancy only if the potential benefit justifies the potential risk to the fetus.

Timolol Maleate: Teratogenicity studies with timolol maleate in mice, rats and rabbits at doses up to 50 mg/kg/day (approximately 40 times* the maximum recommended daily human dose) showed no evidence of fetal malformations. Although delayed fetal ossification was observed at this dose in rats, there were no adverse effects on postnatal development of offspring. Doses of 1000 mg/kg/day (approximately 830 times* the maximum recommended daily human dose) were maternotoxic in mice and resulted in an increased number of fetal resorptions. Increased fetal resorptions were also seen in rabbits at doses of approximately 40 times* the maximum recommended daily human dose, in this case without apparent maternotoxicity.

Hydrochlorothiazide: Studies in which hydrochlorothiazide was orally administered to pregnant mice and rats during their respecitve periods of major organogenesis at doses up to 3000 and 1000 mg hydrochlorothiazide/kg, respectively, provided no evidence of harm to the fetus.

Nonteratogenic Effects.

Hydrochlorothiazide: TIMOLIDE contains hydrochlorothiazide. Thiazides cross the placental barrier and appear in cord blood. The possible hazards to the fetus include fetal or neonatal jaundice, thrombocytopenia, and possibly other adverse reactions which have occurred in the adult.

---

* Based on patient weight of 50 kg

Nursing Mothers

Timolol maleate and thiazides have been detected in human milk. Because of the potential for serious adverse reactions from timolol and hydrochlorothiazide in nursing infants, a decision should be made whether to discontinue nursing or to discontinue the drug, taking into account the importance of the drug to the mother.

Pediatric Use

Safety and effectiveness in pediatric patients have not been established.

ADVERSE REACTIONS

TIMOLIDE is usually well tolerated in properly selected patients. Most adverse effects have been mild and transient. The adverse reactions listed in the following table were spontaneously reported and have been arranged into two groups: (1) incidence greater than 1%; and (2) incidence less than 1%. The incidence was obtained from clinical studies conducted in the United States (257 patients treated with TIMOLIDE).

Incidence Greater Than 1%	*Incidence Less Than 1%*
BODY AS A WHOLE	
fatigue/tiredness (1.9%)	chest pain
	headache
asthenia (1.9%)	
CARDIOVASCULAR	
hypotension (1.6%)	arrhythmia
bradycardia (1.2%)	syncope
	cardiac failure
DIGESTIVE SYSTEM	
none	diarrhea
	dyspepsia
	nausea
	gastrointestinal pain
	constipation
INTEGUMENTARY	
none	rash
	increased pigmentation
	dry mucous membranes
MUSCULOSKELETAL	
none	myalgia
NERVOUS SYSTEM	
dizziness (1.2%)	none
PSYCHIATRIC	
none	insomnia
	decreased libido
	nervousness
	confusion
	trouble concentrating
	somnolence
RESPIRATORY	
bronchial spasm (1.6%)	rales
dyspnea (1.2%)	
UROGENITAL	
none	renal colic

The following additional adverse effects have been reported in clinical experience with the drug: cerebral ischemia, cerebral vascular accident, gout, muscle cramps, oculogyric crisis, worsening of chronic obstructive pulmonary disease, earache, and impotence.

Other adverse reactions that have been reported with the individual components are listed below:

Timolol Maleate—Body as a Whole: extremity pain, decreased exercise tolerance, weight loss, fever; *Cardiovascular:* cardiac arrest, cerebral vascular accident, worsening of angina pectoris, sinoatrial block, AV block, worsening of arterial insufficiency, Raynaud's phenomenon, claudication, palpitations, vasodilatation, cold hands and feet, edema; *Digestive:* hepatomegaly, elevated liver function tests, vomiting; *Hematologic:* nonthrombocytopenic purpura; *Endocrine:* hyperglycemia, hypoglycemia; *Skin:* skin irritation, pruritus, sweating, alopecia; *Musculoskeletal:* arthralgia; *Nervous System:* local weakness, vertigo, paresthesia, increase in signs and symptoms of myasthenia gravis; *Psychiatric:* depression, nightmares, hallucinations; *Respiratory:* cough; *Special Senses:* visual disturbances, diplopia, ptosis, eye irritation, dry eyes, tinnitus; *Urogenital:* urination difficulties.

There have been reports of retroperitoneal fibrosis in patients receiving timolol maleate and in patients receiving other beta-adrenergic blocking agents. A causal relationship between this condition and therapy with beta-adrenergic blocking agents has not been established.

Hydrochlorothiazide—Body as a Whole: weakness; *Digestive:* anorexia, gastric irritation, vomiting, cramping, jaundice (intrahepatic cholestatic jaundice), pancreatitis, sialadenitis; *Nervous System/Psychiatric:* vertigo, paresthesias, restlessness; *Hematologic:* leukopenia, agranulocytosis, thrombocytopenia, aplastic anemia, hemolytic anemia; *Cardiovascular:* hypotension including orthostatic hypotension (may be aggravated by alcohol, barbiturates, narcotics or antihypertensive drugs); *Hypersensitivity:* purpura, photosensitivity, urticaria, necrotizing angiitis (vasculitis, cutaneous vasculitis), fever, respiratory distress including pneumonitis and pulmonary edema, anaphylactic reactions; *Metabolic:* hyperglycemia, glycosuria, hyperuricemia, electrolyte imbalance (see PRECAUTIONS); *Musculoskeletal:* muscle spasm; *Renal:* renal failure, renal dysfunction, interstitial nephritis (See WARNINGS); *Skin:* erythema multiforme including Stevens-Johnson syndrome, exfoliative dermatitis including toxic epidermal necrolysis, alopecia; *Special Senses:* transient blurred vision, xanthopsia.

Potential Adverse Effects: In addition, a variety of adverse effects not observed in clinical trials with timolol maleate, but reported with other beta-adrenergic blocking agents, should be considered potential adverse effects of timolol maleate: *Nervous System:* reversible mental depression progressing to catatonia; an acute reversible syndrome characterized by disorientation for time and place, short-term memory loss, emotional lability, slightly clouded sensorium, and decreased performance on neuropsychometrics; *Cardiovascular:* intensification of AV block (see CONTRAINDICATIONS); *Digestive:* mesenteric arterial thrombosis, ischemic colitis; *Hematologic:* agranulocytosis, thrombocytopenic purpura; *Allergic:* erythematous rash, fever combined with aching and sore throat, laryngospasm with respiratory distress; *Miscellaneous:* Peyronie's disease.

There have been reports of a syndrome comprising psoriasiform skin rash, conjunctivitis sicca, otitis, and sclerosing serositis attributed to the beta-adrenergic receptor blocking agent, practolol. This syndrome has not been reported with TIMOLIDE or BLOCADREN* (Timolol Maleate).

Clinical Laboratory Test Findings: Clinically important changes in standard laboratory parameters were rarely associated with the administration of TIMOLIDE. The changes in laboratory parameters were not progressive and usually were not associated with clinical manifestations. The most common changes were increases in serum triglycerides and

Continued on next page

Information on the Merck & Co., Inc. products listed on these pages is the full prescribing information from product circulars in use September 30, 1996.

Merck & Co.—Cont.

uric acid and decreases in serum potassium and chloride. Decreases in HDL cholesterol have been reported.

* Registered trademark of MERCK & CO., INC.

OVERDOSAGE

No data are available with regard to overdosage with TIMOLIDE in humans.
Pretreatment of mice with hydrochlorothiazide (5 mg/kg) did not alter the LD_{50} of timolol (1320 mg/kg compared to 1300 mg/kg without pretreatment).
No specific information is available on the treatment of overdosage with TIMOLIDE, and no specific antidote is available. Treatment is symptomatic and supportive. Therapy with TIMOLIDE should be discontinued and the patient observed closely. Suggested measures include induction of emesis and/or gastric lavage, and correction of dehydration, electrolyte imbalance, and hypotension by established procedures.
Timolol Maleate
Overdosage has been reported with Tablets BLOCADREN* (timolol maleate). A 30-year-old female ingested 650 mg of BLOCADREN (maximum recommended daily dose—60 mg) and experienced second and third degree heart block. She recovered without treatment but approximately two months later developed irregular heartbeat, hypertension, dizziness, tinnitus, faintness, increased pulse rate and borderline first degree heart block.
The oral LD_{50} of the drug is 1190 and 900 mg/kg in female mice and female rats, respectively.
An *in vitro* hemodialysis study, using ^{14}C timolol added to human plasma or whole blood, showed that timolol was readily dialyzed from these fluids; however, a study of patients with renal failure showed that timolol did not dialyze readily.
The most common signs and symptoms to be expected with overdosage with a beta-adrenergic receptor blocking agent are symptomatic bradycardia, hypotension, bronchospasm, and acute cardiac failure. If overdosage occurs the following therapeutic measures should be considered:

(1) *Gastric lavage.*

(2) *Symptomatic bradycardia:* Use atropine sulfate intravenously in a dosage of 0.25 mg to 2 mg to induce vagal blockade. If bradycardia persists, intravenous isoproterenol hydrochloride should be administered cautiously. In refractory cases the use of a transvenous cardiac pacemaker may be considered.

(3) *Hypotension:* Use sympathomimetic pressor drug therapy, such as dopamine, dobutamine or levarterenol. In refractory cases the use of glucagon hydrochloride has been reported to be useful.

(4) *Bronchospasm:* Use isoproterenol hydrochloride. Additional therapy with aminophylline may be considered.

(5) *Acute cardiac failure:* Conventional therapy with digitalis, diuretics, and oxygen should be instituted immediately. In refractory cases the use of intravenous aminophylline is suggested. This may be followed, if necessary, by glucagon hydrochloride which has been reported to be useful.

(6) *Heart block (second or third degree):* Use isoproterenol hydrochloride or a transvenous cardiac pacemaker.

Hydrochlorothiazide
The most common signs and symptoms observed with hydrochlorothiazide overdosage are those caused by electrolyte depletion (hypokalemia, hypochloremia, hyponatremia) and dehydration resulting from excessive diuresis. If digitalis has also been administered, hypokalemia may accentuate cardiac arrhythmias.

* Registered trademark of MERCK & CO., INC.

DOSAGE AND ADMINISTRATION

The recommended starting and maintenance dosage is 1 tablet twice a day or 2 tablets once a day. Patients usually do not require doses in excess of 50 mg of hydrochlorothiazide daily when combined with other antihypertensive agents. If the antihypertensive response is not satisfactory, another nondiuretic antihypertensive agent may be added.

HOW SUPPLIED

No. 3373—Tablets TIMOLIDE 10-25 are light blue, flat, hexagonal-shaped, compressed tablets, with code MSD 67 on one side and TIMOLIDE on the other. Each tablet contains 10 mg of timolol maleate and 25 mg of hydrochlorothiazide. They are supplied as follows:
NDC 0006-0067-68 bottles of 100.
Shown in Product Identification Guide, page 325
Storage
Store at controlled room temperature, 15–30°C (59–86°F). Keep container tightly closed. Protect from light.
7928431 Issued May 1995
COPYRIGHT © MERCK & CO., INC., 1985
All rights reserved

TIMOPTIC® Sterile Ophthalmic Solution 0.25% and 0.5% (Timolol Maleate Ophthalmic Solution), U.S.P. ℞

DESCRIPTION

TIMOPTIC* (Timolol Maleate) Ophthalmic Solution is a non-selective beta-adrenergic receptor blocking agent. Its chemical name is (-)-1-(*tert*-butylamino)-3-[(4-morpholino-1,2,5-thiadiazol-3-yl)oxy]-2-propanol maleate (1:1) (salt). Timolol maleate possesses an asymmetric carbon atom in its structure and is provided as the levo-isomer. The nominal optical rotation of timolol maleate is:

$$[\alpha]^{25^\circ}_{405\ nm} \text{ in 0.1N HCl (C = 5\%)} = -12.2^\circ.$$

Its molecular formula is $C_{13}H_{24}N_4O_3S \cdot C_4H_4O_4$ and its structural formula is:

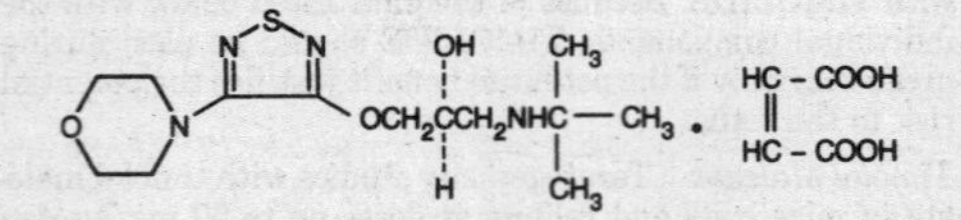

Timolol maleate has a molecular weight of 432.50. It is a white, odorless, crystalline powder which is soluble in water, methanol, and alcohol. TIMOPTIC is stable at room temperature.
TIMOPTIC Ophthalmic Solution is supplied as a sterile, isotonic, buffered, aqueous solution of timolol maleate in two dosage strengths: Each mL of TIMOPTIC 0.25% contains 2.5 mg of timolol (3.4 mg of timolol maleate). Each mL of TIMOPTIC 0.5% contains 5.0 mg of timolol (6.8 mg of timolol maleate). Inactive ingredients: monobasic and dibasic sodium phosphate, sodium hydroxide to adjust pH, and water for injection. Benzalkonium chloride 0.01% is added as preservative.

* Registered trademark of MERCK & CO., INC.

CLINICAL PHARMACOLOGY

Timolol maleate is a $beta_1$ and $beta_2$ (non-selective) adrenergic receptor blocking agent that does not have significant intrinsic sympathomimetic, direct myocardial depressant, or local anesthetic (membrane-stabilizing) activity.
Beta-adrenergic receptor blockade reduces cardiac output in both healthy subjects and patients with heart disease. In patients with severe impairment of myocardial function beta-adrenergic receptor blockade may inhibit the stimulatory effect of the sympathetic nervous system necessary to maintain adequate cardiac function.
Beta-adrenergic receptor blockade in the bronchi and bronchioles results in increased airway resistance from unopposed parasympathetic activity. Such an effect in patients with asthma or other bronchospastic conditions is potentially dangerous.
TIMOPTIC Ophthalmic Solution, when applied topically on the eye, has the action of reducing elevated as well as normal intraocular pressure, whether or not accompanied by glaucoma. Elevated intraocular pressure is a major risk factor in the pathogenesis of glaucomatous visual field loss. The higher the level of intraocular pressure, the greater the likelihood of glaucomatous visual field loss and optic nerve damage.
The onset of reduction in intraocular pressure following administration of TIMOPTIC can usually be detected within one-half hour after a single dose. The maximum effect usually occurs in one to two hours and significant lowering of intraocular pressure can be maintained for periods as long as 24 hours with a single dose. Repeated observations over a period of one year indicate that the intraocular pressure-lowering effect of TIMOPTIC is well maintained.
The precise mechanism of the ocular hypotensive action of TIMOPTIC is not clearly established at this time. Tonography and fluorophotometry studies in man suggest that its predominant action may be related to reduced aqueous formation. However, in some studies a slight increase in outflow facility was also observed. Unlike miotics, TIMOPTIC reduces intraocular pressure with little or no effect on accommodation or pupil size. Thus, changes in visual acuity due to increased accommodation are uncommon, and dim or blurred vision and night blindness produced by miotics are not evident. In addition, in patients with cataracts the inability to see around lenticular opacities when the pupil is constricted is avoided.
In the clinical studies which are reported below, ocular pressure reductions to less than 22 mmHg were used as a reasonable reference point to allow comparisons between treatments. Reduction of ocular pressure to just below 22 mmHg may not be optimal for all patients; therapy should be individualized.
In controlled multiclinic studies in patients with untreated intraocular pressures of 22 mmHg or greater, TIMOPTIC 0.25 percent or 0.5 percent administered twice a day produced a greater reduction in intraocular pressure than 1, 2, 3, or 4 percent pilocarpine solution administered four times a day or 0.5, 1, or 2 percent epinephrine hydrochloride solution administered twice a day.
In the multiclinic studies comparing TIMOPTIC with pilocarpine, 61 percent of patients treated with TIMOPTIC had intraocular pressure reduced to less than 22 mmHg compared to 32 percent of patients treated with pilocarpine. For patients completing these studies, the mean reduction in pressure at the end of the study from pretreatment was 30.7 percent for patients treated with TIMOPTIC and 21.7 percent for patients treated with pilocarpine.
In the multiclinic studies comparing TIMOPTIC with epinephrine, 69 percent of patients treated with TIMOPTIC had intraocular pressure reduced to less than 22 mmHg compared to 42 percent of patients treated with epinephrine. For patients completing these studies, the mean reduction in pressure at the end of the study from pretreatment was 33.2 percent for patients treated with TIMOPTIC and 28.1 percent for patients treated with epinephrine.
In these studies, TIMOPTIC was generally well tolerated and produced fewer and less severe side effects than either pilocarpine or epinephrine. A slight reduction of resting heart rate in some patients receiving TIMOPTIC (mean reduction 2.9 beats/minute standard deviation 10.2) was observed.
TIMOPTIC has also been used in patients with glaucoma wearing conventional (PMMA) hard contact lenses, and has generally been well tolerated. TIMOPTIC has not been studied in patients wearing lenses made with materials other than PMMA. (See PRECAUTIONS, *Information for Patients.*)

INDICATIONS AND USAGE

TIMOPTIC Ophthalmic Solution is indicated in the treatment of elevated intraocular pressure in patients with ocular hypertension or open-angle glaucoma.

CONTRAINDICATIONS

TIMOPTIC is contraindicated in patients with (1) bronchial asthma; (2) a history of bronchial asthma; (3) severe chronic obstructive pulmonary disease (see **WARNINGS**); (4) sinus bradycardia; (5) second or third degree atrioventricular block; (6) overt cardiac failure (see **WARNINGS**); (7) cardiogenic shock; or (8) hypersensitivity to any component of this product.

WARNINGS

As with many topically applied ophthalmic drugs, this drug is absorbed systemically.
The same adverse reactions found with systemic administration of beta-adrenergic blocking agents may occur with topical administration. For example, severe respiratory reactions and cardiac reactions, including death due to bronchospasm in patients with asthma, and rarely death in association with cardiac failure, have been reported following systemic or ophthalmic administration of timolol maleate (see CONTRAINDICATIONS).
Cardiac Failure
Sympathetic stimulation may be essential for support of the circulation in individuals with diminished myocardial contractility, and its inhibition by beta-adrenergic receptor blockade may precipitate more severe failure.
In Patients Without a History of Cardiac Failure continued depression of the myocardium with beta-blocking agents over a period of time can, in some cases, lead to cardiac failure. At the first sign or symptom of cardiac failure TIMOPTIC should be discontinued.
Obstructive Pulmonary Disease
Patients with chronic obstructive pulmonary disease (e.g., chronic bronchitis, emphysema) of mild or moderate severity, bronchospastic disease, or a history of bronchospastic disease (other than bronchial asthma or a history of bronchial asthma, in which TIMOPTIC is contraindicated [see **CONTRAINDICATIONS**]) should, in general, not receive beta-blockers, including TIMOPTIC.
Major Surgery
The necessity or desirability of withdrawal of beta-adrenergic blocking agents prior to major surgery is controversial. Beta-adrenergic receptor blockade impairs the ability of the heart to respond to beta-adrenergically mediated reflex stimuli. This may augment the risk of general anesthesia in surgical procedures. Some patients receiving beta-adrenergic receptor blocking agents have experienced protracted severe hypotension during anesthesia. Difficulty in restarting and maintaining the heartbeat has also been reported. For these reasons, in patients undergoing elective surgery, some authorities recommend gradual withdrawal of beta-adrenergic receptor blocking agents.
If necessary during surgery, the effects of beta-adrenergic blocking agents may be reversed by sufficient doses of adrenergic agonists.

Diabetes Mellitus
Beta-adrenergic blocking agents should be administered with caution in patients subject to spontaneous hypoglycemia or to diabetic patients (especially those with labile diabetes) who are receiving insulin or oral hypoglycemic agents. Beta-adrenergic receptor blocking agents may mask the signs and symptoms of acute hypoglycemia.
Thyrotoxicosis
Beta-adrenergic blocking agents may mask certain clinical signs (e.g., tachycardia) of hyperthyroidism. Patients suspected of developing thyrotoxicosis should be managed carefully to avoid abrupt withdrawal of beta-adrenergic blocking agents that might precipitate a thyroid storm.

PRECAUTIONS

General
Because of potential effects of beta-adrenergic blocking agents on blood pressure and pulse, these agents should be used with caution in patients with cerebrovascular insufficiency. If signs or symptoms suggesting reduced cerebral blood flow develop following initiation of therapy with TIMOPTIC, alternative therapy should be considered.
There have been reports of bacterial keratitis associated with the use of multiple dose containers of topical ophthalmic products. These containers had been inadvertently contaminated by patients who, in most cases, had a concurrent corneal disease or a disruption of the ocular epithelial surface. (See **PRECAUTIONS**, *Information for Patients.*)
Choroidal detachment after filtration procedures has been reported with the administration of aqueous suppressant therapy (e.g. timolol).
Angle-closure glaucoma: In patients with angle-closure glaucoma, the immediate objective of treatment is to reopen the angle. This requires constricting the pupil. Timolol maleate has little or no effect on the pupil. TIMOPTIC should not be used alone in the treatment of angle-closure glaucoma.
Anaphylaxis: While taking beta-blockers, patients with a history of atopy or a history of severe anaphylactic reactions to a variety of allergens may be more reactive to repeated accidental, diagnostic, or therapeutic challenge with such allergens. Such patients may be unresponsive to the usual doses of epinephrine used to treat anaphylactic reactions.
Muscle Weakness: Beta-adrenergic blockade has been reported to potentiate muscle weakness consistent with certain myasthenic symptoms (e.g., diplopia, ptosis, and generalized weakness). Timolol has been reported rarely to increase muscle weakness in some patients with myasthenia gravis or myasthenic symptoms.
As with the use of other antiglaucoma drugs, diminished responsiveness to TIMOPTIC after prolonged therapy has been reported in some patients. However, in one long-term study in which 96 patients have been followed for at least 3 years, no significant difference in mean intraocular pressure has been observed after initial stabilization.
Information for Patients
Patients should be instructed to avoid allowing the tip of the dispensing container to contact the eye or surrounding structures.
Patients should also be instructed that ocular solutions, if handled improperly, can become contaminated by common bacteria known to cause ocular infections. Serious damage to the eye and subsequent loss of vision may result from using contaminated solutions. (See **PRECAUTIONS**, *General.*)
Patients should also be advised that if they develop an intercurrent ocular condition (e.g., trauma, ocular surgery or infection), they should immediately seek their physician's advice concerning the continued use of the present multidose container.
Patients with bronchial asthma, a history of bronchial asthma, severe chronic obstructive pulmonary disease, sinus bradycardia, second or third degree atrioventricular block, or cardiac failure should be advised not to take this product. (See **CONTRAINDICATIONS**.)
The preservative in TIMOPTIC, benzalkonium chloride, may be absorbed by soft contact lenses. Patients wearing soft contact lenses should be instructed to wait at least 15 minutes after instilling TIMOPTIC before they insert their lenses.
Drug Interactions
Although TIMOPTIC used alone has little or no effect on pupil size, mydriasis resulting from concomitant therapy with TIMOPTIC and epinephrine has been reported occasionally.
Beta-adrenergic blocking agents: Patients who are receiving a beta-adrenergic blocking agent orally and TIMOPTIC should be observed for potential additive effects of beta-blockade, both systemic and on intraocular pressure. Patients should not usually receive two topical ophthalmic beta-adrenergic blocking agents concurrently.
Calcium antagonists: Caution should be used in the coadministration of beta-adrenergic blocking agents, such as TIMOPTIC, and oral or intravenous calcium antagonists because of possible atrioventricular conduction disturbances, left ventricular failure, and hypotension. In patients with impaired cardiac function, coadministration should be avoided.
Catecholamine-depleting drugs: Close observation of the patient is recommended when a beta blocker is administered to patients receiving catecholamine-depleting drugs such as reserpine, because of possible additive effects and the production of hypotension and/or marked bradycardia, which may result in vertigo, syncope, or postural hypotension.
Digitalis and calcium antagonists: The concomitant use of beta-adrenergic blocking agents with digitalis and calcium antagonists may have additive effects in prolonging atrioventricular conduction time.
Injectable Epinephrine: (See **PRECAUTIONS**, *General, Anaphylaxis*)
Carcinogenesis, Mutagenesis, Impairment of Fertility
In a two-year oral study of timolol maleate administered orally to rats, there was a statistically significant increase in the incidence of adrenal pheochromocytomas in male rats administered 300 mg/kg/day (approximately 42,000 times the systemic exposure following the maximum recommended human ophthalmic dose). Similar differences were not observed in rats administered oral doses equivalent to approximately 14,000 times the maximum recommended human ophthalmic dose.
In a lifetime oral study in mice, there were statistically significant increases in the incidence of benign and malignant pulmonary tumors, benign uterine polyps and mammary adenocarcinomas in female mice at 500 mg/kg/day (approximately 71,000 times the systemic exposure following the maximum recommended human ophthalmic dose), but not at 5 or 50 mg/kg/day (approximately 700 or 7,000, respectively, times the systemic exposure following the maximum recommended human ophthalmic dose). In a subsequent study in female mice, in which post-mortem examinations were limited to the uterus and the lungs, a statistically significant increase in the incidence of pulmonary tumors was again observed at 500 mg/kg/day.
The increased occurrence of mammary adenocarcinomas was associated with elevations in serum prolactin which occurred in female mice administered oral timolol at 500 mg/kg, but not at doses of 5 or 50 mg/kg/day. An increased incidence of mammary adenocarcinomas in rodents has been associated with administration of several other therapeutic agents that elevate serum prolactin, but no correlation between serum prolactin levels and mammary tumors has been established in humans. Furthermore, in adult human female subjects who received oral dosages of up to 60 mg of timolol maleate (the maximum recommended human oral dosage), there were no clinically meaningful changes in serum prolactin.
Timolol maleate was devoid of mutagenic potential when tested *in vivo* (mouse) in the micronucleus test and cytogenetic assay (doses up to 800 mg/kg) and *in vitro* in a neoplastic cell transformation assay (up to 100 μg/mL). In Ames tests the highest concentrations of timolol employed, 5000 or 10,000 μg/plate, were associated with statistically significant elevations of revertants observed with tester strain TA100 (in seven replicate assays), but not in the remaining three strains. In the assays with tester strain TA100, no consistent dose response relationship was observed, and the ratio of test to control revertants did not reach 2. A ratio of 2 is usually considered the criterion for a positive Ames test.
Reproduction and fertility studies in rats demonstrated no adverse effect on male or female fertility at doses up to 21,000 times the systemic exposure following the maximum recommended human ophthalmic dose.
Pregnancy-Teratogenic effects:
Pregnancy Category C. Teratogenicity studies with timolol in mice, rats, and rabbits at oral doses up to 50 mg/kg/day (7,000 times the systemic exposure following the maximum recommended human ophthalmic dose) demonstrated no evidence of fetal malformations. Although delayed fetal ossification was observed at this dose in rats, there were no adverse effects on postnatal development of offspring. Doses of 1000 mg/kg/day (142,000 times the systemic exposure following the maximum recommended human ophthalmic dose) were maternotoxic in mice and resulted in an increased number of fetal resorptions. Increased fetal resorptions were also seen in rabbits at doses of 14,000 times the systemic exposure following the maximum recommended human ophthalmic dose, in this case without apparent maternotoxicity.
There are no adequate and well-controlled studies in pregnant women. TIMOPTIC should be used during pregnancy only if the potential benefit justifies the potential risk to the fetus.
Nursing Mothers
Timolol maleate has been detected in human milk following oral and ophthalmic drug administration. Because of the potential for serious adverse reactions from TIMOPTIC in nursing infants, a decision should be made whether to discontinue nursing or to discontinue the drug, taking into account the importance of the drug to the mother.
Pediatric Use
Safety and effectiveness in pediatric patients have not been established.

ADVERSE REACTIONS

The most frequently reported adverse experiences have been burning and stinging upon instillation (approximately one in eight patients).
The following additional adverse experiences have been reported less frequently with ocular administration of this or other timolol maleate formulations:
BODY AS A WHOLE
Headache, asthenia/fatigue, and chest pain.
CARDIOVASCULAR
Bradycardia, arrhythmia, hypotension, hypertension, syncope, heart block, cerebral vascular accident, cerebral ischemia, cardiac failure, worsening of angina pectoris, palpitation, cardiac arrest, and pulmonary edema.
DIGESTIVE
Nausea, diarrhea, dyspepsia, anorexia, and dry mouth.
IMMUNOLOGIC
Systemic lupus erythematosus.
NERVOUS SYSTEM/PSYCHIATRIC
Dizziness, depression, increase in signs and symptoms of myasthenia gravis, paresthesia, behavioral changes including confusion, hallucinations, anxiety, disorientation, nervousness, somnolence, and other psychic disturbances.
SKIN
Hypersensitivity, including localized and generalized rash; urticaria, alopecia.
RESPIRATORY
Bronchospasm (predominantly in patients with pre-existing bronchospastic disease), respiratory failure, dyspnea, nasal congestion, cough and upper respiratory infections.
ENDOCRINE
Masked symptoms of hypoglycemia in diabetic patients (see **WARNINGS**).
SPECIAL SENSES
Signs and symptoms of ocular irritation including conjunctivitis, blepharitis, keratitis, ocular pain, discharge (e.g., crusting), foreign body sensation, and itching and tearing; ptosis; decreased corneal sensitivity; cystoid macular edema; visual disturbances including refractive changes and diplopia; pseudopemphigoid; and choroidal detachment following filtration surgery (see **PRECAUTIONS**, *General*).
UROGENITAL
Retroperitoneal fibrosis and impotence.
The following additional adverse effects have been reported in clinical experience with ORAL timolol maleate or other ORAL beta-blocking agents and may be considered potential effects of ophthalmic timolol maleate: *Allergic:* Erythematous rash, fever combined with aching and sore throat, laryngospasm with respiratory distress; *Body as a Whole:* Extremity pain, decreased exercise tolerance, weight loss; *Cardiovascular:* Edema, worsening of arterial insufficiency, Raynaud's phenomenon, vasodilatation; *Digestive:* Gastrointestinal pain, hepatomegaly, vomiting, mesenteric arterial thrombosis, ischemic colitis; *Hematologic:* Nonthrombocytopenic purpura; thrombocytopenic purpura, agranulocytosis; *Endocrine:* Hyperglycemia, hypoglycemia; *Skin:* Pruritus, skin irritation, increased pigmentation, sweating, cold hands and feet; *Musculoskeletal:* Arthralgia, claudication; *Nervous System/Psychiatric:* Vertigo, local weakness, decreased libido, nightmares, insomnia, diminished concentration, reversible mental depression progressing to catatonia, an acute reversible syndrome characterized by disorientation for time and place, short-term memory loss, emotional lability, slightly clouded sensorium, and decreased performance on neuropsychometrics; *Respiratory:* Rales, bronchial obstruction; *Special Senses:* Tinnitus, dry eyes; *Urogenital:* Urination difficulties, Peyronie's disease.

OVERDOSAGE

There have been reports of inadvertent overdosage with TIMOPTIC Ophthalmic Solution resulting in systemic effects similar to those seen with systemic beta-adrenergic blocking agents such as dizziness, headache, shortness of breath, bradycardia, bronchospasm, and cardiac arrest (see also **ADVERSE REACTIONS**).
Overdosage has been reported with Tablets BLOCADREN* (Timolol Maleate). A 30 year old female ingested 650 mg of BLOCADREN (maximum recommended oral daily dose is 60 mg) and experienced second and third degree heart block. She recovered without treatment but approximately two months later developed irregular heartbeat, hypertension, dizziness, tinnitus, faintness, increased pulse rate, and borderline first degree heart block.
Significant lethality was observed in female rats and female mice after a single dose of 900 and 1190 mg/kg (5310 and 3570 mg/m^2) of timolol, respectively.

Continued on next page

Information on the Merck & Co., Inc. products listed on these pages is the full prescribing information from product circulars in use September 30, 1996.

Merck & Co.—Cont.

An *in vitro* hemodialysis study, using[14]C timolol added to human plasma or whole blood, showed that timolol was readily dialyzed from these fluids; however, a study of patients with renal failure showed that timolol did not dialyze readily.

---

* Registered trademark of MERCK & CO., INC.

DOSAGE AND ADMINISTRATION

TIMOPTIC Ophthalmic Solution is available in concentrations of 0.25 and 0.5 percent. The usual starting dose is one drop of 0.25 percent TIMOPTIC in the affected eye(s) twice a day. If the clinical response is not adequate, the dosage may be changed to one drop of 0.5 percent solution in the affected eye(s) twice a day.

Since in some patients the pressure-lowering response to TIMOPTIC may require a few weeks to stabilize, evaluation should include a determination of intraocular pressure after approximately 4 weeks of treatment with TIMOPTIC.

If the intraocular pressure is maintained at satisfactory levels, the dosage schedule may be changed to one drop once a day in the affected eye(s). Because of diurnal variations in intraocular pressure, satisfactory response to the once-a-day dose is best determined by measuring the intraocular pressure at different times during the day.

Dosages above one drop of 0.5 percent TIMOPTIC twice a day generally have not been shown to produce further reduction in intraocular pressure. If the patient's intraocular pressure is still not at a satisfactory level on this regimen, concomitant therapy with pilocarpine and other miotics, and/or epinephrine, and/or systemically administered carbonic anhydrase inhibitors, such as acetazolamide, can be instituted.

When a patient is transferred from another topical ophthalmic beta-adrenergic blocking agent, that agent should be discontinued after proper dosing on one day and treatment with TIMOPTIC started on the following day with 1 drop of 0.25 percent TIMOPTIC in the affected eye(s) twice a day. The dose may be increased to one drop of 0.5 percent TIMOPTIC twice a day if the clinical response is not adequate.

When a patient is transferred from a single antiglaucoma agent, other than a topical ophthalmic beta-adrenergic blocking agent, continue the agent already being used and add one drop of 0.25 percent TIMOPTIC in the affected eye(s) twice a day. On the following day, discontinue the previously used antiglaucoma agent completely and continue with TIMOPTIC. If a higher dosage of TIMOPTIC is required, substitute one drop of 0.5 percent solution in the affected eye(s) twice a day.

When a patient is transferred from several concomitantly administered antiglaucoma agents, individualization is required. If any of the agents is an ophthalmic beta-adrenergic blocker, it should be discontinued before starting TIMOPTIC. Additional adjustments should involve one agent at a time and usually should be made at intervals of not less than one week. A recommended approach is to continue the agents being used and to add one drop of 0.25 percent TIMOPTIC in the affected eye(s) twice a day. On the following day, discontinue one of the other antiglaucoma agents. The remaining antiglaucoma agents may be decreased or discontinued according to the patient's response to treatment. If a higher dosage of TIMOPTIC is required, substitute one drop of 0.5 percent solution in the affected eye(s) twice a day. The physician may be able to discontinue some or all of the other antiglaucoma agents.

HOW SUPPLIED

Sterile Ophthalmic Solution TIMOPTIC is a clear, colorless to light yellow solution.

No. 3366—TIMOPTIC Ophthalmic Solution, 0.25% timolol equivalent, is supplied in a white, opaque, plastic OCUMETER* ophthalmic dispenser with a controlled drop tip as follows:

NDC 0006-3366-32, 2.5 mL
NDC 0006-3366-03, 5 mL
(6505-01-069-6518, 0.25% 5 mL)
NDC 0006-3366-10, 10 mL
(6505-01-093-5458, 0.25% 10 mL)
NDC 0006-3366-12, 15 mL.

No. 3367—TIMOPTIC Ophthalmic Solution, 0.5% timolol equivalent, is supplied in a white, opaque, plastic OCUMETER ophthalmic dispenser with a controlled drop tip as follows:

NDC 0006-3367-32, 2.5 mL
NDC 0006-3367-03, 5 mL
(6505-01-069-6519, 0.5% 5 mL)
NDC 0006-3367-10, 10 mL
(6505-01-092-0422, 0.5% 10 mL)
NDC 0006-3367-12, 15 mL.

Storage
Store at controlled room temperature, 15–30°C (59–86°F). Protect from freezing. Protect from light.

---

*Registered trademark of MERCK & CO., INC.
7950438 Issued December 1995
COPYRIGHT © MERCK & CO., INC., 1985, 1995
All rights reserved

TIMOPTIC® ℞
0.25% and 0.5%
(Timolol Maleate Ophthalmic Solution)
in OCUDOSE® (Dispenser), U.S.P.
Preservative-Free Sterile Ophthalmic Solution
in a Sterile Ophthalmic Unit Dose Dispenser

DESCRIPTION

Timolol maleate is a non-selective beta-adrenergic receptor blocking agent. Its chemical name is (-)-1-(*tert*-butylamino)-3-[(4-morpholino-1,2,5-thiadiazol-3-yl)oxy]-2-propanol maleate (1:1) (salt). Timolol maleate possesses an asymmetric carbon atom in its structure and is provided as the levo-isomer. The nominal optical rotation of timolol maleate is $[\alpha]^{25°}_{405\ nm}$ in 0.1N HCl (C = 5%) = −12.2°.

Its molecular formula is $C_{13}H_{24}N_4O_3S \cdot C_4H_4O_4$ and its structural formula is:

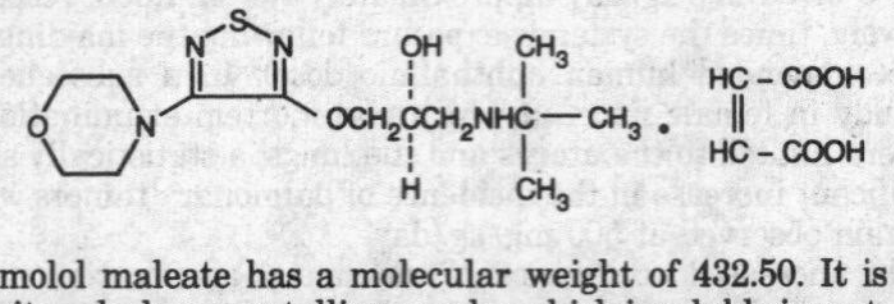

Timolol maleate has a molecular weight of 432.50. It is a white, odorless, crystalline powder which is soluble in water, methanol, and alcohol. Timolol maleate is stable at room temperature.

Timolol maleate ophthalmic solution is supplied in two formulations: Ophthalmic Solution TIMOPTIC* (Timolol Maleate), which contains the preservative benzalkonium chloride; and Ophthalmic Solution TIMOPTIC* (Timolol Maleate), the preservative-free formulation.

Preservative-free Ophthalmic Solution TIMOPTIC is supplied in OCUDOSE*, a unit dose container, as a sterile, isotonic, buffered, aqueous solution of timolol maleate in two dosage strengths: Each mL of Preservative-free TIMOPTIC in OCUDOSE 0.25% contains 2.5 mg of timolol (3.4 mg of timolol maleate). Each mL of Preservative-free TIMOPTIC in OCUDOSE 0.5% contains 5.0 mg of timolol (6.8 mg of timolol maleate). Inactive ingredients: monobasic and dibasic sodium phosphate, sodium hydroxide to adjust pH, and water for injection.

---

*Registered trademark of MERCK & CO., INC.

CLINICAL PHARMACOLOGY

Timolol maleate is a $beta_1$ and $beta_2$ (non-selective) adrenergic receptor blocking agent that does not have significant intrinsic sympathomimetic, direct myocardial depressant, or local anesthetic (membrane-stabilizing) activity.

Beta-adrenergic receptor blockade reduces cardiac output in both healthy subjects and patients with heart disease. In patients with severe impairment of myocardial function beta-adrenergic receptor blockade may inhibit the stimulatory effect of the sympathetic nervous system necessary to maintain adequate cardiac function.

Beta-adrenergic receptor blockade in the bronchi and bronchioles results in increased airway resistance from unopposed parasympathetic activity. Such an effect in patients with asthma or other bronchospastic conditions is potentially dangerous.

TIMOPTIC (Timolol Maleate), when applied topically on the eye, has the action of reducing elevated as well as normal intraocular pressure, whether or not accompanied by glaucoma. Elevated intraocular pressure is a major risk factor in the pathogenesis of glaucomatous visual field loss. The higher the level of intraocular pressure, the greater the likelihood of glaucomatous visual field loss and optic nerve damage.

The onset of reduction in intraocular pressure following administration of TIMOPTIC (Timolol Maleate) can usually be detected within one-half hour after a single dose. The maximum effect usually occurs in one to two hours and significant lowering of intraocular pressure can be maintained for periods as long as 24 hours with a single dose. Repeated observations over a period of one year indicate that the intraocular pressure-lowering effect of TIMOPTIC (Timolol Maleate) is well maintained.

The precise mechanism of the ocular hypotensive action of TIMOPTIC (Timolol Maleate) is not clearly established at this time. Tonography and fluorophotometry studies in man suggest that its predominant action may be related to reduced aqueous formation. However, in some studies a slight increase in outflow facility was also observed. Unlike miotics, TIMOPTIC (Timolol Maleate) reduces intraocular pressure with little or no effect on accommodation or pupil size. Thus, changes in visual acuity due to increased accommodation are uncommon, and dim or blurred vision and night blindness produced by miotics are not evident. In addition, in patients with cataracts the inability to see around lenticular opacities when the pupil is constricted is avoided.

Clinical studies have shown that the mean percent reductions in intraocular pressure with Preservative-free TIMOPTIC and TIMOPTIC (Timolol Maleate) were similar. Preservative-free TIMOPTIC was generally well tolerated.

In the clinical studies which are reported below, ocular pressure reductions to less than 22 mmHg were used as a reasonable reference point to allow comparisons between treatments. Reduction of ocular pressure to just below 22 mmHg may not be optimal for all patients; therapy should be individualized.

In controlled multiclinic studies in patients with untreated intraocular pressures of 22 mmHg or greater, TIMOPTIC (Timolol Maleate) 0.25 percent or 0.5 percent administered twice a day produced a greater reduction in intraocular pressure than 1, 2, 3, or 4 percent pilocarpine solution administered four times a day or 0.5, 1, or 2 percent epinephrine hydrochloride solution administered twice a day.

In the multiclinic studies comparing TIMOPTIC (Timolol Maleate) with pilocarpine, 61 percent of patients treated with TIMOPTIC (Timolol Maleate) had intraocular pressure reduced to less than 22 mmHg compared to 32 percent of patients treated with pilocarpine. For patients completing these studies, the mean reduction in pressure at the end of the study from pretreatment was 30.7 percent for patients treated with TIMOPTIC (Timolol Maleate) and 21.7 percent for patients treated with pilocarpine.

In the multiclinic studies comparing TIMOPTIC (Timolol Maleate) with epinephrine, 69 percent of patients treated with TIMOPTIC (Timolol Maleate) had intraocular pressure reduced to less than 22 mmHg compared to 42 percent of patients treated with epinephrine. For patients completing these studies, the mean reduction in pressure at the end of the study from pretreatment was 33.2 percent for patients treated with TIMOPTIC (Timolol Maleate) and 28.1 percent for patients treated with epinephrine.

In these studies, TIMOPTIC (Timolol Maleate) was generally well tolerated and produced fewer and less severe side effects than either pilocarpine or epinephrine. A slight reduction of resting heart rate in some patients receiving TIMOPTIC (Timolol Maleate) (mean reduction 2.9 beats/minute standard deviation 10.2) was observed.

TIMOPTIC (Timolol Maleate) has also been used in patients with glaucoma wearing conventional (PMMA) hard contact lenses, and has generally been well tolerated. TIMOPTIC (Timolol Maleate) has not been studied in patients wearing lenses made with materials other than PMMA.

INDICATIONS AND USAGE

Preservative-free TIMOPTIC in OCUDOSE is indicated in the treatment of elevated intraocular pressure in patients with ocular hypertension or open-angle glaucoma.

Preservative-free TIMOPTIC in OCUDOSE may be used when a patient is sensitive to the preservative in TIMOPTIC (Timolol Maleate), benzalkonium chloride, or when use of a preservative-free topical medication is advisable.

CONTRAINDICATIONS

Preservative-free TIMOPTIC in OCUDOSE is contraindicated in patients with (1) bronchial asthma; (2) a history of bronchial asthma; (3) severe chronic obstructive pulmonary disease (see **WARNINGS**); (4) sinus bradycardia; (5) second or third degree atrioventricular block; (6) overt cardiac failure (see **WARNINGS**); (7) cardiogenic shock; or (8) hypersensitivity to any component of this product.

WARNINGS

As with many topically applied ophthalmic drugs, this drug is absorbed systemically.

The same adverse reactions found with systemic administration of beta-adrenergic blocking agents may occur with topical administration. For example, severe respiratory reactions and cardiac reactions, including death due to bronchospasm in patients with asthma, and rarely death in association with cardiac failure, have been reported following systemic or ophthalmic administration of timolol maleate (see CONTRAINDICATIONS).

Cardiac Failure
Sympathetic stimulation may be essential for support of the circulation in individuals with diminished myocardial contractility, and its inhibition by beta-adrenergic receptor blockade may precipitate more severe failure.

In Patients Without a History of Cardiac Failure continued depression of the myocardium with beta-blocking agents over a period of time can, in some cases, lead to cardiac failure. At the first sign or symptom of cardiac failure Preservative-free TIMOPTIC in OCUDOSE should be discontinued.

Obstructive Pulmonary Disease

Patients with chronic obstructive pulmonary disease (e.g., chronic bronchitis, emphysema) of mild or moderate severity, bronchospastic disease, or a history of bronchospastic disease (other than bronchial asthma or a history of bronchial asthma, in which TIMOPTIC in OCUDOSE is contraindicated [see **CONTRAINDICATIONS**]) should, in general, not receive beta-blockers, including Preservative-free TIMOPTIC in OCUDOSE.

Major Surgery

The necessity or desirability of withdrawal of beta-adrenergic blocking agents prior to major surgery is controversial. Beta-adrenergic receptor blockade impairs the ability of the heart to respond to beta-adrenergically mediated reflex stimuli. This may augment the risk of general anesthesia in surgical procedures. Some patients receiving beta-adrenergic receptor blocking agents have experienced protracted severe hypotension during anesthesia. Difficulty in restarting and maintaining the heartbeat has also been reported. For these reasons, in patients undergoing elective surgery, some authorities recommend gradual withdrawal of beta-adrenergic receptor blocking agents.

If necessary during surgery, the effects of beta-adrenergic blocking agents may be reversed by sufficient doses of adrenergic agonists.

Diabetes Mellitus

Beta-adrenergic blocking agents should be administered with caution in patients subject to spontaneous hypoglycemia or to diabetic patients (especially those with labile diabetes) who are receiving insulin or oral hypoglycemic agents. Beta-adrenergic receptor blocking agents may mask the signs and symptoms of acute hypoglycemia.

Thyrotoxicosis

Beta-adrenergic blocking agents may mask certain clinical signs (e.g., tachycardia) of hyperthyroidism. Patients suspected of developing thyrotoxicosis should be managed carefully to avoid abrupt withdrawal of beta-adrenergic blocking agents that might precipitate a thyroid storm.

PRECAUTIONS

General

Because of potential effects of beta-adrenergic blocking agents on blood pressure and pulse, these agents should be used with caution in patients with cerebrovascular insufficiency. If signs or symptoms suggesting reduced cerebral blood flow develop following initiation of therapy with Preservative-free TIMOPTIC in OCUDOSE, alternative therapy should be considered.

Choroidal detachment after filtration procedures has been reported with the administration of aqueous suppressant therapy (e.g. timolol).

Angle-closure glaucoma: In patients with angle-closure glaucoma, the immediate objective of treatment is to reopen the angle. This requires constricting the pupil. Timolol maleate has little or no effect on the pupil. TIMOPTIC in OCUDOSE should not be used alone in the treatment of angle-closure glaucoma.

Anaphylaxis: While taking beta-blockers, patients with a history of atopy or a history of severe anaphylactic reactions to a variety of allergens may be more reactive to repeated accidental, diagnostic, or therapeutic challenge with such allergens. Such patients may be unresponsive to the usual doses of epinephrine used to treat anaphylactic reactions.

Muscle Weakness: Beta-adrenergic blockade has been reported to potentiate muscle weakness consistent with certain myasthenic symptoms (e.g., diplopia, ptosis, and generalized weakness). Timolol has been reported rarely to increase muscle weakness in some patients with myasthenia gravis or myasthenic symptoms.

As with the use of other antiglaucoma drugs, diminished responsiveness to TIMOPTIC (Timolol Maleate) after prolonged therapy has been reported in some patients. However, in one long-term study in which 96 patients have been followed for at least 3 years, no significant difference in mean intraocular pressure has been observed after initial stabilization.

Information for Patients

Patients should be instructed about the use of Preservative-free TIMOPTIC in OCUDOSE.

Since sterility cannot be maintained after the individual unit is opened, patients should be instructed to use the product immediately after opening, and to discard the individual unit and any remaining contents immediately after use.

Patients with bronchial asthma, a history of bronchial asthma, severe chronic obstructive pulmonary disease, sinus bradycardia, second or third degree atrioventricular block, or cardiac failure should be advised not to take this product. (See **CONTRAINDICATIONS**.)

Drug Interactions

Although TIMOPTIC (Timolol Maleate) used alone has little or no effect on pupil size, mydriasis resulting from concomitant therapy with TIMOPTIC (Timolol Maleate) and epinephrine has been reported occasionally.

Beta-adrenergic blocking agents: Patients who are receiving a beta-adrenergic blocking agent orally and Preservative-free TIMOPTIC in OCUDOSE should be observed for potential additive effects of beta-blockade, both systemic and on intraocular pressure. Patients should not usually receive two topical ophthalmic beta-adrenergic blocking agents concurrently.

Calcium antagonists: Caution should be used in the coadministration of beta-adrenergic blocking agents, such as Preservative-free TIMOPTIC in OCUDOSE, and oral or intravenous calcium antagonists, because of possible atrioventricular conduction disturbances, left ventricular failure, and hypotension. In patients with impaired cardiac function, coadministration should be avoided.

Catecholamine-depleting drugs: Close observation of the patient is recommended when a beta blocker is administered to patients receiving catecholamine-depleting drugs such as reserpine, because of possible additive effects and the production of hyotension and/or marked bradycardia, which may result in vertigo, syncope, or postural hypotension.

Digitalis and calcium antagonists: The concomitant use of beta-adrenergic blocking agents with digitalis and calcium antagonists may have additive effects in prolonging atrioventricular conduction time.

Injectable Epinephrine: (See **PRECAUTIONS**, *General, Anaphylaxis*)

Carcinogenesis, Mutagenesis, Impairment of Fertility

In a two-year oral study of timolol maleate administered orally to rats, there was a statistically significant increase in the incidence of adrenal pheochromocytomas in male rats administered 300 mg/kg/day (approximately 42,000 times the systemic exposure following the maximum recommended human ophthalmic dose). Similar differences were not observed in rats administered oral doses equivalent to approximately 14,000 times the maximum recommended human ophthalmic dose.

In a lifetime oral study in mice, there were statistically significant increases in the incidence of benign and malignant pulmonary tumors, benign uterine polyps and mammary adenocarcinomas in female mice at 500 mg/kg/day (approximately 71,000 times the systemic exposure following the maximum recommended human ophthalmic dose), but not at 5 or 50 mg/kg/day (approximately 700 or 7,000 times, respectively, the systemic exposure following the maximum recommended human ophthalmic dose). In a subsequent study in female mice, in which post-mortem examinations were limited to the uterus and the lungs, a statistically significant increase in the incidence of pulmonary tumors was again observed at 500 mg/kg/day.

The increased occurrence of mammary adenocarcinomas was associated with elevations in serum prolactin which occurred in female mice administered oral timolol at 500 mg/kg, but not at doses of 5 or 50 mg/kg/day. An increased incidence of mammary adenocarcinomas in rodents has been associated with administration of several other therapeutic agents that elevate serum prolactin, but no correlation between serum prolactin levels and mammary tumors has been established in humans. Furthermore, in adult human female subjects who received oral dosages of up to 60 mg of timolol maleate (the maximum recommended human oral dosage), there were no clinically meaningful changes in serum prolactin.

Timolol maleate was devoid of mutagenic potential when tested *in vivo* (mouse) in the micronucleus test and cytogenetic assay (doses up to 800 mg/kg) and *in vitro* in a neoplastic cell transformation assay (up to 100 μg/mL). In Ames tests the highest concentrations of timolol employed, 5000 or 10,000 μg/plate, were associated with statistically significant elevations of revertants observed with tester strain TA 100 (in seven replicate assays), but not in the remaining three strains. In the assays with tester strain TA 100, no consistent dose response relationship was observed, and the ratio of test to control revertants did not reach 2. A ratio of 2 is usually considered the criterion for a positive Ames test.

Reproduction and fertility studies in rats demonstrated no adverse effect on male or female fertility at doses up to 21,000 times the systemic exposure following the maximum recommended human ophthalmic dose.

Pregnancy-Teratogenic effects:

Pregnancy Category C. Teratogenicity studies with timolol in mice, rats and rabbits at oral doses up to 50 mg/kg/day (7,000 times the systemic exposure following the maximum recommended human ophthalmic dose) demonstrated no evidence of fetal malformations. Although delayed fetal ossification was observed at this dose in rats, there were no adverse effects on postnatal development of offspring. Doses of 1000 mg/kg/day (142,000 times the systemic exposure following the maximum recommended human ophthalmic dose) were maternotoxic in mice and resulted in an increased number of fetal resorptions. Increased fetal resorptions were also seen in rabbits at doses of 14,000 times the systemic exposure following the maximum recommended human ophthalmic dose, in this case without apparent maternotoxicity.

There are no adequate and well-controlled studies in pregnant women. Preservative-free TIMOPTIC in OCUDOSE should be used during pregnancy only if the potential benefit justifies the potential risk to the fetus.

Nursing Mothers

Timolol maleate has been detected in human milk following oral and ophthalmic drug administration. Because of the potential for serious adverse reactions from timolol in nursing infants, a decision should be made whether to discontinue nursing or to discontinue the drug, taking into account the importance of the drug to the mother.

Pediatric Use

Safety and effectiveness in pediatric patients have not been established.

ADVERSE REACTIONS

The most frequently reported adverse experiences have been burning and stinging upon instillation (approximately one in eight patients).

The following additional adverse experiences have been reported less frequently with ocular administration of this or other timolol maleate formulations:

BODY AS A WHOLE

Headache, asthenia/fatigue, and chest pain.

CARDIOVASCULAR

Bradycardia, arrhythmia, hypotension, hypertension, syncope, heart block, cerebral vascular accident, cerebral ischemia, cardiac failure, worsening of angina pectoris, palpitation, cardiac arrest, and pulmonary edema.

DIGESTIVE

Nausea, diarrhea, dyspepsia, anorexia, and dry mouth.

IMMUNOLOGIC

Systemic lupus erythematosus.

NERVOUS SYSTEM/PSYCHIATRIC

Dizziness, depression, increase in signs and symptoms of myasthenia gravis, paresthesia, behavioral changes including confusion, hallucinations, anxiety, disorientation, nervousness, somnolence, and other psychic disturbances.

SKIN

Hypersensitivity, including localized and generalized rash; urticaria, alopecia.

RESPIRATORY

Bronchospasm (predominantly in patients with pre-existing bronchospastic disease), respiratory failure, dyspnea, nasal congestion, cough and upper respiratory infections.

ENDOCRINE

Masked symptoms of hypoglycemia in diabetic patients (see **WARNINGS**).

SPECIAL SENSES

Signs and symptoms of ocular irritation including conjunctivitis, blepharitis, keratitis, ocular pain, discharge (e.g., crusting), foreign body sensation, and itching and tearing; ptosis; decreased corneal sensitivity; cystoid macular edema; visual disturbances including refractive changes and diplopia; pseudopemphigoid; and choroidal detachment following filtration surgery (see **PRECAUTIONS**, *General*).

UROGENITAL

Retroperitoneal fibrosis and impotence.

The following additional adverse effects have been reported in clinical experience with ORAL timolol maleate or other ORAL beta blocking agents, and may be considered potential effects of ophthalmic timolol maleate: *Allergic:* Erythematous rash, fever combined with aching and sore throat, laryngospasm with respiratory distress; *Body as a Whole:* Extremity pain, decreased exercise tolerance, weight loss; *Cardiovascular:* Edema, worsening of arterial insufficiency, Raynaud's phenomenon, vasodilatation; *Digestive:* Gastrointestinal pain, hepatomegaly, vomiting, mesenteric arterial thrombosis, ischemic colitis; *Hematologic:* Nonthrombocytopenic purpura; thrombocytopenic purpura; agranulocytosis; *Endocrine:* Hyperglycemia, hypoglycemia; *Skin:* Pruritus, skin irritation, increased pigmentation, sweating, cold hands and feet; *Musculoskeletal:* Arthralgia, claudication; *Nervous System/Psychiatric:* Vertigo, local weakness, decreased libido, nightmares, insomnia, diminished concentration, reversible mental depression progressing to catatonia; an acute reversible syndrome characterized by disorientation for time and place, short term memory loss, emotional lability, slightly clouded sensorium, and decreased performance on neuropsychometrics; *Respiratory:* Rales, bronchial obstruction; *Special Senses:* Tinnitus, dry eyes; *Urogenital:* Urination difficulties, Peyronie's disease.

Continued on next page

Information on the Merck & Co., Inc. products listed on these pages is the full prescribing information from product circulars in use September 30, 1996.

Merck & Co.—Cont.

OVERDOSAGE

There have been reports of inadvertent overdosage with Ophthalmic Solution TIMOPTIC (Timolol Maleate) resulting in systemic effects similar to those seen with systemic beta-adrenergic blocking agents such as dizziness, headache, shortness of breath, bradycardia, bronchospasm, and cardiac arrest (see also **ADVERSE REACTIONS**).

Overdosage has been reported with Tablets BLOCADREN* (Timolol Maleate). A 30 year old female ingested 650 mg of BLOCADREN (maximum recommended oral daily dose is 60 mg) and experienced second and third degree heart block. She recovered without treatment but approximately two months later developed irregular heartbeat, hypertension, dizziness, tinnitus, faintness, increased pulse rate, and borderline first degree heart block.

Significant lethality was observed in female rats and female mice after a single dose of 900 and 1190 mg/kg (5310 and 3570 mg/m²) of timolol, respectively.

An *in vitro* hemodialysis study, using ^{14}C timolol added to human plasma or whole blood, showed that timolol was readily dialyzed from these fluids; however, a study of patients with renal failure showed that timolol did not dialyze readily.

*Registered trademark of MERCK & CO., Inc.

DOSAGE AND ADMINISTRATION

Preservative-free TIMOPTIC in OCUDOSE is a sterile solution that does not contain a preservative. The solution from one individual unit is to be used immediately after opening for administration to one or both eyes. Since sterility cannot be guaranteed after the individual unit is opened, the remaining contents should be discarded immediately after administration.

Preservative-free TIMOPTIC in OCUDOSE is available in concentrations of 0.25 and 0.5 percent. The usual starting dose is one drop of 0.25 percent Preservative-free TIMOPTIC in OCUDOSE in the affected eye(s) administered twice a day. Apply enough gentle pressure on the individual container to obtain a single drop of solution. If the clinical response is not adequate, the dosage may be changed to one drop of 0.5 percent solution in the affected eye(s) administered twice a day. Since in some patients the pressure-lowering response to Preservative-free TIMOPTIC in OCUDOSE may require a few weeks to stabilize, evaluation should include a determination of intraocular pressure after approximately 4 weeks of treatment with Preservative-free TIMOPTIC in OCUDOSE.

If the intraocular pressure is maintained at satisfactory levels, the dosage schedule may be changed to one drop once a day in the affected eye(s). Because of diurnal variations in intraocular pressure, satisfactory response to the once-a-day dose is best determined by measuring the intraocular pressure at different times during the day.

Dosages above one drop of 0.5 percent TIMOPTIC (Timolol Maleate) twice a day generally have not been shown to produce further reduction in intraocular pressure. If the patient's intraocular pressure is still not at a satisfactory level on this regimen, concomitant therapy with pilocarpine and other miotics, and/or epinephrine, and/or systemically administered carbonic anhydrase inhibitors, such as acetazolamide, can be instituted taking into consideration that the preparation(s) used concomitantly may contain one or more preservatives.

When a patient is transferred from another topical ophthalmic beta-adrenergic blocking agent, that agent should be discontinued after proper dosing on one day and treatment with Preservative-free TIMOPTIC in OCUDOSE started on the following day with one drop of 0.25 percent Preservative-free TIMOPTIC in OCUDOSE in the affected eye(s) twice a day. The dose may be increased to one drop of 0.5 percent Preservative-free TIMOPTIC in OCUDOSE twice a day if the clinical response is not adequate.

When a patient is transferred from a single antiglaucoma agent, other than a topical ophthalmic beta-adrenergic blocking agent, continue the agent already being used and add one drop of 0.25 percent Preservative-free TIMOPTIC in OCUDOSE in the affected eye(s) twice a day. On the following day, discontinue the previously used antiglaucoma agent completely and continue with Preservative-free TIMOPTIC in OCUDOSE. If a higher dosage of Preservative-free TIMOPTIC in OCUDOSE is required, substitute one drop of 0.5 percent solution in the affected eye(s) twice a day.

When a patient is transferred from several concomitantly administered antiglaucoma agents, individualization is required. If any of the agents is an ophthalmic beta-adrenergic blocker, it should be discontinued before starting Preservative-free TIMOPTIC in OCUDOSE. Additional adjustments should involve one agent at a time and usually should be made at intervals of not less than one week. A recommended approach is to continue the agents being used and to add one drop of 0.25 percent Preservative-free TIMOPTIC in OCUDOSE in the affected eye(s) twice a day. On the following day, discontinue one of the other antiglaucoma agents. The remaining antiglaucoma agents may be decreased or discontinued according to the patient's response to treatment. If a higher dosage of Preservative-free TIMOPTIC in OCUDOSE is required, substitute one drop of 0.5 percent solution in the affected eye(s) twice a day. The physician may be able to discontinue some or all of the other antiglaucoma agents.

HOW SUPPLIED

Preservative-free Sterile Ophthalmic Solution TIMOPTIC in OCUDOSE is a clear, colorless to light yellow solution.

No. 3542—Preservative-free TIMOPTIC, 0.25% timolol equivalent, is supplied in OCUDOSE, a clear polyethylene unit dose container. Each individual unit contains 0.45 mL of solution, and is available in a foil laminate overwrapped pouch as follows:

NDC 0006-3542-60; 60 Individual Unit Doses (6505-01-316-8791, 0.25% 60 Individual Unit Doses).

No. 3543—Preservative-free TIMOPTIC, 0.5% timolol equivalent, is supplied in OCUDOSE, a clear polyethylene unit dose container. Each individual unit contains 0.45 mL of solution, and is available in a foil laminate overwrapped pouch as follows:

NDC 0006-3543-60; 60 Individual Unit Doses (6505-01-284-5154, 0.5% 60 Individual Unit Doses).

Storage

Store at controlled room temperature, 15-30°C (59-86°F). Protect from freezing. Protect from light.

Because evaporation can occur through the unprotected polyethylene unit dose container and prolonged exposure to direct light can modify the product, the unit dose container should be kept in the protective foil overwrap and used within one month after the foil package has been opened.

Mgf. by:
MERCK & CO, INC., West Point, PA 19486, USA
Filled by:
PACO
LAKEWOOD, NJ 08701, USA
      7950513   Issued December 1995

TIMOPTIC-XE®   ℞
0.25% and 0.5%
Sterile Ophthalmic Gel Forming Solution
(Timolol Maleate Ophthalmic Gel Forming Solution), U.S.P.

DESCRIPTION

TIMOPTIC-XE* (timolol maleate ophthalmic gel forming solution) is a non-selective beta-adrenergic receptor blocking agent. Its chemical name is (-)-1-(*tert*-butyl-amino)-3-[(4-morpholino-1,2,5-thiadiazol-3-yl)oxy]-2-propanol maleate (1:1) (salt). Timolol maleate possesses an asymmetric carbon atom in its structure and is provided as the levo-isomer. The nominal optical rotation of timolol maleate is:

$$[\alpha]^{25°}_{405\ nm} \text{ in 0.1N HCl (C=5\%)} = -12.2°.$$

Its molecular formula is $C_{13}H_{24}N_4O_3S \cdot C_4H_4O_4$ and its structural formula is:

Timolol maleate has a molecular weight of 432.50. It is a white, odorless, crystalline powder which is soluble in water, methanol, and alcohol.

TIMOPTIC-XE Sterile Ophthalmic Gel Forming Solution is supplied as a sterile, isotonic, buffered, aqueous solution of timolol maleate in two dosage strengths. Each mL of TIMOPTIC-XE 0.25% contains 2.5 mg of timolol (3.4 mg of timolol maleate). Each mL of TIMOPTIC-XE 0.5% contains 5.0 mg of timolol (6.8 mg of timolol maleate). Inactive ingredients: GELRITE* gellan gum, tromethamine, mannitol, and water for injection. Preservative: benzododecinium bromide 0.012%.

GELRITE is a purified anionic heteropolysaccharide derived from gellan gum. An aqueous solution of GELRITE, in the presence of a cation, has the ability to gel. Upon contact with the precorneal tear film, TIMOPTIC-XE forms a gel that is subsequently removed by the flow of tears.

* Registered trademark of Merck & Co., Inc.

CLINICAL PHARMACOLOGY

Mechanism of Action

Timolol maleate is a beta₁ and beta₂ (non-selective) adrenergic receptor blocking agent that does not have significant intrinsic sympathomimetic, direct myocardial depressant, or local anesthetic (membrane-stabilizing) activity.

TIMOPTIC-XE, when applied topically on the eye, has the action of reducing elevated, as well as normal intraocular pressure, whether or not accompanied by glaucoma. Elevated intraocular pressure is a major risk factor in the pathogenesis of glaucomatous visual field loss and optic nerve damage.

The precise mechanism of the ocular hypotensive action of TIMOPTIC-XE is not clearly established at this time. Tonography and fluorophotometry studies of TIMOPTIC* (timolol maleate ophthalmic solution) in man suggest that its predominant action may be related to reduced aqueous formation. However, in some studies, a slight increase in outflow facility was also observed.

Beta-adrenergic receptor blockade reduces cardiac output in both healthy subjects and patients with heart disease. In patients with severe impairment of myocardial function beta-adrenergic receptor blockade may inhibit the stimulatory effect of the sympathetic nervous system necessary to maintain adequate cardiac function.

Beta-adrenergic receptor blockade in the bronchi and bronchioles results in increased airway resistance from unopposed parasympathetic activity. Such an effect in patients with asthma or other bronchospastic conditions is potentially dangerous.

Pharmacokinetics

In a study of plasma drug concentration in six subjects, the systemic exposure to timolol was determined following once daily administration of TIMOPTIC-XE 0.5% in the morning. The mean peak plasma concentration following this morning dose was 0.28 ng/mL.

Clinical Studies

In controlled, double-masked, multicenter clinical studies, comparing TIMOPTIC-XE 0.25% to TIMOPTIC 0.25% and TIMOPTIC-XE 0.5% to TIMOPTIC 0.5%, TIMOPTIC-XE administered once a day was shown to be equally effective in lowering intraocular pressure as the equivalent concentration of TIMOPTIC administered twice a day. The effect of timolol in lowering intraocular pressure was evident for 24 hours with a single dose of TIMOPTIC-XE. Repeated observations over a period of six months indicate that the intraocular pressure-lowering effect of TIMOPTIC-XE was consistent. The results from the largest U.S. and international clinical trials comparing TIMOPTIC-XE 0.5% to TIMOPTIC 0.5% are shown in Figure 1.

Figure 1

Mean IOP and Std Deviation (mm Hg) by Treatment Group

U.S. Study

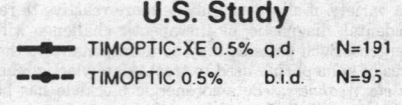

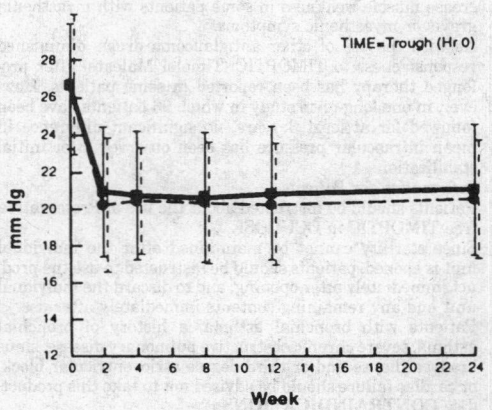

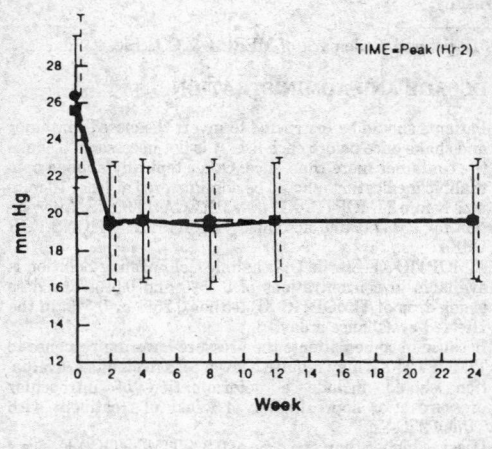

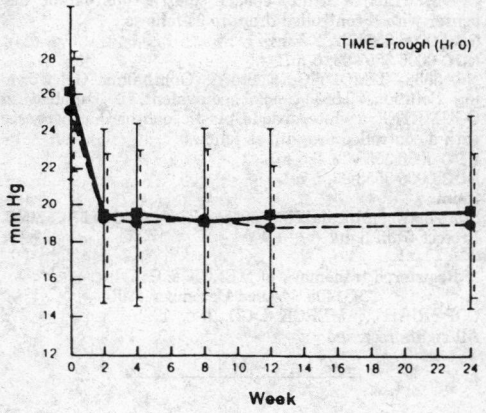

International Study

— TIMOPTIC-XE 0.5% q.d.   N=226
— TIMOPTIC 0.5% b.i.d.   N=116

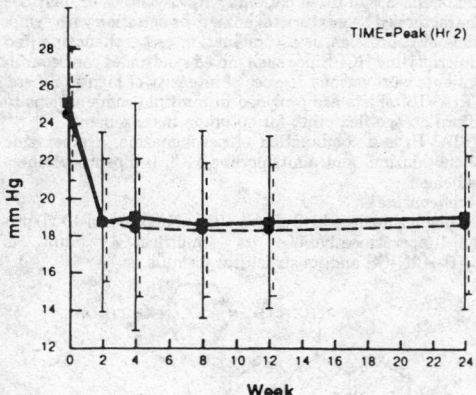

TIMOPTIC-XE administered once daily had a safety profile similar to that of an equivalent concentration of TIMOPTIC administered twice daily. Due to the physical characteristics of the formulation, there was a higher incidence of transient blurred vision in patients administered TIMOPTIC-XE. A slight reduction in resting heart rate was observed in some patients receiving TIMOPTIC-XE 0.5% (mean reduction 24 hours post-dose 0.8 beats/minute, mean reduction 2 hours post-dose 3.8 beats/minute). (See **ADVERSE REACTIONS.**)

TIMOPTIC-XE has not been studied in patients wearing contact lenses.

———

* Registered trademark of MERCK & CO., INC.

INDICATIONS AND USAGE

TIMOPTIC-XE Sterile Ophthalmic Gel Forming Solution is indicated in the treatment of elevated intraocular pressure in patients with ocular hypertension or open-angle glaucoma.

CONTRAINDICATIONS

TIMOPTIC-XE is contraindicated in patients with (1) bronchial asthma; (2) a history of bronchial asthma; (3) severe chronic obstructive pulmonary disease (see WARNINGS); (4) sinus bradycardia; (5) second or third degree atrioventricular block; (6) overt cardiac failure (see WARNINGS); (7) cardiogenic shock; or (8) hypersensitivity to any component of this product.

WARNINGS

As with many topically applied ophthalmic drugs, this drug is absorbed systemically.
The same adverse reactions found with systemic administration of beta-adrenergic blocking agents may occur with topical ophthalmic administration. For example, severe respiratory reactions and cardiac reactions, including death due to bronchospasm in patients with asthma, and rarely death in association with cardiac failure, have been reported following systemic or ophthalmic administration of timolol maleate. (See CONTRAINDICATIONS.)
Cardiac Failure
Sympathetic stimulation may be essential for support of the circulation in individuals with diminished myocardial contractility, and its inhibition by beta-adrenergic receptor blockade may precipitate more severe failure.
In Patients Without a History of Cardiac Failure, continued depression of the myocardium with beta-blocking agents over a period of time can, in some cases, lead to cardiac failure. At the first sign or symptom of cardiac failure, TIMOPTIC-XE should be discontinued.
Obstructive Pulmonary Disease
Patients with chronic obstructive pulmonary disease (e.g., chronic bronchitis, emphysema) of mild or moderate severity, bronchospastic disease, or a history of bronchospastic disease (other than bronchial asthma or a history of bronchial asthma, in which TIMOPTIC-XE is contraindicated [see **CONTRAINDICATIONS**]) should, in general, not receive beta-blockers, including TIMOPTIC-XE.
Major Surgery
The necessity or desirability of withdrawal of beta-adrenergic blocking agents prior to major surgery is controversial. Beta-adrenergic receptor blockade impairs the ability of the heart to respond to beta-adrenergically mediated reflex stimuli. This may augment the risk of general anesthesia in surgical procedures. Some patients receiving beta-adrenergic receptor blocking agents have experienced protracted, severe hypotension during anesthesia. Difficulty in restarting and maintaining the heartbeat has also been reported. For these reasons, in patients undergoing elective surgery, some authorities recommend gradual withdrawal of beta-adrenergic receptor blocking agents.
If necessary during surgery, the effects of beta-adrenergic blocking agents may be reversed by sufficient doses of adrenergic agonists.
Diabetes Mellitus
Beta-adrenergic blocking agents should be administered with caution in patients subject to spontaneous hypoglycemia or to diabetic patients (especially those with labile diabetes) who are receiving insulin or oral hypoglycemic agents. Beta-adrenergic receptor blocking agents may mask the signs and symptoms of acute hypoglycemia.
Thyrotoxicosis
Beta-adrenergic blocking agents may mask certain clinical signs (e.g., tachycardia) of hyperthyroidism. Patients suspected of developing thyrotoxicosis should be managed carefully to avoid abrupt withdrawal of beta-adrenergic blocking agents that might precipitate a thyroid storm.

PRECAUTIONS

General
Because of potential effects of beta-adrenergic blocking agents on blood pressure and pulse, these agents should be used with caution in patients with cerebrovascular insufficiency. If signs or symptoms suggesting reduced cerebral blood flow develop following initiation of therapy with TIMOPTIC-XE, alternative therapy should be considered. There have been reports of bacterial keratitis associated with the use of multiple dose containers of topical ophthalmic products. These containers had been inadvertently contaminated by patients who, in most cases, had a concurrent corneal disease or a disruption of the ocular epithelial surface. (See **PRECAUTIONS**, *Information for Patients.*)
Choroidal detachment after filtration procedures has been reported with the administration of aqueous suppressant therapy (e.g. timolol).
Angle-closure glaucoma: In patients with angle-closure glaucoma, the immediate objective of treatment is to reopen the angle. This may require constricting the pupil. Timolol maleate has little or no effect on the pupil. TIMOPTIC-XE should not be used alone in the treatment of angle-closure glaucoma.
Anaphylaxis: While taking beta-blockers, patients with a history of atopy or a history of severe anaphylactic reactions to a variety of allergens may be more reactive to repeated accidental, diagnostic, or therapeutic challenge with such allergens. Such patients may be unresponsive to the usual doses of epinephrine used to treat anaphylactic reactions.
Muscle Weakness: Beta-adrenergic blockade has been reported to potentiate muscle weakness consistent with certain myasthenic symptoms (e.g., diplopia, ptosis, and generalized weakness). Timolol has been reported rarely to increase muscle weakness in some patients with myasthenia gravis or myasthenic symptoms.
Information for Patients
Patients should be instructed to avoid allowing the tip of the dispensing container to contact the eye or surrounding structures.
Patients should also be instructed that ocular solutions, if handled improperly, can become contaminated by common bacteria known to cause ocular infections. Serious damage to the eye and subsequent loss of vision may result from using contaminated solutions. (See **PRECAUTIONS**, *General.*)
Patients should also be advised that if they develop an intercurrent ocular condition (e.g., trauma, ocular surgery, or infection), they should immediately seek their physician's advice concerning the continued use of the present multidose container.
Patients should be instructed to invert the closed container and shake once before each use. It is not necessary to shake the container more than once.
Patients requiring concomitant topical ophthalmic medications should be instructed to administer these at least 10 minutes before instilling TIMOPTIC-XE.
Patients with bronchial asthma, a history of bronchial asthma, severe chronic obstructive pulmonary disease, sinus bradycardia, second or third degree atrioventricular block, or cardiac failure should be advised not to take this product. (See **CONTRAINDICATIONS.**)
Drug Interactions
Beta-adrenergic blocking agents: Patients who are receiving a beta-adrenergic blocking agent orally and TIMOPTIC-XE should be observed for potential additive effects of beta-blockade, both systemic and on intraocular pressure. Patients should not usually receive two topical ophthalmic beta-adrenergic blocking agents concurrently.
Calcium antagonists: Caution should be used in the coadministration of beta-adrenergic blocking agents, such as TIMOPTIC-XE, and oral or intravenous calcium antagonists because of possible atrioventricular conduction disturbances, left ventricular failure, or hypotension. In patients with impaired cardiac function, coadministration should be avoided.
Catecholamine-depleting drugs: Close observation of the patient is recommended when a beta blocker is administered to patients receiving catecholamine-depleting drugs such as reserpine, because of possible additive effects and the production of hypotension and/or marked bradycardia, which may result in vertigo, syncope, or postural hypotension.
Digitalis and calcium antagonists: The concomitant use of beta-adrenergic blocking agents with digitalis and calcium antagonists may have additive effects in prolonging atrioventricular conduction time.
Injectable Epinephrine: (See **PRECAUTIONS**, *General, Anaphylaxis:*)
Carcinogenesis, Mutagenesis, Impairment of Fertility
In a two-year study of timolol maleate administered orally to rats, there was a statistically significant increase in the incidence of adrenal pheochromocytomas in male rats administered 300 mg/kg/day (approximately 42,000 times the systemic exposure following the maximum recommended human ophthalmic dose). Similar differences were not observed in rats administered oral doses equivalent to approximately

Continued on next page

———

Information on the Merck & Co., Inc. products listed on these pages is the full prescribing information from product circulars in use September 30, 1996.

Merck & Co.—Cont.

14,000 times the maximum recommended human ophthalmic dose.

In a lifetime oral study in mice, there were statistically significant increases in the incidence of benign and malignant pulmonary tumors, benign uterine polyps, and mammary adenocarcinomas in female mice at 500 mg/kg/day (approximately 71,000 times the systemic exposure following the maximum recommended human ophthalmic dose), but not at 5 or 50 mg/kg/day (approximately 700 or 7,000, respectively, times the systemic exposure following the maximum recommended human ophthalmic dose). In a subsequent study in female mice, in which post-mortem examinations were limited to the uterus and the lungs, a statistically significant increase in the incidence of pulmonary tumors was again observed at 500 mg/kg/day.

The increased occurrence of mammary adenocarcinomas was associated with elevations in serum prolactin, which occurred in female mice administered oral timolol at 500 mg/kg, but not at oral doses of 5 or 50 mg/kg/day. An increased incidence of mammary adenocarcinomas in rodents has been associated with administration of several other therapeutic agents that elevate serum prolactin, but no correlation between serum prolactin levels and mammary tumors has been established in humans. Furthermore, in adult human female subjects who received oral dosages of up to 60 mg of timolol maleate (the maximum recommended human oral dosage), there were no clinically meaningful changes in serum prolactin.

Timolol maleate was devoid of mutagenic potential when tested *in vivo* (mouse) in the micronucleus test and cytogenetic assay (doses up to 800 mg) and *in vitro* in a neoplastic cell transformation assay (up to 100 μg/mL). In Ames tests, the highest concentrations of timolol employed, 5,000 or 10,000 μg/plate, were associated with statistically significant elevations of revertants observed with tester strain TA100 (in seven replicate assays), but not in the remaining three strains. In the assays with tester strain TA100, no consistent dose response relationship was observed, and the ratio of test to control revertants did not reach 2. A ratio of 2 is usually considered the criterion for a positive Ames test.

Reproduction and fertility studies in rats demonstrated no adverse effect on male or female fertility at doses up to 21,000 times the systemic exposure following the maximum recommended human ophthalmic dose.

Pregnancy—Teratogenic effects:

Pregnancy Category C. Teratogenicity studies with timolol in mice and rabbits at oral doses up to 50 mg/kg/day (7,000 times the systemic exposure following the maximum recommended human ophthalmic dose) demonstrated no evidence of fetal malformations. Although delayed fetal ossification was observed at this dose in rats, there were no adverse effects on postnatal development of offspring. Doses of 1000 mg/kg/day (142,000 times the systemic exposure following the maximum recommended human ophthalmic dose) were maternotoxic in mice and resulted in an increased number of fetal resorptions. Increased fetal resorptions were also seen in rabbits at doses of 14,000 times the systemic exposure following the maximum recommended human ophthalmic dose, in this case without apparent maternotoxicity.

There are no adequate and well-controlled studies in pregnant women. TIMOPTIC-XE should be used during pregnancy only if the potential benefit justifies the potential risk to the fetus.

Nursing Mothers

Timolol maleate has been detected in human milk following oral and ophthalmic drug administration. Because of the potential for serious adverse reactions from TIMOPTIC-XE in nursing infants, a decision should be made whether to discontinue nursing or to discontinue the drug, taking into account the importance of the drug to the mother.

Pediatric Use

Safety and effectiveness in pediatric patients have not been established.

Geriatric Use

Of the total number of patients in clinical studies of TIMOPTIC-XE, 46% were 65 years of age and over, while 14% were 75 years of age and over. No overall differences in effectiveness or safety were observed between these patients and younger patients, but greater sensitivity of some older individuals to the product cannot be ruled out.

ADVERSE REACTIONS

In clinical trials, transient blurred vision upon instillation of the drop was reported in approximately one in three patients (lasting from 30 seconds to 5 minutes). Less than 1% of patients discontinued from the studies due to blurred vision. The frequency of patients reporting burning and stinging upon instillation was comparable between TIMOPTIC-XE and TIMOPTIC (approximately one in eight patients).

Adverse experiences reported in 1–5% of patients were:

Ocular: Pain, conjunctivitis, discharge (e.g. crusting), foreign body sensation, itching and tearing;

Systemic: Headache, dizziness, and upper respiratory infections.

The following additional adverse experiences have been reported with the ocular administration of other timolol maleate formulations:

BODY AS A WHOLE

Asthenia/fatigue, and chest pain.

CARDIOVASCULAR

Bradycardia, arrhythmia, hypotension, hypertension, syncope, heart block, cerebral vascular accident, cerebral ischemia, cardiac failure, worsening of angina pectoris, palpitation, cardiac arrest, and pulmonary edema.

DIGESTIVE

Nausea, diarrhea, dyspepsia, anorexia, and dry mouth.

IMMUNOLOGIC

Systemic lupus erythematosus.

NERVOUS SYSTEM/PSYCHIATRIC

Depression, increase in signs and symptoms of myasthenia gravis, paresthesia, behavioral changes including confusion, hallucinations, anxiety, disorientation, nervousness, somnolence, and other psychic disturbances.

SKIN

Hypersensitivity, including localized and generalized rash; urticaria; alopecia.

RESPIRATORY

Bronchospasm (predominantly in patients with preexisting bronchospastic disease), respiratory failure, dyspnea, nasal congestion, and cough.

ENDOCRINE

Masked symptoms of hypoglycemia in diabetic patients (see **WARNINGS**).

SPECIAL SENSES

Signs and symptoms of ocular irritation including blepharitis and keratitis; ptosis; decreased corneal sensitivity; cystoid macular edema; visual disturbances including refractive changes and diplopia; pseudopemphigoid; and choroidal detachment following filtration surgery (see PRECAUTIONS, *General*).

UROGENITAL

Retroperitoneal fibrosis, impotence.

The following additional adverse effects have been reported in clinical experience with ORAL timolol maleate or other ORAL beta-blocking agents and may be considered potential effects of ophthalmic timolol maleate: *Allergic:* Erythematous rash, fever combined with aching and sore throat, laryngospasm with respiratory distress; *Body as a Whole:* Extremity pain, decreased exercise tolerance, weight loss; *Cardiovascular:* Edema, worsening of arterial insufficiency, Raynaud's phenomenon, vasodilatation; *Digestive:* Gastrointestinal pain, hepatomegaly, vomiting, mesenteric arterial thrombosis, ischemic colitis; *Hematologic:* Nonthrombocytopenic purpura, thrombocytopenic purpura, agranulocytosis; *Endocrine:* Hyperglycemia, hypoglycemia; *Skin:* Pruritus, skin irritation, increased pigmentation, sweating, cold hands and feet; *Musculoskeletal:* Arthralgia, claudication; *Nervous System/Psychiatric:* Vertigo, local weakness, decreased libido, nightmares, insomnia, diminished concentration, reversible mental depression progressing to catatonia, an acute reversible syndrome characterized by disorientation for time and place, short term memory loss, emotional lability, slightly clouded sensorium, and decreased performance on neuropsychometrics; *Respiratory:* Rales, bronchial obstruction; *Special Senses:* Tinnitus, dry eyes; *Urogenital:* Urination difficulties, Peyronie's disease.

OVERDOSAGE

No data are available in regard to human overdosage with or accidental oral ingestion of TIMOPTIC-XE.

There have been reports of inadvertent overdosage with TIMOPTIC Ophthalmic Solution resulting in systemic effects similar to those seen with systemic beta-adrenergic blocking agents such as dizziness, headache, shortness of breath, bradycardia, bronchospasm, and cardiac arrest (see also ADVERSE REACTIONS).

Overdosage has been reported with Tablets BLOCADREN* (Timolol Maleate). A 30 year old female ingested 650 mg of BLOCADREN (maximum recommended oral daily dose is 60 mg) and experienced second and third degree heart block. She recovered without treatment but approximately two months later developed irregular heartbeat, hypertension, dizziness, tinnitus, faintness, increased pulse rate, and borderline first degree heart block.

Significant lethality was observed in female rats and female mice after a single oral dose of 900 and 1190 mg/kg (5310 and 3570 mg/m^2) of timolol, respectively.

An *in vitro* hemodialysis study, using ^{14}C timolol added to human plasma or whole blood, showed that timolol was readily dialyzed from these fluids; however, a study of patients with renal failure showed that timolol did not dialyze readily.

*Registered trademark of MERCK & CO., Inc.

DOSAGE AND ADMINISTRATION

Patients should be instructed to invert the closed container and shake once before each use. It is not necessary to shake the container more than once. Other topically applied ophthalmic medications should be administered at least 10 minutes before TIMOPTIC-XE. (See **PRECAUTIONS,** *Information for Patients* and accompanying INSTRUCTIONS FOR USE.)

TIMOPTIC-XE Sterile Ophthalmic Gel Forming Solution is available in concentrations of 0.25% and 0.5%. The dose is one drop of TIMOPTIC-XE (either 0.25% or 0.5%) in the affected eye(s) once a day.

Because in some patients the pressure-lowering response to TIMOPTIC-XE may require a few weeks to stabilize, evaluation should include a determination of intraocular pressure after approximately 4 weeks of treatment with TIMOPTIC-XE.

Dosages higher than one drop of 0.5% TIMOPTIC-XE once a day have not been studied. If the patient's intraocular pressure is still not at a satisfactory level on this regimen, concomitant therapy can be considered.

When patients have been switched from therapy with TIMOPTIC administered twice daily to TIMOPTIC-XE administered once daily, the ocular hypotensive effect has remained consistent.

HOW SUPPLIED

TIMOPTIC-XE Sterile Ophthalmic Gel Forming Solution is a colorless to nearly colorless, slightly opalescent, and slightly viscous solution.

No. 3557—TIMOPTIC-XE Sterile Ophthalmic Gel Forming Solution, 0.25% timolol equivalent, is supplied in OCUMETER*, a white, opaque, plastic, ophthalmic dispenser with a controlled drop tip as follows:

NDC 0006-3557-32, 2.5 mL

NDC 0006-3557-03, 5 mL

No. 3558—TIMOPTIC-XE Sterile Ophthalmic Gel Forming Solution, 0.5% timolol equivalent, is supplied in OCUMETER, a white, opaque, plastic, ophthalmic dispenser with a controlled drop tip as follows:

NDC 0006-3558-32, 2.5 mL

NDC 0006-3558-03, 5 mL

Storage

Store between 15° and 25°C (59° and 77°F). **AVOID FREEZING.** Protect from light.

* Registered trademark of MERCK & CO., INC.

7931405 Issued December 1995

COPYRIGHT© MERCK & CO., INC., 1993
All rights reserved

TRIAVIL® Tablets ℞
(Perphenazine-Amitriptyline HCl), U.S.P.

DESCRIPTION

TRIAVIL* (Perphenazine-Amitriptyline HCl), a broad-spectrum psychotherapeutic agent for the management of outpatients and hospitalized patients with psychoses or neuroses characterized by mixtures of anxiety or agitation with symptoms of depression, is a combination of perphenazine and amitriptyline HCl. Since such mixed syndromes can occur in patients with various degrees of intensity of mental illness, TRIAVIL tablets are provided in multiple combinations to afford dosage flexibility for optimum management.

TRIAVIL is a combination of perphenazine, a piperazine phenothiazine, and amitriptyline HCl, a dibenzocycloheptadiene.

Perphenazine

Perphenazine is 4-[3-(2-chloro-10*H*-phenothiazin-10-yl)-propyl]-1-piperazineethanol. Its empirical formula is $C_{21}H_{26}ClN_3OS$ and its structural formula is:

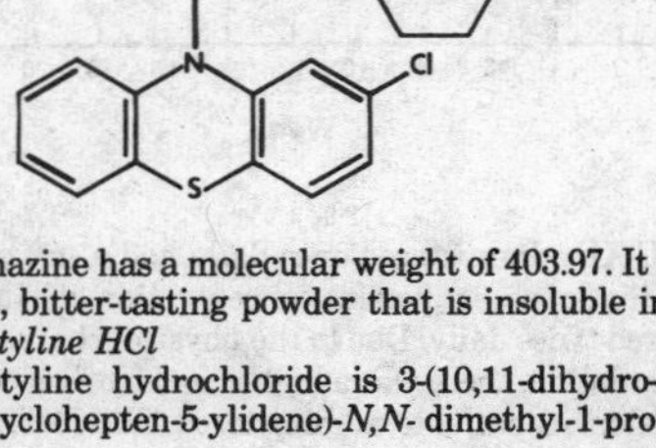

Perphenazine has a molecular weight of 403.97. It is a white, odorless, bitter-tasting powder that is insoluble in water.

Amitriptyline HCl

Amitriptyline hydrochloride is 3-(10,11-dihydro-5*H*-dibenzo[*a,d*]cyclohepten-5-ylidene)-*N,N*-dimethyl-1-propanamine

hydrochloride. Its empirical formula is $C_{20}H_{23}N \cdot HCl$ and its structural formula is:

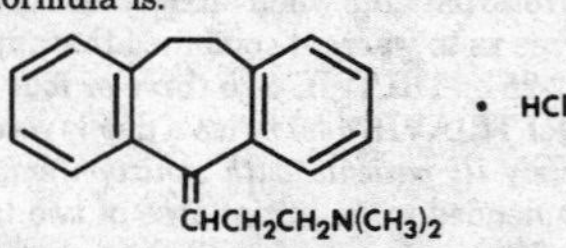

Amitriptyline HCl, a dibenzocycloheptadiene derivative, has a molecular weight of 313.87. It is a white, odorless, crystalline compound which is freely soluble in water.

Tablets TRIAVIL are supplied in 5 potencies:

TRIAVIL 2-10, containing 2 mg of perphenazine and 10 mg of amitriptyline HCl.

TRIAVIL 2-25, containing 2 mg of perphenazine and 25 mg of amitriptyline HCl.

TRIAVIL 4-10, containing 4 mg of perphenazine and 10 mg of amitriptyline HCl.

TRIAVIL 4-25, containing 4 mg of perphenazine and 25 mg of amitriptyline HCl.

TRIAVIL 4-50, containing 4 mg of perphenazine and 50 mg of amitriptyline HCl.

Inactive ingredients are calcium phosphate, cellulose, hydroxypropyl cellulose, hydroxypropyl methylcellulose, lactose, magnesium stearate, starch, talc, and titanium dioxide. TRIAVIL 2-10 also contains FD&C Blue 1. TRIAVIL 2-25 and 4-50 also contain FD&C Yellow 6. TRIAVIL 4-10 also contains iron oxide. TRIAVIL 4-25 also contains D&C Yellow 10 and FD&C Yellow 6.

*Registered trademark of MERCK & CO., INC.

ACTIONS

Perphenazine—In common with all members of the piperazine group of phenothiazine derivatives, perphenazine has greater behavioral potency than phenothiazine derivatives of other groups without a corresponding increase in autonomic, hematologic, or hepatic side effects.

Extrapyramidal effects, however, may occur more frequently. These effects are interpreted as neuropharmacologic. They usually regress after discontinuation of the drug.

Perphenazine is a potent tranquilizer and also a potent antiemetic. Orally, its milligram potency is about five or six times that of chlorpromazine with respect to behavorial effects. It is capable of alleviating symptoms of anxiety, tension, psychomotor excitement, and other manifestations of emotional stress without apparent dulling of mental acuity.

Amitriptyline HCl is an antidepressant with sedative effects. Its mechanism of action in man is not known. It is not a monoamine oxidase inhibitor and it does not act primarily by stimulation of the central nervous system.

INDICATIONS

TRIAVIL is recommended for treatment of (1) patients with *moderate to severe anxiety and/or agitation and depressed mood,* (2) patients with *depression in whom anxiety and/or agitation are severe,* and (3) patients with *depression and anxiety in association with chronic physical disease.* In many of these patients anxiety masks the depressive state so that, although therapy with a tranquilizer appears to be indicated, the administration of a tranquilizer alone will not be adequate.

Schizophrenic patients who have associated depressive symptoms should be considered for therapy with TRIAVIL.

Many patients presenting symptoms such as agitation, anxiety, insomnia, psychomotor retardation, functional somatic complaints, a feeling of tiredness, loss of interest, and anorexia have responded well to therapy with TRIAVIL.

CONTRAINDICATIONS

TRIAVIL is contraindicated in depression of the central nervous system from drugs (barbiturates, alcohol, narcotics, analgesics, antihistamines); in the presence of evidence of bone marrow depression; and in patients known to be hypersensitive to phenothiazines or amitriptyline.

It should not be given concomitantly with monoamine oxidase inhibitors. Hyperpyretic crises, severe convulsions, and deaths have occurred in patients receiving tricyclic antidepressants and monoamine oxidase inhibitors simultaneously. When it is desired to replace a monoamine oxidase inhibitor with TRIAVIL, a minimum of 14 days should be allowed to elapse after the former is discontinued. TRIAVIL should then be initiated cautiously with gradual increase in dosage until optimum response is achieved.

Amitriptyline HCl is not recommended for use during the acute recovery phase following myocardial infarction.

WARNINGS

Tardive dyskinesia

Tardive dyskinesia, a syndrome consisting of potentially irreversible, involuntary dyskinetic movements may develop in patients treated with neuroleptic (antipsychotic) drugs. Although the prevalence of the syndrome appears to be highest among the elderly, especially elderly women, it is impossible to rely upon prevalence estimates to predict, at the inception of neuroleptic treatment, which patients are likely to develop the syndrome. Whether neuroleptic drug products differ in their potential to cause tardive dyskinesia is unknown.

Both the risk of developing the syndrome and the likelihood that it will become irreversible are believed to increase as the duration of treatment and the total cumulative dose of neuroleptic drugs administered to the patient increase. However, the syndrome can develop, although much less commonly, after relatively brief treatment periods at low doses.

There is no known treatment for established cases of tardive dyskinesia, although the syndome may remit, partially or completely, if neuroleptic treatment is withdrawn. Neuroleptic treatment, itself, however, may suppress (or partially suppress) the signs and symptoms of the syndrome and thereby may possibly mask the underlying disease process. The effect that symptomatic suppression has upon the long-term course of the syndrome is unknown.

Given these considerations, neuroleptics should be prescribed in a manner that is most likely to minimize the occurrence of tardive dyskinesia. Chronic neuroleptic treatment should generally be reserved for patients who suffer from a chronic mental illness that, 1) is known to respond to neuroleptic drugs, and, 2) for whom alternative, equally effective, but potentially less harmful treatments are *not* available or appropriate. In patients who do require chronic treatment, the smallest dose and the shortest duration of treatment producing a satisfactory clinical response should be sought. The need for continued treatment should be reassessed periodically.

If signs and symptoms of tardive dyskinesia appear in a patient on neuroleptics, drug discontinuation should be considered. However, some patients may require treatment despite the presence of the syndrome.

(For further information about the description of tardive dyskinesia and its clinical detection, please refer to the section on ADVERSE REACTIONS).

Neuroleptic Malignant Syndrome (NMS)

A potentially fatal symptom complex sometimes referred to as Neuroleptic Malignant Syndrome (NMS) has been reported in association with antipsychotic drugs. Clinical manifestations of NMS are hyperpyrexia, muscle rigidity, altered mental status and evidence of autonomic instability (irregular pulse or blood pressure, tachycardia, diaphoresis, and cardiac dysrhythmias).

The diagnostic evaluation of patients with this syndrome is complicated. In arriving at a diagnosis, it is important to identify cases where the clinical presentation includes both serious medical illness (e.g., pneumonia, systemic infection, etc.) and untreated or inadequately treated extrapyramidal signs and symptoms (EPS). Other important considerations in the differential diagnosis include central anticholinergic toxicity, heat stroke, drug fever and primary central nervous system (CNS) pathology.

The management of NMS should include 1) immediate discontinuation of antipsychotic drugs and other drugs not essential to concurrent therapy, 2) intensive symptomatic treatment and medical monitoring, and 3) treatment of any concomitant serious medical problems for which specific treatments are available. There is no general agreement about specific pharmacological treatment regimens for uncomplicated NMS.

If a patient requires antipsychotic drug treatment after recovery from NMS, the potential reintroduction of drug therapy should be carefully considered. The patient should be carefully monitored, since recurrences of NMS have been reported.

General

TRIAVIL should not be given concomitantly with guanethidine or similarly acting compounds, since amitriptyline, like other tricyclic antidepressants, may block the antihypertensive effect of these compounds.

Because of the atropine-like activity of amitriptyline, TRIAVIL should be used with caution in patients with a history of urinary retention, or with angle-closure glaucoma or increased intraocular pressure. In patients with angle-closure glaucoma, even average doses may precipitate an attack.

It should be used with caution also in patients with convulsive disorders. Dosage of anticonvulsive agents may have to be increased.

Patients with cardiovascular disorders should be watched closely. Tricyclic antidepressants, including amitriptyline HCl, particularly when given in high doses, have been reported to produce arrhythmias, sinus tachycardia, and prolongation of the conduction time. Myocardial infarction and stroke have been reported with drugs of this class.

Close supervision is required when amitriptyline HCl is given to hyperthyroid patients or those receiving thyroid medication.

TRIAVIL may enhance the response to alcohol and the effects of barbiturates and other CNS depressants. In patients who may use alcohol excessively, it should be borne in mind that the potentiation may increase the danger inherent in any suicide attempt or overdosage. Delirium has been reported with concurrent administration of amitriptyline and disulfiram.

Usage in Pregnancy—TRIAVIL is not recommended for use in pregnant patients or in nursing mothers at this time. Reproduction studies in rats have shown no fetal abnormalities; however, clinical experience and follow-up in pregnancy have been limited, and the possibility of adverse effects on fetal development must be considered.

Usage in Children—Since dosage for children has not been established, TRIAVIL is not recommended for use in children.

PRECAUTIONS

General

The possibility of suicide in depressed patients remains during treatment and until significant remission occurs. Such patients should not have access to large quantities of this drug.

Perphenazine

As with all phenothiazine compounds, perphenazine should not be used indiscriminately. Caution should be observed in giving it to patients who have previously exhibited severe adverse reactions to other phenothiazines.

Some of the untoward actions of perphenazine tend to appear more frequently when high doses are used. However, as with other phenothiazine compounds, patients receiving perphenazine in any dosage should be kept under close supervision.

The antiemetic effect of perphenazine may obscure signs of toxicity due to overdosage of other drugs, or render more difficult the diagnosis of disorders such as brain tumors or intestinal obstruction.

A significant, not otherwise explained, rise in body temperature may suggest individual intolerance to perphenazine, in which case TRIAVIL should be discontinued.

Neuroleptic drugs elevate prolactin levels; the elevation persists during chronic administration. Tissue culture experiments indicate that approximately one third of human breast cancers are prolactin dependent *in vitro*, a factor of potential importance if the prescription of these drugs is contemplated in a patient with a previously detected breast cancer. Although disturbances such as galactorrhea, amenorrhea, gynecomastia, and impotence have been reported, the clinical significance of elevated serum prolactin levels is unknown for most patients. An increase in mammary neoplasms has been found in rodents after chronic administration of neuroleptic drugs. Neither clinical studies nor epidemiologic studies conducted to date, however, have shown an association between chronic administration of these drugs and mammary tumorigenesis; the available evidence is considered too limited to be conclusive at this time.

Amitriptyline HCl

Depressed patients, particularly those with known manic depressive illness, may experience a shift to mania or hypomania. Patients with paranoid symptomatology may have an exaggeration of such symptoms. The tranquilizing effect of TRIAVIL seems to reduce the likelihood of these effects.

Concurrent administration of amitriptyline HCl and electroshock therapy may increase the hazards associated with such therapy. Such treatment should be limited to patients for whom it is essential.

Discontinue the drug several days before elective surgery if possible.

Both elevation and lowering of blood sugar levels have been reported.

Amitriptyline HCl should be used with caution in patients with impaired liver function.

Information for Patients

While on therapy with TRIAVIL, patients should be advised as to the possible impairment of mental and/or physical abilities required for performance of hazardous tasks, such as operating machinery or driving a motor vehicle.

Drug Interactions

Perphenazine

If hypotension develops, epinephrine should not be employed, as its action is blocked and partially reversed by perphenazine.

Phenothiazines may potentiate the action of central nervous system depressants (opiates, analgesics, antihistamines, barbiturates, alcohol) and atropine. In concurrent therapy with any of these, TRIAVIL should be given in reduced dosage. Phenothiazines also may potentiate the action of heat and phosphorous insecticides.

Continued on next page

Information on the Merck & Co., Inc. products listed on these pages is the full prescribing information from product circulars in use September 30, 1996.

Merck & Co.—Cont.

Amitriptyline HCl

When amitriptyline HCl is given with anticholinergic agents or sympathomimetic drugs, including epinephrine combined with local anesthetics, close supervision and careful adjustment of dosages are required.

Hyperpyrexia has been reported when amitriptyline HCl is administered with anticholinergic agents or with neuroleptic drugs, particularly during hot weather.

Paralytic ileus may occur in patients taking tricyclic antidepressants in combination with anticholinergic-type drugs.

Cimetidine is reported to reduce hepatic metabolism of certain tricyclic antidepressants, thereby delaying elimination and increasing steady-state concentrations of these drugs. Clinically significant effects have been reported with the tricyclic antidepressants when used concomitantly with cimetidine. Increases in plasma levels of tricyclic antidepressants, and in the frequency and severity of side effects, particularly anticholinergic, have been reported when cimetidine was added to the drug regimen. Discontinuation of cimetidine in well-controlled patients receiving tricyclic antidepressants and cimetidine may decrease the plasma levels and efficacy of the antidepressants.

Caution is advised if patients receive large doses of ethchlorvynol concurrently. Transient delirium has been reported in patients who were treated with 1 g of ethchlorvynol and 75-150 mg of amitriptyline HCl.

ADVERSE REACTIONS

To date, clinical evaluation of TRIAVIL has not revealed any adverse reactions peculiar to the combination. The adverse reactions that occurred were limited to those that have been reported previously for perphenazine and amitriptyline. Treatment with TRIAVIL is commonly associated with sedation, hypotension, neurological impairments, and dry mouth.

Perphenazine

The common acute neurological effects of neuroleptic drugs, including perphenazine, consist of dystonia, akathisia or motor restlessness, and pseudoparkinsonism.

More chronic use of neuroleptics may be associated with the development of tardive dyskinesia. The salient features of this syndrome are described in the WARNINGS section and below.

The following adverse reactions have been reported and, within each category, are listed in order of decreasing severity.

Neurological:

Tardive dyskinesia:

The syndrome is characterized by involuntary choreoathetoid movements which variously involve the tongue, face, mouth, lips, or jaw (e.g., protrusion of the tongue, puffing of cheeks, puckering of the mouth, chewing movements), trunk and extremities. The severity of the syndrome and the degree of impairment produced vary widely.

The syndrome may become clinically recognizable either during treatment, upon dosage reduction, or upon withdrawal of treatment. Movements may decrease in intensity and may disappear altogether if further treatment with neuroleptics is withheld. It is generally believed that reversibility is more likely after short rather than long term neuroleptic exposure. Consequently, early detection of tardive dyskinesia is important. To increase the likelihood of detecting the syndrome at the earliest possible time, the dosage of neuroleptic drug should be reduced periodically (if clinically possible) and the patient observed for signs of the disorder. It has been suggested that fine vermicular movements of the tongue may be an early sign of the syndrome, and that the full-blown syndrome may not develop if medication is stopped when lingual vermiculation appears.

1. Dystonia

This may present as acute, reversible torticollis, opisthotonos, carpopedal spasm, trismus, dysphagia, respiratory difficulty, oculogyric crisis, and protrusion of the tongue. Treatment consists of the parenteral administration of either an anticholinergic antiparkinsonian agent or diphenhydramine.

2. Akathisia

Akathisia presents as constant motor restlessness. The patient with akathisia often complains, *when asked*, about his/her inability to stop moving. Akathisia should *not* be treated with an increased dose of neuroleptic; rather, the dose of antipsychotic may be lowered until the motor restlessness has subsided. The efficacy of anticholinergic treatment of this side effect is unestablished.

3. Pseudoparkinsonism

Pseudoparkinsonism refers to a drug-induced state similar to the classic syndrome. Generally, anticholinergic antiparkinsonian agents (i.e., benztropine, biperiden, procyclidine, or trihexphenidyl) and amantadine are helpful in alleviating symptoms that cannot be managed by neuroleptic dose reduction. The value of prophylactic antiparkinsonian drug

therapy has not been established. The need for continued use of antiparkinsonian medication should be re-evaluated periodically.

Cardiovascular: Hypotension, hypertension, tachycardia, peripheral edema, occasional change in pulse rate, ECG abnormalities (quinidine-like effect), reversed epinephrine effect.

CNS and Neuromuscular: Neuroleptic malignant syndrome (see WARNINGS); extrapyramidal symptoms, including acute dyskinesia (see *Neurological*); reactivation of psychoses and production of catatonic-like states; paradoxical excitement; ataxia; muscle weakness; hypnotic effects; mild insomnia; lassitude; headache; hyperflexia; altered cerebrospinal fluid proteins.

Autonomic: Urinary frequency or incontinence, dry mouth or salivation, nasal congestion.

Allergic: Anaphylactoid reactions, laryngeal edema, asthma, angioneurotic edema.

Hematologic: Blood dyscrasias including pancytopenia, agranulocytosis, leukopenia, thrombocytopenic purpura, eosinophilia.

Gastrointestinal: Liver damage (jaundice, biliary stasis), obstipation, vomiting, nausea, constipation, anorexia.

Dermatologic: Eczema up to exfoliative dermatitis, urticaria, erythema, itching, photosensitivity.

Ophthalmic: Pigmentation of the cornea and lens, blurred vision.

Endocrine: Lactation, galactorrhea, hyperglycemia, gynecomastia, disturbances in menstrual cycle.

Other: False-positive pregnancy tests, including immunologic.

Other adverse reactions that should be considered because they have been reported with various phenothiazine compounds, but not with perphenazine, include:

CNS and Neuromuscular: Grand mal convulsions, cerebral edema.

Gastrointestinal: Polyphagia.

Dermatologic: Photophobia, pigmentation.

Ophthalmic: Pigmentary retinopathy.

Endocrine: Failure of ejaculation.

Amitriptyline HCl

Within each category the following adverse reactions are listed in order of decreasing severity. Included in the listing are a few adverse reactions which have not been reported with this specific drug. However, pharmacological similarities among the tricyclic antidepressant drugs require that each of the reactions be considered when amitriptyline is administered.

Cardiovascular: Myocardial infarction; stroke; heart block; arrhythmias; hypotension, particularly orthostatic hypotension; hypertension; tachycardia; palpitation.

CNS and Neuromuscular: Coma; seizures; hallucinations; delusions; confusional states; disorientation; incoordination; ataxia; tremors; peripheral neuropathy; numbness, tingling, and paresthesias of the extremities; extrapyramidal symptoms; dysarthria; disturbed concentration; excitement; anxiety; insomnia; restlessness; nightmares; drowsiness; dizziness; weakness; fatigue; headache; syndrome of inappropriate ADH (antidiuretic hormone) secretion; tinnitus; alteration in EEG patterns.

Anticholinergic: Paralytic ileus; hyperpyrexia; urinary retention, dilatation of the urinary tract; constipation; blurred vision, disturbance of accommodation, increased intraocular pressure, mydriasis; dry mouth.

Allergic: Skin rash; urticaria; photosensitization; edema of face and tongue.

Hematologic: Bone marrow depression including agranulocytosis, leukopenia, thrombocytopenia; purpura; eosinophilia.

Gastrointestinal: Rarely hepatitis (including altered liver function and jaundice); nausea; epigastric distress; vomiting; anorexia; stomatitis; peculiar taste; diarrhea; parotid swelling; black tongue.

Endocrine: Testicular swelling and gynecomastia in the male; breast enlargement and galactorrhea in the female; increased or decreased libido; elevation and lowering of blood sugar levels.

Other: Alopecia; edema; weight gain or loss; urinary frequency; increased perspiration.

Withdrawal Symptoms: After prolonged administration, abrupt cessation of treatment may produce nausea, headache, and malaise. Gradual dosage reduction has been reported to produce within two weeks, transient symptoms including irritability, restlessness, and dream and sleep disturbance. These symptoms are not indicative of addiction. Rare instances have been reported of mania or hypomania occurring within 2-7 days following cessation of chronic therapy with tricyclic antidepressants.

DOSAGE AND ADMINISTRATION

Since dosage for children has not been established, TRIAVIL is not recommended for use in children.

The total daily dose of TRIAVIL should not exceed four tablets of the 4-50 or eight tablets of any other dosage strength.

Initial Dosage

In psychoneurotic patients when anxiety and depression are of such a degree as to warrant combined therapy, one tablet of TRIAVIL 2-25 or TRIAVIL 4-25 three or four times a day or one tablet of TRIAVIL 4-50 twice a day is recommended.

In more severely ill patients with schizophrenia, TRIAVIL 4-25 is recommended in an initial dose of two tablets three times a day. If necessary, a fourth dose may be given at bedtime.

In elderly patients and adolescents, and some other patients in whom anxiety tends to predominate, TRIAVIL 4-10 may be administered three or four times a day initially, then adjusted as required for subsequent adequate therapy.

Maintenance Dosage

Depending on the condition being treated, therapeutic response may take from a few days to a few weeks or even longer. After a satisfactory response is noted, dosage should be reduced to the smallest amount necessary to obtain relief from the symptoms for which TRIAVIL is being administered. A useful maintenance dosage is one tablet of TRIAVIL 2-25 or 4-25 two to four times a day or one tablet of TRIAVIL 4-50 twice a day. TRIAVIL 2-10 and 4-10 can be used to increase flexibility in adjusting maintenance dosage to the lowest amount consistent with relief of symptoms. In some patients, maintenance dosage is required for many months.

OVERDOSAGE

Manifestations—High doses may cause temporary confusion, disturbed concentration, or transient visual hallucinations. Overdosage may cause drowsiness; hypothermia; tachycardia and other arrhythmic abnormalities, such as bundle branch block; ECG evidence of impaired conduction; congestive heart failure; dilated pupils; disorders of ocular motility; convulsions; severe hypotension; stupor; and coma. Other symptoms may be agitation, hyperactive reflexes, muscle rigidity, vomiting, hyperpyrexia, or any of the adverse reactions listed for perphenazine or amitriptyline.

Levarterenol (norepinephrine) may be used to treat hypotension, but not epinephrine.

All patients suspected of having taken an overdosage should be admitted to a hospital as soon as possible. *Treatment* is symptomatic and supportive. Empty the stomach as quickly as possible by emesis followed by gastric lavage upon arrival at the hospital. Saline emetics should not be used as the antiemetic effect of perphenazine may cause retention of the saline load and subsequent hypernatremia. Following gastric lavage, activated charcoal may be administered. Twenty to 30 g of activated charcoal may be given every four to six hours during the first 24 to 48 hours after ingestion. An ECG should be taken and close monitoring of cardiac function instituted if there is any sign of abnormality. Maintain an open airway and adequate fluid intake; regulate body temperature.

The intravenous administration of 1–3 mg of physostigmine salicylate is reported to reverse the symptoms of tricyclic antidepressant poisoning. Because physostigmine is rapidly metabolized, the dosage of physostigmine should be repeated as required particularly if life threatening signs such as arrhythmias, convulsions, and deep coma recur or persist after the initial dosage of physostigmine. On this basis, in severe overdosage with perphenazine-amitriptyline combinations, symptomatic treatment of central anticholinergic effects with physostigmine salicylate should be considered. Because physostigmine itself may be toxic, it is not recommended for routine use.

Standard measures should be used to manage circulatory shock and metabolic acidosis. Cardiac arrhythmias may be treated with neostigmine, pyridostigmine, or propranolol. Should cardiac failure occur, the use of digitalis should be considered. Close monitoring of cardiac function for not less than five days is advisable.

Anticonvulsants may be given to control convulsions. Amitriptyline and perphenazine increase the CNS depressant action but not the anticonvulsant action of barbiturates; therefore, an inhalation anesthetic, diazepam, or paraldehyde is recommended for control of convulsions. The management of acute symptoms of parkinsonism resulting from perphenazine intoxication may be treated with appropriate doses of COGENTIN* (Benztropine Mesylate) or diphenhydramine hydrochloride.**

Dialysis is of no value because of low plasma concentrations of the drug.

Since overdosage is often deliberate, patients may attempt suicide by other means during the recovery phase.

Deaths by deliberate or accidental overdosage have occurred with this class of drugs.

* Registered trademark of MERCK & CO., INC.
** BENADRYL® (Diphenhydramine Hydrochloride), Parke, Davis & Co.

HOW SUPPLIED

No. 3328—Tablets TRIAVIL 2-10 are blue, triangular, film coated tablets, coded MSD 914. They are supplied as follows:
NDC 0006-0914-68 bottles of 100
NDC 0006-0914-28 unit dose package of 100
NDC 0006-0914-74 bottles of 500.
Shown in Product Identification Guide, page 325
No. 3311—Tablets TRIAVIL 2-25 are orange, triangular, film coated tablets, coded MSD 921. They are supplied as follows:
NDC 0006-0921-68 bottles of 100
NDC 0006-0921-28 unit dose package of 100
NDC 0006-0921-74 bottles of 500.
(6505-01-210-4467 500's)
Shown in Product Identification Guide, page 325
No. 3310—Tablets TRIAVIL 4-10 are salmon, triangular, film coated tablets, coded MSD 934. They are supplied as follows:
NDC 0006-0934-68 bottles of 100
NDC 0006-0934-74 bottles of 500.
Shown in Product Identification Guide, page 325
No. 3312—Tablets TRIAVIL 4-25 are yellow, triangular, film coated tablets, coded MSD 946. They are supplied as follows:
NDC 0006-0946-68 bottles of 100
(6505-01-210-4468 100's)
NDC 0006-0946-28 unit dose package of 100
NDC 0006-0946-74 bottles of 500.
Shown in Product Identification Guide, page 325
No. 3364—Tablets TRIAVIL 4-50 are orange, diamond shaped, film coated tablets, coded MSD 517. They are supplied as follows:
NDC 0006-0517-60 bottles of 60
NDC 0006-0517-68 bottles of 100.
Shown in Product Identification Guide, page 325
Storage
Store Tablets TRIAVIL in a well-closed container. Avoid storage at temperatures above 40°C (104°F). In addition, Tablets TRIAVIL 2-10 must be protected from light and stored in a well-closed, light-resistant container.
A.H.F.S. Categories: 28:16:04, 28:16:08
DC 7398431 Issued September 1990
COPYRIGHT © MERCK & CO., INC., 1985
All rights reserved

TRUSOPT® Sterile Ophthalmic Solution 2% ℞
(Dorzolamide Hydrochloride Ophthalmic Solution)

DESCRIPTION

TRUSOPT* (dorzolamide hydrochloride ophthalmic solution) is a carbonic anhydrase inhibitor formulated for topical ophthalmic use.
Dorzolamide hydrochloride is described chemically as: (4*S-trans*)-4-(ethylamino)-5,6-dihydro-6-methyl-4*H*-thieno [2,3-b]thiopyran-2-sulfonamide 7,7-dioxide monohydrochloride. Dorzolamide hydrochloride is optically active. The specific rotation is

$$\alpha^{25°}_{405} \text{ (C = 1, water) } = \sim -17°.$$

Its empirical formula is $C_{10}H_{16}N_2O_4S_3 \cdot HCl$ and its structural formula is:

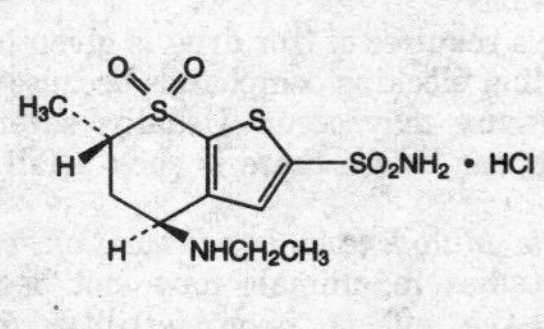

Dorzolamide hydrochloride has a molecular weight of 360.9 and a melting point of about 264°C. It is a white to off-white, crystalline powder, which is soluble in water and slightly soluble in methanol and ethanol.
TRUSOPT Sterile Ophthalmic Solution is supplied as a sterile, isotonic, buffered, slightly viscous, aqueous solution of dorzolamide hydrochloride. The pH of the solution is approximately 5.6. Each mL of TRUSOPT 2% contains 20 mg dorzolamide (22.3 mg of dorzolamide hydrochloride). Inactive ingredients are hydroxyethyl cellulose, mannitol, sodium citrate dihydrate, sodium hydroxide (to adjust pH) and water for injection. Benzalkonium chloride 0.0075% is added as a preservative.

---
* Registered trademark of MERCK & CO., Inc., Whitehouse Station, NJ, USA

CLINICAL PHARMACOLOGY

Mechanism of Action
Carbonic anhydrase (CA) is an enzyme found in many tissues of the body including the eye. It catalyzes the reversible reaction involving the hydration of carbon dioxide and the dehydration of carbonic acid. In humans, carbonic anhydrase exists as a number of isoenzymes, the most active being carbonic anhydrase II (CA-II), found primarily in red blood cells (RBCs), but also in other tissues. Inhibition of carbonic anhydrase in the ciliary processes of the eye decreases aqueous humor secretion, presumably by slowing the formation of bicarbonate ions with subsequent reduction in sodium and fluid transport. The result is a reduction in intraocular pressure (IOP).
TRUSOPT Ophthalmic Solution contains dorzolamide hydrochloride, an inhibitor of human carbonic anhydrase II. Following topical ocular administration, TRUSOPT reduces elevated intraocular pressure. Elevated intraocular pressure is a major risk factor in the pathogenesis of optic nerve damage and glaucomatous visual field loss.
Pharmacokinetics/Pharmacodynamics
When topically applied, dorzolamide reaches the systemic circulation. To assess the potential for systemic carbonic anhydrase inhibition following topical administration, drug and metabolite concentrations in RBCs and plasma and carbonic anhydrase inhibition in RBCs were measured. Dorzolamide accumulates in RBCs during chronic dosing as a result of binding to CA-II. The parent drug forms a single N-desethyl metabolite, which inhibits CA-II less potently than the parent drug but also inhibits CA-I. The metabolite also accumulates in RBCs where it binds primarily to CA-I. Plasma concentrations of dorzolamide and metabolite are generally below the assay limit of quantitation (15nM). Dorzolamide binds moderately to plasma proteins (approximately 33%). Dorzolamide is primarily excreted unchanged in the urine; the metabolite also is excreted in urine. After dosing is stopped, dorzolamide washes out of RBCs nonlinearly, resulting in a rapid decline of drug concentration initially, followed by a slower elimination phase with a half-life of about four months.
To simulate the systemic exposure after long-term topical ocular administration, dorzolamide was given orally to eight healthy subjects for up to 20 weeks. The oral dose of 2 mg b.i.d. closely approximates the amount of drug delivered by topical ocular administration of TRUSOPT 2% t.i.d. Steady state was reached within 8 weeks. The inhibition of CA-II and total carbonic anhydrase activities was below the degree of inhibition anticipated to be necessary for a pharmacological effect on renal function and respiration in healthy individuals.
Clinical Studies
The efficacy of TRUSOPT was demonstrated in clinical studies in the treatment of elevated intraocular pressure in patients with glaucoma or ocular hypertension (baseline IOP ≥ 23 mmHg). The IOP-lowering effect of TRUSOPT was approximately 3 to 5 mmHg throughout the day and this was consistent in clinical studies of up to one year duration.
The efficacy of TRUSOPT when dosed less frequently than three times a day (alone or in combination with other products) has not been established.

INDICATIONS AND USAGE

TRUSOPT Ophthalmic Solution is indicated in the treatment of elevated intraocular pressure in patients with ocular hypertension or open-angle glaucoma.

CONTRAINDICATIONS

TRUSOPT is contraindicated in patients who are hypersensitive to any component of this product.

WARNINGS

TRUSOPT is a sulfonamide and although administered topically is absorbed systemically. Therefore, the same types of adverse reactions that are attributable to sulfonamides may occur with topical administration with TRUSOPT. Fatalities have occurred, although rarely, due to severe reactions to sulfonamides including Stevens-Johnson syndrome, toxic epidermal necrolysis, fulminant hepatic necrosis, agranulocytosis, aplastic anemia, and other blood dyscrasias. Sensitization may recur when a sulfonamide is readministered irrespective of the route of administration. If signs of serious reactions or hypersensitivity occur, discontinue the use of this preparation.

PRECAUTIONS

General
Carbonic anhydrase activity has been observed in both the cytoplasm and around the plasma membranes of the corneal endothelium. The effect of continued administration of TRUSOPT on the corneal endothelium has not been fully evaluated.
The management of patients with acute angle-closure glaucoma requires therapeutic interventions in addition to ocular hypotensive agents. TRUSOPT has not been studied in patients with acute angle-closure glaucoma.
TRUSOPT has not been studied in patients with severe renal impairment (CrCl < 30 mL/min). Because TRUSOPT and its metabolite are excreted predominantly by the kidney, TRUSOPT is not recommended in such patients.
TRUSOPT has not been studied in patients with hepatic impairment and should therefore be used with caution in such patients.
In clinical studies, local ocular adverse effects, primarily conjunctivitis and lid reactions, were reported with chronic administration of TRUSOPT. Many of these reactions had the clinical appearance and course of an allergic-type reaction that resolved upon discontinuation of drug therapy. If such reactions are observed, TRUSOPT should be discontinued and the patient evaluated before considering restarting the drug. (See **ADVERSE REACTIONS**.)
There is a potential for an additive effect on the known systemic effects of carbonic anhydrase inhibition in patients receiving an oral carbonic anhydrase inhibitor and TRUSOPT. The concomitant administration of TRUSOPT and oral carbonic anhydrase inhibitors is not recommended.
There have been reports of bacterial keratitis associated with the use of multiple dose containers of topical ophthalmic products. These containers had been inadvertently contaminated by patients who, in most cases, had a concurrent corneal disease or a disruption of the ocular epithelial surface.
The preservative in TRUSOPT Ophthalmic Solution, benzalkonium chloride, may be absorbed by soft contact lenses. TRUSOPT should not be administered while wearing soft contact lenses.
Information for Patients
TRUSOPT is a sulfonamide and although administered topically is absorbed systemically. Therefore the same types of adverse reactions that are attributable to sulfonamides may occur with topical administration. Patients should be advised that if serious or unusual reactions or signs of hypersensitivity occur, they should discontinue the use of the product (see **WARNINGS**).
Patients should be advised that if they develop any ocular reactions, particularly conjunctivitis and lid reactions, they should discontinue use and seek their physician's advice.
Patients should be instructed to avoid allowing the tip of the dispensing container to contact the eye or surrounding structures.
Patients should also be instructed that ocular solutions, if handled improperly or if the tip of the dispensing container contacts the eye or surrounding structures, can become contaminated by common bacteria known to cause ocular infections. Serious damage to the eye and subsequent loss of vision may result from using contaminated solutions.
Patients also should be advised that if they develop an intercurrent ocular condition (e.g., trauma, ocular surgery or infection), they should immediately seek their physician's advice concerning the continued use of the present multidose container.
If more than one topical ophthalmic drug is being used, the drugs should be administered at least ten minutes apart.
Drug Interactions
Although acid-base and electrolyte disturbances were not reported in the clinical trials with TRUSOPT, these disturbances have been reported with oral carbonic anhydrase inhibitors and have, in some instances, resulted in drug interactions (e.g., toxicity associated with high-dose salicylate therapy). Therefore, the potential for such drug interactions should be considered in patients receiving TRUSOPT.
Carcinogenesis, Mutagenesis, Impairment of Fertility
In a two-year study of dorzolamide hydrochloride administered orally to male and female Sprague-Dawley rats, urinary bladder papillomas were seen in male rats in the highest dosage group of 20 mg/kg/day (250 times the recommended human ophthalmic dose). Papillomas were not seen in rats given oral doses equivalent to approximately 12 times the recommended human ophthalmic dose. No treatment-related tumors were seen in a 21-month study in female and male mice given oral doses up to 75 mg/kg/day (~900 times the recommended human ophthalmic dose).
The increased incidence of urinary bladder papillomas seen in the high-dose male rats is a class-effect of carbonic anhydrase inhibitors in rats. Rats are particularly prone to developing papillomas in response to foreign bodies, compounds causing crystalluria, and diverse sodium salts.
No changes in bladder urothelium were seen in dogs given oral dorzolamide hydrochloride for one year at 2 mg/kg/day

Continued on next page

Information on the Merck & Co., Inc. products listed on these pages is the full prescribing information from product circulars in use September 30, 1996.

Consult 1997 supplements and future editions for revisions

Merck & Co.—Cont.

(25 times the recommended human ophthalmic dose) or monkeys dosed topically to the eye at 0.4 mg/kg/day (~5 times the recommended human ophthalmic dose) for one year. The following tests for mutagenic potential were negative: (1) *in vivo* (mouse) cytogenetic assay; (2) *in vitro* chromosomal aberration assay; (3) alkaline elution assay; (4) V-79 assay; and (5) Ames test.

In reproduction studies of dorzolamide hydrochloride in rats, there were no adverse effects on the reproductive capacity of males or females at doses up to 188 or 94 times, respectively, the recommended human ophthalmic dose.

Pregnancy

Teratogenic Effects. Pregnancy Category C. Developmental toxicity studies with dorzolamide hydrochloride in rabbits at oral doses of ≥2.5 mg/kg/day (31 times the recommended human ophthalmic dose) revealed malformations of the vertebral bodies. These malformations occurred at doses that caused metabolic acidosis with decreased body weight gain in dams and decreased fetal weights. No treatment-related malformations were seen at 1.0 mg/kg/day (13 times the recommended human ophthalmic dose). There were no treatment-related fetal malformations in developmental toxicity studies with dorzolamide hydrochloride in rats at oral doses up to 10 mg/kg/day (125 times the recommended human ophthalmic dose). There are no adequate and well-controlled studies in pregnant women. TRUSOPT should be used during pregnancy only if the potential benefit justifies the potential risk to the fetus.

Nursing Mothers

In a study of dorzolamide hydrochloride in lactating rats, decreases in body weight gain of 5 to 7% in offspring at an oral dose of 7.5 mg/kg/day (94 times the recommended human ophthalmic dose) were seen during lactation. A slight delay in postnatal development (incisor eruption, vaginal canalization and eye openings), secondary to lower fetal body weight, was noted.

It is not known whether this drug is excreted in human milk. Because many drugs are excreted in human milk and because of the potential for serious adverse reactions in nursing infants from TRUSOPT, a decision should be made whether to discontinue nursing or to discontinue the drug, taking into account the importance of the drug to the mother.

Pediatric Use

Safety and effectiveness in pediatric patients have not been established.

Geriatric Use

Of the total number of patients in clinical studies of TRUSOPT, 44% were 65 years of age and over, while 10% were 75 years of age and over. No overall differences in effectiveness or safety were observed between these patients and younger patients, but greater sensitivity of some older individuals to the product cannot be ruled out.

ADVERSE REACTIONS

In clinical studies, the most frequent adverse events associated with TRUSOPT were ocular burning, stinging, or discomfort immediately following ocular administration (approximately one-third of patients). Approximately one-quarter of patients noted a bitter taste following administration. Superficial punctate keratitis occurred in 10–15% of patients and signs and symptoms of ocular allergic reaction in approximately 10%. Events occurring in approximately 1–5% of patients were blurred vision, tearing, dryness, and photophobia. Other ocular events and systemic events were reported infrequently, including headache, nausea, asthenia/fatigue; and, rarely, skin rashes, urolithiasis, and iridocyclitis.

The following adverse reactions have been reported in post-marketing experience:

Hypersensitivity: signs and symptoms of systemic allergic reactions including angioedema, pruritus, and urticaria;
Nervous System: dizziness, paresthesia;
Ocular: transient myopia, which resolved upon discontinuation of treatment.

OVERDOSAGE

Although no human data are available, electrolyte imbalance, development of an acidotic state, and possible central nervous system effects may occur. Serum electrolyte levels (particularly potassium) and blood pH levels should be monitored.

Significant lethality was observed in female rats and mice after single oral doses of dorzolamide hydrochloride 1927 mg/kg and 1320 mg/kg, respectively.

DOSAGE AND ADMINISTRATION

The dose is one drop of TRUSOPT Ophthalmic Solution in the affected eyes(s) three times daily.

TRUSOPT may be used concomitantly with other topical ophthalmic drug products to lower intraocular pressure. If more than one topical ophthalmic drug is being used, the drugs should be administered at least ten minutes apart.

HOW SUPPLIED

TRUSOPT Ophthalmic Solution is a slightly opalescent, nearly colorless, slightly viscous solution.

No. 3519—TRUSOPT Ophthalmic Solution 2% is supplied in OCUMETER®*, a white, opaque, plastic ophthalmic dispenser with a controlled drop tip as follows:

NDC 0006-3519-03, 5 mL
NDC 0006-3519-10, 10 mL
(6505-01-416-4328)
NDC 0006-3519-34, 3×5 mL.

Storage

Store TRUSOPT Ophthalmic Solution at 15–30°C (59–86°F). Protect from light.

---

* Registered trademark of MERCK & CO., Inc., Whitehouse Station, NJ, USA

7879002   Issued May 1996
COPYRIGHT© MERCK & CO., Inc., 1994

URECHOLINE® Tablets   ℞
(Bethanechol Chloride), U.S.P.
URECHOLINE® Injection   ℞
(Bethanechol Chloride), U.S.P.

DESCRIPTION

URECHOLINE* (Bethanechol Chloride), a cholinergic agent, is a synthetic ester which is structurally and pharmacologically related to acetylcholine.

It is designated chemically as 2-[(aminocarbonyl)oxy]-*N, N, N*-trimethyl-1-propanaminium chloride. Its empirical formula is $C_7H_{17}ClN_2O_2$ and its structural formula is:

$$\left[\begin{array}{c} CH_3CH-CH_2N^+(CH_3)_3 \\ | \\ OCONH_2 \end{array} \right] Cl^-$$

It is a white, hygroscopic crystalline compound having a slight amine-like odor, freely soluble in water, and has a molecular weight of 196.68.

URECHOLINE is supplied as 5 mg, 10 mg, 25 mg, and 50 mg tablets for oral use. Inactive ingredients in the tablets are calcium phosphate, lactose, magnesium stearate, and starch. Tablets URECHOLINE 10 mg also contain FD&C Red 3 and FD&C Red 40. Tablets URECHOLINE 25 mg and 50 mg also contain D&C Yellow 10 and FD&C Yellow 6.

URECHOLINE is also supplied as a sterile solution **for subcutaneous use only**. The sterile solution is essentially neutral. Each milliliter contains bethanechol chloride, 5 mg, and Water for Injection, q.s., 1 mL. It may be autoclaved at 120°C for 20 minutes without discoloration or loss of potency.

---

* Registered trademark of MERCK & CO., INC.

CLINICAL PHARMACOLOGY

Bethanechol chloride acts principally by producing the effects of stimulation of the parasympathetic nervous system. It increases the tone of the detrusor urinae muscle, usually producing a contraction sufficiently strong to initiate micturition and empty the bladder. It stimulates gastric motility, increases gastric tone, and often restores impaired rhythmic peristalsis.

Stimulation of the parasympathetic nervous system releases acetylcholine at the nerve endings. When spontaneous stimulation is reduced and therapeutic intervention is required, acetylcholine can be given, but it is rapidly hydrolyzed by cholinesterase, and its effects are transient. Bethanechol chloride is not destroyed by cholinesterase and its effects are more prolonged than those of acetylcholine.

Effects on the GI and urinary tracts sometimes appear within 30 minutes after oral administration of bethanechol chloride, but more often 60–90 minutes are required to reach maximum effectiveness. Following oral administration, the usual duration of action of bethanechol is one hour, although large doses (300–400 mg) have been reported to produce effects for up to six hours. Subcutaneous injection produces a more intense action on bladder muscle than does oral administration of the drug.

Because of the selective action of bethanechol, nicotinic symptoms of cholinergic stimulation are usually absent or minimal when orally or subcutaneously administered in therapeutic doses, while muscarinic effects are prominent. Muscarinic effects usually occur within 5–15 minutes after subcutaneous injection, reach a maximum in 15–30 minutes, and disappear within two hours. Doses that stimulate micturition and defecation and increase peristalsis do not ordinarily stimulate ganglia or voluntary muscles. Therapeutic test doses in normal human subjects have little effect on heart rate, blood pressure, or peripheral circulation. Bethanechol chloride does not cross the blood-brain barrier because of its charged quaternary amine moiety. The metabolic fate and mode of excretion of the drug have not been elucidated.

A clinical study* was conducted on the relative effectiveness of oral and subcutaneous doses of bethanechol chloride on the stretch response of bladder muscle in patients with urinary retention. Results showed that 5 mg of the drug given subcutaneously stimulated a response that was more rapid in onset and of larger magnitude than an oral dose of 50 mg, 100 mg, or 200 mg. All the oral doses, however, had a longer duration of effect than the subcutaneous dose. Although the 50 mg oral dose caused little change in intravesical pressure in this study, this dose has been found in other studies to be clinically effective in the rehabilitation of patients with decompensated bladders.

---

*Diokno, A. C.; Lapides, J., Urol. *10:* 23–24, July 1977.

INDICATIONS AND USAGE

For the treatment of acute postoperative and postpartum nonobstructive (functional) urinary retention and for neurogenic atony of the urinary bladder with retention.

CONTRAINDICATIONS

Hypersensitivity to URECHOLINE tablets or to any component of URECHOLINE injection, hyperthyroidism, peptic ulcer, latent or active bronchial asthma, pronounced bradycardia or hypotension, vasomotor instability, coronary artery disease, epilepsy, and parkinsonism.

URECHOLINE should not be employed when the strength or integrity of the gastrointestinal or bladder wall is in question, or in the presence of mechanical obstruction; when increased muscular activity of the gastrointestinal tract or urinary bladder might prove harmful, as following recent urinary bladder surgery, gastrointestinal resection and anastomosis, or when there is possible gastrointestinal obstruction; in bladder neck obstruction, spastic gastrointestinal disturbances, acute inflammatory lesions of the gastrointestinal tract, or peritonitis; or in marked vagotonia.

WARNING

The sterile solution is for subcutaneous use only. It should never be given intramuscularly or intravenously. Violent symptoms of cholinergic over-stimulation, such as circulatory collapse, fall in blood pressure, abdominal cramps, bloody diarrhea, shock, or sudden cardiac arrest are likely to occur if the drug is given by either of these routes. Although rare, these same symptoms have occurred after subcutaneous injection, and may occur in cases of hypersensitivity or overdosage.

PRECAUTIONS

General

In urinary retention, if the sphincter fails to relax as URECHOLINE contracts the bladder, urine may be forced up the ureter into the kidney pelvis. If there is bacteriuria, this may cause reflux infection.

Information for Patients

URECHOLINE tablets should preferably be taken one hour before or two hours after meals to avoid nausea or vomiting. Dizziness, lightheadedness or fainting may occur, especially when getting up from a lying or sitting position.

Drug Interactions

Special care is required if this drug is given to patients receiving ganglion blocking compounds because a critical fall in blood pressure may occur. Usually, severe abdominal symptoms appear before there is such a fall in the blood pressure.

Carcinogenesis, Mutagenesis, Impairment of Fertility

Long-term studies in animals have not been performed to evaluate the effects upon fertility, mutagenic or carcinogenic potential of URECHOLINE.

Pregnancy

Pregnancy Category C. Animal reproduction studies have not been conducted with URECHOLINE. It is also not known whether URECHOLINE can cause fetal harm when administered to a pregnant woman or can affect reproduction capacity. URECHOLINE should be given to a pregnant woman only if clearly needed.

Nursing Mothers

It is not known whether this drug is secreted in human milk. Because many drugs are secreted in human milk and because of the potential for serious adverse reactions from URECHOLINE in nursing infants, a decision should be made whether to discontinue nursing or to discontinue the drug, taking into account the importance of the drug to the mother.

Pediatric Use
Safety and effectiveness in children have not been established.

ADVERSE REACTIONS

Adverse reactions are rare following oral administration of bethanechol, but are more common following subcutaneous injection. Adverse reactions are more likely to occur when dosage is increased.
The following adverse reactions have been observed: *Body as a Whole:* malaise; *Digestive:* abdominal cramps or discomfort, colicky pain, nausea and belching, diarrhea, borborygmi, salivation; *Renal:* urinary urgency; *Nervous System:* headache; *Cardiovascular:* a fall in blood pressure with reflex tachycardia, vasomotor response; *Skin:* flushing producing a feeling of warmth, sensation of heat about the face, sweating; *Respiratory:* bronchial constriction, asthmatic attacks; *Special Senses:* lacrimation, miosis.
Causal Relationship Unknown: The following adverse reactions have been reported, and a causal relationship to therapy with URECHOLINE has not been established: *Body as a Whole:* hypothermia: *Nervous System:* seizures.

OVERDOSAGE

Early signs of overdosage are abdominal discomfort, salivation, flushing of the skin ("hot feeling"), sweating, nausea and vomiting.
Atropine is a specific antidote. The recommended dose for adults is 0.6 mg (1/100 grain). Repeat doses can be given every two hours, according to clinical response. The recommended dosage in infants and children up to 12 years of age is 0.01 mg/kg (to a maximum single dose of 0.4 mg) repeated every two hours as needed until the desired effect is obtained, or adverse effects of atropine preclude further usage.
Subcutaneous injection of atropine is preferred except in emergencies when the intravenous route may be employed.
When URECHOLINE is administered subcutaneously, a syringe containing a dose of atropine sulfate should always be available to treat symptoms of toxicity.
The oral LD_{50} of bethanechol chloride is 1510 mg/kg in the mouse.

DOSAGE AND ADMINISTRATION

Dosage and route of administration must be individualized, depending on the type and severity of the condition to be treated.
Preferably give the drug when the stomach is empty. If taken soon after eating, nausea and vomiting may occur.
Oral—The usual adult dosage is 10 to 50 mg three or four times a day. The minimum effective dose is determined by giving 5 or 10 mg initially and repeating the same amount at hourly intervals until satisfactory response occurs or until a maximum of 50 mg has been given. The effects of the drug sometimes appear within 30 minutes and usually within 60 to 90 minutes. They persist for about an hour.
Subcutaneous—The usual dose is 1 mL (5 mg), although some patients respond satisfactorily to as little as 0.5 mL (2.5 mg). The minimum effective dose is determined by injecting 0.5 mL (2.5 mg) initially and repeating the same amount at 15 to 30 minute intervals to a maximum of four doses until satisfactory response is obtained, unless disturbing reactions appear. The minimum effective dose may be repeated thereafter three or four times a day as required.
Rarely, single doses up to 2 mL (10 mg) may be required. Such large doses may cause severe reactions and should be used only after adequate trial of single doses of 0.5 to 1 mL (2.5 to 5 mg) has established that smaller doses are not sufficient.
URECHOLINE is usually effective in 5 to 15 minutes after subcutaneous injection.
If necessary, the effects of the drug can be abolished promptly by atropine (see OVERDOSAGE).
Parenteral drug products should be inspected visually for particulate matter and discoloration prior to administration, whenever solution and container permit.

HOW SUPPLIED

Tablets URECHOLINE are round, compressed tablets, scored on one side. They are supplied as follows:
No. 7785—5 mg, white in color, coded MSD 403.
NDC 0006-0403-68 in bottles of 100.
Shown in Product Identification Guide, page 325
No. 7787—10 mg, pink in color, coded MSD 412.
NDC 0006-0412-68 in bottles of 100
(6505-00-616-7856 10 mg 100's).
Shown in Product Identification Guide, page 325
No. 7788—25 mg, yellow in color, coded MSD 457.
NDC 0006-0457-68 in bottles of 100
(6505-00-912-7440 25 mg, 100's).
Shown in Product Identification Guide, page 325
No. 7790 — 50 mg, yellow in color, coded MSD 460.
NDC 0006-0460-68 in bottles of 100.
Shown in Product Identification Guide, page 325
No. 7786—Injection URECHOLINE, 5 mg per mL, is a clear, colorless solution, and is supplied as follows:
NDC 0006-7786-29 in box of 6 × 1 mL vials
(6505-00-616-8947 in box of 6 × 1 mL vials).
Storage
Store Tablets URECHOLINE in a tightly-closed container. Avoid storage at temperatures above 40°C (104°F).
Avoid storage of Injection URECHOLINE at temperatures below −20°C (−4°F) and above 40°C (104°F).
7399332 Issued May 1992
COPYRIGHT © MERCK & CO., INC., 1984
All rights reserved

VAQTA® ℞
(Hepatitis A Vaccine, Inactivated)

DESCRIPTION

VAQTA* [Hepatitis A Vaccine, Inactivated] is an inactivated whole virus vaccine derived from hepatitis A virus (HAV) grown in cell culture in human MRC-5 diploid fibroblasts. It contains inactivated virus of a strain which was originally derived by further serial passage of a proven attenuated strain. The virus is grown, harvested, purified by a combination of physical and high performance liquid chromatographic techniques developed at the Merck Research Laboratories, formalin inactivated, and then adsorbed onto aluminum hydroxide. One milliliter of the vaccine contains approximately 50 units (U) of hepatitis A virus antigen, which is purified and formulated without a preservative. Within the limits of current assay variability, the 50U dose of VAQTA contains less than 0.1 mcg of non-viral protein, less than 4×10^{-6} mcg of DNA, less than 10^{-4} mcg of bovine albumin, and less than 0.8 mcg of formaldehyde. Other process chemical residuals are less than 10 parts per billion (ppb).
VAQTA is a sterile suspension for intramuscular injection. VAQTA is supplied in two formulations:
Pediatric/Adolescent Formulation: each 0.5 mL dose contains approximately 25U of hepatitis A virus antigen adsorbed onto approximately 0.225 mg of aluminum provided as aluminum hydroxide, and 35 mcg of sodium borate as a pH stabilizer, in 0.9% sodium chloride.
Adult Formulation: each 1 mL dose contains approximately 50U of hepatitis A virus antigen adsorbed onto approximately 0.45 mg of aluminum provided as aluminum hydroxide, and 70 mcg of sodium borate as a pH stabilizer, in 0.9% sodium chloride.

*Registered trademark of MERCK & CO., Inc.

CLINICAL PHARMACOLOGY

Hepatitis A Disease
Hepatitis A virus is one of several hepatitis viruses that cause a systemic infection with pathology in the liver. The incubation period ranges from approximately 20 to 50 days. While the course of the disease is generally benign and does not result in chronic hepatitis, infection with hepatitis A virus remains an important cause of morbidity and occasional fulminant hepatitis and death.[1]
Hepatitis A is transmitted most often by the fecal-oral route, with infection occurring primarily within private households. Common-source outbreaks due to contaminated food and water supplies have occurred following consumption of certain foods such as raw shellfish, and uncooked foods prepared by an infected food-handler or otherwise contaminated prior to ingestion (salads, sandwiches, frozen raspberries, etc.) Bloodborne transmission, while uncommon, is possible via blood transfusion, contaminated blood products, or from needles shared with an infected viremic individual. Sexual transmission has also been reported.[1-14,16]
The disease burden due to hepatitis A in the United States has been estimated to be approximately 143,000 infections per year, of which 75,800 result in clinical hepatitis A disease, 11,400 hospitalizations, and 80 deaths due to fulminant hepatitis. Worldwide, it has been estimated that 1.4 million cases are reported annually.[2] The clinical manifestations of hepatitis A infection often pass unrecognized in children ≤2 years of age whereas overt hepatitis A develops in the majority of infected older children and adults. Symptoms and signs of hepatitis A infection are similar to those associated with other types of viral hepatitis and include anorexia, nausea, fever/chills, jaundice, dark urine, light-colored stools, abdominal pain, malaise, and fatigue.[1]
Clinical Trials
Clinical trials conducted worldwide with several formulations of the vaccine in 9181 healthy individuals ranging from 2 to 85 years of age have demonstrated that VAQTA is highly immunogenic and generally well tolerated.
Protection from hepatitis A disease has been shown to be related to the presence of antibody; an anamnestic antibody response occurs in healthy individuals with a history of infection who are subsequently re-exposed to hepatitis A virus.[3] Similarly, protection after vaccination with VAQTA has been associated with the onset of seroconversion (≥10 mIU/mL of hepatitis A antibody, measured by a modification of the HAVAB** radioimmunoassay [RIA][15]) and with an anamnestic antibody response following booster vaccination with VAQTA.
Immunology
In combined clinical studies, 97% of 1214 healthy children and adolescents 2 through 17 years of age seroconverted with a geometric mean titer (GMT) of 43 mIU/mL within 4 weeks after a single ~25U/0.5 mL intramuscular dose of VAQTA. Similarly, 95% of 1428 adults ≥18 years of age seroconverted with a GMT of 37 mIU/mL within 4 weeks after a single ~50U/1.0 mL intramuscular dose of VAQTA. Furthermore, at 2 weeks post-vaccination, 69% (n=744) of adults seroconverted with a GMT of 16 mIU/mL after a single dose of VAQTA.[18] Immune memory was demonstrated by an anamnestic antibody response in individuals who received a booster dose (see *Persistence*).
While a study evaluating VAQTA alone in a post-exposure setting has not been conducted, the concurrent use of VAQTA (~50U) and immune globulin (IG, 0.06 mL/kg) was evaluated in a clinical study involving healthy adults 18 to 39 years of age. Table 1 provides seroconversion rates and GMT at 4 and 24 weeks after the first dose in each treatment group and at one month after a booster dose of VAQTA (administered at 24 weeks).

Table 1
Seroconversion Rates (%) and Geometric Mean Titers (GMT) after Vaccination with VAQTA plus IG, VAQTA Alone, and IG Alone

Weeks	VAQTA plus IG	VAQTA	IG
	Seroconversion Rate GMT (mIU/mL)		
4	100% 42 (n=129)	96% 38 (n=135)	87% 19 (n=30)
24	92% 83 (n=125)	97% 137 (n=132)	0% 5 (n=28)
28	100% 4872 (n=114)	100% 6498 (n=128)	N/A

*The seroconversion rate and the GMT in the group receiving VAQTA alone were significantly higher than in the group receiving VAQTA plus IG (p=0.05, p<0.001, respectively).
N/A=Not Applicable

Efficacy
A very high degree of protection has been demonstrated after a single dose of VAQTA in children and adolescents.[19] The protective efficacy, immunogenicity and safety of VAQTA were evaluated in a randomized, double-blind, placebo-controlled study involving 1037 susceptible healthy children and adolescents 2 through 16 years of age in a U.S. community with recurrent outbreaks of hepatitis A (The Monroe Efficacy Study). Each child received an intramuscular dose of VAQTA (~25U) or placebo. Among those individuals who were initially seronegative (by modified HAVAB), seroconversion was achieved in >99% of vaccine recipients within 4 weeks after vaccination. The onset of seroconversion following a single dose of VAQTA was shown to parallel the onset of protection against clinical hepatitis A disease. Because of the long incubation period of the disease (approximately 20 to 50 days, or longer in children[22]), the primary endpoint was based on clinically confirmed cases*** of hepatitis A occurring ≥50 days after vaccination in order to exclude any children incubating the infection before vaccination. In subjects who were initially seronegative, the protective efficacy of a single dose of VAQTA was observed to be 100% with 21 cases of clinically confirmed hepatitis A occurring in the placebo group and none in the vaccine group (p<0.001). A secondary endpoint was pre-defined as the number of clinically confirmed cases of hepatitis A ≥30 days. With this secondary endpoint, 28 cases of clinically confirmed hepatitis A occurred in the placebo group while none occurred in the vaccine group ≥30 days after vaccination. In addition, it was observed in this trial that no cases of clinically confirmed hepatitis A occurred in the vaccine group after day 16.† Following demonstration of protection with a single dose and termination of the study, a booster

Continued on next page

Information on the Merck & Co., Inc. products listed on these pages is the full prescribing information from product circulars in use September 30, 1996.

Merck & Co.—Cont.

dose was administered to a subset of vaccinees 6, 12, or 18 months after the primary dose.

Persistence

The total duration of the protective effect of VAQTA in healthy vaccinees is unknown at present. However, seropositivity was shown to persist up to 18 months after a single ~25U dose in a cohort of 35 out of 39 children and adolescents who participated in the Monroe Efficacy Study; 95% of this cohort responded anamnestically following a booster at 18 months. To date, no cases of clinically confirmed hepatitis A disease ≥ 50 days after vaccination have occurred in those vaccinees from The Monroe Efficacy Study monitored for up to 4 years.

The effectiveness of VAQTA for use in community outbreak control has been demonstrated by the fact that, although cases of imported infection have occurred, the study community has remained free of outbreaks. In contrast, three nearby sister communities to Monroe have continued to experience outbreaks.[18-20]

In adults, seropositivity has been shown to persist up to 6 months after a single ~50U dose. Studies are ongoing to evaluate longer-term persistence and the need, if any, for additional booster doses. Persistence of immunologic memory was demonstrated with an anamnestic antibody response to a booster dose of ~25U given 6 to 18 months after the primary dose in children and adolescents (Table 2), and to a booster dose of ~50U given 6 months after the primary dose to adults (Table 3).

Table 2
Children/Adolescents
Seroconversion Rates (%) and Geometric Mean Titers (GMT) for Cohorts of Initially Seronegative Vaccinees at the Time of the Booster (~25U) and 4 Weeks Later

Weeks Following Initial ~25U Dose	Cohort* (n=949) 0 and 6 Months	Cohort* (n=35) 0 and 12 Months	Cohort* (n=39) 0 and 18 Months
	Seroconversion Rate GMT (mIU/mL)		
24	97% 109	—	—
28	100% 10609	—	—
52	—	91% 48	—
56	—	100% 12308	—
78	—	—	90% 50
82	—	—	100% 9591

*Blood samples taken at both time points.

Table 3
Adults
Seroconversion Rates (%) and Geometric Mean Titers (GMT) for a Cohort of Vaccinees After a Booster Dose (~50U) of VAQTA Administered at 6 Months

Weeks Following Initial ~50U Dose	Cohort (n=1152) 0 and 6 Months
	Seroconversion Rate GMT (mIU/mL)
24	98% 134
28	100% 6010

** Trademark of Abbott Laboratories
*** The clinical case definition included all of the following occurring at the same time: 1) one or more typical clinical signs or symptoms of hepatitis A (e.g., jaundice, malaise, fever ≥ 38.3℃), 2) elevation of hepatitis A IgM antibody (HAVAB-M), 3) elevation of alanine transferase (ALT) ≥ 2 times the upper limit of normal.
† One vaccinee did not meet the pre-defined criteria for clinically confirmed hepatitis A but did have positive hepatitis A IgM and borderline liver enzyme (ALT) elevations on days 34, 50, and 58 after vaccination with mild clinical symptoms observed on days 49 and 50.

INDICATIONS AND USAGE

VAQTA is indicated for active pre-exposure prophylaxis against disease caused by hepatitis A virus in persons 2 years of age and older. Primary immunization should be given at least 2 weeks prior to expected exposure to HAV.
Individuals who are or will be at increased risk of infection by HAV include:[2-14,16,17]
TRAVELERS
Persons traveling to areas of higher endemicity for hepatitis A. These areas include, but are not limited to, Africa, Asia (except Japan), the Mediterranean basin, Eastern Europe, the Middle East, Central and South America, Mexico, and parts of the Caribbean. Current CDC (Centers for Disease Control and Prevention) advisories should be consulted with regard to specific locales.
MILITARY PERSONNEL
PEOPLE LIVING IN, OR RELOCATING TO, AREAS OF HIGH ENDEMICITY
CERTAIN ETHNIC AND GEOGRAPHIC POPULATIONS THAT EXPERIENCE CYCLIC HEPATITIS A EPIDEMICS SUCH AS:
Native peoples of Alaska and the Americas.
OTHERS
Persons engaging in high-risk sexual activity (such as homosexually active males); users of illicit injectable drugs; residents of a community experiencing an outbreak of hepatitis A.
Hemophiliacs and other recipients of therapeutic blood products (see PRECAUTIONS and DOSAGE AND AMINISTRATION).
Although the epidemiology of hepatitis A does not permit the identification of other specific populations at high risk of disease, outbreaks of hepatitis A or exposure to hepatitis A virus have been described in a variety of populations in which VAQTA may be useful:
—Certain institutional workers (e.g., caretakers for the developmentally challenged)
—Employees of child day-care centers
—Laboratory workers who handle live hepatitis A virus
—Handlers of primate animals that may be harboring HAV
PEOPLE EXPOSED TO HEPATITIS A
For those requiring both immediate and long-term protection, VAQTA may be administered concomitantly with IG.

Revaccination
See DOSAGE AND ADMINISTRATION, *DOSAGE.*
Use With Other Vaccines
Data to recommend concurrent use with other vaccines are limited.
Use With Immune Globulin
For individuals requiring either post-exposure prophylaxis or combined immediate and longer-term protection (e.g., travelers departing on short notice to endemic areas), VAQTA may be administered concomitantly with IG using separate sites and syringes (see CLINICAL PHARMACOLOGY and DOSAGE AND ADMINISTRATION).
VAQTA IS NOT RECOMMENDED FOR USE IN INFANTS YOUNGER THAN 2 YEARS OF AGE SINCE DATA ON USE IN THIS AGE GROUP ARE NOT CURRENTLY AVAILABLE.

CONTRAINDICATIONS
Hypersensitivity to any component of the vaccine.

WARNINGS
Individuals who develop symptoms suggestive of hypersensitivity after an injection of VAQTA should not receive further injections of the vaccine (see CONTRAINDICATIONS).
If VAQTA is used in individuals with malignancies or those receiving immunosuppressive therapy or who are otherwise immunocompromised, the expected immune response may not be obtained.

PRECAUTIONS
General
VAQTA will not prevent hepatitis caused by infectious agents other than hepatitis A virus. Because of the long incubation period (approximately 20 to 50 days) for hepatitis A, it is possible for unrecognized hepatitis A infection to be present at the time the vaccine is given. The vaccine may not prevent hepatitis A in such individuals.
As with any vaccine, adequate treatment provisions, including epinephrine, should be available for immediate use should an anaphylactic or anaphylactoid reaction occur.
VAQTA should be administered with caution to people with bleeding disorders who are at risk of hemorrhage following intramuscular injection (see DOSAGE AND ADMINISTRATION).
As with any vaccine, vaccination with VAQTA may not result in a protective response in all susceptible vaccinees.
An acute infection or febrile illness may be reason for delaying use of VAQTA except when, in the opinion of the physician, withholding the vaccine entails a greater risk.
Carcinogenesis, Mutagenesis, Impairment of Fertility
VAQTA has not been evaluated for its carcinogenic or mutagenic potential, or its potential to impair fertility.
Pregnancy
Pregnancy Category C: Animal reproduction studies have not been conducted with VAQTA. It is also not known whether VAQTA can cause fetal harm when administered to a pregnant woman or can affect reproduction capacity. VAQTA should be given to a pregnant woman only if clearly needed.
Nursing Mothers
It is not known whether VAQTA is excreted in human milk. Because many drugs are excreted in human milk, caution should be exercised when VAQTA is administered to a woman who is breast feeding.
Pediatric Use
VAQTA has been shown to be generally well tolerated and highly immunogenic in individuals 2 through 17 years of age. See DOSAGE AND ADMINISTRATION for the recommended dosage schedule.
Safety and effectiveness in infants below 2 years of age have not been established.

ADVERSE REACTIONS
In combined clinical trials, 16,252 doses of VAQTA were administered to 9181 healthy children, adolescents, and adults. VAQTA was generally well tolerated.
No serious vaccine-related adverse experiences were observed during clinical trials.

The Monroe Efficacy Study
In this study, 1037 healthy children and adolescents, 2 through 16 years of age, received a primary dose of ~25U of hepatitis A vaccine and a booster 6, 12, or 18 months later, or placebo. Subjects were observed during a 5-day period for fever and local complaints and during a 14-day period for systemic complaints. Injection-site complaints, generally mild and transient[19], were the most frequently reported complaints. Table 4 summarizes the local and systemic complaints (≥ 1%) reported in this study, without regard to causality. There were no significant differences in the rates of any complaints between vaccine and placebo recipients after Dose 1. [See Table 4 at left.]

Children/Adolescents — 2 through 17 Years of Age
In combined clinical trials (including Monroe Efficacy Study participants) involving 2595 healthy children and adoles-

Table 4
Local and Systemic Complaints (≥ 1%) in Healthy Children and Adolescents from The Monroe Efficacy Study

Reaction	VAQTA Dose 1*	VAQTA Booster	Placebo*†
Injection-Site Complaints			
Pain	6.4% (33/515)	3.4% (16/475)	6.3% (32/510)
Tenderness	4.9% (25/515)	1.7% (8/475)	6.1% (31/510)
Erythema	1.9% (10/515)	0.8% (4/475)	1.8% (9/510)
Swelling	1.7% (9/515)	1.5% (7/475)	1.6% (8/510)
Warmth	1.7% (9/515)	0.6% (3/475)	1.6% (8/510)
Systemic Complaints			
Abdominal Pain	1.2% (6/519)	1.1% (5/475)	1.0% (5/518)
Pharyngitis	1.2% (6/519)	0% (0/475)	0.8% (4/518)
Headache	0.4% (2/519)	0.8% (4/475)	1.0% (5/518)

* No statistically significant differences between the two groups.
† Second injection of placebo not administered because code for the trial was broken.

cents who received one or more ∼25U doses of hepatitis A vaccine, fever and local complaints were observed during a 5-day period following vaccination and systemic complaints during a 14-day period following vaccination. Injection-site complaints, generally mild and transient, were the most frequently reported complaints. Listed below are the complaints (≥1%) reported, without regard to causality, in decreasing order of frequency within each body system.

LOCALIZED INJECTION-SITE REACTIONS (generally mild and transient)
Pain (18.7%); tenderness (16.8%); warmth (8.6%); erythema (7.5%); swelling (7.3%); ecchymosis (1.3%).
BODY AS A WHOLE
Fever (≥102°F, Oral) (3.1%); abdominal pain (1.6%).
DIGESTIVE SYSTEM
Diarrhea (1.0%); vomiting (1.0%).
NERVOUS SYSTEM/PSYCHIATRIC
Headache (2.3%).
RESPIRATORY SYSTEM
Pharyngitis (1.5%); upper respiratory infection (1.1%); cough (1.0%).
LABORATORY FINDINGS
Very few laboratory abnormalities were reported and included isolated reports of elevated liver function tests, eosinophilia, and increased urine protein.

Adults—18 Years of Age and Older
In combined clinical trials involving 1529 healthy adults who received one or more ∼50U doses of hepatitis A vaccine, fever and local complaints were observed during a 5-day period following vaccination and systemic complaints during a 14-day period following vaccination. Injection-site complaints, generally mild and transient, were the most frequently reported complaints. Listed below are the complaints (≥1%) reported, without regard to causality, in decreasing order of frequency within each body system.

LOCALIZED INJECTION-SITE REACTIONS (generally mild and transient)
Tenderness (52.6%); pain (51.1%); warmth (17.3%); swelling (13.6%); erythema (12.9%); ecchymosis (1.5%); pain/soreness (1.2%).
BODY AS A WHOLE
Asthenia/fatigue (3.9%); fever (≥101°F, Oral) (2.6%); abdominal pain (1.3%).
DIGESTIVE SYSTEM
Diarrhea (2.4%); nausea (2.3%).
MUSCULOSKELETAL SYSTEM
Myalgia (2.0%); arm pain (1.3%); back pain (1.1%); stiffness (1.0%).
NERVOUS SYSTEM/PSYCHIATRIC
Headache (16.1%).
RESPIRATORY SYSTEM
Pharyngitis (2.7%); upper respiratory infection (2.8%); nasal congestion (1.1%).
UROGENITAL SYSTEM
Menstruation disorder (1.1%).

Allergic Reactions
Local and/or systemic allergic reactions that occurred in <1% of children/adolescents or adults in clinical trials regardless of causality included:
LOCAL
Injection site pruritus and/or rash.
SYSTEMIC
Bronchial constriction; asthma; wheezing; edema/swelling; rash; generalized erythema; urticaria; pruritus; eye irritation/itching; dermatitis. (See CONTRAINDICATIONS and WARNINGS.)
As with any vaccine, there is the possibility that use of VAQTA in very large populations might reveal adverse experiences not observed in clinical trials.

DOSAGE AND ADMINISTRATION

Do not inject intravenously, intradermally, or subcutaneously. VAQTA is for intramuscular injection. The *deltoid muscle* is the preferred site for intramuscular injection.
DOSAGE
The vaccination regimen consists of one primary dose and one booster dose for healthy children, adolescents, and adults, as follows:
Pediatric/Adolescent
Individuals 2 through 17 years of age should receive a single 0.5 mL (∼25U) dose of vaccine at elected date and a booster dose of 0.5 mL (∼25U) 6 to 18 months later.
Adult
Adults 18 years of age and older should receive a single 1.0 mL (∼50U) dose of vaccine at elected date and a booster dose of 1.0 mL (∼50U) 6 months later.
Use With Immune Globulin
VAQTA may be administered concomitantly with IG using separate sites and syringes. The vaccination regimen for VAQTA should be followed as stated above. Consult the manufacturer's product circular for the appropriate dosage of IG. A booster dose of VAQTA should be administered at the appropriate time as outlined above.

ADMINISTRATION
Known or Presumed Exposure to HAV/Travel to Endemic Areas
For individuals requiring either post-exposure prophylaxis or combined immediate and longer term protection (e.g., travelers departing on short notice to endemic areas), VAQTA may be administered concomitantly with IG using separate sites and syringes (see CLINICAL PHARMACOLOGY and DOSAGE AND ADMINISTRATION, *Use With Immune Globulin*).
Injection must be accomplished with a needle long enough to ensure intramuscular deposition of the vaccine. The Advisory Committee on Immunization Practices (ACIP) has recommended that "For all intramuscular injections, the needle should be long enough to reach the muscle mass and prevent vaccine from seeping into subcutaneous tissue, but not so long as to endanger underlying neurovascular structures or bone." For toddlers and older children they further state that "... the deltoid may be used if the muscle mass is adequate. The needle size can range from 22 to 25 gauge and from 5/8 to 1¼ inches, based on the size of the muscle... the anterolateral thigh may be used, but the needle should be longer—generally ranging from 7/8 to 1¼ inches." For adults they state that "... the deltoid is recommended for routine intramuscular vaccination among adults... The suggested needle size is 1 to 1½ inches and 20 to 25 gauge."[21]
For individuals with bleeding disorders who are at risk of hemorrhage following intramuscular injection, the ACIP recommends that when any intramuscular vaccine is indicated for such patients, "... it should be administered intramuscularly if, in the opinion of a physician familiar with the patient's bleeding risk, the vaccine can be administered with reasonable safety by this route. If the patient receives antihemophilia or other similar therapy, intramuscular vaccination can be scheduled shortly after such therapy is administered. A fine needle (≤23 gauge) can be used for the vaccination and firm pressure applied to the site (without rubbing) for at least two minutes. The patient or family should be instructed concerning the risk of hematoma from the injection."[21]
The vaccine should be used as supplied; no reconstitution is necessary.
Shake well before withdrawal and use. Thorough agitation is necessary to maintain suspension of the vaccine. Discard if the suspension does not appear homogenous.
Parenteral drug products should be inspected visually for extraneous particulate matter and discoloration prior to administration whenever solution and container permit. After thorough agitation, VAQTA is a slightly opaque, white suspension.
It is important to use a separate sterile syringe and needle for each individual to prevent transmission of infectious agents from one person to another.

HOW SUPPLIED

PEDIATRIC/ADOLESCENT FORMULATION
Vials
No. 4831—VAQTA for pediatric/adolescent use is supplied as 25U/0.5 mL of hepatitis A virus protein in a 0.5 mL single-dose vial, **NDC** 0006-4831-00.
No. 4831—VAQTA for pediatric/adolescent use is supplied as 25U/0.5 mL of hepatitis A virus protein in a 0.5 mL single-dose vial, in a box of 5 single-dose vials, **NDC** 0006-4831-38.
Syringes
No. 4845—VAQTA for pediatric/adolescent use is supplied as 25U/0.5 mL of hepatitis A virus protein in a 0.5 mL single-dose prefilled syringe, **NDC** 0006-4845-00.
No. 4845—VAQTA for pediatric/adolescent use is supplied as 25U/0.5 mL of hepatitis A virus protein in a 0.5 mL single-dose prefilled syringe, in a box of 5 single-dose prefilled syringes, **NDC** 0006-4845-38.
ADULT FORMULATION
Vials
No. 4841—VAQTA for adult use is supplied as 50U/1 mL of hepatitis A virus protein in a 1 mL single-dose vial, **NDC** 0006-4841-00.
No. 4841—VAQTA for adult use is supplied as 50U/1 mL of hepatitis A virus protein in a 1 mL single-dose vial, in a box of 5 single-dose vials, **NDC** 0006-4841-38.
Syringes
No. 4844—VAQTA for adult use is supplied as 50U/1 mL of hepatitis A virus protein in a 1 mL single-dose prefilled syringe, **NDC** 0006-4844-00.
No. 4844—VAQTA for adult use is supplied as 50U/1 mL of hepatitis A virus protein in a 1 mL single-dose prefilled syringe, in a box of 5 single-dose, prefilled syringes, **NDC** 0006-4844-38.
Storage
Store vaccine at 2–8°C (36–46°F).
DO NOT FREEZE since freezing destroys potency.

REFERENCES

1. Lemon, S.M.: Type A viral hepatitis, new developments in an old disease, NEJM *313*(17): 1059–1067, 1985.
2. Hadler, S.C.: Global impact of hepatitis A virus infection changing patterns, in "Viral Hepatitis and Liver Disease", F.B. Hollinger, S.M. Lemon, and H. Margolis (eds), Williams & Wilkins, 14–20, 1991.
3. Villarejos, V.M., et al: Hepatitis A virus infection in households, Am J Epidemiol *115*(4): 577–586, 1982.
4. Vernon, A.A., et al: A large outbreak of hepatitis A in a day-care center: association with non-toilet trained children and persistence of IgM antibody to hepatitis A virus, Am J Epidemiol *115*(3): 325–331, 1982.
5. Desencios, J-C.A., et al: Community wide outbreak of hepatitis A linked to children in daycare centres and with increased transmission in young adult men in Florida 1988–9, J Epidemiol Comm Health *47*: 269–273, 1993.
6. Nickolic, P., et al: A virologically studied epidemic of type A hepatitis in a school for the mentally retarded, Am J Epidemiol *114*(2): 260–266, 1981.
7. Yao, G,: Clinical spectrum and natural history of viral hepatitis A in a 1988 Shanghai epidemic, in "Viral Hepatitis and Liver Disease", F.B. Hollinger, S.M. Lemon, and H. Margolis (eds), Williams & Wilkins, 76–78, 1990.
8. Carl, M., et al: Food-borne hepatitis A: recommendations for control, J Infect Dis *148*: 1133–1135, 1983.
9. Reid, T.M.S., et al: Frozen raspberries and hepatitis A, Epidemiol Infect *98*: 109–112, 1987.
10. Rosenblum, L.S., et al: A multifocal outbreak of hepatitis A traced to commercially distributed lettuce, AJPH *80*(9): 1075–1079, 1990.
11. Centers for Disease Control, Food-borne hepatitis A—Alaska, Florida, North Carolina, Washington, MMWR *39*(14): 228–232, 1990.
12. Hepatitis A among homosexual men—United States, Canada, and Australia, JAMA *267*(12): 1587–1588, 1992.
13. Centers for Disease Control, Hepatitis A among drug abusers, MMWR *37*(19): 297–305, 1988.
14. Hollinger, F.B., et al: Postransfusion hepatitis type A, JAMA *250*(17): 2313–2317, 1983.
15. Miller, W.J., et al: Sensitive assays for hepatitis A antibodies, J Med Virol *41*: 201–204, 1993.
16. Mannucci, P.M., et al: Transmission of hepatitis A to patients with hemophilia by factor VIII concentrates treated with organic solvent and detergent to inactivate viruses. Ann Intern Med *120*(1): 1–7, 1994.
17. Bancroft, W.H., et al: Hepatitis A from the military perspective, in "Hepatitis A", R.J. Gerety (ed), Academic Press, Inc., 81–100, 1984.
18. Data on file at Merck Research Laboratories.
19. Werzberger, A., et al: A Controlled trial of a formalin-inactivated hepatitis A vaccine in healthy children, NEJM *327*(7): 453–457, 1992.
20. Werzberger, A., et al: Anatomy of a trial: a historical view of the Monroe inactivated hepatitis A protective efficacy trial, J Hepatol, *18*(Suppl. 2): S46–S50, 1993.
21. Recommendations of the Advisory Committee on Immunization Practices (ACIP); General Recommendations on Immunization, MMWR *43*(RR-1): June 23, 1994.
22. Ward, R., et al: Infectious Hepatitis, Studies of Its Natural History and Prevention, NEJM *258*(9): 407–416, February 27, 1958.

Syringes of VAQTA are also filled by:
Evans Medical Ltd.
Gaskill Road, Speke, Liverpool L24 9GR, England
7977500 Issued March 1996

VARIVAX® ℞
[Varicella Virus Vaccine Live (Oka/Merck)]

DESCRIPTION

VARIVAX* [Varicella Virus Vaccine Live (Oka/Merck)] is a preparation of the Oka/Merck strain of live, attenuated varicella virus. The virus was initially obtained from a child with natural varicella, then introduced into human embryonic lung cell cultures, adapted to and propagated in embryonic guinea pig cell cultures and finally propagated in human diploid cell cultures (WI-38). Further passage of the virus for varicella vaccine was performed at Merck Research Laboratories (MRL) in human diploid cell cultures (MRC-5) that were free of adventitious agents. This live, attenuated varicella vaccine is a lyophilized preparation containing sucrose, phosphate, glutamate, and processed gelatin as stabilizers. VARIVAX, when reconstituted as directed, is a sterile preparation for subcutaneous administration. Each 0.5 mL dose contains the following: a minimum of 1350 PFU (plaque

Continued on next page

Information on the Merck & Co., Inc. products listed on these pages is the full prescribing information from product circulars in use September 30, 1996.

Merck & Co.—Cont.

forming units) of Oka/Merck varicella virus when reconstituted and stored at room temperature for 30 minutes, approximately 25 mg of sucrose, 12.5 mg hydrolyzed gelatin, 3.2 mg sodium chloride, 0.5 mg monosodium L-glutamate, 0.45 mg of sodium phosphate dibasic, 0.08 mg of potassium phosphate monobasic, 0.08 mg of potassium chloride; residual components of MRC-5 cells including DNA and protein; and trace quantities of sodium phosphate monobasic, EDTA, neomycin, and fetal bovine serum. The product contains no preservative.

To maintain potency, the lyophilized vaccine must be kept frozen at an average temperature of −15°C (+5°F) or colder and must be used before the expiration date (see HOW SUPPLIED, *Stability and Storage*). Storage in a frost-free freezer with an average temperature of −15°C (+5°F) or colder is acceptable.

---

*Registered trademark of MERCK & CO., Inc.

CLINICAL PHARMACOLOGY

Varicella is a highly communicable disease in children, adolescents, and adults caused by the varicella-zoster virus. The disease usually consists of 300 to 500 maculopapular and/or vesicular lesions accompanied by a fever (oral temperature ≥100°F) in up to 70% of individuals.[1,2] Approximately 3.5 million cases of varicella occurred annually from 1980–1994 in the United States with the peak incidence occurring in children five to nine years of age.[3] The incidence rate of chickenpox is 8.3–9.1% per year in children 1-9 years of age.[4] The attack rate of natural varicella following household exposure among healthy susceptible children was shown to be 87%.[2] Although it is generally a benign, self-limiting disease, varicella may be associated with serious complications (e.g., bacterial superinfection, pneumonia, encephalitis, Reye's Syndrome), and/or death.

Evaluation of Clinical Efficacy Afforded by VARIVAX
Clinical Data in Children
In combined clinical trials[5] of VARIVAX at doses ranging from 1,000–17,000 PFU, the majority of subjects who received VARIVAX and were exposed to wild-type virus were either completely protected from chickenpox or developed a milder form (for clinical description see below) of the disease. The protective efficacy of VARIVAX was evaluated in three different ways: 1) by comparing chickenpox rates in vaccinees versus historical controls, 2) by assessment of protection from disease following household exposure, and 3) by a placebo-controlled, double-blind clinical trial.

In early clinical trials,[5] a total of 4142 children received 1000–1625 PFU of attenuated virus per dose of VARIVAX and have been followed for up to six years post single-dose vaccination. In this group there was considerable variation in chickenpox rates among studies and study sites, and much of the reported data were acquired by passive follow-up. It was observed that 2.1%–3.6% of vaccinees per year reported chickenpox (called breakthrough cases). This represents an approximate 67% (57–77%) decrease from the total number of cases expected based on attack rates in children aged 1–9 over this same period (8.3–9.1%).[4,6] In those who developed breakthrough chickenpox postvaccination, the majority experienced mild disease (median number of lesions <50). In one study, a total of 47% (27/58) of breakthrough cases had <50 lesions compared with 8% (7/92) in unvaccinated individuals, and 7% (4/58) of breakthrough cases had >300 lesions compared with 50% (46/92) in unvaccinated individuals.[7] In studies of vaccinated children who contracted chickenpox after a household exposure, 57% (31/54) of the cases reported <50 lesions, while 1.9% (1/54) reported >300 lesions with an oral temperature above 100°F.

In later clinical trials[5] with the current vaccine, a total of 1164 children received 2900–9000 PFU of attenuated virus per dose of VARIVAX and have been followed for up to three years post single-dose vaccination. It was observed that 0.2%–1.0% of vaccinees per year reported breakthrough chickenpox for up to three years post single-dose vaccination. This represents an approximate 93% decrease from the total number of cases expected based on attack rates in children aged 1–9 over this same period (8.3%–9.1%).[3,26] In those who developed breakthrough chickenpox postvaccination, the majority experienced mild disease.

Among a subset of vaccinees who were actively followed, 259 were exposed to an individual with chickenpox in a household setting. There were no reports of breakthrough chickenpox in 80% of exposed children; 20% reported a mild form of chickenpox.[5] This represents a 77% reduction in the expected number of cases when compared to the historical attack rate of varicella following household exposure to chickenpox of 87% in unvaccinated individuals.[2]

Although no placebo-controlled trial was carried out with VARIVAX using the current vaccine, a placebo-controlled trial was conducted using a formulation containing 17,000 PFU per dose.[4,8] In this trial, a single dose of VARIVAX protected 96–100% of children against chickenpox over a two-year period. The study enrolled healthy individuals 1 to 14 years of age (n=491 vaccine, n=465 placebo). In the first year, 8.5% of placebo recipients contracted chickenpox, while no vaccine recipient did, for a calculated protection rate of 100% during the first varicella season. In the second year, when only a subset of individuals agreed to remain in the blinded study (n=163 vaccine, n=161 placebo), 96% protective efficacy was calculated for the vaccine group as compared to placebo.

There are insufficient data to assess the rate of protection against the complications of chickenpox (e.g., encephalitis, hepatitis, pneumonia) in children.

Clinical Data in Adolescents and Adults
Although no placebo-controlled trial was carried out in adolescents and adults, efficacy was determined by evaluation of protection when vaccinees received 2 doses of VARIVAX 4 or 8 weeks apart and were subsequently exposed to chickenpox in a household setting.[5] In up to two years of active follow-up, 17 of 64 (27%) vaccinees reported breakthrough chickenpox following household exposure; of the 17 cases, 12 (71%) reported <50 lesions, 5 reported 50–300 lesions, and none reported >300 lesions with an oral temperature above 100°F. In combined clinical studies of adolescents and adults (n=1019) who received two doses of VARIVAX and later developed breakthrough chickenpox (42 of 1019), 25 of 42 (60%) reported <50 lesions, 16 of 42 (38%) reported 50–300 lesions, and 1 of 42 (2%) reported >300 lesions and an oral temperature above 100°F.[5]

The attack rate of unvaccinated adults exposed to a single contact in a household has not been previously studied. When compared to the previously reported attack rate of natural varicella of 87% following household exposure among unvaccinated children, this represents an approximate 70% reduction in the expected number of cases in the household setting.[2]

There are insufficient data to assess the rate of protection of VARIVAX against the serious complications of chickenpox in adults (e.g., encephalitis, hepatitis, pneumonitis) and during pregnancy (congenital varicella syndrome).

Immunogenicity of VARIVAX
Clinical trials with several formulations of the vaccine containing attenuated virus ranging from 1000 to 17,000 PFU per dose have demonstrated that VARIVAX induces detectable immune responses in a high proportion of individuals and is generally well tolerated in healthy individuals ranging from 12 months to 55 years of age.[4,5,9–15]

Seroconversion as defined by the acquisition of any detectable varicella antibodies (gpELISA > 0.3, a highly sensitive assay which is not commercially available) was observed in 97% of vaccinees at approximately 4–6 weeks postvaccination in 6889 susceptible children 12 months to 12 years of age. Rates of breakthrough disease were significantly lower among children with varicella antibody titers ≥5 compared to children with titers <5. Titers ≥5 were induced in approximately 76% of children vaccinated with a single dose of vaccine at 1000–17,000 PFU per dose. In a multicenter study involving susceptible adolescents and adults 13 years of age and older, two doses of VARIVAX administered four to eight weeks apart induced a seroconversion rate (gpELISA > 0.3) of approximately 75% in 539 individuals four weeks after the first dose and of 99% in 479 individuals four weeks after the second dose. The average antibody response in vaccinees who received the second dose eight weeks after the first dose was higher than that in those, who received the second dose four weeks after the first dose. In another multicenter study involving adolescents and adults, two doses of VARIVAX administered eight weeks apart induced a seroconversion rate (gpELISA > 0.3) of 94% in 142 individuals six weeks after the first dose and 99% in 122 individuals six weeks after the second dose.[5]

VARIVAX also induces cell-mediated immune responses in vaccinees. The relative contributions of humoral immunity and cell-mediated immunity to protection from chickenpox are unknown.

Persistence of Immune Response
Studies in vaccinees examining chickenpox breakthrough rates over 5 years showed the lowest rates (0.2–2.9%) in the first two years postvaccination, with somewhat higher but stable rates in the third through fifth year. The severity of reported breakthrough chickenpox, as measured by number of lesions and maximum temperature, appeared not to increase with time since vaccination.[5]

In clinical studies involving healthy children who received 1 dose of vaccine, detectable varicella antibodies (gpELISA > 0.3) were present in 98.8% (3775/3822) at 1 year, 98.9% (1057/1069) at 2 years, 97.5% (548/562) at 3 years, and 99.5% (220/221) at 4 years postvaccination. Antibody levels were present at least one year in 97.2% (423/435) of healthy adolescents and adults who received two doses of live varicella vaccine separated by 4 to 8 weeks. A boost in antibody levels has been observed in vaccinees following exposure to natural varicella which could account for the apparent long-term persistence of antibody levels after vaccination in these studies. The duration of protection from varicella obtained using VARIVAX in the absence of wild-type boosting is unknown.

VARIVAX also induces cell-mediated immune responses in vaccinees. The relative contributions of humoral immunity and cell-mediated immunity to protection from chickenpox are unknown.

Transmission
In the placebo-controlled trial, transmission of vaccine virus was assessed in household settings (during the 8-week post-vaccination period) in 416 susceptible placebo recipients who were household contacts of 445 vaccine recipients. Of the 416 placebo recipients, three developed chickenpox and seroconverted, nine reported a varicella-like rash and did not seroconvert, and six had no rash but seroconverted. If vaccine virus transmission occurred, it did so at a very low rate and possibly without recognizable clinical disease in contacts. These cases may represent either natural varicella from community contacts or a low incidence of transmission of vaccine virus from vaccinated contacts (see PRECAUTIONS, *Transmission*).[4,16] Post-marketing experience suggests that transmission of vaccine virus may occur rarely between healthy vaccinees who develop a varicella-like rash and healthy susceptible contacts. Transmission of vaccine virus from vaccinees without a varicella-like rash been reported but has not been confirmed.

Herpes Zoster
Overall, 9454 healthy children (12 months to 12 years of age) and 1648 adolescents and adults (13 years of age and older) have been vaccinated with Oka/Merck live attenuated varicella vaccine in clinical trials. Eight cases of herpes zoster have been reported in children during 44,994 person years of follow-up in clinical trials, resulting in a calculated incidence of at least 18 cases per 100,000 person years. The completeness of this reporting has not been determined. One case of herpes zoster has been reported in the adolescent and adult age group during 7826 person years of follow-up in clinical trials resulting in a calculated incidence of 12.8 cases per 100,000 person years.[5]

All nine cases were mild and without sequelae. Two cultures (one child and one adult) obtained from vesicles were positive for wild-type varicella zoster virus as confirmed by restriction endonuclease analysis.[5,17] The long-term effect of VARIVAX on the incidence of herpes zoster, particularly in those vaccinees exposed to natural varicella, is unknown at present.

In children, the reported rate of zoster in vaccine recipients appears not to exceed that previously determined in a population-based study of healthy children who had experienced natural varicella.[5,18,19] The incidence of zoster in adults who have had natural varicella infection is higher than that in children.[20]

Reye's Syndrome
Reye's Syndrome has occurred in children and adolescents following natural varicella infection, the majority of whom had received salicylates.[21] In clinical studies in healthy children and adolescents in the United States, physicians advised varicella vaccine recipients not to use salicylates for six weeks after vaccination. There were no reports of Reye's Syndrome in varicella vaccine recipients during these studies.

Studies with Other Vaccines
In combined clinical studies involving 1080 children 12 to 36 months of age, 653 received VARIVAX and M-M-R*II (Measles, Mumps, and Rubella Virus Vaccine Live) concomitantly at separate sites and 427 received the vaccines six weeks apart. Seroconversion rates and antibody levels were comparable between the two groups at approximately six weeks postvaccination to each of the virus vaccine components. No differences were noted in adverse reactions reported in those who received VARIVAX concomitantly with M-M-R II (Measles, Mumps, and Rubella Virus Vaccine Live) at separate sites and those who received VARIVAX and M-M-R II (Measles, Mumps, and Rubella Virus Vaccine Live) at different times (see PRECAUTIONS, *Drug Interactions, Use with Other Vaccines*).[5]

In a clinical study involving 318 children 12 months to 42 months of age, 160 received an investigational vaccine (a formulation combining measles, mumps, rubella, and varicella in one syringe) concomitantly with booster doses of DTaP (diphtheria, tetanus, acellular pertussis) and OPV (oral poliovirus vaccine) while 144 received M-M-R II (Measles, Mumps, and Rubella Virus Vaccine Live) concomitantly with booster doses of DTaP and OPV followed by VARIVAX 6 weeks later. At six weeks postvaccination, seroconversion rates for measles, mumps, rubella, and varicella and the percentage of vaccinees whose titers were boosted for diphtheria, tetanus, pertussis, and polio were comparable between the two groups, but anti-varicella levels were decreased when the investigational vaccine containing varicella was administered concomitantly with DTaP. No clinically significant differences were noted in adverse reactions between the two groups.[5]

In another clinical study involving 307 children 12 to 18 months of age, 150 received an investigational vaccine (a formulation combining measles, mumps, rubella, and varicella in one syringe) concomitantly with a booster dose of PedvaxHIB* [Haemophilus b Conjugate Vaccine (Meningococcal Protein Conjugate)] while 130 received M-M-R II

(Measles, Mumps, and Rubella Virus Vaccine Live) concomitantly with a booster dose of PedvaxHIB followed by VARIVAX 6 weeks later. At six weeks postvaccination, seroconversion rates for measles, mumps, rubella, and varicella, and geometric mean titers for PedvaxHIB were comparable between the two groups, but anti-varicella levels were decreased when the investigational vaccine containing varicella was administered concomitantly with PedvaxHIB. No clinically significant differences in adverse reactions were seen between the two groups.[5]

VARIVAX is recommended for subcutaneous administration. However, during clinical trials, some children received VARIVAX intramuscularly resulting in seroconversion rates similar to those in children who received the vaccine by the subcutaneous route.[22] Persistence of antibody and efficacy in those receiving intramuscular injections have not been defined.

---

* Registered trademark of MERCK & Co., Inc.

INDICATIONS AND USAGE

VARIVAX is indicated for vaccination against varicella in individuals 12 months of age and older.
Revaccination
The duration of protection of VARIVAX is unknown at present and the need for booster doses is not defined. However, a boost in antibody levels has been observed in vaccinees following exposure to natural varicella as well as following a booster dose of VARIVAX administered four to six years postvaccination.[5]
In a highly vaccinated population, immunity for some individuals may wane due to lack of exposure to natural varicella as a result of shifting epidemiology. Post-marketing surveillance studies are ongoing to evaluate the need and timing for booster vaccination.
Vaccination with VARIVAX may not result in protection of all healthy, susceptible children, adolescents, and adults (see CLINICAL PHARMACOLOGY).

CONTRAINDICATIONS

A history of hypersensitivity to any component of the vaccine, including gelatin.
A history of anaphylactoid reaction to neomycin (each dose of reconstituted vaccine contains trace quantities of neomycin).
Individuals with blood dyscrasias, leukemia, lymphomas of any type, or other malignant neoplasms affecting the bone marrow or lymphatic systems.
Individuals receiving immunosuppressive therapy. Individuals who are on immunosuppressant drugs are more susceptible to infections than healthy individuals. Vaccination with live attenuated varicella vaccine can result in a more extensive vaccine-associated rash or disseminated disease in individuals on immunosuppressant doses of corticosteroids.
Individuals with primary and acquired immunodeficiency states, including those who are immunosuppressed in association with AIDS or other clinical manifestations of infection with human immunodeficiency virus;[23] cellular immune deficiencies; and hypogammaglobulinemic and dysgammaglobulinemic states.
A family history of congenital or hereditary immunodeficiency, unless the immune competence of the potential vaccine recipient is demonstrated.
Active untreated tuberculosis.
Any febrile respiratory illness or other active febrile infection.
Pregnancy; the possible effects of the vaccine on fetal development are unknown at this time. However, natural varicella is known to sometimes cause fetal harm. If vaccination of postpubertal females is undertaken, pregnancy should be avoided for three months following vaccination. (See PRECAUTIONS, *Pregnancy*).

WARNINGS

Children and adolescents with acute lymphoblastic leukemia (ALL) in remission can receive the vaccine under an investigational protocol. More information is available by contacting the VARIVAX coordinating center, Bio-Pharm Clinical Services, Inc., 4 Valley Square, Blue Bell, PA 19422 (215) 283-0897.

PRECAUTIONS

General
Adequate treatment provisions, including epinephrine injection (1:1000), should be available for immediate use should an anaphylactoid reaction occur.
The duration of protection from varicella infection after vaccination with VARIVAX is unknown.
It is not known whether VARIVAX given immediately after exposure to natural varicella virus will prevent illness.

Vaccination should be deferred for at least 5 months following blood or plasma transfusions, or administration of immune globulin or varicella zoster immune globulin (VZIG).[24] Following administration of VARIVAX, any immune globulin including VZIG should not be given for 2 months thereafter unless its use outweighs the benefits of vaccination.[24]
Vaccine recipients should avoid use of salicylates for 6 weeks after vaccination with VARIVAX as Reye's Syndrome has been reported following the use of salicylates during natural varicella infection (see CLINICAL PHARMACOLOGY, *Reye's Syndrome*).
The safety and efficacy of VARIVAX have not been established in children and young adults who are known to be infected with human immunodeficiency viruses with and without evidence of immunosuppression (see also CONTRAINDICATIONS).
Care is to be taken by the health care provider for safe and effective use of VARIVAX.
The health care provider should question the patient, parent, or guardian about reactions to a previous dose of VARIVAX or a similar product.
The health care provider should obtain the previous immunization history of the vaccinee.
VARIVAX should not be injected into a blood vessel.
Vaccination should be deferred in patients with a family history of congenital or hereditary immunodeficiency until the patient's own immune system has been evaluated.
A separate sterile needle and syringe should be used for administration of each dose of VARIVAX to prevent transfer of infectious diseases.
Needles should be disposed of properly and should not be recapped.
Transmission
Post-marketing experience suggests that transmission of vaccine virus may occur rarely between healthy vaccinees who develop a varicella-like rash and healthy susceptible contacts. Transmission of vaccine virus from vaccinees without a varicella-like rash has been reported but has not been confirmed.
Therefore, vaccine recipients should attempt to avoid, whenever possible, close association with susceptible high-risk individuals for up to six weeks. In circumstances where contact with high-risk individuals is unavoidable, the potential risk of transmission of vaccine virus should be weighed against the risk of acquiring and transmitting natural varicella virus. Susceptible high-risk individuals include:
- immunocompromised individuals
- pregnant women without documented history of chickenpox or laboratory evidence of prior infection
- newborn infants of mothers without documented history of chickenpox or laboratory evidence of prior infection
Information for Patients
The health care provider should inform the patient, parent or guardian of the benefits and risks of VARIVAX.
Patients, parents, or guardians should be instructed to report any adverse reactions to the health care provider.
The U.S. Department of Health and Human Services has established a Vaccine Adverse Event Reporting System (VAERS) to accept all reports of suspected adverse events after the administration of any vaccine, including but not limited to the reporting of events required by the National Childhood Vaccine Injury Act of 1986.[25] The VAERS toll-free number for VAERS forms and information is 1-800-822-7967. Pregnancy should be avoided for three months following vaccination.
Drug Interactions
See PRECAUTIONS, *General*, regarding the administration of immune globulins, salicylates, and transfusions.
Drug Interactions, Use with Other Vaccines
Results from clinical studies indicate that VARIVAX can be administered concomitantly with M-M-R II (Measles, Mumps, and Rubella Virus Vaccine Live).
Limited data from an experimental product containing varicella vaccine suggest that VARIVAX can be administered

concomitantly with DTaP (diphtheria, tetanus, acellular pertussis) and PedvaxHIB using separate sites and syringes (see CLINICAL PHARMACOLOGY, *Studies with Other Vaccines*).[5] However, there are no data relating to simultaneous administration of VARIVAX with DTP or OPV.
Carcinogenesis, Mutagenesis, Impairment of Fertility
VARIVAX has not been evaluated for its carcinogenic or mutagenic potential, or its potential to impair fertility.
Pregnancy
Pregnancy Category C: Animal reproduction studies have not been conducted with VARIVAX. It is also not known whether VARIVAX can cause fetal harm when administered to a pregnant woman or can affect reproduction capacity. Therefore, VARIVAX should not be administered to pregnant females; furthermore, pregnancy should be avoided for three months following vaccination (see CONTRAINDICATIONS).
Nursing Mothers
It is not known whether varicella vaccine virus is secreted in human milk. Therefore, because some viruses are secreted in human milk, caution should be exercised if VARIVAX is administered to a nursing woman.
Pediatric Use
No clinical data are available on safety or efficacy of VARIVAX in children less than one year of age and administration to infants under twelve months of age is not recommended.

ADVERSE REACTIONS

In clinical trials,[4,5,9–15] VARIVAX was administered to 11,102 healthy children, adolescents, and adults. VARIVAX was generally well tolerated.
In a double-blind placebo controlled study among 914 healthy children and adolescents who were serologically confirmed to be susceptible to varicella, the only adverse reactions that occurred at a significantly (p < 0.05) greater rate in vaccine recipients than in placebo recipients were pain and redness at the injection site.[4]
Children 1 to 12 Years of Age
In clinical trials involving healthy children monitored for up to 42 days after a single dose of VARIVAX, the frequency of fever, injection-site complaints, or rashes were reported as follows:
[See table 1 above.]
In addition, the most frequently (≥1%) reported adverse experiences, without regard to causality, are listed in decreasing order of frequency: upper respiratory illness, cough, irritability/nervousness, fatigue, disturbed sleep, diarrhea, loss of appetite, vomiting, otitis, diaper rash/contact rash, headache, teething, malaise, abdominal pain, other rash, nausea, eye complaints, chills, lymphadenopathy, myalgia, lower respiratory illness, allergic reactions (including allergic rash, hives), stiff neck, heat rash/prickly heat, arthralgia, eczema/dry skin/dermatitis, constipation, itching.
Pneumonitis has been reported rarely (<1%) in children vaccinated with VARIVAX; a causal relationship has not been established.
Febrile seizures have occurred rarely (<0.1%) in children vaccinated with VARIVAX; a causal relationship has not been established.
Adolescents and Adults 13 Years of Age and Older
In clinical trials involving healthy adolescents and adults, the majority of whom received two doses of VARIVAX and were monitored for up to 42 days after any dose, the fre-

Continued on next page

Table 1
Fever, Local Reactions, or Rashes (%) in Children
0 to 42 Days Postvaccination

Reaction	N	Post dose 1	Peak Occurrence in Postvaccination Days
Fever ≥ 102°F (39°C) Oral	8827	14.7%	0-42
Injection-site complaints (pain/ soreness, swelling and/or erythema, rash, pruritus, hematoma, induration, stiffness)	8916	19.3%	0–2
Varicella-like rash (injection site) Median number of lesions	8916	3.4% 2	8–19
Varicella-like rash (generalized) Median number of lesions	8916	3.8% 5	5–26

Merck & Co.—Cont.

quency of fever, injection-site complaints, or rashes were reported as follows:
[See table 2 below.]
In addition, the most frequently (≥1%) reported adverse experiences, without regard to causality, are listed in decreasing order of frequency: upper respiratory illness, headache, fatigue, cough, myalgia, disturbed sleep, nausea, malaise, diarrhea, stiff neck, irritability/nervousness, lymphadenopathy, chills, eye complaints, abdominal pain, loss of appetite, arthralgia, otitis, itching, vomiting, other rashes, constipation, lower respiratory illness, allergic reactions (including allergic rash, hives), contact rash, cold/canker sore.
As with any vaccine, there is the possibility that broad use of the vaccine could reveal adverse reactions not observed in clinical trials.
The following additional adverse reactions have been reported since the vaccine has been marketed:
Body As A Whole
  Anaphylaxis.
Nervous/Psychiatric
  Encephalitis; ataxia.
Respiratory
  Pharyngitis.
Skin
  Herpes zoster; erythema multiforme.

DOSAGE AND ADMINISTRATION

FOR SUBCUTANEOUS ADMINISTRATION

Do not inject intravenously
Children 12 months to 12 years of age should receive a single 0.5 mL dose administered subcutaneously.
Adolescents and adults 13 years of age and older should receive a 0.5 mL dose administered subcutaneously at elected date and a second 0.5 mL dose 4 to 8 weeks later.
VARIVAX is for subcutaneous administration. The outer aspect of the upper arm (deltoid) is the preferred site of injection.
VARIVAX **SHOULD BE STORED FROZEN** at an average temperature of −15°C (+5°F) or colder until it is reconstituted for injection (see HOW SUPPLIED, *Storage*). Any freezer (e.g. chest, frost-free) that reliably maintains an average temperature of −15°C and has a separate sealed freezer door is acceptable for storing VARIVAX. The diluent should be stored separately at room temperature or in the refrigerator. To reconstitute the vaccine, first withdraw 0.7 mL of diluent into the syringe to be used for reconstitution. Inject all the diluent in the syringe into the vial of lyophilized vaccine and gently agitate to mix thoroughly. Withdraw the entire contents into a syringe, change the needle, and inject the total volume (about 0.5 mL) of reconstituted vaccine subcutaneously, preferably into the outer aspect of the upper arm (deltoid) or the anterolateral thigh. **IT IS RECOMMENDED THAT THE VACCINE BE ADMINISTERED IMMEDIATELY AFTER RECONSTITUTION, TO MINIMIZE LOSS OF POTENCY. DISCARD IF RECONSTITUTED VACCINE IS NOT USED WITHIN 30 MINUTES.**
CAUTION: A sterile syringe free of preservatives, antiseptics, and detergents should be used for each injection and/or reconstitution of VARIVAX because these substances may inactivate the vaccine virus.
It is important to use a separate sterile syringe and needle for each patient to prevent transmission of infectious agents from one individual to another.

To reconstitute the vaccine, use only the diluent supplied, since it is free of preservatives or other anti-viral substances which might inactivate the vaccine virus.
Do not freeze reconstituted vaccine.
Do not give immune globulin including Varicella Zoster Immune Globulin concurrently with VARIVAX (see also PRECAUTIONS).
Parenteral drug products should be inspected visually for particulate matter and discoloration prior to administration, whenever solution and container permit. VARIVAX when reconstituted is a clear, colorless to pale yellow liquid.

HOW SUPPLIED

No. 4826/4309—VARIVAX is supplied as follows: (1) a single-dose vial of lyophilized vaccine, **NDC** 0006-4826-00 (package A); and (2) a box of 10 vials of diluent (package B).
No. 4827/4309—VARIVAX is supplied as follows: (1) a box of 10 single-dose vials of lyophilized vaccine (package A), **NDC** 0006-4827-00; and (2) a box of 10 vials of diluent (package B).
(6505-01-413-1331, Ten Pack)
Stability
VARIVAX retains a potency level of 1500 PFU or higher per dose for at least 18 months in a frost-free freezer with an average temperature of −15°C (+5°F) or colder.
VARIVAX has a minimum potency level of approximately 1350 PFU 30 minutes after reconstitution at room temperature (20–25°C, 68–77°F).
Prior to reconstitution, VARIVAX retains potency when stored for up to 72 continuous hours at refrigerator temperature (2-8°C, 36-46°F).
For information regarding stability under conditions other than those recommended, call 1-800-9-VARIVAX.
Storage
During shipment, to ensure that there is no loss of potency, the vaccine must be maintained at a temperature of −20°C (−4°F) or colder.
Before reconstitution, store the lyophilized vaccine in a freezer at an average temperature of − 15°C (+5°F) or colder. Any freezer (e.g. chest, frost-free) that reliably maintains an average temperature of –15°C and has a separate sealed freezer door is acceptable for storing VARIVAX.
VARIVAX may be stored at refrigerator temperature (2-8°C, 36-46°F) for up to 72 continuous hours prior to reconstitution. Vaccine stored at 2-8°C which is not used within 72 hours of removal from –15°C storage should be discarded.
Before reconstitution, protect from light.
The diluent should be stored separately at room temperature (20-25°C, 68-77°F), or in the refrigerator.

REFERENCES

1. Balfour, H.H.; et al.: Acyclovir treatment of varicella in otherwise healthy children, Pediatr., *116:* 633–639, 1990.
2. Ross, A.H.: Modification of chickenpox in family contacts by administration of gamma globulin, N. Engl. J. Med. *267:* 369–376, 1962.
3. Preblud, S.R.: Varicella: Complications and Costs, Pediatrics, *78* (4 Pt 2):728–735, 1986.
4. Weibel, R.E.; et al.: Live Attenuated Varicella Virus Vaccine, N. Engl. J. Med. *310* (22):1409–1415, 1984.
5. Unpublished data; files of Merck Research Laboratories.
6. Wharton, M.; et al.: Health Impact of Varicella in the 1980's. Thirtieth Interscience Conference on Antimicrobial Agents and Chemotherapy, (Abstract #1138), 1990.
7. Berhstein, H.H.; et al.: Clinical Survey of Natural Varicella Compared with Breakthrough Varicella After Immunization with Live Attenuated Oka/Merck Varicella Vaccine. Pediatrics *92:* 833–837, 1993.
8. Kuter, B.J.; et al.: Oka/Merck Varicella Vaccine in Healthy Children: Final Report of a 2-Year Efficacy Study and 7-Year Follow-up Studies, Vaccine, *9:* 643–647, 1991.
9. Arbeter, A.M.; et al.: Varicella Vaccine Trials in Healthy Children, A Summary of Comparative and Follow-up Studies, AJDC *138:* 434–438, 1984.
10. Weibel, R.E.; et al.: Live Oka/Merck Varicella Vaccine in Healthy Children, JAMA *254* (17): 2435–2439, 1985.
11. Chartrand, D.M.; et al.: New Varicella Vaccine Production Lots in Healthy Children and Adolescents, Abstracts of the 1988 Inter-Science Conference Antimicrobial Agents and Chemotherapy: *237* (Abstract #731).
12. Johnson, C.E.; et al.: Live Attenuated Vaccine in Healthy 12 to 24 month old Children, Pediatrics *81:* 512–518, 1988.
13. Gershon, A.A.; et al.: Immunization of Healthy Adults with Live Attenuated Varicella Vaccine, Journal of Infectious Diseases, *158* (1):132–137, 1988.
14. Gershon, A.A.; et al.: Live Attenuated Varicella Vaccine: Protection in Healthy Adults Compared with Leukemic Children, Journal of Infectious Diseases, *161:* 661–666, 1990.
15. White, C.J.; et al.: Varicella Vaccine (VARIVAX) in Healthy Children and Adolescents: Results From Clinical Trials, 1987 to 1989, Pediatrics, *87* (5):604–610, 1991.
16. Asano, Y.; et al.: Contact Infection from Live Varicella Vaccine Recipients, Lancet *1* (7966):965, 1976.
17. Hammerschlag, M.R.; et al.: Herpes Zoster in an Adult Recipient of Live Attenuated Varicella Vaccine, J Infect Dis *160* (3):535–537, 1989.
18. White, C.J.: Letters to the Editor, Pediatrics *318:* 354, 1992.
19. Guess, H.A.; et al.: Epidemiology of Herpes Zoster in Children and Adolescents: A Population Based Study, Pediatrics *76* (4):512–517, 1985.
20. Ragozzino, M.; et al.: Population-Based Study of Herpes Zoster and Its Sequelae, Medicine *61* (5):310–316, 1982.
21. Morbidity and Mortality Weekly Report *34* (1):13–16, Jan. 11, 1985.
22. Dennehy, P.H.; et al.: Immunogenicity of Subcutaneous Versus Intramuscular Oka/Merck Varicella Vaccination in Healthy Children, Pediatrics *88* (3):604–607, 1991.
23. Center for Disease Control: Immunization of Children Infected with Human T-Lymphotropic Virus Type III/Lymphadenopathy-Associated Virus, Annals of Internal Medicine, *106:* 75–78, 1987.
24. Recommendations of the Advisory Committee on Immunization Practices (ACIP): General Recommendations on Immunization, MMWR*43* (No.RR-1):15–18, January 28, 1994.
25. Vaccine Adverse Event Reporting System-United States, MMWR *39* (41):730–733, 1990.

7999902   Issued May 1996

VASERETIC® Tablets
(Enalapril Maleate-Hydrochlorothiazide)   ℞

USE IN PREGNANCY
When used in pregnancy during the second and third trimesters, ACE inhibitors can cause injury and even death to the developing fetus. When pregnancy is detected, VASERETIC should be discontinued as soon as possible. See WARNINGS, *Pregnancy, Enalapril Maleate, Fetal/Neonatal Morbidity and Mortality.*

DESCRIPTION

VASERETIC* (Enalapril Maleate-Hydrochlorothiazide) combines an angiotensin converting enzyme inhibitor, enalapril maleate, and a diuretic, hydrochlorothiazide. Enalapril maleate is the maleate salt of enalapril, the ethyl ester of a long-acting angiotensin converting enzyme inhibitor, enalaprilat. Enalapril maleate is chemically described as (*S*)-1-[*N*-[1-(ethoxycarbonyl)-3-phenylpropyl]-L-alanyl]-L-proline, (*Z*)-2-butenedioate salt (1:1). Its empirical formula is $C_{20}H_{28}N_2O_5 \cdot C_4H_4O_4$, and its structural formula is:

Table 2
Fever, Local Reactions, or Rashes (%) in Adolescents and Adults

0 to 42 Days Postvaccination

Reaction	N	Post Dose 1	Peak Occurrence in Postvaccination Days	N	Post Dose 2	Peak Occurrence in Postvaccination Days
Fever ≥100°F (37.7°C) Oral	1584	10.2%		956	9.5%	0-42
Injection-site complaints (soreness, erythema, swelling, rash, pruritus, pyrexia, hematoma, induration, numbness)	1606	24.4%	0–2	955	32.5%	0–2
Varicella-like rash (injection site)	1606	3%	6–20	955	1%	0–6
Median number of lesions		2			2	
Varicella-like rash (generalized)	1606	5.5%	7–21	955	0.9%	0–23
Median number of lesions		5			5.5	

Enalapril maleate is a white to off-white crystalline powder with a molecular weight of 492.53. It is sparingly soluble in water, soluble in ethanol, and freely soluble in methanol.
Enalapril is a pro-drug; following oral administration, it is bioactivated by hydrolysis of the ethyl ester to enalaprilat, which is the active angiotensin converting enzyme inhibitor.
Hydrochlorothiazide is 6-chloro-3,4-dihydro-2*H*-1,2,4-benzothiadiazine-7-sulfonamide 1,1-dioxide. Its empirical formula is $C_7H_8ClN_3O_4S_2$ and its structural formula is:

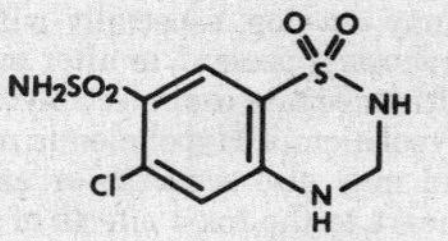

It is a white, or practically white, crystalline powder with a molecular weight of 297.72, which is slightly soluble in water, but freely soluble in sodium hydroxide solution.
VASERETIC is available in two tablet combinations of enalapril maleate with hydrochlorothiazide: VASERETIC 5–12.5, containing 5 mg enalapril maleate and 12.5 mg hydrochlorothiazide and VASERETIC 10–25, containing 10 mg enalapril maleate and 25 mg hydrochlorothiazide. Inactive ingredients are: iron oxides, lactose, magnesium stearate, starch and other ingredients.

* Registered trademark of MERCK & CO., INC.

CLINICAL PHARMACOLOGY

As a result of its diuretic effects, hydrochlorothiazide increases plasma renin activity, increases aldosterone secretion, and decreases serum potassium. Administration of enalapril maleate blocks the renin-angiotensin-aldosterone axis and tends to reverse the potassium loss associated with the diuretic.
In clinical studies, the extent of blood pressure reduction seen with the combination of enalapril maleate and hydrochlorothiazide was approximately additive. The antihypertensive effect of VASERETIC was usually sustained for at least 24 hours.
Concomitant administration of enalapril maleate and hydrochlorothiazide has little, or no effect on the bioavailability of either drug. The combination tablet is bioequivalent to concomitant administration of the separate entities.
Enalapril Maleate
Mechanism of Action: Enalapril, after hydrolysis to enalaprilat, inhibits angiotensin-converting enzyme (ACE) in human subjects and animals. ACE is a peptidyl dipeptidase that catalyzes the conversion of angiotensin I to the vasoconstrictor substance, angiotensin II. Angiotensin II also stimulates aldosterone secretion by the adrenal cortex. Inhibition of ACE results in decreased plasma angiotensin II, which leads to decreased vasopressor activity and to decreased aldosterone secretion. Although the latter decrease is small, it results in small increases of serum potassium. In hypertensive patients treated with enalapril maleate alone for up to 48 weeks, mean increases in serum potassium of approximately 0.2 mEq/L were observed. In patients treated with enalapril maleate plus a thiazide diuretic, there was essentially no change in serum potassium. (See PRECAUTIONS.)
Removal of angiotensin II negative feedback on renin secretion leads to increased plasma renin activity.
ACE is identical to kininase, an enzyme that degrades bradykinin. Whether increased levels of bradykinin, a potent vasodepressor peptide, play a role in the therapeutic effects of enalapril remains to be elucidated.
While the mechanism through which enalapril lowers blood pressure is believed to be primarily suppression of the renin-angiotensin-aldosterone system, enalapril is antihypertensive even in patients with low-renin hypertension. Although enalapril was antihypertensive in all races studied, black hypertensive patients (usually a low-renin hypertensive population) had a smaller average response to enalapril maleate monotherapy than non-black patients. In contrast, hydrochlorothiazide was more effective in black patients than enalapril. Concomitant administration of enalapril maleate and hydrochlorothiazide was equally effective in black and non-black patients.
Pharmacokinetics and Metabolism: Following oral administration of enalapril maleate, peak serum concentrations of enalapril occur within about one hour. Based on urinary recovery, the extent of absorption of enalapril is approximately 60 percent. Enalapril absorption is not influenced by the presence of food in the gastrointestinal tract. Following absorption, enalapril is hydrolyzed to enalaprilat, which is a more potent angiotensin converting enzyme inhibitor than enalapril; enalaprilat is poorly absorbed when administered orally. Peak serum concentrations of enalaprilat occur three to four hours after an oral dose of enalapril maleate. Excretion of enalaprilat and enalapril is primarily renal. Approximately 94 percent of the dose is recovered in the urine and feces as enalaprilat or enalapril. The principal components in urine are enalaprilat, accounting for about 40 percent of the dose, and intact enalapril. There is no evidence of metabolites of enalapril, other than enalaprilat.
The serum concentration profile of enalaprilat exhibits a prolonged terminal phase, apparently representing a small fraction of the administered dose that has been bound to ACE. The amount bound does not increase with dose, indicating a saturable site of binding. The effective half-life for accumulation of enalaprilat following multiple doses of enalapril maleate is 11 hours.
The disposition of enalapril and enalaprilat in patients with renal insufficiency is similar to that in patients with normal renal function until the glomerular filtration rate is 30 mL/min or less. With glomerular filtration rate ≤30 mL/min, peak and trough enalaprilat levels increase, time to peak concentration increases and time to steady state may be delayed. The effective half-life of enalaprilat following multiple doses of enalapril maleate is prolonged at this level of renal insufficiency. Enalaprilat is dialyzable at the rate of 62 mL/min.
Studies in dogs indicate that enalapril crosses the blood-brain barrier poorly, if at all; enalaprilat does not enter the brain. Multiple doses of enalapril maleate in rats do not result in accumulation in any tissues. Milk of lactating rats contains radioactivity following administration of ^{14}C enalapril maleate. Radioactivity was found to cross the placenta following administration of labeled drug to pregnant hamsters.
Pharmacodynamics: Administration of enalapril maleate to patients with hypertension of severity ranging from mild to severe results in a reduction of both supine and standing blood pressure usually with no orthostatic component. Symptomatic postural hypotension is infrequent with enalapril alone but it can be anticipated in volume-depleted patients, such as patients treated with diuretics. In clinical trials with enalapril and hydrochlorothiazide administered concurrently, syncope occurred in 1.3 percent of patients. (See WARNINGS and DOSAGE AND ADMINISTRATION.)
In most patients studied, after oral administration of a single dose of enalapril maleate, onset of antihypertensive activity was seen at one hour with peak reduction of blood pressure achieved by four to six hours.
At recommended doses, antihypertensive effects of enalapril maleate monotherapy have been maintained for at least 24 hours. In some patients the effects may diminish toward the end of the dosing interval; this was less frequently observed with concomitant administration of enalapril maleate and hydrochlorothiazide.
Achievement of optimal blood pressure reduction may require several weeks of enalapril therapy in some patients.
The antihypertensive effects of enalapril have continued during long term therapy. Abrupt withdrawal of enalapril has not been associated with a rapid increase in blood pressure.
In hemodynamic studies in patients with essential hypertension, blood pressure reduction produced by enalapril was accompanied by a reduction in peripheral arterial resistance with an increase in cardiac output and little or no change in heart rate. Following administration of enalapril maleate, there is an increase in renal blood flow; glomerular filtration rate is usually unchanged. The effects appear to be similar in patients with renovascular hypertension.
In a clinical pharmacology study, indomethacin or sulindac was administered to hypertensive patients receiving enalapril maleate. In this study there was no evidence of a blunting of the antihypertensive action of enalapril maleate.
Hydrochlorothiazide
The mechanism of the antihypertensive effect of thiazides is unknown. Thiazides do not usually affect normal blood pressure. Hydrochlorothiazide is a diuretic and antihypertensive. It affects the distal renal tubular mechanism of electrolyte reabsorption. Hydrochlorothiazide increases excretion of sodium and chloride in approximately equivalent amounts. Natriuresis may be accompanied by some loss of potassium and bicarbonate. After oral use diuresis begins within two hours, peaks in about four hours and lasts about 6 to 12 hours. Hydrochlorothiazide is not metabolized but is eliminated rapidly by the kidney. When plasma levels have been followed for at least 24 hours, the plasma half-life has been observed to vary between 5.6 and 14.8 hours. At least 61 percent of the oral dose is eliminated unchanged within 24 hours. Hydrochlorothiazide crosses the placental but not the blood-brain barrier.

INDICATIONS AND USAGE

VASERETIC is indicated for the treatment of hypertension. These fixed dose combinations are not indicated for initial treatment (see DOSAGE AND ADMINISTRATION).
In using VASERETIC, consideration should be given to the fact that another angiotensin converting enzyme inhibitor, captopril, has caused agranulocytosis, particularly in patients with renal impairment or collagen vascular disease, and that available data are insufficient to show that enalapril does not have a similar risk. (See WARNINGS.)
In considering use of VASERETIC, it should be noted that black patients receiving ACE inhibitor monotherapy have been reported to have a higher incidence of angioedema compared to non-blacks. (See WARNINGS, *Angioedema*.)

CONTRAINDICATIONS

VASERETIC is contraindicated in patients who are hypersensitive to any component of this product and in patients with a history of angioedema related to previous treatment with an angiotensin converting enzyme inhibitor. Because of the hydrochlorothiazide component, this product is contraindicated in patients with anuria or hypersensitivity to other sulfonamide-derived drugs.

WARNINGS

General
Enalapril Maleate
Hypotension: Excessive hypotension was rarely seen in uncomplicated hypertensive patients but is a possible consequence of enalapril use in severely salt/volume depleted persons such as those treated vigorously with diuretics or patients on dialysis.
Syncope has been reported in 1.3 percent of patients receiving VASERETIC. In patients receiving enalapril alone, the incidence of syncope is 0.5 percent. The overall incidence of syncope may be reduced by proper titration of the individual components. (See PRECAUTIONS, *Drug Interactions*, ADVERSE REACTIONS and DOSAGE AND ADMINISTRATION.)
In patients with severe congestive heart failure, with or without associated renal insufficiency, excessive hypotension has been observed and may be associated with oliguria and/or progressive azotemia, and rarely with acute renal failure and/or death. Because of the potential fall in blood pressure in these patients, therapy should be started under very close medical supervision. Such patients should be followed closely for the first two weeks of treatment and whenever the dose of enalapril and/or diuretic is increased. Similar considerations may apply to patients with ischemic heart or cerebrovascular disease, in whom an excessive fall in blood pressure could result in a myocardial infarction or cerebrovascular accident.
If hypotension occurs, the patient should be placed in the supine position and, if necessary, receive an intravenous infusion of normal saline. A transient hypotensive response is not a contraindication to further doses, which usually can be given without difficulty once the blood pressure has increased after volume expansion.
Anaphylactoid and Possibly Related Reactions:
Presumably because angiotensin-converting enzyme inhibitors affect the metabolism of eicosanoids and polypeptides, including endogenous bradykinin, patients receiving ACE inhibitors (including VASERETIC) may be subject to a variety of adverse reactions, some of them serious.
Angioedema: Angioedema of the face, extremities, lips, tongue, glottis and/or larynx has been reported in patients treated with angiotensin converting enzyme inhibitors, including enalapril. This may occur at any time during treatment. In such cases VASERETIC should be promptly discontinued and appropriate therapy and monitoring should be provided until complete and sustained resolution of signs and symptoms has occurred. In instances where swelling has been confined to the face and lips the condition has generally resolved without treatment, although antihistamines have been useful in relieving symptoms. Angioedema associated with laryngeal edema may be fatal. **Where there is involvement of the tongue, glottis or larynx, likely to cause airway obstruction, appropriate therapy, e.g., subcutaneous epinephrine solution 1:1000 (0.3 mL to 0.5 mL) and/or measures necessary to ensure a patent airway, should be promptly provided.** (See ADVERSE REACTIONS.)
Patients with a history of angioedema unrelated to ACE inhibitor therapy may be at increased risk of angioedema while receiving an ACE inhibitor (see also INDICATIONS AND USAGE and CONTRAINDICATIONS).
Anaphylactoid reactions during desensitization: Two patients undergoing desensitizing treatment with hymenoptera venom while receiving ACE inhibitors sustained life-threatening anaphylactoid reactions. In the same patients, these reactions were avoided when ACE inhibitors were temporarily withheld, but they reappeared upon inadvertent rechallenge.
Anaphylactoid reactions during membrane exposure: Anaphylactoid reactions have been reported in patients dialyzed with high-flux membranes and treated concomitantly with an ACE inhibitor. Anaphylactoid reactions have also been

Continued on next page

Information on the Merck & Co., Inc. products listed on these pages is the full prescribing information from product circulars in use September 30, 1996.

Merck & Co.—Cont.

reported in patients undergoing low-density lipoprotein apheresis with dextran sulfate absorption (a procedure dependent upon devices not approved in the United States).

Neutropenia/Agranulocytosis: Another angiotensin converting enzyme inhibitor, captopril, has been shown to cause agranulocytosis and bone marrow depression, rarely in uncomplicated patients but more frequently in patients with renal impairment especially if they also have a collagen vascular disease. Available data from clinical trials of enalapril are insufficient to show that enalapril does not cause agranulocytosis at similar rates. Marketing experience has revealed several cases of neutropenia or agranulocytosis in which a causal relationship to enalapril cannot be excluded. Periodic monitoring of white blood cell counts in patients with collagen vascular disease and renal disease should be considered.

Hepatic Failure: Rarely, ACE inhibitors have been associated with a syndrome that starts with cholestatic jaundice and progresses to fulminant hepatic necrosis, and (sometimes) death. The mechanism of this syndrome is not understood. Patients receiving ACE inhibitors who develop jaundice or marked elevations of hepatic enzymes should discontinue the ACE inhibitor and receive appropriate medical follow-up.

Hydrochlorothiazide

Thiazides should be used with caution in severe renal disease. In patients with renal disease, thiazides may precipitate azotemia. Cumulative effects of the drug may develop in patients with impaired renal function.

Thiazides should be used with caution in patients with impaired hepatic function or progressive liver disease, since minor alterations of fluid and electrolyte balance may precipitate hepatic coma.

Sensitivity reactions may occur in patients with or without a history of allergy or bronchial asthma.

The possibility of exacerbation or activation of systemic lupus erythematosus has been reported.

Lithium generally should not be given with thiazides (see PRECAUTIONS, *Drug Interactions, Enalapril Maleate* and *Hydrochlorothiazide*).

Pregnancy
Enalapril-Hydrochlorothiazide

There was no teratogenicity in rats given up to 90 mg/kg/day of enalapril (150 times the maximum human dose) in combination with 10 mg/kg/day of hydrochlorothiazide (2½ times the maximum human dose) or in mice given up to 30 mg/kg/day of enalapril (50 times the maximum human dose) in combination with 10 mg/kg/day of hydrochlorothiazide (2½ times the maximum human dose). At these doses, fetotoxicity expressed as a decrease in average fetal weight occurred in both species. No fetotoxicity occurred at lower doses; 30/10 mg/kg/day of enalapril-hydrochlorothiazide in rats and 10/10 mg/kg/day of enalapril-hydrochlorothiazide in mice.

When used in pregnancy during the second and third trimesters, ACE inhibitors can cause injury and even death to the developng fetus. When pregnancy is detected, VASERETIC should be discontinued as soon as possible. (See *Enalapril Maleate, Fetal/Neonatal Morbidity and Mortality,* below.)

Enalapril Maleate
Fetal/Neonatal Morbidity and Mortality: ACE inhibitors can cause fetal and neonatal morbidity and death when administered to pregnant women. Several dozen cases have been reported in the world literature. When pregnancy is detected, ACE inhibitors should be discontinued as soon as possible.

The use of ACE inhibitors during the second and third trimesters of pregnancy has been associated with fetal and neonatal injury, including hypotension, neonatal skull hypoplasia, anuria, reversible or irreversible renal failure, and death. Oligohydramnios has also been reported, presumably resulting from decreased fetal renal function; oligohydramnios in this setting has been associated with fetal limb contractures, craniofacial deformation, and hypoplastic lung development. Prematurity, intrauterine growth retardation, and patent ductus arteriosus have also been reported, although it is not clear whether these occurrences were due to the ACE-inhibitor exposure.

These adverse effects do not appear to have resulted from intrauterine ACE-inhibitor exposure that has been limited to the first trimester. Mothers whose embryos and fetuses are exposed to ACE inhibitors only during the first trimester should be so informed. Nonetheless, when patients become pregnant, physicians should make every effort to discontinue the use of VASERETIC as soon as possible.

Rarely (probably less often than once in every thousand pregnancies), no alternative to ACE inhibitors will be found. In these rare cases, the mothers should be apprised of the potential hazards to their fetuses, and serial ultrasound examinations should be performed to assess the intraamniotic environment.

If oligohydramnios is observed, VASERETIC should be discontinued unless it is considered lifesaving for the mother.

Contraction stress testing (CST), a non-stress test (NST), or biophysical profiling (BPP) may be appropriate, depending upon the week of pregnancy. Patients and physicians should be aware, however, that oligohydramnios may not appear until after the fetus has sustained irreversible injury.

Infants with histories of *in utero* exposure to ACE inhibitors should be closely observed for hypotension, oliguria, and hyperkalemia. If oliguria occurs, attention should be directed toward support of blood pressure and renal perfusion. Exchange transfusion or dialysis may be required as means of reversing hypotension and/or substituting for disordered renal functon. Enalapril, which crosses the placenta, has been removed from neonatal circulation by peritoneal dialysis with some clinical benefit, and theoretically may be removed by exchange transfusion, although there is no experience with the latter procedure.

No teratogenic effects of enalapril were seen in studies of pregnant rats, and rabbits. On a mg/kg basis, the doses used were up to 333 times (in rats), and 50 times (in rabbits) the maximum recommended human dose.

Hydrochlorothiazide
Teratogenic Effects: Reproduction studies in the rabbit, the mouse and the rat at doses up to 100 mg/kg/day (50 times the human dose) showed no evidence of external abnormalities of the fetus due to hydrochlorothiazide. Hydrochlorothiazide given in a two-litter study in rats at doses of 4–5.6 mg/kg/day (approximately 1–2 times the usual daily human dose) did not impair fertility or produce birth abnormalities in the offspring. Thiazides cross the placental barrier and appear in cord blood.

Nonteratogenic Effects: These may include fetal or neonatal jaundice, thrombocytopenia, and possibly other adverse reactions which have occurred in the adult.

PRECAUTIONS

General
Enalapril Maleate
Impaired Renal Function: As a consequence of inhibiting the renin-angiotensin-aldosterone system, changes in renal function may be anticipated in susceptible individuals. In patients with severe congestive heart failure whose renal function may depend on the activity of the renin-angiotensin-aldosterone system, treatment with angiotensin converting enzyme inhibitors, including enalapril, may be associated with oliguria and/or progressive azotemia and rarely with acute renal failure and/or death.

In clinical studies in hypertensive patients with unilateral or bilateral renal artery stenosis, increases in blood urea nitrogen and serum creatinine were observed in 20 percent of patients. These increases were almost always reversible upon discontinuation of enalapril and/or diuretic therapy. In such patients renal function should be monitored during the first few weeks of therapy.

Some patients with hypertension or heart failure with no apparent pre-existing renal vascular disease have developed increases in blood urea and serum creatinine, usually minor and transient, especially when enalapril has been given concomitantly with a diuretic. This is more likely to occur in patients with pre-existing renal impairment. Dosage reduction of enalapril and/or discontinuation of the diuretic may be required.

Evaluation of the hypertensive patient should always include assessment of renal function.

Hyperkalemia: Elevated serum potassium (greater than 5.7 mEq/L) was observed in approximately one percent of hypertensive patients in clinical trials treated with enalapril alone. In most cases these were isolated values which resolved despite continued therapy, although hyperkalemia was a cause of discontinuation of therapy in 0.28 percent of hypertensive patients. Hyperkalemia was less frequent (approximately 0.1 percent) in patients treated with enalapril plus hydrochlorothiazide. Risk factors for the development of hyperkalemia include renal insufficiency, diabetes mellitus, and the concomitant use of potassium-sparing diuretics, potassium supplements and/or potassium-containing salt substitutes, which should be used cautiously, if at all, with enalapril. (See *Drug Interactions.*)

Cough: Presumably due to the inhibition of the degradation of endogenous bradykinin, persistent nonproductive cough has been reported with all ACE inhibitors, always resolving after discontinuation of therapy. ACE inhibitor-induced cough should be considered in the differential diagnosis of cough.

Surgery/Anesthesia: In patients undergoing major surgery or during anesthesia with agents that produce hypotension, enalapril may block angiotensin II formation secondary to compensatory renin release. If hypotension occurs and is considered to be due to this mechanism, it can be corrected by volume expansion.

Hydrochlorothiazide

Periodic determination of serum electrolytes to detect possible electrolyte imbalance should be performed at appropriate intervals. All patients receiving thiazide therapy should be observed for clinical signs of fluid or electrolyte imbal-

ance: namely hyponatremia, hypochloremic alkalosis, and hypokalemia. Serum and urine electrolyte determinations are particularly important when the patient is vomiting excessively or receiving parenteral fluids. Warning signs or symptoms of fluid and electrolyte imbalance, irrespective of cause, include dryness of mouth, thirst, weakness, lethargy, drowsiness, restlessness, confusion, seizures, muscle pains or cramps, muscular fatigue, hypotension, oliguria, tachycardia, and gastrointestinal disturbances such as nausea and vomiting.

Hypokalemia may develop, especially with brisk diuresis, when severe cirrhosis is present, or after prolonged therapy. Interference with adequate oral electrolyte intake will also contribute to hypokalemia. Hypokalemia may cause cardiac arrhythmia and may also sensitize or exaggerate the response of the heart to the toxic effects of digitalis (e.g., increased ventricular irritability). Because enalapril reduces the production of aldosterone, concomitant therapy with enalapril attenuates the diuretic-induced potassium loss (see *Drug Interactions, Agents Increasing Serum Potassium*). Although any chloride deficit is generally mild and usually does not require specific treatment except under extraordinary circumstances (as in liver disease or renal disease), chloride replacement may be required in the treatment of metabolic alkalosis.

Dilutional hyponatremia may occur in edematous patients in hot weather; appropriate therapy is water restriction, rather than administration of salt except in rare instances when the hyponatremia is life-threatening. In actual salt depletion, appropriate replacement is the therapy of choice.

Hyperuricemia may occur or frank gout may be precipitated in certain patients receiving thiazide therapy.

In diabetic patients dosage adjustments of insulin or oral hypoglycemic agents may be required. Hyperglycemia may occur with thiazide diuretics. Thus latent diabetes mellitus may become manifest during thiazide therapy.

The antihypertensive effects of the drug may be enhanced in the postsympathectomy patient.

If progressive renal impairment becomes evident consider withholding or discontinuing diuretic therapy.

Thiazides have been shown to increase the urinary excretion of magnesium; this may result in hypomagnesemia.

Thiazides may decrease urinary calcium excretion. Thiazides may cause intermittent and slight elevation of serum calcium in the absence of known disorders of calcium metabolism. Marked hypercalcemia may be evidence of hidden hyperparathyroidism. Thiazides should be discontinued before carrying out tests for parathyroid function.

Increases in cholesterol and triglyceride levels may be associated with thiazide diuretic therapy.

Information for Patients
Angioedema: Angioedema, including laryngeal edema, may occur at any time during treatment with angiotensin converting enzyme inhibitors, including enalapril. Patients should be so advised and told to report immediately any signs or symptoms suggesting angioedema (swelling of face, extremities, eyes, lips, tongue, difficulty in swallowing or breathing) and to take no more drug until they have consulted with the prescribing physician.

Hypotension: Patients should be cautioned to report lightheadedness especially during the first few days of therapy. If actual syncope occurs, the patients should be told to discontinue the drug until they have consulted with the prescribing physician.

All patients should be cautioned that excessive perspiration and dehydration may lead to an excessive fall in blood pressure because of reduction in fluid volume. Other causes of volume depletion such as vomiting or diarrhea may also lead to a fall in blood pressure; patients should be advised to consult with the physician.

Hyperkalemia: Patients should be told not to use salt substitutes containing potassium without consulting their physician.

Neutropenia: Patients should be told to report promptly any indication of infection (e.g., sore throat, fever) which may be a sign of neutropenia.

Pregnancy: Female patients of childbearing age should be told about the consequences of second- and third-trimester exposure to ACE inhibitors, and they should also be told that these consequences do not appear to have resulted from intrauterine ACE-inhibitor exposure that has been limited to the first trimester. These patients should be asked to report pregnancies to their physicians as soon as possible.

NOTE: As with many other drugs, certain advice to patients being treated with VASERETIC is warranted. This information is intended to aid in the safe and effective use of this medication. It is not a disclosure of all possible adverse or intended effects.

Drug Interactions
Enalapril Maleate
Hypotension —Patients on Diuretic Therapy: Patients on diuretics and especially those in whom diuretic therapy was recently instituted, may occasionally experience an excessive reduction of blood pressure after initiation of therapy with enalapril. The possibility of hypotensive effects with enalapril can be minimized by either discontinuing the di-

uretic or increasing the salt intake prior to initiation of treatment with enalapril. If it is necessary to continue the diuretic, provide medical supervision for at least two hours and until blood pressure has stabilized for at least an additional hour. (See WARNINGS, and DOSAGE AND ADMINISTRATION.)

Agents Causing Renin Release: The antihypertensive effect of enalapril is augmented by antihypertensive agents that cause renin release (e.g., diuretics).

Other Cardiovascular Agents: Enalapril has been used concomitantly with beta adrenergic-blocking agents, methyldopa, nitrates, calcium-blocking agents, hydralazine and prazosin without evidence of clinically significant adverse interactions.

Agents Increasing Serum Potassium: Enalapril attenuates diuretic-induced potassium loss. Potassium-sparing diuretics (e.g., spironolactone, triamterene, or amiloride), potassium supplements, or potassium-containing salt substitutes may lead to significant increases in serum potassium. Therefore, if concomitant use of these agents is indicated because of demonstrated hypokalemia they should be used with caution and with frequent monitoring of serum potassium.

Lithium: Lithium toxicity has been reported in patients receiving lithium concomitantly with drugs which cause elimination of sodium, including ACE inhibitors. A few cases of lithium toxicity have been reported in patients receiving concomitant enalapril and lithium and were reversible upon discontinuation of both drugs. It is recommended that serum lithium levels be monitored frequently if enalapril is administered concomitantly with lithium.

Hydrochlorothiazide

When administered concurrently the following drugs may interact with thiazide diuretics:

Alcohol, barbiturates, or narcotics —potentiation of orthostatic hypotension may occur.

Antidiabetic drugs (oral agents and insulin)—dosage adjustment of the antidiabetic drug may be required.

Other antihypertensive drugs —additive effect or potentiation.

Cholestyramine and colestipol resins —Absorption of hydrochlorothiazide is impaired in the presence of anionic exchange resins. Single doses of either cholestyramine or colestipol resins bind the hydrochlorothiazide and reduce its absorption from the gastrointestinal tract by up to 85 and 43 percent, respectively.

Corticosteroids, ACTH —intensified electrolyte depletion, particularly hypokalemia.

Pressor amines (e.g., norepinephrine) —possible decreased response to pressor amines but not sufficient to preclude their use.

Skeletal muscle relaxants, nondepolarizing (e.g., tubocurarine) —possible increased responsiveness to the muscle relaxant.

Lithium —should not generally be given with diuretics. Diuretic agents reduce the renal clearance of lithium and add a high risk of lithium toxicity. Refer to the package insert for lithium preparations before use of such preparations with VASERETIC.

Non-steroidal Anti-inflammatory Drugs —In some patients, the administration of a non-steroidal anti-inflammatory agent can reduce the diuretic, natriuretic, and antihypertensive effects of loop, potassium-sparing and thiazide diuretics. Therefore, when VASERETIC and non-steroidal anti-inflammatory agents are used concomitantly, the patient should be observed closely to determine if the desired effect of the diuretic is obtained.

Carcinogenesis, Mutagenesis, Impairment of Fertility

Enalapril in combination with hydrochlorothiazide was not mutagenic in the Ames microbial mutagen test with or without metabolic activation. Enalapril-hydrochlorothiazide did not produce DNA single strand breaks in an *in vitro* alkaline elution assay in rat hepatocytes or chromosomal aberrations in an *in vivo* mouse bone marrow assay.

Enalapril Maleate

There was no evidence of a tumorigenic effect when enalapril was administered for 106 weeks to rats at doses up to 90 mg/kg/day (150 times* the maximum daily human dose). Enalapril has also been administered for 94 weeks to male and female mice at doses up to 90 and 180 mg/kg/day, respectively, (150 and 300 times* the maximum daily dose for humans) and showed no evidence of carcinogenicity.

Neither enalapril maleate nor the active diacid was mutagenic in the Ames microbial mutagen test with or without metabolic activation. Enalapril was also negative in the following genotoxicity studies: rec-assay, reverse mutation assay with *E. coli*, sister chromatid exchange with cultured mammalian cells, and the micronucleus test with mice, as well as in an *in vivo* cytogenic study using mouse bone marrow.

There were no adverse effects on reproductive performance in male and female rats treated with 10 to 90 mg/kg/day of enalapril.

*Based on patient weight of 50 kg

Hydrochlorothiazide

Two-year feeding studies in mice and rats conducted under the auspices of the National Toxicology Program (NTP) uncovered no evidence of a carcinogenic potential of hydrochlorothiazide in female mice (at doses of up to approximately 600 mg/kg/day) or in male and female rats (at doses of up to approximately 100 mg/kg/day). The NTP, however, found equivocal evidence for hepatocarcinogenicity in male mice.

Hydrochlorothiazide was not genotoxic *in vitro* in the Ames mutagenicity assay of *Salmonella typhimurium* strains TA 98, TA 100, TA 1535, TA 1537, and TA 1538 and in the Chinese Hamster Ovary (CHO) test for chromosomal aberrations, or *in vivo* in assays using mouse germinal cell chromosomes, Chinese hamster bone marrow chromosomes, and the *Drosophila* sex-linked recessive lethal trait gene. Positive test results were obtained only in the *in vitro* CHO Sister Chromatid Exchange (clastogenicity) and in the Mouse Lymphoma Cell (mutagenicity) assays, using concentrations of hydrochlorothiazide from 43 to 1300 μg/mL, and in the *Aspergillus nidulans* non-disjunction assay at an unspecified concentration.

Hydrochlorothiazide had no adverse effects on the fertility of mice and rats of either sex in studies wherein these species were exposed, via their diet, to doses of up to 100 and 4 mg/kg, respectively, prior to conception and throughout gestation.

Pregnancy

Pregnancy Categories C (first trimester) *and D* (second and third trimesters). See WARNINGS, *Pregnancy, Enalapril Maleate, Fetal/Neonatal Morbidity and Mortality.*

Nursing Mothers

Enalapril and enalaprilat are detected in human milk in trace amounts. Thiazides do appear in human milk. Because of the potential for serious reactions in nursing infants from either drug, a decision should be made whether to discontinue nursing or to discontinue VASERETIC, taking into account the importance of the drug to the mother.

Pediatric Use

Safety and effectiveness in children have not been established.

ADVERSE REACTIONS

VASERETIC has been evaluated for safety in more than 1500 patients, including over 300 patients treated for one year or more. In clinical trials with VASERETIC no adverse experiences peculiar to this combination drug have been observed. Adverse experiences that have occurred, have been limited to those that have been previously reported with enalapril or hydrochlorothiazide.

The most frequent clinical adverse experiences in controlled trials were: dizziness (8.6 percent), headache (5.5 percent), fatigue (3.9 percent) and cough (3.5 percent). Generally, adverse experiences were mild and transient in nature. Adverse experiences occurring in greater than two percent of patients treated with VASERETIC in controlled clinical trials are shown below.

	Percent of Patients in Controlled Studies	
	VASERETIC (n=1580) Incidence (discontinuation)	Placebo (n=230) Incidence
Dizziness	8.6 (0.7)	4.3
Headache	5.5 (0.4)	9.1
Fatigue	3.9 (0.8)	2.6
Cough	3.5 (0.4)	0.9
Muscle Cramps	2.7 (0.2)	0.9
Nausea	2.5 (0.4)	1.7
Asthenia	2.4 (0.3)	0.9
Orthostatic Effects	2.3 (<0.1)	0.0
Impotence	2.2 (0.5)	0.5
Diarrhea	2.1 (<0.1)	1.7

Clinical adverse experiences occurring in 0.5 to 2.0 percent of patients in controlled trials included: *Body As A Whole:* Syncope, chest pain, abdominal pain; *Cardiovascular:* Orthostatic hypotension, palpitation, tachycardia; *Digestive:* Vomiting, dyspepsia, constipation, flatulence, dry mouth; *Nervous/Psychiatric:* Insomnia, nervousness, paresthesia, somnolence, vertigo; *Skin:* Pruritus, rash; *Other:* Dyspnea, gout, back pain, arthralgia, diaphoresis, decreased libido, tinnitus, urinary tract infection.

Angioedema: Angioedema has been reported in patients receiving VASERETIC, with an incidence higher in black than in non-black patients. Angioedema associated with laryngeal edema may be fatal. If angioedema of the face, extremities, lips, tongue, glottis and/or larynx occurs, treatment with VASERETIC should be discontinued and appropriate therapy instituted immediately. (See WARNINGS.)

Hypotension: In clinical trials, adverse effects relating to hypotension occurred as follows: hypotension (0.9 percent), orthostatic hypotension (1.5 percent), other orthostatic effects (2.3 percent). In addition syncope occurred in 1.3 percent of patients. (See WARNINGS.)

Cough: See PRECAUTIONS, *Cough.*

Clinical Laboratory Test Findings

Serum Electrolytes: See PRECAUTIONS.

Creatinine, Blood Urea Nitrogen: In controlled clinical trials minor increases in blood urea nitrogen and serum creatinine, reversible upon discontinuation of therapy, were observed in about 0.6 percent of patients with essential hypertension treated with VASERETIC. More marked increases have been reported in other enalapril experience. Increases are more likely to occur in patients with renal artery stenosis. (See PRECAUTIONS.)

Serum Uric Acid, Glucose, Magnesium, and Calcium: See PRECAUTIONS.

Hemoglobin and Hematocrit: Small decreases in hemoglobin and hematocrit (mean decreases of approximately 0.3 g percent and 1.0 vol percent, respectively) occur frequently in hypertensive patients treated with VASERETIC but are rarely of clinical importance unless another cause of anemia coexists. In clinical trials, less than 0.1 percent of patients discontinued therapy due to anemia.

Liver Function Tests: Rarely, elevations of liver enzymes and/or serum bilirubin have occurred (see WARNINGS, *Hepatic Failure*).

Other adverse reactions that have been reported with the individual components are listed below and, within each category, are in order of decreasing severity.

Enalapril Maleate —Enalapril has been evaluated for safety in more than 10,000 patients. In clinical trials adverse reactions which occurred with enalapril were also seen with VASERETIC. However, since enalapril has been marketed, the following adverse reactions have been reported: *Body As A Whole:* Anaphylactoid reactions (see WARNINGS, *Anaphylactoid reactions during membrane exposure*); *Cardiovascular:* Cardiac arrest; myocardial infarction or cerebrovascular accident, possibly secondary to excessive hypotension in high risk patients (see WARNINGS, *Hypotension*); pulmonary embolism and infarction; pulmonary edema; rhythm disturbances including atrial tachycardia and bradycardia, atrial fibrillation; hypotension; angina pectoris; *Digestive:* Ileus, pancreatitis, hepatic failure, hepatitis (hepatocellular [proven on rechallenge] or cholestatic jaundice) (see WARNINGS, *Hepatic Failure*), melena, anorexia, glossitis, stomatitis, dry mouth; *Hematologic:* Rare cases of neutropenia, thrombocytopenia and bone marrow depression. Hemolytic anemia, including cases of hemolysis in patients with G-6-PD deficiency, has been reported; a causal relationship to enalapril cannot be excluded. *Nervous System/Psychiatric:* Depression, confusion, ataxia, peripheral neuropathy (e.g., paresthesia, dysesthesia); *Urogenital:* Renal failure, oliguria, renal dysfunction, (see PRECAUTIONS and DOSAGE AND ADMINISTRATION), flank pain, gynecomastia; *Respiratory:* Pulmonary infiltrates, bronchospasm, pneumonia, bronchitis, rhinorrhea, sore throat and hoarseness, asthma, upper respiratory infection; *Skin:* Exfoliative dermatitis, toxic epidermal necrolysis, Stevens-Johnson syndrome, herpes zoster, erythema multiforme, urticaria, pemphigus, alopecia, flushing, photosensitivity; *Special Senses:* Blurred vision, taste alteration, anosmia, conjunctivitis, dry eyes, tearing.

Miscellaneous: A symptom complex has been reported which may include a positive ANA, an elevated erythrocyte sedimentation rate, arthralgia/arthritis, myalgia/myositis, fever, serositis, vasculitis, leukocytosis, eosinophilia, photosensitivity, rash and other dermatologic manifestations.

Fetal/Neonatal Morbidity and Mortality: See WARNINGS, *Pregnancy, Enalapril Maleate, Fetal/Neonatal Morbidity and Mortality.*

Hydrochlorothiazide—Body as a Whole: Weakness; *Digestive:* Pancreatitis, jaundice (intrahepatic cholestatic jaundice), sialadenitis, cramping, gastric irritation, anorexia; *Hematologic:* Aplastic anemia, agranulocytosis, leukopenia, hemolytic anemia, thrombocytopenia; *Hypersensitivity:* Purpura, photosensitivity, urticaria, necrotizing angiitis (vasculitis and cutaneous vasculitis), fever, respiratory distress including pneumonitis and pulmonary edema, anaphylactic reactions; *Musculoskeletal:* Muscle spasm; *Nervous system/Psychiatric:* Restlessness; *Renal:* Renal failure, renal dysfunction, interstitial nephritis (see WARNINGS); *Skin:* Erythema multiforme including Stevens-Johnson syndrome, exfoliative dermatitis including toxic epidermal necrolysis, alopecia; *Special Senses:* Transient blurred vision, xanthopsia.

Continued on next page

Information on the Merck & Co., Inc. products listed on these pages is the full prescribing information from product circulars in use September 30, 1996.

Merck & Co.—Cont.

OVERDOSAGE

No specific information is available on the treatment of overdosage with VASERETIC. Treatment is symptomatic and supportive. Therapy with VASERETIC should be discontinued and the patient observed closely. Suggested measures include induction of emesis and/or gastric lavage, and correction of dehydration, electrolyte imbalance and hypotension by established procedures.
Enalapril Maleate—The oral LD_{50} of enalapril is 2000 mg/kg in mice and rats. The most likely manifestation of overdosage would be hypotension, for which the usual treatment would be intravenous infusion of normal saline solution. Enalaprilat may be removed from general circulation by hemodialysis and has been removed from neonatal circulation by peritoneal dialysis.
Hydrochlorothiazide—The oral LD_{50} of hydrochlorothiazide is greater than 10.0 g/kg in both mice and rats. The most common signs and symptoms observed are those caused by electrolyte depletion (hypokalemia, hypochloremia, hyponatremia) and dehydration resulting from excessive diuresis. If digitalis has also been administered, hypokalemia may accentuate cardiac arrhythmias.

DOSAGE AND ADMINISTRATION

Enalapril and hydrochlorothiazide are effective treatments for hypertension. The usual dosage range of enalapril is 10 to 40 mg per day administered in a single or two divided doses; hydrochlorothiazide is effective in doses of 25 to 100 mg daily. The side effects (see WARNINGS) of enalapril are generally rare and apparently independent of dose; those of hydrochlorothiazide are a mixture of dose-dependent phenomena (primarily hypokalemia) and dose-independent phenomena (e.g., pancreatitis), the former much more common than the latter. Therapy with any combination of enalapril and hydrochlorothiazide will be associated with both sets of dose-independent side effects but the addition of enalapril in clinicial trials blunted the hypokalemia normally seen with diuretics. To minimize dose-independent side effects, it is usually appropriate to begin combination therapy only after a patient has failed to achieve the desired effect with monotherapy.
Dose Titration Guided by Clinical Effect: A patient whose blood pressure is not adequately controlled with either enalapril or hydrochlorothiazide monotherapy may be given VASERETIC 5-12.5 or VASERETIC 10-25. Further increases of enalapril, hydrochlorothiazide or both depend on clinical response. The hydrochlorothiazide dose should generally not be increased until 2–3 weeks have elapsed. In general, patients do not require doses in excess of 20 mg of enalapril or 50 mg of hydrochlorothiazide. The daily dosage should not exceed four tablets of VASERETIC 5-12.5 or two tablets of VASERETIC 10-25.
Replacement Therapy: The combination may be substituted for the titrated components.
Use in Renal Impairment: The usual regimens of therapy with VASERETIC need not be adjusted as long as the patient's creatinine clearance is > 30 mL/min/1.73 m^2 (serum creatinine approximately ≤ 3 mg/dL or 265 μmol/L). In patients with more severe renal impairment, loop diuretics are preferred to thiazides, so enalapril maleate-hydrochlorothiazide is not recommended (see WARNINGS, *Anaphylactoid reactions during membrane exposure*).
Use in Elderly: Clinical studies in VASERETIC did not include sufficient numbers of patients aged 65 and over to determine whether they respond differently from younger patients. In general, dose selection for an elderly patient should be cautious, usually starting at the low end of the dosing range.

HOW SUPPLIED

No. 3644—Tablets VASERETIC 5-12.5 are green, squared capsule-shaped compressed tablets, coded MSD on one side and 173 on the other. Each tablet contains 5 mg of enalapril maleate and 12.5 mg of hydrochlorothiazide. They are supplied as follows:
NDC 0006-0173-68 bottles of 100 (with desiccant).
Shown in Product Identification Guide, page 325
No. 3418—Tablets VASERETIC 10-25, are rust, squared capsule-shaped, compressed tablets, coded MSD 720 on one side and VASERETIC on the other. Each tablet contains 10 mg of enalapril maleate and 25 mg of hydrochlorothiazide. They are supplied as follows:
NDC 0006-0720-68 bottles of 100 (with desiccant).
Shown in Product Identification Guide, page 325
Storage
Store below 30°C (86°F) and avoid transient temperatures above 50°C (122°F). Keep container tightly closed. Protect from moisture.
Dispense in a tight container, if product package is subdivided.

7843629 Issued July 1995

VASOTEC® I.V. Injection ℞
(Enalaprilat)

> **USE IN PREGNANCY**
> **When used in pregnancy during the second and third trimesters, ACE inhibitors can cause injury and even death to the developing fetus.** When pregnancy is detected, VASOTEC I.V. should be discontinued as soon as possible. See WARNINGS. *Fetal/Neonatal Morbidity and Mortality.*

DESCRIPTION

VASOTEC* I.V. (Enalaprilat) is a sterile aqueous solution for intravenous administration. Enalaprilat is an angiotensin converting enzyme inhibitor. It is chemically described as (*S*)-1-[*N*-(1-carboxy-3-phenylpropyl)-L-alanyl]-L-proline dihydrate. Its empirical formula is $C_{18}H_{24}N_2O_5 \cdot 2H_2O$ and its structural formula is:

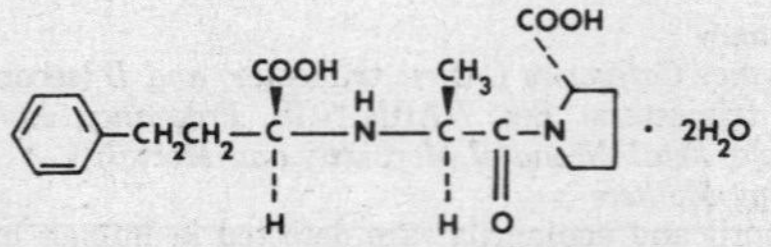

Enalaprilat is a white to off-white, crystalline powder with a molecular weight of 384.43. It is sparingly soluble in methanol and slightly soluble in water.
Each milliliter of VASOTEC I.V. contains 1.25 mg enalaprilat (anhydrous equivalent); sodium chloride to adjust tonicity; sodium hydroxide to adjust pH; water for injection, q.s.; with benzyl alcohol, 9 mg, added as a preservative.

*Registered trademark of MERCK & CO., INC.

CLINICAL PHARMACOLOGY

Enalaprilat, an angiotensin-converting enzyme (ACE) inhibitor when administered intravenously, is the active metabolite of the orally administered pro-drug, enalapril maleate. Enalaprilat is poorly absorbed orally.
Mechanism of Action
Intravenous enalaprilat, or oral enalapril, after hydrolysis to enalaprilat, inhibits ACE in human subjects and animals. ACE is a peptidyl dipeptidase that catalyzes the conversion of angiotensin I to the vasoconstrictor substance, angiotensin II. Angiotensin II also stimulates aldosterone secretion by the adrenal cortex. Inhibition of ACE results in decreased plasma angiotensin II, which leads to decreased vasopressor activity and to decreased aldosterone secretion. Although the latter decrease is small, it results in small increases of serum potassium. In hypertensive patients treated with enalapril alone for up to 48 weeks, mean increases in serum potassium of approximately 0.2 mEq/L were observed. In patients treated with enalapril plus a thiazide diuretic, there was essentially no change in serum potassium. (See PRECAUTIONS.) Removal of angiotensin II negative feedback on renin secretion leads to increased plasma renin activity. ACE is identical to kininase, an enzyme that degrades bradykinin. Whether increased levels of bradykinin, a potent vasodepressor peptide, play a role in the therapeutic effects of enalaprilat remains to be elucidated.
While the mechanism through which enalaprilat lowers blood pressure is believed to be primarily suppression of the renin-angiotensin-aldosterone system, enalaprilat has antihypertensive activity even in patients with low-renin hypertension. In clinical studies, black hypertensive patients (usually a low-renin hypertensive population) had a smaller average response to enalaprilat monotherapy than non-black patients.
Pharmacokinetics and Metabolism
Following intravenous administration of a single dose, the serum concentration profile of enalaprilat is polyexponential with a prolonged terminal phase, apparently representing a small fraction of the administered dose that has been bound to ACE. The amount bound does not increase with dose, indicating a saturable site of binding. The effective half-life for accumulation of enalaprilat, as determined from oral administration of multiple doses of enalapril maleate, is approximately 11 hours. Excretion of enalaprilat is primarily renal with more than 90 percent of an administered dose recovered in the urine as unchanged drug within 24 hours. Enalaprilat is poorly absorbed following oral administration. The disposition of enalaprilat in patients with renal insufficiency is similar to that in patients with normal renal function until the glomerular filtration rate is 30 mL/min or less. With glomerular filtration rate ≤ 30 mL/min, peak and trough enalaprilat levels increase, time to peak concentration increases and time to steady state may be delayed. The effective half-life of enalaprilat is prolonged at this level of renal insufficiency. (See DOSAGE AND ADMINISTRATION.) Enalaprilat is dialyzable at the rate of 62 mL/min. Studies in dogs indicate that enalaprilat does not enter the brain, and that enalapril crosses the blood-brain barrier poorly, if at all. Multiple doses of enalapril maleate in rats do not result in accumulation in any tissues. Milk in lactating rats contains radioactivity following administration of ^{14}C enalapril maleate. Radioactivity was found to cross the placenta following administration of labeled drug to pregnant hamsters.
Pharmacodynamics
VASOTEC I.V. results in the reduction of both supine and standing systolic and diastolic blood pressure, usually with no orthostatic component. Symptomatic postural hypotension is therefore infrequent, although it might be anticipated in volume-depleted patients (see WARNINGS). The onset of action usually occurs within fifteen minutes of administration with the maximum effect occurring within one to four hours. The abrupt withdrawal of enalaprilat has not been associated with a rapid increase in blood pressure.
The duration of hemodynamic effects appears to be dose-related. However, for the recommended dose, the duration of action in most patients is approximately six hours.
Following administration of enalapril, there is an increase in renal blood flow; glomerular filtration rate is usually unchanged. The effects appear to be similar in patients with renovascular hypertension.

INDICATIONS AND USAGE

VASOTEC I.V. is indicated for the treatment of hypertension when oral therapy is not practical.
VASOTEC I.V. has been studied with only one other antihypertensive agent, furosemide, which showed approximately additive effects on blood pressure. Enalapril, the pro-drug of enalaprilat, has been used extensively with a variety of other antihypertensive agents, without apparent difficulty except for occasional hypotension.
In using VASOTEC I.V., consideration should be given to the fact that another angiotensin converting enzyme inhibitor, captopril, has caused agranulocytosis, particularly in patients with renal impairment or collagen vascular disease, and that available data are insufficient to show that VASOTEC I.V. does not have a similar risk. (See WARNINGS.)
In considering use of VASOTEC I.V., it should be noted that in controlled clinical trials ACE inhibitors have an effect on blood pressure that is less in black patients than in non-blacks. In addition, it should be noted that black patients receiving ACE inhibitor monotherapy have been reported to have a higher incidence of angioedema compared to non-blacks. (See WARNINGS, *Angioedema.*)

CONTRAINDICATIONS

VASOTEC I.V. is contraindicated in patients who are hypersensitive to any component of this product and in patients with a history of angioedema related to previous treatment with an angiotensin converting enzyme inhibitor.

WARNINGS

Hypotension
Excessive hypotension is rare in uncomplicated hypertensive patients but is a possible consequence of the use of enalaprilat especially in severely salt/volume depleted persons such as those treated vigorously with diuretics or patients on dialysis. Patients at risk for excessive hypotension, sometimes associated with oliguria and/or progressive azotemia, and rarely with acute renal failure and/or death, include those with the following conditions or characteristics: heart failure, hyponatremia, high dose diuretic therapy, recent intensive diuresis or increase in diuretic dose, renal dialysis, or severe volume and/or salt depletion of any etiology. It may be advisable to eliminate the diuretic, reduce the diuretic dose or increase salt intake cautiously before initiating therapy with VASOTEC I.V. in patients at risk for excessive hypotension who are able to tolerate such adjustment. (See PRECAUTIONS, *Drug Interactions,* ADVERSE REACTIONS, and DOSAGE AND ADMINISTRATION.) In patients with heart failure, with or without associated renal insufficiency, excessive hypotension has been observed and may be associated with oliguria and/or progressive azotemia, and rarely with acute renal failure and/or death. Because of the potential for an excessive fall in blood pressure especially in these patients, therapy should be followed closely whenever the dose of enalaprilat is adjusted and/or diuretic is increased. Similar consideration may apply to

patients with ischemic heart or cerebrovascular disease, in whom an excessive fall in blood pressure could result in a myocardial infarction or cerebrovascular accident.

If hypotension occurs, the patient should be placed in the supine position and, if necessary, receive an intravenous infusion of normal saline. A transient hypotensive response is not a contraindication to further doses, which usually can be given without difficulty once the blood pressure has increased after volume expansion.

Anaphylactoid and Possibly Related Reactions

Presumably because angiotensin-converting enzyme inhibitors affect the metabolism of eicosanoids and polypeptides, including endogenous bradykinin, patients receiving ACE inhibitors (including VASOTEC I.V.) may be subject to a variety of adverse reactions, some of them serious.

Angioedema: Angioedema of the face, extremities, lips, tongue, glottis and/or larynx has been reported in patients treated with angiotensin converting enzyme inhibitors, including enalaprilat. This may occur at any time during treatment. In such cases VASOTEC I.V. should be promptly discontinued and appropriate therapy and monitoring should be provided until complete and sustained resolution of signs and symptoms has occurred. In instances where swelling has been confined to the face and lips the condition has generally resolved without treatment, although antihistamines have been useful in relieving symptoms. Angioedema associated with laryngeal edema may be fatal. **Where there is involvement of the tongue, glottis or larynx, likely to cause airway obstruction, appropriate therapy, e.g., subcutaneous epinephrine solution 1:1000 (0.3 mL to 0.5 mL) and/or measures necessary to ensure a patent airway, should be promptly provided.** (See ADVERSE REACTIONS.)

Patients with a history of angioedema unrelated to ACE inhibitor therapy may be at increased risk of angioedema while receiving an ACE inhibitor (see also INDICATIONS AND USAGE and CONTRAINDICATIONS).

Anaphylactoid reactions during desensitization: Two patients undergoing desensitizing treatment with hymenoptera venom while receiving ACE inhibitors sustained life-threatening anaphylactoid reactions. In the same patients, these reactions were avoided when ACE inhibitors were temporarily withheld, but they reappeared upon inadvertent rechallenge.

Anaphylactoid reactions during membrane exposure: Anaphylactoid reactions have been reported in patients dialyzed with high-flux membranes and treated concomitantly with an ACE inhibitor. Anaphylactoid reactions have also been reported in patients undergoing low-density lipoprotein apheresis with dextran sulfate absorption (a procedure dependent upon devices not approved in the United States).

Neutropenia/Agranulocytosis

Another angiotensin converting enzyme inhibitor, captopril, has been shown to cause agranulocytosis and bone marrow depression, rarely in uncomplicated patients but more frequently in patients with renal impairment especially if they also have a collagen vascular disease. Available data from clinical trials of enalapril are insufficient to show that enalapril does not cause agranulocytosis in similar rates. Marketing experience has revealed several cases of neutropenia, or agranulocytosis in which a causal relationship to enalapril cannot be excluded. Periodic monitoring of white blood cell counts in patients with collagen vascular disease and renal disease should be considered.

Hepatic Failure

Rarely, ACE inhibitors have been associated with a syndrome that starts with cholestatic jaundice and progresses to fulminant hepatic necrosis, and (sometimes) death. The mechanism of this syndrome is not understood. Patients receiving ACE inhibitors who develop jaundice or marked elevations of hepatic enzymes should discontinue the ACE inhibitor and receive appropriate medical follow-up.

Fetal/Neonatal Morbidity and Mortality

ACE inhibitors can cause fetal and neonatal morbidity and death when administered to pregnant women. Several dozen cases have been reported in the world literature. When pregnancy is detected, ACE inhibitors should be discontinued as soon as possible.

The use of ACE inhibitors during the second and third trimesters of pregnancy has been associated with fetal and neonatal injury, including hypotension, neonatal skull hypoplasia, anuria, reversible or irreversible renal failure, and death. Oligohydramnios has also bee reported, presumably resulting from decreased fetal renal function: oligohydramnois in this setting has been associated with fetal limb contractures, craniofacial deformation, and hypoplastic lung development. Prematurity, intrauterine growth retardation, and patent ductus arteriosus have also been reported, although it is not clear whether these occurrences were due to the ACE-inhibitor exposure.

These adverse effects do not appear to have resulted from intrauterine ACE-inhibitor exposure that has been limited to the first trimester. Mothers whose embryos and fetuses are exposed to ACE inhibitors only during the first trimester should be so informed. Nonetheless, when patients become pregnant, physicians should make every effort to discontinue the use of VASOTEC I.V. as soon as possible.

Rarely (probably less often than once in every thousand pregnancies), no alternative to ACE inhibitors will be found. In these rare cases, the mothers should be apprised of the potential hazards to their fetuses, and serial ultrasound examinations should be performed to assess the intraamniotic environment.

If oligohydramnois is observed, VASOTEC I.V. should be discontinued unless it is considered lifesaving for the mother. Contraction stress testing (CST, a non-stress test (NST), or biophysical profiling (BPP) may be appropriate, depending upon the week of pregnancy. Patients and physicians should be aware, however, that oligohydramnois may not appear until after the fetus has sustained irreversible injury.

Infants with histories of *in utero* exposure to ACE inhibitors should be closely observed for hypotension, oliguria, and hyperkalemia. If oliguria occurs, attention should be directed toward support of blood pressure and renal perfusion. Exchange transfusion or dialysis may be required as means of reversing hypotension and/or substituting for disordered renal function. Enalapril, which crosses the placenta, has been removed from neonatal circulation by peritoneal dialysis with some clinical benefit, and theoretically may be removed by exchange transfusion, although there is no experience with the latter procedure.

No teratogenic effects of oral enalapril were seen in studies of pregnant rats and rabbits. On a mg/kg basis, the doses used were up to 333 times (in rats) and 50 times (in rabbits) the maximum recommended human dose.

PRECAUTIONS

General

Impaired Renal Function: As a consequence of inhibiting the renin-angiotensin-aldosterone system, changes in renal function may be anticipated in susceptible individuals. In patients with severe heart failure whose renal function may depend on the activity of the renin-angiotensin-aldosterone system, treatment with angiotensin converting enzyme inhibitors, including enalapril or enalaprilat, may be associated with oliguria and/or progressive azotemia and rarely with acute renal failure and/or death.

In clinical studies in hypertensive patients with unilateral or bilateral renal artery stenosis, increases in blood urea nitrogen and serum creatinine were observed in 20 percent of patients receiving enalapril. These increases were almost always reversible upon discontinuation of enalapril or enalaprilat and/or diuretic therapy. In such patients renal function should be monitored during the first few weeks of therapy.

Some hypertensive patients with no apparent pre-existing renal vascular disease have developed increases in blood urea and serum creatinine, usually minor and transient, especially when enalaprilat has been given concomitantly with a diuretic. This is more likely to occur in patients with pre-existing renal impairment. Dosage reduction of enalaprilat and/or discontinuation of the diuretic may be required.

Evaluation of the hypertensive patient should always include assessment of renal function. (See DOSAGE AND ADMINISTRATION.)

Hyperkalemia: Elevated serum potassium (greater than 5.7 mEq/L) was observed in approximately one percent of hypertensive patients in clinical trials receiving enalapril. In most cases these were isolated values which resolved despite continued therapy. Hyperkalemia was a cause of discontinuation of therapy in 0.28 percent of hypertensive patients. Risk factors for the development of hyperkalemia include renal insufficiency, diabetes mellitus, and the concomitant use of potassium-sparing agents or potassium supplements, which should be used cautiously, if at all, with VASOTEC I.V. (See *Drug Interactions.*)

Cough: Presumably due to the inhibition of the degradation of endogenous bradykinin, persistent nonproductive cough has been reported with all ACE inhibitors, always resolving after discontinuation of therapy. ACE inhibitor-induced cough should be considered in the differential diagnosis of cough.

Surgery/Anesthesia: In patients undergoing major surgery or during anesthesia with agents that produce hypotension, enalapril may block angiotensin II formation secondary to compensatory renin release. If hypotension occurs and is considered to be due to this mechanism, it can be corrected by volume expansion.

Drug Interactions

Hypotension—Patients on Diuretic Therapy: Patients on diuretics and especially those in whom diuretic therapy was recently instituted, may occasionally experience an excessive reduction of blood pressure after initiation of therapy with enalaprilat. The possibility of hypotensive effects with enalaprilat can be minimized by administration of an intravenous infusion of normal saline, discontinuing the diuretic or increasing the salt intake prior to initiation of treatment with enalaprilat. If it is necessary to continue the diuretic, provide close medical supervision for at least one hour after the initial dose of enalaprilat. (See WARNINGS.)

Agents Causing Renin Release: The antihypertensive effect of VASOTEC I.V. appears to be augmented by antihypertensive agents that cause renin release (e.g., diuretics.)

Other Cardiovascular Agents: VASOTEC I.V. has been used concomitantly with digitalis, beta adrenergic-blocking agents, methyldopa, nitrates, calcium-blocking agents, hydralazine and prazosin without evidence of clinically significant adverse interactions.

Agents Increasing Serum Potassium: VASOTEC I.V. attenuates potassium loss caused by thiazide-type diuretics. Potassium-sparing diuretics (e.g., spironolactone, triamterene, or amiloride), potassium supplements, or potassium-containing salt substitutes may lead to significant increases in serum potassium. Therefore, if concomitant use of these agents is indicated because of demonstrated hypokalemia, they should be used with caution and with frequent monitoring of serum potassium.

Lithium: Lithium toxicity has been reported in patients receiving lithium concomitantly with drugs which cause elimination of sodium, including ACE inhibitors. A few cases of lithium toxicity have been reported in patients receiving concomitant enalapril and lithium and were reversible upon discontinuation of both drugs. It is recommended that serum lithium levels be monitored frequently if enalapril is administered concomitantly with lithium.

Carcinogenesis, Mutagenesis, Impairment of Fertility

Carcinogenicity studies have not been done with VASOTEC I.V.

VASOTEC I.V. is the bioactive form of its ethyl ester, enalapril maleate. There was no evidence of a tumorigenic effect when enalapril was administered orally for 106 weeks to rats at doses up to 90 mg/kg/day (150 times* the maximum daily human dose). Enalapril has also been administered for 94 weeks to male and female mice at oral doses up to 90 and 180 mg/kg/day, respectively (150 and 300 times* the maximum oral daily dose for humans), and showed no evidence of carcinogenicity.

VASOTEC I.V. was not mutagenic in the Ames microbial mutagen test with or without metabolic activation. Enalapril showed no drug-related changes in the following genotoxicity studies: rec-assay, reverse mutation assay with *E. coli*, sister chromatid exchange with cultured mammalian cells, the micronucleus test with mice, and in an *in vivo* cytogenic study using mouse bone marrow. There were no adverse effects on reproductive performance in male and female rats treated with 10 to 90 mg enalapril/kg/day.

*Based on patient weight of 50 kg

Pregnancy

Pregnancy Categories C (first trimester) and *D* (second and third trimesters). See WARNINGS, *Fetal/Neonatal Morbidity and Mortality.*

Nursing Mothers

Enalapril and enalaprilat are detected in human milk in trace amounts. Caution should be exercised when VASOTEC I.V. is given to a nursing mother.

Pediatric Use

Safety and effectiveness in children have not been established.

ADVERSE REACTIONS

VASOTEC I.V. has been found to be generally well tolerated in controlled clinical trials involving 349 patients (168 with hypertension, 153 with congestive heart failure and 28 with coronary artery disease). The most frequent clinically significant adverse experience was hypotension (3.4 percent), occurring in eight patients (5.2 percent) with congestive heart failure, three (1.8 percent) with hypertension and one with coronary artery disease. Other adverse experiences occurring in greater than one percent of patients were: headache (2.9 percent) and nausea (1.1 percent).

Adverse experiences occurring in 0.5 to 1.0 percent of patients in controlled clinical trials included: myocardial infarction, fatigue, dizziness, fever, rash and constipation.

Angioedema: Angioedema has been reported in patients receiving enalaprilat, with an incidence higher in black than in non-black patients. Angioedema associated with laryngeal edema may be fatal. If angioedema of the face, extremities, lips, tongue, glottis and/or larynx occurs, treatment with enalaprilat should be discontinued and appropriate therapy instituted immediately. (See WARNINGS.)

Continued on next page

Information on the Merck & Co., Inc. products listed on these pages is the full prescribing information from product circulars in use September 30, 1996.

Merck & Co.—Cont.

Cough: See PRECAUTIONS, *Cough.*
Enalapril Maleate
Since enalapril is converted to enalaprilat, those adverse experiences associated with enalapril might also be expected to occur with VASOTEC I.V.
The following adverse experiences have been reported with enalapril and, within each category, are listed in order of decreasing severity.
Body As A Whole: Syncope, orthostatic effects, anaphylactoid reactions (see WARNINGS, *Anaphylactoid reactions during membrane exposure*), chest pain, abdominal pain, asthenia.
Cardiovascular: Cardiac arrest; myocardial infarction or cerebrovascular accident, possibly secondary to excessive hypotension in high risk patients (see WARNINGS, *Hypotension*); pulmonary embolism and infarction; pulmonary edema; rhythm disturbances including atrial tachycardia and bradycardia; atrial fibrillation; orthostatic hypotension; angina pectoris; palpitation.
Digestive: Ileus, pancreatitis, hepatic failure, hepatitis (hepatocellular [proven on rechallenge] or cholestatic jaundice) (see WARNINGS, *Hepatic Failure*), melena, diarrhea, vomiting, dyspepsia, anorexia, glossitis, stomatitis, dry mouth.
Hematologic: Rare cases of neutropenia, thrombocytopenia and bone marrow depression.
Musculoskeletal: Muscle cramps.
Nervous/Psychiatric: Depression, vertigo, confusion, ataxia, somnolence, insomnia, nervousness, peripheral neuropathy (e.g. paresthesia, dysesthesia).
Respiratory: Bronchospasm, dyspnea, pneumonia, bronchitis, cough, rhinorrhea, sore throat and hoarseness, asthma, upper respiratory infection, pulmonary infiltrates.
Skin: Exfoliative dermatitis, toxic epidermal necrolysis, Stevens-Johnson syndrome, pemphigus, herpes zoster, erythema multiforme, urticaria, pruritus, alopecia, flushing, diaphoresis, photosensitivity.
Special Senses: Blurred vision, taste alteration, anosmia, tinnitus, conjunctivitis, dry eyes, tearing.
Urogenital: Renal failure, oliguria, renal dysfunction (see PRECAUTIONS and DOSAGE AND ADMINISTRATION), urinary tract infection, flank pain, gynecomastia, impotence.
Miscellaneous: A symptom complex has been reported which may include a positive ANA, an elevated erythrocyte sedimentation rate, arthralgia/arthritis, myalgia/myositis, fever, serositis, vasculitis, leukocytosis, eosinophilia, photosensitivity, rash and other dermatologic manifestations.
Hypotension: Combining the results of clinical trials in patients with hypertension or congestive heart failure, hypotension (including postural hypotension, and other orthostatic effects) was reported in 2.3 percent of patients following the initial dose of enalapril or during extended therapy. In the hypertensive patients, hypotension occurred in 0.9 percent and syncope occurred in 0.5 percent of patients. Hypotension or syncope was a cause for discontinuation of therapy in 0.1 percent of hypertensive patients. (See WARNINGS.)
Fetal/Neonatal Morbidity and Mortality: See WARNINGS, *Fetal/Neonatal Morbidity and Mortality.*
Clinical Laboratory Test Findings
Serum Electrolytes: Hyperkalemia (see PRECAUTIONS), hyponatremia.
Creatinine, Blood Urea Nitrogen: In controlled clinical trials minor increases in blood urea nitrogen and serum creatinine, reversible upon discontinuation of therapy, were observed in about 0.2 percent of patients with essential hypertension treated with enalapril alone. Increases are more likely to occur in patients receiving concomitant diuretics or in patients with renal artery stenosis. (See PRECAUTIONS.)
Hematology: Small decreases in hemoglobin and hematocrit (mean decreases of approximately 0.3 g percent and 1.0 vol percent, respectively) occur frequently in hypertensive patients treated with enalapril but are rarely of clinical importance unless another cause of anemia coexists. In clinical trials, less than 0.1 percent of patients discontinued therapy due to anemia. Hemolytic anemia, including cases of hemolysis in patients with G-6-PD deficiency, has been reported; a causal relationship to enalapril cannot be excluded.
Liver Function Tests: Elevations of liver enzymes and/or serum bilirubin have occurred (see WARNINGS, *Hepatic Failure*).

OVERDOSAGE

In clinical studies, some hypertensive patients received a maximum dose of 80 mg of enalaprilat intravenously over a fifteen minute period. At this high dose, no adverse effects beyond those as associated with the recommended dosages were observed.
The intravenous LD_{50} of enalaprilat is 3740–5890 mg/kg in female mice.
The most likely manifestation of overdosage would be hypotension, for which the usual treatment would be intravenous infusion of normal saline solution.
Enalaprilat may be removed from general circulation by hemodialysis and has been removed from neonatal circulation by peritoneal dialysis.

DOSAGE AND ADMINISTRATION

FOR INTRAVENOUS ADMINISTRATION ONLY
The dose in hypertension is 1.25 mg every six hours administered intravenously over a five minute period. A clinical response is usually seen within 15 minutes. Peak effects after the first dose may not occur for up to four hours after dosing. The peak effects of the second and subsequent doses may exceed those of the first.
No dosage regimen for VASOTEC I.V. has been clearly demonstrated to be more effective in treating hypertension than 1.25 mg every six hours. However, in controlled clinical studies in hypertension, doses as high as 5 mg every six hours were well tolerated for up to 36 hours. There has been inadequate experience with doses greater than 20 mg per day.
In studies of patients with hypertension, VASOTEC I.V. has not been administered for periods longer than 48 hours. In other studies, patients have received VASOTEC I.V. for as long as seven days.
The dose for patients being converted to VASOTEC I.V. from oral therapy for hypertension with enalapril maleate is 1.25 mg every six hours. For conversion from intravenous to oral therapy, the recommended initial dose of Tablets VASOTEC (Enalapril Maleate) is 5 mg once a day with subsequent dosage adjustments as necessary.
Patients on Diuretic Therapy
For patients on diuretic therapy the recommended starting dose for hypertension is 0.625 mg administered intravenously over a five minute period. A clinical response is usually seen within 15 minutes. Peak effects after the first dose may not occur for up to four hours after dosing, although most of the effect is usually apparent within the first hour. If after one hour there is an inadequate clinical response, the 0.625 mg dose may be repeated. Additional doses of 1.25 mg may be administered at six hour intervals.
For conversion from intravenous to oral therapy, the recommended initial dose of Tablets VASOTEC (Enalapril Maleate) for patients who have responded to 0.625 mg of enalaprilat every six hours is 2.5 mg once a day with subsequent dosage adjustment as necessary.
Dosage Adjustment in Renal Impairment
The usual dose of 1.25 mg of enalaprilat every six hours is recommended for patients with a creatinine clearance >30 mL/min (serum creatinine of up to approximately 3 mg/dL). For patients with creatinine clearance ≤30 mL/min (serum creatinine ≥3 mg/dL), the initial dose is 0.625 mg. (See WARNINGS.)
If after one hour there is an inadequate clinical response, the 0.625 mg dose may be repeated. Additional doses of 1.25 mg may be administered at six hour intervals.
For dialysis patients, see below, *Patients at Risk of Excessive Hypotension.*
For conversion from intravenous to oral therapy, the recommended initial dose of Tablets VASOTEC (Enalapril Maleate) is 5 mg once a day for patients with creatinine clearance >30 mL/min and 2.5 mg once daily for patients with creatinine clearance ≤30 mL/min. Dosage should then be adjusted according to blood pressure response.
Patients at Risk of Excessive Hypotension
Hypertensive patients at risk of excessive hypotension include those with the following concurrent conditions or characteristics: heart failure, hyponatremia, high dose diuretic therapy, recent intensive diuresis or increase in diuretic dose, renal dialysis, or severe volume and/or salt depletion of any etiology (see WARNINGS). Single doses of enalaprilat as low as 0.2 mg have produced excessive hypotension in normotensive patients with these diagnoses. Because of the potential for an extreme hypotensive response in these patients, therapy should be started under very close medical supervision. The starting dose should be no greater than 0.625 mg administered intravenously over a period of no less than five minutes and preferably longer (up to one hour).
Patients should be followed closely whenever the dose of enalaprilat is adjusted and/or diuretic is increased.
Administration
VASOTEC I.V. should be administered as a slow intravenous infusion, as indicated above, over at least five minutes. It may be administered as provided or diluted with up to 50 mL of a compatible diluent.
Parenteral drug products should be inspected visually for particulate matter and discoloration prior to use whenever solution and container permit.
Compatibility and Stability
VASOTEC I.V. as supplied and mixed with the following intravenous diluents has been found to maintain full activity for 24 hours at room temperature:
5 percent Dextrose Injection
0.9 percent Sodium Chloride Injection
0.9 percent Sodium Chloride Injection in 5 percent Dextrose
5 percent Dextrose in Lactated Ringer's Injection
McGaw ISOLYTE* E.

* Registered trademark of American Hospital Supply Corporation.

HOW SUPPLIED

No. 3508—VASOTEC I.V., 1.25 mg per mL, is a clear, colorless solution and is supplied in vials containing 1 mL and 2 mL.
NDC 0006-3508-01, 1 mL vials
(6505-01-356-8505, 1 mL vial)
NDC 0006-3508-04, 2 mL vials
(6505-01-305-6988, 2 mL vial).
Storage
Store below 30°C (86°F).
7875725 Issued July 1995
COPYRIGHT © MERCK & CO., INC., 1989, 1991, 1992
All rights reserved

VASOTEC® Tablets ℞
(Enalapril Maleate), U.S.P.

USE IN PREGNANCY
When used in pregnancy during the second and third trimesters, ACE inhibitors can cause injury and even death to the developing fetus. When pregnancy is detected, VASOTEC should be discontinued as soon as possible. See WARNINGS. *Fetal/Neonatal Morbidity and Mortality.*

DESCRIPTION

VASOTEC* (Enalapril Maleate) is the maleate salt of enalapril, the ethyl ester of a long-acting angiotensin converting enzyme inhibitor, enalaprilat. Enalapril maleate is chemically described as (*S*)-1-[*N*-[1-(ethoxycarbonyl)-3-phenylpropyl]-L-alanyl]-L-proline, (*Z*)-2-butenedioate salt (1:1). Its empirical formula is $C_{20}H_{28}N_2O_5 \cdot C_4H_4O_4$, and its structural formula is:

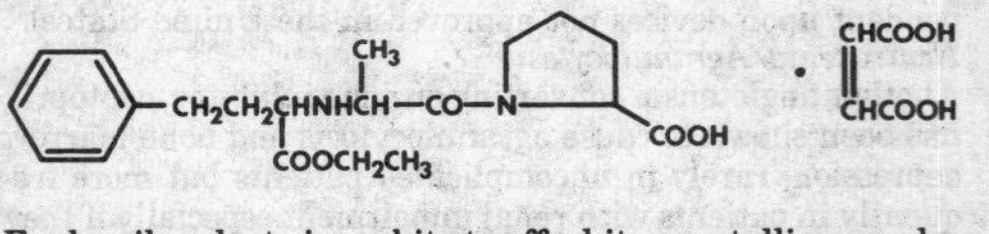

Enalapril maleate is a white to off-white, crystalline powder with a molecular weight of 492.53. It is sparingly soluble in water, soluble in ethanol, and freely soluble in methanol.
Enalapril is a pro-drug; following oral administration, it is bioactivated by hydrolysis of the ethyl ester to enalaprilat, which is the active angiotensin converting enzyme inhibitor.
Enalapril maleate is supplied as 2.5 mg, 5 mg, 10 mg, and 20 mg tablets for oral administration. In addition to the active ingredient enalapril maleate, each tablet contains the following inactive ingredients: lactose, magnesium stearate, starch, and other ingredients. The 2.5 mg, 10 mg and 20 mg tablets also contain iron oxides.

* Registered trademark of MERCK & CO., INC.

CLINICAL PHARMACOLOGY

Mechanism of Action
Enalapril, after hydrolysis to enalaprilat, inhibits angiotensin-converting enzyme (ACE) in human subjects and animals. ACE is a peptidyl dipeptidase that catalyzes the conversion of angiotensin I to the vasoconstrictor substance, angiotensin II. Angiotensin II also stimulates aldosterone secretion by the adrenal cortex. The beneficial effects of enalapril in hypertension and heart failure appear to result primarily from suppression of the renin-angiotensin-aldosterone system. Inhibition of ACE results in decreased plasma angiotensin II, which leads to decreased vasopressor activity and to decreased aldosterone secretion. Although the latter decrease is small, it results in small increases of serum potassium. In hypertensive patients treated with VASOTEC alone for up to 48 weeks, mean increases in serum potassium of approximately 0.2 mEq/L were observed. In patients treated with VASOTEC plus a thiazide diuretic, there was essentially no change in serum potassium. (See PRECAUTIONS.)
Removal of angiotensin II negative feedback on renin secretion leads to increased plasma renin activity.
ACE is identical to kininase, an enzyme that degrades bradykinin. Whether increased levels of bradykinin, a potent vasodepressor peptide, play a role in the therapeutic effects of VASOTEC remains to be elucidated.

While the mechanism through which VASOTEC lowers blood pressure is believed to be primarily suppression of the renin-angiotensin-aldosterone system, VASOTEC is antihypertensive even in patients with low-renin hypertension. Although VASOTEC was antihypertensive in all races studied, black hypertensive patients (usually a low-renin hypertensive population) had a smaller average response to enalapril monotherapy than non-black patients.

Pharmacokinetics and Metabolism

Following oral administration of VASOTEC, peak serum concentrations of enalapril occur within about one hour. Based on urinary recovery, the extent of absorption of enalapril is approximately 60 percent. Enalapril absorption is not influenced by the presence of food in the gastrointestinal tract. Following absorption, enalapril is hydrolyzed to enalaprilat, which is a more potent angiotensin converting enzyme inhibitor than enalapril; enalaprilat is poorly absorbed when administered orally. Peak serum concentrations of enalaprilat occur three to four hours after an oral dose of enalapril maleate. Excretion of VASOTEC is primarily renal. Approximately 94 percent of the dose is recovered in the urine and feces as enalaprilat or enalapril. The principal components in urine are enalaprilat, accounting for about 40 percent of the dose, and intact enalapril. There is no evidence of metabolites of enalapril, other than enalaprilat. The serum concentration profile of enalaprilat exhibits a prolonged terminal phase, apparently representing a small fraction of the administered dose that has been bound to ACE. The amount bound does not increase with dose, indicating a saturable site of binding. The effective half-life for accumulation of enalaprilat following multiple doses of enalapril maleate is 11 hours.

The disposition of enalapril and enalaprilat in patients with renal insufficiency is similar to that in patients with normal renal function until the glomerular filtration rate is 30 mL/min or less. With glomerular filtration rate ≤30 mL/min, peak and trough enalaprilat levels increase, time to peak concentration increases and time to steady state may be delayed. The effective half-life of enalaprilat following multiple doses of enalapril maleate is prolonged at this level of renal insufficiency. (See DOSAGE AND ADMINISTRATION.) Enalaprilat is dialyzable at the rate of 62 mL/min. Studies in dogs indicate that enalapril crosses the blood-brain barrier poorly, if at all; enalaprilat does not enter the brain. Multiple doses of enalapril maleate in rats do not result in accumulation in any tissues. Milk of lactating rats contains radioactivity following administration of ^{14}C enalapril maleate. Radioactivity was found to cross the placenta following administration of labeled drug to pregnant hamsters.

Pharmacodynamics and Clinical Effects

Hypertension: Administration of VASOTEC to patients with hypertension of severity ranging from mild to severe results in a reduction of both supine and standing blood pressure usually with no orthostatic component. Symptomatic postural hypotension is therefore infrequent, although it might be anticipated in volume-depleted patients. (See WARNINGS.)

In most patients studied, after oral administration of a single dose of enalapril, onset of antihypertensive activity was seen at one hour with peak reduction of blood pressure achieved by four to six hours.

At recommended doses, antihypertensive effects have been maintained for at least 24 hours. In some patients the effects may diminish toward the end of the dosing interval (see DOSAGE AND ADMINISTRATION).

In some patients achievement of optimal blood pressure reduction may require several weeks of therapy.

The antihypertensive effects of VASOTEC have continued during long term therapy. Abrupt withdrawal of VASOTEC has not been associated with a rapid increase in blood pressure.

In hemodynamic studies in patients with essential hypertension, blood pressure reduction was accompanied by a reduction in peripheral arterial resistance with an increase in cardiac output and little or no change in heart rate. Following administration of VASOTEC, there is an increase in renal blood flow; glomerular filtration rate is usually unchanged. The effects appear to be similar in patients with renovascular hypertension.

When given together with thiazide-type diuretics, the blood pressure lowering effects of VASOTEC are approximately additive.

In a clinical pharmacology study, indomethacin or sulindac was administered to hypertensive patients receiving VASOTEC. In this study there was no evidence of a blunting of the antihypertensive action of VASOTEC.

Heart Failure: In trials in patients treated with digitalis and diuretics, treatment with enalapril resulted in decreased systemic vascular resistance, blood pressure, pulmonary capillary wedge pressure and heart size, and increased cardiac output and exercise tolerance. Heart rate was unchanged or slightly reduced, and mean ejection fraction was unchanged or increased. There was a beneficial effect on severity of heart failure as measured by the New York Heart Association (NYHA) classification and on symptoms of dys-

pnea and fatigue. Hemodynamic effects were observed after the first dose, and appeared to be maintained in uncontrolled studies lasting as long as four months. Effects on exercise tolerance, heart size, and severity and symptoms of heart failure were observed in placebo-controlled studies lasting from eight weeks to over one year.

Heart Failure, Mortality Trials: In a multicenter, placebo-controlled clinical trial, 2,569 patients with all degrees of symptomatic heart failure and ejection fraction ≤35 percent were randomized to placebo or enalapril and followed for up to 55 months (SOLVD-Treatment). Use of enalapril was associated with an 11 percent reduction in all-cause mortality and a 30 percent reduction in hospitalization for heart failure. Diseases that excluded patients from enrollment in the study included severe stable angina (>2 attacks/day), hemodynamically significant valvular or outflow tract obstruction, renal failure (creatinine >2.5 mg/dL), cerebral vascular disease (e.g., significant carotid artery disease), advanced pulmonary disease, malignancies, active myocarditis and constrictive pericarditis. The mortality benefit associated with enalapril does not appear to depend upon digitalis being present.

A second multicenter trial used the SOLVD protocol for study of asymptomatic or minimally symptomatic patients. SOLVD-Prevention patients, who had left ventricular ejection fraction ≤35% and no history of symptomatic heart failure, were randomized to placebo (n=2117) or enalapril (n=2111) and followed for up to 5 years. The majority of patients in the SOLVD-Prevention trial had a history of ischemic heart disease. A history of myocardial infarction was present in 80 percent of patients, current angina pectoris in 34 percent, and a history of hypertension in 37 percent. No statistically significant mortality effect was demonstrated in this population. Enalapril-treated subjects had 32% fewer first hospitalizations for heart failure, and 32% fewer total heart failure hospitalizations. Compared to placebo, 32 percent fewer patients receiving enalapril developed symptoms of overt heart failure. Hospitalizations for cardiovascular reasons were also reduced. There was an insignificant reduction in hospitalizations for any cause in the enalapril treatment group (for enalapril vs. placebo, respectively, 1166 vs. 1201 first hospitalizations, 2649 vs. 2840 total hospitalizations), although the study was not powered to look for such an effect.

The SOLVD-Prevention trial was not designed to determine whether treatment of asymptomatic patients with low ejection fraction would be superior, with respect to preventing hospitalization, to closer follow-up and use of enalapril at the earliest sign of heart failure. However, under the conditions of follow-up in the SOLVD-Prevention trial (every 4 months at the study clinic; personal physician as needed), 68% of patients on placebo who were hospitalized for heart failure had no prior symptoms recorded which would have signaled initiation of treatment.

The SOLVD-Prevention trial was also not designed to show whether enalapril modified the progression of underlying heart disease.

In another multicenter, placebo-controlled trial (CONSENSUS) limited to patients with NYHA class IV congestive heart failure and radiographic evidence of cardiomegaly, use of enalapril was associated with improved survival. The results are shown in the following table.

	SURVIVAL (%)	
	Six Months	One Year
VASOTEC (n=127)	74	64
Placebo (n=126)	56	48

In both CONSENSUS and SOLVD-Treatment trials, patients were also usually receiving digitalis, diuretics or both.

INDICATIONS AND USAGE

Hypertension

VASOTEC is indicated for the treatment of hypertension. VASOTEC is effective alone or in combination with other antihypertensive agents, especially thiazide-type diuretics. The blood pressure lowering effects of VASOTEC and thiazides are approximately additive.

Heart Failure

VASOTEC is indicated for the treatment of symptomatic congestive heart failure, usually in combination with diuretics and digitalis. In these patients VASOTEC improves symptoms, increases survival, and decreases the frequency of hospitalization (see CLINICAL PHARMACOLOGY, *Heart Failure, Mortality Trials* for details and limitations of survival trials).

Asymptomatic Left Ventricular Dysfunction

In clinically stable asymptomatic patients with left ventricular dysfunction (ejection fraction ≤35 percent), VASOTEC decreases the rate of development of overt heart failure and decreases the incidence of hospitalization for heart failure. (See CLINICAL PHARMACOLOGY, *Heart Failure, Mortality Trials* for details and limitations of survival trials.)

In using VASOTEC consideration should be given to the fact that another angiotensin converting enzyme inhibitor, captopril, has caused agranulocytosis, particularly in patients

with renal impairment or collagen vascular disease, and that available data are insufficient to show that VASOTEC does not have a similar risk. (See WARNINGS.)

In considering use of VASOTEC, it should be noted that in controlled clinical trials ACE inhibitors have an effect on blood pressure that is less in black patients than in non-blacks. In addition, it should be noted that black patients receiving ACE inhibitor monotherapy have been reported to have a higher incidence of angioedema compared to non-blacks. (See WARNINGS, *Angioedema.*)

CONTRAINDICATIONS

VASOTEC is contraindicated in patients who are hypersensitive to this product and in patients with a history of angioedema related to previous treatment with an angiotensin converting enzyme inhibitor.

WARNINGS

Anaphylactoid and Possibly Related Reactions

Presumably because angiotensin-converting enzyme inhibitors affect the metabolism of eicosanoids and polypeptides, including endogenous bradykinin, patients receiving ACE inhibitors (including VASOTEC) may be subject to a variety of adverse reactions, some of them serious.

Angioedema: Angioedema of the face, extremities, lips, tongue, glottis and/or larynx has been reported in patients treated with angiotensin converting enzyme inhibitors, including VASOTEC. This may occur at any time during treatment. In such cases VASOTEC should be promptly discontinued and appropriate therapy and monitoring should be provided until complete and sustained resolution of signs and symptoms has occurred. In instances where swelling has been confined to the face and lips the condition has generally resolved without treatment, although antihistamines have been useful in relieving symptoms. Angioedema associated with laryngeal edema may be fatal. **Where there is involvement of the tongue, glottis or larynx, likely to cause airway obstruction, appropriate therapy, e.g., subcutaneous epinephrine solution 1:1000 (0.3 mL to 0.5 mL) and/or measures necessary to ensure a patent airway, should be promptly provided.** (See ADVERSE REACTIONS.)

Patients with a history of angioedema unrelated to ACE inhibitor therapy may be at increased risk of angioedema while receiving an ACE inhibitor (see also INDICATIONS AND USAGE and CONTRAINDICATIONS).

Anaphylactoid reactions during desensitization: Two patients undergoing desensitizing treatment with hymenoptera venom while receiving ACE inhibitors sustained life-threatening anaphylactoid reactions. In the same patients, these reactions were avoided when ACE inhibitors were temporarily withheld, but they reappeared upon inadvertent rechallenge.

Anaphylactoid reactions during membrane exposure: Anaphylactoid reactions have been reported in patients dialyzed with high-flux membranes and treated concomitantly with an ACE inhibitor. Anaphylactoid reactions have also been reported in patients undergoing low-density lipoprotein apheresis with dextran sulfate absorption (a procedure dependent upon devices not approved in the United States).

Hypotension

Excessive hypotension is rare in uncomplicated hypertensive patients treated with VASOTEC alone. Patients with heart failure given VASOTEC commonly have some reduction in blood pressure, especially with the first dose, but discontinuation of therapy for continuing symptomatic hypotension usually is not necessary when dosing instructions are followed; caution should be observed when initiating therapy. (See DOSAGE AND ADMINISTRATION.) Patients at risk for excessive hypotension, sometimes associated with oliguria and/or progressive azotemia, and rarely with acute renal failure and/or death, include those with the following conditions or characteristics: heart failure, hyponatremia, high dose diuretic therapy, recent intensive diuresis or increase in diuretic dose, renal dialysis, or severe volume and/or salt depletion of any etiology. It may be advisable to eliminate the diuretic (except in patients with heart failure), reduce the diuretic dose or increase salt intake cautiously before initiating therapy with VASOTEC in patients at risk for excessive hypotension who are able to tolerate such adjustments. (See PRECAUTIONS, *Drug Interactions* and ADVERSE REACTIONS.) In patients at risk for excessive hypotension, therapy should be started under very close medical supervision and such patients should be followed closely for the first two weeks of treatment and whenever the dose of enalapril and/or diuretic is increased. Similar considerations may apply to patients with ischemic heart or cerebro-

Continued on next page

Information on the Merck & Co., Inc. products listed on these pages is the full prescribing information from product circulars in use September 30, 1996.

Merck & Co.—Cont.

vascular disease, in whom an excessive fall in blood pressure could result in a myocardial infarction or cerebrovascular accident.

If excessive hypotension occurs, the patient should be placed in the supine position and, if necessary, receive an intravenous infusion of normal saline. A transient hypotensive response is not a contraindication to further doses of VASOTEC, which usually can be given without difficulty once the blood pressure has stabilized. If symptomatic hypotension develops, a dose reduction or discontinuation of VASOTEC or concomitant diuretic may be necessary.

Neutropenia/Agranulocytosis

Another angiotensin converting enzyme inhibitor, captopril, has been shown to cause agranulocytosis and bone marrow depression, rarely in uncomplicated patients but more frequently in patients with renal impairment especially if they also have a collagen vascular disease. Available data from clinical trials of enalapril are insufficient to show that enalapril does not cause agranulocytosis at similar rates. Marketing experience has revealed several cases of neutropenia or agranulocytosis in which a causal relationship to enalapril cannot be excluded. Periodic monitoring of white blood cell counts in patients with collagen vascular disease and renal disease should be considered.

Hepatic Failure

Rarely, ACE inhibitors have been associated with a syndrome that starts with cholestatic jaundice and progresses to fulminant hepatic necrosis, and (sometimes) death. The mechanism of this syndrome is not understood. Patients receiving ACE inhibitors who develop jaundice or marked elevations of hepatic enzymes should discontinue the ACE inhibitor and receive appropriate medical follow-up.

Fetal/Neonatal Morbidity and Mortality

ACE inhibitors can cause fetal and neonatal morbidity and death when administered to pregnant women. Several dozen cases have been reported in the world literature. When pregnancy is detected, ACE inhibitors should be discontinued as soon as possible.

The use of ACE inhibitors during the second and third trimesters of pregnancy has been associated with fetal and neonatal injury, including hypotension, neonatal skull hypoplasia, anuria, reversible or irreversible renal failure, and death. Oligohydramnios has also been reported, presumably resulting from decreased fetal renal function: oligohydramnois in this setting has been associated with fetal limb contractures, craniofacial deformation, and hypoplastic lung development. Prematurity, intrauterine growth retardation, and patent ductus arteriosus have also been reported, although it is not clear whether these occurrences were due to the ACE-inhibitor exposure.

These adverse effects do not appear to have resulted from intrauterine ACE-inhibitor exposure that has been limited to the first trimester. Mothers whose embryos and fetuses are exposed to ACE inhibitors only during the first trimester should be so informed. Nonetheless, when patients become pregnant, physicians should make every effort to discontinue the use of VASOTEC as soon as possible.

Rarely (probably less often than once in every thousand pregnancies), no alternative to ACE inhibitors will be found. In these rare cases, the mothers should be apprised of the potential hazards to their fetuses, and serial ultrasound examinations should be performed to assess the intraamniotic environment.

If oligohydramnois is observed, VASOTEC should be discontinued unless it is considered lifesaving for the mother. Contraction stress testing (CST, a non-stress test (NST), or biophysical profiling (BPP) may be appropriate, depending upon the week of pregnancy. Patients and physicians should be aware, however, that oligohydramnois may not appear until after the fetus has sustained irreversible injury.

Infants with histories of *in utero* exposure to ACE inhibitors should be closely observed for hypotension, oliguria, and hyperkalemia. If oliguria occurs, attention should be directed toward support of blood pressure and renal perfusion. Exchange transfusion or dialysis may be required as means of reversing hypotension and/or substituting for disordered renal function. Enalapril, which crosses the placenta, has been removed from neonatal circulation by peritoneal dialysis with some clinical benefit, and theoretically may be removed by exchange transfusion, although there is no experience with the latter procedure.

No teratogenic effects of oral enalapril were seen in studies of pregnant rats and rabbits. On a mg/kg basis, the doses used were up to 333 times (in rats), and 50 times (in rabbits) the maximum recommended human dose.

PRECAUTIONS

General

Impaired Renal Function: As a consequence of inhibiting the renin-angiotensin-aldosterone system, changes in renal function may be anticipated in susceptible individuals. In patients with severe heart failure whose renal function may depend on the activity of the renin-angiotensin-aldosterone system, treatment with angiotensin converting enzyme inhibitors, including VASOTEC, may be associated with oliguria and/or progressive azotemia and rarely with acute renal failure and/or death.

In clinical studies in hypertensive patients with unilateral or bilateral renal artery stenosis, increases in blood urea nitrogen and serum creatinine were observed in 20 percent of patients. These increases were almost always reversible upon discontinuation of enalapril and/or diuretic therapy. In such patients renal function should be monitored during the first few weeks of therapy.

Some patients with hypertension or heart failure with no apparent pre-existing renal vascular disease have developed increases in blood urea and serum creatinine, usually minor and transient, especially when VASOTEC has been given concomitantly with a diuretic. This is more likely to occur in patients with pre-existing renal impairment. Dosage reduction and/or discontinuation of the diuretic and/or VASOTEC may be required.

Evaluation of patients with hypertension or heart failure should always include assessment of renal function. (See DOSAGE AND ADMINISTRATION.)

Hyperkalemia: Elevated serum potassium (greater than 5.7 mEq/L) was observed in approximately one percent of hypertensive patients in clinical trials. In most cases these were isolated values which resolved despite continued therapy. Hyperkalemia was a cause of discontinuation of therapy in 0.28 percent of hypertensive patients. In clinical trials in heart failure, hyperkalemia was observed in 3.8 percent of patients but was not a cause for discontinuation.

Risk factors for the development of hyperkalemia include renal insufficiency, diabetes mellitus, and the concomitant use of potassium-sparing diuretics, potassium supplements and/or potassium-containing salt substitutes, which should be used cautiously, if at all, with VASOTEC. (See *Drug Interactions.*)

Cough: Presumably due to the inhibition of the degradation of endogenous bradykinin, persistent nonproductive cough has been reported with all ACE inhibitors, always resolving after discontinuation of therapy. ACE inhibitor-induced cough should be considered in the differential diagnosis of cough.

Surgery/Anesthesia: In patients undergoing major surgery or during anesthesia with agents that produce hypotension, enalapril may block angiotensin II formation secondary to compensatory renin release. If hypotension occurs and is considered to be due to this mechanism, it can be corrected by volume expansion.

Information for Patients

Angioedema: Angioedema, including laryngeal edema, may occur at any time during treatment with angiotensin converting enzyme inhibitors, including enalapril. Patients should be so advised and told to report immediately any signs or symptoms suggesting angioedema (swelling of face, extremities, eyes, lips, tongue, difficulty in swallowing or breathing) and to take no more drug until they have consulted with the prescribing physician.

Hypotension: Patients should be cautioned to report lightheadedness, especially during the first few days of therapy. If actual syncope occurs, the patients should be told to discontinue the drug until they have consulted with the prescribing physician.

All patients should be cautioned that excessive perspiration and dehydration may lead to an excessive fall in blood pressure because of reduction in fluid volume. Other causes of volume depletion such as vomiting or diarrhea may also lead to a fall in blood pressure; patients should be advised to consult with the physician.

Hyperkalemia: Patients should be told not to use salt substitutes containing potassium without consulting their physician.

Neutropenia: Patients should be told to report promptly any indication of infection (e.g., sore throat, fever) which may be a sign of neutropenia.

Pregnancy: Female patients of childbearing age should be told about the consequences of second- and third-trimester exposure to ACE inhibitors, and they should also be told that these consequences do not appear to have resulted from intrauterine ACE-inhibitor exposure that has been limited to the first trimester. These patients should be asked to report pregnancies to their physicians as soon as possible.

NOTE: As with many other drugs, certain advice to patients being treated with enalapril is warranted. This information is intended to aid in the safe and effective use of this medication. It is not a disclosure of all possible adverse or intended effects.

Drug Interactions

Hypotension—Patients on Diuretic Therapy: Patients on diuretics and especially those in whom diuretic therapy was recently instituted, may occasionally experience an excessive reduction of blood pressure after initiation of therapy with enalapril. The possibility of hypotensive effects with enalapril can be minimized by either discontinuing the diuretic or increasing the salt intake prior to initiation of treatment with enalapril. If it is necessary to continue the diuretic, provide close medical supervision after the initial dose for at least two hours and until blood pressure has stabilized for at least an additional hour. (See WARNINGS and DOSAGE AND ADMINISTRATION.)

Agents Causing Renin Release: The antihypertensive effect of VASOTEC is augmented by antihypertensive agents that cause renin release (e.g., diuretics).

Other Cardiovascular Agents: VASOTEC has been used concomitantly with beta adrenergic-blocking agents, methyldopa, nitrates, calcium-blocking agents, hydralazine, prazosin and digoxin without evidence of clinically significant adverse interactions.

Agents Increasing Serum Potassium: VASOTEC attenuates potassium loss caused by thiazide-type diuretics. Potassium-sparing diuretics (e.g., spironolactone, triamterene, or amiloride), potassium supplements, or potassium-containing salt substitutes may lead to significant increases in serum potassium. Therefore, if concomitant use of these agents is indicated because of demonstrated hypokalemia, they should be used with caution and with frequent monitoring of serum potassium. Potassium sparing agents should generally not be used in patients with heart failure receiving VASOTEC.

Lithium: Lithium toxicity has been reported in patients receiving lithium concomitantly with drugs which cause elimination of sodium, including ACE inhibitors. A few cases of lithium toxicity have been reported in patients receiving concomitant VASOTEC and lithium and were reversible upon discontinuation of both drugs. It is recommended that serum lithium levels be monitored frequently if enalapril is administered concomitantly with lithium.

Carcinogenesis, Mutagenesis, Impairment of Fertility

There was no evidence of a tumorigenic effect when enalapril was administered for 106 weeks to rats at doses up to 90 mg/kg/day (150 times* the maximum daily human dose). Enalapril has also been administered for 94 weeks to male and female mice at doses up to 90 and 180 mg/kg/day, respectively, (150 and 300 times* the maximum daily dose for humans) and showed no evidence of carcinogenicity.

Neither enalapril maleate nor the active diacid was mutagenic in the Ames microbial mutagen test with or without metabolic activation. Enalapril was also negative in the following genotoxicity studies: rec-assay, reverse mutation assay with *E. coli*, sister chromatid exchange with cultured mammalian cells, and the micronucleus test with mice, as well as in an *in vivo* cytogenic study using mouse bone marrow.

There were no adverse effects on reproductive performance in male and female rats treated with 10 to 90 mg/kg/day of enalapril.

---

*Based on patient weight of 50 kg

Pregnancy

Pregnancy Categories C (first trimester) and *D* (second and third trimesters). See WARNINGS, *Fetal/Neonatal Morbidity and Mortality.*

Nursing Mothers

Enalapril and enalaprilat are detected in human milk in trace amounts. Caution should be exercised when VASOTEC is given to a nursing mother.

Pediatric Use

Safety and effectiveness in children have not been established.

ADVERSE REACTIONS

VASOTEC has been evaluated for safety in more than 10,000 patients, including over 1000 patients treated for one year or more. VASOTEC has been found to be generally well tolerated in controlled clinical trials involving 2987 patients.

For the most part, adverse experiences were mild and transient in nature. In clinical trials, discontinuation of therapy due to clinical adverse experiences was required in 3.3 percent of patients with hypertension and in 5.7 percent of patients with heart failure. The frequency of adverse experiences was not related to total daily dosage within the usual dosage ranges. In patients with hypertension the overall percentage of patients treated with VASOTEC reporting adverse experiences was comparable to placebo.

HYPERTENSION

Adverse experiences occurring in greater than one percent of patients with hypertension treated with VASOTEC in controlled clinical trials are shown below. In patients treated with VASOTEC, the maximum duration of therapy was three years; in placebo treated patients the maximum duration of therapy was 12 weeks.

	VASOTEC (n = 2314) Incidence (discontinuation)	Placebo (n = 230) Incidence
Body As A Whole		
Fatigue	3.0 (<0.1)	2.6
Orthostatic Effects	1.2 (<0.1)	0.0
Asthenia	1.1 (0.1)	0.9

Digestive		
Diarrhea	1.4 (<0.1)	1.7
Nausea	1.4 (0.2)	1.7
Nervous/Psychiatric		
Headache	5.2 (0.3)	9.1
Dizziness	4.3 (0.4)	4.3
Respiratory		
Cough	1.3 (0.1)	0.9
Skin		
Rash	1.4 (0.4)	0.4

HEART FAILURE

Adverse experiences occurring in greater than one percent of patients with heart failure treated with VASOTEC are shown below. The incidences represent the experiences from both controlled and uncontrolled clinical trials (maximum duration of therapy was approximately one year). In the placebo treated patients, the incidences reported are from the controlled trials (maximum duration of therapy is 12 weeks). The percentage of patients with severe heart failure (NYHA Class IV) was 29 percent and 43 percent for patients treated with VASOTEC and placebo, respectively.

	VASOTEC (n = 673) Incidence (discontinuation)	Placebo (n = 339) Incidence
Body As A Whole		
Orthostatic Effects	2.2 (0.1)	0.3
Syncope	2.2 (0.1)	0.9
Chest Pain	2.1 (0.0)	2.1
Fatigue	1.8 (0.0)	1.8
Abdominal Pain	1.6 (0.4)	2.1
Asthenia	1.6 (0.1)	0.3
Cardiovascular		
Hypotension	6.7 (1.9)	0.6
Orthostatic Hypotension	1.6 (0.1)	0.3
Angina Pectoris	1.5 (0.1)	1.8
Myocardial Infarction	1.2 (0.3)	1.8
Digestive		
Diarrhea	2.1 (0.1)	1.2
Nausea	1.3 (0.1)	0.6
Vomiting	1.3 (0.0)	0.9
Nervous/Psychiatric		
Dizziness	7.9 (0.6)	0.6
Headache	1.8 (0.1)	0.9
Vertigo	1.6 (0.1)	1.2
Respiratory		
Cough	2.2 (0.0)	0.6
Bronchitis	1.3 (0.0)	0.9
Dyspnea	1.3 (0.1)	0.4
Pneumonia	1.0 (0.0)	2.4
Skin		
Rash	1.3 (0.0)	2.4
Urogenital		
Urinary Tract Infection	1.3 (0.0)	2.4

Other serious clinical adverse experiences occurring since the drug was marketed or adverse experiences occurring in 0.5 to 1.0 percent of patients with hypertension or heart failure in clinical trials are listed below and, within each category, are in order of decreasing severity.

Body As A Whole: Anaphylactoid reactions (see WARNINGS, *Anaphylactoid and Possibly Related Reactions*).

Cardiovascular: Cardiac arrest; myocardial infarction or cerebrovascular accident, possibly secondary to excessive hypotension in high risk patients (see WARNINGS, *Hypotension*); pulmonary embolism and infarction; pulmonary edema; rhythm disturbances including atrial tachycardia and bradycardia; atrial fibrillation; palpitation.

Digestive: Ileus, pancreatitis, hepatic failure, hepatitis (hepatocellular [proven on rechallenge] or cholestatic jaundice) (see WARNINGS, *Hepatic Failure*), melena, anorexia, dyspepsia, constipation, glossitis, stomatitis, dry mouth.

Hematologic: Rare cases of neutropenia, thrombocytopenia and bone marrow depression.

Musculoskeletal: Muscle cramps.

Nervous/Psychiatric: Depression, confusion, ataxia, somnolence, insomnia, nervousness, peripheral neuropathy (e.g., paresthesia, dysesthesia).

Respiratory: Bronchospasm, rhinorrhea, sore throat and hoarseness, asthma, upper respiratory infection, pulmonary infiltrates.

Skin: Exfoliative dermatitis, toxic epidermal necrolysis, Stevens-Johnson syndrome, pemphigus, herpes zoster, erythema multiforme, urticaria, pruritus, alopecia, flushing, diaphoresis, photosensitivity.

Special Senses: Blurred vision, taste alteration, anosmia, tinnitus, conjunctivitis, dry eyes, tearing.

Urogenital: Renal failure, oliguria, renal dysfunction (see PRECAUTIONS and DOSAGE AND ADMINISTRATION), flank pain, gynecomastia, impotence.

Miscellaneous: A symptom complex has been reported which may include a positive ANA, an elevated erythrocyte sedimentation rate, arthralgia/arthritis, myalgia/myositis, fever, serositis, vasculitis, leukocytosis, eosinophilia, photosensitivity, rash and other dermatologic manifestations.

Angioedema: Angioedema has been reported in patients receiving VASOTEC, with an incidence higher in black than in non-black patients. Angioedema associated with laryngeal edema may be fatal. If angioedema of the face, extremities, lips, tongue, glottis and/or larynx occurs, treatment with VASOTEC should be discontinued and appropriate therapy instituted immediately. (See WARNINGS.)

Hypotension: In the hypertensive patients, hypotension occurred in 0.9 percent and syncope occurred in 0.5 percent of patients following the initial dose or during extended therapy. Hypotension or syncope was a cause for discontinuation of therapy in 0.1 percent of hypertensive patients. In heart failure patients, hypotension occurred in 6.7 percent and syncope occurred in 2.2 percent of patients. Hypotension or syncope was a cause for discontinuation of therapy in 1.9 percent of patients with heart failure. (See WARNINGS.)

Fetal/Neonatal Morbidity and Mortality: See WARNINGS, *Fetal/Neonatal Morbidity and Mortality.*

Cough: See PRECAUTIONS, *Cough.*

Clinical Laboratory Test Findings

Serum Electrolytes: Hyperkalemia (see PRECAUTIONS), hyponatremia.

Creatinine, Blood Urea Nitrogen: In controlled clinical trials minor increases in blood urea nitrogen and serum creatinine, reversible upon discontinuation of therapy, were observed in about 0.2 percent of patients with essential hypertension treated with VASOTEC alone. Increases are more likely to occur in patients receiving concomitant diuretics or in patients with renal artery stenosis. (See PRECAUTIONS.) In patients with heart failure who were also receiving diuretics with or without digitalis increases in blood urea nitrogen or serum creatinine, usually reversible upon discontinuation of VASOTEC and/or other concomitant diuretic therapy, were observed in about 11 percent of patients. Increases in blood urea nitrogen or creatinine were a cause for discontinuation in 1.2 percent of patients.

Hematology: Small decreases in hemoglobin and hematocrit (mean decreases of approximately 0.3 g percent and 1.0 vol percent, respectively) occur frequently in either hypertension or congestive heart failure patients treated with VASOTEC but are rarely of clinical importance unless another cause of anemia coexists. In clinical trials, less than 0.1 percent of patients discontinued therapy due to anemia. Hemolytic anemia, including cases of hemolysis in patients with G-6-PD deficiency, has been reported; a causal relationship to enalapril cannot be excluded.

Liver Function Tests: Elevations of liver enzymes and/or serum bilirubin have occurred (see WARNINGS, *Hepatic Failure*).

OVERDOSAGE

Limited data are available in regard to overdosage in humans.

The oral LD_{50} of enalapril is 2000 mg/kg in mice and rats. The most likely manifestation of overdosage would be hypotension, for which the usual treatment would be intravenous infusion of normal saline solution.

Enalaprilat may be removed from general circulation by hemodialysis and has been removed from neonatal circulation by peritoneal dialysis.

DOSAGE AND ADMINISTRATION

Hypertension

In patients who are currently being treated with a diuretic, symptomatic hypotension occasionally may occur following the initial dose of VASOTEC. The diuretic should, if possible, be discontinued for two to three days before beginning therapy with VASOTEC to reduce the likelihood of hypotension. (See WARNINGS.) If the patient's blood pressure is not controlled with VASOTEC alone, diuretic therapy may be resumed.

If the diuretic cannot be discontinued an initial dose of 2.5 mg should be used under medical supervision for at least two hours and until blood pressure has stabilized for at least an additional hour. (See WARNINGS and PRECAUTIONS, *Drug Interactions.*)

The recommended initial dose in patients not on diuretics is 5 mg once a day. Dosage should be adjusted according to blood pressure response. The usual dosage range is 10 to 40 mg per day administered in a single dose or two divided doses. In some patients treated once daily, the antihypertensive effect may diminish toward the end of the dosing interval. In such patients, an increase in dosage or twice daily administration should be considered. If blood pressure is not controlled with VASOTEC alone, a diuretic may be added.

Concomitant administration of VASOTEC with potassium supplements, potassium salt substitutes, or potassium-sparing diuretics may lead to increases of serum potassium (see PRECAUTIONS).

Dosage Adjustment in Hypertensive Patients with Renal Impairment

The usual dose of enalapril is recommended for patients with a creatinine clearance > 30 mL/min (serum creatinine of up to approximately 3 mg/dL). For patients with creatinine clearance ≤ 30 mL/min (serum creatinine ≥ 3 mg/dL), the first dose is 2.5 mg once daily. The dosage may be titrated upward until blood pressure is controlled or to a maximum of 40 mg daily.

Renal Status	Creatinine-Clearance mL/min	Initial Dose mg/day
Normal Renal Function	> 80 mL/min	5 mg
Mild Impairment	≤ 80 > 30 mL/min	5 mg
Moderate to Severe Impairment	≤ 30 mL/min	2.5 mg
Dialysis Patients*	—	2.5 mg on dialysis days**

*See WARNINGS, *Anaphylactoid reactions during membrane exposure.*

**Dosage on nondialysis days should be adjusted depending on the blood pressure response.

Heart Failure

VASOTEC is indicated for the treatment of symptomatic heart failure, usually in combination with diuretics and digitalis. In the placebo-controlled studies that demonstrated improved survival, patients were titrated as tolerated up to 40 mg, administered in two divided doses.

The recommended initial dose is 2.5 mg. The recommended dosing range is 2.5 to 20 mg given twice a day. Doses should be titrated upward, as tolerated, over a period of a few days or weeks. The maximum daily dose administered in clinical trials was 40 mg in divided doses.

After the initial dose of VASOTEC, the patient should be observed under medical supervision for at least two hours and until blood pressure has stabilized for at least an additional hour. (See WARNINGS and PRECAUTIONS, *Drug Interactions.*) If possible, the dose of any concomitant diuretic should be reduced which may diminish the likelihood of hypotension. The appearance of hypotension after the initial dose of VASOTEC does not preclude subsequent careful dose titration with the drug, following effective management of the hypotension.

Asymptomatic Left Ventricular Dysfunction

In the trial that demonstrated efficacy, patients were started on 2.5 mg twice daily and were titrated as tolerated to the targeted daily dose of 20 mg (in divided doses).

After the initial dose of VASOTEC, the patient should be observed under medical supervision for at least two hours and until blood pressure has stabilized for at least an additional hour. (See WARNINGS and PRECAUTIONS, *Drug Interactions.*) If possible, the dose of any concomitant diuretic should be reduced which may diminish the likelihood of hypotension. The appearance of hypotension after the initial dose of VASOTEC does not preclude subsequent careful dose titration with the drug, following effective management of the hypotension.

Dosage Adjustment in Patients with Heart Failure and Renal Impairment or Hyponatremia

In patients with heart failure who have hyponatremia (serum sodium less than 130 mEq/L) or with serum creatinine greater than 1.6 mg/dL, therapy should be initiated at 2.5 mg daily under close medical supervision. (See DOSAGE AND ADMINISTRATION, *Heart Failure,* WARNINGS and PRECAUTIONS, *Drug Interactions.*) The dose may be increased to 2.5 mg b.i.d., then 5 mg b.i.d. and higher as needed, usually at intervals of four days or more if at the time of dosage adjustment there is not excessive hypotension or significant deterioration of renal function. The maximum daily dose is 40 mg.

HOW SUPPLIED

No. 3411—Tablets VASOTEC, 2.5 mg, are yellow, biconvex barrel shaped, scored, compressed tablets with code MSD 14 on one side and VASOTEC on the other. They are supplied as follows:

NDC 0006-0014-94 unit of use bottles of 90 (with desiccant)

NDC 0006-0014-68 bottles of 100 (with desiccant)
(6505-01-351-3157, 2.5 mg 100's)

NDC 0006-0014-28 unit dose packages of 100

NDC 0006-0014-98 unit of use bottles of 180 (with desiccant)

Continued on next page

Information on the Merck & Co., Inc. products listed on these pages is the full prescribing information from product circulars in use September 30, 1996.

Merck & Co.—Cont.

NDC 0006-0014-82 bottles of 1,000 (with desiccant)
NDC 0006-0014-87 bottles of 10,000 (with desiccant).

Shown in Product Identification Guide, page 325

No. 3412—Tablets VASOTEC, 5 mg. are white, barrel shaped, scored, compressed tablets, with code MSD 712 on one side and VASOTEC on the other. They are supplied as follows:

NDC 0006-0712-94 unit of use bottles of 90 (with desiccant)
NDC 0006-0712-68 bottles of 100 (with desiccant)
(6505-01-236-8880, 5 mg 100's)
NDC 0006-0712-28 unit dose packages of 100
(6505-01-244-4811, 5 mg individually sealed 100's)
NDC 0006-0712-98 unit of use bottles of 180 (with desiccant)
NDC 0006-0712-82 bottles of 1,000 (with desiccant)
NDC 0006-0712-81 bottles of 4,000 (with desiccant)
(6505-01-319-9526, 5 mg 4,000's)
NDC 0006-0712-87 bottles of 10,000 (with desiccant)
(6505-01-379-5575, 5 mg 10,000's).

Shown in Product Identification Guide, page 325

No. 3413—Tablets VASOTEC, 10 mg, are salmon, barrel shaped, compressed tablets, with code MSD 713 on one side and VASOTEC on the other. They are supplied as follows:

NDC 0006-0713-94 unit of use bottles of 90 (with desiccant)
NDC 0006-0713-68 bottles of 100 (with desiccant)
(6505-01-236-8881, 10 mg 100's)
NDC 0006-0713-28 unit dose packages of 100
(6505-01-314-6028, 10 mg individually sealed 100's)
NDC 0006-0713-98 unit of use bottles of 180 (with desiccant)
NDC 0006-0713-82 bottles of 1,000 (with desiccant)
NDC 0006-0713-81 bottles of 4,000 (with desiccant)
(6505-01-320-4728, 10 mg 4,000's)
NDC 0006-0713-87 bottles of 10,000 (with desiccant)
(6505-01-378-8022, 10 mg 10,000's).

Shown in Product Identification Guide, page 325

No. 3414—Tablets VASOTEC, 20 mg, are peach, barrel shaped, compressed tablets, with code MSD 714 on one side and VASOTEC on the other. They are supplied as follows:

NDC 0006-0714-94 unit of use bottles of 90 (with desiccant)
NDC 0006-0714-68 bottles of 100 (with desiccant)
(6505-01-237-0545, 20 mg 100's)
NDC 0006-0714-28 unit dose packages of 100
(6505-01-318-0465, 20 mg individually sealed 100's)
NDC 0006-0714-82 bottles of 1,000 (with desiccant)
NDC 0006-0714-87 bottles of 10,000 (with desiccant)
(6505-01-378-8780, 20 mg 10,000's).

Shown in Product Identification Guide, page 325

Storage
Store below 30°C (86°F) and avoid transient temperatures above 50°C (122°F). Keep container tightly closed. Protect from moisture.
Dispense in a tight container, if product package is subdivided.

7825152 Issued July 1995

COPYRIGHT © MERCK & CO., INC., 1988, 1989, 1992, 1993
All rights reserved

VIVACTIL® Tablets ℞
(Protriptyline HCl), U.S.P.

DESCRIPTION

Protriptyline HCl is *N*-methyl-5*H*-dibenzo[*a,d*]-cycloheptene-5-propanamine hydrochloride. Its empirical formula is $C_{19}H_{21}N \cdot HCl$ and its structural formula is:

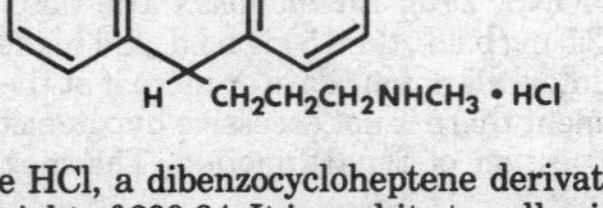
H
CH₂CH₂CH₂NHCH₃ • HCl

Protriptyline HCl, a dibenzocycloheptene derivative, has a molecular weight of 299.84. It is a white to yellowish powder that is freely soluble in water and soluble in dilute HCl.
VIVACTIL* (Protriptyline HCl) is supplied as 5 mg and 10 mg film coated tablets. Inactive ingredients are calcium phosphate, cellulose, guar gum, hydroxypropyl cellulose, hydroxypropyl methylcellulose, lactose, magnesium stearate, starch, talc, and titanium dioxide. Tablets VIVACTIL 5 mg and 10 mg also contain FD&C Yellow 6. Tablets VIVACTIL 10 mg also contain D&C Yellow 10.

---

*Registered trademark of MERCK & CO., INC.

ACTIONS

VIVACTIL is an antidepressant agent. The mechanism of its antidepressant action in man is not known. It is not a monoamine oxidase inhibitor, and it does not act primarily by stimulation of the central nervous system.
VIVACTIL has been found in some studies to have a more rapid onset of action than imipramine or amitriptyline. The initial clinical effect may occur within one week. Sedative and tranquilizing properties are lacking. The rate of excretion is slow.

INDICATIONS

VIVACTIL is indicated for the treatment of symptoms of mental depression in patients who are under close medical supervision. Its activating properties make it particularly suitable for withdrawn and anergic patients.

CONTRAINDICATIONS

VIVACTIL is contraindicated in patients who have shown prior hypersensitivity to it.
It should not be given concomitantly with a monoamine oxidase inhibiting compound. Hyperpyretic crises, severe convulsions, and deaths have occurred in patients receiving tricyclic antidepressant and monoamine oxidase inhibiting drugs simultaneously. When it is desired to substitute VIVACTIL for a monoamine oxidase inhibitor, a minimum of 14 days should be allowed to elapse after the latter is discontinued. VIVACTIL should then be initiated cautiously with gradual increase in dosage until optimum response is achieved.
This drug should not be used during the acute recovery phase following myocardial infarction.

WARNINGS

VIVACTIL may block the antihypertensive effect of guanethidine or similarly acting compounds.
VIVACTIL should be used with caution in patients with a history of seizures, and, because of its autonomic activity, in patients with a tendency to urinary retention, or increased intraocular tension.
Tachycardia and postural hypotension may occur more frequently with VIVACTIL than with other antidepressant drugs. VIVACTIL should be used with caution in elderly patients and patients with cardiovascular disorders; such patients should be observed closely because of the tendency of the drug to produce tachycardia, hypotension, arrhythmias, and prolongation of the conduction time. Myocardial infarction and stroke have occurred with drugs of this class.
On rare occasions, hyperthyroid patients or those receiving thyroid medication may develop arrhythmias when this drug is given.
In patients who may use alcohol excessively, it should be borne in mind that the potentiation may increase the danger inherent in any suicide attempt or overdosage.

Usage in Children
This drug is not recommended for use in children because safety and effectiveness in the pediatric age group have not been established.

Usage in Pregnancy
Safe use in pregnancy and lactation has not been established; therefore, use in pregnant women, nursing mothers or women who may become pregnant requires that possible benefits be weighed against possible hazards to mother and child.
In mice, rats, and rabbits, doses about ten times greater than the recommended human doses had no apparent adverse effects on reproduction.

PRECAUTIONS

General
When protriptyline HCl is used to treat the depressive component of schizophrenia, psychotic symptoms may be aggravated. Likewise, in manic-depressive psychosis, depressed patients may experience a shift toward the manic phase if they are treated with an antidepressant drug. Paranoid delusions, with or without hostility, may be exaggerated. In any of these circumstances, it may be advisable to reduce the dose of VIVACTIL or to use a major tranquilizing drug concurrently.
Symptoms, such as anxiety or agitation, may be aggravated in overactive or agitated patients.
The possibility of suicide in depressed patients remains during treatment and until significant remission occurs. This type of patient should not have access to large quantities of the drug.
Concurrent administration of VIVACTIL and electroshock therapy may increase the hazards of therapy. Such treatment should be limited to patients for whom it is essential.
Discontinue the drug several days before elective surgery, if possible.
Both elevation and lowering of blood sugar levels have been reported.

Information for Patients
While on therapy with VIVACTIL, patients should be advised as to the possible impairment of mental and/or physical abilities required for performance of hazardous tasks, such as operating machinery or driving a motor vehicle.

Drug Interactions
When VIVACTIL is given with anticholinergic agents or sympathomimetic drugs, including epinephrine combined with local anesthetics, close supervision and careful adjustment of dosages are required.
Hyperpyrexia has been reported when tricyclic antidepressants are administered with anticholinergic agents or with neuroleptic drugs, particularly during hot weather.
Cimetidine is reported to reduce hepatic metabolism of certain tricyclic antidepressants, thereby delaying elimination and increasing steady-state concentrations of these drugs. Clinically significant effects have been reported with the tricyclic antidepressants when used concomitantly with cimetidine. Increases in plasma levels of tricyclic antidepressants, and in the frequency and severity of side effects, particularly anticholinergic, have been reported when cimetidine was added to the drug regimen. Discontinuation of cimetidine in well-controlled patients receiving tricyclic antidepressants and cimetidine may decrease the plasma levels and efficacy of the antidepressants.
It may enhance the response to alcohol and the effects of barbiturates and other CNS depressants.
Drugs Metabolized by Cytochrome P450 2D6: The biochemical activity of the drug-metabolizing isozyme, cytochrome P450 2D6 (debrisoquine hydroxylase), is reduced in a subset of the Caucasian population (about 7–10% of Caucasians are so called "poor metabolizers"); reliable estimates of the prevalence of reduced P450 2D6 isozyme activity among Asian, African, and other populations are not yet available. Poor metabolizers have higher than expected plasma concentrations of tricyclic antidepressants (TCAs) when given usual doses. Depending on the fraction of drug metabolized by P450 2D6, the increase in plasma concentration may be small or quite large (8-fold increase in plasma AUC of the TAC).
In addition, certain drugs inhibit the activity of this isozyme and make normal metabolizers resemble poor metabolizers. An individual who is stable on a given dose of TCA may become abruptly toxic when given one of these inhibiting drugs as concomitant therapy. The drugs that inhibit cytochrome P450 2D6 include some that are not metabolized by the enzyme (quinidine; cimetidine) and many that are substrates for P450 2D6 (many other antidepressants, phenothiazines, and the Type 1C antiarrhythmics, propafenone and flecainide). While all the selective serotonin reuptake inhibitors (SSRIs), e.g., fluoxetine, sertraline, and paroxetine, inhibit P450 2D6, they may vary in the extent of inhibition. The extent to which SSRI-TCA interactions may pose clinical problems will depend on the degree of inhibition and the pharmacokinetics of the SSRI involved. Nevertheless, caution is indicated in the coadministration of TCAs with any of the SSRIs, and also in switching from one class to the other. Of particular importance, sufficient time must elapse before initiating TCA treatment in a patient being withdrawn from fluoxetine, given the long half-life of the parent and active metabolite (at least 5 weeks may be necessary).
Concomitant use of tricyclic antidepressants with drugs that can inhibit cytochrome P450 2D6 may require lower doses than usually prescribed for either the tricyclic antidepressant or the other drug. Furthermore, whenever one of these other drugs is withdrawn from co-therapy, an increased dose of tricyclic antidepressant may be required. It is desirable to monitor TCA plasma levels whenever a TCA is going to be coadministered with another drug known to be an inhibitor of P450 2D6.

ADVERSE REACTIONS

Within each category the following adverse reactions are listed in order of decreasing severity. Included in the listing are a few adverse reactions which have not been reported with this specific drug. However, the pharmacological similarities among the tricyclic antidepressant drugs require that each of the reactions be considered when protriptyline is administered. VIVACTIL is more likely to aggravate agitation and anxiety and produce cardiovascular reactions such as tachycardia and hypotension.
Cardiovascular: Myocardial infarction; stroke; heart block; arrhythmias; hypotension, particularly orthostatic hypotension; hypertension; tachycardia; palpitation.
Psychiatric: Confusional states (especially in the elderly) with hallucinations, disorientation, delusions, anxiety, restlessness, agitation; hypomania; exacerbation of psychosis; insomnia, panic, and nightmares.
Neurological: Seizures; incoordination; ataxia; tremors; peripheral neuropathy; numbness, tingling, and paresthesias of extremities; extrapyramidal symptoms; drowsiness; dizziness; weakness and fatigue; headache; syndrome of inappropriate ADH (antidiuretic hormone) secretion; tinnitus; alteration in EEG patterns.
Anticholinergic: Paralytic ileus; hyperpyrexia; urinary retention, delayed micturition, dilatation of the urinary tract; constipation; blurred vision, disturbance of accommo-

dation, increased intraocular pressure, mydriasis; dry mouth and rarely associated sublingual adenitis.
Allergic: Drug fever; petechiae, skin rash, urticaria, itching, photosensitization (avoid excessive exposure to sunlight); edema (general, or of face and tongue).
Hematologic: Agranulocytosis; bone marrow depression; leukopenia; thrombocytopenia; purpura; eosinophilia.
Gastrointestinal: Nausea and vomiting; anorexia; epigastric distress; diarrhea; peculiar taste; stomatitis; abdominal cramps; black tongue.
Endocrine: Impotence, increased or decreased libido; gynecomastia in the male; breast enlargement and galactorrhea in the female; testicular swelling; elevation or depression of blood sugar levels.
Other: Jaundice (simulating obstructive); altered liver function; parotid swelling; alopecia; flushing; weight gain or loss, urinary frequency, nocturia; perspiration.
Withdrawal Symptoms: Though not indicative of addiction, abrupt cessation of treatment after prolonged therapy may produce nausea, headache, and malaise.

DOSAGE AND ADMINISTRATION

Dosage should be initiated at a low level and increased gradually, noting carefully the clinical response and any evidence of intolerance.

Usual Adult Dosage—Fifteen to 40 mg a day divided into 3 or 4 doses. If necessary, dosage may be increased to 60 mg a day. Dosages above this amount are not recommended. Increases should be made in the morning dose.

Adolescent and Elderly Patients—In general, lower dosages are recommended for these patients. Five mg 3 times a day may be given initially, and increased gradually if necessary. In elderly patients, the cardiovascular system must be monitored closely if the daily dose exceeds 20 mg.

When satisfactory improvement has been reached, dosage should be reduced to the smallest amount that will maintain relief of symptoms.
Minor adverse reactions require reduction in dosage. Major adverse reactions or evidence of hypersensitivity require prompt discontinuation of the drug.
Usage in Children—This drug is not recommended for use in children because safety and effectiveness in the pediatric age group have not been established.

OVERDOSAGE

Deaths may occur from overdosage with this class of drugs. Multiple drug ingestion (including alcohol) is common in deliberate tricyclic antidepressant overdose. As management of overdose is complex and changing, it is recommended that the physician contact a poison control center for current information on treatment. Signs and symptoms of toxicity develop rapidly after tricyclic antidepressant overdose, therefore, hospital monitoring is required as soon as possible.
MANIFESTATIONS
Critical manifestations of overdosage include: cardiac dysrhythmias, severe hypotension, convulsions, and CNS depression, including coma. Changes in the electrocardiogram, particularly in QRS axis or width, are clinically significant indicators of tricyclic antidepressant toxicity.
Other signs of overdose may include: confusion, disturbed concentration, transient visual hallucinations, dilated pupils, agitation, hyperactive reflexes, stupor, drowsiness, muscle rigidity, vomiting, hypothermia, hyperpyrexia, or any of the symptoms listed under ADVERSE REACTIONS.
MANAGEMENT
General
Obtain an ECG and immediately initiate cardiac monitoring. Protect the patient's airway, establish an intravenous line and initiate gastric decontamination. A minimum of six hours of observation with cardiac monitoring and observation for signs of CNS or respiratory depression, hypotension, cardiac dysrhythmias and/or conduction blocks, and seizures is necessary. If signs of toxicity occur at any time during this period, extended monitoring is required. There are case reports of patients succumbing to fatal dysrhythmias late after overdose. These patients had clinical evidence of significant poisoning prior to death and most received inadequate gastrointestinal decontamination. Monitoring of plasma drug levels should not guide management of the patient.
Gastrointestinal Decontamination
All patients suspected of a tricyclic antidepressant overdose should receive gastrointestinal decontamination. This should include large volume gastric lavage followed by activated charcoal. If consciousness is impaired, the airway should be secured prior to lavage. Emesis is contraindicated.
Cardiovascular
A maximal limb-lead QRS duration of ≥ 0.10 seconds may be the best indication of the severity of the overdose. Serum alkalinization, to a pH of 7.45 to 7.55, using intravenous sodium bicarbonate and hyperventilation (as needed), should be instituted for patients with dysrhythmias and/or QRS widening. A pH > 7.60 or a pCO2 < 20 mmHg is undesirable. Dysrhythmias unresponsive to sodium bicarbonate therapy/hyperventilation may respond to lidocaine, bretylium or phenytoin. Type 1A and 1C antiarrhythmics are generally contraindicated (e.g., quinidine, disopyramide, and procainamide).
In rare instances, hemoperfusion may be beneficial in acute refractory cardiovascular instability in patients with acute toxicity. However, hemodialysis, peritoneal dialysis, exchange transfusions, and forced diuresis generally have been reported as ineffective in tricyclic antidepressant poisoning.
CNS
In patients with CNS depression, early intubation is advised because of the potential for abrupt deterioration. Seizures should be controlled with benzodiazepines or, if these are ineffective, other anticonvulsants (e.g., phenobarbital, phenytoin). Physostigmine is not recommended except to treat life-threatening symptoms that have been unresponsive to other therapies, and then only in close consultation with a poison control center.
PSYCHIATRIC FOLLOW-UP
Since overdosage is often deliberate, patients may attempt suicide by other means during the recovery phase. Psychiatric referral may be appropriate.
PEDIATRIC MANAGEMENT
The principles of management of child and adult overdosages are similar. It is strongly recommended that the physician contact the local poison control center for specific pediatric treatment.

HOW SUPPLIED

No. 3313—Tablets VIVACTIL, 5 mg, are orange, oval, film coated tablets, coded MSD 26. They are supplied as follows:
NDC 0006-0026-68 bottles of 100
(6505-00-369-7297, 5 mg 100).
Shown in Product Identification Guide, page 325
No. 3314—Tablets VIVACTIL, 10 mg, are yellow, oval, film coated tablets, coded MSD 47. They are supplied as follows:
NDC 0006-0047-68 bottles of 100
(6505-00-462-7353, 10 mg 100's)
NDC 0006-0047-28 unit dose packages of 100.
Shown in Product Identification Guide, page 325
Storage
Store Tablets VIVACTIL in a tightly closed container. Avoid storage at temperatures above 40°C (104°F).

METABOLISM

Metabolic studies indicate that protriptyline is well absorbed from the gastrointestinal tract and is rapidly sequestered in tissues. Relatively low plasma levels are found after administration, and only a small amount of unchanged drug is excreted in the urine of dogs and rabbits. Preliminary studies indicate that demethylation of the secondary amine moiety occurs to a significant extent, and that metabolic transformation probably takes place in the liver. It penetrates the brain rapidly in mice and rats, and moreover that which is present in the brain is almost all unchanged drug.
Studies on the disposition of radioactive protriptyline in human test subjects showed significant plasma levels within 2 hours, peaking at 8 to 12 hours, then declining gradually. Urinary excretion studies in the same subjects showed significant amounts of radioactivity in 2 hours. The rate of excretion was slow. Cumulative urinary excretion during 16 days accounted for approximately 50% of the drug. The fecal route of excretion did not seem to be important.

7904022 Issued January 1996

ZOCOR® Tablets ℞
(Simvastatin)

DESCRIPTION

ZOCOR* (Simvastatin) is a cholesterol lowering agent that is derived synthetically from a fermentation product of *Aspergillus terreus.* After oral ingestion, simvastatin, which is an inactive lactone, is hydrolyzed to the corresponding β-hydroxyacid form. This is an inhibitor of 3-hydroxy-3-methylglutaryl-coenzyme A (HMG-CoA) reductase. This enzyme catalyzes the conversion of HMG-CoA to mevalonate, which is an early and rate-limiting step in the biosynthesis of cholesterol.
Simvastatin is butanoic acid, 2,2-dimethyl-, 1,2,3,7,8,8a-hexahydro-3,7-dimethyl-8-[2-(tetrahydro-4-hydroxy-6-oxo-2*H*-pyran-2-yl) ethyl]-1-napthalenyl ester, [1*S*-[1α,3α,7β,8β(2*S**,4*S**),-8aβ]]. The empirical formula of simvastatin is $C_{25}H_{38}O_5$ and its molecular weight is 418.57. Its structural formula is:
[See chemical structure at top of next column.]

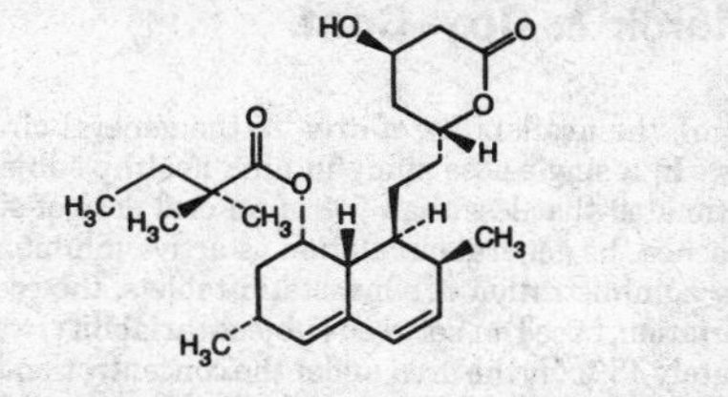

Simvastatin is a white to off-white, nonhygroscopic, crystalline powder that is practically insoluble in water, and freely soluble in chloroform, methanol and ethanol.
Tablets ZOCOR for oral administration contain either 5 mg, 10 mg, 20 mg or 40 mg of simvastatin and the following inactive ingredients: cellulose, hydroxypropyl cellulose, hydroxypropyl methylcellulose, iron oxides, lactose, magnesium stearate, starch, talc, titanium dioxide and other ingredients. Butylated hydroxyanisole is added as a preservative.

---

* Registered trademark of MERCK & CO., INC.

CLINICAL PHARMACOLOGY

The involvement of low-density lipoprotein (LDL) cholesterol in atherogenesis has been well-documented in clinical and pathological studies, as well as in many animal experiments. Epidemiological studies have established that high LDL (low-density lipoprotein) cholesterol and low HDL (high-density lipoprotein) cholesterol are both risk factors for coronary heart disease. In the Scandinavian Simvastatin Survival Study (4S), the effect of improving lipoprotein levels with ZOCOR on total mortality was assessed in 4444 patients with coronary heart disease (CHD) and baseline total cholesterol 212–309 mg/dL (5.5–8.0 mmol/L). The patients were followed for a median of 5.4 years. In this multicenter, randomized, double-blind, placebo-controlled study, ZOCOR significantly reduced the risk of mortality by 30% (11.5% vs 8.2%, placebo vs ZOCOR); of CHD mortality by 42% (8.5% vs 5.0%); and of having a hospital-verified non-fatal myocardial infarction by 37% (19.6% vs 12.9%). Furthermore, ZOCOR significantly reduced the risk for undergoing myocardial revascularization procedures (coronary artery bypass grafting or percutaneous transluminal coronary angioplasty) by 37% (17.2% vs 11.4%) [see CLINICAL PHARMACOLOGY, *Clinical Studies*].
ZOCOR has been shown to reduce both normal and elevated LDL cholesterol concentrations. LDL is formed from very-low-density lipoprotein (VLDL) and is catabolized predominantly by the high affinity LDL receptor. The mechanism of the LDL-lowering effect of ZOCOR may involve both reduction of VLDL cholesterol concentration, and induction of the LDL receptor, leading to reduced production and/or increased catabolism of LDL cholesterol. Apolipoprotein B also falls substantially during treatment with ZOCOR. Since each LDL particle contains one molecule of apolipoprotein B, and since little apolipoprotein B is found in other lipoproteins, this strongly suggests that ZOCOR does not merely cause cholesterol to be lost from LDL, but also reduces the concentration of circulating LDL particles. In addition, ZOCOR modestly reduces VLDL cholesterol and plasma triglycerides and can produce increases of variable magnitude in HDL cholesterol. The effects of ZOCOR on Lp(a), fibrinogen, and certain other independent biochemical risk markers for coronary heart disease are unknown.
ZOCOR is a specific inhibitor of HMG-CoA reductase, the enzyme that catalyzes the conversion of HMG-CoA to mevalonate. The conversion of HMG-CoA to mevalonate is an early step in the biosynthetic pathway for cholesterol.
Pharmacokinetics
Simvastatin is a lactone that is readily hydrolyzed *in vivo* to the corresponding β-hydroxyacid, a potent inhibitor of HMG-CoA reductase. Inhibition of HMG-CoA reductase is the basis for an assay in pharmacokinetic studies of the β-hydroxyacid metabolites (active inhibitors) and, following base hydrolysis, active plus latent inhibitors (total inhibitors) in plasma following administration of simvastatin.
Following an oral dose of ^{14}C-labeled simvastatin in man, 13% of the dose was excreted in urine and 60% in feces. The latter represents absorbed drug equivalents excreted in bile, as well as any unabsorbed drug. Plasma concentrations of total radioactivity (simvastatin plus ^{14}C-metabolites) peaked at 4 hours and declined rapidly to about 10% of peak by 12 hours postdose. Absorption of simvastatin, estimated relative to an intravenous reference dose, in each of two animal species tested, averaged about 85% of an oral dose. In animal studies, after oral dosing, simvastatin achieved substantially higher concentrations in the liver than in nontarget tissues. Simvastatin undergoes extensive first-pass extraction in the liver, its primary site of action, with subsequent excretion of drug equivalents in the bile. As a consequence of extensive hepatic extraction of simvastatin (estimated to be > 60% in

Continued on next page

Information on the Merck & Co., Inc. products listed on these pages is the full prescribing information from product circulars in use September 30, 1996.

Merck & Co.—Cont.

man), the availability of drug to the general circulation is low. In a single-dose study in nine healthy subjects, it was estimated that less than 5% of an oral dose of simvastatin reaches the general circulation as active inhibitors. Following administration of simvastatin tablets, the coefficient of variation, based on between-subject variability, was approximately 48% for the area under the concentration-time curve (AUC) for total inhibitory activity in the general circulation. Both simvastatin and its β-hydroxyacid metabolite are highly bound (approximately 95%) to human plasma proteins. Animal studies have not been performed to determine whether simvastatin crosses the blood-brain and placental barriers. However, when radiolabeled simvastatin was administered to rats, simvastatin-derived radioactivity crossed the blood-brain barrier.

The major active metabolites of simvastatin present in human plasma are the β-hydroxyacid of simvastatin and its 6'--hydroxy, 6'-hydroxy methyl, and 6'-exomethylene derivatives. Peak plasma concentrations of both active and total inhibitors were attained within 1.3 to 2.4 hours postdose. While the recommended therapeutic dose range is 5 to 40 mg/day, there was no substantial deviation from linearity of AUC of inhibitors in the general circulation with an increase in dose to as high as 120 mg. Relative to the fasting state, the plasma profile of inhibitors was not affected when simvastatin was administered immediately before an A.H.A. recommended low-fat meal.

Kinetic studies with another reductase inhibitor, having a similar principal route of elimination, have suggested that for a given dose level higher systemic exposure may be achieved in patients with severe renal insufficiency (as measured by creatinine clearance).

Clinical Studies
ZOCOR has been shown to be highly effective in reducing total and LDL cholesterol in heterozygous familial and non-familial forms of hypercholesterolemia and in mixed hyperlipidemia. A marked response was seen within 2 weeks, and the maximum therapeutic response occurred within 4–6 weeks. The response was maintained during chronic therapy. Furthermore, improving lipoprotein levels with ZOCOR improved survival in patients with CHD and hypercholesterolemia treated with 20–40 mg per day for a median of 5.4 years.

In a multicenter, double-blind, placebo-controlled, dose-response study in patients with familial or non-familial hypercholesterolemia, ZOCOR given as a single-dose in the evening (the recommended dosing) was similarly effective as when given on a twice-daily basis. ZOCOR consistently and significantly decreased total plasma cholesterol (TOTAL-C), LDL cholesterol (LDL-C), total cholesterol/HDL cholesterol (TOTAL-C/HDL-C) ratio, and LDL cholesterol/HDL cholesterol (LDL-C/HDL-C) ratio. ZOCOR also modestly decreased triglycerides (TRIG) and produced increases of variable magnitude in HDL cholesterol (HDL-C).

The results of a dose response study in patients with primary hypercholesterolemia are presented in Table I.
[See table below.]

In the Scandinavian Simvastatin Survival Study (4S), the effect of therapy with ZOCOR on total mortality was assessed in 4444 patients with coronary heart disease (CHD) and baseline total cholesterol 212–309 mg/dL (5.5–8.0 mmol/L). In this multicenter, randomized, double-blind, placebo-controlled study, patients were treated with standard care, including diet, and either ZOCOR 20–40 mg daily (n=2221) or placebo (n=2223) for a median duration of 5.4 years. Over the course of the study, treatment with ZOCOR led to mean reductions in total cholesterol, LDL cholesterol and triglycerides of 25%, 35%, and 10%, respectively, and a mean increase in HDL cholesterol of 8%. ZOCOR significantly reduced the risk of mortality (Figure 1) by 30%, (p=0.0003, 182 deaths in the ZOCOR group vs 256 deaths in the placebo group). The risk of CHD mortality was significantly reduced by 42%, (p=0.00001, 111 vs 189). There was no statistically significant difference between groups in non-cardiovascular mortality. ZOCOR also significantly decreased the risk of having major coronary events (CHD mortality plus hospital-verified and silent non-fatal MI) (Figure 2) of 34%, (p <0.00001, 431 patients vs 622 patients with one or more events). The risk of having a hospital-verified non-fatal MI was reduced by 37%. Furthermore, ZOCOR significantly

reduced the risk for undergoing mycocardial revascularization procedures (coronary artery bypass grafting or percutaneous transluminal coronary angioplasty) by 37%, (p <0.00001, 252 patients vs 383 patients). ZOCOR reduced the risk of major coronary events to a similar extent across the range of baseline total and LDL cholesterol levels. The risk of mortality was significantly reduced in patients ≥60 years of age by 27% and in patients <60 years of age by 37%. Because there were only 53 female deaths, the effect of ZOCOR on mortality in women could not be adequately assessed. However, ZOCOR significantly lessened the risk of having major coronary events by 34% (60 women vs 91 women with one or more event). The randomization was stratified by angina alone (21% of each treatment group) or a previous myocardial infarction (MI). Because there were only 57 deaths among the patients with angina alone at baseline, the effect of ZOCOR on mortality in this subgroup could not be adequately assessed. However, trends in reduced coronary mortality, major coronary events and revascularization procedures were consistent between this group and the total study cohort.

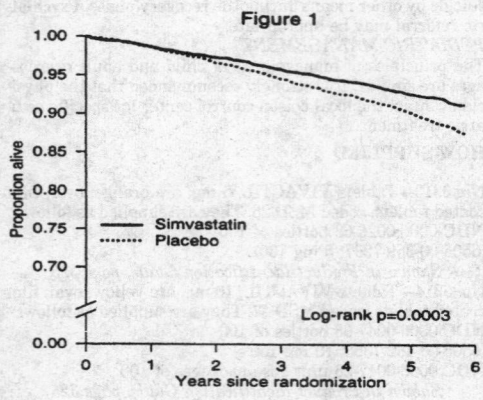

Figure 1

Log-rank p=0.0003

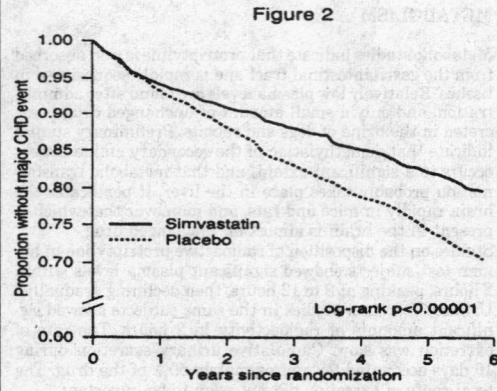

Figure 2

Log-rank p<0.00001

In the Multicenter Anti-Atheroma Study, the effect of therapy with simvastatin on atherosclerosis was assessed by quantitative coronary angiography in hypercholesterolemic men and women with coronary heart disease. In this randomized, double-blind, controlled trial, patients with a mean baseline total cholesterol value of 245 mg/dL (6.4 mmol/L) and a mean baseline LDL value of 170 mg/dL (4.4 mmol/L) were treated with conventional measures and with simvastatin 20 mg/d or placebo. Angiograms were evaluated at baseline, two and four years. A total of 347 patients had a baseline angiogram and at least one follow-up angiogram. The co-primary endpoints of the trial were mean changes per-patient in minimum and mean lumen diameters, indicating focal and diffuse disease, respectively. Simvastatin significantly slowed the progression of lesions as measured in the final angiogram by both these parameters (mean changes in

minimum lumen diameter: −0.04 mm with simvastatin vs −0.12 mm with placebo; mean changes in mean lumen diameter: −0.03 mm with simvastatin vs −0.08 mm with placebo), as well as by change from baseline in percent diameter stenosis (0.9% simvastatin vs 3.6% placebo). After four years, the groups also differed significantly in the proportions of patients categorized with disease progression (23% simvastatin vs 33% placebo) and disease regression (18% simvastatin vs 12% placebo). In addition, simvastatin significantly decreased the proportion of patients with new lesions (13% simvastatin vs 24% placebo) and with new total occlusions (5% vs 11%). The mean change per-patient in mean and minimum lumen diameters calculated by comparing angiograms in the subset of 274 patients who had matched angiographic projections at baseline, two and four years is presented below (Figures 3 and 4).

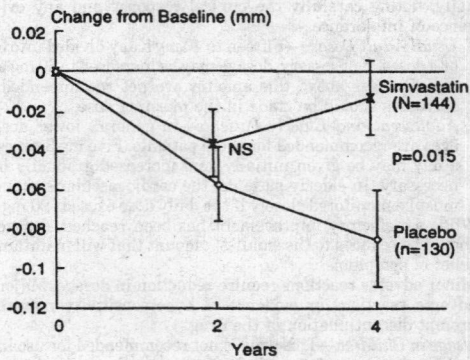

Figure 3

Mean Lumen Diameter
(Mean and Standard Error)

Change from Baseline (mm)

NS

Simvastatin (N=144)

p=0.015

Placebo (n=130)

Years

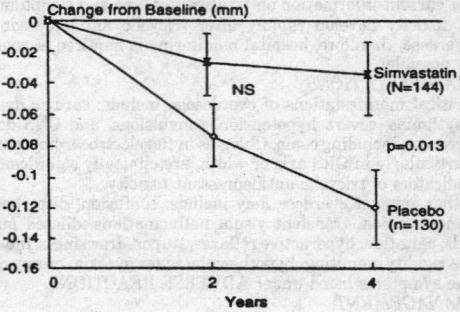

Figure 4

Minimum Lumen Diameter
(Mean and Standard Error)

Change from Baseline (mm)

NS

Simvastatin (N=144)

p=0.013

Placebo (n=130)

Years

In a study designed to evaluate the possible effects of simvastatin on reproductive hormones and sperm characteristics in men with familial hypercholesterolemia, there was a small decrease in the mean percentage of vital sperm and a small increase in the mean percentage of abnormal forms, with these changes achieving statistical significance at week 14. However, there was no effect on numbers or concentration of motile sperm. Simvastatin had no effect on basal reproductive hormone levels (prolactin, luteinizing hormone, follicle-stimulating hormone, and plasma testosterone). Provocative testing (HCG stimulation) was not done. Treatment with another HMG-CoA reductase inhibitor resulted in a statistically significant decrease in plasma testosterone response to HCG.

In a study to evaluate the effect of simvastatin on adrenocortical function in patients with Type II hypercholesterolemia, simvastatin had no effect on basal adrenocortical function as assessed by determination of morning plasma cortisol levels, urine free cortisol, and urinary excretion of 17-hydroxy steroids. Simvastatin also had no effect on adrenocortical reserve as evaluated by the plasma cortisol response to ACTH stimulation and insulin-induced hypoglycemia.

TABLE I
Dose Response in Patients with Primary Hypercholesterolemia
(Mean Percent Change from Baseline After 8 Weeks)

TREATMENT	N	TOTAL-C	LDL-C	HDL-C	LDL-C/HDL-C	TOTAL-C/HDL-C	TRIG.
Placebo	28	−3	−4	+2	−4	−3	+7
ZOCOR							
5 mg q.p.m.	28	−17	−24	+7	−27	−22	−10
10 mg q.p.m.	27	−24	−33	+9	−37	−29	−10
20 mg q.p.m.	26	−25	−33	+11	−36	−30	−19
40 mg q.p.m.	29	−28	−40	+12	−46	−36	−19

INDICATIONS AND USAGE

Therapy with lipid-altering agents should be a component of multiple risk factor intervention in those individuals at significantly increased risk for atherosclerotic vascular disease due to hypercholesterolemia. Lipid-altering agents should be used in addition to a diet restricted in saturated fat and cholesterol when the response to diet and other nonpharmacological measures alone has been inadequate (see NCEP Guidelines, below).

Coronary Heart Disease

In patients with coronary heart disease and hypercholesterolemia, ZOCOR is indicated to:

- Reduce the risk of total mortality by reducing coronary death;
- Reduce the risk of non-fatal myocardial infarction;
- Reduce the risk for undergoing myocardial revascularization procedures.

(For a discussion of efficacy results by gender and other predefined subgroups, see CLINICAL PHARMACOLOGY, *Clinical Studies.)*

Hypercholesterolemia

ZOCOR is indicated for the reduction of elevated total and LDL cholesterol levels in patients with primary hypercholesterolemia (Types IIa and IIb**).

General Recommendations

Prior to initiating therapy with simvastatin, secondary causes for hypercholesterolemia (e.g., poorly controlled diabetes mellitus, hypothyroidism, nephrotic syndrome, dysproteinemias, obstructive liver disease, other drug therapy, alcoholism) should be excluded, and a lipid profile performed to measure TOTAL-C, HDL-C, and triglycerides (TG). For patients with TG less than 400 mg/dL (<4.5 mmol/L), LDL-C can be estimated using the following equation:

LDL-C = Total cholesterol − [0.20 × (triglycerides) + HDL-C]

For TG levels >400 mg/dL (>4.5 mmol/L), this equation is less accurate and LDL-C concentrations should be determined by ultracentrifugation. In many hypertriglyceridemic patients, LDL-C may be low or normal despite elevated TOTAL-C. In such cases, ZOCOR is not indicated.

Lipid determinations should be performed at intervals of no less than four weeks and dosage adjusted according to the patient's response to therapy.

The National Cholesterol Education Program (NCEP) Treatment Guidelines are summarized below:

Definite Atherosclerotic Disease†	Two or More Other Risk Factors††	LDL-Cholesterol mg/dL (mmol/L) Initiation Level	Goal
NO	NO	≥190 (≥4.9)	<160 (<4.1)
NO	YES	≥160 (≥4.1)	<130 (<3.4)
YES	YES or NO	≥130 (≥3.4)	≤100 (≤2.6)

† Coronary heart disease or peripheral vascular disease (including symptomatic carotid artery disease).

†† Other risk factors for coronary heart disease (CHD) include: age (males: ≥45 years; females: ≥55 years or premature menopause without estrogen replacement therapy); family history of premature CHD; current cigarette smoking; hypertension; confirmed HDL-C <35 mg/dL (<0.91 mmol/L); and diabetes mellitus. Subtract one risk factor if HDL-C is ≥60 mg/dL (≥1.6 mmol/L).

Since the goal of treatment is to lower LDL-C, the NCEP recommends that LDL-C levels be used to initiate and assess treatment response. Only if LDL-C levels are not available, should the TOTAL-C be used to monitor therapy.

Although ZOCOR may be useful to reduce elevated LDL cholesterol levels in patients with combined hypercholesterolemia and hypertriglyceridemia where hypercholesterolemia is the major abnormality (Type IIb hyperlipoproteinemia), it has not been studied in conditions where the major abnormality is elevation of chylomicrons, VLDL or IDL (i.e., hyperlipoproteinemia types I, III, IV, or V).**

**Classification of Hyperlipoproteinemias

Type	Lipoproteins elevated	Lipid Elevations major	minor
I (rare)	chylomicrons	TG	→C
IIa	LDL	C	—
IIb	LDL, VLDL	C	TG
III (rare)	IDL	C/TG	—
IV	VLDL	TG	→C
V (rare)	chylomicrons, VLDL	TG	→C

C = cholesterol, TG = triglycerides,
LDL = low-density lipoprotein,
VLDL = very-low-density lipoprotein,
IDL = intermediate-density lipoprotein.

CONTRAINDICATIONS

Hypersensitivity to any component of this medication.

Active liver disease or unexplained persistent elevations of serum transaminases (see WARNINGS).

Pregnancy and lactation. Atherosclerosis is a chronic process and the discontinuation of lipid-lowering drugs during pregnancy should have little impact on the outcome of long-term therapy of primary hypercholesterolemia. Moreoever, cholesterol and other products of the cholesterol biosynthesis pathway are essential components for fetal development, including synthesis of steroids and cell membranes. Because of the ability of inhibitors of HMG-CoA reductase such as ZOCOR to decrease the synthesis of cholesterol and possibly other products of the cholesterol biosynthesis pathway, ZOCOR may cause fetal harm when administered to a pregnant woman. Therefore, simvastatin is contraindicated during pregnancy and in nursing mothers. **Simvastatin should be administered to women of childbearing age only when such patients are highly unlikely to conceive.** If the patient becomes pregnant while taking this drug, simvastatin should be discontinued and the patient should be apprised of the potential hazard to the fetus.

WARNINGS

Liver Dysfunction

Persistent increases (to more than 3 times the upper limit of normal) in serum transaminases have occurred in 1% of patients who received simvastatin in clinical trials. When drug treatment was interrupted or discontinued in these patients, the transaminase levels usually fell slowly to pretreatment levels. The increases were not associated with jaundice or other clinical signs or symptoms. There was no evidence of hypersensitivity.

It is recommended that liver function tests be performed before the initiation of treatment, at 6 and 12 weeks after initiation of therapy or elevation in dose, and periodically thereafter (e.g., semiannually). Patients who develop increased transaminase levels should be monitored with a second liver function evaluation to confirm the finding and be followed thereafter with frequent liver function tests until the abnormality (ies) return to normal. Should an increase in AST or ALT of three times the upper limit of normal or greater persist, withdrawal of therapy with ZOCOR is recommended.

The drug should be used with caution in patients who consume substantial quantities of alcohol and/or have a past history of liver disease. Active liver diseases or unexplained transaminase elevations are contraindications to the use of simvastatin.

As with other lipid-lowering agents, moderate (less than three times the upper limit of normal) elevations of serum transaminases have been reported following therapy with simvastatin. These changes appeared soon after initiation of therapy with simvastatin, were often transient, were not accompanied by any symptoms and did not require interruption of treatment.

Skeletal Muscle

Rare cases of rhabdomyolysis with acute renal failure secondary to myoglobinuria have been associated with simvastatin therapy. Rhabdomyolysis has also been associated with other HMG-CoA reductase inhibitors when they were administered alone or concomitantly with 1) immunosuppressive therapy, including cyclosporine in cardiac transplant patients; 2) gemfibrozil or lipid-lowering doses (≥1 g/day) of nicotinic acid in non-transplant patients, or 3) erythromycin in seriously ill patients. Some of the patients who had rhabdomyolysis in association with the reductase inhibitors had preexisting renal insufficiency, usually as a consequence of long-standing diabetes. In most subjects who have had an unsatisfactory lipid response to either simvastatin or gemfibrozil alone, the possible benefits of combined therapy with these drugs are not considered to outweigh the risk of severe myopathy, rhabdomyolysis, and acute renal failure. While it is not known whether this interaction occurs with fibrates other than gemfibrozil, myopathy and rhabdomyolysis have occasionally been associated with the use of other fibrates alone, including clofibrate. Therefore, the combined use of simvastatin with other fibrates should generally be avoided.

Muscle weakness accompanied by marked elevation of creatine phosphokinase was observed in a renal transplant patient on cyclosporine and simvastatin following the initiation of therapy with the systemic antifungal agent itraconazole. Rhabdomyolysis with renal failure has been reported in a renal transplant patient receiving cyclosporine and another HMG-CoA reductase inhibitor shortly after a dose increase in the systemic itraconazole. The HMG-CoA reductase inhibitors and the azole derivative antifungal agents inhibit cholesterol biosynthesis at different points in the biosynthetic pathway. In patients receiving cyclosporine, simvastatin should be temporarily discontinued if systemic azole derivative antifungal therapy is required; patients not taking cyclosporine should be carefully monitored if systemic azole derivative antifungal therapy is required.

Physicians contemplating combined therapy with simvastatin and lipid-lowering doses of nicotinic acid, or with immunosuppressive drugs should carefully weigh the potential benefits and risks and should carefully monitor patients for any signs and symptoms of muscle pain, tenderness, or weakness, particularly during the initial months of therapy and during any periods of upward dosage titration of either drug. Periodic creatine phosphokinase (CPK) determinations may be considered in such situations, but there is no assurance that such monitoring will prevent the occurrence of severe myopathy.

Because of an apparent relationship between increased plasma levels of active metabolites derived from other HMG-CoA reductase inhibitors and myopathy, in patients taking cyclosporine, the daily dosage should not exceed 10 mg/day (see DOSAGE AND ADMINISTRATION).

Simvastatin therapy should be temporarily withheld or discontinued in any patient with an acute, serious condition suggestive of a myopathy or having a risk factor predisposing to the development of renal failure secondary to rhabdomyolysis, (e.g., severe acute infection, hypotension, major surgery, trauma, severe metabolic, endocrine and electrolyte disorders, and uncontrolled seizures).

Myopathy should be considered in any patient with diffuse myalgias, muscle tenderness or weakness, and/or marked elevation of CPK. Patients should be advised to report promptly unexplained muscle pain, tenderness or weakness, particularly if accompanied by malaise or fever. Simvastatin therapy should be discontinued if markedly elevated CPK levels occur or myopathy is diagnosed or suspected.

PRECAUTIONS

General

Before instituting therapy with ZOCOR, an attempt should be made to control hypercholesterolemia with appropriate diet, exercise, and weight reduction in obese patients, and to treat other underlying medical problems (see INDICATIONS AND USAGE).

Simvastatin may cause elevation of creatine phosphokinase and transaminase levels (see WARNINGS and ADVERSE REACTIONS). This should be considered in the differential diagnosis of chest pain in a patient on therapy with simvastatin.

Homozygous Familial Hypercholesterolemia

ZOCOR is less effective in patients with the rare homozygous familial hypercholesterolemia, possibly because these patients have few functional LDL receptors.

Information for Patients

Patients should be advised to report promptly unexplained muscle pain, tenderness, or weakness, particularly if accompanied by malaise or fever.

Drug Interactions

Immunosuppressive Drugs, Itraconazole, Gemfibrozil, Niacin (Nicotinic Acid), Erythromycin: See WARNINGS, *Skeletal Muscle.*

Antipyrine: Because simvastatin had no effect on the pharmacokinetics of antipyrine, interactions with other drugs metabolized via the same cytochrome isozymes are not expected.

Propranolol: In healthy male volunteers there was a significant decrease in mean C_{max}, but no change in AUC, for simvastatin total and active inhibitors with concomitant administration of single doses of ZOCOR and propranolol. The clinical relevance of this finding is unclear. The pharmacokinetics of the enantiomers of propranolol were not affected.

Digoxin: Concomitant administration of a single dose of digoxin in healthy male volunteers receiving simvastatin resulted in a slight elevation (less than 0.3 ng/mL) in digoxin concentrations in plasma (as measured by a radioimmunoassay) compared to concomitant administration of placebo and digoxin. Patients taking digoxin should be monitored appropriately when simvastatin is initiated.

Warfarin: In two clinical studies, one in normal volunteers and the other in hypercholesterolemic patients, simvastatin 20–40 mg/day modestly potentiated the effect of coumarin anticoagulants: the prothrombin time, reported as International Normalized Ratio (INR), increased from a baseline of 1.7 to 1.8 and from 2.6 to 3.4 in the volunteer and patient studies, respectively. With other reductase inhibitors, clinically evident bleeding and/or increased prothrombin time has been reported in a few patients taking coumarin anticoagulants concomitantly. In such patients, prothrombin time should be determined before starting simvastatin and frequently enough during early therapy to insure that no signif-

Continued on next page

Information on the Merck & Co., Inc. products listed on these pages is the full prescribing information from product circulars in use September 30, 1996.

Consult 1997 supplements and future editions for revisions

Merck & Co.—Cont.

icant alteration of prothrombin time occurs. Once a stable prothrombin time has been documented, prothrombin times can be monitored at the intervals usually recommended for patients on coumarin anticoagulants. If the dose of simvastatin is changed or discontinued, the same procedure should be repeated. Simvastatin therapy has not been associated with bleeding or with changes in prothrombin time in patients not taking anticoagulants.

Other Concomitant Therapy: Although specific interaction studies were not performed, in clinical studies, simvastatin was used concomitantly with angiotensin-converting enzyme (ACE) inhibitors, beta blockers, calcium-channel blockers, diuretics and nonsteroidal anti-inflammatory drugs (NSAIDs) without evidence of clinically significant adverse interactions. The effect of cholestyramine on the absorption and kinetics of simvastatin has not been determined.

Endocrine Function

HMG-CoA reductase inhibitors interfere with cholesterol synthesis and as such might theoretically blunt adrenal and/ or gonadal steroid production. However, clinical studies have shown that simvastatin does not reduce basal plasma cortisol concentration or impair adrenal reserve, and does not reduce basal plasma testosterone concentration (see CLINICAL PHARMACOLOGY, *Clinical Studies*). Another HMG-CoA reductase inhibitor has been shown to reduce the plasma testosterone response to HCG; the effect of simvastatin on HCG-stimulated testosterone secretion has not been studied.

Results of clinical trials with drugs in this class have been inconsistent with regard to drug effects on basal and reserve steroid levels. The effects of HMG-CoA reductase inhibitors on male fertility have not been studied in adequate numbers of male patients. The effects, if any, on the pituitary-gonadal axis in pre-menopausal women are unknown. Patients treated with simvastatin who develop clinical evidence of endocrine dysfunction should be evaluated appropriately. Caution should also be exercised if an HMG-CoA reductase inhibitor or other agent used to lower cholesterol levels is administered to patients also receiving other drugs (e.g., ketoconazole, spironolactone, cimetidine) that may decrease the levels or activity of endogenous steroid hormones.

CNS Toxicity

Optic nerve degeneration was seen in clinically normal dogs treated with simvastatin for 14 weeks at 180 mg/kg/day, a dose that produced mean plasma drug levels about 44 times higher than the mean drug level in humans taking 40 mg/ day.

A chemically similar drug in this class also produced optic nerve degeneration (Wallerian degeneration of retinogeniculate fibers) in clinically normal dogs in a dose-dependent fashion starting at 60 mg/kg/day, a dose that produced mean plasma drug levels about 30 times higher than the mean drug level in humans taking the highest recommended dose (as measured by total enzyme inhibitory activity). This same drug also produced vestibulocochlear Wallerian-like degeneration and retinal ganglion cell chromatolysis in dogs treated for 14 weeks at 180 mg/kg/day, a dose that resulted in a mean plasma drug level similar to that seen with the 60 mg/kg/day dose.

CNS vascular lesions, characterized by perivascular hemorrhage and edema, mononuclear cell infiltration of perivascular spaces, perivascular fibrin deposits and necrosis of small vessels were seen in dogs treated with simvastatin at a dose of 360 mg/kg/day, a dose that produced plasma drug levels that were about 50 times higher than the mean drug levels in humans taking 40 mg/day. Similar CNS vascular lesions have been observed with several other drugs of this class. There were cataracts in female rats after two years of treatment with 50 and 100 mg/kg/day (110 and 120 times the human AUC at 40 mg/day) and in dogs in three month studies at 90 and 360 mg/kg/day and at two years at 50 mg/kg/ day. These treatment levels represented plasma drug levels (AUC) of approximately 42, 40, and 26 times the mean human plasma drug exposure after a 40 milligram daily dose.

Carcinogenesis, Mutagenesis, Impairment of Fertility

In a 72-week carcinogenicity study, mice were administered daily doses of simvastatin of 25, 100, and 400 mg/kg body weight, which resulted in mean plasma drug levels approximately 3, 15, and 33 times higher than the mean human plasma drug concentration (as total inhibitory activity) after a 40 mg oral dose. Liver carcinomas were significantly increased in high-dose females and mid- and high-dose males with a maximum incidence of 90 percent in males. The incidence of adenomas of the liver was significantly increased in mid- and high-dose females. Drug treatment also significantly increased the incidence of lung adenomas in mid- and high-dose males and females. Adenomas of the Harderian gland (a gland of the eye of rodents) were significantly higher in high-dose mice than in controls. No evidence of a tumorigenic effect was observed at 25 mg/kg/day. Although mice were given up to 500 times the human dose (HD) on a mg/ kg/body weight basis, blood levels of HMG-CoA reductase inhibitory activity were only 3–33 times higher in mice than in humans given 40 mg of ZOCOR.

In a separate 92-week carcinogenicity study in mice at doses up to 25 mg/kg/day, no evidence of a tumorigenic effect was observed. Although mice were given up to 31 times the human dose on a mg/kg basis, plasma drug levels were only 2–4 times higher than in humans given 40 mg simvastatin as measured by AUC.

In a two-year study in rats, there was a statistically significant increase in the incidence of thyroid follicular adenomas in female rats exposed to approximately 45 times higher levels of simvastatin than in humans given 40 mg simvastatin (as measured by AUC).

A second two-year rat carcinogenicity study with doses of 50 and 100 mg/kg/day produced hepatocellular adenomas and carcinomas (in female rats at both doses and in males at 100 mg/kg/day). Thyroid follicular cell adenomas were increased in males and females at both doses; thyroid follicular cell carcinomas were increased in females at 100 mg/kg/day. The increased incidence of thyroid neoplasms appears to be consistent with findings from other HMG-CoA reductase inhibitors. These treatment levels represented plasma drug levels (AUC) of approximately 35 and 75 times (males) and 110 and 120 times (females) the mean human plasma drug exposure after a 40 milligram daily dose.

No evidence of mutagenicity was observed in a microbial mutagen test using mutant strains of *Salmonella typhimurium* with or without rat or mouse liver metabolic activation. In addition, no evidence of damage to genetic material was noted in an *in vitro* alkaline elution assay using rat hepatocytes, a V-79 mammalian cell forward mutation study, an *in vitro* chromosome aberration study in CHO cells, or an *in vivo* chromosomal aberration assay in mouse bone marrow. There was decreased fertility in male rats treated with simvastatin for 34 weeks at 25 mg/kg body weight (15 times the maximum human exposure level, based on AUC, in patients receiving 40 mg/day); however, this effect was not observed during a subsequent fertility study in which simvastatin was administered at this same dose level to male rats for 11 weeks (the entire cycle of spermatogenesis including epididymal maturation). No microscopic changes were observed in the testes of rats from either study. At 180 mg/kg/day, (which produces exposure levels 44 times higher than those in humans taking 40 mg/day), seminiferous tubule degeneration (necrosis and loss of spermatogenic epithelium) was observed. In dogs, there was drug-related testicular atrophy, decreased spermatogenesis, spermatocytic degeneration and giant cell formation at 10 mg/kg/day (approximately 7 times the human exposure level, based on AUC, at 40 mg/ day). The clinical significance of these findings is unclear.

Pregnancy

Pregnancy Category X

See CONTRAINDICATIONS.

Safety in pregnant women has not been established. Simvastatin was not teratogenic in rats at doses of 25 mg/kg/day or in rabbits at doses up to 10 mg/kg daily. These doses resulted in 6 times (rat) or 4 times (rabbit) the human exposure based on mg/m² surface area. However, in studies with another structurally-related HMG-CoA reductase inhibitor, skeletal

malformations were observed in rats and mice. Rare reports of congenital anomalies have been received following intrauterine exposure to HMG-CoA reductase inhibitors. There has been one report of severe congenital bony deformity, tracheo-esophageal fistula, and anal atresia (VATER association) in a baby born to a woman who took another HMG-CoA reductase inhibitor with dextroamphetamine sulfate during the first trimester of pregnancy. Simvastatin should be administered to women of child-bearing potential only when such patients are highly unlikely to conceive and have been informed of the potential hazards. If the woman becomes pregnant while taking simvastatin, it should be discontinued and the patient advised again as to the potential hazards to the fetus.

Nursing Mothers

It is not known whether simvastatin is excreted in human milk. Because a small amount of another drug in this class is excreted in human milk and because of the potential for serious adverse reactions in nursing infants, women taking simvastatin should not nurse their infants (see CONTRAINDICATIONS).

Pediatric Use

Safety and effectiveness in children and adolescents have not been established. Because children and adolescents are not likely to benefit from cholesterol lowering for at least a decade and because experience with this drug is limited (no studies in subjects below the age of 20 years), treatment of children or adolescents with simvastatin is not recommended at this time.

ADVERSE REACTIONS

In the pre-marketing controlled clinical studies and their open extensions (2423 patients with mean duration of follow-up of approximately 18 months), 1.4% of patients were discontinued due to adverse experiences attributable to ZOCOR. Adverse reactions have usually been mild and transient. ZOCOR has been evaluated for serious adverse reactions in more than 21,000 patients and is generally well-tolerated.

Clinical Adverse Experiences

Adverse experiences occurring at an incidence of 1 percent or greater in patients treated with ZOCOR, regardless of causality, in controlled clinical studies are shown in the table below:

[See table below.]

In the Scandinavian Simvastatin Survival Study (4S) (see CLINICAL PHARMACOLOGY, *Clinical Studies*) involving 4444 patients treated with 20–40 mg/day of ZOCOR (n=2221) or placebo (n=2223), the safety and tolerability profiles were comparable between groups over the median 5.4 years of the study.

The following effects have been reported with drugs in this class. Not all effects listed below have necessarily been associated with simvastatin therapy.

Skeletal: muscle cramps, myalgia, myopathy, rhabdomyolysis, arthralgias.

Neurological: dysfunction of certain cranial nerves (including alteration of taste, impairment of extra-ocular movement, facial paresis), tremor, dizziness, vertigo, memory loss, paresthesia, peripheral neuropathy, peripheral nerve palsy, psychic disturbances, anxiety, insomnia, depression.

Hypersensitivity Reactions: An apparent hypersensitivity syndrome has been reported rarely which has included one or more of the following features: anaphylaxis, angioedema, lupus erythematous-like syndrome, polymyalgia rheumatica, vasculitis, purpura, thrombocytopenia, leukopenia, hemolytic anemia, positive ANA, ESR increase, eosinophilia, arthritis, arthralgia, urticaria, asthenia, photosensitivity, fever, chills, flushing, malaise, dyspnea, toxic epidermal necrolysis, erythema multiforme, including Stevens-Johnson syndrome.

Gastrointestinal: pancreatitis, hepatitis, including chronic active hepatitis, cholestatic jaundice, fatty change in liver, and, rarely, cirrhosis, fulminant hepatic necrosis, and hepatoma; anorexia, vomiting.

Skin: alopecia, pruritus. A variety of skin changes (e.g., nodules, discoloration, dryness of skin/mucous membranes, changes to hair/nails) has been reported.

Reproductive: gynecomastia, loss of libido, erectile dysfunction.

Eye: progression of cataracts (lens opacities), ophthalmoplegia.

Laboratory Abnormalities: elevated transaminases, alkaline phosphatase, γ-glutamyl transpeptidase, and bilirubin; thyroid function abnormalities.

Laboratory Tests

Marked persistent increases of serum transaminases have been noted (see WARNINGS, *Liver Dysfunction*). About 5% of patients had elevations of creatine phosphokinase (CPK) levels of 3 or more times the normal value on one or more occasions. This was attributable to the noncardiac fraction of CPK. Muscle pain or dysfunction usually was not reported (see WARNINGS, *Skeletal Muscle*).

	ZOCOR (N=1583)	Placebo (N=157)	Cholestyramine (N=179)	Probucol (N=81)
	%	%	%	%
Body as a Whole				
Abdominal pain	3.2	3.2	8.9	2.5
Asthenia	1.6	2.5	1.1	1.2
Gastrointestinal				
Constipation	2.3	1.3	29.1	1.2
Diarrhea	1.9	2.5	7.8	3.7
Dyspepsia	1.1	—	4.5	3.7
Flatulence	1.9	1.3	14.5	6.2
Nausea	1.3	1.9	10.1	2.5
Nervous System/Psychiatric				
Headache	3.5	5.1	4.5	3.7
Respiratory				
Upper respiratory infection	2.1	1.9	3.4	6.2

Concomitant Therapy

In controlled clinical studies in which simvastatin was administered concomitantly with cholestyramine, no adverse reactions peculiar to this concomitant treatment were observed. The adverse reactions that occurred were limited to those reported previously with simvastatin or cholestyramine. The combined use of simvastatin with fibrates should generally be avoided (see WARNINGS, *Skeletal Muscle*).

OVERDOSAGE

Significant lethality was observed in mice after a single oral dose of 9 g/m². No evidence of lethality was observed in rats or dogs treated with doses of 30 and 100 g/m², respectively. No specific diagnostic signs were observed in rodents. At these doses the only signs seen in dogs were emesis and mucoid stools.

A few cases of overdosage with ZOCOR have been reported; no patients had any specific symptoms, and all patients recovered without sequelae. The maximum dose taken was 450 mg. Until further experience is obtained, no specific treatment of overdosage with ZOCOR can be recommended. The dialyzability of simvastatin and its metabolites in man is not known at present.

DOSAGE AND ADMINISTRATION

The patient should be placed on a standard cholesterol–lowering diet before receiving ZOCOR and should continue on this diet during treatment with ZOCOR (see NCEP Treatment Guidelines for details on dietary therapy).

The recommended starting dose is 5–10 mg once a day in the evening. The recommended dosing range is 5–40 mg/day as a single dose in the evening; the maximum recommended dose is 40 mg/day. Doses should be individualized according to baseline LDL-C levels, the recommended goal of therapy (see NCEP Guidelines) and the patient's response. Patients requiring reductions in LDL cholesterol of 20% or more to achieve their goal (see INDICATIONS AND USAGE) should be started on 10 mg/day of ZOCOR. A starting dose of 5 mg should be considered for patients requiring smaller reductions and for the elderly. Adjustments of dosage should be made at intervals of 4 weeks or more.

Cholesterol levels should be monitored periodically and consideration should be given to reducing the dosage of ZOCOR if cholesterol falls significantly below the targeted range.

In the Scandinavian Simvastatin Survival Study (4S) [see CLINICAL PHARMACOLOGY, *Clinical Studies*], patients with coronary heart disease and hypercholesterolemia were treated with a starting dose of 20 mg of ZOCOR given as a single dose in the evening.

General Recommendations

In the elderly, maximum reductions in LDL cholesterol may be achieved with daily doses of 20 mg of ZOCOR or less.

In patients taking immunosuppressive drugs concomitantly with simvastatin (see WARNINGS, *Skeletal Muscle*), therapy should begin with 5 mg of ZOCOR and should not exceed 10 mg/day.

Concomitant Therapy

ZOCOR is effective alone or when used concomitantly with bile-acid sequestrants. Use of ZOCOR with fibrate-type drugs such as gemfibrozil or clofibrate should generally be avoided (see WARNINGS, *Skeletal Muscle*).

Dosage in Patients with Renal Insufficiency

Because ZOCOR does not undergo significant renal excretion, modification of dosage should not be necessary in patients with mild to moderate renal insufficiency. However, caution should be exercised when ZOCOR is administered to patients with severe renal insufficiency; such patients should be started at 5 mg/day and be closely monitored (see CLINICAL PHARMACOLOGY, *Pharmacokinetics* and WARNINGS, *Skeletal Muscle*).

HOW SUPPLIED

No. 3588—Tablets ZOCOR 5 mg are buff, shield-shaped, film-coated tablets, coded MSD 726 on one side and ZOCOR on the other. They are supplied as follows:
NDC 0006-0726-61 unit of use bottles of 60
(6505-01-354-4549, 5 mg 60's)
NDC 0006-0726-54 unit of use bottles of 90
(6505-01-354-4548, 5 mg 90's)
NDC 0006-0726-28 unit dose packages of 100.
Shown in Product Identification Guide, page 325
No. 3589—Tablets ZOCOR 10 mg are peach, shield-shaped, film-coated tablets, coded MSD 735 on one side and ZOCOR on the other. They are supplied as follows:
NDC 0006-0735-61 unit of use bottles of 60
(6505-01-354-4545, 10 mg 60's)
NDC 0006-0735-54 unit of use bottles of 90
(6505-01-354-4544 10 mg 90's)
NDC 0006-0735-28 unit dose packages of 100
(6505-01-354-4543, 10 mg individually sealed 100's)
NDC 0006-0735-82 bottles of 1000
(6505-01-373-7290, 10 mg 1000's)

NDC 0006-0735-87 bottles of 10,000
(6505-01-378-8058, 10 mg 10,000's).
Shown in Product Identification Guide, page 325
No. 3590—Tablets ZOCOR 20 mg are tan, shield-shaped, film-coated tablets, coded MSD 740 on one side and ZOCOR on the other. They are supplied as follows:
NDC 0006-0740-61 unit of use bottles of 60
(6505-01-354-4547, 20 mg 60's)
NDC 0006-0740-82 bottles of 1000
NDC 0006-0740-87 bottles of 10,000
(6505-01-378-8771, 20 mg 10,000's).
Shown in Product Identification Guide, page 325
No. 3591—Tablets ZOCOR 40 mg are brick-red, shield-shaped, film-coated tablets, coded MSD 749 on one side and ZOCOR on the other. They are supplied as follows:
NDC 0006-0749-61 unit of use bottles of 60
(6505-01-354-4546, 40 mg 60's).
Shown in Product Identification Guide, page 325
Storage
Store between 5–30°C (41–86°F).
7825419 Issued November 1995
COPYRIGHT © MERCK & CO., INC., 1991, 1995
All rights reserved

Mericon Industries, Inc.
8819 N. PIONEER ROAD
PEORIA, IL 61615

Direct Inquiries to:
William R. Connelly
(309) 693-2150
FAX: (309) 693-2158

FLORICAL®   OTC
[*flor ĭ cal*]
(fluoride and calcium supplement)

ACTIVE INGREDIENTS
Florical® contains 3.75 mg fluoride (as sodium fluoride), 145 mg calcium (as calcium carbonate)

DIRECTIONS
Take one tablet or capsule daily, or as recommended by physician.

HOW SUPPLIED
Florical® is supplied as tablets or capsules in bottles of 100 or 500.
NDC 00394-0102 (100) and NDC 00394-0100-05

MONOCAL®   OTC
[*mon ŏ cal*]
(fluoride and calcium supplement)

ACTIVE INGREDIENTS
Monocal® contains 3 mg fluoride (as monofluorophosphate) and 250 mg calcium (as calcium carbonate)

DIRECTIONS
Take one tablet daily, or as recommended by physician.

HOW SUPPLIED
Monocal® is supplied as tablets in bottles of 100.
NDC 00394-0105-02

EDUCATIONAL MATERIAL

1. SAMPLES
2. "A RANDOMIZED, CONTROLLED STUDY OF THE CHANGES IN BONE DENSITY IN RESPONSE TO MONOFLUOROPHOSPHATE AND CALCIUM IN OSTEOPOROTIC PATIENTS"
AMY E. SHAW M.D., PEGGY J. JENNINGS Ph.D, JENIFER JOWSEY Ph.D, ROBERT B. MIMS M.D. JAMES K. GUDE M.D.

Merz Pharmaceuticals
DIVISION OF MERZ, INC.
4215 TUDOR LANE (27410)
P.O. Box 18806
GREENSBORO, NC 27419
(formerly Mayrand Pharmaceuticals)

Direct Inquiries to:
Dr. Robert P. Halliday
(910) 856-2003
FAX: (910) 856-0107

For Medical Information Contact:
In Emergencies:
Dr. Robert P. Halliday
(910) 856-2003
FAX: (910) 856-0107
(formerly Mayrand Pharmaceuticals)

ANATUSS® DM SYRUP   OTC

DESCRIPTION
Each 5 ml of ANATUSS DM SYRUP for oral administration contains:

Guaifenesin	100 mg
Pseudoephedrine Hydrochloride	30 mg
Dextromethorphan Hydrobromide	10 mg

In a good tasting cherry flavored vehicle.

HOW SUPPLIED
ANATUSS DM SYRUP is supplied in pints NDC #0259-0383-16, 4 oz bottles NDC #0259-0383-04.

ANATUSS® DM TABLETS   OTC

DESCRIPTION
Each orange, oval European scored ANATUSS DM TABLET for oral administration contains:

Guaifenesin	400 mg
Pseudoephedrine Hydrochloride	60 mg
Dextromethorphan Hydrobromide	20 mg

HOW SUPPLIED
ANATUSS DM TABLETS are available as orange, oval shaped caplets, deep-scored on one side with an "M" appearing on the left of the score and an "P" appearing on the right of the score and 0382 appearing on the bottom side of the tablet.
In bottles of 100: NDC #0259-0382-01, in bottles of 20: NDC #0259-0382-21.

ANATUSS® LA TABLETS   ℞

DESCRIPTION
Each off-white European scored Anatuss LA Tablet for oral administration contains:

Guaifenesin	400 mg
Pseudoephedrine Hydrochloride	120 mg

Guaifenesin, 3-(2-methoxyphenoxy)-1,2-Propanediol, a white odorless, crystalline material with a slightly bitter aromatic taste. Pseudoephedrine Hydrochloride, [1-(methylamino) ethyl]benzenemethanol, a white crystalline, almost odorless powder with a bitter taste.

HOW SUPPLIED
Anatuss LA Tablets are available as off-white oval-shaped tablets, deep-scored on one side with an "M" appearing on the left of the score and an "R" appearing on the right of the score and 0379 appearing on the bottom side of the tablet.
In bottles of 100: NDC #0259-0379-01.

ELDERCAPS®   ℞

DESCRIPTION
Each capsule contains: Vitamin A Acetate, 4000 I.U.; Vitamin D₂, 400 I.U.; Vitamin E, 25 I.U.; Ascorbic Acid, 200 mg.; Thiamine Mononitrate, 10 mg.; Riboflavin, 5 mg.; Pyridoxine HCl, 2 mg.; Niacinamide, 25 mg.; d-Calcium Pantothenate, 10 mg.; Zinc Sulfate, 110 mg.; Magnesium Sulfate, 70 mg.; Manganese Sulfate, 5 mg.; Folic Acid, 1 mg.

HOW SUPPLIED
ELDERCAPS are supplied in bottles of 100: NDC #0259-1337-01.

Continued on next page

Merz Pharmaceuticals—Cont.

ELDERTONIC® OTC

DESCRIPTION
Each 45 ml. contains: Thiamine HCl, 1.5 mg.; Riboflavin, 1.7 mg. (as Riboflavin 5'-Phosphate Sodium); Pyridoxine HCl, 2.0 mg.; Cyanocobalamin, 6.0 mcg.; Dexpanthenol, 10.0 mg.; Niacinamide, 20.0 mg.; Zinc, 15 mg. (as zinc sulfate); Manganese, 2.0 mg. (as manganese sulfate); Magnesium (minimum content as added magnesium), 2.0 mg. (as magnesium sulfate); Alcohol, 13.5%.
In a special sherry wine base.

INDICATIONS
B-complex vitamins with minerals for nutritional supplementation.

DOSAGE
Adults: one tablespoonful three times a day with meals.

WARNING
Do not exceed recommended dosage unless directed by a physician.

USAGE IN PREGNANCY
Safe use of this product in pregnancy has not been established.

CAUTION
Keep out of the reach of children.

HOW SUPPLIED
ELDERTONIC available in 8 oz. bottles: NDC #0259-0351-08, Pint bottles: NDC #0259-0351-16, Quart bottles: NDC #0259-0351-32, Gallons: NDC #0259-0351-28.

MAY–VITA® ELIXIR R

DESCRIPTION
Each 45 ml. contains: Dexpanthenol, 10 mg; Niacinamide, 40 mg.; Pyridoxine HCl (B-6), 4 mg.; Cyanocobalamin (B-12), 12 mcg.; Folic Acid, 1 mg.; Iron, 36 mg. (as polysaccharide iron complex); Zinc, 15 mg. (as zinc sulfate); Manganese, 4 mg. (as manganese sulfate); Alcohol, 13%.

INDICATIONS
For vitamin and mineral replacement therapy in deficiency states and for treatment of iron deficiency anemia and/or nutritional megaloblastic anemias due to inadequate diet.

WARNINGS
Folic acid alone is improper therapy in the treatment of pernicious anemia and other megaloblastic anemias where vitamin B_{12} is deficient.

PRECAUTIONS
Folic acid, especially in doses above 0.1 mg. daily, may obscure pernicious anemia, in that hematologic remission may occur while neurological manifestations remain progressive.

ADVERSE REACTIONS
Allergic sensitization has been reported following both oral and parenteral administration of folic acid.

USE IN PREGNANCY
Safe use of this product in pregnancy has not been established.

DOSAGE
Usual adult dosage is one tablespoonful three times daily with meals. Do not exceed recommended dosage unless directed by a physician.

HOW SUPPLIED
MAY-VITA ELIXIR is supplied in Pint bottles: NDC #0259-0366-16.

NU-IRON® 150 CAPSULES OTC
(polysaccharide-iron complex)
NU-IRON® ELIXIR (polysaccharide-iron complex)
Sugar Free

DESCRIPTION
NU-IRON is a highly water soluble complex of iron and a low molecular weight polysaccharide.
Each NU-IRON 150 Capsule contains:
Iron (elemental) .... 150 mg.
(as Polysaccharide Iron Complex)
Each 5 ml. of NU-IRON Elixir contains:
Iron (elemental) .... 100 mg.
(as Polysaccharide Iron Complex)
Alcohol 10%

ACTION AND USES
NU-IRON is a non-ionic, easily assimilated, relatively non-toxic form of iron. Full therapeutic doses may be achieved with virtually no gastrointestinal side effects. There is no metallic aftertaste and no staining of teeth.

INDICATIONS
For treatment of uncomplicated iron deficiency anemia.

CONTRAINDICATIONS
Hemochromatosis, hemosiderosis or a known hypersensitivity to any of the ingredients.

DOSAGE
ADULTS: One or two NU-IRON 150 Capsules daily, or one or two teaspoonsful NU-IRON Elixir daily. CHILDREN; 6 to 12 years old; one teaspoonful NU-IRON Elixir daily. For younger children consult physician.

HOW SUPPLIED
NU-IRON 150 CAPSULES in bottles of 100: NDC #0259-0291-01, in bottles of 500: NDC #0259-0291-50.
NU-IRON ELIXIR in 8 oz bottles: NDC #0259-0292-08.

NU–IRON® PLUS ELIXIR R
(polysaccharide-iron complex)
Sugar Free

DESCRIPTION
Each 5 ml of NU-IRON PLUS ELIXIR contains:
Iron (elemental) (as Polysaccharide Iron Complex)	100 mg
Folic Acid	1 mg
Vitamin B12	25 mcg
Alcohol	10%

HOW SUPPLIED
NU-IRON PLUS ELIXIR is supplied in 8 oz bottles: NDC #0259-0342-08.

NU–IRON® V TABLETS R
(polysaccharide-iron complex with vitamins)

DESCRIPTION
Each maroon film-coated tablet contains:
IRON, ELEMENTAL (As a polysaccharide-iron complex) 60 mg; Folic Acid 1 mg; Ascorbic Acid 50 mg. (as sodium ascorbate); Cyanocobalamin (Vitamin B-12) 3 mcg.; Vitamin A 4000 I.U.; Vitamin D-2 400 I.U.; Thiamine Mononitrate 3 mg.; Riboflavin 3 mg.; Pyridoxine Hydrochloride 2 mg.; Niacinamide 10 mg.; Calcium Carbonate 312 mg.

HOW SUPPLIED
NU-IRON V TABLETS are available as maroon film-coated capsule-shaped tablets. In bottles of 100: NDC #0259-0331-01.

SEDAPAP® TABLETS R
(Butalbital and Acetaminophen Tablets)
50 mg/650 mg

DESCRIPTION
Butalbital and acetaminophen is supplied in tablet form for oral administration.
Butalbital (5-allyl-5-isobutylbarbituric acid), a slightly bitter, white, odorless, crystalline powder, is a short to intermediate-acting barbiturate. It has the following structural formula:

$C_{11}H_{16}N_2O_3$ MW = 224.26

Acetaminophen (4'-hydroxyacetanalide), a slightly bitter, white, odorless, crystalline powder, is a non-opiate, non-salicylate analgesic and antipyretic. It has the following structural formula:

$C_8H_9NO_2$ MW = 151.16

Each tablet contains:
Butalbital, USP .... 50 mg
Warning: May be habit forming
Acetaminophen, USP .... 650 mg

In addition each tablet contains the following inactive ingredients: Corn Starch, Gelatin, Magnesium Stearate, Microcrystalline Cellulose, Pregelatinized Starch, Sodium Starch Glycolate.

CLINICAL PHARMACOLOGY
This combination drug product is intended as a treatment for tension headache.
It consists of a fixed combination of butalbital and acetaminophen. The role each component plays in the relief of the complex of symptoms known as tension headache is incompletely understood.
Pharmacokinetics: The behavior of the individual components is described below.
Butalbital: Butalbital is well absorbed from the gastrointestinal tract and is expected to distribute to most tissues in the body. Barbiturates in general may appear in breast milk and readily cross the placental barrier. They are bound to plasma and tissue proteins to a varying degree and binding increases directly as a function of lipid solubility.
Elimination of butalbital is primarily via the kidney (59% to 88% of the dose) as unchanged drug or metabolites. The plasma half-life is about 35 hours. Urinary excretion products include parent drug (about 3.6% of the dose), 5-isobutyl-5-(2,3-dihydroxypropyl) barbituric acid (about 24% of the dose), 5-allyl-5-(3-hydroxy-2-methyl-1-propyl) barbituric acid (about 4.8% of the dose), products with the barbituric acid ring hydrolyzed with excretion of urea (about 14% of the dose), as well as unidentified materials. Of the material excreted in the urine, 32% is conjugated.
See OVERDOSAGE for toxicity information.
Acetaminophen: Acetaminophen is rapidly absorbed from the gastrointestinal tract and is distributed throughout most body tissues. The plasma half-life is 1.25 to 3 hours, but may be increased by liver damage and following overdosage. Elimination of acetaminophen is principally by liver metabolism (conjugation) and subsequent renal excretion of metabolites. Approximately 85% of an oral dose appears in the urine within 24 hours of administration, most as the glucuronide conjugate, with small amounts of other conjugates and unchanged drug.
See OVERDOSAGE for toxicity information.

INDICATIONS AND USAGE
Butalbital and acetaminophen tablets are indicated for the relief of the symptom complex of tension (or muscle contraction) headache.
Evidence supporting the efficacy and safety of this combination product in the treatment of multiple recurrent headaches is unavailable. Caution in this regard is required because butalbital is habit-forming and potentially abusable.

CONTRAINDICATIONS
This product is contraindicated under the following conditions:
- Hypersensitivity or intolerance to any component of the product.
- Patients with porphyria.

WARNINGS
Butalbital is habit-forming and potentially abusable. Consequently, the extended use of this product is not recommended.

PRECAUTIONS
General: Butalbital and acetaminophen tablets should be prescribed with caution in certain special-risk patients, such as the elderly or debilitated, and those with severe impairment of renal or hepatic function, or acute abdominal conditions.
Information for Patients: This product may impair mental and/or physical abilities required for the performance of potentially hazardous tasks such as driving a car or operating machinery. Such tasks should be avoided while taking this product.
Alcohol and other CNS depressants may produce an additive CNS depression, when taken with this combination product, and should be avoided.
Butalbital may be habit-forming. Patients should take the drug only for as long as it is prescribed, in the amounts prescribed, and no more frequently than prescribed.
Laboratory Tests: In patients with severe hepatic or renal disease, effects of therapy should be monitored with serial liver and/or renal function tests.

DRUG INTERACTIONS
The CNS effects of butalbital may be enhanced by monoamine oxidase (MAO) inhibitors.
Butalbital and acetaminophen may enhance the effects of: other narcotic analgesics, alcohol, general anesthetics, tranquilizers such as chlordiazepoxide, sedative-hypnotics, or other CNS depressants, causing increased CNS depression.
Drug/Laboratory Test Interactions: Acetaminophen may produce false-positive test results for urinary 5-hydroxyindoleacetic acid.

Carcinogenesis, Mutagenesis, Impairment of Fertility: No adequate studies have been conducted in animals to determine whether acetaminophen or butalbital have a potential for carcinogenesis, mutagenesis or impairment of fertility.

Pregnancy: *Teratogenic Effects:* Pregnancy Category C: Animal reproduction studies have not been conducted with this combination product. It is also not known whether butalbital and acetaminophen can cause fetal harm when administered to a pregnant woman or can affect reproduction capacity. This product should be given to a pregnant woman only when clearly needed.

Nonteratogenic Effects: Withdrawal seizures were reported in a two-day-old male infant whose mother had taken butalbital-containing drug during the last two months of pregnancy. Butalbital was found in the infant's serum. The infant was given phenobarbital 5 mg/kg, which was tapered without further seizure or other withdrawal symptoms.

Nursing Mothers: Barbiturates and acetaminophen are excreted in breast milk in small amounts, but the significance of their effects on nursing infants is not known. Because of potential for serious adverse reactions in nursing infants from butalbital and acetaminophen, a decision should be made whether to discontinue nursing or to discontinue the drug, taking into account the importance of the drug to the mother.

Pediatric Use: Safety and effectiveness in children below the age of 12 have not been established.

ADVERSE REACTIONS

Frequently Observed: The most frequently reported adverse reactions are drowsiness, lightheadedness, dizziness, sedation, shortness of breath, nausea, vomiting, abdominal pain, and intoxicated feeling.

Infrequently Observed: All adverse events tabulated below are classified as infrequent.

Central Nervous: headache, shaky feeling, tingling, agitation, fainting, fatigue, heavy eyelids, high energy, hot spells, numbness, sluggishness, seizure. Mental confusion, excitement or depression can also occur due to intolerance, particularly in elderly or debilitated patients, or due to overdosage of butalbital.

Autonomic Nervous: dry mouth, hyperhidrosis.

Gastrointestinal: difficulty swallowing, heartburn, flatulence, constipation.

Cardiovascular: tachycardia.

Musculoskeletal: leg pain, muscle fatigue.

Genitourinary: diuresis.

Miscellaneous: pruritus, fever, earache, nasal congestion, tinnitus, euphoria, allergic reactions.

Several cases of dermatological reactions, including toxic epidermal necrolysis and erythema multiforme, have been reported.

The following adverse drug events may be borne in mind as potential effects of the components of this product. Potential effects of high dosage are listed in the OVERDOSAGE section.

Acetaminophen: allergic reactions, rash, thrombocytopenia, agranulocytosis.

DRUG ABUSE AND DEPENDENCE

Abuse and Dependence: Butalbital: *Barbiturates may be habit-forming:* Tolerance, psychological dependence, and physical dependence may occur especially following prolonged use of high doses of barbiturates. The average daily dose for the barbiturate addict is usually about 1500 mg. As tolerance to barbiturates develops, the amount needed to maintain the same level of intoxication increases; tolerance to a fatal dosage, however, does not increase more than two-fold. As this occurs, the margin between an intoxication dosage and fatal dosage becomes smaller. The lethal dose of a barbiturate is far less if alcohol is also ingested. Major withdrawal symptoms (convulsions and delirium) may occur within 16 hours and last up to 5 days after abrupt cessation of these drugs. Intensity of withdrawal symptoms gradually declines over a period of approximately 15 days. Treatment of barbiturate dependence consists of cautious and gradual withdrawal of the drug. Barbiturate-dependent patients can be withdrawn by using a number of different withdrawal regimens. One method involves initiating treatment at the patient's regular dosage level and gradually decreasing the daily dosage as tolerated by the patient.

OVERDOSAGE

Following an acute overdosage of butalbital and acetaminophen, toxicity may result from the barbiturate or the acetaminophen.

Signs and Symptoms: Toxicity from barbiturate poisoning include drowsiness, confusion, and coma; respiratory depression; hypotension; and hypovolemic shock.

In acetaminophen overdosage: dose-dependent, potentially fatal hepatic necrosis is the most serious adverse effect. Renal tubular necroses, hypoglycemic coma and thrombocytopenia may also occur. Early symptoms following a potentially hepatotoxic overdose may include: nausea, vomiting, diaphoresis and general malaise. Clinical and laboratory evidence of hepatic toxicity may not be apparent until 48 to 72 hours post-ingestion. In adults hepatic toxicity has rarely been reported with acute overdoses of less than 10 grams, or fatalities with less than 15 grams.

Treatment: A single or multiple overdose with this combination product is a potentially lethal polydrug overdose, and consultation with a regional poison control center is recommended.

Immediate treatment includes support of cardiorespiratory function and measures to reduce drug absorption. Vomiting should be induced mechanically, or with syrup of ipecac, if the patient is alert (adequate pharyngeal and laryngeal reflexes). Oral activated charcoal (1 g/kg) should follow gastric emptying. The first dose should be accompanied by an appropriate cathartic. If repeated doses are used, the cathartic might be included with alternate doses as required. Hypotension is usually hypovolemic and should respond to fluids. Pressors should be avoided. A cuffed endotracheal tube should be inserted before gastric lavage of the unconscious patient and, when necessary, to provide assisted respiration. If renal function is normal, forced diuresis may aid in the elimination of the barbiturate. Alkalinization of the urine increases renal excretion of some barbiturates, especially phenobarbital.

Meticulous attention should be given to maintaining adequate pulmonary ventilation. In severe cases of intoxication, peritoneal dialysis, or preferably hemodialysis may be considered. If hypoprothrombinemia occurs due to acetaminophen overdose, vitamin K should be administered intravenously.

If the dose of acetaminophen may have exceeded 140 mg/kg, acetylcysteine should be administered as early as possible. Serum acetaminophen levels should be obtained, since levels four or more hours following ingestion help predict acetaminophen toxicity. Do not await acetaminophen assay results before initiating treatment. Hepatic enzymes should be obtained initially, and repeated at 24-hour intervals. Methemoglobinemia over 30% should be treated with methylene blue by slow intravenous administration.

Toxic Doses (for adults):

Butalbital: toxic dose 1 g	(20 tablets)
Acetaminophen: toxic dose 10 g	(15 tablets)

DOSAGE AND ADMINISTRATION

One tablet every four hours. Total daily dosage should not exceed 6 tablets.

Extended and repeated use of this product is not recommended because of the potential for physical dependence.

HOW SUPPLIED

SEDAPAP TABLETS [Butalbital 50 mg (WARNING: May be habit forming) and Acetaminophen 650 mg] are available as white capsule shaped tablets scored on one side with an "M" appearing on the left side of the score, and an "R" appearing on the right side of the score and "1278" on the other. In bottles of 100, NDC #0259-1278-01.

Rev. 2/96

STERAPRED® 5 mg UNIPAK   ℞
STERAPRED® 5 mg 12 Day UNIPAK

DESCRIPTION

Each white tablet contains:
Prednisone .... 5 mg.

HOW SUPPLIED

STERAPRED 5 mg UNIPAK available in 21 tablet tapered dose dispensing pack. NDC #0259-0390-21.
STERAPRED 5 mg 12 DAY UNIPAK available in 48 tablet tapered dose dispensing pack. NDC #0259-0391-48

STERAPRED® DS UNIPAK   ℞
STERAPRED® DS 12 DAY UNIPAK

DESCRIPTION

Each white tablet contains:
Prednisone .... 10 mg.

HOW SUPPLIED

STERAPRED DS UNIPAK available in 21 tablet tapered dose dispensing pack: NDC #0259-0364-21.
STERAPRED DS 12 DAY UNIPAK available in 48 tablet tapered dose dispensing pack: NDC #0259-0389-48.

For information on over-the-counter drugs, consult **PDR For Nonprescription Drugs**

Miles Inc.
Pharmaceutical Division
Allergy Products
Biological Products
400 MORGAN LANE
WEST HAVEN, CT 06516

Due to a corporate name change, please see Bayer Corporation.

Milex Products, Inc.
5915 NORTHWEST HIGHWAY
CHICAGO, IL 60631

Direct Inquiries to:
(312) 631-6484

AMINO-CERV™   ℞
[ah-me'no-serv]
pH 5.5 Cervical Creme

ACTIVE INGREDIENTS

Urea 8.34%, Sodium Propionate 0.50%, Methionine 0.83%, Cystine 0.35%, Inositol 0.83%, Benzalkonium Chloride 0.000004%. Buffered to pH of 5.5 in a water-miscible creme base.

DESCRIPTION

An AMINO-ACID and UREA creme specifically formulated for cervical treatment: Cervicitis (mild), postpartum cervicitis, postpartum cervical tears, post surgical cervical procedures.

ADVANTAGES

METHIONINE and CYSTINE are amino-acids necessary for wound healing and forming of epithelial tissue. INOSITOL acts as an essential growth factor and promotes epithelialization.

UREA aids in debridement, dissolves the coagulum and promotes epithelialization. Its solvent action on fibroblasts prevents the formation of excessive tissue—thus preventing stenosis when used as directed.

BENZALKONIUM CHLORIDE serves to lower surface tension and thus aids in spreading the medication. Along with SODIUM PROPIONATE it also exerts a bacteriostatic effect.

AMINO-CERV is geared to the higher pH of the healthy cervix in contrast with pH 4 vaginal preparations. With its pH factor of 5.5 Amino-Cerv promotes faster healing of the cervix, yet will not adversely affect a healthy vagina.

DIRECTIONS

When immediate postpartum bleeding has subsided (usually from 24 to 48 hours after delivery), one Milex Jector full of AMINO-CERV creme should be applied nightly for four weeks. In mild cervicitis (not requiring cautery or cryosurgery) one applicatorful of AMINO-CERV should be injected in the vagina nightly upon retiring for 2 weeks. A small amount of AMINO-CERV should be applied immediately following a surgical cervical procedure with the exception of a cold coning procedure. One applicatorful should be injected nightly upon retiring for 2 to 4 weeks (the duration of treatment depends on extent of the surgical procedure). In each of the post surgical visits, the physician should again apply a small amount of AMINO-CERV with a probe or applicator. The canal is to be completely probed on the last visit.

After COLD CONING, one applicatorful should be injected upon retiring about 24 hours after surgery and nightly thereafter for four weeks. During the four weekly office visits following cold coning, a small amount of AMINO-CERV should be applied with a probe or applicator into the canal by the physician. The canal is to be completely probed on the last visit.

Reasons For Variation of Directions
(1) After most surgical procedures, cauterization, cryosurgery and laser surgery, immediate use of AMINO-CERV is indicated to aid in dissolving dead or burned tissue.
(2) After cold coning, there is no dead tissue to slough off. Therefore, a wait of 24 hours or longer is desirable for normal healing to take place and for some fibroblasts to be laid down before applying the AMINO-CERV (which has a solvent action on both the fibroblasts and the absorbable sutures). When NONABSORBABLE sutures are used, AMINO-CERV can be used immediately.

Continued on next page

Milex—Cont.

CONTRAINDICATIONS
Deleterious side effects have not been a problem at the doses recommended. The usual precautions against allergic reactions should be observed.

STORAGE
Store at room temperature.

PACKAGING
$2^3/_4$ oz. tube with MILEX-JECTOR (2 weeks supply, 14 applications).

Mission Pharmacal Company
10999 IH 10 WEST
SUITE 1000
SAN ANTONIO, TX 78230-1355

Direct Inquiries to:
PO Box 786099
San Antonio, TX 78278–6099
(210) 696-8400
FAX: (210) 696-6010
For Medical Information Contact:
In Emergencies:
George Alexandrides
(210) 533-7118
FAX: (210) 533-4487

CITRACAL®   OTC
[*sit'ra-cal*]
ultradense calcium citrate

ACTIVE INGREDIENTS
CITRACAL® is supplied in an ultra-dense tablet formulation, each containing 950 mg. calcium citrate.

OTHER INGREDIENTS
Polyethylene glycol, povidone, croscarmellose, carnauba wax, bee's wax, magnesium stearate.

SENSITIVE PATIENTS
CITRACAL® is synthesized as a small, easily swallowed tablet, free of gluten (wheat) and dairy products.

ONE TABLET PROVIDES
200 mg. calcium (elemental), equaling 20% of the U.S. recommended daily allowance for adults and children 4 or more years of age.

FOUR TABLETS PROVIDE
800 mg. calcium (elemental), equaling 80% of the U.S. recommended daily allowance for adults and children 4 or more years of age.

DIRECTIONS
Take 1 to 2 tablets twice daily or as recommended by a physician.

HOW SUPPLIED
CITRACAL® is available in bottles of 100. **NDC** 0178-0800-01and bottles of 200 **NDC** 0178-0800-20.

CITRACAL® Caplets + D   OTC
[*sit'ra-cal*]
ultradense calcium citrate

ACTIVE INGREDIENTS
CITRACAL® Caplets + D are supplied in an ultra-dense caplet formulation, each containing 1500 mg. calcium citrate and 200 USPU Vitamin D_3.

HOW SUPPLIED
CITRACAL® Caplets + D are available in bottles of 60. **NDC** 0178-0815-60. And bottles of 120 NDC 0178-0815-12

CITRACAL® LIQUITAB®   OTC
[*sit'ra-cal*]

ACTIVE INGREDIENTS: CITRACAL® LIQUITAB® is supplied as effervescent tablets each containing 2376 mg. of calcium citrate.

This product contains NutraSweet®.

HOW SUPPLIED
CITRACAL® LIQUITAB® is available in bottles of 30 tablets. **NDC** 0178-0811-30.

CALCET®   OTC
[*kăl'cet*]
Calcium Supplement
NDC-0178-0251-01

HOW SUPPLIED
CALCET® tablets are supplied as yellow, bolus shaped, coated tablets in bottles of 100 tablets.

CALCET PLUS®   OTC
[*kăl'cet*]
Calcium-Iron-Zinc-Multivitamin
NDC 0178-0252-60

HOW SUPPLIED
CALCET PLUS tablets are supplied as white, oval shaped, coated tablets in bottles of 60's.

FOSFREE®   OTC
[*fos'frē*]
Calcium—Vitamins—Iron
NDC 0178-0031-60
NDC 0178-0031-12

HOW SUPPLIED
FOSFREE® is supplied as yellow, elliptical shaped, coated tablets in bottles of either 60 or 120 tablets.

IROMIN-G®   OTC
[*i'rŏ-min*]
Hematinic Supplement
NDC-0178-0081-01

HOW SUPPLIED
IROMIN-G® is supplied as red bolus shaped coated tablets in bottles of 100 tablets.

MISSION PRENATAL SERIES

MISSION PRENATAL®   OTC
Vitamins—Iron—Calcium—.4 mg. Folic Acid
NDC 0178-0132-01

MISSION PRENATAL® F.A   OTC
Vitamins—Iron—Calcium—.8 mg. Folic Acid and Zinc
NDC 0178-0153-01

MISSION PRENATAL® H.P.   OTC
Vitamins—Iron—Calcium—0.8 mg. Folic Acid
NDC 0178-0161-01

HOW SUPPLIED
MISSION® PRENATAL is supplied as pink, bolus-shaped, sugar-coated tablets in bottles of 100.
MISSION® PRENATAL F.A. is supplied as blue, bolus-shaped, sugar coated tablets in bottles of 100.
MISSION® PRENATAL H.P. is supplied as green, bolus-shaped, sugar-coated tablets in bottles of 100.

MISSION PRENATAL® Rx   ℞
Prenatal Supplement with
Vitamins and Minerals
NDC 0178-0007-01

HOW SUPPLIED
MISSION PRENATAL Rx is supplied as pink, oval shape, film-coated tablets in bottles of 100.

MISSION PHARMACAL UROLOGICALS

UROCIT®-K   ℞
[*yu'ro-cĭt kay*]
Potassium Citrate

DESCRIPTION
Urocit®-K is a citrate salt of potassium. Its empirical formula is $K_3C_6H_5O_7 \cdot H_2O$, and its structural formula is:

$$HO-\overset{\displaystyle CH_2-COOK}{\underset{\displaystyle CH_2-COOK}{\overset{|}{\underset{|}{C}}}}-COOK \cdot H_2O$$

Potassium citrate is a white granular powder that is soluble in water at 154 g/100 ml, almost insoluble in alcohol, and insoluble in organic solvents.
Urocit®-K is supplied as wax matrix tablets, containing 5 meq (540 mg) potassium citrate and 10 meq (1080 mg) potassium citrate each, for oral administration.

CLINICAL PHARMACOLOGY
When Urocit®-K is given orally, the metabolism of absorbed citrate produces an alkaline load. The induced alkaline load in turn increases urinary pH and raises urinary citrate by augmenting citrate clearance without measurably altering ultrafilterable serum citrate. Thus, Urocit®-K therapy appears to increase urinary citrate principally by modifying the renal handling of citrate, rather than by increasing the filtered load of citrate. The increased filtered load of citrate may play some role, however, as in small comparisons of oral citrate and oral bicarbonate, citrate had a greater effect on urinary citrate.
In addition to raising urinary pH and citrate, Urocit®-K increases urinary potassium by approximately the amount contained in the medication. In some patients, Urocit®-K causes a transient reduction in urinary calcium.
The changes induced by Urocit®-K produce a urine that is less conducive to the crystallization of stone-forming salts (calcium oxalate, calcium phosphate and uric acid). Increased citrate in the urine, by complexing with calcium, decreases calcium ion activity and thus the saturation of calcium oxalate. Citrate also inhibits the spontaneous nucleation of calcium oxalate and calcium phosphate (brushite). The increase in urinary pH also decreases calcium ion activity by increasing calcium complexation to dissociated anions. The rise in urinary pH also increases the ionization of uric acid to more soluble urate ion.
Urocit®-K therapy does not alter the urinary saturation of calcium phosphate, since the effect of increased citrate complexation of calcium is opposed by the rise in pH-dependent dissociation of phosphate. Calcium phosphate stones are more stable in alkaline urine.
In the setting of normal renal function, the rise in urinary citrate following a single dose begins by the first hour and lasts for 12 hours. With multiple doses the rise in citrate excretion reaches its peak by the third day and averts the normally wide circadian fluctuation in urinary citrate, thus maintaining urinary citrate at a higher, more constant level throughout the day. When the treatment is withdrawn, urinary citrate begins to decline toward the pre-treatment level on the first day.
The rise in citrate excretion is directly dependent on the Urocit®-K dosage. Following long-term treatment, Urocit®-K at a dosage of 60 meq/day raises urinary citrate by approximately 400 mg/day and increases urinary pH by approximately 0.7 units.
In patients with severe renal tubular acidosis or chronic diarrheal syndrome where urinary citrate may be very low (<100 mg/day), Urocit®-K may be relatively ineffective in raising urinary citrate. A higher dose of Urocit®-K may therefore be required to produce a satisfactory citraturic response. In patients with renal tubular aciidosis in whom urinary pH may be high, Urocit®-K produces a relatively small rise in urinary pH.

INDICATIONS AND USAGE
Potassium citrate is indicated for the management of renal tubular acidosis (RTA) with calcium stones, hypocitraturic calcium oxalate nephrolithiasis of any etiology, and uric acid lithiasis with or without calcium stones.

CONTRAINDICATIONS
Urocit®-K is contraindicated in patients with hyperkalemia (or who have conditions predisposing them to hyperkalemia), as a further rise in serum potassium concentration may produce cardiac arrest. Such conditions include: chronic renal failure, uncontrolled diabetes mellitus, acute dehydration, strenuous physical exercise in unconditioned individuals, adrenal insufficiency, extensive tissue breakdown, or the administration of a potassium-sparing agent (such as triamterene, spironolactone or amiloride).
Urocit®-K is contraindicated in patients in whom there is cause for arrest or delay in tablet passage through the gastrointestinal tract, such as those suffering from delayed gastric emptying, esophageal compression, intestinal obstruction or stricture or those taking anticholinergic medication.

Because of its ulcerogenic potential, Urocit®-K should not be given to patients with peptic ulcer disease.

Urocit®-K is contraindicated in patients with active urinary tract infection (with either urea-splitting or other organisms, in association with either calcium or struvite stones). The ability of Urocit®-K to increase urinary citrate may be attenuated by bacterial enzymatic degradation of citrate. Moreover, the rise in urinary pH resulting from Urocit®-K therapy might promote further bacterial growth. Urocit®-K is contraindicated in patients with renal insufficiency (glomerular filtration rate of less than 0.7 ml/kg/min), because of the danger of soft tissue calcification and increased risk for the development of hyperkalemia.

WARNINGS

HYPERKALEMIA: In patients with impaired mechanisms for excreting potassium, Urocit®-K administration can produce hyperkalemia and cardiac arrest. Potentially fatal hyperkalemia can develop rapidly and be asymptomatic. The use of Urocit®-K in patients with chronic renal failure, or any other condition which impairs potassium excretion such as severe myocardial damage or heart failure, should be avoided.

INTERACTION WITH POTASSIUM-SPARING DIURETICS

Concomitant administration of Urocit®-K and a potassium-sparing diuretic (such as triamterene, spironolactone or amiloride) should be avoided, since the simultaneous administration of these agents can produce severe hyperkalemia.

GASTROINTESTINAL LESIONS

Because of reports of upper gastrointestinal mucosal lesions following administration of potassium chloride (wax-matrix), and endoscopic examination of the upper gastrointestinal mucosa was performed in 30 normal volunteers after they had taken glycopyrrolate 2 mg. p.o. t.i.d., Urocit®-K 95 meq/day, wax-matrix potassium chloride 96 meq/day or wax matrix placebo, in thrice daily schedule in the fasting state for one week. Urocit®-K and the wax-matrix formulation of potassium chloride were indistinguishable but both were significantly more irritating than the wax-matrix placebo. In a subsequent similar study, lesions were less severe when glycopyrrolate was omitted.

Solid dosage forms of potassium chloride have produced stenotic and/or ulcerative lesions of the small bowel and deaths. These lesions are caused by a high local concentration of potassium ions in the region of the dissolving tablets, which injured the bowel. In addition, perhaps because wax-matrix preparations are not enteric-coated and release some of their potassium content in the stomach, there have been reports of upper gastrointestinal bleeding associated with these products. The frequency of gastrointestinal lesions with wax-matrix potassium chloride products is estimated at one per 100,000 patient-years. Experience with Urocit®-K is limited, but a similar frequency of gastrointestinal lesions should be anticipated.

If there is severe vomiting, abdominal pain or gastro-intestinal bleeding, Urocit®-K should be discontinued immediately and the possibility of bowel perforation or obstruction investigated.

PRECAUTIONS

Information For Patients:
Physicians should consider reminding the patient of the following:

To take each dose without crushing, chewing or sucking the tablet.

To take this medicine only as directed. This is especially important if the patient is also taking both diuretics and digitalis preparations.

To check with physician if there is trouble swallowing tablets or if the tablet seems to stick in the throat.

To check with the doctor at once if tarry stools or other evidence of gastrointestinal bleeding is noticed.

Laboratory Tests: Regular serum potassium determinations are recommended. Careful attention should be paid to acid-base balance, other serum electrolyte levels, the electrocardiogram, and the clinical status of the patient, particularly in the presence of cardiac disease, renal disease or acidosis.

Drug Interactions: POTASSIUM-SPARING DIURETICS: See WARNINGS section.

DRUGS THAT SLOW GASTROINTESTINAL TRANSIT TIME (such as anticholinergics) can be expected to increase the gastrointestinal irritation produced by potassium salts. (See CONTRAINDICATIONS section).

Carcinogenesis, Mutagenesis, Impairment Of Fertility: Long-term carcinogenicity studies in animals have not been performed.

Pregnancy Category C: Animal reproduction studies have not been conducted with Urocit®-K. It is also not known whether Urocit®-K can cause fetal harm when administered to a pregnant woman or can affect reproduction capacity. Urocit®-K should be given to a pregnant woman only if clearly needed.

Nursing Mothers: The normal potassium ion content of human milk is about 13 meq/l. It is not known if Urocit®-K has an effect on this content. Caution should be exercised when Urocit®-K is administered to a nursing woman.

Pediatric Use: Safety and effectiveness in children have not been established.

ADVERSE REACTIONS

Some patients may develop minor gastrointestinal complaints during Urocit®-K therapy, such as abdominal discomfort, vomiting, diarrhea, loose bowel movements or nausea. These symptoms are due to the irritation of the gastrointestinal tract, and may be alleviated by taking the dose with meals or snack, or by reducing the dosage. Patients may find intact matrices in feces. (See also CONTRAINDICATIONS, WARNINGS)

OVERDOSAGE

The administration of potassium salts to persons without predisposing conditions for hyperkalemia (see CONTRAINDICATIONS) rarely causes serious hyperkalemia at recommended dosages. It is important to recognize that hyperkalemia is usually asymptomatic and may be manifested only by an increased serum potassium concentration and characteristic electrocardiographic changes (peaking of T-wave, loss of P-wave, depression of S-T segment and prolongation of the QT interval). Late manifestations include muscle paralysis and cardiovascular collapse from cardiac arrest.

Treatment measures for hyperkalemia include the following: (1) elimination of potassium-rich foods, medications containing potassium, and of potassium-sparing diuretics, (2) intravenous administration of 300–500 ml/hr of 10% dextrose solution containing 10–20 units of insulin/1000 ml, (3) correction of acidosis, if present, with intravenous sodium bicarbonate, and (4) use of exchange resins, hemodialysis or peritoneal dialysis.

In treating hyperkalemia, it should be recalled that in patients who have been stabilized on digitalis, too rapid a lowering of the serum potassium concentration can produce digitalis toxicity.

DOSAGE AND ADMINISTRATION

Treatment with Urocit®-K should be added to a regimen that limits salt intake (avoidance of foods with high salt content and of added salt at the table) and encourages high fluid intake (urine volume should be at least two liters per day). The objective of treatment with Urocit®-K is to provide Urocit®-K in sufficient dosage to restore normal urinary citrate (greater than 320 mg/day and as close to the normal mean of 640 mg/day as possible), and to increase urinary pH to a level of 6.0 to 7.0.

In patients with severe hypocitraturia (urinary citrate of less than 150 mg/day), therapy should be initiated at a dosage of 60 meq/day (20 meq three times/day or 15 meq four times/day with meals or within 30 minutes after meals or bedtime snack). In patients with mild-moderate hypocitraturia (> 150 mg/day), Urocit®-K should be initiated at a dosage of 30 meq/day (10 meq three times/day with meals). Twenty-four hour urinary citrate and/or urinary pH measurements should be used to determine the adequacy of the initial dosage and to evaluate the effectiveness of any dosage change. In addition, urinary citrate and/or pH should be measured every four months.

Doses of Urocit®-K greater than 100 meq/day have not been studied and should be avoided.

Serum electrolytes (sodium, potassium, chloride and carbon dioxide), serum creatinine, and complete blood count should be monitored every four months. Treatment should be discontinued if there is hyperkalemia, a significant rise in serum creatinine, or a significant fall in blood hematocrit or hemoglobin.

HOW SUPPLIED

Urocit®-K is available for oral administration in tablet form in the following sizes: (NDC 0178-0600-01) 5 meq potassium citrate and (NDC 0178-0610-01) 10 meq potassium citrate, packaged in bottles of 100 each.

Store in a cool, dry place.

CAUTION: Federal law prohibits dispensing without a prescription.

Rev. 02890

Mission
PHARMACAL COMPANY
San Antonio, TX 78296-1676

LITHOSTAT® ℞
[lith 'o-stat]
Acetohydroxamic Acid (AHA)

DESCRIPTION

Acetohydroxamic acid (AHA) is a stable, synthetic compound derived from hydroxylamine and ethyl acetate. Its molecular structure is similar to urea:

[See chemical structure at top of next column.]

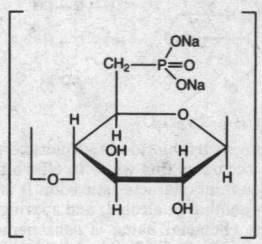

ACETOHYDROXAMIC ACID (AHA)

AHA is weakly acidic, highly soluble in water, and chelates metals - notably iron. The molecular weight is 75.068. AHA has a PKA of 9.32 and a melting point of 89–91°C. Available as 250 mg tablets.

HOW SUPPLIED

LITHOSTAT®, NDC 0178-0500-01, is available for oral administration as 250 mg scored tablets, in unit of use packages of 100 tablets.

THIOLA™ ℞
[thi-ól-a]
Tiopronin Tablets

DESCRIPTION

THIOLA™ (Tiopronin) is a reducing and complexing thiol compound. Tiopronin is N-(2-Mercaptopropionyl) glycine and has the following structure:

$$CH_3\text{-}CH\text{-}CONHCH_2\text{-}COOH$$
$$\mid$$
$$SH$$

Tiopronin has the empirical formula $C_5H_9NO_3S$ and a molecular weight of 163.20. It has one asymmetric center and therefore exists as dl (racemic) mixture.

Tiopronin is a white crystalline powder which is freely soluble in water.

THIOLA™ tablets are white sugar coated tablets, each containing 100 mg. of Tiopronin and are taken orally.

HOW SUPPLIED

THIOLA™ (NDC 0178-0900-01), is available for oral administration as 100 mg. round, white, sugar coated tablets in bottles of 100 tablets each.

For product information call: 1-800-531-3333
In Texas call: 1-800-292-7364

CALCIBIND® ℞
[kal 'sē-bīnd]
Cellulose Sodium Phosphate
Oral Powder

DESCRIPTION

Cellulose Sodium Phosphate (CSP), the active ingredient in CALCIBIND®, is a synthetic compound made by phosphorylation of cellulose and has the following structural formula:

Where n indicates the degree of polymerization and has an average value of approximately 3000. The molecular weight of CSP monomer is 286.1 and the average molecular weight of the polymer is 858,000.

It has an inorganic bound phosphate of 31–36%, free phosphate of 3.5%, sodium content of approximately 11% and a calcium binding capacity of 1.8 mmol of Ca per gram of the oral powder. It has excellent ion exchange properties, the sodium ion exchanging for calcium. When taken orally, CSP binds calcium, the complex of calcium and cellulose phosphate being excreted in feces. The dosage of CALCIBIND® is powder for oral administration.

HOW SUPPLIED

CALCIBIND® NDC 0178-0255-30 is available for oral administration in bottles of 300 grams of CSP bulk powder.

Continued on next page

Mission Pharamcal—Cont.

THERA-GESIC® OTC

[ther 'a-jē-zik]

Analgesic Creme Balm

Methyl Salicylate and Menthol

DESCRIPTION

THERA-GESIC® contains Methyl Salicylate and Menthol in a rapidly absorbed greaseless base.

ACTIONS

Topical analgesic, counterirritant.

INDICATIONS

For the temporary relief of pain associated with musculoskeletal soreness and discomfort; additionally, as a topical adjunct in arthritis, rheumatism, and bursitis.

HOW SUPPLIED

NDC-0178-0320-03	Tubes–3 oz.
NDC-0178-0320-05	Tubes–5 oz.
NDC-0178-0320-25	Pouches–¼ oz.

Monarch Pharmaceuticals

355 BEECHAM STREET
BRISTOL, TN 37620

Direct Inquiries to:
800-776-3637
FAX: 423-989-6279

Medical Emergency Contact:
Dr. Henry Richards, M.D.
800-546-4906
FAX: 423-989-6137

TUSSEND® CIII

DESCRIPTION

Each teaspoonful (5 mL) contains:

Hydrocodone Bitartrate*, USP:	2.5 mg
(*WARNING: May be habit forming)	
Pseudoephedrine Hydrochloride, USP	30 mg
Chlorpheniramine Maleate, USP	2 mg
Alcohol, USP	5%

Hydrocodone bitartrate is an opioid analgesic and antitussive and occurs as fine white, crystals or as crystalline powder. It is affected by light. The chemical name is 4,5α-epoxy-3-methoxy-17-methylmorphinan-6-one-tartrate (1:1) hydrate (2:5). Its structural formula is as follows:

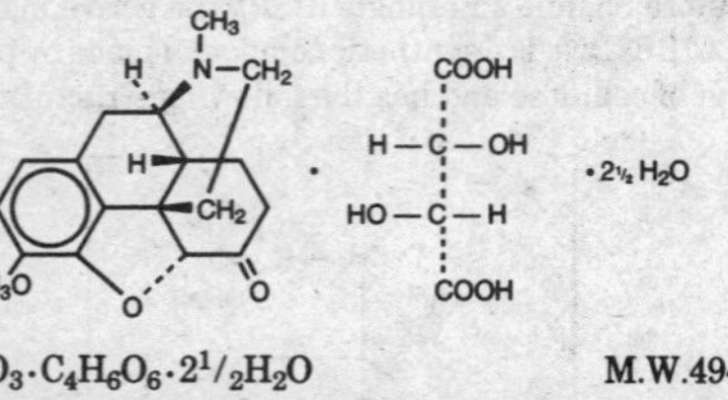

$C_{18}H_{21}NO_3 \cdot C_4H_6O_6 \cdot 2^1/_2H_2O$ M.W.494.50

Pseudoephedrine hydrochloride is an adrenergic (vasoconstrictor) which occurs as fine white to off-white crystals or powder, having a faint characteristic odor. It is very soluble in water, freely soluble in alcohol, and sparingly soluble in chloroform. The chemcial name is benzenemethanol, α[1-(methylamino)ethyl]-. [S-(R*,R*)]-hydrochloride. Its structural formula is as follows:

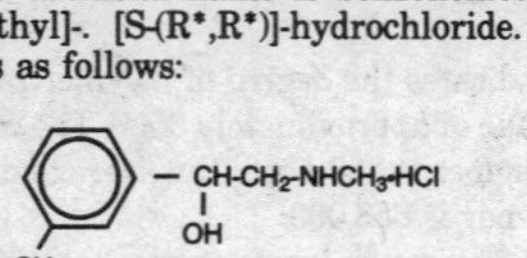

$C_{10}H_{15}NO$ HC1 M.W.201.70

Chlorpheniramine maleate is an antihistaminic that occurs as white, odorless, crystalline powder. Its solutions have a pH between 4 and 5. It is freely soluble in water, soluble in alcohol and in chloroform, and slightly soluble in ether and benzene. The chemical name is 2-pyridinepropanamine, α-(4-chlorophenyl)-N, N-dimethyl-(Z)-2-butenedioate (1:1). Its structural formula is as follows:

[See structure on top of next column.]

TUSSEND® also contains: High Fructose Corn Syrup, Sucrose, Propylene Glycol, Flavor, Methylparaben, Saccharin Sodium, Propylparaben, FD&C Yellow No. 6, and Purified Water, USP.

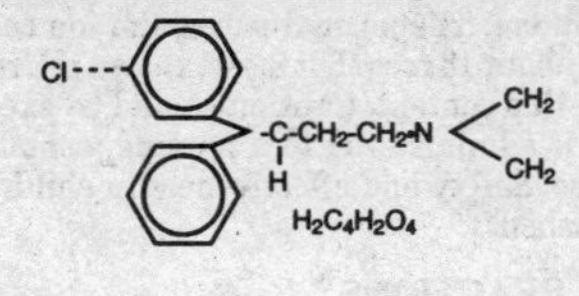

$C_{16}H_{19}ClN_2C_4H_4O_4$ M.W.390.87

CLINICAL PHARMACOLOGY

Hydrocodone is a semi-synthetic narcotic antitussive with multiple actions qualitatively similar to those of codeine. Most of these involve the central nervous system and smooth muscle. The precise mechanism of action of hydrocodone and other opiates is not known; however, hydrocodone is believed to act directly on the cough center. In excessive doses, hydrocodone, like other opium derivatives, will depress respiration. The effects of hydrocodone in therapeutic doses on the cardiovascular system are insignificant. Hydrocodone can produce miosis, euphoria, physical and physiological dependence.

Following a 10 mg oral dose of hydrocodone administered to five adult male subjects, the mean peak concentration was 23.6 +/− 5.2 ng/mL. Maximum serum levels were achieved at 1.3 +/− 0.3 hours and the half-life was determined to be 3.8 +/− 0.3 hours. Hydrocodone exhibits a complex pattern of metabolism including O-demethylation, N-demethylation and 6-keto reduction to the corresponding 6-α- and 6-β-hydroxymetabolites.

Pseudoephedrine acts as an indirect sympathomimetic agent by stimulating sympathetic (adrenergic) nerve endings to release norepinephrine. Norepinephrine in turn stimulates alpha and beta receptors throughout the body. The action of pseudoephedrine hydrochloride is apparently more specific for the blood vessels of the upper respiratory tract and less specific for the blood vessels of the systemic circulation. The vasoconstriction elicited at these sites results in the shrinkage of swollen tissues in the sinuses and nasal passages.

Pseudoephedrine is rapidly and almost completely absorbed from the gastrointestinal tract. Considerable variation in half-life has been observed (from about 45 to 10 hours) which is attributed to differences in absorption and excretion. Excretion rates are also altered by urine pH, increasing with acidification and decreasing with alkalinization. As a result, mean half-life falls to about 4 hours at pH 5 and increases to about 12 to 13 hours at pH 8. After administration of a 60 mg tablet, 87 to 97% of the pseudoephedrine is cleared from the body within 24 hours. The drug is distributed to body tissues and fluids, including fetal tissue, breast milk, and the central nervous system.

About 55% to 75% of an administered dose is excreted unchanged in the urine; the remainder is apparently metabolized in the liver to inactive compounds by N-demethylation, parahydroxylation, and oxidative deamination.

Chlorpheniramine is an antihistamine that possesses anticholinergic and sedative effects. It is considered one of the most effective and least toxic of the histamine antagonists. Chlorpheniramine is a H, receptor antagonist. It antagonizes many of the pharmacologic actions of histamine. It prevents released histamine from dilating capillaries and causing edema of the respiratory mucosa Chlorpheniramine is well absorbed and has a duration of action 4 to 6 hours. Its half-life in serum is 12 to 16 hours. Degradation products of chlorpheniramine's metabolic transformation by the liver are almost completely excreted in 24 hours.

INDICATIONS

TUSSEND® syrup is indicated for relief of cough and congestion due to colds, acute respiratory infections, laryngeal and pulmonary tuberculosis, acute and chronic bronchitis and hay fever. In addtion TUSSEND® syrup helps relieve the sneezing and itching associated with hay fever.

CONTRAINDICATIONS

Hypersensitivity to any of the ingredients. Patients known to be hypersensitive to other sympathomimetic amines may exhibit cross sensitivity with pseudoephedrine. Sympathomimetic amines are contraindicated in patients with severe coronary artery disease, and patients on monoamine oxidase (MAO) inhibitor therapy.

Antihistamines are contraindicated in patients with narrow-angle glaucoma, urinary retention, peptic ulcer, during an asthmatic attack and in patients receiving MAO inhibitors. TUSSEND® syrup should not be administered to pre-mature or full-term infants. TUSSEND® syrup is contraindicated in nursing mothers because of the higher than usual risk for infants from sympathomimetic amines.

WARNINGS

General: Sympathomimetic amines should be used with caution in patients with hypertension, ischemic heart disease, diabetes mellitus, increased intraocular pressure, hyperthyroidism, or prostatic hypertrophy. Sympathomimetics may produce central nervous system stimulation with convulsions or cardiovascular collapse with accompanying hypotension. DO NOT EXCEED RECOMMENDED DOSAGE.

Hypertensive crises can occur with concurrent use of pseudoephedrine and monoamine oxidase (MAO) inhibitors, indomethacin, or with beta blockers and methyldopa. If a hypertensive crises occurs, these drugs should be discontinued immediately and therapy to lower blood pressure should be instituted. Fever should be managed by means of external cooling.

Chlorpheniramine has an atropine-like action and should be used with caution in patients with increased intraocular pressure, cardiovascular disease, hypertension or in patients with a history of bronchial asthma.

Head Injury and Increased Intracranial Pressure: The respiratory depressant effects of narcotics and their capacity to elevate cerebrospinal fluid pressure may be markedly exaggerated in the presence of head injury, other intracranial lesions or a pre-existing increase in intracranial pressure. Furthermore, narcotics produce adverse reactions which may obscure the clinical course of patients with head injuries.

Acute Abdominal Conditions: The administration of narcotics may obscure the diagnosis or clinical course of patients with acute abdominal conditions.

PRECAUTIONS

Special Risk Patients: As with any narcotic, TUSSEND® syrup should be used with caution in elderly or debilitated patients and those with severe impairment of hepatic or renal function, hypothyroidism, Addison's disease, prostatic hypertrophy or urethral stricture. The usual precautions should be observed and the possiblity of respiratory depression should be kept in mind.

Information for Patients: Narcotics and antihistamines may impair the mental and physical abilities required for the performance of potentially hazardous tasks, such as driving a vehicle or operating machinery. Patients should also be warned about the possible additive effects with alcohol and other central nervous system depressants (hypnotics, sedatives, tranquilizers)

Drug Interactions: Patients receiving other narcotics, antipsychotics, antianxiety agents or other CNS depressants (including alcohol) concomitantly with TUSSEND® syrup may exhibit additive CNS depression. When combined therapy is contemplated, the dose of one or both agents should be reduced.

The use of MAO inhibitors or tricyclic antidepressants with hydrocodone preparations may increase the effect of either the antidepressant or hydrocodone.

The concurrent use of anticholinergics with hydrocodone may produce paralytic ileus. Beta-adrenergic blockers and MAO inhibitors may potentiate the pressor effects of pseudoephedrine. Concurrent use of digitalis glycosides may increase the possibility of cardia arrhythmias. Sympathomimetics may reduce the hypotensive effects of guanethidine, mecamylamine, methyldopa, reserpine, and veratrum alkaloids. Concurrent use of tricyclic antidepressants may antagonize the effects of pseudoephedrine.

Laboratory Test Interactions: Antihistamines may suppress the wheal and flare reactions to antigen skin testing. Considerable interindividual variation in the extent and duration of suppression have been reported, depending on the antigen and test technique, antihistamine and dosage regimen, time since the last dose and individual response to testing. In one study, usual oral dosages of chlorpheniramine suppressed the wheal response for about 2 days after the last dose. Whenever possible antihistamines should be discontinued about 4 days prior to skin testing procedures since they may prevent otherwise positive reactions to dermal reactivity indicators.

Carcinogenesis, Mutagenesis and Impairment of Fertility: No long term or reproduction studies in animals have been performed with TUSSEND® syrup to evaluate its carcinogenic, mutagenic and impairment of fertility potential.

Usage In Pregnancy: Teratogenic Effects: Pregnancy Category C. Hydrocodone has been shown to be teratogenic in hamsters when given in doses 700 times the human dose. There are no adequate and well-controlled studies in pregnant women. TUSSEND® syrup should be used during pregnancy only if the potential benefit justifies the potential risk to the fetus.

Nonteratogenic Effects: Babies born to mothers who have been taking opioids regularly prior to delivery will be physically dependent. The withdrawal signs include irritability and excessive crying, tremors, hyperactive reflexes, increased respiratory rate, increased stools, sneezing, yawning, vomiting and fever. The intensity of syndrome does not always correlate with the duration of maternal opioid use or dose. There is no consensus on the best method of managing withdrawal. Chlorpromazine 0.7–1.0 mg/kg q6h, and paregoric 2–4 drops q4h, have been used to treat withdrawal symptoms in infants. The duration of therapy is 4 to 28 days, with doseage decreased as tolerated.

Labor and Delivery: As with all narcotics administration of TUSSEND® syrup to the mother shortly before delivery may result in some degree of respiratory depression in the newborn, especially if higher doses are used.

Nursing Mothers: TUSSEND® syrup is contraindicated in nursing mothers because of the higher than usual risk infants with sympathomimetic amines.

Pediatric Use: Antihistamines may cause excitability, especially in children. Do not exceed recommended dosage because at higher doses nervousness, dizziness or sleeplessness may occur. In young children, as well as adults, the respiratory center is sensitive to the depressant action of narcotic cough suppressants in a dose-dependent manner. Benefit to risk ratio should be carefully considered especially in children with respiratory embarrassment (e.g., croup).

Use in the Elderly: The elderly (60 years and older) are more likely to have adverse reactions to sympathomimetics. Overdose of sympathomimetics in this age group may cause hallucinations, convulsions, CNS depression and death.

ADVERSE REACTIONS

Hydrocodone Bitartrate: The most frequently observed adverse reactions include lightheadedness, dizziness, sedation, nausea and vomiting. These effects seem to be more prominent in ambulatory patients than in nonambulatory patients and some of these adverse reactions may be alleviated if the patient lies down. Other adverse reactions include:

Central Nervous System: Drowsiness, mental clouding, lethargy, impairment of mental and physical performance, anxiety, fear, dysphoria, psychic dependence, mood changes.

Gastrointestinal System: Prolonged administration may produce constipation.

Genitourinary System: Ureteral spasm, spasm of vesical sphincters and urinary retention have been reported.

Pseudoephedrine Hydrochloride: Pseudoephedrine may cause mild central nervous system stimulation, especially in those patients who are hypersensitive to sympathomimetic drugs. Nervousness, excitability, restlessness, dizziness, weakness and insomnia may also occur. Headache and drowsiness have also been reported. Large doses may cause lightheadedness, nausea and/or vomiting. Sympathomimetic drugs have also been associated with certain untoward reactions including fear, anxiety, tenseness, restlessness, tremor, weakness, pallor respiratory difficulty, dysuria, insomnia, hallucination, convulsion, CNS depression, arrhythmias and cardiovascular collapse with hypotension.

Chlorpheniramine Maleate: Slight to moderate drowsiness may occur and is the most frequent side effect.

Other possible side effects of antihistamines in general include:

General: Urticaria, drug rash, anaphylactic shock, photosensitivity, excessive perspiration, chills, dryness of the mouth, nose and throat.

Cardiovascular: Hypotension, headache, palpitation, tachycardia extrasystoles.

Hematological: Hemolytic anemia, thrombocytopenia agranulocytosis.

CNS: Sedation, dizziness, disturbed coordination, fatigue, confusion, restlessness, excitation, nervousness, tremor, irritability, insomnia, euphoria, paresthesia, blurred vision, dipiopia, vertigo, tinnitus, hysteria, neuritis, convulsion.

Gastrointestinal: Epigastric distress, anorexia, nausea, vomiting, diarrhea, constipation.

Genitourinary: Urinary frequency, difficult urination, urinary retention, early menses.

Respiratory: Thickening of bronchial secretions, tightness of chest, wheezing and nasal stuffiness.

DRUG ABUSE AND DEPENDENCE

TUSSEND® syrup is subject to the Federal Controlled Substances Act (Schedule III).

Psychic dependence and tolerance may develop upon repeated administration of narcotics; therefore, TUSSEND® syrup should be prescribed and administered with caution. However, psychic dependence is unlikely to develop when TUSSEND® syrup is used for a short time.

Physical dependence, the condition in which continued administration of the drug is required to prevent the appearance of a withdrawal syndrome, assumes clinically significant proportions only after several weeks of continued narcotic use, although some mild degree of physical dependence may develop after a few days of narcotic therapy. Tolerance, in which increasingly large doses are required to produce the same degree of effectiveness, is manifested initially by a shortened duration of effect, and subsequently by decreases in the intensity of the effect. The rate of development of tolerance varies among patients.

OVERDOSAGE

Signs and Symptoms: Hydrocodone: Serious overdosage with hydrocodone is characterized by respiratory depression (a decrease in respiratory rate and/or tidal volume. Cheyne Stokes respiration, cyanosis), extreme somnolence progressing to stupor or coma, skeletal muscle flaccidity, cold and clammy skin, and sometimes bradycardia and hypotension. In severe overdosage, apnea, circulatory collapse, cardiac arrest and death may occur.

Pseudoephedrine: Overdosage with pseudoephedrine can cause excessive central nervous system stimulation resulting in excitement, nervousness, anxiety, tremor, restlessness and insomnia. Other effects include tachycardia, hypertension, pallor, mydriasis, hyperglycemia and urinary retention. Severe overdosage may cause tachypnea, or hyperpnea, hallucinations, convulsion, or delirium, but in some individuals there may be central nervous system depression with somnolence, stupor, or respiratory depression. Arrythmias (including ventricular fibrillation) may lead to hypotension and circulatory collapse. Severe hypokalemia can occur, probably due to compartmental shift rather than depletion of potassium. No organ damage or significant metabolic arrangement is associated with pseudoephedrine overdosage. The toxic and lethal concentration in human biologic fluids are not known. Excretion rates increase with urine acidification and decrease with alkaninization. Few reports of toxicity due to pseudoephedrine have been published, and no case of fatal overdosage is known.

Chlorpheniramine: Manifestations of antihistamine overdosage may vary from central nervous system depression (sedation, apnea, cardiovascular collapse) to stimulation (insomnia, hallucinations, tremors or convulsions). Other signs and symptoms may be dizziness, tinnitus, ataxia, blurred vision and hypotension. Stimulation is particularly likely in children, as are atropine-like signs and symptoms (drymouth, dilated pupils, flushing, hyperthermia, and gastrointestinal symptoms).

Treatment: Primary attention should be given to the reestablishment of adequate respiratory exchange through provision of a patent airway and the institution of assisted or controlled ventilation. The narcotic antagonist naloxone is a specific antidote against respiratory depression which may result from overdosage or unusual sensitivity to narcotics including hydrocodone. Therefore, an appropriate dose of naloxone hydrochloride (see package insert) should be administered, preferably by the intravenous route and simultaneously with efforts at respiratory resuscitation. Since the duration of action of hydrocodone may exceed that of the antagonist, the patient should be kept under continued surveillance and repeated doses of the antagonist should be administered as needed to maintain adequate respiration.

An antagonist should not be administered in the absence of clinically significant respiratory or cardiovascular depression. Oxygen, intravenous fluids, vasopressors and other supportive measures should be employed as indicated.

Gastric emptying may be useful in removing unabsorbed drug.

The patient should be induced to vomit even if emesis has occurred spontaneously; however, vomiting should not be induced in patients with impaired consciousness. Precautions against aspiration should be taken, especially in infants and children.

Ipecac syrup is the preferred method for inducing vomiting. The action of ipecac is facillitated by physical activity and the administration of eight to twelve fluid ounces of water. If emesis does not occur within fifteen minutes, the dose of ipecac should be repeated. Following emesis, any drug remaining in the stomach may be absorbed by activated charcoal administered as a slurry with water.

If vomiting is unsuccessful or contraindicated, gastric lavage should be performed. Isotonic and one-half isotonic saline are the lavage solution of choice. Saline cathartics, such as milk of magnesia, draw water into the bowel by osmosis and, therefore, may be valuable for their action in rapid dilution of bowel content.

Treatment of the signs and symptoms of overdosage is symptomatic and supportive. Vasopressors may be used to treat hypotension. Short-acting barbiturates diazepam or paraldehyde may be administered to control seizures. Hyperpyrexia, especially in children, may require treatment with tepid water sponge baths or a hypothermic blanket. Apnea is treated with ventilatory support. Stimulants (analeptic agents) should not be used.

DOSAGE AND ADMINISTRATION

ADULTS: Two teaspoonfuls (10 mL) every 4-6 hours. **CHILDREN: 6-12 years:** One teaspoonful (5 mL) every 4-6 hours. Do not exceed four doses in a 24 hour period.

HOW SUPPLIED

TUSSEND® syrup is supplied as a clear yellow liquid, banana-flavored, in bottles of one pint (16 fl. oz.). NDC 61570-004-16.

Storage: Store at controlled room temperature, 15°-30°C (59°-86°F).

Dispense in a tight, light-resistant container as described in USP.

CAUTION

Federal (USA) law prohibits dispensing without prescription.

A Schedule CIII Controlled Substance.

Manufactured for Monarch Pharmaceuticals, Bristol, TN 37620

0932406

Revised 9/95

Shown in Product Identification Guide, page 325

TUSSEND®
EXPECTORANT

2.5 mg hydrocodone bitartrate* (*Warning: May be habit forming), 30 mg pseudoephedrine hydrochloride, and 100 mg guaifenesin per teaspoonful.

DESCRIPTION

Each teaspoonful (5 mL) of TUSSEND® EXPECTORANT contains:

Hydrocodone Bitartrate*, USP .... 2.5 mg
(*WARNING: May be habit forming)
Pseudoephedrine Hydrochloride, USP .... 30 mg
Guaifenesin, USP .... 100 mg
Alcohol, USP 5%

Also contains: citric acid anhydrous, glucose liquid, methylparaben, propylene glycol, propylparaben, purified water, saccharin sodium, sorbitol solution, sucrose, FD&C Red #40, natural and artificial flavoring.

Hydrocodone bitartrate is an antitussive. Chemically it is 4,5α-epoxy-3-methoxy-17-methylmorphinan-6-one tartrate (1:1) hydrate (2:5) with the following structure:

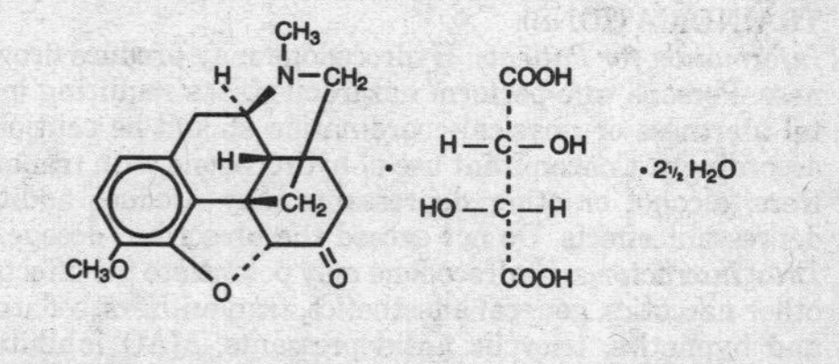

Pseudoephedrine hydrochloride is a nasal decongestant. Chemically it is [S-(R*,R*)]-α-[1-(methylamino)ethyl] benzene methanol hydrochloride with the following structure:

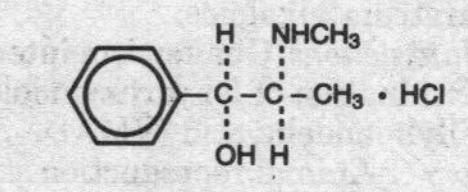

Guaifenesin is an expectorant. Chemically it is 3-(0-methoxyphenoxy)-1,2 propanediol with the following structure:

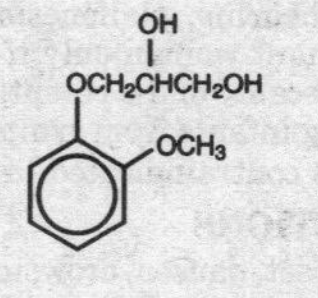

CLINICAL PHARMACOLOGY

Hydrocodone is a semisynthetic narcotic analgesic and antitussive with multiple actions qualitatively similar to those of codeine. Most of these involve the central nervous system and smooth muscle. Hydrocodone suppresses the cough reflex by depressing the medullary cough center. The precise mechanism of action of hydrocodone and other opiates is not known, although it is believed to relate to the existence of opiate receptors in the central nervous system.

Pseudoephedrine hydrochloride is an orally effective nasal decongestant that acts on α-adrenergic receptors in the mucosa of the respiratory tract producing vasoconstriction. Pseudoephedrine shrinks swollen nasal mucous membranes, reduces tissue hyperemia, edema and nasal congestion and increases nasal airway patency. Drainage of sinus secretions is increased and obstructed Eustachian ostia may be opened. Pseudoephedrine produces little if any rebound congestion.

Guaifenesin is an expectorant which enhances the flow of respiratory tract secretions. The enhanced flow of less viscid secretions lubricates irritated respiratory tract membranes, promotes cilliary action and facilitates the removal of inspissated mucus. As a result, sinus and bronchial drainage is improved and nonproductive coughs become more productive and less frequent.

INDICATIONS AND USAGE

For exhausting, nonproductive cough accompanying respiratory tract congestion associated with the common cold, influenza, sinusitis and bronchitis.

CONTRAINDICATIONS

TUSSEND® EXPECTORANT is contraindicated in patients with severe hypertension, severe coronary artery disease, and in patients on MAO inhibitor therapy.

Hypersensitivity: Contraindicated in patients with hypersensitivity or idiosyncrasy to sympathomimetic amines, phenanthrene derivatives, or to any formula ingredients.

Nursing Mothers: Contraindicated because of the higher than usual risk for infants for sympathomimetic amines.

Continued on next page

Monarch —Cont.

WARNINGS
Hydrocodone should be prescribed and administered with the same degree of caution as all oral medications containing a narcotic analgesic. Extreme caution should be exercised in the use of hydrocodone in patients with severe respiratory impairment or patients with impaired respiratory drive.
If sympathomimetic amines are used in patients with hypertension, diabetes mellitus, ischemic heart disease, hyperthyroidism, increased intraocular pressure or prostatic hypertrophy, judicious caution should be exercised (see CONTRAINDICATIONS).
Use in Elderly: The elderly (60 years and older) are more likely to have adverse reactions to sympathomimetics. Overdosage of sympathomimetics in this age group may cause hallucinations, convulsions, CNS depression and death.

PRECAUTIONS
General: Caution should be exercised if used in patients with diabetes, hypertension, cardiovascular diseases, hyperreactivity to ephedrine, or decreased respiratory drive (see CONTRAINDICATIONS).
Information for Patients: Hydrocodone may produce drowsiness. Persons who perform hazardous tasks requiring mental alertness or physical coordination should be cautioned accordingly. Concomitant use of hydrocodone with tranquilizers, alcohol or other depressants may produce additive depressant effects. Do not exceed the prescribed dosage.
Drug Interactions: Hydrocodone may potentiate the effects of other narcotics, general anesthetics, tranquilizers, sedatives and hypnotics, tricyclic antidepressants, MAO inhibitors, alcohol, and other CNS depressants. Beta-adrenergic blockers and MAO inhibitors potentiate the sympathomimetic effects of pseudoephedrine. Sympathomimetics may reduce the antihypertensive effects of methyldopa, mecamylamine, reserpine and veratrum alkaloids.
Laboratory Test Interactions: Guaifenesin interferes with the colorimetric determination of 5-hydroxyindoleacetic acid (5-HIAA) and Vanillylmandelic acid (VMA).
Pregnancy Category C: Animal reproduction studies have not been conducted with pseudoephedrine, guaifenesin, or hydrocodone. It is also not known whether pseudoephedrine, guaifenesin or hydrocodone, can cause fetal harm when administered to a pregnant women or can affect reproduction capacity. Pseudoephedrine, guaifenesin or hydrocodone may be given to a pregnant woman only if clearly needed.
Nursing Mothers: Because of the potential for serious adverse reactions in nursing infants from sympathomimetic amines, pseudoephedrine is contraindicated in nursing mothers.

ADVERSE REACTIONS
Gastrointestinal upset, nausea, drowsiness and constipation. A slight elevation in serum transaminase levels has been noted.
Individuals hyperreactive to pseudoephedrine may display ephedrine-like reactions such as tachycardia, palpitations, headache, dizziness or nausea. Sympathomimetic drugs have been associated with certain untoward reactions including fear, anxiety, tenseness, restlessness, tremor, weakness, pallor, respiratory difficulty, dysuria, insomnia, hallucinations, convulsions, CNS depression, arrhythmias, and cardiovascular collapse with hypotension. Patient idiosyncrasy to adrenergic agents may be manifested by insomnia, dizziness, weakness, tremor or arrhythmias.

DRUG ABUSE AND DEPENDENCE
Controlled Substance: Hydrocodone in TUSSEND® EXPECTORANT is controlled by the Drug Enforcement Administration. TUSSEND® EXPECTORANT is a Schedule III controlled substance.
Abuse: Hydrocodone is a narcotic drug related to codeine with similar abuse potential.
Dependence: Hydrocodone can produce drug dependence of the morphine type. Psychic dependence, physical dependence and tolerance may develop if dosage recommendations are greatly exceeded over a prolonged period of time.

OVERDOSAGE
Acute overdosage with TUSSEND® EXPECTORANT may produce variable clinical signs as hydrocodone produces CNS depression and cardiovascular depression while pseudoephedrine produces CNS stimulation and variable cardiovascular effects Hydrocodone is likely to be responsible for most of the severe reactions from overdosage. Pressor amines should be used with great caution when taking pseudoephedrine. Patients with signs of stimulation should be treated conservatively and depressant medications should be avoided if possible because of potential drug interaction with hydrocodone.

DOSAGE AND ADMINISTRATION
ADULTS: Two teaspoonfuls (10 mL) every 4–6 hours. **CHILDREN 6–12 Years:**
One teaspoonful (5 mL) every 4–6 hours. May be given four times a day as needed. May be taken with meals.

CAUTION:
Federal (USA) law prohibits dispensing without prescription.

HOW SUPPLIED
TUSSEND® EXPECTORANT is a red-colored, fruit punch-flavored liquid supplied in bottles of one pint (16 fl. oz.), NDC 61570-005-16.
Storage: Store at controlled room temperature, 15°–30°C (59°–86°F). Dispense in a tight, light-resistant container as described in USP
Manufactured for: Monarch Pharmaceuticals, Bristol, TN 37620

Revised 6/95
0932361

Shown in Product Identification Guide, page 325

Muro Pharmaceutical, Inc.
890 EAST STREET
TEWKSBURY, MA 01876-1496

Direct Inquiries to:
Professional Service Department
(800) 225-0974
(508) 851-5981

BROMFED® CAPSULES ℞
[*brōm 'fĕd*]

A light green and clear capsule containing white beads. Extended-Release.
Each capsule contains:

Brompheniramine maleate	12 mg
Pseudoephedrine hydrochloride	120 mg

in a specially prepared base to provide prolonged action.

BROMFED-PD® CAPSULES ℞
A dark green and clear capsule containing white beads. Extended-Release.
Each capsule contains:

Brompheniramine maleate	6 mg
Pseudoephedrine hydrochloride	60 mg

in a specially prepared base to provide prolonged action.

BROMFED® and **BROMFED-PD® CAPSULES** also contain inactive ingredients: benzyl alcohol, butyl paraben, carboxymethylcellulose sodium, D & C yellow #10, edetate calcium disodium, FD&C blue #1, FD&C yellow #6, gelatin, methyl paraben, pharmaceutical glaze, propyl paraben, sodium lauryl sulfate, sodium propionate, starch, sucrose and other ingredients.

BROMFED® TABLETS ℞
A white scored tablet.
Each tablet contains:

Brompheniramine maleate	4 mg
Pseudoephedrine hydrochloride	60 mg

Also contains as inactive ingredients colloidal silicon dioxide, lactose, magnesium stearate, microcrystalline cellulose and sodium starch glycolate.

BROMFED® contains ingredients of the following therapeutic classes: antihistamine and nasal decongestant.

CLINICAL PHARMACOLOGY
Brompheniramine maleate is an alkylamine type antihistamine. This group of antihistamines are among the most active histamine antagonists and are generally effective in relatively low doses. The drugs are not so prone to produce drowsiness and are among the most suitable agents for day time use; but again, a significant proportion of patients do experience this effect. Pseudoephedrine hydrochloride is a sympathomimetic which acts predominently on alpha receptors and has little action on beta receptors. It therefore functions as an oral nasal decongestant with minimal CNS stimulation.

INDICATIONS
For the temporary relief of symptoms of seasonal and perennial allergic rhinitis, and vasomotor rhinitis, including nasal obstruction (congestion).

CONTRAINDICATIONS
Hypersensitivity to any of the ingredients. Also contraindicated in patients with severe hypertension, severe coronary artery disease, patients on MAO inhibitor therapy, patients with narrow-angle glaucoma, urinary retention, peptic ulcer and during an asthmatic attack.

WARNINGS
Considerable caution should be exercised in patients with hypertension, diabetes mellitus, ischemic heart disease, hyperthyroidism, increased intraocular pressure and prostatic hypertrophy. The elderly (60 years or older) are more likely to exhibit adverse reactions.
Antihistamines may cause excitability, especially in children. At dosages higher than the recommended dose, nervousness, dizziness or sleeplessness may occur.

PRECAUTIONS
General: Caution should be exercised in patients with high blood pressure, heart disease, diabetes or thyroid disease. The antihistamine in this product may exhibit additive effects with other CNS depressants, including alcohol.
Information for Patients: Antihistamine may cause drowsiness and ambulatory patients who operate machinery or motor vehicles should be cautioned accordingly.
Drug Interactions: MAO inhibitors and beta adrenergic blockers increase the effects of sympathomimetics. Sympathomimetics may reduce the antihypertensive effects of methyldopa, mecamylamine, reserpine and veratrum alkaloids. Concomitant use of antihistamines with alcohol and other CNS depressants may have an additive effect.
Pregnancy: The safety of use of this product in pregnancy has not been established.

ADVERSE REACTIONS
Adverse reactions include drowsiness, lassitude, nausea, giddiness, dryness of mouth, blurred vision, cardiac palpitations, flushing, increased irritability or excitement (especially in children).

DOSAGE AND ADMINISTRATION
BROMFED® CAPSULES Adults and children 12 years of age and over: 1 capsule every 12 hours.
BROMFED-PD® CAPSULES Adults and children 12 years of age and over: 1 or 2 capsules every 12 hours. Children 6 to under 12 years of age: 1 capsule every 12 hours.
BROMFED® TABLETS Adults and children 12 years of age and over: One tablet every 4 hours not to exceed 6 doses in 24 hours. Children 6 to under 12 years of age: One-half tablet every 4 hours not to exceed 6 doses in 24 hours. Do not give to children under 6 years except under the advice and supervision of a physician.

HOW SUPPLIED
BROMFED® CAPSULES. Bottle of 100 (NDC 0451-4000-50) and 500 (NDC 0451-4000-60). Each capsule is coded "BROMFED" "MURO 12-120".
BROMFED-PD® CAPSULES. Bottle of 100 (NDC 0451-4001-50) and 500 (NDC 0451-4001-60). Each capsule is coded "BROMFED-PD" "MURO 6-60".
BROMFED® TABLETS. Bottle of 100 (NDC 0451-4060-50). Each tablet is coded "MURO 4060" on one side and scored on the reverse side.
Dispense in tight child-resistant containers as defined in USP/NF. Store at controlled room temperature.

BROMFED® SYRUP OTC
[*brōm 'fĕd*]

(See PDR For Nonprescription Drugs.)

BROMFED–DM® COUGH SYRUP ℞
[*brōm 'fĕd*]

DESCRIPTION
BROMFED-DM® Cough Syrup is a cherry flavored red syrup.
Each 5 mL (1 teaspoonful) contains:

Brompheniramine Maleate, USP	2 mg
Pseudoephedrine Hydrochloride, USP	30 mg
Dextromethorphan Hydrobromide, USP	10 mg

Inactive Ingredients: Citric Acid, FD&C Red 40, FD&C blue #1, Wild Cherry Flavor, Glycerin, Saccharin Sodium, Sodium Benzoate, Sorbitol, Sucrose, Methylparaben, Purified Water.
Antihistamine/Nasal Decongestant/Antitussive syrup for oral administration.

CLINICAL PHARMACOLOGY
Brompheniramine maleate is a histamine antagonist, specifically an H_1-receptor-blocking agent belonging to the alkylamine class of antihistamines. Antihistamines appear to compete with histamine for receptor sites on effector cells. Brompheniramine also has anticholinergic (drying) and sedative effects. Among the antihistaminic effects, it antagonizes the allergic response (vasodilatation, increased vascular permeability, increased mucus secretion) of nasal tissue. Brompheniramine is well absorbed from the gastrointestinal tract, with peak plasma concentration after single, oral dose of 4 mg reached in 5 hours; urinary excretion is the major route of elimination, mostly as products of biodegradation; the liver is assumed to be the main site of metabolic transformation.
Pseudoephedrine acts on sympathetic nerve endings and also on smooth muscle, making it useful as a nasal decongestant. The nasal decongestant effect is mediated by the action of pseudoephedrine on α-sympathetic receptors, producing

vasoconstriction of the dilated nasal arterioles. Following oral administration, effects are noted within 30 minutes with peak activity occurring at approximately one hour.

Dextromethorphan acts centrally to elevate the threshold for coughing. It has no analgesic or addictive properties. The onset of antitussive action occurs in 15 to 30 minutes after administration and is of long duration.

INDICATIONS AND USAGE

For relief of coughs and upper respiratory symptoms, including nasal congestion, associated with allergy or the common cold.

CONTRAINDICATIONS

Hypersensitivity to any of the ingredients. Do not use in the newborn, in premature infants, in nursing mothers, in patients with severe hypertension or severe coronary artery disease, or in those receiving monoamine oxidase (MAO) inhibitors.

Antihistamines should not be used to treat lower respiratory tract conditions including asthma.

WARNINGS

Especially in infants and small children, antihistamines in overdosage may cause hallucinations, convulsions, and death.

Antihistamines may diminish mental alertness. In the young child, they may produce excitation.

PRECAUTIONS

General: Because of its antihistamine component, **BROMFED-DM® Cough Syrup** should be used with caution in patients with a history of bronchial asthma, narrow angle glaucoma, gastrointestinal obstruction, or urinary bladder neck obstruction. Because of its sympathomimetic component, **BROMFED-DM® Cough Syrup** should be used with caution in patients with diabetes, hypertension, heart disease, or thyroid disease.

Information for Patients: Patients should be warned about engaging in activities requiring mental alertness, such as driving a car or operating dangerous machinery.

Drug Interactions: Antihistamines have additive effects with alcohol and other CNS depressants (hypnotics, sedatives, tranquilizers, antianxiety agents, etc.) MAO inhibitors prolong and intensify the anticholinergic (drying) effects of antihistamines. MAO inhibitors may enhance the effect of pseudoephedrine. Sympathomimetics may reduce the effects of antihypertensive drugs.

Carcinogenesis, Mutagenesis, Impairment of Fertility: Animal studies of **BROMFED-DM® Cough Syrup** to assess the carcinogenic and mutagenic potential of the effect on fertility have not been performed.

Pregnancy

Teratogenic Effects—Pregnancy Category C

Animal reproduction studies have not been conducted with **BROMFED-DM® Cough Syrup.** It is also not known whether **BROMFED-DM® Cough Syrup** can cause fetal harm when administered to a pregnant woman or can affect reproduction capacity. **BROMFED-DM® Cough Syrup** should be given to a pregnant woman only if clearly needed.

Reproduction studies of brompheniramine maleate (a component of **BROMFED-DM® Cough Syrup**) in rats and mice at doses up to 16 times the maximum human dose have revealed no evidence of impaired fertility or harm to the fetus.

Nursing Mothers: Because of the higher risk of intolerance of anithistamines in small infants generally, and in newborns and prematures in particular, **BROMFED-DM® Cough Syrup** is contraindicated in nursing mothers.

ADVERSE REACTIONS

The most frequent adverse reaction to **BROMFED-DM® Cough Syrup** are: sedation, dryness of mouth, nose and throat; thickening of bronchial secretions; dizziness. Other adverse reactions may include:

Dermatologic: Urticaria, drug rash, photosensitivity, pruritus.

Cardiovascular System: Hypotension, hypertension, cardiac arrhythmias, palpitation.

CNS: Disturbed coordination, tremor, irritability, insomnia, visual disturbances, weakness, nervousness, convulsions, headache, euphoria, and dysphoria.

G.U. System: Urinary frequency, difficult urination.

G.I. System: Epigastric discomfort, anorexia, nausea, vomiting, diarrhea, constipation.

Respiratory System: Tightness of chest and wheezing, shortness of breath.

Hematologic System: Hemolytic anemia, thrombocytopenia, agranulocytosis.

OVERDOSAGE

Signs and Symptoms: Central nervous system effects from overdosage of brompheniramine may vary from depression to stimulation, especially in children. Anticholinergic effects may be noted. Toxic doses of pseudoephedrine may result in CNS stimulation, tachycardia, hypertension, and cardiac arrhythmias; signs of CNS depression may occasionally be seen. Dextromethorphan in toxic doses will cause drowsiness, ataxia, nystagmus, opisthotonos, and convulsive seizures.

Toxic Doses: Data suggest that individuals may respond in an unexpected manner to apparently small amounts of a particular drug. A 2½-year old child survived the ingestion of 21 mg/kg of dextromethorphan exhibiting only ataxia, drowsiness, and fever, but seizures have been reported in 2 children following the ingestion of 13–17 mg/kg. Another 2½-year old child survived a dose of 300–900 mg of brompheniramine. The toxic dose of pseudoephedrine should be less than that of ephedrine, which is estimated to be 50 mg/kg.

Treatment: Induce emesis if patient is alert and is seen prior to 6 hours following ingestion. Precautions against aspiration must be taken, especially in infants and small children. Gastric lavage may be carr;ed out, although in some instances tracheostomy may be necessary prior to lavage. Naloxone hydrochloride 0.005 mg/kg intravenously may be of value in reversing the CNS depression that may occur from an overdose of dextromethorphan. CNS stimulants may counter CNS depression. Should CNS hyperactivity or convulsive seizures occur, intravenous short-acting barbiturates may be indicated. Hypertensive responses and/or tachycardia should be treated appropriately. Oxygen, intravenous fluids, and other supportive measures should be employed as indicated.

DOSAGE AND ADMINISTRATION

Adults and children 12 years of age and over: 2 teaspoonfuls every 4 hours. Children 6 to under 12 years: 1 teaspoonful every 4 hours. Children 2 to under 6 years: ½ teaspoonful every 4 hours. Children 6 months to under 2 years: Dosage to be established by physician.

Do not exceed 6 doses during a 24-hour period.

HOW SUPPLIED

BROMFED-DM® Cough Syrup is a red syrup containing in each 5 mL (1 teaspoonful) brompheniramine maleate 2 mg, pseudoephedrine hydrochloride 30 mg and dextromethorphan hydrobromide 10 mg, available in Bottles of 16 fl. oz. (NDC #0451-4101-16.)

Store at controlled room temperature, between 15°C and 30°C (59°F and 86°F).

Dispense in tight, light-resistant, and child-resistant containers as defined in U.S.P./NF.

GUAIFED® CAPSULES ℞

[gwī'ah-fed]

A white opaque and clear capsule containing white beads.
Extended-Release
Each capsule contains:
Pseudoephedrine hydrochloride .... 120 mg
in a specially prepared base to provide prolonged action.
Guaifenesin .... 250 mg
designed for immediate release to provide rapid action.

GUAIFED–PD® CAPSULE ℞

A blue and clear capsule containing white beads.
Extended-Release
Each capsule contains:
Pseudoephedrine hydrochloride .... 60 mg
in a specially prepared base to provide prolonged action.
Guaifenesin .... 300 mg
designed for immediate release to provide rapid action.

GUAIFED® and GUAIFED–PD® CAPSULES also contain as inactive ingredients: Benzyl Alcohol, Butyl Paraben, Edetate Calcium Disodium, Gelatin, Methyl Paraben, Pharmaceutical Glaze, Propyl Paraben, Sodium Lauryl Sulfate, Sodium Propionate, Starch, Sucrose, Titanium Dioxide, FD&C Blue #1 (GUAIFED-PD® only) and other ingredients.

GUAIFED® and GUAIFED–PD® contains ingredients of the following therapeutic classes: nasal decongestant and expectorant.

CLINICAL PHARMACOLOGY

Pseudoephedrine hydrochloride is a sympathomimetic which acts predominantly on alpha adrenergic receptors in the mucosa of the respiratory tract, producing vasoconstriction and has little action on beta receptors. It therefore functions as an oral nasal decongestant with minimal CNS stimulation. Pseudoephedrine hydrochloride also increases sinus drainage and secretions. Guaifenesin is an expectorant which increases the output of phlegm (sputum) and bronchial secretions by reducing adhesiveness and surface tension. The increased flow of less viscid secretions promotes ciliary action and changes a dry, unproductive cough to one that is more productive and less frequent.

INDICATIONS

For temporary relief of nasal congestion and dry non-productive cough associated with the common cold and other respiratory allergies. Helps drainage of the bronchial tubes by thinning the mucus.

CONTRAINDICATIONS

This product is contraindicated in patients with a known hypersensitivity to any of its ingredients. Also contraindicated in patients with severe hypertension, severe coronary artery disease and patients on MAO inhibitor therapy. Should not be used during pregnancy or in nursing mothers. Considerable caution should be exercised in patients with hypertension, diabetes mellitus, ischemic heart disease, hyperthyroidism, increased intraocular pressure and prostatic hypertrophy. The elderly (60 years or older) are more likely to exhibit adverse reactions. At dosages higher than the recommended dose, nervousness, dizziness or sleeplessness may occur.

WARNINGS

Do not take this product for persistent or chronic cough such as occurs with smoking, asthma, or emphysema, or where cough is accompanied by excessive secretions except under the advice and supervision of a physician. This medication should be taken a few hours prior to bedtime to minimize the possibility of sleeplessness. Take this medication with a glass of water after each dose, to help loosen mucus in the lungs.

PRECAUTIONS

General: Caution should be exercised in patients with high blood pressure, heart disease, diabetes or thyroid disease and in patients who exhibit difficulty in urination due to enlargement of the prostate gland. Check with a physician if symptoms do not improve within 7 days or if accompanied by high fever, rash or persistent headache.

Drug Interactions: Do not take this product if you are presently taking a prescription drug for high blood pressure or depression, without first consulting a physician. MAO inhibitors and beta adrenergic blockers may increase the effect of sympathomimetics. Sympathomimetics may reduce the antihypertensive effects of methyldopa, mecamylamine, reserpine and veratrum alkaloids. Pseudoephedrine hydrochloride may increase the possibility of cardiac arrhythmias in patients presently taking digitalis glycosides.

Pregnancy: Pregnancy Catagory B. It has been shown that pseudoephedrine hydrochloride can cause reduced average weight, length, and rate of skeletal ossification in the animal fetus.

Nursing Mothers: Pseudoephedrine is excreted in breast milk; use by nursing mother is not recommended because of the higher than usual risk of side effects from sympathomimetic amines for infants, especially newborn and premature infants.

Geriatrics: Pseudoephedrine should be used with caution in the elderly because they may be more sensitive to the effects of the sympathomimetics.

ADVERSE REACTIONS

Adverse reactions include nausea, cardiac palpitations, increased irritability or excitement, headache, dizziness, tachycardia, diarrhea, drowsiness, stomach pain, seizures, slowed heart rate, shortness of breath and/or troubled breathing.

OVERDOSAGE

KEEP THIS AND ALL DRUGS OUT OF THE REACH OF CHILDREN. IN CASE OF SUSPECTED OVERDOSE, IMMEDIATELY CALL YOUR REGIONAL POISON CONTROL CENTER and/or SEEK PROFESSIONAL ASSISTANCE.

Symptoms of overdosage may be caused by pseudoephedrine. Symptoms of overdosage with pseudoephedrine include anxiety, tenseness, respiratory difficulty, headache and awareness of the slow forceful heartbeat.

TREATMENT OF OVERDOSE

The stomach should be emptied promptly by emetics and/or gastric lavage. The installation of activated charcoal also should be considered. Cardiac function and serum electrolytes should be monitored and treatment instigated if indicated. If convulsions or marked CNS excitement occurs, diazepam may be used.

DOSAGE AND ADMINISTRATION

GUAIFED® CAPSULES Adults and children 12 years of age and over: 1 capsule every 12 hours.

GUAIFED–PD® CAPSULES Adults and children 12 years of age and over: 1 or 2 capsules every 12 hours. Children 6 to under 12 years of age: 1 capsule every 12 hours.

HOW SUPPLIED

GUAIFED® CAPSULES Bottle of 100 (NDC 0451-4002-50). Bottle of 500 (NDC 0451-4002-60). Each capsule is coded "GUAIFED" "MURO 120-250".

GUAIFED–PD® CAPSULES Bottle of 100 (NDC 0451-4003-50). Bottle of 500 (NDC 0451-4003-60). Each capsule is coded "GUAIFED-PD" "MURO 60-300".

Dispense in tight, child-resistant containers as defined in USP/NF. Store at controlled room temperature, between 15°–30°C (59°–86°F).

Keep this and all drugs out of reach of children.

Continued on next page

Muro—Cont.

GUAIFED® SYRUP OTC

(See PDR For Nonprescription Drugs.)

LIQUID PRED® SYRUP ℞

Each teaspoonful contains:
Prednisone 5mg/5mL

HOW SUPPLIED
NDC-0451-1201-04–4 fl. oz. (120 mL)
NDC-0451-1201-08–8 fl. oz. (240 mL)

PRELONE® SYRUP ℞
(Prednisolone Syrup, USP 15 mg per 5 mL)

DESCRIPTION
Prednisolone syrup contains prednisolone which is a glucocorticoid. Glucocorticoids are adrenocortical steroids, both naturally occurring and synthetic, which are readily absorbed from the gastrointestinal tract. Prednisolone is a white to practically white, odorless, crystalline powder. It is very slightly soluble in water, slightly soluble in alcohol, in chloroform, in dioxane, and in methanol.
The chemical name for Prednisolone is pregna-1,4-diene-3, 20-dione, 11, 17, 21-tridihydroxy. Its molecular weight is 360.45. The molecular formula is $C_{21}H_{28}O_5$, and the structural formula is:

PRELONE® Syrup contains 15 mg of prednisolone in each 5 mL Benzoic acid, 0.1% is added as a preservative. It also contains alcohol 5%, citric acid, edetate disodium, glycerin, propylene glycol, purified water, sodium saccharin, sucrose, artificial wild cherry flavor, FD&C blue #1 and red #40.

CLINICAL PHARMACOLOGY
Naturally occurring glucocorticoids (hydrocortisone and cortisone), which also have salt-retaining properties, are used as replacement therapy in adrenocortical deficiency states. Their synthetic analogs such as prednisolone are primarily used for their potent anti-inflammatory effects in disorders of many organ systems.
Glucocorticoids such as prednisolone cause profound and varied metabolic effects. In addition, they modify the body's immune responses to diverse stimuli.

INDICATIONS AND USAGE
PRELONE® Syrup is indicated in the following conditions:

1. **Endocrine Disorders**
   Primary or secondary adrenocortical insufficiency (hydrocortisone or cortisone is the first choice; synthetic analogs may be used in conjunction with mineralocorticoids where applicable; in infancy mineralocorticoid supplementation is of particular importance.)
   Congenital adrenal hyperplasia
   Nonsuppurative thyroiditis
   Hypercalcemia associated with cancer
2. **Rheumatic Disorders**
   As adjunctive therapy for short-term administration (to tide the patient over an acute episode or exacerbation) in:
   Psoriatic arthritis
   Rheumatoid arthritis, including juvenile rheumatoid arthritis (selected cases may require low-dose maintenance therapy)
   Ankylosing spondylitis
   Acute and subacute bursitis
   Acute nonspecific tenosynovitis
   Acute gouty arthritis
   Post-traumatic osteoarthritis
   Synovitis of osteoarthritis
   Epicondylitis
3. **Collagen Diseases**
   During an exacerbation or as maintenance therapy in selected cases of:
   Systemic lupus erythematosus
   Acute rheumatic carditis
4. **Dermatologic Diseases**
   Pemphigus
   Bullous dermatitis herpetiformis
   Severe erythema multiforme
   (Stevens-Johnson syndrome)
   Exfoliative dermatitis
   Mycosis fungoides
   Severe psoriasis
   Severe seborrheic dermatitis
5. **Allergic States**
   Control of severe or incapacitating allergic conditions intractable to adequate trials of conventional treatment:
   Seasonal or perennial allergic rhinitis
   Bronchial asthma
   Contact dermatitis
   Atopic dermatitis
   Serum sickness
   Drug hypersensitivity reactions
6. **Ophthalmic Diseases**
   Severe actue and chronic allergic and inflammatory processes involving the eye and its adnexa such as:
   Allergic corneal marginal ulcers
   Herpes zoster ophthalmicus
   Anterior segment inflammation
   Diffuse posterior uveitis and choroiditis
   Sympathetic ophthalmia
   Allergic conjunctivitis
   Keratitis
   Chorioretinitis
   Optic neuritis
   Iritis and iridocyclitis
7. **Respiratory Diseases**
   Symptomatic sarcoidosis
   Loeffler's syndrome not manageable by other means
   Berylliosis
   Fulminating or disseminated pulmonary tuberculosis when used concurrently with appropriate antituberculous chemotherapy
   Aspiration pneumonitis
8. **Hematologic Disorders**
   Idiopathic thrombocytopenic purpura in adults
   Secondary thrombocytopenia in adults
   Acquired (autoimmune) hemolytic anemia
   Erythroblastopenia (RBC anemia)
   Congenital (erythroid) hypoplastic anemia
9. **Neoplastic Diseases**
   For palliative management of:
   Leukemias and lymphomas in adults
   Acute leukemia of childhood
10. **Edematous States**
    To induce a diuresis or remission of proteinuria in the nephrotic syndrome, without uremia, of the idiopathic type or that due to lupus erythematosus.
11. **Gastrointestinal Diseases**
    To tide the patient over a critical period of the disease in:
    Ulcerative colitis
    Regional enteritis
12. **Miscellaneous**
    Tuberculous meningitis with subarachnoid block or impending block used concurrently with appropriate antituberculous chemotherapy. Trichinosis with neurologic or myocardial involvement.

In addition to the above indicatons *PRELONE® Syrup* is indicated for systemic dermatomyositis (polymyositis).

CONTRAINDICATIONS
Systemic fungal infections.

WARNINGS
In patients on corticosteroid therapy subjected to unusual stress, increased dosage of rapidly acting corticosteroids before, during, and after the stressful situation is indicated.
Corticosteroids may mask some signs of infection, and new infections may appear during their use. There may be decreased resistance and inability to localize infection when corticosteroids are used.
Prolonged use of corticosteroids may produce posterior subcapsular cataracts, glaucoma with possible damage to the optic nerves, and may enhance the establishment of secondary ocular infections due to fungi or viruses.
Use in pregnancy: Since adequate human reproduction studies have not been done with corticosteroids, the use of these drugs in pregnancies, nursing mothers or women of childbearing potential requires that the possible benefits of the drug be weighed against the potential hazards to the mother and embryo or fetus. Infants born of mothers who have received substantial doses of corticosteroids during pregnancy should be carefully observed for signs of hypoadrenalism.
Average and large doses of hydrocortisone or cortisone can cause elevation of blood pressure, salt and water retention, and increased excretion of potassium. These effects are less likely to occur with the synthetic derivaties except when used in large doses. Dietary salt restriction and potassium supplementation may be necessary. All corticosteroids increase calcium excretion.
While on corticosteroid therapy, patients should not be vaccinated against smallpox. Other immunizaton procedures should not be undertaken in patients who are on corticosteroids, especially on high dose, because of possible hazards of neurological complications and a lack of antibody response.
Children who are on drugs which suppress the immune system are more susceptible to infections than healthy children. Chickenpox and measles, for example, can have a more serious or even fatal course in non-immune children or adults on corticosteroids. In such children or adults who have not had these diseases, particular care should be taken to avoid exposure. How the dose, route and duration of corticosteroid administration affects the risk of developing a disseminated infection is not known. The contribution of the underlying disease and/or prior corticosteroid treatment to the risk is also not known. If exposed to chickenpox, prophylaxis with varicella zoster immune globulin (VZIG) may be indicated. If exposed to measles, prophylaxis with pooled intravenous immunoglobulin (IVIG) may be indicated. (See the respective package inserts for complete VZIG and IVIG prescribing information.) If chickenpox develops, treatment with antiviral agents may be considered.
Similarly, corticosteroids should be used with great care in patients with known or suspected Strongyloides (threadworm) infestation. In such patients, corticosteroid-induced immunosuppression may lead to Strongyloides hyperinfection and dissemination with widespread larval migration, often accompanied by severe enterocolitis and potentially fatal gram-negative septicemia.
The use of *PRELONE® Syrup* in active tuberculosis should be restricted to those cases of fulminating or disseminated tuberculosis in which the corticosteroid is used for the management of the disease in conjunction with an appropriate antituberculous regimen.
If corticosteroids are indicated in patients with latent tuberculosis or tuberculin reactivity, close observation is necessary as reactivation of the disease may occur. During the prolonged corticosteroid therapy, these patients should receive chemoprophylaxis.

PRECAUTIONS
Information for patients: Patients who are on immunosuppressant doses of corticosteroids should be warned to avoid exposure to chickenpox or measles. Patients should also be advised that if they are exposed, medical advice should be sought without delay.
GENERAL: Drug-induced secondary adrenocortical insufficiency may be minimized by gradual reduction of dosage. This type of relative insufficiency may persist for months after discontinuation of therapy; therefore, in any situation of stress occurring during that period, hormone therapy should be reinstituted. Since mineralocorticoid secretion may be impaired, salt and/or a mineralocorticoid should be administered concurrently.
There is an enhanced effect of corticosteroids on patients with hypothyroidism and in those with cirrhosis.
Corticosteroids should be used cautiously in patients with ocular herpes simplex because of possible corneal perforation.
The lowest possible dose of corticosteroid should be used to control the condition under treatment, and when reduction in dosage is possible, the reduction should be gradual.
Psychic derangements may appear when corticosteroids are used, ranging from euphoria, insomnia, mood swings, personality changes, and severe depression, to frank psychotic manifestations. Also, existing emotional instability or psychotic tendencies may be aggravated by cortiosteroids.
Aspirin should be used cautiously in conjunction with corticosteroids in hypoprothrombinemia.
Steroids should be used with caution in nonspecific Ulcerative Colitis, if there is a probability of impending perforation, abscess or other pyogenic infections: diverticulitis; fresh intestinal anastomoses; active or latent peptic ulcer; renal insufficiency; hypertension; osteoporosis; and myasthenia gravis.
Growth and development of infants and children on prolonged corticosteroid therapy should be carefully observed.

ADVERSE REACTIONS
Fluid and Electrolyte Disturbances
   Sodium retention
   Fluid retention
   Congestive heart failure in susceptible patients
   Potassium loss
   Hypokalemic alkalosis
   Hypertension
Musculoskeletal
   Muscle weakness
   Steroid myopathy
   Loss of muscle mass
   Osteoporosis
   Vertebral compression fractures
   Aseptic necrosis of femoral and humeral heads
   Pathologic fracture of long bones
Gastrointestinal
   Peptic ulcer with possible perforation and hemorrhage
   Pancreatitis
   Abdominal distention
   Ulcerative esophagitis

Dermatologic
Impaired wound healing
Thin fragile skin
Petechiae and ecchymoses
Facial erythema
Increased sweating
May suppress reactions to skin tests

Neurological
Convulsions
Increased intracranial pressure with papilledema (pseudo-tumor cerebri) usually after treatment
Vertigo
Headache

Endocrine
Menstrual irregularities
Development of Cushingoid state
Suppression of growth in children
Secondary adrenocortical and pituitary unresponsiveness, particularly in times of stress, as in trauma, surgery or illness
Decreased carbohydrate tolerance
Manifestations of latent diabetes mellitus
Increased requirements for insulin or oral hypoglycemic agents in diabetics

Ophthalmic
Posterior subcapsular cataracts
Increased intraocular pressure
Glaucoma
Exophthalmos

Metabolic
Negative nitrogen balance due to protein catabolism

DOSAGE AND ADMINISTRATION

Dosage of *PRELONE® Syrup* should be individualized according to the severity of the disease and the response of the patient. For infants and children, the recommended dosage should be governed by the same considerations rather than strict adherence to the ratio indicated by age or body weight. Hormone therapy is an adjunct to and not a replacement for conventional therapy.

Dosage should be decreased or discontinued gradually when the drug has been administered for more than a few days. The severity, prognosis, expected duration of the disease, and the reaction of the patient to medication are primary factors in determining dosage.

If a period of spontaneous remission occurs in a chronic condition, treatment should be discontinued.

Blood pressure, body weight, routine laboratory studies, including two-hour postprandial blood glucose and serum potassium, and a chest X-ray should be obtained at regular intervals during prolonged therapy. Upper GI X-rays are desirable in patients with known or suspected peptic ulcer disease.

The initial dosage of *PRELONE® Syrup* may vary from 5 mg to 60 mg per day depending on the specific disease entity being treated. In situations of less severity lower doses will generally suffice while in selected patients higher initial doses may be required. The initial dosage should be maintained or adjusted until a satisfactory response is noted. If after a reasonable period of time there is a lack of satisfactory clinical response, *PRELONE® Syrup* should be discontinued and the patient transferred to other appropriate therapy. **IT SHOULD BE EMPHASIZED THAT DOSAGE REQUIREMENTS ARE VARIABLE AND MUST BE INDIVIDUALIZED ON THE BASIS OF THE DISEASE UNDER TREATMENT AND THE RESPONSE OF THE PATIENT.**

After a favorable response is noted, the proper maintenance dosage should be determined by decreasing the initial drug dosage in small decrements at appropriate time intervals until the lowest dosage which will maintain an adequate clinical response is reached. It should be kept in mind that constant monitoring is needed in regard to drug dosage. Included in the situations which may make dosage adjustments necessary are changes in clincial status secondary to remissions or exacerbations in the disease process, the patient's individual drug responsiveness, and the effect of patient exposure to stressful situations not directly related to the disease entity under treatment. In this latter situation it may be necessary to increase the dosage of *PRELONE® Syrup* for a period of time consistent with the patient's condition. If after long-term therapy the drug is to be stopped, it is recommended that it be withdrawn gradually rather than abruptly.

HOW SUPPLIED

PRELONE® Syrup is a cherry flavored red liquid containing 15 mg of Prednisolone in each 5 mL (teaspoonful) and is supplied in 240 mL bottles (NDC #0451-1500-08) and 480 mL bottles (0451-1500-16).

Pharmacist: Dispense with a suitable calibrated measuring device to assure proper measuring of dose.

Dose/Volume Chart

15 mg prednisolone = 1 teaspoon
10 mg prednisolone = 2/3 teaspoon
7.5 mg prednisolone = 1/2 teaspoon
5 mg prednisolone = 1/3 teaspoon

Dispense in tight, light-resistant and child-resistant containers as defined in USP/NF.
Store at room temperature. Do Not Refrigerate.
CAUTION: Federal law prohibits dispensing without prescription.

SALINEX® NASAL MIST AND DROPS   OTC
[sal'i-něx]
(Buffered isotonic sodium chloride solution)

(See PDR For Nonprescription Drugs.)

VOLMAX®   ℞
(albuterol sulfate)
Extended-Release Tablets

DESCRIPTION

Volmax® (albuterol sulfate) Extended-Release Tablets contain albuterol sulfate, the racemic form of albuterol and a relatively selective beta$_2$-adrenergic bronchodilator, in an extended-release formulation. Albuterol sulfate has the chemical name ($\pm$) α'-[(*tert*-butylamino)methyl]-4-hydroxy-*m*-xylene-α,α'-diol sulfate (2:1)(salt), and the following chemical structure:

$$\left[\text{HOCH}_2-\text{HO}-\bigcirc-\text{CHCH}_2\text{NHC(CH}_3)_3 \atop \text{OH} \right]_2 \cdot \text{H}_2\text{SO}_4$$

Albuterol sulfate has a molecular weight of 576.7, and the molecular formula is $(C_{13}H_{21}NO_3)_2 \cdot H_2SO_4$. Albuterol sulfate is a white crystalline powder, soluble in water and slightly soluble in ethanol.

The World Health Organization recommended name for albuterol base is salbutamol.

Each Volmax® Extended-Release Tablet for oral administration contains 4 or 8 mg of albuterol as 4.8 or 9.6 mg, respectively, of albuterol sulfate in a nondeformable cellulosic material that serves as the rate-controlling membrane. Each tablet also contains the inactive ingredients cellulose acetate, croscarmellose sodium, FD&C Blue No. 1 (4-mg tablet only), hydroxypropyl cellulose (8-mg tablet only), hydroxypropyl methylcellulose, magnesium stearate, povidone, silica, sodium chloride, and titanium dioxide.

CLINICAL PHARMACOLOGY

In vitro studies and *in vivo* pharmacologic studies have demonstrated that albuterol has a preferential effect on beta$_2$-adrenergic receptors compared with isoproterenol. While it is recognized that beta$_2$-adrenergic receptors are the predominant receptors in bronchial smooth muscle, recent data indicate that there is a population of beta$_2$-receptors in the human heart existing in a concentration between 10% and 50%. The precise function of these, however, is not yet established.

The pharmacologic effects of beta-adrenergic agonist drugs, including albuterol, are at least in part attributable to stimulation through beta-adrenergic receptors on intracellular adenyl cyclase, the enzyme that catalyzes the conversion of adenosine triphosphate (ATP) to cyclic-3', 5'-adenosine monophosphate (cyclic AMP). Increased cyclic AMP levels are associated with relaxation of bronchial smooth muscle and inhibition of release of mediators of immediate hypersensitivity from cells, especially from mast cells.

Albuterol has been shown in most controlled clinical trials to have more effect on the respiratory tract, in the form of bronchial smooth muscle relaxation, than cardiovascular effect at comparable doses while producing fewer cardiovascular effects.

Albuterol is longer acting than isoproterenol in most patients by any route of administration because it is not a substrate for the cellular uptake processes for catecholamines nor for catechol-*O*-methyl transferase.

Animal studies show that albuterol does not pass the blood-brain barrier.

Recent studies in laboratory animals (minipigs, rodents, and dogs) recorded the occurrence of cardiac arrhythmias and sudden death (with histologic evidence of myocardial necrosis) when beta-agonists and methylxanthines were administered concurrently. The significance of these findings when applied to humans is currently unknown.

In a single-dose study comparing one 8-mg Volmax® Extended-Release Tablet with two 4-mg immediate-release Ventolin® (albuterol sulfate, USP) Tablets in 17 normal volunteers, the extent of availability of Volmax® Extended-Release Tablets was shown to be about 80% of Ventolin® Tablets with or without food. In addition, lower mean peak plasma concentration and longer time to reach the peak

level were observed with Volmax® Extended-Release Tablets as compared with Ventolin® Tablets. (However, bioequivalence between Ventolin® Tablets [4 mg q6h] and Volmax® Extended-Release Tablets [8 mg b.i.d.] was shown in a multiple-dose, steady-state study in fed condition.) The single-dose study results also showed that food decreases the rate of absorption of albuterol from Volmax® Extended-Release Tablets without altering the extent of bioavailability. In addition, the study indicated that food causes a more gradual increase in the fraction of the available dose absorbed from the extended-release formulation as compared with the fasting condition.

In another single-dose study, 8- and 4-mg Volmax® Extended-Release Tablets were shown to be bioequivalent in the fasting state. Definitive studies for the effect of food on 4-mg Volmax® Extended-Release Tablets have not been conducted. However, since food lowers the rate of absorption of 8-mg Volmax® Extended-Release Tablets, it is expected that food reduces the rate of absorption of 4-mg Volmax® Extended-Release Tablets also.

Volmax® Extended-Release Tablets have been formulated to provide duration of action of up to 12 hours. In an 8-day, multiple-dose, crossover study, 15 normal male volunteers were given 8-mg Volmax® Extended-Release Tablets every 12 hours or 4-mg Ventolin® (albuterol sulfate, USP) Tablets every 6 hours. Each dose of Volmax® Extended-Release Tablets and the corresponding doses of Ventolin® Tablets were administered in the post-prandial state. Steady-state plasma concentrations were reached within 2 days for both formulations. Fluctuations (C_{max}-C_{min}/$C_{average}$) in plasma concentrations were similar for Volmax® Extended-Release Tablets administered at 12-hour intervals and Ventolin® Tablets administered every 6 hours. In addition, the relative bioavailability of Volmax® Extended-Release Tablets was approximately 100% of the immediate-release tablet at steady state. A summary of these results is shown in the following table:

Mean Values at Steady State

	C_{max} (ng/mL)	C_{min} (ng/mL)	T_{max} (h)	$T_{1/2}$ (h)	AUC (ng-h/mL)
Volmax®	14.3	8.1	6.0	9.3	134
Ventolin®	14.5	8.1	2.6	7.2	132

The mean plasma albuterol concentration versus time data at steady state after the administration of Volmax® Extended-Release Tablets 8 mg q12h are displayed in the following graph.

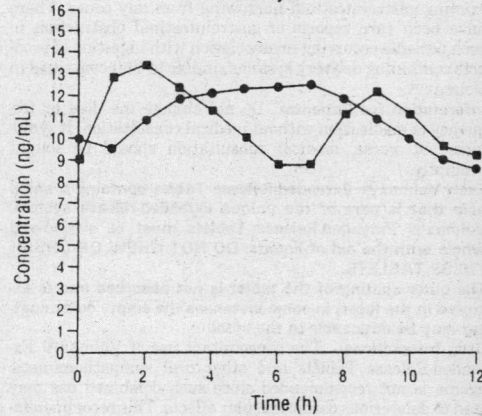

Mean Plasma Albuterol Concentration at Day 8

■ Ventolin® Tablets 4 mg q6h
● Volmax® Extended-Release Tablets 8 mg q12h

INDICATIONS AND USAGE

Volmax® Extended-Release Tablets are indicated for the relief of bronchospasm in patients with reversible obstructive airway disease.

CONTRAINDICATIONS

Volmax® Extended-Release Tablets are contraindicated in patients with a history of hypersensitivity to any of their components.

WARNINGS

Immediate hypersensitivity reactions may occur after administration of albuterol, as demonstrated by rare cases of urticaria, angioedema, rash, bronchospasm, and oropharyngeal edema.

Continued on next page

Muro—Cont.

Controlled clinical studies and other clinical experience have shown that albuterol, like other beta-adrenergic agonists, can produce a significant cardiovascular effect in some patients, as measured by pulse rate, blood pressure, symptoms, and/or electrocardiographic changes.

As with other beta-agonists, cardiac arrhythmias and sudden death have been reported in patients receiving Volmax®. Whether these adverse events are directly related to Volmax® administration is unclear.

PRECAUTIONS

General: Albuterol, as with all sympathomimetic amines, should be used with caution in patients with cardiovascular disorders, especially coronary insufficiency, cardiac arrhythmias, and hypertension; in patients with convulsive disorders, hyperthyroidism, or diabetes mellitus; and in patients who are unusually responsive to sympathomimetic amines.

In controlled clinical trials, increases in SGPT were more frequent among patients treated with Volmax® Extended-Release Tablets (12 of 247 patients, 4.9%) than among the theophylline (6 to 188 patients, 3.2%) and placebo (1 of 138 patients, 0.7%) groups. Increases in serum glucose concentration were also more frequent among patients treated with Volmax® Extended-Release Tablets (23 of 234 patients, 9.8%) than among the theophylline (11 of 173 patients 6.45%) and placebo (3 of 129 patients, 2.3%) groups. Increases in SGOT were also more frequent among patients treated with Volmax® Extended-Release Tablets (10 of 248 patients, 4%) and theophylline (5 of 193, 2.6%) than among patients treated with placebo. Decreases in white blood cell counts were more frequent in patients treated with Volmax® Extended-Release Tablets (10 of 247 patients, 4%) compared with patients receiving theophylline (2 of 185 patients, 1.1%) and patients receiving placebo (1 of 141 patients, 0.7%). Decreases in hemoglobin and hematocrit were more frequent in patients receiving Volmax® Extended-Release Tablets (16 of 228 patients, 7.0%, and 17 of 230 patients, 7.4%, respectively) than in patients receiving theophylline (5 of 171 patients, 2.9%, and 9 of 173 patients, 5.2%, respectively) and patients receiving placebo (5 of 129 patients, 3.9%, and 3 of 132 patients, 2.3%, respectively). The clinical significance of these results is unknown.

Large doses of intravenous albuterol have been reported to aggravate pre-existing diabetes mellitus and ketoacidosis. As with other beta-agonists, albuterol may produce significant hypokalemia in some patients, possibly through intracellular shunting, which has the potential to produce adverse cardiovascular effects.

As with any other nondeformable material, caution should be used when administering Volmax® to patients with preexisting gastrointestinal narrowing from any cause. There have been rare reports of gastrointestinal obstruction in such patients occurring in association with ingestion of products containing delivery systems similar to that contained in Volmax®.

Information for Patients: Do not change the dose or frequency of medication without medical consultation. If symptoms get worse, medical consultation should be sought promptly.

Each Volmax® Extended-Release Tablet contains a small hole that is part of the unique extended-release system. Volmax® Extended-Release Tablets must be swallowed whole with the aid of liquids. DO NOT CHEW OR CRUSH THESE TABLETS.

The outer coating of the tablet is not absorbed and is excreted in the feces; in some instances the empty outer coating may be noticeable in the stool.

Drug Interactions: The concomitant use of Volmax® Extended-Release Tablets and other oral sympathomimetic agents is not recommended since such combined use may lead to deleterious cardiovascular effects. This recommendation does not preclude the judicious use of an aerosol bronchodilator of the adrenergic stimulant type in patients receiving Volmax® Extended-Release Tablets. Such concomitant use, however, should be individualized.

Albuterol should be administered with extreme caution to patients being treated with monoamine oxidase inhibitors or tricyclic antidepressants because the action of albuterol on the vascular system may be potentiated.

Beta-receptor blocking agents and albuterol inhibit the effect of each other.

Carcinogenesis, Mutagenesis, Impairment or Fertility: Safety margins are adjusted to take account of differences in surface area to body weight ratio between test species and man. Albuterol sulfate, like other agents in its class, caused a significant dose-related increased incidence of mesovarium, leiomyomas in a 24-month dietary study in Sprague-Dawley rats. Doses of 2, 10, and 50 mg/kg, corresponding to 1, 4, and 18 times the maximum oral dose for a 50-kg human, were associated with incidences of mesovarium, leiomyomas of 2.4%, 18.6%, and 27.0%, respectively. In a second 24-month dietary study in the same strain, no leiomyomas occurred at 2 mg/kg, and those induced at 20 mg/kg were blocked by coadministration of 33 mg/kg of propranolol. The relevance of these findings to man is not known. There was no evidence of tumorigenicity after dietary administration to CD-1 mice for 18 months or to hamsters for 23 months at doses of 500 and 50 mg/kg, 89 and 14 times the maximum oral dose for a 50-kg human, respectively. *In vitro* studies with albuterol revealed no evidence of mutagenicity at concentrations between 0.5 and 8 mg/plate. A reproduction study in Wistar rats revealed no evidence of impaired fertility in either of two successive generations treated orally with doses up to 50 mg/kg (15 times the maximum oral dose for a 50-kg human) throughout the periods of gametogenesis, mating, pregnancy, and lactation.

Pregnancy: ***Teratogenic Effects: Pregnancy Category C:*** There are no adequate or well-controlled studies in pregnant women. Albuterol should be used during pregnancy only if the potential benefit to the patient justifies the potential risk to the fetus. A reproduction study in CD-1 mice given albuterol subcutaneously at 0.025, 0.25, or 2.5 mg/kg showed a dose-related incidence of cleft palate (0/124, 5/111, and 10/108 fetuses, respectively). Cleft palate occurred in 31% of fetuses exposed to the nonspecific beta-agonist isoproterenol at the maternal dose of 2.5 mg/kg. An oral reproduction study in Stride Dutch rabbits revealed cranioschisis in 7/19 (37%) fetuses at 50 mg/kg, 31 times the maximum oral dose for a 50-kg human.

Labor and Delivery: Oral albuterol has been shown to delay preterm labor in some reports; there are no well-controlled studies that demonstrate that it will stop preterm labor or prevent labor at term. Cautious use of Volmax® Extended-Release Tablets is required in pregnant patients when given for relief of bronchospasm so as to avoid interference with uterine contractility. Use in such patients should be restricted to those in whom the benefits clearly outweigh the risks.

Nursing Mothers: It is not known whether albuterol is excreted in human milk. Because of the potential for tumorigenicity shown for albuterol in animal studies, a decision should be made whether to discontinue nursing or to discontinue the drug, taking into account the importance of the drug to the mother.

Pediatric Use: Safety and effectiveness in children below 12 years of age have not been established.

ADVERSE REACTIONS

The adverse reactions to albuterol are similar in nature to reactions to other sympathomimetic agents. The most frequent adverse reactions to albuterol are nervousness, tremor, headache, tachycardia, and palpitations.

Less frequent adverse reactions are muscle cramps, insomnia, nausea, weakness, dizziness, drowsiness, flushing, restlessness, irritability, chest discomfort, and difficulty in micturition.

Rare cases of urticaria, angioedema, rash, bronchospasm, and oropharyngeal edema have been reported after the use of albuterol.

In addition, albuterol, like other sympathomimetic agents, can cause adverse reactions such as hypertension, angina, vomiting, vertigo, central nervous system stimulation, unusual taste, and drying or irritation of the oropharynx.

In controlled clinical trials conducted in the United States, the following incidence of adverse events was reported:

[See table below.]

A trend was observed among patients treated with Volmax® Extended-Release Tablets toward increasing frequency of muscle cramps with increasing patient age (12–20 years, 1.2%; 21–30 years, 2.6%; 31–40 years, 6.9%; 41–50 years, 6.9%), compared with no such events in the placebo group. Also observed was an increasing frequency of tremor with increasing patient age (12–20 years, 29.4%; 21–30 years, 29.9%; 31–40 years, 27.6%; 41–50 years, 37.9%), compared to 2.9% or less in the placebo group.

The reactions are generally transient in nature, and it is usually not necessary to discontinue treatment with Volmax® Extended-Release Tablets.

OVERDOSAGE

Manifestations of overdosage may include seizures, anginal pain, hypertension, hypokalemia, tachycardia with rates up to 200 beats per minute, and exaggeration of the pharmacologic effects listed in ADVERSE REACTIONS.

Oral administration to male and female mice and rats caused no significant lethality at 2,000 mg/kg. Intravenous administration to male and female mice and rats caused significant lethality at 60–70 mg/kg.

There is insufficient evidence to determine if dialysis is beneficial for overdosage of Volmax® Extended-Release Tablets.

DOSAGE AND ADMINISTRATION

The following dosages of Volmax® Extended-Release Tablets are expressed in terms of albuterol base.

Usual Dosage: The usual recommended dosage for adults and adolescents 12 years of age and older is 8 mg every 12 hours. In some patients, 4 mg every 12 hours may be sufficient.

Alternatively, patients currently maintained on Ventolin® (albuterol sulfate, USP) Tablets or Ventolin® (albuterol sulfate) Syrup can be switched to Volmax® Extended-Release Tablets. For example, the administration of one 4-mg Volmax® Extended-Release Tablet every 12 hours is equivalent to one 2-mg Ventolin® Tablet every 6 hours. Multiples of this regimen up to the maximum recommended daily dose also apply.

Dosage Adjustment: In unusual circumstances, such as adults of low body weight, it may be desirable to use a starting dosage of 4 mg every 12 hours and progress to 8 mg every 12 hours according to response.

Where control of airway obstruction is not achieved with the recommended doses, the doses may be cautiously increased under the control of the supervising physician to a maximum dose of 32 mg per day in divided doses (i.e., q12h) in adults.

Each Volmax® Extended-Release Tablet contains a small hole that is part of the unique extended-release system. Volmax® Extended-Release Tablets must be swallowed whole with the aid of liquids. DO NOT CHEW OR CRUSH THESE TABLETS.

HOW SUPPLIED

Volmax® Extended-Release Tablets, 4 mg of albuterol as the sulfate, are light blue, hexagonal tablets printed with "VOLMAX®" on one side and the number "4" on the other in dark blue ink. They are supplied in HDPE bottles with child-resistant closures of 100 tablets (NDC 0451-0398-50).

Volmax® Extended-Release Tablets, 8 mg of albuterol as the sulfate, are white, hexagonal tablets printed with "VOLMAX®" on one side and the number "8" on the other in dark blue ink. They are supplied in HPDE bottles with child-resistant closures of 100 tablets (NDC 0451-0399-50).

Store between 2° and 30°C (36° and 86°F).

*Ventolin® is a registered trademark of Allen & Hanburys

Event	Volmax® (n=330)	Theophylline (n=197)	Other β-Agonists (n=20)	Placebo (n=178)
Nervousness	8.5%	5.1%	10.0%	2.8%
Tremor	24.2%	6.1%	35.0%	1.1%
Headache	18.8%	26.9%	35.0%	20.8%
Tachycardia	2.7%	0.5%	5.0%	0%
Palpitations	2.4%	0.5%	0%	1.1%
Muscle cramps	2.7%	0.5%	5.0%	0.6%
Insomnia	2.4%	6.1%	0%	1.7%
Nausea/vomiting	4.2%	19.8%	5.0%	3.9%
Dizziness	1.5%	2.0%	0%	5.1%
Somnolence	0.3%	1.0%	0%	0.6%

Mylan Pharmaceuticals Inc.

781 CHESTNUT RIDGE ROAD
P.O. BOX 4310
MORGANTOWN, WV 26504-4310

Direct Inquiries to:
(304) 599-2595
For Medical Information Contact:
Pharmacy Affairs Department
(800) 82-MYLAN
Sales and Ordering:
Sales Department
(800) RX-MYLAN

The following list of Mylan products is provided to facilitate identification. It includes the color(s) and identification codes for all tablets and capsules.

PRODUCT GENERIC NAME Description *Color(s)*	IDENTIFICATION CODE (Front/Back*)
ACEBUTOLOL HYDROCHLORIDE Capsules, 200 mg. ℞ *Med. Orange & Med. Orange*	MYLAN 1200

ACEBUTOTOL HYDROCHLORIDE	MYLAN 1400
Capsules, 400 mg. ℞	
Med. Orange & Med. Orange	
ALBUTEROL	M255/Blank
Tablets, USP, 2 mg. ℞	
White	
ALBUTEROL	M572/Blank
Tablets, USP, 4 mg. ℞	
White	
ALLOPURINOL	M31/Blank
Tablets, USP, 100 mg. ℞	
White	
ALLOPURINOL	M71/Blank
Tablets, USP, 300 mg. ℞	
White	
ALPRAZOLAM	MYLAN A/Scored
Tablets, USP, 0.25 mg. ℂ/℞	
White	
ALPRAZOLAM	MYLAN A3/Scored
Tablets, USP, 0.5 mg. ℂ/℞	
Peach	
ALPRAZOLAM	MYLAN A1/Scored
Tablets, USP, 1 mg. ℂ/℞	
Blue	
ALPRAZOLAM	MYLAN A4/Scored
Tablets, USP, 2 mg. ℂ/℞	
White	
AMILORIDE HYDROCHLORIDE and	M577/Blank
HYDROCHLOROTHIAZIDE	
Tablets, USP, 5 mg./50 mg. ℞	
Lt. Orange	
AMITRIPTYLINE HYDROCHLORIDE	M77/Blank
Tablets, USP, 10 mg. ℞	
White	
AMITRIPTYLINE HYDROCHLORIDE	M51/Blank
Tablets, USP, 25 mg. ℞	
Lt. Green	
AMITRIPTYLINE HYDROCHLORIDE	M36/Blank
Tablets, USP, 50 mg. ℞	
Brown	
AMITRIPTYLINE HYDROCHLORIDE	M37/Blank
Tablets, USP, 75 mg. ℞	
Blue	
AMITRIPTYLINE HYDROCHLORIDE	M38/Blank
Tablets, USP, 100 mg. ℞	
Orange	
AMITRIPTYLINE HYDROCHLORIDE	M39/Blank
Tablets, USP, 150 mg. ℞	
Flesh	
AMOXICILLIN TRIHYDRATE	MYLAN 204
Capsules, USP, 250 mg. ℞	
Buff & Caramel	
AMOXICILLIN TRIHYDRATE	MYLAN 1204
Capsules, USP, 250 mg. ℞	
Normal Yellow & Normal Yellow	
AMOXICILLIN TRIHYDRATE	MYLAN 205
Capsules, USP, 500 mg. ℞	
Buff & Buff	
AMOXICILLIN TRIHYDRATE	MYLAN 1205
Capsules, USP, 500 mg ℞	
Normal Yellow & Normal Yellow	
AMOXICILLIN TRIHYDRATE	—
Powders for Oral Suspension, USP, 125 mg./5 mL. ℞	
AMOXICILLIN TRIHYDRATE	—
Powders for Oral Suspension, USP, 250 mg./5 mL. ℞	
AMPICILLIN TRIHYDRATE	MYLAN 115
Capsules, USP, 250 mg. ℞	
Gray & Scarlet	
AMPICILLIN TRIHYDRATE	MYLAN 2115
Capsules, USP, 250 mg ℞	
White & White	
AMPICILLIN TRIHYDRATE	MYLAN 116
Capsules, USP, 500 mg. ℞	
Gray & Scarlet	
AMPICILLIN TRIHYDRATE	MYLAN 2116
Capsules, USP, 500 mg ℞	
White & White	
AMPICILLIN TRIHYDRATE	—
Powders for Oral Suspension, USP, 125 mg./5 mL. ℞	
AMPICILLIN TRIHYDRATE	—
Powders for Oral Suspension, USP, 250 mg./5 mL. ℞	
ATENOLOL	M/231
Tablets, 50 mg. ℞	
White	
ATENOLOL	M/757
Tablets, 100 mg. ℞	
White	
ATENOLOL and CHLORTHALIDONE	M63/Blank
Tablets, 50 mg./25 mg. ℞	
White	
ATENOLOL and CHLORTHALIDONE	M64/Blank
Tablets, 100 mg./25 mg. ℞	
White	
BUMETANIDE	MYLAN/245
Tablets, USP, 0.5 mg. ℞	
Lt. Green	
BUMETANIDE	MYLAN/370
Tablets, USP, 1 mg. ℞	
Yellow	
BUMETANIDE	MYLAN/417
Tablets, USP, 2 mg. ℞	
Peach	
CAPTOPRIL	MC1/Scored
Tablets, USP, 12.5 mg. ℞	
White	
CAPTOPRIL	MC2/Scored
Tablets, USP, 25 mg. ℞	
White	
CAPTOPRIL	MC3/Blank
Tablets, USP, 50 mg. ℞	
White	
CAPTOPRIL	MC4/Blank
Tablets, USP, 100 mg. ℞	
White	
CEFACLOR	MYLAN 7250
Capsules, USP, 250 mg. ℞	
Pink & White	
CEFACLOR	MYLAN 7500
Capsules, USP, 500 mg. ℞	
Pink & Gray	
CEFACLOR	—
Powders for Oral Suspension, USP, 125 mg./5 mL. ℞	
CEFACLOR	—
Powders for Oral Suspension, USP, 187 mg./5 mL. ℞	
CEFACLOR	—
Powders for Oral Suspension, USP, 250 mg./5 mL. ℞	
CEFACLOR	—
Powders for Oral Suspension, USP, 375 mg./5 mL. ℞	
CEPHALEXIN	MYLAN 6025
Capsules, USP, 250 mg. ℞	
Dark Blue & White	
CEPHALEXIN	MYLAN 6050
Capsules, USP, 500 mg. ℞	
Dark Blue & Lt. Blue	
CEPHALEXIN	—
Powders for Oral Suspension, USP, 125 mg./5 mL. ℞	
CEPHALEXIN	—
Powders for Oral Suspension, USP, 250 mg./5 mL. ℞	
CHLORDIAZEPOXIDE and	MYLAN/211
AMITRIPTYLINE HYDROCHLORIDE	
Tablets, USP, 5 mg./12.5 mg. ℂ/℞	
Green	
CHLORDIAZEPOXIDE and	MYLAN/277
AMITRIPTYLINE HYDROCHLORIDE	
Tablets, USP, 10 mg./25 mg. ℂ/℞	
White	
CHLOROTHIAZIDE	M50/Blank
Tablets, USP, 250 mg. ℞	
White	
CHLOROTHIAZIDE	MYLAN 162/Blank
Tablets, USP, 500 mg. ℞	
White	
CHLORPROPAMIDE	MYLAN 197/100
Tablets, USP, 100 mg. ℞	
Green	
CHLORPROPAMIDE	MYLAN 210/250
Tablets, USP, 250 mg. ℞	
Green	
CHLORTHALIDONE	M35/Blank
Tablets, USP, 25 mg. ℞	
Lt. Yellow	
CHLORTHALIDONE	M75/Blank
Tablets, USP, 50 mg. ℞	
Lt. Green	
CIMETIDINE	M/53
Tablets, USP, 200 mg. ℞	
Green	
CIMETIDINE	M/317
Tablets, USP, 300 mg. ℞	
Green	
CIMETIDINE	M/372
Tablets, USP, 400 mg. ℞	
Green	
CIMETIDINE	M541/Blank
Tablets, USP, 800 mg. ℞	
Green	
CLONIDINE HYDROCHLORIDE	MYLAN 152/Blank
Tablets, USP, 0.1 mg. ℞	
White	
CLONIDINE HYDROCHLORIDE	MYLAN 186/Blank
Tablets, USP, 0.2 mg. ℞	
White	
CLONIDINE HYDROCHLORIDE	MYLAN 199/Blank
Tablets, USP, 0.3 mg. ℞	
White	
CLONIDINE HYDROCHLORIDE and	M1/Blank
CHLORTHALIDONE	
Tablets, USP, 0.1 mg./15 mg. ℞	
Yellow	
CLONIDINE HYDROCHLORIDE and	M27/Blank
CHLORTHALIDONE	
Tablets, USP, 0.2 mg./15 mg. ℞	
Yellow	
CLONIDINE HYDROCHLORIDE and	M72/Blank
CHLORTHALIDONE	
Tablets, USP, 0.3 mg./15 mg. ℞	
Yellow	
CLORAZEPATE DIPOTASSIUM	M30/Blank
Tablets, 3.75 mg. ℂ/℞	
Blue	
CLORAZEPATE DIPOTASSIUM	M40/Blank
Tablets, 7.5 mg. ℂ/℞	
Peach	
CLORAZEPATE DIPOTASSIUM	M70/Blank
Tablets, 15 mg. ℂ/℞	
White	
CYCLOBENZAPRINE HYDROCHLORIDE	M/751
Tablets, USP, 10 mg. ℞	
Butterscotch Yellow	
DIAZEPAM	MYLAN 271/Scored
Tablets, USP, 2 mg. ℂ/℞	
White	
DIAZEPAM	MYLAN 345/Scored
Tablets, USP, 5 mg. ℂ/℞	
Orange	
DIAZEPAM	MYLAN 477/Scored
Tablets, USP, 10 mg. ℂ/℞	
Green	
DILTIAZEM HYDROCHLORIDE	M23/Blank
Tablets, USP, 30 mg. ℞	
White	
DILTIAZEM HYDROCHLORIDE	M45/Scored
Tablets, USP, 60 mg. ℞	
White	
DILTIAZEM HYDROCHLORIDE	M135/Scored
Tablets, USP, 90 mg. ℞	
White	
DILTIAZEM HYDROCHLORIDE	M525/Scored
Tablets, USP, 120 mg. ℞	
White	
DIPHENOXYLATE HYDRO-	M15/Blank
CHLORIDE and ATROPINE SULFATE	
Tablets, USP, 2.5 mg./0.025 mg. ℂ/℞	
White	
DOXEPIN HYDROCHLORIDE	MYLAN 1049
Capsules, USP, 10 mg. ℞	
Buff & Buff	
DOXEPIN HYDROCHLORIDE	MYLAN 3125
Capsules, USP, 25 mg. ℞	
White & Ivory	
DOXEPIN HYDROCHLORIDE	MYLAN 4250
Capsules, USP, 50 mg. ℞	
Ivory & Ivory	
DOXEPIN HYDROCHLORIDE	MYLAN 5375
Capsules, USP, 75 mg. ℞	
Lt. Green & Lt. Green	
DOXEPIN HYDROCHLORIDE	MYLAN 6410
Capsules, USP, 100 mg. ℞	
White & Lt. Green	
DOXYCYCLINE HYCLATE	MYLAN 145
Capsules, USP, 50 mg. ℞	
White & Aqua Blue	
DOXYCYCLINE HYCLATE	MYLAN 148
Capsules, USP, 100 mg. ℞	
Aqua Blue & Aqua Blue	
DOXYCYCLINE HYCLATE	MYLAN 167/100
Tablets, USP, 100 mg. ℞	
Beige	
ERYTHROMYCIN ETHYLSUCCINATE	M400/Blank
Tablets, USP, 400 mg. ℞	
Beige	
ERYTHROMYCIN STEARATE	MYLAN 106/250
Tablets, USP, 250 mg. ℞	
Yellow	
ERYTHROMYCIN STEARATE	MYLAN 107/500
Tablets, USP, 500 mg. ℞	
Yellow	
FENOPROFEN CALCIUM	M471/Scored
Tablets, USP, 600 mg. ℞	
Lt. Orange	
FLUPHENAZINE HYDROCHLORIDE	M/4
Tablets, USP, 1 mg. ℞	
White	
FLUPHENAZINE HYDROCHLORIDE	M/9
Tablets, USP, 2.5 mg. ℞	
Yellow	
FLUPHENAZINE HYDROCHLORIDE	M/74
Tablets, USP, 5 mg. ℞	
Green	
FLUPHENAZINE HYDROCHLORIDE	M/97
Tablets, USP, 10 mg. ℞	
Orange	

Continued on next page

Mylan—Cont.

FLURAZEPAM HYDROCHLORIDE	MYLAN 4415
Capsules, USP, 15 mg. ℂ/℞	
White & Powder Blue	
FLURAZEPAM HYDROCHLORIDE	MYLAN 4430
Capsules, USP, 30 mg. ℂ/℞	
Powder Blue & Powder Blue	
FLURBIPROFEN	M76/Blank
Tablets, USP, 50 mg. ℞	
Beige	
FLURBIPROFEN	M93/Blank
Tablets, USP, 100 mg. ℞	
Beige	
FUROSEMIDE	M2/Blank
Tablets, USP, 20 mg. ℞	
White	
FUROSEMIDE	MYLAN 216/40
Tablets, USP, 40 mg. ℞	
White	
FUROSEMIDE	MYLAN 232/80
Tablets, USP, 80 mg. ℞	
White	
GEMFIBROZIL	MYLAN/517
Tablets, 600 mg. ℞	
White	
GLIPIZIDE	MYLAN G1/Blank
Tablets, USP, 5 mg. ℞	
White	
GLIPIZIDE	MYLAN G2/Blank
Tablets, USP, 10 mg. ℞	
White	
HALOPERIDOL	MYLAN 351/Scored
Tablets, USP, 0.5 mg. ℞	
Orange	
HALOPERIDOL	MYLAN 257/Scored
Tablets, USP, 1 mg. ℞	
Orange	
HALOPERIDOL	MYLAN 214/Scored
Tablets, USP, 2 mg. ℞	
Orange	
HALOPERIDOL	MYLAN 327/Scored
Tablets, USP, 5 mg. ℞	
Orange	
IBUPROFEN	MYLAN 1401/Blank
Tablets, USP, 400 mg. ℞	
White	
IBUPROFEN	MYLAN 1601/Blank
Tablets, USP, 600 mg. ℞	
White	
IBUPROFEN	MYLAN 1801/Blank
Tablets, USP, 800 mg. ℞	
White	
INDAPAMIDE	M/80
Tablets, USP, 2.5 mg. ℞	
White	
INDOMETHACIN	MYLAN 143
Capsules, USP, 25 mg. ℞	
Lt. Green & Lt. Green	
INDOMETHACIN	MYLAN 147
Capsules, USP, 50 mg. ℞	
Lt. Green & Lt. Green	
LOPERAMIDE HYDROCHLORIDE	MYLAN 2100
Capsules, USP, 2 mg. ℞	
Lt. Brown & Lt. Brown	
LORAZEPAM	M/321
Tablets, USP, 0.5 mg. ℂ/℞	
White	
LORAZEPAM	MYLAN 457/Blank
Tablets, USP, 1 mg. ℂ/℞	
White	
LORAZEPAM	MYLAN 777/Blank
Tablets, USP, 2 mg. ℂ/℞	
White	
MAPROTILINE HYDROCHLORIDE	M/60
Tablets, USP, 25 mg. ℞	
White	
MAPROTILINE HYDROCHLORIDE	M/87
Tablets, USP, 50 mg. ℞	
Blue	
MAPROTILINE HYDROCHLORIDE	M/92
Tablets, USP, 75 mg. ℞	
White	
MECLOFENAMATE SODIUM	MYLAN 2150
Capsules, USP, 50 mg. ℞	
Coral & Coral	
MECLOFENAMATE SODIUM	MYLAN 3000
Capsules, USP, 100 mg. ℞	
White & Coral	
METHOTREXATE	M14/Blank
Tablets, USP, 2.5 mg. ℞	
Orange	

METHYCLOTHIAZIDE	M29/Blank
Tablets, USP, 5 mg. ℞	
Blue	
METHYLDOPA	MYLAN/611
Tablets, USP, 250 mg. ℞	
Beige	
METHYLDOPA	MYLAN/421
Tablets, USP, 500 mg. ℞	
Beige	
METHYLDOPA	MYLAN/507
and HYDROCHLOROTHIAZIDE	
Tablets, USP, 250 mg./15 mg. ℞	
Green	
METHYLDOPA	MYLAN/711
and HYDROCHLOROTHIAZIDE	
Tablets, USP, 250 mg./25 mg. ℞	
White	
METOPROLOL TARTRATE	M32/Scored
Tablets, USP, 50 mg. ℞	
Pink	
METOPROLOL TARTRATE	M47/Scored
Tablets, USP, 100 mg. ℞	
Lt. Blue	
NADOLOL	M28/Blank
Tablets, USP, 20 mg. ℞	
Yellow	
NADOLOL	M171/Blank
Tablets, USP, 40 mg. ℞	
Yellow	
NADOLOL	M132/Blank
Tablets, USP, 80 mg. ℞	
Yellow	
NAPROXEN	MYLAN/377
Tablets, USP, 250 mg. ℞	
White	
NAPROXEN	MYLAN/555
Tablets, USP, 375 mg. ℞	
White	
NAPROXEN	MYLAN/451
Tablets, USP, 500 mg. ℞	
White	
NAPROXEN SODIUM	M/537
Tablets, USP, 275 mg. ℞	
Lt. Blue	
NAPROXEN SODIUM	MYLAN/733
Tablets, USP, 550 mg. ℞	
Lt. Blue	
NICARDIPINE	MYLAN 1020
Capsules, USP, 20 mg. ℞	
Blue Green & Ivory	
NICARDIPINE	MYLAN 1430
Capsules, USP, 30 mg. ℞	
Blue Green & Yellow	
NITROGLYCERIN TRANSDERMAL	Nitroglycerin
SYSTEM	0.2 mg/hr
Patches, 0.2 mg./hr. ℞	
NITROGLYCERIN TRANSDERMAL	Nitroglycerin
SYSTEM	0.4 mg/hr
Patches, 0.4 mg./hr. ℞	
NITROGLYCERIN TRANSDERMAL	Nitroglycerin
SYSTEM	0.6 mg/hr
Patches, 0.6 mg./hr. ℞	
NORTRIPTYLINE HYDROCHLORIDE	MYLAN 1410
Capsules, USP, 10 mg. ℞	
Swedish Orange & Swedish Orange	
NORTRIPTYLINE HYDROCHLORIDE	MYLAN 2325
Capsules, USP, 25 mg. ℞	
Orange & Swedish Orange	
NORTRIPTYLINE HYDROCHLORIDE	MYLAN 3250
Capsules, USP, 50 mg. ℞	
Yellow & Swedish Orange	
NORTRIPTYLINE HYDROCHLORIDE	MYLAN 4175
Capsules, USP, 75 mg. ℞	
Brown & Swedish Orange	
PENICILLIN V POTASSIUM	M11/Blank
Tablets (Oval), USP, 250 mg. ℞	
White	
PENICILLIN V POTASSIUM	M95/Blank
Tablets (Round), USP, 250 mg. ℞	
White	
PENICILLIN V POTASSIUM	M273/Blank
Tablets (Round), USP, 250 mg. ℞	
White	
PENICILLIN V POTASSIUM	M98/Blank
Tablets (Oval), USP, 500 mg. ℞	
White	
PENICILLIN V POTASSIUM	M12/Blank
Tablets (Round), USP, 500 mg. ℞	
White	
PENICILLIN POTASSIUM	M275/Scored
Tablets (Capsule Shaped), USP, 500 mg. ℞	
White	
PERPHENAZINE and AMITRIPTYLINE	MYLAN/330
HYDROCHLORIDE	
Tablets, USP, 2 mg./10 mg. ℞	
White	

PERPHENAZINE and AMITRIPTYLINE	MYLAN/442
HYDROCHLORIDE	
Tablets, USP, 2 mg./25 mg. ℞	
Purple	
PERPHENAZINE and AMITRIPTYLINE	MYLAN/727
HYDROCHLORIDE	
Tablets, USP, 4 mg./10 mg. ℞	
Blue	
PERPHENAZINE and AMITRIPTYLINE	MYLAN/574
HYDROCHLORIDE	
Tablets, USP, 4 mg./25 mg. ℞	
Orange	
PERPHENAZINE and AMITRIPTYLINE	MYLAN/73
HYDROCHLORIDE	
Tablets, USP, 4 mg./50 mg. ℞	
Purple	
PINDOLOL	M52/Blank
Tablets, USP, 5 mg. ℞	
White	
PINDOLOL	M127/Blank
Tablets, USP, 10 mg. ℞	
White	
PIROXICAM	MYLAN 1010
Capsules, USP, 10 mg. ℞	
Olive & Dark Green	
PIROXICAM	MYLAN 2020
Capsules, USP, 20 mg. ℞	
Medium Green & Medium Green	
PRAZOSIN HYDROCHLORIDE	MYLAN 1101
Capsules, USP, 1 mg. ℞	
Dk. Green & Brown	
PRAZOSIN HYDROCHLORIDE	MYLAN 2302
Capsules, USP, 2 mg. ℞	
Dk. Brown & Brown	
PRAZOSIN HYDROCHLORIDE	MYLAN 3205
Capsules, USP, 5 mg. ℞	
Lt. Blue & Brown	
PROBENECID	MYLAN 156/500
Tablets, USP, 500 mg. ℞	
Yellow	
PROPOXYPHENE COMPOUND	MYLAN 131
Capsules, USP, 65 mg. ℂ/℞	
Gray & Red	
PROPOXYPHENE HYDROCHLORIDE	MYLAN 129
Capsules, USP, 65 mg. ℂ/℞	
Pink & Pink	
PROPOXYPHENE HYDROCHLORIDE	MYLAN/130
and ACETAMINOPHEN	
Tablets, USP, 65 mg./650 mg. ℂ/℞	
Orange	
PROPOXYPHENE NAPSYLATE	MYLAN/155
and ACETAMINOPHEN	
Tablets, USP, 100 mg./650 mg. ℂ/℞	
Pink	
PROPOXYPHENE NAPSYLATE	MYLAN/1155
and ACETAMINOPHEN	
Tablets, USP, 100 mg./650 mg. ℂ/℞	
White	
PROPRANOLOL HYDROCHLORIDE	MYLAN 182/10
Tablets, USP, 10 mg. ℞	
Orange	
PROPRANOLOL HYDROCHLORIDE	MYLAN 183/20
Tablets, USP, 20 mg. ℞	
Blue	
PROPRANOLOL HYDROCHLORIDE	MYLAN 184/40
Tablets, USP, 40 mg. ℞	
Green	
PROPRANOLOL HYDROCHLORIDE	MYLAN 185/80
Tablets, USP, 80 mg. ℞	
Yellow	
PROPRANOLOL HYDROCHLO-	MYLAN 731/Scored
RIDE and HYDROCHLOROTHIAZIDE	
Tablets, USP, 40 mg./25 mg. ℞	
White	
PROPRANOLOL HYDROCHLO-	MYLAN 347/Scored
RIDE and HYDROCHLOROTHIAZIDE	
Tablets, USP, 80 mg./25 mg. ℞	
White	
RESERPINE and CHLOROTHIAZIDE	M33/Blank
Tablets, USP, 0.125 mg./250 mg. ℞	
Lt. Orange	
RESERPINE and CHLOROTHIAZIDE	M43/Blank
Tablets, USP, 0.125 mg./500 mg. ℞	
Lt. Orange	
SPIRONOLACTONE	MYLAN 146/25
Tablets, USP, 25 mg. ℞	
White	
SPIRONOLACTONE and	M41/Blank
HYDROCHLOROTHIAZIDE	
Tablets, USP, 25 mg./25 mg. ℞	
Ivory	
SULINDAC	MYLAN/427
Tablets, USP, 150 mg. ℞	
Yellow-Orange	

SULINDAC	MYLAN 531/Blank
Tablets, USP, 200 mg. ℞	
Yellow-Orange	
TEMAZEPAM	MYLAN 4010
Capsules, USP, 15 mg. ℂ/℞	
Peach & Peach	
TEMAZEPAM	MYLAN 5050
Capsules, USP, 30 mg. ℂ/℞	
Yellow & Yellow	
TETRACYCLINE HYDROCHLORIDE	MYLAN 101
Capsules, USP, 250 mg. ℞	
Yellow & Orange	
TETRACYCLINE HYDROCHLORIDE	MYLAN 102
Capsules, USP, 500 mg. ℞	
Yellow & Black	
THIORIDAZINE HYDROCHLORIDE	M54/10
Tablets, USP, 10 mg. ℞	
Orange	
THIORIDAZINE HYDROCHLORIDE	M58/25
Tablets, USP, 25 mg. ℞	
Orange	
THIORIDAZINE HYDROCHLORIDE	M59/50
Tablets, USP, 50 mg. ℞	
Orange	
THIORIDAZINE HYDROCHLORIDE	M61/100
Tablets, USP, 100 mg. ℞	
Orange	
THIOTHIXENE	MYLAN 1001
Capsules, USP, 1 mg. ℞	
Caramel & Powder Blue	
THIOTHIXENE	MYLAN 2002
Capsules, USP, 2 mg. ℞	
Caramel & Yellow	
THIOTHIXENE	MYLAN 3005
Capsules, USP, 5 mg. ℞	
White & Caramel	
THIOTHIXENE	MYLAN 5010
Capsules, USP, 10 mg. ℞	
Caramel & Peach	
TIMOLOL MALEATE	M55/Blank
Tablets, USP, 5 mg. ℞	
Green	
TIMOLOL MALEATE	M221/Blank
Tablets, USP, 10 mg. ℞	
Green	
TIMOLOL MALEATE	M715/Blank
Tablets, USP, 20 mg. ℞	
Green	
TOLAZAMIDE	MYLAN 217/250
Tablets, USP, 250 mg. ℞	
White	
TOLAZAMIDE	MYLAN 551/Blank
Tablets, USP, 500 mg. ℞	
White	
TOLBUTAMIDE	M13/Blank
Tablets, USP, 500 mg. ℞	
White	
TOLMETIN SODIUM	MYLAN 5200
Capsules, USP, 400 mg. ℞	
Lt. Blue & Lt. Blue	
TOLMETIN SODIUM	M313/Blank
Tablets, USP, 600 mg. ℞	
Beige	
TRIAMTERENE and	MYLAN 2537
HYDROCHLOROTHIAZIDE	
Capsules, USP, 37.5 mg./25 mg. ℞	
Olive & Yellow	
VERAPAMIL HYDROCHLORIDE	MYLAN 512/Blank
Tablets, USP, 80 mg. ℞	
White	
VERAPAMIL HYDROCHLORIDE	MYLAN 772/Blank
Tablets, USP, 120 mg. ℞	
White	
VERAPAMIL HYDROCHLORIDE	M411/Blank
Extended-Release Tablets, 240 mg. ℞	
Blue	

*Front/Back Side for Tablets
or Both Cap and Body
for Capsules.

IDENTIFICATION PROBLEM?
Turn to the **Product Identification** Guide,
where you'll find more than
1600 products pictured in actual
size and full color.

NABI®
P.O. Box 310701
BOCA RATON, FL 33431-0701

For Medical Information Contact:
Generally:
Immunotherapy Customer Service
(800) 458-HBIG (4244)
(305) 625-5303
FAX: (305) 625-0925
In Emergencies:
Immunotherapy Customer Service
(800) 458-HBIG (4244)
FAX: (305) 625-0925

H-BIG® ℞
(Hepatitis B Immune Globulin [Human])

½ ml syringe	(NDC 59730399-11)
1 ml vial	(NDC 59730399-01)
5 ml vial	(NDC 59730399-05)

Manufactured by:
Abbott Laboratories
North Chicago, IL 60064, U.S.A.
Distributed by:
NABI®
P.O. Box 310701
Boca Raton, FL 33431-0701

Rhₒ (D) IMMUNE GLOBULIN INTRAVENOUS (HUMAN) ℞
WinRho SD®
[*wiñ rō s d*]

Prescribing information for the suppression of Rh isoimmunization is presented below. Refer to the immune thrombocytopenic purpura section (see other side) for additional prescribing information.

DESCRIPTION
Rh_o (D) Immune Globulin Intravenous (Human) (Rh_o (D) IGIV)—WinRho SD®—is a sterile, freeze-dried gamma globulin (IgG) fraction containing antibodies to Rh_o (D). For use in the suppression of Rh isoimmunization, WinRho SD® may be administered either intramuscularly or intravenously. The manufacturing process includes a solvent detergent treatment step (using tri-n-butyl phosphate and Triton X-100) that is effective in inactivating lipid enveloped viruses such as hepatitis B, hepatitis C, and HIV.[1] This process is designed to increase product safety by reducing the risk of lipid enveloped virus transmission. This product contains approximately 2 µg IgA per 1,500 International Units (IU)* (300 µg).[2]
WinRho SD® is prepared from human plasma by an anion-exchange column chromatography method.[3–5]
The product potency is expressed in international units by comparison to the World Health Organization (WHO) standard. A 1,500 International Unit (IU)* (300 µg) vial contains sufficient anti-Rh_o (D) to effectively suppress the immunizing potential of approximately 17 mL of Rh_o (D) positive red blood cells.
The product is stabilized with 0.1 M glycine and 0.15 M sodium chloride. It contains no preservative.

CLINICAL PHARMACOLOGY
Suppression of Rh Isoimmunization
WinRho SD®, Rh_o (D) Immune Globulin Intravenous (Human), is used to suppress the immune response of non-sensitized Rh_o (D) negative individuals following Rh_o (D) positive red blood cell exposure by fetomaternal hemorrhage during delivery of an Rh_o (D) positive infant, abortion (spontaneous or induced), amniocentesis, abdominal trauma, or mismatched transfusion.[6–8] The mechanism of action is not completely understood.
WinRho SD®, when administered within 72 hours of a full-term delivery of an Rh_o (D) positive infant by an

---
* In the past, a full dose of Rh_o (D) Immune Globulin (Human) has traditionally been referred to as a "300 µg" dose. Potency and dosing recommendations are now expressed in IU by comparison to the WHO Anti-D standard. The conversion of "µg" to "IU" is 1 µg = 5 IU.

Rh_o (D) negative mother, will reduce the incidence of Rh isoimmunization from 12–13% to 1–2%. The 1–2% is, for the most part, due to isoimmunization during the last trimester of pregnancy. When treatment is given both antenatally at 28 weeks gestation and postpartum, the Rh immunization rate drops to about 0.1%.[9–12]
When 600 IU (120 µg) of Rh_o (D) IGIV is administered to pregnant women, passive anti-Rh_o (D) antibodies are not detectable in the circulation for more than six weeks and

therefore a dose of 1,500 IU (300 µg) should be used for antenatal administration.
In a clinical study with Rh_o (D) negative volunteers (nine males and one female), Rh_o (D) positive red cells were completely cleared from the circulation within eight hours of intravenous administration of Rh_o (D) IGIV. There was no indication of Rh isoimmunization of these subjects at six months after the clearance of the Rh_o (D) positive red cells.
Pharmacokinetics—IM versus IV Administration
In a clinical study involving Rh_o (D) negative volunteers, two subjects were administered 600 IU (120 µg) Rh_o (D) IGIV by intramuscular administration and two subjects were administered this dose by intravenous administration. Peak levels (36 to 48 ng/mL) were reached within two hours of intravenous administration and peak levels (18 to 19 ng/mL) were reached at five to 10 days after intramuscular administration. The areas under the curve were the same for both routes of administration. The $t_{1/2}$ for anti-Rh_o (D) was about 24 days following IV administration and about 30 days following IM administration.

INDICATIONS AND CLINICAL USE
Pregnancy and Other Obstetric Conditions
WinRho SD®, Rh_o (D) Immune Globulin Intravenous (Human), is recommended for the suppression of Rh isoimmunization in non-sensitized Rh_o (D) negative women within 72 hours after spontaneous or induced abortions, amniocentesis, chorionic villus sampling, ruptured tubal pregnancy, abdominal trauma or transplacental hemorrhage or in the normal course of pregnancy unless the blood type of the fetus or father is known to be Rh_o (D) negative. In the case of maternal bleeding due to threatened abortion, WinRho SD® should be administered as soon as possible. Suppression of Rh isoimmunization reduces the likelihood of hemolytic disease in an Rh_o (D) positive fetus in present and future pregnancies.
The criteria for an Rh-incompatible pregnancy requiring administration of WinRho SD® at 28 weeks gestation and within 72 hours after delivery are:
- the mother must be Rh_o (D) negative,
- the mother is carrying a child whose father is either Rh_o (D) positive or Rh_o (D) unknown,
- the baby is either Rh_o (D) positive or Rh_o (D) unknown, and
- the mother must not be previously sensitized to the Rh_o (D) factor.

In a clinical trial of 1,186 non-sensitized, Rh_o (D) negative pregnant women in cases in which the blood types of the fathers were either Rh_o (D) negative or unknown, Rh_o (D) IGIV was administered according to one of three regimens: 1) 93 women received 600 IU (120 µg) at 28 weeks; 2) 131 women received 1200 IU (240 µg) each at 28 and 34 weeks; 3) 962 women received 1200 IU (240 µg) at 28 weeks. All women received a postnatal administration of 600 IU (120 µg) if the newborn was found to be Rh_o (D) positive. Of 1,186 women who received antenatal Rh_o (D) IGIV, 806 were given Rh_o (D) IGIV postnatally following the delivery of an Rh_o (D) positive infant, of which 325 women underwent testing at six months after delivery for evidence of Rh isoimmunization. Of these 325 women, 23 would have been expected to display signs of Rh isoimmunization; however, none was observed (p < 0.001 in a Chi-square test of significance of difference between observed and expected isoimmunization in the absence of Rh_o (D) IGIV).
Transfusion
WinRho SD®, Rh_o (D) Immune Globulin Intravenous (Human), is recommended for the suppression of Rh isoimmunization in Rh_o (D) negative female children and female adults in their childbearing years transfused with Rh_o (D) positive red blood cells or blood components containing Rh_o (D) positive red blood cells. Treatment should be initiated within 72 hours of exposure. Treatment should be given (without preceding exchange transfusion) only if the transfused Rh_o (D) positive blood represents less than 20% of the total circulating red cells. A 1,500 IU (300 µg) dose will suppress the immunizing potential of approximately 17 mL of Rh_o (D) positive red blood cells.

CONTRAINDICATIONS
Individuals known to have had an anaphylactic or severe systemic reaction to human globulin should not receive WinRho SD® or any other Rh_o (D) Immune Globulin (Human). WinRho SD® contains trace amounts of IgA (approximately 2 µg per 1,500 IU [300 µg] vial). Individuals who are deficient in IgA may have the potential for developing IgA antibodies and have anaphylactic reactions. The physician must weigh the potential benefit of treatment with WinRho SD® against the potential for hypersensitivity reactions.

WARNINGS
For the suppression of Rh isoimmunization in the mother, do not administer to the infant.

Continued on next page

NABI—Cont.

PRECAUTIONS

Suppression of Rh Isoimmunization

WinRho SD®, Rh_o (D) Immune Globulin Intravenous (Human), should not be administered to Rh_o (D) negative individuals who are Rh immunized as evidenced by standard manual Rh antibody screening tests.

A large fetomaternal hemorrhage late in pregnancy or following delivery may cause a weak mixed field positive D^u test result. Such an individual should be assessed for a large fetomaternal hemorrhage and the dose of WinRho SD® adjusted accordingly. WinRho SD® should be administered if there is any doubt about the mother's blood type.

Laboratory Tests

The presence of passively administered anti-Rh_o (D) in maternal or fetal blood can lead to a false positive direct antiglobulin test. If there is an uncertainty about mother's Rh group or immune status, WinRho SD® should be administered to the mother.

Drug Interactions

Administration of WinRho SD® with other drugs has not been evaluated. Refer to Dosage and Administration section for information on drug compatibility.

Pregnancy Category C

Animal reproduction studies have not been conducted with WinRho SD®. It is not known whether WinRho SD® can cause fetal harm when administered to a pregnant woman or can affect reproductive capacity. WinRho SD® should be given to a pregnant woman only if clearly needed.

ADVERSE REACTIONS

Adverse reactions to WinRho SD® are infrequent in Rh_o (D) negative individuals. In the clinical trial of 1,186 Rh_o (D) negative pregnant women, no adverse events were attributed to Rh_o (D) IGIV. Discomfort and slight swelling at the site of injection and slight elevation in temperature have been reported in a small number of cases. As is the case with all drugs of this nature, there is a remote chance of anaphylactic reaction with WinRho SD® in individuals with hypersensitivity to blood products. There was one report of an Rh_o (D) negative patient, who had received one unit of Rh_o (D) positive blood, reporting chills, shaking, nausea, myalgia, vomiting, drowsiness, disorientation, and lethargy after receiving 6,000 IU (1,200 μg) of Rh_o (D) IGIV.

A post-marketing survey conducted since the Canadian licensure of Rh_o (D) IGIV in 1980 for this indication included data obtained from 31,059 injections (25,068 for routine Rh prophylaxis and 5,991 following abortions, amniocentesis, chorionic villus sampling and antepartum hemorrhage). There were 9,905 Rh_o (D) negative women who delivered Rh_o (D) positive infants, almost all of whom had received antenatal as well as postnatal prophylaxis. Of the patients followed in this survey, there were 26 reported treatment failures that resulted in the development of Rh_o (D) antibodies. There were no adverse experiences related to Rh_o (D) IGIV reported in this survey.

SYMPTOMS AND TREATMENT OF OVERDOSAGE

There are no reports of known overdoses in patients being treated for Rh isoimmunization. In clinical studies with nonpregnant Rh_o (D) positive patients with ITP (n=141) treated with 600 to 32,500 IU (120 to 6,500 μg) of Rh_o (D) IGIV, there were no signs or symptoms that warranted medical intervention. However, these same doses were associated with a mild, transient hemolytic anemia.

DOSAGE AND ADMINISTRATION

WinRho SD®, Rh_o (D) Immune Globulin Intravenous (Human), may be given by intravenous or intramuscular administration for the suppression of Rh isoimmunization. WinRho SD® should be reconstituted only with 0.9% Sodium Chloride Injection. It should not be administered with other products.

Pregnancy

The same dosage, as described below, is to be administered by either the intramuscular or intravenous routes.

A 1,500 IU (300 μg) dose of WinRho SD® should be administered at 28 weeks gestation. If WinRho SD® is administered early in the pregnancy, it is recommended that WinRho SD® be administered at 12-week intervals in order to maintain an adequate level of passively acquired anti-Rh.

A 600 IU (120 μg) dose should be administered as soon as possible after delivery of a confirmed Rh_o (D) positive baby and normally no later than 72 hours after delivery. In the event that the Rh status of the baby is not known at 72 hours, WinRho SD® should be administered to the mother at 72 hours after delivery. If more than 72 hours have elapsed, WinRho SD® should not be withheld, but administered as soon as possible up to 28 days after delivery.

Other Obstetric Conditions

The same dosage, as described below, is to be administered by either the intramuscular or intravenous routes.

A 600 IU (120 μg) dose of WinRho SD® should be administered immediately after abortion, amniocentesis (after 34 weeks gestation) or any other manipulation late in pregnancy (after 34 weeks gestation) associated with increased risk of Rh isoimmunization. Administration should take place within 72 hours after the event.

A 1,500 IU (300 μg) dose of WinRho SD® should be administered immediately after amniocentesis before 34 weeks gestation or after chorionic villus sampling. This dose should be repeated every 12 weeks while the woman is pregnant. In the case of threatened abortion, WinRho SD® should be administered as soon as possible.

Transfusion

WinRho SD®, Rh_o (D) Immune Globulin Intravenous (Human), should be administered within 72 hours after exposure for treatment of incompatible blood transfusions or massive fetal hemorrhage as outlined in the table below.

Route of Administration	Dose and Frequency	WinRho SD® Dosage: Rh+Blood	WinRho SD® Dosage: Rh+red cells
Intravenous	3,000 IU (600 μg) every 8 hours until the total dose is administered	45 IU (9 μg)/ mL Blood	90 IU (18 μg)/ mL Cells
Intramuscular	6,000 IU (1,200 μg) every 12 hours until the total dose is administered	60 IU (12 μg) mL Blood	120 IU (24 μg)/ mL Cells

Reconstitution

Intravenous Administration

Aseptically reconstitute the product shortly before use with 2.5 mL of 0.9% Sodium Chloride Injection (see the next table). Inject the diluent slowly onto the inside wall of the vial and wet the pellet by gently swirling until dissolved. Do not shake.

Intramuscular Administration

Aseptically reconstitute the product shortly before use with 1.25 mL of 0.9% Sodium Chloride Injection (see the next table). Inject the diluent slowly onto the inside wall of the vial and wet the pellet by gently swirling until dissolved. Do not shake.

Vial Size	Volume of Diluent to be Added to Vial	Approximate Available Volume	Nominal Concentration per mL
Intravenous Injection			
600 IU (120 μg)	2.5 mL	2.4 mL	240 IU (48 μg)/mL
1,500 IU (300 μg)	2.5 mL	2.4 mL	600 IU (120 μg)/mL
Intramuscular Injection			
600 IU (120 μg)	1.25 mL	1.2 mL	480 IU (96 μg)/mL
1,500 IU (300 μg)	1.25 mL	1.2 mL	1,200 IU (240 μg)/mL

Injection

Parenteral products such as WinRho SD® should be inspected for particulate matter and discoloration prior to administration. Use the product within four hours of reconstitution. Discard any unused portion.

Intravenous Administration

Infuse into a suitable vein over three to five minutes. WinRho SD® should be administered separately from other drugs.

Intramuscular Administration

Administer into the deltoid muscle of the upper arm or the anterolateral aspects of the upper thigh. Due to the risk of sciatic nerve injury, the gluteal region should not be used as a routine injection site. If the gluteal region is used, use only the upper, outer quadrant.

HOW SUPPLIED

WinRho SD®, Rh_o (D) Immune Globulin Intravenous (Human), is available in packages containing:

NDC Number	Contents
60492-0081-1	10 boxes each containing a single dose vial of 600 IU (120 μg) anti-Rh_o (D) IGIV, a single dose vial of 2.5 mL 0.9% Sodium Chloride Injection, and a package insert
60492-0082-1	10 boxes each containing a single dose vial of 1,500 IU (300 μg) anti-Rh_o (D) IGIV, a single dose vial of 2.5 mL 0.9% Sodium Chloride Injection, and a package insert

STORAGE

Store at 2 to 8°C (35 to 46°F). Do not freeze. Do not use after expiration date.

If the reconstituted product is not used immediately, store it at room temperature for no longer than four hours. Do not freeze the reconstituted product. Discard the product if not administered within four hours.

CAUTION

U.S. federal law prohibits dispensing without prescription.

REFERENCES

1. Horowitz, B: Investigations into the application of tri(n-butyl)phosphate/detergent mixtures to blood derivatives. Morgenthaler J (ed): *Virus Inactivation in Plasma Products, Curr. Stud. Hematol. Blood. Transfus.* 1989; 56:83-96.
2. Laschinger, C, et al.: Fluctuating levels of serum IgA in individuals with selective IgA deficiency. *Vox Sang.* 1984; 47:60-67.
3. Bowman JM, et al.: Low protein Rh immune globulin (Rh IgG)-purity, stability, activity and prophylactic value. *Vox Sang* 1973; 24:301-316.
4. Bowman, JM, et al.: WinRho: Rh immune globulin prepared by ion exchange for intravenous use. *Can. Med. Assoc. J.* 1980; 123:1121-1125.
5. Friesen, AD, et al.: Column ion-exchange preparation and characterization of an Rh immune globulin (WinRho) for intravenous use. *J. Appl. Biochem.* 1981; 3:164-175.
6. Chown, B, et al.: The effect of anti-D IgG on D-positive recipients. *Can. Med. Assoc. J.* 1970; 102:1161-1164.
7. Bowman, JM and Chown, B: Prevention of Rh immunization after massive Rh-positive transfusion. *Can. Med. Assoc. J.* 1968; 99:385-388.
8. Bowman, JM: Suppression of Rh isoimmunization: a review. *Obstet. & Gynec.* 1978; 52:385-393.
9. Bowman, JM, et al.: Rh isoimmunization during pregnancy: antenatal prophylaxis. *Can. Med. Assoc. J.* 1978; 118:623-627.
10. Bowman, JM, and Pollock, JM: Antenatal prophylaxis of Rh isoimmunization: 28 weeks'-gestation service program. *Can. Med. Assoc. J.* 1978; 118:627-630.
11. Bowman, JM, and Pollock, JM: Failures of intravenous Rh immune globulin prophylaxis: An analysis of the reasons for such failures. *Trans. Med. Rev.* 1987; 1:101-112.
12. Bowman, JM: Antenatal suppression of Rh alloimmunization. *Clin Obstet. & Gynec.* 1991; 34:296-303.

Manufactured by:
Cangene Corporation
Winnipeg, Canada R3T 5Y3
U.S. License No. 1201
Distributed by:
NABI®
Boca Raton, Florida 33431-0701
NABI Code No. 00371-80-GEN-280696

Rh_o (D) IMMUNE GLOBULIN INTRAVENOUS (HUMAN) ℞

WinRho SD®

[wiñ rō s d]

Prescribing information for the treatment of immune thrombocytopenic purpura is presented below. Refer to the Rh isoimmunization section (see other side) for additional prescribing information.

DESCRIPTION

Rh_o (D) Immune Globulin Intravenous (Human) (Rh_o (D) IGIV)—WinRho SD®—is a sterile, freeze-dried gamma globulin (IgG) fraction containing antibodies to Rh_o (D). For use in the treatment of immune thrombocytopenic purpura (ITP), WinRho SD® must be administered intravenously. The manufacturing process includes a solvent detergent treatment step (using tri-n-butyl phosphate and Triton X-100) that is effective in inactivating lipid enveloped viruses such as hepatitis B, hepatitis C, and HIV.[1] This process is designed to increase product safety by reducing the risk of lipid enveloped virus transmission. This product contains approximately 2 μg IgA per 1,500 International Units (IU)* (300 μg).[2]

WinRho SD® is prepared from human plasma by an anion-exchange column chromatography method.[3–5]

The product potency is expressed in international units by comparison to the World Health Organization (WHO) standard. A 1,500 International Unit (IU)* (300 μg) vial contains sufficient anti-Rh_o (D) to effectively suppress the immunizing potential of approximately 17 mL of Rh_o (D) positive red blood cells.

The product is stabilized with 0.1 M glycine and 0.15 M sodium chloride. It contains no preservative.

CLINICAL PHARMACOLOGY

WinRho SD®, Rh$_o$ (D) Immune Globulin Intravenous (Human), has been shown to increase platelets in ITP patients. Platelet counts usually rise within one to two days and peak within seven to 14 days after initiation of therapy. The duration of response is variable; however, the average duration is approximately 30 days. The mechanism of action is not completely understood.

* In the past, a full dose of Rh$_o$ (D) Immune Globulin (Human) has traditionally been referred to as a "300 μg" dose. Potency and dosing recommendations are now expressed in IU by comparison to the WHO Anti-D standard. The conversion of "μg" to "IU" is 1 μg=5 IU.

INDICATIONS AND CLINICAL USE

WinRho SD®, Rh$_o$ (D) Immune Globulin Intravenous (Human), is recommended for the treatment of nonsplenectomized Rh$_o$ (D) positive

- children with chronic or acute ITP,
- adults with chronic ITP, or
- children and adults with ITP secondary to HIV infection

in clinical situations requiring an increase in platelet count to prevent excessive hemorrhage.

Childhood Chronic ITP

In an open-label, single arm, multicenter study, 24 children with ITP of greater than six months duration were treated initially with 250 IU (50 μg)/kg Rh$_o$ (D) Immune Globulin Intravenous (Human) (125 IU [25 μg]/kg on days 1 and 2), with subsequent doses ranging from 125 to 275 IU (25 to 55 μg)/kg. Response was defined as a platelet increase to at least 50,000/mm³ and a doubling of the baseline. Nineteen of 24 patients responded for an overall response rate of 79%, an overall mean peak platelet count of 229,400/mm³ (range 43,300 to 456,000), and a mean duration of response of 36.5 days (range 6 to 84).[6-7]

Childhood Acute ITP

A multicenter, randomized, controlled trial comparing Rh$_o$ (D) IGIV to high dose and low dose Immune Globulin Intravenous (Human) and prednisone was conducted in 146 children with acute ITP and platelet counts less than 20,000/mm³. Of 38 patients receiving Rh$_o$ (D) IGIV (125 IU [25 μg]/kg on days 1 and 2), 32 patients (84%) responded (platelet count ≥50,000/mm³) with a mean peak platelet count of 319,500/mm³ (range 61,000 to 892,000), with no statistically significant differences compared to other treatment arms. The mean times to achieving ≥20,000/mm³ or ≥50,000/mm³ platelets for patients receiving Rh$_o$ (D) IGIV were 1.9 and 2.8 days, respectively. When comparing the different therapies for time to platelet count ≥20,000/mm³ or ≥50,000/mm³, no statistically significant differences among treatment groups were detected, with a range of 1.3 to 1.9 days and 2.0 to 3.2 days, respectively.[8-9]

Adult Chronic ITP

Twenty-four adults with ITP of greater than six months duration and platelet counts <30,000/mm³ or requiring therapy were enrolled in a single-arm, open-label trial and treated with 100 to 375 IU (20 to 75 μg)/kg Rh$_o$ (D) IGIV (mean dose 231 IU [46.2 μg]/kg). Twenty-one of 24 patients responded (increase ≥20,000/mm³) during the first two courses of therapy for an overall response rate of 88% with a mean peak platelet count of 92,300/mm³ (range 8,000 to 229,000).[10-11]

ITP Secondary to HIV Infection

Eleven children and 52 adults with all Walter Reed classes of HIV infection and ITP, with initial platelet counts of ≤30,000/mm³ or requiring therapy, were treated with 100 to 375 IU (20 to 75 μg)/kg Rh$_o$ (D) IGIV in an open label trial. Rh$_o$ (D) IGIV was administered for an average of 7.3 courses (range 1 to 57) over a mean period of 407 days (range 6 to 1,952). Fifty-seven of 63 patients responded (increase ≥20,000/mm³) during the first six courses of therapy for an overall response rate of 90%. The overall mean change in platelet count for six courses was 60,900/mm³ (range -2,000 to 565,000), and the mean peak platelet count was 81,700/mm³ (range 16,000 to 593,000).[11-13]

CONTRAINDICATIONS

Individuals known to have had an anaphylactic or severe systemic reaction to human globulin should not receive WinRho SD® or any other Rh$_o$ (D) Immune Globulin (Human). WinRho SD®, Rh$_o$ (D) Immune Globulin Intravenous (Human), contains trace amounts of IgA (approximately 2 μg per 1,500 IU [300 μg] vial). Individuals who are deficient in IgA may have the potential for developing IgA antibodies and have anaphylactic reactions. The physician must weigh the potential benefit of treatment with WinRho SD® against the potential for hypersensitivity reactions.

WARNINGS

WinRho SD® must be administered via the intravenous route for the treatment of ITP as its efficacy has not been established by the intramuscular or subcutaneous routes. WinRho SD® should not be administered to Rh$_o$ (D) negative or splenectomized individuals as its efficacy in these patients has not been demonstrated.

PRECAUTIONS

If the patient has a lower than normal hemoglobin level (less than 10 g/dL), a reduced dose of 125 to 200 IU (25 to 40 μg)/kg body weight should be given to minimize the risk of increasing the severity of anemia in the patient. WinRho SD®, Rh$_o$ (D) Immune Globulin Intravenous (Human), must be used with extreme caution in patients with a hemoglobin level that is less than 8 g/dL due to the risk of increasing the severity of the anemia.

Drug Interactions

Administration of WinRho SD® with other drugs has not been evaluated. Refer to Dosage and Administration section for information on drug compatibility.

Pregnancy Category C

Animal reproduction studies have not been conducted with WinRho SD®. It is not known whether WinRho SD® can cause fetal harm when administered to a pregnant woman or can affect reproductive capacity. WinRho SD® should be given to a pregnant woman only if clearly needed.

ADVERSE REACTIONS

WinRho SD®, Rh$_o$ (D) Immune Globulin Intravenous (Human), is administered to Rh$_o$ (D) positive patients with ITP. Therefore, side effects related to the destruction of Rh$_o$ (D) positive red cells, such as decreased hemoglobin, can be expected. At the recommended initial intravenous dose of 250 IU (50 μg)/kg, the mean maximum decrease in hemoglobin was 1.70 g/dL (range +0.40 to −6.1 g/dL). At a reduced dose, ranging from 125 to 200 IU (25 to 40 μg)/kg, the mean maximum decrease in hemoglobin was 0.81 g/dL (range +0.65 to −1.9 g/dL). Only 5/137 (3.7%) of patients had a maximum decrease in hemoglobin of greater than 4 g/dL. In trials in subjects (n=161) with childhood acute ITP, adults and children with chronic ITP, and adults and children with ITP secondary to HIV, 60/848 (7%) of infusions were associated with at least one adverse event that was considered to be related to the study medication. The most common adverse events were headache (19 infusions; 2%), chills (14 infusions; <2%), and fever (nine infusions; 1%). All are expected adverse events associated with infusions of immunoglobulins.

One child with chronic ITP who received an initial dose of 250 IU (50 μg)/kg Rh$_o$ (D) IGIV followed by 175 IU (35 μg)/kg on day 15 had a drop in hemoglobin from 12.4 g/dL to 7.6 g/dL after the second course of treatment. Rh$_o$ (D) IGIV was subsequently withheld.[6]

SYMPTOMS AND TREATMENT OF OVERDOSAGE

There are no reports of known overdoses in patients being treated for Rh isoimmunization or ITP. In clinical studies with nonpregnant Rh$_o$ (D) positive patients with ITP (n=141) treated with 600 to 32,500 IU (120 to 6,500 μg) of Rh$_o$ (D) IGIV there were no signs or symptoms that warranted medical intervention. However, these same doses were associated with a mild, transient hemolytic anemia.

DOSAGE AND ADMINISTRATION

WinRho SD®, Rh$_o$ (D) Immune Globulin Intravenous (Human), must be given by intravenous administration for the treatment of ITP.

WinRho SD® should be reconstituted only with 0.9% Sodium Chloride Injection. It should not be administered with other products. An initial dose of 250 IU (50 μg)/kg body weight is recommended for the treatment of ITP. If the patient has a hemoglobin level that is less than 10 g/dL, a reduced dose of 125 to 200 IU (25 to 40 μg)/kg should be given to minimize the risk of increasing the severity of anemia in the patient. The initial dose may be administered as a single dose or in two divided doses given on separate days. All patients should be monitored to determine clinical response by assessing platelet counts, red cell counts, hemoglobin, and reticulocyte levels.

If subsequent therapy is required to elevate platelet counts, an intravenous dose of 125 to 300 IU (25 to 60 μg)/kg of WinRho SD®, Rh$_o$ (D) Immune Globulin Intravenous (Human), is recommended. The frequency and dose used in maintenance therapy should be determined by the patient's clinical response by assessing platelet counts, red cell counts, hemoglobin, and reticulocyte levels.

Reconstitution for Intravenous Administration

Aseptically reconstitute shortly before use with 2.5 mL of 0.9% Sodium Chloride Injection. Inject the diluent slowly onto the inside wall of the vial and wet the pellet by gently swirling until dissolved. Do not shake.

Vial Size	Volume of Diluent to be Added to Vial	Approximate Available Volume	Nominal Concentration per mL
600 IU (120 μg)	2.5 mL	2.4 mL	240 IU (48 μg)/mL
1,500 IU (300 μg)	2.5 mL	2.4 mL	600 IU (120 μg)/mL

Injection

Parenteral products such as WinRho SD® should be inspected for particulate matter and discoloration prior to administration. Use the product within four hours of reconstitution. Discard any unused portion.

Infuse into a suitable vein over three to five minutes. WinRho SD® should be administered separately from other drugs.

HOW SUPPLIED

WinRho SD®, Rh$_o$ (D) Immune Globulin Intravenous (Human), is available in packages containing:

NDC Number	Contents
60492-0081-1	10 boxes each containing a single dose vial of 600 IU (120 μg) anti-Rh$_o$ (D) IGIV, a single dose vial of 2.5 mL 0.9% Sodium Chloride Injection, and a package insert
60492-0082-1	10 boxes each containing a single dose vial of 1,500 IU (300 μg) anti-Rh$_o$ (D) IGIV, a single dose vial of 2.5 mL 0.9% Sodium Chloride Injection, and a package insert

STORAGE

Store WinRho SD®, Rh$_o$ (D) Immune Globulin Intravenous (Human) at 2 to 8°C (35 to 46°F). Do not freeze. Do not use after expiration date.

If the reconstituted product is not used immediately, store it at room temperature for no longer than four hours. Do not freeze the reconstituted product. Discard the product if not administered within four hours.

CAUTION

U.S. federal law prohibits dispensing without prescription.

REFERENCES

1. Horowitz, B: Investigations into the application of tri(n-butyl)phosphate/detergent mixtures to blood derivatives. Morgenthaler J (ed): *Virus Inactivation in Plasma Products, Curr. Stud. Hematol. Blood. Transfus.* 1989; 56:83-96.
2. Laschinger, C. et al.: Fluctuating levels of serum IgA in individuals with selective IgA deficiency. *Vox Sang.* 1984; 47:60-67.
3. Bowman, JM, et al.: Low protein Rh immune globulin (Rh IgG)-purity, stability, activity and prophylactic value. *Vox Sang* 1973; 24:301-316.
4. Bowman, JM, et al.: WinRho: Rh immune globulin prepared by ion exchange for intravenous use. *Can. Med. Assoc. J.* 1980; 123:1121-1125.
5. Friesen, AD, et al.: Column ion-exchange preparation and characterization of an Rh immune globulin (WinRho) for intravenous use. *J. Appl. Biochem.* 1981; 3:164-175.
6. Unpublished data on file, CITP Report, May 1993.
7. Andrew, M, et al.: A multicenter study of the treatment of childhood chronic idiopathic thrombocytopenic purpura with anti-D. *J Pediatrics* 120:522-527, 1992.
8. Unpublished data on file, AITP Report, May 1993.
9. Blanchette, V, et al.: Randomised trial of intravenous immunoglobulin G, intravenous anti-D, and oral prednisone in childhood acute immune thrombocytopenic purpura. *Lancet* 344: 703-707, 1994.
10. Unpublished data on file, BITP-2 Report, May 1993.
11. Bussel, JB, et al.: Intravenous anti-D treatment of immune thrombocytopenic purpura: Analysis of efficacy, toxicity, and mechanism of effect. *Blood* 77:1884-1893, 1991.
12. Unpublished data on file, BITP-1 Report, May 1993.
13. Bussel, JB, et al.: IV anti-D treatment of ITP: Results in 210 cases. Abstract, *The American Society of Hematology*, Anaheim, CA, December, 1992.

Manufactured by:
Cangene Corporation
Winnipeg, Canada R3T 5Y3
U.S. License No. 1201
Distributed by:
NABI®
Boca Raton, Florida 33431-0701
NABI Code No. 00371-80-GEN-280696

For information on over-the-counter drugs, consult **PDR For Nonprescription Drugs**

Neutrogena Dermatologics
5760 WEST 96th STREET
LOS ANGELES, CA 90045

Direct Inquiries to:
Mitchell S. Wortzman, Ph.D.
(310) 642-1150
FAX: (310) 337-2156
For Medical Information Contact:
In Emergencies:
Mitchell S. Wortzman, Ph.D.
(310) 642-1150
FAX: (310) 337-2156

MELANEX® ℞
Topical Solution
(Hydroquinone USP, 3.0%)
FOR EXTERNAL USE ONLY

CAUTION: Federal law prohibits dispensing without prescription.

DESCRIPTION
Each milliliter of Melanex® Topical Solution contains 30 mg of hydroquinone in a hydroalcoholic base of purified water, SD Alcohol 40 (45%), Laureth-4, Isopropyl Alcohol (4%), Propylene Glycol, Ascorbic Acid.

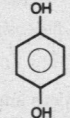

$C_6H_6O_2$ 110.11
1,4 DIHYDROXYBENZENE
Hydroquinone

CLINICAL PHARMACOLOGY
It has been suggested the primary action of hydroquinone is directed at tyrosinase.[1] The selective inhibition of the enzyme affects melanogenesis in the melanocytes resulting in cessation of melanin formation and subsequent reduction in pigmentation. Additional studies indicate hydroquinone acts on the essential subcellular metabolic processes of melanocytes with resultant cytolysis, i.e., non-enzyme-mediated depigmentation.[2]

INDICATIONS AND USAGE
Melanex® is indicated in the temporary depigmentation of hyperpigmented skin conditions such as chloasma, melasma, freckles, senile lentigines, and other forms of melanin hyperpigmentation.

DOSAGE AND ADMINISTRATION
Apply to affected areas twice daily, in the morning and before bedtime. During the day, an effective broad spectrum sunscreen like Neutrogena® Sunblock SPF 15 or SPF 30 should be used and unnecessary solar exposure avoided, or protective clothing should be worn to cover the treated area in order to prevent repigmentation from occurring.

CONTRAINDICATIONS
Melanex® is contraindicated in persons who have shown hypersensitivity to hydroquinone or any of the other ingredients. The safety of topical treatment with hydroquinone during pregnancy has not been established.

PRECAUTIONS
Concurrent use of Melanex® with peroxide products may result in transient dark staining of skin areas so treated. This is due to the oxidation of hydroquinone by the peroxide. This transient staining can be removed by discontinuing concurrent usage and normal soap cleansing.
FOR EXTERNAL USE ONLY
Hydroquinone preparations may produce skin irritation in susceptible individuals and have a slight potential to produce allergic response. Therefore, the physician should use appropriate caution. If rash or irritation develops, discontinue use and consult physician. Do not use on children under 12 years.
If no improvement is seen after two months of treatment, use of product should be discontinued. Avoid contact with eyes. In case of accidental contact, patient should rinse eyes thoroughly with water and contact physician. A bitter taste and anesthetic effect may occur if applied to lips. Keep out of reach of children. Use of Melanex® in paranasal and infraorbital areas increases the chance of irritation (see **ADVERSE REACTIONS**).

ADVERSE REACTIONS
The following have been reported: dryness and fissuring of the paranasal and infraorbital areas, erythema, and sting-

ing. Hydroquinone has been known to produce irritation and sensitization in susceptible individuals.
HOW SUPPLIED: 1 fl. oz. (30 ML) bottle with plastic rod and Appliderm® Applicator unit.
NOTE: Slight darkening of the Melanex® solution is normal and will not affect potency. See expiration date on bottle.

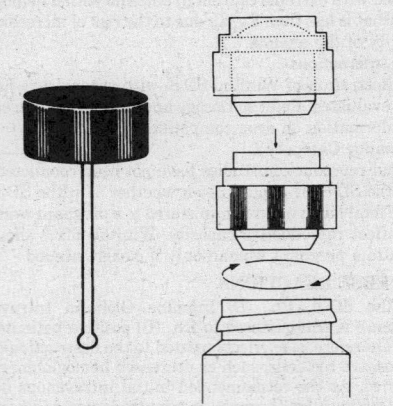

Store at room temperature or below. Avoid excessive heat.
(1) JIMBOW K., OBATHA H., PATHAK M., FITZPATRICK T.B. Mechanism and Depigmentation of Hydroquinone, Journal of Investigative Dermatology 1974, 62:436–449.
(2) op. cit.
For additional information please call:
Neutrogena Technical Department toll-free (800) 421-6857; in California call (800) 649-1150.
NDC #10812-930-01
Distributed by
Neutrogena Dermatologics
5760 W. 96th St.
Los Angeles, CA 90045
Shown in Product Identification Guide, page 325

NeXstar Pharmaceuticals, Inc.
650 CLIFFSIDE DRIVE
SAN DIMAS, CA 91773 USA

For Medical Inquiries:
800-403-3945
Customer Service
800-403-3945

DAUNOXOME® ℞
(daunorubicin citrate liposome injection)

WARNINGS
1. Cardiac function should be monitored regularly in patients receiving DaunoXome because of the potential risk for cardiac toxicity and congestive heart failure. Cardiac monitoring is advised especially in those patients who have received prior anthracyclines or who have pre-existing cardiac disease.
2. Severe myelosuppression may occur.
3. DaunoXome should be administered only under the supervision of a physician who is experienced in the use of cancer chemotherapeutic agents.
4. Dosage should be reduced in patients with impaired hepatic function. **(See DOSAGE AND ADMINISTRATION)**
5. A triad of back pain, flushing, and chest tightness has been reported in 13.8% of the patients (16/116) treated with DaunoXome in the Phase III clinical trial, and in 2.7% of treatment cycles (27/994). This triad generally occurs during the first five minutes of the infusion, subsides with interruption of the infusion, and generally does not recur if the infusion is then resumed at a slower rate.

DESCRIPTION
DaunoXome is a sterile, pyrogen-free, preservative-free product in a single use vial for intravenous infusion.
DaunoXome contains an aqueous solution of the citrate salt of daunorubicin encapsulated within lipid vesicles (liposomes) composed of a lipid bilayer of distearoylphosphatidylcholine and cholesterol (2:1 molar ratio), with a mean diameter of about 45 nm. The lipid to drug weight ratio is 18.7:1

(total lipid:daunorubicin base), equivalent to a 10:5:1 molar ratio of distearoylphosphatidylcholine:cholesterol:-daunorubicin. Daunorubicin is an anthracycline antibiotic with antineoplastic activity, originally obtained from *Streptomyces peucetius*. Daunorubicin has a 4-ring anthracycline moiety linked by a glycosidic bond to daunosamine, an amino sugar. Daunorubicin may also be isolated from *Streptomyces coeruleorubidus* and has the following chemical name: (8S-cis)-8-acetyl-10-[(3-amino-2,3,6-trideoxy-α-L-lyxo-hexopyranosyl)oxy]-7,8,9,10-tetrahydro-6,8,11-trihydroxy-1-methoxy-5,12-naphthacenedione hydrochloride.
Daunorubicin citrate has the following chemical structure:

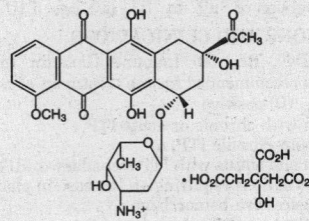

DSPC (distearoylphosphatidylcholine) has the following chemical structure:

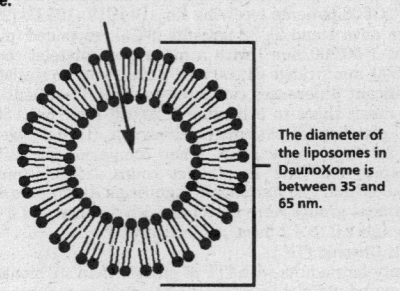

The following represents the idealized, spherical morphology of a liposome:

This represents the aqueous core that contains daunorubicin citrate.

The diameter of the liposomes in DaunoXome is between 35 and 65 nm.

represents a molecule of DSPC.

Note: Liposomal encapsulation can substantially affect a drug's functional properties relative to those of the unencapsulated drug.

In addition, different liposomal drug products may vary from one another in the chemical composition and physical form of the liposomes. Such differences can substantially affect the functional properties of liposomal drug products.

Each vial contains daunorubicin citrate equivalent to 50 mg of daunorubicin base, encapsulated in liposomes consisting of 701 mg distearoylphosphatidylcholine and 171 mg cholesterol. The liposomes encapsulating daunorubicin are dispersed in an aqueous medium containing 2, 125 mg sucrose, 94 mg glycine, and 7 mg calcium chloride dihydrate in a total volume of 25 mL/vial. The pH of the dispersion is between 4.9 and 6.0. The liposome dispersion should appear red and translucent.

CLINICAL PHARMACOLOGY
Mechanism of Action
DaunoXome is a liposomal preparation of daunorubicin formulated to maximize the selectivity of daunorubicin for solid tumors *in situ*. While in the circulation, the DaunoXome formulation helps to protect the entrapped daunorubicin from chemical and enzymatic degradation, minimizes protein binding, and generally decreases uptake by normal (non-reticuloendothelial system) tissues. The specific mechanism by which DaunoXome is able to deliver daunorubicin to solid tumors *in situ* is not known. However, it is believed to be a function of increased permeability of the tumor neovasculature to some particles in the size range of DaunoXome. In animal studies, daunorubicin has been shown to accumulate in tumors to a greater extent when administered as DaunoXome than when administered as daunorubicin. Once within the tumor environment, daunorubicin is released over time enabling it to exert its antineoplastic activity.

Pharmacokinetics

Following intravenous injection of DaunoXome, plasma clearance of daunorubicin shows monoexponential decline. The pharmacokinetic parameter values for total daunorubicin following a single 40 mg/m^2 dose of DaunoXome administered over a 30–60 minute period to patients with AIDS-related Kaposi's sarcoma and following a single rapid intravenous, 80 mg/m^2 dose of conventional daunorubicin to patients with disseminated solid malignancies are shown in Table 1.

TABLE 1
PHARMACOKINETIC PARAMETERS OF DAUNOXOME IN AIDS PATIENTS WITH KAPOSI'S SARCOMA AND REPORTED PARAMETERS FOR CONVENTIONAL DAUNORUBICIN

Parameter (units)	[a]DaunoXome	[b]Conventional Daunorubicin
Plasma Clearance (mL/min)	17.3 ± 6.1	[c]236 ± 181
Volume of Distribution (L)	6.4 ± 1.5	1006 ± 622
Distribution Half-Life (h)	4.41 ± 2.33	0.77 ± 0.3
Elimination Half-Life (h)	—	55.4 ± 13.7

[a]N = 30, [b]N = 4, [c]Calculated

The plasma pharmacokinetics of DaunoXome differ significantly from the results reported for conventional daunorubicin hydrochloride. DaunoXome has a small steady-state volume of distribution 6.4 L, (probably because it is confined to vascular fluid volume), and clearance of 17 mL/min. These differences in the volume of distribution and clearance result in a higher daunorubicin exposure (in terms of plasma AUC) from DaunoXome than with conventional daunorubicin hydrochloride. The apparent elimination half-life of DaunoXome is 4.4 hours, far shorter than that of daunorubicin, and probably represents a distribution half-life. Although preclinical biodistribution data in animals suggest that DaunoXome crosses the normal blood-brain barrier, it is unknown whether DaunoXome crosses the blood-brain barrier in humans.

Metabolism: Daunorubicinol, the major active metabolite of daunorubicin, was detected at low levels in the plasma following intravenous administration of DaunoXome.

No formal assessments of pharmacokinetic drug-drug interactions between DaunoXome and other agents have been conducted.

Special Populations: The pharmacokinetics of DaunoXome have not been evaluated in women, in different ethnic groups, or in subjects with renal and hepatic insufficiency.

Clinical Study

In an open-label, randomized, controlled clinical study conducted at 13 centers in the U.S.A. and Canada in advanced (25 or more mucocutaneous lesions; the development of 10 or more lesions in a one month period of time; symptomatic visceral involvement; or tumor-associated edema) HIV-related Kaposi's sarcoma, two treatment regimens were compared as first line cytotoxic therapy: DaunoXome 40 mg/m^2 and ABV (doxorubicin (Adriamycin®*) 10 mg/m^2, bleomycin 15 U, and vincristine 1.0 mg). All drugs were administered intravenously every 2 weeks. Responses were assessed using the AIDS Clinical Trials Group Oncology Committee of the National Institute of Allergy and Infectious Diseases (ACTG) criteria (a response required at least one of any of the following for at least 28 days; a. ≥50% reduction in the number; b. ≥50% reduction in the sums of the products of the largest perpendicular diameters of bidimensionally measurable marker lesions; or c. complete flattening of ≥50% of all previously raised lesions). Table II summarizes the efficacy results.

*Andriamycin is a registered trademark of Adria Laboratories, Columbus, OH.

TABLE II
EFFICACY DATA
FIRST LINE CYTOTOXIC THERAPY FOR ADVANCED KAPOSI'S SARCOMA

	DaunoXome n = 116	ABV n = 111
Response Rate	23%*	30%
Duration of Response, Median	110 days**	113 days
Time to Progression, Median	92 days***	105 days
Survival	342 days****	291 days

* The 95% confidence interval for difference in the response rates (ABV - DaunoXome) was [−5%, 18%]

** The hazard ratio (ABV/DaunoXome) for duration of response was 0.80, and the 95% confidence intervals were (0.44, 1.46)

*** The hazard ratio (ABV/DaunoXome) for time to progression was 0.78, and the 95% confidence intervals were (0.57, 1.07)

**** The hazard ratio for mortality (ABV/DaunoXome) was 1.29, and 95% confidence intervals were (0.92, 1.79)

Twenty of the 33 ABV responders responded to therapy by criteria more stringent than flattening of lesions (i.e., shrinkage of lesions and/or reduction in the number of lesions). Eleven of the 27 DaunoXome responders responded to therapy by criteria other than flattening of lesions. Photographic evidence of tumor response to DaunoXome and ABV was comparable across all anatomic sites (e.g., face, oral cavity, trunk, legs, and feet).

INDICATIONS AND USAGE

DaunoXome is indicated as a first line cytotoxic therapy for advanced HIV-associated Kaposi's sarcoma. DaunoXome is not recommended in patients with less than advanced HIV-related Kaposi's sarcoma.

CONTRAINDICATIONS

Therapy with DaunoXome is contraindicated in patients who have experienced a serious hypersensitivity reaction to previous doses of DaunoXome or to any of its constituents.

WARNINGS

DaunoXome is intended for administration under the supervision of a physician who is experienced in the use of cancer chemotherapeutic agents.

The primary toxicity of DaunoXome is myelosuppression, especially of the granulocytic series, which may be severe, with much less marked effects on the platelets and erythroid series. Careful hematologic monitoring is required and since patients with HIV infection are immunocompromised, patients must be observed carefully for evidence of intercurrent or opportunistic infections.

Special attention must be given to the potential cardiac toxicity of DaunoXome, particularly in patients who have received prior anthracyclines or who have pre-existing cardiac disease. Although there is no reliable means of predicting congestive heart failure, cardiomyopathy induced by anthracyclines is usually associated with a decrease of the left ventricular ejection fraction (LVEF). Cardiac function should be evaluated in each patient by means of a history and physical examination before each course of DaunoXome and determination of LVEF should be performed at total cumulative doses of DaunoXome of 320 mg/m^2, 480 mg/m^2 and every 240 mg/m^2 thereafter.

A triad of back pain, flushing, and chest tightness has been reported in 13.8% of the patients (16/116) treated with DaunoXome in the randomized clinical trial and in 2.7% of treatment cycles (27/994). This triad generally occurs during the first five minutes of the infusion, subsides with interruption of the infusion, and generally does not recur if the infusion is then resumed at a slower rate. This combination of symptoms appears to be related to the lipid component of DaunoXome, as a similar set of signs and symptoms has been observed with other liposomal products not containing daunorubicin.

Daunorubicin has been associated with local tissue necrosis at the site of drug extravasation. Although no such local tissue necrosis has been observed with DaunoXome, care should be taken to ensure that there is no extravasation of drug when DaunoXome is administered.

Dosage should be reduced in patients with impaired hepatic function. (See **DOSAGE AND ADMINISTRATION**)

Pregnancy Category D

DaunoXome can cause fetal harm when administered to a pregnant woman. DaunoXome was administered to rats on gestation days 6 through 15 at 0.3, 1.0 or 2.0 mg/kg/day, (about 1/20th, 1/6th, or 1/3rd the recommended human dose on a mg/m^2 basis). DaunoXome produced severe maternal toxicity and embryolethality at 2.0 mg/kg/day and was embryotoxic and caused fetal malformations (anophthalmia, microphthalmia, incomplete ossification) at 0.3 mg/kg/day. Embryotoxicity was characterized by increased embryo-fetal deaths, reduced number of litters, and reduced litter sizes. There are no studies of DaunoXome in pregnant women. If DaunoXome is used during pregnancy, or if the patient becomes pregnant while taking DaunoXome, the patient must be warned of the potential hazard to the fetus. Patients should be advised to avoid becoming pregnant while taking DaunoXome.

PRECAUTIONS

Drug Interactions

In the patient population studied, DaunoXome has been administered to patients receiving a variety of concomitant medications (e.g., antiretroviral agents, antiviral agents, anti-infective agents). Although interactions of DaunoXome with other drugs have not been observed, no systematic studies of interactions have been conducted.

Carcinogenesis, Mutagenesis, and Impairment of Fertility

No carcinogenesis, mutagenesis, or impairment of fertility studies were conducted with DaunoXome.

Carcinogenesis: Carcinogenicity and mutagenicity studies have been conducted with daunorubicin, the active component of DaunoXome. A high incidence of mammary tumors was observed about 120 days after a single intravenous dose of 12.5 mg/kg daunorubicin in rats (about 2 times the human dose on a mg/m^2 basis). Mutagenesis: Daunorubicin was mutagenic in *in vitro* tests (Ames assay, V79 hamster cell assay), and clastogenic in *in vitro* (CCRFCEM human lymphoblasts) and in *in vivo* (SCE assay in mouse bone marrow) tests. Impairment of Fertility: Daunorubicin intravenous doses of 0.25 mg/kg/day (about 8 times the human dose on a mg/m^2 basis) in male dogs caused testicular atrophy and total aplasia of spermatocytes in the seminiferous tubules.

Pregnancy

Pregnancy "Category D". See WARNINGS Section.

Pediatric Use

Safety and effectiveness in pediatric patients have not been established.

Use in the Elderly

Safety and effectiveness in the elderly have not been established.

Special Populations

Safety has not been established in patients with pre-existing hepatic or renal dysfunction.

ADVERSE REACTIONS

DaunoXome contains daunorubicin, encapsulated within a liposome. Conventional daunorubicin has acute myelosuppression as its dose limiting side effect, with the greatest effect on the granulocytic series. In addition, daunorubicin causes alopecia, and nausea and vomiting in a significant number of patients treated. Extravasation of conventional daunorubicin can cause severe local tissue necrosis. Chronic therapy at total doses above 300 mg/m^2 causes a cumulative-dose-related cardiomyopathy with congestive heart failure. Administered as DaunoXome, daunorubicin has substantially altered pharmacokinetics and some differences in toxicity. The most important acute toxicity of DaunoXome remains myelosuppression, principally of the granulocytic series, with much less marked effects on the platelets and erythroid series.

In an open-label, randomized, controlled clinical trial conducted in 13 centers in the U.S.A. and Canada in advanced HIV-related Kaposi's sarcoma, two treatment regimens were compared as first line cytotoxic therapy: DaunoXome and ABV (doxorubicin (Adriamycin®*), bleomycin, and vincristine). All drugs were administered intravenously every 2 weeks. The safety data presented below include all reported or observed adverse experiences, including those not considered to be drug related. Patients with advanced HIV-associated Kaposi's sarcoma are seriously ill due to their underlying infection and are receiving several concomitant medications including potentially toxic antiviral and antiretroviral agents. The contribution of the study drugs to the adverse experience profile is therefore difficult to establish.

Table III summarizes the important safety data.

TABLE III
SUMMARY OF IMPORTANT SAFETY DATA

	DaunoXome (N=116) % of patients	ABV (N=111) % of patients
Neutropenia (<1000 cells/mm^3)	36%	35%
Neutropenia (<500 cells/mm^3)	15%	5%
Opportunistic Infections/ Illnesses, % of patients	40%	27%
Median time to first Opportunistic Infections/ Illnesses	214 days	412 days**
Number of cases with absolute reduction in ejection fraction of 20–25%*	3	1
Number of cases removed from therapy due to cardiac causes*	2	0
Alopecia All grades % of patients	8%	36%***
Neuropathy All grades % of patients	13%	41%***

* The denominator is uncertain since there were several instances of missing repeat cardiac evaluations

** p = 0.21

*** p < 0.001

Continued on next page

NeXstar—Cont.

A triad of back pain, flushing and chest tightness was reported in 13.8% of the patients (16/116) treated with DaunoXome in the Phase III clinical trial and in 2.7% of treatment cycles (27/994). Most of the episodes were mild to moderate in severity (12% of patients and 2.5% of treatment cycles).

Mild alopecia was reported in 6% of patients treated with DaunoXome and moderate alopecia in 2% of patients. Mild nausea was reported in 35% of DaunoXome patients, moderate nausea in 16% of patients and severe nausea in 3% of patients. For patients treated with DaunoXome, mild vomiting was reported in 10%, moderate in 10%, and severe in 3% of patients. Although grade 3–4 injection site inflammation was reported in 2 patients treated with DaunoXome, no instances of local tissue necrosis were observed with extravasation.

Table IV is a listing of all the mild-moderate and severe adverse events reported on both treatment arms in Protocol 103-09 in ≥5% of DaunoXome patients.

TABLE IV
ADVERSE EXPERIENCES:
PROTOCOL 103–09

| | DaunoXome (N=116) | | ABV (N=111) | |
	Mild Moderate	Severe	Mild Moderate	Severe
Nausea	51%	3%	45%	5%
Fatigue	43%	6%	44%	7%
Fever	42%	5%	49%	5%
Diarrhea	34%	4%	29%	6%
Cough	26%	2%	19%	0%
Dyspnea	23%	3%	17%	3%
Headache	22%	3%	23%	2%
Allergic Reactions	21%	3%	19%	2%
Abdominal Pain	20%	3%	23%	4%
Anorexia	21%	2%	26%	2%
Vomiting	20%	3%	26%	2%
Rigors	19%	0%	23%	0%
Back Pain	16%	0%	8%	0%
Increased Sweating	12%	2%	12%	0%
Neuropathy	12%	1%	38%	3%
Rhinitis	12%	0%	6%	0%
Edema	9%	2%	8%	1%
Chest Pain	9%	1%	7%	0%
Depression	7%	3%	6%	0%
Malaise	9%	1%	11%	1%
Stomatitis	9%	1%	8%	0%
Alopecia	8%	0%	36%	0%
Dizziness	8%	0%	9%	0%
Sinusitis	8%	0%	5%	1%
Arthralgia	7%	0%	6%	0%
Constipation	7%	0%	18%	0%
Myalgia	7%	0%	12%	0%
Pruritus	7%	0%	14%	0%
Insomnia	6%	0%	14%	0%
Influenza-like symptoms	5%	0%	5%	0%
Tenesmus	4%	1%	1%	0%
Abnormal vision	3%	2%	3%	0%

The following adverse events were reported in ≤5% of patients treated with DaunoXome, tabulated by body system.

Body As A Whole: Infection site inflammation
Cardiovascular: Hot flushes, hypertension, palpitation, syncope, tachycardia
Digestive: Increased appetite, dysphagia, GI hemorrhage, gastritis, gingival bleeding, hemorrhoids, hepatomegaly, melena, dry mouth, tooth caries
Hemic and Lymphatic: Lymphadenopathy, splenomegaly
Metabolic and Nutritional: Dehydration, thirst
Nervous: Amnesia, anxiety, ataxia, confusion, convulsions, emotional liability, abnormal gait, hallucination, hyperkinesia, hypertonia, meningitis, somnolence, abnormal thinking, tremor
Respiratory: Hemoptysis, hiccups, pulmonary infiltration, increased sputum
Skin: Folliculitis, seborrhea, dry skin
Special Senses: Conjunctivitis, deafness, earache, eye pain, taste perversion, tinnitus
Urogenital: Dysuria, nocturia, polyuria

OVERDOSAGE

The symptoms of acute overdosage are increased severities of the observed dose-limiting toxicities of therapeutic doses of DaunoXome, myelosuppression (especially granulocytopenia), fatigue, and nausea and vomiting.

DOSAGE AND ADMINISTRATION

DaunoXome should be administered intravenously over a 60 minute period at a dose of 40 mg/m², with doses repeated every two weeks. Blood counts should be repeated prior to each dose, and therapy withheld if the absolute granulocyte count is less than 750 cells/mm³. Treatment should be continued until there is evidence of progressive disease (e.g., based on best response achieved: new visceral sites of involvement, or progression of visceral disease; development of 10 or more new, cutaneous lesions or a 25% increase in the number of lesions compared to baseline; a change in the character of 25% or more of all previously counted flat lesions to raised; increase in surface area of the indicator lesions), or until other intercurrent complications of HIV disease preclude continuation of therapy.

Patients with Impaired Hepatic and Renal Function
Limited clinical experience exists in treating hepatically and renally impaired patients with DaunoXome.

Therefore, based on experience with daunorubicin HCl, it is recommended that the dosage of DaunoXome *be reduced* if the bilirubin or creatinine is elevated as follows: Serum bilirubin 1.2 to 3 mg/dL, give ³/₄ the normal dose; serum bilirubin or creatinine >3 mg/dL, give ¹/₂ the normal dose.
Do not mix DaunoXome with other drugs.

Preparation Of Solution
DaunoXome should be diluted 1:1 with 5% Dextrose Injection (D5W) before administration. Each vial of DaunoXome contains daunorubicin citrate equivalent to 50 mg daunorubicin base, at a concentration of 2 mg/mL. The recommended concentration after dilution is 1 mg daunorubicin/mL of solution.

Use aseptic technique.
Aseptic technique must be strictly observed in all handling, since no preservative or bacteriostatic agent is present in DaunoXome or in the materials recommended for dilution. Withdraw the calculated volume of DaunoXome from the vial into a sterile syringe, and transfer it into a sterile infusion bag containing an equivalent amount of D5W. Administer diluted DaunoXome immediately. If not used immediately, diluted DaunoXome should be stored refrigerated at 2°–8°C (36°–46°F) for a maximum of 6 hours.

Caution: The only fluid which may be mixed with DaunoXome is D5W; DaunoXome must not be mixed with saline, bacteriostatic agents such as benzyl alcohol, or any other solution.
Do not use an in-line filter for the intravenous infusion of DaunoXome.
All parenteral drug products should be inspected visually for particulate matter and discoloration prior to administration, whenever solution and container permit. DaunoXome is a translucent dispersion of liposomes that scatters light to some degree. Do not use DaunoXome if it appears opaque, or has precipitate or foreign matter present.
Procedures for proper handling and disposal of anticancer drugs should be followed.[1-7]

HOW SUPPLIED

DaunoXome is a translucent, red, liposomal dispersion supplied in single use vials, each sealed with a synthetic rubber stopper and aluminum sealing ring with a plastic cap. DaunoXome provides daunorubicin citrate equivalent to 50 mg of daunorubicin base, at a concentration of 2 mg/mL. DaunoXome is supplied under NDC 56146-0301-1 for a single unit pack, NDC 56146-0301-4 for a 4-unit pack, and NDC 56146-0301-0 for a 10-unit pack.
Storage
Store DaunoXome in a refrigerator, 2°–8°C (36°–46°F). Do not freeze. Protect from light.

U.S. PATENT NUMBERS
The United States Patent Numbers applicable to DaunoXome are: 5,441,745; 5,435,989; 5,019,369; 4,946,683; 4,753,788; and additional patents pending.

REFERENCES
1. Recommendations for the Safe Handling of Parenteral Antineoplastic Drugs. NIH Publication No. 83-2621. For sale by the Superintendent of Documents, US Government Printing Office, Washington, DC 20402.
2. AMA Council Report, Guidelines for Handling Parenteral Antineoplastics. JAMA 1985; 253(11): 1590-1592.
3. National Study Commission on Cytotoxic Exposure–Recommendations for Handling Cytotoxic Agents. Available from Louis P. Jeffrey, Sc.D., Chairman, National Study Commission on Cytotoxic Exposure Massachusetts College of Pharmacy and Allied Health Sciences, 179 Longwood Avenue, Boston, Massachusetts 02115.
4. Clinical Oncological Society of Australia. Guidelines and Recommendations for Safe Handling of Antineoplastic Agents. Med. J. Australia 1983; 1: 426-428.
5. Jones RB, et al; Safe Handling of Chemotherapeutic Agents: A report from the Mount Sinai Medical Center. CA-A Cancer Journal for Clinicians 1983; (Sept/Oct) 258-263.
6. American Society of Hospital Pharmacists Technical Assistance Bulletin on Handling Cytotoxic and Hazardous Drugs. Am. J. Hosp. Pharm. 1990; 47: 1033-1049.
7. OSHA Work-Practice Guidelines for Personnel Dealing with Cytotoxic (Antineoplastic) Drugs. Am. J. Hosp. Pharm. 1986; 43: 1193-1204.

NEXSTAR P0098
Pharmaceuticals, Inc. rev. 4/96
NeXstar Pharmaceuticals, Inc.
650 Cliffside Drive ● San Dimas, CA 91773 USA

DaunoXome is a registered trademark of NeXstar Pharmaceuticals, Inc.
Shown in Product Identification Guide, page 325

Niché Pharmaceuticals, Inc.
P.O. BOX 449
200 N. OAK STREET
ROANOKE, TX 76262

Direct Inquiries to:
Steve F. Brandon
(817) 491-2770
FAX: (817) 491-3533

For Medical Information Contact:
In Emergencies:
Gerald L. Beckloff, M.D.
(817) 491-2770
FAX: (817) 491-3533

MAGTAB® SR ℞
[măg-tăb]
(Magnesium L-lactate dihydrate)
Sustained release Magnesium Supplement

DESCRIPTION

MagTab® SR is a sustained release oral magnesium supplement. Each pale yellow caplet contains 7mEq (84 Mg) magnesium as magnesium lactate in a wax matrix.

INGREDIENTS

Each caplet contains 7mEq (84 Mg) elemental magnesium as magnesium L.Lactate dihydrate (835 Mg) in a sustained release wax matrix formulation. Inactive ingredients: polyethylene glycol, microcrystalline cellulose, carnauba wax, stearic acid, calcium stearate, and D & C yellow No. 10.

INDICATIONS/USES

As a dietary supplement, MagTab® SR is indicated for patients with, or at risk for, magnesium deficiency. Hypomagnesemia and/or magnesium deficiency can result from inadequate nutritional intake or absorption, magnesium depleting drugs such as diuretics, or alcoholism.

WARNINGS

Patients with renal disease should not take magnesium supplements without the advice and direct supervision of a physician.

SIDE EFFECTS

Excessive dosage of magnesium can cause loose stools or diarrhea.

DOSAGE

As a dietary supplement, take 1 or 2 caplets b.i.d. or as directed by a physician. Four caplets of MagTab® SR will meet the USRDA range for average adult males and females (300–350 mg) where magnesium depleting drugs are being used, supplementation with higher dosages may be required and should be considered.

HOW SUPPLIED

MagTab® SR is available for oral administration as uncoated yellow caplets, coded Niche/420. Caplets are supplied as follows:

59016-42016	Bottles of 60
59016-42017	Bottles of 100

Store at 15°–30°C (59°–86°F)
U.S. Patent Number: 5,002,774

UNIFIBER®   OTC
[uni fi' ber]
(Powdered Cellulose)
3 grams Fiber per tablespoon

DESCRIPTION

Unifiber is unique in the fiber field with many patient advantages. It's an all natural insoluble bulk fiber supplement that promotes normal bowel function by adding needed bulk to the diet. Unifiber contains powdered cellulose 75%, water 5%, corn syrup 19%, and xanthan gum 1%. Unifiber mixes easily with liquids or soft foods, and is tasteless, non-gelling, and pleasant to take. One tablespoon of Unifiber provides 3 grams of concentrated dietary fiber.

NUTRITION INFORMATION

Each 4 gram (1T) serving of Unifiber contains 3 grams of fiber, 4 calories, 0% fat, 0% cholesterol, 0% protein, and is free of all electrolytes.

INDICATION/USES

As a dietary supplement, Unifiber is indicated for patients needing a concentrated source of fiber to help maintain and promote normal bowel function. Because Unifiber is electrolyte free, it is an ideal fiber supplement for patients on a restricted diet, such as the OB patient, kidney patients on dialysis, or the diabetic patient.

CONTRADICTION

Intestinal obstruction or fecal impaction.

DOSAGE

Stir one to two tablespoons once or twice daily into a glass of fruit juice, milk, coffee, or water. An advantage of Unifiber is that it can be easily mixed with soft food such as mashed potatoes, applesauce, or pudding. Unifiber may also be administered to tube feeders. Best results are normally seen in 7–10 days. Liquids should be included in the daily diet.

HOW SUPPLIED

Unifiber is available over the counter in powder containers of 5 oz (35 servings), 9 oz (63 servings), or 16 oz (113 servings)

Northampton Medical, Inc.
(See UCB Pharma, Inc.)

Novo Nordisk Pharmaceuticals Inc.
SUITE 200
100 OVERLOOK CENTER
PRINCETON, NJ 08540-7810

Direct Inquiries to:
Professional Services
(609) 987-5800

For Medical Information Contact:
In Emergencies:
Professional Services
(609) 987-5800

HUMAN INSULIN   OTC
NOVOLIN® 70/30
70% NPH, Human Insulin Isophane Suspension and
30% Regular, Human Insulin Injection
(recombinant DNA origin)
100 units/ml

WARNING

ANY CHANGE OF INSULIN SHOULD BE MADE CAUTIOUSLY AND ONLY UNDER MEDICAL SUPERVISION. CHANGES IN PURITY, STRENGTH, BRAND (MANUFACTURER), TYPE (REGULAR, NPH, LENTE®, ETC.), SPECIES (BEEF, PORK, BEEF-PORK, HUMAN) AND/OR METHOD OF MANUFACTURE (RECOMBINANT DNA VERSUS ANIMAL-SOURCE INSULIN) MAY RESULT IN THE NEED FOR A CHANGE IN DOSAGE.
SPECIAL CARE SHOULD BE TAKEN WHEN THE TRANSFER IS FROM A STANDARD BEEF OR MIXED SPECIES INSULIN TO A PURIFIED PORK OR HUMAN INSULIN. IF A DOSAGE ADJUSTMENT IS NEEDED, IT WILL USUALLY BECOME APPARENT EITHER IN THE FIRST FEW DAYS OR OVER A PERIOD OF SEVERAL WEEKS. ANY CHANGE IN TREATMENT SHOULD BE CAREFULLY MONITORED. PLEASE READ THE SECTIONS "INSULIN REACTION AND SHOCK" AND "DIABETIC KETOACIDOSIS AND COMA" FOR SYMPTOMS OF HYPOGLYCEMIA (LOW BLOOD GLUCOSE) AND HYPERGLYCEMIA (HIGH BLOOD GLUCOSE).

INSULIN USE IN DIABETES

Your physician has explained that you have diabetes and that your treatment involves injections of insulin. Insulin is normally produced by the pancreas, a gland that lies behind the stomach. Without insulin, glucose (a simple sugar made from digested food) is trapped in the bloodstream and cannot enter the cells of the body. Some patients who don't make enough of their own insulin, or who cannot use the insulin they do make properly, must take insulin by injection in order to control their blood glucose levels.

Each case of diabetes is different and requires direct and continued medical supervision. Your physician has told you the type, strength and amount of insulin you should use and the time(s) at which you should inject it, and has also discussed with you a diet and exercise schedule. You should contact your physician if you experience any difficulties or if you have questions.

TYPES OF INSULINS

Standard and purified animal insulins as well as human insulins are available. Standard and purified insulins differ in their degree of purification and content of noninsulin material. Standard and purified insulins also vary in species source: they may be of beef, pork, or mixed beef and pork origin. Human insulin is identical in structure to the insulin produced by the human pancreas, and thus differs from animal insulins. Insulins vary in time of action and in strength; see PRODUCT DESCRIPTION and SYRINGES for additional information.

Your physician has prescribed the insulin that is right for you; be sure you have purchased the correct insulin and check it carefully before you use it.

PRODUCT DESCRIPTION

This vial contains Novolin® 70/30 which is a mixture of 70% NPH, Human Insulin Isophane Suspension (recombinant DNA origin) and 30% Regular, Human Insulin Injection (recombinant DNA origin) USP. The concentration of this product is 100 units of insulin per milliliter. It is a cloudy or milky suspension of human insulin with protamine and zinc. The insulin substance (the cloudy material) settles at the bottom of the vial, therefore, the vial must be gently agitated or rotated so that the contents are uniformly mixed before a dose is withdrawn. Novolin® 70/30 has an intermediate duration of action. The effect of Novolin® 70/30 begins approximately ½ hour after injection. The effect is maximal between 2 and approximately 12 hours. The full duration of action may last up to 24 hours after injection. The time course of action of any insulin may vary considerably in different individuals, or at different times in the same individual. Because of this variation, the time periods listed here should be considered as general guidelines only.

This human insulin (recombinant DNA origin) is structurally identical to the insulin produced by the human pancreas. This human insulin is produced by recombinant DNA technology utilziing Saccharomyces cerevisiae (bakers' yeast) as the production organism.

STORAGE

Insulin should be stored in a cold place, preferably in a refrigerator, but not in the freezing compartment. Do not let it freeze. Keep the insulin vial in its carton so that it will stay clean and protected from light. If refrigeration is not possible, the bottle of insulin which you are currently using can be kept unrefrigerated as long as it is kept as cool as possible and away from heat and sunlight.

Never use Novolin® 70/30 if the precipitate (the white deposit at the bottom of the vial) has become lumpy or granular in appearance or has formed a deposit of solid particles on the wall of the vial. This insulin should not be used if the liquid in the vial remains clear after the vial has been gently agitated.

Never use insulin after the expiration date which is printed on the vial label and carton.

SYRINGES

Use the Correct Syringe

Doses of insulin are measured in units. Some insulins are available in two strengths: U-100 and U-40. One milliliter (ml) of U-100 contains 100 units of insulin. One milliliter (ml) of U-40 contains 40 units of insulin. Be sure to use the proper syringe for the strength of the insulin prescribed for you. Syringes are clearly marked "For use with U-100 insulin" or "For use with U-40 insulin". Low dose U-100 syringes are also available. Failure to use the proper syringe can lead to mistakes in dosage.

Disposable Syringes

Disposable syringes and needles require no sterilization provided the package is intact. They should be used only once and discarded.

Reusable Syringes

Reusable syringes and needles must be sterilized before each use.

1. Boil the syringe parts and needles in a pan of water for at least five minutes. Keep a special pan for this purpose. Heavily chlorinated water should not be used; distilled water is preferable.
   If boiling is not possible, the syringe parts and needles may be sterilized by immersion in 70% ethyl alcohol or 91% isopropyl alcohol for at least five minutes. Do not use bathing, rubbing or medicated alcohol for sterilization.
2. Assemble the syringe and fit the needle on the tip of the syringe being careful not to touch the surface of the plunger or needle.
3. Push the plunger in and out several times until the water (or alcohol) has been completely expelled. (The syringe should be thoroughly dried before its use.)

NEEDLE-FREE INJECTORS

This product may not be suitable for use with all needle-free injectors. You should consult the needle-free injector device manufacturer before using the device with this product.

IMPORTANT

Failure to comply with the above and the following antiseptic measures may lead to infections at the injection site.

PREPARING THE INJECTION

1. Clean your hands and the injection site with soap and water or with alcohol. Wipe the rubber stopper with an alcohol swab. (Note: remove the tamper-resistant cap at first use. If the cap has already been removed, do not use this product, return it to your pharmacy.)
2. For insulin suspensions, roll the vial of insulin gently in your hands to mix it. Vigorous shaking immediately before the dose is drawn into the syringe may result in the formation of bubbles or froth which could cause dosage errors.
3. Pull back the plunger until the black tip reaches the marking for the number of units you will inject.
4. Push the needle through the rubber stopper into the vial.
5. Push the plunger all the way in. This inserts air into the bottle.
6. Turn the vial and syringe upside down and slowly pull the plunger back to a few units beyond the correct dose.
7. If there are air bubbles, flick the syringe firmly with your finger to raise the air bubbles to the needle, then slowly push the plunger to the correct unit marking.
8. Lift the vial off the syringe.

GIVING THE INJECTION

1. The following areas are suitable for subcutaneous insulin injection: thighs, upper arms, buttocks, abdomen. Do not change areas without consulting your physician. The actual point of injection should be changed each time; injection sites should be about an inch apart.
2. The injection site should be clean and dry. Pinch up skin area to be injected and hold it firmly.
3. Hold the syringe like a pencil and push the needle quickly and firmly into the pinched-up area. If you go straight in it will probably sting less. Pull back the plunger slightly. If blood comes into the syringe, the needle has entered a blood vessel. Remove the needle and make the injection in another spot.
4. If blood does not appear in the syringe, release skin and push plunger all the way in to inject insulin beneath the skin. Do not inject into a muscle unless your physician has advised it. You should never inject insulin into a vein.
5. Remove needle. If slight bleeding occurs, press lightly with a dry cotton swab for a few seconds—do not rub.

Note:
The dose should be injected over 2–4 seconds. Preparations of insulin suspensions which are injected slowly may clog the tip of the needle, resulting in an inability to complete the

Continued on next page

Novo Nordisk—Cont.

injection. Syringe plugging does not occur when the drug is injected more rapidly.

MIXING INSULIN

Novolin® 70/30 is a premixed insulin containing 70% NPH, Human Insulin Isophane Suspension, recombinant DNA origin (**Novolin® N**) and 30% Regular, Human Insulin Injection, recombinant DNA origin (**Novolin® R**). You should not attempt to change the ratio of this product by adding additional NPH or Regular insulin to this vial. If your physician has prescribed insulin mixed in a proportion other than 70% NPH and 30% Regular, you should use the separate insulin formulations (**Novolin® N** and **Novolin® R**) in the amounts recommended by your physician.

USAGE IN PREGNANCY

It is particularly important to maintain good control of your diabetes during pregnancy and special attention must be paid to your diet, exercise and insulin regimens. If you are pregnant or nursing a baby, consult your physician or nurse educator.

INSULIN REACTION AND SHOCK

Insulin reaction ("hypoglycemia") occurs when the blood glucose falls very low. This can happen if you take too much insulin, miss or delay a meal, exercise more than usual or work too hard without eating, or become ill (especially with vomiting or fever). The first symptoms of an insulin reaction usually come on suddenly. They may include a cold sweat, fatigue, nervousness or shakiness, rapid heartbeat, or nausea. Personality change or confusion may also occur. If you drink or eat something right away (a glass of milk or orange juice, or several sugar candies), you can often stop the progression of symptoms. If symptoms persist, call your physician — an insulin reaction can lead to unconsciousness. If a reaction results in loss of consciousness, emergency medical care should be obtained immediately. If you have had repeated reactions or if an insulin reaction has led to a loss of consciousness, contact your physician. Severe hypoglycemia can result in temporary or permanent impairment of brain function and death.

In certain cases, the nature and intensity of the warning symptoms of hypoglycemia may change. A few patients have reported that after being transferred to human insulin, the early warning symptoms of hypoglycemia were less pronounced than they had been with animal-source insulin.

DIABETIC KETOACIDOSIS AND COMA

Diabetic ketoacidosis may develop if your body has too little insulin. The most common causes are acute illness or infection or failure to take enough insulin by injection. If you are ill you should check your urine for ketones. The symptoms of diabetic ketoacidosis usually come on gradually, over a period of hours or days, and include a drowsy feeling, flushed face, thirst and loss of appetite. Notify your physician right away if the urine test is positive for ketones (acetone) or if you have any of these symptoms. Fast, heavy breathing and rapid pulse are more severe symptoms and you should have medical attention right away. Severe, sustained hyperglycemia may result in diabetic coma and death.

ADVERSE REACTIONS

A few people with diabetes develop red, swollen and itchy skin where the insulin has been injected. This is called a "local reaction" and it may occur if the injection is not properly made, if the skin is sensitive to the cleansing solution, or if you are allergic to the insulin being used. If you have a local reaction, tell your physician.

Generalized insulin allergy occurs rarely, but when it does it may cause a serious reaction, including skin rash over the body, shortness of breath, fast pulse, sweating, and a drop in blood pressure. If any of these symptoms develop, you should seek emergency medical care.

If severe allergic reactions to insulin have occurred (i.e., generalized rash, swelling or breathing difficulties) you should be skin-tested with **each** new insulin preparation before it is used.

IMPORTANT NOTES

1. A change in the type, strength, species or purity of insulin could require a dosage adjustment. Any change in insulin should be made under medical supervision.
2. You may have learned how to test your urine or your blood for glucose. It is important to do these tests regularly and to record the results for review with your physician or nurse educator.
3. If you have an acute illness, especially with vomiting or fever, continue taking your insulin. If possible, stay on your regular diet. If you have trouble eating, drink fruit juices, regular soft drinks, or clear soups; if you can, eat small amounts of bland foods. Test your urine for glucose and ketones and, if possible, test your blood glucose. Note the results and contact your physician for possible insulin dose adjustment. If you have severe and prolonged vomiting, seek emergency medical care.
4. You should always carry identification which states that you have diabetes.

Always consult your physician if you have any questions about your condition or the use of insulin.

Helpful information for people with diabetes is published by American Diabetes Association, 1660 Duke Street, Alexandria, VA 22314.

For information contact: Novo Nordisk Pharmaceuticals Inc., Princeton, NJ 08540

Manufactured by Novo Nordisk A/S, DK-2880 Bagsvaerd, Denmark

HOW SUPPLIED

Vials, U-100, 100 units/mL, 10 mL, (List No. 183711) (1's)
Novolin 70/30 Prefilled™ Syringe, U-100, 100 units/mL, 1.5 mL, (List No. 001771) (5's)
Novolin® 70/30 PenFill®, U-100, 100 units/mL, 1.5 mL, (List No. 183717) (5's)

HUMAN INSULIN **OTC**

NOVOLIN® L

Lente®, Human Insulin Zinc Suspension (recombinant DNA origin)
100 units/ml

DESCRIPTION

Novolin® L is commonly known as Lente® Human Insulin Zinc Suspension (recombinant DNA origin). The concentration of this product is 100 units of insulin per milliliter. It is a cloudy or milky suspension of 70% crystalline and 30% amorphous human insulin. The insulin substance (the cloudy material) settles at the bottom of the vial, therefore, the vial must be gently agitated or rotated so that the contents are uniformly mixed before a dose is withdrawn. **Novolin® L** has an intermediate duration of action. The effect of **Novolin® L** begins approximately 2½ hours after injection. The effect is maximal between 7 and 15 hours and ends approximately 22 hours after injection. The time course of action of any insulin may vary considerably in different individuals or at different times in the same individual. Because of this variation, the periods listed here should be considered as general guidelines only.

This human insulin (recombinant DNA origin) is structurally identical to the insulin produced by the human pancreas. This human insulin is produced by recombinant DNA technology utilizing *Saccharomyces cerevisiae* (bakers' yeast) as the production organism.

STORAGE

Insulin should be stored in a cold place, preferably in a refrigerator, but not in the freezing compartment. **Do not let it freeze.** Keep the insulin vial in its carton so that it will stay clean and protected from light. If refrigeration is not possible, the bottle of insulin which you are currently using can be kept unrefrigerated as long as it is kept as cool as possible and away from heat and sunlight.

Never use **Novolin® L** if the precipitate (the white deposit at the bottom of the vial) has become lumpy or granular in appearance or has formed a deposit of solid particles on the wall of the vial. This insulin should not be used if the liquid in the vial remains clear after the vial has been gently agitated.

Never use insulin after the expiration date which is printed on the vial label and carton.

MIXING TWO TYPES OF INSULIN—SEE NOVOLIN® N

SEE NOVOLIN® 70/30 for complete package insert information on Warning: Insulin Use in Diabetes: Types of Insulins: Syringes: Needle-Free Injectors: Important Statement: Preparing the Injection: Giving the Injection: Usage in Pregnancy: Insulin Reaction and Shock: Diabetic Ketoacidosis and Coma: Adverse Reactions: Important Notes.

HOW SUPPLIED

Vials, U-100, 100 units/mL, 10 mL, (List No. 183511) (1's)

NOVOLIN® N **OTC**

NPH, Human Insulin Isophane Suspension (recombinant DNA origin)
100 units/ml

DESCRIPTION

Novolin® N is commonly known as NPH, Human Insulin Isophane Suspension (recombinant DNA origin). The concentration of this product is 100 units of insulin per milliliter. It is a cloudy or milky suspension of human insulin with protamine and zinc. The insulin substance (the cloudy material) settles at the bottom of the vial, therefore, the vial must be gently agitated or rotated so that the contents are uniformly mixed before a dose is withdrawn. **Novolin® N** has an intermediate duration of action. The effect of **Novolin® N** begins approximately 1½ hours after injection. The effect is maximal between 4 and 12 hours. The full duration of action may last up to 24 hours after injection. The time course of action of any insulin may vary considerably in different individuals, or at different times in the same individual. Because of this variation, the periods listed here should be considered as general guidelines only.

This human insulin (recombinant DNA origin) is structurally identical to the insulin produced by the human pancreas. This human insulin is produced by recombinant DNA technology utilizing *Saccharomyces cerevisiae* (bakers' yeast) as the production organism.

STORAGE

Insulin should be stored in a cold place, preferably in a refrigerator, but not in the freezing compartment. **Do not let it freeze.** Keep the insulin vial in its carton so that it will stay clean and protected from light. If refrigeration is not possible, the bottle of insulin which you are currently using can be kept unrefrigerated as long as it is kept as cool as possible and away from heat and sunlight.

Never use **Novolin® N** if the precipitate (the white deposit at the bottom of the vial) has become lumpy or granular in appearance or has formed a deposit of solid particles on the wall of the vial. This insulin should not be used if the liquid in the vial remains clear after the vial has been gently agitated.

Never use insulin after the expiration date which is printed on the vial label and carton.

MIXING TWO TYPES OF INSULIN

Different insulins should be mixed only under instruction from a physician. Hypodermic syringes may vary in the amount of space between the bottom line and the needle ("dead space"), so if you are mixing two types of insulin be sure to discuss any change in the model and brand of syringe you are using with your physician or pharmacist. When you are mixing two types of insulin, always draw the Regular (clear) insulin into the syringe first.

SEE NOVOLIN® 70/30 for complete package insert information on Warning: Insulin Use in Diabetes: Types of Insulin: Syringes: Needle-Free Injectors: Important Statement: Preparing the Injection: Giving the Injection: Usage in Pregnancy: Insulin Reaction and Shock: Diabetic Ketoacidosis and Coma: Adverse Reactions: Important Notes.

HOW SUPPLIED

Vials, U-100, 100 units/mL, 10 mL, (List No. 183411) (1's)
Novolin N Prefilled™ Syringe, U-100, 100 units/mL, 1.5 mL, (List No. 004571) (5's)
Novolin® N PenFill®, U-100, 100 units/mL, 1.5 mL, (List No. 183417) (5's)

NOVOLIN® R **OTC**

Regular, Human Insulin Injection (recombinant DNA origin) USP
100 units/ml

DESCRIPTION

Novolin® R is commonly known as Regular, Human Insulin Injection (recombinant DNA origin) USP. The concentration of this product is 100 units of insulin per milliliter. It is a clear, colorless solution which has a short duration of action. The effect of **Novolin® R** begins approximately ½ hour after injection. The effect is maximal between 2½ and 5 hours and ends approximately 8 hours after injection. The time course of action of any insulin may vary considerably in different individuals or at different times in the same individual. Because of this variation, the time periods listed here should be considered as general guidelines only.

This human insulin (recombinant DNA origin) is structurally identical to the insulin produced by the human pancreas. This human insulin is produced by recombinant DNA technology utilizing *Saccharomyces cerevisiae* (bakers' yeast) as the production organism.

STORAGE

Insulin should be stored in a cold place, preferably in a refrigerator, but not in the freezing compartment. **Do not let it freeze.** Keep the insulin vial in its carton so that it will stay clean and protected from light. If refrigeration is not possible, the bottle of insulin which you are currently using can be kept unrefrigerated as long as it is kept as cool as possible and away from heat and sunlight.

Never use **Novolin® R** if it becomes viscous (thickened) or cloudy; use it only if it is clear and colorless.

Never use insulin after the expiration date which is printed on the vial label and carton.

MIXING TWO TYPES OF INSULIN—SEE NOVOLIN® N.

IMPORTANT NOTES

1. Due to risk of precipitation in some pump catheters, Novolin® R is not recommended for use in insulin pumps.

2. A change in the type, strength, species or purity of insulin could require a dosage adjustment. Any change in insulin should be made under medical supervision.
3. You may have learned how to test your urine or your blood for glucose. It is important to do these tests regularly and to record the results for review with your physician or nurse educator.
4. If you have an acute illness, especially with vomiting or fever, continue taking your insulin. If possible, stay on your regular diet. If you have trouble eating, drink fruit juices, regular soft drinks, or clear soups; if you can, eat small amounts of bland foods. Test your urine for glucose and ketones and, if possible, test your blood glucose. Note the results and contact your physician for possible insulin dose adjustment. If you have severe and prolonged vomiting, seek emergency medical care.
5. You should always carry identification which states that you have diabetes.

See Novolin® 70/30 for complete package insert information on Warning: Insulin use in Diabetes: Types of Insulin: Syringes: Needle-Free Injectors: Important Statement: Preparing the Injection: Giving the Injection: Usage in Pregnancy: Insulin Reaction and Shock: Diabetic Ketoacidosis and Coma: Adverse Reactions.

HOW SUPPLIED

Vials, U-100, 100 units/mL, 10 mL, (List No. 183311) (1's)
Novolin R Prefilled™ Syringe, U-100, 100 units/mL, 1.5 mL, (List No. 004471) (5's)
Novolin® R PenFill®, U-100, 100 units/mL, 1.5 mL, (List No. 183317) (5's)

VELOSULIN® BR — OTC

Buffered Regular
Human Insulin Injection
(semi-synthetic)
100 units/ml

FOR USE IN EXTERNAL INSULIN INFUSION PUMPS OR WITH U-100 INSULIN SYRINGES
Please read this leaflet carefully.

WARNING

Any change of insulin should be made cautiously and only under medical supervision. Changes in purity, strength (U-40, U-100), brand (manufacturer), type (Lente®, NPH, regular etc.) and/or species source (beef, pork, beef/pork, human) may result in the need for a change in dosage. Adjustment may be needed with the first dose or over a period of several weeks. Be aware that symptoms of hypoglycemia (low blood glucose) or hyperglycemia (high blood glucose) may indicate the need for dosage adjustment. Please read sections entitled "Insulin Reaction" and "Diabetic Ketoacidosis and Coma".

Velosulin® BR should not be mixed with Lente®-type insulin products because the buffering agent in Velosulin® BR may interact with the other insulin and result in a change of activity. This change could lead to an unpredictable effect on blood glucose. When used with an external insulin infusion pump Velosulin® BR should not be mixed with any other insulin.

Velosulin® BR has been tested only in MiniMed® Model 504-S pumps, using the accompanying Model MMT-103 syringe as well as both MiniMed® Model MMT-106 Polyfin™ and MiniMed® Model 111 Sofset™ infusion sets. MiniMed® Model 504-S and Model 506 pumps are equivalent.

Change the catheter tubing and the insulin in the reservoir every 48 hours.

INSULIN USE IN DIABETES

Your physician has explained that you have diabetes and that your treatment involves injections of insulin. Insulin is normally produced by the pancreas, a gland that lies behind the stomach. Without insulin, glucose (a simple sugar made from digested food) is trapped in the bloodstream and cannot enter the cells of the body. Some patients who don't make enough of their own insulin, or who cannot use the insulin they do make properly, must take insulin by injection in order to control their blood glucose levels.

Each case of diabetes is different and requires direct and continued medical supervision. Your physician has told you the type, strength and amount of insulin you should use and the time(s) at which you should inject it, and has also discussed with you a diet and exercise schedule. You should contact your physician if you experience any difficulties or if you have questions.

TYPES OF INSULINS

Standard and purified animal insulins as well as human insulins are available. Standard and purified insulins differ in their degree of purification and content of noninsulin material.

Standard and purified insulins also vary in species source: they may be of beef, pork, or mixed beef and pork origin. Human insulin is identical in structure to the insulin produced by the human pancreas, and thus differs from animal insulins. Insulins vary in time of action and in strength; see PRODUCT DESCRIPTION and SYRINGES for additional information.

Your physician has prescribed the insulin that is right for you; be sure you have purchased the correct insulin and check it carefully before you use it.

PRODUCT DESCRIPTION

Velosulin® BR is a clear solution of insulin in a phosphate buffer. This human insulin is structurally identical to the insulin produced by the pancreas in the human body. This structural identity is obtained by enzymatic conversion of purified pork insulin. When a U-100 insulin syringe is used to deliver the insulin, Velosulin® BR has a rapid onset of action, approximately ½ hour after the injection. The effect lasts up to approximately 8 hours with a maximal effect between the 1st and 3rd hour.

The time course of action of any insulin may vary considerably in different individuals, or at different times in the same individual, or if using an external insulin infusion pump to deliver the insulin.

Because of this variation, the time periods listed here should be considered as general guidelines only when using U-100 insulin syringes to deliver the insulin.

STORAGE

Insulin should be stored in a cold place, preferably in a refrigerator, but not in the freezing compartment. Do not let it freeze. Keep the insulin vial in its carton so that it will stay clean and protected from light. If refrigeration is not possible, the bottle of insulin which you are currently using can be kept unrefrigerated as long as it is kept as cool as possible and away from heat and sunlight.

Do not use the preparation if the color has become other than water clear or if the liquid has become viscous (thickened).

Never use insulin after expiration date which is printed on the vial label and carton.

EXTERNAL INSULIN INFUSION PUMPS

Read and follow the instructions that accompany your insulin infusion pump. It is important to follow the instructions from the manufacturer of the pump that you use.

Use the correct reservoir and catheter for the pump that you are using. Catheter clogging with insulin crystals has been known to occur.

You should change the catheter tubing and the insulin in the reservoir every 48 hours. Failure to do so may affect the amount of insulin you receive. This can cause serious problems for you, such as too little or too much glucose in the blood.

When used with an external insulin infusion pump, Velosulin® BR should not be mixed with any other insulin.

SYRINGES

Use the correct syringe

The volume of the dose depends on the number of units of insulin per ml. Velosulin® BR is only available in the U-100 strength (100 units per ml). Make sure that you understand the markings on your syringe and use only syringe marked for U-100.

Novo Nordisk insulin vials are intended for use with standard insulin syringes. Novo Nordisk has not evaluated the use of these vials with other devices for insulin delivery or with devices intended to aid in giving injections. Consult your doctor and the manufacturer of these devices before use with this product.

Disposable Syringes

Disposable syringes and needles require no sterilization provided the package is intact. They should be used only once and discarded.

Reusable Syringes

Reusable syringes and needles must be sterile when used. The best method of sterilization is to boil the syringe, plunger and needle in water for 5 minutes. If this is not possible, as when travelling, the parts may be sterilized by immersion for at least 5 minutes in a sterilizing liquid like ethyl alcohol, 70%. Do not use bathing, rubbing or medicated alcohol for sterilization.

Remove all liquid from the syringe by pushing the plunger in and out several times and leave it to dry if alcohol has been used for sterilization.

IMPORTANT

Failure to comply with the above and the following antiseptic measures may lead to infections at the injection site.

PREPARING THE INJECTION

1. Clean your hands and the injection site with soap and water or with alcohol.
   Wipe the rubber stopper with an alcohol swab. (Note: remove the tamper-resistant cap at first use. If the cap has already been removed, do not use this product, return it to your pharmacy.)
2. Pull back the plunger until the black tip reaches the marking for the number of units you will inject.
3. Push the needle through the rubber stopper into the vial.
4. Push the plunger all the way in. This inserts air into the bottle.
5. Turn the vial and syringe upside down and slowly pull the plunger back to a few units beyond the correct dose.
6. If there are air bubbles, flick the syringe firmly with your finger to raise the air bubbles to the needle, then slowly push the plunger to the correct unit marking.
7. Life the vial off the syringe.

GIVING THE INJECTION

1. The following areas are suitable for subcutaneous insulin injection: thighs, upper arms, buttocks, abdomen. Do not change areas without consulting your physician. The actual point of injection should be changed each time; injection sites should be about an inch apart.
2. The injection site should be clean and dry. Pinch up skin area to be injected and hold it firmly.
3. Hold the syringe like a pencil and push the needle quickly and firmly into the pinched-up area.
4. Release the skin and push plunger all the way in to inject insulin beneath the skin. Do not inject into a muscle unless your physician has advised it. You should never inject insulin into a vein.
5. Remove the needle. If slight bleeding occurs, press lightly with a dry cotton swab for a few seconds—do not rub.

MIXING TWO TYPES OF INSULIN (IN SYRINGES ONLY)

When using U-100 Insulin Syringes, different insulins should be mixed only under instruction from a physician. Hypodermic syringes may vary in the amount of space between the bottom line and the needle ("dead space"), so if you are mixing two types of insulin be sure to discuss any change in the model and brand of syringe you are using with your physician or pharmacist. When you are mixing two types of insulin, always draw the Regular (clear) insulin into the syringe first.

Velosulin® BR should not be mixed with Lente®-type insulin products because the buffering agent in Velosulin® BR may interact with the other insulin and result in a change of activity. This change could lead to an unpredictable effect on blood glucose. When used with an external insulin infusion pump Velosulin® BR should not be mixed with any other insulin.

USAGE IN PREGNANCY

It is particularly important to maintain good control of your diabetes during pregnancy and special attention must be paid to your diet, exercise and insulin regimens. If you are pregnant or nursing a baby, consult your physician or nurse educator.

INSULIN REACTION

Insulin reaction (too little sugar in the blood, also called hypoglycemia) can occur if you take too much insulin, miss a meal or exercise or work harder than normal. The symptoms, which usually come on suddenly, are hunger, dizziness, and sweating. Personality change or confusion may also occur. Eating sugar or a sugar-sweetened product will normally correct the condition.

If symptoms persist, call a physician; an insulin reaction can lead to unconsciousness. If a reaction results in loss of consciousness, emergency medical care should be obtained immediately. If you have had repeated reactions or if an insulin reaction had led to a loss of consciousness, contact your physician. Severe hypoglycemia can result in temporary or permanent impairment of brain function and death.

In certain cases, the nature and intensity of the warning symptoms of hypoglycemia may change. A few patients have reported that after being transferred to human insulin, the early warning symptoms of hypoglycemia were less pronounced than they had been with animal-source insulin.

DIABETIC KETOACIDOSIS AND COMA

Diabetic ketoacidosis may develop if your body has too little insulin. The most common causes are acute illness, infection or failure to take enough insulin by injection or catheter clogging when used with an external insulin infusion pump. If you are ill, you should check your urine for ketones. The symptoms of diabetic ketoacidosis usually come on gradually, over a period of hours or days, and include a drowsy feeling, fluschned face, thrist and loss of appetite. Notify a physician immediately if the urine test is positive for ketones (acetone) or if you have any of these symptoms. More severe symptoms are fast, heavy breathing and rapid pulse; if these symptoms occur, you should have medical attention right away. Severe, sustained hyperglycemia may result in diabetic coma and death.

ADVERSE REACTIONS

Insulin allergy occurs very rarely, but when it does, it may cause a serious reaction including a general skin rash over

Continued on next page

Novo Nordisk—Cont.

the body, shortness of breath, fast pulse, sweating and a drop in blood pressure. If any of these symptoms develop you should seek emergency medical care.

In a very few diabetics, the skin where insulin has been injected may become red, swollen and itchy. This is called a local reaction. It may occur if the injection is not properly made, if the skin is sensitive to the cleansing solution or if the patient is allergic to insulin. If you have a local reaction, notify your physician.

Patients with severe systemic allergic reactions to insulin (i.e. generalized urticaria, angioedema, anaphylaxis) should be skin tested with each new preparation to be used prior to initiation of therapy with that preparation.

IMPORTANT NOTES

1. A change in the type, strength, species or purity of insulin could require a dosage adjustment. Any change in insulin should be made under medical supervision.

2. You may have learned how to test your urine or your blood for glucose. It is important to do these tests regularly and to record the results for review with your physician or nurse educator.

3. If you have an illness, especially with vomiting or fever, continue taking your insulin. If possible, stay on your regular diet. If you have trouble eating, drink fruit juices, regular soft drinks, or clear soups; if you can, eat small amounts of bland foods. Test your urine for glucose and ketones and, if possible, test your blood glucose. Note the results and contact your physician for possible insulin dose adjustment. If you have severe and prolonged vomiting, seek emergency medical care.

4. You should always carry identification which states that you have diabetes.

Always consult your physician if you have any questions about your condition or the use of insulin.

Helpful information for people with diabetes is published by American Diabetes Association, 1660 Duke St., Alexandria, VA 22314.

Novo Nordisk™, Velosulin® and Lente® are trademarks of Novo Nordisk A/S

MiniMed®, Polyfin™ and Sofset™ are trademarks of MiniMed Inc.

For information contact: Novo Nordisk Pharmaceuticals Inc. Princeton, NJ 08540

Manufactured by: Novo Nordisk A/S, 2880 Bagsvaerd, Denmark

Date of issue: January 1995

HUMAN INSULIN DELIVERY SYSTEMS

There are two types of Human Insulin Delivery Systems available from Novo Nordisk Pharmaceuticals Inc.:

DURABLE INSULIN DELIVERY SYSTEM

For the durable insulin delivery system you will need the following items, which are sold separately:
1) NovoPen® 1.5 injection device
2) Novolin® PenFill® Cartridges
3) NovoFine® 30 Disposable Needles

DISPOSABLE INSULIN DELIVERY SYSTEM

For the disposable insulin delivery system you will need the following items, which are sold separately:
1) Novolin Prefilled® Syringes
2) NovoFine® 30 Disposable Needles

HUMAN INSULIN   OTC
NOVOLIN® 70/30 PenFill®
70% NPH, Human Insulin Isophane Suspension and
30% Regular, Human Insulin Injection
(recombinant DNA origin)
100 units/ml

Please read this leaflet carefully before using this product. Please note the special directions under "PREPARING THE INJECTION".

Novolin® 70/30 PenFill® is for use with NovoPen® and NovolinPen® Insulin Delivery Devices specifically designed for this cartridge.

PenFill® cartridge is for single person use only.

See Important Notes section.

WARNING

ANY CHANGE OF INSULIN SHOULD BE MADE CAUTIOUSLY AND ONLY UNDER MEDICAL SUPERVISION. CHANGES IN PURITY, STRENGTH, BRAND (MANUFACTURER), TYPE (REGULAR, NPH, LENTE®, ETC.), SPECIES (BEEF, PORK, BEEF-PORK, HUMAN), AND/OR METHOD OF

MANUFACTURE (RECOMBINANT DNA VERSUS ANIMAL-SOURCE INSULIN) MAY RESULT IN THE NEED FOR A CHANGE IN DOSAGE.

SPECIAL CARE SHOULD BE TAKEN WHEN THE TRANSFER IS FROM A STANDARD BEEF OR MIXED SPECIES INSULIN TO A PURIFIED PORK OR HUMAN INSULIN. IF A DOSAGE ADJUSTMENT IS NEEDED, IT WILL USUALLY BECOME APPARENT EITHER IN THE FIRST FEW DAYS OR OVER A PERIOD OF SEVERAL WEEKS. ANY CHANGE IN TREATMENT SHOULD BE CAREFULLY MONITORED. PLEASE READ THE SECTIONS "INSULIN REACTION AND SHOCK" AND "DIABETIC KETOACIDOSIS AND COMA" FOR SYMPTOMS OF HYPOGLYCEMIA (LOW BLOOD GLUCOSE) AND HYPERGLYCEMIA (HIGH BLOOD GLUCOSE).

INSULIN USE IN DIABETES

Your physician has explained that you have diabetes and that your treatment involves injections of insulin. Insulin is normally produced by the pancreas, a gland that lies behind the stomach. Without insulin, glucose (a simple sugar made from digested food) is trapped in the bloodstream and cannot enter the cells of the body. Some patients who don't make enough of their own insulin, or who cannot use properly the insulin they do make, must take insulin by injection in order to control their blood glucose levels. Each case of diabetes is different and requires direct and continued medical supervision. Your physician has told you the type, strength and amount of insulin you should use and the time(s) at which you should inject it, and has also discussed with you a diet and exercise schedule. You should contact your physician if you experience any difficulties or if you have questions.

TYPES OF INSULINS

Standard and purified animal insulins as well as human insulins are available. Standard and purified insulins differ in their degree of purification and content of noninsulin material. Standard and purified insulins also vary in species source: they may be of beef, pork, or mixed beef and pork origin. Human insulin is identical in structure to the insulin produced by the human pancreas, and thus differs from animal insulins. Insulins vary in time of action; see PRODUCT DESCRIPTION for additional information.

Your physician has prescribed the insulin that is right for you; be sure you have purchased the correct insulin and check it carefully before you use it.

PRODUCT DESCRIPTION

This package contains five (5) Novolin® 70/30 PenFill® cartridges. Novolin® 70/30 is a mixture of 70% NPH, Human Insulin Isophance Suspension (recombinant DNA origin) and 30% Regular, Human Insulin Injection (recombinant DNA origin) USP. The concentration of this product is 100 units of insulin per milliliter. It is a cloudy or milky suspension of human insulin with protamine and zinc. The insulin substance (the cloudy material) settles at the bottom of the cartridge, therefore, the cartridge must be rotated up and down as described under "PREPARING THE INJECTION" so that the contents are uniformly mixed before the dose is given.

Novolin® 70/30 has an intermediate duration of action. The effect of Novolin® 70/30 begins approximately ½ hour after injection. The effect is maximal between 2 and approximately 12 hours. The full duration of action may last up to 24 hours after injection.

The time course of action of any insulin may vary considerably in different individuals, or at different times in the same individual. Because of this variation, the time periods listed here should be considered as general guidelines only.

This human insulin (recombinant DNA origin) is structurally identical to the insulin produced by the human pancreas. This human insulin is produced by recombinant DNA technology utilizing Saccharomyces cerevisiae (bakers' yeast) as the production organism.

INSULIN DELIVERY DEVICES

These Novolin® cartridges are for use with the NovoPen® 1.5 Dial-A-Dose Insulin Delivery Device specifically designed for these cartridges.

STORAGE

Insulin should be stored in a cold place, preferably in a refrigerator, but not in the freezing compartment. **Do not let it freeze.** Keep Novolin® 70/30 PenFill® cartridges in the carton so that they will stay clean and protected from light. Novolin® 70/30 PenFill® cartridges can be kept unrefrigerated for one (1) week. Unrefrigerated cartridges must be used within this time period or discarded. Be sure to protect cartridges from sunlight and extreme heat or cold.

Never use any Novolin® 70/30 PenFill® cartridge if the precipitate (the white deposit), has become lumpy or granular in appearance or has formed a deposit of solid particles on the wall of the cartridge. This insulin should not be used if the liquid in the cartridge remains clear after it has been mixed.

Never use insulin after the expiration date which is printed on the label and carton.

IMPORTANT

Failure to comply with the following antiseptic measures may lead to infections at the injection site.

—NovoFine® 30 disposable needles are for single use; they should be used only once and destroyed.
—Clean your hands and the injection site with soap and water or with alcohol.
—Wipe the rubber stopper on the insulin cartridge with an alcohol swab.

PREPARING THE INJECTION

Never place a NovoFine® 30 disposable single-use needle on your insulin delivery device until you are ready to give an injection, and remove it immediately after each injection. If the needle is not removed, some liquid may be expelled from the cartridge causing a change in the insulin concentration (strength).

The cloudy material in an insulin suspension will settle to the bottom of the cartridge, so the contents must be mixed before injection. These Novolin® PenFill® cartridges contain a glass ball to aid mixing.

When using a new cartridge, turn the cartridge up and down between positions A and B—See Figure 1. Do this at least 10 times until the liquid appears uniformly white and cloudy.

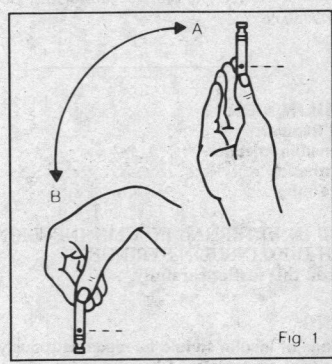
Fig. 1

Assemble your insulin delivery device following the directions in your instruction manual.

For subsequent injections when a cartridge is already in the device, turn the device up and down between positions A and B—See Figure 2. Do this at least 10 times until the liquid appears uniformly white and cloudy. Follow the directions in your insulin delivery device instruction manual.

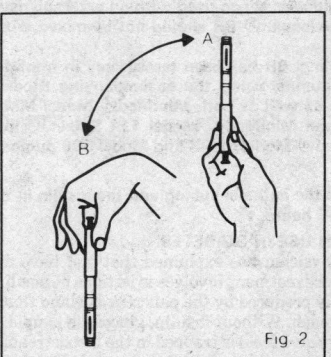
Fig. 2

Always be sure there is sufficient insulin in the cartridge to complete the injection. In order to help you estimate the amount of insulin in the cartridge, the width of the black band corresponds to 12 units of insulin.

Note: Never initiate a new injection unless there is sufficient insulin in the cartridge to ensure proper mixing (the glass ball needs adequate room for movement to mix the suspension). When using a NovoPen® device, never initiate a new injection once the leading edge of the plunger has passed the top edge of the black band.

GIVING THE INJECTION

1. The following areas are suitable for subcutaneous insulin injection: thighs, upper arms, buttocks, abdomen. Do not change areas without consulting your physician. The actual point of injection should be changed each time; injection sites should be about an inch apart.
2. The injection site should be clean and dry. Pinch up skin area to be injected and hold it firmly.
3. Hold the device like a pencil and push the needle quickly and firmly into the pinched-up area. If you go straight in it will probably sting less.
4. Follow the directions for use of your insulin delivery device.
5. Do not inject into a muscle unless your physician has advised it. You should never inject insulin into a vein.
6. Remove needle. If slight bleeding occurs, press lightly with a dry cotton swab for a few seconds—**do not rub.**

USAGE IN PREGNANCY

It is particularly important to maintain good control of your diabetes during pregnancy and special attention must be paid to your diet, exercise and insulin regimens. If you are pregnant or nursing a baby, consult your physician or nurse educator.

INSULIN REACTION AND SHOCK

Insulin reaction (hypoglycemia) occurs when the blood glucose falls very low. This can happen if you take too much insulin, miss or delay a meal, exercise more than usual or work too hard without eating, or become ill (especially with vomiting or fever). The first symptoms of an insulin reaction usually come on suddenly. They may include a cold sweat, fatigue, nervousness or shakiness, rapid heartbeat, or nausea. Personality change or confusion may also occur. If you drink or eat something right away (a glass of milk or orange juice, or several sugar candies), you can often stop the progression of symptoms. If symptoms persist, call your physician—an insulin reaction can lead to unconsciousness. If a reaction results in loss of consciousness, emergency medical care should be obtained immediately. If you have had repeated reactions or if an insulin reaction has led to a loss of consciousness, contact your physician. Severe hypoglycemia can result in temporary or permanent impairment of brain function and death.

In certain cases, the nature and intensity of the warning symptoms of hypoglycemia may change. A few patients have reported that after being transferred to human insulin, the early warning symptoms of hypoglycemia were less pronounced than they had been with animal-source insulin.

DIABETIC KETOACIDOSIS AND COMA

Diabetic ketoacidosis may develop if your body has too little insulin. The most common causes are acute illness or infection or failure to take enough insulin by injection. If you are ill you should check your urine for ketones. The symptoms of diabetic ketoacidosis usually come on gradually, over a period of hours or days, and include a drowsy feeling, flushed face, thirst and loss of appetite. Notify your physician right away if the urine test is positive for ketones (acetone) or if you have any of these symptoms. Fast, heavy breathing and rapid pulse are more severe symptoms and you should have medical attention right away. Severe, sustained hyperglycemia may result in diabetic coma and death.

ADVERSE REACTIONS

A few people with diabetes develop red, swollen and itchy skin where the insulin has been injected. This is called a "local reaction" and it may occur if the injection is not properly made, if the skin is sensitive to the cleansing solution, or if you are allergic to the insulin being used. If you have a local reaction, tell your physican.

Generalized insulin allergy occurs rarely, but when it does it may cause a serious reaction, including skin rash over the body, shortness of breath, fast pulse, sweating, and a drop in blood pressure. If any of these symptoms develop, you should seek emergency medical care.

If severe allergic reactions to insulin have occured (i.e., generalized rash, swelling or breathing difficulties) you should be skin-tested with **each** new insulin preparation before it is used.

IMPORTANT NOTES

1. A change in the type, strength, species or purity of insulin could require a dosage adjustment. Any change in insulin should be made under medical supervision.
2. To avoid possible transmission of disease, PenFill® cartridge is for single person use only.
3. You may have learned how to test your urine or your blood for glucose. It is important to do these tests regularly and to record the results for review with your physician or nurse educator.
4. If you have an acute illness, especially with vomiting or fever, continue taking your insulin. If possible, stay on your regular diet. If you have trouble eating, drink fruit jucies, regular soft drinks, or clear soups; if you can, eat small amounts of bland foods. Test your urine for glucose and ketones and, if possible, test your blood glucose. Note the results and contact your physician for possible insulin dose adjustment. If you have severe and prolonged vomiting, seek emergency medical care.
5. You should always carry identification which states that you have diabetes.

Always consult your physician if you have any questions about your conditon or the use of insulin.

Helpful information for people with diabetes is published by American Diabetes Association, 1660 Duke Street, Alexandria, VA 22314

For information contact:
Novo Nordisk Pharmaceuticals Inc.,
Princeton, NJ 08540
Manufactured by
Novo Nordisk A/S
DK-2880 Bagsvaerd, Denmark
Novo Nordisk™, Novolin® PenFill®, NovoPen®, NovolinPen®, PenNeedle® and Lente® are trademarks owned by Novo Nordisk A/S
Date of issue: December 1992

HOW SUPPLIED

Novolin® 70/30 PenFill® cartridges, U-100, 100 units/mL, 1.5 mL, (List No. 183717) (5's)

NOVOLIN® N PenFill® — OTC

NPH, Human Insulin Isophane Suspension (recombinant DNA origin)
100 units/ml

Please read the leaflet carefully before using this product. Please note the special directions under "PREPARING THE INJECTION".

Novolin® N PenFill® is for use with the NovoPen® 1.5 Dial-A-Dose Insulin Delivery Device specifically designed for this cartridge. PenFill® cartridge is for single person use only. See Important Notes section.

DESCRIPTION

Novolin® N PenFill® cartridges contain **Novolin® N**, commonly known as NPH, Human Insulin Isophane Suspension (recombinant DNA origin). The concentration of this product is 100 units of insulin per milliliter. It is a cloudy or milky suspension of human insulin with protamine and zinc. The insulin substance (the cloudy material) settles at the bottom of the cartridge; therefore, the cartridge must be turned up and down at least 10 times or until the liquid appears uniformly white and cloudy (a glass ball inside the cartridge facilitates mixing).

Novolin® N has an intermediate duration of action. The effect of **Novolin® N** begins approximately $1\frac{1}{2}$ hours after injection. The effect is maximal between 4 and 12 hours. The full duration of action may last up to 24 hours after injection. The time course of action of any insulin may vary considerably in different individuals, or at different times in the same individual. Because of this variation, the time periods listed here should be considered as general guidelines only.

This human insulin (recombinant DNA origin) is structurally identical to the insulin produced by the human pancreas. This human insulin is produced by recombinant DNA technology utilizing *Saccharomyces cerevisiae* (bakers' yeast) as the production organism.

STORAGE

Insulin should be stored in a cold place, preferably in a refrigerator, but not in the freezing compartment. **Do not let it freeze.** Keep the **Novolin® N PenFill®** cartridges in the carton so that they will stay clean and protected from light. **Novolin® N PenFill®** cartridges can be kept unrefrigerated for one (1) week. Unrefrigerated cartridges must be used within this time period or discarded. Be sure to protect cartridges from sunlight and extreme heat or cold.

Never use any **Novolin® N PenFill®** cartridge if the precipitate (the white deposit) has become lumpy or granular in appearance or has formed a deposit of solid particles on the wall of the cartridge. This insulin should not be used if the liquid in the cartridge remains clear after it has been mixed.

Never use insulin after the expiration date which is printed on the cartridge label and carton.

See NOVOLIN® 70/30 PenFill® for package insert information on Warning: Insulin use in Diabetes: Types of Insulin: Insulin Delivery Devices: Important Statement: Preparing the Injection: Giving the Injection: Usage in Pregnancy: Insulin Reaction and Shock: Diabetic Ketoacidosis and Coma: Adverse Reactions: Important Notes.

HOW SUPPLIED

Novolin® N PenFill® cartridges, U-100, 100 units/mL, 1.5 mL, (List No. 183417) (5's)

NOVOLIN® R PenFill® — OTC

Regular, Human Insulin Injection (recombinant DNA origin)
100 units/ml

Please read the leaflet carefully before using this product. Novlin® R PenFill® is for use with the NovoPen® 1.5 Dial-A-Dose Insulin Delivery Device specifically designed for this cartridge.

PenFill® cartridge is for single person use only.

See Important Notes section.

DESCRIPTION

Novolin® R PenFill® cartridges contain **Novolin® R**, commonly known as Regular, Human Insulin Injection (recombinant DNA origin). The concentration of this product is 100 units of insulin per milliliter. It is a clear, colorless solution which has a short duration of action. The effect of **Novolin® R** begins approximately $^1/_2$ hour after injection. The effect is maximal between $2^1/_2$ and 5 hours and ends approximately 8 hours after injection. The time course of action of any insulin may vary considerably in different individuals, or at different times in the same individual. Because of this variation, the time periods listed here should be considered as general guidelines only.

This human insulin (recombinant DNA origin) is structurally identical to the insulin produced by the human pancreas. This human insulin is produced by recombinant DNA technology utilizing *Saccharomyces cerevisiae* (bakers' yeast) as the production organism.

STORAGE

Insulin should be stored in a cold place, preferably in a refrigerator, but not in the freezing compartment. **Do not let it freeze.** Keep **Novolin® R PenFill®** cartridges in the carton so they will stay clean and protected from light. **Novolin® R PenFill®** cartridges can be kept unrefrigerated for one (1) month. Unrefrigerated cartridges must be used within this time period or discarded. Be sure to protect cartridges from sunlight and extreme heat or cold.

Never use any **Novolin® PenFill®** if it becomes viscous (thickened) or cloudy; use it only if it is clear and colorless.

Never use insulin after the expiration date which is printed on the cartridge label and carton.

PREPARING THE INJECTION

Place a single-use **PenNeedle®** on the device. Be sure there is sufficient insulin in the cartridge to complete the injection. Refer to the instruction manual for your insulin delivery device for assistance in estimating the amount of insulin remaining in the cartridge.

See Novolin® 70/30 PenFill® for package insert information on Warning: Insulin Use in Diabetes: Types of Insulins: Insulin Delivery Devices: Important Statement: Giving the Injection: Usage in Pregnancy: Insulin Reaction and Shock: Diabetic Ketoacidosis and Coma: Adverse Reactions: Important Notes.

HOW SUPPLIED

Novolin® R PenFill® cartridges, U-100, 100 units/mL, 1.5 mL, (List No. 183317) (5's)

NovoFine® 30 — ℞

Disposable Needle

DESCRIPTION

The self contained disposable needle consists of a protective plastic outer cap, a smooth plastic needle cap and a protective tab. (The needle should not be used if the protective tab is missing or damaged.)

Each **NovoFine® 30** is 30 gauge, one-third (⅓) inch (8mm) in length and is intended for single use only. Each **NovoFine® 30** is cut to a sharp, low-angle point and coated with silicone for easier penetration.

NovoFine® 30 is specifically designed to be used with all Novo Nordisk insulin delivery systems.

Continued on next page

Novo Nordisk—Cont.

HUMAN INSULIN
NOVOLIN 70/30 PREFILLED™ OTC
70% NPH, Human Insulin Isophane Suspension and 30% Regular,
Human Insulin Injection
(recombinant DNA origin)
in a 1.5 ml Prefilled Syringe
100 units/ml

NOVOLIN N PREFILLED™
NPH, Human Insulin Isophane
Suspension (recombinant DNA origin)
in a 1.5 ml Prefilled Syringe
100 units/ml

NOVOLIN R PREFILLED™
Regular, Human Insulin Injection
(recombinant DNA origin)
in a 1.5 ml Prefilled Syringe
100 units/ml

Insulin Information For The Patient
Please read both sides of this leaflet carefully before using this product.
Novolin Prefilled™ syringe is for single person use only. See Important Notes section.

WARNING

ANY CHANGE OF INSULIN SHOULD BE MADE CAUTIOUSLY AND ONLY UNDER MEDICAL SUPERVISION. CHANGES IN PURITY, STRENGTH, BRAND (MANUFACTURER), TYPE (REGULAR, NPH, LENTE® ETC.), SPECIES (BEEF, PORK, BEEF-PORK, HUMAN) AND/OR METHOD OF MANUFACTURE (RECOMBINANT DNA VERSUS ANIMAL-SOURCE INSULIN) MAY RESULT IN THE NEED FOR A CHANGE IN DOSAGE.
SPECIAL CARE SHOULD BE TAKEN WHEN THE TRANSFER IS FROM A STANDARD BEEF OR MIXED SPECIES INSULIN TO A PURIFIED PORK OR HUMAN INSULIN. IF A DOSAGE ADJUSTMENT IS NEEDED, IT WILL USUALLY BECOME APPARENT EITHER IN THE FIRST FEW DAYS OR OVER A PERIOD OF SEVERAL WEEKS. ANY CHANGE IN TREATMENT SHOULD BE CAREFULLY MONITORED.
PLEASE READ THE SECTIONS "INSULIN REACTION AND SHOCK" AND "DIABETIC KETOACIDOSIS AND COMA" FOR SYMPTOMS OF HYPOGLYCEMIA (LOW BLOOD GLUCOSE) AND HYPERGLYCEMIA (HIGH BLOOD GLUCOSE).

INSULIN USE IN DIABETES
Your physician has explained that you have diabetes and that your treatment involves injections of insulin. Insulin is normally produced by the pancreas, a gland that lies behind the stomach. Without insulin, glucose (a simple sugar made from digested food) is trapped in the bloodstream and cannot enter the cells of the body. Some patients who don't make enough of their own insulin, or who cannot properly use the insulin they do make, must take insulin by injection in order to control their blood glucose levels.
Each case of diabetes is different and requires direct and continued medical supervision. Your physician has told you the type, strength and amount of insulin you should use and the time(s) at which you should inject it, and has also discussed with you a diet and exercise schedule. You should contact your physician if you experience any difficulties or if you have questions.

TYPES OF INSULIN
Standard and purified animal insulin as well as human insulin are available. Standard and purified insulin differ in their degree of purification and content of noninsulin material. Standard and purified insulin also vary in species source: they may be of beef, pork, or mixed beef and pork origin. Human insulin is identical in structure to the insulin produced by the human pancreas, and thus differs from animals insulin. Insulin Products vary in time of action; see PRODUCT DESCRIPTION for additional information.
Your physician has prescribed the insulin that is right for you; be sure you have purchased the correct insulin and check it carefully before you use it.

PRODUCT DESCRIPTION

A package contains five (5) **Novolin Prefilled™** insulin syringes.
This human insulin (recombinant DNA origin) is structurally identical to the insulin produced by the human pancreas. This human insulin is produced by recombinant DNA technology utilizing *Saccharomyces cerevisiae* (bakers' yeast) as the production organism.
The time course of action of any insulin may vary considerably in different individuals, or at different times in the same individual. Because of the variation, the time periods listed here should be considered as general guidelines only.
Novolin 70/30 Prefilled™ contains Novolin® 70/30, a mixture of 70% NPH, Human Insulin Isophane Suspension (recombinant DNA origin) and 30% Regular, Human Insulin Injection (recombinant DNA origin). The concentration of this product is 100 units of insulin per milliliter. It is a cloudy or milky suspension of human insulin with protamine and zinc. The insulin substance (the cloudy material) settles to the bottom of the insulin reservoir, therefore, the syringe must be rotated up and down so that the contents are uniformly mixed before a dose is given. Novolin® 70/30 has an intermediate duration of action. The effect of Novolin® 70/30 begins approximately 1/2 hours after injection. The effect is maximal between 2 and approximately 12 hours. The full duration of action may last up to 24 hours after injection.
Novolin N Prefilled™ contains NPH, Human Insulin Isophane Suspension (recombinant DNA origin). The concentration of this product is 100 units of insulin per milliliter. It is a cloudy or milky suspension of human insulin with protamine and zinc. The insulin substance (the cloudy material) settles to the bottom of the insulin reservoir, therefore, the syringe must be rotated up and down so that the contents are uniformly mixed before a dose is given. Novolin® N has an intermediate duration of action. The effect of Novolin® N begins approximately 1 1/2 hours after injection. The effect is maximal between 4 and approximately 12 hours. The full duration of action may last up to 24 hours after injection.
Novolin R Prefilled™ contains Regular, Human Insulin Injection (recombinant DNA origin). The concentration of this product is 100 units of insulin per milliliter. It is a clear, colorless solution which has a short duration of action. The effect of Novolin® R begins approximately 1/2 hour after injection. The effect is maximal between 2 1/2 and 5 hours and ends approximately 8 hours after injection.

STORAGE

Novolin Prefilled™ insulin syringes should be stored in a cold place, preferably in a refrigerator, but not in the freezing compartment. **Do no let it freeze.** Keep **Novolin Prefilled™** in the carton so that they will stay clean and protected from light. **Novolin 70/30 Prefilled™** and **Novolin N Prefilled™** can be kept unrefrigerated for one (1) week. **Novolin R Prefilled™** can be kept unrefrigerated for (1) month. *Unrefrigerated syringes must be used within this time period or discarded. Be sure to protect syringes from sunlight and extreme heat or cold.
Never use any **Novolin R Prefilled™** if the insulin becomes viscous (thickend or cloudy); use it only if it is clear and colorless. Never use any **Novolin 70/30 Prefilled™ or Novolin N Prefilled™** if the precipitate (the white deposit) has become lumpy or granular in appearance or has formed a deposit of solid particles on the wall of the insulin reservoir. This insulin should not be used if the liquid in the insulin reservoir remains clear after it has been mixed.
Never use insulin after the expiration date which is printed on the label and carton.

IMPORTANT
Failure to comply with the following antiseptic measures may lead to infections at the injection site.
—Disposable needles are for single use; they should be used only once and discarded properly.
—Clean your hands and the injection site with soap and water or with alcohol.
—Wipe the rubber stopper with an alcohol swab.

PREPARING THE INJECTION
Never place a single-use needle on your insulin delivery device until you are ready to give an injection, and remove it immediately after each injection. If the needle is not removed, some liquid may be expelled from the syringe causing a change in the insulin concentration (strength).
The cloudy material in an insulin suspension will settle to the bottom of the insulin reservoir, so the contents must be mixed before injection. These syringes contain a glass ball to aid mixing.
Rotate the syringe up and down so that the contents are uniformly mixed before the dose is given.
Follow the directions for use of this syringe on the reverse side of this insert.

GIVING THE INJECTION
1. The following areas are suitable for subcutaneous insulin injection: thighs, upper arms, buttocks, abdomen. Do not change areas without consulting your physician. The actual point of injection should be changed each time; injection sites should be about an inch apart.
2. The injection site should be clean and dry. Pinch up skin area to be injected and hold it firmly.
3. Hold the device like a pencil and push the needle quickly and firmly into the pinched-up area. If you go straight in it will probably sting less.
4. Do not inject into a muscle unless your physician has advised it. You should never inject insulin into a vein.
5. Remove needle. If slight bleeding occurs, press lightly with a dry cotton swab for a few seconds—**do not rub.**

USAGE IN PREGNANCY

It is particularly important to maintain good control of your diabetes during pregnancy and special attention must be paid to your diet, exercise and insulin regimens. If you are pregnant or nursing a baby, consult your physician or nurse educator.

INSULIN REACTION AND SHOCK
Insulin reaction (hypoglycemia) occurs when the blood glucose falls very low. This can happen if you take too much insulin, miss or delay a meal, exercise more than usual or work too hard without eating, or become ill (especially with vomiting or fever). The first symptoms of an insulin reaction usually come on suddenly. They may include a cold sweat, fatigue, nervousness or shakiness, rapid heartbeat, or nausea. Personality change or confusion may also occur. If you drink or eat something right away (a glass of milk or orange juice, or several sugar candies), you can often stop the progression of symptoms. If symptoms persist, call your physician-an insulin reaction can lead to unconsciousness. If a reaction results in loss of consciousness, emergency medical care should be obtained immediately. If you have had repeated reactions or if an insulin reaction has led to a loss of consciousness, contact your physician. Severe hypoglycemia can result in temporary or permanent impairment of brain function and death.
In certain cases, the nature and intensity of the warning symptoms of hypoglycemia may change. A few patients have reported that after being transferred to human insulin, the early warning symptoms of hypoglycemia were less pronounced than they had been with animal-source insulin.

DIABETIC KETOACIDOSIS AND COMA
Diabetic ketoacidosis may develop if your body has too little insulin. The most common causes are acute illness or infection or failure to take enough insulin by injection. If you are ill you should check your urine for ketones. The symptoms of diabetic ketoacidosis usually come on gradually, over a period of hours or days, and include a drowsy feeling, flushed face, thirst and loss of appetite. Notify your physician right away if the urine test is positive for ketones (acetone) or if you have any of these symptoms. Fast, heavy breathing and rapid pulse are more severe symptoms and you should have medical attention right away. Severe sustained hyperglycemia may result in diabetic coma and death.

ADVERSE REACTIONS

A few people with diabetes develop red, swollen and itchy skin where the insulin has been injected. This is called a "local reaction" and it may occur if the injection is not properly made, if the skin is sensitive to the cleaning solution or if you are allergic to the insulin being used. If you have a local reaction, tell your physician.
Generalized insulin allergy occurs rarely, but when it does it may cause a serious reaction, including skin rash over the body, shortness of breath, fast pulse, sweating, and a drop in blood pressure. If any of these symptoms develop, you should seek emergency medical care.
If severe reactions to insulin have occurred (i.e. generalized rash, swelling or breathing difficulties) you should be skin-tested with each new insulin preparation before it is used.

IMPORTANT NOTES

1. A change in the type, strength, species or purity of insulin could require a dosage adjustment. Any change in insulin should be made under medical supervision.
2. To avoid possible transmission of disease, **Novolin Prefilled™** syringe is for single person use only.
3. You may have learned how to test your urine or your blood for glucose. It is important to do these tests regularly and to record the results for review with your physician or nurse educator.
4. If you have an acute illness, especially with vomiting or fever, continue taking your insulin. If possible, stay on your regular diet. If you have trouble eating, drink fruit juices, regular soft drinks, or clear soups; if you can, eat small amounts of bland foods. Test your urine for glucose and ketones and, if possible, test your blood glucose. Note the results and contact your physician for possible insulin dose adjustment. If you have severe and prolonged vomiting, seek emergency medical care.
5. You should always carry identification which states that you have diabetes.

Always consult your physician if you have any questions about your condition or the use of insulin.

HOW SUPPLIED

Novolin 70/30 Prefilled™ Syringe, U-100, 100 units/ml, 1.5 ml, (List No. 001771) (5's)
Novolin N Prefilled™ Syringe, U-100, 100 units/ml, 1.5 ml, (List No. 004571) (5's)
Novolin R Prefilled™ Syringe, U-100, 100 units/ml, 1.5 ml, (List No. 004471) (5's)
Helpful information for people with diabetes is published by American Diabetes Association, 1600 Duke Street, Alexandria, VA 22314.
Novolin Prefilled™, Novolin®, NovoFine® 30, and PenNeedle® are trademarks of Novo Nordisk A/S
® 1994 Novo Nordisk Pharmaceuticals, Inc. 604-9
Printed in the USA

Prefilled syringe directions for use
This is a disposable dial-a-dose insulin delivery system able to deliver 2–58 units in increments of 2 units. **Novolin**

Prefilled™ syringe must only be used with **NovoFine® 30** disposable needle or other products specifically recommended by Novo Nordisk. **Novolin Prefilled™** syringe is not recommended for the blind or visually impaired without the assistance of a sighted individual trained in the proper use of this product.

Please read these instructions completely before using this device.

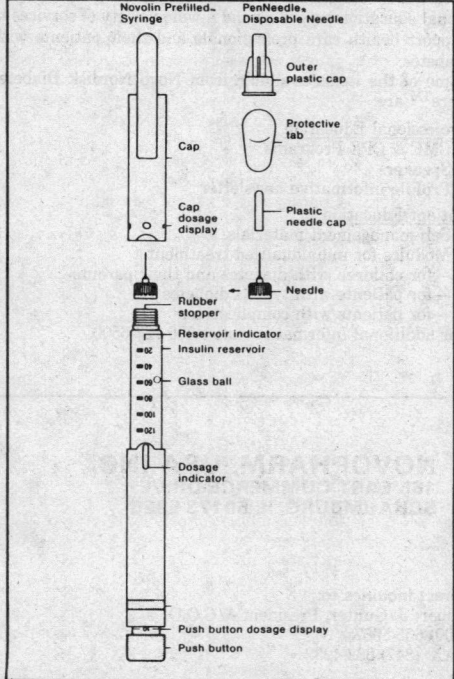

1. Preparing the Syringe
Pull off the cap.

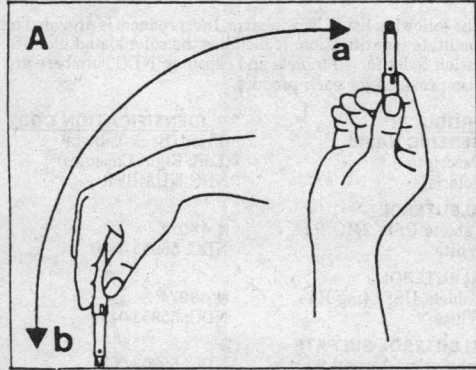

A. Turn the syringe up and down between **a** and **b** so the glass ball is moved from one end of the insulin reservoir to the other. Do this at least 10 times, until the liquid appears uniformly white and cloudy. Wipe rubber stopper with an alcohol swab. This step is not necessary with Novolin R Prefilled™.

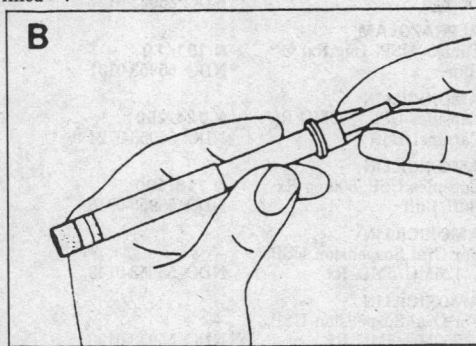

B. Remove the protective tab from disposable needle and screw the needle onto the syringe. Never place a disposable needle on your syringe until you are ready to give an injection. Remove the needle immediately after use. If the needle is not removed, some liquid may be expelled from the syringe causing a change in insulin concentration (strength).

Giving the air shot prior to each injection:
Small amounts of air may collect in the needle and insulin reservoir during normal use.
To avoid the injection of air and ensure proper dosing, hold the syringe with the needle upwards and tap the syringe gently with your finger so any air bubbles collect in the top of the reservoir. Remove both the plastic outer cap and the needle cap.

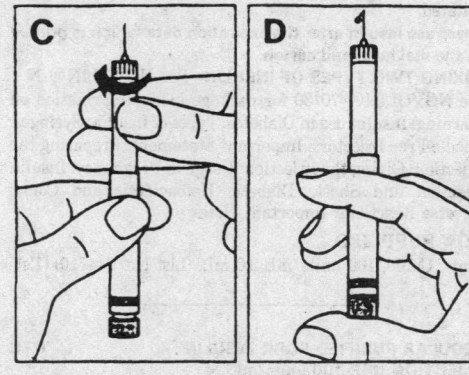

C. Holding the syringe with the needle pointing upwards, **slowly** turn the insulin reservoir clockwise (in the direction of the arrow, fig. C) to the first notch where resistance is felt ($^1/_5$ of a full rotation).
D. Still with the needle pointing upwards, press the push button as far as it will go and see if a drop of insulin appears at the needle tip (Fig. D).
If not, repeat the procedure until insulin appears. A small air bubble may remain but it will not be injected because the operating mechanism prevents the reservoir from being completely emptied.

2. Setting the dose

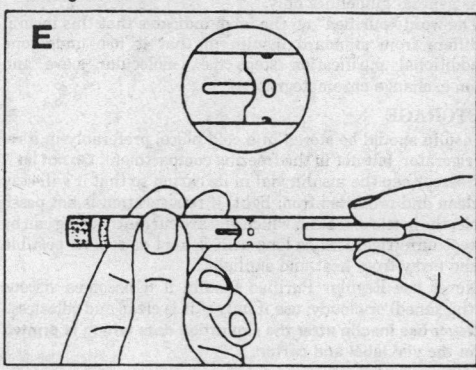

E. Replace the cap, so **0** is opposite the dosage indicator.

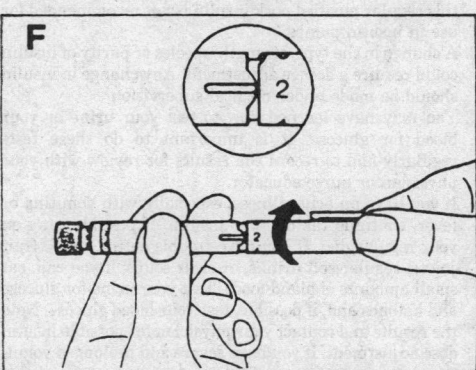

F. Hold the syringe horizontally and turn the cap in the direction of the arrow to set the required dose. Do not put your hand over the push button when dialing the dose. If the button is not allowed to rise freely, insulin will be pushed out of the needle. The dosage display on the cap shows 0, 2, 4, 6 and 8 units.
[See Figure **G** at top of next column.]
G. As the cap is turned, the push button rises. The dosage display below the push button shows 10, 20, 30, 40 and 50 units. Every time you fully turn the cap, 10 units will be set.
To check the dose set, add the figure on the cap opposite the dosage indicator to the highest number showing on the push button display.

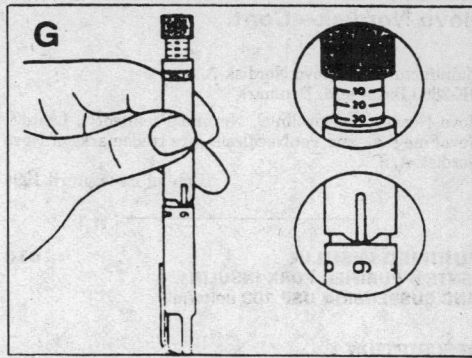

Dosage examples
- **8 units:**
  Turn the cap until 8 is opposite the dosage indicator.
- **36 units:**
  Turn the cap 3 full turns so **0** is opposite the dosage indicator. The 30-line will show on the push button display. Continue turning until 6 is opposite the dosage indicator (see **G**).

If you have set a wrong dose, simply turn the cap forwards or backwards until the right number of units has been set.
58 units is the maximum dose. If you attempt to set a higher dose, insulin will be expelled from the needle and the dose will be wrong. If you set more than 58 units, turn the cap back as far as you can until resistance is felt and the push button is fully depressed. If the dosage indicator is not lined up with **0** when resistance is felt, remove the cap and replace it with **0** opposite the dosage indicator. Now start again, remembering that **58** units is the maximum dose. After the dose is set, remove the cap.

3. Giving the injection
Use the injection technique recommended by your doctor. Check that you have set the proper dose and depress the push button as far as it will go. When depressing the push button you may hear a clicking sound. Do not rely on this clicking sound as a means of determining or confirming your dose. After making the injection, replace the plastic outer cap. Unscrew the needle and discard appropriately. Replace the cap with **0** opposite the dosing indicator.
For additional information see **GIVING THE INJECTION** on the reverse side of this insert.

4. Subsequent Injections
Always check that the push button is fully depressed before using the syringe again. If not, turn the cap until the push button is completely down. Then proceed as stated under steps 1–3.
The numbers on the insulin reservoir can be used to estimate the amount of insulin left in the syringe. These numbers **are not** used for measuring the insulin dose.
You cannot set a dose greater then the number of units remaining in the reservoir.
If you are using Novolin N Prefilled™ or Novolin 70/30 Prefilled™ there must be at least 12 units left in the reservoir to give the glass ball space to move when mixing the insulin. If your dose is less than 12 units — and the reservoir is nearly empty — first dial up to 12 (to check that 12 units are left) and then set the desired dose. If 12 cannot be dialed, change to a new syringe. Discard the used syringe carefully, without the needle attached.

5. Important Notes
- Remember to perform an air shot before each injection. See Figures C and D.
- Care should be taken not to drop the syringe or subject it to impact.
- The compact size of this prefilled syringe makes it easy to use and convenient to carry. Remember to keep it with you; don't leave it in a car or other location where extremes of temperature can occur.
- Novolin Prefilled™ is for use with NovoFine® 30 or PenNeedle® disposable needles.
- Never place a disposable needle on this syringe until you are ready to use it. Remove the needle immediately after use. If the needle is not removed, some liquid may leak from the syringe causing a change in insulin concentration (strength) of Novolin 70/30 and Novolin N insulin.
- Always carry a spare Novolin Prefilled™ syringe with you in case your prefilled syringe is damaged or lost.
- Novo Nordisk cannot be held responsible for adverse reactions occurring as a consequence of using this insulin delivery system with products that are not recommended by Novo Nordisk.
- Keep this syringe out of the reach of children.

Call 800-727-6500 for additional information.

Novo Nordisk Pharmaceuticals Inc.,
Princeton, NJ 08540

Continued on next page

Novo Nordisk—Cont.

Manufactured by Novo Nordisk A/S,
DK-2880 Bagsvaerd, Denmark

Novo Nordisk™ Novolin®, Novolin Prefilled™, Lente®
NovoFine®30, and PenNeedles®, are trademarks of Novo
Nordisk A/S.

Date of issue: April 1994

PURIFIED INSULIN   OTC
LENTE® PURIFIED PORK INSULIN
ZINC SUSPENSION USP 100 units/ml

DESCRIPTION

Lente® Purified Pork Insulin Zinc Suspension, USP,
100 units of insulin per milliliter, is a cloudy or milky suspension of 70% crystalline and 30% amorphous purified
pork insulin. The insulin substance (the cloudy material)
settles at the bottom of the vial, therefore, the vial must be
gently agitated or rotated so that the contents are uniformly
mixed before a dose is withdrawn. **Lente® Purified Insulin**
has an intermediate duration of action. The effect of **Lente®
Purified Insulin** begins approximately 2½ hours after injection. The effect is maximal between 7 and 15 hours and ends
approximately 22 hours after injection. The time course of
action of any insulin may vary considerably in different individuals, or at different times in the same individual. Because
of this variation, the time periods listed here should be
considered as general guidelines only.
The word "purified" on the label indicates that this insulin
differs from standard insulin in that it has undergone
additional purification steps (i.e., molecular sieve and
ion-exchange chromatography).

STORAGE

Insulin should be stored in a cold place, preferably in a refrigerator, but not in the freezing compartment. **Do not let it
freeze.** Keep the insulin vial in its carton so that it will stay
clean and protected from light. If refrigeration is not possible, the bottle of insulin which you are currently using can be
kept unrefrigerated as long as it is kept as cool as possible
and away from heat and sunlight.
Never use **Lente® Purified Insulin** if the precipitate (the
white deposit at the bottom of the vial) has become lumpy or
granular in appearance or has formed a deposit of solid particles on the wall of the vial. This insulin should not be used if
the liquid in the vial remains clear after the vial has been
gently agitated.
**Never use insulin after the expiration date which is printed
on the vial label and carton.**
MIXING TWO TYPES OF INSULIN—See NOVOLIN® N
See NOVOLIN® 70/30 for package insert information on
Warning: Insulin use in Diabetes: Types of Insulin: Syringes:
Needle-Free Injectors: Important Statement: Preparing the
Injection: Giving the Injection; Usage in Pregnancy: Insulin
Reaction and Shock: Diabetic Ketoacidosis and Coma:
Adverse Reactions: Important Notes.

HOW SUPPLIED

Vials, U-100, 100 units/mL, 10 mL, (List No. 244210) (1's)

NPH PURIFIED PORK ISOPHANE   OTC
INSULIN SUSPENSION USP 100 units/ml

DESCRIPTION

NPH Purified Pork Isophane Insulin Suspension, USP,
100 units of insulin per milliliter, is a cloudy or milky suspension of purified pork insulin with protamine and zinc.
The insulin substance (the cloudy material) settles at the
bottom of the vial, therefore, the vial must be gently agitated
or rotated so that the contents are uniformly mixed before a
dose is withdrawn. **NPH Purified Insulin** has an intermediate
duration of action. The effect of **NPH Purified Insulin** begins
approximately 1½ hours after injection. The effect is maximal between 4 and 12 hours and ends approximately 24
hours after injection. The time course of action of any insulin
may vary considerably in different individuals, or at different times in the same individual. Because of this variation,
the time periods listed here should be considered as general
guidelines only.
The word "purified" on the label indicates that this insulin
differs from standard insulin in that it has undergone additional purification steps (i.e., molecular sieve and ion-exchange chromatography).

STORAGE

Insulin should be stored in a cold place, preferably in a refrigerator, but not in the freezing compartment. **Do not let it
freeze.** Keep the insulin vial in its carton so that it will stay
clean and protected from light. If refrigeration is not possi-

ble, the bottle of insulin which you are currently using can be
kept unrefrigerated as long as it is kept as cool as possible
and away from heat and sunlight.
Never use **NPH Purified Insulin** if the precipitate (the white
deposit at the bottom of the vial) has become lumpy or granular in appearance or has formed a deposit of solid particles on
the wall of the vial. This insulin should not be used if the
liquid in the vial remains clear after the vial has been gently
agitated.
**Never use insulin after the expiration date which is printed
on the vial label and carton.**
MIXING TWO TYPES OF INSULIN—See NOVOLIN® N
See NOVOLIN® 70/30 for package insert information on
Warning: Insulin use in Diabetes: Types of Insulin: Syringes:
Needle-Free Injectors: Important Statement: Preparing the
Injection: Giving the Injection: Usage in Pregnancy: Insulin
Reaction and Shock: Diabetic Ketoacidosis and Coma:
Adverse Reactions: Important Notes.

HOW SUPPLIED

Vials, U-100, 100 units/mL, 10 mL, (List No. 244710) (1's)

REGULAR PURIFIED PORK INSULIN   OTC
INJECTION USP 100 units/ml

DESCRIPTION

Regular Purified Pork Insulin Injection, USP, 100 units
of insulin per milliliter, is a clear, colorless solution which
has a short duration of action. The effect of **Regular Purified
Insulin** begins approximately ½ hour after injection. The
effect is maximal between 2½ and 5 hours and ends approximately 8 hours after injection. The time course of action of
any insulin may vary considerably in different individuals,
or at different times in the same individual. Because of this
variation, the time periods listed here should be considered
as general guidelines only.
The word "purified" on the label indicates that this insulin
differs from standard insulin in that it has undergone
additional purification steps (i.e., molecular sieve and
ion-exchange chromatography).

STORAGE

Insulin should be stored in a cold place, preferably in a refrigerator, but not in the freezing compartment. **Do not let it
freeze.** Keep the insulin vial in its carton so that it will stay
clean and protected from light. If refrigeration is not possible, the bottle of insulin which you are currently using can be
kept unrefrigerated as long as it is kept as cool as possible
and away from heat and sunlight.
Never use Regular Purified Insulin if it becomes viscous
(thickened) or cloudy; use it only if it is clear and colorless.
**Never use insulin after the expiration date which is printed
on the vial label and carton.**

IMPORTANT NOTES

1. Due to the risk of precipitation in some pump catheters,
   this regular purified pork insulin is not recommended for
   use in insulin pumps.
2. A change in the type, strength, species or purity of insulin
   could require a dosage adjustment. Any change in insulin
   should be made under medical supervision.
3. You may have learned how to test your urine or your
   blood for glucose. It is important to do these tests
   regularly and to record the results for review with your
   physician or nurse educator.
4. If you have an acute illness, especially with vomiting or
   fever, continue taking your insulin. If possible, stay on
   your regular diet. If you have trouble eating, drink fruit
   juices, regular soft drinks, or clear soups; if you can, eat
   small amounts of bland foods. Test your urine for glucose
   and ketones and, if possible, test your blood glucose. Note
   the results and contact your physician for possible insulin
   dose adjustment. If you have severe and prolonged vomiting, seek emergency medical care.
5. You should always carry identification which states that
   you have diabetes.
**Always consult your physician if you have any questions
about your condition or the use of insulin.**
MIXING TWO TYPES OF INSULIN—See NOVOLIN® N
See NOVOLIN® 70/30 for package insert information on
Warning: Insulin use in Diabetes: Types of Insulin: Syringes:
Needle-Free Injectors: Important Statement: Preparing the
Injection: Giving the Injection: Usage in Pregnancy: Insulin
Reaction and Shock: Diabetic Ketoacidosis and Coma:
Adverse Reactions.

HOW SUPPLIED

Vials, U-100, 100 units/mL, 10 mL, (List No. 244010) (1's)

EDUCATIONAL MATERIAL

PATIENT EDUCATION MATERIALS
NOVO NORDISK DIABETES CARE™
SERVICE PROGRAMS THAT
EDUCATE AND SUPPORT
Novo Nordisk Diabetes Care™ is a comprehensive service
program encompassing patient education materials, profes-
sional education programs and a wide variety of services to
support health care professionals and their patients with
diabetes.
Some of the items available from Novo Nordisk Diabetes
Care™ are:

Professional Education
● CME & CPE Programs
● Speakers
● ProFile informative newsletter

Patient Education
● Self-management materials
● Modules for individualized treatment
  —for children with diabetes and their parents
  —for patients with type II diabetes
  —for patients with complications
For additional information call 1-800-727-6500.

NOVOPHARM, USA INC.
165 EAST COMMERCE DRIVE
SCHAUMBURG, IL 60173-5326

Direct Inquiries to:
Robert J. Gunter, President & C.O.O.
(800) 635-5067
FAX: (847) 882-4232

The following list of Novopharm, Inc. products is provided to
facilitate identification. It includes the color(s) and identification codes for all tablets and capsules. NDC Numbers are
also provided for each product.

PRODUCT	IDENTIFICATION CODE
GENERIC NAME	(Front/Back-Tablets)
Description	(Left/Right-Capsules)
Color(s)	NDC NUMBER
ALBUTEROL	
Tablets USP, 2MG Rx	N 480/2
White	NDC: 55953-0480
ALBUTEROL	
Tablets USP, 4mg Rx	N 499/4
White	NDC: 55953-0499
ALBUTEROL SULFATE	
Inhalation Aerosol 90 mcg	NDC: 55953-0051
ALPRAZOLAM	
Tablets USP, .25mg Rx, ℃	N 126/.25
White	NDC: 55953-0126
ALPRAZOLAM	
Tablets USP, .5mg Rx, ℃	N 127/.5
Orange	NDC: 55953-0127
ALPRAZOLAM	
Tablets USP, 1mg Rx, ℃	N 131/1.0
Blue	NDC: 55953-0131
AMOXICILLIN	
Capsules USP, 250MG Rx	N 724/250
Caramel/Buff	NDC: 55953-0724
AMOXICILLIN	
Capsules USP, 500mg Rx	N 716/500
Buff/Buff	NDC: 55953-0716
AMOXICILLIN	
For Oral Suspension USP,	—
125MG/5ML, Rx	NDC: 55953-0149
AMOXICILLIN	
For Oral Suspension USP,	—
250MG/5ML, Rx	NDC: 55953-0130
ATENOLOL	
Tablets, 50mg Rx	N 039/50
White	NDC: 55953-0039
ATENOLOL	
Tablets, 100mg Rx	N 401/100
White	NDC: 55953-0401

CAPTOPRIL TABLETS
White
12.5 mg	N 132/12.5 55953–0132
25 mg	N 133/25 55953–0133
50 mg	N 134/50 55953–0134
100 mg	N 135/100 55953–0135

CEPHALEXIN
Capsules USP, 250mg Rx N 084/250
Gray/Swedish Orange NDC: 55953-0084

CEPHALEXIN
Capsules USP, 500mg Rx N 114/500
Swedish Orange/ NDC: 55953-114
Swedish Orange

CEPHALEXIN
For Oral Suspension USP —
125MG/5ML Rx NDC: 55953-0106

CEPHALEXIN
For Oral Suspension USP —
250MG/5ML Rx NDC: 55953-0092

CIMETIDINE
Tablets USP, 200mg Rx N 181/200
Green NDC: 55953-0181

CIMETIDINE
Tablets USP, 300mg Rx N 192/300
Green NDC: 55953-0192

CIMETIDINE
Tablets USP, 400mg Rx N 204/400
Green NDC: 55953-0204

CIMETIDINE
Tablets USP, 800mg Rx N 235/800
Green NDC: 55953-0235

CLOFIBRATE
Capsules, USP, 500MG Rx N382
Yellow NDC: 55953-0382

FLURBIPROFEN
Tablets, USP, 50mg Rx N 573/50
White NDC: 55953-0573

FLURBIPROFEN
Tablets, USP, 100mg Rx N 577/100
Deep Blue NDC: 55953-0577

GLYBURIDE
Tablets, USP, 1.25mg Rx N 342/1.25
White NDC: 55953-0342

GLYBURIDE
Tablets, USP, 2.5mg Rx N 343/2.5
Peach NDC: 55953-0343

GLYBURIDE
Tablets USP, 5mg Rx N 344/5
Lt. Green NDC: 55953-0344

INDOMETHACIN
Capsules USP, 25MG Rx N 420/25
Light Green/Light Green NDC: 55953-0420

INDOMETHACIN
Capsules USP, 50MG Rx N 439/50
Light Green/Light Green NDC: 55953-0439

LOPERAMIDE HYDROCHLORIDE
Capsules USP, 2MG Rx N 020/2
White Opaque/White Opaque NDC: 55953-0020

METHYLDOPA
Tablets USP, 125MG Rx N/463
White NDC: 55953-0463

METHYLDOPA
Tablets USP, 250MG Rx N/471
White NDC: 55953-0471

METHYLDOPA
Tablets USP, 500MG Rx N/498
White NDC: 55953-0498

METHYLPHENIDATE TABLES/Ⓒ
5 mg
pale yellow MD/531 55953-0137
10 mg
pale blue MD/530 55953-0140
20 mg
pale orange MD/532 55953-0146
20 mg ER
white MD/562 55953-0148

METOPROLOL TARTRATE
Tablets, USP 50mg, Rx N 727/50
White NDC: 55953-0727

METOPROLOL TARTRATE
Tablets, USP 100mg, Rx N 734/100
White NDC: 55953-0734

MEXILETINE
Capsules, USP 150mg Rx N 739/150
Lt. Orange/Tan NDC: 55953-0739

MEXILETINE
Capsules, USP 200mg Rx N 740/200
Lt. Orange/Lt. Orange NDC: 55953-0740

MEXILETINE
Capsules, USP 250mg Rx N 741/250
Lt. Orange/Dk. Green NDC: 55953-0741

NAPROXEN
Tablets USP, 250mg Rx N 517/250
Yellow/Peach NDC: 55953-0517

NAPROXEN
Tablets USP, 375mg Rx N 518/375
Pink NDC: 55953-0518

NAPROXEN
Tablets USP, 500mg Rx N 520/500
Yellow/Peach NDC: 55953-0520

NAPROXEN SODIUM
Tablets USP, 275mg Rx N 531/275
Lt. Blue NDC: 55953-0531

NAPROXEN SODIUM
Tablets USP, 550mg Rx N 533/550
Lt. Blue NDC: 55953-0533

NIFEDIPINE
Capsules USP, 10MG Rx N 171/10
Brown NDC: 55953-0171

NIFEDIPINE
Capsules USP, 20MG Rx 530/Blank
Reddish Brown NDC: 55953-0045

PINDOLOL
Tablets USP, 5mg Rx N 088/5
White NDC: 55953-0088

PINDOLOL
Tablets USP, 10mg Rx N 093/10
White NDC: 55953-0093

PIROXICAM
Capsules USP, 10mg Rx N 617/10
Dk. Green/Lt. Grey NDC: 55953-0617

PIROXICAM
Capsules USP, 20mg Rx N 640/20
Dk. Green/Dk. Green NDC: 55953-0640

TIMOLOL MALEATE
Tablets USP, 5MG Rx N 961/5
White NDC: 55953-0961

TIMOLOL MALEATE
Tablets USP, 10MG Rx N-972/10
White NDC: 55953-0972

TIMOLOL MALEATE
Tablets USP, 20MG Rx N 984/20
White NDC: 55953-0984

TOLMETIN SODIUM
Capsules USP, 400MG Rx N 815/400
Opaque Red/Opaque Red NDC: 55953-0815

Oclassen Pharmaceuticals, Inc.
100 PELICAN WAY
SAN RAFAEL, CA 94901

Direct Inquiries to:
Marketing Department
(800) 288-4508

For Medical Information Contact:
In Emergencies:
Director, Clinical Operations
(800) 288-4508

CONDYLOX® ℞
[con 'de-lox]
(podofilox)
0.5% topical solution

DESCRIPTION
Condylox® is the brand name of podofilox, an antimitotic drug which can be chemically synthesized or purified from the plant families *Coniferae* and *Berberidaceae* (e.g. species of *Juniperus* and *Podophyllum*). Condylox® 0.5% solution is formulated for topical administration. Each milliliter of solution contains 5 mg of podofilox, in a vehicle containing lactic acid and sodium lactate in alcohol 95%, USP.
Podofilox has a molecular weight of 414.4 daltons, and is soluble in alcohol and sparingly soluble in water. Its chemical name is 5,8,8a,9-Tetrahydro-9-hydroxy-5- (3,4,5-trimethoxylphenyl)furo [3',4':6,7] naphtho [2,3,d] -1,3-dioxol-6(5aH)-one. Podofilox has the following structural formula:
[See chemical structure at top of next column.]

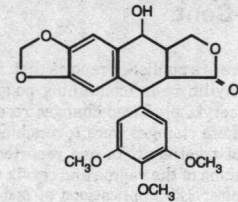

CLINICAL PHARMACOLOGY
Mechanism of Action
Treatment of genital warts with podofilox results in necrosis of visible wart tissue. The exact mechanism of action is unknown.
Pharmacokinetics
In systemic absorption studies in 52 patients, topical applications of 0.05 mL of 0.5% podofilox solution to external genitalia did not result in detectable serum levels. Applications of 0.1 to 1.5 mL resulted in peak serum levels of 1 to 17 ng/mL one to two hours after application. The elimination half-life ranged from 1.0 to 4.5 hours. The drug was not found to accumulate after multiple treatments.

CLINICAL STUDIES
In clinical studies with Condylox® Solution, the test product and its vehicle were applied in a double-blind fashion to comparable patient groups. Patients were treated for two to four weeks, and reevaluated at a two-week follow-up examination. Although the number of patients and warts evaluated at each time period varied, the results among investigators were relatively consistent.
The following table represents the responses noted in terms of frequency of response by lesions treated and the overall response by patients. Data are presented for the 2-week follow-up only for those patients evaluated at that time point.

Responses in Treated Patients

	Initially Cleared*	Recurred after Clearing*	Cleared at 2-Week Follow-Up*
% Warts (n=524)	79% (412/524)	35% (146/412)	60% (269/449)
% Patients (n=70)	50% (35/70)	60% (21/35)	25% (14/57)

* Cleared and clearing mean no visible wart tissue remained at the treated sites

INDICATIONS AND USAGE
Condylox® 0.5% solution is indicated for the topical treatment of external genital warts (Condyloma acuminatum). This product is *not* indicated in the treatment of perianal or mucous membrane warts (see PRECAUTIONS).
Diagnosis
Although genital warts have a characteristic appearance, histopathologic confirmation should be obtained if there is any doubt of the diagnosis. Differentiating warts from squamous cell carcinoma (so-called "Bowenoid papulosis") is of particular concern. Squamous cell carcinoma may also be associated with human papillomavirus but should not be treated with Condylox® 0.5% solution.

CONTRAINDICATIONS
Condylox® 0.5% solution is contraindicated for patients who develop hypersensitivity or intolerance to any component of the formulation.

WARNINGS
Correct diagnosis of the lesions to be treated is essential. See the "Diagnosis" subsection of the INDICATIONS AND USAGE statement.
Condylox® 0.5% solution is intended for cutaneous use only. **Avoid contact with the eye. If eye contact occurs, patients should immediately flush the eye with copious quantities of water and seek medical advice.**

PRECAUTIONS
General
Data are not available on the safe and effective use of this product for treatment of warts occurring in the perianal area or mucous membranes of the genital area (including the urethra, rectum and vagina). The recommended method of application, frequency of application, and duration of usage should not be exceeded (see DOSAGE AND ADMINISTRATION).
Information for Patients
The patient should be provided with a Patient Information leaflet when a Condylox® prescription is filled.
Carcinogenesis, Mutagenesis and Impairment of Fertility
Reports of lifetime carcinogenicity studies in mice are not available. Published animal studies, in general, have not shown the drug substance, podofilox, to be carcino-

Continued on next page

Oclassen—Cont.

genic.[1,2,3,4,5] There are published reports that, in mouse studies, crude podophyllin resin (containing podofilox) applied topically to the cervix produced changes resembling carcinoma *in situ*.[6] These changes were reversible at five weeks after cessation of treatment. In one reported experiment, epidermal carcinoma of the vagina and cervix was found in 1 out of 18 mice after 120 applications of podophyllin[7] (the drug was applied twice weekly over a 15-month period).
Podofilox was not mutagenic in the Ames plate reverse mutation assay at concentrations up to 5 mg/plate, with and without metabolic activation. No cell transformation related to potential oncogenicity was observed in BALB/3T3 cells after exposure to podofilox at concentrations up to 0.008 μg/mL without metabolic activation and 12 μg/mL podofilox with metabolic activation. Results from the mouse micronucleus *in vivo* assay using podofilox 0.5% solution in concentrations up to 25 mg/kg, indicate that podofilox should be considered a potential clastogen (a chemical that induces disruption and breakage of chromosomes).
Daily topical applications of Condylox® 0.5% Solution at doses up to the equivalent of 0.2 mg/kg (5 times the recommended maximum human dose) to rats throughout gametogenesis, mating, gestation, parturition and lactation for two generations demonstrated no impairment of fertility.

Pregnancy

Pregnancy Category C: Podofilox was not teratogenic in the rabbit following topical application of up to 0.21 mg/kg (5 times the maximum human dose) once daily for 13 days. The scientific literature contains references that podofilox is embryotoxic in rats when administered systemically in a dose approximately 250 times the recommended maximum human dose.[8,9] Teratogenicity and embryotoxicity have not been studied with intravaginal application. Many antimitotic drug products are known to be embryotoxic. There are no adequate and well-controlled studies in pregnant women. Podofilox should be used in pregnancy only if the potential benefit justifies the potential risk to the fetus.

Nursing Mothers

It is not known whether this drug is excreted in human milk. Because of the potential for serious adverse reactions in nursing infants from podofilox, a decision should be made whether to discontinue nursing or to discontinue the drug, taking into account the importance of the drug to the mother.

Pediatric Use

Safety and effectiveness in children have not been established.

ADVERSE REACTIONS

In clinical trials, the following local adverse reactions were reported at some point during treatment.

Adverse Experience	Males	Females
Burning	64%	78%
Pain	50%	72%
Inflammation	71%	63%
Erosion	67%	67%
Itching	50%	65%

Reports of burning and pain were more frequent and of greater severity in women than in men.
Adverse effects reported in less than 5% of the patients included pain with intercourse, insomnia, tingling, bleeding, tenderness, chafing, malodor, dizziness, scarring, vesicle formation, crusting, edema, dryness/peeling, foreskin irretraction, hematuria, vomiting and ulceration.

OVERDOSAGE

Topically applied podofilox may be absorbed systemically (see CLINICAL PHARMACOLOGY section). Toxicity reported following systemic administration of podofilox in investigational use for cancer treatment included: nausea, vomiting, fever, diarrhea, bone marrow depression, and oral ulcers. Following 5 to 10 daily intravenous doses of 0.5 to 1 mg/kg/day, significant hematological toxicity occurred but was reversible. Other toxicities occurred at lower doses. Toxicity reported following systemic administration of podophyllum resin included: nausea, vomiting, fever, diarrhea, peripheral neuropathy, altered mental status, lethargy, coma, tachypnea, respiratory failure, leukocytosis, pancytosis, hematuria, renal failure, and seizures. Treatment of topical overdosage should include washing the skin free of any remaining drug and symptomatic and supportive therapy.

DOSAGE AND ADMINISTRATION

In order to ensure that the patient is fully aware of the correct method of therapy and to identify which specific warts should be treated, the technique for initial application of the medication should be demonstrated by the prescriber.
Apply twice daily morning and evening (every 12 hours), for 3 consecutive days, then withhold use for 4 consecutive days. This one week cycle of treatment may be repeated up to four times until there is no visible wart tissue. **If there is incomplete response after four treatment weeks, alternative treatment should be considered. Safety and effectiveness of more than four treatment weeks have not been established.**
Condylox® 0.5% solution is applied to the warts with a cotton-tipped applicator supplied with the drug. The drug-dampened applicator should be touched to the wart to be treated, applying the minimum amount of solution necessary to cover the lesion. **Treatment should be limited to less than 10 cm² of wart tissue and to no more than 0.5 mL of the solution per day.** There is no evidence to suggest that more frequent application will increase efficacy, but additional applications would be expected to increase the rate of local adverse reactions and systemic absorption.
Care should be taken to allow the solution to dry before allowing the return of opposing skin surfaces to their normal positions. After each treatment, the used applicator should be carefully disposed of and the patient should wash his or her hands.

HOW SUPPLIED

3.5 mL of Condylox® 0.5% solution is supplied as a clear liquid in amber glass bottles with child-resistant screw caps. NDC #55515-101-01. Store at controlled room temperature between 15° and 30°C (59° and 86°F). **Avoid excessive heat. Do not freeze.**
Caution—Federal law prohibits dispensing without prescription.

REFERENCES

1. Berenblum, 1951. J. Natl. Cancer Inst. *11:* 839–841
2. H.A. Kaminetsky and M. Swerdlow, 1965. Am. J. Obst. Gyn. *93:* 486–490
3. E.A. McGrew and H.A. Kaminetsky. 1961. Am J. Clin. Pathol. *35:* 538–545
4. F.J.C. Roe and M.H. Salaman, 1955. Brit. J. Cancer. *9:* 177–203
5. H.S. Taper, 1977. Z. Kerbsforsch, *90:* 197–210
6. H.A. Kaminetsky and E.A. McGrew, and R.L. Phillips, 1959. Am. J. Obst. Gyn. *14:* 1–3
7. H.A. Kaminetsky and E.A. McGrew, 1963. Arch. Path. *73:* 481–485
8. K. Didcock, D. Jackson, and J.M. Robson, 1956. Brit. J. Pharmacol. *11:* 437–441
9. J. Thiersch, 1963. Soc. Exptl. Biol. Med. Proc. *113:* 124–127

Revised: Dec., 1990
Mfd. for
OCLASSEN
Pharmaceuticals, Inc.
San Rafael, CA 94901
By Abbott Laboratories
N. Chicago, IL 60064

01-2428-R1

Shown in Product Identification Guide, page 325

CORDRAN®, Flurandrenolide Lotion, USP, 0.05% ℞

[*kōr'drăn*]

DESCRIPTION

Cordran® (Flurandrenolide, USP) is a potent corticosteroid intended for topical use. It occurs as white to off-white, fluffy, crystalline powder and is odorless. Flurandrenolide is practically insoluble in water and in ether. One g dissolves in 72 mL of alcohol and in 10 mL of chloroform. The molecular weight of Cordran is 436.52.
The chemical name of flurandrenolide is pregn-4-ene-3,20-dione, 6-fluoro-11,21-dihydroxy-16,17-[(1-methylethylidene)-bis (oxy)]-, (6α, 11β, 16α)-; its empirical formula is $C_{24}H_{33}FO_6$. The structure is as follows:

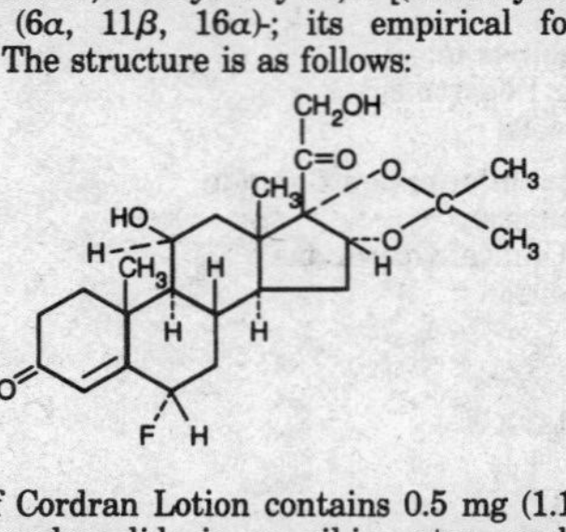

Each mL of Cordran Lotion contains 0.5 mg (1.145 μmol) (0.05%) flurandrenolide in an oil-in-water emulsion base composed of glycerin, cetyl alcohol, stearic acid, glyceryl monostearate, mineral oil, polyoxyl 40 stearate, menthol, benzyl alcohol, and purified water.

CLINICAL PHARMACOLOGY

Cordran is primarily effective because of its anti-inflammatory, antipruritic, and vasoconstrictive actions.
The mechanism of the anti-inflammatory effect of topical corticosteroids is not completely understood. Various laboratory methods, including vasoconstrictor assays, are used to compare and predict potencies and/or clinical efficacies of the topical corticosteroids. There is some evidence to suggest that a recognizable correlation exists between vasoconstrictor potency and therapeutic efficacy in man. Corticosteroids with anti-inflammatory activity may stabilize cellular and lysosomal membranes. There is also the suggestion that the effect on the membranes of lysosomes prevents the release of proteolytic enzymes and, thus, plays a part in reducing inflammation.
Evaporation of water from the lotion vehicle produces a cooling effect, which is often desirable in the treatment of acutely inflamed or weeping lesions.
Pharmacokinetics—The extent of percutaneous absorption of topical corticosteroids is determined by many factors, including the vehicle, the integrity of the epidermal barrier, and the use of occlusive dressings.
Topical corticosteroids can be absorbed from normal intact skin. Inflammation and/or other disease processes in the skin increase percutaneous absorption. Occlusive dressings substantially increase the percutaneous absorption of topical corticosteroids. Thus, occlusive dressings may be a valuable therapeutic adjunct for treatment of resistant dermatoses (*see* Dosage and Administration).
Once absorbed through the skin, topical corticosteroids are handled through pharmacokinetic pathways similar to those of systematically administered corticosteroids. Corticosteroids are bound to plasma proteins in varying degrees. They are metabolized primarily in the liver and then excreted in the kidneys. Some of the topical corticosteroids and their metabolites are also excreted into the bile.

INDICATIONS AND USAGE

Cordran is indicated for the relief of the inflammatory and pruritic manifestations of corticosteroid-responsive dermatoses.

CONTRAINDICATIONS

Topical corticosteroids are contraindicated in patients with a history of hypersensitivity to any of the components of these preparations.

PRECAUTIONS

General—Systemic absorption of topical corticosteroids has produced reversible hypothalamic-pituitary-adrenal (HPA) axis suppression, manifestations of Cushing's syndrome, hyperglycemia, and glucosuria in some patients.
Conditions that augment systemic absorption include application of the more potent steroids, use over large surface areas, prolonged use, and the addition of occlusive dressings.
Therefore, patients receiving a large dose of a potent topical steroid, applied to a large surface area or under an occlusive dressing should be evaluated periodically for evidence of HPA axis suppression using urinary-free cortisol and ACTH stimulation tests. If HPA axis suppression is noted, an attempt should be made to withdraw the drug, to reduce the frequency of application, or to substitute a less potent steroid.
Recovery of HPA axis function is generally prompt and complete on discontinuation of the drug. Infrequently, signs and symptoms of steroid withdrawal may occur, so that supplemental systemic corticosteroids are required.
Children may absorb proportionately large amounts of topical corticosteroids and thus be more susceptible to systemic toxicity (*see* Usage in Children under Precautions).
If irritation develops, topical corticosteroids should be discontinued and appropriate therapy instituted.
In the presence of dermatologic infections, the use of an appropriate antifungal or antibacterial agent should be instituted. If a favorable response does not occur promptly, Cordran should be discontinued until the infection has been adequately controlled.
Information for the Patient—Patients using topical corticosteroids should receive the following information and instructions:

1. This medication is to be used as directed by the physician. It is for external use only. Avoid contact with the eyes.
2. Patients should be advised not to use this medication for any disorder other than that for which it was prescribed.
3. The treated skin area should not be bandaged or otherwise covered or wrapped in order to be occlusive unless the patient is directed to do so by the physician.
4. Patients should report any signs of local adverse reactions, especially under occlusive dressing.
5. Parents of pediatric patients should be advised not to use tight-fitting diapers or plastic pants on a child being treated in the diaper area, because these garmets may constitute occlusive dressings.

Laboratory Tests—The following tests may be helpful in evaluating the HPA axis suppression:
Urinary-free cortisol test
ACTH stimulation test
Carcinogenesis, Mutagenesis, and Impairment of Fertility—Long-term animal studies have not been performed to evaluate the carcinogenic potential or the effect on fertility of topical corticosteroids.
Studies to determine mutagenicity with prednisolone and hydrocortisone have revealed negative results.
Usage in Pregnancy—Pregnancy Category C—Corticosteroids are generally teratogenic in laboratory animals when administered systemically at relatively low dosage levels. The more potent corticosteroids have been shown to be teratogenic after dermal application in laboratory animals. There are no adequate and well-controlled studies in pregnant

women on teratogenic effects from topically applied corticosteroids. Therefore, topical corticosteroids should be used during pregnancy only if the potential benefit justifies the potential risk to the fetus. Drugs of this class should not be used extensively for pregnant patients or in large amounts or for prolonged periods of time.

Nursing Mothers—It is not known whether topical administration of corticosteroids could result in sufficient systemic absorption to produce detectable quantities in breast milk. Systemically administered corticosteroids are secreted into breast milk in quantities *not* likely to have a deleterious effect on the infant. Nevertheless, caution should be exercised when topical corticosteroids are administered to a nursing woman.

Usage in Children—Pediatric patients may demonstrate greater susceptibility to topical corticosteroid-induced HPA axis suppression and Cushing's syndrome than do mature patients because of a larger skin surface area to body weight ratio.

Hypothalamic-pituitary-adrenal (HPA) axis suppression, Cushing's syndrome, and intracranial hypertension have been reported in children receiving topical corticosteroids. Manifestations of adrenal suppression in children include linear growth retardation, delayed weight gain, low plasma cortisol levels, and absence of response to ACTH stimulation. Manifestations of intracranial hypertension include bulging fontanelles, headaches, and bilateral papilledema.

Administration of topical corticosteroids to children should be limited to the least amount compatible with an effective therapeutic regimen. Chronic corticosteroid therapy may interfere with the growth and development of children.

ADVERSE REACTIONS

The following local adverse reactions are reported infrequently with topical corticosteroids but may occur more frequently with the use of occlusive dressings. These reactions are listed in an approximate decreasing order of occurrence:

- Burning
- Itching
- Irritation
- Dryness
- Folliculitis
- Hypertrichosis
- Acneform eruptions
- Hypopigmentation
- Perioral dermatitis
- Allergic contact dermatitis

The following may occur more frequently with occlusive dressings:

- Maceration of the skin
- Secondary infection
- Skin atrophy
- Striae
- Miliaria

OVERDOSAGE

Topically applied corticosteroids can be absorbed in sufficient amounts to produce systemic effects (*see* Precautions).

DOSAGE AND ADMINISTRATION

Topical corticosteroids are generally applied to the affected area as a thin film 1 to 4 times daily, depending on the severity of the condition.

A small quantity of Cordran Lotion should be rubbed gently into the affected area 2 or 3 times daily.

Occlusive dressings may be used for the management of psoriasis or recalcitrant conditions.

If an infection develops, the use of occlusive dressings should be discontinued and appropriate antimicrobial therapy instituted.

Use With Occlusive Dressings

The technique of occlusive dressings (for management of psoriasis and other persistant dermatoses) is as follows:

1. Remove as much as possible of the superficial scaling before applying Cordran Lotion. Soaking in a bath will help soften the scales and permit easier removal by brushing, picking, or rubbing.
2. Rub the lotion thoroughly into the affected areas.
3. Cover with an occlusive plastic film, such as polyethylene, Saran Wrap™, or Handi-Wrap®. (Added moisture may be provided by placing a slightly dampened cloth or gauze over the lesion before the plastic film is applied.)
4. Seal the edges to adjacent normal skin with tape or hold in place by a gauze wrapping.
5. For convenience, the patient may remove the dressing during the day. The dressing should then be reapplied each night.
6. For daytime therapy, the condition may be treated by rubbing Cordran Lotion sparingly into the affected areas.
7. In more resistant cases, leaving the dressing in place for 3 to 4 days at a time may result in a better response.
8. Thin polyethylene gloves are suitable for treatment of the hands and fingers; plastic garment bags may be utilized for treating lesions on the trunk or buttocks. A tight shower cap is useful in treating lesions on the scalp.

Occlusive Dressings Have the Following Advantages—

1. Percutaneous penetration of the corticosteroid is enhanced.
2. Medication is concentrated on the areas of skin where it is most needed.
3. This method of administration frequently is more effective in very resistant dermatoses than is the conventional application of Cordran.

Precautions to Be Observed in Therapy With Occlusive Dressings—Treatment should be continued for at least a few days after clearing of the lesions. If it is stopped too soon, a relapse may occur. Reinstitution of treatment frequently will cause remission.

Because of the increased hazard of secondary infection from resistant strains of staphylococci among hospitalized patients, it is suggested that the use of occlusive plastic films for corticosteroid therapy in such cases be restricted.

Generally, occlusive dressings should not be used on weeping, or exudative, lesions.

When large areas of the body are covered, thermal homeostasis may be impaired. If elevation of body temperature occurs, use of the occlusive dressing should be discontinued.

Rarely, a patient may develop miliaria, folliculitis, or a sensitivty to either the particular dressing material or a combination of Cordran and the occlusive dressing. If miliaria or folliculitis occurs, use of the occlusive dressing should be discontinued. Treatment by inunction with Codran Lotion may be continued. If the sensitivity is caused by the particular material of the dressing, substitution of a different material may be tried.

Warnings—Some plastic films are readily flammable. Patients should be cautioned against the use of any such material.

When plastic films are used on infants and children, the persons caring for the patients must be reminded of the danger of suffocation if the plastic material accidentally covers the face.

HOW SUPPLIED

Lotion (Plastic squeeze bottles):
0.05% (UC 5352)—(15 mL) NDC 55515-052-15; (60 mL) NDC 55515-052-60

Literature issued September 25, 1992
PA5080UCP

Mfd. for
OCLASSEN
Pharmaceuticals, Inc.
San Rafael, CA 94901
by Eli Lily and Company
Indianapolis, IN 46285, U.S.A.

Shown in Product Identification Guide, page 325

CORDRAN® TAPE ℞

[kōr′drăn]
Flurandrenolide Tape, USP

DESCRIPTION

Cordran® Tape (Flurandrenolide Tape, USP) is a transparent, inconspicuous, plastic surgical tape, impervious to moisture. It contains Cordran® (Flurandrenolide, USP), a potent corticosteroid for topical use. Flurandrenolide occurs as white to off-white, fluffy crystalline powder and is odorless. Flurandrenolide is practically insoluble in water and in ether. One g dissolves in 72 mL of alcohol and in 10 mL of chloroform. The molecular weight of flurandrenolide is 436.52.

The chemical name of flurandrenolide is Pregn-4-ene-3,20-dione, 6-fluoro-11,21-dihydroxy-16,17-[(1-methylethylidene)-bis (oxy)]-, (6α, 11β, 16α)-; its empirical formula is $C_{24}H_{33}FO_6$. The structure is as follows:

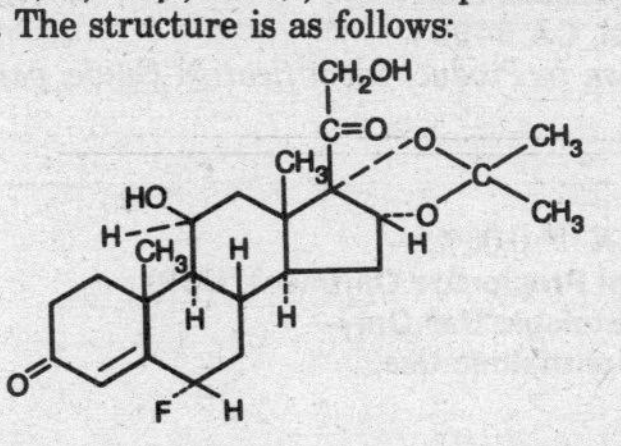

Each square centimeter contains 4 μg (0.00916 μmol) flurandrenolide uniformly distributed in the adhesive layer. The tape is made of a thin, matte-finish polyethylene film that is slightly elastic and highly flexible.

The adhesive is a synthetic copolymer of acrylate ester and acrylic acid that is free from substances of plant origin. The pressure-sensitive adhesive surface is covered with a protective paper liner to permit handling and trimming before application.

CLINICAL PHARMACOLOGY

Cordran is primarily effective because of its anti-inflammatory, antipruritic, and vasoconstrictive actions.

The mechanism of the anti-inflammatory effect of topical corticosteroids is not completely understood. Various laboratory methods, including vasoconstrictor assays, are used to compare and predict potencies and/or clinical efficacies of the topical corticosteroids. There is some evidence to suggest that a recognizable correlation exists between vasoconstrictor potency and therapeutic efficacy in man. Corticosteroids with anti-inflammatory activity may stabilize cellular and lysosomal membranes. There is also the suggestion that the effect on the membranes of lysosomes prevents the release of proteolytic enzymes and, thus, plays a part in reducing inflammation.

The tape serves as both a vehicle and an occlusive dressing. Retention of insensible perspiration by the tape results in hydration of the stratum corneum and improved diffusion of the medication. The skin is protected from scratching, rubbing, desiccation, and chemical irritation. The tape acts as a mechanical splint to fissured skin. Since it prevents removal of the medication by washing or the rubbing action of clothing, the tape formulation provides a sustained action.

Pharmacokinetics—The extent of percutaneous absorption of topical corticosteroids is determined by many factors, including the vehicle, the integrity of the epidermal barrier, and the use of occlusive dressings.

Topical corticosteroids can be absorbed from normal intact skin. Inflammation and/or other disease processes in the skin increase percutaneous absorption. Occlusive dressings substantially increase the percutaneous absorption of topical corticosteroids. Thus, occlusive dressings may be a valuable therapeutic adjunct for treatment of resistant dermatoses (*see* Dosage and Administration).

Once absorbed through the skin, topical corticosteroids are handled through pharmacokinetic pathways similar to those of systematically administered corticosteroids. Corticosteroids are bound to plasma proteins in varying degrees. They are metabolized primarily in the liver and then excreted in the kidneys. Some of the topical corticosteroids and their metabolites are also excreted into the bile.

INDICATIONS AND USAGE

For relief of the inflammatory and pruritic manifestations of corticosteroid-responsive dermatoses, particularly dry, scaling localized lesions.

CONTRAINDICATIONS

Topical corticosteroids are contraindicated in patients with a history of hypersensitivity to any of the components of these preparations.

Use of Cordran Tape is not recommended for lesions exuding serum or in intertriginous areas.

PRECAUTIONS

General—Systemic absorption of topical corticosteroids has produced reversible hypothalamic-pituitary-adrenal (HPA) axis suppression, manifestations of Cushing's syndrome, hyperglycemia, and glucosuria in some patients.

Conditions that augment systemic absorption include application of the more potent steroids, use over large surface areas, prolonged use, and the addition of occlusive dressings. Therefore, patients receiving a large dose of a potent topical steroid applied to a large surface area or under an occlusive dressing should be evaluated periodically for evidence of HPA axis suppression using urinary-free cortisol and ACTH stimulation tests. If HPA axis suppression is noted, an attempt should be made to withdraw the drug, to reduce the frequency of application, or to substitute a less potent steroid.

Recovery of HPA axis function is generally prompt and complete on discontinuation of the drug. Infrequently, signs and symptoms of steroid withdrawal may occur, so that supplemental systemic corticosteroids are required.

Children may absorb proportionately large amounts of topical corticosteroids and thus be more susceptible to systemic toxicity (*see* Usage in Children under Precautions).

If irritation develops, topical corticosteroids should be discontinued and appropriate therapy instituted.

In the presence of dermatologic infections, the use of an appropriate antifungal or antibacterial agent should be instituted. If a favorable response does not occur promptly, Cordran should be discontinued until the infection has been adequately controlled.

Information for the Patient—Patients using topical corticosteroids should receive the following information and instructions:

1. This medication is to be used as directed by the physician. It is for external use only. Avoid contact with the eyes.
2. Patients should be advised not to use this medication for any disorder other than that for which it was prescribed.
3. The treated skin area should not be bandaged or otherwise covered or wrapped in order to be occlusive unless the patient is directed to do so by the physician.
4. Patients should report any signs of local adverse reactions, especially under occlusive dressing.
5. Parents of pediatric patients should be advised not to use tight-fitting diapers or plastic pants on a child being

Continued on next page

Oclassen—Cont.

treated in the diaper area, because these garments may constitute occlusive dressings.

Laboratory Tests—The following tests may be helpful in evaluating the HPA axis suppression:

Urinary-free cortisol test

ACTH stimulation test

Carcinogenesis, Mutagenesis, and Impairment of Fertility—Long-term animal studies have not been performed to evaluate the carcinogenic potential or the effect on fertility of topical corticosteroids.

Studies to determine mutagenicity with prednisolone and hydrocortisone have revealed negative results.

Usage in Pregnancy—Pregnancy Category C—Corticosteroids are generally teratogenic in laboratory animals when administered systemically at relatively low dosage levels. The more potent corticosteroids have been shown to be teratogenic after dermal application in laboratory animals. There are no adequate and well-controlled studies in pregnant women on teratogenic effects from topically applied corticosteroids. Therefore, topical corticosteroids should be used during pregnancy only if the potential benefit justifies the potential risk to the fetus. Drugs of this class should not be used extensively for pregnant patients or in large amounts or for prolonged periods of time.

Nursing Mothers—It is not known whether topical administration of corticosteroids could result in sufficient systemic absorption to produce detectable quantities in breast milk. Systemically administered corticosteroids are secreted into breast milk in quantities *not* likely to have a deleterious effect on the infant. Nevertheless, caution should be exercised when topical corticosteroids are administered to a nursing woman.

Usage in Children—Pediatric patients may demonstrate greater susceptibility to topical corticosteroid-induced HPA axis suppression and Cushing's syndrome than do mature patients because of a larger skin surface area to body weight ratio.

Hypothalamic-pituitary-adrenal (HPA) axis suppression, Cushing's syndrome, and intracranial hypertension have been reported in children receiving topical corticosteroids. Manifestations of adrenal suppression in children include linear growth retardation, delayed weight gain, low plasma-cortisol levels, and absence of response to ACTH stimulation. Manifestations of intracranial hypertension include bulging fontanelles, headaches, and bilateral papilledema.

Administration of topical corticosteroids to children should be limited to the least amount compatible with an effective therapeutic regimen. Chronic corticosteroid therapy may interfere with the growth and development of children.

ADVERSE REACTIONS

The following local adverse reactions are reported infrequently with topical corticosteroids but may occur more frequently with the use of occlusive dressings. These reactions are listed in an approximate decreasing order of occurrence:

Burning
Itching
Irritation
Dryness
Folliculitis
Hypertrichosis
Acneform eruptions
Hypopigmentation
Perioral dermatitis
Allergic contact dermatitis

The following may occur more frequently with occlusive dressings:

Maceration of the skin
Secondary infection
Skin atrophy
Striae
Miliaria

OVERDOSAGE

Topically applied corticosteroids can be absorbed in sufficient amounts to produce systemic effects (*see* Precautions).

DOSAGE AND ADMINISTRATION

Occlusive dressings may be used for the management of psoriasis or recalcitrant conditions.

If an infection develops, the use of Cordran Tape and other occlusive dressings should be discontinued and appropriate antimicrobial therapy instituted.

Replacement of the tape every 12 hours produces the lowest incidence of adverse reactions, but it may be left in place for 24 hours if it is well tolerated and adheres satisfactorily. When necessary, the tape may be used at night only and removed during the day.

If ends of the tape loosen prematurely, they may be trimmed off and replaced with fresh tape.

The directions given below are included on a separate package insert for the patient to follow unless otherwise instructed by the physician.

APPLICATION OF CORDRAN TAPE

IMPORTANT: Skin should be clean and dry before tape is applied. Tape should always be cut, never torn.

DIRECTIONS FOR USE:

1. Prepare skin as directed by your physician or as follows: Gently clean the area to be covered to remove scales, crusts, dried exudates, and any previously used ointments or creams. A germicidal soap or cleanser should be used to prevent the development of odor under the tape. Shave or clip the hair in the treatment area to allow good contact with the skin and comfortable removal. If shower or tub bath is to be taken, it should be completed before the tape is applied. The skin should be dry before application of the tape.
2. Remove tape from package and cut a piece slightly larger than area to be covered. Round off corners.
3. Pull white paper from transparent tape. Be careful that tape does not stick to itself.
4. Apply tape, keeping skin smooth; press tape into place.

REPLACEMENT OF TAPE.

Unless instructed otherwise by your physician, replace tape after 12 hours. Cleanse skin and allow it to dry for 1 hour before applying new tape.

IF IRRITATION OR INFECTION DEVELOPS, REMOVE TAPE AND CONSULT PHYSICIAN.

HOW SUPPLIED

Tape:

4 mcg/sq cm (UC 5350)—12 patches, each 2 in × 3 in (5.1 cm × 7.5 cm) NDC 55515-014-12

4 mcg/sq cm (UC 5350)—small roll, 24 in × 3 in (60 cm × 7.5 cm)
NDC 55515-014-24

4 mcg/sq cm (UC 5350)—large roll, 80 in × 3 in (200 cm × 7.5 cm)
NDC 55515-014-80

Directions for the patient are included in each package.

REFERENCES

Bard JW: Flurandrenolide tape in the treatment of lichen simplex chronicus. *J Ky Med Assoc* 1969;67:668.

Baxter DL, Stoughton RB: Mitotic index of psoriatic lesions treated with anthralin, glucocorticosteroid and occlusion only. *J Invest Dermatol* 1970;54:410.

Compilation of clinical reports on Cordran Tape received by Eli Lilly and Company.

Halprin KM, Fukui K, Ohkawara A: Flurandrenolone (Cordran) tape and carbohydrate metabolizing enzymes. *Arch Dermatol* 1969;100:336.

Labow TA, Eisert J, Sanders SL: Flurandrenolide tape in treatment of psoriasis. *NY State J Med* 1969;69:3138.

Ronchese F: Flurandrenolone tape therapy. *RI Med J* 1969;52:389.

Sellers FM: Investigative study of flurandrenolone tape in a series of ambulatory outpatients. *J Indiana State Med Assoc* 1970;63:34.

Weiner MA: Flurandrenolone tape, a new preparation for occlusive therapy, *J Invest Dermatol* 1966;47:63.

Caution: Federal law prohibits dispensing without prescription

Literature revised January 18, 1995 PA2032UCP

Mfd. for Eli Lilly and Company
Indianapolis, IN 46285, USA
by Minnesota Mining and Manufacturing Company
St. Paul, Minnesota 55101
Dist. by
OCLASSEN
Pharmaceuticals, Inc.
San Rafael, CA 94901

Shown in Product Identification Guide, page 325

CORMAX™ 0.05% ℞

(Clobetasol Propionate Ointment, USP)
For Dermatologic Use Only—
Not For Ophthalmic Use.

DESCRIPTION

Cormax™ (Clobetasol Propionate Ointment, USP) contains the active compound clobetasol propionate, a synthetic corticosteroid, for topical dermatologic use. Clobetasol, an analog of prednisolone, has a high degree of glucocorticoid activity and a slight degree of mineralocorticoid activity.

Chemically, clobetasol propionate is 21-chloro-9-fluoro-11β, 17-dihydroxy-16β-methylpregna-1, 4-diene-3,20-dione, 17-propionate, and it has the following structural formula:

[See chemical structure at top of next column.]

Clobetasol propionate has the molecular formula $C_{25}H_{32}ClFO_5$ and a molecular weight of 467. It is a white to cream-colored crystalline powder insoluble in water.

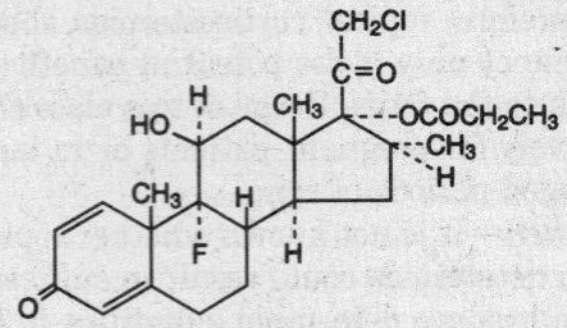

Each gram of Cormax™ (Clobetasol Propionate Ointment, USP) contains 0.5 mg clobetasol propionate in a base composed of propylene glycol, sorbitan sesquioleate, and white petrolatum.

CLINICAL PHARMACOLOGY

The corticosteroids are a class of compounds comprising steroid hormones secreted by the adrenal cortex and their synthetic analogs. In pharmacologic doses, corticosteroids are used primarily for their anti-inflammatory and/or immunosuppressive effects. Topical corticosteroids such as clobetasol propionate are effective in the treatment of corticosteroid-responsive dermatoses primarily because of their anti-inflammatory, antipruritic, and vasoconstrictive actions. However, while the physiologic, pharmacologic, and clinical effects of the corticosteroids are well known, the exact mechanisms of their actions in each disease are uncertain.

Clobetasol propionate, a corticosteroid, has been shown to have topical (dermatologic) and systemic pharmacologic and metabolic effects characteristic of this class of drugs.

Pharmacokinetics: The extent of percutaneous absorption of topical corticosteroids, including clobetasol propionate, is determined by many factors inclding the vehicle, the integrity of the epidermal barrier, and the use of occlusive dressings (see **DOSAGE AND ADMINISTRATION**).

As with all topical corticosteroids, clobetasol propionate can be absorbed from normal intact skin. Inflammation and/or other disease processes in the skin may increase percutaneous absorption. Occlusive dressings substantially increase the percutaneous absorption of topical corticosteroids (see **DOSAGE AND ADMINISTRATION**).

Once absorbed through the skin, topical corticosteroids enter pharmacokinetic pathways similarly to systemically administered corticosteroids.

Corticosteroids are bound to plasma proteins in varying degrees. Corticosteroids are metabolized primarily in the liver and are then excreted by the kidneys. Some of the topical corticosteroids, including clobetasol propionate and its metabolites, are also excreted into the bile.

Clobetasol propionate ointment has been shown to depress the plasma levels of adrenal cortical hormones following repeated nonocclusive application to diseased skin in patients with psoriasis and eczematous dermatitis. These effects have been shown to be transient and reversible upon completion of a two-week course of treatment.

INDICATIONS AND USAGE

Cormax™ (Clobetasol Propionate Ointment, USP) is indicated for short-term treatment of inflammatory and pruritic manifestations of moderate to severe corticosteroid-responsive dermatoses. Treatment beyond two consecutive weeks is not recommended, and the total dosage should not exceed 50 g per week because of the potential for the drug to suppress the hypothalamic-pituitary-adrenal (HPA) axis.

This product is not recommended for use in children under 12 years of age.

CONTRAINDICATIONS

Cormax™ (Clobetasol Propionate Ointment, USP) is contraindicated in patients who are hypersensitive to clobetasol propionate, to other corticosteroids, or to any ingredient in this preparation.

PRECAUTIONS

General: Clobetasol propionate is a highly potent topical corticosteroid that has been shown to suppress the HPA axis at doses as low as 2 g per day. Systemic absorption of topical corticosteroids has resulted in reversible HPA axis supression, manifestations of Cushing's syndrome, hyperglycemia, and glucosuria in some patients.

Conditions that augment systemic absorption include the application of more potent corticosteroids, use over large surface areas, prolonged use, and the addition of occlusive dressings. Therefore, patients receiving a large dose of a potent topical steroid applied to a large surface area should be evaluated periodically for evidence of HPA axis' suppression by using the urinary free cortisol and ACTH stimulation tests. If HPA axis suppression is noted, an attempt should be made to withdraw the drug, to reduce the frequency of application, or to substitute a less potent steroid.

Recovery of HPA axis function is generally prompt and complete upon discontiuation of the drug. Infrequently, signs and symptoms of steroid withdrawal may occur, requiring supplemental systemic corticosteroids.

Children may absorb proportionally larger amounts of topical corticoteroids and thus be more susceptible to systemic toxicity (see **PRECAUTIONS: Pediatric Use**).

If irritation develops, topical corticosteroids should be discontinued and appropriate therapy instituted.
In the presence of dermatologic infections, the use of an appropriate antifungal or antibacterial agent should be instituted. If a favorable response does not occur promptly, the corticosteroid should be discontinued until the infection has been adequately controlled.
Certain areas of the body, such as the face, groin, and axilae, are more prone to atrophic changes than other areas of the body following treatment with corticosteroids. Frequent observations of the patient is important if these areas are to be treated.
As with other potent topical corticosteroids, Cormax™ (Clobetasol Propionate Ointment, USP) should not be used in the treatment of rosacea and perioral dermatitis. Topical corticosteroids in general should not be used in the treatment of acne or as a sole therapy in widespread plaque psoriasis.
Information for patients: Patients using Cormax™ (Clobetasol Propionate Ointment, USP) should receive the following information and instructions:
1. This medication is to be used as directed by the physician and should not be used longer than the prescribed time period. It is for external use only. Avoid contact with the eyes.
2. This medication should not be used for any disorder other than that for which it is prescribed.
3. The treated skin area should not be bandaged or otherwise covered or wrapped so as to be occlusive.
4. Patients should report any signs of local adverse reactions to the physician.
Laboratory Tests: The following tests may be helpful in evaluating HPA axis suppression:
Urinary free cortisol test
ACTH stimulation test
Carcinogenesis, Mutagenesis, Impairment of Fertility:
Long-term animal studies have not been performed to evaluate the carcinogenic potential or the effect on fertility of topical corticosteroids.
Studies to determine mutagenicity with prednisolone have revealed negative results.
Pregnancy: Teratogenic Effects: Pregnancy Category C: The more potent corticosteroids have been shown to be teratogenic in animals after dermal application. Clobetasol propionate has not been tested for teratogenicity by this route; however, it is absorbed percutaneously, and when administered subcutaneously it was a significant teratogen in both the rabbit and the mouse. Clobetasol propionate has greater teratogenic potential than steroids that are less potent.
There are no adequate and well-controlled studies of the teratogenic effects of topically applied corticosteroids, including clobetasol, in pregnant women. Therefore, clobetasol and other topical corticosteroids should be used during pregnancy only if the potential benefit justifies the potential risk to the fetus, and they should not be used extensively on pregnant patients, in large amounts, or for prolonged periods of time.
Nursing Mothers: It is not known whether topical administration of corticosteroids could result in sufficient systemic absorption to produce detectable quantities in breast milk. Systemically administered corticosteroids are secreted into breast milk in quantities not likely to have a deleterious effect on the infant. Nevertheless, caution should be exercised when topical corticosteroids are prescribed for a nursing woman.
Pediatric use: Use of Cormax™ (Clobetasol Propionate Ointment, USP) in children under 12 years of age is not recommended.
Pediatric patients may demonstrate greater susceptibility to topical corticosteroid-induced HPA axis suppression and Cushing's syndrome than mature patients because of a larger skin surface area to body weight ratio.
HPA axis suppression, Cushing's syndrome and intracranial hypertension have been reported in children receiving topical corticosteroids. Manifestations of adrenal suppression in children include linear growth retardation, delayed weight gain, low plasma cortisol levels, and absence of response to ACTH stimulation. Manifestations of intracranial hypertension include bulging fontanelles, headaches, and bilateral papilledema.

ADVERSE REACTIONS

Comax™ (Clobetasol Propionate Ointment, USP) is generally well tolerated when used for two-week treatment periods. The most frequent adverse reactions reported for clobetasol propionate ointment have been local and have included burning sensation, irritation, and itching. These occurred in approximately 0.5% of the patients. Less frequent adverse reactions wers stinging, cracking, erythema, folliculitis, numbness of fingers, skin atrophy, and telangiectasia, which occurred in approximately 0.3% of the patients.
The following local adverse reactions are reported infrequently when topical corticosteroids are used as recommended. These reactions are listed in an approximately decreasing order of occurrence: burning, itching, irritation, dryness, folliculitis, hypetrichosis, acneiform eruptions, hypopigmentation, perioral dermatitis, allergic contact dermatitis, maceration of the skin, secondary infection, skin atrophy, striae, miliaria. Systemic absorption of topical corticosteroids has produced reversible HPA axis suppression, manifestations of Cushing's syndrome, hyperglycemia, and glucosuria in some patients. In rare instances, treatment (or withdrawal of treatment) of psoriasis with corticosteroids is thought to have exacerbated the disease or provoked the pustular form of the disease, so careful patient supervision is recommended.

OVERDOSAGE

Topically applied Cormax™ (Clobetasol Propionate Ointment, USP) can be absorbed in sufficient amounts to produce systemic effects (**see PRECAUTIONS**).

DOSAGE AND ADMINISTRATION

A thin layer of Cormax™ (Clobetasol Propionate Ointment, USP) should be applied with gentle rubbing to the affected skin area twice daily, once in the morning and once at night. Cormax™ is potent: therefore, **treatment must be limited to two consecutive weeks, and amounts greater than 50 g per week should not be used. Cormax™ (Clobetasol Propionate Ointment, USP) is not to be used with occlusive dressings.**

HOW SUPPLIED

Cormax™ (Clobetasol Propionate Ointment, USP) 0.05% is supplied in 15 g (NDC 55515-410-15) and 45 g (NDC 55515-410-45) tubes.
Store at controlled room temperature 15°–30°C (59°–86°F).
Caution: Federal (U.S.A.) law prohibits dispensing without prescription.
Mfd. for
OCLASSEN
Pharmaceuticals, Inc.
San Rafael, CA 94901
by DPT Laboratories, Inc.
San Antonio, TX 78215
Revised March, 1996
126995-0396

Shown in Product Identification Guide, page 325

CORMAX™ ℞
Scalp Application, 0.05% w/w
(Clobetasol Propionate Topical Solution, USP)
For Dermatologic Use Only
Not for Ophthalmic Use

DESCRIPTION

Cormax™ Scalp Application (Clobetasol Propionate Topical Solution, USP) contains the active compound clobetasol propionate, a synthetic corticosteroid, for topical dermatologic use. Clobetasol, an analog of prednisolone, has a high degree of glucocorticoid activity and a slight degree of mineralocorticoid activity.
Chemically, clobetasol propionate is 21-chloro-9-fluoro-11β, 17-dihydroxy-16β-methylpregna-1, 4-diene-3,20-dione 17-propionate, and it has the following structural formula:

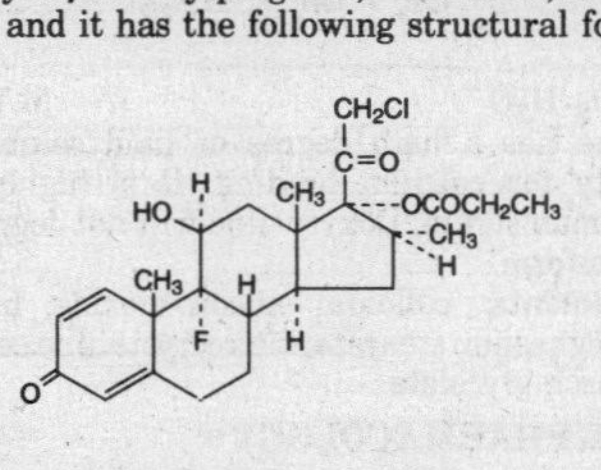

Clobetasol propionate has the molecular formula $C_{25}H_{32}ClFO_5$ and a molecular weight of 467. It is a white to cream-colored crystalline powder insoluble in water.
Each gram of Cormax™ Scalp Application (Clobetasol Propionate Topical Solution, USP) contains 0.5 mg clobetasol propionate in a base composed of purified water, isopropyl alcohol (40% w/w), carbomer 934P, and sodium hydroxide.

CLINICAL PHARMACOLOGY

The corticosteroids are a class of compounds comprising steroid hormones secreted by the adrenal cortex and their synthetic analogs. In pharmacologic doses, corticosteroids are used primarily for their anti-inflammatory and/or immunosuppressive effects. Topical corticosteroids such as clobetasol propionate are effective in the treatment of corticosteroid-responsive dermatoses primarily because of their anti-inflammatory, antipruritic, and vasconstrictive actions. However, while the physiologic, pharmacologic, and clinical effects of the corticosteroids are well known, the exact mechanisms of their actions in each disease are uncertain.
Clobetasol propionate, a corticosteroid, has been shown to have topical (dermatologic) and systemic pharmacologic and metabolic effects characteristic of this class of drugs.
Pharmacokinetics
The extent of percutaneous absorption of topical corticosteroids, including clobetasol propionate, is determined by many factors, including the vehicle, the integrity of the epidermal barrier, and the use of occlusive dressings (see **DOSAGE AND ADMINISTRATION**).
As with all topical corticosteroids, clobetasol propionate can be absorbed from normal intact skin. Inflammation and/or other disease processes in the skin may increase percutaneous absorption. Occlusive dressings substantially increase the percutaneous absorption of topical corticosteroids (see **DOSAGE AND ADMINISTRATION**).
As with all topical corticosteroids, clobetasol propionate can be absorbed from normal intact skin. Inflammation and/or other disease processes in the skin may increase percutaneous absorption. Occlusive dressings substantially increase the percutanous absorption of topical corticosteroids (see **DOSAGE AND ADMINISTRATION**).
Once absorbed through the skin, topical corticosteroids enter pharmacokinetic pathways similarly to systemically administered corticosteroids. Corticosteroids are bound to plasma proteins in varying degrees. Corticosteroids are metabolized primarily in the liver and are then excreted by the kidneys. Some of the topical corticosteroids, including clobetasol propionate and its metabolites, are also excreted in the bile.
Following repeated nonocclusive application in the treatment of scalp psoriasis, there is some evidence that Cormax™ Scalp Application (Clobetasol Propionate Topical Solution, USP) has the potential to depress plasma cortisol levels in some patients. However, hypothalamic-pituitary-adrenal (HPA) axis effects produced by systemically absorbed clobetasol propionate have been shown to be transient and reversible upon completion of a two-week course of treatment.

INDICATIONS AND USAGE

Cormax™ Scalp Application is indicated for short-term topical treatment of inflammatory and pruritic manifestations of moderate to severe corticosteroid-responsive dermatoses of the scalp. Treatment beyond two consecutive weeks is not recommended, and the total dosage should not exceed 50 mL per week because of the potential for the drug to suppress the HPA axis.
This product is not recommended for use in children under 12 years of age.

CONTRAINDICATIONS

Cormax™ Scalp Application (Clobetasol Propionate Topical Solution, USP) is contraindicated in patients with primary infections of the scalp, or in patients who are hypersensitive to clobetasol propionate, to other corticosteroids, or to any ingredient in this preparation.

PRECAUTIONS

General
Clobetasol propionate is a highly potent topical corticosteroid that has been shown to suppress the HPA axis at doses as low as 2 g (of ointment) per day. Systemic absorption of topical corticosteroids has resulted in reversible HPA axis suppression, manifestations of Cushing's syndrome, hyperglycemia, and glucosuria in some patients.
Conditions that augment systemic absorption include the application of the more potent corticosteroids, use over large surface areas, prolonged use and the addition of occlusive dressings. Therefore, patients receiving a large dose of potent topical steroid applied to a large surface area should be evaluated periodically for evidence of HPA axis suppression by using the urinary free cortisol and ACTH stimulation tests. If HPA axis suppression is noted, an attempt should be made to withdraw the drug, to reduce the frequency of application, or to substitute a less potent steroid.
Recovery of HPA axis function is generally prompt and complete upon discontinuation of the drug. Infrequently, signs and symptoms of steroid withdrawal may occur, requiring supplemental systemic corticosteroids.
Children may absorb proportionally larger amounts of topical corticosteroids and thus be more susceptible to systemic toxicity (see **PRECAUTIONS: Pediatric Use**).
If irritation develops, topical corticosteroids should be discontinued and appropriate therapy instituted. Irritation is possible if Cormax™ Scalp Application (Clobetasol Propionate Topical Solution, USP) contacts the eye. If that should occur, immediate flushing of the eye with a large volume of water is recommended.
In the presence of dermatologic infections, the use of an appropriate antifungal or antibacterial agent should be instituted. If a favorable response does not occur promptly, the corticosteroid should be discontinued until the infection has been adequately controlled.
Although Cormax™ Scalp Application (Clobetasol Propionate Topical Solution, USP) is intended for the treatment of inflammatory conditions of the scalp, it should be noted that certain areas of the body, such as the face, groin, and axillae, are more prone to atrophic changes than other areas of the body following treatment with corticosteroids. Frequent observation of the patient is important if these areas are to be treated.

Continued on next page

Oclassen—Cont.

As with other potent topical corticosteroids, Cormax™ Scalp Application should not be used in the treatment of rosacea and perioral dermatitis. Topical corticosteroids in general should not be used in the treatment of acne or as sole therapy in widespread plaque psoriasis.

Information for Patients

Patients using Cormax™ Scalp Application should receive the following information and instructions:

1. This medication is to be used as directed by the physician and should not be used longer than the prescribed time period. It is for external use only. Avoid contact with the eyes.
2. This medication should not be used for any disorder other than that for which it is prescribed.
3. The treated skin area should not be bandaged or otherwise covered or wrapped so as to be occlusive.
4. Patients should report any signs of local adverse reactions to the physician.

Laboratory Tests

The following tests may be helpful in evaluating HPA axis suppression:

Urinary free cortisol test

ACTH stimulation test

Carcinogenesis, Mutagenesis, Impairment of Fertility

Long-term animal studies have not been performed to evaluate the carcinogenic potential or the effect on fertility of topical corticosteroids.

Studies to determine mutagenicity with prednisolone have revealed negative results.

Pregnancy: Teratogenic Effects: Pregnancy Category C

The more potent corticosteroids have been shown to be teratogenic in animals after dermal application. Clobetasol propionate has not been tested for teratogenicity by this route; however, it is absorbed percutaneously, and when administered subcutaneously it was a significant teratogen in both the rabbit and the mouse. Clobetasol propionate has greater teratogenic potential than steroids that are less potent.

There are no adequate and well-controlled studies of the teratogenic effects of topically applied corticosteroids, including clobetasol, in pregnant women. Therefore, clobetasol and other topical corticosteroids should be used during pregnancy only if the potential benefit justifies the potential risk to the fetus, and they should not be used extensively on pregnant patients, in large amounts, or for prolonged periods of time.

Nursing Mothers

It is not known whether topical administration of corticosteroids could result in sufficient systemic absorption to produce detectable quantities in breast milk. Systemically administered corticosteroids are secreted into breast milk in quantities not likely to have a deleterious effect on the infant. Nevertheless, caution should be exercised when topical corticosteroids are prescribed for a nursing woman.

Pediatric Use

Use of Cormax™ Scalp Application (Clobetasol Propionate Topical Solution, USP) in pediatric patients under 12 years of age is not recommended.

Pediatric patients may demonstrate greater susceptibility to topical corticosteroids-induced HPA axis suppression and Cushing's syndrome than mature patients because of a larger skin surface area to body weight ratio.

HPA axis suppression, Cushing's syndrome and intracranial hypertension have been reported in children receiving topical corticosteroids. Manifestations of adrenal suppression in children include linear growth retardation, delayed weight gain, low plasma cortisol levels, and absence of response to ACTH stimulation. Manifestations of intercranial hypertension include bulging fontanelles, headaches, and bilateral papilledema.

ADVERSE REACTIONS

Cormax™ Scalp Application (Clobetasol Propionate Topical Solution, USP) is generally well tolerated when used for two-week treatment periods.

The most frequent adverse events reported have been local and have included burning and/or stinging sensation, which occurred in approximately 10% of the patients; scalp pustules, which occurred in approximately 1% of the patients; and tingling, and folliculitis, each of which occurred in approximately 0.6% of the patients. Less frequent adverse events were itching and tightness of the scalp, dermatitis, tenderness, headache, hair loss, and eye irritation, each of which occurred in approximately 0.3% of the patients.

The following local adverse reactions are reported infrequently when topical corticosteroids are used as recommended. These reactions are listed in an approximately decreasing order of occurrence: burning, itching, irritation, dryness, folliculitis, hypertrichosis, acneiform eruptions, hypopigmentation, perioral dermatitis, allergic contact dermatitis, maceration of the skin, secondary infection, skin atrophy, striae and miliaria. Systemic absorption of topical corticosteroids has produced reversible HPA axis suppression, manifestations of Cushing's syndrome, hyperglycemia, and glucosuria in some patients. In rare instances, treatment (or withdrawal of treatment) of psoriasis with corticosteroids is thought to have exacerbated the disease or provoked the pustular form of the disease, so careful patient supervision is recommended.

OVERDOSAGE

Topically applied Cormax™ Scalp Application (Clobetasol Propionate Topical Solution, USP) can be absorbed in sufficient amounts to produce systemic effects (see **PRECAUTIONS**).

DOSAGE AND ADMINISTRATION

Cormax™ Scalp Application should be applied to the affected scalp areas twice daily, once in the morning and once at night. Cormax™ Scalp Application is potent; therefore, **treatment must be limited to two consecutive weeks and amounts greater than 50mL per week should not be used. Cormax™ Scalp Application is not be used with occlusive dressings.**

HOW SUPPLIED

Cormax™ Scalp Application (Clobetasol Propionate Topical Solution, USP), 0.05% w/w is supplied in plastic squeeze bottles of 25 mL (NDC 55515-430-50). Store at controlled room temperature 15°–30° C (59°–86°F). Do not refrigerate. Do not use near an open flame.

Caution: Federal (U.S.A.) law prohibits dispensing without prescription.

Mfd for

OCLASSEN

Pharmaceuticals, Inc.

San Rafael, CA 94901

by DPT Laboratories, Inc.

San Antonio, TX 78215

Revised: November, 1995

126984-1195

Shown in Product Identification Guide, page 325

MONODOX® ℞

DOXYCYCLINE MONOHYDRATE CAPSULES

[mon 'o-dox]

DESCRIPTION

Doxycycline is a broad-spectrum antibiotic synthetically derived from oxytetracycline. Monodox® 100 mg and 50 mg capsules contain doxycycline monohydrate equivalent to 100 mg or 50 mg of doxycycline for oral administration. The chemical designation of the light-yellow crystalline powder is alpha-6-deoxy-5-oxytetracycline.

Structural formula:

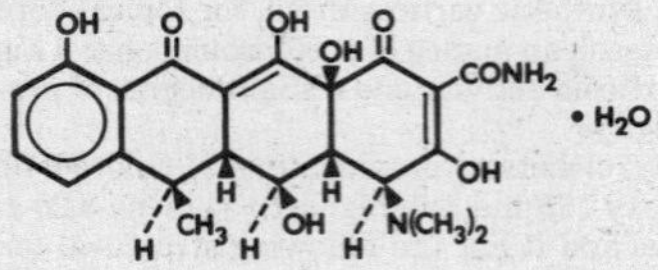

$C_{22}H_{24}N_2O_8 \cdot H_2O$ M.W. = 462.46

Doxycycline has a high degree of lipid solubility and a low affinity for calcium binding. It is highly stable in normal human serum. Doxycycline will not degrade into an epianhydro form.

Inert Ingredients: colloidal silicon dioxide; hard gelatin capsule; magnesium stearate; microcrystalline cellulose; and sodium starch glycolate.

CLINICAL PHARMACOLOGY

Tetracyclines are readily absorbed and are bound to plasma proteins in varying degrees. They are concentrated by the liver in the bile and excreted in the urine and feces at high concentrations in a biologically active form. Doxycycline is virtually completely absorbed after oral administration.

Following a 200 mg dose of doxycycline monohydrate, 24 normal adult volunteers averaged the following serum concentration values:

[See table below.]

	Average Observed Values
Maximum Concentration	3.61 mcg/mL (± 0.9 sd)
Time of Maximum Concentration	2.60 hr (± 1.10 sd)
Elimination Rate Constant	0.049 per hr (± 0.030 sd)
Half-Life	16.33 hr (± 4.53 sd)

Excretion of doxycycline by the kidney is about 40%/72 hours in individuals with normal function (creatinine clearance about 75 mL/min). This percentage excretion may fall as low as 1-5%/72 hours in individuals with severe renal insufficiency (creatinine clearance below 10 mL/min). Studies have shown no significant difference in serum half-life of doxycycline (range 18-22 hours) in individuals with normal and severely impaired renal function.

Hemodialysis does not alter serum half-life.

Microbiology: The tetracyclines are primarily bacteriostatic and are thought to exert their antimicrobial effect by the inhibition of protein synthesis. The tetracyclines, including doxycycline, have a similar antimicrobial spectrum of activity against a wide range of gram-positive and gram-negative organisms. Cross-resistance of these organisms to tetracyclines is common.

While *in vitro* studies have demonstrated the susceptibility of most strains of the following microorganisms, clinical efficacy for infections other than those included in the INDICATIONS AND USAGE section has not been documented.

GRAM-NEGATIVE BACTERIA:

- *Neisseria gonorrhoeae*
- *Haemophilus ducreyi*
- *Haemophilus influenzae*
- *Yersinia pestis* (formerly *Pasteurella pestis*)
- *Francisella tularensis* (formerly *Pasteurella tularensis*)
- *Vibrio cholerae* (formerly *Vibrio comma*)
- *Bartonella bacilliformis*
- *Brucella* species

Because many strains of the following groups of gram-negative microorganisms have been shown to be resistant to tetracyclines, culture and susceptibility testing are recommended:

- *Escherichia coli*
- *Klebsiella* species
- *Enterobacter aerogenes*
- *Shigella* species
- *Acinetobacter* species (formerly *Mima* species and *Herellea* species)
- *Bacteroides* species

GRAM-POSITIVE BACTERIA:

Because many strains of the following groups of gram-positive microorganisms have been shown to be resistant to tetracyclines, culture and susceptibility testing are recommended. Up to 44 percent of strains of *Streptococcus pyogenes* and 74 percent of *Streptococcus faecalis* have been found to be resistant to tetracycline drugs. Therefore, tetracyclines should not be used to treat streptococcal infections unless the organism has been demonstrated to be susceptible.

- *Streptococcus pyogenes*
- *Streptococcus pneumoniae*
- *Enterococcus* group (*Streptococcus faecalis* and *Streptococcus faecium*)
- *Alpha-hemolytic streptococci* (*viridans* group)

OTHER MICROORGANISMS:

- *Chlamydia psittaci*
- *Chlamydia trachomatis*
- *Ureaplasma urealyticum*
- *Borrelia recurrentis*
- *Treponema pallidum*
- *Treponema pertenue*
- *Clostridium* species
- *Fusobacterium fusiforme*
- *Actinomyces* species
- *Bacillus anthracis*
- *Propionibacterium acnes*
- *Entamoeba* species
- *Balantidium coli*

Susceptibility tests: Diffusion Techniques: Quantitative methods that require measurement of zone diameters give the most precise estimate of the susceptibility of bacteria to antimicrobial agents.

One such standard procedure[1] which has been recommended for use with disks to test susceptibility of organisms to doxycycline uses the 30-mcg tetracycline-class disk or the 30-mcg doxycycline disk. Interpretation involves the correlation of the diameter obtained in the disk test with the minimum inhibitory concentration (MIC) for tetracycline or doxycycline, respectively.

Reports from the laboratory giving results of the standard single-disk susceptibility test with a 30-mcg tetracycline-class disk or the 30-mcg doxycycline disk should be interpreted according to the following criteria.

Zone Diameter (mm)		Interpretation
tetracycline	doxycycline	
≥ 19	≥ 16	Susceptible
15–18	13–15	Intermediate
≤ 14	≤ 12	Resistant

A report of "susceptible" indicates that the pathogen is likely to be inhibited by generally achievable blood levels. A report of "intermediate" suggests that the organism would be susceptible if a high dosage is used or if the infection is confined to tissues and fluids in which high antimicrobial levels are attained. A report of "resistant" indicates that achievable concentrations are unlikely to be inhibitory, and other therapy should be selected.

Time (hr):	0.5	1.0	1.5	2.0	3.0	4.0	8.0	12.0	24.0	48.0	72.0
Conc. (mcg/mL)	1.02	2.26	2.67	3.01	3.16	3.03	2.03	1.62	0.95	0.37	0.15

Standardized procedures require the use of laboratory control organisms. The 30-mcg tetracycline-class disk or the 30-mcg doxycycline disk should give the following zone diameters:

Organism	Zone Diameter	
	tetracycline	doxycycline
E. coli ATCC 25922	18–25	18–24
S. aureus ATCC 25923	19–28	23–29

Dilution Techniques:
Use a standardized dilution method[2] (broth, agar, microdilution) or equivalent with tetracycline powder. The MIC values obtained should be interpreted according to the following criteria:

MIC (mcg/mL)	Interpretation
≤ 4	Susceptible
8	Intermediate
≥ 16	Resistant

As with standard diffusion techniques, dilution methods require the use of laboratory control organisms. Standard tetracycline powder should provide the following MIC values:

Organism	MIC (mcg/mL)
S. aureus ATCC 29213	0.25–1
E. faecalis ATCC 29212	8–32
E. coli ATCC 25922	1–4
P. aeruginosa ATCC 27853	8–32

INDICATIONS AND USAGE

Doxycycline is indicated for the treatment of the following infections:
Rocky mountain spotted fever, typhus fever and the typhus group, Q fever, rickettsialpox, and tick fevers caused by Rickettsiae.
Respiratory tract infections caused by *Mycoplasma pneumoniae.*
Lymphogranuloma venereum caused by *Chlamydia trachomatis.*
Psittacosis (ornithosis) caused by *Chlamydia psittaci.*
Trachoma caused by *Chlamydia trachomatis,* although the infectious agent is not always eliminated as judged by immunofluorescence.
Inclusion conjunctivitis caused by *Chlamydia trachomatis.*
Uncomplicated urethral, endocervical or rectal infections in adults caused by *Chlamydia trachomatis.*
Nongonococcal urethritis caused by *Ureaplasma urealyticum.*
Relapsing fever due to *Borrelia recurrentis.*
Doxycycline is also indicated for the treatment of infections caused by the following gram-negative microorganisms:
Chancroid caused by *Haemophilus ducreyi.*
Plague due to *Yersinia pestis* (formerly *Pasteurella pestis*).
Tularemia due to *Francisella tularensis* (formerly *Pasteurella tularensis*).
Cholera caused by *Vibrio cholerae* (formerly *Vibrio comma*).
Campylobacter fetus infections caused by *Campylobacter fetus* (formerly *Vibrio fetus*).
Brucellosis due to *Brucella* species (in conjunction with streptomycin).
Bartonellosis due to *Bartonella bacilliformis.*
Granuloma inguinale caused by *Calymmatobacterium granulomatis.*
Because many strains of the following groups of microorganisms have been shown to be resistant to doxycycline, culture and susceptibility testing are recommended.
Doxycycline is indicated for treatment of infections caused by the following gram-negative microorganisms, when bacteriologic testing indicates appropriate susceptibility to the drug:
Escherichia coli
Enterobacter aerogenes (formerly *Aerobacter aerogenes*)
Shigella species
Acinetobacter species (formerly *Mima* species and *Herellea* species)
Respiratory tract infections caused by *Haemophilus influenzae.*
Respiratory tract and urinary tract infections caused by *Klebsiella* species.
Doxycycline is indicated for treatment of infections caused by the following gram-positive microorganisms when bacteriologic testing indicates appropriate susceptibility to the drug:
Upper respiratory infections caused by *Streptococcus pneumoniae* (formerly *Diplococcus pneumoniae*).
Skin and skin structure infections caused by *Staphylococcus aureus.* Doxycycline is not the drug of choice in the treatment of any type of staphylococcal infections.
When penicillin is contraindicated, doxycycline is an alternative drug in the treatment of the following infections:
Uncomplicated gonorrhea caused by *Neisseria gonorrhoeae.*
Syphilis caused by *Treponema pallidum.*
Yaws caused by *Treponema pertenue.*
Listeriosis due to *Listeria monocytogenes.*
Anthrax due to *Bacillus anthracis.*
Vincent's infection caused by *Fusobacterium fusiforme.*

Actinomycosis caused by *Actinomyces israelii.*
Infections caused by *Clostridium* species.
In acute intestinal amebiasis, doxycycline may be a useful adjunct to amebicides.
In severe acne, doxycycline may be useful adjunctive therapy.

CONTRAINDICATIONS

This drug is contraindicated in persons who have shown hypersensitivity to any of the tetracyclines.

WARNINGS

THE USE OF DRUGS OF THE TETRACYCLINE CLASS DURING TOOTH DEVELOPMENT (LAST HALF OF PREGNANCY, INFANCY, AND CHILDHOOD TO THE AGE OF 8 YEARS) MAY CAUSE PERMANENT DISCOLORATION OF THE TEETH (YELLOW-GRAY-BROWN).
This adverse reaction is more common during long term use of the drugs but has been observed following repeated short-term courses. Enamel hypoplasia has also been reported. TETRACYCLINE DRUGS, THEREFORE, SHOULD NOT BE USED IN THIS AGE GROUP UNLESS OTHER DRUGS ARE NOT LIKELY TO BE EFFECTIVE OR ARE CONTRAINDICATED.
All tetracyclines form a stable calcium complex in any bone-forming tissue. A decrease in the fibula growth rate has been observed in prematures given oral tetracycline in doses of 25 mg/kg every six hours. This reaction was shown to be reversible when the drug was discontinued.
Results of animal studies indicate that tetracyclines cross the placenta, are found in fetal tissues, and can have toxic effects on the developing fetus (often related to retardation of skeletal development). Evidence of embryo toxicity has been noted in animals treated early in pregnancy. If any tetracycline is used during pregnancy or if the patient becomes pregnant while taking these drugs, the patient should be apprised of the potential hazard to the fetus.
The antianabolic action of the tetracyclines may cause an increase in BUN. Studies to date indicate that this does not occur with the use of doxycycline in patients with impaired renal function.
Photosensitivity manifested by an exaggerated sunburn reaction has been observed in some individuals taking tetracyclines. Patients apt to be exposed to direct sunlight or ultraviolet light should be advised that this reaction can occur with tetracycline drugs, and treatment should be discontinued at the first evidence of skin erythema.

PRECAUTIONS

General:
As with other antibiotic preparations, use of this drug may result in overgrowth of non-susceptible organisms, including fungi. If superinfection occurs, the antibiotic should be discontinued and appropriate therapy instituted.
Bulging fontanels in infants and benign intracranial hypertension in adults have been reported in individuals receiving tetracyclines. These conditions disappeared when the drug was discontinued.
Incision and drainage or other surgical procedures should be performed in conjunction with antibiotic therapy when indicated.
Laboratory tests: In venereal disease when coexistent syphilis is suspected, a dark-field examination should be done before treatment is started and the blood serology repeated monthly for at least four months.
In long-term therapy, periodic laboratory evaluations of organ systems, including hematopoietic, renal, and hepatic studies should be performed.
Drug interactions: Because tetracyclines have been shown to depress plasma prothrombin activity, patients who are on anticoagulant therapy may require downward adjustment of their anticoagulant dosage.
Since bacteriostatic drugs may interfere with the bactericidal action of penicillin, it is advisable to avoid giving tetracyclines in conjunction with penicillin.
Absorption of tetracyclines is impaired by antacids containing aluminum, calcium, or magnesium, and iron-containing preparations.
Barbiturates, carbamazepine, and phenytoin decrease the half-life of doxycycline.
The concurrent use of tetracycline and methoxyflurane has been reported to result in fatal renal toxicity.
Concurrent use of tetracycline may render oral contraceptives less effective.
Drug/laboratory test interactions: False elevations of urinary catecholamine levels may occur due to interference with the fluorescence test.
Carcinogenesis, mutagenesis, impairment of fertility: Long-term studies in animals to evaluate the carcinogenic potential of doxycycline have not been conducted. However, there has been evidence of oncogenic activity in rats in studies with related antibiotics, oxytetracycline (adrenal and pituitary tumors) and minocycline (thyroid tumors). Likewise, although mutagenicity studies of doxycycline have not been conducted, positive results in *in vitro* mammalian cell assays have been reported for related antibiotics (tetracycline, oxytetracycline). Doxycycline administered orally at dosage

levels as high as 250 mg/kg/day had no apparent effect on the fertility of female rats. Effect on male fertility has not been studied.
Pregnancy: Pregnancy Category D. (See WARNINGS).
Labor and Delivery: The effect of tetracyclines on labor and delivery is unknown.
Nursing mothers: Tetracyclines are present in the milk of lactating women who are taking a drug in this class. Because of the potential for serious adverse reactions in nursing infants from the tetracyclines, a decision should be made whether to discontinue nursing or discontinue the drug, taking into account the importance of the drug to the mother. (See WARNINGS).
Pediatric Use: See Warnings and Dosage and Administration sections.

ADVERSE REACTIONS

Due to oral doxycycline's virtually complete absorption, side effects to the lower bowel, particularly diarrhea, have been infrequent. The following adverse reactions have been observed in patients receiving tetracyclines.
Gastrointestinal: Anorexia, nausea, vomiting, diarrhea, glossitis, dysphagia, enterocolitis, and inflammatory lesions (with monilial overgrowth) in the anogenital region. These reactions have been caused by both the oral and parenteral administration of tetracyclines. Rare instances of esophagitis and esophageal ulcerations have been reported in patients receiving capsule and tablet forms of drugs in the tetracycline class. Most of these patients took medications immediately before going to bed. (See DOSAGE AND ADMINISTRATION).
Skin: Maculopapular and erythematous rashes. Exfoliative dermatitis has been reported but is uncommon. Photosensitivity is discussed above. (See WARNINGS.)
Renal toxicity: Rise in BUN has been reported and is apparently dose related. (See WARNINGS.)
Hypersensitivity reactions: urticaria, angioneurotic edema, anaphylaxis, anaphylactoid purpura, pericarditis, and exacerbation of systemic lupus erythematosus.
Blood: Hemolytic anemia, thrombocytopenia, neutropenia, and eosinophilia have been reported with tetracyclines.
Other: Bulging fontanels in infants and intracranial hypertension in adults. (See PRECAUTIONS—General.)
When given over prolonged periods, tetracyclines have been reported to produce brown-black microscopic discoloration of the thyroid gland. No abnormalities of thyroid function are known to occur.

OVERDOSAGE

In case of overdosage, discontinue medication, treat symptomatically and institute supportive measures. Dialysis does not alter serum half-life, and it would not be of benefit in treating cases of overdosage.

DOSAGE AND ADMINISTRATION

THE USUAL DOSAGE AND FREQUENCY OF ADMINISTRATION OF DOXYCYCLINE DIFFERS FROM THAT OF THE OTHER TETRACYCLINES. EXCEEDING THE RECOMMENDED DOSAGE MAY RESULT IN AN INCREASED INCIDENCE OF SIDE EFFECTS.
Adults: The usual dose of oral doxycycline is 200 mg on the first day of treatment (administered 100 mg every 12 hours or 50 mg every 6 hours) followed by a maintenance dose of 100 mg/day. The maintenance dose may be administered as a single dose or as 50 mg every 12 hours. In the management of more severe infections (particularly chronic infections of the urinary tract), 100 mg every 12 hours is recommended.
For children above eight years of age: The recommended dosage schedule for children weighing 100 pounds or less is 2 mg/lb of body weight divided into two doses on the first day of treatment, followed by 1 mg/lb of body weight given as a single daily dose or divided into two doses, on subsequent days. For more severe infections, up to 2 mg/lb of body weight may be used. For children over 100 lbs the usual adult dose should be used.
Uncomplicated gonococcal infections in adults (except anorectal infections in men): 100 mg by mouth, twice a day for 7 days. As an alternate single visit dose, administer 300 mg stat followed in one hour by a second 300 mg dose.
Acute epididymo-orchitis caused by *N. gonorrhoeae*: 100 mg, by mouth, twice a day for at least 10 days.
Primary and secondary syphilis: 300 mg a day in divided doses for at least 10 days.
Uncomplicated urethral, endocervical, or rectal infection in adults caused by *Chlamydia trachomatis*: 100 mg, by mouth, twice a day for at least 7 days.
Nongonococcal urethritis caused by *C. trachomatis* and *U. urealyticum*: 100 mg, by mouth, twice a day for at least 7 days.
Acute epididymo-orchitis caused by *C. trachomatis*: 100 mg, by mouth, twice a day for at least 10 days.
When used in streptococcal infections, therapy should be continued for 10 days.
Administration of adequate amounts of fluid along with capsule and tablet forms of drugs in the tetracycline class is

Continued on next page

Oclassen—Cont.

recommended to wash down the drugs and reduce the risk of esophageal irritation and ulceration. (See ADVERSE REACTIONS). If gastric irritation occurs, doxycycline may be given with food. Ingestion of a high fat meal has been shown to delay the time to peak plasma concentrations by an average of one hour and 20 minutes. However, in the same study, food enhanced the average peak concentration by 7.5% and the area under the curve by 5.7%.

HOW SUPPLIED

MONODOX® 50 mg Capsules have a white opaque body with a yellow opaque cap. The capsule bears the inscription "MONODOX 50" in brown and "M 260" in brown. Each capsule contains doxycycline monohydrate equivalent to 50 mg of doxycycline.

MONODOX® 50 mg is available in: Bottles of 100 capsules, NDC 55515-260-06. MONODOX® 100 mg Capsules have a yellow opaque body with a brown opaque cap. The capsule bears the inscription "MONODOX 100" in white and "M 259" in brown. Each capsule contains doxycycline monohydrate equivalent to 100 mg of doxycycline. MONODOX® 100 mg is available in: Bottles of 50 capsules, NDC 55515-259-04 and in bottles of 250 capsules, NDC 55515-259-07.
STORE AT CONTROLLED ROOM TEMPERATURE 15°–30°C (59°–86°F). PROTECT FROM LIGHT.

ANIMAL PHARMACOLOGY AND ANIMAL TOXICOLOGY

Hyperpigmentation of the thyroid has been produced by members of the tetracycline class in the following species: in rats by oxytetracycline, doxycycline, tetracycline PO_4, and methacycline; in minipigs by doxycycline, minocycline, tetracycline PO_4, and methacycline; in dogs by doxycycline and minocycline; in monkeys by minocycline.

Minocycline, tetracycline PO_4, methacycline, doxycycline, tetracycline base, oxytetracycline HCl and tetracycline HCl were goitrogenic in rats fed a low iodine diet. This goitrogenic effect was accompanied by high radioactive iodine uptake. Administration of minocycline also produced a large goiter with high radioiodine uptake in rats fed a relatively high iodine diet.

Treatment of various animal species with this class of drugs has also resulted in the induction of thyroid hyperplasia in the following: in rats and dogs (minocycline), in chickens (chlortetracycline) and in rats and mice (oxytetracycline). Adrenal gland hyperplasia has been observed in goats and rats treated with oxytetracycline.

References:
1. National Committee for Clinical Laboratory Standards, *Performance Standards for Antimicrobial Disk Susceptibility Tests*, Fourth Edition. Approved Standard NCCLS Document M2-A4, Vol. 10, No. 7 NCCLS, Villanova, PA, April 1990.
2. National Committee for Clinical Laboratory Standards, *Methods for Dilution Antimicrobial Susceptibility Tests for Bacteria That Grow Aerobically*, Second Edition. Approved Standard NCCLS Document M7-A2, Vol. 10, No. 8 NCCLS, Villanova, PA, April 1990.

Caution: Federal law prohibits dispensing without prescription.
Manufactured for
OCLASSEN
Pharmaceuticals, Inc.
San Rafael, CA 94901
by Vintage Pharmaceuticals, Inc., Charlotte, N.C.
Revised May 1995   02-18391/R4
Shown in Product Identification Guide, page 325

Odyssey Nutriceutical Sciences, Inc.
60 HAMILTON STREET
CAMBRIDGE, MA 02139
617-497-5100
800-790-8378
FAX 617-497-6990

Direct Inquiries to:
(617) 497-5100
(800) 790-8378
FAX: (617) 497-6990

HEALTHY HEART™   OTC
Dietary Supplement

Healthy Heart™ is a dietary supplement containing several nutrients intended to improve cardiovascular health by lowering serum homocysteine (Boushey, C., *et al*, 1995) and reducing oxidative damage (Hoffman, R. *et al*, 1995).

Each dose contains:
- Vitamin C (ascorbic acid)   600 mg
- Vitamin E (α-tocopherol)   400 I.U.
- Vitamin B_6 (pyridoxine)   50 mg
- Folic Acid   800 mcg
- Vitamin B_{12} (cobalamin)   500 mcg

INDICATION
Dietary supplementation for lowering and/or maintaining low levels of serum homocysteine, and reducing and/or preventing oxidative damage due to free radicals. This product is intended to be used in conjunction with a complete program of education, nutrition and exercise for optimal cardiovascular health. Laboratory testing to evaluate and monitor patients using this product is recommended.

RECOMMENDED INTAKE
One dose taken daily preferably with a meal.

HOW SUPPLIED
Healthy Heart™ is supplied in tablet form. Each daily dose is contained in two tablets.

CAUTION
Each daily dose of Healthy Heart exceeds the Recommended Daily Allowance (RDA) of those nutrients included in the product. Taking more than the recommended amount of these nutrients may cause adverse reactions. Do not use if pregnant or nursing. Please consult your physician prior to taking this product.
The Food and Drug Administration (FDA) has not evaluated any labeling and or health claims that accompany this product. This product is not intended to diagnose, treat, cure or prevent any disease.

REFERENCES
Boushey, CJ, *et al*, JAMA, **274(13)**:1049-1057, 1995
Hoffman, RM, *et al*, Arch Int Med, **155**:241-246, 1995

Ohmeda
Pharmaceutical Products Division Inc.
110 ALLEN ROAD
BOX 804
LIBERTY CORNER, NJ 07938-0804

Direct Inquires to:
Professional Services Department
(800) ANA DRUG
(800) 262-3784

For Medical Information Contact:
In Emergencies:
Lawrence McKay, M.D.
Vice President, Clinical Development
(800) ANA-DRUG
(800) 262-3784

Sales and Ordering:
To place an order between 8:00 AM and 4:00 PM:
(800) 345-2700

BREVIBLOC® INJECTION   ℞
[brĕ vĭ-blok]
(esmolol HCl)

BRIEF SUMMARY
10 mL Ampul-2500 mg
NOT FOR DIRECT INTRAVENOUS INJECTION. AMPUL MUST BE DILUTED PRIOR TO ITS INFUSION—SEE DOSAGE AND ADMINISTRATION SECTION OF COMPLETE PRESCRIBING INFORMATION.
10 mL Single Dose Vial—100 mg

INDICATIONS AND USAGE
Supraventricular Tachycardia
BREVIBLOC® (esmolol HCl) is indicated for the rapid control of ventricular rate in patients with atrial fibrillation or atrial flutter in perioperative, postoperative, or other emergent circumstances where short term control of ventricular rate with a short-acting agent is desirable. BREVIBLOC® is also indicated in noncompensatory sinus tachycardia where, in the physician's judgment, the rapid heart rate requires specific intervention. BREVIBLOC® is not intended for use in chronic settings where transfer to another agent is anticipated.
Intraoperative and Postoperative Tachycardia and/or Hypertension
BREVIBLOC® (esmolol HCl) is indicated for the treatment of tachycardia and hypertension that occur during induction and tracheal intubation, during surgery, on emergence from anesthesia, and in the postoperative period, when in the physician's judgment such specific intervention is considered indicated.

Use of BREVIBLOC® to prevent such events is not recommended.

CONTRAINDICATIONS
BREVIBLOC® (esmolol HCl) is contraindicated in patients with sinus bradycardia, heart block greater than first degree, cardiogenic shock or overt heart failure (see WARNINGS).

WARNINGS
Hypotension: In clinical trials 20–50% of patients treated with BREVIBLOC® (esmolol HCl) have experienced hypotension, generally defined as systolic pressure less than 90 mmHg and/or diastolic pressure less than 50 mmHg. About 12% of the patients have been symptomatic (mainly diaphoresis or dizziness). Hypotension can occur at any dose but is dose-related so that doses beyond 200 mcg/kg/min (0.2 mg/kg/min) are not recommended. Patients should be closely monitored, especially if pretreatment blood pressure is low. Decrease of dose or termination of infusion reverses hypotension, usually within 30 minutes.
Cardiac Failure: Sympathetic stimulation is necessary in supporting circulatory function in congestive heart failure, and beta blockade carries the potential hazard of further depressing myocardial contractility and precipitating more severe failure. Continued depression of the myocardium with beta blocking agents over a period of time can, in some cases, lead to cardiac failure. At the first sign or symptom of impending cardiac failure, BREVIBLOC® (esmolol HCl) should be withdrawn. Although withdrawal may be sufficient because of the short elimination half-life of BREVIBLOC®, specific treatment may also be considered (see OVERDOSAGE). The use of BREVIBLOC® for control of ventricular response in patients with supraventricular arrhythmias should be undertaken with caution when the patient is compromised hemodynamically or is taking other drugs that decrease any or all of the following: peripheral resistance, myocardial filling, myocardial contractility, or electrical impulse propagation in the myocardium. Despite the rapid onset and offset of the effects of BREVIBLOC®, several cases of death have been reported in complex clinical states where BREVIBLOC® was presumably being used to control ventricular rate.
Intraoperative and Postoperative Tachycardia and/or Hypertension: BREVIBLOC® (esmolol HCl) should not be used as the treatment for hypertension in patients in whom the increased blood pressure is primarily due to the vasoconstriction associated with hypothermia.
Bronchospastic Diseases: PATIENTS WITH BRONCHOSPASTIC DISEASES SHOULD, IN GENERAL, NOT RECEIVE BETA BLOCKERS. Because of its relative beta$_1$ selectivity and titratability, BREVIBLOC® (esmolol HCl) may be used with caution in patients with bronchospastic diseases. However, since beta$_1$ selectivity is not absolute, BREVIBLOC® should be carefully titrated to obtain the lowest possible effective dose. In the event of bronchospasm, the infusion should be terminated immediately; a beta$_2$ stimulating agent may be administered if conditions warrant but should be used with particular caution as patients already have rapid ventricular rates.
Diabetes Mellitus and Hypoglycemia: BREVIBLOC® (esmolol HCl) should be used with caution in diabetic patients requiring a beta blocking agent. Beta blockers may mask tachycardia occurring with hypoglycemia, but other manifestations such as dizziness and sweating may not be significantly affected.

PRECAUTIONS
General
Infusion concentrations of 20 mg/mL were associated with more serious venous irritation, including thrombophlebitis, than concentrations of 10 mg/mL. Extravasation of 20 mg/mL may lead to a serious local reaction and possible skin necrosis. Concentrations greater than 10 mg/mL or infusion into small veins or through a butterfly catheter should be avoided.
Because the acid metabolite of BREVIBLOC® is primarily excreted unchanged by the kidney, BREVIBLOC® (esmolol HCl) should be administered with caution to patients with impaired renal function. The elimination half-life of the acid metabolite was prolonged ten-fold and the plasma level was considerably elevated in patients with end-stage renal disease.
Care should be taken in the intravenous administration of BREVIBLOC® as sloughing of the skin and necrosis have been reported in association with infiltration and extravasation of intravenous infusions.
Drug Interactions
Catecholamine-depleting drugs, e.g., reserpine, may have an additive effect when given with beta blocking agents. Patients treated concurrently with BREVIBLOC® (esmolol HCl) and a catecholamine depletor should therefore be closely observed for evidence of hypotension or marked bradycardia, which may result in vertigo, syncope, or postural hypotension.
A study of interaction between BREVIBLOC® and warfarin showed that concomitant administration of BREVIBLOC®

and warfarin does not alter warfarin plasma levels. BREVIBLOC® concentrations were equivocally higher when given with warfarin, but this is not likely to be clinically important.

When digoxin and BREVIBLOC® were concomitantly administered intravenously to normal volunteers, there was a 10–20% increase in digoxin blood levels at some time points. Digoxin did not affect BREVIBLOC® pharmacokinetics. When intravenous morphine and BREVIBLOC® were concomitantly administered in normal subjects, no effect on morphine blood levels was seen, but BREVIBLOC® steady-state blood levels were increased by 46% in the presence of morphine. No other pharmacokinetic parameters were changed.

The effect of BREVIBLOC® on the duration of succinylcholine-induced neuromuscular blockade was studied in patients undergoing surgery. The onset of neuromuscular blockade by succinylcholine was unaffected by BREVIBLOC®, but the duration of neuromuscular blockade was prolonged from 5 minutes to 8 minutes.

Although the interactions observed in these studies do not appear to be of major clinical importance, BREVIBLOC® should be titrated with caution in patients being treated concurrently with digoxin, morphine, succinylcholine or warfarin.

While taking beta blockers, patients with a history of severe anaphylactic reaction to a variety of allergens may be more reactive to repeated challenge, either accidental, diagnostic, or therapeutic. Such patients may be unresponsive to the usual doses of epinephrine used to treat allergic reaction.

Caution should be exercised when considering the use of BREVIBLOC® and verapamil in patients with depressed myocardial function. Fatal cardiac arrests have occurred in patients receiving both drugs. Additionally, BREVIBLOC® should not be used to control supraventricular tachycardia in the presence of agents which are vasoconstrictive and inotropic such as dopamine, epinephrine, and norepinephrine because of the danger of blocking cardiac contractility when systemic vascular resistance is high.

Carcinogenesis, Mutagenesis, Impairment of Fertility

Because of its short term usage no carcinogenicity, mutagenicity or reproductive performance studies have been conducted with BREVIBLOC® (esmolol HCl).

Pregnancy Category C

Teratogenicity studies in rats at intravenous dosages of BREVIBLOC® (esmolol HCl) up to 3000 mcg/kg/min (3 mg/kg/min) (ten times the maximum human maintenance dosage) for 30 minutes daily produced no evidence of maternal toxicity, embryotoxicity or teratogenicity, while a dosage of 10,000 mcg/kg/min (10 mg/kg/min) produced maternal toxicity and lethality. In rabbits, intravenous dosages up to 1000 mcg/kg/min (1 mg/kg/min) for 30 minutes daily produced no evidence of maternal toxicity, embryotoxicity or teratogenicity, while 2500 mcg/kg/min (2.5 mg/kg/min) produced minimal maternal toxicity and increased fetal resorptions.

Although there are no adequate and well-controlled studies in pregnant women, use of esmolol in the last trimester of pregnancy or during labor or delivery has been reported to cause fetal bradycardia, which continued after termination of drug infusion. BREVIBLOC® should be used during pregnancy only if the potential benefit justifies the potential risk to the fetus.

Nursing Mothers

It is not known whether BREVIBLOC® (esmolol HCl) is excreted in human milk; however, caution should be exercised when BREVIBLOC® is administered to a nursing woman.

Pediatric Use

The safety and effectiveness of BREVIBLOC® (esmolol HCl) in children have not been established.

ADVERSE REACTIONS

The following adverse reaction rates are based on use of BREVIBLOC® (esmolol HCl) in clinical trials involving 369 patients with supraventricular tachycardia and over 600 intraoperative and postoperative patients enrolled in clinical trials. Most adverse effects observed in controlled clinical trial settings have been mild and transient. The most important adverse effect has been hypotension (see WARNINGS). Deaths have been reported in post-marketing experience occurring during complex clinical states where BREVIBLOC® was presumably being used simply to control ventricular rate (see WARNINGS/Cardiac Failure).

Cardiovascular—Symptomatic hypotension (diaphoresis, dizziness) occurred in 12% of patients, and therapy was discontinued in about 11%, about half of whom were symptomatic. Asymptomatic hypotension occurred in about 25% of patients. Hypotension resolved during BREVIBLOC® (esmolol HCl) infusion in 63% of these patients and within 30 minutes after discontinuation of infusion in 80% of the remaining patients. Diaphoresis accompanied hypotension in 10% of patients. Peripheral ischemia occurred in approximately 1% of patients. Pallor, flushing, bradycardia (heart rate less than 50 beats per minute), chest pain, syncope, pulmonary edema and heart block have each been reported in less than 1% of patients. In two patients without supraventricular tachycardia but with serious coronary artery disease (post inferior myocardial infarction or unstable angina), severe bradycardia/sinus pause/asystole has developed, reversible in both cases with discontinuation of treatment.

Central Nervous System—Dizziness has occurred in 3% of patients; somnolence in 3%; confusion, headache, and agitation in about 2%; and fatigue in about 1% of patients. Paresthesia, asthenia, depression, abnormal thinking, anxiety, anorexia, and lightheadedness were reported in less than 1% of patients. Seizures were also reported in less than 1% of patients, with one death.

Respiratory—Bronchospasm, wheezing, dyspnea, nasal congestion, rhonchi, and rales have each been reported in less than 1% of patients.

Gastrointestinal—Nausea was reported in 7% of patients. Vomiting has occurred in about 1% of patients. Dyspepsia, constipation, dry mouth, and abdominal discomfort have each occurred in less than 1% of patients. Taste perversion has also been reported.

Skin (Infusion Site)—Infusion site reactions including inflammation and induration were reported in about 8% of patients. Edema, erythema, skin discoloration, burning at the infusion site, thrombophlebitis, and local skin necrosis from extravasation have each occurred in less than 1% of patients.

Miscellaneous—Each of the following has been reported in less than 1% of patients: Urinary retention, speech disorder, abnormal vision, midscapular pain, rigors, and fever.

OVERDOSAGE

Acute Toxicity

Overdoses of BREVIBLOC® (esmolol HCl) can cause cardiac arrest. In addition, overdoses can produce bradycardia, hypotension, electromechanical dissociation and loss of consciousness. Cases of massive accidental overdoses of BREVIBLOC® have occurred due to dilution errors. Some of these overdoses have been fatal while others resulted in permanent disablility. Bolus doses in the range of 625 mg to 2.5 g (12.5–50 mg/kg) have been fatal. Patients have recovered completely from overdoses as high as 1.75 g given over one minute or doses of 7.5 g given over one hour for cardiovascular surgery. The patients who survived appear to be those whose circulation could be supported until the effects of BREVIBLOC® resolved.

Because of its approximately 9-minute elimination half-life, the first step in the management of toxicity should be to discontinue the BREVIBLOC® infusion. Then, based on the observed clinical effects, the following general measures should also be considered.

Bradycardia: Intravenous administration of atropine or another anticholinergic drug.

Bronchospasm: Intravenous administration of beta$_2$ stimulating agent and/or a theophylline derivative.

Cardiac Failure: Intravenous administration of a diuretic and/or digitalis glycoside. In shock resulting from inadequate cardiac contractility, intravenous administration of dopamine, dobutamine, isoproterenol, or amrinone may be considered.

Symptomatic Hypotension: Intravenous administration of fluids and/or pressor agents.

DOSAGE AND ADMINISTRATION

2500 mg AMPUL

THE 2500 mg AMPUL IS NOT FOR DIRECT INTRAVENOUS INJECTION. THIS DOSAGE FORM IS A CONCENTRATED, POTENT DRUG WHICH MUST BE DILUTED PRIOR TO ITS INFUSION. BREVIBLOC® SHOULD NOT BE ADMIXED WITH SODIUM BICARBONATE. BREVIBLOC® SHOULD NOT BE MIXED WITH OTHER DRUGS PRIOR TO DILUTION IN A SUITABLE INTRAVENOUS FLUID.

(See Compatability Section below.)

Dilution: Aseptically prepare a 10 mg/mL infusion by adding two 2500 mg ampuls to a 500 mL container or one 2500 mg ampul to a 250 mL container of a compatible intravenous solution listed below. (Remove overage prior to dilution as appropriate.) This yields a final concentration of 10 mg/mL. The diluted solution is stable for at least 24 hours at room temperature. Note: Concentrations of BREVIBLOC® (esmolol HCl) greater than 10 mg/mL are likely to produce irritation on continued infusion (see PRECAUTIONS). BREVIBLOC® has, however, been well tolerated when administered via a central vein.

100 mg VIAL

This dosage form is prediluted to provide a ready-to-use 10 mg/mL concentration recommended for BREVIBLOC® intravenous administration. It may be used to administer the appropriate BREVIBLOC® (esmolol HCl) loading dosage infusions by hand-held syringe while the maintenance infusion is being prepared.

When using the 100 mg vial, a loading dose of 0.5 mg/kg/min for a 70 kg patient would be 3.5 mL.

Supraventricular Tachycardia

In the treatment of supraventricular tachycardia, responses to BREVIBLOC® (esmolol HCl) usually (over 95%) occur within the range of 50 to 200 mcg/kg/min (0.05 to 0.2 mg/kg/min). The average effective dosage is approximately 100 mcg/kg/min (0.1 mg/kg/min) although dosages as low as 25 mcg/kg/min (0.025 mg/kg/min) have been adequate in some patients. Dosages as high as 300 mcg/kg/min (0.3 mg/kg/min) have been used, but these provide little added effect and an increased rate of adverse effects, and are not recommended. Dosage of BREVIBLOC® in supraventricular tachycardia must be individualized by titration in which each step consists of a loading dosage followed by a maintenance dosage.

To initiate treatment of a patient with supraventricular tachycardia, administer a loading infusion of 500 mcg/kg/min (0.5 mg/kg/min) over one minute followed by a four-minute maintenance infusion of 50 mcg/kg/min (0.05 mg/kg/min). If an adequate therapeutic effect is observed over the five minutes of drug administration, maintain the maintenance infusion dosage with periodic adjustments up or down as needed. If an adequate therapeutic effect is not observed, the same loading dosage is repeated over one minute followed by an increased maintenance infusion rate of 100 mcg/kg/min (0.1 mg/kg/min).

Continue titration procedure as above, repeating the original loading infusion of 500 mcg/kg/min (0.5 mg/kg/min) over 1 minute, but increasing the maintenance infusion rate over the subsequent four minutes by 50 mcg/kg/min (0.05 mg/kg/min) increments. As the desired heart rate or blood pressure is approached, omit subsequent loading doses and titrate the maintenance dosage up or down to endpoint. Also, if desired, increase the interval between steps from 5 to 10 minutes.

	Loading Dose (over 1 minute)		Maintenance Dose (over 4 minutes)	
Time (minutes)	mcg/kg/min	mg/kg/min	mcg/kg/min	mg/kg/min
0–1	500	0.5		
1–5			50	0.05
5–6	500	0.5		
6–10			100	0.1
10–11	500	0.5		
11–15			150	0.15
15–16	•	•		
16–20			* 200	*0.2
20–(24 hrs)			Maintenance dose titrated to heart rate or other clinical endpoint.	

* As the desired heart rate or endpoint is approached, the loading infusion may be omitted and the maintenance infusion titrated to 300 mcg/kg/min (0.3 mg/kg/min) or downward as appropriate. Maintenance dosages above 200 mcg/kg/min (0.2 mg/kg/min) have not been shown to have significantly increased benefits. The interval between titration steps may be increased.

This specific dosage regimen has not been studied intraoperatively and, because of the time required for titration, may not be optimal for intraoperative use.

The safety of dosages above 300 mcg/kg/min (0.3 mg/kg/min) has not been studied.

In the event of an adverse reaction, the dosage of BREVIBLOC® may be reduced or discontinued. If a local infusion site reaction develops, an alternate infusion site should be used and caution should be taken to prevent extravasation. The use of butterfly needles should be avoided.

Abrupt cessation of BREVIBLOC® in patients has not been reported to produce the withdrawal effects which may occur with abrupt withdrawal of beta blockers following chronic use in coronary artery disease (CAD) patients. However, caution should still be used in abruptly discontinuing infusions of BREVIBLOC® in CAD patients.

After achieving an adequate control of the heart rate and a stable clinical status in patients with supraventricular tachycardia, transition to alternative antiarrhythmic agents such as propranolol, digoxin, or verapamil, may be accomplished. A recommended guideline for such a transition is given below but the physician should carefully consider the labeling instructions for the alternative agent selected.

Alternative Agent	Dosage
Propranolol hydrochloride	10–20 mg q 4–6 hrs
Digoxin	0.125–0.5 mg q 6 hrs (p.o. or i.v.)
Verapamil	80 mg q 6 hrs

The dosage of BREVIBLOC® (esmolol HCl) should be reduced as follows:

1. Thirty minutes following the first dose of the alternative agent, reduce the infusion rate of BREVIBLOC® by one-half (50%).
2. Following the second dose of the alternative agent, monitor the patient's response and if satisfactory control is maintained for the first hour, discontinue BREVIBLOC®.

The use of infusions of BREVIBLOC® up to 24 hours has been well documented; in addition, limited data from 24–48

Continued on next page

Ohmeda—Cont.

hrs (N = 48) indicate that BREVIBLOC® is well tolerated up to 48 hours.

Intraoperative and Postoperative Tachycardia and/or Hypertension

In the intraoperative and postoperative settings it is not always advisable to slowly titrate the dose of BREVIBLOC® (esmolol HCl) to a therapeutic effect. Therefore, two dosing options are presented: immediate control dosing and a gradual control when the physician has time to titrate.

1. Immediate Control

For intraoperative treatment of tachycardia and/or hypertension give an 80 mg (approximately 1 mg/kg) bolus dose over 30 seconds followed by a 150 mcg/kg/min infusion, if necessary. Adjust the infusion rate as required up to 300 mcg/kg/min to maintain desired heart rate and/or blood pressure.

2. Gradual Control

For postoperative tachycardia and hypertension, the dosing schedule is the same as that used in supraventricular tachycardia. To initiate treatment, administer a loading dosage infusion of 500 mcg/kg/min of BREVIBLOC® for one minute followed by a four-minute maintenance infusion of 50 mcg/kg/min. If an adequate therapeutic effect is not observed within five minutes, repeat the same loading dosage and follow with a maintenance infusion increased to 100 mcg/kg/min (see above Supraventricular Tachycardia).

Note: Higher dosages (250–300 mcg/kg/min) may be required for adequate control of blood pressure than those required for the treatment of atrial fibrillation, flutter and sinus tachycardia. One third of the postoperative hypertensive patients required these higher doses.

Compatibility with Commonly Use Intravenous Fluids

BREVIBLOC® INJECTION was tested for compatibility with ten commonly used intravenous fluids at a final concentration of 10 mg esmolol HCl per mL. BREVIBLOC® INJECTION was found to be compatible with the following solutions and was stable for at least 24 hours at controlled room temperature or under refrigeration:

Dextrose (5%) Injection, USP

Dextrose (5%) in Lactated Ringer's Injection

Dextrose (5%) in Ringer's Injection

Dextrose (5%) and Sodium Chloride (0.45%) Injection, USP

Dextrose (5%) and Sodium Chloride (0.9%) Injection, USP

Lactated Ringer's Injection, USP

Potassium Chloride (40 mEq/liter) in Dextrose (5%) Injection, USP

Sodium Chloride (0.45%) Injection, USP

Sodium Chloride (0.9%) Injection, USP

BREVIBLOC® INJECTION was NOT compatible with Sodium Bicarbonate (5%) Injection, USP.

Note: Parenteral drug products should be inspected visually for particulate matter and discoloration prior to administration, whenever solution and container permit.

HOW SUPPLIED

NDC 10019-015-71, 100 mg—10 mL vial, Box of 20

NDC 10019-025-18, 2500 mg—10 mL ampul, Box of 10

400-277-02   Rev. 7-95

STORE AT CONTROLLED ROOM TEMPERATURE (59°–86° F, 15°–30° C). Freezing does not adversely affect the product, but exposure to elevated temperatures should be avoided.

95-084

© 1995 Ohmeda Pharmaceutical Products Division Inc
110 Allen Road
PO Box 804
Liberty Corner NJ 07938 0804
1 800 ANA DRUG

DIZAC™   ℞ ©
(diazepam injectable emulsion) CIV

For I.V. Administration Only

Before prescribing, please consult complete product information, a summary of which follows:

INDICATIONS AND USAGE

Dizac is indicated for the management of anxiety disorders or for the short-term relief of the symptoms of anxiety. Anxiety or tension associated with the stress of everyday life usually does not require treatment with an anxiolytic.

In acute alcohol withdrawal Dizac may be useful in the symptomatic relief of acute agitation, tremor, impending or acute delirium tremens and hallucinosis.

As an adjunct prior to endoscopic procedures if apprehension, anxiety or acute stress reactions are present, and to diminish the patient's recall of the procedures. (See WARNINGS.)

Dizac is a useful adjunct for the relief of skeletal muscle spasm due to reflex spasm to local pathology (such as inflammation of the muscles or joints, or secondary to trauma); spasticity caused by upper motor neuron disorders (such as cerebral palsy and paraplegia); athetosis; stiff-man syndrome; and tetanus.

Dizac is a useful adjunct in status epilepticus and severe recurrent convulsive seizures.

Dizac is a useful premedication for relief of anxiety and tension in patients who are to undergo surgical procedures. Intravenously, prior to cardioversion for the relief of anxiety and tension and to diminish the patient's recall of the procedure.

CONTRAINDICATIONS

Dizac is contraindicated in patients with a known hypersensitivity to this drug; acute narrow angle glaucoma; and open angle glaucoma unless patients are receiving appropriate therapy. Because the Dizac emulsion vehicle contains soybean oil, Dizac should not be used in patients with known hypersensitivity to soy protein.

WARNINGS

When used intravenously, the following procedures should be undertaken to reduce the possibility of venous thrombosis, phlebitis, local irritation, swelling, and, rarely, vascular impairment. The emulsion should be injected slowly, taking at least one minute for each 5 mg (1 mL) given; do not use small veins, such as those on the dorsum of the hand or wrist; extreme care should be taken to avoid intra-arterial administration or extravasation of complete prescribing information.

Do not mix or dilute Dizac with other solutions or drugs in syringe or infusion container. If it is not feasible to administer Dizac directly I.V., it may be injected slowly through the infusion tubing as close as possible to the vein insertion.

Extreme care must be used in administering Dizac by the I.V. route to the elderly, to very ill patients and to those with limited pulmonary reserve because of the possibility that apnea and/or cardiac arrest may occur. Concomitant use of barbiturates, alcohol, or other central nervous system depressants increases depression with increased risk of apnea. Resuscitive equipment including that necessary to support respiration should be rapidly available.

When Dizac is used with a narcotic analgesic, the dosage of the narcotic should be reduced by at least one-third and administered in small increments. In some cases the use of a narcotic may not be necessary.

Dizac should not be administered to patients in shock, coma, or in acute alcoholic intoxication with depression of vital signs. As is true of most CNS-acting drugs, patients receiving dizapam should be cautioned against engaging in hazardous occupations requiring complete mental alertness, such as operating machinery or driving a motor vehicle.

Tonic status epilepticus has been precipitated in patients treated with I.V. diazepam for petit mal status or petit mal variant status.

Pregnancy: An increased risk of congenital malformation associated with the use of minor tranquilizers (diazepam, meprobamate and chlordiazepoxide) during the first trimester of pregnancy has been suggested in several studies. Because use of these drugs is rarely a matter of urgency, their use during this period should almost always be avoided. The possibility that a woman of childbearing potential may be pregnant at the time of institution of therapy should be considered. Patients should be advised that if they become pregnant during therapy or intend to become pregnant they should communicate with their physicians about the desirability of discontinuing the drug.

In humans, measurable amounts of diazepam were found in maternal and cord blood, indicating placental transfer of the drug. Until additional information is available, Dizac is not recommended for obstetrical use.

Pediatric use: Efficacy and safety of parenteral diazepam has not been established in the neonate (30 days or less of age).

Prolonged central nervous system depression has been observed in neonates, apparently due to inability to bio-transform diazepam into inactive metabolites.

In pediatric use, in order to obtain maximal clinical effect with the minimum amount of drug and thus to reduce the risk of hazardous side effects, such as apnea or prolonged periods of somnolence, it is recommended that the drug be given slowly over a three-minute period in a dosage not to exceed 0.25 mg/kg. After an interval of 15 to 30 minutes the initial dosage can be safely repeated. If, however, relief of symptoms is not obtained after a third administration, adjunctive therapy appropriate to the condition being treated is recommended.

Withdrawal symptoms of the barbiturate type have occurred after the discontinuation of benzodiazepines. (See DRUG ABUSE AND DEPENDENCE section.)

PRECAUTIONS

Although seizures may be brought under control promptly, a significant proportion of patients experience a return to seizure activity, presumably due to the short-lived effect of diazepam after I.V. administration. The physician should be prepared to readminister the drug. However, diazepam is not recommended for maintenance, and once seizures are brought under control, consideration should be given to the administration of agents useful in longer term control of seizures.

If Dizac is to be combined with other psychotropic agents or anticonvulsant drugs, careful consideration should be given to the pharmacology of the agents to be employed—particularly with known compounds which may potentiate the action of diazepam, such as phenothiazines, narcotics, barbiturates, MAO inhibitors and other antidepressants. In highly anxious patients with evidence of accompanying depression, particularly those who may have suicidal tendencies, protective measures may be necessary. The usual precautions in treating patients with impaired hepatic function should be observed. Metabolites of diazepam are excreted by the kidney; to avoid their excess accumulation, caution should be exercised in the administration to patients with compromised kidney function.

Since an increase in cough reflex and laryngospasm may occur with peroral endoscopic procedures, the use of a topical anesthetic agent and the availability of necessary countermeasures are recommended.

Injectable diazepam has produced hypotension or muscular weakness in some patients particularly when used with narcotics, barbiturates or alcohol.

Lower doses (usually 2 mg to 5 mg) should be used for elderly and debilitated patients.

The clearance of diazepam and certain other benzodiazepines can be delayed in association with Tagamet (cimetidine) administration. The clinical significance of this is unclear.

Labor and Delivery: In humans, measurable amounts of diazepam were found in maternal and cord blood, indicating placental transfer of the drug. Until additional information is available, injectable diazepam is not recommended for obstetrical use.

ADVERSE REACTIONS

Side effects most commonly reported were drowsiness, fatigue and ataxia. Other adverse reactions less frequently reported include: *CNS:* confusion, depression, dysarthria, headache, hypoactivity, slurred speech, syncope, tremor, vertigo. *G.I.:* constipation, nausea. *G.U.:* incontinence, changes in libido, urinary retention. *Cardiovascular:* bradycardia, cardiovascular collapse, hypotension, venous thrombosis, and phlebitis at site of injection. *EENT:* blurred vision, diplopia, nystagmus. *Skin:* urticaria, skin rash. *Other:* hiccups, changes in salivation, neutropenia, jaundice. Paradoxical reactions such as acute hyperexcited status, anxiety, hallucinations, increased muscle spasticity, insomnia, rage, sleep disturbances and stimulation have been reported; should these occur, use of the drug should be discontinued. Minor change in EEG patterns, usually low-voltage fast activity, have been observed in patients during and after diazepam therapy and are of no known significance.

In peroral endoscopic procedures, coughing, depressed respiration, dyspnea, hyperventilation, laryngospasm and pain in throat or chest have been reported.

Because of isolated reports of neutropenia and jaundice, periodic blood counts and liver function tests are advisable during long-term therapy.

DRUG ABUSE AND DEPENDENCE

Controlled substance: Diazepam is a controlled substance listed in Schedule IV by the Drug Enforcement Administration.

Dependence: Withdrawal symptoms, similar in character to those noted with barbiturates and alcohol (convulsions, tremor, abdominal and muscle cramps, vomiting and sweating), have occurred following abrupt discontinuance of diazepam. The more severe withdrawal symptoms have usually been limited to those patients who had received excessive doses over an extended period of time. Generally milder withdrawal symptoms (e.g., dysphoria and insomnia) have been reported following abrupt discontinuance of benzodiazepines taken continuously at therapeutic levels for several months. Consequently, after extended therapy, abrupt discontinuation should generally be avoided and a gradual dosage tapering schedule followed. Addiction-prone individuals (such as drug addicts or alcoholics) should be under careful surveillance when receiving diazepam or other psychotropic agents because of the predisposition of such patients to habituation and dependence.

OVERDOSAGE

Manifestations of diazepam overdosage include sonmolence, confusion, coma, and diminished reflexes. Respiration, pulse and blood pressure should be monitored, as in all cases of drug overdosage, although, in general, these effects have been minimal. General supportive measures should be employed, along with intravenous fluids, and an adequate airway maintained. Hypotension may be combated by the use of norepinephrine or metaraminol. Dialysis is of limited value.

DOSAGE AND ADMINISTRATION

FOR INTRAVENOUS USE ONLY: Dizac is intended for intravenous use only and should <u>NOT</u> be administered intramuscularly or subcutaneously. Dosage should be individualized for maximum beneficial effect. The usual recommended dose in older children and adults ranges from 2 mg to 20 mg I.V., depending on the indication and its severity.

In some conditions, e.g., tetanus, larger doses may be required. (See dosage for specific indications): complete Prescribing Information. There are data comparing intravenously administered Dizac in females and males that are suggestive of (1) a slightly lower bioavailability of diazepam for females compared to males, and (2) for younger patients (age 20–55), a relative potency for females compared to males of roughly 2/3. In acute conditions the injection may be repeated within one hour although an interval of 3 to 4 hours is usually satisfactory. Lower doses (usually 2 mg to 5 mg) and slow increase in dosage should be used for elderly or debilitated patients and when other sedative drugs are administered. (See WARNINGS and ADVERSE REACTIONS.)

For dosage in infants above the age of 30 days and children, see the specific indications in complete Prescribing Information. Facilities for respiratory assistance should be readily available.

Intravenous use: (See WARNINGS, particularly for use in children.) The emulsion should be injected slowly, taking at least one minute for each 5 mg (1 mL) given. Do not use small veins, such as those on the dorsum of the hand or wrist. Extreme care should be taken to avoid intra-arterial administration or extravasation.

Do not add Dizac to infusion sets containing polyvinylchloride. Dizac is compatible with polyethylene-lined or glass infusion sets and polyethylene/polypropylene plastic syringes. Dizac is incompatible with morphine and glycopyrrolate.

Do not mix or dilute Dizac with other solutions or drugs in syringe or infusion container. If it is not feasible to administer Dizac directly I.V., it may be injected slowly through the infusion tubing as close as possible to the vein insertion. Once the acute symptomatology has been properly controlled with Dizac, the patient may be placed on therapy with an appropriate oral agent if further treatment is required.

Prior to use, refer to the DOSAGE AND ADMINISTRATION section in complete Prescribing Information.

HOW SUPPLIED

Dizac™ (diazepam injectable emulsion) For I.V. Administration Only, containing diazepam 5 mg per mL of emulsion (10mg/2mL), is available as follows:

2 mL single-dose ampul (10mg/2mL) packaged in 10s (NDC 10019-850-21)

Contains no preservatives. Discard unused portion.

Storage: Store at or below 25°C (77°F). Do not freeze. It has been demonstrated that Dizac can be exposed to temperature changes between 5°C and 30°C for a period of not more than 4 hours at least 20 times without deterioration of the emulsion quality. **PROTECT FROM LIGHT.**

REFERENCES

1. Data on file, Ohmeda Pharmaceutical Products Division. 2. Schou Olesen A. Huttel MG. Local reactions to i.v. diazepam in three different formulations. *Br J Anaesth.* 1960; 52:609-611. 3. Kawar P. Dundee JW. Frequency of pain on injection and venous sequelae following the i.v. administration of certain anesthetics and sedatives. *Br J Anaesth.* 1962; 54:935-939.

Manufactured for:
Ohmeda PPD Inc.
Liberty Corner, NJ 07938 USA
1 800 ANA DRUG
By:
Pharmacia AB
S-171-97 Stockholm, Sweden   330-701 A
DIZAC
TM of Pharmacia AB   (Rev. 12/95)

ENLON® ℞
[*ĕn'lŏn*]
(edrophonium chloride injection, USP)

ENLON-PLUS® ℞
[*ĕn'-lŏn' plŭs*]
(edrophonium chloride, USP and
atropine sulfate, USP) Injection

ETHRANE® ℞
[*ĕ'thrān*]
(enflurane, USP)
Liquid For Inhalation

FORANE® ℞
[*for'ān*]
(isoflurane, USP)
Liquid for Inhalation

REVEX® ℞
(nalmefene hydrochloride injection)

DESCRIPTION

REVEX® (nalmefene hydrochloride injection), an opioid antagonist, is a 6-methylene analogue of naltrexone. The chemical structure is shown below:

Molecular Formula: $C_{21}H_{25}NO_3 \cdot HCl$
Molecular Weight: 375.9, CAS # 58895-64-0
Chemical Name: 17-(Cyclopropylmethyl)-4,5α-epoxy-6-methylenemorphinan-3,14-diol, hydrochloride salt.

Nalmefene hydrochloride is a white to off-white crystalline powder which is freely soluble in water up to 130 mg/mL and slightly soluble in chloroform up to 0.13 mg/mL, with a pK_a of 7.6.

REVEX® is available as a sterile solution for intravenous, intramuscular, and subcutaneous administration in two concentrations, containing 100 μg or 1.0 mg of nalmefene free base per mL. The 100 μg/mL concentration contains 110.8μg of nalmefene hydrochloride and the 1.0 mg/mL concentration contains 1.108 mg of nalmefene hydrochloride per mL. Both concentrations contain 9.0 mg of sodium chloride per mL and the pH is adjusted to 3.9 with hydrochloric acid. Concentrations and dosages of REVEX® are expressed as the free base equivalent of nalmefene.

CLINICAL PHARMACOLOGY

Pharmacodynamics

REVEX® prevents or reverses the effects of opioids, including respiratory depression, sedation, and hypotension. Pharmacodynamic studies have shown that REVEX® has a longer duration of action than naloxone at fully reversing doses. REVEX® has no opioid agonist activity.

REVEX® is not known to produce respiratory depression, psychotomimetic effects, or pupillary constriction. No pharmacological activity was observed when REVEX® was administered in the absence of opioid agonists.

REVEX® has not been shown to produce tolerance, physical dependence, or abuse potential.

REVEX® can produce acute withdrawal symptoms in individuals who are opioid dependent.

Pharmacokinetics

Nalmefene exhibited dose proportional pharmacokinetics following intravenous administration of 0.5 mg to 2.0 mg. Pharmacokinetic parameters for nalmefene after a 1 mg intravenous administration in adult male volunteers are listed in Table 1.

**Table 1:   Mean (CV%) Nalmefene
Pharmacokinetic Parameters
In Adult Males Following a 1 mg Intravenous Dose**

Parameter	Young, N = 18	Elderly, N = 11
Age	19–32	62–80
C_p at 5 min. (ng/mL)	3.7 (29)	5.8 (38)
V_{dss} (L/kg)	8.6 (19)	8.6 (29)
V_c (L/kg)	3.9 (29)	2.8 (41)
$AUC_{o\text{-inf}}$ (ng-hr/mL)	16.6 (27)	17.3 (14)
Terminal $T_{1/2}$ (hr)	10.8 (48)	9.4 (49)
Cl_{plasma} (L/hr/kg)	0.8 (23)	0.8 (18)

Absorption

Nalmefene was completely bioavailable following intramuscular or subcutaneous administration in 12 male volunteers relative to intravenous nalmefene. The relative bioavailabilities of intramuscular and subcutaneous routes of administration were 101.5% ± 8.1% (Mean ± SD) and 99.7% ± 6.9%, respectively. Nalmefene will be administered primarily as an intravenous bolus, however, nalmefene can be given intramuscularly (IM) or subcutaneously (SC) if venous access cannot be established. While the time to maximum plasma nalmefene concentration was 2.3 ± 1.1 hours following intramuscular and 1.5 ± 1.2 hours following subcutaneous adminstrations, therapeutic plasma concentrations are likely to be reached within 5–15 minutes after a 1 mg dose in an emergency. Because of the variability in the speed of absorption for IM & SC dosing, and the inability to titrate to effect, great care should be taken if repeated doses must be given by these routes.

Distribution

Following a 1 mg parenteral dose, nalmefene was rapidly distributed. In a study of brain receptor occupancy, a 1 mg dose of nalmefene blocked over 80% of brain opioid receptors within 5 minutes after administration. The apparent volumes of distribution centrally (V_c) and at steady-state (V_{dss}) are 3.9 ± 1.1 L/kg and 8.6 ± 1.7 L/kg, respectively. Ultrafiltration studies of nalmefene have demonstrated that 45% (CV 4.1%) is bound to plasma proteins over a concentration range of 0.1 to 2μg/mL. An *in vitro* determination of the distribution of nalmefene in human blood demonstated that nalmefene distributed 67% (CV 8.7%) into red blood cells and 39% (CV 6.4%) into plasma. The whole blood to plasma ratio was 1.3 (CV 6.6%) over the nominal concentration range in whole blood from 0.376 to 30 ng/mL.

Metabolism

Nalmefene is metabolized by the liver, primarily by glucuronide conjugation, and excreted in the urine. Nalmefene is also metabolized to trace amounts of an N-dealkylated metabolite. Nalmefene glucuronide is inactive and the N-dealkylated metabolite has minimal pharmacological activity. Less than 5% of nalmefene is excreted in the urine unchanged. Seventeen percent (17%) of the nalmefene dose is excreted in the feces. The plasma concentration-time profile in some subjects suggests that nalmefene undergoes enterohepatic recycling.

Elimination

After intravenous administration of 1 mg REVEX® to normal males (ages 19–32), plasma concentrations declined biexponentially with a redistribution and a terminal elimination half-life of 41± 34 minutes and 10.8 ± 5.2 hours, respectively. The systemic clearance of nalmefene is 0.8 ± 0.2 L/hr/kg and the renal clearance is 0.08 ± 0.04 L/hr/kg.

Special Populations
Elderly

Dose proportionality was observed in nalmefene $AUC_{0\text{-inf}}$ following 0.5 to 2 mg intravenous administration to elderly male subjects. Following a 1 mg intravenous nalmefene dose, there were no significant differences between young (19–32 years) and elderly (62–80 years) adult male subjects with respect to plasma clearance, steady-state volume of distribution, or half-life. There was an apparent age-related decrease in the central volume of distribution (young: 3.9 ± 1.1 L/kg, elderly: 2.8 ± 1.1 L/kg) that resulted in a greater initial nalmefene concentration in the elderly group. While initial nalmefene plasma concentrations were transiently higher in the elderly, it would not be anticipated that this population would require dosing adjustment. No clinical adverse events were noted in the elderly following the 1 mg intravenous nalmefene dose.

Patients with Hepatic Impairment

Subjects with hepatic disease, when compared to matched normal controls, had a 28.3% decrease in plasma clearance of nalmefene (0.56 ± 0.21 L/hr/kg versus 0.78 ± 0.24 L/hr/kg, respectively). Elimination half-life increased from 10.2 ± 2.2 hours to 11.9 ± 2.0 hours in the hepatically impaired. No dosage adjustment is recommended since nalmefene will be administered as an acute course of therapy.

Patients with Renal Impairment

There was a statistically significant 27% decrease in plasma clearance of nalmefene in the end-stage renal disease (ESRD) population during interdialysis (0.57 ± 0.20 L/hr/kg) and a 25% decreased plasma clearance in the ESRD population during intradialysis (0.59 ± 0.18 L/hr/kg) compared to normals (0.79 ± 0.24 L/hr/kg). The elimination half-life was prolonged in ESRD patients from 10.2 ± 2.2 hours in normals to 26.1 ± 9.9 hours. (See **DOSAGE AND ADMINISTRATION**.)

Gender Differences

There has not been sufficient pharmacokinetic study to make a definitive statement as to whether the pharmacokinetics of nalmefene differs between the genders.

CLINICAL TRIALS

REVEX® has been administered to reverse the effects of opioids after general anesthesia and in the treatment of

Continued on next page

Ohmeda—Cont.

overdose. It has also been used to reverse the systemic effects of intrathecal opioids.

Reversal of Postoperative Opioid Depression
REVEX® (N=326) was studied in 5 controlled trials in patients who had received morphine or fentanyl intraoperatively. The primary efficacy criterion was the reversal of respiratory depression. A positive reversal was defined as both an increase in respiratory rate by 5 breaths per minute and a minimum respiratory rate of 12 breaths per minute. Five minutes after administration, initial single REVEX® doses of 0.1, 0.25, 0.5, or 1.0 μg/kg had effectively reversed respiratory depression in a dose-dependent manner. Twenty minutes after initial administration, respiratory depression had been effectively reversed in most patients receiving cumulative doses within the recommended range (0.1 to 1.0 μg/kg). Total doses of REVEX® above 1.0 μg/kg did not increase the therapeutic response. The postoperative administration of REVEX® at the recommended doses did not prevent the analgesic response to subsequently administered opioids.

Reversal of The Effect of Intrathecally Administered Opioids
Intravenous REVEX® at doses of 0.5 and 1.0 μg/kg was administered to 47 patients given intrathecal morphine. One to 2 doses of 0.5 and 1.0 μg/kg REVEX® reversed respiratory depression in most patients. The administration of REVEX® at the recommended doses did not prevent the analgesic response to subsequently administered opioids.

Management of Known or Suspected Opioid Overdose
REVEX® (N=284) at doses of 0.5 mg to 2.0 mg was studied in 4 trials of patients who were presumed to have taken an opioid overdose. REVEX® doses of 0.5 mg to 1.0 mg effectively reversed respiratory depression within 2 to 5 minutes in most patients subsequently confirmed to have opioid overdose. A total dose greater than 1.5 mg did not increase the therapeutic response.

INDICATIONS AND USAGE
REVEX® is indicated for the complete or partial reversal of opioid drug effects, including respiratory depression, induced by either natural or synthetic opioids.
REVEX® is indicated in the management of known or suspected opioid overdose.

CONTRAINDICATIONS
REVEX® is contraindicated in patients with a known hypersensitivity to the product.

WARNINGS
Use of REVEX® in Emergencies
REVEX®, like all drugs in this class, is not the primary treatment for ventilatory failure. In most emergency settings, treatment with REVEX® should follow, not precede, the establishment of a patent airway, ventilatory assistance, administration of oxygen, and establishment of circulatory access.

Risk of Recurrent Respiratory Depression
Accidental overdose with long-acting opioids [such as methadone and *levo*-alpha-acetylmethadol (LAAM)] may result in prolonged respiratory depression. Respiratory depression in both the postoperative and overdose setting may be complex and involve the effects of anesthetic agents, neuromuscular blockers, and other drugs. While REVEX® has a longer duration of action than naloxone in fully reversing doses, the physician should be aware that a recurrence of respiratory depression is possible, even after an apparently adequate initial response to REVEX® treatment.

Patients treated with REVEX® should be observed until, in the opinion of the physician, there is no reasonable risk of recurrent respiratory depression.

PRECAUTIONS
General
Cardiovascular Risks with Narcotic Antagonists
Pulmonary edema, cardiovascular instability, hypotension, hypertension, ventricular tachycardia, and ventricular fibrillation have been reported in connection with opioid reversal in both postoperative and emergency department settings. In many cases, these effects appear to be the result of abrupt reversal of opioid effects.
Although REVEX® has been used safely in patients with pre-existing cardiac disease, all drugs of this class should be used with caution in patients at high cardiovascular risk or who have received potentially cardiotoxic drugs. (See **DOSAGE AND ADMINISTRATION**.)

Risk Of Precipitated Withdrawal
REVEX®, like other opioid antagonists, is known to produce acute withdrawal symptoms and, therefore, should be used with extreme caution in patients with known physical dependence on opioids or following surgery involving high doses of opioids. Imprudent use or excessive doses of opioid antagonists in the postoperative setting has been associated with hypertension, tachycardia, and excessive mortality in patients at high risk for cardiovascular complications. (See **PRECAUTIONS**.)

Incomplete Reversal Of Buprenorphine
Preclinical studies have shown that nalmefene at doses up to 10 mg/kg (437 times the maximum recommended human dose) produced incomplete reversal of buprenorphine-induced analgesia in animal models. This appears to be a consequence of a high affinity and slow displacement of buprenorphine from the opioid receptors. Hence, REVEX® may not completely reverse buprenorphine-induced respiratory depression.

Drug Interactions
REVEX® has been administered after benzodiazepines, inhalational anesthetics, muscle relaxants, and muscle relaxant antagonists administered in conjunction with general anesthesia. It also has been administered in outpatient settings, both in trials in conscious sedation and in the emergency management of overdose following a wide variety of agents. No deleterious interactions have been observed.
Preclinical studies have shown that both flumazenil and nalmefene can induce seizures in animals. The coadministration of both flumazenil and nalmefene produced fewer seizures than expected in a study in rodents, based on the expected effects of each drug alone. Based on these data, an adverse interaction from the coadministration of the two drugs is not expected, but physicians should remain aware of the potential risk of seizures from agents in these classes.

Carcinogenesis, Mutagenesis, Impairment of Fertility
Nalmefene did not have mutagenic activity in the Ames test with five bacterial strains or the mouse lymphoma assay. Clastogenic activity was not observed in the mouse micronucleus test or in the cytogenic bone marrow assay in rats. However, nalmefene did exhibit a weak but significant clastogenic activity in the human lymphocyte metaphase assay in the absence but not in the presence of exogenous metabolic activation. Oral administration of nalmefene up to 1200 mg/m²/day did not affect fertility, reproductive performance, and offspring survival in rats.

Use in Pregnancy
PREGNANCY CATEGORY B
Reproduction studies have been performed in rats (up to 1200 mg/m²/day) and rabbits (up to 2400 mg/m²/day) by oral administration of nalmefene and in rabbits by intravenous administration up to 96 mg/m²/day (114 times the human dose). There was no evidence of impaired fertility or harm to the fetus. There are, however, no adequate and well-controlled studies in pregnant women. Because animal reproduction studies are not always predictive of human response, this drug should be used during pregnancy only if clearly needed.

Nursing Mothers
Nalmefene and its metabolites were secreted into rat milk, reaching concentrations approximately three times those in plasma at one hour and decreasing to about half the corresponding plasma concentrations by 24 hours following bolus administration. As no clinical information is available, caution should be exercised when REVEX® is administered to a nursing woman.

Use in Children
Safety and effectiveness of REVEX® in children have not been established.

Use in Neonates
The safety and effectiveness of REVEX® in neonates have not been established in clinical studies. In a preclinical study, nalmefene was administered by subcutaneous injection to rat pups at doses up to 205 mg/m²/day throughout maternal lactation without producing adverse effects. A preclinical study evaluating the irritancy of the dosage form following arterial and venous administration in animals showed no vascular irritancy.
REVEX® should only be used in the resuscitation of the newborn when, in the opinion of the treating physician, the expected benefits outweigh the risks.

ADVERSE REACTIONS
Adverse event information was obtained following administration of REVEX® to 152 normal volunteers and in controlled clinical trials to 1127 patients for the treatment of opioid overdose or for postoperative opioid reversal.
Nalmefene was well tolerated and showed no serious toxicity during experimental administration to healthy individuals, even when given at 15 times the highest recommended dose. In a small number of subjects, at doses exceeding the recommended REVEX® dose, nalmefene produced symptoms suggestive of reversal of endogenous opioids; such as have been reported for other narcotic antagonist drugs. These symptoms (nausea, chills, myalgia, dysphoria, abdominal cramps, and joint pain) were usually transient and occurred at very low frequency.
Such symptoms of precipitated opioid withdrawal at the recommended clinical doses were seen in both postoperative and overdose patients who were later found to have had histories of covert opioid use. Symptoms of precipitated withdrawal were similar to those seen with other opioid antagonists, were transient following the lower doses used in the postoperative setting, and more prolonged following the administration of the larger doses used in the treatment of overdose.

Tachycardia and nausea following the use of nalmefene in the postoperative setting were reported at the same frequencies as for naloxone at equivalent doses. The risk of both these adverse events was low at doses giving partial opioid reversal and increased with increases in dose. Thus, total doses larger than 1.0 μg/kg in the postoperative setting and 1.5 mg/70 kg in the treatment of overdose are not recommended.

Relative Frequencies of Common Adverse Reactions
With an Incidence Greater Than 1%
(all patients, all clinical settings)

Adverse Event	Nalmefene N=1127	Naloxone N=369	Placebo N=77
Nausea	18%	18%	6%
Vomiting	9%	7%	4%
Tachycardia	5%	8%	—
Hypertension	5%	7%	—
Postoperative pain	4%	4%	N/A
Fever	3%	4%	—
Dizziness	3%	4%	1%
Headache	1%	1%	4%
Chills	1%	1%	—
Hypotension	1%	1%	—
Vasodilatation	1%	1%	—

Incidence less than 1%
Cardiovascular: Bradycardia, arrhythmia
Digestive: Diarrhea, dry mouth
Nervous System: Somnolence, depression, agitation, nervousness, tremor, confusion, withdrawal syndrome, myoclonus
Respiratory: Pharyngitis
Skin: Pruritus
Urogenital: Urinary retention

The incidence of adverse events was highest in patients who received more than the recommended dose of REVEX®. Laboratory findings: Transient increases in CPK were reported as adverse events in 0.5% of the postoperative patients studied. These increases were believed to be related to surgery and not believed to be related to the administration of REVEX®. Increases in AST were reported as adverse events in 0.3% of the patients receiving either nalmefene or naloxone. The clinical significance of this finding is unknown. No cases of hepatitis or hepatic injury due to either nalmefene or naloxone were observed in the clinical trials.

DRUG ABUSE AND DEPENDENCE
REVEX® is an opioid antagonist with no agonist activity. It has no demonstrated abuse potential, is not addictive, and is not a controlled substance.

OVERDOSAGE
Intravenous doses of up to 24 mg of nalmefene, administered to healthy volunteers in the absence of opioid agonists, produced no serious adverse reactions, severe sign or symptoms, or clinically significant laboratory abnormalities. As with all opioid antagonists, use in patients physically dependent on opioids can result in precipitated withdrawal reactions that may result in symptoms that require medical attention. Treatment of such cases should be symptomatic and supportive. Administration of large amounts of opioids to patients receiving opioid antagonists in an attempt to overcome a full blockade has resulted in adverse respiratory and circulatory reactions.

DOSAGE AND ADMINISTRATION
IMPORTANT INFORMATION – DOSAGE FORMS
REVEX® is supplied in two concentrations that can be identified by their color coded container labels: a concentration suitable for postoperative use (100 μg/mL) in a blue labeled ampul containing ONE (1) mL and a concentration suitable for the management of overdose (1 mg/mL, 10 times as concentrated, 20 times as much drug) in a green labeled ampul and syringe, both containing TWO (2) mL. Proper steps should be taken to prevent use of the incorrect concentration.

General Principles
REVEX® should be titrated to reverse the undesired effects of opioids. Once adequate reversal has been established, additional administration is not required and may actually be harmful due to unwanted reversal of analgesia or precipitated withdrawal.

Duration of Action
The duration of action of REVEX® is as long as most opioid analgesics. The apparent duration of action of REVEX® will vary, however, depending on the half-life and plasma concentration of the narcotic being reversed, the presence or absence of other drugs affecting the brain or muscles of respiration, and the dose of REVEX® administered. Partially reversing doses of REVEX® (1 μg/kg) lose their effect as the drug is redistributed through the body, and the effects of these low doses may not last more than 30-60 minutes in the presence of persistent opioid effects. Fully reversing doses (1 mg/70 kg) have been shown to last many hours in both experimental and clinical studies, but may complicate the management of patients who are in pain, at high cardiovascular risk, or who are physically dependent on opioids.

The recommended doses represent a compromise between a desirable controlled reversal and the need for prompt response and adequate duration of action. Using higher dosages or shorter intervals between incremental doses is likely to increase the incidence and severity of symptoms related to acute withdrawal such as nausea, vomiting, elevated blood pressure, and anxiety.

Patients Tolerant To Or Physically Dependent On Opioids

REVEX® may cause acute withdrawal symptoms in individuals who have some degree of tolerance to and dependence on opioids. These patients should be closely observed for symptoms of withdrawal following administration of the initial and subsequent injections of REVEX®. Subsequent doses should be administered with intervals of at least 2-5 minutes between doses to allow the full effect of each incremental dose of REVEX® to be reached.

Recommended Doses for Reversal of Postoperative Opioid Depression

Use 100 μg/mL dosage strength (blue label) and see Table 2 for initial doses.

The goal of treatment with REVEX® in the postoperative setting is to achieve reversal of excessive opioid effects without inducing a complete reversal and acute pain. This is best accomplished with an initial dose of 0.25 μg/kg followed by 0.25 μg/kg incremental doses at 2-5 minute intervals, stopping as soon as the desired degree of opioid reversal is obtained. A cumulative total dose above 1.0 μg/kg does not provide additional therapeutic effect.

Table 2: Reversal of Postoperative Opioid Depression

Body Weight	mL of REVEX® 100 μg/mL Solution
50 kg	0.125
60 kg	0.150
70 kg	0.175
80 kg	0.200
90 kg	0.225
100 kg	0.250

In cases where the patient is known to be at increased cardiovascular risk, it may be desirable to dilute REVEX® 1:1 with saline or sterile water and use smaller initial and incremental doses of 0.1 μg/kg.

Management of Known or Suspected Opioid Overdose

Use 1.0 mg/mL dosage strength (green label).

The recommended initial dose of REVEX® for non-opioid dependent patients is 0.5 mg/70 kg. If needed, this may be followed by a second dose of 1.0 mg/70 kg, 2-5 minutes later. If a total dose of 1.5 mg/70 kg has been administered without clinical response, additional REVEX® is unlikely to have an effect. Patients should not be given more REVEX® than is required to restore the respiratory rate to normal, thus minimizing the likelihood of cardiovascular stress and precipitated withdrawal syndrome.

If there is a reasonable suspicion of opioid dependency, a challenge dose of REVEX® 0.1 mg/70 kg should be administered initially. If there is no evidence of withdrawal in 2 minutes, the recommended dosing should be followed.

REVEX® had no effect in cases where opioids were not responsible for sedation and hypoventilation. Therefore, patients should only be treated with REVEX® when the likelihood of an opioid overdose is high, based on a history of opioid overdose or the clinical presentation of respiratory depression with concurrent pupillary constriction.

Repeated Dosing

REVEX® is the longest acting of the currently available parenteral opioid antagonists. If recurrence of respiratory depression does occur, the dose should again be titrated to clinical effect using incremental doses to avoid over-reversal.

Hepatic and Renal Disease

Hepatic disease and renal failure substantially reduce the clearance of nalmefene (see **Pharmacokinetics**). For single episodes of opioid antagonism, adjustment of REVEX® dosage is not required. However, in patients with renal failure, the incremental doses should be delivered slowly (over 60 seconds) to minimize the hypertension and dizziness reported following the abrupt administration of nalmefene to such patients.

Loss of Intravenous Access

Should intravenous access be lost or not readily obtainable, a pharmacokinetic study has shown that a single dose of REVEX® should be effective within 5-15 minutes after intramuscular or subcutaneous doses of 1.0 mg. (See **Pharmacokinetics**.)

SAFETY AND HANDLING

REVEX® is distributed in sealed ampuls which represent no known risk to health care workers. REVEX® is also distributed in a disposable syringe. To insure patient safety, the needle should be handled with care and should be destroyed and discarded if damaged in any manner. If the cannula is bent, no attempt should be made to straighten it. To prevent needlestick injuries, needles should not be recapped, purposely bent, or broken by hand.

As with all parenterals, care should be taken to prevent the generation and inhalation of aerosols during preparation and use. Dermal absorption of spilled REVEX® should be prevented by prompt removal of contaminated clothing and rinsing the skin thoroughly with cool water.

HOW SUPPLIED

REVEX® (nalmefene hydrochloride injection) is available in the following presentations:

An ampul containing 1 mL of 100 μg/mL nalmefene base (Blue Label) Box of 10 (NDC 10019-315-21)

An ampul containing 2 mL of 1 mg/mL nalmefene base (Green Label) Box of 10 (NDC 10019-311-22)

A syringe containing 2 mL of 1 mg/mL nalmefene base (Green Label) (NDC 10019-311-32)

Syringe is supplied with 22 gauge × 1 1/4" needle. See the REVEX® Syringe Carton for "Directions for Use of the Syringe".

Store at controlled room temperature.

Manufactured for:
Ohmeda Pharmaceutical Products Division Inc,
Liberty Corner NJ 07938

Manufactured by:
Akorn Manufacturing Co.,
Decatur, IL 62525

REVEX® is a registered trademark of Baker Norton Pharmaceuticals, Inc.

For Product Inquiry 1 - 800 - ANA - DRUG
U.S. Pats 4,535,157 and 3,896,226
400 - 477 - 05 3-96

SUPRANE® ℞

[sū 'prān]
(desflurane, USP)

Suprane® (desflurane, USP) Volatile liquid for Inhalation.
The following is a Brief Summary, please see complete prescribing information before prescribing.

INDICATIONS AND USAGE

SUPRANE® (desflurane, USP) is indicated as an inhalation agent for induction and/or maintenance of anesthesia for inpatient and outpatient surgery in adults (see PRECAUTIONS).

SUPRANE® (desflurane, USP) is not recommended for induction of anesthesia in pediatric patients because of a high incidence of moderate to severe upper airway adverse events (see WARNINGS). After induction of anesthesia with agents other than SUPRANE®, and tracheal intubation, SUPRANE® is indicated for maintenance of anesthesia in infants and children.

CONTRAINDICATIONS

SUPRANE® (desflurane, USP) should not be used in patients with a known or suspected genetic susceptibility to malignant hyperthermia.

WARNINGS

Pediatric Use: SUPRANE® (desflurane, USP) is not recommended for induction of general anesthesia via mask in infants or children because of the high incidence of moderate to severe laryngospasm in 50% of patients, coughing 72%, breathholding 68%, increase in secretions 21% and oxyhemoglobin desaturation 26%.

SUPRANE® (desflurane, USP) should be administered only by persons trained in the administration of general anesthesia, using a vaporizer specifically designed and designated for use with desflurane. Facilities for maintenance of a patent airway, artificial ventilation, oxygen enrichment, and circulatory resuscitation must be immediately available.

Hypotension and respiratory depression increase as anesthesia is deepened

SUPRANE® (desflurane, USP) may present an increased risk in patients with a known sensitivity to halogenated anesthetic agents.

PRECAUTIONS

During the maintenance of anesthesia, increasing concentrations of SUPRANE® (desflurane, USP) produce dose-dependent decreases in blood pressure. Excessive decreases in blood pressure may be related to depth of anesthesia and in such instances may be corrected by decreasing the inspired concentration of SUPRANE®.

Concentrations of desflurane exceeding 1 MAC may increase heart rate. Thus an increased heart rate may not be a sign of inadequate anesthesia.

In patients with intracranial space occupying lesions, SUPRANE® (desflurane, USP) should be administered at 0.8 MAC or less, in conjunction with a barbiturate induction and hyperventilation (hypocapnia). Appropriate measures should be taken to maintain cerebral perfusion pressure (see CLINICAL STUDIES, Neurosurgery).

In patients with coronary artery disease, maintenance of normal hemodynamics is important to the avoidance of myocardial ischemia. Desflurane should not be used as the sole agent for anesthetic induction in patients with coronary artery disease or patients where increases in heart rate or blood pressure are undesirable. It should be used with other medications, preferably intravenous opioids and hypnotics (see CLINICAL TRIALS, Cardiovascular Surgery in complete Prescribing Information).

Inspired concentrations of SUPRANE® (desflurane, USP) greater than 12% have been safely administered to patients, particularly during induction of anesthesia. Such concentrations will proportionately dilute the concentration of oxygen; therefore, maintenance of an adequate concentration of oxygen may require a reduction of nitrous oxide or air if these gases are used concurrently.

The recovery from general anesthesia should be assessed carefully before patients are discharged from the post anesthesia care unit (PACU).

SUPRANE® (desflurane, USP), like some other inhalational anesthetics, can react with desiccated carbon dioxide (CO_2) absorbents to produce carbon monoxide which may result in elevated levels of carboxyhemoglobin in some patients. Case reports suggest that barium hydroxide lime and soda lime become desiccated when fresh gases are passed through the CO_2 absorber cannister at high flow rates over many hours or days. When a clinician suspects that CO_2 absorbent may be desiccated, it should be replaced before the administration of SUPRANE® (desflurane, USP).

Drug Interactions

No clinically significant adverse interactions with commonly used preanesthetic drugs, or drugs used during anesthesia (muscle relaxants, intravenous agents, and local anesthetic agents) were reported in clinical trials. The effect of desflurane on the disposition of other drugs has not been determined.

Like isoflurane, desflurane does not predispose to premature ventricular arrhythmias in the presence of exogenously infused epinephrine in swine.

BENZODIAZEPINES and OPIOIDS (MAC Reduction):

Benzodiazepines (midazolam 25–50 μg/kg) decrease the MAC of desflurane by 16% as do the opioids (fentanyl 3–6 μg/kg) by 50% (see DOSAGE AND ADMINISTRATION in complete Prescribing Information).

NEUROMUSCULAR BLOCKING AGENTS:

Anesthetic concentrations of desflurane at equilibrium (administered for 15 or more minutes before testing) reduced the ED_{95} of succinylcholine by approximately 30% and that of atracurium and pancuronium by approximately 50% compared to N_2O/opioid anesthesia. The effect of desflurane on duration of nondepolarizing neuromuscular blockade has not been studied.

DOSAGE OF MUSCLE RELAXANT CAUSING 95% DEPRESSION IN NEUROMUSCULAR BLOCKADE

Desflurane Concentration	Pancuronium	Mean ED_{95} (μg/kg) Atracurium	Succinylcholine
0.65 MAC 60% N_2O/O_2	26	123	—
1.25 MAC 60% N_2O/O_2	18	91	—
1.25 MAC O_2	22	120	362

Dosage reduction of neuromuscular blocking agents during induction of anesthesia may result in delayed onset of conditions suitable for endotracheal intubation or inadequate muscle relaxation, because potentiation of neuromuscular blocking agents requires equilibration of muscle with the delivered partial pressure of desflurane.

Among nondepolarizing drugs, only pancuronium and atracurium interactions have been studied. In the absence of specific guidelines:

1. For endotracheal intubation, do not reduce the dose of nondepolarizing muscle relaxants or succinylcholine.
2. During maintenance of anesthesia, the dose of nondepolarizing muscle relaxants is likely to be reduced compared to that during N_2O/opioid anesthesia. Administration of supplemental doses of muscle relaxants should be guided by the response to nerve stimulation.

Malignant Hyperthermia: In susceptible individuals, potent inhalation anesthetic agents may trigger a skeletal muscle hypermetabolic state leading to high oxygen demand and the clinical syndrome known as malignant hyperthermia. In genetically susceptible pigs, desflurane induced malignant hyperthermia. The clinical syndrome is signalled by hypercapnia, and may include muscle rigidity, tachycardia, tachypnea, cyanosis, arrhythmias, and/or unstable blood pressure. Some of these nonspecific signs may also appear during light anesthesia; acute hypoxia, hypercapnia, and hypovolemia.

Treatment of malignant hyperthermia includes discontinuation of triggering agents, administration of intravenous dantrolene sodium, and application of supportive therapy. (Consult prescribing information for dantrolene sodium intravenous for additional information on patient management.)

Continued on next page

Ohmeda—Cont.

Renal failure may appear later, and urine flow should be monitored and sustained if possible.

Renal or Hepatic Insufficiency
Nine patients receiving SUPRANE® (desflurane, USP) (N=9) were compared to 9 patients receiving isoflurane, all with chronic renal insufficiency (serum creatinine 1.5–6.9 mg/dL). No differences in hematological or biochemical tests, including renal function evaluation, were seen between the two groups. Similarly, no differences were found in a comparison of patients receiving either SUPRANE® (desflurane, USP) (N=28) or isoflurane (N=30) undergoing renal transplant.

Eight patients receiving SUPRANE® (desflurane, USP) were compared to six patients receiving isoflurane, all with chronic hepatic disease (viral hepatitis, alcoholic hepatitis, or cirrhosis). No differences in hematological or biochemical tests, including hepatic enzymes and hepatic function evaluation, were seen.

Carcinogenesis, Mutagenesis, Impairment of Fertility
Animal carcinogenicity studies have not been performed with SUPRANE® (desflurane, USP). *In vitro* and *in vivo* genotoxicity studies did not demonstrate mutagenicity or chromosomal damage by SUPRANE®. Tests for genotoxicity included the Ames mutation assay, the metaphase analysis of human lymphocytes, and the mouse micronucleus assay.
Fertility was not affected after 1 MAC-Hour per day exposure (cumulative 63 and 14 MAC-Hours for males and females, respectively). At higher doses, parental toxicity (mortalities and reduced weight gain) was observed which could affect fertility.
Teratogenic Effects: No teratogenic effect was observed at approximately 10 and 13 cumulative MAC-Hour exposures at 1 MAC-Hour per day during organogenesis in rats or rabbits. At higher doses increased incidences of post-implantation loss and maternal toxicity were observed. However, at 10 MAC-Hours cumulative exposure in rats, about 6% decrease in the weight of male pups was observed at preterm caesarean delivery.
Pregnancy Category B: There are no adequate and well-controlled studies in pregnant women. SUPRANE® (desflurane, USP) should be used during pregnancy only if the potential benefit justifies the potential risk to the fetus.
Rats exposed to desflurane at 1 MAC-hour per day from gestation day 15 to lactation day 21, did not show signs of dystocia. Body weight of pups delivered by these dams at birth and during lactation were comparable to that of control pups. No treatment related behavioral changes were reported in these pups during lactation.
Labor and Delivery: The safety of desflurane during labor or delivery has not been demonstrated.
Nursing Mothers: The concentrations of desflurane in milk are probably of no clinical importance 24 hours after anesthesia. Because of rapid washout, desflurane concentrations in milk are predicted to be below those found with other volatile potent anesthetics.
Geriatric Use: The average MAC for SUPRANE® (desflurane, USP) in a 70 year old patient is two-thirds the MAC for a 20 year old patient (see DOSAGE AND ADMINISTRATION).
Pediatric Use: SUPRANE® (desflurane, USP) is not recommended for induction of general anesthesia via mask in infants or children because of the high incidence of moderate to severe laryngospasm, coughing, breathholding and increase in secretions and oxyhemoglobin desaturation (see WARNINGS).
Neurosurgical Use: SUPRANE® (desflurane, USP) may produce a dose-dependent increase in cerebrospinal fluid pressure (CSFP) when administered to patients with intracranial space occupying lesions. Desflurane should be administered at 0.8 MAC or less, and in conjunction with a barbiturate induction and hyperventilation (hypocapnia) until cerebral decompression in patients with known or suspected increases in CSFP. Appropriate attention must be paid to maintain cerebral perfusion pressure (see CLINICAL STUDIES, Neurosurgery in full Prescribing Information).

ADVERSE REACTIONS

Adverse event information is derived from controlled clinical trials, the majority of which were conducted in the United States. The studies were conducted using a variety of premedications, other anesthetics, and surgical procedures of varying length. Most adverse events reported were mild and transient, and may reflect the surgical procedures, patient characteristics (including disease) and/or medications administered.
Of the 1,843 patients exposed to SUPRANE® (desflurane, USP) in clinical trials, 370 adults and 152 children were induced with desflurane alone and 687 patients were maintained principally with desflurane. The frequencies given reflect the percent of patients with the event. Each patient was counted once for each type of adverse event. They are presented in alphabetical order according to body system.

PROBABLY CAUSALLY RELATED: Incidence greater than 1%
Induction (use as a mask inhalation agent):

Adult patients (N=370):	Coughing 34%, breathholding 30%, apnea 15%, increased secretions*, laryngospasm*, oxyhemoglobin desaturation ($SpO_2 < 90\%$)*, pharyngitis*.
Pediatric patients (N=152):	Coughing 72%, breathholding 68%, laryngospasm 50%, oxyhemoglobin desaturation ($SpO_2 < 90\%$) 26%, increased secretions 21%, bronchospasm*. (See WARNINGS)

Maintenance or Recovery
Adult and pediatric patients (N=687):

Body as a Whole	Headache.
Cardiovascular:	Bradycardia, hypertension, nodal arrhythmia, tachycardia.
Digestive:	Nausea 27%, vomiting 16%.
Nervous system:	Increased Salivation.
Respiratory:	Apnea*, breathholding, cough increased*, laryngospasm*, pharyngitis.
Special Senses:	Conjunctivitis (conjunctival hyperemia).

*Incidence of events: 3%–10%

PROBABLY CAUSALLY RELATED: Incidence less than 1% and reported in 3 or more patients, regardless of severity (N=1,843)

Cardiovascular:	Arrhythmia, bigeminy, abnormal electrocardiogram myocardial ischemia, vasodilation.
Nervous System:	Agitation, dizziness.
Respiratory:	Asthma, dyspnea, hypoxia.

CAUSAL RELATIONSHIP UNKNOWN: Incidence less than 1% and reported in 3 or more patients, regardless of severity (N=1,843)

Body as a Whole:	Fever.
Cardiovascular:	Hemorrhage, myocardial infarct.
Metabolic and Nutrition:	Increased creatinine phosphokinase.
Musculoskeletal System:	Myalgia.
Skin and Appendages:	Pruritis.

See PRECAUTIONS for information regarding pediatric use and malignant hyperthermia.
Laboratory Findings: Transient elevations in glucose and white blood cell count may occur as with use of other anesthetic agents.

OVERDOSAGE

In the event of overdosage, or suspected overdosage, take the following actions: discontinue administration of SUPRANE® (desflurane, USP), maintain a patent airway, initiate assisted or controlled ventilation with oxygen, and maintain adequate cardiovascular function.

SAFETY AND HANDLING

Occupational Caution: There is no specific work exposure limit established for SUPRANE® (desflurane, USP). However, the National Institute for Occupational Safety and Health Administration has recommended an 8-hr, time-weighted average limit of 2 ppm for halogenated anesthetic agents in general (0.5 ppm when coupled with exposure to N_2O).
The predicted effects of acute overexposure by inhalation of SUPRANE® (desflurane, USP) include headache, dizziness or (in extreme cases) unconsciousness.
There are no documented adverse effects of chronic exposure to halogenated anesthetic vapors (Waste Anesthetic Gases or WAGs) in the workplace. Although results of some epidemiological studies suggest a link between exposure to halogenated anesthetics and increased health problems (particularly spontaneous abortion), the relationship is not conclusive. Since exposure to WAGs is one possible factor in the findings for these studies, operating room personnel, and pregnant women in particular, should minimize exposure. Precautions include adequate general ventilation in the operating room, the use of a well-designated and well-maintained scavenging system, work practices to minimize leaks and spills while the anesthetic agent is in use, and routine equipment maintenance to minimize leaks.

STORAGE

Store at room temperature, 15°–30°C (59°–86°F).
©1996 Ohmeda Pharmaceutical Products Division Inc
Manufactured By: Ohmeda Caribe Inc, Guayama, PR 00784
For: Ohmeda Pharmaceutical Products Division Inc, Liberty Corner NJ 07938   Rev. 7-95

110 Allen Road
PO Box 804
Liberty Corner NJ 07938 0804
1 800 ANA DRUG   96-005

Organon Inc.
375 MT. PLEASANT AVE.
WEST ORANGE, NJ 07052

Direct Inquiries to:
(201) 325-4500

Currently available products are listed below. For complete product line information and price lists, direct inquiries to Organon Inc. Customer Service. For specific product information, contact Organon Inc. Medical Services Department.

ARDUAN®   ℞
(pipecuronium bromide) for injection

HOW SUPPLIED
10 mL vials/10 mg—boxes of 6 vials—NDC-0052-0446-36

TICE® BCG   ℞
BCG VACCINE USP
(for Intravesical or Percutaneous use)

Distributed by Organon Inc.
(See page 1881 for complete product information.)

CALDEROL®   ℞
[*kal-dah 'rol*]
(calcifediol capsules, USP)

HOW SUPPLIED
20 µg (white, soft elastic capsules) bottle of 60
50 µg (orange, soft elastic capsules) bottle of 60
Shown in Product Identification Guide, page 325

CORTROSYN®   ℞

Cosyntropin is α 1–24 corticotropin, a synthetic subunit of ACTH.

HOW SUPPLIED
Box containing: 10 Vials of Cortrosyn® (cosyntropin) for injection 0.25 mg
10 ampuls of solvent (sodium chloride for injection, USP)

COTAZYM®   ℞
[*kōt 'a zīm*]
(pancrelipase capsules, USP)

DESCRIPTION
Cotazym® (pancrelipase capsules, USP) is a powder containing enzymes, principally lipase, with amylase and protease obtained from the pancreas of the hog. Each capsule contains not less than:
Lipase—8,000 USP Units
Protease—30,000 USP Units
Amylase—30,000 USP Units
Precipitated calcium carbonate 25 mg.
Each capsule also contains the inactive ingredients: cornstarch, gelatin, magnesium stearate, talc, FD&C green #3, FD&C yellow #10 as coloring and titanium dioxide.

INDICATIONS AND USAGE

It is indicated in conditions where pancreatic enzymes are either absent or deficient with resultant inadequate fat digestion. Such conditions include but are not limited to chronic pancreatitis, pancreatectomy, cystic fibrosis and steatorrhea of diverse etiologies.

CONTRAINDICATIONS

Known hypersensitivity to pork protein.

PRECAUTIONS

In the event that capsules are opened for any reason care should be taken so that powder is not inhaled or spilled on hands since it may prove irritating to the skin or mucous membranes.

ADVERSE REACTIONS

No adverse reactions have been reported. It should be noted, however, that extremely high doses of exogenous pancreatic enzymes have been associated with hyperuricosuria and hyperuricemia.

DOSAGE AND ADMINISTRATION

One to three capsules just prior to each meal or snack. Individual cases may require higher dosage and dietery adjustment.

STORAGE

Not to exceed 25°C (77°F). Store in dry place when opened.

DISPENSE

In tight container as defined in the USP.

SUPPLIED

Cotazym capsules (regular) bottles of 100 and 500. NDC # 0052-0381-91, NDC # 0052-0381-95.
Shown in Product Identification Guide, page 325

COTAZYM®-S ℞
[kōt 'a zĭm-s]
(pancrelipase, USP)
Enteric coated spheres

Each capsule contains not less than:

5,000	USP Units of Lipase
20,000	USP Units of Protease
20,000	USP Units of Amylase

HOW SUPPLIED

Bottles of 100 capsules
Bottles of 500 capsules
Shown in Product Identification Guide, page 325

DECA-DURABOLIN® Ⓒ ℞
(nandrolone decanoate injection, USP)

HOW SUPPLIED

50 mg/mL—2 mL vials—NDC-0052-0696-02
100 mg/mL—2 mL vials—NDC-0052-0697-02
200 mg/mL—1 mL vials—NDC-0052-0698-01

DESOGEN® ℞
(desogestrel and ethinyl estradiol) Tablets

PATIENTS SHOULD BE COUNSELED THAT THIS PRODUCT DOES NOT PROTECT AGAINST HIV INFECTION (AIDS) AND OTHER SEXUALLY TRANSMITTED DISEASES.

Caution: Federal law prohibits dispensing without prescription.

[See chemical structure at top of next column.]

DESCRIPTION

Desogen® 28 Tablets provide an oral contraceptive regimen of 21 white round tablets each containing 0.15 mg desogestrel (13-ethyl-11- methylene-18,19-dinor-17 alpha-pregn-4-en- 20-yn-17-ol) and 0.03 mg ethinyl estradiol (19-nor-17 alpha-pregna-1,3,5 (10)-trien-20-yne-3,17-diol). Inactive ingredients include vitamin E, corn starch, povidone, stearic acid, colloidal silicon dioxide, lactose, hydroxypropyl methylcellulose, polyethylene glycol, titanium dioxide and talc. Desogen® 28 also contains 7 green round tablets containing the following inactive ingredients: lactose, corn starch, magnesium stearate, FD&C Blue No. 2 aluminum lake, ferric oxide, hydroxypropyl methylcellulose, polyethylene glycol, titanium dioxide and talc.

DESOGESTREL

ETHINYL ESTRADIOL

CLINICAL PHARMACOLOGY

Pharmacodynamics

Combination oral contraceptives act by suppression of gonadotropins. Although the primary mechanism of this action is inhibition of ovulation, other alterations include changes in the cervical mucus, which increase the difficulty of sperm entry into the uterus, and changes in the endometrium which reduce the likelihood of implantation.

Receptor binding studies, as well as studies in animals and humans, have shown that 3-keto-desogestrel, the biologically active metabolite of desogestrel, combines high progestational activity with minimal intrinsic androgenicity (91,92). Desogestrel, in combination with ethinyl estradiol, does not counteract the estrogen-induced increase in SHBG, resulting in lower serum levels of free testosterone (96–99).

Pharmacokinetics

Desogestrel is rapidly and almost completely absorbed and converted into 3-keto-desogestrel, its biologically active metabolite. Following oral administration, the relative bioavailability of desogestrel, as measured by serum levels of 3-keto-desogestrel, is approximately 84%.

In the third cycle of use after a single dose of Desogen®, maximum concentrations of 3-keto-desogestrel of $2,805\pm1,203$ pg/mL (mean$\pm$SD) are reached at 1.4 ± 0.8 hours. The area under the curve ($AUC_{0-\infty}$) is $33,858\pm11,043$ pg/mL·hr after a single dose. At steady state, attained from at least day 19 onwards, maximum concentrations of $5,840\pm1,667$ pg/mL are reached at 1.4 ± 0.9 hours. The minimum plasma levels of 3-keto-desogestrel at steady state are $1,400\pm560$ pg/mL. The AUC_{0-24} at steady state is $52,299\pm17,878$ pg/mL·hr. The mean $AUC_{0-\infty}$ for 3-keto-desogestrel at single dose is significantly lower than the mean AUC_{0-24} at steady state. This indicates that the kinetics of 3-keto-desogestrel are non-linear due to an increase in binding of 3-keto-desogestrel to sex hormone-binding globulin in the cycle, attributed to increased sex hormone-binding globulin levels which are induced by the daily administration of ethinyl estradiol. Sex hormone-binding globulin levels increased significantly in the third treatment cycle from day 1 (150 ± 64 nmol/L) to day 21 (230 ± 59 nmol/L).

The elimination half-life for 3-keto-desogestrel is approximately 38 ± 20 hours at steady state. In addition to 3-keto-desogestrel, other phase I metabolites are 3α-OH-desogestrel, 3β-OH-desogestrel, and 3α-OH-5α-H-desogestrel. These other metabolites are not known to have any pharmacologic effects, and are further converted in part by conjugation (phase II metabolism) into polar metabolites, mainly sulfates and glucuronides.

Ethinyl estradiol is rapidly and almost completely absorbed. In the third cycle of use after a single dose of Desogen®, the relative bioavailability is approximately 83%.

In the third cycle of use after a single dose of Desogen®, maximum concentrations of ethinyl estradiol of 95 ± 34 pg/mL are reached at 1.5 ± 0.8 hours. The $AUC_{0-\infty}$ is $1,471\pm268$ pg/mL·hr after a single dose. At steady state, attained from at least day 19 onwards, maximum ethinyl estradiol concentrations of 141 ± 48 pg/mL are reached at about 1.4 ± 0.7 hours. The minimum serum levels of ethinyl estradiol at steady state are 24 ± 8.3 pg/mL. The AUC_{0-24}, at steady state is $1,117\pm302$ pg/mL·hr. The mean $AUC_{0-\infty}$ for ethinyl estradiol following a single dose during treatment cycle 3 does not significantly differ from the mean AUC_{0-24} at steady state. This finding indicates linear kinetics for ethinyl estradiol.

The elimination half-life is 26 ± 6.8 hours at steady state. Ethinyl estradiol is subject to a significant degree of presystemic conjugation (phase II metabolism). Ethinyl estradiol escaping gut wall conjugation undergoes phase I metabolism and hepatic conjugation (phase II metabolism). Major phase I metabolites are 2-OH-ethinyl estradiol and 2-methoxy-ethinyl estradiol. Sulfate and glucuronide conjugates of both ethinyl estradiol and phase I metabolites, which are excreted in bile, can undergo enterohepatic circulation.

INDICATIONS AND USAGE

Desogen® Tablets are indicated for the prevention of pregnancy in women who elect to use oral contraceptives as a method of contraception.

Oral contraceptives are highly effective. Table I lists the typical accidental pregnancy rates for users of combination oral contraceptives and other methods of contraception. The efficacy of these contraceptive methods, except sterilization, depends upon the reliability with which they are used. Correct and consistent use of these methods can result in lower failure rates.

TABLE I: LOWEST EXPECTED AND TYPICAL FAILURE RATES (%) DURING THE FIRST YEAR OF USE OF A CONTRACEPTIVE METHOD

Method	Lowest* Expected*	Typical**
Oral Contraceptives		3
combined	0.1	N/A
progestin only	0.5	N/A
Diaphragm with spermicidal		
cream or jelly	6	18
Spermicides alone (foam, creams, jellies and vaginal suppositories)	3	21
Vaginal Sponge		
nulliparous	6	18
parous	9	28
IUD (medicated)	2	3
Implant		
capsules	0.04	0.04
rods	0.03	0.03
Condom without spermicide	2	12
Cervical Cap	6	18
Periodic abstinence (all methods)	1–9	20
Female sterilization	0.2	0.4
Male sterilization	0.1	0.15
No contraception (planned pregnancy)	85	85

Adapted from J. Trussell, et al. Table 1, ref. #1.
N/A—Data not available.
* The author's best estimate of the percentage of women expected to experience an accidental pregnancy among couples who initiate a method (not necessarily for the first time) who use it consistently and correctly during the first year, if they do not stop for any other reason.
** This term represents "typical" couples who initiate use of a method (not necessarily for the first time), who experience an accidental pregnancy during the first year, if they do not stop use for any other reason.

In clinical trials with Desogen®, 2,004 subjects completed 19,181 cycles and a total of 12 pregnancies were reported. This represents an overall user-efficacy pregnancy rate of 0.81 woman-years. This rate includes patients who did not take the drug correctly.

CONTRAINDICATIONS

Oral contraceptives should not be used in women who currently have the following conditions:
- Thrombophlebitis or thromboembolic disorders
- A past history of deep vein thrombophlebitis or thromboembolic disorders
- Cerebral vascular or coronary artery disease
- Known or suspected carcinoma of the breast
- Carcinoma of the endometrium or other known or suspected estrogen-dependent neoplasia
- Undiagnosed abnormal genital bleeding
- Cholestatic jaundice of pregnancy or jaundice with prior pill use
- Hepatic adenomas or carcinomas
- Known or suspected pregnancy

WARNINGS

> **Cigarette smoking increases the risk of serious cardiovascular side effects from oral contraceptive use. This risk increases with age and with heavy smoking (15 or more cigarettes per day) and is quite marked in women over 35 years of age. Women who use oral contraceptives should be strongly advised not to smoke.**

The use of oral contraceptives is associated with increased risks of several serious conditions including myocardial infarction, thromboembolism, stroke, hepatic neoplasia, and gallbladder disease, although the risk of serious morbidity or mortality is very small in healthy women without underlying risk factors. The risk of morbidity and mortality in-

Continued on next page

Organon—Cont.

creases significantly in the presence of other underlying risk factors such as hypertension, hyperlipidemias, obesity and diabetes.

Practitioners prescribing oral contraceptives should be familiar with the following information relating to these risks.

The information contained in this package insert is principally based on studies carried out in patients who used oral contraceptives with formulations of higher doses of estrogens and progestogens than those in common use today. The effect of long term use of the oral contraceptives with formulations of lower doses of both estrogens and progestogens remains to be determined.

Throughout this labeling, epidemiological studies reported are of two types: retrospective or case control studies and prospective or cohort studies. Case control studies provide a measure of the relative risk of a disease, namely, a ratio of the incidence of a disease among oral contraceptive users to that among nonusers. The relative risk does not provide information on the actual clinical occurrence of a disease. Cohort studies provide a measure of attributable risk, which is the *difference* in the incidence of disease between oral contraceptive users and nonusers. The attributable risk does provide information about the actual occurrence of a disease in the population (Adapted from refs. 2 and 3 with the author's permission). For further information, the reader is referred to a text on epidemiological methods.

1. THROMBOEMBOLIC DISORDERS AND OTHER VASCULAR PROBLEMS

a. Myocardial infarction

An increased risk of myocardial infarction has been attributed to oral contraceptive use. This risk is primarily in smokers or women with other underlying risk factors for coronary artery disease such as hypertension, hypercholesterolemia, morbid obesity, and diabetes. The relative risk of heart attack for current oral contraceptive users has been estimated to be two to six (4-10). The risk is very low in women under the age of 30.

Smoking in combination with oral contraceptive use has been shown to contribute substantially to the incidence of myocardial infarctions in women in their mid-thirties or older with smoking accounting for the majority of excess cases (11). Mortality rates associated with circulatory disease have been shown to increase substantially in smokers, especially in those 35 years of age and older among women who use oral contraceptives. (See Table II)

TABLE II: Circulatory disease mortality rates per 100,000 women-years by age, smoking status and oral contraceptive use

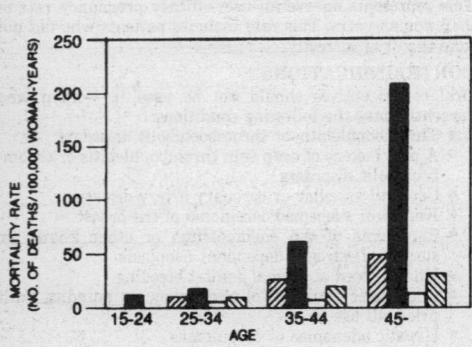

(Adapted from P.M. Layde and V. Beral, ref #12.)

Oral contraceptives may compound the effects of well-known risk factors, such as hypertension, diabetes, hyperlipidemias, age and obesity (13). In particular, some progestogens are known to decrease HDL cholesterol and cause glucose intolerance, while estrogens may create a state of hyperinsulinism (14-18). Oral contraceptives have been shown to increase blood pressure among users (see section 9 in Warnings). Similar effects on risk factors have been associated with an increased risk of heart disease. Oral contraceptives must be used with caution in women with cardiovascular disease risk factors.

b. Thromboembolism

An increased risk of thromboembolic and thrombotic disease associated with the use of oral contraceptives is well established. Case control studies have found the relative risk of users compared to nonusers to be 3 for the first episode of superficial venous thrombosis, 4 to 11 for deep vein thrombosis or pulmonary embolism, and 1.5 to 6 for women with predisposing conditions for venous thromboembolic disease (2,3,19-24). Cohort studies have shown the relative risk to be somewhat lower, about 3 for new cases and about 4.5 for new cases requiring hospitalization (25). The risk of thromboembolic disease associated with oral contraceptives is not related to length of use and disappears after pill use is stopped (2).

A two to four-fold increase in relative risk of postoperative thromboembolic complications has been reported with the use of oral contraceptives (9). The relative risk of venous thrombosis in women who have predisposing conditions is twice that of women without such medical conditions (26). If feasible, oral contraceptives should be discontinued at least four weeks prior to and for two weeks after elective surgery of a type associated with an increase in risk of thromboembolism and during and following prolonged immobilization. Since the immediate postpartum period is also associated with an increased risk of thromboembolism, oral contraceptives should be started no earlier than four weeks after delivery in women who elect not to breast feed.

c. Cerebrovascular diseases

Oral contraceptives have been shown to increase both the relative and attributable risks of cerebrovascular events (thrombotic and hemorrhagic strokes), although, in general, the risk is greatest among older (>35 years), hypertensive women who also smoke. Hypertension was found to be a risk factor for both users and nonusers, for both types of strokes, and smoking interacted to increase the risk of stroke (27-29).

In a large study, the relative risk of thrombotic strokes has been shown to range from 3 for normotensive users to 14 for users with severe hypertension (30). The relative risk of hemorrhagic stroke is reported to be 1.2 for non-smokers who used oral contraceptives, 2.6 for smokers who did not use oral contraceptives, 7.6 for smokers who used oral contraceptives, 1.8 for normotensive users and 25.7 for users with severe hypertension (30). The attributable risk is also greater in older women (3).

d. Dose-related risk of vascular disease from oral contraceptives

A positive association has been observed between the amount of estrogen and progestogen in oral contraceptives and the risk of vascular disease (31-33). A decline in serum high density lipoproteins (HDL) has been reported with many progestational agents (14-16). A decline in serum high density lipoproteins has been associated with an increased incidence of ischemic heart disease. Because estrogens increase HDL cholesterol, the net effect of an oral contraceptive depends on a balance achieved between doses of estrogen and progestogen and the nature and absolute amount of progestogens used in the contraceptives. The amount of both hormones should be considered in the choice of an oral contraceptive.

Minimizing exposure to estrogen and progestogen is in keeping with good principles of therapeutics. For any particular estrogen/progestogen combination, the dosage regimen prescribed should be one which contains the least amount of estrogen and progestogen that is compatible with a low failure rate and the needs of the individual patient. New acceptors of oral contraceptive agents should be started on preparations containing 0.035 mg or less of estrogen.

e. Persistence of risk of vascular disease

There are two studies which have shown persistence of risk of vascular disease for ever-users of oral con-

traceptives. In a study in the United States, the risk of developing myocardial infarction after discontinuing oral contraceptives persists for at least 9 years for women 40-49 years old who had used oral contraceptives for five or more years, but this increased risk was not demonstrated in other age groups (8). In another study in Great Britain, the risk of developing cerebrovascular disease persisted for at least 6 years after discontinuation of oral contraceptives, although excess risk was very small (34). However, both studies were performed with oral contraceptive formulations containing 0.050 mg or higher of estrogens.

2. ESTIMATES OF MORTALITY FROM CONTRACEPTIVE USE

One study gathered data from a variety of sources which have estimated the mortality rate associated with different methods of contraception at different ages (Table III). These estimates include the combined risk of death associated with contraceptive methods plus the risk attributable to pregnancy in the event of method failure. Each method of contraception has its specific benefits and risks. The study concluded that with the exception of oral contraceptive users 35 and older who smoke and 40 and older who do not smoke, mortality associated with all methods of birth control is low and below that associated with childbirth.

The observation of an increase in risk of mortality with age for oral contraceptive users is based on data gathered in the 1970's (35). Current clinical recommendation involves the use of lower estrogen dose formulations and a careful consideration of risk factors. In 1989, the Fertility and Maternal Health Drugs Advisory Committee was asked to review the use of oral contraceptives in women 40 years of age and over. The committee concluded that although cardiovascular disease risk may be increased with oral contraceptive use after age 40 in healthy non-smoking women (even with the newer low-dose formulations), there are also greater potential health risks associated with pregnancy in older women and with the alternative surgical and medical procedures which may be necessary if such women do not have access to effective and acceptable means of contraception. The Committee recommended that the benefits of low-dose oral contraceptive use by healthy non-smoking women over 40 may outweigh the possible risks.

Of course, older women, as all women who take oral contraceptives, should take an oral contraceptive which contains the least amount of estrogen and progestogen that is compatible with a low failure rate and individual patient needs.

[See table III below.]

3. CARCINOMA OF THE REPRODUCTIVE ORGANS AND BREASTS

Numerous epidemiological studies have been performed on the incidence of breast, endometrial, ovarian and cervical cancer in women using oral contraceptives. While there are conflicting reports most studies suggest that the use of oral contraceptives is not associated with an overall increase in the risk of developing breast cancer. Some studies have reported an increased relative risk of developing breast cancer, particularly at a younger age. This increased relative risk appears to be related to duration of use (36-43, 79-89).

Some studies suggest that oral contraceptive use has been associated with an increase in the risk of cervical intraepithelial neoplasia in some populations of women (45-48). However, there continues to be controversy about the extent to which such findings may be due to differences in sexual behavior and other factors.

4. HEPATIC NEOPLASIA

Benign hepatic adenomas are associated with oral contraceptive use, although the incidence of benign tumors is rare in the United States. Indirect calculations have estimated the attributable risk to be in the range of 3.3 cases/100,000 for users, a risk that increases after four or more years of use with oral contraceptives of higher dose (49). Rupture of rare, benign, hepatic adenomas may cause death through intra-abdominal hemorrhage (50,51).

TABLE III: ANNUAL NUMBER OF BIRTH-RELATED OR METHOD-RELATED DEATHS ASSOCIATED WITH CONTROL OF FERTILITY PER 100,000 NON-STERILE WOMEN, BY FERTILITY CONTROL METHOD ACCORDING TO AGE

Method of control and outcome	15–19	20–24	25–29	30–34	35–39	40–44
No fertility control methods*	7.0	7.4	9.1	14.8	25.7	28.2
Oral contraceptives non-smoker**	0.3	0.5	0.9	1.9	13.8	31.6
Oral contraceptives smoker**	2.2	3.4	6.6	13.5	51.1	117.2
IUD**	0.8	0.8	1.0	1.0	1.4	1.4
Condom*	1.1	1.6	0.7	0.2	0.3	0.4
Diaphragm/spermicide*	1.9	1.2	1.2	1.3	2.2	2.8
Periodic abstinence*	2.5	1.6	1.6	1.7	2.9	3.6

* Deaths are birth related
** Deaths are method related

(Adapted from H.W. Ory, ref. #35.)

Studies from Britain have shown an increased risk of developing hepatocellular carcinoma (52–54) in long-term (>8 years) oral contraceptive users. However, these cancers are rare in the U.S. and the attributable risk (the excess incidence) of liver cancers in oral contraceptive users approaches less than one per million users

5. OCULAR LESIONS

There have been clinical case reports of retinal thrombosis associated with the use of oral contraceptives. Oral contraceptives should be discontinued if there is unexplained partial or complete loss of vision; onset of proptosis or diplopia; papilledema; or retinal vascular lesions. Appropriate diagnostic and therapeutic measures should be undertaken immediately.

6. ORAL CONTRACEPTIVE USE BEFORE OR DURING EARLY PREGNANCY

Extensive epidemiological studies have revealed no increased risk of birth defects in women who have used oral contraceptives prior to pregnancy (56-57). The majority of recent studies also do not indicate a teratogenic effect, particularly in so far as cardiac anomalies and limb reduction defects are concerned (55, 56, 58, 59), when oral contraceptives are taken inadvertently during early pregnancy.

The administration of oral contraceptives to induce withdrawal bleeding should not be used as a test for pregnancy. Oral contraceptives should not be used during pregnancy to treat threatened or habitual abortion.

It is recommended that for any patient who has missed two consecutive periods, pregnancy should be ruled out before continuing oral contraceptive use. If the patient has not adhered to the prescribed schedule, the possibility of pregnancy should be considered at the time of the first missed period. Oral contraceptive use should be discontinued until pregnancy is ruled out.

7. GALLBLADDER DISEASE

Earlier studies have reported an increased lifetime relative risk of gallbladder surgery in users of oral contraceptives and estrogens (60,61). More recent studies, however, have shown that the relative risk of developing gallbladder disease among oral contraceptive users may be minimal (62-64). The recent findings of minimal risk may be related to the use of oral contraceptive formulations containing lower hormonal doses of estrogens and progestogens.

8. CARBOHYDRATE AND LIPID METABOLIC EFFECTS

Oral contraceptives have been shown to cause a decrease in glucose tolerance in a significant percentage of users (17). This effect has been shown to be directly related to estrogen dose (65). In general, progestogens increase insulin secretion and create insulin resistance, this effect varying with different progestational agents (17,66). In the nondiabetic woman, oral contraceptives appear to have no effect on fasting blood glucose (67). Because of these demonstrated effects, prediabetic and diabetic women should be carefully monitored while taking oral contraceptives.

A small proportion of women will have persistent hypertriglyceridemia while on the pill. As discussed earlier (see WARNINGS 1.a. and 1.d.), changes in serum triglycerides and lipoprotein levels have been reported in oral contraceptive users.

9. ELEVATED BLOOD PRESSURE

An increase in blood pressure has been reported in women taking oral contraceptives (68) and this increase is more likely in older oral contraceptive users (69) and with extended duration of use (61).

Data from the Royal College of General Practitioners (12) and subsequent randomized trials have shown that the incidence of hypertension increases with increasing progestational activity.

Women with a history of hypertension or hypertension-related diseases, or renal disease (70) should be encouraged to use another method of contraception. If women elect to use oral contraceptives, they should be monitored closely and if significant elevation of blood pressure occurs, oral contraceptive should be discontinued. For most women, elevated blood pressure will return to normal after stopping oral contraceptives (69), and there is no difference in the occurrence of hypertension among former and never users (68,70,71).

10. HEADACHE

The onset or exacerbation of migraine or development of headache with a new pattern which is recurrent, persistent or severe requires discontinuation of oral contraceptives and evaluation of the cause.

11. BLEEDING IRREGULARITIES

Breakthrough bleeding and spotting are sometimes encountered in patients on oral contraceptives, especially during the first three months of use. Nonhormonal causes should be considered and adequate diagnostic measures taken to rule out malignancy or pregnancy in the event of breakthrough bleeding, as in the case of any abnormal vaginal bleeding. If pathology has been excluded, time or a change to another formulation may

solve the problem. In the event of amenorrhea, pregnancy should be ruled out.

Some women may encounter post-pill amenorrhea or oligomenorrhea, especially when such a condition was pre-existent.

12. ECTOPIC PREGNANCY

Ectopic as well as intrauterine pregnancy may occur in contraceptive failures.

PRECAUTIONS

1. PHYSICAL EXAMINATION AND FOLLOW UP

It is good medical practice for all women to have annual history and physical examinations, including women using oral contraceptives. The physical examination, however, may be deferred until after initiation of oral contraceptives if requested by the woman and judged appropriate by the clinician. The physical examination should include special reference to blood pressure, breasts, abdomen and pelvic organs, including cervical cytology, and relevant laboratory tests. In case of undiagnosed, persistent or recurrent abnormal vaginal bleeding, appropriate measures should be conducted to rule out malignancy. Women with a strong family history of breast cancer or who have breast nodules should be monitored with particular care.

2. LIPID DISORDERS

Women who are being treated for hyperlipidemias should be followed closely if they elect to use oral contraceptives. Some progestogens may elevate LDL levels and may render the control of hyperlipidemias more difficult.

3. LIVER FUNCTION

If jaundice develops in any woman receiving such drugs, the medication should be discontinued. Steroid hormones may be poorly metabolized in patients with impaired liver function.

4. FLUID RETENTION

Oral contraceptives may cause some degree of fluid retention. They should be prescribed with caution, and only with careful monitoring, in patients with conditions which might be aggravated by fluid retention.

5. EMOTIONAL DISORDERS

Women with a history of depression should be carefully observed and the drug discontinued if depression recurs to a serious degree.

6. CONTACT LENSES

Contact lens wearers who develop visual changes or changes in lens tolerance should be assessed by an ophthalmologist.

7. DRUG INTERACTIONS

Reduced efficacy and increased incidence of breakthrough bleeding and menstrual irregularities have been associated with concomitant use of rifampin. A similar association, though less marked, has been suggested with barbiturates, phenylbutazone, phenytoin sodium, carbamazepine and possibly with griseofulvin, ampicillin and tetracyclines (72).

8. INTERACTIONS WITH LABORATORY TESTS

Certain endocrine and liver function tests and blood components may be affected by oral contraceptives:

a. Increased prothrombin and factors VII, VIII, IX and X; decreased antithrombin 3; increased norepinephrine-induced platelet aggregability.

b. Increased thyroid binding globulin (TBG) leading to increased circulating total thyroid hormone, as measured by protein-bound iodine (PBI), T4 by column or by radioimmunoassay. Free T3 resin uptake is decreased, reflecting the elevated TBG; free T4 concentration is unaltered.

c. Other binding proteins may be elevated in serum.

d. Sex-hormone binding globulins are increased and result in elevated levels of total circulating sex steroids; however, free or biologically active levels either decrease or remain unchanged.

e. High-density lipoprotein cholesterol (HDL-C) and triglycerides may be increased, while low-density lipoprotein cholesterol (LDL-C) and total cholesterol (Total-C) may be decreased or unchanged.

f. Glucose tolerance may be decreased.

g. Serum folate levels may be depressed by oral contraceptive therapy. This may be of clinical significance if a woman becomes pregnant shortly after discontinuing oral contraceptives.

9. CARCINOGENESIS

See WARNINGS section.

10. PREGNANCY

Pregnancy Category X. See CONTRAINDICATIONS and WARNINGS sections.

11. NURSING MOTHERS

Small amounts of oral contraceptive steroids have been identified in the milk of nursing mothers and a few adverse effects on the child have been reported, including jaundice and breast enlargement. In addition, oral contraceptives given in the postpartum period may interfere with lactation by decreasing the quantity and quality of breast milk. If possible, the nursing mother should

be advised not to use oral contraceptives but to use other forms of contraception until she has completely weaned her child.

12. GENERAL

PATIENTS SHOULD BE COUNSELED THAT THIS PRODUCT DOES NOT PROTECT AGAINST HIV INFECTION (AIDS) AND OTHER SEXUALLY TRANSMITTED DISEASES.

INFORMATION FOR THE PATIENT

See Patient Labeling Printed Below

ADVERSE REACTIONS

An increased risk of the following serious adverse reactions has been associated with the use of oral contraceptives (see WARNINGS section):

- Thrombophlebitis and venous thrombosis with or without embolism
- Arterial thromboembolism
- Pulmonary embolism
- Myocardial infarction
- Cerebral hemorrhage
- Cerebral thrombosis
- Hypertension
- Gallbladder disease
- Hepatic adenomas or benign liver tumors

The following adverse reactions have been reported in patients receiving oral contraceptives and are believed to be drug-related:

- Nausea
- Vomiting
- Gastrointestinal symptoms (such as abdominal cramps and bloating)
- Breakthrough bleeding
- Spotting
- Change in menstrual flow
- Amenorrhea
- Temporary infertility after discontinuation of treatment
- Edema
- Melasma which may persist
- Breast changes: tenderness, enlargement, secretion
- Change in weight (increase or decrease)
- Change in cervical erosion and secretion
- Diminution in lactation when given immediately postpartum
- Cholestatic jaundice
- Migraine
- Rash (allergic)
- Mental depression
- Reduced tolerance to carbohydrates
- Vaginal candidiasis
- Change in corneal curvature (steepening)
- Intolerance to contact lenses

The following adverse reactions have been reported in users of oral contraceptives and the association has been neither confirmed nor refuted:

- Pre-menstrual syndrome
- Cataracts
- Changes in appetite
- Cystitis-like syndrome
- Headache
- Nervousness
- Dizziness
- Hirsutism
- Loss of scalp hair
- Erythema multiforme
- Erythema nodosum
- Hemorrhagic eruption
- Vaginitis
- Porphyria
- Impaired renal function
- Hemolytic uremic syndrome
- Acne
- Changes in libido
- Colitis
- Budd-Chiari Syndrome

OVERDOSAGE

Serious ill effects have not been reported following acute ingestion of large doses of oral contraceptives by young children. Overdosage may cause nausea, and withdrawal bleeding may occur in females.

NON-CONTRACEPTIVE HEALTH BENEFITS

The following non-contraceptive health benefits related to the use of oral contraceptives are supported by epidemiological studies which largely utilized oral contraceptive formulations containing estrogen doses exceeding 0.035 mg of ethinyl estradiol or 0.05 mg of mestranol (73-78). Effects on menses:

- increased menstrual cycle regularity
- decreased blood loss and decreased incidence of iron deficiency anemia
- decreased incidence of dysmenorrhea

Continued on next page

Organon—Cont.

Effects related to inhibition of ovulation:
- decreased incidence of functional ovarian cysts
- decreased incidence of ectopic pregnancies

Effects from long-term use:
- decreased incidence of fibroadenomas and fibrocystic disease of the breast
- decreased incidence of acute pelvic inflammatory disease
- decreased incidence of endometrial cancer
- decreased incidence of ovarian cancer

DESOGEN®

DOSAGE AND ADMINISTRATION

To achieve maximum contraceptive effectiveness, Desogen® must be taken exactly as directed and at intervals not exceeding 24 hours. Desogen® may be initiated using either a Sunday start or a Day 1 start.

NOTE: Each cycle pack dispenser is preprinted with the days of the week, starting with Sunday, to facilitate a Sunday start regimen. Six different "day label strips" are provided with each cycle pack dispenser in order to accommodate a Day 1 start regimen. In this case, the patient should place the self-adhesive "day label strip" that corresponds to her starting day over the preprinted days.

IMPORTANT: The possibility of ovulation and conception prior to initiation of use of Desogen® should be considered. The use of Desogen® for contraception may be initiated 4 weeks postpartum in women who elect not to breast feed. When the tablets are administered during the postpartum period, the increased risk of thromboembolic disease associated with the postpartum period must be considered. (See CONTRAINDICATIONS and WARNINGS concerning thromboembolic disease. See also PRECAUTIONS for "Nursing Mothers".)

If the patient starts on Desogen® postpartum, and has not yet had a period, she should be instructed to use another method of contraception until a white tablet has been taken daily for 7 days.

SUNDAY START

When initiating a Sunday start regimen, another method of contraception should be used until after the first 7 consecutive days of administration.

Using a Sunday start, tablets are taken without interruption as follows: The first white tablet should be taken on the first Sunday after menstruation begins (if menstruation begins on Sunday, the first white tablet is taken on that day). One white tablet is taken daily for 21 days, followed by 1 green (inert) tablet daily for 7 days. For all subsequent cycles, the patient then begins a new 28-tablet regimen on the next day (Sunday) after taking the last green tablet. [If switching from a Sunday start oral contraceptive, the first Desogen tablet should be taken on the second Sunday after the last tablet of a 21 day regimen or should be taken on the first Sunday after the last inactive tablet of a 28 day regimen.]

If a patient misses 1 white tablet, she should take the missed tablet as soon as she remembers. If the patient misses 2 consecutive white tablets in Week 1 or Week 2, the patient should take 2 tablets the day she remembers and 2 tablets the next day; thereafter, the patient should keep taking 1 tablet daily until she finishes the cycle pack. The patient should be instructed to use a back-up method of birth control if she has intercourse in the 7 days after missing pills. If the patient misses 2 consecutive white tablets in the third week or misses 3 or more white tablets in a row at anytime during the cycle, the patient should keep taking 1 white tablet daily until the next Sunday. On Sunday the patient should throw out the rest of that cycle pack and start a new cycle pack that same day. The patient should be instructed to use a back-up method of birth control if she has intercourse in the 7 days after missing pills.

DAY 1 START

Counting the first day of menstruation as "Day 1", tablets are taken without interruption as follows: One white tablet daily for 21 days, then one green (inert) tablet daily for 7 days. For all subsequent cycles, the patient then begins a new 28-tablet regimen on the next day after taking the last green tablet. [If switching directly from another oral contraceptive, the first white tablet should be taken on the first day of menstruation which begins after the last ACTIVE tablet of the previous product.]

If a patient misses 1 white tablet, she should take the missed tablet as soon as she remembers. If the patient misses 2 consecutive white tablets in Week 1 or Week 2, the patient should take 2 tablets the day she remembers and 2 tablets the next day; thereafter, the patient should resume taking 1 tablet daily until she finishes the cycle pack. The patient should be instructed to use a back-up method of birth control if she has intercourse in the 7 days after missing pills. If the patient misses 2 consecutive white tablets in the third week or misses 3 or more white tablets in a row at anytime during the cycle, the patient should throw out the rest of that cycle pack and start a new cycle pack that same day. The patient should be instructed to use a back-up method of birth control if she has intercourse in the 7 days after missing pills.

ALL ORAL CONTRACEPTIVES

Breakthrough bleeding, spotting, and amenorrhea are frequent reasons for patients discontinuing oral contraceptives. In breakthrough bleeding, as in all cases of irregular bleeding from the vagina, nonfunctional causes should be borne in mind. In undiagnosed persistent or recurrent abnormal bleeding from the vagina, adequate diagnostic measures are indicated to rule out pregnancy or malignancy. If both pregnancy and pathology have been excluded, time or a change to another preparation may solve the problem. Changing to an oral contraceptive with a higher estrogen content, while potentially useful in minimizing menstrual irregularity, should be done only if necessary since this may increase the risk of thromboembolic disease.

Use of oral contraceptives in the event of a missed menstrual period:

1. If the patient has not adhered to the prescribed schedule, the possibility of pregnancy should be considered at the time of the first missed period and oral contraceptive use should be discontinued until pregnancy is ruled out.
2. If the patient has adhered to the prescribed regimen and misses two consecutive periods, pregnancy should be ruled out before continuing oral contraceptive use.

HOW SUPPLIED

Desogen® 28 contains 21 round white tablets and 7 round green tablets in a blister card within a recyclable plastic dispenser. Each white tablet (debossed with "TR5" on one side and "Organon" on the other side) contains 0.15 mg desogestrel and 0.03 mg ethinyl estradiol. Each green tablet (debossed with "KH2" on one side and "Organon" on the other side) contains inert ingredients.

Boxes of 6 NDC#0052-0261-06.

STORAGE: Store below 86°F (30°C)

CAUTION: Federal law prohibits dispensing without a prescription.

REFERENCES

1. Reproduced with permission of the Population Council from J. Trussell and K. Kost: Contraceptive failure in the United States: A critical review of the literature. Studies in Family Planning, 18 (5), September–October 1987. **2.** Stadel BV. Oral contraceptives and cardiovascular disease. (Pt.1). N Engl J Med 1981; 305: 612–618. **3.** Stadel BV. Oral contraceptives and cardiovascular disease. (Pt. 2). N Engl J Med 1981; 305: 672–677. **4.** Adam SA, Thorogood M. Oral contraception and myocardial infarction revisited: the effects of new preparations and prescribing patterns. Br J Obstet and Gynecol 1981; 88: 838–845. **5.** Mann JI, Inman WH. Oral contraceptives and death from myocardial infarction. Br Med J 1975; 2(5965):245–248. **6.** Mann JI, Vessey MP, Thorogood M, Doll R. Myocardial infarction in young women with special reference to oral contraceptive practice. Br Med J 1975 2(5956):241–245. **7.** Royal College of General Practitioners' Oral Contraception Study: Further analyses of mortality in oral contraceptive users. Lancet 1981 1:541–546. **8.** Sloan D, Shapiro S, Kaufman DW, Rosenberg L, Miettinen OS, Stolley PD. Risk of myocardial infarction in relation to current and discontinued use of oral contraceptives. N Engl J Med 1981; 305:420–424. **9.** Vessey MP. Female hormones and vascular disease-an epidemiological overview. Br J Fam Plann 1980; 6:1–12. **10.** Russell-Briefel RG, Ezzati TM, Fulwood R, Perlman JA, Murphy RS. Cardiovascular risk status and oral contraceptive use, United States, 1976-80. Prevent Med 1986; 15:352–362. **11.** Goldbaum GM, Kendrick JS, Hogelin GC, Gentry EM. The relative impact of smoking and oral contraceptive use on women in the United States. JAMA 1987 258:1339–1342. **12.** Layde PM, Beral V. Further analyses of mortality in oral contraceptive users: Royal College General Practitioners' Oral Contraception Study. (Table 5) Lancet 1981; 1:541–546. **13.** Knopp RH. Arteriosclerosis risk: the roles of oral contraceptives and postmenopausal estrogens. J Reprod Med 1986; 31(9) (Supplement):913–921. **14.** Krauss RM, Roy S, Mishell DR, Casagrande J, Pike MC. Effects of two low-dose oral contraceptives on serum lipids and lipoproteins: Differential changes in high-density lipoproteins subclasses. Am J Obstet 1983; 145:446–452. **15.** Wahl P, Walden C, Knopp R, Hoover J, Wallace R, Heiss G, Rifkind B. Effect of estrogen/progestin potency on lipid/lipoprotein cholesterol. N Engl J Med 1983; 308: 862–867. **16.** Wynn V, Niththyananthan R. The effect of progestin in combined oral contraceptives on serum lipids with special reference to high-density lipoproteins. Am J Obstet Gynecol 1982; 142:766–771. **17.** Wynn V, Godsland I. Effects of oral contraceptives and carbohydrate metabolism. J Reprod Med 1986; 31 (9) (Supplement):892–897. **18.** LaRosa JC. Atherosclerotic risk factors in cardiovascular disease. J Reprod Med 1986; 31 (9) (Supplement):906–912. **19.** Inman WH, Vessey MP. Investigation of death from pulmonary, coronary, and cerebral thrombosis and embolism in women of child-bearing age. Br Med J 1968; 2 (5599):193–199. **20.** Maguire MG, Tonascia J, Sartwell PE, Stolley PD, Tockman MS. Increased risk of thrombosis due to oral contraceptives: a further report. Am J Epidemiol 1979; 110 (2):188–195. **21.** Pettiti DB, Wingerd J, Pellegrin F, Ramacharan S. Risk of vascular disease in women: smoking, oral contraceptives, noncontraceptive estrogens, and other factors. JAMA 1979; 242:1150–1154. **22.** Vessey MP, Doll R. Investigation of relation between use of oral contraceptives and thromboembolic disease. Br Med J 1968; 2 (5599):199–205. **23.** Vessey MP, Doll R. Investigation of relation between use of oral contraceptives and thromboembolic disease. A further report. Br Med J 1969; 2 (5658):651–657. **24.** Porter JB, Hunter JR, Danielson DA, Jick H, Stergachis A. Oral contraceptives and non-fatal vascular disease-recent experience. Obstet Gynecol 1982; 59 (3):299–302. **25.** Vessey M, Doll R, Peto R, Johnson B, Wiggins P. A long-term follow-up study of women using different methods of contraception: an interim report. Biosocial Sci 1976; 8: 375–427. **26.** Royal College of General Practitioners: Oral contraceptives, venous thrombosis, and varicose veins. J Royal Coll Gen Pract 1978; 28:393–399. **27.** Collaborative Group for the Study of Stroke in Young Women: Oral contraception and increased risk of cerebral ischemia or thrombosis. N Engl J Med 1973; 288:871–878. **28.** Petitti DB, Wingerd J. Use of oral contraceptives, cigarette smoking, and risk of subarachnoid hemorrhage. Lancet 1978; 2:234–236. **29.** Inman WH. Oral contraceptives and fatal subarachnoid hemorrhage. Br Med J 1979; 2 (6203):1468–70. **30.** Collaborative Group for the Study of Stroke in Young Women: Oral contraceptives and stroke in young women: associated risk factors. JAMA 1975; 231:718–722. **31.** Inman WH, Vessey MP, Westerholm B, Engelund A. Thromboembolic disease and the steroidal content of oral contraceptives. A report to the Committee on Safety of Drugs. Br Med J 1970; 2:203–209. **32.** Meade TW, Greenberg G, Thompson SG. Progestogens and cardiovascular reactions associated with oral contraceptives and a comparison of the safety of 50- and 35-mcg oestrogen preparations. Br Med J 1980; 280 (6224):1157–1161. **33.** Kay CR. Progestogens and arterial disease-evidence from the Royal College of General Practitioners' Study. Am J Obstet Gynecol 1982; 142:762–765. **34.** Royal College of General Practitioners: Incidence of arterial disease among oral contraceptive users. J Royal Coll Gen Pract 1983; 33:75–82. **35.** Ory HW. Mortality associated with fertility and fertility control: 1983. Family Planning Perspectives 1983; 15: 50–56. **36.** The Cancer and Steroid Hormone Study of the Centers for Disease Control and the National Institute of Child Health and Human Development: Oral-contraceptive use and the risk of breast cancer. N Engl J Med 1986; 315:405–411. **37.** Pike MC, Henderson BE, Krailo MD, Duke A, Roy S. Breast cancer risk in young women and use of oral contraceptives: possible modifying effect of formulation and age at use. Lancet 1983; 2:926–929. **38.** Paul C, Skegg DG, Spears GFS, Kaldor JM. Oral contraceptives and breast cancer: A national study. Br Med J 1986; 293: 723–725. **39.** Miller DR, Rosenberg L, Kaufman DW, Schottenfeld D, Stolley PD, Shapiro S. Breast cancer risk in relation to early oral contraceptive use. Obstet Gynecol 1986; 68:863–868. **40.** Olson H, Olson KL, Moller TR, Ranstam J, Holm P. Oral contraceptive use and breast cancer in young women in Sweden (letter). Lancet 1985; 2:748–749. **41.** McPherson K, Vessey M, Neil A, Doll R, Jones L, Roberts M. Early contraceptive use and breast cancer: Results of another case-control study. Br J Cancer 1987; 56:653–660. **42.** Huggins GR, Zucker PF. Oral contraceptives and neoplasia: 1987 update. Fertil Steril 1987; 47:733–761. **43.** McPherson K, Drife JO. The pill and breast cancer: why the uncertainty? Br Med J 1986; 293:709–710. **44.** Shapiro S. Oral contraceptives—time to take stock. N Engl J Med 1987; 315:450–451. **45.** Ory H, Naib Z, Conger SB, Hatcher RA, Tyler CW. Contraceptive choice and prevalence of cervical dysplasia and carcinoma in situ. Am J Obstet Gynecol 1976; 124:573–577. **46.** Vessey MP, Lawless M, McPherson K, Yeates D. Neoplasia of the cervix uteri and contraception: a possible adverse effect of the pill. Lancet 1983; 2:930. **47.** Brinton LA, Huggins GR, Lehman HF, Malli K, Savitz DA, Trapido E, Rosenthal J, Hoover R. Long term use of oral contraceptives and risk of invasive cervical cancer. Int J Cancer 1986; 38:339–344. **48.** WHO Collaborative Study of Neoplasia and Steroid Contraceptives: Invasive cervical cancer and combined oral contraceptives. Br Med J 1985; 290:961–965. **49.** Rooks JB, Ory HW, Ishak KG, Strauss LT, Greenspan JR, Hill AP, Tyler CW. Epidemiology of hepatocellular adenoma: the role of oral contraceptive use. JAMA 1979; 242:644–648. **50.** Bein NN, Goldsmith HS. Recurrent massive hemorrhage from benign hepatic tumors secondary to oral contraceptives. Br J Surg 1977; 64:433–435. **51.** Klatskin G. Hepatic tumors: possible relationship to use of oral contraceptives. Gastroenterology 1977; 73:386–394. **52.** Henderson BE, Preston-Martin S, Edmondson HA, Peters RL, Pike MC. Hepatocellular carcinoma and oral contraceptives. Br J Cancer 1983; 48:437–440. **53.** Neuberger J, Forman D, Doll R, Williams R. Oral contraceptives and hepatocellular carcinoma. Br Med J 1986; 292:1355–1357. **54.** Forman D, Vincent TJ, Doll R. Cancer of the liver and oral contraceptives. Br Med J 1986; 292: 1357–1361. **55.** Harlap S, Eldor J. Births following oral contraceptive failures. Obstet Gynecol 1980; 55:447–452. **56.** Savolainen E, Saksela E, Saxen L. Teratogenic hazards of oral contraceptives analyzed in a national malformation register. Am J Obstet Gynecol 1981;

140:521–524. **57.** Janerich DT, Piper JM, Glebatis DM. Oral contraceptives and birth defects. Am J Epidemiol 1980; 112:73–79. **58.** Ferencz C, Matanoski GM, Wilson PD, Rubin JD, Neill CA, Gutberlet R. Maternal hormone therapy and congenital heart disease. Teratology 1980; 21:225–239. **59.** Rothman KJ, Fyler DC, Goldbatt A, Kreidberg MB. Exogenous hormones and other drug exposures of children with congenital heart disease. Am J Epidemiol 1979; 109:433–439. **60.** Boston Collaborative Drug Surveillance Program: Oral contraceptives and venous thromboembolic disease, surgically confirmed gallbladder disease, and breast tumors. Lancet 1973; 1:1399–1404. **61.** Royal College of General Practitioners: Oral contraceptives and health. New York, Pittman, 1974. **62.** Layde PM, Vessey MP, Yeates D. Risk of gallbladder disease: a cohort study of young women attending family planning clinics. J Epidemiol Community Health 1982; 36: 274–278. **63.** Rome Group for the Epidemiology and Prevention of Cholelithiasis (GREPCO): Prevalence of gallstone disease in an Italian adult female population. Am J Epidemiol 1984; 119:796–805. **64.** Strom BL, Tamragouri RT, Morse ML, Lazar EL, West SL, Stolley PD, Jones JK. Oral contraceptives and other risk factors for gallbladder disease. Clin Pharmacol Ther 1986; 39:335–341. **65.** Wynn V, Adams PW, Godsland IF, Melrose J, Niththyananthan R, Oakley NW, Seedj A. Comparison of effects of different combined oral-contraceptive formulations on carbohydrate and lipid metabolism. Lancet 1979; 1:1045–1049. **66.** Wynn V. Effect of progesterone and progestins on carbohydrate metabolism. In Progesterone and Progestin. Edited by Bardin CW, Milgrom E,Mauvis-Jarvis P. New York, Raven Press, 1983 pp. 395–410. **67.** Perlman JA, Roussell-Briefel RG, Ezzati TM, Lieberknecht G. Oral glucose tolerance and the potency of oral contraceptive progestogens. J Chronic Dis 1985; 38:857–864. **68.** Royal College of General Practitioners' Oral Contraception Study: Effect on hypertension and benign breast disease of progestogen component incombined oral contraceptives. Lancet 1977; 1:624. **69.** Fisch IR, Frank J. Oral contraceptives and blood pressure. JAMA 1977; 237:2499–2503. **70.** Laragh AJ. Oral contraceptive induced hypertension-nine years later. Am J Obstet Gynecol 1976; 126:141–147. **71.** Ramcharan S, Peritz E, Pellegrin FA, Williams WT. Incidence of hypertension in the Walnut Creek Contraceptive Drug Study cohort. In Pharmacology of Steroid Contraceptive Drugs. Garattini S, Berendes HW. Eds. New York, Raven Press, 1977 pp. 277–288. (Monographs of the Mario Negri Institute for Pharmacological Research, Milan). **72.** Stockley I. Interactions with oral contraceptives. J Pharm 1976; 216:140–143. **73.** The Cancer and Steroid Hormone Study of the Centers for Disease Control and the National Institute of Child Health and Human Development: Oral contraceptive use and the risk of ovarian cancer. JAMA 1983; 249:1596–1599. **74.** The Cancer and Steroid Hormone Study of the Centers for Disease Control and the National Institute of Child Health and Human Development: Combination oral contraceptive use and the risk of endometrial cancer. JAMA 1987; 257: 796–800. **75.** Ory HW. Functional ovarian cysts and oral contraceptives: negative association confirmed surgically. JAMA 1974; 228: 68–69. **76.** Ory HW, Cole P, Macmahon B, Hoover R. Oral contraceptives and reduced risk of benign breast disease. N Engl J Med 1976; 294:419–422. **77.** Ory HW. The noncontraceptive health benefits from oral contraceptive use. Fam Plann Perspect 1982;14:182–184. **78.** Ory HW, Forrest JD, Lincoln R. Making Choices: Evaluating the health risks and benefits of birth control methods. New York, The Alan Guttmacher Institute, 1983; p. 1. **79.** Schlesselman J, Stadel BV, Murray P, Lai S. Breast Cancer in relation to early use of oral contraceptives 1988; 259:1828–1833. **80.** Hennekens CH, Speizer FE, Lipnick RJ, Rosner B, Bain C, Belanger C, Stampfer MJ, Willett W, Peto R. A case-controlled study of oral contraceptive use and breast cancer. JNCI 1984;72:39–42. **81.** LaVecchia C, Decarli A, Fasoli M, Franceschi S, Gentile A, Negri E, Parazzini F, Tognoni G. Oral contraceptives and cancers of the breast and of the female genital tract. Interim results from a case-control study. Br. J. Cancer 1986; 54:311–317. **82.** Meirik O, Lund E, Adami H, Bergstrom R, Christoffersen T, Bergsjo P. Oral contraceptive use in breast cancer in young women. A Joint National Case-control study in Sweden and Norway. Lancet 1986; 11:650–654. **83.** Kay CR, Hannaford PC. Breast cancer and the pill-A further report from the Royal College of General Practitioners' oral contraception study. Br. J. Cancer 1988; 58:675–680. **84.** Stadel BV, Lai S, Schlesselman JJ, Murray P. Oral contraceptives and premenopausal breast cancer in nulliparous women. Contraception 1988; 38:287–299. **85.** Miller DR, Rosenberg L, Kaufman DW, Stolley P, Warshauer ME, Shapiro S. Breast cancer before age 45 and oral contraceptive use: New Findings. Am. J. Epidemiol 1989; 129:269–280. **86.** The UK National Case-Control Study Group, Oral contraceptive use and breast cancer risk in young women. Lancet 1989; 1:973–982. **87.** Schlesselman JJ. Cancer of the breast and reproductive tract in relation to use of oral contraceptives. Contraception 1989; 40:1–38. **88.** Vessey MP, McPherson K, Villard-Mackintosh L, Yeates D. Oral contraceptives and breast cancer: latest findings in a large cohert study. Br. J. Cancer 1989; 59:613–617. **89.** Jick SS, Walker AM, Stergachis A, Jick H. Oral contraceptives and breast cancer. Br. J. Cancer 1989; 59:618–621. **90.** Godsland, I et al. The effects of different formulations of oral contraceptive agents on lipid and carbohydrate metabolism. N Engl J Med 1990;323:1375–81. **91.** Kloosterboer, HJ et al. Selectivity in progesterone and androgen receptor binding of progestogens used in oral contraception. Contraception, 1988;38:325–32. **92.** Van der Vies, J and de Visser, J. Endocrinological studies with desogestrel. Arzneim. Forsch./Drug Res., 1983;33(I),2:231–6. **93.** Data on file, Organon Inc.. **94.** Fotherby, K. Oral contraceptives, lipids and cardiovascular diseases. Contraception, 1985; Vol. 31; 4:367–94. **95.** Lawrence, DM et al. Reduced sex hormone binding globulin and derived free testosterone levels in women with severe acne. Clinical Endocrinology, 1981;15:87–91. **96.** Cullberg, G et al. Effects of a low-dose desogestrel-ethinyl estradiol combination on hirsutism, androgens and sex hormone binding globulin in women with a polycystic ovary syndrome. Acta Obstet Gynecol Scand, 1985;64:195–202. **97.** Jung-Hoffmann, C and Kuhl, H. Divergent effects of two low-dose oral contraceptives on sex hormone-binding globulin and free testosterone. AJOG, 1987;156:199–203. **98.** Hammond, G et al. Serum steroid binding protein concentrations, distribution of progestogens, and bioavailability of testosterone during treatment with contraceptives containing desogestrel or levonorgestrel. Fertil. Steril., 1984;42:44–51. **99.** Palatsi, R et al. Serum total and unbound testosterone and sex hormone binding globulin (SHBG) in female acne patients treated with two different oral contraceptives. Acta Derm Venereol, 1984; 64:517-23.

BRIEF SUMMARY

PATIENT PACKAGE INSERT

THIS PRODUCT (LIKE ALL ORAL CONTRACEPTIVES) IS INTENDED TO PREVENT PREGNANCY. IT DOES NOT PROTECT AGAINST HIV INFECTION (AIDS) AND OTHER SEXUALLY TRANSMITTED DISEASES.

Oral contraceptives, also known as "birth control pills" or "the pill", are taken to prevent pregnancy, and when taken correctly, have a failure rate of about 1% per year when used without missing any pills. The typical failure rate of large numbers of pill users is less than 3% per year when women who miss pills are included. For most women, oral contraceptives are also free of serious or unpleasant side effects. However, forgetting to take pills considerably increases the chances of pregnancy.

For the majority of women, oral contraceptives can be taken safely. But there are some women who are at high risk of developing certain serious diseases that can be life-threatening or may cause temporary or permanent disability. The risks associated with taking oral contraceptives increase significantly if you:

- smoke
- have high blood pressure, diabetes, high cholesterol
- have or have had clotting disorders, heart attack, stroke, angina pectoris, cancer of the breast or sex organs, jaundice or malignant or benign liver tumors

Although cardiovascular disease risks may be increased with oral contraceptive use after age 40 in healthy, non-smoking women (even with the newer low-dose formulations), there are also greater potential health risks associated with pregnancy in older women.

You should not take the pill if you suspect you are pregnant or have unexplained vaginal bleeding.

Cigarette smoking increases the risk of serious cardiovascular side effects from oral contraceptive use. This risk increases with age and with heavy smoking (15 or more cigarettes per day) and is quite marked in women over 35 years of age. Women who use oral contraceptives are strongly advised not to smoke.

Most side effects of the pill are not serious. The most common such effects are nausea, vomiting, bleeding between menstrual periods, weight gain, breast tenderness, headache, and difficulty wearing contact lenses. These side effects, especially nausea and vomiting, may subside within the first three months of use.

The serious side effects of the pill occur very infrequently, especially if you are in good health and are young. However, you should know that the following medical conditions have been associated with or made worse by the pill:

1. Blood clots in the legs (thrombophlebitis) or lungs (pulmonary embolism), stoppage or rupture of a blood vessel in the brain (stroke), blockage of blood vessels in the heart (heart attack or angina pectoris) or other organs of the body. As mentioned above, smoking increases the risk of heart attacks and strokes, and subsequent serious medical consequences.
2. Liver tumors, which may rupture and cause severe bleeding. A possible but not definite association has been found with the pill and liver cancer. However, liver cancers are extremely rare. The chance of developing liver cancer from using the pill is thus even rarer.
3. High blood pressure, although blood pressure usually returns to normal when the pill is stopped.

The symptoms associated with these serious side effects are discussed in the detailed patient labeling given to you with your supply of pills. Notify your doctor or clinic if you notice any unusual physical disturbances while taking the pill. In addition, drugs such as rifampin, as well as some anticonvulsants and some antibiotics may decrease oral contraceptive effectiveness.

There is conflict among studies regarding breast cancer and oral contraceptive use. Some studies have reported an increase in the risk of developing breast cancer, particularly at a younger age. This increased risk appears to be related to duration of use. The majority of studies have found no overall increase in the risk of developing breast cancer. Some studies have found an increase in the incidence of cancer of the cervix in women who use oral contraceptives. However, this finding may be related to factors other than the use of oral contraceptives. There is insufficient evidence to rule out the possibility that pills may cause such cancers.

Taking the combination pill provides some important non-contraceptive benefits. These include less painful menstruation, less menstrual blood loss and anemia, fewer pelvic infections, and fewer cancers of the ovary and the lining of the uterus.

Be sure to discuss any medical condition you may have with your doctor or clinic. Your doctor or clinic will take a medical and family history before prescribing oral contraceptives and will examine you. The physical examination may be delayed to another time if you request it and your doctor or clinic believes that it is a good medical practice to postpone it. You should be reexamined at least once a year while taking oral contraceptives. The detailed patient information labeling gives you further information which you should read and discuss with your doctor or clinic.

DETAILED PATIENT LABELING

THIS PRODUCT (LIKE ALL ORAL CONTRACEPTIVES) IS INTENDED TO PREVENT PREGNANCY. IT DOES NOT PROTECT AGAINST HIV INFECTION (AIDS) AND OTHER SEXUALLY TRANSMITTED DISEASES.

PLEASE NOTE: This labeling is revised from time to time as important new medical information becomes available. Therefore, please review this labeling carefully.

The following oral contraceptive product contains a combination of progestogen and estrogen, the two kinds of female hormones:

Desogen® 28 Day Regimen

Each white tablet contains 0.15 mg desogestrel and 0.030 mg ethinyl estradiol. Each green tablet contains inert ingredients.

INTRODUCTION

Any woman who considers using oral contraceptives (the birth control pill or the pill) should understand the benefits and risks of using this form of birth control. This patient labeling will give you much of the information you will need to make this decision and will also help you determine if you are at risk of developing any of the serious side effects of the pill. It will tell you how to use the pill properly so that it will be as effective as possible. However, this labeling is not a replacement for a careful discussion between you and your doctor or clinic. You should discuss the information provided in this labeling with him or her, both when you first start taking the pill and during your revisits. You should also follow your doctor's or clinic's advice with regard to regular check-ups while you are on the pill.

EFFECTIVENESS OF ORAL CONTRACEPTIVES

Oral contraceptives or "birth control pills" or "the pill" are used to prevent pregnancy and are more effective than other non-surgical methods of birth control. When they are taken correctly, the chance of becoming pregnant is less than 1% (1 pregnancy per 100 women per year of use) when used perfectly, without missing any pills. Typical failure rates are actually 3% per year. The chance of becoming pregnant increases with each missed pill during a menstrual cycle.

In comparison, typical failure rates for other non-surgical methods of birth control during the first year of use are as follows:

IUD: 3%
Diaphragm with spermicides: 18%
Spermicides alone: 21%
Vaginal sponge: 18 to 28%
Implant: 0.03%
Condom alone: 12%
Periodic abstinence: 20%
No methods: 85%

WHO SHOULD NOT TAKE ORAL CONTRACEPTIVES

Cigarette smoking increases the risk of serious cardiovascular side effects from oral contraceptive use. This risk increases with age and with heavy smoking (15 or more cigarettesper day) and is quite marked in women over 35 years of age. Women who use oral contraceptives are strongly advised not to smoke.

Continued on next page

Organon—Cont.

Some women should not use the pill. For example, you should not take the pill if you are pregnant or think you may be pregnant. You should also not use the pill if you have any of the following conditions:

- A history of heart attack or stroke
- Blood clots in the legs (thrombophlebitis), lungs (pulmonary embolism), or eyes
- A history of blood clots in the deep veins of your legs
- Chest pain (angina pectoris)
- Known or suspected breast cancer or cancer of the lining of the uterus, cervix or vagina
- Unexplained vaginal bleeding (until a diagnosis is reached by your doctor)
- Yellowing of the whites of the eyes or of the skin (jaundice) during pregnancy or during previous use of the pill
- Liver tumor (benign or cancerous)
- Known or suspected pregnancy

Tell your doctor or clinic if you have ever had any of these conditions. Your doctor or clinic can recommend a safer method of birth control.

OTHER CONSIDERATIONS BEFORE TAKING ORAL CONTRACEPTIVES

Tell your doctor or clinic if you have or have had:

- Breast nodules, fibrocystic disease of the breast, an abnormal breast x-ray or mammogram
- Diabetes
- Elevated cholesterol or triglycerides
- High blood pressure
- Migraine or other headaches or epilepsy
- Mental depression
- Gallbladder, heart or kidney disease
- History of scanty or irregular menstrual periods

Women with any of these conditions should be checked often by their doctor or clinic if they choose to use oral contraceptives.

Also, be sure to inform your doctor or clinic if you smoke or are on any medications.

RISKS OF TAKING ORAL CONTRACEPTIVES

1. Risk of developing blood clots

Blood clots and blockage of blood vessels are one of the most serious side effects of taking oral contraceptives and can cause death or serious disability. In particular, a clot in one of the legs can cause thrombophlebitis and a clot that travels to the lungs can cause a sudden blocking of the vessel carrying blood to the lungs. Rarely, clots occur in the blood vessels of the eye and may cause blindness, double vision, or impaired vision.

If you take oral contraceptives and need elective surgery, need to stay in bed for a prolonged illness or have recently delivered a baby, you may be at risk of developing blood clots. You should consult your doctor or clinic about stopping oral contraceptives three to four weeks before surgery and not taking oral contraceptives for two weeks after surgery or during bed rest. You should also not take oral contraceptives soon after delivery of a baby. It is advisable to wait for at least four weeks after delivery if you are not breast feeding or four weeks after a second trimester abortion. If you are breast feeding, you should wait until you have weaned your child before using the pill. (See also the section on Breast Feeding in General Precautions.)

The risk of circulatory disease in oral contraceptive users may be higher in users of high dose pills and may be greater with longer duration of oral contraceptive use. In addition, some of these increased risks may continue for a number of years after stopping oral contraceptives. The risk of abnormal blood clotting increases with age in both users and nonusers of oral contraceptives, but the increased risk from the oral contraceptive appears to be present at all ages. For women aged 20 to 44 it is estimated that about 1 in 2,000 using oral contraceptives will be hospitalized each year because of abnormal clotting. Among nonusers in the same age group, about 1 in 20,000 would be hospitalized each year. For oral contraceptive users in general, it has been estimated that in women between the ages of 15 and 34 the risk of death due to a circulatory disorder is about 1 in 12,000 per year, whereas for nonusers the rate is about 1 in 50,000 per year. In the age group 35 to 44, the risk is estimated to be about 1 in 2,500 per year for oral contraceptive users and about 1 in 10,000 per year for nonusers.

2. Heart attacks and strokes

Oral contraceptives may increase the tendency to develop strokes (stoppage or rupture of blood vessels in the brain) and angina pectoris and heart attacks (blockage of blood vessels in the heart). Any of these conditions can cause death or serious disability.

Smoking greatly increases the possibility of suffering heart attacks and strokes. Furthermore, smoking and the use of oral contraceptives greatly increase the chances of developing and dying of heart disease.

3. Gallbladder disease

Oral contraceptive users probably have a greater risk than nonusers of having gallbladder disease, although this risk may be related to pills containing high doses of estrogens.

4. Liver tumors

In rare cases, oral contraceptives can cause benign but dangerous liver tumors. These benign liver tumors can rupture and cause fatal internal bleeding. In addition, a possible but not definite association has been found with the pill and liver cancers in two studies, in which a few women who developed these very rare cancers were found to have used oral contraceptives for long periods. However, liver cancers are rare.

5. Cancer of the reproductive organs and breasts

There is conflict among studies regarding breast cancer and oral contraceptive use. Some studies have reported an increase in the risk of developing breast cancer, particularly at a younger age. This increased risk appears to be related to duration of use. The majority of studies have found no overall increase in the risk of developing breast cancer.

Some studies have found an increase in the incidence of cancer of the cervix in women who use oral contraceptives. However, this finding may be related to factors other than the use of oral contraceptives. There is insufficient evidence to rule out the possibility that pills may cause such cancers.

ESTIMATED RISK OF DEATH FROM A BIRTH CONTROL METHOD OR PREGNANCY

All methods of birth control and pregnancy are associated with a risk of developing certain diseases which may lead to disability or death. An estimate of the number of deaths associated with different methods of birth control and pregnancy has been calculated and is shown in the following table.

[See table below.]

In the above table, the risk of death from any birth control method is less than the risk of childbirth, except for oral contraceptive users over the age of 35 who smoke and pill users over the age of 40 even if they do not smoke. It can be seen in the table that for women aged 15 to 39, the risk of death was highest with pregnancy (7-26 deaths per 100,000 women, depending on age). Among pill users who do not smoke, the risk of death was always lower than that associated with pregnancy for any age group, although over the age of 40, the risk increases to 32 deaths per 100,000 women, compared to 28 associated with pregnancy at that age. However, for pill users who smoke and are over the age of 35, the estimated number of deaths exceeds those for other methods of birth control. If a woman is over the age of 40 and smokes, her estimated risk of death is four times higher (117/100,000 women) than the estimated risk associated with pregnancy (28/100,000 women) in that age group.

The suggestion that women over 40 who do not smoke should not take oral contraceptives is based on information from older, higher-dose pills. An Advisory Committee of the FDA discussed this issue in 1989 and recommended that the benefits of low-dose oral contraceptive use by healthy, non-smoking women over 40 years of age may outweigh the possible risks.

ANNUAL NUMBER OF BIRTH-RELATED OR METHOD-RELATED DEATHS ASSOCIATED WITH CONTROL OF FERTILITY PER 100,000 NON-STERILE WOMEN, BY FERTILITY CONTROL METHOD ACCORDING TO AGE

Method of control and outcome	15-19	20-24	25-29	30-34	35-39	40-44
No fertility control methods*	7.0	7.4	9.1	14.8	25.7	28.2
Oral contraceptives non-smoker**	0.3	0.5	0.9	1.9	13.8	31.6
Oral contraceptives smoker**	2.2	3.4	6.6	13.5	51.1	117.2
IUD**	0.8	0.8	1.0	1.0	1.4	1.4
Condom*	1.1	1.6	0.7	0.2	0.3	0.4
Diaphragm/spermicide*	1.9	1.2	1.2	1.3	2.2	2.8
Periodic abstinence*	2.5	1.6	1.6	1.7	2.9	3.6

* Deaths are birth related
** Deaths are method related

WARNING SIGNALS

If any of these adverse effects occur while you are taking oral contraceptives, call your doctor or clinic immediately:

- Sharp chest pain, coughing of blood, or sudden shortness of breath (indicating a possible clot in the lung)
- Pain in the calf (indicating a possible clot in the leg)
- Crushing chest pain or heaviness in the chest (indicating a possible heart attack)
- Sudden severe headache or vomiting, dizziness or fainting, disturbances of vision or speech, weakness, or numbness in an arm or leg (indicating a possible stroke)
- Sudden partial or complete loss of vision (indicating a possible clot in the eye)
- Breast lumps (indicating possible breast cancer or fibrocystic disease of the breast; ask your doctor or clinic to show you how to examine your breasts)
- Severe pain or tenderness in the stomach area (indicating a possibly ruptured liver tumor)
- Difficulty in sleeping, weakness, lack of energy, fatigue, or change in mood (possibly indicating severe depression)
- Jaundice or a yellowing of the skin or eyeballs, accompanied frequently by fever, fatigue, loss of appetite, dark colored urine, or light colored bowel movements (indicating possible liver problems)

SIDE EFFECTS OF ORAL CONTRACEPTIVES

1. Vaginal bleeding

Irregular vaginal bleeding or spotting may occur while you are taking the pills. Irregular bleeding may vary from slight staining between menstrual periods to breakthrough bleeding which is a flow much like a regular period. Irregular bleeding occurs most often during the first few months of oral contraceptive use, but may also occur after you have been taking the pill for some time. Such bleeding may be temporary and usually does not indicate any serious problems. It is important to continue taking your pills on schedule. If the bleeding occurs in more than one cycle or lasts for more than a few days, talk to your doctor or clinic.

2. Contact lenses

If you wear contact lenses and notice a change in vision or an inability to wear your lenses, contact your doctor or clinic.

3. Fluid retention

Oral contraceptives may cause edema (fluid retention) with swelling of the fingers or ankles and may raise your blood pressure. If you experience fluid retention, contact your doctor or clinic.

4. Melasma

A spotty darkening of the skin is possible, particularly of the face, which may persist.

5. Other side effects

Other side effects may include nausea and vomiting, change in appetite, headache, nervousness, depression, dizziness, loss of scalp hair, rash, and vaginal infections.

If any of these side effects bother you, call your doctor or clinic.

GENERAL PRECAUTIONS

1. Missed periods and use of oral contraceptives before or during early pregnancy

There may be times when you may not menstruate regularly after you have completed taking a cycle of pills. If you have taken your pills regularly and miss one menstrual period, continue taking your pills for the next cycle but be sure to inform your doctor or clinic before doing so. If you have not taken the pills daily as instructed and missed a menstrual period, you may be pregnant. If you missed two consecutive menstrual periods, you may be pregnant. Check with your doctor or clinic immediately to determine whether you are pregnant. Do not continue to take oral contraceptives until you are sure you are not pregnant, but continue to use another method of contraception.

There is no conclusive evidence that oral contraceptive use is associated with an increase in birth defects, when taken inadvertently during early pregnancy. Previously, a few studies had reported that oral contraceptives might be associated with birth defects, but these findings have not been seen in more recent studies. Nevertheless, oral contraceptives or any other drugs should not be used during pregnancy unless clearly necessary and prescribed by your doctor or clinic. You should check with your doctor or clinic about risks to your unborn child of any medication taken during pregnancy.

2. While breast feeding

If you are breast feeding, consult your doctor or clinic before starting oral contraceptives. Some of the drug will be passed on to the child in the milk. A few adverse effects on the child have been reported, including yellowing of the skin (jaundice) and breast enlargement. In addition, oral contraceptives may decrease the amount and quality of your milk. If possible, do not use oral contraceptives while breast feeding. You should use another method of contraception since breast feeding provides only partial protection from becoming pregnant and this partial protection decreases significantly as you breast feed for longer periods of time. You should con-

sider starting oral contraceptives only after you have weaned your child completely.

3. Laboratory tests

If you are scheduled for any laboratory tests, tell your doctor or clinic you are taking birth control pills. Certain blood tests may be affected by birth control pills.

4. Drug interactions

Certain drugs may interact with birth control pills to make them less effective in preventing pregnancy or cause an increase in breakthrough bleeding. Such drugs include rifampin, drugs used for epilepsy such as barbiturates (for example, phenobarbital), anticonvulsants such as carbamazepine (Tegretol is one brand of this drug), phenytoin (Dilantin is one brand of this drug), phenylbutazone (Butazolidin is one brand), and possibly certain antibiotics. You may need to use additional contraception when you take drugs which can make oral contraceptives less effective.

THIS PRODUCT (LIKE ALL ORAL CONTRACEPTIVES) IS INTENDED TO PREVENT PREGNANCY. IT DOES NOT PROTECT AGAINST TRANSMISSION OF HIV (AIDS) AND OTHER SEXUALLY TRANSMITTED DISEASES SUCH AS CHLAMYDIA, GENITAL HERPES, GENITAL WARTS, GONORRHEA, HEPATITIS B, AND SYPHILIS.

HOW TO TAKE THE PILL

IMPORTANT POINTS TO REMEMBER

BEFORE YOU START TAKING YOUR PILLS:

1. BE SURE TO READ THESE DIRECTIONS:
   Before you start taking your pills.
   Anytime you are not sure what to do.
2. THE RIGHT WAY TO TAKE THE PILL IS TO TAKE ONE PILL EVERY DAY AT THE SAME TIME.
   If you miss pills you could get pregnant. This includes starting the pack late.
   The more pills you miss, the more likely you are to get pregnant.
3. MANY WOMEN HAVE SPOTTING OR LIGHT BLEEDING, OR MAY FEEL SICK TO THEIR STOMACH DURING THE FIRST 1–3 PACKS OF PILLS.
   If you feel sick to your stomach, do not stop taking the pill. The problem will usually go away. If it doesn't go away, check with your doctor or clinic.
4. MISSING PILLS CAN ALSO CAUSE SPOTTING OR LIGHT BLEEDING, even when you make up these missed pills. On the days you take 2 pills to make up for missed pills, you could also feel a little sick to your stomach.
5. IF YOU HAVE VOMITING OR DIARRHEA, for any reason, or IF YOU TAKE SOME MEDICINES, including some antibiotics, your pills may not work as well.
   Use a back-up method (such as condoms, foam, or sponge) until you check with your doctor or clinic.
6. IF YOU HAVE TROUBLE REMEMBERING TO TAKE THE PILL, talk to your doctor or clinic about how to make pill-taking easier or about using another method of birth control.
7. IF YOU HAVE ANY QUESTIONS OR ARE UNSURE ABOUT THE INFORMATION IN THIS LEAFLET, call your doctor or clinic.

BEFORE YOU START TAKING YOUR PILLS:

1. DECIDE WHAT TIME OF DAY YOU WANT TO TAKE YOUR PILL. It is important to take it at about the same time every day.
2. LOOK AT YOUR PILL PACK TO SEE IF IT HAS 21 OR 28 PILLS:
   The **21-pill pack** has 21 "active" [white] pills (with hormones) to take for 3 weeks, followed by 1 week without pills.
   The **28-pill pack** has 21 "active" [white] pills (with hormones) to take for 3 weeks, followed by 1 week of reminder [green] pills (without hormones).
3. ALSO FIND:
   1) where on the pack to start taking the pills,
   2) in what order to take the pills (follow the arrows) and
   3) the week numbers printed on the pack.
4. BE SURE YOU HAVE READY AT ALL TIMES:
   ANOTHER KIND OF BIRTH CONTROL (such as condoms, foam or sponge) to use as a back-up in case you miss pills.
   AN EXTRA, FULL PILL PACK.

WHEN TO START THE FIRST PACK OF PILLS:

You have a choice of which day to start taking your first pack of pills. Decide with your doctor or clinic which is the best day for you. Pick a time of day which will be easy to remember.

DAY 1 START:

1. Pick the day label strip that starts with the first day of your period (this is the day you start bleeding or spotting, even if it is almost midnight when the bleeding begins.)
2. Place this day label strip in the cycle tablet dispenser over the area that has the days of the week (starting with Sunday) imprinted in the plastic.
   Note: If the first day of your period is a Sunday, you can skip steps #1 and #2.
3. Take the first "active" [white] pill of the first pack during the first 24 hours of your period.
4. You will not need to use a back-up method of birth control, since you are starting the pill at the beginning of your period.

SUNDAY START:

1. Take the first "active" [white] pill of the first pack on the Sunday after your period starts, even if you are still bleeding. If your period begins on Sunday, start the pack that same day.
2. Use another method of birth control as a back-up method if you have sex anytime from the Sunday you start your first pack until the next Sunday (7 days). Condoms, foam or the sponge are good back-up methods of birth control.

WHAT TO DO DURING THE MONTH:

1. **TAKE ONE PILL AT THE SAME TIME EVERY DAY UNTIL THE PACK IS EMPTY.**
   Do not skip pills even if you are spotting or bleeding between monthly periods or feel sick to your stomach (nausea).
   Do not skip pills even if you do not have sex very often.
2. **WHEN YOU FINISH A PACK OR SWITCH YOUR BRAND OF PILLS:**
   21 pills: Wait 7 days to start the next pack. You will probably have your period during that week. Be sure that no more than 7 days pass between 21-day packs.
   28 pills: Start the next pack on the day after your last "reminder" pill. Do not wait any days between packs.

WHAT TO DO IF YOU MISS PILLS:

If you **MISS 1** [white] "active" pill:

1. Take it as soon as you remember. Take the next pill at your regular time. This means you take 2 pills in 1 day.
2. You do not need to use a back-up birth control method if you have sex.

If you **MISS 2** [white] "active" pills in a row in **WEEK 1 OR WEEK 2** of your pack:

1. Take 2 pills on the day you remember and 2 pills the next day.
2. Then take 1 pill a day until you finish the pack.
3. You MAY BECOME PREGNANT if you have sex in the **7 days** after you miss pills. You MUST use another birth control method (such as condoms, foam, or sponge) as a back-up method for those 7 days.

If you **MISS 2** [white] "active" pills in a row in **THE 3RD WEEK:**

1. ***If you are a Day 1 Starter:***
   THROW OUT the rest of the pill pack and start a new pack that same day.
   If you are a Sunday Starter:
   Keep taking 1 pill every day until Sunday.
   On Sunday, THROW OUT the rest of the pack and start a new pack of pills that same day.
2. You may not have your period this month but this is expected. However, if you miss your period 2 months in a row, call your doctor or clinic because you might be pregnant.
3. You MAY BECOME PREGNANT if you have sex in the **7 days** after you miss pills.
   You MUST use another birth control method (such as condoms, foam, or sponge) as a back-up method for those 7 days.

If you **MISS 3** OR MORE [white] "active" pills in a row (during the first 3 weeks).

1. ***If you are a Day 1 Starter:***
   THROW OUT the rest of the pill pack and start a new pack that same day.
   If you are a Sunday Starter:
   Keep taking 1 pill every day until Sunday.
   On Sunday, THROW OUT the rest of the pack and start a new pack of pills that same day.
2. You may not have your period this month but this is expected. However, if you miss your period 2 months in a row, call your doctor or clinic because you might be pregnant.
3. You MAY BECOME PREGNANT if you have sex in the **7 days** after you miss pills.
   You MUST use another birth control method (such as condoms, foam, or sponge) as a back-up method for those 7 days.

A REMINDER FOR THOSE ON 28-DAY PACKS:

If you forget any of the 7 [green] "reminder" pills in Week 4:
THROW AWAY the pills you missed.
Keep taking 1 pill each day until the pack is empty.
You do not need a back-up method.

FINALLY, IF YOU ARE STILL NOT SURE WHAT TO DO ABOUT THE PILLS YOU HAVE MISSED:

Use a BACK-UP METHOD anytime you have sex.
KEEP TAKING ONE [WHITE] "ACTIVE" PILL EACH DAY until you can reach your doctor or clinic.

PREGNANCY DUE TO PILL FAILURE

The incidence of pill failure resulting in pregnancy is approximately one percent (i.e., one pregnancy per 100 women per year) if taken every day as directed, but more typical failure rates are about 3%. If failure does occur, the risk to the fetus is minimal.

PREGNANCY AFTER STOPPING THE PILL

There may be some delay in becoming pregnant after you stop using oral contraceptives, especially if you had irregular menstrual cycles before you used oral contraceptives. It may be advisable to postpone conception until you begin menstruating regularly once you have stopped taking the pill and desire pregnancy.

There does not appear to be any increase in birth defects in newborn babies when pregnancy occurs soon after stopping the pill.

OVERDOSAGE

Serious ill effects have not been reported following ingestion of large doses of oral contraceptives by young children. Overdosage may cause nausea and withdrawal bleeding in females. In case of overdosage, contact your doctor, clinic or pharmacist.

OTHER INFORMATION

Your doctor or clinic will take a medical and family history before prescribing oral contraceptives and will examine you. The physical examination may be delayed to another time if you request it and your doctor or clinic believes that it is a good medical practice to postpone it. You should be reexamined at least once a year. Be sure to inform your doctor or clinic if there is a family history of any of the conditions listed previously in this leaflet. Be sure to keep all appointments with your doctor or clinic because this is a time to determine if there are early signs of side effects of oral contraceptive use.

Do not use the drug for any condition other than the one for which it was prescribed. This drug has been prescribed specifically for you; do not give it to others who may want birth control pills.

HEALTH BENEFITS FROM ORAL CONTRACEPTIVES

In addition to preventing pregnancy, use of combination oral contraceptives may provide certain benefits. They are:

- menstrual cycles may become more regular
- blood flow during menstruation may be lighter and less iron may be lost. Therefore, anemia due to iron deficiency is less likely to occur.
- pain or other symptoms during menstruation may be encountered less frequently.
- ectopic (tubal) pregnancy may occur less frequently.
- noncancerous cysts or lumps in the breast may occur less frequently.
- acute pelvic inflammatory disease may occur less frequently.
- oral contraceptive use may provide some protection against developing two forms of cancer: cancer of the ovaries and cancer of the lining of the uterus.

If you want more information about birth control pills, ask your doctor, clinic or pharmacist. They have a more technical leaflet called the Professional Labeling, which you may wish to read. The Professional Labeling is also published in a book entitled *Physicians' Desk Reference,* available in many book stores and public libraries.

 5310130 Revised 12/94

Shown in Product Identification Guide, page 325

DURABOLIN® Ⓒ℞
(nandrolone phenpropionate injection, USP)

HOW SUPPLIED

25 mg/mL—5 mL vials.
50 mg/mL—2 mL vials.

HUMEGON™ ℞
(menotropins for injection, USP)
FOR INTRAMUSCULAR INJECTION

DESCRIPTION

Humegon™ (menotropins for injection, USP) is a purified preparation of gonadotropins. Menotropins are extracted from the urine of postmenopausal females and possess follicle-stimulating hormone (FSH) and luteinizing hormone (LH) activity. The ratio of FSH bioactivity and LH bioactivity in menotropins is adjusted to approximate unity by the addition of human chorionic gonadotropin purified from the urine of pregnant women. Each vial of Humegon™ contains 75 IU or 150 IU of follicle-stimulating hormone activity and 75 IU or 150 IU of luteinizing hormone activity, respectively, plus 10.5 mg lactose, hydrous NF; 0.25 mg monosodium phosphate, monohydrate USP; 0.25 mg disodium phosphate, anhydrous USP; sodium hydroxide NF or phosphoric acid NF to adjust pH; in a sterile, lyophilized form. Humegon™ is administered by intramuscular injection.

Continued on next page

Organon—Cont.

Humegon™ is biologically standardized for FSH and LH gonadotropin activities and the potencies are based on the results of *in vivo* bioassays, which are in agreement with the recommendations of the World Health Organization Expert Committee on Biological Standardization (1982).
Both FSH and LH as well as hCG are glycoproteins that are acidic and water soluble.
Therapeutic class: Infertility.

CLINICAL PHARMACOLOGY

The geometric mean absolute bioavailability of FSH from the 150 IU intramuscular (IM) dose compared to the 150 IU intravenous (IV) dose was 76%. Following single dose IM injections of 75, 150, and 300 IU Humegon™ to healthy male volunteers. FSH dose response was less than proportional between the 75 and 150 IU doses and between the 150 and 300 IU doses. The mean FSH elimination half-lives of 75, 150, and 300 IU IM were 37 hrs, 30 hrs, and 36 hrs, respectively, and 31 hrs following 150 IU IV administration.
Repeated daily IM administration of 150 IU Humegon™ to seven women on 8 consecutive days led to a gradual accumulation of FSH levels which plateaued in 3–4 days. It took 4–5 days for the elevated FSH levels to return to pretreatment levels. These findings underline the importance of very careful and frequent monitoring of the patient in order to reduce the danger of ovarian hyperstimulation.

Women:
Humegon™ administered for seven to twelve days produces ovarian follicular growth in women who do not have primary ovarian failure. Treatment with Humegon™ in most instances results only in follicular growth and maturation. In order to induce ovulation, human chorionic gonadotropin (hCG) must be given following the administration of Humegon™ when clinical assessment of the patient indicates that sufficient follicular maturation has occurred.

Men:
Humegon™ administered concomitantly with human chorionic gonadotropin (hCG) for at least three months induces spermatogenesis in men with primary or secondary pituitary hypofunction who have achieved adequate masculinization with prior hCG therapy.

INDICATIONS AND USAGE

Women:
Humegon™ and hCG given in a sequential manner are indicated for the induction of ovulation and pregnancy in the anovulatory infertile patient, in whom the cause of anovulation is functional and is not due to primary ovarian failure.
Humegon™ and hCG may also be used to stimulate the development of multiple follicles in ovulatory patients participating in an *in vitro* fertilization program.

Men:
Humegon™ with concomitant hCG is indicated for the stimulation of spermatogenesis in men who have primary or secondary hypogonadotropic hypogonadism, and idiopathic infertility.
Humegon™ with concomitant hCG has proven effective in inducing spermatogenesis in men with primary hypogonadotropic hypogonadism due to a congenital factor or prepubertal hypophysectomy and in men with secondary hypogonadotropic hypogonadism due to hypophysectomy, craniopharyngioma, cerebral aneurysm, or chromophobe adenoma.

SELECTION OF PATIENTS

Women:

1. Before treatment with Humegon™ is instituted, a thorough gynecologic and endocrinologic evaluation must be performed. Except for those patients enrolled in an *in vitro* fertilization program, this should include a hysterosalpingogram (to rule out uterine and tubal pathology) and documentation of anovulation by means of basal body temperature, serial vaginal smears, examination of cervical mucus, determination of serum (or urinary) progesterone, urinary pregnanediol, and endometrial biopsy. Patients with tubal pathology should receive Humegon™ only if enrolled in an *in vitro* fertilization program.
2. Primary ovarian failure should be excluded by the determination of gonadotropin levels.
3. Careful examination should be made to rule out the presence of an early pregnancy.
4. Patients in late reproductive life have a greater predilection to endometrial carcinoma as well as a higher incidence of anovulatory disorders. Cervical dilation and curettage should always be done for diagnosis before starting Humegon™ therapy in such patients who demonstrate abnormal uterine bleeding or other signs of endometrial abnormalities.
5. Evaluation of the partner's fertility potential should be included in the workup.

Men:
Patient selection should be made based on a documented lack of pituitary function. Prior to hormonal therapy, these patients will have low testosterone levels and low or absent gonadotropin levels. Patients with primary hypogonadotropic hypogonadism will have a subnormal development of masculinization, and those with secondary hypogonadotropic hypogonadism will have decreased masculinization.

CONTRAINDICATIONS

Women:
Humegon™ is contraindicated in women who have:

1. A high FSH level indicating primary ovarian failure.
2. Uncontrolled thyroid and adrenal dysfunction.
3. An organic intracranial lesion such as a pituitary tumor.
4. The presence of any cause of infertility other than anovulation, unless they are candidates for *in vitro* fertilization.
5. Abnormal bleeding of undetermined origin.
6. Ovarian cysts or enlargement not due to polycystic ovary syndrome.
7. Prior hypersensitivity to menotropins.
8. Humegon™ is contraindicated in women who are pregnant and may cause fetal harm. There are limited human data on the effects of Humegon™ when administered during pregnancy.

Men:
Humegon™ is contraindicated in men who have:

1. Normal gonadotropin levels indicating normal pituitary function.
2. Elevated gonadotropin levels indicating primary testicular failure.
3. Infertility disorders other than hypogonadotropic hypogonadism.

WARNINGS

Humegon™ is a drug that should only be used by physicians who are thoroughly familiar with infertility problems. It is a potent gonadotropic substance capable of causing mild to severe adverse reactions in women. Gonadotropin therapy requires a certain time commitment by physicians and supportive health professionals, and its use requires the availability of appropriate monitoring facilities (see "Precautions—Laboratory Tests"). In female patients it must be used with a great deal of care.

Overstimulation of the Ovary During Humegon™ Therapy:
Ovarian Enlargement: Mild to moderate uncomplicated ovarian enlargement which may be accompanied by abdominal distension and/or abdominal pain occurs in approximately 20% of those treated with Humegon™ and hCG, and generally regresses without treatment within two or three weeks.
In order to minimize the hazard associated with the occasional abnormal ovarian enlargement which may occur with Humegon™-hCG therapy, the lowest dose consistent with expectation of good results should be used. Careful monitoring of ovarian response can further minimize the risk of overstimulation.
If the ovaries are abnormally enlarged on the last day of Humegon™ therapy, hCG should not be administered in this course of therapy; this will reduce the chances of development of the Ovarian Hyperstimulation Syndrome.
The Ovarian Hyperstimulation Syndrome (OHSS): OHSS is a medical event distinct from uncomplicated ovarian enlargement. OHSS may progress rapidly to become a serious medical event. It is characterized by an apparent dramatic increase in vascular permeability which can result in a rapid accumulation of fluid in the peritoneal cavity, thorax, and potentially, the pericardium. The early warning signs of development of OHSS are severe pelvic pain, nausea, vomiting, and weight gain. The following symptomatology has been seen with cases of OHSS: abdominal pain, abdominal distension, gastrointestinal symptoms including nausea, vomiting and diarrhea, severe ovarian enlargement, weight gain, dyspnea, and oliguria. Clinical evaluation may reveal hypovolemia, hemoconcentration, electrolyte imbalances, ascites, hemoperitoneum, pleural effusions, hydrothorax, acute pulmonary distress, and thromboembolic events (see "Pulmonary and Vascular Complications" below).
OHSS occurs in approximately 0.4% of patients when the recommended dose is administered and in 1.3% of patients when higher than recommended doses are administered. Cases of OHSS are more common, more severe and more protracted if pregnancy occurs. OHSS develops rapidly; therefore patients should be followed for at least two weeks after hCG administration. Most often, OHSS occurs after treatment has been discontinued and reaches its maximum at about seven to ten days following treatment. Usually, OHSS resolves spontaneously with the onset of menses. If there is evidence that OHSS may be developng prior to hCG administration (see "Precautions—Laboratory Tests"), the hCG should be withheld.
If OHSS occurs, treatment should be stopped and the patient hospitalized. Treatment is primarily symptomatic, consisting of bed rest, fluid and electrolyte management, and analgesics if needed. The phenomenon of hemoconcentration associated with fluid loss into the peritoneal cavity, pleural cavity, and the pericardial cavity has been seen to occur and should be thoroughly assessed in the following manner: 1) fluid intake and output, 2) weight, 3) hematocrit, 4) serum and urinary electrolytes, 5) urine specific gravity, 6) BUN and creatinine, and 7) abdominal girth. These determinations are to be performed daily or more often if the need arises.
With OHSS there is an increased risk of injury to the ovary. The ascitic, pleural, and pericardial fluid should not be removed unless absolutely necessary to relieve symptoms such as pulmonary distress or cardiac tamponade. Pelvic examination may cause rupture of an ovarian cyst, which may result in hemoperitoneum, and should therefore be avoided. If this does occur, and if bleeding becomes such that surgery is required, the surgical treatment should be designed to control bleeding and to retain as much ovarian tissue as possible. Intercourse should be prohibited in those patients in whom significant ovarian enlargement occurs after ovulation because of the danger of hemoperitoneum resulting from ruptured ovarian cysts.
The management of OHSS may be divided into three phases; an acute, a chronic, and a resolution phase. Because the use of diuretics can accentuate the diminished intravascular volume, diuretics should be avoided except in the late phase of resolution as described below.
Acute Phase: Management during the acute phase should be designed to prevent hemoconcentration due to loss of intravascular volume to the third space and to minimize the risk of thromboembolic phenomena and kidney damage. Treatment is designed to normalize electrolytes while maintaining an acceptable but somewhat reduced intravascular volume. Full correction of the intravascular volume deficit may lead to an unacceptable increase in the amount of third space fluid accumulation. Management includes administration of limited intravenous fluids, electrolytes, and human serum albumin. Monitoring for the development of hyperkalemia is recommended.
Chronic Phase: After stabilizing the patient during the acute phase, excessive fluid accumulation in the third space should be limited by instituting severe potassium, sodium, and fluid restriction.
Resolution Phase: A fall in hematocrit and an increasing urinary output without an increased intake are observed due to the return of third space fluid to the intravascular compartment. Peripheral and/or pulmonary edema may result if the kidneys are unable to excrete third space fluid as rapidly as it is mobilized. Diuretics may be indicated during the resolution phase if necessary to combat pulmonary edema.

Pulmonary and Vascular Complications: Serious pulmonary conditions (e.g., atelectasis, acute respiratory distress syndrome) have been reported. In addition, thromboembolic events both in association with, and separate from, the Ovarian Hyperstimulation Syndrome have been reported following Humegon™ therapy. Intravascular thrombosis, which may originate in venous or arterial vessels, can result in reduced blood flow to vital organs or the extremities. Sequelae of such events have included venous thrombophlebitis, pulmonary embolism, pulmonary infarction, cerebral vascular occlusion (stroke), and arterial occlusion resulting in loss of limb. In rare cases, pulmonary complications and/or thromboembolic events have resulted in death.

Multiple Births: Data from a clinical trial revealed the following results regarding multiple births: Of the pregnancies following therapy with Humegon™ and hCG, 80% resulted in single births. The patient and her partner should be advised of the frequency and potential hazards of multiple gestation before starting treatment.

PRECAUTIONS

General: Careful attention should be given to diagnosis in the selection of candidates for Humegon™ therapy (see "Indications and Usage—Selection of Patients").

Information for Patients: Prior to therapy with Humegon™, patients should be informed of the duration of treatment and the monitoring of their condition that will be required. Possible adverse reactions (see "Adverse Reactions" section) and the risk of multiple births should also be discussed.

Laboratory Tests:
Women:
Treatment for Induction of Ovulation
In most instances, treatment with Humegon™ results only in follicular growth and maturation. In order to induce ovulation, hCG must be given following the administration of Humegon™ when clinical assessment of the patient indicates that sufficient follicular maturation has occurred. This may be directly estimated by measuring serum (or urinary) estrogen levels and sonographic visualization of the ovaries. The combination of both estradiol levels and ultrasonography is useful for monitoring the growth and development of follicles, timing hCG administration, as well as minimizing the risk of the Ovarian Hyperstimulation Syndrome and multiple gestation.
Other clinical parameters which may have potential use for monitoring menotropins therapy include:
a) Changes in vaginal cytology;
b) Appearance and volume of cervical mucus;

c) Spinnbarkeit; and
d) Ferning of cervical mucus.

The above clinical indices provide an indirect estimate of the estrogenic effect upon the target organs, and therefore should only be used adjunctively with more direct estimates of follicular development, i.e., serum estradiol and ultrasonography.

The clinical confirmation of ovulation, with the exception of pregnancy, is obtained by direct and indirect indices of progesterone production. The indices most generally used are as follows:

a) A rise in basal body temperature;
b) Increase in serum progesterone; and
c) Menstruation following the shift in basal body temperature.

When used in conjunction with indices of progesterone production, sonographic visualization of the ovaries will assist in determining if ovulation has occurred. Sonographic evidence of ovulation may include the following:

a) Fluid in the cul-de-sac;
b) Ovarian stigmata; and
c) Collapsed follicle.

Because of the subjectivity of the various tests for the determination of follicular maturation and ovulation, it cannot be overemphasized that the physician should choose the test(s) with which he/she is thoroughly familiar.

Drug Interactions: No clinically significant drug/drug or drug/food adverse interactions have been reported during Humegon™ therapy.

Carcinogenesis and Mutagenesis: Long-term toxicity studies in animals have not been performed to evaluate the carcinogenic potential of Humegon™.

Pregnancy: Pregnancy Category X. See "Contraindications".

Males: No animal studies have been performed that examine the potential teratogenic effect associated with Humegon™ therapy when prescribed for male infertility.

Nursing Mothers: It is not known whether this drug is excreted in human milk. Because many drugs are excreted in human milk, caution should be exercised if Humegon™ is administered to a nursing woman.

ADVERSE REACTIONS

Women:

The following adverse reactions, reported during Humegon™ therapy, are listed in decreasing order of potential severity:

1. Pulmonary and vascular complications (see "Warnings")
2. Ovarian Hyperstimulation Syndrome (see "Warnings")
3. Hemoperitoneum
4. Adnexal torsion (as a complication of ovarian enlargement)
5. Mild to moderate ovarian enlargement
6. Ovarian cysts
7. Abdominal pain
8. Sensitivity to Humegon™
   Febrile reactions after the administration of Humegon™ have occurred. It is not clear whether or not these were pyrogenic responses or possible allergic reactions. In addition, reports of "flu-like symptoms" including fever, chills, musculoskeletal aches, joint pains, nausea, headache and malaise have been received.
9. Gastrointestinal symptoms (nausea, vomiting, diarrhea, abdominal cramps, bloating)
10. Pain, rash, swelling and/or irritation at the site of injection
11. Body rashes
12. Dizziness, tachycardia, dyspnea, tachypnea

The following medical events have been reported subsequent to pregnancies resulting from Humegon™ therapy:

1. Ectopic pregnancy
2. Congenital abnormalities
   From a large clinical trial comprising of 6,096 cycles (2,166 women) with 594 babies examined, the incidence of congenital malformation with Humegon™/hCG therapy was 1.7%. Of the major malformations (nine babies, 1.5%) there were two cases each of anencephaly and harelip, and one each of cleft palate, polydactyly, umbilical hernia, congenital dislocation of hip and equinovarus. There was one case (0.2%) of minor malformation (anomaly of auricle). The congenital anomaly rate after Humegon™ therapy is then no higher than that expected for the general population.

There have been infrequent reports of ovarian neoplasms, both benign and malignant, in women who have undergone multiple drug regimens for ovulation induction; however, a causal relationship has not been established.

Men:

Gynecomastia, breast pain, mastitis, nausea, abnormal lipoprotein fraction, abnormal SGOT and SGPT may occur occasionally during Humegon™- hCG therapy.

DRUG ABUSE AND DEPENDENCE

There have been no reports of abuse or dependence with Humegon™.

OVERDOSAGE

Aside from possible ovarian hyperstimulation (see "Warnings"), little is known concerning the consequences of acute overdosage with Humegon™.

DOSAGE AND ADMINISTRATION

Women:

1. Dosage:

The dose of Humegon™ to produce maturation of the follicle must be individualized for each patient. It is recommended that the initial dose to any patient should be 75 IU of FSH/LH per day, **ADMINISTERED INTRAMUSCULARLY**, for seven to twelve days followed by hCG, 5,000 U to 10,000 U, one day after the last dose of Humegon™. Administration of Humegon™ should not exceed 12 days in a single course of therapy. The patient should be treated until indices of estrogenic activity, as indicated under "Precautions" above, are equivalent to or greater than those of the normal individual. If serum or urinary estradiol determinations or ultrasonographic visualizations are available, they may be useful as a guide to therapy. If the ovaries are abnormally enlarged on the last day of Humegon™ therapy, hCG should not be administered in this course of therapy; this will reduce the chances of development of the Ovarian Hyperstimulation Syndrome. If there is evidence of ovulation but no pregnancy, repeat this dosage regime for at least two more courses before increasing the dose of Humegon™ to 150 IU of FSH/LH per day for seven to twelve days. As before, this dose should be followed by 5,000 U to 10,000 U of hCG one day after the last dose of Humegon™. A Humegon™ dose of 150 IU of FSH/LH per day has proven to be the most effective dose especially for *in vitro* fertilization. If evidence of ovulation is present, but pregnancy does not ensue, repeat the same dose for two more courses. Doses larger than this are not routinely recommended.

During treatment with both Humegon™ and hCG and during a two-week post-treatment period, patients should be examined at least every other day for signs of excessive ovarian stimulation. It is recommended that Humegon™ administration be stopped if the ovaries become abnormally enlarged or abdominal pain occurs. Most of the Ovarian Hyperstimulation Syndrome occurs after treatment has been discontinued and reaches its maximum at about seven to ten days post-ovulation. Patients should be followed for at least two weeks after hCG administration. For ovulation induction, the couple should be encouraged to have intercourse daily, beginning on the day prior to the administration of hCG until ovulation becomes apparent from the indices employed for the determination of progestational activity. Care should be taken to insure insemination. In the light of the foregoing indices and parameters mentioned, it should become obvious that, unless a physician is willing to devote considerable time to these patients and be familiar with and conduct the necessary laboratory studies, he/she should not use Humegon™.

2. Administration:

Dissolve the contents of one vial of Humegon™ in one to two mL of sterile saline and **ADMINISTER INTRAMUSCULARLY** immediately. Any unused reconstituted material should be discarded. Parenteral drug products should be inspected visually for particulate matter and discoloration prior to administration, whenever solution and container permit.

Men:

1. Dosage:

Prior to concomitant therapy with Humegon™ and hCG, pretreatment with hCG alone (5,000 U three times a week) is required. Treatment should continue for a period sufficient to achieve serum testosterone levels within the normal range and masculinization as judged by the appearance of secondary sex characteristics. Such pretreatment may require four to six months, then the recommended dose of Humegon™ is 75 IU FSH/LH **ADMINISTERED INTRAMUSCULARLY, three times** a week and the recommended dose of hCG is 2,000 U **twice** a week. Therapy should be carried on for a minimum of four more months to insure detecting spermatozoa in the ejaculate, as it takes 74 $\pm$ 4 days in the human male for germ cells to reach the spermatozoa stage.

If the patient has not responded with evidence of increased spermatogenesis at the end of four months of therapy, treatment may continue with 75 IU FSH/LH **three times** a week, or the dose can be increased to 150 IU FSH/LH **three times** a week, with the hCG dose unchanged.

2. Administration:

Dissolve the contents of one vial of Humegon™ in one to two mL of sterile saline and **ADMINISTER INTRAMUSCULARLY** immediately. Any unused reconstituted material should be discarded. Parenteral drug products should be inspected visually for particulate matter and discoloration prior to administration, whenever solution and container permit.

HOW SUPPLIED

Humegon™ is supplied in sterile lyophilized form as a white to off-white powder in vials containing 75 IU or 150 IU FSH/LH activity. The following package combinations are available:

—1 vial 75 IU Humegon™ and 1 vial 2 mL Sodium Chloride Injection, USP.
NDC 0052-0300-17

- 5 vials 75 IU Humegon™ and 5 vials 2 mL Sodium Chloride Injection, USP.
NDC 0052-0300-22

—1 vial 150 IU Humegon™ and 1 vial 2 mL Sodium Chloride Injection, USP.
NDC 0052-0304-17

By biological assay, one IU of LH for the Second International Reference Preparation (2nd-IRP) for hMG is biologically equivalent to approximately $^1/_2$ U of hCG.

Lyophilized powder may be stored refrigerated or at room temperature 2°–30°C (35°–86°F). Protect from light. Use immediately after reconstitution. Discard unused material.

CLINICAL STUDIES

Women:

The Induction of Ovulation

Results of clinical experience and effectiveness from the administration of Humegon™ to 2,682 patients in 7,204 courses of therapy are summarized below:

Patients Ovulating	73.2%†
Clinical Pregnancies	26.2%
Patients Aborting	22%*
Multiple Pregnancies	19.5%

† Data reported for 2,409 out of 2,682 patients
* Data reported for 678 out of 704 clinical pregnancies

IVF, GIFT, ZIFT

Results of clinical experience and effectiveness from the administration of Humegon™ in 1,081 cycles of therapy are summarized below:

%Cycles with Oocyte Retrieval	85†
%Cycles with Transfers	65.6*
#Clinical Pregnancies	182
%Clinical Pregnancy/Cycle	16.8
%Clincial Pregnancy/Retrieval	19.8
%Clinical Pregnancy/Transfer	25.6
%Abortion	32.7§

† Data reported for 773 cycles
* Data reported for 791 cycles
§ Data reported for 174 out of 182 clinical pregnancies

Men:

Clinical results of treatment of men with hypogonadotropic hypogonadism and idiopathic infertility were summarized from the medical literature. Efficacy was evaluated in 246 patients, 22 with hypogonadotropic hypogonadism and 224 with idiopathic infertility. Treatment generally consisted of Humegon™, with or without concomitant administration of hCG 500–2,500 IU, two or three times per week for up to 48 months. Sperm count improved in 16 of 22 evaluable (73%) hypogonadotropic hypogonadism patients and in 86 of 224 evaluable (38%) idiopathic infertility patients. Overall, seven of 14 (50%) evaluable hypogonadotropic hypogonadism patients and 26 of 224 (12%) idiopathic infertility patients impregnated their partners following Humegon™ treatment.

Caution: Federal law prohibits dispensing without prescription.

Organon Inc.
West Orange, New Jersey 07052
©Organon Incorporated

5310119 Iss. 9/94

Shown in Product Identification Guide, page 325

NORCURON® ℞
(vecuronium bromide) for injection

THIS DRUG SHOULD BE ADMINISTERED BY ADEQUATELY TRAINED INDIVIDUALS FAMILIAR WITH ITS ACTIONS, CHARACTERISTICS, AND HAZARDS.

DESCRIPTION

NORCURON® (vecuronium bromide) for injection is a nondepolarizing neuromuscular blocking agent of intermediate duration, chemically designated as piperidinium, 1-[(2β, 3α, 5α, 16β, 17β)-3, 17-bis(acetyloxy)-2-(1- piperidinyl) androstan-16-yl]-1-methyl-, bromide. The structural formula is:

[See chemical structure at top of next column.]

Continued on next page

Organon—Cont.

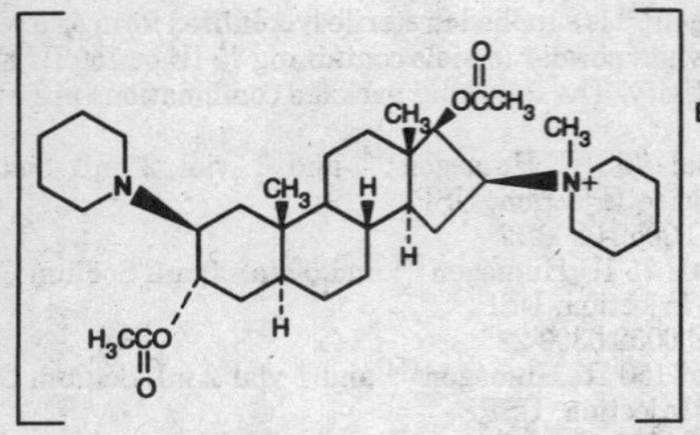

Its chemical formula is $C_{34}H_{57}BrN_2O_4$ with molecular weight 637.74.

Norcuron® is supplied as a sterile nonpyrogenic freeze-dried buffered cake of very fine microscopic crystalline particles for intravenous injection only. Each 10 mL vial contains 10 mg vecuronium bromide, 20.75 mg citric acid anhydrous, 16.25 mg sodium phosphate dibasic anhydrous, 97 mg mannitol (to adjust tonicity), sodium hydroxide and/or phosphoric acid to buffer and adjust to a pH of 4. Each 20 mL vial contains 20 mg of vecuronium bromide, 41.5 mg citric acid anhydrous, 32.5 mg sodium phosphate dibasic anhydrous, 194 mg mannitol (to adjust tonicity), sodium hydroxide and/or phosphoric acid to buffer and adjust to a pH of 4. Bacteriostatic water for injection, USP, when supplied, contains 0.9% w/v BENZYL ALCOHOL, WHICH IS NOT FOR USE IN NEWBORNS.

CLINICAL PHARMACOLOGY

Norcuron® (vecuronium bromide) for injection is a nondepolarizing neuromuscular blocking agent possessing all of the characteristic pharmacological actions of this class of drugs (curariform). It acts by competing for cholinergic receptors at the motor end-plate. The antagonism to acetylcholine is inhibited and neuromuscular block is reversed by acetylcholinesterase inhibitors such as neostigmine, edrophonium, and pyridostigmine. Norcuron® is about ⅓ more potent than pancuronium; the duration of neuromuscular blockade produced by Norcuron® is shorter than that of pancuronium at initially equipotent doses. The time to onset of paralysis decreases and the duration of maximum effect increases with increasing Norcuron® doses. The use of a peripheral nerve stimulator is recommended in assessing the degree of muscular relaxation with all neuromuscular blocking drugs. The ED_{90} (dose required to produce 90% suppression of the muscle twitch response with balanced anesthesia) has averaged 0.057 mg/kg (0.049 to 0.062 mg/kg in various studies). An initial Norcuron® dose of 0.08 to 0.10 mg/kg generally produces first depression of twitch in approximately 1 minute, good or excellent intubation conditions within 2.5 to 3 minutes, and maximum neuromuscular blockade within 3 to 5 minutes of injection in most patients.
Under balanced anesthesia, the time to recovery to 25% of control (clinical duration) is approximately 25 to 40 minutes after injection and recovery is usually 95% complete approximately 45–65 minutes after injection of intubating dose.
The neuromuscular blocking action of Norcuron® is slightly enhanced in the presence of potent inhalation anesthetics. If Norcuron® is first administered more than 5 minutes after the start of the inhalation of enflurane, isoflurane, or halothane, or when steady state has been achieved, the intubating dose of Norcuron® may be decreased by approximately 15% (see **DOSAGE AND ADMINISTRATION** section).
Prior administration of succinylcholine may enhance the neuromuscular blocking effect of Norcuron® and its duration of action. With succinylcholine as the intubating agent, initial doses of 0.04–0.06 mg/kg of Norcuron® will produce complete neuromuscular block with clinical duration of action of 25–30 minutes. If succinylcholine is used prior to Norcuron®, the administration of Norcuron® should be delayed until the patient starts recovering from succinylcholine-induced neuromuscular blockade. The effect of prior use of other nondepolarizing neuromuscular blocking agents on the activity of Norcuron® has not been studied (see **Drug Interactions**).
Repeated administration of maintenance doses of Norcuron® has little or no cumulative effect on the duration of neuromuscular blockade. Therefore, repeat doses can be administered at relatively regular intervals with predictable results. After an initial dose of 0.08 to 0.10 mg/kg under balanced anesthesia, the first maintenance dose (suggested maintenance dose is 0.010 to 0.015 mg/kg) is generally required within 25 to 40 minutes; subsequent maintenance doses, if required, may be administered at approximately 12 to 15 minute intervals. Halothane anesthesia increases the clinical duration of the maintenance dose only slightly. Under enflurane a maintenance dose of 0.010 mg/kg is approximately equal to 0.015 mg/kg dose under balanced anesthesia.
The recovery index (time from 25% to 75% recovery) is approximately 15–25 minutes under balanced or halothane anesthesia. When recovery from Norcuron® neuromuscular blocking effect begins, it proceeds more rapidly than recovery from pancuronium. Once spontaneous recovery has started, the neuromuscular block produced by Norcuron® is readily reversed with various anticholinesterase agents, e.g. pyridostigmine, neostigmine, or edrophonium in conjunction with an anticholinergic agent such as atropine or glycopyrrolate. Rapid recovery is a finding consistent with Norcuron®'s short elimination half-life, although there have been occasional reports of prolonged neuromuscular blockade in patients in the intensive care unit (See **PRECAUTIONS**).
The administration of clinical doses of Norcuron® is not characterized by laboratory or clinical signs of chemically mediated histamine release. This does not preclude the possibility of rare hypersensitivity reactions (See ADVERSE REACTIONS).

Pharmacokinetics: At clinical doses of 0.04–0.10 mg/kg, 60–80% of Norcuron® is usually bound to plasma protein. The distribution half-life following a single intravenous dose (range 0.025–0.280 mg/kg) is approximately 4 minutes. Elimination half-life over this same dosage range is approximately 65–75 minutes in healthy surgical patients and in renal failure patients undergoing transplant surgery.
In late pregnancy, elimination half-life may be shortened to approximately 35–40 minutes. The volume of distribution at steady state is approximately 300–400 mL/kg; systemic rate of clearance is approximately 3–4.5 mL/minute/kg. In man, urine recovery of Norcuron® varies from 3–35% within 24 hours. Data derived from patients requiring insertion of a T-tube in the common bile duct suggests that 25–50% of a total intravenous dose of vecuronium may be excreted in bile within 42 hours. Only unchanged vecuronium has been detected in human plasma following use during surgery. In addition, one metabolite, 3-desacetyl vecuronium, has been rarely detected in human plasma following prolonged clinical use in the I.C.U. (See **PRECAUTIONS: Long Term Use in I.C.U.**). The 3-desacetyl vecuronium metabolite has been recovered in the urine of some patients in quantities that account for up to 10% of injected dose; 3-desacetyl vecuronium has also been recovered by T-tube in some patients accounting for up to 25% of the injected dose.
This metabolite has been judged by animal screening (dogs and cats) to have 50% or more of the potency of Norcuron®; equipotent doses are of approximately the same duration as Norcuron® in dogs and cats. Biliary excretion accounts for about half the dose of Norcuron® within 7 hours in the anesthetized rat. Circulatory bypass of the liver (cat preparation) prolongs recovery from Norcuron®. Limited data derived from patients with cirrhosis or cholestasis suggests that some measurements of recovery may be doubled in such patients. In patients with renal failure, measurements of recovery do not differ significantly from similar measurements in healthy patients.
Studies involving routine hemodynamic monitoring in good risk surgical patients reveal that the administration of Norcuron® in doses up to three times that needed to produce clinical relaxation (0.15 mg/kg) did not produce clinically significant changes in systolic, diastolic or mean arterial pressure. The heart rate, under similar monitoring, remained unchanged in some studies and was lowered by a mean of up to 8% in other studies. A large dose of 0.28 mg/kg administered during a period of no stimulation, while patients were being prepared for coronary artery bypass grafting, was not associated with alterations in rate-pressure-product or pulmonary capillary wedge pressure. Systemic vascular resistance was lowered slightly and cardiac output was increased insignificantly. (The drug has not been studied in patients with hemodynamic dysfunction secondary to cardiac valvular disease). Limited clinical experience with use of Norcuron® during surgery for pheochromocytoma has shown that administration of this drug is not associated with changes in blood pressure or heart rate.
Unlike other nondepolarizing skeletal muscle relaxants, Norcuron® has no clinically significant effects on hemodynamic parameters. Norcuron® will not counteract those hemodynamic changes or known side effects produced by or associated with anesthetic agents, other drugs or various other factors known to alter hemodynamics.

INDICATIONS AND USAGE

Norcuron® is indicated as an adjunct to general anesthesia, to facilitate endotracheal intubation and to provide skeletal muscle relaxation during surgery or mechanical ventilation.

CONTRAINDICATIONS

Norcuron® is contraindicated in patients known to have a hypersensitivity to it.

WARNINGS

NORCURON® SHOULD BE ADMINISTERED IN CAREFULLY ADJUSTED DOSAGE BY OR UNDER THE SUPERVISION OF EXPERIENCED CLINICIANS WHO ARE FAMILIAR WITH ITS ACTIONS AND THE POSSIBLE COMPLICATIONS THAT MIGHT OCCUR FOLLOWING ITS USE. THE DRUG SHOULD NOT BE ADMINISTERED UNLESS FACILITIES FOR INTUBATION, ARTIFICIAL RESPIRATION, OXYGEN THERAPY, AND REVERSAL AGENTS ARE IMMEDIATELY AVAILABLE. THE CLINICIAN MUST BE PREPARED TO ASSIST OR CONTROL RESPIRATION. TO REDUCE THE POSSIBILITY OF PROLONGED NEUROMUSCULAR BLOCKADE AND OTHER POSSIBLE COMPLICATIONS THAT MIGHT OCCUR FOLLOWING LONG-TERM USE IN THE ICU, NORCURON® OR ANY OTHER NEUROMUSCULAR BLOCKING AGENT SHOULD BE ADMINISTERED IN CAREFULLY ADJUSTED DOSES BY OR UNDER THE SUPERVISION OF EXPERIENCED CLINICIANS WHO ARE FAMILIAR WITH ITS ACTIONS AND WHO ARE FAMILIAR WITH APPROPRIATE PERIPHERAL NERVE STIMULATOR MUSCLE MONITORING TECHNIQUES (see **PRECAUTIONS**). In patients who are known to have myasthenia gravis or the myasthenic (Eaton-Lambert) syndrome, small doses of Norcuron® may have profound effects. In such patients, a peripheral nerve stimulator and use of a small test dose may be of value in monitoring the response to administration of muscle relaxants.

PRECAUTIONS

Renal Failure: Norcuron® is well tolerated without clinically significant prolongation of neuromuscular blocking effect in patients with renal failure who have been optimally prepared for surgery by dialysis. Under emergency conditions in anephric patients some prolongation of neuromuscular blockade may occur; therefore, if anephric patients cannot be prepared for non-elective surgery, a lower initial dose of Norcuron® should be considered.

Altered Circulation Time: Conditions associated with slower circulation time in cardiovascular disease, old age, edematous states resulting in increased volume of distribution may contribute to a delay in onset time, therefore, dosage should not be increased.

Hepatic Disease: Experience in patients with cirrhosis or cholestasis has revealed prolonged recovery time in keeping with the role the liver plays in Norcuron® metabolism and excretion (**see Pharmacokinetics**). Data currently available do not permit dosage recommendations in patients with impaired liver function.

Long-term Use in I.C.U.: In the intensive care unit, long-term use of neuromuscular blocking drugs to facilitate mechanical ventilation may be associated with prolonged paralysis and/or skeletal muscle weakness, that may be first noted during attempts to wean such patients from the ventilator. Typically, such patients receive other drugs such as broad spectrum antibiotics, narcotics and/or steroids and may have electrolyte imbalance and diseases which lead to electrolyte imbalance, hypoxic episodes of varying duration, acid-base imbalance and extreme debilitation, any of which may enhance the actions of a neuromuscular blocking agent. Additionally, patients immobilized for extended periods frequently develop symptoms consistent with disuse muscle atrophy. The recovery picture may vary from regaining movement and strength in all muscles to initial recovery of movement of the facial and small muscles of the extremities then to the remaining muscles. In rare cases recovery may be over an extended period of time and may even, on occasion, involve rehabilitation. Therefore, when there is a need for long-term mechanical ventilation, the benefits-to-risk ratio of neuromuscular blockade must be considered.
Continuous infusion or intermittent bolus dosing to support mechanical ventilation, has not been studied sufficiently to support dosage recommendations. IN THE INTENSIVE CARE UNIT, APPROPRIATE MONITORING, WITH THE USE OF A PERIPHERAL NERVE STIMULATOR TO ASSESS THE DEGREE OF NEUROMUSCULAR BLOCKADE IS RECOMMENDED TO HELP PRECLUDE POSSIBLE PROLONGATION OF THE BLOCKADE. WHENEVER THE USE OF NORCURON® OR ANY NEUROMUSCULAR BLOCKING AGENT IS CONTEMPLATED IN THE ICU, IT IS RECOMMENDED THAT NEUROMUSCULAR TRANSMISSION BE MONITORED CONTINUOUSLY DURING ADMINISTRATION AND RECOVERY WITH THE HELP OF A NERVE STIMULATOR. ADDITIONAL DOSES OF NORCURON® OR ANY OTHER NEUROMUSCULAR BLOCKING AGENT SHOULD NOT BE GIVEN BEFORE THERE IS A DEFINITE RESPONSE TO T_1 OR TO THE FIRST TWITCH. IF NO RESPONSE IS ELICITED, INFUSION ADMINISTRATION SHOULD BE DISCONTINUED UNTIL A RESPONSE RETURNS.

Severe Obesity or Neuromuscular Disease: Patients with severe obesity or neuromuscular disease may pose airway and/or ventilatory problems requiring special care before, during and after the use of neuromuscular blocking agents such as Norcuron®.

Malignant Hyperthermia: Many drugs used in anesthetic practice are suspected of being capable of triggering a potentially fatal hypermetabolism of skeletal muscle known as malignant hyperthermia. There are insufficient data derived from screening in susceptible animals (swine) to establish whether or not Norcuron® is capable of triggering malignant hyperthermia.

C.N.S.: Norcuron® has no known effect on consciousness, the pain threshold or cerebration. Administration must be accompanied by adequate anesthesia or sedation.

Drug Interactions: Prior administration of succinylcholine may enhance the neuromuscular blocking effect of Norcuron® (vecuronium bromide) for injection and its duration of action. If succinycholine is used before Norcuron® the administration of Norcuron® should be delayed until the succinylcholine effect shows signs of wearing off. With succinylcholine as the intubating agent, initial doses of 0.04–0.06 mg/kg of Norcuron® may be administered to produce complete neuromuscular block with clinical duration of action of 25–30 minutes (see **CLINICAL PHARMACOLOGY**). The use of Norcuron® before succinylcholine, in order to attenuate some of the side effects of succinylcholine, has not been sufficiently studied.

Other nondepolarizing neuromuscular blocking agents (pancuronium, d-tubocurarine, metocurine, and gallamine) act in the same fashion as does Norcuron®, therefore, these drugs and Norcuron® may manifest an additive effect when used together. There are insufficient data to support concomitant use of Norcuron® and other competitive muscle relaxants in the same patient.

Inhalational Anesthetics: Use of volatile inhalational anesthetics such as enflurane, isoflurane, and halothane with Norcuron® will enhance neuromuscular blockade. Potentiation is most prominent with use of enflurane and isoflurane. With the above agents the initial dose of Norcuron® may be the same as with balanced anesthesia unless the inhalational anesthetic has been administered for a sufficient time at a sufficient dose to have reached clinical equilibrium (see **CLINICAL PHARMACOLOGY**).

Antibiotics: Parenteral/intraperitoneal administration of high doses of certain antibiotics may intensify or produce neuromuscular block on their own. The following antibiotics have been associated with various degrees of paralysis: aminoglycosides (such as neomycin, streptomycin, kanamycin, gentamicin, and dihydrostreptomycin); tetracyclines; bacitracin; polymyxin B; colistin; and sodium colistimethate. If these or other newly introduced antibiotics are used in conjunction with Norcuron®, unexpected prolongation of neuromuscular block should be considered a possibility.

Other: Experience concerning injection of quinidine during recovery from use of other muscle relaxants suggests that recurrent paralysis may occur. This possibility must also be considered for Norcuron®. Norcuron® induced neuromuscular blockade has been counteracted by alkalosis and enhanced by acidosis in experimental animals (cat). Electrolyte imbalance and diseases which lead to electrolyte imbalance, such as adrenal cortical insufficiency, have been shown to alter neuromuscular blockade. Depending on the nature of the imbalance, either enhancement or inhibition may be expected. Magnesium salts, administered for the management of toxemia of pregnancy may enhance the neuromuscular blockade.

Drug/laboratory test interactions: None known

Carcinogenesis, Mutagensis, Impairment of Fertility: Long-term studies in animals have not been performed to evaluate carcinogenic or mutagenic potential or impairment of fertility.

Pregnancy: Pregnancy Category C: Animal reproduction studies have not been conducted with Norcuron®. It is also not known whether Norcuron® can cause fetal harm when administered to a pregnant woman or can affect reproduction capacity. Norcuron® should be given to a pregnant woman only if clearly needed.

Pediatric Use: Infants under 1 year of age but older than 7 weeks also tested under halothane anesthesia, are moderately more sensitive to Norcuron® on a mg/kg basis than adults and take about 1½ times as long to recover. Information presently available does not permit recommendations for usage in neonates.

ADVERSE REACTIONS

The most frequent adverse reaction to nondepolarizing blocking agents as a class consists of an extension of the drug's pharmacological action beyond the time period needed. This may vary from skeletal muscle weakness to profound and prolonged skeletal muscle paralysis resulting in respiration insufficiency or apnea.

Inadequate reversal of the neuromuscular blockade is possible with Norcuron® as with all curariform drugs. These adverse reactions are managed by manual or mechanical ventilation until recovery is judged adequate. Little or no increase in intensity of blockade or duration of action with Norcuron® is noted from the use of thiobarbiturates, narcotic analgesics, nitrous oxide, or droperidol. See **OVERDOSAGE** for discussion of other drugs used in anesthetic practice which also cause respiratory depression.

Prolonged to profound extensions of paralysis and/or muscle weakness as well as muscle atrophy have been reported after long-term use to support mechanical ventilation in the intensive care unit (see **PRECAUTIONS**). The administration of Norcuron® has been associated with rare instances of hypersensitivity reactions (bronchospasm, hypotension and/or tachycardia, sometimes associated with acute urticaria or erythema); (see also **CLINICAL PHARMACOLOGY**).

OVERDOSAGE

The possibility of iatrogenic overdosage can be minimized by carefully monitoring muscle twitch response to peripheral nerve stimulation.

Excessive doses of Norcuron® produced enhanced pharmacological effects. Residual neuromuscular blockade beyond the time period needed may occur with Norcuron® as with other neuromuscular blockers. This may be manifested by skeletal muscle weakness, decreased respiratory reserve, low tidal volume, or apnea. A peripheral nerve stimulator may be used to assess the degree of residual neuromuscular blockade from other causes of decreased respiratory reserve.

Respiratory depression may be due either wholly or in part to other drugs used during the conduct of general anesthesia such as narcotics, thiobarbiturates and other central nervous system depressants. Under such circumstances the primary treatment is maintenance of a patent airway and manual or mechanical ventilation until complete recovery of normal respiration is assured. Regonol® (pyridostigmine bromide) injection, neostigmine, or edrophonium, in conjunction with atropine or glycopyrrolate will usually antagonize the skeletal muscle relaxant action of Norcuron®. Satisfactory reversal can be judged by adequacy of skeletal muscle tone and by adequacy of respiration. A peripheral nerve stimulator may also be used to monitor restoration of twitch height. Failure of prompt reversal (within 30 minutes) may occur in the presence of extreme debilitation, carcinomatosis, and with concomitant use of certain broad spectrum antibiotics, or anesthetic agents and other drugs which enhance neuromuscular blockade or cause respiratory depression of their own. Under such circumstances the management is the same as that of prolonged neuromuscular blockade. Ventilation must be supported by artificial means until the patient has resumed control of his respiration. Prior to the use of reversal agents, reference should be made to the specific package insert of the reversal agent.

DOSAGE AND ADMINISTRATION

Norcuron® (vecuronium bromide) for injection is for intravenous use only.

This drug should be administered by or under the supervision of experienced clinicians familar with the use of neuromuscular blocking agents. Dosage must be individualized in each case. The dosage information which follows is derived from studies based upon units of drug per unit of body weight and is intended to serve as a guide only, especially regarding enhancement of neuromuscular blockade of Norcuron® by volatile anesthetics and by prior use of succinylcholine (see **PRECAUTIONS/Drug Interactions**). Parenteral drug products should be inspected visually for particulate matter and discoloration prior to administration whenever solution and container permit.

To obtain maximum clinical benefits of Norcuron® and to minimize the possibility of overdosage, the monitoring of muscle twitch response to peripheral nerve stimulation is advised.

The recommended initial dose of Norcuron® is 0.08 to 0.10 mg/kg (1.4 to 1.75 times the ED_{90}) given as an intravenous bolus injection. This dose can be expected to produce good or excellent non-emergency intubation conditions in 2.5 to 3 minutes after injection. Under balanced anesthesia, clinically required neuromuscular blockade lasts approximately 25–30 minutes, with recovery to 25% of control achieved approximately 25 to 40 minutes after injection and recovery to 95% of control achieved approximately 45–65 minutes after injection. In the presence of potent inhalation anesthetics, the neuromuscular blocking effect of Norcuron® is enhanced. If Norcuron® is first administered more than 5 minutes after the start of inhalation agent or when steady-state has been achieved, the initial Norcuron® dose may be reduced by approximately 15%, i.e., 0.060 to 0.085 mg/kg.

Prior administration of succinylcholine may enhance the neuromuscular blocking effect and duration of action of Norcuron®. If intubation is performed using succinylcholine, a reduction of initial dose of Norcuron® to 0.04–0.06 mg/kg with inhalation anesthesia and 0.05–0.06 mg/kg with balanced anesthesia may be required.

During prolonged surgical procedures, maintenance doses of 0.010 to 0.015 mg/kg of Norcuron® are recommended; after the initial Norcuron® injection, the first maintenance dose will generally be required within 25 to 40 minutes. However, clinical criteria should be used to determine the need for maintenance doses.

Since Norcuron® lacks clinically important cumulative effects, subsequent maintenance doses, if required, may be administered at relatively regular intervals for each patient, ranging approximately from 12 to 15 minutes under balanced anesthesia, slightly longer under inhalation agents. (If less frequent administration is desired, higher maintenance doses may be administered.)

Should there be reason for the selection of larger doses in individual patients, initial doses ranging from 0.15 mg/kg up to 0.28 mg/kg have been administered during surgery under halothane anesthesia without ill effects to the cardiovascular system being noted as long as ventilation is properly maintained (see **CLINICAL PHARMACOLOGY**).

Use by Continuous Infusion: After an intubating dose of 80–100 μg/kg, a continuous infusion of 1 μg/kg/min can be initiated approximately 20–40 min later. Infusion of Norcuron® should be initiated only after early evidence of spontaneous recovery from the bolus dose. Long-term intravenous infusion to support mechanical ventilation in the intensive care unit has not been studied sufficiently to support dosage recommendations. (see **PRECAUTIONS**).

The infusion of Norcuron® should be individualized for each patient. The rate of administration should be adjusted according to the patient's twitch response as determined by peripheral nerve stimulation. An initial rate of 1 μg/kg/min is recommended, with the rate of the infusion adjusted thereafter to maintain a 90% suppression of twitch response. Average infusion rates may range from 0.8 to 1.2 μg/kg/min.

Inhalation anesthetics, particularly enflurane and isoflurane may enhance the neuromuscular blocking action of nondepolarizing muscle relaxants. In the presence of steady-state concentrations of enflurane or isoflurane, it may be necessary to reduce the rate of infusion 25–60 percent, 45–60 min after the intubating dose. Under halothane anesthesia it may not be necessary to reduce the rate of infusion.

Spontaneous recovery and reversal of neuromuscular blockade following discontinuation of Norcuron® infusion may be expected to proceed at rates comparable to that following a single bolus dose (see **CLINICAL PHARMACOLOGY**).

Infusion solutions of Norcuron® can be prepared by mixing Norcuron® with an appropriate infusion solution such as 5% glucose in water, 0.9% NaCl, 5% glucose in saline, or Lactated Ringers. Unused portions of infusion solutions should be discarded.

Infusion rates of Norcuron® can be individualized for each patient using the following table:

Drug Delivery Rate (μg/kg/min)	Infusion Delivery Rate (mL/kg/min) 0.1 mg/mL*	0.2 mg/mL†
0.7	0.007	0.0035
0.8	0.008	0.0040
0.9	0.009	0.0045
1.0	0.010	0.0050
1.1	0.011	0.0055
1.2	0.012	0.0060
1.3	0.013	0.0065

* 10 mg of Norcuron® in 100 mL solution

† 20 mg of Norcuron® in 100 mL solution

The following table is a guideline for mL/min delivery for a solution of 0.1 mg/mL (10 mg in 100 mL) with an infusion pump.

NORCURON® INFUSION RATE —mL/MIN

Amount of Drug μg/kg/min	Patient Weight—kg 40	50	60	70	80	90	100
0.7	0.28	0.35	0.42	0.49	0.56	0.63	0.70
0.8	0.32	0.40	0.48	0.56	0.64	0.72	0.80
0.9	0.36	0.45	0.54	0.63	0.72	0.81	0.90
1.0	0.40	0.50	0.60	0.70	0.80	0.90	1.00
1.1	0.44	0.55	0.66	0.77	0.88	0.99	1.10
1.2	0.48	0.60	0.72	0.84	0.96	1.08	1.20
1.3	0.52	0.65	0.78	0.91	1.04	1.17	1.30

NOTE: If a concentration of 0.2 mg/mL is used (20 mg in 100 mL), the rate should be decreased by one-half.

Dosage in Children: Older children (10 to 17 years of age) have approximately the same dosage requirements (mg/kg) as adults and may be managed the same way. Younger children (1 to 10 years of age) may require a slightly higher initial dose and may also require supplementation slightly more often than adults.

Infants under one year of age but older than 7 weeks are moderately more sensitive to Norcuron® on a mg/kg basis than adults and take about 1½ times as long to recover. See also subsection of **PRECAUTIONS** titled **Pediatric Use**. Information presently available does not permit recommendation on usage in neonates (see **PRECAUTIONS**). There are insufficient data concerning continuous infusion of vecuronium in children, therefore, no dosing recommendations can be made.

Continued on next page

Organon—Cont.

COMPATIBILITY

Norcuron® is compatible in solution with:
0.9% NaCl solution
5% glucose in water
Sterile water for injection
5% glucose in saline
Lactated Ringers
Use within 24 hours of mixing with the above solutions.
Parenteral drug products should be inspected visually for particulate matter and discoloration prior to administration whenever solution and container permit.

HOW SUPPLIED

10 mL vials (10 mg of vecuronium bromide) and 10 mL prefilled syringes of diluent (bacteriostatic water for injection, USP) 22g 1¼" needle.
Boxes of 10   NDC No. 0052-0441-60
10 mL vials (10 mg vecuronium bromide) and 10 mL vials of diluent (bacteriostatic water for injection, USP).
Boxes of 10   NDC No. 0052-0441-17
10 mL vials (10 mg vecuronium bromide) only; DILUENT NOT SUPPLIED.
Boxes of 10   NDC No. 0052-0441-15
20 mL vials (20 mg vecuronium bromide) only; DILUENT NOT SUPPLIED.
Boxes of 10   NDC No. 0052-0442-46

STORAGE

15–30°C (59–86°F). Protect from light.

AFTER RECONSTITUTION

- When reconstituted with supplied bacteriostatic water for injection: CONTAINS BENZYL ALCOHOL, WHICH IS NOT INTENDED FOR USE IN NEWBORNS. Use within 5 days. May be stored at room temperature or refrigerated.
- When reconstituted with sterile water for injection or other compatible I.V. solutions: Refrigerate vial. Use within 24 hours. Single use only. Discard unused portion.

Caution: Federal law prohibits dispensing without prescription.

ORGANON INC.
WEST ORANGE, NEW JERSEY 07052
5310125 REVISED 7/93

PAVULON® ℞
[pāv-u-lon]
(pancuronium bromide) injection

HOW SUPPLIED

2 mL ampuls—2 mg/mL—boxes of 25—NDC-0052-0444-26
5 mL ampuls—2 mg/mL—boxes of 25—NDC-0052-0444-25
10 mL vials—1 mg/mL—boxes of 25—NDC-0052-0443-25

PREGNYL® ℞
(chorionic gonadotropin for injection, U.S.P.)

DESCRIPTION

Human chorionic gonadotropin (HCG), a polypeptide hormone produced by the human placenta, is composed of an alpha and a beta sub-unit. The alpha sub-unit is essentially identical to the alpha sub-units of the human pituitary gonadotropins, luteinizing hormone (LH) and follicle-stimulating hormone (FSH), as well as to the alpha sub-unit of human thyroid-stimulating hormone (TSH). The beta sub-units of these hormones differ in amino acid sequence.

PREGNYL® (chorionic gonadotropin for injection, USP) is a highly purified pyrogen-free preparation obtained from the urine of pregnant females. It is standardized by a biological assay procedure. It is available for intramuscular injection in multiple dose vials containing 10,000 USP Units of sterile dried powder with 5 mg. monobasic sodium phosphate and 4.4 mg. dibasic sodium phosphate. If required, pH is adjusted with sodium hydroxide and/or phosphoric acid. Each package also contains a 10 mL vial of solvent (water for injection with 0.56% sodium chloride and 0.9% benzyl alcohol). If required, pH is adjusted with sodium hydroxide and/or hydrochloric acid.

CLINICAL PHARMACOLOGY

The action of HCG is virtually identical to that of pituitary LH although HCG appears to have a small degree of FSH activity as well. It stimulates production of gonadal steroid hormones by stimulating the interstitial cells, (Leydig cells) of the testis to produce androgens and the corpus luteum of the ovary to produce progesterone.

Androgen stimulation in the male leads to the development of secondary sex characteristics and may stimulate testicular descent when no anatomical impediment to descent is present. This descent is usually reversible when HCG is discontinued. During the normal menstrual cycle, LH partici-

pates with FSH in the development and maturation of the normal ovarian follicle and the mid-cycle LH surge triggers ovulation. HCG can substitute for LH in this function. During a normal pregnancy, HCG secreted by the placenta maintains the corpus luteum after LH secretion decreases, supporting continued secretion of estrogen and progesterone and preventing menstruation. HCG HAS NO KNOWN EFFECT ON FAT MOBILIZATION, APPETITE OR SENSE OF HUNGER, OR BODY FAT DISTRIBUTION.

INDICATIONS

HCG HAS NOT BEEN DEMONSTRATED TO BE EFFECTIVE ADJUNCTIVE THERAPY IN THE TREATMENT OF OBESITY. THERE IS NO SUBSTANTIAL EVIDENCE THAT IT INCREASES WEIGHT LOSS BEYOND THAT RESULTING FROM CALORIC RESTRICTION, THAT IT CAUSES A MORE ATTRACTIVE OR "NORMAL" DISTRIBUTION OF FAT, OR THAT IT DECREASES THE HUNGER AND DISCOMFORT ASSOCIATED WITH CALORIE-RESTRICTED DIETS.

1. Prepubertal cryptorchidism not due to anatomical obstruction. In general, HCG is thought to induce testicular descent in situations when descent would have occurred at puberty. HCG thus may help predict whether or not orchiopexy will be needed in the future. Although, in some cases, descent following HCG administration is permanent, in most cases, the response is temporary. Therapy is usually instituted between the ages 4 and 9.
2. Selected cases of hypogonadotropic hypogonadism (hypogonadism secondary to a pituitary deficiency) in males.
3. Induction of ovulation and pregnancy in the anovulatory, infertile woman in whom the cause of anovulation is secondary and not due to primary ovarian failure and who has been appropriately pretreated with human menotropins.

CONTRAINDICATIONS

Precocious puberty, prostatic carcinoma or other androgen-dependent neoplasm, prior allergic reaction to HCG.

WARNINGS

HCG should be used in conjunction with human menopausal gonadotropins only by physicians experienced with infertility problems who are familiar with the criteria for patient selection, contraindications, warnings, precautions and adverse reactions described in the package insert for menotropins.

The principal serious adverse reactions during this use are: (1) Ovarian hyperstimulation, a syndrome of sudden ovarian enlargement, ascites with or without pain, and/or pleural effusion, (2) Rupture of ovarian cysts with resultant hemoperitoneum, (3) Multiple births, and (4) Arterial thromboembolism.

PRECAUTIONS

1. Induction of androgen secretion by HCG may induce precocious puberty in patients treated for cryptorchidism. Therapy should be discontinued if signs of precocious puberty occur.
2. Since androgens may cause fluid retention, HCG should be used with caution in patients with cardiac or renal disease, epilepsy, migraine, or asthma.

ADVERSE REACTIONS

Headache, irritability, restlessness, depression, fatigue, edema, precocious puberty, gynecomastia, pain at the site of injection.

DOSAGE AND ADMINISTRATION

(For Intramuscular Use Only): The dosage regimen employed in any particular case will depend upon the indication for use, the age and weight of the patient, and the physician's preference. The following regimens have been advocated by various authorities:

Prepubertal cryptorchidism not due to anatomical obstruction.
1. 4,000 U.S.P. Units three times weekly for three weeks.
2. 5,000 U.S.P. Units every second day for four injections.
3. 15 injections of 500 to 1,000 U.S.P. Units over a period of six weeks.
4. 500 U.S.P. Units three times weekly for four to six weeks. If this course of treatment is not successful, another series is begun one month later, giving 1,000 U.S.P. Units per injection.

Selected cases of hypogonadotropic hypogonadism in males.
1. 500 to 1,000 U.S.P. Units three times a week for three weeks, followed by the same dose twice a week for three weeks.
2. 4,000 U.S.P. Units three times weekly for six to nine months, following which the dosage may be reduced to 2,000 U.S.P. Units three times weekly for an additional three months.

Induction of ovulation and pregnancy in the anovulatory, infertile woman in whom the cause of anovulation is secondary and not due to primary ovarian failure and who has been appropriately pre-treated with human menotropins. (See prescribing information for menotropins for dosage and administration for that drug product.)

5,000 to 10,000 USP Units one day following the last dose of menotropins. (A dosage of 10,000 U.S.P. Units is recommended in the labeling for menotropins).

IMPORTANT: USE COMPLETELY AFTER RECONSTITUTION. RECONSTITUTED SOLUTION IS STABLE FOR 60 DAYS WHEN REFRIGERATED.

HOW SUPPLIED

Two-vial package containing:
1–10 mL lyophilized multiple dose vial containing:
    10,000 USP Units chorionic gonadotropin per vial (NDC 0052-0315-10)
1–10 mL vial of solvent containing:
    water for injection with 0.56% sodium chloride and 0.9% benzyl alcohol (NDC 0052-0325-10.)

When reconstituted, each 10 mL vial contains:

Chorionic gonadotropin	10,000 USP Units
Monobasic sodium phosphate	5 mg.
Dibasic sodium phosphate	4.4 mg.
Sodium chloride	0.56%
Benzyl alcohol	0.9%

If required pH adjusted with sodium hydroxide and/or phosphoric acid.

STORAGE

Store at 15°–30°C (59°–86°F). Reconstituted material will remain stable for 60 days when refrigerated.

CAUTION

Federal law prohibits dispensing without prescription.

DIRECTIONS FOR RECONSTITUTION

Two vial package: Withdraw sterile air from lyophilized vial and inject into diluent. Remove 1–10 mL from diluent and add to lyophilized vial; agitate gently until powder is completely dissolved in solution.

Parenteral drug products should be inspected visually for particulate matter and discoloration prior to administration, whenever solution and container permit.

Revised 12/90

REGONOL® ℞
[re-gō-nol]
(pyridostigmine bromide) injection, USP

HOW SUPPLIED

5 mg/mL: 2 mL ampuls—boxes of 25—NDC-0052-0460-02
5 mg/mL: 5 mL vials—   boxes of 25—NDC-0052-0460-05

REMERON™ ℞
(mirtazapine) Tablets

5310140 4/96

DESCRIPTION

REMERON™ (mirtazapine) is an antidepressant for oral administration. It has a tetracyclic chemical structure unrelated to selective serotonin reuptake inhibitors, tricyclics or monoamine oxidase inhibitors (MAOI). Mirtazapine belongs to the piperazino-azepine group of compounds. It is designated 1,2,3,4,10,14b-hexahydro-2-methylpyrazino [2,1-a]pyrido [2,3-c]benzazepine and has the empirical formula of $C_{17}H_{19}N_3$. Its molecular weight is 265.36. The structural formula is the following and it is the racemic mixture:

Mirtazapine is a white to creamy white crystalline powder which is slightly soluble in water.

REMERON™ is supplied for oral administration as scored film-coated tablets containing 15 or 30 mg of mirtazapine. Each tablet also contains corn starch, hydroxypropyl cellulose, magnesium stearate, colloidal silicon dioxide, lactose and other inactive ingredients.

CLINICAL PHARMACOLOGY

Pharmacodynamics

The mechanism of action of REMERON™ (mirtazapine), as with other antidepressants, is unknown.

Evidence gathered in preclinical studies suggests that mirtazapine enhances central noradrenergic and serotonergic activity. These studies have shown that mirtazapine acts as an antagonist at central presynaptic α_2 adrenergic inhibitory autoreceptors and heteroreceptors, an action that is postulated to result in an increase in central noradrenergic and serotonergic activity.

Mirtazapine is a potent antagonist of 5-HT$_2$ and 5-HT$_3$ receptors. Mirtazapine has no significant affinity for the 5-HT$_{1A}$ and 5-HT$_{1B}$ receptors.

Mirtazapine is a potent antagonist of histamine (H_1) receptors, a property that may explain its prominent sedative effects.

Mirtazapine is a moderate peripheral α_1 adrenergic antagonist, a property that may explain the occasional orthostatic hypotension reported in association with its use.

Mirtazapine is a moderate antagonist at muscarinic receptors, a property that may explain the relatively low incidence of anticholinergic side effects associated with its use.

Pharmacokinetics

REMERON™ (mirtazapine) is rapidly and completely absorbed following oral administration and has a half-life of about 20–40 hours. Peak plasma concentrations are reached within about 2 hours following an oral dose. The presence of food in the stomach has a minimal effect on both the rate and extent of absorption and does not require a dosage adjustment.

Mirtazapine is extensively metabolized after oral administration. Major pathways of biotransformation are demethylation and hydroxylation followed by glucuronide conjugation. In vitro data from human liver microsomes indicate that cytochrome 2D6 and 1A2 are involved in the formation of the 8-hydroxy metabolite of mirtazapine, whereas cytochrome 3A is considered to be responsible for the formation of the N-desmethyl and N-oxide metabolite. Mirtazapine has an absolute bioavailability of about 50%. It is eliminated predominantly via urine (75%) with 15% in feces. Several unconjugated metabolites possess pharmacological activity but are present in the plasma at very low levels. The (−) enantiomer has an elimination half-life that is approximately twice as long as the (+) enantiomer and therefore achieves plasma levels that are about three times as high as that of the (+) enantiomer.

Plasma levels are linearly related to dose over a dose range of 15 to 80 mg. The mean elimination half-life of mirtazapine after oral administration ranges from approximately 20–40 hours across age and gender subgroups, with females of all ages exhibiting significantly longer elimination half-lives than males (mean half-life of 37 hours for females *vs.* 26 hours for males). Steady state plasma levels of mirtazapine are attained within 5 days, with about 50% accumulation (accumulation ratio = 1.5).

Mirtazapine is approximately 85% bound to plasma proteins over a concentration range of 0.01 to 10 μg/mL.

Population Subgroups

Liver Disease—Following a single 15 mg oral dose of mirtazapine, the oral clearance of mirtazapine was decreased by approximately 30% in hepatically impaired patients compared to subjects with normal hepatic function. Caution is indicated in administering REMERON™ (mirtazapine) to patients with compromised hepatic function (see PRECAUTIONS and DOSAGE AND ADMINISTRATION).

Renal Disease—Following a single 15 mg oral dose of mirtazapine, patients with moderate [glomerular filtration rate (GFR) = 11–39 mL/min/1.73 m^2] and severe [GFR <10 mL/min/1.73 m^2] renal impairment had reductions in mean oral clearance of mirtazapine of about 30% and 50%, respectively, compared to normal subjects. Caution is indicated in administering REMERON™ to patients with compromised renal function (see PRECAUTIONS and DOSAGE AND ADMINISTRATION).

Elderly Patients—Following oral administration of mirtazapine 20 mg/day for 7 days to subjects of varying ages (range, 25–74), oral clearance of mirtazapine was reduced in the elderly compared to the younger subjects. The differences were most striking in males, with a 40% lower clearance in elderly males compared to younger males, while the clearance in elderly females was only 10% lower compared to younger females. Caution is indicated in administering REMERON™ to elderly patients (see PRECAUTIONS and DOSAGE AND ADMINISTRATION).

Clinical Trials Showing Effectiveness

The efficacy of REMERON™ (mirtazapine) as a treatment for depression was established in four placebo-controlled, 6-week trials in adult outpatients meeting DSM-III criteria for major depression. Patients were titrated with mirtazapine from a dose range of 5 mg up to 35 mg/day. Overall, these studies demonstrated mirtazapine to be superior to placebo on at least three of the following four measures: 21-Item Hamilton Depression Rating Scale (HDRS) total score; HDRS Depressed Mood Item; CGI Severity score; and Montgomery and Asberg Depression Rating Scale (MADRS). Superiority of mirtazapine over placebo was also found for certain factors of the HDRS including anxiety/somatization factor and sleep disturbance factor. The mean mirtazapine dose for patients who completed these four studies ranged from 21 to 32 mg/day. A fifth study of similar design utilized a higher dose (up to 50 mg) per day and also showed effectiveness.

Examination of age and gender subsets of the population did not reveal any differential responsiveness on the basis of these subgroupings.

INDICATIONS AND USAGE

REMERON™ (mirtazapine) Tablets are indicated for the treatment of depression.

The efficacy of REMERON™ in the treatment of depression was established in six week controlled trials of outpatients whose diagnoses corresponded most closely to the Diagnostic and Statistical Manual of Mental Disorders–3rd edition (DSM-III) category of major depressive disorder (see CLINICAL PHARMACOLOGY).

A major depressive episode (DSM-IV) implies a prominent and relatively persistent (nearly every day for at least 2 weeks) depressed or dysphoric mood that usually interferes with daily functioning, and includes at least five of the following nine symptoms: depressed mood, loss of interest in usual activities, significant change in weight and/or appetite, insomnia or hypersomnia, psychomotor agitation or retardation, increased fatigue, feelings of guilt or worthlessness, slowed thinking or impaired concentration, a suicide attempt or suicidal ideation.

The antidepressant effectiveness of REMERON™ (mirtazapine) in hospitalized depressed patients has not been adequately studied.

The effectiveness of REMERON™ in long-term use, that is, for more than 6 weeks, has not been systematically evaluated in controlled trials. Therefore, the physician who elects to use REMERON™ for extended periods should periodically evaluate the long-term usefulness of the drug for the individual patient.

CONTRAINDICATIONS

REMERON™ (mirtazapine) Tablets are contraindicated in patients with a known hypersensitivity to mirtazapine.

WARNINGS

Agranulocytosis

In premarketing clinical trials, two (one with Sjögren's Syndrome) out of 2,796 patients treated with REMERON™ (mirtazapine) Tablets developed agranulocytosis [absolute neutrophil count (ANC) <500/mm³ with associated signs and symptoms, e.g., fever, infection, etc.] and a third patient developed severe neutropenia [ANC <500/mm³ without any associated symptoms]. For these three patients, onset of severe neutropenia was detected on days 61, 9, and 14 of treatment, respectively. All three patients recovered after REMERON™ was stopped. These three cases yield a crude incidence of severe neutropenia (with or without associated infection) of approximately 1.1 per thousand patients exposed, with a very wide 95% confidence interval, i.e., 2.2 cases per 10,000 to 3.1 cases per 1000. If a patient develops a sore throat, fever, stomatitis or other signs of infection, along with a low WBC count, treatment with REMERON™ should be discontinued and the patient should be closely monitored.

MAO Inhibitors

In patients receiving other antidepressants in combination with a monoamine oxidase inhibitor (MAOI) and in patients who have recently discontinued an antidepressant drug and then are started on an MAOI, there have been reports of serious, and sometimes fatal, reactions, e.g., including nausea, vomiting, flushing, dizziness, tremor, myoclonus, rigidity, diaphoresis, hyperthermia, autonomic instability with rapid fluctuations of vital signs, seizures, and mental status changes ranging from agitation to coma. Although there are no human data pertinent to such an interaction with REMERON™ (mirtazapine), it is recommended that REMERON™ not be used in combination with an MAOI, or within 14 days of initiating or discontinuing therapy with an MAOI.

PRECAUTIONS

General

Somnolence

In U.S. controlled studies, somnolence was reported in 54% of patients treated with REMERON™ (mirtazapine), compared to 18% for placebo and 60% for amitriptyline. In these studies, somnolence resulted in discontinuation for 10.4% of REMERON™ treated patients, compared to 2.2% for placebo. It is unclear whether or not tolerance develops to the somnolent effects of REMERON™. Because of REMERON™'s potentially significant effects on impairment of performance, patients should be cautioned about engaging in activities requiring alertness until they have been able to assess the drug's effect on their own psychomotor performance (see Information for Patients).

Dizziness

In U.S. controlled studies, dizziness was reported in 7% of patients treated with REMERON™ (mirtazapine), compared to 3% for placebo and 14% for amitriptyline. It is unclear whether or not tolerance develops to the dizziness observed in association with the use of REMERON™.

Increased Appetite/Weight Gain

In U.S. controlled studies, appetite increase was reported in 17% of patients treated with REMERON™ (mirtazapine), compared to 2% for placebo and 6% for amitriptyline. In these same trials, weight gain of ≥7% of body weight was reported in 7.5% of patients treated with mirtazapine, compared to 0% for placebo and 5.9% for amitriptyline. In a pool of premarketing U.S. studies, including many patients in long-term, open label treatment, 8% of patients receiving REMERON™ discontinued for weight gain.

Cholesterol/Triglycerides

In U.S. controlled studies, nonfasting cholesterol increases to ≥20% above the upper limits of normal were observed in 15% of patients treated with REMERON™ (mirtazapine), compared to 7% for placebo and 8% for amitriptyline. In these same studies, nonfasting triglyceride increases to ≥500 mg/dL were observed in 6% of patients treated with mirtazapine, compared to 3% for placebo and 3% for amitriptyline.

Transaminase Elevations

Clinically significant ALT (SGPT) elevations (≥3 times the upper limit of the normal range) were observed in 2.0% (8/424) of patients exposed to REMERON™ (mirtazapine) in a pool of short-term U.S. controlled trials, compared to 0.3% (1/328) of placebo patients and 2.0% (3/181) of amitriptyline patients. Most of these patients with ALT increases did not develop signs or symptoms associated with compromised liver function. While some patients were discontinued for the ALT increases, in other cases, the enzyme levels returned to normal despite continued REMERON™ treatment. Mirtazapine should be used with caution in patients with impaired hepatic function (see Pharmacokinetics section of CLINICAL PHARMACOLOGY, and DOSAGE AND ADMINISTRATION).

Activation of Mania/Hypomania

Mania/hypomania occurred in approximately 0.2% (3/1,299 patients) of REMERON™ (mirtazapine) treated patients in U.S. studies. Although the incidence of mania/hypomania was very low during treatment with mirtazapine, it should be used carefully in patients with a history of mania/hypomania.

Seizure

In premarketing clinical trials only one seizure was reported among the 2,796 U.S. and non-U.S. patients treated with REMERON™ (mirtazapine). However, no controlled studies have been carried out in patients with a history of seizures. Therefore, care should be exercised when mirtazapine is used in these patients.

Suicide

Suicidal ideation is inherent in depression and may persist until significant remission occurs. As with any patient receiving antidepressants, high-risk patients should be closely supervised during initial drug therapy. Prescriptions of REMERON™ (mirtazapine) should be written for the smallest quantity consistent with good patient management, in order to reduce the risk of overdose.

Use in Patients with Concomitant Illness

Clinical experience with REMERON™ (mirtazapine) in patients with concomitant systemic illness is limited. Accordingly, care is advisable in prescribing mirtazapine for patients with diseases or conditions that affect metabolism or hemodynamic responses.

Mirtazapine has not been systematically evaluated or used to any appreciable extent in patients with a recent history of myocardial infarction or other significant heart disease. Mirtazapine was not associated with clinically significant ECG abnormalities in U.S. and non-U.S. placebo controlled trials. Mirtazapine was associated with significant orthostatic hypotension in early clinical pharmacology trials with normal volunteers. Orthostatic hypotension was infrequently observed in clinical trials with depressed patients. REMERON™ should be used with caution in patients with known cardiovascular or cerebrovascular disease that could be exacerbated by hypotension (history of myocardial infarction, angina, or ischemic stroke) and conditions that would predispose patients to hypotension (dehydration, hypovolemia, and treatment with antihypertensive medication).

Mirtazapine clearance is decreased in patients with moderate [glomerular filtration rate (GFR) = 11–39 mL/min/1.73 m^2] and severe [GFR <10 mL/min/1.73 m^2] renal impairment, and also in patients with hepatic impairment (see Pharmacokinetics subsection of CLINICAL PHARMACOLOGY). Caution is indicated in administering REMERON™ to such patients (see DOSAGE AND ADMINISTRATION).

Information for Patients

Physicians are advised to discuss the following issues with patients for whom they prescribe REMERON™ (mirtazapine):

Agranulocytosis

Patients who are to receive REMERON™ (mirtazapine) should be warned about the risk of developing agranulocytosis. Patients should be advised to contact their physician if they experience any indication of infection such as fever, chills, sore throat, mucous membrane ulceration or other possible signs of infection. Particular attention should be paid to any flu-like complaints or other symptoms that might suggest infection.

Interference with Cognitive and Motor Performance

REMERON™ (mirtazapine) may impair judgement, thinking, and, particularly, motor skills, because of its prominent sedative effect. The drowsiness associated with mirtazapine use may impair a patient's ability to drive, use machines or perform tasks that require alertness. Thus, patients should

Continued on next page

Organon—Cont.

be cautioned about engaging in hazardous activities until they are reasonably certain that REMERON™ therapy does not adversely affect their ability to engage in such activities.

Completing Course of Therapy

While patients may notice improvement with REMERON™ (mirtazapine) therapy in 1 to 4 weeks, they should be advised to continue therapy as directed.

Concomitant Medication

Patients should be advised to inform their physician if they are taking, or intend to take, any prescription or over-the-counter drugs since there is a potential for REMERON™ (mirtazapine) to interact with other drugs.

Alcohol

The impairment of cognitive and motor skills produced by REMERON™ (mirtazapine) has been shown to be additive with those produced by alcohol. Accordingly, patients should be advised to avoid alcohol while taking mirtazapine.

Pregnancy

Patients should be advised to notify their physician if they become pregnant or intend to become pregnant during REMERON™ (mirtazapine) therapy.

Nursing

Patients should be advised to notify their physician if they are breast-feeding an infant.

Laboratory Tests

There are no routine laboratory tests recommended.

Drug Interactions

As with other drugs, the potential for interaction by a variety of mechanisms (e.g., pharmacodynamic, pharmacokinetic inhibition or enhancement, etc.) is a possibility (see CLINICAL PHARMACOLOGY).

Drugs Affecting Hepatic Metabolism

The metabolism and pharmacokinetics of REMERON™ (mirtazapine) may be affected by the induction or inhibition of drug-metabolizing enzymes.

Drugs that are Metabolized by and/or Inhibit Cytochrome P450 Enzymes

Many drugs are metabolized by and/or inhibit various cytochrome P450 enzymes, e.g., 2D6, 1A2, 3A4, etc. In vitro studies have shown that REMERON™ (mirtazapine) is a substrate for several of these enzymes, including 2D6, 1A2, and 3A4. While in vitro studies have shown that mirtazapine is not a potent inhibitor of any of these enzymes, an indication that mirtazapine is not likely to have a clinically significant inhibitory effect on the metabolism of other drugs that are substrates for these cytochrome P450 enzymes, the concomitant use of mirtazapine with most other drugs metabolized by these enzymes has not been formally studied. Consequently, it is not possible to make any definitive statements about the risks of coadministration of mirtazapine with such drugs.

Alcohol

Concomitant administration of alcohol (equivalent to 60 g) had a minimal effect on plasma levels of REMERON™ (mirtazapine) (15 mg) in 6 healthy male subjects. However, the impairment of cognitive and motor skills produced by REMERON™ were shown to be additive with those produced by alcohol. Accordingly, patients should be advised to avoid alcohol while taking REMERON™.

Diazepam

Concomitant administration of diazepam (15 mg) had a minimal effect on plasma levels of mirtazapine (15 mg) in 12 healthy subjects. However, the impairment of motor skills produced by REMERON™ (mirtazapine) has been shown to be additive with those caused by diazepam. Accordingly, patients should be advised to avoid diazepam and other similar drugs while taking REMERON™.

Carcinogenesis, Mutagenesis, Impairment of Fertility

Carcinogenesis

Carcinogenicity studies were conducted with REMERON™ (mirtazapine) given in the diet at doses of 2, 20, and 200 mg/kg/day to mice and 2, 20, and 60 mg/kg/day to rats. The highest doses used are approximately 20 and 12 times the maximum recommended human dose (MRHD) of 45 mg/day on a mg/m² basis in mice and rats, respectively. There was an increased incidence of hepatocellular adenoma and carcinoma in male mice at the high dose. In rats, there was an increase in hepatocellular adenoma in females at the mid and high doses and in hepatocellular tumors and thyroid follicular adenoma/cystadenoma and carcinoma in males at the high dose. The data suggest that the above effects could possibly be mediated by non-genotoxic mechanisms, the relevance of which to humans is not known.

The doses used in the mouse study may not have been high enough to fully characterize the carcinogenic potential of REMERON™.

Mutagenesis

REMERON™ (mirtazapine) was not mutagenic or clastogenic and did not induce general DNA damage as determined in several genotoxicity tests: Ames test, in vitro gene mutation assay in Chinese hamster V 79 cells, in vitro sister chromatid exchange assay in cultured rabbit lymphocytes, in vivo bone marrow micronucleus test in rats, and unscheduled DNA synthesis assay in HeLa cells.

Impairment of Fertility

In a fertility study in rats, REMERON™ (mirtazapine) was given at doses up to 100 mg/kg (20 times the maximum recommended human dose (MRHD) on a mg/m² basis). Mating and conception were not affected by the drug, but estrous cycling was disrupted at doses that were 3 or more times the MRHD and pre-implantation losses occurred at 20 times the MRHD.

Pregnancy

Teratogenic Effects–Pregnancy Category C

Reproduction studies in pregnant rats and rabbits at doses up to 100 mg/kg and 40 mg/kg, respectively (20 and 17 times the maximum recommended human dose (MRHD) on a mg/m² basis, respectively), have revealed no evidence of teratogenic effects. However, in rats, there was an increase in post-implantation losses in dams treated with REMERON™ (mirtazapine). There was an increase in pup deaths during the first 3 days of lactation and a decrease in pup birth weights. The cause of these deaths is not known. These effects occurred at doses that were 20 times the MRHD, but not at 3 times the MRHD, on a mg/m² basis. There are no adequate and well controlled studies in pregnant women. Because animal reproduction studies are not always predictive of human response, this drug should be used during pregnancy only if clearly needed.

Nursing Mothers

It is not known whether mirtazapine is excreted in human milk. Because many drugs are excreted in human milk, caution should be exercised when REMERON™ (mirtazapine) Tablets are administered to nursing women.

Pediatric Use

Safety and effectiveness in children have not been established.

Geriatric Use

Approximately 190 elderly individuals (≥65 years of age) participated in clinical studies with REMERON™ (mirtazapine). No unusual adverse age-related phenomena were identified in this group. Pharmacokinetic studies revealed a decreased clearance in the elderly. Caution is indicated in administering REMERON™ to elderly patients (see CLINICAL PHARMACOLOGY and DOSAGE AND ADMINISTRATION).

ADVERSE REACTIONS

Associated with Discontinuation of Treatment

Approximately 16 percent of the 453 patients who received REMERON™ (mirtazapine) in U.S. 6-week controlled clinical trials discontinued treatment due to an adverse experience, compared to 7 percent of 361 placebo-treated patients in those studies. The most common events (≥1%) associated with discontinuation and considered to be drug related (i.e., those events associated with dropout at a rate at least twice that of placebo) included:

Common Adverse Events Associated with Discontinuation of Treatment in 6-Week U.S. REMERON™ Trials

Adverse Event	Percentage of Patients Discontinuing with Adverse Event: REMERON™ (n=453)	Placebo (n=361)
Somnolence	10.4%	2.2%
Nausea	1.5%	0%

Commonly Observed Adverse Events in U.S. Controlled Clinical Trials

The most commonly observed adverse events associated with the use of REMERON™ (mirtazapine) (incidence of 5% or greater) and not observed at an equivalent incidence among placebo-treated patients (REMERON™ incidence at least twice that for placebo) were:

Common Treatment-Emergent Adverse Events Associated with the Use of REMERON™ in 6-Week U.S. Trials

Adverse Event	Percentage of Patients Reporting Adverse Event: REMERON™ (n=453)	Placebo (n=361)
Somnolence	54%	18%
Increased Appetite	17%	2%
Weight Gain	12%	2%
Dizziness	7%	3%

Adverse Events Occurring at an Incidence of 1% or More Among REMERON™ Treated Patients

The table that follows enumerates adverse events that occurred at an incidence of 1% or more, and were more frequent than in the placebo group, among REMERON™ (mirtazapine)-treated patients who participated in short-term U.S. placebo-controlled trials in which patients were dosed in a range of 5 to 60 mg/day. This table shows the percentage of patients in each group who had at least one episode of an event at some time during their treatment. Reported adverse events were classified using a standard COSTART-based dictionary terminology.

The prescriber should be aware that these figures cannot be used to predict the incidence of side effects in the course of usual medical practice where patient characteristics and other factors differ from those which prevailed in the clinical trials. Similarly, the cited frequencies cannot be compared with figures obtained from other investigations involving different treatments, uses and investigators. The cited figures, however, do provide the prescribing physician with some basis for estimating the relative contribution of drug and non-drug factors to the side effect incidence rate in the population studied.

INCIDENCE OF ADVERSE CLINICAL EXPERIENCES[1] (≥1%) IN SHORT-TERM U.S. CONTROLLED STUDIES

Body System / Adverse Clinical Experience	REMERON™ (n=453)	Placebo (n=361)
Body as a Whole		
Asthenia	8%	5%
Flu Syndrome	5%	3%
Back Pain	2%	1%
Digestive System		
Dry Mouth	25%	15%
Increased Appetite	17%	2%
Constipation	13%	7%
Metabolic and Nutritional Disorders		
Weight Gain	12%	2%
Peripheral Edema	2%	1%
Edema	1%	0%
Musculoskeletal System		
Myalgia	2%	1%
Nervous System		
Somnolence	54%	18%
Dizziness	7%	3%
Abnormal Dreams	4%	1%
Thinking Abnormal	3%	1%
Tremor	2%	1%
Confusion	2%	0%
Respiratory System		
Dyspnea	1%	0%
Urogenital System		
Urinary Frequency	2%	1%

[1] Events reported by at least 1% of patients treated with REMERON™ (mirtazapine) are included, except the following events which had an incidence on placebo ≥REMERON™: headache, infection, pain, chest pain, palpitation, tachycardia, postural hypotension, nausea, dyspepsia, diarrhea, flatulence, insomnia, nervousness, libido decreased, hypertonia, pharyngitis, rhinitis, sweating, amblyopia, tinnitus, taste perversion.

ECG Changes

In an analysis of ECGs obtained in U.S. placebo-controlled clinical trials, REMERON™ (mirtazapine) and placebo-treated patients had a similar incidence of abnormal changes from baseline at 6–8 weeks of approximately 3%. The abnormalities were generally not considered clinically significant.

Other Adverse Events Observed During the Premarketing Evaluation of REMERON™

During its premarketing assessment, multiple doses of REMERON™ (mirtazapine) were administered to 2,796 patients in clinical studies. The conditions and duration of exposure to mirtazapine varied greatly, and included (in overlapping categories) open and double-blind studies, uncontrolled and controlled studies, inpatient and outpatient studies, fixed dose and titration studies. Untoward events associated with this exposure were recorded by clinical investigators using terminology of their own choosing. Consequently, it is not possible to provide a meaningful estimate of the proportion of individuals experiencing adverse events without first grouping similar types of untoward events into a smaller number of standardized event categories.

In the tabulations that follow, reported adverse events were classified using a standard COSTART-based dictionary terminology. The frequencies presented, therefore, represent the proportion of the 2,796 patients exposed to multiple doses of REMERON™ who experienced an event of the type cited on at least one occasion while receiving REMERON™. All reported events are included except those already listed in the previous table, those adverse experiences subsumed under COSTART terms that are either overly general or

excessively specific so as to be uninformative, and those events for which a drug cause was very remote.

It is important to emphasize that, although the events reported occurred during treatment with REMERON™, they were not necessarily caused by it.

Events are further categorized by body system and listed in order of decreasing frequency according to the following definitions: frequent adverse events are those occurring on one or more occasions in at least 1/100 patients; infrequent adverse events are those occurring in 1/100 to 1/1000 patients; rare events are those occurring in fewer than 1/1000 patients. Only those events not already listed in the previous table appear in this listing. Events of major clinical importance are also described in the WARNINGS and PRECAUTIONS sections.

Body as a Whole: *frequent:* malaise, abdominal pain, abdominal syndrome acute; *infrequent:* chills, fever, face edema, ulcer, photosensitivity reaction, neck rigidity, neck pain, abdomen enlarged; *rare:* cellulitis, chest pain substernal.

Cardiovascular System: *frequent:* hypertension, vasodilatation; *infrequent:* angina pectoris, myocardial infarction, bradycardia, ventricular extrasystoles, syncope, migraine, hypotension; *rare:* atrial arrhythmia, bigeminy, vascular headache, pulmonary embolus, cerebral ischemia, cardiomegaly, phlebitis, left heart failure.

Digestive System: *frequent:* vomiting, anorexia; *infrequent:* eructation, glossitis, cholecystitis, nausea and vomiting, gum hemorrhage, stomatitis, colitis, liver function tests abnormal; *rare:* tongue discoloration, ulcerative stomatitis, salivary gland enlargement, increased salivation, intestinal obstruction, pancreatitis, aphthous stomatitis, cirrhosis of liver, gastritis, gastroenteritis, oral moniliasis, tongue edema.

Endocrine System: *rare:* goiter, hypothyroidism.

Hemic and Lymphatic System: *rare:* lymphadenopathy, leukopenia, petechia, anemia, thrombocytopenia, lymphocytosis, pancytopenia.

Metabolic and Nutritional Disorders: *frequent:* thirst; *infrequent:* dehydration, weight loss; *rare:* gout, SGOT increased, healing abnormal, acid phosphatase increased, SGPT increased, diabetes mellitus.

Musculoskeletal System: *frequent:* myasthenia, arthralgia; *infrequent:* arthritis, tenosynovitis; *rare:* pathological fracture, osteoporosis fracture, bone pain, myositis, tendon rupture, arthrosis, bursitis.

Nervous System: *frequent:* hypesthesia, apathy, depression, hypokinesia, vertigo, twitching, agitation, anxiety, amnesia, hyperkinesia, paresthesia; *infrequent:* ataxia, delirium, delusions, depersonalization, dyskinesia, extrapyramidal syndrome, libido increased, coordination abnormal, dysarthria, hallucinations, manic reaction, neurosis, dystonia, hostility, reflexes increased, emotional lability, euphoria, paranoid reaction; *rare:* aphasia, nystagmus, akathisia, stupor, dementia, diplopia, drug dependence, paralysis, grand mal convulsion, hypotonia, myoclonus, psychotic depression, withdrawal syndrome.

Respiratory System: *frequent:* cough increased, sinusitis; *infrequent:* epistaxis, bronchitis, asthma, pneumonia; *rare:* asphyxia, laryngitis, pneumothorax, hiccup.

Skin and Appendages: *frequent:* pruritus, rash; *infrequent:* acne exfoliative dermatitis, dry skin, herpes simplex, alopecia; *rare:* urticaria, herpes zoster, skin hypertrophy, seborrhea, skin ulcer.

Special Senses: *infrequent:* eye pain, abnormality of accommodation, conjunctivitis, deafness, keratoconjunctivitis, lacrimation disorder, glaucoma, hyperacusis, ear pain; *rare:* blepharitis, partial transitory deafness, otitis media, taste loss, parosmia.

Urogenital System: *frequent:* urinary tract infection; *infrequent:* kidney calculus, cystitis, dysuria, urinary incontinence, urinary retention, vaginitis, hematuria, breast pain, amenorrhea, dysmenorrhea, leukorrhea, impotence; *rare:* polyuria, urethritis, metrorrhagia, menorrhagia, abnormal ejaculation, breast engorgement, breast enlargement, urinary urgency.

DRUG ABUSE AND DEPENDENCE

Controlled Substance Class

REMERON™ (mirtazapine) Tablets are not a controlled substance.

Physical and Psychological Dependence

REMERON™ (mirtazapine) has not been systematically studied in animals or humans for its potential for abuse, tolerance or physical dependence. While clinical trials did not reveal any tendency for any drug-seeking behavior, these observations were not systematic and it is not possible to predict on the basis of this limited experience the extent to which a CNS-active drug will be misused, diverted and/or abused once marketed. Consequently, patients should be evaluated carefully for history of drug abuse, and such patients should be observed closely for signs of mirtazapine misuse or abuse (e.g., development of tolerance, incrementations of dose, drug-seeking behavior).

OVERDOSAGE

Human Experience

There is very limited experience with REMERON™ (mirtazapine) overdose. In premarketing clinical studies, there were eight reports of mirtazapine overdose alone or in combination with other pharmacological agents. The only drug overdose death reported while taking REMERON™ Tablets was in combination with amitriptyline and chlorprothixene in a non-U.S. clinical study. Based on plasma levels, the REMERON™ dose taken was 30–45 mg, while plasma levels of amitriptyline and chlorprothixene were found to be at toxic levels. All other premarketing overdose cases resulted in full recovery. Signs and symptoms reported in association with overdose included disorientation, drowsiness, impaired memory, and tachycardia. There were no reports of ECG abnormalities, coma or convulsions following overdose with REMERON™ alone.

Overdose Management

Treatment should consist of those general measures employed in the management of overdose with any antidepressant. There are no specific antidotes for REMERON™ (mirtazapine). If the patient is unconscious, establish and maintain an airway to ensure adequate oxygenation and ventilation. Gastric evacuation either by the induction of emesis or lavage or both should be considered. Activated charcoal should also be considered in treatment of overdose. Cardiac and vital signs monitoring is recommended along with general symptomatic and supportive measures.

In managing overdosage, consider the possibility of multiple-drug involvement. The physician should consider contacting a poison control center for additional information on the treatment of any overdose.

DOSAGE AND ADMINISTRATION

Initial Treatment

The recommended starting dose for REMERON™ (mirtazapine) is 15 mg/day, administered in a single dose, preferably in the evening prior to sleep. In the controlled clinical trials establishing the antidepressant efficacy of REMERON™, the effective dose range was generally 15–45 mg/day. While the relationship between dose and antidepressant response for REMERON™ has not been adequately explored, patients not responding to the initial 15 mg dose may benefit from dose increases up to a maximum of 45 mg/day. REMERON™ has an elimination half-life of approximately 20–40 hours; therefore, dose changes should not be made at intervals of less than one to two weeks in order to allow sufficient time for evaluation of the therapeutic response to a given dose.

Elderly and Patients with Renal or Hepatic Impairment

The clearance of mirtazapine is reduced in elderly patients and in patients with moderate to severe renal or hepatic impairment. Consequently, the prescriber should be aware that plasma mirtazapine levels may be increased in these patient groups, compared to levels observed in younger adults without renal or hepatic impairment (see Pharmacokinetics subsection of CLINICAL PHARMACOLOGY).

Maintenance/Extended Treatment

There is no body of evidence available from controlled trials to indicate how long the depressed patient should be treated with REMERON™ (mirtazapine). It is generally agreed, however, that pharmacological treatment for acute episodes of depression should continue for up to six months or longer. Whether the dose of antidepressant needed to induce remission is identical to the dose needed to maintain euthymia is unknown.

Switching Patients To or From a Monoamine Oxidase Inhibitor

At least 14 days should elapse between discontinuation of an MAOI and initiation of therapy with REMERON™ (mirtazapine). In addition, at least 14 days should be allowed after stopping REMERON™ before starting an MAOI.

HOW SUPPLIED

REMERON™ (mirtazapine) Tablets are supplied as:

15 mg Tablets—oval, scored, yellow, coated, with "Organon" embossed on one side and "TZ3" on the other side.

Bottles of 30	NDC# 0052-0105-30
Unit Dose, Box of 100	NDC# 0052-0105-90*

30 mg Tablets—oval, scored, red-brown, coated, with "Organon" embossed on one side and "TZ5" on the other side.

Bottles of 30	NDC# 0052-0107-30
Unit Dose, Box of 100	NDC# 0052-0107-90*

* Unit dose packs are provided as a blisterpack with 10 strips, each of which contains 10 tablets.

Store at controlled Room Temperature
20°–25°C (68°–77°F)

Dispense in a tight, light resistant container.

Caution: Federal law prohibits dispensing without prescription.

Organon
Manufactured for Organon Inc.
West Orange, NJ 07052
by N.V.Organon, OSS, Holland

Shown in Product Identification Guide, page 326

REVERSOL® ℞

(edrophonium chloride) injection, USP

HOW SUPPLIED

10 mg/mL: 10 mL Multiple Dose Vials-boxes of 25-NDC-0052-0466-34

SUCCINYLCHOLINE CHLORIDE INJECTION, USP ℞

HOW SUPPLIED

20 mg/mL: 10 mL vials-boxes of 25-NDC-0052-0445-10

TICE® BCG ℞

BCG VACCINE USP

(for Intravesical or Percutaneous use)

DESCRIPTION

TICE® BCG, a BCG Vaccine for intravesical or percutaneous use, is an attenuated, live culture preparation of the Bacillus of Calmette and Guerin (BCG) strain ***Mycobacterium bovis.***[1] The TICE strain was developed at the University of Illinois from a strain originated at the Pasteur Institute.

The medium in which the BCG organism is grown for preparation of the freeze-dried cake is composed of the following ingredients: glycerin, asparagine, citric acid, potassium phosphate, magnesium sulfate, and iron ammonium citrate. The final preparation prior to freeze-drying also contains lactose. The freeze-dried BCG preparation is delivered in glass-sealed ampules, each containing 1 to 8 $\times 10^8$ colony forming units (CFU) of TICE BCG which is equivalent to approximately 50 mg wet weight.

No preservatives have been added.

CLINICAL PHARMACOLOGY

Intravesical Use for Carcinoma In Situ of the Bladder. TICE BCG induces a granulomatous reaction at the local site of administration.[2] Intravesical TICE BCG has been used as a therapy for and prophylaxis against recurrent tumors in patients with carcinoma in situ (CIS) of the bladder. The precise mechanism of action is unknown. A variety of different treatment regimens have been used with the TICE[3–6] and other BCG substrains.[7–12]

An evaluation of intravesical administration of TICE BCG in patients with carcinoma in situ of the urinary bladder was recently completed. Bladder cancer patients were identified who had been treated with TICE BCG under six different Investigational New Drug (IND) applications in which the most important shared aspect was the use of an induction plus maintenance schedule. Comparison of demographic data between the six INDs revealed uniformity. Among these six studies were 119 evaluable patients who received intravesical treatment of CIS of the bladder. Patients with biopsy-proven CIS received TICE BCG (50 mg; 1–8 $\times 10^8$ CFU) intravesically, once weekly for at least 6 weeks and once monthly thereafter for up to 12 months. A longer maintenance was given in some cases. Follow-up cystoscopies were performed at 3 month intervals, as were urine cytologies for most patients (71 of 119). Urine cytology was obtained at the time of the 1989 follow-up for all patients who responded to TICE BCG *treatment, (CR and CRNC, see below).* The median time post treatment for these follow-up cytologies was 47 months.

The study population consisted of 153 patients; 132 males, 19 females and 2 unidentified as to gender. Thirty patients lacking baseline documentation of CIS and 4 patients lost to follow-up were not evaluable for treatment response. Therefore, 119 patients with biopsy or cystoscopy proven CIS prior to TICE BCG administration were available for efficacy evaluation. Some of these patients had undergone transurethral resection (TUR) one or more weeks prior to BCG, primarily for the treatment of papillomatous disease. The mean age for the CIS population was 68.8 ± 9.7 years s.d. (range: 38–97 years).

Sixty-three evaluable patients had received intravesical chemotherapy treatment for their bladder malignancy prior to TICE BCG treatment and had been diagnosed as treatment failures. The treatment had been as follows: thiotepa (30), mitomycin C (10), doxorubicin (1), mitomycin C and thiotepa (14), doxorubicin and thiotepa (1), doxorubicin and mitomycin C (1), thiotepa, mitomycin C and doxorubicin (2), interferon (1), interferon and thiotepa (1), cyclophosphamide IV (1), and cisplatin and thiotepa (1).

For the 119 patients with biopsy or cystoscopy proven CIS, the TICE BCG induction dosage consisted of a mean of 6.6 instillations (± 1.5 standard error of the mean). These patients also received a mean of 10.0 maintenance instillations after completing the induction phase. Twenty patients (16.8%) required TICE BCG reinduction at some point in the

Continued on next page

Organon—Cont.

study. Nine patients in one of the six studies received a percutaneous dose along with intravesical instillation. Data from a recent study show that a percutaneous dose with CIS is unnecessary.[13]

Clinical response criteria were defined as follows:

Complete Histological Response (CR): Complete resolution of carcinoma in situ documented by biopsy or, if a biopsy was not obtained, then by negative cystoscopy. All patients in this category were required to have urine cytology tests that were negative upon examination.

Complete Clinical Response Without Cytology (CRNC): Patients in this category had an apparent complete disappearance of tumor that was not confirmed by urine cytology tests. Complete resolution of carcinoma in situ documented by a biopsy or, if a biopsy was not obtained, then by negative cystoscopy.

Failure/Progression: Patients in this category had urine cytology tests that were found to be positive, although biopsy or cystoscopy was negative. This category also includes patients who continued to have evidence of malignant lesions, or a progression to a higher stage or grade; the appearance of new lesions; reappearance of old lesions.

A 75.6 percent response rate was reported for 119 evaluable patients (Table 1).

TABLE 1: RESPONSE OF PATIENTS TO TICE BCG IN CIS BLADDER CANCER

	Entered	Evaluable	CR	CRNC	Overall Response
No. of Patients	153	119	54	36	90
% Response		—	45.4%	30.2%	75.6%

The median duration of follow-up for the 1989 update, presented in Table 2, is 47 months. Of the 54 patients classified as CR in 1987, 30 remained without evidence of disease (CR) in 1989, whereas 6 patients died of unrelated disease and 18 relapsed. The 15 of 36 patients classified as CRNC in 1987 who remained without evidence of disease in 1989 were all found to meet the criteria of CR status on the basis of negative cytologies. In the interim, 4 CRNC patients died of unrelated diseases, 2 died of unknown causes, and 15 relapsed. Therefore, of the 90 overall responders (75.6%), 36.7 percent of patients relapsed, 13.3 percent died of other diseases, and 50 percent remained in CR. In addition, two patients who relapsed were reinduced in complete response by a second course of TICE BCG.

TABLE 2: THERAPEUTIC EFFICACY OF TICE BCG IN CIS BLADDER CANCER 1989 STATUS OF 90 RESPONDERS (CR OR CRNC)

Response	1987/CR n = 54	1987/CRNC n = 36	1987 Response n = 90	Percent
CR	30	15	45	50.0
CRNC	0	0	0	0.0
Unrelated Deaths	6	6	12	13.3
Failure	18	15	33	36.7

Among the 119 evaluable patients there was no significant difference in response rates between patients with or without prior intravesical chemotherapy: 45 of 63 (71%) versus 45 of 56 (80%), $p > .05$. Similarly, for the patients remaining in CR at the time of the 1989 evaluation, there was no significant difference between those with or without prior chemotherapy.

The median duration of response, calculated from the Kaplan-Meier curve as median time to recurrence, is estimated at 4 years or greater. The median duration of follow-up was 47 months. Of the total 90 responders, 45 patients (50%) remained without evidence of disease.

At a median follow-up of 47 months, 85 (71.4%) of the 119 evaluable patients remain alive. Thirteen patients (10.9%) died from causes unrelated to bladder cancer: cardiovascular disease (6 patients), second primary cancer (3 patients), and other (4 patients). Three patients died from unknown causes and bladder cancer cannot be ruled out. The bladder cancer related deaths were 18 (15%) of the 119. Historical data prior to the use of BCG, in a series of CIS patients treated usually with electrofulguration, indicate 82% of the patients recurred, 60% of the patients developed invasive cancer, and 34% of the patients died of their disease within 5 years.[14]

The incidence of cystectomy for 90 patients who achieved a complete response (CR or CRNC) with TICE BCG was 11%. For 29 patients who did not achieve CR or CRNC, the incidence of cystectomy was 55%, which is consistent with cystectomy rates reported in the literature for CIS patients who were not treated with intravesical therapies.[15]

The median time to cystectomy in patients who achieved a complete response (CR or CRNC) exceeded 74 months, whereas the median time to cystectomy for non-responders was 31 months.

Percutaneous Use for Immunization Against Tuberculosis. Immunization with BCG vaccine lowers the risk of serious complications of primary tuberculosis in children.[16–19] Estimates of efficacy from observational studies in areas where vaccination is performed at birth show that the incidence of tuberculous meningitis and miliary tuberculosis is 52%–100% lower and that the incidence of pulmonary tuberculosis is 2%–80% lower in vaccinated children less than 15 years of age than in unvaccinated controls.[16–21] However, estimates of vaccine efficacy may be distorted because of the following: vaccination was not allocated randomly in observational studies; there were differences in BCG strains, methods, and routes of administration; and there were differences in the characteristics of the populations and environments in which the vaccines have been studied.[22]

INDICATIONS AND USAGE

Intravesical Use for Carcinoma In Situ of the Bladder. Intravesical instillation of TICE BCG is indicated for the treatment of carcinoma in situ of the bladder in the following situations: (1) primary treatment in the absence of an associated invasive cancer without papillary tumors or with papillary tumors after TUR, (2) secondary treatment in the absence of an associated invasive cancer, in patients failing to respond or relapsing after intravesical chemotherapy with other agents, (3) primary or secondary treatment in the absence of invasive cancer for patients with medical contraindications to radical surgery. TICE BCG is not indicated for the treatment of papillary tumors occurring alone.

Percutaneous Use for Immunization Against Tuberculosis.
Exposed tuberculin skin test-negative infants and children: BCG vaccination is recommended for infants and children with negative tuberculin skin test who are (1) at high risk to intimate and prolonged exposure to persistently untreated or ineffectively treated patients with infectious pulmonary tuberculosis and who cannot be removed from the source of exposure and cannot be placed on long-term preventive therapy, or (2) continuously exposed to persons with tuberculosis who have bacilli resistant to isoniazid and rifampin.[22]

Groups with an excessive rate of new infections: BCG vaccination is also recommended for tuberculin-negative infants and children in groups in which the rate of new infections exceeds 1% per year and for whom the usual surveillance and treatment programs have been attempted but are not operationally feasible. These groups include persons without regular access to health care, those for whom usual health care is culturally or socially unacceptable, or groups who have demonstrated an inability to effectively use existing accessible care.

The US Immunization Practices Advisory Committee (ACIP) no longer recommends the use of BCG vaccination of health care workers at risk of repeated exposure to tuberculosis but recommends that these individuals be under tuberculin skin testing surveillance and receive isoniazid prophylaxis in case of tuberculin skin test conversion.[22]

For international travelers, the Centers for Disease Control (CDC) recommends that BCG vaccination be considered only for travelers with insignificant reaction to tuberculin skin test who will be in a high-risk environment for prolonged periods of time without access to tuberculin skin test surveillance.[22]

CONTRAINDICATIONS

Intravesical Use for Carcinoma In Situ of the Bladder. TICE BCG should not be used in immunosuppressed patients or persons with congenital or acquired immune deficiencies, whether due to concurrent disease (e.g., AIDS, leukemia, lymphoma) or cancer therapy (e.g., cytotoxic drugs, radiation). TICE BCG should be avoided in asymptomatic carriers with a positive HIV serology and in patients receiving steroids at immunosuppressive doses or other immunosuppressive therapies because of the possibility of the vaccine establishing a systemic infection.

Treatment should be postponed until resolution of a concurrent febrile illness, urinary tract infection, or gross hematuria. Seven to fourteen days should elapse before BCG is administered following biopsy, TUR, or traumatic catheterization.

A positive Mantoux test is a contraindication only if there is evidence of an active tuberculosis infection.

In the absence of safety data, intravesical TICE BCG should not be given to pregnant or lactating women.

Percutaneous Use for Immunization Against Tuberculosis. TICE BCG Vaccine for the prevention of tuberculosis should not be given to persons with impaired immune responses, whether they be congenital, disease produced, drug or therapy induced (i.e., cytotoxic drugs and radiation used in cancer therapy). The concurrent use of steroids requires caution because of the possibility of the vaccine establishing a systemic infection. If necessary, the infection can be treated with anti-tuberculous drugs.

WARNINGS

***Intravesical Use for Carcinoma In Situ of the Bladder.* TICE BCG is not a vaccine for the prevention of cancer.** There are currently no data on the effectiveness of intravesical installation of TICE BCG in the treatment of invasive bladder cancer.

The use of TICE BCG may cause tuberculin sensitivity. Since this is a valuable aid in the diagnosis of tuberculosis, it may therefore be useful to determine the tuberculin reactivity by PPD skin testing before treatment.

Intravesical instillations should be postponed in the presence of fever, suspected infection, or during treatment with antibiotics, since antimicrobial therapy may interfere with the effectiveness of TICE BCG.

Instillation of TICE BCG onto a bleeding mucosa may promote systemic BCG infection.[23] Death has been reported as a result of systemic BCG infection and sepsis. Patients should be monitored for the presence of symptoms and signs of toxicity after each intravesical treatment. Febrile episodes with flu-like symptoms lasting more than 48 hours, fever ≥ 103°F, systemic manifestations increasing in intensity with repeated instillations, or persistent abnormalities of liver function tests suggest systemic BCG infection and require anti-tuberculous therapy (see **ADVERSE REACTIONS** section).

Small bladder capacity has been associated with increased risk of severe local reactions and should be considered in deciding to use TICE BCG therapy.

Percutaneous Use for Immunization Against Tuberculosis. Administration should be percutaneous with the multiple puncture disc as described below. DO NOT INJECT INTRAVENOUSLY, SUBCUTANEOUSLY, OR INTRADERMALLY. TICE BCG Vaccine should not be used in infants, children, or adults with severe immune deficiency syndromes. Children with family history of immune deficiency disease should not be vaccinated. If they are, an infectious disease specialist should be consulted and anti-tuberculous therapy[24] administered if clinically indicated.

PRECAUTIONS

General: TICE BCG contains live bacteria and should be used with aseptic technique. All equipment, supplies, and receptacles in contact with TICE BCG should be handled and disposed of as biohazardous.

The possibility of allergic reactions should be assessed. TICE BCG administration should not be attempted in individuals with severe immune deficiency disease. TICE BCG Vaccine should be administered with caution to persons in groups at high risk for HIV infection.

Intravesical Use for Carcinoma In Situ of the Bladder.
General: Care should be taken not to traumatize the urinary tract or to introduce contaminants into the urinary system. Seven to fourteen days should elapse before BCG is administered following TUR, biopsy, or traumatic catheterization.

Information For Patients: TICE BCG is retained in the bladder 2 hours and then voided. Patients should void while seated for safety reasons following instillation of suspension. Within 6 hours after treatment, urine voided should be disinfected for 15 minutes with an equal volume of household bleach before flushing. Patients should be instructed to increase fluid intake to "flush" the bladder in the hours following BCG treatment. Patients may experience burning with the first void after treatment. Patients should be attentive to side effects, such as fever, chills, malaise, flu-like symptoms, or increased fatigue. If patient experiences severe urinary side effects, such as burning or pain on urination, urgency, frequency of urination, blood in urine, joint pain, cough, or skin rash, the physician should be notified.

Drug Interaction: Drug combinations containing immunosuppressants and/or bone marrow depressants and/or radiation interfere with the development of the immune response and should not be used in combination with TICE BCG. Antimicrobial therapy for other infections may interfere with the effectiveness of TICE BCG therapy.

Pregnancy Category C: Animal reproduction studies have not been conducted with TICE BCG. It is also not known whether TICE BCG can cause fetal harm when administered to a pregnant woman or can affect reproductive capacity. TICE BCG should be given to a pregnant woman only if clearly needed. Women should be advised not to become pregnant while on therapy.

Nursing Mothers: It is not known whether TICE BCG is excreted in human milk. Because many drugs are excreted in human milk and because of the potential for serious adverse reactions from TICE BCG in nursing infants, a decision should be made whether to discontinue nursing or to discontinue the drug, taking into account the importance of the drug to the mother.

Pediatric Use: Safety and effectiveness of carcinoma in situ of the urinary bladder in children have not been established.

Percutaneous Use for Immunization Against Tuberculosis.
Normal Reaction: The intensity and duration of the local reaction depends on the depth of penetration of the multiple-puncture disc and individual variations in patients' tissue reactions. The initial skin lesions usually appear within 10–14 days and consist of small red papules at the site. The papules reach maximum diameter (about 3 mm) after 4 to 6 weeks, after which they may scale and then slowly subside.

Six months afterward there is usually no visible sign of the vaccination, but on occasion a faintly discernible pattern of the disc points may be visible. On people whose skin tends to keloid formation, there may be slightly more visible evidence of the vaccination.

Vaccination is recommended only for those who are tuberculin negative to a recent skin test with 5 tuberculin units (5TU). Otherwise, vaccination of persons highly sensitive to mycobacterial antigens can result in hypersensitivity reactions including fever, anorexia, myalgia, and neuralgia, which last a few days.

After TICE BCG vaccination, it is usually not possible to clearly distinguish between a tuberculin reaction caused by persistent postvaccination sensitivity and one caused by a virulent suprainfection. Caution is advised in attributing a positive skin test to TICE BCG vaccination. A sharp rise in the tuberculin reaction since the latest test should be further investigated (except in the immediate postvaccination period).

Information For Patients: Keep the vaccination site clean until the local reaction has disappeared.

Drug Interaction: Antimicrobial or immunosuppressive agents may interfere with the development of the immune response and should be used only under medical supervision.

Pregnancy Category C: Animal reproduction studies have not been conducted with TICE BCG. It is also not known whether TICE BCG can cause fetal harm when administered to a pregnant woman or can affect reproduction capacity. TICE BCG should be given to a pregnant woman only if clearly needed.

Nursing Mothers: It is not known whether TICE BCG is excreted in human milk. Because many drugs are excreted in human milk and because of the potential for serious adverse reactions in nursing infants from TICE BCG, a decision should be made whether to discontinue nursing or not to vaccinate, taking into account the importance of tuberculosis vaccination to the mother.

Pediatric Use: See **Treatment and Schedule** under **DOSAGE AND ADMINISTRATION** section. Precautions should be taken with respect to infants vaccinated with BCG and exposed to persons with active tuberculosis.[25]

ADVERSE REACTIONS

Intravesical Use for Carcinoma In Situ of the Bladder. Adverse reactions are often localized to the bladder but may be accompanied by systemic manifestations. Symptoms of bladder irritability, related to the inflammatory response induced by intravesical TICE BCG, are reported in 60 percent of cases. They begin 3–4 hours after instillation and last 24–72 hours. The urinary side effects are usually seen after the third treatment and tend to increase in severity after each administration. There were, however, no long-term urinary complications in this group of patients.

A summary of adverse reactions seen with 674 patients with superficial bladder cancer, including 153 CIS patients treated intravesically with TICE BCG is shown in Table 3.[26]

Irritative bladder adverse effects associated with BCG administration can be managed symptomatically with pyridium, propantheline bromide or oxybutynin chloride, and acetaminophen or ibuprofen.[27] Systemic adverse effects such as malaise, fever, and chills may reflect hypersensitivity reactions and can be treated with antihistamines.[27] The "flu-like" syndrome of 1–2 days' duration that frequently accompanies intravesical BCG administration should be managed by standard symptomatic treatment. Symptoms persisting longer than 2 days suggest continued infection, and consideration should be given to therapy with isoniazid. Localized (e.g., prostatitis, epididymitis) as well as systemic infection can occur with intravesical BCG administration. For systemic infection, an infectious diseases specialist should be consulted and the patient promptly treated with anti-tuberculous therapy as advised.[28] At least two deaths have been reported as a result of systemic BCG infection and sepsis.[27] There have been two cases of nephrogenic adenoma, a benign lesion of bladder epithelium, associated with intravesical BCG therapy.[29] In general, the adverse effects of BCG therapy in bladder carcinoma have been of short duration and moderate morbidity.

Percutaneous Use for Immunization Against Tuberculosis. Occasionally, lymphadenopathy of the regional lymph node, which spontaneously resolves itself, is seen in young children. Only rarely does the node create a fistula followed by a short period of drainage. The usual treatment is to maintain cleanliness of the site of drainage and allow the lesion to heal spontaneously without medical intervention.

Other rare events are osteomyelitis, lupoid reactions, disseminated BCG infection, and death. Osteomyelitis has been reported to occur at a rate of about 1 per 1,000,000 vaccinees.[22] Disseminated BCG infection and death are very rare (about 1 per 5,000,000 vaccinees)[30] and occur almost exclusively in children with impaired immune responses. [See table 3 above.]

OVERDOSAGE

Intravesical Use for Carcinoma In Situ of the Bladder. Overdosage occurs if more than one ampule of TICE BCG is administered per instillation. The patient should be closely monitored for signs of systemic BCG infection and treated with anti-tuberculous medication (see **ADVERSE REACTIONS** section).

TABLE 3: SUMMARY OF ADVERSE EFFECTS SEEN IN 674 PATIENTS WITH SUPERFICIAL BLADDER CANCER, INCLUDING 153 WITH CARCINOMA IN SITU

Local Adverse Effects	Number of Patients	Percent (%)	Toxicity by Grade (%)* Mild	Moderate	Severe	Not Stated
Dysuria	401	59.5	28.2	18.1	10.7	2.5
Urinary Frequency	272	40.4	17.2	15.7	7.4	—
Hematuria	175	26.0	8.2	9.6	7.4	0.8
Cystitis	40	5.9	1.6	2.4	1.9	—
Urgency	39	5.8	1.2	1.8	1.3	1.5
Nocturia	30	4.5	1.3	1.8	0.6	0.7
Cramps/Pain	27	4.0	0.9	1.3	0.9	0.9
Urinary Incontinence	16	2.4	0.4	0.9	—	1.2
Urinary Debris	15	2.2	0.2	1.0	0.4	0.6
Genital Inflammation/ Abscess	12	1.8	0.3	0.4	0.4	0.6
Urinary Tract Infection	10	1.5	0.2	0.3	0.9	0.2
Urethritis	8	1.2	0.3	0.6	—	0.3
Pyuria	5	0.7	0.2	0.1	0.1	0.3
Epididymitis/Prostatitis	2	0.3	—	—	—	0.3
Urinary Obstruction	2	0.3	—	—	—	0.3
Contracted Bladder	1	0.2	—	—	—	0.2
Orchitis	1	0.2	—	—	—	0.2
Systemic Adverse Effects	**Number of Patients**	**Percent (%)**	**Toxicity by Grade (%)* Mild**	**Moderate**	**Severe**	**Not Stated**
Flu-like Syndrome**	224	33.2	9.3	10.9	9.0	4.0
Fever	134	19.9	6.1	5.3	7.6	0.9
Malaise/Fatigue	50	7.4	2.7	3.1	—	1.6
Shaking Chills	22	3.3	0.2	1.5	1.0	0.6
Nausea/Vomiting	20	3.0	1.0	1.6	0.3	—
Arthritis/Myalgia	18	2.7	0.3	1.0	0.4	0.9
Headache/Dizziness	16	2.4	0.3	0.9	—	1.2
Anorexia/Weight Loss	15	2.2	0.4	1.3	0.1	0.5
Allergic	14	2.1	0.6	0.7	0.4	0.3
Cardiac	13	1.9	—	0.3	1.3	0.3
Respiratory (Unclassified)	11	1.6	0.4	0.4	0.2	0.6
Abdominal Pain	10	1.5	—	0.6	0.6	0.3
Anemia	9	1.3	0.2	0.6	0.4	0.1
Diarrhea	8	1.2	0.2	0.6	0.1	0.3
Pneumonitis	8	1.2	0.2	—	0.6	0.4
Gastrointestinal (Unclassified)	7	1.0	0.2	0.1	—	0.7
Neurologic	6	0.9	0.1	—	0.3	0.4
Rash	4	0.6	—	0.4	0.2	—
BCG Sepsis	3	0.4	—	—	0.4	—
Coagulopathy	2	0.3	—	—	0.3	—
Leukopenia	2	0.3	0.2	0.1	—	—
Thrombocytopenia	2	0.3	0.2	0.1	—	—
Hepatic Granuloma	1	0.2	—	—	0.2	—
Hepatitis	1	0.2	—	—	0.2	—

*Grade was determined using ECOG scale of toxicity criteria, Mild = Grade 1, Moderate = Grade 2, Severe = Grade 3 or 4.
**Flu-like syndrome includes fever, shaking chills, malaise and myalgia.

Percutaneous Use of Immunization Against Tuberculosis. Accidental overdosages if treated immediately with anti-tuberculous drugs have not led to complications.[31] If the vaccination response is allowed to progress it can still be treated successfully with anti-tuberculous drugs but complications can include regional adenitis, lupus vulgaris, subcutaneous cold abscesses, ocular lesions, and others.[32]

DOSAGE AND ADMINISTRATION

Intravesical Use for Carcinoma In Situ of the Bladder. The intravesical dose consists of one ampule of TICE BCG suspended in 50 mL preservative-free saline. **Preparation of Agent:** The preparation of the TICE BCG suspension should be done using sterile technique. The pharmacist or individual responsible for mixing the agent should wear gloves, mask, and gown to avoid inadvertent exposure of open sores or inhalation of BCG organisms. Draw 1 mL of sterile, preservative-free saline (0.9% Sodium Chloride Injection USP) at 4°–25°C, into a small (e.g., 3 mL) syringe and add to one ampule of TICE BCG to resuspend. Draw the mixture into the syringe and gently expel back into the ampule three times to ensure thorough mixing. This mixing minimizes the clumping of the mycobacteria. Dispense the cloudy BCG suspension into the top end of a catheter-tip syringe which contains 49 mL saline diluent bringing the total volume to 50 mL. Gently rotate the syringe. The suspended TICE BCG should be used immediately after preparation. Discard after 2 hours.

Note: DO NOT filter the contents of the TICE BCG ampule. Precautions should be taken to avoid exposing the TICE BCG to light. Bacteriostatic solutions must be avoided. In addition, use only sterile preservative-free saline, 0.9% Sodium Chloride Injection USP, as diluent and perform all mixing operations in sterile glass or thermosetting plastic containers and syringes.

Treatment and Schedule: Allow 7–14 days to elapse after bladder biopsy or TUR before TICE BCG is administered. Patients should not drink fluids for 4 hours before treatment and should empty their bladder prior to TICE BCG administration. The reconstituted TICE BCG is instilled into the bladder by gravity flow via the catheter. DO NOT depress plunger and force the flow of the TICE BCG. The TICE BCG is retained in the bladder 2 hours and then voided. Patients unable to retain the suspension for 2 hours should be allowed to void sooner, if necessary. While the TICE BCG is retained in the bladder, the patient may be repositioned from left side to right side and also may alternately lie upon the back and the abdomen, changing these positions every 15 minutes to maximize bladder surface exposure to the agent.

A standard treatment schedule consists of one intravesical instillation per week for 6 weeks. This schedule may be repeated once if tumor remission has not been achieved and if the clinical circumstances warrant. Thereafter, intravesical TICE BCG administration should continue at approximately monthly intervals for at least 6–12 months.

Percutaneous Use for Immunization Against Tuberculosis. **Preparation of Agent:** Using sterile methods, 1 mL of sterile water for injection, USP at 4°–25°C, is added to one ampule of vaccine (see **Pediatric Dose** below for pediatric use). Draw the mixture into a syringe and expel it back into the ampule three times to ensure thorough mixing.

Parenteral drug products should be inspected visually for particulate matter and discoloration prior to administration, whenever solution and container permit. Reconstitution should result in a uniform suspension of the bacilli.

Treatment and Schedule: The vaccine is to be administered after fully explaining the risks and benefits to the vaccinee, parent, or guardian. After the vaccine is prepared, the immunizing dose of 0.2–0.3 mL is dropped on the cleansed surface of the skin, and the vaccine is administered percutaneously utilizing a sterile multiple-puncture disc. The multiple-puncture disc is a thin wafer-like stainless steel plate $^7/_8'' \times 1^1/_8''$, from which 36 points protrude. The disc is held by a magnet type holder. In this method a drop of vaccine is placed on the arm and spread with the wide edge of disc. The

Continued on next page

Organon—Cont.

disc is placed gently over the vaccine and the magnet is centered. The arm is grasped firmly from underneath, tensing the skin appreciably. Downward pressure is applied on the magnet so the points of the disc are well buried in skin. With pressure still exerted, the disc is rocked forward and backward and from side to side several times. Pressure underneath the arm is then released and the magnetic is slid off the disc. In a successful procedure, the points remain in the skin. If the points are on top of the skin, the procedure must be repeated. Remove the disc after successful puncture and spread vaccine evenly over the puncture area with the wide edge of the disc. Discs should only be used once and discarded after autoclaving. Between individual vaccinations the magnet should be sterilized (see instructions for use provided with the device). Discs may be purchased separately from Organon Teknika Corporation, telephone number (800) 662-6842. After vaccination the vaccine should flow into the wounds and dry. No dressing is required; however, it is recommended that the site be kept dry for 24 hours. The patient should be advised that the vaccine contains live organisms. Although the vaccine will not survive in a dry state, infection of others is possible.
Reconstituted vaccine should be kept refrigerated, protected from exposure to light, and used within 2 hours. Vaccination should be repeated for those who remain tuberculin negative to 5TU of tuberculin after 2–3 months.

Pediatric Dose: In infants less than 1 month old the dosage of vaccine should be reduced by one half, by using 2 mL of sterile water when reconstituting. If a vaccinated infant remains tuberculin negative to 5TU on skin testing, and if indications for vaccination persist, the infant should receive a full dose after 1 year of age.

HOW SUPPLIED

TICE BCG vaccine is supplied in a box of one 2 mL ampule of TICE BCG. Each ampule contains 1 to 8 $\times$ 10^8 CFU, which is equivalent to approximately 50 mg (wet weight), as lyophilized (freeze-dried) powder, NDC 0052-0601-01.

STORAGE

Storage of the intact ampules of TICE BCG should be at refrigerated temperatures of 2–8°C (36–46°F). This agent contains live bacteria and should be protected from light. The product should not be used after the expiration date printed on the label.

REFERENCES

1. Guerin C: The history of BCG. In: Rosenthal SR (ed); BCG Vaccine: Tuberculosis-Cancer. Littleton, MA, PSG Publishing Co., Inc. 1980, pp. 35–43.
2. Kelley DR, Haaff E, Becich M, et al.: Prognostic value of purified protein derivative skin test and granuloma formation in patients treated with intravesical bacillus Calmette-Guerin. J Urol 1986; 135:268–271.
3. Brosman SA: The use of bacillus Calmette-Guerin in the therapy of bladder carcinoma in situ. J Urol 1985; 134:36–39.
4. DeKernion JB, Huang M. Linder A, et al.: The management of superficial bladder tumors and carcinoma in situ with intravesical bacillus Calmette-Guerin. J Urol 1985; 133:598–601.
5. Guinan P, Batenhorst R: BCG in the treatment of superficial bladder cancer (Abstract). J Urol 1987; 137:180A.
6. Soloway M, Perry A: Bacillus Calmette-Guerin for treatment of superficial transitional cell carcinoma of the bladder in patients who have failed thiotepa and/or mitomycin C. J Urol 1987; 137:871–873.
7. Morales A: Long-term results and complications of intracavitary bacillus Calmette-Guerin therapy for bladder cancer. J Urol 1984; 132:457–459.
8. Haaff E, Dresner SM, Ratliff TL, Catalona WJ: Two courses of intravesical bacillus Calmette-Guerin for transitional cell carcinoma of the bladder. J Urol 1986; 136:820–824.
9. Herr HW, Pinsky CM, Whitmore WF, et al.: Effect of intravesical bacillus Calmette-Guerin (BCG) on carcinoma in situ. Cancer 1983; 51:1323–1326.
10. Kelley DR, Ratliff T, Catalona WJ, et al.: Intravesical bacillus Calmette-Guerin therapy for superficial bladder cancer. Effect of bacillus Calmette-Guerin viability on treatment results. J Urol 1985; 134:48–53.
11. Schellhammer PF, Ladaga LE, Fillion MB: Bacillus Calmette-Guerin for therapy of superficial transitional cell carcinoma of the bladder. J Urol 1986; 135:261–264.
12. Lamm DL: BCG immunotherapy in bladder cancer. In: Urology Annual 1987. Vol. 1, Appleton & Lange, Norwalk, CT, 1987; pp. 67–86.
13. Lamm DL, Sarosdy MS, DeHaven JI: Percutaneous, oral, or intravesical BCG administration: What is the optimal route? EORTC Genitourinary Group Monograph 6: BCG in Superficial Bladder Cancer. Alan R. Liss, Inc., New York, NY, 1989; pp. 301–310.
14. Utz DC, Hanash KA, Farrow GM: The plight of the patient with carcinoma in situ of the bladder. J Urol 1970; 103: 160–164.
15. Herr HW, Pinsky CM, Whitmore WF Jr., et al.: Long-term effect of intravesical bacillus Calmette-Guerin on flat carcinoma in situ of the bladder. J Urol 1986; 135:265–267.
16. Romanus V: Tuberculosis in bacillus Calmette-Guerin immunized and unimmunized children in Sweden: a ten-year evaluation following the cessation of general bacillus Calmette-Guerin immunization of the newborn in 1975. Pediatr Infect Dis 1987; 6:272–280.
17. Smith PG: Case-control studies of the efficacy of BCG against tuberculosis. In: International Union Against Tuberculosis, Proceedings of the XXXVIth IUAT World Conference on Tuberculosis and Respiratory Diseases, Singapore. Professional Postgraduate Services, International, Japan, 1987; 73–79.
18. Padungchan S, Konjanart S, Kasiratta S, et al.: The effectiveness of BCG vaccination of the newborn against childhood tuberculosis in Bangkok. Bull WHO 1986; 64:247–258.
19. Tidjani O, Amedone A, ten Dam HG: The protective effect of BCG vaccination of the newborn against childhood tuberculosis in an African community. Tubercle 1986; 67:269–281.
20. Young TK, Hershfield ES: A case-control study to evaluate the effectiveness of mass neonatal BCG vaccination among Canadian Indians. Am J Public Health 1986; 76:783–786.
21. Shapiro C, Cook N, Evans D, et al.: A case-control study of BCG and childhood tuberculosis in Cali, Columbia. Int H Epidemiol 1985; 14:441–446.
22. Morbidity and Mortality Weekly Report 37, No. 43 1988; pp. 663–675.
23. Rawls WH, Lamm DL, Eyolfson MF: Septic complications in the use of bacillus Calmette-Guerin (BCG) for noninvasive transitional cell carcinoma. Presented at: 1988 Annual Meeting, American Urological Association, Boston, MA.
24. Lorin MI, Hsu KHK, Jacob SC: Treatment of tuberculosis in children. In: Symposium on anti-infective therapy. Pediatric Clinics of North America, 1983; 30:333–348.
25. Report of the Committee on the Control of Infectious Diseases. American Academy of Pediatrics 1988; 21st Edition.
26. Data on file. Organon Teknika Corporation/Biotechnology Research Institute, Rockville, MD.
27. Lamm DL, Steg A, Boccon-Gibod L, et al.: Complications of bacillus Calmette-Guerin immunotherapy: Review of 2602 patients and comparison of chemotherapy complications. EORTC Genitourinary Group Monograph 6: BCG in Superficial Bladder Cancer. Alan R. Liss, Inc., New York, NY, 1989; pp. 335–355.
28. Standard Therapy for Tuberculosis, 1985. Presented at: National Consensus Conference on Tuberculosis. Chest, 1985; 87 (Suppl):117S–124S.
29. Oates R, Siroky M: Nephrogenic adenoma of urinary bladder due to intravesical BCG therapy. J Urol 1986; 135:186.
30. Mande R: BCG Vaccination. Dawsons, London, 1968.
31. Griffith AH: Ten cases of BCG overdose treated with isoniazid. Tubercle 1963; 44:247–250.
32. Watkins SM: Unusual complications of BCG vaccination. Brit Med J 1971; 1:442.

Manufactured by: Organon Teknika Corporation
100 Akzo Avenue
Durham, NC 27704
Distributed by: Organon Inc.
West Orange, NJ 07052
U.S. License
No. 956
TICE® is a trademark licensed from the University of Illinois.
RM 034.2 Issue Date: March, 1994

Shown in Product Identification Guide, page 326

WIGRAINE® ℞
(ergotamine tartrate and caffeine tablets, USP)

DESCRIPTION

Wigraine® Tablet: Each tablet contains the following:
Ergotamine Tartrate, USP .... 1 mg
Caffeine, USP .... 100 mg
Each tablet also contains: Lactose, Magnesium Stearate, Microcrystalline Cellulose, Purified Water and Starch as inactive ingredients.
Wigraine® tablets are uncoated and prepared to insure rapid disintegration (by an exclusive manufacturing process) and facilitate quick absorption. Rapid onset of effect is important for the satisfactory treatment of acute attacks of vascular headaches.
Wigraine® Suppository: Each suppository contains the following:
Ergotamine tartrate, USP .... 2 mg
Caffeine, USP .... 100 mg
Tartaric Acid .... 21.5 mg
Wigraine® suppositories contain the active ingredients in a synthetic cocoa butter base which melts rapidly at body temperature.

CLINICAL PHARMACOLOGY

Ergotamine is an alpha adrenergic blocking agent with a direct stimulating effect on the smooth muscle of peripheral and cranial blood vessels and produces depression of central vasomotor centers. The compound also has the properties of serotonin antagonism. In comparison to hydrogenated ergotamine, the adrenergic blocking actions are less pronounced and vasoconstrictive actions are greater. Caffeine, also a cranial vasoconstrictor is added to further enhance the vasoconstrictive effect without the necessity of increasing ergotamine dosage.

INDICATIONS AND USAGE

Wigraine® is indicated as therapy to abort or prevent vascular headaches such as migraine, migraine variants, or so-called histamine cephalgia.

CONTRAINDICATIONS

Wigraine® can cause fetal harm when administered to a pregnant women. It can produce prolonged uterine contractions which can result in abortion. Wigraine® is contraindicated in women who are or may become pregnant. If this is used during pregnancy, or if the patient becomes pregnant while taking this drug, the patient should be advised of the potential hazard to the fetus.
Peripheral vascular disease, coronary heart disease, hypertension, impaired hepatic or renal function, sepsis, and hypersensitivity to any of the components.

PRECAUTIONS

Although signs and symptoms of ergotism rarely develop even after long term intermittent use of the orally or rectally administered drugs, care should be exercised to remain within the limits of recommended dosage.

Pregnancy Category X. See Contraindications section.

Nursing Mothers. It is not known whether the ergotamine tartrate in Wigraine® is excreted in human milk. Because some ergot alkaloids have been found in the milk of nursing mothers resulting in symptoms of ergotism in their children, a decision should be made whether to discontinue nursing or to discontinue the drug, taking into account the importance of the drug to the mother.

Pediatric Usage. Safety and effectiveness in children have not been established.

ADVERSE REACTIONS

In order of decreasing severity: precordial distress and pain, muscle pains in the extremities, numbness and tingling in fingers and toes, transient tachycardia or bradycardia, vomiting, nausea, weakness in the legs, diarrhea, localized edema and itching.

DOSAGE AND ADMINISTRATION

Best results are obtained if the tablets or suppositories are administered at the first sign of an attack. Wigraine® tablet: the average adult dose is 2 tablets at the start of a vascular headache (migraine) attack; followed by 1 additional tablet every 1/2 hour if needed, up to 6 tablets per attack. Total weekly dosage should not exceed 10 tablets. Wigraine® suppository: the maximum adult dose is 2 suppositories for an individual attack. In carefully selected patients, with due consideration of maximum dosage recommendations, administration of the drug at bedtime may be an appropriate short-term preventive measure.

OVERDOSAGE

The toxic effects of an acute overdosage of Wigraine® are due primarily to the ergotamine component. The amount of caffeine is such that its toxic effects will be overshadowed by those of ergotamine. Symptoms include vomiting, numbness, tingling, pain and cyanosis of the extremities associated with diminished or absent peripheral pulses, hypertension or hypotension, drowsiness, stupor, coma, convulsions and shock. Treatment consists of removal of the offending drug by induction of emesis, gastric lavage and catharsis. Maintenance of adequate pulmonary ventilation, correction of hypotension, and control of convulsions are important considerations. Treatment of peripheral vasospasm should consist of warmth, but not heat, and protection of the ischemic limbs. Vasodilators may be used with benefit but caution must be exercised to avoid aggravating an already existing hypotension. The LD50 limits of the various components as outlined in NIOSH 1978 Registry of Toxic Effects of Chemical Substances, published by U.S. Department of Health, Education and Welfare are as follows: Ergotamine Tartrate IV LD50 in rats = 80mg/Kg, Caffeine IV LD50 in rats = 105mg/Kg.

HOW SUPPLIED

Wigraine® tablets are white tablets embossed with "ORGANON 542" on one side. They are individually foil stripped

and packaged in boxes of 20's NDC #0052-0542-20 and 100's NDC #0052-0542-91.

STORAGE

Wigraine® tablets should be stored at a maximum of 30°C (86°F) and the suppositories should be refrigerated at 2°–8°C (36°–46°F).

CAUTION

Federal law prohibits dispensing without prescription.

Revised 1/93

Shown in Product Identification Guide, page 326

ZEMURON™ ℞
(rocuronium bromide) injection

THIS DRUG SHOULD BE ADMINISTERED BY ADEQUATELY-TRAINED INDIVIDUALS FAMILIAR WITH ITS ACTIONS, CHARACTERISTICS, AND HAZARDS.

DESCRIPTION

ZEMURON™ (rocuronium bromide) Injection is a nondepolarizing neuromuscular blocking agent with a rapid to intermediate onset depending on dose and intermediate duration. Rocuronium bromide is chemically designated as 1-[17β-(acetyloxy)-3α-hydroxy-2β-(4-morpholinyl)-5α-androstan-16β-yl]-1-(2-propenyl)pyrrolidinium bromide. The structural formula is:

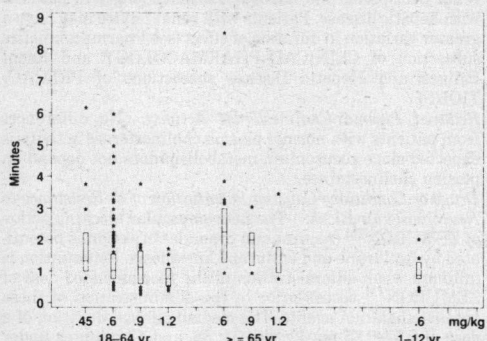

The chemical formula is $C_{32}H_{53}BrN_2O_4$ with a molecular weight of 609.70. The partition coefficient of rocuronium bromide in n-octanol/water is 0.5 at 20°C.

ZEMURON™ (rocuronium bromide) Injection is supplied as a sterile, nonpyrogenic, isotonic solution for intravenous injection only. Each mL contains 10 mg rocuronium bromide and 2 mg sodium acetate. The aqueous solution is adjusted to isotonicity with sodium chloride and to a pH of 4 with acetic acid and/or sodium hydroxide.

CLINICAL PHARMACOLOGY

ZEMURON™ (rocuronium bromide) Injection is a nondepolarizing neuromuscular blocking agent with a rapid to intermediate onset depending on dose and intermediate duration. It acts by competing for cholinergic receptors at the motor end-plate. This action is antagonized by acetylcholinesterase inhibitors, such as neostigmine and edrophonium.

Pharmacodynamics: The ED_{95} (dose required to produce 95% suppression of the first [T_1] mechanomyographic [MMG] response of the adductor pollicis muscle [thumb]) to indirect supramaximal train-of-four stimulation of the ulnar nerve) during opioid/nitrous oxide/oxygen anesthesia is approximately 0.3 mg/kg. Patient variability around the ED_{95} dose suggests that 50% of patients will exhibit T_1 depression of 91–97%.

Table 1 presents intubating conditions in patients with intubation initiated at 60 to 70 seconds.

[See first table above.]

Table 2 presents the time to onset and clinical duration for the initial dose of ZEMURON™ (rocuronium bromide) under opioid/nitrous oxide/oxygen anesthesia in adults and geriatric patients, and under halothane anesthesia in children. [See second table above.]

The time to ≥80% block and clinical duration as a function of dose are presented in Figures 1 and 2.

Table 1. Intubating Conditions in Patients with Intubation Initiated at 60 to 70 seconds. Percent, Median (Range)

ZEMURON™ Dose (mg/kg) Administered over 5 sec	Percent of patients with excellent or good intubating conditions	Time to completion of intubation (min)
Adults* 18–64 yr		
0.45 (n=43)	86%	1.6 (1.0–7.0)
0.6 (n=51)	96%	1.6 (1.0–3.2)
Pediatric 3 mo–1 yr		
0.6 (n=18)	100%	1.0 (1.0–1.5)
Pediatric 1–12 yr		
0.6 (n=12)	100%	1.0 (0.5–2.3)

*Excludes patients undergoing cesarean section

Excellent intubating conditions = jaw relaxed, vocal cords apart and immobile, no diaphragmatic movement.
Good intubating conditions = same as excellent but with some diaphragmatic movement.

Table 2. Time to Onset and Clinical Duration following Initial (intubating) Dose during Opioid/Nitrous Oxide/Oxygen Anesthesia (Adults) and Halothane Anesthesia (Children), Median (Range)

ZEMURON™ Dose (mg/kg) Administered over 5 sec	Time to ≥ 80% Block (min)	Time to Maximum Block (min)	Clinical Duration (min)
Adults 18–64 yr			
0.45 (n=50)	1.3 (0.8–6.2)	3.0 (1.3–8.2)	22 (12–31)
0.6 (n=142)	1.0 (0.4–6.0)	1.8 (0.6–13.0)	31 (15–85)
0.9 (n=20)	1.1 (0.3–3.8)	1.4 (0.8–6.2)	58 (27–111)
1.2 (n=18)	0.7 (0.4–1.7)	1.0 (0.6–4.7)	67 (38–160)
Geriatric ≥ 65 yr			
0.6 (n=31)	2.3 (1.0–8.3)	3.7 (1.3–11.3)	46 (22–73)
0.9 (n=5)	2.0 (1.0–3.0)	2.5 (1.2–5.0)	62 (49–75)
1.2 (n=7)	1.0 (0.8–3.5)	1.3 (1.2–4.7)	94 (64–138)
Pediatric 3 mo–1 yr			
0.6 (n=17)	—	0.8 (0.3–3.0)	41 (24–68)
0.8 (n=9)	—	0.7 (0.5–0.8)	40 (27–70)
Pediatric 1–12 yr			
0.6 (n=27)	0.8 (0.4–2.0)	1.0 (0.5–3.3)	26 (17–39)
0.8 (n=18)	—	0.5 (0.3–1.0)	30 (17–56)

n = the number of patients who had Time to Maximum Block recorded.
Clinical duration = time until return to 25% of control T_1. Patients receiving doses of 0.45 mg/kg who achieved less than 90% block (16% of these patients) had about 12 to 15 minutes to 25% recovery.

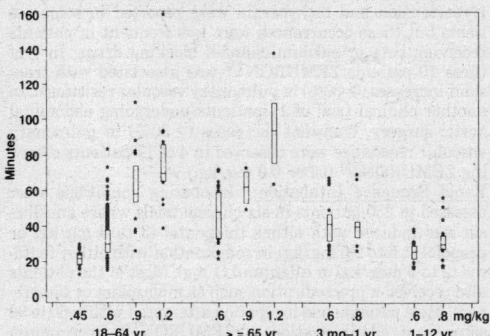

Figure 2. Duration of Clinical Effect *vs.* Initial Dose of ZEMURON™ By Age Group (Median, 25th and 75th percentile, and individual values).

The clinical durations for the first five maintenance doses, in patients receiving five or more maintenance doses are represented in Figure 3 (see also Maintenance Dosing subsection of DOSAGE AND ADMINISTRATION).

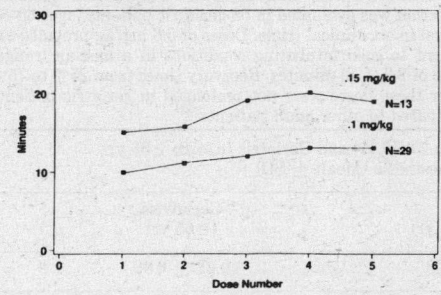

Figure 3. Duration of Clinical Effect *vs.* Number of ZEMURON™ Maintenance Doses, by Dose.

Once spontaneous recovery has reached 25% of control T_1, the neuromuscular block produced by ZEMURON™ is readily reversed with anticholinesterase agents, e.g., edrophonium or neostigmine.

The median spontaneous recovery from 25 to 75% T_1 was 13 minutes in adult patients. When neuromuscular block was reversed in 36 adults at a T_1 of 22–27%, recovery to a T_1 of 89 (50–132)% and T_4/T_1 of 69 (38–92)% was achieved within 5 minutes. Only five of 320 adults reversed received an additional dose of reversal agent. The median (range) dose of neostigmine was 0.04 (0.01 to 0.09) mg/kg and the median (range) dose of edrophonium was 0.5 (0.3 to 1.0) mg/kg.

In geriatric patients (n=51) reversed with neostigmine, the median T_4/T_1 increased from 40 to 88% in 5 minutes. Children (n=27) who received 0.5 mg/kg edrophonium had increases in the median T_4/T_1 from 37% at reversal to 93% after 2 minutes. Children (n=58) who received 1 mg/kg edrophonium had increases in the median T_4/T_1 from 72% at reversal to 100% after 2 minutes. Infants (n=10) who were reversed with 0.03 mg/kg neostigmine recovered from 25 to 75% T_1 within 4 minutes.

There were no reports of less than satisfactory clinical recovery of neuromuscular function.

The neuromuscular blocking action of ZEMURON™ may be enhanced in the presence of potent inhalation anesthetics (see Inhalation Anesthetics subsection of PRECAUTIONS).

Hemodynamics: There were no dose-related effects on the incidence of changes from baseline (≥ 30%) in mean arterial blood pressure (MAP) or heart rate associated with ZEMURON™ (rocuronium bromide) Injection administration over the dose range of 0.12 to 1.2 mg/kg (4 × ED_{95}) within 5 minutes after ZEMURON™ administration and prior to intubation. Increases or decreases in MAP were observed in 2–5% of geriatric and other adult patients, and in about 1% of pediatric patients. Heart rate changes (≥ 30%) occurred in 0–2% of geriatric and other adult patients. Tachycardia (≥ 30%) occurred in 12 of 127 children. Most of the children developing tachycardia were from a single study where the patients were anesthetized with halothane and who did not receive atropine for induction (see Pediatric subsection of Clinical Trials). In U.S. studies, laryngoscopy and tracheal intubation following ZEMURON™ administration were accompanied by transient tachycardia (≥ 30% increases) in about one-third of adult patients under opioid/nitrous oxide/oxy-

Figure 1. Time to ≥80% Block *vs.* Initial Dose of ZEMURON™ By Age Group (Median, 25th and 75th percentile, and individual values).

Continued on next page

Organon—Cont.

gen anesthesia. Animal studies have indicated that the ratio of vagal:neuromuscular block following ZEMURON™ administration is less than vecuronium but greater than pancuronium. The tachycardia observed in some patients may result from this vagal blocking activity.

Histamine Release: In studies of histamine release, clinically significant concentrations of plasma histamine occurred in 1 of 88 patients. Clinical signs of histamine release (flushing, rash, or bronchospasm) associated with the administration of ZEMURON™ (rocuronium bromide) Injection were assessed in clinical trials and reported in 9 of 1137 (0.8%) patients.

Pharmocokinetics: *In an effort to maximize the information gathered in the in vivo pharmacokinetic studies the data from the studies was used to develop population estimates of the parameters for the subpopulations represented (e.g., geriatric, pediatric, renal, and hepatic insufficiency). These population based estimates and a measure of the estimate variability are contained in the following section.*

Following IV administration of ZEMURON™ (rocuronium bromide) Injection, plasma levels of rocuronium follow a three compartment open model. The rapid distribution half-life is 1–2 minutes and the slower distribution half-life is 14–18 minutes. Rocuronium is approximately 30% bound to human plasma proteins. In geriatric and other adult surgical patients undergoing either opioid/nitrous oxide/oxygen or inhalational anesthesia the observed pharmacokinetic profile was essentially unchanged.

[See table 3 below.]

In general, studies with normal adult subjects did not reveal any differences in the pharmacokinetics of rocuronium due to gender.

Studies of distribution, metabolism, and excretion in cats and dogs indicate that rocuronium is eliminated primarily by the liver. The rocuronium analog 17-desacetyl-rocuronium, a metabolite, has been rarely observed in the plasma or urine of humans administered single doses of 0.5–1 mg/kg with or without a subsequent infusion (for up to 12 hr) of rocuronium. In the cat, 17-desacetyl-rocuronium has approximately one-twentieth the neuromuscular blocking potency of rocuronium. The effects of renal failure and hepatic disease on the pharmacokinetics and pharmacodynamics of rocuronium in humans are consistent with these findings.

In general, patients undergoing cadaver kidney transplant have a small reduction in clearance which is offset pharmacokinetically by a corresponding increase in volume, such that the net effect is an unchanged plasma half-life. Patients with demonstrated liver cirrhosis have a marked increase in their volume of distribution resulting in a plasma half-life approximately twice that of patients with normal hepatic function. Table 4 shows the pharmacokinetic parameters in subjects with either impaired renal or hepatic function.

[See table 4 above.]

The net result of these findings is that subjects with renal failure have clinical durations that are similar to but somewhat more variable than the duration that one would expect in subjects with normal renal function. Hepatically impaired patients, due to the large increase in volume, may demonstrate clinical durations approaching 1.5 times that of subjects with normal hepatic function. In both populations the clinician should individualize the dose to the needs of the patient (see INDIVIDUALIZATION OF DOSAGE).

Tissue redistribution accounts for most (about 80%) of the initial amount of rocuronium administered. As tissue compartments fill with continued dosing (4–8 hours), less drug is redistributed away from the site of action and, for an infusion-only dose, the rate to maintain neuromuscular blockade falls to about 20% of the initial infusion rate. The use of a loading dose and a smaller infusion rate reduces the need for adjustment of dose.

Special Populations—Pediatrics: The clinical duration of effects of ZEMURON™ (rocuronium bromide) Injection did not vary with age in patients 4 months to 8 years of age. The terminal half-life and other pharmacokinetic parameters of rocuronium in these children are presented in Table 5.

[See table 5 at top of next page.]

Table 4. Pharmacokinetic Parameters in Adults with Normal Renal and Hepatic Function (n=10, ages 23–65), Renal Transplant Patients (n=10, ages 21–45) and Hepatic Dysfunction Patients (n=9, ages 31–67) During Isoflurane Anesthesia (Mean ± SD)

PK Parameters	Normal Renal and Hepatic Function	Renal Transplant Patients	Hepatic Dysfunction Patients
Clearance (L/kg/hr)	0.16 ± 0.05*	0.13 ± 0.04	0.13 ± 0.06
Volume of Distribution at Steady State (L/kg)	0.26 ± 0.03	0.34 ± 0.11	0.53 ± 0.14
$T_{1/2}$ β Elimination (hr)	2.4 ± 0.8*	2.4 ± 1.1	4.3 ± 2.6

*Differences in the calculated $T_{1/2}$ β and Cl between this study and the study in young adults vs. geriatrics (≥65 years) is related to the different sample populations and anesthetic techniques.

Clinical Trials

In U.S. clinical trials a total of 1,137 patients received ZEMURON™ (rocuronium bromide) Injection including 176 pediatric, 140 geriatric, 55 obstetric, and 766 other adults. Most patients (90%) were ASA physical status I or II, about 9% were ASA III, and 10 patients (undergoing coronary artery bypass grafting or valvular surgery) were ASA IV. In European clinical trials, a total of 1,394 patients received ZEMURON™ including 52 pediatric, 128 geriatric (≥65 years) and 1,214 other adults.

Adult Patients: Intubation using doses of ZEMURON™ (rocuronium bromide) Injection 0.6 to 0.85 mg/kg was evaluated in 203 adults in 11 clinical trials. Excellent to good intubating conditions were generally achieved within 2 minutes and maximum block occurred within 3 minutes in most patients. Doses within this range provide clinical relaxation for a median (range) time of 33 (14–85) minutes under opioid/nitrous oxide/oxygen anesthesia. Larger doses (0.9 and 1.2 mg/kg) were evaluated in two trials with 19 and 16 patients under opioid/nitrous oxide/oxygen anesthesia and provided 58 (27–111) and 67 (38–160) minutes of clinical relaxation, respectively.

Cardiovascular Disease: In one clinical trial, 10 patients with clinically significant cardiovascular disease undergoing coronary artery bypass graft received an initial dose of 0.6 mg/kg ZEMURON™ (rocuronium bromide) Injection. Neuromuscular block was maintained during surgery with bolus maintenance doses of 0.3 mg/kg. Following induction, continuous 0.008 mg/kg/min infusion of ZEMURON™ produced relaxation sufficient to support mechanical ventilation for 6 to 12 hours in the surgical intensive care unit (SICU) while the patients were recovering from surgery. Hypertension and tachycardia were reported in some patients but these occurrences were less frequent in patients receiving beta or calcium channel blocking drugs. In 7 of these 10 patients ZEMURON™ was associated with transient increases (≥30%) in pulmonary vascular resistance. In another clinical trial of 17 patients undergoing abdominal aortic surgery, transient increases (≥30%) in pulmonary vascular resistance were observed in 4 of 17 patients receiving ZEMURON™ 0.6 or 0.9 mg/kg.

Rapid Sequence Intubation: Intubating conditions were assessed in 230 patients in six clinical trials where anesthesia was induced with either thiopental (3 to 6 mg/kg) or propofol (1.5 to 2.5 mg/kg) in combination with either fentanyl (2 to 5 mcg/kg) or alfentanil (1 mg). Most of the patients also received a premedication such as midazolam or temazepam. Most patients had intubation attempted within 60 to 90 seconds of administration of ZEMURON™ (rocuronium bromide) Injection 0.6 mg/kg or succinylcholine 1 to 1.5 mg/kg. Excellent or good intubating conditions were achieved in 119/120 (99% [95% confidence interval 95–99.9%]) patients receiving ZEMURON™ and in 108/110 (98% [94–99.8%]) patients receiving succinylcholine. The duration of action of ZEMURON™ 0.6 mg/kg is longer than succinylcholine and at this dose is approximately equivalent to the duration of other intermediate acting neuromuscular blocking drugs.

Geriatric Patients: ZEMURON™ (rocuronium bromide) Injection was evaluated in 55 geriatric patients (ages 65–80 years) in six clinical trials. Doses of 0.6 mg/kg provided excellent to good intubating conditions in a median (range) time of 2.3 (1–8) minutes. Recovery times from 25% to 75% after these doses were not prolonged in geriatric patients compared to other adult patients.

Table 3. Pharmacokinetic Parameters in Adults (n=22; ages 27–58 yr) and Geriatric (n=20; ≥65 yr) During Opioid/Nitrous Oxide/Oxygen Anesthesia (Mean ± SD)

PK Parameters	Adults (Ages 27–58 yr)	Geriatrics (≥65 yr)
Clearance (L/kg/hr)	0.25 ± 0.08	0.21 ± 0.06
Volume of Distribution at Steady State (L/kg)	0.25 ± 0.04	0.22 ± 0.03
$T_{1/2}$ βElimination (hr)	1.4 ± 0.4	1.5 ± 0.4

Pediatric Patients: ZEMURON™ (rocuronium bromide) Injection 0.6 or 0.8 mg/kg was evaluated for intubation in 75 pediatric patients (n=28; age 3–12 months, n=47; age 1–12 years) in three trials using halothane (1–5%) nitrous oxide (60–70%) in oxygen. Of the children anesthetized with halothane who did not receive atropine for induction, about 80% experienced a transient increase (≥30%) in heart rate after intubation. One of the 19 infants anesthetized with halothane and fentanyl who received atropine for induction experienced this magnitude of change.

Obese Patients: ZEMURON™ (rocuronium bromide) Injection was dosed according to actual body weight (ABW) in most clinical trials. The administration of ZEMURON™ in the 47 of 330 (14%) patients who were at least 30% or more above their ideal body weight (IBW) was not associated with clinically significant differences in the onset, duration, recovery, or reversal of ZEMURON™-induced neuromuscular block.

In one clinical trial in obese patients, ZEMURON™ 0.6 mg/kg was dosed according to ABW (n=12) or IBW (n=11). Obese patients dosed according to IBW had a longer time to maximum block, a shorter clinical duration of 25 (14–29) minutes, and did not achieve intubating conditions comparable to those dosed based on ABW. These results support the recommendation that obese patients be dosed based on actual body weight.

Obstetric Patients: ZEMURON™ (rocuronium bromide) Injection 0.6 mg/kg was administered with thiopental, 3–4 mg/kg (n=13) or 4–6 mg/kg (n=42), for rapid sequence induction of anesthesia for cesarean section. No neonate had APGAR scores <7 at 5 minutes. The umbilical venous plasma concentrations were 18% of maternal concentrations at delivery. Intubating conditions were poor or inadequate in 5 of 13 women receiving 3–4 mg/kg thiopental when intubation was attempted 60 seconds after drug injection. Therefore, ZEMURON™ is not recommended for rapid sequence induction in cesarean section patients.

INDIVIDUALIZATION OF DOSAGE

DOSES OF ZEMURON™ (rocuronium bromide) INJECTION SHOULD BE INDIVIDUALIZED AND A PERIPHERAL NERVE STIMULATOR SHOULD BE USED TO MEASURE NEUROMUSCULAR FUNCTION DURING ZEMURON™ ADMINISTRATION IN ORDER TO MONITOR DRUG EFFECT, DETERMINE THE NEED FOR ADDITIONAL DOSES, AND CONFIRM RECOVERY FROM NEUROMUSCULAR BLOCK.

Based on the known actions of ZEMURON™, the following factors should be considered when administering ZEMURON™:

Renal or Hepatic Impairment: No differences from patients with normal hepatic and kidney function were observed for onset time at a dose of 0.6 mg/kg ZEMURON™ (rocuronium bromide) Injection. When compared to patients with normal renal and hepatic function, the mean clinical duration is similar in patients with end-stage renal disease undergoing renal transplant, and is about 1.5 times longer in patients with hepatic disease. Patients with renal failure may have a greater variation in duration of effect (see Pharmacokinetics subsection of CLINICAL PHARMACOLOGY and Renal Failure and Hepatic Disease subsections of PRECAUTIONS).

Reduced Plasma Cholinesterase Activity: No differences from patients with normal plasma cholinesterase activity is expected since rocuronium metabolism does not depend on plasma cholinesterase.

Drugs or Conditions Causing Potentiation of or Resistance to Neuromuscular Block: The neuromuscular blocking action of ZEMURON™ (rocuronium bromide) Injection is potentiated by isoflurane and enflurane anesthesia. Potentiation is minimal when administration of the recommended dose of ZEMURON™ occurs prior to the administration of these potent inhalation agents. The median clinical duration of a dose of 0.57–0.85 mg/kg was 34, 38, and 42 minutes under opioid/nitrous oxide/oxygen, enflurane and isoflurane maintenance anesthesia, respectively. During 1–2 hr of infusion, the infusion rate of ZEMURON™ required to maintain about 95% block was decreased by as much as 40% under

enflurane and isoflurane anesthesia (see Inhalation Anesthetics subsection of PRECAUTIONS).

When ZEMURON™ is administered to patients chronically receiving anticonvulsant agents such as carbamazepine or phenytoin, shorter durations of neuromuscular block may occur and infusion rates may be higher due to the development of resistance to nondepolarizing muscle relaxants (see Anticonvulsants subsection of PRECAUTIONS).

Pulmonary Hypertension: ZEMURON™ (rocuronium bromide) Injection may be associated with increased pulmonary vascular resistance so caution is appropriate in patients with pulmonary hypertension or valvular heart disease (see Clinical Trials subsection of CLINICAL PHARMACOLOGY).

Obesity: In obese patients, the initial dose of ZEMURON™ (rocuronium bromide) Injection 0.6 mg/kg should be based upon the patient's actual body weight (see Obese Patients subsection of Clinical Trials).

Based on the known actions of other nondepolarizing neuromuscular blocking agents the following additional factors should be considered when administering ZEMURON™:

Drugs or Conditions Causing Potentiation of or Resistance to Neuromuscular Block: Resistance to nondepolarizing agents, consistent with up-regulation of skeletal muscle acetylcholine receptors, is associated with burns, disuse atrophy, denervation, and direct muscle trauma. Receptor up-regulation may also contribute to the resistance to nondepolarizing muscle relaxants which sometimes develops in patients with cerebral palsy, patients chronically receiving anticonvulsant agents such as carbamazepine or phenytoin or with chronic exposure to nondepolarizing agents (see PRECAUTIONS).

Other nondepolarizing neuromuscular blocking agents have been found to exhibit profound neuromuscular blocking effects in cachectic or debilitated patients, patients with neuromuscular diseases, and patients with carcinomatosis. In these or other patients in whom potentiation of neuromuscular block or difficulty with reversal may be anticipated, a decrease from the recommended initial dose should be considered.

Certain antibiotics, magnesium salts, lithium, local anesthetics, procainamide, and quinidine have been shown to increase the duration of neuromuscular block and decrease infusion requirements of other neuromuscular blocking agents. In patients in whom potentiation of neuromuscular block may be anticipated, a decrease from the recommended initial dose should be considered (see Antibiotics and Other subsections of PRECAUTIONS).

Severe acid-base and/or electrolyte abnormalities may potentiate or cause resistance to the neuromuscular blocking action of ZEMURON™ (rocuronium bromide) Injection (see Other subsection of PRECAUTIONS). No data are available in such patients and no dosing recommendations can be made.

Burns: Patients with burns are known to develop resistance to nondepolarizing neuromuscular blocking agents, probably due to up-regulation of post-synaptic skeletal muscle cholinergic receptors (see INDIVIDUALIZATION OF DOSAGE).

INDICATIONS AND USAGE

ZEMURON™ (rocuronium bromide) Injection is a nondepolarizing neuromuscular blocking agent with a rapid to intermediate onset depending on dose and intermediate duration and is indicated for inpatients and outpatients as an adjunct to general anesthesia to facilitate both rapid sequence and routine tracheal intubation, and to provide skeletal muscle relaxation during surgery or mechanical ventilation.

CONTRAINDICATIONS

ZEMURON™ (rocuronium bromide) Injection is contraindicated in patients known to have hypersensitivity to rocuronium bromide.

WARNINGS

ZEMURON™ (rocuronium bromide) INJECTION SHOULD BE ADMINISTERED IN CAREFULLY ADJUSTED DOSAGES BY OR UNDER THE SUPERVISION OF EXPERIENCED CLINICIANS WHO ARE FAMILIAR WITH THE DRUG'S ACTIONS AND THE POSSIBLE COMPLICATIONS OF ITS USE. THE DRUG SHOULD NOT BE ADMINISTERED UNLESS FACILITIES FOR INTUBATION, ARTIFICIAL RESPIRATION, OXYGEN THERAPY, AND AN ANTAGONIST ARE IMMEDIATELY AVAILABLE. IT IS RECOMMENDED THAT CLINICIANS ADMINISTERING NEUROMUSCULAR BLOCKING AGENTS SUCH AS ZEMURON™ EMPLOY A PERIPHERAL NERVE STIMULATOR TO MONITOR DRUG RESPONSE, NEED FOR ADDITIONAL RELAXANT, AND ADEQUACY OF SPONTANEOUS RECOVERY OR ANTAGONISM.

ZEMURON™ HAS NO KNOWN EFFECT ON CONSCIOUSNESS, PAIN THRESHOLD, OR CEREBRATION. THEREFORE, ITS ADMINISTRATION MUST BE ACCOMPANIED BY ADEQUATE ANESTHESIA OR SEDATION.

In patients with myasthenia gravis or myasthenic (Eaton-Lambert) syndrome, small doses of nondepolarizing neuromuscular blocking agents may have profound effects. In such patients, a peripheral nerve stimulator and use of a small test dose may be of value in monitoring the response to administration of muscle relaxants.

ZEMURON™, which has an acid pH, should not be mixed with alkaline solutions (e.g., barbiturate solutions) in the same syringe or administered simultaneously during intravenous infusion through the same needle.

Table 5. Pharmacokinetic Parameters of Rocuronium in Pediatric Patients (ages 3-<12 mo, n=6; 1-<3 yr, n=5; 3-<8 yr, n=7) During Halothane Anesthesia (Mean ±SD)

PK Parameters	Patient Age Range 3-<12 mo	1-<3 yr	3-<8 yr
Clearance (L/kg/hr)	0.35 ± 0.08	0.32 ± 0.07	0.44 ± 0.16
Volume of Distribution at Steady State (L/kg)	0.30 ± 0.04	0.26 ± 0.06	0.21 ± 0.03
$T_{1/2}$ β Elimination (hr)	1.3 ± 0.5	1.1 ± 0.7	0.8 ± 0.3

PRECAUTIONS

Long-term Use in I.C.U.: ZEMURON™ (rocuronium bromide) Injection has not been studied for long-term use in the I.C.U. As with other nondepolarizing neuromuscular blocking drugs, apparent tolerance to ZEMURON™ may develop rarely during chronic administration in the I.C.U. While the mechanism for development of this resistance is not known, receptor up-regulation may be a contributing factor. It is STRONGLY RECOMMENDED THAT NEUROMUSCULAR TRANSMISSION BE MONITORED CONTINUOUSLY DURING ADMINISTRATION AND RECOVERY WITH THE HELP OF A NERVE STIMULATOR. ADDITIONAL DOSES OF ZEMURON™ OR ANY OTHER NEUROMUSCULAR BLOCKING AGENT SHOULD NOT BE GIVEN UNTIL THERE IS A DEFINITE RESPONSE (ONE TWITCH OF THE TRAIN-OF-FOUR) TO NERVE STIMULATION. Prolonged paralysis and/or skeletal muscle weakness may be noted during initial attempts to wean from the ventilator patients who have chronically received neuromuscular blocking drugs in the I.C.U. Therefore, ZEMURON™ should only be used in this setting if, in the opinion of the prescribing physician, the specific advantages of the drug outweigh the risk.

Labor and Delivery: The use of ZEMURON™ (rocuronium bromide) Injection in cesarean section has been studied in a limited number of patients. ZEMURON™ is not recommended for rapid sequence induction in cesarean section patients (see Clinical Trials subsection of CLINICAL PHARMACOLOGY).

Hepatic Disease: Since ZEMURON™ (rocuronium bromide) Injection is primarily excreted by the liver it should be used with caution in patients with clinically significant hepatic disease. ZEMURON™ 0.6 mg/kg has been studied in a limited number of patients (n=9) with clinically significant hepatic disease under steady-state isoflurane anesthesia. After ZEMURON™ 0.6 mg/kg, the median (range) clinical duration of 60 (35–166) minutes was moderately prolonged compared to 42 minutes in patients with normal hepatic function. The median recovery time of 53 minutes was also prolonged in patients with cirrhosis compared to 20 minutes in patients with normal hepatic function. Four of eight patients with cirrhosis, who received ZEMURON™ 0.6 mg/kg under opioid/nitrous oxide/oxygen anesthesia, did not achieve complete block. These findings are consistent with the increase in volume of distribution at steady state observed in patients with significant hepatic disease (see Pharmacokinetics subsection of CLINICAL PHARMACOLOGY). If used for rapid sequence induction in patients with ascites, an increased initial dosage may be necessary to assure complete block. Duration will be prolonged in these cases. The use of doses higher than 0.6 mg/kg has not been studied.

Renal Failure: Due to the limited role of the kidney in the excretion of ZEMURON™ (rocuronium bromide) Injection, usual dosing guidelines should be adequate. ZEMURON™ 0.6 mg/kg has been evaluated in three single center trials (n=30, ages 19–61 years) in patients undergoing renal transplant surgery, or shunt procedures in preparation for dialysis. After ZEMURON™ 0.6 mg/kg, the time to maximum block was about 1–2 minutes and was not different from patients without renal dysfunction. The mean ± SD clinical duration of 54 ± 22 minutes was not considered prolonged compared to 46 ± 12 minutes in normal patients; however, there was substantial variation (range, 22–90 minutes). The spontaneous recovery rate from 25 to 75% of control in renal dysfunction patients of 27 ± 11 minutes was similar to 28 ± 20 minutes in normal patients (see Pharmacokinetics subsection of CLINICAL PHARMACOLOGY).

Malignant Hyperthermia (MH): In an animal study in MH-susceptible swine, the administration of ZEMURON™ (rocuronium bromide) Injection did not appear to trigger malignant hyperthermia. ZEMURON™ has not been studied in MH-susceptible patients. Because ZEMURON™ is always used with other agents, and the occurrence of malignant hyperthermia during anesthesia is possible even in the absence of known triggering agents, clinicians should be familiar with early signs, confirmatory diagnosis and treatment of malignant hyperthermia prior to the start of any anesthetic.

Altered Circulation Time: Conditions associated with slower circulation time, e.g., cardiovascular disease or advanced age, may be associated with a delay in onset time. Because higher doses of ZEMURON™ (rocuronium bromide) Injection produce a longer duration of action, the initial dosage should usually not be increased in these patients to reduce onset time; instead, when feasible, more time should be allowed for the drug to achieve onset of effect.

Drug Interactions: The use of ZEMURON™ (rocuronium bromide) Injection before succinylcholine, for the purpose of attenuating some of the side effects of succinylcholine, has not been studied.

If ZEMURON™ is administered following administration of succinylcholine, it should not be given until recovery from succinylcholine has been observed. The median duration of action of ZEMURON™ 0.6 mg/kg administered after a 1 mg/kg dose of succinylcholine when T_1 returned to 75% of control was 36 minutes (range 14–57, n=12) *vs.* 28 minutes (17–51, n=12) without succinylcholine.

There are no controlled studies documenting the use of ZEMURON™ before or after other nondepolarizing muscle relaxants. Interactions have been observed when other nondepolarizing muscle relaxants have been administered in succession.

Inhalation Anesthetics: Use of inhalation anesthetics has been shown to enhance the activity of other neuromuscular blocking agents, enflurane > isoflurane > halothane.

Isoflurane and enflurane may also prolong the duration of action of initial and maintenance doses of ZEMURON™ (rocuronium bromide) Injection and decrease the average infusion requirement of ZEMURON™ by 40% compared to opioid/nitrous oxide/oxygen anesthesia. No definite interaction between ZEMURON™ and halothane has been demonstrated. In one study, use of enflurane in 10 patients resulted in a 20% increase in mean clinical duration of the initial intubating dose, and a 37% increase in the duration of subsequent maintenance doses, when compared in the same study to 10 patients under opioid/nitrous oxide/oxygen anesthesia. The clinical duration of initial doses of ZEMURON™ of 0.57–0.85 mg/kg under enflurane or isoflurane anesthesia, as used clinically, was increased by 11% and 23%, respectively. The duration of maintenance doses was affected to a greater extent, increasing by 30 to 50% under either enflurane or isoflurane anesthesia. Potentiation by these agents is also observed with respect to the infusion rates of ZEMURON™ required to maintain approximately 95% neuromuscular block. Under isoflurane and enflurane anesthesia, the infusion rates are decreased by approximately 40% compared to opioid/nitrous oxide/oxygen anesthesia. The median spontaneous recovery time (from 25 to 75% of control T_1) is not affected by halothane, but is prolonged by enflurane (15% longer) and isoflurane (62% longer). Reversal-induced recovery of ZEMURON™ neuromuscular block is minimally affected by anesthetic technique.

Intravenous Anesthetics: The use of propofol for induction and maintenance of anesthesia does not alter the clinical duration or recovery characteristics following recommended doses of ZEMURON™ (rocuronium bromide) Injection.

Anticonvulsants: In 2 of 4 patients receiving chronic anticonvulsant therapy apparent resistance to the effects of ZEMURON™ (rocuronium bromide) Injection was observed in the form of diminished magnitude of neuromuscular block, or shortened clinical duration. As with other nondepolarizing neuromuscular blocking drugs, if ZEMURON™ is administered to patients chronically receiving anticonvulsant agents such as carbamazepine or phenytoin, shorter durations of neuromuscular block may occur and infusion rates may be higher due to the development of resistance to nondepolarizing muscle relaxants. While the mechanism for development of this resistance is not known, receptor up-regulation may be a contributing factor (see INDIVIDUALIZATION OF DOSAGE).

Continued on next page

Organon—Cont.

Antibiotics: Drugs which may enhance the neuromuscular blocking action of nondepolarizing agents such as ZEMURON™ (rocuronium bromide) Injection include certain antibiotics (e.g., aminoglycosides; vancomycin; tetracyclines; bacitracin; polymyxins; colistin; and sodium colistimethate). If these antibiotics are used in conjunction with ZEMURON™, prolongation of neuromuscular block should be considered a possibility.

Other: Experience concerning injection of quinidine during recovery from use of other muscle relaxants suggests that recurrent paralysis may occur. This possibility must also be considered for ZEMURON™ (rocuronium bromide) Injection.

ZEMURON™-induced neuromuscular blockade was modified by alkalosis and acidosis in experimental pigs. Both respiratory and metabolic acidosis prolonged the recovery time. The potency of ZEMURON™ was significantly enhanced in metabolic acidosis and alkalosis, but was reduced in respiratory alkalosis. In addition, experience with other drugs has suggested that acute (e.g., diarrhea) or chronic (e.g., adrenocortical insufficiency) electrolyte imbalance may alter neuromuscular blockade. Since electrolyte imbalance and acid-base imbalance are usually mixed, either enhancement or inhibition may occur. Magnesium salts, administered for the management of toxemia of pregnancy, may enhance neuromuscular blockade.

A local tolerance study in rabbits demonstrated that ZEMURON™ was well tolerated following intravenous, intra-arterial and perivenous administration with only a slight irritation of surrounding tissues observed after perivenous administration. In humans, if extravasation occurs it may be associated with signs or symptoms of local irritation; the injection or infusion should be terminated immediately and restarted in another vein (see DOSAGE AND ADMINISTRATION).

Drug/Laboratory Test Interactions: None known.

Carcinogenesis, Mutagenesis, Impairment of Fertility: Studies in animals have not been performed to evaluate carcinogenic potential or impairment of fertility. Mutagenicity studies (Ames test, analysis of chromosomal aberrations in mammalian cells, and micronucleus test) conducted with ZEMURON™ (rocuronium bromide) Injection did not suggest mutagenic potential.

Pregnancy Category B: A teratogenicity study has been conducted in rats using intravenously administered doses of ZEMURON™ (rocuronium bromide) Injection approximating the clinical dose in humans (0.3 mg/kg). No teratogenic effects were observed in this study. There are no adequate and well-controlled studies in pregnant women. ZEMURON™ should be used during pregnancy only if the potential benefit justifies the potential risk to the fetus.

Pediatric Use: The use of ZEMURON™ (rocuronium bromide) Injection in children less than 3 months of age has not been studied. See Pharmacodynamics subsection of CLINICAL PHARMACOLOGY and Use in Pediatrics subsection of DOSAGE AND ADMINISTRATION for clinical experience and recommendations for use in infants and children 3 months to 14 years of age.

ADVERSE REACTIONS

Clinical studies in the U.S. (n=1,137) and Europe (n=1,394) totaled 2,531 patients. Prolonged neuromuscular block is associated with neuromuscular blockers as a class. Prolonged neuromuscular block (166 minutes) occurred after 0.6 mg/kg ZEMURON™ (rocuronium bromide) Injection in an obese 67 year-old female with hepatic dysfunction who had received gentamicin before surgery. The patients exposed in the U.S. clinical studies provide the basis for calculation of adverse reaction rates. The following adverse experiences were reported in patients administered ZEMURON™ (all events judged by investigators during the clinical trials to have a possible causal relationship):

Adverse experiences in greater than 1% patients:—NONE
Adverse experiences in less than 1% of patients Probably Related or Relationship Unknown:

Cardiovascular:	arrhythmia, abnormal electrocardiogram, tachycardia
Digestive:	nausea, vomiting
Respiratory:	asthma (bronchospasm, wheezing, or rhonchi), hiccup
Skin and Appendages:	rash, injection site edema, pruritus

In the European studies, the most commonly reported adverse experiences were transient hypotension (2%) and hypertension (2%); it is in greater frequency than the U.S. studies (0.1% and 0.1%). Changes in heart rate and blood pressure were defined differently from the U.S. studies in which changes in cardiovascular parameters were not considered as adverse events unless judged by the investigator as unexpected, clinically significant, or thought to be histamine related.

Table 6. Infusion Rates Using ZEMURON™ Injection (0.5 mg/mL)*

Patient Weight		Drug Delivery Rate (μg/kg/min)									
(kg)	(Lbs)	4	5	6	7	8	9	10	12	14	16
		Infusion Delivery Rate (mL/hr)									
10	22	4.8	6.0	7.2	8.4	9.6	10.8	12.0	14.4	16.8	19.2
15	33	7.2	9.0	10.8	12.6	14.4	16.2	18.0	21.6	25.2	28.8
20	44	9.6	12.0	14.4	16.8	19.2	21.6	24.0	28.8	33.6	38.4
25	55	12.0	15.0	18.0	21.0	24.0	27.0	30.0	36.0	42.0	48.0
35	77	16.8	21.0	25.2	29.4	33.6	37.8	42.0	50.4	58.8	67.2
50	110	24.0	30.0	36.0	42.0	48.0	54.0	60.0	72.0	84.0	96.0
60	132	28.8	36.0	43.2	50.4	57.6	64.8	72.0	86.4	100.8	115.2
70	154	33.6	42.0	50.4	58.8	67.2	75.6	84.0	100.8	117.6	134.4
80	176	38.4	48.0	57.6	67.2	76.8	86.4	96.0	115.2	134.4	153.6
90	198	43.2	54.0	64.8	75.6	86.4	97.2	108.0	129.6	151.2	172.8
100	220	48.0	60.0	72.0	84.0	96.0	108.0	120.0	144.0	168.0	192.0

Table 7. Infusion Rates Using ZEMURON™ Injection (1 mg/mL)**

Patient Weight		Drug Delivery Rate (μg/kg/min)									
(kg)	(Lbs)	4	5	6	7	8	9	10	12	14	16
		Infusion Delivery Rate (mL/hr)									
10	22	2.4	3.0	3.6	4.2	4.8	5.4	6.0	7.2	8.4	9.6
15	33	3.6	4.5	5.4	6.3	7.2	8.1	9.0	10.8	12.6	14.4
20	44	4.8	6.0	7.2	8.4	9.6	10.8	12.0	14.4	16.8	19.2
25	55	6.0	7.5	9.0	10.5	12.0	13.5	15.0	18.0	21.0	24.0
35	77	8.4	10.5	12.6	14.7	16.8	18.9	21.0	25.2	29.4	33.6
50	110	12.0	15.0	18.0	21.0	24.0	27.0	30.0	36.0	42.0	48.0
60	132	14.4	18.0	21.6	25.2	28.8	32.4	36.0	43.2	50.4	57.6
70	154	16.8	21.0	25.2	29.4	33.6	37.8	42.0	50.4	58.8	67.2
80	176	19.2	24.0	28.8	33.6	38.4	43.2	48.0	57.6	67.2	76.8
90	198	21.6	27.0	32.4	37.8	43.2	48.6	54.0	64.8	75.6	86.4
100	220	24.0	30.0	36.0	42.0	48.0	54.0	60.0	72.0	84.0	96.0

*50 mg ZEMURON™ in 100 mL solution
**100 mg ZEMURON™ in 100 mL solution

OVERDOSAGE

No cases of significant accidental or intentional overdose with ZEMURON™ (rocuronium bromide) Injection have been reported. Overdosage with neuromuscular blocking agents may result in neuromuscular block beyond the time needed for surgery and anesthesia. The primary treatment is maintenance of a patent airway and controlled ventilation until recovery of normal neuromuscular function is assured. Once evidence of recovery from neuromuscular block is observed, further recovery may be facilitated by administration of an anticholinesterase agent (e.g., neostigmine, edrophonium) in conjunction with an appropriate anticholinergic agent (see Antagonism of Neuromuscular Blockade).

Antagonism of Neuromuscular Blockade
ANTAGONISTS (SUCH AS NEOSTIGMINE) SHOULD NOT BE ADMINISTERED PRIOR TO THE DEMONSTRATION OF SOME SPONTANEOUS RECOVERY FROM NEUROMUSCULAR BLOCKADE. THE USE OF A NERVE STIMULATOR TO DOCUMENT RECOVERY AND ANTAGONISM OF NEUROMUSCULAR BLOCKADE IS RECOMMENDED.
Patients should be evaluated for adequate clinical evidence of antagonism, e.g., 5 sec head lift, adequate phonation, ventilation, and upper airway maintenance. Ventilation must be supported until no longer required.
Antagonism may be delayed in the presence of debilitation, carcinomatosis, and concomitant use of certain broad spectrum antibiotics, or anesthetic agents and other drugs which enhance neuromuscular blockade or separately cause respiratory depression. Under such circumstances the management is the same as that of prolonged neuromuscular blockade.

DOSAGE AND ADMINISTRATION

ZEMURON™ (rocuronium bromide) INJECTION IS FOR INTRAVENOUS USE ONLY. THIS DRUG SHOULD BE ADMINISTERED BY OR UNDER THE SUPERVISION OF EXPERIENCED CLINICIANS FAMILIAR WITH THE USE OF NEUROMUSCULAR BLOCKING AGENTS. INDIVIDUALIZATION OF DOSAGE SHOULD BE CONSIDERED IN EACH CASE (see INDIVIDUALIZATION OF DOSAGE).
The dosage information which follows is derived from studies based upon units of drug per unit of body weight. It is expressed in this section in units of mg/kg to assist the clinician in calculating individual patient dosage requirements relative to the product as supplied for clinical use. It is intended to serve as an initial guide to clinicians familiar with other neuromuscular blocking agents to acquire experience with ZEMURON™. The monitoring of twitch response is recommended to evaluate recovery from ZEMURON™ and decrease the hazards of overdosage if additional doses are administered (see Pharmacodynamics subsection of CLINICAL PHARMACOLOGY and Maintenance Dosing subsection).
It is recommended that clinicians administering neuromuscular blocking agents such as ZEMURON™ employ a peripheral nerve stimulator to monitor drug response, determine the need for additional relaxant and adequacy of spontaneous recovery or antagonism.

Rapid Sequence Intubation: In appropriately premedicated and adequately anesthetized patients, ZEMURON™ (rocuronium bromide) Injection 0.6–1.2 mg/kg will provide excellent or good intubating conditions in most patients in less than 2 minutes (see Clinical Trials subsection of CLINICAL PHARMACOLOGY).

Dose for Tracheal Intubation: The recommended initial dose regardless of anesthetic technique is 0.6 mg/kg. Neuromuscular block sufficient for intubation (≥80% block) is attained in a median (range) time of 1 (0.4–6) minute(s) and most patients have intubation completed within 2 minutes. Maximum blockade is achieved in most patients in less than 3 minutes. This dose may be expected to provide 31 (15–85) minutes of clinical relaxation under opioid/nitrous oxide/oxygen anesthesia. Under halothane, isoflurane, and enflurane anesthesia, some extension of the period of clinical relaxation should be expected (see Inhalation Anesthetics subsection of PRECAUTIONS).
A lower dose of ZEMURON™ (rocuronium bromide) Injection (0.45 mg/kg) may be used. Neuromuscular block sufficient for intubation (≥80% block) is attained in a median (range) time of 1.3 (0.8–6.2) minute(s) and most patients have intubation completed within 2 minutes. Maximum blockade is achieved in most patients in less than 4 minutes. This dose may be expected to provide 22 (12–31) minutes of clinical relaxation under opioid/nitrous oxide/oxygen anesthesia. Patients receiving this low dose of 0.45 mg/kg who achieve less than 90% block (about 16% of these patients) may have a more rapid time to 25% recovery, 12–15 minutes.
Should there be reason for the selection of a larger bolus dose in individual patients, initial doses of 0.9 or 1.2 mg/kg can be administered during surgery under opioid/nitrous oxide/oxygen anesthesia without adverse effects to the cardiovascular system. These doses will provide ≥80% block in most patients in less than 2 minutes, with maximum blockade occurring in most patients in less than 3 minutes. Doses of 0.9 and 1.2 mg/kg may be expected to provide 58 (27–111) and 67 (38–160) minutes, respectively, of clinical relaxation under opioid/nitrous oxide/oxygen anesthesia.

Maintenance Dosing: Maintenance doses of 0.1, 0.15, and 0.2 mg/kg ZEMURON™ (rocuronium bromide) Injection, administered at 25% recovery of control T_1 (defined as 3 twiches of train-of-four), provide a median (range) of 12 (2–31), 17 (6–50) and 24 (7–69) minutes of clinical duration under opioid/nitrous oxide/oxygen anesthesia (see Pharmacodynamics subsection of CLINICAL PHARMACOLOGY). In all cases, dosing should be guided based on the clinical duration following initial dose or prior maintenance dose and not administered until recovery of neuromuscular function is evident. A clinically insignificant cumulation of effect with repetitive maintenance dosing has been observed (see Pharmacodynamics subsection of CLINICAL PHARMACOLOGY).

Use by Continuous Infusion: Infusion at an initial rate of 0.01 to 0.012 mg/kg/min of ZEMURON™ (rocuronium bromide) Injection should be initiated only after early evidence of spontaneous recovery from an intubating dose. Due to rapid redistribution (see Pharmacokinetics subsection of CLINICAL PHARMACOLOGY) and the associated rapid spontaneous recovery, initiation of the infusion after substantial return of neuromuscular function (more than 10% of control T_1), may necessitate additional bolus doses to maintain adequate block for surgery.

Upon reaching the desired level of neuromuscular block, the infusion of ZEMURON™ must be individualized for each patient. The rate of administration should be adjusted according to the patient's twitch response as monitored with the use of a peripheral nerve stimulator. In clinical trials, infusion rates have ranged from 0.004 to 0.016 mg/kg/min. Inhalation anesthetics, particularly enflurane and isoflurane may enhance the neuromuscular blocking action of nondepolarizing muscle relaxants. In the presence of steady-state concentrations of enflurane or isoflurane, it may be necessary to reduce the rate of infusion by 30 to 50%, at 45–60 minutes after the intubating dose.

Spontaneous recovery and reversal of neuromuscular blockade following discontinuation of ZEMURON™ infusion may be expected to proceed at rates comparable to that following comparable total doses administered by repetitive bolus injections (see Pharmacodynamics subsection of CLINICAL PHARMACOLOGY).

Infusion solutions of ZEMURON™ can be prepared by mixing ZEMURON™ with an appropriate infusion solution such as 5% glucose in water or Lactated Ringers (see Compatibility). Unused portions of infusion solutions should be discarded.

Infusion rates of ZEMURON™ can be individualized for each patient using the following tables as guidelines: [See tables 6 and 7 on top of preceding page.]

Use in Pediatrics: Initial doses of 0.6 mg/kg in children under halothane anesthesia produce excellent to good intubating conditions within 1 minute. The median (range) time to maximum block was 1 (0.5–3.3) minute(s). This dose will provide a median (range) time of clinical relaxation of 41 (24–68) minutes in 3 months–1 year pediatric patients and 27 (17–41) minutes in 1–12 year-old children. Maintenance doses of 0.075–0.125 mg/kg, administered upon return of T_1 to 25% of control, provide clinical relaxation for 7–10 minutes.

Spontaneous recovery proceeds at approximately the same rate in pediatric patients (3 months–1 year) as in adults, but is more rapid in pediatric patients (1–12 years) than adults (see Tables 2 and 4 in Pharmacodynamics subsection of CLINICAL PHARMACOLOGY). A continuous infusion of ZEMURON™ (rocuronium bromide) Injection initiated at a rate of 0.012 mg/kg/min upon return of T_1 to 10% of control (one twitch present in the train-of-four), may also be used to maintain neuromuscular blockade in children. The infusion of ZEMURON™ must be individualized for each patient. The rate of administration should be adjusted according to the patient's twitch response as monitored with the use of a peripheral nerve stimulator. Spontaneous recovery and reversal of neuromuscular blockade following discontinuation of ZEMURON™ infusion may be expected to proceed at rates comparable to that following similar total exposure to single bolus doses (see Pharmacodynamics subsection of CLINICAL PHARMACOLOGY).

Use in Obese Patients: An analysis across all U.S. controlled clinical studies indicates that the pharmacodynamics of ZEMURON™ (rocuronium bromide) Injection are not different between obese and non-obese patients when dosed based upon their actual body weight.

Use in Geriatrics: Geriatric patients ($\geq$ 65 year) exhibited a slightly prolonged median (range) clinical duration of 46 (22–73), 62 (49–75), and 94 (64–138) minutes under opioid/nitrous oxide/oxygen anesthesia following doses of 0.6, 0.9 and 1.2 mg/kg, respectively. Maintenance doses of 0.1 and 0.15 mg/kg ZEMURON™ (rocuronium bromide) Injection, administered at 25% recovery of T_1, provide approximately 13 and 33 minutes of clinical duration under opioid/nitrous oxide/oxygen anesthesia. The median (range) rate of spontaneous recovery of T_1 from 25 to 75% in geriatric patients is 17 (7–56) minutes which is not different from that in other

adults (see Pharmacokinetics and Pharmacodynamics subsections of CLINICAL PHARMACOLOGY).

Compatibility: ZEMURON™ (rocuronium bromide) Injection is compatible in solution with:

0.9% NaCl solution   Sterile water for injection
5% glucose in water   Lactated Ringers
5% glucose in saline

Use within 24 hours of mixing with the above solutions. Parenteral drug products should be inspected visually for particulate matter and clarity prior to administration whenever solution and container permit. Do not use solution if particulate matter is present.

Safety and Handling: There is no specific work exposure limit for ZEMURON™ (rocuronium bromide) Injection. In case of eye contact, flush with water for at least 10 minutes.

HOW SUPPLIED
ZEMURON™ (rocuronium bromide) Injection is available in the following forms:
ZEMURON™ 5 mL multiple dose vials containing 50 mg rocuronium bromide injection (10 mg/mL)
Boxes of 10   NDC No. 0052-0450-15
ZEMURON™ 10 mL multiple dose vials containing 100 mg rocuronium bromide injection (10 mg/mL)
Boxes of 10   NDC No. 0052-0450-16
Storage: ZEMURON™ (rocuronium bromide) Injection should be stored under refrigeration, 2 to 8°C (36 to 46°F). DO NOT FREEZE. Upon removal from refrigeration to room temperature storage conditions (25°C/77°F), use ZEMURON™ Injection within 30 days.
Caution: Federal law prohibits dispensing without prescription.
ORGANON INC. WEST ORANGE, NEW JERSEY 07052
     5310153   12/94
Shown in Product Identification Guide, page 326

ZYMASE®   ℞
(pancrelipase, USP)
enteric coated spheres

DESCRIPTION
Zymase® capsules contain enteric coated spheres of pancrelipase, a substance containing enzymes, principally lipase, with amylase and protease obtained from the pancreas of the hog. Each capsule contains not less than:
Lipase—12,000 USP Units
Protease—24,000 USP Units
Amylase—24,000 USP Units
Each capsule also contains: Gelatin, purified water, starch, talc, titanium dioxide, FD&C Green #3, FD&C Yellow #10, and other inactive ingredients.

CLINICAL PHARMACOLOGY
Zymase® is protected against inactivation by gastric acidity, and active enzymes are released in the duodenum. The enzymes promote hydrolysis of fats into glycerol and fatty acids, protein into proteases and derived substances, and starch into dextrans and sugars.

INDICATIONS AND USAGE
Zymase® is indicated in conditions where pancreatic enzymes are either absent or deficient with resultant inadequate fat digestion. Such conditions include but are not limited to chronic pancreatitis, pancreatectomy, cystic fibrosis and steatorrhea of diverse etiologies.

CONTRAINDICATIONS
Known hypersensitivity to pork protein.

PRECAUTIONS
To maintain enteric coating integrity, do not chew or crush spheres.

ADVERSE REACTIONS
No adverse reactions have been reported. It should be noted, however, that extremely high doses of exogenous pancreatic enzymes have been associated with hyperuricosuria and hyperuricemia.

DOSAGE AND ADMINISTRATION
One to two capsules with each meal or snack. Individual cases may require higher dosage and dietary adjustment. Where swallowing of capsules is difficult, capsules may be opened and the spheres taken with liquids or soft foods which do not require chewing.

STORAGE
Not to exceed 25°C (77°F). Store in dry place when opened.

DISPENSE
In tight container as defined in the USP.
       Revised 4/93
Shown in Product Identification Guide, page 326

Ortho Biotech Inc.
RARITAN, NJ 08869-0602

Direct Inquiries to:
Customer Services
(800) 325-7504
FAX: (908) 526-6457

LEUSTATIN®   ℞
(cladribine) Injection
For Intravenous Infusion Only

WARNING
LEUSTATIN (cladribine) Injection should be administered under the supervision of a qualified physician experienced in the use of antineoplastic therapy. Suppression of bone marrow function should be anticipated. This is usually reversible and appears to be dose dependent. Serious neurological toxicity (including irreversible paraparesis and quadraparesis) has been reported in patients who received LEUSTATIN Injection by continuous infusion at high doses (4 to 9 times the recommended dose for Hairy Cell Leukemia). Neurologic toxicity appears to demonstrate a dose relationship; however, severe neurological toxicity has been reported rarely following treatment with standard cladribine dosing regimens.
Acute nephrotoxicity has been observed with high doses of LEUSTATIN (4 to 9 times the recommended dose for Hairy Cell Leukemia), especially when given concomitantly with other nephrotoxic agents/therapies.

DESCRIPTION
LEUSTATIN (cladribine) Injection (also commonly known as 2-chloro-2'-deoxy-β-D-adenosine) is a synthetic antineoplastic agent for continuous intravenous infusion. It is a clear, colorless, sterile, preservative-free, isotonic solution. LEUSTATIN Injection is available in single-use vials containing 10 mg (1 mg/mL) of cladribine, a chlorinated purine nucleoside analog. Each milliliter of LEUSTATIN Injection contains 1 mg of the active ingredient and 9 mg (0.15 mEq) of sodium chloride as an inactive ingredient. The solution has a pH range of 5.5 to 8.0. Phosphoric acid and/or dibasic sodium phosphate may have been added to adjust the pH to 6.3 ± 0.3. The chemical name for cladribine is 2-chloro-6-amino-9-(2-deoxy-β-D-erythropento-furanosyl) purine and the structure is represented below:

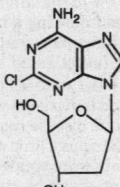

cladribine   MW 285.7

CLINICAL PHARMACOLOGY
Cellular Resistance and Sensitivity:
The selective toxicity of 2-chloro-2'-deoxy-β-D-adenosine towards certain normal and malignant lymphocyte and monocyte populations is based on the relative activities of deoxycytidine kinase, deoxynucleotidase and adenosine deaminase. In cells with a high ratio of deoxycytidine kinase to deoxynucleotidase, 2-chloro-2'-deoxy-β-D-adenosine, a purine nucleoside analog, passively crosses the cell membrane. It is phosphorylated by deoxycytidine kinase to 2-chloro-2'-deoxy-β-D-adenosine monophosphate (2-CdAMP). Since 2-chloro-2'-deoxy-β-D-adenosine is resistant to deamination by adenosine deaminase and there is little deoxynucleotide deaminase in lymphocytes and monocytes, 2-CdAMP accumulates intracellularly and is subsequently converted into the active triphosphate deoxynucleotide, 2-chloro-2'-deoxy-β-D-adenosine triphosphate (2-CdATP). It is postulated that cells with high deoxycytidine kinase and low deoxynucleotidase activities will be selectively killed by 2-chloro-2'-deoxy-β-D-adenosine as toxic deoxynucleotides accumulate intracellularly.
Cells containing high concentrations of deoxynucleotides are unable to properly repair single-strand DNA breaks. The broken ends of DNA activate the enzyme poly (ADP-ribose) polymerase resulting in NAD and ATP depletion and disruption of cellular metabolism. There is evidence, also, that

Continued on next page

Ortho Biotech—Cont.

2-CdATP is incorporated into the DNA of dividing cells, resulting in impairment of DNA synthesis. Thus, 2-chloro-2'-deoxy-β-D-adenosine can be distinguished from other chemotherapeutic agents affecting purine metabolism in that it is cytotoxic to both actively dividing and quiescent lymphocytes and monocytes, inhibiting both DNA synthesis and repair.

HUMAN PHARMACOLOGY

In a clinical investigation, 17 patients with Hairy Cell Leukemia and normal renal function were treated for 7 days with the recommended treatment regimen of LEUSTATIN Injection (0.09 mg/kg/day) by continuous intravenous infusion. The mean steady-state serum concentration was estimated to be 5.7 ng/mL with an estimated systemic clearance of 663.5 mL/h/kg when LEUSTATIN was given by continuous infusion over 7 days. Accumulation of LEUSTATIN over the seven day treatment period was not noted. In Hairy Cell Leukemia patients, there does not appear to be a relationship between serum concentrations and ultimate clinical outcome.

In another study, 8 patients with hematologic malignancies received a two (2) hour infusion of LEUSTATIN Injection (0.12 mg/kg). The mean end-of-infusion plasma LEUSTATIN concentration was 48±19 ng/mL. For 5 of these patients, the disappearance of LEUSTATIN could be described by either a biphasic or triphasic decline. For these patients with normal renal function, the mean terminal half-life was 5.4 hours. Mean values for clearance and steady-state volume of distribution were 978±422 mL/h/kg and 4.5±2.8 L/kg, respectively.

Plasma concentrations are reported to decline multi-exponentially after intravenous infusions with terminal half-lives ranging from approximately 3–22 hours. In general, the apparent volume of distribution of cladribine is very large (mean approximately 9 L/kg), indicating an extensive distribution of cladribine in body tissues. The mean half-life of cladribine in leukemic cells has been reported to be 23 hours. Cladribine penetrates into cerebrospinal fluid. One report indicates that concentrations are approximately 25% of those in plasma.

LEUSTATIN is bound approximately 20% to plasma proteins.

Except for some understanding of the mechanism of cellular toxicity, no other information is available on the metabolism or route of excretion of LEUSTATIN in humans. In a pilot study in rats treated with radiolabeled cladribine, approximately 41% to 44% of the administered label was recovered in the urine in the first 6 hours from a 1 mg/kg bolus or infusion. Only small amounts of radioactivity were recovered after 6 hours. Less than 1% of the administered radioactivity was excreted in the feces following a bolus dose to rats. The effect of renal and hepatic impairment on the elimination of cladribine has not been investigated in humans.

Two single-center open label studies of LEUSTATIN (cladribine) have been conducted in patients with Hairy Cell Leukemia with evidence of active disease requiring therapy. In the study conducted at the Scripps Clinic and Research Foundation (Study A), 89 patients were treated with a single course of LEUSTATIN Injection given by continuous intravenous infusion for 7 days at a dose of 0.09 mg/kg/day. In the study conducted at the M.D. Anderson Cancer Center (Study B), 35 patients were treated with a 7-day continuous intravenous infusion of LEUSTATIN Injection at a comparable dose of 3.6 mg/m²/day. A complete response (CR) required clearing of the peripheral blood and bone marrow of hairy cells and recovery of the hemoglobin to 12 g/dL, platelet count to 100×10^9/L, and absolute neutrophil count to 1500×10^6/L. A good partial response (GPR) required the same hematologic parameters as a complete response, and that fewer than 5% hairy cells remain in the bone marrow. A partial response (PR) required that hairy cells in the bone marrow be decreased by at least 50% from baseline and the same response for hematologic parameters as for complete response.

A pathologic relapse was defined as an increase in bone marrow hairy cells to 25% of pretreatment levels. A clinical relapse was defined as the recurrence of cytopenias, specifically, decreases in hemoglobin ≥2 g/dL, ANC ≥25% or platelet counts ≥50,000. Patients who met the criteria for a complete response but subsequently were found to have evidence of bone marrow hairy cells (<25% of pretreatment levels) were reclassified as partial responses and were not considered to be complete responses with relapse.

Among patients evaluable for efficacy (N=106), using the hematologic and bone marrow response criteria described above, the complete response rates in patients treated with LEUSTATIN Injection were 65% and 68% for Study A and Study B, respectively, yielding a combined complete response rate of 66%. Overall response rates (i.e., Complete plus Good Partial plus Partial Responses) were 89% and 86% in Study A and Study B, respectively, for a combined overall response rate of 88% in evaluable patients treated with LEUSTATIN Injection.

Using an intent-to-treat analysis (N=123) and further requiring no evidence of splenomegaly as a criterion for CR (i.e., no palpable spleen on physical examination and ≤13 cm on CT scan), the complete response rates for Study A and Study B, were 54% and 53%, respectively, giving a combined CR rate of 54%. The overall response rates (CR + GPR + PR) were 90% and 85%, for Studies A and B, respectively, yielding a combined overall response rate of 89%.

RESPONSE RATES TO LEUSTATIN TREATMENT IN PATIENTS WITH HAIRY CELL LEUKEMIA

	CR	Overall
Evaluable Patients N=106	66%	88%
Intent-to-treat Population N=123	54%	89%

In these studies, 60% of the patients had not received prior chemotherapy for Hairy Cell Leukemia or had undergone splenectomy as the only prior treatment and were receiving LEUSTATIN as a first-line treatment. The remaining 40% of the patients received LEUSTATIN as a second-line treatment, having been treated previously with other agents, including α-interferon and/or deoxycoformycin. The overall response rate for patients without prior chemotherapy was 92%, compared with 84% for previously treated patients. LEUSTATIN is active in previously treated patients; however, retrospective analysis suggests that the overall response rate is decreased in patients previously treated with splenectomy or deoxycoformycin and in patients refractory to α-interferon.

OVERALL RESPONSE RATES (CR + GPR + PR) TO LEUSTATIN TREATMENT IN PATIENTS WITH HAIRY CELL LEUKEMIA

	OVERALL RESPONSE (N=123)	NR + RELAPSE
No Prior Chemotherapy	68/74 92%	6 + 4 14%
Any Prior Chemotherapy	41/49 84%	8 + 3 22%
Previous Splenectomy	32/41* 78%	9 + 1 24%
Previous Interferon	40/48 83%	8 + 3 23%
Interferon Refractory	6/11* 55%	5 + 2 64%
Previous Deoxycoformycin	3/6* 50%	3 + 1 66%

NR = No Response
* $P < 0.05$

After a reversible decline, normalization of peripheral blood counts (Hemoglobin >12.0 g/dL, Platelets $>100 \times 10^9$/L, Absolute Neutrophil Count (ANC) $>1500 \times 10^6$/L) was achieved by 92% of evaluable patients. The median time to normalization of peripheral counts was 9 weeks from the start of treatment (Range: 2 to 72). The median time to normalization of Platelet Count was 2 weeks, the median time to normalization of ANC was 5 weeks and the median time to normalization of Hemoglobin was 8 weeks. With normalization of Platelet Count and Hemoglobin, requirements for platelet and RBC transfusions were abolished after Months 1 and 2, respectively, in those patients with complete response.

Platelet recovery may be delayed in a minority of patients with severe baseline thrombocytopenia. Corresponding to normalization of ANC, a trend toward a reduced incidence of infection was seen after the third month, when compared to the months immediately preceding LEUSTATIN therapy. (see also WARNINGS, PRECAUTIONS and ADVERSE REACTIONS).

LEUSTATIN TREATMENT IN PATIENTS WITH HAIRY CELL LEUKEMIA TIME TO NORMALIZATION OF PERIPHERAL BLOOD COUNTS

Parameter	Median Time to Normalization of Count*
Platelet Count	2 weeks
Absolute Neutrophil Count	5 weeks
Hemoglobin	8 weeks
ANC, Hemoglobin and Platelet Count	9 weeks

* Day 1 = First day of infusion

For patients achieving a complete response, the median time to response (i.e., absence of hairy cells in bone marrow and peripheral blood together with normalization of peripheral blood parameters), measured from treatment start, was approximately 4 months. Since bone marrow aspiration and biopsy were frequently not performed at the time of peripheral blood normalization, the median time to complete response may actually be shorter than that which was recorded. At the time of data cut-off, the median duration of complete response was greater than 8 months and ranged to 25+ months. Among 93 responding patients, seven had shown evidence of disease progression at the time of the data cut-off. In four of these patients, disease was limited to the bone marrow without peripheral blood abnormalities (pathologic progression), while in three patients there were also peripheral blood abnormalities (clinical progression). Seven patients who did not respond to a first course of LEUSTATIN received a second course of therapy. In the five patients who had adequate follow-up, additional courses did not appear to improve their overall response.

INDICATIONS FOR USE

LEUSTATIN Injection is indicated for the treatment of active Hairy Cell Leukemia as defined by clinically significant anemia, neutropenia, thrombocytopenia or disease-related symptoms.

CONTRAINDICATIONS

LEUSTATIN Injection is contraindicated in those patients who are hypersensitive to this drug or any of its components.

WARNINGS

Severe bone marrow suppression, including neutropenia, anemia and thrombocytopenia, has been commonly observed in patients treated with LEUSTATIN, especially at high doses. At initiation of treatment, most patients in the clinical studies had hematologic impairment as a manifestation of active Hairy Cell Leukemia. Following treatment with LEUSTATIN, further hematologic impairment occurred before recovery of peripheral blood counts began. During the first two weeks after treatment initiation, mean Platelet Count, ANC, and Hemoglobin concentration declined and subsequently increased with normalization of mean counts by Day 12, Week 5 and Week 8, respectively. The myelosuppressive effects of LEUSTATIN were most notable during the first month following treatment. Forty-four percent (44%) of patients received transfusions with RBCs and 14% received transfusions with platelets during Month 1. Careful hematologic monitoring, especially during the first 4 to 8 weeks after treatment with LEUSTATIN Injection, is recommended. (see PRECAUTIONS)

Fever (T ≥100°F) was associated with the use of LEUSTATIN in approximately two-thirds of patients (131/196) in the first month of therapy. Virtually all of these patients were treated empirically with parenteral antibiotics. Overall, 47% (93/196) of all patients had fever in the setting of neutropenia (ANC ≤1000), including 62 patients (32%) with severe neutropenia (i.e., ANC ≤500).

In a Phase I investigational study using LEUSTATIN in high doses (4 to 9 times the recommended dose for Hairy Cell Leukemia) as part of a bone marrow transplant conditioning regimen, which also included high dose cyclophosphamide and total body irradiation, acute nephrotoxicity and delayed onset neurotoxicity were observed. Thirty-one (31) poor-risk patients with drug-resistant acute leukemia in relapse (29 cases) or non-Hodgkin's Lymphoma (2 cases) received LEUSTATIN for 7 to 14 days prior to bone marrow transplantation. During infusion, 8 patients experienced gastrointestinal symptoms. While the bone marrow was initially cleared of all hematopoietic elements, including tumor cells, leukemia eventually recurred in all treated patients. Within 7 to 13 days after starting treatment with LEUSTATIN, 6 patients (19%) developed manifestations of renal dysfunction (e.g., acidosis, anuria, elevated serum creatinine, etc.) and 5 required dialysis. Several of these patients were also being treated with other medications having known nephrotoxic potential. Renal dysfunction was reversible in 2 of these patients. In the 4 patients whose renal function had not recovered at the time of death, autopsies were performed; in 2 of these, evidence of tubular damage was noted. Eleven (11) patients (35%) experienced delayed onset neurologic toxicity. In the majority, this was characterized by

progressive irreversible motor weakness (paraparesis/quadriparesis), of the upper and/or lower extremities, first noted 35 to 84 days after starting high dose therapy with LEUSTATIN. Non-invasive testing (electromyography and nerve conduction studies) was consistent with demyelinating disease. Severe neurologic toxicity has also been noted with high doses of another drug in this class.

Axonal peripheral polyneuropathy was observed in a dose escalation study at the highest dose levels (approximately 4 times the recommended dose for Hairy Cell Leukemia) in patients not receiving cyclophosphamide or total body irradiation. Severe neurological toxicity has been reported rarely following treatment with standard cladribine dosing regimens.

In patients with Hairy Cell Leukemia treated with the recommended treatment regimen (0.09 mg/kg/day for 7 consecutive days), there have been no reports of neurologic toxicities.

Of the 196 Hairy Cell Leukemia patients entered in the two trials, there were 8 deaths following treatment. Of these, 6 were of infectious etiology, including 3 pneumonias, and 2 occurred in the first month following LEUSTATIN therapy. Of the 8 deaths, 6 occurred in previously treated patients who were refractory to α-interferon.

Benzyl alcohol is a constituent of the recommended diluent for the 7-day infusion solution. Benzyl alcohol has been reported to be associated with a fatal "Gasping Syndrome" in premature infants. (see DOSAGE AND ADMINISTRATION)

Pregnancy Category D: LEUSTATIN Injection should not be given during pregnancy.

Cladribine is teratogenic in mice and rabbits and consequently has the potential to cause fetal harm when administered to a pregnant woman. A significant increase in fetal variations was observed in mice receiving 1.5 mg/kg/day (4.5 mg/m^2) and increased resorptions, reduced litter size and increased fetal malformations were observed when mice received 3.0 mg/kg/day (9 mg/m^2). Fetal death and malformations were observed in rabbits that received 3.0 mg/kg/day (33.0 mg/m^2). No fetal effects were seen in mice at 0.5 mg/kg/day (1.5 mg/m^2) or in rabbits at 1.0 mg/kg/day (11.0 mg/m^2).

Although there is no evidence of teratogenicity in humans due to LEUSTATIN, other drugs which inhibit DNA synthesis (e.g., methotrexate and aminopterin) have been reported to be teratogenic in humans. LEUSTATIN has been shown to be embryotoxic in mice when given at doses equivalent to the recommended dose.

There are no adequate and well controlled studies in pregnant women. If LEUSTATIN is used during pregnancy, or if the patient becomes pregnant while taking this drug, the patient should be apprised of the potential hazard to the fetus. Women of childbearing age should be advised to avoid becoming pregnant.

PRECAUTIONS

General: LEUSTATIN Injection is a potent antineoplastic agent with potentially significant toxic side effects. It should be administered only under the supervision of a physician experienced with the use of cancer chemotherapeutic agents. Patients undergoing therapy should be closely observed for signs of hematologic and non-hematologic toxicity. Periodic assessment of peripheral blood counts, particularly during the first 4 to 8 weeks post-treatment, is recommended to detect the development of anemia, neutropenia and thrombocytopenia and for early detection of any potential sequelae (e.g., infection or bleeding). As with other potent chemotherapeutic agents, monitoring of renal and hepatic function is also recommended, especially in patients with underlying kidney or liver dysfunction. (see WARNINGS and ADVERSE REACTIONS)

Fever was a frequently observed side effect during the first month on study. Since the majority of fevers occurred in neutropenic patients, patients should be closely monitored during the first month of treatment and empiric antibiotics should be initiated as clinically indicated. Although 69% of patients developed fevers, less than $^1/_3$ of febrile events were associated with documented infection. Given the known myelosuppressive effects of LEUSTATIN, practitioners should carefully evaluate the risks and benefits of administering this drug to patients with active infections. (see WARNINGS and ADVERSE REACTIONS)

The kidney has not been established as the organ of excretion for LEUSTATIN. There are inadequate data on dosing of patients with renal or hepatic insufficiency. Development of acute renal insufficiency in some patients receiving high doses of LEUSTATIN has been described. Until more information is available, caution is advised when administering the drug to patients with known or suspected renal or hepatic insufficiency. (see WARNINGS)

Rare cases of tumor lysis syndrome have been reported in patients treated with cladribine with other hematologic malignancies having a high tumor burden.

LEUSTATIN Injection must be diluted in designated intravenous solutions prior to administration. (see DOSAGE AND ADMINISTRATION)

Laboratory Tests: During and following treatment, the patient's hematologic profile should be monitored regularly to determine the degree of hematopoietic suppression. In the clinical studies, following reversible declines in all cell counts, the mean Platelet Count reached 100 × 10^9/L by Day 12, the mean Absolute Neutrophil Count reached 1500 × 10^6/L by Week 5 and the mean Hemoglobin reached 12 g/dL by Week 8. After peripheral counts have normalized, bone marrow aspiration and biopsy should be performed to confirm response to treatment with LEUSTATIN. Febrile events should be investigated with appropriate laboratory and radiologic studies. Periodic assessment of renal function and hepatic function should be performed as clinically indicated.

Drug Interactions: There are no known drug interactions with LEUSTATIN Injection. Caution should be exercised if LEUSTATIN Injection is administered before, after, or in conjunction with other drugs known to cause immunosuppression or myelosuppression. (See WARNINGS)

Carcinogenesis: No animal carcinogenicity studies have been conducted with cladribine.

Mutagenesis: As expected for compounds in this class, the actions of cladribine have been shown to yield DNA damage. In mammalian cells in culture, cladribine has been shown to cause an imbalance of intracellular deoxyribonucleotide triphosphate pools. This imbalance results in the inhibition of DNA synthesis and DNA repair, yielding DNA strand breaks and subsequently cell death. Inhibition of thymidine incorporation into human lymphoblastic cells was 90% at concentrations of 0.3μM. Cladribine was also incorporated into DNA of these cells. Cladribine was not mutagenic to bacteria and did not induce unscheduled DNA synthesis in primary rat hepatocyte cultures.

Impairment of Fertility: When administered intravenously to Cynomolgus monkeys, cladribine has been shown to cause suppression of rapidly generating cells, including testicular cells. The effect on human fertility is unknown.

Pregnancy: Pregnancy Category D: (see WARNINGS)

Nursing Mothers: It is not known whether this drug is excreted in human milk. Because many drugs are excreted in human milk and because of the potential for serious adverse reactions in nursing infants from cladribine, a decision should be made whether to discontinue nursing or discontinue the drug, taking into account the importance of the drug for the mother.

Pediatric Use: Safety and effectiveness in children has not been established. In a Phase I study involving patients 1–21 years old with relapsed acute leukemia, LEUSTATIN was given by continuous intravenous infusion in doses ranging from 3 to 10.7 mg/m^2/day for 5 days (one-half to twice the dose recommended in Hairy Cell Leukemia). In this study, the dose-limiting toxicity was severe myelosuppression with profound neutropenia and thrombocytopenia. At the highest dose (10.7 mg/m^2/day), 3 of 7 patients developed irreversible myelosuppression and fatal systemic bacterial or fungal infections. No unique toxicities were noted in this study.[1] (see WARNINGS and ADVERSE REACTIONS)

ADVERSE REACTIONS

Safety data are based on 196 patients with Hairy Cell Leukemia: the original cohort of 124 patients plus an additional 72 patients enrolled at the same two centers after the original enrollment cutoff. In Month 1 of the Hairy Cell Leukemia clinical trials, severe neutropenia was noted in 70% of patients, fever in 69%, and infection was documented in 28%. Other adverse experiences reported frequently during the first 14 days after initiating treatment included: fatigue (45%), nausea (28%), rash (27%), headache (22%) and injection site reactions (19%). Most non-hematologic adverse experiences were mild to moderate in severity.

Myelosuppression was frequently observed during the first month after starting treatment. Neutropenia (ANC < 500 × 10^6/L) was noted in 70% of patients, compared with 26% in whom it was present initially. Severe anemia (Hemoglobin < 8.5 g/dL) developed in 37% of patients, compared with 10% initially and thrombocytopenia (Platelets < 20 × 10^9/L) developed in 12% of patients, compared to 4% in whom it was noted initially.

During the first month, 54 of 196 patients (28%) exhibited documented evidence of infection. Serious infections (e.g., septicemia, pneumonia) were reported in 6% of all patients; the remainder were mild or moderate. Several deaths were attributable to infection and/or complications related to the underlying disease. During the second month, the overall rate of documented infection was 6%; these infections were mild to moderate and no severe systemic infections were seen. After the third month, the monthly incidence of infection was either less than or equal to that of the months immediately preceding LEUSTATIN therapy.

During the first month, 11% of patients experienced severe fever (i.e., ≥ 104°F). Documented infections were noted in fewer than one-third of febrile episodes. Of the 196 patients studied, 19 were noted to have a documented infection in the month prior to treatment. In the month following treatment, there were 54 episodes of documented infection: 23 (42%) were bacterial, 11 (20%) were viral and 11 (20%) were fungal. Seven (7) of 8 documented episodes of herpes zoster occurred during the month following treatment. Fourteen (14) of 16 episodes of documented fungal infections occurred in the first two months following treatment. Virtually all of these patients were treated empirically with antibiotics. (see WARNINGS and PRECAUTIONS)

Analysis of lymphocyte subsets indicates that treatment with cladribine is associated with prolonged depression of the CD4 counts. Prior to treatment, the mean CD4 count was 766/μL. The mean CD4 count nadir, which occurred 4 to 6 months following treatment, was 272/μL. Fifteen (15) months after treatment, mean CD4 counts remained below 500/μL. CD8 counts behaved similarly, though increasing counts were observed after 9 months. The clinical significance of the prolonged CD4 lymphopenia is unclear.

Another event of unknown clinical significance includes the observation of prolonged bone marrow hypocellularity. Bone marrow cellularity of < 35% was noted after 4 months in 42 of 124 patients (34%) treated in the two pivotal trials. This hypocellularity was noted as late as day 1010. It is not known whether the hypocellularity is the result of disease related marrow fibrosis or if it is the result of cladribine toxicity. There was no apparent clinical effect on the peripheral blood counts.

The vast majority of rashes were mild and occurred in patients who were receiving or had recently been treated with other medications (e.g., allopurinol or antibiotics) known to cause rash.

Most episodes of nausea were mild, not accompanied by vomiting, and did not require treatment with antiemetics. In patients requiring antiemetics, nausea was easily controlled, most frequently with chlorpromazine.

Adverse reactions reported during the first 2 weeks following treatment initiation (regardless of relationship to drug) by > 5% of patients included:

Body as a Whole: fever (69%), fatigue (45%), chills (9%), asthenia (9%), diaphoresis (9%), malaise (7%), trunk pain (6%)

Gastrointestinal: nausea (28%), decreased appetite (17%), vomiting (13%), diarrhea (10%), constipation (9%), abdominal pain (6%)

Hemic/Lymphatic: purpura (10%), petechiae (8%), epistaxis (5%)

Nervous System: headache (22%), dizziness (9%), insomnia (7%)

Cardiovascular System: edema (6%), tachycardia (6%)

Respiratory System: abnormal breath sounds (11%), cough (10%), abnormal chest sounds (9%), shortness of breath (7%)

Skin/Subcutaneous Tissue: rash (27%), injection site reactions (19%), pruritis (6%), pain (6%), erythema (6%)

Musculoskeletal System: myalgia (7%), arthralgia (5%)

Adverse experiences related to intravenous administration included: injection site reaction (9%) (i.e., redness, swelling, pain), thrombosis (2%), phlebitis (2%) and a broken catheter (1%). These appear to be related to the infusion procedure and/or indwelling catheter, rather than the medication or the vehicle. From Day 15 to the last follow-up visit, the only events reported by > 5% of patients were: fatigue (11%), rash (10%), headache (7%), cough (7%), and malaise (5%).

For a description of adverse reactions associated with use of high doses in non-Hairy Cell Leukemia patients, see WARNINGS.

The following additional adverse events have been reported since the drug became commercially available. These adverse events have been reported primarily in patients who received multiple courses of LEUSTATIN Injection:

Hematologic: bone marrow suppression with prolonged pancytopenia, including some reports of aplastic anemia; hemolytic anemia, which was reported in patients with lymphoid malignancies, occurring within the first few weeks following treatment.

Hepatic: reversible, generally mild increases in bilirubin and transamiases.

Nervous System: Neurological toxicity; however, severe neurotoxicity has been reported rarely following treatment with standard cladribine dosing regimens.

Respiratory System: pulmonary interstitial infiltrates; in most cases, an infectious etiology was identified.

Opportunistic infections have occurred in the acute phase of treatment due to the immunosuppression mediated by LEUSTATIN Injection.

OVERDOSAGE

High doses of LEUSTATIN have been associated with: irreversible neurologic toxicity (paraparesis/quadriparesis), acute nephrotoxicity, and severe bone marrow suppression resulting in neutropenia, anemia and thrombocytopenia. (see WARNINGS) There is no known specific antidote to overdosage. Treatment of overdosage consists of discontinuation of LEUSTATIN, careful observation and appropriate supportive measures. It is not known whether the drug can be removed from the circulation by dialysis or hemofiltration.

Continued on next page

Ortho Biotech—Cont.

DOSAGE AND ADMINISTRATION

Usual Dose:

The recommended dose and schedule of LEUSTATIN Injection for active Hairy Cell Leukemia is as a single course given by continuous infusion for 7 consecutive days at a dose of 0.09 mg/kg/day. Deviations from this dosage regimen are not advised. If the patient does not respond to the initial course of LEUSTATIN Injection for Hairy Cell Leukemia, it is unlikely that they will benefit from additional courses. Physicians should consider delaying or discontinuing the drug if neurotoxicity or renal toxicity occurs. (see WARNINGS)

Specific risk factors predisposing to increased toxicity from LEUSTATIN have not been defined. In view of the known toxicities of agents of this class, it would be prudent to proceed carefully in patients with known or suspected renal insufficiency of severe bone marrow impairment of any etiology. Patients should be monitored closely for hematologic and non-hematologic toxicity. (see WARNINGS and PRECAUTIONS)

Preparation and Administration of Intravenous Solutions:

LEUSTATIN Injection must be diluted with the designated diluent prior to administration. Since the drug product does not contain any anti-microbial preservative or bacteriostatic agent, **aseptic technique and proper environmental precautions must be observed in preparation of LEUSTATIN Injection solutions.**

To prepare a single daily dose: Add the calculated dose (0.09 mg/kg or 0.09 mL/kg) of LEUSTATIN Injection to an infusion bag containing 500 mL of 0.9% Sodium Chloride Injection, USP. Infuse continuously over 24 hours. Repeat daily for a total of 7 consecutive days. **The use of 5% dextrose as a diluent is not recommended because of increased degradation of cladribine.** Admixures of LEUSTATIN Injection are chemically and physically stable for at least 24 hours at room temperature under normal room fluorescent light in Baxter Viaflex®† PVC infusion containers. **Since limited compatibility data are available, adherence to the recommended diluents and infusion systems is advised.**

[See table below.]

To prepare a 7-day infusion: The 7-day infusion solution should only be prepared with Bacteriostatic 0.9% Sodium Chloride Injection, USP (0.9% benzyl alcohol preserved). In order to minimize the risk of microbial contamination, both LEUSTATIN Injection and the diluent should be passed through a sterile 0.22μ disposable hydrophilic syringe filter as each solution is being introduced into the infusion reservoir. First add the calculated dose of LEUSTATIN Injection (7 days × 0.09 mg/kg or mL/kg) to the infusion reservoir through the sterile filter. Then add a calculated amount of Bacteriostatic 0.9% Sodium Chloride Injection, USP (0.9% benzyl alcohol preserved) also through the filter to bring the total volume of the solution to 100 mL. After completing solution preparation, clamp off the line, disconnect and discard the filter. Aseptically aspirate air bubbles from the reservoir as necessary using the syringe and a dry second sterile filter or a sterile vent filter assembly. Reclamp the line and discard the syringe and filter assembly. Infuse continuously over 7 days. Solutions prepared with Bacteriostatic Sodium Chloride Injection for individuals weighing more than 85 kg may have reduced preservative effectiveness due to greater dilution of the benzyl alcohol preservative. Admixtures for the 7-day infusion have demonstrated acceptable chemical and physical stability for at least 7 days in the Sims Deltec MEDICATION CASSETTES™ Reservoir‡.

[See table above.]

Since limited compatibility data are available, adherence to the recommended diluents and infusion systems is advised.

Solutions containing LEUSTATIN Injection should not be mixed with other intravenous drugs or additives or infused simultaneously via a common intravenous line, since compatibility testing has not been performed. Preparations containing benzyl alcohol should not be used in neonates. (see WARNINGS)

Care must be taken to assure the sterility of prepared solutions. Once diluted, solutions of LEUSTATIN Injection should be administered promptly or stored in the refrigerator (2° to 8° C) for no more than 8 hours prior to start of administration. Vials of LEUSTATIN Injection are for single-use only. Any unused portion should be discarded in an appropriate manner. (see Handling and Disposal)

Parenteral drug products should be inspected visually for particulate matter and discoloration prior to administration, whenever solution and container permit. A precipitate may occur during the exposure of LEUSTATIN Injection to low temperatures; it may be resolubilized by allowing the solution to warm naturally to room temperature and by shaking vigorously. **DO NOT HEAT OR MICROWAVE.**

	Dose of LEUSTATIN Injection	Recommended Diluent	Quantity of Diluent
24-hour infusion method	1 (day) × 0.09 mg/kg	0.9% Sodium Chloride Injection, USP	500 mL

	Dose of LEUSTATIN Injection	Recommended Diluent	Quantity of Diluent
7-day infusion method (use sterile 0.22μ filter when preparing infusion solution)	7 (days) × 0.09 mg/kg	Bacteriostatic 0.9% Sodium Chloride Injection, USP (0.9% benzyl alcohol)	q.s. to 100 mL

Chemical Stability of Vials:

When stored in refrigerated conditions between 2° to 8°C (36° to 46°F) protected from light, unopened vials of LEUSTATIN Injection are stable until the expiration date indicated on the package. Freezing does not adversely affect the solution. If freezing occurs, thaw naturally to room temperature. DO NOT heat or microwave. Once thawed, the vial of LEUSTATIN Injection is stable until expiry if refrigerated. DO NOT refreeze. Once diluted, solutions containing LEUSTATIN Injection should be administered promptly or stored in the refrigerator (2° to 8°C) for no more than 8 hours prior to administration.

Handling and Disposal:

The potential hazards associated with cytotoxic agents are well established and proper precautions should be taken when handling, preparing, and administering LEUSTATIN Injection. The use of disposable gloves and protective garments is recommended. If LEUSTATIN Injection contacts the skin or mucous membranes, wash the involved surface immediately with copious amounts of water. Several guidelines on this subject have been published.[2–8] There is no general agreement that all of the procedures recommended in the guidelines are necessary or appropriate. Refer to your Institution's guidelines and all applicable state/local regulations for disposal of cytotoxic waste.

HOW SUPPLIED

LEUSTATIN Injection is supplied as a sterile, preservative-free, isotonic solution containing 10 mg (1 mg/mL) of cladribine as 10 mL filled into a single-use clear flint glass 20 mL vial. LEUSTATIN Injection is supplied in 10 mL (1 mg/mL) single-use vials (NDC 59676-201-01) available in a treatment set (case) of seven vials.

Store refrigerated 2° to 8°C (36° to 46°F). Protect from light during storage.

REFERENCES

1. Santana VM, Mirro J, Harwood FC, *et al:* A phase I clinical trial of 2-Chloro-deoxyadenosine in pediatric patients with acute leukemia. *J. Clin. Onc.*, **9**:416 (1991).
2. Recommendations for the Safe Handling of Parenteral Antineoplastic Drugs. NIH Publication No. 83-2621. For sale by the Superintendent of Documents, U.S. Government Printing Office, Washington, D.C. 20402.
3. AMA Council Report. Guidelines for Handling Parenteral Antineoplastics, *JAMA*, March 15 (1985).
4. National Study Commission on Cytotoxic Exposure—Recommendations for Handling Cytotoxic Agents. Available from Louis P. Jeffrey, Sc.D., Chairman, National Study Commission on Cytotoxic Exposure, Massachusetts College of Pharmacy and Allied Health Sciences, 179 Longwood Avenue, Boston, Massachusetts 02115.
5. Clinical Oncological Society of Australia: Guidelines and Recommendations for Safe Handling of Antineoplastic Agents. *Med. J. Australia* **1**:425 (1983).
6. Jones RB, *et al.* Safe Handling of Chemotherapeutic Agents: A Report from the Mount Sinai Medical Center. *Ca—A Cancer Journal for Clinicians*, Sept/Oct. 258–263 (1983).
7. American Society of Hospital Pharmacists Technical Assistance Bulletin on Handling Cytotoxic Drugs in Hospitals. *Am. J. Hosp. Pharm.*, **42**:131 (1985).
8. OSHA Work-Practice Guidelines for Personnel Dealing with Cytotoxic (antineoplastic) Drugs. *Am. J. Hosp. Pharm.*, **43**:1193 (1986).

CAUTION: Federal law prohibits dispensing without prescription.

†Viaflex® containers, manufactured by Baxter Healthcare Corporation—Code No. 2B8013 (tested in 1991)

‡MEDICATION CASSETTE™ Reservoir, manufactured by Sims Deltec, Inc.—Recorder No. 602100A (tested in 1991)

ORTHO BIOTECH INC.
Raritan, New Jersey 08869

 638-10-940-4

Revised December 1995

ORTHOCLONE OKT® 3 Sterile Solution ℞

(muromonab-CD3)

For Intravenous Use Only

WARNING

Only physicians experienced in immunosuppressive therapy and management of solid organ transplant patients should use ORTHOCLONE OKT3 (muromonab-CD3).

Anaphylactic or anaphylactoid reactions may occur following administration of any dose or course of ORTHOCLONE OKT3. Serious and occasionally life-threatening systemic, cardiovascular, and central nervous system reactions have been reported following administration of ORTHOCLONE OKT3. These have included: pulmonary edema, especially in patients with volume overload; shock; cardiovascular collapse; cardiac or respiratory arrest; seizures; and coma. Hence, a patient being treated with ORTHOCLONE OKT3 must be managed in a facility equipped and staffed for cardiopulmonary resuscitation. (see: WARNINGS: Cytokine Release Syndrome, Neuro-Psychiatric Events, Anaphylactic Reactions)

DESCRIPTION

ORTHOCLONE OKT3 (muromonab-CD3) Sterile Solution is a murine monoclonal antibody to the CD3 antigen of human T cells which functions as an immunosuppressant. It is for intravenous use only. The antibody is a biochemically purified IgG_{2a} immunoglobulin with a heavy chain of approximately 50,000 daltons and a light chain of approximately 25,000 daltons. It is directed to a glycoprotein with a molecular weight of 20,000 in the human T cell surface which is essential for T cell functions. Because it is a monoclonal antibody preparation, ORTHOCLONE OKT3 Sterile Solution is a homogeneous, reproducible antibody product with consistent, measurable reactivity to human T cells.

Each 5 mL ampule of ORTHOCLONE OKT3 Sterile Solution contains 5 mg (1 mg/mL) of muromonab-CD3 in a clear colorless solution which may contain a few fine translucent protein particles. Each ampule contains a buffered solution (pH 7.0 ±0.5) of monobasic sodium phosphate (2.25 mg), dibasic sodium phosphate (9.0 mg), sodium chloride (43 mg), and polysorbate 80 (1.0 mg) in water for injection.

The proper name, muromonab-CD3, is derived from the descriptive term murine monoclonal antibody. The CD3 designation identifies the specificity of the antibody as the Cell Differentiation (CD) cluster 3 defined by the First International Workshop on Human Leukocyte Differentiation Antigens.

CLINICAL PHARMACOLOGY

ORTHOCLONE OKT3 reverses graft rejection, most probably by blocking the function of all T cells which play a major role in acute allograft rejection. ORTHOCLONE OKT3 reacts with and blocks the function of a 20,000 dalton molecule (CD3) in the membrane of human T cells that has been associated *in vitro* with the antigen recognition structure of T cells and is essential for signal transduction. In *in vitro* cytolytic assays, ORTHOCLONE OKT3 blocks both the generation and function of effector cells. Binding of ORTHOCLONE OKT3 to T lymphocytes results in early activation of T cells, which leads to cytokine release, followed by blocking T cell functions. After termination of ORTHOCLONE OKT3 therapy, T cell function usually returns to normal within one week.

In vivo, ORTHOCLONE OKT3 reacts with most peripheral blood T cells and T cells in body tissues, but has not been found to react with other hematopoietic elements or other tissues of the body.

A rapid and concomitant decrease in the number of circulating CD2 positive, CD3 positive, CD4 positive, and CD8 positive T cells has been observed in patients studied within minutes after the administration of ORTHOCLONE OKT3. This decrease in the number of CD3 positive T cells results from the specific interaction between ORTHOCLONE OKT3 and the CD3 antigen on the surface of all T lymphocytes. T cell activation results in the release of numerous cytokines/lymphokines, which are felt to be responsible for many of the acute clinical manifestations seen following ORTHOCLONE OKT3 administration. (see: WARNINGS: Cytokine Release Syndrome, Neuro-Psychiatric Events)

While CD3 positive cells are not detectable between days two and seven, increasing numbers of circulating CD4 and CD8

positive cells have been observed. The presence of these CD4 and CD8 positive cells has not been shown to affect reversal of rejection. After termination of ORTHOCLONE OKT3 therapy, CD3 positive cells reappear rapidly and reach pre-treatment levels within a week. In some patients however, increasing numbers of CD3 positive cells have been observed prior to termination of ORTHOCLONE OKT3 therapy. This reappearance of CD3 positive cells has been attributed to the development of neutralizing antibodies to ORTHOCLONE OKT3, which in turn block its ability to bind to the CD3 antigen on T lypmphocytes. (see: PRECAUTIONS: Sensitization)
In the initial clinical trials using low doses of prednisone and azathioprine during ORTHOCLONE OKT3 therapy for renal allograft rejection, antibodies to ORTHOCLONE OKT3 were observed with an incidence of 21% (n=43) for IgM, 86% (n=43) for IgG and 29% (n=35) for IgE. The mean time of appearance of IgG antibodies was 20±2 (mean ±SD) days. Early IgG antibodies appeared towards the end of the second week of treatment in 3% (n=86) of the patients.
Subsequent clinical experience has shown that the dose, duration, and type of immunosuppressive medications used in combination with ORTHOCLONE OKT3 may affect both the incidence and magnitude of the host antibody response. Furthermore, immunosuppressive agents used concomitantly with ORTHOCLONE OKT3 (i.e., steroids, azathioprine, prednisone, or cyclosporine) have altered the time course of anti-mouse antibody development and the specificity of the antibodies formed (i.e., idiotypic, isotypic, allotypic).
Serum levels of ORTHOCLONE OKT3 are measurable using an enzyme-linked immunosorbent assay (ELISA). During the initial clinical trials in renal allograft rejection, in patients treated with 5 mg per day for 14 days, mean serum trough levels of the drug rose over the first three days and then averaged 900 ng/mL on days 3 to 14. Subsequent clinical experience has demonstrated that circulating serum levels greater than or equal to 800 ng/mL of ORTHOCLONE OKT3 blocks the function of cytotoxic T cells *in vitro* and *in vivo*. (see: PRECAUTIONS: Laboratory Tests)
Following administration of ORTHOCLONE OKT3 *in vivo*, leukocytes have been observed in cerebrospinal and peritoneal fluids. The mechanism for this effect is not completely understood, but probably is related to cytokines altering membrane permeability, rather than an active inflammatory process (see: WARNINGS: Cytokine Release Syndrome, Neuro-Psychiatric Events)

INDICATIONS AND USAGE

ORTHOCLONE OKT3 is indicated for the treatment of acute allograft rejection in renal transplant patients.
ORTHOCLONE OKT3 is also indicated for the treatment of steroid-resistant acute allograft rejection in cardiac and hepatic transplant patients.

Acute Renal Rejection:
In a controlled randomized clinical trial, ORTHOCLONE OKT3 was significantly more effective than conventional high-dose steroid therapy in reversing acute renal allograft rejection. In this trial, 122 evaluable patients undergoing acute rejection of cadaveric renal transplants were treated either with ORTHOCLONE OKT3 daily for a mean of 14 days, with concomitant lowering of the dosage of azathioprine and maintenance steroids (62 patients), or with conventional high-dose steroids (60 patients). ORTHOCLONE OKT3 reversed 94% of the rejections compared to a 75% reversal rate obtained with conventional high-dose steroid treatment (p=0.006). The one year Kaplan-Meier (actuarial) estimates of graft survival rates for these patients who had acute rejection were 62% and 45% for ORTHOCLONE OKT3 and steroid-treated patients, respectively (p=0.04). At two years the rates were 56% and 42%, respectively (p=0.06).
One- and two-year patient survivals were not significantly different between the two groups, being 85% and 75% for ORTHOCLONE OKT3 treated patients and 90% and 85% for steroid-treated patients.
In additional open clinical trials, the observed rate of reversal of acute renal allograft rejection was 92% (n=126) for ORTHOCLONE OKT3 therapy. ORTHOCLONE OKT3 was also effective in reversing acute renal allograft rejections in 65% (n=225) of cases where steroids and lymphocyte immune globulin preparations were contraindicated or were not successful (rescue).

Acute Cardiac or Hepatic Allograft Rejection:
ORTHOCLONE OKT3 has also been shown to be effective in reversing acute cardiac and hepatic allograft rejection in patients who are unresponsive to high-doses of steroids. Controlled randomized trials have not been conducted to evaluate the effectiveness of ORTHOCLONE OKT® 3 (muromonab-CD-3) compared to conventional therapy as first line treatment for acute cardiac and hepatic allograft rejection.
The rate of reversal in acute cardiac allograft rejection was 90% (n=61) and was 83% for hepatic allograft rejection (n=124) in patients unresponsive to treatment with steroids.
The dosage of other immunosuppressive agents used in conjunction with ORTHOCLONE OKT3 should be reduced to the lowest level compatible with an effective therapeutic response. (see: WARNINGS and ADVERSE REACTIONS: Infections, Neoplasia; DOSAGE AND ADMINISTRATION)

CONTRAINDICATIONS

ORTHOCLONE OKT3 should not be given to patients who:
- are hypersensitive to this or any other product of murine origin;
- have anti-mouse antibody titers ≥1:1000;
- are in (uncompensated) heart failure or in fluid overload, as evidenced by chest X-ray or a greater than 3 percent weight gain within the week prior to planned ORTHOCLONE OKT3 administration;
- have a history of seizures, or are predisposed to seizures;
- are determined and/or suspected to be pregnant, or who are breast-feeding. (see: PRECAUTIONS: Pregnancy, Nursing Mothers)

WARNINGS

SEE BOXED WARNING

Cytokine Release Syndrome

Temporarily associated with the administration of the first few doses of ORTHOCLONE OKT3 (particularly, the first two to three doses), most patients have developed an acute clinical syndrome [i.e., Cytokine Release Syndrome (CRS)] that has been attributed to the release of cytokines by activated lymphocytes or monocytes. This clinical syndrome has ranged from a more frequently reported mild, self-limited, "flu-like" illness to a less frequently reported severe, life-threatening, shock-like reaction, which may include serious cardiovascular and central nervous system manifestations. The syndrome typically begins approximately 30 to 60 minutes after administration of a dose of ORTHOCLONE OKT3 (but may occur later) and may persist for several hours. The frequency and severity of this symptom complex is usually greatest with the first dose. With each successive dose of ORTHOCLONE OKT3, both the frequency and severity of the Cytokine Release Syndrome tends to diminish. Increasing the amount of a dose or resuming treatment after a hiatus may result in a reappearance of the CRS.
Common clinical manifestations of the Cytokine Release Syndrome may include: high (often spiking, up to 107°F) fever, chills/rigors, headache, tremor, nausea/vomiting, diarrhea, abdominal pain, malaise, muscle/joint aches and pains, and generalized weakness. Less frequently reported adverse experiences include: minor dermatologic reactions (e.g., rash, pruritus, etc.) and a spectrum of often serious, occasionally fatal, cardiorespiratory and neuro-psychiatric adverse experiences. (see: WARNINGS, PRECAUTIONS, and ADVERSE REACTIONS: Neuro-Psychiatric Events)
Cardiorespiratory findings may include: dyspnea, shortness of breath, bronchospasm/wheezing, tachypnea, respiratory arrest/failure/distress, cardiovascular collapse, cardiac arrest, angina/myocardial infarction, chest pain/tightness, tachycardia, (including ventricular) hypertension, hemodynamic instability, hypotension including profound shock, heart failure, pulmonary edema (cardiogenic and non-cardiogenic), adult respiratory distress syndrome, hypoxemia, apnea, and arrhythmias. (see: BOXED WARNING; PRECAUTIONS; ADVERSE REACTIONS)
In the initial renal rejection studies, the most serious post-dose reaction-potentially fatal, severe *pulmonary edema*-occurred in 4.7% of the initial 107 patients. Fluid overload was present before treatment in all of these cases. However, it occurred in 0.0% of the subsequent 311 patients treated with first-dose volume/weight restrictions. In subsequent trials and in post-marketing experience, severe pulmonary edema has occurred in patients who appeared to be euvolemic. The pathogenesis of pulmonary edema may involve all or some of the following: volume overload; increased pulmonary vascular permeability; and/or reduced left ventricular compliance/contractility.
During the first 1 to 3 days of ORTHOCLONE OKT3 therapy, some patients have experienced an acute and transient decline in the glomerular filtration rate (GFR) and diminished urine output with a resulting *increase in the level of serum creatinine*. Massive release of cytokines appears to lead to reversible renal functional impairment and/or delayed renal allograft function.
Similarly, transient elevations in hepatic transaminases have been reported following administration of the first few doses of ORTHOCLONE OKT® 3 (muromonab-CD3).
Patients at risk for more serious complications of the Cytokine Release Syndrome may include those with the following conditions: unstable angina; recent myocardial infarction or symptomatic ischemic heart disease; heart failure of any etiology; pulmonary edema of any etiology; any form of chronic obstructive pulmonary disease; intravascular volume overload or depletion of any etiology (e.g., excessive dialysis, recent intensive diuresis, blood loss, etc.); cerebrovascular disease; patients with advanced symptomatic vascular disease or neuropathy; a history of seizures; and septic shock. Efforts should be made to correct or stabilize background conditions prior to the initiation of therapy.
Prior to administration of ORTHOCLONE OKT3, the patient's volume (fluid) status should be assessed carefully. It is imperative, especially prior to the first few doses, that there be no clinical evidence of volume overload or uncompensated heart failure, including a clear chest X-ray and weight restriction of ≤3% above the patient's minimum weight during the week prior to injection.
Manifestations of the Cytokine Release Syndrome may be prevented or minimized by pretreatment with 8 mg/kg of methylprednisolone (i.e., high-dose steroids), given 1 to 4 hours prior to administration of the first dose of ORTHOCLONE OKT3, and by closely following recommendations for dosage and treatment duration. (see: DOSAGE AND ADMINISTRATION)
The administration of ORTHOCLONE OKT3 should be performed in a facility that is equipped and staffed for cardiopulmonary resuscitation and where a patient can be closely monitored for an appropriate period based on the patient's status.
If any of the more serious presentations of the Cytokine Release Syndrome occur, intensive treatment including oxygen, intravenous fluids, corticosteroids, pressor amines, antihistamines, intubation, etc., may be required.

Anaphylactic Reactions

Serious and occasionally fatal, immediate (usually within 10 minutes) hypersensitivity (anaphylactic) reactions have been reported in patients treated with ORTHOCLONE OKT3. **Manifestations of anaphylaxis may appear similar to manifestations of the Cytokine Release Syndrome (described above). It may be impossible to determine the mechanism responsible for any systemic reaction(s).** Reactions attributed to hypersensitivity have been reported less frequently than those attributed to cytokine release. Acute hypersensitivity reactions may be characterized by: cardiovascular collapse, cardiorespiratory arrest, loss of consciousness, hypotension/shock, tachycardia, tingling, angioedema (including laryngeal, pharyngeal, or facial edema), airway obstruction, bronchospasm, dyspnea, urticaria, and pruritus.
Serious allergic events, including anaphylactic or anaphylactoid reactions, have been reported in patients re-exposed to ORTHOCLONE OKT3 subsequent to their initial course of therapy. Pretreatment with antihistamines and/or steroids may not reliably prevent anaphylaxis in this setting. Possible allergic hazards of retreatment should be weighed against expected therapeutic benefits and alternatives. If retreatment with ORTHOCLONE OKT3 is employed, epinephrine and other emergency life-support equipment should be available, and the patient should be monitored closely.
If hypersensitivity is suspected, discontinue the drug immediately, do not resume therapy or re-expose the patient to ORTHOCLONE OKT3. Serious acute hypersensitivity reactions may require emergency treatment with 0.3 mL to 0.5 mL aqueous epinephrine (1:1000 dilution) subcutaneously and other resuscitative measures including oxygen, intravenous fluids, antihistamines, corticosteroids, pressor amines, and airway management, as clinically indicated. (see: PRECAUTIONS: Cytokine Release Syndrome vs. Anaphylactic Reactions; ADVERSE REACTIONS: Hypersensitivity Reactions)

Neuro-Psychiatric Events

Seizures, encephalopathy, cerebral edema, aseptic meningitis, and headache have been reported, even following the first dose, during therapy with ORTHOCLONE OKT3, resulting in part from T cell activation and subsequent systemic release of cytokines.
Seizures, some accompanied by loss of consciousness or cardiorespiratory arrest, or death, have occurred independently or in conjunction with any of the neurologic syndromes described below. Patients predisposed to seizures may include those with the following conditions: acute tubular necrosis/uremia, fever, infection, a precipitous fall in serum calcium, fluid overload, hypertension, hypoglycemia, history of seizures, and electrolyte imbalances or those who are taking a medication concomitantly that may, by itself, cause seizures. Between 1987 and 1992, 75 post-marketing reports described seizures, averaging about 12 per year, and including 23 fatalities. More than two-thirds of these reports (53) were of domestic spontaneous origin, and their age and sex distributions were broad. Post-licensure reports generally do not provide sufficient basis for estimation of actual risks (incidence rates for specific adverse events), due to the typically substantial but unknown extent of under-ascertainment of incident events. Nonetheless, the number and regularity of seizure reports with ORTHOCLONE OKT® 3 (muromonab-CD3) indicate that this hazard appears not to be rare. Convulsions should be anticipated clinically with appropriate patient monitoring.
Manifestations of encephalopathy may include: impaired cognition, confusion, obtundation, altered mental status, disorientation, auditory/visual hallucinations, psychosis (delirium, paranoia), mood changes (e.g., mania, agitation, combativeness, etc.), diffuse hypotonus, hyperreflexia, myoclonus, tremor, asterixis, involuntary movements, major motor seizures, lethargy/stupor/coma, and diffuse weakness. Approximately one-third of patients with a diagnosis of en-

Continued on next page

Ortho Biotech—Cont.

cephalopathy may have had coexisting aseptic meningitis syndrome.

Cerebral edema (and other signs of increased vascular permeability e.g., otitis media, nasal and ear stuffiness, etc.) has been seen in patients treated with ORTHOCLONE OKT3 and may accompany some of the other neurologic manifestations.

Signs and symptoms of the *aseptic meningitis syndrome* described in association with the use of ORTHOCLONE OKT3 have included: fever, headache, meningismus (stiff neck), and photophobia. In a post-marketing survey involving 214 renal transplant patients, the incidence of this syndrome was 6%. Fever (89%), headache (44%), neck stiffness (14%), and photophobia (10%) were the most commonly reported symptoms; a combination of these four symptoms occurred in 5% of patients. Diagnosis is confirmed by cerebrospinal fluid (CSF) analysis demonstrating leukocytosis with pleocytosis, elevated protein and normal or decreased glucose, with negative viral, bacterial and fungal cultures. In any immunosuppressed transplant patient with clinical findings suggesting meningitis, the possibility of infection should be evaluated. Approximately one-third of the patients with a diagnosis of aseptic meningitis had coexisting signs and symptoms of encephalopathy. Most patients with the aseptic meningitis syndrome had a benign course and recovered without any permanent sequelae during therapy or subsequent to its completion or discontinuation.

Headache is frequently seen after any of the first few doses and may occur in any of the aforementioned neurologic syndromes or by itself.

The following additional neurologic events have each been reported occasionally in post-licensure reports: irreversible blindness, impaired vision, quadri- or paraparesis/plegia, cerebrovascular accident (hemiparesis/plegia), aphasia, transient ischemic attack, subarachnoid hemorrhage, palsy of the VI cranial nerve, and hearing loss.

Signs or symptoms of encephalopathy, meningitis, seizures, and cerebral edema, with or without headache, have typically been reversible. Headache, aseptic meningitis, seizures, and less severe forms of encephalopathy resolved in most patients despite continued treatment. However, some events have been irreversible.

Other neurologic events observed in patients treated with ORTHOCLONE OKT3 include: post-therapy encephalopathy with or without coexisting metabolic disturbances, post-therapy meningitis, CNS lymphoproliferative disorders and infections. Since these patients usually had both serious and multiple coexisting medical conditions and were also receiving multiple concomitant medications, the association of these events with ORTHOCLONE OKT3 treatment is unclear.

Patients who may be at greater risk for CNS adverse experiences include those: with known or suspected CNS disorders (e.g., history of seizure disorder, etc.); with cerebrovascular disease (small or large vessel); with conditions having associated neurologic problems (e.g., head trauma, uremia, etc.); with underlying vascular diseases; or who are receiving a medication concomitantly that may, by itself, affect the central nervous system. (see: WARNINGS, PRECAUTIONS and ADVERSE REACTIONS: Cytokine Release Syndrome; PRECAUTIONS: Drug Interactions)

Consequences of Immunosuppression

Serious and sometimes fatal infections and neoplasias have been reported in association with all immunosuppressive therapies, including those regimens containing ORTHOCLONE OKT® 3 (muromonab-CD-3).

Infections: ORTHOCLONE OKT3 is usually added to immunosuppressive therapeutic regimens, thereby augmenting the degree of immunosuppression. This increase in the total burden of immunosuppression may alter the spectrum of infections observed and increase the risk, the severity, and the potential gravity (morbidity) of infectious complications.

During the first month post-transplant, patients are at greatest risk for the following infections: (1) those present prior to transplant, perhaps exacerbated by post-transplant immunosuppression; (2) infection conveyed by the donor organ; and (3) the usual post-operative urinary tract, intravenous line-related, wound, or pulmonary infections due to bacterial pathogens.

Approximately one to six months post-transplant, patients are at risk for viral infections [e.g., Cytomegalovirus (CMV), Epstein-Barr Virus (EBV), Herpes simplex virus (HSV), etc.] which produce serious systemic disease and which also increase the overall state of immunosuppression. Clinically significant infections (e.g., pneumonia, sepsis, etc.) may occur with any microorganisms including: *Pneumocystis carinii, Listeria monocytogenes, Aspergillus* species, *Candida* species, *Nocardia asteroides, Legionella*, mycobacteria, gram-negative rods, and gram-positive cocci (staphylococci and streptococci), etc. Opportunistic infections, related to decreased T cell function, are associated with all immunosuppressive modalities employed to treat transplant rejection.

Multiple or intensive courses of any anti-T cell antibody preparation, including ORTHOCLONE OKT3, which produce profound impairment of cell-mediated immunity, further increase the risk of (opportunistic) infection, especially with the Herpes viruses (HSV, CMV, EBV) and fungi.

Reactivation (1 to 4 months post-transplant) of EBV and CMV has been reported. Infectious syndromes due to CMV have included: fever of unknown origin, pneumonia, viremia, hepatitis, liver/renal dysfunction, gastritis or gastrointestinal ulcerations, pancreatitis, chorioretinitis, leukopenia, and thrombocytopenia. When administration of an antilymphocyte antibody, including ORTHOCLONE OKT3, is followed by an immunosuppressive regimen including cyclosporine, there is an increased risk of reactivating CMV and impaired ability to limit its proliferation, resulting in symptomatic and disseminated disease. EBV infection, either primary or reactivated, may play an important role in the development of post-transplant lymphoproliferative disorders. (see: WARNINGS and ADVERSE REACTIONS: Neoplasia)

Anti-infective prophylaxis may reduce the morbidity associated with certain potential pathogens and should be considered for high-risk patients. Judicious use of immunosuppressive drugs, including type, dosage, and duration, may limit the risk and seriousness of some opportunistic infections. It is also possible to reduce the risk of serious CMV or EBV infection by avoiding transplantation of a CMV-seropositive (donor) and/or EBV-seropositive (donor) organ into a seronegative patient.

Neoplasia: As a result of depressed cell-mediated immunity, organ transplant patients have an increased risk of developing malignancies. This risk is evidenced almost exclusively by the occurrence of lymphoproliferative disorders (LPD), lymphomas, and skin cancers. In immunosuppressed patients, T cell cytotoxicity is impaired allowing for transformation and proliferation of EBV-infected B lymphocytes. Transformed B lymphocytes are thought to initiate the oncogenic process that ultimately culminates in the development of most post-transplant lymphoproliferative disorders. (see: ADVERSE REACTIONS: Neoplasia)

Following the initiation of ORTHOCLONE OKT3 therapy, patients should be continuously monitored for evidence of LPD, through physical examination and histological evaluation of any suspect lymphoid tissue. Vigilant surveillance is advised, since early detection with subsequent reduction of total immunosuppression may result in regression of some of these lymphoproliferative disorders. Since the potential for the development of LPD is related to the duration and extent (intensity) of total immunosuppression, physicians are advised: to adhere to the recommended dosage and duration of ORTHOCLONE OKT3 therapy; to limit the number of courses of ORTHOCLONE OKT3 and other anti-T lymphocyte antibody preparations administered within a short period of time; and, if appropriate, to reduce the dosage(s) of immunosuppressive drugs used concomitantly to the lowest level compatible with an effective therapeutic response. (see: DOSAGE AND ADMINISTRATION)

The long-term risk of neoplastic events in patients being treated with ORTHOCLONE OKT3 has not been determined.

PRECAUTIONS

General

Prior to Treatment with ORTHOCLONE OKT® 3 (muromonab-CD3)

Fluid Status: The patient's volume (fluid) status should be assessed carefully. It is imperative, especially prior to the first few doses, that there be no clinical evidence of volume overload, uncontrolled hypertension, or uncompensated heart failure, including a clear chest X-ray and weight restriction of $\leq 3\%$ above the patient's minimum weight during the week prior to injection.

Fever: If the temperature of the patient exceeds 37.8°C (100°F), it should be lowered by antipyretics before administration of each dose of ORTHOCLONE OKT3. The possibility of infection should be evaluated.

Blood Tests: Periodic assessment of organ system functions (renal, hepatic, and hematopoietic) should be performed.

During therapy with ORTHOCLONE OKT3: Periodic monitoring to ensure plasma ORTHOCLONE OKT3 levels (≥ 800 ng/mL) or T cell clearance (CD3 positive T cells < 25 cells/mm^3) is recommended.

Severe Cytokine Release Syndrome Versus Anaphylactic Reactions: **It may be very difficult, even impossible, to distinguish between an acute hypersensitivity reaction (e.g., anaphylaxis, angioedema, etc.) and the Cytokine Release Syndrome. Potentially serious signs and symptoms having an immediate onset (usually within 10 minutes) following administration of ORTHOCLONE OKT3 are more likely due to acute hypersensitivity; discontinue the drug immediately. If hypersensitivity is suspected, do not resume therapy or re-expose the patient** to ORTHOCLONE OKT3. Clinical manifestations beginning approximately 30 to 60 minutes (or later) following administration of ORTHOCLONE OKT3, are more likely cytokine-mediated. (see: WARNINGS: Cytokine Release Syndrome, Anaphylactic Reactions)

Neuro-Psychiatric Events: Since some seizures (and other serious central nervous system events) following ORTHOCLONE OKT3 administration have been life-threatening, anti-seizure precautions (e.g., an airway ready for use, if needed) should be taken. (see: WARNINGS and ADVERSE REACTIONS: Neuro-Psychiatric Events)

Infection/Viral-Induced Lymphoproliferative Disorders: Patients must be observed carefully for any signs and symptoms suggesting infection or viral-induced lymphoproliferative disorders (LPD). Anti-infective prophylaxis should be considered for patients at high risk. If infection or viral-induced LPD occur, culture or biopsy as soon as possible, institute promptly appropriate anti-infective therapy, and (if possible) reduce/discontinue immunosuppressive therapy.

When using combinations of immunosuppressive agents, the dose of each agent, including ORTHOCLONE OKT3, should be reduced to the lowest level compatible with an effective therapeutic response so as to reduce the potential for and severity of infections and malignant transformations (see: WARNINGS: Infections, Neoplasia)

Low Protein-Binding Filter: Use a low protein-binding 0.2 or 0.22 micrometer (μm) filter to prepare the injections. (see: ADMINISTRATION INSTRUCTIONS)

Sensitization: ORTHOCLONE OKT3 is a mouse (immunoglobulin) protein that can induce human anti-mouse antibody production (i.e., sensitization) in patients following exposure (See: CLINICAL PHARMACOLOGY). Monitoring for human antibody titers after ORTHOCLONE OKT3 therapy is strongly recommended. (see: CONTRAINDICATIONS)

Reduced T cell clearance or impaired ability to maintain adequate ORTHOCLONE OKT3 levels provides a basis for adjusting ORTHOCLONE OKT3 dosage or for discontinuing therapy. (see: WARNINGS: Anaphylactic Reactions; PRECAUTIONS: Laboratory Tests; ADVERSE REACTIONS: Hypersensitivity Reactions)

Intravascular Thrombosis: As with other immunosuppressive therapies, arterial or venous thromboses of allografts and other vascular beds (e.g., heart, lungs, brain, bowel, etc.) have been reported in patients treated with ORTHOCLONE OKT3. In addition, microangiopathic changes (e.g., platelet microthrombi) in the renal allograft associated in some patients with microangiopathic hemolytic anemia have been reported. This was observed in 5 of 93 (5%) patients receiving doses above the recommended dose (10 mg/day) Because a few cases have also been reported with the recommended dose, the relationship to dose remains uncertain. However, the relative risk appears to be greater with doses above the recommended dose. The decision to use ORTHOCLONE OKT3 in patients with a history of thrombotic events or underlying vascular disease should take these findings into consideration. Concomitant use of prophylactic anti-thrombotic interventions (e.g., mini-dose heparin, etc.) should be considered. (see: ADVERSE REACTIONS)

Information for Patients: Patients should be advised:

- of the signs and symptoms associated with the Cytokine Release Syndrome, including the potentially serious nature of this symptom complex (e.g., systemic, cardiovascular, neuro-psychiatric events).
- to seek medical attention at the first sign of skin rash, urticaria, rapid heartbeat, difficulty in swallowing and breathing, or any swelling that may suggest angioedema, or other allergic reaction.
- to know how they might react to ORTHOCLONE OKT® 3 (muromonab-CD-3) before operating an automobile or machinery, or engaging in activities requiring mental alertness and coordination.
- of the potential benefits and other risks attendant to the use of ORTHOCLONE OKT3. (see: BOXED WARNING; WARNINGS; PRECAUTIONS; ADVERSE REACTIONS)

Drug Interactions: The following medications are frequently used with ORTHOCLONE OKT3 and the information provided below may be helpful in evaluating any adverse events reported in ORTHOCLONE OKT3 treated patients.

With *indomethacin:* Encephalopathy and other CNS effects have been reported in patients treated with indomethacin alone and in conjunction with ORTHOCLONE OKT3. The mechanism of these effects is unknown.

With *corticosteroids:* Psychosis and infections have been seen in patients treated with corticosteroids alone and in conjunction with ORTHOCLONE OKT3.

With *azathioprine:* Infections or malignancies have been reported with azathioprine alone and in conjunction with ORTHOCLONE OKT3.

With *cyclosporine:* Seizures, encephalopathy, infections, malignancies, and thrombotic events have been reported in patients receiving cyclosporine alone and in conjunction with ORTHOCLONE OKT3.

Laboratory Tests: As with many potent drugs, periodic assessment of organ system functions should be performed during treatment with ORTHOCLONE OKT3.

The following tests should be monitored prior to and during ORTHOCLONE OKT3 therapy:

- Renal: BUN, serum creatinine, etc.:
- Hepatic: transaminases, alkaline phosphatase, bilirubin;

- Hematopoietic: WBCs and differential, platelet count, etc.;
- Chest X-ray within 24 hours <u>before</u> initiating ORTHO-CLONE OKT3 treatment. *Recommendation: chest X-ray should be free of any evidence of heart failure or fluid overload.*

One of the following immunologic tests should be monitored during ORTHOCLONE OKT3 therapy:

- Plasma ORTHOCLONE OKT3 levels (as determined by an ELISA); *target ORTHOCLONE OKT3 levels should be* ≥ 800 ng/mL; or
- Quantitative T lymphocyte surface phenotyping (CD3, CD4, CD8); target CD3 positive T cells < 25 cells/mm³.

Testing for human-mouse antibody titers is strongly recommended; *a titer ≥ 1:1000 is a contraindication for use.* (see: CONTRAINDICATIONS; PRECAUTIONS: Sensitization)

Carcinogenesis: Long-term studies have not been performed in laboratory animals to evaluate the carcinogenic potential of ORTHOCLONE OKT3. (see: WARNINGS and ADVERSE REACTIONS: Neoplasia)

Pregnancy Category C: Animal reproductive studies have not been conducted with ORTHOCLONE OKT3. It is also not known whether ORTHOCLONE OKT3 can cause fetal harm when administered to a pregnant woman or can affect reproduction capacity. However, ORTHOCLONE OKT3 is an IgG antibody and may cross the human placenta. The effect on the fetus of the release of cytokines and/or immunosuppression after treatment with ORTHOCLONE OKT3 is not known. If this drug is used during pregnancy, or the patient becomes pregnant while taking this drug, the patient should be apprised of the potential hazard to the fetus. (see: CONTRAINDICATIONS, WARNINGS, and ADVERSE REACTIONS)

Nursing Mothers: It is not known whether ORTHOCLONE OKT3 is excreted in human milk. Because many drugs are excreted in human milk and because of the potential for serious adverse reactions/oncogenesis shown for ORTHOCLONE OKT3 in human studies, a decision should be made to discontinue nursing or to discontinue the drug, taking into account the importance of the drug to the mother. (see: CONTRAINDICATIONS)

Pediatric Use: Safety and effectiveness in children have not been established. No adequately controlled clinical studies have been conducted in children. Published literature[4,10] has reported the use of ORTHOCLONE OKT 3 (muromonab-CD-3) infants/children, beginning with a dose of ≤5 mg. Based on immunologic monitoring, the dosage has been adjusted accordingly (See: PRECAUTIONS: Laboratory Tests). Pediatric recipients are reported to be significantly immunosuppressed for a prolonged period of time and therefore, require close monitoring post-therapy for opportunistic infections, particularly varicella (VZV), which poses an infectious complication unique to this population. Gastrointestinal fluid loss secondary to diarrhea and/or vomiting resulting from the Cytokine Release Syndrome may be significant when treating small children and may require parenteral hydration. It is unknown whether there may be significant long-term sequelae (e.g., neurodevelopmental language difficulties in infants under 1 year of age) related to the occurrence of seizures, high fever, CNS infections, aseptic meningitis, etc., following ORTHOCLONE OKT3 treatment. In cases where administration of ORTHOCLONE OKT3 would be deemed medically appropriate, more vigilant and frequent monitoring is required for children than in adults. (see: BOXED WARNING; WARNINGS; PRECAUTIONS; ADVERSE REACTIONS)

ADVERSE REACTIONS

Cytokine Release Syndrome

In controlled clinical trials for treatment of acute renal allograft rejection, patients treated with ORTHOCLONE OKT3 plus concomitant low-dose immunosuppressive therapy (primarily azathioprine and corticosteroids) were observed to have an increased incidence of adverse experiences during the first two days of treatment, as compared with the group of patients receiving azathioprine and high-dose steroid therapy. During this period the majority of patients experienced pyrexia (90%), of which 19% were 40.0°C (104°F) or above, and chills (59%). In addition, other adverse experiences occurring in 8% or more of the patients during the first two days of ORTHOCLONE OKT3 therapy included: dyspnea (21%), nausea (19%), vomiting (19%), chest pain (14%), diarrhea (14%), tremor (13%), wheezing (13%), headache (11%), tachycardia (10%), rigor (8%), and hypertension (8%). A similar spectrum of clinical manifestations has been observed in open clinical studies and in post-marketing experience involving patients treated with ORTHOCLONE OKT3 for rejection following renal, cardiac, and hepatic transplantation.

Additional serious and occasionally fatal cardiorespiratory manifestations have been reported following any of the first few doses. (see: WARNINGS: Cytokine Release Syndrome; ADVERSE REACTIONS: Cardiovascular, Respiratory)

In the acute renal allograft rejection trials, potentially fatal pulmonary edema had been reported following the first two doses in less than 2% of the patients treated with ORTHOCLONE OKT3. Pulmonary edema was usually associated with fluid overload. However, post-marketing experience revealed that pulmonary edema has occurred in patients who appeared to be euvolemic, presumably as a consequence of cytokine-mediated increased vascular permeability ("leaky capillaries") and/or reduced myocardial contractility/compliance (i.e., left ventricular dysfunction). (see: WARNINGS: Cytokine Release Syndrome; DOSAGE AND ADMINISTRATION)

Infections

In the controlled randomized renal rejection trial conducted during the pre-cyclosporine era, the most common infections during the first 45 days of ORTHOCLONE OKT3 therapy were due to Herpes simplex (27%) and cytomegalovirus (19%). Other severe and life-threatening infections were *Staphylococcus epidermidis* (4.8%), *Pneumocystis carinii* (3.1%), *Legionella* (1.6%), *Cryptococcus* (1.6%), *Serratia* (1.6%) and gram-negative bacteria (1.6%). The incidence of infections was similar in patients treated with ORTHOCLONE OKT3 and in patients treated with high-dose steroids.

In a clinical trial of acute hepatic rejection refractory to conventional treatment, the most common infections reported in patients treated with ORTHOCLONE OKT® 3 (muromonab-CD-3) during the first 45 days of the study were cytomegalovirus (15.7% of patients, of which 43% of infections were severe), fungal infections (14.9% of patients, of which 30% were severe), and Herpes simplex (7.5% of patients, of which 10% were severe). Other severe and life-threatening infections were gram-positive infections (9.0% of patients), gram-negative infections (7.5% of patients), viral infections (1.5% of patients), and *Legionella* (0.7% of patients). In another hepatic rejection trial the incidence of fungal infections was 34% and infections with the Herpes simplex virus was 31%. In a clinical trial of acute cardiac rejection refractory to conventional treatment, the most common infections reported in the ORTHOCLONE OKT® 3 (muromonab-CD3) group during the first 45 days of the study were Herpes simplex (5% of patients, of which 20% were severe), fungal infections (4% of patients, of which 75% were severe), and cytomegalovirus (3% of patients, of which 33% were severe). No other severe or life-threatening infections were reported during this period.

Clinically significant infections (e.g., pneumonia, sepsis, etc.) due to the following pathogens have been reported:

Bacterial: *Clostridium* species (including perfringens), *Corynebacterium*, Enterococcus, *Enterobacter aerogenes*, *Escherichia coli*, *Klebsiella* species, *Lactobacillus*, *Legionella*, Listeria monocytogenes, *Mycobacteria* species, *Nocardia asteroides*, *Proteus* species, *Providencia* species, *Pseudomonas aeruginosa*, *Serratia* species, *Staphylococcus* species, *Streptococcus* species, *Yersinia enterocolitica*, and other gram-negative bacteria.

*Fungal:** *Aspergillus*, *Candida*, Cryptococcal, Dermatophytes.

Protozoa: *Pneumocystis carinii, Toxoplasma gondii.*

Viral: Cytomegalovirus* (CMV), Epstein-Barr virus* (EBV), Herpes simplex virus* (HSV), Hepatitis viruses, Varicella zoster virus (VZV).

As a consequence of being a potent immunosuppressive, the incidence and severity of infections with designated(*) pathogens, especially the Herpes family of viruses, may be increased. (see: WARNINGS: Infections)

Neoplasia

In patients treated with ORTHOCLONE OKT3 post-transplant lymphoproliferative disorders (LPD) reported have ranged from lymphadenopathy or benign polyclonal B cell hyperplasias to malignant and often fatal monoclonal B cell lymphomas. In post-marketing experience, approximately one-third of the lymphoproliferations reported were benign, and two-thirds were malignant. Classification of these lymphomas has induced: B cell, large cell, polyclonal, non-Hodgkin's, lymphocytic, T cell, Burkitt's; the majority have not been classified histologically. When malignant lymphomas have been reported, they have appeared to develop early after transplantation, the majority within the first four months post-treatment. Many of these have been rapidly progressive, some fulminant involving the allografted organ, widely disseminated at time of diagnosis, and fatal. Carcinomas of the skin have included: basal cell, squamous cell, Kaposi's sarcoma, malanoma, and keratocanthoma. Other neoplasms infrequently reported include: multiple myeloma, leukemia, carcinoma of the breast, adenocarcinoma, cholangiocarcinoma, and recurrences of pre-existing hepatoma and renal cell carcinoma. (see: WARNINGS: Neoplasia)

Hypersensitivity Reactions

Reported adverse reactions resulting from the formation of antibodies to ORTHOCLONE OKT3 have inlcuded antigen-antibody (immune complex) mediated syndromes and IgE-mediated reactions. Reported hypersensitivity reactions have ranged from a mild, self-limited rash or pruritus to severe, life-threatening anaphylactic reactions/shock or angioedema (including: swelling of lips, eyelids, laryngeal spasm and airway obstruction with hypoxia). (see: WARNINGS: Anaphylactic Reactions)

Other hypersensitivity reactions have included: ineffectiveness of treatment, serum sickness, arthritis, allergic interstitial nephritis, immune complex deposition resulting in glomerulonephritis, vasculitis, and temporal arteritis, and eosinophilia.

Clinical adverse events occurring in clinical trials and post-marketing experience are listed below by body system:

Body as a Whole: fever (including, spiking temperatures as high as 107°F), chills/rigors, flu-like syndrome, fatigue/malaise, generalized weakness, anorexia.

Cardiovascular: cardiac arrest, hypotension/shock, heart failure, cardiovascular collapse, angina/myocardial infarction, tachycardia, bradycardia, hemodynamic instability, hypertension, left ventricular dysfunction, arrhythmias, chest pain/tightness.

Respiratory: respiratory arrest, adult respiratory distress syndrome (ARDS), respiratory failure, pulmonary edema (cardiogenic or noncardiogenic), apnea, dyspnea, bronchospasm, wheezing, shortness of breath, hypoxemia, tachypnea/hyperventilation, abnormal chest sounds, and pneumonia/pneumonitis (bacterial, viral, *P. carinii*, etc.).

Dermatologic: rash, Stevens-Johnson syndrome, urticaria, pruritus, erythema, flushing, diaphoresis.

Gastrointestinal: diarrhea, nausea/vomiting, abdominal pain, bowel infarction, gastrointestinal hemorrhage.

Hematopoietic: pancytopenia, aplastic anemia, neutropenia, leukopenia, thrombocytopenia, lymphopenia, leukocytosis, lymphadenopathy; arterial and venous thrombosis of allografts and other vascular beds (e.g., heart, lung, brain, bowel, etc.); disturbances of coagulation, including disseminated intravascular coagulation; microangiopathic changes (e.g., platelet microthrombi); microangiopathic hemolytic anemia.

Hepatobiliary: increases in transaminases (SGOT, SGPT, etc.); hepato/splenomegaly or hepatitis, usually secondary to viral infection or lymphoma.

Neuro-Psychiatric: seizures, lethargy/stupor/coma, encephalopathy, psychotic reactions (delirium), encephalitis, meningitis, cerebral edema, headache, dizziness, tremor, aphasia, quadri- or paraparesis/plegia, obtundation, confusion, altered mental status (e.g., paranoia, etc.), impaired cognition, disorientation, auditory and visual hallucinations, agitation/combativeness, mood changes (e.g., mania, etc.), hypotonus, hyperreflexia, myoclonus, asterixis, involuntary movements, CNS infections, CNS malignancies, cerebrovascular accident/hemiparesis/plegia, transient ischemic attack, subarachnoid hemorrhage.

Musculoskeletal: arthralgia, arthritis, myalgia, stiffness/aches/pains.

Special Senses: blindness, blurred vision, diplopia, hearing loss, otitis media, tinnitus, vertigo, VI cranial nerve palsy, photophobia, conjunctivitis, nasal and ear stuffiness.

Renal: anuria/oliguria; delayed graft function; renal insufficiency/renal failure, usually transient and reversible, and occasionally in association with cytokine release syndrome; abnormal urinary cytology including exfoliation of damaged lymphocytes, collecting duct cells and cellular casts.

OVERDOSAGE

Symptoms of overdose with ORTHOCLONE OKT® 3 (muromonab-CD3) may include hyperthermia, severe chills, myalgia, vomiting, diarrhea, edema, oliguria, pulmonary edema and acute renal failure. A high incidence (5%) of microangiopathic hemolytic anemia/HUS syndrome in patients receiving 10 mg per day of ORTHOCLONE OKT3 was also reported. In the event of acute overdosage with ORTHOCLONE OKT3, the patient should be carefully observed and given symptomatic and supportive treatment.

DOSAGE AND ADMINISTRATION

The recommended dose of ORTHOCLONE OKT3 for the treatment of acute renal, steroid-resistant cardiac, or steroid-resistant hepatic allograft rejection is 5 mg per day in a single (**bolus**) intravenous injection for 10 to 14 days. For acute renal rejection, treatment should begin upon diagnosis. For steroid-resistant cardiac or hepatic allograft rejection, treatment should begin when the treating physician deems a rejection has not been reversed by an adequate course of corticosteroid therapy. (see: CLINICAL PHARMACOLOGY; PRECAUTIONS: Sensitization, Laboratory Tests)

For the first few doses, patients should be monitored in a facility equipped and staffed for cardiopulmonary resuscitation with frequent determinations of vital signs. With subsequent doses, the patient should be monitored following ORTHOCLONE OKT3 therapy in a facility equipped and staffed for CPR for an appropriate period of time based on the patient's clinical status. Since the Cytokine Release Syndrome may also occur following a treatment hiatus and resumption of therapy, as with the first few doses, exercise vigilant care.

Prior to the administration of any dose of ORTHOCLONE OKT3, the patient's temperature should be lowered to < 37.8°C (100°F).

Prior to administration of ORTHOCLONE OKT3, the patient's volume status should be assessed carefully. It is imperative, especially prior to the first few doses, that there be

Continued on next page

Ortho Biotech—Cont.

no clinical evidence of volume overload or uncompensated heart failure, including a clear chest X-ray and weight restriction of ≤3% above the patient's minimum weight during the week prior to injection. (see: WARNINGS and ADVERSE REACTIONS: Cytokine Release Syndrome)
Intravenous methylprednisolone sodium succinate 8.0 mg/kg given 1 to 4 hours prior to administering the first dose of ORTHOCLONE OKT3 is strongly recommended to decrease the incidence and severity of reactions to the first dose, which have been attributed to the ORTHOCLONE OKT3 mediated Cytokine Release Syndrome.

Acetaminophen and antihistamines given concomitantly with ORTHOCLONE OKT® 3 (muromonab-CD-3) may also help to reduce some early reactions. (see: WARNINGS and ADVERSE REACTIONS: Cytokine Release Syndrome)
When using concomitant immunosuppressive drugs, the dose of each should be reduced to the lowest level compatible with an effective therapeutic response in order to reduce the potential for malignant transformations and the incidence and/or severity of infections. Maintenance immunosuppression should be resumed approximately three days prior to the cessation of ORTHOCLONE OKT3 therapy. (see: WARNINGS and ADVERSE REACTIONS: Infection, Neoplasia).

ADMINISTRATION INSTRUCTIONS

1. Prior to administration, parenteral drug products should be inspected visually for particulate matter and discoloration. Because ORTHOCLONE OKT3 is a protein solution, it may develop a few fine translucent particles which have been shown not to affect its potency.
2. No bacteriostatic agent is present in this product; adherence to aseptic technique is advised. Once the ampule is opened, use immediately and discard the unused portion.
3. Prepare ORTHOCLONE OKT3 for injection by drawing solution into a syringe through a low protein-binding 0.2 or 0.22 micrometer (μm) filter. Discard filter and attach a new needle for intravenous bolus injection.
4. Since no data is available on compatibility of ORTHOCLONE OKT3 with other intravenous substances or additives, other medications/substances should not be added or infused simultaneously through the same intravenous line. If the same intravenous line is used for sequential infusion of several different drugs, the line should be flushed with saline before and after infusion of ORTHOCLONE OKT3.
5. Administer ORTHOCLONE OKT3 as an intravenous bolus in less than one minute. Do not administer by intravenous infusion or in conjunction with other drug solutions.

HOW SUPPLIED

ORTHOCLONE OKT3 is supplied as a sterile solution in packages of 5 ampules (NDC 59676-101-01). Each 5 mL ampule contains 5 mg of muromonab-CD3.
Storage: Store in a refrigerator at 2° to 8°C (36° to 46°F). DO NOT FREEZE OR SHAKE.

REFERENCES

1. Adair JC, Woodley SL, O'Connell JB, et al. Aseptic Meningitis following Cardiac Transplantation: Clinical Characteristics and Relationship to Immunosuppressive Regimen. Neurology 41:249–252, 1991.
2. Chatenoud L, Legendre C, Ferran C, et al. Corticosteroid Inhibition of the OKT3–Induced Cytokine-Related Syndrome-Dosage and Kinetics Prerequisites. Transplantation 51:334–338, 1991.
3. Cockfield SM, Preiksaitis J, Harvey E, Jones C, Herbert D, Keown P, and Halloran PF. Is Sequential Use of ALG and OKT3 in Renal Transplants Associated With an Increased Incidence of Fulminant Post Transplant Lymphoproliferative Disorders? Transplant. Proc. 23:1106–1107, 1991.
4. Ettenger RB, Marik J. Rosenthal JT, et al. OKT3 for Rejection Reversal in Pediatric Renal Transplantation. Clin. Transplantation 2:180–184, 1988.
5. Gaston RS, Deierhoi MH, Patterson T, et al. OKT3 First-Dose Reaction: Association with T Cell Subsets and Cytokine Release. Kid. International 39:141–148, 1991.
6. Goldman M, Abramowicz D, DePauw L, et al. OKT3-Induced Cytokine Released Attenuation by High-Dose Methylprednisolone. Lancet 2:802–803, 1989.
7. Ortho Multicenter Transplant Study Group. A Randomized Clinical Trial of OKT3 Monoclonal Antibody for Acute Rejection of Cadaveric Renal Transplants. N. Engl. J. Med 313:337–342, 1985.
8. Penn I. The Changing Patterns of Posttransplant Malignancies. Transplant Proc. 23:1101–1103, 1991.
9. Rubin RH and Tolkoff-Rubin NE. The Impact of Infection on the Outcome of Transplantation. Transplant Proc. 23:2068–2074, 1991.
10. Schroeder TJ, Ryckman FC, Hurtubise PE, et al. Immunological Monitoring during and following OKT3 Therapy in Children. Clin. Transplantation 5:191–196, 1991.

ORTHO BIOTECH INC.
Raritan, New Jersey 08869
U.S.A.
©OBI 1986
631-10-191-9
Revised June 1995

PROCRIT®
EPOETIN ALFA
PROCRIT registered trademark of distributor
FOR INJECTION
℞

DESCRIPTION

Erythropoietin is a glycoprotein which stimulates red blood cell production. It is produced in the kidney and stimulates the division and differentiation of committed erythroid progenitors in the bone marrow. PROCRIT (Epoetin alfa), a 165 amino acid glycoprotein manufactured by recombinant DNA technology, has the same biological effects as endogenous erythropoietin.[1] It has a molecular weight of 30,400 daltons and is produced by mammalian cells into which the human erythropoietin gene has been introduced. The product contains the identical amino acid sequence of isolated natural erythropoietin.

PROCRIT is formulated as a sterile, colorless, liquid in an isotonic sodium chloride/sodium citrate buffered solution for intravenous (IV) or subcutaneous (SC) administration.
Single-Dose, Preservative-Free Vial: Each 1 mL of solution contains 2,000, 3,000, 4,000 or 10,000 units of Epoetin alfa, 2.5 mg Albumin (Human), 5.8 mg sodium citrate, 5.8 mg sodium chloride, and 0.06 mg citric acid in Water for Injection, USP (pH 6.9±0.3). This formulation contains no preservative.

Multidose, Preserved Vial: 2 mL (20,000 units, 10,000 Units/mL). Each 1 mL of solution contains 10,000 units of Epoetin alfa, 2.5 mg Albumin (Human), 1.3 mg sodium citrate, 8.2 mg sodium chloride, 0.11 mg citric acid, and 1% benzyl alcohol as preservative in Water for Injection, USP (pH 6.1±0.3).

CLINICAL PHARMACOLOGY

Chronic Renal Failure Patients

Endogenous production of erythropoietin is normally regulated by the level of tissue oxygenation. Hypoxia and anemia generally increase the production of erythropoietin, which in turn stimulates erythropoiesis.[2] In normal subjects, plasma erythropoietin levels range from 0.01 to 0.03 Units/mL,[2,3] and increase up to 100- to 1000-fold during hypoxia or anemia.[2,3] In contrast, in patients with chronic renal failure (CRF), production of erythropoietin is impaired, and this erythropoietin deficiency is the primary cause of their anemia.[3,4]

Chronic renal failure is the clinical situation in which there is a progressive and usually irreversible decline in kidney function. Such patients may manifest the sequelae of renal dysfunction, including anemia, but do not necessarily require regular dialysis. Patients with end-stage renal disease (ESRD) are those patients with CRF who require regular dialysis or kidney transplantation for survival.

PROCRIT has been shown to stimulate erythropoiesis in anemic patients with CRF, including both patients on dialysis and those who do not require regular dialysis.[4-13] The first evidence of a response to the three times weekly (T.I.W.) administration of PROCRIT is an increase in the reticulocyte count within 10 days, followed by increases in the red cell count, hemoglobin, and hematocrit, usually within 2–6 weeks.[4,5] Because of the length of time required for erythropoiesis—several days for erythroid progenitors to mature and be released into the circulation—a clinically significant increase in hematocrit is usually not observed in less than 2 weeks and may require up to 6 weeks in some patients. Once the hematocrit reaches the suggested target range (30–36%), that level can be sustained by PROCRIT therapy in the absence of iron deficiency and concurrent illnesses.

The rate of hematocrit increase varies between patients and is dependent upon the dose of PROCRIT, within a therapeutic range of approximately 50-300 Units/kg (T.I.W.).[4] A greater biologic response is not observed at doses exceeding 300 Units/kg (T.I.W.).[6] Other factors affecting the rate and extent of response include availability of iron stores, the baseline hematocrit, and the presence of concurrent medical problems.

Zidovudine-treated HIV-infected Patients

Responsiveness to PROCRIT in HIV-infected patients is dependent upon the endogenous serum erythropoietin level prior to treatment. Patients with endogenous serum erythropoietin levels ≤500 mUnits/mL, and who are receiving a dose of zidovudine ≤4,200 mg/week, may respond to PROCRIT therapy. Patients with endogenous serum erythropoietin levels >500 mUnits/mL do not appear to respond to PROCRIT therapy. In a series of four clinical trials involving 255 patients, 60% to 80% of HIV-infected patients treated with zidovudine had endogenous serum erythropoietin levels ≤500 mUnits/mL.

Response to PROCRIT in zidovudine-treated HIV-infected patients is manifested by reduced transfusion requirements and increased hematocrit.

Cancer Patients on Chemotherapy

Anemia in cancer patients may be related to the disease itself or the effect of concomitantly administered chemotherapeutic agents. PROCRIT has been shown to increase hematocrit and decrease transfusion requirements after the first month of therapy (months 2 and 3), in anemic cancer patients undergoing chemotherapy.

A series of clinical trials enrolled 131 anemic cancer patients who were receiving cyclic cisplatin- or non cisplatin-containing chemotherapy. Endogenous baseline serum erythropoietin levels varied among patients in these trials with approximately 75% (N=83/110) having endogenous serum erythropoietin levels ≤132 mUnits/mL, and approximately 4% (N=4/110) of patients having endogenous serum erythropoietin levels >500 mUnits/mL. In general, patients with lower baseline serum erythropoietin levels responded more vigorously to PROCRIT than patients with higher baseline erythropoietin levels. Although no specific serum erythropoietin level can be stipulated above which patients would be unlikely to respond to PROCRIT therapy, treatment of patients with grossly elevated serum erythropoietin levels (e.g., >200 mUnits/mL) is not recommended.

Pharmacokinetics

Intravenously administered PROCRIT is eliminated at a rate consistent with first order kinetics with a circulating half-life ranging from approximately 4 to 13 hours in patients with CRF. Within the therapeutic dose range, detectable levels of plasma erythropoietin are maintained for at least 24 hours.[7] After subcutaneous administration of PROCRIT to patients with CRF, peak serum levels are achieved within 5–24 hours after administration and decline slowly thereafter. There is no apparent difference in half-life between patients not on dialysis whose serum creatinine levels were greater than 3, and patients maintained on dialysis.

In normal volunteers, the half-life of intravenously administered PROCRIT is approximately 20% shorter than the half-life in CRF patients. The pharmacokinetics of PROCRIT have not been studied in HIV-infected patients.

INDICATIONS AND USAGE

Treatment of Anemia of Chronic Renal Failure Patients

PROCRIT is indicated in the treatment of anemia associated with chronic renal failure, including patients on dialysis (end-stage renal disease) and patients not on dialysis. PROCRIT is indicated to elevate or maintain the red blood cell level (as manifested by the hematocrit or hemoglobin determinations) and to decrease the need for transfusions in these patients.

PROCRIT is not intended for patients who require immediate correction of severe anemia. PROCRIT may obviate the need for maintenance transfusions but is not a substitute for emergency transfusion.

Prior to initiation of therapy, the patient's iron stores, including transferrin saturation and serum ferritin, should be evaluated. Transferrin saturation should be at least 20% and ferritin at least 100 ng/mL. Blood pressure should be adequately controlled prior to initiation of PROCRIT therapy, and must be closely monitored and controlled during therapy. Non-dialysis patients with symptomatic anemia considered for therapy should have a hematocrit less than 30%. All patients on PROCRIT therapy should be regularly monitored (see "PRECAUTIONS").

PROCRIT should be administered under the guidance of a qualified physician (see "Dosage and Administration").

Treatment of Anemia in Zidovudine-treated HIV-Infected Patients

PROCRIT is indicated for the treatment of anemia related to therapy with zidovudine in HIV-infected patients. PROCRIT is indicated to elevate or maintain the red blood cell level (as manifested by the hematocrit or hemoglobin determinations) and to decrease the need for transfusions in these patients. PROCRIT is not indicated for the treatment of anemia in HIV-infected patients due to other factors such as iron or folate deficiencies, hemolysis or gastrointestinal bleeding, which should be managed appropriately.

PROCRIT, at a dose of 100 Units/kg three times per week, is effective in decreasing the transfusion requirement and increasing the red blood cell level of anemic, HIV-infected patients treated with zidovudine, when the endogenous serum erythropoietin level is ≤500 mUnits/mL and when patients are receiving a dose of zidovudine ≤4,200 mg/week.

Treatment of Anemia in Cancer Patients on Chemotherapy

PROCRIT is indicated for the treatment of anemia in patients with non-myeloid malignancies where anemia is due to the effect of concomitantly administered chemotherapy. PROCRIT is indicated to decrease the need for transfusions in patients who will be receiving concomitant chemotherapy for a minimum of 2 months. PROCRIT is not indicated for the treatment of anemia in cancer patients due to other factors such as iron or folate deficiencies, hemolysis or gastrointestinal bleeding which should be managed appropriately.

Clinical Experience: Response to PROCRIT
Chronic Renal Failure Patients

Response to PROCRIT was consistent across all studies. In the presence of adequate iron stores (see "Pre-Therapy Iron Evaluation"), the time to reach the target hematocrit is a function of the baseline hematocrit and the rate of hematocrit rise.

The rate of increase in hematocrit is dependent upon the dose of PROCRIT administered and individual patient variation. In clinical trials at starting doses of 50–150 Units/kg (T.I.W.), patients responded with an average rate of hematocrit rise of:

HEMATOCRIT INCREASE

STARTING DOSE (T.I.W. IV)	POINTS/DAY	POINTS/2 WEEKS
50 Units/kg	0.11	1.5
100 Units/kg	0.18	2.5
150 Units/kg	0.25	3.5

Over this dose range, approximately 95% of all patients responded with a clinically significant increase in hematocrit, and by the end of approximately 2 months of therapy virtually all patients were transfusion-independent. Changes in the quality of life of patients treated with PROCRIT were assessed as part of a Phase III clinical trial.[5,8] Once the target hematocrit (32-38%) was achieved, statistically significant improvements were demonstrated for most quality of life parameters measured, including energy and activity level, functional ability, sleep and eating behavior, health status, satisfaction with health, sex life, well-being, psychological effect, life satisfaction, and happiness. Patients also reported improvement in their disease symptoms. They showed a statistically significant increase in exercise capacity (VO_2 max), energy, and strength with a significant reduction in aching, dizziness, anxiety, shortness of breath, muscle weakness, and leg cramps.[8,14]

Patients On Dialysis: Thirteen clinical studies were conducted, involving intravenous administration to a total of 1,010 anemic patients on dialysis for 986 patient-years of PROCRIT therapy. In the three largest of these clinical trials, the median maintenance dose necessary to maintain the hematocrit between 30-36% was approximately 75 Units/kg (T.I.W.). In the U.S. multicenter Phase III study, approximately 65% of the patients required doses of 100 Units/kg (T.I.W.), or less, to maintain their hematocrit at approximately 35%. Almost 10% of patients required a dose of 25 Units/kg, or less, and approximately 10% required a dose of more than 200 Units/kg (T.I.W.) to maintain their hematocrit at this level.

A multicenter unit dose study was also conducted in 119 patients receiving peritoneal dialysis who self-administered PROCRIT subcutaneously for approximately 109 patient-years of experience. Patients responded to PROCRIT administered subcutaneously in a manner similar to patients receiving intravenous administration.[15]

Patients With CRF Not Requiring Dialysis: Four clinical trials were conducted in patients with CRF not on dialysis involving 181 patients treated with PROCRIT for approximately 67 patient-years of experience. These patients responded to PROCRIT therapy in a manner similar to that observed in patients on dialysis. Patients with CRF not on dialysis demonstrated a dose-dependent and sustained increase in hematocrit when PROCRIT was administered by either an intravenous (IV) or subcutaneous (SC) route, with similar rates of rise of hematocrit when PROCRIT was administered by either route. Moreover, PROCRIT doses of 75–150 Units/kg per week have been shown to maintain hematocrits of 36-38% for up to six months. Correcting the anemia of progressive renal failure will allow patients to remain active even though their renal function continues to decrease.[16–18]

Zidovudine-treated HIV-Infected Patients

PROCRIT has been studied in four placebo-controlled trials enrolling 297 anemic (hematocrit<30%) HIV-infected (AIDS) patients receiving concomitant therapy with zidovudine, (all patients were treated with Epoetin alfa manufactured by Amgen Inc.) In the subgroup of patients (89/125 PROCRIT, and 88/130 placebo) with prestudy endogenous serum erythropoietin levels ≤500 mUnits/mL (normal endogenous serum erythropoietin levels are 4–26 mUnits/mL), PROCRIT reduced the mean cumulative number of units of blood transfused per patient by approximately 40%, as compared to the placebo group.[19] Among those patients who required transfusions at baseline, 43% of patients treated with PROCRIT versus 18% of placebo-treated patients were transfusion-independent during the second and third months of therapy. PROCRIT therapy also resulted in significant increases in hematocrit in comparison to placebo. When examining the results according to the weekly dose of zidovudine received during Month 3 of therapy, there was a statistically significant (p <0.003) reduction in transfusion requirements in patients treated with PROCRIT (N=51) compared to placebo-treated patients (N=54) whose mean weekly zidovudine dose was ≤4,200 mg/week.[19] Approximately 17% of the patients with endogenous serum erythropoietin levels ≤500 mUnits/mL receiving PROCRIT in doses from 100–200 Units/kg three times weekly (T.I.W.) achieved a hematocrit of 38% without administration of transfusions or a significant reduction in zidovudine dose. In the subgroup of patients whose prestudy endogenous serum erythropoietin levels were >500 mUnits/mL, PROCRIT therapy did not reduce transfusion requirements or increase hematocrit, compared to the corresponding responses in placebo-treated patients.

In a six month open label PROCRIT study, patients responded with decreased transfusion requirements and sustained increases in hematocrit and hemoglobin with doses of PROCRIT up to 300 Units/kg (T.I.W.).[18–20]

Responsiveness to PROCRIT therapy may be blunted by intercurrent infectious/inflammatory episodes and by an increase in zidovudine dosage. Consequently, the dose of PROCRIT must be titrated based on these factors to maintain the desired erythropoietic response.

Cancer Patients on Chemotherapy

PROCRIT has been studied in a series of placebo-controlled, double-blind trials in a total of 131 anemic cancer patients. Within this group, 72 patients were treated with concomitant noncisplatin-containing chemotherapy regimens and 59 patients were treated with concomitant cisplatin-containing chemotherapy regimens. Patients were randomized to PROCRIT 150 Units/kg or placebo subcutaneously (T.I.W.) for 12 weeks.

PROCRIT therapy was associated with a significantly (p <0.008) greater hematocrit response than in the corresponding placebo-treated patients (see TABLE).[19]

HEMATOCRIT (%): MEAN CHANGE FROM BASELINE TO FINAL VALUE[a]

STUDY	PROCRIT	PLACEBO
Chemotherapy	7.6	1.3
Cisplatin	6.9	0.6

[a] Significantly higher in PROCRIT patients than in placebo patients (p <0.008)

In the two types of chemotherapy studies [utilizing a PROCRIT dose of 150 Units/kg (T.I.W.)]the mean number of units of blood transfused per patient after the first month of therapy was significantly (p <0.02) lower in patients treated with PROCRIT (0.71 units in Months 2, 3) than in corresponding placebo-treated patients (1.84 units in Months 2, 3). Moreover, the proportion of patients transfused during Months 2 and 3 of therapy combined was significantly (p <0.03) lower in the patients treated with PROCRIT than in the corresponding placebo-treated patients (22% versus 43%).[19]

Comparable intensity of chemotherapy in the PROCRIT and placebo groups in the chemotherapy trials was suggested by a similar area under the neutrophil time curve in patients treated with PROCRIT and placebo-treated patients as well as by a similar proportion of patients in groups treated with PROCRIT and placebo-treated groups whose absolute neutrophil counts fell below 1,000 cells/μL. Available evidence suggests that patients with lymphoid and solid cancers respond equivalently to PROCRIT therapy, and that patients with or without tumor infiltration of the bone marrow respond equivalently to PROCRIT therapy.

CONTRAINDICATIONS

PROCRIT is contraindicated in patients with:
1) Uncontrolled hypertension.
2) Known hypersensitivity to mammalian cell-derived products.
3) Known hypersensitivity to Albumin (Human).

WARNINGS
Chronic Renal Failure Patients

Hypertension: Patients with uncontrolled hypertension should not be treated with PROCRIT; blood pressure should be controlled adequately before initiation of therapy. Up to 80% of patients with CRF have a history of hypertension.[21] Although there does not appear to be any direct pressor effects of PROCRIT, blood pressure may rise during PROCRIT therapy. During the early phase of treatment when the hematocrit is increasing, approximately 25% of patients on dialysis may require initiation of, or increases in, antihypertensive therapy. Hypertensive encephalopathy and seizures have been observed in patients with CRF treated with PROCRIT.

Special care should be taken to closely monitor and aggressively control blood pressure in patients treated with PROCRIT. Patients should be advised as to the importance of compliance with antihypertensive therapy and dietary restrictions. If blood pressure is difficult to control by initiation of appropriate measures, the hematocrit may be reduced by decreasing or withholding the dose of PROCRIT. A clinically significant decrease in hematocrit may not be observed for several weeks.

It is recommended that the dose of PROCRIT be decreased if the hematocrit increase exceeds 4 points in any two-week period, because of the possible association of excessive rate of rise of hematocrit with an exacerbation of hypertension.

Seizures: Seizures have occurred in patients with CRF participating in PROCRIT clinical trials.

In patients on dialysis, there was a higher incidence of seizures during the first 90 days of therapy (occurring in approximately 2.5% of patients) as compared with later timepoints.

Given the potential for an increased risk of seizures during the first 90 days of therapy, blood pressure and the presence of premonitory neurologic symptoms should be monitored closely. Patients should be cautioned to avoid potentially hazardous activities such as driving or operating heavy machinery during this period.

While the relationship between seizures and the rate of rise of hematocrit is uncertain, it is recommended that the dose of PROCRIT be decreased if the hematocrit increase exceeds 4 points in any two-week period.

Thrombotic Events: During hemodialysis, patients treated with PROCRIT may require increased anticoagulation with heparin to prevent clotting of the artificial kidney. A relationship has not been established with statistical certainty between a rise in hematocrit and the rate of thrombotic events (including thrombosis of vascular access). In clinical trials, clotting of the vascular access (A-V shunt) has occurred at an annualized rate of about 0.25 events per patient-year on PROCRIT therapy, a rate which appears to be no higher than that seen in untreated patients on dialysis. Overall, for patients with CRF (whether on dialysis or not), other thrombotic events (e.g., myocardial infarction, cerebrovascular accident, transient ischemic attack) have occurred in clinical trials at an annualized rate of less than 0.04 events per patient-year of PROCRIT therapy. Patients with pre-existing vascular disease should be monitored closely. See "ADVERSE REACTIONS" for more information about thrombotic events.

Zidovudine-treated HIV-Infected Patients

In contrast to CRF patients, PROCRIT therapy has not been linked to exacerbation of hypertension, seizures, and thrombotic events in HIV-infected patients.

Miscellaneous: The multidose preserved formulation contains benzyl alcohol. Benzyl alcohol has been reported to be associated with an increased incidence of neurological and other complications in premature infants which are sometimes fatal.

PRECAUTIONS
Chronic Renal Failure Patients, Zidovudine-treated HIV-infected Patients and Cancer Patients on Chemotherapy

General: The parenteral administration of any biologic product should be attended by appropriate precautions in case allergic or other untoward reactions occur (see "Contraindications"). In clinical trials, while transient rashes were occasionally observed concurrently with PROCRIT therapy, no serious allergic or anaphylactic reactions were reported. See "ADVERSE REACTIONS" for more information regarding allergic reactions.

The safety and efficacy of PROCRIT therapy have not been established in patients with a known history of a seizure disorder or underlying hematologic disease (e.g., sickle cell anemia, myelodysplastic syndromes, or hypercoagulable disorders).

In some female patients, menses have resumed following PROCRIT therapy; the possibility of pregnancy should be discussed and the need for contraception evaluated.

Hematology: Exacerbation of porphyria has been observed rarely in patients with CRF treated with PROCRIT. However, PROCRIT has not caused increased urinary excretion of porphyrin metabolites in normal volunteers, even in the presence of a rapid erythropoietic response. Nevertheless, PROCRIT should be used with caution in patients with known porphyria.

In pre clinical studies in dogs and rats, but not in monkeys, PROCRIT therapy was associated with subclinical bone marrow fibrosis. Bone marrow fibrosis is a known complication of CRF in humans and may be related to secondary hyperparathyroidism or unknown factors. The incidence of bone marrow fibrosis was not increased in a study of patients on dialysis who were treated with PROCRIT for 12–19 months, compared to the incidence of bone marrow fibrosis in a matched group of patients who had not been treated with PROCRIT.

Hematocrit in CRF patients should be measured twice a week; zidovudine-treated HIV-infected and cancer patients should have hematocrit measured once a week until hematocrit has been stabilized, and measured periodically thereafter.

Delayed or Diminished Response: If the patient fails to respond or to maintain a response to doses within the recommended dosing range, the following etiologies should be considered and evaluated:

Continued on next page

Ortho Biotech—Cont.

1) Iron deficiency: Virtually all patients will eventually require supplemental iron therapy. (See "*Iron Evaluation*").
2) Underlying infectious, inflammatory, or malignant processes.
3) Occult blood loss.
4) Underlying hematologic diseases (i.e., thalassemia, refractory anemia, or other myelodysplastic disorders).
5) Vitamin deficiencies: folic acid or vitamin B12.
6) Hemolysis.
7) Aluminum intoxication.
8) Osteitis fibrosa cystica.

Iron Evaluation: During PROCRIT therapy, absolute or functional iron deficiency may develop. Functional iron deficiency, with normal ferritin levels but low transferrin saturation, is presumably due to the inability to mobilize iron stores rapidly enough to support increased erythropoiesis. Transferrin saturation should be at least 20% <u>and</u> ferritin should be at least 100 ng/mL.
Prior to and during PROCRIT therapy, the patient's iron status, including transferrin saturation (serum iron divided by iron binding capacity) and serum ferritin, should be evaluated. Virtually all patients will eventually require supplemental iron to increase or maintain transferrin saturation to levels which will adequately support erythropoiesis stimulated by PROCRIT.

Drug Interactions: No evidence of interaction of PROCRIT with other drugs was observed in the course of clinical trials.

Carcinogenesis, Mutagenesis, and Impairment of Fertility: Carcinogenic potential of PROCRIT has not been evaluated. PROCRIT does not induce bacterial gene mutation (Ames Test), chromosomal aberrations in mammalian cells, micronuclei in mice, or gene mutation at the HGPRT locus. In female rats treated intravenously with PROCRIT, there was a trend for slightly increased fetal wastage at doses of 100 and 500 Units/kg.

Pregnancy Category C: PROCRIT has been shown to have adverse effects in rats when given in doses five times the human dose. There are no adequate and well-controlled studies in pregnant women. PROCRIT should be used during pregnancy only if potential benefit justifies the potential risk to the fetus.
In studies in female rats, there were decreases in body weight gain, delays in appearance of abdominal hair, delayed eyelid opening, delayed ossification, and decreases in the number of caudal vertebrae in the F1 fetuses of the 500 Units/kg group. In female rats treated intravenously, there was a trend for slightly increased fetal wastage at doses of 100 and 500 Units/kg. PROCRIT has not shown any adverse effect at doses as high as 500 Units/kg in pregnant rabbits (from day 6 to 18 of gestation).

Nursing Mothers: Postnatal observations of the live offspring (F1 generation) of female rats treated with PROCRIT during gestation and lactation revealed no effect of PROCRIT at doses of up to 500 Units/kg. There were, however, decreases in body weight gain, delays in appearance of abdominal hair, eyelid opening, and decreases in the number of caudal vertebrae in the F1 fetuses of the 500 Units/kg group. There were no effects related to PROCRIT on the F2 generation fetuses.
It is not known whether PROCRIT is excreted in human milk. Because many drugs are excreted in human milk, caution should be exercised when PROCRIT is administered to a nursing woman.

Pediatric Use: The safety and effectiveness of PROCRIT in children have not been established (See WARNINGS).

Chronic Renal Failure Patients

Patients with CRF Not Requiring Dialysis: Blood pressure and hematocrit should be monitored no less frequently than for patients maintained on dialysis. Renal function and fluid and electrolyte balance should be closely monitored, as an improved sense of well-being may obscure the need to initiate dialysis in some patients.

Hematology: Sufficient time should be allowed to determine a patient's responsiveness to a dosage of PROCRIT before adjusting the dose. Because of the time required for erythropoiesis and the red cell half-life, an interval of 2–6 weeks may occur between the time of a dose adjustment (initiation, increase, decrease, or discontinuation) and a significant change in hematocrit.
In order to avoid reaching the suggested target hematocrit too rapidly, or exceeding the suggested target range (hematocrit of 30–36%), the guidelines for dose and frequency of dose adjustments (see "Dosage and Administration") should be followed.
For patients who respond to PROCRIT with a rapid increase in hematocrit (e.g., more than 4 points in any two-week period), the dose of PROCRIT should be reduced because of the possible association of excessive rate of rise of hematocrit with an exacerbation of hypertension.

	PERCENT OF PATIENTS REPORTING EVENT	
Event	Patients Treated with PROCRIT (N = 200)	PLACEBO-TREATED Patients (N = 135)
Hypertension	24%	19%
Headache	16%	12%
Arthralgias	11%	6%
Nausea	11%	9%
Edema	9%	10%
Fatigue	9%	14%
Diarrhea	9%	6%
Vomiting	8%	5%
Chest Pain	7%	9%
Skin Reaction (Administration Site)	7%	12%
Asthenia	7%	12%
Dizziness	7%	13%
Clotted Access	7%	2%
Seizure	1.1%	1.1%
CVA/TIA	0.4%	0.6%
MI	0.4%	1.1%
Death	0	1.7%

The elevated bleeding time characteristic of CRF decreases toward normal after correction of anemia in patients treated with PROCRIT. Reduction of bleeding time also occurs after correction of anemia by transfusion.

Laboratory Monitoring: The hematocrit should be determined twice a week until it has stabilized in the suggested target range and the maintenance dose has been established. After any dose adjustment, the hematocrit should also be determined twice weekly for at least 2–6 weeks until it has been determined that the hematocrit has stabilized in response to the dose change. The hematocrit should then be monitored at regular intervals.
A complete blood count with differential and platelet count should be performed regularly. During clinical trials, modest increases were seen in platelets and white blood cell counts. While these changes were statistically significant, they were not clinically significant and the values remained within normal ranges.
In patients with CRF, serum chemistry values [including blood urea nitrogen (BUN), uric acid, creatinine, phosphorus, and potassium] should be monitored regularly. During clinical trials in patients on dialysis, modest increases were seen in BUN, creatinine, phosphorus, and potassium. In some patients with CRF not on dialysis, treated with PROCRIT, modest increases in serum uric acid and phosphorus were observed. While changes were statistically significant, the values remained within the ranges normally seen in patients with CRF.

Diet: As the hematocrit increases and patients experience an improved sense of well-being and quality of life, the importance of compliance with dietary and dialysis prescriptions should be reinforced. In particular, hyperkalemia is not uncommon in patients with CRF. In U.S. studies in patients on dialysis, hyperkalemia has occurred at an annualized rate of approximately 0.11 episodes per patient-year of PROCRIT therapy, often in association with poor compliance to medication, dietary and/or dialysis prescriptions.

Dialysis Management: Therapy with PROCRIT results in an increase in hematocrit and a decrease in plasma volume which could affect dialysis efficiency. In studies to date, the resulting increase in hematocrit did not appear to adversely affect dialyzer function[9,10] or the efficiency of high flux hemodialysis.[11] During hemodialysis, patients treated with PROCRIT may require increased anticoagulation with heparin to prevent clotting of the artificial kidney.
Patients who are marginally dialyzed may require adjustments in their dialysis prescription. As with all patients on dialysis, the serum chemistry values [including blood urea nitrogen (BUN), creatinine, phosphorus, and potassium] in patients treated with PROCRIT should be monitored regularly to assure the adequacy of the dialysis prescription.

Information for Patients: In those situations in which the physician determines that a home dialysis patient can safely and effectively self-administer PROCRIT, the patient should be instructed as to the proper dosage and administration. Home dialysis patients should be referred to the full "Information for Home Dialysis Patients" section attached; it is not a disclosure of all possible effects. Patients should be informed of the signs and symptoms of allergic drug reaction and advised of appropriate actions. If home use is prescribed for a home dialysis patient, the patient should be thoroughly instructed in the importance of proper disposal and cautioned against the reuse of needles, syringes, or drug product. A puncture-resistant container for the disposal of used syringes and needles should be available to the patient. The full container should be disposed of according to the directions provided by the physician.

Renal Function: In patients with CRF not on dialysis, renal function and fluid and electrolyte balance should be closely monitored, as an improved sense of well-being may obscure the need to initiate dialysis in some patients. In patients with CRF not on dialysis, placebo-controlled studies of progression of renal dysfunction over periods of greater than one year have not been completed. In shorter-term trials in patients with CRF not on dialysis, changes in creatinine and creatinine clearance were not significantly different in patients treated with PROCRIT, compared with placebo-treated patients. Analysis of the slope of 1/serum creatinine vs. time plots in these patients indicates no significant change in the slope after the initiation of PROCRIT therapy.

Zidovudine-treated HIV-Infected Patients

Hypertension: Exacerbation of hypertension has not been observed in zidovudine-treated HIV-infected patients treated with PROCRIT. However, PROCRIT should be withheld in these patients if pre-existing hypertension is uncontrolled, and should not be started until blood pressure is controlled. In double-blind studies, a single seizure has been experienced by a patient treated with PROCRIT.[19]

Cancer Patients on Chemotherapy

Hypertension: Hypertension, associated with a significant increase in hematocrit, has been noted rarely in cancer patients treated with PROCRIT. Nevertheless, blood pressure in patients treated with PROCRIT should be monitored carefully, particularly in patients with an underlying history of hypertension or cardiovascular disease.

Seizures: In double-blind, placebo-controlled trials, 3.2% (N=2/63) of patients treated with PROCRIT and 2.9% (N=2/68) of placebo-treated patients had seizures. Seizures in 1.6% (N=1/63) of patients treated with PROCRIT occurred in the context of a significant increase in blood pressure and hematocrit from baseline values. However, both patients treated with PROCRIT also had underlying CNS pathology which may have been related to seizure activity.

Thrombotic Events: In double-blind, placebo-controlled trials, 3.2% (N=2/63) of patients treated with PROCRIT and 11.8% (N=8/68) of placebo-treated patients had thrombotic events (e.g. pulmonary embolism, cerebrovascular accident).

Growth Factor Potential: PROCRIT is a growth factor that primarily stimulates red cell production. However, the possibility that PROCRIT can act as a growth factor for any tumor type, particularly myeloid malignancies, cannot be excluded.

ADVERSE REACTIONS

Chronic Renal Failure Patients
Studies analyzed to date indicate that PROCRIT is generally well-tolerated. The adverse events reported are frequent sequelae of CRF and are not necessarily attributable to PROCRIT therapy. In double-blind, placebo-controlled studies involving over 300 patients with CRF, the events reported in greater than 5% of patients treated with PROCRIT during the blinded phase were:
[See first table above.]
Significant adverse events of concern in patients with CRF treated in double-blinded, placebo-controlled trials occurred in the following percent of patients during the blinded phase of the studies:
[See second table above.]
In the U.S. PROCRIT studies in patients on dialysis (over 567 patients), the incidence (number of events per patient-year) of the most frequently reported adverse events were: hypertension (0.75), headache (0.40), tachycardia (0.31), nausea/vomiting (0.26), clotted vascular access (0.25), shortness of breath (0.14), hyperkalemia (0.11), and diarrhea (0.11). Other

reported events occurred at a rate of less than 0.10 events per patient per year.

Events reported to have occurred within several hours of administration of PROCRIT were rare, mild, and transient, and included injection site stinging in dialysis patients and flu-like symptoms such as arthralgias and myalgias.

In all studies analyzed to date, PROCRIT administration was generally well-tolerated, irrespective of the route of administration.

Hypertension: Increases in blood pressure have been reported in clinical trials, often during the first 90 days of therapy. On occasion, hypertensive encephalopathy and seizures have been observed in patients with CRF treated with PROCRIT. When data from all patients in the U.S. Phase III multicenter trial were analyzed, there was an apparent trend of more reports of hypertensive adverse events in patients on dialysis with a faster rate of rise of hematocrit (greater than 4 hematocrit points in any two-week period). However, in a double-blind, placebo-controlled trial, hypertensive adverse events were not reported at an increased rate in the group treated with PROCRIT (150 Units/kg (T.I.W.) relative to the placebo group.

Seizures: There have been 47 seizures in 1,010 patients on dialysis treated with PROCRIT in clinical trials, with an exposure of 986 patient-years for a rate of approximately 0.048 events per patient-year. However, there appeared to be a higher rate of seizures during the first 90 days of therapy (occurring in approximately 2.5% of patients) when compared to subsequent 90-day periods. The baseline incidence of seizures in the untreated dialysis population is difficult to determine; it appears to be in the range of 5-10% per patient-year.[22-24]

Thrombotic Events: In clinical trials, clotting of the vascular access has occurred at an annualized rate of about 0.25 events per patient-year on PROCRIT therapy. Overall, for patients with CRF (whether on dialysis or not), other thrombotic events (e.g., myocardial infarction, cerebrovascular accident, transient ischemic attack) have occurred at an annualized rate of less than 0.04 events per patient-year of PROCRIT therapy.

In over 125,000 patients treated with commercial PROCRIT, there have been rare reports of serious or unusual thrombo-embolic events including migratory thrombophlebitis, microvascular thrombosis pulmonary embolus, and thrombosis of the retinal artery, and temporal and renal veins. Collectively, these events have been reported in < 0.0001 events per patient-year; in no case has a casual relationship been established.

Allergic Reactions: There have been no reports of serious allergic reactions or anaphylaxis associated with PROCRIT administration during clinical trials. Skin rashes and urticaria have been observed rarely and when reported have generally been mild and transient in nature.

In over 125,000 patients treated with commercial PROCRIT, there have been rare reports of potentially serious allergic reactions including urticaria with associated respiratory symptoms or circumoral edema (< 0.0001 events per patient-year), or urticaria alone (< 0.0001 events per patient-year). Most reactions occurred in situations where a casual relationship could not be established. Many of these patients resumed PROCRIT therapy without recurrence of symptoms, some in conjunction with antihistamine pretreatment. However, symptoms recurred with rechallenge in a few instances, suggesting that allergic reactivity, although rare, may occasionally be associated with PROCRIT therapy. There has been no evidence for development of antibodies to erythropoietin in patients tested to date, including those receiving PROCRIT for over 4 years. Nevertheless, if an anaphylactoid reaction occurs, PROCRIT should be immediately discontinued and appropriate therapy initiated.

Percent of Patients Reporting Event

Event	Patients Treated with PROCRIT (N = 144)	PLACEBO-Treated Patients (N = 153)
Pyrexia	38%	29%
Fatigue	25%	31%
Headache	19%	14%
Cough	18%	14%
Diarrhea	16%	18%
Rash	16%	8%
Congestion, Respiratory	15%	10%
Nausea	15%	12%
Shortness of Breath	14%	13%
Asthenia	11%	14%
Skin Reaction, (Administration Site)	10%	7%
Dizziness	9%	10%

Zidovudine-treated HIV-infected Patients

Adverse events reported in clinical trials with PROCRIT in zidovudine-treated HIV-infected patients were consistent with the progression of HIV infection. In double-blind, placebo-controlled studies of three-months duration involving approximately 300 zidovudine-treated HIV-infected patients, adverse events with an incidence of ≥ 10% in either patients treated with PROCRIT or placebo-treated patients were:

[See table above.]

There were no statistically significant differences between treatment groups in the incidence of the above events.

In the 297 patients studied, PROCRIT was not associated with significant increases in opportunistic infections or mortality.[19] In 71 patients from this group treated with PROCRIT at 150 Units/kg (T.I.W.), serum p24 antigen levels did not appear to increase.[20] Preliminary data showed no enhancement of HIV replication in infected cell lines *in vitro*.[19]

Peripheral white blood cell and platelet counts are unchanged following PROCRIT therapy.

Allergic Reactions: Two zidovudine-treated HIV-infected patients had urticarial reactions within 48 hours of their first exposure to study medication. One patient was treated with PROCRIT and one was treated with placebo (PROCRIT vehicle alone). Both patients had positive immediate skin tests against their study medication with a negative saline control. The basis for this apparent pre-existing hypersensitivity to components of the PROCRIT formulation is unknown, but may be related to HIV-induced immunosuppression or prior exposure to blood products.

Seizures: In double-blind and open label trials of PROCRIT in zidovudine-treated HIV-infected patients, ten patients have experienced seizures.[19] In general, these seizures appear to be related to underlying pathology such as meningitis or cerebral neoplasms, not PROCRIT therapy.

Cancer Patients on Chemotherapy

Adverse experiences reported in clinical trials with PROCRIT in cancer patients were consistent with the underlying disease state. In double-blind, placebo-controlled studies of up to 3-months duration involving 131 cancer patients, adverse events with an incidence > 10% in either patients treated with PROCRIT or placebo-treated patients were as indicated below.

[See table below.]

Although some statistically significant differences between patients treated with PROCRIT and placebo-treated patients were noted, the overall safety profile of PROCRIT appeared to be consistent with the disease process of advanced cancer. During double-blind and subsequent open-label therapy in which patients (N = 72 for total exposure to PROCRIT) were treated for up to 32 weeks with doses as high as 927 Units/kg, the adverse experience profile of PROCRIT was consistent with the progression of advanced cancer.

Based on comparable survival data and on the percentage of patients treated with PROCRIT and placebo-treated patients who discontinued therapy due to death, disease progression or adverse experiences (22% and 13%, respectively; p =0.25), the clinical outcome in patients treated with PROCRIT and placebo-treated patients appeared to be similar. Available data from animal tumor models and measurement of proliferation of solid tumor cells from clinical biopsy specimens in response to PROCRIT suggest that PROCRIT does not potentiate tumor growth. Nevertheless, as a growth factor, the possibility that PROCRIT may potentiate growth of some tumors, particularly myeloid tumors, cannot be excluded. A randomized controlled Phase IV study is currently ongoing to further evaluate this issue.

The mean peripheral white blood cell count was unchanged following PROCRIT therapy compared to the corresponding value in the placebo-treated group.

OVERDOSAGE

The maximum amount of PROCRIT that can be safely administered in single or multiple doses has not been determined. Doses of up to 1,500 Units/kg (T.I.W.) for three to four weeks have been administered without any direct toxic effects of PROCRIT itself.[6] Therapy with PROCRIT can result in polycythemia if the hematocrit is not carefully monitored and the dose appropriately adjusted. If the suggested target range is exceeded, PROCRIT may be temporarily withheld until the hematocrit returns to the suggested target range; PROCRIT therapy may then be resumed using a lower dose (see "Dosage and Administration"). If polycythemia is of concern, phlebotomy may be indicated to decrease the hematocrit.

DOSAGE AND ADMINISTRATION

Chronic Renal Failure Patients

Starting doses of PROCRIT over the range of 50-100 Units/kg three times weekly (T.I.W.) have been shown to be safe and effective in increasing hematocrit and eliminating transfusion dependency in patients with CRF (see "Clinical Experience"). The dose of PROCRIT should be reduced as the hematocrit approaches 36% or increases by more than 4 points in any 2-week period. The dosage of PROCRIT must be individualized to maintain the hematocrit within the suggested target range. At the physician's discretion, the suggested target hematocrit range may be expanded to achieve maximal patient benefit.

PROCRIT may be given either as an intravenous (IV) or subcutaneous (SC) injection. In patients on hemodialysis, PROCRIT usually has been administered as an IV bolus (T.I.W.). While the administration of PROCRIT is independent of the dialysis procedure, PROCRIT may be administered into the venous line at the end of the dialysis procedure to obviate the need for additional venous access. In patients with CRF not on dialysis, PROCRIT may be given either as an IV or SC injection.

Home hemodialysis patients who have been judged competent by their physicians to self-administer PROCRIT without medical or other supervision may give themselves either an IV or SC injection. Home peritoneal dialysis patients who have been judged competent by their physicians to self-administer PROCRIT without medical or other supervision may give themselves a SC injection. The table below provides general therapeutic guidelines for patients with CRF:

[See table at bottom of next page.]

During therapy, hematological parameters should be monitored regularly (see "Laboratory Monitoring").

Percent of Patients Reporting Event

Events	Patients Treated with PROCRIT (N = 63)	PLACEBO-Treated Patients (N = 68)
Pyrexia	29%	19%
Diarrhea	21%[a]	7%
Nausea	17%[b]	32%
Vomiting	17%	15%
Edema	17%[c]	1%
Astheria	13%	16%
Fatigue	13%	15%
Shortness of Breath	13%	9%
Paresthesia	11%	6%
Upper Respiratory Infection	11%	4%
Dizziness	5%	12%
Trunk Pain	3%[d]	16%

[a] p = 0.041
[b] p = 0.069
[c] p = 0.0016
[d] p = 0.017

Continued on next page

Ortho Biotech—Cont.

Pre-Therapy Iron Evaluation: Prior to and during PROCRIT therapy, the patient's iron stores, including transferrin saturation (serum iron divided by iron binding capacity) and serum ferritin, should be evaluated. Transferrin saturation should be at least 20%, and ferritin should be at least 100 ng/mL. Virtually all patients will eventually require supplemental iron to increase or maintain transferrin saturation to levels that will adequately support erythropoiesis stimulated by PROCRIT.

Dose Adjustment: Following PROCRIT therapy, a period of time is required for erythroid progenitors to mature and be released into circulation resulting in an eventual increase in hematocrit. Additionally, red blood cell survival time affects hematocrit and may vary due to uremia. As a result, the time required to elicit a clinically significant change in hematocrit (increase or decrease) following any dose adjustment may be 2–6 weeks.

Dose adjustment should not be made more frequently than once a month, unless clinically indicated. After any dose adjustment, the hematocrit should be determined twice weekly for at least 2–6 weeks (see "Laboratory Monitoring").

- If the hematocrit is increasing and approaching 36%, the dose should be reduced to maintain the suggested target hematocrit range. If the reduced dose does not stop the rise in hematocrit, and it exceeds 36%, doses should be temporarily withheld until the hematocrit begins to decrease, at which point therapy should be reinitiated at a lower dose.
- At any time, if the hematocrit increases by more than 4 points in a 2-week period, the dose should be immediately decreased. After the dose reduction, the hematocrit should be monitored twice weekly for 2–6 weeks, and further dose adjustments should be made as outlined in "Maintenance Dose."
- If a hematocrit increase of 5–6 points is not achieved after an 8-week period and iron stores are adequate (see "Delayed or Diminished Response"), the dose of PROCRIT may be incrementally increased. Further increases may be made at 4–6 week intervals until the desired response is attained.

Maintenance Dose: The maintenance dose must be individualized for each patient on dialysis. In the U.S. Phase III multicenter trial in patients on hemodialysis, the median maintenance dose was 75 Units/kg (T.I.W.), with a range from 12.5 to 525 Units/kg (T.I.W.). Almost 10% of the patients required a dose of 25 Units/kg, or less, and approximately 10% of the patients required more than 200 Units/kg (T.I.W.) to maintain their hematocrit in the suggested target range.

If the hematocrit remains below, or falls below, the suggested target range, iron stores should be re-evaluated. If the transferrin saturation is less than 20%, supplemental iron should be administered. If the transferrin saturation is greater than 20%, the dose of PROCRIT may be increased. Such dose increases should not be made more frequently than once a month, unless clinically indicated, as the response time of the hematocrit to a dose increase can be 2–6 weeks. Hematocrit should be measured twice weekly for 2–6 weeks following dose increases. In patients with CRF not on dialysis, the maintenance dose must also be individualized. PROCRIT doses of 75–150 Units/kg per week have been shown to maintain hematocrits of 36–38% for up to 6 months.

Delayed or Diminished Response: Over 95% of patients with CRF responded with clinically significant increases in hematocrit, and virtually all patients were transfusion-independent within approximately two months of initiation of PROCRIT therapy.

If a patient fails to respond or maintain a response, other etiologies should be considered and evaluated as clinically indicated. See "PRECAUTIONS" section for discussion of delayed or diminished response.

Zidovudine-treated HIV-Infected Patients

Prior to beginning PROCRIT, it is recommended that the endogenous serum erythropoietin level be determined (prior to transfusion). Available evidence suggests that patients receiving zidovudine with endogenous serum erythropoietin levels > 500 mUnits/mL are unlikely to respond to therapy with PROCRIT.

Starting Dose: For patients with serum erythropoietin levels ≤ 500 mUnits/mL who are receiving a dose of zidovudine ≤ 4,200 mg/week, the recommended starting dose of PROCRIT is 100 Units/kg as an intravenous or subcutaneous injection three times weekly (T.I.W.) for 8 weeks.

Increase Dose: During the dose adjustment phase of therapy, the hematocrit should be monitored weekly. If the response is not satisfactory in terms of reducing transfusion requirements or increasing hematocrit after 8 weeks of therapy, the dose of PROCRIT can be increased by 50–100 Units/kg (T.I.W.). Response should be evaluated every 4–8 weeks thereafter and the dose adjusted accordingly by 50–100 Units/kg increments (T.I.W.). If patients have not responded satisfactorily to a PROCRIT dose of 300 Units/kg (T.I.W.), it is unlikely that they will respond to higher doses of PROCRIT.

Maintenance Dose: After attainment of the desired response (i.e., reduced transfusion requirements or increased hematocrit), the dose of PROCRIT should be titrated to maintain the response based on factors such as variations in zidovudine dose and the presence of intercurrent infectious or inflammatory episodes. If the hematocrit exceeds 40%, the dose should be discontinued until the hematocrit drops to 36%. The dose should be reduced by 25% when treatment is resumed and then titrated to maintain the desired hematocrit.

Cancer Patients on Chemotherapy

Baseline endogenous serum erythropoietin levels varied among patients in these trials with approximately 75% (N=83/110) having endogenous serum erythropoietin levels <132 mUnits/mL, and approximately 4% (N=4/110) of patients having endogenous serum erythropoietin levels >500 mUnits/mL. In general, patients with lower baseline serum erythropoietin levels responded more vigorously to PROCRIT than patients with higher erythropoietin levels. Although no specific serum erythropoietin level can be stipulated above which patients would be unlikely to respond to PROCRIT therapy, treatment of patients with grossly elevated serum erythropoietin levels (e.g., > 200 mUnits/mL) is not recommended. The hematocrit should be monitored on a weekly basis in patients receiving PROCRIT therapy until hematocrit becomes stable.

Starting Dose: The recommended starting dose of PROCRIT is 150 Units/kg subcutaneously (T.I.W.).

Dose Adjustment: If the response is not satisfactory in terms of reducing transfusion requirements or increasing hematocrit after 8 weeks of therapy, the dose of PROCRIT can be increased up to 300 Units/kg (T.I.W.). If patients have not responded satisfactorily to a PROCRIT dose of 300 Units/kg (T.I.W.), it is unlikely that they will respond to higher doses of PROCRIT. If the hematocrit exceeds 40%, the dose of PROCRIT should be withheld until the hematocrit falls to 36%. The dose of PROCRIT should be reduced by 25% when treatment is resumed and titrated to maintain the desired hematocrit. If the initial dose of PROCRIT includes a very rapid hematocrit response (e.g., an increase of more than 4 percentage points in any 2-week period), the dose of PROCRIT should be reduced.

PREPARATION AND ADMINISTRATION OF PROCRIT

1. DO NOT SHAKE. It is not necessary to shake PROCRIT. Prolonged vigorous shaking may denature any glycoprotein, rendering it biologically inactive.
2. Parenteral drug products should be inspected visually for particulate matter and discoloration prior to administration. Do not use any vials exhibiting particulate matter or discoloration.
3. Using aseptic techniques, attach a sterile needle to a sterile syringe. Remove the flip top from the vial containing PROCRIT, and wipe the septum with a disinfectant. Insert the needle into the vial, and withdraw into the syringe an appropriate volume of solution.
4. **Single-dose** 1 mL vial contains no preservative. Use one dose per vial; do not re-enter vial. Discard unused portions. **Multidose** 2 mL vial contains preservative. Store at 2 to 8°C after initial entry and between doses. Discard 21 days after initial entry.
5. Do not dilute or administer in conjunction with other drug solutions. However, at the time of subcutaneous administration, PROCRIT may be admixed in a syringe with bacteriostatic 0.9% sodium chloride injection, USP, with benzyl alcohol 0.9% (bacteriostatic saline) at a 1:1 ratio using aseptic technique. The benzyl alcohol in the bacteriostatic saline acts as a local anesthetic which may ameliorate subcutaneous injection site discomfort.

Starting Dose	Reduce Dose When	Increase Dose If	Maintenance Dose	Suggested Target Hct. Range
50–100 Units/kg T.I.W.; IV or SC	1) Hct. approaches 36%, or 2) Hct. increases >4 points in any 2-week period	Hct. does not increase by 5–6 points after 8 weeks of therapy, and hct. is below suggested target range	Individually titrate	30–36%

HOW SUPPLIED

PROCRIT, containing Epoetin alfa, is available in vials containing color coded labels.

1 mL **Single-Dose, Preservative-Free** Solution

Each dosage form is supplied in the following packages:

Cartons containing six (6) **single-dose** vials:
- 2,000 Units/mL (NDC 59676-302-01) (Purple)
- 3,000 Units/mL (NDC 59676-303-01) (Magenta)
- 4,000 Units/mL (NDC 59676-304-01) (Green)
- 10,000 Units/mL (NDC 59676-310-01) (Red)

Trays containing twenty-five (25) **single-dose** vials:
- 2,000 Units/mL (NDC 59676-302-02) (Purple)
- 3,000 Units/mL (NDC 59676-303-02) (Magenta)
- 4,000 Units/mL (NDC 59676-304-02) (Green)
- 10,000 Units/mL (NDC 59676-310-02) (Red)

2 mL **Multidose, Preserved** Solution

Cartons containing six (6) **multidose** vials:
- 10,000 Units/mL (NDC 59676-312-01) (Blue)

STORAGE

Store at 2° to 8° C (36° to 46° F). Do not freeze or shake.

REFERENCES

1. Egrie JC, Strickland TW, Lane J, et al., (1986). "Characterization and Biological Effects of Recombinant Human Erythropoietin."*Immunobiol.* 72:213-224.
2. Graber SE and Krantz SB, (1978). "Erythropoietin and the Control of Red Cell Production."*Ann. Rev. Med.* 29:51-66.
3. Eschbach JW and Adamson JW, (1985). "Anemia of End-Stage Renal Disease (ESRD)."*Kidney Intl.* 28:1-5.
4. Eschbach JW, Egrie JC, Downing MR, Browne JK, and Adamson JW, (1987). "Correction of the Anemia of End-Stage Renal Disease with Recombinant Human Erythropoietin."*NEJM* 316:73-78.
5. Eschbach JW, Abdulhadi MH, Browne JK, et al., (1989). "Recombinant Human Erythropoietin in Anemic Patients with End-Stage Renal Disease."*Ann. Intern. Med.* 111:12.
6. Eschbach JW, Egrie JC, Downing MR, Browne JK, Adamson JW, (1989). "The Use of Recombinant Human Erythropoietin (r-HuEPO): Effect in End-Stage Renal Disease (ESRD),"*Prevention Of Chronic Uremia,* (Friedman, Beyer, DeSanto, Giordano, eds.), Field and Wood Inc., Philadelphia, PA, pp 148-155.
7. Egrie JC, Eschbach JW, McGuire T, and Adamson JW, (1988). "Pharmacokinetics of Recombinant Human Erythropoietin (r-HuEPO) Administered to Hemodialysis (HD) Patients."*Kidney Intl.* 33:262.
8. Evans RW, Radar B, Manninen DL, et al., (1990). "The Quality of Life of Hemodialysis Recipients Treated with Recombinant Human Erythropoietin."*JAMA* 263:6.
9. Paganini E, Garcia J, Ellis P, Bodnar D, and Magnussen M, (1988). "Clinical Sequelae of Correction of Anemia with Recombinant Human Erythropoietin (r-HuEPO); Urea Kinetics, Dialyzer Function and Reuse."*Am. J. Kid. Dis.* 11:16.
10. Delano BG, Lundin AP, Golansky R, Quinn RM, Rao TKS, and Friedman EA, (1988). "Dialyzer Urea and Creatinine Clearances Not Significantly Changed in r-HuEPO Treated Maintenance Hemodialysis (MD) Patients."*Kidney Intl.* 33:219.
11. Stivelman J, Van Wyck D, and Ogden D, (1988). "Use of Recombinant Erythropoietin (r-HuEPO) with High Flux Dialysis (HFD) Does Not Worsen Azotemia or Shorten Access Survival."*Kidney Intl.* 33:239.
12. Lim VS, DeGowin RL, Zavala D, Kirchner PT, Abels R, Perry P, and Fangman J, (1989). "Recombinant Human Erythropoietin Treatment in Pre-Dialysis Patients: A Double-Blind Placebo-Controlled Trial."*Ann. Int. Med.* 110:108-114.
13. Stone WJ, Graber SE, Krantz SB, et al., (1988). "Treatment of the Anemia of Pre-Dialysis Patients with Recombinant Human Erythropoietin: A Randomized, Placebo-Controlled Trial."*Am. J. Med. Sci.* 296:171-179.
14. Lundin AP, Akerman MJH, Chesler RM, Delano BG, Goldberg N, Stein RA, and Friedman EA, (1991). "Exercise in Hemodialysis Patients after Treatment with Recombinant Human Erythropoietin"*Nephron,*. 58:315-319.
15. Data on file, Amgen Inc.
16. Eschbach JW, Kelly MR, Galey NR, Abels RI and Adamson JU (1989). "Treatment of the Anemia of Progressive Renal Failure with Recombinant Human Erythropoietin,-'*NEJM* 321:158-163.
17. The US Recombinant Human Erythropoietin Predialysis Study Group (1991). "Double-Blind, Placebo-Controlled Study of the Therapeutic Use of Recombinant Human Eryth-

ropoietin for Anemia Associated with Chronic Renal Failure in Predialysis Patients,"*Am. J. Kid. Dis.* 18(1):50-59.

18. Danna RP, Rudnick SA, Abels RI, (1990). "Erythropoietin Therapy for the Anemia Associated with AIDS and AIDS Therapy and Cancer."*Erythropoietin in Clinical Applications—An International Perspective,* (MB Garnick, ed.), Marcel Dekker, New York, NY, pp. 301-324.

19. Data on file, Ortho Biologics, Inc.

20. Fischl M, Galpin JE, Levine JD, et al., (1990). "Recombinant Human Erythropoietin for Patients with AIDS Treated with Zidovudine."*NEJM* 322:1488-1493.

21. Kerr DN, (1979). "Chronic Renal Failure,"*Cecil Textbook of Medicine,* (Beeson PB, McDermott W, Wyngaarden JB, eds.), W.B. Saunders, Philadelphia, PA, pp 1351-1367.

22. Raskin NH and Fishman RA, (1976). "Neurologic Disorders in Renal Failure (First of Two Parts)."*NEJM* 294:143-148.

23. Raskin NH and Fishman RA, (1976). "Neurologic Disorder in Renal Failure (Second of Two Parts)."*NEJM* 294:204-210.

24. Messing RO and Simon RP, (1986). "Seizures as a Manifestation of Systemic Disease."*Neurologic Clinics* 4: 563-584.

Manufactured by:
Amgen Inc.
U.S. Lic. # 1080
Thousand Oaks, California 91320-1789
Distributed by:
Ortho Biotech Inc.
Raritan, New Jersey 08869-0670
©OBI 1990   Revised May 1995
Printed in U.S.A.

PROCRIT®   ℞
EPOETIN ALFA

INFORMATION FOR HOME DIALYSIS PATIENTS
PROCRIT and Chronic Renal Failure

PROCRIT (Epoetin alfa) has been prescribed for you by your doctor because you:
1) Have anemia due to your kidney disease.
2) Are able to dialyze at home.
3) Have been determined to be able to administer PROCRIT without direct medical or other supervision.

A lack of energy or feeling of tiredness is the major symptom of anemia. Additional symptoms include shortness of breath, chest pain, and feeling cold all the time. The reason for these symptoms is that there is a lack of red blood cells. Red blood cells carry oxygen, which is important for all of the body's functions. When there are fewer red blood cells, the body does not get all the oxygen it needs.

Kidneys remove toxins from the blood; they also measure the amount of oxygen in the blood. If there is not enough oxygen, the kidneys will produce a hormone called erythropoietin. Erythropoietin is released into the bloodstream and travels to the bone marrow where red blood cells are made. Erythropoietin signals the bone marrow to make more oxygen-carrying red blood cells.

As the kidneys fail, they stop cleansing toxins from your body. They also make less erythropoietin than they should. Therefore, the bone marrow does not receive a strong-enough signal to make the oxygen-carrying red blood cells. Fewer red blood cells are produced so the muscles, brain, and other parts of the body do not get the oxygen they need to function properly.

PROCRIT is a copy of human erythropoietin. PROCRIT replaces the erythropoietin that the failed kidneys can no longer produce, and signals the bone marrow to make the oxygen-carrying red blood cells once again.

The effectiveness of PROCRIT is measured by the increase in hematocrit (the amount of red blood cells in the blood) that results from PROCRIT therapy. The rise in hematocrit is not immediate. It usually takes about two to six weeks before the hematocrit starts to rise. The amount of time it takes, and the dose of PROCRIT that is needed to make the hematocrit increase, varies from patient to patient.

Most patients treated with PROCRIT no longer need blood transfusions. However, certain medical conditions, or unexpected blood loss, may result in the need for a transfusion. In those situations where your doctor has determined that you, as a home dialysis patient, can self-administer PROCRIT, you will receive instruction on how much PROCRIT to use, how to inject it, how often you should inject it, and how you should dispose of the unused portions of each vial.

You will be instructed to monitor your blood pressure carefully every day and to report any changes outside of the guidelines that your doctor has given you. When the number of red blood cells increases, your blood pressure can also increase, so your doctor may prescribe some new or additional blood pressure medication. Be sure to follow your doctor's orders. You may also be instructed to have certain laboratory tests, such as additional hematocrit or iron level measurements, done more frequently. You may be asked to report these tests to your doctor or dialysis center. Also, your doctor may prescribe additional iron for you to take. Be sure to comply with your doctor's orders.

Continue to check your access, as your doctor or nurse has shown you, to make sure it is working. Be sure to let your health care professional know right away if there is a problem.

When you receive your PROCRIT from the dialysis center, doctor's office or home dialysis supplier, always check to see that:
1) The name PROCRIT appears on the carton and bottle label.
2) You will be able to use PROCRIT before the expiration date stamped on the package.

PROCRIT
PROCRIT is produced in mammalian cells that have been genetically altered by the addition of a gene for the natural substance erythropoietin.

The PROCRIT solution in the vial should always be clear and colorless. Do not use PROCRIT if the contents of the vial appear discolored or cloudy, or if the vial appears to contain lumps, flakes, or particles. In addition, if the vial has been shaken vigorously, the solution may appear to be frothy and should not be used. Therefore, care should be taken not to shake the PROCRIT vial vigorously before use.

Single-dose vial: 2000, 3000, 4000 and 10,000 Unit vials of PROCRIT are for single use only. Any unused portions of these vials should be discarded.

Multi-dose Vial: Vials of PROCRIT marked with a blue "M"on the label (10,000 Units/mL- 20,000 Units in a vial) contain a preserved solution and may be entered multiple times. Multidose vials should be stored in the refrigerator between uses and thrown away 21 days after the first use. Carefully follow the instructions for "Preparing the Dose" each time you enter the multidose vial.
Follow your dialysis center's instructions on what to do with the used vials.
Storage:
PROCRIT should be stored in the refrigerator, but not in the freezing compartment. Do not let the vial freeze and do not leave it in direct sunlight. Do not use a vial of PROCRIT that has been frozen or after the expiration date that is stamped on the label. If you have any questions about the safety of a vial of PROCRIT that has been subjected to temperature extremes, be sure to check with your dialysis unit staff.

USE THE CORRECT SYRINGE
Your doctor has instructed you on how to give yourself the correct dosage of PROCRIT. This dosage will usually be measured in units per milliliter or ccs. It is important to use a syringe that is marked in tenths of milliliters (for example, 0.1, 0.2, etc.) mL or cc). Failure to use the proper syringe can lead to a mistake in dosage, and you may receive too much or too little PROCRIT. Too little PROCRIT may not be effective in increasing your hematocrit, and too much PROCRIT may lead to a hematocrit that is too high. Only use disposable syringes and needles as they do not require sterilization; they should be used once and disposed of as instructed by your doctor.

IMPORTANT: TO HELP AVOID CONTAMINATION AND POSSIBLE INFECTION, FOLLOW THESE INSTRUCTIONS EXACTLY.

PREPARING THE DOSE:

1. Wash your hands thoroughly with soap and water before preparing the medication.

2. Check the date on the PROCRIT vial to be sure that the drug has not expired.

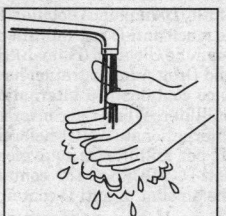

3. Remove the vial of PROCRIT from the refrigerator and allow it to reach room temperature. It is not necessary to shake PROCRIT. Prolonged vigorous shaking may damage the product. Assemble the other supplies you will need for your injection.

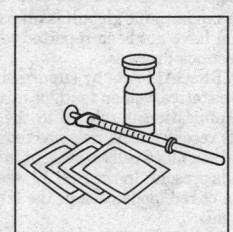

4. Hemodialysis patients should wipe off the venous port of the hemodialysis tubing with an antiseptic swab. Peritoneal dialysis patients should cleanse the skin with an antiseptic swab where the injection is to be made.

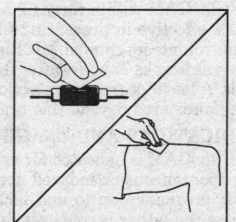

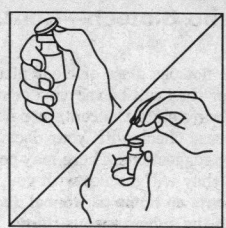

5. Flip off the red protective cap but do not remove the gray rubber stopper. Wipe the top of the gray rubber stopper with an antiseptic swab.

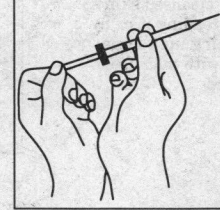

6. Using a syringe and needle designed for subcutaneous injection, draw air into the syringe by pulling back on the plunger. The amount of air should be equal to your PROCRIT dose.

7. Carefully remove the needle cover. Put the needle through the gray rubber stopper of the PROCRIT vial.

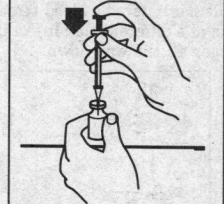

8. Push the plunger into discharge air into the vial. The air injected into the vial will allow PROCRIT to be easily withdrawn into the syringe.

9. Turn the vial and syringe upside down in one hand. Be sure the tip of the needle is in the PROCRIT solution. Your other hand will be free to move the plunger. Draw back on the plunger slowly to draw the correct dose of PROCRIT into the syringe.

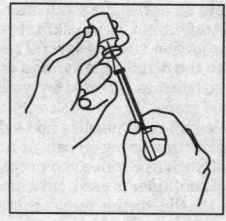

10. Check for air bubbles. The air is harmless, but too large an air bubble will reduce the PROCRIT dose. To remove air bubbles, gently tap the syringe to move the air bubbles to the top of the syringe, then use the plunger to push the solution and the air back into the vial. Then re-measure your correct dose of PROCRIT.

11. Double check your dose. Remove the needle from the vial. Do not lay the syringe down or allow the needle to touch anything.

INJECTING THE DOSE
Patients on home hemodialysis using the intravenous injection route:

1. Insert the needle of the syringe into the previously cleansed venous port and inject the PROCRIT.

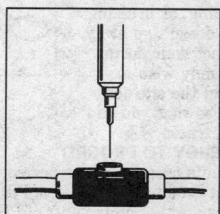

2. Remove the syringe and dispose of the whole unit. **Use the disposable syringe only once.** Dispose of syringes and needles as directed by your doctor, by following these simple steps:
—Place all used needles and syringes in a hard plastic container with a screw-on-cap, or a metal container with a plastic lid, such as a coffee can properly labeled as to content. If a metal container is used, cut a small hole in the plastic lid and tape the lid to the metal container. If a hard-plastic container is used, always screw the cap on tightly after each use. When the container is full, tape around the cap or lid, and dispose of according to your doctor's instructions.

Continued on next page

Ortho Biotech—Cont.

—Do not use glass or clear plastic containers, or any container that will be recycled or returned to a store.
—Always store the container out of the reach of children.
—Please check with your doctor, nurse, or pharmacist for other suggestions. There may be special state and local laws that they will discuss with you.

Patients on home peritoneal dialysis or home hemodialysis using the subcutaneous route:

1. With one hand, stabilize the previously cleansed skin by spreading it or by pinching up a large area with your free hand.

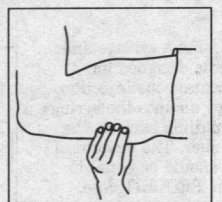

2. Hold the syringe with the other hand, as you would a pencil. Double check that the correct amount of PROCRIT is in the syringe. Insert the needle straight into the skin (90 degree angle). Pull the plunger back slightly. If blood comes into the syringe, do not inject PROCRIT, as the needle has entered a blood vessel; withdraw the syringe and inject at a different site. Inject the PROCRIT by pushing the plunger all the way down.

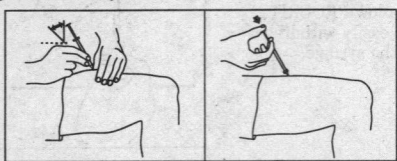

3. Hold an antiseptic swab near the needle and pull the needle straight out of the skin. Press the antiseptic swab over the injection site for several seconds.
4. Use the disposable syringe only once. Dispose of syringes and needles as directed by your doctor, by following these simple steps:
—Place all used needles and syringes in a hard plastic container with a screw-on-cap, or a metal container with a plastic lid, such as a coffee can properly labeled as to content. If a metal container is used, cut a small hole in the plastic lid and tape the lid to the metal container. If a hard-plastic container isused, always screw the cap on tightly after each use. When the container is full, tape around the cap or lid, and dispose ofaccording to your doctor's instructions.
—Do not use glass or clear plastic containers, or any container that will be recycled or returned to a store.
—Always store the container out of the reach of children.
—Please check with your doctor, nurse, or pharmacist for other suggestions. There may be special state and local laws that they will discuss with you.

5. Always change the site for each injection as directed. Occasionally a problem may develop at the injection site. If you notice a lump, swelling, or bruising that doesn't go away, contact your doctor. You may wish to record the site just used so that you can keep track.

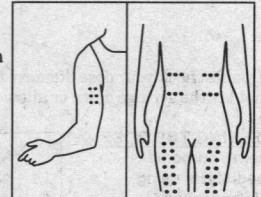

ALLERGY TO PROCRIT

Patients occasionally experience redness, swelling, or itching at the site of injection of PROCRIT. This may indicate an allergy to the components of PROCRIT, or it may indicate a local reaction. If you have a local reaction, consult your doctor. A potentially more serious reaction would be a generalized allergy to PROCRIT which could cause a rash over the whole body, shortness of breath, wheezing, reduction in blood pressure, fast pulse, or sweating.
Severe cases of generalized allergy may be life-threatening. If you think you are having a generalized allergic reaction, stop taking PROCRIT and notify a physician or emergency medical personnel immediately.

IMPORTANT NOTES

Since you are a home dialysis patient and your doctor allows you to self-administer PROCRIT, please note the following:
1. Always follow the instructions of your doctor concerning the dosage and administration of PROCRIT. Do not change the dose or instructions for administration of PROCRIT without consulting your doctor.

2. Your doctor will tell you what to do if you miss a dose of PROCRIT. Always keep a spare syringe and needle on hand.
3. Always consult your doctor if you notice anything unusual about your condition or your use of PROCRIT.

USAGE IN PREGNANCY

If you are pregnant or nursing a baby, consult your physician before using PROCRIT.
Manufactured by:
Amgen Inc.
U. S. LIC. # 1080
Thousand Oaks, California 91320-1789
Distributed by:
Ortho Biotech Inc.
Raritan, New Jersey 08869-0670
©OBI 1994   Revised May 1995
Printed in U.S.A
Shown in Product Identification Guide, page 326

Ortho Diagnostic Systems Inc.
A Johnson & Johnson Company
1001 U.S. HWY 202
RARITAN, NEW JERSEY 08869-0606

Direct Inquiries to:
Customer Service
(800) 322-6374 (ODSI)

MICRhoGAM™   ℞
[*mike 'ro-gam*]
Rh₀ (D) Immune Globulin (Human)
For Intramuscular Injection Only

Micro-Dose for use *only* after spontaneous or induced abortion or termination of ectopic pregnancy up to and including 12 weeks' gestation.

DESCRIPTION

MICRhoGAM Rh₀(D) Immune Globulin (Human) is a sterile solution containing IgG anti-Rh₀(D) for use in preventing Rh immunization in Rh negative individuals exposed to Rh positive red blood cells. A single dose of MICRhoGAM contains sufficient anti-Rh₀(D) (approximately 50 μg)† to suppress the immune response to 2.5 mL (or less) of Rh positive red blood cells.
All donors are carefully screened to eliminate those in high risk groups for disease transmission. Fractionation of the plasma is done by a modification of the cold alcohol procedure. Glycine (15 mg/mL) is included in the final product as a stabilizer. The final product contains 5% ± 1% globulin, 2.9 mg/mL sodium chloride, 0.01% polysorbate 80 and 0.003% thimerosal (mercury derivative).
This product is for intramuscular injection only.
† A full dose of Rh₀(D) Immune Globulin (Human) has traditionally been referred to as a "300 μg" dose and this usage is employed here for convenience in terminology. *It should not be construed as the actual anti-D content.* Each full dose of Rh₀(D) Immune Globulin (Human) must contain at least as much anti-D as 1 milliliter of the U.S. Reference Rh₀(D) Immune Globulin (Human). Studies performed at the Food and Drug Administration have shown that the U.S. Reference contains 820 international units (IU) of anti-D per milliliter. When the conversion factor determined for the International (WHO) Reference Preparation is used, 820 IU per milliliter is equivalent to 164 μg per milliliter of anti-D. MICRhoGAM contains approximately one-sixth the amount of anti-D contained in the full dose.

CLINICAL PHARMACOLOGY

Human immune globulins prepared by cold alcohol fractionation have not been reported to transmit hepatitis or other infectious diseases.
MICRhoGAM acts by suppressing the immune response of Rh negative women to Rh positive red blood cells. The risk of immunization is related to the number of Rh positive red cells received. The risk was found to be 3% when 0.1 mL of fetal red blood cells is present in the mother and 65% when 5 mL is present. In the first 12 weeks of gestation the total volume of red blood cells in the fetus is estimated at less than 2.5 mL.
Clinical studies demonstrated that administration of MICRhoGAM within three (3) hours following abortion was 100% effective in preventing Rh immunization. Studies in male volunteers showed MICRhoGAM to be effective when given as long as 72 hours after the infusion of Rh positive red cells. A lesser degree of protection is afforded if the antibody is administered beyond this time period.

INDICATIONS AND USAGE

MICRhoGAM is indicated for an Rh negative woman following spontaneous or induced abortion or termination of ectopic pregnancy up to and including 12 weeks' gestation, unless the father is conclusively shown to be Rh negative.

CONTRAINDICATIONS

MICRhoGAM must not be used for genetic amniocentesis at 15 to 18 weeks' gestation or antepartum prophylaxis at 28 weeks' gestation. RhoGAM™ Rh₀(D) Immune Globulin (Human) is recommended for any indication beyond 12 weeks' gestation.
Individuals known to have had an anaphylactic or severe systemic reaction to human globulin should not receive MICRhoGAM or any other Rh₀(D) Immune Globulin (Human).

WARNINGS

Do not inject intravenously.

PRECAUTIONS

Pregnancy Category C—Animal reproduction studies have not been conducted with MICRhoGAM. It is also not known whether Rh₀(D) Immune Globulin (Human) can cause fetal harm when administered to a pregnant woman or can affect reproduction capacity. Rh₀(D) Immune Globulin (Human) should be given to a pregnant woman only if clearly needed.

ADVERSE REACTIONS

Systemic reactions associated with administration of MICRhoGAM are extremely rare. Discomfort at the site of injection has been reported and a small number of women have noted a slight elevation in temperature.

DOSAGE AND ADMINISTRATION

Parenteral drug products should be inspected visually for particulate matter and discoloration prior to administration, whenever solution and container permit.
A single dose (approximately 50 μg) of MICRhoGAM will completely suppress the immune response to 2.5 mL of Rh positive red blood cells (packed cells, not whole blood).
Administer a single dose of MICRhoGAM intramuscularly as soon as possible after termination of a pregnancy up to and including 12 weeks' gestation. At or beyond 13 weeks' gestation it is recommended that a single dose of RhoGAM Rh₀(D) Immune Globulin (Human) (approximately 300 μg)† be given instead of MICRhoGAM.
Since there is no lot number and expiration date on the prefilled syringes, they should not be removed from the protective pouch until immediately before use.
† See footnote under Description.

HOW SUPPLIED

—5 prefilled single-dose syringes of MICRhoGAM (Product code 780800) NDC 0562-8080-80
—package insert
—5 control forms
—5 patient identification cards
            and
—25 prefilled single-dose syringes of MICRhoGAM (Product code 780820) NDC 0562-8080-82
—package insert
—25 control forms
—25 patient identification cards

STORAGE

Store at 2 to 8°C. DO NOT FREEZE.

RhoGAM™   ℞
[*ro 'gam*]
Rh₀ (D) Immune Globulin (Human)
For Intramuscular Injection Only

DESCRIPTION

RhoGAM Rh₀(D) Immune Globulin (Human) is a sterile solution containing IgG anti-Rh₀(D) for use in preventing Rh immunization. Each single dose of RhoGAM contains sufficient anti-Rh₀(D) (approximately 300 μg)† to suppress the immune response to 15 mL (or less) of Rh positive red blood cells.
All donors are carefully screened to eliminate those in high risk groups for disease transmission. Fractionation of the plasma is done by a modification of the cold alcohol procedure. The final product contains 5% ± 1% globulin, 2.9 mg/mL sodium chloride, 0.01% polysorbate 80 and 0.003% thimerosal (mercury derivative), with glycine (15 mg/mL) as a stabilizer.
This product is for intramuscular injection only.
† A full dose of Rh₀(D) Immune Globulin (Human) has traditionally been referred to as a "300 μg" dose and this usage is employed here for convenience in terminology. *It should not be construed as the actual anti-D content.* Each full dose of Rh₀(D) Immune Globulin (Human) must contain at least as much anti-D as 1 milliliter of the U.S. Reference Rh₀(D) Immune Globulin (Human). Studies performed at the Food and Drug Administration have shown that the U.S. Reference contains 820 international units (IU) of anti-D per milliliter. When the conversion factor determined for the International (WHO) Reference Preparation is used, 820 IU per milliliter is equivalent to 164 μg per milliliter of anti-D.

CLINICAL PHARMACOLOGY

Human immune globulins prepared by cold alcohol fractionation have not been reported to transmit hepatitis or other infectious diseases.

RhoGAM acts by suppressing the immune response of Rh negative individuals to Rh positive red blood cells.

The obstetrical patient may be exposed to red blood cells from her Rh positive fetus during the normal course of pregnancy. Clinical studies proved that the incidence of Rh immunization as a result of pregnancy was reduced to 1% to 2% from 12% to 13% when RhoGAM was given within 72 hours following delivery. Further studies in which patients received Rh immune globulin, antepartum at 28 to 32 weeks and postpartum, reduced the risk of immunization to less than 0.1%.

An Rh negative individual transfused with one unit of Rh positive red blood cells has about an 80% likelihood of producing anti-Rh$_o$(D). Protection from Rh immunization is accomplished by administering the appropriate dose of RhoGAM.

INDICATIONS AND USAGE

Pregnancy and Other Obstetric Conditions
RhoGAM is indicated whenever it is known or suspected that fetal red cells have entered the circulation of an Rh negative mother unless the fetus or the father can be shown conclusively to be Rh negative.

Transfusion
RhoGAM is indicated for any Rh negative female of childbearing age who receives any Rh positive red blood cells or component such as platelets or granulocytes prepared from Rh positive blood.

CONTRAINDICATIONS

Individuals known to have had an anaphylactic or severe systemic reaction to human globulin should not receive RhoGAM or any other Rh$_o$(D) Immune Globulin (Human).

WARNINGS

Do not inject intravenously.
Do not inject infant.

PRECAUTIONS

The presence of passively acquired anti-Rh$_o$(D) in the maternal serum may cause a positive antibody screening test. This does not preclude further antepartum or postpartum prophylaxis.

Some babies born of women given Rh$_o$(D) Immune Globulin (Human) antepartum have weakly positive direct antiglobulin tests at birth.

Late in pregnancy or following delivery there may be sufficient fetal red blood cells in the maternal circulation to cause a positive result if one tests for the Rh$_o$(D) variant known as D^u. When there is any doubt as to the patient's Rh type, RhoGAM should be administered.

Pregnancy Category C
Animal reproduction studies have not been conducted with RhoGAM. It is also not known whether Rh$_o$(D) Immune Globulin (Human) can cause fetal harm when administered to a pregnant woman or can affect reproduction capacity. Rh$_o$(D) Immune Globulin (Human) should be given to a pregnant woman only if clearly needed. However, use of Rh antibody during the third trimester in full doses of antibody has been reported to produce no evidence of hemolysis in the infant.

ADVERSE REACTIONS

Systemic reactions associated with administration of RhoGAM are extremely rare. Discomfort at the site of injection has been reported and a small number of women have noted a slight elevation in temperature.

About one-quarter of a group of 22 individuals who were given multiple doses of RhoGAM to treat mismatched transfusions noted fever, myalgia and lethargy. Bilirubin levels of 0.4 to 6.8 mg/dL were observed in some of the treated individuals and one had splenomegaly.

DOSAGE AND ADMINISTRATION

Parenteral drug products should be inspected visually for particulate matter and discoloration prior to administration, whenever solution and container permit.

A single dose (approximately 300 μg)† is contained in each prefilled syringe of RhoGAM. This is the usual dose for the indications associated with pregnancy unless there is clinical or laboratory evidence of a fetal-maternal hemorrhage in excess of 15 mL of Rh positive red blood cells. The indications and recommended dosage for RhoGAM are summarized in the following table.

Indications and Recommended Dosage

Indication	Dose (approximately)
Threatened abortion at any stage of gestation with continuation of pregnancy	300 μg†
Abortion or termination of pregnancy at or beyond 13 weeks' gestation**	300 μg
Genetic amniocentesis, chorionic villus sampling (CVS) and percutaneous umbilical blood sampling (PUBS)	300 μg
Abdominal trauma	300 μg
Antepartum prophylaxis at 26 to 28 weeks' gestation††	300 μg
Postpartum (if newborn Rh positive)	300 μg

†See footnote under Description
**If abortion or termination of pregnancy occurs up to and including 12 weeks' gestation, a single dose of MICRhoGAM™ Rh$_o$(D) Immune Globulin (Human) (approximately 50 μg)† may be used instead of RhoGAM.
††If antepartum prophylaxis is indicated, it is essential that the mother receive a postpartum dose if the infant is Rh positive.

If an adverse event requires the administration of RhoGAM early in the pregnancy, there is an obligation to maintain a level of passively acquired anti-Rh$_o$(D) by administration of RhoGAM at 12-week intervals. RhoGAM should be given within 72 hours after delivery if the baby is Rh positive. If delivery occurs within three weeks after the last antepartum dose, the postpartum dose may be withheld, but a test for fetal-maternal hemorrhage (FMH) should still be performed to determine a bleed greater than 15 mL of packed red blood cells.

Whenever there is a fetal-maternal hemorrhage in excess of 15 mL of Rh positive red blood cells, multiple doses of RhoGAM are required. A fetal-maternal hemorrhage of this magnitude is unlikely prior to the last trimester of pregnancy. Patients who may need multiple doses of RhoGAM can be identified by a fetal-maternal hemorrhage screening test. If the test is positive, the volume of the fetal-maternal hemorrhage should be determined by a quantitative method. A single dose of RhoGAM should be administered for every 15 mL of fetal red blood cells. If the dose calculation results in a fraction, administer the next number of whole syringes of RhoGAM.

Multiple doses of RhoGAM are usual for indications associated with transfusion. For every 15 mL of Rh positive red blood cells transfused, the patient should receive a single dose of RhoGAM. If multiple doses are required, consult your pharmacy for pooling directions.

Administer RhoGAM intramuscularly. Do not inject intravenously. Multiple doses may be administered at the same time or at spaced intervals, as long as the total dose is administered within three days of exposure.

Since there is no lot number and expiration date on the prefilled syringes, they should not be removed from the protective pouch until immediately before use.

HOW SUPPLIED

RhoGAM is available in packages containing:
—25 prefilled single-dose syringes of RhoGAM (Product code 780720) NDC 0562-8070-20
—25 package inserts
—25 control forms
—25 patient identification cards
      and
—100 prefilled single-dose syringes of RhoGAM (Product code 780790) NDC 0562-8070-90
—100 package inserts
—100 control forms
—100 patient identification cards

STORAGE

Store at 2 to 8°C. DO NOT FREEZE.

Ortho Pharmaceutical Corporation
RARITAN, NJ 08869-0602

For Medical Information Contact:
Generally:
(800) 682-6532
In Emergencies:
(908) 218-7325

ACI–JEL® Therapeutic Vaginal Jelly ℞

DESCRIPTION

ACI-JEL Vaginal Jelly is a bland, non-irritating, water-dispersible, buffered acid jelly for intravaginal use. ACI-JEL is classified as a Vaginal Therapeutic Jelly. ACI-JEL contains 0.921% glacial acetic acid ($C_2H_4O_2$), 0.025% oxyquinoline sulfate ($C_{18}H_{16}N_2O_6S$), 0.7% ricinoleic acid ($C_{18}H_{34}O_3$), and 5% glycerin ($C_3H_8O_3$) compounded with tragacanth, acacia, propylparaben, potassium hydroxide, stannous chloride, egg albumen, potassium bitartrate, perfume and purified water. ACI-JEL is formulated to pH 3.9–4.1.

CLINICAL PHARMACOLOGY

ACI-JEL acts to restore and maintain normal vaginal acidity through its buffer action.

INDICATIONS AND USAGE

ACI-JEL is indicated as adjunctive therapy in those cases where restoration and maintenance of vaginal acidity are desirable.

CONTRAINDICATIONS

None known.

WARNINGS

No serious adverse reactions or potential safety hazards have been reported with the use of ACI-JEL.

PRECAUTIONS

General: No special care is required for the safe and effective use of ACI-JEL. *Drug Interactions:* No incidence of drug interactions have been reported with concomitant use of ACI-JEL and any other medications. *Laboratory Tests:* The monitoring of vaginal acidity (pH) may be helpful in following the patient's response. (The normal vaginal pH has been shown to be in the range of 4.0 to 5.0.) *Carcinogenesis:* No long-term studies in animals have been performed to evaluate carcinogenic potential. *Pregnancy:* Pregnancy Category C. Animal reproduction studies have not been conducted with ACI-JEL. It is also not known whether ACI-JEL can cause fetal harm when administered to a pregnant woman or can affect reproduction capacity. ACI-JEL should be given to a pregnant woman only if clearly needed. *Nursing Mothers:* It is not known whether this drug is excreted in human milk. Because many drugs are excreted in human milk, caution should be exercised when ACI-JEL is administered to a nursing woman.

ADVERSE REACTIONS

Occasional cases of local stinging and burning have been reported.

DOSAGE AND ADMINISTRATION

The usual dose is one applicatorful, administered intravaginally, morning and evening. Duration of treatment may be determined by the patient's response to therapy.

HOW SUPPLIED

85g Tube (NDC 0062-5421-01) with ORTHO® Measured-Dose Applicator.
Issued July 1984   643-10-310-1

DIENESTROL Cream ℞

(See ORTHO® Dienestrol Cream.)

MICRONOR® Tablets ℞
(norethindrone)

Patients should be counseled that this product does not protect against HIV infection (AIDS) and other sexually transmitted diseases.

DESCRIPTION

MICRONOR® 28 Day Regimen
Each tablet contains 0.35 mg norethindrone. Inactive ingredients include D&C Green No. 5, D&C Yellow No. 10, lactose, magnesium stearate, povidone and starch.

norethindrone

CLINICAL PHARMACOLOGY

1. MODE OF ACTION
MICRONOR progestin-only oral contraceptives prevent conception by suppressing ovulation in approximately half of users, thickening the cervical mucus to inhibit sperm penetration, lowering the midcycle LH and FSH peaks, slowing the movement of the ovum through the fallopian tubes, and altering the endometrium.
2. PHARMACOKINETICS
Serum progestin levels peak about two hours after oral administration, followed by rapid distribution and elimination. By 24 hours after drug ingestion, serum levels are near baseline, making efficacy dependent upon rigid adherence to the dosing schedule. There are large variations in serum levels

Continued on next page

Ortho—Cont.

among individual users. Progestin-only administration results in lower steady-state serum progestin levels and a shorter elimination half-life than concomitant administration with estrogens.

INDICATIONS AND USAGE

1. Indications
Progestin-only oral contraceptives are indicated for the prevention of pregnancy.
2. Efficacy
If used perfectly, the first-year failure rate for progestin-only oral contraceptives is 0.5%. However, the typical failure rate is estimated to be closer to 5%, due to late or omitted pills. Table 1 lists the pregnancy rates for users of all major methods of contraception.

Table 1. Comparison of reversible contraceptive methods: Percent of women experiencing a contraceptive failure (pregnancy) during the first year of use.

Percent of Women Experiencing a Pregnancy within the First year of Use

Method	Average Use	Perfect Use
No contraception	85	85
Spermicides	21	6
Periodic abstinence	20	1-9[1]
Withdrawal	19	4
Cervical caps		
Given birth	36	26
Never given birth	18	9
Diaphragms	18	6
Condoms		
Female	21	5
Male	12	3
Pills	3	—
Progestin-only	—	0.5
Combined	—	0.1
IUDs		
Progesterone	2	1.5
Copper T 380A	0.8	0.6
Injectables	0.3	0.3
Implant	0.09	0.09

Adapted with permission[2].
1. Depending on method (calendar, ovulation, sympto-thermal, post-ovulation).
2. Hatcher RA, Trussell J, Stewart F. et al. Contraceptive Technology 1994-1996. New York, NY: Irvington Publishers 1994.

CONTRAINDICATIONS

Progestin-only oral contraceptives (POPs) should not be used by women who currently have the following conditions:
- Known or suspected pregnancy
- Known or suspected carcinoma of the breast
- Undiagnosed abnormal genital bleeding
- Hypersensitivity to any component of this product
- Benign or malignant liver tumors
- Acute liver disease

WARNINGS

Cigarette smoking increases the risk of serious cardiovascular disease. Women who use oral contraceptives should be strongly advised not to smoke.
MICRONOR does not contain estrogen and, therefore, this insert does not discuss the serious health risks that have been associated with the estrogen component of combined oral contraceptives (COCs). The health care provider is referred to the prescribing information of combined oral contraceptives for a discussion of those risks. The relationship between progestin-only oral contraceptives and these risks is not fully defined. The physician should remain alert to the earliest manifestation of symptoms of any serious disease and discontinue oral contraceptive therapy when appropriate.
1. Ectopic Pregnancy
The incidence of ectopic pregnancies for progestin-only oral contraceptive users is 5 per 1000 women-years. Up to 10% of pregnancies reported in clinical studies of progestin-only oral contraceptive users are extrauterine. Although symptoms of ectopic pregnancy should be watched for, a history of ectopic pregnancy need not be considered a contraindication to use of this contraceptive method. Health providers should be alert to the possibility of an ectopic pregnancy in women who become pregnant or complain of lower abdominal pain while on progestin-only oral contraceptives.
2. Delayed Follicular Atresia/Ovarian Cysts
If follicular development occurs, atresia of the follicle is sometimes delayed and the follicle may continue to grow beyond the size it would attain in a normal cycle. Generally these enlarged follicles disappear spontaneously. Often they are asymptomatic; in some cases they are associated with mild abdominal pain. Rarely they may twist or rupture, requiring surgical intervention.
3. Irregular Genital Bleeding
Irregular menstrual patterns are common among women using progestin-only oral contraceptives. If genital bleeding is suggestive of infection, malignancy, or other abnormal conditions, such nonpharmacologic causes should be ruled out. If prolonged amenorrhea occurs, the possibility of pregnancy should be evaluated.
4. Carcinoma of the Breast and Reproductive Organs
Some epidemiologic studies of oral contraceptive users have reported an increased relative risk of developing breast cancer, particularly at a younger age and apparently related to duration of use. These studies have predominantly involved combined oral contraceptives and there is insufficient data to determine whether the use of POPs similarly increases the risk. Women with breast cancer should not use oral contraceptives because the role of female hormones in breast cancer has not been fully determined.
Some studies suggest that oral contraceptive use has been associated with an increase in the risk of cervical intraepithelial neoplasia in some populations of women. However, there continues to be controversy about the extent to which such findings may be due to differences in sexual behavior and other factors. There is insufficient data to determine whether the use of POPs increases the risk of developing cervical intraepithelial neoplasia.
5. Hepatic Neoplasia
Benign hepatic adenomas are associated with combined oral contraceptive use, although the incidence of benign tumors is rare in the United States. Rupture of benign, hepatic adenomas may cause death through intraabdominal hemorrhage.
Studies from Britain and the U.S. have shown an increased risk of developing hepatocellular carcinoma in combined oral contraceptive users. However, these cancers are rare. There is insufficient data to determine whether POPs increase the risk of developing hepatic neoplasia.

PRECAUTIONS

1. General
Patients should be counseled that this product does not protect against HIV infection (AIDS) and other sexually transmitted diseases.
2. Physical Examination and Follow up
It is considered good medical practice for sexually active women using oral contraceptives to have annual history and physical examinations. The physical examination may be deferred until after initiation of oral contraceptives if requested by the woman and judged appropriate by the clinician.
3. Carbohydrate and Lipid Metabolism
Some users may experience slight deterioration in glucose tolerance, with increases in plasma insulin but women with diabetes mellitus who use progestin-only oral contraceptives do not generally experience changes in their insulin requirements. Nonetheless, prediabetic and diabetic women in particular should be carefully monitored while taking POPs.
Lipid metabolism is occasionally affected in that HDL, HDL_2, and apolipoprotein A-I and A-II may be decreased; hepatic lipase may be increased. There is usually no effect on total cholesterol, HDL_3, LDL, or VLDL.
4. Drug Interactions
The effectiveness of progestin-only pills is reduced by hepatic enzyme-inducing drugs such as the anticonvulsants phenytoin, carbamazepine, and barbiturates, and the antituberculosis drug rifampin. No significant interaction has been found with broad-spectrum antibiotics.
5. Interactions with Laboratory Tests
The following endocrine tests may be affected by progestin-only oral contraceptive use:
- Sex hormone-binding globulin (SHBG) concentrations may be decreased.
- Thyroxine concentrations may be decreased, due to a decrease in thyroid binding globulin (TBG).

6. Carcinogenesis
See WARNINGS section.
7. Pregnancy
Many studies have found no effects on fetal development associated with long-term use of contraceptive doses of oral progestins. The few studies of infant growth and development that have been conducted have not demonstrated significant adverse effects. It is nonetheless prudent to rule out suspected pregnancy before initiating any hormonal contraceptive use.
8. Nursing Mothers
No adverse effects have been found on breastfeeding performance or on the health, growth or development of the infant. Small amounts of progestin pass into the breast milk, resulting in steroid levels in infant plasma of 1–6% of the levels of maternal plasma.
9. Fertility Following Discontinuation
The limited available data indicate a rapid return of normal ovulation and fertility following discontinuation of progestin-only oral contraceptives.
10. Headache
The onset or exacerbation of migraine or development of severe headache with focal neurological symptoms which is recurrent or persistent requires discontinuation of progestin-only contraceptives and evaluation of the cause.

INFORMATION FOR THE PATIENT

1. See Detailed Patient Labeling for detailed information.
2. Counseling issues.
The following points should be discussed with prospective users before prescribing progestin-only oral contraceptives:
- The necessity of taking pills at the same time every day, including throughout all bleeding episodes.
- The need to use a backup method such as condoms and spermicides for the next 48 hours whenever a progestin-only oral contraceptive is taken 3 or more hours late.
- The potential side effects of progestin-only oral contraceptives, particularly menstrual irregularities.
- The need to inform the clinician of prolonged episodes of bleeding, amenorrhea or severe abdominal pain.
- The importance of using a barrier method in addition to progestin-only oral contraceptives if a woman is at risk of contracting or transmitting STDs/HIV.

ADVERSE REACTIONS

Adverse reactions reported with the use of POPs include:
- Menstrual irregularity is the most frequently reported side effect.
- Frequent and irregular bleeding are common, while long duration of bleeding episodes and amenorrhea are less likely.
- Headache, breast tenderness, nausea, and dizziness are increased among progestin-only oral contraceptive users in some studies.
- Androgenic side effects such as acne, hirsutism, and weight gain occur rarely.

OVERDOSAGE

There have been no reports of serious ill effects from overdosage, including ingestion by children.

DOSAGE AND ADMINISTRATION

To achieve maximum contraceptive effectiveness, MICRONOR must be taken exactly as directed. One tablet is taken ever day, at the same time. Administration is continuous, with no interruption between pill packs. See Detailed Patient Labeling for detailed instruction.

HOW SUPPLIED

MICRONOR Tablets are available in a DIALPAK® Tablet Dispenser (NDC 0062-1411-01) containing 28 green tablets (0.35 mg norethindrone).
STORAGE: Store at controlled room temperature (15-30°C; 59-86°F).
CAUTION: Federal law prohibits dispensing without prescription.

REFERENCE

McCann M, and Potter L. Progestin-Only Oral Contraceptives: A Comprehensive Review. Contraception, 50:60 (Suppl. 1), December 1994.

DETAILED PATIENT LABELING

MICRONOR® (norethindrone) **Tablets**

This product (like all oral contraceptives) is used to prevent pregnancy. It does not protect against HIV infection (AIDS) or other sexually transmitted diseases.

DESCRIPTION

MICRONOR® 28 Day Regimen
Each tablet contains 0.35 mg norethindrone. Inactive ingredients include D&C Green No. 5, D&C Yellow No. 10, lactose, magnesium stearate, povidone and starch.

INTRODUCTION

This leaflet is about birth control pills that contain one hormone, a progestin. Please read this leaflet before you begin to take your pills. It is meant to be used along with talking with your doctor or clinic.
Progestin-only pills are often called "POPs" or "the mini-pill". POPs have less progestin than the combined birth control pill (or "the pill") which contains both an estrogen and a progestin.

HOW EFFECTIVE ARE POPs?

About 1 in 200 POP users will get pregnant in the first year if they all take POPs perfectly (that is, on time, every day). About 1 in 20 "typical" POP users (including women who are late taking pills or miss pills) gets pregnant in the first year of use. Table 2 will help you compare the efficacy of different methods.

Table 2. Comparison of reversible contraceptive methods: Percent of women who become pregnant during the first year of use

Percent of Women Experiencing a Pregnancy Within the First Year of Use

Method	Average Use	Perfect Use
No contraception	85	85
Spermicides	21	6

Periodic abstinence	20	1-9[1]
Withdrawal	19	4
Cervical caps		
Given birth	36	26
Never given birth	18	9
Diaphragms	18	6
Condoms		
Female	21	5
Male	12	3
Pills	3	
POPs	—	0.5
Combined pills	—	0.1
IUDs		
Progesterone	2	1.5
Copper T 380A	0.8	0.6
Injectables	0.3	0.3
Implant	0.09	0.09

Adapted with permission[2]

1. Depending on method (calendar, ovulation, sympto-thermal, post-ovulation method).
2. Hatcher RA, Trussell J. et al. Contraceptive Technology 1994-1996. New York, NY: Irvington Publishers 1994.

HOW DO POPs WORK?

POPs can prevent pregnancy in different ways including:
- They make the cervical mucus at the entrance to the womb (the uterus) too thick for the sperm to get through to the egg.
- They prevent ovulation (release of the egg from the ovary) in about half of the cycles.
- They also affect other hormones, the fallopian tubes and the lining of the uterus.

YOU SHOULD NOT TAKE POPs

- If there is any chance you may be pregnant.
- If you have breast cancer.
- If you have bleeding between your periods that has not been diagnosed.
- If you are taking certain drugs for epilepsy (seizures) or for TB. (See "Using POPs with Other Medicines" below.)
- If you are hypersensitive, or allergic, to any component of this product.
- If you have liver tumors, either benign or cancerous.
- If you have acute liver disease.

RISKS OF TAKING POPs

Cigarette smoking greatly increases the possibility of suffering heart attacks and strokes. Women who use oral contraceptives are strongly advised not to smoke.
WARNING: If you have sudden or severe pain in your lower abdomen or stomach area, you may have an ectopic pregnancy or an ovarian cyst. If this happens, you should contact your doctor or clinic immediately.

Ectopic Pregnancy
An ectopic pregnancy is a pregnancy outside the womb. Because POPs protect against pregnancy, the chance of having a pregnancy outside the womb is very low. If you do get pregnant while taking POPs, you have a slightly higher chance that the pregnancy will be ectopic than do users of some other birth control methods.

Ovarian Cysts
These cysts are small sacs of fluid in the ovary. They are more common among POP users than among users of most other birth control methods. They usually disappear without treatment and rarely cause problems.

Cancer of the Reproductive Organs and Breasts
Some studies in women who use combined oral contraceptives that contain both estrogen and a progestin have reported an increase in the risk of developing breast cancer, particularly at a younger age and apparently related to duration of use. There is insufficient data to determine whether the use of POPs similarly increases this risk.
Some studies have found an increase in the incidence of cancer of the cervix in women who use oral contraceptives. However, this finding may be related to factors other than the use of oral contraceptives and there is insufficient data to determine whether the use of POPs increases the risk of developing cancer of the cervix.

Liver Tumors
In rare cases, combined oral contraceptives can cause benign but dangerous liver tumors. These benign liver tumors can rupture and cause fatal internal bleeding. In addition, a possible but not definite association has been found with combined oral contraceptives and liver cancers in studies in which a few women who developed these very rare cancers were found to have used combined oral contraceptives for long periods of time. There is insufficient data to determine whether POPs increase the risk of liver tumors.

Diabetic Women
Diabetic women taking POPs do not generally require changes in the amount of insulin they are taking. However, your physician may monitor you more closely under these conditions.

SEXUALLY TRANSMITTED DISEASES (STDs)

WARNING: POPs do not protect against getting or giving someone HIV (AIDS) or any other STD, such as chlamydia, gonorrhea, genital warts and herpes.

SIDE EFFECTS

Irregular Bleeding:
The most common side effect of POPs is a change in menstrual bleeding. Your periods may be either early or late, and you may have some spotting between periods. Taking pills late or missing pills can result in some spotting or bleeding.

Other Side Effects:
Less common side effects include headaches, tender breasts, nausea and dizziness. Weight gain, acne and extra hair on your face and body have been reported, but are rare.
If you are concerned about any of these side effects, check with your doctor or clinic.

USING POPs WITH OTHER MEDICINES

Before taking a POP, inform your health care provider of any other medication, including over-the-counter medicine, that you may be taking.
These medicines can make POPs less effective:
Medicines for seizures such as:
- Phenytoin (Dilantin)
- Carbamazepine (Tegretol)
- Phenobarbital
Medicine for TB:
- Rifampin (Rifampicin)
Before you begin taking any new medicines be sure your doctor or clinic knows you are taking a progestin-only birth control pill.

HOW TO TAKE POPs

IMPORTANT POINTS TO REMEMBER

- POPs must be taken at the same time every day, so choose a time and then take the pill at that same time every day. Every time you take a pill late, and especially if you miss a pill, you are more likely to get pregnant.
- Start the next pack the day after the last pack is finished. There is no break between packs. Always have your next pack of pills ready.
- You may have some menstrual spotting between periods. Do not stop taking your pills if this happens.
- If you vomit soon after taking a pill, use a backup method (such as a condom and/or a spermicide) for 48 hours.
- If you want to stop taking POPs, you can do so at any time, but, if you remain sexually active and don't wish to become pregnant, be certain to use another birth control method.
- If you are not sure about how to take POPs, ask your doctor or clinic.

STARTING POPs

- It's best to take your first POP on the first day of your menstrual period.
- If you decide to take your first POP on another day, use a backup method (such as a condom and/or spermicide) every time you have sex during the next 48 hours.
- If you have had a miscarriage or an abortion, you can start POPs the next day.

IF YOU ARE LATE OR MISS TAKING YOUR POPs

- If you are more than 3 hours late or you miss one or more POPs:
1) **TAKE** a missed pill as soon as you remember that you missed it,
2) **THEN** go back to taking POPs at your regular time,
3) **BUT** be sure to use a backup method (such as a condom and/or a spermicide) every time you have sex for the next 48 hours.
- If you are not sure what to do about the pills you have missed, keep taking POPs and use a backup method until you can talk to your doctor or clinic.

IF YOU ARE BREASTFEEDING

- If you are fully breastfeeding (not giving your baby any food or formula), you may start your pills 6 weeks after delivery.
- If you are partially breastfeeding (giving your baby some food or formula), you should start taking pills by 3 weeks after delivery.

IF YOU ARE SWITCHING PILLS

- If you are switching from the combined pills to POPs, take the first POP the day after you finish the last active combined pill. Do not take any of the 7 inactive pills from the combined pill pack. You should know that many women

have irregular periods after switching to POPs, but this is normal and to be expected.
- If you are switching from POPs to the combined pills, take the first active combined pill on the first day of your period, even if your POPs pack is not finished.
- If you switch to another brand of POPs, start the new brand anytime.
- If you are breastfeeding, you can switch to another method of birth control at any time, except do not switch to the combined pills until you stop breastfeeding or at least until 6 months after delivery.

PREGNANCY WHILE ON THE PILL

If you think you are pregnant, contact your physician. Even though research has shown that POPs do not cause harm to the unborn baby, it is always best not to take any drugs or medicines that you don't need when you are pregnant. You should get a pregnancy test:
- If your period is late and you took one or more pills late or missed taking them and had sex without a backup method.
- Anytime it has been more than 45 days since the beginning of your last period.

WILL POPs AFFECT YOUR ABILITY TO GET PREGNANT LATER?

If you want to become pregnant, simply stop taking POPs. POPs will not delay your ability to get pregnant.

BREASTFEEDING

If you are breastfeeding, POPs will not affect the quality or amount of your breastmilk or the health of your nursing baby.

OVERDOSE

No serious problems have been reported when many pills were taken by accident, even by a small child, so there is usually no reason to treat an overdose.

OTHER QUESTIONS OR CONCERNS

If you have any questions or concerns, check with your doctor or clinic. You can also ask for the more detailed "Professional Labeling" written for doctors and other health care providers.

HOW TO STORE YOUR POPs

Store your POPs at room temperature (between 59° and 86°F).
ORTHO PHARMACEUTICAL
CORPORATION
Raritan, New Jersey 08869
©OPC 1996
Revised May 1996

635-10-895-2
Shown in Product Identification Guide, page 326

MONISTAT® 3
(miconazole nitrate, 200 mg)
Vaginal Suppositories

℞

DESCRIPTION

MONISTAT 3 Vaginal Suppositories are white to off-white suppositories, each containing the antifungal agent, miconazole nitrate, 1-[2,4-Dichloro-β-[(2,4-dichlorobenzyl)oxy]phenethyl]- imidazole mononitrate, 200 mg, in a hydrogenated vegetable oil base. Miconazole nitrate for vaginal use is also available as MONISTAT 7 Vaginal Cream and MONISTAT 7 Vaginal Suppositories.

MICONAZOLE NITRATE

CLINICAL PHARMACOLOGY

Miconazole nitrate exhibits fungicidal activity *in vitro* against species of the genus *Candida*. The pharmacologic mode of action is unknown. Following intravaginal administration of miconazole nitrate, small amounts are absorbed. Administration of a single dose of miconazole nitrate suppositories (100mg) to healthy subjects resulted in a total recovery from the urine and feces of 0.85% (±0.43%) of the administered dose.
Animal studies indicate that the drug crossed the placenta and doses above those used in humans result in embryo- and fetotoxicity (80 mg/kg, orally), although this has not been reported in human subjects (See PRECAUTIONS).
In multi-center clinical trials in 440 women with vulvovaginal candidiasis, the efficacy of treatment with the MONISTAT 3 Vaginal Suppository for 3 days was compared

Continued on next page

Ortho—Cont.

with treatment for 7 days with MONISTAT 7 Vaginal Cream. The clinical cure rates (free of microbiological evidence and clinical signs and symptoms of candidiasis at 8–10 days and 30–35 days post-therapy) were numerically lower, although not statistically different, with the 3-Day Suppository when compared with the 7-Day Cream.

INDICATIONS AND USAGE

MONISTAT 3 Vaginal Suppositories are indicated for the local treatment of vulvovaginal candidiasis (moniliasis). Effectiveness in pregnancy and in diabetic patients has not been established. As MONISTAT is effective only for candidal vulvovaginitis, the diagnosis should be confirmed by KOH smear and/or cultures. Other pathogens commonly associated with vulvovaginitis (*Trichomonas* and *Haemophilus vaginalis* [*Gardnerella*]) should be ruled out by appropriate laboratory methods.

CONTRAINDICATIONS

Patients known to be hypersensitive to this drug.

PRECAUTIONS

General: Discontinue drug if sensitization or irritation is reported during use. The base contained in the suppository formulation may interact with certain latex products, such as that used in vaginal contraceptive diaphragms. Concurrent use is not recommended. MONISTAT 7 Vaginal Cream may be considered for use under these conditions.

Laboratory Tests: If there is a lack of response to MONISTAT 3 Vaginal Suppositories, appropriate microbiological studies (standard KOH smear and/or cultures) should be repeated to confirm the diagnosis and rule out other pathogens.

Carcinogenesis, Mutagenesis, Impairment of Fertility: Long-term animal studies to determine carcinogenic potential have not been performed.

Fertility (Reproduction): Oral administration of miconazole nitrate in rats has been reported to produce prolonged gestation. However, this effect was not observed in oral rabbit studies. In addition, signs of fetal and embryo toxicity were reported in rat and rabbit studies, and dystocia was reported in rat studies after oral doses at and above 80 mg per kg. Intravaginal administration did not produce these effects in rats.

Pregnancy: Since imidazoles are absorbed in small amounts from the human vagina, they should not be used in the first trimester of pregnancy unless the physician considers it essential to the welfare of the patient.

Clinical studies, during which miconazole nitrate vaginal cream and suppositories were used for up to 14 days, were reported to include 514 pregnant patients. Follow-up reports available in 471 of these patients reveal no adverse effects or complications attributable to miconazole nitrate therapy in infants born to these women.

Nursing Mothers: It is not known whether miconazole nitrate is excreted in human milk. Because many drugs are excreted in human milk, caution should be exercised when miconazole nitrate is administered to a nursing woman.

ADVERSE REACTIONS

During clinical studies with the MONISTAT 3 Vaginal Suppository (miconazole nitrate, 200 mg) 301 patients were treated. The incidence of vulvovaginal burning, itching or irritation was 2%. Complaints of cramping (2%) and headaches (1.3%) were also reported. Other complaints (hives, skin rash) occurred with less than a 0.5% incidence. The therapy-related dropout rate was 0.3%.

OVERDOSE

Overdose of miconazole nitrate in humans has not been reported to date. In mice, rats, guinea pigs and dogs, the oral LD 50 values were found to be 578.1, >640, 275.9 and >160 mg/kg, respectively.

DOSAGE AND ADMINISTRATION

MONISTAT 3 Vaginal Suppositories: One suppository (miconazole nitrate, 200 mg) is inserted intravaginally once daily at bedtime for three consecutive days. Before prescribing another course of therapy, the diagnosis should be reconfirmed by smears and/or cultures to rule out other pathogens.

HOW SUPPLIED

MONISTAT 3 Suppositories (miconazole nitrate, 200 mg) are available as 2.5 gm, elliptically shaped white to off-white suppositories in packages of three (NDC 0062-5437-01) with a vaginal applicator. Store at 59°–86° F (15–30° C).

Shown in Product Identification Guide, page 326

MONISTAT® ℞
(miconazole nitrate)
DUAL-PAK®

3 DAY SUPPOSITORY THERAPY
MONISTAT® 3
(miconazole nitrate, 200 mg)
Vaginal Suppositories

DESCRIPTION

MONISTAT 3 Vaginal Suppositories are white to off-white suppositories, each containing the antifungal agent, miconazole nitrate, 1-[2,4-Dichloro-β-[(2,4-dichlorobenzyl) oxy]phenethyl]-imidazole mononitrate, 200 mg., in a hydrogenated vegetable oil base. Miconazole nitrate for vaginal use is also available as MONISTAT 7 Vaginal Cream and MONISTAT 7 Vaginal Suppositories.

MICONAZOLE NITRATE

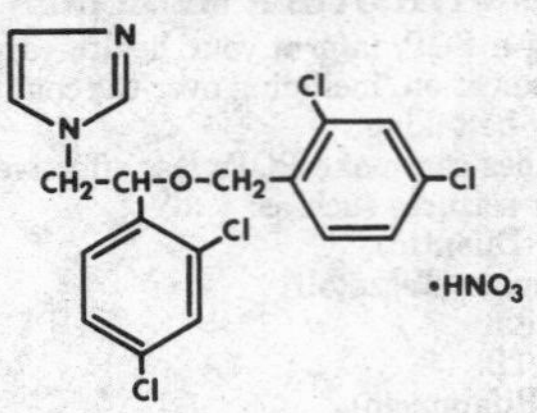

CLINICAL PHARMACOLOGY

Miconazole nitrate exhibits fungicidal activity *in vitro* against species of the genus *Candida*. The pharmacologic mode of action is unknown. Following intravaginal administration of miconazole nitrate, small amounts are absorbed. Administration of a single dose of miconazole nitrate suppositories (100 mg) to healthy subjects resulted in a total recovery from the urine and feces of 0.85% (±0.43%) of the administered dose.

Animal studies indicate that the drug crossed the placenta and doses above those used in humans result in embryo- and feto-toxicity (80 mg/kg, orally), although this has not been reported in human subjects (See PRECAUTIONS).

In multi-center clinical trials in 440 women with vulvovaginal candidiasis, the efficacy of treatment with the MONISTAT 3 Vaginal Suppository for 3 days was compared with treatment for 7 days with MONISTAT 7 Vaginal Cream.

The clinical cure rates (free of microbiological evidence and clinical signs and symptoms of candidiasis at 8–10 days and 30–35 days post-therapy) were numerically lower, although not statistically different, with the 3-Day Suppository when compared with the 7-Day Cream.

INDICATIONS AND USAGE

MONISTAT 3 Vaginal Suppositories are indicated for the local treatment of vulvovaginal candidiasis (moniliasis). Effectiveness in pregnancy and in diabetic patients has not been established. As MONISTAT is effective only for candidal vulvovaginitis, the diagnosis should be confirmed by KOH smear and/or cultures. Other pathogens commonly associated with vulvovaginitis (*Trichomonas* and *Haemophilus vaginalis* [*Gardnerella*]) should be ruled out by appropriate laboratory methods.

CONTRAINDICATIONS

Patients known to be hypersensitive to this drug.

PRECAUTIONS

General: Discontinue drug if sensitization or irritation is reported during use. The base contained in the suppository formulation may interact with certain latex products, such as that used in vaginal contraceptive diaphragms. Concurrent use is not recommended. MONISTAT 7 Vaginal Cream may be considered for use under these conditions.

Laboratory Tests: If there is a lack of response to MONISTAT 3 Vaginal Suppositories, appropriate microbiological studies (standard KOH smear and/or cultures) should be repeated to confirm the diagnosis and rule out other pathogens.

Carcinogenesis, Mutagenesis, Impairment of Fertility: Long-term animal studies to determine carcinogenic potential have not been performed.

Fertility (Reproduction): Oral administration of miconazole nitrate in rats has been reported to produce prolonged gestation. However, this effect was not observed in oral rabbit studies. In addition, signs of fetal and embryo toxicity were reported in rat and rabbit studies, and dystocia was reported in rat studies after oral doses at and above 80 mg per kg. Intravaginal administration did not produce these effects in rats.

Pregnancy: Since imidazoles are absorbed in small amounts from the human vagina, they should not be used in the first trimester of pregnancy unless the physician considers it essential to the welfare of the patient.

Clinical studies, during which miconazole nitrate vaginal cream and suppositories were used for up to 14 days, were reported to include 514 pregnant patients. Follow-up reports available in 471 of these patients reveal no adverse effects or complications attributable to miconazole nitrate therapy in infants born to these women.

Nursing Mothers: It is not known whether miconazole nitrate is excreted in human milk. Because many drugs are excreted in human milk, caution should be exercised when miconazole nitrate is administered to a nursing woman.

ADVERSE REACTIONS

During clinical studies with the MONISTAT 3 Vaginal Suppository (miconazole nitrate, 200 mg) 301 patients were treated. The incidence of vulvovaginal burning, itching or irritation was 2%. Complaints of cramping (2%) and headaches (1.3%) were also reported. Other complaints (hives, skin rash) occurred with less than a 0.5% incidence. The therapy-related dropout rate was 0.3%.

OVERDOSE

Overdose of miconazole nitrate in humans has not been reported to date. In mice, rats, guinea pigs and dogs, the oral LD 50 values were found to be 578.1, >640, 275.9 and >160 mg/kg, respectively.

DOSAGE AND ADMINISTRATION

MONISTAT 3 Vaginal Suppositories: One suppository (miconazole nitrate, 200 mg) is inserted intravaginally once daily at bedtime for three consecutive days. Before prescribing another course of therapy, the diagnosis should be reconfirmed by smears and/or cultures to rule out other pathogens.

HOW SUPPLIED

MONISTAT 3 Suppositories (miconazole nitrate, 200 mg) are available as 2.5 gm, elliptically shaped white to off-white suppositories in packages of three (NDC 0062-5437-01) with a vaginal applicator. Store at 59–86°F (15–30°C).

7 DAY CREAM THERAPY
MONISTAT-DERM®
(miconazole nitrate 2%)
Cream
For Topical Use Only

DESCRIPTION

MONISTAT-DERM (miconazole nitrate 2%) Cream contains miconazole nitrate* 2%, formulated into a water-miscible base consisting of pegoxol 7 stearate, peglicol 5 oleate, mineral oil, benzoic acid, butylated hydroxyanisole and purified water.

ACTIONS

Miconazole nitrate is a synthetic antifungal agent which inhibits the growth of the common dermatophytes, *Trichophyton rubrum, Trichophyton mentagrophytes,* and *Epidermophyton floccosum,* the yeast-like fungus, *Candida albicans,* and the organism responsible for tinea versicolor *(Malassezia furfur).*

INDICATIONS

For topical application in the treatment of tinea pedis (athlete's foot), tinea cruris, and tinea corporis caused by *Trichophyton rubrum, trichophyton mentagrophytes,* and *Epidermophyton floccosum,* in the treatment of cutaneous candidiasis (moniliasis), and in the treatment of tinea versicolor.

CONTRAINDICATIONS

MONISTAT-DERM (miconazole nitrate 2%) Cream has no known contraindications.

PRECAUTIONS

If a reaction suggesting sensitivity or chemical irritation should occur, use of the medication should be discontinued. For external use only. Avoid introduction of MONISTAT-DERM Cream into the eyes.

ADVERSE REACTIONS

There have been isolated reports of irritation, burning, maceration, and allergic contact dermatitis associated with the application of MONISTAT-DERM.

DOSAGE AND ADMINISTRATION

Sufficient MONISTAT-DERM Cream should be applied to cover affected areas twice daily (morning and evening) in patients with tinea pedis, tinea cruris, tinea corporis, and cutaneous candidiasis, and once daily in patients with tinea versicolor. If MONISTAT-DERM Cream is used in intertriginous areas, it should be applied sparingly and smoothed in well to avoid maceration effects.

Early relief of symptoms (2 to 3 days) is experienced by the majority of patients and clinical improvement may be seen fairly soon after treatment is begun; however, *Candida* infections and tinea cruris and corporis should be treated for two weeks and tinea pedis for one month in order to reduce the possibility of recurrence. If a patient shows no clinical improvement after a month of treatment, the diagnosis should be redetermined. Patients with tinea versicolor usually exhibit clinical and mycological clearing after two weeks of treatment.

HOW SUPPLIED

MONISTAT-DERM (miconazole nitrate 2%) Cream containing miconazole nitrate at 2% strength is supplied in 15 g. (NDC 0062-5434-02), 1 oz. (NDC 0062-5434-01) and 3 oz. (NDC 0062-5434-03) tubes.

*Chemical name: 1-[2,4-dichloro-β-{(2,4- dichlorobenzyl) oxy}phenethyl] imidazole mononitrate.

Revised January 1992   643-10-357-6
Shown in Product Identification Guide, page 326

ORTHO-CEPT®   ℞
(desogestrel and ethinyl estradiol) Tablets

Patients should be counseled that this product does not protect against HIV infection (AIDS) and other sexually transmitted diseases.

DESCRIPTION

ORTHO-CEPT 21 and ORTHO-CEPT 28 Tablets provide an oral contraceptive regimen of 21 orange round tablets each containing 0.15 mg desogestrel (13-ethyl-11-methylene-18,19-dinor-17 alpha-pregn-4-en-20-yn-17-ol) and 0.03 mg ethinyl estradiol (19-nor-17 alpha-pregna-1,3,5 (10)-trien-20-yne-3,17,diol). Inactive ingredients include vitamin E, corn starch, povidone, stearic acid, colloidal silicon dioxide, lactose, hydroxypropyl methylcellulose, polyethylene glycol, titanium dioxide, talc and ferric oxide. ORTHO-CEPT 28 also contains 7 green tablets containing the following inactive ingredients: lactose, pregelatinized starch, magnesium stearate, FD&C Blue No. 1 Aluminum Lake, ferric oxide, hydroxypropyl methylcellulose, polyethylene glycol, titanium dioxide and talc.

desogestrel

ethinyl estradiol

CLINICAL PHARMACOLOGY

Pharmacodynamics

Combination oral contraceptives act by suppression of gonadotropins. Although the primary mechanism of this action is inhibition of ovulation, other alterations include changes in the cervical mucus, which increase the difficulty of sperm entry into the uterus, and changes in the endometrium which reduce the likelihood of implantation.

Receptor binding studies, as well as studies in animals and humans, have shown that 3-keto-desogestrel, the biologically active metabolite of desogestrel, combines high progestational activity with minimal intrinsic androgenicity[91,92]. Desogestrel, in combination with ethinyl estradiol, does not counteract the estrogen-induced increases in SHBG, resulting in lower serum levels of free testosterone[96-99].

Pharmacokinetics

Desogestrel is rapidly and almost completely absorbed and converted into 3-keto-desogestrel, its biologically active metabolite. Following oral administration, the relative bioavailability of desogestrel, as measured by serum levels of 3-keto-desogestrel, is approximately 84%.

In the third cycle of use after a single dose of ORTHO-CEPT, maximum concentrations of 3-keto-desogestrel of $2,805\pm1,203$ pg/mL (mean$\pm$SD) are reached at 1.4 ± 0.8 hours. The area under the curve ($AUC_{0-\infty}$) is $33,858\pm11,043$ pg/mL·hr after a single dose. At steady state, attained from at least day 19 onwards, maximum concentrations of $5,840\pm1,667$ pg/mL are reached at 1.4 ± 0.9 hours. The minimum plasma levels of 3-keto-desogestrel at steady state are $1,400\pm560$ pg/mL. The AUC_{0-24} at steady state is $52,299\pm17,878$ pg/mL·hr. The mean $AUC_{0-\infty}$ for 3-keto-desogestrel at single dose is significantly lower than the mean AUC_{0-24} at steady state. This indicates that the kinetics of 3-keto-desogestrel are non-linear due to an increase in binding of 3-keto-desogestrel to sex hormone-binding globulin in the cycle, attributed to increased sex hormone-binding globulin levels which are induced by the daily administration of ethinyl estradiol. Sex hormone-binding globulin levels increased significantly in the third treatment cycle from day 1 (150 ± 64 nmol/L) to day 21 (230 ± 59 nmol/L). The elimination half-life for 3-keto-desogestrel is approximately 38 ± 20 hours at steady state. In addition to 3-keto-

desogestrel, other phase I metabolites are 3α-OH-desogestrel, 3β-OH-desogestrel, and 3α-OH-5α-H-desogestrel. These other metabolites are not known to have any pharmacologic effects, and are further converted in part by conjugation (phase II metabolism) into polar metabolites, mainly sulfates and glucuronides.

Ethinyl estradiol is rapidly and almost completely absorbed. In the third cycle of use after a single dose of ORTHO-CEPT, the relative bioavailability is approximately 83%.

In the third cycle of use after a single dose of ORTHO-CEPT, maximum concentrations of ethinyl estradiol of 95 ± 34 pg/mL are reached at 1.5 ± 0.8 hours. The $AUC_{0-\infty}$ is $1,471\pm268$ pg/mL·hr after a single dose. At steady state, attained from at least day 19 onwards, maximum ethinyl estradiol concentrations of 141 ± 48 pg/mL are reached at about 1.4 ± 0.7 hours. The minimum serum levels of ethinyl estradiol at steady state are 24 ± 8.3 pg/mL. The AUC_{0-24} at steady state is $1,117\pm302$ pg/mL·hr. The mean $AUC_{0-\infty}$ for ethinyl estradiol following a single dose during treatment cycle 3 does not significantly differ from the mean AUC_{0-24} at steady state. This finding indicates linear kinetics for ethinyl estradiol.

The elimination half-life is 26 ± 6.8 hours at steady state. Ethinyl estradiol is subject to a significant degree of presystemic conjugation (phase II metabolism). Ethinyl estradiol escaping gut wall conjugation undergoes phase I metabolism and hepatic conjugation (phase II metabolism). Major phase I metabolites are 2-OH-ethinyl estradiol and 2-methoxy-ethinyl estradiol. Sulfate and glucuronide conjugates of both ethinyl estradiol and phase I metabolites, which are excreted in bile, can undergo enterohepatic circulation.

INDICATIONS AND USAGE

ORTHO-CEPT Tablets are indicated for the prevention of pregnancy in women who elect to use oral contraceptives as a method of contraception.

Oral contraceptives are highly effective. Table I lists the typical accidental pregnancy rates for users of combination oral contraceptives and other methods of contraception. The efficacy of these contraceptive methods, except sterilization, depends upon the reliability with which they are used. Correct and consistent use of these methods can result in lower failure rates.

[See table 1 above.]

In a clinical trial with ORTHO-CEPT, 1,195 subjects completed 11,656 cycles and a total of 10 pregnancies were reported. This represents an overall user-efficacy (typical user-efficacy) pregnancy rate of 1.12 per 100 women-years. This rate includes patients who did not take the drug correctly.

TABLE I: LOWEST EXPECTED AND TYPICAL FAILURE RATES DURING THE FIRST YEAR OF CONTINUOUS USE OF A METHOD
% of Women Experiencing an Accidental Pregnancy in the First Year of Continuous Use

Method	Lowest Expected*	Typical**
(No Contraceptive)	(85)	(85)
Oral Contraceptives		3
combined	0.1	N/A***
progestin only	0.5	N/A***
Diaphragm with spermicidal cream or jelly	6	18
Spermicides alone (foam, creams, gels, jellies, vaginal suppositories, and vaginal film)	6	21
Vaginal Sponge		
nulliparous	9	18
parous	20	36
Implant	0.09	0.09
Injection: depot medroxyprogesterone acetate	0.3	0.3
IUD		
progesterone	1.5	2.0
copper T 380A	0.6	0.8
Condom without spermicides		
female	5	21
male	3	12
Cervical Cap with spermicidal cream or jelly		
nulliparous	9	18
parous	26	36
Periodic abstinence (all methods)	1-9	20
Female sterilization	0.4	0.4
Male sterilization	0.10	0.15

Adapted from RA Hatcher et al, Table 5-2, (1994) ref. #1.
 * The authors' best guess of the percentage of women expected to experience an accidental pregnancy among couples who initiate a method (not necessarily for the first time) and who use it consistently and correctly during the first year if they do not stop for any other reason.
 ** This term represents "typical" couples who initiate use of a method (not necessarily for the first time), who experience an accidental pregnancy during the first year if they do not stop use for any other reason.
 *** N/A—Data not available.

CONTRAINDICATIONS

Oral contraceptives should not be used in women who currently have the following conditions:
- Thrombophlebitis or thromboembolic disorders
- A past history of deep vein thrombophlebitis or thromboembolic disorders
- Cerebral vascular or coronary artery disease
- Known or suspected carcinoma of the breast
- Carcinoma of the endometrium or other known or suspected estrogen-dependent neoplasia
- Undiagnosed abnormal genital bleeding
- Cholestatic jaundice of pregnancy or jaundice with prior pill use
- Hepatic adenomas or carcinomas
- Known or suspected pregnancy

WARNINGS

> Cigarette smoking increases the risk of serious cardiovascular side effects from oral contraceptive use. This risk increases with age and with heavy smoking (15 or more cigarettes per day) and is quite marked in women over 35 years of age. Women who use oral contraceptives should be strongly advised not to smoke.

The use of oral contraceptives is associated with increased risks of several serious conditions including myocardial infarction, thromboembolism, stroke, hepatic neoplasia, and gallbladder disease, although the risk of serious morbidity or mortality is very small in healthy women without underlying risk factors. The risk of morbidity and mortality increases significantly in the presence of other underlying risk factors such as hypertension, hyperlipidemias, obesity and diabetes.

Practitioners prescribing oral contraceptives should be familiar with the following information relating to these risks. The information contained in this package insert is principally based on studies carried out in patients who used oral contraceptives with formulations of higher doses of estrogens and progestogens than those in common use today. The effect of long term use of the oral contraceptives with formulations of lower doses of both estrogens and progestogens remains to be determined.

Throughout this labeling, epidemiological studies reported are of two types: retrospective or case control studies and

Continued on next page

Ortho—Cont.

prospective or cohort studies. Case control studies provide a measure of the relative risk of a disease, namely, a *ratio* of the incidence of a disease among oral contraceptive users to that among nonusers. The relative risk does not provide information on the actual clinical occurrence of a disease. Cohort studies provide a measure of attributable risk, which is the *difference* in the incidence of disease between oral contraceptive users and nonusers. The attributable risk does provide information about the actual occurrence of a disease in the population (Adapted from refs. 2 and 3 with the author's permission). For further information, the reader is referred to a text on epidemiological methods.

1. THROMBOEMBOLIC DISORDERS AND OTHER VASCULAR PROBLEMS

a. Myocardial infarction
An increased risk of myocardial infarction has been attributed to oral contraceptive use. This risk is primarily in smokers or women with other underlying risk factors for coronary artery disease such as hypertension, hypercholesterolemia, morbid obesity, and diabetes. The relative risk of heart attack for current oral contraceptive users has been estimated to be two to six[4–10]. The risk is very low in women under the age of 30.
Smoking in combination with oral contraceptive use has been shown to contribute substantially to the incidence of myocardial infarctions in women in their mid-thirties or older with smoking accounting for the majority of excess cases[11]. Mortality rates associated with circulatory disease have been shown to increase substantially in smokers, especially in those 35 years of age and older among women who use oral contraceptives. (See Table II)

CIRCULATORY DISEASE MORTALITY RATES PER 100,000 WOMAN-YEARS BY AGE, SMOKING STATUS AND ORAL CONTRACEPTIVE USE

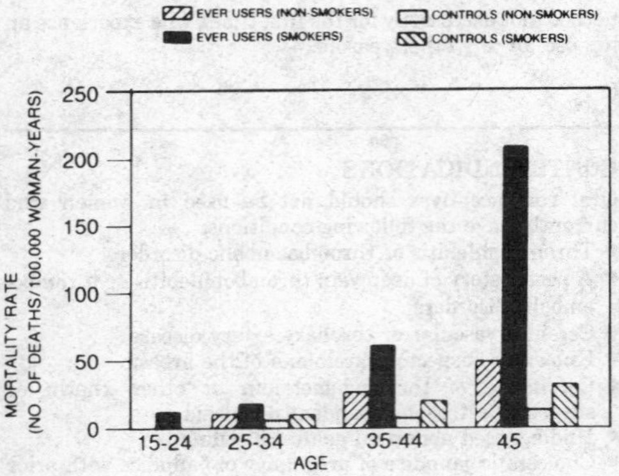

TABLE II. (Adapted from P.M. Layde and V. Beral, ref. #12.)

Oral contraceptives may compound the effects of well-known risk factors, such as hypertension, diabetes, hyperlipidemias, age and obesity.[13] In particular, some progestogens are known to decrease HDL cholesterol and cause glucose intolerance, while estrogens may create a state of hyperinsulinism[14–18]. Oral contraceptives have been shown to increase blood pressure among users (see section 9 in WARNINGS). Similar effects on risk factors have been associated with an increased risk of heart disease. Oral contraceptives must be used with caution in women with cardiovascular disease risk factors.

b. Thromboembolism
An increased risk of thromboembolic and thrombotic disease associated with the use of oral contraceptives is well established. Data from case-control and cohort studies report that oral contraceptives containing desogestral (ORTHO-CEPT contains desogestral) are associated with a two-fold increase in the risk of venous thromboembolic disease as compared to other low-dose (containing less than 50 mcg of estrogen) pills containing other progestins. According to these studies, this two-fold risk increases the yearly occurrence of venous thromboembolic disease by about 10-15 cases per 100,000 women.
Earlier case control studies on older formulations have found the relative risk of users compared to nonusers to be 3 for the first apisode of superficial venous thrombosis, 4 to 11 for deep vein thrombosis or pulmonary embolism, and 1.5 to 6 for women with predisposing conditions for venous thromboembolic disease[2,3,19-24]. Cohort studies have shown the relative risk to be somewhat lower, about 3 for new cases and about 4.5 for new cases requiring hospitalization[25]. The risk of thromboembolic disease associated with oral contraceptives is not related to length of use and disappears after pill use is stopped[2].
A two- to four-fold increase in relative risk of post-operative thromboembolic complications has been reported with the use of oral contraceptives[9]. The relative risk of venous thrombosis in women who have predisposing conditions is twice that of women without such medical conditions[26]. If feasible, oral contraceptives should be discontinued at least four weeks prior to and for two weeks after elective surgery of a type associated with an increase in risk of thromboembolism and during and following prolonged immobilization. Since the immediate postpartum period is also associated with an increased risk of thromboembolism, oral contraceptives should be started no earlier than four weeks after delivery in women who elect not to breast feed.

c. Cerebrovascular diseases
Oral contraceptives have been shown to increase both the relative and attributable risks of cerebrovascular events (thrombotic and hemorrhagic strokes), although, in general, the risk is greatest among older (>35 years), hypertensive women who also smoke. Hypertension was found to be a risk factor for both users and nonusers, for both types of strokes, and smoking interacted to increase the risk of stroke[27–29].
In a large study, the relative risk of thrombotic strokes has been shown to range from 3 for normotensive users to 14 for users with severe hypertension[30]. The relative risk of hemorrhagic stroke is reported to be 1.2 for non-smokers who used oral contraceptives, 2.6 for smokers who did not use oral contraceptives, 7.6 for smokers who used oral contraceptives, 1.8 for normotensive users and 25.7 for users with severe hypertension[30]. The attributable risk is also greater in older women[3].

d. Dose-related risk of vascular disease from oral contraceptives
A positive association has been observed between the amount of estrogen and progestogen in oral contraceptives and the risk of vascular disease[31–33]. A decline in serum high density lipoproteins (HDL) has been reported with many progestational agents[14–16]. A decline in serum high density lipoproteins has been associated with an increased incidence of ischemic heart disease. Because estrogens increase HDL cholesterol, the net effect of an oral contraceptive depends on a balance achieved between doses of estrogen and progestogen and the nature and absolute amount of progestogens used in the contraceptives. The amount of both hormones should be considered in the choice of an oral contraceptive.
Minimizing exposure to estrogen and progestogen is in keeping with good principles of therapeutics. For any particular estrogen/progestogen combination, the dosage regimen prescribed should be one which contains the least amount of estrogen and progestogen that is compatible with a low failure rate and the needs of the individual patient. New acceptors of oral contraceptive agents should be started on preparations containing 0.035 mg or less of estrogen.

e. Persistence of risk of vascular disease
There are two studies which have shown persistence of risk of vascular disease for ever-users of oral contraceptives. In a study in the United States, the risk of developing myocardial infarction after discontinuing oral contraceptives persists for at least 9 years for women 40–49 years old who had used oral contraceptives for five or more years, but this increased risk was not demonstrated in other age groups[8]. In another study in Great Britain, the risk of developing cerebrovascular disease persisted for at least 6 years after discontinuation of oral contraceptives, although excess risk was very small[34]. However, both studies were performed with oral contraceptive formulations containing 0.050 mg or higher of estrogens.

2. ESTIMATES OF MORTALITY FROM CONTRACEPTIVE USE
One study gathered data from a variety of sources which have estimated the mortality rate associated with different methods of contraception at different ages (Table III). These estimates include the combined risk of death associated with contraceptive methods plus the risk attributable to pregnancy in the event of method failure. Each method of contraception has its specific benefits and risks. The study concluded that with the exception of oral contraceptive users 35 and older who smoke and 40 and older who do not smoke, mortality associated with all methods of birth control is low and below that associated with childbirth.
The observation of an increase in risk of mortality with age for oral contraceptive users is based on data gathered in the 1970's[35]. Current clinical recommendation involves the use of lower estrogen dose formulations and a careful consideration of risk factors. In 1989, the Fertility and Maternal Health Drugs Advisory Committee was asked to review the use of oral contraceptives in women 40 years of age and over. The committee concluded that although cardiovascular disease risk may be increased with oral contraceptive use after age 40 in healthy non-smoking women (even with the newer low-dose formulations), there are also greater potential health risks associated with pregnancy in older women and with the alternative surgical and medical procedures which may be necessary if such women do not have access to effective and acceptable means of contraception. The Committee recommended that the benefits of low-dose oral contraceptive use by healthy non-smoking women over 40 may outweigh the possible risks.
Of course, older women, as all women who take oral contraceptives, should take an oral contraceptive which contains the least amount of estrogen and progestogen that is compatible with a low failure rate and individual patient needs.
[See table III below.]

3. CARCINOMA OF THE REPRODUCTIVE ORGANS AND BREASTS
Numerous epidemiological studies have been performed on the incidence of breast, endometrial, ovarian and cervical cancer in women using oral contraceptives. While there are conflicting reports most studies suggest that the use of oral contraceptives is not associated with an overall increase in the risk of developing breast cancer. Some studies have reported an increased relative risk of developing breast cancer, particularly at a younger age. This increased relative risk appears to be related to duration of use[36–43,79–89].
Some studies suggest that oral contraceptive use has been associated with an increase in the risk of cervical intraepithelial neoplasia in some populations of women[45–48]. However, there continues to be controversy about the extent to which such findings may be due to differences in sexual behavior and other factors.

4. HEPATIC NEOPLASIA
Benign hepatic adenomas are associated with oral contraceptive use, although the incidence of benign tumors is rare in the United States. Indirect calculations have estimated the attributable risk to be in the range of 3.3 cases/100,000 for users, a risk that increases after four or more years of use especially with oral contraceptives of higher dose[49]. Rupture of rare, benign, hepatic adenomas may cause death through intra-abdominal hemorrhage[50,51].
Studies from Britain have shown an increased risk of developing hepatocellular carcinoma[52–54] in long-term (>8 years) oral contraceptive users. However, these cancers are rare in the U.S. and the attributable risk (the excess incidence) of

TABLE III—ANNUAL NUMBER OF BIRTH-RELATED OR METHOD-RELATED DEATHS ASSOCIATED WITH CONTROL OF FERTILITY PER 100,000 NON-STERILE WOMEN, BY FERTILITY CONTROL METHOD ACCORDING TO AGE

Method of control and outcome	15–19	20–24	25–29	30–34	35–39	40–44
No fertility control methods*	7.0	7.4	9.1	14.8	25.7	28.2
Oral contraceptives non-smoker**	0.3	0.5	0.9	1.9	13.8	31.6
Oral contraceptives smoker**	2.2	3.4	6.6	13.5	51.1	117.2
IUD**	0.8	0.8	1.0	1.0	1.4	1.4
Condom*	1.1	1.6	0.7	0.2	0.3	0.4
Diaphragm/spermicide*	1.9	1.2	1.2	1.3	2.2	2.8
Periodic abstinence*	2.5	1.6	1.6	1.7	2.9	3.6

* Deaths are birth-related
** Deaths are method-related

Adapted from H.W. Ory, ref. #35.

liver cancers in oral contraceptive users approaches less than one per million users.

5. OCULAR LESIONS
There have been clinical case reports of retinal thrombosis associated with the use of oral contraceptives. Oral contraceptives should be discontinued if there is unexplained partial or complete loss of vision; onset of proptosis or diplopia; papilledema; or retinal vascular lesions. Appropriate diagnostic and therapeutic measures should be undertaken immediately.

6. ORAL CONTRACEPTIVE USE BEFORE OR DURING EARLY PREGNANCY
Extensive epidemiological studies have revealed no increased risk of birth defects in women who have used oral contraceptives prior to pregnancy[56-57]. The majority of recent studies also do not indicate a teratogenic effect, particularly in so far as cardiac anomalies and limb reduction defects are concerned[55,56,58,59], when oral contraceptives are taken inadvertently during early pregnancy.

The administration of oral contraceptives to induce withdrawal bleeding should not be used as a test for pregnancy. Oral contraceptives should not be used during pregnancy to treat threatened or habitual abortion.

It is recommended that for any patient who has missed two consecutive periods, pregnancy should be ruled out before continuing oral contraceptive use. If the patient has not adhered to the prescribed schedule, the possibility of pregnancy should be considered at the time of the first missed period. Oral contraceptive use should be discontinued until pregnancy is ruled out.

7. GALLBLADDER DISEASE
Earlier studies have reported an increased lifetime relative risk of gallbladder surgery in users of oral contraceptives and estrogens[60,61]. More recent studies, however, have shown that the relative risk of developing gallbladder disease among oral contraceptive users may be minimal[62-64]. The recent findings of minimal risk may be related to the use of oral contraceptive formulations containing lower hormonal doses of estrogens and progestogens.

8. CARBOHYDRATE AND LIPID METABOLIC EFFECTS
Oral contraceptives have been shown to cause a decrease in glucose tolerance in a significant percentage of users[17]. This effect has been shown to be directly related to estrogen dose[65]. In general, progestogens increase insulin secretion and create insulin resistance, this effect varying with different progestational agents[17,66]. In the nondiabetic woman, oral contraceptives appear to have no effect on fasting blood glucose[67]. Because of these demonstrated effects, prediabetic and diabetic women should be carefully monitored while taking oral contraceptives.

A small proportion of women will have persistent hypertriglyceridemia while on the pill. As discussed earlier (see WARNINGS 1.a. and 1.d.), changes in serum triglycerides and lipoprotein levels have been reported in oral contraceptive users.

9. ELEVATED BLOOD PRESSURE
An increase in blood pressure has been reported in women taking oral contraceptives[68] and this increase is more likely in older oral contraceptive users[69] and with extended duration of use[61]. Data from the Royal College of General Practitioners[12] and subsequent randomized trials have shown that the incidence of hypertension increases with increasing progestational activity.

Women with a history of hypertension or hypertension-related diseases, or renal disease[70] should be encouraged to use another method of contraception. If women elect to use oral contraceptives, they should be monitored closely and if significant elevation of blood pressure occurs, oral contraceptives should be discontinued. For most women, elevated blood pressure will return to normal after stopping oral contraceptives[69], and there is no difference in the occurrence of hypertension among former and never users[68,70,71].

10. HEADACHE
The onset or exacerbation of migraine or development of headache with a new pattern which is recurrent, persistent or severe requires discontinuation of oral contraceptives and evaluation of the cause.

11. BLEEDING IRREGULARITIES
Breakthrough bleeding and spotting are sometimes encountered in patients on oral contraceptives, especially during the first three months of use. Nonhormonal causes should be considered and adequate diagnostic measures taken to rule out malignancy or pregnancy in the event of breakthrough bleeding, as in the case of any abnormal vaginal bleeding. If pathology has been excluded, time or a change to another formulation may solve the problem. In the event of amenorrhea, pregnancy should be ruled out.

Some women may encounter post-pill amenorrhea or oligomenorrhea, especially when such a condition was pre-existent.

12. ECTOPIC PREGNANCY
Ectopic as well as intrauterine pregnancy may occur in contraceptive failures.

PRECAUTIONS
1. PHYSICAL EXAMINATION AND FOLLOW UP
It is good medical practice for all women to have annual history and physical examinations, including women using oral contraceptives. The physical examination, however, may be deferred until after initiation of oral contraceptives if requested by the woman and judged appropriate by the clinician. The physical examination should include special reference to blood pressure, breasts, abdomen and pelvic organs, including cervical cytology, and relevant laboratory tests. In case of undiagnosed, persistent or recurrent abnormal vaginal bleeding, appropriate measures should be conducted to rule out malignancy. Women with a strong family history of breast cancer or who have breast nodules should be monitored with particular care.

2. LIPID DISORDERS
Women who are being treated for hyperlipidemias should be followed closely if they elect to use oral contraceptives. Some progestogens may elevate LDL levels and may render the control of hyperlipidemias more difficult.

3. LIVER FUNCTION
If jaundice develops in any woman receiving such drugs, the medication should be discontinued. Steroid hormones may be poorly metabolized in patients with impaired liver function.

4. FLUID RETENTION
Oral contraceptives may cause some degree of fluid retention. They should be prescribed with caution, and only with careful monitoring, in patients with conditions which might be aggravated by fluid retention.

5. EMOTIONAL DISORDERS
Women with a history of depression should be carefully observed and the drug discontinued if depression recurs to a serious degree.

6. CONTACT LENSES
Contact lens wearers who develop visual changes or changes in lens tolerance should be assessed by an ophthalmologist.

7. DRUG INTERACTIONS
Reduced efficacy and increased incidence of breakthrough bleeding and menstrual irregularities have been associated with concomitant use of rifampin. A similar association, though less marked, has been suggested with barbiturates, phenylbutazone, phenytoin sodium, carbamazepine and possibly with griseofulvin, ampicillin and tetracyclines[72].

8. INTERACTIONS WITH LABORATORY TESTS
Certain endocrine and liver function tests and blood components may be affected by oral contraceptives:
a. Increased prothrombin and factors VII, VIII, IX and X; decreased antithrombin 3; increased norepinephrine-induced platelet aggregability.
b. Increased thyroid binding globulin (TBG) leading to increased circulating total thyroid hormone, as measured by protein-bound iodine (PBI), T4 by column or by radioimmunoassay. Free T3 resin uptake is decreased, reflecting the elevated TBG; free T4 concentration is unaltered.
c. Other binding proteins may be elevated in serum.
d. Sex hormone binding globulins are increased and result in elevated levels of total circulating sex steroids however, free or biologically active levels either decrease or remain unchanged.
e. High-density lipoprotein (HDL-C) and triglycerides may be increased, while low-density lipoprotein cholesterol (LDL-C) and total cholesterol (Total-C) may be decreased or unchanged.
f. Glucose tolerance may be decreased.
g. Serum folate levels may be depressed by oral contraceptive therapy. This may be of clinical significance if a woman becomes pregnant shortly after discontinuing oral contraceptives.

9. CARCINOGENESIS
See WARNINGS section.

10. PREGNANCY
Pregnancy Category X. See CONTRAINDICATIONS and WARNINGS sections.

11. NURSING MOTHERS
Small amounts of oral contraceptive steroids have been identified in the milk of nursing mothers and a few adverse effects on the child have been reported, including jaundice and breast enlargement. In addition, oral contraceptives given in the postpartum period may interfere with lactation by decreasing the quantity and quality of breast milk. If possible, the nursing mother should be advised not to use oral contraceptives but to use other forms of contraception until she has completely weaned her child.

12. SEXUALLY TRANSMITTED DISEASES
Patients should be counseled that this product does not provide against HIV infection (AIDS) and other sexually transmitted diseases.

INFORMATION FOR THE PATIENT
See Patient Labeling Printed Below

ADVERSE REACTIONS
An increased risk of the following serious adverse reactions has been associated with the use of oral contraceptives (see WARNINGS section).

- Thrombophlebitis and venous thrombosis with or without embolism
- Arterial thromboembolism
- Pulmonary embolism
- Myocardial infarction
- Cerebral hemorrhage
- Cerebral thrombosis
- Hypertension
- Gall bladder disease
- Hepatic adenomas or benign liver tumors

The following adverse reactions have been reported in patients receiving oral contraceptives and are believed to be drug-related:
- Nausea
- Vomiting
- Gastrointestinal symptoms (such as abdominal cramps and bloating)
- Breakthrough bleeding
- Spotting
- Change in menstrual flow
- Amenorrhea
- Temporary infertility after discontinuation of treatment
- Edema
- Melasma which may persist
- Breast changes: tenderness, enlargement, secretion
- Change in weight (increase or decrease)
- Change in cervical erosion and secretion
- Diminution in lactation when given immediately postpartum
- Cholestatic jaundice
- Migraine
- Rash (allergic)
- Mental depression
- Reduced tolerance to carbohydrates
- Vaginal candidiasis
- Change in corneal curvature (steepening)
- Intolerance to contact lenses

The following adverse reactions have been reported in users of oral contraceptives and the association has been neither confirmed nor refuted:
- Pre-menstrual syndrome
- Cataracts
- Changes in appetite
- Cystitis-like syndrome
- Headache
- Nervousness
- Dizziness
- Hirsutism
- Loss of scalp hair
- Erythema multiforme
- Erythema nodosum
- Hemorrhagic eruption
- Vaginitis
- Porphyria
- Impaired renal function
- Hemolytic uremic syndrome
- Acne
- Changes in libido
- Colitis
- Budd-Chiari Syndrome

OVERDOSAGE
Serious ill effects have not been reported following acute ingestion of large doses of oral contraceptives by young children. Overdosage may cause nausea, and withdrawal bleeding may occur in females.

NON-CONTRACEPTIVE HEALTH BENEFITS
The following non-contraceptive health benefits related to the use of oral contraceptives are supported by epidemiological studies which largely utilized oral contraceptive formulations containing estrogen doses exceeding 0.035 mg of ethinyl estradiol or 0.05 mg of mestranol[73-78].
Effects on menses:
- increased menstrual cycle regularity
- decreased blood loss and decreased incidence of iron deficiency anemia
- decreased incidence of dysmenorrhea
Effects related to inhibition of ovulation:
- decreased incidence of functional ovarian cysts
- decreased incidence of ectopic pregnancies
Effects from long-term use:
- decreased incidence of fibroadenomas and fibrocystic disease of the breast
- decreased incidence of acute pelvic inflammatory disease
- decreased incidence of endometrial cancer
- decreased incidence of ovarian cancer

DOSAGE AND ADMINISTRATION
To achieve maximum contraceptive effectiveness, ORTHO-CEPT must be taken exactly as directed and at intervals not exceeding 24 hours. ORTHO-CEPT is available in the DIALPAK® Tablet Dispenser which is preset for a Sunday Start. Day 1 start is also provided.

Continued on next page

Ortho—Cont.

21-Day Regimen (Day 1 Start)

The dosage of ORTHO-CEPT 21 for the initial cycle of therapy is one tablet administered daily from the 1st day through the 21st day of the menstrual cycle, counting the first day of menstrual flow as "Day 1". For subsequent cycles, no tablets are taken for 7 days, then a new course is started of one tablet a day for 21 days. The dosage regimen then continues with 7 days of no medication, followed by 21 days of medication, instituting a three-weeks-on, one-week-off dosage regimen.

The use of ORTHO-CEPT 21 for contraception may be initiated 4 weeks postpartum in women who elect not to breast feed. When the tablets are administered during the postpartum period, the increased risk of thromboembolic disease associated with the postpartum period must be considered. (See CONTRAINDICATIONS and WARNINGS concerning thromboembolic disease. See also PRECAUTIONS for "Nursing Mothers".) If the patient starts on ORTHO-CEPT postpartum, and has not yet had a period, she should be instructed to use another method of contraception until an orange tablet has been taken daily for 7 days. The possibility of ovulation and conception prior to initiation of medication should be considered. If the patient misses one (1) active tablet in Weeks 1, 2, or 3, the tablet should be taken as soon as she remembers. If the patient misses two (2) active tablets in Week 1 or Week 2, the patient should take two (2) tablets the day she remembers and two (2) tablets the next day; and then continue taking one (1) tablet a day until she finishes the pack. The patient should be instructed to use a back-up method of birth control if she has sex in the seven (7) days after missing pills. If the patient misses two (2) active tablets in the third week or misses three (3) or more active tablets in a row, the patient should throw out the rest of the pack and start a new pack that same day. The patient should be instructed to use a back-up method of birth control if she has sex in the seven (7) days after missing pills.

21-Day Regimen (Sunday Start)

When taking ORTHO-CEPT 21, the first orange tablet should be taken on the first Sunday after menstruation begins. If period begins on Sunday, the first orange tablet is taken on that day. If switching directly from another oral contraceptive, the first orange tablet should be taken on the first Sunday after the last ACTIVE tablet of the previous product. One orange tablet is taken daily for 21 days. For subsequent cycles, no tablets are taken for seven days, then a new course is started of one tablet a day for 21 days instituting a 3-weeks-on, one-week-off dosage regimen. When initiating a Sunday start regimen, another method of contraception should be used until after the first 7 consecutive days of administration.

The use of ORTHO-CEPT 21 for contraception may be initiated 4 weeks postpartum in women who elect not to breast feed. When the tablets are administered during the postpartum period, the increased risk of thromboembolic disease associated with the postpartum period must be considered. (See CONTRAINDICATIONS and WARNINGS concerning thromboembolic disease. See also PRECAUTIONS for "Nursing Mothers".) If the patient starts on ORTHO-CEPT postpartum, and has not yet had a period, she should be instructed to use another method of contraception until an orange tablet has been taken daily for 7 days. The possibility of ovulation and conception prior to initiation of medication should be considered. If the patient misses one (1) active tablet in Weeks 1, 2, or 3, the tablet should be taken as soon as she remembers. If the patient misses two (2) active tablets in Week 1 or Week 2, the patient should take two (2) tablets the day she remembers and two (2) tablets the next day; and then continue taking one (1) tablet a day until she finishes the pack. The patient should be instructed to use a back-up method of birth control if she has sex in the seven (7) days after missing pills. If the patient misses two (2) active tablets in the third week or misses three (3) or more tablets in a row, the patient should continue taking one tablet every day until Sunday. On Sunday the patient should throw out the rest of the pack and start a new pack that same day. The patient should be instructed to use a back-up method of birth control if she has sex in the seven (7) days after missing pills.

28-Day Regimen (Day 1 Start)

The dosage of ORTHO-CEPT 28 for the initial cycle of therapy is one tablet administered daily from the 1st day through 21st day of the menstrual cycle, counting the first day of menstrual flow as "Day 1". Tablets are taken without interruption as follows: One orange tablet daily for 21 days, then one green tablet daily for 7 days. After 28 tablets have been taken, a new course is started and an orange tablet is taken the next day.

The use of ORTHO-CEPT 28 for contraception may be initiated 4 weeks postpartum in women who elect not to breast feed. When the tablets are administered during the postpartum period, the increased risk of thromboembolic disease associated with the postpartum period must be considered. (See CONTRAINDICATIONS and WARNINGS concerning thromboembolic disease. See also PRECAUTIONS for "Nursing Mothers".) If the patient starts on ORTHO-CEPT postpartum, and has not yet had a period, she should be instructed to use another method of contraception until an orange tablet has been taken daily for 7 days. The possibility of ovulation and conception prior to initiation of medication should be considered. If the patient misses one (1) active tablet in Weeks 1, 2, or 3, the tablet should be taken as soon as she remembers. If the patient misses two (2) active tablets in Week 1 or Week 2, the patient should take two (2) tablets the day she remembers and two (2) tablets the next day; and then continue taking one (1) tablet a day until she finishes the pack. The patient should be instructed to use a back-up method of birth control if she has sex in the seven (7) days after missing pills. If the patient misses two (2) active tablets in the third week or misses three (3) or more active tablets in a row, the patient should throw out the rest of the pack and start a new pack that same day. The patient should be instructed to use a back-up method of birth control if she has sex in the seven (7) days after missing pills.

28-Day Regimen (Sunday Start)

When taking ORTHO-CEPT 28, the first orange tablet should be taken on the first Sunday after menstruation begins. If period begins on Sunday, the first orange tablet is taken on that day. If switching directly from another oral contraceptive, the first orange tablet should be taken on the first Sunday after the last ACTIVE tablet of the previous product. Tablets are taken without interruption as follows: One orange tablet daily for 21 days, then one green tablet daily for 7 days. After 28 tablets have been taken, a new course is started and an orange tablet is taken the next day (Sunday). When initiating a Sunday start regimen, another method of contraception should be used until after the first 7 consecutive days of administration.

The use of ORTHO-CEPT 28 for contraception may be initiated 4 weeks postpartum. When the tablets are administered during the postpartum period, the increased risk of thromboembolic disease associated with the postpartum period must be considered. (See CONTRAINDICATIONS and WARNINGS concerning thromboembolic disease. See also PRECAUTIONS for "Nursing Mothers".) If the patient starts on ORTHO-CEPT postpartum, and has not yet had a period, she should be instructed to use another method of contraception until an orange tablet has been taken daily for 7 days. The possibility of ovulation and conception prior to initiation of medication should be considered. If the patient misses one (1) active tablet in Weeks 1, 2, or 3, the tablet should be taken as soon as she remembers. If the patient misses two (2) active tablets in Week 1 or Week 2, the patient should take two (2) tablets the day she remembers and two (2) tablets the next day; and then continue taking one (1) tablet a day until she finishes the pack. The patient should be instructed to use a back-up method of birth control if she has sex in the seven (7) days after missing pills. If the patient misses two (2) active tablets in the third week or misses three (3) or more tablets in a row, the patient should continue taking one tablet every day until Sunday. On Sunday the patient should throw out the rest of the pack and start a new pack that same day. The patient should be instructed to use a back-up method of birth control if she has sex in the seven (7) days after missing pills.

ALL ORAL CONTRACEPTIVES

Breakthrough bleeding, spotting, and amenorrhea are frequent reasons for patients discontinuing oral contraceptives. In breakthrough bleeding, as in all cases of irregular bleeding from the vagina, nonfunctional causes should be borne in mind. In undiagnosed persistent or recurrent abnormal bleeding from the vagina, adequate diagnostic measures are indicated to rule out pregnancy or malignancy. If pathology has been excluded, time or a change to another formulation may solve the problem. Changing to an oral contraceptive with a higher estrogen content, while potentially useful in minimizing menstrual irregularity, should be done only if necessary since this may increase the risk of thromboembolic disease.

Use of oral contraceptives in the event of a missed menstrual period:

1. If the patient has not adhered to the prescribed schedule, the possibility of pregnancy should be considered at the time of the first missed period and oral contraceptive use should be discontinued until pregnancy is ruled out.
2. If the patient has adhered to the prescribed regimen and misses two consecutive periods, pregnancy should be ruled out before continuing oral contraceptive use.

HOW SUPPLIED

ORTHO-CEPT® 21 Tablets are available in a DIALPAK® Tablet Dispenser (NDC 0062-1796-15) containing 21 orange tablets (0.15 mg desogestrel and 0.03 mg ethinyl estradiol) which are unscored with "ORTHO" on one side and "D 150" on the opposite side.

ORTHO-CEPT 21 is available for clinic usage in a VERIDATE® Tablet Dispenser (unfilled) and VERIDATE Refills (NDC 0062-1795-20).

ORTHO-CEPT 28 Tablets are available in a DIALPAK Tablet Dispenser (NDC 0062-1796-15) containing 28 tablets, as follows: 21 orange tablets as described under ORTHO-CEPT 21, and 7 green tablets containing inert ingredients.

ORTHO-CEPT 28 is available for clinic usage in a VERIDATE Tablet Dispenser (unfilled) and VERIDATE Refills (NDC 0062-1796-20).

STORAGE: Store before 86° F (30° C).

CAUTION

Federal law prohibits dispensing without prescription.

REFERENCES

1. Hatcher, RA, et al. 1994 Contraceptive Technology. Sixteenth Edition. New York; Irvington Publisher. **2.** Stadel BV. Oral contraceptives and cardiovascular disease. (Pt. 1). N Engl J Med 1981; 305:612–618. **3.** Stadel BV. Oral contraceptives and cardiovascular disease. (Pt. 2). N Engl J Med 1981; 305:672–677. **4.** Adam SA, Thorogood M. Oral contraception and myocardial infarction revisited: the effects of new preparations and prescribing patterns. Br J Obstet and Gynecol 1981; 88:838–845. **5.** Mann JI, Inman WH. Oral contraceptives and death from myocardial infarction. Br Med J 1975; 2(5965):245–248. **6.** Mann JI, Vessey MP, Thorogood M. Doll R. Myocardial infarction in young women with special reference to oral contraceptive practice. Br Med J 1975; 2(5956):241–245. **7.** Royal College of General Practitioners' Oral Contraception Study: Further analyses of mortality in oral contraceptive users. Lancet 1981;1:541–546. **8.** Slone D, Shapiro S, Kaufman DW, Rosenberg L, Miettinen OS, Stolley PD. Risk of myocardial infarction in relation to current and discontinued use of oral contraceptives. N Engl J Med 1981; 305:420–424. **9.** Vessey MP. Female hormones and vascular disease—an epidemiological overview. Br J Fam Plann 1980; 6:1–12. **10.** Russell-Briefel RG, Ezzati TM. Fulwood R, Perlman JA, Murphy RS. Cardiovascular risk status and oral contraceptive use, United States, 1976–80. Prevent Med 1986; 15:352–362. **11.** Goldbaum GM, Kendrick JS, Hogelin GC, Gentry EM. The relative impact of smoking and oral contraceptive use on women in the United States. JAMA 1987; 258:1339–1342. **12.** Layde PM, Beral V. Further analyses of mortality in oral contraceptive users: Royal College General Practitioners' Oral Contraception Study. (Table 5) Lancet 1981; 1:541–546. **13.** Knopp RH. Arteriosclerosis risk: the roles of oral contraceptives and postmenopausal estrogens. J Reprod Med 1986; 31(9) (Supplement):913–921. **14.** Krauss RM, Roy S, Mishell DR, Casagrande J, Pike MC. Effects of two low-dose oral contraceptives on serum lipids and lipoproteins: Differential changes in high-density lipoproteins subclasses. Am J Obstet 1983; 145:446–452. **15.** Wahl P, Walden C, Knopp R, Hoover J, Wallace R, Heiss G, Rifkind B. Effect of estrogen/progestin potency on lipid/lipoprotein cholesterol. N Engl J Med 1983; 308:862–867. **16.** Wynn V, Niththyananthan R. The effect of progestin in combined oral contraceptives on serum lipids with special reference to high-density lipoproteins. Am J Obstet Gynecol 1982; 142:766–771. **17.** Wynn V, Godsland I. Effects of oral contraceptives and carbohydrate metabolism. J Reprod Med 1986; 31 (9) (Supplement):892–897. **18.** LaRosa JC, Atherosclerotic risk factors in cardiovascular disease. J Reprod Med 1986;31 (9) (Supplement):906–912. **19.** Inman WH, Vessey MP. Investigation of death from pulmonary, coronary, and cerebral thrombosis and embolism in women of childbearing age. Br Med J 1968; 2 (5599):193–199. **20.** Maguire MG, Tonascia J, Sartwell PE, Stolley PD, Tockman MS. Increased risk of thrombosis due to oral contraceptives: a further report. Am J Epidemiol 1979; 110(2):188–195. **21.** Pettiti DB, Wingerd J, Pellegrin F, Ramacharan S. Risk of vascular disease in women: smoking, oral contraceptives, noncontraceptive estrogens, and other factors. JAMA 1979; 242:1150–1154. **22.** Vessey MP, Doll R. Investigation of relation between use of oral contraceptives and thromboembolic disease. Br Med J 1968; 2(5599):199–205. **23.** Vessey MP, Doll R. Investigation of relation between use of oral contraceptives and thromboembolic disease. A further report. Br Med J 1969; 2 (5658):651–657. **24.** Porter JB, Hunter JR, Danielson DA, Jick H, Stergachis A. Oral contraceptives and nonfatal vascular disease—recent experience. Obstet Gynecol 1982; 59 (3):299–302. **25.** Vessey M, Doll R, Peto R. Johnson B, Wiggins P. A long-term follow-up study of women using different methods of contraception: an interim report. J Biosocial Sci 1976; 8:375–427. **26.** Royal College of General Practitioners: Oral contraceptives, venous thrombosis, and varicose veins. J Royal Coll Gen Pract 1978; 28:393–399. **27.** Collaborative Group for the Study of Stroke in Young Women: Oral contraception and increased risk of cerebral ischemia or thrombosis. N Engl J Med 1973; 288:871–878. **28.** Petitti DB, Wingerd J. Use of oral contraceptives, cigarette smoking, and risk of subarachnoid hemorrhage. Lancet 1978; 2:234–236. **29.** Inman WH. Oral contraceptives and fatal subarachnoid hemorrhage. Br Med J 1979; 2 (6203):1468–70. **30.** Collaborative Group for the study of Stroke in Young Women: Oral contraceptives and stroke in young women: associated risk factors. JAMA 1975; 231:718–722. **31.** Inman WH, Vessey MP, Westerholm B, Engelund A. Thromboembolic disease and the steroidal con-

tent of oral contraceptives. A report to the Committee on Safety of Drugs. Br Med J 1970; 2:203–209. 32. Meade TW, Greenberg G, Thompson SG. Progestogens and cardiovascular reactions associated with oral contraceptives and a comparison of the safety of 50- and 35-mcg oestrogen preparations. Br Med J 1980; 280 (6224):1157–1161. 33. Kay, CR. Progestogens and arterial disease—evidence from the Royal College of General Practitioners' Study. Am J Obstet Gynecol 1982; 142:762–765. 34. Royal College of General Practitioners: Incidence of arterial disease among oral contraceptive users. J Royal Coll Gen Pract 1983; 33:75–82. 35. Ory HW. Mortality associated with fertility and fertility control: 1983. Family Planning Perspectives 1983; 15:50–56. 36. The Cancer and Steroid Hormone Study of the Centers for Disease Control and the National Institute of Child Health and Human Development: Oral-contraceptive use and the risk of breast cancer. N Engl J Med 1986; 315:405–411. 37. Pike MC, Henderson BE, Krailo MD, Duke A, Roy S. Breast cancer risk in young women and use of oral contraceptives: possible modifying effect of formulation and age at use. Lancet 1983; 2:926–929. 38. Paul C, Skegg DG, Spears GFS, Kaldor JM. Oral contraceptives and breast cancer: A national study. Br Med J 1986; 293:723–725. 39. Miller DR, Rosenberg L, Kaufman DW, Schottenfeld D, Stolley PD, Shapiro S. Breast cancer risk in relation to early oral contraceptive use. Obstet Gynecol 1986; 68:863–868. 40. Olson H, Olson KL, Moller TR, Ranstam J, Holm P. Oral contraceptive use and breast cancer in young women in Sweden (letter). Lancet 1985; 2:748–749. 41. McPherson K, Vessey M, Neil A, Doll R, Jones L, Roberts M. Early contraceptive use and breast cancer: Results of another case-control study. Br J Cancer 1987; 56:653–660. 42. Huggins GR, Zucker PF. Oral contraceptives and neoplasia: 1987 update. Fertil Steril 1987; 47:733–761. 43. McPherson K, Drife JO. The pill and breast cancer: why the uncertainty? Br Med J 1986; 293:709–710. 44. Shapiro S. Oral contraceptives—time to take stock. N Engl J Med 1987; 315:450–451. 45. Ory H, Naib Z, Conger SB, Hatcher RA, Tyler CW. Contraceptive choice and prevalence of cervical dysplasia and carcinoma in situ. Am J Obstet Gynecol 1976;124:573–577. 46. Vessey MP, Lawless M, McPherson K, Yeates D. Neoplasia of the cervix uteri and contraception: a possible adverse effect of the pill. Lancet 1983; 2:930. 47. Brinton LA, Huggins GR, Lehman HF, Malli K, Savitz DA, Trapido E, Rosenthal J, Hoover R. Long term use of oral contraceptives and risk of invasive cervical cancer. Int J Cancer 1986; 38:339–344. 48. WHO Collaborative Study of Neoplasia and Steroid Contraceptives: Invasive cervical cancer and combined oral contraceptives. Br Med J 1985; 290:961–965. 49. Rooks JB, Ory HW, Ishak KG, Strauss LT, Greenspan JR, Hill AP, Tyler CW. Epidemiology of hepatocellular adenoma: the role of oral contraceptive use. JAMA 1979; 242:644–648. 50. Bein NN, Goldsmith HS. Recurrent massive hemorrhage from benign hepatic tumors secondary to oral contraceptives. Br J Surg 1977; 64:433–435. 51. Klatskin G. Hepatic tumors: possible relationship to use of oral contraceptives. Gastroenterology 1977; 73:386–394. 52. Henderson BE, Preston-Martin S, Edmondson HA, Peters RL, Pike MC. Hepatocellular carcinoma and oral contraceptives. Br J Cancer 1983; 48:437–440. 53. Neuberger J, Forman D, Doll R, Williams R. Oral contraceptives and hepatocellular carcinoma. Br Med J 1986; 292:1355–1357. 54. Forman D, Vincent TJ, Doll R. Cancer of the liver and oral contraceptives. Br Med J 1986; 292:1357–1361. 55. Harlap S, Eldor J. Births following oral contraceptive failures. Obstet Gynecol 1980; 55:447–452. 56. Savolainen E, Saksela E, Saxen L. Teratogenic hazards of oral national malformation register. Am J Obstet Gynecol 1981; 140:521–524. 57. Janerich DT, Piper JM, Glebatis DM. Oral contraceptives and birth defects. Am J Epidemiol 1980; 112:73–79. 58. Ferencz C, Matanoski GM, Wilson PD, Rubin JD, Neill CA, Gutberlet R. Maternal hormone therapy and congenital heart disease. Teratology 1980; 21:225–239. 59. Rothman KJ, Fyler DC, Goldblatt A, Kreidberg MB. Exogenous hormones and other drug exposures of children with congenital heart disease. Am J Epidemiol 1979; 109:433–439. 60. Boston Collaborative Drug Surveillance Program: Oral contraceptives and venous thromboembolic disease, surgically confirmed gall-bladder disease, and breast tumors. Lancet 1973; 1:1399–1404. 61. Royal College of General Practitioners: Oral contraceptives and health. New York, Pittman, 1974. 62. Layde PM, Vessey MP, Yeates D. Risk of gall bladder disease: a cohort study of young women attending family planning clinics. J Epidemiol Community Health 1982; 36:274–278. 63. Rome Group for the Epidemiology and Prevention of Cholelithiasis (GREPCO): Prevalence of gallstone disease in an Italian adult female population. Am J Epidemiol 1984; 119:796–805. 64. Strom BL, Tamragouri RT, Morse ML, Lazar EL, West SL, Stolley PD, Jones JK. Oral contraceptives and other risk factors for gall bladder disease. Clin Pharmacol Ther 1986; 39:335–341. 65. Wynn V, Adams PW, Godsland IF, Melrose J, Niththyananthan R, Oakley NW, Seedj A. Comparison of effects of different combined oral-contraceptive formulations on carbohydrate and lipid metabolism. Lancet 1979; 1:1045–1049. 66. Wynn V. Effect of progesterone and progestins on carbohydrate metabolism. In Progesterone and Progestin. Edited by Bardin CW, Milgrom

E, Mauvis-Jarvis P. New York, Raven Press, 1983 pp. 395–410. 67. Perlman JA, Roussell-Briefel RG, Ezzati TM, Lieberknecht G. Oral glucose tolerance and the potency of oral contraceptive progestogens. J Chronic Dis 1985; 38:857–864. 68. Royal College of General Practitioners' Oral Contraception Study: Effect on hypertension and benign breast disease of progestogen component in combined oral contraceptives. Lancet 1977; 1:624. 69. Fisch IR, Frank J. Oral contraceptives and blood pressure. JAMA 1977; 237:2499–2503. 70. Laragh AJ. Oral contraceptive induced hypertension—nine years later. Am J Obstet Gynecol 1976; 126:141–147. 71. Ramcharan S, Peritz E, Pellegrin FA, Williams WT. Incidence of hypertension in the Walnut Creek Contraceptive Drug Study cohort. In Pharmacology of Steroid Contraceptive Drugs. Garattini S, Berendes HW. Eds. New York, Raven Press, 1977 pp. 277–278. (Monographs of the Mario Negri Institute for Pharmacological Research, Milan). 72. Stockley I. Interactions with oral contraceptives. J Pharm 1976; 216:140–143. 73. The Cancer and Steroid Hormone Study of the Centers for Disease Control and the National Institute of Child Health and Human Development: Oral contraceptive use and the risk of ovarian cancer. JAMA 1983; 249:1596–1599. 74. The Cancer and Steroid Hormone Study of the Centers for Disease Control and the National Institute of Child Health and Human Development: Combination oral contraceptive use and the risk of endometrial cancer. JAMA 1987; 257:796–800. 75. Ory HW. Functional ovarian cysts and oral contraceptives: negative association confirmed surgically. JAMA 1974; 228:68–69. 76. Ory HW. Cole P. Macmahon B, Hoover R. Oral contraceptives and reduced risk of benign breast disease. N Engl J Med 1976; 294:419–422. 77. Ory HW. The noncontraceptive health benefits from oral contraceptive use. Fam Plann Perspect 1982; 14:182–184. 78. Ory HW, Forrest JD, Lincoln R. Making Choices: Evaluating the health risks and benefits of birth control methods. New York, The Alan Guttmacher Institute, 1983; p. 1. 79. Schlesselman J, Stadel BV, Murray P, Lai S. Breast Cancer in relation to early use of oral contraceptives 1988; 259:1828–1833. 80. Hennekens CH, Speizer FE, Lipnick RJ, Rosner B, Bain C, Belanger C, Stampfer MJ, Willett W, Peto R. A case-controlled study of oral contraceptive use and breast cancer. JNCI 1984;72:39–42. 81. LaVecchia C, Decarli A, Fasoli M, Franceschi S, Gentile A, Negri E, Parazzini F, Tognoni G. Oral contraceptives and cancers of the breast and of the female genital tract. Interim results from a case-control study. Br J Cancer 1986; 54:311–317. 82. Meirik O, Lund E, Adami H, Bergstrom R, Christoffersen T, Bergsjo P. Oral contraceptive use in breast cancer in young women. A Joint National Case-control study in Sweden and Norway. Lancet 1986; 11:650–654. 83. Kay CR, Hannaford PC. Breast cancer and the pill—A further report from the Royal College of General Practitioners' oral contraception study. Br J Cancer 1988; 58:675–680. 84. Stadel BV, Lai S, Schlesselman JJ, Murray P. Oral contraceptives and premenopausal breast cancer in nulliparous women. Contraception 1988; 38:287–299. 85. Miller DR, Rosenberg L, Kaufman DW, Stolley P, Warshauer ME, Shapiro S. Breast cancer before age 45 and oral contraceptive use: New Findings. Am J Epidemiol 1989; 129:269–280. 86. The UK National Case-Control Study Group, Oral contraceptive use and breast cancer risk in young women. Lancet 1989; 1:973–982. 87. Schlesselman JJ. Cancer of the breast and reproductive tract in relation to use of oral contraceptives. Contraception 1989; 40:1–38. 88. Vessey MP, McPherson K, Villard-Mackintosh L, Yeates D. Oral contraceptives and breast cancer: latest findings in a large cohort study. Br J Cancer 1989; 59:613–617. 89. Jick SS, Walker AM, Stergachis A, Jick H. Oral contraceptives and breast cancer. Br J Cancer 1989; 59:618–621. 90. Godsland, I et al. The effects of different formulations of oral contraceptive agents on lipid and carbohydrate metabolism. N Engl J Med 1990;323:1375–81. 91. Kloosterboer, HJ et al. Selectivity in progesterone and androgen receptor binding of progestogens used in oral contraception. Contraception, 1988;38:325–32. 92. Van der Vies, J and de Visser, J. Endocrinological studies with desogestrel. Arzneim. Forsch./Drug Res., 1983;33(l),2:231–6. 93. Data on file, Organon Inc. 94. Fotherby, K. Oral contraceptives, lipids and cardiovascular diseases. Contraception, 1985; Vol. 31; 4:367–94. 95. Lawrence, DM et al. Reduced sex hormone binding globulin and derived free testosterone levels in women with severe acne. Clinical Endocrinology, 1981; 15:87–91. 96. Cullberg, G et al. Effects of a low-dose desogestrel-ethinyl estradiol combination on hirsutism, androgens and sex hormone binding globulin in women with a polycystic ovary syndrome. Acta Obstet Gynecol Scand, 1985;64:195–202. 97. Jung-Hoffmann, C and Kuhl, H. Divergent effects of two low-dose oral contraceptives on sex hormone-binding globulin and free testosterone. AJOG, 1987; 156:199–203. 98. Hammond, G et al. Serum steroid binding protein concentrations, distribution of progestogens, and bioavailability of testosterone during treatment with contraceptives containing desogestrel or levonorgestrel. Fertil Steril, 1984;42:44–51. 99. Palatsi, R et al. Serum total and unbound testosterone and sex hormone binding globulin (SHBG) in female acne patients treated

with two different oral contraceptives. Acta Derm Venereol, 1984; 64:517–23.

BRIEF SUMMARY PATIENT PACKAGE INSERT

Oral contraceptives, also known as "birth control pills" or "the pill", are taken to prevent pregnancy, and when taken correctly, have a failure rate of about 1% per year when used without missing any pills. The typical failure rate of large numbers of pill users is less than 3% per year when women who miss pills are included. For most women, oral contraceptives are also free of serious or unpleasant side effects. However, forgetting to take pills considerably increases the chances of pregnancy.

For the majority of women, oral contraceptives can be taken safely. But there are some women who are at high risk of developing certain serious diseases that can be life-threatening or may cause temporary or permanent disability. The risks associated with taking oral contraceptives increase significantly if you:

- smoke
- have high blood pressure, diabetes, high cholesterol
- have or have had clotting disorders, heart attack, stroke, angina pectoris, cancer of the breast or sex organs, jaundice or malignant or benign liver tumors

Although cardiovascular disease risks may be increased with oral contraceptive use after age 40 in healthy, non-smoking women (even with the newer low-dose formulations), there are also greater potential health risks associated with pregnancy in older women.

You should not take the pill if you suspect you are pregnant or have unexplained vaginal bleeding.

> **Cigarette smoking increases the risk of serious cardiovascular side effects from oral contraceptive use. This risk increases with age and with heavy smoking (15 or more cigarettes per day) and is quite marked in women over 35 years of age. Women who use oral contraceptives are strongly advised not to smoke.**

Most side effects of the pill are not serious. The most common such effects are nausea, vomiting, bleeding between menstrual periods, weight gain, breast tenderness, headache, and difficulty wearing contact lenses. These side effects, especially nausea and vomiting, may subside within the first three months of use.

The serious side effects of the pill occur very infrequently, especially if you are in good health and are young. However, you should know that the following medical conditions have been associated with or made worse by the pill:

1. Blood clots in the legs (thrombophlebitis) or lungs (pulmonary embolism), stoppage or rupture of a blood vessel in the brain (stroke), blockage of blood vessels in the heart (heart attack or angina pectoris) or other organs of the body. As mentioned above, smoking increases the risk of heart attacks and strokes, and subsequent serious medical consequences.

2. Liver tumors, which may rupture and cause severe bleeding. A possible but not definite association has been found with the pill and liver cancer. However, liver cancers are extremely rare. The chance of developing liver cancer from using the pill is thus even rarer.

3. High blood pressure, although blood pressure usually returns to normal when the pill is stopped.

The symptoms associated with these serious side effects are discussed in the detailed patient labeling given to you with your supply of pills. Notify your doctor or clinic if you notice any unusual physical disturbances while taking the pill. In addition, drugs such as rifampin, as well as some anticonvulsants and some antibiotics may decrease oral contraceptive effectiveness.

There is conflict among studies regarding breast cancer and oral contraceptive use. Some studies have reported an increase in the risk of developing breast cancer, particularly at a younger age. This increased risk appears to be related to duration of use. The majority of studies have found no overall increase in the risk of developing breast cancer. Some studies have found an increase in the incidence of cancer of the cervix in women who use oral contraceptives. However, this finding may be related to factors other than the use of oral contraceptives. There is insufficient evidence to rule out the possibility that pills may cause such cancers.

Taking the pill provides some important non-contraceptive benefits. These include less painful menstruation, less menstrual blood loss and anemia, few pelvic infections, and fewer cancers of the ovary and the lining of the uterus.

Be sure to discuss any medical condition you may have with your doctor or clinic. Your doctor or clinic will take a medical and family history before prescribing oral contraceptives and will examine you. The physical examination may be delayed to another time if you request it and the health care provider believes that it is good medical practice to postpone it. You should be reexamined at least once a year while taking oral contraceptives. The detailed patient information

Continued on next page

Ortho—Cont.

labeling gives you further information which you should read and discuss with your doctor or clinic.

This product (like all oral contraceptives) is intended to prevent pregnancy. It does not protect against transmission of HIV (AIDS) and other sexually transmitted diseases such as chlamydia, genital herpes, genital warts, gonorrhea, hepatitis B, and syphilis.

DETAILED PATIENT LABELING

PLEASE NOTE: This labeling is revised from time to time as important new medical information becomes available. Therefore, please review this labeling carefully.

The following oral contraceptive products contain a combination of a progestogen and estrogen, the two kinds of female hormones:

ORTHO-CEPT® ☐ **21 Day Regimen**
ORTHO-CEPT® ☐ **28 Day Regimen**

Each orange tablet contains 0.15 mg desogestrel and 0.03 mg ethinyl estradiol. Each green tablet in the ORTHO-CEPT 28 day regimen contains inert ingredients.

INTRODUCTION

Any woman who considers using oral contraceptives (the birth control pill or the pill) should understand the benefits and risks of using this form of birth control. This patient labeling will give you much of the information you will need to make this decision and will also help you determine if you are at risk of developing any of the serious side effects of the pill. It will tell you how to use the pill properly so that it will be as effective as possible. However, this labeling is not a replacement for a careful discussion between you and your doctor or clinic. You should discuss the information provided in this labeling with him or her, both when you first start taking the pill and during your revisits. You should also follow your doctor's or clinic's advice with regard to regular check-ups while you are on the pill.

EFFECTIVENESS OF ORAL CONTRACEPTIVES

Oral contraceptives or "birth control pills" or "the pill" are used to prevent pregnancy and are more effective than other non-surgical methods of birth control. When they are taken correctly, the chance of becoming pregnant is less than 1% (1 pregnancy per 100 women per year of use) when used perfectly, without missing any pills. Typical failure rates are actually 3% per year. The chance of becoming pregnant increases with each missed pill during a menstrual cycle.

In comparison, typical failure rates for other non-surgical methods of birth control during the first year of use are as follows:

Implant: <1%
Injection: <1%
IUD: 1 to 2%
Diaphragm with spermicides: 18%
Spermicides alone: 21%
Vaginal sponge: 18 to 36%
Cervical Cap: 18 to 36%
Condom alone (male): 12%
Condom alone (female): 21%
Periodic abstinence: 20%
No methods: 85%

WHO SHOULD NOT TAKE ORAL CONTRACEPTIVES

> **Cigarette smoking increases the risk of serious cardiovascular side effects from oral contraceptive use. This risk increases with age and with heavy smoking (15 or more cigarettes per day) and is quite marked in women over 35 years of age. Women who use oral contraceptives are strongly advised not to smoke.**

Some women should not use the pill. For example, you should not take the pill if you are pregnant or think you may be pregnant. You should also not use the pill if you have any of the following conditions:

- A history of heart attack or stroke
- Blood clots in the legs (thrombophlebitis), lungs (pulmonary embolism), or eyes
- A history of blood clots in the deep veins of your legs
- Chest pain (angina pectoris)
- Known or suspected breast cancer or cancer of the lining of the uterus, cervix or vagina
- Unexplained vaginal bleeding (until a diagnosis is reached by your doctor)
- Yellowing of the whites of the eyes or of the skin (jaundice) during pregnancy or during previous use of the pill
- Liver tumor (benign or cancerous)
- Known or suspected pregnancy

Tell your doctor or clinic if you have ever had any of these conditions. Your doctor or clinic can recommend another method of birth control.

OTHER CONSIDERATIONS BEFORE TAKING ORAL CONTRACEPTIVES

Tell your doctor or clinic if you have or have had:

- Breast nodules, fibrocystic disease of the breast, an abnormal breast x-ray or mammogram
- Diabetes
- Elevated cholesterol or triglycerides
- High blood pressure
- Migraine or other headaches or epilepsy
- Mental depression
- Gallbladder, heart or kidney disease
- History of scanty or irregular menstrual periods

Women with any of these conditions should be checked often by their doctor or clinic if they choose to use oral contraceptives.

Also, be sure to inform your doctor or clinic if you smoke or are on any medications.

RISKS OF TAKING ORAL CONTRACEPTIVES

1. Risk of developing blood clots

Blood clots and blockage of blood vessels are one of the most serious side effects of taking oral contraceptives and can cause death or serious disability. In particular, a clot in the legs can cause thrombophlebitis and a clot that travels to the lungs can cause a sudden blocking of the vessel carrying blood to the lungs. Rarely, These risks are greater with desogestrel–containing oral contraceptives, such as ORTHO-CEPT, than with other low-dose pills. Rarely, clots occur in the blood vessels of the eye and may cause blindness, double vision, or impaired vision.

If you take oral contraceptives and need elective surgery, need to stay in bed for a prolonged illness or have recently delivered a baby, you may be at risk of developing blood clots. You should consult your doctor or clinic about stopping oral contraceptives three to four weeks before surgery and not taking oral contraceptives for two weeks after surgery or during bed rest. You should also not take oral contraceptives soon after delivery of a baby. It is advisable to wait for at least four weeks after delivery if you are not breast feeding or four weeks after a second trimester abortion. If you are breast feeding, you should wait until you have weaned your child before using the pill. (See also the section on Breast Feeding in General Precautions.)

The risk of circulatory disease in oral contraceptive users may be higher in users of high dose pills and may be greater with longer duration of oral contraceptive use. In addition, some of these increased risks may continue for a number of years after stopping oral contraceptives. The risk of abnormal blood clotting increases with age in both users and nonusers of oral contraceptives, but the increased risk from the oral contraceptive appears to be present at all ages. For women aged 20 to 44 it is estimated that about 1 in 2,000 using oral contraceptives will be hospitalized each year because of abnormal clotting. Among nonusers in the same age group, about 1 in 20,000 would be hospitalized each year. For oral contraceptive users in general, it has been estimated that in women between the ages of 15 and 34 the risk of death due to a circulatory disorder is about 1 in 12,000 per year, whereas for nonusers the rate is about 1 in 50,000 per year. In the age group 35 to 44, the risk is estimated to be about 1 in 2,500 per year for oral contraceptive users and about 1 in 10,000 per year for nonusers.

2. Heart attacks and strokes

Oral contraceptives may increase the tendency to develop strokes (stoppage or rupture of blood vessels in the brain) and angina pectoris and heart attacks (blockage of blood vessels in the heart). Any of these conditions can cause death or serious disability.

Smoking greatly increases the possibility of suffering heart attacks and strokes. Furthermore, smoking and the use of oral contraceptives greatly increase the chances of developing and dying of heart disease.

3. Gallbladder disease

Oral contraceptive users probably have a greater risk than nonusers of having gallbladder disease, although this risk may be related to pills containing high doses of estrogens.

4. Liver tumors

In rare cases, oral contraceptives can cause benign but dangerous liver tumors. These benign liver tumors can rupture and cause fatal internal bleeding. In addition, a possible but not definite association has been found with the pill and liver cancers in two studies, in which a few women who developed these very rare cancers were found to have used oral contraceptives for long periods. However, liver cancers are rare.

5. Cancer of the reproductive organs and breasts

There is conflict among studies regarding breast cancer and oral contraceptive use. Some studies have reported an increase in the risk of developing breast cancer, particularly at a younger age. This increased risk appears to be related to duration of use. The majority of studies have found no overall increase in the risk of developing breast cancer. Some studies have found an increase in the incidence of cancer of the cervix in women who use oral contraceptives. However, this finding may be related to factors other than the use of oral contraceptives. There is insufficient evidence to rule out the possibility that pills may cause such cancers.

ESTIMATED RISK OF DEATH FROM A BIRTH CONTROL METHOD OR PREGNANCY

All methods of birth control and pregnancy are associated with a risk of developing certain diseases which may lead to disability or death. An estimate of the number of deaths associated with different methods of birth control and pregnancy has been calculated and is shown in the following table. [See table below.]

In the above table, the risk of death from any birth control method is less than the risk of childbirth, except for oral contraceptive users over the age of 35 who smoke and pill users over the age of 40 even if they do not smoke. It can be seen in the table that for women aged 15 to 39, the risk of death was highest with pregnancy (7–26 deaths per 100,000 women, depending on age). Among pill users who do not smoke, the risk of death is always lower than that associated with pregnancy for any age group, although over the age of 40, the risk increases to 32 deaths per 100,000 women, compared to 28 associated with pregnancy at that age. However, for pill users who smoke and are over the age of 35, the estimated number of deaths exceeds those for other methods of birth control. If a woman is over the age of 40 and smokes, her estimated risk of death is four times higher (117/100,000 women) than the estimated risk associated with pregnancy (28/100,000 women) in that age group.

The suggestion that women over 40 who do not smoke should not take oral contraceptives is based on information from older, higher-dose pills. An Advisory Committee of the FDA discussed this issue in 1989 and recommended that the benefits of low-dose oral contraceptive use by healthy, non-smoking women over 40 years of age may outweigh the possible risks.

WARNING SIGNALS

If any of these adverse effects occur while you are taking oral contraceptives, call your doctor or clinic immediately:

- Sharp chest pain, coughing of blood, or sudden shortness of breath (indicating a possible clot in the lung)
- Pain in the calf (indicating a possible clot in the leg)
- Crushing chest pain or heaviness in the chest (indicating a possible heart attack)
- Sudden severe headache or vomiting, dizziness or fainting, disturbances of vision or speech, weakness, or numbness in an arm or leg (indicating a possible stroke)
- Sudden partial or complete loss of vision (indicating a possible clot in the eye)
- Breast lumps (indicating possible breast cancer or fibrocystic disease of the breast; ask your doctor or clinic to show you how to examine your breasts)
- Severe pain or tenderness in the stomach area (indicating a possibly ruptured liver tumor)
- Difficulty in sleeping, weakness, lack of energy, fatigue, or change in mood (possibly indicating severe depression)
- Jaundice or a yellowing of the skin or eyeballs, accompanied frequently by fever, fatigue, loss of appetite, dark colored urine, or light colored bowel movements (indicating possible liver problems)

SIDE EFFECTS OF ORAL CONTRACEPTIVES

1. Vaginal bleeding

Irregular vaginal bleeding or spotting may occur while you are taking the pills. Irregular bleeding may vary from slight

ANNUAL NUMBER OF BIRTH-RELATED OR METHOD-RELATED DEATHS ASSOCIATED WITH CONTROL OF FERTILITY PER 100,000 NONSTERILE WOMEN, BY FERTILITY CONTROL METHOD ACCORDING TO AGE

Method of control and outcome	15–19	20–24	25–29	30–34	35–39	40–44
No fertility control methods*	7.0	7.4	9.1	14.8	25.7	28.2
Oral contraceptives non-smoker**	0.3	0.5	0.9	1.9	13.8	31.6
Oral contraceptives smoker**	2.2	3.4	6.6	13.5	51.1	117.2
IUD**	0.8	0.8	1.0	1.0	1.4	1.4
Condom*	1.1	1.6	0.7	0.2	0.3	0.4
Diaphragm/spermicide*	1.9	1.2	1.2	1.3	2.2	2.8
Periodic abstinence*	2.5	1.6	1.6	1.7	2.9	3.6

* Deaths are birth-related
** Deaths are method-related

staining between menstrual periods to breakthrough bleeding which is a flow much like a regular period. Irregular bleeding occurs most often during the first few months of oral contraceptive use, but may also occur after you have been taking the pill for some time. Such bleeding may be temporary and usually does not indicate any serious problems. It is important to continue taking your pills on schedule. If the bleeding occurs in more than one cycle or lasts for more than a few days, talk to your doctor or clinic.

2. Contact lenses
If you wear contact lenses and notice a change in vision or an inability to wear your lenses, contact your doctor or clinic.

3. Fluid retention
Oral contraceptives may cause edema (fluid retention) with swelling of the fingers or ankles and may raise your blood pressure. If you experience fluid retention, contact your doctor or clinic.

4. Melasma
A spotty darkening of the skin is possible, particularly of the face, which may persist.

5. Other side effects
Other side effects may include nausea and vomiting, change in appetite, headache, nervousness, depression, dizziness, loss of scalp hair, rash, and vaginal infections.
If any of these side effects bother you, call your doctor or clinic.

GENERAL PRECAUTIONS

1. Missed periods and use of oral contraceptives before or during early pregnancy
There may be times when you may not menstruate regularly after you have completed taking a cycle of pills. If you have taken your pills regularly and miss one menstrual period, continue taking your pills for the next cycle but be sure to inform your doctor or clinic before doing so. If you have not taken the pills daily as instructed and missed a menstrual period, you may be pregnant. If you missed two consecutive menstrual periods, you may be pregnant. Check with your doctor or clinic immediately to determine whether you are pregnant. Do not continue to take oral contraceptives until you are sure you are not pregnant, but continue to use another method of contraception.
There is no conclusive evidence that oral contraceptive use is associated with an increase in birth defects, when taken inadvertently during early pregnancy. Previously, a few studies had reported that oral contraceptives might be associated with birth defects, but these findings have not been seen in more recent studies. Nevertheless, oral contraceptives or any other drugs should not be used during pregnancy unless clearly necessary and prescribed by your doctor or clinic. You should check with your doctor or clinic about risks to your unborn child of any medication taken during pregnancy.

2. While breast feeding
If you are breast feeding, consult your doctor or clinic before starting oral contraceptives. Some of the drug will be passed on to the child in the milk. A few adverse effects on the child have been reported, including yellowing of the skin (jaundice) and breast enlargement. In addition, oral contraceptives may decrease the amount and quality of your milk. If possible, do not use oral contraceptives while breast feeding. You should use another method of contraception since breast feeding provides only partial protection from becoming pregnant and this partial protection decreases significantly as you breast feed for longer periods of time. You should consider starting oral contraceptives only after you have weaned your child completely.

3. Laboratory tests
If you are scheduled for any laboratory tests, tell your doctor or clinic you are taking birth control pills. Certain blood tests may be affected by birth control pills.

4. Drug interactions
Certain drugs may interact with birth control pills to make them less effective in preventing pregnancy or cause an increase in breakthrough bleeding. Such drugs include rifampin, drugs used for epilepsy such as barbiturates (for example, phenobarbital), anticonvulsants such as carbamazepine (Tegretol is one brand of this drug), phenytoin (Dilantin is one brand of this drug), phenylbutazone (Butazolidin is one brand), and possibly certain antibiotics. You may need to use additional contraception when you take drugs which can make oral contraceptives less effective.

5. Sexually transmitted diseases
This product (like all oral contraceptives) is intended to prevent pregnancy. It does not protect against transmission of HIV (AIDS) and other sexually transmitted diseases such as chlamydia, genital herpes, genital warts, gonorrhea, hepatitis B, and syphilis.

HOW TO TAKE THE PILL

IMPORTANT POINTS TO REMEMBER

<u>BEFORE</u> YOU START TAKING YOUR PILLS:
1. BE SURE TO READ THESE DIRECTIONS:
Before you start taking your pills.
Anytime you are not sure what to do.
2. THE RIGHT WAY TO TAKE THE PILL IS TO TAKE ONE PILL EVERY DAY AT THE SAME TIME.
If you miss pills you could get pregnant. This includes starting the pack late. The more pills you miss, the more likely you are to get pregnant.
3. MANY WOMEN HAVE SPOTTING OR LIGHT BLEEDING, OR MAY FEEL SICK TO THEIR STOMACH DURING THE FIRST 1–3 PACKS OF PILLS. If you feel sick to your stomach, do not stop taking the pill. The problem will usually go away. If it doesn't go away, check with your doctor or clinic.
4. MISSING PILLS CAN ALSO CAUSE SPOTTING OR LIGHT BLEEDING, even when you make up these missed pills.
On the days you take 2 pills to make up for missed pills, you could also feel a little sick to your stomach.
5. IF YOU HAVE VOMITING OR DIARRHEA, for any reason, or IF YOU TAKE SOME MEDICINES, including some antibiotics, your pills may not work as well.
Use a back-up method (such as condoms, foam, or sponge) until you check with your doctor or clinic.
6. IF YOU HAVE TROUBLE REMEMBERING TO TAKE THE PILL, talk to your doctor or clinic about how to make pill-taking easier or about using another method of birth control.
7. IF YOU HAVE ANY QUESTIONS OR ARE UNSURE ABOUT THE INFORMATION IN THIS LEAFLET, call your doctor or clinic.

<u>BEFORE</u> YOU START TAKING YOUR PILLS

1. DECIDE WHAT TIME OF DAY YOU WANT TO TAKE YOUR PILL.
It is important to take it at about the same time every day.
2. LOOK AT YOUR PILL PACK TO SEE IF IT HAS 21 OR 28 PILLS:
The <u>21-pill pack</u> has 21 "active" orange pills (with hormones) to take for 3 weeks, followed by 1 week without pills.
The <u>28-pill pack</u> has 21 "active" orange pills (with hormones) to take for 3 weeks, followed by 1 week of reminder green pills (without hormones).
3. ALSO FIND:
1) where on the pack to start taking pills,
2) in what order to take the pills.
CHECK PICTURE OF PILL PACK AND ADDITIONAL INSTRUCTIONS FOR USING THIS PACKAGE IN THE BRIEF SUMMARY PATIENT PACKAGE INSERT.
4. BE SURE YOU HAVE READY AT ALL TIMES:
ANOTHER KIND OF BIRTH CONTROL (such as condoms, foam, or sponge) to use as a back-up method in case you miss pills.
AN EXTRA, FULL PILL PACK

WHEN TO START THE <u>FIRST</u> PACK OF PILLS

You have a choice of which day to start taking your first pack of pills. ORTHO-CEPT is available in the DIALPAK® Tablet Dispenser which is preset for a Sunday Start. Day 1 start is also provided. Decide with your doctor or clinic which is the best day for you. Pick a time of day which will be easy to remember.

DAY 1 START:
1. Take the first "active" orange pill of the first pack during the <u>first 24 hours of your period.</u>
2. You will not need to use a back-up method of birth control, since you are starting the pill at the beginning of your period.

SUNDAY START:
1. Take the first "active" orange pill of the first pack on the <u>Sunday after your period starts</u>, even if you are still bleeding. If your period begins on Sunday, start the pack that same day.
2. <u>Use another method of birth control</u> as a back-up method if you have sex anytime from the Sunday you start your first pack until the next Sunday (7 days). Condoms, foam, or the sponge are good back-up methods of birth control.

WHAT TO DO DURING THE MONTH

1. TAKE ONE PILL AT THE SAME TIME EVERY DAY UNTIL THE PACK IS EMPTY.
Do not skip pills even if you are spotting or bleeding between monthly periods or feel sick to your stomach (nausea).
Do not skip pills even if you do not have sex very often.
2. WHEN YOU FINISH A PACK OR SWITCH YOUR BRAND OF PILLS:
<u>21 pills:</u> Wait 7 days to start the next pack. You will probably have your period during that week. Be sure that no more than 7 days pass between 21-day packs.
<u>28 pills:</u> Start the next pack on the day after your last "reminder" pill. Do not wait any days between packs.

WHAT TO DO IF YOU MISS PILLS

If you **MISS 1** orange "active" pill:
1. Take it as soon as you remember. Take the next pill at your regular time. This means you may take 2 pills in 1 day.
2. You do not need to use a back-up birth control method if you have sex.

If you **MISS 2** orange "active" pills in a row in **WEEK 1 OR WEEK 2** of your pack:
1. Take 2 pills on the day you remember and 2 pills the next day.
2. Then take 1 pill a day until you finish the pack.
3. You MAY BECOME PREGNANT if you have sex in the <u>7 days</u> after you miss pills. You MUST use another birth control method (such as condoms, foam, or sponge) as a back-up method for those 7 days.

If you **MISS 2** orange "active" pills in a row in **THE 3RD WEEK:**
1. **If you are a Day 1 Starter:**
THROW OUT the rest of the pill pack and start a new pack that same day.
If you are a Sunday Starter:
Keep taking 1 pill every day until Sunday. On Sunday, THROW OUT the rest of the pack and start a new pack of pills that same day.
2. You may not have your period this month but this is expected. However, if you miss your period 2 months in a row, call your doctor or clinic because you might be pregnant.
3. You MAY BECOME PREGNANT if you have sex in the <u>7 days</u> after you miss pills. You MUST use another birth control method (such as condoms, foam, or sponge) as a back-up method for those 7 days.

If you **MISS 3 OR MORE** orange "active" pills in a row (during the first 3 weeks).
1. **If you are a Day 1 Starter:**
THROW OUT the rest of the pill pack and start a new pack that same day.
If you are a Sunday Starter:
Keep taking 1 pill every day until Sunday. On Sunday THROW OUT the rest of the pack and start a new pack of pills that same day.
2. You may not have your period this month but this is expected. However, if you miss your period 2 months in a row, call your doctor or clinic because you might be pregnant.
3. You MAY BECOME PREGNANT if you have sex in the <u>7 days</u> after you miss pills. You MUST use another birth control method (such as condoms, foam, or sponge) as a back-up method for those 7 days.

A REMINDER FOR THOSE ON 28-DAY PACKS:
If you forget any of the 7 green "reminder" pills in Week 4:
THROW AWAY the pills you missed.
Keep taking 1 pill each day until the pack is empty.
You do not need a back-up method.

FINALLY, IF YOU ARE STILL NOT SURE WHAT TO DO ABOUT THE PILLS YOU HAVE MISSED:
Use a BACK-UP METHOD anytime you have sex.
KEEP TAKING ONE "ACTIVE" PILL EACH DAY until you can reach your doctor or clinic.

PREGNANCY DUE TO PILL FAILURE

The incidence of pill failure resulting in pregnancy is approximately one percent (i.e., one pregnancy per 100 women per year) if taken every day as directed, but more typical failure rates are about 3%. If failure does occur, the risk to the fetus is minimal.

PREGNANCY AFTER STOPPING THE PILL

There may be some delay in becoming pregnant after you stop using oral contraceptives, especially if you had irregular menstrual cycles before you used oral contraceptives. It may be advisable to postpone conception until you begin menstruating regularly once you have stopped taking the pill and desire pregnancy.
There does not appear to be any increase in birth defects in newborn babies when pregnancy occurs soon after stopping the pill.

OVERDOSAGE

Serious ill effects have not been reported following ingestion of large doses of oral contraceptives by young children. Overdosage may cause nausea and withdrawal bleeding in females. In cases of overdosage, contact your doctor, clinic or pharmacist.

OTHER INFORMATION

Your doctor or clinic will take a medical and family history before prescribing oral contraceptives and will examine you. The physical examination may be delayed to another time if you request it and the health care provider believes that it is a good medical practice to postpone it. You should be reexamined at least once a year. Be sure to inform your doctor or clinic if there is a family history of any of the conditions listed previously in this leaflet. Be sure to keep all appoint-

Continued on next page

Ortho—Cont.

ments with your doctor or clinic because this is a time to determine if there are early signs of side effects of oral contraceptive use.

Do not use the drug for any condition other than the one for which it was prescribed. This drug has been prescribed specifically for you; do not give it to others who may want birth control pills.

HEALTH BENEFITS FROM ORAL CONTRACEPTIVES

In addition to preventing pregnancy, use of combination oral contraceptives may provide certain benefits. They are:

- menstrual cycles may become more regular
- blood flow during menstruation may be lighter and less iron may be lost. Therefore, anemia due to iron deficiency is less likely to occur.
- pain or other symptoms during menstruation may be encountered less frequently
- ectopic (tubal) pregnancy may occur less frequently
- noncancerous cysts or lumps in the breast may occur less frequently
- acute pelvic inflammatory disease may occur less frequently
- oral contraceptive use may provide some protection against developing two forms of cancer: cancer of the ovaries and cancer of the lining of the uterus.

If you want more information about birth control pills, ask your doctor, clinic or pharmacist. They have a more technical leaflet called the Professional Labeling, which you may wish to read. The professional labeling is also published in a book entitled *Physicians' Desk Reference*, available in many book stores and public libraries.

Packaged and Distributed by:
ORTHO PHARMACEUTICAL CORPORATION
Raritan, New Jersey 08869 and
Jointly Manufactured by:
ORTHO PHARMACEUTICAL CORPORATION
Raritan, New Jersey 08869 and
DIOSYNTH bv
Oss, The Netherlands
©OPC 1992   REVISED JANUARY 1996   PO7-220
631-10-840-3

Shown in Product Identification Guide, page 326

ORTHO-CYCLEN® Tablets
ORTHO TRI-CYCLEN® Tablets
(norgestimate/ethinyl estradiol)   ℞

Patients should be counseled that this product does not protect against HIV infection (AIDS) and other sexually transmitted diseases.

DESCRIPTION

Each of the following products is a combination oral contraceptive containing the progestational compound norgestimate and the estrogenic compound ethinyl estradiol.
ORTHO-CYCLEN □ 21 Tablets and ORTHO-CYCLEN □ 28 Tablets.

Each blue tablet contains 0.250 mg of the progestational compound norgestimate (18,19-Dinor-17-pregn-4-en-20-yn-3-one,17-(acetyloxy)-13-ethyl-, oxime,(17α)-(+)-) and 0.035 mg of the estrogenic compound, ethinyl estradiol (19-nor-17α-pregna,1,3,5(10)-trien-20-yne-3,17-diol). Inactive ingredients include FD & C Blue No. 2 Aluminum Lake, lactose, magnesium stearate, and pregelatinized starch.

Norgestimate

Ethinyl Estradiol

Each green tablet in the ORTHO-CYCLEN □ 28 package contains only inert ingredients, as follows: D & C Yellow No. 10 Aluminum Lake, FD & C Blue No. 2 Aluminum Lake, lactose, magnesium stearate, microcrystalline cellulose and pregelatinized starch.
ORTHO TRI-CYCLEN □ 21 Tablets and ORTHO TRI-CYCLEN □ 28 Tablets.

Each white tablet contains 0.180 mg of the progestational compound, norgestimate (18,19-Dinor-17-pregn-4-en-20-yn-3-one, 17-(acetyloxy)-13-ethyl-, oxime,(17α)-(+)-) and 0.035 mg of the estrogenic compound, ethinyl estradiol (19-nor-17α-pregna,1,3,5(10)-trien-20-yne-3,17-diol). Inactive ingredients include lactose, magnesium stearate, and pregelatinized starch.

Each light blue tablet contains 0.215 mg of the progestational compound norgestimate (18,19-Dinor-17-pregn-4-en-20-yn-3-one,17-(acetyloxy)-13-ethyl-,oxime,(17α)-(+)-) and 0.035 mg of the estrogenic compound, ethinyl estradiol (19-nor-17α-pregna,1,3,5(10)-trien-20-yne-3,17-diol). Inactive ingredients include FD & C Blue No. 2 Aluminum Lake, lactose, magnesium stearate, and pregelatinized starch.

Each blue tablet contains 0.250 mg of the progestational compound norgestimate (18,19-Dinor-17-pregn-4-en-20-yn-3-one, 17-(acetyloxy)-13-ethyl-,oxime,(17α)-(+)-) and 0.035 mg of the estrogenic compound, ethinyl estradiol (19-nor-17α-pregna,1,3,5(10)-trien-20-yne-3,17-diol). Inactive ingredients include FD & C Blue No. 2 Aluminum Lake, lactose, magnesium stearate, and pregelatinized starch.

Each green tablet in the ORTHO TRI-CYCLEN □ 28 package contains only inert ingredients, as follows: D & C Yellow No. 10 Aluminum Lake, FD & C Blue No. 2 Aluminum Lake, lactose, magnesium stearate, microcrystalline cellulose and pregelatinized starch.

CLINICAL PHARMACOLOGY

Combination oral contraceptives act by suppression of gonadotropins. Although the primary mechanism of this action is inhibition of ovulation, other alterations include changes in the cervical mucus (which increase the difficulty of sperm entry into the uterus) and the endometrium (which reduce the likelihood of implantation).

Receptor binding studies, as well as studies in animals and humans, have shown that norgestimate and 17-deacetyl norgestimate, the major serum metabolite, combine high progestational activity with minimal intrinsic androgenicity.[90-93] Norgestimate, in combination with ethinyl estradiol, does not counteract the estrogen-induced increases in sex hormone binding globulin (SHBG), resulting in lower serum testosterone.[90,91,94]

Norgestimate and ethinyl estradiol are well absorbed following oral administration of ORTHO-CYCLEN and ORTHO TRI-CYCLEN. On the average, peak serum concentrations of norgestimate and ethinyl estradiol are observed within two

hours (0.5–2.0 hr for norgestimate and 0.75–3.0 hr for ethinyl estradiol) after administration followed by a rapid decline due to distribution and elimination. Although norgestimate serum concentrations following single or multiple dosing were generally below assay detection within 5 hours, a major norgestimate serum metabolite, 17-deacetyl norgestimate, (which exhibits a serum half-life ranging from 12 to 30 hours) appears rapidly in serum with concentrations greatly exceeding that of norgestimate. The 17-deacetylated metabolite is pharmacologically active and the pharmacologic profile is similar to that of norgestimate. The elimination half-life of ethinyl estradiol ranged from approximately 6 to 14 hours.

Both norgestimate and ethinyl estradiol are extensively metabolized and eliminated by renal and fecal pathways. Following administration of ^{14}C-norgestimate, 47% (45–49%) and 37% (16–49%) of the administered radioactivity was eliminated in the urine and feces, respectively. Unchanged norgestimate was not detected in the urine. In addition to 17-deacetyl norgestimate, a number of metabolites of norgestimate have been identified in human urine following administration of radiolabeled norgestimate. These include 18,19-Dinor-17-pregn-4-en-20-yn-3-one, 17-hydroxy-13-ethyl, (17α)-(-); 18,19-Dinor-5β-17-pregnan-20-yn,3α, 17β-dihydroxy-13-ethyl,(17α), various hydroxylated metabolites and conjugates of these metabolites. Ethinyl estradiol is metabolized to various hydroxylated products and their glucuronide and sulfate conjugates.

INDICATIONS AND USAGE

ORTHO-CYCLEN and ORTHO TRI-CYCLEN Tablets are indicated for the prevention of pregnancy in women who elect to use oral contraceptives as a method of contraception. Oral contraceptives are highly effective. Table I lists the typical accidental pregnancy rates for users of combination oral contraceptives and other methods of contraception. The efficacy of these contraceptive methods, except sterilization, depends upon the reliability with which they are used. Correct and consistent use of methods can result in lower failure rates.

[See table below.]

In clinical trials with ORTHO-CYCLEN, 1,651 subjects completed 24,272 cycles and a total of 18 pregnancies were reported. This represents an overall use-efficacy (typical user efficacy) pregnancy rate of 0.96 per 100 women-years. This rate includes patients who did not take the drug correctly. In four clinical trials with ORTHO TRI-CYCLEN, the use-efficacy pregnancy rate ranged from 0.68 to 1.47 per 100 women-years. In total, 4,756 subjects completed 45,244 cycles and a total of 42 pregnancies were reported. This represents an overall use-efficacy rate of 1.21 per 100 women-years. One of these 4 studies was a randomized comparative clinical trial in which 4,633 subjects completed 22,312 cycles. Of the 2,312 patients on ORTHO TRI-CYCLEN, 8 pregnan-

TABLE I: LOWEST EXPECTED AND TYPICAL FAILURE RATES DURING THE FIRST YEAR OF CONTINUOUS USE OF A METHOD
% of Women Experiencing an Accidental Pregnancy in the First Year of Continuous Use

Method	Lowest Expected*	Typical**
(No Contraceptive)	(85)	(85)
Oral contraceptives		3
combined	0.1	N/A***
progestin only	0.5	N/A***
Diaphragm with spermicidal cream or jelly	6	18
Spermicides alone (foams, creams, gels, jellies, vaginal suppositories, and vaginal film)	6	21
Vaginal sponge		
nulliparous	9	18
parous	20	36
Implant	0.09	0.09
Injection: depot medroxyprogesterone acetate	0.3	0.3
IUD		
progesterone	1.5	2.0
copper T 380A	0.6	0.8
Condom without spermicides		
female	5	21
male	3	12
Cervical Cap with spermicidal cream or jelly		
nulliparous	9	18
parous	26	36
Periodic abstinence (all methods)	1–9	20
Female sterilization	0.4	0.4
Male sterilization	0.10	0.15

Adapted from RA Hatcher et al, Table 5-2, (1994) ref. #1.

* The authors' best guess of the percentage of women expected to experience an accidental pregnancy among couples who initiate a method (not necessarily for the first time) and who use it consistently and correctly during the first year if they do not stop for any reason.

** This term represents "typical" couples who initiate use of a method (not necessarily for the first time), who experience an accidental pregnancy during the first year if they do not stop use for any other reason.

*** N/A—Data not available.

cies were reported. This represents an overall use-efficacy pregnancy rate of 0.94 per 100 women-years.

CONTRAINDICATIONS

Oral contraceptives should not be used in women who currently have the following conditions:

- Thrombophlebitis or thromboembolic disorders
- A past history of deep vein thrombophlebitis or thromboembolic disorders
- Cerebral vascular or coronary artery disease
- Known or suspected carcinoma of the breast
- Carcinoma of the endometrium or other known or suspected estrogen-dependent neoplasia
- Undiagnosed abnormal genital bleeding
- Cholestatic jaundice of pregnancy or jaundice with prior pill use
- Hepatic adenomas or carcinomas
- Known or suspected pregnancy

WARNINGS

> **Cigarette smoking increases the risk of serious cardiovascular side effects from oral contraceptive use. This risk increases with age and with heavy smoking (15 or more cigarettes per day) and is quite marked in women over 35 years of age. Women who use oral contraceptives should be strongly advised not to smoke.**

The use of oral contraceptives is associated with increased risk of several serious conditions including myocardial infarction, thromboembolism, stroke, hepatic neoplasia, and gallbladder disease, although the risk of serious morbidity or mortality is very small in healthy women without underlying risk factors. The risk of morbidity and mortality increases significantly in the presence of other underlying risk factors such as hypertension, hyperlipidemias, obesity and diabetes.

Practitioners prescribing oral contraceptives should be familiar with the following information relating to these risks. The information contained in this package insert is principally based on studies carried out in patients who used oral contraceptives with higher formulations of estrogens and progestogens than those in common use today. The effect of long-term use of the oral contraceptives with lower formulations of both estrogens and progestogens remains to be determined.

Throughout this labeling, epidemiological studies reported are of two types: retrospective or case control studies and prospective or cohort studies. Case control studies provide a measure of the relative risk of a disease, namely, a *ratio* of the incidence of a disease among oral contraceptive users to that among non-users. The relative risk does not provide information on the actual clinical occurrence of a disease. Cohort studies provide a measure of attributable risk, which is the *difference* in the incidence of disease between oral contraceptive users and non-users. The attributable risk does provide information about the actual occurrence of a disease in the population (adapted from refs. 2 and 3 with the author's permission). For further information, the reader is referred to a text on epidemiological methods.

1. THROMBOEMBOLIC DISORDERS AND OTHER VASCULAR PROBLEMS

a. Myocardial Infarction

An increased risk of myocardial infarction has been attributed to oral contraceptive use. This risk is primarily in smokers or women with other underlying risk factors for coronary artery disease such as hypertension, hypercholesterolemia, morbid obesity, and diabetes. The relative risk of heart attack for current oral contraceptive users has been estimated to be two to six[4–10]. The risk is very low under the age of 30. Smoking in combination with oral contraceptive use has been shown to contribute substantially to the incidence of myocardial infarctions in women in their mid-thirties or older with smoking accounting for the majority of excess

cases[11]. Mortality rates associated with circulatory disease have been shown to increase substantially in smokers, especially in those 35 years of age and older among women who use oral contraceptives.

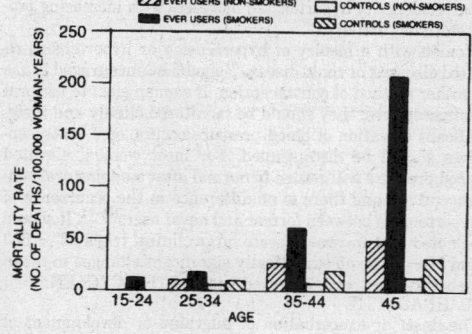

CIRCULATORY DISEASE MORTALITY RATES PER 100,000 WOMEN-YEARS BY AGE, SMOKING STATUS AND ORAL CONTRACEPTIVE USE

EVER USERS (NON-SMOKERS)   CONTROLS (NON-SMOKERS)
EVER USERS (SMOKERS)   CONTROLS (SMOKERS)

TABLE II. (Adapted from P.M. Layde and V. Beral, ref. #12.)

Oral contraceptives may compound the effects of well-known risk factors, such as hypertension, diabetes, hyperlipidemias, age and obesity[13]. In particular some progestogens are known to decrease HDL cholesterol and cause glucose intolerance, while estrogens may create a state of hyperinsulinism[14–18]. Oral contraceptives have been shown to increase blood pressure among users (see Section 9 in WARNINGS). Similar effects on risk factors have been associated with an increased risk of heart disease. Oral contraceptives must be used with caution in women with cardiovascular disease risk factors.

b. Thromboembolism

An increased risk of thromboembolic and thrombotic disease associated with the use of oral contraceptives is well established. Case control studies have found the relative risk of users compared to nonusers to be 3 for the first episode of superficial venous thrombosis, 4 to 11 for deep vein thrombosis or pulmonary embolism, and 1.5 to 6 for women with predisposing conditions for venous thromboembolic disease[2,3,19–24]. Cohort studies have shown the relative risk to be somewhat lower, about 3 for new cases and about 4.5 for new cases requiring hospitalization[25]. The risk of thromboembolic disease associated with oral contraceptives is not related to length of use and disappears after pill use is stopped.[2]

A two- to four-fold increase in relative risk of post-operative thromboembolic complications has been reported with the use of oral contraceptives[9]. The relative risk of venous thrombosis in women who have predisposing conditions is twice that of women without such medical conditions[26]. If feasible, oral contraceptives should be discontinued at least four weeks prior to and for two weeks after elective surgery of a type associated with an increase in risk of thromboembolism and during and following prolonged immobilization. Since the immediate postpartum period is also associated with an increased risk of thromboembolism, oral contraceptives should be started no earlier than four weeks after delivery in women who elect not to breast feed or four weeks after a second trimester abortion.

c. Cerebrovascular diseases

Oral contraceptives have been shown to increase both the relative and attributable risks of cerebrovascular events

(thrombotic and hemorrhagic strokes), although, in general, the risk is greatest among older (> 35 years), hypertensive women who also smoke. Hypertension was found to be a risk factor for both users and nonusers, for both types of strokes, and smoking interacted to increase the risk of stroke[27–29]. In a large study, the relative risk of thrombotic strokes has been shown to range from 3 for normotensive users to 14 for users with severe hypertension[30]. The relative risk of hemorrhagic stroke is reported to be 1.2 for non-smokers who used oral contraceptives, 2.6 for smokers who did not use oral contraceptives, 7.6 for smokers who used oral contraceptives, 1.8 for normotensive users and 25.7 for users with severe hypertension[30]. The attributable risk is also greater in older women[3].

d. Dose-related risk of vascular disease from oral contraceptives

A positive association has been observed between the amount of estrogen and progestogen in oral contraceptives and the risk of vascular disease[31–33]. A decline in serum high density lipoproteins (HDL) has been reported with many progestational agents[14–16]. A decline in serum high density lipoproteins has been associated with an increased incidence of ischemic heart disease. Because estrogens increase HDL cholesterol, the net effect of an oral contraceptive depends on a balance achieved between doses of estrogen and progestogen and the activity of the progestogen used in the contraceptives. The activity and amount of both hormones should be considered in the choice of an oral contraceptive.

Minimizing exposure to estrogen and progestogen is in keeping with good principles of therapeutics. For any particular estrogen/progestogen combination, the dosage regimen prescribed should be one which contains the least amount of estrogen and progestogen that is compatible with a low failure rate and the needs of the individual patient. New acceptors of oral contraceptive agents should be started on preparations containing 0.035 mg or less of estrogen.

e. Persistence of risk of vascular disease

There are two studies which have shown persistence of risk of vascular disease for ever-users of oral contraceptives. In a study in the United States, the risk of developing myocardial infarction after discontinuing oral contraceptives persists for at least 9 years for women 40–49 years who had used oral contraceptives for five or more years, but this increased risk was not demonstrated in other age groups[8]. In another study in Great Britain, the risk of developing cerebrovascular disease persisted for at least 6 years after discontinuation of oral contraceptives, although excess risk was very small[34]. However, both studies were performed with oral contraceptive formulations containing 50 micrograms or higher of estrogens.

2. ESTIMATES OF MORTALITY FROM CONTRACEPTIVE USE

One study gathered data from a variety of sources which have estimated the mortality rate associated with different methods of contraception at different ages (Table III). These estimates include the combined risk of death associated with contraceptive methods plus the risk attributable to pregnancy in the event of method failure. Each method of contraception has its specific benefits and risks. The study concluded that with the exception of oral contraceptive users 35 and older who smoke, and 40 and older who do not smoke, mortality associated with all methods of birth control is low and below that associated with childbirth. The observation of an increase in risk of mortality with age for oral contraceptive users is based on data gathered in the 1970's[35]. Current clinical recommendation involves the use of lower estrogen dose formulations and a careful consideration of risk factors. In 1989, the Fertility and Maternal Health Drugs Advisory Committee was asked to review the use of oral contraceptives in women 40 years of age and over. The Committee concluded that although cardiovascular disease risks may be increased with oral contraceptive use after age 40 in healthy non-smoking women (even with the newer low-dose formulations), there are also greater potential health risks associated with pregnancy in older women and with the alternative surgical and medical procedures which may be necessary if such women do not have access to effective and acceptable means of contraception. The Committee recommended that the benefits of low-dose oral contraceptive use by healthy non-smoking women over 40 may outweigh the possible risks.

Of course, older women, as all women, who take oral contraceptives, should take an oral contraceptive which contains the least amount of estrogen and progestogen that is compatible with a low failure rate and individual patient needs.

[See table III at left.]

3. CARCINOMA OF THE REPRODUCTIVE ORGANS AND BREASTS

Numerous epidemiological studies have been performed on the incidence of breast, endometrial, ovarian, and cervical

TABLE III—ANNUAL NUMBER OF BIRTH-RELATED OR METHOD-RELATED DEATHS ASSOCIATED WITH CONTROL OF FERTILITY PER 100,000 NON-STERILE WOMEN, BY FERTILITY CONTROL METHOD ACCORDING TO AGE

Method of control and outcome	15–19	20–24	25–29	30–34	35–39	40–44
No fertility control methods*	7.0	7.4	9.1	14.8	25.7	28.2
Oral contraceptives non-smoker**	0.3	0.5	0.9	1.9	13.8	31.6
Oral contraceptives smoker**	2.2	3.4	6.6	13.5	51.1	117.2
IUD**	0.8	0.8	1.0	1.0	1.4	1.4
Condom*	1.1	1.6	0.7	0.2	0.3	0.4
Diaphragm/spermicide*	1.9	1.2	1.2	1.3	2.2	2.8
Periodic abstinence*	2.5	1.6	1.6	1.7	2.9	3.6

* Deaths are birth-related
** Deaths are method-related

Adapted from H.W. Ory, ref. #35.

Continued on next page

Ortho—Cont.

cancer in women using oral contraceptives. While there are conflicting reports, most studies suggest that the use of oral contraceptives is not associated with an overall increase in the risk of developing breast cancer. Some studies have reported an increased relative risk of developing breast cancer, particularly at a younger age. This increased relative risk appears to be related to duration of use[36-44],[79-89].

Some studies suggest that oral contraceptive use has been associated with an increase in the risk of cervical intraepithelial neoplasia in some populations of women[45-48]. However, there continues to be controversy about the extent to which such findings may be due to differences in sexual behavior and other factors.

4. HEPATIC NEOPLASIA

Benign hepatic adenomas are associated with oral contraceptive use, although the incidence of benign tumors is rare in the United States. Indirect calculations have estimated the attributable risk to be in the range of 3.3 cases/100,000 for users, a risk that increases after four or more years of use especially with oral contraceptives of higher dose[49]. Rupture of rare, benign, hepatic adenomas may cause death through intra-abdominal hemorrhage[50,51].

Studies from Britain have shown an increased risk of developing hepatocellular carcinoma[52-54] in long-term (> 8 years) oral contraceptive users. However, these cancers are rare in the U.S. and the attributable risk (the excess incidence) of liver cancers in oral contraceptive users approaches less than one per million users.

5. OCULAR LESIONS

There have been clinical case reports of retinal thrombosis associated with the use of oral contraceptives. Oral contraceptives should be discontinued if there is unexplained partial or complete loss of vision; onset of proptosis or diplopia; papilledema; or retinal vascular lesions. Appropriate diagnostic and therapeutic measures should be undertaken immediately.

6. ORAL CONTRACEPTIVE USE BEFORE OR DURING EARLY PREGNANCY

Extensive epidemiological studies have revealed no increased risk of birth defects in women who have used oral contraceptives prior to pregnancy[56,57]. The majority of recent studies also do not indicate a teratogenic effect, particularly in so far as cardiac anomalies and limb reduction defects are concerned[55,56,58,59], when taken inadvertently during early pregnancy.

The administration of oral contraceptives to induce withdrawal bleeding should not be used as a test for pregnancy. Oral contraceptives should not be used during pregnancy to treat threatened or habitual abortion.

It is recommended that for any patient who has missed two consecutive periods, pregnancy should be ruled out before continuing oral contraceptive use. If the patient has not adhered to the prescribed schedule, the possibility of pregnancy should be considered at the time of the first-missed period. Oral contraceptive use should be discontinued until pregnancy is ruled out.

7. GALLBLADDER DISEASE

Earlier studies have reported an increased lifetime relative risk of gallbladder surgery in users of oral contraceptives and estrogens[60,61]. More recent studies, however, have shown that the relative risk of developing gallbladder disease among oral contraceptive users may be minimal[62-64]. The recent findings of minimal risk may be related to the use of oral contraceptive formulations containing lower hormonal doses of estrogens and progestogens.

8. CARBOHYDRATE AND LIPID METABOLIC EFFECTS

Oral contraceptives have been shown to cause a decrease in glucose tolerance in a significant percentage of users[17]. This effect has been shown to be directly related to estrogen dose[65]. Progestogens increase insulin secretion and create insulin resistance, this effect varying with different progestational agents[17,66]. However, in the non-diabetic woman, oral contraceptives appear to have no effect on fasting blood glucose[67]. Because of these demonstrated effects, prediabetic and diabetic women in particular should be carefully monitored while taking oral contraceptives.

A small proportion of women will have persistent hypertriglyceridemia while on the pill. As discussed earlier (see WARNINGS 1a and 1d), changes in serum triglycerides and lipoprotein levels have been reported in oral contraceptive users.

In clinical studies with ORTHO-CYCLEN there were no clinically significant changes in fasting blood glucose levels. No statistically significant changes in mean fasting blood glucose levels were observed over 24 cycles of use. Glucose tolerance tests showed minimal, clinically insignificant changes from baseline to cycles 3, 12, and 24.

In clinical studies with ORTHO TRI-CYCLEN there were no clinically significant changes in fasting blood glucose levels. Minimal statistically significant changes were noted in glu-

cose levels over 24 cycles of use. Glucose tolerance tests showed no clinically significant changes from baseline to cycles 3, 12, and 24.

9. ELEVATED BLOOD PRESSURE

An increase in blood pressure has been reported in women taking oral contraceptives[68] and this increase is more likely in older oral contraceptive users[69] and with extended duration of use[61]. Data from the Royal College of General Practitioners[12] and subsequent randomized trials have shown that the incidence of hypertension increases with increasing progestational activity.

Women with a history of hypertension or hypertension-related diseases, or renal disease[70] should be encouraged to use another method of contraception. If women elect to use oral contraceptives, they should be monitored closely and if significant elevation of blood pressure occurs, oral contraceptives should be discontinued. For most women, elevated blood pressure will return to normal after stopping oral contraceptives, and there is no difference in the occurrence of hypertension between former and never users[68-71]. It should be noted that in two separate large clinical trials (N = 633 and N = 911), no statistically significant changes in mean blood pressure were observed with ORTHO-CYCLEN.

10. HEADACHE

The onset or exacerbation of migraine or development of headache with a new pattern which is recurrent, persistent or severe requires discontinuation of oral contraceptives and evaluation of the cause.

11. BLEEDING IRREGULARITIES

Breakthrough bleeding and spotting are sometimes encountered in patients on oral contraceptives, especially during the first three months of use. Nonhormonal causes should be considered and adequate diagnostic measures taken to rule out malignancy or pregnancy in the event of breakthrough bleeding as in the case of any abnormal vaginal bleeding. If pathology has been excluded, time or a change to another formulation may solve the problem. In the event of amenorrhea, pregnancy should be ruled out.

Some women may encounter post-pill amenorrhea or oligomenorrhea, especially when such a condition was preexistent.

12. ECTOPIC PREGNANCY

Ectopic as well as intrauterine pregnancy may occur in contraceptive failures.

PRECAUTIONS

1. PHYSICAL EXAMINATION AND FOLLOW UP

It is good medical practice for all women to have annual history and physical examinations, including women using oral contraceptives. The physical examination, however, may be deferred until after initiation of oral contraceptives if requested by the woman and judged appropriate by the clinician. The physical examination should include special reference to blood pressure, breasts, abdomen and pelvic organs, including cervical cytology, and relevant laboratory tests. In case of undiagnosed, persistent or recurrent abnormal vaginal bleeding, appropriate measures should be conducted to rule out malignancy. Women with a strong family history of breast cancer or who have breast nodules should be monitored with particular care.

2. LIPID DISORDERS

Women who are being treated for hyperlipidemias should be followed closely if they elect to use oral contraceptives. Some progestogens may elevate LDL levels and may render the control of hyperlipidemias more difficult.

3. LIVER FUNCTION

If juandice develops in any woman receiving such drugs, the medication should be discontinued. Steroid hormones may be poorly metabolized in patients with impaired liver function.

4. FLUID RETENTION

Oral contraceptives may cause some degree of fluid retention. They should be prescribed with caution, and only with careful monitoring, in patients with conditions which might be aggravated by fluid retention.

5. EMOTIONAL DISORDERS

Women with a history of depression should be carefully observed and the drug discontinued if depression recurs to a serious degree.

6. CONTACT LENSES

Contact lens wearers who develop visual changes or changes in lens tolerance should be assessed by an ophthalmologist.

7. DRUG INTERACTIONS

Reduced efficacy and increased incidence of breakthrough bleeding and menstrual irregularities have been associated with concomitant use of rifampin. A similar association, though less marked, has been suggested with barbiturates, phenylbutazone, phenytoin sodium, carbamazepine, and possibly with griseofulvin, ampicillin and tetracyclines[72].

8. INTERACTIONS WITH LABORATORY TESTS

Certain endocrine and liver function tests and blood components may be affected by oral contraceptives:
a. Increased prothrombin and factors VII, VIII, IX, and X; decreased antithrombin 3; increased norepinephrine-induced platelet aggregability.

b. Increased thyroid binding globulin (TBG) leading to increased circulating total thyroid hormone, as measured by protein-bound iodine (PBI), T4 by column or by radioimmunoassay. Free T3 resin uptake is decreased, reflecting the elevated TBG, free T4 concentration is unaltered.
c. Other binding proteins may be elevated in serum.
d. Sex hormone binding globulins are increased and result in elevated levels of total circulating sex steroids: however, free or biologically active levels either decrease or remain unchanged.
e. High-density lipoprotein (HDL-C) and total cholesterol (Total-C) may be increased, low density lipoprotein (LDL-C) may be increased or decreased, while LDL-C/HDL-C ratio may be decreased and triglycerides may be unchanged.
f. Glucose tolerance may be decreased.
g. Serum folate levels may be depressed by oral contraceptive therapy. This may be of clinical significance if a woman becomes pregnant shortly after discontinuing oral contraceptives.

9. CARCINOGENESIS
See WARNINGS section.

10. PREGNANCY
Pregnancy Category X. See CONTRAINDICATIONS and WARNINGS Sections.

11. NURSING MOTHERS
Small amounts of oral contraceptive steroids have been identified in the milk of nursing mothers and a few adverse effects on the child have been reported, including jaundice and breast enlargement. In addition, oral contraceptives given in the postpartum period may interfere with lactation by decreasing the quantity and quality of breast milk. If possible, the nursing mother should be advised not to use oral contraceptives but to use other forms of contraception until she has completely weaned her child.

12. SEXUALLY TRANSMITTED DISEASES
Patients should be counseled that this product does not protect against HIV infection (AIDS) and other sexually transmitted diseases.

INFORMATION FOR THE PATIENT
See Patient Labeling Printed Below

ADVERSE REACTIONS
An increased risk of the following serious adverse reactions has been associated with the use of oral contraceptives (see WARNINGS Section).
- Thrombophlebitis and venous thrombosis with or without embolism
- Arterial thromboembolism
- Pulmonary embolism
- Myocardial infarction
- Cerebral hemorrhage
- Cerebral thrombosis
- Hypertension
- Gallbladder disease
- Hepatic adenomas or benign liver tumors

The following adverse reactions have been reported in patients receiving oral contraceptives and are believed to be drug-related:
- Nausea
- Vomiting
- Gastrointestinal symptoms (such as abdominal cramps and bloating)
- Breakthrough bleeding
- Spotting
- Change in menstrual flow
- Amenorrhea
- Temporary infertility after discontinuation of treatment
- Edema
- Melasma which may persist
- Breast changes: tenderness, enlargement, secretion
- Change in weight (increase or decrease)
- Change in cervical erosion and secretion
- Diminution in lactation when given immediately postpartum
- Cholestatic jaundice
- Migraine
- Rash (allergic)
- Mental depression
- Reduced tolerance to carbohydrates
- Vaginal candidiasis
- Change in corneal curvature (steepening)
- Intolerance to contact lenses

The following adverse reactions have been reported in users of oral contraceptives and the association has been neither confirmed nor refuted:
- Pre-menstrual syndrome
- Cataracts
- Changes in appetite
- Cystitis-like syndrome
- Headache
- Nervousness
- Dizziness
- Hirsutism
- Loss of scalp hair
- Erythema multiforme

- Erythema nodosum
- Hemorrhagic eruption
- Vaginitis
- Porphyria
- Impaired renal function
- Hemolytic uremic syndrome
- Acne
- Changes in libido
- Colitis
- Budd-Chiari Syndrome

OVERDOSAGE

Serious ill effects have not been reported following acute ingestion of large doses of oral contraceptives by young children. Overdosage may cause nausea and withdrawal bleeding may occur in females.

NON-CONTRACEPTIVE HEALTH BENEFITS

The following non-contraceptive health benefits related to the use of combination oral contraceptives are supported by epidemiological studies which largely utilized oral contraceptive formulations containing estrogen doses exceeding 0.035 mg of ethinyl estradiol or 0.05 mg mestranol[73–78].

Effects on menses:
- increased menstrual cycle regularity
- decreased blood loss and decreased incidence of iron deficiency anemia
- decreased incidence of dysmenorrhea

Effects related to inhibition of ovulation:
- decreased incidence of functional ovarian cysts
- decreased incidence of ectopic pregnancies

Other effects:
- decreased incidence of fibroadenomas and fibrocystic disease of the breast
- decreased incidence of acute pelvic inflammatory disease
- decreased incidence of endometrial cancer
- decreased incidence of ovarian cancer

DOSAGE AND ADMINISTRATION

To achieve maximum contraceptive effectiveness, ORTHO-CYCLEN Tablets and ORTHO TRI-CYCLEN Tablets must be taken exactly as directed and at intervals not exceeding 24 hours. ORTHO-CYCLEN and ORTHO TRI-CYCLEN are available in the DIALPAK® Tablet Dispenser which is preset for a Sunday start. Day 1 start is also provided.

21-Day Regimen (Day 1 Start)

The dosage of ORTHO-CYCLEN ☐ 21 and ORTHO TRI-CYCLEN ☐ 21 for the initial cycle of therapy is one tablet administered daily from the 1st day through the 21st day of the menstrual cycle, counting the first day of menstrual flow as "Day 1". For subsequent cycles, no tablets are taken for 7 days, then a new course is started of one tablet a day for 21 days. The dosage regimen then continues with 7 days of no medication, followed by 21 days of medication, instituting a three-weeks-on, one-week-off dosage regimen.

If the patient misses one (1) active tablet in Weeks 1, 2, or 3, the tablet should be taken as soon as she remembers. If the patient misses two (2) active tablets in Week 1 or Week 2, the patient should take two (2) tablets the day she remembers and two (2) tablets the next day; and then continue taking one (1) tablet a day until she finishes the pack. The patient should be instructed to use a back-up method of birth control if she has sex in the seven (7) days after missing pills. If the patient misses two (2) active tablets in the third week or misses three (3) or more active tablets in a row, the patient should throw out the rest of the pack and start a new pack that same day. The patient should be instructed to use a back-up method of birth control if she has sex in the seven (7) days after missing pills.

Complete instructions to facilitate patient counseling on proper pill usage may be found in the Detailed Patient Labeling ("How to Take the Pill" Section).

21-Day Regimen (Sunday Start)

When taking ORTHO-CYCLEN ☐ 21 and ORTHO TRI-CYCLEN ☐ 21, the first tablet should be taken on the first Sunday after menstruation begins. If period begins on Sunday, the first tablet is taken on that day. One tablet is taken daily for 21 days. For subsequent cycles, no tablets are taken for 7 days, then a new tablet is taken the next day (Sunday). For the first cycle of a Sunday Start regimen, another method of contraception should be used until after the first 7 consecutive days of administration.

If the patient misses one (1) active tablet in Weeks 1, 2, or 3, the tablet should be taken as soon as she remembers. If the patient misses two (2) active tablets in Week 1 or Week 2, the patient should take two (2) tablets the day she remembers and two (2) tablets the next day; and then continue taking one (1) tablet a day until she finishes the pack. The patient should be instructed to use a back-up method of birth control if she has sex in the seven (7) days after missing pills. If the patient misses two (2) active tablets in the third week or misses three (3) or more active tablets in a row, the patient should continue taking one tablet every day until Sunday. On Sunday the patient should throw out the rest of the pack and start a new pack that same day. The patient should be instructed to use a back-up method of birth control if she has sex in the seven (7) days after missing pills.

Complete instructions to facilitate patient counseling on proper pill usage may be found in the Detailed Patient Labeling ("How to Take the Pill" section).

28-Day Regimen (Day 1 Start)

The dosage of ORTHO-CYCLEN ☐ 28 and ORTHO TRI-CYCLEN ☐ 28 for the initial cycle of therapy is one active tablet administered daily from the 1st day through 21st day of the menstrual cycle, counting the first day of menstrual flow as "Day 1" followed by one green tablet daily for 7 days. Tablets are taken without interruption for 28 days. After 28 tablets have been taken, a new course is started the next day.

If the patient misses one (1) active tablet in Weeks 1, 2, or 3, the tablet should be taken as soon as she remembers. If the patient misses two (2) active tablets in Week 1 or Week 2, the patient should take two (2) tablets the day she remembers and two (2) tablets the next day; and then continue taking one (1) tablet a day until she finishes the pack. The patient should be instructed to use a back-up method of birth control if she has sex in the seven (7) days after missing pills. If the patient misses two (2) active tablets in the third week or misses three (3) or more active tablets in a row, the patient should throw out the rest of the pack and start a new pack that same day. The patient should be instructed to use a back-up method of birth control if she has sex in the seven (7) days after missing pills.

Complete instructions to facilitate patient counseling on proper pill usage may be found in the Detailed Patient Labeling ("How to Take the Pill" section).

28-Day Regimen (Sunday Start)

When taking ORTHO-CYCLEN ☐ 28 and ORTHO TRI-CYCLEN ☐ 28, the first tablet should be taken on the first Sunday after menstruation begins. If period begins on Sunday, the first tablet should be taken that day. Take one active tablet daily for 21 days followed by one green tablet daily for 7 days. After 28 tablets have been taken, a new course is started and a blue tablet is taken the next day (Sunday). For the first cycle of a Sunday Start regimen, another method of contraception should be used until after the first 7 consecutive days of administration.

If the patient misses one (1) active tablet in Weeks 1, 2, or 3, the tablet should be taken as soon as she remembers. If the patient misses two (2) active tablets in Week 1 or Week 2, the patient should take two (2) tablets the day she remembers and two (2) tablets the next day; and then continue taking one (1) tablet a day until she finishes the pack. The patient should be instructed to use a back-up method of birth control if she has sex in the seven (7) days after missing pills. If the patient misses two (2) active tablets in the third week or misses three (3) or more active tablets in a row, the patient should continue taking one tablet every day until Sunday. On Sunday the patient should throw out the rest of the pack and start a new pack that same day. The patient should be instructed to use a back-up method of birth control if she has sex in the seven (7) days after missing pills.

Complete instructions to facilitate patient counseling on proper pill usage may be found in the Detailed Patient Labeling ("How to Take the Pill" section).

The use of ORTHO-CYCLEN and ORTHO TRI-CYCLEN for contraception may be initiated 4 weeks postpartum in women who elect not to breast feed. When the tablets are administered during the postpartum period, the increased risk of thromboembolic disease associated with the postpartum period must be considered. (See CONTRAINDICATIONS and WARNINGS concerning thromboembolic disease. See also PRECAUTIONS for "Nursing Mothers.") The possibility of ovulation and conception prior to initiation of medication should be considered.

(See Discussion of Dose-Related Risk of Vascular Disease from Oral Contraceptives.)

ADDITIONAL INSTRUCTIONS FOR ALL DOSING REGIMENS

Breakthrough bleeding, spotting, and amenorrhea are frequent reasons for patients discontinuing oral contraceptives. In breakthrough bleeding, as in all cases of irregular bleeding from the vagina, nonfunctional causes should be borne in mind. In undiagnosed persistent or recurrent abnormal bleeding from the vagina, adequate diagnostic measures are indicated to rule out pregnancy or malignancy. If pathology has been excluded, time or a change to another formulation may solve the problem. Changing to an oral contraceptive with a higher estrogen content, while potentially useful in minimizing menstrual irregularity, should be done only if necessary since this may increase the risk of thromboembolic disease.

Use of oral contraceptives in the event of a missed menstrual period:

1. If the patient has not adhered to the prescribed schedule, the possibility of pregnancy should be considered at the time of the first missed period and oral contraceptive use should be discontinued until pregnancy is ruled out.
2. If the patient has adhered to the prescribed regimen and misses two consecutive periods, pregnancy should be ruled out before continuing oral contraceptive use.

HOW SUPPLIED

ORTHO-CYCLEN ☐ 21 Tablets are available in a DIALPAK® Tablet Dispenser (NDC 0062-1900-15) containing 21 tablets. Each blue tablet contains 0.250 mg of the progestational compound, norgestimate, together with 0.035 mg of the estrogenic compound, ethinyl estradiol which are unscored with "Ortho" and "250" debossed on each side.

ORTHO-CYCLEN ☐ 21 Tablets are available for clinic usage in a VERIDATE® Tablet Dispenser (unfilled) and VERIDATE Refills (NDC 0062-1900-20).

ORTHO-CYCLEN ☐ 28 Tablets are available in a DIALPAK® Tablet Dispenser (NDC 0062-1901-15) containing 28 tablets as follows: 21 blue tablets as described under ORTHO-CYCLEN ☐ 21 Tablets, and 7 green tablets containing inert ingredients.

ORTHO-CYCLEN ☐ 28 Tablets are available for clinic usage in a VERIDATE® Tablet Dispenser (unfilled) and VERIDATE Refills (NDC 0062-1901-20).

ORTHO TRI-CYCLEN ☐ 21 Tablets are available in a DIALPAK® Tablet Dispenser (NDC 0062-1902-15) containing 21 tablets. Each white tablet contains 0.180 mg of the progestational compound, norgestimate, together with 0.035 mg of the estrogenic compound, ethinyl estradiol. Each light blue tablet contains 0.215 mg of the progestational compound, norgestimate, together with 0.035 mg of the estrogenic compound, ethinyl estradiol. Each blue tablet contains 0.250 mg of the progestational compound, norgestimate, together with 0.035 mg of the estrogenic compound, ethinyl estradiol.

The white tablets are unscored, with "Ortho" and "180" debossed on each side; the light blue tablets are unscored with "Ortho" and "215" debossed on each side; the blue tablets are unscored with "Ortho" and "250" debossed on each side.

ORTHO TRI-CYCLEN ☐ 21 Tablets are available for clinic usage in a VERIDATE® Tablet Dispenser (unfilled) and VERIDATE Refills (NDC 0062-1902-20).

ORTHO TRI-CYCLEN ☐ 28 Tablets are available in a DIALPAK® Tablet Dispenser (NDC 0062-1903-15) containing 28 tablets. Each white tablet contains 0.180 mg of the progestational compound, norgestimate, together with 0.035 mg of the estrogenic compound, ethinyl estradiol. Each light blue tablet contains, 0.215 mg of the progestational compound, norgestimate, together with 0.035 mg of the estrogenic compound, ethinyl estradiol. Each blue tablet contains 0.250 mg of the progestational compound, norgestimate, together with 0.035 mg of the estrogenic compound, ethinyl estradiol. Each green tablet contains inert ingredients.

The white tablets are unscored, with "Ortho" and "180" debossed on each side; the light blue tablets are unscored with "Ortho" and "215" debossed on each side; the blue tablets are unscored with "Ortho" and "250" debossed on each side.

ORTHO TRI-CYCLEN ☐ 28 Tablets are available for clinic usage in a VERIDATE® Tablet Dispenser (unfilled) and VERIDATE Refills (NDC 0062-1903-20).

Caution: Federal law prohibits dispensing without prescription

REFERENCES

1. Hatcher RA, et al. 1994. Contraceptive Technology. Sixteenth Edition. New York: Irving Publishers. **2.** Stadel BV. Oral contraceptives and cardiovascular disease. (Pt. 1). N Engl J Med 1981; 305:612–618. **3.** Stadel BV. Oral contraceptives and cardiovascular disease. (Pt. 2). N Engl J Med 1981; 305:672–677. **4.** Adam SA, Thorogood M. Oral contraception and myocardial infarction revisited: the effects of new preparations and prescribing patterns. Br J Obstet Gynaecol 1981; 88:838–845. **5.** Mann JI, Inman WH. Oral contraceptives and death from myocardial infarction. Br Med J 1975; 2(5965):245–248. **6.** Mann JI, Vessey MP, Thorogood M, Doll R. Myocardial infarction in young women with special reference to oral contraceptive practice. Br Med J 1975; 2(5956):241–245. **7.** Royal College of General Practitioners' Oral Contraception Study: Further analyses of mortality in oral contraceptive users. Lancet 1981; 1:541–546. **8.** Slone D, Shapiro S, Kaufman DW, Rosenberg L, Miettinen OS, Stolley PD. Risk of myocardial infarction in relation to current and discontinued use of oral contraceptives. N Engl J Med 1981; 305:420–424. **9.** Vessey MP. Female hormones and vascular disease—an epidemiological overview. Br J Fam Plann 1980; 6(Supplement):1–12. **10.** Russell-Briefel RG, Ezzati TM, Fulwood R, Perlman JA, Murphy RS. Cardiovascular risk status and oral contraceptive use, United States, 1976–80. Prevent Med 1986; 15:352–362. **11.** Goldbaum GM, Kendrick JS, Hogelin GC, Gentry EM. The relative impact of smoking and oral contraceptive use on women in the United States. JAMA 1987; 258:1339–1342. **12.** Layde PM, Beral V. Further analyses of mortality in oral contraceptive users; Royal College of General Practitioners' Oral Contraception Study. (Table 5) Lancet 1981; 1:541–546. **13.** Knopp RH. Arteriosclerosis risk: the roles of oral contraceptives and postmenopausal estrogens. J Reprod Med 1986; 31(9) (Supplement):913–921. **14.** Krauss RM, Roy S, Mishell DR, Casa-

Continued on next page

Ortho—Cont.

grande J, Pike MC. Effects of two low-dose oral contraceptives on serum lipids and lipoproteins: Differential changes in high-density lipoproteins subclasses. Am J Obstet 1983; 145:446–452. **15.** Wahl P, Walden C, Knopp R, Hoover J, Wallace R, Heiss G, Rifkind B. Effect of estrogen/progestin potency on lipid/lipoprotein cholesterol. N Engl J Med 1983; 308:862–867. **16.** Wynn V, Niththyananthan R. The effect of progestin in combined oral contraceptives on serum lipids with special reference to high density lipoproteins. Am J Obstet Gynecol 1982; 142:766–771. **17.** Wynn V, Godsland I. Effects of oral contraceptives on carbohydrate metabolism. J Reprod Med 1986; 31(9)(Supplement):892–897. **18.** La Rosa JC. Atherosclerotic risk factors in cardiovascular disease. J Reprod Med 1986; 31(9)(Supplement):906–912. **19.** Inman WH, Vessey MP. Investigation of death from pulmonary, coronary, and cerebral thrombosis and embolism in women of child-bearing age. Br Med J 1968; 2(5599):193–199. **20.** Maguire MG, Tonascia J, Sartwell PE, Stolley PD, Tockman MS. Increased risk of thrombosis due to oral contraceptives: a further report. Am J Epidemiol 1979; 110(2):188–195. **21.** Petitti DB, Wingerd J, Pellegrin F, Ramacharan S. Risk of vascular disease in women: smoking, oral contraceptives, noncontraceptive estrogens, and other factors. JAMA 1979; 242:1150–1154. **22.** Vessey MP, Doll R. Investigation of relation between use of oral contraceptives and thromboembolic disease. Br Med J 1968; 2(5599):199–205. **23.** Vessey MP, Doll R. Investigation of relation between use of oral contraceptives and thromboembolic disease. A further report. Br Med J 1969; 2(5658):651–657. **24.** Porter JB, Hunter JR, Danielson DA, Jick H, Stergachis A. Oral contraceptives and nonfatal vascular disease—recent experience. Obstet Gynecol 1982; 59(3):299–302. **25.** Vessey M, Doll R, Peto R, Johnson B, Wiggins P. A long-term follow-up study of women using different methods of contraception: an interim report. J Biosocial Sci 1976; 8:375–427. **26.** Royal College of General Practitioners: Oral Contraceptives, venous thrombosis, and varicose veins. J Royal Coll Gen Pract 1978; 28:393–399. **27.** Collaborative Group for the Study of Stroke in Young Women: Oral contraception and increased risk of cerebral ischemia or thrombosis. N Engl J Med 1973; 288:871–878. **28.** Petitti DB, Wingerd J. Use of oral contraceptives, cigarette smoking, and risk of subarachnoid hemorrhage. Lancet 1978; 2:234–236. **29.** Inman WH. Oral contraceptives and fatal subarachnoid hemorrhage. Br Med J 1979; 2(6203):1468–1470. **30.** Collaborative Group for the Study of Stroke in Young Women: Oral Contraceptives and stroke in young women: associated risk factors. JAMA 1975; 231:718–722. **31.** Inman WH, Vessey MP, Westerholm B, Engelund A. Thromboembolic disease and the steroidal content of oral contraceptives. A report to the Committee on Safety of Drugs. Br Med J 1970; 2:203–209. **32.** Meade TW, Greenberg G, Thompson SG. Progestogens and cardiovascular reactions associated with oral contraceptives and a comparison of the safety of 50- and 35-mcg oestrogen preparations. Br Med J 1980; 280(6224):1157–1161. **33.** Kay CR. Progestogens and arterial disease—evidence from the Royal College of General Practitioners' Study. Am J Obstet Gynecol 1982; 142:762–765. **34.** Royal College of General Practitioners: Incidence of arterial disease among oral contraceptive users. J Royal Coll Gen Pract 1983; 33:75–82. **35.** Ory HW. Mortality associated with fertility and fertility control: 1983. Family Planning Perspectives 1983; 15:50–56. **36.** The Cancer and Steroid Hormone Study of the Centers for Disease Control and the National Institute of Child Health and Human Development: Oral contraceptive use and the risk of breast cancer. N Engl J Med 1986; 315:405–411. **37.** Pike MC, Henderson BE, Krailo MD, Duke A, Roy S. Breast cancer in young women and use of oral contraceptives: possible modifying effect of formulation and age at use. Lancet 1983; 2:926–929. **38.** Paul C, Skegg DG, Spears GFS, Kaldor JM. Oral contraceptives and breast cancer: A national study. Br Med J 1986; 293:723–725. **39.** Miller DR, Rosenberg L, Kaufman DW, Schottenfeld D, Stolley PD, Shapiro S. Breast cancer risk in relation to early oral contraceptive use. Obstet Gynecol 1986; 68:863–868. **40.** Olson H, Olson KL, Moller TR, Ranstam J, Holm P. Oral contraceptive use and breast cancer in young women in Sweden (letter). Lancet 1985; 2:748–749. **41.** McPherson K, Vessey M, Neil A, Doll R, Jones L, Roberts M. Early contraceptive use and breast cancer: Results of another case-control study. Br J Cancer 1987; 56:653–660. **42.** Huggins GR, Zucker PF. Oral contraceptives and neoplasia: 1987 update. Fertil Steril 1987; 47:733–761. **43.** McPherson K, Drife JO. The pill and breast cancer: why the uncertainty? Br Med J 1986; 293:709–710. **44.** Shapiro S. Oral contraceptives—time to take stock. N Engl J Med 1987; 315:450–451. **45.** Ory H, Naib Z, Conger SB, Hatcher RA, Tyler CW. Contraceptive choice and prevalence of cervical dysplasia and carcinoma in situ. Am J Obstet Gynecol 1976; 124:573–577. **46.** Vessey MP, Lawless M, McPherson K, Yeates D. Neoplasia of the cervix uteri and contraception: a possible adverse effect of the pill. Lancet 1983; 2:930. **47.** Brinto LA, Huggins GR, Lehman HF, Malli K, Savitz DA, Trapido E, Rosenthal J, Hoover R. Long term use of oral contraceptives and risk of invasive cervical cancer. Int J Cancer 1986; 38:339–344. **48.** WHO Collaborative Study of Neoplasia and Steroid Contraceptives: Invasive cervical cancer and combined oral contraceptives. Br Med J 1985; 290:961–965. **49.** Rooks JB, Ory HW, Ishak KG, Strauss LT, Greenspan JR, Hill AP, Tyler CW. Epidemiology of hepatocellular adenoma: the role of oral contraceptive use. JAMA 1979; 242:644–648. **50.** Bein NN, Goldsmith HS. Recurrent massive hemorrhage from benign hepatic tumors secondary to oral contraceptives. Br J Surg 1977; 64:433–435. **51.** Klatskin G. Hepatic tumors: possible relationship to use of oral contraceptives. Gastroenterology 1977; 73:386–394. **52.** Henderson BE, Preston-Martin S, Edmondson HA, Peters RL, Pike MC. Hepatocellular carcinoma and oral contraceptives. Br J Cancer 1983; 48:437–440. **53.** Neuberger J, Forman D, Doll R, Williams R. Oral contraceptives and hepatocellular carcinoma. Br Med J 1986; 292:1355–1357. **54.** Forman D, Vincent TJ, Doll R. Cancer of the liver and oral contraceptives. Br Med J 1986; 292:1357–1361. **55.** Harlap S, Eldor J. Births following oral contraceptive failures. Obstet Gynecol 1980; 55:447–452. **56.** Savolainen E, Saksela E, Saxen L. Teratogenic hazards of oral contraceptives analyzed in a national malformation register. Am J Obstet Gynecol 1981:140:521–524. **57.** Janerich DT, Piper JM, Glebatis DM. Oral contraceptives and birth defects. Am J Epidemiol 1980; 112:73–79. **58.** Ferencz C, Matanoski GM, Wilson PD, Rubin JD, Neill CA, Gutberlet R. Maternal hormone therapy and congenital heart disease. Teratology 1980; 21:225–239. **59.** Rothman KJ, Fyler DC, Goldblatt A, Kreidberg MB. Exogenous hormones and other drug exposures of children with congenital heart disease. Am J Epidemiol 1979; 109:433–439. **60.** Boston Collaborative Drug Surveillance Program: Oral contraceptives and venous thromboembolic disease, surgically confirmed gallbladder disease, and breast tumors. Lancet 1973; 1:1399–1404. **61.** Royal College of General Practitioners: Oral contraceptives and health. New York, Pittman 1974. **62.** Layde PM, Vessey MP, Yeates D. Risk of gallbladder disease: a cohort study of young women attending family planning clinics. J Epidemiol Community Health 1982; 36:274–278. **63.** Rome Group for Epidemiology and Prevention of Cholelithiasis (GREPCO): Prevalence of gallstone disease in an Italian adult female population. Am J Epidemiol 1984; 119:796–805. **64.** Storm BL, Tamragouri RT, Morse ML, Lazar EL, West SL, Stolley PD, Jones JK. Oral contraceptives and other risk factors for gallbladder disease. Clin Pharmacol Ther 1986; 39:335–341. **65.** Wynn V, Adams PW, Godsland IF, Melrose J, Niththyananthan R, Oakley NW, Seedj A. Comparison of effects of different combined oral contraceptive formulations on carbohydrate and lipid metabolism. Lancet 1979; 1:1045–1049. **66.** Wynn V. Effect of progesterone and progestins on carbohydrate metabolism. In: Progesterone and Progestin. Bardin CW, Milgrom E, Mauvis-Jarvis P. Eds. New York, Raven Press 1983; pp. 395–410. **67.** Perlman JA, Roussell-Briefel RG, Ezzati TM, Lieberknecht G. Oral glucose tolerance and the potency of oral contraceptive progestogens. J Chronic Dis 1985; 38:857–864. **68.** Royal College of General Practitioners' Oral Contraception Study: Effect on hypertension and benign breast disease of progestogen component in combined oral contraceptives. Lancet 1977; 1:624. **69.** Fisch IR, Frank J. Oral contraceptives and blood prssure. JAMA 1977; 237:2499–2503. **70.** Laragh AJ. Oral contraceptive induced hypertension—nine years later. Am J Obstet Gynecol 1976; 126:141–147. **71.** Ramcharan S, Peritz E, Pellegrin FA, Williams WT. Incidence of hypertension in the Walnut Creek Contraceptive Drug Study cohort: In: Pharmacology of steroid contraceptive drugs. Garattini S, Berendes HW. Eds. New York, Raven Press, 1977; pp. 277–288, (Monographs of the Mario Negri Institute for Pharmacological Research Milan.) **72.** Stockley I. Interactions with oral contraceptives. J Pharm 1976; 216:140–143. **73.** The Cancer and Steroid Hormone Study of the Centers for Disease Control and the National Institute of Child Health and Human Development: Oral contraceptive use and the risk of ovarian cancer. JAMA 1983; 249:1596–1599. **74.** The Cancer and Steroid Hormone Study of the Centers for Disease Control and the National Institute of Child Health and Human Development: Combination oral contraceptive use and the risk of endometrial cancer. JAMA 1987; 257:796–800. **75.** Ory HW. Functional ovarian cysts and oral contraceptives: negative association confirmed surgically. JAMA 1974; 228:68–69. **76.** Ory HW, Cole P, MacMahon B, Hoover R. Oral contraceptives and reduced risk of benign breast disease. N Engl J Med 1976;294:419–422. **77.** Ory HW. The noncontraceptive health benefits from oral contraceptive use. Fam Plann Perspect 1982;14:182–184. **78.** Ory HW, Forrest JD, Lincoln R. Making choices: Evaluating the health risks and benefits of birth control methods. New York, The Alan Guttmacher Institute, 1983; p.1. **79.** Schlesselman J, Stadel BV, Murray P, Lai S. Breast cancer in relation to early use of oral contraceptives. JAMA 1988; 259:1828–1833. **80.** Hennekens CH, Speizer FE, Lipnick RJ, Rosner B, Bain C, Belanger C, Stampfer MJ, Willett W, Peto R. A case-control study of oral contraceptive use and breast cancer. JNCI 1984;72:39–42. **81.** LaVecchia C, Decarli A, Fasoli M, Franceschi S, Gentile A, Negri E, Parazzini F, Tognoni G. Oral contraceptives and cancers of the breast and of the female genital tract. Interim results from a case-control study. Br J Cancer 1986; 54:311–317. **82.** Meirik O, Lund E, Adami H, Bergstrom R, Christoffersen T, Bergsjo P. Oral contraceptive use and breast cancer in young women. A Joint National Case-control study in Sweden and Norway. Lancet 1986; II:650–654. **83.** Kay CR, Hannaford PC. Breast cancer and the pill—A further report from the Royal College of General Practitioners' oral contraception study. Br J Cancer 1988; 58:675–680. **84.** Stadel BV, Lai S, Schlesselman JJ, Murray P. Oral contraceptives and premenopausal breast cancer in nulliparous women. Contraception 1988; 38:287–299. **85.** Miller DR, Rosenberg L, Kaufman DW, Stolley P, Warshauer ME, Shapiro S. Breast cancer before age 45 and oral contraceptive use: New Findings. Am J Epidemiol 1989; 129:269–280. **86.** The UK National Case-Control Study Group, Oral contraceptive use and breast cancer risk in young women. Lancet 1989; 1:973–982. **87.** Schlesselman JJ. Cancer of the breast and reproductive tract in relation to use of oral contraceptives. Contraception 1989; 40:1–38. **88.** Vessey MP, McPherson K, Villard-Mackintosh L, Yeates D. Oral contraceptives and breast cancer: latest findings in a large cohort study. Br J Cancer 1989; 59:613–617. **89.** Jick SS, Walker AM, Stergachis A, Jick H. Oral contraceptives and breast cancer. Br J Cancer 1989; 59:618–621. **90.** Anderson FD, Selectivity and minimal androgenicity of norgestimate in monophasic and triphasic oral contraceptives. Acta Obstet Gynecol Scand 1992: 156 (Supplement): 15–21. **91.** Chapdelaine A, Desmans J-L, Derman RJ. Clinical evidence of minimal androgenic activity of norgestimate. Int J Fertil 1989; 34(51):347–352. **92.** Philips A, Demarest K, Hahn DW, Wong F, McGuire JL. Progestational and androgenic receptor binding affinities and in vivo activities of norgestimate and other progestins. Contraception 1989; 41(4):399–409. **93.** Phillips A, Hahn DW, Klimek S, McGuire JL. A comparison of the potencies and activities of progestogens used in contraceptives. Contraception 1987; 36(2):181–192. **94.** Janeud A, Rouffy J, Upmelis D, Dain M-P. A comparison study of lipid and androgen metabolism with triphasic oral contraceptive formulations containing norgestimate or levonorgestrel. Acta Obstet Gynecol Scand 1992; 156 (Supplement):34–38.

BRIEF SUMMARY PATIENT PACKAGE INSERT

Oral contraceptives, also known as "birth control pills" or "the pill", are taken to prevent pregnancy and when taken correctly, have a failure rate of less than 1% per year when used without missing any pills. The typical failure rate of large numbers of pill users is less than 3% per year when women who miss pills are included. For most women oral contraceptives are also free of serious or unpleasant side effects. However, forgetting to take pills considerably increases the chances of pregnancy.

For the majority of women, oral contraceptives can be taken safely. But there are some women who are at high risk of developing certain serious diseases that can be fatal or may cause temporary or permanent disability. The risks associated with taking oral contraceptives increase significantly if you:

- smoke
- have high blood pressure, diabetes, high cholesterol
- have or have had clotting disorders, heart attack, stroke, angina pectoris, cancer of the breast or sex organs, jaundice or malignant or benign liver tumors.

Although cardiovascular disease risks may be increased with oral contraceptive use after age 40 in healthy, non-smoking women (even with the newer low-dose formulations), there are also greater potential health risks associated with pregnancy in older women.

You should not take the pill if you suspect you are pregnant or have unexplained vaginal bleeding.

Cigarette smoking increases the risk of serious cardiovascular side effects from oral contraceptive use. This risk increases with age and with heavy smoking (15 or more cigarettes per day) and is quite marked in women over 35 years of age. Women who use oral contraceptives are strongly advised not to smoke.

Most side effects of the pill are not serious. The most common such effects are nausea, vomiting, bleeding between menstrual periods, weight gain, breast tenderness, and difficulty wearing contact lenses. These side effects, especially nausea and vomiting, may subside within the first three months of use.

The serious side effects of the pill occur very infrequently, especially if you are in good health and are young. However, you should know that the following medical conditions have been associated with or made worse by the pill:

1. Blood clots in the legs (thrombophlebitis), lungs (pulmonary embolism), stoppage or rupture of a blood vessel in the brain (stroke), blockage of blood vessels in the heart (heart attack or angina pectoris) or other organs of the body. As mentioned above, smoking increases the risk of heart attacks and strokes and subsequent serious medical consequences.

2. Liver tumors, which may rupture and cause severe bleeding. A possible but not definite association has been found with the pill and liver cancer. However, liver cancers are extremely rare. The chance of developing liver cancer from using the pill is thus even rarer.
3. High blood pressure, although blood pressure usually returns to normal when the pill is stopped.
The symptoms associated with these serious side effects are discussed in the detailed leaflet given to you with your supply of pills. Notify your doctor or health care provider if you notice any unusual physical disturbances while taking the pill. In addition, drugs such as rifampin, as well as some anticonvulsants and some antibiotics may decrease oral contraceptive effectiveness.
There is conflict among studies regarding breast cancer and oral contraceptive use. Some studies have reported an increase in the risk of developing breast cancer, particularly at a younger age. This increased risk appears to be related to duration of use. The majority of studies have found no overall increase in the risk of developing breast cancer. Some studies have found an increase in the incidence of cancer of the cervix in women who use oral contraceptives. However, this finding may be related to factors other than the use of oral contraceptives. There is insufficient evidence to rule out the possibility pills may cause such cancers.
Taking the combination pill provides some important noncontraceptive benefits. These include less painful menstruation, less menstrual blood loss and anemia, fewer pelvic infections, and fewer cancers of the ovary and the lining of the uterus.
Be sure to discuss any medical condition you may have with your health care provider. Your health care provider will take a medical and family history before prescribing oral contraceptives and will examine you. The physical examination may be delayed to another time if you request it and the health care provider believes it is a good medical practice to postpone it. You should be reexamined at least once a year while taking oral contraceptives. Your pharmacist should have given you the detailed patient information labeling which gives you further information which you should read and discuss with your health care provider.
This product (like all oral contraceptives) is intended to prevent pregnancy. It does not protect against transmission of HIV (AIDS) and other sexually transmitted diseases such as chlamydia, genital herpes, genital warts, gonorrhea, hepatitis B, and syphilis.

DETAILED PATIENT LABELING

PLEASE NOTE: This labeling is revised from time to time as important new medical information becomes available. Therefore, please review this labeling carefully.

ORTHO-CYCLEN ☐ **21** Day Regimen and
ORTHO-CYCLEN ☐ **28** Day Regimen
Each blue tablet contains 0.250 mg norgestimate and 0.035 mg ethinyl estradiol. Each green tablet in ORTHO-CYCLEN ☐ 28 Day Regimen contains inert ingredients.
ORTHO TRI-CYCLEN ☐ **21** Day Regimen and
ORTHO TRI-CYCLEN ☐ **28** Day Regimen
Each white tablet contains 0.180 mg norgestimate and 0.035 mg ethinyl estradiol. Each light blue tablet contains 0.215 mg norgestimate and 0.035 mg ethinyl estradiol. Each blue tablet contains 0.250 mg norgestimate and 0.035 mg ethinyl estradiol. Each green tablet in the ORTHO TRI-CYCLEN ☐ 28 Day Regimen contains inert ingredients.

INTRODUCTION

Any woman who considers using oral contraceptives (the birth control pill or the pill) should understand the benefits and risks of using this form of birth control. This patient labeling will give you much of the information you will need to make this decision and will also help you determine if you are at risk of developing any of the serious side effects of the pill. It will tell you how to use the pill properly so that it will be as effective as possible. However, this labeling is not a replacement for a careful discussion between you and your health care provider. You should discuss the information provided in this labeling with him or her, both when you first start taking the pill and during your revisits. You should also follow your health care provider's advice with regard to regular check-ups while you are on the pill.

EFFECTIVENESS OF ORAL CONTRACEPTIVES

Oral contraceptives or "birth control pills" or "the pill" are used to prevent pregnancy and are more effective than other non-surgical methods of birth control. When they are taken correctly, the chance of becoming pregnant is less than 1% (1 pregnancy per 100 women per year of use) when used perfectly, without missing any pills. Typical failure rates are actually 3% per year. The chance of becoming pregnant increases with each missed pill during a menstrual cycle.
In comparison, typical failure rates for other non-surgical methods of birth control during the first year of use are as follows:
Implant: <1%
Injection <1%
IUD: 1 to 2%
Diaphragm with spermicides: 18%
Spermicides alone: 21%
Vaginal sponge: 18 to 36%
Cervical Cap: 18 to 36%
Condom alone (male): 12%
Condom alone (female): 21%
Periodic abstinence: 20%
No methods: 85%

WHO SHOULD NOT TAKE ORAL CONTRACEPTIVES

Cigarette smoking increases the risk of serious cardiovascular side effects from oral contraceptive use. This risk increases with age and with heavy smoking (15 or more cigarettes per day) and is quite marked in women over 35 years of age. Women who use oral contraceptives are strongly advised not to smoke.

Some women should not use the pill. For example, you should not take the pill if you are pregnant or think you may be pregnant. You should also not use the pill if you have any of the following conditions:
- A history of heart attack or stroke
- Blood clots in the legs (thrombophlebitis), lungs (pulmonary embolism), or eyes
- A history of blood clots in the deep veins of your legs
- Chest pain (angina pectoris)
- Known or suspected breast cancer or cancer of the lining of the uterus, cervix or vagina
- Unexplained vaginal bleeding (until a diagnosis is reached by your doctor)
- Yellowing of the whites of the eyes or the skin (jaundice) during pregnancy or during previous use of the pill
- Liver tumor (benign or cancerous)
- Known or suspected pregnancy

Tell your health care provider if you have ever had any of these conditions. Your health care provider can recommend a safer method of birth control.

OTHER CONSIDERATIONS BEFORE TAKING ORAL CONTRACEPTIVES

Tell your health care provider if you have or have had:
- Breast nodules, fibrocystic disease of the breast, an abnormal breast x-ray or mammogram
- Diabetes
- Elevated cholesterol or triglycerides
- High blood pressure
- Migraine or other headaches or epilepsy
- Mental depression
- Gallbladder, heart or kidney disease
- History of scanty or irregular menstrual periods

Women with any of these conditions should be checked often by their health care provider if they choose to use oral contraceptives.
Also, be sure to inform your doctor or health care provider if you smoke or are on any medications.

RISKS OF TAKING ORAL CONTRACEPTIVES

1. Risk of developing blood clots
Blood clots and blockage of blood vessels are the most serious side effects of taking oral contraceptives and can cause death or serious disability. In particular, a clot in the legs can cause thrombophlebitis and a clot that travels to the lungs can cause a sudden blocking of the vessel carrying blood to the lungs. Rarely, clots occur in the blood vessels of the eye and may cause blindness, double vision, or impaired vision.
If you take oral contraceptives and need elective surgery, need to stay in bed for a prolonged illness or have recently delivered a baby, you may be at risk of developing blood clots. You should consult your doctor about stopping oral contraceptives four weeks before surgery and not taking oral contraceptives for two weeks after surgery or during bed rest. You should also not take oral contraceptives soon after delivery of a baby. It is advisable to wait for at least four weeks after delivery if you are not breast feeding or four weeks after a second trimester abortion. If you are breast feeding, you should wait until you have weaned your child before using the pill. (See also the section on Breast Feeding in General Precautions.)
The risk of circulatory disease in oral contraceptive users may be higher in users of high-dose pills and may be greater with longer duration of oral contraceptive use. In addition, some of these increased risks may continue for a number of years after stopping oral contraceptives. The risk of abnormal blood clotting increases with age in both users and nonusers of oral contraceptives, but the increased risk from the oral contraceptive appears to be present at all ages. For women aged 20 to 44 it is estimated that about 1 in 2,000 using oral contraceptives will be hospitalized each year because of abnormal clotting. Among nonusers in the same age group, about 1 in 20,000 would be hospitalized each year. For oral contraceptive users in general, it has been estimated that in women between the ages of 15 and 34 the risk of death due to a circulatory disorder is about 1 in 12,000 per year, whereas for nonusers the rate is about 1 in 50,000 per year. In the age group 35 to 44, the risk is estimated to be about 1 in 2,500 per year for oral contraceptive users and about 1 in 10,000 per year for nonusers.
2. Heart attacks and strokes
Oral contraceptives may increase the tendency to develop strokes (stoppage or rupture of blood vessels in the brain) and angina pectoris and heart attacks (blockage of blood vessels in the heart). Any of these conditions can cause death or disability.
Smoking greatly increases the possibility of suffering heart attacks and strokes. Furthermore, smoking and the use of oral contraceptives greatly increase the chances of developing and dying of heart disease.
3. Gallbladder disease
Oral contraceptive users probably have a greater risk than nonusers of having gallbladder disease, although this risk may be related to pills containing high doses of estrogens.
4. Liver tumors
In rare cases, oral contraceptives can cause benign but dangerous liver tumors. These benign liver tumors can rupture and cause fatal internal bleeding. In addition, a possible but not definite association has been found with the pill and liver cancers in two studies, in which a few women who developed these very rare cancers were found to have used oral contraceptives for long period. However, liver cancers are rare.
5. Cancer of the reproductive organs and breasts
There is conflict among studies regarding breast cancer and oral contraceptive use. Some studies have reported an increase in the risk of developing breast cancer, particularly at a younger age. This increased risk appears to be related to duration of use. The majority of studies have found no overall increase in the risk of developing breast cancer. Some studies have found an increase in the incidence of cancer of the cervix in women who use oral contraceptives. However, this finding may be related to factors other than the use of oral contraceptives. There is insufficient evidence to rule out the possibility that pills may cause such cancers.

ESTIMATED RISK OF DEATH FROM A BIRTH CONTROL METHOD OR PREGNANCY

All methods of birth control and pregnancy are associated with a risk of developing certain diseases which may lead to disability or death. An estimate of the number of deaths associated with different methods of birth control and pregnancy has been calculated and is shown in the following table.
[See table above.]

ANNUAL NUMBER OF BIRTH-RELATED OR METHOD-RELATED DEATHS ASSOCIATED WITH CONTROL OF FERTILITY PER 100,000 NONSTERILE WOMEN, BY FERTILITY CONTROL METHOD ACCORDING TO AGE

Method of control and outcome	15–19	20–24	25–29	30–34	35–39	40–44
No fertility control methods*	7.0	7.4	9.1	14.8	25.7	28.2
Oral contraceptives non-smoker**	0.3	0.5	0.9	1.9	13.8	31.6
Oral contraceptives smoker**	2.2	3.4	6.6	13.5	51.1	117.2
IUD**	0.8	0.8	1.0	1.0	1.4	1.4
Condom*	1.1	1.6	0.7	0.2	0.3	0.4
Diaphragm/spermicide*	1.9	1.2	1.2	1.3	2.2	2.8
Periodic abstinence*	2.5	1.6	1.6	1.7	2.9	3.6

* Deaths are birth-related
** Deaths are method-related

Adapted from H.W. Ory, ref. #35.

In the above table, the risk of death from any birth control method is less than the risk of childbirth, except for oral contraceptive users over the age of 35 who smoke and pill users over the age of 40 even if they do not smoke. It can be seen in the table that for women aged 15 to 39, the risk of death was highest with pregnancy (7–26 deaths per 100,000 women, depending on age). Among pill users who do not smoke, the risk of death was always lower than that associated with pregnancy for any age group, although over the age of 40, the risk increases to 32 deaths per 100,000 women, compared to

Continued on next page

Ortho—Cont.

28 associated with pregnancy at that age. However, for pill users who smoke and are over the age of 35, the estimated number of deaths exceed those for other methods of birth control. If a woman is over the age of 40 and smokes, her estimated risk of death is four times higher (117/100,000 women) than the estimated risk associated with pregnancy (28/100,000 women) in that age group.

The suggestion that women over 40 who do not smoke should not take oral contraceptives is based on information from older, higher-dose pills. An Advisory Committee of the FDA discussed this issue in 1989 and recommended that the benefits of low-dose oral contraceptive use by healthy, non-smoking women over 40 years of age may outweigh the possible risks.

WARNING SIGNALS

If any of these adverse effects occur while you are taking oral contraceptives, call your doctor immediately:

- Sharp chest pain, coughing of blood, or sudden shortness of breath (indicating a possible clot in the lung)
- Pain in the calf (indicating a possible clot in the leg)
- Crushing chest pain or heaviness in the chest (indicating a possible heart attack)
- Sudden severe headache or vomiting, dizziness or fainting, disturbances of vision or speech, weakness, or numbness in an arm or leg (indicating a possible stroke)
- Sudden partial or complete loss of vision (indicating a possible clot in the eye)
- Breast lumps (indicating possible breast cancer or fibrocystic disease of the breast; ask your doctor or health care provider to show you how to examine your breasts)
- Severe pain or tenderness in the stomach area (indicating a possibly ruptured liver tumor)
- Difficulty in sleeping, weakness, lack of energy, fatigue, or change in mood (possibly indicating severe depression)
- Jaundice or yellowing of the skin or eyeballs, accompanied frequently by fever, fatigue, loss of appetite, dark colored urine, or light colored bowel movements (indicating possible liver problems)

SIDE EFFECTS OF ORAL CONTRACEPTIVES

1. Vaginal bleeding

Irregular vaginal bleeding or spotting may occur while you are taking the pills. Irregular bleeding may vary from slight staining between menstrual periods to breakthrough bleeding which is a flow much like a regular period. Irregular bleeding occurs most often during the first few months of oral contraceptive use, but may also occur after you have been taking the pill for some time. Such bleeding may be temporary and usually does not indicate any serious problems. It is important to continue taking your pills on schedule. If the bleeding occurs in more than one cycle or lasts for more than a few days, talk to your doctor or health care provider.

2. Contact lenses

If you wear contact lenses and notice a change in vision or an inability to wear your lenses, contact your doctor or health care provider.

3. Fluid retention

Oral contraceptives may cause edema (fluid retention) with swelling of the fingers or ankles and may raise your blood pressure. If you experience fluid retention, contact your doctor or health care provider.

4. Melasma

A spotty darkening of the skin is possible, particularly of the face, which may persist.

5. Other side effects

Other side effects may include nausea and vomiting, change in appetite, headache, nervousness, depression, dizziness, loss of scalp hair, rash, and vaginal infections.

If any of these side effects bother you, call your doctor or health care provider.

GENERAL PRECAUTIONS

1. Missed periods and use of oral contraceptives before or during early pregnancy

There may be times when you may not menstruate regularly after you have completed taking a cycle of pills. If you have taken your pills regularly and miss one menstrual period, continue taking your pills for the next cycle but be sure to inform your health care provider before doing so. If you have not taken the pills daily as instructed and missed a menstrual period, you may be pregnant. If you missed two consecutive menstrual periods, you may be pregnant. Check with your health care provider immediately to determine whether you are pregnant. Do not continue to take oral contraceptives until you are sure you are not pregnant, but continue to use another method of contraception.

There is no conclusive evidence that oral contraceptive use is associated with an increase in birth defects, when taken inadvertently during early pregnancy. Previously, a few studies had reported that oral contraceptives might be associated with birth defects, but these findings have not been seen in more recent studies. Nevertheless, oral contraceptives or

any other drugs should not be used during pregnancy unless clearly necessary and prescribed by your doctor. You should check with your doctor about risks to your unborn child of any medication taken during pregnancy.

2. While breast feeding

If you are breast feeding, consult your doctor before starting oral contraceptives. Some of the drug will be passed on to the child in the milk. A few adverse effects on the child have been reported, including yellowing of the skin (jaundice) and breast enlargement. In addition, oral contraceptives may decrease the amount and quality of your milk. If possible, do not use oral contraceptives while breast feeding. You should use another method of contraception since breast feeding provides only partial protection from becoming pregnant and this partial protection decreases significantly as you breast feed for longer periods of time. You should consider starting oral contraceptives only after you have weaned your child completely.

3. Laboratory tests

If you are scheduled for any laboratory tests, tell your doctor you are taking birth control pills. Certain blood tests may be affected by birth control pills.

4. Drug interactions

Certain drugs may interact with birth control pills to make them less effective in preventing pregnancy or cause an increase in breakthrough bleeding. Such drugs include rifampin, drugs used for epilepsy such as barbiturates (for example, phenobarbital) anticonvulsants such as carbamazepine (Tergretol is one brand of this drug), phenytoin (Dilantin is one brand of this drug), phenylbutazone (Butazolidin is one brand) and possibly certain antibiotics. You may need to use additional contraception when you take drugs which can make oral contraceptives less effective.

5. Sexually transmitted diseases

This product (like all oral contraceptives) is intended to prevent pregnancy. It does not protect against transmission of HIV (AIDS) and other sexually transmitted diseases such as chlamydia, genital herpes, genital warts, gonorrhea, hepatitis B, and syphilis.

HOW TO TAKE THE PILL

IMPORTANT POINTS TO REMEMBER

BEFORE YOU START TAKING YOUR PILLS:
1. BE SURE TO READ THESE DIRECTIONS:
Before you start taking your pills.
Anytime you are not sure what to do.
2. THE RIGHT WAY TO TAKE THE PILL IS TO TAKE ONE PILL EVERY DAY AT THE SAME TIME.
If you miss pills you could get pregnant. This includes starting the pack late. The more pills you miss, the more likely you are to get pregnant.
3. MANY WOMEN HAVE SPOTTING OR LIGHT BLEEDING, OR MAY FEEL SICK TO THEIR STOMACH DURING THE FIRST 1–3 PACKS OF PILLS.
If you feel sick to your stomach, do not stop taking the pill. The problem will usually go away. If it doesn't go away, check with your doctor or clinic.
4. MISSING PILLS CAN ALSO CAUSE SPOTTING OR LIGHT BLEEDING, even when you make up these missed pills.
On the days you take 2 pills to make up for missed pills, you could also feel a little sick to your stomach.
5. IF YOU HAVE VOMITING OR DIARRHEA, for any reason, or IF YOU TAKE SOME MEDICINES, including some antibiotics, your pills may not work as well. Use a back-up method (such as condoms, foam, or sponge) until you check with your doctor or clinic.
6. IF YOU HAVE TROUBLE REMEMBERING TO TAKE THE PILL, talk to your doctor or clinic about how to make pill-taking easier or about using another method of birth control.
7. IF YOU HAVE ANY QUESTIONS OR ARE UNSURE ABOUT THE INFORMATION IN THIS LEAFLET, call your doctor or clinic.

BEFORE YOU START TAKING YOUR PILLS

1. DECIDE WHAT TIME OF DAY YOU WANT TO TAKE YOUR PILL. It is important to take it at about the same time every day.
2. LOOK AT YOUR PILL PACK TO SEE IF IT HAS 21 OR 28 PILLS:
The 21-pill pack has 21 "active" pills (with hormones) to take for 3 weeks. This is followed by 1 week without pills.
The 28-pill pack has 21 "active" pills (with hormones) to take for 3 weeks. This is followed by 1 week of "reminder" green pills (without hormones).
ORTHO-CYCLEN: There are 21 blue "active" pills.
ORTHO TRI-CYCLEN: There are 7 white "active" pills, 7 light blue "active" pills, and 7 blue "active" pills.

3. ALSO FIND:
1) where on the pack to start taking pills,
2) in what order to take the pills.
CHECK PICTURE OF PILL PACK AND ADDITIONAL INSTRUCTIONS FOR USING THIS PACKAGE IN THE BRIEF SUMMARY PATIENT PACKAGE INSERT.
4. BE SURE YOU HAVE READY AT ALL TIMES:
ANOTHER KIND OF BIRTH CONTROL (such as condoms, foam, or sponge) to use as a back-up in case you miss pills.
AN EXTRA, FULL PILL PACK.

WHEN TO START THE FIRST PACK OF PILLS

You have a choice of which day to start taking your first pack of pills. ORTHO-CYCLEN and ORTHO TRI-CYCLEN are available in the DIALPAK® Tablet Dispenser which is preset for a Sunday Start. Day 1 Start is also provided. Decide with your doctor or clinic which is the best day for you. Pick a time of day which will be easy to remember.

DAY 1 START:
ORTHO-CYCLEN: Take the first "active" blue pill of the first pack during the first 24 hours of your period.
ORTHO TRI-CYCLEN: Take the first "active" white pill of the first pack during the first 24 hours of your period.
You will not need to use a back-up method of birth control, since you are starting the pill at the beginning of your period.

SUNDAY START:
ORTHO-CYCLEN: Take the first "active" blue pill of the first pack on the Sunday after your period starts, even if you are still bleeding. If your period begins on Sunday, start the pack that same day.
ORTHO TRI-CYCLEN: Take the first "active" white pill of the first pack on the Sunday after your period starts, even if you are still bleeding. If your period begins on Sunday, start the pack that same day.
Use another method of birth control as a back-up method if you have sex anytime from the Sunday you start your first pack until the next Sunday (7 days). Condoms, foam, or the sponge are good back-up methods of birth control.

WHAT TO DO DURING THE MONTH

1. TAKE ONE PILL AT THE SAME TIME EVERY DAY UNTIL THE PACK IS EMPTY.
Do not skip pills even if you are spotting or bleeding between monthly periods or feel sick to your stomach (nausea).
Do not skip pills even if you do not have sex very often.
2. WHEN YOU FINISH A PACK OR SWITCH YOUR BRAND OF PILLS: 21 pills: Wait 7 days to start the next pack. You will probably have your period during that week. Be sure that no more than 7 days pass between 21-day packs.
28 pills: Start the next pack on the day after your last "reminder" pill. Do not wait any days between packs.

WHAT TO DO IF YOU MISS PILLS

ORTHO-CYCLEN:
If you **MISS 1** blue "active" pill:
1. Take it as soon as you remember. Take the next pill at your regular time. This means you may take 2 pills in 1 day.
2. You do not need to use a back-up birth control method if you have sex.
If you **MISS 2** blue "active" pills in a row in **WEEK 1 OR WEEK 2** of your pack:
1. Take 2 pills on the day you remember and 2 pills the next day.
2. Then take 1 pill a day until you finish the pack.
3. You MAY BECOME PREGNANT if you have sex in the 7 days after you miss pills. You MUST use another birth control method (such as condoms, foam, or sponge) as a back-up for those 7 days.
If you **MISS 2** blue "active" pills in a row THE 3RD WEEK:
1. If you are a Day 1 Starter:
THROW OUT the rest of the pill pack and start a new pack that same day.
If you are a Sunday Starter:
Keep taking 1 pill every day until Sunday. On Sunday, THROW OUT the rest of the pack and start a new pack of pills that same day.
2. You may not have your period this month but this is expected. However, if you miss your period 2 months in a row, call your doctor or clinic because you might be pregnant.
3. You MAY BECOME PREGNANT if you have sex in the 7 days after you miss pills. You MUST use another birth control method (such as condoms, foam, or sponge) as a back-up for those 7 days.
If you **MISS 3 OR MORE** blue "active" pills in a row (during the first 3 weeks):
1. If you are a Day 1 Starter:
THROW OUT the rest of the pill pack and start a new pack that same day.
If you are a Sunday Starter:
Keep taking 1 pill every day until Sunday. On Sunday, THROW OUT the rest of the pack and start a new pack of pills that same day.

2. You may not have your period this month but this is expected. However, if you miss your period 2 months in a row, call your doctor or clinic because you might be pregnant.

3. You MAY BECOME PREGNANT if you have sex in the 7 days after you miss pills. You MUST use another birth control method (such as condoms, foam, or sponge) as a back-up for those 7 days.

ORTHO TRI-CYLEN:
If you MISS 1 white, light blue or blue "active" pill:
1. Take it as soon as you remember. Take the next pill at your regular time. This means you may take 2 pills in 1 day.
2. You do not need to use a back-up birth control method if you have sex.

If you MISS 2 white or light blue "active" pills in a row in WEEK 1 OR WEEK 2 of your pack:
1. Take 2 pills on the day you remember and 2 pills the next day.
2. Then take 1 pill a day until you finish the pack.
3. You MAY BECOME PREGNANT if you have sex in the 7 days after you miss pills. You MUST use another birth control method (such as condoms, foam, or sponge) as a back-up method for those 7 days.

If you MISS 2 blue "active" pills in a row in THE 3RD WEEK:
1. If you are a Day 1 Starter:
THROW OUT the rest of the pill pack and start a new pack that same day.
If you are a Sunday Starter:
Keep taking 1 pill every day until Sunday. On Sunday, THROW OUT the rest of the pack and start a new pack of pills that same day.
2. You may not have your period this month but this is expected. However, if you miss your period 2 months in a row, call your doctor or clinic because you might be pregnant.
3. You MAY BECOME PREGNANT if you have sex in the 7 days after you miss pills. You MUST use another birth control method (such as condoms, foam, or sponge) as a back-up method for those 7 days.

If you MISS 3 OR MORE white, light blue or blue "active" pills in a row (during the first 3 weeks):
1. If you are a Day 1 Starter:
THROW OUT the rest of the pill pack and start a new pack that same day.
If you are a Sunday Starter:
Keep taking 1 pill every day until Sunday. On Sunday, THROW OUT the rest of the pack and start a new pack of pills that same day.
2. You may not have your period this month but this is expected. However, if you miss your period 2 months in a row, call your doctor or clinic because you might be pregnant.
3. You MAY BECOME PREGNANT if you have sex in the 7 days after you miss pills. You MUST use another birth control method (such as condoms, foam, or sponge) as a back-up method for those 7 days.

A REMINDER FOR THOSE ON 28-DAY PACKS:
If you forget any of the 7 green "reminder" pills in Week 4: THROW AWAY the pills you missed.
Keep taking 1 pill each day until the pack is empty.
You do not need a back-up method.

FINALLY, IF YOU ARE STILL NOT SURE WHAT TO DO ABOUT THE PILLS YOU HAVE MISSED:
Use a BACK-UP METHOD anytime you have sex.
KEEP TAKING ONE ACTIVE PILL EACH DAY until you can reach your doctor or clinic.

PREGNANCY DUE TO PILL FAILURE
The incidence of pill failure resulting in pregnancy is approximately one percent (i.e., one pregnancy per 100 women per year) if taken every day as directed, but more typical failure rates are about 3%. If failure does occur, the risk to the fetus is minimal.

PREGNANCY AFTER STOPPING THE PILL
There may be some delay in becoming pregnant after you stop using oral contraceptives, especially if you had irregular menstrual cycles before you used oral contraceptives. It may be advisable to postpone conception until you begin menstruating regularly once you have stopped taking the pill and desire pregnancy.
There does not appear to be any increase in birth defects in newborn babies when pregnancy occurs soon after stopping the pill.

OVERDOSAGE
Serious ill effects have not been reported following ingestion of large doses of oral contraceptives by young children. Overdosage may cause nausea and withdrawal bleeding in females. In case of overdosage, contact your health care provider or pharmacist.

OTHER INFORMATION
Your health care provider will take a medical and family history before prescribing oral contraceptives and will examine you. The physical examination may be delayed to another time if you request it and the health care provider believes that it is a good medical practice to postpone it. You should be reexamined at least once a year. Be sure to inform your health care provider if there is a family history of any of the conditions listed previously in this leaflet. Be sure to keep all appointments with your health care provider, because this is a time to determine if there are early signs of side effects of oral contraceptive use.
Do not use the drug for any condition other than the one for which it was prescribed. This drug has been prescribed specifically for you; do not give it to others who may want birth control pills.

HEALTH BENEFITS FROM ORAL CONTRACEPTIVES
In addition to preventing pregnancy, use of combination oral contraceptives may provide certain benefits. They are:
- menstrual cycles may become more regular
- blood flow during menstruation may be lighter and less iron may be lost. Therefore, anemia due to iron deficiency is less likely to occur
- pain or other symptoms during menstruation may be encountered less frequently
- ectopic (tubal) pregnancy may occur less frequently
- noncancerous cysts or lumps in the breast may occur less frequently
- acute pelvic inflammatory disease may occur less frequently
- oral contraceptive use may provide some protection against developing two forms of cancer: cancer of the ovaries and cancer of the lining of the uterus.
If you want more information about birth control pills, ask your doctor/health care provider or pharmacist. They have a more technical leaflet called the Professional Labeling, which you may wish to read. The professional labeling is also published in a book entitled *Physicians' Desk Reference*, available in many book stores and public libraries.
ORTHO PHARMACEUTICAL CORPORATION
Raritan, New Jersey 08869
©OPC 1993   REVISED August 1994   631-10-900-3
Shown in Product Identification Guide, page 326

ORTHO® DIAPHRAGM KITS   ℞

DESCRIPTION
ORTHO Diaphragm Kits include three different types in a variety of sizes.
1. The ALL-FLEX® Arcing Spring Diaphragm is a molded, buff-colored, natural rubber vaginal diaphragm containing a distortion-free, dual spring-within-a-spring which provides unique arcing action no matter where the rim is compressed. It is appropriate not only where ordinary diaphragms are indicated, but also in patients with mild cystocele, rectocele or retroversion.
2. The ORTHO® Coil Spring Diaphragm is a molded natural rubber vaginal diaphragm. The rim encases a tension-adjusted, cadmium-plated coil spring.
3. The ORTHO-WHITE® Flat Spring Diaphragm is a molded, pure white, natural rubber vaginal diaphragm containing a flat, watch-type spring which allows compressibility in one plane only, thus facilitating insertion.
ORTHO Diaphragms are used in conjunction with spermicides, e.g., GYNOL II® Original Formula Contraceptive Jelly, or ORTHO-CREME® Contraceptive Cream in conception control.

ACTION
These Diaphragms when properly fitted serve two purposes:
a. To stop the sperm from entering the cervical canal;
b. To hold the spermicide.

INDICATIONS
ORTHO Diaphragms, in conjunction with an appropriate spermicide, are indicated for the prevention of pregnancy in women who elect to use diaphragms as a method of contraception.

CONTRAINDICATIONS
Known hypersensitivity to natural rubber products and prior history of Toxic Shock Syndrome (TSS).

WARNINGS
An association has been reported between diaphragm use and toxic shock syndrome (TSS), a serious condition which can be fatal.
For contraceptive effectiveness, the diaphragm should remain in place for six hours after intercourse and should be removed as soon as possible thereafter.
Continuous wearing of a contraceptive diaphragm for more than twenty-four hours is not recommended. Removal of the diaphragm before six hours may increase the risk of becoming pregnant. Retention of the diaphragm for any period of time may encourage the growth of certain bacteria in the vaginal tract. It has been suggested that under certain as yet unestablished conditions, overgrowth of these bacteria may lead to symptoms of toxic shock syndrome. Primary symptoms of TSS are sudden high fever (usually 102° or more), and vomiting, diarrhea, fainting or near fainting when standing up, dizziness or a rash that looks like sunburn. There may also be other signs of TSS such as aching of muscles and joints, redness of the eyes, sore throat and weakness. Patients should be instructed that if they experience sudden high fever and one or more of the other symptoms, they should remove the diaphragm and consult their physician immediately.

PRECAUTIONS
Diaphragm users should be instructed to consult their physician or health care provider:
1. If they are not sure about the insertion and placement of the diaphragm.
2. If they or their partner feel or are made uncomfortable by the presence of the diaphragm.
3. If the diaphragm slips out of place when walking, coughing, or straining.
4. If the diaphragm no longer fits snugly above the pubic bone.
5. If at times other than menstruation there is blood on the diaphragm when it is removed.
6. If there are any holes, tears or other deterioration of the diaphragm.
7. If unable to remove the diaphragm.
8. IMPORTANT—For contraceptive effectiveness, the diaphragm should remain in place for six hours after intercourse and should be removed as soon as possible thereafter. Continuous wearing of a contraceptive diaphragm for more than twenty-four hours is not recommended. Removal of the diaphragm before six hours may increase the risk of becoming pregnant. Retention of the diaphragm for any period of time may encourage the growth of certain bacteria in the vaginal tract. It has been suggested that under certain as yet unestablished conditions, overgrowth of these bacteria may lead to symptoms of toxic shock syndrome. Primary symptoms of TSS are sudden high fever (usually 102° or more), and vomiting, diarrhea, fainting or near fainting when standing up, dizziness or a rash that looks like a sunburn. There may also be other signs of TSS such as aching of muscles and joints, redness of the eyes, sore throat and weakness. If the patient has a sudden high fever and one or more of the other symptoms, the diaphragm should be removed immediately and TSS should be considered.
9. Diaphragm users should have another diaphragm fitting if they have lost or gained more than ten pounds, have had the diaphragm for more than a year, or have had a baby or an abortion. As a matter of routine, each time a pelvic examination is performed, refitting should be done. The size and shape of the vagina changes and this may require a new size diaphragm. Even if the diaphragm size does not change, it is advisable to replace the diaphragm every two years or sooner.
10. Diaphragms may increase the risk of urinary tract infections especially if not properly fitted. Patients should be instructed to consult their physician if they experience any of the signs or symptoms of this type of infection which include pain on urination, blood in the urine, elevated temperature, frequent urination, or a sensation of obstruction while urinating.
11. Persons sensitive to natural rubber may have an allergic reaction to diaphragm use.
12. Persons sensitive to spermicides used with the diaphragm should discontinue use.

INSTRUCTIONS
1. Proper placement of the diaphragm is vital for effectiveness.
2. To be fully effective the diaphragm should never be used without contraceptive cream or jelly. The contraceptive cream or jelly must be spread around the inner surface of the diaphragm as well as around the rim.
3. To avoid pregnancy the diaphragm must be used every time there is intercourse.
4. The diaphragm may be inserted up to six hours before intercourse. If more than six hours has elapsed between insertion of the diaphragm and intercourse, additional contraceptive jelly or cream must be inserted. The diaphragm should not be removed to insert this additional cream or jelly.
The following Patient Instructions for insertion and removal are contained in the booklet "After Your Doctor Prescribes your Ortho Diaphragm" which is included in each Ortho Diaphragm Kit.
Preparing for insertion
1. It is recommended that you urinate and wash your hands before inserting the diaphragm.
2. Prior to inserting your diaphragm, put an applicatorful (about a teaspoon) of contraceptive jelly into the cup of the dome of the diaphragm. You may elect to simply squeeze the

Continued on next page

Ortho—Cont.

tube or use the applicator provided with the starter kit of contraceptive cream or jelly.

3. Spread a small amount around the edge with your fingertip, (if the amount applied to the rim is excessive, it will be difficult to control the diaphragm during insertion) then insert.

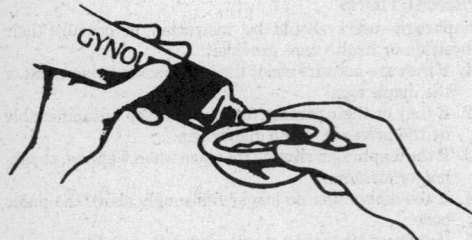

4. You can insert the diaphragm while you are standing with one leg up, squatting, or lying down. The position of the cervix and the walls of the vagina will be different depending on your position. If you are used to one position and then change to another, take extra care in positioning the diaphragm to be sure the cervix is covered.

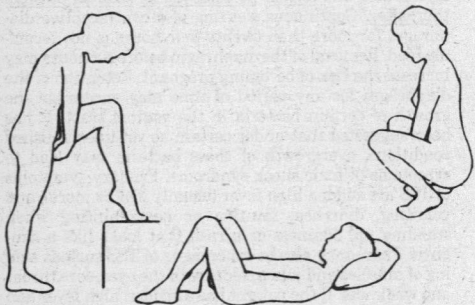

Inserting the diaphragm

1. Hold the diaphragm with the dome down (spermicide up) and press the opposite sides of the rim together between your thumb and third finger (A-1 and A-2). The diaphragm can be held from above or below.

2. Spread the lips of your vagina with your free hand. Hold the compressed diaphragm dome down (spermicide up) and push it gently inward along the rear wall of the vagina as far as it can go. Your index finger, kept on the outer rim of the diaphragm, helps you guide the diaphragm into place (B-1 and B-2).

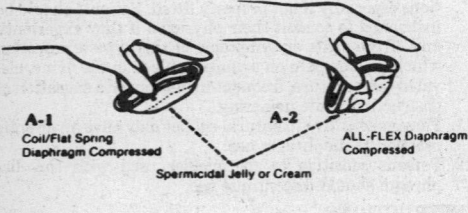

A-1 Coil/Flat Spring Diaphragm Compressed

A-2 ALL-FLEX Diaphragm Compressed

Spermicidal Jelly or Cream

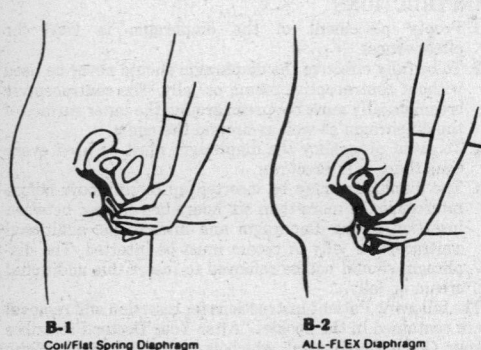

B-1 Coil/Flat Spring Diaphragm Being Introduced

B-2 ALL-FLEX Diaphragm Being Introduced

3. With your index finger, push the front rim of the the diaphragm up until it is locked in place just above the pubic bone (C).

4. Check with your index finger to be sure the diaphragm is in place and is holding the contraceptive jelly or cream over the cervix. It is important that the cervix be covered by the diaphragm and spermicide and that the diaphragm be locked in place between the upper edge of the pubic bone and the

rear wall of the vagina. You should be able to feel your cervix through the rubber shield. You can feel the front rim of the diaphragm above the pubic bone, but you may not be able to follow the rim all the way around since your fingers may not be long enough (D).

5. If, after some practice, you still find insertion awkward or difficult, vary your body and hand positions slightly until you can insert the diaphragm comfortably.

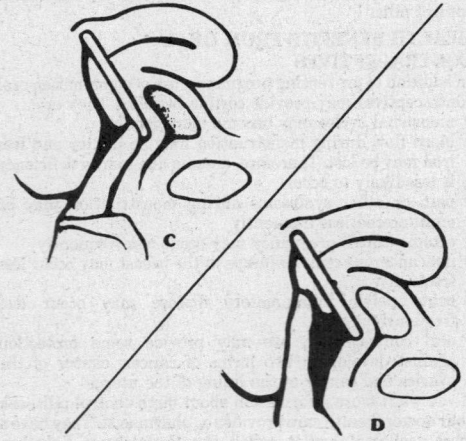

Removing the diaphragm

To remove the diaphragm, put your index finger behind the front rim (E) and pull the diaphragm down and out (F).

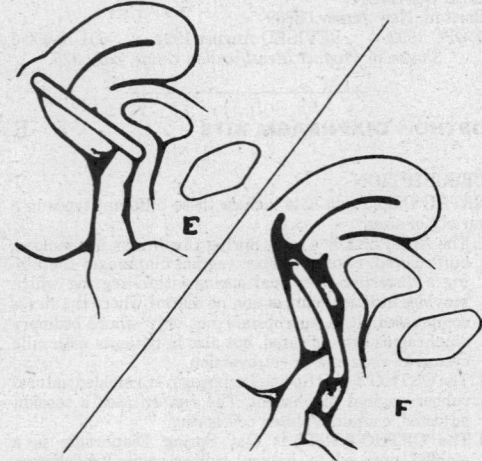

HOW SUPPLIED

All ORTHO Diaphragm Kits are available individually and contain a tube of GYNOL II Original Formula Contraceptive Jelly. Each diaphragm is contained in an attractive plastic compact.

1. The ALL-FLEX Arcing Spring Diaphragm is available in sizes 55mm through 95mm in 5mm increments.

2. The ORTHO Coil Spring Diaphragm is available in sizes 55mm through 100mm in 5mm increments.

3. The ORTHO-WHITE Flat Spring Diaphragm is available in sizes 55mm through 95mm in 5mm increments.

HOW TO FIT ORTHO DIAPHRAGMS

1. To measure for diaphragm size:
Hold index and middle fingers together and insert into vagina up to the posterior fornix. Raise hand to bring surface of index finger to contact with pubic arch.
Use tip of thumb to mark the point directly beneath the inferior margin of the pubic bone and withdraw finger in this position.

2. To determine diaphragm size:
Place one end of rim of fitting diaphragm or ring on tip of middle finger. The opposite end should lie just in front of the thumb tip. This is the approximate diameter of the diaphragm needed.
Insert a fitting diaphragm or ring of the appropriate size into the vagina.
Try both a larger and a smaller size before making a decision.

3. The proper size will fit snugly in the posterior fornix and behind the pubic arch without undue pressure.
Revised June 1996

Shown in Product Identification Guide, page 326

ORTHO® Dienestrol Cream   R

1. **ESTROGENS HAVE BEEN REPORTED TO INCREASE THE RISK OF ENDOMETRIAL CARCINOMA.**

Three independent case control studies have shown an increased risk of endometrial cancer in postmenopausal women exposed to exogenous estrogens for prolonged periods.[1–3] This risk was independent of the other known risk factors for endometrial cancer. These studies are further supported by the finding that incidence rates of endometrial cancer have increased sharply since 1969 in eight different areas of the United States with population-based cancer reporting systems, an increase which may be related to the rapidly expanding use of estrogens during the last decade.[4]

The three case control studies reported that the risk of endometrial cancer in estrogen users was about 4.5 to 13.9 times greater than in nonusers. The risk appears to depend on both duration of treatment[1] and on estrogen dose.[3] In view of these findings, when estrogens are used for the treatment of menopausal symptoms, the lowest dose that will control symptoms should be utilized and medication should be discontinued as soon as possible. When prolonged treatment is medically indicated, the patient should be reassessed on at least a semiannual basis to determine the need for continued therapy. Although the evidence must be considered preliminary, one study suggests that cyclic administration of low doses of estrogen may carry less risk than continuous administration;[3] it therefore appears prudent to utilize such a regimen.

Close clinical surveillance of all women taking estrogens is important. In all cases of undiagnosed persistent or recurring abnormal vaginal bleeding, adequate diagnostic measures should be undertaken to rule out malignancy.

There is no evidence at present that "natural" estrogens are more or less hazardous than "synthetic" estrogens at equiestrogenic doses.

2. **ESTROGENS SHOULD NOT BE USED DURING PREGNANCY**

The use of female sex hormones, both estrogens and progestogens, during early pregnancy may seriously damage the offspring. It has been shown that females exposed *in utero* to diethylstilbestrol, a non-steroidal estrogen, have an increased risk of developing in later life a form of vaginal or cervical cancer that ordinarily is extremely rare.[5,6] This risk has been estimated as not greater than 4 per 1000 exposures.[7] Furthermore, a high percentage of such exposed women (from 30 to 90 percent) have been found to have vaginal adenosis,[8–12] epithelial changes of the vagina and cervix. Although these changes are histologically benign, it is not known whether they are precursors of malignancy. Although similar data are not available with the use of other estrogens, it cannot be presumed they would not induce similar changes.

Several reports suggest an association between intrauterine exposure to female sex hormones and congenital anomalies, including congenital heart defects and limb reduction defects.[13–16] One case control study[16] estimated a 4.7 fold increased risk of limb reduction defects in infants exposed in utero to sex hormones (oral contraceptives, hormone withdrawal tests for pregnancy, or attempted treatment for threatened abortion). Some of these exposures were very short and involved only a few days of treatment. The data suggest that the risk of limb reduction defects in exposed fetuses is somewhat less than 1 per 1000.

In the past, female sex hormones have been used during pregnancy in an attempt to treat threatened or habitual abortion. There is considerable evidence that estrogens are ineffective for these indications, and there is no evidence from well controlled studies that progestogens are effective for these uses.

If ORTHO Dienestrol Cream is used during pregnancy, or if the patient becomes pregnant while using this drug, she should be apprised of the potential risks to the fetus, and the advisability of pregnancy continuation.

DESCRIPTION

ORTHO Dienestrol Cream
Cream for Intravaginal use only
Active ingredient: Dienestrol 0.01%.
Dienestrol is a synthetic, non-steroidal estrogen. It is compounded in a cream base suitable for intravaginal use only. The cream base is composed of glyceryl monostearate, peanut oil, glycerin, benzoic acid, glutamic acid, butylated hydroxyanisole, citric acid, sodium chloride and water. The pH is approximately 4.3.
[See chemical structure at top of next column.]

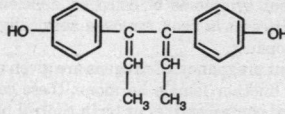

4.4'-(Diethylideneethylene)diphenol

CLINICAL PHARMACOLOGY

Systemic absorption and mode of action of dienestrol are undetermined.

INDICATIONS AND USAGE

ORTHO Dienestrol Cream is indicated in the treatment of atrophic vaginitis and kraurosis vulvae.

ORTHO DIENESTROL CREAM HAS NOT BEEN SHOWN TO BE EFFECTIVE FOR ANY PURPOSE DURING PREGNANCY AND ITS USE MAY CAUSE SEVERE HARM TO THE FETUS (*SEE* BOXED WARNING).

CONTRAINDICATIONS

Estrogens may cause fetal harm when administered to a pregnant woman (see Boxed Warning). Estrogens are contraindicated in women who are or may become pregnant. If this drug is used during pregnancy, or if the patient becomes pregnant while using this drug, the patient should be apprised of the potential hazard to the fetus.

Estrogens should also not be used in women with any of the following conditions:

1. Known or suspected cancer of the breast.
2. Known or suspected estrogen-dependent neoplasia.
3. Undiagnosed abnormal genital bleeding.
4. Active thrombophlebitis or thromboembolic disorders.
5. A past history of thrombophlebitis, thrombosis, or thromboembolic disorders associated with previous estrogen use.

WARNINGS

1. *Induction of malignant neoplasms.* Long-term continuous administration of natural and synthetic estrogens in certain animal species increases the frequency of carcinomas of the breast, cervix, vagina, and liver. There is now evidence that estrogens increase the risk of carcinoma of the endometrium in humans. (*See* Boxed Warning.)

At the present time there is no satisfactory evidence that estrogens given to postmenopausal women increase the risk of cancer of the breast,[18] although a recent long-term followup of a single physician's practice has raised this possibility.[18a] Because of the animal data, there is a need for caution in prescribing estrogens for women with a strong family history of breast cancer or who have breast nodules, fibrocystic disease, or abnormal mammograms.

2. *Gallbladder disease.* A recent study has reported a 2- to 3-fold increase in the risk of surgically confirmed gall bladder disease in women receiving postmenopausal estrogens,[18] similar to the 2-fold increase previously noted in users of oral contraceptives.[19,24] In the case of oral contraceptives the increased risk appeared after two years of use.[24]

3. *Effects similar to those caused by estrogen-progestogen oral contraceptives.* There are several serious adverse effects of oral contraceptives, most of which have not, up to now, been documented as consequences of postmenopausal estrogen therapy. This may reflect the comparatively low doses of estrogen used in postmenopausal women. It would be expected that the larger doses of estrogen used to treat prostatic or breast cancer or postpartum breast engorgement are more likely to result in these adverse effects, and, in fact, it has been shown that there is an increased risk of thrombosis in men receiving estrogens for prostatic cancer and women for postpartum breast engorgement.[20–23]

a. *Thromboembolic disease.* It is now well established that users of oral contraceptives have an increased risk of various thromboembolic and thrombotic vascular diseases, such as thrombophlebitis, pulmonary embolism, stroke, and myocardial infarction.[24–31] Cases of retinal thrombosis, mesenteric thrombosis, and optic neuritis have been reported in oral contraceptive users. There is evidence that the risk of several of these adverse reactions is related to the dose of the drug.[32,33] An increased risk of postsurgery thromboembolic complications has also been reported in users of oral contraceptives.[34,35] If feasible, estrogen should be discontinued at least 4 weeks before surgery of the type associated with an increased risk of thromboembolism, or during periods of prolonged immobilization.

While an increased rate of thromboembolic and thrombotic disease in postmenopausal users of estrogens has not been found,[18,36] this does not rule out the possibility that such an increase may be present or that subgroups of women who have underlying risk factors or who are receiving relatively large doses of estrogens may have increased risk. Therefore estrogens should not be used in persons with active thrombophlebitis or thromboembolic disorders, and they should not be used (except in treatment of malignancy) in persons with a history of such disorders in association with estrogen use. They should be used with caution in patients with cerebral vascular or coronary artery disease and only for those in whom estrogens are clearly needed.

Large doses of estrogen (5 mg conjugated estrogens per day), comparable to those used to treat cancer of the prostate and breast, have been shown in a large prospective clinical trial in men to increase the risk of nonfatal myocardial infarction, pulmonary embolism and thrombophlebitis. When estrogen doses of this size are used, any of the thromboembolic and thrombotic adverse effects associated with oral contraceptive use should be considered a clear risk.

b. *Hepatic adenoma.* Benign hepatic adenomas appear to be associated with the use of oral contraceptives.[38–40] Although benign, and rare, these may rupture and may cause death through intra-abdominal hemorrhage. Such lesions have not yet been reported in association with other estrogen or progestogen preparations but should be considered in estrogen users having abdominal pain and tenderness, abdominal mass, or hypovolemic shock. Hepatocellular carcinoma has also been reported in women taking estrogen-containing oral contraceptives.[39] The relationship of this malignancy to these drugs is not known at this time.

c. *Elevated blood pressure.* Increased blood pressure is not uncommon in women using oral contraceptives. There is now a report that this may occur with use of estrogens during menopause.[41] Blood pressure should be monitored with estrogen use, especially if high doses are used.

d. *Glucose tolerance.* A worsening of glucose tolerance has been observed in a significant percentage of patients on estrogen-containing oral contraceptives. For this reason, diabetic patients should be carefully observed while receiving estrogen.

4. *Hypercalcemia.* Administration of estrogens may lead to severe hypercalcemia in patients with breast cancer and bone metastases. If this occurs, the drug should be stopped and appropriate measures taken to reduce the serum calcium level.

PRECAUTIONS

A. General

1. A complete medical and family history should be taken prior to the initiation of any estrogen therapy. The pretreatment and periodic physical examinations should include special reference to blood pressure, breasts, abdomen, and pelvic organs, and should include a Papanicolaou smear. As a general rule, estrogen should not be prescribed for longer than one year without another physical examination being performed.

2. Fluid retention—Because estrogens may cause some degree of fluid retention, conditions which might be influenced by this factor such as epilepsy, migraine, and cardiac or renal dysfunction, require careful observation.

3. Certain patients may develop undesirable manifestations of excessive estrogenic stimulation, such as abnormal or excessive uterine bleeding, mastodynia, etc.

4. Oral contraceptives appear to be associated with an increased incidence of mental depression.[24] Although it is not clear whether this is due to the estrogenic or progestogenic component of the contraceptive, patients with a history of depression should be carefully observed.

5. Preexisting uterine leiomyomata may increase in size during estrogen use.

6. The pathologist should be advised of estrogen therapy when relevant specimens are submitted.

7. Patients with a past history of jaundice during pregnancy have an increased risk of recurrence of jaundice while receiving estrogen-containing oral contraceptive therapy. If jaundice develops in any patient receiving estrogen, the medication should be discontinued while the cause is investigated.

8. Estrogens may be poorly metabolized in patients with impaired liver function and they should be administered with caution in such patients.

9. Because estrogens influence the metabolism of calcium and phosphorus, they should be used with caution in patients with metabolic bone diseases that are associated with hypercalcemia or in patients with renal insufficiency.

10. Because of the effects of estrogens on epiphyseal closure, they should be used judiciously in young patients in whom bone growth is not complete.

11. The lowest effective dose appropriate for the specific indication should be utilized. Studies of the addition of a progestin for seven or more days of a cycle of estrogen administration have reported a lowered incidence of endometrial hyperplasia. Morphological and biochemical studies of endometrium suggest that 10 to 13 days of progestin are needed to provide maximal maturation of the endometrium and to eliminate any hyperplastic changes. Whether this will provide protection from endometrial carcinoma has not been clearly established. There are possible additional risks which may be associated with the inclusion of progestin in estrogen replacement regimens. The potential risks include adverse effects on carbohydrate and lipid metabolism. The choice of progestin and dosage may be important in minimizing these adverse effects.

B. Information for Patients: See text of Patient Package Information which is reproduced below.

C. Drug/Laboratory Test Interactions

Certain endocrine and liver function tests may be affected by estrogen-containing oral contraceptives. The following similar changes may be expected with larger doses of estrogen:

1. Increased sulfobromophthalein retention.
2. Increased prothrombin and factors VII, VIII, IX and X; decreased antithrombin 3; increased norepinephrine-induced platelet aggregability.
3. Increased thyroid-binding globulin (TBG) leading to increased circulating total thyroid hormone, as measured by PBI, T4 by column, or T4 by radioimmunoassay. Free T3 resin uptake is decreased, reflecting the elevated TBG; free T4 concentration is unaltered.
4. Impaired glucose tolerance.
5. Decreased pregnanediol excretion.
6. Reduced response to metyrapone test.
7. Reduced serum folate concentration.
8. Increased serum triglyceride and phospholipid concentration.

D. Carcinogenesis, Mutagenesis, Impairment of Fertility: See "Warnings" section for information on carcinogenesis, mutagenesis and impairment of fertility.

E. Pregnancy:
Teratogenic Effects.
Pregnancy Category X.
See "Contraindications" section.

F. Nursing Mothers: It is not known whether this drug is excreted in human milk. Because many drugs are excreted in human milk, caution should be exercised when estrogens are administered to a nursing woman.

ADVERSE REACTIONS

(*See* Warnings regarding induction of neoplasia, adverse effects on the fetus, increased incidence of gall bladder disease, and adverse effects similar to those of oral contraceptives, including thromboembolism.) The following additional adverse reactions have been reported with estrogenic therapy, including oral contraceptives:

1. *Genitourinary system.*
Increase in size of uterine fibromyomata.
Vaginal candidiasis.
Breakthrough bleeding, spotting, change in menstrual flow.
Dysmenorrhea.
Premenstrual-like syndrome.
Amenorrhea during and after treatment.
Change in cervical eversion and in degree of cervical secretion.
Cystitis-like syndrome.

2. *Breasts.*
Tenderness, enlargement, secretion.

3. *Gastrointestinal.*
Cholestatic jaundice.
Nausea, vomiting.
Abdominal cramps, bloating.

4. *Skin.*
Erythema multiforme.
Erythema nodosum.
Hemorrhagic eruption.
Loss of scalp hair.
Hirsutism.
Chloasma or melasma which may persist when drug is discontinued.

5. *Eyes.*
Steepening of corneal curvature.
Intolerance to contact lenses.

6. *CNS.*
Mental depression.
Headache, migraine, dizziness.
Chorea.

7. *Miscellaneous.*
Reduced carbohydrate tolerance.
Aggravation of porphyria.
Edema.
Changes in libido.
Increase or decrease in weight.

OVERDOSAGE

Numerous reports of ingestion of large doses of estrogen-containing oral contraceptives by young children indicate that serious ill effects do not occur. Overdosage of estrogen may cause nausea, and withdrawal bleeding may occur in females.

DOSAGE AND ADMINISTRATION

Given cyclically for short term use only:
For treatment of atrophic vaginitis, or kraurosis vulvae associated with the menopause.
The lowest dose that will control symptoms should be chosen and medication should be discontinued as promptly as possible.
Attempts to discontinue or taper medication should be made at 3 to 6 month intervals.
The usual dosage range is one or two applicatorsful per day for one or two weeks, then gradually reduced to one half initial dosage for a similar period. A maintenance dosage of one

Continued on next page

Ortho—Cont.

applicatorful, one to three times a week, may be used after restoration of the vaginal mucosa has been achieved. Treated patients with an intact uterus should be monitored closely for signs of endometrial cancer and appropriate diagnostic measures should be taken to rule out malignancy in the event of persistent or recurring abnormal vaginal bleeding.

HOW SUPPLIED

Available in 2.75 oz. (78g) tubes with or without ORTHO® Measured Dose Applicator.
With applicator: NDC 0062-5450-77
Without applicator: NDC 0062-5450-00
Store at controlled room temperature.

REFERENCES

1. Ziel, H.K. and W.D. Finkle, "Increased Risk of Endometrial Carcinoma Among Users of Conjugated Estrogens," *New England Journal of Medicine*, 293:1167–1170, 1975.
2. Smith, D.C., R. Prentice, D.J. Thompson, and W.L. Hermann, "Association of Exogenous Estrogen and Endometrial Carcinoma," *New England Journal of Medicine*, 293:1164–1167, 1975.
3. Mack, T.M., M.C. Pike, B.E. Henderson, R.I. Pfeffer, V.R. Gerkins, M. Arthur, and S.E. Brown, "Estrogens and Endometrial Cancer in a Retirement Community," *New England Journal of Medicine*, 294:1267–1287, 1976.
4. Weiss, N.S., D.R. Szekely and D.F. Austin, "Increasing Incidence of Endometrial Cancer in the United States," *New England Journal of Medicine*, 294:1259–1262, 1976.
5. Herbst, A.L., H. Ulfelder and D.C. Poskanzer, "Adenocarcinoma of Vagina," *New England Journal of Medicine*, 284:878–881, 1971.
6. Greenwald, P., J. Barlow, P. Nasca, and W. Burnett, "Vaginal Cancer after Maternal Treatment with Synthetic Estrogens," *New England Journal of Medicine*, 285:390–392, 1971.
7. Lanier, A., K. Noller, D. Decker, L. Elveback, and L. Kurland, "Cancer and Stilbestrol. A Follow-up of 1719 Persons Exposed to Estrogens in Utero and Born 1943–1959," *Mayo Clinic Proceedings*, 48:793–799, 1973.
8. Herbst, A., R. Kurman, and R. Scully, "Vaginal and Cervical Abnormalities After Exposure to Stilbestrol In Utero," *Obstetrics and Gynecology*, 40:287–298, 1972.
9. Herbst, A., S. Robboy, G. Macdonald, and R. Scully, "The Effects of Local Progesterone on Stilbestrol-Associated Vaginal Adenosis," *American Journal of Obstetrics and Gynecology* 118:607–615, 1974.
10. Herbst, A., D. Poskanzer, S. Robboy, L. Friedlander, and R. Scully, "Prenatal Exposure to Stilbestrol, A Prospective Comparison of Exposed Female Offspring with Unexposed Controls," *New England Journal of Medicine*, 292:334–339, 1975.
11. Staffi, A., R. Mattingly, D. Foley, and W. Fetherston, "Clinical Diagnosis of Vaginal Adenosis," *Obstetrics and Gynecology*, 43:118–128, 1974.
12. Sherman, A.I., M. Goldrath, A. Berlin, V. Vakhariya, F. Banooni, W. Michaels, P. Goodman, S. Brown, "Cervical-Vaginal Adenosis After *In Utero* Exposure to Synthetic Estrogens," *Obstetrics and Gynecology*, 44:531–545, 1974.
13. Gal, I., B. Kirman, and J. Stern, "Hormone Pregnancy Tests and Congenital Malformation," *Nature*, 216:83, 1967.
14. Levy, E.P., A. Cohen, and F.C. Fraser, "Hormone Treatment During Pregnancy and Congenital Heart Defects," *Lancet*, 1:611, 1973.
15. Nora, J. and A. Nora, "Birth Defects and Oral Contraceptives," *Lancet*, 1:941–942, 1973.
16. Janerich, D.T., J.M. Piper, and D.M. Glebatis, "Oral Contraceptives and Congenital Limb-Reduction Defects," *New England Journal of Medicine*, 291:697–700, 1974.
17. "Estrogens for Oral or Parenteral Use," *Federal Register*, 40:8212, 1975.
18. Boston Collaborative Drug Surveillance Program, "Surgically Confirmed Gall Bladder Disease, Venous Thromboembolism and Breast Tumors in Relation to Post-Menopausal Estrogen Therapy," *New England Journal of Medicine*, 290:15–19, 1974.
18a. Hoover, R., L.A. Gray, Sr., P. Cole, and B. MacMahon, "Menopausal Estrogens and Breast Cancer," *New England Journal of Medicine*, 295:401–405, 1976.
19. Boston Collaborative Drug Surveillance Program, "Oral Contraceptives and Venous Thromboembolic Disease, Surgically Confirmed Gall Bladder Disease, and Breast Tumors," *Lancet* 1:1399–1404, 1973.
20. Daniel, D.G., H. Campbell, and A.C. Turnbull, "Puerperal Thromboembolism and Suppression of Lactation," *Lancet*, 2:287–289, 1967.
21. The Veterans Administration Cooperative Urological Research Group, "Carcinoma of the Prostate: Treatment Comparisons," *Journal of Urology*, 98:516–522, 1967.
22. Bailer, J.C., "Thromboembolism and Oestrogen Therapy," *Lancet*, 2:560, 1967.
23. Blackard, C., R. Doe, G. Mellinger, and D. Byar, "Incidence of Cardiovascular Disease and Death In Patients Receiving Diethylstilbestrol for Carcinoma of the Prostate," *Cancer*, 26:249–256, 1970.
24. Royal College of General Practitioners, "Oral Contraception and Thromboembolic Disease," *Journal of the Royal College of General Practitioners*, 13:267–279, 1967.
25. Inman, W.H.W. and M.P. Vessey, "Investigation of Deaths from Pulmonary, Coronary, and Cerebral Thrombosis and Embolism in Women of Child-Bearing Age," *British Medical Journal*, 2:193–199, 1968.
26. Vessey, M.P. and R. Doll, "Investigation of Relation Between Use of Oral Contraceptives and Thromboembolic Disease, A Further Report," *British Medical Journal*, 2:651–657, 1969.
27. Sartwell, P.E., A.T. Masi, F.G. Arthes, G.R. Greene, and H.E. Smith, "Thromboembolism and Oral Contraceptives: An Epidemiological Case Control Study," *American Journal of Epidemiology*, 90:365–380, 1969.
28. Collaborative Group for the Study of Stroke In Young Women, "Oral Contraception and Increased Risk of Cerebral Ischemia or Thrombosis," *New England Journal of Medicine*, 288:871–878, 1973.
29. Collaborative Group for the Study of Stroke in Young Women, "Oral Contraceptives and Stroke in Young Women: Associated Risk Factors," *Journal of the American Medical Association*, 231:718–722, 1975.
30. Mann, J.I. and W.H.W. Inman, "Oral Contraceptives and Death from Myocardial Infarction," *British Medical Journal*, 2:245–248, 1975.
31. Mann, J.I., M.P. Vessey, M. Thorogood, and R. Doll., "Myocardial Infarction in Young Women with Special Reference to Oral Contraceptive Practice," *British Medical Journal*, 2:241–245, 1975.
32. Inman, W.H.W., V.P. Vessey, B. Westerholm, and A. Engelund, "Thromboembolic Disease and the Steroidal Content of Oral Contraceptives," *British Medical Journal*, 2:203–209, 1970.
33. Stolley, P.D., J.A. Tonascia, M.S. Tockman, P.E. Sartwell, A.H. Rutledge, and M.P. Jacobs, "Thrombosis with Low-Estrogen Oral Contraceptives," *American Journal of Epidemiology*, 102:197–208, 1975.
34. Vessey, M.P., R. Doll, A.S. Fairbairn, and G. Glober, "Post-Operative Thromboembolism and the Use of the Oral Contraceptives," *British Medical Journal*, 3:123–126, 1970.
35. Greene, G.R. and P.E. Sartwell, "Oral Contraceptive Use in Patients with Thromboembolism Following Surgery, Trauma or Infection," *American Journal of Public Health*, 62:680–685, 1972.
36. Rosenberg, L., M.B. Armstrong and H. Jick, "Myocardial Infarction and Estrogen Therapy in Postmenopausal Women," *New England Journal of Medicine*, 294:1256–1259, 1976.
37. Coronary Drug Project Research Group, "The Coronary Drug Project: Initial Findings Leading to Modifications of Its Research Protocol," *Journal of the American Medical Association*, 214:1303–1313, 1970.
38. Baum, J., F. Holtz, J.J. Bookstein, and E.W. Klein, "Possible Association between Benign Hepatomas and Oral Contraceptives," *Lancet*, 2:926–928, 1973.
39. Mays, E.T., W.M. Christopherson, M.M. Mahr, and H.C. Williams, "Hepatic Changes in Young Women Ingesting Contraceptive Steroids, Hepatic Hemorrhage and Primary Hepatic Tumors." *Journal of the American Medical Association*, 235:730–782, 1976.
40. Edmondson, H.A., B. Henderson, and B. Benton, "Liver Cell Adenomas Associated with the Use of Oral Contraceptives," *New England Journal of Medicine*, 294:470–472, 1976.
41. Pfeffer, R.I. and S. Van Den Noore, "Estrogen Use and Stroke Risk in Postmenopausal Women," *American Journal of Epidemiology*, 103:445–456, 1976.

PATIENT INFORMATION ABOUT ESTROGENS

Estrogens are female hormones produced by the ovaries. The ovaries make several different kinds of estrogens. In addition, scientists have been able to make a variety of synthetic estrogens. As far as we know, all these synthetic estrogens have similar properties and therefore much the same usefulness, side effects, and risks. This leaflet is intended to help you understand what estrogens are used for, some of the risks involved in their use, and to help minimize these risks. This leaflet includes important information about estrogens, but not all the information. If you want to know more, you can ask your doctor or pharmacist to let you read the package insert prepared for the doctor.

USES OF ESTROGEN

THERE IS NO PROPER USE OF ESTROGENS IN A PREGNANT WOMAN

Estrogens are prescribed by doctors for a number of purposes, including:

1. To provide estrogen during a period of adjustment when a woman's ovaries no longer produce it, in order to prevent certain uncomfortable symptoms of estrogen deficiency. (All women normally decrease the production of estrogens, generally between the ages of 45 and 55; this is called the menopause.)

2. To prevent symptoms of estrogen deficiency when a woman's ovaries have been removed surgically before the natural menopause.

3. To prevent pregnancy. (Estrogens are given along with a progestogen, another female hormone; these combinations are called oral contraceptives or birth control pills. Patient labeling is available to women taking oral contraceptives and they will not be discussed in this leaflet.)

4. To treat certain cancers in women and men.

5. To prevent painful swelling of the breasts after pregnancy in women who choose not to nurse their babies.

ESTROGENS IN THE MENOPAUSE

In the natural course of their lives, all women eventually experience a decrease in estrogen production. This usually occurs between ages 45 and 55 but may occur earlier or later. Sometimes the ovaries may need to be removed by an operation before natural menopause, producing a "surgical menopause."

When the amount of estrogen in the blood begins to decrease, many women may develop typical symptoms: Feelings of warmth in the face, neck, and chest or sudden intense episodes of heat and sweating throughout the body (called "hot flashes" or "hot flushes"). These symptoms are sometimes very uncomfortable. A few women eventually develop changes in the vagina (called "atrophic vaginitis") which cause discomfort, especially during and after intercourse. Estrogens can be prescribed to treat these symptoms of the menopause. It is estimated that considerably more than half of all women undergoing the menopause have only mild symptoms or no symptoms at all and therefore do not need estrogens. Other women may need estrogens for a few months, while their bodies adjust to lower estrogen levels. Sometimes the need will be for periods longer than six months. In an attempt to avoid over-stimulation of the uterus (womb), estrogens are usually given cyclically during each month of use, that is three weeks of pills followed by one week without pills.

Sometimes women experience nervous symptoms or depression during menopause. There is no evidence that estrogens are effective for such symptoms and they should not be used to treat them, although other treatment may be needed.

You may have heard that taking estrogens for long periods (years) after the menopause will keep your skin soft and supple and keep you feeling young. There is no evidence that this is so, however, and such long-term treatment carries important risks.

ESTROGENS TO PREVENT SWELLING OF THE BREASTS AFTER PREGNANCY

If you do not breast-feed your baby after delivery, your breasts may fill up with milk and become painful and engorged. This usually begins about three to four days after delivery and may last for a few days to up to a week or more. Sometimes the discomfort is severe, but usually it is not and can be controlled by pain-relieving drugs such as aspirin and by binding the breasts up tightly. Estrogens can be used to try to prevent the breasts from filling up. While this treatment is sometimes successful, in many cases the breasts fill up to some degree in spite of treatment. The dose of estrogens needed to prevent pain and swelling of the breasts is much larger than the dose needed to treat symptoms of the menopause and this may increase your chances of developing blood clots in the legs or lungs (see below). Therefore, it is important that you discuss the benefits and the risks of estrogen use with your doctor if you have decided not to breast-feed your baby.

SOME OF THE DANGERS OF ESTROGEN

1. *Cancer of the uterus.* If estrogens are used in the postmenopausal period for more than a year, there is an increased risk of *endometrial cancer* (cancer of the uterus). Women taking estrogens have roughly five to ten times as great a chance of getting this cancer as women who take no estrogens. To put this another way, while a postmenopausal woman not taking estrogens has one chance in 1,000 each year of getting cancer of the uterus, a woman taking estrogens has five to ten chances in 1,000 each year. For this reason *it is important to take estrogens only when you really need them.*

The risk of this cancer is greater the longer estrogens are used and also seems to be greater when larger doses are taken. For this reason *it is important to take the lowest dose of estrogen that will control symptoms and to take it only as long as it is needed.* If estrogens are needed for longer periods of time, your doctor will want to reevaluate your need for estrogens at least every six months.

Women using estrogens should report any irregular vaginal bleeding to their doctors; such bleeding may be of no importance, but it can be an early warning of cancer of the uterus. If you have undiagnosed vaginal bleeding, you should not use estrogens until a diagnosis is made and you are certain there is no cancer of the uterus.

If you have had your uterus completely removed (total hysterectomy), there is no danger of developing cancer of the uterus.

2. *Other possible cancers.* Estrogens can cause development of other tumors in animals, such as tumors of the breast, cervix, vagina, or liver, when given for a long time. At present there is no good evidence that women using estrogen in the menopause have an increased risk of such tumors, but there is no way yet to be sure they do not; and one study raises the possibility that use of estrogens in the menopause may increase the risk of breast cancer many years later. This is a further reason to use estrogens only when clearly needed. While you are taking estrogens, it is important that you go to your doctor at least once a year for a physical examination. Also, if members of your family have had breast cancer or if you have breast nodules or abnormal mammograms (breast x-rays), your doctor may wish to carry out more frequent examinations of your breasts.

3. *Gall bladder disease.* Women who use estrogens after menopause are more likely to develop gall bladder disease needing surgery than women who do not use estrogens. Birth control pills have a similar effect.

4. *Abnormal blood clotting.* Oral contraceptives, some of which contain estrogens, increase the risk of blood clotting in various parts of the body. This can result in a stroke (if the clot is in the brain), a heart attack (clot in a blood vessel of the heart), or a pulmonary embolus (a clot which forms in the legs or pelvis, then breaks off and travels to the lungs). Any of these can be fatal. Blood clots may result in the loss of a limb, paralysis or loss of sight, depending on where the blood clot is formed or lodges if it breaks loose.

The larger doses of estrogen used to prevent swelling of the breasts after pregnancy have been reported to cause clotting in the legs and lungs.

It is recommended that if you have had any blood clotting disorders including clotting in the legs or lungs, or a heart attack or stroke, you should not use estrogens.

SPECIAL WARNING ABOUT PREGNANCY

You should not receive estrogen if you are pregnant. If this should occur, there is a greater than usual chance that the developing child will be born with a birth defect, although the possibility remains fairly small. A female child may have an increased risk of developing cancer of the vagina or cervix later in life (in the teens or twenties). Every possible effort should be made to avoid exposure to estrogens during pregnancy. If exposure occurs, see your doctor.

SOME OTHER EFFECTS OF ESTROGENS

In addition to the serious known risks of estrogens described above, estrogens have the following side effects and potential risks:

1. *Nausea and vomiting.* The most common side effect of estrogen therapy is nausea. Vomiting is less common.
2. *Effects on breasts.* Estrogens may cause breast tenderness or enlargement and may cause the breasts to secrete a liquid.
3. *Effects on the uterus.* Estrogens may cause benign fibroid tumors of the uterus to get larger.

Some women will have menstrual bleeding when estrogens are stopped. But if the bleeding occurs on days you are still taking estrogens you should report this to your doctor.

4. *Effects on liver.* Women taking estrogens develop on rare occasions a tumor of the liver which can rupture and bleed into the abdomen. You should report any swelling or unusual pain or tenderness in the abdomen to your doctor immediately.

Women with a past history of jaundice (yellowing of the skin and white parts of the eyes) may get jaundice again during estrogen use.

5. *Other effects.* Estrogens may cause excess fluid to be retained in the body. This may make some conditions worse, such as epilepsy, migraine, heart disease, or kidney disease.

If any of the above occur, stop taking estrogens and call your doctor.

SUMMARY

Estrogens have important uses, but they have serious risks as well. You must decide, with your doctor, whether the risks are acceptable to you in view of the benefits of treatment. Except where your doctor has prescribed estrogens for use in special cases of cancer of the breast or prostate, you should not use estrogens if you have cancer of the breast or uterus, are pregnant, have undiagnosed abnormal vaginal bleeding, blood clotting disorders including clotting in the legs or lungs, or have had a stroke, heart attack or angina.

You must understand that your doctor will require regular physical examinations while you are taking them and will try to discontinue the drug as soon as possible and use the smallest dose possible. You can help minimize the risk by being alert for signs of trouble including:

1. Abnormal bleeding from the vagina.
2. Pains in the calves or chest or sudden shortness of breath, or coughing blood (indicating possible clots in the legs, heart or lungs).
3. Severe headache, dizziness, faintness, or changes in vision (indicating possible developing clots in the brain or eye).
4. Breast lumps (you should ask your doctor how to examine your own breasts).
5. Jaundice (yellowing of the skin).
6. Mental depression.
7. <u>Any</u> other unusual condition or problem.

Based on his or her assessment of your medical needs, your doctor has prescribed this drug for you. Do not give the drug to anyone else.

HOW SUPPLIED

Available in 2.75 oz. (78g) tubes with or without ORTHO® Measured-Dose Applicator.
With applicator: NDC 0062-5450-77
Without applicator: NDC 0062-5450-00
Store at controlled room temperature.

ORTHO-EST® ℞
(estropipate tablets, USP)

WARNINGS:

1. ESTROGENS HAVE BEEN REPORTED TO INCREASE THE RISK OF ENDOMETRIAL CARCINOMA IN POSTMENOPAUSAL WOMEN.

Close clinical surveillance of all women taking estrogens is important. Adequate diagnostic measures, including endometrial sampling when indicated, should be undertaken to rule out malignancy in all cases of undiagnosed persistent or recurring abnormal vaginal bleeding. There is no evidence that "natural" estrogens are more or less hazardous than "synthetic" estrogens at equi-estrogenic doses.

2. ESTROGENS SHOULD NOT BE USED DURING PREGNANCY.

There is no indication for estrogen therapy during pregnancy or during the immediate postpartum period. Estrogens are ineffective for the prevention or treatment of threatened, or habitual abortion. Estrogens are not indicated for the prevention of postpartum breast engorgement.

Estrogen therapy during pregnancy is associated with an increased risk of congenital defects in the reproductive organs of the fetus, and possibly other birth defects. Studies of women who received diethylstilbestrol (DES) during pregnancy have shown that female offspring have an increased risk of vaginal adenosis, squamous cell dysplasia of the uterine cervix, and clear cell vaginal cancer later in life; male offspring have an increased risk of urogenital abnormalities and possibly testicular cancer later in life. The 1985 DES Task Force concluded that use of DES during pregnancy is associated with a subsequent increased risk of breast cancer in the mothers, although a causal relationship remains unproven and the observed level of excess risk is similar to that for a number of other breast cancer risk factors.

DESCRIPTION

ORTHO-EST (estropipate tablets USP), (formerly piperazine estrone sulfate), is a natural estrogenic substance prepared from purified crystalline estrone, solubilized as the sulfate and stabilized with piperazine. It is appreciably soluble in water and has almost no odor or taste—properties which are ideally suited for oral administration. The amount of piperazine in ORTHO-EST is not sufficient to exert a pharmacological action. Its addition ensures solubility, stability and uniform potency of the estrone sulfate. Chemically, estropipate, molecular weight: 436.56, is represented by estra-1,3,5(10)-trien-17-one, 3-(sulfooxy)-, compound with piperazine (1:1). The structural formula may be represented as follows:

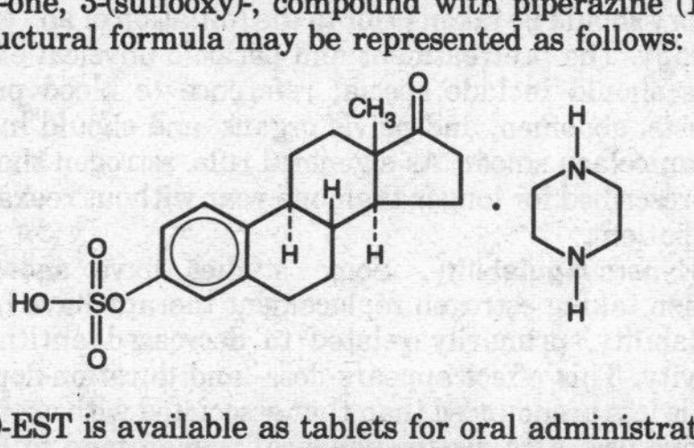

ORTHO-EST is available as tablets for oral administration containing either 0.75 mg (ORTHO-EST .625) or 1.5 mg (ORTHO-EST 1.25) estropipate. (Calculated as sodium estrone sulfate .625 mg and 1.25 mg respectively).

Inactive Ingredients:

Each tablet contains: Lactose, magnesium stearate and pregelatinized starch. ORTHO-EST 1.25 also contains: D&C Red No. 7 Calcium Lake, FD&C Blue No. 2 Aluminium Lake.

CLINICAL PHARMACOLOGY

Estrogen drug products act by regulating the transcription of a limited number of genes. Estrogens diffuse through cell membranes, distribute themselves throughout the cell, and bind to and activate the nuclear estrogen receptor, a DNA-binding protein which is found in estrogen-responsive tissues. The activated estrogen receptor binds to specific DNA sequences, or hormone-response elements, which enhance the transcription of adjacent genes and in turn lead to the observed effects. Estrogen receptors have been identified in tissues of the reproductive tract, breast, pituitary, hypothalamus, liver, and bone of women.

Estrogens are important in the development and maintenance of the female reproductive system and secondary sex characteristics. By a direct action, they cause growth and development of the uterus, Fallopian tubes, and vagina. With other hormones, such as pituitary hormones and progestrone, they cause enlargement of the breasts through promotion of ductal growth, stromal development, and the accretion of fat. Estrogens are intricately involved with other hormones, especially progestrone, in the processes of the ovulatory menstrual cycle and pregnancy, and affect the release of pituitary gonadotropins. They also contribute to the shaping of the skeleton, maintenance of tone and elasticity of urogenital structures, changes in the epiphyses of the long bones that allow for the pubertal growth spurt and its termination, and pigmentation of the nipples and genitals.

Estrogens occur naturally in several forms. The primary source of estrogen in normally cycling adult women is the ovarian follicle, which secretes 70 to 500 micrograms of estradiol daily, depending on the phase of the menstrual cycle. This is converted primarily to estrone, which circulates in roughly equal proportion to estradiol, and to small amounts of estriol. After menopause, most endogenous estrogen is produced by conversion of androstenedione, secreted by the adrenal cortex, to estrone by peripheral tissues. Thus, estrone-especially in its sulfate ester form—is the most abundant circulating estrogen in postmenopausal women. Although circulating estrogens exist in a dynamic equilibrium of metabolic interconversions, estradiol is the principal intracellular human estrogen and is substantially more potent than estrone or estriol at the receptor.

Estrogens used in therapy are well absorbed through the skin, mucous membranes, and gastrointestinal tract. When applied for a local action, absorption is usually sufficient to cause systemic effects. When conjugated with aryl and alkyl groups for parenteral administration, the rate of absorption of oily preparations is slowed with a prolonged duration of action, such that a single intramuscular injection of estradiol valerate or estradiol cypionate is absorbed over several weeks.

Administered estrogens and their esters are handled within the body essentially the same as the endogenous hormones. Metabolic conversion of estrogens occurs primarily in the liver (first pass effect), but also at local target tissue sites. Complex metabolic processes result in a dynamic equilibrium of circulating conjugated and unconjugated estrogenic forms which are continually interconverted, especially between estrone and estradiol and between esterified and unesterified forms. Although naturally-occurring estrogens circulate in the blood largely bound to sex hormone-binding globulin and albumin, only unbound estrogens enter target tissue cells. A significant proportion of the circulating estrogen exists as sulfate conjugates, especially estrone sulfate, which serves as a circulating reservoir for the formation of more active estrogenic species. A certain proportion of the estrogen is excreted into the bile and then reabsorbed from the intestine. During this enterohepatic recirculation, estrogens are desulfated and resulfated and undergo degradation through conversion to less active estrogens (estriol and other estrogens), oxidation to nonestrogenic substances (catecholestrogens, which interact with catecholamine metabolism, especially in the central nervous system), and conjugation with glucuronic acids (which are then rapidly excreted in the urine).

When given orally, naturally-occurring estrogens and their esters are extensively metabolized (first pass effect) and circulate primarily as estrone sulfate, with smaller amounts of other conjugated and unconjugated estrogenic species. This results in limited oral potency. By contrast, synthetic estrogens, such as ethinyl estradiol and the nonsteroidal estrogens, are degraded very slowly in the liver and other tissues, which results in their high intrinsic potency. Estrogen drug products administered by non-oral routes are not subject to first-pass metabolism, but also undergo significant hepatic uptake, metabolism, and enterohepatic recycling.

INDICATIONS AND USAGE

Estrogen drug products are indicated in the:

1. Treatment of moderate to severe vasomotor symptoms associated with the menopause. There is no adequate evidence that estrogens are effective for nervous symptoms or depression which might occur during menopause and they should not be used to treat these conditions.
2. Treatment of vulval and vaginal atrophy.
3. Treatment of hypoestrogenism due to hypogonadism, castration or primary ovarian failure.
4. Prevention of osteoporosis.

Since estrogen administration is associated with risk, selection of patients should ideally be based on prospective identification of risk factors for developing osteoporosis. Unfortunately, there is no certain way to identify those women who

Continued on next page

Ortho—Cont.

will develop osteoporotic fractures. Most prospective studies of efficacy for this indication have been carried out in white menopausal women, without stratification by other risk factors, and tend to show a universally salutary effect on bone. Thus, patient selection must be individualized based on the balance of risks and benefits. A more favorable risk/benefit ratio exists in a hysterectomized woman because she has no risk of endometrial cancer (see BOXED WARNINGS).
Estrogen replacement therapy reduces bone resorption and retards or halts postmenopausal bone loss. Case-control studies have shown an approximately 60 percent reduction in hip and wrist fractures in women whose extrogen replacement was begun within a few years of menopause. Studies also suggest that estrogen reduces the rate of vertebral fractures. Even when started as late as 6 years after menopause, estrogen prevents further loss of bone mass for as long as the treatment is continued. The results of a double-blind, placebo-controlled two-year study have shown that treatment with one tablet of estropipate .75 daily for 25 days (of a 31-day cycle per month) prevents vertebral bone mass loss in postmenopausal women. When estrogen therapy is discontinued, bone mass declines at a rate comparable to the immediate postmenopausal period. There is no evidence that estrogen replacement therapy restores bone mass to premenopausal levels.
At skeletal maturity there are sex and race differences in both the total amount of bone present and its density, in favor of men and blacks. Thus, women are at higher risk than men because they start with less bone mass and, for several years following natural or induced menopause, the rate of bone mass decline is accelerated. White and Asian women are at higher risk than black women.
Early menopause is one of the strongest predictors for the development of osteoporosis. In addition, other factors affecting the skeleton which are associated with osteoporosis include genetic factors (small build, family history), endocrine factors (nulliparity, thyrotoxicosis, hyperparathyroidism, Cushing's syndrome, hyperprolactinemia, Type I diabetes), lifestyle (cigarette smoking, alcohol abuse, sedentary exercise habits) and nutrition (below average body weight, dietary calcium intake).
The mainstays of prevention and management of osteoporosis are estrogen, an adequate lifetime calcium intake, and exercise. Postmenopausal women absorb dietary calcium less efficiently than premenopausal women and require an average of 1500 mg/day of elemental calcium to remain in neutral calcium balance. By comparison, premenopausal women require about 1000 mg/day and the average calcium intake in the USA is 400-600 mg/day. Therefore, when not contraindicated, calcium supplementation may be helpful.
Weight-bearing exercise and nutrition may be important adjuncts to the prevention and management of osteoporosis. Immobilization and prolonged bed rest produce rapid bone loss, while weight-bearing exercise has been shown both to reduce bone loss and to increase bone mass. The optimal type and amount of physical activity that would prevent osteoporosis have not been established, however in two studies an hour of walking and running exercises twice or three times weekly significantly increased lumbar spine bone mass.

CONTRAINDICATIONS

Estrogens should not be used in individuals with any of the following conditions:

1. Known or suspected pregnancy (see BOXED WARNINGS).
   Estrogens may cause fetal harm when administered to a pregnant woman.
2. Undiagnosed abnormal genital bleeding.
3. Known or suspected cancer of the breast except in appropriately selected patients being treated for metastatic disease.
4. Known or suspected estrogen-dependent neoplasia.
5. Active thrombophlebitis or thromboembolic disorders.

WARNINGS

1. ***Induction of malignant neoplasms.***
Endometrial cancer. The reported endometrial cancer risk among unopposed estrogen users is about 2- to 12-fold greater than in nonusers, and appears dependent on duration of treatment and on estrogen dose. Most studies show no significant increased risk associated with use of estrogens for less than one year. The greatest risk appears associated with prolonged use—with increased risks of 15-to 24-fold for five to ten years or more. In three studies, persistence of risk was demonstrated for 8 to over 15 years after cessation of estrogen treatment. In one study a significant decrease in the incidence of endometrial cancer occurred six months after estrogen withdrawal. Concurrent progestin therapy may offset this risk but the overall health impact in postmenopausal women is not known (see PRECAUTIONS).
Breast cancer. While the majority of studies have not shown an increased risk of breast cancer in women who have ever used estrogen replacement therapy, some have reported a moderately increased risk (relative risks of 1.3- 2.0) in those taking higher doses or those taking lower doses for prolonged periods of time, especially in excess of 10 years. Other studies have not shown this relationship.
Congenital lesions with malignant potential. Estrogen therapy during pregnancy is associated with an increased risk of fetal congenital reproductive tract disorders, and possibly other birth defects. Studies of women who received DES during pregnancy have shown that female offspring have an increased risk of vaginal adenosis, squamous cell dysplasia of the uterine cervix, and clear cell vaginal cancer later in life; male offspring have an increased risk of urogenital abnormalities and possibly testicular cancer later in life. Although some of these changes are benign, others are precursors of malignancy.
2. ***Gallbladder disease.*** Two studies have reported a 2- to 4-fold increase in the risk of gallbladder disease requiring surgery in women receiving postmenopausal estrogens.
3. ***Cardiovascular disease.*** Large doses of estrogen (5 mg conjugated estrogens per day), comparable to those used to treat cancer of the prostate and breast, have been shown in a large prospective clinical trial in men to increase the risks of nonfatal myocardial infarction, pulmonary embolism, and thrombophlebitis. These risks cannot necessarily be extrapolated from men to women. However, to avoid the theoretical cardiovascular risk to women caused by high estrogen doses, the dose for estrogen replacement therapy should not exceed the lowest effective dose.
4. ***Elevated blood pressure.*** Occasional blood pressure increases during estrogen replacement therapy have been attributed to idiosyncratic reactions to estrogens. More often, blood pressure has remained the same or has dropped. One study showed that postmenopausal estrogen users have higher blood pressure than nonusers. Two other studies showed slightly lower blood pressure among estrogen users compared to nonusers. Postmenopausal estrogen use does not increase the risk of stroke. Nonetheless, blood pressure should be monitored at regular intervals with estrogen use.
5. ***Hypercalcemia.*** Administration of estrogens may lead to severe hypercalcemia in patients wtih breast cancer and bone metastases. If this occurs, the drug should be stopped and appropriate measures taken to reduce the serum calcium level.

PRECAUTIONS

A. *General*
1. **Addition of a progestin.** Studies of the addition of a progestin for seven or more days of a cycle of estrogen administration have reported a lowered incidence of endometrial hyperplasia which would otherwise be induced by estrogen treatment. Morphological and biochemical studies of endometrium suggest that 10 to 14 days of progestin are needed to provide maximal maturation of the endometrium and to eliminate any hyperplastic changes. There are possible additional risks which may be associated with the inclusion of progestins in estrogen replacement regimens. These include: (1) adverse effects on lipoprotein metaboliosm (lowering HDL and raising LDL) which may diminish the possible cardioprotective effect of estrogen therapy (see PRECAUTIONS, D.4., below); (2) impairment of glucose tolerance; and (3) possible enhancement of mitotic activity in breast epithelial tissue (although few epidemiological data are available to address this point). The choice of progestin, its dose, and its regimen may be important in minimizing these adverse effects, but these issues remain to be clarified.
2. **Physical examination.** A complete medical and family history should be taken prior to the initiation of any estrogen therapy. The pretreatment and periodic physical examinations should include special reference to blood pressure, breasts, abdomen, and pelvic organs, and should include a Papanicolaou smear. As a general rule, estrogen should not be prescribed for longer than one year without reexamining the patient.
3. **Hypercoagulability.** Some studies have shown that women taking estrogen replacement therapy have hypercoagulability, primarily related to decreased antithrombin activity. This effect appears dose- and duration-dependent and is less pronounced than that associated with oral contraceptive use. Also, postmenopausal women tend to have increased coagulation parameters at baseline compared to premenopausal women. There is some suggestion that low dose postmenopausal mestranol may increase the risk of thromboembolism, although the majority of studies (of primarily conjugated estrogens users) report no such increase. There is insufficient information on hypercoagulability in women who have had previous thromboembolic disease.
4. **Familial hyperlipoproteinemia.** Estrogen therapy may be associated with massive elevations of plasma triglycerides leading to pancreatitis and other complications in patients with familial defects of lipoprotein metabolism.
5. **Fluid retention.** Because estrogens may cause some degree of fluid retention, conditions which might be exacerbated by this factor, such as asthma, epilepsy, migraine, and cardiac or renal dysfunction, require careful observation.
6. **Uterine bleeding and mastodynia.** Certain patients may develop undesirable manifestations of estrogenic stimulation, such as abnormal uterine bleeding and mastodynia.
7. **Impaired liver function.** Estrogen may be poorly metabolized in patients with impaired liver function and should be administered with caution.

B. *Information for the Patient.* See text of Patient Package Insert below.
C. *Laboratory Tests.* Estrogen administration should generally be guided by clinical response at the smallest dose, rather than laboratory monitoring, for relief of symptoms for those indications in which symptoms are observable.
D. *Drug/Laboratory Test Interactions.*
1. Accelerated prothrombin time, partial thromboplastin time, and platelet aggregation time; increased platelet count; increased factors II, VII antigen, VIII antigen, VIII coagulant activity, IX, X, XII, VII—X complex, II—VII—X complex, and beta-thromboglobulin; decreased levels of anti-factor Xa and antithrombin III, decreased antithrombin III activity; increased levels of fibrinogen and fibrinogen activity; increased plasminogen antigen and activity.
2. Increased thyroid-binding globulin (TBG) leading to increased circulating total thyroid hormone, as measured by protein-bound iodine (PBI), T4 levels (by column or by radioimmunoassay) or T3 levels by radioimmunoassay. T3 resin uptake is decreased, reflecting the elevated TBG. Free T4 and free T3 concentrations are unaltered.
3. Other binding proteins may be elevated in serum, i.e., corticosteroid binding globulin (CBG), sex hormone-binding globulin (SHBG), leading to increased circulating corticosteroids and sex steroids respectively. Free or biologically active hormone concentrations are unchanged. Other plasma proteins may be increased (angiotensinogen/renin substrate, alpha-I-antitrypsin, ceruloplasmin).
4. Increased plasma HDL and HDL-2 subfraction concentrations, reduced LDL cholesterol concentration, increased triglycerides levels.
5. Impaired glucose tolerance.
6. Reduced response to metyrapone test.
7. Reduced serum folate concentration.

E. *Carcinogenesis, Mutagenesis, and Impairment of Fertility.* Long-term continuous administration of natural and synthetic estrogens in certain animal species increases the frequency of carcinomas of the breast, uterus, cervix, vagina, testis, and liver. See "CONTRAINDICATIONS" and "WARNINGS" sections.
F. *Pregnancy Category X.* Estrogens should not be used during pregnancy. See "CONTRAINDICATIONS" and BOXED WARNING.
G. *Nursing Mothers.* As a general principle, the administration of any drug to nursing mothers should be done only when clearly necessary since many drugs are excreted in human milk. In addition, estrogen administration to nursing mothers has been shown to decrease the quantity and quality of the milk.

ADVERSE REACTIONS

The following additional adverse reactions have been reported with estrogen therapy (see WARNINGS regarding induction of neoplasia, adverse effects on the fetus, increased incidence of gallbladder disease, cardiovascular disease, elevated blood pressure, and hypercalcemia).

1. *Genitourinary system.*
   Changes in vaginal bleeding pattern and abnormal withdrawal bleeding or flow; breakthrough bleeding, spotting.
   Increase in size of uterine leiomyomata.
   Vaginal candidiasis.
   Change in amount of cervical secretion.
2. *Breast.*
   Tenderness, enlargement.
3. *Gastrointestinal.*
   Nausea, vomiting.
   Abdominal cramps, bloating.
   Cholestatic jaundice.
   Increased incidence of gallbladder disease.
4. *Skin.*
   Chloasma or melasma that may persist when drug is discontinued.
   Erythema multiforme.
   Erythema nodosum.
   Hemorrhagic eruption.
   Loss of scalp hair.
   Hirsuitism.
5. *Eyes.*
   Steepening of corneal curvature.
   Intolerance to contact lenses.
6. *Central Nervous System.*
   Headache, migraine, dizziness.
   Mental depression.
   Chorea.
7. *Miscellaneous.*
   Increase or decrease in weight.
   Reduced carbohydrate tolerance.
   Aggravation of porphyria.

Edema.
Changes in libido.

OVERDOSAGE

Serious ill effects have not been reported following acute ingestion of large doses of estrogen-containing oral contraceptives by young children. Overdosage of estrogen may cause nausea and vomiting, and withdrawal bleeding may occur in females.

DOSAGE AND ADMINISTRATION

1. For treatment of moderate to severe vasomotor symptoms, vulval and vaginal atrophy associated with the menopause, the lowest dose and regimen that will control symptoms should be chosen and medication should be discontinued as promptly as possible.
Attempts to discontinue or taper medication should be made at 3-month to 6-month intervals.
Usual dosage ranges:
Vasomotor symptoms—0.75 mg to 6 mg estropipate per day. The lowest dose that will control symptoms should be chosen. If the patient has not menstruated within the last two months or more, cyclic administration is started arbitrarily. If the patient is menstruating, cyclic administration is started on day 5 of bleeding.
Vulval and vaginal atrophy—0.75 mg to 6 mg estropipate daily, depending upon the tissue response of the individual patient. The lowest dose that will control symptoms should be chosen. Administer cyclically.
2. For treatment of female hypoestrogenism due to hypogonadism, castration, or primary ovarian failure.
Usual dosage ranges:
Female hypogonadism—A daily dose of 1.5 mg to 9 mg estropipate may be given for the first three weeks of a theoretical cycle, followed by a rest period of eight to ten days. The lowest dose that will control symptoms should be chosen. If bleeding does not occur by the end of this period, the same dosage schedule is repeated. The number of courses of estrogen therapy necessary to produce bleeding may vary depending on the responsiveness of the endometrium. If satisfactory withdrawal bleeding does not occur, an oral progestogen may be given in addition to estrogen during the third week of the cycle.
Female castration or primary ovarian failure—A daily dose of 1.5 mg to 9 mg estropipate may be given for the first three weeks of a theoretical cycle, followed by a rest period of eight to ten days. Adjust dosage upward or downward according to the severity of symptoms and response of the patient. For maintenance, adjust dosage to lowest level that will provide effective control.
Treated patients with an intact uterus should be monitored closely for signs of endometrial cancer and appropriate diagnostic measures should be taken to rule out malignancy in the event of persistent or recurring abnormal vaginal bleeding.
3. For prevention of osteoporosis. A daily dose of one ORTHO-EST .625 (0.75 mg estropipate) tablet for 25 days of a 31-day cycle per month.

HOW SUPPLIED

ORTHO-EST (estropipate tablets, USP) is supplied as ORTHO-EST .625 (0.75 mg estropipate; calculated as sodium estrone sulfate 0.625 mg), white, diamond-shaped tablets, scored on one side and imprinted with ORTHO 1801 on the other, NDC 0062-1801-01; and ORTHO-EST 1.25 (1.5 mg estropipate; calculated as sodium estrone sulfate 1.25 mg), lavender, diamond-shaped tablets, scored on one side and imprinted with ORTHO 1800 on the other, NDC 0062-1800-01. Both tablet sizes are available in bottles of 100.
Tablets are standardized to provide uniform estrone activity and are scored to provide dosage flexibility.
Dispense in tight, light-resistant containers as defined in the USP.
Store below 30°C (86°F).

PATIENT INFORMATION
WHAT YOU SHOULD KNOW ABOUT ESTROGENS
ORTHO-EST
(estropipate tablets, USP)

INTRODUCTION

This leaflet describes when and how to use estrogens, and the risks and benefits of estrogen treatment.
Estrogens have important benefits but also some risks. You must decide, with your doctor, whether the risks to you of estrogen use are acceptable because of their benefits. If you use estrogens, check with your doctor to be sure you are using the lowest possible dose that works, and that you do not use them longer than necessary. How long you need to use estrogens will depend on the reason for use.

WARNINGS
ESTROGENS INCREASE THE RISK OF CANCER OF THE UTERUS IN WOMEN WHO HAVE HAD THEIR MENOPAUSE ("CHANGE OF LIFE").

If you use any estrogen-containing drug, it is important to visit your doctor regularly and report any unusual

---

vaginal bleeding right away. Vaginal bleeding after menopause may be a warning sign of uterine cancer. Your doctor should evaluate any unusual vaginal bleeding to find out the cause.
ESTROGENS SHOULD NOT BE USED DURING PREGNANCY.
Estrogens do not prevent miscarriage (spontaneous abortion) and are not needed in the days following childbirth. If you take estrogens during pregnancy, your unborn child has a greater than usual chance of having birth defects. The risk of developing these defects is small, but clearly larger than the risk in children whose mothers did not take estrogens during pregnancy. These birth defects may affect the baby's urinary system and sex organs. Daughters born to mothers who took DES (an estrogen drug) have a higher than usual chance of developing cancer of the vagina or cervix when they become teenagers or young adults. Sons may have a higher than usual chance of developing cancer of the testicles when they become teenagers or young adults.

USES OF ESTROGEN

(Not every estrogen drug is approved for every use listed in this section. If you want to know which of these possible uses are approved for the medicine prescribed for you, ask your doctor or pharmacist to show you the professional labeling. You can also look up the specific estrogen product in a book called the "Physicians' Desk Reference", which is available in many book stores and public libraries. Generic drugs carry virtually the same labeling information as their brand name versions.)
● **To reduce moderate or severe menopausal symptoms.** Estrogens are hormones made by the ovaries of normal women. Between ages 45 and 55, the ovaries normally stop making estrogens. This leads to a drop in body estrogen levels which causes the "change of life" or menopause (the end of monthly menstrual periods). If both ovaries are removed during an operation before natural menopause takes place, the sudden drop in estrogen levels causes "surgical menopause".
When the estrogen levels begin dropping, some women develop very uncomfortable symptoms, such as feelings of warmth in the face, neck, and chest, or sudden intense episodes of heat and sweating ("hot flashes" or "hot flushes"). Using estrogen drugs can help the body adjust to lower estrogen levels and reduce these symptoms. Most women have only mild menopausal symptoms or none at all and do not need to use estrogen drugs for these symptoms. Others may need to take estrogens for a few months while their bodies adjust to lower estrogen levels. The majority of women do not need estrogen replacement for longer than six months for these symptoms.
● **To treat vulval and vaginal atrophy** (itching, burning, dryness in or around the vagina, difficulty or burning on urination) associated with menopause.
● **To treat certain conditions in which a young women's ovaries do not produce enough estrogen naturally.**
● **To treat certain types of abnormal vaginal bleeding due to hormonal imbalance** when your doctor has found no serious cause of the bleeding.
● **To treat certain cancers in special situations, in men and women.**
● **To prevent thinning of bones.**
Osteoporosis is a thinning of the bones that makes them weaker and allows them to break more easily. The bones of the spine, wrists and hips break more often in osteoporosis. Both men and women start to lose bone mass after about age 40, but women lose bone mass faster after the menopause. Using estrogens after the menopause slows down bone thinning and may prevent bones from breaking. Lifelong adequate calcium intake, either in the diet (such as dairy products) or by calcium supplements (to reach a total daily intake of 1000 milligrams per day before menopause or 1500 milligrams per day after menopause), may help to prevent osteoporosis. Regular weight-bearing exercise (like walking and running for an hour, two or three times a week) may also help to prevent osteoporosis. Before you change your calcium intake or exercise habits, it is important to discuss these lifestyle changes with your doctor to find out if they are safe for you.
Since estrogen use has some risks, only women who are likely to develop osteoporosis should use estrogens for prevention. Women who are likely to develop osteoporosis often have the following characteristics: white or Asian race, slim, cigarette smokers, and a family history of osteoporosis in a mother, sister, or aunt. Women who have relatively early menopause, often because their ovaries were removed during an operation ("surgical menopause"), are more likely to develop osteoporosis than women whose menopause happens at the average age.

WHO SHOULD NOT USE ESTROGENS

Estrogens should not be used:
● **During pregnancy (see BOXED WARNING).**
If you think you may be pregnant, do not use any form of estrogen-containing drug. Using estrogens while you are

---

pregnant may cause your unborn child to have birth defects. Estrogens do not prevent miscarriage.
● **If you have unusual vaginal bleeding which has not been evaluated by your doctor (see BOXED WARNING).**
Unusual vaginal bleeding can be a warning sign of cancer of the uterus, especially if it happens after menopause. Your doctor must find out the cause of the bleeding so that he or she can recommend the proper treatment. Taking estrogens without visiting your doctor can cause you serious harm if your vaginal bleeding is caused by cancer of the uterus.
● **If you have had cancer.**
Since estrogens increase the risk of certain types of cancer, you should not use estrogens if you have ever had cancer of the breast or uterus, unless your doctor recommends that the drug may help in the cancer treatment. (For certain patients with breast or prostate cancer, estrogens may help.)
● **If you have any circulation problems.**
Estrogen drugs should not be used except in unusually special situations in which your doctor judges that you need estrogen therapy so much that the risks are acceptable. Men and women with abnormal blood clotting conditions should avoid estrogen use (see DANGERS OF ESTROGENS, below).
● **When they do not work.**
During menopause, some women develop nervous symptoms or depression. Estrogens do not relieve these symptoms. You may have heard that taking estrogens for years after menopause will keep your skin soft and supple and keep you feeling young. There is no evidence for these claims and such long-term estrogen use may have serious risks.
● **After childbirth or when breastfeeding a baby.**
Estrogens should not be used to try to stop the breasts from filling with milk after a baby is born. Such treatment may increase the risk of developing blood clots (see DANGERS OF ESTROGENS, below).
If you are breastfeeding, you should avoid using any drugs because many drugs pass through to the baby in the milk. While nursing a baby, you should take drugs only on the advice of your health care provider.

DANGERS OF ESTROGENS

● **Cancer of the uterus.**
Your risk of developing cancer of the uterus gets higher the longer you use estrogens and the larger doses you use. One study showed that after women stop taking estrogens, this higher cancer risk quickly returns to the usual level of risk (as if you had never used estogen therapy). Three other studies showed that the cancer risk stayed high for 8 to more than 15 years after stopping estrogen treatment. **Because of this risk, IT IS IMPORTANT TO TAKE THE LOWEST DOSE THAT WORKS AND TO TAKE IT ONLY AS LONG AS YOU NEED IT.**
Using progestin therapy together with estrogen therapy may reduce the higher risk of uterine cancer related to estrogen use (but see Other Information, below).
If you have had your uterus removed (total hysterectomy), there is no danger of developing cancer of the uterus.
● **Cancer of the breast.**
Most studies have not shown a higher risk of breast cancer in women who have ever used estrogens. However, some studies have reported that breast cancer developed more often (up to twice the usual rate) in women who used estrogens for long periods of time (especially more than 10 years), or who used higher doses for shorter time periods.
Regular breast examinations by a health professional and monthly self-examination are recommended for all women.
● **Gallbladder disease.**
Women who use estrogens after menopause are more likely to develop gallbladder disease needing surgery than women who do not use estrogens.
● **Abnormal blood clotting.**
Taking estrogens may cause changes in your blood clotting system. These changes allow the blood to clot more easily, possibly allowing clots to form in your bloodstream. If blood clots do form in your bloodstream, they can cut off the blood supply to vital organs, causing serious problems. These problems may include a stroke (by cutting off blood to the brain), a heart attack (by cutting off blood to the heart), a pulmonary embolus (by cutting off blood to the lungs), or other problems. Any of these conditions may cause death or serious long-term disability. However, most studies of low dose estrogen usage by women do not show an increased risk of these complications.

SIDE EFFECTS

In addition to the risks listed above, the following side effects have been reported with estrogen use:
Nausea and vomiting
Breast tenderness or enlargement
Enlargement of benign tumors ("fibroids") of the uterus.
Retention of excess fluid. This may make some conditions worsen, such as asthma, epilepsy, migraine, heart disease, or kidney disease.

Continued on next page

Ortho—Cont.

A spotty darkening of the skin, particularly on the face.

REDUCING RISK OF ESTROGEN USE

If you use estrogens, you can reduce your risks by doing these things:

● **See your doctor regularly.** While you are using estrogens, it is important to visit your doctor at least once a year for a check up. If you develop vaginal bleeding while taking estrogens, you may need further evaluation. If members of your family have had breast cancer or if you have ever had breast lumps or an abnormal mammogram (breast X ray), you may need to have more frequent breast examinations.

● **Reassess your need for estrogens.** You and your doctor should reevaluate whether or not you still need estrogens at least every six months.

● **Be alert for signs of trouble.** If any of these warning signals (or any other unusual symptoms) happen while you are using estrogens, call your doctor immediately:
Abnormal bleeding from the vagina (possible uterine cancer).
Pains in the calves or chest, sudden shortness of breath, or coughing blood (possible clot in the legs, heart, or lungs).
Severe headache or vomiting, dizziness, faintness, changes in vision or speech, weakness or numbness of an arm or leg (possible clot in the brain or eye).
Breast lumps (possible breast cancer, ask your doctor or health professional to show you how to examine your breasts monthly).
Yellowing of the skin or eyes (possible liver problem).
Pain, swelling, or tenderness in the abdomen (possible gallbladder problem).

OTHER INFORMATION

Some doctors may choose to prescribe a progestin, a different hormonal drug, for you to take together with your estrogen treatment. Progestins lower your risk of developing endometrial hyperplasia (a possible pre-cancerous condition of the uterus) while using estrogens. Taking estrogens and progestins together may also protect you from the higher risk of uterine cancer, but this has not been clearly established. Combined use of progestin and estrogen treatment may have additional risks, however. The possible risks include unhealthy effects on blood fats (especially a lowering of HDL cholesterol, the "good" blood fat which protects against heart disease risk), unhealthy effects on blood sugar (which might worsen a diabetic condition), and a possible further increase in the breast cancer risk which may be associated with long-term estrogen use. The type of progestin drug used and its dosage schedule may be important in minimizing these effects.
Your doctor has prescribed this drug for you and you alone. Do not give the drug to anyone else.
If you will be taking calcium supplements as part of the treatment to help prevent osteoporosis, check with your doctor about how much to take.
Keep this and all drugs out of the reach of children. In case of overdose, call your doctor, hospital or poison control center immediately.
This leaflet provides a summary of the most important information about estrogens. If you want more information, ask your doctor or pharmacist to show you the professional labeling. The professional labeling is also published in a book called the "Physicians' Desk Reference," which is available in book stores and public libraries. Generic drugs carry virtually the same labeling information as their brand name versions.

HOW SUPPLIED

ORTHO-EST .625 (estropipate tablets USP, 0.75 mg) is a white, diamond-shaped tablet.
ORTHO-EST 1.25 (estropipate tablets USP, 1.5 mg) is a lavender, diamond-shaped tablet.

ORTHO PHARMACEUTICAL CORPORATION
Raritan, New Jersey 08869
© OPC 1993
631-10-181-3   Revised April 1996
Shown in Product Identification Guide, page 326

ORTHO–NOVUM® Tablets ℞
(norethindrone/mestranol) or
(norethindrone/ethinyl estradiol)
and
MODICON® Tablets ℞
(norethindrone/ethinyl estradiol)

Patients should be counseled that this product does not protect against HIV infection (AIDS) and other sexually transmitted diseases.

COMBINATION ORAL CONTRACEPTIVES

Each of the following products is a combination oral contraceptive containing the progestational compound norethindrone and the estrogenic compound ethinyl estradiol:

ORTHO-NOVUM 7/7/7 ☐ 21 Tablets and ORTHO-NOVUM 7/7/7 ☐ 28 Tablets: Each white tablet contains 0.5 mg of norethindrone and 0.035 mg of ethinyl estradiol. Inactive ingredients include lactose, magnesium stearate and pregelatinized starch. Each light peach tablet contains 0.75 mg of norethindrone and 0.035 mg of ethinyl estradiol. Inactive ingredients include FD&C Yellow No. 6, lactose, magnesium stearate and pregelatinized starch. Each peach tablet contains 1 mg of norethindrone and 0.035 mg of ethinyl estradiol. Inactive ingredients include FD&C Yellow No. 6, lactose, magnesium stearate and pregelatinized starch. Each green tablet in the ORTHO-NOVUM 7/7/7 ☐ 28 package contains only inert ingredients, as follows: D&C Yellow No. 10 Aluminum Lake, FD&C Blue No. 2 Aluminum Lake, lactose, magnesium stearate, microcrystalline cellulose and pregelatinized starch.

ORTHO-NOVUM 10/11 ☐ 21 Tablets and ORTHO-NOVUM 10/11 ☐ 28 Tablets: Each white tablet contains 0.5 mg of norethindrone and 0.035 mg of ethinyl estradiol. Inactive ingredients include lactose, magnesium stearate and pregelatinized starch. Each peach tablet contains 1 mg norethindrone and 0.035 mg of ethinyl estradiol. Inactive ingredients include FD&C Yellow No. 6, lactose, magnesium stearate and pregelatinized starch. Each green tablet in the ORTHO-NOVUM 10/11 ☐ 28 package contains only inert ingredients, as listed under green tablets in ORTHO-NOVUM 7/7/7 ☐ 28.

ORTHO-NOVUM 1/35 ☐ 21 Tablets and ORTHO-NOVUM 1/35 ☐ 28 Tablets: Each peach tablet contains 1 mg of norethindrone and 0.035 mg of ethinyl estradiol. Inactive ingredients include FD&C Yellow No. 6, lactose, magnesium stearate and pregelatinized starch. Each green tablet in the ORTHO-NOVUM 1/35 ☐ 28 package contains only inert ingredients, as listed under green tablets in ORTHO-NOVUM 7/7/7 ☐ 28.

MODICON 21 Tablets and MODICON 28 Tablets: Each white tablet contains 0.5 mg of norethindrone and 0.035 mg of ethinyl estradiol. Inactive ingredients include lactose, magnesium stearate and pregelatinized starch. Each green tablet in the MODICON 28 package contains only inert ingredients, as listed under green tablets in ORTHO-NOVUM 7/7/7 ☐ 28.

Each of the following products is a combination oral contraceptive containing the progestational compound norethindrone and the estrogenic compound mestranol:

ORTHO-NOVUM 1/50 ☐ 21 Tablets and ORTHO-NOVUM 1/50 ☐ 28 Tablets: Each yellow tablet contains 1 mg of norethindrone and 0.05 mg of mestranol. Inactive ingredients include D&C Yellow No. 10, lactose, magnesium stearate and pregelatinized starch. Each green tablet in the ORTHO-NOVUM 1/50 ☐ 28 package contains only inert ingredients, as listed under green tablets in ORTHO-NOVUM 7/7/7 ☐ 28.

norethindrone

ethinyl estradiol

mestranol

CLINICAL PHARMACOLOGY
COMBINATION ORAL CONTRACEPTIVES

Combination oral contraceptives act by suppression of gonadotropins. Although the primary mechanism of this action is inhibition of ovulation, other alterations include changes in the cervical mucus (which increase the difficulty of sperm entry into the uterus) and the endometrium (which reduce the likelihood of implantation).

INDICATIONS AND USAGE

ORTHO-NOVUM 7/7/7 ☐ 21, ORTHO-NOVUM 7/7/7 ☐ 28, ORTHO-NOVUM 10/11 ☐ 21, ORTHO-NOVUM 10/11 ☐ 28, ORTHO-NOVUM 1/35 ☐ 21, ORTHO-NOVUM 1/35 ☐ 28, MODICON 21, MODICON 28, ORTHO-NOVUM 1/50 ☐ 21, and ORTHO-NOVUM 1/50 ☐ 28 are indicated for the prevention of pregnancy in women who elect to use this product as a method of contraception.

Oral contraceptives are highly effective. Table I lists the typical accidental pregnancy rates for users of combination oral contraceptives and other methods of contraception. The efficacy of these contraceptive methods, except sterilization, depends upon the reliability with which they are used. Correct and consistent use of methods can result in lower failure rates.

TABLE I: LOWEST EXPECTED AND TYPICAL FAILURE RATES DURING THE FIRST YEAR OF CONTINUOUS USE OF A METHOD
% of Women Experiencing an Accidental Pregnancy in the First Year of Continuous Use

Method	Lowest Expected*	Typical**
(No Contraceptive)	(85)	(85)
Oral contraceptives		3
combined	0.1	N/A***
progestin only	0.5	N/A***
Diaphragm with spermicidal cream or jelly	6	18
Spermicides alone (foams, creams, gels, jellies vaginal suppositories, and vaginal film)	6	21
Vaginal sponge		
nulliparous	9	18
parous	20	36
Implant	0.09	0.09
Injection: depot medroxyprogesterone acetate	0.3	0.3
IUD		
progesterone	1.5	2.0
Copper T 380A	0.6	0.8
Condom without spermicides		
female	5	21
male	3	12
Cervical Cap with spermicidal cream or jelly		
nulliparous	9	18
parous	26	36
Periodic abstinence (all methods)	1–9	20
Female sterilization	0.4	0.4
Male sterilization	0.10	0.15

Adapted from RA Hatcher et al, Table 5–2, (1994) ref. #1.
* The authors' best guess of the percentage of women expected to experience an accidental pregnancy among couples who initiate a method (not necessarily for the first time) and who use it consistently and correctly during the first year if they do not stop for any other reason.
** This term represents "typical" couples who initiate use of a method (not necessarily for the first time), who experience an accidental pregnancy during the first year if they do not stop for any other reason.
*** N/A—Data not available

CONTRAINDICATIONS

Oral contraceptives should not be used in women who currently have the following conditions:
● Thrombophlebitis or thromboembolic disorders
● A past history of deep vein thrombophlebitis or thromboembolic disorders
● Cerebral vascular or coronary artery disease
● Known or suspected carcinoma of the breast
● Carcinoma of the endometrium or other known or suspected estrogen-dependent neoplasia
● Undiagnosed abnormal genital bleeding
● Cholestatic jaundice of pregnancy or jaundice with prior pill use
● Hepatic adenomas or carcinomas
● Known or suspected pregnancy

WARNINGS

Cigarette smoking increases the risk of serious cardiovascular side effects from oral contraceptive use. This risk increases with age and with heavy smoking (15 or more cigarettes per day) and is quite marked in women over 35 years of age. Women who use oral contraceptives should be strongly advised not to smoke.

The use of oral contraceptives is associated with increased risks of several serious conditions including myocardial infarction, thromboembolism, stroke, hepatic neoplasia, and gallbladder disease, although the risk of serious morbidity or mortality is very small in healthy women without underlying factors. The risk of morbidity and mortality increases

significantly in the presence of other underlying risk factors such as hypertension, hyperlipidemias, obesity and diabetes. Practitioners prescribing oral contraceptives should be familiar with the following information relating to these risks. The information contained in this package insert is principally based on studies carried out in patients who used oral contraceptives with higher formulations of estrogens and progestogens than those in common use today. The effect of long term use of the oral contraceptives with lower formulations of both estrogens and progestogens remains to be determined.

Throughout this labeling, epidemiological studies reported are of two types: retrospective or case control studies and prospective or cohort studies. Case control studies provide a measure of the relative risk of a disease, namely, a *ratio* of the incidence of a disease among oral contraceptive users to that among nonusers. The relative risk does not provide information on the actual clinical occurrence of a disease. Cohort studies provide a measure of attributable risk, which is the *difference* in the incidence of disease between oral contraceptive users and nonusers. The attributable risk does provide information about the actual occurrence of a disease in the population (adapted from refs. 2 and 3 with the author's permission). For further information, the reader is referred to a text on epidemiological methods.

1. THROMBOEMBOLIC DISORDERS AND OTHER VASCULAR PROBLEMS

a. Myocardial Infarction

An increased risk of myocardial infarction has been associated with oral contraceptive use. This risk is primarily in smokers or women with other underlying risk factors for coronary artery disease such as hypertension, hypercholesterolemia, morbid obesity, and diabetes. The relative risk of heart attack for current oral contraceptive users has been estimated to be two to six[4–10]. The risk is very low under the age of 30.

Smoking in combination with oral contraceptive use has been shown to contribute substantially to the incidence of myocardial infarctions in women in their mid-thirties or older with smoking accounting for the majority of excess cases[11]. Mortality rates associated with circulatory disease have been shown to increase substantially in smokers, especially in those 35 years of age and older among women who use oral contraceptives.

Table II:

CIRCULATORY DISEASE MORTALITY RATES PER 100,000 WOMAN-YEARS BY AGE, SMOKING STATUS AND ORAL CONTRACEPTIVE USE

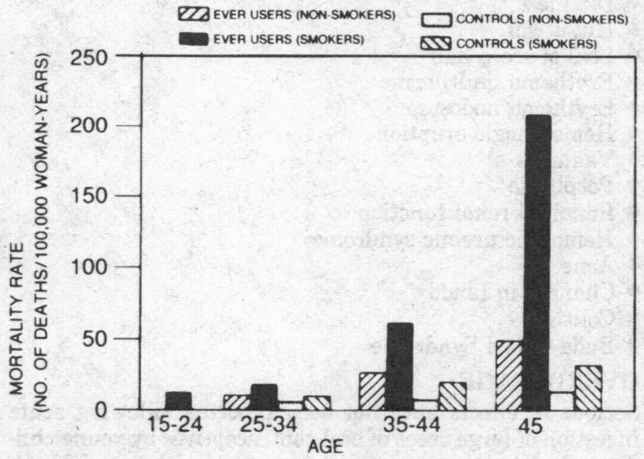

(Adapted from P.M. Layde and V. Beral, ref. #12.)

Oral contraceptives may compound the effects of well-known risk factors, such as hypertension, diabetes, hyperlipidemias, age and obesity[13]. In particular, some progestogens are known to decrease HDL cholesterol and cause glucose intolerance, while estrogens may create a state of hyperinsulinism[14–18]. Oral contraceptives have been shown to increase blood pressure among users (see section 9 in WARNINGS). Similar effects on risk factors have been associated with an increased risk of heart disease. Oral contraceptives must be used with caution in women with cardiovascular disease risk factors.

b. Thromboembolism

An increased risk of thromboembolic and thrombotic disease associated with the use of oral contraceptives is well established. Case control studies have found the relative risk of users compared to non-users to be 3 for the first episode of superficial venous thrombosis, 4 to 11 for deep vein thrombosis or pulmonary embolism, and 1.5 to 6 for women with predisposing conditions for venous thromboembolic disease[2,3,19–24]. Cohort studies have shown the relative risk to be somewhat lower, about 3 for new cases and about 4.5 for new cases requiring hospitalization[25]. The risk of thromboembolic disease associated with oral contraceptives is not related to length of use and disappears after pill use is stopped[2].

A two- to four-fold increase in relative risk of post-operative thromboembolic complications has been reported with the use of oral contraceptives[9]. The relative risk of venous thrombosis in women who have predisposing conditions is twice that of women without such medical conditions[26]. If feasible, oral contraceptives should be discontinued at least four weeks prior to and for two weeks after elective surgery of a type associated with an increase in risk of thromboembolism and during and following prolonged immobilization. Since the immediate postpartum period is also associated with an increased risk of thromboembolism, oral contraceptives should be started no earlier than four weeks after delivery in women who elect not to breast feed or four weeks after a second trimester abortion.

c. Cerebrovascular diseases

Oral contraceptives have been shown to increase both the relative and attributable risks of cerebrovascular events (thrombotic and hemorrhagic strokes), although, in general, the risk is greatest among older (> 35 years), hypertensive women who also smoke. Hypertension was found to be a risk factor for both users and non-users, for both types of strokes, and smoking interacted to increase the risk of stroke[27–29].

In a large study, the relative risk of thrombotic strokes has been shown to range from 3 for normotensive users to 14 for users with severe hypertension[30]. The relative risk of hemorrhagic stroke is reported to be 1.2 for non-smokers who used oral contraceptives, 2.6 for smokers who did not use oral contraceptives, 7.6 for smokers who used oral contraceptives, 1.8 for normotensive users and 25.7 for users with severe hypertension[30]. The attributable risk is also greater in older women[3].

d. Dose-related risk of vascular disease from oral contraceptives

A positive association has been observed between the amount of estrogen and progestogen in oral contraceptives and the risk of vascular disease[31–33]. A decline in serum high density lipoproteins (HDL) has been reported with many progestational agents[14–16]. A decline in serum high density lipoproteins has been associated with an increased incidence of ischemic heart disease. Because estrogens increase HDL cholesterol, the net effect of an oral contraceptive depends on a balance achieved between doses of estrogen and progestogen and the activity of the progestogen used in the contraceptive. The activity and amount of both hormones should be considered in the choice of an oral contraceptive.

Minimizing exposure to estrogen and progestogen is in keeping with good principles of therapeutics. For any particular estrogen/progestogen combination, the dosage regimen prescribed should be one which contains the least amount of estrogen and progestogen that is compatible with a low failure rate and the needs of the individual patient. New acceptors of oral contraceptives agents should be started on preparations containing 0.035 mg or less of estrogen.

e. Persistence of risk of vascular disease

There are two studies which have shown persistence of risk of vascular disease for ever-users of oral contraceptives. In a study in the United States, the risk of developing myocardial infarction after discontinuing oral contraceptives persists for at least 9 years for women 40–49 years who had used oral contraceptives for five or more years, but this increased risk was not demonstrated in other age groups[8]. In another study in Great Britain, the risk of developing cerebrovascular disease persisted for at least 6 years after discontinuation of oral contraceptives, although excess risk was very small[34]. However, both studies were performed with oral contraceptive formulations containing 50 micrograms or higher of estrogens.

2. ESTIMATES OF MORTALITY FROM CONTRACEPTIVE USE

One study gathered data from a variety of sources which have estimated the mortality rate associated with different methods of contraception at different ages (Table III). These estimates include the combined risk of death associated with contraceptive methods plus the risk attributable to pregnancy in the event of method failure. Each method of contraception has its specific benefits and risks. The study concluded that with the exception of oral contraceptive users 35 and older who smoke and 40 and older who do not smoke, mortality associated with all methods of birth control is low and below that associated with childbirth. The observation of an increase in risk of mortality with age for oral contraceptive users is based on data gathered in the 1970's[35]. Current clinical recommendation involves the use of lower estrogen dose formulations and a careful consideration of risk factors. In 1989, the Fertility and Maternal Health Drugs Advisory Committee was asked to review the use of oral contraceptives in women 40 years of age and older. The Committee concluded that although cardiovascular disease risks may be increased with oral contraceptive use after age 40 in healthy non-smoking women (even with the newer low-dose formulations), there are also greater potential health risks associated with pregnancy in older women and with the alternative surgical and medical procedures which may be necessary if such women do not have access to effective and acceptable means of contraception. The Committee recommended that the benefits of low-dose oral contraceptive use by healthy non-smoking women over 40 may outweigh the possible risks.

Of course, older women, as all women who take oral contraceptives, should take an oral contraceptive which contains the least amount of estrogen and progestogen that is compatible with a low failure rate and individual patient needs.

[See table above.]

TABLE III; ANNUAL NUMBER OF BIRTH-RELATED OR METHOD-RELATED DEATHS ASSOCIATED WITH CONTROL OF FERTILITY PER 100,000 NON-STERILE WOMEN, BY FERTILITY CONTROL METHOD ACCORDING TO AGE

Method of control and outcome	15–19	20–24	25–29	30–34	35–39	40–44
No fertility control methods*	7.0	7.4	9.1	14.8	25.7	28.2
Oral contraceptives non-smoker**	0.3	0.5	0.9	1.9	13.8	31.6
Oral contraceptives smoker**	2.2	3.4	6.6	13.5	51.1	117.2
IUD**	0.8	0.8	1.0	1.0	1.4	1.4
Condom*	1.1	1.6	0.7	0.2	0.3	0.4
Diaphragm/ spermacide*	1.9	1.2	1.2	1.3	2.2	2.8
Periodic abstinence*	2.5	1.6	1.6	1.7	2.9	3.6

* Deaths are birth-related
** Deaths are method-related

Adapted from H.W. Ory, ref. #35.

3. CARCINOMA OF THE REPRODUCTIVE ORGANS AND BREASTS

Numerous epidemiological studies have been performed on the incidence of breast, endometrial, ovarian and cervical cancer in women using oral contraceptives. While there are conflicting reports, most studies suggest that use of oral contraceptives is not associated with an overall increase in the risk of developing breast cancer. Some studies have reported an increased relative risk of developing breast cancer, particularly at a younger age. This increased relative risk appears to be related to duration of use[36–44,79–89].

Some studies suggest that oral contraceptive use has been associated with an increase in the risk of cervical intraepithelial neoplasia in some populations of women[45–48]. However, there continues to be controversy about the extent to which such findings may be due to differences in sexual behavior and other factors.

4. HEPATIC NEOPLASIA

Benign hepatic adenomas are associated with oral contraceptive use, although the incidence of benign tumors is rare in the United States. Indirect calculations have estimated the attributable risk to be in the range of 3.3 cases/100,000 for users, a risk that increases after four or more years of use especially with oral contraceptives of higher dose[49]. Rupture of benign, hepatic adenomas may cause death through intra-abdominal hemorrhage[50–51].

Studies from Britain have shown an increased risk of developing hepatocellular carcinoma[52–54] in long-term (> 8 years) oral contraceptive users. However, these cancers are rare in the U.S. and the attributable risk (the excess incidence) of liver cancers in oral contraceptive users approaches less than one per million users.

Continued on next page

Ortho—Cont.

5. OCULAR LESIONS

There have been clincial case reports of retinal thrombosis associated with the use of oral contraceptives. Oral contraceptives should be discontinued if there is unexplained partial or complete loss of vision; onset of proptosis or diplopia; papilledema; or retinal vascular lesions. Appropriate diagnostic and therapeutic measures should be undertaken immediately.

6. ORAL CONTRACEPTIVE USE BEFORE OR DURING EARLY PREGNANCY

Extensive epidemiological studies have revealed no increased risk of birth defects in women who have used oral contraceptives prior to pregnancy[56,57]. The majority of recent studies also do not indicate a teratogenic effect, particularly in so far as cardiac anomalies and limb reduction defects are concerned[55,56,58,59], when taken inadvertently during early pregnancy.

The administration of oral contraceptives to induce withdrawal bleeding should not be used as a test for pregnancy. Oral contraceptives should not be used during pregnancy to treat threatened or habitual abortion.

7. GALLBLADDER DISEASE

Earlier studies have reported an increased lifetime relative risk of gallbladder surgery in users of oral contraceptives and estrogens[60,61]. More recent studies, however, have shown that the relative risk of developing gallbladder disease among oral contraceptive users may be minimal[62-64]. The recent findings of minimal risk may be related to the use of oral contraceptive formulations containing lower hormonal doses of estrogens and progestogens.

8. CARBOHYDRATE AND LIPID METABOLIC EFFECTS

Oral contraceptives have been shown to cause a decrease in glucose tolerance in a significant percentage of users[17]. This effect has been shown to be directly related to estrogen dose[65]. Progestogens increase insulin secretion and create insulin resistance, this effect varying with different progestational agents[17,66]. However, in the non-diabetic woman, oral contraceptives appear to have no effect on fasting blood glucose[67]. Because of these demonstrated effects, prediabetic and diabetic women in particular should be carefully monitored while taking oral contraceptives.

A small proportion of women will have persistent hypertriglyceridemia while on the pill. As discussed earlier (see WARNINGS 1a and 1d), changes in serum triglycerides and lipoprotein levels have been reported in oral contraceptive users.

9. ELEVATED BLOOD PRESSURE

An increase in blood pressure has been reported in women taking oral contraceptives[68] and this increase is more likely in older oral contraceptive users[69] and with extended duration of use[61]. Data from the Royal College of General Practitioners[12] and subsequent randomized trials have shown that the incidence of hypertension increases with increasing progestational activity.

Women with a history of hypertension or hypertension-related diseases, or renal disease[70] should be encouraged to use another method of contraception. If women elect to use oral contraceptives, they should be monitored closely and if significant elevation of blood pressure occurs, oral contraceptives should be discontinued. For most women, elevated blood pressure will return to normal after stopping oral contraceptives, and there is no difference in the occurrence of hypertension between former and never users[68-71].

10. HEADACHE

The onset or exacerbation of migraine or development of headache with a new pattern which is recurrent, persistent or severe requires discontinuation of oral contraceptives and evaluation of the cause.

11. BLEEDING IRREGULARITIES

Breakthrough bleeding and spotting are sometimes encountered in patients on oral contraceptives, especially during the first three months of use. Non-hormonal causes should be considered and adequate diagnostic measures taken to rule out malignancy or pregnancy in the event of breakthrough bleeding, as in the case of any abnormal vaginal bleeding. If pathology has been excluded, time or a change to another formulation may solve the problem. In the event of amenorrhea, pregnancy should be ruled out.

An alteration in menstrual patterns is likely to occur in women using progestogen-only contraceptives. The amount and duration of flow, cycle length, breakthrough bleeding, spotting and amenorrhea will probably be quite variable. Bleeding irregularities occur more frequently with the use of progestogen-only oral contraceptives than with the combinations and the dropout rate due to such conditions is higher.

Some women may encounter post-pill amenorrhea or oligomenorrhea, especially when such a condition was preexistent.

12. ECTOPIC PREGNANCY

Ectopic as well as intrauterine pregnancy may occur in contraceptive failures. However, in progestogen-only oral contraceptive failures, the ratio of ectopic to intrauterine pregnancies is higher than in women who are not receiving oral contraceptives, since the drugs are more effective in preventing intrauterine than ectopic pregnancies.

PRECAUTIONS

1. PHYSICAL EXAMINATION AND FOLLOW UP

It is good medical practice for all women to have annual history and physical examinations, including women using oral contraceptives. The physical examination, however, may be deferred until after initiation of oral contraceptives if requested by the woman and judged appropriately by the clinician. The physical examination should include special reference to blood pressure, breasts, abdomen and pelvic organs, including cervical cytology, and relevant laboratory tests. In case of undiagnosed, persistent or recurrent abnormal vaginal bleeding, appropriate diagnostic measures should be conducted to rule out malignancy. Women with a strong family history of breast cancer or who have breast nodules should be monitored with particular care.

2. LIPID DISORDERS

Women who are being treated for hyperlipidemias should be followed closely if they elect to use oral contraceptives. Some progestogens may elevate LDL levels and may render the control of hyperlipidemias more difficult.

3. LIVER FUNCTION

If jaundice develops in any woman receiving such drugs, the medication should be discontinued. Steroid hormones may be poorly metabolized in patients with impaired liver function.

4. FLUID RETENTION

Oral contraceptives may cause some degree of fluid retention. They should be prescribed with caution, and only with careful monitoring, in patients with conditions which might be aggravated by fluid retention.

5. EMOTIONAL DISORDERS

Women with a history of depression should be carefully observed and the drug discontinued if depression recurs to a serious degree.

6. CONTACT LENSES

Contact lens wearers who develop visual changes or changes in lens tolerance should be assessed by an ophthalmologist.

7. DRUG INTERACTIONS

Reduced efficacy and increased incidence of breakthrough bleeding and menstrual irregularities have been associated with concomitant use of rifampin. A similar assocation, though less marked, has been suggested with barbiturates, phenylbutazone, phenytoin sodium, carbamazepine and possibly with griseofulvin, ampicillin and tetracyclines[72].

8. INTERACTIONS WITH LABORATORY TESTS

Certain endocrine and liver function tests and blood components may be affected by oral contraceptives:

a. Increased prothrombin and factors VII, VIII, IX, and X; decreased antithrombin 3; increased norepinephrine-induced platelet aggregability.

b. Increased thyroid binding globulin (TBG) leading to increased circulating total thyroid hormone, as measured by protein-bound iodine (PBI), T4 by column or by radio-immunoassay. Free T3 resin uptake is decreased, reflecting the elevated TBG, free T4 concentration is unaltered.

c. Other binding proteins may be elevated in serum.

d. Sex-binding globulins are increased and result in elevated levels of total circulating sex steroids and corticoids; however, free or biologically active levels remain unchanged.

e. Triglycerides may be increased.

f. Glucose tolerance may be decreased.

g. Serum folate levels may be depressed by oral contraceptive therapy. This may be of clinical significance if a woman becomes pregnant shortly after discontinuing oral contraceptives.

9. CARCINOGENESIS

See WARNINGS section.

10. PREGNANCY

Pregnancy Category X. See CONTRAINDICATIONS and WARNINGS sections.

11. NURSING MOTHERS

Small amounts of oral contraceptive steroids have been identified in the milk of nursing mothers and a few adverse effects on the child have been reported, including jaundice and breast enlargement. In addition, oral contraceptives given in the postpartum period may interfere with lactation by decreasing the quantity and quality of breast milk. If possible, the nursing mother should be advised not to use oral contraceptives but to use other forms of contraception until she has completely weaned her child.

12. SEXUALLY TRANSMITTED DISEASES

Patients should be counseled that this product does not protect against HIV infection (AIDS) and other sexually transmitted diseases.

INFORMATION FOR THE PATIENT

See Patient Labeling Printed Below

ADVERSE REACTIONS

An increased risk of the following serious adverse reactions has been associated with the use of oral contraceptives (see WARNINGS section).

- Thrombophlebitis and venous thrombosis with or without embolism
- Arterial thromboembolism
- Pulmonary embolism
- Myocardial infarction
- Cerebral hemorrhage
- Cerebral thrombosis
- Hypertension
- Gallbladder disease
- Hepatic adenomas or benign liver tumors

The following adverse reactions have been reported in patients receiving oral contraceptives and are believed to be drug-related:

- Nausea
- Vomiting
- Gastrointestinal symptoms (such as abdominal cramps and bloating)
- Breakthrough bleeding
- Spotting
- Change in menstrual flow
- Amenorrhea
- Temporary infertility after discontinuance of treatment
- Edema
- Melasma which may persist
- Breast changes: tenderness, enlargement, secretion
- Change in weight (increase or decrease)
- Change in cervical erosion and secretion
- Diminution in lactation when given immediately postpartum
- Cholestatic jaundice
- Migraine
- Rash (allergic)
- Mental depression
- Reduced tolerance to carbohydrates
- Vaginal candidiasis
- Change in corneal curvature (steepening)
- Intolerance to contact lenses

The following adverse reactions have been reported in users of oral contraceptives and the association has been neither confirmed nor refuted:

- Pre-menstrual syndrome
- Cataracts
- Changes in appetite
- Cystitis-like syndrome
- Headache
- Nervousness
- Dizziness
- Hirsutism
- Loss of scalp hair
- Erythema multiforme
- Erythema nodosum
- Hemorrhagic eruption
- Vaginitis
- Porphyria
- Impaired renal function
- Hemolytic uremic syndrome
- Acne
- Changes in libido
- Colitis
- Budd-Chiari Syndrome

OVERDOSAGE

Serious ill effects have not been reported following acute ingestion of large doses of oral contraceptives by young children. Overdosage may cause nausea, and withdrawal bleeding may occur in females.

NON-CONTRACEPTIVE HEALTH BENEFITS

The following non-contraceptive health benefits related to the use of combination oral contraceptives are supported by epidemiological studies which largely utilized oral contraceptive formulations containing estrogen doses exceeding 0.035 mg of estrogen or 0.05 mg mestranol.[73-78]

Effects on menses:

- increased menstrual cycle regularity
- decreased blood loss and decreased incidence of iron deficiency anemia
- decreased incidence of dysmenorrhea

Effects related to inhibition of ovulation:

- decreased incidence of functional ovarian cysts
- decreased incidence of ectopic pregnancies

Other effects:

- decreased incidence of fibroadenomas and fibrocystic disease of the breast
- decreased incidence of acute pelvic inflammatory disease
- decreased incidence of endometrial cancer
- decreased incidence of ovarian cancer

DOSAGE AND ADMINISTRATION

To achieve maximum contraceptive effectiveness, ORTHO-NOVUM Tablets, and MODICON Tablets must be taken exactly as directed and at intervals not exceeding 24 hours. ORTHO-NOVUM Tablets and MODICON Tablets are available in the DIALPAK® Tablet Dispenser which is preset for a Sunday Start. Day 1 Start is also available.

21-Day Regimen (Sunday Start)
When taking ORTHO-NOVUM 7/7/7 ☐ 21, ORTHO-NOVUM 10/11 ☐ 21, ORTHO-NOVUM 1/35 ☐ 21, MODICON 21, and ORTHO-NOVUM 1/50 ☐ 21, the first tablet should be taken on the first Sunday after menstruation begins. If period begins on Sunday, the first tablet is taken on that day. One tablet is taken daily for 21 days. For subsequent cycles, no tablets are taken for 7 days, then a tablet is taken the next day (Sunday). For the first cycle of a Sunday Start regimen, another method of contraception should be used until after the first 7 consecutive days of administration.
If the patient misses one (1) active tablet in Weeks 1, 2, or 3, the tablet should be taken as soon as she remembers. If the patient misses two (2) active tablets in Week 1 or Week 2, the patient should take two (2) tablets the day she remembers and two (2) tablets the next day; and then continue taking one (1) tablet a day until she finishes the pack. The patient should be instructed to use a back-up method of birth control if she has sex in the seven (7) days after missing pills. If the patient misses two (2) active tablets in the third week or misses three (3) or more active tablets in a row, the patient should continue taking one tablet every day until Sunday. On Sunday, the patient should throw out the rest of the pack and start a new pack that same day. The patient should be instructed to use a back-up method of birth control if she has sex in the seven (7) days after missing pills.
Complete instructions to facilitate patient counseling on proper pill usage may be found in the Detailed Patient Labeling ("How to Take the Pill" section).

21-Day Regimen (Day 1 Start)
The dosage of ORTHO-NOVUM 7/7/7 ☐ 21, ORTHO-NOVUM 10/11 ☐ 21, ORTHO-NOVUM 1/35 ☐ 21, MODICON 21, and ORTHO-NOVUM 1/50 ☐ 21, for the initial cycle of therapy is one tablet administered daily from the 1st day through the 21st day of the menstrual cycle, counting the first day of menstrual flow as "Day 1." For subsequent cycles, no tablets are taken for 7 days, then a new course is started of one tablet a day for 21 days. The dosage regimen then continues with 7 days of no medication, followed by 21 days of medication, instituting a three-weeks-on, one-week-off dosage regimen.
If the patient misses one (1) active tablet in Weeks 1, 2, or 3, the tablet should be taken as soon as she remembers. If the patient misses two (2) active tablets in Week 1 or Week 2, the patient should take two (2) tablets the day she remembers and two (2) tablets the next day; and then continue taking one (1) tablet a day until she finishes the pack. The patient should be instructed to use a back-up method of birth control if she has sex in the seven (7) days after missing pills. If the patient misses two (2) active tablets in the third week or misses three (3) or more active tablets in a row, the patient should throw out the rest of the pack and start a new pack that same day. The patient should be instructed to use a back-up method of birth control if she has sex in the seven (7) days after missing pills.
Complete instructions to facilitate patient counseling on proper pill usage may be found in the Detailed Patient Labeling ("How to Take the Pill" section).

28-Day Regimen (Sunday Start)
When taking ORTHO-NOVUM 7/7/7 ☐ 28, ORTHO-NOVUM 10/11 ☐ 28, ORTHO-NOVUM 1/35 ☐ 28, MODICON 28, and ORTHO-NOVUM 1/50 ☐ 28, the first tablet should be taken on the first Sunday after menstruation begins. If period begins on Sunday, the first tablet should be taken that day. Take one active tablet daily for 21 days followed by one green placebo tablet daily for 7 days. After 28 tablets have been taken, a new course is started the next day (Sunday). For the first cycle of a Sunday Start regimen, another method of contraception should be used until after the first 7 consecutive days of administration.
If the patient misses one (1) active tablet in Weeks 1, 2, or 3, the tablet should be taken as soon as she remembers. If the patient misses two (2) active tablets in Week 1 or Week 2, the patient should take two (2) tablets the day she remembers and two (2) tablets the next day; and then continue taking one (1) tablet a day until she finishes the pack. The patient should be instructed to use a back-up method of birth control if she has sex in the seven (7) days after missing pills. If the patient misses two (2) active tablets in the third week or misses three (3) or more active tablets in a row, the patient should continue taking one tablet every day until Sunday. On Sunday, the patient should throw out the rest of the pack and start a new pack that same day. The patient should be instructed to use a back-up method of birth control if she has sex in the seven (7) days after missing pills.
Complete instructions to facilitate patient counseling on proper pill usage may be found in the Detailed Patient Labeling ("How to Take the Pill" section).

28-Day Regimen (Day 1 Start)
The dosage of ORTHO-NOVUM 7/7/7 ☐ 28, ORTHO-NOVUM 10/11 ☐ 28, ORTHO-NOVUM 1/35 ☐ 28, MODICON 28, and ORTHO-NOVUM 1/50 ☐ 28, for the initial cycle of therapy is one active tablet administered daily from the 1st through the 21st day of the menstrual cycle, counting the first day of menstrual flow as "Day 1" followed by one green tablet daily for 7 days. Tablets are taken without interruption for 28 days. After 28 tablets have been taken, a new course is started the next day.
If the patient misses one (1) active tablet in Weeks 1, 2, or 3, the tablet should be taken as soon as she remembers. If the patient misses two (2) active tablets in Week 1 or Week 2, the patient should take two (2) tablets the day she remembers and two (2) tablets the next day; and then continue taking one (1) tablet a day until she finishes the pack. The patient should be instructed to use a back-up method of birth control if she has sex in the seven (7) days after missing pills. If the patient misses two (2) active tablets in the third week or misses three (3) or more active tablets in a row, the patient should throw out the rest of the pack and start a new pack that same day. The patient should be instructed to use a back-up method of birth control if she has sex in the seven (7) days after missing pills.
Complete instructions to facilitate patient counseling on proper pill usage may be found in the Detailed Patient Labeling ("How to Take the Pill" section).
The use of ORTHO-NOVUM 7/7/7, ORTHO-NOVUM 10/11, ORTHO-NOVUM 1/35, MODICON and ORTHO-NOVUM 1/50 for contraception may be initiated 4 weeks postpartum in women who elect not to breast feed. When the tablets are administered during the postpartum period, the increased risk of thromboembolic disease associated with the postpartum period must be considered. (See CONTRAINDICATIONS and WARNINGS concerning thromboembolic disease. See also PRECAUTIONS for "Nursing Mothers.") The possibility of ovulation and conception prior to initiation of medication should be considered.
(See Discussion of Dose-Related Risk of Vascular Disease from Oral Contraceptives.)

ADDITIONAL INSTRUCTIONS FOR ALL DOSING REGIMENS
Breakthrough bleeding, spotting, and amenorrhea are frequent reasons for patients discontinuing oral contraceptives. In breakthrough bleeding, as in all cases of irregular bleeding from the vagina, nonfunctional causes should be borne in mind. In undiagnosed persistent or recurrent abnormal bleeding from the vagina, adequate diagnostic measures are indicated to rule out pregnancy or malignancy. If pathology has been excluded, time or a change to another formulation may solve the problem. Changing to an oral contraceptive with a higher estrogen content, while potentially useful in minimizing menstrual irregularity, should be done only if necessary since this may increase the risk of thromboembolic disease.
Use of oral contraceptives in the event of a missed menstrual period:
1. If the patient has not adhered to the prescribed schedule, the possibility of pregnancy should be considered at the time of the first missed period and oral contraceptive use should be discontinued until pregnancy is ruled out.
2. If the patient has adhered to the prescribed regimen and misses two consecutive periods, pregnancy should be ruled out before continuing oral contraceptive use.

HOW SUPPLIED
ORTHO-NOVUM 7/7/7 ☐ 21 Tablets are available in a DIALPAK® Tablet Dispenser (NDC 0062-1780-15) containing 21 tablets, as follows: 7 white tablets (0.5 mg norethindrone and 0.035 mg ethinyl estradiol), 7 light peach tablets (0.75 mg norethindrone and 0.035 mg ethinyl estradiol) and 7 peach tablets (1 mg norethindrone and 0.035 mg ethinyl estradiol). The white tablets are unscored with "Ortho" and "535" debossed on each side; the light peach tablets are unscored with "Ortho" and "75" debossed on each side; the peach tablets are unscored with "Ortho" and "135" debossed on each side.
ORTHO-NOVUM 7/7/7 ☐ 21 is available for clinic usage in a VERIDATE® Tablet Dispenser (unfilled) and VERIDATE Refills (NDC 0062-1780-20).
ORTHO-NOVUM 7/7/7 ☐ 28 Tablets are available in a DIALPAK Tablet Dispenser (NDC 0062-1781-15) containing 28 tablets as follows: 7 white, 7 light peach and 7 peach tablets as described under ORTHO-NOVUM 7/7/7 ☐ 21, and 7 green tablets containing inert ingredients.
ORTHO-NOVUM 7/7/7 ☐ 28 is available for clinic usage in a VERIDATE Tablet Dispenser (unfilled) and VERIDATE Refills (NDC 0062-1781-20).
ORTHO-NOVUM 10/11 ☐ 21 Tablets are available in a DIALPAK Tablet Dispenser (NDC 0062-1770-15) containing 21 tablets, as follows: 10 white tablets (0.5 mg norethindrone and 0.035 mg ethinyl estradiol) and 11 peach tablets (1 mg norethindrone and 0.035 mg ethinyl estradiol). The white tablets are unscored with "Ortho" and "535" debossed on each side; the peach tablets are unscored with "Ortho" and "135" debossed on each side.
ORTHO-NOVUM 10/11 ☐ 28 Tablets are available in a DIALPAK Tablet Dispenser (NDC 0062-1771-15) containing 28 tablets, as follows: 10 white and 11 peach tablets as described under ORTHO-NOVUM 10/11 ☐ 21, and 7 green tablets containing inert ingredients.
ORTHO-NOVUM 10/11 ☐ 28 is available for clinic usage in a VERIDATE Tablet Dispenser (unfilled) and VERIDATE Refills (NDC 0062-1771-20).
ORTHO-NOVUM 1/35 ☐ 21 Tablets are available in a DIALPAK Tablet Dispenser (NDC 0062-1760-15) containing 21 peach tablets (1 mg norethindrone and 0.035 mg ethinyl estradiol) which are unscored with "Ortho" and "135" debossed on each side.
ORTHO-NOVUM 1/35 ☐ 21 is available for clinic usage in a VERIDATE Tablet Dispenser (unfilled) and VERIDATE Refills (NDC 0062-1760-20).
ORTHO-NOVUM 1/35 ☐ 28 Tablets are available in a DIALPAK Tablet Dispenser (NDC 0062-1761-15) containing 28 tablets, as follows: 21 peach tablets as described under ORTHO-NOVUM 1/35 ☐ 21, and 7 green tablets containing inert ingredients.
ORTHO-NOVUM 1/35 ☐ 28 is available for clinic usage in a VERIDATE Tablet Dispenser (unfilled) and VERIDATE Refills (NDC 0062-1761-20).
MODICON 21 Tablets are available in a DIALPAK Tablet Dispenser (NDC 0062-1712-15) containing 21 white tablets (0.5 mg norethindrone and 0.035 mg ethinyl estradiol) which are unscored with "Ortho" and "535" debossed on each side.
MODICON 28 Tablets are available in a DIALPAK Tablet Dispenser (NDC 0062-1714-15) containing 28 tablets, as follows: 21 white tablets as described under MODICON 21, and 7 green tablets containing inert ingredients.
MODICON 28 is available for clinic usage in a VERIDATE Tablet Dispenser (unfilled) and VERIDATE Refills (NDC 0062-1714-20).
ORTHO-NOVUM 1/50 ☐ 21 Tablets are available in a DIALPAK Tablet Dispenser (NDC 0062-1331-15) containing 21 yellow tablets (1 mg norethindrone and 0.05 mg mestranol) which are unscored with "Ortho" and "150" debossed on each side.
ORTHO-NOVUM 1/50 ☐ 21 is available for clinic usage in a VERIDATE Tablet Dispenser (unfilled) and VERIDATE Refills (NDC 0062-1331-20).
ORTHO-NOVUM 1/50 ☐ 28 Tablets are available in a DIALPAK Tablet Dispenser (NDC 0062-1332-15) containing 28 tablets, as follows: 21 yellow tablets as described under ORTHO-NOVUM 1/50 ☐ 21, and 7 green tablets containing inert ingredients.
ORTHO-NOVUM 1/50 ☐ 28 is available for clinic usage in a VERIDATE Tablet Dispenser (unfilled) and VERIDATE Refills (NDC 0062-1332-20).

REFERENCES
1. Hatcher RA, et al. 1994. Contraceptive Technology. Sixteenth Edition. New York: Irvington Publishers.
2. Stadel BV. Oral contraceptives and cardiovascular disease. (Pt. 1). N Engl J Med 1981; 305:612–618. **3.** Stadel BV. Oral contraceptives and cardiovascular disease. (Pt. 2). N Engl J Med 1981; 305:672–677. **4.** Adam SA, Thorogood M. Oral contraception and myocardial infarction revisted: the effects of new preparations and prescribing patterns. Br J Obstet Gynecol 1981; 88:838–845. **5.** Mann JI, Inman WH. Oral contraceptives and death from myocardial infarction. Br Med J 1975; 2(5965):245–248. **6.** Mann JI, Vessel MP, Thorogood M, Doll R. Myocardial infarction in young women with special reference to oral contraceptive practice. Br Med J 1975; 2(5956):241–245. **7.** Royal College of General Practitioners' Oral Contraception Study: Further analyses of mortality in oral contraceptive users. Lancet 1981; 1:541–546. **8.** Slone D, Shapiro S, Kaufman DW, Rosenberg L, Miettinen OS, Stolley PD. Risk of myocardial infarction in relation to current and discontinued use of oral contraceptives. N Engl J Med 1981; 305:420–424. **9.** Vessey MP. Female hormones and vascular disease-an epidemiological overview. Br J Fam Plann 1980; 6(Supplement):1–12. **10.** Russell-Briefel RG, Ezzati TM, Fulwood R, Perlman JA, Murphy RS. Cardiovascular risk status and oral contraceptive use, United States, 1976–80. Prevent Med 1986; 15:352–362. **11.** Goldbaum GM, Kendrick JS, Hogelin GC, Gentry EM. The relative impact of smoking and oral contraceptive use on women in the United States. JAMA 1987; 258:1339–1342. **12.** Layde PM, Beral V. Further analyses of mortality in oral contraceptive users: Royal College of General Practitioners' Oral Contraception Study. (Table 5) Lancet 1981; 1:541–546. **13.** Knopp RH. Arteriosclerosis risk: the roles of oral contraceptives and postmenopausal estrogens. J Reprod Med 1986; 31(9) (Supplement):913–921. **14.** Krauss RM, Roy S. Mishell DR, Casagrande J, Pike MC. Effects of two low-dose oral contraceptives on serum lipids and lipoproteins: Differential changes in high-density lipoproteins subclasses. Am J Obstet 1983; 145:446–452. **15.** Wahl P, Walden C, Knopp R. Hoover J, Wallace R, Heiss G, Rifkind B. Effect of estrogen/progestin potency on lipid/lipoprotein cholesterol. N Engl J Med 1983; 308:862–867. **16.** Wynn V. Niththyananthan R. The effect of progestin in combined oral contraceptives on serum lipids with special reference to high density lipoproteins. Am J Obstet Gynecol 1982; 142:766–771. **17.** Wynn V, Godsland I. Effects of oral contraceptives on carbohydrate metabolism. J

Continued on next page

Ortho—Cont.

Reprod Med 1986; 31(9)(Supplement):892–897. **18.** La Rosa JC. Atherosclerotic risk factors in cardiovascular disease. J. Reprod Med 1986; 31(9)(Supplement):906–912. **19.** Inman WH, Vessey MP. Investigation of death from pulmonary, coronary, and cerebral thrombosis and embolism in women of child-bearing age. Br Med J 1968; 2(5599):193–199. **20.** Maquire MG, Tonascia J, Sartwell PE, Stolley PD, Tockman MS. Increased risk of thrombosis due to oral contraceptives: a further report. Am J Epidemiol 1979; 110(2):188–195. **21.** Petitti DB, Wingerd J, Pellegrin F, Ramacharan S. Risk of vascular disease in women: smoking, oral contraceptives, noncontraceptive estrogens, and other factors. JAMA 1979; 242:1150–1154. **22.** Vessey MP, Doll R. Investigation of relation between use of oral contraceptives and thromboembolic disease. Br Med J 1968; 2(5599):199–205. **23.** Vessey MP, Doll R. Investigation of relation between use of oral contraceptives and thromboembolic disease. A further report. Br Med J 1969; 2(5658):651–657. **24.** Porter JB, Hunter JR, Danielson DA, Jick H. Stergachis A. Oral contraceptives and nonfatal vascular disease-recent experience. Obstet Gynecol 1982; 59(3):299–302. **25.** Vessey M, Doll R, Peto R, Johnson B, Wiggins P. A long-term follow-up study of women using different methods of contraception: an interim report. J Biosocial Sci 1976; 8:375–427. **26.** Royal College of General Practitioners: Oral Contraceptives, venous thrombosis, and varicose veins. J Royal Coll Gen Pract 1978; 28:393–399. **27.** Collaborative Group for the Study of Stroke in Young Women: Oral contraception and increased risk of cerebral ischemia or thrombosis. N Engl J Med 1973; 288:871–878.
28. Petitti DB, Wingerd J. Use of oral contraceptives, cigarette smoking, and risk of subarachnoid hemorrhage. Lancet 1978; 2:234–236. **29.** Inman WH. Oral contraceptives and fatal subarachnoid hemorrhage. Br Med J 1979; 2(6203):1468–1470. **30.** Collaborative Group for the Study of Stroke in Young Women: Oral Contraceptives and stroke in young women: associated risk factors. JAMA 1975; 231:718–722. **31.** Inman WH, Vessey MP, Westerholm B, Engelund A. Thromboembolic disease and the steroidal content of oral contraceptives. A report to the Committee on Safety of Drugs. Br Med J 1970; 2:203–209. **32.** Meade TW, Greenberg G, Thompson SG. Progestogens and cardiovascular reactions associated with oral contraceptives and a comparison of the safety of 50- and 35-mcg oestrogen preparations. Br Med J 1980; 280(6224):1157–1161. **33.** Kay CR. Progestogens and arterial disease-evidence from the Royal College of General Practitioners' Study. Am J Obstet Gynecol 1982; 142:762–765. **34.** Royal College of General Practitioners: Incidence of arterial disease among oral contraceptive users. J Royal Coll Gen Pract 1983; 33:75–82. **35.** Ory HW. Mortality associated with fertility and fertility control: 1983. Family Planning Perspectives 1983; 15:50–56. **36.** The Cancer and Steroid Hormone Study of the Centers for Disease Control and the National Institute of Child Health and Human Development: Oral contraceptive use and the risk of breast cancer. N Engl J Med 1986; 315:405–411. **37.** Pike MC, Henderson BE, Krailo MD, Duke A, Roy S. Breast cancer in young women and use of oral contraceptives: possible modifying effect of formulation and age at use. Lancet 1983; 2:926–929. **38.** Paul C, Skegg DG, Spears GFS, Kaldor JM. Oral contraceptives and breast cancer: A national study. Br Med J 1986; 293:723–725. **39.** Miller DR, Rosenberg L, Kaufman DW, Schottenfeld D, Stolley PD, Shapiro S. Breast cancer risk in relation to early oral contraceptive use. Obstet Gynecol 1986; 68:863–868. **40.** Olson H, Olson KL, Moller TR, Ranstam J, Holm P. Oral contraceptive use and breast cancer in young women in Sweden (letter). Lancet 1985; 2:748–749. **41.** McPherson K, Vessey M, Neil A, Doll R, Jones L, Roberts M. Early contraceptive use and breast cancer: Results of another case-control study. Br J Cancer 1987; 56:653–660. **42.** Huggins GR, Zucker PF. Oral contraceptives and neoplasia: 1987 update. Fertil Steril 1987; 47:733–761. **43.** McPherson K, Drife JO. The pill and breast cancer: why the uncertainty? Br Med J 1986; 293:709–710. **44.** Shapiro S. Oral contraceptives-time to take stock. N Engl J Med 1987; 315:450–451, **45.** Ory H, Naib Z, Conger SB, Hatcher RA, Tyler CW. Contraceptive choice and prevalence of cervical dysplasia and carcinoma in situ. Am J Obstet Gynecol 1976; 124:573–577. **46.** Vessey MP, Lawless M, McPherson K, Yeates D. Neoplasia of the cervix uteri and contraception: a possible adverse effect of the pill. Lancet 1983; 2:930. **47.** Brinton LA, Huggins GR, Lehman HF, Malli K, Savitz DA, Trapido E, Rosenthal J, Hoover R. Long term use of oral contraceptives and risk of invasive cervical cancer. Int J Cancer 1986; 38:339–344. **48.** WHO Collaborative Study of Neoplasia and Steroid Contraceptives: Invasive cervical cancer and combined oral contraceptives. Br Med J 1985; 290:961–965. **49.** Rooks JB, Ory HW, Ishak KG, Strauss LT, Greenspan JR, Hill AP, Tyler CW. Epidemiology of hepatocellular adenoma: the role of oral contraceptive use. JAMA 1979; 242:644–648. **50.** Bein NN, Goldsmith HS. Recurrent massive hemorrhage from benign hepatic tumors secondary to oral contraceptives. Br J Surg 1977; 64:433–435. **51.** Klatskin G, Hepatic tumors: possible relationship to use of oral contraceptives. Gastroenterology 1977; 73:386–394. **52.** Henderson BE, Preston-Martin S, Edmondson HA, Peters RL, Pike MC. Hepatocellular carcinoma and oral contraceptives. Br J Cancer 1983; 48:437–440. **53.** Neuberger J, Forman D, Doll R, Williams R. Oral contraceptives and hepatocellular carcinoma. Br Med J 1986; 292:1355–1357. **54.** Forman D, Vincent TJ, Doll R. Cancer of the liver and oral contraceptives. Br Med J 1986; 292:1357–1361. **55.** Harlap S, Eldor J. Births following oral contraceptive failures. Obstet Gyncecol 1980; 55:447–452. **56.** Savolainen E, Saksela E, Saxen L. Teratogenic hazards of oral contraceptives analyzed in a national malformation register. Am J Obstet Gynecol 1981: 140:521–524. **57.** Janerich DT, Piper JM, Glebatis DM. Oral contraceptives and birth defects. Am J Epidemiol 1980; 112:73–79. **58.** Ferencz C, Matanoski GM, Wilson PD, Rubin JD, Neill CA, Gutberlet R. Maternal hormone therapy and congenital heart disease. Teratology 1980; 21:225–239. **59.** Rothman KJ, Fyler DC, Goldblatt A, Kreidberg MB. Exogenous hormones and other drug exposures of children with congenital heart disease. Am J Epidemiol 1979; 109:433–439. **60.** Boston Collaborative Drug Surveillance Program: Oral contraceptives and venous thromboembolic disease, surgically confirmed gallbladder disease, and breast tumors. Lancet 1973; 1:1399–1404. **61.** Royal College of General Practitioners: Oral contraceptives and health. New York, Pittman 1974. **62.** Layde PM, Vessey MP, Yeates D. Risk of gallbladder disease: a cohort study of young women attending family planning clinics. J Epidemiol Community Health 1982; 36:274–278. **63.** Rome Group for Epidemiology and Prevention of Cholelithiasis (GREPCO): Prevalence of gallstone disease in an Italian adult female population. Am J Epidemiol 1984; 119:796–805. **64.** Storm BL, Tamragouri RT, Morse ML, Lazar EL, West SL, Stolley PD, Jones JK. Oral contraceptives and other risk factors for gall bladder disease. Clin Pharmacol Ther 1986; 39:335–341. **65.** Wynn V, Adams PW, Godsland IF, Melrose J, Niththyananthan R, Oakley NW, Seedj A. Comparison of effects of different combined oral contraceptive formulations on carbohydrate and lipid metabolism. Lancet 1979; 1:1045–1049. **66.** Wynn V. Effect of progesterone and progestins on carbohydrate metabolism. In: Progesterone and Progestin. Bardin CW, Milgrom E, Mauvis-Jarvis P. eds. New York, Raven Press 1983; pp. 395–410. **67.** Perlman JA, Roussell-Briefel RG, Ezzati TM, Lieberknecht G. Oral glucose tolerance and the potency of oral contraceptive progestogens. J Chronic Dis 1985: 38:857–864. **68.** Royal College of General Practitioners' Oral Contraception Study: Effect on hypertension and benign breast disease of progestogen component in combined oral contraceptives. Lancet 1977; 1:624. **69.** Fisch IR, Frank J. Oral contraceptives and blood pressure. JAMA 1977; 237:2499–2503. **70.** Laragh AJ. Oral contraceptive induced hypertension–nine years later. Am J Obstet Gynecol 1976; 126:141–147. **71.** Ramcharan S, Peritz E, Pellegrin FA, Williams WT. Incidence of hypertension in the Walnut Creek Contraceptive Drug Study cohort: In: Pharmacology of steroid contraceptive drugs. Garattini S, Berendes HW. Eds. New York, Raven Press, 1977; pp. 277–288, (Monographs of the Mario Negri Institute for Pharmacological Research Milan). **72.** Stockley I. Interactions with oral contraceptives. J Pharm 1976; 216:140–143. **73.** The Cancer and Steroid Hormone Study of the Centers for Disease Control and the National Institute of Child Health and Human Development: Oral contraceptive use and the risk of ovarian cancer. JAMA 1983; 249:1596–1599. **74.** The Cancer and Steroid Hormone Study of the Centers for Disease Control and the National Institute of Child Health and Human Development: Combination oral contraceptive use and the risk of endometrial cancer. JAMA 1987; 257:796–800. **75.** Ory HW. Functional ovarian cysts and oral contraceptives: negative association confirmed surgically. JAMA 1974; 228:68–69. **76.** Ory WH, Cole P, MacMahon B, Hoover R. Oral contraceptives and reduced risk of benign breast disease. N Engl J Med 1976; 294:419–422. **77.** Ory HW. The noncontraceptive health benefits from oral contraceptive use. Fam Plann Perspect 1982; 14:182–184. **78.** Ory HW, Forrest JD, Lincoln R. Making choices: Evaluating the health risks and benefits of birth control methods. New York, The Alan Guttmacher Institute, 1983; p. 1. **79.** Schlesselman J, Stadel BV, Murray P, Lai S. Breast cancer in relation to early use of oral contraceptives. JAMA 1988; 259:1828–1833. **80.** Hennekens CH, Speizer FE, Lipnick RJ, Rosner B, Bain C, Belanger C, Stampfer MJ, Willett W, Peto R. A case-control study of oral contraceptive use and breast cancer. JNCI 1984; 72:39–42. **81.** LaVecchia C, DeCarli A, Fasoli M, Franceschi S, Gentile A, Negri E, Parazzini F, Tognoni G. Oral contraceptives and cancers of the breast and of the female genital tract. Interim results from a case-control study. Br J Cancer 1986; 54:311–317. **82.** Meirik O, Lund E, Adami H, Bergstrom R, Christoffersen T, Bergsjo P. Oral contraceptive use and breast cancer in young women. A Joint National Case-control study in Sweden and Norway. Lancet 1986; 11:650–654. **83.** Kay CR, Hannaford PC. Breast cancer and the pill-A further report from the Royal College of General Practitioners' oral contraception study. Br J Cancer 1988; 58:675–680. **84.** Stadel BV, Lai S, Schlesselman JJ, Murray P. Oral contraceptives and premenopausal breast cancer in nulliparous women. Contraception 1988; 38:287–299. **85.** Miller DR, Rosenberg L, Kaufman DW, Stolley P, Warshauer ME, Shapiro S. Breast cancer before age 45 and oral contraceptive use: New Findings. Am J Epidemiol 1989; 129:269–280. **86.** The UK National Case-Control Study Group, Oral contraceptive use and breast cancer risk in young women. Lancet 1989; 1:973–982. **87.** Schlesselman JJ. Cancer of the breast and reproductive tract in relation to use of oral contraceptives. Contraception 1989; 40:1–38. **88.** Vessey MP, McPherson K, Villard-Mackintosh L, Yeates D. Oral contraceptives and breast cancer; latest findings in a large cohort study. Br J Cancer 1989; 59: 613–617. **89.** Jick SS, Walker AM, Stergachis A, Jick H. Oral contraceptives and breast cancer. Br J Cancer 1989; 59:618–621.

BRIEF SUMMARY PATIENT PACKAGE INSERT

Oral contraceptives, also known as "birth control pills" or "the pill", are taken to prevent pregnancy and when taken correctly, have a failure rate of less than 1% per year when used without missing any pills. The typical failure rate of large numbers of pill users is less than 3% per year when women who miss pills are included. For most women oral contraceptives are also free of serious or unpleasant side effects. However, forgetting to take pills considerably increases the chances of pregnancy.

For the majority of women, oral contraceptives can be taken safely. But there are some women who are at high risk of developing certain serious diseases that can be fatal or may cause temporary or permanent disability. The risks associated with taking oral contraceptives increase significantly if you:

- smoke
- have high blood pressure, diabetes, high cholesterol
- have or have had clotting disorders, heart attack, stroke, angina pectoris, cancer of the breast or sex organs, jaundice or malignant or benign liver tumors.

Although cardiovascular disease risks may be increased with oral contraceptive use after age 40 in healthy, non-smoking women (even with the newer low-dose formulations), there are also greater health risks associated with pregnancy in older women.

You should not take the pill if you suspect you are pregnant or have unexplained vaginal bleeding.

Cigarette smoking increases the risk of serious cardiovascular side effects from oral contraceptive use. This risk increases with age and with heavy smoking (15 or more cigarettes per day) and is quite marked in women over 35 years of age. Women who use oral contraceptives are strongly advised not to smoke.

Most side effects of the pill are not serious. The most common such effects are nausea, vomiting, bleeding between menstrual periods, weight gain, breast tenderness, and difficulty wearing contact lenses. These side effects, especially nausea and vomiting, may subside within the first three months of use.

The serious side effects of the pill occur very infrequently, especially if you are in good health and are young. However, you should know that the following medical conditions have been associated with or made worse by the pill:

1. Blood clots in the legs (thrombophlebitis), lungs (pulmonary embolism), stoppage or rupture of a blood vessel in the brain (stroke), blockage of blood vessels in the heart (heart attack or angina pectoris) or other organs of the body. As mentioned above, smoking increases the risk of heart attacks and strokes and subsequent serious medical consequences.
2. Liver tumors, which may rupture and cause severe bleeding. A possible but not definite association has been found with the pill and liver cancer. However, liver cancers are extremely rare. The chance of developing liver cancer from using the pill is thus even rarer.
3. High blood pressure, although blood pressure usually returns to normal when the pill is stopped.

The symptoms associated with these serious side effects are discussed in the detailed leaflet given to you with your supply of pills. Notify your doctor or health care provider if you notice any unusual physical disturbances while taking the pill. In addition, drugs such as rifampin, as well as some anticonvulsants and some antibiotics may decrease oral contraceptive effectiveness.

There is conflict among studies regarding breast cancer and oral contraceptive use. Some studies have reported an increase in the risk of developing breast cancer, particularly at a younger age. This increased risk appears to be related to duration of use. The majority of studies have found no overall increase in the risk of developing breast cancer. Some studies have found an increase in the incidence of cancer of the cervix in women who use oral contraceptives. However, this finding may be related to factors other than the use of oral contraceptives. There is insufficient evidence to rule out the possibility pills may cause such cancers.

Taking the combination pill provides some important noncontraceptive benefits. These include less painful menstruation, less menstrual blood loss and anemia, fewer pelvic infections, and fewer cancers of the ovary and the lining of the uterus.

Be sure to discuss any medical condition you may have with your health care provider. Your health care provider will take a medical and family history before prescribing oral contraceptives and will examine you. The physical examination may be delayed to another time if you request it and the health care provider believes that it is a good medical practice to postpone it. You should be reexamined at least once a year while taking oral contraceptives. Your pharmacist should have given you the detailed patient information labeling which gives you further information which you should read and discuss with your health care provider.

This product (like all oral contraceptives) is intended to prevent pregnancy. It does not protect against transmission of HIV (AIDS) and other sexually transmitted diseases such as chlamydia, genital herpes, genital warts, gonorrhea, hepatitis B, and syphilis.

DETAILED PATIENT LABELING

PLEASE NOTE: This labeling is revised from time to time as important new medical information becomes available. Therefore, please review this labeling carefully.

The following oral contraceptive products contain a combination of an estrogen and progestogen, the two kinds of female hormones:

ORTHO-NOVUM 7/7/7 □ 21 Day Regimen and ORTHO-NOVUM 7/7/7 □ 28 Day Regimen

Each white tablet contains 0.5 mg norethindrone and 0.035 mg ethinyl estradiol. Each light peach tablet contains 0.75 mg norethindrone and 0.035 mg ethinyl estradiol. Each peach tablet contains 1 mg norethindrone and 0.035 mg ethinyl estradiol. Each green tablet in ORTHO-NOVUM 7/7/7 □ 28 Day Regimen contains inert ingredients.

ORTHO-NOVUM 10/11 □ 21 Day Regimen and ORTHO-NOVUM 10/11 □ 28 Day Regimen

Each white tablet contains 0.5 mg norethindrone and 0.035 mg ethinyl estradiol. Each peach tablet contains 1 mg norethindrone and 0.035 mg ethinyl estradiol. Each green tablet in ORTHO-NOVUM 10/11 □ 28 Day Regimen contains inert ingredients.

ORTHO-NOVUM 1/35 □ 21 Day Regimen and ORTHO-NOVUM 1/35 □ 28 Day Regimen

Each peach tablet contains 1 mg norethindrone and 0.035 mg ethinyl estradiol. Each green tablet in ORTHO-NOVUM 1/35 □ 28 Day Regimen contains inert ingredients.

MODICON 21 Day Regimen and MODICON 28 Day Regimen

Each white tablet contains 0.5 mg norethindrone and 0.035 mg ethinyl estradiol. Each green tablet in MODICON 28 Day Regimen contains inert ingredients.

ORTHO-NOVUM 1/50 □ 21 Day Regimen and ORTHO-NOVUM 1/50 □ 28 Day Regimen

Each yellow tablet contains 1 mg norethindrone and 0.05 mg mestranol. Each green tablet in ORTHO-NOVUM 1/50 □ 28 Day Regimen contains inert ingredients.

INTRODUCTION

Any woman who considers using oral contraceptives (the birth control pill or the pill) should understand the benefits and risks of using this form of birth control. This patient labeling will give you much of the information you will need to make this decision and will also help you determine if you are at risk of developing any of the serious side effects of the pill. It will tell you how to use the pill properly so that it will be as effective as possible. However, this labeling is not a replacement for a careful discussion between you and your health care provider. You should discuss the information provided in this labeling with him or her, both when you first start taking the pill and during your revisits. You should also follow your health care provider's advice with regard to regular check-ups while you are on the pill.

EFFECTIVENESS OF ORAL CONTRACEPTIVES

Oral contraceptives or "birth control pills" or "the pill" are used to prevent pregnancy and are more effective than other non-surgical methods of birth control. When they are taken correctly, the chance of becoming pregnant is less than 1% (1 pregnancy per 100 women per year of use) when used perfectly, without missing any pills. Typical failure rates are actually 3% per year. The chance of becoming pregnant increases with each missed pill during a menstrual cycle.

In comparison, typical failure rates for other non-surgical methods of birth control during the first year of use are as follows:

Implant: <1%
Injectable: <1%
IUD: 1 to 2%
Diaphragm with spermicides: 18%
Spermicides alone: 21%
Vaginal sponge: 18% to 36%
Cervical Cap: 18 to 36%
Condom Alone (male): 12%
Condom alone (female): 21%
Periodic abstinence: 20%
No methods: 85%

ANNUAL NUMBER OF BIRTH-RELATED OR METHOD-RELATED DEATHS ASSOCIATED WITH CONTROL OF FERTILITY PER 100,000 NONSTERILE WOMEN, BY FERTILITY CONTROL METHOD ACCORDING TO AGE

Method of control and outcome	15–19	20–24	25–29	30–34	35–39	40–44
No fertility control methods*	7.0	7.4	9.1	14.8	25.7	28.2
Oral contraceptives, non-smoker**	0.3	0.5	0.9	1.9	13.8	31.6
Oral contraceptives, smoker**	2.2	3.4	6.6	13.5	51.1	117.2
IUD**	0.8	0.8	1.0	1.0	1.4	1.4
Condom*	1.1	1.6	0.7	0.2	0.3	0.4
Diaphragm/spermicide*	1.9	1.2	1.2	1.3	2.2	2.8
Periodic abstinence*	2.5	1.6	1.6	1.7	2.9	3.6

* Deaths are birth-related
** Deaths are method-related

WHO SHOULD NOT TAKE ORAL CONTRACEPTIVES

Cigarette smoking increases the risk of serious cardiovascular side effects from oral contraceptive use. This risk increases with age and with heavy smoking (15 or more cigarettes per day) and is quite marked in women over 35 years of age. Women who use oral contraceptives are strongly advised not to smoke.

Some women should not use the pill. For example, you should not take the pill if you are pregnant or think you may be pregnant. You should also not use the pill if you have any of the following conditions:

- A history of heart attack or stroke
- Blood clots in the legs (thrombophlebitis), lungs (pulmonary embolism), or eyes
- A history of blood clots in the deep veins of your legs
- Chest pain (angina pectoris)
- Known or suspected breast cancer or cancer of the lining of the uterus, cervix or vagina
- Unexplained vaginal bleeding (until a diagnosis is reached by your doctor)
- Yellowing of the whites of the eyes or of the skin (jaundice) during pregnancy or during previous use of the pill
- Liver tumor (benign or cancerous)
- Known or suspected pregnancy

Tell your health care provider if you have ever had any of these conditions. Your health care provider can recommend a safer method of birth control.

OTHER CONSIDERATIONS BEFORE TAKING ORAL CONTRACEPTIVES

Tell your health care provider if you have or have had:

- Breast nodules, fibrocystic disease of the breast, an abnormal breast x-ray or mammogram
- Diabetes
- Elevated cholesterol or triglycerides
- High blood pressure
- Migraine or other headaches or epilepsy
- Mental depression
- Gallbladder, heart or kidney disease
- History of scanty or irregular menstrual periods

Women with any of these conditions should be checked often by their health care provider if they choose to use oral contraceptives.

Also, be sure to inform your doctor or health care provider if you smoke or are on any medications.

RISKS OF TAKING ORAL CONTRACEPTIVES

1. Risk of developing blood clots

Blood clots and blockage of blood vessels are one of the most serious side effects of taking oral contraceptives and can cause death or serious disability. In particular, a clot in the legs can cause thrombophlebitis and a clot that travels to the lungs can cause a sudden blocking of the vessel carrying blood to the lungs. Rarely, clots occur in the blood vessels of the eye and may cause blindness, double vision, or impaired vision.

If you take oral contraceptives and need elective surgery, need to stay in bed for a prolonged illness or have recently delivered a baby, you may be at risk of developing blood clots. You should consult your doctor about stopping oral contraceptives three to four weeks before surgery and not taking oral contraceptives for two weeks after surgery or during bed rest. You should also not take oral contraceptives soon after delivery of a baby. It is advisable to wait for at least four weeks after delivery if you are not breast feeding or four weeks after a second trimester abortion. If you are breast feeding, you should wait until you have weaned your child before using the pill. (See also the section on Breast Feeding in General Precautions.)

The risk of circulatory disease in oral contraceptive users may be higher in users of high dose pills and may be greater with longer duration of oral contraceptive use. In addition, some of these increased risks may continue for a number of years after stopping oral contraceptives. The risk of abnormal blood clotting increases with age in both users and nonusers of oral contraceptives, but the increased risk from the oral contraceptive appears to be present at all ages. For women aged 20 to 44, it is estimated that about 1 in 2,000 using oral contraceptives will be hospitalized each year because of abnormal clotting. Among nonusers in the same age group, about 1 in 20,000 would be hospitalized each year. For oral contraceptive users in general, it has been estimated that in women between the ages of 15 and 34 the risk of death due to a circulatory disorder is about 1 in 12,000 per year, whereas for nonusers the rate is about 1 in 50,000 per year. In the age group 35 to 44, the risk is estimated to be about 1 in 2,500 per year for oral contraceptive users and about 1 in 10,000 per year for nonusers.

2. Heart attacks and strokes

Oral contraceptives may increase the tendency to develop strokes (stoppage or rupture of blood vessels in the brain) and angina pectoris and heart attacks (blockage of blood vessels in the heart). Any of these conditions can cause death or serious disability.

Smoking greatly increases the possibility of suffering heart attacks and strokes. Furthermore, smoking and the use of oral contraceptives greatly increase the chances of developing and dying of heart disease.

3. Gallbladder disease

Oral contraceptive users probably have a greater risk than nonusers of having gallbladder disease, although this risk may be related to pills containing high doses of estrogens.

4. Liver tumors

In rare cases, oral contraceptives can cause benign but dangerous liver tumors. These benign liver tumors can rupture and cause fatal internal bleeding. In addition, a possible but not definite association has been found with the pill and liver cancers in two studies, in which a few women who developed these very rare cancers were found to have used oral contraceptives for long periods. However, liver cancers are rare.

5. Cancer of the reproductive organs

There is conflict among studies regarding breast cancer and oral contraceptive use. Some studies have reported an increase in the risk of developing breast cancer, particularly at a younger age. This increased risk appears to be related to duration of use. The majority of studies have found no overall increase in the risk of developing breast cancer. Some studies have found an increase in the incidence of cancer of the cervix in women who use oral contraceptives. However, this finding may be related to factors other than the use of oral contraceptives. There is insufficient evidence to rule out the possibility that pills may cause such cancers.

ESTIMATED RISK OF DEATH FROM A BIRTH CONTROL METHOD OR PREGNANCY

All methods of birth control and pregnancy are associated with a risk of developing certain diseases which may lead to disability or death. An estimate of the number of deaths associated with different methods of birth control and pregnancy has been calculated and is shown in the following table.

[See table above.]

In the above table, the risk of death from any birth control method is less than the risk of childbirth, except for oral contraceptive users over the age of 35 who smoke and pill users over the age of 40 even if they do not smoke. It can be seen in the table that for women aged 15 to 39, the risk of death was highest with pregnancy (7–26 deaths per 100,000 women, depending on age). Among pill users who do not smoke, the risk of death was always lower than that associated with pregnancy for any age group, although over the age of 40, the risk increases to 32 deaths per 100,000 women, compared to 28 associated with pregnancy at that age. However, for pill

Continued on next page

Ortho—Cont.

users who smoke and are over the age of 35, the estimated number of deaths exceeds those for other methods of birth control. If a woman is over the age of 40 and smokes, her estimated risk of death is four times higher (117/100,000 women) than the estimated risk associated with pregnancy (28/100,000 women) in that age group.
The suggestion that women over 40 who do not smoke should not take oral contraceptives is based on information from older, higher-dose pills. An Advisory Committee of the FDA discussed this issue in 1989 and recommended that the benefits of low-dose oral contraceptive use by healthy, non-smoking women over 40 years of age may outweigh the possible risks.

WARNING SIGNALS

If any of these adverse effects occur while you are taking oral contraceptives, call your doctor immediately:

- Sharp chest pain, coughing of blood, or sudden shortness of breath (indicating a possible clot in the lung)
- Pain in the calf (indicating a possible clot in the leg)
- Crushing chest pain or heaviness in the chest (indicating a possible heart attack)
- Sudden severe headache or vomiting, dizziness or fainting, disturbances of vision or speech, weakness, or numbness in an arm or leg (indicating a possible stroke)
- Sudden partial or complete loss of vision (indicating a possible clot in the eye)
- Breast lumps (indicating possible breast cancer or fibrocystic disease of the breast; ask your doctor or health care provider to show you how to examine your breasts)
- Severe pain or tenderness in the stomach area (indicating a possibly ruptured liver tumor)
- Difficulty in sleeping, weakness, lack of energy, fatigue, or change in mood (possibly indicating severe depression)
- Jaundice or a yellowing of the skin or eyeballs, accompanied frequently by fever, fatigue, loss of appetite, dark colored urine, or light colored bowel movements (indicating possible liver problems)

SIDE EFFECTS OF ORAL CONTRACEPTIVES

1. Vaginal bleeding
Irregular vaginal bleeding or spotting may occur while you are taking the pills. Irregular bleeding may vary from slight staining between menstrual periods to breakthrough bleeding which is a flow much like a regular period. Irregular bleeding occurs most often during the first few months of oral contraceptive use, but may also occur after you have been taking the pill for some time. Such bleeding may be temporary and usually does not indicate any serious problems. It is important to continue taking your pills on schedule. If the bleeding occurs in more than one cycle or lasts for more than a few days, talk to your doctor or health care provider.

2. Contact lenses
If you wear contact lenses and notice a change in vision or an inability to wear your lenses, contact your doctor or health care provider.

3. Fluid retention
Oral contraceptives may cause edema (fluid retention) with swelling of the fingers or ankles and may raise your blood pressure. If you experience fluid retention, contact your doctor or health care provider.

4. Melasma
A spotty darkening of the skin is possible, particularly of the face, which may persist.

5. Other side effects
Other side effects may include nausea and vomiting, change in appetite, headache, nervousness, depression, dizziness, loss of scalp hair, rash, and vaginal infections.
If any of these side effects bother you, call your doctor or health care provider.

GENERAL PRECAUTIONS

1. Missed periods and use of oral contraceptives before or during early pregnancy
There may be times when you may not menstruate regularly after you have completed taking a cycle of pills. If you have taken your pills regularly and miss one menstrual period, continue taking your pills for the next cycle but be sure to inform your health care provider before doing so. If you have not taken the pills daily as instructed and missed a menstrual period, you may be pregnant. If you missed two consecutive menstrual periods, you may be pregnant. Check with your health care provider immediately to determine whether you are pregnant. Do not continue to take oral contraceptives until you are sure you are not pregnant, but continue to use another method of contraception.
There is no conclusive evidence that oral contraceptive use is associated with an increase in birth defects, when taken inadvertently during early pregnancy. Previously, a few studies had reported that oral contraceptives might be associated with birth defects, but these findings have not been seen in more recent studies. Nevertheless, oral contraceptives or any other drugs should not be used during pregnancy unless clearly necessary and prescribed by your doctor. You should check with your doctor about risks to your unborn child of any medication taken during pregnancy.

2. While breast feeding
If you are breast feeding, consult your doctor before starting oral contraceptives. Some of the drug will be passed on to the child in the milk. A few adverse effects on the child have been reported, including yellowing of the skin (jaundice) and breast enlargement. In addition, oral contraceptives may decrease the amount and quality of your milk. If possible, do not use oral contraceptives while breast feeding. You should use another method of contraception since breast feeding provides only partial protection from becoming pregnant and this partial protection decreases significantly as you breast feed for longer periods of time. You should consider starting oral contraceptives only after you have weaned your child completely.

3. Laboratory tests
If you are scheduled for any laboratory tests, tell your doctor you are taking birth control pills. Certain blood tests may be affected by birth control pills.

4. Drug interactions
Certain drugs may interact with birth control pills to make them less effective in preventing pregnancy or cause an increase in breakthrough bleeding. Such drugs include rifampin, drugs used for epilepsy such as barbiturates (for example, phenobarbital) anticonvulsants such as carbamazepine (Tegretol is one brand of this drug), phenytoin (Dilantin is one brand of this drug), phenylbutazone (Butazolidin is one brand) and possibly certain antibiotics. You may need to use additional contraception when you take drugs which can make oral contraceptives less effective.

5. Sexually transmitted diseases
This product (like all oral contraceptives) is intended to prevent pregnancy. It does not protect against transmission of HIV (AIDS) and other sexually transmitted diseases such as chlamydia, genital herpes, genital warts, gonorrhea, hepatitis B, and syphilis.

HOW TO TAKE THE PILL

IMPORTANT POINTS TO REMEMBER

BEFORE YOU START TAKING THE PILLS:
1. BE SURE TO READ THESE DIRECTIONS:
Before you start taking your pills.
Anytime you are not sure what to do.
2. THE RIGHT WAY TO TAKE THE PILL IS TO TAKE ONE PILL EVERY DAY AT THE SAME TIME.
If you miss pills you could get pregnant. This includes starting the pack late.
The more pills you miss, the more likely you are to get pregnant.
3. MANY WOMEN HAVE SPOTTING OR LIGHT BLEEDING, OR MAY FEEL SICK TO THEIR STOMACH DURING THE FIRST 1–3 PACKS OF PILLS. If you feel sick to your stomach, do not stop taking the pill. The problem will usually go away. If it doesn't go away, check with your doctor or clinic.
4. MISSING PILLS CAN ALSO CAUSE SPOTTING OR LIGHT BLEEDING, even when you make up these missed pills.
On the days you take 2 pills to make up for missed pills, you could also feel a little sick to your stomach.
5. IF YOU HAVE VOMITING OR DIARRHEA, for any reason, or IF YOU TAKE SOME MEDICINES, including some antibiotics, your pills may not work as well. Use a back-up method (such as condoms, foam, or sponge) until you check with your doctor or clinic.
6. IF YOU HAVE TROUBLE REMEMBERING TO TAKE THE PILL, talk to your doctor or clinic about how to make pill-taking easier or about using another method of birth control.
7. IF YOU HAVE ANY QUESTIONS OR ARE UNSURE ABOUT THE INFORMATION IN THIS LEAFLET, call your doctor or clinic.

BEFORE YOU START TAKING YOUR PILLS

1. DECIDE WHAT TIME OF DAY YOU WANT TO TAKE YOUR PILL.
It is important to take it at about the same time every day.
2. LOOK AT YOUR PILL PACK TO SEE IF IT HAS 21 OR 28 PILLS.
The 21-pill pack has 21 "active" pills (with hormones) to take for 3 weeks. This is followed by 1 week without pills.
The 28-pill pack has 21 "active" pills (with hormones) to take for 3 weeks. This is followed by 1 week of reminder green pills (without hormones).
ORTHO-NOVUM 7/7/7: There are 7 white "active" pills, 7 light peach "active" pills, and 7 peach "active" pills.
ORTHO-NOVUM 10/11: There are 10 white "active" pills and 11 peach "active" pills.
ORTHO-NOVUM 1/35: There are 21 peach "active" pills.
MODICON: There are 21 white "active" pills.
ORTHO-NOVUM 1/50: There are 21 yellow "active" pills.
3. ALSO FIND:
1) where on the pack to start taking pills.
2) in what order to take the pills
CHECK PICTURE OF PILL PACK AND ADDITIONAL INSTRUCTIONS FOR USING THIS PACKAGE IN THE BRIEF SUMMARY PATIENT PACKAGE INSERT.
4. BE SURE YOU HAVE READY AT ALL TIMES:
ANOTHER KIND OF BIRTH CONTROL (such as condoms, foam, or sponge) to use as a back-up method in case you miss pills.
AN EXTRA, FULL PILL PACK.

WHEN TO START THE FIRST PACK OF PILLS

You have a choice of which day to start taking your first pack of pills. ORTHO-NOVUM 7/7/7, ORTHO-NOVUM 10/11, ORTHO-NOVUM 1/35, ORTHO-NOVUM 1/50, and MODICON are available in the DIALPAK® Tablet Dispenser which is preset for a Sunday Start. Day 1 start is also provided. Decide with your doctor or clinic which is the best day for you. Pick a time of day which will be easy to remember.

SUNDAY START:
ORTHO-NOVUM 7/7/7: Take the first "active" white pill of the first pack on the Sunday after your period starts, even if you are still bleeding. If your period begins on Sunday, start the pack the same day.
ORTHO-NOVUM 10/11: Take the first "active" white pill of the first pack on the Sunday after your period starts, even if you are still bleeding. If your period begins on Sunday, start the pack the same day.
ORTHO-NOVUM 1/35: Take the first "active" peach pill of the first pack on the Sunday after your period starts, even if you are still bleeding. If your period begins on Sunday, start the pack the same day.
MODICON: Take the first "active" white pill of the first pack on the Sunday after your period starts, even if you are still bleeding. If your period begins on Sunday, start the pack the same day.
ORTHO-NOVUM 1/50: Take the first "active" yellow pill of the first pack on the Sunday after your period starts, even if you are still bleeding. If your period begins on Sunday, start the pack the same day.
Use another method of birth control as a back-up method if you have sex anytime from the Sunday you start your first pack until the next Sunday (7 days). Condoms, foam, or the sponge are good back-up methods of birth control.

DAY 1 START:
ORTHO-NOVUM 7/7/7: Take the first "active" white pill of the first pack during the first 24 hours of your period.
ORTHO-NOVUM 10/11: Take the first "active" white pill of the first pack during the first 24 hours of your period.
ORTHO-NOVUM 1/35: Take the first "active" peach pill of the first pack during the first 24 hours of your period.
MODICON: Take the first "active" white pill of the first pack during the first 24 hours of your period.
ORTHO-NOVUM 1/50: Take the first "active" yellow pill of the first pack during the first 24 hours of your period.

WHAT TO DO DURING THE MONTH:

Do not skip pills even if you are spotting or bleeding between monthly periods or feel sick to your stomach (nausea).
Do not skip pills even if you do not have sex very often.
2. WHEN YOU FINISH A PACK OR SWITCH YOUR BRAND OF PILLS:
21 pills: Wait 7 days to start the next pack. You will probably have your period during that week. Be sure that no more than 7 days pass between 21-day packs.
28 pills: Start the next pack on the day after your last "reminder" pill. Do not wait any days between packs.

WHAT TO DO IF YOU MISS PILLS

ORTHO-NOVUM 7/7/7:
If you MISS 1 white, light peach, or peach "active" pill:
1. Take it as soon as you remember. Take the next pill at your regular time. This means you may take 2 pills in 1 day.
2. You do not need to use a back-up birth control method if you have sex.
If you MISS 2 white or light peach "active" pills in a row in WEEK 1 or WEEK 2 of your pack:
1. Take 2 pills on the day you remember and 2 pills the next day.
2. Then take 1 pill a day until you finish the pack.
3. You MAY BECOME PREGNANT if you have sex in the 7 days after you miss pills. You MUST use another birth control method (such as condoms, foam, or sponge) as a back-up method for those 7 days.
If you MISS 2 peach "active" pills in a row in THE 3RD WEEK:
1. **If you are a Sunday Starter:**
Keep taking 1 pill every day until Sunday. On Sunday, THROW OUT the rest of the pack and start a new pack of pills that same day.

If you are a Day 1 Starter:

THROW OUT the rest of the pill pack and start a new pack that same day.

2. You may not have your period this month but this is expected. However, if you miss your period 2 months in a row, call your doctor or clinic because you might be pregnant.

3. You MAY BECOME PREGNANT if you have sex in the 7 days after you miss pills. You MUST use another birth control method (such as condoms, foam, or sponge) as a back-up method for those 7 days.

If you MISS 3 OR MORE white, light peach, or peach "active" pills in a row (during the first 3 weeks):

1. If you are a Sunday Starter:

Keep taking 1 pill every day until Sunday. On Sunday, THROW OUT the rest of the pack and start a new pack of pills that same day.

If you are a Day 1 Starter:

THROW OUT the rest of the pill pack and start a new pack of pills that same day.

2. You may not have your period this month but this is expected. However, if you miss your period 2 months in a row, call your doctor or clinic because you might be pregnant.

3. You MAY BECOME PREGNANT if you have sex in the 7 days after you miss pills. You MUST use another birth control method (such as condoms, foam, or sponge) as a back-up method for those 7 days.

ORTHO-NOVUM 10/11:

If you MISS 1 white or peach "active" pill:

1. Take it as soon as you remember. Take the next pill at your regular time. This means you may take 2 pills in 1 day.

2. You do not need to use a back-up birth control method if you have sex.

If you MISS 2 white or peach "active" pills in a row in WEEK 1 or WEEK 2 of your pack:

1. Take 2 pills on the day you remember and 2 pills the next day.

2. Then take 1 pill a day until you finish the pack.

3. You MAY BECOME PREGNANT if you have sex in the 7 days after you miss pills. You MUST use another birth control method (such as condoms, foam, or sponge) as a back-up method for those 7 days.

If you MISS 2 peach "active" pills in a row in THE 3RD WEEK:

1. If you are a Sunday Starter:

Keep taking 1 pill every day until Sunday. On Sunday, THROW OUT the rest of the pack and start a new pack of pills that same day.

If you are a Day 1 Starter:

THROW OUT the rest of the pill pack and start a new pack that same day.

2. You may not have your period this month but this is expected. However, if you miss your period 2 months in a row, call your doctor or clinic because you might be pregnant.

3. You MAY BECOME PREGNANT if you have sex in the 7 days after you miss pills. You MUST use another birth control method (such as condoms, foam, or sponge) as a back-up method for those 7 days.

If you MISS 3 OR MORE white or peach "active" pills in a row (during the first 3 weeks):

1. If you are a Sunday Starter:

Keep taking 1 pill every day until Sunday. On Sunday, THROW OUT the rest of the pack and start a new pack of pills that same day.

If you are a Day 1 Starter:

THROW OUT the rest of the pill pack and start a new pack of pills that same day.

2. You may not have your period this month but this is expected. However, if you miss your period 2 months in a row, call your doctor or clinic because you might be pregnant.

3. You MAY BECOME PREGNANT if you have sex in the 7 days after you miss pills. You MUST use another birth control method (such as condoms, foam, or sponge) as a back-up method for those 7 days.

ORTHO-NOVUM 1/35:

If you MISS 1 peach "active" pill:

1. Take it as soon as you remember. Take the next pill at your regular time. This means you may take 2 pills in 1 day.

2. You do not need to use a back-up birth control method if you have sex.

If you MISS 2 peach "active" pills in a row in WEEK 1 or WEEK 2 of your pack:

1. Take 2 pills on the day you remember and 2 pills the next day.

2. Then take 1 pill a day until you finish the pack.

3. You MAY BECOME PREGNANT if you have sex in the 7 days after you miss pills. You MUST use another birth control method (such as condoms, foam, or sponge) as a back-up method for those 7 days.

If you MISS 2 peach "active" pills in a row in THE 3RD WEEK:

1. If you are a Sunday Starter:

Keep taking 1 pill every day until Sunday. On Sunday, THROW OUT the rest of the pack and start a new pack of pills that same day.

If you are a Day 1 Starter:

THROW OUT the rest of the pill pack and start a new pack of pills that same day.

2. You may not have your period this month but this is expected. However, if you miss your period 2 months in a row, call your doctor or clinic because you might be pregnant.

3. You MAY BECOME PREGNANT if you have sex in the 7 days after you miss pills. You MUST use another birth control method (such as condoms, foam, or sponge) as a back-up method for those 7 days.

If you MISS 3 OR MORE peach "active" pills in a row (during the first 3 weeks):

1. If you are a Sunday Starter:

Keep taking 1 pill every day until Sunday. On Sunday, THROW OUT the rest of the pack and start a new pack of pills that same day.

If you are a Day 1 Starter:

THROW OUT the rest of the pill pack and start a new pack of pills that same day.

2. You may not have your period this month but this is expected. However, if you miss your period 2 months in a row, call your doctor or clinic because you might be pregnant.

3. You MAY BECOME PREGNANT if you have sex in the 7 days after you miss pills. You MUST use another birth control method (such as condoms, foam, or sponge) as a back-up method for those 7 days.

MODICON:

If you MISS 1 white "active" pill:

1. Take it as soon as you remember. Take the next pill at your regular time. This means you may take 2 pills in 1 day.

2. You do not need to use a back-up birth control method if you have sex.

If you MISS 2 white "active" pills in a row in WEEK 1 or WEEK 2 of your pack:

1. Take 2 pills on the day you remember and 2 pills the next day.

2. Then take 1 pill a day until you funish the pack.

3. You MAY BECOME PREGNANT if you have sex in the 7 days after you miss pills. You MUST use another birth control method (such as condoms, foam, or sponge) as a back-up method for those 7 days.

If you MISS 2 white "active" pills in a row in THE 3RD WEEK:

1. If you are a Sunday Starter:

Keep taking 1 pill every day until Sunday. On Sunday, THROW OUT the rest of the pack and start a new pack of pills that same day.

If you are a Day 1 Starter:

THROW OUT the rest of the pill pack and start a new pack that same day.

2. You may not have your period this month but this is expected. However, if you miss your period 2 months in a row, call your doctor or clinic because you might be pregnant.

3. You MAY BECOME PREGNANT if you have sex in the 7 days after you miss pills. You MUST use another birth control method (such as condoms, foam, or sponge) as a back-up method for those 7 days.

If you MISS 3 OR MORE white "active" pills in a row (during the first 3 weeks):

1. If you are a Sunday Starter:

Keep taking 1 pill every day until Sunday. On Sunday, THROW OUT the rest of the pack and start a new pack of pills that same day.

If you are a Day 1 Starter:

THROW OUT the rest of the pill pack and start a new pack of pills that same day.

2. You may not have your period this month but this is expected. However, if you miss your period 2 months in a row, call your doctor or clinic because you might be pregnant.

3. You MAY BECOME PREGNANT if you have sex in the 7 days after you miss pills. You MUST use another birth control method (such as condoms, foam, or sponge) as a back-up method for those 7 days.

ORTHO-NOVUM 1/50:

If you MISS 1 yellow "active" pill:

1. Take it as soon as you remember. Take the next pill at your regular time. This means you may take 2 pills in 1 day.

2. You do not need to use a back-up birth control method if you have sex.

If you MISS 2 yellow "active" pills in a row in WEEK 1 or WEEK 2 of your pack:

1. Take 2 pills on the day you remember and 2 pills the next day.

2. Then take 1 pill a day until you finish the pack.

3. You MAY BECOME PREGNANT if you have sex in the 7 days after you miss pills. You MUST use another birth control method (such as condoms, foam, or sponge) as a back-up method for those 7 days.

If you MISS 2 yellow "active" pills in a row in THE 3RD WEEK:

1. If you are a Sunday Starter:

Keep taking 1 pill every day until Sunday. On Sunday, THROW OUT the rest of the pack and start a new pack of pills that same day.

If you are a Day 1 Starter:

THROW OUT the rest of the pill pack and start a new pack that same day.

2. You may not have your period this month but this is expected. However, if you miss your period 2 months in a row, call your doctor or clinic because you might be pregnant.

3. You MAY BECOME PREGNANT if you have sex in the 7 days after you miss pills. You MUST use another birth control method (such as condoms, foam, or sponge) as a back-up method for those 7 days.

If you MISS 3 OR MORE yellow "active" pills in a row (during the first 3 weeks):

1. If you are a Sunday Starter:

Keep taking 1 pill every day until Sunday. On Sunday, THROW OUT the rest of the pack and start a new pack of pills that same day.

If you are a Day 1 Starter:

THROW OUT the rest of the pill pack and start a new pack of pills that same day.

2. You may not have your period this month but this is expected. However, if you miss your period 2 months in a row, call your doctor or clinic because you might be pregnant.

3. You MAY BECOME PREGNANT if you have sex in the 7 days after you miss pills. You MUST use another birth control method (such as condoms, foam, or sponge) as a back-up method for those 7 days.

A REMINDER FOR THOSE ON 28-DAY PACKS:

If you forget any of the 7 green "reminder" pills in Week 4: THROW AWAY the pills you missed.

Keep taking 1 pill each day until the pack is empty.

You do not need a back-up method.

FINALLY, IF YOU ARE STILL NOT SURE WHAT TO DO ABOUT THE PILLS YOU HAVE MISSED:

Use a BACK-UP METHOD anytime you have sex.

KEEP TAKING ONE "ACTIVE" PILL EACH DAY until you can reach your doctor or clinic.

PREGNANCY DUE TO PILL FAILURE

Combination Oral Contraceptives

The incidence of pill failure resulting in pregnancy is approximately one percent (i.e., one pregnancy per 100 women per year) if taken every day as directed, but more typical failure rates are about 3%. If failure does occur, the risk to the fetus is minimal.

PREGNANCY AFTER STOPPING THE PILL

There may be some delay in becoming pregnant after you stop using oral contraceptives, especially if you had irregular menstrual cycles before you used oral contraceptives. It may be advisable to postpone conception until you begin menstruating regularly once you have stopped taking the pill and desire pregnancy.

There does not appear to be any increase in birth defects in newborn babies when pregnancy occurs soon after stopping the pill.

OVERDOSAGE

Serious ill effects have not been reported following ingestion of large doses of oral contraceptives by young children. Overdosage may cause nausea and withdrawal bleeding in females. In case of overdosage, contact your health care provider or pharmacist.

OTHER INFORMATION

Your health care provider will take a medical and family history before prescribing oral contraceptives and will examine you. The physical examination may be delayed to another time if you request it and the health care provider believes that it is a good medical practice to postpone it. You should be reexamined at least once a year. Be sure to inform your health care provider if there is a family history of any of the conditions listed previously in this leaflet. Be sure to keep all appointments with your health care provider, because this is a time to determine if there are early signs of side effects of oral contraceptive use.

Do not use the drug for any condition other than the one for which it was prescribed. This drug has been prescribed specifically for you; do not give it to others who may want birth control pills. contraceptives >

HEALTH BENEFITS FROM ORAL CONTRACEPTIVES

In addition to preventing pregnancy, use of combination oral contraceptives may provide certain benefits. They are:

- menstrual cycles may become more regular
- blood flow during menstruation may be lighter and less iron may be lost. Therefore, anemia due to iron deficiency is less likely to occur.
- pain or other symptoms during menstruation may be encountered less frequently
- ectopic (tubal) pregnancy may occur less frequently
- noncancerous cysts or lumps in the breast may occur less frequently

Continued on next page

Consult 1997 supplements and future editions for revisions

Ortho—Cont.

- acute pelvic inflammatory disease may occur less frequently
- oral contraceptive use may provide some protection against developing two forms of cancer: cancer of the ovaries and cancer of the lining of the uterus.

If you want more information about birth control pills, ask your doctor or pharmacist. They have a more technical leaflet called the Professional Labeling, which you may wish to read. The Professional Labeling is also published in a book entitled *Physicians' Desk Reference*, available in many book stores and public libraries.

ORTHO PHARMACEUTICAL
CORPORATION
Raritan, New Jersey 08869
Revised June 1996

TRADEMARK
635-10-030-3

Shown in Product Identification Guide, pages 326 and 327

PARAGARD® T 380A

Intrauterine Copper Contraceptive

Patients should be counseled that this product does not protect against HIV Infection (AIDS) and other sexually transmitted diseases.

CAUTION: Federal law prohibits dispensing without prescription.

NOTICE

You have received a Patient Package Insert that Federal Regulations (21 CFR 310.502) require you to furnish to each patient who is considering the use of the ParaGard® T 380A.

The Patient Package Insert contains information on the safety and efficacy of the ParaGard® T 380A. Before inserting the ParaGard® T 380A:

- You should read the physician prescription labeling and be familiar with all the information it contains.
- You should counsel the patient and answer her questions about contraception, the ParaGard® T 380A, and the information in the Patient Package Insert.
- You and the patient should read each section of the Patient Package Insert, and if the patient agrees, she may sign a consent form provided for your convenience.

The Patient Package Insert is also available in Spanish and other foreign languages. Address requests to Ortho Pharmaceutical Corporation Inc. or telephone 1-800-322-4966.

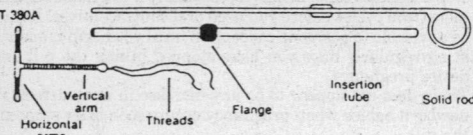

DESCRIPTION

The polyethylene body of the ParaGard® T 380A is wound with approximately 176 mg of copper wire and carries a copper collar of approximately 68.7 mg of copper on each of its transverse arms. The exposed surface areas of copper are 380 ± 23 mm². The dimensions of the ParaGard® T 380A are 36 mm in the vertical direction and 32 mm in the horizontal direction. The tip of the vertical arm of the ParaGard® T 380A is enlarged to form a bulb having a diameter of 3 mm. The ParaGard® T 380A is equipped with a monofilament polyethylene thread which is tied through the bulb, resulting in two threads at the tip to aid in removal of the IUD. The ParaGard® T 380A contains barium sulfate to render it radiopaque.

The ParaGard® T 380A is packaged together with an insertion tube and solid rod in a Tyvek®-polyethylene pouch and then sterilized. The insertion tube is equipped with a movable flange to aid in gauging the depth to which the insertion tube is inserted through the cervical canal and into the uterine cavity.

CLINICAL PHARMACOLOGY

Available data indicate that the contraceptive effectiveness of the ParaGard® T 380A is enhanced by copper being released continuously from the copper coil and sleeves into the uterine cavity. The exact mechanism by which metallic copper enhances the contraceptive effect of an IUD has not been conclusively demonstrated. Various hypotheses have been advanced, including interference with sperm transport, fertilization, and implantation. Clinical studies with copper-bearing IUDs also suggest that fertilization is prevented either due to an altered number or lack of viability of spermatozoa.[1]

INDICATIONS AND USAGE

The ParaGard® T 380A is indicated for intrauterine contraception. ParaGard® T 380A is highly effective. Table II and Table III list an expected pregnancy rate for one year between 0.7 and 0.5, respectively. ParaGard® T 380A should not be kept in place longer than 10 years.

RECOMMENDED PATIENT PROFILE

The ParaGard® T 380A is recommended for women who have had at least one child, are in a stable, mutually monogamous relationship, and have no history of pelvic inflammatory disease.

CONTRAINDICATIONS

The ParaGard® T 380A should not be inserted when one or more of the following conditions exist:

1. Pregnancy or suspicion of pregnancy.
2. Abnormalities of the uterus resulting in distortion of the uterine cavity.
3. Acute pelvic inflammatory disease or a history of pelvic inflammatory disease.
4. Postpartum endometritis or infected abortion in the past 3 months.
5. Known or suspected uterine or cervical malignancy, including unresolved, abnormal "Pap" smear.
6. Genital bleeding of unknown etiology.
7. Untreated acute cervicitis or vaginitis, including bacterial vaginosis, until infection is controlled.
8. Copper-containing IUDs should not be inserted in the presence of diagnosed Wilson's disease.
9. Known allergy to copper.
10. Patient or her partner has multiple sexual partners.
11. Conditions associated with increased susceptibility to infections with micro-organisms. Such conditions include, but are not limited to, leukemia, acquired immune deficiency syndrome (AIDS), and I.V. drug abuse.
12. Genital actinomycosis.
13. A previously inserted IUD that has not been removed.

WARNINGS

1. PREGNANCY

Effects on the offspring when pregnancy occurs with the ParaGard® T 380A in place are unknown.

a. Septic Abortion

Reports indicate an increased incidence of septic abortion with septicemia, septic shock, and death in patients becoming pregnant with an IUD in place. Most of these reports have been associated with, but not limited to, the mid-trimester of pregnancy. In some cases, the initial symptoms have been insidious and not easily recognized. If pregnancy should occur with an IUD *in situ*, the IUD should be removed if the string is visible and removal is easily accomplished. Of course, manipulation may result in spontaneous abortion. If removal proves to be difficult, or if threads are not visible, interruption of the pregnancy should be considered and offered as an option.

b. Continuation of Pregnancy

If the patient elects to maintain the pregnancy and the IUD remains *in situ*, she should be warned that there is an increased risk of spontaneous abortion and sepsis. In addition, she is at increased risk of premature labor and delivery. As a consequence of premature birth, the fetus is at increased risk of damage. She should be followed more closely than the usual obstetrical patient. The patient must be advised to report immediately all abnormal symptoms, such as flu-like syndrome, fever, abdominal cramping or pain, bleeding or vaginal discharge, because generalized symptoms of septicemia may be insidious.

2. ECTOPIC PREGNANCY

a. Patients with a history of ectopic pregnancy are at an increased risk of subsequent pregnancies being ectopic. Although current data indicate that there is no increased risk of ectopic pregnancy in patients using the ParaGard® T 380A and some data suggest there may be a lower risk than the general population using no method of contraception, a pregnancy which occurs with the ParaGard® T 380A in place is more likely to be ectopic than a pregnancy occurring without the ParaGard® T 380A[2–4]. Therefore, patients who become pregnant while using the ParaGard® T 380A should be carefully evaluated for the possibility of an ectopic pregnancy.

b. Special attention should be directed to patients with delayed menses, slight metrorrhagia and/or unilateral pelvic pain, and to those patients who wish to terminate a pregnancy because of IUD failure, to determine whether ectopic pregnancy has occurred.

3. PELVIC INFECTION (PELVIC INFLAMMATORY DISEASE, PID)

The ParaGard® T 380A is contraindicated in the presence of PID or in women with a history of PID. Use of all IUDs, including the ParaGard® T 380A, has been associated with an increased incidence of PID. Therefore, a decision to use the ParaGard® T 380A must include consideration of the risks of PID. The highest rate of PID has been reported to occur after insertion and up to four months thereafter. A study suggests that the highest incidence occurs within 20 days postinsertion, then falls, remaining constant thereafter.[5] Administration of prophylactic antibiotics has been reported, although studies do not confirm the utility of this prophylactic measure in reducing PID. PID can necessitate hysterectomy and can also lead to tubo-ovarian abscesses, tubal occlusion and infertility, and tubal damage that can predispose to ectopic pregnancy. PID can result in peritonitis and, infrequently, in death. The effect of PID on fertility is especially important for women who may wish to have children at a later date.

a. Women at special risk of PID

The risk of PID appears to be greater for women who have multiple sexual partners and also for those women whose sexual partners have multiple sexual partners, as PID is most frequently caused by sexually transmitted diseases.

b. PID warning to ParaGard® T 380A users

All women who choose the ParaGard® T 380A must be informed prior to insertion that IUD use has been associated with an increased incidence of PID and that PID can necessitate hysterectomy, can cause tubal damage leading to ectopic pregnancy or infertility or, in infrequent cases, can cause death. Patients must be taught to recognize and report to their physician promptly any symptoms of pelvic inflammatory disease. These symptoms include development of menstrual disorders (prolonged or heavy bleeding), unusual vaginal discharge, abdominal or pelvic pain or tenderness, dyspareunia, chills, and fever.

c. Asymptomatic PID

PID may be asymptomatic but still result in tubal damage and its sequelae.[6,7]

d. Treatment of PID

Following diagnosis of PID, or suspected PID, bacteriologic specimens should be obtained and antibiotic therapy should be initiated promptly. Removal of the ParaGard® T 380A after initiation of antibiotic therapy is usually appropriate. Time should be allowed for therapeutic blood levels to be reached prior to removal. Guidelines for PID treatment are available from the Center for Disease Control (CDC), Atlanta, Georgia. A copy of the printed guidelines has been provided to you by Ortho Pharmaceutical Corporation Inc. The guidelines were established after deliberation by a group of experts and staff of the CDC, but they should not be construed as rules suitable for use in all patients. Adequate PID treatment requires the application of current standards of therapy prevailing at the time of occurrence of the infection with reference to the prescription labeling of the antibiotic selected.

Genital actinomycosis has been associated primarily with long-term IUD use. If actinomycosis occurs, promptly institute appropriate antibiotic therapy and remove the ParaGard® T 380A.

4. EMBEDMENT

Partial penetration or embedment of the ParaGard® T 380A in the endometrium or myometrium can result in difficult removal. In some cases this can result in breakage of the IUD, necessitating surgical removal.

5. PERFORATION

Partial or total perforation of the uterine wall or cervix may occur with use of the ParaGard® T 380A. The rate of perforation in randomized trials of the ParaGard® T 380A has been 1 in 1,360. Insertions immediately after the expulsion of the placenta are not known to be associated with increased risks of perforation, but insertion later in the first postpartum month, particularly during lactation, has been associated with an increased risk of perforation.[8,9] Thus, unless performed immediately postpartum, insertion should be delayed to the second postpartum month. IUD insertion immediately postabortion in the first trimester is not known to be associated with increased risks of perforation, but insertion after second trimester abortion should be delayed until the second postabortion month.

The possibility of perforation must be kept in mind during insertion and at the time of any subsequent examination. If perforation occurs, the ParaGard® T 380A should be removed as soon as possible. A surgical procedure may be required. Abdominal adhesions, intestinal penetration, intestinal obstruction, and local inflammatory reaction with abscess formation and erosion of adjacent viscera may result if the ParaGard® T 380A is left in the peritoneal cavity. There are reports of migration after insertion.

6. MEDICAL DIATHERMY

The use of medical diathermy (short-wave and microwave) in a patient with a metal-containing IUD may cause heat injury to the surrounding tissue. Therefore, medical diathermy to the abdominal and sacral areas should not be used on patients with a ParaGard® T 380A in place.

7. EFFECTS OF COPPER

Additional amounts of copper available to the body from the ParaGard® T 380A may precipitate symptoms in women with Wilson's disease. The incidence of Wilson's disease is approximately 1 in 200,000. The long-term effects of intrauterine copper to a child conceived in the presence of an IUD are unknown.

8. RISKS OF MORTALITY

The available data from a variety of sources have been analyzed to estimate the risk of death associated with various methods of contraception. The estimates of risk of death include the combined risk of the contraceptive method plus the

risk of pregnancy or abortion in the event of method failure. The findings of the analysis are shown in Table I.[10]
[See table at right.]

TABLE I—Annual Number of Birth-Related or Method-Related Deaths Associated with Control of Fertility per 100,000 Nonsterile Women by Fertility Control Method, by Age.

Methods	Age Group					
	15–19	20–24	25–29	30–34	35–39	40–44
No Birth Control Method/Term	4.7	5.4	4.8	6.3	11.7	20.6
No Birth Control Method/AB	2.1	2.0	1.6	1.9	2.8	5.3
IUD	0.2	0.3	0.2	0.1	0.3	0.6
Periodic Abstinence	1.4	1.3	0.7	1.0	1.0	1.9
Withdrawal	0.9	1.7	0.9	1.3	0.8	1.5
Condom	0.6	1.2	0.6	0.9	0.5	1.0
Diaphragm/Cap	0.6	1.1	0.6	0.9	1.6	3.1
Sponge	0.8	1.5	0.8	1.1	2.2	4.1
Spermicides	1.6	1.9	1.4	1.9	1.5	2.7
Oral Contraceptives	0.8	1.3	1.1	1.8	1.0	1.9
Implants/Injectables	0.2	0.6	0.5	0.8	0.5	0.6
Tubal Sterilization	1.3	1.2	1.1	1.1	1.2	1.3
Vasectomy	0.1	0.1	0.1	0.1	0.1	0.2

PRECAUTIONS

Patients should be counseled that this product does not protect against HIV Infection (AIDS) and other sexually transmitted diseases.

1. Patient Counseling
Prior to insertion, the physician, nurse, or other trained health professional must provide the patient with the Patient Package Insert. The patient should be given the opportunity to read the information and discuss fully any questions she may have concerning the ParaGard® T 380A as well as other methods of contraception.

2. Patient Evaluation and Clinical Considerations

a. A complete medical and social history, including that of the partner, should be obtained to determine conditions that might influence the selection of an IUD. A physical examination should include a pelvic examination, a "Pap" smear, and appropriate tests for any other forms of genital disease, such as gonorrhea and chlamydia laboratory evaluations, if indicated. If actinomyces-like organisms are detected on the Pap smear, they should be cultured to determine whether genital actinomyces is present. The physician should determine that the patient is not pregnant.

b. The uterus should be carefully sounded prior to the insertion to determine the degree of patency of the endocervical canal and the internal os, and the direction and depth of the uterine cavity. In occasional cases, severe cervical stenosis may be encountered. Do not use excessive force to overcome this resistance.

c. The uterus should sound to a depth of 6 to 9 centimeters (cm). Insertion of an IUD into a uterine cavity measuring less than 6.0 cm by sounding may increase the incidence of expulsion, bleeding, pain, perforation, and possibly, pregnancy.

d. Clinicians are cautioned that it is imperative for them to become thoroughly familiar with the instructions for use before attempting placement of the ParaGard® T 380A. To reduce the possibility of insertion in the presence of an existing undetermined pregnancy, the optimal time for insertion is the latter part of the menstrual period, or one or two days thereafter. The ParaGard® T 380A should not be inserted postpartum or postabortion until involution of the uterus is complete. The incidence of perforation and expulsion is greater if involution is not complete. Data also suggest that there may be an increased risk of perforation and expulsion if the woman is lactating.[8,9] Other recent studies report no increased incidence of perforation or expulsion in lactating women.[11,12]
The ParaGard® T 380A should be placed at the fundus of the uterine cavity. Proper placement helps avoid partial or complete expulsion that could result in pregnancy. Contraceptive effectiveness is enhanced by proper placement.

e. Patients experiencing menorrhagia and/or metrorrhagia following IUD insertion may be at risk for the development of hypochromic microcytic anemia. Careful consideration of this risk must be given before insertion in patients with anemia or a history of menorrhagia or hypermenorrhea. Patients receiving anticoagulants or having a coagulopathy may have a greater risk of menorrhagia or hypermenorrhea.

f. Syncope, bradycardia, or other neurovascular episodes may occur during insertion or removal of IUDs, especially in patients with a previous disposition to these conditions or cervical stenosis.

g. Use of an IUD in patients with cervicitis should be postponed until treatment has eradicated the infection.

h. Patients with valvular or congenital heart disease are more prone to develop subacute bacterial endocarditis than patients who do not have valvular or congenital heart disease. Use of an IUD in these patients may represent a potential source of septic emboli. Patients with known congenital heart disease who may be at increased risk should be treated with appropriate antibiotics at the time of insertion.

i. Patients requiring chronic corticosteroid therapy or insulin for diabetes should be monitored with special care for infection.

j. Since the ParaGard® T 380A may be partially or completely expelled, patients should be reexamined and evaluated shortly after the first postinsertion menses, but no later than 3 months afterwards. Thereafter, annual examination with appropriate evaluation, including a "Pap" smear, should be carried out. The ParaGard® T 380A should be kept in place no longer than 10 years.

k. The patient should be told that some bleeding or cramps may occur during the first few weeks after insertion. If these symptoms continue or are severe she should report them to her physician. She should be instructed on how to check to make certain that the threads still protrude from the cervix and cautioned that there is no contraceptive protection if the ParaGard® T 380A has been expelled. She should check frequently, at least after each menstrual period. She should be cautioned not to dislodge the ParaGard® T 380A by pulling on the thread. If a partial expulsion occurs, removal is indicated.

l. Rarely, a copper-induced urticarial allergic skin reaction may develop in women using a copper-containing IUD. If the symptoms of such an allergic response occur, the patient should be instructed to tell the consulting physician that a copper-containing device is being used.

m. The effect of magnetic resonance imaging of the pelvis was investigated in one study[13] in women with the CU-7® (Intrauterine Copper Contraceptive) and the LIPPES LOOP™ IUD. The CU-7® has a different configuration and contains less copper than the ParaGard® T 380A. The results of the study indicate that neither the CU-7® nor the LIPPES LOOP™ were moved under the influence of the magnetic field nor did they heat during the spin-echo sequences usually employed for pelvic imaging.

3. Insertion Prophylaxis
Observe strict asepsis at insertion; clean the endocervix with an antiseptic solution, because the presence of organisms capable of establishing PID cannot be determined by appearance, and because IUD insertion may be associated with introduction of vaginal bacteria into the uterus. Data do not confirm the utility of prophylactic administration of antibiotics in reducing the incidence of PID, and their use in nursing women is not recommended.

4. Requirements for Continuation and Removal

a. The ParaGard® T 380A must be replaced before the end of the tenth year of use. There is no evidence of decreasing contraceptive efficacy with time before ten years, but the contraceptive effectiveness at longer times has not been established; therefore, the patient should be informed of the known duration of contraceptive efficacy and be advised to return in 10 years for removal and possible insertion of a new ParaGard® T 380A.

b. The ParaGard® T 380A should be removed for the following medical reasons: menorrhagia- and/or metrorrhagia-producing anemia; pelvic infection; genital actinomycosis; intractable pelvic pain; dyspareunia; pregnancy; endometrial or cervical malignancy; uterine or cervical perforation; increase in length of the threads extending from the cervix, or any other indication of partial expulsion. Insertions immediately following placental delivery or first trimester abortion may result in threads becoming slightly longer as the uterus involutes and may not represent expulsion or partial expulsion.

c. If the retrieval threads cannot be visualized, they may have retracted into the uterus or have been broken, or the ParaGard® T 380A may have been broken, or the ParaGard® T 380A may have been expelled. Localization may be made by feeling with a probe, X-ray, or sonography. When the physician elects to recover a ParaGard® T 380A with the threads not visible, the removal instructions should be reviewed.

d. Should the patient's relationship cease to be mutually monogamous, or should her partner become HIV positive, or acquire a sexually transmitted disease, she should be instructed to report this change to her clinician immediately. It may be advisable to recommend the use of a barrier method as a partial protection against acquiring sexually transmitted diseases until the ParaGard® T 380A can be removed.

5. Continuing Care of Patients Using ParaGard® T 380A

a. Any inquiries regarding pain, odorous discharge, bleeding, fever, genital lesions or sores, or a missed period should be promptly responded to and prompt examination is recommended.

b. If examination during visits subsequent to insertion reveals that the length of the threads has visibly or palpably changed from their length at time of insertion, the ParaGard® T 380A should be considered displaced and should be removed. A new ParaGard® T 380A may be inserted at that time or during the next menses if it is certain that conception has not occurred. Under no circumstances should reinsertion with an expelled ParaGard® T 380A be attempted. A new ParaGard® T 380A should be inserted.

c. Since the ParaGard® T 380A may be partially or completely expelled, patients should be reexamined and evaluated shortly after the first postinsertion menses, but no later than 3 months afterwards. Thereafter, at least annual examination with appropriate evaluation, including a "Pap" smear, and if indicated, gonococcal and chlamydial laboratory evaluations, should be carried out. The ParaGard® T 380A should be kept in place no longer than 10 years.

d. In the event a pregnancy is confirmed during ParaGard® T 380A use, the following steps should be taken:
- Determine whether pregnancy is ectopic and take appropriate measures if it is.
- Inform patient of the risks of leaving an IUD *in situ* or removing it during pregnancy, and of the lack of data on the long term effects of the ParaGard® T 380A on the offspring of women who have had it *in utero* during conception or gestation (see WARNINGS). This information should include the risk of septic spontaneous abortion with the IUD *in situ*.
- If possible, the ParaGard® T 380A should be removed after the patient has been warned of the risks of removal. If removal is difficult, the patient should be counseled about and offered pregnancy termination.
- If the ParaGard® T 380A is left in place, the patient's course should be followed closely.

ADVERSE REACTIONS

These adverse reactions are not listed in any order of frequency or severity.
Reported adverse reactions with intrauterine contraceptives include: endometritis; spontaneous abortion; septic abortion; septicemia; perforation of the uterus and cervix; embedment; fragmentation of the IUD; pelvic infection; tubo-ovarian abscess; tubal damage; vaginitis; leukorrhea; cervical erosion; pregnancy; ectopic pregnancy; fetal damage; difficult removal; complete or partial expulsion of the IUD, particularly in those patients with uteri measuring less than 6.0 cm by sounding; menstrual spotting; prolongation of menstrual flow; anemia; amenorrhea or delayed menses; pain and cramping; dysmenorrhea; backaches; dyspareunia; neurovascular episodes, including bradycardia and syncope secondary to insertion. Uterine perforation and IUD displacement into the abdomen have been followed by peritonitis, abdominal adhesions, intestinal penetration, intestinal obstruction, and cystic masses in the pelvis. (Certain of these adverse reactions can lead to loss of fertility, partial or total removal of reproductive organs, hormonal imbalance, or death). Urticarial allergic skin reaction may occur.

CLINICAL STUDIES

Different event rates have been reported with the use of different intrauterine contraceptives. Inasmuch as these rates are usually derived from separate studies conducted by different investigators in several populations, they cannot be compared with precision. Considerably different rates are likely to be obtained because event rates per unit of time tend to decrease as studies are extended, since more susceptible subjects discontinue due to expulsions, adverse reactions, or pregnancy, leaving the study population richer in less susceptible subjects. In clinical trials conducted by The Population Council[14,16] and WHO, use-effectiveness of the ParaGard® T 380A as calculated by the life table method was determined through ten (10) years of use.
Data suggest a higher pregnancy rate in women under 20.[14,15,17]
[See table II at top right of next page.]

Continued on next page

Ortho—Cont.

TABLE III
GROSS ANNUAL EVENT RATES PER 100 CONTINUING USERS BY YEAR AND PARITY

	1 Year Parous
Pregnancy	0.5
Expulsion	2.3
Bleeding/Pain	3.4
Infection	0.3
Other Medical	0.5
Planning Pregnancy	0.6
Other Personal	0.7
Continuation	92.1
No. Completed	1842.0

Rates were calculated by combining the experience on a weighted basis from both an international study by the World Health Organization (2110 women) and a U.S. study by GynoPharma Inc. (230 women).

The lowest expected and typical failure rates during the first year of continuous use of all contraceptive methods are listed in Table IV (Adapted from Reference 16).

[See Table IV below.]

Footnotes to Table IV:
1. Among *typical* couples who initiate use of a method (not necessarily for the first time), the percentage who experience an accidental pregnancy during the first year if they do not stop use for any other reason.
2. Among couples who initiate use of a method (not necessarily for the first time) and who use it *perfectly* (both consistently and correctly), the percentage who experience an accidental pregnancy during the first year if they do not stop use for any other reason.
3. Among couples attempting to avoid pregnancy, the percentage who continue to use a method for one year.
4. The percentages failing in columns (2) and (3) are based on data from populations where contraception is not used and from women who cease using contraception in order to become pregnant. Among such populations, about 89% become pregnant within one year. This estimate was lowered slightly (to 85%) to represent the percentage who would become pregnant within 1 year among women now relying on reversible methods of contraception if they abandoned contraception altogether.
5. Foams, creams, gels, vaginal suppositories, and vaginal film.
6. Cervical mucus (ovulation) method supplemented by calendar in the pre-ovulatory and basal body temperature in the post-ovulatory phases.
7. With spermicidal cream or jelly.
8. Without spermicides.
9. The treatment schedule is one dose as soon as possible (but no more than 72 hours) after unprotected intercourse, and a second dose 12 hours after the first dose. The hormones that have been studied in the clinical trials of postcoital hormonal contraception are found in Nordette, Levlen, Lo/Orval (1 dose is 4 pills), Triphasil, Tri-Levlin (1 dose is 4 yellow pills), and Ovral (1 dose is 2 pills).
10. However, to maintain effective protection against pregnancy, another method of contraception must be used as soon as menstruation resumes, the frequency or duration of breastfeeds is reduced, bottle feeds are introduced, or the baby reaches 6 months of age.

HOW SUPPLIED

Available in cartons of one (NDC 54765-380-01) or five (NDC 54765-380-05) sterile units. Each ParaGard® T 380A is packaged in a Tyvek®-polyethylene pouch, together with an insertion tube and solid rod.

INSTRUCTIONS FOR USE
Paragard® T 380A
(Intrauterine Copper Contraceptive)
CLINICIANS SHOULD HAVE DEMONSTRATED CLINICAL COMPETENCE IN PARAGARD® T 380A INSERTIONS RECEIVED UNDER SUPERVISION. PREVIOUS EDUCATION RE: SURGICAL PROCEDURES WILL REQUIRE VARYING LEVELS OF EXPERIENCE.
The ParaGard® T 380A (Intrauterine Copper Contraceptive) represents a different design in intrauterine contraceptives. Physicians are, therefore, cautioned that they should become thoroughly familiar with instructions for insertion before attempting placement of the ParaGard® T 380A. The insertion technique is different in several respects from that employed with other intrauterine contraceptives and the physician should pay particular attention to the drawings and commentary accompanying these instructions.

TABLE II
ParaGard® T 380A
(Intrauterine Copper Contraceptive)
GROSS ANNUAL TERMINATION AND CONTINUATION RATES PER 100* USERS
All Copper T 380A IUD Acceptors
Combined Population Council and WHO Studies

	YEAR									
RATE OF ITEM	1	2	3	4	5	6	7	8	9	10
Pregnancy	0.7	0.3	0.6	0.2	0.3	0.2	0.0	0.4	0.0	0.0
Expulsion	5.7	2.5	1.6	1.2	0.3	0.0	0.6	1.7	0.2	0.4
Bleeding/Pain	11.9	9.8	7.0	3.5	3.7	2.7	3.0	2.5	2.2	3.7
Other Medical	2.5	2.1	1.6	1.7	0.1	0.3	1.0	0.4	0.7	0.3
Continuation	76.8	78.3	81.2	86.2	89.0	91.9	87.9	88.1	92.0	91.8
No. of Women:										
At Start of Year	4932	3149	2018	1121	872	621	563	483	423	325
At End of Year	3149	2018	1121	872	621	563	483	423	325	230

* Rates were calculated by weighing the annual rates by the number of subjects starting each year for each of the Population Council (3536 acceptors) and the World Health Organization (1396 acceptors) trials.

A single ParaGard® T 380A is placed at the fundus of the uterine cavity.
The ParaGard® T 380A may be inserted at any time during the cycle. However, it is essential that pregnancy be ruled out before insertion.
The ParaGard® T 380A is indicated for use up to 10 years. Therefore, the ParaGard® T 380A must be removed and a new one inserted on or before 10 years from the date of insertion.

PRELIMINARY PREPARATION AND INSERTION
1. Before insertion, you and the patient will want to review the Patient Package Insert. If the patient agrees, she may sign the Consent Form provided for your records.
2. Take a medical and social history.
3. Refer to CONTRAINDICATIONS, WARNINGS, and PRECAUTIONS.
4. Pelvic examination is to be performed prior to insertion of the ParaGard® T 380A, including a cervical "Pap" smear, and gonococcal and chlamydial evaluations, if indicated, and any other necessary specific tests.
5. If appropriate, commence antibiotic prophylaxis one hour before insertion.
6. Use of aseptic technique during insertion is essential.
7. The endocervix should be cleansed with an antiseptic solution and a tenaculum applied to the cervix with downward traction for correction of the angulation as well as stabilization of the cervix.

8. With a speculum in place, gently insert a sterile sound to determine the depth and direction of the uterine canal. Be sure to determine the position of the uterus before insertion.

CAUTION
Any intrauterine procedure can result in severe pain, bradycardia, and syncope.
It is generally believed that perforations, if they occur, are encountered at the time of insertion, although the perforation may not be detected until some time later. The position of the uterus should be determined during the preinsertion examination. Great care must be exercised during the preinsertion sounding and subsequent insertion. No attempt should be made to force the insertion.

HOW TO LOAD AND INSERT ParaGard® T 380A
STEP 1
To minimize chance of introducing contamination, do not remove the ParaGard® T 380A from the inserter tube prior to placement in the uterus. Do not bend the arms of the ParaGard® T 380A earlier than 5 minutes before it is to be introduced into the uterus.
In the absence of sterile gloves, this can be accomplished without destroying sterility by folding the arms in the partially opened package. Place the partially opened package on a flat surface and pull the solid rod partially from the package so it will not interfere with assembly. Place thumb and index finger on top of package on ends of the horizontal

TABLE IV— Percentage of women experiencing a contraceptive failure during the first year of typical use and the first year of perfect use and the percentage continuing use at the end of the first year, United States.[16]

Method	% of Women Experiencing an Accidental Pregnancy Within the First Year of Use		% of Women Continuing Use at One Year[3]
	Typical Use[1]	Perfect Use[2]	
Chance[4]	85	85	
Spermicides[6]	21	6	43
Periodic Abstinence	20		67
Calendar		9	
Ovulation Method		3	
Sympto-Thermal[6]		2	
Post-Ovulation		1	
Withdrawal	19	4	
Cap[7]			
Parous Women	36	26	45
Nulliparous Women	18	9	58
Sponge			
Parous Women	36	20	45
Nulliparous Women	18	9	58
Diaphragm[7]	18	6	58
Condom[8]			
Female (Reality)	21	5	56
Male	12	3	63
Pill	3		72
Progestin Only		0.5	
Combined		0.1	
IUD			
Progesterone T	2.0	1.5	81
Copper T 380A			
(ParaGard® T 380A)	0.8	0.6	78
Depo-Provera®	0.3	0.3	70
Norplant® (6 Capsules)	0.09	0.09	85
Female Sterilization	0.4	0.4	100
Male Sterilization	0.15	0.10	100

Emergency Contraceptive Pills: Treatment initiated within 72 hours after unprotected intercourse reduces the risk of pregnancy by at least 75%[9].
Lactational Amenorrhea Method: LAM is a highly effective temporary method of contraception.[10]

arms. Push insertion tube against arms of ParaGard® T 380A as indicated by arrow in Fig. 1A to start arms folding.

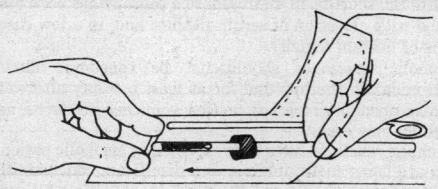

Fig. 1A

Complete the bending by bringing thumb and index finger together while using the other hand to maneuver the insertion tube to pick up the arms of the ParaGard® T 380A (Fig. 1B). Insert no further than necessary to insure retention of the arms. Introduce the solid rod into the insertion tube from the bottom alongside the threads until it touches the bottom of the ParaGard® T 380A.

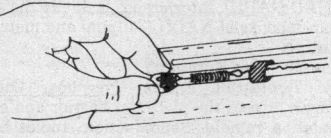

Fig. 1B

STEP 2
Adjust the movable flange so that it indicates the depth to which the ParaGard® T 380A should be inserted and the direction in which the arms of the ParaGard® T 380A will open. At this point, make certain that the horizontal arms of the ParaGard® T 380A and the long axis of the flange lie in the same horizontal plane. Introduce the loaded insertion tube through the cervical canal and upwards until the ParaGard® T 380A lies in contact with the fundus. The movable flange should be at the cervix (Fig. 2).
DO NOT FORCE THE INSERTION.

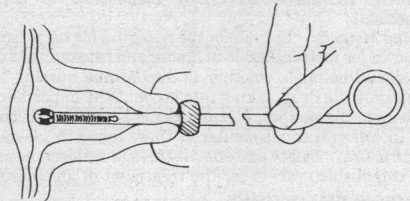

Fig. 2

STEP 3
To release the arms of the ParaGard® T 380A, withdraw the insertion tube not more than $1/2$ inch while the solid rod is not permitted to move. This releases the arms of the ParaGard® T 380A (Fig. 3).

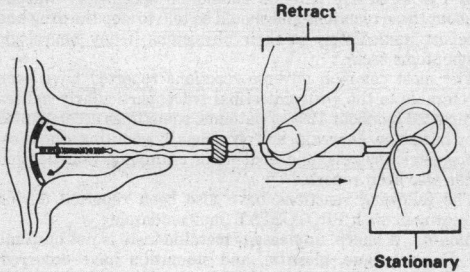

Retract

Stationary

Fig. 3

STEP 4
After the arms are released, the insertion tube should be moved upward gently until the resistance of the fundus is felt. This will assure placement of the T at the highest possible position within the endometrial cavity (Fig. 4).

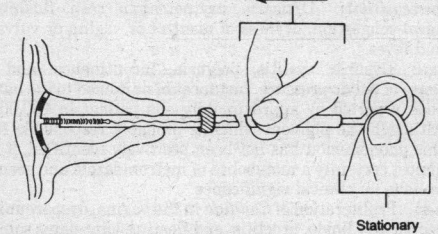

Stationary

Fig. 4

STEP 5
Withdraw the solid rod while holding the insertion tube stationary (Fig. 5).

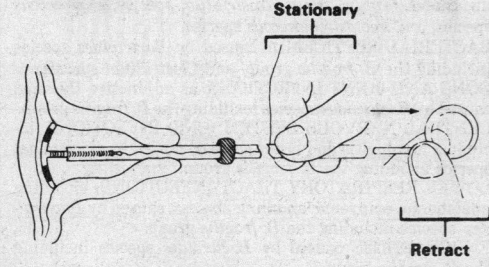

Stationary

Retract

Fig. 5

STEP 6
Withdraw the insertion tube from the cervix. Be sure sufficient length of the threads are visible (approximately 1 in. or 2.5 cm.) to facilitate checking for the presence of the ParaGard® T 380A (Fig. 6). Notation of length of the threads should be made in patient record.

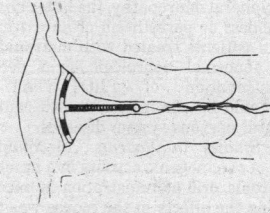

Fig. 6

HOW TO REMOVE ParaGard® T 380A
To remove the ParaGard® T 380A, pull gently on the exposed threads. The arms of the ParaGard® T 380A will fold upwards as it is withdrawn from the uterus. Even if removal proves difficult, the ParaGard® T 380A should not remain in the uterus after 10 years.

REFERENCES
1. Alvarez F et al: New insights on the mode of action on intrauterine contraceptives in women. *Fertil Steril* 1988; 49:768–773.
2. World Health Organization's Special Programme of Research, Development and Research Training in Human Reproduction: A multinational case-control study of ectopic pregnancy. *Clin Reprod Fertil* 1985; 3:131–143.
3. Ory HW, Women's Health Study: Ectopic pregnancy and intrauterine contraceptive devices: New perspectives. *Obstet Gynecol* 1981; 57:137–144.
4. Marchbanks PA et al: Risk factors for ectopic pregnancy: A population-based study. *JAMA* 1988; 259:1823–1827.
5. Farley TMM et al: Intrauterine devices and pelvic inflammatory disease: An international perspective. *Lancet* 1992; 339:785–788.
6. Cramer DW et al: Tubal infertility and the intrauterine device. *N Engl J Med* 1985; 312:941–947.
7. Daling JR et al: Primary tubal infertility in relation to the use of an intrauterine device. *N Engl J Med* 1985; 312:937–941.
8. Heartwell SF, Schlesselman S: Risk of uterine perforation among users of intrauterine devices. *Obstet Gynecol* 1983; 61:31–36.
9. Chi I-C, Kelly E: Is lactation a risk factor of IUD and sterilization-related uterine perforations? A hypothesis. *Int J Gynaecol Obstet* 1984; 22:315–317.
10. Harlap S, Kost K, Forrest JD: Preventing pregnancy, protecting health: a new look at birth control choices in the United States. The Alan Guttmacher Institute 1991:1–129.
11. Chi I-C et al: Performance of the Copper T 380A Intrauterine device in breast feeding women. *Contraception* 1989; 39:603–618.
12. Farr G. Rivera R: Interactions between intrauterine contraceptive device use and breast-feeding status at time of intrauterine contraceptive device insertion. Analysis of TCu-380A acceptors in developing countries. *Am J Obstet Gynecol* 1992; 167:144–151.
13. Mark AS, Hricak H: Intrauterine contraceptive devices: MR imaging. *Radiology* 1987; 311–314.
14. Sivin, I, Stern J: Long-acting, more effective Copper T IUDs: A summary of US experience, 1970–1975, *Stud Fam Plann* 1979; 10:263–281.
15. Sivin I, Schmidt F: Effectiveness of IUDs: A review. *Contraception* 1987; 36:55–84.
16. Trussell J: The Essentials of Contraception, in R.A. Hatcher, et al: *Contraceptive Technology*, 16th Revised Ed., New York, Irvington, 1994, 113–114.
17. World Health Organization (WHO): Mechanism of action, safety, and efficacy of intrauterine devices. Report of a WHO Scientific Group. Technical Report Series 753. Geneva; World Health Organization, 1987, p. 22.

Manufactured for
ORTHO PHARMACEUTICAL CORPORATION
Raritan, New Jersey 08869
by FEI Products, Inc.
N. Tonawanda, New York 14120
© OPC 1995
Revised January 1996
Code #631-40-410-2
Shown in Product Identification Guide, page 327

PROTOSTAT® ℞
(metronidazole) Tablets

> **WARNING**
> Metronidazole has been shown to be carcinogenic in mice and rats. *(See Warnings.)* Unnecessary use of this drug should be avoided. Its use should be reserved for the conditions described in the *Indications And Usage* section below.

DESCRIPTION
PROTOSTAT (metronidazole) is a 1-(β-hydroxyethyl)-2-methyl-5-nitroimidazole. Both the 250 mg and 500 mg tablets include the following inactive ingredients: Lactose, magnesium stearate, microcrystalline cellulose, povidone, sodium starch glycolate, and stearic acid. Metronidazole is classified therapeutically as an antiprotozoal *(Trichomonas),* and antibacterial (antianaerobic) agent. It occurs as pale yellow crystals that are slightly soluble in water and alcohol. Metronidazole has the following structural formula:

$$O_2N\text{—}\underset{N}{\overset{CH_2CH_2OH}{\diagup}}\text{—}CH_3$$

CLINICAL PHARMACOLOGY
Metronidazole is usually well absorbed after oral administration, with peak plasma concentrations occurring between one and two hours. An average elimination half-life is 8 hours in healthy humans. Plasma concentrations of metronidazole are proportional to the administered dose. Oral administration of 250 mg., 500 mg., or 2,000 mg. produced peak plasma concentrations of 6 mcg/ml, 12 mcg/ml, and 40 mcg/ml, respectively. Studies reveal no significant bioavailability differences between males and females; however, because of weight differences, the resulting plasma levels in males are generally lower.

Metronidazole is the major component appearing in the plasma, with lesser quantities of the 2-hydroxymethyl metabolite also being present. Less than 20% of the circulating metronidazole is bound to plasma proteins. Both the parent compound and the metabolite possess *in vitro* trichomonacidal activity and *in vitro* bactericidal activity against most strains of anaerobic bacteria.

The major route of elimination of metronidazole and its metabolites is via the urine (60-80% of the dose), with fecal excretion accounting for 6-15% of the dose. The metabolites that appear in the urine result primarily from side-chain oxidation [1-(β-hydroxyethyl)-2-hydroxymethyl-5-nitroimidazole and 2-methyl-5-nitroimidazole-1-yl-acetic acid] and glucuronide conjugation, with unchanged metronidazole accounting for approximately 20% of the total. Renal clearance of metronidazole is approximately 10 ml/min/1.73m^2.

Decreased renal function does not alter the single-dose pharmacokinetics of metronidazole. However, plasma clearance of metronidazole is decreased in patients with decreased liver function.

Metronidazole appears in cerebrospinal fluid, saliva, and breast milk in concentrations similar to those found in plasma. Bactericidal concentrations of metronidazole have also been detected in pus from hepatic abscesses.

Microbiology: Metronidazole possesses direct trichomonacidal and amoebicidal activity against *Trichomonas Vaginalis* and *Entamoeba histolytica.* The *in vitro* minimal inhibitory concentration (MIC) for most strains of these organisms is 1 mcg/ml or less. Metronidazole's mechanism of antiprotozoal action is unknown.

Anaerobic Bacteria: Metronidazole is active *in vitro* against obligate anaerobes, but does not appear to possess any clinically relevant activity against facultative anaerobes or obligate aerobes. Against susceptible organisms, metronidazole is generally bactericidal at concentrations equal to or

Continued on next page

Ortho—Cont.

slightly higher than the minimal inhibitory concentrations (MIC). Metronidazole has been shown to have *in vitro* and clinical activity against the following organisms:

Anaerobic gram-negative bacilli, including:

Bacteroides species, including the *Bacteroides fragilis* group *(B. fragilis, B. distasonis, B. ovatus, B. thetaiotaomicron, B. vulgatus)*

Fusobacterium species

Anaerobic gram-positive bacilli, including:

Clostridium species and susceptible strains of *Eubacterium*

Anaerobic gram-positive cocci, including:

Peptococcus species

Peptostreptococcus species

Susceptibility tests: Bacteriologic studies should be performed to determine the causative organisms and their susceptibility to metronidazole; however, the rapid, routine susceptibility testing of individual isolates of anaerobic bacteria is not always practical, and therapy may be started while awaiting these results.

Quantitative methods give the most precise estimates of susceptibility to antibacterial drugs. A standardized agar dilution method and a broth microdilution method are recommended.[1]

Control strains are recommended for standardized susceptibility testing. Each time the test is performed, one or more of the following strains should be included: *Clostridium perfringens* ATCC 13124, *Bacteroides fragilis* ATCC 25285, and *Bacteroides thetaiotaomicron* ATCC 29741. The mode metronidazole MIC's for those three strains are reported to be 0.25, 0.25, and 0.5 mcg/ml, respectively.

A clinical laboratory is considered under acceptable control if the results of the control strains are within one doubling dilution of the mode MIC's reported for metronidazole.

A bacterial isolate may be considered susceptible if the MIC value for metronidazole is not more than 16 mcg/ml. An organism is considered resistant if the MIC is greater than 16 mcg/ml. A report of "resistant" from the laboratory indicates that the infecting organism is not likely to respond to therapy.

INDICATIONS AND USAGE

Symptomatic Trichomoniasis: PROTOSTAT is indicated for the treatment of symptomatic trichomoniasis in females and males when the presence of trichomonad has been confirmed by appropriate laboratory procedures (wet smears and/or cultures).

Asymptomatic Trichomoniasis: PROTOSTAT is indicated in the treatment of asymptomatic females when the organism is associated with endocervicitis, cervicitis, or cervical erosion. Since there is evidence that presence of the trichomonad can interfere with accurate assessment of abnormal cytological smears, additional smears should be performed after eradication of the parasite.

Treatment of Asymptomatic Consorts: *T. vaginalis* infection is a venereal disease. Therefore, asymptomatic sexual partners of treated patients should be treated simultaneously if the organism has been found to be present in order to prevent reinfection of the partner. The decision as to whether to treat an asymptomatic male partner with a negative culture or one in whom no culture has been attempted is an individual one. In making this decision, it should be noted that there is evidence that women may become reinfected if the consort is not treated. Also, since there can be considerable difficulty in isolating the organism from the asymptomatic male carrier, negative smears and cultures cannot be relied upon in this regard. In any event, the consort should be treated with PROTOSTAT in cases of reinfection.

Amebiasis: PROTOSTAT is indicated in the treatment of acute intestinal amebiasis (amebic dysentery) and amebic liver abscess.

In amebic liver abscess, PROTOSTAT therapy does not obviate the need for aspiration or drainage of pus.

Anaerobic Bacterial Infections: PROTOSTAT is indicated in the treatment of serious infections caused by susceptible anaerobic bacteria. Indicated surgical procedures should be performed in conjunction with PROTOSTAT therapy. In a mixed aerobic and anaerobic infection, antibiotics appropriate for the treatment of aerobic infection should be used in addition to PROTOSTAT. In the treatment of most serious anaerobic infections the intravenous form of metronidazole is usually administered initially. This may be followed by oral therapy with PROTOSTAT at the discretion of the physician.

INTRA-ABDOMINAL INFECTION, including peritonitis, intra-abdominal abscess, and liver abscess, caused by *Bacteroides* species including the *B. fragilis* group *(B. fragilis, B. distasonis, B. ovatus, B. thetaiotaomicron, B. vulgatus), Clostridium* species, *Eubacterium* species, *Peptococcus* species, and *Peptostreptococcus* species.

SKIN AND SKIN STRUCTURE INFECTIONS caused by *Bacteroides* species including the *B. fragilis* group, *Clostridium* species, *Peptococcus* species, *Peptostreptococcus* species, and *Fusobacterium* species.

GYNECOLOGIC INFECTIONS, including endometritis, endomyometritis, tubo-ovarian abscess, and post-surgical vaginal cuff infection, caused by *Bacteroides* species including the *B. fragilis* group, *Clostridium* species, *Peptococcus* species, and *Peptostreptococcus* species.

BACTERIAL SEPTICEMIA caused by *Bacteroides* species including the *B. fragilis* group, and *Clostridium* species.

BONE AND JOINT INFECTIONS, as adjunctive therapy, caused by *Bacteroides* species including the *B. fragilis* group.

CENTRAL NERVOUS SYSTEM (CNS) INFECTIONS, including meningitis and brain abscess, caused by *Bacteroides* species including the *B. fragilis* group.

LOWER RESPIRATORY TRACT INFECTIONS, including pneumonia, empyema, and lung abscess, caused by *Bacteroides* species including the *B. fragilis* group.

ENDOCARDITIS caused by *Bacteroides* species including the *B. fragilis* group.

CONTRAINDICATIONS

PROTOSTAT is contraindicated in patients with a prior history of hypersensitivity to metronidazole or other nitroimidazole derivatives. PROTOSTAT is contraindicated during the first trimester of pregnancy. (*See Warnings.*)

WARNINGS

Convulsive Seizures and Peripheral Neuropathy: Convulsive seizures and peripheral neuropathy, the latter characterized mainly by numbness or paresthesia of an extremity, have been reported in patients treated with metronidazole. The appearance of abnormal neurologic signs demands the prompt discontinuation of PROTOSTAT therapy. PROTOSTAT should be administered with caution to patients with central nervous system diseases.

Tumorigenicity Studies in Rodents: Metronidazole has shown evidence of carcinogenic activity in a number of studies involving chronic, oral administration in mice and rats. Prominent among the effects in the mouse was the promotion of pulmonary tumorigenesis. This has been observed in all six reported studies in that species, including one study in which the animals were dosed on an intermittent schedule (administration during every fourth week only). At very high dose levels (approx. 500mg/kg/day) there was a statistically significant increase in the incidence of malignant liver tumors in males. Also, the published results of one of the mouse studies indicated an increase in the incidence of malignant lymphomas as well as pulmonary neoplasms associated with lifetime feeding of the drug. All these effects are statistically significant.

Several long-term oral dosing studies in the rats have been completed. There was a statistically significant increase in the incidence of various neoplasms, particularly in mammary and hepatic tumors, among female rats administered metronidazole over those noted in the concurrent female control groups.

Two lifetime tumorigenicity studies in hamsters have been performed and reported to be negative.

Mutagenicity Studies: Although metronidazole has shown mutagenic activity in a number of *in vitro* assay systems, studies in mammals (*in vivo*) have failed to demonstrate a potential for genetic damage.

PRECAUTIONS

General: Patients with severe hepatic disease metabolize metronidazole slowly, with resultant accumulation of metronidazole and its metabolites in the plasma. Accordingly, for such patients, doses below those usually recommended should be administered cautiously.

Known or previously unrecognized candidiasis may present more prominent symptoms during therapy with PROTOSTAT and requires treatment with a candicidal agent.

Information for Patients: Alcoholic beverages should be avoided while taking metronidazole and at least one day afterward. (*See Drug Interactions.*)

Laboratory Tests: PROTOSTAT (metronidazole) is a nitroimidazole and should be used with care in patients with evidence of, or history of, blood dyscrasia. A mild leukopenia has been observed during its administration; however, no persistent hematologic abnormalities attributable to metronidazole have been observed in clinical studies. Total and differential leukocyte counts are recommended before and after therapy for trichomoniasis and amebiasis, especially if a second course of therapy is necessary, and before and after therapy for anaerobic infection.

Drug Interactions: Metronidazole has been reported to potentiate the anticoagulant effect of coumarin and warfarin resulting in a prolongation of prothrombin time. This possible drug interaction should be considered when PROTOSTAT is prescribed for patients on this type of anticoagulant therapy.

The simultaneous administration of drugs that induce microsomal liver enzymes, such as phenytoin or phenobarbital may accelerate the elimination of metronidazole, resulting in reduced plasma levels; impaired clearance of phenytoin has also been reported.

The simultaneous administration of drugs that decrease microsomal liver enzyme activity, such as cimetidine,

may prolong the half-life and decrease plasma clearance of metronidazole. In patients stabilized on relatively high doses of lithium, short-term metronidazole therapy has been associated with elevation of serum lithium and, in a few cases, signs of lithium toxicity.

Alcoholic beverages should not be consumed during metronidazole therapy and for at least one day afterward because abdominal cramps, nausea, vomiting, headache, and flushing may occur.

Psychotic reactions have been reported in alcoholic patients who are using metronidazole and disulfiram concurrently. Metronidazole should not be given to patients who have taken disulfiram within the last two weeks.

Drug/Laboratory Test Interactions: Metronidazole may interfere with certain types of determinations of serum chemistry values, such as aspartate aminotransferase (AST, SGOT), alanine aminotransferase (ALT, SGPT), lactate dehydrogenase (LDH), triglycerides, and hexokinase glucose. Values of zero may be observed. All of the assays in which interference has been reported involve enzymatic coupling of the assay to oxidation-reduction of nicotine adenine dinucleotide (NAD NADH). Interference is due to the similarity in absorbance peaks of NADH (340 nm) and metronidazole (322 nm) at pH 7.

Carcinogenesis: (*See Warnings.*)

Pregnancy: Teratogenic Effects—Pregnancy Category B. Metronidazole crosses the placental barrier and enters the fetal circulation rapidly. Reproduction studies have been performed in rats at doses up to five times the human dose and have revealed no evidence of impaired fertility or harm to the fetus due to metronidazole. Metronidazole administered intraperitoneally to pregnant mice at approximately the human dose caused fetotoxicity; administered orally to pregnant mice, no fetotoxicity was observed. There are, however, no adequate and well-controlled studies in pregnant women. Because animal reproduction studies are not always predictive of human response, and because metronidazole is a carcinogen in rodents, this drug should be used during pregnancy only if clearly needed (see Contraindications). Use of PROTOSTAT for trichomoniasis in the second and third trimesters should be restricted to those in whom local palliative treatment has been inadequate to control symptoms.

Nursing Mothers: Because of the potential for tumorigenicity shown for metronidazole in mouse and rat studies, a decision should be made whether to discontinue nursing or to discontinue the drug, taking into account the importance of the drug to the mother. Metronidazole is secreted in breast milk in concentrations similar to those found in plasma.

Pediatric Use: Safety and effectiveness in children have not been established, except for the treatment of amebiasis.

ADVERSE REACTIONS

The two most serious adverse reactions reported in patients treated with PROTOSTAT (metronidazole) have been convulsive seizures and peripheral neuropathy, the latter characterized mainly by numbness or paresthesia of an extremity. Since persistent peripheral neuropathy has been reported in some patients receiving prolonged administration of PROTOSTAT, patients should be specifically warned about these reactions and should be told to stop the drug and report immediately to their physicians if any neurologic symptoms occur.

The most common adverse reactions reported have been referable to the gastrointestinal tract, particularly nausea reported by about 12% of patients, sometimes accompanied by headache, anorexia, and occasionally vomiting; diarrhea; epigastric distress; and abdominal cramping. Constipation has also been reported.

The following reactions have also been reported during treatment with PROTOSTAT (metronidazole):

Mouth: A sharp, unpleasant metallic taste is not unusual. Furry tongue, glossitis, and stomatitis have occurred; these may be associated with a sudden overgrowth of *Candida* which may occur during effective therapy.

Hematopoietic: Reversible neutropenia (leukopenia); rarely, reversible thrombocytopenia.

Cardiovascular: Flattening of the T-wave may be seen in electrocardiographic tracings.

Central Nervous System: Convulsive seizures, peripheral neuropathy, dizziness, vertigo, incoordination, ataxia, confusion, irritability, depression, weakness, and insomnia.

Hypersensitivity: Urticaria, erythematous rash, flushing, nasal congestion, dryness of mouth (or vagina or vulva), and fever.

Renal: Dysuria, cystitis, polyuria, incontinence, and a sense of pelvic pressure. Instances of darkened urine have been reported by approximately one patient in 100,000. Although the pigment which is probably responsible for this phenomenon has not been positively identified, it is almost certainly a metabolite of metronidazole and seems to have no clinical significance.

Other: Proliferation of *Candida* in the vagina, dyspareunia, decrease of libido, proctitis, and fleeting joint pains sometimes resembling "serum sickness." If patients receiving PROTOSTAT drink alcoholic beverages, they may experi-

ence abdominal distress, nausea, vomiting, flushing, or headache. A modification of the taste of alcoholic beverages has also been reported.

Crohn's disease patients are known to have an increased incidence of gastrointestinal and certain extraintestinal cancers. There have been some reports in the medical literature of breast and colon cancer in Crohn's disease patients who have been treated with metronidazole at high doses for extended periods of time. A cause and effect relationship has not been established. Crohn's disease is not an approved indication for metronidazole.

OVERDOSAGE

Single oral doses of metronidazole, up to 15 g, have been reported in suicide attempts and accidental overdoses. Symptoms reported include nausea, vomiting, and ataxia. Oral metronidazole has been studied as a radiation sensitizer in the treating of malignant tumors. Neurotoxic effects, including seizures and peripheral neuropathy, have been reported after 5 to 7 days of doses of 6 to 10.4 g every other day.

Treatment: There is no specific antidote for PROTOSTAT overdose; therefore, management of the patient should consist of symptomatic and supportive therapy.

DOSAGE AND ADMINISTRATION

Trichomoniasis:

In The Female: One-day treatment — two grams of PROTOSTAT given either as a single dose or in two divided doses of one gram each given in the same day.

Seven-day course of treatment—250 mg three times daily for seven consecutive days. There is some indication from controlled comparative studies that cure rates as determined by vaginal smears, signs and symptoms, may be higher after a seven-day course of treatment than after a one-day treatment regimen.

The dosage regimen should be individualized. Single-dose treatment can assure compliance, especially if administered under supervision, in those patients who cannot be relied on to continue the seven-day regimen.

A seven-day course of treatment may minimize reinfection of the female long enough to treat sexual contacts. Further, some patients may tolerate one course of therapy better than the other.

Pregnant patients should not be treated during the first trimester with either regimen. If treated during the second or third trimester, the one-day course of therapy should not be used, as it results in higher serum levels which reach the fetal circulation. *(See Contraindications and Precautions.)*

When repeated courses of the drug are required, it is recommended that an interval of four to six weeks elapse between courses and that the presence of the trichomonad be reconfirmed by appropriate laboratory measures. Total and differential leukocyte counts should be made before and after treatment.

In The Male: Treatment should be individualized as for the female.

Amebiasis: Adults: For Acute Intestinal Amebiasis (Acute Amebic Dysentery):

750 mg. orally 3 times daily for 5 to 10 days.

For Amebic Liver Abscess: 500 mg or 750 mg orally 3 times daily for 5 to 10 days.

Children: 35 to 50 mg/kg of body weight/24 hours divided into 3 doses, orally for 10 days.

Anaerobic Bacterial Infections: In the treatment of most serious anaerobic infections the intravenous form of metronidazole is usually administered initially.

Following intravenous therapy, oral metronidazole may be used when conditions warrant based upon the severity of the disease and the response of the patient to intravenous treatment.

The usual adult *oral* dosage is 7.5 mg/kg every six hours (approximately 500 mg for a 70 kg adult). A maximum of 4.0 g should not be exceeded during a 24-hour period.

The usual duration of therapy is 7 to 10 days; however, infections of the bone and joint, lower respiratory tract, and endocardium may require longer treatment.

Patients with severe hepatic disease metabolize metronidazole slowly, with resultant accumulation of metronidazole and its metabolites in the plasma. Accordingly, for such patients, doses below those usually recommended should be administered cautiously. Close monitoring of plasma metronidazole levels[2] and toxicity is recommended.

The dose of PROTOSTAT should not be specifically reduced in anuric patients since accumulated metabolites may be rapidly removed by dialysis.

HOW SUPPLIED

Available in tablets containing 250 mg and 500 mg of metronidazole, USP. PROTOSTAT 250 mg is a white to off-white capsule-shaped, convex tablet. Each 250 mg PROTOSTAT Tablet is scored on one side and imprinted with ORTHO 1570 on the other side, packaged in a bottle of 100 tablets (NDC 0062-1570-01). PROTOSTAT 500 mg is a white to off-white capsule-shaped, convex tablet. Each 500 mg PROTOSTAT Tablet is scored on one side and imprinted with ORTHO 1571 on the other side, packaged in a bottle of 50 tablets (NDC 0062-1571-01).

Dispense in well-closed, light-resistant containers as defined in the USP.

Store below 86°F (30°C).

1. Proposed standard: PSM-11—Proposed Reference Dilution Procedure for Antimicrobic Susceptibility Testing of Anaerobic Bacteria, National Committee for Clinical Laboratory Standards, and Sutter, et al: Collaborative Evaluation of a Proposed Reference Dilution Method of Susceptibility Testing of Anaerobic Bacteria, Antimicrob. Agents Chemother. *16*:495-502 (Oct.) 1979; and Talley, et al: *In Vitro* Activity of Thienamycin Antimicrob. Agents Chemother. *14*:436–438 (Sept.) 1978.

2. Ralph, E.D., and Kirby, W.M.M.: Bioassay of Metronidazole With Either Anaerobic or Aerobic Incubation, J. Infect. Dis. *132*:587–591 (Nov.) 1975; or Gulaid, et al: Determination of Metronidazole and Its Major Metabolites in Biological Fluids by High Pressure Liquid Chromatography, Br. J. Clin. Pharmacol. *6*:430–432, 1978.

Revised January 1992

631-10-680-3

Shown in Product Identification Guide, page 327

SULTRIN® Triple Sulfa Cream ℞
(sulfathiazole/sulfacetamide/ sulfabenzamide)

SULTRIN® Triple Sulfa Vaginal Tablets ℞
(sulfathiazole/sulfacetamide/ sulfabenzamide)

DESCRIPTION

SULTRIN Cream contains sulfathiazole (Benzenesulfonamide,4-amino-N-2-thiazolyl-N[1]-2-thiazolylsulfanilamide) 3.42%, sulfacetamide (Acetamide,N-[(4-aminophenyl) sulfonyl]-N-Sulfanilylacetamide) 2.86%, and sulfabenzamide (Benzamide,N-[(4-aminophenyl) sulfonyl]-N-Sulfanilylbenzamide) 3.7%, compounded with cetyl alcohol 2%, cholesterol, diethylaminoethyl stearamide, glyceryl monostearate, lanolin, lecithin, methylparaben, peanut oil, phosphoric acid, propylene glycol, propylparaben, purified water, stearic acid and urea.

Each SULTRIN Tablet contains sulfathiazole (Benzenesulfonamide,4-amino-N -2- thiazolyl-N[1]-2-thiazolylsulfanilamide) 172.5 mg, sulfacetamide (Acetamide,N-[(4-aminophenyl)sulfonyl] -N- Sulfanilylacetamide) 143.75 mg and sulfabenzamide (Benzamide,N-[(4-aminophenyl)sulfonyl]-N-Sulfanilylbenzamide) 184.0 mg, compounded with guar gum, lactose, magnesium stearate, starch and urea.

SULTRIN Cream and SULTRIN Tablets are topical antibacterial preparations available for intravaginal administration.

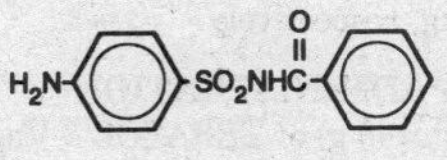

Sulfabenzamide

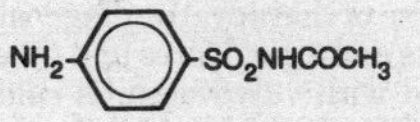

Sulfacetamide

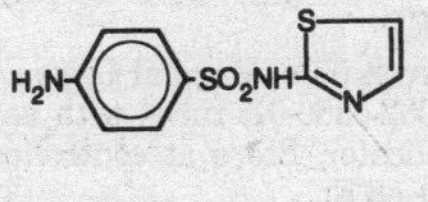

Sulfathiazole

CLINICAL PHARMACOLOGY

The mode of action of SULTRIN is not completely known. SULTRIN Cream and SULTRIN Tablets are topical antibacterial preparations used intravaginally against *Haemophilus (Gardnerella) vaginalis* bacteria. Indirect effects, such as lowering the vaginal pH, may be equally important mechanisms.

INDICATIONS AND USAGE

SULTRIN Cream and SULTRIN Tablets are indicated for the treatment of vaginitis caused by *Haemophilus (Gardnerella) vaginalis* bacteria.

The diagnosis of a *Haemophilus (Gardnerella) vaginalis* vaginitis should be firmly established before initiation of treatment with SULTRIN.

CONTRAINDICATIONS

SULTRIN is contraindicated in the following circumstances: kidney disease; hypersensitivity to sulfonamides; in pregnancy at term and during the nursing period because sulfonamides cross the placenta, are excreted in breast milk and may cause Kernicterus.

WARNINGS

Deaths associated with the administration of sulfonamides have been reported from hypersensitivity reactions, agranulocytosis, aplastic anemia and other blood dyscrasias.

The presence of clinical signs such as sore throat, fever, pallor, purpura or jaundice may be early indications of serious blood disorders.

PRECAUTIONS

Because sulfonamides may be absorbed from the vaginal mucosa, the usual precautions for oral sulfonamides apply. Patients should be observed for skin rash or evidence of systemic toxicity, and if these develop, the medications should be discontinued.

Laboratory tests: Standard office diagnostic procedures for vaginitis are usually sufficient to establish the diagnosis of *Haemophilus (Gardnerella) vaginalis* and to rule out a trichomonal or monilial infection. These include noting a fish-like odor upon addition of 10% KOH to vaginal discharge and microscopic identification of "clue cells" in a wet mount preparation. If cultures are obtained, care must be taken to use appropriate media and methods for *Haemophilus (Gardnerella) vaginalis.*

Carcinogenesis, mutagenesis, impairment of fertility: The sulfonamides bear certain chemical similarities to some goitrogens. Rats appear to be especially susceptible to the goitrogenic effects of sulfonamides, and long-term administration has produced thyroid malignancies in this species.

Pregnancy:

Teratogenic Effects: Pregnancy Category C: The safe use of sulfonamides in pregnancy has not been established. The teratogenicity potential of most sulfonamides has not been thoroughly investigated in either animals or humans. However, a significant increase in the incidence of cleft palate and other bony abnormalities of offspring has been observed when certain sulfonamides of the short, intermediate and long-acting types were given to pregnant rats and mice at high oral doses (7 to 25 times the human therapeutic dose).

Nursing Mothers: Because of the potential for serious adverse reactions in nursing infants from SULTRIN, a decision should be made whether to discontinue nursing or to discontinue the drug, taking into account the importance of the drug to the mother. See CONTRAINDICATIONS.

Pediatric use: Safety and effectiveness in children have not been established.

ADVERSE REACTIONS

There has been one reported case of Agranulocytosis in a patient receiving SULTRIN Cream. The most frequent adverse reactions to SULTRIN are localized irritation and/or allergy including rare reports of Stevens Johnson syndrome which may be fatal.

DOSAGE AND ADMINISTRATION

SULTRIN Cream. One full applicator intravaginally twice daily for four to six days. This course of therapy may be repeated if necessary; the dosage may be reduced one-half to one-quarter.

SULTRIN Vaginal Tablets. One tablet intravaginally before retiring and again in the morning for ten days. This course may be repeated, if necessary.

HOW SUPPLIED

Cream—78 g tubes with the ORTHO* Measured-Dose Applicator.

Vaginal Tablets (as white, capsule-shaped tablets with the Ortho Shield and the word "Ortho" debossed on one side)—Package of twenty foil-wrapped tablets with vaginal applicator.

NDC 0062-5440-77; SULTRIN Cream
NDC 0062-5441-64; SULTRIN Tablets
REVISED June 1992 643-10-380-6

TERAZOL® 3 ℞
VAGINAL CREAM 0.8%
(terconazole)

DESCRIPTION

TERAZOL® 3 (terconazole) Vaginal Cream 0.8% is a white to off-white, water washable cream for intravaginal administration containing 0.8% of the antifungal agent terconazole, *cis* -1-[*p*-[[2-(2,4-Dichlorophenyl)-2-(1H-1,2.4-triazol-1-ylmethyl)-1,3-dioxolan-4-yl] methoxy] phenyl]-4-isopropylpiperazine, compounded in a cream base consisting of butylated hydroxyanisole, cetyl alcohol, isopropyl myristate, polysorbate 60, polysorbate 80, propylene glycol, stearyl alcohol, and purified water.

The structural formula of terconazole is as follows:
[See chemical structure at top of next column.]

Terconazole, a triazole derivative, is a white to almost white powder with a molecular weight of 532.47. It is insoluble in water; sparingly soluble in ethanol; and soluble in butanol.

Continued on next page

Ortho—Cont.

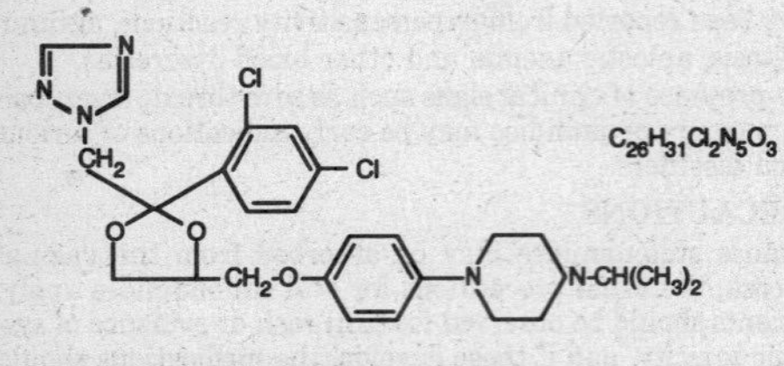

$C_{26}H_{31}Cl_2N_5O_3$

CLINICAL PHARMACOLOGY

Following daily intravaginal administration of 0.8% terconazole 40 mg (0.8% cream × 5 g) for seven days to normal humans, plasma concentrations were low and gradually rose to a daily peak (mean of 5.9 ng/mL or 0.006 mcg/mL) at 6.6 hours. Results from similar studies in patients with vulvovaginal candidiasis indicate that the slow rate of absorption, the lack of accumulation, and the mean peak plasma concentration of terconazole was not different from that observed in healthy women. The absorption characteristics of terconazole 0.8% in pregnant or non-pregnant patients with vulvovaginal candidiasis were also similar to those found in normal volunteers.

Following oral (30 mg) administration of ^{14}C-labelled terconazole, the harmonic half-life of elimination from the blood for the parent terconazole was 6.9 hours (range 4.0–11.3). Terconazole is extensively metabolized; the plasma AUC for terconazole compared to the AUC for total radioactivity was 0.6%. Total radioactivity was eliminated from the blood with a harmonic half-life of 52.2 hours (range 44–60). Excretion of radioactivity was both by renal (32–56%) and fecal (47–52%) routes.

In vitro, terconazole is highly protein bound (94.9%) and the degree of binding is independent of the drug concentration.

Photosensitivity reactions were observed in some normal volunteers following repeated dermal application of terconazole 2.0% and 0.8% creams under conditions of filtered artificial ultraviolet light. Photosensitivity reactions have not been observed in U.S. and foreign clinical trials in patients who were treated with terconazole 0.8% vaginal cream.

Microbiology: Terconazole exhibits fungicidal activity *in vitro* against *Candida albicans*. Antifungal activity also has been demonstrated against other fungi. The MIC values for terconazole against most species of lactic acid bacteria typically found in the human vagina were ≥128 mcg/mL. The exact pharmacologic mode of action of terconazole is uncertain; however, it may exert its antifungal activity by the disruption of normal fungal cell membrane permeability. No resistance to terconazole has developed during successive passages of *C. albicans*.

INDICATIONS AND USAGE

TERAZOL 3 Vaginal Cream is indicated for the local treatment of vulvovaginal candidiasis (moniliasis). As TERAZOL 3 Vaginal Cream is effective only for vulvovaginitis caused by the genus *Candida*, the diagnosis should be confirmed by KOH smears and/or cultures.

CONTRAINDICATIONS

Patients known to be hypersensitive to terconazole or to any of the components of the cream.

WARNINGS

None.

PRECAUTIONS

General: Discontinue use and do not retreat with terconazole if sensitization, irritation, fever, chills or flu-like symptoms are reported during use.

Laboratory Tests: If there is lack of response to TERAZOL 3 Vaginal Cream, appropriate microbiologic studies (standard KOH smear and/or cultures) should be repeated to confirm the diagnosis and rule out other pathogens.

Drug Interactions: The levels of estradiol (E2) and progesterone did not differ significantly when 0.8% terconazole vaginal cream was administered to healthy female volunteers established on a low dose oral contraceptive.

Carcinogenesis, Mutagenesis, Impairment of Fertility:

Carcinogenesis: Studies to determine the carcinogenic potential of terconazole have not been performed.

Mutagenicity: Terconazole was not mutagenic when tested *in vitro* for induction of microbial point mutations (Ames test) or for inducing cellular transformation, or *in vivo* for chromosome breaks (micronucleus test) or dominant lethal mutations in mouse germ cells.

Impairment of Fertility: No impairment of fertility occurred when female rats were administered terconazole orally up to 40 mg/kg/day for a three month period.

PREGNANCY: Teratogenic Effects.

Pregnancy Category C.

There was no evidence of teratogenicity when terconazole was administered orally up to 40 mg/kg/day or subcutaneously up to 20 mg/kg/day in rats. Dosages at or below 10 mg/kg/day produced no embryotoxicity; however, there was a delay in fetal ossification at 10 mg/kg/day in rats. There was some evidence of embryotoxicity in rabbits and rats at 20–40 mg/kg. In rats, this was reflected as a decrease in litter size and number of viable young and reduced fetal weight. There was also delay in ossification and an increased incidence of skeletal variants. The no-effect oral dose of 10/mg/kg/day resulted in a mean peak plasma level of terconazole in pregnant rats of 0.176 mcg/mL which exceeds by 30 times the mean peak plasma level (0.006 mcg/mL) seen in normal subjects after intravaginal administration of terconazole 0.8% vaginal cream. This safety assessment does not account for possible exposure of the fetus through direct transfer of terconazole from the irritated vagina by diffusion across amniotic membranes. Since terconazole is absorbed from the human vagina, it should not be used in the first trimester of pregnancy unless the physician considers it essential to the welfare of the patient.

Nursing Mothers: It is not known whether this drug is excreted in human milk. Animal studies have shown that rat offspring exposed via the milk of treated (40 mg/kg/orally) dams showed decreased survival during the first few post-partum days, but overall pup weight and weight gain were comparable to or greater than controls throughout lactation. Because many drugs are excreted in human milk, and because of the potential for adverse reaction in nursing infants from terconazole, a decision should be made whether to discontinue nursing or to discontinue the drug, taking into account the importance of the drug to the mother.

Pediatric Use: Safety and efficacy in children have not been established.

ADVERSE REACTIONS

During controlled clinical studies conducted in the United States, patients with vulvovaginal candidiasis were treated with terconazole 0.8% vaginal cream for three days. Based on comparative analyses with placebo and a standard agent, the adverse experiences considered most likely related to terconazole 0.8% vaginal cream were headache (21% vs. 16% with placebo) and dysmenorrhea (6% vs. 2% with placebo). Genital complaints in general, and burning and itching in particular, occurred less frequently in the terconazole 0.8% vaginal cream 3 day regimen (5% vs. 6%–9% with placebo). Other adverse experiences reported with terconazole 0.8% vaginal cream were abdominal pain (3.4% vs. 1% with placebo) and fever (1% vs. 0.3% with placebo). The therapy related dropout rate was 2.0% for the terconazole 0.8% vaginal cream. The adverse drug experience most frequently causing discontinuation of therapy was vulvovaginal itching, 0.7% with the terconazole 0.8% vaginal cream group and 0.3% with the placebo group.

OVERDOSAGE

Overdose of terconazole in humans has not been reported to date. In the rat, the oral LD 50 values were found to be 1741 and 849 mg/kg for the male and female, respectively. The oral LD 50 values for the male and female dog were ≃1280 and ≥640 mg/kg, respectively.

DOSAGE AND ADMINISTRATION

One full applicator (5 g) of TERAZOL 3 Vaginal Cream (40 mg terconazole) should be administered intravaginally once daily at bedtime for three consecutive days. Before prescribing another course of therapy, the diagnosis should be reconfirmed by smears and/or cultures and other pathogens commonly associated with vulvovaginitis ruled out. The therapeutic effect of TERAZOL 3 Vaginal Cream is not affected by menstruation.

HOW SUPPLIED

TERAZOL 3 (terconazole) Vaginal Cream 0.8% is available in 20 g (NDC 0062-5356-01) tubes with an ORTHO® Measured-Dose Applicator. Store at controlled room temperature 15–30°C (59–86°F).

Caution: Federal (U.S.A.) law prohibits dispensing without prescription.

631-11-314-3 Revised March 1995

Shown in Product Identification Guide, page 327

TERAZOL® 3 ℞

Vaginal Suppositories 80 mg
(terconazole)

DESCRIPTION

TERAZOL 3 Vaginal Suppositories are white to off-white suppositories for intravaginal administration containing 80 mg of the antifungal agent terconazole, *cis*-1-[*p*-[[2-(2,4-Dichlorophenyl)-2-(1H-1,2,4-triazol-1-ylmethyl)-1,3-dioxolan-4-yl]methoxy]phenyl]-4-isopropylpiperazine, in triglycerides derived from coconut and/or palm kernel oil (a base of hydrogenated vegetable oils) and butylated hydroxyanisole.

[See chemical structure at top of next column.]

TERCONAZOLE

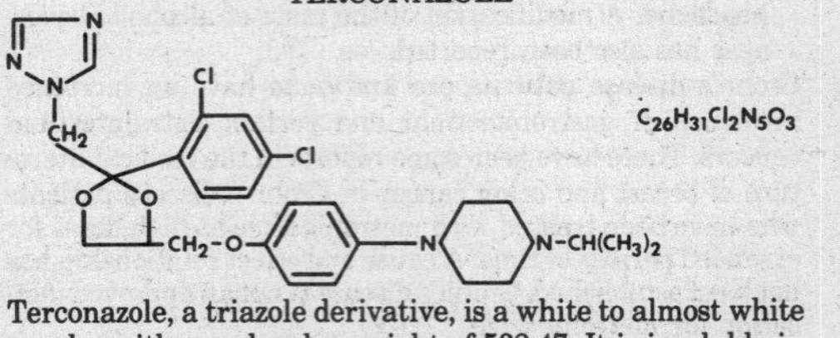

$C_{26}H_{31}Cl_2N_5O_3$

Terconazole, a triazole derivative, is a white to almost white powder with a molecular weight of 532.47. It is insoluble in water; sparingly soluble in ethanol; and soluble in butanol.

CLINICAL PHARMACOLOGY

Microbiology: Terconazole exhibits fungicidal activity *in vitro* against *Candida albicans*. The MIC values for terconazole against most species of lactic acid bacteria typically found in the human vagina were ≥128 mcg/mL, therefore, these beneficial bacteria are not affected by drug treatment. The exact pharmacologic mode of action of terconazole is uncertain; however, it may exert its antifungal activity by the disruption of normal fungal cell membrane permeability. No resistance to terconazole has developed during successive passages of *C. albicans*.

Human Pharmacology: Following intravaginal administration of terconazole in humans, absorption ranged from 5–8% in three hysterectomized subjects and 12–16% in two non-hysterectomized subjects with tubal ligations. Following oral (30 mg) administration of ^{14}C-labelled terconazole, the half-life of elimination from the blood for the parent terconazole was 6.9 hours (range 4.0–11.3). Terconazole is extensively metabolized; the plasma AUC for terconazole compared to the AUC for total radioactivity was 0.6%. Total radioactivity was eliminated from the blood with a half-life of 52.2 hours (range 44–60). Excretion of radioactivity was both by renal (32–56%) and fecal (47–52%) routes.

Photosensitivity reactions were observed in some normal volunteers following repeated dermal application of terconazole 2.0% and 0.8% creams under conditions of filtered artificial ultraviolet light.

Photosensitivity reactions have not been observed in U.S. and foreign clinical trials in patients who were treated vaginally with terconazole suppositories or cream.

INDICATIONS AND USAGE

TERAZOL 3 Vaginal Suppositories are indicated for the local treatment of vulvovaginal candidiasis (moniliasis). As TERAZOL 3 Vaginal Suppositories are effective only for vulvovaginitis caused by the genus *Candida*, the diagnosis should be confirmed by KOH smears and/or cultures.

CONTRAINDICATIONS

Patients known to be hypersensitive to terconazole or to any components of the suppository.

WARNINGS

None.

PRECAUTIONS

General: Discontinue use and do not retreat with terconazole if sensitization, irritation, fever, chills or flu-like symptoms are reported during use. The base contained in the suppository formulation may interact with certain rubber or latex products, such as those used in vaginal contraceptive diaphragms, therefore concurrent use is not recommended.

If there is lack of response to TERAZOL 3 Vaginal Suppositories, appropriate microbiological studies (standard KOH smear and/or cultures) should be repeated to confirm the diagnosis and rule out other pathogens.

Drug Interactions: The therapeutic effect of TERAZOL 3 Vaginal Suppositories is not affected by oral contraceptive usage.

Carcinogenesis, Mutagenesis, Impairment of Fertility

Carcinogenesis: Studies to determine the carcinogenic potential of terconazole have not been performed.

Mutagenicity: Terconazole was not mutagenic when tested *in vitro* for induction of microbial point mutations (Ames test), or for inducing cellular transformation, or *in vivo* for chromosome breaks (micronucleus test) or dominant lethal mutations in mouse germ cells.

Impairment of Fertility: No impairment of fertility occurred when female rats were administered terconazole orally up to 40 mg/kg/day.

Pregnancy: Pregnancy Category C

There was no evidence of teratogenicity when terconazole was administered orally up to 40 mg/kg/day (25 × the recommended intravaginal human dose) in rats, or 20 mg/kg/day in rabbits, or subcutaneously in rats up to 20 mg/kg/day. Dosages at or below 10 mg/kg/day produced no embryotoxicity; however, there was a delay in fetal ossification at 10 mg/kg/day in rats. There was some evidence of embryotoxicity in rabbits and rats at 20–40 mg/kg. In rats this was reflected as a decrease in litter size and number of viable young and reduced fetal weight. There was also delay in ossification and an increased incidence of skeletal variants.

The no-effect oral dose of 10 mg/kg/day resulted in a mean peak plasma level of terconazole in pregnant rats of 0.176

mcg/mL which exceeds by 44 times the mean peak plasma level (0.004 mcg/mL) seen in normal subjects after intravaginal administration of terconazole. This assessment does not account for possible exposure of the fetus through direct transfer of terconazole from the irritated vagina to the fetus by diffusion across amniotic membranes.
Since terconazole is absorbed from the human vagina, it should not be used in the first trimester of pregnancy unless the physician considers it essential to the welfare of the patient.

Nursing Mothers: It is not known whether terconazole is excreted in human milk. Animal studies have shown that rat off-spring exposed via the milk of treated (40 mg/kg/orally) dams showed decreased survival during the first few postpartum days. Because many drugs are excreted in human milk, and because of the potential for adverse reaction in nursing infants from terconazole, a decision should be made whether to discontinue nursing or to discontinue the drug, taking into account the importance of the drug to the mother.

Pediatric Use: Safety and efficacy in children have not been established.

ADVERSE REACTIONS

During controlled clinical studies conducted in the United States, 284 patients with vulvovaginal candidiasis were treated with terconazole 80 mg vaginal suppositories. Based on comparative analyses with placebo (295 patients) the adverse experiences considered adverse reactions most likely related to terconazole 80 mg vaginal suppositories were headache (30.3% vs 20.7% with placebo) and pain of the female genitalia (4.2% vs 0.7% with placebo). Adverse reactions that were reported but were not statistically significantly different from placebo were burning (15.2% vs 11.2% with placebo) and body pain (3.9% vs 1.7% with placebo). Fever (2.8% vs 1.4% with placebo) and chills (1.8% vs 0.7% with placebo) have also been reported. The therapy-related dropout rate was 3.5% and the placebo therapy-related dropout rate was 2.7%. The adverse drug experience on terconazole most frequently causing discontinuation was burning (2.5% vs 1.4% with placebo) and pruritus (1.8% vs 1.4% with placebo).

DOSAGE AND ADMINISTRATION

One TERAZOL 3 Vaginal Suppository (80 mg terconazole) is administered intravaginally once daily at bedtime for three consecutive days. Before prescribing another course of therapy, the diagnosis should be reconfirmed by smears and/or cultures and other pathogens commonly associated with vulvovaginitis ruled out. The therapeutic effect of TERAZOL 3 Vaginal Suppositories is not affected by menstruation.

HOW SUPPLIED

TERAZOL 3 (terconazole) Vaginal Suppositories 80 mg are available as 2.5 g, elliptically shaped white to off-white suppositories in packages of three (NDC 0062-5351-01) with a vaginal applicator. Store at Controlled Room Temperature 15°-30°C (59°-86°F)
Caution: Federal (USA) law prohibits dispensing without a prescription.
631-11-303-7 REVISED March 1995
Shown in Product Identification Guide, page 327

TERAZOL® 7 ℞
Vaginal Cream 0.4%
(terconazole)

DESCRIPTION

TERAZOL 7 Vaginal Cream is a white to off-white, water washable cream for intravaginal administration containing 0.4% of the antifungal agent terconazole, *cis*-1-[*p*-[[2-(2,4-Dichlorophenyl)-2-(1H-1, 2, 4-triazol-1-ylmethyl)-1,3-dioxolan-4-yl]methoxy]phenyl]-4-isopropylpiperazine, compounded in a cream base consisting of butylated hydroxyanisole, cetyl alcohol, isopropyl myristate, polysorbate 60, polysorbate 80, propylene glycol, stearyl alcohol, and purified water.

TERCONAZOLE

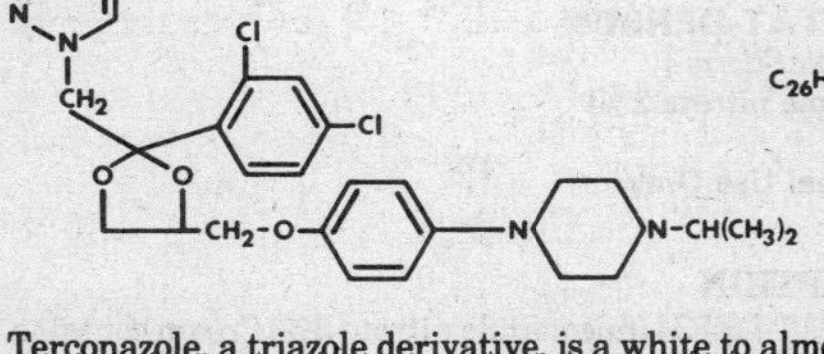

$C_{26}H_{31}Cl_2N_5O_3$

Terconazole, a triazole derivative, is a white to almost white powder with a molecular weight of 532.47. It is insoluble in water; sparingly soluble in ethanol; and soluble in butanol.

CLINICAL PHARMACOLOGY

Microbiology: Terconazole exhibits fungicidal activity *in vitro* against *Candida albicans.* Antifungal activity also has been demonstrated against other fungi. The MIC values for terconazole against most species of lactic acid bacteria typically found in the human vagina were ≥ 128 mcg/mL, therefore these beneficial bacteria are not affected by drug treatment.
The exact pharmacologic mode of action of terconazole is uncertain; however, it may exert its antifungal activity by the disruption of normal fungal cell membrane permeability. No resistance to terconazole has developed during successive passages of *C. albicans.*

Human Pharmacology: Following intravaginal administration of terconazole in humans, absorption ranged from 5–8% in three hysterectomized subjects and 12–16% in two nonhysterectomized subjects with tubal ligations.
Following oral (30 mg) administration of ^{14}C-labelled terconazole, the half-life of elimination from the blood for the parent terconazole was 6.9 hours (range 4.0–11.3). Terconazole is extensively metabolized; the plasma AUC for terconazole compared to the AUC for total radioactivity was 0.6%. Total radioactivity was eliminated from the blood with a half-life of 52.2 hours (range 44–60). Excretion of radioactivity was both by renal (32–56%) and fecal (47–52%) routes.
Photosensitivity reactions were observed in some normal volunteers following repeated dermal application of terconazole 2.0% and 0.8% creams under conditions of filtered artificial ultraviolet light. Photosensitivity reactions have not been observed in U.S. and foreign clinical trials in patients who were treated with terconazole 0.4% vaginal cream.

INDICATIONS AND USAGE

TERAZOL 7 Vaginal Cream is indicated for the local treatment of vulvovaginal candidiasis (moniliasis). As TERAZOL 7 Vaginal Cream is effective only for vulvovaginitis caused by the genus *Candida,* the diagnosis should be confirmed by KOH smears and/or cultures.

CONTRAINDICATIONS

Patients known to be hypersensitive to terconazole or to any of the components of the cream.

WARNINGS

None.

PRECAUTIONS

General: Discontinue use and do not retreat with terconazole if sensitization, irritation, fever, chills or flu-like symptoms are reported during use. If there is lack of response toTERAZOL 7 Vaginal Cream, appropriate microbiological studies (standard KOH smear and/or cultures) should be repeated to confirm the diagnosis and rule out other pathogens.

Drug Interactions: The therapeutic effect of TERAZOL 7 Vaginal Cream is not affected by oral contraceptive usage.

Carcinogenesis, Mutagenesis, Impairment of Fertility:

Carcinogenesis: Studies to determine the carcinogenic potential of terconazole have not been performed.

Mutagenicity: Terconazole was not mutagenic when tested *in vitro* for induction of microbial point mutations (Ames test) or for inducing cellular transformation, or *in vivo* for chromosome breaks (micronucleus test) or dominant lethal mutations in mouse germ cells.

Impairment of Fertility: No impairment of fertility occurred when female rats were administered terconazole orally up to 40 mg/kg/day.

Pregnancy: Pregnancy Category C.
There was no evidence of teratogenicity when terconazole was administered orally up to 40 mg/kg/day (100 × the recommended intravaginal human dose) in rats, or 20 mg/kg/day in rabbits, or subcutaneously in rats up to 20 mg/kg/day.
Dosages at or below 10 mg/kg/day produced no embryotoxicity; however, there was a delay in fetal ossification at 10 mg/kg/day in rats. There was some evidence of embryotoxicity in rabbits and rats at 20–40 mg/kg. In rats this was reflected as a decrease in litter size and number of viable young and reduced fetal weight. There was also delay in ossification and an increased incidence of skeletal variants.
The no-effect oral dose of 10 mg/kg/day resulted in a mean peak plasma level of terconazole in pregnant rats of 0.176 mcg/mL which exceeds by 44 times the mean peak plasma levels (0.004 mcg/mL) seen in normal subjects after intravaginal administration of terconazole. This safety assessment does not account for possible exposure of the fetus through direct transfer of terconazole from the irritated vagina to the fetus by diffusion across amniotic membranes.
Since terconazole is absorbed from the human vagina, it should not be used in the first trimester of pregnancy unless the physician considers it essential to the welfare of the patient.

Nursing Mothers: It is not known whether this drug is excreted in human milk. Animal studies have shown that rat off-spring exposed via the milk of treated (40 mg/kg/orally) dams showed decreased survival during the first few postpartum days, but overall pup weight and weight gain were comparable to or greater than controls throughout lactation. Because many drugs are excreted in human milk, and because of the potential for adverse reaction in nursing infants from terconazole, a decision should be made whether to discontinue nursing or to discontinue the drug, taking into account the importance of the drug to the mother.

Pediatric Use: Safety and efficacy in children have not been established.

ADVERSE REACTIONS

During controlled clinical studies conducted in the United States, 521 patients with vulvovaginal candidiasis were treated with terconazole 0.4% vaginal cream. Based on comparative analyses with placebo, the adverse experiences considered most likely related to terconazole 0.4% vaginal cream were headaches (26% *vs* 17% with placebo) and body pain (2.1% *vs* 0% with placebo). Vulvovaginal burning (5.2%), itching (2.3%) or irritation (3.1%) occurred less frequently with terconazole 0.4% vaginal cream than with the vehicle placebo. Fever (1.7% *vs* 0.5% with placebo) and chills (0.4% *vs* 0.0% with placebo) have also been reported. The therapy-related dropout rate was 1.9%. The adverse drug experience on terconazole most frequently causing discontinuation was vulvovaginal itching (0.6%), which was lower than the incidence for placebo (0.9%).

OVERDOSAGE

Overdose of terconazole in humans has not been reported to date. In the rat, the oral LD 50 values were found to be 1741 and 849 mg/kg for the male and female, respectively. The oral LD 50 values for the male and female dog were ≃1280 and ≥ 640 mg/kg, respectively.

DOSAGE AND ADMINISTRATION

One full applicator (5 g) of TERAZOL 7 Vaginal Cream (20 mg terconazole) is administered intravaginally once daily at bedtime for seven consecutive days. Before prescribing another course of therapy, the diagnosis should be reconfirmed by smears and/or cultures and other pathogens commonly associated with vulvovaginitis ruled out. The therapeutic effect of TERAZOL 7 Vaginal Cream is not affected by menstruation.

HOW SUPPLIED

TERAZOL® 7 (terconazole) Vaginal Cream 0.4% is available in 45 g (NDC 0062-5350-01) tubes with an ORTHO® Measured-Dose Applicator. Store at controlled room temperature 15°–30°C (59°–86°F).
Caution: Federal (USA) law prohibits dispensing without a prescription.
631-11-301-5 Revised March 1995
Shown in Product Identification Guide, page 327

Ortho Pharmaceutical Corporation
DERMATOLOGICAL DIVISION
1000 U.S. HWY. ROUTE 202
P.O. BOX 300
RARITAN, NJ 08869-0602

For Medical Information Contact:
Dermatological Medical Information
(800) 426-7762

ERYCETTE® ℞
[*ə'ris-ət*]
(erythromycin 2%)
TOPICAL SOLUTION

DESCRIPTION

Erythromycin is an antibiotic produced from a strain of *Streptomyces erythraeus.* It is basic and readily forms salts with acids. Each ml of ERYCETTE (erythromycin 2%) Topical Solution contains 20 mg of erythromycin base in a vehicle consisting of alcohol (66%) and propylene glycol. It may contain citric acid to adjust pH. Each pledget is filled to contain 0.8 ml. ERYCETTE is not USP with regard to minimum volume.

ACTIONS

Although the mechanism by which ERYCETTE Solution acts in reducing inflammatory lesions of acne vulgaris is unknown, it is presumably due to its antibiotic action.

INDICATIONS

ERYCETTE Solution is indicated for the topical control of acne vulgaris.

CONTRAINDICATIONS

ERYCETTE Solution is contraindicated in persons who have shown hypersensitivity to any of its ingredients.

Continued on next page

Ortho—Cont.

PRECAUTIONS

General: The use of antibiotic agents may be associated with the overgrowth of antibiotic-resistant organisms. If this occurs, administration of this drug should be discontinued and appropriate measures taken.

Information for Patients: ERYCETTE Solution is for external use only and should be kept away from the eyes, nose, mouth, and other mucous membranes. Concomitant topical acne therapy should be used with caution because a cumulative irritant effect may occur, especially with the use of peeling, desquamating, or abrasive agents. Each pledget should be used once and discarded.

Carcinogenesis, Mutagenesis, Impairment of Fertility: Long-term animal studies to evaluate carcinogenic potential, mutagenicity, or the effect on fertility of erythromycin have not been performed.

Pregnancy: Pregnancy Category C. Animal reproduction studies have not been conducted with erythromycin. It is also not known whether erythromycin can cause fetal harm when administered to a pregnant woman or can affect reproduction capacity. Erythromycin should be given to a pregnant woman only if clearly needed.

Nursing Mothers: It is not known whether erythromycin is excreted in human milk after topical application. However, this is reported to occur with oral and parenteral administration. Therefore, caution should be exercised when erythromycin is administered to a nursing woman.

ADVERSE REACTIONS

Adverse conditions reported include dryness, tenderness, pruritis, desquamation, erythema, oiliness, and burning sensation. Irritation of the eyes has also been reported. A case of generalized urticarial reaction, possibly related to the drug, which required the use of systemic steroid therapy has been reported.

DOSAGE AND ADMINISTRATION

The ERYCETTE pledget should be rubbed over the affected area twice a day after the skin is thoroughly washed with warm water and soap and patted dry. Acne lesions on the face, neck, shoulders, chest and back may be treated in this manner. Additional pledgets may be used, if needed. Each pledget should be used once and discarded.

HOW SUPPLIED

ERYCETTE (erythromycin 2%) Topical Solution is supplied as foil-covered saturated pledgets (swabs) in boxes of 60 (NDC 0062-1185-01).

Store at controlled room temperature 15–30°C (59°–86°F).

Shown in Product Identification Guide, page 326

GRIFULVIN V ® ℞

[gri'fulvən]
(griseofulvin tablets) microsize
Tablets 250 mg or 500 mg
(griseofulvin oral suspension) microsize
Suspension 125 mg/5 mL

DESCRIPTION

Griseofulvin is an antibiotic derived from a species of *Penicillium*. Each GRIFULVIN V Tablet contains either 250 mg or 500 mg of griseofulvin microsize, and also contains calcium stearate, colloidal silicon dioxide, starch, and wheat gluten. Additionally, the 250 mg tablet also contains dibasic calcium phosphate. Each 5 mL of GRIFULVIN V Suspension contains 125 mg of griseofulvin microsize and also contains alcohol 0.2%, docusate sodium, FD&C Red No. 40, FD&C Yellow No. 6, flavors, magnesium aluminium silicate, menthol, methylparaben, propylene glycol, propylparaben, saccharin sodium, simethicone emulsion, sodium alginate, sucrose, and purified water.

CLINICAL PHARMACOLOGY

GRIFULVIN V (griseofulvin microsize) acts systemically to inhibit the growth of *Trichophyton, Microsporum* and *Epidermophyton* genera of fungi. Fungistatic amounts are deposited in the keratin, which is gradually exfoliated and replaced by noninfected tissue.

Griseofulvin absorption from the gastrointestinal tract varies considerably among individuals, mainly because of insolubility of the drug in aqueous media of the upper G.I. tract. The peak serum level found in fasting adults given 0.5 g occurs at about four hours and ranges between 0.5 and 2.0 mcg/mL.

It should be noted that some individuals are consistently "poor absorbers" and tend to attain lower blood levels at all times. This may explain unsatisfactory therapeutic results in some patients. Better blood levels can probably be attained in most patients if the tablets are administered after a meal with a high fat content.

INDICATIONS AND USAGE

Major indications for GRIFULVIN V are:
  Tinea capitis (ringworm of the scalp)
  Tinea corporis (ringworm of the body)
  Tinea pedis (athlete's foot)
  Tinea unguium (onychomycosis; ringworm of the nails):
  Tinea cruris (ringworm of the thigh)
  Tinea barbae (barber's itch)

GRIFULVIN V inhibits the growth of those genera of fungi that commonly cause ringworm infections of the hair, skin, and nails, such as:

Trichophyton rubrum
Trichophyton tonsurans
Trichophyton mentagrophytes
Trichophyton interdigitalis
Trichophyton verrucosum
Trichophyton sulphureum
Trichophyton schoenleini
Microsporum audouini
Microsporum canis
Microsporum gypseum
Epidermophyton floccosum
Trichophyton megnini
Trichophyton gallinae
Trichophyton crateriform

Note: Prior to therapy, the type of fungi responsible for the infection should be identified. The use of the drug is not justified in minor or trivial infections which will respond to topical antifungal agents alone.

It is *not* effective in:
  Bacterial infections
  Candidiasis (Moniliasis)
  Histoplasmosis
  Actinomycosis
  Sporotrichosis
  Chromoblastomycosis
  Coccidioidomycosis
  North American Blastomycosis
  Cryptococcosis (Torulosis)
  Tinea versicolor
  Nocardiosis

CONTRAINDICATIONS

This drug is contraindicated in patients with porphyria, hepatocellular failure, and in individuals with a history of hypersensitivity to griseofulvin.

Two cases of conjoined twins have been reported in patients taking griseofulvin during the first trimester of pregnancy. Griseofulvin should not be prescribed to pregnant patients.

WARNINGS

Prophylactic Usage: Safety and efficacy of prophylactic use of this drug have not been established.

Chronic feeding of griseofulvin, at levels ranging from 0.5-2.5% of the diet, resulted in the development of liver tumors in several strains of mice, particularly in males. Smaller particle sizes result in an enhanced effect. Lower oral dosage levels have not been tested. Subcutaneous administration of relatively small doses of griseofulvin once a week during the first three weeks of life has also been reported to induce hepatomata in mice. Although studies in other animal species have not yielded evidence of tumorigenicity, these studies were not of adequate design to form a basis for conclusions in this regard.

In subacute toxicity studies, orally administered griseofulvin produced hepatocellular necrosis in mice, but this has not been seen in other species. Disturbances in porphyrin metabolism have been reported in griseofulvin-treated laboratory animals. Griseofulvin has been reported to have a colchicine-like effect on mitosis and cocarcinogenicity with methylcholanthrene in cutaneous tumor induction in laboratory animals.

Reports of animal studies in the Soviet literature state that a griseofulvin preparation was found to be embryotoxic and teratogenic on oral administration to pregnant Wistar rats. Rat reproduction studies done thus far in the United States and Great Britain have been inconclusive in this regard, and additional animal reproduction studies are underway. Pups with abnormalities have been reported in the litters of a few bitches treated with griseofulvin.

Suppression of spermatogenesis has been reported to occur in rats but investigation in man failed to confirm this.

PRECAUTIONS

Patients on prolonged therapy with any potent medication should be under close observation. Periodic monitoring of organ system function, including renal, hepatic and hemopoietic, should be done.

Since griseofulvin is derived from species of penicillin, the possibility of cross sensitivity with penicillin exists; however, known penicillin-sensitive patients have been treated without difficulty.

Since a photosensitivity reaction is occasionally associated with griseofulvin therapy, patients should be warned to avoid exposure to intense natural or artificial sunlight.

Should a photosensitivity reaction occur, lupus erythematosus may be aggravated.

Drug Interactions: Patients on warfarin-type anticoagulant therapy may require dosage adjustment of the anticoagulant during and after griseofulvin therapy. Concomitant use of barbiturates usually depresses griseofulvin activity and may necessitate raising the dosage.

The concomitant administration of griseofulvin has been reported to reduce the efficacy of oral contraceptives and to increase the incidence of breakthrough bleeding.

ADVERSE REACTIONS

When adverse reactions occur, they are most commonly of the hypersensitivity type such as skin rashes, urticaria and rarely, angioneurotic edema, and may necessitate withdrawal of therapy and appropriate countermeasures. Paresthesias of the hands and feet have been reported rarely after extended therapy. Other side effects reported occasionally are oral thrush, nausea, vomiting, epigastric distress, diarrhea, headache, fatigue, dizziness, insomnia, mental confusion and impairment of performance of routine activities. Proteinuria and leukopenia have been reported rarely. Administration of the drug should be discontinued if granulocytopenia occurs.

When rare, serious reactions occur with griseofulvin, they are usually associated with high dosages, long periods of therapy, or both.

DOSAGE AND ADMINISTRATION

Accurate diagnosis of the infecting organism is essential. Identification should be made either by direct microscopic examination of a mounting of infected tissue in a solution of potassium hydroxide or by culture on an appropriate medium.

Medication must be continued until the infecting organism is completely eradicated as indicated by appropriate clinical or laboratory examination. Representative treatment periods are tinea capitis, 4 to 6 weeks; tinea corporis, 2 to 4 weeks; tinea pedis, 4 to 8 weeks; tinea unguium—depending on rate of growth—fingernails, at least 4 months; toenails, at least 6 months.

General measures in regard to hygiene should be observed to control sources of infection or reinfection. Concomitant use of appropriate topical agents is usually required, particularly in treatment of tinea pedis since in some forms of athlete's foot, yeasts and bacteria may be involved. Griseofulvin will not eradicate the bacterial or monilial infection.

Adults: A daily dose of 500 mg. will give a satisfactory response in most patients with tinea corporis, tinea cruris, and tinea capitis.

For those fungus infections more difficult to eradicate such as tinea pedis and tinea unguium, a daily dose of 1.0 g is recommended.

Children: Approximately 5 mg per pound of body weight per day is an effective dose for most children. On this basis the following dosage schedule for children is suggested:

  Children weighing 30 to 50 pounds—125 mg to 250 mg daily.

  Children weighing over 50 pounds—250 mg to 500 mg daily.

HOW SUPPLIED

GRIFULVIN V 250 mg Tablets in bottles of 100 (NDC 0062-0211-60) (white, scored, imprinted "ORTHO 211").

GRIFULVIN V 500 mg Tablets in bottles of 100 (NDC 0062-0214-60) and 500 (NDC 0062-0214-70) (white, scored, imprinted "ORTHO 214").

  Dispense GRIFULVIN V Tablets in a tight container as defined in the USP.

GRIFULVIN V Suspension 125 mg per 5 mL in bottles of 4 fl oz (120mL) (NDC 0062-0206-04).

  Dispense GRIFULVIN V Suspension in tight, light-resistant container as defined in the USP.

STORE AT ROOM TEMPERATURE
Revised November 1992
631-10-560-1

Shown in Product Identification Guide, page 326

MONISTAT-DERM® ℞

['män ə-stat-dərm]
(miconazole nitrate 2%)
Cream
For Topical Use Only

DESCRIPTION

MONISTAT-DERM (miconazole nitrate 2%) Cream contains miconazole nitrate* 2%, formulated into a water-miscible base consisting of pegoxol 7 stearate, peglicol 5 oleate, mineral oil, benzoic acid, and butylated hydroxyanisole and purified water.

*Chemical name: 1-[2,4-dichloro-β-{(2,4-dichlorobenzyl)oxy} phenethyl] imidazole mononitrate.

ACTIONS

Miconazole nitrate is a synthetic antifungal agent which inhibits the growth of the common dermatophytes, *Trichophyton rubrum, Trichophyton mentagrophytes,* and *Epidermophyton floccosum,* the yeast-like fungus, *Candida albicans,* and the organism responsible for tinea versicolor (*Malassezia furfur*).

INDICATIONS

For topical application in the treatment of tinea pedis (athlete's foot), tinea cruris, and tinea corporis caused by *Trichophyton rubrum, Trichophyton mentagrophytes,* and *Epidermophyton floccosum,* in the treatment of cutaneous candidiasis (moniliasis), and in the treatment of tinea versicolor.

CONTRAINDICATIONS

MONISTAT-DERM (miconazole nitrate 2%) Cream has no known contraindications.

PRECAUTIONS

If a reaction suggesting sensitivity or chemical irritation should occur, use of the medication should be discontinued. For external use only. Avoid introduction of MONISTAT-DERM Cream into the eyes.

ADVERSE REACTIONS

There have been isolated reports of irritation, burning, maceration, and allergic contact dermatitis associated with application of MONISTAT-DERM.

DOSAGE AND ADMINISTRATION

Sufficient MONISTAT-DERM Cream should be applied to cover affected areas twice daily (morning and evening) in patients with tinea pedis, tinea cruris, tinea corporis, and cutaneous candidiasis, and once daily in patients with tinea versicolor. If MONISTAT-DERM Cream is used in intertriginous areas, it should be applied sparingly and smoothed in well to avoid maceration effects.

Early relief of symptoms (2 to 3 days) is experienced by the majority of patients and clinical improvement may be seen fairly soon after treatment is begun; however, *Candida* infections and tinea cruris and corporis should be treated for two weeks and tinea pedis for one month in order to reduce the possibility of recurrence. If a patient shows no clinical improvement after a month of treatment, the diagnosis should be redetermined. Patients with tinea versicolor usually exhibit clinical and mycological clearing after two weeks of treatment.

HOW SUPPLIED

MONISTAT-DERM (miconazole nitrate 2%) Cream containing miconazole nitrate at 2% strength is supplied in 15 g. (NDC 0062-5434-02), 1 oz. (NDC 0062-5434-01) and 3 oz. (NDC 0062-5434-03) tubes.

Shown in Product Identification Guide, page 326

RENOVA®   ℞
(TRETINOIN EMOLLIENT CREAM)
0.05%
FOR TOPICAL USE ON THE FACE ONLY

Prescribing Information

DESCRIPTION

RENOVA (tretinoin emollient cream) 0.05% contains the active ingredient tretinoin (a retinoid) in an emollient cream base. Tretinoin is a yellow to light orange crystalline powder having a characteristic floral odor. Tretinoin is soluble in dimethylsulfoxide, slightly soluble in polyethylene glycol 400, octanol, and 100% ethanol. It is practically insoluble in water and mineral oil, and it is insoluble in glycerin. The chemical name for tretinoin is (all-E)-3,7-dimethyl-9-(2,6,6-trimethyl-1-cyclonexen-1-yl)-2,4,6,8- nonatetraenoic acid. Tretinoin is also referred to as all-*trans*-retinoic acid and has a molecular weight of 300.44. The structural formula is represented below.

TRETINOIN

Tretinoin is available as RENOVA at a concentration of 0.05% w/w in a water in oil emulsion formulation consisting of light mineral oil, NF; sorbitol solution, USP; hydroxyoctacosanyl hydroxystearate; methoxy PEG-22/dodecyl glycol copolymer; PEG-45/dodecyl glycol copolymer; stearoxytrimethylsilane and stearyl alcohol; dimethicone 50 cs; fragrance; methylparaben, NF; edetate disodium, USP; quaternium-15; butylated hydroxytoluene, NF; citric acid monohydrate, USP; and purified water, USP.

CLINICAL PHARMACOLOGY

The exact mechanism of action of tretinoin is unknown although retinoids are believed to exert an effect on the growth and differentiation of various epithelial cells. When applied topically, however, there was no noted increase in desmosine, hydroxyproline, or elastin mRNA in human skin. In addition, the role of the irritative nature of this product in effecting the positive effects attributed to this product for its indication has not yet been fully determined.

The transdermal absorption of tretinoin from various topical formulations ranged from 1% to 31% of applied dose, depending on whether it was applied to healthy skin or dermatitic skin. When percutaneous absorption of RENOVA was assessed in healthy male subjects (n=14) after a single application, as well as after repeated daily applications for 28 days, the absorption of tretinoin was less than 2% and endogenous concentrations of tretinoin and its major metabolites were unaltered.

INDICATIONS AND USAGE
(To understand fully the indication for this product, please read the entire INDICATIONS AND USAGE section of the labeling.)
RENOVA (tretinoin emollient cream) 0.05% is indicated as an adjunctive agent (see second bullet point below) for use in the mitigation (palliation) of <u>fine</u> wrinkles, mottled hyperpigmentation, and tactile roughness of facial skin in patients who do not achieve such palliation using comprehensive skin care and sun avoidance programs alone (see bullet point 3 for populations in which effectiveness has not been established). **RENOVA DOES NOT ELIMINATE WRINKLES, REPAIR SUN DAMAGED SKIN, REVERSE PHOTOAGING, or RESTORE A MORE YOUTHFUL or YOUNGER DERMAL HISTOLOGIC PATTERN.** Many patients achieve desired palliative effects on fine wrinkling, mottled hyperpigmentation, and tactile roughness of facial skin with the use of comprehensive skin care and sun avoidance programs including sunscreens, protective clothing, and emollient creams <u>NOT</u> containing tretinoin.
- RENOVA has demonstrated NO MITIGATING EFFECT on significant signs of chronic sun exposure such as <u>coarse</u> or <u>deep</u> wrinkling, skin yellowing, lentigines, telangiectasia, skin laxity, keratinocytic atypia, melanocytic atypia, or dermal elastosis.
- RENOVA should be used under medical supervision as an adjunct to a comprehensive skin care and sun avoidance program that includes the use of effective sunscreens (minimum SPF of 15) and protective clothing when desired results on fine wrinkles, mottled hyperpigmentation, and roughness of facial skin have not been achieved with a comprehensive skin care and sun avoidance program alone.
- The effectiveness of RENOVA in the mitigation of fine wrinkles, mottled hyperpigmentation, and tactile roughness of facial skin has not been established in people greater than 50 years of age OR in people with moderately to heavily pigmented skin. In addition, patients with visible actinic keratoses and patients with a history of skin cancer were excluded from clinical trials of RENOVA. Thus the effectiveness and safety of RENOVA in these populations are not known at this time. (See **WARNINGS** section.)
- Neither the safety nor the effectiveness of RENOVA for the prevention or treatment of actinic keratoses or skin neoplasms has been established.
- Neither the safety nor the efficacy of using RENOVA daily for greater than 48 weeks has been established, and daily use beyond 48 weeks has not been systematically and histologically investigated in adequate and well-controlled trials. (See **WARNINGS** section.)

CLINICAL TRIALS DATA:
Two adequate and well-controlled trials were conducted involving a total of 161 evaluable patients treated with RENOVA and 154 evaluable patients treated with the vehicle emollient cream on the face for 24 weeks as an adjunct to a comprehensive skin care and sun avoidance program, to assess the effects on fine wrinkling, mottled hyperpigmentation, and tactile skin roughness. Patients were evaluated at baseline on a 10 point scale and changes from that baseline rating were categorized as follows:

No Improvement: No change or an increase of 1 unit or more.
Minimal Improvement: Reduction of 1 unit.
Moderate Improvement: Reduction of 2 units or more.

In these trials, the fine wrinkles, mottled hyperpigmentation, and tactile roughness of the facial skin were thought to be caused by multiple factors which included intrinsic aging or environmental factors, such as chronic sun exposure. The results of these assessments are as follows:
[See table above.]
Most of the improvement in these signs was noted during the first 24 weeks of therapy. Thereafter, therapy primarily maintained the improvement realized during the first 24 weeks.

A majority of patients will lose most mitigating effects of RENOVA on fine wrinkles, mottled hyperpigmentation, and tactile roughness of facial skin with discontinuation of a comprehensive skin care and sun avoidance program including RENOVA; however, the safety and effectiveness of using RENOVA daily for greater than 48 weeks have <u>not</u> been established.

CONTRAINDICATIONS

This drug is contraindicated in individuals with a history of sensitivity reactions to any of its components. It should be discontinued if hypersensitivity to any of its ingredients is noted.

WARNINGS

- RENOVA is a dermal irritant, and the results of continued irritation of the skin for greater than 48 weeks are not known. There is evidence of atypical changes in melanocytes and keratinocytes, and of increased dermal elastosis in some patients treated with RENOVA for longer than 48 weeks. The significance of these findings is unknown.
- Safety and effectiveness of RENOVA in individuals with moderately or heavily pigmented skin have not been established.

- RENOVA should not be administered if the patient is also taking drugs known to be photosensitizers (e.g., thiazides, tetracyclines, fluoroquinolones, phenothiazines, sulfonamides) because of the possibility of augmented phototoxicity.
- Safety and effectiveness of RENOVA in individuals older than 50 years of age have not been established.

This product should <u>only</u> be used under medical supervision as part of a comprehensive skin care and sun avoidance program. (See **INDICATIONS AND USAGE** section.) It should only be applied before retiring at night. Because of heightened burning susceptibility, exposure to sunlight (including sunlamps) should be avoided or minimized during use of RENOVA. Patients must be warned to use sunscreens (minimum SPF of 15) and protective clothing when using RENOVA. Patients with sunburn should be advised not to

FINE WRINKLING

	NO IMPROVEMENT	MINIMAL IMPROVEMENT	MODERATE IMPROVEMENT
RENOVA + CSP*	36%	40%	24%
Vehicle + CSP	62%	30%	8%

MOTTLED HYPERPIGMENTATION

	NO IMPROVEMENT	MINIMAL IMPROVEMENT	MODERATE IMPROVEMENT
RENOVA + CSP	35%	27%	38%
Vehicle +CSP	53%	21%	27%

TACTILE SKIN ROUGHNESS

	NO IMPROVEMENT	MINIMAL IMPROVEMENT	MODERATE IMPROVEMENT
RENOVA + CSP	49%	35%	16%
Vehicle + CSP	67%	23%	10%

*CSP = Comprehensive skin protection and sun avoidance programs including use of sunscreens, protective clothing, and emollient cream.

Continued on next page

Ortho—Cont.

use RENOVA until fully recovered. Patients who may have considerable sun exposure due to their occupation and those patients with inherent sensitivity to sunlight should exercise particular caution when using RENOVA and assure that the precautions outlined in the Information for Patients subsection are observed.

RENOVA should be kept out of the eyes, mouth, angles of the nose, and mucous membranes. Topical use may cause severe local erythema, pruritus, burning, stinging, and peeling at the site of application. If the degree of local irritation warrants, patients should be directed to use less medication, decrease the frequency of application, discontinue use temporarily, or discontinue use altogether.

Tretinoin has been reported to cause severe irritation on eczematous skin and should be used only with utmost caution in patients with this condition.

Application of larger amounts of medication than recommended will not lead to more rapid or better results, and marked redness, peeling, or discomfort may occur.

PRECAUTIONS

General: RENOVA should only be used as an adjunct to a comprehensive skin care and sun avoidance program. (See **INDICATIONS AND USAGE** section.)

If a drug sensitivity, chemical irritation, or a sytemic adverse reaction develops, use of RENOVA should be discontinued. Weather extremes, such as wind or cold, may be more irritating to patients using RENOVA.

Information for Patients: A patient information leaflet has been prepared and is included with each package of RENOVA. In addition, patients should be instructed:

- That RENOVA is not a cosmetic preparation and should be applied only as an adjunct to a comprehensive skin care and sun avoidance program,
- Never to use more RENOVA than instructed and never use RENOVA more often than instructed as application of larger amounts of medication than recommended will not lead to more rapid or better results, and marked redness, peeling, or discomfort may occur,
- Only to apply RENOVA before retiring at night,
- To use a sunscreen with a minimum SPF of 15 during the day when being treated with RENOVA. Following discontinuation of RENOVA, continued avoidance of the sun and use of a sunscreen with a minimum SPF of 15 is recommended,
- To avoid direct sun exposure as much as possible whenever using RENOVA, and to avoid sunlamps totally while using RENOVA,
- NOT to use RENOVA if pregnant or attempting to become pregnant or at high risk of pregnancy,
- NOT to use RENOVA if sunburned or if the patient has eczema or other chronic skin condition(s),
- NOT to use RENOVA if inherently sensitive to sunlight,
- NOT to use RENOVA if also taking other drugs that increase sensitivity to sunlight,
- To use RENOVA with caution if also using other topical agents with a strong skin drying effect, products with high concentrations of alcohol, astringents, spices or lime, medicated soaps or shampoos, permanent wave solutions, electrolysis, hair depilatories or waxes, or other preparations or processes that might dry or irritate the skin, unless otherwise instructed by their health care practitioner,
- To discontinue use of RENOVA and consult their health care provider if sensitivity or increased chemical irritation occurs,
- That a majority of patients will lose most mitigating effects on fine wrinkles, mottled hyperpigmentation, and tactile roughness of facial skin with discontinuation of a comprehensive skin care and sun avoidance program including RENOVA; however, the safety and effectiveness of using RENOVA daily for greater than 48 weeks have not been established,
- That most of the improvement noted with RENOVA is seen during the first 24 weeks of therapy. Thereafter, therapy primarily maintained the improvement realized during the first 24 weeks.

Drug Interactions: Concomitant topical medications, medicated or abrasive soaps, shampoos, cleansers, cosmetics with a strong drying effect, products with high concentrations of alcohol, astringents, spices or lime, permanent wave solutions, electrolysis, hair depilatories or waxes, and products that may irritate the skin should be used with caution in patients being treated with RENOVA because they may increase irritation with RENOVA.

RENOVA should not be administered if the patient is also taking drugs known to be photosensitizers (e.g., thiazides, tetracyclines, fluoroquinolones, phenothiazines, sulfonamides) because of the possibility of augmented phototoxicity.

Carcinogenesis, Mutagenesis, Impairment of Fertility: In a life-time dermal study in CD-1 mice, at 100 and 200 times the average recommended human topical clinical dose, a few skin tumors in the female mice and liver tumors in male mice were observed. The biological significance of these find-

ings is not clear because they occurred at doses that exceeded the dermal maximally tolerated dose (MTD) of tretinoin and because they were within the background natural occurrence rate for these tumors in this strain of mice. There was no evidence of carcinogenic potential when tretinoin was administered topically at a dose 5 times the average recommended human topical clinical dose. For purposes of comparisons of the animal exposure to human exposure, the "recommended human topical clinical dose" is defined as 500 mg of 0.05% RENOVA applied daily to a 50 kg person.

In a chronic, two-year bioassay of Vitamin A acid in mice performed by Tsubura and Yamamoto, generalized amyloid deposition was reported in all groups in the basal layer of the Vitamin A treated skin. In CD-1 mice, a similar study reported hyalinization at the treated skin sites and the incidence of this finding was 0/50, 3/50, 3/50, and 2/50 in male mice and 1/50, 0/50, 4/50, and 2/50 in female mice from the vehicle control, 0.25 mg/kg, 0.5 mg/kg, and 1 mg/kg groups, respectively.

Studies in hairless albino mice suggest that tretinoin may enhance the tumorigenic potential of carcinogenic doses of UVB and UVA light from a solar simulator. In other studies, when lightly pigmented hairless mice treated with tretinoin were exposed to carcinogenic doses of UVB light, the incidence and rate of development of skin tumors were either reduced or no effect was seen. Due to significantly different experimental conditions, no strict comparison of these disparate data is possible at this time. Although the significance of these studies to humans is not clear, patients should minimize exposure to sun.

The mutagenic potential of tretinoin was evaluated in the Ames assay and in the *in vivo* mouse micronucleus assay, both of which were negative.

Dermal Segment I and III studies with RENOVA have not been performed in any species. In oral Segment I and Segment III studies in rats with tretinoin, decreased survival of neonates and growth retardation were observed at doses in excess of 2 mg/kg/day (>400 times the average recommended human topical clinical dose).

Pregnancy:

Teratogenic effects: Pregnancy Category C.

ORAL tretinoin has been shown to be teratogenic in rats, mice, rabbits, hamsters, and subhuman primates. It was teratogenic and fetotoxic in rats when given orally in doses 1000 times the average recommended human topical clinical dose. However, variations in teratogenic doses among various strains of rats have been reported. In the cynomolgus monkey, which, metabolically, is closer to humans for tretinoin than the other species examined, fetal malformations were reported at doses of 10 mg/kg/day or greater, but none were observed at 5 mg/kg/day (1000 times the average recommended human topical clinical dose), although increased skeletal variations were observed at all doses. A dose-related increased embryolethality and abortion was reported. Similar results have also been reported in pigtail macaques.

TOPICAL tretinoin in animal teratogenicity tests has generated equivocal results. There is evidence for teratogenicity (shortened or kinked tail) of topical tretinoin in Wistar rats at doses greater than 1 mg/kg/day (200 times the recommended human topical clinical dose). Anomalies (humerus: short 13%, bent 6%, os parietal incompletely ossified 14%) have also been reported when 10 mg/kg/day was dermally applied.

There are other reports in New Zealand White rabbits with doses of approximately 80 times the recommended human topical clinical dose of an increased incidence of domed head and hydrocephaly, typical of retinoid-induced fetal malformations in this species.

In contrast, several well-controlled animal studies have shown that dermally applied tretinoin was not teratogenic at doses of 100 and 200 times the recommended human topical clinical dose, in rats and rabbits, respectively.

With widespread use of any drug, a small number of birth defect reports associated temporally with the administration of the drug would be expected by chance alone. Thirty cases of temporally-associated congenital malformations have been reported during two decades of clinical use of another formulation of topical tretinoin (Retin-A). Although no definite pattern of teratogenicity and no causal association has been established from these cases, 5 of the reports describe the rare birth defect category holoprosencephaly (defects associated with incomplete midline development of the forebrain). The significance of these spontaneous reports in terms of risk to the fetus is not known.

Non-teratogenic effects:

Dermal tretinoin has been shown to be fetotoxic in rabbits when administered in doses 100 times the recommended topical human clinical dose. Oral tretinoin has been shown to be fetotoxic in rats when administered in doses 500 times the recommended topical human clinical dose.

There are, however, no adequate and well-controlled studies in pregnant women. RENOVA should not be used during pregnancy.

Nursing Mothers: It is not known whether this drug is excreted in human milk. Because many drugs are excreted in

human milk, caution should be exercised when RENOVA is administered to a nursing woman.

Pediatric Use: Safety and effectiveness in patients less than 18 years of age have not been established.

Geriatric Use: Safety and effectiveness in individuals older than 50 years of age have not been established.

ADVERSE REACTIONS

(See **BOXED WARNING, WARNINGS,** and **PRECAUTIONS** sections.)

In double-blind, vehicle-controlled studies involving 179 patients who applied RENOVA to their face, adverse reactions associated with the use of RENOVA were limited primarily to the skin. During these trials, 4% of patients had to discontinue use of RENOVA because of adverse reactions. These discontinuations were due to skin irritation or related cutaneous adverse reactions.

Local reactions such as peeling, dry skin, burning, stinging, erythema, and pruritus were reported by almost all subjects during therapy with RENOVA. These signs and symptoms were usually of mild to moderate severity and generally occurred early in therapy. In most patients the dryness, peeling, and redness recurred after an initial (24 week) decline.

OVERDOSAGE

Application of larger amounts of medication than recommended will not lead to more rapid or better results, and marked redness, peeling, or discomfort may occur. Oral ingestion of the drug may lead to the same side effects as those associated with excessive oral intake of Vitamin A.

DOSAGE AND ADMINISTRATION

- Do NOT use RENOVA if the patient is pregnant or is attempting to become pregnant or is at high risk of pregnancy,
- Do NOT use RENOVA if the patient is sunburned or if the patient has eczema or other chronic skin condition(s),
- Do NOT use RENOVA if the patient is inherently sensitive to sunlight,
- Do NOT use RENOVA if the patient is also taking drugs known to be photosensitizers (e.g., thiazides, tetracyclines, fluoroquinolones, phenothiazines, sulfonamides) because of the possibility of augmented phototoxicity.

RENOVA is not a cosmetic product. It should only be used with care under medical supervision as an adjunct to a comprehensive skin care and sun avoidance program that includes the use of sunscreens (minimum SPF of 15) and protective clothing when desired results on fine wrinkles, mottled hyperpigmentation, and tactile roughness of facial skin have not been achieved with a comprehensive skin care and sun avoidance program alone. Patients require detailed instruction to obtain maximal benefits and to understand all the precautions necessary to use this product with greatest safety. (See **INDICATIONS AND USAGE** section, **Information for Patients** subsection, and the **PATIENT PACKAGE INSERT**.)

RENOVA should be applied to the face once a day before retiring using only enough to cover the entire affected area lightly. Patients should gently wash their face with a mild soap, pat the skin dry, and wait 20 to 30 minutes before applying RENOVA. The patient should apply a pea-sized amount of cream to cover the entire face lightly. Special caution should be taken when applying the cream to avoid the eyes, ears, nostrils, and mouth.

Application of RENOVA may cause a transitory feeling of warmth or slight stinging.

Mitigation (palliation) of facial fine wrinkling, mottled hyperpigmentation and tactile roughness may occur gradually over the course of therapy. Up to six months of therapy may be required before the effects are seen. Most of the improvement noted with RENOVA is seen during the first 24 weeks of therapy. Thereafter, therapy primarily maintains the improvement realized during the first 24 weeks.

With discontinuation of RENOVA therapy, a majority of patients will lose most mitigating effects of RENOVA on fine wrinkles, mottled hyperpigmentation, and tactile roughness of facial skin; however, the safety and effectiveness of using RENOVA daily for greater than 48 weeks have not been established.

Application of larger amounts of medication than recommended will not lead to more rapid or better results, and marked redness, peeling, or discomfort may occur.

Patients treated with RENOVA may use cosmetics but the areas to be treated should be cleansed thoroughly before the medication is applied. (See **PRECAUTIONS** section.)

HOW SUPPLIED

RENOVA is available in tubes containing 40 grams (NDC 0062-0185-05) and 60 grams (NDC 0062-0185-03).

Storage: Store between 15° and 25°C (59° and 77°F). DO NOT FREEZE.

QUESTIONS: Physicians and Pharmacists can call 1-800-426-7762, from 8:30 a.m. to 4:30 p.m. Eastern Time, Monday through Friday.

Caution: Federal law prohibits dispensing without prescription.

DERMATOLOGICAL DIVISION
ORTHO PHARMACEUTICAL CORPORATION
Raritan, New Jersey 08869
 Revised January 1996
U.S. Patents 4,603,146, 4,423,041 and 4,877,805
651-10-870-2
Shown in Product Identification Guide, page 326

RETIN-A® ℞

['ret in-ā]
(tretinoin)
Liquid • Cream • Gel
For Topical Use Only

DESCRIPTION

RETIN-A Gel, Cream and Liquid, containing tretinoin are used for the topical treatment of acne vulgaris. RETIN-A Gel contains tretinoin (retinoic acid, vitamin A acid) in either of two strengths. 0.025% or 0.01% by weight, in a gel vehicle of butylated hydroxytoluene, hydroxypropyl cellulose and alcohol (denatured with *tert*-butyl alcohol and brucine sulfate) 90% w/w. RETIN-A (tretinoin) Cream contains tretinoin in either of three strengths, 0.1%, 0.05%, or 0.025% by weight, in a hydrophilic cream vehicle of stearic acid, isopropyl myristate, polyoxyl 40 stearate, stearyl alcohol, xanthan gum, sorbic acid, butylated hydroxytoluene, and purified water. RETIN-A Liquid contains tretinoin 0.05% by weight, polyethylene glycol 400, butylated hydroxytoluene and alcohol (denatured with *tert*-butyl alcohol and brucine sulfate) 55%. Chemically, tretinoin is *all-trans*-retinoic acid and has the following structure:

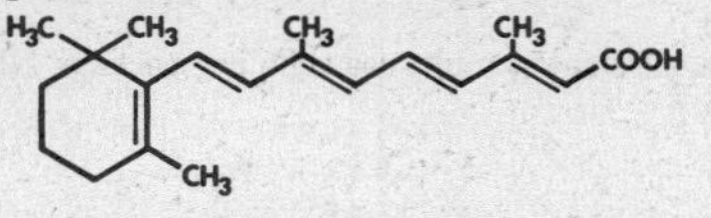

CLINICAL PHARMACOLOGY

Although the exact mode of action of tretinoin is unknown, current evidence suggests that topical tretinoin decreases cohesiveness of follicular epithelial cells with decreased microcomedo formation. Additionally, tretinoin stimulates mitotic activity and increased turnover of follicular epithelial cells causing extrusion of the comedones.

INDICATIONS AND USAGE

RETIN-A is indicated for topical application in the treatment of acne vulgaris. The safety and efficacy of the long-term use of this product in the treatment of other disorders have not been established.

CONTRAINDICATIONS

Use of the product should be discontinued if hypersensitivity to any of the ingredients is noted.

PRECAUTIONS

General: If a reaction suggesting sensitivity or chemical irritation occurs, use of the medication should be discontinued. Exposure to sunlight, including sunlamps, should be minimized during the use of RETIN-A, and patients with sunburn should be advised not to use the product until fully recovered because of heightened susceptibility to sunlight as a result of the use of tretinoin. Patients who may be required to have considerable sun exposure due to occupation and those with inherent sensitivity to the sun should exercise particular caution. Use of sunscreen products and protective clothing over treated areas is recommended when exposure cannot be avoided. Weather extremes, such as wind or cold, also may be irritating to patients under treatment with tretinoin.
RETIN-A (tretinoin) acne treatment should be kept away from the eyes, the mouth, angles of the nose, and mucous membranes. Topical use may induce severe local erythema and peeling at the site of application. If the degree of local irritation warrants, patients should be directed to use the medication less frequently, discontinue use temporarily, or discontinue use altogether. Tretinoin has been reported to cause severe irritation on eczematous skin and should be used with utmost caution in patients with this condition.
Drug Interactions: Concomitant topical medication, medicated or abrasive soaps and cleansers, soaps and cosmetics that have a strong drying effect, and products with high concentrations of alcohol, astringents, spices or lime should be used with caution because of possible interaction with tretinoin. Particular caution should be exercised in using preparations containing sulfur, resorcinol, or salicylic acid with RETIN-A. It also is advisable to "rest" a patient's skin until the effects of such preparations subside before use of RETIN-A is begun.
Carcinogenesis: Long-term animal studies to determine the carcinogenic potential of tretinoin have not been performed. Studies in hairless albino mice suggest that tretinoin may accelerate the tumorigenic potential of weakly carcinogenic light from a solar simulator. In other studies, when lightly pigmented hairless mice treated with tretinoin were exposed to carcinogenic doses of UVB light, the incidence and rate of development of skin tumors was reduced. Due to significantly different experimental conditions, no strict comparison of these disparate data is possible. Although the significance of these studies to man is not clear, patients should avoid or minimize exposure to sun.
Pregnancy: Teratogenic effects. Pregnancy Category C. *Oral* tretinoin has been shown to be teratogenic in rats when given in doses 1000 times the topical human dose. Oral tretinoin has been shown to be fetotoxic in rats when given in doses 500 times the topical human dose. *Topical* tretinoin has not been shown to be teratogenic in rats and rabbits when given in doses of 100 and 320 times the topical human dose, respectively (assuming a 50 kg adult applies 250 mg of 0.1% cream topically). However, at these topical doses, delayed ossification of a number of bones occurred in both species. These changes may be considered variants of normal development and are usually corrected after weaning. There are no adequate and well-controlled studies in pregnant women. Tretinoin should be used during pregnancy only if the potential benefit justifies the potential risk to the fetus.
Nursing mothers: It is not known whether this drug is excreted in human milk. Because many drugs are excreted in human milk, caution should be exercised when RETIN-A is administered to a nursing woman.

GELS ARE FLAMMABLE. Note: Keep away from heat and flame. Keep tube tightly closed.

ADVERSE REACTIONS

The skin of certain sensitive individuals may become excessively red, edematous, blistered, or crusted. If these effects occur, the medication should either be discontinued until the integrity of the skin is restored, or the medication should be adjusted to a level the patient can tolerate. True contact allergy to topical tretinoin is rarely encountered. Temporary hyper- or hypopigmentation has been reported with repeated application of RETIN-A. Some individuals have been reported to have heightened susceptibility to sunlight while under treatment with RETIN-A. To date, all adverse effects of RETIN-A have been reversible upon discontinuance of therapy (see Dosage and Administration Section).

OVERDOSAGE

If medication is applied excessively, no more rapid or better results will be obtained and marked redness, peeling, or discomfort may occur. Oral ingestion of the drug may lead to the same side effects as those associated with excessive oral intake of Vitamin A.

DOSAGE AND ADMINISTRATION

RETIN-A Gel, Cream or Liquid should be applied once a day, before retiring, to the skin where acne lesions appear, using enough to cover the entire affected area lightly. Liquid: The liquid may be applied using a fingertip, gauze pad or cotton swab. If gauze or cotton is employed, care should be taken not to oversaturate it to the extent that the liquid would run into areas where treatment is not intended. Gel: Excessive application results in "pilling" of the gel, which minimizes the likelihood of overapplication by the patient.
Application may cause a transitory feeling of warmth or slight stinging. In cases where it has been necessary to temporarily discontinue therapy or to reduce the frequency of application, therapy may be resumed or frequency of application increased when the patients become able to tolerate the treatment.
Alterations of vehicle, drug concentration, or dose frequency should be closely monitored by careful observation of the clinical therapeutic response and skin tolerance.
During the early weeks of therapy, an *apparent* exacerbation of inflammatory lesions may occur. This is due to the action of the medication on deep, previously unseen lesions and should not be considered a reason to discontinue therapy.
Therapeutic results should be noticed after two to three weeks but more than six weeks of therapy may be required before definite beneficial effects are seen.
Once the acne lesions have responded satisfactorily, it may be possible to maintain the improvement with less frequent applications, or other dosage forms.
Patients treated with RETIN-A (tretinoin) acne treatment may use cosmetics, but the areas to be treated should be cleansed thoroughly before the medication is applied. (See **Precautions**)

HOW SUPPLIED

RETIN-A (tretinoin) is supplied as:
RETIN-A Cream

NDC Code	RETIN-A Strength/Form	RETIN-A Qty.
0062-0165-01	0.025% Cream	20g
0062-0165-02	0.025% Cream	45g
0062-0175-12	0.05% Cream	20g
0062-0175-13	0.05% Cream	45g
0062-0275-23	0.1% Cream	20g
0062-0275-01	0.1% Cream	45g

RETIN-A Gel

NDC Code	RETIN-A Strength/Form	RETIN-A Qty.
0062-0575-44	0.01% Gel	15g
0062-0575-46	0.01% Gel	45g
0062-0475-42	0.025% Gel	15g
0062-0475-45	0.025% Gel	45g

RETIN-A Liquid

NDC Code	RETIN-A Strength/Form	RETIN-A Qty.
0062-0075-07	0.05% Liquid	28 ml

Storage Conditions: RETIN-A Liquid, 0.05%, and RETIN-A Gel, 0.025% and 0.01%: store below 86°F. RETIN-A Cream, 0.1%, 0.05%, and 0.025%: store below 80°F.
Revised September 1993 643-11-339-1
Shown in Product Identification Guide, page 326

SPECTAZOLE® ℞

['spek-ti-zōl]
(econazole nitrate 1%)
Cream
For Topical Use Only

DESCRIPTION

SPECTAZOLE Cream contains the antifungal agent, econazole nitrate 1%, in a water-miscible base consisting of pegoxol 7 stearate, peglicol 5 oleate, mineral oil, benzoic acid, butylated hydroxyanisole and purified water. The white to off-white soft cream is for topical use only.
Chemically, econazole nitrate is 1-[2-{(4-chlorophenyl) methoxy}-2-(2,4-dichlorophenyl)ethyl]-1H-imidazole mononitrate. Its structure is as follows:

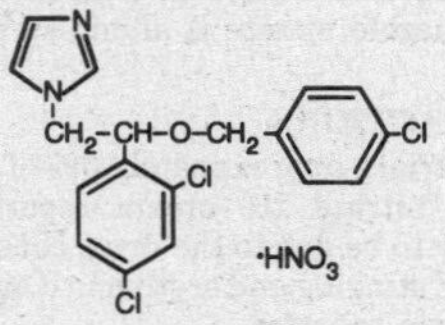

CLINICAL PHARMACOLOGY

After topical application to the skin of normal subjects, systemic absorption of econazole nitrate is extremely low. Although most of the applied drug remains on the skin surface, drug concentrations were found in the stratum corneum which, by far, exceeded the minimum inhibitory concentration for dermatophytes. Inhibitory concentrations were achieved in the epidermis and as deep as the middle region of the dermis. Less than 1% of the applied dose was recovered in the urine and feces.
Microbiology: Econazole nitrate has been shown to be active against most strains of the following microorganisms, both *in vitro* and in clinical infections as described in the INDICATIONS AND USAGE section.

Dermatophytes	**Yeasts**
Epidermophyton floccosum	*Candida albicans*
Microsporum audouini	*Malassezia furfur*
Microsporum canis	
Microsporum gypseum	
Trichophyton mentagrophytes	
Trichophyton rubrum	
Trichophyton tonsurans	

Econazole nitrate exhibits broad-spectrum antifungal activity against the following organisms *in vitro*, but the clinical significance of these data is unknown.

Dermatophytes	**Yeasts**
Trichophyton verrucosum	*Candida guillermondii*
	Candida parapsilosis
	Candida tropicalis

INDICATIONS AND USAGE

SPECTAZOLE Cream is indicated for topical application in the treatment of tinea pedis, tinea cruris, and tinea corporis caused by *Trichophyton rubrum, Trichophyton mentagrophytes, Trichophyton tonsurans, Microsporum canis, Microsporum audouini, Microsporum gypseum,* and *Epidermophyton floccosum,* in the treatment of cutaneous candidiasis, and in the treatment of tinea versicolor.

CONTRAINDICATIONS

SPECTAZOLE Cream is contraindicated in individuals who have shown hypersensitivity to any of its ingredients.

Continued on next page

Ortho—Cont.

WARNINGS
SPECTAZOLE is not for ophthalmic use.

PRECAUTIONS
General: If a reaction suggesting sensitivity or chemical irritation should occur, use of the medication should be discontinued.

For external use only. Avoid introduction of SPECTAZOLE Cream into the eyes.

Carcinogenicity Studies: Long-term animal studies to determine carcinogenic potential have not been performed.

Fertility (Reproduction): Oral administration of econazole nitrate in rats has been reported to produce prolonged gestation. Intravaginal administration in humans has not shown prolonged gestation or other adverse reproductive effects attributable to econazole nitrate therapy.

Pregnancy: Pregnancy Category C. Econazole nitrate has not been shown to be teratogenic when administered orally to mice, rabbits or rats. Fetotoxic or embryotoxic effects were observed in Segment I oral studies with rats receiving 10 to 40 times the human dermal dose. Similar effects were observed in Segment II or Segment III studies with mice, rabbits and/or rats receiving oral doses 80 or 40 times the human dermal dose.

Econazole nitrate should be used in the first trimester of pregnancy only when the physician considers it essential to the welfare of the patient. The drug should be used during the second and third trimesters of pregnancy only if clearly needed.

Nursing Mothers: It is not known whether econazole nitrate is excreted in human milk. Following oral administration of econazole nitrate to lactating rats, econazole and/or metabolites were excreted in milk and were found in nursing pups. Also, in lactating rats receiving large oral doses (40 or 80 times the human dermal dose), there was a reduction in postpartum viability of pups and survival to weaning; however, at these high doses, maternal toxicity was present and may have been a contributing factor. Caution should be exercised when econazole nitrate is administered to a nursing woman.

ADVERSE REACTIONS
During clinical trials, approximately 3% of patients treated with econazole nitrate 1% cream reported side effects thought possibly to be due to the drug, consisting mainly of burning, itching, stinging and erythema. One case of pruritic rash has also been reported.

OVERDOSE
Overdosage of econazole nitrate in humans has not been reported to date. In mice, rats, guinea pigs and dogs, the oral LD 50 values were found to be 462, 668, 272, and > 160 mg/kg, respectively.

DOSAGE AND ADMINISTRATION
Sufficient SPECTAZOLE Cream should be applied to cover affected areas once daily in patients with tinea pedis, tinea cruris, tinea corporis, and tinea versicolor, and twice daily (morning and evening) in patients with cutaneous candidiasis.

Early relief of symptoms is experienced by the majority of patients and clinical improvement may be seen fairly soon after treatment is begun; however, candidal infections and tinea cruris and corporis should be treated for two weeks and tinea pedis for one month in order to reduce the possibility of recurrence. If a patient shows no clinical improvement after the treatment period, the diagnosis should be redetermined. Patients with tinea versicolor usually exhibit clinical and mycological clearing after two weeks of treatment.

HOW SUPPLIED
SPECTAZOLE (econazole nitrate 1%) Cream is supplied in tubes of 15 grams (NDC 0062-5460-02), 30 grams (NDC 0062-5460-01), and 85 grams (NDC 0062-5460-03).
Store SPECTAZOLE Cream below 86°F.
Revised March 1994   631-10-331-8
Shown in Product Identification Guide, page 326

For EMERGENCY telephone numbers,
consult the **Manufacturers Index.**

Paddock Laboratories, Inc.
**3940 QUEBEC AVENUE NORTH
MINNEAPOLIS, MN 55427**

Direct Inquiries to:
(800) 328-5113

For Medical Information Contact:
Medical Department
(800) 328-5113

ACTIDOSE with SORBITOL™   OTC
[*act 'ĭ –dose*]
(Activated Charcoal with Sorbitol Suspension)

DESCRIPTION
Actidose with Sorbitol is supplied in bottles and tubes. Each 120 mL package contains 25 grams of activated charcoal in suspension and 48 grams of sorbitol. Each 240 mL package contains 50 grams of activated charcoal in suspension and 96 grams of sorbitol. Each milliliter contains 208 mg (0.208 gram) activated in charcoal and 400 mg (0.4 gram) sorbitol.

HOW SUPPLIED
25 g unit-of-use bottle NDC 0574-0120-04
50 g unit-of-use bottle NDC 0574-0120-08
25 g unit-of-use tube NDC 0574-0120-74
50 g unit-of-use tube NDC 0574-0120-76

ACTIDOSE-AQUA™   OTC
[*act 'ĭ 'dose a–qua*]
(Activated Charcoal Suspension)

DESCRIPTION
Actidose-Aqua is supplied in bottles and tubes. Each 72 mL package contains 15 grams of activated charcoal in suspension, each 120 mL package contains 25 grams of activated charcoal in suspension and each 240 mL package contains 50 grams of activated charcoal in suspension. Each milliliter contains 208 mg (0.208 gram) activated charcoal.

HOW SUPPLIED
15 g unit-of-use bottle NDC 0574-0120-25
25 g unit-of-use bottle NDC 0574-0120-04
50 g unit-of-use bottle NDC 0574-0120-08
25 g unit-of-use tube NDC 0574-0120-74
50 g unit-of-use tube NDC 0574-0120-76

CLINDA-DERM™   ℞
[*clĭ n'dă-dĕrm*]
(Clindamycin Phosphate Topical Solution, USP, 1%)

DESCRIPTION
Clindamycin phosphate is a water-soluble ester of a semi-synthetic antibiotic produced from lincomycin. Clinda-Derm™ contains clindamycin phosphate equivalent to 10 mEq of clindamycin per ml. in a clear solution vehicle of 51.5% v/v isopropyl alcohol, propylene glycol, sodium hydroxide, and purified water.

HOW SUPPLIED
Bottles of 2 fl. oz. (60 ml.) Store at controlled room temperature 15–30°C (59–86°F)
NDC 0574-0016-02

DIABE-TUSS DM™ Syrup   OTC
(Dextromethorphan Hydrobromide USP)

DESCRIPTION
Cherry flavored cough suppressant in an alcohol-free, sugar-free, dye-free base. Each teaspoonful (5 mL) contains dextromethorphan hydrobromide USP 15 mg.

INDICATIONS
Temporarily relieves cough due to minor throat and bronchial irritation associated with the common cold.

DOSAGE AND ADMINISTRATION
(See dosage below. Do not exceed four doses in a 24-hour period)
Adults and children over 12 years: 2 teaspoonfuls every 6 hours.
Children 6 to 12 years: 1 teaspoonful every 6 hours.
Children 2 to 6 years: ½ teaspoonful every 6 hours.
Children under 2: Consult a doctor.

HOW SUPPLIED
DIABE-TUSS DM is available in 118 mL (4 Fl Oz) bottles.
NDC: 0574-0022-04

ERYTHRA-DERM™   ℞
(Erythromycin Topical Solution USP, 2%)

DESCRIPTION
Erythromycin is an antibiotic produced from a strain of *Streptomyces erythraeus*. It is basic and readily forms salts with acids. ERYTHRA-DERM contains 20 mg/ml erythromycin base in a clear solution vehicle of 66 percent alcohol, propylene glycol and citric acid.

HOW SUPPLIED
Bottles of 2 fl. oz. (60 ml). Store at controlled room temperature (59°F–86°F). NDC 0574-0014-02

GLUTOSE 15™   OTC
GLUTOSE 45™
(Oral Glucose Gel)

DESCRIPTION
Glutose gel is a lemon-flavored, dye-free oral glucose gel for treatment of insulin reaction or hypoglycemia. Glutose gel contains Dextrose (d-Glucose) 40%.

HOW SUPPLIED
Glutose 15: 3 x 15g unit-of-use tubes per package NDC 0574-0069-30
Glutose 45: 1 x 45g multi-use tube per package NDC 0574-0069-45

GLUTOSE™ Tablets   OTC
(Oral Glucose Chewable Tablets)

DESCRIPTION
Glutose tablets are lemon-flavored chewable tablets for treatment of insulin reaction or hypoglycemia. Each tablet contains 5 grams of Dextrose.

HOW SUPPLIED
Box of 12 tablets NDC 0574-0068-12

NYSTATIN PADDOCK™

NYSTATIN, USP   ℞
**For Extemporaneous Preparation
of Oral Suspension**

DESCRIPTION
Nystatin USP is an antifungal antibiotic obtained from *Streptomyces noursei*. It is known to be a mixture, but the composition has not been completely elucidated. Nystatin A_1 is closely related to amphotericin B. Each is a macrocyclic lactone containing a ketal ring, an all-trans polyene system, and a mycosamine (3-amino-3-deoxy-rhamnose) moiety.

Nystatin USP is a ready-to-use, non-sterile powder for oral administration which contains no excipients or preservatives. It is available in containers of 50 million, 150 million, 500 million, 1 billion, 2 billion, and 5 billion units. Each mg contains not less than 5,000 units.

HOW SUPPLIED

Product Code (NDC)	Size (units)	Approx. Weight (grams)
0574-0404-05	50 million	8.3 – 10
0574-0404-15	150 million	25 – 30
0574-0404-50	500 million	83 – 100
0574-0404-01	1 billion	167 – 200
0574-0404-02	2 billion	333 – 400
0574-0404-00	5 billion	833 – 1,000

Storage: Store in a refrigerator. 2°–8°C (36°–46°F) protect from light.

07-95

NYSTOP™   ℞
**Nystatin Topical Powder USP
For topical use only.
Not for ophthalmic use.**

DESCRIPTION
Nystatin Topical Powder USP is for dermatologic use. Nystatin Topical Powder USP provides, in each gram, 100,000 USP nystatin units dispersed in talc.

CLINICAL PHARMACOLOGY

Nystatin is an antifungal antibiotic which is both fungistatic and fungicidal *in vitro* against a wide variety of yeasts and yeast-like fungi. It probably acts by binding to sterols in the cell membrane of the fungus with a resultant change in membrane permeability allowing leakage of intracellular components. Nystatin is a polyene antibiotic of undetermined structural formula that is obtained from *Streptomyces noursei*, and is the first well tolerated antifungal antibiotic of dependable efficacy for the treatment of cutaneous, oral and intestinal infections caused by *Candida* (Monilia) *albicans* and other Candida species. It exhibits no appreciable activity against bacteria.

Nystatin provides specific therapy for all localized forms of candidiasis. Symptomatic relief is rapid, often occurring within 24 to 72 hours after the initiation of treatment. Cure is effected both clinically and mycologically in most cases of localized candidiasis.

INDICATIONS AND USAGE

Nystatin Topical Powder is indicated in the treatment of cutaneous or mucocutaneous mycotic infections caused by *Candida* (Monilia) *albicans* and other Candida species.

CONTRAINDICATIONS

Nystatin Topical Powder is contraindicated in patients with a history of hypersensitivity to any of its components.

PRECAUTIONS

Should a reaction of hypersensitivity occur the drug should be immediately withdrawn and appropriate measures taken. This preparation is not for ophthalmic use.

ADVERSE REACTIONS

Nystatin is virtually nontoxic and nonsensitizing and is well tolerated by all age groups including debilitated infants, even on prolonged administration. If irritation on topical application should occur, discontinue medication.

DOSAGE AND ADMINISTRATION

The powder should be applied to candidal lesions two or three times daily until lesions have healed. For fungal infection of the feet caused by Candida species, the powder should be dusted freely on the feet as well as in shoes and socks. Nystatin Topical Powder does not stain skin or mucous membranes and provides a simple, convenient means of treatment. The cream is usually preferred to the ointment in candidiasis involving intertriginous areas; very moist lesions, however, are best treated with topical dusting powder.

HOW SUPPLIED

Nystatin Topical Powder USP is supplied in 15 gram plastic squeeze bottles providing, in each gram, 100,000 USP nystatin units.

Nystatin Topical Powder USP 15 grams NDC 0574-2008-15

Keep tightly closed. Store at controlled room temperature 15°-30° C (59°-86° F); avoid excessive heat (40° C, 104° F).

CAUTION: FEDERAL LAW PROHIBITS DISPENSING WITHOUT A PRESCRIPTION.

PODOCON-25™   ℞
(25% podophyllin in benzoin tincture)

DESCRIPTION

Podocon-25™ is composed of Podophyllin (Podophyllum Resin, American) 25% in Benzoin Tincture. Podophyllum Resin is the powdered mixture of resins removed from the May apple or Mandrake (*Podophyllum peltatum Linne'*), a perennial plant of northern and middle United States[1]. The podophyllum resin used in this product is exclusively the American podophyllin (rather than the Indian resin). American podophyllin typically has a reduced level of podophyllotoxin (see below).

CLINICAL PHARMACOLOGY

Podophyllin is a cytotoxic agent that has been used topically in the treatment of genital warts. It arrests mitosis in metaphase, an effect it shares with other cytotoxic agents such as the vinca alkaloids[2]. The active agent is podophyllotoxin, whose concentration varies with the type of podophyllin used; the American source normally containing one-fourth the amount of podophyllotoxin as the Indian source[3].
NOTE: PODOCON-25 IS TO BE APPLIED ONLY BY A PHYSICIAN. IT IS NOT TO BE DISPENSED TO THE PATIENT.

INDICATIONS

Podocon-25 (25% podophyllin in benzoin tincture) is indicated for the removal of soft genital (venereal) warts (condylomata acuminata)[4].

CONTRAINDICATIONS

Podocon-25 is contraindicated in diabetics, patients using steroids or with poor blood circulation. Podocon-25 should not be used on bleeding warts, moles, birthmarks or unusual warts with hair growing from them. It is recommended that Podocon-25 not be used during pregnancy (see Pregnancy warning below).

WARNINGS

Podophyllin is a powerful caustic and severe irritant. Keep away from the eyes; if eye contact occurs, flush with copious amounts of warm water and consult physician or poison control center immediately for advice.

PRECAUTIONS

Do not use Podocon-25 if wart or surrounding tissue is inflamed or irritated. Do not use on bleeding warts, moles, birthmarks or unusual warts with hair growing from them.

ADVERSE REACTIONS

The use of topical podophyllin has been known to result in paresthesia, polyneuritis, paralytic ileus, pyrexia leukopenia, thrombocytopenia, coma and death[5].
Pregnancy: There have been reports of complications associated with the topical use of podophyllin on condylomas of pregnant patients including birth defects, fetal death and still birth[6]. In the absence of controlled saftety studies, podophyllin remains contraindicated for use on pregnant patients.
Nursing Mothers: It is not known whether podophyllin is excreted in human milk following topical application. In the absence of controlled safety studies, podophyllin remains contraindicated for use on nursing patients.

DOSAGE AND ADMINISTRATION

PODOCON-25 IS TO BE APPLIED ONLY BY A PHYSICIAN. IT IS NOT TO BE DISPENSED TO THE PATIENT. Thoroughly cleanse affected area. Use supplied applicator to apply Podocon-25 sparingly to lesion. Avoid contact with healthy tissue. Allow to dry thoroughly. Only intact (no bleeding) lesions should be treated. As podophyllin is a powerful caustic and severe irritant, it is recommended the first application of Podocon-25 be left in contact for only a short time (30 to 40 minutes) to determine patient's sensitivity. To avoid systemic absorption, time of contact should be minimum time necessary to produce the desired result (1 to 4 hours, depending on condititon of lesion and of patient), the physician developing his own experience and technique. Large areas or numerous warts should not be treated at once. After treatment time has elapsed, remove dried Podocon-25 thoroughly with alcohol or soap and water.

HOW SUPPLIED

Podocon-25 is available in 15-ml bottles with tapered tip applicator attached inside cap. NDC 0574-0601-15
Store at room temperature 15°-30° C (59°-86° F) in tight, light-resistant containers.
Caution: Federal law prohibits dispensing without prescription.
1) Blumgarten, A.F.: Text Book of Materia Medica, Pharmacology and Therapeutics; Ed. 7, New York, The Macmillan Company, 1937, pp. 220 and 223.
2) Green, L.K., Klima, M, Burns, T.; Arch Dermatol. Vol 124, Nov 1988, p. 1718.
3) Martindale, 28th Ed. London, 1982. pp. 1366, 1367.
4) Medical Letter; Vol 26, New Rochelle, N.Y., 1984, p10.
5) Fisher: Severe Systemic and Local Reactions to Topical Podophyllum Resins; Cutis, Volume 28, 1981
6) Zackheim: Hazards of Topical Mitotic-Blocking Agents; Arch. Dermat. Volume 113, 1977.

Palisades Pharmaceuticals, Inc.
64 NORTH SUMMIT STREET
TENAFLY, NEW JERSEY 07670

Secondary to a merger, the products of Palisades Pharmaceuticals, Inc. are now listed under Glenwood-Palisades.

NOTICE
Before prescribing or administering
any product described in
PHYSICIANS' DESK REFERENCE.
check the PDR Supplements
for revised information.

Par Pharmaceutical, Inc.
ONE RAM RIDGE ROAD
SPRING VALLEY, NY 10977

Direct Inquiries to:
Customer Service
(800) 828-9393
(914) 425-7100

NOTE: PRODUCT NAME CHANGE

Silver Sulfadiazine Cream, 1%
(NDC #49884-521)
is now marketed under

THERMAZENE® CREAM, 1%
(NDC #49884-459)

The following is a listing of products currently available from Par Pharmaceutical, Inc.

NDC # 49884-	Product
411	Albuterol Sulfate Syrup 2 mg/5 mL
104	Allopurinol Tablets 100 mg
105	Allopurinol Tablets 300 mg
448	Alprazolam Tablets 0.25 mg
449	Alprazolam Tablets 0.5 mg
450	Alprazolam Tablets 1 mg
117	Amiloride HCl Tablets 5 mg
456	Atenolol Tablets 50 mg
457	Atenolol Tablets 100 mg
164	Benztropine Mesylate Tablets 0.5 mg
165	Benztropine Mesylate Tablets 1 mg
166	Benztropine Mesylate Tablets 2 mg
444	Captopril 12.5 mg
445	Captopril 25 mg
446	Captopril 50 mg
447	Captopril 100 mg
246	Carisoprodol and Aspirin Tablets 200 mg/325 mg
016	Chlorzoxazone Tablets 250 mg
405	Cimetidine Tablets 300 mg
406	Cimetidine Tablets 400 mg
407	Cimetidine Tablets 800 mg
113	Clonidine HCl and Chlorthalidone Tablets 0.1 mg/15 mg
115	Clonidine HCl and Chlorthalidone Tablets 0.2 mg/15 mg
116	Clonidine HCl and Chlorthalidone Tablets 0.3 mg/15 mg
043	Cyproheptadine HCl Tablets 4 mg
083	Dexamethasone Tablets 0.25 mg
084	Dexamethasone Tablets 0.5 mg
085	Dexamethasone Tablets 0.75 mg
086	Dexamethasone Tablets 1.5 mg
087	Dexamethasone Tablets 4 mg
129	Dexamethasone Tablets 6 mg
217	Doxepin HCl Capsules 10 mg
218	Doxepin HCl Capsules 25 mg
219	Doxepin HCl Capsules 50 mg
220	Doxepin HCl Capsules 75 mg
221	Doxepin HCl Capsules 100 mg
222	Doxepin HCl Capsules 150 mg
061	Fluphenazine HCl Tablets 1 mg
062	Fluphenazine HCl Tablets 2.5 mg
076	Fluphenazine HCl Tablets 5 mg
064	Fluphenazine HCl Tablets 10 mg
193	Flurazepam HCl Capsules 15 mg
194	Flurazepam HCl Capsules 30 mg
451	Glipizide Tablets 5 mg
452	Glipizide Tablets 10 mg
223	Haloperidol Tablets 0.5 mg
224	Haloperidol Tablets 1 mg
225	Haloperidol Tablets 2 mg
226	Haloperidol Tablets 5 mg
227	Haloperidol Tablets 10 mg
029	Hydralazine HCl Tablets 10 mg
027	Hydralazine HCl Tablets 25 mg
028	Hydralazine HCl Tablets 50 mg
121	Hydralazine HCl Tablets 100 mg
143	Hydra-Zide (Hydralazine HCl and Hydrochlorothiazide) Capsules 25 mg/25 mg
144	Hydra-Zide (Hydralazine HCl and Hydrochlorothiazide) Capsules 50 mg/50 mg

Continued on next page

Par—Cont.

145	Hydra-Zide (Hydralazine HCl and Hydrochloro-thiazide) Capsules 100 mg/50 mg
200	Ibuprofen Tablets 200 mg
162	Ibuprofen Tablets 400 mg
467	Ibuprofen Tablets 400 mg
163	Ibuprofen Tablets 600 mg
468	Ibuprofen Tablets 600 mg
216	Ibuprofen Tablets 800 mg
469	Ibuprofen Tablets 800 mg
054	Imipramine HCl Tablets 10 mg
055	Imipramine HCl Tablets 25 mg
056	Imipramine HCl Tablets 50 mg
020	Isosorbide Dinitrate Tablets 5 mg
021	Isosorbide Dinitrate Tablets 10 mg
022	Isosorbide Dinitrate Tablets 20 mg
009	Isosorbide Dinitrate Tablets 30 mg
034	Meclizine HCl Tablets 12.5 mg
035	Meclizine HCl Tablets 25 mg
015	Meclizine HCl Tablets 50 mg
289	Megestrol Acetate Tablets 20 mg
290	Megestrol Acetate Tablets 40 mg
478	Melatonin 1.5 mg
479	Melatonin 500 mcg
482	Melatonin SR
258	Metaproterenol Sulfate Tablets 10 mg
259	Metaproterenol Sulfate Tablets 20 mg
249	Methocarbamol and Aspirin Tablets 400 mg/325 mg
186	Methyldopa and Hydrochlorothiazide Tablets 250 mg/15 mg
187	Methyldopa and Hydrochlorothiazide Tablets 250 mg/25 mg
188	Methyldopa and Hydrochlorothiazide Tablets 500 mg/30 mg
189	Methyldopa and Hydrochlorothiazide Tablets 500 mg/50 mg
412	Metoprolol Tartrate Tablets 50 mg
413	Metoprolol Tartrate Tablets 100 mg
095	Metronidazole Compressed Tablets 250 mg
114	Metronidazole Compressed Tablets 500 mg
256	Minoxidil Tablets 2.5 mg
257	Minoxidil Tablets 10 mg
119	Nystatin Tablets 500,000 Units
442	Pindolol Tablets 5 mg
443	Pindolol Tablets 10 mg
440	Piroxicam Capsules 10 mg
441	Piroxicam Capsules 20 mg
240	Temazepam Capsules 15 mg
241	Temazepam Capsules 30 mg
459	Thermazene Cream 1% (Silver Sulfadiazine Cream 1%)
279	Triamterene and Hydrochlorothiazide Tablets 75 mg/50 mg
017	Triamterene and Hydrochlorothiazide Tablets 75 mg/50 mg
453	Triazolam Tablets 0.125 mg
454	Triazolam Tablets 0.25 mg

LOOKING FOR A SPECIFIC PRODUCT?
Whatever name you use, you'll
find it listed in the **Brand and Generic
Name Index** (PINK section).

QUESTION ABOUT AN ACTIVE INGREDIENT?
Look in the
Brand and Generic Name Index
(PINK section)
to find products that contain it.

LOOKING FOR A PARTICULAR TYPE OF DRUG?
Consult the **Product Category Index**
(BLUE section)
to locate a drug by
its classification.

Parke-Davis
**Division of Warner-Lambert Company
201 TABOR ROAD
MORRIS PLAINS, NEW JERSEY 07950**

**For Medical Information Contact:
Generally:**
Customer Service
Product/Medical Information
(800) 223-0432
FAX: (201) 540-2248
After Hours and Weekend Emergencies:
(201) 540-6089

PARCODE®
(Parke-Davis Accurate Recognition Code)

Code Number	Product Name
001-	
006	*Unassigned*
007	**Dilantin® Infatabs®** Each tablet contains 50 mg phenytoin, USP.
008-	
165	*Unassigned*
166	**Mandelamine® Tablets** Each tablet contains 0.5 gram methenamine mandelate, USP.
167	**Mandelamine® Tablets** Each tablet contains 1 gram methenamine mandelate, USP.
168-	
180	*Unassigned*
181	**Pyridium® Tablets** Each tablet contains 200 mg phenazopyridine hydrochloride, USP.
182-	
210	*Unassigned*
211	**Choledyl® Tablets** Each tablet contains 200 mg oxtriphylline, USP.
212-	
220	*Unassigned*
221	**Choledyl® SA Tablets** Each sustained-action tablet contains 600 mg oxtriphylline, USP.
222-	
236	*Unassigned*
237	**Zarontin® Capsules** Each capsule contains 250 mg ethosuximide, USP.
238-	
269	*Unassigned*
270	**Nardil® Tablets** Each tablet contains 15 mg phenelzine sulfate, USP.
271-	
361	*Unassigned*
362	**Dilantin® Kapseals®** Each Kapseal contains 100 mg extended phenytoin sodium, USP. The Kapseal is a No. 3 capsule with Orange band. (The Orange band on White capsule is a trademark registered in the US Patent Office.)
363-	
364	*Unassigned*
365	**Dilantin® Kapseals®** Each Kapseal contains 30 mg extended phenytoin sodium, USP. The Kapseal is a No. 4 capsule with Pink opaque band.
366-	
489	*Unassigned*
490	**Easprin® Enteric Coated Tablets** Each tablet contains 15 grains (975 mg) aspirin, USP.
491-	
524	*Unassigned*
525	**Celontin® Kapseals®** Each Kapseal contains 300 mg methsuximide, USP. The Kapseal is a Yellow Tint No. 2 capsule with Orange band.
526	*Unassigned*
527	**Accupril® Tablets** Each tablet contains quinapril hydrochloride equivalent to 5 mg quinapril.
528	*Unassigned*
529	**Humatin® Capsules** Each capsule contains paromomycin sulfate, USP, equivalent to 250 mg paromomycin.
530	**Accupril® Tablets** Each tablet contains quinapril hydrochloride equivalent to 10 mg quinapril.
531	*Unassigned*
532	**Accupril® Tablets** Each tablet contains quinapril hydrochloride equivalent to 20 mg quinapril.
533-	
534	*Unassigned*
535	**Accupril® Tablets** Each tablet contains quinapril hydrochloride equivalent to 40 mg quinapril.
536-	
539	*Unassigned*
540	**Ponstel® Kapseals®** Each Kapseal contains 250 mg mefenamic acid. The Kapseal is an Ivory opaque No. 1 capsule with Light Blue opaque band. The blue band on ivory capsule combination is a Parke-Davis trademark.
541-	
621	*Unassigned*
622	**Ferrous Fumarate Tablets** Each tablet contains 75 mg ferrous fumarate.
623-	
695	*Unassigned*
696	**ERYC® Capsules** Each capsule contains 250 mg erythromycin, USP.
697-	
736	*Unassigned*
737	**Lopid® Tablets** Each tablet contains 600 mg gemfibrozil.
738-	
914	*Unassigned*
915	**Loestrin® 1/20 Tablets** Each tablet contains norethindrone acetate, 1 mg; ethinyl estradiol, 20 mcg.
916	**Loestrin® 1.5/30 Tablets** Each tablet contains norethindrone acetate, 1.5 mg; ethinyl estradiol, 30 mcg.
917-	
999	*Unassigned*

ACCUPRIL® ℞
(Quinapril Hydrochloride Tablets)

USE IN PREGNANCY
When used in pregnancy during the second and third trimesters, ACE inhibitors can cause injury and even death to the developing fetus. When pregnancy is detected, ACCUPRIL should be discontinued as soon as possible. See WARNINGS, Fetal/Neonatal Morbidity and Mortality.

DESCRIPTION
ACCUPRIL® (quinapril hydrochloride) is the hydrochloride salt of quinapril, the ethyl ester of a nonsulfhydryl, angiotensin-converting enzyme (ACE) inhibitor, quinaprilat. Quinapril hydrochloride is chemically described as [3S-[2[R*(R*)], 3R*]]-2-[2-[[1-(ethoxycarbonyl)-3-phenylpropyl] amino] -1- oxopropyl]-1,2,3,4- tetrahydro -3- isoquinolinecar-

boxylic acid, monohydrochloride. Its empirical formula is $C_{25}H_{30}N_2O_5 \cdot HCl$.

Quinapril hydrochloride is a white to off-white amorphous powder that is freely soluble in aqueous solvents.

ACCUPRIL tablets contain 5 mg, 10 mg, 20 mg, or 40 mg of quinapril for oral administration. Each tablet also contains candelilla wax, crospovidone, gelatin, lactose, magnesium carbonate, magnesium stearate, synthetic red iron oxide, and titanium dioxide.

CLINICAL PHARMACOLOGY

Mechanism of Action: Quinapril is deesterified to the principal metabolite, quinaprilat, which is an inhibitor of ACE activity in human subjects and animals. ACE is a peptidyl dipeptidase that catalyzes the conversion of angiotensin I to the vasoconstrictor, angiotensin II. The effect of quinapril in hypertension and in congestive heart failure (CHF) appears to result primarily from the inhibition of circulating and tissue ACE activity, thereby reducing angiotensin II formation. Quinapril inhibits the elevation in blood pressure caused by intravenously administered angiotensin I, but has no effect on the pressor response to angiotensin II, norepinephrine or epinephrine. Angiotensin II also stimulates the secretion of aldosterone from the adrenal cortex, thereby facilitating renal sodium and fluid reabsorption. Reduced aldosterone secretion by quinapril may result in a small increase in serum potassium. In controlled hypertension trials, treatment with ACCUPRIL alone resulted in mean increases in potassium of 0.07 mmol/L (see PRECAUTIONS). Removal of angiotensin II negative feedback on renin secretion leads to increased plasma renin activity (PRA).

While the principal mechanism of antihypertensive effect is thought to be through the renin-angiotensin-aldosterone system, quinapril exerts antihypertensive actions even in patients with low renin hypertension. ACCUPRIL was an effective antihypertensive in all races studied, although it was somewhat less effective in blacks (usually a predominantly low renin group) than in nonblacks. ACE is identical to kininase II, an enzyme that degrades bradykinin, a potent peptide vasodilator; whether increased levels of bradykinin play a role in the therapeutic effect of quinapril remains to be elucidated.

Pharmacokinetics and Metabolism: Following oral administration, peak plasma quinapril concentrations are observed within one hour. Based on recovery of quinapril and its metabolites in urine, the extent of absorption is at least 60%. The rate and extent of quinapril absorption are diminished moderately (approximately 25–30%) when ACCUPRIL tablets are administered during a high-fat meal. Following absorption, quinapril is deesterified to its major active metabolite, quinaprilat (about 38% of oral dose), and to other minor inactive metabolites. Following multiple oral dosing of ACCUPRIL, there is an effective accumulation half-life of quinaprilat of approximately 3 hours, and peak plasma quinaprilat concentrations are observed approximately 2 hours post-dose. Quinaprilat is eliminated primarily by renal excretion, up to 96% of an IV dose, and has an elimination half-life in plasma of approximately 2 hours and a prolonged terminal phase with a half-life of 25 hours. The pharmacokinetics of quinapril and quinaprilat are linear over a single-dose range of 5–80 mg doses and 40–160 mg in multiple daily doses. Approximately 97% of either quinapril or quinaprilat circulating in plasma is bound to proteins.

In patients with renal insufficiency, the elimination half-life of quinaprilat increases as creatinine clearance decreases. There is a linear correlation between plasma quinaprilat clearance and creatinine clearance. In patients with end-stage renal disease, chronic hemodialysis or continuous ambulatory peritoneal dialysis has little effect on the elimination of quinapril and quinaprilat. Elimination of quinaprilat may be reduced in elderly patients (≥ 65 years) and in those with heart failure; this reduction is attributable to decrease in renal function (see DOSAGE AND ADMINISTRATION). Quinaprilat concentrations are reduced in patients with alcoholic cirrhosis due to impaired deesterification of quinapril. Studies in rats indicate that quinapril and its metabolites do not cross the blood-brain barrier.

Pharmacodynamics and Clinical Effects

Hypertension: Single doses of 20 mg of ACCUPRIL provide over 80% inhibition of plasma ACE for 24 hours. Inhibition of the pressor response to angiotensin I is shorter-lived, with a 20 mg dose giving 75% inhibition for about 4 hours, 50% inhibition for about 8 hours, and 20% inhibition at 24 hours. With chronic dosing, however, there is substantial inhibition of angiotensin II levels at 24 hours by doses of 20–80 mg. Administration of 10 to 80 mg of ACCUPRIL to patients with mild to severe hypertension results in a reduction of sitting and standing blood pressure to about the same extent with minimal effect on heart rate. Symptomatic postural hypotension is infrequent although it can occur in patients who are salt- and/or volume-depleted (see WARNINGS). Antihypertensive activity commences within 1 hour with peak effects usually achieved by 2 to 4 hours after dosing. During chronic therapy, most of the blood pressure lowering effect of a given dose is obtained in 1–2 weeks. In multiple-dose studies, 10–80 mg per day in single or divided doses lowered sys-

tolic and diastolic blood pressure throughout the dosing interval, with a trough effect of about 5–11/3–7 mm Hg. The trough effect represents about 50% of the peak effect. While the dose-response relationship is relatively flat, doses of 40–80 mg were somewhat more effective at trough than 10–20 mg, and twice daily dosing tended to give a somewhat lower trough blood pressure than once daily dosing with the same total dose. The antihypertensive effect of ACCUPRIL continues during long-term therapy, with no evidence of loss of effectiveness.

Hemodynamic assessments in patients with hypertension indicate that blood pressure reduction produced by quinapril is accompanied by a reduction in total peripheral resistance and renal vascular resistance with little or no change in heart rate, cardiac index, renal blood flow, glomerular filtration rate, or filtration fraction.

Use of ACCUPRIL with a thiazide diuretic gives a blood-pressure lowering effect greater than that seen with either agent alone.

In patients with hypertension, ACCUPRIL 10–40 mg was similar in effectiveness to captopril, enalapril, propranolol, and thiazide diuretics.

Therapeutic effects appear to be the same for elderly (≥ 65 years of age) and younger adult patients given the same daily dosages, with no increase in adverse events in elderly patients.

Heart Failure: In a placebo-controlled trial involving patients with congestive heart failure treated with digitalis and diuretics, parenteral quinaprilat, the active metabolite of quinapril, reduced pulmonary capillary wedge pressure and systemic vascular resistance and increased cardiac output/index. Similar favorable hemodynamic effects were seen with oral quinapril in baseline-controlled trials, and such effects appeared to be maintained during chronic oral quinapril therapy. Quinapril reduced renal hepatic vascular resistance and increased renal and hepatic blood flow with glomerular filtration rate remaining unchanged.

A significant dose response relationship for improvement in maximal exercise tolerance has been observed with ACCUPRIL therapy. Beneficial effects on the severity of heart failure as measured by New York Heart Association (NYHA) classification and Quality of Life and on symptoms of dyspnea, fatigue, and edema were evident after 6 months in a double blind, placebo controlled study. Favorable effects were maintained for up to two years of open label therapy. The effects of quinapril on long-term mortality in heart failure have not been evaluated.

INDICATIONS AND USAGE

Hypertension

ACCUPRIL is indicated for the treatment of hypertension. It may be used alone or in combination with thiazide diuretics.

Heart Failure

ACCUPRIL is indicated in the management of heart failure as adjunctive therapy when added to conventional therapy including diuretics and/or digitalis.

In using ACCUPRIL, consideration should be given to the fact that another angiotensin converting enzyme inhibitor, captopril, has caused agranulocytosis, particularly in patients with renal impairment or collagen vascular disease. Available data are insufficient to show that ACCUPRIL does not have a similar risk (see WARNINGS).

Angioedema in black patients:

Black patients receiving ACE inhibitor monotherapy have been reported to have a higher incidence of angioedema compared to non-blacks. It should also be noted that in controlled clinical trials ACE inhibitors have an effect on blood pressure that is less in black patients than in non-blacks.

CONTRAINDICATIONS

ACCUPRIL is contraindicated in patients who are hypersensitive to this product and in patients with a history of angioedema related to previous treatment with an ACE inhibitor.

WARNINGS

Anaphylactoid and Possibly Related Reactions

Presumably because angiotensin-converting inhibitors affect the metabolism of eicosanoids and polypeptides, including endogenous bradykinin, patients receiving ACE inhibitors (including Accupril) may be subject to a variety of adverse reactions, some of them serious.

Angioedema: Angioedema of the face, extremities, lips, tongue, glottis, and larynx has been reported in patients treated with ACE inhibitors and has been seen in 0.1% of patients receiving ACCUPRIL.

In two similarly sized U.S. postmarketing trials that, combined, enrolled over 3,000 black patients and over 19,000 non-blacks, angioedema was reported in 0.30% and 0.55% of blacks (in study 1 and 2 respectively) and 0.39% and 0.17% of non-blacks.

Angioedema associated with laryngeal edema can be fatal. If laryngeal stridor or angioedema of the face, tongue, or glottis occurs, treatment with ACCUPRIL should be discontinued immediately, the patient treated in accordance with accepted medical care, and carefully observed until the swelling disappears. In instances where swelling is confined to the face and lips, the condition generally resolves without treat-

ment; antihistamines may be useful in relieving symptoms. Where there is involvement of the tongue, glottis, or larynx likely to cause airway obstruction, emergency therapy including, but not limited to, subcutaneous epinephrine solution 1:1000 (0.3 to 0.5 mL) should be promptly administered (see ADVERSE REACTIONS).

Patients with a history of angioedema: Patients with a history of angioedema unrelated to ACE inhibitor therapy may be at increased risk of angioedema while receiving an ACE inhibitor (see also CONTRAINDICATIONS).

Anaphylactoid reactions during desensitization: Two patients undergoing desensitizing treatment with hymenoptera venom while receiving ACE inhibitors sustained life-threatening anaphylactoid reactions. In the same patients, these reactions were avoided when ACE inhibitors were temporarily withheld, but they reappeared upon inadvertent rechallenge.

Anaphylactoid reactions during membrane exposure: Anaphylactoid reactions have been reported in patients dialyzed with high-flux membranes and treated concomitantly with an ACE inhibitor. Anaphylactoid reactions have also been reported in patients undergoing low-density lipoprotein apheresis with dextran sulfate absorption (a procedure dependent upon devices not approved in the United States).

Hepatic Failure: Rarely, ACE inhibitors have been associated with a syndrome that starts with cholestatic jaundice and progresses to fulminant hepatic necrosis and (sometimes) death. The mechanism of this syndrome is not understood. Patients receiving ACE inhibitors who develop jaundice or marked elevations of hepatic enzymes should discontinue the ACE inhibitor and receive appropriate medical follow-up.

Hypotension: Excessive hypotension is rare in patients with uncomplicated hypertension treated with ACCUPRIL alone. Patients with heart failure given ACCUPRIL commonly have some reduction in blood pressure, but discontinuation of therapy because of continuing symptomatic hypotension usually is not necessary when dosing instructions are followed. Caution should be observed when initiating therapy in patients with heart failure (see DOSAGE AND ADMINISTRATION). In controlled studies, syncope was observed in 0.4% of patients (N=3203); this incidence was similar to that observed for captopril (1%) and enalapril (0.8%).

Patients at risk of excessive hypotension, sometimes associated with oliguria and/or progressive azotemia, and rarely with acute renal failure and/or death, include patients with the following conditions or characteristics: heart failure, hyponatremia, high dose diuretic therapy, recent intensive diuresis or increase in diuretic dose, renal dialysis, or severe volume and/or salt depletion of any etiology. It may be advisable to eliminate the diuretic (except in patients with heart failure), reduce the diuretic dose or cautiously increase salt intake (except in patients with heart failure) before initiating therapy with ACCUPRIL in patients at risk for excessive hypotension who are able to tolerate such adjustments.

In patients at risk of excessive hypotension, therapy with ACCUPRIL should be started under close medical supervision. Such patients should be followed closely for the first two weeks of treatment and whenever the dose of ACCUPRIL and/or diuretic is increased. Similar considerations may apply to patients with ischemic heart or cerebrovascular disease in whom an excessive fall in blood pressure could result in a myocardial infarction or a cerebrovascular accident.

If excessive hypotension occurs, the patient should be placed in the supine position and, if necessary, receive an intravenous infusion of normal saline. A transient hypotensive response is not a contraindication to further doses of ACCUPRIL, which usually can be given without difficulty once the blood pressure has stabilized. If symptomatic hypotension develops, a dose reduction or discontinuation of ACCUPRIL or concomitant diuretic may be necessary.

Neutropenia/Agranulocytosis: Another ACE inhibitor, captopril, has been shown to cause agranulocytosis and bone marrow depression rarely in patients with uncomplicated hypertension, but more frequently in patients with renal impairment, especially if they also have a collagen vascular disease, such as systemic lupus erythematosus or scleroderma. Agranulocytosis did occur during ACCUPRIL treatment in one patient with a history of neutropenia during previous captopril therapy. Available data from clinical trials of ACCUPRIL are insufficient to show that, in patients without prior reactions to other ACE inhibitors, ACCUPRIL does not cause agranulocytosis at similar rates. As with other ACE inhibitors, periodic monitoring of white blood cell

Continued on next page

This product information was prepared in August 1996. On these and other Parke-Davis Products, information may be obtained by addressing PARKE-DAVIS, Division of Warner-Lambert Company, Morris Plains, New Jersey 07950.

Parke-Davis—Cont.

counts in patients with collagen vascular disease and/or renal disease should be considered.

Fetal/Neonatal Morbidity and Mortality: ACE inhibitors can cause fetal and neonatal morbidity and death when administered to pregnant women. Several dozen cases have been reported in the world literature. When pregnancy is detected, ACE inhibitors should be discontinued as soon as possible.

The use of ACE inhibitors during the second and third trimesters of pregnancy has been associated with fetal and neonatal injury, including hypotension, neonatal skull hypoplasia, anuria, reversible or irreversible renal failure, and death. Oligohydramnios has also been reported, presumably resulting from decreased fetal renal function; oligohydramnios in this setting has been associated with fetal limb contractures, craniofacial deformation, and hypoplastic lung development. Prematurity, intrauterine growth retardation, and patent ductus arteriosus have also been reported, although it is not clear whether these occurrences were due to the ACE inhibitor exposure.

These adverse effects do not appear to have resulted from intrauterine ACE inhibitor exposure that has been limited to the first trimester. Mothers whose embryos and fetuses are exposed to ACE inhibitors only during the first trimester should be so informed. Nonetheless, when patients become pregnant, physicians should make every effort to discontinue the use of ACCUPRIL as soon as possible.

Rarely (probably less often than once in every thousand pregnancies), no alternative to ACE inhibitors will be found. In these rare cases, the mothers should be apprised of the potential hazards to their fetuses, and serial ultrasound examinations should be performed to assess the intraamniotic environment.

If oligohydramnios is observed, ACCUPRIL should be discontinued unless it is considered life-saving for the mother. Contraction stress testing (CST), a non-stress test (NST), or biophysical profiling (BPP) may be appropriate, depending upon the week of pregnancy. Patients and physicians should be aware, however, that oligohydramnios may not appear until after the fetus has sustained irreversible injury.

Infants with histories of *in utero* exposure to ACE inhibitors should be closely observed for hypotension, oliguria, and hyperkalemia. If oliguria occurs, attention should be directed toward support of blood pressure and renal perfusion. Exchange transfusion or dialysis may be required as a means of reversing hypotension and/or substituting for disordered renal function. Removal of ACCUPRIL, which crosses the placenta, from the neonatal circulation is not significantly accelerated by these means.

No teratogenic effects of ACCUPRIL were seen in studies of pregnant rats and rabbits. On a mg/kg basis, the doses used were up to 180 times (in rats) and one time (in rabbits) the maximum recommended human dose.

PRECAUTIONS

General

Impaired renal function: As a consequence of inhibiting the renin-angiotensin-aldosterone system, changes in renal function may be anticipated in susceptible individuals. In patients with severe heart failure whose renal function may depend on the activity of the renin-angiotensin-aldosterone system, treatment with ACE inhibitors, including ACCUPRIL, may be associated with oliguria and/or progressive azotemia and rarely acute renal failure and/or death.

In clinical studies in hypertensive patients with unilateral or bilateral renal artery stenosis, increases in blood urea nitrogen and serum creatinine have been observed in some patients following ACE inhibitor therapy. These increases were almost always reversible upon discontinuation of the ACE inhibitor and/or diuretic therapy. In such patients, renal function should be monitored during the first few weeks of therapy.

Some patients with hypertension or heart failure with no apparent preexisting renal vascular disease have developed increases in blood urea and serum creatinine, usually minor and transient, especially when ACCUPRIL has been given concomitantly with a diuretic. This is more likely to occur in patients with preexisting renal impairment. Dosage reduction and/or discontinuation of any diuretic and/or ACCUPRIL may be required.

Evaluation of patients with hypertension or heart failure should always include assessment of renal function (see DOSAGE AND ADMINISTRATION).

Hyperkalemia and potassium-sparing diuretics: In clinical trials, hyperkalemia (serum potassium ≥5.8 mmol/L) occurred in approximately 2% of patients receiving ACCUPRIL. In most cases, elevated serum potassium levels were isolated values which resolved despite continued therapy. Less than 0.1% of patients discontinued therapy due to hyperkalemia. Risk factors for the development of hyperkalemia include renal insufficiency, diabetes mellitus, and the concomitant use of potassium-sparing diuretics, potassium supplements, and/or potassium-containing salt substitutes,

which should be used cautiously, if at all, with ACCUPRIL (see PRECAUTIONS, Drug Interactions).

Cough: Presumably due to the inhibition of the degradation of endogenous bradykinin, persistent nonproductive cough has been reported with all ACE inhibitors, always resolving after discontinuation of therapy. ACE inhibitor-induced cough should be considered in the differential diagnosis of cough.

Surgery/anesthesia: In patients undergoing major surgery or during anesthesia with agents that produce hypotension, ACCUPRIL will block angiotensin II formation secondary to compensatory renin release. If hypotension occurs and is considered to be due to this mechanism, it can be corrected by volume expansion.

Information for Patients

Pregnancy: Female patients of childbearing age should be told about the consequences of second- and third-trimester exposure to ACE inhibitors, and they should also be told that these consequences do not appear to have resulted from intrauterine ACE-inhibitor exposure that has been limited to the first trimester. These patients should be asked to report pregnancies to their physicians as soon as possible.

Angioedema: Angioedema, including laryngeal edema, can occur with treatment with ACE inhibitors, especially following the first dose. Patients should be so advised and told to report immediately any signs or symptoms suggesting angioedema (swelling of face, extremities, eyes, lips, tongue, difficulty in swallowing or breathing) and to stop taking the drug until they have consulted with their physician (see WARNINGS).

Symptomatic hypotension: Patients should be cautioned that lightheadedness can occur, especially during the first few days of ACCUPRIL therapy, and that it should be reported to a physician. If actual syncope occurs, patients should be told to not take the drug until they have consulted with their physician (see WARNINGS).

All patients should be cautioned that inadequate fluid intake or excessive perspiration, diarrhea, or vomiting can lead to an excessive fall in blood pressure because of reduction in fluid volume, with the same consequences of lightheadedness and possible syncope.

Patients planning to undergo any surgery and/or anesthesia should be told to inform their physician that they are taking an ACE inhibitor.

Hyperkalemia: Patients should be told not to use potassium supplements or salt substitutes containing potassium without consulting their physician (see PRECAUTIONS).

Neutropenia: Patients should be told to report promptly any indication of infection (eg, sore throat, fever) which could be a sign of neutropenia.

NOTE: As with many other drugs, certain advice to patients being treated with ACCUPRIL is warranted. This information is intended to aid in the safe and effective use of this medication. It is not a disclosure of all possible adverse or intended effects.

Drug Interactions

Concomitant diuretic therapy: As with other ACE inhibitors, patients on diuretics, especially those on recently instituted diuretic therapy, may occasionally experience an excessive reduction of blood pressure after initiation of therapy with ACCUPRIL. The possibility of hypotensive effects with ACCUPRIL may be minimized by either discontinuing the diuretic or cautiously increasing salt intake prior to initiation of treatment with ACCUPRIL. If it is not possible to discontinue the diuretic, the starting dose of quinapril should be reduced (see DOSAGE AND ADMINISTRATION).

Agents increasing serum potassium: Quinapril can attenuate potassium loss caused by thiazide diuretics and increase serum potassium when used alone. If concomitant therapy of ACCUPRIL with potassium-sparing diuretics (eg, spironolactone, triamterene, or amiloride), potassium supplements, or potassium-containing salt substitutes is indicated, they should be used with caution along with appropriate monitoring of serum potassium (see PRECAUTIONS).

Tetracycline and other drugs that interact with magnesium: Simultaneous administration of tetracycline with ACCUPRIL reduced the absorption of tetracycline by approximately 28% to 37%, possibly due to the high magnesium content in ACCUPRIL tablets. This interaction should be considered if coprescribing ACCUPRIL and tetracycline or other drugs that interact with magnesium.

Lithium: Increased serum lithium levels and symptoms of lithium toxicity have been reported in patients receiving concomitant lithium and ACE inhibitor therapy. These drugs should be coadministered with caution and frequent monitoring of serum lithium levels is recommended. If a diuretic is also used, it may increase the risk of lithium toxicity.

Other agents: Drug interaction studies of ACCUPRIL with other agents showed:

● Multiple dose therapy with propranolol or cimetidine has no effect on the pharmacokinetics of single doses of ACCUPRIL.

● The anticoagulant effect of a single dose of warfarin (measured by prothrombin time) was not significantly changed by quinapril coadministration twice-daily.

● ACCUPRIL treatment did not affect the pharmacokinetics of digoxin.

● No pharmacokinetic interaction was observed when single doses of ACCUPRIL and hydrochlorothiazide were administered concomitantly.

Carcinogenesis, Mutagenesis, Impairment of Fertility

Quinapril hydrochloride was not carcinogenic in mice or rats when given in doses up to 75 or 100 mg/kg/day (50 to 60 times the maximum human daily dose, respectively, on an mg/kg basis and 3.8 to 10 times the maximum human daily dose when based on an mg/m² basis) for 104 weeks. Female rats given the highest dose level had an increased incidence of mesenteric lymph node hemangiomas and skin/subcutaneous lipomas. Neither quinapril nor quinaprilat were mutagenic in the Ames bacterial assay with or without metabolic activation. Quinapril was also negative in the following genetic toxicology studies: *in vitro* mammalian cell point mutation, sister chromatid exchange in cultured mammalian cells, micronucleus test with mice, *in vitro* chromosome aberration with V79 cultured lung cells, and in an *in vivo* cytogenetic study with rat bone marrow. There were no adverse effects on fertility or reproduction in rats at doses up to 100 mg/kg/day (60 and 10 times the maximum daily human dose when based on mg/kg and mg/m², respectively).

Pregnancy

Pregnancy Categories C (first trimester) and D (second and third trimesters): See WARNINGS, Fetal/Neonatal Morbidity and Mortality.

Nursing Mothers

It is not known if quinapril or its metabolites are secreted in human milk. Quinapril is secreted to a limited extent, however, in milk of lactating rats (5% or less of the plasma drug concentration was found in rat milk). Because many drugs are secreted in human milk, caution should be exercised when ACCUPRIL is given to a nursing mother.

Geriatric Use

Elderly patients exhibited increased area under the plasma concentration time curve (AUC) and peak levels for quinaprilat compared to values observed in younger patients; this appeared to relate to decreased renal function rather than to age itself. In controlled and uncontrolled studies of ACCUPRIL where 918 (21%) patients were 65 years and older, no overall differences in effectiveness or safety were observed between older and younger patients. However, greater sensitivity of some older individual patients cannot be ruled out.

Pediatric Use

The safety and effectiveness of ACCUPRIL in children have not been established.

ADVERSE REACTIONS

Hypertension

ACCUPRIL has been evaluated for safety in 4960 subjects and patients. Of these, 3203 patients, including 655 elderly patients, participated in controlled clinical trials. ACCUPRIL has been evaluated for long-term safety in over 1400 patients treated for 1 year or more.

Adverse experiences were usually mild and transient.

In placebo-controlled trials, discontinuation of therapy because of adverse events was required in 4.7% of patients with hypertension.

Adverse experiences probably or possibly related to therapy or of unknown relationship to therapy occurring in 1% or more of the 1563 patients in placebo-controlled hypertension trials who were treated with ACCUPRIL are shown below.

Adverse Events in Placebo-Controlled Trials

	Accupril (N=1563) Incidence (Discontinuance)	Placebo (N=579) Incidence (Discontinuance)
Headache	5.6 (0.7)	10.9 (0.7)
Dizziness	3.9 (0.8)	2.6 (0.2)
Fatigue	2.6 (0.3)	1.0
Coughing	2.0 (0.5)	0.0
Nausea and/or Vomiting	1.4 (0.3)	1.9 (0.2)
Abdominal Pain	1.0 (0.2)	0.7

Heart Failure

Accupril has been evaluated for safety in 1222 ACCUPRIL treated patients. Of these, 632 patients participated in controlled clinical trials. In placebo-controlled trials, discontinuation of therapy because of adverse events was required in 6.8% of patients with congestive heart failure.

Adverse experiences probably or possibly related or of unknown relationship to therapy occurring in 1% or more of the 585 patients in placebo-controlled congestive heart failure trials who were treated with ACCUPRIL are shown below.

	Accupril (N=585) Incidence (Discontinuance)	Placebo (N=295) Incidence (Discontinuance)
Dizziness	7.7 (0.7)	5.1 (1.0)
Coughing	4.3 (0.3)	1.4
Fatigue	2.6 (0.2)	1.4
Nausea and/or Vomiting	2.4 (0.2)	0.7
Chest Pain	2.4	1.0
Hypotension	2.9 (0.5)	1.0
Dyspnea	1.9 (0.2)	2.0
Diarrhea	1.7	1.0
Headache	1.7	1.0 (0.3)
Myalgia	1.5	2.0
Rash	1.4 (0.2)	1.0
Back Pain	1.2	0.3

See PRECAUTIONS. Cough.

Hypertension and/or Heart Failure

Clinical adverse experiences probably, possibly, or definitely related, or of uncertain relationship to therapy occurring in 0.5% to 1.0% (except as noted) of the patients with CHF or hypertension treated with ACCUPRIL (with or without concomitant diuretic) in controlled or uncontrolled trials (N=4847) and less frequent, clinically significant events seen in clinical trials or post-marketing experience (the rarer events are in italics) include (listed by body system):

General: back pain, malaise, *viral infections*

Cardiovascular: palpitation, vasodilation, tachycardia, *heart failure, hyperkalemia, myocardial infarction, cerebrovascular accident, hypertensive crisis, angina pectoris, orthostatic hypotension, cardiac rhythm disturbances, cardiogenic shock*

Hematology: *hemolytic anemia*

Gastrointestinal: dry mouth or throat, constipation, *gastrointestinal hemorrhage, pancreatitis, abnormal liver function tests*

Nervous/Psychiatric: somnolence, vertigo, syncope, nervousness, depression, insomnia, paresthesia

Integumentary: alopecia, increased sweating, pemphigus, pruritus, *exfoliative dermatitis, photosensitivity reaction, dermatopolymyositis*

Urogenital: impotence, *acute renal failure, worsening renal failure*

Other: amblyopia, pharyngitis, *agranulocytosis, hepatitis, thrombocytopenia*

Fetal/Neonatal Morbidity and Mortality

See WARNINGS, Fetal/Neonatal Morbidity and Mortality.

Angioedema

Angioedema has been reported in patients receiving ACCUPRIL (0.1%). Angioedema associated with laryngeal edema may be fatal. If angioedema of the face, extremities, lips, tongue, glottis, and/or larynx occurs, treatment with ACCUPRIL should be discontinued and appropriate therapy instituted immediately. (See WARNINGS.)

Clinical Laboratory Test Findings

Hematology: (See WARNINGS)

Hyperkalemia: (See PRECAUTIONS)

Creatinine and Blood Urea Nitrogen: Increases (>1.25 times the upper limit of normal) in serum creatinine and blood urea nitrogen were observed in 2% and 2%, respectively, of all patients treated with ACCUPRIL alone. Increases are more likely to occur in patients receiving concomitant diuretic therapy than in those on ACCUPRIL alone. These increases often remit on continued therapy. In controlled studies of heart failure, increases in blood urea nitrogen and serum creatinine were observed in 11% and 8%, respectively, of patients treated with ACCUPRIL; most often these patients were receiving diuretics with or without digitalis.

OVERDOSAGE

No data are available with respect to overdosage in humans. Doses of 1440 to 4280 mg/kg of quinapril cause significant lethality in mice and rats.

The most likely clinical manifestation would be symptoms attributable to severe hypotension.

Laboratory determinations of serum levels of quinapril and its metabolites are not widely available, and such determinations have, in any event, no established role in the management of quinapril overdose.

No data are available to suggest physiological maneuvers (eg, maneuvers to change pH of the urine) that might accelerate elimination of quinapril and its metabolites.

Hemodialysis and peritoneal dialysis have little effect on the elimination of quinapril and quinaprilat. Angiotensin II could presumably serve as a specific antagonist-antidote in the setting of quinapril overdose, but angiotensin II is essentially unavailable outside of scattered research facilities. Because the hypotensive effect of quinapril is achieved through vasodilation and effective hypovolemia, it is reasonable to treat quinapril overdose by infusion of normal saline solution.

DOSAGE AND ADMINISTRATION

Hypertension

Monotherapy: The recommended initial dosage of ACCUPRIL in patients not on diuretics is 10 mg once daily. Dosage should be adjusted according to blood pressure response measured at peak (2–6 hours after dosing) and trough (predosing). Generally, dosage adjustments should be made at intervals of at least 2 weeks. Most patients have required dosages of 20, 40, or 80 mg/day, given as a single dose or in two equally divided doses. In some patients treated once daily, the antihypertensive effect may diminish toward the end of the dosing interval. In such patients an increase in dosage or twice daily administration may be warranted. In general, doses of 40–80 mg and divided doses give a somewhat greater effect at the end of the dosing interval.

Concomitant Diuretics: If blood pressure is not adequately controlled with ACCUPRIL monotherapy, a diuretic may be added. In patients who are currently being treated with a diuretic, symptomatic hypotension occasionally can occur following the initial dose of ACCUPRIL. To reduce the likelihood of hypotension, the diuretic should, if possible, be discontinued 2 to 3 days prior to beginning therapy with ACCUPRIL (see WARNINGS). Then, if blood pressure is not controlled with ACCUPRIL alone, diuretic therapy should be resumed.

If the diuretic cannot be discontinued, an initial dose of 5 mg ACCUPRIL should be used with careful medical supervision for several hours and until blood pressure has stabilized. The dosage should subsequently be titrated (as described above) to the optimal response (see WARNINGS, PRECAUTIONS, and Drug Interactions).

Renal Impairment: Kinetic data indicate that the apparent elimination half-life of quinaprilat increases as creatinine clearance decreases. Recommended starting doses, based on clinical and pharmacokinetic data from patients with renal impairment, are as follows:

Creatinine Clearance	Maximum Recommend Initial Dose
>60 mL/min	10 mg
30–60 mL/min	5 mg
10–30 mL/min	2.5 mg
<10 mL/min	Insufficient data for dosage recommendation

Patients should subsequently have their dosage titrated (as described above) to the optimal response.

Elderly (≥65 years): The recommended initial dosage of ACCUPRIL in elderly patients is 10 mg given once daily followed by titration (as described above) to the optimal response.

Heart Failure

ACCUPRIL is indicated as adjunctive therapy when added to conventional therapy including diuretics and/or digitalis. The recommended starting dose is 5 mg twice daily. This dose may improve symptoms of heart failure, but increases in exercise duration have generally required higher doses. Therefore, if the initial dosage of ACCUPRIL is well tolerated, patients should then be titrated at weekly intervals until an effective dose, usually 20 to 40 mg daily given in two equally divided doses, is reached or undesirable hypotension, orthostasis, or azotemia (see WARNINGS) prohibit reaching this dose.

Following the initial dose of ACCUPRIL, the patient should be observed under medical supervision for at least two hours for the presence of hypotension or orthostasis and, if present, until blood pressure stabilizes. The appearance of hypotension, orthostasis, or azotemia early in dose titration should not preclude further careful dose titration. Consideration should be given to reducing the dose of concomitant diuretics.

DOSE ADJUSTMENTS IN PATIENTS WITH HEART FAILURE AND RENAL IMPAIRMENT OR HYPONATREMIA

Pharmacokinetic data indicate that quinapril elimination is dependent on level of renal function. In patients with heart failure and renal impairment, the recommended initial dose of ACCUPRIL is 5 mg in patients with a creatinine clearance above 30 mL/min and 2.5 mg in patients with a creatinine clearance of 10 to 30 mL/min. There is insufficient data for dosage recommendation in patients with a creatinine clearance less than 10 mL/min. (SEE DOSAGE AND ADMINISTRATION, Heart Failure, WARNINGS, and PRECAUTIONS, Drug Interactions.)

If the initial dose is well tolerated, ACCUPRIL may be administered the following day as a twice daily regimen. In the absence of excessive hypotension or significant deterioration of renal function, the dose may be increased at weekly intervals based on clinical and hemodynamic response.

HOW SUPPLIED

ACCUPRIL tablets are supplied as follows:

5-mg tablets: brown, film-coated, elliptical, scored tablets, coded "PD 527" on one side and "5" on the other.
N0071-0527-23 bottles of 90 tablets
N0071-0527-40 10 × 10 unit dose blisters

10-mg tablets: brown, film-coated, triangular tablets, coded "PD 530" on one side and "10" on the other.
N0071-0530-23 bottles of 90 tablets
N0071-0530-40 10 × 10 unit dose blisters

20-mg tablets: brown, film-coated, round tablets, coded "PD 532" on one side and "20" on the other.
N0071-0532-23 bottles of 90 tablets
N0071-0532-40 10 × 10 unit dose blisters

40-mg tablets: brown, film-coated, elliptical tablets, coded "PD 535" on one side and "40" on the other.
N0071-0535-23 bottles of 90 tablets

Dispense in well-closed containers as defined in the USP.

Storage: Store at controlled room temperature 15°–30°C (59°–86°F). Protect from light.

Caution—Federal law prohibits dispensing without prescription.

© 1996, Warner-Lambert Co.

Revised March 1996

PARKE-DAVIS
Div of Warner-Lambert Co
Morris Plains, NJ 07950 USA
Revised October 1994   0527G073

Shown in Product Identification Guide, page 327

ANUSOL–HC® 2.5%   ℞
(Hydrocortisone Cream, USP)

Caution—Federal law prohibits dispensing without prescription.

DESCRIPTION

The topical corticosteroids constitute a class of primarily synthetic steroids used as antiinflammatory and antipruritic agents. Anusol-HC 2.5% (Hydrocortisone Cream, USP) is a topical corticosteroid with hydrocortisone 2.5% (active ingredient) in a water-washable cream containing the following inactive ingredients: benzyl alcohol, petrolatum, stearyl alcohol, propylene glycol, isopropyl myristate, polyoxyl 40 stearate, carbomer 934, sodium lauryl sulfate, edetate disodium, sodium hydroxide to adjust the pH, and purified water.

Hydrocortisone has the chemical name Pregn-4-ene-3,20-dione, 11,17,21, trihydroxy-,(11β).

MOLECULAR FORMULA $C_{21}H_{30}O_5$
MOLECULAR WEIGHT 362.47
CAS REGISTRY NUMBER 50-23-7

CLINICAL PHARMACOLOGY

Topical corticosteroids share antiinflammatory, antipruritic and vasoconstrictive actions.

The mechanism of antiinflammatory activity of the topical corticosteroids is unclear. Various laboratory methods, including vasoconstrictor assays, are used to compare and predict potencies and/or clinical efficacies of the topical corticosteroids. There is some evidence to suggest that a recognizable correlation exists between vasoconstrictor potency and therapeutic efficacy in man.

Pharmacokinetics: The extent of percutaneous absorption of topical corticosteroids is determined by many factors including the vehicle, the integrity of the epidermal barrier, and the use of occlusive dressings.

Topical corticosteroids can be absorbed from normal intact skin. Inflammation and/or other disease processes in the skin increase percutaneous absorption. Occlusive dressings substantially increase the percutaneous absorption of topical corticosteroids. Thus, occlusive dressings may be a valuable therapeutic adjunct for treatment of resistant dermatoses (see DOSAGE AND ADMINISTRATION).

Once absorbed through the skin, topical corticosteroids are handled through pharmacokinetic pathways similar to systemically administered corticosteroids. Corticosteroids are bound to plasma proteins in varying degrees. Corticosteroids are metabolized primarily in the liver and are then excreted by the kidneys. Some of the topical corticosteroids and their metabolites are also excreted into the bile.

INDICATIONS AND USAGE

Topical corticosteroids are indicated for the relief of the inflammatory and pruritic manifestations of corticosteroid-responsive dermatoses.

Continued on next page

This product information was prepared in August 1996. On these and other Parke-Davis Products, information may be obtained by addressing PARKE-DAVIS, Division of Warner-Lambert Company, Morris Plains, New Jersey 07950.

Parke-Davis—Cont.

CONTRAINDICATIONS
Topical corticosteroids are contraindicated in those patients with a history of hypersensitivity to any of the components of the preparation.

PRECAUTIONS
General: Systemic absorption of topical corticosteroids has produced reversible hypothalamic-pituitary-adrenal (HPA) axis suppression, manifestations of Cushing's syndrome, hyperglycemia, and glucosuria in some patients.

Conditions which augment systemic absorption include the application of the more potent steroids, use over large surface areas, prolonged use, and the addition of occlusive dressings.

If HPA axis suppression is noted (by using the urinary free cortisol and ACTH stimulation tests) an attempt should be made to withdraw the drug or to reduce the frequency of application.

Recovery of HPA axis function is generally prompt and complete upon discontinuation of the drug. Infrequently, signs and symptoms of steroid withdrawal may occur, requiring supplemental systemic corticosteroids.

Children may absorb proportionally larger amounts of topical corticosteroids and thus be more susceptible to systemic toxicity (see PRECAUTIONS—Pediatric Use).

If irritation develops, topical corticosteroids should be discontinued and appropriate therapy instituted. In the presence of dermatological infections, the use of an appropriate antifungal or antibacterial agent should be instituted. If a favorable response does not occur promptly, the corticosteroid should be discontinued until the infection has been adequately controlled.

Information for the Patient: Patients using topical corticosteroids should receive the following information and instructions:

1. This medication is to be used as directed by the physician. It is for external use only. Avoid contact with the eyes.
2. Patients should be advised not to use this medication for any disorder other than for which it has been prescribed.
3. The treated skin area should not be bandaged or otherwise covered or wrapped as to be occlusive unless directed by the physician.
4. Patients should report any signs of local adverse reactions especially under occlusive dressing.
5. Parents of pediatric patients should be advised not to use tight-fitting diapers or plastic pants on a child being treated in the diaper area, as these garments may constitute occlusive dressings.

Laboratory Tests: The urinary free cortisol test and the ACTH stimulation test may be helpful in evaluating the HPA axis suppression.

Carcinogenesis, Mutagenesis, and Impairment of Fertility: Long-term animal studies have not been performed to evaluate the carcinogenic potential or the effect on fertility of topical corticosteroids. Studies to determine mutagenicity with hydrocortisone have revealed negative results.

Pregnancy Category C: Corticosteroids are generally teratogenic in laboratory animals when administered systemically at relatively low dosage levels. The more potent corticosteroids have been shown to be teratogenic after dermal application in laboratory animals. There are no adequate and well-controlled studies in pregnant women on teratogenic effects from topically applied corticosteroids.

Therefore, topical corticosteroids should be used during pregnancy only if the potential benefit justifies the potential risk to the fetus. Drugs of this class should not be used extensively on pregnant patients, in large amounts, or for prolonged periods of time.

Nursing Mothers: It is not known whether topical administration of corticosteroids could result in sufficient systemic absorption to produce detectable quantities in breast milk. Systemically administered corticosteroids are secreted into breast milk in quantities not likely to have a deleterious effect on the infant. Nevertheless, caution should be exercised when topical corticosteroids are administered to a nursing woman.

Pediatric Use: PEDIATRIC PATIENTS MAY DEMONSTRATE GREATER SUSCEPTIBILITY TO TOPICAL CORTICOSTEROID-INDUCED HPA AXIS SUPPRESSION AND CUSHING'S SYNDROME THAN MATURE PATIENTS BECAUSE OF A LARGER SKIN SURFACE AREA TO BODY WEIGHT RATIO.

Hypothalamic-pituitary-adrenal (HPA) axis suppression, Cushing's syndrome, and intracranial hypertension have been reported in children receiving topical corticosteroids. Manifestations of adrenal suppression in children include linear growth retardation, delayed weight gain, low plasma cortisol levels, and absence of response to ACTH stimulation. Manifestations of intracranial hypertension include bulging fontanelles, headaches, and bilateral papilledema.

Administration of topical corticosteroids to children should be limited to the least amount compatible with an effective therapeutic regimen. Chronic corticosteroid therapy may interfere with the growth and development of children.

ADVERSE REACTIONS
The following local adverse reactions are reported infrequently with topical corticosteroids, but may occur more frequently with the use of occlusive dressings. These reactions are listed in an approximate decreasing order of occurrence:

Burning
Itching
Irritation
Dryness
Folliculitis
Hypertrichosis
Acneiform eruptions
Hypopigmentation
Perioral dermatitis
Allergic contact dermatitis
Maceration of the skin
Secondary infection
Skin atrophy
Striae
Miliaria

OVERDOSAGE
Topically applied corticosteroids can be absorbed in sufficient amounts to produce systemic effects. (See PRECAUTIONS).

DOSAGE AND ADMINISTRATION
Anusol-HC 2.5% (Hydrocortisone Cream, USP) should be applied to the affected area two to four times daily depending on the severity of the condition.

Occlusive dressings may be used for the management of psoriasis or recalcitrant conditions. If an infection develops, the use of occlusive dressings should be discontinued and appropriate antimicrobial therapy instituted.

HOW SUPPLIED
Anusol-HC 2.5% (Hydrocortisone Cream, USP) is supplied in 30 gram tubes (N 0071-3131-13).

Store at controlled room temperature 15°–30°C (59°–86°F). Store away from heat. Protect from freezing.
Revised July 1993
Manufactured by
Allergan Herbert
Skin Care Division of Allergan, Inc.
Irvine, CA 92713 USA
Distributed by
PARKE-DAVIS
Div of Warner-Lambert Co   70221 30-6/S
Morris Plains, NJ 07950 USA   **3131G012**
Shown in Product Identification Guide, page 327

ANUSOL–HC® 25–mg SUPPOSITORIES   ℞
[ăn 'ū-sōl ″]
(Hydrocortisone Acetate)

DESCRIPTION
Each Anusol-HC 25-mg Suppository contains 25 mg hydrocortisone acetate in a hydrogenated cocoglyceride base. Hydrocortisone acetate is a corticosteroid. Chemically, hydrocortisone acetate is pregn-4-ene-3,20-dione, 21-(acetyloxy)-11,17-dihydroxy-,(11β)-.

CLINICAL PHARMACOLOGY
In normal subjects, about 26 percent of hydrocortisone acetate is absorbed when the hydrocortisone acetate suppository is applied to the rectum. Absorption of hydrocortisone acetate may vary across abraded or inflamed surfaces.

Topical steroids are primarily effective because of their anti-inflammatory, antipruritic and vasoconstrictive action.

INDICATIONS AND USAGE
For use in inflamed hemorrhoids, post irradiation (factitial) proctitis, as an adjunct in the treatment of chronic ulcerative colitis, cryptitis, other inflammatory conditions of the anorectum, and pruritus ani.

CONTRAINDICATION
Anusol-HC suppositories are contraindicated in those patients with a history of hypersensitivity to any of the components.

PRECAUTIONS
Do not use unless adequate proctologic examination is made. If irritation develops, the product should be discontinued and appropriate therapy instituted.

In the presence of an infection, the use of an appropriate antifungal or antibacterial agent should be instituted. If a favorable response does not occur promptly, the corticosteroid should be discontinued until the infection has been adequately controlled.

No long-term studies in animals have been performed to evaluate the carcinogenic potential of corticosteroid suppositories.

Information for Patients
Staining of fabric may occur with use of the suppository. Precautionary measures are recommended.

Pregnancy Category C
In laboratory animals, topical steroids have been associated with an increase in the incidence of fetal abnormalities when gestating females have been exposed to rather low dosage levels. There are no adequate and well-controlled studies in pregnant women. Anusol-HC suppositories should only be used during pregnancy if the potential benefit justifies the risk to the fetus. Drugs of this class should not be used extensively on pregnant patients, in large amounts, or for prolonged periods of time.

It is not known whether this drug is excreted in human milk, and because many drugs are excreted in human milk and because of the potential for serious adverse reactions in nursing infants from Anusol-HC suppositories, a decision should be made whether to discontinue nursing or to discontinue the drug, taking into account the importance of the drug to the mother.

ADVERSE REACTIONS
The following local adverse reactions have been reported with corticosteroid suppositories:

1. Burning
2. Itching
3. Irritation
4. Dryness
5. Folliculitis
6. Hypopigmentation
7. Allergic Contact Dermatitis
8. Secondary infection

DRUG ABUSE AND DEPENDENCE
Drug abuse and dependence have not been reported in patients treated with Anusol-HC suppositories.

OVERDOSAGE
If signs and symptoms of systemic overdosage occur discontinue use.

DOSAGE AND ADMINISTRATION
Usual dosage: One suppository in the rectum morning and night for two weeks in nonspecific proctitis. In more severe cases, one suppository three times daily; or two suppositories twice daily. In factitial proctitis, recommended therapy is six to eight weeks or less, according to response.

OPENING INSTRUCTIONS

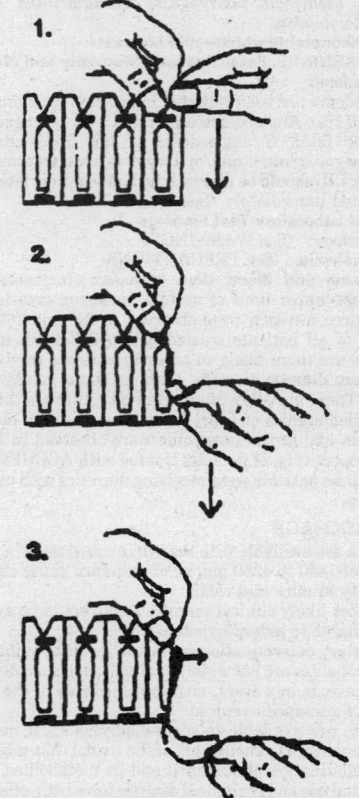

Avoid excessive handling of the suppository. It is designed to melt at body temperature.
1. Tear at the "V" cut and peel the foil in a downward motion.
2. Continue tearing downward to almost the full length of the suppository.
3. Gently remove the suppository from the foil packet.

HOW SUPPLIED

Anusol-HC 25-mg Suppositories are off-white, smooth surfaced, rod shaped with one rounded end. Package of 12 suppositories (N0071-1726-07) and package of 24 suppositories (N0071-1726-13).
Store below 30° C (86° F). Protect from freezing.
Revised September 1993
Caution—Federal law prohibits dispensing without prescription.
Manufactured by: ABLE LABORATORIES, INC.
South Plainfield, NJ 07080
For PARKE-DAVIS
Div. of Warner-Lambert Co.
Morris Plains, NJ 07950 USA
Manufacturer's Code 53265   1726G061
Shown in Product Identification Guide, page 327

BENADRYL®   ℞

[bĕ′nă-dril]
(Diphenhydramine Hydrochloride Injection, USP)

DESCRIPTION

Benadryl (diphenhydramine hydrochloride) is an antihistamine drug having the chemical name 2-(Diphenylmethoxy)-N, N-dimethylethylamine hydrochloride. It occurs as a white, crystalline powder, is freely soluble in water and alcohol and has a molecular weight of 291.82. The molecular formula is $C_{17}H_{21}NO \cdot HCl$.
Benadryl in the parenteral form is a sterile, pyrogen-free solution available in a concentration of 50 mg of diphenhydramine hydrochloride per mL. The solutions for parenteral use have been adjusted to a pH between 5.0 and 6.0 with either sodium hydroxide or hydrochloric acid. The multidose Steri-Vials® contain 0.1 mg/mL benzethonium chloride as a germicidal agent.

CLINICAL PHARMACOLOGY

Diphenhydramine hydrochloride is an antihistamine with anticholinergic (drying) and sedative side effects. Antihistamines appear to compete with histamine for cell receptor sites on effector cells.
Benadryl in the injectable form has a rapid onset of action. Diphenhydramine hydrochloride is widely distributed throughout the body, including the CNS. A portion of the drug is excreted unchanged in the urine, while the rest is metabolized via the liver. Detailed information on the pharmacokinetics of Diphenhydramine Hydrochloride Injection is not available.

INDICATIONS AND USAGE

Benadryl in the injectable form is effective for the following conditions when Benadryl in the oral form is impractical.
Antihistaminic: For amelioration of allergic reactions to blood or plasma, in anaphylaxis as an adjunct to epinephrine and other standard measures after the acute symptoms have been controlled, and for other uncomplicated allergic conditions of the immediate type when oral therapy is impossible or contraindicated.
Motion Sickness: For active treatment of motion sickness.
Antiparkinsonism: For use in parkinsonism, when oral therapy is impossible or contraindicated, as follows: parkinsonism in the elderly who are unable to tolerate more potent agents, mild cases of parkinsonism in other age groups, and in other cases of parkinsonism in combination with centrally acting anticholinergic agents.

CONTRAINDICATIONS

Use in Newborn or Premature Infants
This drug should *not* be used in newborn or premature infants.

Use in Nursing Mothers
Because of the higher risk of antihistamines for infants generally, and for newborns and prematures in particular, antihistamine therapy is contraindicated in nursing mothers.

Use as a Local Anesthetic
Because of the risk of local necrosis, this drug should not be used as a local anesthetic.

Antihistamines are also contraindicated in the following conditions:
Hypersensitivity to diphenhydramine hydrochloride and other antihistamines of similar chemical structure.

WARNINGS

Antihistamines should be used with considerable caution in patients with narrow-angle glaucoma, stenosing peptic ulcer, pyloroduodenal obstruction, symptomatic prostatic hypertrophy, or bladder-neck obstruction.

Use in Children
In infants and children, especially, antihistamines in *overdosage* may cause hallucinations, convulsions, or death.

As in adults, antihistamines may diminish mental alertness in children. In the young child, particularly, they may produce excitation.
Use in the Elderly (approximately 60 years or older)
Antihistamines are more likely to cause dizziness, sedation, and hypotension in elderly patients.

PRECAUTIONS

General: Diphenhydramine hydrochloride has an atropine-like action and, therefore, should be used with caution in patients with a history of bronchial asthma, increased intraocular pressure, hyperthyroidism, cardiovascular disease or hypertension. Use with caution in patients with lower respiratory disease including asthma.
Information for Patients: Patients taking diphenhydramine hydrochloride should be advised that this drug may cause drowsiness and has an additive effect with alcohol. Patients should be warned about engaging in activities requiring mental alertness such as driving a car or operating appliances, machinery, etc.
Drug Interactions: Diphenhydramine hydrochloride has additive effects with alcohol and other CNS depressants (hypnotics, sedatives, tranquilizers, etc.).
MAO inhibitors prolong and intensify the anticholinergic (drying) effects of antihistamines.
Carcinogenesis, Mutagenesis, Impairment of Fertility: Long-term studies in animals to determine mutagenic and carcinogenic potential have not been performed.
Pregnancy: Pregnancy Category B. Reproduction studies have been performed in rats and rabbits at doses up to 5 times the human dose and have revealed no evidence of impaired fertility or harm to the fetus due to diphenhydramine hydrochloride. There are, however, no adequate and well-controlled studies in pregnant women. Because animal reproduction studies are not always predictive of human response, this drug should be used during pregnancy only if clearly needed.

ADVERSE REACTIONS

The most frequent adverse reactions are underscored.
1. *General:* Urticaria, drug rash, anaphylactic shock, photosensitivity, excessive perspiration, chills, dryness of mouth, nose, and throat
2. *Cardiovascular System:* Hypotension, headache, palpitations, tachycardia, extrasystoles
3. *Hematologic System:* Hemolytic anemia, thrombocytopenia, agranulocytosis
4. *Nervous System:* Sedation, sleepiness, dizziness, disturbed coordination, fatigue, confusion, restlessness, excitation, nervousness, tremor, irritability, insomnia, euphoria, paresthesia, blurred vision, diplopia, vertigo, tinnitus, acute labyrinthitis, neuritis, convulsions
5. *GI System:* Epigastric distress, anorexia, nausea, vomiting, diarrhea, constipation
6. *GU System:* Urinary frequency, difficult urination, urinary retention, early menses
7. *Respiratory System:* Thickening of bronchial secretions, tightness of chest and wheezing, nasal stuffiness

OVERDOSAGE

Antihistamine overdosage reactions may vary from central nervous system depression to stimulation. Stimulation is particularly likely in children. Atropine-like signs and symptoms, dry mouth; fixed, dilated pupils; flushing, and gastrointestinal symptoms may also occur.
Stimulants should not be used.
Vasopressors may be used to treat hypotension.

DOSAGE AND ADMINISTRATION

Benadryl in the injectable form is indicated when the oral form is impractical.
Parenteral drug products should be inspected visually for particulate matter and discoloration prior to administration, whenever solution and container permit.
DOSAGE SHOULD BE INDIVIDUALIZED ACCORDING TO THE NEEDS AND THE RESPONSE OF THE PATIENT.
Children: 5 mg/kg/24 hr or 150 mg/m²/24 hr. Maximum daily dosage is 300 mg. Divide into four doses, administered intravenously or deeply intramuscularly.
Adults: 10 to 50 mg intravenously or deeply intramuscularly; 100 mg if required; maximum daily dosage is 400 mg.

HOW SUPPLIED

Benadryl in parenteral form is supplied as:
Benadryl Steri-Vials®—Sterile, pyrogen-free solution containing 50 mg diphenhydramine hydrochloride in each milliliter of solution with 0.1 mg/mL benzethonium chloride as a germicidal agent. Available in 10-mL (N-0071-4402-10) Steri-Vials.
Benadryl Steri-Dose®—sterile, pyrogen-free solution containing 50 mg diphenhydramine hydrochloride in a 1-mL disposable syringe (Steri-Dose). Available in packages of ten syringes (N 0071-4259-45).
Benadryl Ampoule—sterile, pyrogen-free solution containing 50 mg diphenhydramine hydrochloride in a 1-mL ampoule. Available in packages of ten (N 0071-4259-03).

WARNING: Manufactured with CFC-12, a substance which harms public health and environment by destroying ozone in the upper atmosphere.

STORAGE CONDITIONS

Store at controlled room temperature 15°–30°C (59°–86°F). Protect from freezing and light.
Caution—Federal law prohibits dispensing without prescription.
Revised January 1996   4259G440
                                              129

CELONTIN® KAPSEALS®   ℞

[cĕ″lŏn′tĭn]
(methsuximide capsules, USP)

DESCRIPTION

Celontin (methsuximide) is an anticonvulsant succinimide, chemically designated as N,2-Dimethyl-2-phenylsuccinimide.
Each Celontin capsule contains 150 mg or 300 mg methsuximide, USP. Also contains starch, NF. The capsule and band contain citric acid, USP; colloidal silicon dioxide, NF; D&C yellow No. 10; FD&C red No. 3; FD&C yellow No. 6 (Sunset Yellow); gelatin, NF; glyceryl monooleate; sodium benzoate, NF; sodium lauryl sulfate NF. The 150-mg capsule and band also contain FD&C blue No. 1; titanium dioxide, USP. The 300-mg capsule and band also contain polyethylene glycol 200.

ACTION

Methsuximide suppresses the paroxysmal three cycle per second spike and wave activity associated with lapses of consciousness which is common in absence (petit mal) seizures. The frequency of epileptiform attacks is reduced, apparently by depression of the motor cortex and elevation of the threshold of the central nervous system to convulsive stimuli.

INDICATION

Celontin is indicated for the control of absence (petit mal) seizures that are refractory to other drugs.

CONTRAINDICATION

Methsuximide should not be used in patients with a history of hypersensitivity to succinimides.

WARNINGS

Blood dyscrasias, including some with fatal outcome, have been reported to be associated with the use of succinimides; therefore, periodic blood counts should be performed. Should signs and/or symptoms of infection (eg sore throat, fever) develop, blood counts should be considered at that point.
It has been reported that succinimides have produced morphological and functional changes in animal liver. For this reason, methsuximide should be administered with extreme caution to patients with known liver or renal disease. Periodic urinalysis and liver function studies are advised for all patients receiving the drug.
Cases of systemic lupus erythematosus have been reported with the use of succinimides. The physician should be alert to this possibility.

USAGE IN PREGNANCY

Reports suggest an association between the use of anticonvulsant drugs by women with epilepsy and an elevated incidence of birth defects in children born to these women. Data are more extensive with respect to phenytoin and phenobarbital, but these are also the most commonly prescribed anticonvulsants; less systematic or anecdotal reports suggest a possible similar association with the use of all known anticonvulsant drugs.
The reports suggesting an elevated incidence of birth defects in children of drug-treated epileptic women cannot be regarded as adequate to prove a definite cause and effect relationship. There are intrinsic methodologic problems in obtaining adequate data on drug teratogenicity in humans; the possibility also exists that other factors, eg, genetic factors or the epileptic condition itself, may be more important than drug therapy in leading to birth defects. The great majority of mothers on anticonvulsant medication deliver normal infants. It is important to note that anticonvulsant drugs should not be discontinued in patients in whom the drug is administered to prevent major seizures because of the strong possibility of precipitating status epilepticus with attendant hypoxia and threat to life. In individual cases where the severity and frequency of the seizure disorder are such that the removal of medication does not pose a serious threat to the

Continued on next page

This product information was prepared in August 1996. On these and other Parke-Davis Products, information may be obtained by addressing PARKE-DAVIS, Division of Warner-Lambert Company, Morris Plains, New Jersey 07950.

Parke-Davis—Cont.

patient, discontinuation of the drug may be considered prior to and during pregnancy, although it cannot be said with any confidence that even minor seizures do not pose some hazard to the developing embryo or fetus.

The prescribing physician will wish to weigh these considerations in treating or counseling epileptic women of childbearing potential.

PRECAUTIONS

General:

It is recommended that the physician withdraw the drug slowly on the appearance of unusual depression, aggressiveness, or other behavioral alterations.

As with other anticonvulsants, it is important to proceed slowly when increasing or decreasing dosage, as well as when adding or eliminating other medication. Abrupt withdrawal of anticonvulsant medication may precipitate absence (petit mal) status.

Methsuximide, when used alone in mixed types of epilepsy, may increase the frequency of grand mal seizures in some patients.

Information for Patients:

Methsuximide may impair the mental and/or physical abilities required for the performance of potentially hazardous tasks, such as driving a motor vehicle or other such activity requiring alertness, therefore, the patient should be cautioned accordingly.

Patients taking methsuximide should be advised of the importance of adhering strictly to the prescribed dosage regimen.

Patients should be instructed to promptly contact their physician if they develop signs and/or symptoms suggesting an infection (eg sore throat, fever).

ADVICE TO THE PHARMACIST AND PATIENT: Since methsuximide has a relatively low melting temperature (124°F), storage conditions which may promote high temperatures (closed cars, delivery vans, or storage near steam pipes) should be avoided. Do not dispense or use capsules that are not full or in which contents have melted. Effectiveness may be reduced. Protect from excessive heat (104°F).

Drug Interactions:

Since Celontin (methsuximide) may interact with concurrently administered antiepileptic drugs, periodic serum level determinations of these drugs may be necessary (eg methsuximide may increase the plasma concentrations of phenytoin and phenobarbital).

Pregnancy:

See WARNINGS.

ADVERSE REACTIONS

Gastrointestinal System: Gastrointestinal symptoms occur frequently and have included nausea or vomiting, anorexia, diarrhea, weight loss, epigastric and abdominal pain, and constipation.

Hemopoietic System: Hemopoietic complications associated with the administration of methsuximide have included eosinophilia, leukopenia, monocytosis, and pancytopenia with or without bone marrow suppression.

Nervous System: Neurologic and sensory reactions reported during therapy with methsuximide have included drowsiness, ataxia or dizziness, irritability and nervousness, headache, blurred vision, photophobia, hiccups, and insomnia. Drowsiness, ataxia, and dizziness have been the most frequent side effects noted. Psychologic abnormalities have included confusion, instability, mental slowness, depression, hypochondriacal behavior, and aggressiveness. There have been rare reports of psychosis, suicidal behavior, and auditory hallucinations.

Integumentary System: Dermatologic manifestations which have occurred with the administration of methsuximide have included urticaria, Stevens-Johnson syndrome, and pruritic erythematous rashes.

Cardiovascular: Hyperemia.

Genitourinary system: Proteinuria, microscopic hematuria

Body as a Whole: Periorbital edema.

OVERDOSAGE

Acute overdoses may produce nausea, vomiting, and CNS depression including coma with respiratory depression. Methsuximide poisoning may follow a biphasic course. Following an initial comatose state, patients have awakened and then relapsed into a coma within 24 hours. It is believed that an active metabolite of methsuximide, N-desmethylmethsuximide, is responsible for this biphasic profile. It is important to follow plasma levels of N-desmethylmethsuximide in methsuximide poisonings. Levels greater than 40 µg/mL have caused toxicity and coma has been seen at levels of 150 µg/mL.

Treatment:

Treatment should include emesis (unless the patient is or could rapidly become obtunded, comatose, or convulsing) or gastric lavage, activated charcoal, cathartics, and general supportive measures. Charcoal hemoperfusion may be useful in removing the N-desmethyl metabolite of methsuximide. Forced diuresis and exchange transfusions are ineffective.

DOSAGE AND ADMINISTRATION

Optimum dosage of Celontin must be determined by trial. A suggested dosage schedule is 300 mg per day for the first week. If required, dosage may be increased thereafter at weekly intervals by 300 mg per day for the three weeks following to a daily dosage of 1.2 g. Because therapeutic effect and tolerance vary among patients, therapy with Celontin must be individualized according to the response of each patient. Optimal dosage is that amount of Celontin which is barely sufficient to control seizures so that side effects may be kept to a minimum. The smaller capsule (150 mg) facilitates administration to small children.

Celontin may be administered in combination with other anticonvulsants when other forms of epilepsy coexist with absence (petit mal).

HOW SUPPLIED

N 0071-0525-24 (P-D 525)—Celontin Kapseals, #1 capsule each containing 300 mg methsuximide; bottles of 100.

N 0071-0537-24 (P-D 537)—Celontin Kapseals, Half Strength, #4 capsule each containing 150 mg methsuximide, bottles of 100.

Store at controlled room temperature 15°–30°C (59°–86°F).
Protect from light and moisture.

Protect from excessive heat (104°F).

CAUTION—Federal law prohibits dispensing without prescription.

©1995 Warner-Lambert Co.

Revised May 1995 0537G091

Shown in Product Identification Guide, page 327

CEREBYX® ℞

(Fosphenytoin Sodium Injection)

DESCRIPTION

Cerebyx® (fosphenytoin sodium injection) is a prodrug intended for parenteral administration; its active metabolite is phenytoin. Each Cerebyx vial contains 75 mg/mL fosphenytoin sodium (hereafter referred to as fosphenytoin) **equivalent to 50 mg/mL phenytoin sodium** after administration. Cerebyx is supplied in vials as a ready-mixed solution in Water for Injection, USP, and Tromethamine, USP (TRIS), buffer adjusted to pH 8.6 to 9.0 with either Hydrochloric Acid, NF, or Sodium Hydroxide, NF. Cerebyx is a clear, colorless to pale yellow, sterile solution.

The chemical name of fosphenytoin is 5,5-diphenyl-3-[(phosphonooxy)methyl]-2,4-imidazolidinedione disodium salt. The molecular structure of fosphenytoin is:

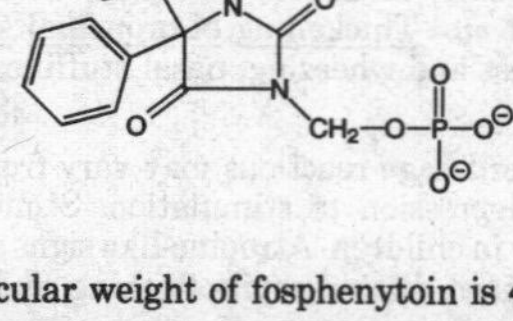

The molecular weight of fosphenytoin is 406.24.

IMPORTANT NOTE: Throughout all Cerebyx® product labeling, the amount and concentration of fosphenytoin is expressed in terms of phenytoin sodium equivalents (PE). Fosphenytoin's weight is expressed as phenytoin sodium equivalents to avoid the need to perform molecular weight-based adjustments when converting between fosphenytoin and phenytoin sodium doses. Cerebyx should always be prescribed and dispensed in phenytoin sodium equivalent units (PE) (see DOSAGE AND ADMINISTRATION).

CLINICAL PHARMACOLOGY

Introduction

Following parenteral administration of Cerebyx, fosphenytoin is converted to the anticonvulsant phenytoin. For every mmol of fosphenytoin administered, one mmol of phenytoin is produced. The pharmacological and toxicological effects of fosphenytoin include those of phenytoin. However, the hydrolysis of fosphenytoin to phenytoin yields two metabolites, phosphate and formaldehyde. Formaldehyde is subsequently converted to formate, which is in turn metabolized via a folate dependent mechanism. Although phosphate and formaldehyde (formate) have potentially important biological effects, these effects typically occur at concentrations considerably in excess of those obtained when Cerebyx is administered under conditions of use recommended in this labeling.

Mechanism of Action

Fosphenytoin is a prodrug of phenytoin and accordingly, its anticonvulsant effects are attributable to phenytoin.

After IV administration to mice, fosphenytoin blocked the tonic phase of maximal electroshock seizures at doses equivalent to those effective for phenytoin. In addition to its ability to suppress maximal electroshock seizures in mice and rats, phenytoin exhibits anticonvulsant activity against kindled seizures in rats, audiogenic seizures in mice, and seizures produced by electrical stimulation of the brainstem in rats. The cellular mechanisms of phenytoin thought to be responsible for its anticonvulsant actions include modulation of voltage-dependent sodium channels of neurons, inhibition of calcium flux across neuronal membranes, modulation of voltage-dependent calcium channels of neurons, and enhancement of the sodium-potassium ATPase activity of neurons and glial cells. The modulation of sodium channels may be a primary anticonvulsant mechanism because this property is shared with several other anticonvulsants in addition to phenytoin.

Pharmacokinetics and Drug Metabolism

Fosphenytoin

Absorption/Bioavailability: *Intravenous:* When Cerebyx is administered by IV infusion, maximum plasma fosphenytoin concentrations are achieved at the end of the infusion. Fosphenytoin has a half-life of approximately 15 minutes.

Intramuscular: Fosphenytoin is completely bioavailable following IM administration of Cerebyx. Peak concentrations occur at approximately 30 minutes postdose. Plasma fosphenytoin concentrations following IM administration are lower but more sustained than those following IV administration due to the time required for absorption of fosphenytoin from the injection site.

Distribution: Fosphenytoin is extensively bound (95% to 99%) to human plasma proteins, primarily albumin. Binding to plasma proteins is saturable with the result that the percent bound decreases as total fosphenytoin concentrations increase. Fosphenytoin displaces phenytoin from protein binding sites. The volume of distribution of fosphenytoin increases with Cerebyx dose and rate. and ranges from 4.3 to 10.8 liters.

Metabolism and Elimination: The conversion half-life of fosphenytoin to phenytoin is approximately 15 minutes. The mechanism of fosphenytoin conversion has not been determined, but phosphatases probably play a major role. Fosphenytoin is not excreted in urine. Each mmol of fosphenytoin is metabolized to 1 mmol of phenytoin, phosphate, and formate (see CLINICAL PHARMACOLOGY, Introduction and PRECAUTIONS, Phosphate Load for Renally Impaired Patients).

Phenytoin (after Cerebyx administration)

In general, IM administration of Cerebyx generates systemic phenytoin concentrations that are similar enough to oral phenytoin sodium to allow essentially interchangeable use.

The pharmacokinetics of fosphenytoin following IV administration of Cerebyx, however, are complex, and when used in an emergency setting (eg, status epilepticus), differences in rate of availability of phenytoin could be critical. Studies have therefore empirically determined an infusion rate for Cerebyx that gives a rate and extent of phenytoin systemic availability similar to that of a 50 mg/min phenytoin sodium infusion.

A dose of 15 to 20 mg PE/kg of Cerebyx infused at 100 to 150 mg PE/min yields plasma free phenytoin concentrations over time that approximate those achieved when an equivalent dose of phenytoin sodium (eg, parenteral Dilantin®) is administered at 50 mg/min (see DOSAGE AND ADMINISTRATION, WARNINGS).

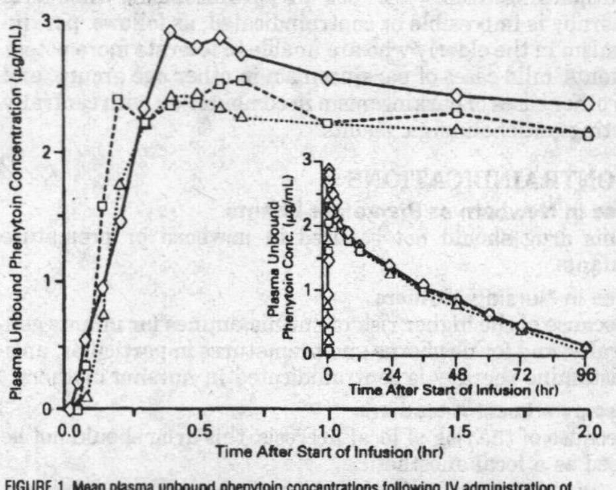

FIGURE 1. Mean plasma unbound phenytoin concentrations following IV administration of 1200 mg PE Cerebyx infused at 100 mg PE/min (triangles) or 150 mg PE/min (squares) and 1200 mg Dilantin infused at 50 mg/min (diamonds) to healthy subjects (N = 12). Inset shows time course for the entire 96-hour sampling period.

Following administration of single IV Cerebyx doses of 400 to 1200 mg PE, mean maximum total phenytoin concentrations increase in proportion to dose, but do not change appreciably with changes in infusion rate. In contrast, mean maximum unbound phenytoin concentrations increase with both dose and rate.

Absorption/Bioavailability: Fosphenytoin is completely converted to phenytoin following IV administration, with a half-life of approximately 15 minutes. Fosphenytoin is also completely converted to phenytoin following IM administra-

tion and plasma total phenytoin concentrations peak in approximately 3 hours.

Distribution: Phenytoin is highly bound to plasma proteins, primarily albumin, although to a lesser extent than fosphenytoin. In the absence of fosphenytoin, approximately 12% of total plasma phenytoin is unbound over the clinically relevant concentration range. However, fosphenytoin displaces phenytoin from plasma protein binding sites. This increases the fraction of phenytoin unbound (up to 30% unbound) during the period required for conversion of fosphenytoin to phenytoin (approximately 0.5 to 1 hour postinfusion).

Metabolism and Elimination: Phenytoin derived from administration of Cerebyx is extensively metabolized in the liver and excreted in urine primarily as 5-(p-hydroxyphenyl)-5-phenythydantoin and its glucuronide; little unchanged phenytoin (1%-5% of the Cerebyx dose) is recovered in urine. Phenytoin hepatic metabolism is saturable, and following administration of single IV Cerebyx doses of 400 to 1200 mg PE, total and unbound phenytoin AUC values increase disproportionately with dose. Mean total phenytoin half-life values (12.0 to 28.9 hr) following Cerebyx administration at these doses are similar to those after equal doses of parenteral Dilantin and tend to be greater at higher plasma phenytoin concentrations.

Special Populations

Patients with Renal or Hepatic Disease: Due to an increased fraction of unbound phenytoin in patients with renal or hepatic disease, or in those with hypoalbuminemia, the interpretation of total phenytoin plasma concentrations should be made with caution (see DOSAGE AND ADMINISTRATION). Unbound phenytoin concentrations may be more useful in these patient populations. After IV administration of Cerebyx to patients with renal and/or hepatic disease, or in those with hypoalbuminemia, fosphenytoin clearance to phenytoin may be increased without similar increase in phenytoin clearance. This has the potential to increase the frequency and severity of adverse events (see PRECAUTIONS).

Age: The effect of age was evaluated in patients 5 to 98 years of age. Patient age had no significant impact on fosphenytoin pharmacokinetics. Phenytoin clearance tends to decrease with increasing age (20% less in patients over 70 years of age relative to that in patients 20–30 years of age). Phenytoin dosing requirements are highly variable and must be individualized (see DOSAGE AND ADMINISTRATION).

Gender and Race: Gender and race have no significant impact on fosphenytoin or phenytoin pharmacokinetics.

Pediatrics: Only limited pharmacokinetic data are available in children (N=8; age 5 to 10 years). In these patients with status epilepticus who received loading doses of Cerebyx, the plasma fosphenytoin, total phenytoin, and unbound phenytoin concentration-time profiles did not signal any major differences from those in adult patients with status epilepticus receiving comparable doses.

Clinical Studies

Infusion tolerance was evaluated in clinical studies. One double-blind study assessed infusion-site tolerance of equivalent loading doses (15–20 mg PE/kg) of Cerebyx infused at 150 mg PE/min or phenytoin infused at 50 mg/min. The study demonstrated better local tolerance (pain and burning at the infusion site), fewer disruptions of the infusion, and a shorter infusion period for Cerebyx-treated patients (Table 1).

TABLE 1. Infusion Tolerance of Equivalent Loading Doses of IV Cerebyx and IV Phenytoin

	IV Cerebyx N=90	IV Phenytoin N=22
Local Intolerance	9%[a]	90%
Infusion Disrupted	21%	67%
Average Infusion Time	13 min	44 min

[a] Percent of patients.

Cerebyx-treated patients, however, experienced more systemic sensory disturbances (see PRECAUTIONS, Sensory Disturbances).

Infusion disruptions in Cerebyx-treated patients were primarily due to systemic burning, pruritus, and/or paresthesia while those in phenytoin-treated patients were primarily due to pain and burning at the infusion site (see Table 1).

In a double-blind study investigating temporary substitution of Cerebyx for oral phenytoin, IM Cerebyx was as well-tolerated as IM placebo. IM Cerebyx resulted in a slight increase in transient, mild to moderate local itching (23% of patients vs 11% of IM placebo-treated patients at any time during the study). This study also demonstrated that equimolar doses of IM Cerebyx may be substituted for oral phenytoin sodium with no dosage adjustments needed when initiating IM or returning to oral therapy. In contrast, switching between IM and oral phenytoin requires dosage adjustments because of slow and erratic phenytoin absorption from muscle.

INDICATIONS AND USAGE

Cerebyx is indicated for short-term parenteral administration when other means of phenytoin administration are unavailable, inappropriate, or deemed less advantageous. The safety and effectiveness of Cerebyx in this use has not been systematically evaluated for more than 5 days.

Cerebyx can be used for the control of generalized convulsive status epilepticus and prevention and treatment of seizures occurring during neurosurgery. It can also be substituted, short-term, for oral phenytoin.

CONTRAINDICATIONS

Cerebyx is contraindicated in patients who have demonstrated hypersensitivity to Cerebyx or its ingredients, or to phenytoin or other hydantoins.

Because of the effect of parenteral phenytoin on ventricular automaticity, Cerebyx is contraindicated in patients with sinus bradycardia, sino-atrial block, second and third degree A-V block, and Adams-Strokes syndrome.

WARNINGS

DOSES OF CEREBYX ARE EXPRESSED AS THEIR PHENYTOIN SODIUM EQUIVALENTS IN THIS LABELING (PE= phenytoin sodium equivalent).

DO NOT, THEREFORE, MAKE ANY ADJUSTMENT IN THE RECOMMENDED DOSES WHEN SUBSTITUTING CEREBYX FOR PHENYTOIN SODIUM OR VICE VERSA.

The following warnings are based on experience with Cerebyx or phenytoin.

Status Epilepticus Dosing Regimen

- **Do not administer Cerebyx at a rate greater than 150 mg PE/min.**

The dose of IV Cerebyx (15 to 20 mg PE/kg) that is used to treat status epilepticus is administered at a maximum rate of 150 mg PE/min. The typical Cerebyx infusion administered to a 50 kg patient would take between 5 and 7 minutes. Note that the delivery of an identical molar dose of phenytoin using parenteral Dilantin or generic phenytoin sodium injection cannot be accomplished in less than 15 to 20 minutes because of the untoward cardiovascular effects that accompany the direct intravenous administration of phenytoin at rates greater than 50 mg/min.

If rapid phenytoin loading is a primary goal, IV administration of Cerebyx is preferred because the time to achieve therapeutic plasma phenytoin concentrations is greater following IM than that following IV administration (see DOSAGE AND ADMINISTRATION).

Withdrawal Precipitated Seizure, Status Epilepticus

Antiepileptic drugs should not be abruptly discontinued because of the possibility of increased seizure frequency, including status epilepticus. When, in the judgement of the clinician, the need for dosage reduction, discontinuation, or substitution of alternative medication arises, this should be done gradually. However, in the event of an allergic or hypersensitivity reaction, rapid substitution of alternative therapy may be necessary. In this case, alternative therapy should be an antiepileptic drug not belonging to the hydantoin chemical class.

Cardiovascular Depression

Hypotension may occur, especially after IV administration at high doses and high rates of administration. Following administration of phenytoin, severe cardiovascular reactions and fatalities have been reported with atrial and ventricular conduction depression and ventricular fibrillation. Severe complications are most commonly encountered in elderly or gravely ill patients. Therefore, careful cardiac monitoring is needed when administering IV loading doses of Cerebyx. Reduction in rate of administration or discontinuation of dosing may be needed.

Cerebyx should be used with caution in patients with hypotension and severe myocardial insufficiency.

Rash

Cerebyx should be discontinued if a skin rash appears. If the rash is exfoliative, purpuric, or bullous, or if lupus erythematosus, Stevens-Johnson syndrome, or toxic epidermal necrolysis is suspected, use of this drug should not be resumed and alternative therapy should be considered. If the rash is of a milder type (measles-like scarlatiniform), therapy may be resumed after the rash has completely disappeared. If the rash recurs upon reinstitution, further Cerebyx or phenytoin administration is contraindicated.

Hepatic Injury

Cases of acute hepatotoxicity, including infrequent cases of acute hepatic failure, have been reported with phenytoin. These incidents have been associated with a hypersensitivity syndrome characterized by fever, skin eruptions, and lymphadenopathy, and usually occur within the first 2 months of treatment. Other common manifestations include jaundice, hepatomegaly, elevated serum transaminase levels, leukocytosis, and eosinophilia. The clinical course of acute phenytoin hepatotoxicity ranges from prompt recovery to fatal outcomes. In these patients with acute hepatotoxicity, Cerebyx should be immediately discontinued and not readministered.

Hemopoietic System

Hemopoietic complications, some fatal, have occasionally been reported in association with administration of phenytoin. These have included thrombocytopenia, leukopenia, granulocytopenia, agranulocytosis, and pancytopenia with or without bone marrow suppression.

There have been a number of reports that have suggested a relationship between phenytoin and the development of lymphadenopathy (local or generalized), including benign lymph node hyperplasia, pseudolymphoma, lymphoma, and Hodgkin's disease. Although a cause and effect relationship has not been established, the occurrence of lymphadenopathy indicates the need to differentiate such a condition from other types of lymph node pathology. Lymph node involvement may occur with or without symptoms and signs resembling serum sickness, eg, fever, rash, and liver involvement. In all cases of lymphadenopathy, follow-up observation for an extended period is indicated and every effort should be made to achieve seizure control using alternative antiepileptic drugs.

Alcohol Use

Acute alcohol intake may increase plasma phenytoin concentrations while chronic alcohol use may decrease plasma concentrations.

Usage in Pregnancy

Clinical:

A. *Risks to Mother.* An increase in seizure frequency may occur during pregnancy because of altered phenytoin pharmacokinetics. Periodic measurements of plasma phenytoin concentrations may be valuable in the management of pregnant women as a guide to appropriate adjustment of dosage (see PRECAUTIONS, Laboratory Tests). However, postpartum restoration of the original dosage will probably be indicated.

B. *Risks to the Fetus.* If this drug is used during pregnancy, or if the patient becomes pregnant while taking the drug, the patient should be apprised of the potential harm to the fetus.

Prenatal exposure to phenytoin may increase the risks for congenital malformations and other adverse developmental outcomes. Increased frequencies of major malformations (such as orofacial clefts and cardiac defects), minor anomalies (dysmorphic facial features, nail and digit hypoplasia), growth abnormalities (including microcephaly), and mental deficiency have been reported among children born to epileptic women who took phenytoin alone or in combination with other antiepileptic drugs during pregnancy. There have also been several reported cases of malignancies, including neuroblastoma, in children whose mothers received phenytoin during pregnancy. The overall incidence of malformations for children of epileptic women treated with antiepileptic drugs (phenytoin and/or others) during pregnancy is about 10%, or two-to three-fold that in the general population. However, the relative contributions of antiepileptic drugs and other factors associated with epilepsy to this increased risk are uncertain and in most cases it has not been possible to attribute specific developmental abnormalities to particular antiepileptic drugs.

Patients should consult with their physicians to weigh the risks and benefits of phenytoin during pregnancy.

C. *Postpartum Period.* A potentially life-threatening bleeding disorder related to decreased levels of vitamin K-dependent clotting factors may occur in newborns exposed to phenytoin *in utero*. This drug-induced condition can be prevented with vitamin K administration to the mother before delivery and to the neonate after birth.

Preclinical: Increased frequencies of malformations (brain, cardiovascular, digit, and skeletal anomalies), death, growth retardation, and functional impairment (chromodacryorrhea, hyperactivity, circling) were observed among the offspring of rats receiving fosphenytoin during pregnancy. Most of the adverse effects of embryo-fetal development occurred at doses of 33 mg PE/kg or higher (approximately 30% of the maximum human loading dose or higher on a mg/m^2 basis), which produced peak maternal plasma phenytoin concentrations of approximately 20 $\mu g/mL$ or greater. Maternal toxicity was often associated with these doses and plasma concentrations, however, there is no evidence to suggest that the developmental effects were secondary to the maternal effects. The single occurrence of a rare brain malformation at a non-maternotoxic dose of 17 mg PE/kg (approximately 10% of the maximum human loading dose on a mg/m^2 basis) was also considered drug-induced. The developmental effects of fosphenytoin in rats were similar to those which have been reported following administration of phenytoin to pregnant rats.

Continued on next page

This product information was prepared in August 1996. On these and other Parke-Davis Products, information may be obtained by addressing PARKE-DAVIS, Division of Warner-Lambert Company, Morris Plains, New Jersey 07950.

Parke-Davis—Cont.

No effects on embryo-fetal development were observed when rabbits were given up to 33 mg PE/kg of fosphenytoin (approximately 50% of the maximum human loading dose on a mg/m² basis) during pregnancy. Increased resorption and malformation rates have been reported following administration of phenytoin doses of 75 mg/kg or higher (approximately 120% of the maximum human loading dose or higher on a mg/m² basis) to pregnant rabbits.

PRECAUTIONS
General: (Cerebyx specific)
Sensory Disturbances
Severe burning, itching, and/or paresthesia were reported by 7 of 16 normal volunteers administered IV Cerebyx at a dose of 1200 mg PE at the maximum rate of administration (150 mg PE/min). The severe sensory disturbance lasted from 3 to 50 minutes in 6 of these subjects and for 14 hours in the seventh subject. In some cases, milder sensory disturbances persisted for as long as 24 hours. The location of the discomfort varied among subjects with the groin mentioned most frequently as an area of discomfort. In a separate cohort of 16 normal volunteers (taken from 2 other studies) who were administered IV Cerebyx at a dose of 1200 mg PE at the maximum rate of administration (150 mg PE/min), none experienced severe disturbances, but most experienced mild to moderate itching or tingling.
Patients administered Cerebyx at doses of 20 mg PE/kg at 150 mg PE/min are expected to experience discomfort of some degree. The occurrence and intensity of the discomfort can be lessened by slowing or temporarily stopping the infusion.
The effect of continuing infusion unaltered in the presence of these sensations is unknown. No permanent sequelae have been reported thus far. The pharmacologic basis for these positive sensory phenomena is unknown, but other phosphate ester drugs, which deliver smaller phosphate loads, have been associated with burning, itching, and/or tingling predominantly in the groin area.
Phosphate Load
The phosphate load provided by Cerebyx (0.0037 mmol phosphate/mg PE Cerebyx) should be considered when treating patients who require phosphate restriction, such as those with severe renal impairment.
IV Loading in Renal and/or Hepatic Disease or in Those With Hypoalbuminemia
After IV administration to patients with renal and/or hepatic disease, or in those with hypoalbuminemia, fosphenytoin clearance to phenytoin may be increased without a similar increase in phenytoin clearance. This has the potential to increase the frequency and severity of adverse events (see CLINICAL PHARMACOLOGY: Special Populations, and DOSAGE AND ADMINISTRATION: Dosing in Special Populations).
General: (phenytoin associated)
Cerebyx is *not* indicated for the treatment of *absence seizures*. A small percentage of individuals who have been treated with phenytoin have been shown to metabolize the drug slowly. *Slow metabolism* may be due to limited enzyme availability and lack of induction; it appears to be genetically determined.
Phenytoin and other hydantoins are contraindicated in patients who have experienced phenytoin hypersensitivity. Additionally, caution should be exercised if using structurally similar (eg, barbiturates, succinimides, oxazolidinediones, and other related compounds) in these same patients. Phenytoin has been infrequently associated with the exacerbation of *porphyria*. Caution should be exercised when Cerebyx is used in patients with this disease.
Hyperglycemia, resulting from phenytoin's inhibitory effect on insulin release, has been reported. Phenytoin may also raise the serum glucose concentrations in diabetic patients. Plasma concentrations of phenytoin sustained above the optimal range may produce confusional states referred to as "delirium," "psychosis," or "encephalopathy," or rarely, irreversible cerebellar dysfunction. Accordingly, at the first sign of *acute toxicity,* determination of plasma phenytoin concentrations is recommended (see PRECAUTIONS: Laboratory Tests). Cerebyx dose reduction is indicated if phenytoin concentrations are excessive, if symptoms persist, administration of Cerebyx should be discontinued.
The liver is the primary site of biotransformation of phenytoin; patients with impaired liver function, elderly patients, or those who are gravely ill may show early signs of toxicity. Phenytoin and other hydantoins are not indicated for seizures due to hypoglycemic or other metabolic causes. Appropriate diagnostic procedures should be performed as indicated.
Phenytoin has the potential to lower serum folate levels.
Laboratory Tests
Phenytoin doses are usually selected to attain therapeutic plasma total phenytoin concentrations of 10 to 20 μg/mL, (unbound phenytoin concentrations of 1 to 2 μg/mL). Following Cerebyx administration, it is recommended that pheny-

toin concentrations <u>not</u> be monitored until conversion to phenytoin is essentially complete. This occurs within approximately 2 hours after the end of IV infusion and 4 hours after IM injection.
Prior to complete conversion, commonly used immunoanalytical techniques, such as TDx®/TDxFLx™ (fluorescence polarization) and Emit® 2000 (enzyme multiplied), may significantly overestimate plasma phenytoin concentrations because of cross-reactivity with fosphenytoin. The error is dependent on plasma phenytoin and fosphenytoin concentration (influenced by Cerebyx dose, route and rate of administration, and time of sampling relative to dosing), and analytical method. Chromatographic assay methods accurately quantitate phenytoin concentrations in biological fluids in the presence of fosphenytoin. Prior to complete conversion, blood samples for phenytoin monitoring should be collected in tubes containing EDTA as an anticoagulant to minimize *ex vivo* conversion of fosphenytoin to phenytoin. However, even with specific assay methods, phenytoin concentrations measured before conversion of fosphenytoin is complete will not reflect phenytoin concentrations ultimately achieved.
Drug Interactions
No drugs are known to interfere with the conversion of fosphenytoin to phenytoin. Conversion could be affected by alterations in the level of phosphatase activity, but given the abundance and wide distribution of phosphatases in the body it is unlikely that drugs would affect this activity enough to affect conversion of fosphenytoin to phenytoin. Drugs highly bound to albumin could increase the unbound fraction of fosphenytoin. Although, it is unknown whether this could result in clinically significant effects, caution is advised when administering Cerebyx with other drugs that significantly bind to serum albumin.
The pharmacokinetics and protein binding of fosphenytoin, phenytoin, and diazepam were not altered when diazepam and Cerebyx were concurrently administered in single submaximal doses.
The most significant drug interactions following administration of Cerebyx are expected to occur with drugs that interact with phenytoin. Phenytoin is extensively bound to serum plasma proteins and is prone to competitive displacement. Phenytoin is metabolized by hepatic cytochrome P450 enzymes and is particularly susceptible to inhibitory drug interactions because it is subject to saturable metabolism. Inhibition of metabolism may produce significant increases in circulating phenytoin concentrations and enhance the risk of drug toxicity. Phenytoin is a potent inducer of hepatic drug-metabolizing enzymes.
The most commonly occurring drug interactions are listed below:
- Drugs that may increase plasma phenytoin concentrations include: acute alcohol intake, amiodarone, chloramphenicol, chlordiazepoxide, cimetidine, diazepam, dicumarol, disulfiram, estrogens, ethosuximide, fluoxetine, H₂-antagonists, halothane, isoniazid, methylphenidate, phenothiazines, phenylbutazone, salicylates, succinimides, sulfonamides, tolbutamide, trazodone.
- Drugs that may decrease plasma phenytoin concentrations include: carbamazepine, chronic alcohol abuse, reserpine.
- Drugs that may either increase or decrease plasma phenytoin concentrations include: phenobarbital, valproic acid, and sodium valproate. Similarly, the effects of phenytoin on phenobarbital, valproic acid and sodium plasma valproate concentrations are unpredictable.
- Although not a true drug interaction, tricyclic antidepressants may precipitate seizures in susceptible patients and Cerebyx dosage may need to be adjusted.
- Drugs whose efficacy is impaired by phenytoin include: anticoagulants, corticosteroids, coumarin, digitoxin, doxycycline, estrogens, furosemide, oral contraceptives, rifampin, quinidine, theophylline, vitamin D.
Monitoring of plasma phenytoin concentrations may be helpful when possible drug interactions are suspected (see Laboratory Tests).
Drug/Laboratory Test Interactions
Phenytoin may decrease serum concentrations of T₄. It may also produce artifactually low results in dexamethasone or metyrapone tests. Phenytoin may also cause increased serum concentrations of glucose, alkaline phosphatase, and gamma glutamyl transpeptidase (GGT).
Care should be taken when using immunoanalytical methods to measure plasma phenytoin concentrations following Cerebyx administration (see Laboratory Tests).
Carcinogenesis, Mutagenesis, Impairment of Fertility
The carcinogenic potential of fosphenytoin has not been studied. Assessment of the carcinogenic potential of phenytoin in mice and rats is ongoing.
Structural chromosome aberration frequency in cultured V79 Chinese hamster lung cells was increased by exposure to fosphenytoin in the presence of metabolic activation. No evidence of mutagenicity was observed in bacteria (Ames test) or Chinese hamster lung cells *in vitro*, and no evidence for clastogenic activity was observed in an *in vivo* mouse bone marrow micronucleus test.

No effects on fertility were noted in rats of either sex given fosphenytoin. Maternal toxicity and altered estrous cycles, delayed mating, prolonged gestation length, and developmental toxicity were observed following administration of fosphenytoin during mating, gestation, and lactation at doses of 50 mg PE/kg or higher (approximately 40% of the maximum human loading dose or higher on a mg/m² basis).

Pregnancy-Category D: (see WARNINGS)
Use in Nursing Mothers
It is not known whether fosphenytoin is excreted in human milk.
Following administration of Dilantin, phenytoin appears to be excreted in low concentrations in human milk. Therefore, breast-feeding is not recommended for women receiving Cerebyx.

Pediatric Use
The safety of Cerebyx in pediatric patients has not been established.

Geriatric Use
No systematic studies in geriatric patients have been conducted. Phenytoin clearance tends to decrease with increasing age (see CLINICAL PHARMACOLOGY: Special Populations).

ADVERSE REACTIONS
The more important adverse clinical events caused by the IV use of Cerebyx or phenytoin are cardiovascular collapse and/or central nervous system depression. Hypotension can occur when either drug is administered rapidly by the IV route. The rate of administration is very important; for Cerebyx, it should not exceed 150 mg PE/min.
The adverse clinical events most commonly observed with the use of Cerebyx in clinical trials were nystagmus, dizziness, pruritus, paresthesia, headache, somnolence, and ataxia. With two exceptions, these events are commonly associated with the administration of IV phenytoin. Paresthesia and pruritus, however, were seen much more often following Cerebyx administration and occurred more often with IV Cerebyx administration than with IM Cerebyx administration. These events were dose and rate related; most alert patients (41 of 64; 64%) administered doses of ≥15 mg PE/kg at 150 mg PE/min experienced discomfort of some degree. These sensations, generally described as itching, burning, or tingling, were usually not at the infusion site. The location of the discomfort varied with the groin mentioned most frequently as a site of involvement. The paresthesia and pruritus were transient events that occurred within several minutes of the start of infusion and generally resolved within 10 minutes after completion of Cerebyx infusion. Some patients experienced symptoms for hours. These events did not increase in severity with repeated administration.
Concurrent adverse events or clinical laboratory change suggesting an allergic process were not seen (see PRECAUTIONS, Sensory Disturbances).
Approximately 2% of the 859 individuals who received Cerebyx in premarketing clinical trials discontinued treatment because of an adverse event. The adverse events most commonly associated with withdrawal were pruritus (0.5%), hypotension (0.3%), and bradycardia (0.2%).
Dose and Rate Dependency of Adverse Events Following IV Cerebyx: The incidence of adverse events tended to increase as both dose and infusion rate increased. In particular, at doses of ≥15 mg PE/kg and rates ≥150 mg PE/min, transient pruritus, tinnitus, nystagmus, somnolence, and ataxia occurred 2 to 3 times more often than at lower doses or rates.

Incidence in Controlled Clinical Trials
All adverse events were recorded during the trials by the clinical investigators using terminology of their own choosing. Similar types of events were grouped into standardized categories using modfied COSTART dictionary terminology. These categories are used in the tables and listings below with the frequencies representing the proportion of individuals exposed to Cerebyx or comparative therapy.
The prescriber should be aware that these figures cannot be used to predict the frequency of adverse events in the course of usual medical practice where patient characteristics and other factors may differ from those prevailing during clinical studies. Similarly, the cited frequencies cannot be directly compared with figures obtained from other clinical investigations involving different treatments, uses or investigators. An inspection of these frequencies, however, does provide the prescribing physician with one basis to estimate the relative contribution of drug and nondrug factors to the adverse event incidences in the population studied.
Incidence in Controlled Clinical Trials-IV Administration To Patients With Epilepsy or Neurosurgical Patients: Table 2 lists treatment-emergent adverse events that occurred in at least 2% of patients treated with IV Cerebyx at the maximum dose and rate in a randomized, double-blind, controlled clinical trial where the rates for phenytoin and Cerebyx administration would have resulted in equivalent systemic exposure to phenytoin.

TABLE 2. Treatment-Emergent Adverse Event Incidence Following IV Administration at the Maximum Dose and Rate to Patients With Epilepsy or Neurosurgical Patients

(Events in at Least 2% of Cerebyx-Treated Patients)

BODY SYSTEM Adverse Event	IV Cerebyx N=90	IV Phenytoin N=22
BODY AS A WHOLE		
Pelvic Pain	4.4	0.0
Asthenia	2.2	0.0
Back Pain	2.2	0.0
Headache	2.2	4.5
CARDIOVASCULAR		
Hypotension	7.7	9.1
Vasodilatation	5.6	4.5
Tachycardia	2.2	0.0
DIGESTIVE		
Nausea	8.9	13.6
Tongue Disorder	4.4	0.0
Dry Mouth	4.4	4.5
Vomiting	2.2	9.1
NERVOUS		
Nystagmus	44.4	59.1
Dizziness	31.1	27.3
Somnolence	20.0	27.3
Ataxia	11.1	18.2
Stupor	7.7	4.5
Incoordination	4.4	4.5
Paresthesia	4.4	0.0
Extrapyramidal Syndrome	4.4	0.0
Tremor	3.3	9.1
Agitation	3.3	0.0
Hypesthesia	2.2	9.1
Dysarthria	2.2	0.0
Vertigo	2.2	0.0
Brain Edema	2.2	4.5
SKIN AND APPENDAGES		
Pruritus	48.9	4.5
SPECIAL SENSES		
Tinnitus	8.9	9.1
Diplopia	3.3	0.0
Taste Perversion	3.3	0.0
Amblyopia	2.2	9.1
Deafness	2.2	0.0

Incidence in Controlled Trials-IM Administration to Patients With Epilepsy. Table 3 lists treatment-emergent adverse events that occurred in at least 2% of Cerebyx-treated patients in a double-bind, randomized controlled clinical trial of adult epilepsy patients receiving either IM Cerebyx substituted for oral Dilantin or continuing oral Dilantin. Both treatments were administered for 5 days.

TABLE 3. Treatment-Emergent Adverse Event Incidence Following Substitution of IM Cerebyx for Oral Dilantin in Patients With Epilepsy

(Events in at Least 2% of Cerebyx-Treated Patients)

BODY SYSTEM Adverse Event	IM Cerebyx N=179	Oral Dilantin N=61
BODY AS A WHOLE		
Headache	8.9	4.9
Asthenia	3.9	3.3
Accidental Injury	3.4	6.6
DIGESTIVE		
Nausea	4.5	0.0
Vomiting	2.8	0.0
HEMATOLOGIC AND LYMPHATIC		
Ecchymosis	7.3	4.9
NERVOUS		
Nystagmus	15.1	8.2
Tremor	9.5	13.1
Ataxia	8.4	8.2
Incoordination	7.8	4.9
Somnolence	6.7	9.8
Dizziness	5.0	3.3
Paresthesia	3.9	3.3
Reflexes Decreased	2.8	4.9
SKIN AND APPENDAGES		
Pruritus	2.8	0.0

Adverse Events During All Clinical Trials
Cerebyx has been administered to 859 individuals during all clinical trials. All adverse events seen at least twice are listed in the following, except those already included in previous tables and listings. Events are further classified within body system categories and enumerated in order of decreasing frequency using the following definitions: frequent adverse events are defined as those occurring in greater than 1/100 individuals; infrequent adverse events are those occurring in 1/100 to 1/1000 individuals.

Body As a Whole: *Frequent:* fever, injection-site reaction, infection, chills, face edema, injection-site pain; *Infrequent:* sepsis, injection-site inflammation, injection-site edema, injection-site hemorrhage, flu syndrome, malaise, generalized edema, shock, photosensitivity reaction, cachexia, cryptococcosis.

Cardiovascular: *Frequent:* hypertension; *Infrequent:* cardiac arrest, migraine, syncope, cerebral hemorrhage, palpitation, sinus bradycardia, atrial flutter, bundle branch block, cardiomegaly, cerebral infarct, postural hypotension, pulmonary embolus. QT interval prolongation, thrombophlebitis, ventricular extrasystoles, congestive heart failure.

Digestive: *Frequent:* constipation; *Infrequent:* dyspepsia, diarrhea, anorexia, gastrointestinal hemorrhage, increased salivation, liver function tests abnormal, tenesmus, tongue edema, dysphagia, flatulence, gastritis, ileus.

Endocrine: *Infrequent:* diabetes insipidus.

Hematologic and Lymphatic: *Infrequent:* thrombocytopenia, anemia, leukocytosis, cyanosis, hypochromic anemia, leukopenia, lymphadenopathy, petachia.

Metabolic and Nutritional: *Frequent:* hypokalemia; *Infrequent:* hyperglycemia, hypophosphatemia, alkalosis, acidosis, dehydration, hyperkalemia, ketosis.

Musculoskeletal: *Frequent:* myasthenia; *Infrequent:* myopathy, leg cramps, arthralgia, myalgia.

Nervous: *Frequent:* reflexes increased, speech disorder, dysarthria, intracranial hypertension, thinking abnormal, nervousness, hypesthesia; *Infrequent:* confusion, twitching, Babinski sign positive, circumoral paresthesia, hemiplegia, hypotonia, convulsion, extrapyramidal syndrome, insomnia, meningitis, depersonalization, CNS depression, depression, hypokinesia, hyperkinesia, brain edema, paralysis, psychosis, aphasia, emotional lability, coma, hyperesthesia, myoclonus, personality disorder, acute brain syndrome, encephalitis, subdural hematoma, emcephalopathy, hostility, akathisia, amnesia, neurosis.

Respiratory: *Frequent:* pneumonia; *Infrequent:* pharyngitis, sinusitis, hyperventilation, rhinitis, apnea, aspiration pneumonia, asthma, dyspnea, atelectasis, cough increased, sputum increased, epistaxis, hypoxia, pneumothorax, hemoptysis, bronchitis.

Skin and Appendages: *Frequent:* rash; *Infrequent:* maculopapular rash, urticaria, sweating, skin discoloration, contact dermatitis, pustular rash, skin nodule.

Special Senses: *Frequent:* taste perversion; *Infrequent:* deafness, visual field defect, eye pain, conjunctivitis, photophobia, hyperacusis, mydriasis, parosmia, ear pain, taste loss.

Urogenital: *Infrequent:* urinary retention, oliguria, dysuria, vaginitis, albuminuria, genital edema, kidney failure, polyuria, urethral pain, urinary incontinence, vaginal moniliasis.

OVERDOSAGE

There is no experience with Cerebyx overdosage in humans. The median lethal dose of fosphenytoin given intravenously in mice and rats was 156 mg PE/kg and approximately 250 mg PE/kg, or about 0.6 and 2 times, respectively, the maximum human loading dose on a mg/m² basis. Signs of acute toxicity in animals included ataxia, labored breathing, ptosis, and hypoactivity.

Because Cerebyx is a prodrug of phenytoin, the following information may be helpful. Initial symptoms of acute phenytoin toxicity are nystagmus, ataxia, and dysarthria. Other signs include tremor, hyperreflexia, lethargy, slurred speech, nausea, vomiting, coma, and hypotension. Depression of respiratory and circulatory systems leads to death. There are marked variations among individuals with respect to plasma phenytoin concentrations where toxicity occurs. Lateral gaze nystagmus usually appears at 20 μg/mL, ataxia at 30 μg/mL, and dysarthria and lethargy appear when the plasma concentration is over 40 μg/mL. However, phenytoin concentrations as high as 50 μg/mL have been reported without evidence of toxicity. As much as 25 times the therapeutic phenytoin dose has been taken, resulting in plasma phenytoin concentrations over 100 μg/mL, with complete recovery.

Treatment is nonspecific since there is no known antidote to Cerebyx or phenytoin overdosage. The adequacy of the respiratory and circulatory systems should be carefully observed, and appropriate supportive measures employed. Hemodialysis can be considered since phenytoin is not completely bound to plasma proteins. Total exchange transfusion has been used in the treatment of severe intoxication in children. In acute overdosage the possibility of other CNS depressants, including alcohol, should be borne in mind.

Formate and phosphate are metabolites of fosphenytoin and therefore may contribute to signs of toxicity following overdosage. Signs of formate toxicity are similar to those of methanol toxicity and are associated with severe anion-gap metabolic acidosis. Large amounts of phosphate, delivered rapidly, could potentially cause hypocalcemia with paresthesia, muscle spasms, and seizures. Ionized free calcium levels can be measured and, if low, used to guide treatment.

DOSAGE AND ADMINISTRATION

The dose, concentration in dosing solutions, and infusion rate of IV Cerebyx is expressed as phenytoin sodium equivalents (PE) to avoid the need to perform molecular weight-based adjustments when converting between fosphenytoin and phenytoin sodium doses. Cerebyx should always be prescribed and dispensed in phenytoin sodium equivalent units (PE). Cerebyx has important differences in administration from those for parenteral phenytoin sodium (see below). Products with particulate matter or discoloration should not be used. Prior to IV infusion, dilute Cerebyx in 5% dextrose or 0.9% saline solution for injection to a concentration ranging from 1.5 to 25 mg PE/mL.

Status Epilepticus
- The loading dose of Cerebyx is 15 to 20 mg PE/kg administered at 100 to 150 mg PE/min.
- Because of the risk of hypotension, fosphenytoin should be administered no faster than 150 mg PE/min. Continuous monitoring of the electrocardiogram, blood pressure, and respiratory function is essential and the patient should be observed throughout the period where maximal serum phenytoin concentrations occur, approximately 10 to 20 minutes after the end of Cerebyx infusions.
- Because the full antiepileptic effect of phenytoin, whether given as Cerebyx or parenteral phenytoin is not immediate, other measures, including concomitant administration of an IV benzodiazepine, will usually be necessary for the control of status epilepticus.
- The loading dose should be followed by maintenance doses of Cerebyx, or phenytoin either orally or parenterally.

If administration of Cerebyx does not terminate seizures, the use of other anticonvulsants and other appropriate measures should be considered.

IM Cerebyx should not be used in the treatment of status epilepticus because therapeutic phenytoin concentrations may not be reached as quickly as with IV administration. If IV access is impossible, loading doses of Cerebyx have been given by the IM route for other indications.

Nonemergent Loading and Maintenance Dosing
The loading dose of Cerebyx is 10-20 mg PE/kg given IV or IM. The rate of administration for IV Cerebyx should be no greater than 150 mg PE/min. Continuous monitoring of the electrocardiogram, blood pressure, and respiratory function is essential and the patient should be observed throughout the period where maximal serum phenytoin concentrations occur, approximately 10 to 20 minutes after the end of Cerebyx infusions.

The initial daily maintenance dose of Cerebyx is 4-6 mg PE/kg/day.

IM or IV Substitution For Oral Phenytoin Therapy
Cerebyx can be substituted for oral phenytoin sodium therapy at the same total daily dose.

Dilantin capsules are approximately 90% bioavailable by the oral route. Phenytoin, supplied as Cerebyx, is 100% bioavailable by both the IM and IV routes. For this reason, plasma phenytoin concentrations may increase modestly when IM or IV Cerebyx is substituted for oral phenytoin sodium therapy.

The rate of administration for IV Cerebyx should be no greater than 150 mg PE/min.

In controlled trials, IM Cerebyx was administered as a single daily dose utilizing either 1 or 2 injection sites. Some patients may require more frequent dosing.

Dosing in Special Populations
Patients with Renal or Hepatic Disease: Due to an increased fraction of unbound phenytoin in patients with renal or hepatic disease, or in those with hypoalbuminemia, the interpretation of total phenytoin plasma concentrations should be made with caution (see CLINICAL PHARMACOLOGY: Special Populations). Unbound phenytoin concentrations may be more useful in these patient populations. After IV Cerebyx administration to patients with renal and/or hepatic disease, or in those with hypoalbuminemia, fosphenytoin clearance to phenytoin may be increased without a similar increase in phenytoin clearance. This has the potential to increase the frequency and severity of adverse events (see PRECAUTIONS).

Elderly Patients: Age does not have a significant impact on the pharmacokinetics of fosphenytoin following Cerebyx administration. Phenytoin clearance is decreased slightly in elderly patients and lower or less frequent dosing may be required.

Pediatric: The safety of Cerebyx in pediatric patients has not been established.

Continued on next page

This product information was prepared in August 1996. On these and other Parke-Davis Products, information may be obtained by addressing PARKE-DAVIS, Division of Warner-Lambert Company, Morris Plains, New Jersey 07950.

Parke-Davis—Cont.

HOW SUPPLIED

Cerebyx Injection is supplied as follows:

10 mL per vial—Each vial contains fosphenytoin sodium 750 mg equivalent to 500 mg of phenytoin sodium: N 0071-4008-10 Packages of 10.

2 mL per vial—Each vial contains fosphenytoin sodium 150 mg equivalent to 100 mg of phenytoin sodium: N 0071-4007-05. Packages of 25.

Both sizes of vials contain Tromethamine, USP (TRIS), Hydrochloric Acid, NF, or Sodium Hydroxide, NF, and Water for Injection, USP

Cerebyx should always be prescribed in phenytoin sodium equivalent units (PE) (see DOSAGE AND ADMINISTRATION).

Storage

Store under refrigeration at 2°C to 8°C (36°F to 46°F). The product should not be stored at room temperature for more than 48 hours. Vials that develop particulate matter should not be used.

Caution: Federal law prohibits dispensing without prescription.

© 1996, Warner-Lambert Co.

Issued date: July 1996

PARKE-DAVIS

Div of Warner-Lambert Co.

Morris Plains, NJ 07950 USA   4007G030

CHLOROMYCETIN®   ℞
[chlō"rō-my-cē'tin sŭc'cĭ-nāte"]
SODIUM SUCCINATE
(sterile chloramphenicol
sodium succinate, USP)
FOR INTRAVENOUS ADMINISTRATION

> **WARNING**
>
> Serious and fatal blood dyscrasias (aplastic anemia, hypoplastic anemia, thrombocytopenia, and granulocytopenia) are known to occur after the administration of chloramphenicol. In addition, there have been reports of aplastic anemia attributed to chloramphenicol which later terminated in leukemia. Blood dyscrasias have occurred after both short-term and prolonged therapy with this drug. Chloramphenicol must not be used when less potentially dangerous agents will be effective, as described in the Indications section. *It must not be used in the treatment of trivial infections or where it is not indicated, as in colds, influenza, infections of the throat; or as a prophylactic agent to prevent bacterial infections.*
>
> **Precautions:** It is essential that adequate blood studies be made during treatment with the drug. While blood studies may detect early peripheral blood changes, such as leukopenia, reticulocytopenia, or granulocytopenia, before they become irreversible, such studies cannot be relied on to detect bone marrow depression prior to development of aplastic anemia. To facilitate appropriate studies and observation during therapy, it is desirable that patients be hospitalized.

IMPORTANT CONSIDERATIONS IN PRESCRIBING INJECTABLE CHLORAMPHENICOL SODIUM SUCCINATE CHLORAMPHENICOL SODIUM SUCCINATE IS INTENDED FOR INTRAVENOUS USE ONLY. IT HAS BEEN DEMONSTRATED TO BE INEFFECTIVE WHEN GIVEN INTRAMUSCULARLY.

1. Chloramphenicol sodium succinate must be hydrolyzed to its microbiologically active form and there is a lag in achieving adequate blood levels compared with the base given intravenously.
2. The oral form of chloramphenicol is readily absorbed and adequate blood levels are achieved and maintained on the recommended dosage.
3. Patients started on intravenous chloramphenicol sodium succinate should be changed to the oral form as soon as practicable.

DESCRIPTION

Chloramphenicol is an antibiotic that is clinically useful for, *and should be reserved for,* serious infections caused by organisms susceptible to its antimicrobial effects when less potentially hazardous therapeutic agents are ineffective or contraindicated. Sensitivity testing is essential to determine its indicated use, but may be performed concurrently with therapy initiated on clinical impression that one of the indicated conditions exists (see Indications section).

Each gram (10 ml of a 10% solution) of chloramphenicol sodium succinate contains approximately 52 mg (2.25 mEq) of sodium.

ACTIONS AND PHARMACOLOGY

In vitro chloramphenicol exerts mainly a bacteriostatic effect on a wide range of gram-negative and gram-positive bacteria and is active *in vitro* against rickettsias, the lymphogranuloma-psittacosis group, and *Vibrio cholerae*. It is particularly active against *Salmonella typhi* and *Hemophilus influenzae*. The mode of action is through interference or inhibition of protein synthesis in intact cells and in cell-free systems.

Chloramphenicol administered orally is absorbed rapidly from the intestinal tract. In controlled studies in adult volunteers using the recommended dosage of 50 mg/kg/day, a dosage of 1 g every 6 hours for 8 doses was given. Using the microbiological assay method, the average peak serum level was 11.2 mcg/ml one hour after the first dose. A cumulative effect gave a peak rise to 18.4 mcg/ml after the fifth dose of 1 g. Mean serum levels ranged from 8 to 14 mcg/ml over the 48-hour period. Total urinary excretion of chloramphenicol in these studies ranged from a low of 68% to a high of 99% over a three-day period. From 8 to 12% of the antibiotic excreted is in the form of free chloramphenicol; the remainder consists of microbiologically inactive metabolites, principally the conjugate with glucuronic acid. Since the glucuronide is excreted rapidly, most chloramphenicol detected in the blood is in the microbiologically active free form. Despite the small proportion of unchanged drug excreted in the urine, the concentration of free chloramphenicol is relatively high, amounting to several hundred mcg/ml in patients receiving divided doses of 50 mg/kg/day. Small amounts of active drug are found in bile and feces. Chloramphenicol diffuses rapidly, but its distribution is not uniform. Highest concentrations are found in liver and kidney, and lowest concentrations are found in brain and cerebrospinal fluid. Chloramphenicol enters cerebrospinal fluid even in the absence of meningeal inflammation, appearing in concentrations about half of those found in the blood. Measurable levels are also detected in pleural and in ascitic fluids, saliva, milk, and in the aqueous and vitreous humors. Transport across the placental barrier occurs with somewhat lower concentration in cord blood of newborn infants than in maternal blood.

INDICATIONS

In accord with the concepts in the warning box and this Indications section, chloramphenicol must be used only in those serious infections for which less potentially dangerous drugs are ineffective or contraindicated. However, chloramphenicol may be chosen to initiate antibiotic therapy on the clinical impression that one of the conditions below is believed to be present; *in vitro* sensitivity tests should be performed concurrently so that the drug may be discontinued as soon as possible if less potentially dangerous agents are indicated by such tests. The decision to continue use of chloramphenicol rather than another antibiotic when both are suggested by *in vitro* studies to be effective against a specific pathogen should be based upon severity of the infection, susceptibility of the pathogen to the various antimicrobial drugs, efficacy of the various drugs in the infection, and the important additional concepts contained in the Warning Box above:

1. **Acute infections caused by *Salmonella typhi****
It is not recommended for the routine treatment of the typhoid carrier state.
2. **Serious infections caused by susceptible strains in accordance with the concepts expressed above:**
   a. *Salmonella* species
   b. *H. influenzae*, specifically meningeal infections
   c. Rickettsia
   d. Lymphogranuloma-psittacosis group
   e. Various gram-negative bacteria causing bacteremia, meningitis, or other serious gram-negative infections
   f. Other susceptible organisms which have been demonstrated to be resistant to all other appropriate antimicrobial agents.
3. **Cystic fibrosis regimens**

---

*In the treatment of typhoid fever, some authorities recommend that chloramphenicol be administered at therapeutic levels for 8 to 10 days after the patient has become afebrile to lessen the possibility of relapse.

CONTRAINDICATIONS

Chloramphenicol is contraindicated in individuals with a history of previous hypersensitivity and/or toxic reaction to it. *It must not be used in the treatment of trivial infections or where it is not indicated, as in colds, influenza, infections of the throat; or as a prophylactic agent to prevent bacterial infection.*

PRECAUTIONS

1. Baseline blood studies should be followed by periodic blood studies approximately every two days during therapy. The drug should be discontinued upon appearance of reticulocytopenia, leukopenia, thrombocytopenia, anemia, or any other blood study findings attributable to chloramphenicol. However, it should be noted that such studies do not exclude

the possible later appearance of the irreversible type of bone marrow depression.

2. Repeated courses of the drug should be avoided if at all possible. Treatment should not be continued longer than required to produce a cure with little or no risk of relapse of the disease.
3. Concurrent therapy with other drugs that may cause bone marrow depression should be avoided.
4. Excessive blood levels may result from administration of the recommended dose to patients with impaired liver or kidney function, including that due to immature metabolic processes in the infant. The dosage should be adjusted accordingly or, preferably, the blood concentration should be determined at appropriate intervals.
5. There are no studies to establish the safety of this drug in pregnancy.
6. Since chloramphenicol readily crosses the placental barrier, caution in use of the drug is particularly important during pregnancy at term or during labor because of potential toxic effects on the fetus (gray syndrome).
7. Precaution should be used in therapy of premature and full-term infants to avoid "gray syndrome" toxicity (see Adverse Reactions). Serum drug levels should be carefully followed during therapy of the newborn infant.
8. Precaution should be used in therapy during lactation because of the possibility of toxic effects on the nursing infant.
9. The use of this antibiotic, as with other antibiotics, may result in an overgrowth of nonsusceptible organisms, including fungi. If infections caused by nonsusceptible organisms appear during therapy, appropriate measures should be taken.

ADVERSE REACTIONS

1. Blood Dyscrasias
The most serious adverse effect of chloramphenicol is bone marrow depression. Serious and fatal blood dyscrasias (aplastic anemia, hypoplastic anemia, thrombocytopenia, and granulocytopenia) are known to occur after the administration of chloramphenicol. An irreversible type of marrow depression leading to aplastic anemia with a high rate of mortality is characterized by the appearance weeks or months after therapy of bone marrow aplasia or hypoplasia. Peripherally, pancytopenia is most often observed, but in a small number of cases only one or two of the three major cell types (erythrocytes, leukocytes, platelets) may be depressed. A reversible type of bone marrow depression, which is dose-related, may occur. This type of marrow depression is characterized by vacuolization of the erythroid cells, reduction of reticulocytes, and leukopenia, and responds promptly to the withdrawal of chloramphenicol.
An exact determination of the risk of serious and fatal blood dyscrasias is not possible because of lack of accurate information regarding (1) the size of the population at risk, (2) the total number of drug-associated dyscrasias, and (3) the total number of nondrug-associated dyscrasias.
In a report to the California State Assembly by the California Medical Association and the State Department of Public Health in January 1967, the risk of fatal aplastic anemia was estimated at 1:24,200 to 1:40,500 based on two dosage levels. There have been reports of aplastic anemia attributed to chloramphenicol which later terminated in leukemia. Paroxysmal nocturnal hemoglobinuria has also been reported.
2. Gastrointestinal Reactions
Nausea, vomiting, glossitis and stomatitis, diarrhea, and enterocolitis may occur in low incidence.
3. Neurotoxic Reactions
Headache, mild depression, mental confusion, and delirium have been described in patients receiving chloramphenicol. Optic and peripheral neuritis have been reported, usually following long-term therapy. If this occurs, the drug should be promptly withdrawn.
4. Hypersensitivity Reactions
Fever, macular and vesicular rashes, angio- edema, urticaria, and anaphylaxis may occur. Herxheimer's reactions have occurred during therapy for typhoid fever.
5. "Gray Syndrome"
Toxic reactions including fatalities have occurred in the premature and newborn; the signs and symptoms associated with these reactions have been referred to as the gray syndrome. One case of "gray syndrome" has been reported in an infant born to a mother having received chloramphenicol during labor. One case has been reported in a 3-month-old infant. The following summarizes the clinical and laboratory studies that have been made on these patients:
   a) In most cases, therapy with chloramphenicol had been instituted within the first 48 hours of life.
   b) Symptoms first appeared after 3 to 4 days of continued treatment with high doses of chloramphenicol.
   c) The symptoms appeared in the following order:
      (1) abdominal distention with or without emesis;
      (2) progressive pallid cyanosis;
      (3) vasomotor collapse, frequently accompanied by irregular respiration;

(4) death within a few hours of onset of these symptoms.

d) The progression of symptoms from onset to exitus was accelerated with higher dose schedules.

e) Preliminary blood serum level studies revealed unusually high concentrations of chloramphenicol (over 90 mcg/ml after repeated doses).

f) Termination of therapy upon early evidence of the associated symptomatology frequently reversed the process with complete recovery.

ADMINISTRATION

Chloramphenicol, like other potent drugs, should be prescribed at recommended doses known to have therapeutic activity. Administration of 50 mg/kg/day in divided doses will produce blood levels of the magnitude to which the majority of susceptible microorganisms will respond.

As soon as feasible, an oral dosage form of chloramphenicol should be substituted for the intravenous form because adequate blood levels are achieved with chloramphenicol by mouth.

The following method of administration is recommended: Intravenously as a 10% (100 mg/ml) solution to be injected over at least a one-minute interval. This is prepared by the addition of 10 ml of an aqueous diluent, such as water for injection or 5% dextrose injection.

DOSAGE

Adults

Adults should receive 50 mg/kg/day in divided doses at 6-hour intervals. In exceptional cases, patients with infections due to moderately resistant organisms may require increased dosage up to 100 mg/kg/day to achieve blood levels inhibiting the pathogen, but these high doses should be decreased as soon as possible. Adults with impairment of hepatic or renal function or both may have reduced ability to metabolize and excrete the drug. In instances of impaired metabolic processes, dosages should be adjusted accordingly. (See discussion under Newborn Infants.) Precise control of concentration of the drug in the blood should be carefully followed in patients with impaired metabolic processes by the available microtechniques (information available on request).

Children

Dosage of 50 mg/kg/day divided into 4 doses at 6-hour intervals yields blood levels in the range effective against most susceptible organisms. Severe infections (eg, bacteremia or meningitis), especially when adequate cerebrospinal fluid concentrations are desired, may require dosage up to 100 mg/kg/day; however, it is recommended that dosage be reduced to 50 mg/kg/day as soon as possible. Children with impaired liver or kidney function may retain excessive amounts of the drug.

Newborn Infants

(See section titled "Gray Syndrome" under Adverse Reactions.)

A total of 25 mg/kg/day in 4 equal doses at 6-hour intervals usually produces and maintains concentrations in blood and tissues adequate to control most infections for which the drug is indicated. Increased dosage in these individuals, demanded by severe infections, should be given only to maintain the blood concentration within a therapeutically effective range. After the first two weeks of life, full-term infants ordinarily may receive up to a total of 50 mg/kg/day equally divided into 4 doses at 6-hour intervals. *These dosage recommendations are extremely important because blood concentration in all premature infants and full-term infants under two weeks of age differs from that of other infants. This difference is due to variations in the maturity of the metabolic functions of the liver and the kidneys.*

When these functions are immature (or seriously impaired in adults), high concentrations of the drug are found which tend to increase with succeeding doses.

Infants and Children with Immature Metabolic Processes

In young infants and other children in whom immature metabolic functions are suspected, a dose of 25 mg/kg/day will usually produce therapeutic concentrations of the drug in the blood. In this group particularly, the concentration of the drug in the blood should be carefully followed by microtechniques. (Information available on request.)

HOW SUPPLIED

N 0071-4057-03—(Steri-Vial® No. 57) Chloromycetin Sodium Succinate is freeze-dried in the vial and supplied in Steri-Vials (rubber diaphragm-capped vials). When reconstituted as directed, each vial contains a sterile solution equivalent to 100 mg of chloramphenicol per mL (1 g/10 mL). Available in packages of 10 vials.

Chloromycetin, brand of chloramphenicol, Reg US Pat Off

Store between 15° and 25°C (59° and 77°F).

Caution: Federal law prohibits dispensing without prescription. Revised August 1994

4057G021

COGNEX® ℞
(Tacrine Hydrochloride Capsules)

DESCRIPTION

Cognex® (tacrine hydrochloride) is a reversible cholinesterase inhibitor, known chemically as 1,2,3,4-tetrahydro-9-acridinamine monohydrochloride monohydrate. Tacrine hydrochloride is commonly referred to in the clinical and pharmacological literature as THA. It has an empirical formula of $C_{13}H_{14}N_2 \cdot HCl \cdot H_2O$ and a molecular weight of 252.74.

Tacrine hydrochloride is a white solid and is freely soluble in distilled water, 0.1N hydrochloric acid, acetate buffer (pH 4.0), phosphate buffer (pH 7.0 to 7.4), methanol, dimethylsulfoxide (DMSO), ethanol, and propylene glycol. The compound is sparingly soluble in linoleic acid and PEG 400.

Each capsule of Cognex® contains tacrine as the hydrochloride. Inactive ingredients are hydrous lactose, magnesium stearate, and microcrystalline cellulose. The hard gelatin capsules contain gelatin, NF; silicon dioxide, NF; sodium lauryl sulfate, NF; and the following dyes: 10 mg: D&C Yellow #10, FD&C Green #3, titanium dioxide; 20 mg: D&C Yellow #10, FD&C Blue #1, titanium dioxide; 30 mg: D&C Yellow #10, FD&C Blue #1, FD&C Red #40, titanium dioxide; 40 mg: D&C Yellow #10, FD&C Blue #1, FD&C Red #40, D&C Red #28, titanium dioxide.

Each 10-, 20-, 30-, and 40-mg Cognex® capsule for oral administration contains 12.75, 25.50, 38.25, and 51.00 mg of tacrine HCl, respectively.

CLINICAL PHARMACOLOGY

Although widespread degeneration of multiple CNS neuronal systems eventually occurs, early pathological changes in Alzheimer's Disease involve, in a relatively selective manner, cholinergic neuronal pathways that project from the basal forebrain to the cerebral cortex and hippocampus. The resulting deficiency of cortical acetylcholine is believed to account for some of the clinical manifestations of mild to moderate dementia. Tacrine, an orally bioavailable, centrally active, reversible cholinesterase inhibitor, presumably acts by elevating acetylcholine concentrations in the cerebral cortex by slowing the degradation of acetylcholine released by still intact cholinergic neurons. If this theoretical mechanism of action is correct, tacrine's effects may lessen as the disease process advances and fewer cholinergic neurons remain functionally intact. There is no evidence that tacrine alters the course of the underlying dementing process.

Clinical Trial Data

The conclusion that Cognex® is an effective treatment for Alzheimer's Disease derives from two adequate and well controlled clinical investigations that evaluated tacrine's effects in patients with probable Alzheimer's disease of mild to moderate severity (NINCDS criteria, Mini-Mental State Examination (MMSE) of Folstein, Folstein and McHugh scores of 10 to 26).

In each study, outcomes during treatment with tacrine and placebo were assessed on two primary measures: (1) the cognitive subscale of the Alzheimer's Disease Assessment Scale (ADAS cog) of Rosen, Mohs, and Davis and (2) a clinician's rated clinical global impression of change.

Study Endpoints

The ADAS cog is a multi-item test battery administered by a psychometrician that examines aspects of memory, attention, praxis, reason, and language. The worst possible score is 70. Elderly, normal adults may score as low as 0 or 1 unit, but individuals judged not to be demented can score higher. The mean score of patients entering each study was approximately 28 units (range 7 to 62). The ADAS cog score is reported to deteriorate at a rate of about 6 to 10 units per year for untreated patients at this stage of dementia.

The clinician's global assessments used in the two studies relied on a clinician's judgment about the overall clinical change observed in patients over the course of the study. Although the conditions for obtaining the clinical assessment differed in each study, the global assessment was rated on a 7-point scale in both studies. A rating of four (4) represents no change; lower ratings indicate improvement from baseline and higher ratings deterioration.

Twelve-Week Study

In one study of 12 weeks duration, patients were randomized to sequences that provided a comparison between placebo, 20, 40, and 80 mg/day by study's end. Statistically significant drug-placebo differences were detected on both primary outcome measures for the group titrated to 80 mg/day. Estimates of the size of the treatment effect varied between 2 and 4 ADAS cog units. The imprecision in these estimates reflects the fact that different analyses, conducted in attempts to account for the effects of the failure of a substantial fraction of the patients randomized to complete the full 12 weeks of the study, yielded different results.

The placebo-80 mg/day comparison also achieved statistical significance on the clinician's global impression of change (CGIC) with a 0.3 to 0.4 unit mean difference. The following diagram illustrates the percentages of patients falling into each global category at trial's end for the patients given placebo or 80 mg/day.

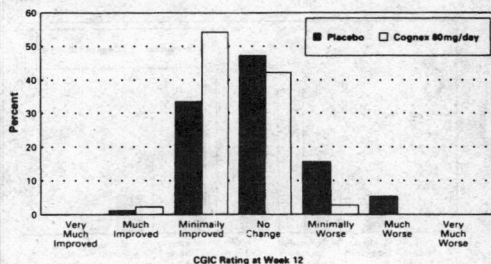

FIGURE 1. Percent of Patients in Each of the Seven Outcome Categories on the Clinician-Rated CGIC for Patients Completing 12 Weeks of Treatment (83% of patients randomized to placebo completed 12 weeks of treatment and are represented above; 56% of those randomized to the 80 mg/day Cognex® sequence completed 12 weeks)

Thirty-Week Study

The second study was 30 weeks long. Six hundred sixty-three patients were randomized to 4 treatment sequences (placebo and 3 drug groups) that called for the daily dose of tacrine to be increased at 6-week intervals, starting with a 40-mg/day dose. By study's end, a comparison between placebo, 80, 120, and 160 mg/day was possible. Patients in the 160 mg group received this dose for the final 12 weeks; the 120 mg group received that dose for 18 weeks.

The study showed statistically significant drug-placebo differences for the 80 and 120 mg/day groups at 18 weeks and for the 120 and 160 mg/day groups at 30 weeks on both a performance-based test of cognitive function (the ADAS cog) and a clinician's assessment of global change (Clinician Interview Based Impression: CIBI). Because many patients failed to complete 30 weeks on treatment, analyses that used each patient's last on-study value or retrieved patients' (see below) 30-week value, even if they were no longer in the study ("intent-to-treat" analysis) were also carried out. All analyses confirmed the effectiveness of tacrine, although the estimated mean treatment effect was different in each analysis.

Effects on ADAS Cog: The results for the ADAS cog are shown in Figure 2 for the subset of patients actually completing the full 30 weeks of the study. They show that individual patients, whether assigned to tacrine or to placebo, had a wide range of responses. This variability in response is illustrated in the display that follows (Figure 2).

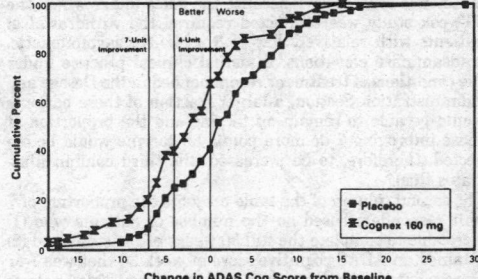

FIGURE 2. Cumulative Percent of Patients Completing 30 Weeks of Treatment Who Attained a Change in ADAS Cog Score From Baseline at Least as Large as the Value on the X Axis. The display is based on scores obtained from a subset of patients (ie, 64% of the 184 randomized to placebo and 27% of the 239 randomized to the 160 mg/day treatment group).

Figure 2 presents the cumulative percentage (Y axis) of patients assigned to placebo or 160 mg/day who actually completed 30 weeks on treatment and who attained a change in ADAS cog score from baseline at least as large as the ADAS cog change score value given on the X axis. A negative change from baseline represents improvement; a positive change deterioration. Thus, in a display of this type, the curve for an effective treatment is shifted to the left of the curve for placebo. The frequency in each group of any response, e.g., an improvement of 7 ADAS cog units, can be found by plotting the change on the X axis, then reading upward along the Y axis. The variability of response is apparent from the fact that the distribution of responses under both treatment conditions range from large negative to large positive values. Nonetheless, the mean drug-placebo ADAS cog difference for the 30-week 160 mg/day completer patients is 4.8 units, a statistically significant difference.

Effects on CIBI: The results on the CIBI are shown in Figure 3.

[See Figure at top of next column.]

Continued on next page

This product information was prepared in August 1996. On these and other Parke-Davis Products, information may be obtained by addressing PARKE-DAVIS, Division of Warner-Lambert Company, Morris Plains, New Jersey 07950.

Parke-Davis—Cont.

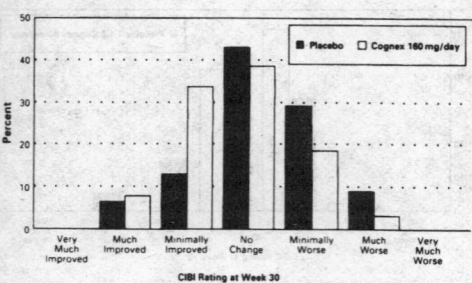

FIGURE 3 Percent of Patients in Each of the Seven Outcome Categories of the CIBI Among Those Completing 30 Weeks. The display is based on scores obtained from the same subset of patients as Figure 2

Figure 3 is a histogram of the frequency distribution of CIBI scores attained by patients assigned to placebo or to the 160 mg/day tacrine dose group who actually completed the full 30 weeks of the study. The mean tacrine-placebo difference for this group of patients on the CIBI was 0.5 units and was statistically significant.

Expected Responses in Newly Treated Patients: Although the results described clearly document tacrine's effectiveness, they are based on only a fraction of the patients initially randomized to tacrine, those who could tolerate tacrine and remain on treatment uninterrupted for the full 30 weeks. In considering the expected outcome in a group of patients newly started on tacrine, account must be taken both of the likelihood of staying on therapy and the responses in patients who do so.

Table 1 provides 3 different estimates of the proportion of patients assigned to treatment with tacrine at 160 mg a day or with placebo who attained a particular measure of improvement (i.e., a 7 point improvement from baseline in ADAS cog score). The criterion has been chosen entirely for illustrative purposes.

[See table 1 below.]

The first column of the table is based on all patients participating in the study. The proportion provides an estimate of the likelihood that a patient entering the study will (1) still be on his or her assigned treatment at week 30 **and** (2) will improve 7 or more ADAS cognitive points over his or her baseline score. The estimate of response derived in this manner is conservative because the rules under which the 30-week study was conducted required the withdrawal of patients with relatively low ($> 3 \times$ ULN), asymptomatic, transaminase elevations. In actual clinical practice under the conditions of treatment recommended in the Dosage and Administration Section, a larger fraction of these patients would be able to remain on tacrine and the proportion of those improving 7 or more points on tacrine would be expected, therefore, to be increased (the third column illustrates this).

The second column of the table presents the proportion of 7 unit responders based on the number of patients who (1) were able to complete the full 30 weeks of the study and (2) attained an ADAS cognitive score at week 30 that was 7 or more points better than their baseline score. This analysis provides an optimistic estimate of tacrine's effects because it reflects experience gained only with the minority of patients who were able to remain on treatment to the study's end. The comparison between the proportions of placebo and 160 mg patients attaining a 7 or more point improvement is complicated further by the fact that a larger proportion of tacrine assigned patients withdrew prematurely.

The third column of the table presents the proportion of patients who had evaluations made at 30 weeks and had a 7-point or greater response. The analysis includes data from patients still on their assigned treatment at week 30 as well as patients who withdrew from the study prior to that time, but were retrieved for a week 30 evaluation. Because patients who withdrew prior to week 30 were permitted to receive tacrine under "open label" conditions, retrieved patients included in this analysis could be receiving either no treatment or treatment with tacrine. In this analysis, patients are considered under the treatment to which they were randomized, regardless of the treatment they were

actually receiving at week 30. Thus, some placebo patients could have received tacrine and some tacrine patients could have been receiving no tacrine. Like the analysis based on percent randomized (column I), this analysis, therefore, tends to provide a conservative view of the expected effects of tacrine treatment.

Effects of Cognex® Over Time: Figure 4 shows for each dose group the time course of change from baseline in ADAS cog scores for patients completing 30 weeks of treatment. There appears to be a persistent difference between groups, but all groups, after initial improvement, deteriorate with time.

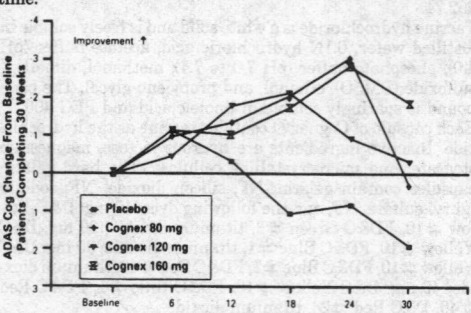

FIGURE 4 ADAS Cog Change From Baseline Over Time for the Subset of Patients Completing 30 Weeks of Treatment. In all tacrine treatment groups dosing was initiated at 40 mg/day and increased in increments of 40 mg every 6 weeks until the target dose was achieved.

Patient age, gender, and other baseline patient characteristics were not found to predict clinical outcome.

Clinical Pharmacokinetics (Absorption, Distribution, Metabolism, and Elimination)

Absorption: Cognex® is rapidly absorbed after oral administration; maximal plasma concentrations occur within 1 to 2 hours. The rate and extent of tacrine absorption following administration of tacrine capsules and solution are virtually indistinguishable. Absolute bioavailability of tacrine is approximately 17 (SD ± 13) %. Food reduces tacrine bioavailability by approximately 30–40%; however, there is no food effect if tacrine is administered at least an hour before meals. The effect of achlorhydria on the absorption of tacrine is unknown.

Distribution: Mean volume of distribution of tacrine is approximately 349 (SD ± 193) L. Tacrine is about 55% bound to plasma proteins. The extent and degree of tacrine's distribution within various body compartments has not been systematically studied. However, 336 hours after the administration of a single radiolabeled dose, approximately 25% of the radiolabel was not recovered in a mass balance study, suggesting the possibility that tacrine and/or one or more of its metabolites may be retained.

Metabolism: Tacrine is extensively metabolized by the cytochrome P450 system to multiple metabolites, not all of which have been identified. The vast majority of radiolabeled species present in the plasma following a single dose of ^{14}C radiolabeled tacrine are unidentified (ie, only 5% of radioactivity in plasma has been identified [tacrine and 3-hydroxylated metabolites; 1-, 2-, and 4-hydroxytacrine]). Studies utilizing human liver preparations demonstrated that cytochrome P450 IA2 is the principal isozyme involved in tacrine metabolism. These findings are consistent with the observation that tacrine and/or one of its metabolites inhibits the metabolism of theophylline in humans (see PRECAUTIONS: Drug-Drug Interactions: theophylline). Results from a study utilizing quinidine to inhibit cytochrome P450 IID6 indicate that tacrine is not metabolized extensively by this enzyme system.

Following aromatic ring hydroxylation, tacrine's metabolites undergo glucuronidation. Whether tacrine and/or its metabolites undergo biliary excretion or entero-hepatic circulation is unknown.

Special Populations: Age: Based on pooled pharmacokinetic studies (n = 192), there is no clinically relevant influence of age (50 to 84 years) on tacrine clearance. *Gender:* Average tacrine plasma concentrations are approximately 50% higher in females than in males. This is not explained by differences in body surface area or elimination half-life. The difference is probably due to higher systemic availability after oral dosing and may reflect the known lower activity of

cytochrome P450 IA2 in women. *Race:* The effect of race on tacrine clearance has not been studied. *Smoking:* Mean plasma tacrine concentrations in current smokers are approximately one third the concentrations in nonsmokers. Cigarette smoking is known to induce cytochrome P450 IA2. *Renal disease:* Renal disease does not appear to affect the clearance of tacrine. *Liver disease:* Although studies in patients with liver disease have not been done, it is likely that functional hepatic impairment will reduce the clearance of tacrine and its metabolites.

Presystemic Clearance/Elimination/Excretion: Tacrine undergoes presystemic clearance (ie, first pass metabolism). The extent of this first pass metabolism depends upon the dose of tacrine administered. Because the enzyme system involved can be saturated at relatively low doses, a larger fraction of a high dose of tacrine will escape first pass elimination than of a smaller dose. Thus, when a 40 mg daily dose is increased by 40 mg, the average plasma concentration will be increased by approximately 6 ng/mL. However, when a daily dose of 80 or 120 mg is increased by 40 mg, the increment in average plasma concentration is approximately 10 ng/mL.

Elimination of tacrine from the plasma, however, is not dose dependent (ie, the half-life is independent of dose or plasma concentration). The elimination half-life is approximately 2 to 4 hours. Following initiation of therapy or a change in daily dose, steady state tacrine plasma concentration should be attained within 24 to 36 hours.

Drug Interactions (See PRECAUTIONS)

INDICATIONS AND USAGE

Cognex® (tacrine hydrochloride capsules) is indicated for the treatment of mild to moderate dementia of the Alzheimer's type.

Evidence of Cognex®'s effectiveness in the treatment of dementia of the Alzheimer's type derives from results of two adequate and well-controlled clinical investigations that compared tacrine and placebo on both a performance based measure of cognition and a clinician's global assessment of change. (See CLINICAL PHARMACOLOGY Section: Clinical Trial Data.)

CONTRAINDICATIONS

Cognex® is contraindicated in patients with known hypersensitivity to tacrine or acridine derivatives.

Cognex® is contraindicated in patients previously treated with Cognex® who developed treatment-associated jaundice confirmed by elevated total bilirubin greater than 3.0 mg/dL.

WARNINGS

Anesthesia

Cognex®, as a cholinesterase inhibitor, is likely to exaggerate succinylcholine-type muscle relaxation during anesthesia.

Cardiovascular Conditions

Because of its cholinomimetic action, Cognex® may have vagotonic effects on the heart rate (eg, bradycardia). This action may be particularly important to patients with conduction abnormalities, bradyarrhythmia, or a sick sinus syndrome.

Gastrointestinal Disease and Dysfunction

Cognex® is an inhibitor of cholinesterase and may be expected to increase gastric acid secretion due to increased cholinergic activity. Therefore, patients at increased risk for developing ulcers—eg, those with a history of ulcer disease or those receiving concurrent nonsteroidal anti-inflammatory drugs (NSAIDs)—should be monitored closely for symptoms of active or occult gastrointestinal bleeding.

Cognex®, also as a predictable consequence of its pharmacological properties, can cause nausea, vomiting, and loose stools at recommended doses.

Liver Injury

Cognex® should be prescribed with care in patients with current evidence or history of abnormal liver function indicated by significant abnormalities in serum transaminase (ALT/SGPT; AST/SGOT), bilirubin, and gamma-glutamyl transpeptidase (GGT) levels (see PRECAUTIONS and DOSAGE AND ADMINISTRATION sections).

The use of tacrine in patients without a prior history of liver disease is commonly associated with serum aminotransferase elevations, some to levels ordinarily considered to indicate clinically important hepatic injury (see Table 2).

Experience gained in more than 8000 patients who received tacrine in clinical studies and the treatment IND program indicates that if tacrine is promptly withdrawn following detection of these elevations, clinically evident signs and symptoms of liver injury are rare.

Long-term follow up of patients who experience transaminase elevations, however, is limited and it is impossible, therefore, to exclude, with certainty, the possibility of chronic sequelae.

Controlled Clinical Trials, Treatment IND and Post Marketing Experience:

Experience with tacrine in controlled trials and in a large, less closely monitored experience (a treatment IND) is summarized below:

Table 1. Proportion of Patients Attaining ≥ 7 Unit Improvement on the ADAS Cog at the Week 30 Assessment

Treatment Group N Randomized	I N (%) of Those Randomized	II N (%) of Those Completing Week 30	III N (%) of Those With Week 30 Assessments
Placebo (N = 184)	10/184 (5.4)	10/117 (8.5)	11/143[1] (7.7)
160 mg/day (N = 239)	13/239 (5.4)	13/64 (20.3)	25/172[2] (14.5)

[1]: 13 of the 143 were receiving tacrine when evaluated.
[2]: 41 of the 172 were not receiving tacrine when evaluated.

Clinically evident liver toxicity: One of more than 8000 patients exposed to tacrine in clinical studies and the treatment IND program had documented elevated bilirubin (5.3 × Upper Limit of Normal, ULN) and jaundice with transaminase levels (AST/SGOT) nearly 20 × ULN.

Rare cases of liver toxicity associated with jaundice, raised serum bilirubin, pyrexia, hepatitis and liver failure have been reported in post-marketing experience. Most of these cases have been reversible but some deaths have occurred. Since there was multiple pathology including infection, gallstones and carcinoma it was not possible to clearly establish the relationship to Cognex® treatment.

Blood chemistry signs of liver injury: Experience from the 30-week clinical study (described earlier) provides a representative estimate of the frequency of ALT/SGPT elevations expected for patients whose transaminase levels are monitored weekly and who receive Cognex® according to the recommended regimen for dose introduction and titration (Table 2). A dosing regimen employing a more rapid escalation of the daily dose of tacrine may be associated with more serious clinical events (see *Monitoring of Liver function and the Management of the patient who develops transaminase elevations*).

Table 2. Cumulative Incidence of ALT/SGPT Elevations Based on Maximum Values with Weekly Monitoring During the 30-Week Study
[Number and (%) of Patients]

Maximum ALT	Males N=229	Females N=250	Total N=479
Within Normal Limits	121(53)	100(40)	221(46)
>ULN	108(47)	150(60)	258(54)
>2 times ULN	77(34)	104(42)	181(38)
>3 times ULN	58(25)	81(32)	139(29)
>10 times ULN	12 (5)	19 (8)	31 (6)
>20 times ULN	3 (1)	6 (2)	9 (2)

Experience in 2446 patients who participated in all clinical trials, including the 30-week study, indicates approximately 50% of patients treated with Cognex® can be expected to have at least 1 ALT/SGPT level above ULN; approximately 25% of patients are likely to develop elevations >3 × ULN, and about 7% of patients may develop elevations >10 × ULN. Data collected from the treatment IND program were consistent with those obtained during clinical studies, and showed 3% of 5665 patients experiencing an ALT/SGPT elevation >10 × ULN.

In clinical trials where transaminases were monitored weekly, the median time to onset of the first ALT/SGPT elevation above ULN was approximately 6 weeks, with maximum ALT/SGPT occurring 1 week later, even in instances when Cognex® treatment was stopped. Under the conditions of forced slow upwards dose titration (increases of 40 mg a day every 6 weeks) employed in clinical studies, 95% of transaminase elevations >3 × ULN occurred within the first 18 weeks of Cognex® therapy, and 99% of the 10-fold elevations occurred by the 12th week and on not more than 80 mg; note, however, that for most patients ALT was monitored weekly and Cognex® was stopped when liver enzymes exceeded 3 × ULN. A total of 276 patients were monitored for ALT/SGPT levels every other week in two double-blind clinical studies, an open-label study, and amended treatment IND. The incidence, severity, time to onset, peak and recovery of ALT/SGPT levels were similar to weekly monitoring. With less frequent monitoring than every other week or the less stringent discontinuation criteria recommended below (see DOSAGE AND ADMINISTRATION), it is possible that marked elevations might be more common. It must also be appreciated that experience with prolonged exposure to the high dose (160 mg/day) is limited. In all cases, transaminase levels returned to within normal limits upon discontinuation of Cognex® treatment or following dosage reduction, usually within 4 to 6 weeks.

This relatively benign experience may be the consequence of careful laboratory monitoring that facilitated the discontinuation of patients early on after the onset of their transaminase elevations. Consequently, frequent monitoring of serum transaminase levels is recommended (see DOSAGE AND ADMINISTRATION, WARNINGS: Liver Injury: Monitoring of Liver Function and the Management of the Patient Who Develops Transaminase Elevations, and PRECAUTIONS: Laboratory Tests).

Liver biopsy experience: Liver biopsy results in 7 patients who received tacrine (1 in a Parke-Davis sponsored study and 6 in studies reported in the literature) revealed hepatocellular necrosis in 6 patients, and granulomatous changes in the seventh. In all cases, liver function tests returned to normal with no evidence of persisting hepatic dysfunction.

Experience with the Rechallenge of Patients with Transaminase Elevations following recovery: Two hundred and twelve patients among the 866 patients assigned to tacrine in the 12 and 30 week studies were withdrawn because they developed transaminase elevations >3 × ULN. One hundred and forty-five of these patients were subsequently rechallenged with weekly monitoring of ALT/SGPT. During their initial exposure to tacrine, 20 of these 145 had experienced initial elevations >10 times ULN, while the remainder had experienced elevations between 3 and 10 × ULN. Upon rechallenge with an initial dose of 40 mg/day, only 48 (33%) of the 145 patients developed transaminase elevations greater than 3 × ULN. Of these patients, 44 had elevations that were between 3 and 10 × ULN and 4 had elevations that were >10 × ULN.

The mean time to onset of elevations occurred earlier on rechallenge than on initial exposure (22 versus 48 days). Of the 145 patients rechallenged, 127 (88%) were able to continue Cognex® treatment, and 91 of these 127 patients titrated to doses higher than those associated with the initial transaminase elevation.

Predictors of the risk of transaminase elevations: The incidence of transaminase elevations is higher among females. There are no other known predictors of the risk of hepatocellular injury.

Monitoring of Liver function and the Management of the patient who develops transaminase elevations. (See also DOSAGE AND ADMINISTRATION and PRECAUTIONS: Laboratory Tests.)

Blood chemistries: Serum transaminase levels (specifically ALT/SGPT) should be monitored every other week for at least the first 16 weeks following initiation of Cognex® treatment after which monitoring may be decreased to monthly for 2 months and every 3 months thereafter. For patients who develop ALT/SGPT elevations greater than two times the upper limit of normal, the dose and monitoring should be modified as described in Table 4 (see DOSAGE AND ADMINISTRATION).

A full monitoring sequence should be repeated in the event that a patient suspends treatment with tacrine for more than 4 weeks.

If ALT/SGPT elevations occur, the frequency of monitoring and the dose of Cognex® should be modified according to the table shown below in DOSAGE AND ADMINISTRATION.

Rechallenge: **Patients with clinical jaundice confirmed by a significant elevation in total bilirubin (>3 mg/dL) and/or those exhibiting clinical signs and/or symptoms of hypersensitivity (e.g. rash or fever) in association with ALT/SGPT elevations should immediately and permanently discontinue Cognex® and not be rechallenged.** Other patients who are required to discontinue Cognex® treatment because of ALT/SGPT elevations may be rechallenged once ALT/SGPT levels return to within normal limits. (See DOSAGE AND ADMINISTRATION.)

Rechallenge of patients with ALT/SGPT elevations less than 10 × ULN has not resulted in serious liver injury. However, because experience in the rechallenge of patients who had elevations greater than 10 × ULN is limited, the risks associated with the rechallenge of these patients are not well characterized. Careful, frequent (weekly) monitoring of serum ALT/SGPT should be undertaken when rechallenging such patients.

If rechallenged, patients should be given an initial dose of 40 mg/day (10 mg QID) and ALT/SGPT levels monitored weekly. If, after 6 weeks on 40 mg/day, the patient is tolerating the dosage with no unacceptable elevations in ALT/SGPT, recommended dose-titration may be resumed. Weekly monitoring of the ALT/SGPT levels should continue for a total of 16 weeks after which monitoring may be decreased to monthly for 2 months and every 3 months thereafter.

Liver biopsy: Liver biopsy is not indicated in cases of uncomplicated transaminase elevation.

Genitourinary
Cholinomimetics may cause bladder outflow obstruction.

Neurological Conditions
Seizures: Cholinomimetics are believed to have some potential to cause generalized convulsions; seizure activity may, however, also be a manifestation of Alzheimer's disease.

Sudden worsening of the degree of cognitive impairment: Worsening of cognitive function has been reported following abrupt discontinuation of Cognex® or after a large reduction in total daily dose (80 mg/day or more).

Pulmonary Conditions
Because of its cholinomimetic action, Cognex® should be prescribed with care to patients with a history of asthma.

PRECAUTIONS
General
Liver Injury: see WARNINGS
Hematology
An absolute neutrophil count (ANC) less than 500/μL occurred in 4 patients who received Cognex® during the course of clinical trials. Three of the 4 patients had concurrent medical conditions commonly associated with a low ANC; 2 of these patients remained on Cognex®. The fourth patient, who had a history of hypersensitivity (penicillin allergy), withdrew from the study as a result of a rash and also developed an ANC <500/μL, which returned to normal; this patient was not rechallenged and, therefore, the role played by Cognex® in this reaction is unknown.

Six patients had an absolute neutrophil count ≤1500/μL, associated with an elevation of ALT/SGPT.

The total clinical experience in more than 8000 patients does not indicate a clear association between Cognex® treatment and serious white blood cell abnormalities.

Information for Patients and Caregivers
Patients and caregivers should be advised that the effect of Cognex® (brand of tacrine hydrochloride) therapy is thought to depend upon its administration at regular intervals, as directed.

The caregiver should be advised about the possibility of adverse effects. Two types should be distinguished: (1) those occurring in close temporal association with the initiation of treatment or an increase in dose (eg, nausea, vomiting, loose stools, diarrhea, etc) and (2) those with a delayed onset (eg, rash, jaundice, changes in the color of stool—black, very dark or light [ie, acholic]).

Patients and caregivers should be encouraged to inform the physician about the emergence of new events or any increase in the severity of existing adverse clinical events.

Caregivers should be advised that abrupt discontinuation of Cognex® or a large reduction in total daily dose (80 mg/day or more) may cause a decline in cognitive function and behavioral disturbances. Unsupervised increases in the dose of tacrine may also have serious consequences. Consequently, changes in dose should not be undertaken in the absence of direct instruction of a physician.

Laboratory Tests (see WARNINGS: Liver Injury and DOSAGE AND ADMINISTRATION)
Serum transaminase levels (specifically ALT/SGPT) should be monitored in patients given Cognex® (see WARNINGS: Liver Injury).

Drug-Drug Interactions
Possible metabolic basis for interactions: Tacrine is primarily eliminated by hepatic metabolism via cytochrome P450 drug metabolizing enzymes. Drug-drug interactions may occur when Cognex® is given concurrently with agents such as theophylline that undergo extensive metabolism via cytochrome P450 IA2.

Theophylline. **Coadministration of tacrine with theophylline increased theophylline elimination half-life and average plasma theophylline concentrations by approximately 2-fold. Therefore, monitoring of plasma theophylline concentrations and appropriate reduction of theophylline dose are recommended in patients receiving tacrine and theophylline concurrently. The effect of theophylline on tacrine pharmacokinetics has not been assessed.**

Cimetidine. Cimetidine increased the Cmax and AUC of tacrine by approximately 54% and 64%, respectively.

Anticholinergics. Because of its mechanism of action, Cognex® has the potential to interfere with the activity of anticholinergic medications.

Cholinomimetics and Cholinesterase Inhibitors. A synergistic effect is expected when Cognex® is given concurrently with succinylcholine (see WARNINGS), cholinesterase inhibitors, or cholinergic agonists such as bethanechol.

Other Interactions. Rate and extent of tacrine absorption were not influenced by the coadministration of an antacid containing magnesium and aluminum. Tacrine had no major effect on digoxin or diazepam pharmacokinetics or the anticoagulant activity of warfarin.

Carcinogenesis, Mutagenesis, Impairment of Fertility
Tacrine was mutagenic to bacteria in the Ames test. Unscheduled DNA synthesis was induced in rat and mouse hepatocytes *in vitro*. Results of cytogenetic (chromosomal aberration) studies were equivocal. Tacrine was not mutagenic in an *in vitro* mammalian mutation test. Overall, the results of these tests, along with the fact that tacrine belongs to a chemical class (acridines) containing some members which are animal carcinogens, suggest that tacrine may be carcinogenic.

Studies of the effects of tacrine on fertility have not been performed.

Pregnancy
Category C: Animal reproduction studies have not been conducted with tacrine. It is also not known whether Cognex® can cause fetal harm when administered to a pregnant woman or can affect reproductive capacity.

Nursing Mothers
It is not known whether this drug is excreted in human milk.

Pediatric Use
There are no adequate and well-controlled trials to document the safety and efficacy of tacrine in any dementing illness occurring in children.

Continued on next page

This product information was prepared in August 1996. On these and other Parke-Davis Products, information may be obtained by addressing PARKE-DAVIS, Division of Warner-Lambert Company, Morris Plains, New Jersey 07950.

Parke-Davis—Cont.

ADVERSE REACTIONS

Common Adverse Events Leading to Discontinuation

In clinical trials, approximately 17% of the 2706 patients who received Cognex® and 5% of the 1886 patients who received placebo withdrew permanently because of adverse events. It should be noted that some of the placebo-treated patients were exposed to Cognex® prior to receiving placebo due to the variety of study designs used, including crossover studies. Transaminase elevations were the most common reason for withdrawals during Cognex® treatment (8% of all Cognex®-treated patients, or 212 of 456 patients withdrawn). The controlled clinical trial protocols required that any patient with an ALT/SGPT elevation >3 × ULN be withdrawn, because of concern about potential hepatotoxicity. Apart from withdrawals due to transaminase elevations, 244 patients (9%) withdrew for adverse events while receiving Cognex®.

Other adverse events that most frequently led to the withdrawal of tacrine-treated patients in clinical trials were nausea and/or vomiting (1.5%), agitation (0.9%), rash (0.7%), anorexia (0.7%), and confusion (0.5%). These adverse events also most frequently led to the withdrawal of placebo-treated patients, although at lower frequencies (0.1% to 0.2%).

Most Frequent Adverse Clinical Events Seen in Association With the Use of Tacrine

The events identified here are those that occurred at an absolute incidence of at least 5% of patients treated with Cognex®, and at a rate at least 2-fold higher in patients treated with Cognex® than placebo.

The most common adverse events associated with the use of Cognex® were elevated transaminases, nausea and/or vomiting, diarrhea, dyspepsia, myalgia, anorexia, and ataxia. Of these events, nausea and/or vomiting, diarrhea, dyspepsia, and anorexia appeared to be dose-dependent.

Adverse Events Reported in Controlled Trials

The events cited in the tables below reflect experience gained under closely monitored conditions of clinical trials with a highly selective patient population. In actual clinical practice or in other clinical trials, these frequency estimates may not apply, as the conditions of use, reporting behavior, and the kinds of patients treated may differ.

Table 3 lists treatment-emergent signs and symptoms that occurred in at least 2% of patients with Alzheimer's disease in placebo-controlled trials and who received the recommended regimen for dose introduction and titration of Cognex® (see DOSAGE AND ADMINISTRATION).

Table 3. Adverse Events Occurring in at Least 2% of Patients Receiving Cognex® Using the Recommended Regimen for Dose Introduction and Titration in Controlled Clinical Trials
[Number (%) of Patients]

BODY SYSTEM/ Adverse Events	Cognex® N = 634		Placebo N = 342	
LABORATORY DEVIATIONS				
Elevated Transaminase[a]	184	(29)	5	(2)
BODY AS A WHOLE				
Headache	67	(11)	52	(15)
Fatigue	26	(4)	9	(3)
Chest Pain	24	(4)	18	(5)
Weight Decrease	21	(3)	4	(1)
Back Pain	15	(2)	14	(4)
Asthenia	15	(2)	7	(2)
DIGESTIVE SYSTEM				
Nausea and/or Vomiting	178	(28)	29	(9)
Diarrhea	99	(16)	18	(5)
Dyspepsia	57	(9)	22	(6)
Anorexia	54	(9)	11	(3)
Abdominal Pain	48	(8)	24	(7)
Flatulence	22	(4)	5	(2)
Constipation	24	(4)	8	(2)
HEMIC AND LYMPHATIC SYSTEM				
Purpura	15	(2)	8	(2)
MUSCULOSKELETAL SYSTEM				
Myalgia	54	(9)	18	(5)
NERVOUS SYSTEM				
Dizziness	73	(12)	39	(11)
Confusion	42	(7)	24	(7)
Ataxia	36	(6)	12	(4)
Insomnia	37	(6)	18	(5)
Somnolence	22	(4)	11	(3)
Tremor	14	(2)	2	(<1)
PSYCHOBIOLOGIC FUNCTION				
Agitation	43	(7)	30	(9)
Depression	22	(4)	14	(4)
Thinking Abnormal	17	(3)	14	(4)
Anxiety	16	(3)	7	(2)
Hallucination	15	(2)	12	(4)
Hostility	15	(2)	5	(2)

RESPIRATORY SYSTEM				
Rhinitis	51	(8)	22	(6)
Upper Respiratory Infection	18	(3)	11	(3)
Coughing	17	(3)	18	(5)
SKIN AND APPENDAGES				
Rash[b]	46	(7)	18	(5)
Facial Flushing, Skin Flushing	16	(3)	3	(<1)
UROGENITAL SYSTEM				
Urination Frequency	21	(3)	12	(4)
Urinary Tract Infection	21	(3)	20	(6)
Urinary Incontinence	16	(3)	9	(3)

[a] ALT or AST value of approximately 3 × ULN or greater or that resulted in a change in patient management. Patients were monitored weekly.

[b] Includes COSTART terms: rash, rash-erythematous, rash-maculopapular, urticaria, petechial rash, rash-vesiculobullous, and pruritus.

Other Adverse Events Observed During All Clinical Trials

Cognex® has been administered to 2706 individuals during clinical trials. A total of 1471 patients were treated for at least 3 months, 1137 for at least 6 months, and 773 for at least 1 year. Any untoward reactions that occurred during these trials were recorded as adverse events by the clinical investigators using terminology of their own choosing. To provide a meaningful estimate of the proportion of individuals having similar types of events, the events were grouped into a smaller number of standardized categories using a modified COSTART dictionary. These categories are used in the listing below. The frequencies represent the proportion of the 2706 individuals exposed to Cognex® who experienced that event while receiving Cognex®. All adverse events are included except those already listed on the previous table and those COSTART terms too general to be informative. Events are further classified by body system categories and listed using the following definitions: frequent adverse events are defined as those occurring in at least 1/100 patients; infrequent adverse events are those occurring in 1/100 to 1/1000 patients; and rare adverse events are those occurring in less than 1/1000 patients. These adverse events are not necessarily related to Cognex® treatment. Only rare adverse events deemed to be potentially important are included.

Body As a Whole: *Frequent:* Chill, fever, malaise, peripheral edema. *Infrequent:* Face edema, dehydration, weight increase, cachexia, edema (generalized), lipoma. *Rare:* Heat exhaustion, sepsis, cholingeric crisis, death.

Cardiovascular System: *Frequent:* Hypotension, hypertension. *Infrequent:* Heart failure, myocardial infarction, angina pectoris, cerebrovascular accident, transient ischemic attack, phlebitis, venous insufficiency, abdominal aortic aneurysm, atrial fibrillation or flutter, palpitation, tachycardia, bradycardia, pulmonary embolus, migraine, hypercholesterolemia. *Rare:* Heart arrest, premature atrial contractions, A-V block, bundle branch block.

Digestive System: *Infrequent:* Glossitis, gingivitis, mouth or throat dry, stomatitis, increased salivation, dysphagia, esophagitis, gastritis, gastroenteritis, GI hemorrhage, stomach ulcer, hiatal hernia, hemorrhoids, stools bloody, diverticulitis, fecal impaction, fecal incontinence, hemorrhage (rectum), cholelithiasis, cholecystitis, increased appetite. *Rare:* Duodenal ulcer, bowel obstruction.

Endocrine System: *Infrequent:* Diabetes. *Rare:* Hyperthyroid, hypothyroid.

Hemic and Lymphatic: *Infrequent:* Anemia, lymphadenopathy. *Rare:* Leukopenia, thrombocytopenia, hemolysis, pancytopenia.

Musculoskeletal: *Frequent:* Fracture, arthralgia, arthritis, hypertonia. *Infrequent:* Osteoporosis, tendinitis, bursitis, gout. *Rare:* Myopathy.

Nervous System: *Frequent:* Convulsions, vertigo, syncope, hyperkinesia, paresthesia. *Infrequent:* Dreaming abnormal, dysarthria, aphasia, amnesia, wandering, twitching, hypesthesia, delirium, paralysis, bradykinesia, movement disorder, cogwheel rigidity, paresis, neuritis, hemiplegia, Parkinson's disease, neuropathy, extrapyramidal syndrome, reflexes decreased/absent. *Rare:* Tardive dyskinesia, dysesthesia, dystonia, encephalitis, coma, apraxia, oculogyric crisis, akathisia, oral facial dyskinesia, Bell's palsy, exacerbation of Parkinson's disease.

Psychobiologic Function: *Frequent:* Nervousness. *Infrequent:* Apathy, increased libido, paranoia, neurosis. *Rare:* Suicidal, psychosis, hysteria.

Respiratory System: *Frequent:* Pharyngitis, sinusitis, bronchitis, pneumonia, dyspnea. *Infrequent:* Epistaxis, chest congestion, asthma, hyperventilation, lower respiratory infection. *Rare:* Hemoptysis, lung edema, lung cancer, acute epiglottitis.

Skin and Appendages: *Frequent:* Sweating increased. *Infrequent:* Acne, alopecia, dermatitis, eczema, skin dry, herpes zoster, psoriasis, cellulitis, cyst, furunculosis, herplex simplex, hyperkeratosis, basal cell carcinoma, skin cancer. *Rare:* Desquamation, seborrhea, squamous cell carcinoma, ulcer (skin), skin necrosis, melanoma.

Urogenital System: *Infrequent:* Hematuria, renal stone, kidney infection, glycosuria, dysuria, polyuria, nocturia, pyuria, cystitis, urinary retention, urination urgency, vaginal hemorrhage, pruritus (genital), breast pain, impotence, prostate cancer. *Rare:* Bladder tumor, renal tumor, renal failure, urinary obstruction, breast cancer, epididymitis, carcinoma (ovary).

Special Senses: *Frequent:* Conjunctivitis. *Infrequent:* Cataract, eyes dry, eye pain, visual field defect, diplopia, amblyopia, glaucoma, hordeolum, deafness, earache, tinnitus, inner ear infection, otitis media, unusual taste. *Rare:* Vision loss, ptosis, blepharitis, labyrinthitis, inner ear disturbance.

Postintroduction Reports

Voluntary reports of adverse events temporally associated with Cognex® that have been received since market introduction, that are not listed above, and that may have no causal relationship with the drug include the following: pancreatitis, perforated duodenal ulcer.

OVERDOSAGE

As in any case of overdose, general supportive measures should be utilized. Overdosage with cholinesterase inhibitors can cause a cholinergic crisis characterized by severe nausea/vomiting, salivation, sweating, bradycardia, hypotension, collapse, and convulsions. Increasing muscle weakness is a possibility and may result in death if respiratory muscles are involved.

Tertiary anticholinergics such as atropine may be used as an antidote for Cognex® overdosage. Intravenous atropine sulfate titrated to effect is recommended: in adults, initial dose of 1.0 to 2.0 mg IV with subsequent doses based on clinical response. In children, the usual IM or IV dose is 0.05 mg/kg, repeated every 10–30 minutes until muscarinic signs and symptoms subside and repeated if they reappear. Atypical increases in blood pressure and heart rate have been reported with other cholinomimetics when coadministered with quaternary anticholinergics such as glycopyrrolate.

It is not known whether Cognex® or its metabolites can be eliminated by dialysis (hemodialysis, peritoneal dialysis, or hemofiltration).

The estimated median lethal dose of tacrine following a single oral dose in rats is 40 mg/kg, or approximately 12 times the maximum recommended human dose of 160 mg/day. Dose-related signs of cholinergic stimulation were observed in animals and included vomiting, diarrhea, salivation, lacrimation, ataxia, convulsions, tremor, and stereotypic head and body movements.

DOSAGE AND ADMINISTRATION

The recommendations for dose titration are based on experience from clinical trials. The rate of dose escalation may be slowed if a patient is intolerant to the titration schedule recommended below. It is not advisable, however, to accelerate the dose incrementation plan.

Following initiation of therapy, or any dosage increase, patients should be observed carefully for adverse effects. Cognex® should be taken between meals whenever possible; however, if minor GI upset occurs, Cognex® may be taken with meals to improve tolerability. Taking Cognex® with meals can be expected to reduce plasma levels approximately 30% to 40%.

Initiation of Treatment

The initial dose of Cognex® brand of tacrine hydrochloride is 40 mg/day (10 mg QID). This dose should be maintained for a minimum of 6 weeks with every-other-week monitoring of transaminase levels. It is important that the dose not be increased during this period because of the potential for delayed onset of transaminase elevations.

Dose Titration

Following 6 weeks of treatment at 40 mg/day, the dose of Cognex® should then be increased to 80 mg/day (20 mg QID), providing there are no significant transaminase elevations and the patient is tolerating treatment. Patients should be titrated to higher doses (120 and 160 mg/day, in divided doses on a QID schedule) at 6-week intervals on the basis of tolerance.

Dose Adjustment

Serum ALT/SGPT should be monitored every other week for at least the first 16 weeks following initiation of Cognex® treatment, after which monitoring may be decreased to monthly for every 2 months and every 3 months thereafter. For patients who develop ALT/SGPT elevations greater than two times in the upper limit of normal, the dose and monitoring regimen should be modified as described in Table 4.

A full monitoring and dose titration sequence must be repeated in the event that a patient suspends treatment with tacrine for more than 4 weeks.

Table 4. Recommended Dose amd Monitoring Regimen Modification in Response to ALT/SGPT Elevations

ALT/SGPT Level	Treatment and Monitoring Regimen
≤2 × ULN	Continue treatment according to recommended titration and monitoring schedule.

>2 to ≤3 × ULN	Continue treatment according to recommended titration. Monitor ALT/SGPT levels weekly until levels return to normal limits.
>3 to ≤5 × ULN	Reduce the daily dose of Cognex® by 40 mg/day. Monitor ALT/SGPT levels weekly. Resume dose titration and every other week monitoring when the levels of the ALT/SGPT return to normal limits.
>5 × ULN	Stop Cognex® treatment. Monitor the patient closely for signs and symptoms associated with hepatitis and follow ALT/SGPT levels until within normal limits. See Rechallenge section below. Experience is limited in patients with ALT/SGPT >10 × ULN. The risk of rechallenge must be considered against demonstrated clinical benefit. **Patients with clinical jaundice confirmed by a significant elevation in total bilirubin (>3 mg/dL) and/or those exhibiting clinical signs and/or symptoms of hypersensitivity (e.g. rash or fever) in association with ALT/SGPT elevations should immediately and permanently discontinue Cognex® and not be rechallenged.**

Rechallenge
Patients who are required to discontinue Cognex® treatment because of ALT/SGPT elevations may be rechallenged once ALT/SGPT levels return to normal limits.
Rechallenge of patients exposed to ALT/SGPT elevations less than 10 × ULN has not resulted in serious liver injury. However, because experience in the rechallenge of patients who had elevations greater than 10 × ULN is limited, the risks associated with the rechallenge of these patients are not well characterized. Careful, frequent (weekly) monitoring of serum ALT/SGPT should be undertaken when rechallenging such patients.
If rechallenged, patients should be given an initial dose of 40 mg/day (10 mg QID) and ALT/SGPT levels monitored weekly. If, after 6 weeks on 40 mg/day, the patient is tolerating the dosage with no unacceptable elevations in ALT/SGPT, the recommended dose-titration may be resumed. Weekly monitoring of the ALT/SGPT levels should continue for a total of 16 weeks after which monitoring may be decreased to monthly for 2 months and every 3 months thereafter.

HOW SUPPLIED
Cognex® is supplied as capsules of tacrine hydrochloride containing 10, 20, 30, and 40 mg of tacrine. The capsule logo is Cognex®, with the strength (eg, 10, 20, 30, or 40) printed underneath.

10 mg (yellow/dark green)	Bottles of 120 (N 0071-0096-25) Unit-dose package of 100 (10 × 10) (N 0071-0096-40)
20 mg (yellow/light blue)	Bottles of 120 (N 0071-0097-25) Unit-dose package of 100 (10 × 10) (N 0071-0097-40)
30 mg (yellow/swedish orange)	Bottles of 120 (N 0071-0095-25) Unit-dose package of 100 (10 × 10) (N 0071-0095-40)
40 mg (yellow/lavender)	Bottles of 120 (N 0071-0098-25) Unit-dose package of 100 (10 × 10) (N 0071-0098-40)

Storage
Store at controlled room temperature 15°C to 30°C (59°F to 86°F) away from moisture.
Caution—Federal law prohibits dispensing without prescription.

April 1995 **0096G022**
Shown in Product Identification Guide, page 327

COLY-MYCIN® S OTIC ℞
[*cō"ly-my'cĭn s ō'tĭc*]
with Neomycin and Hydrocortisone (colistin sulfate—neomycin sulfate—thonzonium bromide—hydrocortisone acetate otic suspension)

DESCRIPTION
Coly-Mycin S Otic with Neomycin and Hydrocortisone (colistin sulfate-neomycin sulfate-thonzonium bromide-hydrocortisone acetate otic suspension) is a sterile aqueous suspension containing in each ml: Colistin base activity, 3 mg (as the sulfate); Neomycin base activity, 3.3 mg (as the sulfate); Hydrocortisone acetate, 10 mg (1%); Thonzonium bromide, 0.5 mg (0.05%); Polysorbate 80, acetic acid, and sodium acetate in a buffered aqueous vehicle. Thimerosal (mercury derivative), 0.002%, added as a preservative. It is a non-viscous liquid, buffered at pH 5, for instillation into the canal of the external ear or direct application to the affected aural skin.

CLINICAL PHARMACOLOGY
1. Colistin sulfate—an antibiotic with bactericidal action against most gram-negative organisms, notably *Pseudomonas aeruginosa, E. coli.*, and *Klebsiella-Aerobacter.*
2. Neomycin sulfate—a broad-spectrum antibiotic, bactericidal to many pathogens, notably *Staph aureus* and *Proteus* sp.
3. Hydrocortisone acetate—a corticosteroid that controls inflammation, edema, pruritus and other dermal reactions.
4. Thonzonium bromide—a surface-active agent that promotes tissue contact by dispersion and penetration of the cellular debris and exudate.

INDICATIONS AND USAGE
For the treatment of superficial bacterial infections of the external auditory canal, caused by organisms susceptible to the action of the antibiotics; and for the treatment of infections of mastoidectomy and fenestration cavities, caused by organisms susceptible to the antibiotics.

CONTRAINDICATIONS
This product is contraindicated in those individuals who have shown hypersensitivity to any of its components, and in herpes simplex, vaccinia and varicella.

WARNINGS
As with other antibiotic preparations, prolonged treatment may result in overgrowth of nonsusceptible organisms and fungi.
If the infection is not improved after one week, cultures and susceptibility tests should be repeated to verify the identity of the organism and to determine whether therapy should be changed.
Patients who prefer to warm the medication before using should be cautioned against heating the solution above body temperature, in order to avoid loss of potency.

PRECAUTIONS
General: If sensitization or irritation occurs, medication should be discontinued promptly.
This drug should be used with care in cases of perforated eardrum and in longstanding cases of chronic otitis media because of the possibility of ototoxicity caused by neomycin.
Treatment should not be continued for longer than ten days.
Allergic cross-reactions may occur which could prevent the use of any or all of the following antibiotics for the treatment of future infections: kanamycin, paromomycin, streptomycin, and possibly gentamicin.

ADVERSE REACTIONS
Neomycin is a not uncommon cutaneous sensitizer. There are articles in the current literature that indicate an increase in the prevalence of persons sensitive to neomycin.

DOSAGE AND ADMINISTRATION
The external auditory canal should be thoroughly cleansed and dried with a sterile cotton applicator.
When using the calibrated dropper:
For adults, 5 drops of the suspension should be instilled into the affected ear 3 or 4 times daily. For infants and children, 4 drops are suggested because of the smaller capacity of the ear canal.
This dosage correlates to the 4 drops (for adults) and 3 drops (for children) recommended when using the dropper-bottle container for this product.
The patient should lie with the affected ear upward and then the drops should be instilled. This position should be maintained for 5 minutes to facilitate penetration of the drops into the ear canal. Repeat, if necessary, for the opposite ear.
If preferred, a cotton wick may be inserted into the canal and then the cotton may be saturated with the suspension. The wick should be kept moist by adding further solution every 4 hours. The wick should be replaced at least once every 24 hours.

HOW SUPPLIED
Coly-Mycin S Otic is supplied as:
N 0071-3141-35—5-mL bottle with dropper
N 0071-3141-36—10-mL bottle with dropper
Each ml contains: Colistin sulfate equivalent to 3 mg of colistin base, Neomycin sulfate equivalent to 3.3 mg neomycin base, Hydrocortisone acetate 10 mg (1%), Thonzonium bromide 0.5 mg (0.05%), and Polysorbate 80 in an aqueous vehicle buffered with acetic acid and sodium acetate. Thimerosal (mercury derivative) 0.002% added as a preservative.
Shake well before using.
A sterilized dropper-cap assembly for use on the bottle of suspension is included in the package.
Store at controlled room temperature 15°-30°C (59°-86°F). Stable for 18 months at room temperature; prolonged exposure to higher temperatures should be avoided.
3141G035
165
Caution—Federal law prohibits dispensing without prescription.
WARNING: Manufactured with CFC-12, a substance which harms public health and environment by destroying ozone in the upper atmosphere.
Revised September 1994

KAPSEALS® DILANTIN® ℞
[*dī-lăn'tĭn"*]
(Extended Phenytoin Sodium Capsules, USP)

DESCRIPTION
Phenytoin Sodium is an antiepileptic drug. Phenytoin sodium is related to the barbiturates in chemical structure, but has a five-membered ring. The chemical name is sodium 5,5-diphenyl-2,4-imidazolidinedione.
Each Dilantin—*Extended Phenytoin Sodium Capsule* USP contains 30 mg or 100 mg phenytoin sodium USP. Also contains lactose, NF; sucrose, NF; talc, USP; and other ingredients. The capsule shell and band contain colloidal silicon dioxide, NF; FD&C red No. 3; gelatin, NF; glyceryl monooleate; sodium lauryl sulfate, NF. The Dilantin 30-mg capsule shell and band also contain citric acid, USP; FD&C blue No. 1; sodium benzoate, NF; titanium dioxide, USP. The Dilantin 100-mg capsule shell and band also contain FD&C yellow No. 6; hydrogen peroxide 3%; polyethylene glycol 200. Product *in vivo* performance is characterized by a slow and extended rate of absorption with peak blood concentrations expected in 4 to 12 hours as contrasted to *Prompt Phenytoin Sodium Capsules* USP with a rapid rate of absorption with peak blood concentration expected in 1½ to 3 hours.

CLINICAL PHARMACOLOGY
Phenytoin is an antiepileptic drug which can be useful in the treatment of epilepsy. The primary site of action appears to be *the motor cortex* where spread of seizure activity is inhibited. Possibly by promoting sodium efflux from neurons, phenytoin tends to *stabilize* the threshold against hyperexcitability caused by excessive stimulation or environmental changes capable of reducing membrane sodium gradient. This includes the reduction of posttetanic potentiation at synapses. Loss of posttetanic potentiation prevents cortical seizure foci from detonating adjacent cortical areas. Phenytoin reduces the maximal activity of brain stem centers responsible for the tonic phase of tonic-clonic (grand mal) seizures.
The plasma half-life in man after oral administration of phenytoin averages 22 hours, with a range of 7 to 42 hours. Steady-state therapeutic levels are achieved 7 to 10 days after initiation of therapy with recommended doses of 300 mg/day.
When serum level determinations are necessary, they should be obtained at least 5-7 half-lives after treatment initiation, dosage change, or addition or subtraction of another drug to the regimen so that equilibrium or steady-state will have been achieved. Trough levels provide information about clinically effective serum level range and confirm patient compliance and are obtained just prior to the patient's next scheduled dose. Peak levels indicate an individual's threshold for emergence of dose-related side effects and are obtained at the time of expected peak concentration. For Dilantin Kapseals peak serum levels occur 4-12 hours after administration.
Optimum control without clinical signs of toxicity occurs more often with serum levels between 10 and 20 mcg/ml, although some mild cases of tonic-clonic (grand mal) epilepsy may be controlled with lower serum levels of phenytoin.
In most patients maintained at a steady dosage, stable phenytoin serum levels are achieved. There may be wide interpatient variability in phenytoin serum levels with equivalent dosages. Patients with unusually low levels may be noncompliant or hypermetabolizers of phenytoin. Unusually high levels result from liver disease, congenital enzyme deficiency or drug interactions which result in metabolic interference. The patient with large variations in phenytoin plasma levels, despite standard doses, presents a difficult clinical problem. Serum level determinations in such patients may be particularly helpful. As phenytoin is highly protein bound,

Continued on next page

This product information was prepared in August 1996. On these and other Parke-Davis Products, information may be obtained by addressing PARKE-DAVIS, Division of Warner-Lambert Company, Morris Plains, New Jersey 07950.

Parke-Davis—Cont.

free phenytoin levels may be altered in patients whose protein binding characteristics differ from normal.

Most of the drug is excreted in the bile as inactive metabolites which are then reabsorbed from the intestinal tract and excreted in the urine. Urinary excretion of phenytoin and its metabolites occurs partly with glomerular filtration but more importantly, by tubular secretion. Because phenytoin is hydroxylated in the liver by an enzyme system which is saturable at high plasma levels, small incremental doses may increase the half-life and produce very substantial increases in serum levels, when these are in the upper range. The steady-state level may be disproportionately increased, with resultant intoxication, from an increase in dosage of 10% or more.

INDICATIONS AND USAGE

Dilantin is indicated for the control of generalized tonic-clonic (grand mal) and complex partial (psychomotor, temporal lobe) seizures and prevention and treatment of seizures occurring during or following neurosurgery.

Phenytoin serum level determinations may be necessary for optimal dosage adjustments (see Dosage and Administration and Clinical Pharmacology sections).

CONTRAINDICATIONS

Phenytoin is contraindicated in those patients who are hypersensitive to phenytoin or other hydantoins.

WARNINGS

Abrupt withdrawal of phenytoin in epileptic patients may precipitate status epilepticus. When, in the judgment of the clinician, the need for dosage reduction, discontinuation, or substitution of alternative antiepileptic medication arises, this should be done gradually. However, in the event of an allergic or hypersensitivity reaction, rapid substitution of alternative therapy may be necessary. In this case, alternative therapy should be an antiepileptic drug not belonging to the hydantoin chemical class.

There have been a number of reports suggesting a relationship between phenytoin and the development of lymphadenopathy (local or generalized) including benign lymph node hyperplasia, pseudolymphoma, lymphoma, and Hodgkin's Disease. Although a cause and effect relationship has not been established, the occurrence of lymphadenopathy indicates the need to differentiate such a condition from other types of lymph node pathology. Lymph node involvement may occur with or without symptoms and signs resembling serum sickness, eg, fever, rash and liver involvement.

In all cases of lymphadenopathy, follow-up observation for an extended period is indicated and every effort should be made to achieve seizure control using alternative antiepileptic drugs.

Acute alcoholic intake may increase phenytoin serum levels while chronic alcoholic use may decrease serum levels.

In view of isolated reports associating phenytoin with exacerbation of porphyria, caution should be exercised in using this medication in patients suffering from this disease.

Usage in Pregnancy:

A number of reports suggests an association between the use of antiepileptic drugs by women with epilepsy and a higher incidence of birth defects in children born to these women. Data are more extensive with respect to phenytoin and phenobarbital, but these are also the most commonly prescribed antiepileptic drugs; less systematic or anecdotal reports suggest a possible similar association with the use of all known antiepileptic drugs.

The reports suggesting a higher incidence of birth defects in children of drug-treated epileptic women cannot be regarded as adequate to prove a definite cause and effect relationship. There are intrinsic methodologic problems in obtaining adequate data on drug teratogenicity in humans; genetic factors or the epileptic condition itself may be more important than drug therapy in leading to birth defects. The great majority of mothers on antiepileptic medication deliver normal infants. It is important to note that antiepileptic drugs should not be discontinued in patients in whom the drug is administered to prevent major seizures, because of the strong possibility of precipitating status epilepticus with attendant hypoxia and threat to life. In individual cases where the severity and frequency of the seizure disorder are such that the removal of medication does not pose a serious threat to the patient, discontinuation of the drug may be considered prior to and during pregnancy, although it cannot be said with any confidence that even minor seizures do not pose some hazard to the developing embryo or fetus. The prescribing physician will wish to weigh these considerations in treating or counseling epileptic women of childbearing potential.

In addition to the reports of increased incidence of congenital malformation, such as cleft lip/palate and heart malformations in children of women receiving phenytoin and other antiepileptic drugs, there have more recently been reports of a fetal hydantoin syndrome. This consists of prenatal growth deficiency, microcephaly and mental deficiency in children born to mothers who have received phenytoin, barbiturates, alcohol, or trimethadione. However, these features are all interrelated and are frequently associated with intrauterine growth retardation from other causes.

There have been isolated reports of malignancies, including neuroblastoma, in children whose mothers received phenytoin during pregnancy.

An increase in seizure frequency during pregnancy occurs in a high proportion of patients, because of altered phenytoin absorption or metabolism. Periodic measurement of serum phenytoin levels is particularly valuable in the management of a pregnant epileptic patient as a guide to an appropriate adjustment of dosage. However, postpartum restoration of the original dosage will probably be indicated.

Neonatal coagulation defects have been reported within the first 24 hours in babies born to epileptic mothers receiving phenobarbital and/or phenytoin. Vitamin K has been shown to prevent or correct this defect and has been recommended to be given to the mother before delivery and to the neonate after birth.

PRECAUTIONS

General:

The liver is the chief site of biotransformation of phenytoin; patients with impaired liver function, elderly patients, or those who are gravely ill may show early signs of toxicity.

A small percentage of individuals who have been treated with phenytoin have been shown to metabolize the drug slowly. Slow metabolism may be due to limited enzyme availability and lack of induction; it appears to be genetically determined.

Phenytoin should be discontinued if a skin rash appears (see "Warnings" section regarding drug discontinuation). If the rash is exfoliative, purpuric, or bullous or if lupus erythematosus, Stevens-Johnson syndrome, or toxic epidermal necrolysis is suspected, use of the drug should not be resumed and alternative therapy should be considered. (See ADVERSE REACTIONS section.) If the rash is of a milder type (measles-like or scarlatiniform), therapy may be resumed after the rash has completely disappeared. If the rash recurs upon reinstitution of therapy, further phenytoin medication is contraindicated.

Phenytoin and other hydantoins are contraindicated in patients who have experienced phenytoin hypersensitivity. Additionally, caution should be exercised if using structurally similar compounds (eg, barbiturates, succinimides, oxazolidinediones and other related compounds) in these same patients.

Hyperglycemia, resulting from the drug's inhibitory effects on insulin release, has been reported. Phenytoin may also raise the serum glucose level in diabetic patients.

Osteomalacia has been associated with phenytoin therapy and is considered to be due to phenytoin's interference with Vitamin D metabolism.

Phenytoin is not indicated for seizures due to hypoglycemic or other causes. Appropriate diagnostic procedures should be performed as indicated.

Phenytoin is not effective for absence (petit mal) seizures. If tonic-clonic (grand-mal) and absence (petit mal) seizures are present, combined drug therapy is needed.

Serum levels of phenytoin sustained above the optimal range may produce confusional states referred to as "delirium," "psychosis," or "encephalopathy," or rarely irreversible cerebellar dysfunction. Accordingly, at the first sign of acute toxicity, plasma levels are recommended. Dose reduction of phenytoin therapy is indicated if plasma levels are excessive; if symptoms persist, termination is recommended. (See Warnings section.)

Information for Patients:

Patients taking phenytoin should be advised of the importance of adhering strictly to the prescribed dosage regimen, and of informing the physician of any clinical condition in which it is not possible to take the drug orally as prescribed, eg, surgery, etc.

Patients should also be cautioned on the use of other drugs or alcoholic beverages without first seeking the physician's advice.

Patients should be instructed to call their physician if skin rash develops.

The importance of good dental hygiene should be stressed in order to minimize the development of gingival hyperplasia and its complications.

Laboratory Tests:

Phenytoin serum level determinations may be necessary to achieve optimal dosage adjustments.

Drug Interactions:

There are many drugs which may increase or decrease phenytoin levels or which phenytoin may affect. Serum level determinations for phenytoin are especially helpful when possible drug interactions are suspected. The most commonly occurring drug interactions are listed below.

1. Drugs which may increase phenytoin serum levels include: acute alcohol intake, amiodarone, chloramphenicol, chlordiazepoxide, diazepam, dicumarol, disulfiram, estrogens, H_2-antagonists, halothane, isoniazid, methylphenidate, phenothiazines, phenylbutazone, salicylates, succinimides, sulfonamides, tolbutamide, trazodone.
2. Drugs which may decrease phenytoin levels include: carbamazepine, chronic alcohol abuse, reserpine, and sucralfate. Moban® brand of molindone hydrochloride contains calcium ions which interfere with the absorption of phenytoin. Ingestion times of phenytoin and antacid preparations containing calcium should be staggered in patients with low serum phenytoin levels to prevent absorption problems.
3. Drugs which may either increase or decrease phenytoin serum levels include: phenobarbital, sodium valproate, and valproic acid. Similarly, the effect of phenytoin on phenobarbital, valproic acid and sodium valproate serum levels is unpredictable.
4. Although not a true drug interaction, tricyclic antidepressants may precipitate seizures in susceptible patients and phenytoin dosage may need to be adjusted.
5. Drugs whose efficacy is impaired by phenytoin include: corticosteroids, coumarin anticoagulants, digitoxin, doxycycline, estrogens, furosemide, oral contraceptives, quinidine, rifampin, theophylline, vitamin D.

Drug/Laboratory Test Interactions:

Phenytoin may cause decreased serum levels of protein-bound iodine (PBI). It may also produce lower than normal values for dexamethasone or metyrapone tests. Phenytoin may cause increased serum levels of glucose, alkaline phosphatase, and gamma glutamyl transpeptidase (GGT).

Carcinogenesis:

See 'Warnings' section for information on carcinogenesis.

Pregnancy:

See WARNINGS section.

Nursing Mothers:

Infant breast feeding is not recommended for women taking this drug because phenytoin appears to be secreted in low concentrations in human milk.

ADVERSE REACTIONS

Central Nervous System: The most common manifestations encountered with phenytoin therapy are referable to this system and are usually dose-related. These include nystagmus, ataxia, slurred speech, decreased coordination, and mental confusion. Dizziness, insomnia, transient nervousness, motor twitchings, and headaches have also been observed. There have also been rare reports of phenytoin induced dyskinesias, including chorea, dystonia, tremor and asterixis, similar to those induced by phenothiazine and other neuroleptic drugs.

A predominantly sensory peripheral polyneuropathy has been observed in patients receiving long-term phenytoin therapy.

Gastrointestinal System: Nausea, vomiting, constipation, toxic hepatitis and liver damage.

Integumentary System: Dermatological manifestations sometimes accompanied by fever have included scarlatiniform or morbilliform rashes. A morbilliform rash (measles-like) is the most common; other types of dermatitis are seen more rarely. Other more serious forms which may be fatal have included bullous, exfoliative or purpuric dermatitis, lupus erythematosus, Stevens-Johnson syndrome, and toxic epidermal necrolysis (see Precautions section).

Hemopoietic System: Hemopoietic complications, some fatal, have occasionally been reported in association with administration of phenytoin. These have included thrombocytopenia, leukopenia, granulocytopenia, agranulocytosis, and pancytopenia with or without bone marrow suppression. While macrocytosis and megaloblastic anemia have occurred, these conditions usually respond to folic acid therapy. Lymphadenopathy including benign lymph node hyperplasia, pseudolymphoma, lymphoma, and Hodgkin's Disease have been reported (see WARNINGS section).

Connective Tissue System: Coarsening of the facial features, enlargement of the lips, gingival hyperplasia, hypertrichosis, and Peyronie's Disease.

Cardiovascular: Periarteritis nodosa.

Immunologic: Hypersensitivity syndrome (which may include, but is not limited to, symptoms such as arthralgias, eosinophilia, fever, liver dysfunction, lymphadenopathy or rash), systemic lupus erythematosus, immunoglobulin abnormalities.

OVERDOSAGE

The lethal dose in children is not known. The lethal dose in adults is estimated to be 2 to 5 grams. The initial symptoms are nystagmus, ataxia, and dysarthria. Other signs are tremor, hyperflexia, lethargy, slurred speech, nausea, vomiting. The patient may become comatose and hypotensive. Death is due to respiratory and circulatory depression.

There are marked variations among individuals with respect to phenytoin plasma levels where toxicity may occur. Nystagmus, on lateral gaze, usually appears at 20 mcg/ml, ataxia at 30 mcg/ml, dysarthria and lethargy appear when the plasma concentration is over 40 mcg/ml, but as high a concentration as 50 mcg/ml has been reported without evidence of toxicity. As much as 25 times the therapeutic dose has been taken to result in a serum concentration over 100 mcg/ml with complete recovery.

Treatment:

Treatment is nonspecific since there is no known antidote. The adequacy of the respiratory and circulatory systems should be carefully observed and appropriate supportive measures employed. Hemodialysis can be considered since phenytoin is not completely bound to plasma proteins. Total exchange transfusion has been used in the treatment of severe intoxication in children.

In acute overdosage, the possibility of other CNS depressants, including alcohol, should be borne in mind.

DOSAGE AND ADMINISTRATION

Serum concentrations should be monitored in changing from extended Phenytoin Sodium Capsules USP (Dilantin) to Prompt Phenytoin Sodium Capsules USP, and from the sodium salt to the free acid form.

Dilantin® Kapseals® and Dilantin Parenteral are formulated with the sodium salt of phenytoin. The free acid form of phenytoin is used in Dilantin-125 Suspension and Dilantin Infatabs. Because there is approximately an 8% increase in drug content with the free acid form over that of the sodium salt, dosage adjustments and serum level monitoring may be necessary when switching from a product formulated with the free acid to a product formulated with the sodium salt and vice versa.

General:

Dosage should be individualized to provide maximum benefit. In some cases, serum blood level determinations may be necessary for optimal dosage adjustments—the clinically effective serum level is usually 10-20 mcg/ml. With recommended dosage, a period of seven to ten days may be required to achieve steady-state blood levels with phenytoin and changes in dosage (increase or decrease) should not be carried out at intervals shorter than seven to ten days.

Adult Dosage:

Divided Daily Dosage

Patients who have received no previous treatment may be started on one 100-mg Dilantin (Extended Phenytoin Sodium Capsule) three times daily and the dosage then adjusted to suit individual requirements. For most adults, the satisfactory maintenance dosage will be one capsule three to four times a day. An increase up to two capsules three times a day may be made, if necessary.

Once-a-Day Dosage:

In adults, if seizure control is established with divided doses of three 100 mg Dilantin capsules daily, once-a-day dosage with 300 mg of extended phenytoin sodium capsules may be considered. Studies comparing divided doses of 300 mg with a single daily dose of this quantity indicated absorption, peak plasma levels, biologic half-life, difference between peak and minimum values, and urinary recovery were equivalent. Once-a-day dosage offers a convenience to the individual patient or to nursing personnel for institutionalized patients and is intended to be used only for patients requiring this amount of drug daily. A major problem in motivating noncompliant patients may also be lessened when the patient can take this drug once a day. However, patients should be cautioned not to miss a dose, inadvertently.

Only extended phenytoin sodium capsules are recommended for once-a-day dosing. Inherent differences in dissolution characteristics and resultant absorption rates of phenytoin due to different manufacturing procedures and/or dosage forms preclude such recommendation for other phenytoin products. When a change in the dosage form or brand is prescribed, careful monitoring of phenytoin serum levels should be carried out.

Loading Dose:

Some authorities have advocated use of an oral loading dose of phenytoin in adults who require rapid steady-state serum levels and where intravenous administration is not desirable. This dosing regimen should be reserved for patients in a clinic or hospital setting where phenytoin serum levels can be closely monitored. Patients with a history of renal or liver disease should not receive the oral loading regimen.

Initially, one gram of phenytoin capsules is divided into 3 doses (400 mg, 300 mg, 300 mg) and administered at two-hourly intervals. Normal maintenance dosage is then instituted 24 hours after the loading dose, with frequent serum level determinations.

Pediatric Dosage:

Initially, 5 mg/kg/day in two or three equally divided doses, with subsequent dosage individualized to a maximum of 300 mg daily. A recommended daily maintenance dosage is usually 4 to 8 mg/kg. Children over 6 years old may require the minimum adult dose (300 mg/day).

HOW SUPPLIED

N 0071-0362 (Kapseal 362, transparent #3 capsule with an orange band)—Dilantin 100 mg; in 100's, 1,000's, and unit dose 100's.

N 0071-0365 (Kapseal 365, transparent #4 capsule with a pink band)—Dilantin 30 mg; in 100's.

Store below 30°C (86°F). Protect from light and moisture.

Also available as:

N 0071-2214—Dilantin-125® Suspension 125 mg phenytoin/5 ml with a maximum alcohol content not greater than 0.6 percent, available in 8-oz bottles. The minimum sales unit is 100 pouches.

N 0071-0007 (Tablet 7)—Dilantin Infatabs® each contain 50 mg phenytoin, 100's and unit dose 100's.

For Parenteral Use:

N 0071-4488-47 (Steri-Dose® 4488)-Dilantin ready-mixed solution containing 50 mg phenytoin sodium per milliliter is supplied in a 2-mL sterile disposable syringe (22 gauge × 1¼ inch needle). Packages of ten syringes.

N 0071-4488-45 Dilantin ready-mixed solution containing 50 mg phenytoin sodium per milliliter is supplied in 2-mL Steri-Vials.® Packages of twenty-five.

N 0071-4475-45 Dilantin ready-mixed solution containing 50 mg phenytoin sodium per milliliter is supplied in 5-mL Steri-Vials.® Packages of twenty-five.

Store below 30°C (86°F). Protect from light and moisture.

© 1995, Warner-Lambert Co.

Revised August 1995   0362G286

Shown in Product Identification Guide, page 327

INFATABS®
DILANTIN®   ℞
[dī-lăn'tĭn" ĭn'fă-tăbs"]
(Phenytoin Tablets, USP)

NOT FOR ONCE A DAY DOSING

DESCRIPTION

Dilantin is an antiepileptic drug.

Dilantin (phenytoin) is related to the barbiturates in chemical structure, but has a five-membered ring. The chemical name is 5,5-diphenyl-2,4-imidazolidinedione.

Each Dilantin Infatab, for oral administration, contains 50 mg phenytoin, USP. Also contains: D&C yellow No. 10, Al lake; FD&C yellow No. 6, Al lake flavor; saccharin sodium, USP; sucrose, NF; talc, USP; and other ingredients.

CLINICAL PHARMACOLOGY

Phenytoin is an antiepileptic drug which can be useful in the treatment of epilepsy. The primary site of action appears to be the motor cortex where spread of seizure activity is inhibited. Possibly by promoting sodium efflux from neurons, phenytoin tends to stabilize the threshold against hyperexcitability caused by excessive stimulation or environmental changes capable of reducing membrane sodium gradient. This includes the reduction of posttetanic potentiation at synapses. Loss of posttetanic potentiation prevents cortical seizure foci from detonating adjacent cortical areas. Phenytoin reduces the maximal activity of brain stem centers responsible for the tonic phase of tonic-clonic (grand mal) seizures.

Clinical studies using Dilantin Infatabs have shown an average plasma half-life of 14 hours with a range of 7 to 29 hours. Steady-state therapeutic levels are achieved at least 7 to 10 days (5-7 half-lives) after initiation of therapy with recommended doses of 300 mg/day.

When serum level determinations are necessary, they should be obtained at least 5-7 half-lives after treatment initiation, dosage change, or addition or subtraction of another drug to the regimen so that equilibrium or steady-state will have been achieved. Trough levels provide information about clinically effective serum level range and confirm patient compliance and are obtained just prior to the patient's next scheduled dose. Peak levels indicate an individual's threshold for emergence of dose-related side effects and are obtained at the time of expected peak concentration. For Dilantin Infatabs peak levels occur 1½-3 hours after administration.

Optimum control without clinical signs of toxicity occurs more often with serum levels between 10 and 20 mcg/ml, although some mild cases of tonic-clonic (grand mal) epilepsy may be controlled with lower serum levels of phenytoin.

In most patients maintained at a steady dosage, stable phenytoin serum levels are achieved. There may be wide interpatient variability in phenytoin serum levels with equivalent dosages. Patients with unusually low levels may be noncompliant or hypermetabolizers of phenytoin. Unusually high levels result from liver disease, congenital enzyme deficiency or drug interactions which result in metabolic interference. The patient with large variations in phenytoin plasma levels, despite standard doses, presents a difficult clinical problem. Serum level determinations in such patients may be particularly helpful. As phenytoin is highly protein bound, free phenytoin levels may be altered in patients whose protein binding characteristics differ from normal.

Most of the drug is excreted in the bile as inactive metabolites which are then reabsorbed from the intestinal tract and excreted in the urine. Urinary excretion of phenytoin and its metabolites occurs partly with glomerular filtration but more importantly, by tubular secretion. Because phenytoin is hydroxylated in the liver by an enzyme system which is saturable at high plasma levels small incremental doses may increase the half-life and produce very substantial increases in serum levels, when these are in the upper range. The steady-state level may be disproportionately increased, with resultant intoxication, from an increase in dosage of 10% or more.

Clinical studies show that chewed and unchewed Dilantin Infatabs are bioequivalent, yield approximately equivalent plasma levels, and are more rapidly absorbed than 100-mg Dilantin Kapseals.®

INDICATIONS AND USAGE

Dilantin Infatabs (Phenytoin Tablets, USP) are indicated for the control of generalized tonic-clonic (grand mal) and complex partial (psychomotor, temporal lobe) seizures and prevention and treatment of seizures occurring during or following neurosurgery. Phenytoin serum level determinations may be necessary for optimal dosage adjustments (see Dosage and Administration and Clinical Pharmacology sections).

CONTRAINDICATIONS

Phenytoin is contraindicated in those patients who are hypersensitive to phenytoin or other hydantoins.

WARNINGS

Abrupt withdrawal of phenytoin in epileptic patients may precipitate status epilepticus. When, in the judgment of the clinician, the need for dosage reduction, discontinuation, or substitution of alternative antiepileptic medication arises, this should be done gradually. However, in the event of an allergic or hypersensitivity reaction, rapid substitution of alternative therapy may be necessary. In this case, alternative therapy should be an antiepileptic drug not belonging to the hydantoin chemical class.

There have been a number of reports suggesting a relationship between phenytoin and the development of lymphadenopathy (local or generalized) including benign lymph node hyperplasia, pseudolymphoma, lymphoma, and Hodgkin's Disease. Although a cause and effect relationship has not been established, the occurrence of lymphadenopathy indicates the need to differentiate such a condition from other types of lymph node pathology. Lymph node involvement may occur with or without symptoms and signs resembling serum sickness eg, fever, rash and liver involvement. In all cases of lymphadenopathy, follow-up observation for an extended period is indicated and every effort should be made to achieve seizure control using alternative antiepileptic drugs. Acute alcoholic intake may increase phenytoin serum levels while chronic alcoholic use may decrease serum levels.

In view of isolated reports associating phenytoin with exacerbation of porphyria, caution should be exercised in using this medication in patients suffering from this disease.

Usage in Pregnancy

A number of reports suggest an association between the use of antiepileptic drugs by women with epilepsy and a higher incidence of birth defects in children born to these women. Data are more extensive with respect to phenytoin and phenobarbital, but these are also the most commonly prescribed antiepileptic drugs; less systematic or anecdotal reports suggest a possible similar association with the use of all known antiepileptic drugs.

The reports suggesting a higher incidence of birth defects in children of drug-treated epileptic women cannot be regarded as adequate to prove a definite cause and effect relationship. There are intrinsic methodologic problems in obtaining adequate data on drug teratogenicity in humans: genetic factors or the epileptic condition itself, may be more important than drug therapy in leading to birth defects. The great majority of mothers on antiepileptic medication deliver normal infants. It is important to note that antiepileptic drugs should not be discontinued in patients in whom the drug is administered to prevent major seizures, because of the strong possibility of precipitating status epilepticus with attendant hypoxia and threat to life. In individual cases where the severity and frequency of the seizure disorder are such that the removal of medication does not pose a serious threat to the patient, discontinuation of the drug may be considered prior to and during pregnancy, although it cannot be said with any confidence that even minor seizures do not pose some hazard to the developing embryo or fetus. The prescribing physician will wish to weigh these considerations in treating or counseling epileptic women of childbearing potential.

In addition to the reports of increased incidence of congenital malformations, such as cleft lip/palate and heart malformations in children of women receiving phenytoin and other antiepileptic drugs, there have more recently been reports of a fetal hydantoin syndrome. This consists of prenatal growth deficiency, microcephaly and mental deficiency in children born to mothers who have received phenytoin, barbiturates, alcohol, or trimethadione. However, these features are all

Continued on next page

This product information was prepared in August 1996. On these and other Parke-Davis Products, information may be obtained by addressing PARKE-DAVIS, Division of Warner-Lambert Company, Morris Plains, New Jersey 07950.

Parke-Davis—Cont.

interrelated and are frequently associated with intrauterine growth retardation from other causes.

There have been isolated reports of malignancies, including neuroblastoma, in children whose mothers received phenytoin during pregnancy.

An increase in seizure frequency during pregnancy occurs in a high proportion of patients, because of altered phenytoin absorption or metabolism. Periodic measurement of serum phenytoin levels is particularly valuable in the management of a pregnant epileptic patient as a guide to an appropriate adjustment of dosage. However, postpartum restoration of the original dosage will probably be indicated.

Neonatal coagulation defects have been reported within the first 24 hours in babies born to epileptic mothers receiving phenobarbital and/or phenytoin. Vitamin K has been shown to prevent or correct this defect and has been recommended to be given to the mother before delivery and to the neonate after birth.

PRECAUTIONS

General

The liver is the chief site of biotransformation of phenytoin; patients with impaired liver function, elderly patients, or those who are gravely ill may show early signs of toxicity. A small percentage of individuals who have been treated with phenytoin have been shown to metabolize the drug slowly. Slow metabolism may be due to limited enzyme availability and lack of induction; it appears to be genetically determined.

Phenytoin should be discontinued if a skin rash appears (see "Warnings" section regarding drug discontinuation). If the rash is exfoliative, purpuric, or bullous or if lupus erythematosus, Stevens-Johnson syndrome, or toxic epidermal necrolysis is suspected, use of this drug should not be resumed, and alternative therapy should be considered (see Adverse Reactions). If the rash is of a milder type (measles-like or scarlatiniform), therapy may be resumed after the rash has completely disappeared. If the rash recurs upon reinstitution of therapy, further phenytoin medication is contraindicated. Phenytoin and other hydantoins are contraindicated in patients who have experienced phenytoin hypersensitivity. Additionally, caution should be exercised if using structurally similar (eg barbiturates, succinimides, oxazolidinediones and other related compounds) in these same patients.

Hyperglycemia, resulting from the drug's inhibitory effects on insulin release, has been reported. Phenytoin may also raise the serum glucose level in diabetic patients.

Osteomalacia has been associated with phenytoin therapy and is considered to be due to phenytoin's interference with Vitamin D metabolism.

Phenytoin is not indicated for seizures due to hypoglycemic or other metabolic causes. Appropriate diagnostic procedures should be performed as indicated.

Phenytoin is not effective for absence (petit mal) seizures. If tonic-clonic (grand-mal) and absence (petit mal) seizures are present, combined drug therapy is needed.

Serum levels of phenytoin sustained above the optimal range may produce confusional states referred to as "delirium," "psychosis," or "encephalopathy," or rarely irreversible cerebellar dysfunction. Accordingly, at the first sign of acute toxicity, plasma levels are recommended. Dose reduction of phenytoin therapy is indicated if plasma levels are excessive; if symptoms persist, termination is recommended. (See Warnings).

Information for Patients

Patients taking phenytoin should be advised of the importance of adhering strictly to the prescribed dosage regimen, and of informing the physician of any clinical condition in which it is not possible to take the drug orally as prescribed, eg, surgery, etc.

Patients should also be cautioned on the use of other drugs or alcoholic beverages without first seeking the physician's advice.

Patients should be instructed to call their physician if skin rash develops.

The importance of good dental hygiene should be stressed in order to minimize the development of gingival hyperplasia and its complications.

Laboratory Tests

Phenytoin serum level determinations may be necessary to achieve optimal dosage adjustments.

Drug Interactions

There are many drugs which may increase or decrease phenytoin levels or which phenytoin may affect. Serum level determinations for phenytoin are especially helpful when possible drug interactions are suspected. The most commonly occurring drug interactions are listed below:

1. Drugs which may increase phenytoin serum levels include: acute alcohol intake, amiodarone, chloramphenicol, chlordiazepoxide, diazepam, dicumarol, disulfiram, estrogens, H_2-antagonists, halothane, isoniazid, methylphenidate, phenothiazines, phenylbutazone, salicylates, succinimides, sulfonamides, tolbutamide, trazodone.

2. Drugs which may decrease phenytoin serum levels include: carbamazepine, chronic alcohol abuse, reserpine, and sucralfate. Moban® brand of Molindone Hydrochloride contains calcium ions which interfere with the absorption of phenytoin. Ingestion times of phenytoin and antacid preparations containing calcium should be staggered in patients with low serum phenytoin levels to prevent absorption problems.

3. Drugs which may either increase or decrease phenytoin serum levels include: phenobarbital, sodium valproate, and valproic acid. Similarly, the effect of phenytoin on phenobarbital, valproic acid and sodium valproate serum levels is unpredictable.

4. Although not a true drug interaction, tricyclic antidepressants may precipitate seizures in susceptible patients and phenytoin dosage may need to be adjusted.

5. Drugs whose efficacy is impaired by phenytoin include: corticosteroids, coumarin anticoagulants, digitoxin, doxycycline, estrogens, furosemide, oral contraceptives, quinidine, rifampin, theophylline, vitamin D.

Drug/Laboratory Test Interactions

Phenytoin may cause decreased serum levels of protein-bound iodine (PBI). It may also produce lower than normal values for dexamethasone or metyrapone tests. Phenytoin may cause increased serum levels of glucose, alkaline phosphatase, and gamma glutamyl transpeptidase (GGT).

Carcinogenesis

See 'Warnings' section for information on carcinogenesis.

Pregnancy

See Warnings Section.

Nursing Mothers

Infant breast-feeding is not recommended for women taking this drug because phenytoin appears to be secreted in low concentrations in human milk.

ADVERSE REACTIONS

Central Nervous System: The most common manifestations encountered with phenytoin therapy are referable to this system and are usually dose-related. These include nystagmus, ataxia, slurred speech, decreased coordination and mental confusion. Dizziness, insomnia, transient nervousness, motor twitchings, and headache have also been observed.

There have also been rare reports of phenytoin induced dyskinesias, including chorea, dystonia, tremor and asterixis, similar to those induced by phenothiazine and other neuroleptic drugs.

A predominantly sensory peripheral polyneuropathy has been observed in patients receiving long-term phenytoin therapy.

Gastrointestinal System: Nausea, vomiting, constipation, toxic hepatitis and liver damage.

Integumentary System: Dermatological manifestations sometimes accompanied by fever have included scarlatiniform or morbilliform rashes. A morbilliform rash (measles-like) is the most common; other types of dermatitis are seen more rarely. Other more serious forms which may be fatal have included bullous, exfoliative or purpuric dermatitis, lupus erythematosus, Stevens-Johnson syndrome, and toxic epidermal necrolysis (see Precautions section).

Hemopoietic System: Hemopoietic complications, some fatal, have occasionally been reported in association with administration of phenytoin. These have included thrombocytopenia, leukopenia, granulocytopenia, agranulocytosis, and pancytopenia with or without bone marrow suppression. While macrocytosis and megaloblastic anemia have occurred, these conditions usually respond to folic acid therapy. Lymphadenopathy including benign lymph node hyperplasia, pseudolymphoma, lymphoma, and Hodgkin's Disease have been reported (see Warnings section).

Connective Tissue System: Coarsening of the facial features, enlargement of the lips, gingival hyperplasia, hypertrichosis, and Peyronie's Disease.

Cardiovascular: Periarteritis nodosa.

Immunologic: Hypersensitivity syndrome (which may include, but is not limited to, symptoms such as arthralgias, eosinophilia, fever, liver dysfunction, lymphadenopathy or rash), systemic lupus erythematosus, and immunoglobulin abnormalities.

OVERDOSAGE

The lethal dose in children is not known. The lethal dose in adults is estimated to be 2 to 5 grams. The initial symptoms are nystagmus, ataxia, and dysarthria. Other signs are tremor, hyperflexia, lethargy, slurred speech, nausea, vomiting. The patient may become comatose and hypotensive. Death is due to respiratory and circulatory depression.

There are marked variations among individuals with respect to phenytoin plasma levels where toxicity may occur. Nystagmus on lateral gaze usually appears at 20 mcg/ml, ataxia at 30 mcg/ml, dysarthria and lethargy appear when the plasma concentration is over 40 mcg/ml, but as high a concentration as 50 mcg/ml has been reported without evidence of toxicity. As much as 25 times the therapeutic dose has been taken to result in a serum concentration over 100 mcg/ml with complete recovery.

Treatment

Treatment is nonspecific since there is no known antidote. The adequacy of the respiratory and circulatory systems should be carefully observed and appropriate supportive measures employed. Hemodialysis can be considered since phenytoin is not completely bound to plasma proteins. Total exchange transfusion has been used in the treatment of severe intoxication in children.

In acute overdosage the possibility of other CNS depressants, including alcohol, should be borne in mind.

DOSAGE AND ADMINISTRATION

When given in equal doses, Dilantin Infatabs yield higher plasma levels than Dilantin Kapseals.® For this reason serum concentrations should be monitored and care should be taken when switching a patient from the sodium salt to the free acid form.

Dilantin® Kapseals,® Dilantin Parenteral, and Dilantin with Phenobarbital are formulated with the sodium salt of phenytoin. The free acid form of phenytoin is used in Dilantin-30 Pediatric and Dilantin-125 Suspensions and Dilantin Infatabs. Because there is approximately an 8% increase in drug content with the free acid form over that of the sodium salt, dosage adjustments and serum level monitoring may be necessary when switching from a product formulated with the free acid to a product formulated with the sodium salt and vice versa.

General

Not for once a day dosing.

Dosage should be individualized to provide maximum benefit. In some cases, serum blood level determinations may be necessary for optimal dosage adjustments—the clinically effective serum level is usually 10–20 mcg/ml. With recommended dosage, a period of seven to ten days may be required to achieve steady-state blood levels with phenytoin and changes in dosage (increase or decrease) should not be carried out at intervals shorter than seven to ten days.

Dilantin Infatabs can be either chewed thoroughly before being swallowed or swallowed whole.

Adult Dosage

Patients who have received no previous treatment may be started on two Infatabs three times daily, and the dose is then adjusted to suit individual requirements. For most adults, the satisfactory maintenance dosage will be six to eight Infatabs daily; an increase to twelve Infatabs daily may be made, if necessary.

Pediatric Dosage

Initially, 5 mg/kg/day in two or three equally divided doses, with subsequent dosage individualized to a maximum of 300 mg daily. A recommended daily maintenance dosage is usually 4 to 8 mg/kg. Children over 6 years old may require the minimum adult dose (300 mg/day). If the daily dosage cannot be divided equally, the larger dose should be given before retiring.

HOW SUPPLIED

Dilantin Infatabs are supplied as:

N 0071-0007-24—Bottle of 100.

Store at a room temperature below 30°C (86°F).

N 0071-0007-40—Unit dose (10/10's).

Store at controlled room temperature 15°–30°C (59°–86°F). Protect from moisture.

Each tablet contains 50 mg phenytoin in a yellow triangular scored chewable tablet.

Shown in Product Identification Guide, page 327

Dilantin is also supplied in the following forms:

N 0071-0362-24—Bottle of 100.

N 0071-0362-32—Bottle of 1000.

N 0071-0362-40—Unit dose (10/10's).

Each Kapseal® contains 100 mg phenytoin sodium.

N 0071-0365-24—Bottle of 100.

Each Kapseal® contains 30 mg phenytoin sodium.

N 0071-2214-20—8 oz bottle.

N 0071-2214-40—Unit dose pouches (5 ml × 100).

Each 5 ml of suspension contains 125 mg phenytoin with a maximum alcohol content not greater than 0.6 percent.

N 0071-4488-47—2-ml prefilled Steri-Dose® syringes.

A sterile solution for parenteral use containing 50 mg phenytoin sodium per mL in a disposable syringe (22 gauge × 1¹/₄ inch needle). Supplied in packages of ten.

N 0071-4488-45 Dilantin ready-mixed solution containing 50 mg phenytoin sodium per milliliter is supplied in 2-mL Steri-Vials.® Packages of twenty-five.

N 0071-4475-45 Dilantin ready-mixed solution containing 50 mg phenytoin sodium per milliliter is supplied in 5 mL Steri-Vials.® Packages of twenty-five.

Caution—Federal law prohibits dispensing without prescription.

© 1995, Warner-Lambert Co.

Revised May 1995   0007G164

Shown in Product Identification Guide, page 327

DILANTIN-125® ℞
[*dī-lăn'tĭn*]
(Phenytoin Oral Suspension, USP)

DESCRIPTION

Dilantin (phenytoin) is related to the barbiturates in chemical structure, but has a five-membered ring. The chemical name is 5,5-diphenyl-2,4 imidazolidinedione.

Each teaspoonful of suspension contains 125 mg of phenytoin, USP with a maximum alcohol content not greater than 0.6 percent. Also contains carboxymethylcellulose sodium, USP; citric acid, anhydrous, USP; flavors; glycerin, USP; magnesium aluminum silicate, NF; polysorbate 40, NF; purified water, USP; sodium benzoate, NF; sucrose, NF; vanillin, NF; and FD&C yellow No. 6.

CLINICAL PHARMACOLOGY

Phenytoin is an antiepileptic drug which can be useful in the treatment of epilepsy. The primary site of action appears to be *the motor cortex* where spread of seizure activity is inhibited. Possibly by promoting sodium efflux from neurons, phenytoin tends to *stabilize* the threshold against hyperexcitability caused by excessive stimulation or environmental changes capable of reducing membrane sodium gradient. This includes the reduction of posttetanic potentiation at synapses. Loss of posttetanic potentiation prevents cortical seizure foci from detonating adjacent cortical areas. Phenytoin reduces the maximal activity of brain stem centers responsible for the tonic phase of tonic-clonic (grand mal) seizures.

The plasma half-life in man after oral administration of phenytoin averages 22 hours, with a range of 7 to 42 hours. Steady-state therapeutic levels are achieved at least 7 to 10 days (5–7 half-lives) after initiation of therapy with recommended doses of 300 mg/day.

When serum level determinations are necessary, they should be obtained at least 5–7 half-lives after treatment initiation, dosage change, or addition or subtraction of another drug to the regimen so that equilibrium or steady-state will have been achieved. Trough levels provide information about clinically effective serum level range and confirm patient compliance and are obtained just prior to the patient's next scheduled dose. Peak levels indicate an individual's threshold for emergence of dose-related side effects and are obtained at the time of expected peak concentration. For Dilantin-125 Suspension peak levels occur 1½–3 hours after administration.

Optimum control without clinical signs of toxicity occurs more often with serum levels between 10 and 20 mcg/mL, although some mild cases of tonic-clonic (grand mal) epilepsy may be controlled with lower serum levels of phenytoin.

In most patients maintained at a steady dosage, stable phenytoin serum levels are achieved. There may be wide interpatient variability in phenytoin serum levels with equivalent dosages. Patients with unusually low levels may be noncompliant or hypermetabolizers of phenytoin. Unusually high levels result from liver disease, congenital enzyme deficiency or drug interactions which result in metabolic interference. The patient with large variations in phenytoin plasma levels, despite standard doses, presents a difficult clinical problem. Serum level determinations in such patients may be particularly helpful. As phenytoin is highly protein bound, free phenytoin levels may be altered in patients whose protein binding characteristics differ from normal.

Most of the drug is excreted in the bile as inactive metabolites which are then reabsorbed from the intestinal tract and excreted in the urine. Urinary excretion of phenytoin and its metabolites occurs partly with glomerular filtration but more importantly, by tubular secretion. Because phenytoin is hydroxylated in the liver by an enzyme system which is saturable at high plasma levels small incremental doses may increase the half-life and produce very substantial increases in serum levels, when these are in the upper range. The steady-state level may be disproportionately increased, with resultant intoxication, from an increase in dosage of 10% or more.

INDICATIONS AND USAGE

Dilantin (phenytoin) is indicated for the control of tonic-clonic (grand mal) and psychomotor (temporal lobe) seizures.

Phenytoin serum level determinations may be necessary for optimal dosage adjustments (see Dosage and Administration and Clinical Pharmacology sections).

CONTRAINDICATIONS

Dilantin is contraindicated in those patients with a history of hypersensitivity to phenytoin or other hydantoins.

WARNINGS

Abrupt withdrawal of phenytoin in epileptic patients may precipitate status epilepticus. When in the judgment of the clinician the need for dosage reduction, discontinuation, or substitution of alternative anticonvulsant medication arises, this should be done gradually. In the event of an allergic or hypersensitivity reaction, more rapid substitution of alternative therapy may be necessary. In this case, alternative therapy should be an anticonvulsant not belonging to the hydantion chemical class.

There have been a number of reports suggesting a relationship between phenytoin and the development of lymphadenopathy (local or generalized) including benign lymph node hyperplasia, pseudolymphoma, lymphoma, and Hodgkin's Disease. Although a cause and effect relationship has not been established, the occurrence of lymphadenopathy indicates the need to differentiate such a condition from other types of lymph node pathology. Lymph node involvement may occur with or without symptoms and signs resembling serum sickness eg, fever, rash and liver involvement.

In all cases of lymphadenopathy, follow-up observation for an extended period is indicated and every effort should be made to achieve seizure control using alternative antiepileptic drugs.

Acute alcoholic intake may increase phenytoin serum levels while chronic alcoholic use may decrease serum levels.

In view of isolated reports associating phenytoin with exacerbation of porphyria, caution should be exercised in using this medication in patients suffering from this disease.

Usage in Pregnancy: A number of reports suggests an association between the use of antiepileptic drugs by women with epilepsy and a higher incidence of birth defects in children born to these women. Data are more extensive with respect to phenytoin and phenobarbital, but these are also the most commonly prescribed antiepileptic drugs; less systematic or anecdotal reports suggest a possible similar association with the use of all known antiepileptic drugs.

The reports suggesting a higher incidence of birth defects in children of drug-treated epileptic women cannot be regarded as adequate to prove a definite cause and effect relationship. There are intrinsic methodologic problems in obtaining adequate data on drug teratogenicity in humans; genetic factors or the epileptic condition itself may be more important than drug therapy in leading to birth defects. The great majority of mothers on antiepileptic medication deliver normal infants. It is important to note that antiepileptic drugs should not be discontinued in patients in whom the drug is administered to prevent major seizures, because of the strong possibility of precipitating status epilepticus with attendant hypoxia and threat to life. In individual cases where the severity and frequency of the seizure disorder are such that the removal of medication does not pose a serious threat to the patient, discontinuation of the drug may be considered prior to and during pregnancy, although it cannot be said with any confidence that even minor seizures do not pose some hazards to the developing embryo or fetus. The prescribing physician will wish to weigh these considerations in treating and counseling epileptic women of childbearing potential.

In addition to the reports of increased incidence of congenital malformation, such as cleft lip/palate and heart malformations in children of women receiving phenytoin and other antiepileptic drugs, there have more recently been reports of a fetal hydantoin syndrome. This consists of prenatal growth deficiency, microcephaly and mental deficiency in children born to mothers who have received phenytoin, barbiturates, alcohol, or trimethadione. However, these features are all interrelated and are frequently associated with intrauterine growth retardation from other causes.

There have been isolated reports of malignancies, including neuroblastoma, in children whose mothers received phenytoin during pregnancy.

An increase in seizure frequency during pregnancy occurs in a high proportion of patients, because of altered phenytoin absorption or metabolism. Periodic measurement of serum phenytoin levels is particularly valuable in the management of a pregnant epileptic patient as a guide to an appropriate adjustment of dosage. However, postpartum restoration of the original dosage will probably be indicated.

Neonatal coagulation defects have been reported within the first 24 hours in babies born to epileptic mothers receiving phenobarbital and/or phenytoin. Vitamin K has been shown to prevent or correct this defect and has been recommended to be given to the mother before delivery and the neonate after birth.

PRECAUTIONS

General: The liver is the chief site of biotransformation of phenytoin; patients with impaired liver function, elderly patients, or those who are gravely ill may show early signs of toxicity.

A small percentage of individuals who have been treated with phenytoin have been shown to metabolize the drug slowly. Slow metabolism may be due to limited enzyme availability and lack of induction; it appears to be genetically determined.

Phenytoin should be discontinued if a skin rash appears (see "Warnings" section regarding drug discontinuation). If the rash is exfoliative, purpuric, or bullous or if lupus erythematosus, Stevens-Johnson syndrome, or toxic epidermal necrolysis is suspected, use of this drug should not be resumed and alternative therapy should be considered. (See Adverse Reactions section). If the rash is of a milder type (measles-like or scarlatiniform), therapy may be resumed after the rash has completely disappeared. If the rash recurs upon reinstitution of therapy, further phenytoin medication is contraindicated.

Phenytoin and other hydantoins are contraindicated in patients who have experienced phenytoin hypersensitivity. Additionally, caution should be exercised if using structurally similar (eg, barbiturates, succinamides, oxazolidinediones and other related compounds) in these same patients.

Hyperglycemia, resulting from the drug's inhibitory effects on insulin release, has been reported. Phenytoin may also raise the serum glucose level in diabetic patients.

Osteomalacia has been associated with phenytoin therapy and is considered to be due to phenytoin's interference with Vitamin D metabolism.

Phenytoin is not indicated for seizures due to hypoglycemic or other metabolic causes. Appropriate diagnostic procedures should be performed as indicated.

Phenytoin is not effective for absence (petit mal) seizures. If tonic-clonic (grand mal) and absence (petit mal) seizures are present, combined drug therapy is needed.

Serum levels of phenytoin sustained above the optimal range may produce confusional states referred to as "delirium," "psychosis" or "encephalopathy," or rarely irreversible cerebellar dysfunction. Accordingly, at the first sign of acute toxicity, plasma levels are recommended. Dose reduction of phenytoin therapy is indicated if plasma levels are excessive; if symptoms persist, termination is recommended. (See Warnings section).

Information for Patients: Patients taking phenytoin should be advised of the importance of adhering strictly to the prescribed dosage regimen, and of informing the physician of any clinical condition in which it is not possible to take the drug orally as prescribed, eg, surgery, etc. Patients should be instructed to use an accurately calibrated measuring device when using this medication to ensure accurate dosing.

Patients should also be cautioned on the use of other drugs or alcoholic beverages without first seeking the physician's advice.

Patients should be instructed to call their physician if skin rash develops.

The importance of good dental hygiene should be stressed in order to minimize the development of gingival hyperplasia and its complications.

Laboratory Tests: Phenytoin serum level determinations may be necessary to achieve optimal dosage adjustments.

Drug Interactions: There are many drugs which may increase or decrease phenytoin levels or which phenytoin may affect. Serum level determinations for phenytoin are especially helpful when possible drug interactions are suspected.

The most commonly occurring drug interactions are:

1. Drugs which may increase phenytoin serum levels include: acute alcohol intake, amiodarone, chloramphenicol, chlordiazepoxide, diazepam, dicumarol, disulfiram, estrogens, ethosuximide, fluoxetine, H_2-antagonists, halothane, isoniazid, methylphenidate, phenothiazines, phenylbutazone, salicylates, succinimides, sulfonamides, tolbutamide, trazodone.
2. Drugs which may decrease phenytoin levels include: carbamazepine, chronic alcohol abuse, reserpine and sucralfate. Moban® brand of molindone hydrochloride contains calcium ions which interfere with the absorption of phenytoin. Ingestion times of phenytoin and antacid preparations containing calcium should be staggered in patients with low serum phenytoin levels to prevent absorption problems.
3. Drugs which may either increase or decrease phenytoin serum levels include: phenobarbital, sodium valproate, and valproic acid. Similarly, the effect of phenytoin on phenobarbital, valproic acid and sodium valproate serum levels is unpredictable.
4. Although not a true drug interaction, tricyclic antidepressants may precipitate seizures in susceptible patients and phenytoin dosage may need to be adjusted.
5. Drugs whose efficacy is impaired by phenytoin include: corticosteroids, coumarin anticoagulants, digitoxin, doxycycline, estrogens, furosemide, oral contraceptives, quinidine, rifampin, theophylline, vitamin D.

Drug/Laboratory Test Interactions: Phenytoin may cause decreased serum levels of protein-bound iodine (PBI). It may also produce lower than normal values for dexamethasone or metyrapone tests. Phenytoin may cause increased serum levels of glucose, alkaline phosphatase, and gamma glutamyl transpeptidase (GGT).

Carcinogenesis: See 'Warnings' section for information on carcinogenesis.

Continued on next page

This product information was prepared in August 1996. On these and other Parke-Davis Products, information may be obtained by addressing PARKE-DAVIS, Division of Warner-Lambert Company, Morris Plains, New Jersey 07950.

Parke-Davis—Cont.

Pregnancy: See Warnings section.
Nursing Mothers: Infant breast feeding is not recommended for women taking this drug because phenytoin appears to be secreted in low concentrations in human milk.

ADVERSE REACTIONS

Central Nervous System: The most common manifestations encountered with phenytoin therapy are referable to this system and are usually dose-related. These include nystagmus, ataxia, slurred speech, decreased coordination, and mental confusion. Dizziness, insomnia, transient nervousness, motor twitchings, and headaches have also been observed. There have also been rare reports of phenytoin induced dyskinesias, including chorea, dystonia, tremor and asterixis, similar to those induced by phenothiazine and other neuroleptic drugs.
A predominantly sensory peripheral polyneuropathy has been observed in patients receiving long-term phenytoin therapy.
Gastrointestinal System: Nausea, vomiting, constipation, toxic hepatitis and liver damage.
Integumentary System: Dermatological manifestations sometimes accompanied by fever have included scarlatiniform or morbilliform rashes. A morbilliform rash (measles-like) is the most common; other types of dermatitis are seen more rarely. Other more serious forms which may be fatal have included bullous, exfoliative or purpuric dermatitis, lupus erythematosus, Stevens-Johnson syndrome, and toxic epidermal necrolysis (see Precautions section).
Hemopoietic System: Hemopoietic complications, some fatal, have occasionally been reported in association with administration of phenytoin. These have included thrombocytopenia, leukopenia, granulocytopenia, agranulocytosis, and pancytopenia with or without bone marrow suppression. While macrocytosis and megaloblastic anemia have occurred, these conditions usually respond to folic acid therapy. Lymphadenopathy including benign lymph node hyperplasia, pseudolymphoma, lymphoma, and Hodgkin's Disease have been reported (see Warnings section).
Connective Tissue System: Coarsening of the facial features, enlargement of the lips, gingival hyperplasia, hypertrichosis, and Peyronie's Disease.
Cardiovascular: Periarteritis nodosa.
Immunologic: Hypersensitivity syndrome (which may include, but is not limited to, symptoms such as arthralgias, eosinophilia, fever, liver dysfunction, lymphadenopathy or rash), systemic lupus erythematosus, and immunoglobulin abnormalities.

OVERDOSAGE

The lethal dose in children is not known. The lethal dose in adults is estimated to be 2 to 5 grams. The initial symptoms are nystagmus, ataxia, and dysarthria. Other signs are tremor, hyperflexia, lethargy, slurred speech, nausea, vomiting. The patient may become comatose and hypotensive. Death is due to respiratory and circulatory depression.
There are marked variations among individuals with respect to phenytoin plasma levels where toxicity may occur. Nystagmus, on lateral gaze, usually appears at 20 mcg/mL, ataxia at 30 mcg/mL, dysarthria and lethargy appear when the plasma concentration is over 40 mcg/mL, but as high a concentration as 50 mcg/mL has been reported without evidence of toxicity. As much as 25 times the therapeutic dose has been taken to result in a serum concentration over 100 mcg/mL with complete recovery.
Treatment: Treatment is nonspecific since there is no known antidote.
The adequacy of the respiratory and circulatory systems should be carefully observed and appropriate supportive measures employed. Hemodialysis can be considered since phenytoin is not completely bound to plasma proteins. Total exchange transfusion has been used in the treatment of severe intoxication in children.
In acute overdosage the possibility of other CNS depressants, including alcohol, should be borne in mind.

DOSAGE AND ADMINISTRATION

Serum concentrations should be monitored and care should be taken when switching a patient from the sodium salt to the free acid form.
Dilantin® Kapseals®, Dilantin Parenteral, and Dilantin with Phenobarbital are formulated with the sodium salt of phenytoin. The free acid form of phenytoin is used in Dilantin-125 Suspension and Dilantin Infatabs. Because there is approximately an 8% increase in drug content with the free acid form over that of the sodium salt, dosage adjustments and serum level monitoring may be necessary when switching from a product formulated with the free acid to a product formulated with the sodium salt and vice versa.
General: Dosage should be individualized to provide maximum benefit. In some cases serum blood level determinations may be necessary for optimal dosage adjustments—the clinically effective serum level is usually 10–20 mcg/mL. With recommended dosage, a period of seven to ten days may be required to achieve steady-state blood levels with phenytoin and changes in dosage (increase or decrease) should not be carried out at intervals shorter than seven to ten days.
Adult Dose: Patients who have received no previous treatment may be started on one teaspoonful (5 mL) of Dilantin-125 Suspension three times daily, and the dose is then adjusted to suit individual requirements. An increase to five teaspoonfuls daily may be made, if necessary.
Pediatric Dose: Initially, 5 mg/kg/day in two or three equally divided doses, with subsequent dosage individualized to a maximum of 300 mg daily. A recommended daily maintenance dosage is usually 4 to 8 mg/kg. Children over 6 years may require the minimum adult dose (300 mg/day).

HOW SUPPLIED

N 0071-2214—Dilantin-125® Suspension (phenytoin oral suspension, USP), 125 mg phenytoin/5 mL with a maximum alcohol content not greater than 0.6 percent, an orange suspension with an orange-vanilla flavor; available in 8-oz bottles and individual unit dose foil pouches which deliver 5 mL (125 mg phenytoin). The minimum sales unit is 100 pouches.
Store below 30°C (86°F). Protect from freezing and light.
Also available as:
N 0071-0362 (Kapseal® 362)—Dilantin (extended phenytoin sodium capsules, USP) 100 mg; in 100's, 1000's, unit dose 100's.
N 0071-0365 (Kapseal® 365)—Dilantin (extended phenytoin sodium capsules, USP) 30 mg, in 100's.
N 0071-0007 (Tablet 7)—Dilantin Infatabs® (phenytoin tablets, USP) each contain 50 mg phenytoin; 100's and unit dose 100's.
For Parenteral Use:
N 0071-4488-47 (Steri-Dose® 4488)-Dilantin ready-mixed solution containing 50 mg phenytoin sodium per milliliter is supplied in a 2-mL sterile disposable syringe (22 gauge × 1¼ inch needle). Packages of ten syringes.
N 0071-4488-45 Dilantin ready-mixed solution containing 50 mg phenytoin sodium per milliliter is supplied in 2 mL Steri-Vials.® Packages of twenty-five.
N 0071-4475-45 Dilantin ready-mixed solution containing 50 mg phenytoin sodium per milliliter is supplied in 5 mL Steri-Vials.® Packages of twenty-five.
Storage: Store below 30° C (86° F). Protect from freezing and light.
Caution—Federal law prohibits dispensing without prescription.
© 1995, Warner-Lambert Co.
Revised April 1995   2214G127

DORYX®   ℞
(Coated Doxycycline Hyclate Pellets)

DESCRIPTION

DORYX® Capsules contain specially coated pellets of doxycycline hyclate for oral administration. Also contains lactose, NF; microcrystalline cellulose, NF; povidone, USP. The capsule shell and/or band contains FD and C blue No. 1; FD and C yellow No. 6; D and C yellow No. 10; gelatin, NF; silicon dioxide; sodium lauryl sulfate, NF; titanium dioxide, USP. Doxycycline is a broad-spectrum antibiotic synthetically derived from oxytetracycline and available as doxycycline hyclate. The chemical designation of this light-yellow crystalline powder is alpha-6-desoxy-5-oxytetracycline. Doxycycline has a high degree of lipoid solubility and a low affinity for calcium binding. It is highly stable in normal human serum. Doxycycline will not degrade into an epianhydro form.

CLINICAL PHARMACOLOGY

Tetracyclines are readily absorbed and are bound to plasma proteins in varying degree. They are concentrated by the liver in the bile, and excreted in the urine and feces at high concentrations and in a biologically active form.
Doxycycline is virtually completely absorbed after oral administration. Following a 200 mg dose, normal adult volunteers averaged peak serum levels of 2.6 mcg/mL of doxycycline at 2 hours decreasing to 145 mcg/mL at 24 hours. Excretion of doxycycline by the kidney is about 40%/72 hours in individuals with normal function (creatinine clearance about 75 mL/min). This percentage excretion may fall as low as 1–5%/72 hours in individuals with severe renal insufficiency (creatinine clearance below 10 mL/min). Studies have shown no significant difference in serum half-life of doxycycline (range 18–22 hours) in individuals with normal and severely impaired renal function.
Hemodialysis does not alter serum half-life.
Microbiology: Doxycycline is primarily bacteriostatic and is thought to exert its antimicrobial effect by the inhibition of protein synthesis. Doxycycline is active against a wide range of gram-positive and gram-negative organisms. The drugs in the tetracycline class have closely similar antimicrobial spectra and cross resistance among them is common.

Susceptibility Tests: Diffusion Techniques: The use of antibiotic disc susceptibility test methods which measure zone diameter gives an accurate estimation of susceptibility of organisms to DORYX: One such standard procedure[1] has been recommended for use with discs for testing antimicrobials. Doxycycline 30 mcg discs should be used for the determination of the susceptibility of organisms to doxycycline.
With this type of procedure, a report of "susceptible" from the laboratory indicates that the infecting organism is likely to respond to therapy. A report of "intermediate susceptibility" suggests that the organism would be susceptible if high dosage is used or if the infection is confined to tissue and fluids (e.g., urine) in which high antibiotic levels are obtained. A report of "resistant" indicates that the infecting organism is not likely to respond to therapy. With the doxycycline disc, a zone of 16 mm or greater indicates susceptibility, zone sizes of 12 mm or less indicate resistance, and zone sizes of 13 to 15 mm indicate intermediate susceptibility.
Standardized procedures require the use of laboratory control organisms. The 30 mcg tetracycline disc should give zone diameters between 19 and 28 mm for *S.aureus* ATCC 25923 and between 18 and 25 mm for *E.coli* ATCC 25922. The 30 mcg doxycycline disc should give zone diameters between 23 and 29 mm for *S.aureus* ATCC 25923, and between 18 and 24 mm for *E.coli* ATCC 25922.
Dilution Techniques: A bacterial isolate may be considered susceptible if the MIC (minimal inhibitory concentration) value for doxycycline is less than 4 mcg/mL. Organisms are considered resistant if the MIC is greater than 12.5 mcg/mL. MICs greater than 4.0 mcg/mL and less than 12.5 mcg/mL indicate intermediate susceptibility.
As with standard diffusion methods, dilution procedures require the use of laboratory control mechanisms. Standard doxycycline powder should give MIC values in the range of 0.25 mcg/mL and 1.0 mcg/mL for *S.aureus* ATCC 25923. For *E.coli* ATCC 25922 the MIC range should be between 1.0 mcg/mL and 4.0 mcg/mL.

INDICATIONS AND USAGE

Doxycycline is indicated in infections caused by the following microorganisms:
Rickettsiae (Rocky Mountain spotted fever, typhus fever and the typhus group, Q fever, rickettsialpox and tick fevers).
Mycoplasma pneumoniae (PPLO, Eaton's agent).
Agents of psittacosis and ornithosis.
Agents of lymphogranuloma venereum and granuloma inguinale.
The spirochetal agent of relapsing fever (*Borrelia recurrentis*).
The following gram-negative microorganisms:
Haemophilus ducreyi (chancroid)
Yersinia pestis (formerly *Pasteurella pestis*)
Francisella tularensis (formerly *Pasteurella tularensis*)
Bartonella bacilliformis
Bacteroides species
Vibrio cholerae (formerly *Vibrio comma*)
Campylobacter fetus (formerly *Vibrio fetus*)
Brucella species (in conjunction with streptomycin)
Because many strains of the following groups of microorganisms have been shown to be resistant to tetracyclines, culture and susceptibility testing are recommended.
Doxycycline is indicated for treatment of infections caused by the following gram-negative microorganisms, when bacteriological testing indicates appropriate susceptibility to the drug:
Escherichia coli
Enterobacter aerogenes (formerly *Aerobacter aerogenes*)
Shigella species
Mima species and *Herellea* species
Haemophilus influenzae (respiratory infections)
Klebsiella species (respiratory and urinary infections)
Doxycycline is indicated for treatment of infections caused by the following gram-positive microorganisms when bacteriological testing indicates appropriate susceptibility to the drug:
Streptococcus species:
Up to 44 percent of strains of *Streptococcus pyogenes* and 74 percent of *Streptococcus faecalis* have been found to be resistant to tetracycline drugs. Therefore, tetracyclines should not be used for streptococcal disease unless the organism has been demonstrated to be susceptible.
For upper respiratory infections due to group A beta-hemolytic streptococci, penicillin is the usual drug of choice, including prophylaxis of rheumatic fever.
Diplococcus pneumoniae.
Staphylococcus aureus, (respiratory, skin and soft-tissue infections). Tetracyclines are not the drug of choice in the treatment of any type of staphylococcal infection.
When penicillin is contraindicated, doxycycline is an alternative drug in the treatment of infections due to:
Treponema pallidum and *Treponema pertenue* (syphilis and yaws)
Listeria monocytogenes
Clostridium species
Bacillus anthracis

Fusobacterium fusiforme (Vincent's infection)
Actinomyces species

In acute intestinal amebiasis doxycycline may be a useful adjunct to amebicides.

In severe acne doxycycline may be useful adjunctive therapy.

Doxycycline is indicated in the treatment of trachoma, although the infectious agent is not always eliminated, as judged by immunofluorescence.

Inclusion conjunctivitis may be treated with oral doxycycline alone or with a combination of topical agents.

Doxycycline is indicated for the treatment of uncomplicated urethral, endocervical or rectal infections in adults caused by *Chlamydia trachomatis*.[2]

Doxycycline is indicated for the treatment of nongonococcal urethritis caused by *Chlamydia trachomatis* and *Ureaplasma urealyticum* and for the treatment of acute epididymo-orchitis caused by *Chlamydia trachomatis*.[2]

Doxycycline is indicated for the treatment of uncomplicated gonococcal infections in adults (except for anorectal infections in men), the gonococcal arthritis-dermatitis syndrome and acute epididymo-orchitis caused by *N. gonorrhoeae*.[2]

CONTRAINDICATIONS

The drug is contraindicated in persons who have shown hypersensitivity to any of the tetracyclines.

WARNINGS

THE USE OF DRUGS OF THE TETRACYCLINE CLASS DURING TOOTH DEVELOPMENT (LAST HALF OF PREGNANCY, INFANCY AND CHILDHOOD TO THE AGE OF 8 YEARS) MAY CAUSE PERMANENT DISCOLORATION OF THE TEETH (YELLOW-GRAY-BROWN). This adverse reaction is more common during long term use of the drugs but has been observed following repeated short term courses. Enamel hypoplasia has also been reported. TETRACYCLINE DRUGS, THEREFORE, SHOULD NOT BE USED IN THIS AGE GROUP UNLESS OTHER DRUGS ARE NOT LIKELY TO BE EFFECTIVE OR ARE CONTRAINDICATED.

Results of animal studies indicate that tetracyclines cross the placenta, are found in fetal tissues and can have toxic effects on the developing fetus (often related to retardation of skeletal development). Evidence of embryotoxicity has been noted in animals treated early in pregnancy. If any tetracycline is used during pregnancy or if the patient becomes pregnant while taking these drugs, the patient should be apprised of potential hazard to the fetus.

As with other tetracyclines, doxycycline forms a stable calcium complex in any bone-forming tissue. A decrease in the fibula growth rate has been observed in prematures given oral tetracycline in doses of 25 mg/kg every six hours. This reaction was shown to be reversible when the drug was discontinued.

Photosensitivity manifested by an exaggerated sunburn reaction has been observed in some individuals taking tetracyclines. Patients apt to be exposed to direct sunlight or ultraviolet light should be advised that this reaction can occur with tetracycline drugs, and treatment should be discontinued at the first evidence of skin erythema.

The antianabolic action of the tetracyclines may cause an increase in BUN. Studies to date indicate that this does not occur with the use of doxycycline in patients with impaired renal function.

PRECAUTIONS

As with other antibiotic preparations, use of this drug may result in overgrowth of nonsusceptible organisms, including fungi. If superinfection occurs, the antibiotic should be discontinued and appropriate therapy instituted.

All infections due to group A beta-hemolytic streptococci should be treated for at least 10 days.

Laboratory tests: In venereal disease when coexistent syphilis is suspected, dark-field examination should be done before treatment is started and the blood serology repeated monthly for at least 4 months.

In long term therapy, periodic laboratory evaluation of organ systems, including hematopoietic, renal and hepatic studies should be performed.

Drug interactions: Because tetracyclines have been shown to depress plasma prothrombin activity, patients who are on anticoagulant therapy may require downward adjustment of their anticoagulant dosage.

Since bacteriostatic drugs may interfere with the bactericidal action of penicillin, it is advisable to avoid giving tetracyclines in conjunction with penicillin.

For concomitant therapy with antacids or iron-containing preparations and food see "Dosage and Administration" section.

Carcinogenesis, mutagenesis, impairment of fertility: Long term studies are currently being conducted to determine whether tetracyclines have carcinogenic potential. Animal studies conducted in rats and mice have not provided conclusive evidence that tetracyclines may be carcinogenic or that they impair fertility. In two mammalian cell assays (L51784 mouse lymphoma and Chinese hamster lung cells *in vitro*) positive responses for mutagenicity occurred at concentra-

tions of 60 and 10 mcg/mL respectively. In humans no association between tetracyclines and these effects have been made.

Pregnancy: Pregnancy Category D (See Warnings section).

Nursing mothers: Tetracyclines are present in the milk of lactating women who are taking a drug in this class. Because of the potential for serious adverse reactions in nursing infants from the tetracyclines, a decision should be made whether to discontinue nursing or discontinue the drug, taking into account the importance of the drug to the mother (see Warnings section).

Pediatric use: See Warnings and Dosage and Administration sections.

ADVERSE REACTIONS

Due to oral doxycycline's virtually complete absorption, side effects to the lower bowel, particularly diarrhea, have been infrequent. The following adverse reactions have been observed in patients receiving tetracyclines:

Gastrointestinal: Anorexia, nausea, vomiting, diarrhea, glossitis, dysphagia, enterocolitis, and inflammatory lesions (with monilial overgrowth) in the anogenital region. These reactions have been caused by both the oral and parenteral administration of tetracyclines. Rare instances of esophagitis and esophageal ulcerations have been reported in patients receiving capsule and tablet forms of drugs in the tetracycline class. Most of these patients took medications immediately before going to bed. (See Dosage and Administration section.)

Skin: Maculopapular and erythematous rashes. Exfoliative dermatitis has been reported but is uncommon. Photosensitivity is discussed above (see Warnings section.)

Renal toxicity: Rise in BUN has been reported and is apparently dose related. (See Warnings section.)

Hypersensitivity reactions: Urticaria, angioneurotic edema, anaphylaxis, anaphylactoid purpura, pericarditis, and exacerbation of systemic lupus erythematosus.

Bulging fontanels in infants and benign intracranial hypertension in adults have been reported in individuals receiving tetracyclines. These conditions disappeared when the drug was discontinued.

Blood: Hemolytic anemia, thrombocytopenia, neutropenia, and eosinophilia have been reported with tetracyclines.

When given over prolonged periods, tetracyclines have been reported to produce brown-black microscopic discoloration of thyroid glands. No abnormalities of thyroid function are known to occur.

DOSAGE AND ADMINISTRATION

THE USUAL DOSAGE AND FREQUENCY OF ADMINISTRATION OF DOXYCYCLINE DIFFERS FROM THAT OF THE OTHER TETRACYCLINES. EXCEEDING THE RECOMMENDED DOSAGE MAY RESULT IN AN INCREASED INCIDENCE OF SIDE EFFECTS.

Adults: The usual dose of oral doxycycline is 200 mg on the first day of treatment (administered 100 mg every 12 hours) followed by a maintenance dose of 100 mg/day. The maintenance dose may be administered as a single dose or as 50 mg every 12 hours. In the management of more severe infections (particularly chronic infections of the urinary tract), 100 mg every 12 hours is recommended.

For children above eight years of age: The recommended dosage schedule for children weighing 100 pounds or less is 2 mg/lb of body weight divided into two doses on the first day of treatment, followed by 1 mg/lb of body weight given as a single daily dose or divided into two doses on subsequent days. For more severe infections up to 2 mg/lb of body weight may be used. For children over 100 pounds, the usual adult dose should be used.

Uncomplicated gonococcal infections in adults (except ano-rectal infections in men): 100 mg, by mouth, twice-a-day for 7 days.[2] As an alternate single visit dose, administer 300 mg stat followed in one hour by a second 300 mg dose. The dose may be administered with food, including milk or carbonated beverage, as required.

Acute epididymo-orchitis caused by *N. gonorrhoeae:* 100 mg, by mouth, twice-a-day for at least 10 days.[2]

Primary and secondary syphilis: 300 mg a day in divided doses for at least 10 days.

Uncomplicated urethral, endocervical, or rectal infection in adults caused by *Chlamydia trachomatis:* 100 mg by mouth, twice-a-day for at least 7 days.[2]

Nongonococcal urethritis caused by *C. trachomatis* and *U. urealyticum:* 100 mg, by mouth, twice-a-day for at least 7 days.[2]

Acute epididymo-orchitis caused by *C. trachomatis:* 100 mg, by mouth, twice-a-day for at least 10 days.[2]

The therapeutic antibacterial serum activity will usually persist for 24 hours following recommended dosage.

When used in streptococcal infections, therapy should be continued for 10 days.

Administration of adequate amounts of fluid along with capsule and tablet forms of drugs in the tetracycline class is recommended to wash down the drugs and reduce the risk of esophageal irritation and ulceration (see Adverse Reactions).

If gastric irritation occurs, it is recommended that doxycycline be given with food or milk. The absorption of doxycycline is not markedly influenced by simultaneous ingestion of food or milk.

Concomitant therapy: Antacids containing aluminum, calcium or magnesium, sodium bicarbonate, and iron-containing preparations should not be given to patients taking oral tetracyclines.

Studies to date have indicated that administration of doxycycline at the usual recommended doses does not lead to excessive accumulation of the antibiotic in patients with renal impairment.

HOW SUPPLIED

DORYX® Capsules have a yellow transparent body with light blue opaque cap; the capsule bearing the inscription "DORYX" in white. Pellets are colored yellow. Each capsule contains specially coated pellets of doxycycline hyclate equivalent to 100 mg of doxycycline, supplied in:

Bottles of 50 capsules ....N 0071-0838-19

STORAGE CONDITIONS

Store at controlled room temperature below 25° C (77° F).

References:

1. NCCLS Approved Standard:
   M2-A3, Vol. 4, Performance Standards for Antimicrobial Disk Susceptibility Tests, Third Edition: available from the National Committee for Clinical Laboratory Standards, 771 East Lancaster Avenue, Villanova, Pa. 19085
2. CDC Sexually Transmitted Diseases Treatment Guidelines 1982

Caution—Federal law prohibits dispensing without prescription.

Manufactured by
Faulding Pharmaceutical/DBL
A Division of F.H. Faulding & Co. Limited
1538 Main North Road
Salisbury, South Australia 5108
Distributed by
PARKE-DAVIS
Div of Warner-Lambert Co
Morris Plains, NJ 07950 USA
Revised June 1994   0838G025
Shown in Product Identification Guide, page 327

EASPRIN®   ℞
[*ēas'prĭn''*]
(Aspirin Delayed-release Tablets, USP)
Enteric Coated Tablets

Caution—Federal law prohibits dispensing without prescription.

DESCRIPTION

Easprin (Aspirin Delayed-release Tablets, USP) enteric coated tablets contain 15 grains (975 mg) aspirin for oral administration. Also contains: candelilla wax; colloidal silicon dioxide, NF; corn starch 1500; dusty rose Opaspray; hydroxypropyl methylcellulose, USP (15 cps); methylparaben, NF; microcrystalline cellulose, NF; mistron spray talc; polyethylene glycol 3350, NF; propylparaben, NF; stearic acid powder; vanillin, NF; zinc stearate, USP. The enteric coating is designed to prevent the release of aspirin in the stomach and thereby reduce gastric irritation and total occult blood loss. The pharmacologic effects of aspirin include analgesia, antipyresis, antiinflammatory activity, and antirheumatic activity.

CLINICAL PHARMACOLOGY

Aspirin is a salicylate that has demonstrated antiinflammatory, analgesic, antipyretic, and antirheumatic activity.

Aspirin's mode of action as an antiinflammatory and antirheumatic agent may be due to inhibition of synthesis and release of prostaglandins.

Aspirin appears to produce analgesia by virtue of both a peripheral and CNS effect. Peripherally, aspirin acts by inhibiting the synthesis and release of prostaglandins. Acting centrally, it would appear to produce analgesia at a hypothalamic site in the brain, although the mode of action is not known.

Aspirin also acts on the hypothalamus to produce antipyresis; heat dissipation is increased as a result of vasodilation and increased peripheral blood flow. Aspirin's antipyretic activity may also be related to inhibition of synthesis and release of prostaglandins.

In a crossover study, Easprin at a dose of one tablet (15 grains) three times a day produced an average fecal blood

Continued on next page

This product information was prepared in August 1996. On these and other Parke-Davis Products, information may be obtained by addressing PARKE-DAVIS, Division of Warner-Lambert Company, Morris Plains, New Jersey 07950.

Parke-Davis—Cont.

loss of 1.54 ml per day. Uncoated aspirin at a dosage of three 5 grain tablets given three times a day caused an average fecal blood loss of 4.33 ml per day.

Easprin Tablets are enteric coated. This coating acts to prevent the release of aspirin in the stomach but permits the tablet to dissolve with resultant absorption in the upper portion of the small intestine. This reduces any gastric irritation that may occur with uncoated aspirin but does delay the onset of action. Aspirin is rapidly hydrolyzed primarily in the liver to salicylic acid, which is conjugated with glycine (forming salicyluric acid) and glucuronic acid and excreted largely in the urine. As a result of the rapid hydrolysis, plasma concentrations of aspirin are always low and rarely exceed 20 mcg/ml at ordinary therapeutic doses. The peak salicylate level for uncoated aspirin occurs in about 2 hours; however with enteric coated aspirin tablets this is delayed. A direct correlation between salicylate plasma levels and clinical analgesic effectiveness has not been definitely established, but effective analgesia is usually achieved at plasma levels of 15 to 30 mg per 100 ml. Effective antiinflammatory activity is usually achieved at salicylate plasma levels of 20 to 30 mg per 100 ml. There is also poor correlation between toxic symptoms and plasma salicylate concentrations, but most patients exhibit symptoms of salicylism at plasma salicylate levels of 35 mg per 100 ml. The plasma half-life for aspirin is approximately 15 minutes; that for salicylate lengthens as the dose increases: Doses of 300 to 650 mg have a half-life of 3.1 to 3.2 hours; with doses of 1 gram, the half-life is increased to 5 hours and with 2 grams it is increased to about 9 hours.

Salicylates are excreted mainly by the kidney. Studies in man indicate that salicylate is excreted in the urine as free salicylic acid (10%), salicyluric acid (75%), salicylic phenolic (10%), and acyl (5%) glucuronides and gentisic acid (< 1%).

INDICATIONS AND USAGE

Easprin is indicated in patients who need the higher 15 grain dose of aspirin in the long-term palliative treatment of mild to moderate pain and inflammation of arthritic and other inflammatory conditions.

CONTRAINDICATIONS

Easprin should not be used in patients who have previously exhibited hypersensitivity to aspirin and/or nonsteroidal antiinflammatory agents.

Easprin should not be given to patients with a recent history of gastrointestinal bleeding or in patients with bleeding disorders (eg, hemophilia).

WARNINGS

Easprin Tablets should be used with caution when anticoagulants are prescribed concurrently, for aspirin may depress the concentration of prothrombin in plasma and thereby increase bleeding time. Large doses of salicylates have a hypoglycemic action and may enhance the effect of the oral hypoglycemics. Consequently, they should not be given concomitantly; if however, this is necessary, the dosage of the hypoglycemic agent must be reduced while the salicylate is given. This hypoglycemic action may also affect the insulin requirements of diabetics.

Although salicylates in large doses are uricosuric agents, smaller amounts may decrease the uricosuric effects of probenecid, sulfinpyrazone, and phenylbutazone.

> Reye Syndrome may develop in individuals who have chicken pox, influenza, or flu symptoms. Some studies suggest a possible association between the development of Reye Syndrome and the use of medicines containing salicylate or aspirin. Easprin is not recommended for use in patients with chicken pox, influenza or flu symptoms.

PRECAUTIONS

General: Easprin Tablets should be administered with caution to patients with asthma, nasal polyps, or nasal allergies.

In patients receiving large doses of aspirin and/or prolonged therapy, mild salicylate intoxication (salicylism) may develop that may be reversed by reduction in dosage.

Although the fecal blood loss with Easprin is less than that with uncoated aspirin tablets, Easprin Tablets should be administered with caution to patients with a history of gastric distress, ulcer, or bleeding problems. Occult gastrointestinal bleeding occurs in many patients but is not correlated with gastric distress. The amount of blood lost is usually insignificant clinically, but with prolonged administration, it may result in iron deficiency anemia.

Sodium excretion produced by spironolactone may be decreased in the presence of salicylates.

Salicylates can produce changes in thyroid function tests.

Salicylates should be used with caution in patients with severe hepatic damage, preexisting hypoprothrombinemia, or Vitamin K deficiency, and in those undergoing surgery.

DRUG INTERACTIONS

Anticoagulants: See Warnings section.

Hypoglycemic Agents: See Warnings section.

Uricosuric Agents: Aspirin may decrease the effects of probenecid, sulfinpyrazone, and phenylbutazone.

Spironolactone: See general precautions section.

Alcohol: Has a synergistic effect with aspirin in causing gastrointestinal bleeding.

Corticosteroids: Concomitant administration with aspirin may increase the risk of gastrointestinal ulceration and may reduce serum salicylate levels.

Pyrazolone Derivatives (phenylbutazone, oxyphenbutazone, and possibly dipyrone): Concomitant administration with aspirin may increase the risk of gastrointestinal ulceration.

Nonsteroidal Antiinflammatory Agents: Aspirin is contraindicated in patients who are hypersensitive to nonsteroidal antiinflammatory agents.

Urinary Alkalinizers: Decrease aspirin effectiveness by increasing the rate of salicylate renal excretion.

Phenobarbital: Decreases aspirin effectiveness by enzyme induction.

Phenytoin: Serum phenytoin levels may be increased by aspirin.

Propranolol: May decrease aspirin's antiinflammatory action by competing for the same receptors.

Antacids: Easprin should not be given concurrently with antacids, since an increase in the pH of the stomach may affect the enteric coating of the tablets.

Usage in Pregnancy: It has been reported that adverse effects were increased in the mother and fetus following chronic ingestion of aspirin. Prolonged pregnancy and labor with increased bleeding before and after delivery, as well as decreased birth weight and increased rate of stillbirth were correlated with high blood salicylate levels. Because of possible adverse effects on the neonate and the potential for increased maternal blood loss, aspirin should be avoided during the last three months of pregnancy.

ADVERSE REACTIONS

Gastrointestinal: Dyspepsia, thirst, nausea, vomiting, diarrhea, acute reversible heptatotoxicity, gastrointestinal bleeding, and/or ulceration.

Special Senses: Tinnitus, vertigo, reversible hearing loss and dimness of vision.

Hematologic: Prolongation of bleeding time, leukopenia, thrombocytopenia, purpura, decreased plasma iron concentration and shortened erythrocyte survival time.

Dermatologic and Hypersensitivity: Urticaria, angioedema, pruritus, sweating, various skin eruptions, asthma, and anaphylaxis.

Neurologic: Mental confusion, drowsiness and dizziness.

Body as a whole: Headache and fever.

OVERDOSAGE

Overdosage of 200 to 500 mg/kg is in the fatal range. Early symptoms are CNS stimulation with vomiting, hyperpnea, hyperactivity, and possibly convulsions. This progresses quickly to depression, coma, respiratory failure, and collapse. These symptoms are accompanied by severe electrolyte disturbances.

In the treatment of salicylate overdosage, intensive supportive therapy should be instituted immediately. Plasma salicylate levels should be measured in order to determine the severity of the poisoning and to provide a guide for therapy. Emptying of the stomach should be accomplished as soon as possible with ipecac syrup unless the patient is depressed. In depressed patients use airway protected gastric lavage. Delay absorption with activated charcoal and give a saline cathartic. Proceed according to Standard Reference Procedures for Salicylate Intoxication.

DOSAGE AND ADMINISTRATION

Usual Adult Dosage: One tablet 3 to 4 times daily.

Patients who have displayed no significant adverse effects on a long term qid regimen and who receive a total daily dosage of aspirin no greater than 3.9 grams may be considered for a bid regimen (2 tablets of Easprin twice daily). Patients on the bid Easprin regimen should be closely monitored for serum salicylate levels, increased incidence of CNS-related adverse effects, increased fecal blood loss, or any other signs or symptoms suggestive of significant blood loss.

If necessary, dosage may be increased until relief is obtained, but dosage should be maintained slightly below that which produces tinnitus. Plasma salicylate levels may also be helpful in determining proper dosage (see CLINICAL PHARMACOLOGY section).

HOW SUPPLIED

Easprin enteric coated tablets each containing 15 grains (975 mg) aspirin are available:
N 0071-0490-24—Bottles of 100

Storage: Store at controlled room temperature 15° to 30°C (59° to 86°F).

Revised May 1994

0490G018

Shown in Product Identification Guide, page 327

ERYC® ℞

[*ĕ'ryc*]

(Erythromycin Delayed-Release Capsules, USP)

DESCRIPTION

ERYC Capsules contain enteric-coated pellets of erythromycin base for oral administration. Erythromycin is produced by a strain of *Streptomyces erythraeus* and belongs to the macrolide group of antibiotics. It is basic and readily forms salts with acids, but it is the base which is microbiologically active. Each ERYC Capsule contains 250 milligrams of erythromycin base. Also contains: lactose, NF; povidone, USP; FD&C Yellow No. 6 . The capsule shell contains gelatin, NF; titanium dioxide, USP; FD&C Yellow No. 6.

Erythromycin base is (3*R**, 4*S**, 5*S**, 6*R**, 7*R**, 9*R**, 11*R**, 12*R**, 13*S**, 14*R**) -4-[(2,6-Dideoxy-3-*C* -methyl -3-*O*-methyl-α-L- *ribo*-hexopyranosyl)-oxy]-14-ethyl -7,12,13-trihydroxy-3, 5,7,9,11,13-hexamethyl-6-[[3,4,6-trideoxy-3-(dimethylamino)-β -D - *xylo* - hexopyranosyl]oxy]oxacyclotetradecane - 2, 10 - dione.

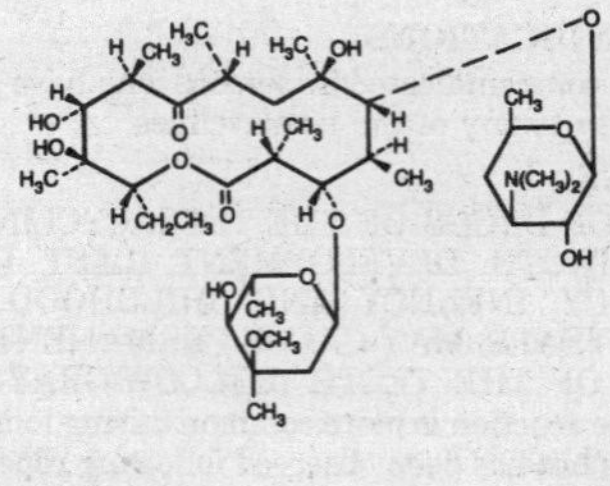

$C_{37}H_{67}NO_{13}$ MW733.94

CLINICAL PHARMACOLOGY

Orally administered erythromycin base and its salts are readily absorbed in the microbiologically active form. Interindividual variations in the absorption of erythromycin are, however, observed, and some patients do not achieve acceptable serum levels. Erythromycin is largely bound to plasma proteins, and the freely dissociating bound fraction after administration of erythromycin base represents 90% of the total erythromycin absorbed. After absorption, erythromycin diffuses readily into most body fluids. In the absence of meningeal inflammation, low concentrations are normally achieved in the spinal fluid, but the passage of the drug across the blood-brain barrier increases in meningitis. Erythromycin is excreted in breast milk. The drug crosses the placental barrier, but fetal plasma levels are low. Erythromycin is not removed by peritoneal dialysis or hemodialysis.

In the presence of normal hepatic function erythromycin is concentrated in the liver and is excreted in the bile; the effect of hepatic dysfunction on biliary excretion of erythromycin is not known. After oral administration, less than 5% of the administered dose can be recovered in the active form in the urine.

The enteric coating of pellets in ERYC Capsules protects the erythromycin base from inactivation by gastric acidity. Because of their small size and enteric coating, the pellets readily pass intact from the stomach to the small intestine and dissolve efficiently to allow absorption of erythromycin in a uniform manner. After administration of a single dose of a 250-mg ERYC capsule, peak serum levels in the range of 1.13 to 1.68 mcg/mL are attained in approximately 3 hours and decline to 0.30–0.42 mcg/mL in 6 hours. Optimal conditions for stability in the presence of gastric secretion and for complete absorption are attained when ERYC is taken on an empty stomach.

Microbiology: Erythromycin acts by inhibition of protein synthesis by binding 50 S ribosomal subunits of susceptible organisms. It does not affect nucleic acid synthesis. Antagonism has been demonstrated *in vitro* between erythromycin, clindamycin, lincomycin, and chloramphenicol. Many strains of *Haemophilus influenzae* are resistant to erythromycin alone, but are susceptible to erythromycin and sulfonamides together. Staphylococci resistant to erythromycin may emerge during a course of erythromycin therapy. Specimens should be obtained for culture and susceptibility testing.

Erythromycin is usually active against the following organisms *in vitro* and in clinical infections:

- *Streptococcus pyogenes* (group A beta-hemolytic streptococci)
- Alpha-hemolytic streptococci (viridans group)
- *Staphylococcus aureus* (Resistant organisms may emerge during treatment.)
- *Streptococcus pneumoniae*
- *Mycoplasma pneumoniae*
- *Treponema pallidum*
- *Corynebacterium diphtheriae*
- *Corynebacterium minutissimum*
- *Entamoeba histolytica*
- *Listeria monocytogenes*

Neisseria gonorrhoeae
Bordetella pertussis
Legionella pneumophila (agent of Legionnaires' disease)
Ureaplasma urealyticum
Chlamydia trachomatis

Susceptibility Testing: Quantitative methods that require measurement of zone diameters give the most precise estimates of antibiotic susceptibility. One such standardized single disc procedure has been recommended for use with discs to test susceptibility to erythromycin.[1] Interpretation involves correlation of the zone diameters obtained in the disc test with minimum inhibitory concentration (MIC) values for erythromycin.

Reports from the laboratory giving results of the standardized single-disc susceptibility test using a 15-mcg erythromycin disc should be interpreted according to the following criteria:

Susceptible organisms produce zones of 18 mm or greater indicating that the tested organism is likely to respond to therapy.

Resistant organisms produce zones of 13 mm or less, indicating that other therapy should be selected.

Organisms of intermediate susceptibility produce zones of 14 to 17 mm. The "intermediate" category provides a "buffer zone" which should prevent small uncontrolled technical factors from causing major discrepancies in interpretations; thus when a zone diameter falls within the "intermediate" range, the results may be considered equivocal. If alternate drugs are not available, confirmation by dilution tests may be indicated.

Standardized procedures require the use of control organisms. The 15-mcg erythromycin disc should give some diameter between 22 and 30 mm for *S aureus* ATCC 25923 control strain.

A bacterial isolate may be considered susceptible if the MIC value[2] for erythromycin is not more than 2 mcg/mL. Organisms are considered resistant if the MIC is 8 mcg/mL or higher.

The MIC of erythromycin for *S aureus* ATCC 29213 control strain should be between 0.12 and 0.5 mcg/mL.

INDICATIONS AND USAGE

ERYC is indicated in the treatment of infections caused by susceptible strains of the designated microorganisms in the diseases listed below:

Upper respiratory tract infections of mild to moderate degree caused by *Streptococcus pyogenes* (group A beta-hemolytic streptococci); *Streptococcus pneumoniae (Diplococcus pneumoniae); Haemophilus influenzae* (when used concomitantly with adequate doses of sulfonamides, since many strains of *H influenzae* are susceptible at the erythromycin concentrations ordinarily achieved). (See appropriate sulfonamide labeling for prescribing information.)

Lower respiratory tract infections of mild to moderate severity caused by *Streptococcus pyogenes* (group A beta-hemolytic streptococci); *Streptococcus pneumoniae (Diplococcus pneumoniae).*

Respiratory tract infections due to *Mycoplasma pneumoniae.*

Pertussis (whooping cough) caused by *Bordetella pertussis.* Erythromycin is effective in eliminating the organism from the nasopharynx of infected individuals, rendering them noninfectious. Some clinical studies suggest that erythromycin may be helpful in the prophylaxis of pertussis in exposed susceptible individuals.

Diphtheria—As an adjunct to antitoxin in infections due to *Corynebacterium diphtheriae,* to prevent establishment of carriers and to eradicate the organism in carriers.

Erythrasma—In the treatment of infections due to *Corynebacterium minutissimum.*

Intestinal amebiasis caused by *Entamoeba histolytica* (oral erythromycins only). Extraenteric amebiasis requires treatment with other agents.

Acute pelvic inflammatory disease caused by *Neisseria gonorrhoeae.* Erythromycin lactobionate for injection, USP followed by erythromycin base orally, as an alternative drug in treatment of acute inflammatory disease caused by *N gonorrhoeae* in female patients with a history of sensitivity to penicillin. Before treatment of gonorrhoeae, patients who are suspected of also having syphilis should have a microscopic examination for *Treponema pallidum* (by immunofluorescence or dark field) before receiving erythromycin and monthly serologic tests for a minimum of 4 months thereafter.

Infections due to *Listeria monocytogenes.*

Skin and soft tissue infections of mild to moderate severity caused by *Streptococcus pyogenes* and *Staphylococcus aureus* (resistant staphylococci may emerge during treatment).

Primary syphilis caused by *Treponema pallidum.* Erythromycin (oral forms only) is an alternate choice of treatment for primary syphilis in patients allergic to the penicillins. In treatment of primary syphilis, spinal fluid should be examined before treatment and as part of the follow-up after therapy.

Erythromycins are indicated for treatment of the following infections caused by *Chlamydia trachomatis:* conjunctivitis of the newborn, pneumonia of infancy, urogenital infections during pregnancy. When tetracyclines are contraindicated or not tolerated, erythromycin is indicated for the treatment of uncomplicated urethral, endocervical, or rectal infections in adults due to *Chlamydia trachomatis.*[3]

Erythromycin is indicated for the treatment of nongonococcal urethritis caused by *Ureaplasma urealyticum* when tetracyclines are contraindicated or not tolerated.[3]

Legionnaires' disease caused by *Legionella pneumophila.* Although no controlled clinical efficacy studies have been conducted, *in vitro* and limited preliminary clinical data suggest that erythromycin may be effective in treating Legionnaires' disease.

Therapy with erythromycin should be monitored by bacteriological studies and by clinical response (see CLINICAL PHARMACOLOGY—Microbiology section).

Prevention of Initial Attacks of Rheumatic Fever: Penicillin is considered by the American Heart Association to be the drug of choice in the prevention of initial attacks of rheumatic fever (treatment of group A beta-hemolytic streptococcal infections of the upper respiratory tract).[4] Erythromycin is indicated for the treatment of penicillin-allergic patients. The therapeutic dose should be administered for 10 days.

Prevention of Recurrent Attacks of Rheumatic Fever: Penicillin or sulfonamides are considered by the American Heart Association to be the drug of choice in the prevention of recurrent attacks of rheumatic fever. In patients allergic to penicillin and sulfonamides, oral erythromycin is recommended by the American Heart Association in the long-term prophylaxis of streptococcal pharyngitis (for the prevention of recurrent attacks of rheumatic fever).[4]

Prevention of Bacterial Endocarditis: Although no controlled clinical efficacy trials have been conducted, oral erythromycin has been recommended by the American Heart Association for the prevention of bacterial endocarditis in penicillin-allergic patients with most congenital cardiac malformations, rheumatic or other acquired valvular dysfunction, idiopathic hypertrophic subaortic stenosis (HSS), previous history of bacterial endocarditis and mitral valve prolapse with insufficiency when they undergo dental procedures and surgical procedures of the upper respiratory tract.[5]

CONTRAINDICATIONS

ERYC is contraindicated in patients with known hypersensitivity to this antibiotic.

Erythromycin is contraindicated in patients taking terfenadine. (See PRECAUTIONS-Drug Interactions.)

WARNINGS

There have been reports of hepatic dysfunction, with or without jaundice, occurring in patients receiving oral erythromycin products.

PRECAUTIONS

General: Erythromycin is principally excreted by the liver. Caution should be exercised when erythromycin is administered to patients with impaired hepatic function. (See CLINICAL PHARMACOLOGY and WARNINGS sections.)

Prolonged or repeated use of erythromycin may result in an overgrowth of nonsusceptible bacteria or fungi. If superinfection occurs, erythromycin should be discontinued and appropriate therapy instituted.

When indicated, incision and drainage or other surgical procedures should be performed in conjunction with antibiotic therapy.

Laboratory Tests: Erythromycin interferes with the fluorometric determination of urinary catecholamines.

Drug Interactions: Erythromycin use in patients who are receiving high doses of theophylline may be associated with an increase of serum theophylline levels and potential theophylline toxicity. In cases of theophylline toxicity and/or elevated serum theophylline levels, the dose of theophylline should be reduced while the patient is receiving concomitant erythromycin therapy.

Concomitant administration of erythromycin and digoxin has been reported to result in elevated digoxin serum levels.

There have been reports of increased anticoagulant effects when erythromycin and oral anticoagulants were used concomitantly.

Concurrent use of erythromycin and ergotamine or dihydroergotamine has been associated in some patients with acute ergot toxicity characterized by severe vasospasm and dysethesia.

Erythromycin has been reported to decrease the clearance of triazolam and thus may increase the pharmacologic effect of triazolam.

The use of erythromycin in patients concurrently taking drugs metabolized by the cytochrome P450 system may be associated with elevations in serum levels of these other drugs. There have been reports of interactions of erythromycin with carbamazepine, cyclosporine, hexobarbital and phenytoin. Serum concentrations of drugs metabolized by the cytochrome P450 system should be monitored closely in patients concurrently receiving erythromycin.

Erythromycin significantly alters the metabolism of terfenadine when taken concomitantly. Rare cases of serious cardiovascular adverse events, including death, cardiac arrest, torsades de pointes, and other ventricular arrhythmias, have been observed. (See CONTRAINDICATIONS.)

Carcinogenesis, Mutagenesis, and Impairment of Fertility: Long-term (20-month) oral studies conducted in rats with erythromycin base did not provide evidence of tumorigenicity. Mutagenicity studies have not been conducted. There was no apparent effect on male or female fertility in rats fed erythromycin (base) at levels up to 0.25 percent of diet.

Pregnancy: Pregnancy Category B: There is no evidence of teratogenicity or any other adverse effect on reproduction in female rats fed erythromycin base (up to 0.25 percent of diet) prior to and during mating, during gestation, and through weaning of two successive litters. There are, however, no adequate and well-controlled studies in pregnant women. Because animal reproduction studies are not always predictive of human response, this drug should be used during pregnancy only if clearly needed. Erythromycin has been reported to cross the placental barrier in humans, but fetal plasma levels are generally low.

Labor and Delivery: The effect of erythromycin on labor and delivery is unknown.

Nursing Mothers: Erythromycin is excreted in breast milk; therefore, caution should be exercised when erythromycin is administered to a nursing woman.

Pediatric Use: See INDICATIONS AND USAGE and DOSAGE AND ADMINISTRATION sections.

ADVERSE REACTIONS

The most frequent side effects of oral erythromycin preparations are gastrointestinal and are dose-related. They include nausea, vomiting, abdominal pain, diarrhea, and anorexia. Symptoms of hepatic dysfunction and/or abnormal liver function test results may occur (see WARNINGS section).

Pseudomembranous colitis has been rarely reported in association with erythromycin therapy.

Allergic reactions ranging from urticaria and mild eruptions to anaphylaxis have occurred.

There have been isolated reports of reversible hearing loss occurring chiefly in patients with renal insufficiency and in patients receiving high doses of erythromycin.

OVERDOSAGE

In case of overdosage, erythromycin should be discontinued. Overdosage should be handled with the prompt elimination of unabsorbed drug and all other appropriate measures.

Erythromycin is not removed by peritoneal dialysis or hemodialysis.

DOSAGE AND ADMINISTRATION

ERYC is well absorbed and may be given without regard to meals. Optimum blood levels are obtained in a fasting state (administration at least one half hour and preferably two hours before or after a meal); however, blood levels obtained upon administration of enteric-coated erythromycin products in the presence of food are still above minimum inhibitory concentrations (MICs) of most organisms for which erythromycin is indicated.

ADULTS: The usual dose is 250 mg every 6 hours taken one hour before meals. If twice-a-day dosage is desired, the recommended dose is 500 mg every 12 hours. Dosage may be increased up to 4 grams per day, according to the severity of the infection. Twice-a-day dosing is not recommended when doses larger than 1 gram daily are administered.

CHILDREN: Age, weight, and severity of the infection are important factors in determining the proper dosage. The usual dosage is 30 to 50 mg/kg/day in divided doses. For the treatment of more severe infections, this dose may be doubled.

Streptococcal infections: A therapeutic dosage of oral erythromycin should be administered for at least 10 days. For continuous prophylaxis against recurrences of streptococcal infections in persons with a history of rheumatic heart disease, the dose is 250 mg twice a day.

For the prevention of bacterial endocarditis in penicillin-allergic patients with valvular heart disease who are to undergo dental procedures or surgical procedures of the upper respiratory tract, the adult dose is 1 gram orally (20 mg/kg for children) one hour prior to the procedure and then 500 mg (10 mg/kg for children) orally 6 hours later[5] (see INDICATIONS AND USAGE section).

Primary syphilis: 30–40 grams given in divided doses over a period of 10–15 days.

Continued on next page

This product information was prepared in August 1996. On these and other Parke-Davis Products, information may be obtained by addressing PARKE-DAVIS, Division of Warner-Lambert Company, Morris Plains, New Jersey 07950.

Parke-Davis—Cont.

Intestinal amebiasis: 250 mg four times daily for 10 to 14 days for adults; 30 to 50 mg/kg/day in divided doses for 10 to 14 days for children.

Legionnaires' disease: Although optimal doses have not been established, doses utilized in reported clinical data were those recommended above (1 to 4 grams daily in divided doses).

Urogenital infections during pregnancy due to *Chlamydia trachomatis:* Although the optimal dose and duration of therapy have not been established, the suggested treatment is erythromycin 500 mg, by mouth, 4 times a day on an empty stomach for at least 7 days. For women who cannot tolerate this regimen, a decreased dose of 250 mg, by mouth, 4 times a day should be used for at least 14 days.[3]

For adults with uncomplicated urethral, endocervical, or rectal infections caused by *Chlamydia trachomatis* in whom tetracyclines are contraindicated or not tolerated: 500 mg, by mouth, 4 times a day for at least 7 days.[3]

Pertussis: Although optimum dosage and duration of therapy have not been established, doses of erythromycin utilized in reported clinical studies were 40–50 mg/kg/day, given in divided doses for 5 to 14 days.

Nongonococcal urethritis due to *Ureaplasma urealyticum:* When tetracycline is contraindicated or not tolerated: 500 mg of erythromycin, orally, 4 times daily for at least 7 days.[3]

Acute pelvic inflammatory disease due to *N gonorrhoeae:* 500 mg IV of erythromycin lactobionate for injection, USP every 6 hours for 3 days followed by 250 mg of erythromycin, orally, every 6 hours for 7 days.

HOW SUPPLIED

ERYC (Capsule 696), clear and orange opaque capsules, each containing 250 mg erythromycin as enteric-coated pellets, are available as follows:

N 0071-0696-24 Bottles of 100

Storage Conditions: Store at room temperature below 30°C (86°F).

REFERENCES

1. Approved Standard ASM-2 "Performance Standards for Antimicrobial Disc Susceptibility Test." National Committee for Clinical Laboratory Standards, 771 East Lancaster Avenue, Villanova, PA 19085.
2. Ericson, H.M. and Sherris, J.C. "Antibiotic Sensitivity Testing Report of an International Collaborative Study." *Acta Pathologica et Microbiologica Scandinavica,* Section B, Supp. 217, 1971, pp. 1–90.
3. CDC Sexually Transmitted Diseases Treatment Guidelines 1985.
4. Committee on Rheumatic Fever and Infective Endocarditis of the Council on Cardiovascular Disease of the Young: Prevention of Rheumatic Fever, Circulation 70(6): 1118A–1122A, December 1984.
5. Committee on Rheumatic Fever and Infective Endocarditis of the Council on Cardiovascular Disease of the Young: Prevention of Bacterial Endocarditis, Circulation 70(6): 1123A–1127A, December 1984.

Caution—Federal law prohibits dispensing without prescription.

June 1994

Manufactured by
Faulding Pharmaceutical/DBL
A Division of F.H. Faulding & Co. Limited
1538 Main North Road
Salisbury, South Australia 5108
Distributed by
PARKE-DAVIS
Div of Warner-Lambert Co
Morris Plains, NJ 07950 USA

0696G390

Shown in Product Identification Guide, page 327

LOPID®   ℞
[lō'pĭd]
(Gemfibrozil Tablets, USP)

DESCRIPTION

Lopid® (gemfibrozil tablets, USP) is a lipid regulating agent. It is available as tablets for oral administration. Each tablet contains 600 mg gemfibrozil. Each also contains calcium stearate, NF; candelilla wax FCC; microcrystalline cellulose, NF; hydroxypropyl cellulose, NF; hydroxypropyl methylcellulose, USP; methylparaben, NF; Opaspray white; polyethylene glycol, NF; polysorbate 80, NF; propylparaben, NF; colloidal silicon dioxide, NF; pregelatinized starch, NF. The chemical name is 5-(2,5-dimethylphenoxy)-2,2-dimethylpentanoic acid.

The empirical formula is $C_{15}H_{22}O_3$ and the molecular weight is 250.35; the solubility in water and acid is 0.0019% and in dilute base it is greater than 1%. The melting point is 58°–61°C. Gemfibrozil is a white solid which is stable under ordinary conditions.

CLINICAL PHARMACOLOGY

Lopid (gemfibrozil tablets, USP) is a lipid regulating agent which decreases serum triglycerides and very low density lipoprotein (VLDL) cholesterol, and increases high density lipoprotein (HDL) cholesterol. While modest decreases in total and low density lipoprotein (LDL) cholesterol may be observed with Lopid therapy, treatment of patients with elevated triglycerides due to Type IV hyperlipoproteinemia often results in a rise in LDL-cholesterol. LDL-cholesterol levels in Type IIb patients with elevations of both serum LDL-cholesterol and triglycerides are, in general, minimally affected by Lopid treatment; however, Lopid usually raises HDL-cholesterol significantly in this group. Lopid increases levels of high density lipoprotein (HDL) subfractions HDL_2 and HDL_3, as well as apolipoproteins AI and AII. Epidemiological studies have shown that both low HDL-cholesterol and high LDL-cholesterol are independent risk factors for coronary heart disease.

In the primary prevention component of the Helsinki Heart Study (refs. 1,2), in which 4081 male patients between the ages of 40 and 55 were studied in a randomized, double-blind, placebo-controlled fashion, Lopid therapy was associated with significant reductions in total plasma triglycerides and a significant increase in high density lipoprotein cholesterol. Moderate reductions in total plasma cholesterol and low density lipoprotein cholesterol were observed for the Lopid treatment group as a whole, but the lipid response was heterogeneous, especially among different Fredrickson types. The study involved subjects with serum non-HDL-cholesterol of over 200 mg/dL and no previous history of coronary heart disease. Over the 5-year study period, the Lopid group experienced a 1.4% absolute (34% relative) reduction in the rate of serious coronary events (sudden cardiac deaths plus fatal and nonfatal myocardial infarctions) compared to placebo, p = 0.04 (see Table I). There was a 37% relative reduction in the rate of nonfatal myocardial infarction compared to placebo, equivalent to a treatment-related difference of 13.1 events per thousand persons. Deaths from any cause during the double-blind portion of the study totaled 44 (2.2%) in the Lopid randomization group and 43 (2.1%) in the placebo group.

[See table 1 below.]

Among Fredrickson types, during the 5-year double-blind portion of the primary prevention component of the Helsinki Heart Study, the greatest reduction in the incidence of serious coronary events occurred in Type IIb patients who had elevations of both LDL-cholesterol and total plasma triglycerides. This subgroup of Type IIb gemfibrozil group patients had a lower mean HDL-cholesterol level at baseline than the Type IIa subgroup that had elevations of LDL-cholesterol and normal plasma triglycerides. The mean increase in HDL-cholesterol among the Type IIb patients in this study was 12.6% compared to placebo. The mean change in LDL-cholesterol among Type IIb patients was −4.1% with Lopid compared to a rise of 3.9% in the placebo subgroup. The Type IIb subjects in the Helsinki Heart Study had 26 fewer coronary events per thousand persons over 5 years in the gemfibrozil group compared to placebo. The difference in coronary events was substantially greater between Lopid and placebo for that subgroup of patients with the triad of LDL-cholesterol > 175 mg/dL (> 4.5 mmol), triglycerides > 200 mg/dL (> 2.2 mmol), and HDL-cholesterol < 35 mg/dL (< 0.90 mmol) (see Table I).

Further information is available from a 3.5 year (8.5 year cumulative) follow-up of all subjects who had participated in the Helsinki Heart Study. At the completion of the Helsinki Heart study, subjects could choose to start, stop, or continue to receive Lopid; without knowledge of their own lipid values or double-blind treatment, 60% of patients originally randomized to placebo began therapy with Lopid and 60% of patients originally randomized to Lopid continued medica-

tion. After approximately 6.5 years following randomization, all patients were informed of their original treatment group and lipid values during the 5 years of the double-blind treatment. After further elective changes in Lopid treatment status, 61% of patients in the group originally randomized to Lopid were taking drug; in the group originally randomized to placebo, 65% were taking Lopid. The event rate per 1000 occurring during the open-label follow-up period is detailed in Table II.

Table II
Cardiac Events and All-Cause Mortality (events per 1000 patients) Occurring during the 3.5 Year Open-Label Follow-up to the Helsinki Heart Study[1]

Group:	PDrop N=215	PN N=494	PL N=1283	LDrop N=221	LN N=574	LL N=1207
Cardiac Events	38.8	22.9	22.5	37.2	28.3	25.4
All-Cause Mortality	41.9	22.3	15.6	72.3	19.2	24.9

[1] The six open-label groups are designated first by the original randomization (P = placebo, L = Lopid) and then by the drug taken in the follow-up period (N = Attend clinic but took no drug, L = Lopid, Drop = No attendance at clinic during open-label).

Cumulative mortality through 8.5 years showed a 20% relative excess of deaths in the group originally randomized to Lopid versus the originally randomized placebo group and a 20% relative decrease in cardiac events in the group originally randomized to Lopid versus the originally randomized placebo group (see Table III). This analysis of the originally randomized "intent-to-treat" population neglects the possible complicating effects of treatment switching during the open-label phase. Adjustment of hazard ratios taking into account open-label treatment status from years 6.5 to 8.5 could change the reported hazard ratios for mortality toward unity.

Table III
Cardiac Events, Cardiac Deaths, Non-Cardiac Deaths and All-Cause Mortality in the Helsinki Heart Study, Year 0–8.5.[1]

Event	Lopid at Study Start	Placebo at Study Start	Lopid: Placebo Hazard Ratio[2]	Cl Hazard[3] Ratio
Cardiac Events[4]	110	131	0.80	0.62–1.03
Cardiac Deaths	36	38	0.98	0.63–1.54
Non-Cardiac Deaths	65	45	1.40	0.95–2.05
All-Cause Mortality	101	83	1.20	0.90–1.61

[1] Intention-to-Treat Analysis of originally randomized patients neglecting the open-label treatment switches and exposure to study conditions.
[2] Hazard ratio for risk of event in the group originally randomized to Lopid compared to the group originally randomized to placebo neglecting open-label treatment switch and exposure to study condition.
[3] 95% confidence intervals of Lopid:placebo group hazard ratio.
[4] Fatal and non-fatal myocardial infarctions plus sudden cardiac deaths over the 8.5 year period.

It is not clear to what extent the findings of the primary prevention component of the Helsinki Heart Study can be extrapolated to other segments of the dyslipidemic population not studied (such as women, younger or older males, or those with lipid abnormalities limited solely to HDL-cholesterol) or to other lipid-altering drugs.

Table I
Reduction in CHD Rates (events per 1000 patients) by Baseline Lipids[1] in the Helsinki Heart Study, Years 0–5[2]

	All Patients			LDL-C > 175; HDL-C > 46.4			LDL-C > 175; TG > 177			LDL-C > 175; TG > 200; HDL-C < 35		
	P	L	Dif[3]	P	L	Dif	P	L	Dif	P	L	Dif
Incidence of Evidents[4]	41	27	14	32	29	3	71	44	27	149	64	85

[1] lipid values in mg/dL at baseline
[2] P=placebo group; L=Lopid group
[3] difference in rates between placebo and Lopid groups
[4] fatal and nonfatal myocardial infarctions plus sudden cardiac deaths (events per 1000 patients over 5 years)

The secondary prevention component of the Helsinki Heart Study was conducted over 5 years in parallel and at the same centers in Finland in 628 middle-aged males excluded from the primary prevention component of the Helsinki Heart Study because of a history of angina, myocardial infarction or unexplained ECG changes (ref. 3). The primary efficacy endpoint of the study was cardiac events (the sum of fatal and non-fatal myocardial infarctions and sudden cardiac deaths). The hazard ratio (Lopid:placebo) for cardiac events was 1.47 (95% confidence limits 0.88–2.48, p = 0.14). Of the 35 patients in the Lopid group who experienced cardiac events, 12 patients suffered events after discontinuation from the study. Of the 24 patients in the placebo group with cardiac events, 4 patients suffered events after discontinuation from the study. There were 17 cardiac deaths in the Lopid group and 8 in the placebo group (hazard ratio 2.18; 95% confidence limits 0.94–5.05, p = 0.06). Ten of these deaths in the Lopid group and 3 in the placebo group occurred after discontinuation from therapy. In this study of patients with known or suspected coronary heart disease, no benefit from Lopid treatment was observed in reducing cardiac events or cardiac deaths. Thus, Lopid has shown benefit only in selected dyslipidemic patients *without* suspected or established coronary heart disease. Even in patients with coronary heart disease and the triad of elevated LDL-cholesterol, elevated triglycerides, plus low HDL-cholesterol, the possible effect of Lopid on coronary events has not been adequately studied.

No efficacy in the patients with established coronary heart disease was observed during the Coronary Drug Project with the chemically and pharmacologically related drug, clofibrate. The Coronary Drug Project was a 6-year randomized, double-blind study involving 1000 clofibrate, 1000 nicotinic acid, and 3000 placebo patients with known coronary heart disease. A clinically and statistically significant reduction in myocardial infarctions was seen in the concurrent nicotinic acid group compared to placebo; no reduction was seen with clofibrate.

The mechanism of action of gemfibrozil has not been definitely established. In man, Lopid has been shown to inhibit peripheral lipolysis and to decrease the hepatic extraction of free fatty acids, thus reducing hepatic triglyceride production. Lopid inhibits synthesis and increases clearance of VLDL carrier apolipoprotein B, leading to a decrease in VLDL production.

Animal studies suggest that gemfibrozil may, in addition to elevating HDL-cholesterol, reduce incorporation of long-chain fatty acids into newly formed triglycerides, accelerate turnover and removal of cholesterol from the liver, and increase excretion of cholesterol in the feces. Lopid is well absorbed from the gastrointestinal tract after oral administration. Peak plasma levels occur in 1 to 2 hours with a plasma half-life of 1.5 hours following multiple doses. Plasma levels appear proportional to dose and do not demonstrate accumulation across time following multiple doses.

Lopid mainly undergoes oxidation of a ring methyl group to successively form a hydroxymethyl and a carboxyl metabolite. Approximately seventy percent of the administered human dose is excreted in the urine, mostly as the glucuronide conjugate, with less than 2% excreted as unchanged gemfibrozil. Six percent of the dose is accounted for in the feces.

INDICATIONS AND USAGE

Lopid (gemfibrozil tablets, USP) is indicated as adjunctive therapy to diet for:
1. Treatment of adult patients with very high elevations of serum triglyceride levels (Types IV and V hyperlipidemia) who present a risk of pancreatitis and who do not respond adequately to a determined dietary effort to control them. Patients who present such risk typically have serum triglycerides over 2000 mg/dL and have elevations of VLDL-cholesterol as well as fasting chylomicrons (Type V hyperlipidemia). Subjects who consistently have total serum or plasma triglycerides below 1000 mg/dL are unlikely to present a risk of pancreatitis. Lopid therapy may be considered for those subjects with triglyceride elevations between 1000 and 2000 mg/dL who have a history of pancreatitis or of recurrent abdominal pain typical of pancreatitis. It is recognized that some Type IV patients with triglycerides under 1000 mg/dL may, through dietary or alcoholic indiscretion, convert to a Type V pattern with massive triglyceride elevations accompanying fasting chylomicronemia, but the influence of Lopid therapy on the risk of pancreatitis in such situations has not been adequately studied. Drug therapy is not indicated for patients with Type I hyperlipoproteinemia, who have elevations of chylomicrons and plasma triglycerides, but who have normal levels of very low density lipoprotein (VLDL). Inspection of plasma refrigerated for 14 hours is helpful in distinguishing Types I, IV, and V hyperlipoproteinemia (ref. 4).
2. Reducing the risk of developing coronary heart disease only in Type IIb patients without history of or symptoms of existing coronary heart disease who have had an inadequate response to weight loss, dietary therapy, exercise,

and other pharmacologic agents (such as bile acid sequestrants and nicotinic acid, known to reduce LDL- and raise HDL-cholesterol **and** who have the following triad of lipid abnormalities: low HDL-cholesterol levels in addition to elevated LDL-cholesterol and elevated triglycerides (see WARNINGS, PRECAUTIONS, and CLINICAL PHARMACOLOGY). The National Cholesterol Education Program has defined a serum HDL-cholesterol value that is consistently below 35 mg/dL as constituting an independent risk factor for coronary heart disease (ref. 5). Patients with significantly elevated triglycerides should be closely observed when treated with gemfibrozil. In some patients with high triglyceride levels, treatment with gemfibrozil is associated with a significant increase in LDL-cholesterol. BECAUSE OF POTENTIAL TOXICITY SUCH AS MALIGNANCY, GALLBLADDER DISEASE, ABDOMINAL PAIN LEADING TO APPENDECTOMY AND OTHER ABDOMINAL SURGERIES, AN INCREASED INCIDENCE IN NONCORONARY MORTALITY, AND THE 44% RELATIVE INCREASE DURING THE TRIAL PERIOD IN AGE-ADJUSTED ALL-CAUSE MORTALITY SEEN WITH THE CHEMICALLY AND PHARMACOLOGICALLY RELATED DRUG, CLOFIBRATE, THE POTENTIAL BENEFIT OF GEMFIBROZIL IN TREATING TYPE IIA PATIENTS WITH ELEVATIONS OF LDL-CHOLESTEROL ONLY IS NOT LIKELY TO OUTWEIGH THE RISKS. LOPID IS ALSO NOT INDICATED FOR THE TREATMENT OF PATIENTS WITH LOW HDL-CHOLESTEROL AS THEIR ONLY LIPID ABNORMALITY.

In a subgroup analysis of patients in the Helsinki Heart Study with above-median HDL-cholesterol values at baseline (greater than 46.4 mg/dL), the incidence of serious coronary events was similar for gemfibrozil and placebo subgroups (see Table I).

The initial treatment for dyslipidemia is dietary therapy specific for the type of lipoprotein abnormality. Excess body weight and excess alcohol intake may be important factors in hypertriglyceridemia and should be managed prior to any drug therapy. Physical exercise can be an important ancillary measure, and has been associated with rises in HDL-cholesterol. Diseases contributory to hyperlipidemia such as hypothyroidism or diabetes mellitus should be looked for and adequately treated. Estrogen therapy is sometimes associated with massive rises in plasma triglycerides, especially in subjects with familial hypertriglyceridemia. In such cases, discontinuation of estrogen therapy may obviate the need for specific drug therapy of hypertriglyceridemia. The use of drugs should be considered only when reasonable attempts have been made to obtain satisfactory results with nondrug methods. If the decision is made to use drugs, the patient should be instructed that this does not reduce the importance of adhering to diet.

CONTRAINDICATIONS

1. Hepatic or severe renal dysfunction, including primary biliary cirrhosis.
2. Preexisting gallbladder disease (see WARNINGS).
3. Hypersensitivity to gemfibrozil.

WARNINGS

1. Because of chemical, pharmacological, and clinical similarities between gemfibrozil and clofibrate, the adverse findings with clofibrate in two large clinical studies may also apply to gemfibrozil. In the first of those studies, the Coronary Drug Project, 1000 subjects with previous myocardial infarction were treated for 5 years with clofibrate. There was no difference in mortality between the clofibrate-treated subjects and 3000 placebo-treated subjects, but twice as many clofibrate-treated subjects developed cholelithiasis and cholecystitis requiring surgery. In the other study, conducted by the World Health Organization (WHO), 5000 subjects without known coronary heart disease were treated with clofibrate for 5 years and followed one year beyond. There was a statistically significant, 44%, higher age-adjusted total mortality in the clofibrate-treated than in a comparable placebo-treated control group during the trial period. The excess mortality was due to a 33% increase in noncardiovascular causes, including malignancy, post-cholecystectomy complications, and pancreatitis. The higher risk of clofibrate-treated subjects for gallbladder disease was confirmed.

Because of the more limited size of the Helsinki Heart Study, the observed difference in mortality from any cause between the Lopid and placebo group is not statistically significantly different from the 29% excess mortality reported in the clofibrate group in the separate WHO study at the 9 year follow-up (see CLINICAL PHARMACOLOGY). Noncoronary heart disease related mortality showed an excess in the group originally randomized to Lopid primarily due to cancer deaths observed during the open-label extension.

During the 5 year primary prevention component of the Helsinki Heart Study mortality from any cause was 44 (2.2%) in the Lopid group and 43 (2.1%) in the placebo group; including the 3.5 year follow-up period since the

trial was completed, cumulative mortality from any cause was 101 (4.9%) in the Lopid group and 83 (4.1%) in the group originally randomized to placebo (hazard ratio 1.20 in favor of placebo). Because of the more limited size of the Helsinki Heart Study, the observed difference in mortality from any cause between the Lopid and placebo groups at year-5 or at year-8.5 is not statistically significantly different from the 29% excess mortality reported in the clofibrate group in the separate WHO study at the 9 year follow-up. Noncoronary heart disease related mortality showed an excess in the group originally randomized to Lopid at the 8.5 year follow-up (65 Lopid versus 45 placebo noncoronary deaths).

The incidence of cancer (excluding basal cell carcinoma) discovered during the trial and in the 3.5 years after the trial was completed was 51 (2.5%) in both originally randomized groups. In addition, there were 16 basal cell carcinomas in the group originally randomized to Lopid and 9 in the group randomized to placebo (p = 0.22). There were 30 (1.5%) deaths attributed to cancer in the group originally randomized to Lopid and 18 (0.9%) in the group originally randomized to placebo (p = 0.11). Adverse outcomes, including coronary events, were higher in gemfibrozil patients in a corresponding study in men with a history of known or suspected coronary heart disease in the secondary prevention component of the Helsinki Heart Study. (See CLINICAL PHARMACOLOGY.)

2. A gallstone prevalence substudy of 450 Helsinki Heart Study participants showed a trend toward a greater prevalence of gallstones during the study within the Lopid treatment group (7.5% vs 4.9% for the placebo group, a 55% excess for the gemfibrozil group). A trend toward a greater incidence of gallbladder surgery was observed for the Lopid group (17 vs 11 subjects, a 54% excess). This result did not differ statistically from the increased incidence of cholecystectomy observed in the WHO study in the group treated with clofibrate. Both clofibrate and gemfibrozil may increase cholesterol excretion into the bile leading to cholelithiasis. If cholelithiasis is suspected, gallbladder studies are indicated. Lopid therapy should be discontinued if gallstones are found.

3. Since a reduction of mortality from coronary heart disease has not been demonstrated and because liver and interstitial cell testicular tumors were increased in rats, Lopid should be administered only to those patients described in the INDICATIONS AND USAGE section. If a significant serum lipid response is not obtained, Lopid should be discontinued.

4. Concomitant Anticoagulants—Caution should be exercised when anticoagulants are given in conjunction with Lopid. The dosage of the anticoagulant should be reduced to maintain the prothrombin time at the desired level to prevent bleeding complications. Frequent prothrombin determinations are advisable until it has been definitely determined that the prothrombin level has stabilized.

5. Concomitant therapy with Lopid and Mevacor® (lovastatin) has been associated with rhabdomyolysis, markedly elevated creatine kinase (CK) levels and myoglobinuria, leading in a high proportion of cases to acute renal failure. IN VIRTUALLY ALL PATIENTS WHO HAVE HAD AN UNSATISFACTORY LIPID RESPONSE TO EITHER DRUG ALONE, ANY POTENTIAL LIPID BENEFIT OF COMBINED THERAPY WITH LOVASTATIN AND GEMFIBROZIL DOES NOT OUTWEIGH THE RISKS OF SEVERE MYOPATHY, RHABDOMYOLYSIS, AND ACUTE RENAL FAILURE (see Drug Interactions). The use of fibrates alone, including Lopid, may occasionally be associated with myositis. Patients receiving Lopid and complaining of muscle pain, tenderness, or weakness should have prompt medical evaluation for myositis, including serum creatine kinase level determination. If myositis is suspected or diagnosed, Lopid therapy should be withdrawn.

6. Cataracts—Subcapsular bilateral cataracts occurred in 10% and unilateral in 6.3% of male rats treated with gemfibrozil at 10 times the human dose.

PRECAUTIONS

1. **Initial Therapy**—Laboratory studies should be done to ascertain that the lipid levels are consistently abnormal. Before instituting Lopid therapy, every attempt should be made to control serum lipids with appropriate diet, exercise, weight loss in obese patients, and control of any medical problems such as diabetes mellitus and hypothyroidism that are contributing to the lipid abnormalities.

Continued on next page

This product information was prepared in August 1996. On these and other Parke-Davis Products, information may be obtained by addressing PARKE-DAVIS, Division of Warner-Lambert Company, Morris Plains, New Jersey 07950.

Parke-Davis—Cont.

2. **Continued Therapy**—Periodic determination of serum lipids should be obtained, and the drug withdrawn if lipid response is inadequate after 3 months of therapy.

3. **Drug Interactions**—(A) **HMG-CoA reductase inhibitors:** Rhabdomyolysis has occurred with combined gemfibrozil and lovastatin therapy. It may be seen as early as 3 weeks after initiation of combined therapy or after several months. In most subjects who have had an unsatisfactory lipid response to either drug alone, the possible benefit of combined therapy with lovastatin (or other HMG-CoA reductase inhibitors) and gemfibrozil does not outweigh the risks of severe myopathy, rhabdomyolysis, and acute renal failure. There is no assurance that periodic monitoring of creatine kinase will prevent the occurrence of severe myopathy and kidney damage.

(B) **Anticoagulants:** CAUTION SHOULD BE EXERCISED WHEN ANTICOAGULANTS ARE GIVEN IN CONJUNCTION WITH LOPID. THE DOSAGE OF THE ANTICOAGULANT SHOULD BE REDUCED TO MAINTAIN THE PROTHROMBIN TIME AT THE DESIRED LEVEL TO PREVENT BLEEDING COMPLICATIONS. FREQUENT PROTHROMBIN DETERMINATIONS ARE ADVISABLE UNTIL IT HAS BEEN DEFINITELY DETERMINED THAT THE PROTHROMBIN LEVEL HAS STABILIZED.

4. **Carcinogenesis, Mutagenesis, Impairment of Fertility**—Long-term studies have been conducted in rats at 0.2 and 2 times the human dose (based on surface area, mg/meter^2). Based on two-week toxicokinetic studies, exposure (AUC) of the dose groups was estimated to be 0.2 and 1.3 times the human exposure. The incidence of benign liver nodules and liver carcinomas was significantly increased in high dose male rats. The incidence of liver carcinomas increased also in low dose males, but this increase was not statistically significant (p=0.1). Male rats had a dose-related and statistically significant increase of benign Leydig cell tumors. The higher dose female rats had a significant increase in the combined incidence of benign and malignant liver neoplasms.

Long-term studies have been conducted in mice at 0.1 and 1 times the human dose (based on surface area). Based on two-week toxicokinetic studies, exposure (AUC) of the two dose groups was estimated to be 0.1 and 0.7 times the human exposure. There were no statistically significant differences from controls in the incidence of liver tumors, but the doses tested were lower than those shown to be carcinogenic with other fibrates. Electron microscopy studies have demonstrated a florid hepatic peroxisome proliferation following Lopid administration to the male rat. An adequate study to test for peroxisome proliferation has not been done in humans, but changes in peroxisome morphology have been observed. Peroxisome proliferation has been shown to occur in humans with either of two other drugs of the fibrate class when liver biopsies were compared before and after treatment in the same individual.

Administration of approximately 0.6 and 2 times the human dose (based on surface area) to male rats for 10 weeks resulted in a dose-related decrease of fertility. Subsequent studies demonstrated that this effect was reversed after a drug-free period of about eight weeks, and it was not transmitted to the offspring.

5. **Pregnancy Category C**—Lopid has been shown to produce adverse effects in rats and rabbits at doses between 0.5 and 3 times the human dose (based on surface area) but no developmental toxicity or teratogenicity among offspring of either species. There are no adequate and well-controlled studies in pregnant women. Lopid should be used during pregnancy only if the potential benefit justifies the potential risk to the fetus.

Administration of Lopid to female rats at 0.6 and 2 times the human dose (based on surface area) before and throughout gestation caused a dose-related decrease in conception rate and, at the high dose, an increase in stillborns and a slight reduction in pup weight during lactation. There were also dose-related increased skeletal variations. Anophthalmia occurred, but rarely.

Administration of 0.6 and 2 times the human dose (based on surface area) of Lopid to female rats from gestation day 15 through weaning caused dose-related decreases in birth weight and suppressions of pup growth during lactation.

Administration of 1 and 3 times the human dose (based on surface area) of Lopid to female rabbits during organogenesis caused a dose-related decrease in litter size and, at the high dose, an increased incidence of parietal bone variations.

6. **Nursing Mothers**—It is not known whether this drug is excreted in human milk. Because many drugs are excreted in human milk and because of the potential for tumorigenicity shown for Lopid in animal studies, a decision should be made whether to discontinue nursing or to discontinue the drug, taking into account the importance of the drug to the mother.

7. **Hematologic Changes**—Mild hemoglobin, hematocrit and white blood cell decreases have been observed in occasional patients following initiation of Lopid therapy. However, these levels stabilize during long-term administration. Rarely, severe anemia, leukopenia, thrombocytopenia, and bone marrow hypoplasia have been reported. Therefore, periodic blood counts are recommended during the first 12 months of Lopid administration.

8. **Liver Function**—Abnormal liver function tests have been observed occasionally during Lopid administration, including elevations of AST (SGOT), ALT (SGPT), LDH, bilirubin, and alkaline phosphatase. These are usually reversible when Lopid is discontinued. Therefore periodic liver function studies are recommended and Lopid therapy should be terminated if abnormalities persist.

9. **Kidney Function**—There have been reports of worsening renal insufficiency upon the addition of Lopid therapy in individuals with baseline plasma creatinine > 2.0 mg/dL. In such patients, the use of alternative therapy should be considered against the risks and benefits of a lower dose of Lopid.

10. **Use in Children**—Safety and efficacy in children have not been established.

ADVERSE REACTIONS

In the double-blind controlled phase of the primary prevention component of the Helsinki Heart Study, 2046 patients received Lopid for up to 5 years. In that study, the following adverse reactions were statistically more frequent in subjects in the Lopid group:

	LOPID (N = 2046)	PLACEBO (N = 2035)
	Frequency in percent of subjects	
Gastrointestinal reactions	34.2	23.8
Dyspepsia	19.6	11.9
Abdominal pain	9.8	5.6
Acute appendicitis (histologically confirmed in most cases where data were available)	1.2	0.6
Atrial fibrillation	0.7	0.1

Adverse events reported by more than 1% of subjects, but without a significant difference between groups:

Diarrhea	7.2	6.5
Fatigue	3.8	3.5
Nausea/Vomiting	2.5	2.1
Eczema	1.9	1.2
Rash	1.7	1.3
Vertigo	1.5	1.3
Constipation	1.4	1.3
Headache	1.2	1.1

Gallbladder surgery was performed in 0.9% of Lopid and 0.5% of placebo subjects in the primary prevention component, a 64% excess, which is not statistically different from the excess of gallbladder surgery observed in the clofibrate compared to the placebo group of the WHO study. Gallbladder surgery was also performed more frequently in the Lopid group compared to placebo (1.9% vs 0.3%, p = 0.07) in the secondary prevention component. A statistically significant increase in appendectomy in the gemfibrozil group was seen also in the secondary prevention component (6 on gemfibrozil vs 0 on placebo, p = 0.014).

Nervous system and special senses adverse reactions were more common in the Lopid group. These included hypesthesia, paresthesias, and taste perversion. Other adverse reactions that were more common among Lopid treatment group subjects but where a causal relationship was not established include cataracts, peripheral vascular disease, and intracerebral hemorrhage.

From other studies it seems probable that Lopid is causally related to the occurrence of MUSCULOSKELETAL SYMPTOMS (see WARNINGS), and to ABNORMAL LIVER FUNCTION TESTS and HEMATOLOGIC CHANGES (see PRECAUTIONS).

Reports of viral and bacterial infections (common cold, cough, urinary tract infections) were more common in gemfibrozil treated patients in other controlled clinical trials of 805 patients. Additional adverse reactions that have been reported for gemfibrozil are listed below by system. These are categorized according to whether a causal relationship to treatment with Lopid is probable or not established: [See table at left.]

DOSAGE AND ADMINISTRATION

The recommended dose for adults is 1200 mg administered in two divided doses 30 minutes before the morning and evening meal.

OVERDOSAGE

There have been reported cases of overdosage with Lopid. In one case a 7 year old child recovered after ingesting up to 9

	CAUSAL RELATIONSHIP PROBABLE	CAUSAL RELATIONSHIP NOT ESTABLISHED
General:		weight loss
Cardiac:		extrasystoles
Gastrointestinal:	cholestatic jaundice	pancreatitis
		hepatoma
		colitis
Central Nervous System:	dizziness	confusion
	somnolence	convulsions
	paresthesia	syncope
	peripheral neuritis	
	decreased libido	
	depression	
	headache	
Eye:	blurred vision	retinal edema
Genitourinary:	impotence	decreased male fertility
		renal dysfunction
Musculoskeletal:	myopathy	
	myasthenia	
	myalgia	
	painful extremities	
	arthralgia	
	synovitis	
	rhabdomyolysis (see WARNINGS and Drug Interactions under PRECAUTIONS)	
Clinical Laboratory:	increased creatine phosphokinase	positive antinuclear antibody
	increased bilirubin	
	increased liver transaminases (AST [SGOT], ALT [SGPT])	
	increased alkaline phosphatase	
Hematopoietic:	anemia	thrombocytopenia
	leukopenia	
	bone marrow hypoplasia	
	eosinophilia	
Immunologic:	angioedema	anaphylaxis
	laryngeal edema	Lupus-like syndrome
	urticaria	vasculitis
Integumentary:	exfoliative dermatitis	alopecia
	rash	
	dermatitis	
	pruritus	

grams of Lopid. Symptomatic supportive measures should be taken should an overdose occur.

HOW SUPPLIED

Lopid (Tablet 737), white, elliptical, film-coated, scored tablets, each containing 600 mg gemfibrozil, are available as follows:

N 0071-0737-20: Bottles of 60
N 0071-0737-30: Bottles of 500
N 0071-0737-40: Unit dose packages of 100 (10 strips of 10 tablets each)

Parcode No. 737
Storage: Store below 30°C (86°F).

REFERENCES

1. Frick MH, Elo O, Haapa K, et al: Helsinki Heart Study: Primary prevention trial with gemfibrozil in middle-aged men with dyslipidemia. *N Engl J Med* 1987; 317:1237-1245.
2. Manninen V, Elo O, Frick MH, et al: Lipid alterations and decline in the incidence of coronary heart disease in the Helsinki Heart Study. *JAMA* 1988; 260:641-651.
3. Frick MH, Heinonen OP, et al: Efficacy of Gemfibrozil in Dyslipidemic Subjects with Suspected Heart Disease. An Ancillary Study in the Helsinki Heart Study Frame Population. *Annals of Medicine* 1993; 25:41-45.
4. Nikkila EA: Familial lipoprotein lipase deficiency and related disorders of chylomicron metabolism. In Stanbury J.B. et al. (eds.): *The Metabolic Basis of Inherited Disease*, 5th ed., McGraw-Hill, 1983, Chap. 30, pp. 622-642.
5. Report of the National Cholesterol Education Program Expert Panel on Detection, Evaluation, and Treatment of High Blood Cholesterol. *Arch Int Med* 1988;148:36-69.

Caution—Federal law prohibits dispensing without prescription.

Revised June 1994   0737G019
Shown in Product Identification Guide, page 327

NARDIL®   ℞
(Phenelzine Sulfate Tablets, USP)

DESCRIPTION

Nardil® (phenelzine sulfate) belongs to the class of drugs known as monoamine oxidase (MAO) inhibitors. Chemically, it is phenethylhydrazine sulfate, a hydrazine derivative.
Each Nardil tablet for oral administration contains phenelzine sulfate equivalent to 15 mg of phenelzine base. Also contains: acacia, NF; calcium carbonate; carnauba wax, NF; corn-starch, NF; FD and C yellow No. 6; gelatin, NF; kaolin, USP; magnesium stearate, NF; mannitol, USP; pharmaceutical glaze, NF; povidone, USP; sucrose, NF; talc, USP; white wax, NF; white wheat flour.

CLINICAL PHARMACOLOGY

Monoamine oxidase is a complex enzyme system, widely distributed throughout the body. Drugs that inhibit monoamine oxidase in the laboratory are associated with a number of clinical effects. Thus, it is unknown whether MAO inhibition per se, other pharmacologic actions, or an interaction of both is responsible for the clinical effects observed. Therefore, the physician should become familiar with all the effects produced by drugs of this class.

INDICATIONS AND USAGE

Nardil has been found to be effective in depressed patients clinically characterized as "atypical," "nonendogenous," or "neurotic." These patients often have mixed anxiety and depression and phobic or hypochondriacal features. There is less conclusive evidence of its usefulness with severely depressed patients with endogenous features.
Nardil should rarely be the first antidepressant drug used. Rather, it is more suitable for use with patients who have failed to respond to the drugs more commonly used for these conditions.

CONTRAINDICATIONS

Nardil is contraindicated in patients with known sensitivity to the drug, pheochromocytoma, congestive heart failure, a history of liver disease, or abnormal liver function tests.
The potentiation of sympathomimetic substances and related compounds by MAO inhibitors may result in hypertensive crises (see WARNINGS). Therefore, patients being treated with Nardil should not take sympathomimetic drugs (including amphetamines, cocaine, methylphenidate, dopamine, epinephrine and norepinephrine) or related compounds (including methyldopa, L-dopa, L-tryptophan, L-tyrosine, and phenylalanine). Hypertensive crises during Nardil therapy may also be caused by the ingestion of foods with a high concentration of tyramine or dopamine. Therefore, patients being treated with Nardil should avoid high protein food that has undergone protein breakdown by aging, fermentation, pickling, smoking, or bacterial contamination; patients should also avoid cheeses (especially aged varieties), pickled herring, beer, wine, liver, yeast extract (including brewer's yeast in large quantities), dry sausage (including Genoa salami, hard salami, pepperoni, and Lebanon bologna), pods of broad beans (fava beans), and yogurt. Excessive

amounts of caffeine and chocolate may also cause hypertensive reactions.
Nardil should not be used in combination with dextromethorphan or with CNS depressants such as alcohol and certain narcotics. Excitation, seizures, delirium, hyperpyrexia, circulatory collapse, coma, and death have been reported in patients receiving MAOI therapy who have been given a single dose of meperidine. Nardil should not be administered together with or in rapid succession to other MAO inhibitors because HYPERTENSIVE CRISES and convulsive seizures, fever, marked sweating, excitation, delirium, tremor, coma, and circulatory collapse may occur.

List of MAO Inhibitors

Generic Name	Trademark
pargyline hydrochloride	Eutonyl® (Abbot Laboratories)
pargyline hydrochloride and methylclothiazide	Eutron® (Abbot Laboratories)
furazolidone	Furoxone® (Roberts Pharmaceutical Corp)
isocarboxazid	Marplan® (Roche Laboratories)
procarbazine	Mutalane® (Roche Laboratories)
tranylcypromine	Parnate® (SmithKline Beecham Pharmaceuticals)

Nardil should also not be used in combination with buspirone HCl, since several cases of elevated blood pressure have been reported in patients taking MAO inhibitors who were then given buspirone HCl. At least 10 days should elapse between the discontinuation of Nardil and the institution of another antidepressant or buspirone HCl, or the discontinuation of another MAO inhibitor and the institution of Nardil.
There have been reports of serious reactions (including hyperthermia, rigidity, myoclonic movements and death) when fluoxetine has been combined with an MAO inhibitor. Therefore, Nardil should not be used in combination with fluoxetine. Allow at least five weeks between discontinuation of fluoxetine and initiation of Nardil and at least 10 days between discontinuation of Nardil and initiation of fluoxetine. The combination of MAO inhibitors and tryptophan has been reported to cause behavioral and neurologic syndromes including disorientation, confusion, amnesia, delirium, agitation, hypomanic signs, ataxia, myoclonus, hyperreflexia, shivering, ocular oscillations, and Babinski signs.
The concurrent administration of an MAO inhibitor and bupropion hydrochloride (Wellbutrin®) is contraindicated. At least 14 days should elapse between discontinuation of an MAO inhibitor and initiation of treatment with bupropion hydrochloride.
Patients taking Nardil should not undergo elective surgery requiring general anesthesia. Also, they should not be given cocaine or local anesthesia containing sympathomimetic vasoconstrictors. The possible combined hypotensive effects of Nardil and spinal anesthesia should be kept in mind. Nardil should be discontinued at least 10 days prior to elective surgery.
MAO inhibitors, including Nardil, are contraindicated in patients receiving guanethidine.

WARNINGS

The most serious reactions to Nardil involve changes in blood pressure.
Hypertensive Crises: The most important reaction associated with Nardil administration is the occurrence of hypertensive crises, which have sometimes been fatal.
These crises are characterized by some or all of the following symptoms: occipital headache which may radiate frontally, palpitation, neck stiffness or soreness, nausea, vomiting, sweating (sometimes with fever and sometimes with cold, clammy skin), dilated pupils, and photophobia. Either tachycardia or bradycardia may be present and can be associated with constricting chest pain.
NOTE: Intracranial bleeding has been reported in association with the increase in blood pressure.
Blood pressure should be observed frequently to detect evidence of any pressor response in all patients receiving Nardil. Therapy should be discontinued immediately upon the occurrence of palpitation or frequent headaches during therapy.
Recommended treatment in hypertensive crisis: If a hypertensive crisis occurs, Nardil should be discontinued immediately and therapy to lower blood pressure should be instituted immediately. On the basis of present evidence, phentolamine is recommended. (The dosage reported for phentolamine is 5 mg intravenously.) Care should be taken to administer this drug slowly in order to avoid producing an excessive hypotensive effect. Fever should be managed by means of external cooling.
Warning to the Patient: All patients should be warned that the following foods, beverages, and medications must be avoided while taking Nardil, and for two weeks after discontinuing use.

Foods and Beverages To Avoid
Meat and Fish
Pickled herring
Liver
Dry sausage (including Genoa salami, hard salami, pepperoni, and Lebanon bologna)
Vegetables
Broad bean pods (fava bean pods)
Sauerkraut
Dairy Products
Cheese (cottage cheese and cream cheese are allowed)
Yogurt
Beverages
Beer and wine
Alcohol-free and reduced-alcohol beer and wine products
Miscellaneous
Yeast extract (including brewer's yeast in large quantities)
Meat extract
Excessive amounts of chocolate and caffeine
Also, any spoiled or improperly refrigerated, handled, or stored protein-rich foods such as meats, fish, and dairy products, including foods that may have undergone protein changes by aging, pickling, fermentation, or smoking to improve flavor should be avoided.
OTC Medications To Avoid
Cold and cough preparations (including those containing dextromethorphan)
Nasal decongestants (tablets, drops, or spray)
Hay-fever medications
Sinus medications
Asthma inhalant medications
Antiappetite medicines
Weight-reducing preparations
"Pep" pills
L-tryptophan containing preparations
Also, certain prescription drugs should be avoided. Therefore, patients under the care of another physician or dentist should inform him/her they are taking Nardil.
Patients should be warned that the use of the above foods, beverages, or medications may cause a reaction characterized by headache and other serious symptoms due to a rise in blood pressure, with the exception of dextromethorphan which may cause reactions similar to those seen with meperidine. Also, there has been a report of an interaction between Nardil and dextromethorphan (ingested as a lozenge) causing drowsiness and bizarre behavior.
Patients should be instructed to report promptly the occurrence of headache or other unusual symptoms.
Concomitant Use with Dibenzazepine Derivative Drugs
If the decision is made to administer Nardil concurrently with other antidepressant drugs, or within less than 10 days after discontinuation of antidepressant therapy, the patient should be cautioned by the physician regarding the possibility of adverse drug interaction.

List of Dibenzazepine Derivative Drugs

Generic Name	Trademark
nortriptyline hydrochloride	Aventyl® (Eli Lilly & Co)
amitriptyline hydrochloride	Elavil® (Stuart Pharmaceuticals)
amitriptyline hydrochloride	Endep® (Roche)
perphenazine and amitriptyline hydrochloride	Etrafon® (Schering Corporation)
perphenazine and amitriptyline hydrochloride	Triavil® (Merck Sharp & Dohme)
clomipramine hydrochloride	Anafranil® (CIBA-Geigy)
desipramine hydrochloride	Norpramin® (Marion Merrill-Dow)
desipramine hydrochloride	Pertofrane® (USV)
imipramine hydrochloride	Tofranil® (Geigy)
doxepin	Adapin® (Pennwalt)
doxepin	Sinequan® (Pfizer)
carbamazepine	Tegretol® (Geigy)
cyclobenzaprine HCl	Flexeril® (Merck Sharp & Dohme)
amoxapine	Asendin® (Lederle)

Continued on next page

This product information was prepared in August 1996. On these and other Parke-Davis Products, information may be obtained by addressing PARKE-DAVIS, Division of Warner-Lambert Company, Morris Plains, New Jersey 07950.

Parke-Davis—Cont.

maprotiline HCl	Ludiomil® (CIBA)
trimipramine maleate	Surmontil® (Wyeth-Ayerst)
protriptyline HCl	Vivactil® (Merck Sharp & Dohme)

Nardil should be used with caution in combination with antihypertensive drugs, including thiazide diuretics and β-blockers, since exaggerated hypotensive effects may result.

Use in Pregnancy: The safe use of Nardil during pregnancy or lactation has not been established. The potential benefit of this drug, if used during pregnancy, lactation, or in women of childbearing age, should be weighed against the possible hazard to the mother or fetus.

Doses of Nardil in pregnant mice well exceeding the maximum recommended human dose have caused a significant decrease in the number of viable offspring per mouse. In addition, the growth of young dogs and rats has been retarded by doses exceeding the maximum human dose.

Use in Children: Nardil is not recommended for patients under 16 years of age, since there are no controlled studies of safety in this age group. Nardil, as with other hydrazine derivatives, has been reported to induce pulmonary and vascular tumors in an uncontrolled lifetime study in mice.

PRECAUTIONS

In depressed patients, the possibility of suicide should always be considered and adequate precautions taken. It is recommended that careful observations of patients undergoing Nardil treatment be maintained until control of depression is achieved. If necessary, additional measures (ECT, hospitalization, etc) should be instituted.

All patients undergoing treatment with Nardil should be closely followed for symptoms of postural hypotension. Hypotensive side effects have occurred in hypertensive as well as normal and hypotensive patients. Blood pressure usually returns to pretreatment levels rapidly when the drug is discontinued or the dosage is reduced.

Because the effect of Nardil on the convulsive threshold may be variable, adequate precautions should be taken when treating epileptic patients.

Of the more severe side effects that have been reported with any consistency, hypomania has been the most common. This reaction has been largely limited to patients in whom disorders characterized by hyperkinetic symptoms coexist with, but are obscured by, depressive affect; hypomania usually appeared as depression improved. If agitation is present, it may be increased with Nardil. Hypomania and agitation have also been reported at higher than recommended doses or following long-term therapy.

Nardil may cause excessive stimulation in schizophrenic patients; in manic-depressive states it may result in a swing from a depressive to a manic phase.

MAO inhibitors, including Nardil, potentiate hexobarbital hypnosis in animals. Therefore, barbiturates should be given at a reduced dose with Nardil.

MAO inhibitors inhibit the destruction of serotonin and norepinephrine, which are believed to be released from tissue stores by rauwolfia alkaloids. Accordingly, caution should be exercised when rauwolfia is used concomitantly with an MAO inhibitor, including Nardil.

There is conflicting evidence as to whether or not MAO inhibitors affect glucose metabolism or potentiate hypoglycemic agents. This should be kept in mind if Nardil is administered to diabetics.

ADVERSE REACTIONS

Nardil is a potent inhibitor of monoamine oxidase. Because this enzyme is widely distributed throughout the body, diverse pharmacologic effects can be expected to occur. When they occur, such effects tend to be mild or moderate in severity (see below), often subside as treatment continues, and can be minimized by adjusting dosage; rarely is it necessary to institute counteracting measures or to discontinue Nardil.

Common side effects include:

Nervous System—Dizziness, headache, drowsiness, sleep disturbances (including insomnia and hypersomnia), fatigue, weakness, tremors, twitching, myoclonic movements, hyperreflexia.

Gastrointestinal—Constipation, dry mouth, gastrointestinal disturbances, elevated serum transaminases (without accompanying signs and symptoms).

Metabolic—Weight gain.

Cardiovascular—Postural hypotension, edema.

Genitourinary—Sexual disturbances, ie, anorgasmia and ejaculatory disturbances.

Less common mild to moderate side effects (some of which have been reported in a single patient or by a single physician) include:

Nervous System—Jitteriness, palilalia, euphoria, nystagmus, paresthesias.

Genitourinary—Urinary retention.

Metabolic—Hypernatremia.

Dermatologic—Skin rash, sweating.

Special Senses—Blurred vision, glaucoma.

Although reported less frequently, and sometimes only once, additional severe side effects include:

Nervous System—Ataxia, shock-like coma, toxic delirium, manic reaction, convulsions, acute anxiety reaction, precipitation of schizophrenia, transient respiratory and cardiovascular depression following ECT.

Gastrointestinal—To date, fatal progressive necrotizing hepatocellular damage has been reported in a very few patients. Reversible jaundice.

Hematologic—Leukopenia.

Immunologic—Lupus-like syndrome.

Metabolic—Hypermetabolic syndrome (which may include, but is not limited to, hyperpyrexia, tachycardia, tachypnea, muscular rigidity, elevated CK levels, metabolic acidosis, hypoxia, coma and may resemble an overdose).

Respiratory—Edema of the glottis.

General—Fever associated with increased muscle tone.

Withdrawal may be associated with nausea, vomiting, and malaise.

An uncommon withdrawal syndrome following abrupt withdrawal of Nardil has been infrequently reported. Signs and symptoms of this syndrome generally commence 24 to 72 hours after drug discontinuation and may range from vivid nightmares with agitation to frank psychosis and convulsions. This syndrome generally responds to reinstitution of low-dose Nardil therapy followed by cautious downward titration and discontinuation.

DOSAGE AND ADMINISTRATION

Initial dose: The usual starting dose of Nardil is one tablet (15 mg) three times a day.

Early phase treatment: Dosage should be increased to at least 60 mg per day at a fairly rapid pace consistent with patient tolerance. It may be necessary to increase dosage up to 90 mg per day to obtain sufficient MAO inhibition. Many patients do not show a clinical response until treatment at 60 mg has been continued for at least 4 weeks.

Maintenance dose: After maximum benefit from Nardil is achieved, dosage should be reduced slowly over several weeks. Maintenance dose may be as low as one tablet, 15 mg, a day or every other day, and should be continued for as long as is required.

OVERDOSAGE

Note—For management of *hypertensive crises* see WARNINGS section.

Accidental or intentional overdosage may be more common in patients who are depressed. It should be remembered that multiple drugs and/or alcohol may have been ingested.

Depending on the amount of overdosage with Nardil, a varying and mixed clinical picture may develop, involving signs and symptoms of central nervous system and cardiovascular stimulation and/or depression. Signs and symptoms may be absent or minimal during the initial 12-hour period following ingestion and may develop slowly thereafter, reaching a maximum in 24–48 hours. Death has been reported following overdosage. Therefore, immediate hospitalization, with continuous patient observation and monitoring throughout this period, is essential.

Signs and symptoms of overdosage may include, alone or in combination, any of the following: drowsiness, dizziness, faintness, irritability, hyperactivity, agitation, severe headache, hallucinations, trismus, opisthotonus, rigidity, convulsions, and coma; rapid and irregular pulse, hypertension, hypotension, and vascular collapse; precordial pain, respiratory depression and failure, hyperpyrexia, diaphoresis, and cool, clammy skin.

Intensive symptomatic and supportive treatment may be required. Induction of emesis or gastric lavage with instillation of charcoal slurry may be helpful in early poisoning, provided the airway has been protected against aspiration. Signs and symptoms of central nervous system stimulation, including convulsions, should be treated with diazepam, given slowly intravenously. Phenothiazine derivatives and central nervous system stimulants should be avoided. Hypotension and vascular collapse should be treated with intravenous fluids and, if necessary, blood pressure titration with an intravenous infusion of dilute pressor agent. It should be noted that adrenergic agents may produce a markedly increased pressor response.

Respiration should be supported by appropriate measures, including management of the airway, use of supplemental oxygen, and mechanical ventilatory assistance, as required.

Body temperature should be monitored closely. Intensive management of hyperpyrexia may be required. Maintenance of fluid and electrolyte balance is essential.

There are no data on the lethal dose in man. The pathophysiologic effects of massive overdosage may persist for several days, since the drug acts by inhibiting physiologic enzyme systems. With symptomatic and supportive measures, recovery from *mild* overdosage may be expected within 3 to 4 days.

Hemodialysis, peritoneal dialysis, and charcoal hemoperfusion may be of value in massive overdosage, but sufficient data are not available to recommend their routine use in these cases.

Toxic blood levels of phenelzine have not been established, and assay methods are not practical for clinical or toxicological use.

HOW SUPPLIED

Each Nardil tablet is orange, biconvex, glossy sugar-coated, and imprinted with "P-D 270" in brown ink and contains phenelzine sulfate equivalent to 15 mg of phenelzine base.

N 0071-0270-24 Bottles of 100

Store between 15°-30° C (59°-86°F).

Caution: Federal law prohibits dispensing without prescription.

US Patent 3,314,855

Revised July 1995 0270G054

Shown in Product Identification Guide, page 327

NEURONTIN® ℞
(Gabapentin Capsules)

DESCRIPTION

Neurontin® (gabapentin capsules) is supplied as imprinted hard shell capsules containing 100 mg, 300 mg, and 400 mg of gabapentin. The inactive ingredients are lactose, corn starch, and talc. The 100-mg capsule shell contains gelatin and titanium dioxide. The 300-mg capsule shell contains gelatin, titanium dioxide, and yellow iron oxide. The 400-mg capsule shell contains gelatin, red iron oxide, titanium dioxide, and yellow iron oxide. The imprinting ink contains FD&C Blue No. 2 and titanium dioxide.

Gabapentin is described as 1-(aminomethyl)cyclohexaneacetic acid with an empirical formula of $C_9H_{17}NO_2$ and a molecular weight of 171.24. The molecular structure of gabapentin is:

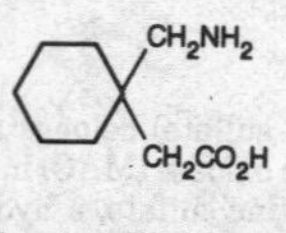

Gabapentin is a white to off-white crystalline solid. It is freely soluble in water and both basic and acidic aqueous solutions.

CLINICAL PHARMACOLOGY

Mechanism of Action

The mechanism by which gabapentin exerts its anticonvulsant action is unknown, but in animal test systems designed to detect anticonvulsant activity, gabapentin prevents seizures as do other marketed anticonvulsants. Gabapentin exhibits antiseizure activity in mice and rats in both the maximal electroshock and pentylenetetrazole seizure models and other preclinical models (e.g., strains with genetic epilepsy, etc.) The relevance of these models to human epilepsy is not known.

Gabapentin is structurally related to the neurotransmitter GABA (gamma-aminobutyric acid) but it does not interact with GABA receptors, it is not converted metabolically into GABA or a GABA agonist, and it is not an inhibitor of GABA uptake or degradation. Gabapentin was tested in radioligand binding assays at concentrations up to 100 μM and did not exhibit affinity for a number of other common receptor sites, including benzodiazepine, glutamate, N-methyl-D-aspartate (NMDA), quisqualate, kainate, stychnine-insensitive or strychnine-sensitive glycine, alpha 1, alpha 2, or beta adrenergic, adenosine A1 or A2, cholinergic, muscarinic or nicotinic, dopamine D1 or D2, histamine H1, serotonin S1 or S2, opiate mu, delta or kappa, voltage-sensitive calcium channel sites labeled with nitrendipine or diltiazem, or at voltage-sensitive sodium channel sites with batrachotoxinin A 20-alpha-benzoate.

Several test systems ordinarily used to assess activity at the NMDA receptor have been examined. Results are contradictory. Accordingly, no general statement about the effects, if any, of gabapentin at the NMDA receptor can be made.

In vitro studies with radiolabeled gabapentin have revealed a gabapentin binding site in areas of rat brain including neocortex and hippocampus. The identity and function of this binding site remain to be elucidated.

Pharmacokinetics and Drug Metabolism

All pharmacological actions following gabapentin administration are due to the activity of the parent compound; gabapentin is not appreciably metabolized in humans.

Oral Bioavailability: Gabapentin bioavailability is not dose proportional; i.e., as dose is increased, bioavailability decreases. A 400-mg dose, for example, is about 25% less bioavailable than a 100-mg dose. Over the recommended dose range of 300 to 600 mg T.I.D., however, the differences in bioavailability are not large, and bioavailability is about 60 percent. Food has no effect on the rate and extent of absorption of gabapentin.

Distribution: Gabapentin circulates largely unbound (<3%) to plasma protein. The apparent volume of distribution of gabapentin after 150 mg intravenous administration is 58±6 L (Mean ±SD). In patients with epilepsy, steady-state predose (Cmin) concentrations of gabapentin in cerebrospinal fluid were approximately 20% of the corresponding plasma concentrations.

Elimination: Gabapentin is eliminated from the systemic circulation by renal excretion as unchanged drug. Gabapentin is not appreciably metabolized in humans.

Gabapentin elimination half-life is 5 to 7 hours and is unaltered by dose or following multiple dosing. Gabapentin elimination rate constant, plasma clearance, and renal clearance are directly proportional to creatinine clearance (see Special Populations: Patients With Renal Insufficiency, below). In elderly patients, and in patients with impaired renal function, gabapentin plasma clearance is reduced. Gabapentin can be removed from plasma by hemodialysis.

Dosage adjustment in patients with compromised renal function or undergoing hemodialysis is recommended (see DOSAGE AND ADMINISTRATION, Table 2).

Special Populations: *Patients With Renal Insufficiency:* Subjects (N=60) with renal insufficiency (mean creatinine clearance ranging from 13–114 mL/min) were administered single 400-mg oral doses of gabapentin. The mean gabapentin half-life ranged from about 6.5 hours (patients with creatinine clearance >60 mL/min) to 52 hours (creatinine clearance <30 mL/min) and gabapentin renal clearance from about 90 mL/min (>60 mL/min group) to about 10 mL/min (<30 mL/min). Mean plasma clearance (CL/F) decreased from approximately 190 mL/min to 20 mL/min.

Dosage adjustment in patients with compromised renal function is necessary (see DOSAGE AND ADMINISTRATION).

Hemodialysis: In a study in anuric subjects (N=11), the apparent elimination half-life of gabapentin on nondialysis days was about 132 hours; dialysis three times a week (4 hours duration) lowered the apparent half-life of gabapentin by about 60%, from 132 hours to 51 hours. Hemodialysis thus has a significant effect on gabapentin elimination in anuric subjects.

Dosage adjustment in patients undergoing hemodialysis is necessary (see DOSAGE AND ADMINISTRATION).

Hepatic Disease: Because gabapentin is not metabolized, no study was performed in patients with hepatic impairment.

Age: The effect of age was studied in subjects 20–80 years of age. Apparent oral clearance (CL/F) of gabapentin decreased as age increased, from about 225 mL/min in those under 30 years of age to about 125 mL/min in those over 70 years of age. Renal clearance (CLr) and CLr adjusted for body surface area also declined with age; however, the decline in the renal clearance of gabapentin with age can largely be explained by the decline in renal function. Reduction of gabapentin dose may be required in patients who have age related compromised renal function. (See PRECAUTIONS, Geriatric Use, and DOSAGE AND ADMINISTRATION.)

Pediatric: No pharmacokinetic data are available in children below the age of 18 years.

Gender: Although no formal study has been conducted to compare the pharmacokinetics of gabapentin in men and women, it appears that the pharmacokinetic parameters for males and females are similar and there are no significant gender differences.

Race: Pharmacokinetic differences due to race have not been studied. Because gabapentin is primarily renally excreted and there are no important racial differences in creatinine clearance, pharmacokinetic differences due to race are not expected.

Clinical Studies

The effectiveness of Neurontin® as adjunctive therapy (added to other antiepileptic drugs) was established in three multicenter placebo-controlled, double-blind, parallel-group clinical trials in 705 adults with refractory partial seizures. The patients enrolled had a history of at least 4 partial seizures per month in spite of receiving one or more antiepileptic drugs at therapeutic levels and were observed on their established antiepileptic drug regimen during a 12-week baseline period. In patients continuing to have at least 2 (or 4 in some studies) seizures per month, Neurontin® or placebo was then added on to the existing therapy during a 12-week treatment period. Effectiveness was assessed primarily on the basis of the percent of patients with a 50% or greater reduction in seizure frequency from baseline to treatment (the "responder rate") and a derived measure called response ratio, a measure of change defined as (T − B)/(T + B), where B is the patient's baseline seizure frequency and T is the patient's seizure frequency during treatment. Response ratio is distributed within the range −1 to +1. A zero value indicates no change while complete elimination of seizures would give a value of −1; increased seizure rates would give positive values. A response ratio of −0.33 corresponds to a 50% reduction in seizure frequency. The results given below are for all partial seizures in the intent-to-treat (all patients who received any doses of treatment) population in each study, unless otherwise indicated.

One study compared Neurontin® 1200 mg/day T.I.D. with placebo. Responder rate was 23% (14/61) in the Neurontin® group and 9% (6/66) in the placebo group; the difference between groups was statistically significant. Response ratio was also better in the Neurontin® group (−0.199) than in the placebo group (−0.044), a difference that also achieved statistical significance.

A second study compared primarily 1200 mg/day T.I.D. Neurontin® (N=101) with placebo (N=98). Additional smaller Neurontin® dosage groups (600 mg/day, N=53; 1800 mg/day, N=54) were also studied for information regarding dose response. Responder rate was higher in the Neurontin® 1200 mg/day group (16%) than in the placebo group (8%), but the difference was not statistically significant. The responder rate at 600 mg (17%) was also not significantly higher than in the placebo, but the responder rate in the 1800 mg group (26%) was statistically significantly superior to the placebo rate. Response ratio was better in the Neurontin® 1200 mg/day group (−0.103) than in the placebo group (−0.022); but this difference was also not statistically significant (p = 0.224). A better response was seen in the Neurontin® 600 mg/day group (−0.105) and 1800 mg/day group (−0.222) than in the 1200 mg/day group, with the 1800 mg/day group achieving statistical significance compared to the placebo group.

A third study compared Neurontin® 900 mg/day T.I.D. (N = 111) and placebo (N = 109). An additional Neurontin® 1200 mg/day dosage group (N = 52) provided dose-response data. A statistically significant difference in responder rate was seen in the Neurontin® 900 mg/day group (22%) compared to that in the placebo group (10%). Response ratio was also statistically significantly superior in the Neurontin® 900 mg/day group (− 0.119) compared to that in the placebo group (= 0.027), as was response ratio in 1200 mg/day Neurontin® (−0.184) compared to placebo.

Analyses were also performed in each study to examine the effect of Neurontin® on preventing secondarily generalized tonic-clonic seizures. Patients who experienced a secondarily generalized tonic-clonic seizure in either the baseline or in the treatment period in all three placebo-controlled studies were included in these analyses. There were several response ratio comparisons that showed a statistically significant advantage for Neurontin® compared to placebo and favorable trends for almost all comparisons.

Analysis of responder rate using combined data from all three studies and all doses (N=162, Neurontin® ; N=89, placebo) also showed a significant advantage for Neurontin® over placebo in reducing the frequency of secondarily generalized tonic-clonic seizures.

In two of the three controlled studies, more than one dose of Neurontin® was used. Within each study the results did not show a consistently increased response to dose. However, looking across studies, a trend toward increasing efficacy with increasing dose is evident (see Figure 1).

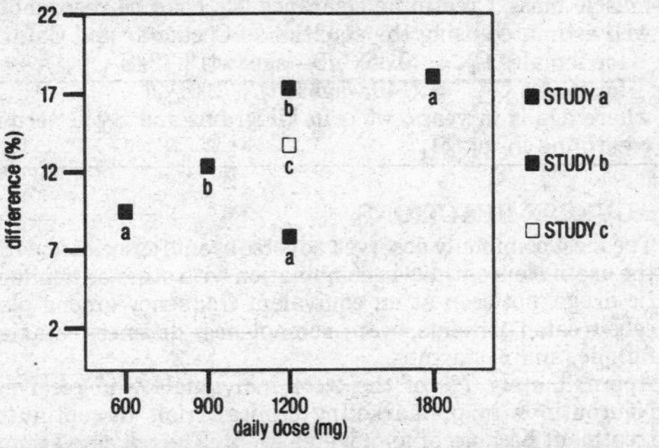

FIGURE 1. Responder Rate in Patients Receiving Neurontin® Expressed as a Difference from Placebo by Dose and Study

In the figure, treatment effect magnitude, measured on the Y axis in terms of the difference in the proportion of gabapentin and placebo assigned patients attaining a 50% or greater reduction in seizure frequency from baseline, is plotted against the daily dose of gabapentin administered (X axis).

Although no formal analysis by gender has been performed, estimates of response (Response Ratio) derived from clinical trials (398 men, 307 women) indicate no important gender differences exist. There was no consistent pattern indicating that age had any effect on the response to Neurontin® . There were insufficient numbers of patients of races other than Caucasian of permit a comparison of efficacy among racial groups.

INDICATIONS AND USAGE

Neurontin® (gabapentin) is indicated as adjunctive therapy in the treatment of partial seizures with and without secondary generalization in adults with epilepsy.

CONTRAINDICATIONS

Neurontin® is contraindicated in patients who have demonstrated hypersensitivity to the drug or its ingredients.

WARNINGS

Withdrawal Precipitated Seizure, Status Epilepticus

In the placebo-controlled studies, the incidence of status epilepticus in patients receiving Neurontin® was 0.6% (3 of 543) versus 0.5% in patients receiving placebo (2 of 378).

In the placebo-controlled studies, the incidence of status epilepticus in patients receiving Neurontin® was 0.6% (5 of 543) versus 0.5% in patients receiving placebo (2 of 378). Among the 2074 patients treated with Neurontin® across all studies (controlled and uncontrolled) 31 (1.5%) had status epilepticus. Of these, 14 patients had no prior history of status epilepticus either before treatment or while on other medications. Because adequate historical data are not available, it is impossible to say whether or not treatment with Neurontin® is associated with a higher or lower rate of status epilepticus than would be expected to occur in a similar population not treated with Neurontin®.

Tumorigenic Potential

In standard preclinical *in vivo* lifetime carcinogenicity studies, an unexpectedly high incidence of pancreatic acinar adenocarcinomas was indentified in male, but not female, rats. (See PRECAUTIONS: Carcinogenesis, Mutagenesis, Impairment of Fertility.) The clinical significance of this finding is unknown. Clinical experience during gabapentin's premarketing development provides no direct means to assess its potential for inducing tumors in humans.

In clinical studies comprising 2085 patient-years of exposure, new tumors were reported in 10 patients (2 breast, 3 brain, 2 lung, 1 adrenal, 1 non-Hodgkin's lymphoma, 1 endometrial carcinoma *in situ*), and preexisting tumors worsened in 11 patients (9 brain, 1 breast, 1 prostate) during or up to 2 years following discontinuation of Neurontin®. Without knowledge of the background incidence and recurrence in a similar population not treated with Neurontin®, it is impossible to know whether the incidence seen in this cohort is or is not affected by treatment.

Sudden and Unexplained Deaths

During the course of premarketing development of Neurontin®, 8 sudden and unexplained deaths were recorded among a cohort of 2203 patients treated (2103 patient-years of exposure).

Some of these could represent seizure-related deaths in which the seizure was not observed, e.g., at night. This represents an incidence of 0.0038 deaths per patient-year. Although this rate exceeds that expected in a healthy population matched for age and sex, it is within the range of estimates for the incidence of sudden unexplained deaths in patients with epilepsy not receiving Neurontin® (ranging from 0.0005 for the general population of epileptics, to 0.003 for a clinical trial population similar to that in the Neurontin® program, to 0.005 for patients with refractory epilepsy). Consequently, whether these figures are reassuring or raise further concern depends on comparability of the populations reported upon to the Neurontin® cohort and the accuracy of the estimates provided.

PRECAUTIONS

Information for Patients

Patients should be instructed to take Neurontin® only as prescribed.

Patients should be advised that Neurontin® may cause dizziness, somnolence and other symptoms and signs of CNS depression. Accordingly, they should be advised neither to drive a car nor to operate other complex machinery until they have gained sufficient experience on Neurontin® to gauge whether or not it affects their mental and/or motor performance adversely.

Laboratory Tests

Clinical trials data do not indicate that routine monitoring of clinical laboratory parameters is necessary for the safe use of Neurontin®. The value of monitoring Neurontin® blood concentrations has not been established. Neurontin® may be used in combination with other antiepileptic drugs without concern for alteration of the blood concentrations of gabapentin or of other antiepileptic drugs.

Drug Interactions

Gabapentin is not appreciably metabolized nor does it interfere with the metabolism of commonly coadministered antiepileptic drugs.

The drug interaction data described in this section were obtained from studies involving healthy adults and patients with epilepsy.

Phenytoin: In a single and multiple dose study of Neurontin® (400 mg T.I.D.) in epileptic patients (N=8) maintained on phenytoin monotherapy for at least 2 months, gabapentin had no effect on the steady-state trough plasma concentra-

Continued on next page

This product information was prepared in August 1996. On these and other Parke-Davis Products, information may be obtained by addressing PARKE-DAVIS, Division of Warner-Lambert Company, Morris Plains, New Jersey 07950.

Parke-Davis—Cont.

tions of phenytoin and phenytoin had no effect on gabapentin pharmacokinetics.

Carbamazepine: Steady-state trough plasma carbamazepine and carbamazepine 10, 11 epoxide concentrations were not affected by concomitant gabapentin (400 mg T.I.D.; N=12) administration. Likewise, gabapentin pharmacokinetics were unaltered by carbamazepine administration.

Valproic Acid: The mean steady-state trough serum valproic acid concentrations prior to and during concomitant gabapentin administration (400 mg T.I.D.; N=17) were not different and neither were gabapentin pharmacokinetics parameters affected by valproic acid.

Phenobarbital: Estimates of steady-state pharmacokinetic parameters for phenobarbital or gabapentin (300 mg T.I.D.; N=12) are identical whether the drugs are administered alone or together.

Cimetidine: In the presence of cimetidine at 300 mg Q.I.D. (N=12) the mean apparent oral clearance of gabapentin fell by 14% and creatinine clearance fell by 10%. Thus cimetidine appeared to alter the renal excretion of both gabapentin and creatinine, an endogenous marker of renal function. This small decrease in excretion of gabapentin by cimetidine is not expected to be of clinical importance. The effect of gabapentin on cimetidine was not evaluated.

Oral Contraceptive: Based on AUC and half-life, multiple-dose pharmacokinetic profiles of norethindrone and ethinyl estradiol following administration of tablets containing 2.5 mg of norethindrone acetate and 50 mcg of ethinyl estradiol were similar with and without coadministration of gabapentin (400 mg T.I.D.; N=13). The Cmax of norethindrone was 13% higher when it was coadministered with gabapentin; this interaction is not expected to be of clinical importance.

Antacid (Maalox®): Maalox reduced the bioavailability of gabapentin (N=16) by about 20%. This decrease in bioavailability was about 5% when gabapentin was administered 2 hours after Maalox. It is recommended that gabapentin be taken at least 2 hours following Maalox administration.

Effect of Probenecid: Probenecid is a blocker of renal tubular secretion. Gabapentin pharmacokinetic parameters without and with probenecid were comparable. This indicates that gabapentin does not undergo renal tubular secretion by the pathway that is blocked by probenecid.

Drug/Laboratory Tests Interactions

Because false positive readings were reported with the Ames N-Multistix SG® dipstick test for urinary protein when gabapentin was added to the other antiepileptic drugs, the more specific sulfosalicylic acid precipitation procedure is recommended to determine the presence of urine protein.

Carcinogenesis, Mutagenesis, Impairment of Fertility

Gabapentin was given in the diet to mice at 200, 600, and 2000 mg/kg/day and to rats at 250, 1000, and 2000 mg/kg/day for 2 years. A statistically significant increase in the incidence of pancreatic acinar cell adenomas and carcinomas was found in male rats receiving the high dose; the no-effect dose for the occurrence of carcinomas was 1000 mg/kg/day. Peak plasma concentrations of gabapentin in rats receiving the high dose of 2000 mg/kg were 10 times higher than plasma concentrations in humans receiving 3600 mg per day, and in rats receiving 1000 mg/kg/day peak plasma concentrations were 6.5 times higher than in humans receiving 3600 mg/day. The pancreatic acinar cell carcinomas did not affect survival, did not metastasize and were not locally invasive. Studies to attempt to define a mechanism by which this relatively rare tumor type is occurring are in progress. The relevance of this finding to carcinogenic risk in humans is unclear.

Gabapentin did not demonstrate mutagenic or genotoxic potential in three *in vitro* and two *in vivo* assays. It was negative in the Ames test and the *in vitro* HGPRT forward mutation assay in Chinese hamster lung cells; it did not produce significant increases in chromosomal aberrations in the *in vitro* Chinese hamster lung cell assay; it was negative in the *in vivo* chromosomal aberration assay and in the *in vivo* micronucleus test in Chinese hamster bone marrow.

No adverse effects on fertility or reproduction were observed in rats at doses up to 2000 mg/kg (approximately 5 times the maximum recommended human dose on an mg/m^2 basis).

Pregnancy

Pregnancy Category C: Gabapentin has beeen shown to be fetotoxic in rodents, causing delayed ossification of several bones in the skull, vertebrae, forelimbs, and hindlimbs. These effects occurred when pregnant mice received oral doses of 1000 or 3000 mg/kg/day during the period of organogeneis, or approximately 1 to 4 times the maximum dose of 3600 mg/day given to epileptic patients on a mg/m^2 basis. The no-effect level was 500 mg/kg/day or approximately ½ of the human dose on a mg/m^2 basis.

When rats were dosed prior to and during mating, and throughout gestation, pups from all dose groups (500, 1000 and 2000 mg/kg/day) were affected. These doses are equivalent to less than approximately 1 to 5 times the maximum human dose on a mg/m^2 basis. There was an increased incidence of hydroureter and/or hydronephrosis in rats in a study of fertility and general reproductive performance at 2000 mg/kg/day with no effect at 1000 mg/kg/day, in a teratology study at 1500 mg/kg/day with no effect at 300 mg/kg/day, and in a perinatal and postnatal study at all doses studied (500, 1000 and 2000 mg/kg/day). The doses at which the effects occurred are approximately 1 to 5 times the maximum human dose of 3600 mg/day on a mg/m^2 basis; the no-effect doses were approximately 3 times (Fertility and General Reproductive Performance study) and approximately equal to (Teratogenicity study) the maximum human dose on a mg/m^2 basis. Other than hydroureter and hydronephrosis, the etiologies of which are unclear, the incidence of malformations was not increased compared to controls in offspring of mice, rats, or rabbits given doses up to 50 times (mice), 30 times (rats), and 25 times (rabbits) the human daily dose on a mg/kg basis, or 4 times (mice), 5 times (rats), or 8 times (rabbits) the human daily dose on a mg/m^2 basis.

In a teratology study in rabbits, an increased incidence of postimplantation fetal loss occurred in dams exposed to 60, 300 and 1500 mg/kg/day, or less than approximately ¼ to 8 times the maximum human dose on a mg/m^2 basis. There are no adequate and well-controlled studies in pregnant women. Because animal reproduction studies are not always predictive of human response, this drug should be used during pregnancy only if the potential benefit justifies the potential risk to the fetus.

Use in Nursing Mothers

It is not known if gabapentin is excreted in human milk and the effect on the nursing infant is unknown. However, because many drugs are excreted in human milk, Neurontin® should be used in women who are nursing only if the benefits clearly outweigh the risks.

Pediatric Use

Safety and effectiveness in children below the age of 12 years have not been established.

Geriatric Use

No systematic studies in geriatric patients have been conducted. Adverse clinical events reported among 59 Neurontin® exposed patients over age 65 did not differ in kind from those reported for younger individuals. The small number of older individuals evaluated, however, limits the strength of any conclusions reached about the influence, if any, of age on the kind and incidence of adverse events or laboratory abnormality associated with the use of Neurontin®.

Because Neurontin® is eliminated primarily by renal excretion, the dose of Neurontin® should be adjusted as noted in DOSAGE AND ADMINISTRATION (Table 2) for elderly patients with compromised renal function. Creatinine clearance is difficult to measure in outpatients and serum creatinine may be reduced in the elderly because of decreased muscle mass. Creatinine clearance (C_{Cr}) can be reasonably well estimated using the equation of Cockcroft and Gault:

for females $C_{Cr} = (0.85)(140-\text{age})(\text{wt})/[(72)(S_{Cr})]$

for males $C_{Cr} = (140-\text{age})(\text{wt})/[(72)(S_{Cr})]$

where age is in years, wt is in kilograms and S_{Cr} is serum creatinine in mg/dL.

ADVERSE REACTIONS

The most commonly observed adverse events associated with the use of Neurontin® in combination with other antiepileptic drugs, not seen at an equivalent frequency among placebo-treated patients, were somnolence, dizziness, ataxia, fatique, and nystagmus.

Approximately 7% of the 2074 individuals who received Neurontin® in premarketing clinical trials discontinued treatment because of an adverse event. The adverse events most commonly associated with withdrawal were somnolence (1.2%), ataxia (0.8%), fatique (0.6%), nausea and/or vomiting (0.6%), and dizziness (0.6%).

Incidence in Controlled Clinical Trials

Table 1 lists treatment-emergent signs and symptoms that occurred in at least 1% of Neurontin®-treated patients with epilepsy participating in placebo-controlled trials and were numerically more common in the Neurontin® group. In these studies, either Neurontin® or placebo was added to the patient's current antiepileptic drug therapy. Adverse events were usually mild to moderate in intensity.

The prescriber should be aware that these figures, obtained when Neurontin® was added to concurrent antiepileptic drug therapy, cannot be used to predict the frequency of adverse events in the course of usual medical practice where patient characteristics and other factors may differ from those prevailing during clinical studies. Similarly, the cited frequences cannot be directly compared with figures obtained from other clinical investigations involving different treatments, uses, or investigators. An inspection of these frequencies, however, does provide the prescribing physician with one basis to estimate the relative contribution of drug and nondrug factors to the adverse event incidences in the population studied.

TABLE 1. Treatment-Emergent Adverse Event Incidence in Controlled Add-On Trials (Events in at least 1% of Neurontin patients and numerically more frequent than in the placebo group)

Body System/ Adverse Event	Neurontin®[a] N=543 %	Placebo[a] N=378 %
Body As A Whole		
Fatique	11.0	5.0
Weight Increase	2.9	1.6
Back Pain	1.8	0.5
Peripheral Edema	1.7	0.5
Cardiovascular		
Vasodilatation	1.1	0.3
Digestive System		
Dyspepsia	2.2	0.5
Mouth or Throat Dry	1.7	0.5
Constipation	1.5	0.8
Dental Abnormalities	1.5	0.3
Increased Appetite	1.1	0.8
Hematologic and Lymphatic Systems		
Leukopenia	1.1	0.5
Musculoskeletal System		
Myalgia	2.0	1.9
Fracture	1.1	0.8
Nervous System		
Somnolence	19.3	8.7
Dizziness	17.1	6.9
Ataxia	12.5	5.6
Nystagmus	8.3	4.0
Tremor	6.8	3.2
Nervousness	2.4	1.9
Dysarthria	2.4	0.5
Amnesia	2.2	0.0
Depression	1.8	1.1
Thinking Abnormal	1.7	1.3
Twitching	1.3	0.5
Coordination Abnormal	1.1	0.3
Respiratory System		
Rhinitis	4.1	3.7
Pharyngitis	2.8	1.6
Coughing	1.8	1.3
Skin and Appendages		
Abrasion	1.3	0.0
Pruritus	1.3	0.5
Urogenital System		
Impotence	1.5	1.1
Special Senses		
Diplopia	5.9	1.9
Amblyopia[b]	4.2	1.1
Laboratory Deviations		
WBC Decreased	1.1	0.5

[a]Plus background antiepileptic drug therapy
[b]Amblyopia was often described as blurred vision.

Other events in more than 1% of patients but equally or more frequent in the placebo group included: headache, viral infection, fever, nausea and/or vomiting, abdominal pain, diarrhea, convulsions, confusion, insomnia, emotional lability, rash, acne.

Among the treatment-emergent adverse events occurring at an incidence of at least 10% of Neurontin-treated patients, somnolence and ataxia appeared to exhibit a positive dose-response relationship.

The overall incidence of adverse events and the types of adverse events seen were similar among men and women treated with Neurontin®. The incidence of adverse events increased slightly with increasing age in patients treated with either Neurontin® or placebo. Because only 3% of patients (28/921) in placebo-controlled studies were identified as nonwhite (black or other), there are insufficient data to support a statement regarding the distribution of adverse events by race.

Other Adverse Events Observed During All Clinical Trials

Neurontin® has been administered to 2074 individuals during all clinical trials, only some of which were placebo-controlled. During these trials, all adverse events were recorded by the clinical investigators using terminology of their own choosing. To provide a meaningful estimate of the proportion of individuals having adverse events, similar types of events were grouped into a smaller number of standardized categories using modified COSTART dictionary terminology. These categories are used in the listing below. The frequencies presented represent the proportion of the 2074 individuals exposed to Neurontin® who experienced an event of the type cited on at least one occasion while receiving Neurontin®. All reported events are included except those already listed in the previous table, those too general to be informative, and those not reasonably associated with the use of the drug. Events are further classified within body system categories and enumerated in order of decreasing frequency using the following definitions: frequent adverse events are defined as those occurring in at least 1/100 patients; infrequent adverse events are those occurring in 1/100 to 1/1000 patients;

rare events are those occurring in fewer than 1/1000 patients.

Body As A Whole: *Frequent:* asthenia, malaise, face edema; *Infrequent:* allergy, generalized edema, weight decrease, chill; *Rare:* strange feelings, lassitude, alcohol intolerance, hangover effect.

Cardiovascular System: *Frequent:* hypertension; *Infrequent:* hypotension, angina pectoris, peripheral vascular disorder, palpitation, tachycardia, migraine, murmur; *Rare:* atrial fibrillation, heart failure, thrombophlebitis, deep thrombophlebitis, myocardial infarction, cerebrovascular accident, pulmonary thrombosis, ventricular extrasystoles, bradycardia, premature atrial contraction, pericardial rub, heart block, pulmonary embolus, hyperlipidemia, hypercholesterolemia, pericardial effusion, pericarditis.

Digestive System: *Frequent:* anorexia, flatulence, gingivitis; *Infrequent:* glossitis, gum hemorrhage, thirst, stomatitis, increased salivation, gastroenteritis, hemorrhoids, bloody stools, fecal incontinence, hepatomegaly; *Rare:* dysphagia, eructation, pancreatitis, peptic ulcer, colitis, blisters in mouth, tooth discolor, perleche, salivary gland enlarged, lip hemorrhage, esophagitis, hiatal hernia, hematemesis, proctitis, irritable bowel syndrome, rectal hemorrhage, esophageal spasm.

Endocrine System: *Rate:* hyperthyroid, hypothyroid, goiter, hypoestrogen, ovarian failure, epididymitis, swollen testicle, cushingoid appearance.

Hematologic and Lymphatic System: *Frequent:* purpura most often described as bruises resulting from physical trauma; *Infrequent:* anemia, thrombocytopenia, lymphadenopathy; *Rare:* WBC count increased, lymphocytosis, non-Hodgkin's lymphoma, bleeding time increased.

Musculoskeletal System: *Frequent:* arthralgia; *Infrequent:* tendinitis, arthritis, joint stiffness, joint swelling, positive Romberg test; *Rare:* costochondritis, osteoporosis, bursitis, contracture.

Nervous System: *Frequent:* vertigo, hyperkinesia, paresthesia, decreased or absent reflexes, increased reflexes, anxiety, hostility; *Infrequent:* CNS tumors, syncope, dreaming abnormal, aphasia, hypesthesia, intracranial hemorrhage, hypotonia, dysesthesia, paresis, dystonia, hemiplegia, facial paralysis, stupor, cerebellar dysfunction, positive Babinski sign, decreased position sense, subdural hematoma, apathy, hallucination, decrease or loss of libido, agitation, paranoia, depersonalization, euphoria, feeling high, doped-up sensation, suicidal, psychosis; *Rare:* choreoathetosis, orofacial dyskinesia, encephalopathy, nerve palsy, personality disorder, increased libido, subdued temperament, apraxia, fine motor control disorder, meningismus, local myoclonus, hyperesthesia, hypokinesia, mania, neurosis, hysteria, antisocial reaction, suicide gesture.

Respiratory System: *Frequent:* pneumonia; *Infrequent:* epistaxis, dyspnea, apnea; *Rare:* mucositis, aspiration pneumonia, hyperventilation, hiccup, laryngitis, nasal obstruction, snoring, bronchospasm, hypoventilation, lung edema.

Dermatological: *Infrequent:* alopecia, eczema, dry skin, increased sweating, urticaria, hirsutism, seborrhea, cyst, herpes simplex; *Rare:* herpes zoster, skin discolor skin papules photosensitive reaction, leg ulcer, scalp seborrhea, psoriasis, desquamation, maceration, skin nodules, subcutaneous nodule, melanosis, skin necrosis, local swelling.

Urogenital System: *Infrequent:* hematuria, dysuria, urination frequency, cystitis urinary retention, urinary incontinence, vaginal hemorrhage, amenorrhea, dysmenorrhea, menorrhagia, breast cancer, unable to climax, ejaculation abnormal; *Rare:* kidney pain, leukorrhea, pruritus genital, renal stone, acute renal failure, anuria, glycosuria, nephrosis, nocturia, pyuria, urination urgency, vaginal pain, breast pain, testicle pain.

Special Senses: *Frequent:* abnormal vision; *Infrequent:* cataract, conjunctivitis, eyes dry, eye pain, visual field defect, photophobia, bilateral or unilateral ptosis, eye hemorrhage, hordeolum, hearing loss, earache, tinnitus, inner ear infection, otitis, taste loss, unusual taste, eye twitching, ear fullness; *Rare:* eye itching, abnormal accommodation, perforated ear drum, sensitivity to noise, eye focusing problem, watery eyes, retinopathy, glaucoma, iritis, corneal disorders, lacrimal dysfunction, degenerative eye changes, blindness, retinal degeneration, miosis, chorioretinitis, strabismus, eustachian tube dysfunction, labyrinthitis, otitis externa, odd smell.

DRUG ABUSE AND DEPENDENCE

The abuse and dependence potential of Neurontin® has not been evaluated in human studies.

OVERDOSAGE

A lethal dose of gabapentin was not identified in mice and rats receiving single oral doses as high as 8000 mg/kg. Signs of acute toxicity in animals included ataxia, labored breathing, ptosis, sedation, hypoactivity, or excitation.

Acute oral overdoses of Neurontin® up to 49 grams have been reported. In these cases, double vision, slurred speech, drowsiness, lethargy and diarrhea were observed. All patients recovered with supportive care.

Gabapentin can be removed by hemodialysis. Although hemodialysis has not been performed in the few overdose cases reported, it may be indicated by the patient's clinical state or in patients with significant renal impairment.

DOSAGE AND ADMINISTRATION

Neurontin® is recommended for add-on therapy in patients over 12 years of age. Evidence bearing on its safety and effectiveness in children is not available.

Neurontin® is given orally with or without food.

The effective dose of Neurontin® is 900 to 1800 mg/day and given in divided doses (three times a day) using 300– or 400–mg capsules. Titration to an effective dose can take place rapidly, over a few days, giving 300 mg on Day 1, 300 mg twice a day on Day 2, and 300 mg three times a day on Day 3. To minimize potential side effects, especially somnolence, dizziness, fatigue, and ataxia, the first dose on Day 1 may be administered at bedtime. If necessary, the dose may be increased using 300– or 400–mg capsules three times a day up to 1800 mg/day. Dosages up to 2400 mg/day have been well tolerated in long-term clinical studies. Doses of 3600 mg/day have also been administered to a small number of patients for a relatively short duration, and have been well tolerated. The maximum time between doses in the T.I.D. schedule should not exceed 12 hours.

It is not necessary to monitor gabapentin plasma concentrations to optimize Neurontin® therapy. Further, because there are no significant pharmacokinetic interactions among Neurontin® and other commonly used antiepileptic drugs, the addition of Neurontin® does not alter the plasma levels of these drugs appreciably.

If Neurontin® is discontinued and/or alternate anticonvulsant medication is added to the therapy, this should be done gradually over a minimum of 1 week.

Dosage adjustment in patients with compromised renal function or undergoing hemodialysis is recommended as follows:

TABLE 2. Neurontin® Dosage Based on Renal Function

Renal Function Creatinine Clearance (mL/min)	Total Daily Dose (mg/day)	Dose Regimen (mg)
<60	1200	400 T.I.D
30—60	600	300 B.I.D
15—30	300	300 Q.D
<15	150	300 Q.O.D.[a]
Hemodialysis	—	200–300[b]

[a] Every other day

[b] Loading dose of 300 to 400 mg in patients who have never received Neurontin®, then 200 to 300 mg Neurontin® following each 4 hours of hemodialysis

HOW SUPPLIED

Neurontin® (gabapentin capsules) are supplied as follows:

100-mg capsules;
White hard gelatin capsules printed with "PD" on one side and "Neurontin®/100 mg" on the other; available in:
Bottles of 100: N 0071–0803–24
Unit dose 50's: N 0071–0803–40

300-mg capsules;
Yellow hard gelatin capsules printed with "PD" on one side and "Neurontin®/300 mg" on the other; available in:
Bottles of 100: N 0071–0805–24
Unit dose 50's: N 0071–0805–40

400-mg capsules;
Orange hard gelatin capsules printed with "PD" on one side and "Neurontin®/400 mg" on the other; available in:
Bottles of 100: N 0071–0806–24
Unit dose 50's: N 0071–0806–40

Storage

Store at controlled room temperature 15°–30°C (59°–86°F).

Caution: Federal law prohibits dispensing without prescription.

Issued December 1994 0803G021

Shown in Product Identification Guide, page 327

NITROSTAT® ℞

(Nitroglycerin Tablets, USP)

DESCRIPTION

Nitrostat is a stabilized sublingual nitroglycerin tablet manufactured by a patented process* which prevents the migration of nitroglycerin by adding the nonvolatile fixing agent polyethylene glycol 3350. This stabilized formulation has been shown to be more stable and more uniform than conventional molded tablets. Nitrostat tablets contain 0.3 mg (1/200 grain), 0.4 mg (1/150 grain) and 0.6 mg (1/100 grain) nitroglycerin. Also contains lactose, NF; polyethylene glycol 3350, NF; sucrose, NF.

Nitroglycerin, an organic nitrate, is a vasodilating agent.

CLINICAL PHARMACOLOGY

Relaxation of vascular smooth muscle is the principal pharmacologic action of nitroglycerin. The mechanism by which nitroglycerin produces relaxation of smooth muscle is unknown. Although venous effects predominate, nitroglycerin produces, in a dose-related manner, dilation of both arterial and venous beds. Dilation of the postcapillary vessels, including large veins, promotes peripheral pooling of blood and decreases venous return to the heart, reducing left ventricular end-diastolic pressure (preload). Arteriolar relaxation reduces systemic vascular resistance and arterial pressure (afterload). Myocardial oxygen consumption or demand (as measured by the pressure-rate product, tension-time index and stroke-work index) is decreased by both the arterial and venous effects of nitroglycerin, and a more favorable supply-demand ratio can be achieved.

Nitroglycerin also dilates large epicardial coronary arteries; however, the extent to which this effect contributes to the relief of exertional angina is unclear.

Therapeutic doses of nitroglycerin may reduce systolic, diastolic and mean arterial blood pressure. Effective coronary perfusion pressure is usually maintained, but can be compromised if blood pressure falls excessively or increased heart rate decreases diastolic filling time.

Elevated central venous and pulmonary capillary wedge pressures, pulmonary vascular resistance and systemic vascular resistance are also reduced by nitroglycerin therapy. Heart rate is usually slightly increased, presumably a reflex response to the fall in blood pressure. Cardiac index may be increased, decreased, or unchanged. Patients with elevated left ventricular filling pressure and systemic vascular resistance values in conjunction with a depressed cardiac index are likely to experience an improvement in cardiac index. On the other hand, when filling pressures and cardiac index are normal, cardiac index may be slightly reduced by intravenous nitroglycerin.

Mechanism of Action

Nitroglycerin forms free radical nitric oxide (NO) which activates guanylate cyclase, resulting in an increase of guanosine 3'5' monophosphate (cyclic GMP) in smooth muscle and other tissues. This eventually leads to dephosphorylation of the light chain of myosin, which regulates the contractile state in smooth muscle, resulting in vasodilation.

Pharmacokinetics and Metabolism

Nitroglycerin is rapidly absorbed following sublingual administration. Its onset of action is approximately one to three minutes. Significant pharmacologic effects are present for 30 to 60 minutes following administration by the above route.

Nitroglycerin is rapidly metabolized to dinitrates and mononitrates, with a short half-life, estimated at 1 to 4 minutes. A liver reductase enzyme is of primary importance in the metabolism of nitroglycerin to glycerol nitrate metabolites and organic nitrate. Two active major metabolites 1,2- and 1,3-dinitroglycerols are less potent vasodilators and have longer half-lives than the parent compound. Dinitrates are metabolized to mononitrates and ultimately glycerol. The monohydrate is not considered biologically active with respect to cardiovascular effects.

At plasma concentrations of between 50 and 500 ng/mL, the binding of nitroglycerin to plasma proteins is approximately 60%, while that of 1,2 dinitroglycerin and 1,3 dinitroglycerin is 60% and 30%, respectively. The activity and half-life of 1,2 dinitroglycerin and 1,3 dinitroglycerin are not well characterized. The mononitrate is not active.

INDICATIONS AND USAGE

Nitroglycerin is indicated for the acute relief of an attack or prophylaxis of angina pectoris due to coronary artery disease.

CONTRAINDICATIONS

Sublingual nitroglycerin therapy is contraindicated in patients with early myocardial infarction, severe anemia, increased intracranial pressure and those with a known hypersensitivity to nitroglycerin.

WARNINGS

The use of nitroglycerin during the early course of acute myocardial infarction requires particular attention to hemodynamic monitoring and clinical status.

PRECAUTIONS

General: Only the smallest dose required for effective relief of the acute anginal attack should be used. Excessive use may lead to the development of tolerance. Nitrostat tablets are intended for sublingual or buccal administration and should not be swallowed.

Severe hypotension, particularly with upright posture, may occur even with small doses of nitroglycerin. The drug should be used cautiously in patients with volume depletion or low systolic blood pressure.

Continued on next page

This product information was prepared in August 1996. On these and other Parke-Davis Products, information may be obtained by addressing PARKE-DAVIS, Division of Warner-Lambert Company, Morris Plains, New Jersey 07950.

Parke-Davis—Cont.

Paradoxical bradycardia and increased angina pectoris may accompany nitroglycerin-induced hypotension.

Nitrate therapy may aggravate angina caused by hypertrophic cardiomyopathy.

Tolerance to the vascular and antianginal effects of nitroglycerin and cross-tolerance to other nitrates and nitrites may occur.

The drug should be discontinued if blurring of vision or drying of the mouth occurs. Excessive dosage of nitroglycerin may produce severe headaches.

Information for Patients: If possible, patients should sit down when taking Nitrostat tablets. This eliminates the possibility of falling due to lightheadedness or dizziness. Nitroglycerin may produce a burning or tingling sensation when administered sublingually; however, the ability to produce a burning or tingling sensation should not be considered a reliable method for determining the potency of the tablets.

Nitroglycerin should be kept in the original glass container, tightly capped. The cotton should be discarded once the bottle is opened.

Drug Interactions: Concomitant use of nitrates and alcohol may cause hypotension. Patients receiving antihypertensive drugs, beta-adrenergic blockers or phenothiazines and nitrates should be observed for possible additive hypotensive effects. Marked orthostatic hypotension has been reported when calcium channel blockers and organic nitrates were used concomitantly. Dose adjustment of either class of agent may be necessary.

Aspirin may decrease the clearance and enhance the hemodynamic effects of sublingual nitroglycerin.

A decrease in the therapeutic effect of sublingual nitroglycerin may result from use of long-acting nitrates.

Drug/Laboratory Test Interactions: Nitrates may interfere with the Zlatkis-Zak color reaction causing a false report of decreased serum cholesterol.

Carcinogenesis, Mutagenesis, Impairment of Fertility: No long-term studies in animals were performed to evaluate the carcinogenic potential of nitroglycerin.

Pregnancy Category C: Animal reproduction studies have not been conducted with nitroglycerin. It is also not known whether nitroglycerin can cause fetal harm when administered to a pregnant woman or can affect reproduction capacity. Nitroglycerin should be given to a pregnant woman only if clearly needed.

Nursing Mother: It is not known whether nitroglycerin is excreted in human milk. Because many drugs are excreted in human milk, caution should be exercised when intravenous nitroglycerin is administered to a nursing woman.

Pediatric Use: The safety and effectiveness of nitroglycerin in pediatric patients have not been established.

ADVERSE REACTIONS

Headache which may be severe and persistent may occur immediately after use. Vertigo, weakness, palpitation and other manifestations of postural hypotension may develop occasionally, particularly in erect, immobile patients. Marked sensitivity to the hypotensive effects of nitrates (manifested by nausea, vomiting, weakness, diaphoresis, pallor and collapse) may occur at therapeutic doses. Syncope due to nitrate vasodilation has been reported. Flushing, drug rash, and exfoliative dermatitis have been reported in patients receiving nitrate therapy.

OVERDOSAGE

Nitrate overdose may result in: severe hypotension, tachycardia, bradycardia, heart block, palpitation, death due to circulatory collapse, syncope, persistent throbbing headache, vertigo, visual disturbance, increased intracranial pressure, paralysis and coma followed by convulsions, flushing and diaphoresis, nausea and vomiting, colic and diarrhea, dyspnea and methemoglobinemia.

Since hypotension from nitroglycerin overdosage results from venodilation and arterial hypovolemia, therapy should be directed toward central volume expansion. Elevation of extremities may be sufficient, but intravenous infusion may also be necessary. Use of arterial vasoconstrictors may do more harm than good. Management of nitroglycerin overdose in patients with renal disease or congestive heart failure may require invasive monitoring.

If methemoglobinemia is present, intravenous administration of methylene blue 1–2 mg/kg of body weight may be required.

DOSAGE AND ADMINISTRATION

One tablet should be dissolved under the tongue or in the buccal pouch at the first sign of an acute anginal attack. The dose may be repeated approximately every five minutes, until relief is obtained. If the pain persists after a total of 3 tablets in a 15-minute period, prompt medical attention is recommended. Nitrostat may be used prophylactically 5 to 10 minutes prior to engaging in activities which might precipitate an acute attack.

During administration the patient should rest, preferably in the sitting position.

No dosage adjustment is required in patients with renal failure.

HOW SUPPLIED

Nitrostat is supplied in three strengths in bottles containing 100 tablets each, with color-coded labels, and in color-coded Patient Convenience Packages of four bottles of 25 tablets each.

0.3 mg ($^1/_{200}$ grain): N 0071-0569-24—Bottle of 100 tablets
0.4 mg ($^1/_{150}$ grain): N 0071-0570-13—Convenience Package
N 0071-0570-24—Bottle of 100 tablets
0.6 mg ($^1/_{100}$ grain): N 0071-0571-24—Bottle of 100 tablets

Store at controlled room temperature 15°–30°C (59°–86°F). Protect from moisture.

*US Patent No. 3,789,119

Caution—Federal law prohibits dispensing without prescription.

©1995, Warner-Lambert Co.
Revised November 1995

PARKE-DAVIS 0569G270
Div of Warner-Lambert Co
Morris Plains, NJ 07950 USA
Shown in Product Identification Guide, page 327

PONSTEL® ℞
[pŏn 'stĕl"]
(mefenamic acid)

DESCRIPTION

Ponstel (mefenamic acid) is N-(2,3-xylyl)-anthranilic acid. It is an analgesic agent for oral administration. Ponstel is available in capsules containing 250 mg of mefenamic acid. Each capsule also contains lactose, NF. The capsule shell and/or band contains citric acid, USP; D&C yellow No. 10; FD&C blue No. 1; FD&C red No. 3; FD&C yellow No. 6; gelatin, NF; glycerol monooleate; silicon dioxide, NF; sodium benzoate, NF; sodium lauryl sulfate, NF; titanium dioxide, USP.

It is a white powder with a melting point of 230–231° C, molecular weight 241.28, and water solubility of 0.004% at pH 7.1.

CLINICAL PHARMACOLOGY

Ponstel is a nonsteroidal agent with demonstrated antiinflammatory, analgesic, and antipyretic activity in laboratory animals.[1,2] The mode of action is not known. In animal studies, Ponstel was found to inhibit prostaglandin synthesis and to compete for binding at the prostaglandin receptor site.[3] Pharmacologic studies show Ponstel did not relieve morphine abstinence signs in abstinent, morphine-habituated monkeys.[1]

Following a single 1-gram oral dose, peak plasma levels of 10 μg/ml occurred in 2 to 4 hours with a half-life of 2 hours. Following multiple doses, plasma levels are proportional to dose with no evidence of drug accumulation. One gram of Ponstel given four times daily produces peak blood levels of 20 μg/ml by the second day of administration.[4]

Following a single dose, sixty-seven percent of the total dose is excreted in the urine as unchanged drug or as one of two metabolites. Twenty to twenty-five percent of the dose is excreted in the feces during the first three days.[4]

In controlled, double-blind, clinical trials, Ponstel was evaluated for the treatment of primary spasmodic dysmenorrhea. The parameters used in determining efficacy included pain assessment by both patient and investigator; the need for concurrent analgesic medication; and evaluation of change in frequency and severity of symptoms characteristic of spasmodic dysmenorrhea. Patients received either Ponstel, 500 mg (2 capsules) as an initial dose and 250 mg every 6 hours, or placebo at onset of bleeding or of pain, whichever began first. After three menstrual cycles, patients were crossed over to the alternate treatment for an additional three cycles. Ponstel was significantly superior to placebo in all parameters, and both treatments (drug and placebo) were equally tolerated.

INDICATIONS AND USAGE

Ponstel is indicated for the relief of moderate pain[5] when therapy will not exceed one week. Ponstel is also indicated for the treatment of primary dysmenorrhea.[5,6]

Studies in children under 14 years of age have been inadequate to evaluate the safety and effectiveness of Ponstel.

CONTRAINDICATIONS

Ponstel should not be used in patients who have previously exhibited hypersensitivity to it.

Because the potential exists for cross-sensitivity to aspirin or other nonsteroidal antiinflammatory drugs, Ponstel should not be given to patients in whom these drugs induce symptoms of bronchospasm, allergic rhinitis, or urticaria.

Ponstel is contraindicated in patients with active ulceration or chronic inflammation of either the upper or lower gastrointestinal tract.

Ponstel should be avoided in patients with preexisting renal disease.

WARNINGS

If diarrhea occurs, the dosage should be reduced or temporarily suspended (see Adverse Reactions and Dosage and Administration). Certain patients who develop diarrhea may be unable to tolerate the drug because of recurrence of the symptoms on subsequent exposure.

Risk of GI Ulceration, Bleeding and Perforation with NSAID Therapy: Serious gastrointestinal toxicity such as bleeding, ulceration, and perforation, can occur at any time, with or without warning symptoms, in patients treated chronically with NSAID therapy. Although minor upper gastrointestinal problems, such as dyspepsia, are common, usually developing early in therapy, physicians should remain alert for ulceration and bleeding in patients treated chronically with NSAIDs even in the absence of previous GI tract symptoms. In patients observed in clinical trials of several months to two years duration, symptomatic upper GI ulcers, gross bleeding or perforation appear to occur in approximately 1% of patients treated for 3–6 months, and in about 2–4% of patients treated for one year. Physicians should inform patients about the signs and/or symptoms of serious GI toxicity and what steps to take if they occur.

Studies to date have not identified any subset of patients not at risk of developing peptic ulceration and bleeding. Except for a prior history of serious GI events and other risk factors known to be associated with peptic ulcer disease, such as alcoholism, smoking, etc., no risk factors (eg, age, sex) have been associated with increased risk. Elderly or debilitated patients seem to tolerate ulceration or bleeding less well than other individuals and most spontaneous reports of fatal GI events are in this population. Studies to date are inconclusive concerning the relative risk of various NSAIDs in causing such reactions. High doses of any NSAID probably carry a greater risk of these reactions, although controlled clinical trials showing this do not exist in most cases. In considering the use of relatively large doses (within the recommended dosage range), sufficient benefit should be anticipated to offset the potential increased risk of GI toxicity.

PRECAUTIONS

If rash occurs, administration of the drug should be stopped. A false-positive reaction for urinary bile, using the diazo tablet test, may result after mefenamic acid administration. If biliuria is suspected, other diagnostic procedures, such as the Harrison spot test, should be performed.

Renal Effects: As with other nonsteroidal antiinflammatory drugs, long-term administration of mefenamic acid to animals has resulted in renal papillary necrosis and other abnormal renal pathology. In humans, there have been reports of acute interstitial nephritis with hematuria, proteinuria and occasionally nephrotic syndrome.

A second form of renal toxicity has been seen in patients with prerenal conditions leading to a reduction in renal blood flow or blood volume, where the renal prostaglandins have a supportive role in the maintenance of renal perfusion. In these patients administration of an NSAID may cause a dose-dependent reduction in prostaglandin formation and may precipitate overt renal decompensation. Patients at greatest risk of this reaction are those with impaired renal function, heart failure, liver dysfunction, those taking diuretics, and the elderly Discontinuation of NSAID therapy is typically followed by recovery to the pretreatment state. Since Ponstel is eliminated primarily by the kidneys, the drug should not be administered to patients with significantly impaired renal functions.

As with other nonsteroidal antiinflammatory drugs, borderline elevations of one or more liver tests may occur in some patients. These abnormalities may progress, may remain essentially unchanged, or may be transient with continued therapy. The SGPT (ALT) test is probably the most sensitive indicator of liver dysfunction. Meaningful (3 times the upper limit of normal) elevations of SGPT or SGOT (AST) occurred in controlled clinical trials in less than 1% of patients. A patient with symptoms and/or signs suggesting liver dysfunction, or in whom an abnormal liver test has occurred, should be evaluated for evidence of the development of more severe hepatic reaction while on therapy with Ponstel. Severe hepatic reactions, including jaundice and cases of fatal hepatitis, have been reported with other nonsteroidal antiinflammatory drugs. Although such reactions are rare, if abnormal liver tests persist or worsen, if clinical signs and symptoms consistent with liver disease develop, or if systemic manifestations occur (eg eosinophilia, rash, etc), Ponstel should be discontinued.

Information for Patients: Patients should be advised that if rash, diarrhea or other digestive problems arise, they should stop the drug and consult their physician.

Patients in whom aspirin or other nonsteroidal antiinflammatory drugs induce symptoms of bronchospasm, allergic

rhinitis, or urticaria should be made aware that the potential exists for cross-sensitivity to Ponstel.

The long-term effects, if any, of intermittent Ponstel therapy for dysmenorrhea are not known. Women on such therapy should consult their physician if they should decide to become pregnant.

Ponstel, like other drugs of its class, is not free of side effects. The side effects of these drugs can cause discomfort and, rarely, there are more serious side effects, such as gastrointestinal bleeding, which may result in hospitalization and even fatal outcomes.

NSAIDs (nonsteroidal antiinflammatory drugs) are often essential agents in the management of arthritis and have a major role in the treatment of pain, but they also may be commonly employed for conditions which are less serious.

Physicians may wish to discuss with their patients the potential risks (see WARNINGS, PRECAUTIONS, and ADVERSE REACTIONS sections) and likely benefits of NSAID treatment, particularly when the drugs are used for less serious conditions where treatment without NSAIDs may represent an acceptable alternative to both the patient and physician.

Laboratory Tests: Because serious GI tract ulceration and bleeding can occur without warning symptoms, physicians should follow chronically treated patients for the signs and symptoms of ulceration and bleeding and should inform them of the importance of this follow-up (see Risk of GI Ulcerations, Bleeding and Perforation with NSAID Therapy).

Drug Interactions: Ponstel may prolong prothrombin time.[5] Therefore, when the drug is administered to patients receiving oral anticoagulant drugs, frequent monitoring of prothrombin time is necessary.

Use in Pregnancy: Pregnancy Category C. Reproduction studies have been performed in rats, rabbits and dogs. Rats given up to 10 times the human dose showed decreased fertility, delay in parturition, and a decreased rate of survival to weaning. Rabbits at 2.5 times the human dose showed an increase in the number of resorptions. There were no fetal anomalies observed in these studies nor in dogs at up to 10 times the human dose.[5]

There are no adequate and well-controlled studies in pregnant women. Because animal reproduction studies are not always predictive of human response, this drug should be used only if clearly needed.

The use of Ponstel in late pregnancy is not recommended because of the effects on the fetal cardiovascular system of drugs of this class.

Nursing Mothers: Trace amounts of Ponstel may be present in breast milk and transmitted to the nursing infant[7]; thus Ponstel should not be taken by the nursing mother because of the effects on the infant cardiovascular system of drugs of this class.

Use in Children: Safety and effectiveness in children below the age of 14 have not been established.

ADVERSE REACTIONS

Gastrointestinal: The most frequently reported adverse reactions associated with the use of Ponstel involve the gastrointestinal tract. In controlled studies for up to eight months, the following disturbances were reported in decreasing order of frequency: diarrhea (approximately 5% of patients), nausea with or without vomiting, other gastrointestinal symptoms, and abdominal pain.

In certain patients, the diarrhea was of sufficient severity to require discontinuation of medication. The occurrence of the diarrhea is usually dose related, generally subsides on reduction of dosage, and rapidly disappears on termination of therapy.

Other gastrointestinal reactions less frequently reported were anorexia, pyrosis, flatulence, and constipation.

Gastrointestinal ulceration with and without hemorrhage has been reported.

Hematopoietic: Cases of autoimmune hemolytic anemia have been associated with the continuous administration of Ponstel for 12 months or longer. In such cases the Coombs test results are positive with evidence of both accelerated RBC production and RBC destruction. The process is reversible upon termination of Ponstel administration.

Decreases in hematocrit have been noted in 2–5% of patients and primarily in those who have received prolonged therapy. Leukopenia, eosinophilia, thrombocytopenic purpura, agranulocytosis, pancytopenia, and bone marrow hypoplasia have also been reported on occasion.

Nervous System: Drowsiness, dizziness, nervousness, headache, blurred vision, and insomnia have occurred.

Integumentary: Urticaria, rash, and facial edema have been reported.

Renal: As with other nonsteroidal antiinflammatory agents, renal failure, including papillary necrosis, has been reported. In elderly patients renal failure has occurred after taking Ponstel for 2–6 weeks. The renal damage may not be completely reversible. Hematuria and dysuria have also been reported with Ponstel.

Other: Eye irritation, ear pain, perspiration, mild hepatic toxicity, and increased need for insulin in a diabetic have been reported. There have been rare reports of palpitation, dyspnea, and reversible loss of color vision.

OVERDOSAGE

Although doses up to 6000 mg/day have been given, no specific information is available on the management of acute massive overdosage.

Should accidental overdosage occur, the stomach should be emptied by inducing emesis or by careful gastric lavage followed by the administration of activated charcoal.[8] Laboratory studies indicate that Ponstel should be absorbed from the gastrointestinal tract by activated charcoal.[4] Vital functions should be monitored and supported. Because mefenamic acid and its metabolities are firmly bound to plasma proteins, hemodialysis and peritoneal dialysis may be of little value.[4]

DOSAGE AND ADMINISTRATION

Administration is by the oral route, preferably with food. The recommended regimen in acute pain for adults and children over 14 years of age is 500 mg as an initial dose followed by 250 mg every six hours as needed, usually not to exceed one week.[5]

For the treatment of primary dysmenorrhea, the recommended dosage is 500 mg as an initial dose followed by 250 mg every 6 hours, starting with the onset of bleeding and associated symptoms. Clinical studies indicate that effective treatment can be initiated with the start of menses and should not be necessary for more than 2 to 3 days.[6]

HOW SUPPLIED

N 0071-0540-24 (P-D 540) Ponstel (mefenamic acid) is available as 250 mg capsules in bottles of 100.

REFERENCES

1. Winder CV, et al: Antiinflammatory, antipyretic and antinociceptive properties of N-(2,3-xylyl) anthranilic acid (mefenamic acid). *J Pharmacol Exp Ther* 138: 405–413, 1962.
2. Wax J, et al: Comparative activities, tolerances and safety of nonsteroidal antiinflammatory agents in rats. *J Pharmacol Exp Ther* 192: 172–178, 1975.
3. Ferreira SH, Vane JR: Aspirin and prostaglandins, in *The Prostaglandins*, Ramwell PW Ed, Plenum Press, NY, vol. 2, 1974, pp 1–47.
4. Glazko AJ: Experimental observations of flufenamic, mefenamic, and meclofenamic acids. Part III. Metabolic disposition, in *Fenamates in Medicine.* A Symposium, London 1966; *Annals of Physical Medicine*, supplement, pp 23–36, 1967.
5. Data on file, Medical Affairs Dept, Parke-Davis.
6. Budoff PW: Use of mefenamic acid in the treatment of primary dysmenorrhea. *JAMA* 241: 2713–2716, 1979.
7. Buchanan RA, et al: The breast milk excretion of mefenamic acid. *Curr Ther Res* 10:592, 1968.
8. Corby DG, Decker WJ: Management of acute poisoning with activated charcoal. *Pediatrics* 54:324, 1974.

0540G152

Caution—Federal law prohibits dispensing without prescription.

Revised May 1995

Shown in Product Identification Guide, page 327

PROCANBID™ ℞

(Procainamide Hydrochloride Extended-Release Tablets*)
***Procanbid is not USP for dissolution.**

> **WARNINGS:**
> Positive ANA Titer: The prolonged administration of procainamide often leads to the development of a positive antinuclear antibody (ANA) test, with or without symptoms of a lupus erythematosus-like syndrome. If a positive ANA titer develops, the benefits versus risks of continued procainamide therapy should be assessed.

DESCRIPTION

Procanbid (Procainamide Hydrochloride Extended-Release Tablets), a Group 1A cardiac antiarrhythmic drug, is p-amino-N[2-(diethylamino) ethyl]benzamide monohydrochloride, molecular weight 271.79.

Procainamide hydrochloride differs from procaine which is the p-aminobenzoyl ester of 2-(diethylamino)-ethanol. Procainamide as the free base has a pK_a of 9.24; the monohydrochloride is very soluble in water.

Procanbid (Procainamide Hydrochloride Extended-Release Tablets) contains 500 mg or 1000 mg of procainamide hydrochloride for oral administration. The release of procainamide hydrochloride is controlled by 2 mechanisms using T-Kote™ technology. The core of the tablet consists of a wax matrix which is then coated with a polymeric, control-release layer. Both strengths of Procanbid contain black iron oxide; candelilla wax, FCC; carnauba wax, NF; colloidal silicon dioxide, NF; hydroxypropyl cellulose, NF; hydroxypropylmethyl cellulose; magnesium stearate, NF; polyacrylate dispersion; polyethylene glycol 3350, NF; polyethylene glycol 8000, NF; propylene glycol; simethicone emulsion, USP; talc, USP; and titanium dioxide. The 500-mg tablet additionally contains FD&C blue No. 1 aluminum lake. The 1000-mg tablet additionally contains polysorbate 80.

CLINICAL PHARMACOLOGY

Mechanism of Action: Procainamide (PA) increases the effective refractory period of the atria, and to a lesser extent the bundle of His-Purkinje system and ventricles of the heart. It reduces impulse conduction velocity in the atria, His-Purkinje fibers, and ventricular muscle, but has variable effects on the atrioventricular (A-V) node, a direct slowing action and a weaker vagolytic effect that may speed A-V conduction slightly. Myocardial excitability is reduced in the atria, Purkinje fibers, papillary muscles, and ventricles by an increase in the threshold for excitation, combined with inhibition of ectopic pacemaker activity by retardation of the slow phase of diastolic depolarization, thus decreasing automatically especially in ectopic sites. Contractility of the undamaged heart is usually not affected by therapeutic concentrations, although slight reduction of cardiac output may occur, and may be significant in the presence of myocardial damage. Therapeutic levels of PA may exert vagolytic effects and produce slight acceleration of heart rate, while high or toxic concentrations may prolong A-V conduction time or induce A-V block, or even cause abnormal automaticity and spontaneous firing, by unknown mechanisms.

The electrocardiogram may reflect these effects by showing slight sinus tachycardia (due to the anticholinergic action) and widened QRS complexes and, less regularly, prolonged Q-T and P-R intervals (due to longer systole and slower conduction), as well as some decrease in QRS and T wave amplitude. These direct effects of PA on electrical activity, conduction, responsiveness, excitability, and automaticity are characteristic of a Group 1A antiarrhythmic agent, the prototype for which is quinidine; PA effects are very similar. However, PA has weaker vagal blocking action than does quinidine, does not induce alpha-adrenergic blockade, and is less depressing to cardiac contractility.

Pharmacokinetics and Drug Metabolism

Absorption/Bioavailability: PA is well absorbed following oral administration. The absolute bioavailability from immediate-release PA HCl capsules is approximately 85% in patients and healthy subjects. Bioavailability of Procanbid is similar to that of PA HCl extended-release tablets, USP (Procan®SR) which have been shown to be similar to that of immediate-release PA.

The Procanbid T-Kote™ delivery system is designed to control the rate of PA release such that absorption is sustained throughout a 12-hour dosing interval. After administration of Procanbid with a high-fat meal, the extent of PA absorption was increased by about 20%. Peak, trough, and average plasma PA concentrations following twice daily administration of Procanbid to healthy subjects are similar to those achieved when Procan SR is administered 4 times daily (Figure 1). In patients with frequent ventricular premature depolarizations (VPDs), peak and steady-state average PA concentrations following administration of Procanbid every 12 hours are bioequivalent to those following administration of an equivalent daily dose of Procan SR. While corresponding minimum concentrations are slightly lower than those for Procan SR, they remain within the acceptable therapeutic range of 3 to 10 mcg/mL.

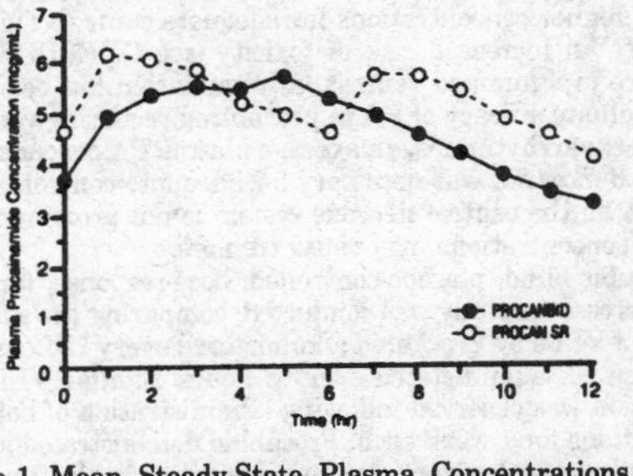

Figure 1. Mean Steady-State Plasma Concentrations Following Administration of Two 1000-mg Procanbid Tablets Every 12 Hours or One 1000-mg Procan SR Tablet Every 6 Hours to Patients with VPDs.

Twice-daily administration of two 1000-mg Procanbid tablets to patients with frequent VPDs produced a mean plasma PA concentration of 4.6 mcg/mL. Average peak and trough levels are within the generally accepted therapeutic range of 3 to 10 mcg/mL. Relative proportions of PA and N-acetyl-

Continued on next page

This product information was prepared in August 1996. On these and other Parke-Davis Products, information may be obtained by addressing PARKE-DAVIS, Division of Warner-Lambert Company, Morris Plains, New Jersey 07950.

Parke-Davis—Cont.

procainamide (NAPA) during administration of Procanbid are similar to those following administration of immediate-release PA or Procan SR.

Distribution: Plasma protein binding of PA is insignificant, approximately 20%. The apparent volume of distribution is approximately 2 L/kg. It is not known if PA crosses the placenta.

Metabolism/Excretion: The elimination half-life of PA is 3 to 4 hours in patients with normal renal function, but reduced renal function prolongs the half-life (see Special Populations). PA is mainly eliminated intact by the kidneys. The only metabolite of any significance is N-acetylprocainamide (NAPA). Renal excretion accounts for > 80% of the elimination of NAPA. Approximately 16 to 21% of PA is metabolized to NAPA in "slow acetylators"; in "rapid acetylators" the range is 24 to 33%. In white and black populations the numbers of rapid and slow acetylators are about 50%. The plasma concentration of NAPA is lower than the PA concentration in most individuals. The reverse may occur in individuals forming more of the metabolite while also having reduced kidney function. NAPA has significant antiarrhythmic activity.

An average of 65% of the dose was recovered as intact drug in the urine after intravenous administration of PA. The renal clearance of PA ranged from 400 to 600 mL/min. Active renal secretion ranged from 300 to 500 mL/min, and is thus the major elimination pathway for PA. The tubular secretion utilizes the base-secreting system also responsible for secretion of metformin, cimetidine, ranitidine, triamterene, and flecainide. Thus there is a potential for drug-drug interactions at this level.

Special Populations: *Patients with Renal Disease:* Decline in renal function, such as that occurring with advancing age or renal disease, increases the PA elimination half-life which can result in relatively high plasma concentrations of PA (see WARNINGS). Accumulation of NAPA due to impaired renal function can be more extensive than accumulation of PA.

Patients with Congestive Heart Failure: PA clearance is reduced in patients with severe heart failure, in part due to decreased renal perfusion (see WARNINGS).

Age, Gender, and Race: PA clearance decreases with increasing patient age, in part due to concurrent decreases in renal function. However, the pharmacokinetis of PA and NAPA are similar in young healthy subjects (mean age 32 yr) and patients with frequent VPDs (mean age 60 yr) following administration of Procanbid every 12 hours. Steady state plasma procainamide concentrations in women receiving Procanbid are 30 percent higher than those seen in men receiving the same dosing regimen. When corrected for body surface area this difference is only 16 percent. Concentrations of N-acetylprocainamide are not significantly different among men and women whether corrected for body surface area or not. Procanbid tablets produce similar PA and NAPA concentrations in black and caucasian individuals.

Pharmacodynamics: While therapeutic plasma PA concentrations have been reported to be 3 to 10 mcg/mL, patients such as those with sustained ventricular tachycardia may need higher concentrations for adequate control. This may justify an increased risk of toxicity (see OVERDOSAGE). Where programmed ventricular stimulation has been used to evaluate efficacy of PA in preventing recurring ventricular tachyarrhythmias, an average plasma PA concentration of 13.6 mcg/mL was necessary for adequate control. Action of PA on the central nervous system is not prominent, but high concentrations may cause tremors.

A double-blind, placebo-controlled, dose-response, formulation-crossover study was conducted, comparing the suppression of VPDs by Procanbid administered every 12 hours and Procan SR administered every 6 hours. Similar VPD suppression was observed following administration of both formulations for 1 week each. Procanbid demonstrated significant pharmacologic activity (mean percent change from base line in VPDs) compared with placebo, and a significant linear dose-response relationship was observed. VPD suppression was maintained throughout the dosing interval.

In this study, VPD rate tended to decrease with increasing concentration of PA and NAPA; however, PA concentration alone was a poor predictor of antiarrhythmic effect. The concentration-effect relationship for administration of Procanbid every 12 hours was indistinguishable from that for administration of Procan SR every 6 hours.

INDICATIONS AND USAGE

Procanbid tablets are indicated for the treatment of documented ventricular arrhythmias, such as sustained ventricular tachycardia, that in the judgment of the physician are life-threatening. Because of the proarrhythmic effects of procainamide, its use with lesser arrhythmias is generally not recommended. Treatment of patients with asymptomatic ventricular premature depolarizations should be avoided.

Initiation of procainamide treatment, as with other antiarrhythmic agents used to treat life-threatening arrhythmias, should be carried out in the hospital.

Antiarrhythmic drugs have not been shown to enhance survival in patients with ventricular arrhythmias.

Because procainamide has the potential to produce serious hematologic disorders (0.5%), particularly leukopenia or agranulocytosis (sometimes fatal), its use should be reserved for patients in whom, in the opinion of the physician, the benefits of treatment clearly outweigh the risks. (See WARNINGS and Boxed Warning.)

CONTRAINDICATIONS

Complete Heart Block: Procainamide should not be administered to patients with complete heart block because of its effects in suppressing nodal or ventricular pacemakers and the hazard of asystole. It may be difficult to recognize complete heart block in patients with ventricular tachycardia, but if significant slowing of ventricular rate occurs during PA treatment without evidence of A-V conduction appearing, PA should be stopped. In cases of second degree A-V block or various types of hemiblock, PA should be avoided or discontinued because of the possibility of increased severity of block unless the ventricular rate is controlled by an electrical pacemaker.

Idiosyncratic Hypersensitivity: In patients sensitive to procaine or other ester-type local anesthetics, cross sensitivity to PA is unlikely; however, it should be borne in mind, and PA should not be used if it produces acute allergic dermatitis, asthma, or anaphylactic symptoms.

Lupus Erythematosus: An established diagnosis of systemic lupus erythematosus is a contraindication to PA therapy, since aggravation of symptoms is highly likely.

Torsades De Pointes: In the unusual ventricular arrhythmia called "les torsades de pointes" (twisting of the points), characterized by alternation of 1 or more ventricular premature beats in the directions of the QRS complexes on ECG in persons with prolonged Q-T and often enhanced U waves, Group 1A antiarrhythmic drugs are contraindicated. Administration of PA in such cases may aggravate this special type of ventricular extrasystole or tachycardia instead of suppressing it.

WARNINGS

Mortality: In the National Heart, Lung, and Blood Institute's Cardiac Arrhythmia Suppression Trial (CAST), a long-term, multi-centered, randomized, double-blind study in patients with asymptomatic non-life-threatening ventricular arrhythmias who had a myocardial infarction more than 6 days but less than 2 years previously, an excessive mortality or non-fatal cardiac arrest rate (7.7%) was seen in patients treated with encainide or flecainide compared with that seen in patients assigned to carefully matched placebo-treated groups (3.0%). The average duration of treatment with encainide or flecainide in this study was 10 months.

The applicability of the CAST results to other populations (eg, those without recent myocardial infarction) is uncertain. Considering the known proarrhythmic properties of procainamide and the lack of evidence of improved survival for any antiarrhythmic drug in patients without life-threatening arrhythmias, the use of Procanbid as well as other antiarrhythmic agents should be reserved for patients with life-threatening ventricular arrhythmias.

BLOOD DYSCRASIAS: Agranulocytosis, bone marrow depression, neutropenia, hypoplastic anemia, and thrombocytopenia have been reported in patients receiving procainamide hydrochloride at a rate of approximately 0.5%. Most of these patients received procainamide hydrochloride within the recommended dosage range. Fatalities have occurred (with approximately 20%–25% mortality in reported cases of agranulocytosis). Since most of these events have been noted during the first 12 weeks of therapy, it is recommended that complete blood counts including white cell, differential, and platelet counts be performed at weekly intervals for the first 3 months of therapy, and periodically thereafter. Complete blood counts should be performed promptly if the patient develops any signs of infection (such as fever, chills, sore throat, or stomatitis), bruising, or bleeding. If any of these hematologic disorders are identified, procainamide hydrochloride should be discontinued. Blood counts usually return to normal within 1 month of discontinuation. Caution should be used in patients with pre-existing marrow failure or cytopenia of any type (see ADVERSE REACTIONS).

Digitalis Intoxication: Caution should be exercised in the use of procainamide in arrhythmias associated with digitalis intoxication. Procainamide can suppress digitalis-induced arrhythmias; however, if there is concomitant marked disturbance of atrioventricular conduction, additional depression of conduction and ventricular asystole or fibrillation may result. Therefore, use of procainamide should be considered only if discontinuation of digitalis, and therapy with potassium, lidocaine, or phenytoin are ineffective.

First Degree Heart Block: Caution should be exercised also if the patient exhibits or develops first degree heart block while taking PA, and dosage reduction is advised in such cases. If the block persists despite dosage reduction, continuation of PA administration must be evaluated on the basis of current benefit versus risk of increased heart block.

Predigitalization for Atrial Flutter or Fibrillation: Patients with atrial flutter or fibrillation should be cardioverted or digitalized prior to PA administration to avoid enhancement of A-V conduction which may result in ventricular rate acceleration beyond tolerable limits. Adequate digitalization reduces but does not eliminate the possibility of sudden increase in ventricular rate as the atrial rate is slowed by PA in these arrhythmias.

Congestive Heart Failure: For patients in congestive heart failure, and those with acute ischemic heart disease or cardiomyopathy, caution should be used in PA therapy, since even slight depression of myocardial contractility may further reduce the cardiac output of the damaged heart.

Concurrent Other Antiarrhythmic Agents: Concurrent use of PA with other Group 1A antiarrhythmic agents such as quinidine or disopyramide may produce enhanced prolongation of conduction or depression of contractility and hypotension, especially in patients with cardiac decompensation. Such use should be reserved for patients with serious arrhythmias unresponsive to a single drug and employed only if close observation is possible.

Renal Insufficiency: Renal insufficiency may lead to accumulation of high plasma concentrations of PA and/or NAPA from conventional oral doses of PA, with effects similar to those of overdosage (see OVERDOSAGE), unless dosage is adjusted for the individual patient.

Myasthenia Gravis: Patients with myasthenia gravis may show worsening of symptoms from PA due to its procaine-like effect on diminishing acetylcholine release at skeletal muscle motor nerve endings, so that PA administration may be hazardous without optimal adjustment of anticholinesterase medications and other precautions.

PRECAUTIONS

General: Immediately after initiation of PA therapy, patients should be closely observed for possible hypersensitivity reactions, especially if procaine or local anesthetic sensitivity is suspected, and for muscular weakness if myasthenia gravis is a possibility.

In conversion of atrial fibrillation to normal sinus rhythm by any means, dislodgment of mural thrombi may lead to embolization, which should be kept in mind.

Based upon the approximate half-life of 3 hours for PA, pharmacokinetic steady state would be reached within 1 day. After achieving and maintaining therapeutic plasma concentrations and satisfactory electrocardiographic and clinical responses, continued frequent periodic monitoring of vital signs and electrocardiograms is advised. If evidence of QRS widening of more than 25% or marked prolongation of the Q-T interval occurs, concern for overdosage is appropriate, and reduction in dosage is advisable if a 50% increase occurs. Elevated serum creatinine or urea nitrogen, reduced creatinine clearance, or history of renal insufficiency, as well as use in older patients (over age 50), provide grounds to anticipate that less than the usual dosage may suffice, since the urinary elimination of PA and NAPA may be reduced, leading to gradual accumulation beyond normally predicted amounts. If facilities are available for measurement of plasma PA and NAPA, or acetylation capability, individual dose adjustment for optimal therapeutic concentrations may be easier, but close observation of clinical effectiveness is the most important criterion.

In the longer term, periodic complete blood counts are useful to detect possible idiosyncratic hematologic effects of PA on neutrophil, platelet, or red cell homeostatis; agranulocytosis has been reported to occur occasionally in patients on long-term PA therapy. A rising titer of serum ANA may precede clinical symptoms of the lupoid syndrome (see Boxed Warning and ADVERSE REACTIONS). If the lupus erythematosus-like syndrome develops in a patient with recurrent life-threatening arrhythmias not controlled by other agents, corticosteroid suppressive therapy may be used concomitantly with PA. Since the PA-induced lupoid syndrome rarely includes dangerous pathologic renal changes, PA therapy may not necessarily have to be stopped unless the symptoms of serositis and the possibility of further lupoid effects are of greater risk than the benefit of PA in controlling arrhythmias. Patients with rapid acetylation capability are less likely to develop the lupoid syndrome after prolonged PA therapy.

Information for Patients: The physician is advised to explain to the patient that close cooperation in adhering to the prescribed dosage schedule is of great importance in controlling the cardiac arrhythmia safely. The patient should understand clearly that more medication is not necessarily

better and may be dangerous, that skipping doses or increasing intervals between doses to suit personal convenience may lead to loss of control of the heart problem, and that "making up" missed doses by doubling up later may be hazardous.

The patient should be encouraged to disclose any past history of drug sensitivity, especially to procaine or other local anesthetic agents, and to report any history of kidney disease, congestive heart failure, myasthenia gravis, liver disease, or lupus erythematosus.

The patient should be counseled to report promptly any symptoms of arthralgia, myalgia, fever, chills, skin rash, easy bruising, sore throat or sore mouth, infections, dark urine or icterus, wheezing, muscular weakness, chest or abdominal pain, palpitations, nausea, vomiting, anorexia, diarrhea, hallucinations, dizziness, or depression.

The patient should be advised not to break or chew the tablet as this would interfere with designed dissolution characteristics. The tablet matrix of Procanbid may be seen in the stool since it does not disintegrate following release of procainamide.

Laboratory Tests: Laboratory tests such as complete blood count (CBC), electrocardiogram, and serum creatinine or urea nitrogen may be indicated, depending on the clinical situation, and periodic rechecking of the CBC and ANA may be helpful in early detection of untoward reactions.

Drug Interactions: If other antiarrhythmic drugs are being used, additive effects on the heart may occur with PA administration, and dosage reduction may be necessary (see WARNINGS).

Anticholinergic drugs administered concurrently with PA may produce additive antivagal effects on A-V nodal conduction, although this is not as well documented for PA as for quinidine.

Coadministration of cimetidine decreases renal clearance of PA, potentially leading to clinically significant increases in plasma concentrations. Large (> 300 mg/day) doses of ranitidine possibly have this effect also. Plasma PA concentrations higher than those for administration of PA alone have been reported for coadministration with either amiodarone or trimethoprim. Alcohol (ethanol) consumption tends to decrease the half-life of PA in the blood through induction of its acetylation to NAPA.

Patients taking PA who require neuromuscular blocking agents such as succinylcholine may require less than usual doses of the latter, due to PA effects of reducing acetylcholine release.

Drug/Laboratory Test Interactions: Suprapharmacologic concentrations of lidocaine and meprobamate may inhibit fluorescence of PA and NAPA, and propranolol shows a native fluorescence close to the PA/NAPA peak wavelengths, so that tests which depend on fluorescence measurement may be affected.

Carcinogenesis, Mutagenesis, Impairment of Fertility: Long-term studies in animals have not been performed.

Pregnancy Category C: Animal reproduction studies have not been conducted with PA. It also is not known whether PA can cause fetal harm when administered to a pregnant woman or can affect reproduction capacity. PA should be given to a pregnant woman only if clearly needed.

Nursing Mothers: Both PA and NAPA are excreted in human milk, and absorbed by the nursing infant. Because of the potential for serious adverse reactions in nursing infants, a decision to discontinue nursing or the drug should be made, taking into account the importance of the drug to the mother.

Pediatric Use: Safety and effectiveness in pediatric patients have not been established.

ADVERSE REACTIONS

Cardiovascular System: Hypotension following oral PA administration is rare. Hypotension and serious disturbances of cardiac rhythm such as ventricular asystole or fibrillation are more common after intravenous administration (see OVERDOSAGE, WARNINGS). Second degree heart block has been reported in 2 of almost 500 patients taking PA orally.

Multisystem Effects: A lupus erythematosus-like syndrome of arthralgia, pleural or abdominal pain, and sometimes arthritis, pleural effusion, pericarditis, fever, chills, myalgia, and possibly related hematologic or skin lesions (see below) is fairly common after prolonged PA administration, perhaps more often in patients who are slow acetylators (see Boxed Warning and PRECAUTIONS). While some studies have reported less than 1 in 500, others have reported the syndrome in up to 30% of patients on long-term oral PA therapy. If discontinuation of PA does not reverse the lupoid symptoms, corticosteroid treatment may be effective.

Hematologic System: Neutropenia, thrombocytopenia, or hemolytic anemia may rarely be encountered. Agranulocytosis has occured after repeated use of PA, and deaths have been reported (see WARNINGS and Boxed Warning).

Skin: Angioneurotic edema, urticaria, pruritus, flushing, and maculopapular rash have also occurred occasionally.

Gastrointestinal System: Anorexia, nausea, vomiting, abdominal pain, bitter taste, or diarrhea may occur in 3% to

4% of patients taking oral procainamide. Hepatomegaly with increased serum aminotransferase activity has been reported after a single oral dose.

Nervous System: Dizziness or giddiness, weakness, mental depression, and psychosis with hallucinations have been reported occasionally.

OVERDOSAGE

Progressive widening of the QRS complex, prolonged Q-T and P-R intervals, lowering of the R and T waves, as well as increasing A-V block, may be seen with doses which are excessive for a given patient. Increased ventricular extrasystoles or even ventricular tachycardia or fibrillation may occur. After intravenous administration but seldom after oral therapy, transient high plasma concentrations of PA may induce hypotension, affecting systolic more than diastolic pressures, especially in hypertensive patients. Such high levels may also produce central nervous depression, tremor, and even respiratory depression.

Plasma levels above 10 mcg/mL are increasingly associated with toxic findings, which are seen occasionally in the 10 to 12 mcg/mL range, more often in the 12 to 15 mcg/mL range, and commonly in patients with plasma levels greater than 15 mcg/mL. A single oral dose of IR PA 2000 mg may produce overdosage symptoms, while 3000 mg of IR PA may be dangerous, especially if the patient is a slow acetylator, has decreased renal function, or underlying organic heart disease.

Treatment of overdosage or toxic manifestations includes general supportive measures, close observation, monitoring of vital signs and possibly intravenous pressor agents, and mechanical cardiorespiratory support. If available, PA and NAPA plasma levels may be helpful in assessing the potential degree of toxicity and response to therapy. Both PA and NAPA are removed from the circulation by hemodialysis but not peritoneal dialysis. No specific antidote for PA is known.

DOSAGE AND ADMINISTRATION

The dose should be adjusted for the individual patient, based on clinical assessment of the degree of underlying myocardial disease, the patient's age, and renal function. For patients who have been receiving another formulation of procainamide, the dose of the other formulation can function as a general guide, but re-titration with Procanbid is recommended.

As a general guide, for younger patients with normal renal function, an initial total daily oral dose of up to 50 mg/kg of body weight of Procanbid tablets may be used, given in 2 divided doses, every 12 hours, to maintain therapeutic blood concentrations. For older patients, especially those over 50 years of age, or for patients with renal, hepatic, or cardiac insufficiency, lesser amounts or longer intervals may produce adequate blood concentrations, and decrease the probability of occurrence of dose-related adverse reactions.

CARE SHOULD BE TAKEN WHEN DISPENSING PROCANBID TO ASSURE THE BID DOSAGE FORM HAS BEEN PRESCRIBED AND DISPENSED. Procanbid tablets should be swallowed whole and should not be bitten or cut.

To provide up to 50 mg/kg of body weight per day*

Patients Weighing	Dose
88–110 lb (40–50 kg)	1000 mg q12 hrs
132–154 lb (60–70 kg)	1500 mg q12 hrs
176–198 lb (80–90 kg)	2000 mg q12 hrs
> 220 lb (>100 kg)	2500 mg q12 hrs

*Initial dosage schedule guide only, to be adjusted for each patient individually, based on age, cardiorenal function, blood concentration (if available), and clinical response.

HOW SUPPLIED

Procanbid tablets are supplied as follows:
500 mg: Blue, film-coated, elliptical tablets, coded "PROCANBID" on one side and "500" on the other.
N 0071-0562-20   Bottles of 60
N 0071-0562-40   Unit dose packages of 100 (10 strips of 10 tablets each).
1000 mg: Gray, film-coated, elliptical tablets, coded "PROCANBID" on one side and "1000" on the other.
N 0071-0564-20   Bottles of 60
N 0071-0564-40   Unit dose packages of 100 (10 strips of 10 tablets each).
Dispense in well-closed containers as defined in the USP.
Store at 20°–25°C (68°–77°F) [see USP].
Caution—Federal law prohibits dispensing without prescription.
September 1995
©1995, Warner-Lambert Co.
PARKE-DAVIS
Div of Warner-Lambert Co
Morris Plains, NJ 07950 USA   0562G020
Shown in Product Identification Guide, page 327

PYRIDIUM® ℞
[py "rĭ'dĭ-ŭm]
(Phenazopyridine Hydrochloride Tablets, USP)

DESCRIPTION

Pyridium (phenazopyridine hydrochloride) is chemically designated 2,6-Pyridinediamine, 3-(phenylazo), monohydrochloride. It is a urinary tract analgesic agent for oral administration. Pyridium tablets contain the following ACTIVE INGREDIENTS: 100 mg or 200 mg phenazopyridine hydrochloride. INACTIVE INGREDIENTS: Acacia, Confectioners Sugar, Corn Starch, Dusting Powder, Gelatin, Hydrogenated Vegetable Oil, Lactose, Magnesium Stearate, Opalux Maroon (includes FD&C Red #40 and FD&C Blue #2), Povidone, Sodium Benzoate, Sodium Starch Glycolate, Sucrose, Titanium Dioxide, Polishing Wax.

CLINICAL PHARMACOLOGY

Pyridium is excreted in the urine where it exerts a topical analgesic effect on the mucosa of the urinary tract. This action helps to relieve pain, burning, urgency and frequency. The precise mechanism of action is not known.
The pharmacokinetic properties of Pyridium have not been determined. Phenazopyridine is rapidly excreted by the kidneys, with as much as 65% of an oral dose being excreted unchanged in the urine.

INDICATIONS AND USAGE

Pyridium is indicated for the symptomatic relief of pain, burning, urgency, frequency, and other discomforts arising from irritation of the lower urinary tract mucosa caused by infection, trauma, surgery, endoscopic procedures, or the passage of sounds or catheters. The use of Pyridium for relief of symptoms should not delay definitive diagnosis and treatment of causative conditions. Because it provides only symptomatic relief, prompt appropriate treatment of the cause of pain must be instituted and Pyridium should be discontinued when symptoms are controlled.
The analgesic action may reduce or eliminate the need for systemic analgesics or narcotics. It is, however, compatible with antibacterial therapy and can help to relieve pain and discomfort during the interval before antibacterial therapy controls the infection. Treatment of a urinary tract infection with Pyridium should not exceed 2 days because there is a lack of evidence that the combined administration of Pyridium and an antibacterial provides greater benefit than administration of the antibacterial alone after 2 days. (See DOSAGE AND ADMINISTRATION section.)

CONTRAINDICATIONS

Pyridium should not be used in patients who have previously exhibited hypersensitivity to it. The use of Pyridium is contraindicated in patients with renal insufficiency.

PRECAUTIONS

General: A yellowish tinge of the skin or sclera may indicate accumulation due to impaired renal excretion and the need to discontinue therapy.
The decline in renal function associated with advanced age should be kept in mind.
Information for Patients: Pyridium produces an orange to red color in the urine and may stain fabric. Staining of contact lenses has been reported.
Laboratory Test Interactions: Due to its properties as an azo dye, Pyridium may interfere with urinalysis based on spectrometry or color reactions.
Carcinogenesis, Mutagenesis, Impairment of Fertility: Long-term administration of phenazopyridine hydrochloride has induced neoplasia in rats (large intestine) and mice (liver). Although no association between phenazopyridine hydrochloride and human neoplasia has been reported, adequate epidemiological studies along these lines have not been conducted.
Pregnancy Category B: Reproduction studies have been performed in rats at doses up to 50 mg/kg/day and have revealed no evidence of impaired fertility or harm to the fetus due to Pyridium. There are, however, no adequate and well controlled studies in pregnant women. Because animal reproduction studies are not always predictive of human response, this drug should be used during pregnancy only if clearly needed.
Nursing Mothers: No information is available on the appearance of Pyridium or its metabolites in human milk.

ADVERSE REACTIONS

Headache, rash, pruritus and occasional gastrointestinal disturbance. An anaphylactoid-like reaction has been described. Methemoglobinemia, hemolytic anemia, renal and

Continued on next page

This product information was prepared in August 1996. On these and other Parke-Davis Products, information may be obtained by addressing PARKE-DAVIS, Division of Warner-Lambert Company, Morris Plains, New Jersey 07950.

Parke-Davis—Cont.

hepatic toxicity have been reported, usually at overdosage levels (see OVERDOSAGE section).

OVERDOSAGE

Exceeding the recommended dose in patients with good renal function or administering the usual dose to patients with impaired renal function (common in elderly patients) may lead to increased serum levels and toxic reactions. Methemoglobinemia generally follows a massive, acute overdose. Methylene blue, 1 to 2 mg/kg body weight intravenously or ascorbic acid 100 to 200 mg given orally should cause prompt reduction of the methemoglobinemia and disappearance of the cyanosis which is an aid in diagnosis. Oxidative Heinz body hemolytic anemia may also occur, and "bite cells" (degmacytes) may be present in a chronic overdosage situation. Red blood cell G-6-PD deficiency may predispose to hemolysis. Renal and hepatic impairment and occasional failure, usually due to hypersensitivity, may also occur.

DOSAGE AND ADMINISTRATION

100 mg tablets: Adult dosage is two tablets 3 times a day after meals. 200 mg tablets: Adult dosage is one tablet 3 times a day after meals.

When used concomitantly with an antibacterial agent for the treatment of a urinary tract infection, the administration of Pyridium should not exceed 2 days.

HOW SUPPLIED

N 0071-0180-24 100-mg tablets
Bottles of 100

Tablets are dark maroon, coated, round and coded P-D 180.

N 0071-0181-24 200-mg tablets
Bottles of 100

Tablets are dark maroon, coated, round and coded P-D 181.

Store at controlled room temperature 15°–30° C (59°–86° F).

Revised August 1994

Manufactured by:
ABLE LABORATORIES, INC.
South Plainfield, NJ 07080
For: **PARKE-DAVIS**
Div. of Warner-Lambert Co.
Morris Plains, NJ 07950 USA
Manufacturer's Code 53265 **0180G251**

Shown in Product Identification Guide, page 327

ZARONTIN® ℞

[*ză″rŏn′tĭn*]
(ethosuximide, USP)
Capsules

DESCRIPTION

Zarontin (ethosuximide) is an anticonvulsant succinimide, chemically designated as alpha-ethyl-alpha-methyl-succinimide, with the following structural formula:

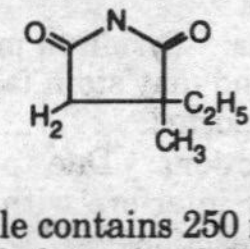

Each Zarontin capsule contains 250 mg ethosuximide, USP. Also contains: polyethylene glycol 400, NF. The capsule contains D&C yellow No. 10; FD&C red No. 3; gelatin, NF; glycerin, USP; and sorbitol.

CLINICAL PHARMACOLOGY

Ethosuximide suppresses the paroxysmal three cycle per second spike and wave activity associated with lapses of consciousness which is common in absence (petit mal) seizures. The frequency of epileptiform attacks is reduced, apparently by depression of the motor cortex and elevation of the threshold of the central nervous system to convulsive stimuli.

INDICATIONS AND USAGE

Zarontin is indicated for the control of absence (petit mal) epilepsy.

CONTRAINDICATION

Ethosuximide should not be used in patients with a history of hypersensitivity to succinimides.

WARNINGS

Blood dyscrasias, including some with fatal outcome, have been reported to be associated with the use of ethosuximide; therefore, periodic blood counts should be performed. Should signs and/or symptoms of infection (eg, sore throat, fever) develop, blood counts should be considered at that point.

Ethosuximide is capable of producing morphological and functional changes in the animal liver. In humans, abnormal liver and renal function studies have been reported.

Ethosuximide should be administered with extreme caution to patients with known liver or renal diseases. Periodic urinalysis and liver function studies are advised for all patients receiving the drug.

Cases of systemic lupus erythematosus have been reported with the use of ethosuximide. The physician should be alert to this possibility.

Usage in Pregnancy: Reports suggest an association between the use of anticonvulsant drugs by women with epilepsy and an elevated incidence of birth defects in children born to these women. Data are more extensive with respect to phenytoin and phenobarbital, but these are also the most commonly prescribed anticonvulsants; less systematic or anecdotal reports suggest a possible similar association with the use of all known anticonvulsant drugs.

The reports suggesting an elevated incidence of birth defects in children of drug-treated epileptic women cannot be regarded as adequate to prove a definite cause and effect relationship. There are intrinsic methodological problems in obtaining adequate data on drug teratogenicity in humans; the possibility also exists that other factors, eg, genetic factors or the epileptic condition itself, may be more important than drug therapy in leading to birth defects. The great majority of mothers on anticonvulsant medication deliver normal infants. It is important to note that anticonvulsant drugs should not be discontinued in patients in whom the drug is administered to prevent major seizures because of the strong possibility of precipitating status epilepticus with attendant hypoxia and threat to life. In individual cases where the severity and frequency of the seizure disorder are such that the removal of medication does not pose a serious threat to the patient, discontinuation of the drug may be considered prior to and during pregnancy, although it cannot be said with any confidence that even minor seizures do not pose some hazard to the developing embryo or fetus.

The prescribing physician will wish to weigh these considerations in treating or counseling epileptic women of childbearing potential.

PRECAUTIONS

General

Ethosuximide, when used alone in mixed types of epilepsy, may increase the frequency of grand mal seizures in some patients.

As with other anticonvulsants, it is important to proceed slowly when increasing or decreasing dosage, as well as when adding or eliminating other medication. Abrupt withdrawal of anticonvulsant medication may precipitate absence (petit mal) status.

Information for Patients

Ethosuximide may impair the mental and/or physical abilities required for the performance of potentially hazardous tasks, such as driving a motor vehicle or other such activity requiring alertness; therefore, the patient should be cautioned accordingly.

Patients taking ethosuximide should be advised of the importance of adhering strictly to the prescribed dosage regimen.

Patients should be instructed to promptly contact their physician if they develop signs and/or symptoms (eg, sore throat, fever) suggesting an infection.

Drug Interactions

Since Zarontin (ethosuximide) may interact with concurrently administered antiepileptic drugs, periodic serum level determinations of these drugs may be necessary (eg, ethosuximide may elevate phenytoin serum levels and valproic acid has been reported to both increase and decrease ethosuximide levels).

Pregnancy

See WARNINGS.

ADVERSE REACTIONS

Gastrointestinal System: Gastrointestinal symptoms occur frequently and include anorexia, vague gastric upset, nausea and vomiting, cramps, epigastric and abdominal pain, weight loss, and diarrhea. There have been reports of gum hypertrophy and swelling of the tongue.

Hemopoietic System: Hemopoietic complications associated with the administration of ethosuximide have included leukopenia, agranulocytosis, pancytopenia, with or without bone marrow suppression, and eosinophilia.

Nervous System: Neurologic and sensory reactions reported during therapy with ethosuximide have included drowsiness, headache, dizziness, euphoria, hiccups, irritability, hyperactivity, lethargy, fatigue, and ataxia. Psychiatric or psychological aberrations associated with ethosuximide administration have included disturbances of sleep, night terrors, inability to concentrate, and aggressiveness. These effects may be noted particularly in patients who have previously exhibited psychological abnormalities. There have been rare reports of paranoid psychosis, increased libido, and increased state of depression with overt suicidal intentions.

Integumentary System: Dermatologic manifestations which have occurred with the administration of ethosuximide have included urticaria, Stevens-Johnson syndrome, systemic lupus erythematosus, pruritic erythematous rashes, and hirsutism.

Special Senses: Myopia.

Genitourinary System: Vaginal bleeding, microscopic hematuria.

OVERDOSAGE

Acute overdoses may produce nausea, vomiting, and CNS depression including coma with respiratory depression. A relationship between ethosuximide toxicity and its plasma levels has not been established. The therapeutic range of serum levels is 40 mcg/mL to 100 mcg/mL, although levels as high as 150 mcg/mL have been reported without signs of toxicity.

Treatment:

Treatment should include emesis (unless the patient is or could rapidly become obtunded, comatose, or convulsing) or gastric lavage, activated charcoal, cathartics and general supportive measures. Hemodialysis may be useful to treat ethosuximide overdose. Forced diuresis and exchange transfusions are ineffective.

DOSAGE AND ADMINISTRATION

Zarontin is administered by the oral route. The *initial* dose for patients 3 to 6 years of age is one capsule (250 mg) per day; for patients 6 years of age and older, 2 capsules (500 mg) per day. The dose thereafter must be individualized according to the patient's response. Dosage should be increased by small increments. One useful method is to increase the daily dose by 250 mg every four to seven days until control is achieved with minimal side effects. Dosages exceeding 1.5 g daily, in divided doses, should be administered only under the strictest supervision of the physician. The *optimal* dose for most children is 20 mg/kg/day. This dose has given average plasma levels within the accepted therapeutic range of 40 to 100 mcg/mL. Subsequent dose schedules can be based on effectiveness and plasma level determinations.

Zarontin may be administered in combination with other anticonvulsants when other forms of epilepsy coexist with absence (petit mal). The *optimal* dose for most children is 20 mg/kg/day.

HOW SUPPLIED

Zarontin is supplied as:

N 0071-0237-24 Bottles of 100. Each capsule contains 250 mg ethosuximide.

Store at controlled room temperature 15°–30°C (59°–86°F).

Zarontin is also supplied as:

N 0071-2418-23—1 pint bottles. Each 5 mL of syrup contains 250 mg ethosuximide in a raspberry flavored base.

Caution—Federal law prohibits dispensing without prescription.

Revised May 1995 **0237G027**

Shown in Product Identification Guide, page 327

ZARONTIN® ℞

[*ză″rŏn′tĭn*]
(ethosuximide)
Syrup

DESCRIPTION

Zarontin (ethosuximide) is an anticonvulsant succinimide, chemically designated as alpha-ethyl-alpha-methyl-succinimide, with the following structural formula:

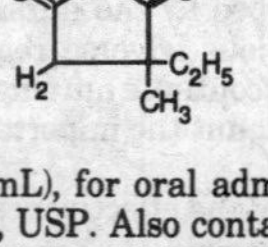

Each teaspoonful (5 mL), for oral administration, contains 250 mg ethosuximide, USP. Also contains citric acid; anhydrous, USP; FD&C red No. 40; FD&C yellow No. 6; flavor; glycerin, USP; purified water, USP; saccharin sodium, USP; sodium benzoate, NF; sodium citrate, USP; sucrose, NF.

CLINICAL PHARMACOLOGY

Ethosuximide suppresses the paroxysmal three cycle per second spike and wave activity associated with lapses of consciousness which is common in absence (petit mal) seizures. The frequency of epileptiform attacks is reduced, apparently by depression of the motor cortex and elevation of the threshold of the central nervous system to convulsive stimuli.

INDICATION AND USAGE

Zarontin is indicated for the control of absence (petit mal) epilepsy.

CONTRAINDICATIONS

Ethosuximide should not be used in patients with a history of hypersensitivity to succinimides.

WARNINGS

Blood dyscrasias, including some with fatal outcome, have been reported to be associated with the use of ethosuximide; therefore, periodic blood counts should be performed. Should signs and/or symptoms of infection (eg, sore throat, fever) develop, blood counts should be considered at that point. Ethosuximide is capable of producing morphological and functional change in the animal liver. In humans, abnormal liver and renal function studies have been reported. Ethosuximide should be administered with extreme caution to

patients with known liver or renal disease. Periodic urinalysis and liver function studies are advised for all patients receiving the drug.

Cases of systemic lupus erythematosus have been reported with the use of ethosuximide. The physician should be alert to this possibility.

Usage in Pregnancy: Reports suggest an association between the use of anticonvulsant drugs by women with epilepsy and an elevated incidence of birth defects in children born to these women. Data are more extensive with respect to phenytoin and phenobarbital, but these are also the most commonly prescribed anticonvulsants; less systematic or anecdotal reports suggest a possible similar association with the use of all known anticonvulsant drugs.

The reports suggesting an elevated incidence of birth defects in children of drug-treated epileptic women cannot be regarded as adequate to prove a definite cause and effect relationship. There are intrinsic methodologic problems in obtaining adequate data on drug teratogenicity in humans; the possibility also exists that other factors, eg. genetic factors or the epileptic condition itself, may be more important than drug therapy in leading to birth defects. The great majority of mothers on anticonvulsant medication deliver normal infants. It is important to note that anticonvulsant drugs should not be discontinued in patients in whom the drug is administered to prevent major seizures because of the strong possibility of precipitating status epilepticus with attendant hypoxia and threat to life. In individual cases where the severity and frequency of the seizure disorder are such that the removal of medication does not pose a serious threat to the patient, discontinuation of the drug may be considered prior to and during pregnancy, although it cannot be said with any confidence that even minor seizures do not pose some hazard to the developing embryo or fetus.

The prescribing physician will wish to weigh these considerations in treating or counseling epileptic women of childbearing potential.

PRECAUTIONS

General: Ethosuximide, when used alone in mixed types of epilepsy, may increase the frequency of grand mal seizures in some patients.

As with other anticonvulsants, it is important to proceed slowly when increasing or decreasing dosage, as well as when adding or eliminating other medication. Abrupt withdrawal of anticonvulsant medication may precipitate absence (petit mal) status.

Information for Patients: Ethosuximide may impair the mental and/or physical abilities required for the performance of potentially hazardous tasks such as driving a motor vehicle or other such activity requiring alertness; therefore, the patient should be cautioned accordingly.

Patients taking ethosuximide should be advised of the importance of adhering strictly to the prescribed dosage regimen. Patients should be instructed to promptly contact their physician when they develop signs and/or symptoms suggesting an infection (eg, sore throat, fever).

Drug Interactions: Since Zarontin (ethosuximide) may interact with concurrently administered antiepileptic drugs, periodic serum level determinations of both drugs are recommended (ethosuximide may elevate phenytoin serum levels and valproic acid has been reported to both increase and decrease ethosuximide levels).

Pregnancy: See WARNINGS

ADVERSE REACTIONS

Gastrointestinal System: Gastrointestinal symptoms occur frequently and include anorexia, vague gastric upset, nausea and vomiting, cramps, epigastric and abdominal pain, weight loss, and diarrhea. There have been reports of gum hypertrophy and swelling of the tongue.

Hemopoietic System: Hemopoietic complications associated with the administration of ethosuximide have included leukopenia, agranulocytosis, pancytopenia with or without bone marrow suppression, and eosinophilia.

Nervous System: Neurologic and sensory reactions reported during therapy with ethosuximide have included drowsiness, headache, dizziness, euphoria, hiccups, irritability, hyperactivity, lethargy, fatigue, and ataxia.

Psychiatric or psychological aberrations associated with ethosuximide administration have included disturbances of sleep, night terrors, inability to concentrate, and aggressiveness. These effects may be noted particularly in patients who have previously exhibited psychological abnormalities. There have been rare reports of paranoid psychosis, increased libido, and increased state of depression with overt suicidal intentions.

Integumentary System: Dermatologic manifestations which have occurred with the administration of ethosuximide have included urticaria, Stevens-Johnson syndrome, systemic lupus erythematosus, pruritic erythematous rashes, and hirsutism.

Special Senses: Myopia.

Genitourinary System: Vaginal bleeding, microscopic hematuria.

DOSAGE AND ADMINISTRATION

Zarontin is administered by the oral route. The *initial* dose for patients 3 to 6 years of age is one teaspoonful (250 mg) per day; for patients 6 years of age and older, 2 teaspoonfuls (500 mg) per day. The dose thereafter must be individualized according to the patient's response. Dosage should be increased by small increments. One useful method is to increase the daily dose by 250 mg every four to seven days until control is achieved with minimal side effects. Dosages exceeding 1.5 g daily, in divided doses, should be administered only under the strictest supervision of the physician. The *optimal* dose for most children is 20 mg/kg/day. This dose has given average plasma levels within the accepted therapeutic range of 40 to 100 mcg/mL. Subsequent dose schedules can be based on effectiveness and plasma level determinations.

Zarontin may be administered in combination with other anticonvulsants when other forms of epilepsy coexist with absence (petit mal). The optimal dose for most children is 20 mg/kg/day.

OVERDOSAGE

Acute overdoses produce CNS depression including coma with respiratory depression. A relationship between ethosuximide toxicity and its plasma levels has not been established. The therapeutic range of serum levels is 40 mcg/mL to 100 mcg/mL, although levels as high as 150 mcg/mL have been reported without signs of toxicity.

Treatment: Treatment should include emesis (unless the patient is, or could rapidly become, obtunded, comatose, or convulsing) or gastric lavage, activated charcoal, cathartics, and general supportive measures. Hemodialysis may be useful to treat ethosuximide overdose. Forced diuresis and exchange transfusions are ineffective.

HOW SUPPLIED

Zarontin is supplied as:
N0071-2418-23—1 pint bottles. Each 5 ml of syrup contains 250 mg ethosuximide in a raspberry flavored base.
Store below 30°C (86°F). Protect from freezing and light.
Zarontin is also supplied in the following form:
N0071-0237-24—Bottles of 100. Each capsule contains 250 mg ethosuximide.
Store at controlled room temperature 15°–30°C (59°–86°F).
Caution—Federal law prohibits dispensing without prescription.
Revised May 1994   2418G026

Pedinol Pharmacal Inc.
30 BANFI PLAZA NORTH
FARMINGDALE, N.Y. 11735

Direct Inquiries to:
Director of Professional Services
(516) 293-9500

BREEZEE MIST® FOOT POWDER   OTC

DESCRIPTION
Cooling formula soothes and helps keep feet dry and odor free.

HOW SUPPLIED
4 oz. (113g) aerosol can. 0884 0659-04
Store at controlled room temperature 15°–30°C (59°–86°F)

CASTELLANI PAINT Modified   OTC
CASTELLANI PAINT Modified–Colorless   OTC

DESCRIPTION
Castellani Paint Modified is a first aid antiseptic and drying agent. Care should be taken to avoid spilling. Guard against staining as Castellani Paint Modified will stain skin and clothing.

HOW SUPPLIED

Bottle Size 1 oz. (29.57 mL)	1 pt. (453.6 mL)
Color NDC 0884-2893-01	NDC 0884-2893-16
Colorless NDC 0884-2993-01	NDC 0884-2993-16

Store at controlled room temperature 15°–30°C (59°–86°F)

CITRADERM™   OTC
[*sitra-durm*]
L-Ascorbic Acid USP 10%

DESCRIPTION
FACIAL COMPLEX—The highest level of stable Vitamin C (L-Ascorbic Acid) available in a super emollient, quick absorbing, non-greasy formula.

DIRECTIONS
Apply sparingly and feather into skin as directed by your Dermatologist. Apply moisturizer or TI-SCREEN Sunscreen SPF 15 as usual.
Cap tightly after use.
CAUTION: FOR EXTERNAL USE ONLY. KEEP OUT OF THE REACH OF CHILDREN.
Keep away from open flame. Store in a cool, dry place, away from sunlight.

HOW SUPPLIED
FACIAL COMPLEX CREAM 0.5 oz   0884-5996-15

DERMACIN™ CREME   R
(FLUOCINONIDE CREAM USP, 0.05%)

DESCRIPTION
The topical corticosteroids constitute a class of primarily synthetic steroids used as anti-inflammatory and antipruritic agents. The steroids in this class include fluocinonide. Fluocinonide is designed chemically as pregna-1,4-diene-3,20-dione, 21-(acetyloxy)-6,9-difluoro-11-hydroxy-16, 17-[(1-methylethylidene)bis(oxy)]-, (6a,11B,16a)-.
Each gram of Fluocinonide Cream USP, 0.05% contains 0.5 mg of Fluocinonide in PGEA™ cream base, a specially formulated cream base consisting of ethoxylated alcohol (Beheneth-20), polyethylene glycol 8000, sorbitan monostearate, stearic acid, propylene glycol and citric acid, anhydrous.
The cream is white, non-staining greaseless, anhydrous and water washable.

HOW SUPPLIED
Available in a 30 gram (1.06 oz) tube. NDC 0884-5793-01

FORMALYDE-10® SPRAY   R

DESCRIPTION
Formalyde-10 Spray is a topical solution containing Formaldehyde 10% to safeguard against offensive odor and dry excessive moisture of the feet. Drying agent for pre & post-surgical removal of warts where dryness is required.

HOW SUPPLIED
Available in 2 oz. (59.14 mL) plastic spray bottle.
NDC 0884 4789-02
Store at controlled room temperature 15°–30°C (59°–86°F)

FUNGOID® CREME   R

DESCRIPTION
Fungoid Creme (Clotrimazole Cream USP, 1%) is indicated for the topical treatment of candidiasis due to Candida albicans and tinea versicolor due to Malassezia furfur.

HOW SUPPLIED
NDC 0884-2495-45
Fungoid® Creme is available in a 45 gram tube.
Store between 2°-30°C (36°-86°F).

FUNGOID® SOLUTION   R
Antifungal Solution

DESCRIPTION
Undecylenic Acid is chemically 10-hendecenoic acid having an empirical formula $C_{11}H_{20}O_2$ and the chemical bond structure $CH_2=CH(CH_2)_8CO_2H$. Undecylenic Acid is a colorless to pale yellow liquid which is soluble in water, alcohol, chlorform and ether. It is a fungistatic agent employed in the treatment of tinea pedis, (athlete's foot) tinea capitis, ringworm and dermatophytosis. Benzalkonium Chloride, Chloroxylenol and PEG 8 are in the base for their softening effect.

HOW SUPPLIED
NDC 0884-3194-01
Available in a 1 oz (29.57 mL) plastic bottle with controlled dropper.
Store at controlled room temperature 15°–30°C (59°–86°F).

Continued on next page

Pedinol Pharmacal—Cont.

FUNGOID® TINCTURE   OTC

DESCRIPTION

A topical antifungal which is applied as a thin application twice a day (morning and night), to the affected area using the attached brush, **or as recommended by your physician.** Remove Fungoid Tincture from any untreated areas.

HOW SUPPLIED

1 oz. (29.57 mL) bottle with brush applicator NDC 0884-0293-01, 1 pt. (473.12 mL) bottle NDC 0884-0293-16.
FUNGOID TINCTURE TOPICAL ANTIFUNGAL TREATMENT KIT includes: 1 oz. (29.57 mL) FUNGOID TINCTURE, 2 oz. (56.7g) NAIL SCRUB, nail brush. NDC 0884-5493-01.
Store at controlled room temperature 15°–30°C (59°–86°F). Protect from freezing.

G–MYTICIN® CREME 0.1%   ℞
(gentamicin sulfate 0.1%)

DESCRIPTION

G-myticin Creme—each gram contains gentamicin sulfate equivalent to 1 mg. of gentamicin base, and is a topical wide-spectrum antibiotic which provides highly effective treatment in primary and secondary bacterial infections of the skin. *NOTE:* G-myticin Creme is not effective against viruses or fungal skin infections.

HOW SUPPLIED

G-myticin Creme—15 gm tube.
Creme NDC 0884-3684-15.

HYDRISINOL® CREME and LOTION   OTC

DESCRIPTION

Both Hydrisinol Creme and Lotion contain Sulfonated Castor Oil in a Hydrogenated Vegetable Oil Base for application on dry, cracked, calloused skin and are particularly useful after a bath, shower, exposure to the sun or wind to help soften the skin by containing the moisture in the skin.

HOW SUPPLIED

4 oz. (113.4g) 0884 0142-04 and 1 lb. (453.6g) jars 0884-0142-16;
8 oz. (226.8g) plastic bottle 0884-3042-08.

LACTINOL-E® CREME   ℞
LACTINOL® LOTION   ℞

DESCRIPTION

Lactic acid has been reported as an effective naturally occurring humectant in the skin. It has beneficial effects on dry skin and on severe hyperkeratotic conditions. Vitamin E has been used as an aid to control dry or chapped skin. Vitamin E has also found application as an aid in the relief of minor skin disorders such as burns, sunburn, and irritated skin. It has antioxidant properties thus protecting the skin. Lactinol-E Creme and Lactinol Lotion which contain Lactic Acid 10%, is indicated for moisturizing and softening dry, scaly skin (xerosis), ichthyosis vulgaris and itching associated with these conditions.

HOW SUPPLIED

Lactinol-E Creme is available in a 4 oz. (113.4g) plastic jar. NDC 0884-4990-04
Lactinol Lotion is available in an 8 oz. (226.8g) bottle. NDC 0884-5292-08
Store at controlled room temperature 15°–30°C (59°–86°F).

LAZER® CREME   OTC

DESCRIPTION

The moisturizing ingredients Vitamin A and Vitamin E aid in the natural healing process of fissures, keratosis and dryness of the skin, post surgical regeneration of the skin and to revitalize lasered tissue.

HOW SUPPLIED

Available in 2 oz. (56.7g) plastic jar. 0884 3886-02

LAZERFORMALYDE® SOLUTION   ℞

DESCRIPTION

Lazerformalyde Solution is a topical solution containing Formaldehyde 10% as a drying agent for pre and post surgical removal of warts or for non-surgical laser treatment of warts where dryness is required. Safeguards against offensive odor and dries excessive moisture of feet.

HOW SUPPLIED

Available in 3 oz. (88.71 mL) plastic bottle with **roll-on** applicator. NDC 0884 3986-03
Store at controlled room temperature 15°–30°C (59°–86°F).

LAZERSPORIN–C® SOLUTION   ℞

DESCRIPTION

Lazersporin-C Solution is a combination of Neomycin Sulfate USP, Polymixin B Sulfate USP, and Hydrocortisone 1% USP for the treatment of superficial bacterial infections of the external auditory canal caused by organisms susceptible to the action of the antibiotics. **For otic use. Not for ophthalmic use.**

HOW SUPPLIED

10cc bottle with sterile dropper. NDC 0884 4086-10
Store at controlled room temperature 15°–30°C (59°–86°F).

NAIL SCRUB™   OTC

DESCRIPTION

Nail Scrub is a nail rejuvenator, cleanser and bleaching agent which is applied to the nail surface and scrubbed briskly with a nail brush. The nail scrub is then washed off and the nail dried. Nail scrub is useful for smoothing out rough, thickened nails and reduction of discoloration from fungus infections.

HOW SUPPLIED

Available in 2 oz. (56.7g) plastic bottle with applicator tip. 0884 4891-02

OSTIDERM®
OSTIDERM® ROLL ON   OTC

DESCRIPTION

Safeguards against offensive odor and dries excessive moisture of the feet. Provides comfort while absorbing moisture. **NOTE: If contents harden, add hot water and stir.** Not for Roll-On.

HOW SUPPLIED

1.5 oz. (42.5g) jar. 0884 2051-45
3 oz (88.71 mL) Roll 0884-2052-03
Store at Controlled Room Temperature 15–30°C (59°–86°F).

PEDI–BORO® SOAK PAKS   OTC

DESCRIPTION

Pedi-Boro makes a soothing wet dressing of a modified Burow's Solution, Buffered. A mild astringent solution to aid in the relief of minor skin irritations due to allergies, poison ivy, insect bites, or athlete's foot, and as an aid in the relief of swelling associated with minor bruises. Dissolve one or two paks in a pint of water and prepare fresh daily.

HOW SUPPLIED

Box of 12's 0884 1773-27
Box of 100's 0884 1773-10

PEDI–DRI® TOPICAL POWDER   ℞

DESCRIPTION

Pedi-Dri Topical Powder provides in each gram 100,000 USP nystatin units dispersed in a corn starch, kaolin formulation. Nystatin is an antifungal antibiotic which is both fungistatic and fungicidal in vitro against a wide variety of yeasts and yeast-like fungus. It probably acts by binding to sterols in the cell membrane of the fungus with a resultant change in membrane permeability allowing leakage of intracellular compounds. Nystatin is a polyene antibiotic of undetermined structural formula that is obtained from Streptomyces noursei, and is the first well tolerated antifungal antibiotic of dependable efficacy for the treatment of cutaneous, oral and intestinal infections caused by Candida (Monilia) albicans and other candida species. It exhibits no appreciable activity against bacteria. Nystatin provides specific therapy for all localized forms of candidiasis. Symptomatic relief is rapid, often occurring within 24 to 48 hours after the initiation of treatment.
Pedi-Dri Topical Powder (Nystatin) is a topical preparation indicated in the treatment of cutaneous or mucocutaneous mycotic infections caused by Candida albicans and other Candida species. The formulation also safeguards against offensive odor and dries excessive moisture.

HOW SUPPLIED

Available in a 2 oz. plastic bottle (56.7g) with shaker cap. NDC 0884-0394-02
Store at controlled room temperature 15°–30°C (59°–86°F).

PEDI–PRO® TOPICAL POWDER   OTC

DESCRIPTION

PEDI-PRO is an absorbing, drying, deodorizing topical powder

HOW SUPPLIED

2 oz. (56.7g) plastic bottle. 0884 3584-02

SAL–ACID® PLASTER   OTC

DESCRIPTION

Medicated plaster of Salicylic Acid 40%, for the removal of common and plantar warts. The common wart can be easily recognized by the rough, cauliflower-like appearance of the surface. The plantar wart is recognized by its location only on the bottom of the foot, its tenderness and the interruption of the footprint pattern. The specialized gauze pad helps relieve painful pressure, while the SAL-ACID PLASTER medication remedies the wart. To be applied over the wart daily as directed by your physician.

HOW SUPPLIED

SAL-ACID® PLASTER is available in 14 plasters per package, 0884-4393-14.

SALACTIC® FILM   OTC
SAL–PLANT® GEL

DESCRIPTION

Salactic Film and Sal-Plant Gel both contain Salicylic Acid 17% USP in a collodion-like vehicle, for the removal of common warts. The common wart is easily recognized by the rough cauliflower-like appearance of the surface.
For the removal of plantar warts on the bottom of the foot. The plantar wart is recognized by its location only on the bottom of the foot, its tenderness and the interruption of the footprint pattern.

HOW SUPPLIED

Salactic Film available in 0.5 oz (15 mL) bottle with brush applicator. NDC 0884-2592-15
Sal-Plant Gel available in a 0.5 oz (14g) tube with tip applicator. NDC 0884 5192-15

TI–SCREEN®   OTC
SPF 15
SPF 16 (NATURAL AND BABY)
SPF 20
SPF 30
LIP PROTECTANT SPF 15

DESCRIPTION

SPF 15 and SPF 30 are moisturizing sunscreen lotions. SPF 20 is a sportsgel. SPF 16 is a natural moisturizing sunblock.
SPF 15 lip protectant sunscreen.

HOW SUPPLIED

TI-SCREEN SPF 15 Lotion 4 oz. bottle NDC 0884-1596-04
SPF 16 Lotion, 4 oz. bottle NDC 0884-1696-04
SPF 16 Baby 4 oz. bottle NDC 0884-6196-04
SPF 20 Gel 4 oz. bottle NDC 0884-2096-04
SPF 30 Lotion 4 oz. bottle NDC 0884-3096-04
SPF 15 Lip Prot. 0.15 oz. stick NDC 0884-1096-01

UREACIN®–10 LOTION   OTC
UREACIN®–20 CREME   OTC

DESCRIPTION

Ureacin-10 Lotion and Ureacin-20 Creme are topical treatments for rough, dry, cracked, calloused skin.

HOW SUPPLIED

Ureacin®-10, 8 oz. (226.8g) plastic bottle 0884 3249-08, Ureacin®-20, 4 oz. (113.4g) plastic jar 0884-0449-04.
Store at controlled room temperature 15°–30°C (59°–86°F)

Persōn & Covey, Inc.
P.O. Box 25018
GLENDALE, CA 91221-5018

For Additional Information:
(818) 240-1030
(800) 423-2341

AQUANIL HC™ LOTION   OTC
Lipid-free with 1.0% Hydrocortisone
Non-comedogenic

INDICATIONS
AQUANIL HC Lotion contains 1.0% Hydrocortisone an effective anti-itch ingredient, in a gentle, free flowing, lipid-free (oil free), lotion, formulated for sensitive skin. It is indicated for the temporary relief of minor skin irritations, inflammations, itches and rashes due to seborrheic dermatitis, insect bites, eczema, psoriasis, soaps, detergents, cosmetics, jewelry, poison oak, poison ivy and poison sumac. Other uses of this product should be only under the advice and supervision of a physician.

DIRECTIONS
For adults and children 2 years of age and older: Apply to affected area not more than 3 to 4 times daily. For children under 2 years of age there is no recommended dosage except under the advice and supervision of a physician.

WARNINGS
For external use only. Avoid contact with eyes. If condition worsens, or if symptoms persist for more than 7 days or clear up and occur again within a few days, discontinue use of this product and do not begin use of any other hydrocortisone product unless you have consulted a physician. Do not use for diaper rash, consult a physician. Keep this and all drugs out of reach of children. In case of accidental ingestion, seek professional assistance or contact a Poison Control Center immediately.

Store at room temperature.
Shake well before using.

Active Ingredient: Hydrocortisone U.S.P. 1.0% (Micronized). Inactive Ingredients: Purified Water, Glycerin, Cetyl Alcohol, Stearyl Alcohol, Benzyl Alcohol. Sodium Laureth Sulfate, Simethicone, Xanthan Gum.

HOW SUPPLIED
Plastic bottle, 118.3 ml (4 fluid oz.) (NDC 0096-0732-04)

DHS™ Tar Shampoo and   OTC
DHS Tar Gel Shampoo (Scented)
Aids in the control of the scaling of seborrhea (dandruff) and psoriasis of the scalp.

DIRECTIONS
Wet hair thoroughly apply a liberal quantity of DHS Tar Shampoo and massage into a lather. Rinse thoroughly and repeat application. Allow lather to remain on scalp for about 5 minutes. Use DHS Tar Shampoo once or twice weekly, or as directed by your physician.

CONTAINS
Tar, equivalent to 0.5% Coal Tar, TEA-Lauryl Sulfate, Purified Water, U.S.P., Sodium Chloride, PEG-8 Distearate, Cocamide DEA, Cocamide MEA, Citric Acid. DHS Tar Gel Shampoo also contains: Hydroxypropyl Methylcellulose and fragrance.

WARNINGS
For external use only. Avoid contact with eyes. If contact occurs, rinse eyes thoroughly with water. If condition worsens or does not improve after regular use of the product as directed consult a physician. Use caution in exposing skin to sunlight after applying this product. It may increase your tendency to sunburn for up to 24 hours after application. Do not use this product for prolonged periods without consulting a physician. Do not use this product with other forms of psoriasis therapy such as ultraviolet radiation or prescription drugs, unless directed to do so by a physician. If condition covers a large portion of the body, consult your physician before using this product. In rare instances, discoloration of gray, blond, bleach or tinted hair may occur. Store away from direct sunlight. Keep this and all drugs out of the reach of children. In

case of accidental ingestion, seek professional assistance or contact a Poison Control Center immediately.

HOW SUPPLIED
Plastic bottles. DHS Tar Shampoo, 4, 8 and 16 fl. oz. (NDC 0096-0728-04, 0096-0728-08, 0096-0728-16). DHS Tar Gel Shampoo 8 fl. oz. (NDC 0096-0730-08).

DHS Zinc Dandruff Shampoo
2% Zinc Pyrithione
Aids in the control of dandruff/seborrheic dermatitis of the scalp.

DIRECTIONS
Shake well before using. Wet hair thoroughly; apply a liberal quantity of DHS Zinc Shampoo and massage into a lather. Rinse thoroughly and repeat application. Allow lather to remain on scalp for about 5 minutes. Use DHS Zinc Shampoo at least twice weekly for the first two weeks, then regularly thereafter, or as directed by your physician.

CONTAINS
2% Zinc Pyrithione, Purified Water, U.S.P., TEA-Lauryl Sulfate, PEG-8 Distearate, Sodium Chloride, Cocamide DEA, Cocamide MEA, Magnesium Aluminum Silicate, Hydroxypropyl Methylcellulose, fragrance and FD&C yellow #6.

WARNING
For external use only. Avoid contact with eyes. If contact occurs, rinse eyes thoroughly with water. If condition worsens or does not improve after regular use of this product as directed, consult a physician. If condition covers a large portion of the body, consult your physician before using this product. **Keep this and all drugs out of the reach of children.** In case of accidental ingestion, seek professional assistance or contact a Poison Control Center immediately.

HOW SUPPLIED
Plastic bottles, 8 and 12 fl. oz. (NDC 0096-0729-08 , 0096-0729-12).

DHS Sal Shampoo
3% Salicylic Acid USP aids in the control of dandruff, psoriasis and seborrheic dermatitis.

DIRECTIONS
Wet hair thoroughly, apply a liberal amount of DHS Sal and massage into a rich lather. Allow lather to remain on scalp for several minutes. Rinse hair and repeat application. For best results use at least twice a week or as directed by a physician.

WARNINGS
For external use only. Avoid contact with eyes. If contact occurs, rinse eyes thoroughly with water. If condition worsens or does not improve after regular use of this products as directed, consult a physician. If condition covers a large portion of the body, consult your physician before using this product. Keep this and all drugs out of reach of children. In case of accidental ingestion, seek professional assistance or contact a Poison Control Center immediately.
Active Ingredient: 3% Salicylic Acid U.S.P. Other Ingredients: Purified Water, Sodium C14–16, Olefin Sulfonate, Tea-Lauryl Sulfate, Cocamidopropyl Betaine, PEG-8 Distearate, Cocamide DEA, Cocamide MEA, Disodium EDTA.

HOW SUPPLIED
Plastic bottle 4 fl. oz NDC 0096-0731-04

DML™ FACIAL MOISTURIZER   OTC
Moisturizer with Sunscreen (SPF 15)
Hyaluronic Acid
Non-comedogenic
Fragrance Free

INDICATION
Contains special ingredients that help soothe dry, sensitive skin. Contains sunscreen agents with an SPF of 15 to protect from damaging effects of sunlight (UVA & UVB).

DIRECTIONS
Apply to face as needed or as directed by your dermatologist.

CAUTION
For external use only. Avoid contact with eyes. Keep out of reach of children.

CONTENTS
Active: Octyl Methoxycinnamate 7.5%, Oxybenzone USP 4%, Inactive: Purified Water, Propylene Glycol Dioctanoate, Petrolatum USP, Glycerin, Cetyl Phosphate (and) DEA-Cetyl Phosphate, Glyceryl Stearate (and) PEG-100 Stearate, Stearic Acid, Hyaluronic Acid, Benzyl Alcohol, Dimethicone, PVP/Eicosene Copolymer, Sodium Carbomer 941, Disodium EDTA, Magnesium Aluminum Silicate.

HOW SUPPLIED
Plastic tube, 1½ oz.   (NDC 0096-0721-45)

DRYSOL™   ℞

A Solution of:
Aluminum Chloride (Hexahydrate) 20% w/v in Anhydrous Ethyl Alcohol (S.D. Alcohol 40) 93% v/v.

INDICATION
An aid in the management of hyperhidrosis.

DIRECTIONS
Apply Drysol to the affected area once a day, **only at bedtime.** To help prevent irritation, the area should be completely dry prior to application. Do not apply Drysol to broken, irritated or recently shaved skin.

FOR MAXIMUM EFFECT
Your doctor may instruct you to cover the treated area with saran wrap held in place by a snug fitting "T" or body shirt, mitten or sock. (Never hold saran in place with tape.) Wash the treated area the following morning. Excessive sweating may be stopped after two or more treatments. Thereafter, apply Drysol once or twice weekly or as needed.

NOTICE
Drysol may produce a burning or prickling sensation. Keep cap tightly closed when not in use to prevent evaporation.

WARNING
For external use only. Keep out of the reach of children. Avoid contact with the eyes. If irritation or sensitization occurs, discontinue use or consult with a physician. Drysol may be harmful to certain metals and fabrics. Keep away from open flame.

HOW SUPPLIED
37.5 cc polyethylene bottle (NDC 0096-0707-37) 35 cc bottle and Drysol Dab-O-Matic 60 cc (NDC 0096-0707-60) with Dab-O-Matic applicator head (NDC 0096-0707-35).

SOLBAR® SUNSCREENS   OTC

SOLBAR sunscreens are specially formulated to provide maximum protection from the sun's burning and tanning rays. Provides substantial broad spectrum protection from UVA and UVB light for sun sensitive and fair skinned persons. Fragrance-free formulas. Liberal and regular use of these products over the years may help reduce the chance of premature aging of the skin and skin cancer.

SOLBAR® PF ULTRA CREAM SPF 50†*+   OTC
Ultra protection sunscreen
Broad Spectrum UVA and UVB protection

CONTAINS
Oxybenzone U.S.P., Octyl Methoxycinnamate, Octocrylene

INDICATIONS
SOLBAR PF 50 Cream is specially formulated for ultra protection from the sun's burning and tanning rays. Oxybenzone enhances protection from UVA and UVB light which is particularly important to photosensitive or photoallergic people. Waterproof formula maintains sunburn protection up to 80 minutes in water. Liberal and regular use of this product over the years may help reduce the chance of premature aging of the skin and skin cancer.

HOW SUPPLIED
Plastic bottle, 4oz. (NDC 0096-0686-04).

SOLBAR® PF ULTRA LIQUID SPF 30†*+   OTC
Ultra protection sunscreen
Broad Spectrum UVA and UVB protection

CONTAINS
Octocrylene, Octyl Methoxycinnamate, Oxybenzone and SD Alcohol 40.

INDICATIONS
SOLBAR PF 30 LIQUID is specially formulated for oily, acne prone skin ultra protection from the sun's burning and tanning rays. Oxybenzone enhances the protection from long wave ultraviolet which is particularly important to photosensitive or photoallergic people. Liberal and regular use of this product over the years may help reduce the chance of

Continued on next page

Person & Covey, Inc.—Cont.

premature aging of the skin and skin cancer.
WARNING: Keep away from open flame.

HOW SUPPLIED

Plastic bottle, 3.8 oz. (NDC 0096-0685-04)

---

† Directions: Apply liberally on all exposed skin. To ensure maximum protection, reapply after swimming or exercise.
* Caution: If irritation or sensitization occurs, discontinue use and consult a physician. Avoid contact with the eyes.
+ Warning: For external use only. Keep out of the reach of children.

XERAC™ AC   ℞
Aluminum Chloride Hexahydrate in
Anhydrous Ethyl Alcohol

DESCRIPTION

A solution of Aluminum Chloride (Hexahydrate) 6.25% (w/v) in Anhydrous Ethyl Alcohol (S.D. Alcohol 40) 96% (v/v).

INDICATION

For topical application as an antiperspirant (anhidrotic).

DIRECTIONS

Apply Xerac AC to the axillae at bedtime or as directed by physician. To help prevent irritation, the area should be completely dry prior to application. Do not apply Xerac AC to broken or irritated skin. Keep container tightly closed.

ADVERSE REACTIONS

Transient stinging or itching may occur. It is not evidence of contact sensitivity and may be prevented or reduced by applying Xerac AC only to skin which is completely dry or by removing the solution with soap and water.

WARNING

For external use only. Some users of this product will experience skin irritation. If this occurs, discontinue use. Avoid contact with the eyes. This product may be harmful to certain metals and fabrics. Keep the container tightly closed when not in use to prevent evaporation. Keep this and all medication out of the reach of children. Do not use near open flame.

HOW SUPPLIED

In bottles with Dab-O-Matic applicator head. 35 cc (NDC 0096-0709-35) and 60 cc (NDC 0096-0709-60).

Pfizer Inc
Consumer Health Care
Group
235 E. 42nd STREET
NY, NY 10017-5755

Direct Inquiries to:
Address Questions & Comments to:
Consumer Relations
(800) 723-7529

For Medical Emergencies/Information Contact:
(800) 723-7529

BONINE®   OTC
(Meclizine hydrochloride)
Chewable Tablets

ACTION

BONINE (meclizine) is an H_1 histamine receptor blocker of the piperazine side chain group. It exhibits its action by an effect on the Central Nervous System (CNS), possibly by its ability to block muscarinic receptors in the brain.

INDICATIONS

BONINE is effective in the management of nausea, vomiting and dizziness associated with motion sickness.

CONTRAINDICATIONS

Do not take this product, unless directed by a doctor, if you have a breathing problem such as emphysema or chronic bronchitis, or if you have glaucoma or difficulty in urination due to enlargement of the prostate gland.

WARNINGS

May cause drowsiness; alcohol, sedatives and tranquilizers may increase the drowsiness effect. Avoid alcoholic beverages while taking this product. Do not take this product if you are taking sedatives or tranquilizers without first consulting your doctor. Do not drive or operate dangerous machinery while taking this medication.

Usage in Children:
Clinical studies establishing safety and effectiveness in children have not been done; therefore, usage is not recommended in children under 12 years of age.
Usage in Pregnancy:
As with any drug, if you are pregnant or nursing a baby, seek advice of a health care professional before taking this product.

ADVERSE REACTIONS

Drowsiness, dry mouth, and on rare occasions, blurred vision have been reported.

DOSAGE AND ADMINISTRATION

For motion sickness, take one or two tablets of Bonine once daily, one hour before travel starts, for up to 24 hours of protection against motion sickness. The tablet can be chewed with or without water or swallowed whole with water. Thereafter, the dose may be repeated every 24 hours for the duration of the travel.

HOW SUPPLIED

BONINE (meclizine HCl) is available in convenient packets of 8 chewable tablets of 25 mg. meclizine HCl.

INACTIVE INGREDIENTS

FD&C Red #40, Lactose, Magnesium Stearate, Purified Siliceous Earth, Raspberry Flavor, Saccharin Sodium, Starch, Talc.

UNISOM®   OTC
[yu 'na-som]
Nighttime Sleep Aid
(doxylamine succinate)

PRODUCT OVERVIEW

KEY FACTS

Unisom is an ethanolamine antihistamine (doxylamine) which characteristically shows a high incidence of sedation. It produces a reduced latency to end of wakefulness and early onset of sleep.

MAJOR USES

Unisom has been shown to be clinically effective as a sleep aid when 1 tablet is given 30 minutes before retiring.

SAFETY INFORMATION

Unisom is contraindicated in pregnancy and nursing mothers. It is also contraindicated in patients with asthma, glaucoma, and enlargement of the prostate. Caution should be used if taken when alcohol is being consumed. Caution is also indicated when taken concurrently with other medications due to the anticholinergic properties of antihistamines.

PRESCRIBING INFORMATION

UNISOM®   OTC
[yu 'na-som]
Nighttime Sleep Aid
(doxylamine succinate)

DESCRIPTION

Pale blue oval scored tablets containing 25 mg. of doxylamine succinate, 2-[α-(2-dimethylaminoethoxy)α-methylbenzyl]pyridine succinate.

ACTION AND USES

Doxylamine succinate is an antihistamine of the ethanolamine class, which characteristically shows a high incidence of sedation. In a comparative clinical study of over 20 antihistamines on more than 3000 subjects, doxylamine succinate 25 mg. was one of the three most sedating antihistamines, producing a significantly reduced latency to end of wakefulness and comparing favorably with established hypnotic drugs such as secobarbital and pentobarbital in sedation activity. It was chosen as the antihistamine, based on dosage, causing the earliest onset of sleep. In another clinical study, doxylamine succinate 25 mg. scored better than secobarbital 100 mg. as a nighttime hypnotic. Two additional, identical clinical studies, involving a total of 121 subjects demonstrated that doxylamine succinate 25 mg. reduced the sleep latency period by a third, compared to placebo. Duration of sleep was 26.6% longer with doxylamine succinate, and the quality of sleep was rated higher with the drug than with placebo. An EEG study on 6 subjects confirmed the results of these studies. In yet another study, no statistically significant difference was found between doxylamine succinate and flurazepam in the average time required for 200 patients with mild to moderate insomnia to fall asleep over 5 nights following a nightly dose of doxylamine succinate 25 mg. or flurazepam 30 mg., nor was any statistically significant difference found in the total time the 200 patients slept. Patients on doxylamine succinate awoke an average of 1.2 times per night while those on flurazepam awoke an average of 0.9 times per night. In either case the patients awoke rested the following morning. On a rating scale of 1 to 5, doxylamine succinate was given a 3.0, flurazepam a 3.4 by patients rating the degree of restfulness provided by their medication (5 represents "very well rested"). Although statistically significant, the difference between doxylamine succinate 25 mg. and flurazepam 30 mg. in the number of awakenings and degree of restfulness is clinically insignificant.

ADMINISTRATION AND DOSAGE

One tablet 30 minutes before retiring. Not for children under 12 years of age.

SIDE EFFECTS

Occasional anticholinergic effects may be seen.

PRECAUTIONS

Unisom® should be taken only at bedtime.

CONTRAINDICATIONS

Do not take this product, unless directed by a doctor, if you have a breathing problem such as emphysema or chronic bronchitis, or if you have glaucoma or difficulty in urination due to enlargement of the prostate gland. This product should not be taken by pregnant women or those who are nursing a baby.

WARNINGS

Should be taken with caution if alcohol is being consumed. Product should not be taken if patient is concurrently on any other drug, without prior consultation with physician. Should not be taken for longer than two weeks unless approved by physician.

HOW SUPPLIED

Boxes of 8, 16, 32 or 48 tablets.

INACTIVE INGREDIENTS

Dibasic Calcium Phosphate, FD&C Blue #1 Aluminum Lake, Magnesium Stearate, Microcrystalline Cellulose, Sodium Starch Glycolate.

MAXIMUM STRENGTH UNISOM   OTC
SLEEPGELS
Nighttime Sleep Aid

DESCRIPTION

Maximum Strength Unisom SleepGels are liquid-filled, blue soft gelatin capsules.

ACTIVE INGREDIENT

Diphenhydramine Hydrochloride 50 mg.

INACTIVE INGREDIENTS

FD&C Blue No. 1, Gelatin, Glycerin, Pharmaceutical Glaze, Polyethylene Glycol, Propylene Glycol, Purified Water, Sorbitol, Titanium Dioxide.

INDICATIONS

Helps to reduce difficulty falling asleep.

ACTION

Diphenhydramine Hydrochloride is an ethanolamine antihistamine with anticholinergic and sedative effects.

ADMINISTRATION AND DOSAGE

Adults and children 12 years of age and over: Oral dosage is one softgel (50 mg.) at bedtime if needed, or as directed by a doctor.

WARNINGS

Do not take this product if you have asthma, glaucoma, emphysema, chronic pulmonary disease, shortness of breath, difficulty in breathing or difficulty in urination due to enlargement of the prostate gland unless directed by a doctor. Do not take this product if pregnant or nursing a baby.
• Do not give to children under 12 years of age.
• If sleeplessness persists continuously for more than two weeks, consult your doctor. Insomnia may be a symptom of serious underlying medical illness.
• Avoid alcoholic beverages while taking this product. Do not take this product if you are taking sedatives or tranquilizers, without first consulting your doctor.
• Keep this and all drugs out of the reach of children.
• In case of accidental overdose, seek professional assistance or contact a Poison Control Center immediately.

DRUG INTERACTION

Monoamine oxidase (MAO) inhibitors prolong and intensify the anticholinergic effects of antihistamines. The CNS depressant effect is heightened by alcohol and other CNS depressant drugs.

SYMPTOMS OF ORAL OVERDOSAGE

Antihistamine overdosage reactions may vary from central nervous system depression to stimulation.
Stimulation is particularly likely in children. Atropine-like signs and symptoms, such as dry mouth, fixed and dilated pupils, flushing, and gastrointestinal symptoms, may also occur.

ATTENTION

Use only if softgel blister seals are unbroken.

HOW SUPPLIED

Boxes of 16 liquid filled softgels in child resistant blisters and boxes of 8 with non-child resistant packaging. Also in a 32 count easy to open child resistant bottle.
Store between 15° and 30°C (59° and 86°F).

UNISOM® WITH PAIN RELIEF®   OTC
[yu 'na-som]
Nighttime Sleep Aid and Pain Reliever

PRODUCT OVERVIEW

KEY FACTS

Unisom With Pain Relief (diphenhydramine sleep aid/acetaminophen pain relief formula) is a product with a dual antihistamine sleep aid/analgesic action to utilize the sedative effects of an antihistamine and relieve mild to moderate pain that may disturb normal sleep patterns. If patients have difficulty in falling asleep but are not experiencing pain at the same time, regular Unisom Sleep Aid which contains doxylamine succinate or Maximum Strength Unisom Sleep-Gels which contains diphenhydramine is indicated.

MAJOR USES

One Unisom With Pain Relief is indicated 30 minutes before retiring to help reduce difficulty in falling asleep while relieving accompanying minor aches and pains, such as headache, muscle aches or menstrual discomfort.

SAFETY INFORMATION

Do not take this product, unless directed by a doctor, if you have a breathing problem such as emphysema or chronic bronchitis, or if you have glaucoma or difficulty in urination due to enlargement of the prostate gland. Unisom With Pain Relief is contraindicated in pregnancy or in nursing mothers. Excessive dosing may lead to liver damage. Product is intended for patients 12 years and older. Alcoholic beverages should be avoided while taking this product. This product should not be taken without first consulting a physician if sedatives or tranquilizers are being taken.

PRESCRIBING INFORMATION

UNISOM WITH PAIN RELIEF®
[yu 'na-som]
Nighttime Sleep Aid and Pain Reliever

DESCRIPTION

Unisom With Pain Relief® is a pale blue, capsule-shaped, coated tablet.

ACTIVE INGREDIENTS

650 mg. acetaminophen and 50 mg. diphenhydramine HCl per tablet.

INDICATIONS

Unisom With Pain Relief (diphenhydramine sleep aid formula) is indicated to help reduce difficulty in falling asleep while relieving accompanying minor aches and pains such as headache, muscle ache or menstrual discomfort. If there is difficulty in falling asleep, but pain is not being experienced at the same time, regular Unisom sleep aid is indicated which contains doxylamine succinate as its active ingredient.

ADMINISTRATION AND DOSAGE

One tablet at bedtime if needed, or as directed by a physician.

CONTRAINDICATIONS

Do not take this product, unless directed by a doctor, if you have a breathing problem such as emphysema or chronic bronchitis, or if you have glaucoma or difficulty in urination due to enlargement of the prostate gland. Do not take this product if pregnant or nursing a baby.
Do not take this product for treatment of arthritis except under the advice and supervision of a physician.

WARNINGS

Do not exceed recommended dosage because severe liver damage may occur. If symptoms persist continuously for more than ten days, consult your physician. Insomnia may be a symptom of serious underlying medical illness. Avoid alcoholic beverages while taking this product. Do not take this product if you are taking sedatives or tranquilizers, without first consulting your doctor. For adults only. Do not give to children under 12 years of age. Keep this and all medications out of reach of children. IN CASE OF ACCIDENTAL OVERDOSE SEEK PROFESSIONAL ADVICE OR CONTACT A POISON CONTROL CENTER IMMEDIATELY.

CAUTION

This product contains an antihistamine and will cause drowsiness. It should be used only at bedtime.

DRUG INTERACTION

Monoamine oxidase (MAO) inhibitors prolong and intensify the anticholinergic effects of antihistamines. The CNS depressant effect is heightened by alcohol and other CNS depressant drugs.

ATTENTION

Use only if tablet blister seals are unbroken. Child resistant packaging.

HOW SUPPLIED

Boxes of 8 and 16 tablets in child resistant blisters.

INACTIVE INGREDIENTS

Corn starch, FD&C Blue #1 Aluminum Lake, FD&C Blue #2 Aluminum Lake, Hydroxypropyl Methylcellulose, Magnesium Stearate, Polyethylene Glycol, Polysorbate 80, Povidone, Stearic Acid, Titanium Dioxide.

Pfizer Inc
235 EAST 42nd STREET
NEW YORK, NY 10017-5755

For Medical Information Contact:
(800) 438-1985
24 hours a day, seven days a week.

Product Identification Codes

To provide quick and positive identification of Pfizer Inc products, we have either a unique identifying number of the National Drug Code or the product name on all tablets or capsules.
In order that you may quickly identify a product by its code number, we have compiled below a numerical list of code numbers with their corresponding product names. We are also listing the code numbers by alphabetical order of products.

Numerical Listing

Product Ident. Number	Product
035	Spectrobid® (bacampicillin HCl) Tablets, 400 mg, equivalent to 280 mg ampicillin
092	Urobiotic®-250 (oxytetracycline HCl 250 mg with sulfamethizole 250 mg and phenazopyridine 50 mg) Capsules
094	Vibramycin® Hyclate (doxycycline hyclate) Capsules 50 mg
095	Vibramycin® Hyclate (doxycycline hyclate) Capsules 100 mg
099	Vibra-Tabs® (doxycycline hyclate) Film Coated Tablets 100 mg
143	Geocillin® (carbenicillin indanyl sodium) Tablets, equivalent to 382 mg carbenicillin
152	Norvasc® (amlodipine besylate) Tablets 2.5 mg
153	Norvasc® (amlodipine besylate) Tablets 5 mg
154	Norvasc® (amlodipine besylate) Tablets 10 mg
155	Glucotrol XL™ (glipizide) Extended Release Tablets, 5 mg GITS
156	Glucotrol XL™ (glipizide) Extended Release Tablets, 10 mg GITS
159	TAO® (troleandomycin) Capsules, 250 mg
210	Antivert® (meclizine HCl) Tablets, 12.5 mg
211	Antivert® /25 (meclizine HCl) Tablets, 25 mg
214	Antivert® /50 (meclizine HCl) Tablets, 50 mg
254	Marax® (ephedrine sulfate, 25 mg; theophylline, 130 mg; and Atarax® [hydroxyzine HCl], 10 mg) Tablets
260	Procardia® (nifedipine) Capsules, 10 mg
261	Procardia® (nifedipine) Capsules, 20 mg
265	Procardia XL® (nifedipine) Extended Release Tablets, 30 mg GITS
266	Procardia XL® (nifedipine) Extended Release Tablets, 60 mg GITS
267	Procardia XL® (nifedipine) Extended Release Tablets, 90 mg GITS
275	Cardura® (doxazosin mesylate) Tablets, 1 mg
276	Cardura® (doxazosin mesylate) Tablets, 2 mg
277	Cardura® (doxazosin mesylate) Tablets, 4 mg
278	Cardura® (doxazosin mesylate) Tablets, 8 mg
305	Zithromax® (azithromycin) Capsules 250 mg
305	Zithromax® (azithromycin) Z-Pak™ (6 × 250-mg Capsules)
308	Zithromax® (azithromycin) Tablets 600 mg
322	Feldene® (piroxicam) Capsules 10 mg
323	Feldene® (piroxicam) Capsules 20 mg
341	Diflucan® (fluconazole) Tablets, 50 mg
342	Diflucan® (fluconazole) Tablets, 100 mg
343	Diflucan® (fluconazole) Tablets, 200 mg
350	Diflucan® (fluconazole) Tablets, 150 mg
393	Diabinese® (chlorpropamide) Tablets 100 mg
394	Diabinese® (chlorpropamide) Tablets 250 mg
411	Glucotrol® (glipizide) Tablets, 5 mg
412	Glucotrol® (glipizide) Tablets, 10 mg
430	Minizide® 1 Capsules (1 mg prazosin HCl and 0.5 mg polythiazide)
431	Minipress® (prazosin HCl) Capsules 1 mg
432	Minizide® 2 Capsules (2 mg prazosin HCl and 0.5 mg polythiazide)
436	Minizide® 5 Capsules (5 mg prazosin HCl and 0.5 mg polythiazide)
437	Minipress® (prazosin HCl) Capsules 2 mg
438	Minipress® (prazosin HCl) Capsules 5 mg
490	Zoloft™ (sertraline HCl) Tablets, 50 mg
491	Zoloft™ (sertraline HCl) Tablets, 100 mg
534	Sinequan® (doxepin HCl) Capsules 10 mg
535	Sinequan® (doxepin HCl) Capsules 25 mg
536	Sinequan® (doxepin HCl) Capsules 50 mg
537	Sinequan® (doxepin HCl) Capsules 150 mg
538	Sinequan® (doxepin HCl) Capsules 100 mg
539	Sinequan® (doxepin HCl) Capsules 75 mg
541	Vistaril® (hydroxyzine pamoate) Capsules 25 mg
542	Vistaril® (hydroxyzine pamoate) Capsules 50 mg
543	Vistaril® (hydroxyzine pamoate) Capsules 100 mg
550	Zyrtec™ (cetirizine hydrochloride) Tablets 5 mg
551	Zyrtec™ (cetirizine hydrochloride) Tablets 10 mg
560	Atarax® (hydroxyzine HCl) Tablets, 10 mg
561	Atarax® (hydroxyzine HCl) Tablets, 25 mg
562	Atarax® (hydroxyzine HCl) Tablets, 50 mg
563	Atarax® (hydroxyzine HCl) Tablets, 100 mg
571	Navane® (thiothixene) Capsules, 1 mg
572	Navane® (thiothixene) Capsules, 2 mg
573	Navane® (thiothixene) Capsules, 5 mg
574	Navane® (thiothixene) Capsules, 10 mg
577	Navane® (thiothixene) Capsules, 20 mg

Alphabetical Listing

Prod. Ident. Number	Product
210	Antivert® (meclizine HCl) Tablets, 12.5 mg
211	Antivert® /25 (meclizine HCl) Tablets, 25 mg
214	Antivert® /50 (meclizine HCl) Tablets, 50 mg
560	Atarax® (hydroxyzine HCl) Tablets, 10 mg
561	Atarax® (hydroxyzine HCl) Tablets, 25 mg

Continued on next page

Consult 1997 supplements and future editions for revisions

Pfizer Inc—Cont.

562 Atarax® (hydroxyzine HCl) Tablets, 50 mg
563 Atarax® (hydroxyzine HCl) Tablets, 100 mg
275 Cardura® (doxazosin mesylate) Tablets, 1 mg
276 Cardura® (doxazosin mesylate) Tablets, 2 mg
277 Cardura® (doxazosin mesylate) Tablets, 4 mg
278 Cardura® (doxazosin mesylate) Tablets, 8 mg
393 Diabinese® (chlorpropamide) Tablets 100 mg
394 Diabinese® (chlorpropamide) Tablets 250 mg
341 Diflucan® (fluconazole) Tablets 50 mg
342 Diflucan® (fluconazole) Tablets 100 mg
350 Diflucan® (fluconazole) Tablets 150 mg
343 Diflucan® (fluconazole) Tablets 200 mg
322 Feldene® (piroxicam) Capsules 10 mg
323 Feldene® (piroxicam) Capsules 20 mg
143 Geocillin® (carbenicillin indanyl sodium) Tablets equivalent to 382 mg carbenicillin
411 Glucotrol® (glipizide) Tablets 5 mg
412 Glucotrol® (glipizide) Tablets 10 mg
155 Glucotrol XL™ (glipizide) Extended Release Tablets 5 mg GITS
156 Glucotrol XL™ (glipizide) Extended Release Tablets 10 mg GITS
254 Marax® (ephedrine sulfate, 25 mg; theophylline, 130 mg; and Atarax [hydroxyzine HCl], 10 mg) Tablets
431 Minipress® (prazosin HCl) Capsules 1 mg
437 Minipress® (prazosin HCl) Capsules 2 mg
438 Minipress® (prazosin HCl) Capsules 5 mg
430 Minizide® 1 Capsules (1 mg prazosin HCl and 0.5 mg polythiazide)
432 Minizide® 2 Capsules (2 mg prazosin HCl and 0.5 mg polythiazide)
436 Minizide® 5 Capsules (5 mg prazosin HCl and 0.5 mg polythiazide)
571 Navane® (thiothixene) Capsules, 1 mg
572 Navane® (thiothixene) Capsules, 2 mg
573 Navane® (thiothixene) Capsules, 5 mg
574 Navane® (thiothixene) Capsules, 10 mg
577 Navane® (thiothixene) Capsules, 20 mg
152 Norvasc® (amlodipine besylate) Tablets 2.5 mg
153 Norvasc® (amlodipine besylate) Tablets 5 mg
154 Norvasc® (amlodipine besylate) Tablets 10 mg
260 Procardia® (nifedipine) Capsules, 10 mg
261 Procardia® (nifedipine) Capsules, 20 mg
265 Procardia XL® (nifedipine) Extended Release Tablets, 30 mg GITS
266 Procardia XL® (nifedipine) Extended Release Tablets, 60 mg GITS
267 Procardia XL® (nifedipine) Extended Release Tablets, 90 mg GITS
534 Sinequan® (doxepin HCl) Capsules 10 mg
535 Sinequan® (doxepin HCl) Capsules 25 mg
536 Sinequan® (doxepin HCl) Capsules 50 mg
539 Sinequan® (doxepin HCl) Capsules 75 mg
538 Sinequan® (doxepin HCl) Capsules 100 mg
537 Sinequan® (doxepin HCl) Capsules 150 mg

035 Spectrobid® (bacampicillin HCl) Tablets, 400 mg, equivalent to 280 mg ampicillin
159 TAO® (troleandomycin) Capsules, 250 mg
092 Urobiotic®-250 (oxytetracycline HCl 250 mg with sulfamethizole 250 mg and phenazopyridine 50 mg) Capsules
094 Vibramycin® Hyclate (doxycycline hyclate) Capsules 50 mg
095 Vibramycin® Hyclate (doxycycline hyclate) Capsules 100 mg
099 Vibra-Tabs® (doxycycline hyclate) Film Coated Tablets 100 mg
541 Vistaril® (hydroxyzine pamoate) Capsules 25 mg
542 Vistaril® (hydroxyzine pamoate) Capsules 50 mg
543 Vistaril® (hydroxyzine pamoate) Capsules 100 mg
305 Zithromax® (azithromycin) Capsules 250 mg
305 Zithromax® (azithromycin) Z-PAK™ (6 × 250-mg Capsules)
308 Zithromax® (azithromycin) 600 mg Tablets
490 Zoloft™ (sertraline HCl) Tablets, 50 mg
491 Zoloft™ (sertraline HCl) Tablets, 100 mg
550 Zyrtec™ (cetirizine hydrochloride) Tablets 5 mg
551 Zyrtec™ (cetirizine hydrochloride) Tablets 10 mg

ANTIVERT® TABLETS ℞
[än 'tĭ-vert"]
(12.5 mg meclizine HCl)
ANTIVERT®/25 TABLETS ℞
(25 mg meclizine HCl)
ANTIVERT®/50 TABLETS ℞
(50 mg meclizine HCl)

DESCRIPTION

Chemically, Antivert (meclizine HCl) is 1-(p-chloro-α-phenyl-benzyl) -4- (m -methylbenzyl) piperazine dihydrochloride monohydrate.

Inert ingredients for the tablets are: dibasic calcium phosphate; magnesium stearate; polyethylene glycol; starch; sucrose. The 12.5 mg tablets also contain: Blue 1. The 25 mg tablets also contain: Yellow 6 Lake; Yellow 10 Lake. The 50 mg tablets also contain: Blue 1 Lake; Yellow 10 Lake.

ACTIONS

Antivert is an antihistamine which shows marked protective activity against nebulized histamine and lethal doses of intravenously injected histamine in guinea pigs. It has a marked effect in blocking the vasodepressor response to histamine, but only a slight blocking action against acetylcholine. Its activity is relatively weak in inhibiting the spasmogenic action of histamine on isolated guinea pig ileum.

INDICATIONS

Based on a review of this drug by the National Academy of Sciences-National Research Council and/or other information, FDA has classified the indications as follows:
Effective: Management of nausea and vomiting, and dizziness associated with motion sickness.
Possibly Effective: Management of vertigo associated with diseases affecting the vestibular system.
Final classification of the less than effective indications requires further investigation.

CONTRAINDICATIONS

Meclizine HCl is contraindicated in individuals who have shown a previous hypersensitivity to it.

WARNINGS

Since drowsiness may, on occasion, occur with use of this drug, patients should be warned of this possibility and cautioned against driving a car or operating dangerous machinery.
Patients should avoid alcoholic beverages while taking this drug. Due to its potential anticholinergic action, this drug should be used with caution in patients with asthma, glaucoma, or enlargement of the prostate gland.

USAGE IN CHILDREN

Clinical studies establishing safety and effectiveness in children have not been done; therefore, usage is not recommended in children under 12 years of age.

USAGE IN PREGNANCY

Pregnancy Category B. Reproduction studies in rats have shown cleft palates at 25–50 times the human dose. Epidemiological studies in pregnant women, however, do not indicate that meclizine increases the risk of abnormalities when administered during pregnancy. Despite the animal findings, it would appear that the possibility of fetal harm is remote. Nevertheless, meclizine, or any other medication, should be used during pregnancy only if clearly necessary.

ADVERSE REACTIONS

Drowsiness, dry mouth and, on rare occasions, blurred vision have been reported.

DOSAGE AND ADMINISTRATION

Vertigo:
For the control of vertigo associated with diseases affecting the vestibular system, the recommended dose is 25 to 100 mg daily, in divided dosage, depending upon clinical response.
Motion Sickness:
The initial dose of 25 to 50 mg of Antivert should be taken one hour prior to embarkation for protection against motion sickness. Thereafter, the dose may be repeated every 24 hours for the duration of the journey.

HOW SUPPLIED

Antivert—12.5 mg tablets: bottles of 100 (NDC 0662-2100-66), 1000 (NDC 0662-2100-82).
Antivert/25—25 mg tablets: bottles of 100 (NDC 0662-2110-66), 1000 (NDC 0662-2110-82).
Antivert/50—50 mg tablets: bottles of 100 (NDC 0662-2140-66).

69-2148-37-7
Shown in Product Identification Guide, page 327

ATARAX® ℞
[ăt 'ā-raks"]
(hydroxyzine hydrochloride)
TABLETS AND SYRUP

DESCRIPTION

Hydroxyzine hydrochloride is designated chemically as 1-(p-chlorobenzhydryl) 4-[2-(2-hydroxyethoxy)-ethyl] piperazine dihydrochloride.
Inert ingredients for the tablets are: acacia; carnauba wax; dibasic calcium phosphate; gelatin; lactose; magnesium stearate; precipitated calcium carbonate; shellac; sucrose; talc; white wax. The 10 mg tablets also contain: sodium hydroxide; starch; titanium dioxide; Yellow 6 Lake. The 25 mg tablets also contain: starch, velo dark green. The 50 mg tablets also contain: starch; velo yellow. The 100 mg tablets also contain: alginic acid; Blue 1; polyethylene glycol; Red 3.
The inert ingredients for the syrup are: alcohol; menthol; peppermint oil; sodium benzoate; spearmint oil; sucrose; water.

CLINICAL PHARMACOLOGY

Atarax is unrelated chemically to the phenothiazines, reserpine, meprobamate, or the benzodiazepines.
Atarax is not a cortical depressant, but its action may be due to a suppression of activity in certain key regions of the subcortical area of the central nervous system. Primary skeletal muscle relaxation has been demonstrated experimentally. Bronchodilator activity, and antihistaminic and analgesic effects have been demonstrated experimentally and confirmed clinically. An antiemetic effect, both by the apomorphine test and the veriloid test, has been demonstrated. Pharmacological and clinical studies indicate that hydroxyzine in therapeutic dosage does not increase gastric secretion or acidity and in most cases has mild antisecretory activity. Hydroxyzine is rapidly absorbed from the gastrointestinal tract and Atarax's clinical effects are usually noted within 15 to 30 minutes after oral administration.

INDICATIONS

For symptomatic relief of anxiety and tension associated with psychoneurosis and as an adjunct in organic disease states in which anxiety is manifested.
Useful in the management of pruritus due to allergic conditions such as chronic urticaria and atopic and contact dermatoses, and in histamine-mediated pruritus.
As a sedative when used as premedication and following general anesthesia, Hydroxyzine may potentiate meperidine (Demerol®) and barbiturates, so their use in pre-anesthetic adjunctive therapy should be modified on an individual basis. Atropine and other belladonna alkaloids are not affected by the drug. Hydroxyzine is not known to interfere with the action of digitalis in any way and it may be used concurrently with this agent.
The effectiveness of hydroxyzine as an antianxiety agent for long term use, that is more than 4 months, has not been assessed by systematic clinical studies. The physician should

reassess periodically the usefulness of the drug for the individual patient.

CONTRAINDICATIONS

Hydroxyzine, when administered to the pregnant mouse, rat, and rabbit, induced fetal abnormalities in the rat and mouse at doses substantially above the human therapeutic range. Clinical data in human beings are inadequate to establish safety in early pregnancy. Until such data are available, hydroxyzine is contraindicated in early pregnancy. Hydroxyzine is contraindicated for patients who have shown a previous hypersensitivity to it.

WARNINGS

Nursing Mothers: It is not known whether this drug is excreted in human milk. Since many drugs are so excreted, hydroxyzine should not be given to nursing mothers.
For Tablets Only: This product is manufactured with 1,1,1-trichloroethane, a substance which harms public health and the environment by destroying ozone in the upper atmosphere.

PRECAUTIONS

THE POTENTIATING ACTION OF HYDROXYZINE MUST BE CONSIDERED WHEN THE DRUG IS USED IN CONJUNCTION WITH CENTRAL NERVOUS SYSTEM DEPRESSANTS SUCH AS NARCOTICS, NON-NARCOTIC ANALGESICS AND BARBITURATES. Therefore when central nervous system depressants are administered concomitantly with hydroxyzine their dosage should be reduced. Since drowsiness may occur with use of this drug, patients should be warned of this possibility and cautioned against driving a car or operating dangerous machinery while taking Atarax. Patients should be advised against the simultaneous use of other CNS depressant drugs, and cautioned that the effect of alcohol may be increased.

ADVERSE REACTIONS

Side effects reported with the administration of Atarax (hydroxyzine hydrochloride) are usually mild and transitory in nature.
Anticholinergic: Dry mouth.
Central Nervous System: Drowsiness is usually transitory and may disappear in a few days of continued therapy or upon reduction of the dose. Involuntary motor activity including rare instances of tremor and convulsions have been reported, usually with doses considerably higher than those recommended. Clinically significant respiratory depression has not been reported at recommended doses.

OVERDOSAGE

The most common manifestation of Atarax overdosage is hypersedation. As in the management of overdosage with any drug, it should be borne in mind that multiple agents may have been taken.
If vomiting has not occurred spontaneously, it should be induced. Immediate gastric lavage is also recommended. General supportive care, including frequent monitoring of the vital signs and close observation of the patient, is indicated. Hypotension, though unlikely, may be controlled with intravenous fluids and Levophed® (levarterenol), or Aramine® (metaraminol). Do not use epinephrine as Atarax counteracts its pressor action.
There is no specific antidote. It is doubtful that hemodialysis would be of any value in the treatment of overdosage with hydroxyzine. However, if other agents such as barbiturates have been ingested concomitantly, hemodialysis may be indicated. There is no practical method to quantitate hydroxyzine in body fluids or tissue after its ingestion or administration.

DOSAGE

For symptomatic relief of anxiety and tension associated with psychoneurosis and as an adjunct in organic disease states in which anxiety is manifested: in adults, 50–100 mg q.i.d.; children under 6 years, 50 mg daily in divided doses and over 6 years, 50–100 mg daily in divided doses.
For use in the management of pruritus due to allergic conditions such as chronic urticaria and atopic and contact dermatoses, and in histamine-mediated pruritus: in adults, 25 mg t.i.d. or q.i.d.; children under 6 years, 50 mg daily in divided doses and over 6 years, 50–100 mg daily in divided doses.
As a sedative when used as a premedication and following general anesthesia: 50–100 mg in adults, and 0.6 mg/kg in children.
When treatment is initiated by the intramuscular route of administration, subsequent doses may be administered orally.
As with all medications, the dosage should be adjusted according to the patient's response to therapy.

SUPPLY

Atarax Tablets
10 mg—orange tablets: 100's (NDC 0049-5600-66), 500's (NDC 0049-5600-73) Unit Dose 10 × 10's (NDC 0049-5600-41), and Unit of Use 40's (NDC 0049-5600-43)
25 mg—green tablets: 100's (NDC 0049-5610-66), 500's (NDC 0049-5610-73) Unit Dose 10 × 10's (NDC 0049-5610-41), and Unit of Use 40's (NDC 0049-5610-43)

50 mg—yellow tablets: 100's (NDC 0049-5620-66), 500's (NDC 0049-5620-73)
100 mg—red tablets: 100's (NDC 0049-5630-66)
Atarax Syrup
10 mg per teaspoon (5 ml): 1 pint bottles (NDC 0049-5590-93)
Alcohol Content—Ethyl Alcohol—0.5% v/v

BIBLIOGRAPHY

Available on request.
69-0618-00-5   Revised Dec. 1993
Shown in Product Identification Guide, page 327

CARDURA®   ℞
(doxazosin mesylate)
Tablets

DESCRIPTION

CARDURA® (doxazosin mesylate) is a quinazoline compound that is a selective inhibitor of the alpha$_1$ subtype of alpha adrenergic receptors. The chemical name of doxazosin mesylate is 1-(4-amino-6,7-dimethoxy-2-quinazolinyl)-4-(1,4-benzodioxan-2-ylcarbonyl) piperazine methanesulfonate. The empirical formula for doxazosin mesylate is $C_{23}H_{25}N_5O_5 \cdot CH_4O_3S$ and the molecular weight is 547.6. It has the following structure:

CARDURA® (doxazosin mesylate) is freely soluble in dimethylsulfoxide, soluble in dimethylformamide, slightly soluble in methanol, ethanol, and water (0.8% at 25℃), and very slightly soluble in acetone and methylene chloride. CARDURA® is available as colored tablets for oral use and contains 1 mg (white), 2 mg (yellow), 4 mg (orange) and 8 mg (green) of doxazosin as the free base.
The inactive ingredients for all tablets are: microcrystalline cellulose, lactose, sodium starch glycolate, magnesium stearate and sodium lauryl sulfate. The 2 mg tablet contains D & C yellow 10 and FD & C yellow 6; the 4 mg tablet contains FD & C yellow 6; the 8 mg tablet contains FD & C blue 10 and D & C yellow 10.

CLINICAL PHARMACOLOGY

Pharmacodynamics
A. Benign Prostatic Hyperplasia (BPH)
Benign prostatic hyperplasia (BPH) is a common cause of urinary outflow obstruction in aging males. Severe BPH may lead to urinary retention and renal damage. A static and a dynamic component contribute to the symptoms and reduced urinary flow rate associated with BPH. The static component is related to an increase in prostate size caused, in part, by a proliferation of smooth muscle cells in the prostatic stroma. However, the severity of BPH symptoms and the degree of urethral obstruction do not correlate well with the size of the prostate. The dynamic component of BPH is associated with an increase in smooth muscle tone in the prostate and bladder neck. The degree of tone in this area is mediated by the alpha$_1$ adrenoceptor, which is present in high density in the prostatic stroma, prostatic capsule and

bladder neck. Blockade of the alpha$_1$ receptor decreases urethral resistance and may relieve the obstruction and BPH symptoms. In the human prostate, CARDURA® antagonizes phenylephrine (alpha$_1$ agonist)-induced contractions, *in vitro*, and binds with high affinity to the alpha$_{1c}$ adrenoceptor. The receptor subtype is thought to be the predominant functional type in the prostate. CARDURA® acts within 1–2 weeks to decrease the severity of BPH symptoms and improve urinary flow rate. Since alpha$_1$ adrenoceptors are of low density in the urinary bladder (apart from the bladder neck), CARDURA® should maintain bladder contractility.
The efficacy of CARDURA® was evaluated extensively in over 900 patients with BPH in double-blind, placebo-controlled trials. CARDURA® treatment was superior to placebo in improving patient symptoms and urinary flow rate. Significant relief with CARDURA® was seen as early as one week into the treatment regimen, with CARDURA® treated patients (N=173) showing a significant (p<0.01) increase in maximum flow rate of 0.8 mL/sec compared to a decrease of 0.5 mL/sec in the placebo group (N=41). In long term studies improvement was maintained for up to 2 years of treatment. In 66–71% of patients, improvements above baseline were seen in both symptoms and maximum urinary flow rate.
In three placebo-controlled studies of 14–16 weeks duration obstructive symptoms (hesitation, intermittency, dribbling, weak urinary stream, incomplete emptying of the bladder) and irritative symptoms (nocturia, daytime frequency, urgency, burning) of BPH were evaluated at each visit by patient-assessed symptom questionnaires. The bothersomeness of symptoms was measured with a modified Boyarsky questionnaire. Symptom severity/frequency was assessed using a modified Boyarsky questionnaire or an AUA-based questionnaire. Uroflowmetric evaluations were performed at times of peak (2–6 hours post-dose) and/or trough (24 hours post-dose) plasma concentrations of CARDURA®.
The results from the three placebo-controlled studies (N=609) showing significant efficacy with 4 mg and 8 mg doxazosin are summarized in Table 1. In all three studies, CARDURA® resulted in statistically significant relief of obstructive and irritative symptoms compared to placebo. Statistically significant improvements of 2.3–3.3 mL/sec in maximum flow rate were seen with CARDURA® in Studies 1 and 2, compared to 0.1–0.7 mL/sec with placebo.
[See table 1 below.]
In one fixed dose study (study 2) CARDURA® therapy (4–8 mg, once daily) resulted in a significant and sustained improvement in maximum urinary flow rate of 2.3–3.3 mL/sec (Table 1) compared to placebo (0.1 mL/sec). In this study, the only study in which weekly evaluations were made, significant improvement with CARDURA® vs. placebo was seen after one week. The proportion of patients who responded with a maximum flow rate improvement of ≥ 3 mL/sec was significantly larger with CARDURA® (34–42%) than placebo (13–17%). A significantly greater improvement was also seen in average flow rate with CARDURA® (1.6 mL/sec) than with placebo (0.2 mL/sec). The onset and time course of symptom relief and increased urinary flow from study 1 are illustrated in Figure 1.
[See Figure 1 at bottom of next page.]
In BPH patients (N=450) treated for up to 2 years in open-label studies, CARDURA® therapy resulted in significant improvement above baseline in urinary flow rates and BPH

TABLE 1
SUMMARY OF EFFECTIVENESS DATA IN PLACEBO-CONTROLLED TRIALS

	SYMPTOM SCORE[a]			MAXIMUM FLOW RATE (mL/sec)		
	N	MEAN BASELINE	MEAN[b] CHANGE	N	MEAN BASELINE	MEAN[c] CHANGE
STUDY 1 (Titration to maximum dose of 8 mg)[a]						
Placebo	47	15.6	−2.3	41	9.7	+0.7
CARDURA	49	14.5	−4.9**	41	9.8	+2.9**
STUDY 2 (Titration to fixed dose—14 weeks)[d]						
Placebo	37	20.7	−2.5	30	10.6	+0.1
CARDURA 4 mg	38	21.2	−5.0**	32	9.8	+2.3*
CARDURA 8 mg	42	19.9	−4.2*	36	10.5	+3.3**
Study 3 (Titration to fixed dose—12 weeks)						
Placebo	47	14.9	−4.7	44	9.9	+2.1
CARDURA 4 mg	46	16.6	−6.1*	46	9.6	+2.6

[a] AUA questionnaire (range 0–30) in studies 1 and 3.
   Modified Boyarsky Questionnaire (range 7–39) in study 2.
[b] Change is to endpoint.
[c] Change is to fixed-dose efficacy phase, 22–26 hours post-dose for studies 1 and 3 and 2–6 hours post-dose for study 2.
[d] Study in hypertensives with BPH
[e] 36 patients received a dose of 8 mg CARDURA®
*(**) p<0.05 (0.01) compared to placebo mean change.

STUDY 2
Maximum Flow Rate

Maximum Flow Rate: 0.1 (Placebo), 2.3* (4 mg), 3.3** (8 mg)
Symptom Score: −2.5 (Placebo), −5.0** (4 mg), −4.2* (8 mg)

Continued on next page

Pfizer Inc—Cont.

symptoms. The significant effects of CARDURA® were maintained over the entire treatment period.

Although blockade of alpha-1 adrenoceptors also lowers blood pressure in hypertensive patients with increased peripheral vascular resistance, CARDURA® treatment of normotensive men with BPH did not result in a clinically significant blood pressure lowering effect (Table 2). The proportion of normotensive patients with a sitting systolic blood pressure less than 90 mmHg and/or diastolic blood pressure less than 60 mmHg at any time during treatment with CARDURA® 1–8 mg once daily was 6.7% with doxazosin and not significantly different (statistically) from that with placebo (5%).

TABLE 2

Mean Changes in Blood Pressure from Baseline to the Mean of the Final Efficacy Phase in Normotensives (Diastolic BP <90 mmHg) in Two Double-blind, Placebo-controlled U.S. Studies with CARDURA® 1–8 mg once daily.

Sitting BP (mmHg)	PLACEBO (N=85) Baseline	PLACEBO (N=85) Change	CARDURA® (N=183) Baseline	CARDURA® (N=183) Change
Systolic	128.4	−1.4	128.8	−4.9*
Diastolic	79.2	−1.2	79.6	−2.4*
Standing BP (mmHg)	Baseline	Change	Baseline	Change
Systolic	128.5	−0.6	128.5	−5.3*
Diastolic	80.5	−0.7	80.4	−2.6*

* $p \leq 0.05$ compared to placebo

B. Hypertension

The mechanism of action of CARDURA® (doxazosin mesylate) is selective blockade of the $alpha_1$ (postjunctional) subtype of adrenergic receptors. Studies in normal human subjects have shown that doxazosin competitively antagonized the pressor effects of phenylephrine (an $alpha_1$ agonist) and the systolic pressor effect of norepinephrine. Doxazosin and prazosin have similar abilities to antagonize phenylephrine. The antihypertensive effect of CARDURA® results from a decrease in systemic vascular resistance. The parent compound doxazosin is primarily responsible for the antihypertensive activity. The low plasma concentrations of known active and inactive metabolites of doxazosin (2-piperazinyl, 6'- and 7'-hydroxy and 6- and 7-0-desmethyl compounds) compared to parent drug indicate that the contribution of even the most potent compound (6'-hydroxy) to the antihypertensive effect of doxazosin in man is probably small. The 6'- and 7'-hydroxy metabolites have demonstrated antioxidant properties at concentrations of 5 μM, in vitro.

Administration of CARDURA® results in a reduction in systemic vascular resistance. In patients with hypertension there is little change in cardiac output. Maximum reductions in blood pressure usually occur 2–6 hours after dosing and are associated with a small increase in standing heart rate. Like other $alpha_1$-adrenergic blocking agents, doxazosin has a greater effect on blood pressure and heart rate in the standing position.

In a pooled analysis of placebo-controlled hypertension studies with over 300 hypertensive patients per treatment group, doxazosin, at doses of 1–16 mg given once daily, lowered blood pressure at 24 hours by about 10/8 mmHg compared to placebo in the standing position and about 9/5 mmHg in the supine position. Peak blood pressure effects (1–6 hours) were larger by about 50–75% (i.e., trough values were about 55–70% of peak effect), with the larger peak-trough differences seen in systolic pressures. There was no apparent difference in the blood pressure response of Caucasians and blacks or of patients above and below age 65. In these predominantly normocholesterolemic patients doxazosin produced small reductions in total serum cholesterol (2–3%), LDL cholesterol (4%), and a similarly small increase in HDL/total cholesterol ratio (4%). The clinical significance of these findings is uncertain. In the same patient popula-

tion, patients receiving CARDURA® gained a mean of 0.6 kg compared to a mean loss of 0.1 kg for placebo patients.

Pharmacokinetics

After oral administration of therapeutic doses, peak plasma levels of CARDURA® (doxazosin mesylate) occur at about 2–3 hours. Bioavailability is approximately 65%, reflecting first pass metabolism of doxazosin by the liver. The effect of food on the pharmacokinetics of CARDURA® was examined in a crossover study with twelve hypertensive subjects. Reductions of 18% in mean maximum plasma concentration and 12% in the area under the concentration-time curve occurred when CARDURA® was administered with food. Neither of these differences was statistically or clinically significant.

CARDURA® is extensively metabolized in the liver, mainly by O-demethylation of the quinazoline nucleus or hydroxylation of the benzodioxan moiety. Although several active metabolites of doxazosin have been identified, the pharmacokinetics of these metabolites have not been characterized. In a study of two subjects administered radiolabelled doxazosin 2 mg orally and 1 mg intravenously on two separate occasions, approximately 63% of the dose was eliminated in the feces and 9% of the dose was found in the urine. On average only 4.8% of the dose was excreted as unchanged drug in the feces and only a trace of the total radioactivity in the urine was attributed to unchanged drug. At the plasma concentrations achieved by therapeutic doses approximately 98% of the circulating drug is bound to plasma proteins.

Plasma elimination of doxazosin is biphasic, with a terminal elimination half-life of about 22 hours. Steady-state studies in hypertensive patients given doxazosin doses of 2–16 mg once daily showed linear kinetics and dose proportionality. In two studies, following the administration of 2 mg orally once daily, the mean accumulation ratios (steady-state AUC vs first dose AUC) were 1.2 and 1.7. Enterohepatic recycling is suggested by secondary peaking of plasma doxazosin concentrations.

In a crossover study in 24 normotensive subjects, the pharmacokinetics and safety of doxazosin were shown to be similar with morning and evening dosing regimens. The area under the curve after morning dosing was, however, 11% less than that after evening dosing and the time to peak concentration after evening dosing occurred significantly later than that after morning dosing (5.6 hr vs 3.5 hr).

The pharmacokinetics of CARDURA® in young (<65 years) and elderly (≥65 years) subjects were similar for plasma half-life values and oral clearance. Pharmacokinetic studies in elderly patients and patients with renal impairment have shown no significant alterations compared to younger patients with normal renal function. There have, however, been no studies of patients with liver impairment, and there are only limited data on the effects of drugs known to influence hepatic metabolism [e.g., cimetidine (see Precautions)]. Use of doxazosin in patients with altered liver function should be undertaken with particular caution, if at all, as excretion is almost wholly hepatic.

In two placebo-controlled studies, of normotensive and hypertensive BPH patients, in which doxazosin was administered in the morning and the titration interval was two weeks and one week, respectively, trough plasma concentrations of CARDURA® were similar in the two populations. Linear kinetics and dose proportionality were observed.

INDICATIONS AND USAGE

A. Benign Prostatic Hyperplasia (BPH). CARDURA® is indicated for the treatment of both the urinary outflow obstruction and obstructive and irritative symptoms associated with BPH: obstructive symptoms (hesitation, intermittency, dribbling, weak urinary stream, incomplete emptying of the bladder) and irritative symptoms (nocturia, daytime frequency, urgency, burning). CARDURA® may be used in all BPH patients whether hypertensive or normotensive. In patients with hypertension and BPH, both conditions were effectively treated with CARDURA® monotherapy. CARDURA® provides rapid improvement in symptoms and urinary flow rate in 66–71% of patients. Sustained improvements with CARDURA® were seen in patients treated

for up to 14 weeks in double-blind studies and up to 2 years in open-label studies.

B. Hypertension. CARDURA® (doxazosin mesylate) is also indicated for the treatment of hypertension. CARDURA® may be used alone or in combination with diuretics, beta-adrenergic blocking agents, calcium channel blockers or angiotensin-converting enzyme inhibitors.

CONTRAINDICATIONS

CARDURA® is contraindicated in patients with a known sensitivity to quinazolines (e.g. prazosin, terazosin).

WARNINGS

Syncope and "First-dose" Effect: Doxazosin, like other alpha-adrenergic blocking agents, can cause marked hypotension, especially in the upright position, with syncope and other postural symptoms such as dizziness. Marked orthostatic effects are most common with the first dose but can also occur when there is a dosage increase, or if therapy is interrupted for more than a few days. To decrease the likelihood of excessive hypotension and syncope, it is essential that treatment be initiated with the 1 mg dose. The 2, 4, and 8 mg tablets are not for initial therapy. Dosage should then be adjusted slowly (see DOSAGE AND ADMINISTRATION section) with evaluations and increases in dose every two weeks to the recommended dose. Additional antihypertensive agents should be added with caution.

Patients being titrated with doxazosin should be cautioned to avoid situations where injury could result should syncope occur, during both the day and night.

In an early investigational study of the safety and tolerance of increasing daily doses of doxazosin in normotensives beginning at 1 mg/day, only 2 of 6 subjects could tolerate more than 2 mg/day without experiencing symptomatic postural hypotension. In another study of 24 healthy normotensive male subjects receiving initial doses of 2 mg/day of doxazosin, seven (29%) of the subjects experienced symptomatic postural hypotension between 0.5 and 6 hours after the first dose necessitating termination of the study. In this study 2 of the normotensive subjects experienced syncope. Subsequent trials in hypertensive patients always began doxazosin dosing at 1 mg/day resulting in a 4% incidence of postural side effects at 1 mg/day with no cases of syncope.

In multiple dose clinical trials in hypertension involving over 1500 hypertensive patients with dose titration every one to two weeks, syncope was reported in 0.7% of patients. None of these events occurred at the starting dose of 1 mg and 1.2% (8/664) occurred at 16 mg/day.

In placebo-controlled, clinical trials in BPH, 3 out of 665 patients (0.5%) taking doxazosin reported syncope. Two of the patients were taking 1 mg doxazosin, while one patient was taking 2 mg doxazosin when syncope occurred. In the open-label, long-term extension follow-up of approximately 450 BPH patients, there were 3 reports of syncope (0.7%). One patient was taking 2 mg, one patient was taking 8 mg and one patient was taking 12 mg when syncope occurred. In a clinical pharmacology study, one subject receiving 2 mg experienced syncope.

If syncope occurs, the patient should be placed in a recumbent position and treated supportively as necessary.

PRECAUTIONS

General:

Prostate Cancer: Carcinoma of the prostate causes many of the symptoms associated with BPH and the two disorders frequently co-exist. Carcinoma of the prostate should therefore be ruled out prior to commencing therapy with CARDURA®.

Orthostatic Hypotension: While syncope is the most severe orthostatic effect of CARDURA®, other symptoms of lowered blood pressure, such as dizziness, lightheadedness, or vertigo can occur, especially at initiation of therapy or at the time of dose increases.

a) Hypertension

These symptoms were common in clinical trials in hypertension, occurring in up to 23% of all patients treated and causing discontinuation of therapy in about 2%

In placebo-controlled titration trials in hypertension, orthostatic effects were minimized by beginning therapy at 1 mg per day and titrating every two weeks to 2, 4, or 8 mg per day. There was an increased frequency of orthostatic effects in patients given 8 mg or more, 10%, compared to 5% at 1–4 mg and 3% in the placebo group.

b) Benign Prostatic Hyperplasia

In placebo-controlled trials in BPH, the incidence of orthostatic hypotension with doxazosin was 0.3% and did not increase with increasing dosage (to 8 mg/day). The incidence of discontinuations due to hypotension or orthostatic symptoms was 3.3% with doxazosin and 1% with placebo. The titration interval in these studies was one to two weeks.

Patients in occupations in which orthostatic hypotension could be dangerous should be treated with particular caution. As alpha-antagonists can cause orthostatic effects, it is important to evaluate standing blood pressure two minutes after standing and patients should be advised to exercise care when arising from a supine or sitting position.

Figure 1–Study 1

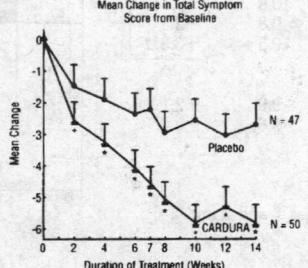

Mean Change in Total Symptom Score from Baseline

Placebo   N = 47
CARDURA   N = 50

Duration of Treatment (Weeks)

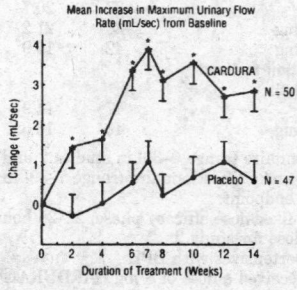

Mean Increase in Maximum Urinary Flow Rate (mL/sec) from Baseline

CARDURA   N = 50
Placebo   N = 47

Duration of Treatment (Weeks)

If hypotension occurs, the patient should be placed in the supine position and, if this measure is inadequate, volume expansion with intravenous fluids or vasopressor therapy may be used. A transient hypotensive response is not a contraindication to further doses of CARDURA® (doxazosin mesylate).

Information for Patients (See Patient Package Insert): Patients should be made aware of the possibility of syncopal and orthostatic symptoms, especially at the initiation of therapy, and urged to avoid driving or hazardous tasks for 24 hours after the first dose, after a dosage increase, and after interruption of therapy when treatment is resumed. They should be cautioned to avoid situations where injury could result should syncope occur during initiation of doxazosin therapy. They should also be advised of the need to sit or lie down when symptoms of lowered blood pressure occur, although these symptoms are not always orthostatic, and to be careful when rising from a sitting or lying position. If dizziness, lightheadedness, or palpitations are bothersome they should be reported to the physician, so that dose adjustment can be considered. Patients should also be told that drowsiness or somnolence can occur with CARDURA® or any selective $alpha_1$ adrenoceptor antagonist, requiring caution in people who must drive or operate heavy machinery.

Drug/Laboratory Test Interactions: CARDURA® does not affect the plasma concentration of prostate specific antigen in patients treated for up to 3 years. Both doxazosin, an $alpha_1$ inhibitor, and finasteride, a 5-alpha reductase inhibitor, are highly protein bound and hepatically metabolized. There is no definitive controlled clinical experience on the concomitant use of $alpha_1$ inhibitors and 5-alpha reductase inhibitors at this time.

Impaired Liver Function: CARDURA® should be administered with caution to patients with evidence of impaired hepatic function or to patients receiving drugs known to influence hepatic metabolism (see CLINICAL PHARMACOLOGY). There is no controlled clinical experience with CARDURA® in patients with these conditions.

Leukopenia/Neutropenia: Analysis of hematologic data from hypertensive patients receiving CARDURA® in controlled hypertension clinical trials showed that the mean WBC (N=474) and mean neutrophil counts (N=419) were decreased by 2.4% and 1.0% respectively, compared to placebo, a phenomenon seen with other alpha blocking drugs. In BPH patients the incidence of clinically significant WBC abnormalities was 0.4% (2/459) with CARDURA® and 0% (0/147) with placebo, with no statistically significant difference between the two treatment groups. A search through a data base of 2400 hypertensive patients and 665 BPH patients revealed 4 hypertensives in which drug-related neutropenia could not be ruled out and one BPH patient in which drug related leukopenia could not be ruled out. Two hypertensives had a single low value on the last day of treatment. Two hypertensives had stable, non-progressive neutrophil counts in the $1000/mm^3$ range over periods of 20 and 40 weeks. One BPH patient had a decrease from WBC count of $4800/mm^3$ to $2700/mm^3$ at the end of the study; there was no evidence of clinical impairment. In cases where follow-up was available the WBCs and neutrophil counts returned to normal after discontinuation of CARDURA®. No patients became symptomatic as a result of the low WBC or neutrophil counts.

Drug Interactions: Most (98%) of plasma doxazosin is protein bound. *In vitro* data in human plasma indicate that CARDURA® has no effect on protein binding of digoxin, warfarin, phenytoin or indomethacin. There is no information on the effect of other highly plasma protein bound drugs on doxazosin binding. CARDURA® has been administered without any evidence of an adverse drug interaction to patients receiving thiazide diuretics, beta-blocking agents, and nonsteroidal anti-inflammatory drugs. In a placebo-controlled trial in normal volunteers, the administration of a single 1 mg dose of doxazosin on day 1 of a four-day regimen of oral cimetidine (400 mg twice daily) resulted in a 10% increase in mean AUC of doxazosin (p=0.006), and a slight but not statistically significant increase in mean C_{max} and mean half-life of doxazosin. The clinical significance of this increase in doxazosin AUC is unknown.

In clinical trials, CARDURA® tablets have been administered to patients on a variety of concomitant medications; while no formal interaction studies have been conducted, no interactions were observed. CARDURA® tablets have been used with the following drugs or drug classes: 1) analgesic/anti-inflammatory (e.g., acetaminophen, aspirin, codeine and codeine combinations, ibuprofen, indomethacin); 2) antibiotics (e.g., erythromycin, trimethoprim and sulfamethoxazole, amoxicillin); 3) antihistamines (e.g., chlorpheniramine); 4) cardiovascular agents (e.g., atenolol, hydrochlorothiazide, propranolol); 5) corticosteroids; 6) gastrointestinal agents (e.g., antacids); 7) hypoglycemics and endocrine drugs; 8) sedatives and tranquilizers (e.g., diazepam); 9) cold and flu remedies.

Cardiac Toxicity in Animals: An increased incidence of myocardial necrosis or fibrosis was displayed by Sprague-Dawley rats after 6 months of dietary administration at concentrations calculated to provide 80 mg doxazosin/kg/day and after 12 months of dietary administration at concentrations calculated to provide 40 mg doxazosin/kg/day (AUC exposure in rats 8 times the human AUC exposure with a 12 mg/day therapeutic dose). Myocardial fibrosis was observed in both rats and mice treated in the same manner with 40 mg doxazosin/kg/day for 18 months (exposure 8 times human AUC exposure in rats and somewhat equivalent to human C_{max} exposure in mice). No cardiotoxicity was observed at lower doses (up to 10 or 20 mg/kg/day, depending on the study) in either species. These lesions were not observed after 12 months of oral dosing in dogs at maximum doses of 20 mg/kg/day [maximum plasma concentrations (C_{max}) in dogs 14 times the C_{max} exposure in humans receiving a 12 mg/day therapeutic dose] and in Wistar rats at doses of 100 mg/kg/day (C_{max} exposures 15 times human C_{max} exposure with a 12 mg/day therapeutic dose). There is no evidence that similar lesions occur in humans.

Carcinogenicity, Mutagenesis and Impairment of Fertility: Chronic dietary administration (up to 24 months) of doxazosin mesylate at maximally tolerated concentrations (highest dose 40 mg/kg/day: 8 times human AUC exposure) revealed no evidence of carcinogenicity in rats. There was no evidence of carcinogenicity in a similarly conducted 18 month oral study in mice. The mouse study, however, was compromised by the failure to use a maximally tolerated dose of doxazosin.

Mutagenicity studies revealed no drug- or metabolite-related effects at either chromosomal or subchromosomal levels.

Studies in rats showed reduced fertility in males treated with doxazosin at oral doses of 20 (but not 5 or 10) mg/kg/day, about 4 times the AUC exposures obtained with a 12 mg/day human dose. This effect was reversible within two weeks of drug withdrawal. There have been no reports of any effects of doxazosin on male fertility in humans.

Pregnancy: Teratogenic Effects, Pregnancy Category C. Studies in pregnant rabbits and rats at daily oral doses of up to 41 and 20 mg/kg, respectively (plasma drug concentrations 10 and 4 times human C_{max} and AUC exposures with a 12 mg/day therapeutic dose), have revealed no evidence of harm to the fetus. A dosage regimen of 82 mg/kg/day in the rabbit was associated with reduced fetal survival. There are no adequate and well-controlled studies in pregnant women. Because animal reproduction studies are not always predictive of human response, CARDURA® should be used during pregnancy only if clearly needed.

Radioactivity was found to cross the placenta following oral administration of labelled doxazosin to pregnant rats.

Nonteratogenic Effects. In peri-postnatal studies in rats, postnatal development at maternal doses of 40 or 50 mg/kg/day of doxazosin (8 times human AUC exposure with a 12 mg/day therapeutic dose) was delayed as evidenced by slower body weight gain and a slightly later appearance of anatomical features and reflexes.

Nursing Mothers: Studies in lactating rats given a single oral dose of 1 mg/kg of [2-^{14}C]-CARDURA® indicate that doxazosin accumulates in rat breast milk with a maximum concentration about 20 times greater than the maternal plasma concentration. It is not known whether this drug is excreted in human milk. Because many drugs are excreted in human milk, caution should be exercised when CARDURA® is administered to a nursing mother.

Pediatric Use: The safety and effectiveness of CARDURA® as an antihypertensive agent have not been established in children.

Use in Elderly: The safety and effectiveness profile of CARDURA® in BPH was similar in the elderly (age ≥65 years) and younger (age <65 years) patients.

ADVERSE REACTIONS

A. *Benign Prostatic Hyperplasia*

The incidence of adverse events has been ascertained from worldwide clinical trials in 965 BPH patients. The incidence rates presented below (Table 3) are based on combined data from seven placebo-controlled trials involving once daily administration of CARDURA® in doses of 1–16 mg in hypertensives and 0.5–8 mg in normotensives. The adverse events when the incidence in the CARDURA® group was at least 1% are summarized in Table 3. No significant difference in the incidence of adverse events compared to placebo was seen except for dizziness, fatigue, hypotension, edema and dyspnea. Dizziness and dyspnea appeared to be dose-related. [See table above.]

TABLE 3
ADVERSE REACTIONS DURING PLACEBO-CONTROLLED STUDIES
BENIGN PROSTATIC HYPERPLASIA

Body System	CARDURA® (N=665)	PLACEBO (N=300)
BODY AS A WHOLE		
Back pain	1.8%	2.0%
Chest pain	1.2%	0.7%
Fatigue	8.0%*	1.7%
Headache	9.9%	9.0%
Influenza-like symptoms	1.1%	1.0%
Pain	2.0%	1.0%
CARDIOVASCULAR SYSTEM		
Hypotension	1.7%*	0.0%
Palpitation	1.2%	0.3%
DIGESTIVE SYSTEM		
Abdominal Pain	2.4%	2.0%
Diarrhea	2.3%	2.0%
Dyspepsia	1.7%	1.7%
Nausea	1.5%	0.7%
METABOLIC AND NUTRITIONAL DISORDERS		
Edema	2.7%*	0.7%
NERVOUS SYSTEM		
Dizziness†	15.6%*	9.0%
Mouth Dry	1.4%	0.3%
Somnolence	3.0%	1.0%
RESPIRATORY SYSTEM		
Dyspnea	2.6%*	0.3%
Respiratory Disorder	1.1%	0.7%
SPECIAL SENSES		
Vision Abnormal	1.4%	0.7%
UROGENITAL SYSTEM		
Impotence	1.1%	1.0%
Urinary Tract Infection	1.4%	2.3%
SKIN & APPENDAGES		
Sweating Increased	1.1%	1.0%
PSYCHIATRIC DISORDERS		
Anxiety	1.1%	0.3%
Insomnia	1.2%	0.3%

*$p \leq 0.05$ for treatment differences

†Includes vertigo

In these placebo-controlled studies of 665 CARDURA® patients, treated for a mean of 85 days, additional adverse reactions have been reported. These are less than 1% and not distinguishable from those that occurred in the placebo group. Adverse reactions with an incidence of less than 1% but of clinical interest are (CARDURA® vs. placebo): *Cardiovascular System:* angina pectoris (0.6% vs. 0.7%), postural hypotension (0.3% vs. 0.3%), syncope (0.5% vs. 0.0%), tachycardia (0.9% vs. 0.0%); *Urogenital System:* dysuria (0.5% vs. 1.3%), and *Psychiatric Disorders:* libido decreased (0.8% vs. 0.3%). The safety profile in patients treated for up to three years was similar to that in the placebo-controlled studies. The majority of adverse experiences with CARDURA® were mild.

B. *Hypertension*

CARDURA® (doxazosin mesylate) has been administered to approximately 4000 hypertensive patients, of whom 1679 were included in the hypertension clinical development program. In that program, minor adverse effects were frequent, but led to discontinuation of treatment in only 7% of patients. In placebo-controlled studies adverse effects occurred in 49% and 40% of patients in the doxazosin and placebo groups, respectively, and led to discontinuation in 2% of patients in each group. The major reasons for discontinuation were postural effects (2%), edema, malaise/fatigue, and some heart rate disturbance, each about 0.7%.

In controlled hypertension clinical trials directly comparing CARDURA® to placebo there was no significant difference in the incidence of side effects, except for dizziness (including postural), weight gain, somnolence and fatigue/malaise. Postural effects and edema appeared to be dose related. The prevalence rates presented below are based on combined data from placebo-controlled studies involving once daily administration of doxazosin at doses ranging from 1–16 mg. Table 4 summarizes those adverse experiences (possibly/probably related) reported for patients in these hypertension studies where the prevalence rate in the doxazosin group was at least 0.5% or where the reaction is of particular interest.

Continued on next page

Pfizer Inc—Cont.

TABLE 4
ADVERSE REACTIONS DURING PLACEBO-CONTROLLED STUDIES

	HYPERTENSION	
	DOXAZOSIN (N = 339)	PLACEBO (N = 336)
CARDIOVASCULAR SYSTEM		
Dizziness	19%	9%
Vertigo	2%	1%
Postural Hypotension	0.3%	0%
Edema	4%	3%
Palpitation	2%	3%
Arrhythmia	1%	0%
Hypotension	1%	0%
Tachycardia	0.3%	1%
Peripheral Ischemia	0.3%	0%
SKIN APPENDAGES		
Rash	1%	1%
Pruritus	1%	1%
MUSCULOSKELETAL SYSTEM		
Arthralgia/Arthritis	1%	0%
Muscle Weakness	1%	0%
Myalgia	1%	0%
CENTRAL & PERIPHERAL N.S.		
Headache	14%	16%
Paresthesia	1%	1%
Kinetic Disorders	1%	0%
Ataxia	1%	0%
Hypertonia	1%	0%
Muscle Cramps	1%	0%
AUTONOMIC		
Mouth Dry	2%	2%
Flushing	1%	0%
SPECIAL SENSES		
Vision Abnormal	2%	1%
Conjunctivitis/Eye Pain	1%	1%
Tinnitus	1%	0.3%
PSYCHIATRIC		
Somnolence	5%	1%
Nervousness	2%	2%
Depression	1%	1%
Insomnia	1%	1%
Sexual Dysfunction	2%	1%
GASTROINTESTINAL		
Nausea	3%	4%
Diarrhea	2%	3%
Constipation	1%	1%
Dyspepsia	1%	1%
Flatulence	1%	1%
Abdominal Pain	0%	2%
Vomiting	0%	1%
RESPIRATORY		
Rhinitis	3%	1%
Dyspnea	1%	1%
Epistaxis	1%	0%
URINARY		
Polyuria	2%	0%
Urinary Incontinence	1%	0%
Micturition Frequency	0%	2%
GENERAL		
Fatigue/Malaise	12%	6%
Chest Pain	2%	2%
Asthenia	1%	1%
Face Edema	1%	0%
Pain	2%	2%

Additional adverse reactions have been reported, but these are, in general, not distinguishable from symptoms that might have occurred in the absence of exposure to doxazosin. The following adverse reactions occurred with a frequency of between 0.5% and 1%: syncope, hypoesthesia, increased sweating, agitation, increased weight. The following additional adverse reactions were reported by <0.5% of 3960 patients who received doxazosin in controlled or open, short- or long-term clinical studies, including international studies. *Cardiovascular System:* angina pectoris, myocardial infarction, cerebrovascular accident; *Autonomic Nervous System:* pallor; *Metabolic:* thirst, gout, hypokalemia; *Hematopoietic:* lymphadenopathy, purpura; *Reproductive System:* breast

pain; *Skin Disorders:* alopecia, dry skin, eczema; *Central Nervous System:* paresis, tremor, twitching, confusion, migraine, impaired concentration; *Psychiatric:* paroniria, amnesia, emotional lability, abnormal thinking, depersonalization; *Special Senses:* parosmia, earache, taste perversion, photophobia, abnormal lacrimation; *Gastrointestinal System:* increased appetite, anorexia, fecal incontinence, gastroenteritis; *Respiratory System:* bronchospasm, sinusitis, coughing, pharyngitis; *Urinary System:* renal calculus; *General Body System:* hot flushes, back pain, infection, fever/rigors, decreased weight, influenza-like symptoms.

CARDURA® has not been associated with any clinically significant changes in routine biochemical tests. No clinically relevant adverse effects were noted on serum potassium, serum glucose, uric acid, blood urea nitrogen, creatinine or liver function tests. CARDURA® has been associated with decreases in white blood cell counts (See Precautions).

OVERDOSAGE

Experience with CARDURA® overdosage is limited. Two adolescents who each intentionally ingested 40 mg CARDURA® with diclofenac or paracetamol, were treated with gastric lavage with activated charcoal and made full recoveries. A two year-old child who accidentally ingested 4 mg CARDURA® was treated with gastric lavage and remained normotensive during the five hour emergency room observation period. A six-month old child accidentally received a crushed 1 mg tablet of CARDURA® and was reported to have been drowsy. A 32 year old female with chronic renal failure, epilepsy and depression intentionally ingested 60 mg CARDURA® (blood level 0.9 μg/mL; normal values in hypertensives = 0.02 μg/mL); death was attributed to a grand mal seizure resulting from hypotension. A 39 year-old female who ingested 70 mg CARDURA®, alcohol and Dalmane® (flurazepam) developed hypotension which responded to fluid therapy.

The oral LD_{50} of doxazosin is greater than 1000 mg/kg in mice and rats. The most likely manifestation of overdosage would be hypotension, for which the usual treatment would be intravenous infusion of fluid. As doxazosin is highly protein bound, dialysis would not be indicated.

DOSAGE AND ADMINISTRATION

DOSAGE MUST BE INDIVIDUALIZED. The initial dosage of CARDURA® in patients with hypertension and/or BPH is 1 mg given once daily in the a.m. or p.m. This starting dose is intended to minimize the frequency of postural hypotension and first dose syncope associated with CARDURA®. Postural effects are most likely to occur between 2 and 6 hours after a dose. Therefore blood pressure measurements should be taken during this time period after the first dose and with each increase in dose. If CARDURA® administration is discontinued for several days, therapy should be restarted using the initial dosing regimen.

A. **BENIGN PROSTATIC HYPERPLASIA 1–8 mg once daily.** The initial dosage of CARDURA® is 1 mg, given once daily in the a.m. or p.m. Depending on the individual patient's urodynamics and BPH symptomatology, dosage may then be increased to 2 mg and thereafter to 4 mg and 8 mg once daily, the maximum recommended dose for BPH. The recommended titration interval is 1–2 weeks. Blood pressure should be evaluated routinely in these patients.

B. **HYPERTENSION 1–16 mg once daily.** The initial dosage of CARDURA® is 1 mg given once daily. Depending on the individual patient's standing blood pressure response (based on measurements taken at 2–6 hours post-dose and 24 hours post-dose), dosage may then be increased to 2 mg and thereafter if necessary to 4 mg, 8 mg and 16 mg to achieve the desired reduction in blood pressure. **Increases in dose beyond 4 mg increase the likelihood of excessive postural effects including syncope, postural dizziness/vertigo and postural hypotension. At a titrated dose of 16 mg once daily the frequency of postural effects is about 12% compared to 3% for placebo.**

HOW SUPPLIED

CARDURA® (doxazosin mesylate) is available as colored tablets for oral administration. Each tablet contains doxazosin mesylate equivalent to 1 mg (white), 2 mg (yellow), 4 mg (orange) or 8 mg (green) of the active constituent, doxazosin.

CARDURA® TABLETS (doxazosin mesylate) are available as 1 mg (white), 2 mg (yellow), 4 mg (orange) and 8 mg (green) scored tablets.

Bottles of 100:

1 mg	(NDC 0049-2750-66)
2 mg	(NDC 0049-2760-66)
4 mg	(NDC 0049-2770-66)
8 mg	(NDC 0049-2780-66)

Unit Dose Packages of 100:

1 mg	(NDC 0049-2750-41)
2 mg	(NDC 0049-2760-41)
4 mg	(NDC 0049-2770-41)
8 mg	(NDC 0049-2780-41)

Recommended Storage: Store below 86°F (30°C).
CAUTION: Federal law prohibits dispensing without prescription.
© **1994 PFIZER INC**
65-4538-44-3

Rev. Dec. 1994

Shown in Product Identification Guide, page 327

CEFOBID® ℞
[*sĕf'ō-bĭd*]
(sterile cefoperazone sodium USP)
and (cefoperazone sodium injection USP)
For Intravenous or Intramuscular Use

DESCRIPTION

CEFOBID® (cefoperazone sodium) is a sterile, semisynthetic, broad-spectrum, parenteral cephalosporin antibiotic for intravenous or intramuscular administration. It is sodium (6R, 7R)-7-[(R)-2-(4-ethyl-2,3-dioxo-1-piperazinecarboxamido)-2-(*p*-hydroxyphenyl)acetamido-3-[[(1-methyl-*H*-tetrazol-5-yl)thio] methyl]-8-oxo-5-thia-1-azabicyclo[4.2.0]oct-2-ene-2-carboxylate. Its molecular formula is $C_{25}H_{26}N_9 NaO_8S_2$ with a molecular weight of 667.65. The structural formula is given below:

CEFOBID contains 34 mg sodium (1.5 mEq) per gram. CEFOBID is a white powder which is freely soluble in water. The pH of a 25% (w/v) freshly reconstituted solution varies between 4.5–6.5 and the solution ranges from colorless to straw yellow depending on the concentration.

CEFOBID in crystalline form is supplied in vials equivalent to 1 g or 2 g of cefoperazone and in Piggyback Units for intravenous administration equivalent to 1 g or 2 g cefoperazone. CEFOBID is also supplied premixed as a frozen, sterile, non-pyrogenic, iso-osmotic solution equivalent to 1 g or 2 g cefoperazone in plastic containers. After thawing, the solution is intended for intravenous use.

The plastic container is fabricated from specially formulated polyvinyl chloride. Solutions in contact with the plastic container can leach out certain of its chemical components in very small amounts within the expiration period, e.g., di-2-ethylhexyl phthalate (DEHP), up to 5 parts per million. However, the safety of the plastic has been confirmed in tests in animals according to the USP biological tests for plastic containers, as well as by tissue culture toxicity studies.

CLINICAL PHARMACOLOGY

High serum and bile levels of CEFOBID are attained after a single dose of the drug. Table 1 demonstrates the serum concentrations of CEFOBID in normal volunteers following either a single 15-minute constant rate intravenous infusion of 1, 2, 3 or 4 grams of the drug, or a single intramuscular injection of 1 or 2 grams of the drug.
[See Table 1 on top of next page.]
The mean serum half-life of CEFOBID is approximately 2.0 hours, independent of the route of administration.

In vitro studies with human serum indicate that the degree of CEFOBID reversible protein binding varies with the serum concentration from 93% at 25 mcg/mL of CEFOBID to 90% at 250 mcg/mL and 82% at 500 mcg/mL.

CEFOBID achieves therapeutic concentrations in the following body tissues and fluids:

Tissue or Fluid	Dose	Concentration
Ascitic Fluid	2 g	64 mcg/mL
Cerebrospinal Fluid (in patients with inflamed meninges)	50 mg/kg	1.8 mcg/mL to 8.0 mcg/mL
Urine	2 g	3,286 mcg/mL
Sputum	3 g	6.0 mcg/mL
Endometrium	2 g	74 mcg/g
Myometrium	2 g	54 mcg/g
Palatine Tonsil	1 g	8 mcg/g
Sinus Mucous Membrane	1 g	8 mcg/g
Umbilical Cord Blood	1 g	25 mcg/mL
Amniotic Fluid	1 g	4.8 mcg/mL
Lung	1 g	28 mcg/g
Bone	2 g	40 mcg/g

CEFOBID is excreted mainly in the bile. Maximum bile concentrations are generally obtained between one and three hours following drug administration and exceed concurrent serum concentrations by up to 100 times. Reported biliary

concentrations of CEFOBID range from 66 mcg/mL at 30 minutes to as high as 6000 mcg/mL at 3 hours after an intravenous bolus injection of 2 grams.
Following a single intramuscular or intravenous dose, the urinary recovery of CEFOBID over a 12-hour period averages 20–30%. No significant quantity of metabolites has been found in the urine. Urinary concentrations greater than 2200 mcg/mL have been obtained following a 15-minute infusion of a 2 g dose. After an IM injection of 2 g, peak urine concentrations of almost 1000 mcg/mL have been obtained, and therapeutic levels are maintained for 12 hours.
Repeated administration of CEFOBID at 12-hour intervals does not result in accumulation of the drug in normal subjects. Peak serum concentrations, areas under the curve (AUC's), and serum half-lives in patients with severe renal insufficiency are not significantly different from those in normal volunteers. In patients with hepatic dysfunction, the serum half-life is prolonged and urinary excretion is increased. In patients with combined renal and hepatic insufficiencies, CEFOBID may accumulate in the serum.
CEFOBID has been used in pediatrics, but the safety and effectiveness in children have not been established. The half-life of CEFOBID in serum is 6–10 hours in low birth-weight neonates.

TABLE 1. Cefoperazone Serum Concentrations

	Mean Serum Concentrations (mcg/mL)						
Dose/Route	**0***	**0.5 hr**	**1 hr**	**2 hr**	**4 hr**	**8 hr**	**12 hr**
1 g IV	153	114	73	38	16	4	0.5
2 g IV	252	153	114	70	32	8	2
3 g IV	340	210	142	89	41	9	2
4 g IV	506	325	251	161	71	19	6
1 g IM	32**	52	65	57	33	7	1
2 g IM	40**	69	93	97	58	14	4

*Hours post-administration, with 0 time being the end of the infusion.
**Values obtained 15 minutes post-injection.

Microbiology
CEFOBID is active *in vitro* against a wide range of aerobic and anaerobic, gram-positive and gram-negative pathogens. The bactericidal action of CEFOBID results from the inhibition of bacterial cell wall synthesis. CEFOBID has a high degree of stability in the presence of beta-lactamases produced by most gram-negative pathogens. CEFOBID is usually active against organisms which are resistant to other beta-lactam antibiotics because of beta-lactamase production. CEFOBID is usually active against the following organisms *in vitro* and in clinical infections:

Gram-Positive Aerobes:
Staphylococcus aureus, penicillinase and non-penicillinase-producing strains
Staphylococcus epidermidis
Streptococcus pneumoniae (formerly *Diplococcus pneumoniae*)
Streptococcus pyogenes (Group A beta-hemolytic streptococci)
Streptococcus agalactiae (Group B beta-hemolytic streptococci)
Enterococcus (*Streptococcus faecalis, S. faecium* and *S. durans*)

Gram-Negative Aerobes:
Escherichia coli
Klebsiella species (including *K. pneumoniae*)
Enterobacter species
Citrobacter species
Haemophilus influenzae
Proteus mirabilis
Proteus vulgaris
Morganella morganii (formerly *Proteus morganii*)
Providencia stuartii
Providencia rettgeri (formerly *Proteus rettgeri*)
Serratia marcescens
Pseudomonas aeruginosa
Pseudomonas species
Some strains of *Acinetobacter calcoaceticus*
Neisseria gonorrhoeae

Anaerobic Organisms:
Gram-positive cocci (including *Peptococcus* and *Peptostreptococcus*)
Clostridium species
Bacteroides fragilis
Other *Bacteroides* species

CEFOBID is also active *in vitro* against a wide variety of other pathogens although the clinical significance is unknown. These organisms include: *Salmonella* and *Shigella* species, *Serratia liquefaciens, N. meningitidis, Bordetella pertussis, Yersinia enterocolitica, Clostridium difficile, Fusobacterium* species, *Eubacterium* species and beta-lactamase producing strains of *H. influenzae* and *N. gonorrhoeae.*

Susceptibility Testing:
Diffusion Technique. For the disk diffusion method of susceptibility testing, a 75 mcg CEFOBID diffusion disk should be used. Organisms should be tested with the CEFOBID 75 mcg disk since CEFOBID has been shown *in vitro* to be active against organisms which are found to be resistant to other beta-lactam antibiotics.
Tests should be interpreted by the following criteria:

Zone Diameter	Interpretation
Greater than or equal to 21 mm	Susceptible
16–20 mm	Moderately Susceptible
Less than or equal to 15 mm	Resistant

Quantitative procedures that require measurement of zone diameters give the most precise estimate of susceptibility. One such method which has been recommended for use with the CEFOBID 75 mcg disk is the NCCLS approved standard. (Performance Standards for Antimicrobic Disk Susceptibility Tests. Second Information Supplement Vol. 2 No. 2 pp. 49–69. Publisher—National Committee for Clinical Laboratory Standards, Villanova, Pennsylvania.)
A report of "susceptible" indicates that the infecting organism is likely to respond to CEFOBID therapy and a report of "resistant" indicates that the infecting organism is not likely to respond to therapy. A "moderately susceptible" report suggests that the infecting organism will be susceptible to CEFOBID if a higher than usual dosage is used or if the infection is confined to tissues and fluids (e.g., urine or bile) in which high antibiotic levels are attained.
Dilution Techniques. Broth or agar dilution methods may be used to determine the minimal inhibitory concentration (MIC) of CEFOBID. Serial twofold dilutions of CEFOBID should be prepared in either broth or agar. Broth should be inoculated to contain 5×10^5 organisms/mL and agar "spotted" with 10^4 organisms.
MIC test results should be interpreted in light of serum, tissue, and body fluid concentrations of CEFOBID. Organisms inhibited by CEFOBID at 16 mcg/mL or less are considered susceptible, while organisms with MIC's of 17–63 mcg/mL are moderately susceptible. Organisms inhibited at CEFOBID concentrations of greater than or equal to 64 mcg/mL are considered resistant, although clinical cures have been obtained in some patients infected by such organisms.

INDICATIONS AND USAGE

CEFOBID is indicated for the treatment of the following infections when caused by susceptible organisms:
Respiratory Tract Infections caused by *S. pneumoniae, H. influenzae, S. aureus* (penicillinase and non-penicillinase producing strains), *S. pyogenes** (Group A beta-hemolytic streptococci), *P. aeruginosa, Klebsiella pneumoniae, E. coli, Proteus mirabilis,* and *Enterobacter* species.
Peritonitis and Other Intra-abdominal Infections caused by *E. coli, P. aeruginosa,** and anaerobic gram-negative bacilli (including *Bacteroides fragilis*).
Bacterial Septicemia caused by *S. pneumoniae, S. agalactiae*, S. aureus, Pseudomonas aeruginosa*, E. coli, Klebsiella* spp.,* Klebsiella pneumoniae* , Proteus species* (indole-positive and indole-negative), *Clostridium* spp.* and anaerobic gram-positive cocci.*
Infections of the Skin and Skin Structures caused by *S. aureus* (penicillinase and non-penicillinase producing strains), *S. pyogenes**, and *P. aeruginosa.*
Pelvic Inflammatory Disease, Endometritis, and Other Infections of the Female Genital Tract caused by *N. gonorrhoeae, S. epidermidis*, S. agalactiae, E. coli, Clostridium* spp.,* *Bacteroides* species (including *Bacteroides fragilis*) and anaerobic gram-positive cocci.
Cefobid,® like other cephalosporins, has no activity against *Chlamydia trachomatis.* Therefore, when cephalosporins are used in the treatment of patients with pelvic inflammatory disease and *C. trachomatis* is one of the suspected pathogens, appropriate anti-chlamydial coverage should be added.
Urinary Tract Infections caused by *Escherichia coli* and *Pseudomonas aeruginosa.*
Enterococcal Infections: Although cefoperazone has been shown to be clinically effective in the treatment of infections caused by enterococci in cases of **peritonitis and other intra-abdominal infections, infections of the skin and skin structures, pelvic inflammatory disease, endometritis and other infections of the female genital tract, and urinary tract infection,*** the majority of clinical isolates of enterococci tested are not susceptible to cefoperazone but fall just at or in the intermediate zone of susceptibilty, and are moderately resistant to cefoperazone. However, *in vitro* susceptibility testing may not correlate directly with *in vivo* results. Despite this, cefoperazone therapy has resulted in clinical cures of enterococcal infections, chiefly in polymicrobial infections. Cefoperazone should be used in enterococcal infections with care and at doses that achieve satisfactory serum levels of cefoperazone.

*Efficacy of this organism in this organ system was studied in fewer than 10 infections.

Susceptibility Testing
Before instituting treatment with CEFOBID, appropriate specimens should be obtained for isolation of the causative organism and for determination of its susceptibility to the drug. Treatment may be started before results of susceptibility testing are available.
Combination Therapy
Synergy between CEFOBID and aminoglycosides has been demonstrated with many gram-negative bacilli. However, such enhanced activity of these combinations is not predictable. If such therapy is considered, *in vitro* susceptibility tests should be performed to determine the activity of the drugs in combination, and renal function should be monitored carefully. (See PRECAUTIONS, and DOSAGE AND ADMINISTRATION sections).

CONTRAINDICATIONS

CEFOBID is contraindicated in patients with known allergy to the cephalosporin-class of antibiotics.

WARNINGS

BEFORE THERAPY WITH CEFOBID IS INSTITUTED, CAREFUL INQUIRY SHOULD BE MADE TO DETERMINE WHETHER THE PATIENT HAS HAD PREVIOUS HYPERSENSITIVITY REACTIONS TO CEPHALOSPORINS, PENICILLINS OR OTHER DRUGS. THIS PRODUCT SHOULD BE GIVEN CAUTIOUSLY TO PENICILLIN-SENSITIVE PATIENTS. ANTIBIOTICS SHOULD BE ADMINISTERED WITH CAUTION TO ANY PATIENT WHO HAS DEMONSTRATED SOME FORM OF ALLERGY, PARTICULARLY TO DRUGS. SERIOUS ACUTE HYPERSENSITIVITY REACTIONS MAY REQUIRE THE USE OF SUBCUTANEOUS EPINEPHRINE AND OTHER EMERGENCY MEASURES.
PSEUDOMEMBRANOUS COLITIS HAS BEEN REPORTED WITH THE USE OF CEPHALOSPORINS (AND OTHER BROAD-SPECTRUM ANTIBIOTICS); THEREFORE, IT IS IMPORTANT TO CONSIDER ITS DIAGNOSIS IN PATIENTS WHO DEVELOP DIARRHEA IN ASSOCIATION WITH ANTIBIOTIC USE.
Treatment with broad-spectrum antibiotics alters normal flora of the colon and may permit overgrowth of clostridia. Studies indicate a toxin produced by *Clostridium difficile* is one primary cause of antibiotic-associated colitis. Cholestyramine and colestipol resins have been shown to bind the toxin *in vitro.*
Mild cases of colitis may respond to drug discontinuance alone.
Moderate to severe cases should be managed with fluid, electrolyte, and protein supplementation as indicated.
When the colitis is not relieved by drug discontinuance or when it is severe, oral vancomycin is the treatment of choice for antibiotic-associated pseudomembranous colitis produced by *C. difficile.* Other causes of colitis should also be considered.

PRECAUTIONS

Although transient elevations of the BUN and serum creatinine have been observed, CEFOBID alone does not appear to cause significant nephrotoxicity. However, concomitant administration of aminoglycosides and other cephalosporins has caused nephrotoxicity.
CEFOBID is extensively excreted in bile. The serum half-life of CEFOBID is increased 2–4 fold in patients with hepatic disease and/or biliary obstruction. In general, total daily dosage above 4 g should not be necessary in such patients. If higher dosages are used, serum concentrations should be monitored.
Because renal excretion is not the main route of elimination of CEFOBID (see CLINICAL PHARMACOLOGY), patients with renal failure require no adjustment in dosage when usual doses are administered. When high doses of CEFOBID are used, concentrations of drug in the serum should be monitored periodically. If evidence of accumulation exists, dosage should be decreased accordingly.
The half-life of CEFOBID is reduced slightly during hemodialysis. Thus, dosing should be scheduled to follow a dialysis period. In patients with both hepatic dysfunction and significant renal disease, CEFOBID dosage should not exceed 1–2 g daily without close monitoring of serum concentrations.
As with other antibiotics, vitamin K deficiency has occurred rarely in patients treated with CEFOBID. The mechanism is most probably related to the suppression of gut flora which normally synthesize this vitamin. Those at risk include pa-

Continued on next page

Pfizer Inc—Cont.

tients with a poor nutritional status, malabsorption states (e.g., cystic fibrosis), alcoholism, and patients on prolonged hyper-alimentation regimens (administered either intravenously or via a naso-gastric tube). Prothrombin time should be monitored in these patients and exogenous vitamin K administered as indicated.

A disulfiram-like reaction characterized by flushing, sweating, headache, and tachycardia has been reported when alcohol (beer, wine) was ingested within 72 hours after CEFOBID administration. Patients should be cautioned about the ingestion of alcoholic beverages following the administration of CEFOBID. A similar reaction has been reported with other cephalosporins.

Prolonged use of CEFOBID may result in the overgrowth of nonsusceptible organisms. Careful observation of the patient is essential. If superinfection occurs during therapy, appropriate measures should be taken.

CEFOBID should be prescribed with caution in individuals with a history of gastrointestinal disease, particularly colitis.

Drug Laboratory Test Interactions
A false-positive reaction for glucose in the urine may occur with Benedict's or Fehling's solution.

Carcinogenesis, Mutagenesis, Impairment of Fertility
Long term studies in animals have not been performed to evaluate carcinogenic potential. The maximum duration of CEFOBID animal toxicity studies is six months. In none of the *in vivo* or *in vitro* genetic toxicology studies did CEFOBID show any mutagenic potential at either the chromosomal or subchromosomal level. CEFOBID produced no impairment of fertility and had no effects on general reproductive performance or fetal development when administered subcutaneously at daily doses up to 500 to 1000 mg/kg prior to and during mating, and to pregnant female rats during gestation. These doses are 10 to 20 times the estimated usual single clinical dose. CEFOBID had adverse effects on the testes of prepubertal rats at all doses tested. Subcutaneous administration of 1000 mg/kg per day (approximately 16 times the average adult human dose) resulted in reduced testicular weight, arrested spermatogenesis, reduced germinal cell population and vacuolation of Sertoli cell cytoplasm. The severity of lesions was dose dependent in the 100 to 1000 mg/kg per day range; the low dose caused a minor decrease in spermatocytes. This effect has not been observed in adult rats. Histologically the lesions were reversible at all but the highest dosage levels. However, these studies did not evaluate subsequent development of reproductive function in the rats. The relationship of these findings to humans is unknown.

Usage in Pregnancy
Pregnancy Category B: Reproduction studies have been performed in mice, rats, and monkeys at doses up to 10 times the human dose and have revealed no evidence of impaired fertility or harm to the fetus due to CEFOBID. There are, however, no adequate and well controlled studies in pregnant women. Because animal reproduction studies are not always predictive of human response, this drug should be used during pregnancy only if clearly needed.

Usage in Nursing Mothers
Only low concentrations of CEFOBID are excreted in human milk. Although CEFOBID passes poorly into breast milk of nursing mothers, caution should be exercised when CEFOBID is administered to a nursing woman.

Pediatric Use
Safety and effectiveness in children have not been established. For information concerning testicular changes in prepubertal rats (see Carcinogenesis, Mutagenesis, Impairment of Fertility).

ADVERSE REACTIONS

In clinical studies the following adverse effects were observed and were considered to be related to CEFOBID therapy or of uncertain etiology:

Hypersensitivity: As with all cephalosporins, hypersensitivity manifested by skin reactions (1 patient in 45), drug fever (1 in 260), or a change in Coombs' test (1 in 60) has been reported. These reactions are more likely to occur in patients with a history of allergies, particularly to penicillin.

Hematology: As with other beta-lactam antibiotics, reversible neutropenia may occur with prolonged administration. Slight decreases in neutrophil count (1 patient in 50) have been reported. Decreased hemoglobins (1 in 20) or hematocrits (1 in 20) have been reported, which is consistent with published literature on other cephalosporins. Transient eosinophilia has occurred in 1 patient in 10.

Hepatic: Of 1285 patients treated with cefoperazone in clinical trials, one patient with a history of liver disease developed significantly elevated liver function enzymes during CEFOBID therapy. Clinical signs and symptoms of nonspecific hepatitis accompanied these increases. After CEFOBID therapy was discontinued, the patient's enzymes returned to pre-treatment levels and the symptomatology resolved. As with other antibiotics that achieve high bile levels, mild

	Final Cefoperazone Concentration	Step 1 Volume of Sterile Water	Step 2 Volume of 2% Lidocaine	Withdrawable Volume*†
1 g vial	333 mg/mL	2.0 mL	0.6 mL	3 mL
	250 mg/mL	2.8 mL	1.0 mL	4 mL
2 g vial	333 mg/mL	3.8 mL	1.2 mL	6 mL
	250 mg/mL	5.4 mL	1.8 mL	8 mL

When a diluent other than Lidocaine HCl Injection (USP) is used reconstitute as follows:

	Cefoperazone Concentration	Volume of Diluent to be Added	Withdrawable Volume*
1 g vial	333 mg/mL	2.6 mL	3 mL
	250 mg/mL	3.8 mL	4 mL
2 g vial	333 mg/mL	5.0 mL	6 mL
	250 mg/mL	7.2 mL	8 mL

* There is sufficient excess present to allow for withdrawal of the stated volume.
† Final lidocaine concentration will approximate that obtained if a 0.5% Lidocaine Hydrochloride Solution is used as diluent.

Controlled Room Temperature (15°–25°C/59°–77°F)
24 Hours — Approximate Concentrations

Bacteriostatic Water for Injection [Benzyl Alcohol or Parabens] (USP)	300 mg/mL
5% Dextrose Injection (USP)	2 mg to 50 mg/mL
5% Dextrose and Lactated Ringer's Injection	2 mg to 50 mg/mL
5% Dextrose and 0.9% Sodium Chloride Injection (USP)	2 mg to 50 mg/mL
5% Dextrose and 0.2% Sodium Chloride Injection (USP)	2 mg to 50 mg/mL
10% Dextrose Injection (USP)	2 mg to 50 mg/mL
Lactated Ringer's Injection (USP)	2 mg/mL
0.5% Lidocaine Hydrochloride Injection (USP)	300 mg/mL
0.9% Sodium Chloride Injection (USP)	2 mg to 300 mg/mL
Normosol® M and 5% Dextrose Injection	2 mg to 50 mg/mL
Normosol® R	2 mg to 50 mg/mL
Sterile Water for Injection	300 mg/mL

Reconstituted CEFOBID solutions may be stored in glass or plastic syringes, or in glass or flexible plastic parenteral solution containers.

Refrigerator Temperature (2°–8°C/36°–46°F)
5 Days — Approximate Concentrations

Bacteriostatic Water for Injection [Benzyl Alcohol or Parabens] (USP)	300 mg/mL
5% Dextrose Injection (USP)	2 mg to 50 mg/mL
5% Dextrose and 0.9% Sodium Chloride Injection (USP)	2 mg to 50 mg/mL
5% Dextrose and 0.2% Sodium Chloride Injection (USP)	2 mg to 50 mg/mL
Lactated Ringer's Injection (USP)	2 mg/mL
0.5% Lidocaine Hydrochloride Injection (USP)	300 mg/mL
0.9% Sodium Chloride Injection (USP)	2 mg to 300 mg/mL
Normosol® M and 5% Dextrose Injection	2 mg to 50 mg/mL
Normosol® R	2 mg to 50 mg/mL
Sterile Water for Injection	300 mg/mL

Reconstituted CEFOBID solutions may be stored in glass or plastic syringes, or in glass or flexible plastic parenteral solution containers.

Freezer Temperature (−20° to −10°C/−4° to 14°F)
3 Weeks — Approximate Concentrations

5% Dextrose Injection (USP)	50 mg/mL
5% Dextrose and 0.9% Sodium Chloride Injection (USP)	2 mg/mL
5% Dextrose and 0.2% Sodium Chloride Injection (USP)	2 mg/mL

5 Weeks

0.9% Sodium Chloride Injection (USP)	300 mg/mL
Sterile Water for Injection	300 mg/mL

Reconstituted CEFOBID solutions may be stored in plastic syringes, or in flexible plastic parenteral solution containers. Frozen samples should be thawed at room temperature before use. After thawing, unused portions should be discarded. Do not refreeze.

---

transient elevations of liver function enzymes have been observed in 5–10% of the patients receiving CEFOBID therapy. The relevance of these findings, which were not accompanied by overt signs or symptoms of hepatic dysfunction, has not been established.

Gastrointestinal: Diarrhea or loose stools has been reported in 1 in 30 patients. Most of these experiences have been mild or moderate in severity and self-limiting in nature. In all cases, these symptoms responded to symptomatic therapy or ceased when cefoperazone therapy was stopped. Nausea and vomiting have been reported rarely.

Symptoms of pseudomembranous colitis can appear during or for several weeks subsequent to antibiotic therapy (see WARNINGS).

Renal Function Tests: Transient elevations of the BUN (1 in 16) and serum creatinine (1 in 48) have been noted.

Local Reactions: CEFOBID is well tolerated following intramuscular administration. Occasionally, transient pain (1 in 140) may follow administration by this route. When CEFOBID is administered by intravenous infusion some patients may develop phlebitis (1 in 120) at the infusion site.

DOSAGE AND ADMINISTRATION

The usual adult daily dose of CEFOBID is 2 to 4 grams per day administered in divided doses every 12 hours.

In severe infections or infections caused by less sensitive organisms, the total daily dose and/or frequency may be increased. Patients have been successfully treated with a total daily dosage of 6–12 grams divided into 2, 3 or 4 administrations ranging from 1.5 to 4 grams per dose.

When treating infections caused by *Streptococcus pyogenes*, therapy should be continued for at least 10 days.

If *C. trachomatis* is a suspected pathogen, appropriate antichlamydial coverage should be added, because cefoperazone has no activity against this organism.

Solutions of CEFOBID and aminoglycoside should not be directly mixed, since there is a physical incompatibility between them. If combination therapy with CEFOBID and an aminoglycoside is contemplated (see INDICATIONS) this can be accomplished by sequential intermittent intravenous infusion provided that separate secondary intravenous tubing is used, and that the primary intravenous tubing is adequately irrigated with an approved diluent between doses. It is also suggested that CEFOBID be administered prior to the aminoglycoside. *In vitro* testing of the effectiveness of drug combination(s) is recommended.

In a pharmacokinetic study, a total daily dose of 16 grams was administered to severely immunocompromised patients by constant infusion without complications. Steady state serum concentrations were approximately 150 mcg/mL in these patients.

RECONSTITUTION

The following solutions may be used for the initial reconstitution of CEFOBID sterile powder:

Table 1. Solutions for Initial Reconstitution.
5% Dextrose Injection (USP)
5% Dextrose and 0.9% Sodium Chloride Injection (USP)
5% Dextrose and 0.2% Sodium Chloride Injection (USP)
10% Dextrose Injection (USP)
Bacteriostatic Water for Injection [Benzyl Alcohol or Parabens] (USP)*†
0.9% Sodium Chloride Injection (USP)
Normosol® M and 5% Dextrose Injection
Normosol® R
Sterile Water for Injection*

* Not to be used as a vehicle for intravenous infusion
† Preparations containing Benzyl Alcohol should not be used in neonates.

General Reconstitution Procedures
CEFOBID sterile powder for intravenous or intramuscular use may be initially reconstituted with any compatible solution mentioned above in Table 1. Solutions should be allowed to stand after reconstitution to allow any foaming to dissipate to permit visual inspection for complete solubilization. Vigorous and prolonged agitation may be necessary to solubilize CEFOBID in higher concentrations (above 333 mg cefoperazone/mL). The maximum solubility of CEFOBID sterile powder is approximately 475 mg cefoperazone/mL of compatible diluent.

Preparation For Intravenous Use
General. CEFOBID concentrations between 2 mg/mL and 50 mg/mL are recommended for intravenous administration.

Preparation of Vials. Vials of CEFOBID sterile powder may be initially reconstituted with a minimum of 2.8 mL per gram of cefoperazone of any compatible reconstituting solution appropriate for intravenous administration listed above in Table 1. For ease of reconstitution the use of 5 mL of compatible solution per gram of CEFOBID is recommended. The entire quantity of the resulting solution should then be withdrawn for further dilution and administration using any of the following vehicles for intravenous infusion:

Table 2. Vehicles for Intravenous Infusion.
- 5% Dextrose Injection (USP)
- 5% Dextrose and Lactated Ringer's Injection
- 5% Dextrose and 0.9% Sodium Chloride Injection (USP)
- 5% Dextrose and 0.2% Sodium Chloride Injection (USP)
- 10% Dextrose Injection (USP)
- Lactated Ringer's Injection (USP)
- 0.9% Sodium Chloride Injection (USP)
- Normosol® M and 5% Dextrose Injection
- Normosol® R

Preparation of Piggy Back Units. CEFOBID sterile powder in Piggy Back Units for intravenous use may be prepared by adding between 20 mL and 40 mL of any appropriate diluent listed in Table 2 per gram of cefoperazone. If 5% Dextrose and Lactated Ringer's Injection or Lactated Ringer's Injection (USP) is the chosen vehicle for administration the CEFOBID sterile powder should initially be reconstituted using 2.8–5 mL per gram of any compatible reconstituting solution listed in Table 1 prior to the final dilution.
The resulting intravenous solution should be administered in one of the following manners:
Intermittent Infusion: Solutions of CEFOBID should be administered over a 15–30 minute time period.
Continuous Infusion: CEFOBID can be used for continuous infusion after dilution to a final concentration of between 2 and 25 mg cefoperazone per mL.

Preparation For Intramuscular Injection
Any suitable solution listed above may be used to prepare CEFOBID sterile powder for intramuscular injection. When concentrations of 250 mg/mL or more are to be administered, a lidocaine solution should be used. These solutions should be prepared using a combination of Sterile Water for Injection and 2% Lidocaine Hydrochloride Injection (USP) that approximates a 0.5% Lidocaine Hydrochloride Solution. A two-step dilution process as follows is recommended: First, add the required amount of Sterile Water for Injection and agitate until CEFOBID powder is completely dissolved. Second, add the required amount of 2% lidocaine and mix.
[See first table on top of preceding page.]

DIRECTIONS FOR USE OF CEFOBID (cefoperazone sodium) INJECTION IN PLASTIC CONTAINERS
CEFOBID supplied premixed as a frozen, sterile, iso-osmotic solution in plastic containers is to be administered either as continuous or intermittent infusion.
Thaw container at room temperature. After thawing, check for minute leaks by squeezing bag firmly. If leaks are found, discard solution as sterility may be impaired. Additives should not be introduced into this solution. Do not use if the solution is cloudy or precipitated or if the seal is not intact. After thawing, the solution is stable for 10 days if stored under refrigeration (5°C) and for 48 hours at room temperature. DO NOT REFREEZE. Use sterile equipment.
CAUTION: Do not use plastic container in series connections. Such use could result in air embolism due to residual air being drawn from the primary container before administration of the fluid from the secondary container is complete.

Preparation for administration
1. Suspend container from eyelet support.
2. Remove plastic protector from outlet port at bottom of container.
3. Attach administration set. Refer to complete directions accompanying set.

Storage and Stability: CEFOBID sterile powder is to be stored at or below 25°C (77°F) and protected from light prior to reconstitution. After reconstitution, protection from light is not necessary.
The following parenteral diluents and approximate concentrations of CEFOBID provide stable solutions under the following conditions for the indicated time periods. (After the indicated time periods, unused portions of solutions should be discarded.)
[See second table on top of preceding page.]

HOW SUPPLIED
CEFOBID sterile powder is available in vials containing cefoperazone sodium equivalent to 1 gram cefoperazone × 10 (NDC 0049-1201-83), and 2 gram cefoperazone × 10 (NDC 0049-1202-83) for intramuscular and intravenous administration.
CEFOBID sterile powder is available in Piggyback Units containing cefoperazone sodium equivalent to 1 gram cefoperazone × 10 (NDC 0049-1211-83), and 2 gram cefoperazone × 10 (NDC 0049-1212-83) for intravenous administration.
CEFOBID (cefoperazone sodium) injection is supplied premixed as a frozen, sterile, nonpyrogenic, iso-osmotic solution in plastic containers. Each 50 mL unit contains cefoperazone sodium equivalent to 1 g cefoperazone with approximately 2.3 g dextrose hydrous USP added (NDC 0049-1216-18) or 2 g cefoperazone with approximately 1.8 g dextrose hydrous USP added (NDC 0049-1215-18). The solution is iso-osmotic (approximately 300 mOsmol/L), and solution pH may have been adjusted with sodium hydroxide and/or hydrochloric acid. Do not store above −20°C.
CEFOBID supplied as a frozen, sterile, nonpyrogenic, iso-osmotic solution in 50 ml plastic containers is manufactured for Roerig Division of Pfizer Pharmaceuticals by Baxter Healthcare Corporation, Deerfield, IL 60015.
Revised Jan. 1995 70-4169-00-5

CEFOBID® ℞
[*sĕf'ō-bĭd*]
Sterile Cefoperazone Sodium, USP
PHARMACY BULK PACKAGE
NOT FOR DIRECT INFUSION

DESCRIPTION
CEFOBID (cefoperazone sodium) is a sterile, semisynthetic, broad-spectrum, parenteral cephalosporin antibiotic for intravenous or intramuscular administration. It is the sodium salt of 7-[(*R*)-2-(4-ethyl-2,3-dioxo-1-piperazinecarboxamido)-2-(*p*-hydroxyphenyl)acetamido-3-[[(l-methyl-*H*-tetrazol-5-yl)thio]methyl]-8-oxo-5-thia-1-azabicyclo[4.2.0]oct-2-ene-2-carboxylate. Its chemical formula is $C_{25}H_{26}N_9NaO_8S_2$ with a molecular weight of 667.65. The structural formula is given below:

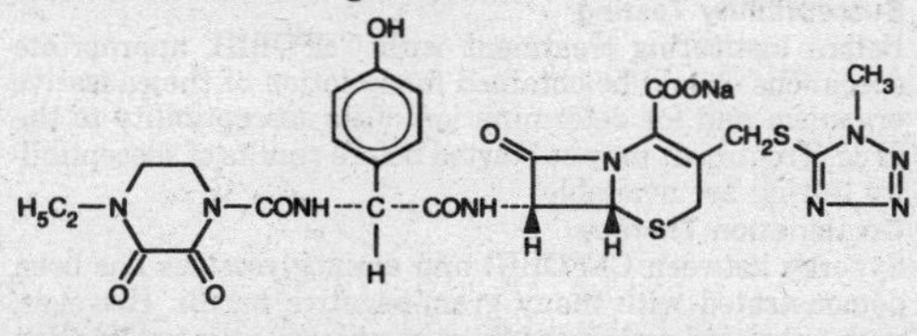

CEFOBID contains 34 mg sodium (1.5 mEq) per gram. CEFOBID is a white powder which is freely soluble in water. The pH of a 25% (w/v) freshly reconstituted solution varies between 4.5–6.5 and the solution ranges from colorless to straw yellow depending on the concentration. CEFOBID in crystalline form is supplied in vials equivalent to 1 g or 2 g of cefoperazone and in Piggyback Units for intravenous administration equivalent to 1 g or 2 g cefoperazone. CEFOBID is also supplied premixed as a frozen, sterile, nonpyrogenic, iso-osmotic solution equivalent to 1 g or 2 g cefoperazone in plastic containers. After thawing, the solution is intended for intravenous use.
The plastic container is fabricated from specially formulated polyvinyl chloride. Solutions in contact with the plastic container can leach out certain of its chemical components in very small amounts within the expiration period, e.g., di 2-ethylhexyl phthalate (DEHP), up to 5 parts per million. However, the safety of the plastic has been confirmed in tests in animals according to the USP biological tests for plastic containers, as well as by tissue culture toxicity studies.
A pharmacy bulk package is a container of a sterile preparation for parenteral use that contains many single doses. This Pharmacy Bulk Package is for use in a pharmacy admixture service; it provides many single doses of cefoperazone for addition to suitable parenteral fluids in the preparation of admixtures for intravenous infusion. (See DOSAGE AND ADMINISTRATION, and DIRECTIONS FOR PROPER USE OF PHARMACY BULK PACKAGE).

CLINICAL PHARMACOLOGY
High serum and bile levels of CEFOBID are attained after a single dose of the drug. Table 1 demonstrates the serum concentrations of CEFOBID in normal volunteers following either a single 15-minute constant rate intravenous infusion of 1, 2, 3 or 4 grams of the drug, or a single intramuscular injection of 1 or 2 grams of the drug.
[See table 1 below.]
The mean serum half-life of CEFOBID is approximately 2.0 hours, independent of the route of administration.
In vitro studies with human serum indicate that the degree of CEFOBID reversible protein binding varies with the serum concentration from 93% at 25 mcg/mL of CEFOBID to 90% at 250 mcg/mL and 82% at 500 mcg/mL.
CEFOBID achieves therapeutic concentrations in the following body tissues and fluids:

Tissue or Fluid	Dose	Concentration
Ascitic Fluid	2 g	64 mcg/mL
Cerebrospinal Fluid (in patients with inflamed meninges)	50 mg/kg	1.8 mcg/mL to 8.0 mcg/mL
Urine	2 g	3,286 mcg/mL
Sputum	3 g	6.0 mcg/mL
Endometrium	2 g	74 mcg/g
Myometrium	2 g	54 mcg/g
Palatine Tonsil	1 g	8 mcg/g
Sinus Mucous Membrane	1 g	8 mcg/g
Umbilical Cord Blood	1 g	25 mcg/mL
Amniotic Fluid	1 g	4.8 mcg/mL
Lung	1 g	28 mcg/g
Bone	2 g	40 mcg/g

CEFOBID is excreted mainly in the bile. Maximum bile concentrations are generally obtained between one and three hours following drug administration and exceed concurrent serum concentrations by up to 100 times. Reported biliary concentrations of CEFOBID range from 66 mcg/mL at 30 minutes to as high as 6000 mcg/mL at 3 hours after an intravenous bolus injection of 2 grams.
Following a single intramuscular or intravenous dose, the urinary recovery of CEFOBID over a 12-hour period averages 20–30%. No significant quantity of metabolites has been found in the urine. Urinary concentrations greater than 2200 mcg/mL have been obtained following a 15-minute infusion of a 2 g dose. After an IM injection of 2 g, peak urine concentrations of almost 1000 mcg/mL have been obtained, and therapeutic levels are maintained for 12 hours.
Repeated administration of CEFOBID at 12-hour intervals does not result in accumulation of the drug in normal subjects. Peak serum concentrations, areas under the curve (AUC's), and serum half-lives in patients with severe renal insufficiency are not significantly different from those in normal volunteers. In patients with hepatic dysfunction, the serum half-life is prolonged and urinary excretion is increased. In patients with combined renal and hepatic insufficiencies, CEFOBID may accumulate in the serum.
CEFOBID has been used in pediatrics, but the safety and effectiveness in children have not been established. The half-life of CEFOBID in serum is 6–10 hours in low birth-weight neonates.

Microbiology
CEFOBID is active *in vitro* against a wide range of aerobic and anaerobic, gram-positive and gram-negative pathogens. The bactericidal action of CEFOBID results from the inhibition of bacterial cell wall synthesis. CEFOBID has a high degree of stability in the presence of beta-lactamases produced by most gram-negative pathogens. CEFOBID is usually active against organisms which are resistant to other beta-lactam antibiotics because of beta-lactamase produc-

TABLE 1. Cefoperazone Serum Concentrations

Dose/Route	Mean Serum Concentrations (mcg/ml) 0*	0.5 hr	1 hr	2 hr	4 hr	8 hr	12 hr
1 g IV	153	114	73	38	16	4	0.5
2 g IV	252	153	114	70	32	8	2
3 g IV	340	210	142	89	41	9	2
4 g IV	506	325	251	161	71	19	6
1 g IM	32**	52	65	57	33	7	1
2 g IM	40**	69	93	97	58	14	4

*Hours post-administration, with 0 time being the end of the infusion.
**Values obtained 15 minutes post-injection.

Continued on next page

Pfizer Inc—Cont.

tion. CEFOBID is usually active against the following organisms *in vitro* and in clinical infections:

Gram-Positive Aerobes:
Staphylococcus aureus, penicillinase and non-penicillinase-producing strains
Staphylococcus epidermidis
Streptococcus pneumoniae (formerly *Diplococcus pneumoniae*)
Streptococcus pyogenes (Group A beta-hemolytic streptococci)
Streptococcus agalactiae (Group B beta-hemolytic streptococci)
Enterococcus (*Streptococcus faecalis, S. faecium* and *S. durans*)

Gram-Negative Aerobes:
Escherichia coli
Klebsiella species (including *K. pneumoniae*)
Enterobacter species
Citrobacter species
Haemophilus influenzae
Proteus mirabilis
Proteus vulgaris
Morganella morganii (formerly *Proteus morganii*)
Providencia stuartii
Providencia rettgeri (formerly *Proteus rettgeri*)
Serratia marcescens
Pseudomonas aeruginosa
Pseudomonas species
Some strains of *Acinetobacter calcoaceticus*
Neisseria gonorrhoeae

Anaerobic Organisms:
Gram-positive cocci (including *Peptococcus* and *Peptostreptococcus*)
Clostridium species
Bacteroides fragilis
Other *Bacteroides* species

CEFOBID is also active *in vitro* against a wide variety of other pathogens although the clinical significance is unknown. These organisms include: *Salmonella* and *Shigella* species, *Serratia liquefaciens, N. meningitidis, Bordetella pertussis, Yersinia enterocolitica, Clostridium difficile, Fusobacterium* species, *Eubacterium* species and beta-lactamase producing strains of *H. influenzae* and *N. gonorrhoeae.*

SUSCEPTIBILITY TESTING

Diffusion Technique. For the disk diffusion method of susceptibility testing, a 75 mcg CEFOBID diffusion disk should be used. Organisms should be tested with the CEFOBID 75 mcg disk since CEFOBID has been shown *in vitro* to be active against organisms which are found to be resistant to other beta-lactam antibiotics.

Tests should be interpreted by the following criteria:

Zone Diameter	Interpretation
Greater than or equal to 21 mm	Susceptible
16–20 mm	Moderately Susceptible
Less than or equal to 15 mm	Resistant

Quantitative procedures that require measurement of zone diameters give the most precise estimate of susceptibility. One such method which has been recommended for use with the CEFOBID 75 mcg disk is the NCCLS approved standard. (Performance Standards for Antimicrobic Disk Susceptibility Tests. Second Information Supplement Vol. 2 No. 2 pp. 49–69. Publisher—National Committee for Clinical Laboratory Standards, Villanova, Pennsylvania.)

A report of "susceptible" indicates that the infecting organism is likely to respond to CEFOBID therapy and a report of "resistant" indicates that the infecting organism is not likely to respond to therapy. A "moderately susceptible" report suggests that the infecting organism will be susceptible to CEFOBID if a higher than usual dosage is used or if the infection is confined to tissues and fluids (e.g., urine or bile) in which high antibiotic levels are attained.

Dilution Techniques. Broth or agar dilution methods may be used to determine the minimal inhibitory concentration (MIC) of CEFOBID. Serial twofold dilutions of CEFOBID should be prepared in either broth or agar. Broth should be inoculated to contain 5×10^5 organisms/mL and agar "spotted" with 10^4 organisms.

MIC test results should be interpreted in light of serum, tissue, and body fluid concentrations of CEFOBID. Organisms inhibited by CEFOBID at 16 mcg/mL or less are considered susceptible, while organisms with MIC's of 17–63 mcg/mL are moderately susceptible. Organisms inhibited at CEFOBID concentrations of greater than or equal to 64 mcg/mL are considered resistant, although clinical cures have been obtained in some patients infected by such organisms.

INDICATIONS AND USAGE

CEFOBID is indicated for the treatment of the following infections when caused by susceptible organisms:

Respiratory Tract Infections caused by *S. pneumoniae, H. influenzae, S. aureus* (penicillinase and non-penicillinase producing strains), *S. pyogenes** (Group A beta-hemolytic streptococci), *P. aeruginosa, Klebsiella pneumoniae, E. coli, Proteus mirabilis,* and *Enterobacter* species.

Peritonitis and Other Intra-abdominal Infections caused by *E. coli, P. aeruginosa,** and anaerobic gram-negative bacilli (including *Bacteroides fragilis*).

Bacterial Septicemia caused by *S. pneumoniae, S. agalactiae,* S. aureus, Pseudomonas aeruginosa,* E. coli, Klebsiella* spp.,* *Klebsiella pneumoniae,* Proteus* species* (indole-positive and indole-negative), *Clostridium* spp.* and anaerobic gram-positive cocci.*

Infections of the Skin and Skin Structures caused by *S. aureus* (penicillinase and non-penicillinase producing strains), *S. pyogenes,** and *P. aeruginosa.*

Pelvic Inflammatory Disease, Endometritis, and Other Infections of the Female Genital Tract caused by *N. gonorrhoeae, S. epidermidis,* S. agalactiae, E. coli, Clostridium* spp.,* *Bacteroides* species (including *Bacteroides fragilis*) and anaerobic gram-positive cocci.

Cefobid,® like other cephalosporins, has no activity against *Chlamydia trachomatis.* Therefore, when cephalosporins are used in the treatment of patients with pelvic inflammatory disease and *C. trachomatis* is one of the suspected pathogens, appropriate anti-chlamydial coverage should be added.

Urinary Tract Infections caused by *Escherichia coli,* and *Pseudomonas aeruginosa.*

Enterococcal Infections: Although cefoperazone has been shown to be clinically effective in the treatment of infections caused by enterococci in cases of **peritonitis and other intra-abdominal infections, infections of the skin and skin structures, pelvic inflammatory disease, endometritis and other infections of the female genital tract, and urinary tract infection,*** the majority of clinical isolates of enterococci tested are not susceptible to cefoperazone but fall just at or in the intermediate zone of susceptibilty, and are moderately resistant to cefoperazone. However, *in vitro* susceptibility testing may not correlate directly with *in vivo* results. Despite this, cefoperazone therapy has resulted in clinical cures of enterococcal infections, chiefly in polymicrobial infections. Cefoperazone should be used in enterococcal infections with care and at doses that achieve satisfactory serum levels of cefoperazone.

*Efficacy of this organism in this organ system was studied in fewer than 10 infections.

Susceptibility Testing
Before instituting treatment with CEFOBID, appropriate specimens should be obtained for isolation of the causative organism and for determination of its susceptibility to the drug. Treatment may be started before results of susceptibility testing are available.

Combination Therapy
Synergy between CEFOBID and aminoglycosides has been demonstrated with many gram-negative bacilli. However, such enhanced activity of these combinations is not predictable. If such therapy is considered, *in vitro* susceptibility tests should be performed to determine the activity of the drugs in combination, and renal function should be monitored carefully. (See PRECAUTIONS, and DOSAGE AND ADMINISTRATION sections).

CONTRAINDICATIONS

CEFOBID is contraindicated in patients with known allergy to the cephalosporin-class of antibiotics.

WARNINGS

BEFORE THERAPY WITH CEFOBID IS INSTITUTED, CAREFUL INQUIRY SHOULD BE MADE TO DETERMINE WHETHER THE PATIENT HAS HAD PREVIOUS HYPERSENSITIVITY REACTIONS TO CEPHALOSPORINS, PENICILLINS OR OTHER DRUGS. THIS PRODUCT SHOULD BE GIVEN CAUTIOUSLY TO PENICILLIN-SENSITIVE PATIENTS. ANTIBIOTICS SHOULD BE ADMINISTERED WITH CAUTION TO ANY PATIENT WHO HAS DEMONSTRATED SOME FORM OF ALLERGY, PARTICULARLY TO DRUGS. SERIOUS ACUTE HYPERSENSITIVITY REACTIONS MAY REQUIRE THE USE OF SUBCUTANEOUS EPINEPHRINE AND OTHER EMERGENCY MEASURES.

PSEUDOMEMBRANOUS COLITIS HAS BEEN REPORTED WITH THE USE OF CEPHALOSPORINS (AND OTHER BROAD-SPECTRUM ANTIBIOTICS); THEREFORE, IT IS IMPORTANT TO CONSIDER ITS DIAGNOSIS IN PATIENTS WHO DEVELOP DIARRHEA IN ASSOCIATION WITH ANTIBIOTIC USE.

Treatment with broad-spectrum antibiotics alters normal flora of the colon and may permit overgrowth of clostridia. Studies indicate a toxin produced by *Clostridium difficile* is one primary cause of antibiotic-associated colitis. Cholestyramine and colestipol resins have been shown to bind the toxin *in vitro.*

Mild cases of colitis may respond to drug discontinuance alone.

Moderate to severe cases should be managed with fluid, electrolyte, and protein supplementation as indicated.

When the colitis is not relieved by drug discontinuance or when it is severe, oral vancomycin is the treatment of choice for antibiotic-associated pseudomembranous colitis produced by *C. difficile.* Other causes of colitis should also be considered.

PRECAUTIONS

Although transient elevations of the BUN and serum creatinine have been observed, CEFOBID alone does not appear to cause significant nephrotoxicity. However, concomitant administration of aminoglycosides and other cephalosporins has caused nephrotoxicity.

CEFOBID is extensively excreted in bile. The serum half-life of CEFOBID is increased 2–4 fold in patients with hepatic disease and/or biliary obstruction. In general, total daily dosage above 4 g should not be necessary in such patients. If higher dosages are used, serum concentrations should be monitored.

Because renal excretion is not the main route of elimination of CEFOBID (see CLINICAL PHARMACOLOGY), patients with renal failure require no adjustment in dosage when usual doses are administered. When high doses of CEFOBID are used, concentrations of drug in the serum should be monitored periodically. If evidence of accumulation exists, dosage should be decreased accordingly.

The half-life of CEFOBID is reduced slightly during hemodialysis. Thus, dosing should be scheduled to follow a dialysis period. In patients with both hepatic dysfunction and significant renal disease, CEFOBID dosage should not exceed 1–2 g daily without close monitoring of serum concentrations.

As with other antibiotics, vitamin K deficiency has occurred rarely in patients treated with CEFOBID. The mechanism is most probably related to the suppression of gut flora which normally synthesize this vitamin. Those at risk include patients with a poor nutritional status, malabsorption states (e.g., cystic fibrosis), alcoholism, and patients on prolonged hyper-alimentation regimens (administered either intravenously or via a naso-gastric tube). Prothrombin time should be monitored in these patients and exogenous vitamin K administered as indicated.

A disulfiram-like reaction characterized by flushing, sweating, headache, and tachycardia has been reported when alcohol (beer, wine) was ingested within 72 hours after CEFOBID administration. Patients should be cautioned about the ingestion of alcoholic beverages following the administration of CEFOBID. A similar reaction has been reported with other cephalosporins.

Prolonged use of CEFOBID may result in the overgrowth of nonsusceptible organisms. Careful observation of the patient is essential. If superinfection occurs during therapy, appropriate measures should be taken.

CEFOBID should be prescribed with caution in individuals with a history of gastrointestinal disease, particularly colitis.

Drug Laboratory Test Interactions
A false-positive reaction for glucose in the urine may occur with Benedict's or Fehling's solution.

Carcinogenesis, Mutagenesis, Impairment of Fertility
Long-term studies in animals have not been performed to evaluate carcinogenic potential. The maximum duration of CEFOBID animal toxicity studies is six months. In none of the *in vivo* or *in vitro* genetic toxicology studies did CEFOBID show any mutagenic potential at either the chromosomal or subchromosomal level. CEFOBID produced no impairment of fertility and had no effects on general reproductive performance or fetal development when administered subcutaneously at daily doses up to 500 to 1000 mg/kg prior to and during mating, and to pregnant female rats during gestation. These doses are 10 to 20 times the estimated usual single clinical dose. CEFOBID had adverse effects on the testes of prepubertal rats at all doses tested. Subcutaneous administration of 1000 mg/kg per day (approximately 16 times the average adult human dose) resulted in reduced testicular weight, arrested spermatogenesis, reduced germinal cell population and vacuolation of Sertoli cell cytoplasm. The severity of lesions was dose dependent in the 100 to 1000 mg/kg per day range; the low dose caused a minor decrease in spermatocytes. This effect has not been observed in adult rats. Histologically the lesions were reversible at all but the highest dosage levels. However, these studies did not evaluate subsequent development of reproductive function in the rats. The relationship of these findings to humans is unknown.

Usage in Pregnancy
Pregnancy Category B: Reproduction studies have been performed in mice, rats, and monkeys at doses up to 10 times the human dose and have revealed no evidence of impaired fertility or harm to the fetus due to CEFOBID. There are, however, no adequate and well controlled studies in pregnant women. Because animal reproduction studies are not always predictive of human response, this drug should be used during pregnancy only if clearly needed.

Usage in Nursing Mothers
Only low concentrations of CEFOBID are excreted in human milk. Although CEFOBID passes poorly into breast milk of nursing mothers, caution should be exercised when CEFOBID is administered to a nursing woman.

Pediatric Use
Safety and effectiveness in children have not been established. For information concerning testicular changes in prepubertal rats, see Carcinogenesis, Mutagenesis, Impairment of Fertility.

ADVERSE REACTIONS

In clinical studies the following adverse effects were observed and were considered to be related to CEFOBID therapy or of uncertain etiology:

Hypersensitivity: As with all cephalosporins, hypersensitivity manifested by skin reactions (1 patient in 45), drug fever (1 in 260), or a change in Coombs' test (1 in 60) has been reported. These reactions are more likely to occur in patients with a history of allergies, particularly to penicillin.

Hematology: As with other beta-lactam antibiotics, reversible neutropenia may occur with prolonged administration. Slight decreases in neutrophil count (1 patient in 50) have been reported. Decreased hemoglobins (1 in 20) or hematocrits (1 in 20) have been reported, which is consistent with published literature on other cephalosporins. Transient eosinophilia has occurred in 1 patient in 10.

Hepatic: Of 1285 patients treated with cefoperazone in clinical trials, one patient with a history of liver disease developed significantly elevated liver function enzymes during CEFOBID therapy. Clinical signs and symptoms of nonspecific hepatitis accompanied these increases. After CEFOBID therapy was discontinued, the patient's enzymes returned to pre-treatment levels and the symptomatology resolved. As with other antibiotics that achieve high bile levels, mild transient elevations of liver function enzymes have been observed in 5–10% of the patients receiving CEFOBID therapy. The relevance of these findings, which were not accompanied by overt signs or symptoms of hepatic dysfunction, has not been established.

Gastrointestinal: Diarrhea or loose stools has been reported in 1 in 30 patients. Most of these experiences have been mild or moderate in severity and self-limiting in nature. In all cases, these symptoms responded to symptomatic therapy or ceased when cefoperazone therapy was stopped. Nausea and vomiting have been reported rarely.
Symptoms of pseudomembranous colitis can appear during or for several weeks subsequent to antibiotic therapy (see WARNINGS).

Renal Function Tests: Transient elevations of the BUN (1 in 16) and serum creatinine (1 in 48) have been noted.

Local Reactions: CEFOBID is well tolerated following intramuscular administration. Occasionally, transient pain (1 in 140) may follow administration by this route. When CEFOBID is administered by intravenous infusion some patients may develop phlebitis (1 in 120) at the infusion site.

DOSAGE AND ADMINISTRATION

Sterile cefoperazone sodium can be administered by IM or IV injection (following dilution). However, the intent of this pharmacy bulk package is for the preparation of solutions for IV infusion only.

The usual adult daily dose of CEFOBID is 2 to 4 grams per day administered in equally divided doses every 12 hours.
In severe infections or infections caused by less sensitive organisms, the total daily dose and/or frequency may be increased. Patients have been successfully treated with a total daily dosage of 6–12 grams divided into 2, 3 or 4 administrations ranging from 1.5 to 4 grams per dose.
When treating infections caused by *Streptococcus pyogenes*, therapy should be continued for at least 10 days.
If *C. trachomatis* is a suspected pathogen, appropriate antichlamydial coverage should be added, because cefoperazone has no activity against this organism.
Solutions of CEFOBID and aminoglycoside should not be directly mixed, since there is a physical incompatibility between them. If combination therapy with CEFOBID and an aminoglycoside is contemplated (see INDICATIONS) this can be accomplished by sequential intermittent intravenous infusion provided that separate secondary intravenous tubing is used, and that the primary intravenous tubing is adequately irrigated with an approved diluent between doses. It is also suggested that CEFOBID be administered prior to the aminoglycoside. *In vitro* testing of the effectiveness of drug combination(s) is recommended.
In a pharmacokinetic study, a total daily dose of 16 grams was administered to severely immunocompromised patients by constant infusion without complications. Steady state serum concentrations were approximately 150 mcg/ml in these patients.

RECONSTITUTION

The following solutions may be used for the initial reconstitution of CEFOBID sterile powder:

Table 1. Solutions for Initial Reconstitution
- 5% Dextrose Injection (USP)
- 5% Dextrose and 0.9% Sodium Chloride Injection (USP)
- 5% Dextrose and 0.2% Sodium Chloride Injection (USP)
- 10% Dextrose Injection (USP)
- Bacteriostatic Water for Injection [Benzyl Alcohol or Parabens] (USP)*†
- 0.9% Sodium Chloride Injection (USP)
- Normosol® M and 5% Dextrose Injection
- Normosol® R
- Sterile Water for Injection*

* Not to be used as a vehicle for intravenous infusion.
† Preparations containing Benzyl Alcohol should not be used in neonates.

General Reconstitution Procedures
CEFOBID sterile powder for intravenous or intramuscular use may be initially reconstituted with any compatible solution mentioned above in Table 1. Solutions should be allowed to stand after reconstitution to allow any foaming to dissipate to permit visual inspection for complete solubilization. Vigorous and prolonged agitation may be necessary to solubilize CEFOBID in higher concentrations (above 333 mg cefoperazone/mL). The maximum solubility of CEFOBID sterile powder is approximately 475 mg cefoperazone/mL of compatible diluent.

Preparation For Intravenous Use
General. CEFOBID concentrations between 2 mg/mL and 50 mg/mL are recommended for intravenous administration.

Table 2. Vehicles for Intravenous Infusion
- 5% Dextrose Injection (USP)
- 5% Dextrose and Lactated Ringer's Injection
- 5% Dextrose and 0.9% Sodium Chloride Injection (USP)
- 5% Dextrose and 0.2% Sodium Chloride Injection(USP)
- 10% Dextrose Injection (USP)
- Lactated Ringer's Injection (USP)
- 0.9% Sodium Chloride Injection (USP)
- Normosol® M and 5% Dextrose Injection
- Normosol® R

DIRECTIONS FOR PROPER USE OF PHARMACY BULK PACKAGE

The 10 gram vial should be reconstituted with 95 mL of sterile water for injection in two separate aliquots in a suitable work area such as a laminar flow hood. Add 45 mL of solution, shake to dissolve and add 50 mL, shake for final solution. The resulting solution will contain 100 mg/mL of cefoperazone. This closure may be penetrated only one time after reconstitution, if needed, using a suitable sterile transfer device or dispensing set which allows measured dispensing of the contents.
Discard unused solution within 24 hours of initial entry.

Reconstituted Bulk Solutions Should Not Be Used For Direct Infusion.

Although after reconstitution of the Pharmacy Bulk Package, no significant loss of potency occurs for 24 hours at room temperature and for 5 days if refrigerated, transfer individual dose to appropriate intravenous infusion solutions as soon as possible following reconstituion of the bulk package. Discard unused portions of solution held longer than these recommended periods at room temperature or under refrigeration. The stability of the solution which has been transferred into a container varies according to diluent and concentration. (See STORAGE AND STABILITY.)
The 10 gram vials may be further diluted with the parenteral diluents listed under **Table 2. Vehicles for Intravenous Infusion.** The parenteral diluents and approximate concentrations of CEFOBID that provide stable solutions are presented under STORAGE AND STABILITY.
Parenteral drug products should be inspected visually for particulate matter and discoloration prior to administration, whenever solution and container permit.

DIRECTIONS FOR USE OF CEFOBID (cefoperazone sodium) INJECTION IN PLASTIC CONTAINERS
CEFOBID supplied premixed as a frozen, sterile, iso-osmotic solution in plastic containers is to be administered either as continuous or intermittent infusion.
Thaw container at room temperature. After thawing, check for minute leaks by squeezing bag firmly. If leaks are found, discard solution as sterility may be impaired. Additives should not be introduced into this solution. Do not use if the solution is cloudy or precipitated or if the seal is not intact.
After thawing, the solution is stable for 10 days if stored under refrigeration (5°C) and for 48 hours at room temperature. DO NOT REFREEZE. Use sterile equipment.
CAUTION: Do not use plastic container in series connections. Such use could result in air embolism due to residual air being drawn from the primary container before administration of the fluid from the secondary container is complete.

Preparation for Administration
1. Suspend container from eyelet support.
2. Remove plastic protector from outlet port at bottom of container.
3. Attach administration set. Refer to complete directions accompanying set.

STORAGE AND STABILITY

CEFOBID sterile powder is to be stored at or below 25°C (77°F) and protected from light prior to reconstitution. After reconstitution, protection from light is not necessary.
The following parenteral diluents and approximate concentrations of CEFOBID provide stable solutions under the following conditions for the indicated time periods. (After the indicated time periods, unused portions of solutions should be discarded.)
[See table at left.]

Controlled Room Temperature (15°–25°C/59°–77°F) 24 Hours	Approximate Concentrations
Bacteriostatic Water for Injection [Benzyl Alcohol or Parabens] (USP)	300 mg/mL
5% Dextrose Injection (USP)	2 mg to 50 mg/mL
5% Dextrose and Lactated Ringer's Injection	2 mg to 50 mg/mL
5% Dextrose and 0.9% Sodium Chloride Injection (USP)	2 mg to 50 mg/mL
5% Dextrose and 0.2% Sodium Chloride Injection (USP)	2 mg to 50 mg/mL
10% Dextrose Injection (USP)	2 mg to 50 mg/mL
Lactated Ringer's Injection (USP)	2 mg/mL
0.5% Lidocaine Hydrochloride Injection (USP)	300 mg/mL
0.9% Sodium Chloride Injection (USP)	2 mg to 300 mg/mL
Normosol® M and 5% Dextrose Injection	2 mg to 50 mg/mL
Normosol® R	2 mg to 50 mg/mL
Sterile Water for Injection	100 mg to 300 mg/mL

Reconstituted CEFOBID solutions may be stored in glass or plastic syringes, or in glass or flexible plastic parenteral solution containers.

Refrigerator Temperature (2°–8°C/36°–46°F) 5 Days	Approximate Concentrations
Bacteriostatic Water for Injection [Benzyl Alcohol or Parabens] (USP)	300 mg/mL
5% Dextrose Injection (USP)	2 mg to 50 mg/mL
5% Dextrose and 0.9% Sodium Chloride Injection (USP)	2 mg to 50 mg/mL
5% Dextrose and 0.2% Sodium Chloride Injection (USP)	2 mg to 50 mg/mL
Lactated Ringer's Injection (USP)	2 mg/mL
0.5% Lidocaine Hydrochloride Injection (USP)	300 mg/mL
0.9% Sodium Chloride Injection (USP)	2 mg to 300 mg/mL
Normosol® M and 5% Dextrose Injection	2 mg to 50 mg/mL
Normosol® R	2 mg to 50 mg/mL
Sterile Water for Injection	100 mg to 300 mg/mL

Reconstituted CEFOBID solutions may be stored in glass or plastic syringes, or in glass or flexible plastic parenteral solution containers.

Freezer Temperature (−20° to −10°C/−4° to 14°F)	Approximate Concentrations
3 Weeks	
5% Dextrose Injection (USP)	50 mg/mL
5% Dextrose and 0.9% Sodium Chloride Injection (USP)	2 mg/mL
5% Dextrose and 0.2% Sodium Chloride Injection (USP)	2 mg/mL
5 Weeks	
0.9% Sodium Chloride Injection (USP)	300 mg/mL
Sterile Water for Injection	300 mg/mL

Reconstituted CEFOBID solutions may be stored in plastic syringes, or in flexible plastic parenteral solution containers. Frozen samples should be thawed at room temperature before use. After thawing, unused portions should be discarded. Do not refreeze.

Continued on next page

Pfizer Inc—Cont.

HOW SUPPLIED

CEFOBID sterile powder is available in Pharmacy Bulk Package containing cefoperazone sodium equivalent to 10 g cefoperazone × 1 (NDC 0049-1219-28).

OTHER SIZE PACKAGES AVAILABLE

CEFOBID sterile powder is available in vials containing cefoperazone sodium equivalent to 1 g cefoperazone × 10 (NDC 0049-1201-83) and 2 g cefoperazone × 10 (NDC 0049-1202-83) for intramuscular and intravenous administration.

CEFOBID sterile powder is available in Piggyback Units containing cefoperazone sodium equivalent to 1 gram cefoperazone × 10 (NDC 0049-1211-83), and 2 g cefoperazone × 10 (NDC 0049-1212-83).

CEFOBID (cefoperazone sodium) injection is supplied premixed as a frozen, sterile, nonpyrogenic, iso-osmotic solution in plastic containers. Each 50 mL unit contains cefoperazone sodium equivalent to 1 g cefoperazone with approximately 2.3 g dextrose hydrous USP added (NDC 0049-1216-18) or 2 g cefoperazone with approximately 1.8 g dextrose hydrous USP added (NDC 0049-1215-18). The solution is iso-osmotic (approximately 300 mOsmol/L), and solution pH may have been adjusted with sodium hydroxide and/or hydrochloric acid. Do not store above −20°C.

CEFOBID supplied as a frozen, sterile, nonpyrogenic, iso-osmotic solution in 50 ml plastic containers is manufactured for Roerig Division of Pfizer Pharmaceuticals by Baxter Healthcare Corporation, Deerfield, IL 60015.

70-4482-00-5 Revised April 1995

DIABINESE® ℞

[dī-ab 'in-ees]
(chlorpropamide)
Tablets, USP
For Oral Use

DESCRIPTION

DIABINESE (chlorpropamide), is an oral blood-glucose-lowering drug of the sulfonylurea class. Chlorpropamide is 1-[(p-Chlorophenyl) sulfonyl]-3-propylurea, $C_{10}H_{13}ClN_2O_3S$, and has the structural formula:

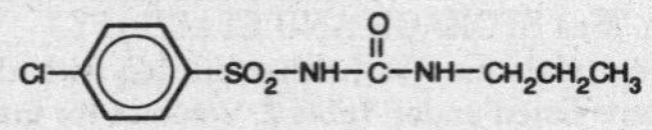

Chlorpropamide is a white crystalline powder, that has a slight odor. It is practically insoluble in water at pH 7.3 (solubility at pH 6 is 2.2 mg/ml). It is soluble in alcohol and moderately soluble in chloroform. The molecular weight of chlorpropamide is 276.74. DIABINESE is available as 100 mg and 250 mg tablets.

Inert ingredients are: alginic acid; Blue 1 Lake; hydroxypropyl cellulose; magnesium stearate; precipitated calcium carbonate; sodium lauryl sulfate; starch.

CLINICAL PHARMACOLOGY

DIABINESE appears to lower the blood glucose acutely by stimulating the release of insulin from the pancreas, an effect dependent upon functioning beta cells in the pancreatic islets. The mechanism by which DIABINESE lowers blood glucose during long-term administration has not been clearly established. Extra-pancreatic effects may play a part in the mechanism of action of oral sulfonylurea hypoglycemic drugs. While chlorpropamide is a sulfonamide derivative, it is devoid of antibacterial activity.

DIABINESE may also prove effective in controlling certain patients who have experienced primary or secondary failure to other sulfonylurea agents.

A method developed which permits easy measurement of the drug in blood is available on request.

Chlorpropamide does not interfere with the usual tests to detect albumin in the urine.

DIABINESE is absorbed rapidly from the gastrointestinal tract. Within one hour after a single oral dose, it is readily detectable in the blood, and the level reaches a maximum within two to four hours. It undergoes metabolism in humans and it is excreted in the urine as unchanged drug and as hydroxylated or hydrolyzed metabolites. The biological half-life of chlorpropamide averages about 36 hours. Within 96 hours, 80–90% of a single oral dose is excreted in the urine. However, long-term administration of therapeutic doses does not result in undue accumulation in the blood, since absorption and excretion rates become stabilized in about 5 to 7 days after the initiation of therapy.

DIABINESE exerts a hypoglycemic effect in normal humans within one hour, becoming maximal at 3 to 6 hours and persisting for at least 24 hours. The potency of chlorpropamide is approximately six times that of tolbutamide. Some experimental results suggest that its increased duration of action may be the result of slower excretion and absence of significant deactivation.

INDICATIONS AND USAGE

DIABINESE is indicated as an adjunct to diet to lower the blood glucose in patients with non-insulin-dependent diabetes mellitus (type II) whose hyperglycemia cannot be controlled by diet alone.

In initiating treatment for non-insulin-dependent diabetes, diet should be emphasized as the primary form of treatment. Caloric restriction and weight loss are essential in the obese diabetic patient. Proper dietary management alone may be effective in controlling the blood glucose and symptoms of hyperglycemia. The importance of regular physical activity should also be stressed, and cardiovascular risk factors should be identified and corrective measures taken where possible.

If this treatment program fails to reduce symptoms and/or blood glucose, the use of an oral sulfonylurea or insulin should be considered. Use of DIABINESE must be viewed by both the physician and patient as a treatment in addition to diet, and not as a substitute for diet or as a convenient mechanism for avoiding dietary restraint. Furthermore, loss of blood glucose control on diet alone may be transient, thus requiring only short-term administration of DIABINESE.

During maintenance programs, DIABINESE should be discontinued if satisfactory lowering of blood glucose is no longer achieved. Judgments should be based on regular clinical and laboratory evaluations.

In considering the use of DIABINESE in asymptomatic patients, it should be recognized that controlling the blood glucose in non-insulin-dependent diabetes, has not been definitely established to be effective in preventing the long-term cardiovascular or neural complications of diabetes.

CONTRAINDICATIONS

DIABINESE is contraindicated in patients with:

1. Known hypersensitivity to the drug.
2. Diabetic ketoacidosis, with or without coma. This condition should be treated with insulin.

WARNINGS

SPECIAL WARNING ON INCREASED RISK OF CARDIOVASCULAR MORTALITY

The administration of oral hypoglycemic drugs has been reported to be associated with increased cardiovascular mortality as compared to treatment with diet alone or diet plus insulin. This warning is based on the study conducted by the University Group Diabetes Program (UGDP), a long-term prospective clinical trial designed to evaluate the effectiveness of glucose-lowering drugs in preventing or delaying vascular complications in patients with non-insulin-dependent diabetes. The study involved 823 patients who were randomly assigned to one of four treatment groups (*Diabetes,* 19 (supp. 2): 747–830, 1970.)

UGDP reported that patients treated for 5 to 8 years with diet plus a fixed dose of tolbutamide (1.5 grams per day) had a rate of cardiovascular mortality approximately 2½ times that of patients treated with diet alone. A significant increase in total mortality was not observed, but the use of tolbutamide was discontinued based on the increase in cardiovascular mortality, thus limiting the opportunity for the study to show an increase in over-all mortality. Despite controversy regarding the interpretation of these results, the findings of the UGDP study provide an adequate basis for this warning. The patient should be informed of the potential risks and advantages of DIABINESE and of alternative modes of therapy.

Although only one drug in the sulfonylurea class (tolbutamide) was included in this study, it is prudent from a safety standpoint to consider that this warning may also apply to other oral hypoglycemic drugs in this class, in view of their close similarities in mode of action and chemical structure.

PRECAUTIONS

General

Hypoglycemia: All sulfonylurea drugs are capable of producing severe hypoglycemia. Proper patient selection, dosage, and instructions are important to avoid hypoglycemic episodes. Renal or hepatic insufficiency may cause elevated blood levels of DIABINESE and the latter may also diminish gluconeogenic capacity, both of which increase the risk of serious hypoglycemic reactions. Elderly, debilitated or malnourished patients, and those with adrenal or pituitary insufficiency are particularly susceptible to the hypoglycemic action of glucose-lowering drugs. Hypoglycemia may be difficult to recognize in the elderly, and in people who are taking beta-adrenergic blocking drugs. Hypoglycemia is more likely to occur when caloric intake is deficient, after severe or prolonged exercise, when alcohol is ingested, or when more than one glucose-lowering drug is used.

Because of the long half-life of chlorpropamide, patients who become hypoglycemic during therapy require careful supervision of the dose and frequent feedings for at least 3 to 5 days. Hospitalization and intravenous glucose may be necessary.

Loss of control of blood glucose: When a patient stabilized on any diabetic regimen is exposed to stress such as fever, trauma, infection, or surgery, a loss of control may occur. At such times, it may be necessary to discontinue DIABINESE and administer insulin.

The effectiveness of any oral hypoglycemic drug, including DIABINESE, in lowering blood glucose to a desired level decreases in many patients over a period of time, which may be due to progression of the severity of the diabetes or to diminished responsiveness to the drug. This phenomenon is known as secondary failure, to distinguish it from primary failure in which the drug is ineffective in an individual patient when first given.

INFORMATION FOR PATIENTS

Patients should be informed of the potential risks and advantages of DIABINESE and of alternative modes of therapy. They should also be informed about the importance of adherence to dietary instructions, of a regular exercise program, and of regular testing of urine and/or blood glucose.

The risks of hypoglycemia, its symptoms and treatment, and conditions that predispose to its development should be explained to patients and responsible family members. Primary and secondary failure should also be explained.

Patients should be instructed to contact their physician promptly if they experience symptoms of hypoglycemia or other adverse reactions.

LABORATORY TESTS

Blood and urine glucose should be monitored periodically. Measurement of glycosylated hemoglobin may be useful.

DRUG INTERACTIONS

The hypoglycemic action of sulfonylurea may be potentiated by certain drugs including nonsteroidal anti-inflammatory agents and other drugs that are highly protein bound, salicylates, sulfonamides, chloramphenicol, probenecid, coumarins, monoamine oxidase inhibitors, and beta adrenergic blocking agents. When such drugs are administered to a patient receiving DIABINESE, the patient should be observed closely for hypoglycemia. When such drugs are withdrawn from a patient receiving DIABINESE, the patient should be observed closely for loss of control.

Certain drugs tend to produce hyperglycemia and may lead to loss of control. These drugs include the thiazides and other diuretics, corticosteroids, phenothiazines, thyroid products, estrogens, oral contraceptives, phenytoin, nicotinic acid, sympathomimetics, calcium channel blocking drugs, and isoniazid. When such drugs are administered to a patient receiving DIABINESE, the patient should be closely observed for loss of control. When such drugs are withdrawn from a patient receiving DIABINESE, the patient should be observed closely for hypoglycemia.

Since animal studies suggest that the action of barbiturates may be prolonged by therapy with chlorpropamide, barbiturates should be employed with caution. In some patients, a disulfiram-like reaction may be produced by the ingestion of alcohol.

A potential interaction between oral miconazole and oral hypoglycemic agents leading to severe hypoglycemia has been reported. Whether this interaction also occurs with the intravenous, topical, or vaginal preparations of miconazole is not known.

Carcinogenesis, Mutagenesis, Impairment of Fertility: Chronic toxicity studies have been carried out in dogs and rats. Dogs treated for 6, 13, or 20 months with doses of DIABINESE greater than 20 times the human dose, have not shown any gross histological or pathological abnormalities. After treatment with 100 mg/kg of DIABINESE for 20 months, a dog showed no histopathological liver changes.

Rats treated with continuous DIABINESE therapy for 6 to 12 months showed varying degrees of suppression of spermatogenesis at higher dosage levels (up to 125 mg/kg). The extent of suppression seemed to follow that of growth retardation associated with chronic administration of high-dose DIABINESE in rats.

Pregnancy

Teratogenic Effects:

Pregnancy Category C. Animal reproductive studies have not been conducted with DIABINESE. It is also not known whether DIABINESE can cause fetal harm when administered to a pregnant woman or can affect reproduction capacity. DIABINESE should be given to a pregnant woman only if clearly needed.

Because recent information suggests that abnormal blood glucose levels during pregnancy are associated with a higher incidence of congenital abnormalities, many experts recommend that insulin be used during pregnancy to maintain blood glucose levels as close to normal as possible.

Nonteratogenic Effects:

Prolonged severe hypoglycemia (4 to 10 days) has been reported in neonates born to mothers who were receiving a sulfonylurea drug at the time of delivery. This has been reported more frequently with the use of agents with prolonged half-lives. If DIABINESE is used during pregnancy, it should be discontinued at least one month before the expected delivery date.

Strength	Tablet Description	Tablet Code	NDC	Package Size
DIABINESE (chlorpropamide) 100 mg	Blue, D-shaped, scored	393	0663-3930-66 0069-3930-66	100's
			0663-3930-73 0069-3930-73	500's
			0663-3930-41 0069-3930-41	100 (10 × 10) unit dose
DIABINESE (chlorpropamide) 250 mg	Blue, D-shaped, scored	394	0663-3940-66 0069-3940-66	100's
			0663-3940-71 0069-3940-71	250's
			0663-3940-82 0069-3940-82	1000's
			0663-3940-41 0069-3940-41	100 (10 × 10) unit dose

Nursing Mothers: An analysis of a composite of two samples of human breast milk, each taken five hours after ingestion of 500 mg of chlorpropamide by a patient, revealed a concentration of 5 mcg/ml. For reference, the normal peak blood level of chlorpropamide after a single 250 mg dose is 30 mcg/ml. Therefore, it is not recommended that a woman breast feed while taking this medication.

Use in Children: Safety and effectiveness in children have not been established.

ADVERSE REACTIONS

Hypoglycemia: See PRECAUTIONS and OVERDOSAGE sections.

Gastrointestinal Reactions: Cholestatic jaundice may occur rarely; DIABINESE should be discontinued if this occurs. Gastrointestinal disturbances are the most common reactions; nausea has been reported in less than 5% of patients, and diarrhea, vomiting, anorexia, and hunger in less than 2%. Other gastrointestinal disturbances have occurred in less than 1% of patients including proctocolitis. They tend to be dose related and may disappear when dosage is reduced.

Dermatologic Reactions: Pruritus has been reported in less than 3% of patients. Other allergic skin reactions, e.g., urticaria and maculopapular eruptions have been reported in approximately 1% or less of patients. These may be transient and may disappear despite continued use of DIABINESE; if skin reactions persist the drug should be discontinued.

Porphyria cutanea tarda and photosensitivity reactions have been reported with sulfonylureas.

Skin eruptions rarely progressing to erythema multiforme and exfoliative dermatitis have also been reported.

Hematologic Reactions: Leukopenia, agranulocytosis, thrombocytopenia, hemolytic anemia, aplastic anemia, pancytopenia, and eosinophilia have been reported with sulfonylureas.

Metabolic Reactions: Hepatic porphyria and disulfiram-like reactions have been reported with DIABINESE. See DRUG INTERACTIONS section.

Endocrine Reactions: On rare occasions, chlorpropamide has caused a reaction identical to the syndrome of inappropriate antidiuretic hormone (ADH) secretion. The features of this syndrome result from excessive water retention and include hyponatremia, low serum osmolality, and high urine osmolality. This reaction has also been reported for other sulfonylureas.

OVERDOSAGE

Overdosage of sulfonylureas including DIABINESE can produce hypoglycemia. Mild hypoglycemic symptoms without loss of consciousness or neurologic findings should be treated aggressively with oral glucose and adjustments in drug dosage and/or meal patterns. Close monitoring should continue until the physician is assured that the patient is out of danger. Severe hypoglycemic reactions with coma, seizure, or other neurological impairment occur infrequently, but constitute medical emergencies requiring immediate hospitalization. If hypoglycemic coma is diagnosed or suspected, the patient should be given a rapid intravenous injection of concentrated (50%) glucose solution. This should be followed by a continuous infusion of a more dilute (10%) glucose solution at a rate that will maintain the blood glucose at a level above 100 mg/dL. Patients should be closely monitored for a minimum of 24 to 48 hours since hypoglycemia may recur after apparent clinical recovery.

DOSAGE AND ADMINISTRATION

There is no fixed dosage regimen for the management of diabetes mellitus with DIABINESE or any other hypoglycemic agent. In addition to the usual monitoring of urinary glucose, the patient's blood glucose must also be monitored periodically to determine the minimum effective dose for the patient; to detect primary failure, i.e., inadequate lowering of blood glucose at the maximum recommended dose of medication; and to detect secondary failure, i.e., loss of an adequate blood glucose lowering response after an initial period of effectiveness. Glycosylated hemoglobin levels may also be of value in monitoring the patient's response to therapy.

Short-term administration of DIABINESE may be sufficient during periods of transient loss of control in patients usually controlled well on diet.

The total daily dosage is generally taken at a single time each morning with breakfast. Occasionally cases of gastrointestinal intolerance may be relieved by dividing the daily dosage. A LOADING OR PRIMING DOSE IS NOT NECESSARY AND SHOULD NOT BE USED.

Initial Therapy: 1. The mild to moderately severe, middle-aged, stable, non-insulin-dependent diabetic patient should be started on 250 mg daily. In elderly patients, debilitated or malnourished patients, and patients with impaired renal or hepatic function, the initial and maintenance dosing should be conservative to avoid hypoglycemic reactions (see PRECAUTIONS section). Older patients should be started on smaller amounts of DIABINESE, in the range of 100 to 125 mg daily.

2. No transition period is necessary when transferring patients from other oral hypoglycemic agents to DIABINESE. The other agent may be discontinued abruptly and chlorpropamide started at once. In prescribing chlorpropamide, due consideration must be given to its greater potency.

Many mild to moderately severe, middle-aged, stable non-insulin-dependent diabetic patients receiving insulin can be placed directly on the oral drug and their insulin abruptly discontinued. For patients requiring more than 40 units of insulin daily, therapy with DIABINESE may be initiated with a 50 per cent reduction in insulin for the first few days, with subsequent further reductions dependent upon the response.

During the initial period of therapy with chlorpropamide, hypoglycemic reactions may occasionally occur, particularly during the transition from insulin to the oral drug. Hypoglycemia within 24 hours after withdrawal of the intermediate or long-acting types of insulin will usually prove to be the result of insulin carry-over and not primarily due to the effect of chlorpropamide.

During the insulin withdrawal period, the patient should test his urine for sugar and ketone bodies at least three times daily and report the results frequently to his physician. If they are abnormal, the physician should be notified immediately. In some cases, it may be advisable to consider hospitalization during the transition period.

Five to seven days after the initial therapy, the blood level of chlorpropamide reaches a plateau. Dosage may subsequently be adjusted upward or downward by increments of not more than 50 to 125 mg at intervals of three to five days to obtain optimal control. More frequent adjustments are usually undesirable.

Maintenance Therapy: Most moderately severe, middle-aged, stable non-insulin-dependent diabetic patients are controlled by approximately 250 mg daily. Many investigators have found that some milder diabetics do well on daily doses of 100 mg or less. Many of the more severe diabetics may require 500 mg daily for adequate control. PATIENTS WHO DO NOT RESPOND COMPLETELY TO 500 MG DAILY WILL USUALLY NOT RESPOND TO HIGHER DOSES. MAINTENANCE DOSES ABOVE 750 mg DAILY SHOULD BE AVOIDED.

HOW SUPPLIED

[See table above.]

RECOMMENDED STORAGE

Store below 86°F (30°C).

CAUTION

Federal law prohibits dispensing without prescription.

69-2141-00-1 Revised April 1995

Shown in Product Identification Guide, page 327

DIFLUCAN® ℞

(Fluconazole Tablets)
(Fluconazole Injection–for intravenous infusion only)
(Fluconazole for Oral Suspension)

DESCRIPTION

DIFLUCAN® (fluconazole), the first of a new subclass of synthetic triazole antifungal agents, is available as tablets for oral administration, as a powder for oral suspension and as a sterile solution for intravenous use in glass and in Viaflex® Plus plastic containers.

Fluconazole is designated chemically as 2,4-difluoro-α,α[1]-bis(1H-1,2,4-triazol-1-ylmethyl) benzyl alcohol with an empirical formula of $C_{13}H_{12}F_2N_6O$ and molecular weight 306.3. The structural formula is:

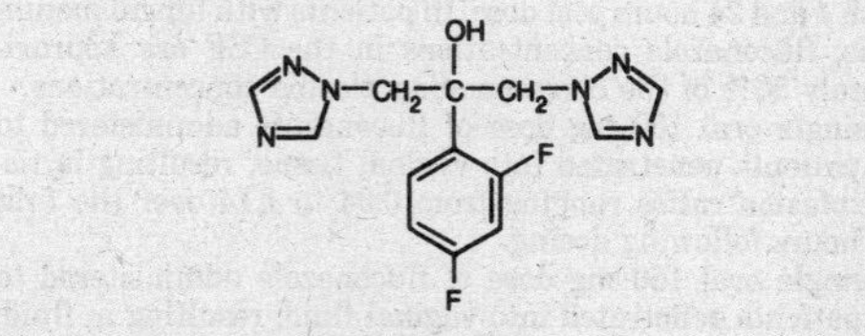

Fluconazole is a white crystalline solid which is slightly soluble in water and saline.

DIFLUCAN tablets contain 50, 100, 150, or 200 mg of fluconazole and the following inactive ingredients: microcrystalline cellulose, dibasic calcium phosphate anhydrous, povidone, croscarmellose sodium, FD&C Red No. 40 aluminum lake dye, and magnesium stearate.

DIFLUCAN for oral suspension contains 350 mg or 1400 mg of fluconazole and the following inactive ingredients: sucrose, sodium citrate dihydrate, citric acid anhydrous, sodium benzoate, titanium dioxide, colloidal silicon dioxide, xanthan gum and natural orange flavor. After reconstitution with 24 mL of distilled water or Purified Water (USP), each mL of reconstituted suspension contains 10 mg or 40 mg of fluconazole.

DIFLUCAN injection is an iso-osmotic, sterile, nonpyrogenic solution of fluconazole in a sodium chloride or dextrose diluent. Each mL contains 2 mg of fluconazole and 9 mg of sodium chloride or 56 mg of dextrose, hydrous. The pH ranges from 4.0 to 8.0 in the sodium chloride diluent and from 3.5 to 6.5 in the dextrose diluent. Injection volumes of 100 mL and 200 mL are packaged in glass and in Viaflex® Plus plastic containers.

The Viaflex® Plus plastic container is fabricated from a specially formulated polyvinyl chloride (PL 146® Plastic) (Viaflex and PL 146 are registered trademarks of Baxter International, Inc.). The amount of water that can permeate from inside the container into the overwrap is insufficient to affect the solution significantly. Solutions in contact with the plastic container can leach out certain of its chemical components in very small amounts within the expiration period, e.g. di-2-ethylhexylphthalate (DEHP), up to 5 parts per million. However, the suitability of the plastic has been confirmed in tests in animals according to USP biological tests for plastic containers as well as by tissue culture toxicity studies.

CLINICAL PHARMACOLOGY

Mode of Action

Fluconazole is a highly selective inhibitor of fungal cytochrome P-450 sterol C-14 alpha-demethylation. Mammalian cell demethylation is much less sensitive to fluconazole inhibition. The subsequent loss of normal sterols correlates with the accumulation of 14 alpha-methyl sterols in fungi and may be responsible for the fungistatic activity of fluconazole.

Pharmacokinetics and Metabolism

The pharmacokinetic properties of fluconazole are similar following administration by the intravenous or oral routes. In normal volunteers, the bioavailability of orally administered fluconazole is over 90% compared with intravenous administration. Bioequivalence was established between the 100 mg tablet and both suspension strengths when administered as a single 200 mg dose.

Peak plasma concentrations (Cmax) in fasted normal volunteers occur between 1 and 2 hours with a terminal plasma elimination half-life of approximately 30 hours (range 20–50 hours) after oral administration.

In fasted normal volunteers, administration of a single oral 400 mg dose of DIFLUCAN (fluconazole) leads to a mean Cmax of 6.72 μg/mL (range: 4.12 to 8.08 μg/mL) and after single oral doses of 50–400 mg, fluconazole plasma concentrations and AUC (area under the plasma concentration-time curve) are dose proportional.

Administration of a single oral 150 mg tablet of DIFLUCAN (fluconazole) to ten lactating women resulted in a mean Cmax of 2.61 μg/mL (range: 1.57 to 3.65 μg/mL).

Steady-state concentrations are reached within 5–10 days following oral doses of 50–400 mg given once daily. Administration of a loading dose (on day 1) of twice the usual daily dose results in plasma concentrations close to steady-state by the second day. The apparent volume of distribution of fluconazole approximates that of total body water. Plasma

Continued on next page

Pfizer Inc—Cont.

protein binding is low (11–12%). Following either single- or multiple-oral doses for up to 14 days, fluconazole penetrates into all body fluids studied (see table below). In normal volunteers, saliva concentrations of fluconazole were equal to or slightly greater than plasma concentrations regardless of dose, route, or duration of dosing. In patients with bronchiectasis, sputum concentrations of fluconazole following a single 150 mg oral dose were equal to plasma concentrations at both 4 and 24 hours post dose. In patients with fungal meningitis, fluconazole concentrations in the CSF are approximately 80% of the corresponding plasma concentrations.
A single oral 150 mg dose of fluconazole administered to 27 patients penetrated into vaginal tissue, resulting in tissue:plasma ratios ranging from 0.94 to 1.14 over the first 48 hours following dosing.
A single oral 150 mg dose of fluconazole administered to 14 patients penetrated into vaginal fluid, resulting in fluid: plasma ratios ranging from 0.36 to 0.71 over the first 72 hours following dosing.

Tissue or Fluid	Ratio of Fluconazole Tissue (Fluid)/Plasma Concentration*
Cerebrospinal fluid†	.5–.9
Saliva	1
Sputum	1
Blister fluid	1
Urine	10
Normal skin	10
Nails	1
Blister skin	2
Vaginal tissue	1
Vaginal fluid	0.4–0.7

* Relative to concurrent concentrations in plasma in subjects with normal renal function.
† Independent of degree of meningeal inflammation.

In normal volunteers, fluconazole is cleared primarily by renal excretion, with approximately 80% of the administered dose appearing in the urine as unchanged drug. About 11% of the dose is excreted in the urine as metabolites.
The pharmacokinetics of fluconazole are markedly affected by reduction in renal function. There is an inverse relationship between the elimination half-life and creatinine clearance. The dose of DIFLUCAN may need to be reduced in patients with impaired renal function. (See DOSAGE AND ADMINISTRATION.) A 3-hour hemodialysis session decreases plasma concentrations by approximately 50%.
In normal volunteers, DIFLUCAN administration (doses ranging from 200 mg to 400 mg once daily for up to 14 days) was associated with small and inconsistent effects on testosterone concentrations, endogenous corticosteroid concentrations, and the ACTH-stimulated cortisol response.

Pharmacokinetics in Children

In children, the following pharmacokinetic data {Mean (%cv)} have been reported:
[See table below.]

Age Studied	Dose (mg/kg)	Clearance (mL/min/kg)	Half-life (Hours)	Cmax (µg/mL)	Vdss (L/kg)
9 Months-13 years	Single-Oral 2 mg/kg	0.40 (38%) N=14	25.0	2.9 (22%) N=16	—
9 Months-13 years	Single-Oral 8 mg/kg	0.51 (60%) N=15	19.5	9.8 (20%) N=15	—
5–15 years	Multiple i.v. 2 mg/kg	0.49 (40%) N=4	17.4	5.5 (25%) N=5	0.722 (36%) N=4
5–15 years	Multiple i.v. 4 mg/kg	0.59 (64%) N=5	15.2	11.4 (44%) N=6	0.729 (33%) N=5
5–15 years	Multiple i.v. 8 mg/kg	0.66 (31%) N=7	17.6	14.1 (22%) N=8	1.069 (37%) N=7

Clearance corrected for body weight was not affected by age in these studies. Mean body clearance in adults is reported to be 0.23 (17%) mL/min/kg.
In premature newborns (gestational age 26 to 29 weeks), the mean (%cv) clearance within 36 hours of birth was 0.180 (35%, N=7) mL/min/kg, which increased with time to a mean of 0.218 (31%, N=9) mL/min/kg six days later and 0.333 (56%, N=4) mL/min/kg 12 days later. Similarly, the half-life was 73.6 hours, which decreased with time to a mean of 53.2 hours six days later and 46.6 hours 12 days later.

Drug Interaction Studies

Oral contraceptives: Oral contraceptives were administered as a single dose both before and after the oral administration of DIFLUCAN 50 mg once daily for 10 days in 10 healthy women. There was no significant difference in ethinyl estradiol or levonorgestrel AUC after the administration of 50 mg of DIFLUCAN. The mean increase in ethinyl estradiol AUC was 6% (range: −47 to 108%) and levonorgestrel AUC increased 17% (range: −33 to 141%).
Twenty-five normal females received daily doses of both 200 mg of DIFLUCAN tablets or placebo for two, ten-day periods. The treatment cycles were one month apart with all subjects receiving DIFLUCAN during one cycle and placebo during the other. The order of study treatment was random. Single doses of an oral contraceptive tablet containing levonorgestrel and ethinyl estradiol were administered on the final treatment day (day 10) of both cycles. Following administration of 200 mg of DIFLUCAN, the mean percentage increase of AUC for levonorgestrel compared to placebo was 25% (range: −12 to 82%) and the mean percentage increase for ethinyl estradiol compared to placebo was 38% (range: −11 to 101%). Both of these increases were statistically significantly different from placebo.
Cimetidine: DIFLUCAN 100 mg was administered as a single oral dose alone and two hours after a single dose of cimetidine 400 mg to six healthy male volunteers. After the administration of cimetidine, there was a significant decrease in fluconazole AUC and Cmax. There was a mean ± SD decrease in fluconazole AUC of 13% ± 11% (range: −3.4 to −31%) and Cmax decreased 19% ± 14% (range: −5 to −40%). However, the administration of cimetidine 600 mg to 900 mg intravenously over a four hour period (from one hour before to 3 hours after a single oral dose of DIFLUCAN 200 mg) did not affect the bioavailability or pharmacokinetics of fluconazole in 24 healthy male volunteers.
Antacid: Administration of Maalox® (20 mL) to 14 normal male volunteers immediately prior to a single dose of DIFLUCAN 100 mg had no effect on the absorption or elimination of fluconazole.
Hydrochlorothiazide: Concomitant oral administration of 100 mg DIFLUCAN and 50 mg hydrochlorothiazide for 10 days in 13 normal volunteers resulted in a significant increase in fluconazole AUC and Cmax compared to DIFLUCAN given alone. There was a mean ± SD increase in fluconazole AUC and Cmax of 45% ± 31% (range: 19 to 114%) and 43% ± 31% (range: 19 to 122%), respectively. These changes are attributed to a mean ± SD reduction in renal clearance of 30% ± 12% (range: −10 to −50%).
Rifampin: Administration of a single oral 200 mg dose of DIFLUCAN after 15 days of rifampin administered as 600 mg daily in eight healthy male volunteers resulted in a significant decrease in fluconazole AUC and a significant increase in apparent oral clearance of fluconazole. There was a mean ± SD reduction in fluconazole AUC of 23% ± 9% (range: −13 to −42%). Apparent oral clearance of fluconazole increased 32% ± 17% (range: 16 to 72%). Fluconazole half-life decreased from 33.4 ± 4.4 hours to 26.8 ± 3.9 hours. (See PRECAUTIONS.)
Warfarin: There was a significant increase in prothrombin time response (area under the prothrombin time-time curve) following a single dose of warfarin (15 mg) administered to 13 normal male volunteers following oral DIFLUCAN 200 mg administered daily for 14 days as compared to the administration of warfarin alone. There was a mean ± SD increase in the prothrombin time response (area under the prothrombin time-time curve) of 7% ± 4% (range: −2 to 13 %). (See PRECAUTIONS.) Mean is based on data from 12 subjects as one of 13 subjects experienced a 2-fold increase in his prothrombin time response.
Phenytoin: Phenytoin AUC was determined after 4 days of phenytoin dosing (200 mg daily, orally for 3 days followed by 250 mg intravenously for one dose) both with and without the administration of fluconazole (oral DIFLUCAN 200 mg daily for 16 days) in 10 normal male volunteers. There was a significant increase in phenytoin AUC. The mean ± SD increase in phenytoin AUC was 88% ± 68% (range: 16 to 247%). The absolute magnitude of this interaction is unknown because of the intrinsically nonlinear disposition of phenytoin. (See PRECAUTIONS.)
Cyclosporine: Cyclosporine AUC and Cmax were determined before and after the administration of fluconazole 200 mg daily for 14 days in eight renal transplant patients who had been on cyclosporine therapy for at least 6 months and on a stable cyclosporine dose for at least 6 weeks. There was a significant increase in cyclosporine AUC, Cmax, Cmin (24 hour concentration), and a significant reduction in apparent oral clearance following the administration of fluconazole. The mean ± SD increase in AUC was 92% ± 43% (range: 18 to 147%). The Cmax increased 60% ± 48% (range: −5 to 133%). The Cmin increased 157% ± 96% (range: 33 to 360%). The apparent oral clearance decreased 45% ± 15% (range: −15 to −60%). (See PRECAUTIONS.)
Zidovudine: Plasma zidovudine concentrations were determined on two occasions (before and following fluconazole 200 mg daily for 15 days) in 13 volunteers with AIDS or ARC who were on a stable zidovudine dose for at least two weeks. There was a significant increase in zidovudine AUC following the administration of fluconazole. The mean ± SD increase in AUC was 20% ± 32% (range: −27 to 104%). The metabolite, GZDV, to parent drug ratio significantly decreased after the administration of fluconazole, from 7.6 ± 3.6 to 5.7 ± 2.2.
Theophylline: The pharmacokinetics of theophylline were determined from a single intravenous dose of aminophylline (6 mg/kg) before and after the oral administration of fluconazole 200 mg daily for 14 days in 16 normal male volunteers. There were significant increases in theophylline AUC, Cmax, and half-life with a corresponding decrease in clearance. The mean ± SD theophylline AUC increased 21% ± 16% (range: −5 to 48%). The Cmax increased 13% ± 17% (range: −13 to 40%). Theophylline clearance decreased 16% ± 11% (range: −32 to 5%). The half-life of theophylline increased from 6.6 ± 1.7 hours to 7.9 ± 1.5 hours.
Terfenadine: Six healthy volunteers received terfenadine 60 mg BID for 15 days. Fluconazole 200 mg was administered daily from days 9 through 15. Fluconazole did not affect terfenadine plasma concentrations. Terfenadine acid metabolite AUC increased 36% ± 36% (range: 7 to 102%) from day 8 to day 15 with the concomitant administration of fluconazole. There was no change in cardiac repolarization as measured by Holter QTc intervals. (See PRECAUTIONS.)
Oral hypoglycemics: The effects of fluconazole on the pharmacokinetics of the sulfonylurea oral hypoglycemic agents tolbutamide, glipizide, and glyburide were evaluated in three placebo-controlled studies in normal volunteers. All subjects received the sulfonylurea alone as a single dose and again as a single dose following the administration of DIFLUCAN 100 mg daily for 7 days. In these three studies 22/46 (47.8%) of DIFLUCAN treated patients and 9/22 (40.1%) of placebo treated patients experienced symptoms consistent with hypoglycemia. (See PRECAUTIONS.)
Tolbutamide: In 13 normal male volunteers, there was significant increase in tolbutamide (500 mg single dose) AUC and Cmax following the administration of fluconazole. There was a mean ± SD increase in tolbutamide AUC of 26% ± 9% (range: 12 to 39%). Tolbutamide Cmax increased 11% ± 9% (range: −6 to 27%). (See PRECAUTIONS.)
Glipizide: The AUC and Cmax of glipizide (2.5 mg single dose) were significantly increased following the administration of fluconazole in 13 normal male volunteers. There was a mean ± SD increase in AUC of 49% ± 13% (range: 27 to 73%) and an increase in Cmax of 19% ± 23% (range: −11 to 79%). (See PRECAUTIONS.)
Glyburide: The AUC and Cmax of glyburide (5 mg single dose) were significantly increased following the administration of fluconazole in 20 normal male volunteers. There was a mean ± SD increase in AUC of 44% ± 29% (range: −13 to 115%) and Cmax increased 19% ± 19% (range: −23 to 62%). Five subjects required oral glucose following the ingestion of glyburide after 7 days of fluconazole administration. (See PRECAUTIONS.)

Microbiology

Fluconazole exhibits *in vitro* activity against *Cryptococcus neoformans* and *Candida* spp. Fungistatic activity has also been demonstrated in normal and immunocompromised animal models for systemic and intracranial fungal infections due to *Cryptococcus neoformans* and for systemic infections due to *Candida albicans*.
In common with other azole antifungal agents, most fungi show a higher apparent sensitivity to fluconazole *in vivo* than *in vitro*. Fluconazole administered orally and/or intravenously was active in a variety of animal models of fungal infection using standard laboratory strains of fungi. Activity has been demonstrated against fungal infections caused by *Aspergillus flavus* and *Aspergillus fumigatus* in normal mice. Fluconazole has also been shown to be active in animal models of endemic mycoses, including one model of *Blastomyces dermatitidis* pulmonary infections in normal mice; one model of *Coccidioides immitis* intracranial infections in normal mice; and several models of *Histoplasma capsulatum* pulmonary infection in normal and immunosuppressed mice. The clinical significance of results obtained in these studies is unknown.
Oral fluconazole has been shown to be active in an animal model of vaginal candidiasis.
Concurrent administration of fluconazole and amphotericin B in infected normal and immunosuppressed mice showed the following results: a small additive antifungal effect in systemic infection with *C. albicans*, no interaction in intra-

cranial infection with *Cr. neoformans*, and antagonism of the two drugs in systemic infection with *Asp. fumigatus*. The clinical significance of results obtained in these studies is unknown.

There have been reports of cases of superinfection with Candida species other than *C. albicans*, which are often inherently not susceptible to DIFLUCAN (e.g., *Candida krusei*). Such cases may require alternative antifungal therapy.

INDICATIONS AND USAGE

DIFLUCAN (fluconazole) is indicated for the treatment of:

1. Vaginal Candidiasis (vaginal yeast infections due to *Candida*).
2. Oropharyngeal and esophageal candidiasis. In open noncomparative studies of relatively small numbers of patients, DIFLUCAN was also effective for the treatment of Candida urinary tract infections, peritonitis, and systemic Candida infections including candidemia, disseminated candidiasis, and pneumonia.
3. Cryptococcal meningitis. Before prescribing DIFLUCAN (fluconazole) for AIDS patients with cryptococcal meningitis, please see CLINICAL STUDIES section. Studies comparing DIFLUCAN to amphotericin B in non-HIV infected patients have not been conducted.

Prophylaxis. DIFLUCAN is also indicated to decrease the incidence of candidiasis in patients undergoing bone marrow transplantation who receive cytotoxic chemotherapy and/or radiation therapy.

Specimens for fungal culture and other relevant laboratory studies (serology, histopathology) should be obtained prior to therapy to isolate and identify causative organisms. Therapy may be instituted before the results of the cultures and other laboratory studies are known; however, once these results become available, anti-infective therapy should be adjusted accordingly.

CLINICAL STUDIES

Cryptococcal meningitis: In a multicenter study comparing DIFLUCAN (200 mg/day) to amphotericin B (0.3 mg/kg/day) for treatment of cryptococcal meningitis in patients with AIDS, a multivariate analysis revealed three pretreatment factors that predicted death during the course of therapy: abnormal mental status, cerebrospinal fluid cryptococcal antigen titer greater than 1:1024, and cerebrospinal fluid white blood cell count of less than 20 cells/mm^3. Mortality among high risk patients was 33% and 40% for amphotericin B and DIFLUCAN patients, respectively (p=0.58), with overall deaths 14% (9 of 63 subjects) and 18% (24 of 131 subjects) for the 2 arms of the study (p=0.48). Optimal doses and regimens for patients with acute cryptococcal meningitis and at high risk for treatment failure remain to be determined. (Saag, *et al.* N Engl J Med 1992; 326:83–9)

Vaginal candidiasis: Two adequate and well-controlled studies were conducted in the U.S. using the 150 mg tablet. In both, the results of the fluconazole regimen were comparable to the control regimen (clotrimazole or miconazole intravaginally for 7 days) both clinically and statistically at the one month post-treatment evaluation.

The therapeutic cure rate, defined as a complete resolution of signs and symptoms of vaginal candidiasis (clinical cure), along with a negative KOH examination and negative culture for *Candida* (microbiologic eradication), was 55% in both the fluconazole group and the vaginal products group.

	Fluconazole PO 150 mg tablet	Vaginal Product qhs x 7 days
Enrolled	448	422
Evaluable at Late Follow-up	347 (77%)	327 (77%)
Clinical cure	239/347 (69%)	235/327 (72%)
Mycologic erad.	213/347 (61%)	196/327 (60%)
Therapeutic cure	190/347 (55%)	179/327 (55%)

Approximately three-fourths of the enrolled patients had acute vaginitis (<4 episodes/12 months) and achieved 80% clinical cure, 67% mycologic eradication and 59% therapeutic cure when treated with a 150 mg DIFLUCAN tablet administered orally. These rates were comparable to control products. The remaining one-fourth of enrolled patients had recurrent vaginitis (≥4 episodes/12 months) and achieved 57% clinical cure, 47% mycologic eradication and 40% therapeutic cure. The numbers are too small to make meaningful clinical or statistical comparisons with vaginal products in the treatment of patients with recurrent vaginitis.

Substantially more gastrointestinal events were reported in the fluconazole group compared to the vaginal product group. Most of the events were mild to moderate. Because fluconazole was given as a single dose, no discontinuations occurred.

Parameter	Fluconazole PO	Vaginal Products
Evaluable patients	448	422
With any adverse event	141 (31%)	112 (27%)
Nervous System	90 (20%)	69 (16%)
Gastrointestinal	73 (16%)	18 (4%)
With drug-related event	117 (26%)	67 (16%)
Nervous System	61 (14%)	29 (7%)
Headache	58 (13%)	28 (7%)
Gastrointestinal	68 (15%)	13 (3%)
Abdominal pain	25 (6%)	7 (2%)
Nausea	30 (7%)	3 (1%)
Diarrhea	12 (3%)	2 (<1%)
Application site event	0 (0%)	19 (5%)
Taste Perversion	6 (1%)	0 (0%)

Pediatric Studies

Oropharyngeal candidiasis: An open-label, comparative study of the efficacy and safety of DIFLUCAN (2–3 mg/kg/day) and oral nystatin (400,000 I.U. 4 times daily) in immunocompromised children with oropharyngeal candidiasis was conducted. Clinical and mycological response rates were higher in the children treated with fluconazole.

Clinical cure at the end of treatment was reported for 86% of fluconazole treated patients compared to 46% of nystatin treated patients. Mycologically, 76% of fluconazole treated patients had the infecting organism eradicated compared to 11% for nystatin treated patients.

	Fluconazole	Nystatin
Enrolled	96	90
Clinical Cure	76/88 (86%)	36/78 (46%)
Mycological eradication*	55/72 (76%)	6/54 (11%)

*Subjects without follow-up cultures for any reason were considered nonevaluable for mycological response.

The proportion of patients with clinical relapse 2 weeks after the end of treatment was 14% for subjects receiving DIFLUCAN and 16% for subjects receiving nystatin. At 4 weeks after the end of treatment the percentages of patients with clinical relapse were 22% for DIFLUCAN and 23% for nystatin.

CONTRAINDICATIONS

DIFLUCAN (fluconazole) is contraindicated in patients who have shown hypersensitivity to fluconazole or to any of its excipients. There is no information regarding cross hypersensitivity between fluconazole and other azole antifungal agents. Caution should be used in prescribing DIFLUCAN to patients with hypersensitivity to other azoles.

WARNINGS

(1) Hepatic injury: DIFLUCAN has been associated with rare cases of serious hepatic toxicity, including fatalities primarily in patients with serious underlying medical conditions. In cases of DIFLUCAN associated hepatotoxicity, no obvious relationship to total daily dose, duration of therapy, sex or age of the patient has been observed. DIFLUCAN hepatotoxicity has usually, but not always, been reversible on discontinuation of therapy. Patients who develop abnormal liver function tests during DIFLUCAN therapy should be monitored for the development of more severe hepatic injury. DIFLUCAN should be discontinued if clinical signs and symptoms consistent with liver disease develop that may be attributable to DIFLUCAN.

(2) Anaphylaxis: In rare cases, anaphylaxis has been reported.

(3) Dermatologic: Patients have rarely developed exfoliative skin disorders during treatment with DIFLUCAN. In patients with serious underlying diseases (predominantly AIDS and malignancy), these have rarely resulted in a fatal outcome. Patients who develop rashes during treatment with DIFLUCAN should be monitored closely and the drug discontinued if lesions progress.

PRECAUTIONS

General

Single Dose

The convenience and efficacy of the single dose oral tablet of fluconazole regimen for the treatment of vaginal yeast infections should be weighed against the acceptability of a higher incidence of drug related adverse events with DIFLUCAN (26%) versus intravaginal agents (16%) in U.S. comparative clinical studies. (See ADVERSE REACTIONS and CLINICAL STUDIES.)

Drug Interactions: (See CLINICAL PHARMACOLOGY and PRECAUTIONS-General)

Clinically or potentially significant drug interactions between DIFLUCAN and the following agents/classes have been observed. These are described in greater detail below:

Oral hypoglycemics
Coumarin-type anticoagulants
Phenytoin
Cyclosporine
Rifampin
Theophylline
Terfenadine

Oral hypoglycemics: Clinically significant hypoglycemia may be precipitated by the use of DIFLUCAN with oral hypoglycemic agents; one fatality has been reported from hypoglycemia in association with combined DIFLUCAN and glyburide use. DIFLUCAN reduces the metabolism of tolbutamide, glyburide, and glipizide and increases the plasma concentration of these agents. When DIFLUCAN is used concomitantly with these or other sulfonylurea oral hypoglycemic agents, blood glucose concentrations should be carefully monitored and the dose of the sulfonylurea should be adjusted as necessary.

Coumarin-type anticoagulants: Prothrombin time may be increased in patients receiving concomitant DIFLUCAN and coumarin-type anticoagulants. Careful monitoring of prothrombin time in patients receiving DIFLUCAN and coumarin-type anticoagulants is recommended.

Phenytoin: DIFLUCAN increases the plasma concentrations of phenytoin. Careful monitoring of phenytoin concentrations in patients receiving DIFLUCAN and phenytoin is recommended.

Cyclosporine: DIFLUCAN may significantly increase cyclosporine levels in renal transplant patients with or without renal impairment. Careful monitoring of cyclosporine concentrations and serum creatinine is recommended in patients receiving DIFLUCAN and cyclosporine.

Rifampin: Rifampin enhances the metabolism of concurrently administered DIFLUCAN. Depending on clinical circumstances, consideration should be given to increasing the dose of DIFLUCAN when it is administered with rifampin.

Theophylline: DIFLUCAN increases the serum concentrations of theophylline. Careful monitoring of serum theophylline concentrations in patients receiving DIFLUCAN and theophylline is recommended.

Terfenadine: Because of the occurrence of serious cardiac dysrhythmias secondary to prolongation of the QTc interval in patients receiving other azole antifungals in conjunction with terfenadine, interaction studies have been performed. One study at a 200 mg daily dose of fluconazole failed to demonstrate a prolongation of QTc intervals. (See Drug Interaction Studies.) Definitive interaction studies at higher doses of DIFLUCAN have not been conducted.

The use of fluconazole in patients concurrently taking drugs metabolized by the cytochrome P450 system (i.e., terfenadine, cisapride and astemizole) may be associated with elevations in serum levels of these other drugs. In the absence of definitive information at higher doses of fluconazole, the coadministration of DIFLUCAN and such agents should be carefully monitored.

Fluconazole tablets coadministered with ethinyl estradiol- and levonorgestrel-containing oral contraceptives produced an overall mean increase in ethinyl estradiol and levonorgestrel levels; however, in some patients there were decreases up to 47% and 33% of ethinyl estradiol and levonorgestrel levels. (See Drug Interaction Studies.) The data presently available indicate that the decreases in some individual ethinyl estradiol and levonorgestrel AUC values with fluconazole treatment are likely the result of random variation. While there is evidence that fluconazole can inhibit the metabolism of ethinyl estradiol and levonorgestrel, there is no evidence that fluconazole is a net inducer of ethinyl estradiol or levonorgestrel metabolism. The clinical significance of these effects is presently unknown.

Physicians should be aware that interaction studies with medications other than those listed in the CLINICAL PHARMACOLOGY section have not been conducted, but such interactions may occur.

Carcinogenesis, Mutagenesis and Impairment of Fertility

Fluconazole showed no evidence of carcinogenic potential in mice and rats treated orally for 24 months at doses of 2.5, 5 or 10 mg/kg/day (approximately 2–7x the recommended human dose). Male rats treated with 5 and 10 mg/kg/day had an increased incidence of hepatocellular adenomas.

Fluconazole, with or without metabolic activation, was negative in tests for mutagenicity in 4 strains of *S. typhimurium*, and in the mouse lymphoma L5178Y system. Cytogenetic studies *in vivo* (murine bone marrow cells, following oral administration of fluconazole) and *in vitro* (human lymphocytes exposed to fluconazole at 1000 μg/mL) showed no evidence of chromosomal mutations.

Fluconazole did not affect the fertility of male or female rats treated orally with daily doses of 5, 10 or 20 mg/kg or with parenteral doses of 5, 25 or 75 mg/kg, although the onset of parturition was slightly delayed at 20 mg/kg p.o. In an intravenous perinatal study in rats at 5, 20 and 40 mg/kg, dystocia and prolongation of parturition were observed in a few dams at 20 mg/kg (approximately 5–15x the recommended human dose) and 40 mg/kg, but not at 5 mg/kg. The disturbances in parturition were reflected by a slight increase in the number of still-born pups and decrease of neonatal survival at these dose levels. The effects on parturition in rats are consistent with the species specific estrogen-lowering property produced by high doses of fluconazole. Such a hormone change has not been observed in women treated with fluconazole. (See CLINICAL PHARMACOLOGY.)

Pregnancy

Teratogenic Effects. Pregnancy Category C: Fluconazole was administered orally to pregnant rabbits during organogenesis in two studies, at 5, 10 and 20 mg/kg and at 5, 25, and 75 mg/kg, respectively. Maternal weight gain was impaired at all dose levels, and abortions occurred at 75 mg/kg (approximately 20–60x the recommended human dose); no adverse fetal effects were detected. In several studies in which

Continued on next page

Pfizer Inc—Cont.

pregnant rats were treated orally with fluconazole during organogenesis, maternal weight gain was impaired and placental weights were increased at 25 mg/kg. There were no fetal effects at 5 or 10 mg/kg; increases in fetal anatomical variants (supernumerary ribs, renal pelvis dilation) and delays in ossification were observed at 25 and 50 mg/kg and higher doses. At doses ranging from 80 mg/kg (approximately 20–60x the recommended human dose) to 320 mg/kg embryolethality in rats was increased and fetal abnormalities included wavy ribs, cleft palate and abnormal craniofacial ossification. These effects are consistent with the inhibition of estrogen synthesis in rats and may be a result of known effects of lowered estrogen on pregnancy, organogenesis and parturition.

There are no adequate and well controlled studies in pregnant women. There have been reports of multiple congenital abnormalities in infants whose mothers were being treated for 3 or more months with high dose (400–800 mg/day) fluconazole therapy for coccidioidomycosis (an unindicated use). The relationship between fluconazole use and these events is unclear. DIFLUCAN should be used in pregnancy only if the potential benefit justifies the possible risk to the fetus.

Nursing Mothers
Fluconazole is secreted in human milk at concentrations similar to plasma. Therefore, the use of DIFLUCAN in nursing mothers is not recommended.

Pediatric Use
An open-label, randomized, controlled trial has shown DIFLUCAN to be effective in the treatment of oropharyngeal candidiasis in children 6 months to 13 years of age. (See CLINICAL STUDIES.)

The use of DIFLUCAN in children with cryptococcal meningitis, Candida esophagitis, or systemic Candida infections is supported by the efficacy shown for these indications in adults and by the results from several small noncomparative pediatric clinical studies. In addition, pharmacokinetic studies in children (see CLINICAL PHARMACOLOGY), have established a dose proportionality between children and adults. (See DOSAGE AND ADMINISTRATION.)

In a noncomparative study of children with serious systemic fungal infections, most of which were candidemia, the effectiveness of DIFLUCAN was similar to that reported for the treatment of candidemia in adults. Of 17 subjects with culture-confirmed candidemia, 11 of 14 (79%) with baseline symptoms (3 were asymptomatic) had a clinical cure; 13/15 (87%) of evaluable patients had a mycologic cure at the end of treatment but two of these patients relapsed at 10 and 18 days, respectively, following cessation of therapy.

The efficacy of DIFLUCAN for the suppression of cryptococcal meningitis was successful in 4 of 5 children treated in a compassionate-use study of fluconazole for the treatment of life-threatening or serious mycosis. There is no information regarding the efficacy of fluconazole for primary treatment of cryptococcal meningitis in children.

The safety profile of DIFLUCAN in children has been studied in 577 children ages 1 day to 17 years who received doses ranging from 1 to 15 mg/kg/day for 1 to 1,616 days. (See ADVERSE REACTIONS.)

Efficacy of DIFLUCAN has not been established in infants less than 6 months of age. (See CLINICAL PHARMACOLOGY.) A small number of patients (29) ranging in age from 1 day to 6 months have been treated safely with DIFLUCAN.

ADVERSE REACTIONS

In Patients Receiving a Single Dose for Vaginal Candidiasis:
During comparative clinical studies conducted in the United States, 448 patients with vaginal candidiasis were treated with DIFLUCAN, 150 mg single dose. The overall incidence of side effects possibly related to DIFLUCAN was 26%. In 422 patients receiving active comparative agents, the incidence was 16%. The most common treatment-related adverse events reported in the patients who received 150 mg single dose fluconazole for vaginitis were headache (13%), nausea (7%), and abdominal pain (6%). Other side effects reported with an incidence equal to or greater than 1% included diarrhea (3%), dyspepsia (1%), dizziness (1%), and taste perversion (1%). Most of the reported side effects were mild to moderate in severity. Rarely, angioedema and anaphylactic reaction have been reported in marketing experience.

In Patients Receiving Multiple Doses for Other Infections:
Sixteen percent of over 4000 patients treated with DIFLUCAN (fluconazole) in clinical trials of 7 days or more experienced adverse events. Treatment was discontinued in 1.5% of patients due to adverse clinical events and in 1.3% of patients due to laboratory test abnormalities.
Clinical adverse events were reported more frequently in HIV infected patients (21%) than in non-HIV infected patients (13%); however, the patterns in HIV infected and non-HIV infected patients were similar. The proportions of patients discontinuing therapy due to clinical adverse events were similar in the two groups (1.5%).

The following treatment-related clinical adverse events occurred at an incidence of 1% or greater in 4048 patients receiving DIFLUCAN for 7 or more days in clinical trials: nausea 3.7%, headache 1.9%, skin rash 1.8%, vomiting 1.7%, abdominal pain 1.7%, and diarrhea 1.5%.

The following adverse events have occurred under conditions where a causal association is probable:

Hepatobiliary: In combined clinical trials and marketing experience, there have been rare cases of serious hepatic reactions during treatment with DIFLUCAN. (See WARNINGS.) The spectrum of these hepatic reactions has ranged from mild transient elevations in transaminases to clinical hepatitis, cholestasis and fulminant hepatic failure, including fatalities. Instances of fatal hepatic reactions were noted to occur primarily in patients with serious underlying medical conditions (predominantly AIDS or malignancy) and often while taking multiple concomitant medications. Transient hepatic reactions, including hepatitis and jaundice, have occurred among patients with no other identifiable risk factors. In each of these cases, liver function returned to baseline on discontinuation of DIFLUCAN.

In two comparative trials evaluating the efficacy of DIFLUCAN for the suppression of relapse of cryptococcal meningitis, a statistically significant increase was observed in median AST (SGOT) levels from a baseline value of 30 IU/L to 41 IU/L in one trial and 34 IU/L to 66 IU/L in the other. The overall rate of serum transaminase elevations of more than 8 times the upper limit of normal was approximately 1% in fluconazole-treated patients in clinical trials. These elevations occurred in patients with severe underlying disease, predominantly AIDS or malignancies, most of whom were receiving multiple concomitant medications, including many known to be hepatotoxic. The incidence of abnormally elevated serum transaminases was greater in patients taking DIFLUCAN concomitantly with one or more of the following medications: rifampin, phenytoin, isoniazid, valproic acid, or oral sulfonylurea hypoglycemic agents.

Immunologic: In rare cases, anaphylaxis has been reported. The following adverse events have occurred under conditions where a causal association is uncertain:

Central Nervous System: seizures.
Dermatologic: Exfoliative skin disorders including Stevens-Johnson Syndrome and toxic epidermal necrolysis (see WARNINGS), alopecia.
Hematopoietic and *Lymphatic:* leukopenia, including neutropenia and agranulocytosis, thrombocytopenia.
Metabolic: hypercholesterolemia, hypertriglyceridemia, hypokalemia.

Adverse Reactions in Children:
In Phase 2/3 clinical trials conducted in the United States and in Europe, 577 pediatric patients, ages 1 day to 17 years were treated with DIFLUCAN at doses up to 15 mg/kg/day for up to 1,616 days. Thirteen percent of children experienced treatment related adverse events. The most commonly reported events were vomiting (5%), abdominal pain (3%), nausea (2%), and diarrhea (2%). Treatment was discontinued in 2.3% of patients due to adverse clinical events and in 1.4% of patients due to laboratory test abnormalities. The majority of treatment-related laboratory abnormalities were elevations of transaminases or alkaline phosphatase.

Percentage of Patients With Treatment-Related Side Effects

	Fluconazole (N=577)	Comparative Agents (N=451)
With any side effect	13.0	9.3
Vomiting	5.4	5.1
Abdominal pain	2.8	1.6
Nausea	2.3	1.6
Diarrhea	2.1	2.2

OVERDOSAGE
There has been one reported case of overdosage with DIFLUCAN (fluconazole). A 42-year-old patient infected with human immunodeficiency virus developed hallucinations and exhibited paranoid behavior after reportedly ingesting 8200 mg of DIFLUCAN. The patient was admitted to the hospital, and his condition resolved within 48 hours.
In the event of overdose, symptomatic treatment (with supportive measures and gastric lavage if clinically indicated) should be instituted.
Fluconazole is largely excreted in urine. A three hour hemodialysis session decreases plasma levels by approximately 50%.
In mice and rats receiving very high doses of fluconazole, clinical effects in both species included decreased motility and respiration, ptosis, lacrimation, salivation, urinary incontinence, loss of righting reflex and cyanosis; death was sometimes preceded by clonic convulsions.

DOSAGE AND ADMINISTRATION
Dosage and Administration in Adults:
Single Dose
Vaginal candidiasis: The recommended dosage of DIFLUCAN for vaginal candidiasis is 150 mg as a single oral dose.

Multiple Dose
SINCE ORAL ABSORPTION IS RAPID AND ALMOST COMPLETE, THE DAILY DOSE OF DIFLUCAN (FLUCONAZOLE) IS THE SAME FOR ORAL (TABLETS AND SUSPENSION) AND INTRAVENOUS ADMINISTRATION. In general, a loading dose of twice the daily dose is recommended on the first day of therapy to result in plasma concentrations close to steady-state by the second day of therapy.
The daily dose of DIFLUCAN for the treatment of infections other than vaginal candidiasis should be based on the infecting organism and the patient's response to therapy. Treatment should be continued until clinical parameters or laboratory tests indicate that active fungal infection has subsided. An inadequate period of treatment may lead to recurrence of active infection. Patients with AIDS and cryptococcal meningitis or recurrent oropharyngeal candidiasis usually require maintenance therapy to prevent relapse.
Oropharyngeal candidiasis: The recommended dosage of DIFLUCAN for oropharyngeal candidiasis is 200 mg on the first day, followed by 100 mg once daily. Clinical evidence of oropharyngeal candidiasis generally resolves within several days, but treatment should be continued for at least 2 weeks to decrease the likelihood of relapse.
Esophageal candidiasis: The recommended dosage of DIFLUCAN for esophageal candidiasis is 200 mg on the first day, followed by 100 mg once daily. Doses up to 400 mg/day may be used, based on medical judgment of the patient's response to therapy. Patients with esophageal candidiasis should be treated for a minimum of three weeks and for at least two weeks following resolution of symptoms.
Systemic Candida infections: For systemic Candida infections including candidemia, disseminated candidiasis, and pneumonia, optimal therapeutic dosage and duration of therapy have not been established. In open, noncomparative studies of small numbers of patients, doses of up to 400 mg daily have been used.
Urinary tract infection and peritonitis: For the treatment of Candida urinary tract infections and peritonitis, daily doses of 50–200 mg have been used in open, noncomparative studies of small numbers of patients.
Cryptococcal meningitis: The recommended dosage for treatment of acute cryptococcal meningitis is 400 mg on the first day, followed by 200 mg once daily. A dosage of 400 mg once daily may be used, based on medical judgment of the patient's response to therapy. The recommended duration of treatment for initial therapy of cryptococcal meningitis is 10–12 weeks after the cerebrospinal fluid becomes culture negative. The recommended dosage of DIFLUCAN for suppression of relapse of cryptococcal meningitis in patients with AIDS is 200 mg once daily.
Prophylaxis in patients undergoing bone marrow transplantation: The recommended DIFLUCAN daily dosage for the prevention of candidiasis of patients undergoing bone marrow transplantation is 400 mg, once daily. Patients who are anticipated to have severe granulocytopenia (less than 500 neutrophils per cu mm) should start DIFLUCAN prophylaxis several days before the anticipated onset of neutropenia, and continue for 7 days after the neutrophil count rises above 1000 cells per cu mm.
Dosage and Administration in Children:
The following dose equivalency scheme should generally provide equivalent exposure in pediatric and adult patients:

Pediatric Patients	Adults
3 mg/kg	100 mg
6 mg/kg	200 mg
12* mg/kg	400 mg

* Some older children may have clearances similar to that of adults. Absolute doses exceeding 600 mg/day are not recommended.

Experience with DIFLUCAN in neonates is limited to pharmacokinetic studies in premature newborns. (See CLINICAL PHARMACOLOGY.) Based on the prolonged half-life seen in premature newborns (gestational age 26 to 29 weeks), these children, in the first two weeks of life, should receive the same dosage (mg/kg) as in older children, but administered every 72 hours. After the first two weeks, these children should be dosed once daily. No information regarding DIFLUCAN pharmacokinetics in full-term newborns is available.
Oropharyngeal candidiasis: The recommended dosage of DIFLUCAN for oropharyngeal candidiasis in children is 6 mg/kg on the first day, followed by 3 mg/kg once daily. Treatment should be administered for at least 2 weeks to decrease the likelihood of relapse.
Esophageal candidiasis: For the treatment of esophageal candidiasis, the recommended dosage of DIFLUCAN in children is 6 mg/kg on the first day, followed by 3 mg/kg once daily. Doses up to 12 mg/kg/day may be used based on medical judgment of the patient's response to therapy. Patients with esophageal candidiasis should be treated for a minimum of three weeks and for at least 2 weeks following the resolution of symptoms.

Systemic Candida infections: For the treatment of candidemia and disseminated Candida infections, daily doses of 6–12 mg/kg/day have been used in an open, noncomparative study of a small number of children.

Cryptococcal meningitis: For the treatment of acute cryptococcal meningitis, the recommended dosage is 12 mg/kg on the first day, followed by 6 mg/kg once daily. A dosage of 12 mg/kg once daily may be used, based on medical judgment of the patient's response to therapy. The recommended duration of treatment for initial therapy of cryptococcal meningitis is 10–12 weeks after the cerebrospinal fluid becomes culture negative. For suppression of relapse of cryptococcal meningitis in children with AIDS, the recommended dose of DIFLUCAN is 6 mg/kg once daily.

Dosage In Patients With Impaired Renal Function:
Fluconazole is cleared primarily by renal excretion as unchanged drug. There is no need to adjust single dose therapy for vaginal candidiasis because of impaired renal function. In patients with impaired renal function who will receive multiple doses of DIFLUCAN, an initial loading dose of 50 to 400 mg should be given. After the loading dose, the daily dose (according to indication) should be based on the following table:

Creatinine Clearance (mL/min)	Percent of Recommended Dose
>50	100%
≤50 (no dialysis)	50%
Regular dialysis	100% after each dialysis

These are suggested dose adjustments based on pharmacokinetics following administration of multiple doses. Further adjustment may be needed depending upon clinical condition.

When serum creatinine is the only measure of renal function available, the following formula (based on sex, weight, and age of the patient) should be used to estimate the creatinine clearance in adults:

$$\text{Males: } \frac{\text{Weight (kg)} \times (140-\text{age})}{72 \times \text{serum creatinine (mg/100mL)}}$$

Females: $0.85 \times$ above value

Although the pharmacokinetics of fluconazole has not been studied in children with renal insufficiency, dosage reduction in children with renal insufficiency should parallel that recommended for adults. The following formula may be used to estimate creatinine clearance in children.

$$K \times \frac{\text{linear length or height (cm)}}{\text{serum creatinine (mg/100 mL)}}$$

(Where K=0.55 for children older than 1 year and 0.45 for infants.)

Administration
DIFLUCAN may be administered either orally or by intravenous infusion. DIFLUCAN injection has been used safely for up to fourteen days of intravenous therapy. The intravenous infusion of DIFLUCAN should be administered at a maximum rate of approximately 200 mg/hour, given as a continuous infusion.

DIFLUCAN injections in glass and Viaflex® Plus plastic containers are intended only for intravenous administration using sterile equipment.

Parenteral drug products should be inspected visually for particulate matter and discoloration prior to administration whenever solution and container permit.

Do not use if the solution is cloudy or precipitated or if the seal is not intact.

Directions for Mixing the Oral Suspension
Prepare a suspension at time of dispensing as follows: tap bottle until all the powder flows freely. To reconstitute, add 24 mL of distilled water or Purified Water (USP) to fluconazole bottle and shake vigorously to suspend powder. Each bottle will deliver 35 mL of suspension. The concentrations of the reconstituted suspensions are as follows:

Fluconazole Content per Bottle	Concentration of Reconstituted Suspension
350 mg	10 mg/mL
1400 mg	40 mg/mL

Note: Shake oral suspension well before using. Store reconstituted suspension between 86°F (30°C) and 41°F (5°C) and discard unused portion after 2 weeks. Protect from freezing.

Directions for IV Use of DIFLUCAN in Viaflex® Plus Plastic Containers
Do not remove unit from overwrap until ready for use. The overwrap is a moisture barrier. The inner bag maintains the sterility of the product.

CAUTION: Do not use plastic containers in series connections. Such use could result in air embolism due to residual air being drawn from the primary container before administration of the fluid from the secondary container is completed.

To Open
Tear overwrap down side at slit and remove solution container. Some opacity of the plastic due to moisture absorption during the sterilization process may be observed. This is normal and does not affect the solution quality or safety. The opacity will diminish gradually. After removing overwrap, check for minute leaks by squeezing inner bag firmly. If leaks are found, discard solution as sterility may be impaired.

DO NOT ADD SUPPLEMENTARY MEDICATION.

Preparation for Administration:
1. Suspend container from eyelet support.
2. Remove plastic protector from outlet port at bottom of container.
3. Attach administration set. Refer to complete directions accompanying set.

HOW SUPPLIED

DIFLUCAN® Tablets: Pink trapezoidal tablets containing 50, 100 or 200 mg of fluconazole are packaged in bottles or unit dose blisters. The 150 mg fluconazole tablets are pink and oval shaped, packaged in a single dose unit blister.

DIFLUCAN® Tablets are supplied as follows:

DIFLUCAN® 50 mg Tablets: Engraved with DIFLUCAN® and 50 on the front and ROERIG on the back.
NDC 0049-3410-30 Bottles of 30

DIFLUCAN® 100 mg Tablets: Engraved with DIFLUCAN® and 100 on the front and ROERIG on the back.
NDC 0049-3420-30 Bottles of 30
NDC 0049-3420-41 Unit dose package of 100

DIFLUCAN® 150 mg Tablets: Engraved with DIFLUCAN® and 150 mg on the front and ROERIG on the back.
NDC 0049-3500-79 Unit dose package of 1

DIFLUCAN® 200 mg Tablets: Engraved with DIFLUCAN® and 200 on the front and ROERIG on the back.
NDC 0049-3430-30 Bottles of 30
NDC 0049-3430-41 Unit dose package of 100

Storage: Store tablets below 86°F (30°C).

DIFLUCAN® for Oral Suspension: DIFLUCAN® for oral suspension is supplied as an orange-flavored powder to provide 35 mL per bottle as follows:
NDC 0049-3440-19 Fluconazole 350 mg per bottle
NDC 0049-3450-19 Fluconazole 1400 mg per bottle

Storage: Store dry powder below 86°F (30°C). Store reconstituted suspension between 86°F (30°C) and 41°F (5°C) and discard unused portion after 2 weeks. Protect from freezing.

DIFLUCAN® Injections: DIFLUCAN® injections for intravenous infusion administration are formulated as sterile iso-osmotic solutions containing 2 mg/mL of fluconazole. They are supplied in glass bottles or in Viaflex® Plus plastic containers containing volumes of 100 mL or 200 mL affording doses of 200 mg and 400 mg of fluconazole, respectively. DIFLUCAN® injections in Viaflex® Plus plastic containers are available in both sodium chloride and dextrose diluents.

DIFLUCAN® Injections in Glass Bottles:
NDC 0049-3371-26 Fluconazole in Sodium Chloride Diluent 200 mg/100 mL × 6
NDC 0049-3372-26 Fluconazole in Sodium Chloride Diluent 400 mg/200 mL × 6

Storage: Store between 86°F (30°C) and 41°F (5°C). Protect from freezing.

DIFLUCAN® Injections in Viaflex® Plus Plastic Containers:
NDC 0049-3435-26 Fluconazole in Sodium Chloride Diluent 200 mg/100 mL × 6
NDC 0049-3436-26 Fluconazole in Sodium Chloride Diluent 400 mg/200 mL × 6
NDC 0049-3437-26 Fluconazole in Dextrose Diluent 200 mg/100 mL × 6
NDC 0049-3438-26 Fluconazole in Dextrose Diluent 400 mg/200 mL × 6

Storage: Store between 77°F (25°C) and 41°F (5°C). Brief exposure up to 104°F (40°C) does not adversely affect the product. Protect from freezing.

© 1996 PFIZER INC

69-4526-00-3 Revised May 1996

Shown in Product Identification Guide, pages 327 and 328

EMETE-CON® ℞

[ā-mĕt′ā-kŏn″]
(benzquinamide hydrochloride)
For Intramuscular and Intravenous Use

DESCRIPTION

Benzquinamide is a non-amine-depleting benzoquinolizine derivative, chemically unrelated to the phenothiazines and to other antiemetics.

Chemically, Emete-con (benzquinamide hydrochloride) is N,N-diethyl-1,3,4,6,7,11b-hexahydro-2-hydroxy-9,10-dimethoxy-2H-benzo-[a]quinolizine-3-carboxamide acetate hydrochloride. The empirical formula is $C_{22}H_{32}N_2O_5 \cdot HCl$ and the molecular weight is 441.

[See chemical structure at top of next column.]

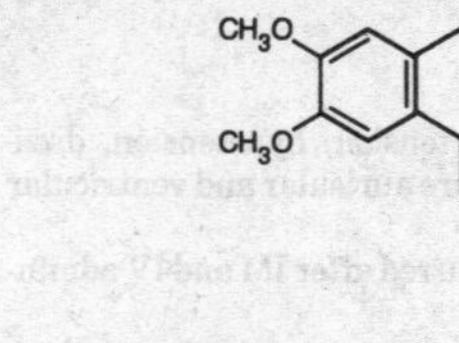

Emete-con for injection contains benzquinamide hydrochloride equivalent to 50 mg/vial of benzquinamide. When reconstituted with 2.2 ml of proper diluent, each vial yields 2 ml of a solution containing benzquinamide hydrochloride equivalent to 25 mg/ml of benzquinamide. When reconstituted this product maintains its potency for 14 days at room temperature.

ACTIONS

Benzquinamide HCl exhibited antiemetic, antihistaminic, mild anticholinergic and sedative action in animals. Studies conducted in dogs and human volunteers have demonstrated suppression of apomorphine-induced vomiting; however, relevance to clinical efficacy has not been established. The mechanism of action in humans is unknown. The onset of antiemetic activity in humans usually occurs within 15 minutes.

Benzquinamide metabolism has been studied in animals and in man. In both species, 5-10% of an administered dose is excreted unchanged in the urine. The remaining drug undergoes metabolic transformation in the liver by at least three pathways to a spectrum of metabolites which are excreted in the urine and in the bile, from which the more polar metabolites are not reabsorbed but are excreted in the feces. The half-life in plasma of Emete-con is about 40 minutes. More than 95% of an administered dose was excreted within 72 hours in animal studies using C14-labeled benzquinamide. In blood, benzquinamide is about 58% bound to plasma protein.

INDICATIONS

Emete-con is indicated for the prevention and treatment of nausea and vomiting associated with anesthesia and surgery.

Since the incidence of postoperative and postanesthetic vomiting has decreased with the adoption of modern techniques and agents, the prophylactic use of Emete-con should be restricted to those patients in whom emesis would endanger the results of surgery or result in harm to the patient.

CONTRAINDICATIONS

Emete-con is contraindicated in individuals who have demonstrated hypersensitivity to the drug.

WARNINGS

Use in Pregnancy
No teratogenic effects of benzquinamide were demonstrated in reproduction studies in chick embryos, mice, rats and rabbits. The relevance of these data to the human is not known. However, safe use of this drug in pregnancy has not been established and its use in pregnancy is not recommended.

Use in Children
As the data available at present are insufficient to establish proper dosage in children, the use of Emete-con in children is not recommended.

Intravenous Use
Sudden increase in blood pressure and transient arrhythmias (premature ventricular and auricular contractions) have been reported following intravenous administration of benzquinamide. Until a more predictable pattern of the effect of intravenous benzquinamide has been established, the intramuscular route of administration is considered preferable. The intravenous route of administration should be restricted to patients without cardiovascular disease and receiving no preanesthetic and/or concomitant cardiovascular drugs.

If patients receiving pressor agents or epinephrine-like drugs are also given benzquinamide, the latter should be given in fractions of the normal dose. Blood pressure should be monitored. Safeguards against hypertensive reactions are particularly important in hypertensive patients.

PRECAUTIONS

Benzquinamide, like other antiemetics, may mask signs of overdosage of toxic drugs or may obscure diagnosis of such conditions as intestinal obstruction and brain tumor.

ADVERSE REACTIONS

The following adverse reactions have been reported in subjects who have received benzquinamide. However, drowsiness appears to be the most common reaction. One case of pronounced allergic reaction has been encountered, characterized by pyrexia and urticaria.

System Affected
Autonomic Nervous System: Dry mouth, shivering, sweating, hiccoughs, flushing, salivation, blurred vision.

Continued on next page

Pfizer Inc—Cont.

Cardiovascular System: Hypertension, hypotension, dizziness, atrial fibrillation, premature auricular and ventricular contractions.
Hypertensive episodes have occurred after IM and IV administration.
Central Nervous System: Drowsiness, insomnia, restlessness, headache, excitement, nervousness.
Gastrointestinal System: Anorexia, nausea.
Musculoskeletal System: Twitching, shaking/tremors, weakness.
Skin: Hives/rash.
Other Systems: Fatigue, shaking chills, increased temperature.

DOSAGE AND ADMINISTRATION

Intramuscular: 50 mg (0.5 mg/kg–1.0 mg/kg)
First dose may be repeated in one hour with subsequent doses every 3-4 hours, as necessary. The precautions applicable to all intramuscular injections should be observed. Emete-con (benzquinamide hydrochloride) should be injected well within the mass of a larger muscle. The deltoid area should be used only if well developed. Injections should not be made into the lower and mid-thirds of the upper arm. Aspiration of the syringe should be carried out to avoid inadvertent intravascular injection.
Therapeutic blood levels and demonstrable antiemetic activity appear within fifteen minutes of intramuscular administration. When the objective of therapy is the prevention of nausea and vomiting, intramuscular administration is recommended at least fifteen minutes prior to emergence from anesthesia.
Intravenous: 25 mg (0.2 mg/kg–0.4 mg/kg as a single dose) administered slowly (1 ml per 0.5 to 1 minute). Subsequent doses should be given intramuscularly.
The intravenous route of administration should be restricted to patients without cardiovascular disease (See WARNINGS). If it is necessary to use Emete-con intravenously in elderly or debilitated patients, benzquinamide should be administered cautiously and the lower dose range is recommended.
This preparation must be initially reconstituted with 2.2 ml of Sterile Water for Injection, Bacteriostatic Water for Injection with benzyl alcohol or with methylparaben and propylparaben. This procedure yields 2 ml of a solution equivalent to 25 mg benzquinamide/ml, which maintains its potency for 14 days at room temperature.

OVERDOSAGE

Manifestations: On the basis of acute animal toxicology studies, gross Emete-con overdosage in humans might be expected to manifest itself as a combination of Central Nervous System stimulant and depressant effects. This speculation is derived from experimental studies in which intravenous doses of benzquinamide, at least 150 times the human therapeutic dose, were administered to dogs.
Treatment: There is no specific antidote for Emete-con overdosage. General supportive measures should be instituted, as indicated. Atropine may be helpful. Although there has been no direct experience with dialysis, it is not likely to be of value, since benzquinamide is extensively bound to plasma protein.

HOW SUPPLIED

Emete-con for IM/IV use is available in a vial containing benzquinamide HCl equivalent to 50 mg of benzquinamide in packages of 10 vials.

CAUTION

Federal law prohibits dispensing without prescription.
May 1977 60-1787-00-4

FELDENE® ℞
[*fĕl 'deen*]
(piroxicam)
CAPSULES
For Oral Use

DESCRIPTION

FELDENE (piroxicam) is 4-Hydroxy-2-methyl-*N*-2-pyridinyl-2*H*-1,2-benzothiazine-3-carboxamide 1,1-dioxide, an oxicam. Members of the oxicam family are not carboxylic acids, but they are acidic by virtue of the enolic 4-hydroxy substituent. FELDENE occurs as a white crystalline solid, sparingly soluble in water, dilute acid and most organic solvents. It is slightly soluble in alcohols and in aqueous alkaline solution. It exhibits a weakly acidic 4-hydroxy proton (pKa 5.1) and a weakly basic pyridyl nitrogen (pKa 1.8). It has the following structure:
[See chemical structure at top of next column.]

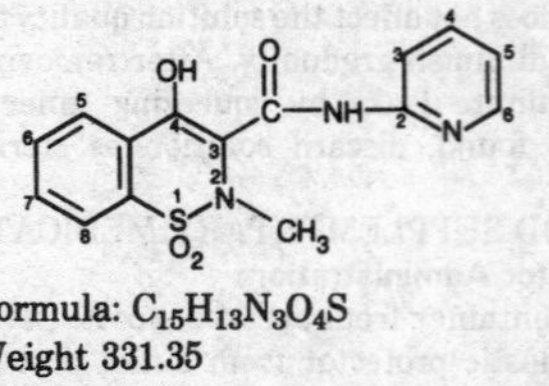

Molecular Formula: $C_{15}H_{13}N_3O_4S$
Molecular Weight 331.35

Inert ingredients in the formulations are: hard gelatin capsules (which may contain Blue 1, Red 3, and other inert ingredients); lactose; magnesium stearate; sodium lauryl sulfate; starch.

CLINICAL PHARMACOLOGY

FELDENE has shown anti-inflammatory, analgesic and antipyretic properties in animals. Edema, erythema, tissue proliferation, fever, and pain can all be inhibited in laboratory animals by the administration of FELDENE. It is effective regardless of the etiology of the inflammation. The mode of action of FELDENE is not fully established at this time. However, a common mechanism for the above effects may exist in the ability of FELDENE to inhibit the biosynthesis of prostaglandins, known mediators of inflammation.
It is established that FELDENE does not act by stimulating the pituitary-adrenal axis.
FELDENE is well absorbed following oral administration. Drug plasma concentrations are proportional for 10 and 20 mg doses, generally peak within three to five hours after medication, and subsequently decline with a mean half-life of 50 hours (range of 30 to 86 hours, although values outside of this range have been encountered).
This prolonged half-life results in the maintenance of relatively stable plasma concentrations throughout the day on once daily doses and to significant drug accumulation upon multiple dosing. A single 20 mg dose generally produces peak piroxicam plasma levels of 1.5 to 2 mcg/mL, while maximum drug plasma concentrations, after repeated daily ingestion of 20 mg FELDENE, usually stabilize at 3–8 mcg/mL. Most patients approximate steady state plasma levels within 7 to 12 days. Higher levels, which approximate steady state at two to three weeks, have been observed in patients in whom longer plasma half-lives of piroxicam occurred.
FELDENE and its biotransformation products are excreted in urine and feces, with about twice as much appearing in the urine as the feces. Metabolism occurs by hydroxylation at the 5 position of the pyridyl side chain and conjugation of this product; by cyclodehydration; and by a sequence of reactions involving hydrolysis of the amide linkage, decarboxylation, ring contraction, and N-demethylation. Less than 5% of the daily dose is excreted unchanged.
Concurrent administration of aspirin (3900 mg/day) and FELDENE (20 mg/day), resulted in a reduction of plasma levels of piroxicam to about 80% of their normal values. The use of FELDENE in conjunction with aspirin is not recommended because data are inadequate to demonstrate that the combination produces greater improvement than that achieved with aspirin alone and the potential for adverse reactions is increased. Concomitant administration of antacids had no effect on FELDENE plasma levels. The effects of impaired renal function or hepatic disease on plasma levels have not been established.
FELDENE, like salicylates and other nonsteroidal anti-inflammatory agents, is associated with symptoms of gastrointestinal tract irritation (see ADVERSE REACTIONS). However, in a study utilizing ^{51}Cr-tagged red blood cells, 20 mg of FELDENE administered as a single dose for four days did not result in a significant increase in fecal blood loss and did not detectably affect the gastric mucosa. In the same study a total daily dose of 3900 mg of aspirin, i.e., 972 mg q.i.d., caused a significant increase in fecal blood loss and mucosal lesions as demonstrated by gastroscopy.
In controlled clinical trials, the effectiveness of FELDENE (piroxicam) has been established for both acute exacerbations and long-term management of rheumatoid arthritis and osteoarthritis.
The therapeutic effects of FELDENE are evident early in the treatment of both diseases with a progressive increase in response over several (8–12) weeks. Efficacy is seen in terms of pain relief and, when present, subsidence of inflammation. Doses of 20 mg/day FELDENE display a therapeutic effect comparable to therapeutic doses of aspirin, with a lower incidence of minor gastrointestinal effects and tinnitus.
FELDENE has been administered concomitantly with fixed doses of gold and corticosteroids. The existence of a "steroid-sparing" effect has not been adequately studied to date.

INDICATIONS AND USAGE

FELDENE is indicated for acute or long-term use in the relief of signs and symptoms of the following:
1. osteoarthritis
2. rheumatoid arthritis
Dosage recommendations for use in children have not been established.

CONTRAINDICATIONS

FELDENE should not be used in patients who have previously exhibited hypersensitivity to it, or in individuals with the syndrome comprised of bronchospasm, nasal polyps, and angioedema precipitated by aspirin or other nonsteroidal anti-inflammatory drugs.

WARNINGS

Risk of GI Ulceration, Bleeding and Perforation with NSAID Therapy
Serious gastrointestinal toxicity such as bleeding, ulceration, and perforation can occur at any time, with or without warning symptoms, in patients treated chronically with NSAID therapy. Although minor upper gastrointestinal problems, such as dyspepsia, are common, usually developing early in therapy, physicians should remain alert for ulceration and bleeding in patients treated chronically with NSAIDs even in the absence of previous GI tract symptoms. In patients observed in clinical trials of several months to two years duration, symptomatic upper GI ulcers, gross bleeding or perforation appear to occur in approximately 1% of patients treated for 3–6 months, and in about 2–4% of patients treated for one year. Physicians should inform patients about the signs and/or symptoms of serious GI toxicity and what steps to take if they occur.
Studies to date have not identified any subset of patients not at risk of developing peptic ulceration and bleeding. Except for a prior history of serious GI events and other risk factors known to be associated with peptic ulcer disease, such as alcoholism, smoking, etc., no risk factors (e.g., age, sex) have been associated with increased risk. Elderly or debilitated patients seem to tolerate ulceration or bleeding less well than other individuals and most spontaneous reports of fatal GI events are in this population. Studies to date are inconclusive concerning the relative risk of various NSAIDs in causing such reactions. High doses of any NSAID probably carry a greater risk of these reactions, although controlled clinical trials showing this do not exist in most cases. In considering the use of relatively large doses (within the recommended dosage range), sufficient benefit should be anticipated to offset the potential increased risk of GI toxicity.

PRECAUTIONS

Renal Effects: As with other nonsteroidal anti-inflammatory drugs, long-term administration of piroxicam to animals has resulted in renal papillary necrosis and other abnormal renal pathology. In humans, there have been reports of acute interstitial nephritis with hematuria, proteinuria, and occasionally, nephrotic syndrome.
A second form of renal toxicity has been seen in patients with prerenal conditions leading to a reduction in renal blood flow or blood volume, where the renal prostaglandins have a supportive role in the maintenance of renal perfusion. In these patients administration of an NSAID may cause a dose-dependent reduction in prostaglandin formation and may precipitate overt renal decompensation. Patients at greatest risk of this reaction are those with impaired renal function, heart failure, liver dysfunction, those taking diuretics, and the elderly. Discontinuation of NSAID therapy is typically followed by recovery to the pretreatment state.
Because of extensive renal excretion of piroxicam and its biotransformation products (less than 5% of the daily dose excreted unchanged, see CLINICAL PHARMACOLOGY), lower doses of piroxicam should be anticipated in patients with impaired renal function, and they should be carefully monitored.
Although other nonsteroidal anti-inflammatory drugs do not have the same direct effects on platelets that aspirin does, all drugs inhibiting prostaglandin biosynthesis do interfere with platelet function to some degree; therefore, patients who may be adversely affected by such an action should be carefully observed when FELDENE is administered.
Because of reports of adverse eye findings with nonsteroidal anti-inflammatory agents, it is recommended that patients who develop visual complaints during treatment with FELDENE have ophthalmic evaluation.
As with other nonsteroidal anti-inflammatory drugs, borderline elevations of one or more liver tests may occur in up to 15% of patients. These abnormalities may progress, may remain essentially unchanged, or may be transient with continued therapy. The SGPT (ALT) test is probably the most sensitive indicator of liver dysfunction. Meaningful (3 times the upper limit of normal) elevations of SGPT or SGOT (AST) occurred in controlled clinical trials in less than 1% of patients. A patient with symptoms and/or signs suggesting liver dysfunction, or in whom an abnormal liver test has occurred, should be evaluated for evidence of the development of more severe hepatic reaction while on therapy with FELDENE. Severe hepatic reactions, including jaundice and cases of fatal hepatitis, have been reported with FELDENE. Although such reactions are rare, if abnormal liver tests persist or worsen, if clinical signs and symptoms consistent with liver disease develop, or if systemic manifestations occur (e.g. eosinophilia, rash, etc.), FELDENE should be discontinued. (See also ADVERSE REACTIONS.)

Although at the recommended dose of 20 mg/day of FELDENE increased fecal blood loss due to gastrointestinal irritation did not occur (see CLINICAL PHARMACOLOGY), in about 4% of the patients treated with FELDENE alone or concomitantly with aspirin, reductions in hemoglobin and hematocrit values were observed. Therefore, these values should be determined if signs or symptoms of anemia occur.

Peripheral edema has been observed in approximately 2% of the patients treated with FELDENE. Therefore, as with other nonsteroidal anti-inflammatory drugs, FELDENE should be used with caution in patients with heart failure, hypertension or other conditions predisposing to fluid retention, since its usage may be associated with a worsening of these conditions.

A combination of dermatological and/or allergic signs and symptoms suggestive of serum sickness have occasionally occurred in conjunction with the use of FELDENE. These include arthralgias, pruritus, fever, fatigue, and rash including vesiculo bullous reactions and exfoliative dermatitis.

Information for Patients

FELDENE, like other drugs of its class, is not free of side effects. The side effects of these drugs can cause discomfort and, rarely, there are more serious side effects, such as gastrointestinal bleeding, which may result in hospitalization and even fatal outcomes.

NSAIDs (Nonsteroidal Anti-Inflammatory Drugs) are often essential agents in the management of arthritis, but they also may be commonly employed for conditions which are less serious.

Physicians may wish to discuss with their patients the potential risks (see WARNINGS, PRECAUTIONS, and ADVERSE REACTIONS sections) and likely benefits of NSAID treatment, particularly when the drugs are used for less serious conditions where treatment without NSAIDs may represent an acceptable alternative to both the patient and physician.

Laboratory Tests

Because serious GI tract ulceration and bleeding can occur without warning symptoms, physicians should follow chronically treated patients for the signs and symptoms of ulceration and bleeding and should inform them of the importance of this follow-up (see Risk of GI Ulceration, Bleeding and Perforation with NSAID Therapy).

Drug Interactions

FELDENE is highly protein bound, and, therefore, might be expected to displace other protein-bound drugs. Although this has not occurred in *in vitro* studies with coumarin-type anticoagulants, interactions with coumarin-type anticoagulants have been reported with FELDENE since marketing, therefore, physicians should closely monitor patients for a change in dosage requirements when administering FELDENE to patients on coumarin-type anticoagulants and other highly protein-bound drugs.

Plasma levels of piroxicam are depressed to approximately 80% of their normal values when FELDENE is administered in conjunction with aspirin (3900 mg/day), but concomitant administration of antacids has no effect on piroxicam plasma levels (see CLINICAL PHARMACOLOGY).

Nonsteroidal anti-inflammatory agents, including FELDENE, have been reported to increase steady state plasma lithium levels. It is recommended that plasma lithium levels be monitored when initiating, adjusting and discontinuing FELDENE.

Carcinogenesis, Chronic Animal Toxicity and Impairment of Fertility

Subacute and chronic toxicity studies have been carried out in rats, mice, dogs, and monkeys.

The pathology most often seen was that characteristically associated with the animal toxicology of anti-inflammatory agents: renal papillary necrosis (see PRECAUTIONS) and gastrointestinal lesions.

In classical studies in laboratory animals piroxicam did not show any teratogenic potential.

Reproductive studies revealed no impairment of fertility in animals.

Pregnancy and Nursing Mothers

Like other drugs which inhibit the synthesis and release of prostaglandins, piroxicam increased the incidence of dystocia and delayed parturition in pregnant animals when piroxicam administration was continued late into pregnancy. Gastrointestinal tract toxicity was increased in pregnant females in the last trimester of pregnancy compared to non-pregnant females or females in earlier trimesters of pregnancy.

FELDENE is not recommended for use in nursing mothers or in pregnant women because of the animal findings and since safety for such use has not been established in humans.

Use in Children

Dosage recommendations and indications for use in children have not been established.

ADVERSE REACTIONS

The incidence of adverse reactions to piroxicam is based on clinical trials involving approximately 2300 patients, about 400 of whom were treated for more than one year and 170 for more than two years. About 30% of all patients receiving daily doses of 20 mg of FELDENE experienced side effects. Gastrointestinal symptoms were the most prominent side effects—occurring in approximately 20% of the patients, which in most instances did not interfere with the course of therapy. Of the patients experiencing gastrointestinal side effects, approximately 5% discontinued therapy with an overall incidence of peptic ulceration of about 1%.

Other than the gastrointestinal symptoms, edema, dizziness, headache, changes in hematological parameters, and rash have been reported in a small percentage of patients. Routine ophthalmoscopy and slit-lamp examinations have revealed no evidence of ocular changes in 205 patients followed from 3 to 24 months while on therapy.

Incidence Greater Than 1% The following adverse reactions occurred more frequently than 1 in 100.

Gastrointestinal: stomatitis, anorexia, epigastric distress*, nausea*, constipation, abdominal discomfort, flatulence, diarrhea, abdominal pain, indigestion

Hematological: decreases in hemoglobin* and hematocrit* (see PRECAUTIONS), anemia, leucopenia, eosinophilia

Dermatologic: pruritus, rash

Central Nervous System: dizziness, somnolence, vertigo

Urogenital: BUN and creatinine elevations (see PRECAUTIONS)

Body as a Whole: headache, malaise

Special Senses: tinnitus

Cardiovascular/Respiratory: edema (see PRECAUTIONS)

*Reactions occurring in 3% to 9% of patients treated with FELDENE. Reactions occurring in 1–3% of patients are unmarked.

Incidence Less Than 1% (Causal Relationship Probable)

The following adverse reactions occurred less frequently than 1 in 100. The probability exists that there is a causal relationship between FELDENE and these reactions.

Gastrointestinal: liver function abnormalities, jaundice, hepatitis (see PRECAUTIONS), vomiting, hematemesis, melena, gastrointestinal bleeding, perforation and ulceration (see WARNINGS), dry mouth

Hematological: thrombocytopenia, petechial rash, ecchymosis, bone marrow depression including aplastic anemia, epistaxis

Dermatologic: sweating, erythema, bruising, desquamation, exfoliative dermatitis, erythema multiforme, toxic epidermal necrolysis, Stevens-Johnson syndrome, vesiculo bullous reaction, photoallergic skin reactions

Central Nervous System: depression, insomnia, nervousness

Urogenital: hematuria, proteinuria, interstitial nephritis, renal failure, hyperkalemia, glomerulitis, papillary necrosis, nephrotic syndrome (see PRECAUTIONS)

Body as a Whole: pain (colic), fever, flu-like syndrome (see PRECAUTIONS)

Special Senses: swollen eyes, blurred vision, eye irritations

Cardiovascular/Respiratory: hypertension, worsening of congestive heart failure (see PRECAUTIONS), exacerbation of angina

Metabolic: hypoglycemia, hyperglycemia, weight increase, weight decrease

Hypersensitivity: anaphylaxis, bronchospasm, urticaria/angioedema, vasculitis, "serum sickness" (see PRECAUTIONS)

Incidence Less Than 1% (Causal Relationship Unknown)

Other adverse reactions were reported with a frequency of less than 1 in 100, but a causal relationship between FELDENE and the reaction could not be determined.

Gastrointestinal: pancreatitis

Dermatologic: onycholysis, loss of hair

Central Nervous System: akathisia, hallucinations, mood alterations, dream abnormalities, mental confusion, paresthesias

Urogenital System: dysuria

Body as a Whole: weakness

Cardiovascular/Respiratory: palpitations, dyspnea

Hypersensitivity: positive ANA

Special Senses: transient hearing loss

Hematological: hemolytic anemia

OVERDOSAGE

In the event treatment for overdosage is required the long plasma half-life (see CLINICAL PHARMACOLOGY) of piroxicam should be considered. The absence of experience with acute overdosage precludes characterization of sequelae and recommendation of specific antidotal efficacy at this time. It is reasonable to assume, however, that the standard measures of gastric evacuation and general supportive therapy would apply. In addition to supportive measures, the use of activated charcoal may effectively reduce the absorption and reabsorption of piroxicam. Experiments in dogs have demonstrated that the use of multiple-dose treatments with activated charcoal could reduce the half-life of piroxicam elimination from 27 hours (without charcoal) to 11 hours and reduce the systemic bioavailability of piroxicam by as much as 37% when activated charcoal is given as late as 6 hours after administration of piroxicam.

ADMINISTRATION AND DOSAGE

Rheumatoid Arthritis, Osteoarthritis

It is recommended that FELDENE therapy be initiated and maintained at a single daily dose of 20 mg. If desired the daily dose may be divided. Because of the long half-life of FELDENE, steady-state blood levels are not reached for 7–12 days. Therefore although the therapeutic effects of FELDENE are evident early in treatment, there is a progressive increase in response over several weeks and the effect of therapy should not be assessed for two weeks.

Dosage recommendations and indications for use in children have not been established.

HOW SUPPLIED

FELDENE Capsules for oral administration
Bottles of 100: 10 mg (NDC 0069-3220-66)
(NDC 0663-3220-66)
(NDC 59012-322-66) maroon and blue # 322
20 mg (NDC 0069-3230-66)
(NDC 59012-323-66) maroon #323
Bottles of 500: 20 mg (NDC 0069-3230-73)
(NDC 0663-3230-73)
(NDC 59012-323-73) maroon #323
Unit dose packages of 100: 20 mg (NDC 0069-3230-41)
(NDC 59012-323-41) maroon #323

© 1982 PFIZER INC

69-4100-32-4 Rev. Oct. 1993

Shown in Product Identification Guide, page 328

GEOCILLIN® ℞

[*gē ′ō-sil-ĭn*]
(carbenicillin indanyl sodium)
TABLETS
For Oral Use

DESCRIPTION

Geocillin, a semisynthetic penicillin, is the sodium salt of the indanyl ester of Geopen® (carbenicillin disodium). The chemical name is:

1-(5-Indanyl)-N-(2-carboxy-3,3-dimethyl-7-oxo-4-thia-1-azabicyclo[3.2.0]hept-6-yl)-2-phenylmalonamate monosodium salt.

The structural formula is:

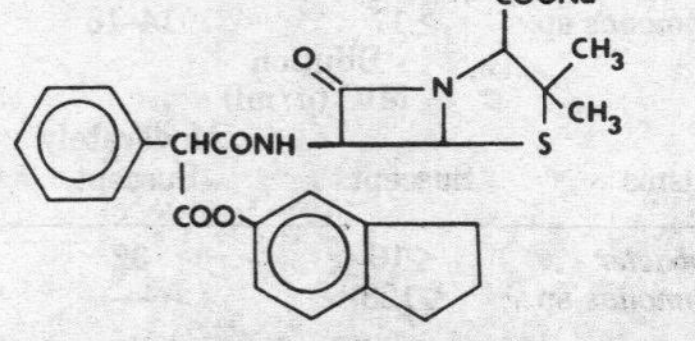

The empirical formula is: $C_{26}H_{25}N_2NaO_6S$ and mol. wt. is 516.55.

Geocillin tablets are yellow, capsule-shaped and film-coated, made of a white crystalline solid. Carbenicillin is freely soluble in water. Each Geocillin tablet contains 382 mg of carbenicillin, 118 mg of indanyl sodium ester. Each Geocillin tablet contains 23 mg of sodium.

Inert ingredients are: glycine; magnesium stearate and sodium lauryl sulfate. May also include the following: hydroxypropyl cellulose; hydroxypropyl methylcellulose; opaspray (which may include Blue 2 Lake, Yellow 6 Lake, Yellow 10 Lake, and other inert ingredients); opadry light yellow (which may contain D&C Yellow 10 Lake, FD&C Yellow 6 Lake and other inert ingredients); opadry clear (which may contain other inert ingredients).

CLINICAL PHARMACOLOGY

Free carbenicillin is the predominant pharmacologically active fraction of Geocillin. Carbenicillin exerts its antibacterial activity by interference with final cell wall synthesis of susceptible bacteria.

Geocillin is acid stable, and rapidly absorbed from the small intestine following oral administration. It provides relatively low plasma concentrations of antibiotic and is primarily excreted in the urine. After absorption, Geocillin is rapidly converted to carbenicillin by hydrolysis of the ester linkage. Following ingestion of a single 500 mg tablet of Geocillin, a peak carbenicillin plasma concentration of approximately 6.5 mcg/ml is reached in 1 hour. About 30% of this dose is excreted in the urine unchanged within 12 hours, with another 6% excreted over the next 12 hours.

In a multiple dose study utilizing volunteers with normal renal function, the following mean urine and serum levels of carbenicillin were achieved:

[See table at bottom of next page.]

Microbiology

The antibacterial activity of Geocillin is due to its rapid conversion to carbenicillin by hydrolysis after absorption. Though Geocillin provides substantial *in vitro* activity against a variety of both gram-positive and gram-negative microorganisms, the most important aspect of its profile is in its antipseudomonal and antiproteal activity. Because of the high urine levels obtained following administration, Geocillin has demonstrated clinical efficacy in urinary infections due to susceptible strains of:

Continued on next page

Pfizer Inc—Cont.

Escherichia coli
Proteus mirabilis
Proteus vulgaris
Morganella morganii (formerly *Proteus morganii*)
Pseudomonas species
Providencia rettgeri (formerly *Proteus rettgeri*)
Enterobacter species
Enterococci (*S. faecalis*)

In addition, *in vitro* data, not substantiated by clinical studies, indicate the following pathogens to be usually susceptible to Geocillin:

Staphylococcus species (nonpenicillinase producing)
Streptococcus species

Resistance
Most *Klebsiella* species are usually resistant to the action of Geocillin. Some strains of *Pseudomonas* species have developed resistance to carbenicillin.

Susceptibility Testing
Geopen (carbenicillin disodium) Susceptibility Powder or 100 ug. Geopen Susceptibility Discs may be used to determine microbial susceptibility to Geocillin using one of the following standard methods recommended by the National Committee for Clinical Laboratory Standards:

M2-A3, "Performance Standards for Antimicrobial Disk Susceptibility Tests"
M7-A, "Methods for Dilution Antimicrobial Susceptibility Tests for Bacteria that Grow Aerobically"
M11-A, "Reference Agar Dilution Procedure for Antimicrobial Susceptibility Testing of Anaerobic Bacteria"
M17-P, "Alternative Methods for Antimicrobial Susceptibility Testing of Anaerobic Bacteria"

Tests should be interpreted by the following criteria:

Disk Diffusion
Zone diameter (mm)

Organisms	Suscept.	Intermed.	Resist.
Enterobacter	≥ 23	18–22	≤ 17
Pseudomonas sp.	≥ 17	14–16	≤ 13

Dilution
MIC (μ/ml)

Organisms	Suscept.	Moderately Suscept.	Resist.
Enterobacter	≤ 16	32	≥ 64
Pseudomonas sp.	≤ 128	—	≥ 156

Interpretations of susceptible, intermediate, and resistant correlate zone size diameters with MIC values. A laboratory report of "susceptible" indicates that the suspected causative microorganism most likely will respond to therapy with carbenicillin. A laboratory report of "resistant" indicates that the infecting microorganism most likely will not respond to therapy. A laboratory report of "moderately susceptible" indicates that the microorganism is most likely susceptible if a high dosage of carbenicillin is used, or if the infection is such that high levels of carbenicillin may be attained in urine. A report of "intermediate" using the disk diffusion method may be considered an equivocal result, and dilution tests may be indicated.

INDICATIONS AND USAGE

Geocillin (carbenicillin indanyl sodium) is indicated in the treatment of acute and chronic infections of the upper and lower urinary tract and in asymptomatic bacteriuria due to susceptible strains of the following organisms:

Escherichia coli
Proteus mirabilis
Morganella morganii
   (formerly *Proteus morganii*)
Providencia rettgeri
   (formerly *Proteus rettgeri*)
Proteus vulgaris
Pseudomonas
Enterobacter
Enterococci

Geocillin is also indicated in the treatment of prostatitis due to susceptible strains of the following organisms:

Escherichia coli
   Enterococcus (*S. faecalis*)
Proteus mirabilis
Enterobacter sp.

WHEN HIGH AND RAPID BLOOD AND URINE LEVELS OF ANTIBIOTIC ARE INDICATED, THERAPY WITH GEOPEN (CARBENICILLIN DISODIUM) SHOULD BE INITIATED BY PARENTERAL ADMINISTRATION FOLLOWED, AT THE PHYSICIAN'S DISCRETION, BY ORAL THERAPY.

NOTE: Susceptibility testing should be performed prior to and during the course of therapy to detect the possible emergence of resistant organisms which may develop.

CONTRAINDICATIONS

Geocillin is ordinarily contraindicated in patients who have a known penicillin allergy.

WARNINGS

Serious and occasionally fatal hypersensitivity (anaphylactic) reactions have been reported in patients on oral penicillin therapy. Although anaphylaxis is more frequent following parenteral therapy, it has occurred in patients on oral penicillins. These reactions are more apt to occur in individuals with a history of penicillin hypersensitivity and/or a history of sensitivity to multiple allergens.

There have been reports of individuals with a history of penicillin hypersensitivity who have experienced severe hypersensitivity reactions when treated with a cephalosporin, and vice versa. Before initiating therapy with a penicillin, careful inquiry should be made concerning previous hypersensitivity reactions to penicillins, cephalosporins, or other allergens. If an allergic reaction occurs, the drug should be discontinued and the appropriate therapy instituted.

SERIOUS ANAPHYLACTOID REACTIONS REQUIRE IMMEDIATE EMERGENCY TREATMENT WITH EPINEPHRINE. OXYGEN, INTRAVENOUS STEROIDS AND AIRWAY MANAGEMENT, INCLUDING INTUBATION, SHOULD ALSO BE ADMINISTERED AS INDICATED.

PRECAUTIONS

General: As with any penicillin preparation, an allergic response, including anaphylaxis, may occur particularly in a hypersensitive individual.

Long term use of Geocillin may result in the overgrowth of nonsusceptible organisms. If superinfection occurs during therapy, appropriate measures should be taken.

Since carbenicillin is primarily excreted by the kidney, patients with severe renal impairment (creatinine clearance of less than 10 ml/min) will not achieve therapeutic urine levels of carbenicillin.

In patients with creatinine clearance of 10–20 ml/min it may be necessary to adjust dosage to prevent accumulation of drug.

Laboratory Tests: As with other penicillins, periodic assessment of organ system function including renal, hepatic, and hematopoietic systems is recommended during prolonged therapy.

Drug Interactions: Geocillin (carbenicillin indanyl sodium) blood levels may be increased and prolonged by concurrent administration of probenecid.

Carcinogenesis, Mutagenesis, Impairment of Fertility: There are no long-term animal or human studies to evaluate carcinogenic potential. Rats fed 250–1000 mg/kg/day for 18 months developed mild liver pathology (e.g., bile duct hyperplasia) at all dose levels, but there was no evidence of drug-related neoplasia. Geocillin administered at daily doses ranging to 1000 mg/kg had no apparent effect on the fertility or reproductive performance of rats.

Pregnancy Category B: Reproduction studies have been performed at dose levels of 1000 or 500 mg/kg in rats, 200 mg/kg in mice, and at 500 mg/kg in monkeys with no harm to fetus due to Geocillin. There are, however, no adequate and well controlled studies in pregnant women. Because animal reproduction studies are not always predictive of human response, this drug should be used during pregnancy only if clearly needed.

Labor and Delivery: It is not known whether the use of Geocillin in humans during labor or delivery has immediate or delayed adverse effects on the fetus, prolongs the duration of labor, or increases the likelihood that forceps delivery or other obstetrical intervention or resuscitation of the newborn will be necessary.

Nursing Mothers: Carbenicillin class antibiotics are excreted in milk although the amounts excreted are unknown; therefore, caution should be exercised if administered to a nursing woman.

Pediatric Use: Since only limited clinical data is available to date in children, the safety of Geocillin administration in this age group has not yet been established.

ADVERSE REACTIONS

The following adverse reactions have been reported as possibly related to Geocillin administration in controlled studies which include 344 patients receiving Geocillin.

Gastrointestinal: The most frequent adverse reactions associated with Geocillin therapy are related to the gastrointestinal tract. Nausea, bad taste, diarrhea, vomiting, flatulence, and glossitis were reported. Abdominal cramps, dry mouth, furry tongue, rectal bleeding, anorexia, and unspecified epigastric distress were rarely reported.

Dermatologic: Hypersensitivity reactions such as skin rash, urticaria, and less frequently pruritus.

Hematologic: As with other penicillins, anemia, thrombocytopenia, leukopenia, neutropenia, and eosinophilia have infrequently been observed. The clinical significance of these abnormalities is not known.

Miscellaneous: Other reactions rarely reported were hyperthermia, headache, itchy eyes, vaginitis, and loose stools.

Abnormalities of Hepatic Function Tests: Mild SGOT elevations have been observed following Geocillin administration.

OVERDOSAGE

Geocillin is generally nontoxic. Geocillin when taken in excessive amounts may produce mild gastrointestinal irritation. The drug is rapidly excreted in the urine and symptoms are transitory. The usual symptoms of anaphylaxis may occur in hypersensitive individuals.

Carbenicillin blood levels achievable with Geocillin are very low, and toxic reactions as a function of overdosage should not occur systematically. The oral LD_{50} in mice is 3,600 mg/kg, in rats 2,000 mg/kg, and in dogs is in excess of 500 mg/kg. The lethal human dose is not known.

Although never reported, the possibility of accumulation of indanyl should be considered when large amounts of Geocillin are ingested. Free indole, which is a phenol derivative, may be potentially toxic. In general 8–15 grams of phenol, and presumably a similar amount of indole, are required orally before toxicity (peripheral vascular collapse) may occur. The metabolic by-products of indole are nontoxic. In patients with hepatic failure it may be possible for unmetabolized indole to accumulate.

The metabolic by-products of Geocillin, indanyl sulfate and glucuronide, as well as free carbenicillin, are dialyzable.

DOSAGE AND ADMINISTRATION

Geocillin is available as a coated tablet to be administered orally.

Usual Adult Dose

URINARY TRACT INFECTIONS	
Escherichia coli, *Proteus* species, and *Enterobacter*	1–2 tablets 4 times daily
Pseudomonas and *Enterococcus*	2 tablets 4 times daily
PROSTATITIS	
Escherichia coli, *Proteus mirabilis*, *Enterobacter* and *Enterococcus*	2 tablets 4 times daily

HOW SUPPLIED

Geocillin is available as film-coated tablets in bottles of 100's (NDC 0049-1430-66), and unit-dose packages of 100 (10 × 10's) (NDC 0049-1430-41). Each tablet contains carbenicillin indanyl sodium equivalent to 382 mg of carbenicillin.

Revised Sept. 1991   69-1970-00-2

Shown in Product Identification Guide, page 328

DRUG	DOSE	Mean Urine Concentration of Carbenicillin mcg/ml Hours After Initial Dose		
		0–3	3–6	6–24
Geocillin	1 tablet q.6 hr	1130	352	292
Geocillin	2 tablets q.6 hr	1428	789	809

Mean serum concentrations of carbenicillin in this study for these dosages are:

DRUG	DOSE	Mean Serum Concentration mcg/ml Hours After Initial Dose								
		$1/2$	1	2	4	6	24	25	26	28
Geocillin	1 tablet q.6 hr	5.1	6.5	3.2	1.9	0.0	0.4	8.8	5.4	0.4
Geocillin	2 tablets q.6 hr	6.1	9.6	7.9	2.6	0.4	0.8	13.2	12.8	3.8

GLUCOTROL® ℞

[*glū 'kă-trōl*]
(glipizide)
TABLETS
For Oral Use

DESCRIPTION

GLUCOTROL (glipizide) is an oral blood-glucose-lowering drug of the sulfonylurea class.
The Chemical Abstracts name of glipizide is 1-cyclohexyl-3-[[p- [2-(5-methylpyrazinecarboxamido)ethyl]phenyl] sulfonyl]urea. The molecular formula is $C_{21}H_{27}N_5O_4S$; the molecular weight is 445.55; the structural formula is shown below:

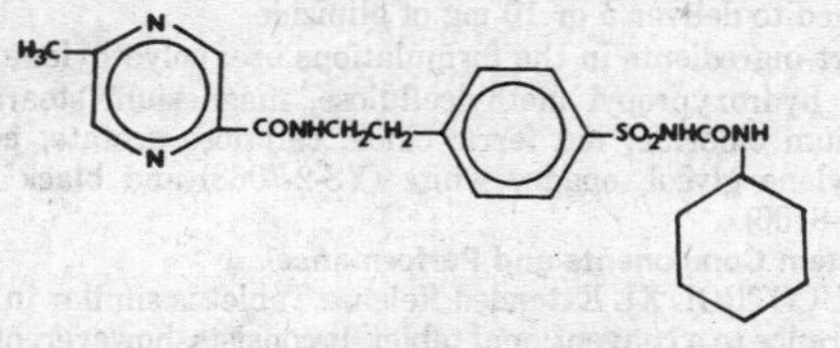

Glipizide is a whitish, odorless powder with a pKa of 5.9. It is insoluble in water and alcohols, but soluble in 0.1 *N* NaOH; it is freely soluble in dimethylformamide. GLUCOTROL tablets for oral use are available in 5 and 10 mg strengths.
Inert ingredients are: colloidal silicon dioxide; lactose; microcrystalline cellulose; starch; stearic acid.

CLINICAL PHARMACOLOGY

Mechanism of Action: The primary mode of action of GLUCOTROL in experimental animals appears to be the stimulation of insulin secretion from the beta cells of pancreatic islet tissue and is thus dependent on functioning beta cells in the pancreatic islets. In humans GLUCOTROL appears to lower the blood glucose acutely by stimulating the release of insulin from the pancreas, an effect dependent upon functioning beta cells in the pancreatic islets. The mechanism by which GLUCOTROL lowers blood glucose during long-term administration has not been clearly established. In man, stimulation of insulin secretion by GLUCOTROL in response to a meal is undoubtedly of major importance. Fasting insulin levels are not elevated even on long-term GLUCOTROL administration, but the postprandial insulin response continues to be enhanced after at least 6 months of treatment. The insulinotropic response to a meal occurs within 30 minutes after an oral dose of GLUCOTROL in diabetic patients, but elevated insulin levels do not persist beyond the time of the meal challenge. Extrapancreatic effects may play a part in the mechanism of action of oral sulfonylurea hypoglycemic drugs.
Blood sugar control persists in some patients for up to 24 hours after a single dose of GLUCOTROL, even though plasma levels have declined to a small fraction of peak levels by that time (see Pharmacokinetics below).
Some patients fail to respond initially, or gradually lose their responsiveness to sulfonylurea drugs, including GLUCOTROL. Alternatively, GLUCOTROL may be effective in some patients who have not responded or have ceased to respond to other sulfonylureas.
Other Effects: It has been shown that GLUCOTROL therapy was effective in controlling blood sugar without deleterious changes in the plasma lipoprotein profiles of patients treated for NIDDM.
In a placebo-controlled, crossover study in normal volunteers, GLUCOTROL had no antidiuretic activity, and, in fact, led to a slight increase in free water clearance.
Pharmacokinetics: Gastrointestinal absorption of GLUCOTROL in man is uniform, rapid, and essentially complete. Peak plasma concentrations occur 1–3 hours after a single oral dose. The half-life of elimination ranges from 2–4 hours in normal subjects, whether given intravenously or orally. The metabolic and excretory patterns are similar with the two routes of administration, indicating that first-pass metabolism is not significant. GLUCOTROL does not accumulate in plasma on repeated oral administration. Total absorption and disposition of an oral dose was unaffected by food in normal volunteers, but absorption was delayed by about 40 minutes. Thus GLUCOTROL was more effective when administered about 30 minutes before, rather than with, a test meal in diabetic patients. Protein binding was studied in serum from volunteers who received either oral or intravenous GLUCOTROL and found to be 98–99% one hour after either route of administration. The apparent volume of distribution of GLUCOTROL after intravenous administration was 11 liters, indicative of localization within the extracellular fluid compartment. In mice no GLUCOTROL or metabolites were detectable autoradiographically in the brain or spinal cord of males or females, nor in the fetuses of pregnant females. In another study, however, very small amounts of radioactivity were detected in the fetuses of rats given labelled drug.
The metabolism of GLUCOTROL is extensive and occurs mainly in the liver. The primary metabolites are inactive hydroxylation products and polar conjugates and are excreted mainly in the urine. Less than 10% unchanged GLUCOTROL is found in the urine.

INDICATIONS AND USAGE

GLUCOTROL is indicated as an adjunct to diet for the control of hyperglycemia and its associated symptomatology in patients with non-insulin-dependent diabetes mellitus (NIDDM; type II), formerly known as maturity-onset diabetes, after an adequate trial of dietary therapy has proved unsatisfactory.
In initiating treatment for non-insulin-dependent diabetes, diet should be emphasized as the primary form of treatment. Caloric restriction and weight loss are essential in the obese diabetic patient. Proper dietary management alone may be effective in controlling the blood glucose and symptoms of hyperglycemia. The importance of regular physical activity should also be stressed, and cardiovascular risk factors should be identified, and corrective measures taken where possible.
If this treatment program fails to reduce symptoms and/or blood glucose, the use of an oral sulfonylurea or insulin should be considered. Use of GLUCOTROL must be viewed by both the physician and patient as a treatment in addition to diet, and not as a substitute for diet or as a convenient mechanism for avoiding dietary restraint. Furthermore, loss of blood glucose control on diet alone also may be transient, thus requiring only short-term administration of GLUCOTROL.
During maintenance programs, GLUCOTROL should be discontinued if satisfactory lowering of blood glucose is no longer achieved. Judgments should be based on regular clinical and laboratory evaluations.
In considering the use of GLUCOTROL in asymptomatic patients, it should be recognized that controlling blood glucose in non-insulin-dependent diabetes has not been definitely established to be effective in preventing the long-term cardiovascular or neural complications of diabetes.

CONTRAINDICATIONS

GLUCOTROL is contraindicated in patients with:
1. Known hypersensitivity to the drug.
2. Diabetic ketoacidosis, with or without coma. This condition should be treated with insulin.

WARNINGS

SPECIAL WARNING ON INCREASED RISK OF CARDIOVASCULAR MORTALITY: The administration of oral hypoglycemic drugs has been reported to be associated with increased cardiovascular mortality as compared to treatment with diet alone or diet plus insulin. This warning is based on the study conducted by the University Group Diabetes Program (UGDP), a long-term prospective clinical trial designed to evaluate the effectiveness of glucose-lowering drugs in preventing or delaying vascular complications in patients with non-insulin-dependent diabetes. The study involved 823 patients who were randomly assigned to one of four treatment groups (*Diabetes,* 19, supp. 2: 747–830, 1970). UGDP reported that patients treated for 5 to 8 years with diet plus a fixed dose of tolbutamide (1.5 grams per day) had a rate of cardiovascular mortality approximately $2^1/_2$ times that of patients treated with diet alone. A significant increase in total mortality was not observed, but the use of tolbutamide was discontinued based on the increase in cardiovascular mortality, thus limiting the opportunity for the study to show an increase in overall mortality. Despite controversy regarding the interpretation of these results, the findings of the UGDP study provide an adequate basis for this warning. The patient should be informed of the potential risks and advantages of GLUCOTROL and of alternative modes of therapy.
Although only one drug in the sulfonylurea class (tolbutamide) was included in this study, it is prudent from a safety standpoint to consider that this warning may also apply to other oral hypoglycemic drugs in this class, in view of their close similarities in mode of action and chemical structure.

PRECAUTIONS

General
Renal and Hepatic Disease: The metabolism and excretion of GLUCOTROL may be slowed in patients with impaired renal and/or hepatic function. If hypoglycemia should occur in such patients, it may be prolonged and appropriate management should be instituted.
Hypoglycemia: All sulfonylurea drugs are capable of producing severe hypoglycemia. Proper patient selection, dosage, and instructions are important to avoid hypoglycemic episodes. Renal or hepatic insufficiency may cause elevated blood levels of GLUCOTROL and the latter may also diminish gluconeogenic capacity, both of which increase the risk of serious hypoglycemic reactions. Elderly, debilitated or malnourished patients, and those with adrenal or pituitary insufficiency are particularly susceptible to the hypoglycemic action of glucose-lowering drugs. Hypoglycemia may be difficult to recognize in the elderly, and in people who are taking beta-adrenergic blocking drugs. Hypoglycemia is more likely to occur when caloric intake is deficient, after severe or prolonged exercise, when alcohol is ingested, or when more than one glucose-lowering drug is used.
Loss of Control of Blood Glucose: When a patient stabilized on any diabetic regimen is exposed to stress such as fever, trauma, infection, or surgery, a loss of control may occur. At such times, it may be necessary to discontinue GLUCOTROL and administer insulin.
The effectiveness of any oral hypoglycemic drug, including GLUCOTROL, in lowering blood glucose to a desired level decreases in many patients over a period of time, which may be due to progression of the severity of the diabetes or to diminished responsiveness to the drug. This phenomenon is known as secondary failure, to distinguish it from primary failure in which the drug is ineffective in an individual patient when first given.
Laboratory Tests: Blood and urine glucose should be monitored periodically. Measurement of glycosylated hemoglobin may be useful.
Information for Patients: Patients should be informed of the potential risks and advantages of GLUCOTROL and of alternative modes of therapy. They should also be informed about the importance of adhering to dietary instructions, of a regular exercise program, and of regular testing of urine and/or blood glucose.
The risks of hypoglycemia, its symptoms and treatment, and conditions that predispose to its development should be explained to patients and responsible family members. Primary and secondary failure should also be explained.
Drug Interactions: The hypoglycemic action of sulfonylureas may be potentiated by certain drugs including nonsteroidal anti-inflammatory agents, some azoles, and other drugs that are highly protein bound, salicylates, sulfonamides, chloramphenicol, probenecid, coumarins, monoamine oxidase inhibitors, and beta-adrenergic blocking agents. When such drugs are administered to a patient receiving GLUCOTROL, the patient should be observed closely for hypoglycemia. When such drugs are withdrawn from a patient receiving GLUCOTROL, the patient should be observed closely for loss of control. *In vitro* binding studies with human serum proteins indicate that GLUCOTROL binds differently than tolbutamide and does not interact with salicylate or dicumarol. However, caution must be exercised in extrapolating these findings to the clinical situation and in the use of GLUCOTROL with these drugs.
Certain drugs tend to produce hyperglycemia and may lead to loss of control. These drugs include the thiazides and other diuretics, corticosteroids, phenothiazines, thyroid products, estrogens, oral contraceptives, phenytoin, nicotinic acid, sympathomimetics, calcium channel blocking drugs, and isoniazid. When such drugs are administered to a patient receiving GLUCOTROL, the patient should be closely observed for loss of control. When such drugs are withdrawn from a patient receiving GLUCOTROL, the patient should be observed closely for hypoglycemia.
A potential interaction between oral miconazole and oral hypoglycemic agents leading to severe hypoglycemia has been reported. Whether this interaction also occurs with the intravenous, topical, or vaginal preparations of miconazole is not known. The effect of concomitant administration of DIFLUCAN (fluconazole) and GLUCOTROL has been demonstrated in a placebo-controlled crossover study in normal volunteers. All subjects received GLUCOTROL alone and following treatment of 100 mg of DIFLUCAN as a single daily oral dose for 7 days. The mean percentage increase in the GLUCOTROL AUC after fluconazole administration was 56.9% (range: 35 to 81).
Carcinogenesis, Mutagenesis, Impairment of Fertility: A twenty month study in rats and an eighteen month study in mice at doses up to 75 times the maximum human dose revealed no evidence of drug-related carcinogenicity. Bacterial and *in vivo* mutagenicity tests were uniformly negative. Studies in rats of both sexes at doses up to 75 times the human dose showed no effects on fertility.
Pregnancy: Pregnancy Category C: GLUCOTROL (glipizide) was found to be mildly fetotoxic in rat reproductive studies at all dose levels (5–50 mg/kg). This fetotoxicity has been similarly noted with other sulfonylureas, such as tolbutamide and tolazamide. The effect is perinatal and believed to be directly related to the pharmacologic (hypoglycemic) action of GLUCOTROL. In studies in rats and rabbits no teratogenic effects were found. There are no adequate and well controlled studies in pregnant women. GLUCOTROL should be used during pregnancy only if the potential benefit justifies the potential risk to the fetus.
Because recent information suggests that abnormal blood glucose levels during pregnancy are associated with a higher incidence of congenital abnormalities, many experts recommend that insulin be used during pregnancy to maintain blood glucose levels as close to normal as possible.
Nonteratogenic Effects: Prolonged severe hypoglycemia (4 to 10 days) has been reported in neonates born to mothers who were receiving a sulfonylurea drug at the time of delivery. This has been reported more frequently with the use of

Continued on next page

Pfizer Inc—Cont.

agents with prolonged half-lives. If GLUCOTROL is used during pregnancy, it should be discontinued at least one month before the expected delivery date.

Nursing Mothers: Although it is not known whether GLUCOTROL is excreted in human milk, some sulfonylurea drugs are known to be excreted in human milk. Because the potential for hypoglycemia in nursing infants may exist, a decision should be made whether to discontinue nursing or to discontinue the drug, taking into account the importance of the drug to the mother. If the drug is discontinued and if diet alone is inadequate for controlling blood glucose, insulin therapy should be considered.

Pediatric Use: Safety and effectiveness in children have not been established.

ADVERSE REACTIONS

In U.S. and foreign controlled studies, the frequency of serious adverse reactions reported was very low. Of 702 patients, 11.8% reported adverse reactions and in only 1.5% was GLUCOTROL discontinued.

Hypoglycemia: See PRECAUTIONS and OVERDOSAGE sections.

Gastrointestinal: Gastrointestinal disturbances are the most common reactions. Gastrointestinal complaints were reported with the following approximate incidence: nausea and diarrhea, one in seventy; constipation and gastralgia, one in one hundred. They appear to be dose-related and may disappear on division or reduction of dosage. Cholestatic jaundice may occur rarely with sulfonylureas: GLUCOTROL should be discontinued if this occurs.

Dermatologic: Allergic skin reactions including erythema, morbilliform or maculopapular eruptions, urticaria, pruritus, and eczema have been reported in about one in seventy patients. These may be transient and may disappear despite continued use of GLUCOTROL; if skin reactions persist, the drug should be discontinued. Porphyria cutanea tarda and photosensitivity reactions have been reported with sulfonylureas.

Hematologic: Leukopenia, agranulocytosis, thrombocytopenia, hemolytic anemia, aplastic anemia, and pancytopenia have been reported with sulfonylureas.

Metabolic: Hepatic porphyria and disulfiram-like reactions have been reported with sulfonylureas. In the mouse, GLUCOTROL pretreatment did not cause an accumulation of acetaldehyde after ethanol administration. Clinical experience to date has shown that GLUCOTROL has an extremely low incidence of disulfiram-like alcohol reactions.

Endocrine Reactions: Cases of hyponatremia and the syndrome of inappropriate antidiuretic hormone (SIADH) secretion have been reported with this and other sulfonylureas.

Miscellaneous: Dizziness, drowsiness, and headache have each been reported in about one in fifty patients treated with GLUCOTROL. They are usually transient and seldom require discontinuance of therapy.

Laboratory Tests: The pattern of laboratory test abnormalities observed with GLUCOTROL was similar to that for other sulfonylureas. Occasional mild to moderate elevations of SGOT, LDH, alkaline phosphatase, BUN and creatinine were noted. One case of jaundice was reported. The relationship of these abnormalities to GLUCOTROL is uncertain, and they have rarely been associated with clinical symptoms.

OVERDOSAGE

There is no well documented experience with GLUCOTROL overdosage. The acute oral toxicity was extremely low in all species tested (LD_{50} greater than 4 g/kg).

Overdosage of sulfonylureas including GLUCOTROL can produce hypoglycemia. Mild hypoglycemic symptoms without loss of consciousness or neurologic findings should be treated aggressively with oral glucose and adjustments in drug dosage and/or meal patterns. Close monitoring should continue until the physician is assured that the patient is out of danger. Severe hypoglycemic reactions with coma, seizure, or other neurological impairment occur infrequently, but constitute medical emergencies requiring immediate hospitalization. If hypoglycemic coma is diagnosed or suspected, the patient should be given a rapid intravenous injection of concentrated (50%) glucose solution. This should be followed by a continuous infusion of a more dilute (10%) glucose solution at a rate that will maintain the blood glucose at a level above 100 mg/dL. Patients should be closely monitored for a minimum of 24 to 48 hours since hypoglycemia may recur after apparent clinical recovery. Clearance of GLUCOTROL from plasma would be prolonged in persons with liver disease. Because of the extensive protein binding of GLUCOTROL, dialysis is unlikely to be of benefit.

DOSAGE AND ADMINISTRATION

There is no fixed dosage regimen for the management of diabetes mellitus with GLUCOTROL or any other hypoglycemic agent. In addition to the usual monitoring of urinary glucose, the patient's blood glucose must also be monitored periodically to determine the minimum effective dose for the patient; to detect primary failure, i.e., inadequate lowering of blood glucose at the maximum recommended dose of medication; and to detect secondary failure, i.e., loss of an adequate blood-glucose-lowering response after an initial period of effectiveness. Glycosylated hemoglobin levels may also be of value in monitoring the patient's response to therapy.

Short-term administration of GLUCOTROL may be sufficient during periods of transient loss of control in patients usually controlled well on diet.

In general, GLUCOTROL should be given approximately 30 minutes before a meal to achieve the greatest reduction in postprandial hyperglycemia.

Initial Dose: The recommended starting dose is 5 mg, given before breakfast. Geriatric patients or those with liver disease may be started on 2.5 mg.

Titration: Dosage adjustments should ordinarily be in increments of 2.5–5 mg, as determined by blood glucose response. At least several days should elapse between titration steps. If response to a single dose is not satisfactory, dividing that dose may prove effective. The maximum recommended once daily dose is 15 mg. Doses above 15 mg should ordinarily be divided and given before meals of adequate caloric content. The maximum recommended total daily dose is 40 mg.

Maintenance: Some patients may be effectively controlled on a once-a-day regimen, while others show better response with divided dosing. Total daily doses above 15 mg should ordinarily be divided. Total daily doses above 30 mg have been safely given on a b.i.d. basis to long-term patients.

In elderly patients, debilitated or malnourished patients, and patients with impaired renal or hepatic function, the initial and maintenance dosing should be conservative to avoid hypoglycemic reactions (see PRECAUTIONS section).

Patients Receiving Insulin: As with other sulfonylurea-class hypoglycemics, many stable non-insulin-dependent diabetic patients receiving insulin may be safely placed on GLUCOTROL. When transferring patients from insulin to GLUCOTROL, the following general guidelines should be considered:

For patients whose daily insulin requirement is 20 units or less, insulin may be discontinued and GLUCOTROL therapy may begin at usual dosages. Several days should elapse between GLUCOTROL titration steps.

For patients whose daily insulin requirement is greater than 20 units, the insulin dose should be reduced by 50% and GLUCOTROL therapy may begin at usual dosages. Subsequent reductions in insulin dosage should depend on individual patient response. Several days should elapse between GLUCOTROL titration steps.

During the insulin withdrawal period, the patient should test urine samples for sugar and ketone bodies at least three times daily. Patients should be instructed to contact the prescriber immediately if these tests are abnormal. In some cases, especially when patient has been receiving greater than 40 units of insulin daily, it may be advisable to consider hospitalization during the transition period.

Patients Receiving Other Oral Hypoglycemic Agents: As with other sulfonylurea-class hypoglycemics, no transition period is necessary when transferring patients to GLUCOTROL. Patients should be observed carefully (1–2 weeks) for hypoglycemia when being transferred from longer half-life sulfonylureas (e.g., chlorpropamide) to GLUCOTROL due to potential overlapping of drug effect.

HOW SUPPLIED

GLUCOTROL tablets are white, dye-free, scored, diamond-shaped, and imprinted as follows:

5 mg–Pfizer 411; 10 mg–Pfizer 412.

5 mg Bottles: 100's (NDC 0049-4110-66)
(NDC 59012-411-66);
500's (NDC 0049-4110-73) (NDC 59012-411-73);
UNIT DOSE 100's (NDC 0049-4110-41) (NDC 59012-411-41).

10 mg Bottles: 100's (NDC 0049-4120-66)
(NDC 59012-412-66);
500's (NDC 0049-4120-73) (NDC 59012-412-73);
UNIT DOSE 100's (NDC 0049-4120-41) (NDC 59012-412-41).

RECOMMENDED STORAGE: Store below 86°F (30°C).

CAUTION: Federal law prohibits dispensing without prescription.

September 1993 69-4227-00-9

Shown in Product Identification Guide, page 328

GLUCOTROL XL® ℞

(glipizide)

Extended Release Tablets

For Oral Use

DESCRIPTION

Glipizide is an oral blood-glucose-lowering drug of the sulfonylurea class.

The Chemical Abstracts name of glipizide is 1-cyclohexyl-3- [[p- [2 -(5-methylpyrazinecarboxamido)ethyl]phenyl]sulfonyl]urea. The molecular formula is $C_{21}H_{27}N_5O_4S$; the molecular weight is 445.55; the structural formula is shown below:

[See structure at top of next column.]

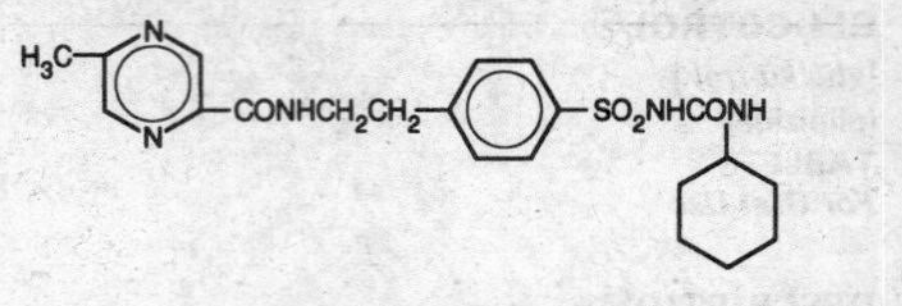

Glipizide is a whitish, odorless powder with a pKa of 5.9. It is insoluble in water and alcohols, but soluble in 0.1 *N* NaOH; it is freely soluble in dimethylformamide. GLUCOTROL XL® is a registered trademark for glipizide GITS. Glipizide GITS (Gastrointestinal Therapeutic System) is formulated as a once-a-day controlled release tablet for oral use and is designed to deliver 5 or 10 mg of glipizide.

Inert ingredients in the formulations are: polyethylene oxide, hydroxypropyl methylcellulose, magnesium stearate, sodium chloride, red ferric oxide, cellulose acetate, polyethylene glycol, opadry white (YS-2-7063) and black ink (S-1-8106).

System Components and Performance

GLUCOTROL XL Extended Release Tablet is similar in appearance to a conventional tablet. It consists, however, of an osmotically active drug core surrounded by a semipermeable membrane. The core itself is divided into two layers: an "active" layer containing the drug, and a "push" layer containing pharmacologically inert (but osmotically active) components. The membrane surrounding the tablet is permeable to water but not to drug or osmotic excipients. As water from the gastrointestinal tract enters the tablet, pressure increases in the osmotic layer and "pushes" against the drug layer, resulting in the release of drug through a small, laser-drilled orifice in the membrane on the drug side of the tablet. The GLUCOTROL XL Extended Release Tablet is designed to provide a controlled rate of delivery of glipizide into the gastrointestinal lumen which is independent of pH or gastrointestinal motility. The function of the GLUCOTROL XL Extended Release Tablet depends upon the existence of an osmotic gradient between the contents of the bi-layer core and fluid in the GI tract. Drug delivery is essentially constant as long as the osmotic gradient remains constant, and then gradually falls to zero. The biologically inert components of the tablet remain intact during GI transit and are eliminated in the feces as an insoluble shell.

CLINICAL PHARMACOLOGY

Mechanism of Action: Glipizide appears to lower blood glucose acutely by stimulating the release of insulin from the pancreas, an effect dependent upon functioning beta cells in the pancreatic islets. Extrapancreatic effects also may play a part in the mechanism of action of oral sulfonylurea hypoglycemic drugs. Two extrapancreatic effects shown to be important in the action of glipizide are an increase in insulin sensitivity and a decrease in hepatic glucose production. However, the mechanism by which glipizide lowers blood glucose during long-term administration has not been clearly established. Stimulation of insulin secretion by glipizide in response to a meal is of major importance. The insulinotropic response to a meal is enhanced with GLUCOTROL XL administration in diabetic patients. The postprandial insulin and C-peptide responses continue to be enhanced after at least 6 months of treatment. In 2 randomized, double-blind, dose-response studies comprising a total of 347 patients, there was no significant increase in fasting insulin in all GLUCOTROL XL-treated patients combined compared to placebo, although minor elevations were observed at some doses. There was no increase in fasting insulin over the long-term.

Some patients fail to respond initially, or gradually lose their responsiveness to sulfonylurea drugs, including glipizide. Alternatively, glipizide may be effective in some patients who have not responded or have ceased to respond to other sulfonylureas.

Effects on Blood Glucose

The effectiveness of GLUCOTROL XL Extended Release Tablets in NIDDM at doses from 5-60 mg once daily has been evaluated in 4 therapeutic clinical trials each with long-term open extensions involving a total of 598 patients. Once daily administration of 5, 10 and 20 mg produced statistically significant reductions from placebo in hemoglobin A_{1C}, fasting plasma glucose and postprandial glucose in mild to severe NIDDM patients. In a pooled analysis of the patients treated with 5 mg and 20 mg, the relationship between dose and GLUCOTROL XL's effect of reducing hemoglobin A_{1C} was not established. However, in the case of fasting plasma glucose patients treated with 20 mg had a statistically significant reduction of fasting plasma glucose compared to the 5 mg-treated group.

The reductions in hemoglobin A_{1C} and fasting plasma glucose were similar in younger and older patients. Efficacy of GLUCOTROL XL was not affected by gender, race or weight (as assessed by body mass index). In long term extension trials, efficacy of GLUCOTROL XL was maintained in 81% of patients for up to 12 months.

In an open, two-way crossover study 132 patients were randomly assigned to either GLUCOTROL XL or

Glucotrol® for 8 weeks and then crossed over to the other drug for an additional 8 weeks. GLUCOTROL XL administration resulted in significantly lower fasting plasma glucose levels and equivalent hemoglobin A_{1C} levels, as compared to Glucotrol.

Other Effects: It has been shown that GLUCOTROL XL therapy is effective in controlling blood glucose without deleterious changes in the plasma lipoprotein profiles of patients treated for NIDDM.

In a placebo-controlled, crossover study in normal volunteers, glipizide had no anti-diuretic activity, and, in fact, led to a slight increase in free water clearance.

Pharmacokinetics and Metabolism: Glipizide is rapidly and completely absorbed following oral administration in an immediate release dosage form. The absolute bioavailability of glipizide was 100% after single oral doses in patients with NIDDM. Beginning 2 to 3 hours after administration of GLUCOTROL XL Extended Release Tablets, plasma drug concentrations gradually rise reaching maximum concentrations within 6 to 12 hours after dosing. With subsequent once daily dosing of GLUCOTROL XL Extended Release Tablets, effective plasma glipizide concentrations are maintained throughout the 24 hour dosing interval with less peak to trough fluctuation than that observed with twice daily dosing of immediate release glipizide. The mean relative bioavailability of glipizide in 21 males with NIDDM after administration of 20 mg GLUCOTROL XL Extended Release Tablets, compared to immediate release Glucotrol (10 mg given twice daily), was 90% at steady state. Steady state plasma concentrations were achieved by at least the fifth day of dosing with GLUCOTROL XL Extended Release Tablets in 21 males with NIDDM and patients younger than 65 years. Approximately 1 to 2 days longer were required to reach steady state in 24 elderly ($\geq$65 years) males and females with NIDDM. No accumulation of drug was observed in patients with NIDDM during chronic dosing with GLUCOTROL XL Extended Release Tablets. Administration of GLUCOTROL XL with food has no effect on the 2 to 3 hour lag time in drug absorption. In a single dose, food effect study in 21 healthy male subjects, the administration of GLUCOTROL XL immediately before a high fat breakfast resulted in a 40% increase in the glipizide mean Cmax value, which was significant, but the effect on the AUC was not significant. There was no change in glucose response between the fed and fasting state. Markedly reduced GI retention times of the GLUCOTROL XL tablets over prolonged periods (e.g., short bowel syndrome) may influence the pharmacokinetic profile of the drug and potentially result in lower plasma concentrations. In a multiple dose study in 26 males with NIDDM, the pharmacokinetics of glipizide were linear over the dose range of 5 to 60 mg of GLUCOTROL XL in that the plasma drug concentrations increased proportionately with dose. In a single dose study in 24 healthy subjects, four 5 mg, two 10 mg, and one 20 mg GLUCOTROL XL Extended Release Tablets were bioequivalent.

Glipizide is eliminated primarily by hepatic biotransformation: less than 10% of a dose is excreted as unchanged drug in urine and feces; approximately 90% of a dose is excreted as biotransformation products in urine (80%) and feces (10%). The major metabolites of glipizide are products of aromatic hydroxylation and have no hypoglycemic activity. A minor metabolite which accounts for less than 2% of a dose, an acetylamino-ethyl benzine derivative, is reported to have $^1/_{10}$ to $^1/_3$ as much hypoglycemic activity as the parent compound. The mean total body clearance of glipizide was approximately 3 liters per hour after single intravenous doses in patients with NIDDM. The mean apparent volume of distribution was approximately 10 liters. Glipizide is 98-99% bound to serum proteins, primarily to albumin. The mean terminal elimination half-life of glipizide ranged from 2 to 5 hours after single or multiple doses in patients with NIDDM. There were no significant differences in the pharmacokinetics of glipizide after single dose administration to older diabetic subjects compared to younger healthy subjects. There is only limited information regarding the effects of renal impairment on the disposition of glipizide, and no information regarding the effects of hepatic disease. However, since glipizide is highly protein bound and hepatic biotransformation is the predominant route of elimination, the pharmacokinetics and/or pharmacodynamics of glipizide may be altered in patients with renal or hepatic impairment.

In mice no glipizide or metabolites were detectable autoradiographically in the brain or spinal cord of males or females, nor in the fetuses of pregnant females. In another study, however, very small amounts of radioactivity were detected in the fetuses of rats given labelled drug.

INDICATIONS AND USAGE

GLUCOTROL XL is indicated as an adjunct to diet for the control of hyperglycemia and its associated symptomatology in patients with non-insulin-dependent diabetes mellitus (NIDDM; type II), formerly known as maturity-onset diabetes, after an adequate trial of dietary therapy has proved unsatisfactory. GLUCOTROL XL is indicated when diet alone has been unsuccessful in correcting hyperglycemia, but even after the introduction of the drug in the patient's regimen, dietary measures should continue to be considered as important. In 12 week, well-controlled studies there was a maximal average net reduction in hemoglobin A_{1C} of 1.7% in absolute units between placebo-treated and GLUCOTROL XL-treated patients.

In initiating treatment for non-insulin-dependent diabetes, diet should be emphasized as the primary form of treatment. Caloric restriction and weight loss are essential in the obese diabetic patient. Proper dietary management alone may be effective in controlling blood glucose and symptoms of hyperglycemia. The importance of regular physical activity should also be stressed, cardiovascular risk factors should be identified, and corrective measures taken where possible.

If this treatment program fails to reduce symptoms and/or blood glucose, the use of an oral sulfonylurea should be considered. If additional reduction of symptoms and/or blood glucose is required, the addition of insulin to the treatment regimen should be considered. Use of GLUCOTROL XL must be viewed by both the physician and patient as a treatment in addition to diet, and not as a substitute for diet or as a convenient mechanism for avoiding dietary restraint. Furthermore, loss of blood glucose control on diet alone also may be transient, thus requiring only short-term administration of glipizide.

During maintenance programs, GLUCOTROL XL should be discontinued if satisfactory lowering of blood glucose is no longer achieved. Judgments should be based on regular clinical and laboratory evaluations. Hemoglobin A_{1C} levels may be useful.

In considering the use of GLUCOTROL XL in asymptomatic patients, it should be recognized that controlling blood glucose in non-insulin-dependent diabetes has not been definitely established to be effective in preventing the long-term cardiovascular or neural complications of diabetes. However, in insulin-dependent diabetes mellitus controlling blood glucose has been effective in slowing the progression of diabetic retinopathy, nephropathy, and neuropathy.

CONTRAINDICATIONS

Glipizide is contraindicated in patients with:

1. Known hypersensitivity to the drug.
2. Diabetic ketoacidosis, with or without coma. This condition should be treated with insulin.

WARNINGS

SPECIAL WARNING ON INCREASED RISK OF CARDIOVASCULAR MORTALITY: The administration of oral hypoglycemic drugs has been reported to be associated with increased cardiovascular mortality as compared to treatment with diet alone or diet plus insulin. This warning is based on the study conducted by the University Group Diabetes Program (UGDP), a long-term prospective clinical trial designed to evaluate the effectiveness of glucose-lowering drugs in preventing or delaying vascular complications in patients with non-insulin-dependent diabetes. The study involved 823 patients who were randomly assigned to one of four treatment groups (*Diabetes*, 19, SUPP. 2: 747-830, 1970).

UGDP reported that patients treated for 5 to 8 years with diet plus a fixed dose of tolbutamide (1.5 grams per day) had a rate of cardiovascular mortality approximately $2^1/_2$ times that of patients treated with diet alone. A significant increase in total mortality was not observed, but the use of tolbutamide was discontinued based on the increase in cardiovascular mortality, thus limiting the opportunity for the study to show an increase in overall mortality. Despite controversy regarding the interpretation of these results, the findings of the UGDP study provide an adequate basis for this warning. The patient should be informed of the potential risks and advantages of glipizide and of alternative modes of therapy.

Although only one drug in the sulfonylurea class (tolbutamide) was included in this study, it is prudent from a safety standpoint to consider that this warning may also apply to other oral hypoglycemic drugs in this class, in view of their close similarities in mode of action and chemical structure.

As with any other non-deformable material, caution should be used when administering GLUCOTROL XL Extended Release Tablets in patients with preexisting severe gastrointestinal narrowing (pathologic or iatrogenic). There have been rare reports of obstructive symptoms in patients with known strictures in association with the ingestion of another drug in this non-deformable sustained release formulation.

PRECAUTIONS

General

Renal and Hepatic Disease: The pharmacokinetics and/or pharmacodynamics of glipizide may be affected in patients with impaired renal or hepatic function. If hypoglycemia should occur in such patients, it may be prolonged and appropriate management should be instituted.

GI Disease: Markedly reduced GI retention times of the GLUCOTROL XL Extended Release Tablets may influence the pharmacokinetic profile and hence the clinical efficacy of the drug.

Hypoglycemia: All sulfonylurea drugs are capable of producing severe hypoglycemia. Proper patient selection, dosage, and instructions are important to avoid hypoglycemic episodes. Renal or hepatic insufficiency may affect the disposition of glipizide and the latter may also diminish gluconeogenic capacity, both of which increase the risk of serious hypoglycemic reactions. Elderly, debilitated or malnourished patients, and those with adrenal or pituitary insufficiency are particularly susceptible to the hypoglycemic action of glucose-lowering drugs. Hypoglycemia may be difficult to recognize in the elderly, and in people who are taking beta-adrenergic blocking drugs. Hypoglycemia is more likely to occur when caloric intake is deficient, after severe or prolonged exercise, when alcohol is ingested, or when more than one glucose-lowering drug is used.

Loss of Control of Blood Glucose: When a patient stabilized on any diabetic regimen is exposed to stress such as fever, trauma, infection, or surgery, a loss of control may occur. At such times, it may be necessary to discontinue glipizide and administer insulin.

The effectiveness of any oral hypoglycemic drug, including glipizide, in lowering blood glucose to a desired level decreases in many patients over a period of time, which may be due to progression of the severity of the diabetes or to diminished responsiveness to the drug. This phenomenon is known as secondary failure, to distinguish it from primary failure in which the drug is ineffective in an individual patient when first given. Adequate adjustment of dose and adherence to diet should be assessed before classifying a patient as a secondary failure.

Laboratory Tests: Blood and urine glucose should be monitored periodically. Measurement of hemoglobin A_{1C} may be useful.

Information for Patients: Patients should be informed that GLUCOTROL XL Extended Release Tablets should be swallowed whole. Patients should not chew, divide or crush tablets. Patients should not be concerned if they occasionally notice in their stool something that looks like a tablet. In the GLUCOTROL XL Extended Release Tablet, the medication is contained within a nonabsorbable shell that has been specially designed to slowly release the drug so the body can absorb it. When this process is completed, the empty tablet is eliminated from the body.

Patients should be informed of the potential risks and advantages of GLUCOTROL XL and of alternative modes of therapy. They should also be informed about the importance of adhering to dietary instructions, of a regular exercise program, and of regular testing of urine and/or blood glucose.

The risks of hypoglycemia, its symptoms and treatment, and conditions that predispose to its development should be explained to patients and responsible family members. Primary and secondary failure also should be explained.

Drug Interactions: The hypoglycemic action of sulfonylureas may be potentiated by certain drugs including nonsteroidal anti-inflammatory agents and other drugs that are highly protein bound, salicylates, sulfonamides, chloramphenicol, probenecid, coumarins, monoamine oxidase inhibitors, and beta-adrenergic blocking agents. When such drugs are administered to a patient receiving glipizide, the patient should be observed closely for hypoglycemia. When such drugs are withdrawn from a patient receiving glipizide, the patient should be observed closely for loss of control. *In vitro* binding studies with human serum proteins indicate that glipizide binds differently than tolbutamide and does not interact with salicylate or dicumarol. However, caution must be exercised in extrapolating these findings to the clinical situation and in the use of glipizide with these drugs.

Certain drugs tend to produce hyperglycemia and may lead to loss of control. These drugs include the thiazides and other diuretics, corticosteroids, phenothiazines, thyroid products, estrogens, oral contraceptives, phenytoin, nicotinic acid, sympathomimetics, calcium channel blocking drugs, and isoniazid. When such drugs are administered to a patient receiving glipizide, the patient should be closely observed for loss of control. When such drugs are withdrawn from a patient receiving glipizide, the patient should be observed closely for hypoglycemia.

A potential interaction between oral miconazole and oral hypoglycemic agents leading to severe hypoglycemia has been reported. Whether this interaction also occurs with the intravenous, topical, or vaginal preparations of miconazole is not known. The effect of concomitant administration of Diflucan® (fluconazole) and Glucotrol has been demonstrated in a placebo-controlled crossover study in normal volunteers. All subjects received Glucotrol alone and following treatment with 100 mg of Diflucan® as a single daily oral dose for 7 days. The mean percentage increase in the Glucotrol AUC after fluconazole administration was 56.9% (range: 35 to 81%).

Carcinogenesis, Mutagenesis, Impairment of Fertility: A twenty month study in rats and an eighteen month study in mice at doses up to 75 times the maximum human dose revealed no evidence of drug-related carcinogenicity. Bacterial

Continued on next page

Pfizer Inc—Cont.

and *in vivo* mutagenicity tests were uniformly negative. Studies in rats of both sexes at doses up to 75 times the human dose showed no effects on fertility.

Pregnancy: Pregnancy Category C: Glipizide was found to be mildly fetotoxic in rat reproductive studies at all dose levels (5–50 mg/kg). This fetotoxicity has been similarly noted with other sulfonylureas, such as tolbutamide and tolazamide. The effect is perinatal and believed to be directly related to the pharmacologic (hypoglycemic) action of glipizide. In studies in rats and rabbits no teratogenic effects were found. There are no adequate and well controlled studies in pregnant women. Glipizide should be used during pregnancy only if the potential benefit justifies the potential risk to the fetus.

Because recent information suggests that abnormal blood glucose levels during pregnancy are associated with a higher incidence of congenital abnormalities, many experts recommend that insulin be used during pregnancy to maintain blood glucose levels as close to normal as possible.

Nonteratogenic Effects: Prolonged severe hypoglycemia (4 to 10 days) has been reported in neonates born to mothers who were receiving a sulfonylurea drug at the time of delivery. This has been reported more frequently with the use of agents with prolonged half-lives. If glipizide is used during pregnancy, it should be discontinued at least one month before the expected delivery date.

Nursing Mothers: Although is is not known whether glipizide is excreted in human milk, some sulfonylurea drugs are known to be excreted in human milk. Because the potential for hypoglycemia in nursing infants may exist, a decision should be made whether to discontinue nursing or to discontinue the drug, taking into account the importance of the drug to the mother. If the drug is discontinued and if diet alone is inadequate for controlling blood glucose, insulin therapy should be considered.

Pediatric Use: Safety and effectiveness in children have not been established.

Geriatric Use: Of the total number of patients in clinical studies of GLUCOTROL XL, 33 percent were 65 and over. No overall differences in effectiveness or safety were observed between these patients and younger patients, but greater sensitivity of some individuals cannot be ruled out. Approximately 1–2 days longer were required to reach steady state in the elderly. (See CLINICAL PHARMACOLOGY and DOSAGE AND ADMINISTRATION).

ADVERSE REACTIONS

In U.S. controlled studies the frequency of serious adverse experiences reported was very low and causal relationship has not been established.

The 580 patients from 31 to 87 years of age who received GLUCOTROL XL Extended Release Tablets in doses from 5 mg to 60 mg in both controlled and open trials were included in the evaluation of adverse experiences. All adverse experiences reported were tabulated independently of their possible causal relation to medication.

Hypoglycemia: See PRECAUTIONS and OVERDOSAGE sections.

Only 3.4% of patients receiving GLUCOTROL XL Extended Release Tablets had hypoglycemia documented by a blood glucose measurement <60 mg/dL and/or symptoms believed to be associated with hypoglycemia. In a comparative efficacy study of GLUCOTROL XL and Glucotrol, hypoglycemia occurred rarely with an incidence of less than 1% with both drugs.

In double-blind, placebo-controlled studies the adverse experiences reported with an incidence of 3% or more in GLUCOTROL XL-treated patients include:

Adverse Effect	GLUCOTROL XL (%) (N=278)	Placebo (%) (N=69)
Asthenia	10.1	13.0
Headache	8.6	8.7
Dizziness	6.8	5.8
Nervousness	3.6	2.9
Tremor	3.6	0.0
Diarrhea	5.4	0.0
Flatulence	3.2	1.4

The following adverse experiences occurred with an incidence of less than 3% in GLUCOTROL XL-treated patients:

Body as a whole—pain
Nervous system—insomnia, paresthesia, anxiety, depression and hypesthesia
Gastrointestinal—nausea, dyspepsia, constipation and vomiting
Metabolic—hypoglycemia
Musculoskeletal—arthralgia, leg cramps and myalgia
Cardiovascular—syncope
Skin—sweating and pruritus
Respiratory—rhinitis
Special senses—blurred vision
Urogenital—polyuria

Other adverse experiences occurred with an incidence of less than 1% in GLUCOTROL XL-treated patients:

Body as a whole—chills
Nervous system—hypertonia, confusion, vertigo, somnolence, gait abnormality and decreased libido
Gastrointestinal—anorexia and trace blood in stool
Metabolic—thirst and edema
Cardiovascular—arrhythmia, migraine, flushing and hypertension
Skin—rash and urticaria
Respiratory—pharyngitis and dyspnea
Special senses—pain in the eye, conjunctivitis and retinal hemorrhage
Urogenital—dysuria

Although these adverse experiences occurred in patients treated with GLUCOTROL XL, a causal relationship to the medication has not been established in all cases.

There have been rare reports of gastrointestinal irritation and gastrointestinal bleeding with use of another drug in this non-deformable sustained release formulation, although causal relationship to the drug is uncertain.

The following are adverse experiences reported with immediate release glipizide and other sulfonylureas, but have not been observed with GLUCOTROL XL:

Hematologic: Leukopenia, agranulocytosis, thrombocytopenia, hemolytic anemia, aplastic anemia, and pancytopenia have been reported with sulfonylureas.

Metabolic: Hepatic porphyria and disulfiram-like reactions have been reported with sulfonylureas. In the mouse, glipizide pretreatment did not cause an accumulation of acetaldehyde after ethanol administration. Clinical experience to date has shown that glipizide has an extremely low incidence of disulfiram-like alcohol reactions.

Endocrine Reactions: Cases of hyponatremia and the syndrome of inappropriate antidiuretic hormone (SIADH) secretion have been reported with glipizide and other sulfonylureas.

Laboratory Tests: The pattern of laboratory test abnormalities observed with glipizide was similar to that for other sulfonylureas. Occasional mild to moderate elevations of SGOT, LDH, alkaline phosphatase, BUN and creatinine were noted. One case of jaundice was reported. The relationship of these abnormalities to glipizide is uncertain, and they have rarely been associated with clinical symptoms.

OVERDOSAGE

There is no well-documented experience with GLUCOTROL XL overdosage in humans. There have been no known suicide attempts associated with purposeful overdosing with GLUCOTROL XL. In nonclinical studies the acute oral toxicity of glipizide was extremely low in all species tested (LD_{50} greater than 4 g/kg). Overdosage of sulfonylureas including glipizide can produce hypoglycemia. Mild hypoglycemic symptoms without loss of consciousness or neurologic findings should be treated aggressively with oral glucose and adjustments in drug dosage and/or meal patterns. Close monitoring should continue until the physician is assured that the patient is out of danger. Severe hypoglycemic reactions with coma, seizure, or other neurological impairment occur infrequently, but constitute medical emergencies requiring immediate hospitalization. If hypoglycemic coma is diagnosed or suspected, the patient should be given rapid intravenous injection of concentrated (50%) glucose solution. This should be followed by a continuous infusion of a more dilute (10%) glucose solution at a rate that will maintain the blood glucose at a level above 100 mg/dL. Patients should be closely monitored for a minimum of 24 to 48 hours since hypoglycemia may recur after apparent clinical recovery. Clearance of glipizide from plasma may be prolonged in persons with liver disease. Because of the extensive protein binding of glipizide, dialysis is unlikely to be of benefit.

DOSAGE AND ADMINISTRATION

There is no fixed dosage regimen for the management of diabetes mellitus with GLUCOTROL XL Extended Release Tablet or any other hypoglycemic agent. Glycemic control should be monitored with hemoglobin A_{1C} and/or blood glucose levels to determine the minimum effective dose for the patient; to detect primary failure, i.e., inadequate lowering of blood glucose at the maximum recommended dose of medication; and to detect secondary failure, i.e., loss of an adequate blood-glucose-lowering response after an initial period of effectiveness. Home blood glucose monitoring may also provide useful information to the patient and physician. Short-term administration of GLUCOTROL XL Extended Release Tablet may be sufficient during periods of transient loss of control in patients usually controlled on diet.

In general, GLUCOTROL XL should be given with breakfast.

Recommended Dosing: The recommended starting dose of GLUCOTROL XL is 5 mg per day, given with breakfast. The recommended dose for geriatric patients is also 5 mg per day. Dosage adjustment should be based on laboratory measures of glycemic control. While fasting blood glucose levels generally reach steady state following initiation or change in GLUCOTROL XL dosage, a single fasting glucose determination may not accurately reflect the response to therapy. In most cases, hemoglobin A_{1C} level measured at three month intervals is the preferred means of monitoring response to therapy.

Hemoglobin A_{1C} should be measured as GLUCOTROL XL therapy is initiated at the 5 mg dose and repeated approximately three months later. If the result of this test suggests that glycemic control over the preceding three months was inadequate, the GLUCOTROL XL dose may be increased to 10 mg. Subsequent dosage adjustments should be made on the basis of hemoglobin A_{1C} levels measured at three month intervals. If no improvement is seen after three months of therapy with a higher dose, the previous dose should be resumed. Decisions which utilize fasting blood glucose to adjust GLUCOTROL XL therapy should be based on at least two or more similar, consecutive values obtained seven days or more after the previous dose adjustment.

Most patients will be controlled with 5 mg or 10 mg taken once daily. However, some patients may require up to the maximum recommended daily dose of 20 mg. While the glycemic control of selected patients may improve with doses which exceed 10 mg, clinical studies conducted to date have not demonstrated an additional group average reduction of hemoglobin A_{1C} beyond what was achieved with the 10 mg dose.

Based on the results of a randomized crossover study patients receiving immediate release glipizide may be switched safely to GLUCOTROL XL Extended Tablets once-a-day at the nearest equivalent total daily dose. Patients receiving immediate release Glucotrol also may be titrated to the appropriate dose of GLUCOTROL XL starting with 5 mg once daily. The decision to switch to the nearest equivalent dose or to titrate should be based on clinical judgement.

In elderly patients, debilitated or malnourished patients, and patients with impaired renal or hepatic function, the initial and maintenance dosing should be conservative to avoid hypoglycemic reactions (see PRECAUTIONS section).

Patients Receiving Insulin: As with other sulfonylurea-class hypoglycemics, many stable non-insulin-dependent diabetic patients receiving insulin may be transferred safely to treatment with GLUCOTROL XL Extended Release Tablets. When transferring patients from insulin to GLUCOTROL XL, the following general guidelines should be considered:

For patients whose daily insulin requirement is 20 units or less, insulin may be discontinued and GLUCOTROL XL therapy may begin at usual dosages. Several days should elapse between titration steps.

For patients whose daily insulin requirement is greater than 20 units, the insulin dose should be reduced by 50% and GLUCOTROL XL therapy may begin at usual dosages. Subsequent reductions in insulin dosage should depend on individual patient response. Several days should elapse between titration steps.

During the insulin withdrawal period, the patient should test urine samples for sugar and ketone bodies at least three times daily. Patients should be instructed to contact the prescriber immediately if these tests are abnormal. In some cases, especially when the patient has been receiving greater than 40 units of insulin daily, it may be advisable to consider hospitalization during the transition period.

Patients Receiving Other Oral Hypoglycemic Agents: As with other sulfonylurea-class hypoglycemics, no transition period is necessary when transferring patients to GLUCOTROL XL Extended Release Tablets. Patients should be observed carefully (1–2 weeks) for hypoglycemia when being transferred from longer half-life sulfonylureas (e.g., chlorpropamide) to GLUCOTROL XL due to potential overlapping of drug effect.

HOW SUPPLIED

GLUCOTROL XL® Extended Release Tablets are supplied as 5 mg and 10 mg round, biconvex, tablets and imprinted with black ink with color-coating as follows:

Bottles of 100:
5 mg, White tablets, (NDC 0049-1550-66)
10 mg, White tablets, (NDC 0049-1560-66)
Bottles of 500:
5 mg, White tablets, (NDC 0049-1550-73)
10 mg, White tablets, (NDC 0049-1560-73)

Recommended Storage: The tablets should be protected from moisture and humidity and stored at controlled room temperature, 59° to 86°F (15° to 30°C).

CAUTION: Federal law prohibits dispensing without prescription.

65-4952-00-2　　　　　　　　　　　Issued February 1995

Shown in Product Identification Guide, page 328

MARAX® ℞

[*mă´rax*]

(ephedrine sulfate, theophylline, hydroxyzine HCl)
TABLETS AND DF SYRUP

CONTENTS

	Each Tablet Contains:	Each Teaspoon (5 ml) Syrup Contains:
Ephedrine Sulfate	25 mg	6.25 mg
Theophylline	130 mg	32.50 mg
Atarax® (hydroxyzine HCl)	10 mg	2.5 mg
Alcohol (Ethyl Alcohol)		5% v/v.

Inert ingredients for tablets are: alginic acid; magnesium stearate; precipitated calcium carbonate; sodium lauryl sulfate.
Inert ingredients for syrup are: alcohol; cherry flavor; hydrochloric acid; sodium benzoate; special flavor compound; sucrose; water.

ACTIONS

The action of ephedrine as a vasoconstrictor is well known. It is therefore of significant benefit in symptomatic relief of the congestion occurring in bronchial asthma. As a bronchodilator, it has a slower onset but longer duration of action than does epinephrine, which, in contrast to ephedrine, is not effective upon oral administration.
The diverse actions of theophylline—bronchospasmolytic, cardiovascular, and diuretic—are well established, and make it a particularly useful drug in the treatment of bronchial asthma, both in the acute attack and in the prophylactic therapy of the disease.
Atarax (hydroxyzine HCl) modifies the central stimulatory action of ephedrine preventing excessive excitation in patients on Marax therapy.
In animal studies Atarax has demonstrated antiserotonin activity and antispasmodic potency of a nonspecific nature.
Marax-DF Syrup produces an expectorant action wherein the tenacity of the sputum is decreased and the ease of expectoration is increased.

INDICATIONS

Based on a review of this drug by the National Academy of Sciences-National Research Council and/or other information, FDA has classified the indications as follows:
"Possibly" Effective: For controlling bronchospastic disorders.
Final classification of the less than effective indication requires further investigation.

CONTRAINDICATIONS

Because of the ephedrine, Marax is contraindicated in cardiovascular disease, hyperthyroidism, and hypertension. This drug is contraindicated in individuals who have shown hypersensitivity to the drug or its components.
Hydroxyzine, when administered to the pregnant mouse, rat, and rabbit induced fetal abnormalities in the rat at doses substantially above the human therapeutic range. Clinical data in human beings are inadequate to establish safety in early pregnancy. Until such data are available, hydroxyzine is contraindicated in early pregnancy.

PRECAUTIONS

Because of the ephedrine component this drug should be used with caution in elderly males or those with known prostatic hypertrophy.
The potentiating action of hydroxyzine, although mild, must be taken into consideration when the drug is used in conjunction with central nervous system depressants; and when other central nervous system depressants are administered concomitantly with hydroxyzine their dosage should be reduced. Patients should be cautioned that hydroxyzine can increase the effect of alcohol.
Patients should be warned—because of the hydroxyzine component—of the possibility of drowsiness occurring and cautioned against driving a car or operating dangerous machinery while taking this drug.

ADVERSE REACTIONS

With large doses of ephedrine, excitation, tremulousness, insomnia, nervousness, palpitation, tachycardia, precordial pain, cardiac arrhythmias, vertigo, dryness of the nose and throat, headache, sweating, and warmth may occur. Because ephedrine is a sympathomimetic agent some patients may develop vesical sphincter spasm and resultant urinary hesitation, and occasionally acute urinary retention. This should be borne in mind when administering preparations containing ephedrine to elderly males or those with known prostatic hypertrophy. At the recommended dose for Marax, a side effect occasionally reported is palpitation, and this can be controlled with dosage adjustment, additional amounts of concurrently administered Atarax (hydroxyzine HCl), or discontinuation of the medication. When ephedrine is given three or more times daily patients may develop tolerance after several weeks of therapy.
Theophylline when given on an empty stomach frequently causes gastric irritation accompanied by upper abdominal discomfort, nausea, and vomiting. Administration of the medication after meals will serve to minimize this side effect. Theophylline may cause diuresis and cardiac stimulation.
The amount of Atarax present in Marax has not resulted in disturbing side effects. When used alone specifically as a tranquilizer in the normal dosage range (25 to 50 mg three or four times a day), side effects are infrequent; even at these higher doses, no serious side effects have been reported and confirmed to date. Those which do occasionally occur when Atarax is used alone are drowsiness, xerostomia and, at extremely high doses, involuntary motor activity, unsteadiness of gait, neuromuscular weakness, all of which may be controlled by reduction of the dosage or discontinuation of the medication.
With the relatively low dose of Atarax in Marax, these effects are not likely to occur. In addition, the ataractic action of Atarax may modify the cardiac stimulatory action of ephedrine, and concurrently, increasing the amount of Atarax may control or abolish this undesirable effect of ephedrine.

DOSAGE AND ADMINISTRATION

The dosage of Marax should be adjusted according to the severity of complaints, and the patient's individual toleration.
Tablets: In general, an adult dose of 1 tablet, 2 to 4 times daily, should be sufficient. Some patients are controlled adequately with 1/2 to 1 tablet at bedtime. The time interval between doses should not be shorter than four hours. The dosage for children over 5 years of age and for adults who are sensitive to ephedrine, is one-half the usual adult dose. Clinical experience to date has been confined to ages above 5 years.
Syrup: The dose for children over 5 years of age is 1 teaspoon (5 ml), 3 to 4 times daily. Dosage for children 2 to 5 years of age is 1/2 to 1 teaspoon (2.5-5 ml), 3 to 4 times daily. Not recommended for children under 2 years of age.

HOW SUPPLIED

Marax Tablets are available as scored, dye free, m-shaped tablets in bottles of 100 (NDC 0049-2540-66) and 500 (NDC 0049-2540-73).
Marax-DF Syrup is available in pints (NDC 0049-2550-93) and gallons (NDC 0049-2550-54) as a colorless syrup, free of all coal tar dyes, and should be dispensed in tight, light-resistant containers (USP).

69-0928-32-7
66-2265-00-4

Shown in Product Identification Guide, page 328

MINIPRESS® CAPSULES ℞

[*mĭn´ē-prĕs*]

(prazosin hydrochloride)
For Oral Use

DESCRIPTION

MINIPRESS® (prazosin hydrochloride), a quinazoline derivative, is the first of a new chemical class of antihypertensives. It is the hydrochloride salt of 1-(4-amino-6,7-dimethoxy-2-quinazolinyl)-4-(2-furoyl) piperazine and its structural formula is:

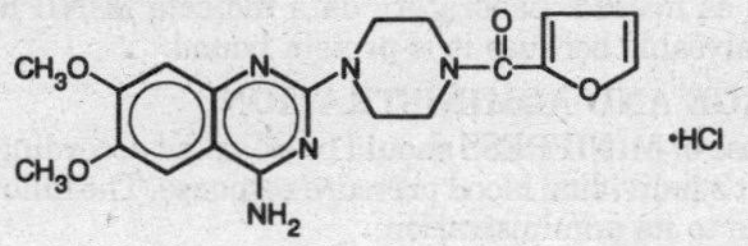

Molecular formula $C_{19}H_{21}N_5O_4 \cdot HCl$

It is a white, crystalline substance, slightly soluble in water and isotonic saline, and has a molecular weight of 419.87. Each 1 mg capsule of MINIPRESS for oral use contains drug equivalent to 1 mg free base.
Inert ingredients in the formulations are: hard gelatin capsules (which may contain Blue 1, Red 3, Red 28, Red 40, and other inert ingredients); magnesium stearate; sodium lauryl sulfate; starch; sucrose.

CLINICAL PHARMACOLOGY

The exact mechanism of the hypotensive action of prazosin is unknown. Prazosin causes a decrease in total peripheral resistance and was originally thought to have a direct relaxant action on vascular smooth muscle. Recent animal studies, however, have suggested that the vasodilator effect of prazosin is also related to blockade of postsynaptic *alpha*-adrenoceptors. The results of dog forelimb experiments demonstrate that the peripheral vasodilator effect of prazosin is confined mainly to the level of the resistance vessels (arterioles). Unlike conventional *alpha*-blockers, the antihypertensive action of prazosin is usually not accompanied by a reflex tachycardia. Tolerance has not been observed to develop in long term therapy.
Hemodynamic studies have been carried out in man following acute single dose administration and during the course of long term maintenance therapy. The results confirm that the therapeutic effect is a fall in blood pressure unaccompanied by a clinically significant change in cardiac output, heart rate, renal blood flow and glomerular filtration rate. There is no measurable negative chronotropic effect.
In clinical studies to date, MINIPRESS (prazosin hydrochloride) has not increased plasma renin activity.
In man, blood pressure is lowered in both the supine and standing positions. This effect is most pronounced on the diastolic blood pressure.
Following oral administration, human plasma concentrations reach a peak at about three hours with a plasma half-life of two to three hours. The drug is highly bound to plasma protein. Bioavailability studies have demonstrated that the total absorption relative to the drug in a 20% alcoholic solution is 90%, resulting in peak levels approximately 65% of that of the drug in solution. Animal studies indicate that MINIPRESS (prazosin hydrochloride) is extensively metabolized, primarily by demethylation and conjugation, and excreted mainly via bile and feces. Less extensive human studies suggest similar metabolism and excretion in man.
In clinical studies in which lipid profiles were followed, there were generally no adverse changes noted between pre- and post-treatment lipid levels.

INDICATIONS AND USAGE

MINIPRESS (prazosin hydrochloride) is indicated in the treatment of hypertension. It can be used alone or in combination with other antihypertensive drugs such as diuretics or beta-adrenergic blocking agents.

CONTRAINDICATIONS

None known.

WARNINGS

MINIPRESS (prazosin hydrochloride) may cause syncope with sudden loss of consciousness. In most cases this is believed to be due to an excessive postural hypotensive effect, although occasionally the syncopal episode has been preceded by a bout of severe tachycardia with heart rates of 120–160 beats per minute. Syncopal episodes have usually occurred within 30 to 90 minutes of the initial dose of the drug; occasionally they have been reported in association with rapid dosage increases or the introduction of another antihypertensive drug into the regimen of a patient taking high doses of MINIPRESS (prazosin hydrochloride). The incidence of syncopal episodes is approximately 1% in patients given an initial dose of 2 mg or greater. Clinical trials conducted during the investigational phase of this drug suggest that syncopal episodes can be minimized by limiting the initial dose of the drug to 1 mg, by subsequently increasing the dosage slowly, and by introducing any additional antihypertensive drugs into the patient's regimen with caution (see DOSAGE AND ADMINISTRATION). Hypotension may develop in patients given MINIPRESS who are also receiving a beta-blocker such as propranolol.
If syncope occurs, the patient should be placed in the recumbent position and treated supportively as necessary. This adverse effect is self-limiting and in most cases does not recur after the initial period of therapy or during subsequent dose titration.
Patients should always be started on the 1 mg capsules of MINIPRESS (prazosin hydrochloride). The 2 and 5 mg capsules are not indicated for initial therapy.
More common than loss of consciousness are the symptoms often associated with lowering of the blood pressure, namely, dizziness and lightheadedness. The patient should be cautioned about these possible adverse effects and advised what measures to take should they develop. The patient should also be cautioned to avoid situations where injury could result should syncope occur during the initiation of MINIPRESS (prazosin hydrochloride) therapy.

PRECAUTIONS

Information for Patients: Dizziness or drowsiness may occur after the first dose of this medicine. Avoid driving or performing hazardous tasks for the first 24 hours after taking this medicine or when the dose is increased. Dizziness, lightheadedness or fainting may occur, especially when rising from a lying or sitting position. Getting up slowly may help lessen the problem. These effects may also occur if you drink alcohol, stand for long periods of time, exercise, or if the weather is hot. While taking MINIPRESS, be careful in the amount of alcohol you drink. Also, use extra care during exercise or hot weather, or if standing for long periods. Check with your physician if you have any questions.

Continued on next page

Pfizer Inc—Cont.

Drug Interactions

MINIPRESS (prazosin hydrochloride) has been administered without any adverse drug interaction in limited clinical experience to date with the following: (1) cardiac glycosides—digitalis and digoxin; (2) hypoglycemics—insulin, chlorpropamide, phenformin, tolazamide, and tolbutamide; (3) tranquilizers and sedatives—chlordiazepoxide, diazepam, and phenobarbital; (4) antigout—allopurinol, colchicine, and probenecid; (5) antiarrhythmics—procainamide, propranolol (see WARNINGS however), and quinidine; and (6) analgesics, antipyretics and anti-inflammatories—propoxyphene, aspirin, indomethacin, and phenylbutazone.

Addition of a diuretic or other antihypertensive agent to MINIPRESS has been shown to cause an additive hypotensive effect. This effect can be minimized by reducing the MINIPRESS dose to 1 to 2 mg three times a day, by introducing additional antihypertensive drugs cautiously and then by retitrating MINIPRESS based on clinical response.

Drug/Laboratory Test Interactions

In a study on five patients given from 12 to 24 mg of prazosin per day for 10 to 14 days, there was an average increase of 42% in the urinary metabolite of norepinephrine and an average increase in urinary VMA of 17%. Therefore, false positive results may occur in screening tests for pheochromocytoma in patients who are being treated with prazosin. If an elevated VMA is found, prazosin should be discontinued and the patient retested after a month.

Laboratory Tests

In clinical studies in which lipid profiles were followed, there were generally no adverse changes noted between pre- and post-treatment lipid levels.

Carcinogenesis, Mutagenesis, Impairment of Fertility:

No carcinogenic potential was demonstrated in an 18 month study in rats with MINIPRESS at dose levels more than 225 times the usual maximum recommended human dose of 20 mg per day. MINIPRESS was not mutagenic in in vivo genetic toxicology studies. In a fertility and general reproductive performance study in rats, both males and females, treated with 75 mg/kg (225 times the usual maximum recommended human dose), demonstrated decreased fertility while those treated with 25 mg/kg (75 times the usual maximum recommended human dose) did not.

In chronic studies (one year or more) of MINIPRESS in rats and dogs, testicular changes consisting of atrophy and necrosis occurred at 25 mg/kg/day (75 times the usual maximum recommended human dose). No testicular changes were seen in rats or dogs at 10 mg/kg/day (30 times the usual maximum recommended human dose). In view of the testicular changes observed in animals, 105 patients on long term MINIPRESS therapy were monitored for 17-ketosteroid excretion and no changes indicating a drug effect were observed. In addition, 27 males on MINIPRESS for up to 51 months did not have changes in sperm morphology suggestive of drug effect.

Usage in Pregnancy:

Pregnancy Category C. MINIPRESS has been shown to be associated with decreased litter size at birth, 1, 4, and 21 days of age in rats when given doses more than 225 times the usual maximum recommended human dose. No evidence of drug-related external, visceral, or skeletal fetal abnormalities were observed. No drug-related external, visceral, or skeletal abnormalities were observed in fetuses of pregnant rabbits and pregnant monkeys at doses more than 225 times and 12 times the usual maximum recommended human dose respectively.

The use of prazosin and a beta-blocker for the control of severe hypertension in 44 pregnant women revealed no drug-related fetal abnormalities or adverse effects. Therapy with prazosin was continued for as long as 14 weeks.[1]

Prazosin has also been used alone or in combination with other hypotensive agents in severe hypertension of pregnancy by other investigators. No fetal or neonatal abnormalities have been reported with the use of prazosin.[2]

There are no adequate and well controlled studies which establish the safety of MINIPRESS (prazosin HCl) in pregnant women. MINIPRESS should be used during pregnancy only if the potential benefit justifies the potential risk to the mother and fetus.

Nursing Mothers:

MINIPRESS has been shown to be excreted in small amounts in human milk. Caution should be exercised when MINIPRESS is administered to a nursing woman.

Usage in Children:

Safety and effectiveness in children have not been established.

ADVERSE REACTIONS

Clinical trials were conducted on more than 900 patients. During these trials and subsequent marketing experience, the most frequent reactions associated with MINIPRESS therapy are: dizziness 10.3%, headache 7.8%, drowsiness 7.6%, lack of energy 6.9%, weakness 6.5%, palpitations 5.3%, and nausea 4.9%. In most instances side effects have disappeared with continued therapy or have been tolerated with no decrease in dose of drug.

Less frequent adverse reactions which are reported to occur in 1–4% of patients are:

Gastrointestinal: vomiting, diarrhea, constipation.

Cardiovascular: edema, orthostatic hypotension, dyspnea, syncope.

Central Nervous System: vertigo, depression, nervousness.

Dermatologic: rash.

Genitourinary: urinary frequency.

EENT: blurred vision, reddened sclera, epistaxis, dry mouth, nasal congestion.

In addition, fewer than 1% of patients have reported the following (in some instances, exact causal relationships have not been established):

Gastrointestinal: abdominal discomfort and/or pain, liver function abnormalities, pancreatitis.

Cardiovascular: tachycardia.

Central Nervous System: paresthesia, hallucinations.

Dermatologic: pruritus, alopecia, lichen planus.

Genitourinary: incontinence, impotence, priapism.

EENT: tinnitus.

Other: diaphoresis, fever, positive ANA titer, arthralgia.

Single reports of pigmentary mottling and serous retinopathy, and a few reports of cataract development or disappearance have been reported. In these instances, the exact causal relationship has not been established because the baseline observations were frequently inadequate.

In more specific slit-lamp and funduscopic studies, which included adequate baseline examinations, no drug-related abnormal ophthalmological findings have been reported. Literature reports exist associating MINIPRESS therapy with a worsening of pre-existing narcolepsy. A causal relationship is uncertain in these cases.

OVERDOSAGE

Accidental ingestion of at least 50 mg of MINIPRESS (prazosin hydrochloride) in a two year old child resulted in profound drowsiness and depressed reflexes. No decrease in blood pressure was noted. Recovery was uneventful.

Should overdosage lead to hypotension, support of the cardiovascular system is of first importance. Restoration of blood pressure and normalization of heart rate may be accomplished by keeping the patient in the supine position. If this measure is inadequate, shock should first be treated with volume expanders. If necessary, vasopressors should then be used. Renal function should be monitored and supported as needed. Laboratory data indicate MINIPRESS is not dialysable because it is protein bound.

DOSAGE AND ADMINISTRATION

The dose of MINIPRESS should be adjusted according to the patient's individual blood pressure response. The following is a guide to its administration:

Initial Dose

1 mg two or three times a day. (See WARNINGS)

Maintenance Dose

Dosage may be slowly increased to a total daily dose of 20 mg given in divided doses. The therapeutic dosages most commonly employed have ranged from 6 mg to 15 mg daily given in divided doses. Doses higher than 20 mg usually do not increase efficacy, however a few patients may benefit from further increases up to a daily dose of 40 mg given in divided doses. After initial titration some patients can be maintained adequately on a twice daily dosage regimen.

Use With Other Drugs

When adding a diuretic or other antihypertensive agent, the dose of MINIPRESS should be reduced to 1 mg or 2 mg three times a day and retitration then carried out.

HOW SUPPLIED

[See table below.]

References

1. Lubbe, WF, and Hodge, JV: *New Zealand Med J* **94** (691) 169–172, 1981.
2. Davey, DA, and Dommisse, J: *S.A. Med J,* Oct 4, 1980 (551–556).

69-2318-37-2   Revised July 1990

Shown in Product Identification Guide, page 328

MINIZIDE® CAPSULES   ℞

[mĭn 'ē-zīd]
(prazosin hydrochloride/polythiazide)
FOR ORAL ADMINISTRATION

> This fixed combination drug is not indicated for initial therapy of hypertension. Hypertension requires therapy titrated to the individual patient. If the fixed combination represents the dose so determined, its use may be more convenient in patient management. The treatment of hypertension is not static, but must be re-evaluated as conditions in each patient warrant.

DESCRIPTION

MINIZIDE is a combination of MINIPRESS® (prazosin hydrochloride) plus RENESE® (polythiazide).

MINIPRESS (prazosin hydrochloride), a quinazoline derivative, is the first of that chemical class of antihypertensives. It is the hydrochloride salt of 1-(4-amino-6, 7-dimethoxy-2-quinazolinyl)-4-(2-furoyl) piperazine and its structural formula is:

It is a white, crystalline substance, slightly soluble in water and isotonic saline, and has a molecular weight of 419.87. Each 1 mg capsule of MINIPRESS contains drug equivalent to 1 mg free base.

RENESE (polythiazide) is an orally effective, nonmercurial diuretic, saluretic, and antihypertensive agent.

It is designated chemically as 2H-1,2,4-Benzothiadiazine-7-sulfonamide,6-chloro-3,4-dihydro -2- methyl -3-[[(2,2,2-trifluoroethyl) thio]methyl]-,1,1-dioxide, and has the following structural formula:

It is a white, crystalline substance insoluble in water, but readily soluble in alkaline solution.

Inert ingredients in the formulations are: hard gelatin capsules (which may contain Blue 1, Green 3, Red 3 and other inert ingredients); magnesium stearate; sodium lauryl sulfate; starch; sucrose.

CLINICAL PHARMACOLOGY

MINIZIDE (prazosin hydrochloride/polythiazide)

Minizide produces a more pronounced antihypertensive response than occurs after either prazosin hydrochloride or polythiazide alone in equivalent doses.

Strength	Capsule Color	Capsule Code	NDC	Package Size
MINIPRESS 1 mg	White	431	0069-4310-71	250's
			0663-4310-82	1000's
			0663-4310-41	100 (10×10) Unit Dose
MINIPRESS 2 mg	Pink and White	437	0663-4370-71	250's
			0663-4370-82	1000's
			0663-4370-41	100 (10×10) Unit Dose
MINIPRESS 5 mg	Blue and White	438	0663-4380-71	250's
			0663-4380-73	500's
			0663-4380-41	100 (10×10) Unit Dose

MINIPRESS (prazosin hydrochloride)

The exact mechanism of the hypotensive action of prazosin is unknown. Prazosin causes a decrease in total peripheral resistance and was originally thought to have a direct relaxant action on vascular smooth muscle. Recent animal studies, however, have suggested that the vasodilator effect of prazosin is also related to blockade of postsynaptic *alpha*-adrenoceptors. The results of dog forelimb experiments demonstrate that the peripheral vasodilator effect of prazosin is confined mainly to the level of the resistance vessels (arterioles). Unlike conventional *alpha*-blockers, the antihypertensive action of prazosin is usually not accompanied by a reflex tachycardia. Tolerance has not been observed to develop in long term therapy.

Hemodynamic studies have been carried out in man following acute single dose administration and during the course of long term maintenance therapy. The results confirm that the therapeutic effect is a fall in blood pressure unaccompanied by a clinically significant change in cardiac output, heart rate, renal blood flow, and glomerular filtration rate. There is no measurable negative chronotropic effect.

In clinical studies to date, MINIPRESS has not increased plasma renin activity.

In man, blood pressure is lowered in both the supine and standing positions. This effect is most pronounced on the diastolic blood pressure.

Following oral administration, human plasma concentrations reach a peak at about three hours with a plasma half-life of two to three hours. The drug is highly bound to plasma protein. Bioavailability studies have demonstrated that the total absorption relative to the drug in a 20% alcoholic solution is 90%, resulting in peak levels approximately 65% of that of the drug in solution. Animal studies indicate that MINIPRESS is extensively metabolized, primarily by demethylation and conjugation, and excreted mainly via bile and feces. Less extensive human studies suggest similar metabolism and excretion in man.

MINIPRESS has been administered without any adverse drug interaction in limited clinical experience to date with the following: (1) cardiac glycosides—digitalis and digoxin; (2) hypoglycemics—insulin, chlorpropamide, phenformin, tolazamide, and tolbutamide; (3) tranquilizers and sedatives—chlordiazepoxide, diazepam, and phenobarbital; (4) antigout—allopurinol, colchicine, and probenecid; (5) antiarrhythmics—procainamide, propranolol (see WARNINGS however), and quinidine; and (6) analgesics, antipyretics and anti-inflammatories—propoxyphene, aspirin, indomethacin, and phenylbutazone.

RENESE (polythiazide)

RENESE is a member of the benzothiadiazine (thiazide) family of diuretic/antihypertensive agents. Its mechanism of action results in an interference with the renal tubular mechanism of electrolyte reabsorption. At maximal therapeutic dosage all thiazides are approximately equal in their diuretic potency. The mechanism whereby thiazides function in the control of hypertension is unknown. Renese is well absorbed, giving peak human plasma concentrations about 5 hours after oral administration. Drug is removed slowly thereafter with a plasma elimination half-life of approximately 27 hours. One fifth of the drug is recovered unchanged in human urine; the remainder is cleared via feces and as metabolites. Animal studies indicate metabolism occurs by rupture of the thiadiazine ring and loss of the side chain.

INDICATIONS AND USAGE

MINIZIDE is indicated in the treatment of hypertension. (See box warning.)

CONTRAINDICATIONS

RENESE is contraindicated in patients with anuria, and in patients known to be sensitive to thiazides or to other sulfonamide derivatives.

WARNINGS

MINIPRESS (prazosin hydrochloride)

MINIPRESS may cause syncope with sudden loss of consciousness. In most cases this is believed to be due to an excessive postural hypotensive effect, although occasionally the syncopal episode has been preceded by a bout of severe tachycardia with heart rates of 120–160 beats per minute. Syncopal episodes have usually occurred within 30 to 90 minutes of the initial dose of the drug; occasionally they have been reported in association with rapid dosage increases or the introduction of another antihypertensive drug into the regimen of a patient taking high doses of MINIPRESS. The incidence of syncopal episodes is approximately 1% in patients given an initial dose of 2 mg or greater. Clinical trials conducted during the investigational phase of this drug suggest that syncopal episodes can be minimized by limiting the initial dose of the drug to 1 mg, by subsequently increasing the dosage slowly, and by introducing any additional antihypertensive drugs into the patient's regimen with caution (see DOSAGE AND ADMINISTRATION). Hypotension may develop in patients given MINIPRESS who are also receiving a beta-blocker such as propranolol.

If syncope occurs, the patient should be placed in the recumbent position and treated supportively as necessary. This adverse effect is self-limiting and in most cases does not recur after the initial period of therapy or during subsequent dose titration.

Patients should always be started on the 1 mg capsules of MINIPRESS. The 2 and 5 mg capsules are not indicated for initial therapy.

More common than loss of consciousness are the symptoms often associated with lowering of the blood pressure, namely, dizziness and lightheadedness. The patient should be cautioned about these possible adverse effects and advised what measures to take should they develop. The patient should also be cautioned to avoid situations where injury could result should syncope occur during the initiation of MINIPRESS therapy.

RENESE (polythiazide)

RENESE should be used with caution in severe renal disease. In patients with renal disease, thiazides may precipitate azotemia. Cumulative effects of the drug may develop in patients with impaired renal function.

Thiazides should be used with caution in patients with impaired hepatic function or progressive liver disease, since minor alterations of fluid and electrolyte balance may precipitate hepatic coma.

Sensitivity reactions may occur in patients with a history of allergy or bronchial asthma.

The possibility of exacerbation or activation of systemic lupus erythematosus has been reported.

Thiazides may be additive or potentiative of the action of other antihypertensive drugs.

Potentiation occurs with ganglionic or peripheral adrenergic blocking drugs.

Periodic determinations of serum electrolytes to detect possible electrolyte imbalance should be performed at appropriate intervals.

All patients receiving thiazide therapy should be observed for clinical signs of fluid or electrolyte imbalance, namely, hyponatremia, hypochloremic alkalosis, and hypokalemia. Serum and urine electrolyte determinations are particularly important when the patient is vomiting excessively or receiving parenteral fluids. Medications such as digitalis may also influence serum electrolytes. Warning signs, irrespective of cause, are: dryness of mouth, thirst, weakness, lethargy, drowsiness, restlessness, muscle pains or cramps, muscular fatigue, hypotension, oliguria, tachycardia, and gastrointestinal disturbances such as nausea and vomiting.

Hypokalemia may develop with thiazides as with any potent diuretic, especially with brisk diuresis, when severe cirrhosis is present, or during concomitant use of corticosteroids or ACTH.

Interference with adequate oral electrolyte intake will also contribute to hypokalemia. Digitalis therapy may exaggerate the metabolic effects of hypokalemia, especially with reference to myocardial activity.

Any chloride deficit is generally mild and usually does not require specific treatment except under extraordinary circumstances (as in hepatic or renal disease). Dilutional hyponatremia may occur in edematous patients in hot weather; appropriate therapy is water restriction rather than administration of salt, except in rare instances when the hyponatremia is life-threatening. In actual salt depletion, appropriate replacement is the therapy of choice.

Hyperuricemia may occur or frank gout may be precipitated in certain patients receiving thiazide therapy.

Insulin requirements in diabetic patients may be either increased, decreased, or unchanged. Latent diabetes mellitus may become manifest during thiazide administration.

Thiazide drugs may increase responsiveness to tubocurarine.

The antihypertensive effects of the drug may be enhanced in the post-sympathectomy patient.

Thiazides may decrease arterial responsiveness to norepinephrine. This diminution is not sufficient to preclude effectiveness of the pressor agent for therapeutic use.

If progressive renal impairment becomes evident, as indicated by a rising nonprotein nitrogen or blood urea nitrogen, a careful reappraisal of therapy is necessary with consideration given to withholding or discontinuing diuretic therapy.

Thiazides may decrease serum protein-bound iodine levels without signs of thyroid disturbance.

PRECAUTIONS

Drug/Laboratory Test Interactions: In a study on five patients given from 12 to 24 mg of prazosin per day for 10 to 14 days, there was an average increase of 42% in the urinary metabolite of norepinephrine and an average increase in urinary VMA of 17%. Therefore, false positive results may occur in screening tests for pheochromocytoma in patients who are being treated with prazosin. If an elevated VMA is found, prazosin should be discontinued and the patient retested after a month.

Carcinogenesis, Mutagenesis, Impairment of Fertility: No carcinogenic or mutagenic studies have been conducted with MINIZIDE. However, no carcinogenic potential was demonstrated in 18 month studies in rats with either MINIPRESS or RENESE at dose levels more than 100 times the usual maximum human doses. MINIPRESS was not mutagenic in *in vivo* genetic toxicology studies.

MINIZIDE produced no impairment of fertility in male or female rats at 50 and 25 mg/kg/day of MINIPRESS and RENESE respectively. In chronic studies (one year or more) of MINIPRESS in rats and dogs, testicular changes consisting of atrophy and necrosis occurred at 25 mg/kg/day (60 times the usual maximum recommended human dose). No testicular changes were seen in rats or dogs at 10 mg/kg/day (24 times the usual maximum recommended human dose). In view of the testicular changes observed in animals, 105 patients on long term MINIPRESS therapy were monitored for 17-ketosteroid excretion and no changes indicating a drug effect were observed. In addition, 27 males on MINIPRESS alone for up to 51 months did not have changes in sperm morphology suggestive of drug effect.

Use in Pregnancy: Pregnancy Category C. MINIZIDE was not teratogenic in either rats or rabbits when administered in oral doses more than 100 times the usual maximum human dose. Studies in rats indicated that the combination of RENESE (40 times the usual maximum recommended human dose) and MINIPRESS (8 times the usual maximum recommended human dose) caused a greater number of stillbirths, a more prolonged gestation, and a decreased survival of pups to weaning than that caused by MINIPRESS alone. There are no adequate and well controlled studies in pregnant women. Therefore, MINIZIDE should be used in pregnancy only if the potential benefit justifies the potential risk to the fetus.

Nursing Mothers: It is not known whether MINIPRESS or RENESE are excreted in human milk. Thiazides appear in breast milk. Thus, if use of the drug is deemed essential the patient should stop nursing.

Pediatric Use: Safety and effectiveness in children has not been established.

ADVERSE REACTIONS

MINIPRESS (prazosin hydrochloride)

The most common reactions associated with MINIPRESS therapy are: dizziness 10.3%, headache 7.8%, drowsiness 7.6%, lack of energy 6.9%, weakness 6.5%, palpitations 5.3%, and nausea 4.9%. In most instances side effects have disappeared with continued therapy or have been tolerated with no decrease in dose of drug.

The following reactions have been associated with MINIPRESS, some of them rarely. (In some instances exact causal relationships have not been established.)

Gastrointestinal: vomiting, diarrhea, constipation, abdominal discomfort and/or pain, liver function abnormalities, pancreatitis.

Cardiovascular: edema, dyspnea, syncope, tachycardia.

Central Nervous System: nervousness, vertigo, depression, paresthesia, hallucinations.

Dermatologic: rash, pruritus, alopecia, lichen planus.

Genitourinary: urinary frequency, incontinence, impotence, priapism.

EENT: blurred vision, reddened sclera, epistaxis, tinnitus, dry mouth, nasal congestion.

Other: diaphoresis, fever.

Single reports of pigmentary mottling and serous retinopathy, and a few reports of cataract development or disappear-

STRENGTH	COMPONENTS	COLOR	CAPSULE CODE	PKG. SIZE
MINIZIDE® 1	1 mg prazosin + 0.5 mg polythiazide (NDC 0663-4300-66) (NDC 0069-4300-66)	Blue-Green	430	100's
MINIZIDE® 2	2 mg prazosin + 0.5 mg polythiazide (NDC 0663-4320-66) (NDC 0069-4320-66)	Blue-Green/Pink	432	100's
MINIZIDE® 5	5 mg prazosin + 0.5 mg polythiazide (NDC 0663-4360-66) (NDC 0069-4360-66)	Blue-Green/Blue	436	100's

Continued on next page

Pfizer Inc—Cont.

ance have been reported. In these instances, the exact causal relationship has not been established because the baseline observations were frequently inadequate.
In more specific slit-lamp and funduscopic studies, which included adequate baseline examinations, no drug-related abnormal ophthalmological findings have been reported.
Literature reports exist associating MINIPRESS therapy with a worsening of pre-existing narcolepsy. A causal relationship is uncertain in these cases.

RENESE (polythiazide)

Gastrointestinal: anorexia, gastric irritation, nausea, vomiting, cramping, diarrhea, constipation, jaundice (intrahepatic cholestatic jaundice), pancreatitis.
Central Nervous System: dizziness, vertigo, paresthesia, headache, xanthopsia.
Hematologic: leukopenia, agranulocytosis, thrombocytopenia, aplastic anemia.
Dermatologic: purpura, photosensitivity, rash, urticaria, necrotizing angiitis, (vasculitis) (cutaneous vasculitis).
Cardiovascular: Orthostatic hypotension may occur and be aggravated by alcohol, barbiturates, or narcotics.
Other: hyperglycemia, glycosuria, hyperuricemia, muscle spasm, weakness, restlessness.

OVERDOSAGE

MINIPRESS (prazosin hydrochloride)

Accidental ingestion of at least 50 mg of MINIPRESS in a two year old child resulted in profound drowsiness and depressed reflexes. No decrease in blood pressure was noted. Recovery was uneventful.
Should overdosage lead to hypotension, support of the cardiovascular system is of first importance. Restoration of blood pressure and normalization of heart rate may be accomplished by keeping the patient in the supine position. If this measure is inadequate, shock should first be treated with volume expanders. If necessary, vasopressors should then be used. Renal function should be monitored and supported as needed. Laboratory data indicate that MINIPRESS is not dialyzable because it is protein bound.

RENESE (polythiazide)

Should overdosage with RENESE occur, electrolyte balance and adequate hydration should be maintained. Gastric lavage is recommended, followed by supportive treatment. Where necessary, this may include intravenous dextrose and saline with potassium and other electrolyte therapy, administered with caution as indicated by laboratory testing at appropriate intervals.

DOSAGE AND ADMINISTRATION

MINIZIDE (prazosin hydrochloride/polythiazide)

Dosage: as determined by individual titration of MINIPRESS (prazosin hydrochloride) and RENESE (polythiazide). (See box warning.)
Usual MINIZIDE dosage is one capsule two or three times daily, the strength depending upon individual requirement following titration.
The following is a general guide to the administration of the individual components of MINIZIDE:

MINIPRESS (prazosin hydrochloride)

Initial Dose: 1 mg two or three times a day. (See WARNINGS.)
Maintenance Dose: Dosage may be slowly increased to a total daily dose of 20 mg given in divided doses. The therapeutic dosages most commonly employed have ranged from 6 mg to 15 mg daily given in divided doses. Doses higher than 20 mg usually do not increase efficacy, however a few patients may benefit from further increases up to a daily dose of 40 mg given in divided doses. After initial titration some patients can be maintained adequately on a twice daily dosage regimen.
Use With Other Drugs: When adding a diuretic or other antihypertensive agent, the dose of MINIPRESS should be reduced to 1 mg or 2 mg three times a day and retitration then carried out.

RENESE

The usual dose of RENESE for antihypertensive therapy is 2 to 4 mg daily.

HOW SUPPLIED

[See table on bottom of preceding page.]

#69-2463-00-7 Revised Oct. 1995

Shown in Product Identification Guide, page 328

NAVANE® ℞

[*nah 'vān*]
(thiothixene) CAPSULES

NAVANE® ℞

(thiothixene hydrochloride) CONCENTRATE

DESCRIPTION

Navane (thiothixene) is a thioxanthene derivative. Specifically, it is the *cis* isomer of N,N-dimethyl-9-[3-(4-methyl-1-piperazinyl)-propylidene] thioxanthene-2-sulfonamide.
[See chemical structure at top of next column.]

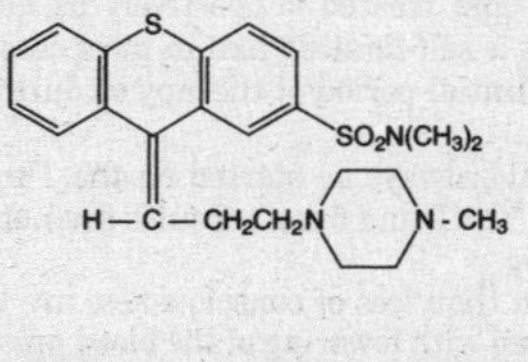

The thioxanthenes differ from the phenothiazines by the replacement of nitrogen in the central ring with a carbon-linked side chain fixed in space in a rigid structural configuration. An N,N-dimethyl sulfonamide functional group is bonded to the thioxanthene nucleus.
Inert ingredients for the capsule formulations are: hard gelatin capsules (which contain gelatin and titanium dioxide; may contain Yellow 10, Yellow 6, Blue 1, Green 3, Red 3, and other inert ingredients); lactose; magnesium stearate; sodium lauryl sulfate; starch.
Inert ingredients for the oral concentrate formulation are: alcohol; cherry flavor; dextrose; passion fruit flavor; sorbitol solution; water.

ACTIONS

Navane is a psychotropic agent of the thioxanthene series. Navane possesses certain chemical and pharmacological similarities to the piperazine phenothiazines and differences from the aliphatic group of phenothiazines.

INDICATIONS

Navane is effective in the management of manifestations of psychotic disorders. Navane has not been evaluated in the management of behavioral complications in patients with mental retardation.

CONTRAINDICATIONS

Navane is contraindicated in patients with circulatory collapse, comatose states, central nervous system depression due to any cause, and blood dyscrasias. Navane is contraindicated in individuals who have shown hypersensitivity to the drug. It is not known whether there is a cross sensitivity between the thioxanthenes and the phenothiazine derivatives, but this possibility should be considered.

WARNINGS

Tardive Dyskinesia—Tardive dyskinesia, a syndrome consisting of potentially irreversible, involuntary, dyskinetic movements may develop in patients treated with neuroleptic (antipsychotic) drugs. Although the prevalence of the syndrome appears to be highest among the elderly, especially elderly women, it is impossible to rely upon prevalence estimates to predict, at the inception of neuroleptic treatment, which patients are likely to develop the syndrome. Whether neuroleptic drug products differ in their potential to cause tardive dyskinesia is unknown.
Both the risk of developing the syndrome and the likelihood that it will become irreversible are believed to increase as the duration of treatment and the total cumulative dose of neuroleptic drugs administered to the patient increase. However, the syndrome can develop, although much less commonly, after relatively brief treatment periods at low doses.
There is no known treatment for established cases of tardive dyskinesia, although the syndrome may remit, partially or completely, if neuroleptic treatment is withdrawn. Neuroleptic treatment, itself, however, may suppress (or partially suppress) the signs and symptoms of the syndrome and thereby may possibly mask the underlying disease process. The effect that symptomatic suppression has upon the long-term course of the syndrome is unknown.
Given these considerations, neuroleptics should be prescribed in a manner that is most likely to minimize the occurrence of tardive dyskinesia. Chronic neuroleptic treatment should generally be reserved for patients who suffer from a chronic illness that, 1) is known to respond to neuroleptic drugs, and 2) for whom alternative, equally effective, but potentially less harmful treatments are *not* available or appropriate. In patients who do require chronic treatment, the smallest dose and the shortest duration of treatment producing a satisfactory clinical response should be sought. The need for continued treatment should be reassessed periodically.
If signs and symptoms of tardive dyskinesia appear in a patient on neuroleptics, drug discontinuation should be considered. However, some patients may require treatment despite the presence of the syndrome.
(For further information about the description of tardive dyskinesia and its clinical detection, please refer to "Information for Patients" in the PRECAUTIONS section, and to the ADVERSE REACTIONS section.)
Neuroleptic Malignant Syndrome (NMS)—A potentially fatal symptom complex sometimes referred to as Neuroleptic Malignant Syndrome (NMS) has been reported in association with antipsychotic drugs. Clinical manifestations of NMS are hyperpyrexia, muscle rigidity, altered mental status and evidence of autonomic instability (irregular pulse or blood pressure, tachycardia, diaphoresis, and cardiac dysrhythmias).
The diagnostic evaluation of patients with this syndrome is complicated. In arriving at a diagnosis, it is important to identify cases where the clinical presentation includes both serious medical illness (e.g., pneumonia, systemic infection, etc.) and untreated or inadequately treated extrapyramidal signs and symptoms (EPS). Other important considerations in the differential diagnosis include central anticholinergic toxicity, heat stroke, drug fever and primary central nervous system (CNS) pathology.
The management of NMS should include 1) immediate discontinuation of antipsychotic drugs and other drugs not essential to concurrent therapy, 2) intensive symptomatic treatment and medical monitoring, and 3) treatment of any concomitant serious medical problems for which specific treatments are available. There is no general agreement about specific pharmacological treatment regimens for uncomplicated NMS.
If a patient requires antipsychotic drug treatment after recovery from NMS, the potential reintroduction of drug therapy should be carefully considered. The patient should be carefully monitored, since recurrences of NMS have been reported.
Usage in Pregnancy—Safe use of Navane during pregnancy has not been established. Therefore, this drug should be given to pregnant patients only when, in the judgment of the physician, the expected benefits from the treatment exceed the possible risks to mother and fetus. Animal reproduction studies and clinical experience to date have not demonstrated any teratogenic effects.
In the animal reproduction studies with Navane, there was some decrease in conception rate and litter size, and an increase in resorption rate in rats and rabbits. Similar findings have been reported with other psychotropic agents. After repeated oral administration of Navane to rats (5 to 15 mg/kg/day), rabbits (3 to 50 mg/kg/day), and monkeys (1 to 3 mg/kg/day) before and during gestation, no teratogenic effects were seen.
Usage in Children—The use of Navane in children under 12 years of age is not recommended because safe conditions for its use have not been established.
As is true with many CNS drugs, Navane may impair the mental and/or physical abilities required for the performance of potentially hazardous tasks such as driving a car or operating machinery, especially during the first few days of therapy. Therefore, the patient should be cautioned accordingly.
As in the case of other CNS-acting drugs, patients receiving Navane (thiothixene) should be cautioned about the possible additive effects (which may include hypotension) with CNS depressants and with alcohol.

PRECAUTIONS

General: An antiemetic effect was observed in animal studies with Navane; since this effect may also occur in man, it is possible that Navane may mask signs of overdosage of toxic drugs and may obscure conditions such as intestinal obstruction and brain tumor.
In consideration of the known capability of Navane and certain other psychotropic drugs to precipitate convulsions, extreme caution should be used in patients with a history of convulsive disorders or those in a state of alcohol withdrawal, since it may lower the convulsive threshold. Although Navane potentiates the actions of the barbiturates, the dosage of the anticonvulsant therapy should not be reduced when Navane is administered concurrently.
Though exhibiting rather weak anticholinergic properties, Navane should be used with caution in patients who might be exposed to extreme heat or who are receiving atropine or related drugs.
Use with caution in patients with cardiovascular disease.
Caution as well as careful adjustment of the dosages is indicated when Navane is used in conjunction with other CNS depressants.
Also, careful observation should be made for pigmentary retinopathy, and lenticular pigmentation (fine lenticular pigmentation has been noted in a small number of patients treated with Navane for prolonged periods). Blood dyscrasias (agranulocytosis, pancytopenia, thrombocytopenic purpura), and liver damage (jaundice, biliary stasis), have been reported with related drugs.
Neuroleptic drugs elevate prolactin levels; the elevation persists during chronic administration. Tissue culture experiments indicate that approximately one-third of human breast cancers are prolactin dependent *in vitro*, a factor of potential importance if the prescription of these drugs is contemplated in a patient with a previously detected breast cancer. Although disturbances such as galactorrhea, amenorrhea, gynecomastia, and impotence have been reported, the clinical significance of elevated serum prolactin levels is unknown for most patients. An increase in mammary neoplasms has been found in rodents after chronic administration of neuroleptic drugs. Neither clinical studies nor epide-

miologic studies conducted to date, however, have shown an association between chronic administration of these drugs and mammary tumorigenesis; the available evidence is considered too limited to be conclusive at this time.

Information for Patients: Given the likelihood that some patients exposed chronically to neuroleptics will develop tardive dyskinesia, it is advised that all patients in whom chronic use is contemplated be given, if possible, full information about this risk. The decision to inform patients and/or their guardians must obviously take into account the clinical circumstances and the competency of the patient to understand the information provided.

ADVERSE REACTIONS

NOTE: Not all of the following adverse reactions have been reported with Navane. However, since Navane has certain chemical and pharmacologic similarities to the phenothiazines, all of the known side effects and toxicity associated with phenothiazine therapy should be borne in mind when Navane is used.

Cardiovascular Effects: Tachycardia, hypotension, lightheadedness, and syncope. In the event hypotension occurs, epinephrine should not be used as a pressor agent since a paradoxical further lowering of blood pressure may result. Nonspecific EKG changes have been observed in some patients receiving Navane. These changes are usually reversible and frequently disappear on continued Navane therapy. The incidence of these changes is lower than that observed with some phenothiazines. The clinical significance of these changes is not known.

CNS Effects: Drowsiness, usually mild, may occur although it usually subsides with continuation of Navane therapy. The incidence of sedation appears similar to that of the piperazine group of phenothiazines but less than that of certain aliphatic phenothiazines. Restlessness, agitation and insomnia have been noted with Navane. Seizures and paradoxical exacerbation of psychotic symptoms have occurred with Navane infrequently.

Hyperreflexia has been reported in infants delivered from mothers having received structurally related drugs.

In addition, phenothiazine derivatives have been associated with cerebral edema and cerebrospinal fluid abnormalities.

Extrapyramidal symptoms, such as pseudo-parkinsonism, akathisia and dystonia have been reported. Management of these extra-pyramidal symptoms depends upon the type and severity. Rapid relief of acute symptoms may require the use of an injectable antiparkinson agent. More slowly emerging symptoms may be managed by reducing the dosage of Navane and/or administering an oral antiparkinson agent.

Persistent Tardive Dyskinesia: As with all antipsychotic agents tardive dyskinesia may appear in some patients on long term therapy or may occur after drug therapy has been discontinued. The syndrome is characterized by rhythmical involuntary movements of the tongue, face, mouth or jaw (e.g., protrusion of tongue, puffing of cheeks, puckering of mouth, chewing movements). Sometimes these may be accompanied by involuntary movements of extremities.

Since early detection of tardive dyskinesia is important, patients should be monitored on an ongoing basis. It has been reported that fine vermicular movement of the tongue may be an early sign of the syndrome. If this or any other presentation of the syndrome is observed, the clinician should consider possible discontinuation of neuroleptic medication. (See WARNINGS section.)

Hepatic Effects: Elevations of serum transaminase and alkaline phosphatase, usually transient, have been infrequently observed in some patients. No clinically confirmed cases of jaundice attributable to Navane (thiothixene) have been reported.

Hematologic Effects: As is true with certain other psychotropic drugs, leukopenia and leucocytosis, which are usually transient, can occur occasionally with Navane. Other antipsychotic drugs have been associated with agranulocytosis, eosinophilia, hemolytic anemia, thrombocytopenia and pancytopenia.

Allergic Reactions: Rash, pruritus, urticaria, photosensitivity and rare cases of anaphylaxis have been reported with Navane. Undue exposure to sunlight should be avoided. Although not experienced with Navane, exfoliative dermatitis and contact dermatitis (in nursing personnel), have been reported with certain phenothiazines.

Endocrine Disorders: Lactation, moderate breast enlargement and amenorrhea have occurred in a small percentage of females receiving Navane. If persistent, this may necessitate a reduction in dosage or the discontinuation of therapy. Phenothiazines have been associated with false positive pregnancy tests, gynecomastia, hypoglycemia, hyperglycemia and glycosuria.

Autonomic Effects: Dry mouth, blurred vision, nasal congestion, constipation, increased sweating, increased salivation and impotence have occurred infrequently with Navane therapy. Phenothiazines have been associated with miosis, mydriasis, and adynamic ileus.

Other Adverse Reactions: Hyperpyrexia, anorexia, nausea, vomiting, diarrhea, increase in appetite and weight, weakness or fatigue, polydipsia, and peripheral edema.

Although not reported with Navane, evidence indicates there is a relationship between phenothiazine therapy and the occurrence of a systemic lupus erythematosus-like syndrome.

Neuroleptic Malignant Syndrome (NMS): Please refer to the text regarding NMS in the WARNINGS section.

NOTE: Sudden deaths have occasionally been reported in patients who have received certain phenothiazine derivatives. In some cases the cause of death was apparently cardiac arrest or asphyxia due to failure of the cough reflex. In others, the cause could not be determined nor could it be established that death was due to phenothiazine administration.

DOSAGE AND ADMINISTRATION

Dosage of Navane should be individually adjusted depending on the chronicity and severity of the condition. In general, small doses should be used initially and gradually increased to the optimal effective level, based on patient response.

Some patients have been successfully maintained on once-a-day Navane therapy.

The use of Navane in children under 12 years of age is not recommended because safe conditions for its use have not been established.

In milder conditions, an initial dose of 2 mg three times daily. If indicated, a subsequent increase to 15 mg/day total daily dose is often effective.

In more severe conditions, an initial dose of 5 mg twice daily. The usual optimal dose is 20 to 30 mg daily. If indicated, an increase to 60 mg/day total daily dose is often effective. Exceeding a total daily dose of 60 mg rarely increases the beneficial response.

OVERDOSAGE

Manifestations include muscular twitching, drowsiness and dizziness. Symptoms of gross overdosage may include CNS depression, rigidity, weakness, torticollis, tremor, salivation, dysphagia, hypotension, disturbances of gait, or coma.

Treatment: Essentially symptomatic and supportive. Early gastric lavage is helpful. Keep patient under careful observation and maintain an open airway, since involvement of the extrapyramidal system may produce dysphagia and respiratory difficulty in severe overdosage. If hypotension occurs, the standard measures for managing circulatory shock should be used (I.V. fluids and/or vasoconstrictors).

If a vasoconstrictor is needed, levarterenol and phenylephrine are the most suitable drugs. Other pressor agents, including epinephrine, are not recommended, since phenothiazine derivatives may reverse the usual pressor action of these agents and cause further lowering of blood pressure.

If CNS depression is marked, symptomatic treatment is indicated. Extrapyramidal symptoms may be treated with antiparkinson drugs.

There are no data on the use of peritoneal or hemodialysis, but they are known to be of little value in phenothiazine intoxication.

HOW SUPPLIED

Navane (thiothixene) Capsules

Bottles of 100's: 1 mg (NDC 0049-5710-66); 2 mg (NDC 0049-5720-66); 5 mg (NDC 0049-5730-66); 10 mg (NDC 0049-5740-66); 20 mg (NDC 0049-5770-66). 1000's: 2 mg (NDC 0049-5720-82); 5 mg (NDC 0049-5730-82); 10 mg (NDC 0049-5740-82). 500's: 20 mg (NDC 0049-5770-73).

Unit Doses of: 10 mg (NDC 0049-5740-41); and 20 mg (NDC 0049-5770-41).

Navane (thiothixene hydrochloride) Concentrate is available in 120 ml (4 oz.) bottles (NDC 0049-5750-47) with an accompanying dropper calibrated at 2 mg, 3 mg, 4 mg, 5 mg, 6 mg, 8 mg, and 10 mg. Each ml. contains thiothixene hydrochloride equivalent to 5 mg of thiothixene. Contains alcohol, U.S.P. 7.0% v/v. (small loss unavoidable).

Revised Jan. 1988 77-1655-00-7

Shown in Product Identification Guide, page 328

NAVANE® ℞

[nah'vān]

(thiothixene hydrochloride)

Intramuscular For Injection

STERILE

DESCRIPTION

Navane (thiothixene hydrochloride) is a thioxanthene derivative. Specifically, thiothixene is the *cis* isomer of N,N-dimethyl-9-[3-(4-methyl-1-piperazinyl)-propylidene]thioxanthene-2-sulfonamide.

The thioxanthenes differ from the phenothiazines by the replacement of nitrogen in the central ring with a carbon-linked side chain fixed in space in a rigid structural configuration. An N,N-dimethyl sulfonamide functional group is bonded to the thioxanthene nucleus.

[See chemical structure at top of next column.]

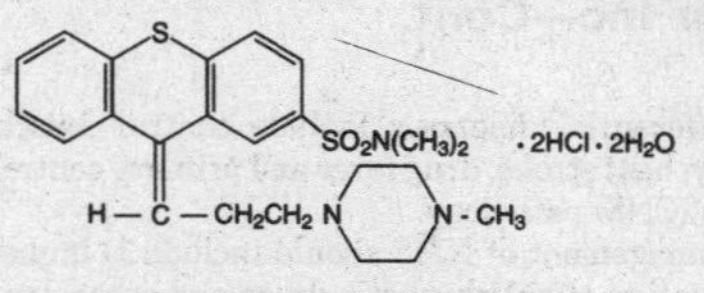

thiothixene hydrochloride

Inert ingredients for the intramuscular for injection formulation are: water; mannitol.

ACTIONS

Navane is a psychotropic agent of the thioxanthene series. Navane possesses certain chemical and pharmacological similarities to the piperazine phenothiazines and differences from the aliphatic group of phenothiazines. Navane's mode of action has not been clearly established.

INDICATIONS

Navane is effective in the management of manifestations of psychotic disorders. Navane has not been evaluated in the management of behavioral complications in patients with mental retardation.

CONTRAINDICATIONS

Navane is contraindicated in patients with circulatory collapse, comatose states, central nervous system depression due to any cause, and blood dyscrasias. Navane is contraindicated in individuals who have shown hypersensitivity to the drug. It is not known whether there is a cross sensitivity between the thioxanthenes and the phenothiazine derivatives, but this possibility should be considered.

WARNINGS

Tardive Dyskinesia—Tardive dyskinesia, a syndrome consisting of potentially irreversible, involuntary, dyskinetic movements may develop in patients treated with neuroleptic (antipsychotic) drugs. Although the prevalence of the syndrome appears to be highest among the elderly, especially elderly women, it is impossible to rely upon prevalence estimates to predict, at the inception of neuroleptic treatment, which patients are likely to develop the syndrome. Whether neuroleptic drug products differ in their potential to cause tardive dyskinesia is unknown.

Both the risk of developing the syndrome and the likelihood that it will become irreversible are believed to increase as the duration of treatment and the total cumulative dose of neuroleptic drugs administered to the patient increase. However, the syndrome can develop, although much less commonly, after relatively brief treatment periods at low doses.

There is no known treatment for established cases of tardive dyskinesia, although the syndrome may remit, partially or completely, if neuroleptic treatment is withdrawn. Neuroleptic treatment, itself, however, may suppress (or partially suppress) the signs and symptoms of the syndrome and thereby may possibly mask the underlying disease process. The effect that symptomatic suppression has upon the long-term course of the syndrome is unknown.

Given these considerations, neuroleptics should be prescribed in a manner that is most likely to minimize the occurrence of tardive dyskinesia. Chronic neuroleptic treatment should generally be reserved for patients who suffer from a chronic illness that, 1) is known to respond to neuroleptic drugs, and, 2) for whom alternative, equally effective, but potentially less harmful treatments are *not* available or appropriate. In patients who do require chronic treatment, the smallest dose and the shortest duration of treatment producing a satisfactory clinical response should be sought. The need for continued treatment should be reassessed periodically.

If signs and symptoms of tardive dyskinesia appear in a patient on neuroleptics, drug discontinuation should be considered. However, some patients may require treatment despite the presence of the syndrome.

(For further information about the description of tardive dyskinesia and its clinical detection, please refer to "Information for Patients" in the PRECAUTIONS section, and to the ADVERSE REACTIONS section.)

Neuroleptic Malignant Syndrome (NMS)—A potentially fatal symptom complex sometimes referred to as Neuroleptic Malignant Syndrome (NMS) has been reported in association with antipsychotic drugs. Clinical manifestations of NMS are hyperpyrexia, muscle rigidity, altered mental status and evidence of autonomic instability (irregular pulse or blood pressure, tachycardia, diaphoresis, and cardiac dysrhythmias).

The diagnostic evaluation of patients with this syndrome is complicated. In arriving at a diagnosis, it is important to identify cases where the clinical presentation includes both serious medical illness (e.g., pneumonia, systemic infection, etc.) and untreated or inadequately treated extrapyramidal signs and symptoms (EPS). Oher important considerations in

Continued on next page

Pfizer Inc—Cont.

the differential diagnosis include central anticholinergic toxicity, heat stroke, drug fever and primary central nervous system (CNS) pathology.

The management of NMS should include 1) immediate discontinuation of antipsychotic drugs and other drugs not essential to concurrent therapy, 2) intensive symptomatic treatment and medical monitoring, and 3) treatment of any concomitant serious medical problems for which specific treatments are available. There is no general agreement about specific pharmacological treatment regimens for uncomplicated NMS.

If a patient requires antipsychotic drug treatment after recovery from NMS, the potential reintroduction of drug therapy should be carefully considered. The patient should be carefully monitored, since recurrences of NMS have been reported.

Usage in Pregnancy—Safe use of Navane during pregnancy has not been established. Therefore, this drug should be given to pregnant patients only when, in the judgment of the physician, the expected benefits from treatment exceed the possible risks to mother and fetus. Animal reproductive studies and clinical experience to date have not demonstrated any teratogenic effects.

In the animal reproduction studies with Navane, there was some decrease in conception rate and litter size, and an increase in resorption rate in rats and rabbits, changes which have been similarly reported with other psychotropic agents. After repeated oral administration of Navane to rats (5 to 15 mg/kg/day), rabbits (3 to 50 mg/kg/day), and monkeys (1 to 3 mg/kg/day) before and during gestation, no teratogenic effects were seen. (See Precautions)

Usage in Children—The use of Navane in children under 12 years of age is not recommended because safety and efficacy in the pediatric age group have not been established.

As is true with many CNS drugs, Navane may impair the mental and/or physical abilities required for the performance of potentially hazardous tasks such as driving a car or operating machinery, especially during the first few days of therapy. Therefore, the patient should be cautioned accordingly.

As in the case of other CNS-acting drugs, patients receiving Navane should be cautioned about the possible additive effects (which may include hypotension) with CNS depressants and with alcohol.

PRECAUTIONS

General: An antiemetic effect was observed in animal studies with Navane (thiothixene hydrochloride); since this effect may also occur in man, it is possible that Navane may mask signs of overdosage of toxic drugs and may obscure conditions such as intestinal obstruction and brain tumor.

In consideration of the known capability of Navane and certain other psychotropic drugs to precipitate convulsions, extreme caution should be used in patients with a history of convulsive disorders, or those in a state of alcohol withdrawal since it may lower the convulsive threshold. Although Navane potentiates the actions of the barbiturates, the dosage of the anticonvulsant therapy should not be reduced when Navane is administered concurrently.

Caution as well as careful adjustment of the dosage is indicated when Navane is used in conjunction with other CNS depressants other than anticonvulsant drugs.

Though exhibiting rather weak anticholinergic properties, Navane should be used with caution in patients who are known or suspected to have glaucoma, or who might be exposed to extreme heat, or who are receiving atropine or related drugs.

Use with caution in patients with cardiovascular disease.

Also, careful observation should be made for pigmentary retinopathy, and lenticular pigmentation (fine lenticular pigmentation has been noted in a small number of patients treated with Navane for prolonged periods). Blood dyscrasias (agranulocytosis, pancytopenia, thrombocytopenic purpura), and liver damage (jaundice, biliary stasis), have been reported with related drugs.

Undue exposure to sunlight should be avoided. Photosensitive reactions have been reported in patients on Navane.

As with all intramuscular preparations, Navane Intramuscular For Injection should be injected well within the body of a relatively large muscle. The preferred sites are the upper outer quadrant of the buttock (i.e., gluteus maximus) and the mid-lateral thigh.

The deltoid area should be used only if well developed such as in certain adults and older children, and then only with caution to avoid radial nerve injury. Intramuscular injections should not be made into the lower and mid-thirds of the upper arm. As with all intramuscular injections, aspiration is necessary to help avoid inadvertent injection into a blood vessel.

Neuroleptic drugs elevate prolactin levels; the elevation persists during chronic administration. Tissue culture experiments indicate that approximately one-third of human breast cancers are prolactin dependent *in vitro*, a factor of potential importance if the prescription of these drugs is contemplated in a patient with a previously detected breast cancer. Although disturbances such as galactorrhea, amenorrhea, gynecomastia, and impotence have been reported, the clinical significance of elevated serum prolactin levels is unknown for most patients. An increase in mammary neoplasms has been found in rodents after chronic administration of neuroleptic drugs. Neither clinical studies nor epidemiologic studies conducted to date, however, have shown an association between chronic administration of these drugs and mammary tumorigenesis; the available evidence is considered too limited to be conclusive at this time.

Information for Patients: Given the likelihood that some patients exposed chronically to neuroleptics will develop tardive dyskinesia, it is advised that all patients in whom chronic use is contemplated be given, if possible, full information about this risk. The decision to inform patients and/or their guardians must obviously take into account the clinical circumstances and the competency of the patient to understand the information provided.

ADVERSE REACTIONS

NOTE: Not all of the following adverse reactions have been reported with Navane. However, since Navane has certain chemical and pharmacologic similarities to the phenothiazines, all of the known side effects and toxicity associated with phenothiazine therapy should be borne in mind when Navane is used.

Cardiovascular Effects: Tachycardia, hypotension, lightheadedness, and syncope. In the event hypotension occurs, epinephrine should not be used as a pressor agent since a paradoxical further lowering of blood pressure may result. Nonspecific EKG changes have been observed in some patients receiving Navane. These changes are usually reversible and frequently disappear on continued Navane therapy. The clinical significance of these changes is not known.

CNS Effects: Drowsiness, usually mild, may occur although it usually subsides with continuation of Navane therapy. The incidence of sedation appears similar to that of the piperazine group of phenothiazines, but less than that of certain aliphatic phenothiazines. Restlessness, agitation and insomnia have been noted with Navane. Seizures and paradoxical exacerbation of psychotic symptoms have occurred with Navane infrequently.

Hyperreflexia has been reported in infants delivered from mothers having received structurally related drugs.

In addition, phenothiazine derivatives have been associated with cerebral edema and cerebrospinal fluid abnormalities. Extrapyramidal symptoms, such as pseudo-parkinsonism, akathisia, and dystonia have been reported. Management of these extrapyramidal symptoms depends upon the type and severity. Rapid relief of acute symptoms may require the use of an injectable antiparkinson agent. More slowly emerging symptoms may be managed by reducing the dosage of Navane and/or administering an oral antiparkinson agent.

Persistent Tardive Dyskinesia: As with all antipsychotic agents tardive dyskinesia may appear in some patients on long term therapy or may occur after drug therapy has been discontinued. The syndrome is characterized by rhythmical involuntary movements of the tongue, face, mouth or jaw (e.g., protrusion of tongue, puffing of cheeks, puckering of mouth, chewing movements). Sometimes these may be accompanied by involuntary movements of extremities.

Since early detection of tardive dyskinesia is important, patients should be monitored on an ongoing basis. It has been reported that fine vermicular movement of the tongue may be an early sign of the syndrome. If this or any other presentation of the syndrome is observed, the clinician should consider possible discontinuation of neuroleptic medication. (See Warnings section.)

Hepatic Effects: Elevations of serum transaminase and alkaline phosphatase, usually transient, have been infrequently observed in some patients. No clinically confirmed cases of jaundice attributable to Navane (thiothixene hydrochloride) have been reported.

Hematologic Effects: As is true with certain other psychotropic drugs, leukopenia and leucocytosis, which are usually transient, can occur occasionally with Navane. Other antipsychotic drugs have been associated with agranulocytosis, eosinophilia, hemolytic anemia, thrombocytopenia and pancytopenia.

Allergic Reactions: Rash, pruritus, urticaria, and rare cases of anaphylaxis have been reported with Navane. Undue exposure to sunlight should be avoided. Although not experienced with Navane, exfoliative dermatitis, contact dermatitis (in nursing personnel), have been reported with certain phenothiazines.

Endocrine Disorders: Lactation, moderate breast enlargement and amenorrhea have occurred in a small percentage of females receiving Navane. If persistent, this may necessitate a reduction in dosage or the discontinuation of therapy. Phenothiazines have been associated with false positive pregnancy tests, gynecomastia, hypoglycemia, hyperglycemia, and glycosuria.

Autonomic Effects: Dry mouth, blurred vision, nasal congestion, constipation, increased sweating, increased salivation, and impotence have occurred infrequently with Navane therapy. Phenothiazines have been associated with miosis, mydriasis, and adynamic ileus.

Other Adverse Reactions: Hyperpyrexia, anorexia, nausea, vomiting, diarrhea, increase in appetite and weight, weakness or fatigue, polydipsia and peripheral edema.

Although not reported with Navane, evidence indicates there is a relationship between phenothiazine therapy and the occurrence of a systemic lupus erythematosus-like syndrome.

Neuroleptic Malignant Syndrome (NMS): Please refer to the text regarding NMS in the WARNINGS section.

NOTE: Sudden deaths have occasionally been reported in patients who have received certain phenothiazine derivatives. In some cases the cause of death was apparently cardiac arrest or asphyxia due to failure of the cough reflex. In others, the cause could not be determined nor could it be established that death was due to phenothiazine administration.

DOSAGE AND ADMINISTRATION

Preparation

Navane (thiothixene hydrochloride) Intramuscular For Injection must be reconstituted with 2.2 ml of sterile water for injection.

For Intramuscular Use Only

Dosage of Navane should be individually adjusted depending on the chronicity and severity of the condition. In general, small doses should be used initially and gradually increased to the optimal effective level, based on patient response.

Usage in children under 12 years of age is not recommended. Where more rapid control and treatment of acute behavior is desirable, the intramuscular form of Navane may be indicated. It is also of benefit where the very nature of the patient's symptomatology, whether acute or chronic, renders oral administration impractical or even impossible.

For treatment of acute symptomatology or in patients unable or unwilling to take oral medication, the usual dose is 4 mg of Navane Intramuscular For Injection administered 2 to 4 times daily. Dosage may be increased or decreased depending on response. Most patients are controlled on a total daily dosage of 16 to 20 mg. The maximum recommended dosage is 30 mg/day. An oral form should supplant the injectable form as soon as possible. It may be necessary to adjust the dosage when changing from the intramuscular to oral dosage forms. Dosage recommendations for Navane Capsules and Concentrate can be found in the Navane oral package insert.

OVERDOSAGE

Manifestations include muscular twitching, drowsiness, and dizziness. Symptoms of gross overdosage may include CNS depression, rigidity, weakness, torticollis, tremor, salivation, dysphagia, hypotension, disturbances of gait, or coma.

Treatment: Essentially symptomatic and supportive. Keep patient under careful observation and maintain an open airway, since involvement of the extrapyramidal system may produce dysphagia and respiratory difficulty in severe overdosage. If hypotension occurs, the standard measures for managing circulatory shock should be used (I.V. fluids and/or vasoconstrictors).

If a vasoconstrictor is needed, levarterenol and phenylephrine are the most suitable drugs. Other pressor agents, including epinephrine, are not recommended, since phenothiazine derivatives may reverse the usual pressor elevating action of these agents and cause further lowering of blood pressure.

If CNS depression is marked, symptomatic treatment is indicated. Extrapyramidal symptoms may be treated with antiparkinson drugs.

There are no data on the use of peritoneal or hemodialysis, but they are known to be of little value in phenothiazine intoxication.

HOW SUPPLIED

Navane (thiothixene hydrochloride) Intramuscular For Injection is available in amber glass vials in packages of 10 vials (NDC 0049-5765-83). When reconstituted with 2.2 ml of STERILE WATER FOR INJECTION, each ml contains thiothixene hydrochloride equivalent to 5 mg of thiothixene, and 59.6 mg of mannitol. The reconstituted solution of Navane Intramuscular For Injection may be stored for 48 hours at room temperature before discarding.

70-4177-00-4
Revised January 1988

NORVASC® ℞
[nor'vask]
(amlodipine besylate)
Tablets

DESCRIPTION

NORVASC® is the besylate salt of amlodipine, a long-acting calcium channel blocker.

NORVASC is chemically described as (R.S.) 3-ethyl-5-methyl -2- (2-aminoethoxymethyl)-4-(2-chlorophenyl) -1,4-dihydro-6-methyl-3,5-pyridinedicarboxylate benzenesulphonate. Its empirical formula is $C_{20}H_{25}ClN_2O_5 \cdot C_6H_6O_3S$, and its structural formula is:

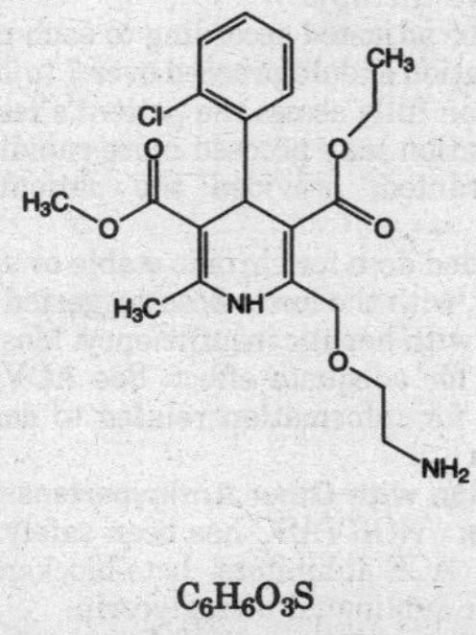

Amlodipine besylate is a white crystalline powder with a molecular weight of 567.1. It is slightly soluble in water and sparingly soluble in ethanol. NORVASC (amlodipine besylate) tablets are formulated as white tablets equivalent to 2.5, 5 and 10 mg of amlodipine for oral administration. In addition to the active ingredient, amlodipine besylate, each tablet contains the following inactive ingredients: microcrystalline cellulose, dibasic calcium phosphate anhydrous, sodium starch glycolate, and magnesium stearate.

CLINICAL PHARMACOLOGY

Mechanism of Action: NORVASC is a dihydropyridine calcium antagonist (calcium ion antagonist or slow channel blocker) that inhibits the transmembrane influx of calcium ions into vascular smooth muscle and cardiac muscle. Experimental data suggest that NORVASC binds to both dihydropyridine and nondihydropyridine binding sites. The contractile processes of cardiac muscle and vascular smooth muscle are dependent upon the movement of extracellular calcium ions into these cells through specific ion channels. NORVASC inhibits calcium ion influx across cell membranes selectively, with a greater effect on vascular smooth muscle cells than on cardiac muscle cells. Negative inotropic effects can be detected *in vitro* but such effects have not been seen in intact animals at therapeutic doses. Serum calcium concentration is not affected by NORVASC. Within the physiologic pH range, NORVASC is an ionized compound (pKa=8.6), and its kinetic interaction with the calcium channel receptor is characterized by a gradual rate of association and dissociation with the receptor binding site, resulting in a gradual onset of effect.

NORVASC is a peripheral arterial vasodilator that acts directly on vascular smooth muscle to cause a reduction in peripheral vascular resistance and reduction in blood pressure.

The precise mechanisms by which NORVASC relieves angina have not been fully delineated, but are thought to include the following:

Exertional Angina: In patients with exertional angina, NORVASC reduces the total peripheral resistance (afterload) against which the heart works and reduces the rate pressure product, and thus myocardial oxygen demand, at any given level of exercise.

Vasospastic Angina: NORVASC has been demonstrated to block constriction and restore blood flow in coronary arteries and arterioles in response to calcium, potassium epinephrine, serotonin, and thromboxane A_2 analog in experimental animal models and in human coronary vessels *in vitro*. This inhibition of coronary spasm is responsible for the effectiveness of NORVASC in vasospastic (Prinzmetal's or variant) angina.

Pharmacokinetics and Metabolism: After oral administration of therapeutic doses of NORVASC, absorption produces peak plasma concentrations between 6 and 12 hours. Absolute bioavailability has been estimated to be between 64 and 90%. The bioavailability of NORVASC is not altered by the presence of food.

NORVASC is extensively (about 90%) converted to inactive metabolites via hepatic metabolism with 10% of the parent compound and 60% of the metabolites excreted in the urine. *Ex vivo* studies have shown that approximately 93% of the circulating drug is bound to plasma proteins in hypertensive patients. Elimination from the plasma is biphasic with a terminal elimination half-life of about 30–50 hours. Steady-state plasma levels of NORVASC are reached after 7 to 8 days of consecutive daily dosing.

The pharmacokinetics of NORVASC are not significantly influenced by renal impairment. Patients with renal failure may therefore receive the usual initial dose.

Elderly patients and patients with hepatic insufficiency have decreased clearance of amlodipine with a resulting increase in AUC of approximately 40–60%, and a lower initial dose may be required. A similar increase in AUC was observed in patients with moderate to severe heart failure.

Pharmacodynamics: *Hemodynamics* Following administration of therapeutic doses to patients with hypertension, NORVASC produces vasodilation resulting in a reduction of supine and standing blood pressures. These deceases in blood pressure are not accompanied by a significant change in heart rate or plasma catecholamine levels with chronic dosing. Although the acute intravenous administration of amlodipine decreases arterial blood pressure and increases heart rate in hemodynamic studies of patients with chronic stable angina, chronic administration of oral amlodipine in clinical trials did not lead to clinically significant changes in heart rate or blood pressures in normotensive patients with angina.

With chronic once daily oral administration, antihypertensive effectiveness is maintained for at least 24 hours. Plasma concentrations correlate with effect in both young and elderly patients. The magnitude of reduction in blood pressure with NORVASC is also correlated with the height of pretreatment elevation; thus, individuals with moderate hypertension (diastolic pressure 105–114 mmHg) had about a 50% greater response than patients with mild hypertension (diastolic pressure 90–104 mmHg). Normotensive subjects experienced no clinically significant change in blood pressure (+1/−2 mmHg).

In hypertensive patients with normal renal function, therapeutic doses of NORVASC resulted in a decrease in renal vascular resistance and an increase in glomerular filtration rate and effective renal plasma flow without change in filtration fraction or proteinuria.

As with other calcium channel blockers, hemodynamic measurements of cardiac function at rest and during exercise (or pacing) in patients with normal ventricular function treated with NORVASC have generally demonstrated a small increase in cardiac index without significant influence on dP/dt or on left ventricular end diastolic pressure or volume. In hemodynamic studies, NORVASC has not been associated with a negative inotropic effect when administered in the therapeutic dose range to intact animals and man, even when co-administered with beta-blockers to man. Similar findings, however, have been observed in normals or well-compensated patients with heart failure with agents possessing significant negative inotropic effects.

Studies in Patients with Congestive Heart Failure: NORVASC has been compared to placebo in four 8–12 week studies of patients with NYHA class II/III heart failure, involving a total of 697 patients. In these studies, there was no evidence of worsened heart failure based on measures of exercise tolerance, NYHA classification, symptoms, or LVEF. In a long-term (follow-up at least 6 months, mean 13.8 months) placebo-controlled mortality/morbidity study of NORVASC 5-10 mg in 1153 patients with NYHA classes III (n=931) or IV (n=222) heart failure on stable doses of diuretics, digoxin, and ACE inhibitors, NORVASC had no effect on the primary endpoint of the study which was the combined endpoint of all-cause mortality and cardiac morbidity (as defined by life-threatening arrhythmia, acute myocardial infarction, or hospitalization for worsened heart failure), or on NYHA classification, or symptoms of heart failure. Total combined all-cause mortality and cardiac morbidity events were 222/571 (39%) for patients on NORVASC and 246/583 (42%) for patients on placebo; the cardiac morbid events represented about 25% of the endpoints in the study.

Electrophysiologic Effects: NORVASC does not change sinoatrial nodal function or atrioventricular conduction in intact animals or man. In patients with chronic stable angina, intravenous administration of 10 mg did not significantly alter A-H and H-V conduction and sinus node recovery time after pacing. Similar results were obtained in patients receiving NORVASC and concomitant beta blockers. In clinical studies in which NORVASC was administered in combination with beta-blockers to patients with either hypertension or angina, no adverse effects on electrocardiographic parameters were observed. In clinical trials with angina patients alone, NORVASC therapy did not alter electrocardiographic intervals or produce higher degrees of AV blocks.

Effects in Hypertension: The antihypertensive efficacy of NORVASC has been demonstrated in a total of 15 double-blind, placebo-controlled, randomized studies involving 800 patients on NORVASC and 538 on placebo. Once daily administration produced statistically significant placebo-corrected reductions in supine and standing blood pressures at 24 hours postdose, averaging about 12/6 mmHg in the standing position and 13/7 mmHg in the supine position in patients with mild to moderate hypertension. Maintenance of the blood pressure effect over the 24 hour dosing interval was observed, with little difference in peak and trough effect. Tolerance was not demonstrated in patients studied for up to 1 year. The 3 parallel, fixed dose, dose response studies showed that the reduction in supine and standing blood pressures was dose-related within the recommended dosing range. Effects on diastolic pressure were similar in young and older patients. The effect on systolic pressure was greater in older patients, perhaps because of greater baseline systolic pressure. Effects were similar in black and white patients.

Effects in Chronic Stable Angina: The effectiveness of 5–10 mg/day of NORVASC in exercise-induced angina has been evaluated in 8 placebo-controlled, double-blind clinical trials of up to 6 weeks duration involving 1038 patients (684 NORVASC, 354 placebo) with chronic stable angina. In 5 of the 8 studies significant increases in exercise time (bicycle or treadmill) were seen with the 10 mg dose. Increases in symptom-limited exercise time averaged 12.8% (63 sec) for NORVASC 10 mg, and averaged 7.9% (38 sec) for NORVASC 5 mg. NORVASC 10 mg also increased time to 1 mm ST segment deviation in several studies and decreased angina attack rate. The sustained efficacy of NORVASC in angina patients has been demonstrated over long-term dosing. In patients with angina there were no clinically significant reductions in blood pressures (4/1 mmHg) or changes in heart rate (+0.3 bpm).

Effects in Vasospastic Angina: In a double-blind, placebo-controlled clinical trial of 4 weeks duration in 50 patients, NORVASC therapy decreased attacks by approximately 4/week compared with a placebo decrease of approximately 1/week ($p<0.01$). Two of 23 NORVASC and 7 of 27 placebo patients discontinued from the study due to lack of clinical improvement.

INDICATIONS AND USAGE

1. Hypertension

NORVASC is indicated for the treatment of hypertension. It may be used alone or in combination with other antihypertensive agents.

2. Chronic Stable Angina

NORVASC is indicated for the treatment of chronic stable angina. NORVASC may be used alone or in combination with other antianginal agents.

3. Vasospastic Angina (Prinzmetal's or Variant Angina)

NORVASC is indicated for the treatment of confirmed or suspected vasospastic angina. NORVASC may be used as monotherapy or in combination with other antianginal drugs.

CONTRAINDICATIONS

NORVASC is contraindicated in patients with known sensitivity to amlodipine.

WARNINGS

Increased Angina and/or Myocardial Infarction: Rarely, patients, particularly those with severe obstructive coronary artery disease, have developed documented increased frequency, duration and/or severity of angina or acute myocardial infarction on starting calcium channel blocker therapy or at the time of dosage increase. The mechanism of this effect has not been elucidated.

PRECAUTIONS

General: Since the vasodilation induced by NORVASC is gradual in onset, acute hypotension has rarely been reported after oral administration of NORVASC. Nonetheless, caution should be exercised when administering NORVASC as with any other peripheral vasodilator particularly in patients with severe aortic stenosis.

Use in Patients with Congestive Heart Failure: In general, calcium channel blockers should be used with caution in patients with heart failure. NORVASC (5–10 mg per day) has been studied in a placebo-controlled trial of 1153 patients with NYHA Class III or IV heart failure (see CLINICAL PHARMACOLOGY) on stable doses of ACE inhibitor, digoxin, and diuretics. Follow-up was at least 6 months, with a mean of about 14 months. There was no overall adverse effect on survival or cardiac morbidity (as defined by life-threatening arrhythmia, acute myocardial infarction, or hospitalization for worsened heart failure). NORVASC has been compared to placebo in four 8-12 week studies of patients with NYHA class II/III heart failure, involving a total of 697 patients. In these studies, there was no evidence of worsened heart failure based on measures of exercise tolerance, NYHA classification, symptoms, or LVEF.

Beta-Blocker Withdrawal: NORVASC is not a beta-blocker and therefore gives no protection against the dangers of abrupt beta-blocker withdrawal; any such withdrawal should be by gradual reduction of the dose of beta-blocker.

Patients with Hepatic Failure: Since NORVASC is extensively metabolized by the liver and the plasma elimination half-life (t 1/2) is 56 hours in patients with impaired hepatic function, caution should be exercised when administering NORVASC to patients with severe hepatic impairment.

Drug Interactions: *In vitro* data in human plasma indicate that NORVASC has no effect on the protein binding of drugs tested (digoxin, phenytoin, warfarin, and indomethacin). Special studies have indicated that the co-administration of NORVASC with digoxin did not change serum digoxin levels or digoxin renal clearance in normal volunteers; that co-administration with cimetidine did not alter the pharmacokinetics of amlodipine; and that co-administration with

Continued on next page

Pfizer Inc—Cont.

warfarin did not change the warfarin prothrombin response time.
In clinical trials, NORVASC has been safely administered with thiazide diuretics, beta-blockers, angiotensin converting enzyme inhibitors, long-acting nitrates, sublingual nitroglycerin, digoxin, warfarin, non-steroidal anti-inflammatory drugs, antibiotics, and oral hypoglycemic drugs.
Drug/Laboratory Test Interactions: None known.
Carcinogenesis, Mutagenesis, Impairment of Fertility: Rats and mice treated with amlodipine in the diet for two years, at concentrations calculated to provide daily dosage levels of 0.5, 1.25, and 2.5 mg/kg/day showed no evidence of carcinogenicity. The highest dose (for mice, similar to, and for rats twice* the maximum recommended clinical dose of 10 mg on a mg/m² basis) was close to the maximum tolerated dose for mice but not for rats.
Mutagenicity studies revealed no drug related effects at either the gene or chromosome levels.
There was no effect on the fertility of rats treated with amlodipine (males for 64 days and females 14 days prior to mating) at doses up to 10 mg/kg/day (8 times* the maximum recommended human dose of 10 mg on a mg/m² basis).
Pregnancy Category C: No evidence of teratogenicity or other embryo/fetal toxicity was found when pregnant rats or rabbits were treated orally with up to 10 mg/kg amlodipine (respectively 8 times* and 23 times* the maximum recommended human dose of 10 mg on a mg/m² basis) during their respective periods of major organogenesis. However, litter size was significantly decreased (by about 50%) and the number of intrauterine deaths was significantly increased (about 5-fold) in rats administered 10 mg/kg amlodipine for 14 days before mating and throughout mating and gestation. Amlodipine has been shown to prolong both the gestation period and the duration of labor in rats at this dose. There are no adequate and well-controlled studies in pregnant women. Amlodipine should be used during pregnancy only if the potential benefit justifies the potential risk to the fetus.
Nursing Mothers: It is not known whether amlodipine is excreted in human milk. In the absence of this information, it is recommended that nursing be discontinued while NORVASC is administered.
Pediatric Use: Safety and effectiveness of NORVASC in children have not been established.
* Based on patient weight of 50 kg.

ADVERSE REACTIONS

NORVASC has been evaluated for safety in more than 11,000 patients in U.S. and foreign clinical trials. In general, treatment with NORVASC was well-tolerated at doses up to 10 mg daily. Most adverse reactions reported during therapy with NORVASC were of mild or moderate severity. In controlled clinical trials directly comparing NORVASC (N=1730) in doses up to 10 mg to placebo (N=1250), discontinuation of NORVASC due to adverse reactions was required in only about 1.5% of patients and was not significantly different from placebo (about 1%). The most common side effects are headache and edema. The incidence (%) of side effects which occurred in a dose related manner are as follows:

Adverse Event	2.5 mg N=275	5.0 mg N=296	10.0 mg N=268	Placebo N=520
Edema	1.8	3.0	10.8	0.6
Dizziness	1.1	3.4	3.4	1.5
Flushing	0.7	1.4	2.6	0.0
Palpitation	0.7	1.4	4.5	0.6

Other adverse experiences which were not clearly dose related but which were reported with an incidence greater than 1.0% in placebo-controlled clinical trials include the following:

Placebo Controlled Studies

	NORVASC (%) (N=1730)	PLACEBO (%) (N=1250)
Headache	7.3	7.8
Fatigue	4.5	2.8
Nausea	2.9	1.9
Abdominal Pain	1.6	0.3
Somnolence	1.4	0.6

For several adverse experiences that appear to be drug and dose related, there was a greater incidence in women than men associated with amlodipine treatment as shown in the following table:

ADR	NORVASC M=% (N=1218)	NORVASC F=% (N=512)	PLACEBO M=% (N=914)	PLACEBO F=% (N=336)
Edema	5.6	14.6	1.4	5.1
Flushing	1.5	4.5	0.3	0.9
Palpitations	1.4	3.3	0.9	0.9
Somnolence	1.3	1.6	0.8	0.3

The following events occurred in ≤1% but >0.1% of patients in controlled clinical trials or under conditions of open trials or marketing experience where a causal relationship is uncertain; they are listed to alert the physician to a possible relationship:
Cardiovascular: arrhythmia (including ventricular tachycardia and atrial fibrillation), bradycardia, chest pain, hypotension, peripheral ischemia, syncope, tachycardia, postural dizziness, postural hypotension.
Central and Peripheral Nervous System: hypoesthesia, paresthesia, tremor, vertigo.
Gastrointestinal: anorexia, constipation, dyspepsia,** dysphagia, diarrhea, flatulence, vomiting, gingival hyperplasia.
General: asthenia,** back pain, hot flushes, malaise, pain, rigors, weight gain.
Musculoskeletal System: arthralgia, arthrosis, muscle cramps,** myalgia.
Psychiatric: sexual dysfunction (male** and female), insomnia, nervousness, depression, abnormal dreams, anxiety, depersonalization.
Respiratory System: dyspnea,** epistaxis.
Skin and Appendages: pruritus,** rash,** rash erythematous, rash maculopapular.
**These events occurred in less than 1% in placebo controlled trials, but the incidence of these side effects was between 1% and 2% in all multiple dose studies.
Special Senses: abnormal vision, conjunctivitis, diplopia, eye pain, tinnitus.
Urinary System: micturition frequency, micturition disorder, nocturia.
Autonomic Nervous System: dry mouth, sweating increased.
Metabolic and Nutritional: thirst.
Hemopoietic: purpura.
The following events occurred in ≤0.1% of patients: cardiac failure, pulse irregularity, extrasystoles, skin discoloration, urticaria, skin dryness, alopecia, dermatitis, muscle weakness, twitching, ataxia, hypertonia, migraine, cold and clammy skin, apathy, agitation, amnesia, gastritis, increased appetite, loose stools, coughing, rhinitis, dysuria, polyuria, parosmia, taste perversion, abnormal visual accommodation, and xerophthalmia.
Other reactions occurred sporadically and cannot be distinguished from medications or concurrent disease states such as myocardial infarction and angina.
NORVASC therapy has not been associated with clinically significant changes in routine laboratory tests. No clinically relevant changes were noted in serum potassium, serum glucose, total triglycerides, total cholesterol, HDL cholesterol, uric acid, blood urea nitrogen, or creatinine.
In postmarketing experience, jaundice and hepatic enzyme elevations (mostly consistent with cholestasis) in some cases severe enough to require hospitalization have been reported in association with use of amlodipine.
NORVASC has been used safely in patients with chronic obstructive pulmonary disease, well compensated congestive heart failure, peripheral vascular disease, diabetes mellitus, and abnormal lipid profiles.

OVERDOSAGE

Single oral doses of 40 mg/kg and 100 mg/kg in mice and rats, respectively, caused deaths. A single oral dose of 4 mg/kg or higher in dogs caused a marked peripheral vasodilation and hypotension.
Overdosage might be expected to cause excessive peripheral vasodilation with marked hypotension and possibly a reflex tachycardia. In humans, experience with intentional overdosage of NORVASC is limited. Reports of intentional overdosage include a patient who ingested 250 mg and was asymptomatic and was not hospitalized; another (120 mg) was hospitalized, underwent gastric lavage and remained normotensive; the third (105 mg) was hospitalized and had hypotension (90/50 mmHg) which normalized following plasma expansion. A patient who took 70 mg amlodipine and an unknown quantity of benzodiazepine in a suicide attempt, developed shock which was refractory to treatment and died the following day with abnormally high benzodiazepine plasma concentration. A case of accidental drug overdose has been documented in a 19 month old male who ingested 30 mg amlodipine (about 2 mg/kg). During the emergency room presentation, vital signs were stable with no evidence of hypotension, but a heart rate of 180 bpm. Ipecac was administered 3.5 hours after ingestion and on subsequent observation (overnight) no sequelae were noted.
If massive overdose should occur, active cardiac and respiratory monitoring should be instituted. Frequent blood pressure measurements are essential. Should hypotension occur, cardiovascular support including elevation of the extremities and the judicious administration of fluids should be initiated. If hypotension remains unresponsive to these conservative measures, administration of vasopressors (such as phenylephrine), should be considered with attention to circulating volume and urine output. Intravenous calcium gluconate may help to reverse the effects of calcium entry blockade. As NORVASC is highly protein bound, hemodialysis is not likely to be of benefit.

DOSAGE AND ADMINISTRATION

The usual initial antihypertensive oral dose of NORVASC is 5 mg once daily with a maximum dose of 10 mg once daily. Small, fragile, or elderly individuals, or patients with hepatic insufficiency may be started on 2.5 mg once daily and this dose may be used when adding NORVASC to other antihypertensive therapy.
Dosage should be adjusted according to each patient's need. In general, titration should proceed over 7 to 14 days so that the physician can fully assess the patient's response to each dose level. Titration may proceed more rapidly, however, if clinically warranted, provided the patient is assessed frequently.
The recommended dose for chronic stable or vasospastic angina is 5–10 mg, with the lower dose suggested in the elderly and in patients with hepatic insufficiency. Most patients will require 10 mg for adequate effect. See ADVERSE REACTIONS section for information related to dosage and side effects.
Co-administration with Other Antihypertensive and/or Antianginal Drugs: NORVASC has been safely administered with thiazides, ACE inhibitors, beta-blockers, long-acting nitrates, and/or sublingual nitroglycerin.

HOW SUPPLIED

NORVASC®—2.5 mg Tablets (amlodipine besylate equivalent to 2.5 mg of amlodipine per tablet) are supplied as white, diamond, flat-faced, beveled edged engraved with "NORVASC" on one side and "2.5" on the other side and supplied as follows:
NDC 0069-1520-66 Bottle of 100
NORVASC®—5 mg Tablets (amlodipine besylate equivalent to 5 mg of amlodipine per tablet) are white, elongated octagon, flat-faced, beveled edged engraved with both "NORVASC" and "5" on one side and plain on the other side and supplied as follows:
NDC 0069-1530-66 Bottle of 100
NDC 0069-1530-41 Unit Dose package of 100
NDC 0069-1530-72 Bottle of 300
NORVASC®—10 mg Tablets (amlodipine besylate equivalent to 10 mg of amlodipine per tablet) are white, round, flat-faced, beveled edged engraved with both "NORVASC" and "10" on one side and plain on the other side and supplied as follows:
NDC 0069-1540-66 Bottle of 100
NDC 0069-1540-41 Unit Dose package of 100
Store bottles at controlled room temperature, 59° to 86°F (15° to 30°C) and dispense in tight, light-resistant containers (USP).

70-4782-00-4 Revised June 1996
Shown in Product Identification Guide, page 328

Buffered
PFIZERPEN® ℞
(penicillin G potassium)
for Injection

DESCRIPTION

Buffered Pfizerpen (penicillin G potassium) for Injection is a sterile, pyrogen-free powder for reconstitution. Buffered Pfizerpen for Injection is an antibacterial agent for intramuscular, continuous intravenous drip, intrapleural or other local infusion, and intrathecal administration.
Each million units contains approximately 6.8 milligrams of sodium (0.3 mEq) and 65.6 milligrams of potassium (1.68 mEq).
Chemically, Pfizerpen is monopotassium 3,3-dimethyl-7-oxo-6-(2-phenylacetamido)-4-thia-1-azabicyclo (3.2.0) heptane-2-carboxylate. It has a molecular weight of 372.48 and the following chemical structure.

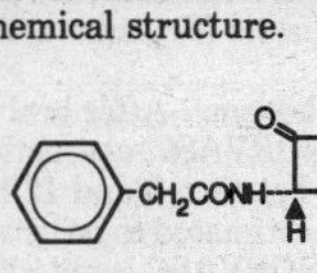

Formula
$C_{16}H_{17}KN_2O_4S$

Penicillin G potassium is a colorless or white crystal, or a white crystalline powder which is odorless, or practically so, and moderately hygroscopic. Penicillin G potassium is very soluble in water. The pH of the reconstituted product is between 6.0–8.5.

CLINICAL PHARMACOLOGY

Aqueous penicillin G is rapidly absorbed following both intramuscular and subcutaneous injection. Initial blood levels following parenteral administration are high but transient. Penicillins bind to serum proteins, mainly albumin. Therapeutic levels of the penicillins are easily achieved under normal circumstances in extracellular fluid and most other body tissues. Penicillins are distributed in varying degrees

into pleural, pericardial, peritoneal, ascitic, synovial, and interstitial fluids. Penicillins are excreted in breast milk. Penetration into the cerebrospinal fluid, eyes, and prostate is poor. Penicillins are rapidly excreted in the urine by glomerular filtration and active tubular secretion, primarily as unchanged drug. Approximately 60 percent of the total dose of 300,000 units is excreted in the urine within this 5 hour period. For this reason high and frequent doses are required to maintain the elevated serum levels desirable in treating certain severe infections in individuals with normal kidney function. In neonates and young infants, and in individuals with impaired kidney function, excretion is considerably delayed.

Microbiology

Penicillin G exerts a bactericidal action against penicillin-susceptible microorganisms during the stage of active multiplication. It acts through the inhibition of biosynthesis of cell wall mucopeptide rendering the cell wall osmotically unstable. It is not active against the penicillinase-producing bacteria, which include many strains of staphylococci. While *in vitro* studies have demonstrated the susceptibility of most strains of the following organisms, clinical efficacy for infections other than those included in the INDICATIONS AND USAGE section has not been documented. Penicillin G exerts high *in vitro* activity against staphylococci (except penicillinase-producing strains), streptococci (groups A, C, G, H, L, and M), and pneumococci. Other organisms susceptible to penicillin G are *N. gonorrhoeae, Corynebacterium diphtheriae, Bacillus anthracis,* Clostridia, *Actinomyces bovis, Streptobacillus moniliformis, Listeria monocytogenes* and Leptospira. *Treponema pallidum* is extremely sensitive to the bactericidal action of penicillin G. Some species of gram-negative bacilli are sensitive to moderate to high concentrations of the drug obtained with intravenous administration. These include most strains of *Escherichia coli;* all strains of *Proteus mirabilis,* Salmonella and Shigella; and some strains of *Aerobacter aerogenes* and *Alcaligenes faecalis.*
Penicillin acts synergistically with gentamicin or tobramycin against many strains of enterococci.

Susceptibility Testing: Penicillin G Susceptibility Powder or 10 units Penicillin G Susceptibility Discs may be used to determine microbial susceptibility to penicillin G using one of the following standard methods recommended by the National Committee for Laboratory Standards:
M2-A3, "Performance Standards for Antimicrobial Disk Susceptibility Tests"
M7-A, "Methods for Dilution Antimicrobial Susceptibility Tests for Bacteria that Grow Aerobically"
M11-A, "Reference Agar Dilution Procedure for Antimicrobial Susceptibility Testing of Anaerobic Bacteria"
M17-P, "Alternative Methods for Antimicrobial Susceptibility Testing of Anaerobic Bacteria"
Tests should be interpreted by the following criteria:

	Zone Diameter, nearest whole mm		
	Susceptible	Moderately Susceptible	Resistant
Staphylococci	≥ 29	—	≤ 28
N. gonorrhoeae	≥ 20	—	≤ 19
Enterococci	—	≥ 15	≤ 14
Non-enterococcal streptococci and *L. monocytogenes*	≥ 28	20–27	≤ 19

	Approximate MIC Correlates	
	Susceptible	Resistant
Staphylococci	≤ 0.1 μg/mL	β-lactamase
N. gonorrhoeae	≤ 0.1 μg/mL	β-lactamase
Enterococci		≥ 16 μg/mL
Non-enterococcal streptococci and *L. monocytogenes*	≤ 0.12 μg/mL	≥ 4 μg/mL

Interpretations of susceptible, intermediate, and resistant correlate zone size diameters with MIC values. A laboratory report of "susceptible" indicates that the suspected causative microorganism most likely will respond to therapy with penicillin G. A laboratory report of "resistant" indicates that the infecting microorganism most likely will not respond to therapy. A laboratory report of "moderately susceptible" indicates that the microorganism is most likely susceptible if a high dosage of penicillin G is used, or if the infection is such that high levels of penicillin G may be attained, as in urine. A report of "intermediate" using the disk diffusion method may be considered an equivocal result, and dilution tests may be indicated.
Control organisms are recommended for susceptibility testing. Each time the test is performed the following organisms should be included. The range for zones of inhibition is shown below;

Control Organism	Zone of Inhibition Range
Staphylococcus aureus (ATCC 25923)	27–35

INDICATIONS AND USAGE

Aqueous penicillin G (parenteral) is indicated in the therapy of severe infections caused by penicillin G-susceptible microorganisms when rapid and high penicillin levels are required in the conditions listed below. Therapy should be guided by bacteriological studies (including susceptibility tests) and by clinical response.
The following infections will usually respond to adequate dosage of aqueous penicillin G (parenteral):
Streptococcal infections.
NOTE: Streptococci in groups A, C, H, G, L, and M are very sensitive to penicillin G. Some group D organisms are sensitive to the high serum levels obtained with aqueous penicillin G.
Aqueous penicillin (parenteral) is the penicillin dosage form of choice for bacteremia, empyema, severe pneumonia, pericarditis, endocarditis, meningitis, and other severe infections caused by sensitive strains of the gram-positive species listed above.
Pneumococcal infections.
Staphylococcal infections —penicillin G sensitive.
Other infections:
Anthrax.
Actinomycosis.
Clostridial infections (including tetanus).
Diphtheria (to prevent carrier state).
Erysipeloid (*Erysipelothrix insidiosa*) endocarditis.
Fusospirochetal infections—severe infections of the oropharynx (Vincent's), lower respiratory tract and genital area due to *Fusobacterium fusiformisans* spirochetes.
Gram-negative bacillary infections (bateremias)—(*E. coli, A. aerogenes, A. faecalis,* Salmonella, Shigella and *P. mirabilis*).
Listeria infections (*Listeria monocytogenes*).
Meningitis and endocarditis.
Pasteurella infections (*Pasteurella multocida*).
Bacteremia and meningitis.
Rat-bite fever (*Spirillum minus* or *Streptobacillus moniliformis*).
Gonorrheal endocarditis and arthritis (*N. gonorrhoeae*).
Syphilis (*T. pallidum*) including congenital syphilis.
Meningococcic meningitis.
Although no controlled clinical efficacy studies have been conducted, aqueous crystalline penicillin G for injection and penicillin G procaine suspension have been suggested by the American Heart Association and the American Dental Association for use as part of a combined parenteral-oral regimen for prophylaxis against bacterial endocarditis in patients with congenital heart disease or rheumatic, or other acquired valvular heart disease when they undergo dental procedures and surgical procedures of the upper respiratory tract.[1] Since it may happen that *alpha* hemolytic streptococci relatively resistant to penicillin may be found when patients are receiving continuous oral penicillin for secondary prevention of rheumatic fever, prophylactic agents other than penicillin may be chosen for these patients and prescribed in addition to their continuous rheumatic fever prophylactic regimen.
NOTE: When selecting antibiotics for the prevention of bacterial endocarditis the physician or dentist should read the full joint statement of the American Heart Association and the American Dental Association.[1]

CONTRAINDICATIONS

A history of a previous hypersensitivity reaction to any penicillin is a contraindication.

WARNINGS

Serious and occasionally fatal hypersensitivity (anaphylactoid) reactions have been reported in patients on penicillin therapy. These reactions are more likely to occur in individuals with a history of penicillin hypersensitivity and/or a history of sensitivity to multiple allergens. There have been reports of individuals with a history of penicillin hypersensitivity who have experienced severe reactions when treated with cephalosporins. Before initiating therapy with any penicillin, careful inquiry should be made concerning previous hypersensitivity reactions to penicillin, cephalosporins, or other allergens. If an allergic reaction occurs, the drug should be discontinued and the appropriate therapy instituted. Serious anaphylactoid reactions require immediate emergency treatment with epinephrine. Oxygen, intravenous steroids, and airway management including intubation, should also be administered as indicated.

PRECAUTIONS

General: Penicillin should be used with caution in individuals with histories of significant allergies and/or asthma.
Intramuscular Therapy: Care should be taken to avoid intravenous or accidental intraarterial administration, or injection into or near major peripheral nerves or blood vessels, since such injections may produce neurovascular damage. Particular care should be taken with IV administration because of the possibility of thrombophlebitis.

In streptococcal infections, therapy must be sufficient to eliminate the organism (10 days minimum) otherwise the sequelae of streptococcal disease may occur. Cultures should be taken following the completion of treatment to determine whether streptococci have been eradicated.
The use of antibiotics may result in overgrowth of nonsusceptible organisms. Constant observation of the patient is essential. If new infections due to bacteria or fungi appear during therapy, the drug should be discontinued and appropriate measures taken. Whenever allergic reactions occur, penicillin should be withdrawn unless, in the opinion of the physician, the condition being treated is life threatening and amenable only to penicillin therapy.
Aqueous penicillin G by the intravenous route in high doses (above 10 million units), should be administered slowly because of the adverse effects of electrolyte imbalance from either the potassium or sodium content of the penicillin. Potassium penicillin G contains 1.7 mEq potassium and 0.3 mEq sodium per million units. The patient's renal, cardiac, and vascular status should be evaluated and if impairment of function is suspected or known to exist a reduction in the total dosage should be considered. Frequent evaluation of electrolyte balance, renal and hematopoietic function is recommended during therapy when high doses of intravenous aqueous penicillin G are used.
Laboratory Tests: In prolonged therapy with penicillin, periodic evaluation of the renal, hepatic, and hematopoietic systems is recommended for organ system dysfunction. This is particularly important in prematures, neonates and other infants, and when high doses are used.
Positive Coomb's tests have been reported after large intravenous doses.
Monitor serum potassium and implement corrective measures when necessary.
When treating gonococcal infections in which primary and secondary syphilis are suspected, proper diagnostic procedures, including dark field examinations, should be done before receiving penicillin and monthly serological tests made for at least four months. All cases of penicillin treated syphilis should receive clinical and serological examinations every six months for two to three years.
In suspected staphylococcal infections, proper laboratory studies, including susceptibility tests, should be performed.
In streptococcal infections, cultures should be taken following completion of treatment to determine whether streptococci have been eradicated. Therapy must be sufficient to eliminate the organism (a minimum of 10 days), otherwise the sequelae of streptococcal disease (e.g., endocarditis, rheumatic fever) may occur.
Drug Interactions: Concurrent administration of bacteriostatic antibiotics (e.g., erythromycin, tetracycline) may diminish the bactericidal effects of penicillins by slowing the rate of bacterial growth. Bactericidal agents work most effectively against the immature cell wall of rapidly proliferating microorganisms. This has been demonstrated *in vitro:* however, the clinical significance of this interaction is not well documented. There are few clinical situations in which the concurrent use of "static" and "cidal" antibiotics are indicated. However, in selected circumstances in which such therapy is appropriate, using adequate doses of antibacterial agents and beginning penicillin therapy first, should minimize the potential for interaction.
Penicillin blood levels may be prolonged by concurrent administration of probenecid which blocks the renal tubular secretion of penicillins.
Displacement of penicillin from plasma protein binding sites will elevate the level of free penicillin in the serum.
Carcinogenesis, Mutagenesis, Impairment of Fertility: No information on long-term studies are available on the carcinogenesis, mutagenesis, or the impairment of fertility with the use of penicillins.
Pregnancy Category B—*Teratogenic Effects:* Reproduction studies performed in the mouse, rat, and rabbit have revealed no evidence of impaired fertility or harm to the fetus due to penicillin G. Human experience with the penicillins during pregnancy has not shown any positive evidence of adverse effects on the fetus. There are, however, no adequate and well controlled studies in pregnant women showing conclusively that harmful effects of these drugs on the fetus can be excluded. Because animal reproduction studies are not always predictive of human response, this drug should be used during pregnancy only if clearly needed.
Nursing Mothers: Penicillins are excreted in human milk. Caution should be exercised when penicillin G is administered to a nursing woman.
Pediatric Use: Penicillins are excreted largely unchanged by the kidney. Because of incompletely developed renal function in infants, the rate of elimination will be slow. Use caution in administering to newborns and evaluate organ system function frequently.

ADVERSE REACTIONS

Penicillin is a substance of low toxicity but does have a significant index of sensitization. The following hypersensitivity

Continued on next page

Pfizer Inc—Cont.

Approx. Desired Concentration (units/ml)	Approx. Volume (ml) 1,000,000 units	Solvent for Vial of 5,000,000 units	Infusion Only 20,000,000 units
50,000	20.0	—	—
100,000	10.0	—	—
250,000	4.0	18.2	75.0
500,000	1.8	8.2	33.0
750,000	—	4.8	—
1,000,000	—	3.2	11.5

reactions have been reported: skin rashes ranging from maculopapular eruptions to exfoliative dermatitis; urticaria; and reactions resembling serum sickness, including chills, fever, edema, arthralgia and prostration. Severe and occasionally fatal anaphylaxis has occurred (see WARNINGS).

Hemolytic anemia, leucopenia, thrombocytopenia, nephropathy, and neuropathy are rarely observed adverse reactions and are usually associated with high intravenous dosage. Patients given continuous intravenous therapy with penicillin G potassium in high dosage (10 million to 100 million units daily) may suffer severe or even fatal potassium poisoning, particularly if renal insufficiency is present. Hyperreflexia, convulsions and coma may be indicative of this syndrome.

Cardiac arrhythmias and cardiac arrest may also occur. (High dosage of penicillin G sodium may result in congestive heart failure due to high sodium intake.)

The Jarisch-Herxheimer reaction has been reported in patients treated for syphilis.

OVERDOSAGE

Neurological adverse reactions, including convulsions, may occur with the attainment of high CSF levels of beta-lactams. In case of overdosage, discontinue medication, treat symptomatically, and institute supportive measures as required. Penicillin G potassium is hemodialyzable.

DOSAGE AND ADMINISTRATION

Severe infections due to Susceptible Strains of Streptococci, Pneumococci and Staphylococci—bacteremia, pneumonia, endocarditis, pericarditis, empyema, meningitis and other severe infections—a minimum of 5 million units daily.

Syphilis—Aqueous penicillin G may be used in the treatment of acquired and congenital syphilis, but because of the necessity of frequent dosage, hospitalization is recommended. Dosage and duration of therapy will be determined by age of patient and stage of the disease.

Gonorrheal endocarditis—a minimum of 5 million units daily.

Meningococcic meningitis—1–2 million units intramuscularly every 2 hours, or continuous IV drip of 20–30 million units/day.

Actinomycosis—1–6 million units/day for cervicofacial cases; 10–20 million units/day for thoracic and abdominal disease.

Clostridial infections—20 million units/day; penicillin is adjunctive therapy to antitoxin.

Fusospirochetal infections—severe infections of oropharynx, lower respiratory tract and genital area—5–10 million units/day.

Rat-bite fever (*Spirillum minus* or *Streptobacillus moniliformis*)—12–15 million units/day for 3–4 weeks.

Listeria infections (*Listeria monocytogenes*).

Neonates—500,000 to 1 million units/day.

Adults with meningitis—15–20 million units/day for 2 weeks.

Adults with endocarditis—15–20 million units/day for 4 weeks.

Pasteurella infections (*Pasteurella multocida*).

Bacteremia and meningitis—4–6 million units/day for 2 weeks.

Erysipeloid (*Erysipelothrix insidiosa*).

Endocarditis—2–20 million units/day for 4–6 weeks.

Gram-negative bacillary infections (*E. coli, Enterobacter aerogenes, A. faecalis,* Salmonella, Shigella and *Proteus mirabilis*).

Bacteremia—20–80 million units/day.

Diphtheria (carrier state): 300,000–400,000 units of penicillin/day in divided doses for 10–12 days.

Anthrax—A minimum of 5 million units of penicillin/day in divided doses until cure is effected.

For prophylaxis against bacterial endocarditis[1] in patients with congenital heart disease or rheumatic, or other acquired valvular heart disease when undergoing dental procedures or surgical procedures of the upper respiratory tract, use a combined parenteral-oral regimen. One million units of aqueous crystalline penicillin G (30,000 units/kg in children) intramuscularly mixed with 600,000 units procaine penicillin G (600,000 units for children) should be given one-half to one hour before the procedure. Oral penicillin V (phenoxymethyl penicillin), 500 mg for adults or 250 mg for children less than 60 lb, should be given every 6 hours for 8 doses. Doses for children should not exceed recommendations for adults for a single dose or for a 24 hour period.

Reconstitution

The following table shows the amount of solvent required for solution of various concentrations.

[See table above.]

When the required volume of solvent is greater than the capacity of the vial, the penicillin can be dissolved by first injecting only a portion of the solvent into the vial, then withdrawing the resultant solution and combining it with the remainder of the solvent in a larger sterile container.

Buffered Pfizerpen (penicillin G potassium) for Injection is highly water soluble. It may be dissolved in small amounts of Water for Injection, or Sterile Isotonic Sodium Chloride Solution for Parenteral Use. All solutions should be stored in a refrigerator. When refrigerated, penicillin solutions may be stored for seven days without significant loss of potency.

Buffered Pfizerpen for Injection may be given intramuscularly or by continuous intravenous drip for dosages of 500,000, 1,000,000, or 5,000,000 units. It is also suitable for intrapleural, intraarticular, and other local instillations.

THE 20,000,000 UNIT DOSAGE MAY BE ADMINISTERED BY INTRAVENOUS INFUSION ONLY.

(1) Intramuscular Injection: Keep total volume of injection small. The intramuscular route is the preferred route of administration. Solutions containing up to 100,000 units of penicillin per ml of diluent may be used with a minimum of discomfort. Greater concentration of penicillin G per ml is physically possible and may be employed where therapy demands. When large dosages are required, it may be advisable to administer aqueous solutions of penicillin by means of continuous intravenous drip.

(2) Continuous Intravenous Drip: Determine the volume of fluid and rate of its administration required by the patient in a 24-hour period in the usual manner for fluid therapy, and add the appropriate daily dosage of penicillin to this fluid. For example, if an adult patient requires 2 liters of fluid in 24 hours and a daily dosage of 10 million units of penicillin, add 5 million units to 1 liter and adjust the rate of flow so that the liter will be infused in 12 hours.

(3) Intrapleural or Other Local Infusion: If fluid is aspirated, give infusion in a volume equal to $^1/_4$ or $^1/_2$ the amount of fluid aspirated, otherwise, prepare as for intramuscular injection.

(4) Intrathecal Use: The intrathecal use of penicillin in meningitis must be highly individualized. It should be employed only with full consideration of the possible irritating effects of penicillin when used by this route. The preferred route of therapy in bacterial meningitides is intravenous, supplemented by intramuscular injection.

Parenteral drug products should be inspected visually for particulate matter and discoloration prior to administration, whenever solution and container permit.

Sterile solution may be left in refrigerator for one week without significant loss of potency.

HOW SUPPLIED

Buffered Pfizerpen (penicillin G potassium) for Injection is available in vials containing respectively 5,000,000 units × 10's (NDC 0049-0520-83), 20,000,000 units × 1's (NDC 0049-0530-28), and a bulk pharmacy package of 20,000,000 units × 10's (NDC 0049-0530-83) of dry powder for reconstitution; buffered with sodium citrate and citric acid to an optimum pH.

Each million units contains approximately 6.8 milligrams of sodium (0.3 mEq) and 65.6 milligrams of potassium (1.68 mEq).

Store the dry powder below 86°F (30°C).

REFERENCE

1. American Heart Association. 1977. Prevention of bacterial endocarditis. Circulation. 56:139A–143A.

Revised April 1987 70-4209-00-5

PROCARDIA® ℞
[pro-car 'dē-ă]
nifedipine
CAPSULES
For Oral Use

DESCRIPTION

PROCARDIA® (nifedipine) is an antianginal drug belonging to a class of pharmacological agents, the calcium channel blockers. Nifedipine is 3,5-pyridinedicarboxylic acid, 1,4-dihydro-2, 6-dimethyl-4-(2-nitrophenyl)-, dimethyl ester, $C_{17}H_{18}N_2O_6$, and has the structural formula:

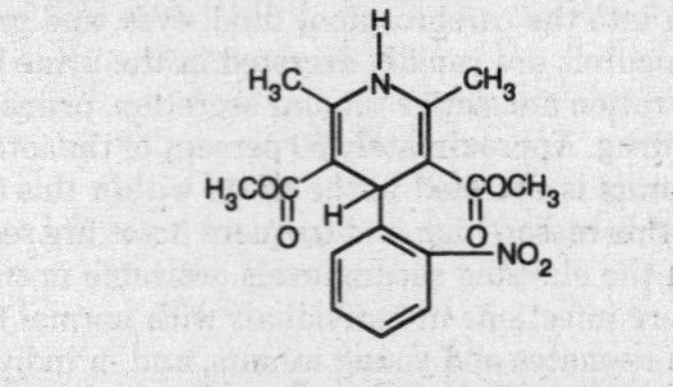

Nifedipine is a yellow crystalline substance, practically insoluble in water but soluble in ethanol. It has a molecular weight of 346.3. PROCARDIA capsules are formulated as soft gelatin capsules for oral administration each containing 10 mg or 20 mg nifedipine.

Inert ingredients in the formulations are: glycerin; peppermint oil; polyethylene glycol; soft gelatin capsules (which contain Yellow 6, and may contain Red Ferric Oxide and other inert ingredients), and water. The 10 mg capsules also contain saccharin sodium.

CLINICAL PHARMACOLOGY

PROCARDIA is a calcium ion influx inhibitor (slow channel blocker or calcium ion antagonist) and inhibits the transmembrane influx of calcium ions into cardiac muscle and smooth muscle. The contractile processes of cardiac muscle and vascular smooth muscle are dependent upon the movement of extracellular calcium ions into these cells through specific ion channels. PROCARDIA selectively inhibits calcium ion influx across the cell membrane of cardiac muscle and vascular smooth muscle without changing serum calcium concentrations.

Mechanism of Action

The precise means by which this inhibition relieves angina has not been fully determined, but includes at least the following two mechanisms:

1) Relaxation and Prevention of Coronary Artery Spasm

PROCARDIA dilates the main coronary arteries and coronary arterioles, both in normal and ischemic regions, and is a potent inhibitor of coronary artery spasm, whether spontaneous or ergonovine-induced. This property increases myocardial oxygen delivery in patients with coronary artery spasm, and is responsible for the effectiveness of PROCARDIA in vasospastic (Prinzmetal's or variant) angina. Whether this effect plays any role in classical angina is not clear, but studies of exercise tolerance have not shown an increase in the maximum exercise rate-pressure product, a widely accepted measure of oxygen utilization. This suggests that, in general, relief of spasm or dilation of coronary arteries is not an important factor in classical angina.

2) Reduction of Oxygen Utilization

PROCARDIA regularly reduces arterial pressure at rest and at a given level of exercise by dilating peripheral arterioles and reducing the total peripheral resistance (afterload) against which the heart works. This unloading of the heart reduces myocardial energy consumption and oxygen requirements and probably accounts for the effectiveness of PROCARDIA in chronic stable angina.

Pharmacokinetics and Metabolism

PROCARDIA is rapidly and fully absorbed after oral administration. The drug is detectable in serum 10 minutes after oral administration, and peak blood levels occur in approximately 30 minutes. Bioavailability is proportional to dose from 10 to 30 mg; half-life does not change significantly with dose. There is little difference in relative bioavailability when PROCARDIA capsules are given orally and either swallowed whole, bitten and swallowed, or, bitten and held sublingually. However, biting through the capsule prior to swallowing does result in slightly earlier plasma concentrations (27 ng/mL 10 minutes after 10 mg) than if capsules are swallowed intact. It is highly bound by serum proteins. PROCARDIA is extensively converted to inactive metabolites and approximately 80 percent of PROCARDIA and metabolites are eliminated via the kidneys. The half-life of nifedipine in plasma is approximately two hours. Since hepatic biotransformation is the predominant route for the disposition of nifedipine, the pharmacokinetics may be altered in patients with chronic liver disease. Patients with hepatic impairment (liver cirrhosis) have a longer disposition half-life and higher bioavailability of nifedipine than healthy volunteers. The degree of serum protein binding of nifedipine is high (92–98%). Protein binding may be greatly reduced in patients with renal or hepatic impairment.

Hemodynamics

Like other slow channel blockers, PROCARDIA exerts a negative inotropic effect on isolated myocardial tissue. This is rarely, if ever, seen in intact animals or man, probably because of reflex responses to its vasodilating effects. In man, PROCARDIA causes decreased peripheral vascular resistance and a fall in systolic and diastolic pressure, usually modest (5–10mm Hg systolic), but sometimes larger. There is usually a small increase in heart rate, a reflex response to vasodilation. Measurements of cardiac function in patients with normal ventricular function have generally found a

small increase in cardiac index without major effects on ejection fraction, left ventricular end diastolic pressure (LVEDP) or volume (LVEDV). In patients with impaired ventricular function, most acute studies have shown some increase in ejection fraction and reduction in left ventricular filling pressure.

Electrophysiologic Effects

Although like other members of its class, PROCARDIA decreases sinoatrial node function and atrioventricular conduction in isolated myocardial preparations, such effects have not been seen in studies in intact animals or in man. In formal electrophysiologic studies, predominantly in patients with normal conduction systems, PROCARDIA has had no tendency to prolong atrioventricular conduction, prolong sinus node recovery time, or slow sinus rate.

INDICATIONS AND USAGE

I. Vasospastic Angina

PROCARDIA (nifedipine) is indicated for the management of vasospastic angina confirmed by any of the following criteria: 1) classical pattern of angina at rest accompanied by ST segment elevation, 2) angina or coronary artery spasm provoked by ergonovine, or 3) angiographically demonstrated coronary artery spasm. In those patients who have had angiography, the presence of significant fixed obstructive disease is not incompatible with the diagnosis of vasospastic angina, provided that the above criteria are satisfied. PROCARDIA may also be used where the clinical presentation suggests a possible vasospastic component but where vasospasm has not been confirmed, e.g., where pain has a variable threshold on exertion or when angina is refractory to nitrates and/or adequate doses of beta blockers.

II. Chronic Stable Angina

(Classical Effort-Associated Angina)

PROCARDIA is indicated for the management of chronic stable angina (effort-associated angina) without evidence of vasospasm in patients who remain symptomatic despite adequate doses of beta blockers and/or organic nitrates or who cannot tolerate those agents.

In chronic stable angina (effort-associated angina) PROCARDIA has been effective in controlled trials of up to eight weeks duration in reducing angina frequency and increasing exercise tolerance, but confirmation of sustained effectiveness and evaluation of long term safety in these patients are incomplete.

Controlled studies in small numbers of patients suggest concomitant use of PROCARDIA and beta blocking agents may be beneficial in patients with chronic stable angina, but available information is not sufficient to predict with confidence the effects of concurrent treatment, especially in patients with compromised left ventricular function or cardiac conduction abnormalities. When introducing such concomitant therapy, care must be taken to monitor blood pressure closely since severe hypotension can occur from the combined effects of the drugs. (See WARNINGS.)

CONTRAINDICATIONS

Known hypersensitivity reaction to PROCARDIA.

WARNINGS

Excessive Hypotension

Although in most patients, the hypotensive effect of PROCARDIA is modest and well tolerated, occasional patients have had excessive and poorly tolerated hypotension. These responses have usually occurred during initial titration or at the time of subsequent upward dosage adjustment. Although patients have rarely experienced excessive hypotension on PROCARDIA alone, this may be more common in patients on concomitant beta-blocker therapy. Although not approved for this purpose, PROCARDIA and other immediate-release nifedipine capsules have been used (orally and sublingually) for acute reduction of blood pressure. Several well-documented reports describe cases of profound hypotension, myocardial infarction, and death when immediate-release nifedipine was used in this way. **PROCARDIA capsules should not be used for the acute reduction of blood pressure.**

PROCARDIA and other immediate-release nifedipine capsules have also been used for the long-term control of essential hypertension, although no properly-controlled studies have been conducted to define an appropriate dose or dose interval for such treatment. **PROCARDIA capsules should not be used for the control of essential hypertension.**

Several well-controlled, randomized trials studied the use of immediate-release nifedipine in patients who had just sustained myocardial infarctions. In none of these trials did immediate-release nifedipine appear to provide any benefit. In some of the trials, patients who received immediate-release nifedipine had significantly worse outcomes than patients who received placebo. **PROCARDIA capsules should not be administered within the first week or two after myocardial infarction, and it should also be avoided in the setting of acute coronary syndrome (when infarction may be imminent).**

Severe hypotension and/or increased fluid volume requirements have been reported in patients receiving PROCARDIA together with a beta blocking agent who un-

derwent coronary artery bypass surgery using high dose fentanyl anesthesia. The interaction with high dose fentanyl appears to be due to the combination of PROCARDIA and a beta blocker, but the possibility that it may occur with PROCARDIA alone, with low doses of fentanyl, in other surgical procedures, or with other narcotic analgesics cannot be ruled out. In PROCARDIA treated patients where surgery using high dose fentanyl anesthesia is contemplated, the physician should be aware of these potential problems and, if the patient's condition permits, sufficient time (at least 36 hours) should be allowed for PROCARDIA to be washed out of the body prior to surgery.

Increased Angina and/or Myocardial Infarction

Rarely, patients, particularly those who have severe obstructive coronary artery disease, have developed well documented increased frequency, duration and/or severity of angina or acute myocardial infarction on starting PROCARDIA or at the time of dosage increase. The mechanism of this effect is not established.

Beta Blocker Withdrawal

Patients recently withdrawn from beta blockers may develop a withdrawal syndrome with increased angina, probably related to increased sensitivity to catecholamines. Initiation of PROCARDIA treatment will not prevent this occurrence and might be expected to exacerbate it by provoking reflex catecholamine release. There have been occasional reports of increased angina in a setting of beta blocker withdrawal and PROCARDIA initiation. It is important to taper beta blockers if possible, rather than stopping them abruptly before beginning PROCARDIA.

Congestive Heart Failure

Rarely, patients, usually receiving a beta blocker, have developed heart failure after beginning PROCARDIA. Patients with tight aortic stenosis may be at greater risk for such an event, as the unloading effect of PROCARDIA would be expected to be of less benefit to these patients, owing to their fixed impedance to flow across the aortic valve.

PRECAUTIONS

General: Hypotension: Because PROCARDIA decreases peripheral vascular resistance, careful monitoring of blood pressure during the initial administration and titration of PROCARDIA is suggested. Close observation is especially recommended for patients already taking medications that are known to lower blood pressure. (See WARNINGS.)

Peripheral Edema: Mild to moderate peripheral edema, typically associated with arterial vasodilation and not due to left ventricular dysfunction, occurs in about one in ten patients treated with PROCARDIA (nifedipine). This edema occurs primarily in the lower extremities and usually responds to diuretic therapy. With patients whose angina is complicated by congestive heart failure, care should be taken to differentiate this peripheral edema from the effects of increasing left ventricular dysfunction.

Laboratory Tests: Rare, usually transient, but occasionally significant elevations of enzymes such as alkaline phosphatase, CPK, LDH, SGOT and SGPT have been noted. The relationship to PROCARDIA therapy is uncertain in most cases, but probable in some. These laboratory abnormalities have rarely been associated with clinical symptoms, however, cholestasis with or without jaundice has been reported. Rare instances of allergic hepatitis have been reported.

PROCARDIA, like other calcium channel blockers, decreases platelet aggregation *in vitro*. Limited clinical studies have demonstrated a moderate but statistically significant decrease in platelet aggregation and increase in bleeding time in some PROCARDIA patients. This is thought to be a function of inhibition of calcium transport across the platelet membrane. No clinical significance for these findings has been demonstrated.

Positive direct Coombs Test with/without hemolytic anemia has been reported but a causal relationship between PROCARDIA administration and positivity of this laboratory test, including hemolysis, could not be determined.

Although PROCARDIA has been used safely in patients with renal dysfunction and has been reported to exert a beneficial effect in certain cases, rare, reversible elevations in BUN and serum creatinine have been reported in patients with pre-existing chronic renal insufficiency. The relationship to PROCARDIA therapy is uncertain in most cases but probable in some.

Drug Interactions: Beta-adrenergic blocking agents: (See INDICATIONS and WARNINGS.) Experience in over 1400 patients in a non-comparative clinical trial has shown that concomitant administration of PROCARDIA and beta-blocking agents is usually well tolerated, but there have been occasional literature reports suggesting that the combination may increase the likelihood of congestive heart failure, severe hypotension or exacerbation of angina.

Long acting nitrates: PROCARDIA may be safely co-administered with nitrates, but there have been no controlled studies to evaluate the antianginal effectiveness of this combination.

Digitalis: Since there have been isolated reports of patients with elevated digoxin levels, and there is a possible interaction between digoxin and nifedipine, it is recommended that

digoxin levels be monitored when initiating, adjusting, and discontinuing nifedipine to avoid possible over- or under-digitalization.

Quinidine: There have been rare reports of an interaction between quinidine and nifedipine (with a decreased plasma level of quinidine).

Coumarin anticoagulants: There have been rare reports of increased prothrombin time in patients taking coumarin anticoagulants to whom PROCARDIA was administered. However, the relationship to PROCARDIA therapy is uncertain.

Cimetidine: A study in six healthy volunteers has shown a significant increase in peak nifedipine plasma levels (80%) and area-under-the-curve (74%) after a one week course of cimetidine at 1000 mg per day and nifedipine at 40 mg per day. Ranitidine produced smaller, non-significant increases. The effect may be mediated by the known inhibition of cimetidine on hepatic cytochrome P-450, the enzyme system probably responsible for the first-pass metabolism of nifedipine. If nifedipine therapy is initiated in a patient currently receiving cimetidine, cautious titration is advised.

Carcinogenesis, Mutagenesis, Impairment of Fertility: Nifedipine was administered orally to rats for two years and was not shown to be carcinogenic. When given to rats prior to mating, nifedipine caused reduced fertility at a dose approximately 30 times the maximum recommended human dose. There is a literature report of reversible reduction in the ability of human sperm obtained from a limited number of infertile men taking recommended doses of nifedipine to bind to and fertilize an ovum *in vitro*. *In vivo* mutagenicity studies were negative.

Pregnancy: Pregnancy Category C: Nifedipine has been shown to produce teratogenic findings in rats and rabbits, including digital anomalies similar to those reported for phenytoin. Digital anomalies have been reported to occur with other members of the dihydropyridine class and are possibly a result of compromised uterine blood flow. Nifedipine administration was associated with a variety of embryotoxic, placentotoxic, and fetotoxic effects, including stunted fetuses (rats, mice, rabbits), rib deformities (mice), cleft palate (mice), small placentas and underdeveloped chorionic villi (monkeys), embryonic and fetal deaths (rats, mice, rabbits), and prolonged pregnancy/decreased neonatal survival (rats; not evaluated in other species). On a mg/kg basis, all of the doses associated with the teratogenic embryotoxic or fetotoxic effects in animals were higher (3.5 to 42 times) than the maximum recommended human dose of 120 mg/day. On a mg/m^2 basis, some doses were higher and some were lower than the maximum recommended human dose but all are within an order of magnitude of it. The doses associated with placentotoxic effects in monkeys were equivalent to or lower than the maximum recommended human dose on mg/m^2 basis.

There are no adequate and well-controlled studies in pregnant women. PROCARDIA should be used during pregnancy only if the potential benefit justifies the potential risk to the fetus.

ADVERSE REACTIONS

In multiple-dose U.S. and foreign controlled studies in which adverse reactions were reported spontaneously, adverse effects were frequent but generally not serious and rarely required discontinuation of therapy or dosage adjustment. Most were expected consequences of the vasodilator effects of PROCARDIA.

Adverse Effect	PROCARDIA (%) (N=226)	Placebo (%) (N=235)
Dizziness, lightheadedness, giddiness	27	15
Flushing, heat sensation	25	8
Headache	23	20
Weakness	12	10
Nausea, heartburn	11	8
Muscle cramps, tremor	8	3
Peripheral edema	7	1
Nervousness, mood changes	7	4
Palpitation	7	5
Dyspnea, cough, wheezing	6	3
Nasal congestion, sore throat	6	8

There is also a large uncontrolled experience in over 2100 patients in the United States. Most of the patients had vasospastic or resistant angina pectoris, and about half had concomitant treatment with beta-adrenergic blocking agents. The most common adverse events were:

Incidence Approximately 10%
Cardiovascular: peripheral edema
Central Nervous System: dizziness or lightheadedness
Gastrointestinal: nausea
Systemic: headache and flushing, weakness
Incidence Approximately 5%
Cardiovascular: transient hypotension

Continued on next page

Pfizer Inc—Cont.

Incidence 2% or Less
Cardiovascular: palpitation
Respiratory: nasal and chest congestion, shortness of breath
Gastrointestinal: diarrhea, constipation, cramps, flatulence
Musculoskeletal: inflammation, joint stiffness, muscle cramps
Central Nervous System: shakiness, nervousness, jitteriness, sleep disturbances, blurred vision, difficulties in balance
Other: dermatitis, pruritus, urticaria, fever, sweating, chills, sexual difficulties.

Incidence Approximately 0.5%
Cardiovascular: syncope (mostly with initial dosing and/or an increase in dose), erythromelalgia.

Incidence Less Than 0.5%
Hematologic: thrombocytopenia, anemia, leukopenia, purpura
Gastrointestinal: allergic hepatitis
Face and Throat: angioedema (mostly oropharyngeal edema with breathing difficulty in a few patients), gingival hyperplasia.
CNS: depression, paranoid syndrome
Special Senses: transient blindness at the peak of plasma level, tinnitus
Urogenital: nocturia, polyuria
Other: arthritis with ANA (+), exfoliative dermatitis, gynecomastia
Musculoskeletal: myalgia

Several of these side effects appear to be dose related. Peripheral edema occurred in about one in 25 patients at doses less than 60 mg per day and in about one patient in eight at 120 mg per day or more. Transient hypotension, generally of mild to moderate severity and seldom requiring discontinuation of therapy, occurred in one of 50 patients at less than 60 mg per day and in one of 20 patients at 120 mg per day or more.

Very rarely, introduction of PROCARDIA therapy was associated with an increase in anginal pain, possibly due to associated hypotension. Transient unilateral loss of vision has also occurred.

In addition, more serious adverse events were observed, not readily distinguishable from the natural history of the disease in these patients. It remains possible, however, that some or many of these events were drug related. Myocardial infarction occurred in about 4% of patients and congestive heart failure or pulmonary edema in about 2%. Ventricular arrhythmias or conduction disturbances each occurred in fewer than 0.5% of patients.

In a subgroup of over 1000 patients receiving PROCARDIA with concomitant beta blocker therapy, the pattern and incidence of adverse experiences was not different from that of the entire group of PROCARDIA (nifedipine) treated patients. (See PRECAUTIONS.)

In a subgroup of approximately 250 patients with a diagnosis of congestive heart failure as well as angina pectoris (about 10% of the total patient population), dizziness or lightheadedness, peripheral edema, headache or flushing each occurred in one in eight patients. Hypotension occurred in about one in 20 patients. Syncope occurred in approximately one patient in 250. Myocardial infarction or symptoms of congestive heart failure each occurred in about one patient in 15. Atrial or ventricular dysrhythmias each occurred in about one patient in 150.

OVERDOSAGE

Experience with nifedipine overdosage is limited. Generally, overdosage with nifedipine leading to pronounced hypotension calls for active cardiovascular support including monitoring of cardiovascular and respiratory function, elevation of extremities, and judicious use of calcium infusion, pressor agents and fluids. Clearance of nifedipine would be expected to be prolonged in patients with impaired liver function. Since nifedipine is highly protein bound, dialysis is not likely to be of any benefit; however, plasmapheresis may be beneficial.

DOSAGE AND ADMINISTRATION

The dosage of PROCARDIA needed to suppress angina and that can be tolerated by the patient must be established by titration. Excessive doses can result in hypotension.

Therapy should be initiated with the 10 mg capsule. The starting dose is one 10 mg capsule, swallowed whole, 3 times/day. The usual effective dose range is 10–20 mg three times daily. Some patients, especially those with evidence of coronary artery spasm, respond only to higher doses, more frequent administration, or both. In such patients, doses of 20–30 mg three or four times daily may be effective. Doses above 120 mg daily are rarely necessary. More than 180 mg per day is not recommended.

In most cases, PROCARDIA titration should proceed over a 7–14 day period so that the physician can assess the response to each dose level and monitor the blood pressure before proceeding to higher doses.

If symptoms so warrant, titration may proceed more rapidly provided that the patient is assessed frequently. Based on the patient's physical activity level, attack frequency, and sublingual nitroglycerin consumption, the dose of PROCARDIA may be increased from 10 mg t.i.d. to 20 mg t.i.d. and then to 30 mg t.i.d. over a three-day period.

In hospitalized patients under close observation, the dose may be increased in 10 mg increments over four to six-hour periods as required to control pain and arrhythmias due to ischemia. A single dose should rarely exceed 30 mg.

No "rebound effect" has been observed upon discontinuation of PROCARDIA. However, if discontinuation of PROCARDIA is necessary, sound clinical practice suggests that the dosage should be decreased gradually with close physician supervision.

Co-Administration with Other Antianginal Drugs
Sublingual nitroglycerin may be taken as required for the control of acute manifestations of angina, particularly during PROCARDIA titration. See **Precautions, Drug Interactions,** for information on co-administration of PROCARDIA with beta blockers or long acting nitrates.

HOW SUPPLIED

PROCARDIA® soft gelatin capsules are supplied in:
Bottles of 100:
10 mg (NDC 0069-2600-66) (NDC 59012-260-66) orange #260;
20 mg (NDC 0069-2610-66) (NDC 59012-261-66) orange and light brown #261
Bottles of 300:
10 mg (NDC 0069-2600-72) (NDC 59012-260-72) orange #260;
20 mg (NDC 0069-2610-72) (NDC 59012-261-72) orange and light brown #261
Unit dose packages of 100:
10 mg (NDC 0069-2600-41) (NDC 59012-260-41) orange #260;
20 mg (NDC 0069-2610-41) (NDC 59012-261-41) orange and light brown #261

The capsules should be protected from light and moisture and stored at controlled room temperature 59° to 77°F (15° to 25°C) in the manufacturer's original container.

Pfizer Labs
Division of Pfizer Inc, NY, NY 10017
69-4990-00-7 Revised February 1996
Shown in Product Identification Guide, page 328

PROCARDIA XL® ℞

[*pro-car 'dē-ă*]
(nifedipine)
Extended Release Tablets
For Oral Use

DESCRIPTION

Nifedipine is a drug belonging to a class of pharmacological agents known as the calcium channel blockers. Nifedipine is 3,5-pyridinedicarboxylic acid, 1,4-dihydro-2,6-dimethyl-4-(2-nitrophenyl)-, dimethyl ester, $C_{17}H_{18}N_2O_6$, and has the structural formula:

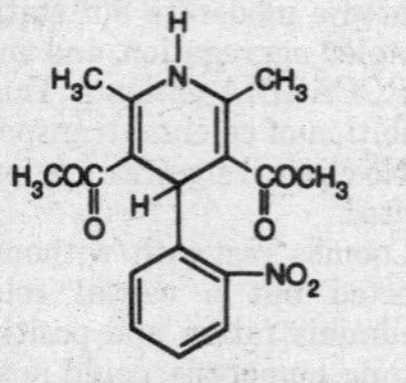

Nifedipine is a yellow crystalline substance, practically insoluble in water but soluble in ethanol. It has a molecular weight of 346.3. PROCARDIA XL is a trademark for Nifedipine GITS. Nifedipine GITS (Gastrointestinal Therapeutic System) Tablet is formulated as a once-a-day controlled-release tablet for oral administration designed to deliver 30, 60, or 90 mg of nifedipine.

Inert ingredients in the formulations are: cellulose acetate; hydroxypropyl cellulose; hydroxypropyl methylcellulose; magnesium stearate; polyethylene glycol; polyethylene oxide; red ferric oxide; sodium chloride; titanium dioxide.

System Components and Performance
PROCARDIA XL Extended Release Tablet is similar in appearance to a conventional tablet. It consists, however, of a semipermeable membrane surrounding an osmotically active drug core. The core itself is divided into two layers: an "active" layer containing the drug, and a "push" layer containing pharmacologically inert (but osmotically active) components. As water from the gastrointestinal tract enters the tablet, pressure increases in the osmotic layer and "pushes" against the drug layer, releasing drug through the precision laser-drilled tablet orifice in the active layer.

PROCARDIA XL Extended Release Tablet is designed to provide nifedipine at an approximately constant rate over 24 hours. This controlled rate of drug delivery into the gastrointestinal lumen is independent of pH or gastrointestinal motility. PROCARDIA XL depends for its action on the existence of an osmotic gradient between the contents of the bi-layer core and fluid in the GI tract. Drug delivery is essentially constant as long as the osmotic gradient remains constant, and then gradually falls to zero. Upon swallowing, the biologically inert components of the tablet remain intact during GI transit and are eliminated in the feces as an insoluble shell.

CLINICAL PHARMACOLOGY

Nifedipine is a calcium ion influx inhibitor (slow-channel blocker or calcium ion antagonist) and inhibits the transmembrane influx of calcium ions into cardiac muscle and smooth muscle. The contractile processes of cardiac muscle and vascular smooth muscle are dependent upon the movement of extracellular calcium ions into these cells through specific ion channels. Nifedipine selectively inhibits calcium ion influx across the cell membrane of cardiac muscle and vascular smooth muscle without altering serum calcium concentrations.

Mechanism of Action

A) Angina
The precise mechanisms by which inhibition of calcium influx relieves angina has not been fully determined, but includes at least the following two mechanisms:

1) Relaxation and Prevention of Coronary Artery Spasm
Nifedipine dilates the main coronary arteries and coronary arterioles, both in normal and ischemic regions, and is a potent inhibitor of coronary artery spasm, whether spontaneous or ergonovine-induced. This property increases myocardial oxygen delivery in patients with coronary artery spasm, and is responsible for the effectiveness of nifedipine in vasospastic (Prinzmetal's or variant) angina. Whether this effect plays any role in classical angina is not clear, but studies of exercise tolerance have not shown an increase in the maximum exercise rate-pressure product, a widely accepted measure of oxygen utilization. This suggests that, in general, relief of spasm or dilation of coronary arteries is not an important factor in classical angina.

2) Reduction of Oxygen Utilization
Nifedipine regularly reduces arterial pressure at rest and at a given level of exercise by dilating peripheral arterioles and reducing the total peripheral vascular resistance (afterload) against which the heart works. This unloading of the heart reduces myocardial energy consumption and oxygen requirements, and probably accounts for the effectiveness of nifedipine in chronic stable angina.

B) Hypertension
The mechanism by which nifedipine reduces arterial blood pressure involves peripheral arterial vasodilatation and the resulting reduction in peripheral vascular resistance. The increased peripheral vascular resistance that is an underlying cause of hypertension results from an increase in active tension in the vascular smooth muscle. Studies have demonstrated that the increase in active tension reflects an increase in cytosolic free calcium.

Nifedipine is a peripheral arterial vasodilator which acts directly on vascular smooth muscle. The binding of nifedipine to voltage-dependent and possibly receptor-operated channels in vascular smooth muscle results in an inhibition of calcium influx through these channels. Stores of intracellular calcium in vascular smooth muscle are limited and thus dependent upon the influx of extracellular calcium for contraction to occur. The reduction in calcium influx by nifedipine causes arterial vasodilation and decreased peripheral vascular resistance which results in reduced arterial blood pressure.

Pharmacokinetics and Metabolism
Nifedipine is completely absorbed after oral administration. Plasma drug concentrations rise at a gradual, controlled rate after a PROCARDIA XL Extended Release Tablet dose and reach a plateau at approximately six hours after the first dose. For subsequent doses, relatively constant plasma concentrations at this plateau are maintained with minimal fluctuations over the 24 hour dosing interval. About a four-fold higher fluctuation index (ratio of peak to trough plasma concentration) was observed with the conventional immediate release Procardia® capsule at t.i.d. dosing than with once daily PROCARDIA XL Extended Release Tablet. At steady-state the bioavailability of the PROCARDIA XL Extended Release Tablet is 86% relative to Procardia capsules. Administration of the PROCARDIA XL Extended Release Tablet in the presence of food slightly alters the early rate of drug absorption, but does not influence the extent of drug bioavailability. Markedly reduced GI retention time over prolonged periods (i.e., short bowel syndrome), however, may influence the pharmacokinetic profile of the drug which could potentially result in lower plasma concentrations. Pharmacokinetics of PROCARDIA XL Extended Release Tablets are linear over the dose range of 30 to 180 mg in that plasma drug concentrations are proportional to dose administered. There was no evidence of dose dumping either in the

presence or absence of food for over 150 subjects in pharmacokinetic studies.

Nifedipine is extensively metabolized to highly water-soluble, inactive metabolites accounting for 60 to 80% of the dose excreted in the urine. The elimination half-life of nifedipine is approximately two hours. Only traces (less than 0.1% of the dose) of unchanged form can be detected in the urine. The remainder is excreted in the feces in metabolized form, most likely as a result of biliary excretion. Thus, the pharmacokinetics of nifedipine are not significantly influenced by the degree of renal impairment. Patients in hemodialysis or chronic ambulatory peritoneal dialysis have not reported significantly altered pharmacokinetics of nifedipine. Since hepatic biotransformation is the predominant route for the disposition of nifedipine, the pharmacokinetics may be altered in patients with chronic liver disease. Patients with hepatic impairment (liver cirrhosis) have a longer disposition half-life and higher bioavailability of nifedipine than healthy volunteers. The degree of serum protein binding of nifedipine is high (92–98%). Protein binding may be greatly reduced in patients with renal or hepatic impairment.

Hemodynamics
Like other slow-channel blockers, nifedipine exerts a negative inotropic effect on isolated myocardial tissue. This is rarely, if ever, seen in intact animals or man, probably because of reflex responses to its vasodilating effects. In man, nifedipine decreases peripheral vascular resistance which leads to a fall in systolic and diastolic pressures, usually minimal in normotensive volunteers (less than 5–10 mm Hg systolic), but sometimes larger. With PROCARDIA XL Extended Release Tablets, these decreases in blood pressure are not accompanied by any significant change in heart rate. Hemodynamic studies in patients with normal ventricular function have generally found a small increase in cardiac index without major effects on ejection fraction, left ventricular end diastolic pressure (LVEDP) or volume (LVEDV). In patients with impaired ventricular function, most acute studies have shown some increase in ejection fraction and reduction in left ventricular filling pressure.

Electrophysiologic Effects
Although, like other members of its class, nifedipine causes a slight depression of sinoatrial node function and atrioventricular conduction in isolated myocardial preparations, such effects have not been seen in studies in intact animals or in man. In formal electrophysiologic studies, predominantly in patients with normal conduction systems, nifedipine has had no tendency to prolong atrioventricular conduction or sinus node recovery time, or to slow sinus rate.

INDICATIONS AND USAGE
I. Vasospastic Angina
PROCARDIA XL is indicated for the management of vasospastic angina confirmed by any of the following criteria: 1) classical pattern of angina at rest accompanied by ST segment elevation, 2) angina or coronary artery spasm provoked by ergonovine, or 3) angiographically demonstrated coronary artery spasm. In those patients who have had angiography, the presence of significant fixed obstructive disease is not incompatible with the diagnosis of vasospastic angina, provided that the above criteria are satisfied. PROCARDIA XL may also be used where the clinical presentation suggests a possible vasospastic component but where vasospasm has not been confirmed, e.g., where pain has a variable threshold on exertion or in unstable angina where electrocardiographic findings are compatible with intermittent vasospasm, or when angina is refractory to nitrates and/or adequate doses of beta blockers.

II. Chronic Stable Angina
(Classical Effort-Associated Angina)
PROCARDIA XL is indicated for the management of chronic stable angina (effort-associated angina) without evidence of vasospasm in patients who remain symptomatic despite adequate doses of beta blockers and/or organic nitrates or who cannot tolerate those agents.
In chronic stable angina (effort-associated angina) nifedipine has been effective in controlled trials of up to eight weeks duration in reducing angina frequency and increasing exercise tolerance, but confirmation of sustained effectiveness and evaluation of long term safety in these patients is incomplete.
Controlled studies in small numbers of patients suggest concomitant use of nifedipine and beta blocking agents may be beneficial in patients with chronic stable angina, but available information is not sufficient to predict with confidence the effects of concurrent treatment, especially in patients with compromised left ventricular function or cardiac conduction abnormalities. When introducing such concomitant therapy, care must be taken to monitor blood pressure closely since severe hypotension can occur from the combined effects of the drugs. (See WARNINGS.)

III. Hypertension
PROCARDIA XL is indicated for the treatment of hypertension. It may be used alone or in combination with other antihypertensive agents.

CONTRAINDICATIONS
Known hypersensitivity reaction to nifedipine.

WARNINGS
Excessive Hypotension
Although in most angina patients the hypotensive effect of nifedipine is modest and well tolerated, occasional patients have had excessive and poorly tolerated hypotension. These responses have usually occurred during initial titration or at the time of subsequent upward dosage adjustment, and may be more likely in patients on concomitant beta blockers. Severe hypotension and/or increased fluid volume requirements have been reported in patients receiving nifedipine together with a beta-blocking agent who underwent coronary artery bypass surgery using high dose fentanyl anesthesia. The interaction with high dose fentanyl appears to be due to the combination of nifedipine and a beta blocker, but the possibility that it may occur with nifedipine alone, with low doses of fentanyl, in other surgical procedures, or with other narcotic analgesics cannot be ruled out. In nifedipine-treated patients where surgery using high dose fentanyl anesthesia is contemplated, the physician should be aware of these potential problems and if the patient's condition permits, sufficient time (at least 36 hours) should be allowed for nifedipine to be washed out of the body prior to surgery.
The following information should be taken into account in those patients who are being treated for hypertension as well as angina:

Increased Angina and/or Myocardial Infarction
Rarely, patients, particularly those who have severe obstructive coronary artery disease, have developed well documented increased frequency, duration and/or severity of angina or acute myocardial infarction on starting nifedipine or at the time of dosage increase. The mechanism of this effect is not established.

Beta Blocker Withdrawal
It is important to taper beta blockers if possible, rather than stopping them abruptly before beginning nifedipine. Patients recently withdrawn from beta blockers may develop a withdrawal syndrome with increased angina, probably related to increased sensitivity to catecholamines. Initiation of nifedipine treatment will not prevent this occurrence and on occasion has been reported to increase it.

Congestive Heart Failure
Rarely, patients usually receiving a beta blocker, have developed heart failure after beginning nifedipine. Patients with tight aortic stenosis may be at greater risk for such an event, as the unloading effect of nifedipine would be expected to be of less benefit to those patients, owing to their fixed impedance to flow across the aortic valve.

PRECAUTIONS
General—Hypotension: Because nifedipine decreases peripheral vascular resistance, careful monitoring of blood pressure during the initial administration and titration of nifedipine is suggested. Close observation is especially recommended for patients already taking medications that are known to lower blood pressure. (See WARNINGS.)
Peripheral Edema: Mild to moderate peripheral edema occurs in a dose dependent manner with an incidence ranging from approximately 10% to about 30% at the highest dose studied (180 mg). It is a localized phenomenon thought to be associated with vasodilation of dependent arterioles and small blood vessels and not due to left ventricular dysfunction or generalized fluid retention. With patients whose angina or hypertension is complicated by congestive heart failure, care should be taken to differentiate this peripheral edema from the effects of increasing left ventricular dysfunction.
Other: As with any other non-deformable material, caution should be used when administering PROCARDIA XL in patients with preexisting severe gastrointestinal narrowing (pathologic or iatrogenic). There have been rare reports of obstructive symptoms in patients with known strictures in association with the ingestion of PROCARDIA XL.
Information for Patients: PROCARDIA XL Extended Release Tablets should be swallowed whole. Do not chew, divide or crush tablets. Do not be concerned if you occasionally notice in your stool something that looks like a tablet. In PROCARDIA XL, the medication is contained within a nonabsorbable shell that has been specially designed to slowly release the drug for your body to absorb. When this process is completed, the empty tablet is eliminated from your body.
Laboratory Tests: Rare, usually transient, but occasionally significant elevations of enzymes such as alkaline phosphatase, CPK, LDH, SGOT and SGPT have been noted. The relationship to nifedipine therapy is uncertain in most cases, but probable in some. These laboratory abnormalities have rarely been associated with clinical symptoms; however, cholestasis with or without jaundice has been reported. A small (5.4%) increase in mean alkaline phosphatase was noted in patients treated with PROCARDIA XL. This was an isolated finding not associated with clinical symptoms and it rarely resulted in values which fell outside the normal range. Rare instances of allergic hepatitis have been reported. In controlled studies, PROCARDIA XL did not adversely affect serum uric acid, glucose, or cholesterol. Serum potassium was unchanged in patients receiving PROCARDIA XL in the absence of concomitant diuretic therapy, and slightly decreased in patients receiving concomitant diuretics.

Nifedipine, like other calcium channel blockers, decreases platelet aggregation in vitro. Limited clinical studies have demonstrated a moderate but statistically significant decrease in platelet aggregation and increase in bleeding time in some nifedipine patients. This is thought to be a function of inhibition of calcium transport across the platelet membrane. No clinical significance for these findings has been demonstrated.

Positive direct Coombs test with/without hemolytic anemia has been reported but a causal relationship between nifedipine administration and positivity of this laboratory test, including hemolysis, could not be determined.

Although nifedipine has been used safely in patients with renal dysfunction and has been reported to exert a beneficial effect in certain cases, rare reversible elevations in BUN and serum creatinine have been reported in patients with preexisting chronic renal insufficiency. The relationship to nifedipine therapy is uncertain in most cases but probable in some.

Drug Interactions: Beta-adrenergic blocking agents: (See INDICATIONS and WARNINGS.) Experience in over 1400 patients with Procardia capsules in a noncomparative clinical trial has shown that concomitant administration of nifedipine and beta-blocking agents is usually well tolerated but there have been occasional literature reports suggesting that the combination may increase the likelihood of congestive heart failure, severe hypotension, or exacerbation of angina.
Long Acting Nitrates: Nifedipine may be safely co-administered with nitrates, but there have been no controlled studies to evaluate the antianginal effectiveness of this combination.
Digitalis: Administration of nifedipine with digoxin increased digoxin levels in nine of twelve normal volunteers. The average increase was 45%. Another investigator found no increase in digoxin levels in thirteen patients with coronary artery disease. In an uncontrolled study of over two hundred patients with congestive heart failure during which digoxin blood levels were not measured, digitalis toxicity was not observed. Since there have been isolated reports of patients with elevated digoxin levels, it is recommended that digoxin levels be monitored when initiating, adjusting, and discontinuing nifedipine to avoid possible over- or underdigitalization.
Coumarin Anticoagulants: There have been rare reports of increased prothrombin time in patients taking coumarin anticoagulants to whom nifedipine was administered. However, the relationship to nifedipine therapy is uncertain.
Cimetidine: A study in six healthy volunteers has shown a significant increase in peak nifedipine plasma levels (80%) and area-under-the-curve (74%), after a one week course of cimetidine at 1000 mg per day and nifedipine at 40 mg per day. Ranitidine produced smaller, non-significant increases. The effect may be mediated by the known inhibition of cimetidine on hepatic cytochrome P-450, the enzyme system probably responsible for the first-pass metabolism of nifedipine. If nifedipine therapy is initiated in a patient currently receiving cimetidine, cautious titration is advised.
Carcinogenesis, Mutagenesis, Impairment of Fertility: Nifedipine was administered orally to rats for two years and was not shown to be carcinogenic. When given to rats prior to mating, nifedipine caused reduced fertility at a dose approximately 30 times the maximum recommended human dose. There is a literature report of reversible reduction in the ability of human sperm obtained from a limited number of infertile men taking recommended doses of nifedipine to bind to and fertilize an ovum in vitro. In vivo mutagenicity studies were negative.
Pregnancy: Pregnancy Category C. Nifedipine has been shown to produce teratogenic findings in rats and rabbits, including digital anomalies similar to those reported for phenytoin. Digital anomalies have been reported to occur with other members of the dihydropyridine class and are possibly a result of compromised uterine blood flow. Nifedipine administration was associated with a variety of embryotoxic, placentotoxic, and fetotoxic effects, including stunted fetuses (rats, mice, rabbits), rib deformities (mice), cleft palate (mice), small placentas and underdeveloped chorionic villi (monkeys), embryonic and fetal deaths (rats, mice, rabbits), and prolonged pregnancy/decreased neonatal survival (rats, not evaluated in other species). On a mg/kg basis, all of the doses associated with the teratogenic embryotoxic or fetotoxic effects in animals were higher (3.5 to 42 times) than the maximum recommended human dose of 120 mg/ day. On a mg/m^2 basis, some doses were higher and some were lower than the maximum recommended human dose but all are within an order of magnitude of it. The doses asso-

Continued on next page

Pfizer Inc—Cont.

ciated with placentotoxic effects in monkeys were equivalent to or lower than the maximum recommended human dose on mg/m^2 basis.
There are no adequate and well-controlled studies in pregnant women. PROCARDIA XL Extended Release Tablets should be used during pregnancy only if the potential benefit justifies the potential risk to the fetus.

ADVERSE EXPERIENCES

Over 1000 patients from both controlled and open trials with PROCARDIA XL Extended Release Tablets in hypertension and angina were included in the evaluation of adverse experiences. All side effects reported during PROCARDIA XL Extended Release Tablet therapy were tabulated independent of their causal relation to medication. The most common side effect reported with PROCARDIA XL was edema which was dose related and ranged in frequency from approximately 10% to about 30% at the highest dose studied (180 mg). Other common adverse experiences reported in placebo-controlled trials include:

Adverse Effect	PROCARDIA XL (%) (N=707)	Placebo (%) (N=266)
Headache	15.8	9.8
Fatigue	5.9	4.1
Dizziness	4.1	4.5
Constipation	3.3	2.3
Nausea	3.3	1.9

Of these, only edema and headache were more common in PROCARDIA XL patients than placebo patients.
The following adverse reactions occurred with an incidence of less than 3.0%. With the exception of leg cramps, the incidence of these side effects was similar to that of placebo alone.
Body as a Whole/Systemic: asthenia, flushing, pain
Cardiovascular: palpitations
Central Nervous System: insomnia, nervousness, paresthesia, somnolence
Dermatologic: pruritus, rash
Gastrointestinal: abdominal pain, diarrhea, dry mouth, dyspepsia, flatulence
Musculoskeletal: arthralgia, leg cramps
Respiratory: chest pain (nonspecific), dyspnea
Urogenital: impotence, polyuria
Other adverse reactions were reported sporadically with an incidence of 1.0% or less. These include:
Body as a Whole/Systemic: face edema, fever, hot flashes, malaise, periorbital edema, rigors
Cardiovascular: arrhythmia, hypotension, increased angina, tachycardia, syncope
Central Nervous System: anxiety, ataxia, decreased libido, depression, hypertonia, hypoesthesia, migraine, paroniria, tremor, vertigo
Dermatologic: alopecia, increased sweating, urticaria, purpura
Gastrointestinal: eructation, gastroesophageal reflux, gum hyperplasia, melena, vomiting, weight increase
Musculoskeletal: back pain, gout, myalgias
Respiratory: coughing, epistaxis, upper respiratory tract infection, respiratory disorder, sinusitis
Special Senses: abnormal lacrimation, abnormal vision, taste perversion, tinnitus
Urogenital/Reproductive: breast pain, dysuria, hematuria, nocturia
Adverse experiences which occurred in less than 1 in 1000 patients cannot be distinguished from concurrent disease states or medications.
The following adverse experiences, reported in less than 1% of patients, occurred under conditions (e.g., open trials, marketing experience) where a causal relationship is uncertain: gastrointestinal irritation, gastrointestinal bleeding.
In multiple-dose U.S. and foreign controlled studies with nifedipine capsules in which adverse reactions were reported spontaneously, adverse effects were frequent but generally not serious and rarely required discontinuation of therapy or dosage adjustment. Most were expected consequences of the vasodilator effects of PROCARDIA.

Adverse Effect	PROCARDIA CAPSULES (%) (N=226)	Placebo (%) (N=235)
Dizziness, lightheadedness, giddiness	27	15
Flushing, heat sensation	25	8
Headache	23	20
Weakness	12	10
Nausea, heartburn	11	8
Muscle cramps, tremor	8	3
Peripheral edema	7	1
Nervousness, mood changes	7	4
Palpitation	7	5
Dyspnea, cough, wheezing	6	3
Nasal congestion, sore throat	6	8

There is also a large uncontrolled experience in over 2100 patients in the United States. Most of the patients had vasospastic or resistant angina pectoris, and about half had concomitant treatment with beta-adrenergic blocking agents. The relatively common adverse events were similar in nature to those seen with PROCARDIA XL.
In addition, more serious adverse events were observed, not readily distinguishable from the natural history of the disease in these patients. It remains possible, however, that some or many of these events were drug related. Myocardial infarction occurred in about 4% of patients and congestive heart failure or pulmonary edema in about 2%. Ventricular arrhythmias or conduction disturbances each occurred in fewer than 0.5% of patients.
In a subgroup of over 1000 patients receiving PROCARDIA with concomitant beta blocker therapy, the pattern and incidence of adverse experiences was not different from that of the entire group of PROCARDIA (nifedipine) treated patients. (See PRECAUTIONS.)
In a subgroup of approximately 250 patients with a diagnosis of congestive heart failure as well as angina, dizziness or lightheadedness, peripheral edema, headache or flushing each occurred in one in eight patients. Hypotension occurred in about one in 20 patients. Syncope occurred in approximately one patient in 250. Myocardial infarction or symptoms of congestive heart failure each occurred in about one patient in 15. Atrial or ventricular dysrhythmias each occurred in about one patient in 150.
In post-marketing experience, there have been rare reports of exfoliative dermatitis caused by nifedipine.

OVERDOSAGE

Experience with nifedipine overdosage is limited. Generally, overdosage with nifedipine leading to pronounced hypotension calls for active cardiovascular support including monitoring of cardiovasular and respiratory function, elevation of extremities, judicious use of calcium infusion, pressor agents and fluids. Clearance of nifedipine would be expected to be prolonged in patients with impaired liver function. Since nifedipine is highly protein-bound, dialysis is not likely to be of any benefit.
There has been one reported case of massive overdosage with PROCARDIA XL Extended Release Tablets. The main effects of ingestion of approximately 4800 mg of PROCARDIA XL in a young man attempting suicide as a result of cocaine-induced depression was initial dizziness, palpitations, flushing, and nervousness. Within several hours of ingestion, nausea, vomiting, and generalized edema developed. No significant hypotension was apparent at presentation, 18 hours post-ingestion. Electrolyte abnormalities consisted of a mild, transient elevation of serum creatinine, and modest elevations of LDH and CPK, but normal SGOT. Vital signs remained stable, no electrocardiographic abnormalities were noted and renal function returned to normal within 24 to 48 hours with routine supportive measures alone. No prolonged sequelae were observed.
The effect of a single 900 mg ingestion of Procardia capsules in a depressed anginal patient also on tricyclic antidepressants was a loss of consciousness within 30 minutes of ingestion, and profound hypotension, which responded to calcium infusion, pressor agents, and fluid replacement. A variety of ECG abnormalities were seen in this patient with a history of bundle branch block, including sinus bradycardia and varying degrees of AV block. These dictated the prophylactic placement of a temporary ventricular pacemaker, but otherwise resolved spontaneously. Significant hyperglycemia was seen initially in this patient, but plasma glucose levels rapidly normalized without further treatment.
A young hypertensive patient with advanced renal failure ingested 280 mg of Procardia capsules at one time, with resulting marked hypotension responding to calcium infusion and fluids. No AV conduction abnormalities, arrhythmias, or pronounced changes in heart rate were noted, nor was there any further deterioration in renal function.

DOSAGE AND ADMINISTRATION

Dosage must be adjusted according to each patient's needs. Therapy for either hypertension or angina should be initiated with 30 or 60 mg once daily. PROCARDIA XL Extended Release Tablets should be swallowed whole and should not be bitten or divided. In general, titration should proceed over a 7–14 day period so that the physician can fully assess the response to each dose level and monitor blood pressure before proceeding to higher doses. Since steady-state plasma levels are achieved on the second day of dosing, if symptoms so warrant, titration may proceed more rapidly provided the patient is assessed frequently. Titration to doses above 120 mg is not recommended.
Angina patients controlled on Procardia capsules alone or in combination with other antianginal medications may be safely switched to PROCARDIA XL Extended Release Tablets at the nearest equivalent total daily dose (e.g., 30 mg t.i.d. of Procardia capsules may be changed to 90 mg once daily of PROCARDIA XL Extended Release Tablets). Subsequent titration to higher or lower doses may be necessary and should be initiated as clinically warranted. Experience with doses greater than 90 mg in patients with angina is limited. Therefore, doses greater than 90 mg should be used with caution and only when clinically warranted.
No "rebound effect" has been observed upon discontinuation of PROCARDIA XL Extended Release Tablets. However, if discontinuation of nifedipine is necessary, sound clinical practice suggests that the dosage should be decreased gradually with close physician supervision.
Care should be taken when dispensing PROCARDIA XL to assure that the extended release dosage form has been prescribed.

Co-Administration with Other Antianginal Drugs
Sublingual nitroglycerin may be taken as required for the control of acute manifestations of angina, particularly during nifedipine titration. See PRECAUTIONS, Drug Interactions, for information on co-administration of nifedipine with beta blockers or long acting nitrates.

HOW SUPPLIED

PROCARDIA XL® Extended Release Tablets are supplied as 30 mg, 60 mg and 90 mg round biconvex, rose-pink, film-coated tablets in:
Bottles of 100:
30 mg (NDC 0069-2650-66) (NDC 59012-265-66)
60 mg (NDC 0069-2660-66) (NDC 59012-266-66)
90 mg (NDC 0069-2670-66) (NDC 59012-267-66)
Bottles of 300:
30 mg (NDC 0069-2650-72) (NDC 59012-265-72)
60 mg (NDC 0069-2660-72) (NDC 59012-266-72)
Bottles of 5000:
30 mg (NDC 0069-2650-94) (NDC 59012-265-94)
60 mg (NDC 0069-2660-94) (NDC 59012-266-94)
Unit dose packages of 100:
30 mg (NDC 0069-2650-41) (NDC 59012-265-41)
60 mg (NDC 0069-2660-41) (NDC 59012-266-41)
90 mg (NDC 0069-2670-41) (NDC 59012-267-41)
Store below 86°F (30°C).
Protect from moisture and humidity.

69-4848-00-3 Revised March 1996
Shown in Product Identification Guide, page 328

SINEQUAN® ℞

[sin 'a-kwon]
(doxepin HCl)
Capsules
Oral Concentrate

DESCRIPTION

SINEQUAN® (doxepin hydrochloride) is one of a class of psychotherapeutic agents known as dibenzoxepin tricyclic compounds. The molecular formula of the compound is $C_{19}H_{21}NO \cdot HCl$ having a molecular weight of 316. It is a white crystalline solid readily soluble in water, lower alcohols and chloroform.
Inert ingredients for the capsule formulations are: hard gelatin capsules (which may contain Blue 1, Red 3, Red 40, Yellow 10, and other inert ingredients); magnesium stearate; sodium lauryl sulfate; starch.
Inert ingredients for the oral concentrate formulation are: glycerin; methylparaben; peppermint oil; propylparaben; water.

CHEMISTRY

SINEQUAN (doxepin HCl) is a dibenzoxepin derivative and is the first of a family of tricyclic psychotherapeutic agents. Specifically, it is an isomeric mixture of: 1-Propanamine, 3-dibenz [*b,e*] oxepin-11(6*H*)ylidene-*N,N* -dimethyl-, hydrochloride.

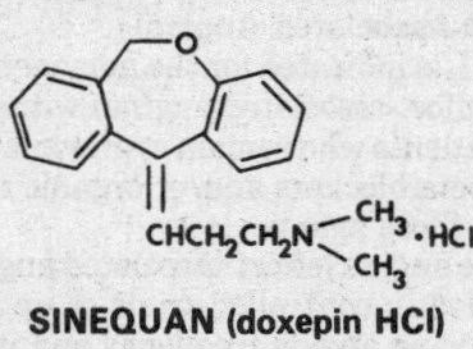

SINEQUAN (doxepin HCl)

ACTIONS

The mechanism of action of SINEQUAN (doxepin HCl) is not definitely known. It is not a central nervous system stimulant nor a monoamine oxidase inhibitor. The current hypothesis is that the clinical effects are due, at least in part, to influences on the adrenergic activity at the synapses so that deactivation of norepinephrine by reuptake into the nerve terminals is prevented. Animal studies suggest that doxepin HCl does not appreciably antagonize the antihypertensive action of guanethidine. In animal studies anticholinergic, antiserotonin and antihistamine effects on smooth muscle have been demonstrated. At higher than usual clinical doses, norepinephrine response was potentiated in animals. This effect was not demonstrated in humans.
At clinical dosages up to 150 mg per day, SINEQUAN can be given to man concomitantly with guanethidine and related compounds without blocking the antihypertensive effect. At

dosages above 150 mg per day blocking of the antihypertensive effect of these compounds has been reported.

SINEQUAN is virtually devoid of euphoria as a side effect. Characteristic of this type of compound, SINEQUAN has not been demonstrated to produce the physical tolerance or psychological dependence associated with addictive compounds.

INDICATIONS

SINEQUAN is recommended for the treatment of:
1. Psychoneurotic patients with depression and/or anxiety.
2. Depression and/or anxiety associated with alcoholism (not to be taken concomitantly with alcohol).
3. Depression and/or anxiety associated with organic disease (the possibility of drug interaction should be considered if the patient is receiving other drugs concomitantly).
4. Psychotic depressive disorders with associated anxiety including involutional depression and manic-depressive disorders.

The target symptoms of psychoneurosis that respond particularly well to SINEQUAN include anxiety, tension, depression, somatic symptoms and concerns, sleep disturbances, guilt, lack of energy, fear, apprehension and worry.

Clinical experience has shown that SINEQUAN is safe and well tolerated even in the elderly patient. Owing to lack of clinical experience in the pediatric population, SINEQUAN is not recommended for use in children under 12 years of age.

CONTRAINDICATIONS

SINEQUAN is contraindicated in individuals who have shown hypersensitivity to the drug. Possibility of cross sensitivity with other dibenzoxepines should be kept in mind. SINEQUAN is contraindicated in patients with glaucoma or a tendency to urinary retention. These disorders should be ruled out, particularly in older patients.

WARNINGS

The once-a-day dosage regimen of SINEQUAN in patients with intercurrent illness or patients taking other medications should be carefully adjusted. This is especially important in patients receiving other medications with anticholinergic effects.

Usage in Geriatrics: The use of SINEQUAN on a once-a-day dosage regimen in geriatric patients should be adjusted carefully based on the patient's condition.

Usage in Pregnancy: Reproduction studies have been performed in rats, rabbits, monkeys and dogs and there was no evidence of harm to the animal fetus. The relevance to humans is not known. Since there is no experience in pregnant women who have received this drug, safety in pregnancy has not been established. There has been a report of apnea and drowsiness occurring in a nursing infant whose mother was taking SINEQUAN.

Usage in Children: The use of SINEQUAN in children under 12 years of age is not recommended because safe conditions for its use have not been established.

PRECAUTIONS

Drug Interactions: *Drugs Metabolized by P450 2D6:* The biochemical activity of the drug metabolizing isozyme cytochrome P450 2D6 (debrisoquin hydroxylase) is reduced in a subset of the Caucasian population (about 7–10% of Caucasians are so-called "poor metabolizers"); reliable estimates of the prevalence of reduced P450 2D6 isozyme activity among Asian, African and other populations are not yet available. Poor metabolizers have higher than expected plasma concentrations of tricyclic antidepressants (TCAs) when given usual doses. Depending on the fraction of drug metabolized by P450 2D6, the increase in plasma concentration may be small, or quite large (8-fold increase in plasma AUC of the TCA).

In addition, certain drugs inhibit the activity of this isozyme and make normal metabolizers resemble poor metabolizers. An individual who is stable on a given dose of TCA may become abruptly toxic when given one of these inhibiting drugs as concomitant therapy. The drugs that inhibit cytochrome P450 2D6 include some that are not metabolized by the enzyme (quinidine; cimetidine) and many that are substrates for P450 2D6 (many other antidepressants, phenothiazines, and the Type 1C antiarrhythmics propafenone and flecainide). While all the selective serotonin reuptake inhibitors (SSRIs), e.g., fluoxetine, sertraline, and paroxetine, inhibit P450 2D6, they may vary in the extent of inhibition. The extent to which SSRI-TCA interactions may pose clinical problems will depend on the degree of inhibition and the pharmacokinetics of the SSRI involved. Nevertheless, caution is indicated in the co-administration of TCAs with any of the SSRIs and also in switching from one class to the other. Of particular importance, sufficient time must elapse before initiating TCA treatment in a patient being withdrawn from fluoxetine, given the long half-life of the parent and active metabolite (at least 5 weeks may be necessary).

Concomitant use of tricyclic antidepressants with drugs that can inhibit cytochrome P450 2D6 may require lower doses than usually prescribed for either the tricyclic antidepressant or the other drug. Furthermore, whenever one of these drugs is withdrawn from co-therapy, an increased dose of

tricyclic antidepressant may be required. It is desirable to monitor TCA plasma levels whenever a TCA is going to be coadministered with another drug known to be an inhibitor of P450 2D6.

MAO Inhibitors: Serious side effects and even death have been reported following the concomitant use of certain drugs with MAO inhibitors. Therefore, MAO inhibitors should be discontinued at least two weeks prior to the cautious initiation of therapy with SINEQUAN. The exact length of time may vary and is dependent upon the particular MAO inhibitor being used, the length of time it has been administered, and the dosage involved.

Cimetidine: Cimetidine has been reported to produce clinically significant fluctuations in steady-state serum concentrations of various tricyclic antidepressants. Serious anticholinergic symptoms (i.e., severe dry mouth, urinary retention and blurred vision) have been associated with elevations in the serum levels of tricyclic antidepressant when cimetidine therapy is initiated. Additionally, higher than expected tricyclic antidepressant levels have been observed when they are begun in patients already taking cimetidine. In patients who have been reported to be well controlled on tricyclic antidepressants receiving concurrent cimetidine therapy, discontinuation of cimetidine has been reported to decrease established steady-state serum tricyclic antidepressant levels and compromise their therapeutic effects.

Alcohol: It should be borne in mind that alcohol ingestion may increase the danger inherent in any intentional or unintentional SINEQUAN overdosage. This is especially important in patients who may use alcohol excessively.

Tolazamide: A case of severe hypoglycemia has been reported in a type II diabetic patient maintained on tolazamide (1 gm/day) 11 days after the addition of doxepin (75 mg/day).

Drowsiness: Since drowsiness may occur with the use of this drug, patients should be warned of the possibility and cautioned against driving a car or operating dangerous machinery while taking the drug. Patients should also be cautioned that their response to alcohol may be potentiated.

Suicide: Since suicide is an inherent risk in any depressed patient and may remain so until significant improvement has occurred, patients should be closely supervised during the early course of therapy. Prescriptions should be written for the smallest feasible amount.

Psychosis: Should increased symptoms of psychosis or shift to manic symptomatology occur, it may be necessary to reduce dosage or add a major tranquilizer to the dosage regimen.

ADVERSE REACTIONS

NOTE: Some of the adverse reactions noted below have not been specifically reported with SINEQUAN use. However, due to the close pharmacological similarities among the tricyclics, the reactions should be considered when prescribing SINEQUAN (doxepin HCl).

Anticholinergic Effects: Dry mouth, blurred vision, constipation, and urinary retention have been reported. If they do not subside with continued therapy, or become severe, it may be necessary to reduce the dosage.

Central Nervous System Effects: Drowsiness is the most commonly noticed side effect. This tends to disappear as therapy is continued. Other infrequently reported CNS side effects are confusion, disorientation, hallucinations, numbness, paresthesias, ataxia, extrapyramidal symptoms, seizures, tardive dyskinesia, and tremor.

Cardiovascular: Cardiovascular effects including hypotension, hypertension, and tachycardia have been reported occasionally.

Allergic: Skin rash, edema, photosensitization, and pruritus have occasionally occurred.

Hematologic: Eosinophilia has been reported in a few patients. There have been occasional reports of bone marrow depression manifesting as agranulocytosis, leukopenia, thrombocytopenia, and purpura.

Gastrointestinal: Nausea, vomiting, indigestion, taste disturbances, diarrhea, anorexia, and aphthous stomatitis have been reported. (See Anticholinergic Effects.)

Endocrine: Raised or lowered libido, testicular swelling, gynecomastia in males, enlargement of breasts and galactorrhea in the female, raising or lowering of blood sugar levels, and syndrome of inappropriate antidiuretic hormone secretion have been reported with tricyclic administration.

Other: Dizziness, tinnitus, weight gain, sweating, chills, fatigue, weakness, flushing, jaundice, alopecia, headache, exacerbation of asthma, and hyperpyrexia (in association with chlorpromazine) have been occasionally observed as adverse effects.

Withdrawal Symptoms: The possibility of development of withdrawal symptoms upon abrupt cessation of treatment after prolonged SINEQUAN administration should be borne in mind. These are not indicative of addiction and gradual withdrawal of medication should not cause these symptoms.

DOSAGE AND ADMINISTRATION

For most patients with illness of mild to moderate severity, a starting daily dose of 75 mg is recommended. Dosage may subsequently be increased or decreased at appropriate inter-

vals and according to individual response. The usual optimum dose range is 75 mg/day to 150 mg/day.

In more severely ill patients higher doses may be required with subsequent gradual increase to 300 mg/day if necessary. Additional therapeutic effect is rarely to be obtained by exceeding a dose of 300 mg/day.

In patients with very mild symptomatology or emotional symptoms accompanying organic disease, lower doses may suffice. Some of these patients have been controlled on doses as low as 25-50 mg/day.

The total daily dosage of SINEQUAN may be given on a divided or once-a-day dosage schedule. If the once-a-day schedule is employed, the maximum recommended dose is 150 mg/day. This dose may be given at bedtime. **The 150 mg capsule strength is intended for maintenance therapy only and is not recommended for initiation of treatment.**

Anti-anxiety effect is apparent before the antidepressant effect. Optimal antidepressant effect may not be evident for two to three weeks.

OVERDOSAGE

Deaths may occur from overdosage with this class of drugs. Multiple drug ingestion (including alcohol) is common in deliberate tricyclic antidepressant overdose. As the management is complex and changing, it is recommended that the physician contact a poison control center for current information on treatment. Signs and symptoms of toxicity develop rapidly after tricyclic antidepressant overdose; therefore, hospital monitoring is required as soon as possible.

Manifestations: Critical manifestations of overdose include: cardiac dysrhythmias, severe hypotension, convulsions, and CNS depression, including coma. Changes in the electrocardiogram, particularly in QRS axis or width, are clinically significant indicators of tricyclic antidepressant toxicity.

Other signs of overdose may include: confusion, distributed concentration, transient visual hallucinations, dilated pupils, agitation, hyperactive reflexes, stupor, drowsiness, muscle rigidity, vomiting, hypothermia, hyperpyrexia, or any of the symptoms listed under ADVERSE REACTIONS.

General Recommendations:

General: Obtain an ECG and immediately initiate cardiac monitoring. Protect the patient's airway, establish an intravenous line and initiate gastric decontamination. A minimum of six hours of observation with cardiac monitoring and observation for signs of CNS or respiratory depression, hypotension, cardiac dysrhythmias and/or conduction blocks, and seizures is strongly advised. If signs of toxicity occur at any time during this period, extended monitoring is recommended. There are case reports of patients succumbing to fatal dysrhythmias late after overdose; these patients had clinical evidence of significant poisoning prior to death and most received inadequate gastrointestinal decontamination. Monitoring of plasma drug levels should not guide management of the patient.

Gastrointestinal Decontamination: All patients suspected of tricyclic antidepressant overdose should receive gastrointestinal decontamination. This should include large volume gastric lavage followed by activated charcoal. If consciousness is impaired, the airway should be secured prior to lavage. Emesis is contraindicated.

Cardiovascular: A maximal limb-lead QRS duration of ≥ 0.10 seconds may be the best indication of the severity of the overdose. Intravenous sodium bicarbonate should be used to maintain the serum pH in the range of 7.45 to 7.55. If the pH response is inadequate, hyperventilation may also be used. Concomitant use of hyperventilation and sodium bicarbonate should be done with extreme caution, with frequent pH monitoring. A pH > 7.60 or a $pCO_2 < 20$ mm Hg is undesirable. Dysrhythmias unresponsive to sodium bicarbonate therapy/hyperventilation may respond to lidocaine, bretylium or phenytoin. Type 1A and 1C antiarrhythmics are generally contraindicated (e.g., quinidine, disopyramide, and procainamide).

In rare instances, hemoperfusion may be beneficial in acute refractory cardiovascular instability in patients with acute toxicity. However, hemodialysis, peritoneal dialysis, exchange tranfusions, and forced diuresis generally have been reported as ineffective in tricyclic antidepressant poisoning.

CNS: In patients with CNS depression, early intubation is advised because of the potential for abrupt deterioration. Seizures should be controlled with benzodiazepines, or if these are ineffective, other anticonvulsants (e.g., phenobarbital, phenytoin). Physostigmine is not recommended except to treat life-threatening symptoms that have been unresponsive to other therapies, and then only in consultation with a poison control center.

Psychiatric Follow-up: Since overdosage is often deliberate, patients may attempt suicide by other means during the recovery phase. Psychiatric referral may be appropriate.

Pediatric Management: The principles of management of child and adult overdosages are similar. It is strongly recommended that the physician contact the local poison control center for specific pediatric treatment.

Continued on next page

Pfizer Inc—Cont.

HOW SUPPLIED

SINEQUAN® is available as capsules containing doxepin HCl equivalent to:

10 mg—100's (NDC 0049-5340-66) (NDC 0662-5340-66), 1000's (NDC 0049-5340-82) (NDC 0662-5340-82)
25 mg—100's (NDC 0049-5350-66) (NDC 0662-5350-66), 1000's (NDC 0049-5350-82) (NDC 0662-5350-82), 5000's (NDC 0049-5350-94) (NDC 0662-5350-94)
50 mg—100's (NDC 0049-5360-66) (NDC 0662-5360-66), 1000's (NDC 0049-5360-82) (NDC 0662-5360-82), 5000's (NDC 0049-5360-94) (NDC 0662-5360-94)
75 mg—100's (NDC 0049-5390-66) (NDC 0662-5390-66), 1000's (NDC 0049-5390-82) (NDC 0662-5390-82)
100 mg—100's (NDC 0049-5380-66) (NDC 0662-5380-66), 1000's (NDC 0049-5380-82) (NDC 0662-5380-82)
150 mg—50's (NDC 0049-5370-50) (NDC 0662-5370-50), 500's (NDC 0049-5370-73) (NDC 0062-5370-73)

SINEQUAN® Oral Concentrate is available in 120 mL bottles (NDC 0049-5100-47) (NDC 0662-5100-47) with an accompanying dropper calibrated at 5 mg, 10 mg, 15 mg, 20 mg, and 25 mg. Each mL contains doxepin HCl equivalent to 10 mg doxepin. Just prior to administration, SINEQUAN® Oral Concentrate should be diluted with approximately 120 mL of water, whole or skimmed milk, or orange, grapefruit, tomato, prune or pineapple juice. SINEQUAN® Oral Concentrate is not physically compatible with a number of carbonated beverages. For those patients requiring antidepressant therapy who are on methadone maintenance, SINEQUAN® Oral Concentrate and methadone syrup can be mixed together with Gatorade®, lemonade, orange juice, sugar water, Tang®, or water; but not with grape juice. Preparation and storage of bulk dilutions is not recommended.

69-2135-00-0 Revised May 1996

Shown in Product Identification Guide, page 328

SPECTROBID® ℞
[spek 'trō-bid]
(bacampicillin HCl)
TABLETS

DESCRIPTION

SPECTROBID® (bacampicillin HCl) is a member of the ampicillin class of semi-synthetic penicillins derived from the basic penicillin nucleus: 6-aminopenicillanic acid. SPECTROBID, as well as ampicillin and other ampicillin analogues, is acid resistant and suitable for oral administration.

SPECTROBID is the hydrochloride salt of 1-ethoxycarbonyloxyethyl ester of ampicillin and is available as a tablet. During the process of absorption from the gastrointestinal tract, SPECTROBID is hydrolyzed rapidly to ampicillin, a well characterized and effective antibacterial agent. Each 400 mg tablet of SPECTROBID is chemically equivalent to 280 mg of ampicillin.

Chemically, SPECTROBID is 1′-ethoxycarbonyloxyethyl - 6 - (D-α aminophenylacetamide) - penicillinate hydrochloride. It has a molecular weight of 501.96 and the following structural formula:

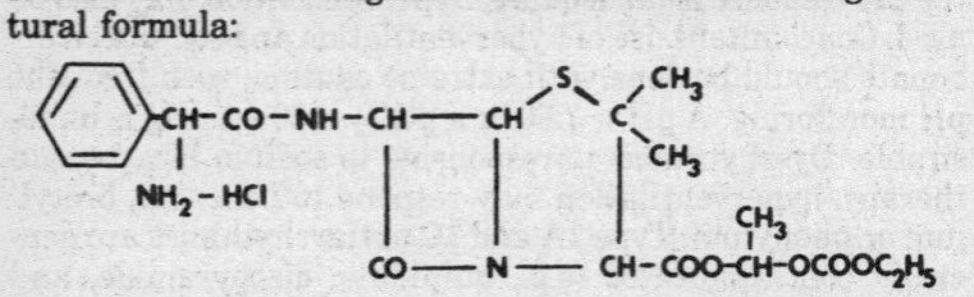

Inert ingredients for the tablets are: microcrystalline cellulose, lactose and magnesium stearate. May also include the following: hydroxypropyl methylcellulose; and opaspray white, opadry white and opadry clear (these components may contain other inert ingredients).

ACTIONS

Clinical Pharmacology

SPECTROBID is characterized by its more complete and more rapid absorption from the GI tract than ampicillin. SPECTROBID tablets of 400 mg, 800 mg, and 1600 mg have provided ampicillin peak serum concentrations of 7.9, 12.9, and 20.1 mcg/mL. These peak levels are approximately three times the levels obtained with administration of equivalent amounts of ampicillin. The areas-under-the-serum-concentration curves obtained during the first 6 hours were 24.8 and 12.9 mcg/mL/hr., when bacampicillin HCl 800 mg and ampicillin 500 mg were administered to adults. (See Graph.)

In fasting adult volunteers, a 400 mg dose of the tablet gave a peak serum ampicillin concentration of 7.2 mcg/mL. In fasting pediatric patients a 12.5 mg/kg dose provided a peak of 8.4 mcg/mL.

After oral administration of SPECTROBID tablet, ampicillin activity in serum peaks at 0.7–0.9 hours (compared to 1.5–2.0 hours after administration of ampicillin). Serum ampicillin half-life is 1.1 hours after either SPECTROBID or ampicillin administration.

Peak tissue and body fluid ampicillin concentrations also are higher after administration of SPECTROBID. Utilizing a special skin window technique to determine ampicillin levels, therapeutic levels in the interstitial fluid were higher and more prolonged after SPECTROBID than after ampicillin administration. SPECTROBID is stable in the presence of gastric acid. Food does not retard absorption of SPECTROBID tablets which may be given without regard to meals. SPECTROBID has been shown to be rapidly and well absorbed after oral administration, with about 75% of a given dose being recoverable in the urine as active ampicillin within 8 hours of administration. Urinary excretion can be delayed by concurrent administration of probenecid. The active moiety of SPECTROBID (i.e., ampicillin) diffuses readily into most body tissues and fluids. In serum, ampicillin is only 20% protein-bound, compared to 60–90% for other penicillins.

Microbiology

SPECTROBID per se has no *in vitro* antibacterial activity and owes its *in vivo* bactericidal activity to the parent compound, ampicillin. The ampicillin class of penicillins (including SPECTROBID) has a broad spectrum of activity against many gram-negative and gram-positive bacteria. Like other penicillins, the ampicillin class of penicillins inhibits the synthesis of cell wall mucopeptide.

Ampicillin class antibiotics are inactivated by β-lactamases produced by certain strains of *Enterobacter, Citrobacter, Haemophilus influenzae,* and *Escherichia coli,* and by most strains of staphylococci and indole-positive *Proteus* spp. Ampicillin class antibiotics are not active against *Pseudomonas, Klebsiella,* or *Serratia* spp.

SUSCEPTIBILITY TESTING

Elution Technique: For the automated method of susceptibility testing (i.e., Autobac™), gram-negative organisms should be tested with the 4.5 mcg ampicillin elution disk, while gram-positive organisms should be tested with the 0.22 mcg disk.

Diffusion Technique: For the Kirby-Bauer method of susceptibility testing, a 10 mcg ampicillin diffusion disk should be used. With this procedure, a laboratory report of "susceptible" indicates that the infecting organism is likely to respond to SPECTROBID therapy, and a report of "resistant" indicates that the infecting organism is not likely to respond to therapy. An "intermediate susceptibility" report suggests that the infecting organism would be susceptible to SPECTROBID if a high dosage is used or if the infection is confined to tissues and fluids (e.g., urine) in which high antibiotic levels are attained.

Dilution Techniques: Broth or agar dilution methods may be used to determine the minimal inhibitory concentration (MIC) value for susceptibility of bacterial isolates to SPECTROBID. Since SPECTROBID per se has no *in vitro* activity, ampicillin powder should be used in a twofold concentration series of the antibiotic prepared in either broth (in tubes) or agar (in petri plates). Tubes should be inoculated to contain 10^4 to 10^5 organisms/mL or plates "spotted" with 10^3 to 10^4 organisms.

INDICATIONS AND USAGE

SPECTROBID is indicated for the treatment of the following infections when caused by ampicillin-susceptible organisms:

1. Upper and Lower Respiratory Tract Infections (including acute exacerbations of chronic bronchitis) due to streptococci (β-hemolytic streptococci, *Streptococcus pyogenes*), pneumococci (*Streptococcus pneumoniae*), nonpenicillinase-producing staphylococci and *H. influenzae;*
2. Urinary Tract Infections due to *E. coli, Proteus mirabilis,* and *Streptococcus faecalis* (enterococci);
3. Skin and Skin Structure Infections due to streptococci and susceptible staphylococci;
4. Gonorrhea (acute uncomplicated urogenital infections) due to *Neisseria gonorrhoeae.*

Bacteriological studies to determine the causative organisms and their susceptibility to SPECTROBID (i.e., ampicillin) should be performed. Therapy may be instituted prior to obtaining results of susceptibility testing. Indicated surgical procedures should be performed.

CONTRAINDICATIONS

The use of ampicillin class antibiotics is contraindicated in individuals with a history of an allergic reaction to any of the penicillin antibiotics and/or cephalosporins.

WARNINGS

Serious and occasional fatal hypersensitivity (anaphylactic) reactions have been reported in patients on penicillin therapy. Although anaphylaxis is more frequent following parenteral therapy, it has occurred in patients on oral penicillins. These reactions are more apt to occur in individuals with a history of penicillin hypersensitivity and/or hypersensitivity to multiple allergens.

There have been reports of individuals with a history of penicillin hypersensitivity who have experienced severe reactions when treated with cephalosporins. Before therapy with a penicillin, careful inquiry should be made concerning previous hypersensitivity reactions to penicillins, cephalosporins, and other allergens.

IF AN ALLERGIC REACTION OCCURS, THE DRUG SHOULD BE DISCONTINUED AND THE APPROPRIATE THERAPY INSTITUTED. SERIOUS ANAPHYLACTOID REACTIONS REQUIRE IMMEDIATE EMERGENCY TREATMENT WITH EPINEPHRINE. OXYGEN, INTRAVENOUS STEROIDS, AND AIRWAY MANAGEMENT, INCLUDING INTUBATION, SHOULD ALSO BE ADMINISTERED AS INDICATED.

PRECAUTIONS

1. General: The possibility of superinfections with mycotic or bacterial pathogens should be kept in mind during therapy. If superinfections occur (usually involving *Aerobacter, Pseudomonas,* or *Candida*), the drug should be discontinued and appropriate therapy instituted.

As with any potent agent, it is advisable to check periodically for organ system dysfunction during prolonged therapy. This includes renal, hepatic, and hematopoietic systems and is particularly important in prematures, neonates, and patients with liver or renal impairments.

A high percentage of patients with mononucleosis who receive ampicillin develop a skin rash. Thus, ampicillin class antibiotics should not be administered to patients with mononucleosis.

2. Clinically Significant Drug Interactions: The concurrent administration of allopurinol and ampicillin increases substantially the incidence of rashes in patients receiving both drugs as compared to patients receiving ampicillin alone. It is not known whether this potentiation of ampicillin rashes is due to allopurinol or the hyperuricemia present in these patients. There are no data available on the incidence of rash in patients treated concurrently with SPECTROBID (bacampicillin HCl) and allopurinol. SPECTROBID should not be co-administered with Antabuse (disulfiram).

3. Drug and Laboratory Test Interactions: When testing for the presence of glucose in urine using Clinitest™, Benedict's Solution, or Fehling's Solution, high urine concentrations of ampicillin may result in false-positive reactions. Therefore, it is recommended that glucose tests based on enzymatic glucose oxidase reactions (such as Clinistix™ or Testape™) be used.

Following administration of ampicillin to pregnant women a transient decrease in plasma concentration of total conjugated estriol, estriol-glucuronide, conjugated estrone and estradiol, has been noted.

4. Pregnancy Category B: Reproduction studies have been performed in mice and rats at SPECTROBID doses of up to 750 mg/kg (more than 25 times the human dose) and have revealed no evidence of impaired fertility or harm to the fetus due to SPECTROBID.

There are, however, no adequate and well controlled studies in pregnant women. Because animal reproduction studies are not always predictive of human response, this drug should be used during pregnancy only if clearly needed.

5. Carcinogenesis, Mutagenesis, Impairment of Fertility: No carcinogenicity or mutagenicity studies were conducted. No impairment of fertility and no significant effect on general reproductive performance was observed in rats administered oral doses of up to 750 mg/kg of bacampicillin HCl per day prior to and during mating and gestation. In addition, bacampicillin HCl caused no drug-related effects on the reproductive organs of rats or dogs receiving daily oral doses of up to 800 and 650 mg/kg respectively for 6 months.

6. Labor and Delivery: Oral ampicillin class antibiotics are generally poorly absorbed during labor. Studies in guinea pigs showed that intravenous administration of ampicillin decreased the uterine tone, frequency of contractions, height of contractions, and duration of contractions. However, it is not known whether use of SPECTROBID in humans during labor or delivery has immediate or delayed adverse effects on the fetus, prolongs the duration of labor, or increases the likelihood that forceps delivery or other obstetrical intervention or resuscitation of the newborn will be necessary.

7. Nursing Mothers: Ampicillin class antibiotics are excreted in milk; therefore, caution should be exercised when ampicillin class antibiotics are administered to a nursing woman.

8. Pediatric Use: SPECTROBID tablets are indicated for children weighing 25 kg or more.

ADVERSE REACTIONS

As with other penicillins, it may be expected that untoward reactions will be essentially limited to sensitivity phenomena. They are more likely to occur in individuals who have previously demonstrated hypersensitivity to penicillins and in those with a history of allergy, asthma, hay fever, or urticaria.

In well controlled clinical trials conducted in the U.S. the most frequent adverse reactions to SPECTROBID were epigastric upset (2%) and diarrhea (2%). Increased dosage may result in an increased incidence of diarrhea. In the same clinical trials the most frequent adverse effects for amoxicillin were diarrhea (4%) and nausea (2%).

The following adverse reactions have been reported for ampicillin.

Gastrointestinal: diarrhea, gastritis, stomatitis, nausea, vomiting, glossitis, black "hairy" tongue, enterocolitis, and pseudomembranous colitis.

Hypersensitivity Reactions: skin rashes, urticaria, erythema multiforme, and an occasional case of exfoliative dermatitis. These reactions may be controlled with antihistamines and, if necessary, systemic corticosteroids. Whenever such reactions occur, the drug should be discontinued, unless the opinion of the physician dictates otherwise.

Serious and occasional fatal hypersensitivity (anaphylactic) reactions can occur with oral penicillins. (See WARNINGS.)

Liver: A moderate rise in serum glutamic oxaloacetic transaminase (SGOT) has been noted in some ampicillin treated patients, but the significance of this finding is unknown. In well controlled clinical trials no difference was noted between ampicillin and SPECTROBID with regard to the incidence of liver function test abnormalities.

Hemic and Lymphatic Systems: Anemia, thrombocytopenia, thrombocytopenic purpura, eosinophilia, leukopenia, and agranulocytosis have been reported during therapy with penicillins. These reactions are usually reversible on discontinuation of therapy and are believed to be hypersensitivity phenomena.

DOSAGE AND ADMINISTRATION

SPECTROBID tablets may be given without regard to meals.
UPPER RESPIRATORY TRACT INFECTIONS (including otitis media) due to streptococci, pneumococci, nonpenicillinase-producing staphylococci and *H. influenzae*;
URINARY TRACT INFECTIONS due to *E. coli, Proteus mirabilis,* and *Streptococcus faecalis;*
SKIN AND SKIN STRUCTURES INFECTIONS due to streptococci and susceptible staphylococci:
Usual Dosage
Adults: 1 × 400 mg tablet every 12 hours (for patients weighing 25 kg or more).
Children: (≥ 25kg) 25 mg/kg per day in 2 equally divided doses at 12 hour intervals.
IN SEVERE INFECTIONS OR THOSE CAUSED BY LESS SUSCEPTIBLE ORGANISMS:
Usual Dosage
Adults: 2 × 400 mg tablets every 12 hours (for patients weighing 25 kg or more).
Children: (≥ 25 kg) 50 mg/kg per day in 2 equally divided doses at 12 hour intervals.
LOWER RESPIRATORY TRACT INFECTIONS due to streptococci, pneumococci, nonpenicillinase-producing staphylococci, and *H. influenzae:*
Usual Dosage
Adults: 2 × 400 mg tablets every 12 hours (for patients weighing 25 kg or more).
Children: (≥ 25 kg) 50 mg/kg per day in 2 equally divided doses at 12 hour intervals.
GONORRHEA—acute uncomplicated urogenital infections due to *N. gonorrhoeae* (males and females):
1.6 grams (4 × 400 mg tablet plus 1 gram probenecid) as a single oral dose.
No pediatric dosage has been established.
Cases of gonorrhea with a suspected lesion of syphilis should have dark field examination before receiving SPECTROBID and monthly serological tests for a minimum of four months. Larger doses may be required for stubborn or severe infections.
It should be recognized that in the treatment of chronic urinary tract infections, frequent bacteriological and clinical appraisals are necessary. Smaller doses than those recommended above should not be used. In stubborn infections, therapy may be required for several weeks. It may be necessary to continue clinical and/or bacteriological follow-up for several months after cessation of therapy. Except for gonorrhea, treatment should be continued for a minimum of 48 to 72 hours beyond the time that the patient becomes asymptomatic or evidence of bacterial eradication has been obtained.
IT IS RECOMMENDED THAT THERE BE AT LEAST 10 DAYS' TREATMENT FOR ANY INFECTION CAUSED BY HEMOLYTIC STREPTOCOCCI TO PREVENT THE OCCURRENCE OF ACUTE RHEUMATIC FEVER OR GLOMERULONEPHRITIS.

HOW SUPPLIED

SPECTROBID® (bacampicillin HCl) Tablets
400 mg (NDC 0049-0350-66): white, film-coated, oblong, unscored are available in bottles of 100.
[See Figure at top of next column.]

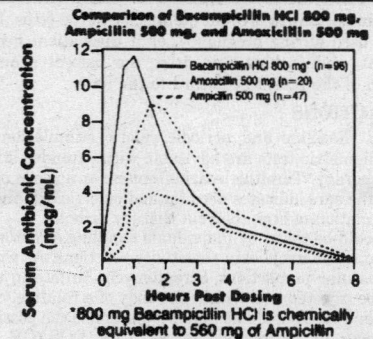

Comparison of Bacampicillin HCl 800 mg, Ampicillin 500 mg, and Amoxicillin 500 mg

*800 mg Bacampicillin HCl is chemically equivalent to 560 mg of Ampicillin

Rev. July 1992   69-4092-00-7
Shown in Product Identification Guide, page 328

STREPTOMYCIN SULFATE Injection, USP ℞
1 g/2.5 mL Ampules
For Intramuscular Use Only

WARNING
THE RISK OF SEVERE NEUROTOXIC REACTIONS IS SHARPLY INCREASED IN PATIENTS WITH IMPAIRED RENAL FUNCTION OR PRE-RENAL AZOTEMIA. THESE INCLUDE DISTURBANCES OF VESTIBULAR AND COCHLEAR FUNCTION. OPTIC NERVE DYSFUNCTION, PERIPHERAL NEURITIS, ARACHNOIDITIS, AND ENCEPHALOPATHY MAY ALSO OCCUR. THE INCIDENCE OF CLINICALLY DETECTABLE, IRREVERSIBLE VESTIBULAR DAMAGE IS PARTICULARLY HIGH IN PATIENTS TREATED WITH STREPTOMYCIN.
RENAL FUNCTION SHOULD BE MONITORED CAREFULLY; PATIENTS WITH RENAL IMPAIRMENT AND/OR NITROGEN RETENTION SHOULD RECEIVE REDUCED DOSAGES. THE PEAK SERUM CONCENTRATION IN INDIVIDUALS WITH KIDNEY DAMAGE SHOULD NOT EXCEED 20 TO 25 MCG/ML.
THE CONCURRENT OR SEQUENTIAL USE OF OTHER NEUROTOXIC AND/OR NEPHROTOXIC DRUGS WITH STREPTOMYCIN SULFATE, INCLUDING NEOMYCIN, KANAMYCIN, GENTAMICIN, CEPHALORIDINE, PAROMOMYCIN, VIOMYCIN, POLYMYXIN B, COLISTIN, TOBRAMYCIN AND CYCLOSPORINE SHOULD BE AVOIDED.
THE NEUROTOXICITY OF STREPTOMYCIN CAN RESULT IN RESPIRATORY PARALYSIS FROM NEUROMUSCULAR BLOCKAGE, ESPECIALLY WHEN THE DRUG IS GIVEN SOON AFTER THE USE OF ANESTHESIA OR OF MUSCLE RELAXANTS.
THE ADMINISTRATION OF STREPTOMYCIN IN PARENTERAL FORM SHOULD BE RESERVED FOR PATIENTS WHERE ADEQUATE LABORATORY AND AUDIOMETRIC TESTING FACILITIES ARE AVAILABLE DURING THERAPY.

DESCRIPTION
Streptomycin is a water-soluble aminoglycoside derived from *Streptomyces griseus.* It is marketed as the sulfate salt of streptomycin. The chemical name of streptomycin sulfate is D-Streptamine, *O*-2-deoxy-2-(methylamino)-α-L-glucopyranosyl-(1→2)-*O*-5-deoxy-3-*C*-formyl-α-L-lyxofuranosyl-(1→4)-*N,N*'-bis(aminoiminomethyl)-, sulfate (2:3) (salt). The empirical formula for Streptomycin Sulfate is $(C_{21}H_{39}N_7O_{12})_2 \cdot 3H_2SO_4$ and the molecular weight is 1457.38. It has the following structure:

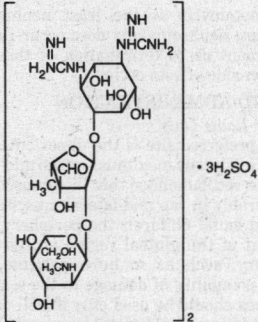

Streptomycin Sulfate Injection, 1 g/2.5 mL (400 mg/mL), is supplied as a sterile, nonpyrogenic solution for intramuscular use.

Each mL contains: Streptomycin sulfate equivalent to 400 mg of streptomycin, sodium citrate dihydrate 12 mg, phenol 0.25% w/v as preservative, sodium metabisulfite 2 mg in Water for Injection. pH range 5.0 to 8.0

CLINICAL PHARMACOLOGY
Following intramuscular injection of 1 g of streptomycin, as the sulfate, a peak serum level of 25 to 50 mcg/mL is reached within 1 hour, diminishing slowly to about 50 percent after 5 to 6 hours.
Appreciable concentrations are found in all organ tissues except the brain. Significant amounts have been found in pleural fluid and tuberculous cavities. Streptomycin passes through the placenta with serum levels in the cord blood similar to maternal levels. Small amounts are excreted in milk, saliva, and sweat.
Streptomycin is excreted by glomerular filtration. In patients with normal kidney function, between 29% and 89% of a single 600 mg dose is excreted in the urine within 24 hours. Any reduction of glomerular function results in decreased excretion of the drug and concurrent rise in serum and tissue levels.
Microbiology
Streptomycin sulfate is a bactericidal antibiotic. It acts by interfering with normal protein synthesis.
Streptomycin has been shown to be active against most strains of the following organisms both *in vitro* and in clinical infection. (See INDICATIONS AND USAGE.):
Brucella (brucellosis),
Calymmatobacterium granulomatis (donovanosis, granuloma inguinale),
Escherichia coli, Proteus spp., *Aerobacter aerogenes, Klebsiella pneumoniae,* and *Enterococcus faecalis* in urinary tract infections,
Francisella tularensis,
Haemophilus ducreyi (chancroid),
Haemophilus influenzae (in respiratory, endocardial, and meningeal infections—concomitantly with another antibacterial agent),
Klebsiella pneumoniae pneumonia (concomitantly with another antibacterial agent),
Mycobacterium tuberculosis,
Pasteurella pestis,
Streptococcus viridans, *Enterococcus faecalis* (in endocardial infections—concomitantly with penicillin).
SUSCEPTIBILITY TESTS: Diffusion Techniques
Quantitative methods that require measurement of zone diameters give the most precise estimate of the susceptibility of bacteria to antimicrobial agents. One such standard procedure[1] which has been recommended for use with disks to test susceptibility of organisms to streptomycin uses the 10 mcg streptomycin disk. Interpretation involves the correlation of the diameter obtained in the disk test with the minimum inhibitory concentration (MIC) for streptomycin.
Reports from the laboratory giving results of the standard single disk susceptibility test with a 10 mcg streptomycin disk should be interpreted according to the following criteria:

Zone Diameter (mm)	Interpretation
≥ 15	(S) Susceptible
11–12	(I) Intermediate
≤ 10	(R) Resistant

A report of "Susceptible" indicates that the pathogen is likely to respond to monotherapy with streptomycin. A report of "Intermediate" indicates that the result be considered equivocal, and, if the organism is not fully susceptible to alternative clinically feasible drugs, the test should be repeated. This category provides a buffer zone which prevents small uncontrolled technical factors from causing major discrepancies in interpretations. A report of "Resistant" indicates that achievable drug concentrations are unlikely to be inhibitory and other therapy should be selected.
Standardized procedures require the use of laboratory control organisms. The 10 mcg streptomycin disk should give the following zone diameter:

Organism	Zone diameter (mm)
E. coli ATCC 25922	12–20
S. aureus ATCC 25923	14–22

Methods Section:
Two standardized *in vitro* susceptibility methods are available for testing streptomycin against *Mycobacterium tuberculosis* organisms. The agar proportion method (CDC or NCCLS M24–P) utilizes middlebrook 7H10 medium impregnated with streptomycin at two final concentrations, 2.0 and 10.0 mcg/mL. MIC_{90} values are calculated by comparing the quantity of organisms growing in the medium containing drug to the control cultures. Mycobacterial growth in the presence of drug ≥ 1% of the control indicates resistance. The radiometric broth method employs the BACTEC 460 machine to compare the growth index from untreated control cultures to cultures grown in the presence of 6.0 mcg/mL of streptomycin. Strict adherence to the manufacturer's

Continued on next page

Pfizer Inc—Cont.

instructions for sample processing and data interpretation is required for this assay.

Susceptibility test results obtained by these two different methods cannot be compared unless equivalent drug concentrations are evaluated.

The clinical relevance of *in vitro* susceptibility test results for mycobacterial species other than *M. tuberculosis* using either the BACTEC or the proportion method has not been determined.

INDICATIONS AND USAGE

Streptomycin is indicated for the treatment of individuals with moderate to severe infections caused by susceptible strains of microorganisms in the specific conditions listed below:

1. Mycobacterium tuberculosis: The Advisory Council for the Elimination of Tuberculosis, the American Thoracic Society, and the Center for Disease Control recommend that either streptomycin or ethambutol be added as a fourth drug in a regimen containing isoniazid (INH), rifampin and pyrazinamide for initial treatment of tuberculosis unless the likelihood of INH or rifampin resistance is very low. The need for a fourth drug should be reassessed when the results of susceptibility testing are known. In the past when the national rate of primary drug resistance to isoniazid was known to be less than 4% and was either stable or declining, therapy with two and three drug regimens was considered adequate. If community rates of INH resistance are currently less than 4%, an initial treatment regimen with less than four drugs may be considered.

Streptomycin is also indicated for therapy of tuberculosis when one or more of the above drugs is contraindicated because of toxicity or intolerance. The management of tuberculosis has become more complex as a consequence of increasing rates of drug resistance and concomitant HIV infection. Additional consultation from experts in the treatment of tuberculosis may be desirable in those settings.

2. Non-tuberculosis infections: The use of streptomycin should be limited to the treatment of infections caused by bacteria which have been shown to be susceptible to the antibacterial effects of streptomycin and which are not amenable to therapy with less potentially toxic agents.
   a. *Pasteurella pestis* (plague),
   b. *Francisella tularensis* (tularemia),
   c. *Brucella*,
   d. *Calymmatobacterium granulomatis* (donovanosis, granuloma inguinale),
   e. *H. ducreyi* (chancroid),
   f. *H. influenzae* (in respiratory, endocardial, and meningeal infections—concomitantly with another antibacterial agent),
   g. *K. pneumoniae* pneumonia (concomitantly with another antibacterial agent),
   h. *E. coli*, *Proteus*, *A. aerogenes*, *K. pneumoniae*, and *Enterococcus faecalis* in urinary tract infections,
   i. *Streptococcus viridans*, *Enterococcus faecalis* (in endocardial infections—concomitantly with penicillin),
   j. Gram-negative bacillary bacteremia (concomitantly with another antibacterial agent).

CONTRAINDICATIONS

A history of clinically significant hypersensitivity to streptomycin is a contraindication to its use. Clinically significant hypersensitivity to other aminoglycosides may contraindicate the use of streptomycin because of the known cross-sensitivity of patients to drugs in this class.

WARNINGS

Ototoxicity: Both vestibular and auditory dysfunction can follow the administration of streptomycin. The degree of impairment is directly proportional to the dose and duration of streptomycin administration, to the age of the patient, to the level of renal function and to the amount of underlying existing auditory dysfunction. The ototoxic effects of the aminoglycosides, including streptomycin, are potentiated by the co-administration of ethacrynic acid, mannitol, furosemide and possibly other diuretics.

The vestibulotoxic potential of streptomycin exceeds that of its capacity for cochlear toxicity. Vestibular damage is heralded by headache, nausea, vomiting and disequilibrium. Early cochlear injury is demonstrated by the loss of high frequency hearing. Appropriate monitoring and early discontinuation of the drug may permit recovery prior to irreversible damage to the sensorineural cells.

Sulfites: Streptomycin contains sodium metabisulfite, a sulfite that may cause allergic type reactions including anaphylactic symptoms and life-threatening or less severe asthmatic episodes in certain susceptible people. The over-all prevalence of sulfite sensitivity in the general population is unknown and probably low. Sulfite sensitivity is seen more frequently in asthmatic than in non-asthmatic people.

Pregnancy: Streptomycin can cause fetal harm when administered to a pregnant woman. Because streptomycin readily crosses the placental barrier, caution in use of the drug is important to prevent ototoxicity in the fetus. If this drug is used during pregnancy, or if the patient becomes pregnant while taking this drug, the patient should be apprised of the potential hazard to the fetus.

PRECAUTIONS

General: Baseline and periodic caloric stimulation tests and audiometric tests are advisable with extended streptomycin therapy. Tinnitus, roaring noises, or a sense of fullness in the ears indicates need for audiometric examination or termination of streptomycin therapy or both.

Care should be taken by individuals handling streptomycin for injection to avoid skin sensitivity reactions. As with all intramuscular prepartions, Streptomycin Sulfate Injection should be injected well within the body of a relatively large muscle and care should be taken to minimize the possibility of damage to peripheral nerves. (See DOSAGE AND ADMINISTRATION.)

Extreme caution must be exercised in selecting a dosage regimen in the presence of pre-existing renal insuffiency. In severely uremic patients a single dose may produce high blood levels for several days and the cumulative effect may produce ototoxic sequelae. When streptomycin must be given for prolonged periods of time alkalinization of the urine may minimize or prevent renal irritation.

A syndrome of apparent central nervous system depression, characterized by stupor and flaccidity, occasionally coma and deep respiratory depression, has been reported in very young infants in whom streptomycin dosage had exceeded the recommended limits. Thus, infants should not receive streptomycin in excess of the recommended dosage.

In the treatment of venereal infections such as granuloma inguinale, and chancroid, if concomitant syphilis is suspected, suitable laboratory procedures such as a dark field examination should be performed before the start of treatment, and monthly serologic tests should be done for at least four months.

As with other antibiotics, use of this drug may result in overgrowth of nonsusceptible organisms, including fungi. If superinfection occurs, appropriate therapy should be instituted.

Drug Interactions: The ototoxic effects of the aminoglycosides, including streptomycin, are potentiated by the co-administration of ethacrynic acid, furosemide, mannitol and possibly other diuretics.

Pregnancy: Category D: See WARNINGS section.

Nursing Mothers: Because of the potential for serious adverse reactions in nursing infants from streptomycin, a decision should be made whether to discontinue nursing or to discontinue the drug, taking into account the importance of the drug to the mother.

Pediatric Use: (See DOSAGE AND AMINISTRATION.)

ADVERSE REACTIONS

The following reactions are common: vestibular ototoxicity (nausea, vomiting, and vertigo); paresthesia of face; rash; fever; urticaria; angioneurotic edema; and eosinophilia.

The following reactions are less frequent: cochlear ototoxicity (deafness); exfoliative dermatitis; anaphylaxis; azotemia; leucopenia; thrombocytopenia, pancytopenia; hemolytic anemia; muscular weakness; and amblyopia.

Vestibular dysfunction resulting from the parenteral administration of streptomycin is cumulatively related to the total daily dose. When 1.8 to 2 g/day are given, symptoms are likely to develop in the large percentage of patients—especially in the elderly or patients with impaired renal function—within four weeks. Therefore, it is recommended that caloric and audiometric tests be done prior to, during, and following intensive therapy with streptomycin in order to facilitate detection of any vestibular dysfunction and/or impairment of hearing which may occur.

Vestibular symptoms generally appear early and usually are reversible with early detection and cessation of streptomycin administration. Two to three months after stopping the drug, gross vestibular symptoms usually disappear, except for the relative inability to walk in total darkness or on very rough terrain.

Although streptomycin is the least nephrotoxic of the aminoglycosides, nephrotoxicity does occur rarely.

Clinical judgment as to termination of therapy must be exercised when side effects occur.

DOSAGE AND ADMINISTRATION

Intramuscular Route Only

Adults: The preferred site is the upper outer quadrant of the buttock, (*i.e.*, gluteus maximus), or the mid-lateral thigh.

Children: It is recommended that intramuscular injections be given preferably in the mid-lateral muscles of the thigh.

In infants and small children the periphery of the upper outer quadrant of the gluteal region should be used only when necessary, such as in burn patients, in order to minimize the possibility of damage to the sciatic nerve.

The deltoid area should be used only if well developed such as in certain adults and older children, and then only with caution to avoid radial nerve injury. Intramuscular injections should not be made into the lower and mid-third of the upper arm. As with all intramuscular injections, aspiration is necessary to help avoid inadvertent injection into a blood vessel.

Injection sites should be alternated. As higher doses or more prolonged therapy with streptomycin may be indicated for more severe or fulminating infections (endocarditis, meningitis, etc.), the physician should always take adequate measures to be immediately aware of any toxic signs or symptoms occurring in the patient as a result of streptomycin therapy.

1. TUBERCULOSIS: The standard regimen for the treatment of drug susceptible tuberculosis has been two months of INH, rifampin and pyrazinamide followed by four months of INH and rifampin (patients with concomitant infection with tuberculosis and HIV may require treatment for a longer period). When streptomycin is added to this regimen because of suspected or proven drug resistance (see INDICATIONS AND USAGE section), the recommended dosing for streptomycin is as follows:

	Daily	Twice Weekly	Thrice Weekly
Children	20–40 mg/kg	25–30 mg/kg	25–30 mg/kg
	Max 1 g	Max 1.5 g	Max 1.5 g
Adults	15 mg/kg	25–30 mg/kg	25–30 mg/kg
	Max 1 g	Max 1.5 g	Max 1.5 g

Streptomycin is usually administered daily as a single intramuscular injection. A total dose of not more than 120 g over the course of therapy should be given unless there are no other therapeutic options. In patients older than 60 years of age the drug should be used at a reduced dosage due to the risk of increased toxicity. (See BOXED WARNING).

Therapy with streptomycin may be terminated when toxic symptoms have appeared, when impending toxicity is feared, when organisms become resistant, or when full treatment effect has been obtained. The total period of drug treatment of tuberculosis is a minimum of 1 year; however, indications for terminating therapy with streptomycin may occur at any time as noted above.

2. TULAREMIA: One to 2 g daily in divided doses for 7 to 14 days until the patient is afebrile for 5 to 7 days.

3. PLAGUE: Two grams of streptomycin daily in two divided doses should be administered intramuscularly. A minimum of 10 days of therapy is recommended.

4. BACTERIAL ENDOCARDITIS:
   a. *Streptococcal endocarditis:* In penicillin-sensitive alpha and non-hemolytic streptococcal endocarditis (penicillin MIC ≤ 0.1 mcg/mL), streptomycin may be used for 2-week treatment concomitantly with penicillin. The streptomycin regimen is 1 g b.i.d. for the first week, and 500 mg b.i.d. for the second week. If the patient is over 60 years of age, the dosage should be 500 mg b.i.d. for the entire 2-week period.
   b. *Enterococcal endocarditis:* Streptomycin in doses of 1 g b.i.d. for 2 weeks and 500 mg b.i.d. for an additional 4 weeks is given in combination with penicillin. Ototoxicity may require termination of the streptomycin prior to completion of the 6-week course of treatment.

5. CONCOMITANT USE WITH OTHER AGENTS: For concomitant use with other agents to which the infecting organism is also sensitive: Streptomycin is considered a second-line agent for the treatment of gram-negative bacillary bacteremia, meningitis, and pneumonia; brucellosis; granuloma inguinale; chancroid, and urinary tract infection.

For adults: 1 to 2 grams in divided doses every six to twelve hours for moderate to severe infections. Doses should generally not exceed 2 grams per day.

For children: 20 to 40 mg/kg/day (8 to 20 mg/lb/day) in divided doses every 6 to 12 hours. (Particular care should be taken to avoid excessive dosage in children.)

Parenteral drug products should be inspected visually for particulate matter and discoloration prior to administration, whenever solution and container permit.

HOW SUPPLIED

Streptomycin Sulfate Injection, USP is supplied in packages of 10 ampules (NDC 0049-0620-33). Each ampule contains streptomycin sulfate equivalent to 1 g of streptomycin in 2.5 mL.

Store under refrigeration at 36° to 46°F (2° to 8°C).

REFERENCES

[1] National Committee for Clinical Laboratory Standards. Performance Standards for Antimicrobial Disk Susceptibility Tests—Fourth Edition. Approved Standard NCCLS Document M2-A4. Vol. 10, No. 7. NCCLS, Villanova, PA 1990.

© 1992 PFIZER INC.

70-4895-00-0   Issued April 1993

TAO® ℞

[tā'ō]

(troleandomycin)

Capsules

DESCRIPTION

TAO (troleandomycin) is a synthetically derived acetylated ester of oleandomycin, an antibiotic elaborated by a species of *Streptomyces antibioticus*. It is a white crystalline compound, insoluble in water, but readily soluble and stable in the presence of gastric juice. The compound has a molecular weight of 814 and corresponds to the empirical formula $C_{41}H_{67}NO_{15}$.

Inert ingredients in the formulation are: hard gelatin capsules (which may contain inert ingredients); lactose; magnesium stearate; sodium lauryl sulfate; starch.

ACTIONS

TAO is an antibiotic shown to be active *in vitro* against the following gram-positive organisms:

Streptococcus pyogenes

Diplococcus pneumoniae

Susceptibility plate testing: If the Kirby-Bauer method of disc sensitivity is used, a 15 mcg. oleandomycin disc should give a zone of over 18 mm when tested against a troleandomycin sensitive bacterial strain.

INDICATIONS

Diplococcus pneumoniae

Pneumococcal pneumonia due to susceptible strains.

Streptococcus pyogenes

Group A beta-hemolytic streptococcal infections of the upper respiratory tract.

Injectable benzathine penicillin G is considered by the American Heart Association to be the drug of choice in the treatment and prevention of streptococcal pharyngitis and in long term prophylaxis of rheumatic fever.

Troleandomycin is generally effective in the eradication of streptococci from the nasopharynx. However, substantial data establishing the efficacy of TAO in the subsequent prevention of rheumatic fever are not available at present.

CONTRAINDICATIONS

Troleandomycin is contraindicated in patients with known hypersensitivity to this antibiotic.

WARNINGS

Usage in Pregnancy: Safety for use in pregnancy has not been established.

The administration of troleandomycin has been associated with an allergic type of cholestatic hepatitis. Some patients receiving troleandomycin for more than two weeks or in repeated courses have shown jaundice accompanied by right upper quadrant pain, fever, nausea, vomiting, eosinophilia, and leukocytosis. These changes have been reversible on discontinuance of the drug. Liver function tests should be monitored in patients on such dosage, and the drug discontinued if abnormalities develop. Reports in the literature have suggested that the concurrent use of ergotamine-containing drugs and troleandomycin may induce ischemic reactions. Therefore, the concurrent use of ergotamine-containing drugs and troleandomycin should be avoided. Troleandomycin should be administered with caution to patients concurrently receiving estrogen containing oral contraceptives.

Studies in chronic asthmatic patients have suggested that the concurrent use of theophylline and troleandomycin may result in elevated serum concentrations of theophylline. Therefore, it is recommended that patients receiving such concurrent therapy be observed for signs of theophylline toxicity, and that therapy be appropriately modified if such signs develop.

PRECAUTIONS

Troleandomycin is principally excreted by the liver.

Caution should be exercised in administering the antibiotic to patients with impaired hepatic function.

ADVERSE REACTIONS

The most frequent side effects of troleandomycin preparations are gastrointestinal, such as abdominal cramping and discomfort, and are dose related. Nausea, vomiting, and diarrhea occur infrequently with usual oral doses.

During prolonged or repeated therapy, there is a possibility of overgrowth of nonsusceptible bacteria or fungi. If such infections occur, the drug should be discontinued and appropriate therapy instituted.

Mild allergic reactions such as urticaria and other skin rashes have occurred. Serious allergic reactions, including anaphylaxis, have been reported.

DOSAGE AND ADMINISTRATION

Clinical judgment based on the type of infection and its severity should determine dosage within the below listed ranges.

Adults: 250 to 500 mg 4 times a day

Children: 125 to 250 mg (3-5 mg/lb or 6.6 to 11 mg/kg) every 6 hours

When used in streptococcal infection, therapy should be continued for ten days.

HOW SUPPLIED

TAO is supplied as:

Capsules 250 mg: Each capsule contains troleandomycin equivalent to 250 mg of oleandomycin; bottles of 100 (NDC 0049-1590-66).

Revised July 1995 69-1800-00-8

TERRA–CORTRIL® ℞

Terramycin ® (oxytetracycline HCl)

—Cortril® (hydrocortisone acetate)

OPHTHALMIC SUSPENSION

DESCRIPTION

Terra-Cortril suspension combines the antibiotic, oxytetracycline HCl ($C_{22}H_{24}N_2O_9 \cdot HCl$) and the adrenocorticoid, hydrocortisone acetate ($C_{23}H_{32}O_6$). **Each ml of Terra-Cortril contains Terramycin (oxytetracycline HCl) equivalent to 5 mg of oxytetracycline, and 15 mg of Cortril (hydrocortisone acetate) incorporated in mineral oil with aluminum tristearate.**

For Ophthalmic Use Only.

CLINICAL PHARMACOLOGY

Corticosteroids suppress the inflammatory response to a variety of agents and they probably delay or slow healing. Since corticoids may inhibit the body's defense mechanism against infection, a concomitant antimicrobial drug may be used when this inhibition is considered to be clinically significant in a particular case.

The anti-infective component in the combination is included to provide action against specific organisms susceptible to it.

Terramycin is considered active against the following microorganisms:

Rickettsiae (Rocky Mountain spotted fever, typhus fever and the typhus group, Q fever, rickettsialpox and tick fevers),

Mycoplasma pneumoniae (PPLO, Eaton Agent),

Agents of psittacosis and ornithosis,

Agents of lymphogranuloma venereum and granuloma inguinale,

The spirochetal agent of relapsing fever (*Borrelia recurrentis*).

The following gram-negative microorganisms:

Haemophilus ducreyi (chancroid),

Pasteurella pestis and *Pasteurella tularensis,*

Bartonella bacilliformis,

Bacteroides species,

Vibrio comma and *Vibrio fetus,*

Brucella species (in conjunction with streptomycin).

Because many strains of the following groups of microorganisms have been shown to be resistant to tetracyclines, culture and susceptibility testing are recommended.

Oxytetracycline is indicated for treatment of infections caused by the following gram-negative microorganisms, when bacteriologic testing indicates appropriate susceptibility to the drug:

Escherichia coli,

Enterobacter aerogenes (formerly *Aerobacter aerogenes*),

Shigella species,

Mima species and *Herellea* species,

Haemophilus influenzae (respiratory infections),

Klebsiella species (respiratory and urinary infections).

Oxytetracycline is indicated for treatment of infections caused by the following gram-positive microorganisms when bacteriologic testing indicates appropriate susceptibility to the drug:

Streptococcus species:

Up to 44 percent of strains of *Streptococcus pyogenes* and 74 percent of *Streptococcus faecalis* have been found to be resistant to tetracycline drugs. Therefore, tetracyclines should not be used for streptococcal disease unless the organism has been demonstrated to be sensitive.

For upper respiratory infections due to Group A beta-hemolytic streptococci, pencillin is the usual drug of choice, including prophylaxis of rheumatic fever.

Diplococcus pneumoniae,

Staphylococcus aureus, skin and soft tissue infections. Oxytetracycline is not the drug of choice in the treatment of any type of staphylococcal infections.

When penicillin is contraindicated, tetracyclines are alternative drugs in the treatment of infections due to:

Neisseria gonorrhoeae,

Treponema pallidum and *Treponema pertenue* (syphilis and yaws),

Listeria monocytogenes,

Clostridium species,

Bacillus anthracis,

Fusobacterium fusiforme (Vincent's infection),

Actinomyces species.

Tetracyclines are indicated in the treatment of trachoma, although the infectious agent is not always eliminated, as judged by immunofluorescence.

Inclusion conjunctivitis may be treated with oral tetracyclines or with a combination of oral and topical agents.

When a decision to administer both a corticoid and an antimicrobial is made, the administration of such drugs in combination has the advantage of greater patient compliance and convenience, with the added assurance that the appropriate dosage of both drugs is administered, plus assured compatibility of ingredients when both types of drug are in the same formulation and, particularly, that the correct volume of drug is delivered and retained.

The relative potency of corticosteroids depends on the molecular structure, concentration, and release from the vehicle.

INDICATIONS AND USAGE

For steroid-responsive inflammatory ocular conditions for which a corticosteroid is indicated and where bacterial infection or risk of bacterial ocular infection exists.

Ocular steroids are indicated in inflammatory conditions of the palpebral and bulbar conjunctiva, cornea, and anterior segment of the globe where the inherent risk of steroid use in certain infective conjunctivitides is accepted to obtain a diminution in edema and inflammation. They are also indicated in chronic anterior uveitis and corneal injury from chemical radiation, thermal burns, or penetration of foreign bodies.

The use of a combination drug with an anti-infective component is indicated where the risk of infection is high or where there is an expectation that potentially dangerous numbers of bacteria will be present in the eye.

The particular anti-infective drug in this product is active against the following common bacterial eye pathogens:

Staphylococcus aureus

Streptococci, including *Streptococcus pneumoniae*

Escherichia coli

Neisseria species

The product does not provide adequate coverage against:

Haemophilus influenzae

Klebsiella/Enterobacter species

Pseudomonas aeruginosa

Serratia marcescens

CONTRAINDICATIONS

Epithelial herpes simplex keratitis (dendritic keratitis), vaccinia, varicella, and many other viral diseases of the cornea and conjunctiva. Mycobacterial infection of the eye. Fungal diseases of ocular structures. Hypersensitivity to a component of the medication. (Hypersensitivity to the antibiotic component occurs at a higher rate than for other components.)

The use of these combinations is always contraindicated after uncomplicated removal of a corneal foreign body.

WARNINGS

Prolonged use may result in glaucoma, with damage to the optic nerve, defects in visual acuity and fields of vision, and posterior subcapsular cataract formation. Prolonged use may suppress the host response and thus increase the hazard of secondary ocular infections. In those diseases causing thinning of the cornea or sclera, perforations have been known to occur with the use of topical steroids. In acute purulent conditions of the eye, steroids may mask infection or enhance existing infection. If these products are used for 10 days or longer, intraocular pressure should be routinely monitored even though it may be difficult in children and uncooperative patients.

Employment of steroid medication in the treatment of herpes simplex requires great caution.

PRECAUTIONS

The initial prescription and renewal of the medication order beyond 20 milliliters should be made by a physician only after examination of the patient with the aid of magnification, such as slit lamp biomicroscopy and, where appropriate, fluorescein staining.

The possibility of persistent fungal infections of the cornea should be considered after prolonged steroid dosing.

ADVERSE REACTIONS

Adverse reactions have occurred with steroid/anti-infective combination drugs which can be attributed to the steroid component, the anti-infective component, or the combination. Exact incidence figures are not available since no denominator of treated patients is available.

Reactions occurring most often from the presence of the anti-infective ingredient are allergic sensitizations. The reactions due to the steroid component in decreasing order of frequency are: elevation of intraocular pressure (IOP) with possible development of glaucoma, and infrequent optic nerve damage; posterior subcapsular cataract formation; and delayed wound healing.

Secondary Infection: The development of secondary infection has occurred after use of combinations containing ste-

Continued on next page

Pfizer Inc—Cont.

roids and antimicrobials. Fungal infections of the cornea are particularly prone to develop coincidentally with long-term applications of steroid. The possibility of fungal invasion must be considered in any persistent corneal ulceration where steroid treatment has been used.
Secondary bacterial ocular infection following suppression of host responses also occurs.

DOSAGE AND ADMINISTRATION

Instill 1 or 2 drops of Terra-Cortril Ophthalmic Suspension into the affected eye three times daily.
Not more than 20 milliliters should be prescribed initially and the prescription should not be refilled without further evaluation as outlined in "Precautions" above.

HOW SUPPLIED

Terra-Cortril Ophthalmic Suspension (NDC 0049-0670-48) is supplied in 5 ml vials with separate sterile dropper.
August 1987 60-2323-00-3

TERRAMYCIN® ℞
(oxytetracycline)
INTRAMUSCULAR SOLUTION*
FOR INTRAMUSCULAR USE ONLY
contains 2% lidocaine

DESCRIPTION

Oxytetracycline is a product of the metabolism of *Streptomyces rimosus* and is one of the family of tetracycline antibiotics.
Oxytetracycline diffuses readily through the placenta into the fetal circulation, into the pleural fluid and, under some circumstances, into the cerebrospinal fluid. It appears to be concentrated in the hepatic system and excreted in the bile, so that it appears in the feces, as well as in the urine, in a biologically active form.

COMPOSITION

[See table below.]

ACTIONS

Oxytetracycline is primarily bacteriostatic and is thought to exert its antimicrobial effect by the inhibition of protein synthesis. Oxytetracycline is active against a wide range of gram-negative and gram-positive organisms.
The drugs in the tetracycline class have closely similar antimicrobial spectra, and cross resistance among them is common. Microorganisms may be considered susceptible if the M.I.C. (minimum inhibitory concentration) is not more than 4.0 mcg/ml and intermediate if the M.I.C. is 4.0 to 12.5 mcg/ml.
Susceptibility plate testing: A tetracycline disc may be used to determine microbial susceptibility to drugs in the tetracycline class. If the Kirby-Bauer method of disc susceptibility testing is used, a 30 mcg tetracycline disc should give a zone of at least 19 mm when tested against an oxytetracycline-susceptible bacterial strain.
Tetracyclines are readily absorbed and are bound to plasma proteins in varying degree. They are concentrated by the liver in the bile and excreted in the urine and feces at high concentrations and in a biologically active form.

INDICATIONS

Oxytetracycline is indicated in infections caused by the following microorganisms:
Rickettsiae (Rocky Mountain spotted fever, typhus fever and the typhus group, Q fever, rickettsialpox and tick fevers),
Mycoplasma pneumoniae (PPLO, Eaton Agent),
Agents of psittacosis and ornithosis,
Agents of lymphogranuloma venereum and granuloma inguinale,
The spirochetal agent of relapsing fever (*Borrelia recurrentis*).
The following gram-negative microorganisms:
Haemophilus ducreyi (chancroid),
Pasteurella pestis, and *Pasteurella tularensis*,
Bartonella bacilliformis,
Bacteroides species,
Vibrio comma and *Vibrio fetus*,
Brucella species (in conjunction with streptomycin).
Because many strains of the following groups of microorganisms have been shown to be resistant to tetracyclines, culture and susceptibility testing are recommended.
Oxytetracycline is indicated for treatment of infections caused by the following gram-negative microorganisms, when bacteriologic testing indicates appropriate susceptibility to the drug:
Escherichia coli,
Enterobacter aerogenes (formerly *Aerobacter aerogenes*),
Shigella species,
Mima species and *Herellea* species,
Haemophilus influenzae (respiratory infections),
Klebsiella species (respiratory and urinary infections).
Oxytetracycline is indicated for treatment of infections caused by the following gram-positive microorganisms when bacteriologic testing indicates appropriate susceptibility to the drug:
Streptococcus species;
Up to 44 percent of strains of *Streptococcus pyogenes* and 74 percent of *Streptococcus faecalis* have been found to be resistant to tetracycline drugs. Therefore, tetracyclines should not be used for streptococcal disease unless the organism has been demonstrated to be sensitive.
For upper respiratory infections due to Group A beta-hemolytic streptococci, penicillin is the usual drug of choice, including prophylaxis of rheumatic fever.
Diplococcus pneumoniae,
Staphylococcus aureus, skin and soft tissue infections. Oxytetracycline is not the drug of choice in the treatment of any type of staphylococcal infections.
When penicillin is contraindicated, tetracyclines are alternative drugs in the treatment of infections due to:
Neisseria gonorrhoeae,
Treponema pallidum and *Treponema pertenue* (syphilis and yaws),
Listeria monocytogenes,
Clostridium species,
Bacillus anthracis,
Fusobacterium fusiforme (Vincent's infection),
Actinomyces species.
In acute intestinal amebiasis, the tetracyclines may be a useful adjunct to amebicides.
Tetracyclines are indicated in the treatment of trachoma, although the infectious agent is not always eliminated, as judged by immunofluorescence.
Inclusion conjunctivitis may be treated with oral tetracyclines or with a combination of oral and topical agents.

CONTRAINDICATIONS

This drug is contraindicated in persons who have shown hypersensitivity to any of the tetracyclines.

WARNINGS

THE USE OF TETRACYCLINES DURING TOOTH DEVELOPMENT (LAST HALF OF PREGNANCY, INFANCY, AND CHILDHOOD TO THE AGE OF 8 YEARS) MAY CAUSE PERMANENT DISCOLORATION OF THE TEETH (YELLOW-GRAY-BROWN). This adverse reaction is more common during long term use of the drugs but has been observed following repeated short term courses. Enamel hypoplasia has also been reported. *TETRACYCLINES, THEREFORE, SHOULD NOT BE USED IN THIS AGE GROUP UNLESS OTHER DRUGS ARE NOT LIKELY TO BE EFFECTIVE OR ARE CONTRAINDICATED.*
If renal impairment exists, even usual oral or parenteral doses may lead to excessive systemic accumulation of the drug and possible liver toxicity. Under such conditions, lower than usual total doses are indicated and, if therapy is prolonged, serum level determinations of the drug may be advisable. This hazard is of particular importance in the parenteral administration of tetracyclines to pregnant or postpartum patients with pyelonephritis. When used under these circumstances, the blood level should not exceed 15 mcg/ml and liver function tests should be made at frequent intervals. Other potentially hepatotoxic drugs should not be prescribed concomitantly.
(In the presence of renal dysfunction, particularly in pregnancy, intravenous tetracycline therapy in daily doses exceeding 2 grams has been associated with deaths due to liver failure.)
Photosensitivity manifested by an exaggerated sunburn reaction has been observed in some individuals taking tetracyclines. Patients apt to be exposed to direct sunlight or ultraviolet light should be advised that this reaction can occur with tetracycline drugs, and treatment should be discontinued at the first evidence of skin erythema.
The antianabolic action of the tetracyclines may cause an increase in BUN. While this is not a problem in those with normal renal function, in patients with significantly impaired function, higher serum levels of this drug may lead to azotemia, hyperphosphatemia, and acidosis.
The product contains sodium formaldehyde sulfoxylate which serves as an antioxidant. Upon oxidation, this compound can form a potential sulfiting agent. Sulfiting agents may cause allergic-type reactions including anaphylactic symptoms and life-threatening or less severe asthmatic episodes in certain susceptible people. The over-all prevalence of sulfite sensitivity in the general population is unknown and probably low. Sulfite sensitivity is seen more frequently in asthmatic than in nonasthmatic people.
Usage in pregnancy. (See above "Warnings" about use during tooth development.)
Results of animal studies indicate that tetracyclines cross the placenta, are found in fetal tissues and can have toxic effects on the developing fetus (often related to retardation of skeletal development). Evidence of embryotoxicity has also been noted in animals treated early in pregnancy.
Usage in newborns, infants, and children. (See above "Warnings" about use during tooth development).
All tetracyclines form a stable calcium complex in any bone-forming tissue. A decrease in the fibula growth rate has been observed in prematures given oral tetracycline in doses of 25 mg/kg every 6 hours. This reaction was shown to be reversible when the drug was discontinued.
Tetracyclines are present in the milk of lactating women who are taking a drug in this class.

PRECAUTIONS

As with all intramuscular preparations, Terramycin (oxytetracycline) Intramuscular Solution should be injected well within the body of a relatively large muscle. ADULTS: The preferred sites are the upper outer quadrant of the buttock, (i.e., gluteus maximus), and the mid-lateral thigh. CHILDREN: It is recommended that intramuscular injections be given preferably in the mid-lateral muscles of the thigh. In infants and small children the periphery of the upper outer quadrant of the gluteal region should be used only when necessary, such as in burn patients, in order to minimize the possibility of damage to the sciatic nerve.
The deltoid area should be used only if well developed such as in certain adults and older children, and then only with caution to avoid radial nerve injury. Intramuscular injections should not be made into the lower and mid-thirds of the upper arm. As with all intramuscular injections, aspiration is necessary to help avoid inadvertent injection into a blood vessel.
As with other antibiotic preparations, use of this drug may result in overgrowth of nonsusceptible organisms, including fungi. If superinfection occurs, the antibiotic should be discontinued and appropriate therapy instituted.
In venereal diseases when coexistent syphilis is suspected, a dark field examination should be done before treatment is started and the blood serology repeated monthly for at least 4 months.
Because tetracyclines have been shown to depress plasma prothrombin activity, patients who are on anticoagulant therapy may require downward adjustment of their anticoagulant dosage.
In long term therapy, periodic laboratory evaluation of organ systems, including hematopoietic, renal and hepatic studies should be performed.
All infections due to Group A beta-hemolytic streptococci should be treated for at least 10 days.
Since bacteriostatic drugs may interfere with the bactericidal action of penicillin, it is advisable to avoid giving tetracycline in conjunction with penicillin.

ADVERSE REACTIONS

Local irritation may be present after intramuscular injection. The injection should be deep, with care taken not to injure the sciatic nerve nor inject intravascularly.
Gastrointestinal: anorexia, nausea, vomiting, diarrhea, glossitis, dysphagia, enterocolitis, and inflammatory lesions (with monilial overgrowth) in the anogenital region. These

Terramycin Intramuscular
contents per ml (w/v)

Ingredient	2 ml Single Dose Ampules 100 mg/2 ml	250 mg/2 ml	10 ml/Vial Multidose 50 mg/ml 10 ml (5 × 2 ml Doses)
oxytetracycline	50 mg	125 mg	50 mg
lidocaine	2.0%	2.0%	2.0%
magnesium chloride hexahydrate	2.5%	6.0%	2.5%
sodium formaldehyde sulfoxylate	0.5%	0.5%	0.3%
α-monothioglycerol	—	—	1.0%
monoethanolamine	approx. 1.7%	approx. 4.2%	approx. 2.6%
citric acid	—	—	1.0%
propyl gallate	—	—	0.02%
propylene glycol	75.2%	67.0%	74.1%
water	18.8%	16.8%	18.5%

reactions have been caused by both the oral and parenteral administration of tetracyclines.

Skin: maculopapular and erythematous rashes. Exfoliative dermatitis has been reported but is uncommon. Photosensitivity is discussed above. (See "Warnings").

Renal toxicity: Rise in BUN has been reported and is apparently dose related. (See "Warnings").

Hypersensitivity reactions: Urticaria, angioneurotic edema, anaphylaxis, anaphylactoid purpura, pericarditis, and exacerbation of systemic lupus erythematosus.

Bulging fontanels in infants and benign intracranial hypertension in adults have been reported in individuals receiving full therapeutic dosages. These conditions disappeared rapidly when the drug was discontinued.

Blood: Hemolytic anemia, thrombocytopenia, neutropenia, and eosinophilia have been reported.

When given over prolonged periods, tetracyclines have been reported to produce brown-black microscopic discoloration of thyroid glands. No abnormalities of thyroid function studies are known to occur.

DOSAGE AND ADMINISTRATION

Intramuscular Administration:

Adults: The usual daily dose is 250 mg administered once every 24 hours or 300 mg given in divided doses at 8 to 12 hour intervals.

For children above eight years of age: 15–25 mg/kg body weight up to a maximum of 250 mg per single daily injection. Dosage may be divided and given at 8 to 12 hour intervals.

Intramuscular therapy should be reserved for situations in which oral therapy is not feasible.

The intramuscular administration of oxytetracycline produces lower blood levels than oral administration in the recommended dosages. Patients placed on intramuscular oxytetracycline should be changed to the oral dosage form as soon as possible. If rapid, high blood levels are needed, oxytetracycline should be administered intravenously.

In patients with renal impairment: (See "Warnings") Total dosage should be decreased by reduction of recommended individual doses and/or by extending time intervals between doses.

HOW SUPPLIED

Terramycin (oxytetracycline) Intramuscular Solution is available as follows:

50 mg/mL—in 10 ml multiple dose vials, packages of 5 (NDC 0049-0750-77).

*U.S. Pat. Nos. 3,017,323 and 3,026,248

Revised March 1987 70-1051-00-2

TERRAMYCIN® ℞
(oxytetracycline HCl with polymyxin B sulfate)
OPHTHALMIC OINTMENT
STERILE

DESCRIPTION

Each gram of sterile ointment contains oxytetracycline HCl equivalent to 5 mg oxytetracycline, 10,000 units of polymyxin B sulfate, white petrolatum, and liquid petrolatum.

ACTIONS

Terramycin® is a widely used antibiotic with clinically proved activity against gram-positive and gram-negative bacteria, rickettsiae, spirochetes, large viruses, and certain protozoa.

Polymyxin B Sulfate, one of a group of related antibiotics derived from *Bacillus polymyxa,* is rapidly bactericidal. This action is exclusively against gram-negative organisms. It is particularly effective against *Pseudomonas aeruginosa (B. pyocyaneus)* and Koch-Weeks bacillus, frequently found in local infections of the eye.

There is thus made available a particularly effective antimicrobial combination of the broad-spectrum antibiotic Terramycin as well as polymyxin B sulfate against primarily causative or secondarily infecting organisms.

INDICATIONS

The sterile preparation, Terramycin with Polymyxin B Sulfate Ophthalmic Ointment, is indicated for the treatment of superficial ocular infections involving the conjunctiva and/or cornea caused by Terramycin with Polymyxin B Sulfate-susceptible organisms.

It may be administered topically alone, or as an adjunct to systemic therapy.

It is effective in infections caused by susceptible strains of staphylococci, streptococci, pneumococci, *Hemophilus influenzae, Pseudomonas aeruginosa,* Koch-Weeks bacillus, and *Proteus.*

CONTRAINDICATIONS

This drug is contraindicated in individuals who have shown hypersensitivity to any of its components.

PRECAUTIONS

As with all antibiotic preparations, use of this drug may result in overgrowth of nonsusceptible organisms, including fungi. If superinfection occurs, the antibiotic should be discontinued and appropriate specific therapy should be instituted.

ADVERSE REACTIONS

Terramycin with Polymyxin B Sulfate Ophthalmic Ointment is well tolerated by the epithelial membranes and other tissues of the eye. Allergic or inflammatory reactions due to individual hypersensitivity are rare.

DOSAGE AND ADMINISTRATION

Approximately 1/2 inch of the ointment is squeezed from the tube onto the lower lid of the affected eye two to four times daily.

The patient should be instructed to avoid contamination of the tip of the tube when applying the ointment.

HOW SUPPLIED

Terramycin with Polymyxin B Sulfate Ophthalmic Ointment is supplied in 1/8 oz (3.5 g) tubes (NDC 0049-0801-08).

August 1987 60-2324-00-1

UNASYN® ℞
(ampicillin sodium/sulbactam sodium)

DESCRIPTION

UNASYN is an injectable antibacterial combination consisting of the semisynthetic antibiotic ampicillin sodium and the beta-lactamase inhibitor sulbactam sodium for intravenous and intramuscular administration.

Ampicillin sodium is derived from the penicillin nucleus, 6-aminopenicillanic acid. Chemically, it is monosodium (2S, 5R, 6R)-6-[(R)-2-amino-2-phenylacetamido]-3,3-dimethyl-7-oxo-4-thia-1-azabicyclo[3.2.0]heptane-2-carboxylate and has a molecular weight of 371.39. Its chemical formula is $C_{16}H_{18}N_3NaO_4S$. The structural formula is:

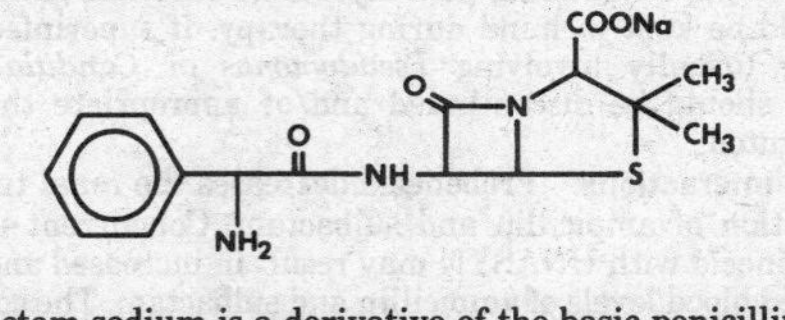

Sulbactam sodium is a derivative of the basic penicillin nucleus. Chemically, sulbactam sodium is sodium penicillinate sulfone; sodium (2S, 5R)-3,3-dimethyl-7-oxo-4-thia-1-azabicyclo[3.2.0]heptane-2-carboxylate 4,4-dioxide. Its chemical formula is $C_8H_{10}NNaO_5S$ with a molecular weight of 255.22. The structural formula is:

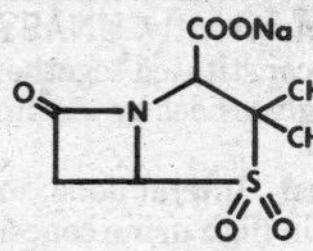

UNASYN, ampicillin sodium/sulbactam sodium parenteral combination, is available as a white to off-white dry powder for reconstitution. UNASYN dry powder is freely soluble in aqueous diluents to yield pale yellow to yellow solutions containing ampicillin sodium and sulbactam sodium equivalent to 250 mg ampicillin per mL and 125 mg sulbactam per mL. The pH of the solutions is between 8.0 and 10.0.

Dilute solutions (up to 30 mg ampicillin and 15 mg sulbactam per mL) are essentially colorless to pale yellow. The pH of dilute solutions remains the same.

1.5 g of UNASYN (1 g ampicillin as the sodium salt plus 0.5 g sulbactam as the sodium salt) parenteral contains approximately 115 mg (5 mEq) of sodium.

3 g of UNASYN (2 g ampicillin as the sodium salt plus 1 g sulbactam as the sodium salt) parenteral contains approximately 230 mg (10 mEq) of sodium.

CLINICAL PHARMACOLOGY

General: Immediately after completion of a 15-minute intravenous infusion of UNASYN, peak serum concentrations of ampicillin and sulbactam are attained. Ampicillin serum levels are similar to those produced by the administration of equivalent amounts of ampicillin alone. Peak ampicillin serum levels ranging from 109 to 150 mcg/mL are attained after administration of 2000 mg of ampicillin plus 1000 mg sulbactam and 40 to 71 mcg/mL after administration of 1000 mg ampicillin plus 500 mg sulbactam. The corresponding mean peak serum levels for sulbactam range from 48 to 88 mcg/mL and 21 to 40 mcg/mL, respectively. After an intramuscular injection of 1000 mg ampicillin plus 500 mg sulbactam, peak ampicillin serum levels ranging from 8 to 37 mcg/mL and peak sulbactam serum levels ranging from 6 to 24 mcg/mL are attained.

The mean serum half-life of both drugs is approximately 1 hour in healthy volunteers.

Approximately 75 to 85% of both ampicillin and sulbactam are excreted unchanged in the urine during the first 8 hours after administration of UNASYN to individuals with normal renal function. Somewhat higher and more prolonged serum levels of ampicillin and sulbactam can be achieved with the concurrent administration of probenecid.

In patients with impaired renal function the elimination kinetics of ampicillin and sulbactam are similarly affected, hence the ratio of one to the other will remain constant whatever the renal function. The dose of UNASYN in such patients should be administered less frequently in accordance with the usual practice for ampicillin (see Dosage and Administration).

Ampicillin has been found to be approximately 28% reversibly bound to human serum protein and sulbactam approximately 38% reversibly bound.

The following average levels of ampicillin and sulbactam were measured in the tissues and fluids listed:

TABLE A
Concentration of UNASYN in Various Body Tissues and Fluids

Fluid or Tissue	Dose (grams) Ampicillin/ Sulbactam	Concentration (mcg/mL or mcg/g) Ampicillin/ Sulbactam
Peritoneal Fluid	0.5/0.5 IV	7/14
Blister Fluid (Cantharides)	0.5/0.5 IV	8/20
Tissue Fluid	1/0.5 IV	8/4
Intestinal Mucosa	0.5/0.5 IV	11/18
Appendix	2/1 IV	3/40

Penetration of both ampicillin and sulbactam into cerebrospinal fluid in the presence of inflamed meninges has been demonstrated after IV administration of UNASYN.

MICROBIOLOGY

Ampicillin is similar to benzyl penicillin in its bactericidal action against susceptible organisms during the stage of active multiplication. It acts through the inhibition of cell wall mucopeptide biosynthesis. Ampicillin has a broad spectrum of bactericidal activity against many gram-positive and gram-negative aerobic and anaerobic bacteria. (Ampicillin is, however, degraded by beta-lactamases and therefore the spectrum of activity does not normally include organisms which produce these enzymes.)

A wide range of beta-lactamases found in microorganisms resistant to penicillins and cephalosporins have been shown in biochemical studies with cell free bacterial systems to be irreversibly inhibited by sulbactam. Although sulbactam alone possesses little useful antibacterial activity except against the *Neisseriaciae,* whole organism studies have shown that sulbactam restores ampicillin activity against beta-lactamase producing strains. In particular, sulbactam has good inhibitory activity against the clinically important plasmid mediated beta-lactamases most frequently responsible for transferred drug resistance. Sulbactam has no effect on the activity of ampicillin against ampicillin susceptible strains.

The presence of sulbactam in the UNASYN formulation effectively extends the antibiotic spectrum of ampicillin to include many bacteria normally resistant to it and to other beta-lactam antibiotics. Thus, UNASYN possesses the properties of a broad-spectrum antibiotic and a beta-lactamase inhibitor.

While *in vitro* studies have demonstrated the susceptibility of most strains of the following organisms, clinical efficacy for infections other than those included in the indications section has not been documented.

Gram-Positive Bacteria: *Staphylococcus aureus* (beta-lactamase and non-beta-lactamase producing), *Staphylococcus epidermidis* (beta-lactamase and non-beta-lactamase producing), *Staphylococcus saprophyticus* (beta-lactamase and non-beta-lactamase producing), *Streptococcus faecalis*† (Enterococcus), *Streptococcus pneumoniae*† (formerly *D. pneumoniae), Streptococcus pyogenes*†, *Streptococcus viridans*†.

Gram-Negative Bacteria: *Hemophilus influenzae* (beta-lactamase and non-beta-lactamase producing). *Moraxella (Branhamella) catarrhalis* (beta-lactamase and non-beta-lactamase producing). *Escherichia coli* (beta-lactamase and non-beta-lactamase producing). *Klebsiella* species (all known strains are beta-lactamase producing). *Proteus mirabilis* (beta-lactamase and non-beta-lactamase producing). *Proteus vulgaris, Providencia rettgeri, Providencia stuartii, Morganella morganii,* and *Neisseria gonorrhoeae* (beta-lactamase and non-beta-lactamase producing).

Anaerobes: *Clostridium* species†, *Peptococcus* species†, *Peptostreptococcus* species, *Bacteroides* species, including *B. fragilis.*

†These are not beta-lactamase producing strains and, therefore, are susceptible to ampicillin alone.

Continued on next page

Pfizer Inc—Cont.

Susceptibility Testing

Diffusion Technique: For the Kirby-Bauer method of susceptibility testing, a 20 mcg (10 mcg ampicillin + 10 mcg sulbactam) diffusion disk should be used. The method is one outlined in the NCCLS publication M2-A4.[1] With this procedure, a report from the laboratory of "Susceptible" indicates that the infecting organism is likely to respond to UNASYN therapy and a report of "Resistant" indicates that the infecting organism is not likely to respond to therapy. An "Intermediate" susceptibility report suggests that the infecting organism would be susceptible to UNASYN if a higher dosage is used or if the infection is confined to tissues or fluids (e.g., urine) in which high antibiotic levels are attained.

Dilution Techniques: Broth or agar dilution methods may be used to determine the minimal inhibitory concentration (MIC) value for susceptibility of bacterial isolates to ampicillin/sulbactam. The method used is one outlined in the NCCLS publication M7-A2.[2] Tubes should be inoculated to contain 10^5 to 10^6 organisms/mL or plates "spotted" with 10^4 organisms.

The recommended dilution method employs a constant ampicillin/sulbactam ratio of 2:1 in all tubes with increasing concentrations of ampicillin. MIC's are reported in terms of ampicillin concentration in the presence of sulbactam at a constant 2 parts ampicillin to 1 part sulbactam.

[See table below.]

INDICATIONS AND USAGE

UNASYN is indicated for the treatment of infections due to susceptible strains of the designated microorganisms in the conditions listed below.

Skin and Skin Structure Infections caused by beta-lactamase producing strains of *Staphylococcus aureus, Escherichia coli,* Klebsiella* spp.* (including *K. pneumoniae*), Proteus mirabilis,* Bacteroides fragilis,* Enterobacter* spp.,* and *Acinetobacter calcoaceticus.**

Intra-Abdominal Infections caused by beta-lactamase producing strains of *Escherichia coli, Klebsiella* spp. (including *K. pneumoniae*), Bacteroides* spp. (including *B. fragilis*), and *Enterobacter* spp.*

Gynecological Infections caused by beta-lactamase producing strains of *Escherichia coli,** and *Bacteroides* spp.* (including *B. fragilis*).*

* Efficacy for this organism in this organ system was studied in fewer than 10 infections.

While UNASYN is indicated only for the conditions listed above, infections caused by ampicillin-susceptible organisms are also amenable to treatment with UNASYN due to its ampicillin content. Therefore, mixed infections caused by ampicillin-susceptible organisms and beta-lactamase producing organisms susceptible to UNASYN should not require the addition of another antibiotic.

Appropriate culture and susceptibility tests should be performed before treatment in order to isolate and identify the organisms causing infection and to determine their susceptibility to UNASYN.

Therapy may be instituted prior to obtaining the results from bacteriological and susceptibility studies, when there is reason to believe the infection may involve any of the beta-lactamase producing organisms listed above in the indicated organ systems. Once the results are known, therapy should be adjusted if appropriate.

CONTRAINDICATIONS

The use of UNASYN is contraindicated in individuals with a history of hypersensitivity reactions to any of the penicillins.

WARNINGS

SERIOUS AND OCCASIONALLY FATAL HYPERSENSITIVITY (ANAPHYLACTIC) REACTIONS HAVE BEEN REPORTED IN PATIENTS ON PENICILLIN THERAPY. THESE REACTIONS ARE MORE APT TO OCCUR IN INDIVIDUALS WITH A HISTORY OF PENICILLIN HYPERSENSITIVITY AND/OR HYPERSENSITIVITY REACTIONS TO MULTIPLE ALLERGENS. THERE HAVE BEEN REPORTS OF INDIVIDUALS WITH A HISTORY OF PENICILLIN HYPERSENSITIVITY WHO HAVE EXPERIENCED SEVERE REACTIONS WHEN TREATED WITH CEPHALOSPORINS. BEFORE THERAPY WITH A PENICILLIN, CAREFUL INQUIRY SHOULD BE MADE CONCERNING PREVIOUS HYPERSENSITIVITY REACTIONS TO PENICILLINS, CEPHALOSPORINS, AND OTHER ALLERGENS. IF AN ALLERGIC REACTION OCCURS, UNASYN SHOULD BE DISCONTINUED AND THE APPROPRIATE THERAPY INSTITUTED.

SERIOUS ANAPHYLACTOID REACTIONS REQUIRE IMMEDIATE EMERGENCY TREATMENT WITH EPINEPHRINE. OXYGEN, INTRAVENOUS STEROIDS, AND AIRWAY MANAGEMENT, INCLUDING INTUBATION, SHOULD ALSO BE ADMINISTERED AS INDICATED.

Pseudomembranous colitis has been reported with nearly all antibacterial agents, including UNASYN, and has ranged in severity from mild to life-threatening. Therefore, it is important to consider this diagnosis in patients who present with diarrhea subsequent to the administration of antibacterial agents.

Treatment with antibacterial agents alters the normal flora of the colon and may permit overgrowth of clostridia. Studies indicate that toxin produced by *Clostridium difficile* is one primary cause of "antibiotic-associated colitis."

Mild cases of pseudomembranous colitis usually respond to drug discontinuation alone. In moderate to severe cases, consideration should be given to management with fluids and electrolytes, protein supplementation and treatment with an antibacterial drug clinically effective against *C. difficile* colitis.

PRECAUTIONS

General: A high percentage of patients with mononucleosis who receive ampicillin develop a skin rash. Thus, ampicillin class antibiotics should not be administered to patients with mononucleosis. In patients treated with UNASYN the possibility of superinfections with mycotic or bacterial pathogens should be kept in mind during therapy. If superinfections occur (usually involving *Pseudomonas* or *Candida*), the drug should be discontinued and/or appropriate therapy instituted.

Drug Interactions: Probenecid decreases the renal tubular secretion of ampicillin and sulbactam. Concurrent use of probenecid with UNASYN may result in increased and prolonged blood levels of ampicillin and sulbactam. The concurrent administration of allopurinol and ampicillin increases substantially the incidence of rashes in patients receiving both drugs as compared to patients receiving ampicillin alone. It is not known whether this potentiation of ampicillin rashes is due to allopurinol or the hyperuricemia present in these patients. There are no data with UNASYN and allopurinol administered concurrently. UNASYN and aminoglycosides should not be reconstituted together due to the *in vitro* inactivation of aminoglycosides by the ampicillin component of UNASYN.

Drug/Laboratory Test Interactions: Administration of UNASYN will result in high urine concentration of ampicillin. High urine concentrations of ampicillin may result in false positive reactions when testing for the presence of glucose in urine using Clinitest™, Benedict's Solution or Fehling's Solution. It is recommended that glucose tests based on enzymatic glucose oxidase reactions (such as Clinistix™ or Testape™) be used. Following administration of ampicillin to pregnant women, a transient decrease in plasma concentration of total conjugated estriol, estriol-glucuronide, conjugated estrone and estradiol has been noted. This effect may also occur with UNASYN.

Recommended ampicillin/sulbactam, Susceptibility Ranges[1,2,3]

	Resistant	Intermediate	Susceptible
Gram(−) and Staphylococcus			
Bauer/Kirby Zone Sizes	≤11 mm	12–13 mm	≥14 mm
MIC (mcg of ampicillin/mL)	≥32	16	≤8
Hemophilus influenzae			
Bauer/Kirby Zone Sizes	≤19	—	≥20
MIC (mcg of ampicillin/mL)	≥4	—	≤2

[1]The non-beta-lactamase producing organisms which are normally susceptible to ampicillin, such as *Streptococci*, will have similar zone sizes as for ampicillin disks.

[2]*Staphylococci* resistant to methicillin, oxacillin, or nafcillin must be considered resistant to UNASYN.

[3]The quality control cultures should have the following assigned daily ranges for ampicillin/sulbactam:

		Disks	Mode MIC (mcg/mL ampicillin/mcg/mL sulbactam)
E. coli	(ATCC 25922)	20–24 mm	2/1
S. aureus	(ATCC 25923)	29–37 mm	0.12/0.06
E. coli	(ATCC 35218)	13–19 mm	8/4

Carcinogenesis, Mutagenesis, Impairment of Fertility: Long-term studies in animals have not been performed to evaluate carcinogenic or mutagenic potential.

Pregnancy

Pregnancy Category B: Reproduction studies have been performed in mice, rats, and rabbits at doses up to ten (10) times the human dose and have revealed no evidence of impaired fertility or harm to the fetus due to UNASYN. There are, however, no adequate and well controlled studies in pregnant women. Because animal reproduction studies are not always predictive of human response, this drug should be used during pregnancy only if clearly needed. (See—Drug/Laboratory Test Interactions.)

Labor and Delivery: Studies in guinea pigs have shown that intravenous administration of ampicillin decreased the uterine tone, frequency of contractions, height of contractions, and duration of contractions. However, it is not known whether the use of UNASYN in humans during labor or delivery has immediate or delayed adverse effects on the fetus, prolongs the duration of labor, or increases the likelihood that forceps delivery or other obstetrical intervention or resuscitation of the newborn will be necessary.

Nursing Mothers: Low concentrations of ampicillin and sulbactam are excreted in the milk; therefore, caution should be exercised when UNASYN is administered to a nursing woman.

Pediatric Use: The efficacy and safety of UNASYN have not been established in infants and children under the age of 12.

ADVERSE REACTIONS

UNASYN is generally well tolerated. The following adverse reactions have been reported.

Local Adverse Reactions

Pain at IM injection site—16%
Pain at IV injection site—3%
Thrombophlebitis—3%

Systemic Adverse Reactions

The most frequently reported adverse reactions were diarrhea in 3% of the patients and rash in less than 2% of the patients.

Additional systemic reactions reported in less than 1% of the patients were: itching, nausea, vomiting, candidiasis, fatigue, malaise, headache, chest pain, flatulence, abdominal distension, glossitis, urine retention, dysuria, edema, facial swelling, erythema, chills, tightness in throat, substernal pain, epistaxis and mucosal bleeding.

Adverse Laboratory Changes

Adverse laboratory changes without regard to drug relationship that were reported during clinical trials were:

Hepatic: Increased AST (SGOT), ALT (SGPT), alkaline phosphatase, and LDH.

Hematologic: Decreased hemoglobin, hematocrit, RBC, WBC, neutrophils, lymphocytes, platelets and increased lymphocytes, monocytes, basophils, eosinophils, and platelets.

Blood Chemistry: Decreased serum albumin and total proteins.

Renal: Increased BUN and creatinine.

Urinalysis: Presence of RBC's and hyaline casts in urine.

The following adverse reactions have been reported with ampicillin-class antibiotics and can also occur with UNASYN.

Gastrointestinal: Gastritis, stomatitis, black "hairy" tongue, and enterocolitis. Onset of pseudomembranous colitis symptoms may occur during or after antibiotic treatment. (See WARNINGS.)

Hypersensitivity Reactions: Urticaria, erythema multiforme, and an occasional case of exfoliative dermatitis have been reported. These reactions may be controlled with antihistamines and, if necessary, systemic corticosteroids. Whenever such reactions occur, the drug should be discontinued, unless the opinion of the physician dictates otherwise. Serious and occasional fatal hypersensitivity (anaphylactic) reactions can occur with a penicillin. (See WARNINGS.)

Hematologic: In addition to the adverse laboratory changes listed above for UNASYN, agranulocytosis has been reported during therapy with penicillins. All of these reactions are usually reversible on discontinuation of therapy and are believed to be hypersensitivity phenomena. Some individuals have developed positive direct Coombs Tests during treatment with UNASYN, as with other beta-lactam antibiotics.

OVERDOSAGE

Neurological adverse reactions, including convulsions, may occur with the attainment of high CSF levels of beta-lactams. Ampicillin may be removed from circulation by hemodialysis. The molecular weight, degree of protein binding and pharmacokinetics profile of sulbactam suggest that this compound may also be removed by hemodialysis.

DOSAGE AND ADMINISTRATION

UNASYN may be administered by either the IV or the IM routes.

For IV administration, the dose can be given by slow intravenous injection over at least 10–15 minutes or can also be de-

Diluent	Maximum Concentration (mg/mL) UNASYN (Ampicillin/Sulbactam)	Use Periods
Sterile Water for Injection	45 (30/15)	8 hrs @ 25°C
	45 (30/15)	48 hrs @ 4°C
	30 (20/10)	72 hrs @ 4°C
0.9% Sodium Chloride Injection	45 (30/15)	8 hrs @ 25°C
	45 (30/15)	48 hrs @ 4°C
	30 (20/10)	72 hrs @ 4°C
5% Dextrose Injection	30 (20/10)	2 hrs @ 25°C
	30 (20/10)	4 hrs @ 4°C
	3 (2/1)	4 hrs @ 4°C
Lactated Ringer's Injection	45 (30/15)	8 hrs @ 25°C
	45 (30/15)	24 hrs @ 4°C
M/6 Sodium Lactate Injection	45 (30/15)	8 hrs @ 25°C
5% Dextrose in 0.45% Saline	45 (30/15)	8 hrs @ 25°C
	3 (2/1)	4 hrs @ 25°C
10% Invert Sugar	15 (10/5)	4 hrs @ 4°C
	3 (2/1)	4 hrs @ 4°C
	30 (20/10)	3 hrs @ 4°C

livered, in greater dilutions with 50–100 mL of a compatible diluent as an intravenous infusion over 15–30 minutes. UNASYN may be administered by deep intramuscular injection. (See Preparation for Intramuscular Injection.) The recommended adult dosage of UNASYN is 1.5 g (1 g ampicillin as the sodium salt plus 0.5 g sulbactam as the sodium salt) to 3 g (2 g ampicillin as the sodium salt plus 1 g sulbactam as the sodium salt) every six hours. This 1.5 to 3 g range represents the total of ampicillin content plus the sulbactam content of UNASYN, and corresponds to a range of 1 g ampicillin/0.5 g sulbactam to 2 g ampicillin/1 g sulbactam. The total dose of sulbactam should not exceed 4 grams per day.

Impaired Renal Function

In patients with impairment of renal function the elimination kinetics of ampicillin and sulbactam are similarly affected, hence the ratio of one to the other will remain constant whatever the renal function. The dose of UNASYN in such patients should be administered less frequently in accordance with the usual practice for ampicillin and according to the following recommendations:

UNASYN Dosage Guide For Patients With Renal Impairment

Creatinine Clearance (mL/min/1.73m²)	Ampicillin/ Sulbactam Half-Life (Hours)	Recommended UNASYN Dosage
≥ 30	1	1.5–3.0 g q 6h–q 8h
15–29	5	1.5–3.0 g q 12h
5–14	9	1.5–3.0 g q 24h

When only serum creatinine is available, the following formula (based on sex, weight, and age of the patient) may be used to convert this value into creatinine clearance. The serum creatinine should represent a steady state of renal function.

$$\text{Males} \quad \frac{\text{weight (kg)} \times (140 - \text{age})}{72 \times \text{serum creatinine}}$$

Females   0.85 × above value

COMPATABILITY, RECONSTITUTION AND STABILITY

UNASYN sterile powder is to be stored at or below 30°C (86°F) prior to reconstitution.

When concomitant therapy with aminoglycosides is indicated, UNASYN and aminoglycosides should be reconstituted and administered separately, due to the *in vitro* inactivation of aminoglycosides by any of the aminopenicillins.

DIRECTIONS FOR USE

General Dissolution Procedures: UNASYN sterile powder for intravenous and intramuscular use may be reconstituted with any of the compatible diluents described in this insert. Solutions should be allowed to stand after dissolution to allow any foaming to dissipate in order to permit visual inspection for complete solubilization.

Preparation for Intravenous Use

1.5 g and 3.0 g Bottles: UNASYN sterile powder in piggyback units may be reconstituted directly to the desired concentrations using any of the following parenteral diluents. Reconstitution of UNASYN, at the specified concentrations, with these diluents provide stable solutions for the time periods indicated in the following table: (After the indicated time periods, any unused portions of solutions should be discarded.) [See table above.]

If piggyback bottles are unavailable, standard vials of UNASYN sterile powder may be used. Initially, the vials may be reconstituted with Sterile Water for Injection to yield solutions containing 375 mg UNASYN per mL (250 mg ampicillin/125 mg sulbactam per mL). An appropriate volume should then be immediately diluted with a suitable parenteral diluent to yield solutions containing 3 to 45 mg UNASYN per mL (2 to 30 mg ampicillin/1 to 15 mg sulbactam per mL).

1.5 g ADD-Vantage® Vials: UNASYN in the ADD-Vantage® system is intended as a single dose for intravenous administration after dilution with the ADD-Vantage® Flexible Diluent Container containing 50 mL, 100 mL or 250 mL of 0.9% Sodium Chloride Injection, USP.

3 g ADD-Vantage® Vials: UNASYN in the ADD-Vantage® system is intended as a single dose for intravenous administration after dilution with the ADD-Vantage® Flexible Diluent Container containing 100 mL or 250 mL of 0.9% Sodium Chloride Injection, USP.

UNASYN in the ADD-Vantage® system is to be reconstituted with 0.9% Sodium Chloride Injection, USP only. See INSTRUCTIONS FOR USE OF THE ADD-Vantage® VIAL. Reconstitution of UNASYN, at the specified concentration, with 0.9% Sodium Chloride Injection, USP provides stable solutions for the time period indicated below:

Maximum Concentration (mg/mL)

Diluent	UNASYN (Ampicillin/Sulbactam)	Use Period
0.9% Sodium Chloride Injection	30 (20/10)	8 hrs @ 25°C

In 0.9% Sodium Chloride Injection, USP

The final diluted solution of UNASYN should be completely administered *within 8 hours* in order to assure proper potency.

Preparation for Intramuscular Injection

1.5 g and 3.0 g Standard Vials: Vials for intramuscular use may be reconstituted with Sterile Water for Injection USP, 0.5% Lidocaine Hydrochloride Injection USP or 2% Lidocaine Hydrochloride Injection USP. Consult the following table for recommended volumes to be added to obtain solutions containing 375 mg UNASYN per mL (250 mg ampicillin/125 mg sulbactam per mL). Note: *Use only freshly prepared solutions and administer within one hour after preparation.*

UNASYN Vial Size	Volume of Diluent to be Added	Withdrawal Volume*
1.5 g	3.2 mL	4.0 mL
3.0 g	6.4 mL	8.0 mL

*There is sufficient excess present to allow withdrawal and administration of the stated volumes.

Animal Pharmacology: While reversible glycogenosis was observed in laboratory animals, this phenomenon was dose- and time-dependent and is not expected to develop at the therapeutic doses and corresponding plasma levels attained during the relatively short periods of combined ampicillin/sulbactam therapy in man.

HOW SUPPLIED

UNASYN (ampicillin sodium/sulbactam sodium) is supplied as a sterile off-white dry powder in glass vials and piggyback bottles. The following packages are available:

Vials containing 1.5 g (NDC 0049-0013-83) equivalent of UNASYN (1 g ampicillin as the sodium salt plus 0.5 g sulbactam as the sodium salt)

Vials containing 3 g (NDC 0049-0014-83) equivalent of UNASYN (2 g ampicillin as the sodium salt plus 1 g sulbactam as the sodium salt)

Bottles containing 1.5 g (NDC 0049-0022-83) equivalent of UNASYN (1 g ampicillin as the sodium salt plus 0.5 g sulbactam as the sodium salt)

Bottles containing 3 g (NDC 0049-0023-83) equivalent of UNASYN (2 g ampicillin as the sodium salt plus 1 g sulbactam as the sodium salt)

Pharmacy Bulk Package containing 15 g (NDC 0049-0024-28) equivalent of UNASYN (10 g ampicillin as the sodium salt plus 5 g sulbactam as the sodium salt)

ADD-Vantage® vials containing 1.5 g (NDC 0049-0031-83) equivalent of UNASYN (1 g ampicillin as the sodium salt plus 0.5 g sulbactam as the sodium salt) are distributed by Pfizer Inc.

ADD-Vantage® vials containing 3 g (NDC 0049-0032-83) equivalent of UNASYN (2 g ampicillin as the sodium salt plus 1 g sulbactum as the sodium salt) are distributed by Pfizer Inc.

The 1.5 g UNASYN ADD-Vantage® vials are only to be used with Abbott Laboratories' ADD-Vantage® Flexible Diluent Container containing 0.9% Sodium Chloride Injection, USP, 50 mL, 100 mL, or 250 mL sizes.

The 3 g UNASYN ADD-Vantage® vials are only to be used with Abbott Laboratories' ADD-Vantage® Flexible Diluent Container containing 0.9% Sodium Chloride Injection, USP, 100 mL or 250 mL sizes.

INSTRUCTIONS FOR USE OF THE ADD-Vantage® VIAL

To Open Diluent Container: Peel overwrap from the corner and remove container. Some opacity of the plastic due to moisture absorption during the sterilization process may be observed. This is normal and does not affect the solution quality or safety. The opacity will diminish gradually.

To Assemble Vial and Flexible Diluent Container: (Use Aseptic Technique)

1. Remove the protective covers from the top of the vial and the vial port on the diluent container as follows:

a. To remove the breakaway vial cap, swing the pull ring over the top of the vial and pull down far enough to start the opening (see Figure 1), pull the ring approximately half way around the cap and then pull straight up to remove the cap (see Figure 2).

NOTE: Do not access vial with syringe.

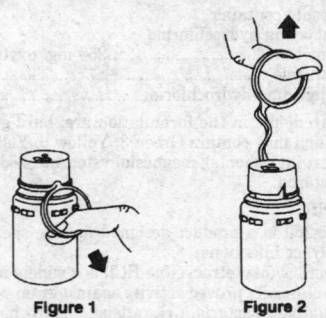

Figure 1   Figure 2

b. To remove the vial port cover, grasp the tab on the pull ring, pull up to break the three tie strings, then pull back to remove the cover. (See Figure 3.)

2. Screw the vial into the vial port until it will go no further. THE VIAL MUST BE SCREWED IN TIGHTLY TO ASSURE A SEAL. This occurs approximately ¹/₂ turn (180°) after the first audible click. (See Figure 4.) The clicking sound does not assure a seal, the vial must be turned as far as it will go.

NOTE: Once vial is sealed, do not attempt to remove. (See Figure 4.)

3. Recheck the vial to assure that it is tight by trying to turn it further in the direction of assembly.

4. Label appropriately.

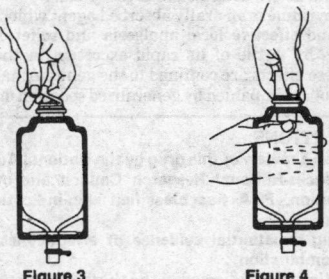

Figure 3   Figure 4

To Prepare Admixture

1. Squeeze the bottom of the diluent container gently to inflate the portion of the container surrounding the end of the drug vial.

2. With the other hand, push the drug vial down into the container telescoping the walls of the container. Grasp the inner cap of the vial through the walls of the container. (See Figure 5.)

3. Pull the inner cap from the drug vial. (See Figure 6.) Verify that the rubber stopper has been pulled out, allowing the drug and diluent to mix.

4. Mix container contents thoroughly and use within the specified time.

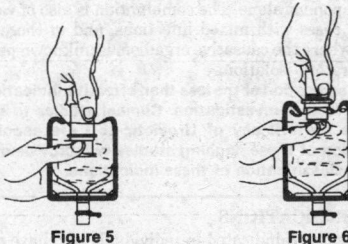

Figure 5   Figure 6

Continued on next page

Pfizer Inc—Cont.

REFERENCES

1. National Committee for Clinical Laboratory Standards, *Performance Standards for Antimicrobial Disk Susceptibility Tests*—Fourth Edition. Approved Standard NCCLS Document M2-A4, Vol. 10, No. 7 NCCLS. Villanova, PA. April 1990.
2. National Committee for Clinical Laboratory Standards, *Methods for Dilution Antimicrobial Susceptibility Tests for Bacteria that Grow Aerobically.* Second Edition. Approved Standard NCCLS Document M7-A2. Vol. 10, No. 8 NCCLS. Villanova, PA. April 1990.

69-4361-00-2 Rev. Jan. 1994

Shown in Product Identification Guide, page 328

UROBIOTIC®-250 ℞

[u ″rō-bī-ot ′ik]

CAPSULES

Each capsule contains

Oxytetracycline hydrochloride equivalent to	250 mg. oxytetracycline
Sulfamethizole	250 mg
Phenazopyridine hydrochloride	50 mg

Inert ingredients in the formulation are: hard gelatin capsules (which may contain Green 3, Yellow 6, Yellow 10 and other inert ingredients); magnesium stearate; sodium lauryl sulfate; starch.

ACTIONS

Urobiotic-250 is a product designed for use specifically in urinary tract infections.

Terramycin® (oxytetracycline HCl) is a widely used antibiotic with clinically proved activity against gram-positive and gram-negative bacteria, rickettsiae, spirochetes, large viruses, and certain protozoa. Terramycin is well tolerated and well absorbed after oral administration. It diffuses readily through the placenta and is present in the fetal circulation. It diffuses into the pleural fluid, and under some circumstances, into the cerebrospinal fluid. Oxytetracycline HCl appears to be concentrated in the hepatic system and is excreted in the bile. It is excreted in the urine and in the feces, in high concentrations, in a biologically active form.

Sulfamethizole is a chemotherapeutic agent active against a number of important gram-positive and gram-negative bacteria. This sulfonamide is well absorbed, has a low degree of acetylation, and is extremely soluble. Because of these features and its rapid renal excretion, sulfamethizole has a low order of toxicity and provides prompt and high concentrations of the active drug in the urinary tract.

Phenazopyridine is an orally absorbed agent which produces prompt and effective local analgesia and relief of urinary symptoms by virtue of its rapid excretion in the urinary tract. These effects are confined to the genitourinary system and are not accompanied by generalized sedation or narcosis.

INDICATIONS

Based on a review of this drug by the National Academy of Sciences-National Research Council and/or other information, FDA has classified the indications as follows:

"Lacking substantial evidence of effectiveness as a fixed combination":

Urobiotic-250 is indicated in the therapy of a number of genitourinary infections caused by susceptible organisms. These infections include the following: pyelonephritis, pyelitis, ureteritis, cystitis, prostatitis, and urethritis.

Since both Terramycin and sulfamethizole provide effective levels in blood, tissue, and urine, Urobiotic-250 provides a multiple antimicrobial approach at the site of infection. Both antibacterial components are active against the most common urinary pathogens, including *Escherichia coli, Pseudomonas aeruginosa, Aerobacter aerogenes, Streptococcus faecalis, Streptococcus hemolyticus, and Micrococcus pyogenes.* Urobiotic-250 is particularly useful in the treatment of infections caused by bacteria more sensitive to the combination than to either component alone. The combination is also of value in those cases with mixed infections, and in those instances where the causative organism is unknown pending laboratory isolation.

Final classification of the less than effective indications requires further investigation. Clinical studies to substantiate the efficacy of Urobiotic-250 are ongoing. Completion of these ongoing studies will provide data for final classification of these indications.

CONTRAINDICATIONS

This drug is contraindicated in individuals who have shown hypersensitivity to any of its components.

This drug, because of the sulfonamide component, should not be used in patients with a history of sulfonamide sensitivities, and in pregnant females at term.

WARNINGS

If renal impairment exists, even usual oral or parenteral doses may lead to excessive systemic accumulation of the drug and possible liver toxicity. Under such conditions, lower than usual doses are indicated and if therapy is prolonged, tetracycline serum level determinations may be advisable.

Oxytetracycline HCl, which is one of the ingredients of Urobiotic-250, may form a stable calcium complex in any bone-forming tissue with no serious harmful effects reported thus far in humans. However, use of oxytetracycline during tooth development (last trimester of pregnancy, neonatal period and early childhood) may cause discoloration of the teeth (yellow-grey-brownish). This effect occurs mostly during long term use of the drug but it also has been observed in usual short treatment courses.

Because of its sulfonamide content, this drug should be used only after critical appraisal in patients with liver damage, renal damage, urinary obstruction, or blood dyscrasias. Deaths have been reported from hypersensitivity reactions, agranulocytosis, aplastic anemia, and other blood dyscrasias associated with sulfonamide administration. When used intermittently, or for a prolonged period, blood counts and liver and kidney function tests should be performed.

Certain hypersensitive individuals may develop a photodynamic reaction precipitated by exposure to direct sunlight during the use of this drug. This reaction is usually of the photoallergic type which may also be produced by other tetracycline derivatives. Individuals with a history of photosensitivity reactions should be instructed to avoid exposure to direct sunlight while under treatment with this or other tetracycline drugs, and treatment should be discontinued at first evidence of skin discomfort.

NOTE: Reactions of a photoallergic nature are exceedingly rare with Terramycin (oxytetracycline HCl). Phototoxic reactions are not believed to occur with Terramycin.

PRECAUTIONS

As with all antibiotic preparations, use of this drug may result in overgrowth of nonsusceptible organisms, including fungi. If superinfection occurs, the antibiotic should be discontinued and appropriate specific therapy should be instituted. This drug should be used with caution in persons having histories of significant allergies and/or asthma.

ADVERSE REACTIONS

Glossitis, stomatitis, proctitis, nausea, diarrhea, vaginitis, and dermatitis, as well as reactions of an allergic nature, may occur during oxytetracycline HCl therapy, but are rare. If adverse reactions, individual idiosyncrasy, or allergy occur, discontinue medication. Rare instances of esophagitis and esophageal ulcerations have been reported in patients receiving capsule forms of drugs in the tetracycline class. Most of these patients took medications immediately before going to bed. (See Dosage and Administration.)

With oxytetracycline therapy bulging fontanels in infants and benign intracranial hypertension in adults have been reported in individuals receiving full therapeutic dosages. These conditions disappeared rapidly when the drug was discontinued.

As in all sulfonamide therapy, the following reactions may occur: nausea, vomiting, diarrhea, hepatitis, pancreatitis, blood dyscrasias, neuropathy, drug fever, skin rash, infection of the conjunctiva and sclera, petechiae, purpura, hematuria and crystalluria. The dosage should be decreased or the drug withdrawn, depending upon the severity of the reaction.

DOSAGE AND ADMINISTRATION

Urobiotic-250 is recommended in adults only. A dose of 1 capsule four times daily is suggested. In refractory cases 2 capsules four times a day may be used.

Therapy should be continued for a minimum of seven days or until bacteriologic cure in acute urinary tract infections.

Administration of adequate amounts of fluid along with capsule forms of drugs in the tetracycline class is recommended to wash down the drugs and reduce the risk of esophageal irritation and ulceration. (See Adverse Reactions.)

To aid absorption of the drug, it should be given at least one hour before or two hours after eating. Aluminum hydroxide gel given with antibiotics has been shown to decrease their absorption and is contraindicated.

SUPPLY

Urobiotic-250 capsules: bottles of 50 (NDC 0049-0920-50), and unit dose packages of 100 (10 × 10's) (NDC 0049-0920-41).

LITERATURE AVAILABLE

Yes.

70-1636-00-9
Revised Dec. 1986

VIBRAMYCIN® Calcium ℞

[vī-brə ′mīs-ən]

doxycycline calcium
oral suspension
SYRUP

VIBRAMYCIN® Hyclate

[vī-brə ′mīs-ən]

doxycycline hyclate
CAPSULES

VIBRAMYCIN® Monohydrate

[vī-brə ′mīs-ən]

doxycycline monohydrate
for ORAL SUSPENSION

VIBRA-TABS®

[vī-brə ′mīs-ən]

doxycycline hyclate
FILM COATED TABLETS

DESCRIPTION

Vibramycin is a broad-spectrum antibiotic synthetically derived from oxytetracycline, and is available as Vibramycin Monohydrate (doxycycline monohydrate); Vibramycin Hyclate and Vibra-Tabs (doxycycline hydrochloride hemiethanolate hemihydrate); and Vibramycin Calcium (doxycycline calcium) for oral administration.

The structural formula of doxycycline monohydrate is

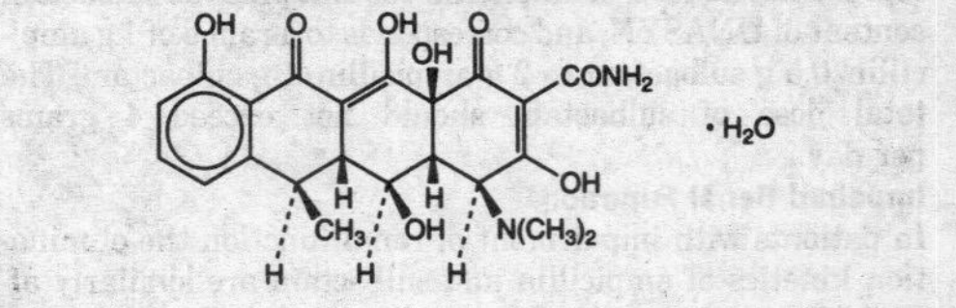

with a molecular formula of $C_{22}H_{24}N_2O_8 \cdot H_2O$ and a molecular weight of 462.46. The chemical designation for doxycycline is 4-(Dimethylamino)-1, 4, 4a, 5, 5a, 6, 11, 12a-octahydro-3, 5, 10, 12, 12a-pentahydroxy-6-methyl-1, 11-dioxo-2-naphthacenecarboxamide monohydrate. The molecular formula for doxycycline hydrochloride hemiethanolate hemihydrate is $(C_{22}H_{24}N_2O_8 \cdot HCl)_2 \cdot C_2H_6O \cdot H_2O$ and the molecular weight is 1025.89. Doxycycline is a light-yellow crystalline powder. Doxycycline hyclate is soluble in water, while doxycycline monohydrate is very slightly soluble in water.

Doxycycline has a high degree of lipoid solubility and a low affinity for calcium binding. It is highly stable in normal human serum. Doxycycline will not degrade into an epianhydro form.

Inert ingredients in the syrup formulation are: apple flavor; butylparaben; calcium chloride; carmine; glycerin; hydrochloric acid; magnesium aluminum silicate; povidone; propylene glycol; propylparaben; raspberry flavor; simethicone emulsion; sodium hydroxide; sodium metabisulfite; sorbitol solution; water.

Inert ingredients in the capsule formulations are: hard gelatin capsules (which may contain Blue 1 and other inert ingredients); magnesium stearate; microcrystalline cellulose; sodium lauryl sulfate.

Inert ingredients for the oral suspension formulation are: carboxymethylcellulose sodium; Blue 1; methylparaben; microcrystalline cellulose; propylparaben; raspberry flavor; Red 28; simethicone emulsion; sucrose.

Inert ingredients for the tablet formulation are: ethylcellulose; hydroxypropyl methylcellulose; magnesium stearate; microcrystalline cellulose; propylene glycol; sodium lauryl sulfate; talc; titanium dioxide; Yellow 6 Lake.

CLINICAL PHARMACOLOGY

Tetracyclines are readily absorbed and are bound to plasma proteins in varying degree. They are concentrated by the liver in the bile, and excreted in the urine and feces at high concentrations and in a biologically active form. Doxycycline is virtually completely absorbed after oral administration.

Following a 200 mg dose, normal adult volunteers averaged peak serum levels of 2.6 mcg/mL of doxycycline at 2 hours decreasing to 1.45 mcg/mL at 24 hours. Excretion of doxycycline by the kidney is about 40%/72 hours in individuals with normal function (creatinine clearance about 75 mL/min.). This percentage excretion may fall as low as 1–5%/72 hours in individuals with severe renal insufficiency (creatinine clearance below 10 mL/min.). Studies have shown no significant difference in serum half-life of doxycycline (range 18–22 hours) in individuals with normal and severely impaired renal function.

Hemodialysis does not alter serum half-life.

Results of animal studies indicate that tetracyclines cross the placenta and are found in fetal tissues.

Microbiology

The tetracyclines are primarily bacteriostatic and are thought to exert their antimicrobial effect by the inhibition of protein synthesis. The tetracyclines, including doxycycline, have a similar antimicrobial spectrum of activity

against a wide range of gram-positive and gram-negative organisms. Cross-resistance of these organisms to tetracyclines is common.

Gram-Negative Bacteria
Neisseria gonorrhoeae
Calymmatobacterium granulomatis
Haemophilus ducreyi
Haemophilus influenzae
Yersinia pestis (formerly *Pasteurella pestis*)
Francisella tularensis (formerly *Pasteurella tularensis*)
Vibrio cholera (formerly *Vibrio comma*)
Bartonella bacilliformis
Brucella species

Because many strains of the following groups of gram-negative microorganisms have been shown to be resistant to tetracyclines, culture and susceptibility testing are recommended:
Escherichia coli
Klebsiella species
Enterobacter aerogenes
Shigella species
Acinetobacter species (formerly *Mima* species and *Herellea* species)
Bacteroides species

Gram-Positive Bacteria
Because many strains of the following groups of gram-positive microorganisms have been shown to be resistant to tetracycline, culture and susceptibility testing are recommended. Up to 44 percent of strains of *Streptococcus pyogenes* and 74 percent of *Streptococcus faecalis* have been found to be resistant to tetracycline drugs. Therefore, tetracycline should not be used for streptococcal disease unless the organism has been demonstrated to be susceptible.
Streptococcus pyogenes
Streptococcus pneumoniae
Enterococcus group (*Streptococcus faecalis* and *Streptococcus faecium*)
Alpha-hemolytic streptococci (viridans group)

Other Microorganisms
Rickettsiae
Chlamydia psittaci
Chlamydia trachomatis
Mycoplasma pneumoniae
Ureaplasma urealyticum
Borrelia recurrentis
Treponema pallidum
Treponema pertenue
Clostridium species
Fusobacterium fusiforme
Actinomyces species
Bacillus anthracis
Propionbacterium acnes
Entamoeba species
Balantidium coli
Plasmodium falciparum

Doxycycline has been found to be active against the asexual erythrocytic forms of *Plasmodium falciparum* but not against the gametocytes of *P. falciparum*. The precise mechanism of action of the drug is not known.

Susceptibility tests: Diffusion techniques: Quantitative methods that require measurement of zone diameters give the most precise estimate of the susceptibility of bacteria to antimicrobial agents. One such standard procedure[1] which has been recommended for use with disks to test susceptibility of organisms to doxycycline uses the 30-mcg tetracycline-class disk or the 30-mcg doxycycline disk. Interpretation involves the correlation of the diameter obtained in the disk test with the minimum inhibitory concentration (MIC) for tetracycline or doxycycline, respectively.

Reports from the laboratory giving results of the standard single-disk susceptibility test with a 30-mcg tetracycline-class disk or the 30-mcg doxycycline disk should be interpreted according to the following criteria:

Zone Diameter (mm)		Interpretation
tetracycline	doxycycline	
≥ 19	≥ 16	Susceptible
15–18	13–15	Intermediate
≤ 14	≤ 12	Resistant

A report of "Susceptible" indicates that the pathogen is likely to be inhibited by generally achievable blood levels. A report of "Intermediate" suggests that the organism would be susceptible if a high dosage is used or if the infection is confined to tissues and fluids in which high antimicrobial levels are attained. A report of "Resistant" indicates that achievable concentrations are unlikely to be inhibitory, and other therapy should be selected.

Standardized procedures require the use of laboratory control organisms. The 30-mcg tetracycline-class disk or the 30-mcg doxycycline disk should give the following zone diameters:

Organism	Zone Diameter (mm)	
	tetracycline	doxycycline
E. coli ATCC 25922	18–25	18–24
S. aureus ATCC 25923	19–28	23–29

Dilution techniques: Use a standardized dilution method[2] (broth, agar, microdilution) or equivalent with tetracycline powder. The MIC values obtained should be interpreted according to the following criteria:

MIC (mcg/mL)	Interpretation
≤ 4	Susceptible
8	Intermediate
≥ 16	Resistant

As with standard diffusion techniques, dilution methods require the use of laboratory control organisms. Standard tetracycline powder should provide the following MIC values:

Organism	MIC (mcg/mL)
E. coli ATCC 25922	1.0–4.0
S. aureus ATCC 29213	0.25–1.0
E. faecalis ATCC 29212	8–32
P. aeruginosa ATCC 27853	8–32

INDICATIONS AND USAGE

Treatment:
Doxycycline is indicated for the treatment of the following infections:

Rocky mountain spotted fever, typhus fever and the typhus group, Q fever, rickettsialpox, and tick fevers caused by Rickettsiae.

Respiratory tract infections caused by *Mycoplasma pneumoniae*.

Lymphogranuloma venereum caused by *Chlamydia trachomatis*.

Psittacosis (ornithosis) caused by *Chlamydia psittaci*.

Trachoma caused by *Chlamydia trachomatis*, although the infectious agent is not always eliminated as judged by immunofluorescence.

Inclusion conjunctivitis caused by *Chlamydia trachomatis*.

Uncomplicated urethral, endocervical or rectal infections in adults caused by *Chlamydia trachomatis*.

Nongonococcal urethritis caused by *Ureaplasma urealyticum*.

Relapsing fever due to *Borrelia recurrentis*.

Doxycycline is also indicated for the treatment of infections caused by the following gram-negative microorganisms:

Chancroid caused by *Haemophilus ducreyi*.

Plague due to *Yersinia pestis* (formerly *Pasteurella pestis*).

Tuleremia due to *Francisella tulerensis* (formerly *Pasteurella tulerensis*).

Cholera caused by *Vibrio cholerae* (formerly *Vibrio comma*).

Campylobacter fetus infections caused by *Campylobacter fetus* (formerly *Vibrio fetus*).

Brucellosis due to *Brucella* species (in conjunction with streptomycin).

Bartonellosis due to *Bartonella bacilliformis*.

Granuloma inguinale caused by *Calymmatobacterium granulomatis*.

Because many strains of the following groups of microorganisms have been shown to be resistant to doxycycline, culture and susceptibility testing are recommended.

Doxycycline is indicated for treatment of infections caused by the following gram-negative microorganisms, when bacteriologic testing indicates appropriate susceptibility to the drug:

Escherichia coli.

Enterobacter aerogenes (formerly *Aerobacter aerogenes*).

Shigella species.

Acinetobacter species (formerly *Mima* species and *Herellea* species).

Respiratory tract infections caused by *Haemophilus influenzae*.

Respiratory tract and urinary tract infections caused by *Klebsiella* species.

Doxycycline is indicated for treatment of infections caused by the following gram-positive microorganisms when bacteriologic testing indicates appropriate susceptibility to the drug:

Upper respiratory infections caused by *Streptococcus pneumoniae* (formerly *Diplococcus pneumoniae*).

When penicillin is contraindicated, doxycycline is an alternative drug in the treatment of the following infections:

Uncomplicated gonorrhea caused by *Neisseria gonorrhoeae*.

Syphilis caused by *Treponema pallidum*.

Yaws caused by *Treponema pertenue*.

Listeriosis due to *Listeria monocytogenes*.

Anthrax due to *Bacillus anthracis*.

Vincent's infection caused by *Fusobacterium fusiforme*.

Actinomycosis caused by *Actinomyces israelii*.

Infections caused by *Clostridium* species.

In acute intestinal amebiasis, doxycycline may be a useful adjunct to amebicides.

In severe acne, doxycycline may be useful adjunctive therapy.

Prophylaxis:
Doxycycline is indicated for the prophylaxis of malaria due to *Plasmodium falciparum* in short-term travelers (< 4 months) to areas with chloroquine and/or pyrimethamine-sulfadoxine resistant strains. See DOSAGE AND ADMINIS-

TRATION section and Information for Patients subsection of the PRECAUTIONS section.

CONTRAINDICATIONS

This drug is contraindicated in persons who have shown hypersensitivity to any of the tetracyclines.

WARNINGS

THE USE OF DRUGS OF THE TETRACYCLINE CLASS DURING TOOTH DEVELOPMENT (LAST HALF OF PREGNANCY, INFANCY AND CHILDHOOD TO THE AGE OF 8 YEARS) MAY CAUSE PERMANENT DISCOLORATION OF THE TEETH (YELLOW-GRAY-BROWN). This adverse reaction is more common during long-term use of the drugs, but has been observed following repeated short-term courses. Enamel hypoplasia has also been reported. TETRACYCLINE DRUGS, THEREFORE, SHOULD NOT BE USED IN THIS AGE GROUP UNLESS OTHER DRUGS ARE NOT LIKELY TO BE EFFECTIVE OR ARE CONTRA-INDICATED.

All tetracyclines form a stable calcium complex in any bone-forming tissue. A decrease in fibula growth rate has been observed in prematures given oral tetracycline in doses of 25 mg/kg every 6 hours. This reaction was shown to be reversible when the drug was discontinued.

Results of animal studies indicate that tetracyclines cross the placenta, are found in fetal tissues, and can have toxic effects on the developing fetus (often related to retardation of skeletal development). Evidence of embryotoxicity has also been noted in animals treated early in pregnancy. If any tetracycline is used during pregnancy or if the patient becomes pregnant while taking this drug, the patient should be apprised of the potential hazard to the fetus.

The antianabolic action of the tetracyclines may cause an increase in BUN. Studies to date indicate that this does not occur with the use of doxycycline in patients with impaired renal function.

Photosensitivity manifested by an exaggerated sunburn reaction has been observed in some individuals taking tetracyclines. Patients apt to be exposed to direct sunlight or ultraviolet light should be advised that this reaction can occur with tetracycline drugs, and treatment should be discontinued at the first evidence of skin erythema.

Vibramycin Syrup contains sodium metabisulfite, a sulfite that may cause allergic-type reactions including anaphylactic symptoms and life-threatening or less severe asthmatic episodes in certain susceptible people. The over-all prevalence of sulfite sensitivity in the general population is unknown and probably low. Sulfite sensitivity is seen more frequently in asthmatic than in non-asthmatic people.

PRECAUTIONS

General
As with other antibiotic preparations, use of this drug may result in overgrowth of nonsusceptible organisms, including fungi. If superinfection occurs, the antibiotic should be discontinued and appropriate therapy instituted.

Bulging fontanels in infants and benign intracranial hypertension in adults have been reported in individuals receiving tetracyclines. These conditions disappeared when the drug was discontinued.

Incision and drainage or other surgical procedures should be performed in conjunction with antibiotic therapy, when indicated.

Doxycycline offers substantial but not complete suppression of the asexual blood stages of *Plasmodium* strains.

Doxycycline does not suppress *P. falciparum's* sexual blood stage gametocytes. Subjects completing this prophylactic regimen may still transmit the infection to mosquitoes outside endemic areas.

Information for Patients
Patients taking doxycycline for malaria prophylaxis should be advised:

—that no present-day antimalarial agent, including doxycycline, guarantees protection against malaria.

—to avoid being bitten by mosquitoes by using personal protective measures that help avoid contact with mosquitoes, especially from dusk to dawn (e.g., staying in well-screened areas, using mosquito nets, covering the body with clothing, and using an effective insect repellent.)

—that doxycycline prophylaxis:

  —should begin 1–2 days before travel to the malarious area,

  —should be continued daily while in the malarious area and after leaving the malarious area,

  —should be continued for 4 further weeks to avoid development of malaria after returning from an endemic area,

  —should not exceed 4 months.

All patients taking doxycycline should be advised:

—to avoid excessive sunlight or artificial ultraviolet light while receiving doxycycline and to discontinue therapy if phototoxicity (e.g., skin eruption, etc.) occurs. Sunscreen or sunblock should be considered. (See WARNINGS.)

—to drink fluids liberally along with doxycycline to reduce the risk of esophageal irritation and ulceration. (See ADVERSE REACTIONS.)

Continued on next page

Pfizer Inc—Cont.

—that the absorption of tetracyclines is reduced when taken with foods, especially those which contain calcium. However, the absorption of doxycycline is not markedly influenced by simultaneous ingestion of food or milk. (See DRUG INTERACTIONS.)
—that the absorption of tetracyclines is reduced when taking bismuth subsalicylate. (See DRUG INTERACTIONS.)
—that the use of doxycycline might increase the incidence of vaginal candidiasis.

Laboratory Tests
In venereal disease, when co-existent syphilis is suspected, dark field examinations should be done before treatment is started and the blood serology repeated monthly for at least 4 months.
In long-term therapy, periodic laboratory evaluation of organ systems, including hematopoietic, renal, and hepatic studies, should be performed.

Drug Interactions
Because tetracyclines have been shown to depress plasma prothrombin activity, patients who are on anticoagulant therapy may require downward adjustment of their anticoagulant dosage.
Since bacteriostatic drugs may interfere with the bactericidal action of penicillin, it is advisable to avoid giving tetracyclines in conjunction with penicillin.
Absorption of tetracyclines is impaired by antacids containing aluminum, calcium, or magnesium, and iron-containing preparations.
Absorption of tetracyclines is impaired by bismuth subsalicylate.
Barbiturates, carbamazepine, and phenytoin decrease the half-life of doxycycline.
The concurrent use of tetracycline and Penthrane (methoxyflurane) has been reported to result in fatal renal toxicity.
Concurrent use of tetracycline may render oral contraceptives less effective.

Drug/Laboratory Test Interactions
False elevations of urinary catecholamine levels may occur due to interference with the fluorescence test.

Carcinogenesis, Mutagenesis, Impairment of Fertility
Long-term studies in animals to evaluate carcinogenic potential of doxycycline have not been conducted. However, there has been evidence of oncogenic activity in rats in studies with the related antibiotics, oxytetracycline (adrenal and pituitary tumors), and minocycline (thyroid tumors).
Likewise, although mutagenicity studies of doxycycline have not been conducted, positive results in *in vitro* mammalian cell assays have been reported for related antibiotics (tetracycline, oxytetracycline).
Doxycycline administered orally at dosage levels as high as 250 mg/kg/day had no apparent effect on the fertility of female rats. Effect on male fertility has not been studied.

Pregnancy Category
Teratogenic effects: Category "D" — (See WARNINGS).
Nonteratogenic effects: (See WARNINGS).

Labor and Delivery
The effect of tetracyclines on labor and delivery is unknown.

Nursing Mothers
Tetracyclines are excreted in human milk. Because of the potential for serious adverse reactions in nursing infants from doxycycline, a decision should be made whether to discontinue nursing or to discontinue the drug, taking into account the importance of the drug to the mother. (See WARNINGS).

Pediatric Use
See WARNINGS and DOSAGE AND ADMINISTRATION.

ADVERSE REACTIONS

Due to oral doxycycline's virtually complete absorption, side effects of the lower bowel, particularly diarrhea, have been infrequent. The following adverse reactions have been observed in patients receiving tetracyclines:
Gastrointestinal: anorexia, nausea, vomiting, diarrhea, glossitis, dysphagia, enterocolitis, and inflammatory lesions (with monilial overgrowth) in the anogenital region. Hepatotoxicity has been reported rarely. These reactions have been caused by both the oral and parenteral administration of tetracyclines. Rare instances of esophagitis and esophageal ulcerations have been reported in patients receiving capsule and tablet forms of the drugs in the tetracycline class. Most of these patients took medications immediately before going to bed. (See DOSAGE AND ADMINISTRATION.)
Skin: maculopapular and erythematous rashes. Exfoliative dermatitis has been reported but is uncommon. Photosensitivity is discussed above. (See WARNINGS.)
Renal toxicity: Rise in BUN has been reported and is apparently dose related. (See WARNINGS.)
Hypersensitivity reactions: urticaria, angioneurotic edema, anaphylaxis, anaphylactoid purpura, serum sickness, pericarditis, and exacerbation of systemic lupus erythematosus.
Blood: Hemolytic anemia, thrombocytopenia, neutropenia, and eosinophilia have been reported.
Other: bulging fontanels in infants and intracranial hypertension in adults. (See PRECAUTIONS—General.)
When given over prolonged periods, tetracyclines have been reported to produce brown-black microscopic discoloration of the thyroid gland. No abnormalities of thyroid function studies are known to occur.

OVERDOSAGE

In case of overdosage, discontinue medication, treat symptomatically and institute supportive measures. Dialysis does not alter serum half-life and thus would not be of benefit in treating cases of overdosage.

DOSAGE AND ADMINISTRATION

THE USUAL DOSAGE AND FREQUENCY OF ADMINISTRATION OF DOXYCYCLINE DIFFERS FROM THAT OF THE OTHER TETRACYCLINES. EXCEEDING THE RECOMMENDED DOSAGE MAY RESULT IN AN INCREASED INCIDENCE OF SIDE EFFECTS. Adults: The usual dose of oral doxycycline is 200 mg on the first day of treatment (administered 100 mg every 12 hours) followed by a maintenance dose of 100 mg/day. The maintenance dose may be administered as a single dose or as 50 mg every 12 hours.
In the management of more severe infections (particularly chronic infections of the urinary tract), 100 mg every 12 hours is recommended.
For children above eight years of age: The recommended dosage schedule for children weighing 100 pounds or less is 2 mg/lb of body weight divided into two doses on the first day of treatment, followed by 1 mg/lb of body weight given as a single daily dose or divided into two doses, on subsequent days. For more severe infections up to 2 mg/lb of body weight may be used. For children over 100 lb the usual adult dose should be used.
The therapeutic antibacterial serum activity will usually persist for 24 hours following recommended dosage.
When used in streptococcal infections, therapy should be continued for 10 days.
Administration of adequate amounts of fluid along with capsule and tablet forms of drugs in the tetracycline class is recommended to wash down the drugs and reduce the risk of esophageal irritation and ulceration. (See ADVERSE REACTIONS.)
If gastric irritation occurs, it is recommended that doxycycline be given with food or milk. The absorption of doxycycline is not markedly influenced by simultaneous ingestion of food or milk.
Studies to date have indicated that administration of doxycycline at the usual recommended doses does not lead to excessive accumulation of the antibiotic in patients with renal impairment.
Uncomplicated gonococcal infections in adults (except anorectal infections in men): 100 mg, by mouth, twice a day for 7 days. As an alternate single visit dose, administer 300 mg stat followed in one hour by a second 300 mg dose. The dose may be administered with food, including milk or carbonated beverage, as required.
Uncomplicated urethral, endocervical, or rectal infection in adults caused by *Chlamydia trachomatis:* 100 mg by mouth twice a day for 7 days.
Nongonococcal urethritis (NGU) caused by *C. trachomatis* or *U. urealyticum:* 100 mg by mouth twice a day for 7 days.
Syphilis—early: Patients who are allergic to penicillin should be treated with doxycycline 100 mg by mouth twice a day for 2 weeks.
Syphilis of more than one year's duration: Patients who are allergic to penicillin should be treated with doxycycline 100 mg by mouth twice a day for 4 weeks.
Acute epididymo-orchitis caused by *N. gonorrhoeae:* 100 mg, by mouth, twice a day for at least 10 days.
Acute epididymo-orchitis caused by *C. trachomatis:* 100 mg, by mouth, twice a day for at least 10 days.
For prophylaxis of malaria: For adults, the recommended dose is 100 mg daily. For children over 8 years of age, the recommended dose is 2 mg/kg given once daily up to the adult dose. Prophylaxis should begin 1–2 days before travel to the malarious area. Prophylaxis should be continued daily during travel in the malarious area and for 4 weeks after the traveler leaves the malarious area.

HOW SUPPLIED

Vibramycin Hyclate (doxycycline hyclate) is available in capsules containing doxycycline hyclate equivalent to:
50 mg doxycycline
bottles of 50 (NDC 0069-0940-50),
unit-dose pack of 100 (10 × 10's) (NDC 0069-0940-41).
The capsules are white and light blue and are imprinted with "VIBRA" on one half and "PFIZER 094" on the other half.
100 mg doxycycline
bottles of 50 (NDC 0069-0950-50) and 500 (NDC 0069-0950-73),
unit-dose pack of 100 (10 × 10's) (NDC 0069-0950-41).
The capsules are light blue and are imprinted with "VIBRA" on one half and "PFIZER 095" on the other half.
Vibra-Tabs (doxycycline hyclate) is available in salmon colored film-coated tablets containing doxycycline hyclate equivalent to:
100 mg doxycycline
bottles of 50 (NDC 0069-0990-50) and 500 (NDC 0069-0990-73),
The tablets are imprinted on one side with "VIBRA-TABS" and "PFIZER 099" on the other side.
Vibramycin Calcium Syrup (doxycycline calcium oral suspension) is available as a raspberry-apple flavored oral suspension. Each teaspoonful (5 mL) contains doxycycline calcium equivalent to 50 mg of doxycycline: bottles of 1 oz (30 mL) (NDC 0069-0971-51), and 1 pint (473 mL) (NDC 0069-0971-93).
Vibramycin Monohydrate (doxycycline monohydrate) for Oral Suspension is available as a raspberry-flavored, dry powder for oral suspension. When reconstituted, each teaspoonful (5 mL) contains doxycycline monohydrate equivalent to 25 mg of doxycycline: 2 oz (60 mL) bottles (NDC 0069-0970-65).
All products are to be stored below 86°F (30°C) and dispensed in tight, light-resistant containers (USP). The unit dose packs should also be stored in a dry place.

ANIMAL PHARMACOLOGY AND ANIMAL TOXICOLOGY

Hyperpigmentation of the thyroid has been produced by members of the tetracycline class in the following species: in rats by oxytetracycline, doxycycline, tetracycline PO_4, and methacycline; in minipigs by doxycycline, minocycline, tetracycline PO_4, and methacycline; in dogs by doxycycline and minocycline; in monkeys by minocycline.
Minocycline, tetracycline PO_4, methacycline, doxycycline, tetracycline base, oxytetracycline HCl, and tetracycline HCl were goitrogenic in rats fed a low iodine diet. This goitrogenic effect was accompanied by high radioactive iodine uptake. Administration of minocycline also produced a large goiter with high radioiodine uptake in rats fed a relatively high iodine diet.
Treatment of various animal species with this class of drugs has also resulted in the induction of thyroid hyperplasia in the following: in rats and dogs (minocycline); in chickens (chlortetracycline); and in rats and mice (oxytetracycline). Adrenal gland hyperplasia has been observed in goats and rats treated with oxytetracycline.

REFERENCES

1. National Committee for Clinical Laboratory Standards, *Performance Standards for Antimicrobial Disk Susceptibility Tests,* Fourth Edition. Approved Standard NCCLS Document M2-A4, Vol. 10, No. 7 NCCLS, Villanova, PA, April 1990.
2. National Committee for Clinical Laboratory Standards, *Methods for Dilution Antimicrobial Susceptibility Tests for Bacteria that Grow Aerobically,* Second Edition. Approved Standard NCCLS Document M7-A2, Vol. 10, No. 8 NCCLS, Villanova, PA, April 1990.

65-1680-00-5 Revised April 1993

Shown in Product Identification Guide, page 328

VIBRAMYCIN® Hyclate ℞
[*vī″bra-mī′sin*]
doxycycline hyclate for injection
INTRAVENOUS
For Intravenous Use Only

DESCRIPTION

Vibramycin (doxycycline hyclate for injection) Intravenous is a broad-spectrum antibiotic synthetically derived from oxytetracycline, and is available as Vibramycin Hyclate (doxycycline hydrochloride hemiethanolate hemihydrate). The chemical designation of this light-yellow crystalline powder is alpha-6-deoxy-5-oxytetracycline. Doxycycline has a high degree of lipoid solubility and a low affinity for calcium binding. It is highly stable in normal human serum.

ACTIONS

Doxycycline is primarily bacteriostatic and thought to exert its antimicrobial effect by the inhibition of protein synthesis. Doxycycline is active against a wide range of gram-positive and gram-negative organisms.
The drugs in the tetracycline class have closely similar antimicrobial spectra and cross resistance among them is common. Microorganisms may be considered susceptible to doxycycline (likely to respond to doxycycline therapy) if the minimum inhibitory concentration (M.I.C.) is not more than 4.0 mcg/mL. Microorganisms may be considered intermediate (harboring partial resistance) if the M.I.C. is 4.0 to 12.5 mcg/mL and resistant (not likely to respond to therapy) if the M.I.C. is greater than 12.5 mcg/mL.
Susceptibility plate testing: If the Kirby-Bauer method of disc susceptibility testing is used, a 30 mcg doxycycline disc should give a zone of at least 16 mm when tested against a doxycycline-susceptible bacterial strain. A tetracycline disc may be used to determine microbial susceptibility. If the

Kirby-Bauer method of disc susceptibility testing is used, a 30 mcg tetracycline disc should give a zone of at least 19 mm when tested against a tetracycline-susceptible bacterial strain.

Tetracyclines are readily absorbed and are bound to plasma proteins in varying degree. They are concentrated by the liver in the bile, and excreted in the urine and feces at high concentrations and in a biologically active form.

Following a single 100 mg dose administered in a concentration of 0.4 mg/mL in a one-hour infusion, normal adult volunteers average a peak of 2.5 mcg/mL, while 200 mg of a concentration of 0.4 mg/mL administered over two hours averaged a peak of 3.6 mcg/mL.

Excretion of doxycycline by the kidney is about 40 percent/72 hours in individuals with normal function (creatinine clearance about 75 mL/min.). This percentage excretion may fall as low as 1-5 percent/72 hours in individuals with severe renal insufficiency (creatinine clearance below 10 mL/min.). Studies have shown no significant difference in serum half-life of doxycycline (range 18-22 hours) in individuals with normal and severely impaired renal function.

Hemodialysis does not alter this serum half-life of doxycycline.

INDICATIONS

Doxycycline is indicated in infections caused by the following microorganisms:

Rickettsiae (Rocky Mountain spotted fever, typhus fever, and the typhus group, Q fever, rickettsialpox and tick fevers).

Mycoplasma pneumoniae (PPLO, Eaton Agent).

Agents of psittacosis and ornithosis.

Agents of lymphogranuloma venereum and granuloma inguinale.

The spirochetal agent of relapsing fever (*Borrelia recurrentis*).

The following gram-negative microorganisms:

Haemophilus ducreyi (chancroid),
Pasteurella pestis and *Pasteurella tularensis*,
Bartonella bacilliformis,
Bacteroides species,
Vibrio comma and *Vibrio fetus*,
Brucella species (in conjunction with streptomycin).

Because many strains of the following groups of microorganisms have been shown to be resistant to tetracyclines, culture and susceptibility testing are recommended. Doxycycline is indicated for treatment of infections caused by the following gram-negative microorganisms when bacteriologic testing indicates appropriate susceptibility to the drug:

Escherichia coli,
Enterobacter aerogenes (formerly *Aerobacter aerogenes*),
Shigella species,
Mima species and *Herellea* species,
Haemophilus influenzae (respiratory infections),
Klebsiella species (respiratory and urinary infections).

Doxycycline is indicated for treatment of infections caused by the following gram-positive microorganisms when bacteriologic testing indicates appropriate susceptibility to the drug:

Streptococcus species:

Up to 44 percent of strains of *Streptococcus pyogenes* and 74 percent of *Streptococcus faecalis* have been found to be resistant to tetracycline drugs. Therefore, tetracyclines should not be used for streptococcal disease unless the organism has been demonstrated to be sensitive.

For upper respiratory infections due to group A beta-hemolytic streptococci, penicillin is the usual drug of choice, including prophylaxis of rheumatic fever.

Diplococcus pneumoniae,
Staphylococcus aureus, respiratory, skin and soft tissue infections. Tetracyclines are not the drugs of choice in the treatment of any type of staphylococcal infections.

When penicillin is contraindicated, doxycycline is an alternative drug in the treatment of infections due to:

Neisseria gonorrhoeae and *N. meningitidis*,
Treponema pallidum and *Treponema pertenue* (syphilis and yaws),
Listeria monocytogenes,
Clostridium species,
Bacillus anthracis,
Fusobacterium fusiforme (Vincent's infection),
Actinomyces species.

In acute intestinal amebiasis, doxycycline may be a useful adjunct to amebicides.

Doxycycline is indicated in the treatment of trachoma, although the infectious agent is not always eliminated, as judged by immunofluorescence.

CONTRAINDICATIONS

This drug is contraindicated in persons who have shown hypersensitivity to any of the tetracyclines.

WARNINGS

THE USE OF DRUGS OF THE TETRACYCLINE CLASS DURING TOOTH DEVELOPMENT (LAST HALF OF PREGNANCY, INFANCY AND CHILDHOOD TO THE AGE OF 8 YEARS) MAY CAUSE PERMANENT DISCOLORATION OF THE TEETH (YELLOW-GRAY-BROWN). This adverse reaction is more common during long-term use of the drugs but has been observed following repeated short-term courses. Enamel hypoplasia has also been reported. *TETRACYCLINE DRUGS, THEREFORE, SHOULD NOT BE USED IN THIS AGE GROUP UNLESS OTHER DRUGS ARE NOT LIKELY TO BE EFFECTIVE OR ARE CONTRAINDICATED.*

Photosensitivity manifested by an exaggerated sunburn reaction has been observed in some individuals taking tetracyclines. Patients apt to be exposed to direct sunlight or ultraviolet light should be advised that this reaction can occur with tetracycline drugs, and treatment should be discontinued at the first evidence of skin erythema.

The antianabolic action of the tetracyclines may cause an increase in BUN. Studies to date indicate that this does not occur with the use of doxycycline in patients with impaired renal function.

Usage in Pregnancy

(See above WARNINGS about use during tooth development.)

Vibramycin Intravenous has not been studied in pregnant patients. It should not be used in pregnant women unless, in the judgment of the physician, it is essential for the welfare of the patient.

Results of animal studies indicate that tetracyclines cross the placenta, are found in fetal tissues and can have toxic effects on the developing fetus (often related to retardation of skeletal development). Evidence of embryotoxicity has also been noted in animals treated early in pregnancy.

Usage in Children

The use of Vibramycin Intravenous in children under 8 years is not recommended because safe conditions for its use have not been established.

(See above WARNINGS about use during tooth development.)

As with other tetracyclines, doxycycline forms a stable calcium complex in any bone-forming tissue. A decrease in the fibula growth rate has been observed in prematures given oral tetracycline in doses of 25 mg/kg every 6 hours. This reaction was shown to be reversible when the drug was discontinued.

Tetracyclines are present in the milk of lactating women who are taking a drug in this class.

PRECAUTIONS

As with other antibiotic preparations, use of this drug may result in overgrowth of nonsusceptible organisms, including fungi. If superinfection occurs, the antibiotic should be discontinued and appropriate therapy instituted.

In venereal diseases when coexistent syphilis is suspected, a dark field examination should be done before treatment is started and the blood serology repeated monthly for at least 4 months.

Because tetracyclines have been shown to depress plasma prothrombin activity, patients who are on anticoagulant therapy may require downward adjustment of their anticoagulant dosage.

In long-term therapy, periodic laboratory evaluation of organ systems, including hematopoietic, renal, and hepatic studies should be performed.

All infections due to group A beta-hemolytic streptococci should be treated for at least 10 days.

Since bacteriostatic drugs may interfere with the bactericidal action of penicillin, it is advisable to avoid giving tetracycline in conjunction with penicillin.

ADVERSE REACTIONS

Gastrointestinal: anorexia, nausea, vomiting, diarrhea, glossitis, dysphagia, enterocolitis, and inflammatory lesions (with monilial overgrowth) in the anogenital region. Hepatotoxicity has been reported rarely. These reactions have been caused by both the oral and parenteral administration of tetracyclines.

Skin: maculopapular and erythematous rashes. Exfoliative dermatitis has been reported but is uncommon. Photosensitivity is discussed above. (See WARNINGS.)

Renal toxicity: Rise in BUN has been reported and is apparently dose related. (See WARNINGS.)

Hypersensitivity reactions: urticaria, angioneurotic edema, anaphylaxis, anaphylactoid purpura, pericarditis and exacerbation of systemic lupus erythematosus.

Bulging fontanels in infants and benign intracranial hypertension in adults have been reported in individuals receiving full therapeutic dosages. These conditions disappeared rapidly when the drug was discontinued.

Blood: Hemolytic anemia, thrombocytopenia, neutropenia and eosinophilia have been reported.

When given over prolonged periods, tetracyclines have been reported to produce brown-black microscopic discoloration of thyroid glands. No abnormalities of thyroid function studies are known to occur.

DOSAGE AND ADMINISTRATION

Note: Rapid administration is to be avoided. Parenteral therapy is indicated only when oral therapy is not indicated. Oral therapy should be instituted as soon as possible. If intravenous therapy is given over prolonged periods of time, thrombophlebitis may result.

THE USUAL DOSAGE AND FREQUENCY OF ADMINISTRATION OF VIBRAMYCIN I.V. (100-200 MG/DAY) DIFFERS FROM THAT OF THE OTHER TETRACYCLINES (1-2 G/DAY). EXCEEDING THE RECOMMENDED DOSAGE MAY RESULT IN AN INCREASED INCIDENCE OF SIDE EFFECTS.

Studies to date have indicated that Vibramycin at the usual recommended doses does not lead to excessive accumulation of the antibiotic in patients with renal impairment.

Adults: The usual dosage of Vibramycin I.V. is 200 mg on the first day of treatment administered in one or two infusions. Subsequent daily dosage is 100 to 200 mg depending upon the severity of infection, with 200 mg administered in one or two infusions.

In the treatment of primary and secondary syphilis, the recommended dosage is 300 mg daily for at least 10 days. For children above eight years of age: The recommended dosage schedule for children weighing 100 pounds or less is 2 mg/lb of body weight on the first day of treatment, administered in one or two infusions. Subsequent daily dosage is 1 to 2 mg/lb of body weight given as one or two infusions, depending on the severity of the infection. For children over 100 pounds the usual adult dose should be used. (See WARNINGS Section for Usage in Children.)

General: The duration of infusion may vary with the dose (100 to 200 mg per day), but is usually one to four hours. A recommended minimum infusion time for 100 mg of a 0.5 mg/mL solution is one hour. Therapy should be continued for at least 24-48 hours after symptoms and fever have subsided. The therapeutic antibacterial serum activity will usually persist for 24 hours following recommended dosage. Intravenous solutions should not be injected intramuscularly or subcutaneously. Caution should be taken to avoid the inadvertent introduction of the intravenous solution into the adjacent soft tissue.

PREPARATION OF SOLUTION

To prepare a solution containing 10 mg/mL, the contents of the vial should be reconstituted with 10 mL (for the 100 mg/vial container) or 20 mL (for the 200 mg/vial container) of Sterile Water for Injection or any of the ten intravenous infusion solutions listed below. Each 100 mg of Vibramycin (i.e., withdraw entire solution from the 100 mg vial) is further diluted with 100 mL to 1000 mL of the intravenous solutions listed below. Each 200 mg of Vibramycin (i.e., withdraw entire solution from the 200 mg vial) is further diluted with 200 mL to 2000 mL of the following intravenous solutions:

1. Sodium Chloride Injection, USP
2. 5% Dextrose Injection, USP
3. Ringer's Injection, USP
4. Invert Sugar, 10% in Water
5. Lactated Ringer's Injection, USP
6. Dextrose 5% in Lactated Ringer's
7. Normosol-M® in D5-W (Abbott)
8. Normosol-R® in D5-W (Abbott)
9. Plasma-Lyte® 56 in 5% Dextrose (Travenol)
10. Plasma-Lyte® 148 in 5% Dextrose (Travenol)

This will result in desired concentrations of 0.1 to 1.0 mg/mL. Concentrations lower than 0.1 mg/mL or higher than 1.0 mg/mL are not recommended.

Stability

Vibramycin IV is stable for 48 hours in solution when diluted with Sodium Chloride Injection, USP, or 5% Dextrose Injection, USP, to concentrations between 1.0 mg/mL and 0.1 mg/mL and stored at 25°C. Vibramycin IV in these solutions is stable under fluorescent light for 48 hours, but must be protected from direct sunlight during storage and infusion. Reconstituted solutions (1.0 to 0.1 mg/mL) may be stored up to 72 hours prior to start of infusion if refrigerated and protected from sunlight and artificial light. Infusion must then be completed within 12 hours. Solutions must be used within these time periods or discarded.

Vibramycin IV, when diluted with Ringer's Injection, USP, or Invert Sugar, 10% in Water, or Normosol-M® in D5-W (Abbott), or Normosol-R®in D5-W (Abbott), or Plasma-Lyte® 56 in 5% Dextrose (Travenol), or Plasma-Lyte® 148 in 5% Dextrose (Travenol) to a concentration between 1.0 mg/mL and 0.1 mg/mL, must be completely infused within 12 hours after reconstitution to ensure adequate stability. During infusion, the solution must be protected from direct sunlight. Reconstituted solutions (1.0 to 0.1 mg/mL) may be stored up to 72 hours prior to start of infusion if refrigerated and protected from sunlight and artifical light. Infusion must then be completed within 12 hours. Solutions must be used within these time periods or discarded.

When diluted with Lactated Ringer's Injection, USP, or Dextrose 5% in Lactated Ringer's, infusion of the solution (ca. 1.0 mg/mL) or lower concentrations (not less than 0.1 mg/

Continued on next page

Pfizer Inc—Cont.

mL) must be completed within six hours after reconstitution to ensure adequate stability. During infusion, the solution must be protected from direct sunlight. Solutions must be used within this time period or discarded.

Solutions of Vibramycin (doxycycline hyclate for injection) at a concentration of 10 mg/mL in Sterile Water for Injection, when frozen immediately after reconstitution are stable for 8 weeks when stored at −20°C. If the product is warmed, care should be taken to avoid heating it after the thawing is complete. Once thawed the solution should not be refrozen.

HOW SUPPLIED

Vibramycin (doxycycline hyclate for injection) Intravenous is available as a sterile powder in a vial containing doxycycline hyclate equivalent to 100 mg of doxycycline with 480 mg of ascorbic acid, packages of 5 (NDC 0049-0960-77).

65-1940-00-2

LITERATURE AVAILABLE

Yes.

VISTARIL®   ℞

[vĭs 'tăr-ĭl]
(hydroxyzine pamoate)
Capsules and Oral Suspension

DESCRIPTION

Hydroxyzine pamoate is designated chemically as 1-(p-chlorobenzhydryl) 4- [2- (2-hydroxyethoxy) ethyl] diethylenediamine salt of 1,1'- methylene bis (2 hydroxy-3-naphthalene carboxylic acid).

Inert ingredients for the capsule formulations are: hard gelatin capsules (which may contain Yellow 10, Green 3, Yellow 6, Red 33, and other inert ingredients); magnesium stearate; sodium lauryl sulfate; starch; sucrose.

Inert ingredients for the oral suspension formulation are: carboxymethylcellulose sodium; lemon flavor; propylene glycol; sorbic acid; sorbitol solution; water.

CLINICAL PHARMACOLOGY

Vistaril® (hydroxyzine pamoate) is unrelated chemically to the phenothiazines, reserpine, meprobamate, or the benzodiazepines.

Vistaril is not a cortical depressant, but its action may be due to a suppression of activity in certain key regions of the subcortical area of the central nervous system. Primary skeletal muscle relaxation has been demonstrated experimentally. Bronchodilator activity, and antihistaminic and analgesic effects have been demonstrated experimentally and confirmed clinically. An antiemetic effect, both by the apomorphine test and the veriloid test, has been demonstrated. Pharmacological and clinical studies indicate that hydroxyzine in therapeutic dosage does not increase gastric secretion or acidity and in most cases has mild antisecretory activity. Hydroxyzine is rapidly absorbed from the gastrointestinal tract and Vistaril's clinical effects are usually noted within 15 to 30 minutes after oral administration.

INDICATIONS

For symptomatic relief of anxiety and tension associated with psychoneurosis and as an adjunct in organic disease states in which anxiety is manifested.

Useful in the management of pruritus due to allergic conditions such as chronic urticaria and atopic and contact dermatoses, and in histamine-mediated pruritus.

As a sedative when used as premedication and following general anesthesia, **Hydroxyzine may potentiate meperidine (Demerol®) and barbiturates,** so their use in pre-anesthetic adjunctive therapy should be modified on an individual basis. Atropine and other belladonna alkaloids are not affected by the drug. Hydroxyzine is not known to interfere with the action of digitalis in any way and it may be used concurrently with this agent.

The effectiveness of hydroxyzine as an antianxiety agent for long–term use, that is, more than 4 months, has not been assessed by systematic clinical studies. The physician should reassess periodically the usefulness of the drug for the individual patient.

CONTRAINDICATIONS

Hydroxyzine, when administered to the pregnant mouse, rat, and rabbit, induced fetal abnormalities in the rat and mouse at doses substantially above the human therapeutic range. Clinical data in human beings are inadequate to establish safety in early pregnancy. Until such data are available, hydroxyzine is contraindicated in early pregnancy. Hydroxyzine pamoate is contraindicated for patients who have shown a previous hypersensitivity to it.

WARNINGS

Nursing Mothers: It is not known whether this drug is excreted in human milk. Since many drugs are so excreted, hydroxyzine should not be given to nursing mothers.

PRECAUTIONS

THE POTENTIATING ACTION OF HYDROXYZINE MUST BE CONSIDERED WHEN THE DRUG IS USED IN CONJUNCTION WITH CENTRAL NERVOUS SYSTEM DEPRESSANTS SUCH AS NARCOTICS, NON-NARCOTIC ANALGESICS AND BARBITURATES. Therefore, when central nervous system depressants are administered concomitantly with hydroxyzine, their dosage should be reduced. Since drowsiness may occur with use of the drug, patients should be warned of this possibility and cautioned against driving a car or operating dangerous machinery while taking Vistaril (hydroxyzine pamoate). Patients should be advised against the simultaneous use of other CNS depressant drugs, and cautioned that the effect of alcohol may be increased.

ADVERSE REACTIONS

Side effects reported with the administration of Vistaril are usually mild and transitory in nature.
Anticholinergic: Dry mouth.
Central Nervous System: Drowsiness is usually transitory and may disappear in a few days of continued therapy or upon reduction of the dose. Involuntary motor activity, including rare instances of tremor and convulsions, has been reported, usually with doses considerably higher than those recommended. Clinically significant respiratory depression has not been reported at recommended doses.

OVERDOSAGE

The most common manifestation of overdosage of Vistaril is hypersedation. As in the management of overdosage with any drug, it should be borne in mind that multiple agents may have been taken.

If vomiting has not occurred spontaneously, it should be induced. Immediate gastric lavage is also recommended. General supportive care, including frequent monitoring of the vital signs and close observation of the patient, is indicated. Hypotension, though unlikely, may be controlled with intravenous fluids and Levophed® (levarterenol) or Aramine® (metaraminol). Do not use epinephrine, as Vistaril counteracts its pressor action. Caffeine and Sodium Benzoate Injection, USP, may be used to counteract central nervous system depressant effects.

There is no specific antidote. It is doubtful that hemodialysis would be of any value in the treatment of overdosage with hydroxyzine. However, if other agents such as barbiturates have been ingested concomitantly, hemodialysis may be indicated. There is no practical method to quantitate hydroxyzine in body fluids or tissue after its ingestion or administration.

DOSAGE

For symptomatic relief of anxiety and tension associated with psychoneurosis and as an adjunct in organic disease states in which anxiety is manifested: in adults, 50–100 mg q.i.d.; children under 6 years, 50 mg daily in divided doses and over 6 years, 50–100 mg daily in divided doses.

For use in the management of pruritus due to allergic conditions such as chronic urticaria and atopic and contact dermatoses, and in histamine-mediated pruritus: in adults, 25 mg t.i.d. or q.i.d.; children under 6 years, 50 mg daily in divided doses and over 6 years, 50–100 mg daily in divided doses.

As a sedative when used as a premedication and following general anesthesia: 50–100 mg in adults, and 0.6 mg/kg in children.

When treatment is initiated by the intramuscular route of administration, subsequent doses may be administered orally.

As with all medications, the dosage should be adjusted according to the patient's response to therapy.

HOW SUPPLIED

Vistaril® Capsules (hydroxyzine pamoate equivalent to hydroxyzine hydrochloride)

25 mg:	100's (NDC 0069-5410-66), 500's (NDC 0069-5410-73), and Unit Dose (10 × 10's) (NDC 0069-5410-41) two-tone green capsules
50 mg:	100's (NDC 0069-5420-66), 500's (NDC 0069-5420-73), and Unit Dose (10 × 10's) (NDC 0069-5420-41) green and white capsules
100 mg:	100's (NDC 0069-5430-66), 500's (NDC 0069-5430-73), and Unit Dose (10 × 10's) (NDC 0069-5430-41) green and gray capsules

Vistaril® Oral Suspension (hydroxyzine pamoate equivalent to 25 mg hydroxyzine hydrochloride per teaspoonful-5 mL): 1 pint (473 mL) bottles (NDC 0069-5440-93) and 4 ounce (120 mL) bottles (NDC 0069-5440-97) in packages of 4.
Shake vigorously until product is completely resuspended.

BIBLIOGRAPHY

Available on request.
69-0846-00-1   Revised November 1994
Shown in Product Identification Guide, page 328

VISTARIL®   ℞
hydroxyzine hydrochloride
Intramuscular Solution
For Intramuscular Use Only

CHEMISTRY

Hydroxyzine hydrochloride is designated chemically as 1-(p-chlorobenzhydryl) 4-[2-(2-hydroxyethoxy) ethyl] piperazine dihydrochloride.

ACTIONS

VISTARIL (hydroxyzine hydrochloride) is unrelated chemically to phenothiazine, reserpine, and meprobamate. Hydroxyzine has demonstrated its clinical effectiveness in the chemotherapeutic aspect of the total management of neuroses and emotional disturbances manifested by anxiety, tension, agitation, apprehension or confusion.

Hydroxyzine has been shown clinically to be a rapid-acting true ataraxic with a wide margin of safety. It induces a calming effect in anxious, tense, psychoneurotic adults and also in anxious, hyperkinetic children without impairing mental alertness. It is not a cortical depressant, but its action may be due to a suppression of activity in certain key regions of the subcortical area of the central nervous system.

Primary skeletal muscle relaxation has been demonstrated experimentally.

Hydroxyzine has been shown experimentally to have antispasmodic properties, apparently mediated through interference with the mechanism that responds to spasmogenic agents such as serotonin, acetylcholine, and histamine.

Antihistaminic effects have been demonstrated experimentally and confirmed clinically.

An antiemetic effect, both by the apomorphine test and the veriloid test, has been demonstrated. Pharmacological and clinical studies indicate that hydroxyzine in therapeutic dosage does not increase gastric secretion or acidity and in most cases provides mild antisecretory benefits.

INDICATIONS

The total management of anxiety, tension, and psychomotor agitation in conditions of emotional stress requires in most instances a combined approach of psychotherapy and chemotherapy. Hydroxyzine has been found to be particularly useful for this latter phase of therapy in its ability to render the disturbed patient more amenable to psychotherapy in long term treatment of the psychoneurotic and psychotic, although it should not be used as the sole treatment of psychosis or of clearly demonstrated cases of depression.

Hydroxyzine is also useful in alleviating the manifestations of anxiety and tension as in the preparation for dental procedures and in acute emotional problems. It has also been recommended for the management of anxiety associated with organic disturbances and as adjunctive therapy in alcoholism and allergic conditions with strong emotional overlay, such as in asthma, chronic urticaria, and pruritus.

VISTARIL (hydroxyzine hydrochloride) Intramuscular Solution is useful in treating the following types of patients when intramuscular administration is indicated:

1. The acutely disturbed or hysterical patient.
2. The acute or chronic alcoholic with anxiety withdrawal symptoms or delirium tremens.
3. As pre- and postoperative and pre- and postpartum adjunctive medication to permit reduction in narcotic dosage, allay anxiety and control emesis.

VISTARIL (hydroxyzine hydrochloride) has also demonstrated effectiveness in controlling nausea and vomiting, excluding nausea and vomiting of pregnancy. (See Contraindications.)

In prepartum states, the reduction in narcotic requirement effected by hydroxyzine is of particular benefit to both mother and neonate.

Hydroxyzine benefits the cardiac patient by its ability to allay the associated anxiety and apprehension attendant to certain types of heart disease. Hydroxyzine is not known to interfere with the action of digitalis in any way and may be used concurrently with this agent.

The effectiveness of hydroxyzine in long term use, that is, more than 4 months, has not been assessed by systematic clinical studies. The physician should reassess periodically the usefulness of the drug for the individual patient.

CONTRAINDICATIONS

Hydroxyzine hydrochloride intramuscular solution is intended only for intramuscular administration and should not, under any circumstances, be injected subcutaneously, intra-arterially, or intravenously.

This drug is contraindicated for patients who have shown a previous hypersensitivity to it.

Hydroxyzine, when administered to the pregnant mouse, rat, and rabbit, induced fetal abnormalities in the rat at doses substantially above the human therapeutic range. Clinical data in human beings are inadequate to establish safety in early pregnancy. Until such data are available, hydroxyzine is contraindicated in early pregnancy.

PRECAUTIONS

THE POTENTIATING ACTION OF HYDROXYZINE MUST BE CONSIDERED WHEN THE DRUG IS USED IN CONJUNCTION WITH CENTRAL NERVOUS SYSTEM DEPRESSANTS SUCH AS NARCOTICS, BARBITURATES, AND ALCOHOL. Rarely, cardiac arrests and death have been reported in association with the combined use of hydroxyzine hydrochloride IM and other CNS depressants. Therefore when central nervous system depressants are administered concomitantly with hydroxyzine their dosage should be reduced up to 50 per cent. The efficacy of hydroxyzine as adjunctive pre- and postoperative sedative medication has also been well established, especially as regards its ability to allay anxiety, control emesis, and reduce the amount of narcotic required.

HYDROXYZINE MAY POTENTIATE NARCOTICS AND BARBITURATES, so their use in preanesthetic adjunctive therapy should be modified on an individual basis. Atropine and other belladonna alkaloids are not affected by the drug. When hydroxyzine is used preoperatively or prepartum, narcotic requirements may be reduced as much as 50 per cent. Thus, when 50 mg of VISTARIL (hydroxyzine hydrochloride) Intramuscular Solution is employed, meperidine dosage may be reduced from 100 mg to 50 mg. The administration of meperidine may result in severe hypotension in the postoperative patient or any individual whose ability to maintain blood pressure has been compromised by a depleted blood volume. Meperidine should be used with great caution and in reduced dosage in patients who are receiving other pre- and/or postoperative medications and in whom there is a risk of respiratory depression, hypotension, and profound sedation or coma occurring. Before using any medications concomitant with hydroxyzine, the manufacturer's prescribing information should be read carefully.

Since drowsiness may occur with the use of this drug, patients should be warned of this possibility and cautioned against driving a car or operating dangerous machinery while taking this drug.

As with all intramuscular preparations, VISTARIL Intramuscular Solution should be injected well within the body of a relatively large muscle. Inadvertent subcutaneous injection may result in significant tissue damage.

ADULTS: The preferred site is the upper outer quadrant of the buttock, (i.e., gluteus maximus), or the mid-lateral thigh.

CHILDREN: It is recommended that intramuscular injections be given preferably in the mid-lateral muscles of the thigh. In infants and small children the periphery of the upper outer quadrant of the gluteal region should be used only when necessary, such as in burn patients, in order to minimize the possibility of damage to the sciatic nerve.

The deltoid area should be used only if well developed such as in certain adults and older children, and then only with caution to avoid radial nerve injury. Intramuscular injections should not be made into the lower and mid-third of the upper arm. As with all intramuscular injections, aspiration is necessary to help avoid inadvertent injection into a blood vessel.

ADVERSE REACTIONS

Therapeutic doses of hydroxyzine seldom produce impairment of mental alertness. However, drowsiness may occur; if so, it is usually transitory and may disappear in a few days of continued therapy or upon reduction of the dose. Dryness of the mouth may be encountered at higher doses. Extensive clinical use has substantiated the absence of toxic effects on the liver or bone marrow when administered in the recommended doses for over four years of uninterrupted therapy. The absence of adverse effects has been further demonstrated in experimental studies in which excessively high doses were administered.

Involuntary motor activity, including rare instances of tremor and convulsions, has been reported, usually with doses considerably higher than those recommended. Continuous therapy with over one gram per day has been employed in some patients without these effects having been encountered.

DOSAGE AND ADMINISTRATION

The recommended dosages for VISTARIL (hydroxyzine hydrochloride) Intramuscular Solution are:

For adult psychiatric and emotional emergencies, including acute alcoholism.	IM: 50–100 mg stat., and q. 4–6h., p.r.n.
Nausea and vomiting excluding nausea and vomiting of pregnancy.	Adults: 25–100 mg IM Children: 0.5 mg/lb body weight IM
Pre- and postoperative adjunctive medication.	Adults: 25–100 mg IM Children: 0.5 mg/lb body weight IM
Pre- and postpartum adjunctive therapy.	25–100 mg IM

As with all potent medications, the dosage should be adjusted according to the patient's response to therapy.

FOR ADDITIONAL INFORMATION OF THE ADMINISTRATION AND SITE OF SELECTION SEE PRECAUTIONS SECTION. NOTE: VISTARIL (hydroxyzine hydrochloride) Intramuscular Solution may be administered without further dilution.

Patients may be started on intramuscular therapy when indicated. They should be maintained on oral therapy whenever this route is practicable.

HOW SUPPLIED

VISTARIL (hydroxyzine hydrochloride) Intramuscular Solution

Multi-Dose Vials

25 mg/mL: 10 mL vials (NDC 0049-5450-74)

50 mg/mL: 10 mL vials (NDC 0049-5460-74)

Unit Dose Vials

50 mg/mL–1 mL fill: packages of 25 vials (NDC 0049-5462-76)

100 mg/2 mL–2 mL fill: packages of 25 vials (NDC 0049-5460-76)

STORAGE

Store below 86° F (30°C).

Protect from freezing.

FORMULA

Dosage Strength	25 mg/1 mL	50 mg/1 mL 100 mg/2 mL
Hydroxyzine hydrochloride	25 mg/mL	50 mg/mL
Benzyl Alcohol	0.9%	0.9%
Sodium hydroxide		to adjust to optimum pH

70-0843-00-5

Revised May 1993

ZITHROMAX® ℞
(azithromycin capsules)
and
(azithromycin for oral suspension)

DESCRIPTION

ZITHROMAX® (azithromycin capsules and azithromycin for oral suspension) contain the active ingredient azithromycin, an azalide, a subclass of macrolide antibiotics, for oral administration. Azithromycin has the chemical name $(2R,3S,4R,5R,8R,10R,11R,12S,13S,14R)$-13-[(2,6-dideoxy-3-$C$-methyl-3-$O$-methyl-$\alpha$-$L$-$ribo$-hexopyranosyl)oxy]-2-ethyl-3,4,10-trihydroxy-3,5,6,8,10,12,14-heptamethyl-11-[[3,4,6-trideoxy-3-(dimethylamino)-β-D-$xylo$-hexopyranosyl]oxy]-1-oxa-6-azacyclopentadecan-15-one. Azithromycin is derived from erythromycin; however, it differs chemically from erythromycin in that a methyl-substituted nitrogen atom is incorporated into the lactone ring. Its molecular formula is $C_{38}H_{72}N_2O_{12}$, and its molecular weight is 749.00. Azithromycin has the following structural formula:

Azithromycin, as the dihydrate, is a white crystalline powder with a molecular formula of $C_{38}H_{72}N_2O_{12}\cdot 2H_2O$ and a molecular weight of 785.0.

ZITHROMAX® capsules contain azithromycin dihydrate equivalent to 250 mg of azithromycin. The capsules are supplied in red opaque hard-gelatin capsules (containing FD&C Red #40). They also contain the following inactive ingredients: anhydrous lactose, corn starch, magnesium stearate, and sodium lauryl sulfate.

It is also supplied as a powder for oral suspension.

ZITHROMAX® for oral suspension is supplied in bottles containing 300 mg, 600 mg, 900 mg, or 1200 mg azithromycin dihydrate powder equivalent to 300 mg, 600 mg, 900 mg, 1200 mg azithromycin per bottle and the following inactive ingredients: sucrose; sodium phosphate, tribasic, anhydrous; hydroxypropyl cellulose; xanthan gum; FD&C Red #40; and spray dried artificial cherry, creme de vanilla, and banana flavors. After constitution, each 5 mL of suspension contains 100 mg or 200 mg of azithromycin.

CLINICAL PHARMACOLOGY

Adult Pharmacokinetics: Following oral administration, azithromycin is rapidly absorbed and widely distributed throughout the body. Rapid distribution of azithromycin into tissues and high concentration within cells result in significantly higher azithromycin concentrations in tissues than in plasma or serum.

The pharmacokinetic parameters of azithromycin capsules in plasma after dosing 500 mg loading dose on day 1 followed by 250 mg q.d. on days 2 through 5 in healthy young adults (age 18–40 years old) are portrayed in the following chart:

Pharmacokinetic Parameters
(Mean)   Total n=12

	Day 1	Day 5
C_{max} (µg/mL)	0.41	0.24
T_{max} (h)	2.5	3.2
AUC_{0-24} (µg·h/mL)	2.6	2.1
C_{min} (µg/mL)	0.05	0.05
Urinary Excret. (% dose)	4.5	6.5

In this study, there was no significant difference in the disposition of azithromycin between male and female subjects. Plasma concentrations of azithromycin declined in a polyphasic pattern resulting in an average terminal half-life of 68 hours. With this regimen, C_{min} and C_{max} remained essentially unchanged from day 2 through day 5 of therapy. However, without a loading dose, azithromycin C_{min} levels required 5 to 7 days to reach steady-state.

When studied in healthy elderly subjects from age 65 to 85 years, the pharmacokinetic parameters of azithromycin in elderly men were similar to those in young adults; however, in elderly women, although higher peak concentrations (increased by 30 to 50%) were observed, no significant accumulation occurred.

The high values in adults for apparent steady-state volume of distribution (31.1 L/kg) and plasma clearance (630 mL/min) suggest that the prolonged half-life is due to extensive uptake and subsequent release of drug from tissues.

Selected tissue (or fluid) concentration and tissue (or fluid) to plasma/serum concentration ratios are shown in the following table:

AZITHROMYCIN CONCENTRATIONS FOLLOWING TWO–250 mg (500 mg) CAPSULES IN ADULTS

TISSUE OR FLUID	TIME AFTER DOSE (h)	TISSUE OR FLUID CONCENTRATION (µg/g or µg/mL)[1]
SKIN	72–96	0.4
LUNG	72–96	4.0
SPUTUM*	2–4	1.0
SPUTUM**	10–12	2.9
TONSIL***	9–18	4.5
TONSIL***	180	0.9
CERVIX****	19	2.8

TISSUE OR FLUID	CORRESPONDING PLASMA OR SERUM LEVEL (µg/mL)	TISSUE (FLUID) PLASMA (SERUM) RATIO[1]
SKIN	0.012	35
LUNG	0.012	>100
SPUTUM*	0.64	2
SPUTUM**	0.1	30
TONSIL***	0.03	>100
TONSIL***	0.006	>100
CERVIX****	0.04	70

[1] High tissue concentrations should not be interpreted to be quantitatively related to clinical efficacy. The antimicrobial activity of azithromycin is pH related. Azithromycin is concentrated in cell lysosomes which have a low intraorganelle pH, at which the drug's activity is reduced. However, the extensive distribution of drug to tissues may be relevant to clinical activity.

* Sample was obtained 2–4 hours after the first dose.

** Sample was obtained 10–12 hours after the first dose.

*** Dosing regimen of 2 doses of 250 mg each, separated by 12 hours.

**** Sample was obtained 19 hours after a single 500 mg dose.

The extensive tissue distribution was confirmed by examination of additional tissues and fluids (bone, ejaculum, prostate, ovary, uterus, salpinx, stomach, liver, and gallbladder). As there are no data from adequate and well-controlled studies of azithromycin treatment of infections in these additional body sites, the clinical significance of these tissue concentration data is unknown.

Continued on next page

Pfizer Inc—Cont.

Only very low concentrations were noted in cerebrospinal fluid (less than 0.01 µg/mL) in the presence of non-inflamed meninges.

The serum protein binding of azithromycin is variable in the concentration range approximating human exposure, decreasing from 51% at 0.02 µg/mL to 7% at 2 µg/mL.

Biliary excretion of azithromycin, predominantly as unchanged drug, is a major route of elimination. Over the course of a week, approximately 6% of the administered dose appears as unchanged drug in urine.

There are no pharmacokinetic data available from studies in hepatically- or renally-impaired individuals.

When azithromycin capsules were administered with food to 11 adult healthy male subjects, the rate of absorption (C_{max}) of azithromycin from the capsule formulation was reduced by 52% and the extent of absorption (AUC) by 43%.

The AUC of azithromycin was unaffected by co-administration of an antacid containing aluminum and magnesium hydroxide with ZITHROMAX® capsules (azithromycin); however, the C_{max} was reduced by 24%. Administration of cimetidine (800 mg) two hours prior to azithromycin had no effect on azithromycin absorption.

The effect of azithromycin on the plasma levels or pharmacokinetics of theophylline administered in multiple doses adequate to reach therapeutic steady-state plasma levels is not known. (See PRECAUTIONS.)

When azithromycin suspension was administered with food to 28 adult healthy male subjects, the rate of absorption (C_{max}) was increased by 56% while the extent of absorption (AUC) was unchanged.

Pediatric Pharmacokinetics:

In two clinical studies, azithromycin for oral suspension was dosed at 10 mg/kg on day 1, followed by 5 mg/kg on days 2 through 5 to two groups of children (aged 1–5 years and 5–15 years, respectively). The mean pharmacokinetic parameters at Day 5 were $C_{max}=0.216$ µg/mL, $T_{max}=1.9$ hours, and $AUC_{0-24}=1.822$ µg·hr/mL for the 1- to 5-year-old group and were $C_{max}=0.383$ µg/mL, $T_{max}=2.4$ hours, and $AUC_{0-24}=3.109$ µg·hr/mL for the 5- to 15-year-old group.

There are no pharmacokinetic data on azithromycin suspension when administered at a dose of 12 mg/kg/day in the presence or absence of food. (For the pediatric pharyngitis/tonsillitis dose, see DOSAGE AND ADMINISTRATION.)

Microbiology: Azithromycin acts by binding to the 50S ribosomal subunit of susceptible microorganisms and, thus, interfering with microbial protein synthesis. Nucleic acid synthesis is not affected.

Azithromycin concentrates in phagocytes and fibroblasts as demonstrated by in vitro incubation techniques. Using such methodology, the ratio of intracellular to extracellular concentration was > 30 after one hour incubation. In vivo studies suggest that concentration in phagocytes may contribute to drug distribution to inflamed tissues.

Azithromycin has been shown to be active against most strains of the following microorganisms, both in vitro and in clinical infections as described in the INDICATIONS AND USAGE section.

Aerobic Gram-Positive Microorganisms

Staphylococcus aureus
Streptococcus agalactiae
Streptococcus pneumoniae
Streptococcus pyogenes

NOTE: Azithromycin demonstrates cross-resistance with erythromycin-resistant gram-positive strains. Most strains of *Enterococcus faecalis* and methicillin-resistant staphylococci are resistant to azithromycin.

Aerobic Gram-Negative Microorganisms

Haemophilus influenzae
Moraxella catarrhalis

"Other" Microorganisms

Chlamydia trachomatis

Beta-lactamase production should have no effect on azithromycin activity.

The following in vitro data are available, but their clinical significance is unknown.

Azithromycin exhibits in vitro minimal inhibitory concentrations (MIC's) of 2.0 µg/mL or less against most (≥90%) strains of the following microorganisms; however, the safety and effectiveness of azithromycin in treating clinical infections due to these microorganisms have not been established in adequate and well-controlled trials.

Aerobic Gram-Positive Microorganisms

Streptococci (Groups C, F, G)
Viridans group streptococci

Aerobic Gram-Negative Microorganisms

Bordetella pertussis
Campylobacter jejuni
Haemophilus ducreyi
Legionella pneumophila

Anaerobic Microorganisms

Bacteroides bivius
Clostridium perfringens
Peptostreptococcus species

"Other" Microorganisms

Borrelia burgdorferi
Mycoplasma pneumoniae
Treponema pallidum
Ureaplasma urealyticum

Susceptibility Tests

The in vitro potency of azithromycin is markedly affected by the pH of the microbiological growth medium during incubation. Incubation in a 10% CO_2 atmosphere will result in lowering of media pH (7.2 to 6.6) within 18 hours and in an apparent reduction of the in vitro potency of azithromycin. Thus, the initial pH of the growth medium should be 7.2–7.4, and the CO_2 content of the incubation atmosphere should be as low as practical.

Azithromycin can be solubilized for in vitro susceptibility testing by dissolving in a minimum amount of 95% ethanol and diluting to working concentration with water.

Dilution Techniques:

Quantitative methods are used to determine antimicrobial minimal inhibitory concentrations (MIC's). These MIC's provide estimates of the susceptibility of bacteria to antimicrobial compounds. The MIC's should be determined using a standardized procedure. Standardized procedures are based on a dilution method[1] (broth or agar) or equivalent with standardized inoculum concentrations and standardized concentrations of azithromycin powder. The MIC values should be interpreted according to the following criteria:

MIC (µg/mL)	Interpretation
≤2	Susceptible (S)
4	Intermediate (I)
≥8	Resistant (R)

A report of "Susceptible" indicates that the pathogen is likely to be inhibited if the antimicrobial compound in the blood reaches the concentrations usually achievable. A report of "Intermediate" indicates that the result should be considered equivocal, and, if the microorganism is not fully susceptible to alternative, clinically feasible drugs, the test should be repeated. This category implies possible clinical applicability in body sites where the drug is physiologically concentrated or in situations where high dosage of drug can be used. This category also provides a buffer zone which prevents small uncontrolled technical factors from causing major discrepancies in interpretation. A report of "Resistant" indicates that the pathogen is not likely to be inhibited if the antimicrobial compound in the blood reaches the concentrations usually achievable; other therapy should be selected. Standardized susceptibility test procedures require the use of laboratory control microorganisms to control the technical aspects of the laboratory procedures. Standard azithromycin powder should provide the following MIC values:

Microorganism	MIC (µg/mL)
Escherichia coli ATCC 25922	2.0–8.0
Enterococcus faecalis ATCC 29212	1.0–4.0
Staphylococcus aureus ATCC 29213	0.25–1.0

Diffusion Techniques:

Quantitative methods that require measurement of zone diameters also provide reproducible estimates of the susceptibility of bacteria to antimicrobial compounds. One such standardized procedure[2] requires the use of standardized inoculum concentrations. This procedure uses paper disks impregnated with 15-µg azithromycin to test the susceptibility of microorganisms to azithromycin.

Reports from the laboratory providing results of the standard single-disk susceptibility test with a 15-µg azithromycin disk should be interpreted according to the following criteria;

Zone Diameter (mm)	Interpretation
≥18	Susceptible (S)
14–17	Intermediate (I)
≤13	Resistant (R)

Interpretation should be as stated above for results using dilution techniques. Interpretation involves correlation of the diameter obtained in the disk test with the MIC for azithromycin.

As with standardized dilution techniques, diffusion methods require the use of laboratory control microorganisms that are used to control the technical aspects of the laboratory procedures. For the diffusion technique, the 15-µg azithromycin disk should provide the following zone diameters in this laboratory test quality control strain:

Microorganism	Zone Diameter (mm)
Staphylococcus aureus ATCC 25923	21–26

INDICATIONS AND USAGE

ZITHROMAX® (azithromycin) is indicated for the treatment of patients with mild to moderate infections (pneumonia: see WARNINGS) caused by susceptible strains of the designated microorganisms in the specific conditions listed below. As recommended dosages, durations of therapy, and applicable patient populations vary among these infections, please see DOSAGE AND ADMINISTRATION for specific dosing recommendations.

Adults:

Acute bacterial exacerbations of chronic obstructive pulmonary disease due to *Haemophilus influenzae*, *Moraxella catarrhalis*, or *Streptococcus pneumoniae*.

Community-acquired pneumonia of mild severity due to *Streptococcus pneumoniae* or *Haemophilus influenzae* in patients appropriate for outpatient oral therapy.

NOTE: Azithromycin should not be used in patients with pneumonia who are judged to be inappropriate for outpatient oral therapy because of moderate to severe illness or risk factors such as any of the following:

patients with nosocomially acquired infections, patients with known or suspected bacteremia, patients requiring hospitalization, elderly or debilitated patients, or patients with significant underlying health problems that may compromise their ability to respond to their illness (including immunodeficiency or functional asplenia).

Pharyngitis/tonsillitis caused by *Streptococcus pyogenes* as an alternative to first-line therapy in individuals who cannot use first-line therapy.

NOTE: Penicillin by the intramuscular route is the usual drug of choice in the treatment of *Streptococcus pyogenes* infection and the prophylaxis of rheumatic fever. ZITHROMAX® is often effective in the eradication of susceptible strains of *Streptococcus pyogenes* from the nasopharynx. Because some strains are resistant to ZITHROMAX,® susceptibility tests should be performed when patients are treated with ZITHROMAX.® Data establishing efficacy of azithromycin in subsequent prevention of rheumatic fever are not available.

Uncomplicated skin and skin structure infections due to *Staphylococcus aureus*, *Streptococcus pyogenes*, or *Streptococcus agalactiae*. Abscesses usually require surgical drainage.

Non-gonococcal urethritis and cervicitis due to *Chlamydia trachomatis*.

ZITHROMAX®, at the recommended dose, should not be relied upon to treat gonorrhea or syphilis. Antimicrobial agents used in high doses for short periods of time to treat non-gonococcal urethritis may mask or delay the symptoms of incubating gonorrhea or syphilis. All patients with sexually-transmitted urethritis or cervicitis should have a serologic test for syphilis and appropriate cultures for gonorrhea performed at the time of diagnosis. Appropriate antimicrobial therapy and follow-up tests for these diseases should be initiated if infection is confirmed.

Appropriate culture and susceptibility tests should be performed before treatment to determine the causative organism and its susceptibility to azithromycin. Therapy with ZITHROMAX® may be initiated before results of these tests are known; once the results become available, antimicrobial therapy should be adjusted accordingly.

Children: (See Pediatric Use and CLINICAL STUDIES IN PEDIATRIC PATIENTS.)

Acute otitis media caused by *Haemophilus influenzae*, *Moraxella catarrhalis* or *Streptococcus pneumoniae*. (For specific dosage recommendation, see DOSAGE AND ADMINISTRATION.)

Pharyngitis/tonsillitis caused by *Streptococcus pyogenes* as an alternative to first line therapy in individuals who cannot use first-line therapy. (For specific dosage recommendation, see DOSAGE AND ADMINISTRATION.)

NOTE: Penicillin by the intramuscular route is the usual drug of choice in the treatment of *Streptococcus pyogenes* infection and the prophylaxis of rheumatic fever. ZITHROMAX® is often effective in the eradication of susceptible strains of *Streptococcus pyogenes* from the nasopharynx. Because some strains are resistant to ZITHROMAX®, susceptibility tests should be performed when patients are treated with ZITHROMAX®. Data establishing efficacy of azithromycin in subsequent prevention of rheumatic fever are not available.

Appropriate culture and susceptibility tests should be performed before treatment to determine the causative organism and its susceptibility to azithromycin. Therapy with ZITHROMAX® may be initiated before results of these tests are known; once the results become available, antimicrobial therapy should be adjusted accordingly.

CONTRAINDICATIONS

ZITHROMAX® is contraindicated in patients with known hypersensitivity to azithromycin, erythromycin, or any macrolide antibiotic.

WARNINGS

Serious allergic reactions, including angioedema and anaphylaxis, have been reported rarely in patients on azithromycin therapy. (See CONTRAINDICATIONS.) Despite initially successful symptomatic treatment of the allergic symptoms, when symptomatic therapy was discontinued, the allergic symptoms recurred soon thereafter in some patients without further azithromycin exposure. These patients required prolonged periods of observation and symptomatic treatment. The relationship of these episodes to the long tissue half-life of azithromycin and subsequent prolonged exposure to antigen is unknown at present.

If an allergic reaction occurs, the drug should be discontinued and appropriate therapy should be instituted. Physicians should be aware that reappearance of the allergic symptoms may occur when symptomatic therapy is discontinued.

In the treatment of pneumonia, azithromycin has only been shown to be safe and effective in the treatment of community-acquired pneumonia of mild severity due to *Streptococcus pneumoniae* or *Haemophilus influenzae* in patients appropriate for outpatient oral therapy. Azithromycin should not be used in patients with pneumonia who are judged to be inappropriate for outpatient oral therapy because of moderate to severe illness or risk factors such as any of the following: patients with nosocomially acquired infections, patients with known or suspected bacteremia, patients requiring hospitalization, elderly or debilitated patients, or patients with significant underlying health problems that may compromise their ability to respond to their illness (including immunodeficiency or functional asplenia).

Pseudomembranous colitis has been reported with nearly all antibacterial agents and may range in severity from mild to life-threatening. Therefore, it is important to consider this diagnosis in patients who present with diarrhea subsequent to the administration of antibacterial agents.

Treatment with antibacterial agents alters the normal flora of the colon and may permit overgrowth of clostridia. Studies indicate that a toxin produced by *Clostridium difficile* is a primary cause of "antibiotic-associated colitis."

After the diagnosis of pseudomembranous colitis has been established, therapeutic measures should be initiated. Mild cases of pseudomembranous colitis usually respond to discontinuation of the drug alone. In moderate to severe cases, consideration should be given to management with fluids and electrolytes, protein supplementation, and treatment with an antibacterial drug clinically effective against *Clostridium difficile* colitis.

PRECAUTIONS

General: Because azithromycin is principally eliminated via the liver, caution should be exercised when azithromycin is administered to patients with impaired hepatic function. There are no data regarding azithromycin usage in patients with renal impairment; thus, caution should be exercised when prescribing azithromycin in these patients.

The following adverse events have not been reported in clinical trials with azithromycin, an azalide; however, they have been reported with macrolide products: ventricular arrhythmias, including ventricular tachycardia and *torsades de pointes,* in individuals with prolonged QT intervals.

There has been a spontaneous report from the post-marketing experience of a patient with previous history of arrhythmias who experienced *torsades de pointes* and subsequent myocardial infarction following a course of azithromycin therapy.

Information for Patients:

Patients should be cautioned to take ZITHROMAX® capsules and ZITHROMAX® suspension at least one hour prior to a meal or at least two hours after a meal. These medications should not be taken with food.

Patients should also be cautioned not to take aluminum- and magnesium-containing antacids and azithromycin simultaneously.

The patient should be directed to discontinue azithromycin immediately and contact a physician if any signs of an allergic reaction occur.

Drug Interactions: Aluminum- and magnesium-containing antacids reduce the peak serum levels (rate) but not the AUC (extent) of azithromycin absorption.

Administration of cimetidine (800 mg) two hours prior to azithromycin had no effect on azithromycin absorption.

Azithromycin did not affect the plasma levels or pharmacokinetics of theophylline administered as a single intravenous dose. The effect of azithromycin on the plasma levels or pharmacokinetics of theophylline administered in multiple doses resulting in therapeutic steady-state levels of theophylline is not known. However, concurrent use of macrolides and theophylline has been associated with increases in the serum concentrations of theophylline. Therefore, until further data are available, prudent medical practice dictates careful monitoring of plasma theophylline levels in patients receiving azithromycin and theophylline concomitantly.

Azithromycin did not affect the prothrombin time response to a single dose of warfarin. However, prudent medical practice dictates careful monitoring of prothrombin time in all patients treated with azithromycin and warfarin concomitantly. Concurrent use of macrolides and warfarin in clinical practice has been associated with increased anticoagulant effects.

The following drug interactions have not been reported in clinical trials with azithromycin; however, no specific drug interaction studies have been performed to evaluate potential drug-drug interaction. Nonetheless, they have been observed with macrolide products. Until further data are developed regarding drug interactions when azithromycin and these drugs are used concomitantly, careful monitoring of patients is advised:

Digoxin—elevated digoxin levels.

Ergotamine or dihydroergotamine—acute ergot toxicity characterized by severe peripheral vasospasm and dysesthesia.

Triazolam—decrease the clearance of triazolam and thus may increase the pharmacologic effect of triazolam.

Drugs metabolized by the cytochrome P^{450} system—elevations of serum carbamazepine, terfenadine, cyclosporine, hexobarbital, and phenytoin levels.

Laboratory Test Interactions: There are no reported laboratory test interactions.

Carcinogenesis, Mutagenesis, Impairment of Fertility: Long-term studies in animals have not been performed to evaluate carcinogenic potential. Azithromycin has shown no mutagenic potential in standard laboratory tests: mouse lymphoma assay, human lymphocyte clastogenic assay, and mouse bone marrow clastogenic assay. No evidence of impaired fertility due to azithromycin was found.

Pregnancy: Teratogenic Effects. Pregnancy Category B: Reproduction studies have been performed in rats and mice at doses up to moderately maternally toxic dose levels (i.e., 200 mg/kg/day). These doses, based on a mg/m^2 basis, are estimated to be 4 to 2 times, respectively, the human daily dose of 500 mg. In the animal studies, no evidence of harm to the fetus due to azithromycin was found. There are, however, no adequate and well-controlled studies in pregnant women. Because animal reproduction studies are not always predictive of human response, azithromycin should be used during pregnancy only if clearly needed.

Nursing Mothers: It is not known whether azithromycin is excreted in human milk. Because many drugs are excreted in human milk, caution should be exercised when azithromycin is administered to a nursing woman.

Pediatric Use: (See **CLINICAL PHARMACOLOGY, INDICATIONS AND USAGE,** and **DOSAGE AND ADMINISTRATION.**)

Acute Otitis Media: Safety and effectiveness in the treatment of children with otitis media (dosage regimen: 10 mg/kg on Day 1 followed by 5 mg/kg on Days 2–5) under 6 months of age have not been established.

Pharyngitis/Tonsillitis: Safety and effectiveness in the treatment of children with pharyngitis/tonsillitis (dosage regimen: 12 mg/kg on Days 1–5) under 2 years of age have not been established.

Studies evaluating the use of repeated courses of therapy have not been conducted. (See CLINICAL PHARMACOLOGY and ANIMAL TOXICOLOGY.)

Geriatric Use: Pharmacokinetic parameters in older volunteers (65–85 years old) were similar to those in younger volunteers (18–40 years old) for the 5-day therapeutic regimen. Dosage adjustment does not appear to be necessary for older patients with normal renal and hepatic function receiving treatment with this dosage regimen. (See **CLINICAL PHARMACOLOGY.**)

ADVERSE REACTIONS

In clinical trials, most of the reported side effects were mild to moderate in severity and were reversible upon discontinuation of the drug. Approximately 0.7% of the patients (adults and children) from the multiple-dose clinical trials discontinued ZITHROMAX® (azithromycin) therapy because of treatment-related side effects. Most of the side effects leading to discontinuation were related to the gastrointestinal tract, e.g., nausea, vomiting, diarrhea, or abdominal pain. Potentially serious side effects of angioedema and cholestatic jaundice were reported rarely.

Clinical:

Adults:

Multiple-dose regimen: Overall, the most common side effects in adult patients receiving a multiple-dose regimen of ZITHROMAX® were related to the gastrointestinal system with diarrhea/loose stools (5%), nausea (3%), and abdominal pain (3%) being the most frequently reported.

No other side effects occurred in patients on the multiple-dose regimen of ZITHROMAX® with a frequency greater than 1%. Side effects that occurred with a frequency of 1% or less included the following:

Cardiovascular: Palpitations, chest pain.

Gastrointestinal: Dyspepsia, flatulence, vomiting, melena, and cholestatic jaundice.

Genitourinary: Monilia, vaginitis, and nephritis.

Nervous System: Dizziness, headache, vertigo, and somnolence.

General: Fatigue.

Allergic: Rash, photosensitivity, and angioedema.

Single 1-gram dose regimen: Overall, the most common side effects in patients receiving a single-dose regimen of 1 gram of ZITHROMAX® were related to the gastrointestinal system and were more frequently reported than in patients receiving the multiple-dose regimen.

Side effects that occurred in patients on the single one-gram dosing regimen of ZITHROMAX® with a frequency of 1% or greater included diarrhea/loose stools (7%), nausea (5%), abdominal pain (5%), vomiting (2%), dyspepsia (1%), and vaginitis (1%).

Children:

Multiple-dose regimens: The types of side effects in children were comparable to those seen in adults, with different incidence rates for the two dosage regimens recommended in children.

Acute Otitis Media: For the recommended dosage regimen of 10 mg/kg on Day 1 followed by 5 mg/kg on Days 2–5, the most frequent side effects were diarrhea/loose stools (2%), abdominal pain (2%), vomiting (1%), and nausea (1%).

Pharyngitis/tonsillitis: For the recommended dosage regimen of 12 mg/kg on Days 1–5, the most frequent side effects were diarrhea/loose stools (6%), vomiting (5%), abdominal pain (3%), nausea (2%), and headache (1%).

With either treatment regimen, no other side effects occurred in children treated with ZITHROMAX® with a frequency of greater than 1%. Side effects that occurred with a frequency of 1% or less included the following:

Cardiovascular: Chest pain.

Gastrointestinal: Dyspepsia, constipation, anorexia, flatulence, and gastritis.

Nervous System: Headache (otitis media dosage), hyperkinesia, dizziness, agitation, nervousness, insomnia.

General: Fever, fatigue, malaise.

Allergic: Rash.

Special Senses: Conjunctivitis.

Laboratory Abnormalities:

Adults:

Significant abnormalities (irrespective of drug relationship) occurring during the clinical trials were reported as follows: with an incidence of 1–2%, elevated serum creatine phosphokinase, potassium, ALT (SGPT), GGT, and AST (SGOT), with an incidence of less than 1%, leukopenia, neutropenia, decreased platelet count, elevated serum alkaline phosphatase, bilirubin, BUN, creatinine, blood glucose, LDH, and phosphate.

When follow-up was provided, changes in laboratory tests appeared to be reversible.

In multiple-dose clinical trials involving more than 3000 patients, 3 patients discontinued therapy because of treatment-related liver enzyme abnormalities and 1 because of a renal function abnormality.

Children:

Significant abnormalities (irrespective of drug relationship) occurring during clinical trials were all reported at a frequency of less than 1%, but were similar in type to the adult pattern.

In multiple-dose clinical trials involving almost 3000 pediatric patients, no patients discontinued therapy because of treatment-related abnormalities.

DOSAGE AND ADMINISTRATION

(See INDICATIONS AND USAGE and CLINICAL PHARMACOLOGY.)

Adults:

The recommended dose of ZITHROMAX® for the treatment of mild to moderate acute bacterial exacerbations of chronic obstructive pulmonary disease, community-acquired pneumonia of mild severity, pharyngitis/tonsillitis (as second-line therapy), and uncomplicated skin and skin structure infections due to the indicated organisms is: 500 mg as a single dose on the first day followed by 250 mg once daily on days 2 through 5.

ZITHROMAX® capsules should be given at least 1 hour before or 2 hours after a meal.

ZITHROMAX® capsules should not be taken with food.

The recommended dose of ZITHROMAX® for the treatment of non-gonococcal urethritis and cervicitis due to *C. trachomatis* is: a single 1 gram (1000 mg) dose of ZITHROMAX®.

Children:

Acute Otitis Media: The recommended dose of ZITHROMAX® for oral suspension for the treatment of children with acute otitis media is 10 mg/kg as a single dose on the first day (not to exceed 500 mg/day) followed by 5 mg/kg on days 2 through 5 (not to exceed 250 mg/day). (See chart below.)

ZITHROMAX® for oral suspension should be given at least 1 hour before or 2 hours after a meal.

ZITHROMAX® for oral suspension should not be taken with food.

PEDIATRIC DOSAGE GUIDELINES FOR OTITIS MEDIA
(Age 6 months and above, see Pediatric Use.)
Based on Body Weight

OTITIS MEDIA

Dosing Calculated on 10 mg/kg on Day 1 dose, followed by 5 mg/kg on Days 2 to 5.

Weight		100 mg/5 mL Suspension		200 mg/5 mL Suspension		Total mL per Treatment Course
Kg	lbs	Day 1	Days 2–5	Day 1	Days 2–5	
10	22	5 mL (1 tsp)	2.5 mL ($^1/_2$ tsp)			15 mL

Continued on next page

Pfizer Inc—Cont.

20	44	5 mL (1 tsp)	2.5 mL (1/2 tsp)	15 mL
30	66	7.5 mL (1 1/2 tsp)	3.75 mL (3/4 tsp)	22.5 mL
40	88	10 mL (2 tsp)	5 mL (1 tsp)	30 mL

Pharyngitis/Tonsillitis: The recommended dose for children with pharyngitis/tonsillitis is 12 mg/kg once a day for 5 days (not to exceed 500 mg/day). (See chart below.)

ZITHROMAX® for oral suspension should be given at least 1 hour before or 2 hours after a meal.

ZITHROMAX® for oral suspension should not be taken with food.

PEDIATRIC DOSAGE GUIDELINES FOR PHARYNGITIS/TONSILLITIS
(Age 2 years and above, see Pediatric Use.)
Based on Body Weight

PHARYNGITIS/TONSILLITIS

Dosing Calculated on 12 mg/kg once daily Days 1 to 5.

Weight Kg	lbs	200 mg/5 mL Suspension Day 1–5	Total mL per Treatment Course
8	18	2.5 mL (1/2 tsp)	12.5 mL
17	37	5 mL (1 tsp)	25 mL
25	55	7.5 mL (1 1/2 tsp)	37.5 mL
33	73	10 mL (2 tsp)	50 mL
40	88	12.5 mL (2 1/2 tsp)	62.5 mL

Constituting instructions for ZITHROMAX® Oral Suspension, 300, 600, 900, 1200 mg bottles. The table below indicates the volume of water to be used for constitution:

Amount of water to be added	Total volume after constitution (azithromycin content)	Azithromycin concentration after constitution
9 mL (300 mg)	15 mL (300 mg)	100 mg/5 mL
9 mL (600 mg)	15 mL (600 mg)	200 mg/5 mL
12 mL (900 mg)	22.5 mL (900 mg)	200 mg/5 mL
15 mL (1200 mg)	30 mL (1200 mg)	200 mg/5 mL

Shake well before each use. Oversized bottle provides shake space. Keep tightly closed.
After mixing, store at 5° to 30°C (41° to 86°F) and use within 10 days. Discard after full dosing is completed.

HOW SUPPLIED

ZITHROMAX® capsules (imprinted with "Pfizer 305") are supplied in red opaque hard-gelatin capsules containing azithromycin dihydrate equivalent to 250 mg of azithromycin. These are packaged in bottles and blister cards of 6 capsules (Z-PAKS™) as follows:

Bottles of 50	NDC 0069-3050-50
Boxes of 3 (Z-PAKS™ of 6)	NDC 0069-3050-34
Unit Dose package of 50	NDC 0069-3050-86

Store capsules below 30°C (86°F).
ZITHROMAX® for oral suspension after constitution contains a flavored suspension.
ZITHROMAX® for oral suspension is supplied in bottles with accompanying calibrated dropper as follows:

Azithromycin contents per bottle	NDC
300 mg	0069-3110-19
600 mg	0069-3120-19
900 mg	0069-3130-19
1200 mg	0069-3140-19

Storage: Store dry powder below 30°C (86°F). Store constituted suspension between 5° to 30°C (41° to 86°F) and discard when full dosing is completed.

CLINICAL STUDIES IN PEDIATRIC PATIENTS (See INDICATIONS AND USAGE and Pediatric Use.)
From the perspective of evaluating pediatric clinical trials, Days 11–14 (6–9 days after completion of the five-day regimen) were considered on-therapy evaluations because of the extended half-life of azithromycin. Day 11–14 data are provided for clinical guidance. Day 30 evaluations were considered the primary test of cure endpoint.

Acute Otitis Media
Efficacy Protocol 1
In a double-blind, controlled clinical study of acute otitis media performed in the United States, azithromycin (10 mg/kg on Day 1 followed by 5 mg/kg on Days 2–5) was compared to an antimicrobial/beta-lactamase inhibitor. In this study, very strict evaluability criteria were used to determine clinical response and safety results were obtained. For the 553 patients who were evaluated for clinical efficacy, the clinical success rate (i.e., cure plus improvement) at the Day 11 visit was 88% for azithromycin and 88% for the control agent. For the 521 patients who were evaluated at the Day 30 visit, the clinical success rate was 73% for azithromycin and 71% for the control agent.
In the safety analysis of the above study, the incidence of adverse events, primarily gastrointestinal, in all patients treated was 9% with azithromycin and 31% with the control agent. The most common side effects were diarrhea/loose stools (4% azithromycin vs. 20% control), vomiting (2% azithromycin vs. 7% control), and abdominal pain (2% azithromycin vs. 5% control).

Efficacy Protocol 2
In a noncomparative clinical and microbiologic trial performed in the United States, where significant rates of beta-lactamase producing organisms (35%) were found, 131 patients were evaluable for clinical efficacy. The combined clinical success rate (i.e., cure and improvement) at the Day 11 visit was 84% for azithromycin. For the 122 patients who were evaluated at the Day 30 visit, the clinical success rate was 70% for azithromycin.
Microbiologic determinations were made at the pre-treatment visit. Microbiology was not reassessed at later visits. The following presumptive bacterial/clinical cure outcomes (i.e., clinical success) were obtained from the evaluable group:

Bacteriological Eradication:

	Day 11 Azithromycin	Day 30 Azithromycin
S. pneumoniae	61/74 (82%)	40/56 (71%)
H. influenzae	43/54 (80%)	30/47 (64%)
M. catarrhalis	28/35 (80%)	19/26 (73%)
S. pyogenes	11/11 (100%)	7/7
Overall	177/217 (82%)	97/137 (73%)

In the safety analysis of this study, the incidence of adverse events, primarily gastrointestinal, in all patients treated was 9%. The most common side effect was diarrhea (4%).
Efficacy Protocol 3
In another controlled comparative clinical and microbiologic study of otitis media performed in the United States, azithromycin was compared to an antimicrobial/beta-lactamase inhibitor. This study utilized two of the same investigators as Efficacy Protocol 2 (above), and these two investigators enrolled 90% of the patients in Efficacy Protocol 3. For this reason, Efficacy Protocol 3 was not considered to be an independent study. Significant rates of beta-lactamase producing organisms (20%) were found. Ninety-two (92) patients were evaluable for clinical and microbiologic efficacy. The combined clinical success rate (i.e., cure and improvement) of those patients with a baseline pathogen at the Day 11 visit was 88% for azithromycin vs. 100% for control; at the Day 30 visit, the clinical success rate was 82% for azithromycin vs. 80% for control.
Microbiologic determinations were made at the pre-treatment visit. Microbiology was not reassessed at later visits. At the Day 11 and Day 30 visits, the following presumptive bacterial/clinical cure outcomes (i.e., clinical success) were obtained from the evaluable group:

Bacteriologic Eradication:

	Day 11 Azithromycin	Day 11 Control	Day 30 Azithromycin	Day 30 Control
S. pneumoniae	25/29 (86%)	26/26 (100%)	22/28 (79%)	18/22 (82%)
H. influenzae	9/11 (82%)	9/9	8/10 (80%)	6/8
M. catarrhalis	7/7	5/5	5/5	2/3
S. pyogenes	2/2	5/5	2/2	4/4
Overall	43/49 (88%)	45/45 (100%)	37/45 (82%)	30/37 (81%)

In the safety analysis of the above study, the incidence of adverse events, primarily gastrointestinal, in all patients treated was 4% with azithromycin and 31% with the control agent. The most common side effect was diarrhea/loose stools (2% azithromycin vs. 29% control).

Pharyngitis/Tonsillitis
In 3 double-blind controlled studies, conducted in the United States, azithromycin (12 mg/kg once a day for 5 days) was compared to penicillin V (250 mg three times a day for 10 days) in the treatment of pharyngitis due to documented Group A *β*-hemolytic streptococci (GABHS or *S. pyogenes*). Azithromycin was clinically and microbiologically statistically superior to penicillin at Day 14 and Day 30 with the following clinical success (i.e., cure and improvement) and bacteriologic efficacy rates (for the combined evaluable patient with documented GABHS):

Three U.S. Streptococcal Pharyngitis Studies
Azithromycin vs. Penicillin V
EFFICACY RESULTS

	Day 14	Day 30
Bacteriologic Eradication:		
Azithromycin	323/340 (95%)	255/330 (77%)
Penicillin V	242/332 (73%)	206/325 (63%)
Clinical Success (Cure plus improvement)		
Azithromycin	336/343 (98%)	310/330 (94%)
Penicillin V	284/338 (84%)	241/325 (74%)

Approximately 1% of azithromycin-susceptible *S. pyogenes* isolates were resistant to azithromycin following therapy.
The incidence of adverse events, primarily gastrointestinal, in all patients treated was 18% on azithromycin and 13% on penicillin. The most common side effects were diarrhea/loose stools (6% azithromycin vs. 2% penicillin), vomiting (6% azithromycin vs. 4% penicillin), and abdominal pain (3% azithromycin vs. 1% penicillin).

ANIMAL TOXICOLOGY

Phospholipidosis (intracellular phospholipid accumulation) has been observed in some tissues of mice, rats, and dogs given multiple doses of azithromycin. It has been demonstrated in numerous organ systems (e.g., eye, dorsal root ganglia, liver, gallbladder, kidney, spleen, and pancreas) in dogs treated with azithromycin at doses which, expressed on a mg/kg basis, are only 2 times greater than the recommended adult human dose and in rats at doses comparable to the recommended adult human dose. This effect has been reversible after cessation of azithromycin treatment. Phospholipidosis has been observed to a similar extent in the tissues of neonatal rats and dogs given daily doses of azithromycin ranging from 10 days to 30 days. Based on the pharmacokinetic data, phospholipidosis has been seen in the rat (30 mg/kg dose) at observed C_{max} value of 1.3 μg/mL (6 times greater than the observed C_{max} of 0.216 μg/mL at the pediatric dose of 10 mg/kg). Similarly, it has been shown in the dog (10 mg/kg dose) at observed C_{max} value of 1.5 μg/mL (7 times greater than the observed same C_{max} and drug dose in the studied pediatric population). On mg/m^2 basis, 30 mg/kg dose in the rat (135 mg/m^2) and 10 mg/kg dose in the dog (79 mg/m^2) are approximately 0.4 and 0.6 times, respectively, the recommended dose in the pediatric patients with an average body weight of 25 kg. This effect, similar to that seen in the adult animals, is reversible after cessation of azithromycin treatment. The significance of these findings for animals and for humans is unknown.

REFERENCES

1. National Committee for Clinical Laboratory Standards. Methods for Dilution Antimicrobial Susceptibility Tests for Bacteria that Grow Aerobically—Third Edition. Approved Standard NCCLS Document M7-A3, Vol. 13, No. 25, NCCLS, Villanova, PA, December 1993.
2. National Committee for Clinical Laboratory Standards. Performance Standards for Antimicrobial Disk Susceptibility Tests—Fifth Edition. Approved Standard NCCLS Document M2-A5, Vol. 13, No. 24, NCCLS, Villanova, PA, December 1993.

Licensed from Pliva
70-5179-00-3 Revised May 1996
Shown in Product Identification Guide, page 328

ZITHROMAX® ℞
(azithromycin capsules)
(azithromycin tablets)
and
(azithromycin for oral suspension)

DESCRIPTION

ZITHROMAX® (azithromycin capsules, azithromycin tablets and azithromycin for oral suspension) contain the active ingredient azithromycin, an azalide, a subclass of macrolide antibiotics, for oral administration. Azithromycin has the chemical name (*2R,3S,4R,5R,8R,10R,11R,12S,13S,14R*)-13-[(2,6-dideoxy-3-*C*-methyl -3- *O*-methyl -*α*- *L*-*ribo*-hexopyranosyl)oxy] -2- ethyl - 3,4,10-trihydroxy - 3,5,6,8,10,12,14 -heptamethyl-11-[[3,4,6-trideoxy-3-(dimethylamino) -*β*-*D*- *xylo*-hexopyranosyl]oxy]-1-oxa-6-azacyclopentadecan-15-one. Azithromycin is derived from erythromycin; however, it differs chemically from erythromycin in that a methyl-substituted nitrogen atom is incorporated into the lactone ring. Its molecular formula is $C_{38}H_{72}N_2O_{12}$, and its molecular weight is 749.0. Azithromycin has the following structural formula:
[See chemical structure at top of next column.]

DOSE/DOSAGE FORM	Subjects	Day No.	C_{max} (μg/ml)	T_{max} (hr)	C_{24} (μg/ml)	AUC (μg·hr/ml)	$T_{1/2}$ (hr)	Urinary Excretion (% of dose)
MEAN (CV%) PK PARAMETER								
500 mg/250 mg capsule	12	Day 1	0.41	2.5	0.05	2.6[a]	—	4.5
and 250 mg on Days 2–5	12	Day 5	0.24	3.2	0.05	2.1[a]	—	6.5
1200 mg/600 mg tablets	12	Day 1	0.66	2.5	0.074	6.8[b]	40	—
			(62%)	(79%)	(49%)	(64%)	(33%)	—

[a]0–24 hr, [b]0–last.

Azithromycin, as the dihydrate, is a white crystalline powder with a molecular formula of $C_{38}H_{72}N_2O_{12}\cdot 2H_2O$ and a molecular weight of 785.0.

ZITHROMAX® capsules contain azithromycin dihydrate equivalent to 250 mg of azithromycin. The capsules are supplied in red opaque hard-gelatin capsules (containing FD&C Red #40). They also contain the following inactive ingredients: anhydrous lactose, corn starch, magnesium stearate, and sodium lauryl sulfate.

ZITHROMAX® tablets contain azithromycin dihydrate equivalent to 600 mg azithromycin. The tablets are supplied as white, modified oval-shaped, film-coated tablets. They also contain the following inactive ingredients: dibasic calcium phosphate anhydrous, pregelatinized starch, sodium croscarmellose, magnesium stearate, sodium lauryl sulfate, and an aqueous film coat consisting of hydroxypropyl methyl cellulose, titanium dioxide, lactose and triacetin.

ZITHROMAX® for oral suspension is supplied in a single dose packet containing azithromycin dihydrate equivalent to 1 g azithromycin. It also contains the following inactive ingredients: colloidal silicon dioxide, sodium phosphate tribasic, anhydrous; spray dried artificial banana flavor, spray dried artificial cherry flavor, and sucrose.

CLINICAL PHARMACOLOGY

Pharmacokinetics: Following oral administration, azithromycin is rapidly absorbed and widely distributed throughout the body. Rapid distribution of azithromycin into tissues and high concentration within cells result in significantly higher azithromycin concentrations in tissues than in plasma or serum. The 1 g single dose packet is bioequivalent to four 250 mg capsules.

The pharmacokinetic parameters of azithromycin in plasma after dosing as per labeled recommendations in healthy young adults (age 18–40 years old) are portrayed in the following chart:
[See table above.]

In these studies (500 mg Day 1, 250 mg Days 2–5), there was no significant difference in the disposition of azithromycin between male and female subjects. Plasma concentrations of azithromycin following single 500 mg oral and i.v. doses declined in a polyphasic pattern resulting in an average terminal half-life of 68 hours. With a regimen of 500 mg on Day 1 and 250 mg/day on Days 2–5, C_{min} and C_{max} remained essentially unchanged from Day 2 through Day 5 of therapy. However, without a loading dose, azithromycin C_{min} levels required 5 to 7 days to reach steady-state.

When azithromycin capsules were administered with food, the rate of absorption (C_{max}) of azithromycin was reduced by 52% and the extent of absorption (AUC) by 43%.

When the oral suspension of azithromycin was administered with food, the C_{max} increased by 46% and the AUC by 14%. The absolute bioavailability of two 600 mg tablets was 34% (CV=56%). Administration of two 600 mg tablets with food increased C_{max} by 31% (CV=43%) while the extent of absorption (AUC) was unchanged (mean ratio of AUCs=1.00; CV=55%).

The AUC of azithromycin in 250 mg capsules was unaffected by coadministration of an antacid containing aluminum and magnesium hydroxide with ZITHROMAX® (azithromycin); however, the C_{max} was reduced by 24%. Administration of cimetidine (800 mg) two hours prior to azithromycin had no effect on azithromycin absorption.

When studied in healthy elderly subjects from age 65 to 85 years, the pharmacokinetic parameters of azithromycin (500 mg Day 1, 250 mg Days 2–5) in elderly men were similar to those in young adults; however, in elderly women, although higher peak concentrations (increased by 30 to 50%) were observed, no significant accumulation occurred.

The high values in adults for apparent steady-state volume of distribution (31.1 L/kg) and plasma clearance (630 mL/min) suggest that the prolonged half-life is due to extensive uptake and subsequent release of drug from tissues. Selected tissue (or fluid) concentration and tissue (or fluid) to plasma/serum concentration ratios are shown in the following table:

AZITHROMYCIN CONCENTRATIONS FOLLOWING TWO 250 mg (500 mg) CAPSULES IN ADULTS

TISSUE OR FLUID	TIME AFTER DOSE (h)	TISSUE OR FLUID CONCENTRATION (μg/g or μg/mL)[1]
SKIN	72–96	0.4
LUNG	72–96	4.0
SPUTUM*	2–4	1.0
SPUTUM**	10–12	2.9
TONSIL***	9–18	4.5
TONSIL***	180	0.9
CERVIX****	19	2.8

TISSUE OR FLUID	CORRESPONDING PLASMA OR SERUM LEVEL (μg/mL)	TISSUE (FLUID) PLASMA (SERUM) RATIO[1]
SKIN	0.012	35
LUNG	0.012	> 100
SPUTUM*	0.64	2
SPUTUM**	0.1	30
TONSIL***	0.03	> 100
TONSIL***	0.006	> 100
CERVIX****	0.04	70

[1] High tissue concentrations should not be interpreted to be quantitatively related to clinical efficacy. The antimicrobial activity of azithromycin is pH related. Azithromycin is concentrated in cell lysosomes which have a low intraorganelle pH, at which the drug's activity is reduced. However, the extensive distribution of drug to tissues may be relevant to clinical activity.
* Sample was obtained 2–4 hours after the first dose.
** Sample was obtained 10–12 hours after the first dose.
*** Dosing regimen of 2 doses of 250 mg each, separated by 12 hours.
**** Sample was obtained 19 hours after a single 500 mg dose.

The extensive tissue distribution was confirmed by examination of additional tissues and fluids (bone, ejaculum, prostate, ovary, uterus, salpinx, stomach, liver, and gallbladder). As there are no data from adequate and well-controlled studies of azithromycin treatment of infections in these additional body sites, the clinical significance of these tissue concentration data is unknown.

Following a regimen of 500 mg on the first day and 250 mg daily for 4 days, only very low concentrations were noted in cerebrospinal fluid (less than 0.01 μg/mL) in the presence of non-inflamed meninges.

Following oral administration of a single 1200 mg dose (two 600 mg tablets), the mean maximum concentration in peripheral leukocytes was 140 μg/mL. Concentrations remained above 32 μg/mL for approximately 60 hr. The mean half-lives for 6 males and 6 females were 34 hr and 57 hr, respectively. Leukocyte to plasma C_{max} ratios for males and females were 258 ($\pm$77%) and 175 ($\pm$60%), respectively, and the AUC ratios were 804 ($\pm$31%) and 541 ($\pm$28%), respectively. The clinical relevance of these findings is unknown. The serum protein binding of azithromycin is variable in the concentration range approximating human exposure, decreasing from 51% at 0.02 μg/mL to 7% at 2 μg/mL. Biliary excretion of azithromycin, predominantly as unchanged drug, is a major route of elimination. Over the course of a week, approximately 6% of the administered dose appears as unchanged drug in urine.

There are no pharmacokinetic data available from studies in hepatically- or renally-impaired individuals.

The effect of azithromycin on the plasma levels or pharmacokinetics of theophylline administered in multiple doses adequate to reach therapeutic steady-state plasma levels is not known. (See PRECAUTIONS.)

Mechanism of Action: Azithromycin acts by binding to the 50S ribosomal subunit of susceptible microorganisms and, thus, interfering with microbial protein synthesis. Nucleic acid synthesis is not affected.

Azithromycin concentrates in phagocytes and fibroblasts as demonstrated by in vitro incubation techniques. Using such methodology, the ratio of intracellular to extracellular concentration was > 30 after one hour incubation. In vivo studies suggest that concentration in phagocytes may contribute to drug distribution to inflamed tissues.

Microbiology:
Azithromycin has been shown to be active against most strains of the following microorganisms, both in vitro and in clinical infections as described in the INDICATIONS AND USAGE section.

Aerobic Gram-Positive Microorganisms
Staphylococcus aureus
Streptococcus agalactiae
Streptococcus pneumoniae
Streptococcus pyogenes
NOTE: Azithromycin demonstrates cross-resistance with erythromycin-resistant gram-positive strains. Most strains of *Enterococcus faecalis* and methicillin-resistant staphylococci are resistant to azithromycin.

Aerobic Gram-Negative Microorganisms
Haemophilus influenzae
Moraxella catarrhalis

"Other" Microorganisms
Chlamydia trachomatis
Beta-lactamase production should have no effect on azithromycin activity.

Azithromycin has been shown to be active in vitro and in the prevention of disease caused by the following microorganisms:

Mycobacteria
Mycobacterium avium complex (MAC) consisting of:
Mycobacterium avium
Mycobacterium intracellulare.
The following in vitro data are available, *but their clinical significance is unknown.*

Azithromycin exhibits in vitro minimal inhibitory concentrations (MICs) of 2.0 μg/mL or less against most ($\geq$ 90%) strains of the following microorganisms; however, the safety and effectiveness of azithromycin in treating clinical infections due to these microorganisms have not been established in adequate and well-controlled trials.

Aerobic Gram-Positive Microorganisms
Streptococci (Groups C, F, G)
Viridans group streptococci

Aerobic Gram-Negative Microorganisms
Bordetella pertussis
Campylobacter jejuni
Haemophilus ducreyi
Legionella pneumophila

Anaerobic Microorganisms
Bacteroides bivius
Clostridium perfringens
Peptostreptococcus species

"Other" Microorganisms
Borrelia burgdorferi
Mycoplasma pneumoniae
Treponema pallidum
Ureaplasma urealyticum

Susceptibility Testing of Bacteria Excluding Mycobacteria
The in vitro potency of azithromycin is markedly affected by the pH of the microbiological growth medium during incubation. Incubation in a 10% CO_2 atmosphere will result in lowering of media pH (7.2 to 6.6) within 18 hours and in an apparent reduction of the in vitro potency of azithromycin. Thus, the initial pH of the growth medium should be 7.2–7.4, and the CO_2 content of the incubation atmosphere should be as low as practical.

Azithromycin can be solubilized for in vitro susceptibility testing by dissolving in a minimum amount of 95% ethanol and diluting to working concentration with water.

Dilution Techniques:
Quantitative methods are used to determine minimal inhibitory concentrations that provide reproducible estimates of the susceptibility of bacteria to antimicrobial compounds. One such standardized procedure uses a standardized dilution method[1] (broth, agar or microdilution) or equivalent with azithromycin powder. The MIC values should be interpreted according to the following criteria:

MIC (μg/mL)	Interpretation
≤ 2	Susceptible (S)
4	Intermediate (I)
≥ 8	Resistant (R)

A report of "Susceptible" indicates that the pathogen is likely to respond to monotherapy with azithromycin. A report of "Intermediate" indicates that the result should be considered equivocal, and, if the microorganism is not fully susceptible to alternative, clinically feasible drugs, the test should be repeated. This category also provides a buffer zone which prevents small uncontrolled technical factors from

Continued on next page

Pfizer Inc—Cont.

causing major discrepancies in interpretation. A report of "Resistant" indicates that usually achievable drug concentrations are unlikely to be inhibitory and that other therapy should be selected.

Measurement of MIC or MBC and achieved antimicrobial compound concentrations may be appropriate to guide therapy in some infections. (See CLINICAL PHARMACOLOGY section for further information on drug concentrations achieved in infected body sites and other pharmacokinetic properties of this antimicrobial drug product.)

Standardized susceptibility test procedures require the use of laboratory control microorganisms. Standard azithromycin powder should provide the following MIC values:

Microorganism	MIC (μg/mL)
Escherichia coli ATCC 25922	2.0–8.0
Enterococcus faecalis ATCC 29212	1.0–4.0
Staphylococcus aureus ATCC 29213	0.25–1.0

Diffusion Techniques:

Quantitative methods that require measurement of zone diameters also provide reproducible estimates of the susceptibility of bacteria to antimicrobial compounds. One such standardized procedure[2] that has been recommended for use with disks to test the susceptibility of microorganisms to azithromycin uses the 15-μg azithromycin disk. Interpretation involves the correlation of the diameter obtained in the disk test with the minimal inhibitory concentration (MIC) for azithromycin.

Reports from the laboratory providing results of the standard single-disk susceptibility test with a 15 μg azithromycin disk should be interpreted according to the following criteria;

Zone Diameter (mm)	Interpretation
≥18	(S) Susceptible
14–17	(I) Intermediate
≤13	(R)Resistant

Interpretation should be as stated above for results using dilution techniques.

As with standardized dilution techniques, diffusion methods require the use of laboratory control microorganisms. The 15-μg azithromycin disk should provide the following zone diameters in these laboratory test quality control strains:

Microorganism	Zone Diameter (mm)
Staphylococcus aureus ATCC 25923	21–26

***In Vitro* Activity of Azithromycin Against Mycobacteria.**

Azithromycin has demonstrated *in vitro* activity against *Mycobacterium avium* complex (MAC) organisms. While gene probe techniques may be used to distinguish *M. avium* species from *M. intracellulare,* many studies only report results on *M. avium* complex (MAC) isolates. Azithromycin has also been shown to be active against phagocytized *M. avium* complex (MAC) organisms in mouse and human macrophage cell cultures as well as in the beige mouse infection model.

Various *in vitro* methodologies employing broth or solid media at different pHs, with and without oleic acid-albumin dextrose-catalase (OADC), have been used to determine azithromycin MIC values for *Mycobacterium avium* complex strains. In general, MIC values decreased 4 to 8 fold as the pH of middlebrook 7H11 agar media increased from 6.6 to 7.4. At pH 7.4, MIC values determined with Mueller-Hinton agar were 4 fold higher than that observed with middlebrook 7H12 media at the same pH. Utilization of oleic acid-albumin-dextrose-catalase (OADC) in these assays has been shown to further alter MIC values. The ability to correlate MIC values and plasma drug levels is difficult as azithromycin concentrates in macrophages and tissues.

A cross resistance relationship between azithromycin and clarithromycin has been observed with some *Mycobacterium avium* complex (MAC) isolates. The various mechanisms of cross resistance between azithromycin and clarithromycin for *M. avium* complex organisms have not been fully characterized. The clinical significance of azithromycin and clarithromycin cross resistance is unknown.

Susceptibility testing for *Mycobacterium avium* complex (MAC):

The disk diffusion techniques and dilution methods for susceptibility testing against gram-positive and gram-negative bacteria should not be used for determining azithromycin MIC values against mycobacteria. *In vitro* susceptibility testing methods and diagnostic products currently available for determining minimal inhibitory concentration (MIC) values against *Mycobacterium avium* complex (MAC) organisms have not been established or validated. Azithromycin MIC values will vary depending on the susceptibility testing method employed, composition and pH of media and the utilization of nutritional supplements. Breakpoints to determine whether clinical isolates of *M. avium* or *M. intracellulare* are susceptible to azithromycin have not been established.

INDICATIONS AND USAGE

ZITHROMAX® (azithromycin) is indicated for the treatment of patients with mild to moderate infections (pneumonia: see WARNINGS) caused by susceptible strains of the designated microorganisms in the specific conditions listed below.

Lower Respiratory Tract:

Acute bacterial exacerbations of chronic obstructive pulmonary disease due to *Haemophilus influenzae, Moraxella catarrhalis,* or *Streptococcus pneumoniae.*

Community-acquired pneumonia of mild severity due to *Streptococcus pneumoniae* or *Haemophilus influenzae* in patients appropriate for outpatient oral therapy.

NOTE: Azithromycin should not be used in patients with pneumonia who are judged to be inappropriate for outpatient oral therapy because of moderate to severe illness or risk factors such as any of the following:

patients with nosocomially acquired infections,
patients with known or suspected bacteremia,
patients requiring hospitalization,
elderly or debilitated patients, or
patients with significant underlying health problems that may compromise their ability to respond to their illness (including immunodeficiency or functional asplenia).

Upper Respiratory Tract:

Streptococcal pharyngitis/tonsillitis—As an alternative to first line therapy of acute pharyngitis/tonsillitis due to *Streptococcus pyogenes* occurring in individuals who cannot use first line therapy.

NOTE: Penicillin is the usual drug of choice in the treatment of *Streptococcus pyogenes* infection and the prophylaxis of rheumatic fever. ZITHROMAX® is often effective in the eradication of susceptible strains of *Streptococcus pyogenes* from the nasopharynx. Data establishing efficacy of azithromycin in subsequent prevention of rheumatic fever are not available.

Skin and Skin Structure

Uncomplicated skin and skin structure infections due to *Staphylococcus aureus, Streptococcus pyogenes,* or *Streptococcus agalactiae.* Abscesses usually require surgical drainage.

Sexually Transmitted Diseases

Non-gonococcal urethritis and cervicitis due to *Chlamydia trachomatis.*

ZITHROMAX®, at the recommended dose, should not be relied upon to treat gonorrhea or syphilis. Anitmicrobial agents used in high doses for short periods of time to treat non-gonococcal urethritis may mask or delay the symptoms of incubating gonorrhea or syphilis. All patients with sexually-transmitted urethritis or cervicitis should have a serologic test for syphilis and appropriate cultures for gonorrhea performed at the time of diagnosis. Appropriate antimicrobial therapy and follow-up tests for these diseases should be initiated if infection is confirmed.

Appropriate culture and susceptibility tests should be performed before treatment to determine the causative organism and its susceptibility to azithromycin. Therapy with ZITHROMAX® may be initiated before results of these tests are known; once the results become available, antimicrobial therapy should be adjusted accordingly.

Disseminated *Mycobacterium Avium* Complex (MAC) Disease

ZITHROMAX®, taken alone or in combination with rifabutin at its approved dose, is indicated for the prevention of disseminated *Mycobacterium avium* complex (MAC) disease in persons with advanced HIV infection. (See Clinical Trials section.)

CONTRAINDICATIONS

ZITHROMAX® is contraindicated in patients with known hypersensitivity to azithromycin, erythromycin, or any macrolide antibiotic.

WARNINGS

Rare serious allergic reactions, including angioedema and anaphylaxis, have been reported rarely in patients on azithromycin therapy. (See CONTRAINDICATIONS.) Despite initially successful symptomatic treatment of the allergic symptoms, when symptomatic therapy was discontinued, the allergic symptoms **recurred soon thereafter in some patients without further azithromycin exposure.** These patients required prolonged periods of observation and symptomatic treatment. The relationship of these episodes to the long tissue half-life of azithromycin and subsequent prolonged exposure to antigen is unknown at present.

If an allergic reaction occurs, the drug should be discontinued and appropriate therapy should be instituted. Physicians should be aware that reappearance of the allergic symptoms may occur when symptomatic therapy is discontinued.

In the treatment of pneumonia, azithromycin has only been shown to be safe and effective in the treatment of community-acquired pneumonia of mild severity due to *Streptococcus pneumoniae* or *Haemophilus influenzae* in patients appropriate for outpatient oral therapy. Azithromycin should not be used in patients with pneumonia who are judged to be inappropriate for outpatient oral therapy because of moderate to severe illness or risk factors such as any of the following: patients with nosocomially acquired infections, patients with known or suspected bacteremia, patients requiring hospitalization, elderly or debilitated patients, or patients with significant underlying health problems that may compromise their ability to respond to their illness (including immunodeficiency or functional asplenia). Pseudomembranous colitis has been reported with nearly all antibacterial agents and may range in severity from mild to life-threatening. Therefore, it is important to consider this diagnosis in patients who present with diarrhea subsequent to the administration of antibacterial agents.

Treatment with antibacterial agents alters the normal flora of the colon and may permit overgrowth of clostridia. Studies indicate that a toxin produced by *Clostridium difficile* is a primary cause of "antibiotic-associated colitis."

After the diagnosis of pseudomembranous colitis has been established, therapeutic measures should be initiated. Mild cases of pseudomembranous colitis usually respond to discontinuation of the drug alone. In moderate to severe cases, consideration should be given to management with fluids and electrolytes, protein supplementation, and treatment with an antibacterial drug clinically effective against *Clostridium difficile* colitis.

PRECAUTIONS

General: Because azithromycin is principally eliminated via the liver, caution should be exercised when azithromycin is administered to patients with impaired hepatic function. There are no data regarding azithromycin usage in patients with renal impairment; thus, caution should be exercised when prescribing azithromycin in these patients.

The following adverse events have not been reported in clinical trials with azithromycin, an azalide; however, they have been reported with macrolide products: ventricular arrhythmias, including ventricular tachycardia and *torsades de pointes,* in individuals with prolonged QT intervals.

Information for Patients:

Patients should be cautioned to take ZITHROMAX® capsules at least one hour prior to a meal or at least two hours after a meal. Azithromycin capsules should not be taken with food.

ZITHROMAX® tablets may be taken with or without food. However, increased tolerability has been observed when tablets are taken with food.

ZITHROMAX® for oral suspension in single 1 g packets can be taken with or without food after constitution.

Patients should also be cautioned not to take aluminum- and magnesium-containing antacids and azithromycin simultaneously.

The patient should be directed to discontinue azithromycin immediately and contact a physician if any signs of an allergic reaction occur.

Drug Interactions: Aluminum- and magnesium-containing antacids reduce the peak serum levels (rate) but not the AUC (extent) of azithromycin (500 mg) absorption.

Administration of cimetidine (800 mg) two hours prior to azithromycin had no effect on azithromycin (500 mg) absorption.

Azithromycin (500 mg Day 1, 250 mg Days 2–5) did not affect the plasma levels or pharmacokinetics of theophylline administered as a single intravenous dose. The effect of azithromycin on the plasma levels or pharmacokinetics of theophylline administered in multiple doses resulting in therapeutic steady-state levels of theophylline is not known. However, concurrent use of macrolides and theophylline has been associated with increases in the serum concentrations of theophylline. Therefore, until further data are available, prudent medical practice dictates careful monitoring of plasma theophylline levels in patients receiving azithromycin and theophylline concomitantly.

Azithromycin (500 mg Day 1, 250 mg Days 2–5) did not affect the prothrombin time response to a single dose of warfarin. However, prudent medical practice dictates careful monitoring of prothrombin time in all patients treated with azithromycin and warfarin concomitantly. Concurrent use of macrolides and warfarin in clinical practice has been associated with increased anticoagulant effects.

Dose adjustments are not indicated when azithromycin and zidovudine are coadministered. When zidovudine (100 mg q3h ×5) was coadministered with daily azithromycin (600 mg, n=5 or 1200 mg. n=7), mean C_{max}, AUC and Clr increased by 26% (CV 54%), 10% (CV 26%) and 38% (CV114%), respectively. The mean AUC of phosphorylated zidovudine increased by 75% (CV 95%), while zidovudine glucuronide C_{max} and AUC increased by less than 10%. In another study, addition of 1 gram azithromycin per week to a regimen of 10 mg/kg daily zidovudine resulted in 25% (CV 70%) and 13% (CV 37%) increases in zidovudine C_{max} and AUC, respectively. Zidovudine glucuronide mean C_{max} and AUC increased by 16% (CV 61%) and 8.0% (CV 32%), respectively.

Doses of 1200 mg/day azithromycin for 14 days in 6 subjects increased C_{max} of concurrently administered didanosine (200 mg *q*.12h) by 44% (54% CV) and AUC by 14% (23% CV).

However, none of these changes were significantly different from those produced in a parallel placebo control group of subjects.

Preliminary data suggest that coadministration of azithromycin and rifabutin did not markedly affect the mean serum concentrations of either drug. Administration of 250 mg azithromycin daily for 10 days (500 mg on the first day) produced mean concentrations of azithromycin 1 day after the last dose of 53 ng/ml when coadministered with 300 mg daily rifabutin and 49 mg/ml when coadministered with placebo. Mean concentrations 5 days after the last dose were 23 ng/ml and 21 ng/ml in the two groups of subjects. Administration of 300 mg rifabutin for 10 days produced mean concentrations of rifabutin one half day after the last dose of 60 mg/ml when coadministered with daily 250 mg azithromycin and 71 mg/ml when coadministered with placebo. Mean concentrations 5 days after the last dose were 8.1 ng/ml and 9.2 ng/ml in the two groups of subjects.

The following drug interactions have not been reported in clinical trials with azithromycin; however, no specific drug interaction studies have been performed to evaluate potential drug-drug interaction. Nonetheless, they have been observed with macrolide products. Until further data are developed regarding drug interactions when azithromycin and these drugs are used concomitantly, careful monitoring of patients is advised:

Digoxin—elevated digoxin levels.

Ergotamine or dihydroergotamine—acute ergot toxicity characterized by severe peripheral vasospasm and dysesthesia.

Triazolam—decrease the clearance of triazolam and thus may increase the pharmacologic effect of triazolam.

Drugs metabolized by the cytochrome P^{450} system —elevations of serum carbamazepine, cyclosporine, hexobarbital, and phenytoin levels.

Laboratory Test Interactions: There are no reported laboratory test interactions.

Carcinogenesis, Mutagenesis, Impairment of Fertility: Long-term studies in animals have not been performed to evaluate carcinogenic potential. Azithromycin has shown no mutagenic potential in standard laboratory tests: mouse lymphoma assay, human lymphocyte clastogenic assay, and mouse bone marrow clastogenic assay.

Pregnancy: Teratogenic Effects. Pregnancy Category B: Reproduction studies have been performed in rats and mice at doses up to moderately maternally toxic dose levels (i.e., 200 mg/kg/day). These doses, based on a mg/m² basis, are estimated to be 4 to 2 times, respectively, the human daily dose of 500 mg.

With regard to the MAC prophylaxis dose of 1200 mg weekly, on a mg/m²/day basis, the doses in rats and mice are approximately 2 and 1 times the human dose, respectively.

No evidence of impaired fertility or harm to the fetus due to azithromycin was found. There are, however, no adequate and well-controlled studies in pregnant women. Because animal reproduction studies are not always predictive of human response, azithromycin should be used during pregnancy only if clearly needed.

Nursing Mothers: It is not known whether azithromycin is excreted in human milk. Because many drugs are excreted in human milk, caution should be exercised when azithromycin is administered to a nursing woman.

Pediatric Use:

In controlled clinical studies, azithromycin has been administered to pediatric patients ranging in age from 6 months to 12 years. For information regarding the use of ZITHROMAX (azithromycin for oral suspension) in the treatment of pediatric patients, please refer to the INDICATIONS AND USAGE and DOSAGE AND ADMINISTRATION sections of the prescribing information for ZITHROMAX (azithromycin for oral suspension) 100 mg/5 mL and 200 mg/5 mL bottles.

Prevention of Disseminated *Mycobacterium avium* complex (MAC) Disease: Safety and efficacy of azithromycin for the prevention of MAC in children have not been established. Limited safety data are available for 24 children 5 months to 14 years of age (mean 4.6 years) who received azithromycin for treatment of opportunistic infections. The mean duration of therapy was 186.7 days (range 13–710 days) at doses of <5 to 20 mg/kg/day. Three children were treated for 6 months or more and 4 children were treated for 1 month or more with a dose of >10 mg/kg/day. Adverse events were similar to those observed in the adult population, most of which involved the gastrointestinal tract. While none of these children prematurely discontinued treatment due to a side effect, one child discontinued due to a laboratory abnormality (eosinophilia). The protocols upon which these data are based specified a daily dose of 10–20 mg/kg/day of azithromycin.

Geriatric Use: Pharmacokinetic parameters in older volunteers (65–85 years old) were similar to those in younger volunteers (18–40 years old) for the 5-day therapeutic regimen. Dosage adjustment does not appear to be necessary for older patients with normal renal and hepatic function receiving treatment with this dosage regimen. (See CLINICAL PHARMACOLOGY.)

Cumulative Incidence Rate, %: Placebo (n=89)

Month	MAC Free and Alive	MAC	Adverse Experience	Lost to Follow-up
6	69.7	13.5	6.7	10.1
12	47.2	19.1	15.7	18.0
18	37.1	22.5	18.0	22.5

Cumulative Incidence Rate, %: Azithromycin (n=85)

Month	MAC Free and Alive	MAC	Adverse Experience	Lost to Follow-up
6	84.7	3.5	9.4	2.4
12	63.5	8.2	16.5	11.8
18	44.7	11.8	25.9	17.6

Cumulative Incidence Rate, %: Ritabutin (n=223)

Month	MAC Free and Alive	MAC	Adverse Experience	Lost to Follow-up
6	83.4	7.2	8.1	1.3
12	60.1	15.2	16.1	8.5
18	40.8	21.5	24.2	13.5

Cumulative Incidence Rate, %: Azithromycin (n=223)

Month	MAC Free and Alive	MAC	Adverse Experience	Lost to Follow-up
6	85.2	3.6	5.8	5.4
12	65.5	7.6	16.1	10.8
18	45.3	12.1	23.8	18.8

Cumulative Incidence Rate, %: Azithromycin/Rifabutin Combination (n=218)

Month	MAC Free and Alive	MAC	Adverse Experience	Lost to Follow-up
6	89.4	1.8	5.5	3.2
12	71.6	2.8	15.1	10.6
18	49.1	6.4	29.4	15.1

ADVERSE REACTIONS

In clinical trials, most of the reported side effects were mild to moderate in severity and were reversible upon discontinuation of the drug. Approximately 0.7% of the patients from the multiple-dose clinical trials discontinued ZITHROMAX® (azithromycin) therapy because of treatment-related side effects. Most of the side effects leading to discontinuation were related to the gastrointestinal tract, e.g., nausea, vomiting, diarrhea, or abdominal pain. Rarely but potentially serious side effects were angioedema and cholestatic jaundice.

Clinical:

Multiple-dose regimen:

Overall, the most common side effects in adult patients receiving a multiple-dose regimen of ZITHROMAX® were related to the gastrointestinal system with diarrhea/loose stools (5%), nausea (3%), and abdominal pain (3%) being the most frequently reported.

No other side effects occurred in patients on the multiple-dose regimen of ZITHROMAX® with a frequency greater than 1%. Side effects that occurred with a frequency of 1% or less included the following:

Cardiovascular: Palpitations, chest pain.

Gastrointestinal: Dyspepsia, flatulence, vomiting, melena, and cholestatic jaundice.

Genitourinary: Monilia, vaginitis, and nephritis.

Nervous System: Dizziness, headache, vertigo, and somnolence.

General: Fatigue.

Allergic: Rash, photosensitivity, and angioedema.

Chronic therapy with 1200 mg weekly regimen: The nature of side effects seen with the 1200 mg weekly dosing regimen for the prevention of *Mycobacterium avium* infection in severely immunocompromised HIV-infected patients were similar to those seen with short term dosing regimens. (See CLINICAL TRIALS).

Single 1-gram dose regimen: Overall, the most common side effects in patients receiving a single-dose regimen of 1 gram of ZITHROMAX® were related to the gastrointestinal system and were more frequently reported than in patients receiving the multiple-dose regimen.

Side effects that occurred in patients on the single one-gram dosing regimen of ZITHROMAX® with a frequency of 1% or greater included diarrhea/loose stools (7%), nausea (5%), abdominal pain (5%), vomiting (2%), dyspepsia (1%), and vaginitis (1%).

Laboratory Abnormalities:

Significant abnormalities (irrespective of drug relationship) occurring during the clinical trials were reported as follows:

With an incidence of 1–2%, elevated serum creatine phosphokinase, potassium, ALT (SGPT), GGT, and AST (SGOT).

With an incidence of less than 1%, leukopenia, neutropenia, decreased platelet count, elevated serum alkaline phosphatase, bilirubin, BUN, creatinine, blood glucose, LDH, and phosphate.

When follow-up was provided, changes in laboratory tests appeared to be reversible.

In multiple-dose clinical trials involving more than 3000 patients, 3 patients discontinued therapy because of treatment-related liver enzyme abnormalities and 1 because of a renal function abnormality.

In a phase I drug interaction study performed in normal volunteers, 1 of 6 subjects given the combination of azithromycin and rifabutin, 1 of 7 given rifabutin alone and 0 of 6 given azithromycin alone developed a clinically significant neutropenia (<500 cells/mm³).

Laboratory abnormalities seen in clinical trials for the prevention of disseminated *Mycobacterium avium* disease in severely immunocompromised HIV-infected patients are presented in the CLINICAL TRIALS section.

DOSAGE AND ADMINISTRATION (See INDICATIONS AND USAGE.)

ZITHROMAX® capsules should be given at least 1 hour before or 2 hours after a meal. ZITHROMAX® capsules should not be mixed with or taken with food. ZITHROMAX® for oral suspension (single dose 1 g packet) can be taken with or without food after constitution. Not for pediatric use. For pediatric suspension, please refer to the INDICATIONS AND USAGE and DOSAGE AND ADMINISTRATION sections of the prescribing information for ZITHROMAX (azithromycin for oral suspension) 100 mg/5 mL and 200 mg/5 mL bottles.

ZITHROMAX® tablets may be taken without regard to food. However, increased tolerability has been observed when tablets are taken with food.

The recommended dose of ZITHROMAX® for the treatment of individuals 16 years of age and older with mild to moderate acute bacterial exacerbations of chronic obstructive pulmonary disease, pneumonia, pharyngitis/tonsillitis (as second line therapy), and uncomplicated skin and skin structure infections due to the indicated organisms is: 500 mg as a single dose on the first day followed by 250 mg once daily on Days 2 through 5 for a total dose of 1.5 grams of ZITHROMAX®.

The recommended dose of ZITHROMAX® for the prevention of disseminated *Mycobacterium avium* complex (MAC) disease is: 1200 mg taken once weekly. This dose of ZITHROMAX® may be combined with the approved dosage regimen of rifabutin.

The recommended dose of ZITHROMAX® for the treatment of non-gonococcal urethritis and cervicitis due to *C. trachomatis* is: a single 1 gram (1000 mg) dose of ZITHROMAX®. This dose can be administered as four 250 mg capsules or as one single dose packet (1 g).

DIRECTIONS FOR ADMINISTRATION OF ZITHROMAX® for oral suspension in the single dose packet (1 g): The entire contents of the packet should be mixed thoroughly with two ounces (approximately 60 mL) of water.

Continued on next page

Pfizer Inc—Cont.

Drink the entire contents immediately; add an additional two ounces of water, mix, and drink to assure complete consumption of dosage. **The single dose packet should not be used to administer doses other than 1000 mg of azithromycin. This packet not for pediatric use.**

HOW SUPPLIED

ZITHROMAX® capsules (imprinted with "Pfizer 305") are supplied in red opaque hard-gelatin capsules containing azithromycin dihydrate equivalent to 250 mg of azithromycin. These are packaged in bottles and blister cards of 6 capsules (Z-PAKS™) as follows:

Bottles of 50   NDC 0069-3050-50
Boxes of 3 (Z-PAKS™ of 6)   NDC 0069-3050-34
Unit Dose package of 50   NDC 0069-3050-86
Store capsules below 30°C (86°F).
ZITHROMAX® 600 mg tablets (engraved on front with "PFIZER" and on back with "308") are supplied as white, modified, oval-shaped, film-coated tablets containing azithromycin dihydrate equivalent to 600 mg azithromycin. These are packaged in bottles of 30 tablets. ZITHROMAX® tablets are supplied as follows:

Bottles of 30   NDC 0069-3080-30
Tablets should be stored at or below 30° C (86°F).
ZITHROMAX® for oral suspension is supplied in single dose packets containing azithromycin dihydrate equivalent to 1 gram of azithromycin as follows:

Boxes of 10 Single Dose
Packets (1 g)   NDC 0069-3051-07
Boxes of 3 Single Dose
Packets (1 g)   NDC 0069-3051-75
Store single dose packets between 5° and 30°C (41° and 86°F).

CLINICAL STUDIES IN PATIENTS WITH ADVANCED HIV INFECTION FOR THE PREVENTION OF DISEASE DUE TO DISSEMINATED *MYCOBACTERIUM AVIUM* COMPLEX (MAC) (See INDICATIONS AND USAGE):

Two randomized, double blind clinical trials were performed in patients with CD4 counts <100 cells/μL. The first study (155) compared azithromycin (1200 mg once weekly) to placebo and enrolled 182 patients with a mean CD4 count of 35 cells/μL. The second study (174) randomized 723 patients to either azithromycin (1200 mg once weekly), rifabutin (300 mg daily) or the combination of both. The mean CD4 count was 51 cells/μL. The primary endpoint in these studies was disseminated MAC disease. Other endpoints included the incidence of clinically significant MAC disease and discontinuations from therapy for drug-related side effects.

MAC bacteremia
In trial 155, 85 patients randomized to receive azithromycin and 89 patients randomized to receive placebo met study entrance criteria. Cumulative incidences at 6, 12 and 18 months of the possible outcomes are in the following table:
[See first table on top of preceding page.]
The difference in the one year cumulative incidence rates of disseminated MAC disease (placebo–azithromycin) is 10.9%. This difference is statistically significant (p=0.037) with a 95% confidence interval for this difference of (0.8%, 20.9%). The comparable number of patients experiencing adverse events and the fewer number of patients lost to follow-up on azithromycin should be taken into account when interpreting the significance of this difference.
In trial 174, 223 patients randomized to receive rifabutin, 223 patients randomized to receive azithromycin, and 218 patients randomized to receive both rifabutin and azithromycin met study entrance criteria. Cumulative incidences at 6, 12 and 18 months of the possible outcomes are recorded in the following table:
[See second table on top of preceding page.]
Comparing the cumulative one year incidence rates, azithromycin monotherapy is at least as effective as rifabutin monotherapy. The difference (rifabutin–azithromycin) in the one year rates (7.6%) is statistically significant (p=0.022) with an adjusted 95% confidence interval (0.9%, 14.3%). Additionally, azithromycin/rifabutin combination therapy is more effective than rifabutin alone. The difference (rifabutin–azithromycin/rifabutin) in the cumulative one year incidence rates (12.5%) is statistically significant (<0.001) with an adjusted 95% confidence interval of (6.6%, 18.4%). The comparable number of patients experiencing adverse events and the fewer number of patients lost to follow-up on rifabutin should be taken into account when interpreting the significance of this difference.
In Study 174, sensitivity testing* was performed on all available MAC isolates from subjects randomized to either azithromycin, rifabutin or the combination. The distribution of MIC values for azithromycin from susceptibility testing of the breakthrough isolates was similar between study arms. As the efficacy of azithromycin in the treatment of disseminated MAC has not been established, the clinical relevance of these *in vitro* MICs as an indicator of susceptibility or resistance is not known. (*Methodology per Inderlied CB, et al. Determination of *In Vitro* Susceptibility of *Mycobacterium avium* Complex Isolates to Antimicrobial Agents by Various Methods. Antimicrob. Agents Chemother 1987; 31: 1697–1702).

INCIDENCE OF ONE OR MORE TREATMENT RELATED* ADVERSE EVENTS** IN HIV INFECTED PATIENTS RECEIVING PROPHYLAXIS FOR DISSEMINATED MAC OVER APPROXIMATELY 1 YEAR

	Study 155		Study 174		
	Placebo (N=91)	Azithromycin 1200 mg weekly (N=89)	Azithromycin 1200 mg weekly (N=233)	Rifabutin 300 mg daily (N=236)	Azithromycin +Rifabutin (N=224)
Mean Duration of Therapy (days)	303.8	402.9	315	296.1	344.4
Discontinuation of Therapy	2.3	8.2	13.5	15.9	22.7
Autonomic Nervous System					
Mouth Dry	0	0	0	3.0	2.7
Central Nervous System					
Dizziness	0	1.1	3.9	1.7	0.4
Headache	0	0	3.0	5.5	4.5
Gastrointestinal					
Diarrhea	15.4	52.8	50.2	19.1	50.9
Loose Stools	6.6	19.1	12.9	3.0	9.4
Abdominal Pain	6.6	27	32.2	12.3	31.7
Dyspepsia	1.1	9	4.7	1.7	1.8
Flatulence	4.4	9	10.7	5.1	5.8
Nausea	11	32.6	27.0	16.5	28.1
Vomiting	1.1	6.7	9.0	3.8	5.8
General					
Fever	1.1	0	2.1	4.2	4.9
Fatigue	0	2.2	3.9	2.1	3.1
Malaise	0	1.1	0.4	0	2.2
Musculoskeletal					
Arthralgia	0	0	3.0	4.2	7.1
Psychiatric					
Anorexia	1.1	0	2.1	2.1	3.1
Skin & Appendages					
Pruritus	3.3	0	3.9	3.4	7.6
Rash	3.2	3.4	8.1	9.4	11.1
Skin discoloration	0	0	0	2.1	2.2
Special Senses					
Tinnitus	4.4	3.4	0.9	1.3	0.9
Hearing Decreased	2.2	1.1	0.9	0.4	0
Uveitis	0	0	0.4	1.3	1.8
Taste Perversion	0	0	1.3	2.5	1.3

* Includes those events considered possibly or probably related to study drug
** >2% adverse event rates for any group (except uveitis).

Prophylaxis Against Disseminated MAC Abnormal Laboratory Values*

		Placebo	Azithromycin 1200 mg weekly	Rifabutin 300 mg daily	Azithromycin & Rifabutin
Hemoglobin	<8 g/dl	1/51 2%	4/170 2%	4/114 4%	8/107 8%
Platelet Count	$<50 \times 10^3/mm^3$	1/71 1%	4/260 2%	2/182 1%	6/181 3%
WBC Count	$<1 \times 10^3/mm^3$	0/8 0%	2/70 3%	2/47 4%	0/43 0%
Neutrophils	<500/mm³	0/26 0%	4/106 4%	3/82 4%	2/78 3%
SGOT	$>5 \times ULN^a$	1/41 2%	8/158 5%	3/121 3%	6/114 5%
SGPT	$>5 \times ULN$	0/49 0%	8/166 5%	3/130 2%	5/117 4%
Alk Phos	$>5 \times ULN$	1/80 1%	4/247 2%	2/172 1%	3/164 2%

a= Upper Limit of Normal
* excludes subjects outside of the relevant normal range at baseline

Clinically Significant Disseminated MAC Disease
In association with the decreased incidence of bacteremia, patients in the groups randomized to either azithromycin alone or azithromycin in combination with rifabutin showed reductions in the signs and symptoms of disseminated MAC disease, including fever or night sweats, weight loss and anemia.

Discontinuations From Therapy For Drug-Related Side Effects
In Study 155, discontinuations for drug-related toxicity occurred in 8.2% of subjects treated with azithromycin and 2.3% of those given placebo (p=0.121). In Study 174, more subjects discontinued from the combination of azithromycin and rifabutin (22.7%) than from azithromycin alone (13.5%; p=0.026) or rifabutin alone (15.9%; p=0.209).

Safety
As these patients with advanced HIV disease were taking multiple concomitant medications and experienced a variety of intercurrent illnesses, it was often difficult to attribute adverse events to study medication. Overall, the nature of side effects seen on the weekly dosage regimen of azithromycin over a period of approximately one year in patients with advanced HIV disease was similar to that previously reported for shorter course therapies.
[See first table above.]
Side effects related to the gastrointestinal tract were seen more frequently in patients receiving azithromycin than in those receiving placebo or rifabutin. In Study 174, 86% of diarrheal episodes were mild to moderate in nature with discontinuation of therapy for this reason occurring in only 9/233 (3.8%) of patients.

Changes in Laboratory Values
In these immunocompromised patients with advanced HIV infection, it was necessary to assess laboratory abnormalities developing on study with additional criteria if baseline values were outside of the relevant normal range.
[See second table above.]

ANIMAL TOXICOLOGY

Phospholipidosis (intracellular phospholipid binding) has been observed in some tissues of mice, rats, and dogs given multiple doses of azithromycin. It has been demonstrated in numerous organ systems (e.g., eye, dorsal root ganglia, liver, gallbladder, kidney, spleen, and pancreas) in dogs administered doses which, based on pharmacokinetics, are as low as 2 times greater than the recommended adult human dose and in rats at doses comparable to the recommended adult human dose. This effect has been reversible after cessation of azithromycin treatment. The significance of these findings for humans is unknown.

REFERENCES

1. National Committee for Clinical Laboratory Standards. Methods for Dilution Antimicrobial Susceptibility Tests for Bacteria that Grow Aerobically—Third Edition. Approved Standard NCCLS Document M7-A3, Vol. 13, No. 25, NCCLS, Villanova, PA, December 1993.

2. National Committee for Clinical Laboratory Standards. Performance Standards for Antimicrobial Disk Susceptibility Tests—Fifth Edition. Approved Standard NCCLS Document M2-A5, Vol. 13, No. 24, NCCLS, Villanova, PA, December 1993.

Licensed from Pliva © **1996 PFIZER INC**
Pfizer **Printed in U.S.A.**
70-4763-00-2 Revised June 1996
Shown in Product Identification Guide, page 328

ZOLOFT® ℞
(sertraline hydrochloride)
Tablets

DESCRIPTION

ZOLOFT® (sertraline hydrochloride) is an antidepressant for oral administration. It is chemically unrelated to tricyclic, tetracyclic, or other available antidepressant agents. It has a molecular weight of 342.7. Sertraline hydrochloride has the following chemical name: (1S-cis)-4-(3,4-dichlorophenyl)-1,2,3,4-tetrahydro-N-methyl-1-naphthalenamine hydrochloride. The empirical formula $C_{17}H_{17}NCl_2 \cdot HCl$ is represented by the following structural formula:

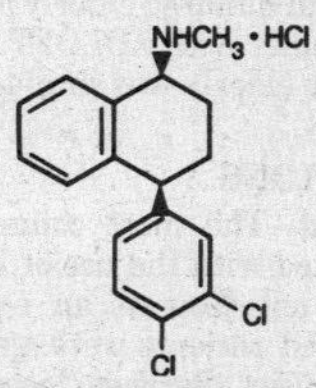

Sertraline hydrochloride is a white crystalline powder that is slightly soluble in water and isopropyl alcohol, and sparingly soluble in ethanol.

ZOLOFT is supplied for oral administration as scored tablets containing sertraline hydrochloride equivalent to 50 and 100 mg of sertraline and the following inactive ingredients: dibasic calcium phosphate dihydrate, FD&C Blue #2 aluminum lake (in 50 mg tablet), hydroxypropyl cellulose, hydroxypropyl methylcellulose, magnesium stearate, microcrystalline cellulose, polyethylene glycol, polysorbate 80, sodium starch glycolate, synthetic yellow iron oxide (in 100 mg tablet), and titanium dioxide.

CLINICAL PHARMACOLOGY

Pharmacodynamics

The mechanism of action of sertraline is presumed to be linked to its inhibition of CNS neuronal uptake of serotonin (5HT). Studies at clinically relevant doses in man have demonstrated that sertraline blocks the uptake of serotonin into human platelets. *In vitro* studies in animals also suggest that sertraline is a potent and selective inhibitor of neuronal serotonin reuptake and has only very weak effects on norepinephrine and dopamine neuronal reuptake. *In vitro* studies have shown that sertraline has no significant affinity for adrenergic ($alpha_1$, $alpha_2$, beta), cholinergic, GABA, dopaminergic, histaminergic, serotonergic ($5HT_{1A}$, $5HT_{1B}$, $5HT_2$), or benzodiazepine receptors; antagonism of such receptors has been hypothesized to be associated with various anticholinergic, sedative, and cardiovascular effects for other psychotropic drugs. The chronic administration of sertraline was found in animals to downregulate brain norepinephrine receptors, as has been observed with other clinically effective antidepressants. Sertraline does not inhibit monoamine oxidase.

Pharmacokinetics

Systemic Bioavailability—In man, following oral once-daily dosing over the range of 50 to 200 mg for 14 days, mean peak plasma concentrations (Cmax) of sertraline occurred between 4.5 to 8.4 hours post-dosing. The average terminal elimination half-life of plasma sertraline is about 26 hours. Based on this pharmacokinetic parameter, steady-state sertraline plasma levels should be achieved after approximately one week of once-daily dosing. Linear dose-proportional pharmacokinetics were demonstrated in a single dose study in which the Cmax and area under the plasma concentration time curve (AUC) of sertraline were proportional to dose over a range of 50 to 200 mg. Consistent with the terminal elimination half-life, there is an approximately two-fold accumulation, compared to a single dose, of sertraline with repeated dosing over a 50 to 200 mg dose range. The single dose bioavailability of sertraline tablets is approximately equal to an equivalent dose of solution.

The effects of food on the bioavailability of sertraline were studied in subjects administered a single dose with and without food. AUC was slightly increased when drug was administered with food but the Cmax was 25% greater, while the time to reach peak plasma concentration decreased from 8 hours post-dosing to 5.5 hours.

Metabolism—Sertraline undergoes extensive first pass metabolism. The principal initial pathway of metabolism for sertraline is N-demethylation. N-desmethylsertraline has a plasma terminal elimination half-life of 62 to 104 hours. Both *in vitro* biochemical and *in vivo* pharmacological testing have shown N-desmethylsertraline to be substantially less active than sertraline. Both sertraline and N-desmethylsertraline undergo oxidative deamination and subsequent reduction, hydroxylation, and glucuronide conjugation. In a study of radiolabeled sertraline involving two healthy male subjects, sertraline accounted for less than 5% of the plasma radioactivity. About 40–45% of the administered radioactivity was recovered in urine in 9 days. Unchanged sertraline was not detectable in the urine. For the same period, about 40–45% of the administered radioactivity was accounted for in feces, including 12–14% unchanged sertraline.

Desmethylsertraline exhibits time-related, dose dependent increases in AUC (0–24 hour), Cmax and Cmin, with about a 5–9 fold increase in these pharmacokinetic parameters between day 1 and day 14.

Protein Binding—*In vitro* protein binding studies performed with radiolabeled ^{3}H-sertraline showed that sertraline is highly bound to serum proteins (98%) in the range of 20 to 500 ng/mL. However, at up to 300 and 200 ng/mL concentrations, respectively, sertraline and N-desmethylsertraline did not alter the plasma protein binding of two other highly protein bound drugs, viz., warfarin and propranolol (see PRECAUTIONS).

Age—Sertraline plasma clearance in a group of 16 (8 male, 8 female) elderly patients treated for 14 days at a dose of 100 mg/day was approximately 40% lower than in a similarly studied group of younger (25 to 32 y.o.) individuals. Steady-state, therefore, should be achieved after 2 to 3 weeks in older patients. The same study showed a decreased clearance of desmethylsertraline in older males, but not in older females.

Liver Disease—As might be predicted from its primary site of metabolism, liver impairment can affect the elimination of sertraline. The elimination half-life of sertraline was prolonged in a single dose study of patients with mild, stable cirrhosis, with a mean of 52 hours compared to 22 hours seen in subjects without liver disease. In hepatically impaired patients, it was observed that the Cmax and AUC were increased by 1.7 and 4.4 fold, respectively, compared to healthy subjects. This suggests that the use of sertraline in patients with liver disease must be approached with caution. If sertraline is administered to patients with liver disease, a lower or less frequent dose should be used (see PRECAUTIONS and DOSAGE AND ADMINISTRATION).

Renal Disease—The pharmacokinetics of sertraline in patients with significant renal dysfunction have not been determined.

INDICATIONS AND USAGE

ZOLOFT (sertraline hydrochloride) is indicated for the treatment of depression. The efficacy of ZOLOFT in the treatment of a major depressive episode was established in six to eight week controlled trials of outpatients whose diagnoses corresponded most closely to the DSM-III category of major depressive disorder.

A major depressive episode implies a prominent and relatively persistent depressed or dysphoric mood that usually interferes with daily functioning (nearly every day for at least 2 weeks); it should include at least 4 of the following 8 symptoms: change in appetite, change in sleep, psychomotor agitation or retardation, loss of interest in usual activities or decrease in sexual drive, increased fatigue, feelings of guilt or worthlessness, slowed thinking or impaired concentration, and a suicide attempt or suicidal ideation.

The antidepressant action of ZOLOFT in hospitalized depressed patients has not been adequately studied.

A study of depressed outpatients who had responded to ZOLOFT during an initial eight-week open treatment phase and were then randomized to continuation on ZOLOFT or placebo demonstrated a significantly lower relapse rate over the next eight weeks for patients taking ZOLOFT compared to those on placebo. However, the effectiveness of ZOLOFT in long-term use, that is, for more than 16 weeks, has not been systematically evaluated in controlled trials. Therefore, the physician who elects to use ZOLOFT for extended periods should periodically reevaluate the long-term usefulness of the drug for the individual patient.

CONTRAINDICATIONS

Concomitant use in patients taking monoamine oxidase inhibitors (MAOIs) is contraindicated (see WARNINGS).

WARNINGS

Cases of serious sometimes fatal reactions have been reported in patients receiving ZOLOFT (sertraline hydrochloride), a selective serotonin reuptake inhibitor (SSRI), in combination with a monoamine oxidase inhibitor (MAOI). Symptoms of a drug interaction between an SSRI and an MAOI include: hyperthermia, rigidity, myoclonus, autonomic instability with possible rapid fluctuations of vital signs, mental status changes that include confusion, irritability, and extreme agitation progressing to delirium and coma. These reactions have also been reported in patients who have recently discontinued an SSRI and have been started on an MAOI. Some cases presented with features resembling neuroleptic malignant syndrome. Therefore, ZOLOFT should not be used in combination with an MAOI, or within 14 days of discontinuing treatment with an MAOI. Similarly, at least 14 days should be allowed after stopping ZOLOFT before starting an MAOI.

Drugs Metabolized by P450 3A4—Terfenadine, astemizole, and cisapride are metabolized by the cytochrome P450 3A4 isozyme. Potent inhibitors of 3A4, such as ketoconazole or erythromycin, block the metabolism of terfenadine, astemizole, and cisapride. As a result, increased plasma concentrations of terfenadine, astemizole, or cisapride may cause QT prolongation and torsades de pointes-type ventricular tachycardia, which is sometimes fatal. Sertraline has been shown to have some inhibition of P450 3A4 *in vitro*, although the clinical significance of this has not been established. Consequently, caution should be used when administering terfenadine, astemizole or cisapride in combination with sertraline.

PRECAUTIONS

General

Activation of Mania/Hypomania—During premarketing testing, hypomania or mania occurred in approximately 0.4% of ZOLOFT (sertraline hydrochloride) treated patients. Activation of mania/hypomania has also been reported in a small proportion of patients with Major Affective Disorder treated with other marketed antidepressants.

Weight Loss—Significant weight loss may be an undesirable result of treatment with sertraline for some patients, but on average, patients in controlled trials had minimal, 1 to 2 pound weight loss, versus smaller changes on placebo. Only rarely have sertraline patients been discontinued for weight loss.

Seizure—ZOLOFT has not been evaluated in patients with a seizure disorder. These patients were excluded from clinical studies during the product's premarket testing. Accordingly, like other antidepressants, ZOLOFT should be introduced with care in epileptic patients.

Suicide—The possibility of a suicide attempt is inherent in depression and may persist until significant remission occurs. Close supervision of high risk patients should accompany initial drug therapy. Prescriptions for ZOLOFT should be written for the smallest quantity of tablets consistent with good patient management, in order to reduce the risk of overdose.

Weak Uricosuric Effect—ZOLOFT is associated with a mean decrease in serum uric acid of approximately 7%. The clinical significance of this weak uricosuric effect is unknown, and there have been no reports of acute renal failure with ZOLOFT.

Use in Patients with Concomitant Illness—Clinical experience with ZOLOFT in patients with certain concomitant systemic illness is limited. Caution is advisable in using ZOLOFT in patients with diseases or conditions that could affect metabolism or hemodynamic responses.

ZOLOFT has not been evaluated or used to any appreciable extent in patients with a recent history of myocardial infarction or unstable heart disease. Patients with these diagnoses were excluded from clinical studies during the product's premarket testing. However, the electrocardiograms of 774 patients who received ZOLOFT in double-blind trials were evaluated and the data indicate that ZOLOFT is not associated with the development of significant ECG abnormalities.

ZOLOFT is extensively metabolized by the liver. In subjects with mild, stable cirrhosis of the liver, the clearance of sertraline was decreased, thus increasing the elimination half-life. A lower or less frequent dose should be used in patients with cirrhosis.

Since ZOLOFT is extensively metabolized, excretion of unchanged drug in urine is a minor route of elimination. However, until the pharmacokinetics of ZOLOFT have been studied in patients with renal impairment and until adequate numbers of patients with severe renal impairment have been evaluated during chronic treatment with ZOLOFT, it should be used with caution in such patients.

Interference with Cognitive and Motor Performance—In controlled studies, ZOLOFT did not cause sedation and did not interfere with psychomotor performance.

Hyponatremia—Several cases of hyponatremia have been reported and appeared to be reversible when ZOLOFT was discontinued. Some cases were possibly due to the syndrome of inappropriate antidiuretic hormone secretion. The majority of these occurrences have been in elderly individuals, some in patients taking diuretics or who were otherwise volume depleted.

Continued on next page

Pfizer Inc—Cont.

Platelet Function—There have been rare reports of altered platelet function and/or abnormal results from laboratory studies in patients taking ZOLOFT. While there have been reports of abnormal bleeding or purpura in several patients taking ZOLOFT, it is unclear whether ZOLOFT had a causative role.

Information for Patients

Physicians are advised to discuss the following issues with patients for whom they prescribe ZOLOFT:

Patients should be told that although ZOLOFT has not been shown to impair the ability of normal subjects to perform tasks requiring complex motor and mental skills in laboratory experiments, drugs that act upon the central nervous system may affect some individuals adversely.

Patients should be told that although ZOLOFT has not been shown in experiments with normal subjects to increase the mental and motor skill impairments caused by alcohol, the concomitant use of ZOLOFT and alcohol in depressed patients is not advised.

Patients should be told that while no adverse interaction of ZOLOFT with over-the-counter (OTC) drug products is known to occur, the potential for interaction exists. Thus, the use of any OTC product should be initiated cautiously according to the directions of use given for the OTC product.

Patients should be advised to notify their physician if they become pregnant or intend to become pregnant during therapy.

Patients should be advised to notify their physician if they are breast feeding an infant.

Laboratory Tests

None.

Drug Interactions

Potential Effects of Coadministration of Drugs Highly Bound to Plasma Proteins—Because sertraline is tightly bound to plasma protein, the administration of ZOLOFT (sertraline hydrochloride) to a patient taking another drug which is tightly bound to protein, (e.g., warfarin, digitoxin) may cause a shift in plasma concentrations potentially resulting in an adverse effect. Conversely, adverse effects may result from displacement of protein bound ZOLOFT by other tightly bound drugs.

In a study comparing prothrombin time AUC (0–120 hr) following dosing with warfarin (0.75 mg/kg) before and after 21 days of dosing with either ZOLOFT (50–200 mg/day) or placebo, there was a mean increase in prothrombin time of 8% relative to baseline for ZOLOFT compared to a 1% decrease for placebo ($p<0.02$). The normalization of prothrombin time for the ZOLOFT group was delayed compared to the placebo group. The clinical significance of this change is unknown. Accordingly, prothrombin time should be carefully monitored when ZOLOFT therapy is initiated or stopped.

Cimetidine—In a study assessing disposition of ZOLOFT (100 mg) on the second of 8 days of cimetidine administration (800 mg daily), there were increases in ZOLOFT mean AUC (50%), Cmax (24%) and half-life (26%) compared to the placebo group. The clinical significance of these changes is unknown.

CNS Active Drugs—In a study comparing the disposition of intravenously administered diazepam before and after 21 days of dosing with either ZOLOFT (50 to 200 mg/day escalating dose) or placebo, there was a 32% decrease relative to baseline in diazepam clearance for the ZOLOFT group compared to a 19% decrease relative to baseline for the placebo group ($p<0.03$). There was a 23% increase in Tmax for desmethyldiazepam in the ZOLOFT group compared to a 20% decrease in the placebo group ($p<0.03$). The clinical significance of these changes is unknown.

In a placebo-controlled trial in normal volunteers, the administration of two doses of ZOLOFT did not significantly alter steady-state lithium levels or the renal clearance of lithium.

Nonetheless, at this time, it is recommended that plasma lithium levels be monitored following initiation of ZOLOFT therapy with appropriate adjustments to the lithium dose.

The risk of using ZOLOFT in combination with other CNS active drugs has not been systematically evaluated. Consequently, caution is advised if the concomitant administration of ZOLOFT and such drugs is required.

There is limited controlled experience regarding the optimal timing of switching from other antidepressants to ZOLOFT. Care and prudent medical judgment should be exercised when switching, particularly from long-acting agents. The duration of an appropriate washout period which should intervene before switching from one selective serotonin reuptake inhibitor (SSRI) to another has not been established.

Monoamine Oxidase Inhibitors—See CONTRAINDICATIONS and WARNINGS.

Drugs Metabolized by P450 3A4—See WARNINGS.

Drugs Metabolized by P450 2D6—Many antidepressants, e.g., the SSRIs, including sertraline, and most tricyclic antidepressants inhibit the biochemical activity of the drug metabolizing isozyme cytochrome P450 2D6 (debrisoquin hydroxylase), and, thus, may increase the plasma concentrations of co-administered drugs that are metabolized by P450 2D6. The drugs for which this potential interaction is of greatest concern are those metabolized primarily by 2D6 and which have a narrow therapeutic index, e.g., the tricyclic antidepressants and the Type 1C antiarrhythmics propafenone and flecainide. The extent to which this interaction is an important clinical problem depends on the extent of the inhibition of P450 2D6 by the antidepressant and the therapeutic index of the co-administered drug. There is variability among the antidepressants in the extent of clinically important 2D6 inhibition, and in fact sertraline at lower doses has a less prominent inhibitory effect on 2D6 than some others in the class. Nevertheless, even sertraline has the potential for clinically important 2D6 inhibition. Consequently, concomitant use of a drug metabolized by P450 2D6 with ZOLOFT may require lower doses than usually prescribed for the other drug. Furthermore, whenever ZOLOFT is withdrawn from co-therapy, an increased dose of the co-administered drug may be required (see Tricyclic Antidepressants under PRECAUTIONS).

Tricyclic Antidepressants (TCAs)—The extent to which SSRI-TCA interactions may pose clinical problems will depend on the degree of inhibition and the pharmacokinetics of the SSRI involved. Nevertheless, caution is indicated in the co-administration of TCAs with ZOLOFT, because sertraline may inhibit TCA metabolism. Plasma TCA concentrations may need to be monitored, and the dose of TCA may need to be reduced, if a TCA is co-administered with ZOLOFT (see Drugs Metabolized by P450 2D6 under PRECAUTIONS).

Hypoglycemic Drugs—In a placebo-controlled trial in normal volunteers, administration of ZOLOFT for 22 days (including 200 mg/day for the final 13 days) caused a statistically significant 16% decrease from baseline in the clearance of tolbutamide following an intravenous 1000 mg dose. ZOLOFT administration did not noticeably change either the plasma protein binding or the apparent volume of distribution of tolbutamide, suggesting that the decreased clearance was due to a change in the metabolism of the drug. The clinical significance of this decrease in tolbutamide clearance is unknown.

Atenolol—ZOLOFT (100 mg) when administered to 10 healthy male subjects had no effect on the beta-adrenergic blocking ability of atenolol.

Digoxin—In a placebo-controlled trial in normal volunteers, administration of ZOLOFT for 17 days (including 200 mg/day for the last 10 days) did not change serum digoxin levels or digoxin renal clearance.

Microsomal Enzyme Induction—Preclinical studies have shown ZOLOFT to induce hepatic microsomal enzymes. In clinical studies, ZOLOFT was shown to induce hepatic enzymes minimally as determined by a small (5%) but statistically significant decrease in antipyrine half-life following administration of 200 mg/day for 21 days. This small change in antipyrine half-life reflects a clinically insignificant change in hepatic metabolism.

Electroconvulsive Therapy—There are no clinical studies establishing the risks or benefits of the combined use of electroconvulsive therapy (ECT) and ZOLOFT.

Alcohol—Although ZOLOFT did not potentiate the cognitive and psychomotor effects of alcohol in experiments with normal subjects, the concomitant use of ZOLOFT and alcohol in depressed patients is not recommended.

Carcinogenesis, Mutagenesis, Impairment of Fertility

Lifetime carcinogenicity studies were carried out in CD-1 mice and Long-Evans rats at doses up to 40 mg/kg in mice (10 times, on a mg/kg basis, and the same, on a mg/m² basis, as the maximum recommended human dose) and at doses up to 40 mg/kg in rats (10 times, on a mg/kg basis, and 2 times, on a mg/m² basis, the maximum recommended human dose). There was a dose-related increase in the incidence of liver adenomas in male mice receiving sertraline at 10–40 mg/kg. No increase was seen in female mice or in rats of either sex receiving the same treatments, nor was there an increase in hepatocellular carcinomas. Liver adenomas have a variable rate of spontaneous occurrence in the CD-1 mouse and are of unknown significance to humans. There was an increase in follicular adenomas of the thyroid in female rats receiving sertraline at 40 mg/kg; this was not accompanied by thyroid hyperplasia. While there was an increase in uterine adenocarcinomas in rats receiving sertraline at 10–40 mg/kg compared to placebo controls, this effect was not clearly drug related.

Sertraline had no genotoxic effects, with or without metabolic activation, based on the following assays: bacterial mutation assay; mouse lymphoma mutation assay; and tests for cytogenetic aberrations *in vivo* in mouse bone marrow and *in vitro* in human lymphocytes.

A decrease in fertility was seen in one of two rat studies at a dose of 80 mg/kg (20 times the maximum human dose on a mg/kg basis and 4 times on a mg/m² basis).

Pregnancy—Pregnancy Category B

Teratogenic Effects—Reproduction studies have been performed in rats and rabbits at doses up to approximately 20 times and 10 times the maximum daily human mg/kg dose (4 to 4.5 times the mg/m² dose), respectively.

There was no evidence of teratogenicity at any dose level. At doses approximately 2.5–10 times the maximum daily human mg/kg dose, sertraline was associated with delayed ossification in fetuses, probably secondary to effects on the dams.

There are no adequate and well-controlled studies in pregnant women. Because animal reproduction studies are not always predictive of human response, this drug should be used during pregnancy only if clearly needed.

Non-teratogenic Effects—There was also decreased neonatal survival following maternal administration of sertraline at doses as low as approximately 5 times the maximum human mg/kg dose. The decrease in pup survival was shown to be most probably due to *in utero* exposure to sertraline. The clinical significance of these effects is unknown.

Labor and Delivery—The effect of ZOLOFT on labor and delivery in humans is unknown.

Nursing Mothers—It is not known whether, and if so in what amount, sertraline or its metabolites are excreted in human milk. Because many drugs are excreted in human milk, caution should be exercised when ZOLOFT is administered to a nursing woman.

Pediatric Use—Safety and effectiveness in children have not been established.

Geriatric Use—Several hundred elderly patients have participated in clinical studies with ZOLOFT. The pattern of adverse reactions in the elderly was similar to that in younger patients.

ADVERSE REACTIONS

Commonly Observed—The most commonly observed adverse events associated with the use of ZOLOFT (sertraline hydrochloride) and not seen at an equivalent incidence among placebo treated patients were: gastrointestinal complaints, including nausea, diarrhea/loose stools and dyspepsia; tremor; dizziness; insomnia; somnolence; increased sweating; dry mouth; and male sexual dysfunction (primarily ejaculatory delay).

Associated with Discontinuation of Treatment—Fifteen percent of 2710 subjects who received ZOLOFT in premarketing multiple dose clinical trials discontinued treatment due to an adverse event. The more common events (reported by at least 1% of subjects) associated with discontinuation included agitation, insomnia, male sexual dysfunction (primarily ejaculatory delay), somnolence, dizziness, headache, tremor, anorexia, diarrhea/loose stools, nausea, and fatigue.

Incidence in Controlled Clinical Trials—The table that follows enumerates adverse events that occurred at a frequency of 1% or more among ZOLOFT patients who participated in controlled trials comparing titrated ZOLOFT with placebo. Most patients received doses of 50 to 200 mg per day. The prescriber should be aware that these figures cannot be used to predict the incidence of side effects in the course of usual medical practice where patient characteristics and other factors differ from those which prevailed in the clinical trials. Similarly, the cited frequencies cannot be compared with figures obtained from other clinical investigations involving different treatments, uses, and investigators. The cited figures, however, do provide the prescribing physician with some basis for estimating the relative contribution of drug and non-drug factors to the side effect incidence rate in the population studied.

Treatment-Emergent Adverse Experience Incidence in Placebo-Controlled Clinical Trials*

Adverse Experience	(Percent of Patients Reporting) ZOLOFT (N=861)	Placebo (N=853)
Autonomic Nervous System Disorders		
Mouth Dry	16.3	9.3
Sweating Increased	8.4	2.9
Cardiovascular		
Palpitations	3.5	1.6
Chest Pain	1.0	1.6
Centr. & Periph. Nerv. System Disorders		
Headache	20.3	19.0
Dizziness	11.7	6.7
Tremor	10.7	2.7
Paresthesia	2.0	1.8
Hypoesthesia	1.7	0.6
Twitching	1.4	0.1
Hypertonia	1.3	0.4
Disorders of Skin and Appendages		
Rash	2.1	1.5
Gastrointestinal Disorders		
Nausea	26.1	11.8
Diarrhea/Loose Stools	17.7	9.3
Constipation	8.4	6.3
Dyspepsia	6.0	2.8
Vomiting	3.8	1.8
Flatulence	3.3	2.5
Anorexia	2.8	1.6
Abdominal Pain	2.4	2.2
Appetite Increased	1.3	0.9

General		
Fatigue	10.6	8.1
Hot Flushes	2.2	0.5
Fever	1.6	0.6
Back Pain	1.5	0.9
Metabolic and Nutritional Disorders		
Thirst	1.4	0.9
Musculoskeletal System Disorders		
Myalgia	1.7	1.5
Psychiatric Disorders		
Insomnia	16.4	8.8
Sexual Dysfunction–Male (1)	15.5	2.2
Somnolence	13.4	5.9
Agitation	5.6	4.0
Nervousness	3.4	1.9
Anxiety	2.6	1.3
Yawning	1.9	0.2
Sexual Dysfunction–Female (2)	1.7	0.2
Concentration Impaired	1.3	0.5
Reproductive		
Menstrual Disorder (2)	1.0	0.5
Respiratory System Disorders		
Rhinitis	2.0	1.5
Pharyngitis	1.2	0.9
Special Senses		
Vision Abnormal	4.2	2.1
Tinnitus	1.4	1.1
Taste Perversion	1.2	0.7
Urinary System Disorders		
Micturition Frequency	2.0	1.2
Micturition Disorder	1.4	0.5

*Events reported by at least 1% of patients treated with ZOLOFT are included.

(1)—Primarily ejaculatory delay; % based on male patients only: 271 ZOLOFT and 271 placebo patients.

(2)—% based on female patients only: 590 ZOLOFT and 582 placebo patients.

Other Events Observed During the Premarketing Evaluation of ZOLOFT (sertraline hydrochloride): During its premarketing assessment, multiple doses of ZOLOFT were administered to approximately 2700 subjects. The conditions and duration of exposure to ZOLOFT varied greatly, and included (in overlapping categories) clinical pharmacology studies, open and double-blind studies, uncontrolled and controlled studies, inpatient and outpatient studies, fixed-dose and titration studies, and studies for indications other than depression. Untoward events associated with this exposure were recorded by clinical investigators using terminology of their own choosing. Consequently, it is not possible to provide a meaningful estimate of the proportion of individuals experiencing adverse events without first grouping similar types of untoward events into a smaller number of standardized event categories.

In the tabulations that follow, a World Health Organization dictionary of terminology has been used to classify reported adverse events. The frequencies presented, therefore, represent the proportion of the approximately 2700 individuals exposed to multiple doses of ZOLOFT who experienced an event of the type cited on at least one occasion while receiving ZOLOFT. All events are included except those already listed in the previous table and those reported in terms so general as to be uninformative. It is important to emphasize that although the events reported occurred during treatment with ZOLOFT, they were not necessarily caused by it.

Events are further categorized by body system and listed in order of decreasing frequency according to the following definitions: frequent adverse events are those occurring on one or more occasions in at least 1/100 patients (only those not already listed in the tabulated results from placebo controlled trials appear in this listing); infrequent adverse events are those occurring in 1/100 to 1/1000 patients; rare events are those occurring in fewer than 1/1000 patients. Events of major clinical importance are also described in the PRECAUTIONS section.

Autonomic Nervous System Disorders—*Infrequent:* flushing, mydriasis, increased saliva, cold clammy skin; *Rare:* pallor.

Cardiovascular—*Infrequent:* postural dizziness, hypertension, hypotension, postural hypotension, edema, dependent edema, periorbital edema, peripheral edema, peripheral ischemia, syncope, tachycardia; *Rare:* precordial chest pain, substernal chest pain, aggravated hypertension, myocardial infarction, varicose veins.

Central and Peripheral Nervous System Disorders—*Frequent:* confusion; *Infrequent:* ataxia, abnormal coordination, abnormal gait, hyperesthesia, hyperkinesia, hypokinesia, migraine, nystagmus, vertigo; *Rare:* local anesthesia, coma, convulsions, dyskinesia, dysphonia, hyporeflexia, hypotonia, ptosis.

Disorders of Skin and Appendages—*Infrequent:* acne, alopecia, pruritus, erythematous rash, maculopapular rash, dry skin; *Rare:* bullous eruption, dermatitis, erythema multiforme, abnormal hair texture, hypertrichosis, photosensitivity reaction, follicular rash, skin discoloration, abnormal skin odor, urticaria.

Endocrine Disorders—*Rare:* exophthalmos, gynecomastia.

Gastrointestinal Disorders—*Infrequent:* dysphagia, eructation; *Rare:* diverticulitis, fecal incontinence, gastritis, gastroenteritis, glossitis, gum hyperplasia, hemorrhoids, hiccup, melena, hemorrhagic peptic ulcer, proctitis, stomatitis, ulcerative stomatitis, tenesmus, tongue edema, tongue ulceration.

General—*Frequent:* asthenia; *Infrequent:* malaise, generalized edema, rigors, weight decrease, weight increase; *Rare:* enlarged abdomen, halitosis, otitis media, aphthous stomatitis.

Hematopoietic and Lymphatic—*Infrequent:* lymphadenopathy, purpura; *Rare:* anemia, anterior chamber eye hemorrhage.

Metabolic and Nutritional Disorders—*Rare:* dehydration, hypercholesterolemia, hypoglycemia.

Musculoskeletal System Disorders—*Infrequent:* arthralgia, arthrosis, dystonia, muscle cramps, muscle weakness; *Rare:* hernia.

Psychiatric Disorders—*Infrequent:* abnormal dreams, aggressive reaction, amnesia, apathy, delusion, depersonalization, depression, aggravated depression, emotional lability, euphoria, hallucination, neurosis, paranoid reaction, suicide ideation and attempt, teeth-grinding, abnormal thinking; *Rare:* hysteria, somnambulism, withdrawal syndrome.

Reproductive—*Infrequent:* dysmenorrhea,(2) intermenstrual bleeding;(2) *Rare:* amenorrhea,(2) balanoposthitis,(1) breast enlargement,(2) female breast pain,(2) leukorrhea,(2) menorrhagia, (2) atrophic vaginitis.(2)

(1)—% based on male subjects only: 1005.

(2)—% based on female subjects only: 1705.

Respiratory System Disorders—*Infrequent:* bronchospasm, coughing, dyspnea, epistaxis; *Rare:* bradypnea, hyperventilation, sinusitis, stridor.

Special Senses—*Infrequent:* abnormal accommodation, conjunctivitis, diplopia, earache, eye pain, xerophthalmia; *Rare:* abnormal lacrimation, photophobia, visual field defect.

Urinary System Disorders—*Infrequent:* dysuria, face edema, nocturia, polyuria, urinary incontinence; *Rare:* oliguria, renal pain, urinary retention.

Laboratory Tests—In man, asymptomatic elevations in serum transaminases (SGOT [or AST] and SGPT [or ALT]) have been reported infrequently (approximately 0.8%) in association with ZOLOFT administration. These hepatic enzyme elevations usually occurred within the first 1 to 9 weeks of drug treatment and promptly diminished upon drug discontinuation.

ZOLOFT therapy was associated with small mean increases in total cholesterol (approximately 3%) and triglycerides (approximately 5%), and a small mean decrease in serum uric acid (approximately 7%) of no apparent clinical importance.

Other Events Observed During the Postmarketing Evaluation of ZOLOFT—Reports of adverse events temporally associated with ZOLOFT that have been received since market introduction, that are not listed above and that may have no causal relationship with the drug include the following: galactorrhea, hyperprolactinemia, neuroleptic malignant syndrome-like events, psychosis, rare reports of pancreatitis, and liver events—clinical features (which in the majority of cases appeared to be reversible with discontinuation of ZOLOFT) occurring in one or more patients include: elevated enzymes, increased bilirubin, hepatomegaly, hepatitis, jaundice, abdominal pain, vomiting, liver failure and death.

DRUG ABUSE AND DEPENDENCE

Controlled Substance Class—ZOLOFT (sertraline hydrochloride) is not a controlled substance.

Physical and Psychological Dependence—ZOLOFT has not been systematically studied, in animals or humans, for its potential for abuse, tolerance, or physical dependence. However, the premarketing clinical experience with ZOLOFT did not reveal any tendency for a withdrawal syndrome or any drug-seeking behavior. As with any new CNS active drug, physicians should carefully evaluate patients for history of drug abuse and follow such patients closely, observing them for signs of ZOLOFT misuse or abuse (e.g., development of tolerance, incrementation of dose, drug-seeking behavior).

OVERDOSAGE

Human Experience—As of November, 1992, there were 79 reports of non-fatal acute overdoses involving ZOLOFT, of which 28 were overdoses of ZOLOFT alone and the remainder involved a combination of other drugs and/or alcohol in addition to ZOLOFT. In those cases of overdose involving only ZOLOFT, the reported doses ranged from 500 mg to 6000 mg. In a subset of 18 of these patients in whom ZOLOFT blood levels were determined, plasma concentrations ranged from <5 ng/mL to 554 ng/mL. Symptoms of overdose with ZOLOFT alone included somnolence, nausea, vomiting, tachycardia, ECG changes, anxiety and dilated pupils. Treatment was primarily supportive and included monitoring and use of activated charcoal, gastric lavage or cathartics and hydration. Although there were no reports of death when ZOLOFT was taken alone, there were 4 deaths involving overdoses of ZOLOFT in combination with other drugs and/or alcohol. Therefore, any overdosage should be treated aggressively.

Management of Overdoses—Establish and maintain an airway, insure adequate oxygenation and ventilation. Activated charcoal, which may be used with sorbitol, may be as or more effective than emesis or lavage, and should be considered in treating overdose.

Cardiac and vital signs monitoring is recommended along with general symptomatic and supportive measures.

There are no specific antidotes for ZOLOFT.

Due to the large volume of distribution of ZOLOFT, forced diuresis, dialysis, hemoperfusion, and exchange transfusion are unlikely to be of benefit.

In managing overdosage, consider the possibility of multiple drug involvement. The physician should consider contacting a poison control center on the treatment of any overdose.

DOSAGE AND ADMINISTRATION

Initial Treatment—ZOLOFT (sertraline hydrochloride) treatment should be initiated with a dose of 50 mg once daily. While a relationship between dose and antidepressant effect has not been established, patients were dosed in a range of 50–200 mg/day in the clinical trials demonstrating the antidepressant effectiveness of ZOLOFT. Consequently, patients not responding to a 50 mg dose may benefit from dose increases up to a maximum of 200 mg/day. Given the 24 hour elimination half-life of ZOLOFT, dose changes should not occur at intervals of less than 1 week.

ZOLOFT should be administered once daily, either in the morning or evening.

As indicated under PRECAUTIONS, a lower or less frequent dosage should be used in patients with hepatic impairment. In addition, particular care should be used in patients with renal impairment.

Maintenance/Continuation/Extended Treatment—There is evidence to suggest that depressed patients responding during an initial 8 week treatment phase will continue to benefit during an additional 8 weeks of treatment. While there are insufficient data regarding any benefits from treatment beyond 16 weeks, it is generally agreed among expert psychopharmacologists that acute episodes of depression require several months or longer of sustained pharmacological therapy. Whether the dose of antidepressant needed to induce remission is identical to the dose needed to maintain and/or sustain euthymia is unknown.

Switching Patients to or from a Monoamine Oxidase Inhibitor—At least 14 days should elapse between discontinuation of an MAOI and initiation of therapy with ZOLOFT. In addition, at least 14 days should be allowed after stopping ZOLOFT before starting an MAOI (see CONTRAINDICATIONS and WARNINGS).

HOW SUPPLIED

ZOLOFT® capsular-shaped scored tablets, containing sertraline hydrochloride equivalent to 50 and 100 mg of sertraline, are packaged in bottles.

ZOLOFT® 50 mg Tablets: light blue film coated tablets engraved on the front with ZOLOFT and on the back scored and engraved with 50 mg.

NDC 0049-4900-66 Bottles of 100
NDC 0049-4900-73 Bottles of 500
NDC 0049-4900-94 Bottles of 5000
NDC 0049-4900-41 Unit Dose Packages of 100

ZOLOFT® 100 mg Tablets: light yellow film coated tablets engraved on the front with ZOLOFT and on the back scored and engraved with 100 mg.

NDC 0049-4910-66 Bottles of 100
NDC 0049-4910-73 Bottles of 500
NDC 0049-4910-94 Bottles of 5000
NDC 0049-4910-41 Unit Dose Packages of 100

Store at controlled room temperature, 59° to 86°F (15° to 30°C).

© 1996 Pfizer Inc

69-4721-00-8 Revised April 1996

Shown in Product Identification Guide, page 328

ZYRTEC™ ℞
(cetirizine hydrochloride)
Tablets
For Oral Use

DESCRIPTION

Cetirizine hydrochloride, the active component of ZYRTEC™ tablets, is an orally active and selective H_1-receptor antagonist. The chemical name is (±)-[2-[4-(p-chloro-α-phenylbenzyl)-1-piperazinyl]ethoxy] acetic acid, dihydrochloride. Cetirizine hydrochloride is a racemic compound with an empirical formula of $C_{21}H_{25}ClN_2O_3 \cdot 2HCl$. The molecular weight is 461.82 and the chemical structure is shown below:

[See chemical structure at top of next column.]

Continued on next page

Pfizer Inc—Cont.

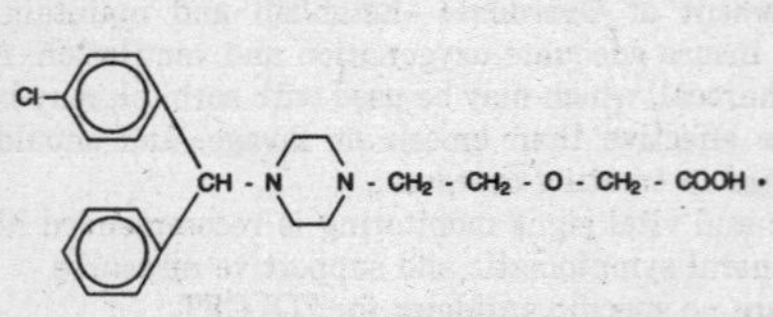

Cetirizine hydrochloride is a white, crystalline powder and is water soluble. ZYRTEC is formulated as a white (dye-free), film-coated, rounded-off rectangular shaped tablet for oral administration and is available in 5 and 10 mg strengths. Inert ingredients are: lactose; magnesium stearate; povidone; titanium dioxide; hydroxypropyl methylcellulose; polyethylene glycol; and corn starch.

CLINICAL PHARMACOLOGY

Mechanism of Actions: Cetirizine, a human metabolite of hydroxyzine, is an antihistamine; its principal effects are mediated via selective inhibition of peripheral H_1 receptors. The antihistaminic activity of cetirizine has been clearly documented in a variety of animal and human models. *In vivo* and *ex vivo* animal models have shown negligible anticholinergic and antiserotonergic activity. In clinical studies, however, dry mouth was more common with cetirizine than with placebo. *In vitro* receptor binding studies have shown no measurable affinity for other than H_1 receptors. Autoradiographic studies with radiolabeled cetirizine in the rat have shown negligible penetration into the brain. *Ex vivo* experiments in the mouse have shown that systemically administered cetirizine does not significantly occupy cerebral H_1 receptors.

Pharmacokinetics: Cetirizine is rapidly absorbed after oral administration of a tablet, which had bioavailability similar to an oral solution. Food had no effect on the extent of cetirizine absorption, but T_{max} was delayed by 1.7 hours and C_{max} was decreased by 23% in the presence of food. A mass balance study in 6 healthy male volunteers indicated that 70% of the administered radioactive dose was recovered in the urine and 10% in the feces, for a combined total recovery of about 80%. Approximately 50% of the administered radioactive dose was excreted in urine as unchanged drug. Most of the rapid increase in peak plasma radioactivity is associated with parent drug indicating low first pass metabolism. Cetirizine is metabolized to a very limited extent by oxidative O-dealkylation to a metabolite with negligible antihistaminic activity.

Cetirizine exhibits linear kinetics over the dosage range of 5 to 60 mg. In pharmacokinetic studies in 146 healthy volunteers, the mean $\pm$SD terminal half-life was 8.3 $\pm$1.8 hours, oral clearance was 54 $\pm$13 mL/min, and the apparent volume of distribution was 0.50 $\pm$0.08 L/kg. No accumulation was observed for cetirizine following daily doses of 10 mg for 10 days. The steady-state maximum plasma concentration was 311 $\pm$40 ng/mL and was achieved within 1.0 $\pm$0.5 hour. Individual histograms of cetirizine C_{max} and AUC showed unimodal distributions with a two- to four-fold variability in healthy subjects. Plasma protein binding of cetirizine is 93 $\pm$0.3% and is independent of concentration in the range of 0.025 to 1.0 mcg/mL; this concentration range covers the therapeutic plasma levels.

Formal pharmacokinetic interaction studies were conducted with cetirizine and pseudoephedrine, antipyrine, ketoconazole, erythromycin, and azithromycin. No pharmacokinetic interactions were observed. In a multiple dose study of theophylline (400 mg once daily) and cetirizine, there was a small (16%) decrease in clearance of cetirizine.

Special Populations

Effect of Age: Following a single 10 mg oral dose, half-life increased by about 50% and clearance decreased by 40% in 16 elderly subjects as compared to the 14 normal subjects. The decrease in cetirizine clearance in these elderly volunteers appeared to be related to their decreased renal function.

Effect of Gender: The effect of gender on cetirizine pharmacokinetics has not been adequately studied.

Effect of Race: No race-related differences were observed in the kinetics of cetirizine between 86 white adult males and 11 black adult males.

Renally Impaired Patients: The kinetics of cetirizine were studied following multiple oral daily doses of 10 mg for 7 days in 7 normal volunteers (creatinine clearance 89–128 mL/min), 8 patients with mild renal function impairment (creatinine clearance 42–77 mL/min) and 7 patients with moderate renal function impairment (creatinine clearance 11–31 mL/min). The pharmacokinetics of the drug were similar in patients with mild impairment and normal volunteers. Moderately renally impaired patients had a 3-fold increase in half-life and 70% decrease in clearance compared to normal volunteers. Patients (N=5) on hemodialysis (creatinine clearance less than 7 mL/min) given a single oral 10 mg dose of cetirizine had a 3-fold increase in half-life and a 70% decrease in clearance compared to normals. Cetirizine was not completely cleared by hemodialysis as less than 10% of the administered dose was removed during the dialysis session. Dosing adjustment is necessary in patients with moderate or severe renal impairment and patients on dialysis. (See also DOSAGE AND ADMINISTRATION.)

Hepatically Impaired Patients: Sixteen patients with chronic liver diseases (hepatocellular, cholestatic, and biliary cirrhosis), given 10 or 20 mg of cetirizine as a single oral dose had a 50% increase in half-life along with a 40% decrease in clearance compared to 16 healthy subjects.

Dosing adjustment may be necessary in hepatically impaired patients. (See also DOSAGE AND ADMINISTRATION.)

Pharmacodynamics: Studies in normal volunteers show that ZYRTEC at doses of 5 and 10 mg strongly inhibits the skin wheal and flare caused by the intradermal injection of histamine. The onset of this activity after a single 10 mg dose occurs within 20 minutes in 50% of subjects and within one hour in 95% of subjects; this activity persists for at least 24 hours. In a 35-day study in children ages 5 to 12, no tolerance to the antihistaminic (suppression of wheal and flare response) effects of ZYRTEC was found. The effects of intradermal injection of various other mediators or histamine releasers are also inhibited by cetirizine, as is response to a cold challenge in patients with cold-induced urticaria. In mildly asthmatic subjects, ZYRTEC at 5 to 20 mg blocked bronchoconstriction due to nebulized histamine, with virtually total blockade after a 20 mg dose. In studies conducted for up to 12 hours following cutaneous antigen challenge, the late phase recruitment of eosinophils, neutrophils and basophils, components of the allergic inflammatory response, was inhibited by ZYRTEC at a dose of 20 mg.

In four clinical studies in healthy adult males, no clinically significant mean increases in QTc were observed in ZYRTEC treated subjects. In the first study, a placebo-controlled crossover trial, ZYRTEC was given at doses up to 60 mg per day, 6 times the maximum clinical dose, for 1 week, and no significant mean QTc prolongation occurred. In the second study, a crossover trial, ZYRTEC 20 mg and erythromycin (500 mg every 8 hours) were given alone and in combination. There was no significant effect on QTc with the combination or with ZYRTEC alone. In the third trial, also a crossover study, ZYRTEC 20 mg and ketoconazole (400 mg per day) were given alone and in combination. ZYRTEC caused a mean increase in QTc of 9.1 msec from baseline after 10 days of therapy. Ketoconazole also increased QTc by 8.3 msec. The combination caused an increase of 17.4 msec, equal to the sum of the individual effects. Thus, there was no significant drug interaction on QTc with the combination of ZYRTEC and ketoconazole. In the fourth study, a placebo-controlled parallel trial, ZYRTEC 20 mg was given alone or in combination with azithromycin (500 mg as a single dose on the first day followed by 250 mg once daily). There was no significant increase in QTc with ZYRTEC 20 mg alone or in combination with azithromycin.

In a six-week, placebo-controlled study of 186 patients with allergic rhinitis and mild to moderate asthma, ZYRTEC 10 mg once daily improved rhinitis symptoms and did not alter pulmonary function. This study supports the safety of administering ZYRTEC to allergic rhinitis patients with mild to moderate asthma.

Clinical Studies: Nine multicenter, randomized, double-blind, clinical trials comparing cetirizine 5 to 20 mg to placebo in patients with seasonal or perennial allergic rhinitis were conducted in the United States. Five of these showed significant reductions in symptoms of allergic rhinitis, 3 in seasonal allergic rhinitis (1 to 4 weeks in duration) and 2 in perennial allergic rhinitis for up to 8 weeks in duration. Two 4-week multicenter, randomized, double-blind, clinical trials comparing cetirizine 5 to 20 mg to placebo in patients with chronic idiopathic urticaria were also conducted and showed significant improvement in symptoms of chronic idiopathic urticaria. In general, the 10 mg dose was more effective than the 5 mg dose and the 20 mg dose gave no added effect. Some of these trials included pediatric patients age 12 to 16 years.

INDICATIONS AND USAGE

Seasonal Allergic Rhinitis: ZYRTEC is indicated for the relief of symptoms associated with seasonal allergic rhinitis due to allergens such as ragweed, grass and tree pollens in adults and children 12 years of age and older. Symptoms treated effectively include sneezing, rhinorrhea, nasal pruritus, ocular pruritus, tearing and redness of the eyes.

Perennial Allergic Rhinitis: ZYRTEC is indicated for the relief of symptoms associated with perennial allergic rhinitis due to allergens such as dust mites, animal dander and molds in adults and children 12 years of age and older. Symptoms treated effectively include sneezing, rhinorrhea, post-nasal discharge, nasal pruritus, ocular pruritus and tearing.

Chronic Urticaria: ZYRTEC is indicated for the treatment of the uncomplicated skin manifestations of chronic idiopathic urticaria in adults and children 12 years of age and older. It significantly reduces the occurrence, severity and duration of hives and significantly reduces pruritus.

CONTRAINDICATIONS

ZYRTEC is contraindicated in those patients with a known hypersensitivity to it or any of its ingredients or hydroxyzine.

PRECAUTIONS

Activities Requiring Mental Alertness: In clinical trials, the occurrence of somnolence has been reported in some patients taking ZYRTEC; due caution should therefore be exercised when driving a car or operating potentially dangerous machinery. Concurrent use of ZYRTEC with alcohol or other CNS depressants should be avoided because additional reductions in alertness and additional impairment of CNS performance may occur.

Drug-drug Interactions: No clinically significant drug interactions have been found with theophylline at a low dose, azithromycin, pseudoephedrine, ketoconazole, or erythromycin. There was a small decrease in the clearance of cetirizine caused by a 400 mg dose of theophylline; it is possible that larger theophylline doses could have a greater effect.

Carcinogenesis, Mutagenesis and Impairment of Fertility: No evidence of carcinogenicity was observed in a 2-year carcinogenicity study in rats at dietary doses up to 20 mg/kg/day (15 times the maximum recommended human dose on a mg/m^2/day basis). An increased incidence of benign liver tumors was found in a 2-year carcinogenicity study in male mice at a dietary dose of 16 mg/kg/day (6 times the maximum recommended human dose on a mg/m^2/day basis). The clinical significance of these findings during long-term use of ZYRTEC is not known. Cetirizine was not mutagenic in the Ames test, and not clastogenic in the human lymphocyte assay, the mouse lymphoma assay, and the *in vivo* micronucleus test in rats. No impairment of fertility was found in a fertility and general reproductive performance study in mice at a dose of 64 mg/kg/day (26 times the maximum recommended human dose on a mg/m^2/day basis).

Pregnancy Category B: Cetirizine was not teratogenic in mice, rats and rabbits at doses up to 96, 225, and 135 mg/kg/day (40, 180, and 216 times the maximum recommended human dose on a mg/m^2/day basis), respectively. There are no adequate and well-controlled studies in pregnant women. Because animal studies are not always predictive of human response, ZYRTEC should be used in pregnancy only if clearly needed.

Nursing Mothers: Retarded pup weight gain was found in mice during lactation when dams were given cetirizine at 96 mg/kg/day (40 times the maximum recommended human dose on a mg/m^2/day basis). Studies in beagle dogs indicate that approximately 3% of the dose is excreted in breast milk. Cetirizine has been reported to be excreted in human breast milk; use of ZYRTEC in nursing mothers is not recommended.

Geriatric Use: In placebo-controlled trials, 186 patients age 65 to 94 years received doses of 5 to 20 mg of ZYRTEC per day. Adverse events were similar in this group to patients under age 65. Subset analysis of efficacy in this group was not done.

Pediatric Use: Safety and effectiveness in children under 12 years of age has not been established.

ADVERSE REACTIONS

Controlled and uncontrolled clinical trials conducted in the United States and Canada included more than 6000 patients, with more than 3900 receiving ZYRTEC at doses of 5 to 20 mg per day. The duration of treatment ranged from 1 week to 6 months, with a mean exposure of 30 days.

Most adverse reactions reported during therapy with ZYRTEC were mild or moderate. In placebo-controlled trials, the incidence of discontinuations due to adverse reactions in patients receiving ZYRTEC 5 mg or 10 mg was not significantly different from placebo (2.9% vs. 2.4%, respectively). The most common adverse reaction that occurred more frequently on cetirizine than placebo was somnolence. The incidence of somnolence associated with ZYRTEC was dose related, 6% in placebo, 11% at 5 mg and 14% at 10 mg. Discontinuations due to somnolence for ZYRTEC were uncommon (1.0% on ZYRTEC vs. 0.6% on placebo). Fatigue and dry mouth also appeared to be treatment-related adverse reactions. There were no differences by age, race, gender or by body weight with regard to the incidence of adverse reactions.

Table 1 lists adverse experiences which were reported for ZYRTEC 5 and 10 mg in controlled clinical trials in the United States and that were more common with ZYRTEC than placebo.

Table 1.
Adverse Experiences Reported in Placebo-Controlled United States ZYRTEC Trials (Maximum Dose of 10 mg) at Rates of 2% or Greater (Percent Incidence)

Adverse Experience	ZYRTEC (N=2034)	Placebo (N=1612)
Somnolence	13.7	6.3
Fatigue	5.9	2.6
Dry Mouth	5.0	2.3
Pharyngitis	2.0	1.9
Dizziness	2.0	1.2

In addition, headache and nausea occurred in more than 2% of the patients, but were more common in placebo patients. The following events were observed infrequently (less than 2%), in 3982 patients who received ZYRTEC in U.S. trials, including an open study of six months duration; a causal relationship with ZYRTEC administration has not been established.

Autonomic Nervous System: anorexia, urinary retention, flushing, increased salivation

Cardiovascular: palpitation, tachycardia, hypertension, cardiac failure

Central and Peripheral Nervous Systems: paresthesia, confusion, hyperkinesia, hypertonia, migraine, tremor, vertigo, leg cramps, ataxia, dysphonia, abnormal coordination, hyperesthesia, hypoesthesia, myelitis, paralysis, ptosis, twitching, visual field defect

Gastrointestinal: increased appetite, dyspepsia, abdominal pain, diarrhea, flatulence, constipation, vomiting, ulcerative stomatitis, aggravated tooth caries, stomatitis, tongue discoloration, tongue edema, gastritis, rectal hemorrhage, hemorrhoids, melena, abnormal hepatic function

Genitourinary: polyuria, urinary tract infection, cystitis, dysuria, hematuria

Hearing and Vestibular: earache, tinnitus, deafness, ototoxicity

Metabolic/Nutritional: thirst, dehydration, diabetes mellitus

Musculoskeletal: myalgia, arthralgia, arthrosis, arthritis, muscle weakness

Psychiatric: insomnia, nervousness, depression, emotional lability, impaired concentration, anxiety, depersonalization, paroniria, abnormal thinking, agitation, amnesia, decreased libido, euphoria

Respiratory System: epistaxis, rhinitis, coughing, bronchospasm, dyspnea, upper respiratory tract infection, hyperventilation, sinusitis, increased sputum, bronchitis, pneumonia

Reproductive: dysmenorrhea, female breast pain, intermenstrual bleeding, leukorrhea, menorrhagia, vaginitis

Reticuloendothelial: lymphadenopathy

Skin: pruritus, rash, dry skin, urticaria, acne, dermatitis, erythematous rash, increased sweating, alopecia, angioedema, furunculosis, bullous eruption, eczema, hyperkeratosis, hypertrichosis, photosensitivity reaction, photosensitivity toxic reaction, maculopapular rash, seborrhea, purpura

Special Senses: taste perversion, taste loss, parosmia

Vision: blindness, loss of accommodation, eye pain, conjunctivitis, xerophthalmia, glaucoma, ocular hemorrhage

Body as a Whole: increased weight, back pain, malaise, fever, asthenia, generalized edema, periorbital edema, peripheral edema, rigors, leg edema, face edema, hot flashes, enlarged abdomen, nasal polyp

Occasional instances of transient, reversible hepatic transaminase elevations have occurred during cetirizine therapy. A single case of possible drug-induced hepatitis with significant transaminase elevation (500 to 1000 IU/L) and elevated bilirubin has been reported.

In foreign marketing experience the following additional rare, but potential severe adverse events have been reported: hemolytic anemia, thrombocytopenia, orofacial dyskinesia, severe hypotension, anaphylaxis, hepatitis, glomerulonephritis, stillbirth, and cholestasis.

DRUG ABUSE AND DEPENDENCE

There is no information to indicate that abuse or dependency occurs with ZYRTEC.

OVERDOSAGE

Overdosage has been reported with ZYRTEC. In one patient who took 150 mg of ZYRTEC, the patient was somnolent but did not display any other clinical signs or abnormal blood chemistry or hematology results. Should overdose occur, treatment should be symptomatic or supportive, taking into account any concomitantly ingested medications. There is no known specific antidote to ZYRTEC. ZYRTEC is not effectively removed by dialysis, and dialysis will be ineffective unless a dialyzable agent has been concomitantly ingested. The minimal lethal oral dose in rodents is approximately 100 times the maximum recommended clinical dose on a mg/m² basis and the liver is the target organ of toxicity.

DOSAGE AND ADMINISTRATION

The recommended initial dose of ZYRTEC is 5 or 10 mg per day in adults and children 12 years and older, depending on symptom severity. Most patients in clinical trials started at 10 mg. ZYRTEC is given as a single daily dose, with or without food. The time of administration may be varied to suit individual patient needs.

In patients with decreased renal function (creatinine clearance 11–31 mL/min), patients on hemodialysis (creatinine clearance less than 7 mL/min), and in hepatically impaired patients, a dose of 5 mg once daily is recommended.

HOW SUPPLIED

ZYRTEC™ tablets are white (dye-free), film-coated, rounded-off rectangular shaped containing 5 mg or 10 mg cetirizine hydrochloride.

5 mg tablets are engraved with "PFIZER" on one side and with "550" on the other.

Bottles of 100: NDC 0069-5500-66

10 mg tablets are engraved with "PFIZER" on one side and with "551" on the other.

Bottles of 100: NDC 0069-5510-66

STORAGE: Store at room temperature 59° to 86°F (15°–30°C).

Cetirizine is licensed from UCB Pharma, Inc.

©1995 PFIZER INC

Pfizer Labs
Division of Pfizer Inc, NY, NY 10017
69-4573-00-0   Issued December 1995
Shown in Product Identification Guide, page 328

EDUCATIONAL MATERIAL

Printed Material

1. Zoloft—These patient education booklets on depression are available from Roerig and Pratt Pharmaceutical representatives in English and Spanish: *Dealing with Depression, Unmasking Depression, Depression and Older People, Depression and Adolescents, and Depression in Women, Depression and the Family, and Depression and HIV.*
2. Cardura—JNC V Patient Education Poster/Pad
   This patient education material is adapted from the JNC V guidelines on managing hypertension. The JNC V recommends lifestyle modifications before starting antihypertensive drug therapy, and this poster and pad make it easy for patients to follow these recommendations. Available from Roerig Pharmaceutical representatives.
3. Diflucan—These booklets are available in English and Spanish:
   Patient Education—HIV
   Patient Education—Cancer
   Patient Education—General
   Patient Education—Vaginitis
4. Norvasc
   1. *High Blood Pressure—What you Should Know.* Available in Spanish and English.
   2. *Norvasc—Know Your Medicine.* These are available from Labs and Pratt Representatives
5. Procardia XL
   1. *Procardia XL—Know Your Medicine.* Available from Labs and Pratt Representatives.
6. Zithromax—These brochures are available from Roerig, Labs, and Specialty Representatives:
   Patient Education—MAC (Spanish & English)-#AC043R96
   Patient Education—1 gram pack (Spanish & English)-#AC105X95 & #AC106X95
   Patient Education—Pediatrics—#ZC023E95
   Patient Education—*Know Your Medicine*—RTI #AD184X95
   Patient Education—*Know Your Medicine*—Pediatrics—#WD106R95
   Patient Education—*Know Your Medicine*—1 gram pack—#WD111R95
   Zithromax Patient tear sheets—#AC195X95
   It is Time to Call the Doctor?—#AI139X95
   Pediatrics—*All About Ears* flip chart—#ZC056W95

Patient Compliance Program

Rhythms is a uncompletely confidential compliance program offered to health care practitioners for use with patients. It includes a multimedia format to provide needed reinforcement and support to patients at each step on their way to recovery from depression.

Audio Tape

1. *Taking Control: A Patient's Guide to High Blood Pressure*—Discussion of the diagnosis and treatment of hypertension by Randall Zusman, MD, Massachusetts General Hospital, Harvard Medical School.

Films/Videos

1. "Say Goodbye to High Blood Pressure"—A one hour patient education video. An informative look at the causes, effects, and treatments plus a daily exercise and relaxation program.
2. *Taking Control of Depression: Mending the Mind*—leading experts in depression speak directly to patients in a reassuring and hopeful tone that can support your efforts. Available for your lending library by Roerig and Pratt Pharmaceutical representatives.

Computer Programs (IBM Compatible)

"Coronary Heart Disease Risk Factor Modification"—Allows calculation of a 10-year CHD risk estimate from the Framingham data base utilizing age, sex, smoking status, left ventricular hypertrophy, diabetes, blood pressure (diastolic or systolic), total cholesterol, and HDL cholesterol. Available from Roerig Representative.

Samples

Cardura® (doxazosin mesylate) Tablets—1 mg, 2 mg, 4 mg
Diflucan® (fluconazole)—100 mg, 150 mg Tablets, 350 mg OS
Glucotrol® and Glucotrol® XL (glipizide) Tablets—5 mg
Norvasc® (amlodipine besylate) Tablets—2.5 mg, 5 mg, 10 mg
Procardia® Capsules (nifedipine)—10 mg
Procardia® XL Tablets—30 mg, 60 mg
Unasyn® (ampicillin sodium/sulbactam sodium) Vials—1.5 g
Zithromax® (azithromycin)—250 mg Capsules, 600 mg Tablets, and 600 mg OS
Zoloft® (sertraline HCl) Tablets—50 mg, 100 mg
Zyrtec® (cetirizine HCl) Tablets—10 mg

Pfizer Labs Division
See Pfizer Inc

Pharmaceutical Associates, Inc.
A Subsidiary of Beach Products, Inc.
201 DELAWARE STREET
GREENVILLE, SC 29605

Direct Inquiries to:
Clete Harmon, Director of Q.A.
PH: (800) 845-8210
      (864) 277-7282
FAX: (864) 277-8045

HOSPITAL UNIT DOSE AND UNIT OF ISSUE

NDC LABELER CODE: 000121

ACETAMINOPHEN AND CODEINE PHOSPHATE ORAL SOLUTION USP   ℂ ℞

Each teaspoonful (5 mL) contains:
Acetaminophen .... 120 mg
Codeine Phosphate .... 12 mg
Alcohol .... 7 %

HOW SUPPLIED
Bottles of 4 oz and 16 oz
Unit Dose of 5 mL, 10 mL, 12.5 mL, and 15 mL

AMANTADINE HYDROCHLORIDE SYRUP USP   ℞

Each teaspoonful (5 mL) contains:
Amantadine Hydrochloride .... 50 mg

HOW SUPPLIED
Bottles of 16 oz
Unit Dose of 10 mL and 20 mL

FLUPHENAZINE HYDROCHLORIDE ELIXIR USP   ℞

Each mL contains:
Fluphenazine hydrochloride .... 0.5 mg

HOW SUPPLIED
Bottles of 60 mL with accompanying dropper
Bottles of 473 mL

Continued on next page

Pharmaceutical Assoc.—Cont.

HALOPERIDOL ORAL SOLUTION USP ℞

Each 1 mL contains:
Haloperidol (as the lactate)............................. 2 mg

HOW SUPPLIED
Bottles of 4 oz with accompanying dropper
Unit Dose of 5 mL and 10 mL

LACTULOSE SOLUTION USP ℞

Each 15 mL contains:
10 g Lactulose (and less than 1.6 g galactose, less than 1.2 g lactose, and 1.2 g or less of other sugars)

HOW SUPPLIED
Bottles of 8 oz
Unit Dose of 30 mL

METOCLOPRAMIDE ORAL SOLUTION USP ℞

Each teaspoonful (5 mL) contains:
Metoclopramide .... 5 mg
(present as the hydrochloride)

HOW SUPPLIED
Bottles of 16 oz
Unit Dose of 10 mL

MILK OF MAGNESIA CASCARA SUSPENSION OTC

Each 2 tablespoonfuls (30 mL) contain:
Magnesium Hydroxide .... 2400 mg
(equivalent to 30 mL Milk of Magnesia)
Aromatic Cascara Fluidextract .... 5 mL
Alcohol .... 3.0–3.3 %

HOW SUPPLIED
Bottles of 4 oz
Unit Dose of 15 mL and 30 mL

SODIUM CITRATE AND CITRIC ACID ORAL SOLUTION USP ℞

Each teaspoonful (5 mL) contains:
Sodium Citrate Dihydrate .... 500 mg
Citric Acid Monohydrate .... 334 mg

HOW SUPPLIED
Bottles of 16 oz
Unit Dose of 15 mL and 30 mL

OTHER PRODUCTS AVAILABLE:

Acetaminophen Elixir (160 mg/5 mL) OTC
  5 mL, 10 mL, 20 mL, and 20.3 mL
Aluminum Hydroxide Gel USP (320 mg/5 mL) OTC
  30 mL, 12 oz, and 16 oz
Aluminum Hydroxide Gel Concentrate OTC
  (600 mg/5 mL)
  30 mL, 6 oz, 12 oz, and 16 oz
Aromatic Cascara Fluidextract USP 5 mL OTC
Chloral Hydrate Syrup USP 500 mg/5 mL ℞ ℂ
Diphenhydramine HCl Elixir (12.5 mg/5 mL) ℞
  5 mL, 10 mL, and 20 mL
Docusate Sodium Liquid (50 mg/5 mL) OTC
  10 mL, 25 mL, and 16 oz
Docusate Sodium Syrup USP (20 mg/5mL) OTC
  25 mL and 16 oz
Docusate Sodium with Casanthranol OTC
  (60 mg/30 mg per 15 mL)
  15 mL, 30 mL, and 16 oz
Ferrous Sulfate Liquid 300 mg/5 mL OTC
Guaifenesin Syrup USP (100 mg/5 mL) OTC
  5 mL, 10 mL, 15 mL, and 4 oz
Guaifenesin Syrup with Codeine OTC ℂ
  (100 mg/10 mg per 5 mL)
  5 mL, 10 mL, 4 oz, and 16 oz
Guaifenesin Syrup with Dextromethorphan OTC
  (100 mg/10 mg per 5 mL)
  5 mL, 10 mL, and 4 oz
Milk of Magnesia USP OTC
  15 mL and 30 mL
Milk of Magnesia Concentrate 10 mL OTC

Milk of Magnesia Cascara Concentrate OTC
  Susp. 15 mL
Mineral Oil USP 30 mL OTC
Phenobarbital Elixir (20 mg/5 mL) ℞ ℂ
  5 mL, 7.5 mL, and 15 mL
Potassium Chloride Oral Soln. USP 10% ℞
  Sugar-Free (20 mEq/15 mL)
  15 mL and 30 mL
Potassium Chloride Oral Soln. USP 20% ℞
  Sugar-Free (40 mEq/15 mL)
  15 mL and 30 mL
Promethazine HCl and Codeine Phosphate Syrup ℞ ℂ
  (6.25 mg/10 mg per 5 mL)
  5 mL and 10 mL
Pseudoephedrine HCl Syrup (30 mg/5 mL) 4 oz OTC
Sorbitol Solution USP (70% w/w) OTC
  15 mL, 30 mL, and 16 oz
Sore Throat Spray (Phenol 1.4%) OTC
  Cherry, Menthol, and Mint Flavors in 6 oz

Pharmacia & Upjohn Company
KALAMAZOO, MI 49001

Direct Inquiries to:
(616) 323-4000

For Medical and Pharmaceutical Information, Including Emergencies, Contact:
(616) 833-8244

PRODUCT IDENTIFICATION

Prescription capsules and tablets manufactured by Pharmacia & Upjohn Company are imprinted with one or a combination of the following: (1) Product trademark, (2) Dosage strength, (3) "Adria," "Pharmacia," "Upjohn," "U," or the code "KP." That portion of the National Drug Code (NDC) number that indicates product and strength.
A list of oral solid dosage forms with NDC product identification numbers is provided below.

Code #	Product	Strength
10	**HALCION®** Tablets (triazolam tablets, USP) *See Product Identification Guide*	0.125 mg
12	**CORTEF®** Tablets (hydrocortisone tablets, USP)	5 mg
14	**HALOTESTIN®** Tablets (fluoxymesterone tablets, USP) *See Product Identification Guide*	2 mg
15	**CORTISONE ACETATE** Tablets, USP	5 mg
17	**HALCION®** Tablets (triazolam tablets, USP) *See Product Identification Guide*	0.25 mg
18	**DIDREX®** Tablets (benzphetamine hydrochloride tablets) *See Product Identification Guide*	50 mg
19	**HALOTESTIN®** Tablets (fluoxymesterone tablets, USP) *See Product Identification Guide*	5 mg
23	**CORTISONE ACETATE** Tablets, USP	10 mg
24	**DIDREX®** Tablets (benzphetamine hydrochloride tablets) *See Product Identification Guide*	50 mg
29	**XANAX®** Tablets (alprazolam tablets, USP) *See Product Identification Guide*	0.25 mg
31	**CORTEF®** Tablets (hydrocortisone tablets, USP)	10 mg
32	**DELTASONE®** Tablets (prednisone tablets, USP) *See Product Identification Guide*	2.5 mg
32	**EMCYT** Capsules (estramustine phosphate sodium)	140 mg
34	**CORTISONE ACETATE** Tablets, USP	25 mg
36	**HALOTESTIN®** Tablets (fluoxymesterone tablets, USP) *See Product Identification Guide*	10 mg
44	**CORTEF®** Tablets (hydrocortisone tablets, USP)	20 mg
45	**DELTASONE®** Tablets (prednisone tablets, USP) *See Product Identification Guide*	5 mg
50	**PROVERA®** Tablets (medroxyprogesterone acetate tablets, USP) *See Product Identification Guide*	10 mg
55	**XANAX®** Tablets (alprazolam tablets, USP) *See Product Identification Guide*	0.5 mg
64	**PROVERA®** Tablets (medroxyprogesterone acetate tablets, USP) *See Product Identification Guide*	2.5 mg
90	**XANAX®** Tablets (alprazolam tablets, USP) *See Product Identification Guide*	1 mg
94	**XANAX®** Tablets (alprazolam tablets, USP) *See Product Identification Guide*	2 mg
100	**ORINASE®** Tablets (tolbutamide tablets, USP)	500 mg
101	**ALBAMYCIN®** Capsules (novobiocin sodium capsules)	250 mg
101	**AZULFIDINE** Tablets (sulfasalazine)	500 mg
102	**AZULFIDINE EN-tabs** (sulfasalazine delayed release)	500 mg
105	**DIPENTUM** Capsules (olsalazine sodium)	250 mg
121	**LONITEN®** Tablets (minoxidil tablets, USP) *See Product Identification Guide*	2.5 mg
131	**MICRONASE®** Tablets (glyburide tablets) *See Product Identification Guide*	1.25 mg
137	**LONITEN®** Tablets (minoxidil tablets, USP) *See Product Identification Guide*	10 mg
141	**MICRONASE®** Tablets (glyburide tablets) *See Product Identification Guide*	2.5 mg
165	**DELTASONE®** Tablets (prednisone tablets, USP) *See Product Identification Guide*	20 mg
171	**MICRONASE®** Tablets (glyburide tablets) *See Product Identification Guide*	5 mg
193	**DELTASONE®** Tablets (prednisone tablets, USP) *See Product Identification Guide*	10 mg
225	**CLEOCIN HCl®** Capsules (clindamycin hydrochloride capsules, USP) *See Product Identification Guide*	150 mg
286	**PROVERA®** Tablets (medroxyprogesterone acetate tablets, USP) *See Product Identification Guide*	5 mg
301	**MYCOBUTIN** (rifabutin capsules)	150 mg
331	**CLEOCIN HCl®** Capsules (clindamycin hydrochloride capsules, USP) *See Product Identification Guide*	75 mg
341	**GLYNASE®** PresTab™ Tablets (micronized glyburide tablets) *See Product Identification Guide*	1.5 mg
352	**GLYNASE®** PresTab™ Tablets (micronized glyburide tablets) *See Product Identification Guide*	3 mg
388	**DELTASONE®** Tablets (prednisone tablets, USP) *See Product Identification Guide*	50 mg
395	**CLEOCIN HCl®** Capsules (clindamycin hydrochloride capsules, USP) *See Product Identification Guide*	300 mg
450	**COLESTID®** Tablets (micronized colestipol hydrochloride)	1 g
500	**LINCOCIN®** Capsules (lincomycin hydrochloride capsules, USP)	500 mg
617	**VANTIN®** Tablets (cefpodoxime proxetil tablets)	100 mg
618	**VANTIN®** Tablets (cefpodoxime proxetil tablets)	200 mg
3449	**GLYNASE®** PresTab Tablets (micronized glyburide tablets)	6 mg
3772	**OGEN®** Tablets (estropipate tablets, USP)	0.75 mg
3773	**OGEN®** Tablets (estropipate tablets, USP)	1.5 mg
3774	**OGEN®** Tablets (estropipate tablets, USP)	3 mg

ADRIAMYCIN RDF® ℞
(Doxorubicin Hydrochloride for Injection, USP)
ADRIAMYCIN PFS® ℞
[adrē'ah-mī-cĭn]
(Doxorubicin Hydrochloride Injection, USP)
FOR INTRAVENOUS USE ONLY

WARNING
1. Severe local tissue necrosis will occur if there is extravasation during administration (See DOSAGE AND

ADMINISTRATION). Doxorubicin must not be given by the intramuscular or subcutaneous route.

2. Myocardial toxicity manifested in its most severe form by potentially fatal congestive heart failure may occur either during therapy or months to years after termination of therapy. The probability of developing impaired myocardial function based on a combined index of signs, symptoms and decline in left ventricular ejection fraction (LVEF) is estimated to be 1 to 2% at a total cumulative dose of 300 mg/m^2 of doxorubicin, 3 to 5% at a dose of 400 mg/m^2, 5 to 8% at 450 mg/m^2 and 6 to 20% at 500 mg/m^2.* The risk of developing CHF increases rapidly with increasing total cumulative doses of doxorubicin in excess of 450 mg/m^2. This toxicity may occur at lower cumulative doses in patients with prior mediastinal irradiation or on concurrent cyclophosphamide therapy or with pre-existing heart disease.
3. Dosage should be reduced in patients with impaired hepatic function.
4. Severe myelosuppression may occur.
5. Doxorubicin should be administered only under the supervision of a physician who is experienced in the use of cancer chemotherapeutic agents.

* Data on file at Pharmacia

DESCRIPTION

Doxorubicin is a cytotoxic anthracycline antibiotic isolated from cultures of *Streptomyces peucetius* var. *caesius*.

Doxorubicin consists of a naphthacenequinone nucleus linked through a glycosidic bond at ring atom 7 to an amino sugar, daunosamine.

Chemically, doxorubicin hydrochloride is:

5,12-Naphthacenedione, 10-[(3-amino-2,3,6-trideoxy-α-L-*lyxo*-hexopyranosyl)oxy]-7,8,9,10-tetrahydro-6,8,11-trihydroxy-8-(hydroxylacetyl)-1-methoxy-, hydrochloride (8*S-cis*)-.

The structural formula is as follows:

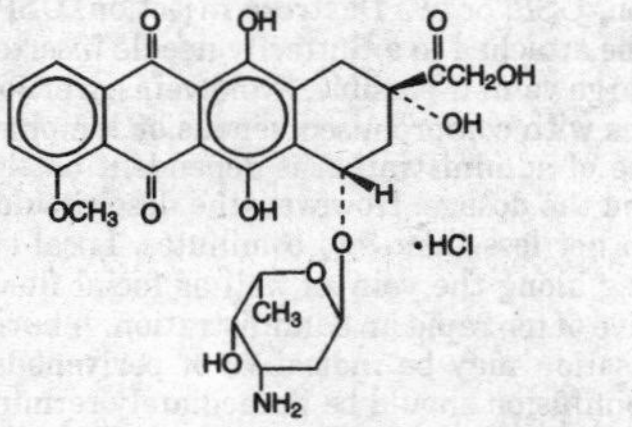

$C_{27}H_{29}NO_{11} \cdot HCl$ M.W. 579.99

Doxorubicin binds to nucleic acids, presumably by specific intercalation of the planar anthracycline nucleus with the DNA double helix. The anthracycline ring is lipophilic, but the saturated end of the ring system contains abundant hydroxyl groups adjacent to the amino sugar, producing a hydrophilic center. The molecule is amphoteric, containing acidic functions in the ring phenolic groups and a basic function in the sugar amino group. It binds to cell membranes as well as plasma proteins.

ADRIAMYCIN RDF® (Doxorubicin Hydrochloride for Injection, USP) a sterile red-orange lyophilized powder for intravenous use only, is available in 10, 20 and 50 mg single dose vials and a 150 mg multidose vial.

Each 10 mg single dose vial contains 10 mg of doxorubicin HCl, USP, 50 mg of lactose, NF (hydrous) and 1 mg of methylparaben, NF (added to enhance dissolution) as a sterile red-orange lyophilized powder.

Each 20 mg single dose vial contains 20 mg of doxorubicin HCl, USP, 100 mg of lactose, NF (hydrous) and 2 mg of methylparaben, NF (added to enhance dissolution) as a sterile red-orange lyophilized powder.

Each 50 mg single dose vial contains 50 mg of doxorubicin HCl, USP, 250 mg of lactose, NF (hydrous) and 5 mg of methylparaben, NF (added to enhance dissolution) as a sterile red-orange lyophilized powder.

Each 150 mg multidose vial contains 150 mg of doxorubicin HCl, USP, 750 mg of lactose, NF (hydrous) and 15 mg of methylparaben, NF (added to enhance dissolution) as a sterile red-orange lyophilized powder.

ADRIAMYCIN PFS® (Doxorubicin Hydrochloride Injection, USP) is a sterile parenteral, isotonic solution for intravenous use only, containing no preservative, available in 5 mL (10 mg), 10 mL (20 mg), 25 mL (50 mg), and 37.5 mL (75 mg) single dose vials and a 100 mL (200 mg) multidose vial.

Each mL contains doxorubicin HCl 2 mg, USP and the following inactive ingredients: sodium chloride 0.9% and water for injection q.s. Hydrochloric acid is used to adjust the pH to a target pH of 3.0.

CLINICAL PHARMACOLOGY

The cytotoxic effect of doxorubicin on malignant cells and its toxic effects on various organs are thought to be related to nucleotide base intercalation and cell membrane lipid binding activities of doxorubicin. Intercalation inhibits nucleotide replication and action of DNA and RNA polymerases. The interaction of doxorubicin with topoisomerase II to form DNA-cleavable complexes appears to be an important mechanism of doxorubicin cytocidal activity. Doxorubicin cellular membrane binding may effect a variety of cellular functions. Enzymatic electron reduction of doxorubicin by a variety of oxidases, reductases and dehydrogenases generate highly reactive species including the hydroxyl free radical OH·. Free radical formation has been implicated in doxorubicin cardiotoxicity by means of Cu (II) and Fe (III) reduction at the cellular level.

Animal studies have shown activity in a spectrum of experimental tumors, immunosuppression, carcinogenic properties in rodents, induction of a variety of toxic effects, including delayed and progressive cardiac toxicity, myelosuppression in all species and atrophy to testes in rats and dogs.

Pharmacokinetic studies, determined in patients with various types of tumors undergoing either single or multi-agent therapy have shown that doxorubicin follows a multiphasic disposition after intravenous injection. The initial distributive half-life of approximately 5.0 minutes suggests rapid tissue uptake of doxorubicin, while its slow elimination from tissues is reflected by a terminal half-life of 20 to 48 hours. Steady-state distribution volumes exceed 20 to 30 L/kg and are indicative of extensive drug uptake into tissues. Plasma clearance is in the range of 8 to 20 mL/min/kg and is predominately by metabolism and biliary excretion. Approximately 40% of the dose appears in the bile in 5 days, while only 5 to 12% of the drug and its metabolites appear in the urine during the same time period. Binding of doxorubicin and its major metabolite, doxorubicinol to plasma proteins is about 74 to 76% and is independent of plasma concentration of doxorubicin up to 2μM. Enzymatic reduction at the 7 position and cleavage of the daunosamine sugar yields aglycones which are accompanied by free radical formation, the local production of which may contribute to the cardiotoxic activity of doxorubicin. Disposition of doxorubicinol (DOX-OL) in patients is formation rate limited. The terminal half-life of DOX-OL is similar to doxorubicin. The relative exposure of DOX-OL, compared to doxorubicin ranges between 0.4 to 0.6. In urine, $<$3% of the dose was recovered as DOX-OL over 7 days. The literature contains no information regarding gender related differences in the pharmacokinetics of doxorubicin and doxorubicinol.

In four patients, dose-independent pharmacokinetics have been shown for doxorubicin in the dose range of 30 to 70 mg/m^2. Systemic clearance of doxorubicin is significantly reduced in obese women with ideal body weight greater than 130%. There was a significant reduction in clearance without any change in volume of distribution in obese patients when compared with normal patients with less than 115% ideal body weight. The clearance of doxorubicin and doxorubicinol was also reduced in patients with impaired hepatic function. Doxorubicin was excreted in the milk of one lactating patient, with peak milk concentration at 24 hours after treatment being approximately 4.4 -fold greater than the corresponding plasma concentration. Doxorubicin was detectable in the milk up to 72 hours after therapy with 70 mg/m^2 of doxorubicin given as a 15 minute intravenous infusion and 100 mg/m^2 of cisplatin as a 26 hour intravenous infusion. The peak concentration of doxorubicinol in milk at 24 hours was 0.2 μM and AUC up to 24 hours was 16.5μM.hr while the AUC for doxorubicin was 9.9μM.hr.

Doxorubicin does not cross the blood brain barrier.

INDICATIONS AND USAGE

ADRIAMYCIN PFS and ADRIAMYCIN RDF have been used successfully to produce regression in disseminated neoplastic conditions such as acute lymphoblastic leukemia, acute myeloblastic leukemia, Wilms' tumor, neuroblastoma, soft tissue and bone sarcomas, breast carcinoma, ovarian carcinoma, transitional cell bladder carcinoma, thyroid carcinoma, gastric carcinoma, Hodgkin's disease, malignant lymphoma and bronchogenic carcinoma in which the small cell histologic type is the most responsive compared to other cell types.

CONTRAINDICATIONS

Doxorubicin therapy should not be started in patients who have marked myelosuppression induced by previous treatment with other antitumor agents or by radiotherapy. Doxorubicin treatment is contraindicated in patients who received previous treatment with complete cumulative doses of doxorubicin, daunorubicin, idarubicin, and/or other anthracyclines and anthracenes.

WARNINGS

Special attention must be given to the cardiotoxicity induced by doxorubicin. Irreversible myocardial toxicity, manifested in its most severe form by life-threatening and potentially fatal congestive heart failure, may occur either during therapy or months to years after termination of therapy. The probability of developing impaired myocardial function, based on a combined index of signs, symptoms and decline in left ventricular ejection fraction (LVEF) is estimated to be 1 to 2% at a total cumulative dose of 300 mg/m^2 of doxorubicin, 3 to 5% at a dose of 400 mg/m^2, 5 to 8% at a dose of 450 mg/m^2 and 6 to 20% at a dose of 500 mg/m^2 given in a schedule of a bolus injection once every 3 weeks (data on file at Pharmacia Adria). In a retrospective review by Von Hoff et al, the probability of developing congestive heart failure was reported to be 5/168 (3%) at a cumulative dose of 430 mg/m^2 of doxorubicin, 8/110 (7%) at 575 mg/m^2 and 3/14 (21%) at 728 mg/m^2. The cumulative incidence of CHF was 2.2%. In a prospective study of doxorubicin in combination with cyclophosphamide, fluorouracil and/or vincristine in patients with breast cancer or small cell lung cancer, the cumulative incidence of congestive heart failure was 5 to 6%. The probability of CHF at various cumulative doses of doxorubicin was 1.5% at 300 mg/m^2, 4.9% at 400 mg/m^2, 7.7% at 450 mg/m^2 and 20.5% at 500 mg/m^2.

Cardiotoxicity may occur at lower doses in patients with prior mediastinal irradiation, concurrent cyclophosphamide therapy and advanced age. Data also suggest that pre-existing heart disease is a co-factor for increased risk of doxorubicin cardiotoxicity. In such cases, cardiac toxicity may occur at doses lower than the respective recommended cumulative dose of doxorubicin. Studies have suggested that concomitant administration of doxorubicin and calcium channel entry blockers may increase the risk of doxorubicin cardiotoxicity. The total dose of doxorubicin administered to the individual patient should also take into account previous or concomitant therapy with related compounds such as daunorubicin, idarubicin and mitoxantrone. Cardiomyopathy and/or congestive heart failure may be encountered several months or years after discontinuation of doxorubicin therapy.

The risk of congestive heart failure and other acute manifestations of doxorubicin cardiotoxicity in children may be as much or lower than in adults. Children appear to be at particular risk for developing delayed cardiac toxicity in that doxorubicin induced cardiomyopathy impairs myocardial growth as children mature, subsequently leading to possible development of congestive heart failure during early adulthood. As many as 40% of children may have subclinical cardiac dysfunction and 5 to 10% of children may develop congestive heart failure on long term follow-up. This late cardiac toxicity may be related to the dose of doxorubicin. The longer the length of follow-up the greater the increase in the detection rate.

Treatment of doxorubicin induced congestive heart failure includes the use of digitalis, diuretics, after load reducers such as angiotensin I converting enzyme (ACE) inhibitors, low salt diet, and bed rest. Such intervention may relieve symptoms and improve the functional status of the patient.

Monitoring Cardiac Function

In adult patients severe cardiac toxicity may occur precipitously without antecedent ECG changes. Cardiomyopathy induced by anthracyclines is usually associated with very characteristic histopathologic changes on an endomyocardial biopsy (EM biopsy), and a decrease of left ventricular ejection fraction (LVEF), as measured by multi-gated radionuclide angiography (MUGA scans) and/or echocardiogram (ECHO), from pretreatment baseline values. However, it has not been demonstrated that monitoring of the ejection fraction will predict when individual patients are approaching their maximally tolerated cumulative dose of doxorubicin. Cardiac function should be carefully monitored during treatment to minimize the risk of cardiac toxicity. A baseline cardiac evaluation with an ECG, LVEF, and/or an echocardiogram (ECHO) is recommended especially in patients with risk factors for increased cardiac toxicity (pre-existing heart disease, mediastinal irradiation, or concurrent cyclophosphamide therapy). Subsequent evaluations should be obtained at a cumulative dose of doxorubicin of at least 400 mg/m^2 and periodically thereafter during the course of therapy. Children are at increased risk for developing delayed cardiotoxicity following doxorubicin administration and therefore a follow-up cardiac evaluation is recommended periodically to monitor for this delayed cardiotoxicity.

In adults, a 10% decline in LVEF to below the lower limit of normal or an absolute LVEF of 45%, or a 20% decline in LVEF at any level is indicative of deterioration in cardiac function. In children, deterioration in cardiac function during or after the completion of therapy with doxorubicin is indicated by a drop in fractional shortening (FS) by an absolute value of 10 percentile units or below 29%, and a decline in LVEF of 10 percentile units or an LVEF below 55%. In general, if test results indicate deterioration in cardiac function associated with doxorubicin, the benefit of continued

Continued on next page

Information on these Pharmacia & Upjohn products is based on labeling in effect June 1, 1996. Further information concerning these and other Pharmacia & Upjohn products may be obtained by direct inquiry to Medical Information, Pharmacia & Upjohn, Kalamazoo, MI 49001.

Pharmacia & Upjohn—Cont.

therapy should be carefully evaluated against the risk of producing irreversible cardiac damage.

Acute life-threatening arrhythmias have been reported to occur during or within a few hours after doxorubicin administration.

There is a high incidence of bone marrow depression, primarily of leukocytes, requiring careful hematologic monitoring. With the recommended dose schedule, leukopenia is usually transient, reaching its nadir 10 to 14 days after treatment with recovery usually occurring by the 21st day. White blood counts as low as $1000/mm^3$ are to be expected during treatment with appropriate doses of doxorubicin. Red blood cell and platelet levels should also be monitored since they may also be depressed. Hematologic toxicity may require dose reduction or suspension or delay of doxorubicin therapy. Persistent severe myelosuppression may result in superinfection or hemorrhage.

Doxorubicin may potentiate the toxicity of other anticancer therapies. Exacerbation of cyclophosphamide induced hemorrhagic cystitis and enhancement of the hepatotoxicity of 6-mercaptopurine have been reported. Radiation induced toxicity to the myocardium, mucosae, skin and liver have been reported to be increased by the administration of doxorubicin.

Since metabolism and excretion of doxorubicin occurs predominantly by the hepatobiliary route, toxicity to recommended doses of doxorubicin can be enhanced by hepatic impairment; therefore, prior to the individual dosing, evaluation of hepatic function is recommended using conventional laboratory tests such as SGOT, SGPT, alkaline phosphatase and bilirubin (See DOSAGE AND ADMINISTRATION).

Necrotizing colitis manifested by typhlitis (cecal inflammation), bloody stools and severe and sometimes fatal infections have been associated with a combination of doxorubicin given by i.v. push daily for 3 days and cytarabine given by continuous infusion daily for 7 or more days.

On intravenous administration of doxorubicin, extravasation may occur with or without an accompanying stinging or burning sensation, even if blood returns well on aspiration of the infusion needle (See DOSAGE AND ADMINISTRATION). If any signs or symptoms of extravasation have occurred, the injection or infusion should be immediately terminated and restarted in another vein.

Pregnancy Category D—Safe use of doxorubicin in pregnancy has not been established. Doxorubicin is embryotoxic and teratogenic in rats and embryotoxic and abortifacient in rabbits. There are no adequate and well-controlled studies in pregnant women. If doxorubicin is to be used during pregnancy, or if the patient becomes pregnant during therapy, the patient should be apprised of the potential hazard to the fetus. Women of childbearing age should be advised to avoid becoming pregnant.

PRECAUTIONS
General
Doxorubicin is not an anti-microbial agent.
Information for Patients
ADRIAMYCIN PFS and ADRIAMYCIN RDF impart a red coloration to the urine for 1 to 2 days after administration, and patients should be advised to expect this during active therapy.
Drug Interactions
Literature contain the following drug interactions with doxorubicin in humans: cyclosporine (Sandimmune) may induce coma and/or seizures, phenobarbital increases the elimination of doxorubicin, phenytoin levels may be decreased by doxorubicin, streptozocin (Zanosar) may inhibit the hepatic metabolism, and administration of live vaccines to immunosuppressed patients, including those undergoing cytotoxic chemotherapy, may be hazardous. Information on other potential drug interactions may be found in the literature.
Laboratory Tests
Initial treatment with doxorubicin requires observation of the patient and periodic monitoring of complete blood counts, hepatic function tests, and radionuclide left vetricular ejection fraction (See WARNINGS section).
Like other cytotoxic drugs, doxorubicin may induce "tumor lysis syndrome" and hyperuricemia in patients with rapidly growing tumors. Appropriate supportive and pharmacologic measures may prevent or alleviate this complication.
Carcinogenesis, Mutagenesis, Impairment of Fertility
Formal long-term carcinogenicity studies have not been conducted with doxorubicin. Doxorubicin and related compounds have been shown to have mutagenic and carcinogenic properties when tested in experimental models (including bacterial systems, mammalian cells in culture, and female Sprague-Dawley rats).
The possible adverse effect on fertility in males and females in humans or experimental animals have not been adequately evaluated. Testicular atrophy was observed in rats and dogs.
A variant of chemotherapy-related acute non-lymphocytic leukemia has been reported to occur infrequently a few years after multiple drug treatment of some neoplasms, which sometimes included doxorubicin. The exact role of doxorubicin has not been elucidated.
Pregnancy Category D
(See WARNINGS section.)
Nursing Mothers:
Because of the potential for serious adverse reactions in nursing infants from doxorubicin, mothers should be advised to discontinue nursing during doxorubicin therapy.

ADVERSE REACTIONS
Dose limiting toxicities of therapy are myelosuppression and cardiotoxicity. Other reactions reported are:
Cardiotoxicity—(See WARNINGS section.)
Cutaneous—Reversible complete alopecia occurs in most cases. Hyperpigmentation of nailbeds and dermal crease, primarily in children, and onycholysis have been reported in a few cases. Recall of skin reaction due to prior radiotherapy has occurred with doxorubicin administration.
Gastrointestinal—Acute nausea and vomiting occurs frequently and may be severe. This may be alleviated by antiemetic therapy. Mucositis (stomatitis and esophagitis) may occur 5 to 10 days after administration. The effect may be severe leading to ulceration and represents a site of origin for severe infections. The dosage regimen consisting of administration of doxorubicin on three successive days results in greater incidence and severity of mucositis. Ulceration and necrosis of the colon, especially the cecum, may occur leading to bleeding or severe infections which can be fatal. This reaction has been reported in patients with acute non-lymphocytic leukemia treated with a 3-day course of doxorubicin combined with cytarabine. Anorexia and diarrhea have been occasionally reported.
Vascular—Phlebosclerosis has been reported especially when small veins are used or a single vein is used for repeated administration. Facial flushing may occur if the injection is given too rapidly.
Local—Severe cellulitis, vesication and tissue necrosis will occur if extravasation of doxorubicin occurs during administration. Erythematous streaking along the vein proximal to the site of injection had been reported (See DOSAGE AND ADMINISTRATION).
Hematologic—The occurrence of secondary acute myeloid leukemia with or without a preleukemic phase has been reported rarely in patients concurrently treated with doxorubicin in association with DNA-damaging antineoplastic agents. Such cases could have a short (1–3 years) latency period.
Hypersensitivity—Fever, chills and urticaria have been reported occasionally. Anaphylaxis may occur. A case of apparent cross sensitivity to lincomycin has been reported.
Other—Conjunctivitis and lacrimation occur rarely.

OVERDOSAGE
Acute overdosage with doxorubicin enhances the toxic effect of mucositis, leukopenia and thrombocytopenia. Treatment of acute overdosage consists of treatment of the severely myelosuppressed patient with hospitalization, antimicrobials, platelet transfusions and symptomatic treatment of mucositis. Use of hemopoietic growth factor (G-CSF, GM-CSF) may be considered.
The 150 mg ADRIAMYCIN RDF and the 100 mL (2 mg/mL) ADRIAMYCIN PFS vials are packaged as multiple dose vials and caution should be exercised to prevent inadvertent overdosage.
Cumulative dosage with doxorubicin increases the risk of cardiomyopathy and resultant congestive heart failure (See WARNINGS Section). Treatment consists of vigorous management of congestive heart failure with digitalis preparations, diuretics, and after-load reducers such as ACE inhibitors.

DOSAGE AND ADMINISTRATION
Care in the administration of ADRIAMYCIN PFS and ADRIAMYCIN RDF will reduce the chance of perivenous infiltration *(See WARNINGS)*. It may also decrease the chance of local reactions such as urticaria and erythematous streaking. On intravenous administration of doxorubicin, extravasation may occur with or without an accompanying burning or stinging sensation, even if blood returns well on aspiration of the infusion needle. If any signs or symptoms of extravasation have occurred, the injection or infusion should be immediately terminated and restarted in another vein. If extravasation is suspected, intermittent application of ice to the site for 15 min. q.i.d. × 3 days may be useful. The benefit of local administration of drugs has not been clearly established. Because of the progressive nature of extravasation reactions, close observation and plastic surgery consultation is recommended. Blistering, ulceration and/or persistent pain are indications for wide excision surgery, followed by split-thickness skin grafting.[1]
The most commonly used dose schedule when used as a single agent is 60 to 75 mg/m² as a single intravenous injection administered at 21-day intervals. The lower dosage should be given to patients with inadequate marrow reserves due to old age, or prior therapy, or neoplastic marrow infiltration.
ADRIAMYCIN PFS and ADRIAMYCIN RDF have been used concurrently with other approved chemotherapeutic agents. Evidence is available that in some types of neoplastic disease combination chemotherapy is superior to single agents. The benefits and risks of such therapy continue to be elucidated. When used in combination with other chemotherapy drugs, the most commonly used dosage of doxorubicin is 40 to 60 mg/m² given as a single intravenous injection every 21 to 28 days. Doxorubicin dosage must be reduced in case of hyperbilirubinemia as follows:

Plasma bilirubin concentration (mg/dL)	Dosage reduction (%)
1.2 – 3.0	50
3.1 – 5.0	75

Reconstitution Directions: ADRIAMYCIN RDF 10 mg, 20 mg, 50 mg, and 150 mg vials should be reconstituted with 5 mL, 10 mL, 25 mL, and 75 mL, respectively, of Sodium Chloride Injection, USP (0.9%), to give a final concentration of 2 mg/mL of doxorubicin hydrochloride. An appropriate volume of air should be withdrawn from the vial during reconstitution to avoid excessive pressure buildup. Bacteriostatic diluents are not recommended.
After adding the diluent, the vial should be shaken and the contents allowed to dissolve. The reconstituted solution is stable for 7 days at room temperature and under normal room light (100 foot-candles) and 15 days under refrigeration (2° to 8°C). It should be protected from exposure to sunlight. Discard any of the unused solution from the 10 mg, 20 mg, and 50 mg single dose vials. Unused solutions of the multiple dose vial remaining beyond the recommended storage times should be discarded.
It is recommended that ADRIAMYCIN PFS and ADRIAMYCIN RDF be slowly administered into the tubing of a freely running intravenous infusion of Sodium Chloride Injection, USP, or 5% Dextrose Injection, USP. The tubing should be attached to a Butterfly needle inserted preferably into a large vein. If possible, avoid veins over joints or in extremities with compromised venous or lymphatic drainage. The rate of administration is dependent on the size of the vein, and the dosage. However, the dose should be administered in not less than 3 to 5 minutes. Local erythematous streaking along the vein as well as facial flushing may be indicative of too rapid an administration. A burning or stinging sensation may be indicative of perivenous infiltration and the infusion should be immediately terminated and restarted in another vein. Perivenous infiltration may occur painlessly.
Doxorubicin should not be mixed with heparin or fluorouracil since it has been reported that these drugs are incompatible to the extent that a precipitate may form. Until specific compatibility data are available, it is not recommended that doxorubicin be mixed with other drugs.
Parenteral drug products should be inspected visually for particulate matter and discoloration prior to administration, whenever solution and container permit.
Handling and Disposal: Skin reactions associated with doxorubicin have been reported. Skin accidently exposed to doxorubicin should be rinsed copiously with soap and warm water, and if the eyes are involved, standard irrigation techniques should be used immediately. The use of goggles, gloves, and protective gowns is recommended during preparation and administration of the drug.
Procedures for proper handling and disposal of anti-cancer drugs should be considered. Several guidelines on this subject have been published.[2–8] There is no general agreement that all the procedures recommended in the guidelines are necessary or appropriate.

HOW SUPPLIED
ADRIAMYCIN RDF® (Doxorubicin Hydrochloride for Injection, USP) is available as follows:
NDC 0013-1086-91 10 mg single dose vial,
                 10 vial packs
NDC 0013-1096-91 20 mg single dose vial,
                 10 vial packs
NDC 0013-1106-79 50 mg single dose vial,
                 single packs
Store at controlled room temperature, 15° to 30°C (59° to 86°F). Protect from light.
Retain in carton until time of use. Contains no preservative. Discard unused portion.
MULTIDOSE VIAL:
NDC 0013-1116-83 150 mg multidose vial,
                 single packs
Store at controlled room temperature, 15° to 30°C (59° to 86°F). Protect from light. Retain in carton until time of use.
RECONSTITUTED SOLUTION STABILITY
After adding the diluent, the vial should be shaken and the contents allowed to dissolve. The reconstituted solution is stable for 7 days at room temperature and under normal room light (100 foot-candles) and 15 days under refrigeration

(2° to 8°C). It should be protected from exposure to sunlight. Discard any unused solution from the 10 mg, 20 mg and 50 mg single dose vials. Unused solutions of the multiple dose vial remaining beyond the recommended storage times should be discarded.

MANUFACTURER:
PHARMACIA S.p.A
MILAN, ITALY

ADRIAMYCIN PFS® (Doxorubicin Hydrochloride Injection, USP)
SINGLE DOSE VIALS:
Sterile single use only, contains no preservative.

NDC 0013-1136-91	10 mg vial, 2 mg/mL, 5 mL, 10 vial packs
NDC 0013-1146-91	20 mg vial, 2 mg/mL, 10 mL, 10 vial packs
NDC 0013-1156-79	50 mg vial, 2 mg/mL, 25 mL, single vial packs
NDC 0013-1176-87	75 mg vial, 2 mg/mL, 37.5 mL, single vial packs

Store under refrigeration, 2° to 8°C (36° to 46°F). Protect from light. Retain in carton until time of use. Discard unused portion.

MULTIDOSE VIAL:
Sterile multidose vial, contains no preservative.

NDC 0013-1166-83	200 mg, 2 mg/mL, 100 mL, multidose vial, single vial packs

Store under refrigeration, 2° to 8°C (36° to 46°F). Protect from light. Retain in carton until contents are used.

MANUFACTURERS:

PHARMACIA S.p.A	Pharmacia Inc.
MILAN, ITALY	Kalamazoo, MI 49001, USA

CAUTION: Federal law prohibits dispensing without prescription.

REFERENCES

1. Rudolph R., Larson DL: Etiology and Treatment of Chemotherapeutic Agent Extravasation Injuries: A Review J. Clin Oncol 5:1116-1126, 1987.
2. Recommendations for the Safe Handling of Parenteral Antineoplastic Drugs. NIH Publication No. 83-2621. For sale by the Superintendent of Documents, US Government Printing Office, Washington, DC 20402.
3. AMA Council Report, Guidelines for Handling Parenteral Antineoplastics, JAMA. 1985; 253 (11): 1590-1592.
4. National Study Commission on Cytotoxic Exposure-Recommendations for Handling Cytotoxic Agents. Available from Louis P. Jeffrey, Sc.D., Chairman, National Study Commission on Cytotoxic Exposure, Massachusetts College of Pharmacy and Allied Health Sciences, 179 Longwood Avenue, Boston, Massachusetts 02115.
5. Clinical Oncological Society of. Australia. Guidelines and Recommendations for Safe Handling of Antineoplastic Agents. Med J Australia. 1983; 1:426-428.
6. Jones RB, et al: Safe Handling of Chemotherapeutic Agents: A Report from the Mount Sinai Medical Center. CA - A Cancer Journal for Clinicians. 1983; (Sept/Oct) 258-263.
7. American Society of Hospital Pharmacists Technical Assistance Bulletin on Handling Cytotoxic and Hazardous Drugs. Am J Hosp Pharm. 1990; 47:1033-1049.
8. OSHA Work-Practice Guidelines for Personnel Dealing with Cytotoxic (Antineoplastic) Drugs. Am J Hosp Pharm. 1986; 43:1193-1204.

Pharmacia & Upjohn Company
042310496 April 1, 1996

AZULFIDINE EN-tabs® ℞
(sulfasalazine delayed release tablets, USP)
Enteric-coated

AZULFIDINE® Tablets ℞
(sulfasalazine tablets, USP)

DESCRIPTION

AZULFIDINE EN-tabs®, (sulfasalazine delayed release tablets, USP), Enteric-coated, 500 mg, for Oral Administration.

AZULFIDINE EN-tabs are film coated with cellulose acetate phthalate to prevent disintegration of the tablet in the stomach and thus reduce possible irritation of the gastric mucosa. Azulfidine® Tablets, (sulfasalazine tablets, USP), 500 mg, for Oral Administration.

Therapeutic classification: Anti-inflammatory agent.

Chemical designation: 5-([p-(2-Pyridylsulfamoyl)phenyl] azo) salicylic acid.

Chemical Structure:

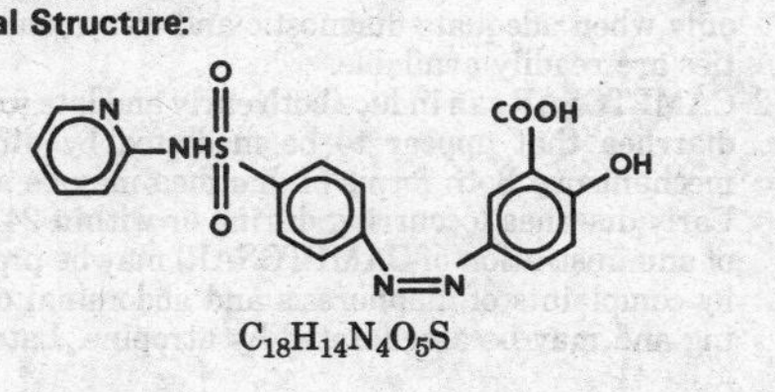

$C_{18}H_{14}N_4O_5S$

CLINICAL PHARMACOLOGY

After oral administration, AZULFIDINE is partially absorbed and extensively metabolized as described below.

About one-third of a given dose of sulfasalazine (SS) is absorbed from the small intestine. The remaining two-thirds pass to the colon where the compound is split (presumably by intestinal bacteria) into its components, 5-aminosalicylic acid (5-ASA) and sulfapyridine (SP). Most of the SP thus liberated is absorbed, whereas only about one-third of the 5-ASA is absorbed, the remainder being excreted in the feces. The distribution, metabolism and excretion of SS and its two components are as follows:

AZULFIDINE EN-tabs Enteric-coated tablets:

Sulfasalazine (SS): Detectable serum concentrations of SS have been found in healthy subjects within 90 minutes after the ingestion of a single 2g dose of AZULFIDINE EN-tabs. Maximum concentrations of SS occur between 3 and 12 hours, with the mean peak concentration (6 mcg/ml) occurring at 6 hours. Small amounts of SS are excreted unchanged in the urine.

Sulfapyridine (SP): Following absorption and distribution, SP is acetylated and hydroxylated in the liver, and then conjugated with glucuronic acid. After ingestion of a single 2g dose of AZULFIDINE EN-tabs by healthy subjects, peak concentrations of SP and its various metabolites appear in the serum between 12 and 24 hours, with peak concentrations (13 mcg/ml) occurring at 12 and lasting until 24 hours. The total recovery of SS and its SP metabolites from the urine of healthy subjects 3 days after the administration of a single 2g dose of AZULFIDINE EN-tabs averaged 81%.

5-aminosalicylic acid (5-ASA): The serum concentration of 5-ASA in patients with ulcerative colitis was found to range from 0 to 4 mcg/ml, and to exist mainly in the form of free 5-ASA. The urinary recovery of this compound was mostly in the acetylated form.

Mean serum concentrations of total SP, i.e. SP and its metabolites, tend to be significantly greater in patients with a slow acetylator phenotype than in those with a fast acetylator phenotype. Total serum sulfapyridine concentrations greater than 50 mcg/ml appear to be associated with an increased incidence of adverse reactions.

The mode of action of AZULFIDINE is still under investigation. It may be related to the immunosuppressant properties that have been observed in animal and **in vitro** models, to its affinity for connective tissue, and/or to the relatively high concentration it reaches in serous fluids, the liver and intestinal walls, as demonstrated in autoradiographic studies in animals. AZULFIDINE has also been described as a highly efficient vehicle for carrying its principal metabolites, SP and 5-ASA, to the colon, where a local action for both of them has been postulated. Recent clinical studies utilizing rectal administration of SS, SP and 5-ASA have indicated that the major therapeutic action may reside in the 5-ASA moiety.

AZULFIDINE Tablets:

Sulfasalazine (SS): Detectable serum concentrations of SS have been found in healthy subjects within 90 minutes after the ingestion of a single 2 g dose of AZULFIDINE Tablets. Maximum concentrations of SS occur between 1.5 and 6 hours, with the mean peak concentration (14 mcg/ml) occurring at 3 hours. Small amounts of SS are excreted unchanged in the urine.

Sulfapyridine (SP): Following absorption and distribution, SP is acetylated and hydroxylated in the liver, and then conjugated with glucuronic acid. After ingestion of a single 2g dose of AZULFIDINE Tablets by healthy subjects, SP and its various metabolites appear in the serum within 3 to 6 hours. Maximum concentrations of total SP occur between 6 and 24 hours, with the mean peak concentration (21 mcg/ml) occurring at 12 hours. The total recovery of SS and its SP metabolites from the urine of healthy subjects 3 days after the administration of a single 2 g dose of AZULFIDINE Tablets averaged 91%.

5-aminosalicylic acid (5-ASA): The serum concentration of 5-ASA in patients with ulcerative colitis was found to range from 0 to 4 mcg/ml, and to exist mainly in the form of free 5-ASA. The urinary recovery of this compound was mostly in the acetylated form.

Mean serum concentrations of total SP, i.e. SP and its metabolites, tend to be significantly greater in patients with a slow acetylator phenotype than in those with a fast acetylator phenotype. Total serum sulfapyridine concentrations greater than 50 mcg/ml appear to be associated with an increased incidence of adverse reactions.

The mode of action of AZULFIDINE is still under investigation. It may be related to the immunosuppressant properties that have been observed in animal and **in vitro** models, to its affinity for connective tissue, and/or to the relatively high concentration it reaches in serous fluids, the liver and intestinal walls, as demonstrated in autoradiographic studies in animals. AZULFIDINE has also been described as a highly efficient vehicle for carrying its principal metabolites, SP and 5-ASA, to the colon, where a local action for both of them has been postulated. Recent clinical studies utilizing rectal administration of SS, SP and 5-ASA have indicated that the major therapeutic action may reside in the 5-ASA moiety.

INDICATIONS AND USAGE

AZULFIDINE is indicated:

a. in the treatment of mild to moderate ulcerative colitis, and as adjunctive therapy in severe ulcerative colitis.

b. for the prolongation of the remission period between acute attacks of ulcerative colitis.

AZULFIDINE EN-tabs are particularly indicated in patients who cannot take the regular AZULFIDINE tablet because of gastrointestinal intolerance, and in whom there is evidence that this intolerance is not primarily due to high blood levels of sulfapyridine and its metabolites, e.g. patients experiencing nausea. vomiting, etc., when taking the first few doses of the drug or patients in whom a reduction in dosage does not alleviate the gastrointestinal side effects.

CONTRAINDICATIONS

Hypersensitivity to sulfasalazine, its metabolites, sulfonamides or salicylates. In infants under two years of age. Intestinal and urinary obstruction. Patients with porphyria should not receive sulfonamides as these drugs have been reported to precipitate an acute attack.

WARNINGS

Only after critical appraisal should AZULFIDINE be used in patients with hepatic or renal damage or blood dyscrasias. Deaths associated with the administration of AZULFIDINE have been reported from hypersensitivity reactions, agranulocytosis, aplastic anemia, other blood dyscrasias, renal and liver damage irreversible neuromuscular and CNS changes, and fibrosing alveolitis. The presence of clinical signs such as sore throat, fever, pallor, purpura or jaundice may be indications of serious blood disorders. Complete blood counts as well as a urinalysis with careful microscopic examination should be done frequently in patients receiving AZULFIDINE. Oligospermia and infertility have been observed in men treated with AZULFIDINE. Withdrawal of the drug appears to reverse these effects.

PRECAUTIONS

General: AZULFIDINE should be given with caution to patients with severe allergy or bronchial asthma. Adequate fluid intake must be maintained in order to prevent crystalluria and stone formation. Patients with glucose-6 phosphate dehydrogenase deficiency should be observed closely for signs of hemolytic anemia. This reaction is frequently dose related. If toxic or hypersensitivity reactions occur, the drug should be discontinued immediately.

Isolated instances have been reported when AZULFIDINE EN-tabs have passed undisintegrated. This may be due to a lack of intestinal esterases in these patients. If this is observed, the administration of AZULFIDINE EN-tabs should be discontinued immediately.

Information for Patients: Patients should be informed of the possibility of adverse reactions and of the need for careful medical supervision. They should also be made aware that ulcerative colitis rarely remits completely, and that the risk of relapse can be substantially reduced by continued administration of AZULFIDINE (at a maintenance dosage). Patients should be instructed to take AZULFIDINE in evenly divided doses perferably after meals. Additionally, patients should be advised that AZULFIDINE may produce an orange-yellow discoloration of the urine or skin.

Laboratory Tests: The progress of the disease during treatment can be evaluated by clinical criteria, including the presence of fever, weight changes, degree and frequency of diarrhea and bleeding as well as by sigmoidoscopy and the evaluation of biopsy samples. The determination of serum sulfapyridine levels may be useful since concentrations greater than 50 mcg/ml appear to be associated with an increased incidence of adverse reactions. Complete blood counts, as well as a urinalysis with careful microscopic examination should be done frequently in patients receiving AZULFIDINE.

Drug Interactions: Reduced absorption of folic acid and digoxin have been reported when administered concomitantly with AZULFIDINE.

Drug/Laboratory Test Interactions: The presence of AZULFIDINE or its metabolites in body fluids has not been reported to interfere with laboratory test procedures.

Carcinogenesis, Mutagenesis, Impairment of Fertility: - There have been no long-term studies of the carcinogenic or mutagenic potential of AZULFIDINE. Impairment of male fertility was observed in reproductive studies performed in rats and rabbits at doses up to six times the human dose. Oligospermia and infertility have been described in men treated

Continued on next page

Information on these Pharmacia & Upjohn products is based on labeling in effect June 1, 1996. Further information concerning these and other Pharmacia & Upjohn products may be obtained by direct inquiry to Medical Information, Pharmacia & Upjohn, Kalamazoo, MI 49001.

Pharmacia & Upjohn—Cont.

with AZULFIDINE. Withdrawal of the drug appears to reverse these effects (see "**WARNINGS**").

Pregnancy:

Teratogenic Effects:

Pregnancy Category B: Reproduction studies have been performed in rats and rabbits at doses up to 6 times the human dose and have revealed no evidence of impaired female fertility or harm to the fetus due to AZULFIDINE.

There are, however, no adequate and well-controlled studies in pregnant women. Because animal reproduction studies are not always predictive of human response, this drug should be used during pregnancy only if clearly needed.

A national survey evaluated the outcome of pregnancies associated with inflammatory bowel disease (IBD). In a group of 186 women treated with AZULFIDINE alone or AZULFIDINE and concomitant steroid therapy, the incidence of fetal morbidity and mortality was comparable to that for 245 untreated IBD pregnancies as well as with population data from the National Center for Health Statistics[1].

Another study of 1,445 pregnancies associated with exposure to sulfonamides in which AZULFIDINE was included indicated that this group of drugs appeared to be devoid of any association with fetal malformation[2]. A review of the medical literature covering 1,155 pregnancies which occurred in women having ulcerative colitis suggested that the outcome was similar to what was expected in the general population[3].

No clinical studies have been performed which indicate the effect of AZULFIDINE on the later growth development and functional maturation of children whose mothers received the drug during pregnancy.

Nonteratogenic Effects: AZULFIDINE and sulfapyridine pass the placental barrier. Although sulfapyridine has been shown to have a poor bilirubin displacing capacity, the potential for kernicterus in newborns should be kept in mind.

A case of agranulocytosis has been reported in an infant whose mother was taking both AZULFIDINE and prednisone throughout pregnancy.

Nursing Mothers: Caution should be exercised when AZULFIDINE is administered to a nursing woman. Sulfonamides are excreted in the milk. In the newborn, they compete with bilirubin for binding sites on the plasma proteins and may thus cause kernicterus. Insignificant amounts of uncleaved sulfasalazine have been found in milk, whereas the sulfapyridine levels in milk are about 30–60 percent of those in the serum. Sulfapyridine has been shown to have a poor bilirubin displacing capacity.

Pediatric Use: Safety and effectiveness in children below the age of two years have not been established.

ADVERSE REACTIONS

The most common adverse reactions associated with AZULFIDINE are anorexia, headache, nausea, vomiting, gastric distress and apparently reversible oligospermia. These occur in about one-third of the patients. Less frequent adverse reactions are skin rash, pruritis, urticaria, fever, Heinz body anemia, hemolytic anemia and cyanosis which may occur at a frequency of one in every thirty patients or less. Experience suggests that with a daily dosage of 4g or more, or total serum sulfapyridine levels above 50 mcg/ml, the incidence of adverse reactions tends to increase.

Although the listing which follows includes a few adverse reactions which have not been reported with this specific drug, the pharmacological similarities among the sulfonamides require that each of these reactions be considered when AZULFIDINE is administered.

Other adverse reactions which occur rarely, in approximately 1 in 1000 patients or less are:

Blood dyscrasias: aplastic anemia, agranulocytosis, leukopenia, megaloblastic (macrocytic) anemia, purpura, thrombocytopenia, hypoprothrombinemia, methemoglobinemia, congenital neutropenia, and myelodysplastic syndrome.

Hypersensitivity reactions: erythema multiforme (Stevens-Johnson syndrome), exfoliative dermatitis, epidermal necrolysis (Lyell's syndrome) with corneal damage, anaphylaxis, serum sickness syndrome, pneumonitis with or without eosinophilia, vasculitis, fibrosing alveolitis, pleuritis, pericarditis with or without tamponade, allergic myocarditis, polyarteritis nodosa, L.E. syndrome, hepatitis and hepatic necrosis with or without immune complexes, parapsoriasis varioliformis acuta (Mucha-Haberman syndrome), rhabdomyolysis, photosensitization, arthralgia, periorbital edema, conjunctival and scleral injection and alopecia.

Gastrointestinal reactions: hepatitis, pancreatitis, bloody diarrhea, impaired folic acid absorption, impaired digoxin absorption, stomatitis, diarrhea, abdominal pains, and neutropenic enterocolitis.

CNS reactions: transverse myelitis, convulsions, meningitis, transient lesions of the posterior spinal column, cauda equina syndrome, Guillain-Barre syndrome, peripheral neuropathy, mental depression, vertigo, hearing loss, insomnia, ataxia, hallucinations, tinnitus and drowsiness.

Renal reactions: toxic nephrosis with oliguria and anuria, nephritis, nephrotic syndrome, hematuria, crystaluria, proteinuria, and hemolytic-uremic syndrome.

Other reactions: urine discoloration and skin discoloration.

The sulfonamides bear certain chemical similarities to some goitrogens, diuretics (acetazolamide and the thiazides), and oral hypoglycemic agents. Goiter production, diuresis and hypoglycemia have occurred rarely in patients receiving sulfonamides. Cross-sensitivity may exist with these agents. Rats appear to be especially susceptible to the goitrogenic effects of sulfonamides and long-term administration has produced thyroid malignancies in this species.

DRUG ABUSE AND DEPENDENCE

None reported.

OVERDOSAGE

There is evidence that the incidence and severity of toxicity are directly related to the total serum sulfapyridine concentration. Symptoms of overdosage may include nausea, vomiting, gastric distress and abdominal pains. In more advanced cases, CNS symptoms such as drowsiness, convulsions, etc. may be observed. Serum sulfapyridine concentrations may be used to monitor the progress of recovery from overdosage.

Experience suggests that with a daily dosage of 4g or more or total serum sulfapyridine levels above 50 mcg/ml the incidence of adverse reactions tends to increase. There are no documented reports of deaths due to ingestion of large single doses of AZULFIDINE.

It has not been possible to determine that oral LD_{50} in laboratory animals such as mice, since the highest daily oral dose which can be given (12 g/Kg) is not lethal. Doses of AZULFIDINE of 16g per day have been given to patients without mortality.

Instructions for overdosage: Gastric lavage or emesis plus catharsis as indicated. Alkalinize urine. If kidney function is normal, force fluids. If anuria is present, restrict fluids and salt, and treat appropriately. Catherization of the ureters may be indicated for complete renal blockage by crystals.

The low molecular weight of AZULFIDINE and its metabolites may facilitate their removal by dialysis. For agranulocytosis, discontinue the drug immediately, hospitalize the patient and institute appropriate therapy.

For hypersensitivity reactions, discontinue treatment immediately. Such reactions may be controlled with antihistamines and, if necessary, systemic corticosteroids. When in the physician's opinion, reinstitution of AZULFIDINE is warranted, regimens modeled upon desensitization procedures may be attempted approximately two weeks after AZULFIDINE has been discontinued and symptoms have disappeared (see "**DOSAGE AND ADMINISTRATION**").

DOSAGE AND ADMINISTRATION

Dosage should be adjusted to each individual's response and tolerance. The drug should be given in evenly divided doses over each 24-hour period; intervals between nighttime doses should not exceed 8 hours, with administration after meals recommended when feasible. Experience suggests that with daily dosages of 4g or more, the incidence of adverse reactions tends to increase; hence, patients receiving these dosages should be instructed about and carefully observed for the appearance of adverse effects.

Various desensitization-like regimens have been reported to be effective in 34 of 53 patients[4], 7 of 8 patients[5] and 19 of 20 patients[6]. Upon reinstituting AZULFIDINE, such regimens comprise a total daily dose of 50 to 250 mg which, every 4 to 7 days thereafter, is doubled until the desired therapeutic level is achieved. If the symptoms of sensitivity recur, AZULFIDINE should be discontinued. Desensitization should not be attempted in patients who have a history of agranulocytosis or who have experienced an anaphylactoid reaction while on previous course of AZULFIDINE therapy.

USUAL DOSAGE

Initial Therapy:

Adults: 3–4g daily in evenly divided doses. In some cases it is advisable to initiate therapy with a smaller dosage, e.g. 1–2g daily, to lessen adverse gastrointestinal effects. If daily doses exceeding 4g are required to achieve desired effects, the increased risk of toxicity should be kept in mind.

Children, two years of age and older: 40–60mg per Kg body weight in each 24-hour period, divided into 3–6 doses.

Maintenance Therapy:

Adults: 2g daily.

Children, two years of age and older: 30 mg per Kg body weight in each 24-hour period, divided into 4 doses.

Response to therapy and adjustment of dosage should be determined by periodic examination. It is often necessary to continue medication, even when clinical symptoms, including diarrhea, have been controlled.

AZULFIDINE EN-tabs Enteric-coated tablets:

When endoscopic examination confirms satisfactory improvement, dosage is reduced to a maintenance level. If diarrhea recurs, dosage should be increased to previously effective levels. If symptoms of gastric intolerance (anorexia, nausea, vomiting, etc.) occur after the first few doses of AZULFIDINE EN-tabs, they are probably due to increased serum levels of total sulfapyridine, and may be alleviated by halving the dose and subsequently increasing it gradually over several days. If symptoms continue, the drug should be stopped for five to seven days, then reinstituted at a lower daily dose.

AZULFIDINE Tablets:

When endoscopic examination confirms satisfactory improvement, dosage is reduced to a maintenance level. If symptoms of gastric intolerance (anorexia, nausea, vomiting, etc.) occur after the first few doses of AZULFIDINE, they are probably due to mucosal irritation and may be alleviated by distributing the total daily dose more evenly over the day or by giving enteric-coated EN-tabs. If diarrhea recurs, dosage should be increased to previously effective levels.

If such symptoms occur after the first few days of treatment with AZULFIDINE, they are probably due to increased serum levels of total sulfapyridine, and may be alleviated by halving the dose and subsequently increasing it gradually over several days. If symptoms continue, the drug should be stopped for five to seven days, then reinstituted at a lower daily dose.

HOW SUPPLIED

AZULFIDINE EN-tabs Enteric-coated tablets:

Elliptical, gold colored, film enteric coated tablets, monogrammed "102" in the following package sizes:

AZULFIDINE EN-tabs 500 mg 100's—NDC No. 00130102-01.

AZULFIDINE EN-tabs 500 mg 500's—NDC No. 00130102-05.

Storage: Room Temperature (15–30°C/59–86°F).

Also Available as:

AZULFIDINE Tablets 500 mg 100's—NDC No. 0013-0101-01.

AZULFIDINE Tablets 500 mg 500's—NDC No. 0013-0101-05.

AZULFIDINE Tablets 500 mg Unit Dose 100's—NDC No. 0013-0101-11.

AZULFIDINE Tablets:

Round, gold colored scored tablets, monogrammed "101" in the following package sizes:

AZULFIDINE Tablets 500 mg 100's—NDC No. 0013-0101-01.

AZULFIDINE Tablets 500 mg 500's—NDC No. 0013-0101-05.

AZULFIDINE Unit Dose Tablets 500 mg 100's—NDC No. 0013-0101-11.

Storage: Room Temperature (15–30°C/59–86°F).

Also Available as:

AZULFIDINE EN-tabs 500 mg 100's—NDC No. 0013-0102-01.

AZULFIDINE EN-tabs 500 mg 500's—NDC No. 0013-0102-05.

REFERENCES

1. Pregnancy in Inflammatory Bowel Disease: Effect of Sulfasalazine and Corticosteroids on Fetal Outcome. Mogadam, M. et al, Gastroenterology, **80**: 72–76, 1981.
2. Birth Defects and Drugs During Pregnancy, David W. Kaufman, Editor, Publishing Sciences Group Inc.
3. Fertility, Sterility and Pregnancy in Chronic Inflammatory Bowel Disease. Jarnerot, G., Scand J. Gastroenterology, **17**: 1–4, 1982.
4. Korelitz B. et al: Gastroenterology **82**: 1104, 1982.
5. Holdsworth, C.G.: Brit. Med. J. **282**: 110, 1981.
6. Taffet, S.L. and Das, K.M.: Amer. J. Med. **73**:520–524, 1982.

CAUTION: Federal Law Prohibits Dispensing Without Prescription.

Pharmacia
Pharmacia Inc.
Columbus, Ohio 43216

110-B-039-20

©1994 Pharmacia Inc. 102000794 Revised: July 1994

Shown in Product Identification Guide, page 328

CAMPTOSAR® ℞

brand of Irinotecan hydrochloride Injection
For Intravenous Use Only

WARNINGS

1. CAMPTOSAR Injection should be administered only under the supervision of a physician who is experienced in the use of cancer chemotherapeutic agents. Appropriate management of complications is possible only when adequate diagnostic and treatment facilities are readily available.
2. CAMPTOSAR can induce both early and late forms of diarrhea that appear to be mediated by different mechanisms. Both forms of diarrhea may be severe. Early diarrhea (occurring during or within 24 hours of administration of CAMPTOSAR) may be preceded by complaints of diaphoresis and abdominal cramping and may be ameliorated by atropine. Late diar-

rhea (occurring more than 24 hours after administration of CAMPTOSAR) can be prolonged, may lead to dehydration and electrolyte imbalance, and can be life-threatening. Late diarrhea should be treated promptly with loperamide; patients with severe diarrhea should be carefully monitored and given fluid and electrolyte replacement if they become dehydrated (see **WARNINGS** section). Administration of CAMPTOSAR should be interrupted if severe diarrhea occurs.

3. Severe myelosuppression may occur (see **WARNINGS** section).

DESCRIPTION

CAMPTOSAR Injection (irinotecan hydrochloride injection) is an antineoplastic agent of the topoisomerase I inhibitor class. Irinotecan hydrochloride was clinically investigated as CPT-11.

CAMPTOSAR is supplied as a sterile, pale yellow, clear, aqueous solution. It is available in 100 mg, single-dose, 5 mL vials. Each milliliter of solution contains 20 mg of irinotecan hydrochloride (on the basis of the trihydrate salt), 45 mg of sorbitol NF powder, and 0.9 mg of lactic acid, USP. The pH of the solution has been adjusted to 3.5 (range, 3.0 to 3.8) with sodium hydroxide or hydrochloric acid. CAMPTOSAR is intended for dilution with 5% Dextrose Injection, USP (D5W), or 0.9% Sodium Chloride Injection, USP, prior to intravenous infusion. The preferred diluent is 5% Dextrose Injection, USP.

Irinotecan hydrochloride is a semisynthetic derivative of camptothecin, an alkaloid extract from plants such as *Camptotheca acuminata.* The chemical name is (4*S*)-4,11-diethyl -4- hydroxy-9-[(4-piperi-dinopiperidino)carbonyloxy]-1*H*-pyrano[3′,4′:6,7]indolizino[1,2-*b*]quinoline -3,14(4*H*,12*H*)-dione hydrochloride. Its structural formula is as follows:

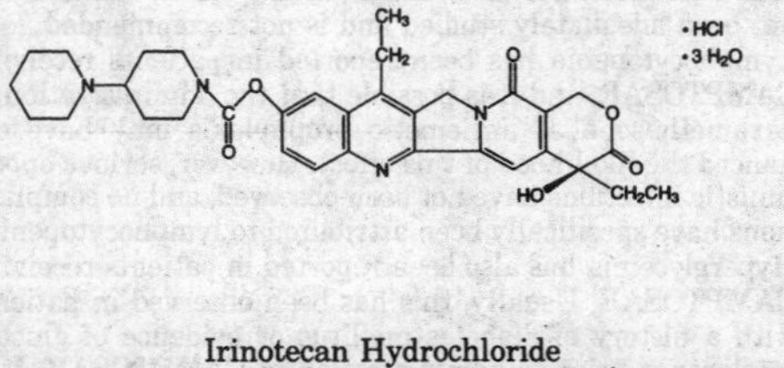

Irinotecan Hydrochloride

Irinotecan hydrochloride is a pale yellow to yellow crystalline powder, with the empirical formula $C_{33}H_{38}N_4O_6 \cdot HCl \cdot 3H_2O$ and a molecular weight of 677.19. It is slightly soluble in water and organic solvents.

CLINICAL PHARMACOLOGY

Irinotecan is a derivative of camptothecin. Camptothecine interact specifically with the enzyme topoisomerase I which relieves torsional strain in DNA by inducing reversible single-strand breaks. Irinotecan and its active metabolite SN-38 bind to the topoisomerase I - DNA complex and prevent religation of these single-strand breaks. Current research suggests that the cytotoxicity of irinotecan is due to double-strand DNA damage produced during DNA synthesis when replication enzymes interact with the ternary complex formed by topoisomerase I, DNA, and either irinotecan or SN-38. Mammalian cells cannot efficiently repair these double-strand breaks.

Irinotecan serves as a water-soluble precursor of the lipophilic metabolite SN-38. SN-38 is formed from irinotecan by carboxylesterase-mediated cleavage of the carbamate bond between the camptothecin moiety and the dipiperidino side chain. SN-38 is approximately 1000 times as potent as irinotecan as an inhibitor of topoisomerase I purified from human and rodent tumor cell lines. In vitro cytotoxicity assays show that the potency of SN-38 relative to irinotecan varies from 2- to 2000-fold. However, the plasma area under the concentration versus time curve (AUC) values for SN-38 are 2% to 8% of irinotecan and SN-38 is 95% bound to plasma proteins compared to approximately 50% bound to plasma proteins for irinotecan (see **Pharmacokinetics**). The precise contribution of SN-38 to the activity of CAMPTOSAR is thus unknown. Both irinotecan and SN-38 exist in an active lactone form and an inactive hydroxy acid anion form. A pH-dependent equilibrium exists between the two forms such that an acid pH promotes the formation of the lactone, while a more basic pH favors the hydroxy acid anion form.

Administration of irinotecan has resulted in anti-tumor activity in mice bearing cancers of rodent origin and in human carcinoma xenografts of various histological types.

Pharmacokinetics

After intravenous infusion of CAMPTOSAR in humans, irinotecan plasma concentrations decline in a multiexponential manner, with a mean terminal elimination half-life of about 6 hours. The mean terminal elimination half-life of the active metabolite SN-38 is about 10 hours. The half-lives of the lactone (active) forms of irinotecan and SN-38 are similar to those of total irinotecan and SN-38, as the lactone and hydroxy acid forms are in equilibrium.

Summary of Mean (± Standard Deviation) Irinotecan and SN–38 Pharmacokinetic Parameters in Patients With Metastatic Carcinoma of the Colon and Rectum

Dose (mg/m^2)	Irinotecan C_{max} (ng/mL)	AUC_{0-24} (ng-hr/mL)	$t_{1/2}$ (hr)	V_{area} (L/m^2)	CL ($L/hr/m^2$)	SN–38 C_{max} (ng/mL)	AUC_{0-24} (ng-hr/mL)	$t_{1/2}$ (hr)
125 (N=64)	1,680 ± 797	10,200 ± 3,270	5.8 ± 0.7	110 ± 48.5	13.3 ± 6.01	26.3 ± 11.9	229 ± 108	10.4 ± 3.1

C_{max}—Maximum plasma concentration.
AUC_{0-24}—Area under the plasma concentration-time curve from time 0 to 24 hours after the end of the 90-minute infusion.
$t_{1/2}$—Terminal elimination half-life.
V_{area}—Volume of distribution of terminal elimination phase.
CL—Total systemic clearance.

Over the dose range of 50 to 350 mg/m^2, the AUC of irinotecan increases linearly with dose; the AUC of SN-38 increases less than proportionally with dose. Maximum concentrations of the active metabolite SN-38 are generally seen within 1 hour following the end of a 90-minute infusion of CAMPTOSAR.

Irinotecan exhibits moderate plasma protein binding (30% to 68% bound) SN-38 is highly bound to human plasma proteins (approximately 95% bound). This plasma protein to which irinotecan and SN-38 predominantly binds is albumin.

[See table above.]

Metabolism and Excretion: The metabolic conversion of irinotecan to the active metabolite SN-38 is mediated by carboxylesterase enzymes and primarily occurs in the liver. SN-38 subsequently undergoes conjugation to form a glucuronide metabolite. SN-38 glucuronide had 1/50 to 1/100 the activity of SN-38 in cytotoxicity assays using two cell lines in vitro. The disposition of irinotecan has not been fully elucidated in humans. The urinary excretion of irinotecan is 11% to 20%; SN-38, <1%; and SN-38 glucuronide, 3%. The cumulative biliary and urinary excretion of irinotecan and its metabolites (SN-38 and SN-38 glucuronide) over a period of 48 hours following administration of CAMPTOSAR in two patients ranged from approximately 25% (100 mg/m^2) to 50% (300 mg/m^2).

Pharmacokinetics in Special Populations

Geriatric: The terminal half-life of irinotecan was 6.0 hours in patients who were 65 years or older and 5.5 hours in patients younger than 65 years. Dose-normalized AUC_{0-24} for SN-38 in patients who were at least 65 years of age was 11% higher than in patients younger than 65 years. No change in dosage and administration is recommended for geriatric patients.

Pediatric: The pharmacokinetics of irinotecan have not been studied in the pediatric population.

Gender: The pharmacokinetics of irinotecan do not appear to be influenced by gender.

Race: The influence of race on the pharmacokinetics of irinotecan has not been evaluated.

Hepatic Insufficiency: The influence of hepatic insufficiency on the pharmacokinetic characteristics of irinotecan and its metabolites has not been formally studied. Among patients with known hepatic tumor involvement (a majority of patients), irinotecan and SN-38 AUC values were somewhat higher than values for patients without liver metastases. For patients having liver metastases without decreased hepatic function, no change in dosage and administration is recommended.

Renal Insufficiency: The influence of renal insufficiency on the pharmacokinetics of irinotecan has not been evaluated.

Drug-Drug Interactions

Possible pharmacokinetic interactions of CAMPTOSAR with other concomitantly administered medications have not been formally investigated.

CLINICAL STUDIES

In phase 1 studies of CAMPTOSAR Injection, the maximum-tolerated dose as a single agent in the treatment of patients with solid tumors was 120 to 150 mg/m^2 when administered once weekly for 4 weeks, followed by a 2-week rest period. The dose-limiting toxicities were diarrhea and neutropenia. In one study, use of granulocyte colony-stimulating factor (G-CSF) appeared to increase the tolerated dose from 120 to 145 mg/m^2.

Data from three open-label, phase 2, single-agent clinical studies, involving a total of 304 patients in 59 centers, support the use of CAMPTOSAR in the treatment of patients with metastatic cancer of the colon or rectum that has recurred or progressed following treatment with fluorouracil (5-FU)-based therapy. These studies were designed to evaluate tumor response rate and do not provide information on actual clinical benefit, such as effect on survival and disease-related symptoms. In each study, CAMPTOSAR was administered in repeated 6-week courses consisting of a 90-minute intravenous infusion once weekly for 4 weeks, followed by a 2-week rest period. Starting doses of CAMPTOSAR in these trials were 100, 125, or 150 mg/m^2, but the 150 mg/m^2 dose proved poorly tolerated (unacceptably high rates of grade 4 late diarrhea and febrile neutropenia). Study 1 enrolled 48 patients and was conducted under the auspices of a single investigator at several regional hospitals. Study 2 was a multicenter study conducted by the North Central Cancer Treatment Group. All 90 patients enrolled in Study 2 received a starting dose of 125 mg/m^2. Study 3 was a multicenter study that enrolled 166 patients from 30 institutions. The initial dose in Study 3 was 125 mg/m^2 but was reduced to 100 mg/m^2 because the toxicity seen at the 125 mg/m^2 dose was perceived to be greater than that seen in previous studies. All patients in these studies had metastatic colorectal cancer, and the majority had disease that recurred or progressed following a 5-FU-based regimen administered for metastatic disease.

The results of the individual studies are shown in the following table:

[See table at bottom of next page.]

In the intent-to-treat analysis of the pooled data across all three studies, 193 of the 304 patients began therapy at the recommended starting dose of 125 mg/m^2. Among these 193 patients, 2 complete and 27 partial responses were observed, for an overall response rate of 15.0% (95% Confidence Interval [CI], 10.0% to 20.1%) at this starting dose. A considerably lower response rate was seen with a starting dose of 100 mg/m^2. The majority of responses were observed within the first two courses of therapy, and all but one of the responses were observed by the fourth course of therapy (one response was observed after the eighth course). The response duration (median) for patients beginning therapy at 125 mg/m^2 was 5.8 months (range, 2.6 to 15.1 months).

Response rates to CAMPTOSAR were similar in males and females and among patients older and younger than 65 years. Rates were also similar in patients with cancer of the colon or cancer of the rectum and in patients with single and multiple metastatic sites. Response rate was 18.5% in patients with a performance status of 0 and 7.6% in patients with a performance status of 1 or 2. Patients with a performance status of 3 or 4 have not been studied. Over half of the patients responding to CAMPTOSAR had not responded to prior 5-FU-based treatment given for metastatic disease.

Patients who had received previous irradiation to the pelvis also responded to CAMPTOSAR at approximately the same rate as those who had not previously received irradiation.

INDICATIONS AND USAGE

CAMPTOSAR Injection is indicated for the treatment of patients with metastatic carcinoma of the colon or rectum whose disease has recurred or progressed following 5-FU-based therapy.

CONTRAINDICATIONS

CAMPTOSAR is contraindicated in patients with a known hypersensitivity to the drug.

WARNINGS

Diarrhea:

CAMPTOSAR Injection can induce both early and late forms of diarrhea that appear to be mediated by different mechanisms. Early diarrhea (occurring during or within 24 hours of administration of CAMPTOSAR) is cholinergic in nature. It can be severe but is usually transient. It may be

Continued on next page

Information on these Pharmacia & Upjohn products is based on labeling in effect June 1, 1996. Further information concerning these and other Pharmacia & Upjohn products may be obtained by direct inquiry to Medical Information, Pharmacia & Upjohn, Kalamazoo, MI 49001.

Pharmacia & Upjohn—Cont.

preceded by complaints of diaphoresis and abdominal cramping. Early diarrhea may be ameliorated by administration of atropine (see PRECAUTIONS, General, for dosing recommendations for atropine).

Late diarrhea (occurring more than 24 hours after administration of CAMPTOSAR) can be prolonged, may lead to dehydration and electrolyte imbalance, and can be life-threatening. Late diarrhea should be treated promptly with loperamide (see PRECAUTIONS, Information for Patients, for dosing recommendations for loperamide). Patients with severe diarrhea should be carefully monitored and given fluid and electrolyte replacement if they become dehydrated. National Cancer Institute (NCI) grade 3 diarrhea is defined as an increase of 7 to 9 stools daily, or incontinence, or severe cramping and NCI grade 4 diarrhea is defined as an increase of $\geq$ 10 stools daily, or grossly bloody stool, or need for parenteral support. If grade 3 or 4 late diarrhea occurs, administration of CAMPTOSAR should be delayed until the patient recovers and subsequent doses should be decreased (see DOSAGE AND ADMINISTRATION).

Myelosuppression:
Deaths due to sepsis following severe myelosuppression have been reported in patients treated with CAMPTOSAR. Therapy with CAMPTOSAR should be temporarily discontinued if neutropenic fever occurs or if the absolute neutrophil count drops below 500/mm^3. The dose of CAMPTOSAR should be reduced if there is a clinically significant decrease in the total white blood cell count ($<$2000/mm^3), neutrophil count ($<$1000/mm^3), hemoglobin ($<$8 gm/dL), or platelet count ($<$100,000/mm^3) (see DOSAGE AND ADMINISTRATION). Routine administration of a colony-stimulating factor (CSF) is not necessary, but physicians may wish to consider CSF use in individual patients experiencing significant neutropenia.

Pregnancy:
CAMPTOSAR may cause fetal harm when administered to a pregnant woman. Radioactivity related to ^{14}C-irinotecan crosses the placenta of rats following intravenous administration of 10 mg/kg (which in separate studies produced an irinotecan C_{max} and AUC about 3 and 0.5 times, respectively, the corresponding values in patients administered 125 mg/m^2). Administration of 6 mg/kg/day intravenous irinotecan to rats (which in separate studies produced an irinotecan C_{max} and AUC about 2 and 0.2 times, respectively, the corresponding values in patients administered 125 mg/m^2) and rabbits (about one-half the recommended human dose on a mg/m^2 basis) during the period of organogenesis, is embryotoxic as characterized by increased post-implantation loss and decreased numbers of live fetuses. Irinotecan was teratogenic in rats at doses greater than 1.2 mg/kg/day (which in separate studies produced an irinotecan C_{max} and AUC about 2/3 and 1/40th, respectively, of the corresponding values in patients administered 125 mg/m^2) and in rabbits at 6.0 mg/kg/day (about one-half the recommended weekly human dose on a mg/m^2 basis). Teratogenic effects included a variety of external, visceral, and skeletal abnormalities. Irinotecan administered to rat dams for the period following organogenesis through weaning at doses of 6 mg/kg/day caused decreased learning ability and decreased female body weights in the offspring. There are no adequate and well-controlled studies of irinotecan in pregnant women. If the drug is used during pregnancy, or if the patient becomes pregnant while receiving this drug, the patient should be apprised of the potential hazard to the fetus. Women of childbearing potential should be advised to avoid becoming pregnant while receiving treatment with CAMPTOSAR.

PRECAUTIONS

General
Care of Intravenous Site:
CAMPTOSAR is administered by intravenous infusion. Care should be taken to avoid extravasation, and the infusion site should be monitored for signs of inflammation. Should extravasation occur, flushing the site with sterile water and application of ice are recommended.

Premedication with Antiemetics:
Irinotecan is emetigenic. It is recommended that patients receive premedication with antiemetic agents. In clinical studies, the majority of patients received 10 mg of dexamethasone given in conjunction with another type of antiemetic agent, such as a 5-HT$_3$ blocker (eg, ondansetron or granisetron). Antiemetic agents should be given on the day of treatment, starting at least 30 minutes before administration of CAMPTOSAR. Physicians should also consider providing patients with an antiemetic regimen (eg, prochlorperazine) for subsequent use as needed.

Treatment of Early Diarrhea:
Administration of 0.25 to 1 mg of intravenous atropine should be considered (unless clinically contraindicated) in patients experiencing diaphoresis, abdominal cramping, or early diarrhea (diarrhea occurring during or within 24 hours following administration of CAMPTOSAR).

Patients at Particular Risk:
Physicians should exercise particular caution in monitoring the effects of CAMPTOSAR in the elderly ($\geq$ 65 years) and in patients who had previously received pelvic/abdominal irradiation (see ADVERSE REACTIONS).

Information for Patients
Patients and patients' caregivers should be informed of the expected toxic effects of CAMPTOSAR, particularly of its gastrointestinal manifestations, such as nausea, vomiting, and diarrhea. Each patient should be instructed to have loperamide readily available and to begin treatment for late diarrhea (occurring more than 24 hours after administration of CAMPTOSAR) at the first episode of poorly formed or loose stools or the earliest onset of bowel movements more frequent than normally expected for the patient. One dosage regimen for loperamide used in clinical trials consisted of the following (Note: This dosage regimen exceeds the usual dosage recommendations for loperamide.): 4 mg at the first onset of late diarrhea and then 2 mg every 2 hours until the patient is diarrhea-free for at least 12 hours. During the night, the patient may take 4 mg of loperamide every 4 hours. The patient should also be instructed to notify the physician if diarrhea occurs. Premedication with loperamide is not recommended.

The use of drugs with laxative properties should be avoided because of the potential for exacerbation of diarrhea. Patients should be advised to contact their physician to discuss any laxative use.

Patients should consult their physician if vomiting occurs, fever or evidence of infection develops, or if symptoms of dehydration, such as fainting, lightheadedness, or dizziness, are noted following therapy with CAMPTOSAR.

Patients should be alerted to the possibility of alopecia.

Laboratory Tests
Careful monitoring of the white blood cell count with differential, hemoglobin, and platelet count is recommended before each dose of CAMPTOSAR.

Drug Interactions
The adverse effects of CAMPTOSAR, such as myelosuppression and diarrhea, would be expected to be exacerbated by other antineoplastic agents having similar adverse effects. Patients who have previously received pelvic/abdominal irradiation are at increased risk of severe myelosuppression following the administration of CAMPTOSAR. The concurrent administration of CAMPTOSAR with irradiation has not been adequately studied and is not recommended.

Lymphocytopenia has been reported in patients receiving CAMPTOSAR, and it is possible that the administration of dexamethasone as antiemetic prophylaxis may have enhanced the likelihood of this effect. However, serious opportunistic infections have not been observed, and no complications have specifically been attributed to lymphocytopenia. Hyperglycemia has also been reported in patients receiving CAMPTOSAR. Usually, this has been observed in patients with a history of diabetes mellitus or evidence of glucose intolerance prior to administration of CAMPTOSAR. It is probable that dexamethasone, given as antiemetic prophylaxis, contributed to hyperglycemia in some patients.

The incidence of akathisia in clinical trials was greater (8.5%, 4/47 patients) when prochlorperazine was administered on the same day as CAMPTOSAR than when these drugs were given on separate days (1.3%, 1/80 patients). The 8.5% incidence of akathisia, however, is within the range reported for use of prochlorperazine when given as a premedication for other chemotherapies.

It would be expected that laxative use during therapy with CAMPTOSAR would worsen the incidence or severity of diarrhea, but this has not been studied.

In view of the potential risk of dehydration secondary to vomiting and/or diarrhea induced by CAMPTOSAR, the physician may wish to withhold diuretics during dosing with CAMPTOSAR and, certainly, during periods of active vomiting or diarrhea.

Drug-Laboratory Test Interactions
There are no known interactions between CAMPTOSAR and laboratory tests.

Carcinogenesis, Mutagenesis & Impairment of Fertility
Long-term carcinogenicity studies with irinotecan were not conducted. Rats were, however, administered intravenous doses of 2 mg/kg or 25 mg/kg irinotecan once per week for 13 weeks (in separate studies, the 25 mg/kg dose produced an irinotecan C_{max} and AUC that were about 7.0 times and 1.3 times the respective values in patients administered 125 mg/m^2) and were then allowed to recover for 91 weeks. Under these conditions, there was a significant linear trend with dose for the incidence of combined uterine horn endometrial stromal polyps and endometrial stromal sarcomas. Neither irinotecan or SN-38 was mutagenic in the in vitro Ames assay. Irinotecan was clastogenic both in vitro (chromosome aberrations in Chinese hamster ovary cells) and in vivo (micronucleus test in mice). No significant adverse effects on fertility and general reproductive performance were observed after intravenous administration of irinotecan in doses of up to 6 mg/kg/day to rats and rabbits. However, atrophy of male reproductive organs was observed after multiple daily irinotecan doses both rodents at 20 mg/kg (which in separate studies produced an irinotecan C_{max} and AUC about 5 and 1 times, respectively, the corresponding values in patients administered 125 mg/m^2) and dogs at 0.4 mg/kg (which in separate studies produced an irinotecan C_{max} and AUC about one-half and 1/15th, respectively, the corresponding values in patients administered 125 mg/m^2).

	Study			
	1	**2**		**3**
Number of Patients	48	90	64	102
Dose (mg/m^2/wk $\times$ 4)	125*	125	125	100
Male (%)	54	64	50	49
Age $<$65 yr (%)	54	54	64	54
Ethnic Origin (%)				
White	79.2	95.6	81.3	91.2
African American	12.5	4.4	10.9	4.9
Hispanic	8.3	0.0	7.8	2.0
Oriental/Asian	0.0	0.0	0.0	2.0
Performance Status 0 (%)	60	38	59	44
Performance Status 1 (%)	38	48	33	51
Performance Status 2 (%)	2	14	8	5
Prior 5-FU Therapy (%)				
For Metastatic Disease	81.3	65.5	73.4	67.7
$\leq$6 months after Adjuvant	14.6	6.7	26.6	27.5
$>$6 months after Adjuvant	2.1	15.6	0.0	2.0
Classification Unknown	2.1	12.2	0.0	2.9
Primary Tumor (%)				
Colon	100	71	89	87
Rectum	0	29	11	8
Number of Courses of CAMPTOSAR (median)	3.5	3.0	3.0	3.0
Median Dose Intensity† (mg/m^2/wk)	62	56	61	54
Objective Response Rate (%)‡	20.8	13.3	14.1	7.8
(95% Cl)	[9.3, 32.3]	[6.3, 20.4]	[5.5, 22.6]	[2.6, 13.1]
Time to Response (median, months)	2.6	2.1	2.8	2.8
Response Duration (median, months)	6.4	5.9	5.6	6.2
Survival (median, months)	10.4	8.1	10.7	9.3

* Nine patients received 150 mg/m^2 as a starting dose; 2 (22.2%) responded to CAMPTOSAR.
† Total dose administered in a course ÷ 6 (number of weeks in a course).
‡ There were 2/304 complete responses; the remainder were partial responses.

Pregnancy

Pregnancy Category D—see WARNINGS.

Nursing Mothers

Radioactivity appeared in rat milk within 5 minutes of intravenous administration of radio-labeled irinotecan and was concentrated up to 65-fold at 4 hours after administration relative to plasma concentrations. Because many drugs are excreted in human milk and because of the potential for serious adverse reactions in nursing infants, it is recommended that nursing be discontinued when receiving therapy with CAMPTOSAR.

Pediatric Use

The safety and effectiveness of CAMPTOSAR in pediatric patients have not been established.

ADVERSE REACTIONS

US Clinical Trials

In three clinical studies, 304 patients with metastatic carcinoma of the colon or rectum that had recurred or progressed following 5-FU-based therapy were treated with CAMPTOSAR. Seventeen of the patients died within 30 days of the administration of CAMPTOSAR; in five cases (1.6%, 5/304), the deaths were potentially drug-related. These five patients experienced a constellation of medical events that included known effects of CAMPTOSAR.

One of these patients died of neutropenic sepsis without fever. Neutropenic fever, defined as NCl grade 4 neutropenia and grade 2 or greater fever, occurred in nine (3.0%) other patients; these patients recovered with supportive care. One hundred and nineteen (39.1%) of the 304 patients were hospitalized a total of 156 times because of adverse events; 81 (26.6%) patients were hospitalized for events judged to be related to administration of irinotecan. The primary reasons for drug-related hospitalization were diarrhea, with or without nausea and/or vomiting (18.4%); neutropenia/leukopenia, with or without diarrhea and/or fever (8.2%); and nausea and/or vomiting (4.9%). Adjustments in the dose of CAMPTOSAR were made during the course of treatment and for subsequent courses based on individual patient tolerance. The first dose of at least one course of CAMPTOSAR was reduced for 67% of patients who began the studies at the 125 mg/m^2 starting dose. Within-course dose reductions were required for 32% of the courses initiated at the 125 mg/m^2 dose level. The most common reasons for dose reduction were late diarrhea, neutropenia, and leukopenia. Thirteen (4.3%) patients discontinued treatment with CAMPTOSAR because of adverse events. The adverse events in the following table are based on the experience of the 304 patients enrolled in the three studies described in the CLINICAL STUDIES section.

Adverse Events Occurring in > 10% of 304 Previously Treated Patients with Metastatic Carcinoma of the Colon or Rectum

Body System & Event	% of Patients Reporting NCI Grades 1–4	NCI Grades 3 & 4
GASTROINTESTINAL		
Diarrhea (late)*	87.8	30.6
7–9 stools/day (grade 3)	—	(16.4)
≥ 10 stools/day (grade 4)	—	(14.1)
Nausea	86.2	16.8
Vomiting	66.8	12.5
Anorexia	54.9	5.9
Diarrhea (early)†	50.7	7.9
Constipation	29.9	2.0
Flatulence	12.2	0
Stomatitis	11.8	0.7
Dyspepsia	10.5	0
HEMATOLOGIC		
Leukopenia	63.2	28.0
Anemia	60.5	6.9
Neutropenia	53.9	26.3
500 to < 1000/mm^3 (grade 3)	—	(14.8)
< 500/mm^3 (grade 4)	—	(11.5)
BODY AS A WHOLE		
Asthenia	75.7	12.2
Abdominal cramping/pain	56.9	16.4
Fever	45.4	0.7
Pain	23.7	2.3
Headache	16.8	0.7
Back pain	14.5	1.6
Chills	13.8	0.3
Minor Infection‡	14.5	0
Edema	10.2	1.3
Abdominal Enlargement	10.2	0.3
METABOLIC & NUTRITIONAL		
↓Body weight	30.3	0.7
Dehydration	14.8	4.3
↑Alkaline phosphatase	13.2	3.9
↑SGOT	10.5	1.3
DERMATOLOGIC		
Alopecia	60.5	NA§
Sweating	16.4	0
Rash	12.8	0.7
RESPIRATORY		
Dyspnea	22.0	3.6
↑Coughing	17.4	0.3
Rhinitis	15.5	0
NEUROLOGIC		
Insomnia	19.4	0
Dizziness	14.8	0
CARDIOVASCULAR		
Vasodilation (Flushing)	11.2	0

* Occurring > 24 hours after administration of CAMPTOSAR.

† Occurring ≤ 24 hours after administration of CAMPTOSAR.

‡ Primarily upper respiratory infections.

§ Not applicable; complete hair loss = NCI grade 2.

STUDIES

Gastrointestinal: Diarrhea, nausea, and vomiting were common adverse events following treatment with CAMPTOSAR and could be severe. These events occurred early (during or within 24 hours of administration of CAMPTOSAR) or late (more than 24 hours after administration of CAMPTOSAR). The median time to onset of late diarrhea was 11 days following administration of CAMPTOSAR. For patients starting treatment at the 125 mg/m^2 dose, the median duration of any grade of diarrhea was 3 days. Among those patients treated at the 125 mg/m^2 dose who experienced grade 3 or 4 diarrhea, the median duration of the entire episode of diarrhea was 7 days. The frequency of grade 3 or 4 late diarrhea was somewhat greater in patients starting treatment at 125 mg/m^2 than in patients given a 100 mg/m^2 starting dose (34% versus 24%). The frequency of grade 3 and 4 late diarrhea was significantly greater in patients ≥ 65 years than in patients < 65 years of age (39.8% versus 23.4%; $p = 0.0025$). In Study 2, the frequency of grade 3 and 4 late diarrhea was significantly greater in male than in female patients (43.1% versus 15.6%; $p = 0.01$). However, there were no gender differences in the frequency of grade 3 and 4 late diarrhea in the other two studies.

Hematology: CAMPTOSAR commonly caused neutropenia, leukopenia (including lymphocytopenia), and anemia. Serious thrombocytopenia was uncommon. Neutropenic fever (concurrent NCl grade 4 neutropenia and fever of grade 2 or greater) occurred in 3.0% of the patients; 5.6% of patients received G-CSF for the treatment of neutropenia. NCl grade 3 or 4 anemia was noted in 6.9% of the patients. Blood transfusions were given to 9.9% of the patients. The frequency of grade 3 and 4 neutropenia was significantly higher in patients who received previous pelvic/abdominal irradiation than in those who had not received irradiation (48.1% versus 24.1%; $p = 0.0356$). There were no significant differences in the frequency of grade 3 and 4 neutropenia by age or gender.

Body as a Whole: Asthenia, fever, and abdominal pain were the most common events of this type.

Hepatic: NCl grade 3 or 4 liver enzyme abnormalities were observed in fewer than 10% of patients. These events typically occurred in patients with known hepatic metastases.

Dermatologic: Alopecia was reported during treatment with CAMPTOSAR. Rashes have also been reported but did not result in discontinuation of treatment.

Respiratory: Severe pulmonary events were infrequent; NCl grade 3 or 4 dyspnea was reported in 3.6% of patients. Over half the patients with dyspnea had lung metastases; the extent to which malignant pulmonary involvement or other preexisting lung disease may have contributed to dyspnea in these patients is unknown.

Neurologic: Insomnia and dizziness were observed, but were not usually considered to be directly related to the administration of CAMPTOSAR. Dizziness may sometimes have represented symptomatic evidence of orthostatic hypotension in patients with dehydration.

Cardiovascular: Vasodilation (flushing) has been observed during administration of CAMPTOSAR but has not required intervention.

Non-US Clinical Trials

Irinotecan has been studied in over 1100 patients in Japan and in over 400 patients in France. Patients in these studies had a variety of tumor types, including cancer of the colon or rectum, and were treated with several different doses and schedules. In general, the types of toxicities observed were similar to those seen in US trials with CAMPTOSAR. There is some information from Japanese trials that patients with considerable ascites or pleural effusions were at increased risk for neutropenia or diarrhea. A potentially life-threatening pulmonary syndrome, consisting or dyspnea, fever, and a reticulondular pattern on chest x-ray, was observed in a small percentage of patients in early Japanese studies. The contribution of irinotecan to these preliminary events was difficult to assess because these patients also had lung tumors and some had preexisting nonmalignant pulmonary disease. As a result of these observations, however, clinical studies in the United States have enrolled few patients with compromised pulmonary function, significant ascites, or pleural effusions.

OVERDOSAGE

In US phase 1 trials, single doses of up to 345 mg/m^2 of irinotecan injection were administered to patients with various cancers. Single doses of up to 750 mg/m^2 of irinotecan have been given in non-US trials. The adverse events in these patients were similar to those reported with the recommended dosage and regimen. There is no known antidote for overdosage of CAMPTOSAR. Maximum supportive care should be instituted to prevent dehydration due to diarrhea and to treat any infectious complications.

Lethality was observed after single intravenous irinotecan doses of approximately 111 mg/kg in mice and 73 mg/kg in rats (approximately 2.6 and 3.4 times the recommended human dose of 125 mg/m^2, respectively). Death was preceded by cyanosis, tremors, respiratory distress, and convulsions.

DOSAGE AND ADMINISTRATION

Starting Dose and Dose Modifications

The recommended starting dose of CAMPTOSAR Injection is 125 mg/m^2. All doses should be administered as an intravenous infusion over 90 minutes (see Preparation of Infusion Solution). The recommended treatment regimen (one treatment course) is 125 mg/m^2 administered once weekly for 4 weeks, followed by a 2-week rest period. Thereafter, additional courses of treatment may be repeated every 6 weeks (4 weeks on therapy, followed by 2 weeks off therapy). Subsequent doses should be adjusted to as high as 150 mg/m^2 or to as low as 50 mg/m^2 in 25 to 50 mg/m^2 increments depending upon individual patient tolerance of treatment (see Recommended Dose Modifications table at right). Provided intolerable toxicity does not develop, treatment with additional courses of CAMPTOSAR may be continued indefinitely in patients who attain a response or in patients whose disease remains stable. Patients should be carefully monitored for toxicity.

The table at right describes the recommended dose modifications during a course of therapy and at the start of each subsequent course of therapy. These recommendations are based on toxicities commonly observed with the administration of CAMPTOSAR. Therapy with CAMPTOSAR should be interrupted when grade 3 or 4 late diarrhea occurs (see PRECAUTIONS, Information for Patients) or when other intolerable toxicity is observed. Dose modifications for hematologic toxicities other than neutropenia (eg, leukopenia, anemia or thrombocytopenia, and platelets) during a course of therapy and at the start of a subsequent course of therapy are the same as recommended for neutropenia.

Dose modifications for nonhematologic toxicities other than diarrhea (nausea, vomiting, etc) during a course of therapy are the same as those recommended for diarrhea. At the start of subsequent course of therapy, the dose of CAMPTOSAR should be decreased by 25 mg/m^2, compared to the initial dose of the previous course, for other NCl grade 2 or by 50 mg/m^2 for other grade 3 or 4 nonhematologic toxicities. All dose modifications should be based on the worst preceding toxicity. A new course of therapy should not begin until the granulocyte count has recovered to ≥ 1500/mm^3 and the platelet count has recovered to ≥ 100,000/mm^3 and treatment-related diarrhea is fully resolved. Treatment should be delayed 1 to 2 weeks to allow for recovery from treatment-related toxicity. If the patient has not recovered after a 2-week delay, consideration should be given to discontinuing CAMPTOSAR.

It is recommended that patients receive premedication with antiemetic agents (see PRECAUTIONS, General).

Preparation & Administration Precautions

As with other potentially toxic anticancer agents, care should be exercised in the handling and preparation of infusion solutions prepared from CAMPTOSAR injection. The use of gloves is recommended. If a solution of CAMPTOSAR contacts the skin, wash the skin immediately and thoroughly with soap and water. If CAMPTOSAR contacts the mucous membranes, flush thoroughly with water. Several published guidelines for handling and disposal of anticancer agents are available.[1–7]

Continued on next page

Information on these Pharmacia & Upjohn products is based on labeling in effect June 1, 1996. Further information concerning these and other Pharmacia & Upjohn products may be obtained by direct inquiry to Medical Information, Pharmacia & Upjohn, Kalamazoo, MI 49001.

Pharmacia & Upjohn—Cont.

Preparation of Infusion Solution

Inspect vial contents for particulate matter and repeat inspection when drug product is withdrawn from vial into syringe.

CAMPTOSAR Injection must be diluted prior to infusion. CAMPTOSAR should be diluted in 5% Dextrose Injection, USP, (preferred) or 0.9% Sodium Chloride Injection, USP, to a final concentration range of 0.12 to 1.1 mg/mL. In most clinical trials, CAMPTOSAR was administered in 500 mL of 5% Dextrose Injection, USP.

The solution is physically and chemically stable for up to 24 hours at room temperature (approximately 25°C) and in ambient fluorescent lighting. Solutions diluted in 5% Dextrose Injection, USP, and stored at refrigerated temperatures (approximately 2° to 8°C), and protected from light are physically and chemically stable for 48 hours. Refrigeration of admixtures using 0.9% Sodium Chloride Injection, USP, is not recommended due to a low and sporadic incidence of visible particulates. Freezing CAMPTOSAR and admixtures of CAMPTOSAR may result in precipitation of the drug and should be avoided. Because of possible microbial contamination during dilution, it is advisable to use the admixture within 24 hours if refrigerated (2° to 8°C, 36° to 46°F) or within 6 hours if kept at room temperature (15° to 30°C, 59° to 86°F).

[See table below.]

Other drugs should not be added to the infusion solution. Parenteral drug products should be inspected visually for particulate matter and discoloration prior to administration whenever solution and container permit.

HOW SUPPLIED

Each mL of CAMPTOSAR Injection contains 20 mg irinotecan (on the basis of the trihydrate salt); 45 mg sorbitol; and 0.9 mg lactic acid. When necessary, pH has been adjusted to 3.5 (range, 3.0 to 3.8) with sodium hydroxide or hydrochloric acid.

CAMPTOSAR Injection is available as single-dose vials in the following package size:

5 mL amber glass vial NDC 0009-7529-01

This is packaged in a backing/plastic blister to protect against inadvertent breakage and leakage. The vial should be inspected for damage and visible signs of leaks before removing the bakcing/plastic blister. If damaged, incinerate the unopened package.

Store at controlled room temperature 15° to 30°C (59° to 86°F). Protect from light. It is recommended that the vial (and backing/plastic blister) should remain in the carton until the time of use.

Caution: Federal law prohibits dispensing without prescription.

REFERENCES

1. Recommendations for the Safe Handling of Parenteral Antineoplastic Drugs. NIH Publication No. 83-2621. For sale by the Superintendent of Documents, US Government Printing Office, Washington, DC 20402.
2. AMA Council Report. Guidelines for handling parenteral antineoplastics. JAMA 1985; 253(11): 1590–2.
3. National Study Commission on Cytotoxic Exposure. Recommendations for handling cytotoxic agents. Available from Louis P. Jeffrey, ScD, Chairman, National Study Commission on Cytotoxic Exposure, Massachusetts College of Pharmacy and Allied Health Sciences, 179 Longwood Avenue, Boston, MA 02115.
4. Clinical Oncological Society of Australia. Guidelines and recommendations for safe handling of antineoplastic agents. Med J Australia 1983;1:426–8.
5. Jones RB, et. al. Safe handling of chemotherapeutic agents: a report from the Mount Sinai Medical Center. CA-A Cancer J for Clinicians, 1983;Sept./Oct. 258–63.
6. American Society of Hospital Pharmacists Technical Assistance Bulletin on handling cytotoxic and hazardous drugs. Am J Hosp Pharm 1990; 47:1033–49.
7. OSHA work-practice guidelines for personnel dealing with cytotoxic (antineoplastic) drugs. Am J Hosp Pharm 1986;43:1193–1204.

Manufactured by Pharmacia & Upjohn Company, Kalamazoo, Michigan 49001, USA
Licensed from Yakult Honsha Co, LTD, Japan, and Daiichi Pharmaceutical Co, LTD, Japan
June 1996

816 907 000
692053

Recommended Dose Modifications†

A new course of therapy should not begin until the granulocyte count has recovered to $\geq 1500/mm^3$, and the platelet count has recovered to $\geq 100,000/mm^3$, and treatment-related diarrhea is fully resolved. Treatment should be delayed 1 to 2 weeks to allow for recovery from treatment-related toxicities. If the patient has not recovered after a 2-week delay, consideration should be given to discontinuing CAMPTOSAR.

Toxicity NCI Grade* (Value)	During a Course of Therapy†	At the Start of the Next Courses of Therapy† (After Adequate Recovery), Compared to the Starting Dose in the Previous Course
No toxicity	Maintain dose level	↑25 mg/m² up to a maximum dose of 150 mg/m²
Neutropenia		
1 (1500 to 1900/mm³)	Maintain dose level	Maintain dose level
2 (1000 to 1400/mm³)	↓25 mg/m²	Maintain dose level
3 (500 to 900/mm³)	Omit dose, then ↓25 mg/m² when resolved to ≤ grade 2	↓25 mg/m²
4 (<500/mm³)	Omit dose, then ↓50 mg/m² when resolved to ≤ grade 2	↓50 mg/m²
Neutropenic fever (grade 4 neutropenia & ≥ grade 2 fever)	Omit dose, then ↓50 mg/m² when resolved	↓50 mg/m²
Other hematologic toxicities	Dose modifications for leukopenia, thrombocytopenia, and anemia during a course of therapy and at the start of subsequent courses of therapy are also based on NCI toxicity criteria and are the same as recommended for neutropenia above.	
Diarrhea		
1 (2–3 stools/day > pretx‡)	Maintain dose level	Maintain dose level
2 (4–6 stools/day > pretx)	↓25 mg/m²	Maintain, if the only grade 2 tox§
3 (7–9 stools/day > pretx)	Omit dose, then ↓25 mg/m² when resolved to ≤ grade 2	↓25 mg/m², if the only grade 3 tox
4 (≥10 stools/day > pretx)	Omit dose, then ↓50 mg/m² when resolved to ≤ grade 2	↓50 mg/m²
Other nonhematologic toxicities		
1	Maintain dose level	Maintain dose level
2	↓25 mg/m²	↓25 mg/m²
3	Omit dose, then ↓25 mg/m² when resolved to ≤ grade 2	↓50 mg/m²
4	Omit dose, then ↓50 mg/m² when resolved to ≤ grade 2	↓50 mg/m²

* National Cancer Institute Common Toxicity Criteria.
† All dose modifications should be based on the worst preceding toxicity.
‡ Pretreatment.
§ Toxicity.

CAVERJECT®
brand of alprostadil for injection
For Intracavernosal Use

℞

DESCRIPTION

CAVERJECT Sterile Powder contains alprostadil as the naturally occurring form of prostaglandin E₁ (PGE₁) and is designated chemically as (11α,13E,15S)-11,15-dihydroxy-9-oxoprost-13-en-1-oic acid. The molecular weight is 354.49. Alprostadil is a white to off-white crystalline powder with a melting point between 115° and 116°C. Its solubility at 35°C is 8000 micrograms per 100 milliliter double distilled water. CAVERJECT is available as a sterile freeze-dried powder for intracavernosal use in two sizes: 10-microgram vial—When reconstituted as directed with 1 milliliter of bacteriostatic water for injection or sterile water, both preserved with benzyl alcohol 0.945% w/v, gives 1.13 milliliters of reconstituted solution. Each milliliter contains 10.5 micrograms alprostadil, 172 milligrams lactose, 47 micrograms sodium citrate, and 8.4 milligrams benzyl alcohol. The deliverable amount of alprostadil in each milliliter is 10 micrograms because approximately 0.5 microgram is lost due to adsorption to the vial and syringe; 20-microgram vial—When reconstituted as directed with 1 milliliter of bacteriostatic water for injection or sterile water, both preserved with benzyl alcohol 0.945% w/v, gives 1.13 milliliters of reconstituted solution. Each milliliter contains 20.5 micrograms alprostadil, 172 milligrams lactose, 47 micrograms sodium citrate, and 8.4 milligrams benzyl alcohol. The deliverable amount of alprostadil in each milliliter is 20 micrograms because approximately 0.5 microgram is lost due to adsorption to the vial and syringe. When necessary, the pH of alprostadil for injection was adjusted with hydrochloric acid and/or sodium hydroxide before lyophilization. The structural formula of alprostadil is represented below:

CLINICAL PHARMACOLOGY

Alprostadil has a wide variety of pharmacological actions; vasodilation and inhibition of platelet aggregation are among the most notable of these effects. In most animal species tested, alprostadil relaxed retractor penis and corpus cavernosum urethrae *in vitro*. Alprostadil also relaxed isolated preparations of human corpus cavernosum and spongiosum, as well as cavernous arterial segments contracted by either noradrenaline or PGF₂α *in vitro*. In pigtail monkeys (*Macaca nemestrina*), alprostadil increased cavernous arterial blood flow *in vivo*. The degree and duration of cavernous smooth muscle relaxation in this animal model was dose-dependent.

Alprostadil induces erection by relaxation of trabecular smooth muscle and by dilation of cavernosal arteries. This leads to expansion of lacunar spaces and entrapment of blood by compressing the venules against the tunica albuginea, a process referred to as the corporal veno-occlusive mechanism.

Pharmacokinetics:

Absorption: For the treatment of erectile dysfunction, alprostadil is administered by injection into the corpora cavernosa. The absolute bioavailibility of alprostadil has not been determined.

Distribution: Following intracavernosal injection of 20 micrograms alprostadil, mean peripheral plasma concentrations of alprostadil at 30 and 60 minutes after injection (89 and 102 picograms/milliliter, respectively) were not significantly greater than baseline levels of endogenous alprostadil (96 picograms/milliliter). Alprostadil is bound in plasma primarily to albumin (81% bound) and to a lesser extent α-globulin IV-4 fraction (55% bound). No significant binding to erythrocytes or white blood cells was observed.

Metabolism: Alprostadil is rapidly converted to compounds which are further metabolized prior to excretion. Following intravenous administration, approximately 80% of circulating alprostadil is metabolized in one pass through the lungs, primarily by *beta*- and *omega*-oxidation. Hence, any alprostadil entering the systemic circulation following intracavernosal injection is very rapidly metabolized. Following intracavernosal injection of 20 micrograms alprostadil, peripheral levels of the major circulating metabolite, 13, 14-dihydro-15-oxo-PGE₁, increased to reach a peak 30 minutes after injection and returned to pre-dose levels by 60 minutes after injection.

Excretion: The metabolites of alprostadil are excreted primarily by the kidney, with almost 90% of an administered intravenous dose excreted in urine within 24 hours postdose. The remainder of the dose is excreted in the feces.

There is no evidence of tissue retention of alprostadil or its metabolites following intravenous administration.

Pharmacokinetics in Special Populations:

Geriatric: The potential effect of age on the pharmacokinetics of alprostadil has not been formally evaluated. In patients with acute respiratory distress syndrome (ARDS), the mean (± SD) pulmonary extraction of alprostadil was 72% ± 15% in 11 elderly patients aged 65 years or older (mean, 71 ± 6 years) and 65% ± 20% in 6 young patients aged 35 years or younger (mean, 28 ± 5 years).

Pediatric: Alprostadil plasma concentrations were measured in 10 neonates (gestational age of 34 weeks in 2 infants and 38 to 40 weeks in 8 infants) receiving steady-state intravenous infusions of alprostadil to treat underlying cardiac malformations. Infusion rates of alprostadil ranged from 5 to 50 (median, 45) nanograms/kilogram/minute, resulting in alprostadil plasma concentrations ranging between 22 and 530 (median, 56) picograms/milliliter. The wide range of alprostadil plasma concentrations in neonates reflects high variability in individual clearances of alprostadil in this patient population.

Gender: The potential influence of gender on the pharmacokinetics of alprostadil has not been formally studied in healthy subjects. Two studies determined the pulmonary extraction of alprostadil following intravascular administration in 23 patients with ARDS. The mean (± SD) pulmonary extraction was 66% ± 20% in 17 male patients and 69% ± 18% in 6 female patients, suggesting that the pharmacokinetics of alprostadil are not influenced by gender.

Race: The potential influence of race on the pharmacokinetics of alprostadil has not been formally evaluated.

Renal and Hepatic Insufficiency: Pulmonary first-pass metabolism is the primary factor influencing the systemic clearance of alprostadil. Although the pharmacokinetics of alprostadil have not been formally examined in patients with renal or hepatic insufficiency, alterations in renal or hepatic function would not be expected to have a major influence on the pharmacokinetics of alprostadil.

Pulmonary Disease: The pulmonary extraction of alprostadil following intravascular administration was reduced by 15% (66 ± 3.2% vs 78 ± 2.4%) in patients with ARDS compared with a control group of patients with normal respiratory function who were undergoing cardiopulmonary bypass surgery. Pulmonary clearance was found to vary as a function of cardiac output and pulmonary intrinsic clearance in a group of 14 patients with ARDS or at risk of developing ARDS following trauma or sepsis. In this study, the extraction efficiency of alprostadil ranged from subnormal (11%) to normal (90%), with an overall mean of 67%.

Drug-Drug Interactions: The potential for pharmacokinetic drug-drug interactions between alprostadil and other agents has not been formally studied.

INDICATION AND USAGE

CAVERJECT is indicated for the treatment of erectile dysfunction due to neurogenic, vasculogenic, psychogenic, or mixed etiology.

Intracavernosal CAVERJECT may be a useful adjunct to other diagnostic tests in the diagnosis of erectile dysfunction.

CONTRAINDICATIONS

CAVERJECT should not be used in patients who have a known hypersensitivity to the drug, in patients who have conditions that might predispose them to priapism, such as sickle cell anemia or trait, multiple myeloma, or leukemia, or in patients with anatomical deformation of the penis, such as angulation, cavernosal fibrosis, or Peyronie's disease. Patients with penile implants should not be treated with CAVERJECT.

CAVERJECT should not be used in women or children and is not for use in newborns.

CAVERJECT should not be used in men for whom sexual activity is inadvisable or contraindicated.

PRECAUTIONS

General Precautions: Priapism (erection lasting over 6 hours) is known to occur following intracavernosal administration of vasoactive substances, including CAVERJECT. The patient should be instructed to immediately report to his physician or, if unavailable, to seek immediate medical assistance for any erection that persists for longer than 6 hours. Treatment of priapism should be according to established medical practice.

The overall incidence of penile fibrosis, including Peyronie's disease, reported in clinical studies with CAVERJECT was 3%. In one self-injection clinical study where duration of use was up to 18 months, the incidence of fibrosis was 7.8%. Regular follow-up of patients, with careful examination of the penis, is strongly recommended to detect signs of penile fibrosis. Treatment with CAVERJECT should be discontinued in patients who develop penile angulation, cavernosal fibrosis, or Peyronie's disease.

Patients on anticoagulants, such as warfarin or heparin, may have increased propensity for bleeding after intracavernosal injection.

Underlying treatable medical causes of erectile dysfunction should be diagnosed and treated prior to initiation of therapy with CAVERJECT.

The safety and efficacy of combinations of CAVERJECT and other vasoactive agents have not been systematically studied. Therefore, the use of such combinations is not recommended.

The patient should be instructed not to re-use or to share needles or syringes. As with all prescription medicines, the patient should not allow anyone else to use his medicine.

Information for the Patient:

To ensure safe and effective use of CAVERJECT, the patient should be thoroughly instructed and trained in the self-injection technique before he begins intracavernosal treatment with CAVERJECT at home. The desirable dose should be established in the physician's office. The instructions for preparation of the solution of CAVERJECT should be carefully followed. Vials with precipitates or discoloration should be discarded. The reconstituted vial is designed for one use only and should be discarded after withdrawal of proper volume of the solution. The content of the reconstituted vial should not be shaken. The needle must be properly discarded after use; it must not be re-used or shared with other persons. Patient instructions for administration are included in each package of CAVERJECT.

The dose of CAVERJECT that is established in the physician's office should not be changed by the patient without consulting the physician. The patient may expect an erection to occur within 5 to 20 minutes. A standard treatment goal is to produce an erection lasting no longer than 1 hour. Generally, CAVERJECT should be used no more than 3 times per week, with at least 24 hours between each use.

Patients should be aware of possible side effects of therapy with CAVERJECT; the most frequently occurring is penile pain after injection, usually mild to moderate in severity. A potentially serious adverse reaction with intracavernosal therapy is priapism. Accordingly, the patient should be instructed to contact the physician's office immediately or, if unavailable, to seek immediate medical assistance if an erection persists for longer than 6 hours.

The patient should report any penile pain that was not present before or that increased in intensity, as well as the occurrence of nodules or hard tissue in the penis to his physician as soon as possible. As with any intravenous injection, an infection is a possibility. Patients should be instructed to report to the physician any penile redness, swelling, tenderness or curvature of the erect penis. The patient must visit the physician's office for regular checkups for assessment of the therapeutic benefit and safety of treatment with CAVERJECT.

Note: Use of intracavernosal CAVERJECT offers no protection from the transmission of sexually transmitted diseases. Individuals who use CAVERJECT should be counseled about the protective measures that are necessary to guard against the spread of sexually transmitted diseases, including the human immunodeficiency virus (HIV).

The injection of CAVERJECT can induce a small amount of bleeding at the site of injection (see ADVERSE REACTIONS section—hematoma, ecchymosis, hemorrhage at the site of injection). In patients infected with blood-borne diseases, this could increase the risk of transmission of blood-borne diseases between partners.

In clinical trials, concomitant use of agents such as antihypertensive drugs, diuretics, antidiabetic agents (including insulin), or non-steroidal anti-inflammatory drugs had no effect on the efficacy or safety of CAVERJECT.

Carcinogenesis, Mutagenesis, and Impairment of Fertility:

Long-term carcinogenicity studies have not been conducted. Rat reproductive studies indicate that alprostadil at doses of up to 0.2 milligram/kilogram/day does not adversely affect or alter rat spermatogenesis, providing a 200-fold margin of safety compared with the usual human doses. The following battery of mutagenicity assays revealed no potential for mutagenesis: bacterial mutation (Ames), alkaline elution, rat micronucleus, sister chromatid exchange, CHO/HGPRT mammalian cell forward gene mutation, and unscheduled DNA synthesis (UDS).

A 1-year irritancy study was conducted in three groups of 5 male Cynomolgus monkeys injected intracavernosally twice weekly with either vehicle or 3 or 8.25 micrograms of alprostadil per injection. An additional two groups of 6 monkeys each were injected with vehicle or with 8.25 micrograms/injection twice weekly as described previously plus they received multiple doses during weeks 44, 48, and 52. Three monkeys from each group were retained for a 4-week recovery period. There was no evidence of drug-related penile irritancy or nonpenile tissue lesions, which could be directly related to alprostadil. The irritancy which was noted for control and treated monkeys was considered to be a result of the injection procedure itself, and any lesions noted were shown to be reversible. At the end of the 4-week recovery period, the histological changes in the penis had regressed.

Pregnancy, Nursing Mothers, and Pediatric Use:

CAVERJECT is not indicated for use in newborns, children, or women.

ADVERSE REACTIONS

Local Adverse Reactions: The following local adverse reaction information was derived from controlled and uncontrolled studies, including an uncontrolled 18-month safety study.

Local Adverse Reactions Reported by ≥ 1% of Patients Treated with CAVERJECT for up to 18 Months*

Event	CAVERJECT N=1861
Penile pain	37%
Prolonged erection	4%
Penile fibrosis**	3%
Injection site hematoma	3%
Penis disorder***	3%
Injection site ecchymosis	2%
Penile rash	1%
Penile edema	1%

* Except for penile pain (2%), no significant local adverse reactions were reported by 294 patients who received 1 to 3 injections of placebo.

** See General Precautions.

*** Includes numbness, yeast infection, irritation, sensitivity, phimosis, pruritus, erythema, venous leak, penile skin tear, strange feeling of penis, discoloration of penile head, itch at tip of penis.

Penile Pain: Penile pain after intracavernosal administration of CAVERJECT was reported at least once by 37% of patients in clinical studies of up to 18 months in duration. In the majority of the cases, penile pain was rated mild or moderate in intensity. Three percent of patients discontinued treatment because of penile pain. The frequency of penile pain was 2% in 294 patients who received 1 to 3 injections of placebo.

Prolonged Erection/Priapism: In clinical trials, prolonged erection was defined as an erection that lasted for 4 to 6 hours; priapism was defined as erection that lasted 6 hours or longer. The frequency of prolonged erection after intracavernosal administration of CAVERJECT was 4%, while the frequency of priapism was 0.4%. In the majority of cases, spontaneous detumescence occurred. To minimize the chances of prolonged erection or priapism, CAVERJECT should be titrated slowly to the lowest effective dose (see DOSAGE AND ADMINISTRATION section). The patient must be instructed to immediately report to his physician or, if unavailable, to seek immediate medical assistance for any erection that persists for longer than 6 hours. If priapism is not treated immediately, penile tissue damage and permanent loss of potency may result.

Hematoma/Ecchymosis: The frequency of hematoma and ecchymosis was 3% and 2%, respectively. In most cases, hematoma/ecchymosis was judged to be a complication of a faulty injection technique. Accordingly, proper instruction of the patient in self-injection is of importance to minimize the potential of hematoma/ecchymosis (see DOSAGE AND ADMINISTRATION).

The following local adverse reactions were reported by fewer than 1% of patients after injection of CAVERJECT: balanitis, injection site hemorrhage, injection site inflammation, injection site itching, injection site swelling, injection site edema, urethral bleeding, penile warmth, numbness, yeast infection, irritation, sensitivity, phimosis, pruritus, erythema, venous leak, painful erection, and abnormal ejaculation.

Systemic Adverse Events: The following systemic adverse event information was derived from controlled and uncontrolled studies, including an uncontrolled 18-month safety study.

Systemic Adverse Events Reported by ≥ 1% of Patients Treated with CAVERJECT for up to 18 Months*

Body System/Reaction	CAVERJECT N=1861
Cardiovascular System	
Hypertension	2%
Central Nervous System	
Headache	2%
Dizziness	1%
Musculoskeletal System	
Back pain	1%
Respiratory System	
Upper respiratory infection	4%
Flu syndrome	2%
Sinusitis	2%
Nasal congestion	1%
Cough	1%

Continued on next page

Information on these Pharmacia & Upjohn products is based on labeling in effect June 1, 1996. Further information concerning these and other Pharmacia & Upjohn products may be obtained by direct inquiry to Medical Information, Pharmacia & Upjohn, Kalamazoo, MI 49001.

Pharmacia & Upjohn—Cont.

Urogenital System	
Prostatic Disorder**	2%
Miscellaneous	
Localized pain***	2%
Trauma****	2%

* No significant adverse events were reported by 294 patients who received 1 to 3 injections of placebo.
** prostatitis, pain, hypertrophy, enlargement
*** pain in various anatomical structures other than injection site
**** injuries, fractures, abrasions, lacerations, dislocations

The following systemic events, which were reported for < 1% of patients in clinical studies, were judged by investigators to be possibly related to use of CAVERJECT: testicular pain, scrotal disorder, scrotal edema, hematuria, testicular disorder, impaired urination, urinary frequency, urinary urgency, pelvic pain, hypotension, vasodilation, peripheral vascular disorder, supraventricular extrasystoles, vasovagal reactions, hypesthesia, non-generalized weakness, diaphoresis, rash, non-application site pruritus, skin neoplasm, nausea, dry mouth, increased serum creatinine, leg cramps, and mydriasis.

Hemodynamic changes, manifested as decreases in blood pressure and increases in pulse rate, were observed during clinical studies, principally at doses above 20 micrograms and above 30 micrograms of alprostadil, respectively, and appeared to be dose-dependent. However, these changes were usually clinically unimportant; only three patients discontinued the treatment because of symptomatic hypotension.

CAVERJECT had no clinically important effect on serum or urine laboratory tests.

OVERDOSAGE

Overdosage was not observed in clinical trials with CAVERJECT. If intracavernous overdose of CAVERJECT occurs, the patient should be under medical supervision until any systemic effects have resolved and/or until penile detumescence has occurred. Symptomatic treatment of any systemic symptoms would be appropriate.

DOSAGE AND ADMINISTRATION

The dose of CAVERJECT should be individualized for each patient by careful titration under supervision by the physician. In clinical studies, patients were treated with CAVERJECT in doses ranging from 0.2 to 140 micrograms; however, since 99% of patients received doses of 60 micrograms or less, doses of greater than 60 micrograms are not recommended. In general, the lowest possible effective dose should always be employed. In clinical studies, over 80% of patients experienced an erection sufficient for sexual intercourse after intracavernosal injection of CAVERJECT. A 1/2-inch, 27- to 30-gauge needle is generally recommended.

Initial Titration in Physician's Office:

Erectile Dysfunction of Vasculogenic, Psychogenic, or Mixed Etiology. Dosage titration should be initiated at 2.5 micrograms of alprostadil. If there is a partial response, the dose may be increased by 2.5 micrograms to a dose of 5 micrograms and then in increments of 5 to 10 micrograms, depending upon erectile response, until the dose that produces an erection suitable for intercourse and not exceeding a duration of 1 hour is reached. If there is no response to the initial 2.5 microgram dose, the second dose may be increased to 7.5 micrograms, followed by increments of 5 to 10 micrograms. The patient must stay in the physician's office until complete detumescence occurs. If there is no response, then the next higher dose may be given within 1 hour. If there is a response, then there should be at least a 1-day interval before the next dose is given.

Erectile Dysfunction of Pure Neurogenic Etiology (Spinal Cord Injury). Dosage titration should be initiated at 1.25 micrograms of alprostadil. The dose may be increased by 1.25 micrograms to a dose of 2.5 micrograms, followed by an increment of 2.5 micrograms to a dose of 5 micrograms, and then in 5-microgram increments until the dose that produces an erection suitable for intercourse and not exceeding a duration of 1 hour is reached. The patient must stay in the physician's office until complete detumescence occurs. If there is no response, then the next higher dose may be given within 1 hour. If there is a response, then there should be at least a 1-day interval before the next dose is given.

The majority of patients (56%) in one clinical study involving 579 patients were titrated to doses of greater than 5 micrograms but less than or equal to 20 micrograms. The mean dose at the end of the titration phase was 17.8 micrograms of alprostadil.

Maintenance Therapy:

The first injections of CAVERJECT must be done at the physician's office by medically trained personnel. Self-injection therapy by the patient can be started only after the patient is properly instructed and well trained in the self-injection technique. The physician should make a careful assessment of the patient's skills and competence with this procedure. The intracavernosal injection must be done under sterile conditions. The site of injection is usually along the dorsolateral aspect of the proximal third of the penis. Visible veins should be avoided. The side of the penis that is injected and the site of injection must be alternated; the injection site must be cleansed with an alcohol swab.

The dose of CAVERJECT that is selected for self-injection treatment should provide the patient with an erection that is satisfactory for sexual intercourse and that is maintained for no longer than 1 hour. If the duration of erection is longer than 1 hour, the dose of CAVERJECT should be reduced. Self-injection therapy for use at home should be initiated at the dose that was determined in the physician's office; however, dose adjustment, if required (up to 57% of patients in one clinical study), should be made only after consultation with the physician. The dose should be adjusted in accordance with the titration guidelines described above. The effectiveness of CAVERJECT for long-term use of up to 6 months has been documented in an uncontrolled, self-injection study. The mean dose of CAVERJECT at the end of 6 months was 20.7 micrograms in this study.

Careful and continuous follow-up of the patient while in the self-injection program must be exercised. This is especially true for the initial self-injections, since adjustments in the dose of CAVERJECT may be needed. The recommended frequency of injection is no more than 3 times weekly, with at least 24 hours between each dose. The reconstituted vial of CAVERJECT is intended for single use only and should be discarded after use. The user should be instructed in the proper disposal of the syringe, needle, and vial.

While on self-injection treatment, it is recommended that the patient visit the prescribing physician's office every 3 months. At that time, the efficacy and safety of the therapy should be assessed, and the dose of CAVERJECT should be adjusted, if needed.

CAVERJECT as an Adjunct to the Diagnosis of Erectile Dysfunction:

In the simplest diagnostic test for erectile dysfunction (pharmacologic testing), patients are monitored for the occurrence of an erection after an intracavernosal injection of CAVERJECT. Extensions of this testing are the use of CAVERJECT as an adjunct to laboratory investigations, such as duplex or Doppler imaging, ^{133}Xenon washout tests, radioisotope penogram, and penile arteriography, to allow visualization and assessment of penile vasculature. For any of these tests, a single dose of CAVERJECT that induces an erection with firm rigidity should be used.

General Procedure for Solution Preparation:

CAVERJECT is packaged in a 5-milliliter glass vial. Bacteriostatic water for injection or sterile water, both preserved with benzyl alcohol 0.945% w/v, must be used as the diluent for reconstitution. After reconstitution with 1 milliliter of diluent, the volume of the resulting solution is 1.13 milliliters. One milliliter of this solution will contain either 10.5 or 20.5 micrograms of alprostadil depending on vial strength, 172 milligrams of lactose, and 47 micrograms of sodium citrate. The deliverable amount of alprostadil is either 10 or 20 micrograms per milliliter because approximately 0.5 microgram is lost due to adsorption to the vial and syringe. After reconstitution, the solution of CAVERJECT should be used immediately and not stored or frozen. Parenteral drug products should be inspected visually for particulate matter and discoloration prior to administration whenever the solution and container permit.

HOW SUPPLIED

CAVERJECT is a dry lyophilized powder and is supplied in vials containing 11.9 micrograms or 23.2 micrograms of alprostadil for intracavernosal administration. Store at 2° to 8° C (36° to 46° F) until dispensed. After dispensing, CAVERJECT may be stored up to 3 months at or below 25° C (77° F). When reconstituted and used as directed, the deliverable amount of alprostadil is 10 and 20 micrograms, respectively. The reconstituted solution should be used immediately and not stored or frozen. Only the accompanying diluent or bacteriostatic water for injection with benzyl alcohol should be used when reconstituting CAVERJECT.

CAVERJECT is available in the following packages:

6—10 microgram vials with diluent syringes	NDC 0009-3778-08
6—20 microgram vials with diluent syringes	NDC 0009-3701-01
Other available packages:	
6—10 microgram vials	NDC 0009-3778-05
6—20 microgram vials	NDC 0009-3701-05

PATIENT INSTRUCTIONS FOR CAVERJECT® STERILE POWDER (alprostadil for injection) AND PRE-FILLED DILUENT (bacteriostatic water for injection) SYRINGE

IMPOTENCE: CAUSES AND TREATMENTS

There are several causes of impotence, a condition known medically as erectile dysfunction. These include: medications that you may be taking for other conditions, impaired blood circulation in the penis, nerve damage, emotional problems, excessive smoking or alcohol use, use of street drugs, and hormonal imbalances. Often, impotence is due to more than one cause.

Treatments for impotence include: switching medications (if you are taking a medication that causes impotence), administration of hormones, penile injections, use of medical devices that produce an erection, surgical procedures to correct blood flow in the penis, penile implants, and psychological counseling. Your doctor has selected CAVERJECT for injection to treat your impotence. Your doctor can also discuss other available treatments. You should not stop taking any prescription medications, unless told to do so by your doctor.

USE OF CAVERJECT

CAVERJECT is injected into a specific area of the penis and should produce an erection in 5 to 20 minutes. The erection should last for about 1 hour. Generally, you should not use CAVERJECT more than 3 times a week, with at least 24 hours between uses.

Who Should Not Use CAVERJECT?

Men who have conditions that might result in long-lasting erections should not use CAVERJECT. Some of these conditions include: sickle cell anemia or trait, leukemia, and tumor of the bone marrow (multiple myeloma). Men with penile implants, or an abnormally formed penis, or who have been advised not to engage in sexual activity should not use CAVERJECT. CAVERJECT should not be used by women or children.

What Are The Risks Of Using CAVERJECT?

Erections that last more than 6 hours can cause serious and permanent damage. **Call your doctor or seek professional help immediately if you still have an erection 6 hours after injection.**

The most common side effect of CAVERJECT is mild to moderate pain after injection. About one-third of patients report this effect.

Call your doctor if you notice any redness, lumps, swelling, tenderness, or curving of the erect penis.

A small amount of bleeding at the injection site may occur. Tell your doctor if you have a condition or are taking a medicine that interferes with blood clotting.

NOTE: CAVERJECT offers no protection from the transmission of sexually transmitted diseases such as HIV (the virus that causes AIDS). Small amounts of bleeding at the injection site can increase the risk of transmission of blood-borne diseases between partners.

There is no approved injectable treatment using multiple drug components or "cocktails" for erectile dysfunction. Moreover, there are no data on the efficacy and safety of these combinations.

STORAGE

1. Unused packs of CAVERJECT may be stored at or below 25°C (77°F) for up to 3 months. Do not freeze.
2. After reconstitution, the solution of CAVERJECT should be used immediately.
3. During travel, care should be taken to avoid allowing the product to freeze or be stored at temperatures above 25°C (77°F). Therefore, do not store in checked luggage during air travel or leave in a closed automobile.

ADDITIONAL INFORMATION

There is a technical leaflet discussion of CAVERJECT written for health-care professionals that your pharmacist can let you read.

More information about erectile dysfunction and its treatment is available from the National Institutes of Health (Washington, DC), the American Foundation for Urological Diseases (Baltimore, MD), or the Impotence Institute of America (Washington, DC).

PREPARING AND INJECTING CAVERJECT

You must be properly instructed and trained in the injection technique by your doctor before using CAVERJECT.

Before using CAVERJECT, talk to your doctor about what to expect when using it, possible side effects, and what to do if side effects occur. Your dose has been selected for your individual needs. Do not change your dose without consulting your doctor. If you are not sure of the volume or dose to be used, talk to your doctor or pharmacist.

Follow these instructions exactly to prepare and inject a sterile dose of CAVERJECT.

Use the needle/syringe, and vial **only once** then safely discard the supplies and any unused solution (see the "Disposal of Injection Materials" section of these instructions).

Supplies Needed

To prepare and inject CAVERJECT you will need a vial of CAVERJECT Sterile Powder, the pre-filled diluent syringe with attached needle, and two alcohol swabs (Figure A). All required materials are provided in the blue plastic case in which CAVERJECT is supplied.

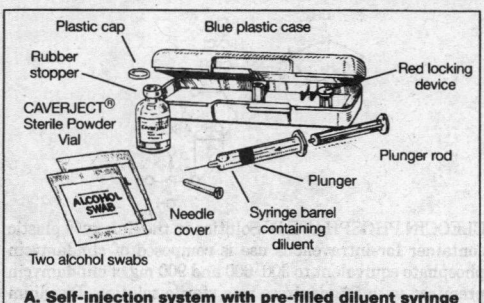

A. Self-injection system with pre-filled diluent syringe

The pre-filled syringe contains the diluent (bacteriostatic water for injection preserved with benzyl alcohol 0.945% w/v) you will use to dissolve the CAVERJECT Sterile Powder. You will use the same syringe to inject the solution of CAVERJECT into your penis.

CAVERJECT comes in both 10 microgram and 20 microgram strengths. **MAKE SURE YOU HAVE THE RIGHT STRENGTH VIAL OF CAVERJECT.**

Prepare the Dose

1. Wash your hands thoroughly, and dry them with a clean towel.

2. Handle the syringe by the syringe barrel only. Do not touch the needle with your hands. Do not allow the needle to touch any surface.

3. Insert plunger rod into open end of syringe barrel. Gently screw threaded end of plunger rod into rubber stopper. Do not overtighten.

4. Remove the plastic cap from the vial of CAVERJECT.

5. Wipe the rubber stopper on the vial of CAVERJECT with one alcohol swab. Discard this alcohol swab.

6. Grasp the syringe barrel (not the plunger) and remove the needle cover. Do not discard the needle cover, you will need to use it again (see step 13). Do not touch the exposed needle. Hold the syringe with the needle pointing up and push the plunger to the 1-cc (mL) mark on the syringe. This is to expel air and excess diluent.

7. Push the needle through the center of the vial's rubber stopper and push the syringe plunger all the way down to expel all the diluent into the vial. Proceed immediately to step 8.

8. Without removing the needle or touching the needle or stopper, gently swirl (do not shake) the vial until all the powder is dissolved in the diluent. Then turn the vial and needle/syringe upside down and **gently** swirl the vial to dissolve any powder in the neck of the vial. **DO NOT USE THE SOLUTION IF IT IS CLOUDY, COLORED OR CONTAINS PARTICLES.**

9. Keeping the needle in the vial, firmly hold the vial and syringe upside down in one hand (see Figure B).

10. Keeping the needle tip below the level of fluid, slowly pull back on the syringe plunger until all the fluid is removed from the vial.

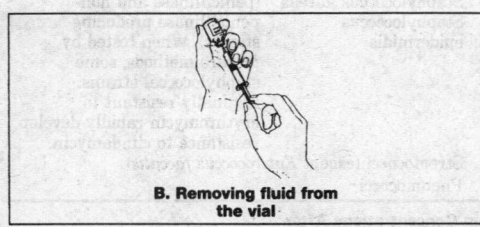

B. Removing fluid from the vial

11. If there are air bubbles, gently tap the syringe barrel until they float to the top of the solution (see Figure C). Holding the syringe upright, push the syringe plunger to the correct volume mark for the dose prescribed by your doctor. This will expel any air and excess solution into the vial.

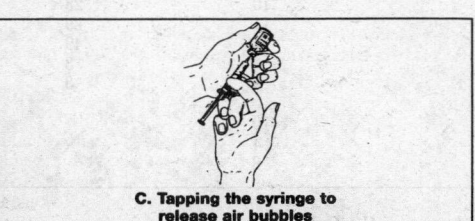

C. Tapping the syringe to release air bubbles

12. Grasp the syringe barrel (not the plunger) and pull the needle/syringe from the vial of CAVERJECT.

13. Place the needle cover over the needle and set the syringe down on a level surface.

Select Injection Site

1. CAVERJECT will be injected into a corpus cavernosum (spongy tissue) of the penis. One corpus cavernosum runs the length of the right side of the penis. Another corpus cavernosum runs the length of the left side of the penis (see Figures D and E).

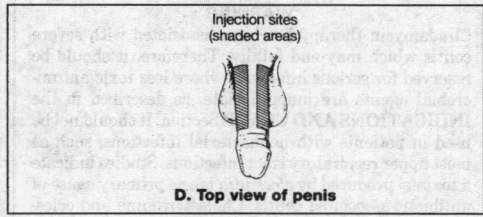

D. Top view of penis

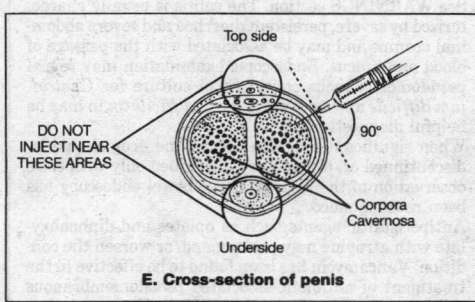

E. Cross-section of penis

2. Choose an injection site on one side of the shaft of the penis as shown in Figure D. AVOID VISIBLE BLOOD VESSELS.

3. WITH EACH USE OF CAVERJECT, ALTERNATE THE SIDE OF THE PENIS AND VARY THE SITE OF THE INJECTION.

Inject Your Dose of CAVERJECT

1. You should be sitting upright or slightly reclined when injecting CAVERJECT.

2. If your penis is not circumcised, pull the foreskin back. Holding the head of your penis with your thumb and forefinger, stretch it lengthwise along your thigh so that you can clearly see the selected injection site.

3. Clean the injection site with a new alcohol swab. Do not discard this swab, you will need to use it again (see step 7).

4. Remove the cover from the needle. Reposition the penis firmly against your thigh as in step 2 to keep it from moving during the injection.

5. Hold the syringe between your thumb and index finger (Figure F). Using a steady motion, push the needle straight into the selected site until the metal part of the needle is almost entirely in the penis.

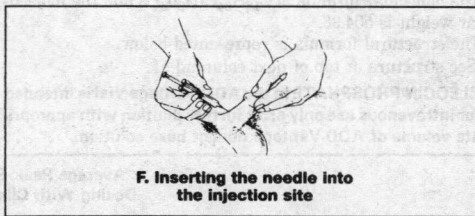

F. Inserting the needle into the injection site

6. Holding the syringe barrel between two fingers, move your thumb or finger to the top of the plunger and, with a steady motion, push down on the plunger so that the entire volume of CAVERJECT is slowly injected (Figure G).

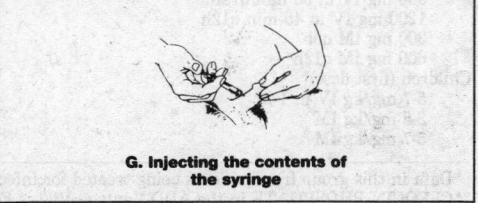

G. Injecting the contents of the syringe

7. Grasp the syringe barrel and pull the needle out of your penis. **APPLY PRESSURE TO THE INJECTION SITE WITH THE ALCOHOL SWAB FOR ABOUT 5 MINUTES OR UNTIL ANY BLEEDING STOPS.**

Disposal of Injection Materials

After use, dispose of all injection materials safely. Your pharmacist may be able to supply a disposal box especially for syringes. If not, the blue plastic case of CAVERJECT may be used as follows:

1. Place the used syringe and vial into the blue plastic case. Then remove the red plastic locking device. Close the case firmly so that it snaps shut (Figure H).

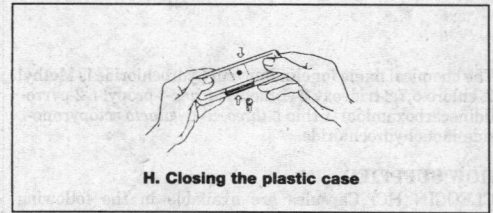

H. Closing the plastic case

2. Remove the perforated center portion of the case label to uncover a keyway. Place the red locking device in the hole in the upper lid of the blue plastic case and push down until completely inserted (Figure I). **Once the locking device is in position, the case will be permanently closed. The case can now be discarded safely. This case, which contains used supplies of CAVERJECT, is not suitable for recycling.**

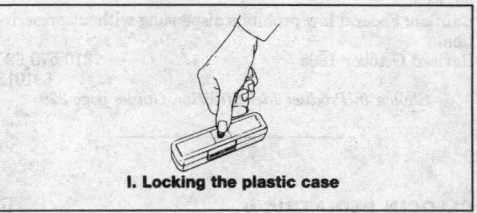

I. Locking the plastic case

3. Do not re-use or share needles or syringes. As with all prescription medicines, do not allow anyone else to use your medicine.

Caution: Federal law prohibits dispensing without prescription.

Revised February 1996   **816 442 001**
                                                       691811
Shown in Product Identification Guide, page 328

CLEOCIN HCl   ℞

Capsules
brand of clindamycin hydrochloride capsules, USP

DESCRIPTION

Clindamycin hydrochloride is the hydrated hydrochloride salt of clindamycin. Clindamycin is a semisynthetic antibiotic produced by a 7(S)-chloro-substitution of the 7(R)-hydroxyl group of the parent compound lincomycin.

CLEOCIN HCl Capsules contain clindamycin hydrochloride equivalent to 75 mg, 150 mg or 300 mg of clindamycin. Inactive ingredients: **75 mg**—corn starch, FD&C blue no. 1, FD&C yellow no. 5, gelatin, lactose, magnesium stearate and talc; **150 mg**—corn starch, FD&C blue no. 1, FD&C yellow no. 5, gelatin, lactose, magnesium stearate, talc and tita-

Continued on next page

Information on these Pharmacia & Upjohn products is based on labeling in effect June 1, 1996. Further information concerning these and other Pharmacia & Upjohn products may be obtained by direct inquiry to Medical Information, Pharmacia & Upjohn, Kalamazoo, MI 49001.

Pharmacia & Upjohn—Cont.

nium dioxide; **300 mg**—corn starch, FD&C blue no. 1, gelatin, lactose, magnesium stearate, talc and titanium dioxide. The structural formula is represented below:

The chemical name for clindamycin hydrochloride is Methyl 7-chloro-6,7,8-trideoxy-6-(1-methyl-*trans*-4-propyl-L-2-pyrrolidinecarboxamido)-1-thio-L-*threo*-α-D-*galacto*-octopyranoside monohydrochloride.

HOW SUPPLIED

CLEOCIN HCl Capsules are available in the following strengths, colors and sizes:

75 mg Green
Bottles of 100   NDC 0009-0331-02
150 mg Light Blue and Green
Bottles of 16   NDC 0009-0225-01
Bottles of 100   NDC 0009-0225-02
Unit dose package of 100   NDC 0009-0225-03
300 mg Light Blue
Bottles of 16   NDC 0009-0395-13
Bottles of 100   NDC 0009-0395-14
Unit dose package of 100   NDC 0009-0395-02
Store at controlled room temperature 15° to 30° C (59° to 86° F).
Caution: Federal law prohibits dispensing without prescription.

Revised October 1995   810 570 620
    691015

Shown in Product Identification Guide, page 329

CLEOCIN PEDIATRIC®   ℞
[*klēo'sin*]
brand of clindamycin palmitate hydrochloride flavored granules (clindamycin palmitate hydrochloride for oral solution, USP)

Not for Injection

DESCRIPTION

Clindamycin palmitate hydrochloride is a water soluble hydrochloride salt of the ester of clindamycin and palmitic acid. Clindamycin is a semisynthetic antibiotic produced by a 7(S)-chloro- substitution of the 7(R)-hydroxyl group of the parent compound lincomycin.
The structural formula is represented below:

The chemical name for clindamycin palmitate hydrochloride is Methyl 7-chloro-6,7,8-trideoxy-6-(1-methyl-*trans*-4-propyl-L-2-pyrro-lidinecarboxamido)-1-thio-L-*threo*-α-D-*galacto*-octopyranoside 2-palmitate monohydrochloride.
CLEOCIN PEDIATRIC Flavored Granules contain clindamycin palmitate hydrochloride for reconstitution. Each 5 mL contains the equivalent of 75 mg clindamycin. Inactive ingredients: artificial cherry flavor, dextrin, ethylparaben, pluronic F68, polymethylsiloxane, sucrose.

HOW SUPPLIED

CLEOCIN PEDIATRIC Flavored Granules for oral solution is available in bottles of 100 mL (NDC 0009-0760-04).
When reconstituted as directed, each bottle yields a solution containing 75 mg of clindamycin per 5 mL.
Caution: Federal law prohibits dispensing without prescription.

Revised March 1991   810 568 011

CLEOCIN PHOSPHATE®   ℞
[*klēō-sin*]
**brand of clindamycin phosphate sterile solution and clindamycin phosphate IV solution
(clindamycin phosphate injection, USP and clindamycin phosphate injection in 5% dextrose)
Sterile Solution is for Intramuscular and Intravenous Use
CLEOCIN PHOSPHATE in the ADD-Vantage™ Vial is For Intravenous Use Only**

WARNING

Clindamycin therapy has been associated with severe colitis which may end fatally. Therefore, it should be reserved for serious infections where less toxic antimicrobial agents are inappropriate, as described in the **INDICATIONS AND USAGE** Section. It should not be used in patients with nonbacterial infections, such as most upper respiratory tract infections. Studies indicate a toxin(s) produced by *clostridia* is one primary cause of antibiotic-associated colitis. Cholestyramine and colestipol resins have been shown to bind the toxin *in vitro*. See WARNINGS section. The colitis is usually characterized by severe, persistent diarrhea and severe abdominal cramps and may be associated with the passage of blood and mucus. Endoscopic examination may reveal pseudomembranous colitis. Stool culture for *Clostridium difficile* and stool assay for *C. difficile* toxin may be helpful diagnostically.

When significant diarrhea occurs, the drug should be discontinued or, if necessary, continued only with close observation of the patient. Large bowel endoscopy has been recommended.

Antiperistaltic agents such as opiates and diphenoxylate with atropine may prolong and/or worsen the condition. Vancomycin has been found to be effective in the treatment of antibiotic-associated pseudomembranous colitis produced by *Clostridium difficile*. The usual adult dosage is 500 milligrams to 2 grams of vancomycin orally per day in three to four divided doses administered for 7 to 10 days. Cholestyramine or colestipol resins bind vancomycin *in vitro*. If both a resin and vancomycin are to be administered concurrently, it may be advisable to separate the time of administration of each drug.

Diarrhea, colitis, and pseudomembranous colitis have been observed to begin up to several weeks following cessation of therapy with clindamycin.

DESCRIPTION

CLEOCIN PHOSPHATE Sterile Solution in vials contains clindamycin phosphate, a water soluble ester of clindamycin and phosphoric acid. Each mL contains the equivalent of 150 mg clindamycin, 0.5 mg disodium edetate and 9.45 mg benzyl alcohol added as preservative in each mL. Clindamycin is a semisynthetic antibiotic produced by a 7(S)-chloro-substitution of the 7(R)-hydroxyl group of the parent compound lincomycin.
The chemical name of clindamycin phosphate is L-*threo*-α-D-*galacto*-Octopyranoside, methyl 7-chloro-6,7,8-trideoxy-6-[[(1-methyl-4-propyl-2-pyrrolidinyl) carbonyl] amino]-1-thio-, 2-(dihydrogen phosphate), (2S-*trans*)-.
The molecular formula is $C_{18}H_{34}ClN_2O_8PS$ and the molecular weight is 504.96.
The structural formula is represented below:
[See structure at top of next column.]

CLEOCIN PHOSPHATE in the ADD-Vantage Vial is intended for intravenous use only after further dilution with appropriate volume of ADD-Vantage diluent base solution.

CLEOCIN PHOSPHATE IV Solution in the Galaxy® plastic container for intravenous use is composed of clindamycin phosphate equivalent to 300, 600 and 900 mg of clindamycin premixed with 5% dextrose as a sterile solution. Disodium edetate has been added at a concentration of 0.04 mg/mL. The pH has been adjusted with sodium hydroxide and/or hydrochloric acid.
The plastic container is fabricated from a specially designed multilayer plastic, PL 2501. Solutions in contact with the plastic container can leach out certain of its chemical components in very small amounts within the expiration period. The suitability of the plastic has been confirmed in tests in animals according to the USP biological tests for plastic containers, as well as by tissue culture toxicity studies.

CLINICAL PHARMACOLOGY

Biologically inactive clindamycin phosphate is rapidly converted to active clindamycin.
By the end of short-term intravenous infusion, peak serum levels of active clindamycin are reached. Biologically inactive clindamycin phosphate disappears rapidly from the serum; the average disappearance half-life is 6 minutes; however, the serum disappearance half-life of active clindamycin is about 3 hours in adults and 2½ hours in children.
After intramuscular injection of clindamycin phosphate, peak levels of active clindamycin are reached within 3 hours in adults and 1 hour in children. Serum level curves may be constructed from IV peak serum levels as given in Table 1 by application of disappearance half-lives listed above.
Serum levels of clindamycin can be maintained above the *in vitro* minimum inhibitory concentrations for most indicated organisms by administration of clindamycin phosphate every 8 to 12 hours in adults and every 6 to 8 hours in children, or by continuous intravenous infusion. An equilibrium state is reached by the third dose.
The disappearance half-life of clindamycin is increased slightly in patients with markedly reduced renal or hepatic function. Hemodialysis and peritoneal dialysis are not effective in removing clindamycin from the serum. Dosage schedules need not be modified in the presence of mild or moderate renal or hepatic disease.
No significant levels of clindamycin are attained in the cerebrospinal fluid even in the presence of inflamed meninges. Serum assays for active clindamycin require an inhibitor to prevent *in vitro* hydrolysis of clindamycin phosphate. [See Table 1 below.]
Microbiology: Although clindamycin phosphate is inactive *in vitro*, rapid *in vivo* hydrolysis converts this compound to the antibacterially active clindamycin.
Clindamycin has been shown to have *in vitro* activity against isolates of the following organisms:
Aerobic gram positive cocci, including:

Staphylococcus aureus	(penicillinase and non-
Staphylococcus epidermidis	penicillinase producing strains). When tested by *in vitro* methods, some staphylococcal strains originally resistant to erythromycin rapidly develop resistance to clindamycin.
Streptococci (except *Enterococcus faecalis*)	
Pneumococci	

Table 1. Average Peak Serum Concentrations After Dosing With Clindamycin Phosphate

Dosage Regimen	Clindamycin mcg/mL	Clindamycin Phosphate mcg/mL
Healthy Adult Males (Post equilibrium)		
300 mg IV in 10 min q8h	7	15
600 mg IV in 20 min q8h**	10	23
900 mg IV in 30 min q12h**	11	29
1200 mg IV in 45 min q12h	14	49
300 mg IM q8h	6	3
600 mg IM q12h*	9	3
Children (first dose)*		
5-7 mg/kg IV in 1 hr	10	
3-5 mg/kg IM	4	
5-7 mg/kg IM	8	

*Data in this group from patients being treated for infection.
**CLEOCIN PHOSPHATE in the ADD-Vantage Vial is For Intravenous Use Only.

Anaerobic gram negative bacilli, including:
  Bacteroides species (including *Bacteroides fragilis* group
  and *Bacteroides melaninogenicus* group)
  Fusobacterium species
Anaerobic gram positive nonsporeforming bacilli, including:
  Propionibacterium
  Eubacterium
  Actinomyces species
Anaerobic and microaerophilic gram positive cocci, including:
  Peptococcus species
  Peptostreptococcus species
  Microaerophilic streptococci

Clostridia: Clostridia are more resistant than most anaerobes to clindamycin. Most *Clostridium perfringens* are susceptible, but other species, e.g., *Clostridium sporogenes* and *Clostridium tertium* are frequently resistant to clindamycin. Susceptibility testing should be done.

Cross resistance has been demonstrated between clindamycin and lincomycin.

Antagonism has been demonstrated between clindamycin and erythromycin.

In vitro Susceptibility Testing

Disk diffusion technique-Quantitative methods that require measurement of zone diameters give the most precise estimates of antibiotic susceptibility. One such procedure[1] has been recommended for use with disks to test susceptibility to clindamycin.

Reports from a laboratory using the standardized single-disk susceptibility test[1] with a 2 mcg clindamycin disk should be interpreted according to the following criteria:

Susceptible organisms produce zones of 17 mm or greater, indicating that the tested organism is likely to respond to therapy.

Organisms of intermediate susceptibility produce zones of 15–16 mm, indicating that the tested organism would be susceptible if a high dosage is used or if the infection is confined to tissues and fluids (e.g., urine), in which high antibiotic levels are attained.

Resistant organisms produce zones of 14 mm or less, indicating that other therapy should be selected.

Standardized procedures require the use of control organisms. The 2 mcg clindamycin disk should give a zone diameter between 24 and 30 mm for *S. aureus* ATCC 25923.

Dilution techniques—A bacterial isolate may be considered susceptible if the minimum inhibitory concentration (MIC) for clindamycin is not more than 1.6 mcg/mL. Organisms are considered moderately susceptible if the MIC is greater than 1.6 mcg/mL and less than or equal to 4.8 mcg/mL. Organisms are considered resistant if the MIC is greater than 4.8 mcg per mL.

The range of MICs for the control strains are as follows:
*S. aureus*ATCC 29213, 0.06—0.25 mcg/mL.
E. faecalis ATCC 29212, 4.0—16 mcg/mL.

For anaerobic bacteria the minimum inhibitory concentration (MIC) of clindamycin can be determined by agar dilution and broth dilution (including microdilution) techniques.[2] If MICs are not determined routinely, the disk broth method is recommended for routine use. THE KIRBY-BAUER DISK DIFFUSION METHOD AND ITS INTERPRETIVE STANDARDS ARE NOT RECOMMENDED FOR ANAEROBES.

INDICATIONS AND USAGE

CLEOCIN PHOSPHATE products are indicated in the treatment of serious infections caused by susceptible anaerobic bacteria.

CLEOCIN PHOSPHATE products are also indicated in the treatment of serious infections due to susceptible strains of streptococci, pneumococci, and staphylococci. Its use should be reserved for penicillin-allergic patients or other patients for whom, in the judgment of the physician, a penicillin is inappropriate. Because of the risk of antibiotic-associated pseudomembranous colitis, as described in the WARNING box, before selecting clindamycin the physician should consider the nature of the infection and the suitability of less toxic alternatives (e.g., erythromycin).

Bacteriologic studies should be performed to determine the causative organisms and their susceptibility to clindamycin. Indicated surgical procedures should be performed in conjunction with antibiotic therapy.

CLEOCIN PHOSPHATE is indicated in the treatment of serious infections caused by susceptible strains of the designated organisms in the conditions listed below:

Lower respiratory tract infections including pneumonia, empyema, and lung abscess caused by anaerobes, *Streptococcus pneumoniae*, other streptococci (except *E. faecalis*), and *Staphylococcus aureus*.

Skin and skin structure infections caused by *Streptococcus pyogenes*, *Staphylococcus aureus*, and anaerobes.

Gynecological infections including endometritis, nongonococcal tubo-ovarian abscess, pelvic cellulitis, and post-surgical vaginal cuff infection caused by susceptible anaerobes.

Intra-abdominal infections including peritonitis and intra-abdominal abscess caused by susceptible anaerobic organisms.

Septicemia caused by *Staphylococcus aureus*, streptococci (except *Enterococcus faecalis*), and susceptible anaerobes.

Bone and joint infections including acute hematogenous osteomyelitis caused by *Staphylococcus aureus* and as adjunctive therapy in the surgical treatment of chronic bone and joint infections due to susceptible organisms.

CONTRAINDICATIONS

This drug is contraindicated in individuals with a history of hypersensitivity to preparations containing clindamycin or lincomycin.

WARNINGS

See WARNING box. Studies indicate a toxin(s) produced by clostridia is one primary cause of antibiotic-associated colitis.[3-7] Cholestyramine and colestipol resins have been shown to bind the toxin *in vitro*. Mild cases of colitis may respond to drug discontinuance alone. Moderate to severe cases should be managed promptly with fluid, electrolyte and protein supplementation as indicated. Vancomycin has been found to be effective in the treatment of antibiotic-associated pseudomembranous colitis produced by *Clostridium difficile*. The usual adult dosage is 500 milligrams to 2 grams of vancomycin orally per day in three to four divided doses administered for 7 to 10 days. Cholestyramine or colestipol resins bind vancomycin *in vitro*. If both a resin and vancomycin are to be administered concurrently, it may be advisable to separate the time of administration of each drug. Systemic corticoids and corticoid retention enemas may help relieve the colitis. Other causes of colitis should also be considered.

A careful inquiry should be made concerning previous sensitivities to drugs and other allergens.

This product contains benzyl alcohol as a preservative. Benzyl alcohol has been associated with a fatal "Gasping Syndrome" in premature infants. (See PRECAUTIONS—Pediatric Use).

Usage in Meningitis—Since clindamycin does not diffuse adequately into the cerebrospinal fluid, the drug should not be used in the treatment of meningitis.

SERIOUS ANAPHYLACTOID REACTIONS REQUIRE IMMEDIATE EMERGENCY TREATMENT WITH EPINEPHRINE. OXYGEN AND INTRAVENOUS CORTICOSTEROIDS SHOULD ALSO BE ADMINISTERED AS INDICATED.

PRECAUTIONS

General

Review of experience to date suggests that a subgroup of older patients with associated severe illness may tolerate diarrhea less well. When clindamycin is indicated in these patients, they should be carefully monitored for change in bowel frequency.

CLEOCIN PHOSPHATE products should be prescribed with caution in individuals with a history of gastrointestinal disease, particularly colitis.

CLEOCIN PHOSPHATE should be prescribed with caution in atopic individuals.

Certain infections may require incision and drainage or other indicated surgical procedures in addition to antibiotic therapy.

The use of CLEOCIN PHOSPHATE may result in overgrowth of nonsusceptible organisms—particularly yeasts. Should superinfections occur, appropriate measures should be taken as indicated by the clinical situation.

CLEOCIN PHOSPHATE should not be injected intravenously undiluted as a bolus, but should be infused over at least 10–60 minutes as directed in the DOSAGE AND ADMINISTRATION section.

Patients with very severe renal disease and/or very severe hepatic disease accompanied by severe metabolic aberrations should be dosed with caution, and serum clindamycin levels monitored during high-dose therapy (see OVERDOSAGE).

Laboratory Tests

During prolonged therapy periodic liver and kidney function tests and blood counts should be performed.

Drug Interactions

Clindamycin has been shown to have neuromuscular blocking properties that may enhance the action of other neuromuscular blocking agents. Therefore, it should be used with caution in patients receiving such agents.

Antagonism has been demonstrated between clindamycin and erythromycin *in vitro*. Because of possible clinical significance, the two drugs should not be administered concurrently.

Pregnancy: Safety for use in pregnancy has not been established.

Nursing Mothers

Clindamycin has been reported to appear in breast milk in the range of 0.7 to 3.8 mcg/mL at dosages of 150 mg orally to 600 mg intravenously. Because of the potential for adverse reactions due to clindamycin in neonates (see Pediatric Use), the decision to discontinue the drug should be made, taking into account the importance of the drug to the mother.

Pediatric Use

When CLEOCIN PHOSPHATE Sterile Solution is administered to newborns, infants, and children, appropriate monitoring of organ system functions is desirable.

Usage in Newborns and Infants

This product contains benzyl alcohol as a preservative. Benzyl alcohol has been associated with a fatal "Gasping Syndrome" in premature infants.

The potential for the toxic effect in children from chemicals that may leach from the single dose premixed IV preparation in plastic has not been evaluated.

ADVERSE REACTIONS

The following reactions have been reported with the use of clindamycin.

Gastrointestinal: Antibiotic-associated colitis (see WARNINGS), abdominal pain, nausea, and vomiting. An unpleasant or metallic taste occasionally has been reported after intravenous administration of the higher doses of clindamycin phosphate.

Hypersensitivity Reactions: Maculopapular rash and urticaria have been observed during drug therapy. Generalized mild to moderate morbilliform-like skin rashes are the most frequently reported of all adverse reactions. Rare instances of erythema multiforme, some resembling Stevens-Johnson syndrome, have been associated with clindamycin. A few cases of anaphylactoid reactions have been reported. If a hypersensitivity reaction occurs, the drug should be discontinued. The usual agents (epinephrine, corticosteroids, antihistamines) should be available for emergency treatment of serious reactions.

Liver: Jaundice and abnormalities in liver function tests have been observed during clindamycin therapy.

Renal: Although no direct relationship of clindamycin to renal damage has been established, renal dysfunction as evidenced by azotemia, oliguria, and/or proteinuria has been observed in rare instances.

Hematopoietic: Transient neutropenia (leukopenia) and eosinophilia have been reported. Reports of agranulocytosis and thrombocytopenia have been made. No direct etiologic relationship to concurrent clindamycin therapy could be made in any of the foregoing.

Local Reactions: Pain, induration and sterile abscess have been reported after intramuscular injection and thrombophlebitis after intravenous infusion. Reactions can be minimized or avoided by giving deep intramuscular injections and avoiding prolonged use of indwelling intravenous catheters.

Musculoskeletal: Rare instances of polyarthritis have been reported.

Cardiovascular: Rare instances of cardiopulmonary arrest and hypotension have been reported following too rapid intravenous administration. (See DOSAGE AND ADMINISTRATION section).

OVERDOSAGE

Hemodialysis and peritoneal dialysis are not effective in removing clindamycin from the serum.

DOSAGE AND ADMINISTRATION

If diarrhea occurs during therapy, this antibiotic should be discontinued (see WARNING box).

Adults: Parenteral (IM or IV Administration): Serious infections due to aerobic gram-positive cocci and the more susceptible anaerobes (NOT generally including *Bacteroides fragilis*, *Peptococcus* species and *Clostridium* species other than *Clostridium perfringens*):
600–1200 mg/day in 2, 3 or 4 equal doses.

More severe infections, particularly those due to proven or suspected *Bacteroides fragilis*, *Peptococcus* species, or *Clostridium* species other than *Clostridium perfringens*:
1200–2700 mg/day in 2, 3 or 4 equal doses.

For more serious infections, these doses may have to be increased. In life-threatening situations due to either aerobes or anaerobes these doses may be increased. Doses of as much as 4800 mg daily have been given intravenously to adults. See Dilution and Infusion Rates section below.

Single intramuscular injections of greater than 600 mg are not recommended.

Alternatively, drug may be administered in the form of a single rapid infusion of the first dose followed by continuous IV infusion as follows:
[See table at bottom of next page.]

Neonates (less than 1 month):
15 to 20 mg/kg/day in 3 to 4 equal doses. The lower dosage may be adequate for small prematures.

Continued on next page

Information on these Pharmacia & Upjohn products is based on labeling in effect June 1, 1996. Further information concerning these and other Pharmacia & Upjohn products may be obtained by direct inquiry to Medical Information, Pharmacia & Upjohn, Kalamazoo, MI 49001.

Pharmacia & Upjohn—Cont.

Children (over 1 month of age): Parenteral (IM or IV) administration: 20 to 40 mg/kg/day in 3 or 4 equal doses. The higher doses would be used for more severe infections. As an alternative to dosing on a body weight basis, children may be dosed on the basis of square meters body surface: 350 mg/m^2/day for serious infections and 450 mg/m^2/day for more severe infections.
Parenteral therapy may be changed to oral CLEOCIN PEDIATRIC® Flavored Granules (clindamycin palmitate hydrochloride) or CLEOCIN HCl® Capsules (clindamycin hydrochloride) when the condition warrants and at the discretion of the physician.
In cases of β-hemolytic streptococcal infections, treatment should be continued for at least 10 days.
Dilution and Infusion Rates: Clindamycin phosphate must be diluted prior to IV administration. The concentration of clindamycin in diluent for infusion should not exceed 18 mg per mL. Infusion rates should not exceed 30 mg per minute. The usual infusion dilutions and rates are as follows:

Dose	Diluent	Time
300 mg	50 mL	10 min
600 mg	50 mL	20 min
900 mg	50–100 mL	30 min
1200 mg	100 mL	40 min

Administration of more than 1200 mg in a single 1-hour infusion is not recommended.
Parenteral drug products should be inspected visually for particulate matter and discoloration prior to administration, whenever solution and container permit.
Dilution and Compatibility: Physical and biological compatibility studies monitored for 24 hours at room temperature have demonstrated no inactivation or incompatibility with the use of CLEOCIN PHOSPHATE Sterile Solution (clindamycin phosphate) in IV solutions containing sodium chloride, glucose, calcium or potassium, and solutions containing vitamin B complex in concentrations usually used clinically. No incompatibility has been demonstrated with the antibiotics cephalothin, kanamycin, gentamicin, penicillin or carbenicillin.
The following drugs are physically incompatible with clindamycin phosphate: ampicillin sodium, phenytoin sodium, barbiturates, aminophylline, calcium gluconate, and magnesium sulfate.
The compatibility and duration of stability of drug admixtures will vary depending on concentration and other conditions. For current information regarding compatibilities of clindamycin phosphate under specific conditions, please contact the Medical Correspondence Unit, The Upjohn Company.
Physico-Chemical Stability of diluted solutions of CLEOCIN PHOSPHATE
Room temperature: 6, 9 and 12 mg/mL (equivalent to clindamycin base) in dextrose injection 5%, sodium chloride injection 0.9%, or Lactated Ringers Injection in glass bottles or minibags, demonstrated physical and chemical stability for at least 16 days at 25° C. Also, 18 mg/mL (equivalent to clindamycin base) in dextrose injection 5%, in minibags, demonstrated physical and chemical stability for at least 16 days at 25° C.
Refrigeration: 6, 9 and 12 mg/mL (equivalent to clindamycin base) in dextrose injection 5%, sodium chloride injection 0.9%, or Lactated Ringers Injection in glass bottles or minibags, demonstrated physical and chemical stability for at least 32 days at 4° C.
IMPORTANT: This chemical stability information in no way indicates that it would be acceptable practice to use this product well after the preparation time. Good professional practice suggests that compounded admixtures should be administered as soon after preparation as is feasible.
Frozen: 6, 9 and 12 mg/mL (equivalent to clindamycin base) in dextrose injection 5%, sodium chloride injection 0.9%, or Lactated Ringers Injection in minibags demonstrated physical and chemical stability for at least eight weeks at −10° C. Frozen solutions should be thawed at room temperature and not refrozen.

DIRECTIONS FOR DISPENSING

Pharmacy Bulk Package—Not for Direct Infusion
The Pharmacy Bulk Package is for use in a Pharmacy Admixture Service only under a laminar flow hood. Entry into the vial should be made with a small diameter sterile transfer set or other small diameter sterile dispensing device, and contents dispensed in aliquots using aseptic technique. Multiple entries with a needle and syringe are not recommended. AFTER ENTRY USE ENTIRE CONTENTS OF VIAL PROMPTLY. ANY UNUSED PORTION MUST BE DISCARDED WITHIN 24 HOURS AFTER INITIAL ENTRY.

DIRECTIONS FOR USE

CLEOCIN PHOSPHATE IV Solution in Galaxy Plastic Container
Premixed CLEOCIN PHOSPHATE IV Solution is for intravenous administration using sterile equipment. Check for minute leaks prior to use by squeezing bag firmly. If leaks are found, discard solution as sterility may be impaired. Do not add supplementary medication. Parenteral drug products should be inspected visually for particulate matter and discoloration prior to administration whenever solution and container permit. Do not use unless solution is clear and seal is intact.
Caution: Do not use plastic containers in series connections. Such use could result in air embolism due to residual air being drawn from the primary container before administration of the fluid from the secondary container is complete.
Preparation for Administration:
1. Suspend container from eyelet support.
2. Remove protector from outlet port at bottom of container.
3. Attach administration set. Refer to complete directions accompanying set.

Preparation of CLEOCIN PHOSPHATE in ADD-Vantage System—For IV Use Only. CLEOCIN PHOSPHATE 600 mg and 900 mg may be reconstituted in 50 mL or 100 mL, respectively, of Dextrose Injection 5% or Sodium Chloride Injection 0.9% in the ADD-diluent container. Refer to separate instructions for ADD-Vantage‡ System.

HOW SUPPLIED

Each mL of CLEOCIN PHOSPHATE Sterile Solution contains clindamycin phosphate equivalent to 150 mg clindamycin; 0.5 mg disodium edetate; 9.45 mg benzyl alcohol added as preservative. When necessary, pH is adjusted with sodium hydroxide and/or hydrochloric acid. CLEOCIN PHOSPHATE is available in the following packages:

25-2 mL vials	NDC 0009-0870-21
25-4 mL vials	NDC 0009-0775-20
25-6 mL vials	NDC 0009-0902-11
1-60 mL Pharmacy Bulk Package	NDC 0009-0728-05

CLEOCIN PHOSPHATE is supplied in ADD-Vantage vials as follows:

NDC	Vial Size	Total Clindamycin Phosphate/vial	Amount of Diluent
0009-3124-01	4 mL	600 mg	50 mL
0009-3447-01	6 mL	900 mg	100 mL

Store at controlled room temperature 15° to 30° C (59° to 86° F).
CLEOCIN PHOSPHATE IV Solution in Galaxy plastic containers is a sterile solution of clindamycin phosphate with 5% dextrose. The single dose Galaxy plastic containers are available as follows:

24-300 mg/50 mL containers	NDC 0009-3381-01
24-600 mg/50 mL containers	NDC 0009-3375-01
24-900 mg/50 mL containers	NDC 0009-3382-01

Exposure of pharmaceutical products to heat should be minimized. It is recommended that Galaxy plastic containers be stored at room temperature (25° C). Avoid temperatures above 30° C.
Caution: Federal law prohibits dispensing without prescription.
Revised March 1996 810 020 031
691273

[1]Bauer AW, Kirby WMM, Sherris JC, Turck M; Antibiotic susceptibility testing by a standardized single disk method. *Am. J. Clin. Path.*, 45:493-496, 1966. Standardized Disk Susceptibility Test, *Federal Register*, 37:20527-29, 1972.
[2]National Committee for Clinical Lab. Standards. Methods for Antimicrobial Susceptibility Testing of Anaerobic Bacteria—Second Edition; Tentative Standard. NCCLS publication M11-T2. Villanova, PA; NCCLS; 1988.
[3]Bartlett JG, et al: Antibiotic associated pseudomembranous colitis due to toxin-producing *Clostridia*. *N Eng J Med* 298(10): 531-534, 1978.
[4]George RH, et al: Identification of *Clostridium difficile* as a cause of pseudomembranous colitis. *Br Med J* 6114:669-671, 1978.
[5]Larson HE, Price AB: Pseudomembranous colitis presence of clostridial toxin. *Lancet* 8052/3:1312-1314, 1977.
[6]Rifkin GD, Fekety FR, Silva J: Antibiotic-induced colitis-implication of a toxin neutralized by *Clostridium sordellii* antitoxin. *Lancet* 8048:1103-1106, 1977.
[7]Bailey WR, Scott EG: Diagnostic Microbiology. The CV Mosby Company, St. Louis, 1978.

‡ADD-Vantage is a registered trademark of Abbott Laboratories.
CLEOCIN PHOSPHATE IV Solution in the Galaxy plastic containers is manufactured for The Upjohn Company by Baxter Healthcare Corporation, Deerfield, IL 60015.
Galaxy® is a registered trademark of Baxter International, Inc.

To maintain serum clindamycin levels	Rapid infusion rate	Maintenance infusion rate
Above 4 mcg/mL	10 mg/min for 30 min	0.75 mg/min
Above 5 mcg/mL	15 mg/min for 30 min	1.00 mg/min
Above 6 mcg/mL	20 mg/min for 30 min	1.25 mg/min

CLEOCIN® ℞

[*klēō-sin*]
brand of clindamycin phosphate vaginal cream
FOR INTRAVAGINAL USE ONLY
NOT FOR OPHTHALMIC, DERMAL, OR ORAL USE

DESCRIPTION

Clindamycin phosphate is a water soluble ester of the semi-synthetic antibiotic produced by a 7(S)-chloro-substitution of the 7(R)-hydroxyl group of the parent antibiotic lincomycin. The chemical name for clindamycin phosphate is methyl 7-chloro-6,7,8-trideoxy-6-(1-methyl-*trans*-4-propyl-L-2-pyrrolidinecarboxamido) -1- thio-L-*threo*-α] -*D*- *galacto*-octopyranoside 2-(dihydrogen phosphate). It has a molecular weight of 504.96, and the molecular formula is $C_{18}H_{34}ClN_2O_8PS$. The structural formula is represented at right:

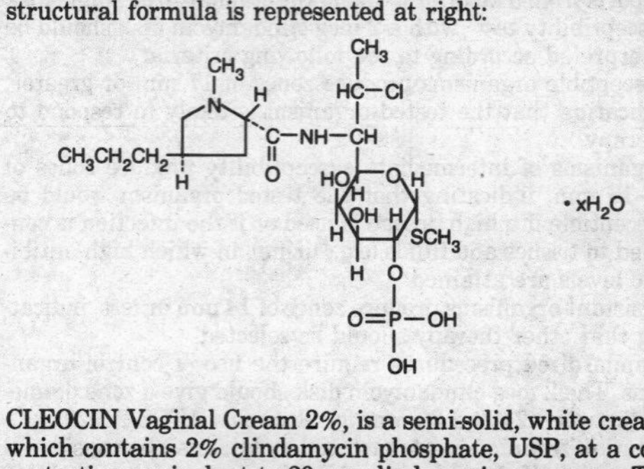

CLEOCIN Vaginal Cream 2%, is a semi-solid, white cream, which contains 2% clindamycin phosphate, USP, at a concentration equivalent to 20 mg clindamycin per gram. The pH of the cream is between 3.0 and 6.0. The cream also contains benzyl alcohol, cetostearyl alcohol, cetyl palmitate, mineral oil, polysorbate 60, propylene glycol, purified water, sorbitan monostearate, and stearic acid.
Each applicatorful of 5 grams of vaginal cream contains approximately 100 mg of clindamycin phosphate.

CLINICAL PHARMACOLOGY

Following a once a day intravaginal dose of 100 mg of clindamycin phosphate vaginal cream 2%, administered to 6 healthy female volunteers for 7 days, approximately 5% (range 0.6% to 11%) of the administered dose was absorbed systemically. The peak serum clindamycin concentration observed on the first day averaged 18 ng/mL (range 4 to 47 ng/mL) and averaged 25 ng/mL (range 6 to 61 ng/mL) on day 7. These peak concentrations were attained in approximately 10 hours post-dosing (range 4-24 hours).
Following a once a day intravaginal dose of 100 mg of clindamycin phosphate vaginal cream 2%, administered for 7 consecutive days to 5 women with bacterial vaginosis, absorption was slower and less variable than that observed in healthy females. Approximately, 5% (range 2% to 8%) of the dose was absorbed systemically. The peak serum clindamycin concentration observed on the first day averaged 13 ng/mL (range 3 to 34 ng/mL) and averaged 16 ng/mL (range 7 to 26 ng/mL) on day 7. These peak concentrations were attained in approximately 16 hours post-dosing (range 8-24 hours).
There was little or no systemic accumulation of clindamycin after repeated vaginal dosing of clindamycin phosphate vaginal cream 2%. The systemic $t_{1/2}$ was 1.5 to 2.6 hours.

MICROBIOLOGY

Clindamycin inhibits bacterial protein synthesis by its action at the bacterial ribosome. The antibiotic binds preferentially to the 50S ribosomal subunit and affects the process of peptide chain initiation. Although clindamycin phosphate is inactive *in vitro*, rapid *in vivo* hydrolysis converts this compound to the antibacterially active clindamycin.
Culture and sensitivity testing of bacteria are not routinely performed to establish the diagnosis of bacterial vaginosis. (See INDICATIONS AND USAGE.) Standard methodology for the susceptibility testing of the potential bacterial vaginosis pathogens, *Gardnerella vaginalis*, *Mobiluncus* spp., or *Mycoplasma hominis*, has not been defined.
Nonetheless, clindamycin is an antimicrobial agent active *in vitro* against most strains of the following organisms that have been reported to be associated with bacterial vaginosis:
Bacteroides spp.
Gardnerella vaginalis
Mobiluncus spp.

Mycoplasma hominis
Peptostreptococcus spp.

INDICATIONS AND USAGE

CLEOCIN Vaginal Cream 2%, is indicated in the treatment of bacterial vaginosis (formerly referred to as *Haemophilus* vaginitis, *Gardnerella* vaginitis, nonspecific vaginitis, *Corynebacterium* vaginitis, or anaerobic vaginosis). CLEOCIN Vaginal Cream 2%, can be used to treat non-pregnant women and pregnant women during the second trimester. (See CLINICAL STUDIES.)

NOTE: For purposes of this indication, a clinical diagnosis of bacterial vaginosis is usually defined by the presence of a homogeneous vaginal discharge that (a) has a pH of greater than 4.5, (b) emits a "fishy" amine odor when mixed with a 10% KOH solution, and (c) contains clue cells on microscopic examination. Gram's stain results consistent with a diagnosis of bacterial vaginosis include (a) markedly reduced or absent *Lactobacillus* morphology, (b) predominance of *Gardnerella* morphotype, and (c) absent or few white blood cells. Other pathogens commonly associated with vulvovaginitis, e.g., *Trichomonas vaginalis, Chlamydia trachomatis, N. gonorrhoeae, Candida albicans*, and *Herpes simplex* virus should be ruled out.

CONTRAINDICATIONS

CLEOCIN Vaginal Cream 2%, is contraindicated in individuals with a history of hypersensitivity to clindamycin, lincomycin, or any of the components of this vaginal cream. CLEOCIN Vaginal Cream 2%, is also contraindicated in individuals with a history of regional enteritis, ulcerative colitis, or a history of "antibiotic-associated" colitis.

WARNINGS

Pseudomembranous colitis has been reported with nearly all antibacterial agents, including clindamycin, and may range in severity from mild to life-threatening. Orally and parenterally administered clindamycin has been associated with severe colitis which may end fatally. Diarrhea, bloody diarrhea, and colitis (including pseudomembranous colitis) have been reported with the use of orally and parenterally administered clindamycin, as well as with topical (dermal) formulations of clindamycin. Therefore, it is important to consider this diagnosis in patients who present with diarrhea subsequent to the administration of clindamycin, even when administered by the vaginal route, because approximately 5% of the clindamycin dose is systemically absorbed from the vagina.

Treatment with antibacterial agents alters the normal flora of the colon and may permit overgrowth of clostridia. Studies indicate that a toxin produced by *Clostridium difficile* is a primary cause of "antibiotic-associated colitis".

After the diagnosis of pseudomembranous colitis has been established, therapeutic measures should be initiated. Mild cases of pseudomembranous colitis usually respond to discontinuation of the drug alone. In moderate to severe cases, consideration should be given to management with fluids and electrolytes, protein supplementation, and treatment with an antibacterial drug clinically effective against *Clostridium difficile* colitis.

Onset of pseudomembranous colitis symptoms may occur during or after antimicrobial treatment.

This cream contains mineral oil. Mineral oil may weaken latex or rubber products such as condoms or vaginal contraceptive diaphragms; therefore, use of such products within 72 hours following treatment with CLEOCIN Vaginal Cream 2%, is not recommended.

PRECAUTIONS

General

CLEOCIN Vaginal Cream 2%, contains ingredients that will cause burning and irritation of the eye. In the event of accidental contact with the eye, rinse the eye with copious amounts of cool tap water.

The use of CLEOCIN (clindamycin phosphate 2%) Vaginal Cream may result in the overgrowth of nonsusceptible organisms in the vagina. Approximately 33% of the pregnant women and 16% of the non-pregnant women developed symptomatic cervicitis/vaginitis with 26% of the pregnant women and 11% of the non-pregnant women developing cervicitis/vaginitis secondary to *Candida albicans*.

Information for the Patient:

The patient should be instructed not to engage in vaginal intercourse during treatment with this product.

Drug Interactions

Clindamycin has been shown to have neuromuscular blocking properties that may enhance the action of other neuromuscular blocking agents. Therefore, it should be used with caution in patients receiving such agents.

Carcinogenesis, Mutagenesis, Impairment of Fertility

Long term studies in animals have not been performed with clindamycin to evaluate carcinogenic potential. Genotoxicity tests performed included a rat micronucleus test and an Ames test. Both tests were negative. Fertility studies in rats treated orally with up to 300 mg/kg/day (31 times the human exposure based on mg/m^2) revealed no effects on fertility or mating ability.

Pregnancy: Teratogenic effects

Pregnancy Category B

Reproduction studies have been performed in rats and mice using oral and parenteral doses of clindamycin up to 600 mg/kg/day (62 and 25 times, respectively, the maximum human exposure based on mg/m^2) and have revealed no evidence of harm to the fetus due to clindamycin. In one mouse strain, cleft palates were observed in treated fetuses; this outcome was not produced in other mouse strains or in other species and is, therefore, considered to be a strain specific effect.

CLEOCIN Vaginal Cream 2%, has been studied in pregnant women during the second trimester. (See INDICATIONS AND USAGE; PRECAUTIONS, General; and ADVERSE REACTIONS.)

There are, however, no adequate and well-controlled studies in pregnant women during the first trimester of pregnancy. Because animal reproduction studies are not always predictive of human response, this drug should be used during the first trimester of pregnancy only if clearly needed.

Nursing Mothers

It is not known if clindamycin is excreted in human milk following the use of vaginally administered clindamycin phosphate. However, after oral or parenteral administration, clindamycin has been detected in human milk.

Because of the potential for serious adverse reactions in nursing infants from clindamycin phosphate, a decision should be made whether to discontinue nursing or to discontinue the drug, taking into account the importance of the drug to the mother.

Pediatric Use

Safety and effectiveness in children have not been established.

ADVERSE REACTIONS

Clinical trials: Non-pregnant women

In clinical trials, approximately 4% of non-pregnant patients treated with CLEOCIN Vaginal Cream 2%, discontinued therapy due to drug-related adverse events. Medical events judged to be related, probably related, or possibly related to vaginally administered clindamycin phosphate vaginal cream 2%, were reported for 249/1020 (24%) non-pregnant patients. Unless percentages are otherwise stipulated, the incidence of individual adverse reactions listed below was less than 1%:

Genital tract:
- Cervicitis/vaginitis, symptomatic (16%):
  - *Candida albicans* (11%)
  - *Trichomonas vaginalis* (1%)
- Vulvar irritation (6%)

Central nervous system:
- Dizziness, headache, vertigo

Dermatologic:
- Rash

Gastrointestinal:
- Heartburn, nausea, vomiting, diarrhea, constipation, abdominal pain

Hypersensitivity:
- Urticaria

Clinical trials: Pregnant women

In a clinical trial of pregnant women during the second trimester, 2% (4/180) discontinued therapy due to drug-related adverse events. Medical events judged to be related, probably related or possibly related to vaginally administered clindamycin phosphate vaginal cream 2% were reported for 22% (40/180) of pregnant patients.

The percent of patients reporting adverse events greater than 2% regardless of their association with treatment are listed below:

Genital Tract
- Cervicitis/Vaginitis, symptomatic (33%)
  - *Candida albicans* infection (26%)

Vulvovaginal irritation (7%)
Preterm Labor (8%)
Amnionitis (6%)
Endometritis (5%)
Labor Disorders (3%)
Preeclampsia (4%)
Labor Induction (2%)
Abruptio placenta (2%)
Oligohydramnios (2%)

Urinary Tract (11%)
- Urinary Tract Infection (8%)
- Pyelonephritis (2%)

Cardiovascular (4%)
- Hypertension of Pregnancy (3%)

Endocrine (4%)
- Gestational Diabetes (3%)

Headache (2%)
Upper Respiratory Infection (3%)
Abdominal Pain (2%)
Pruritus (2%)

Other clindamycin formulations:

Other effects that have been reported in association with the use of topical (dermal) formulations of clindamycin include severe colitis (including pseudomembranous colitis), contact dermatitis, skin irritation (*e.g.*, erythema, peeling and burning), oily skin, gram-negative folliculitis, abdominal pain, and gastrointestinal disturbances.

Clindamycin vaginal cream affords minimal peak serum levels and systemic exposure (A.U.C.'s) of clindamycin compared to 100 mg oral clindamycin dosing. Although these lower levels of exposure are less likely to produce the common reactions seen with oral clindamycin, the possibility of these and other reactions cannot be excluded presently. Data from well-controlled trials directly comparing clindamycin administered orally to clindamycin administered vaginally are not available.

The following adverse reactions and altered laboratory tests have been reported with the oral or parenteral use of clindamycin:

Gastrointestinal: Abdominal pain, esophagitis, nausea, vomiting, and diarrhea. (See WARNINGS.)

Hematopoietic: Transient neutropenia (leukopenia), eosinophilia, agranulocytosis, and thrombocytopenia have been reported. No direct etiologic relationship to concurrent clindamycin therapy could be made in any of these reports.

Hypersensitivity Reactions: Maculopapular rash and urticaria have been observed during drug therapy. Generalized mild to moderate morbilliform-like skin rashes are the most frequently reported of all adverse reactions. Rare instances of erythema multiforme, some resembling Stevens-Johnson syndrome, have been associated with clindamycin. A few cases of anaphylactoid reactions have been reported. If a hypersensitivity reaction occurs, the drug should be discontinued.

Liver: Jaundice and abnormalities in liver function tests have been observed during clindamycin therapy.

Musculoskeletal: Rare instances of polyarthritis have been reported.

Renal: Although no direct relationship of clindamycin to renal damage has been established, renal dysfunction as evidenced by azotemia, oliguria, and/or proteinuria has been observed in rare instances.

OVERDOSAGE

Vaginally applied clindamycin phosphate vaginal cream 2%, could be absorbed in sufficient amounts to produce systemic effects. (See WARNINGS.)

DOSAGE AND ADMINISTRATION

The recommended dose is one applicatorful of clindamycin phosphate vaginal cream 2%, (5 grams containing approximately 100 mg of clindamycin phosphate) intravaginally, preferably at bedtime, for seven consecutive days.

HOW SUPPLIED

CLEOCIN Vaginal Cream 2%, (clindamycin phosphate vaginal cream) is supplied in a 40 g tube (NDC 0009-3448-01) with 7 disposable applicators.

Store at controlled room temperature 15° to 30° C (59° to 86° F). Protect from freezing.

CLINICAL STUDIES

In clinical studies, non-pregnant women and pregnant women during the second trimester who had a diagnosis of bacterial vaginosis were treated with CLEOCIN Vaginal Cream 2% or a control regimen. The diagnosis of bacterial vaginosis was based on the criteria defined in the INDICATIONS AND USAGE section. Clinical cure rates, defined as resolution of all BV signs and symptoms at 4 weeks after the completion of therapy, were seen in approximately one-half of the patients treated with CLEOCIN Vaginal Cream 2%, compared to about one-third of the patients treated with a sulfa preparation and about one-tenth of the patients who received the cream vehicle. The actual results are presented in the table below:

Clinical Cure Rates at One Month

	CLEOCIN % (n/N)	Placebo % (n/N)	Sultrin % (n/N)
Pregnant Women	50% (65/129)	8% (10/119)	—
Non-pregnant Women			
Study 1:	35% (17/48)	9% (5/57)	—
Study 2:	53% (42/80)	—	35% (28/80)

Caution: Federal law prohibits dispensing without prescription.

Revised October 1995 815 255 302
691697

Continued on next page

Information on these Pharmacia & Upjohn products is based on labeling in effect June 1, 1996. Further information concerning these and other Pharmacia & Upjohn products may be obtained by direct inquiry to Medical Information, Pharmacia & Upjohn, Kalamazoo, MI 49001.

Pharmacia & Upjohn—Cont.

DIRECTIONS FOR USE

Seven plastic applicators are provided with this package. They are designed to allow proper vaginal administration of the cream.

Remove cap from cream tube. Screw a plastic applicator on the threaded end of the tube.

Rolling tube from the bottom, squeeze gently and force the medication into the applicator. The applicator is filled when the plunger reaches its predetermined stopping point. Unscrew the applicator from the tube and replace the cap.

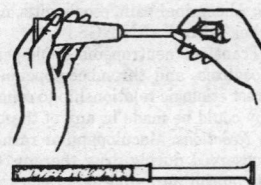

While lying on your back, firmly grasp the applicator barrel and insert into vagina as far as possible without causing discomfort.

Slowly push the plunger until it stops.

Carefully withdraw applicator from vagina, and discard applicator.

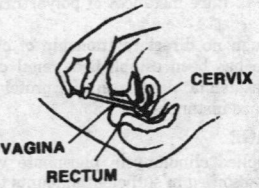

REMEMBER TO APPLY ONE APPLICATORFUL EACH NIGHT BEFORE BEDTIME, OR AS PRESCRIBED BY YOUR DOCTOR.

CLEOCIN T® ℞

[klēō-sin]

brand of clindamycin phosphate topical solution, topical gel and topical lotion

For External Use

DESCRIPTION

CLEOCIN T Topical Solution, CLEOCIN T Topical Gel and CLEOCIN T Topical Lotion contain clindamycin phosphate, USP, at a concentration equivalent to 10 mg clindamycin per milliliter. Each CLEOCIN T Topical Solution pledget applicator contains approximately 1 mL of topical solution.

Clindamycin phosphate is a water soluble ester of the semisynthetic antibiotic produced by a 7(S)-chloro-substitution of the 7(R)-hydroxyl group of the parent antibiotic lincomycin.

The solution contains isopropyl alcohol 50% v/v, propylene glycol, and water.

The gel contains allantoin, carbomer 934P, methylparaben, polyethylene glycol 400, propylene glycol, sodium hydroxide, and purified water.

The lotion contains cetostearyl alcohol (2.5%); glycerin; glyceryl stearate SE (with potassium monostearate); isostearyl alcohol (2.5%); methylparaben (0.3%); sodium lauroyl sarcosinate; stearic acid; and purified water.

The structural formula is represented below:

The chemical name for clindamycin phosphate is Methyl 7-chloro-6,7,8-trideoxy-6-(1-methyl-*trans*-4-propyl-L-2-pyrrolidinecarboxamido)-1-thio-L-*threo*-α-D-*galacto*-octopyranoside 2-(dihydrogen phosphate).

CLINICAL PHARMACOLOGY

Although clindamycin phosphate is inactive *in vitro*, rapid *in vivo* hydrolysis converts this compound to the antibacterially active clindamycin.

Cross resistance has been demonstrated between clindamycin and lincomycin.

Antagonism has been demonstrated between clindamycin and erythromycin.

Following multiple topical applications of clindamycin phosphate at a concentration equivalent to 10 mg clindamycin per mL in an isopropyl alcohol and water solution, very low levels of clindamycin are present in the serum (0-3 ng/mL) and less than 0.2% of the dose is recovered in urine as clindamycin.

Clindamycin activity has been demonstrated in comedones from acne patients. The mean concentration of antibiotic activity in extracted comedones after application of CLEOCIN T Topical Solution for 4 weeks was 597 mcg/g of comedonal material (range 0-1490). Clindamycin *in vitro* inhibits all *Propionibacterium acnes* cultures tested (MICs 0.4 mcg/mL). Free fatty acids on the skin surface have been decreased from approximately 14% to 2% following application of clindamycin.

INDICATIONS AND USAGE

CLEOCIN T Topical Solution, CLEOCIN T Topical Gel and CLEOCIN T Topical Lotion are indicated in the treatment of acne vulgaris. In view of the potential for diarrhea, bloody diarrhea and pseudomembranous colitis, the physician should consider whether other agents are more appropriate. (See CONTRAINDICATIONS, WARNINGS and ADVERSE REACTIONS.)

CONTRAINDICATIONS

CLEOCIN T Topical Solution, CLEOCIN T Topical Gel and CLEOCIN T Topical Lotion are contraindicated in individuals with a history of hypersensitivity to preparations containing clindamycin or lincomycin, a history of regional enteritis or ulcerative colitis, or a history of antibiotic-associated colitis.

WARNINGS

Orally and parenterally administered clindamycin has been associated with severe colitis which may result in patient death. Use of the topical formulation of clindamycin results in absorption of the antibiotic from the skin surface. Diarrhea, bloody diarrhea, and colitis (including pseudomembranous colitis) have been reported with the use of topical and systemic clindamycin.

Studies indicate a toxin(s) produced by clostridia is one primary cause of antibiotic-associated colitis. The colitis is usually characterized by severe persistent diarrhea and severe abdominal cramps and may be associated with the passage of blood and mucus. Endoscopic examination may reveal pseudomembranous colitis. Stool culture for _Clostridium difficile_ and stool assay for C. _difficile_ toxin may be helpful diagnostically.

When significant diarrhea occurs, the drug should be discontinued. Large bowel endoscopy should be considered to establish a definitive diagnosis in cases of severe diarrhea. Antiperistaltic agents such as opiates and diphenoxylate with atropine may prolong and/or worsen the condition. Vancomycin has been found to be effective in the treatment of antibiotic-associated pseudomembranous colitis produced by _Clostridium difficile_. The usual adult dosage is 500 milligrams to 2 grams of vancomycin orally per day in three to four divided doses administered for 7 to 10 days. Cholestyramine or colestipol resins bind vancomycin _in vitro_. If both a resin and vancomycin are to be administered concurrently, it may be advisable to separate the time of administration of each drug.

Diarrhea, colitis, and pseudomembranous colitis have been observed to begin up to several weeks following cessation of oral and parenteral therapy with clindamycin.

PRECAUTIONS

General

CLEOCIN T Topical Solution contains an alcohol base which will cause burning and irritation of the eye. In the event of accidental contact with sensitive surfaces (eye, abraded skin, mucous membranes), bathe with copious amounts of cool tap water. The solution has an unpleasant taste and caution should be exercised when applying medication around the mouth.

CLEOCIN T should be prescribed with caution in atopic individuals.

Drug Interactions

Clindamycin has been shown to have neuromuscular blocking properties that may enhance the action of other neuromuscular blocking agents. Therefore it should be used with caution in patients receiving such agents.

Pregnancy: Teratogenic effects—Pregnancy Category B

Reproduction studies have been performed in rats and mice using subcutaneous and oral doses of clindamycin ranging from 100 to 600 mg/kg/day and have revealed no evidence of impaired fertility or harm to the fetus due to clindamycin. There are, however, no adequate and well-controlled studies in pregnant women. Because animal reproduction studies are not always predictive of human response, this drug should be used during pregnancy only if clearly needed.

Nursing Mothers

It is not known whether clindamycin is excreted in human milk following use of CLEOCIN T. However, orally and parenterally administered clindamycin has been reported to appear in breast milk. Because of the potential for serious adverse reactions in nursing infants, a decision should be made whether to discontinue nursing or to discontinue the drug, taking into account the importance of the drug to the mother.

Pediatric Use

Safety and effectiveness in children under the age of 12 have not been established.

ADVERSE REACTIONS

In 18 clinical studies of various formulations of CLEOCIN T using placebo vehicle and/or active comparator drugs as controls, patients experienced a number of treatment emergent adverse dermatologic events [see table below].

Number of Patients Reporting Events

Treatment Emergent Adverse Event	Solution n=553 (%)	Gel n=148 (%)	Lotion n=160 (%)
Burning	62 (11)	15 (10)	17 (11)
Itching	36 (7)	15 (10)	17 (11)
Burning/Itching	60 (11)	# (–)	# (–)
Dryness	105 (19)	34 (23)	29 (18)
Erythema	86 (16)	10 (7)	22 (14)
Oiliness/Oily Skin	8 (1)	26 (18)	12* (10)
Peeling	61 (11)	# (–)	11 (7)

\# not recorded
* of 126 subjects

Orally and parenterally administered clindamycin has been associated with severe colitis which may end fatally.

Cases of diarrhea, bloody diarrhea and colitis (including pseudomembranous colitis) have been reported as adverse reactions in patients treated with oral and parenteral formulations of clindamycin and rarely with topical clindamycin (see WARNINGS).

Abdominal pain and gastrointestinal disturbances as well as gram-negative folliculitis have also been reported in association with the use of topical formulations of clindamycin.

OVERDOSAGE

Topically applied CLEOCIN T can be absorbed in sufficient amounts to produce systemic effects. (See WARNINGS.)

DOSAGE AND ADMINISTRATION

Apply a thin film of CLEOCIN T Topical Solution, CLEOCIN T Topical Lotion, CLEOCIN T Topical Gel, or use a CLEOCIN T Topical Solution pledget for the application of CLEOCIN T twice daily to affected area. More than one pledget may be used. Each pledget should be used only once and then be discarded.

Lotion: Shake well immediately before using.

Pledget: Remove pledget from foil just before use. Do not use if the seal is broken. Discard after single use.

Keep all liquid dosage forms in containers tightly closed.

HOW SUPPLIED

CLEOCIN T Topical Solution containing clindamycin phosphate equivalent to 10 mg clindamycin per milliliter is available in the following sizes:

30 mL applicator bottle—NDC 0009-3116-01

60 mL applicator bottle—NDC 0009-3116-02

Carton of 60 single-use pledget applicators—NDC 0009-3116-14

CLEOCIN T Topical Gel containing clindamycin phosphate equivalent to 10 mg clindamycin per milliliter is available in the following sizes:

60 gram tube—NDC 0009-3331-01

30 gram tube—NDC 0009-3331-02

CLEOCIN T Topical Lotion containing clindamycin phosphate equivalent to 10 mg clindamycin per milliliter is available in the following size:

60 mL plastic squeeze bottle—NDC 0009-3329-01

Store at controlled room temperature 15° to 30° C (59° to 86° F).

Protect from freezing.

CAUTION

Federal law prohibits dispensing without prescription.

Revised May 1996
811 373 626
691605

Shown in Product Identification Guide, page 329

COLESTID® ℞
[*kō-less-tid*]
brand of micronized colestipol hydrochloride tablets

DESCRIPTION

The active ingredient in COLESTID Tablets is micronized colestipol hydrochloride, which is a lipid lowering agent for oral use. Colestipol is an insoluble, high molecular weight basic anion-exchange copolymer of diethylenetriamine and 1-chloro-2, 3-epoxypropane, with approximately 1 out of 5 amine nitrogens protonated (chloride form). It is a light yellow water-insoluble resin which is hygroscopic and swells when suspended in water or aqueous fluids.

Each COLESTID Tablet contains one gram of micronized colestipol hydrochloride. COLESTID Tablets are light yellow in color and are tasteless and odorless. Inactive ingredients: cellulose acetate phthalate, glyceryl triacetate, carnauba wax, hydroxypropyl methylcellulose, magnesium stearate, povidone, silicon dioxide. COLESTID Tablets contain no calories.

HOW SUPPLIED

COLESTID Tablets are yellow, elliptical, imprinted U, and are supplied as follows:

Bottles of 120 NDC 0009-0450-03
Bottles of 500 NDC 0009-0450-04

Each tablet contains 1 gram of colestipol hydrochloride.
Store at controlled room temperature.
Caution: Federal law prohibits dispensing without prescription.
Revised September 1995 815 838 001
691015

COLESTID® ℞
[*ko-less-tid*]
FLAVORED COLESTID® ℞
brand of colestipol hydrochloride granules (colestipol hydrochloride for oral suspension)

DESCRIPTION

COLESTID Granules and FLAVORED COLESTID Granules contain colestipol hydrochloride, which is a lipid lowering agent for oral use. Colestipol hydrochloride is an insoluble, high molecular weight basic anion-exchange copolymer of diethylenetriamine and 1-chloro-2, 3-epoxypropane, with approximately 1 out of 5 amine nitrogens protonated (chloride form). It is a light yellow water-insoluble resin which is hygroscopic and swells when suspended in water or aqueous fluids.

COLESTID is tasteless and odorless. Inactive ingredient: silicon dioxide. One dose (1 packet or 1 level teaspoon) of COLESTID contains 5 grams of colestipol hydrochloride. FLAVORED COLESTID is orange flavored and light orange in color. One dose (1 packet or 1 level scoopful) of FLAVORED COLESTID is approximately 7.5 grams which contains 5 grams of colestipol hydrochloride. This product also contains the following inactive ingredients: aspartame, beta carotene, citric acid, flavor (natural and artificial), glycerine, maltol, mannitol, and methylcellulose.

CLINICAL PHARMACOLOGY

Cholesterol is the major, and probably the sole precursor of bile acids. During normal digestion, bile acids are secreted via the bile from the liver and gall bladder into the intestines. Bile acids emulsify the fat and lipid materials present in food, thus facilitating absorption. A major portion of the bile acids secreted is reabsorbed from the intestines and returned via the portal circulation to the liver, thus completing the enterohepatic cycle. Only very small amounts of bile acids are found in normal serum.

Colestipol hydrochloride binds bile acids in the intestine forming a complex that is excreted in the feces. This nonsystemic action results in a partial removal of the bile acids from the enterohepatic circulation, preventing their reabsorption. Since colestipol hydrochloride is an anion exchange resin, the chloride anions of the resin can be replaced by other anions, usually those with a greater affinity for the resin than chloride ion.

Colestipol hydrochloride is hydrophilic, but it is virtually water insoluble (99.75%) and it is not hydrolyzed by digestive enzymes. The high molecular weight polymer in colestipol hydrochloride apparently is not absorbed. In humans, less than 0.17% of a single ^{14}C-labeled colestipol hydrochloride dose is excreted in the urine when given following 60 days of chronic dosing of 20 grams of colestipol hydrochloride per day.

The increased fecal loss of bile acids due to colestipol hydrochloride administration leads to an increased oxidation of cholesterol to bile acids. This results in an increase in the number of low-density lipoprotein (LDL) receptors, increased hepatic uptake of LDL and a decrease in beta lipoprotein or low density lipoprotein serum levels, and a decrease in serum cholesterol levels. Although colestipol hydrochloride produces an increase in the hepatic synthesis of cholesterol in man, serum cholesterol levels fall.

There is evidence to show that this fall in cholesterol is secondary to an increased rate of clearance of cholesterol-rich lipoproteins (beta or low density lipoproteins) from the plasma. Serum triglyceride levels may increase or remain unchanged in colestipol hydrochloride treated patients.

The decline in serum cholesterol levels with colestipol hydrochloride treatment is usually evident by one month. When colestipol hydrochloride is discontinued, serum cholesterol levels usually return to baseline levels within one month.

Periodic determinations of serum cholesterol levels as outlined in the National Cholesterol Education Program (NCEP) guidelines should be done to confirm a favorable initial and long-term response[1].

In a large, placebo-controlled, multiclinic study, the LRC-CPPT,[2] hypercholesterolemic subjects treated with cholestyramine, a bile-acid sequestrant with a mechanism of action and an effect on serum cholesterol similar to that of colestipol hydrochloride, had reductions in total and low-density lipoprotein cholesterol (LDL-C). Over the seven-year study period the cholestyramine group experienced a 19% reduction (relative to the incidence in the placebo group) in the combined rate of coronary heart disease death plus non-fatal myocardial infarction (cumulative incidences of 7% cholestyramine and 8.6%, placebo). The subjects included in the study were middle-aged men (age 35–59) with serum cholesterol-levels above 265 mg/dL, LDL-C above 175 mg/dL on a moderate cholesterol-lowering diet, and no history of heart disease. It is not clear to what extent these findings can be extrapolated to other segments of the hypercholesterolemic population not studied.

Treatment with colestipol hydrochloride results in a significant increase in lipoprotein LpAI. Lipoprotein LpAI is one of the two major lipoprotein particles within the high-density lipoprotein (HDL) density range[3], and has been shown in cell culture to promote cholesterol efflux or removal from cells[4]. Although the significance of this finding has not been established in clinical studies, the elevation of the lipoprotein LpAI particle within the HDL fraction is consistent with an antiatherogenic effect of colestipol hydrochloride, even though little change is observed in HDL cholesterol.

In patients with heterozygous familial hypercholesterolemia who have not obtained an optimal response to colestipol hydrochloride alone in maximal doses, the combination of colestipol hydrochloride and nicotinic acid has been shown to further lower serum cholesterol, triglyceride, and LDL cholesterol (LDL-C) values. Simultaneously, HDL cholesterol (HDL-C) values increased significantly. In many such patients it is possible to normalize serum lipid values.[5-7]

Preliminary evidence suggests that the cholesterol-lowering effects of lovastatin and the bile acid sequestrant, colestipol hydrochloride, are additive.

The effect of intensive lipid-lowering therapy on coronary atherosclerosis has been assessed by arteriography in hyperlipidemic patients. In these randomized, controlled clinical trials, patients were treated for two to four years by either conventional measures (diet, placebo, or in some cases low-dose resin), or with intensive combination therapy using diet and COLESTID Granules plus either nicotinic acid or lovastatin. When compared to conventional measures, intensive lipid-lowering combination therapy significantly reduced the frequency of progression and increased the frequency of regression of coronary atherosclerotic lesions in patients with or at risk for coronary artery disease.[8-11]

INDICATIONS AND USAGE

Since no drug is innocuous, strict attention should be paid to the indications and contraindications, particularly when selecting drugs for chronic long-term use.

COLESTID Granules and FLAVORED COLESTID Granules are indicated as adjunctive therapy to diet for the reduction of elevated serum total and low-density lipoprotein (LDL) cholesterol in patients with primary hypercholesterolemia (elevated low density lipoproteins [LDL] cholesterol) who do not respond adequately to diet. Generally, COLESTID and FLAVORED COLESTID have no clinically significant effect on serum triglycerides, but with its use triglyceride levels may be raised in some patients.

Therapy with lipid-altering agents should be a component of multiple risk factor intervention in those individuals at significantly increased risk for atherosclerotic vascular disease due to hypercholesterolemia. Treatment should begin and continue with dietary therapy (see NCEP guidelines). A minimum of six months of intensive dietary therapy and counseling should be carried out prior to initiation of drug therapy. Shorter periods may be considered in patients with severe elevations of LDL-C or with definite CHD.

According to the NCEP guidelines, the goal of treatment is to lower LDL-C, and LDL-C is to be used to initiate and assess treatment response. Only if LDL-C levels are not available, should the Total-C be used to monitor therapy. The NCEP treatment guidelines are shown below.

		LDL-Cholesterol mg/dL (mmol/L)	
Definite Atherosclerotic Disease*	Two or More Other Risk Factors**	Initiation Level	Goal
No	No	≥190 (≥4.9)	<160 (<4.1)
No	Yes	≥160 (≥4.1)	<130 (<3.4)
Yes	Yes or No	≥130 (≥3.4)	≤100 (≤2.6)

* Coronary heart disease or peripheral vascular disease (including symptomatic carotid artery disease).

** Other risk factors for coronary heart disease (CHD) include: age (males: ≥45 years; females: ≥55 years or premature menopause without estrogen replacement therapy); family history of premature CHD; current cigarette smoking; hypertension; confirmed HDL-C <35 mg/dL (0.91 mmol/L); and diabetes mellitus. Subtract one risk factor if HDL-C is ≥60 mg/dL (1.6 mmol/L).

CONTRAINDICATIONS

COLESTID Granules and FLAVORED COLESTID Granules are contraindicated in those individuals who have shown hypersensitivity to any of its components.

WARNINGS

TO AVOID ACCIDENTAL INHALATION OR ESOPHAGEAL DISTRESS, *COLESTID GRANULES* AND *FLAVORED COLESTID GRANULES* SHOULD NOT BE TAKEN IN ITS DRY FORM. ALWAYS MIX *COLESTID* AND *FLAVORED COLESTID* WITH WATER OR OTHER FLUIDS BEFORE INGESTING.

PHENYLKETONURICS: *FLAVORED COLESTID* CONTAINS 18.2 MG PHENYLALANINE PER 7.5-GRAM DOSE.

PRECAUTIONS

Prior to initiating therapy with COLESTID Granules and FLAVORED COLESTID Granules, secondary causes of hypercholesterolemia (e.g., poorly controlled diabetes mellitus, hypothyroidism, nephrotic syndrome, dysproteinemias, obstructive liver disease, other drug therapy, alcoholism), should be excluded, and a lipid profile performed to assess Total cholesterol, HDL-C, and triglycerides (TG). For individuals with TG less than 400 mg/dL (<4.5 mmol/L), LDL-C can be estimated using the following equation:

LDL-C = Total cholesterol-[(Triglycerides/5)+HDL-C]

For TG levels >400 mg/dL, this equation is less accurate and LDL-C concentrations should be determined by ultracentrifugation. In hypertriglyceridemic patients, LDL-C may be low or normal despite elevated Total-C. In such cases COLESTID and FLAVORED COLESTID may not be indicated.

Because it sequesters bile acids, colestipol hydrochloride may interfere with normal fat absorption and thus may reduce absorption of folic acid and fat soluble vitamins such as A, D, and K.

Chronic use of colestipol hydrochloride may be associated with an increased bleeding tendency due to hypoprothrombinemia from vitamin K deficiency. This will usually respond promptly to parenteral vitamin K_1 and recurrences can be prevented by oral administration of vitamin K_1.

Serum cholesterol and triglyceride levels should be determined periodically based on NCEP guidelines to confirm a favorable initial and adequate long-term response.

COLESTID and FLAVORED COLESTID may produce or severely worsen pre-existing constipation. The dosage should be increased gradually in patients to minimize the risk of developing fecal impaction. In patients with pre-existing constipation, the starting dose should be 1 packet or 1 scoop once daily for 5–7 days, increasing to twice daily with monitoring of constipation and of serum lipoproteins, at least twice, 4–6 weeks apart. Increased fluid and fiber intake should be encouraged to alleviate constipation and a stool softener may occasionally be indicated. If the initial dose is well tolerated, the dose may be increased as needed by one dose/day (at monthly intervals) with periodic monitoring of serum lipoproteins. If constipation worsens or the desired therapeutic response is not achieved at one to six doses/day, combination therapy or alternate therapy should be considered. Particular effort should be made to avoid constipation in patients with symptomatic coronary artery disease. Constipation associated with COLESTID and FLAVORED COLESTID may aggravate hemorrhoids.

Continued on next page

Information on these Pharmacia & Upjohn products is based on labeling in effect June 1, 1996. Further information concerning these and other Pharmacia & Upjohn products may be obtained by direct inquiry to Medical Information, Pharmacia & Upjohn, Kalamazoo, MI 49001.

Consult 1997 supplements and future editions for revisions

Pharmacia & Upjohn—Cont.

While there have been no reports of hypothyroidism induced in individuals with normal thyroid function, the theoretical possibility exists, particularly in patients with limited thyroid reserve.

Since colestipol hydrochloride is a chloride form of an anion exchange resin, there is a possibility that prolonged use may lead to the development of hyperchloremic acidosis.

Carcinogenesis, mutagenesis and impairment of fertility

In studies conducted in rats in which cholestyramine resin (a bile acid sequestering agent similar to colestipol hydrochloride) was used as a tool to investigate the role of various intestinal factors, such as fat, bile salts and microbial flora, in the development of intestinal tumors induced by potent carcinogens, the incidence of such tumors was observed to be greater in cholestyramine resin treated rats than in control rats.

The relevance of this laboratory observation from studies in rats with cholestyramine resin to the clinical use of colestipol hydrochloride is not known. In the LRC-CPPT study referred to above, the total incidence of fatal and non-fatal neoplasms was similar in both treatment groups. When the many different categories of tumors are examined, various alimentary system cancers were somewhat more prevalent in the cholestyramine group. The small numbers and the multiple categories prevent conclusions from being drawn. Further follow-up of the LRC-CPPT participants by the sponsors of that study is planned for cause-specific mortality and cancer morbidity.

When colestipol hydrochloride was administered in the diet to rats for 18 months, there was no evidence of any drug related intestinal tumor formation. In the Ames assay, colestipol hydrochloride was not mutagenic.

Use in Pregnancy

Since colestipol hydrochloride is essentially not absorbed systemically (less than 0.17% of the dose), it is not expected to cause fetal harm when administered during pregnancy in recommended dosages. There are no adequate and well controlled studies in pregnant women, and the known interference with absorption of fat soluble vitamins may be detrimental even in the presence of supplementation. The use of COLESTID or FLAVORED COLESTID in pregnancy or by women of childbearing potential requires that the potential benefits of drug therapy be weighed against possible hazards to the mother or child.

Nursing Mother

Caution should be exercised when COLESTID or FLAVORED COLESTID is administered to a nursing mother. The possible lack of proper vitamin absorption described in the "pregnancy" section may have an effect on nursing infants.

Use in Children

Safety and effectiveness in children have not been established.

Drug Interactions

Since colestipol hydrochloride is an anion exchange resin, it may have a strong affinity for anions other than the bile acids. *In vitro* studies have indicated that colestipol hydrochloride binds a number of drugs. Therefore, COLESTID and FLAVORED COLESTID resin may delay or reduce the absorption of concomitant oral medication. The interval between the administration of COLESTID and FLAVORED COLESTID and any other medication should be as long as possible. Patients should take other drugs at least one hour before or four hours after COLESTID and FLAVORED COLESTID to avoid impeding their absorption.

Repeated doses of colestipol hydrochloride given prior to a single dose of propranolol in human trials have been reported to decrease propranolol absorption. However, in a follow-up study in normal subjects, single dose administration of colestipol hydrochloride and propranolol and twice-a-day administration for 5 days of both agents did not effect the extent of propranolol absorption, but had a small yet statistically significant effect on its rate of absorption; the time to reach maximum concentration was delayed 30 minutes. Effects on the absorption of other beta-blockers have not been determined. Therefore, patients on propranolol should be observed when COLESTID or FLAVORED COLESTID is either added or deleted from a therapeutic regimen.

Studies in humans show that the absorption of chlorothiazide as reflected in urinary excretion is markedly decreased even when administered one hour before colestipol hydrochloride. The absorption of tetracycline, furosemide, penicillin G, hydrochlorothiazide, and gemfibrozil was significantly decreased when given simultaneously with colestipol hydrochloride; these drugs were not tested to determine the effect of administration one hour before colestipol hydrochloride.

No depressant effect on blood levels in humans was noted when colestipol hydrochloride was administered with any of the following drugs: aspirin, clindamycin, clofibrate, methyldopa, nicotinic acid (niacin), tolbutamide, phenytoin or warfarin. Particular caution should be observed with digitalis

preparations since there are conflicting results for the effect of colestipol hydrochloride on the availability of digoxin and digitoxin. The potential for binding of these drugs if given concomitantly is present. Discontinuing colestipol hydrochloride could pose a hazard to health if a potentially toxic drug that is significantly bound to the resin has been titrated to a maintenance level while the patient was taking colestipol hydrochloride.

Bile acid binding resins may also interfere with the absorption of oral phosphate supplements and hydrocortisone.

ADVERSE REACTIONS

Gastrointestinal

The most common adverse reactions are confined to the gastrointestinal tract. To achieve minimal GI disturbance with an optimal LDL-cholesterol lowering effect, a gradual increase of dosage starting with one dose/day is recommended. Constipation is the major single complaint and at times is severe. Most instances of constipation are mild, transient, and controlled with standard treatment. Increased fluid intake and inclusion of additional dietary fiber should be the first step; a stool softener may be added if needed. Some patients require decreased dosage or discontinuation of therapy. Hemorrhoids may be aggravated.

Other, less frequent gastrointestinal complaints consist of abdominal discomfort (abdominal pain and cramping), intestinal gas, (bloating and flatulence), indigestion and heartburn, diarrhea and loose stools, and nausea and vomiting. Bleeding hemorrhoids and blood in the stool have been infrequently reported. Peptic ulceration, cholecystitis, and cholelithiasis have been rarely reported in patients receiving colestipol hydrochloride granules, and are not necessarily drug related.

Transient and modest elevations of aspartate aminotransferase (AST, SGOT), alanine aminotransferase (ALT, SGPT) and alkaline phosphatase were observed on one or more occasions in various patients treated with colestipol hydrochloride.

The following non-gastrointestinal adverse reactions have been reported with generally equal frequency in patients receiving COLESTID Granules, FLAVORED COLESTID Granules, or placebo in clinical studies:

Cardiovascular

Chest pain, angina, and tachycardia have been infrequently reported.

Hypersensitivity

Rash has been infrequently reported. Urticaria and dermatitis have been rarely noted in patients receiving colestipol hydrochloride granules.

Musculoskeletal

Musculoskeletal pain, aches and pains in the extremities, joint pains, arthritis, and backache have been reported.

Neurologic

Headache, migraine headache and sinus headache have been reported. Other infrequently reported complaints include dizziness, light-headedness, and insomnia.

Miscellaneous

Anorexia, fatigue, weakness, shortness of breath, and swelling of the hands or feet, have been infrequently reported.

OVERDOSAGE

Overdosage of COLESTID Granules or FLAVORED COLESTID Granules has not been reported. Should overdosage occur, however, the chief potential harm would be obstruction of the gastrointestinal tract. The location of such potential obstruction, the degree of obstruction and the presence or absence of normal gut motility would determine treatment.

DOSAGE AND ADMINISTRATION

One dose (1 packet or 1 level teaspoon) of COLESTID Granules contains 5 grams of colestipol hydrochloride. One dose (1 packet or 1 level scoopful) of FLAVORED COLESTID Granules is approximately 7.5 grams which contains 5 grams of colestipol hydrochloride. The recommended daily adult dose is one to six packets or level scoopfuls given once or in divided doses. Treatment should be started with one dose once or twice daily with an increment of one dose/day at one- or two-month intervals. Appropriate use of lipid profiles as per NCEP guidelines including LDL-cholesterol and triglycerides is advised so that optimal, but not excessive doses are used to obtain the desired therapeutic effect on LDL-cholesterol level. If the desired therapeutic effect is not obtained at one to six doses/day with good compliance and acceptable side effects, combined therapy or alternate treatment should be considered.

To avoid accidental inhalation or esophageal distress, COLESTID and FLAVORED COLESTID should not be taken in its dry form. COLESTID and FLAVORED COLESTID should always be mixed with water or other fluids before ingesting. Patients should take other drugs at least one hour before or four hours after COLESTID or FLAVORED COLESTID to minimize possible interference with their absorption. (See PRECAUTIONS, Drug Interactions.)

Before COLESTID or FLAVORED COLESTID Administration

1. Define the type of hyperlipoproteinemia, as described in NCEP guidelines.

2. Institute a trial of diet and weight reduction.

3. Establish baseline serum total and LDL-cholesterol and triglyceride levels.

During COLESTID or FLAVORED COLESTID Administration

1. The patient should be carefully monitored clinically, including serum cholesterol and triglyceride levels. Periodic determinations of serum cholesterol levels as outlined in the NCEP guidelines should be done to confirm a favorable initial and longer-term response.

2. Failure of total or LDL-cholesterol to fall within the desired range should lead one to first examine dietary and drug compliance. If these are deemed acceptable, combined therapy or alternate treatment should be considered.

3. Significant rise in triglyceride level should be considered as indication for dose reduction, drug discontinuation, or combined or alternate therapy.

Mixing and Administration Guide

COLESTID and FLAVORED COLESTID should always be mixed in a liquid such as water or the beverage of your choice. It may also be taken in soups or with cereals or pulpy fruits. COLESTID or FLAVORED COLESTID *should never be taken in its dry form.*

FLAVORED COLESTID is an orange-flavored product. Although it may be mixed with a variety of liquids or foods, the selection should be based on patient preference.

With Beverages

1. Add the prescribed amount of COLESTID or FLAVORED COLESTID to a glassful (three ounces or more) of water or the beverage of your choice. A heavy or pulpy juice may minimize complaints relative to consistency.

2. Stir the mixture until the medication is completely mixed. (COLESTID and FLAVORED COLESTID will not dissolve in the liquid.) COLESTID and FLAVORED COLESTID may also be mixed with carbonated beverages, slowly stirred in a large glass; however, this mixture may be associated with GI complaints.

Rinse the glass with a small amount of additional beverage to make sure all the medication is taken.

With cereals, soups, and fruits

COLESTID and FLAVORED COLESTID may be taken mixed with milk in hot or regular breakfast cereals, or even mixed in soups that have a high fluid content. It may also be added to fruits that are pulpy such as crushed pineapple, pears, peaches, or fruit cocktail.

HOW SUPPLIED

COLESTID Granules are available as follows:
Cartons of 30 foil packets — NDC 0009-0260-01
Cartons of 90 foil packets — NDC 0009-0260-04
Bottles of 300 grams with scoop — NDC 0009-0260-17
Bottles of 500 grams with scoop — NDC 0009-0260-02
Each packet or level scoop supplies 5 grams of COLESTID.

FLAVORED COLESTID Granules are available as follows:
Cartons of 60 foil packets — NDC 0009-0370-03
Bottles of 450 grams (equivalent to approximately 60 doses) with scoop — NDC 0009-0370-05

Each packet or each level scoopful supplies approximately 7.5 grams of FLAVORED COLESTID containing 5 grams of colestipol hydrochloride.

Store at controlled room temperature 15° to 30° C (59° to 86° F).

REFERENCES

1. Summary of the Second Report of the National Cholesterol Education Program (NCEP) Expert Panel on Detection, Evaluation, and Treatment of High Blood Cholesterol in Adults (Adult Treatment Panel II). *JAMA* 269(23):3015-3023, 1993.

2. Lipid Metabolism-Atherogenesis Branch, National Heart, Lung, and Blood Institute, Bethesda, MD: The Lipid Research Clinics Coronary Primary Prevention Trial Results. I. Reduction in Incidence of Coronary Heart Disease. *JAMA* 251:351-364, 1984.

3. Parra HJ, et al. Differential electroimmunoassay of human LpA-I lipoprotein particles on ready-to-use plates. *Clin. Chem.* 36(8):1431-1435, 1990.

4. Barbaras R, et al. Cholesterol efflux from cultured adipose cells is mediated by LpAI particles but not by LpAI:AII particles. *Biochem. Biophys. Res. Comm.* 142(1):63-69, 1987.

5. Kane JP, et al. Normalization of low-density-lipoprotein levels in heterozygous familial hypercholesterolemia with a combined drug regimen. *N Engl. J. Med.* 304:251-258, 1981.

6. Illingworth DR, et al. Colestipol plus nicotinic acid in treatment of heterozygous familial hypercholesterolemia. *Lancet* 1:296-298, 1981.

7. Kuo PT, et al. Familial type II hyperlipoproteinemia with coronary heart disease:Effect of diet-colestipol-nicotinic acid treatment. *Chest* 79:286-291, 1981.

8. Blankenhorn DH, et al. Beneficial Effects of Combined Colestipol-Niacin Therapy on Coronary Atherosclerosis and Coronary Venous Bypass Grafts. *JAMA* 257(23):3233-3240, 1987.

9. Cashin-Hemphill L, et al. Beneficial Effects of Colestipol-Niacin on Coronary Atherosclerosis: A 4-Year Follow-up. *JAMA* 264:3013-3017, 1990.

10. Brown G, et al. Regression of Coronary Artery Disease as a Result of Intensive Lipid-Lowering Therapy in Men with High Levels of Apolipoprotein B. *N Engl, J. Med* 323:1289-1298, 1990.
11. Kane JP, et al. Regression of Coronary Atherosclerosis During Treatment of Familial Hypercholesterolemia with Combined Drug Regimens. *JAMA* 264:3007-3012, 1990.

Caution: Federal law prohibits dispensing without prescription.

Revised March 1996 816 577 002 691344

CORVERT™ ℞
(brand of ibutilide fumarate injection)
For intravenous infusion only

DESCRIPTION

CORVERT Injection (ibutilide fumarate injection) is an antiarrhythmic drug with predominantly class III (cardiac action potential prolongation) properties according to the Vaughan Williams Classification. Each milliliter of CORVERT Injection contains 0.1 mg of ibutilide fumarate (equivalent to 0.087 mg ibutilide free base), 0.189 mg sodium acetate trihydrate, 8.90 mg sodium chloride, hydrochloric acid to adjust pH to approximately 4.6, and Water for Injection. CORVERT Injection is an isotonic, clear, colorless, sterile aqueous solution.

Ibutilide fumarate has one chiral center, and exists as a racemate of the (+) and (−) enantiomers.

The chemical name for ibutilide fumarate is Methanesulfonamide, N-{4-[4-(ethylheptylamino)-1-hydroxybutyl] phenyl}, (+) (−), (E)-2-butenedioate (1:0.5) (hemifumarate salt). Its molecular formula is $C_{22}H_{38}N_2O_5S$, and its molecular weight is 442.62.

Ibutilide fumarate is a white to off-white powder with an aqueous solubility of over 100 mg/mL at pH 7 or lower.

The structural formula is represented below:

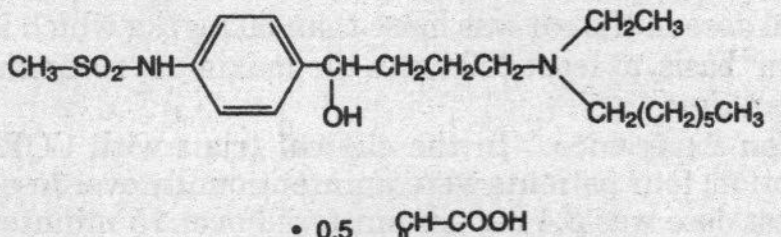

CLINICAL PHARMACOLOGY

Mechanism of Action: CORVERT Injection prolongs action potential duration in isolated adult cardiac myocytes and increases both atrial and ventricular refractoriness *in vivo*, ie, class III electrophysiologic effects. Voltage clamp studies indicate that CORVERT, at nanomolar concentrations, delays repolarization by activation of a slow, inward current (predominantly sodium), rather than by blocking outward potassium currents, which is the mechanism by which most other class III antiarrhythmics act. These effects lead to prolongation of atrial and ventricular action potential duration and refractoriness, the predominant electrophysiologic properties of CORVERT in humans that are thought to be the basis for its antiarrhythmic effect.

Electrophysiologic Effects: CORVERT produces mild slowing of the sinus rate and atrioventricular conduction, CORVERT produces no clinically significant effect on QRS duration at intravenous doses up to 0.03 mg/kg administered over a 10-minute period. Although there is no established relationship between plasma concentration and antiarrhythmic effect, CORVERT produces dose-related prolongation of the QT interval, which is thought to be associated with its antiarrhythmic activity. (See WARNINGS for relationship between QTc prolongation and torsades de pointes-type arrhythmias.) In a study in healthy volunteers, intravenous infusions of CORVERT resulted in prolongation of the QT interval that was directly correlated with ibutilide plasma concentration during and after 10-minute and 8-hour infusions. A steep ibutilide concentration/response (QT prolongation) relationship was shown. The maximum effect was a function of both the dose of CORVERT and the infusion rate.

Hemodynamic Effects: A study of hemodynamic function in patients with ejection fractions both above and below 35% showed no clinically significant effects on cardiac output, mean pulmonary arterial pressure, or pulmonary capillary wedge pressure at doses of CORVERT up to 0.03 mg/kg.

Pharmacokinetics: After intravenous infusion, ibutilide plasma concentrations rapidly decrease in a multiexponential fashion. The pharmacokinetics of ibutilide are highly variable among subjects. Ibutilide has a high systemic plasma clearance that approximates liver blood flow (about 29 mL/min/kg), a large steady-state volume of distribution (about 11 L/kg) in healthy volunteers, and minimal (about 40%) protein binding. Ibutilide is also cleared rapidly and highly distributed in patients being treated for atrial flutter or atrial fibrillation. The elimination half-life averages about 6 hours (range from 2 to 12 hours). The pharmacokinetics of ibutilide are linear with respect to the dose of CORVERT over the dose range of 0.01 mg/kg to 0.10 mg/kg. The enantiomers of ibutilide fumarate have pharmacokinetic properties similar to each other and to ibutilide fumarate. The pharmacokinetics of CORVERT Injection in patients with atrial flutter or atrial fibrillation are similar regardless of the type of arrhythmia, patient age, sex, or the concomitant use of digoxin, calcium channel blockers, or beta blockers.

Metabolism and elimination: In healthy male volunteers, about 82% of a 0.01 mg/kg dose of [^{14}C] ibutilide fumarate was excreted in the urine (about 7% of the dose as unchanged ibutilide) and the remainder (about 19%) was recovered in the feces.

Eight metabolites of ibutilide were detected in metabolic profiling of urine. These metabolites are thought to be formed primarily by ω-oxidation followed by sequential β-oxidation of the heptyl side chain of ibutilide. Of the eight metabolites, only the ω-hydroxy metabolite possesses class III electrophysiologic properties similar to that of ibutilide in an *in vitro* isolated rabbit myocardium model. The plasma concentrations of this active metabolite, however, are less than 10% of that of ibutilide.

Clinical Studies: Treatment with intravenous ibutilide fumarate for acute termination of recent onset atrial flutter/fibrillation was evaluated in 466 patients participating in two randomized, double-blind, placebo-controlled clinical trials. Patients had had their arrhythmias for 3 hours to 90 days, were anticoagulated for at least 2 weeks if atrial fibrillation was present more than 3 days, had serum potassium of at least 4.0 mEq/L and QTc below 440 msec, and were monitored by telemetry for at least 24 hours. Patients could not be on class I or other class III antiarrhythmics (these had to be discontinued at least 5 half-lives prior to infusion) but could be on calcium channel blockers, beta blockers, or digoxin. In one trial, single 10-minute infusions of 0.005 to 0.025 mg/kg were tested in parallel groups (0.3 to 1.5 mg in a 60 kg person). In the second trial, up to two infusions of ibutilide fumarate were evaluated—the first 1.0 mg, the second given 10 minutes after completion of the first infusion, either 0.5 or 1.0 mg. In a third double-blind study, 319 patients with atrial fibrillation or atrial flutter of 3 hours to 45 days duration were randomized to receive single, 10-minute intravenous infusions of either sotalol (1.5 mg/kg) or CORVERT (1 mg or 2 mg). Among patients with atrial flutter, 53% receiving 1 mg ibutilide fumarate and 70% receiving 2 mg ibutilide fumarate converted, compared to 18% of those receiving sotalol. In patients with atrial fibrillation, 22% receiving 1 mg ibutilide fumarate and 43% receiving 2 mg ibutilide fumarate converted compared to 10% of patients receiving sotalol.

Patients in clinical trials were hemodynamically stable. Patients with specific cardiovascular conditions such as symptomatic heart failure, recent acute myocardial infarction, and angina were excluded. About two thirds had cardiovascular symptoms, and the majority of patients had left atrial enlargement, decreased left ventricular ejection fraction, a history of valvular disease, or previous history of atrial fibrillation or flutter. Electrical cardioversion was allowed 90 minutes after the infusion was complete. Patients could be given other antiarrhythmic drugs 4 hours postinfusion.

Results of the first two studies are shown in the tables below. Conversion of atrial flutter/fibrillation usually (70% of those who converted) occurred within 30 minutes of the start of infusion and was dose related. The latest conversion seen was at 90 minutes after the start of the infusion. Most converted patients remained in normal sinus rhythm for 24 hours. Overall responses in these patients, defined as termination of arrhythmias for any length of time during or within 1 hour following completed infusion of randomized dose, were in the range of 43% to 48% at doses above 0.0125 mg/kg (vs 2% for placebo). Twenty-four hour responses were similar. For these atrial arrhythmias, ibutilide was more effective in patients with flutter than fibrillation (≥48% vs ≤40%).

PERCENT OF PATIENTS WHO CONVERTED (First Trial)

			Ibutilide			
		Placebo	0.005 mg/kg	0.01 mg/kg	0.015 mg/kg	0.025 mg/kg
	n	41	41	40	38	40
Both	Initially*	2	12	33	45	48
	At 24 hours†	2	12	28	42	43
Atrial flutter	Initially*	0	14	30	58	55
	At 24 hours†	0	14	30	58	50
Atrial fibrillation	Initially*	5	10	35	32	40
	At 24 hours†	5	10	25	26	35

*Percent of patients who converted within 70 minutes after the start of infusion.
†Percent of patients who remained in sinus rhythm 24 hours after dosing.

PERCENT OF PATIENTS WHO CONVERTED (Second Trial)

			Ibutilide	
		Placebo	1.0 mg/ 0.5 mg	1.0 mg/ 1.0 mg
	n	86	86	94
Both	Initially*	2	43	44
	At 24 hours†	2	34	37
Atrial flutter	Initially*	2	48	63
	At 24 hours†	2	45	59
Atrial fibrillation	Initially*	2	38	25
	At 24 hours†	2	21	17

*Percent of patients who converted within 90 minutes after the start of infusion.
†Percent of patients who remained in sinus rhythm 24 hours after dosing.

The numbers of patients who remained in the converted rhythm at the end of 24 hours were slightly less than those patients who converted initially, but the difference between conversion rates for ibutilide compared to placebo was still statistically significant. In long-term follow-up, approximately 40% of all patients remained recurrence free, usually with chronic prophylactic treatment, 400 to 500 days after acute treatment, regardless of the method of conversion.

Patients with more recent onset of arrhythmia had a higher rate of conversion. Response rates were 42% and 50% for patients with onset of atrial fibrillation/flutter for less than 30 days in the two efficacy studies compared to 16% and 31% in those with more chronic arrhythmias.

Ibutilide was equally effective in patients below and above 65 years of age and in men and women. Female patients constituted about 20% of patients in controlled studies.

INDICATIONS AND USAGE

CORVERT Injection is indicated for the rapid conversion of atrial fibrillation or atrial flutter of recent onset to sinus rhythm. Patients with atrial arrhythmias of longer duration are less likely to respond to CORVERT. The effectiveness of ibutilide has not been determined in patients with arrhythmias of more than 90 days in duration.

LIFE-THREATENING ARRHYTHMIAS
APPROPRIATE TREATMENT ENVIRONMENT

CORVERT can cause potentially fatal arrhythmias, particularly sustained polymorphic ventricular tachycardia, usually in association with QT prolongation (torsades de pointes), but sometimes without documented QT prolongation. In clinical studies, these arrhythmias, which require cardioversion, occurred in 1.7% of treated patients during, or within a number of hours of, use of CORVERT. These arrhythmias can be reversed if treated promptly (see WARNINGS, Proarrhythmia). It is essential that CORVERT be administered in a setting of continuous ECG monitoring and by personnel trained in identification and treatment of acute ventricular arrhythmias, particularly polymorphic ventricular tachycardia. *Patients with atrial fibrillation of more than 2 to 3 days' duration must be adequately anticoagulated, generally for at least 2 weeks.*

CHOICE OF PATIENTS

Patients with chronic atrial fibrillation have a strong tendency to revert after conversion to sinus rhythm (see CLINICAL STUDIES) and treatments to maintain sinus rhythm carry risks. Patients to be treated with CORVERT, therefore, should be carefully selected such that the expected benefits of maintaining sinus rhythm outweigh the immediate risks of CORVERT, and the risks of maintenance therapy, and are likely to offer an advantage compared with alternative management.

CONTRAINDICATIONS

CORVERT Injection is contraindicated in patients who have previously demonstrated hypersensitivity to ibutilide fumarate or any of the other product components.

Continued on next page

Information on these Pharmacia & Upjohn products is based on labeling in effect June 1, 1996. Further information concerning these and other Pharmacia & Upjohn products may be obtained by direct inquiry to Medical Information, Pharmacia & Upjohn, Kalamazoo, MI 49001.

Pharmacia & Upjohn—Cont.

WARNINGS

Proarrhythmia: Like other antiarrhythmic agents, CORVERT Injection can induce or worsen ventricular arrhythmias in some patients. This may have potentially fatal consequences. Torsades de pointes, a polymorphic ventricular tachycardia that develops in the setting of a prolonged QT interval, may occur because of the effect CORVERT has on cardiac repolarization, but CORVERT can also cause polymorphic VT in the absence of excessive prolongation of the QT interval. In general, with drugs that prolong the QT interval, the risk of torsades de pointes is thought to increase progressively as the QT interval is prolonged and may be worsened with bradycardia, a varying heart rate, and hypokalemia. In clinical trials conducted in patients with atrial fibrillation and atrial flutter, those with QTc intervals > 440 msec were not usually allowed to participate, and serum potassium had to be above 4.0 mEq/L. Although change in QTc was dose dependent for ibutilide, there was no clear relationship between risk of serious proarrhythmia and dose in clinical studies, possibly due to the small number of events. In clinical trials of intravenous ibutilide, patients with a history of congestive heart failure (CHF) or low left ventricular ejection fraction appeared to have a higher incidence of sustained polymorphic ventricular tachycardia (VT), than those without such underlying conditions; for sustained polymorphic VT the rate was 5.4% in patients with a history of CHF and 0.8% without it. There was also a suggestion that women had a higher risk of proarrhythmia, but the sex difference was not observed in all studies and was most prominent for nonsustained ventricular tachycardia. The incidence of sustained ventricular arrhythmias was similar in male (1.8%) and female (1.5%) patients, possibly due to the small number of events. CORVERT is not recommended in patients who have previously demonstrated polymorphic ventricular tachycardia (eg, torsades de pointes).

During clinical trials, 1.7% of patients with atrial flutter or atrial fibrillation treated with CORVERT developed sustained polymorphic ventricular tachycardia requiring cardioversion. In these clinical trials, many initial episodes of polymorphic ventricular tachycardia occurred after the infusion of CORVERT was stopped but generally not more than 40 minutes after the start of the first infusion. There were, however, instances of recurrent polymorphic VT that occurred about 3 hours after the initial infusion. In two cases, the VT degenerated into ventricular fibrillation, requiring immediate defibrillation. Other cases were managed with cardiac pacing and magnesium sulfate infusions. Nonsustained polymorphic ventricular tachycardia occurred in 2.7% of patients and nonsustained monomorphic ventricular tachycardias occurred in 4.9% of the patients (see ADVERSE REACTIONS).

Proarrhythmic events must be anticipated. Skilled personnel and proper equipment, including cardiac monitoring equipment, intracardiac pacing facilities, a cardioverter/defibrillator, and medication for treatment of sustained ventricular tachycardia, including polymorphic ventricular tachycardia, must be available during and after administration of CORVERT. Before treatment with CORVERT, hypokalemia and hypomagnesemia should be corrected to reduce the potential for proarrhythmia. Patients should be observed with continuous ECG monitoring for at least 4 hours following infusion or until QTc has returned to baseline. Longer monitoring is required if any arrhythmic activity is noted. Management of polymorphic ventricular tachycardia includes discontinuation of ibutilide, correction of electrolyte abnormalities, especially potassium and magnesium, and overdrive cardiac pacing, electrical cardioversion, or defibrillation. Pharmacologic therapies include magnesium sulfate infusions. Treatment with antiarrhythmics should generally be avoided.

PRECAUTIONS

General

Antiarrhythmics: Class Ia antiarrhythmic drugs (Vaughan Williams Classification), such as disopyramide, quinidine, and procainamide, and other class III drugs, such as amiodarone and sotalol, should not be given concomitantly with CORVERT Injection or within 4 hours postinfusion because of their potential to prolong refractoriness. In the clinical trials, class I or other class III antiarrhythmic agents were withheld for at least 5 half-lives prior to ibutilide infusion and for 4 hours after dosing, but thereafter were allowed at the physician's discretion.

Other drugs that prolong the QT interval: The potential for proarrhythmia may increase with the administration of CORVERT Injection to patients who are being treated with drugs that prolong the QT interval, such as phenothiazines, tricyclic antidepressants, tetracyclic antidepressants, and certain antihistamine drugs (H_1 receptor antagonists).

Heart block: Of the nine (1.5%) ibutilide-treated patients with reports of reversible heart block, five had first degree, three had second degree, and one had complete heart block.

Laboratory Test Interactions: None known.

Drug Interactions: No specific pharmacokinetic or other formal drug interaction studies were conducted.

Digoxin: Supraventricular arrhythmias may mask the cardiotoxicity associated with excessive digoxin levels. Therefore, it is advisable to be particularly cautious in patients whose plasma digoxin levels are above or suspected to be above the usual therapeutic range. Coadministration of digoxin did not have effects on either the safety or efficacy of ibutilide in the clinical trials.

Calcium channel blocking agents: Coadministration of calcium channel blockers did not have any effect on either the safety or efficacy of ibutilide in the clinical trials.

Beta-adrenergic blocking agents: Coadministration of beta-adrenergic blocking agents did not have any effect on either the safety or efficacy of ibutilide in the clinical trials.

Carcinogenesis, Mutagenesis, Impairment of Fertility: No animal studies have been conducted to determine the carcinogenic potential of CORVERT; however, it was not genotoxic in a battery of assays, including the Ames assay, mammalian cell forward gene mutation assay, unscheduled DNA synthesis assay, and mouse micronucleus assay. Similarly, no drug-related effects on fertility or mating were noted in a reproductive study in rats.

Pregnancy: Pregnancy Category C. Ibutilide administered orally was teratogenic (adactyly, cleft palate, scoliosis) and embryocidal in reproduction studies in rats. On a mg/m^2 basis, corrected for the 3% oral bioavailability, the "no adverse effect dose" (5 mg/kg per day given orally) was approximately the same as the maximum recommended human dose (MRHD); the teratogenic dose (20 mg/kg per day given orally) was about four times the MRHD on a mg/m^2 basis, or 16 times the MRHD on a mg/kg basis. CORVERT should not be administered to a pregnant woman unless clinical benefit outweighs potential risk to the fetus.

Nursing Mothers: The excretion of ibutilide into breast milk has not been studied; accordingly, breastfeeding should be discouraged during therapy with CORVERT.

Pediatric Use: Clinical trials with CORVERT in patients with atrial fibrillation and atrial flutter did not include anyone under the age of 18. Safety and effectiveness of ibutilide in pediatric patients has not been established.

Geriatric Use: The mean age of patients in clinical trials was 65. No age-related differences were observed in pharmacokinetic, efficacy, or safety parameters for patients less than 65 compared to patients 65 years and older.

Use in Patients With Hepatic or Renal Dysfunction: The safety, effectiveness, and pharmacokinetics of CORVERT have not been established in patients with hepatic or renal dysfunction. However, it is unlikely that dosing adjustments would be necessary in patients with compromised renal or hepatic function based on the following considerations: (1) CORVERT is indicated for rapid intravenous therapy (duration ≤ 30 minutes) and is dosed to a known, well-defined pharmacologic action (termination of arrhythmia) or to a maximum of two 10-minute infusions; (2) less than 10% of the dose of CORVERT is excreted unchanged in the urine; and (3) drug distribution appears to be one of the primary mechanisms responsible for termination of the pharmacologic effect. Nonetheless, patients with abnormal liver function should be monitored by telemetry for more than the 4-hour period generally recommended.

In 285 patients with atrial fibrillation or atrial flutter who were treated with CORVERT, the clearance of ibutilide was independent of renal function, as assessed by creatinine clearance (range 21 to 140 mL/min).

ADVERSE REACTIONS

CORVERT Injection was generally well tolerated in clinical trials. Of the 586 patients with atrial fibrillation or atrial flutter who received CORVERT in phase II/III studies, 149 (25%) reported medical events related to the cardiovascular system, including sustained polymorphic ventricular tachycardia (1.7%) and nonsustained polymorphic ventricular tachycardia (2.7%).

Other clinically important adverse events with an uncertain relationship to CORVERT include the following (0.2% represents one patient): sustained monomorphic ventricular tachycardia (0.2%), nonsustained monomorphic ventricular tachycardia (4.9%), AV block (1.5%), bundle branch block (1.9%), ventricular extrasystoles (5.1%), supraventricular extrasystoles (0.9%), hypotension/postural hypotension (2.0%), bradycardia/sinus bradycardia (1.2%), nodal arrhythmia (0.7%), congestive heart failure (0.5%), tachycardia/sinus tachycardia/supraventricular tachycardia (2.7%), idioventricular rhythm (0.2%), syncope (0.3%), and renal failure (0.3%). The incidence of these events, except for syncope, was greater in the group treated with CORVERT than in the placebo group.

Another adverse reaction that may be associated with the administration of CORVERT was nausea, which occurred with a frequency greater than 1% more in ibutilide-treated patients than those treated with placebo.

The medical events reported for more than 1% of the placebo-and ibutilide-treated patients are shown in the following Table.

Treatment-Emergent Medical Events With Frequency of More Than 1% and Higher Than That of Placebo

Event	Placebo N=127 Patients n	%	All Ibutilide N=586 Patients n	%
Cardiovascular				
Ventricular extrasystoles	1	0.8	30	5.1
Nonsustained monomorphic VT	1	0.8	29	4.9
Nonsustained polymorphic VT	—	—	16	2.7
Hypotension	2	1.6	12	2.0
Bundle branch block	—	—	11	1.9
Sustained polymorphic VT	—	—	10	1.7
AV block	1	0.8	9	1.5
Hypertension	—	—	7	1.2
QT segment prolonged	—	—	7	1.2
Bradycardia	1	0.8	7	1.2
Palpitation	1	0.8	6	1.0
Tachycardia	1	0.8	16	2.7
Gastrointestinal				
Nausea	1	0.8	11	1.9
Central Nervous System				
Headache	4	3.1	21	3.6

OVERDOSAGE

Acute Experience in Animals: Acute overdose in animals results in CNS toxicity; notably, CNS depression, rapid gasping breathing, and convulsions. The intravenous median lethal dose in the rat was more than 50 mg/kg which is, on a mg/m^2 basis, at least 250 times the maximum recommended human dose.

Human Experience: In the clinical trials with CORVERT Injection, four patients were unintentionally overdosed. The largest dose was 3.4 mg administered over 15 minutes. One patient (0.025 mg/kg) developed increased ventricular ectopy and monomorphic ventricular tachycardia, another patient (0.032 mg/kg) developed AV block—3rd degree and nonsustained polymorphic VT and two patients (0.038 and 0.020 mg/kg) had no medical event reports. Based on known pharmacology, the clinical effects of an overdosage with ibutilide could exaggerate the expected prolongation of repolarization seen at usual clinical doses. Medical events (eg, proarrhythmia, AV block) that occur after the overdosage should be treated with measures appropriate for that condition.

DOSAGE AND ADMINISTRATION

The recommended dose based on controlled trials (see CLINICAL STUDIES) is outlined in the Table below. Ibutilide infusion should be stopped as soon as the presenting arrhythmia is terminated or in the event of sustained or nonsustained ventricular tachycardia, or marked prolongation of QT or QTc.

Recommended Dose of CORVERT Injection

Patient Weight	*Initial Infusion (over 10 minutes)*	*Second Infusion*
60 kg (132 lb) or more	*One vial (1 mg ibutilide fumarate)*	*If the arrhythmia does not terminate within 10 minutes after the end of the initial infusion, a second 10-minute infusion of equal strength may be administered 10 minutes after completion of the first infusion.*
Less than 60 kg (132 lb)	*0.1 mL/kg (0.01 mg/kg Ibutilide fumarate)*	

In a trial comparing ibutilide and sotalol (see CLINICAL STUDIES), 2 mg ibutilide fumarate administered as a single infusion to patients weighing more than 60 kg was also effective in terminating atrial fibrillation or atrial flutter.

Patients should be observed with continuous ECG monitoring for at least 4 hours following infusion or until QTc has returned to baseline. Longer monitoring is required if any arrhythmic activity is noted. Skilled personnel and proper equipment (see WARNINGS, Proarrhythmia), such as a cardioverter/defibrillator, and medication for treatment of sustained ventricular tachycardia, including polymorphic ventricular tachycardia, must be available during administration of CORVERT and subsequent monitoring of the patient.

Dilution: CORVERT Injection may be administered undiluted or diluted in 50 mL of diluent. CORVERT may be

added to 0.9% Sodium Chloride Injection or 5% Dextrose Injection before infusion. The contents of one 10 mL vial (0.1 mg/mL) may be added to a 50 mL infusion bag to form an admixture of approximately 0.017 mg/mL ibutilide fumarate. Parenteral drug products should be inspected visually for particulate matter and discoloration prior to administration whenever solution and container permit.

Compatibility and Stability: The following diluents are compatible with CORVERT Injection (0.1 mg/mL):

5% Dextrose Injection
0.9% Sodium Chloride Injection

The following intravenous solution containers are compatible with admixtures of CORVERT Injection (0.1 mg/mL):

polyvinyl chloride plastic bags
polyolefin bags

Admixtures of the product, with approved diluents, are chemically and physically stable for 24 hours at room temperature (15° to 30°C or 59° to 86°F) and for 48 hours at refrigerated temperatures (2° to 8°C or 36° to 46°F). Strict adherence to the use of aseptic technique during the preparation of the admixture is recommended in order to maintain sterility.

HOW SUPPLIED

CORVERT Injection (ibutilide fumarate injection) is supplied as an acetate-buffered isotonic solution at a concentration of 0.1 mg/mL that has been adjusted to approximately pH 4.6 in 10 mL clear glass, single-dose, flip-top vials.

Single-dose 10 mL vial (0.1 mg/mL) NDC 0009-3794-01

Store at controlled room temperature (20° to 25°C or 68° to 77°F) [see USP]. Store vial in carton until used.

Caution: Federal law prohibits dispensing without prescription.

816 418 001

Revised April 1996 691659

CYTOSAR-U® ℞

Sterile Powder
(brand of sterile cytarabine, USP)
For Intravenous, Intrathecal and Subcutaneous Use Only

> **WARNING**
>
> Only physicians experienced in cancer chemotherapy should use CYTOSAR-U Sterile Powder.
>
> For induction therapy patients should be treated in a facility with laboratory and supportive resources sufficient to monitor drug tolerance and protect and maintain a patient compromised by drug toxicity. The main toxic effect of CYTOSAR-U is bone marrow suppression with leukopenia, thrombocytopenia and anemia. Less serious toxicity includes nausea, vomiting, diarrhea and abdominal pain, oral ulceration, and hepatic dysfunction.
>
> The physician must judge possible benefit to the patient against known toxic effects of this drug in considering the advisability of therapy with CYTOSAR-U. Before making this judgment or beginning treatment, the physician should be familiar with the following text.

DESCRIPTION

CYTOSAR-U (cytarabine) Sterile Powder, commonly known as ara-C, an antineoplastic, is a sterile lyophilized material for reconstitution and intravenous, intrathecal or subcutaneous administration. It is available in multi-dose vials containing 100 mg, 500 mg, 1 g or 2 g sterile cytarabine. The pH of CYTOSAR-U was adjusted, when necessary, with hydrochloric acid and/or sodium hydroxide.

Cytarabine is chemically 4-amino-1-β-D-arabinofuranosyl-2 (1H)-pyrimidinone. The structural formula is:

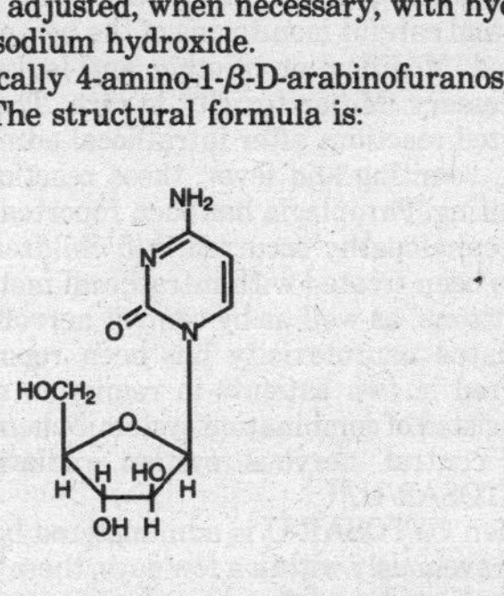

Cytarabine is an odorless, white to off-white, crystalline powder which is freely soluble in water and slightly soluble in alcohol and in chloroform.

PHARMACOLOGY

Cell Culture Studies

Cytarabine is cytotoxic to a wide variety of proliferating mammalian cells in culture. It exhibits cell phase specificity, primarily killing cells undergoing DNA synthesis (S-phase) and under certain conditions blocking the progression of cells from the G_1 phase to the S-phase. Although the mechanism of action is not completely understood, it appears that cytarabine acts through the inhibition of DNA polymerase. A limited, but significant, incorporation of cytarabine into both DNA and RNA has also been reported. Extensive chromosomal damage, including chromatoid breaks, have been produced by cytarabine and malignant transformation of rodent cells in culture has been reported. Deoxycytidine prevents or delays (but does not reverse) the cytotoxic activity. Cell culture studies have shown an antiviral effect.[1] However, efficacy against herpes zoster or smallpox could not be demonstrated in controlled clinical trials.[2-4]

Cellular Resistance and Sensitivity

Cytarabine is metabolized by deoxycytidine kinase and other nucleotide kinases to the nucleotide triphosphate, an effective inhibitor of DNA polymerase; it is inactivated by a pyrimidine nucleoside deaminase, which converts it to the nontoxic uracil derivative. It appears that the balance of kinase and deaminase levels may be an important factor in determining sensitivity or resistance of the cell to cytarabine.

Animal Studies

In experimental studies with mouse tumors, cytarabine was most effective in those tumors with a high growth fraction. The effect was dependent on the treatment schedule; optimal effects were achieved when the schedule (multiple closely spaced doses or constant infusion) ensured contact of the drug with the tumor cells when the maximum number of cells were in the susceptible S-phase. The best results were obtained when courses of therapy were separated by intervals sufficient to permit adequate host recovery.

Human Pharmacology

Cytarabine is rapidly metabolized and is not effective orally; less than 20 percent of the orally administered dose is absorbed from the gastrointestinal tract.

Following rapid intravenous injection of cytarabine labeled with tritium, the disappearance from plasma is biphasic. There is an initial distributive phase with a half-life of about 10 minutes, followed by a second elimination phase with a half-life of about 1 to 3 hours. After the distributive phase, more than 80 percent of plasma radioactivity can be accounted for by the inactive metabolite 1-β-D-arabinofuranosyluracil (ara-U). Within 24 hours about 80 percent of the administered radioactivity can be recovered in the urine, approximately 90 percent of which is excreted as ara-U.

Relatively constant plasma levels can be achieved by continuous intravenous infusion.

After subcutaneous or intramuscular administration of cytarabine labeled with tritium, peak-plasma levels of radioactivity are achieved about 20 to 60 minutes after injection and are considerably lower than those after intravenous administration.

Cerebrospinal fluid levels of cytarabine are low in comparison to plasma levels after single intravenous injection. However, in one patient in whom cerebrospinal levels were examined after 2 hours of constant intravenous infusion, levels approached 40 percent of the steady state plasma level. With intrathecal administration, levels of cytarabine in the cerebrospinal fluid declined with a first order half-life of about 2 hours. Because cerebrospinal fluid levels of deaminase are low, little conversion to ara-U was observed.

Immunosuppressive Action

CYTOSAR-U Sterile Powder is capable of obliterating immune responses in man during administration with little or no accompanying toxicity.[5-6] Suppression of antibody responses to E-coli-VI antigen and tetanus toxoid have been demonstrated. This suppression was obtained during both primary and secondary antibody responses.

CYTOSAR-U also suppressed the development of cell-mediated immune responses such as delayed hypersensitivity skin reaction to dinitrochlorobenzene. However, it had no effect on already established delayed hypersensitivity reactions.

Following 5-day courses of intensive therapy with CYTOSAR-U the immune response was suppressed, as indicated by the following parameters: macrophage ingress into skin windows; circulating antibody response following primary antigenic stimulation; lymphocyte blastogenesis with phytohemagglutinin. A few days after termination of therapy there was a rapid return to normal.[7]

INDICATIONS AND USAGE

CYTOSAR-U in combination with other approved anticancer drugs is indicated for remission induction in acute nonlymphocytic leukemia of adults and pediatric patients. It has also been found useful in the treatment of acute lymphocytic leukemia and the blast phase of chronic myelocytic leukemia. Intrathecal administration of CYTOSAR-U is indicated in the prophylaxis and treatment of meningeal leukemia.

CONTRAINDICATIONS

CYTOSAR-U Sterile Powder is contraindicated in those patients who are hypersensitive to the drug.

WARNINGS (See boxed WARNING)

Cytarabine is a potent bone marrow suppressant. Therapy should be started cautiously in patients with pre-existing drug-induced bone marrow suppression. Patients receiving this drug must be under close medical supervision and, during induction therapy, should have leukocyte and platelet counts performed daily. Bone marrow examinations should be performed frequently after blasts have disappeared from the peripheral blood. Facilities should be available for management of complications, possibly fatal, of bone marrow suppression (infection resulting from granulocytopenia and other impaired body defenses, and hemorrhage secondary to thrombocytopenia). One case of anaphylaxis that resulted in acute cardiopulmonary arrest and required resuscitation has been reported. This occurred immediately after the intravenous administration of CYTOSAR-U Sterile Powder.

Severe and at times fatal CNS, GI and pulmonary toxicity (different from that seen with conventional therapy regimens of CYTOSAR-U) has been reported following some experimental dose schedules for CYTOSAR-U.[8-11] These reactions include reversible corneal toxicity, and hemorrhagic conjunctivitis, which may be prevented or diminished by prophylaxis with a local corticosteroid eye drop; cerebral and cerebellar dysfunction, including personality changes, somnolence and coma, usually reversible; severe gastrointestinal ulceration, including pneumatosis cystoides intestinalis leading to peritonitis; sepsis and liver abscess; pulmonary edema, liver damage with increased hyperbilirubinemia; bowel necrosis; and necrotizing colitis. Rarely, severe skin rash, leading to desquamation has been reported. Complete alopecia is more commonly seen with experimental high dose therapy than with standard treatment programs using CYTOSAR-U. If experimental high dose therapy is used, do not use a diluent containing benzyl alcohol.

Cases of cardiomyopathy with subsequent death have been reported following experimental high dose therapy with cytarabine in combination with cyclophosphamide when used for bone marrow transplant preparation.[12]

A syndrome of sudden respiratory distress, rapidly progressing to pulmonary edema and radiographically pronounced cardiomegaly has been reported following experimental high dose therapy with cytarabine used for the treatment of relapsed leukemia from one institution in 16/72 patients. The outcome of this syndrome can be fatal.[13]

Benzyl alcohol is contained in the diluent for this product. Benzyl alcohol has been reported to be associated with a fatal "Gasping Syndrome" in premature infants.

Two patients with childhood acute myelogenous leukemia who received intrathecal and intravenous CYTOSAR-U at conventional doses (in addition to a number of other concomitantly administered drugs) developed delayed progressive ascending paralysis resulting in death in one of the two patients.[14]

Use in Pregnancy (Category D)

CYTOSAR-U can cause fetal harm when administered to a pregnant woman. (See ANIMAL TOXICOLOGY). There are no adequate and well-controlled studies in pregnant women. If CYTOSAR-U is used during pregnancy, or if the patient becomes pregnant while taking CYTOSAR-U, the patient should be apprised of the potential hazard to the fetus. Women of childbearing potential should be advised to avoid becoming pregnant.

A review of the literature has shown 32 reported cases where CYTOSAR-U was given during pregnancy, either alone or in combination with other cytotoxic agents:

Eighteen normal infants were delivered. Four of these had first trimester exposure. Five infants were premature or of low birth weight. Twelve of the 18 normal infants were followed up at ages ranging from six weeks to seven years, and showed no abnormalities. One apparently normal infant died at 90 days of gastroenteritis.

Two cases of congenital abnormalities have been reported, one with upper and lower distal limb defects,[16] and the other with extremity and ear deformities[17] Both of these cases had first trimester exposure.

There were seven infants with various problems in the neonatal period, including pancytopenia; transient depression of WBC, hematocrit or platelets; electrolyte abnormalities; transient eosinophilia; and one case of increased IgM levels and hyperpyrexia possibly due to sepsis. Six of the seven infants were also premature. The child with pancytopenia died at 21 days of sepsis.

Therapeutic abortions were done in five cases. Four fetuses were grossly normal, but one had an enlarged spleen and another showed Trisomy C chromosome abnormality in the chorionic tissue.

Because of the potential for abnormalities with cytotoxic therapy, particularly during the first trimester, a patient who is or who may become pregnant while on CYTOSAR-U

Continued on next page

Information on these Pharmacia & Upjohn products is based on labeling in effect June 1, 1996. Further information concerning these and other Pharmacia & Upjohn products may be obtained by direct inquiry to Medical Information, Pharmacia & Upjohn, Kalamazoo, MI 49001.

Pharmacia & Upjohn—Cont.

should be apprised of the potential risk to the fetus and the advisability of pregnancy continuation. There is a definite, but considerably reduced risk if therapy is initiated during the second or third trimester. Although normal infants have been delivered to patients treated in all three trimesters of pregnancy, follow-up of such infants would be advisable.

PRECAUTIONS

1. General Precautions
Patients receiving CYTOSAR-U Sterile Powder must be monitored closely. Frequent platelet and leukocyte counts and bone marrow examinations are mandatory. Consider suspending or modifying therapy when drug-induced marrow depression has resulted in a platelet count under 50,000 or a polymorphonuclear granulocyte count under 1000/mm[3]. Counts of formed elements in the peripheral blood may continue to fall after the drug is stopped and reach lowest values after drug-free intervals of 12 to 24 days. When indicated, restart therapy when definite signs of marrow recovery appear (on successive bone marrow studies). Patients whose drug is withheld until "normal" peripheral blood values are attained may escape from control.

When large intravenous doses are given quickly, patients are frequently nauseated and may vomit for several hours post-injection. This problem tends to be less severe when the drug is infused.

The human liver apparently detoxifies a substantial fraction of an administered dose. In particular, patients with renal or hepatic function impairment may have a higher likelihood of CNS toxicity after high-dose CYTOSAR-U treatment.[46,47] Use the drug with caution and possibly at reduced dose in patients whose liver or kidney function is poor.

Periodic checks of bone marrow, liver and kidney functions should be performed in patients receiving CYTOSAR-U.

Like other cytotoxic drugs, CYTOSAR-U may induce hyperuricemia secondary to rapid lysis of neoplastic cells. The clinician should monitor the patient's blood uric acid level and be prepared to use such supportive and pharmacologic measures as might be necessary to control this problem.

Acute pancreatitis has been reported to occur in patients being treated with CYTOSAR-U who have had prior treatment with L=asparaginase.[15]

2. Information for patient
Not applicable

3. Laboratory tests
See General Precautions

4. Drug Interactions
Reversible decreases in steady-state plasma digoxin concentrations and renal glycoside excretion were observed in patients receiving beta-acetyldigoxin and chemotherapy regimens containing cyclophosphamide, vincristine and prednisone with or without CYTOSAR-U or procarbazine.[39] Steady-state plasma digitoxin concentrations did not appear to change. Therefore, monitoring of plasma digoxin levels may be indicated in patients receiving similar combination chemotherapy regimens. The utilization of digitoxin for such patients may be considered as an alternative.

An *in vitro* interaction study between gentamicin and cytarabine showed a cytarabine related antagonism for the susceptibility of *K. pneumoniae* strains. This study suggests that in patients on cytarabine being treated with gentamicin for a *K. pneumoniae* infection, the lack of a prompt therapeutic response may indicate the need for reevaluation of antibacterial therapy.[40]

Clinical evidence in one patient showed possible inhibition of fluorocytosine efficacy during therapy with CYTOSAR-U.[41] This may be due to potential competitive inhibition of its uptake.[42]

5. Carcinogenesis, mutagenesis, impairment of fertility
Extensive chromosomal damage, including chromatoid breaks have been produced by cytarabine and malignant transformation of rodent cells in culture has been reported.

6. Pregnancy
Pregnancy Category D. See WARNINGS.

7. Labor and delivery
Not applicable

8. Nursing mothers
It is not known whether this drug is excreted in human milk. Because many drugs are excreted in human milk and because of the potential for serious adverse reactions in nursing infants from cytarabine, a decision should be made whether to discontinue nursing or to discontinue the drug, taking into account the importance of the drug to the mother.

9. Pediatric use
See INDICATIONS AND USAGE

ADVERSE REACTIONS

Expected Reactions
Because cytarabine is a bone marrow suppressant, anemia, leukopenia, thrombocytopenia, megaloblastosis and reduced reticulocytes can be expected as a result of administration with CYTOSAR-U Sterile Powder. The severity of these reactions are dose and schedule dependent.[18] Cellular changes in the morphology of bone marrow and peripheral smears can be expected.[19]

Following 5-day constant infusions or acute injections of 50 mg/m[2] to 600 mg/m[2], white cell depression follows a biphasic course. Regardless of initial count, dosage level, or schedule, there is an initial fall starting the first 24 hours with a nadir at days 7-9. This is followed by a brief rise which peaks around the twelfth day. A second and deeper fall reaches nadir at days 15-24. Then there is rapid rise to above baseline in the next 10 days. Platelet depression is noticeable at 5 days with a peak depression occurring between days 12-15. Thereupon, a rapid rise to above baseline occurs in the next 10 days.[20]

Infectious Complications
Infection: Viral, bacterial, fungal, parasitic, or saprophytic infections, in any location in the body may be associated with the use of CYTOSAR-U alone or in combination with other immunosuppressive agents following immunosuppressant doses that affect cellular or humoral immunity. These infections may be mild, but can be severe and at times fatal.

The Cytarabine (Ara-C) Syndrome
A cytarabine syndrome has been described by Castleberry.[21] It is characterized by fever, myalgia, bone pain, occasionally chest pain, maculopapular rash, conjunctivitis and malaise. It usually occurs 6-12 hours following drug administration. Corticosteroids have been shown to be beneficial in treating or preventing this syndrome. If the symptoms of the syndrome are deemed treatable, corticosteroids should be contemplated as well as continuation of therapy with CYTOSAR-U.

Most Frequent Adverse Reactions
anorexia
nausea
vomiting
diarrhea
oral and anal inflammation or ulceration
hepatic dysfunction
fever
rash
thrombophlebitis
bleeding (all sites)

Nausea and vomiting are most frequent following rapid intravenous injection.

Less Frequent Adverse Reactions
sepsis
pneumonia
cellulitis at injection site
skin ulceration
urinary retention
renal dysfunction
neuritis
  neural toxicity
sore throat
esophageal ulceration
esophagitis
chest pain
pericarditis
bowel necrosis
abdominal pain
freckling
  jaundice
conjunctivitis (may occur with rash)
dizziness
alopecia
anaphylaxis (See WARNINGS)
allergic edema
pruritus
shortness of breath
urticaria
headache

Experimental Doses
Severe and at times fatal CNS, GI and pulmonary toxicity (different from that seen with conventional therapy regimens of CYTOSAR-U) has been reported following some experimental dose schedules of CYTOSAR-U.[8-11] These reactions include reversible corneal toxicity and hemorrhagic conjunctivitis, which may be prevented or diminished by prophylaxis with a local corticosteroid eye drop; cerebral and cerebellar dysfunction, including personality changes, somnolence and coma, usually reversible; severe gastrointestinal ulceration, including pneumatosis cystoides intestinalis leading to peritonitis; sepsis and liver abscess; pulmonary edema, liver damage with increased hyperbilirubinemia; bowel necrosis; and necrotizing colitis. Rarely, severe skin rash leading to desquamation has been reported. Complete alopecia is more commonly seen with experimental high dose therapy than with standard treatment programs using CYTOSAR-U. If experimental high dose therapy is used, do not use a diluent containing benzyl alcohol.

Cases of cardiomyopathy with subsequent death have been reported following experimental high dose therapy with cytarabine in combination with cyclophosphamide when used for bone marrow transplant preparation.[12] **This cardiac toxicity may be schedule dependent.[45]**

A syndrome of sudden respiratory distress, rapidly progressing to pulmonary edema and radiographically pronounced cardiomegaly has been reported following experimental high dose therapy with cytarabine used for the treatment of relapsed leukemia from one institution in 16/72 patients. The outcome of this syndrome can be fatal.[13]

Two patients with adult acute non-lymphocytic leukemia developed peripheral motor and sensory neuropathies after consolidation with high-dose CYTOSAR-U, daunorubicin, and asparaginase. Patients treated with high-dose CYTOSAR-U should be observed for neuropathy since dose schedule alterations may be needed to avoid irreversible neurologic disorders.[22]

Ten patients treated with experimental intermediate doses of CYTOSAR-U (1 g/m[2]) with and without other chemotherapeutic agents (meta-AMSA, daunorubicin, etoposide) at various dose regimen developed a diffuse interstitial pneumonitis without clear cause that may have been related to the CYTOSAR-U.[43]

Two cases of pancreatitis have been reported following experimental doses of CYTOSAR-U and numerous other drugs. CYTOSAR-U could have been the causative agent.[44]

OVERDOSAGE
There is no antidote for overdosage of CYTOSAR-U. Doses of 4.5 g/m[2] by intravenous infusion over 1 hour every 12 hours for 12 doses has caused an unacceptable increase in irreversible CNS toxicity and death.[9]

Single doses as high as 3 g/m[2] have been administered by rapid intravenous infusion without apparent toxicity.[23]

DOSAGE AND ADMINISTRATION
CYTOSAR-U Sterile Powder is not active orally. The schedule and method of administration varies with the program of therapy to be used. CYTOSAR-U may be given by intravenous infusion or injection, subcutaneously, or intrathecally. Thrombophlebitis has occurred at the site of drug injection or infusion in some patients, and rarely patients have noted pain and inflammation at subcutaneous injection sites. In most instances, however, the drug has been well tolerated. Patients can tolerate higher total doses when they receive the drug by rapid intravenous injection as compared with slow infusion. This phenomenon is related to the drug's rapid inactivation and brief exposure of susceptible normal and neoplastic cells to significant levels after rapid injection. Normal and neoplastic cells seem to respond in somewhat parallel fashion to these different modes of administration and no clear-cut clinical advantage has been demonstrated for either.

In the induction therapy of acute non-lymphocytic leukemia, the usual cytarabine dose in combination with other anticancer drugs is 100 mg/m[2]/day by continuous IV infusion (Days 1–7) or 100 mg/m[2] IV every 12 hours (Days 1–7).

The literature should be consulted for the current recommendations for use in acute lymphocytic leukemia.

Intrathecal Use in Meningeal Leukemia
CYTOSAR-U has been used intrathecally in acute leukemia in doses ranging from 5 mg/m[2] to 75 mg/m[2] of body surface area. The frequency of administration varied from once a day for 4 days to once every 4 days. The most frequently used dose was 30 mg/m[2] every 4 days until cerebrospinal fluid findings were normal, followed by one additional treatment.[24-28] The dosage schedule is usually governed by the type and severity of central nervous system manifestations and the response to previous therapy.

If used intrathecally, do not use a diluent containing benzyl alcohol. Many clinicians reconstitute with autologous spinal fluid or preservative-free 0.9% Sodium Chloride, USP, for Injection and use immediately.

CYTOSAR-U given intrathecally may cause systemic toxicity and careful monitoring of the hemopoietic system is indicated. Modification of other anti-leukemia therapy may be necessary. Major toxicity is rare. The most frequently reported reactions after intrathecal administration were nausea, vomiting and fever; these reactions are mild and self-limiting. Paraplegia has been reported.[29] Necrotizing leukoencephalopathy occurred in 5 children; these patients had also been treated with intrathecal methotrexate and hydrocortisone, as well as by central nervous system radiation.[30] Isolated neurotoxicity has been reported.[31] Blindness occurred in two patients in remission whose treatment had consisted of combination systemic chemotherapy, prophylactic central nervous system radiation and intrathecal CYTOSAR-U.[32]

When CYTOSAR-U is administered both intrathecally and intravenously within a few days, there is an increased risk of spinal cord toxicity, however, in serious life-threatening disease, concurrent use of intravenous and intrathecal CYTOSAR-U is left to the discretion of the treating physician.[48]

Focal leukemic involvement of the central nervous system may not respond to intrathecal CYTOSAR-U and may better be treated with radiotherapy.

The 100 mg vial may be reconstituted with 5 mL of Bacteriostatic Water for Injection with Benzyl Alcohol 0.945% w/v added as preservative. The resulting solution contains 20 mg

of cytarabine per mL. (Do not use Bacteriostatic Water for Injection with Benzyl Alcohol 0.945% w/v as a diluent for intrathecal use. See WARNINGS).

The 500 mg vial may be reconstituted with 10 mL Bacteriostatic Water for Injection with Benzyl Alcohol 0.945% w/v added as preservative. The resulting solution contains 50 mg of cytarabine per mL. (Do not use Bacteriostatic Water for Injection with Benzyl Alcohol 0.945% w/v as a diluent for intrathecal use. See WARNINGS).

The 1 gram vial may be reconstituted with 10 mL of Bacteriostatic Water for Injection with Benzyl Alcohol 0.945% w/v added as preservative. The resulting solution contains 100 mg of cytarabine per mL. (Do not use Bacteriostatic Water for Injection with Benzyl Alcohol 0.945% w/v as a diluent for intrathecal use. See WARNINGS).

The 2 gram vial may be reconstituted with 20 mL of Bacteriostatic Water for Injection with Benzyl Alcohol 0.945% w/v added as preservative. The resulting solution contains 100 mg of cytarabine per mL. (Do not use Bacteriostatic Water for Injection with Benzyl Alcohol 0.945% w/v as a diluent for intrathecal use. See WARNINGS).

If used intrathecally many clinicians reconstitute with preservative-free 0.9% Sodium Chloride for Injection and use immediately.

The pH of the reconstituted solutions is about 5. Solutions reconstituted with Bacteriostatic Water for Injection with Benzyl Alcohol 0.945% w/v may be stored at controlled room temperature, 15° to 30° C (59° to 86° F) for 48 hours. Discard any solutions in which a slight haze develops.

Solutions reconstituted without a preservative should be used immediately.

Chemical Stability of Infusion Solutions:

Chemical stability studies were performed by ultraviolet assay on CYTOSAR-U in infusion solutions. These studies showed that when reconstituted CYTOSAR-U was added to Water for Injection, 5% Dextrose in Water or Sodium Chloride Injection, 94 to 96 percent of the cytarabine was present after 192 hours storage at room temperature.

Parenteral drugs should be inspected visually for particulate matter and discoloration, prior to administration, whenever solution and container permit.

Procedures for proper handling and disposal of anticancer drugs should be considered. Several guidelines on this subject have been published.[33–38]

There is no general agreement that all of the procedures recommended in the guidelines are necessary or appropriate.

HOW SUPPLIED

CYTOSAR-U Sterile Powder (sterile cytarabine) is available in multi-dose vials of four sizes:

100 mg vial, NDC 0009–0373–01
500 mg vial, NDC 0009–0473–01
1 g vial, NDC 0009–3295–01
2 g vial, NDC 0009–3296–01

Store the product at controlled room temperature 15° to 30° C (59° to 86° F).

REFERENCES

1. Zaky DA, Betts RF, Douglas RG, et al: Varicella-Zoster Virus and Subcutaneous Cytarabine: Correlation of In Vitro Sensitivities to Blood Levels. *Antimicrob Agents Chemother* 1975; *7*:229–232.
2. Davis CM, VanDersarl JV, Coltman CA Jr: Failure of Cytarabine in Varicella-Zoster Infections. *JAMA* 1973; *224*: 122–123.
3. Betts RF, Zaky DA, Douglas RG, et al: Ineffectiveness of Subcutaneous Cytosine Arabinoside in Localized Herpes Zoster. *Ann Intern Med* 1975; *82*:778–783.
4. Dennis DT, Doberstyn EB, Awoke S, et al: Failure of Cytosine Arabinoside in Treatment Smallpox; A Double-blind Study, *Lancet* 1974; *2*:377–379.
5. Gray GD: ARA-C and Derivatives as Examples of Immunosuppressive Nucleoside Analogs. *Ann NY Acad Sci* 1975; 255:372–379.
6. Mitchell MS, Wade ME, DeConti RC, et al: Immunosuppressive Effects of Cytosine Arabinoside and Methotrexate in Man. *Ann Intern Med* 1969; *70*:535–547.
7. Frei E, Ho DHW, Bodey GP, et al: Pharmacologic and Cytokinetic Studies of Arabinosyl Cytosine, In *Unifying Concepts of Leukemia. Bibl. Hematol.* No. 39. Karger, Basel 1973, pp 1085–1097.
8. Hopen G, Mondino BJ, Johnson BL, et al: Corneal Toxicity with Systemic Cytarabine. *Am J Ophthalmol* 1981; *91*:500–504.
9. Lazarus HM, Herzig RH, Herzig GP, et al: Central Nervous System Toxicity of High-Dose Systemic Cytosine Arabinoside. *Cancer* 1981; *48*:2577–2582.
10. Slavin RE, Dias MA, Soral R: Cytosine Arabinoside Induced Gastrointestinal Toxic Alterations in Sequential Chemotherapeutic Protocols—A Clinical Pathologic Study of 33 Patients. *Cancer* 1978; *42*:1747–1759.
11. Haupt HM, Hutchins GM, Moore GW: Ara-C Lung: Noncardiogenic Pulmonary Edema Complicating Cytosine Arabinoside Therapy of Leukemia. *Am J Med* 1981; *70*:256–261.
12. Takvorian T, Anderson K, Ritz J: A Fatal Cardiomyopathy Associated with High Dosage Ara-C (HIDAC) and Cyclophosphamide (CTX) in Bone Marrow Transplantation (BMTx). (Abstract submitted for 1985 AACR Meetings in Houston, Texas.)
13. Andersson BS, Cogan B, Keating MJ, Estey EH, et al: Subacute Pulmonary Failure Complicating Therapy with High-Dose Ara-C in Acute Leukemia. *Cancer* 1985; *56*:2181–2184.
14. Dunton SF, Ruprecht N, Spruce W,et al: Progressive Ascending Paralysis Following Administration of Intrathecal and Intravenous Cytosine Arabinoside. *Cancer* 1986; 57:1083–1088.
15. Altman AJ, Dinndorf P, Quinn JJ: Acute Pancreatitis in Association with Cytosine Arabinoside Therapy. *Cancer* 1982; *49*:1384–1386.
16. Shafer AI: Teratogenic Effects of Antileukemic Chemotherapy. *Arch Intern Med* 1981; *141*:514–515.
17. Wagner VM, et al: Congenital Abnormalities in Baby Born to Cytarabine Treated Mother. *Lancet* 1980; *2*:98–99.
18. Frei E III, Bickers JN, Hewlett JS, et al: Dose Schedule and Antitumor Studies of Arabinosyl Cytosine (NSC 63878). *Cancer Res* 1969; *29*:1325–1332.
19. Bell WR, Wang JJ, Carbone PP, et al: Cytogenetic and Morphologic Abnormalities in Human Bone Marrow Cells during Cytosine Arabinoside Therapy. *J Hematol* 1966; *27*:771–781.
20. Burke PJ, Serpick AA, Carbone PP, et al: A Clinical Evaluation of Dose and Schedule of Administration of Cytosine Arabinoside (NSC 63878). *Cancer Res* 1968; *28*:274–279
21. Castleberry RP, Crist WM, Holbrook T, et al: The Cytosine Arabinoside (Ara-C) Syndrome. *Med Pediatr Oncol 1981; 9:257–264.*
22. Powell BL, Capizzi RL, Lyerly EW, et al: Peripheral Neuropathy After High-Dose Cytosine Arabinoside, Daunorubicin, and Asparaginase Consolidation for Acute Nonlymphocytic Leukemia. *J Clin Oncol* 1986; *4* (1):95–97.
23. Rudnick SA, et al: High Dose Cytosine Arabinoside (HDARAC) In Refractory Acute Leukemia. *Cancer* 1979; *44*:1189–1193.
24. Proceedings of the Chemotherapy Conference on ARA-C: Development and Application (Cytosine Arabinoside Hydrochloride—NSC 63878), Oct. 10, 1969
25. Lay HN, Colebatch JH, Ekert H: Experiences with Cytosine Arabinoside in Childhood Leukaemia and Lymphoma. *Med J Aust* 1971; 2:187–192.
26. Halikowski B, Cyklis R, Armata J, et al: Cytosine Arabinoside Administered Intrathecally in Cerebromeningeal Leukemia, *Acta Paediat Scand* 1970; *59*:164–168.
27. Wang JJ, Pratt CB: Intrathecal Arabinosyl Cytosine in Meningeal Leukemia. *Cancer* 1970; *25*:531–534.
28. Band PR, Holland JF, Bernard J, et al: Treatment of Central Nervous System Leukemia with Intrathecal Cytosine Arabinoside. *Cancer* 1973; *32*:744–748.
29. Saiki JH, Thompson S, Smith F, et al: Paraplegia Following Intrathecal Chemotherapy. *Cancer* 1972; *29*:370–374.
30. Rubenstein LJ, Herman MM, Long TF, et al: Disseminated Necrotizing Leukoencephalopathy: A Complication of Treated Central System Leukemia and Lymphoma. *Cancer* 1975; *35*:291–305.
31. Marmont AM, Damasio EE: Neurotoxicity of Intrathecal Chemotherapy for Leukaemia. *Brit Med J* 1973; *4*:47.
32. Margileth DA, Poplack DG, Pizzo PA, et al: Blindness During Remission in Two Patients with Acute Lymphoblastic Leukemia. *Cancer* 1977; *39*:58–61.
33. Recommendations for the Safe Handling of Parenteral Antineoplastic Drugs. NIH Publication No. 83–2621. For sale by the Superintendent of Documents, US Government Printing Office, Washington, DC 20402.
34. AMA Council Report. Guidelines for Handling Parenteral Antineoplastics. *JAMA*, March 15, 1985.
35. National Study Commission on Cytotoxic Exposure-Recommendations for Handling Cytotoxic Agents. Available from Louis P. Jeffrey, ScD, Director of Pharmacy Services, Rhode Island Hospital, 593 Eddy Street, Providence, Rhode Island 02902.
36. Clinical Oncological Society of Australia: Guidelines and recommendations for safe handling of antineoplastic agents. *Med J Australia* 1983; *1*:426–428.
37. Jones, RB, et al: Safe handling of chemotherapeutic agents: A report from the Mount Sinai Medical Center CA-A *Cancer Journal for Clinicians* Sept/Oct., 1983, pp. 258–263.
38. American Society of Hospital Pharmacists Technical assistance bulletin on handling cytotoxic drugs in hospitals *Am J Hosp Pharm* 1985; *42*:131–137.
39. Kuhlman J: Inhibition of Digoxin Absorption but not of Digitoxin During Cytostatic Drug Therapy. *Arzneim Forsch* 1982; *32*:698–704.
40. Moody MR, Morris JJ, Yang VM, et al: Effect of Two Cancer Chemotherapeutic Agents on the Antibacterial Activity of Three Antimicrobial Agents. *Antimicrob Agents Chemother* 1978; *14*:737–742.
41. Holt RJ: Clinical Problems with 5–Fluorocytosine. *Mykosen* 1978; *21*(11):363–369.
42. Polak A, Grenson M: Interference Between the Uptake of Pyrimidines and Purines in Yeasts. *Path Microbiol* 1973; *39*:37–38.
43. Peters WG, Willemze R, Colly LP: Results of Induction and Consolidation Treatment with Intermediate and High-Dose Ara-C and m-AMSA Containing Regimens in Patients with Primarily Failed or Relapsed Acute Leukemia and Non-Hodgkin's Lymphoma. *Scan J Hemat* 1986; *36* (Suppl 44):7-16.
44. Siemers RF, Friedenberg WR, Norfleet RG: High-Dose Cytosine Arabinoside-Associated Pancreatitis. *Cancer* 1985; *56*:1940–1942.
45. Paul S, et al: "High Dose Ara-C Does Not Increase the Cardiotoxicity of cyclophosphamide — Total Body Irradiation Conditioning Regimen for Bone Marrow Transplantation". *Proceeding of ASCO* 1989; *8*:16, abstract 60.
46. Nand S, Messmore HL, Patel R, et al: Neurotoxicity Associated With Systemic High-Dose Cytosine Arabinoside. *J Clin Oncol* 1986; 4 (4):571–575.
47. Damon LE, Mass R, Linker CA: The Association Between High-Dose Cytarabine Neurotoxicity and Renal Insufficiency. *J Clin Oncol* 1989; 7 (10):1563–1568.
48. Watterson J, Toogood I, Nieder M, et al: Excessive Spinal Cord Toxicity from Intensive Central Nervous System-Directed Therapies. *Cancer* 1994; *74*:3034–3041.

ANIMAL TOXICOLOGY

Toxicity of cytarabine in experimental animals, as well as activity, is markedly influenced by the schedule of administration. For example, in mice, the LD_{10} for single intraperitoneal administration is greater than 6000 mg/m². However, when administered as 8 doses, each separated by 3 hours, the LD_{10} is less than 750 mg/m² total dose. Similarly, although a total dose of 1920 mg/m² administered as 12 injections at 6-hour intervals was lethal to beagle dogs (severe bone marrow hypoplasia with evidence of liver and kidney damage), dogs receiving the same total dose administered in 8 injections (again at 6-hour intervals) over a 48–hour period survived with minimal signs of toxicity. The most consistent observation in surviving dogs was elevated transaminase levels. In all experimental species the primary limiting toxic effect is marrow suppression with leukopenia. In addition, cytarabine causes abnormal cerebellar development in the neonatal hamster and is teratogenic to the rat fetus.

Caution: Federal law prohibits dispensing without prescription.

Revised March 1996 810 126 220
691618

DEPO-PROVERA® ℞

[*Dəp-ō-prō-vera*]
Contraceptive Injection
(sterile medroxyprogesterone acetate suspension, USP)

Patients should be counseled that this product does not protect against HIV infection (AIDS) and other sexually transmitted diseases.

DESCRIPTION

DEPO-PROVERA Contraceptive Injection contains medroxyprogesterone acetate, a derivative of progesterone, as its active ingredient. Medroxyprogesterone acetate is active by the parenteral and oral routes of administration. It is a white to off-white, odorless crystalline powder that is stable in air and that melts between 200° C and 210° C. It is freely soluble in chloroform, soluble in acetone and dioxane, sparingly soluble in alcohol and methanol, slightly soluble in ether, and insoluble in water.

The chemical name for medroxyprogesterone acetate is pregn-4-ene-3,20-dione, 17-(acetyloxy)-6-methyl-, (6α)-. The structural formula is as follows:

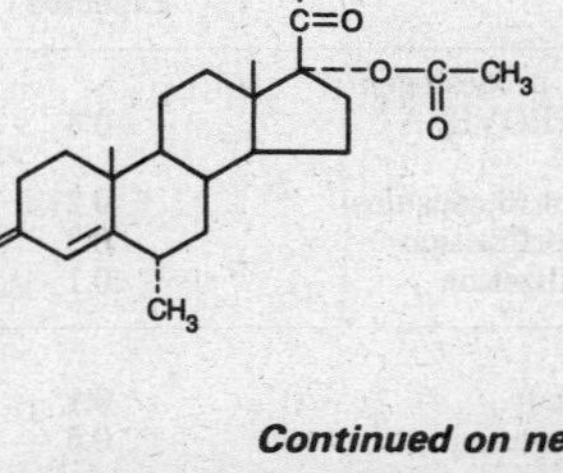

Continued on next page

Information on these Pharmacia & Upjohn products is based on labeling in effect June 1, 1996. Further information concerning these and other Pharmacia & Upjohn products may be obtained by direct inquiry to Medical Information, Pharmacia & Upjohn, Kalamazoo, MI 49001.

Pharmacia & Upjohn—Cont.

DEPO-PROVERA Contraceptive Injection for intramuscular (IM) injection is available in vials and prefilled syringes, each containing 1 mL of medroxyprogesterone acetate sterile aqueous suspension 150 mg/mL.

Each mL contains:

Medroxyprogesterone acetate	150 mg
Polyethylene glycol 3350	28.9 mg
Polysorbate 80	2.41 mg
Sodium chloride	8.68 mg
Methylparaben	1.37 mg
Propylparaben	0.150 mg
Water for injection	qs

When necessary, pH is adjusted with sodium hydroxide or hydrochloric acid, or both.

CLINICAL PHARMACOLOGY

DEPO-PROVERA Contraceptive Injection (medroxyprogesterone acetate), when administered at the recommended dose to women every 3 months, inhibits the secretion of gonadotropins which, in turn, prevents follicular maturation and ovulation and results in endometrial thinning. These actions produce its contraceptive effect.

Following a single 150 mg IM dose of DEPO-PROVERA Contraceptive Injection, medroxyprogesterone acetate concentrations, measured by an extracted radioimmunoassay procedure, increase for approximately 3 weeks to reach peak plasma concentrations of 1 to 7 ng/mL. The levels then decrease exponentially until they become undetectable (<100 pg/mL) between 120 to 200 days following injection. Using an unextracted radioimmunoassay procedure for the assay of medroxyprogesterone acetate in serum, the apparent half-life for medroxyprogesterone acetate following IM administration of DEPO-PROVERA Contraceptive Injection is approximately 50 days.

Women with lower body weights conceive sooner than women with higher body weights after discontinuing DEPO-PROVERA Contraceptive Injection.

The effect of hepatic and/or renal disease on the pharmacokinetics of DEPO-PROVERA Contraceptive Injection is unknown.

INDICATIONS AND USAGE

DEPO-PROVERA Contraceptive Injection is indicated only for the prevention of pregnancy. To ensure that DEPO-PROVERA Contraceptive Injection is not administered inadvertently to a pregnant woman, the first injection must be given ONLY during the first 5 days of a normal menstrual period; ONLY within the first 5-days postpartum if not breast-feeding, and if exclusively breast-feeding, ONLY at the sixth postpartum week. The efficacy of DEPO-PROVERA Contraceptive Injection depends on adherence to the recommended dosage schedule (see DOSAGE AND ADMINISTRATION). It is a long-term injectable contraceptive in women when administered at 3-month (13-week) intervals. Dosage does not need to be adjusted for body weight.

In five clinical studies using DEPO-PROVERA Contraceptive Injection, the 12-month failure rate for the group of women treated with DEPO-PROVERA Contraceptive Injection was zero (no pregnancies reported) to 0.7 by Life-Table method. Pregnancy rates with contraceptive measures are typically reported for only the first year of use as shown in Table 1. Except for intrauterine devices (IUD), implants, sterilization, and DEPO-PROVERA Contraceptive Injection, the efficacy of these contraceptive measures depends in part on the reliability of use. The effectiveness of DEPO-PROVERA Contraceptive Injection is dependent on the patient returning every 3 months (13 weeks) for reinjection.

Table 1
Lowest Expected and Typical Failure Rates[*]
Expressed as Percent of Women Experiencing an Accidental Pregnancy in the First Year of Continuous Use

Method	Lowest Expected	Typical
Injectable progestogen		
DEPO-PROVERA	0.3	0.3
Implants		
Norplant (6 capsules)	0.2[†]	0.2[†]
Female sterilization	0.2	0.4
Male sterilization	0.1	0.15
Pill		3
Combined	0.1	
Progestogen only	0.5	
IUD		3
Progestasert	2	
Copper T 380A	0.8	
Condom	2	12
Diaphragm	6	18
Cap	6	18
Spermicides	3	21
Sponge		
Parous women	9	28
Nulliparous women	6	18
Periodic abstinence	1–9	20
Withdrawal	4	18
No method	85	85

Source: Trussell et al[1]
* Lowest expected—when used exactly as directed.
Typical—includes those not following directions exactly.
† from Norplant® package insert.

CONTRAINDICATIONS

1. Known or suspected pregnancy or as a diagnostic test for pregnancy.
2. Undiagnosed vaginal bleeding.
3. Known or suspected malignancy of breast.
4. Active thrombophlebitis, or current or past history of thromboembolic disorders, or cerebral vascular disease.
5. Liver dysfunction or disease.
6. Known hypersensitivity to DEPO-PROVERA Contraceptive Injection (medroxyprogesterone acetate or any of its other ingredients).

WARNINGS

1. Bleeding Irregularities
Most women using DEPO-PROVERA Contraceptive Injection experience disruption of menstrual bleeding patterns. Altered menstrual bleeding patterns include irregular or unpredictable bleeding or spotting, or rarely, heavy or continuous bleeding. If abnormal bleeding persists or is severe, appropriate investigation should be instituted to rule out the possibility of organic pathology, and appropriate treatment should be instituted when necessary.

As women continue using DEPO-PROVERA Contraceptive Injection, fewer experience irregular bleeding and more experience amenorrhea. By month 12 amenorrhea was reported by 55% of women, and by month 24 amenorrhea was reported by 68% of women using DEPO-PROVERA Contraceptive Injection.[2]

2. Bone Mineral Density Changes
Use of DEPO-PROVERA Contraceptive Injection may be considered among the risk factors for development of osteoporosis. The rate of bone loss is greatest in the early years of use and then subsequently approaches the normal rate of age related fall.

3. Cancer Risks
Long-term case-controlled surveillance of users of DEPO-PROVERA Contraceptive Injection users found slight or no increased overall risk of breast cancer[3] and no overall increased risk of ovarian,[4] liver,[5] or cervical[6] cancer and a prolonged, protective effect of reducing the risk of endometrial[7] cancer in the population of users.

An increased relative risk (RR) of 2.19 (95% CI 1.23 to 3.89)[3] of breast cancer has been associated with use of DEPO-PROVERA Contraceptive Injection in women whose first exposure to drug was within the previous 4 years and who were under 35 years of age [CI = Confidence Interval]. However, the overall RR for ever-users of DEPO-PROVERA Contraceptive Injection was only 1.2 (95% CI 0.96 to 1.52).

[NOTE: A RR of 1.0 indicates neither an increased nor a decreased risk of cancer associated with the use of the drug, relative to no use of the drug. In the case of the subpopulation with a RR of 2.19, the 95% CI is fairly wide and does not include the value of 1.0, thus inferring an increased risk of breast cancer in the defined sub-group relative to nonusers. The value of 2.19 means that women whose first exposure to drug was within the previous 4 years and who are under 35 years of age have a 2.19-fold (95% CI 1.23 to 3.89-fold) increased risk of breast cancer relative to nonusers. The National Cancer Institute[8] reports an average annual incidence rate for breast cancer for US women, all races, age 30 to 34 years of 26.7 per 100,000. A RR of 2.19, thus, increases the possible risk from 26.7 to 58.5 cases per 100,000 women. The attributable risk, thus, is 3.18 per 10,000 women per year.] A statistically insignificant increase in RR estimates of invasive squamous-cell cervical cancer has been associated with the use of DEPO-PROVERA Contraceptive Injection in women who were first exposed before the age of 35 years (RR 1.22 to 1.28 and 95% CI 0.93 to 1.70). The overall, nonsignificant relative rate of invasive squamous-cell cervical cancer in women who ever used DEPO-PROVERA Contraceptive Injection was estimated to be 1.11 (95% CI 0.96 to 1.29). No trends in risk with duration of use or times since initial or most recent exposure were observed.

4. Thromboembolic Disorders
The physician should be alert to the earliest manifestations of thrombotic disorders (thrombophlebitis, pulmonary embolism, cerebrovascular disorders, and retinal thrombosis). Should any of these occur or be suspected, the drug should not be readministered.

5. Ocular Disorders
Medication should not be readministered pending examination if there is a sudden partial or complete loss of vision or if there is a sudden onset of proptosis, diplopia, or migraine. If examination reveals papilledema or retinal vascular lesions, medication should not be readministered.

6. Unexpected Pregnancies
To ensure that DEPO-PROVERA Contraceptive Injection is not administered inadvertently to a pregnant woman, the first injection must be given ONLY during the first 5 days of a normal menstrual period; ONLY within the first 5-days postpartum if not breast-feeding, and if exclusively breast-feeding, ONLY at the sixth postpartum week (see DOSAGE AND ADMINISTRATION).

Infants from unexpected pregnancies that occur 1 to 2 months after injection of DEPO-PROVERA Contraceptive Injection may be at an increased risk of low birth weight, which, in turn, is associated with an increased risk of neonatal death. The attributable risk is low because such pregnancies are uncommon.[9,10]

A significant increase in incidence of polysyndactyly and chromosomal anomalies was observed among infants of users of DEPO-PROVERA Contraceptive Injection, the former being most pronounced in women under 30 years of age. The unrelated nature of these defects, the lack of confirmation from other studies, the distant preconceptual exposure to DEPO-PROVERA Contraceptive Injection, and the chance effects due to multiple statistical comparisons, make a causal association unlikely.[11]

Children exposed to medroxyprogesterone acetate *in utero* and followed to adolescence, showed no evidence of any adverse effects on their health including their physical, intellectual, sexual, or social development.

Several reports suggest an association between intrauterine exposure to progestational drugs in the first trimester of pregnancy and genital abnormalities in male and female fetuses. The risk of hypospadias (five to eight per 1,000 male births in the general population) may be approximately doubled with exposure to these drugs. There are insufficient data to quantify the risk to exposed female fetuses, but because some of these drugs induce mild virilization of the external genitalia of the female fetus and because of the increased association of hypospadias in the male fetus, it is prudent to avoid the use of these drugs during the first trimester of pregnancy.

To ensure that DEPO-PROVERA Contraceptive Injection is not administered inadvertently to a pregnant woman, it is important that the first injection be given only during the first 5 days after the onset of a normal menstrual period within 5 days postpartum if not breast-feeding and if breast-feeding, at the sixth week postpartum (see DOSAGE AND ADMINISTRATION).

7. Ectopic Pregnancy
Health-care providers should be alert to the possibility of an ectopic pregnancy among women using DEPO-PROVERA Contraceptive Injection who become pregnant or complain of severe abdominal pain.

8. Lactation
Detectable amounts of drug have been identified in the milk of mothers receiving DEPO-PROVERA Contraceptive Injection. In nursing mothers treated with DEPO-PROVERA Contraceptive Injection, milk composition, quality, and amount are not adversely affected. Infants exposed to medroxyprogesterone from breast milk have been studied for developmental and behavioral effects through puberty. No adverse effects have been noted.

9. Anaphylaxis and Anaphylactoid Reaction
Anaphylaxis and anaphylactoid reaction have been reported with the use of DEPO-PROVERA Contraceptive Injection. If an anaphylactic reaction occurs appropriate therapy should be instituted. Serious anaphylactic reactions require emergency medical treatment.

PRECAUTIONS

GENERAL

1. Physical Examination
The pretreatment and annual history and physical examination should include special reference to breast and pelvic organs, as well as a Papanicolaou smear.

2. Fluid Retention
Because progestational drugs may cause some degree of fluid retention, conditions that might be influenced by this condition, such as epilepsy, migraine, asthma, and cardiac or renal dysfunction, require careful observation.

3. Weight Changes
There is a tendency for women to gain weight while on therapy with DEPO-PROVERA Contraceptive Injection. From an initial average body weight of 136 lb, women who completed 1 year of therapy with DEPO-PROVERA Contraceptive Injection gained an average of 5.4 lb. Women who completed 2 years of therapy gained an average of 8.1 lb. Women who completed 4 years gained an average of 13.8 lb. Women who completed 6 years gained an average of 16.5 lb. Two percent of women withdrew from a large-scale clinical trial because of excessive weight gain.

4. Return of Fertility
DEPO-PROVERA Contraceptive Injection has a prolonged contraceptive effect. In a large US study of women who discontinued use of DEPO-PROVERA Contraceptive Injection to become pregnant, data are available for 61% of them.

Based on Life-Table analysis of these data, it is expected that 68% of women who do become pregnant may conceive within 12 months, 83% may conceive within 15 months, and 93% may conceive within 18 months from the last injection. The median time to conception for those who do conceive is 10 months following the last injection with a range of 4 to 31 months, and is unrelated to the duration of use. No data are available for 39% of the patients who discontinued DEPO-PROVERA Contraceptive Injection to become pregnant and who were lost to follow-up or changed their mind.

5. CNS Disorders and Convulsions

Patients who have a history of psychic depression should be carefully observed and the drug not be readministered if the depression recurs.

There have been a few reported cases of convulsions in patients who were treated with DEPO-PROVERA Contraceptive Injection. Association with drug use or pre-existing conditions is not clear.

6. Carbohydrate Metabolism

A decrease in glucose tolerance has been observed in some patients on DEPO-PROVERA Contraceptive Injection treatment. The mechanism of this decrease is obscure. For this reason, diabetic patients should be carefully observed while receiving such therapy.

7. Liver Function

If jaundice develops, consideration should be given to not readministering the drug.

8. Protection Against Sexually Transmitted Diseases

Patients should be counseled that this product does not protect against HIV infection (AIDS) and other sexually transmitted diseases.

DRUG INTERACTIONS

Aminoglutethimide administered concomitantly with the DEPO-PROVERA Contraceptive Injection may significantly depress the serum concentrations of medroxyprogesterone acetate.[12] Users of DEPO-PROVERA Contraceptive Injection should be warned of the possibility of decreased efficacy with the use of this or any related drugs.

LABORATORY TEST INTERACTIONS

The pathologist should be advised of progestin therapy when relevant specimens are submitted.

The following laboratory tests may be affected by progestins including DEPO-PROVERA Contraceptive Injection:

(a) Plasma and urinary steroid levels are decreased (eg, progesterone, estradiol, pregnanediol, testosterone, cortisol).
(b) Gonadotropin levels are decreased.
(c) Sex-hormone-binding-globulin concentrations are decreased.
(d) Protein-bound iodine and butanol extractable protein-bound iodine may increase. T_3-uptake values may decrease.
(e) Coagulation test values for prothrombin (Factor II), and Factors VII, VIII, IX, and X may increase.
(f) Sulfobromophthalein and other liver function test values may be increased.
(g) The effects of medroxyprogesterone acetate on lipid metabolism are inconsistent. Both increases and decreases in total cholesterol, triglycerides, low-density lipoprotein (LDL) cholesterol, and high-density lipoprotein (HDL) cholesterol have been observed in studies.

CARCINOGENESIS

See "WARNINGS" section 3.

PREGNANCY

Pregnancy Category X. See "WARNINGS" section 6.

NURSING MOTHERS

See "WARNINGS" section 8.

INFORMATION FOR THE PATIENT

See Patient Labeling.

Patient labeling is included with each single-dose vial and prefilled syringe of DEPO-PROVERA Contraceptive Injection to help describe its characteristics to the patient. It is recommended that prospective users be given this labeling and be informed about the risks and benefits associated with the use of DEPO-PROVERA Contraceptive Injection, as compared with other forms of contraception or with no contraception at all. It is recommended that physicians or other health-care providers responsible for those patients advise them at the beginning of treatment that their menstrual cycle may be disrupted and that irregular and unpredictable bleeding or spotting results, and that this usually decreases to the point of amenorrhea as treatment with DEPO-PROVERA Contraceptive Injection continues, without other therapy being required.

ADVERSE REACTIONS

In the largest clinical trial with DEPO-PROVERA Contraceptive Injection, over 3,900 women, who were treated for up to 7 years, reported the following adverse reactions, which may or may not be related to the use of DEPO-PROVERA Contraceptive Injection.

The following adverse reactions were reported by more than 5% of subjects:

Menstrual irregularities
(bleeding or amenorrhea, or both)
Weight changes
Headache
Nervousness
Abdominal pain or discomfort
Dizziness
Asthenia (weakness or fatigue)

Adverse reactions reported by 1% to 5% of subjects using DEPO-PROVERA Contraceptive Injection were:

Decreased libido or anorgasmia
Backache
Leg cramps
Depression
Nausea
Insomnia
Leukorrhea
Acne
Vaginitis
Pelvic pain
Breast pain
No hair growth or alopecia
Bloating
Rash
Edema
Hot flashes
Arthralgia

Events reported by fewer than 1% of subjects included: galactorrhea, melasma, chloasma, convulsions, changes in appetite, gastrointestinal disturbances, jaundice, genitourinary infections, vaginal cysts, dyspareunia, paresthesia, chest pain, pulmonary embolus, allergic reactions, anemia, drowsiness, syncope, dyspnea and asthma, tachycardia, fever, excessive sweating and body odor, dry skin, chills, increased libido, excessive thirst, hoarseness, pain at injection site, blood dyscrasia, rectal bleeding, changes in breast size, breast lumps or nipple bleeding, axillary swelling, breast cancer, prevention of lactation, sensation of pregnancy, lack of return to fertility, paralysis, facial palsy, scleroderma, osteoporosis, uterine hyperplasia, cervical cancer, varicose veins, dysmenorrhea, hirsutism, unexpected pregnancy, thrombophlebitis, deep vein thrombosis.

In addition, voluntary reports have been received of anaphylaxis and anaphylactoid reaction with use of DEPO-PROVERA Contraceptive Injection.

DOSAGE AND ADMINISTRATION

Both the 1 mL vial and the 1 mL prefilled syringe of DEPO-PROVERA Contraceptive Injection should be vigorously shaken just before use to ensure that the dose being administered represents a uniform suspension.

The recommended dose is 150 mg of DEPO-PROVERA Contraceptive Injection every 3 months (13 weeks) administered by deep, IM injection in the gluteal or deltoid muscle. To ensure the patient is not pregnant at the time of the first injection, the first injection **MUST** be given **ONLY** during the first 5 days of a normal menstrual period; **ONLY** within the first 5-days postpartum if not breast-feeding; and if exclusively breast-feeding, **ONLY** at the sixth postpartum week. If the time interval between injections is greater than 13 weeks, the physician should determine that the patient is not pregnant before administering the drug. The efficacy of DEPO-PROVERA Contraceptive Injection depends on adherence to the dosage schedule of administration.

HOW SUPPLIED

DEPO-PROVERA Contraceptive Injection (medroxyprogesterone acetate sterile aqueous suspension 150 mg/mL) is available as:

NDC 0009-0746-30	1 mL vial
NDC 0009-0746-34	5 × 1 mL vials
NDC 0009-0746-35	25 × 1 mL vials
NDC 0009-7376-01	1 mL prefilled syringe
NDC 0009-7376-02	6 × 1 mL prefilled syringes
NDC 0009-7376-03	24 × 1 mL prefilled syringes

Store at controlled room temperature 15° to 30° C (59° to 86° F).

REFERENCES

1. Trussell J, Hatcher RA, Cates W Jr, Stewart FH, Kost K. A guide to interpreting contraceptive efficacy studies. *Obstet Gynecol.* 1990; *76*:558–567.
2. Schwallie PC, Assenzo JR. Contraceptive use-efficacy study utilizing medroxyprogesterone acetate administered as an intramuscular injection once every 90 days. *Fertil Steril.* 1973; *24*:331–339.
3. WHO Collaborative Study of Neoplasia and Steroid Contraceptives. Breast cancer and depot-medroxyprogesterone acetate: a multi-national study. *Lancet.* 1991; *338*:833–838.
4. WHO Collaborative Study of Neoplasia and Steroid Contraceptives. Depot-medroxyprogesterone acetate (DMPA) and risk of epithelial ovarian cancer. *Int J. Cancer.* 1991; *49*:191–195.
5. WHO Collaborative Study of Neoplasia and Steroid Contraceptives. Depot-medroxyprogesterone acetate (DMPA) and risk of liver cancer. *Int J Cancer.* 1991; *49*:182–185.
6. WHO Collaborative Study of Neoplasia and Steroid Contraceptives. Depot-medroxyprogesterone acetate (DMPA) and risk of invasive squamous-cell cervical cancer. *Contraception.* 1992; *45*:299–312.
7. WHO Collaborative Study of Neoplasia and Steroid Contraceptives. Depot-medroxyprogesterone acetate (DMPA) and risk of endometrial cancer. *Int J Cancer.* 1991; *49*:186–190.
8. Surveillance, Epidemiology, and End Results: Incidence and Mortality Data, 1973–1977. National Cancer Institute Monograph, 57: June 1981. (NIH publication No. 81-2330).
9. Gray RH, Pardthaisong T. *In Utero* exposure to steroid contraceptives and survival during infancy. *Am J Epidemiol.* 1991; *134*:804–811.
10. Pardthaisong T, Gray RH. *In Utero* exposure to steroid contraceptives and outcome of pregnancy. *Am J Epidemiol.* 1991; *134*:795–803.
11. Pardthaisong T, Gray RH, McDaniel EB, Chandacham A. Steroid contraceptive use and pregnancy outcome. *Teratology.* 1988; *38*:51–58.
12. Van Deijk WA, Biljham GH, Mellink WAM, Meulenberg PMM. Influence of aminoglutethimide on plasma levels of medroxyprogesterone acetate: its correlation with serum cortisol. *Cancer Treatment Reports.* 1985; *69*:1, 85–90.

Caution: Federal law prohibits dispensing without prescription.

DEPO-PROVERA Contraceptive Injection 1 mL vials are manufactured by

The Upjohn Company, Kalamazoo, MI 49001, USA

DEPO-PROVERA Contraceptive Injection 1 mL prefilled syringes are manufactured by

N.V. Upjohn S.A., Puurs, Belgium for The Upjohn Company, Kalamazoo, MI 49001, USA

Revised February 1996 815 459 107
691400

DEPO-PROVERA®

Contraceptive Injection

(sterile medroxyprogesterone acetate suspension, USP)

This product is intended to prevent pregnancy. It does not protect against HIV infection (AIDS) and other sexually transmitted diseases.

Patient Labeling

Introduction

Every woman who considers using DEPO-PROVERA Contraceptive Injection needs to understand the benefits and risks of this form of birth control and to discuss them with her health-care provider. This leaflet is intended to give you much of the information you will need in order to decide if DEPO-PROVERA Contraceptive Injection is the right choice for you. Your health-care provider will help you to compare DEPO-PROVERA Contraceptive Injection with other contraceptive methods and will answer any questions you have after you have read this information.

DEPO-PROVERA Contraceptive Injection is given as an intramuscular injection (a shot) in the buttock or upper arm once every 3 months (13 weeks). Promptly at the end of the 3–month interval, you will need to return to your health-care provider for your next injection in order to continue your contraceptive protection.

DEPO-PROVERA Contraceptive Injection contains medroxyprogesterone acetate, a chemical similar to (but not the same as) the natural hormone progesterone that is produced by your ovaries during the second half of your menstrual cycle. DEPO-PROVERA Contraceptive Injection acts by preventing your egg cells from ripening. If an egg is not released from the ovaries during your menstrual cycle, it cannot become fertilized by sperm and result in pregnancy. DEPO-PROVERA Contraceptive Injection also causes changes in the lining of your uterus that make it less likely for pregnancy to occur.

Effectiveness of DEPO-PROVERA Contraceptive Injection

To ensure that DEPO-PROVERA Contraceptive Injection is not administered inadvertently to a pregnant woman, the first injection must be given **ONLY** during the first 5 days of a normal menstrual period; **ONLY** within the first 5-days postpartum if not breast-feeding, and if exclusively breast-feeding, **ONLY** at the sixth postpartum week (see **Administration of DEPO-PROVERA Contraceptive Injection**). The efficacy of DEPO-PROVERA Contraceptive Injection depends on adherence to the recommended dosage schedule.

DEPO-PROVERA Contraceptive Injection is over 99% effective, making it one of the most reliable methods of birth control available. This means that the average annual pregnancy rate is less than one for every 100 women who use DEPO-PROVERA Contraceptive Injection. The effective-

Continued on next page

Information on these Pharmacia & Upjohn products is based on labeling in effect June 1, 1996. Further information concerning these and other Pharmacia & Upjohn products may be obtained by direct inquiry to Medical Information, Pharmacia & Upjohn, Kalamazoo, MI 49001.

Pharmacia & Upjohn—Cont.

ness of most contraceptive methods depends, in part, on how reliably each woman uses the method. The effectiveness of DEPO-PROVERA Contraceptive Injection depends only on the patient returning every 3 months (13 weeks) for her next injection.

The following table shows the percent of women who become pregnant while using different kinds of contraceptive methods. It gives both the lowest expected rate of pregnancy (the rate expected in women who use each method exactly as it should be used) and the typical rate of pregnancy (which includes women who became pregnant because they forgot to use their birth control or because they did not follow the directions exactly).

Percent of Women Experiencing an Accidental Pregnancy in the First Year of Continuous Use

Method	Lowest Expected	Typical
DEPO-PROVERA	0.3	0.3
Implants (Norplant)	0.2*	0.2*
Female sterilization	0.2	0.4
Male sterilization	0.1	0.15
Oral contraceptives (pill)	—	3
Combined	0.1	—
Progestogen only	0.5	—
IUD	—	3
Progestasert	2	—
Copper T 380A	0.8	—
Condom (without spermicide)	2	12
Diaphragm (with spermicide)	6	18
Cervical cap	6	18
Withdrawal	4	18
Periodic abstinence	1–9	20
Spermicide alone	3	21
Vaginal sponge	—	—
used before childbirth	6	18
used after childbirth	9	28
No method	85	85

Source: Trussell et al; Obstet Gynecol 1990;76:558–567.
* From Norplant® package insert.

Who Should Not Use DEPO-PROVERA Contraceptive Injection

Certain women should not use DEPO-PROVERA Contraceptive Injection. You should not use DEPO-PROVERA Contraceptive Injection if you have any of the following conditions:
• if you think you might be pregnant
• if you have any vaginal bleeding without a known reason
• if you have had cancer of the breast
• if you have had a stroke
• if you have or have had blood clots (phlebitis) in your legs
• if you have problems with your liver or liver disease
• if you are allergic to DEPO-PROVERA Contraceptive Injection (medroxyprogesterone acetate or any of its other ingredients)

Other Things to Consider Before Choosing DEPO-PROVERA Contraceptive Injection

Before your doctor prescribes DEPO-PROVERA Contraceptive Injection, you will have a physical examination. It is important to tell your doctor or health-care provider if you have any of the following:
• a family history of cancer of the breast
• an abnormal mammogram (breast X-ray), fibrocystic breast disease, breast nodules or lumps, or bleeding from your nipples
• kidney disease
• irregular or scanty menstrual periods
• high blood pressure
• migraine headaches
• asthma
• epilepsy (convulsions or seizures)
• diabetes or a family history of diabetes
• a history of depression
• if you are taking any prescription or over-the-counter medications

This product is intended to prevent pregnancy. It does not protect against transmission of HIV (AIDS) and other sexually transmitted diseases such as chlamydia, genital herpes, genital warts, gonorrhea, hepatitis B, and syphilis.

Return of Fertility

Because DEPO-PROVERA Contraceptive Injection is a long-acting birth control method, it takes some time after your last injection for its effect to wear off. Based on the results from a large study done in the United States, of those women who stop using DEPO-PROVERA Contraceptive Injection in order to become pregnant, about half of those who become pregnant do so in about 10 months after their last injection; about two-thirds of those who become pregnant do so in about 12 months, about 83% of those who become pregnant do so in about 15 months, and about 93% of those who be-

come pregnant do so in about 18 months after their last injection. The length of time you use DEPO-PROVERA Contraceptive Injection has no effect on how long it takes you to become pregnant after you stop using it.

Risks of Using DEPO-PROVERA Contraceptive Injection

1. Irregular Menstrual Bleeding
The side effect reported most frequently by women who use DEPO-PROVERA Contraceptive Injection for contraception is a change in their normal menstrual cycle. During the first year of using DEPO-PROVERA Contraceptive Injection, you might have one or more of the following changes:
• irregular or unpredictable bleeding or spotting,
• an increase or decrease in menstrual bleeding, or
• no bleeding at all.
Unusually heavy or continuous bleeding, however, is not a usual effect of DEPO-PROVERA Contraceptive Injection and if this happens you should see your health-care provider right away.

With continued use of DEPO-PROVERA Contraceptive Injection, bleeding usually decreases and many women stop having periods completely. In clinical studies of DEPO-PROVERA Contraceptive Injection, 55% of the women studied reported no menstrual bleeding (amenorrhea) after 1 year of use and 68% of the women studied reported no menstrual bleeding after 2 years of use.

The reason that your periods stop is because DEPO-PROVERA Contraceptive Injection causes a resting state in your ovaries. When your ovaries do not release an egg monthly, the regular monthly growth of the lining of your uterus does not occur and, therefore, the bleeding that comes with your normal menstruation does not take place. When you stop using DEPO-PROVERA Contraceptive Injection your menstrual period will usually, in time, return to its normal cycle.

2. Bone Mineral Changes
Use of DEPO-PROVERA Contraceptive Injection may be associated with a decrease in the amount of mineral stored in your bones. This could increase your risk of developing bone fractures. The rate of bone mineral loss is greatest in the early years of DEPO-PROVERA Contraceptive Injection use but, after that, it begins to resemble the normal rate of age-related bone mineral loss.

3. Cancer
Studies of women who have used different forms of contraception found that women who used DEPO-PROVERA Contraceptive Injection for contraception had no increased overall risk of developing cancer of the breast, ovary, uterus, cervix, or liver. However, women under 35 years of age whose first exposure to DEPO-PROVERA Contraceptive Injection was within the previous 4 years may have a slightly increased risk of developing breast cancer similar to that seen with oral contraceptives. You should discuss this with your health-care provider.

4. Unexpected Pregnancy
Because DEPO-PROVERA Contraceptive Injection is such an effective contraceptive method, the risk of unexpected pregnancy for women who get their shots regularly (every 3 months [13 weeks]) is very low. While there have been reports of an increased risk of low birth weight and neonatal infant death or other health problems in infants conceived close to the time of injection, such pregnancies are uncommon. If you think you may have become pregnant while using DEPO-PROVERA Contraceptive Injection for contraception, see your health-care provider as soon as possible.

5. Allergic Reactions
Severe allergic reactions known as anaphylaxis and anaphylactoid reactions have also been reported in some women using DEPO-PROVERA Contraceptive Injection.

6. Other Risks
Women who use hormone-based contraceptives may have an increased risk of blood clots or stroke. Also, if a contraceptive method fails, there is a possibility that the fertilized egg will begin to develop outside of the uterus (ectopic pregnancy). While these events are rare, you should tell your health-care provider if you have any of the Warning Signals listed in the next section.

Warning Signals

If any of these problems occur following an injection of DEPO-PROVERA Contraceptive Injection, call your health-care provider immediately:
• Sharp chest pain, coughing up of blood, or sudden shortness of breath (indicating a possible clot in the lung)
• Sudden severe headache or vomiting, dizziness or fainting, problems with your eyesight or speech, weakness, or numbness in an arm or leg (indicating a possible stroke)
• Severe pain or swelling in the calf (indicating a possible clot in the leg)
• Unusually heavy vaginal bleeding
• Severe pain or tenderness in the lower abdominal area
• Persistent pain, pus, or bleeding at the injection site

Side Effects of DEPO-PROVERA Contraceptive Injection

1. Weight Gain
You may experience a weight gain while you are using DEPO-PROVERA Contraceptive Injection. About two-thirds of the women who used DEPO-PROVERA Contraceptive Injection in the clinical trials reported a weight gain of about

5 pounds during the first year of use. You may continue to gain weight after the first year. Women in one large study who used DEPO-PROVERA Contraceptive Injection for 2 years gained an average total of 8.1 pounds over those 2 years, or approximately 4 pounds per year. Women who continued for 4 years gained an average total of 13.8 pounds over those 4 years, or approximately 3.5 pounds per year. Women who continued for 6 years gained an average total of 16.5 pounds over those 6 years, or approximately 2.75 pounds per year.

2. Other Side Effects
In a clinical study of over 3,900 women who used DEPO-PROVERA Contraceptive Injection for up to 7 years, some women reported the following effects that may or may not have been related to their use of DEPO-PROVERA Contraceptive Injection:
• irregular menstrual bleeding
• amenorrhea
• headache
• nervousness
• abdominal cramps
• dizziness
• weakness or fatigue
• decreased sexual desire
• leg cramps
• nausea
• vaginal discharge or irritation
• breast swelling and tenderness
• bloating
• swelling of the hands or feet
• backache
• depression
• insomnia
• acne
• pelvic pain
• no hair growth or excessive hair loss
• rash
• hot flashes
• joint pain
Other problems were reported by very few of the women in the clinical trials, but some of these could be serious. These include: convulsions, jaundice, urinary tract infections, allergic reactions, fainting, paralysis, osteoporosis, lack of return to fertility, deep vein thrombosis, pulmonary embolus, breast cancer, or cervical cancer. If these or any other problems occur during your use of DEPO-PROVERA Contraceptive Injection, discuss them with your health-care provider.

General Precautions

1. Missed Periods
During the time you are using DEPO-PROVERA Contraceptive Injection for contraception, you may skip a period, or your periods may stop completely. If you have been receiving your injection of DEPO-PROVERA Contraceptive Injection regularly every 3 months (13 weeks), then you are probably not pregnant. However, if you think that you may be pregnant, see your health-care provider.

2. Laboratory Test Interactions
If you are scheduled for any laboratory tests, tell your health-care provider that you are using DEPO-PROVERA Contraceptive Injection for contraception. Certain blood tests are affected by hormones such as DEPO-PROVERA Contraceptive Injection.

3. Drug Interactions
Cytadren (aminoglutethimide) is an anticancer drug that may significantly decrease the effectiveness of DEPO-PROVERA Contraceptive Injection if the two drugs are given during the same time.

4. Nursing Mothers
Although DEPO-PROVERA Contraceptive Injection can be passed to the nursing infant in the breast milk, no harmful effects have been found in these children. DEPO-PROVERA Contraceptive Injection does not prevent the breasts from producing milk, so it can be used by nursing mothers. However, to minimize the amount of DEPO-PROVERA Contraceptive Injection that is passed to the infant in the first weeks after birth, you should wait until 6 weeks after childbirth before you start using DEPO-PROVERA Contraceptive Injection for contraception.

Administration of DEPO-PROVERA Contraceptive Injection

The recommended dose of DEPO-PROVERA Contraceptive Injection is 150 mg every 3 months (13 weeks) given in a single intramuscular injection in the buttock or upper arm. To ensure that you are not pregnant at the time of the first injection, it is essential that the injection be given **ONLY** during the first 5 days of a normal menstrual period. If used following the delivery of a child, the first injection of DEPO-PROVERA Contraceptive Injection **MUST** be given within 5 days after childbirth if you are not breast-feeding, or if you are exclusively breast-feeding, the injection **MUST** be given 6 weeks after childbirth. If you wait longer than 3 months (13 weeks) between injections, or longer than 6 weeks after delivery, your health-care provider should determine that you are not pregnant before giving you your injection of DEPO-PROVERA Contraceptive Injection.

Caution: Federal law prohibits dispensing without prescription.

Revised February 1995 815 459 107
691400

Shown in Product Identification Guide, page 329

DEPO-PROVERA® ℞

[*Dep-ō-prō-vera*]

brand of medroxyprogesterone acetate
sterile aqueous suspension
(sterile medroxyprogesterone acetate suspension, USP)

DESCRIPTION

DEPO-PROVERA Sterile Aqueous Suspension contains medroxyprogesterone acetate, which is a derivative of progesterone and is active by the parenteral and oral routes of administration. It is a white to off-white, odorless crystalline powder, stable in air, melting between 200° and 210° C. It is freely soluble in chloroform, soluble in acetone and in dioxane, sparingly soluble in alcohol and methanol, slightly soluble in ether and insoluble in water.

The chemical name for medroxyprogesterone acetate is Pregn-4-ene-3,20-dione, 17-(acetyloxy)-6-methyl-, (6α)-. The structural formula is:

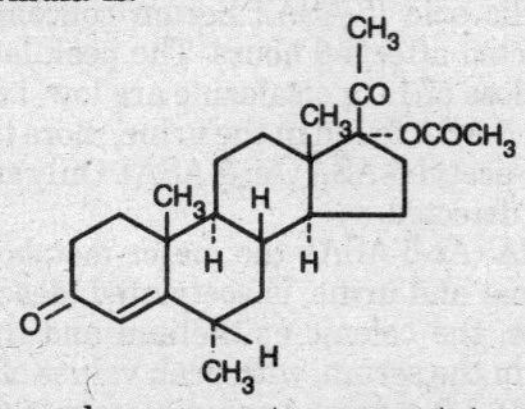

medroxyprogesterone acetate

DEPO-PROVERA for intramuscular injection is available as 400 mg/mL medroxyprogesterone acetate. Each mL of the 400 mg/mL suspension contains:

Medroxyprogesterone acetate	400 mg
Polyethylene glycol 3350	20.3 mg
Sodium sulfate anhydrous	11 mg
with	
Myristyl-gamma-picolinium chloride	1.69 mg

added as preservative

When necessary, pH was adjusted with sodium hydroxide and/or hydrochloric acid.

ACTIONS

Medroxyprogesterone acetate, administered parenterally in the recommended doses to women with adequate endogenous estrogen, transforms proliferative endometrium into secretory endometrium.

Medroxyprogesterone acetate inhibits (in the usual dose range) the secretion of pituitary gonadotropin which, in turn, prevents follicular maturation and ovulation.

Because of its prolonged action and the resulting difficulty in predicting the time of withdrawal bleeding following injection, medroxyprogesterone acetate is not recommended in secondary amenorrhea or dysfunctional uterine bleeding. In these conditions oral therapy is recommended.

INDICATIONS AND USES

Adjunctive therapy and palliative treatment of inoperable, recurrent, and metastatic endometrial or renal carcinoma.

CONTRAINDICATIONS

1. Known or suspected pregnancy or as a diagnostic test for pregnancy
2. Undiagnosed vaginal bleeding
3. Known or suspected malignancy of breast
4. Active thrombophlebitis, or current or past history of thromboembolic disorders, or cerebral vascular disease
5. Liver dysfunction or disease
6. Known sensitivity to DEPO-PROVERA (medroxyprogesterone acetate or any of its other ingredients).

WARNINGS

1. *Pregnancy* The use of progestational drugs during the first four months of pregnancy is not recommended. Progestational agents have been used beginning with the first trimester of pregnancy in attempts to prevent abortion but there is no evidence that such use is effective. Furthermore, the use of progestational agents, with their uterine-relaxant properties, in patients with fertilized defective ova may cause a delay in spontaneous abortion.

2. *Intrauterine Exposure* Several reports suggest an association between intrauterine exposure to progestational drugs in the first trimester of pregnancy and genital abnormalities in male and female fetuses. The risk of hypospadias (5 to 8 per 1,000 male births in the general population) may be approximately doubled with exposure to these drugs. There are insufficient data to quantify the risk to exposed female fetuses, but insofar as some of these drugs induce mild virilization of the external genitalia of the female fetus, and because of the increased association of hypospadias in the male fetus, it is prudent to avoid the use of these drugs during the first trimester of pregnancy.

If the patient is exposed to DEPO-PROVERA Sterile Aqueous Suspension during the first four months of pregnancy or if she becomes pregnant while taking this drug, she should be apprised of the potential risks to the fetus.

3. *Thromboembolic Disorders* The physician should be alert to the earliest manifestations of thrombotic disorder (thrombophlebitis, cerebrovascular disorder, pulmonary embolism, and retinal thrombosis). Should any of these occur or be suspected, the drug should be discontinued immediately.

4. *Ocular Disorders* Medication should be discontinued pending examination if there is a sudden partial or complete loss of vision, or if there is a sudden onset of proptosis, diplopia or migraine. If examination reveals papilledema or retinal vascular lesions, medication should be withdrawn.

5. *Lactation* Detectable amounts of drug have been identified in the milk of mothers receiving progestational drugs. The effect of this on the nursing infant has not been determined.

6. *Multi-dose Use* Multi-dose use of DEPO-PROVERA Sterile Aqueous Suspension from a single vial requires special care to avoid contamination. Although initially sterile, any multi-dose use of vials may lead to contamination unless strict aseptic technique is observed.

PRECAUTIONS

1. *Physical Examination* The pretreatment physical examination should include special reference to breast and pelvic organs, as well as Papanicolaou smear.

2. *Fluid Retention* Because progestational drugs may cause some degree of fluid retention, conditions which might be influenced by this condition, such as epilepsy, migraine, asthma, cardiac or renal dysfunction, require careful observation.

3. *Vaginal Bleeding* In cases of breakthrough bleeding, as in all cases of irregular bleeding per vaginum, nonfunctional causes should be borne in mind and adequate diagnostic measures undertaken.

4. *Depression* Patients who have a history of psychic depression should be carefully observed and the drug discontinued if the depression recurs to a serious degree.

5. *Masking of Climacteric* The age of the patient constitutes no absolute limiting factor although treatment with progestin may mask the onset of the climacteric.

6. *Use with Estrogen* Studies of the addition of a progestin product to an estrogen replacement regimen for seven or more days of a cycle of estrogen administration have reported a lowered incidence of endometrial hyperplasia. Morphological and biochemical studies of endometria suggest that 10–13 days of a progestin are needed to provide maximal maturation of the endometrium and to eliminate any hyperplastic changes. Whether this will provide protection from endometrial carcinoma has not been clearly established.

There are possible risks which may be associated with the inclusion of progestin in estrogen replacement regimen, including adverse effects on carbohydrate and lipid metabolism. The dosage used may be important in minimizing these adverse effects.

A decrease in glucose tolerance has been observed in a small percentage of patients on estrogen-progestin combination treatment. The mechanism of this decrease is obscure. For this reason, diabetic patients should be carefully observed while receiving such therapy.

7. *Prolonged Use* The effect of prolonged use of DEPO-PROVERA Sterile Aqueous Suspension at the recommended doses on pituitary, ovarian, adrenal, hepatic, and uterine function is not known.

8. *Multi-dose Use* When multi-dose vials are used, special care to prevent contamination of the contents is essential. There is some evidence that benzalkonium chloride is not an adequate antiseptic for sterilizing DEPO-PROVERA Sterile Aqueous Suspension multi-dose vials. A povidone-iodine solution or similar product is recommended to cleanse the vial top prior to aspiration of contents. (See WARNINGS)

DRUG INTERACTIONS

Aminoglutethemide administered concomitantly with DEPO-PROVERA Sterile Aqueous Suspension may significantly depress the serum concentrations of medroxyprogesterone acetate. DEPO-PROVERA users should be warned of the possibility of decreased efficacy with the use of this or any related drugs.

LABORATORY TEST INTERACTIONS

The pathologist should be advised of progestin therapy when relevant specimens are submitted. The following laboratory tests may be affected by progestins including DEPO-PROVERA Sterile Aqueous Suspension:

a) Plasma and urinary steroid levels are decreased (e.g. progesterone, estradiol, pregnanediol, testosterone, cortisol).
b) Gonadotropin levels are decreased.
c) Sex-hormone binding globulin concentrations are decreased.
d) Protein bound iodine and butanol extractable protein bound iodine may increase. T_3 uptake values may decrease.
e) Coagulation test values for prothrombin (Factor II), and Factors VII, VIII, IX, and X may increase.
f) Sulfobromophthalein and other liver function test values may be increased.
g) The effects of medroxyprogesterone acetate on lipid metabolism are inconsistent. Both increases and decreases in total cholesterol, triglycerides, low-density lipoprotein (LDL) cholesterol, and high-density lipoprotein (HDL) cholesterol have been observed in studies.

CARCINOGENESIS, MUTAGENESIS, IMPAIRMENT OF FERTILITY

Long-term intramuscular administration of Medroxyprogesterone acetate (MPA) has been shown to produce mammary tumors in beagle dogs. There is no evidence of a carcinogenic effect associated with the oral administration of MPA to rats and mice. Medroxyprogesterone acetate was not mutagenic in a battery of *in vitro* or *in vivo* genetic toxicity assays. Medroxyprogesterone acetate at high doses is an anti-fertility drug and high doses would be expected to impair fertility until the cessation of treatment.

INFORMATION FOR THE PATIENT

See Patient Information at end of insert.

ADVERSE REACTIONS

—(See WARNINGS for possible adverse effects on the fetus)
—breakthrough bleeding
—spotting
—change in menstrual flow
—amenorrhea
—headache
—nervousness
—dizziness
—edema
—change in weight (increase or decrease)
—changes in cervical erosion and cervical secretions
—cholestatic jaundice, including neonatal jaundice
—breast tenderness and galactorrhea
—skin sensitivity reactions consisting of urticaria, pruritus, edema and generalized rash
—acne, alopecia and hirsutism
—rash (allergic) with and without pruritis
—anaphylactoid reactions and anaphylaxis
—mental depression
—pyrexia
—fatigue
—insomnia
—nausea
—somnolence

In a few instances there have been undesirable sequelae at the site of injection, such as residual lump, change in color of skin, or sterile abscess.

A statistically significant association has been demonstrated between use of estrogen-progestin combination drugs and pulmonary embolism and cerebral thrombosis and embolism. For this reason patients on progestin therapy should be carefully observed. There is also evidence suggestive of an association with neuro-ocular lesions, e.g. retinal thrombosis and optic neuritis.

The following adverse reactions have been observed in patients receiving estrogen-progestin combination drugs:
—rise in blood pressure in susceptible individuals
—premenstrual syndrome
—changes in libido
—changes in appetite
—cystitis-like syndrome
—headache
—nervousness
—fatigue
—backache
—hirsutism
—loss of scalp hair
—erythema multiforma
—erythema nodosum
—hemorrhagic eruption
—itching
—dizziness

The following laboratory results may be altered by the use of estrogen-progestin combination drugs:
—increased sulfobromophthalein retention and other hepatic function tests
—coagulation tests: increase in prothrombin factors VII, VIII, IX, and X
—metyrapone test
—pregnanediol determinations
—thyroid function: increase in PBI, and butanol extractable protein bound iodine and decrease in T_3 uptake values

Continued on next page

Information on these Pharmacia & Upjohn products is based on labeling in effect June 1, 1996. Further information concerning these and other Pharmacia & Upjohn products may be obtained by direct inquiry to Medical Information, Pharmacia & Upjohn, Kalamazoo, MI 49001.

Consult 1997 supplements and future editions for revisions

Pharmacia & Upjohn—Cont.

DOSAGE AND ADMINISTRATION

The suspension is intended for intramuscular administration only.

Endometrial or renal carcinoma—doses of 400 mg to 1000 mg of DEPO-PROVERA Sterile Aqueous Suspension per week are recommended initially. If improvement is noted within a few weeks or months and the disease appears stabilized, it may be possible to maintain improvement with as little as 400 mg per month. Medroxyprogesterone acetate is not recommended as primary therapy, but as adjunctive and palliative treatment in advanced inoperable cases including those with recurrent or metastatic disease.

When multi-dose vials are used, special care to prevent contamination of the contents is essential (See WARNINGS).

HOW SUPPLIED

DEPO-PROVERA Sterile Aqueous Suspension is available as 400 mg/mL in 2.5 and 10 mL vials.

The text of the patient insert for progestational drugs is set forth below.

PATIENT INFORMATION

DEPO-PROVERA Sterile Aqueous Suspension is a progestational drug. The information below is required by the U.S. Food and Drug Administration to be provided to all patients taking such products. This information relates only to the risk to the unborn child associated with use of progestational drugs during pregnancy. For further information on the use, side effects, and other risks associated with this product, ask your doctor.

WARNING FOR WOMEN

Progesterone or progesterone-like drugs have been used to prevent miscarriage in the first few months of pregnancy. No adequate evidence is available to show that they are effective for this purpose. Furthermore, most cases of early miscarriage are due to causes which could not be helped by these drugs.

There is an increased risk of minor birth defects in children whose mothers take this drug during the first 4 months of pregnancy. Several reports suggest an association between mothers who take these drugs in the first trimester of pregnancy and genital abnormalities in male and female babies. The risk to the male baby is the possibility of being born with a condition in which the opening of the penis is on the underside rather than the tip of the penis (hypospadias). Hypospadias occurs in about 5 to 8 per 1000 male births and is about doubled with exposure to these drugs. There is not enough information to quantify the risk to exposed female fetuses, but enlargement of the clitoris and fusion of the labia may occur, although rarely.

Therefore, since drugs of this type may induce mild masculinization of the external genitalia of the female fetus, as well as hypospadias in the male fetus, it is wise to avoid using the drug during the first trimester of pregnancy.

These drugs have been used as a test for pregnancy but such use is no longer considered safe because of possible damage to a developing baby. Also, more rapid methods for testing for pregnancy are now available.

If you take DEPO-PROVERA Sterile Aqueous Suspension and later find you were pregnant when you took it, be sure to discuss this with your doctor as soon as possible.

Caution: Federal law prohibits dispensing without prescription.

Kalamazoo, Michigan 49001, U.S.A.

Revised May 1993 810 597 109
691015

DEPO®-TESTOSTERONE Ⓒ℞

[dĕp-ō-tes-tŏsterone]

brand of testosterone cypionate sterile solution (testosterone cypionate injection, USP)

DESCRIPTION

DEPO-Testosterone Sterile Solution, for intramuscular injection, contains testosterone cypionate which is the oil-soluble 17 (beta)- cyclopentylpropionate ester of the androgenic hormone testosterone.

Testosterone cypionate is a white or creamy white crystalline powder, odorless or nearly so and stable in air. It is insoluble in water, freely soluble in alcohol, chloroform, dioxane, ether, and soluble in vegetable oils.

The chemical name for testosterone cypionate is androst-4-en-3-one, 17- (3-cyclopentyl-1-oxopropoxy)-, (17β)-. Its molecular formula is $C_{27}H_{40}O_3$, and the molecular weight 412.61.

The structural formula is represented below:

[See chemical structure at top of next column.]

DEPO-Testosterone is available in two strengths, 100 mg/mL and 200 mg/mL testosterone cypionate.

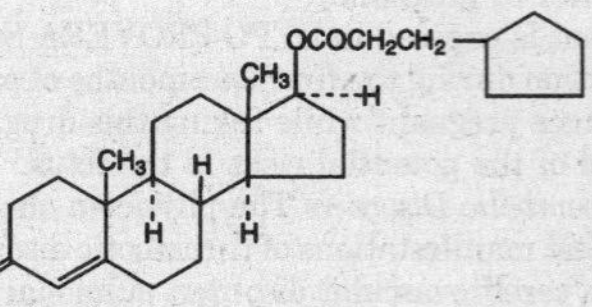

Each mL of the **100 mg/mL** solution contains:

Testosterone cypionate	100 mg
Benzyl benzoate	0.1 mL
Cottonseed oil	736 mg
Benzyl alcohol (as preservative)	9.45 mg

Each mL of the **200 mg/mL** solution contains:

Testosterone cypionate	200 mg
Benzyl benzoate	0.2 mL
Cottonseed oil	560 mg
Benzyl alcohol (as preservative)	9.45 mg

HOW SUPPLIED

DEPO-Testosterone Sterile Solution is available as follows:

100 mg/mL
10 mL vials NDC 0009-0347-02
200 mg/mL
1 mL vials NDC 0009-0417-01
10 mL vials NDC 0009-0417-02

Vials should be stored at controlled room temperature 15°–30° C (59°–86° F) and protected from light.

Caution: Federal law prohibits dispensing without prescription.

Revised March 1992 811 020 108
691272

DIPENTUM® Capsules ℞

[di·pent 'um]
(olsalazine sodium)

DESCRIPTION

The active ingredient in Dipentum® (olsalazine sodium) Capsules is a sodium salt of a salicylate, disodium 3, 3′-azobis (6-hydroxybenzoate) a compound that is effectively bioconverted to 5-aminosalicylic acid (5-ASA), which has anti-inflammatory activity in ulcerative colitis. Its empirical formula is $C_{14}H_8N_2Na_2O_6$ with a molecular weight of 346.21. The structural formula is:

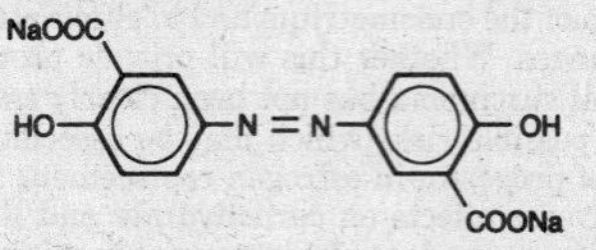

Olsalazine sodium is a yellow crystalline powder which melts with decomposition at 240°C. It is the sodium salt of a weak acid, soluble in water and DMSO, and practically insoluble in ethanol, chloroform and ether. Olsalazine sodium has acceptable stability under acidic or basic conditions.

Dipentum® is supplied in hard gelatin capsules for oral administration. The inert ingredient in each 250 mg capsule of olsalazine sodium is magnesium stearate. The capsule shell has the following inactive ingredients: black iron oxide, caramel, gelatin, and titanium dioxide.

CLINICAL PHARMACOLOGY

After oral administration, olsalazine has limited systemic bioavailability. Based on oral and intravenous dosing studies, approximately 2.4% of a single 1.0 g oral dose is absorbed. Less than 1% of olsalazine is recovered in the urine. The remaining 98-99% of an oral dose will reach the colon where each molecule is rapidly converted into two molecules of 5-aminosalicylic acid (5-ASA) by colonic bacteria and the low prevailing redox potential found in this environment. The liberated 5-ASA is absorbed slowly resulting in very high local concentrations in the colon.

The conversion of olsalazine to mesalamine (5-ASA) in the colon is similar to that of sulfasalazine, which is converted into sulfapyridine and mesalamine. It is thought that the mesalamine component is therapeutically active in ulcerative colitis (A.K. Azad-Kahn et al, *LANCET*, 2: 892-895, 1977). The usual dose of sulfasalazine for maintenance of remission in patients with ulcerative colitis is 2 grams daily, which would provide approximately 0.8 gram of mesalamine to the colon. More than 0.9 gram of mesalamine would usually be made available in the colon from 1 gram of olsalazine.

The mechanism of action of mesalamine (and sulfasalazine) is unknown, but appears to be topical rather than systemic. Mucosal production of arachidonic acid (AA) metabolites, both through the cyclooxygenase pathways, i.e., prostanoids, and through the lipoxygenase pathways, i.e., leukotrienes (LTs) and hydroxyeicosatetraenoic acids (HETEs) is increased in patients with chronic inflammatory bowel disease, and it is possible that mesalamine diminishes inflammation by blocking cyclooxygenase and inhibiting prostaglandin (PG) production in the colon.

<u>Pharmacokinetics</u>

The pharmacokinetics of olsalazine are similar in both healthy volunteers and in patients with ulcerative colitis. Maximum serum concentrations of olsalazine appear after approximately 1 hour, and even after a 1.0 g single dose are low, e.g., 1.6–6.2 umol/L. Olsalazine, has a very short serum half-life, approximately 0.9 hours. Olsalazine is more than 99% bound to plasma proteins. It does not interfere with protein binding of warfarin. The urinary recovery of olsalazine is below 1%. Total recovery of oral 14C-labeled olsalazine in animals and humans ranges from 90 to 97%. Approximately 0.1% of an oral dose of olsalazine is metabolized in the liver to olsalazine-O-sulfate (olsalazine-S). Olsalazine-S, in contrast to olsalazine has a half-life of 7 days. Olsalazine-S accumulates to steady state within 2-3 weeks. Patients on daily doses of 1.0 g olsalazine for 2-4 years show a stable plasma concentration of olsalazine-S (3.3-12.4 umol/L). Olsalazine-S, is more than 99% bound to plasma proteins. Its long half-life is mainly due to slow dissociation from the protein binding site. Less than 1% of both olsalazine and olsalazine-S appears undissociated in plasma.

5-aminosalicylic acid (5-ASA): Serum concentrations of 5-ASA are detected after 4-8 hours. The peak levels of 5-ASA after an oral dose of 1.0 g olsalazine are low, i.e., 0-4.3 umol/L. Of the total 5-ASA found in the urine, more than 90% is in the form on N-acetyl-5-ASA (Ac-5-ASA). Only small amounts of 5-ASA are detected.

N-acetyl-5-ASA (Ac-5-ASA), the major metabolite of 5-ASA found in plasma and urine, is acetylated (deactivated) in at least two sites, the colonic epithelium and the liver. Ac-5-ASA is found in the serum, with peak values of 1.7-8.7 umol/L after a single 1.0 g dose. Approximately 20% of the total 5-ASA is recovered in the urine, where it is found almost exclusively as Ac-5-ASA. The remaining 5-ASA is partially acetylated and is excreted in the feces. From fecal dialysis, the concentration of 5-ASA in the colon following olsalazine has been calculated to be 18-49 mmol/L.

No accumulation of 5-ASA or Ac-5-ASA in plasma has been detected. 5-ASA and Ac-5-ASA are 74 and 81%, respectively, bound to plasma proteins.

ANIMAL TOXICOLOGY

Preclinical subacute and chronic toxicity studies in rats have shown the kidney to be the major target organ of olsalazine toxicity. At an oral daily dose of 400 mg/kg or higher, olsalazine treatment produced nephritis and tubular necrosis, in a 4-week study; interstitial nephritis and tubular calcinosis in a 6-month study, and renal fibrosis, mineralization and transitional cell hyperplasia in a 1 year study.

CLINICAL STUDIES

Two controlled studies have demonstrated the efficacy of olsalazine as maintenance therapy in patients with ulcerative colitis. In the first, ulcerative colitis patients in remission were randomized to olsalazine 500 mg B.I.D. or placebo, and relapse rates for a six month period of time were compared. For the 52 patients randomized to olsalazine, 12 relapses occurred, while for the 49 placebo patients, 22 relapses occurred. This difference in relapse rates was significant ($p < .02$).

In the second study, 164 ulcerative colitis patients in remission were randomized to olsalazine 500 mg B.I.D. or sulfasalazine 1 gram B.I.D., and relapse rates were compared after six months. The relapse rate for olsalazine was 19.5% while that for sulfasalazine was 12.2%, a non-significant difference.

INDICATIONS AND USAGE

Olsalazine is indicated for the maintenance of remission of ulcerative colitis in patients who are intolerant of sulfasalazine.

CONTRAINDICATIONS

Hypersensitivity to salicylates.

PRECAUTIONS

<u>*General*</u>

Overall, approximately 17% of subjects receiving olsalazine in clinical studies reported diarrhea sometime during therapy. This diarrhea resulted in withdrawal of treatment in 6% of patients. This diarrhea appears to be dose related, although it may be difficult to distinguish from the underlying symptoms of the disease.

Exacerbation of the symptoms of colitis thought to have been caused by mesalamine or sulfasalazine has been noted. Although renal abnormalities were not reported in clinical trials with olsalazine, there have been rare reports from post-marketing experience (see under **ADVERSE REACTIONS**). Therefore, the possibility of renal tubular damage due to absorbed mesalamine or its n-acetylated metabolite, as noted in the ANIMAL TOXICOLOGY section must be kept in mind, particularly for patients with pre-existing renal disease. In these patients, monitoring with urinalysis, BUN and creatinine determinations is advised.

Information for Patients

Patients should be instructed to take olsalazine with food. The drug should be taken in evenly divided doses. Patients should be informed that about 17% of subjects receiving olsalazine during clinical studies reported diarrhea some time during therapy. If diarrhea occurs, patients should contact their physician.

Drug interactions.
Increased prothrombin time in patients taking concomitant warfarin has been reported.

Drug/laboratory test interactions.
None known.

Carcinogenesis, Mutagenesis, Impairment of Fertility

In a two year oral rat carcinogenicity study, olsalazine was tested in male and female Wistar rats at daily doses of 200, 400 and 800 mg/kg/day (approximately 10 to 40 times the human maintenance dose, based on a patient weight of 50 kg and a human dose of 1 g). Urinary bladder transitional cell carcinomas were found in three male rats (6%, p=0.022, exact trend test) receiving 40 times the human dose and were not found in untreated male controls. In the same study, urinary bladder transitional cell carcinoma and papilloma occurred in 2 untreated control female rats (2%). No such tumors were found in any of the female rats treated at doses up to 40 times the human dose.

In an eighteen month oral mouse carcinogenicity study, olsalazine was tested in male and female CD-1 mice at daily doses of 500, 1000 and 2000 mg/kg/day (approximately 25 to 100 times the human maintenance dose). Liver hemangiosarcomata were found in two male mice (4%) receiving olsalazine at 100 times the human dose, while no such tumor occurred in the other treated male mice groups or any of the treated female mice. The observed incidence of this tumor is within the 4% incidence in historical controls.

Olsalazine was not mutagenic in in vitro Ames tests, mouse lymphoma cell mutation assays, human lymphocyte chromosomal aberration tests and the in vivo rat bone marrow cell chromosomal aberration test.

Olsalazine in a dose range of 100 to 400 mg/kg/day (approximately 5 to 20 times the human maintenance dose) did not influence the fertility of male or female rats. The oligospermia and infertility in men associated with sulfasalazine have not been reported with olsalazine.

Pregnancy: Teratogenic effects. Pregnancy Category C.

Olsalazine has been shown to produce fetal development toxicity as indicated by reduced fetal weights, retarded ossifications and immaturity of the fetal visceral organs when given during organogenesis to pregnant rats in doses 5 to 20 times the human dose (100 to 400 mg/kg). There are no adequate and well-controlled studies in pregnant women.

Olsalazine should be used during pregnancy only if the potential benefit justifies the potential risk to the fetus.

Nursing Mothers

Oral administration of olsalazine to lactating rats in doses 5 to 20 times the human dose produced growth retardation in their pups. It is not known whether this drug is excreted in human milk. Because many drugs are excreted in human milk, caution should be exercised when olsalazine is administered to a nursing woman.

Pediatric Use

Safety and effectiveness in a pediatric population have not been established.

ADVERSE REACTIONS

Olsalazine has been evaluated in ulcerative colitis patients in remission as well as those with acute disease. Both sulfasalazine-tolerant and intolerant patients have been studied in controlled clinical trials. Overall, 10.4% of patients discontinued olsalazine because of an adverse experience compared with 6.7% of placebo patients. The most commonly reported adverse reactions leading to treatment withdrawal were diarrhea or loose stools (olsalazine 5.9%; placebo 4.8%), abdominal pain and rash or itching (slightly more than 1% of patients receiving olsalazine). Other adverse reactions to olsalazine leading to withdrawal occurred in fewer than 1% of patients (Table 1).

TABLE 1:
Adverse Reactions Resulting in Withdrawal
From Controlled Studies

	Total Olsalazine (N=441)	Placebo (N=208)
Diarrhea/Loose Stools	26 (5.9%)	10 (4.8%)
Nausea	3	2
Abdominal Pain	5 (1.1%)	0
Rash/Itching	5 (1.1%)	0
Headache	3	0
Heartburn	2	0
Rectal Bleeding	1	0
Insomnia	1	0
Dizziness	1	0
Anorexia	1	0
Light Headedness	1	0
Depression	1	0
Miscellaneous	4 (0.9%)	3 (1.4%)
Total Number of Patients Withdrawn	46 (10.4%)	14 (6.7%)

For those controlled studies, the comparative incidences of adverse reactions reported in 1% or more patients treated with olsalazine or placebo are provided in Table 2.

TABLE 2: COMPARATIVE INCIDENCE (%)
OF ADVERSE EFFECTS REPORTED BY
ONE PERCENT OR MORE OF ULCERATIVE
COLITIS PATIENTS TREATED WITH
OLSALAZINE OR PLACEBO IN
DOUBLE BLIND CONTROLLED STUDIES

	OLSALAZINE (N=441) %	PLACEBO (N=208) %
ADVERSE EVENT		
Digestive System		
Diarrhea	11.1	6.7
Abdominal Pain/ Cramps	10.1	7.2
Nausea	5.0	3.9
Dyspepsia	4.0	4.3
Bloating	1.5	1.4
Anorexia	1.3	1.9
Vomiting	1.0	—
Stomatitis	1.0	—
Increased Blood in Stool	—	3.4
CNS/Psychiatric		
Headache	5.0	4.8
Fatigue/Drowsiness/ Lethargy	1.8	2.9
Depression	1.5	—
Vertigo/Dizziness	1.0	—
Insomnia	—	2.4
Skin		
Rash	2.3	1.4
Itching	1.3	—
Musculoskeletal		
Arthralgia/Joint Pain	4.0	2.9
Miscellaneous		
Upper Respiratory Infection	1.5	

Over 2,500 patients have been treated with olsalazine in various controlled and uncontrolled clinical studies. In these as well as in the post-marketing experience, olsalazine was administered mainly to patients intolerant to sulfasalazine. There have been rare reports of the following adverse effects in patients receiving olsalazine. These were often difficult to distinguish from possible symptoms of the underlying disease or from the effects of prior and/or concomitant therapy. A causal relationship to the drug has not been demonstrated for some of these reactions.

Digestive:
Pancreatitis, diarrhea with dehydration, increased blood in stool, rectal bleeding, flare in symptoms, rectal discomfort, epigastric discomfort, flatulence. Rare cases of granulomatous hepatitis and nonspecific, reactive hepatitis have been reported in patients receiving olsalazine. Additionally, a patient developed mild cholestatic hepatitis during treatment with sulfasalazine and experienced the same symptoms two weeks later after the treatment was changed to olsalazine. Withdrawal of olsalazine led to complete recovery in these cases.

Neurologic:
Paresthesia, tremors, insomnia, mood swings, irritability, fever, chills, rigors.

Dermatologic:
Erythema nodosum, photosensitivity, erythema, hot flashes, alopecia.

Musculoskeletal:
Muscle cramps.

Cardiovascular/Pulmonary:
Pericarditis, second degree heart block, interstitial pulmonary disease, hypertension, orthostatic hypotension, peripheral edema, chest pains, tachycardia, palpitations, bronchospasm, shortness of breath.

A patient who developed thyroid disease 9 days after starting Dipentum was given propranolol and radioactive iodine and subsequently developed shortness of breath and nausea. The patient died 5 days later with signs and symptoms of acute diffuse myocarditis.

Genitourinary:
Frequency, dysuria, hematuria, proteinuria, nephrotic syndrome, interstitial nephritis, impotence, menorrhagia.

Hematologic:
Leucopenia, neutropenia, lymphopenia, eosinophilia, thrombocytopenia, anemia, hemolytic anemia, reticulocytosis.

Laboratory:
ALT (SGPT) or AST (SGOT) elevated beyond the normal range.

Special senses:
Tinnitus, dry mouth, dry eyes, watery eyes, blurred vision.

DRUG ABUSE AND DEPENDENCY

Abuse:
None reported.

Dependence:
Drug dependence has not been reported with chronic administration of olsalazine.

OVERDOSAGE

No overdosage has been reported in humans. Maximum single oral doses of 5 g/kg in mice and rats and 2 g/kg in dogs were not lethal. Symptoms of acute toxicity were decreased motor activity and diarrhea in all species tested and in addition, vomiting in dogs.

DOSAGE AND ADMINISTRATION

The usual dosage in adults for maintenance of remission is 1.0 g/day in two divided doses.

HOW SUPPLIED

Beige colored capsules, containing 250 mg olsalazine sodium imprinted with "DIPENTUM® 250 mg" on the capsule shell. Packaged in bottles of 100 (NDC #0013-0105-01).
Storage
Controlled Room Temperature (15-30°C/59-86°F)
Federal law prohibits dispensing without prescription.
111001294

Manufactured by: Pharmacia AB
Uppsala, Sweden
for: Pharmacia Inc.
Columbus, OH 43216

©1994 Pharmacia Inc. Revised: December 1994
11-B-077-07
Shown in Product Identification Guide, page 329

EMCYT® ℞
[em'sit]
(estramustine phosphate sodium)
CAPSULES

DESCRIPTION

Estramustine phosphate sodium, an antineoplastic agent, is an off-white powder readily soluble in water. Emcyt is available as white opaque capsules, each containing estramustine phosphate sodium as the disodium salt monohydrate equivalent to 140 mg estramustine phosphate, for oral administration. Each capsule also contains magnesium stearate, silicon dioxide, sodium lauryl sulfate and talc. Gelatin capsule shells contain the following pigment: titanium dioxide.
Chemically, estramustine phosphate sodium is estra-1,3, 5(10)-triene-3,17-diol (17β) -,3- [bis(2-chloroethyl)carbamate] 17-(dihydrogen phosphate), disodium salt, monohydrate. It is also referred to as estradiol 3-[bis(2-chloroethyl)carbamate] 17-(dihydrogen phosphate), disodium salt, monohydrate. Estramustine phosphate sodium has an empiric formula of $C_{23}H_{30}Cl_2NNa_2O_6P \cdot H_2O$, a calculated molecular weight of 582.4, and the following structural formula:

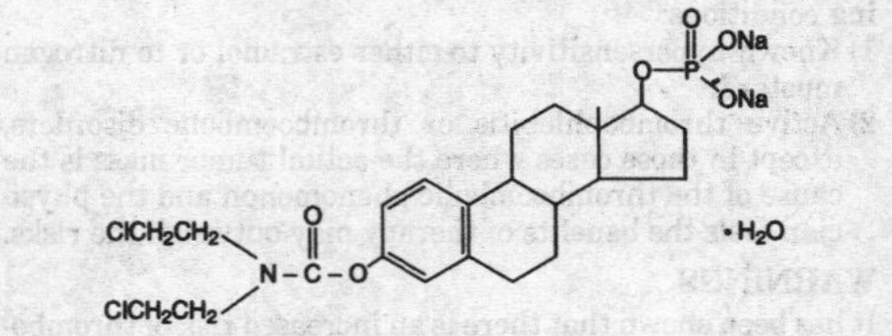

CLINICAL PHARMACOLOGY

Estramustine phosphate (Figure 1) is a molecule combining estradiol and nornitrogen mustard by a carbamate link. The molecule is phosphorylated to make it water soluble.

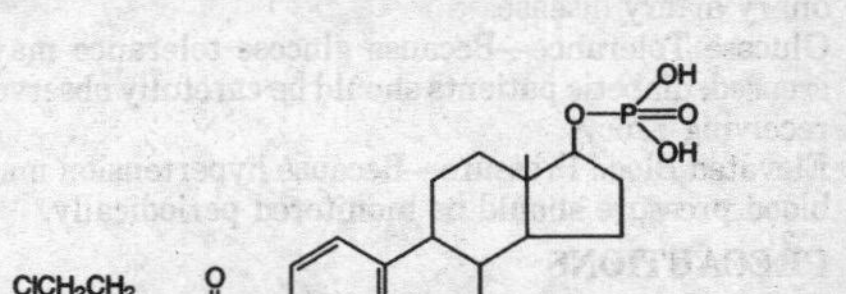

Figure 1. Estramustine Phosphate

Estramustine phosphate taken orally is readily dephosphorylated during absorption, and the major metabolites in plasma are estramustine (Figure 2), the estrone analog (Figure 3), estradiol and estrone.

[See chemical structures at top of next column.]

Continued on next page

Information on these Pharmacia & Upjohn products is based on labeling in effect June 1, 1996. Further information concerning these and other Pharmacia & Upjohn products may be obtained by direct inquiry to Medical Information, Pharmacia & Upjohn, Kalamazoo, MI 49001.

Pharmacia & Upjohn—Cont.

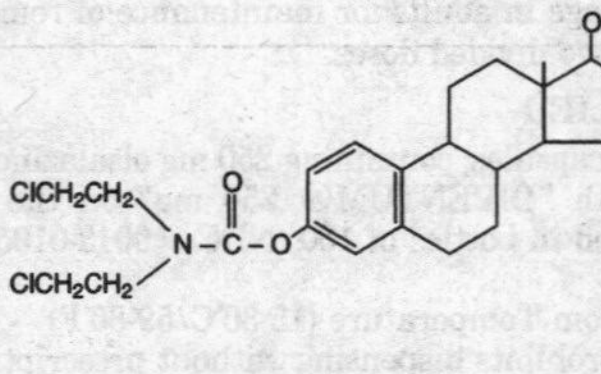

Figure 2. Estramustine

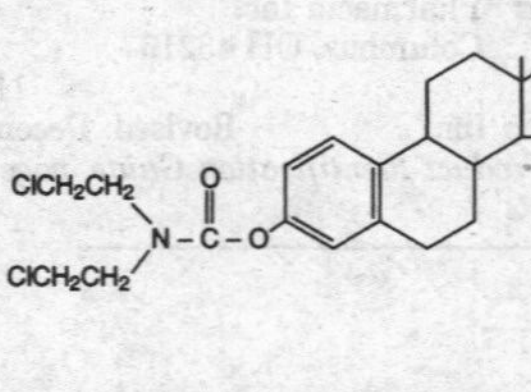

Figure 3. Estrone Analog of Estramustine

Prolonged treatment with estramustine phosphate produces elevated total plasma concentrations of estradiol that fall within ranges similar to the elevated estradiol levels found in prostatic cancer patients given conventional estradiol therapy. Estrogenic effects, as demonstrated by changes in circulating levels of steroids and pituitary hormones, are similar in patients treated with either estramustine phosphate or conventional estradiol.

The metabolic urinary patterns of the estradiol moiety of estramustine phosphate and estradiol itself are very similar, although the metabolites derived from estramustine phosphate are excreted at a slower rate.

INDICATIONS AND USAGE

Emcyt is indicated in the palliative treatment of patients with metastatic and/or progressive carcinoma of the prostate.

CONTRAINDICATIONS

Emcyt should not be used in patients with any of the following conditions:

1) Known hypersensitivity to either estradiol or to nitrogen mustard.
2) Active thrombophlebitis or thromboembolic disorders, except in those cases where the actual tumor mass is the cause of the thromboembolic phenomenon and the physician feels the benefits of therapy may outweigh the risks.

WARNINGS

It has been shown that there is an increased risk of thrombosis, including fatal and nonfatal myocardial infarction, in men receiving estrogens for prostatic cancer. Emcyt should be used with caution in patients with a history of thrombophlebitis, thrombosis or thromboembolic disorders, especially if they were associated with estrogen therapy. Caution should also be used in patients with cerebral vascular or coronary artery disease.

Glucose Tolerance—Because glucose tolerance may be decreased, diabetic patients should be carefully observed while receiving Emcyt.

Elevated Blood Pressure—Because hypertension may occur, blood pressure should be monitored periodically.

PRECAUTIONS

General: Fluid Retention—Exacerbation of preexisting or incipient peripheral edema or congestive heart disease has been seen in some patients receiving Emcyt therapy. Other conditions which might be influenced by fluid retention, such as epilepsy, migraine or renal dysfunction, require careful observation.

Emcyt may be poorly metabolized in patients with impaired liver function and should be administered with caution in such patients.

Because Emcyt may influence the metabolism of calcium and phosphorus it should be used with caution in patients with metabolic bone diseases that are associated with hypercalcemia or in patients with renal insufficiency.

Information for the Patient: Because of the possibility of mutagenic effects, patients should be advised to use contraceptive measures.

Laboratory Tests: Certain endocrine and liver function tests may be affected by estrogen-containing drugs. Abnormalities of hepatic enzymes and of bilirubin have occurred in patients receiving Emcyt, but have seldom been severe enough to require cessation of therapy. Such tests should be done at appropriate intervals during therapy and repeated after the drug has been withdrawn for two months.

Food/Drug Interaction: Milk, milk products and calcium-rich foods or drugs may impair the absorption of Emcyt.

Carcinogenesis, Mutagenesis, Impairment of Fertility: Long-term continuous administration of estrogens in certain animal species increases the frequency of carcinomas of the breast and liver. Compounds structurally similar to Emcyt are carcinogenic in mice. Carcinogenic studies of Emcyt have not been conducted in man. Although testing by the Ames method failed to demonstrate mutagenicity for estramustine phosphate sodium, it is known that both estradiol and nitrogen mustard are mutagenic. For this reason and because some patients who had been impotent while on estrogen therapy have regained potency while taking Emcyt, the patient should be advised to use contraceptive measures.

ADVERSE REACTIONS

In a randomized, double-blind trial comparing therapy with Emcyt in 93 patients (11.5 to 15.9 mg/kg/day) or diethylstilbestrol (DES) in 93 patients (3.0 mg/day), the following adverse effects were reported:

	EMCYT n=93	DES n=93
CARDIOVASCULAR–RESPIRATORY		
Cardiac Arrest	0	2
Cerebrovascular Accident	2	0
Myocardial Infarction	3	1
Thrombophlebitis	3	7
Pulmonary Emboli	2	5
Congestive Heart Failure	3	2
Edema	19	17
Dyspnea	11	3
Leg Cramps	8	11
Upper Respiratory Discharge	1	1
Hoarseness	1	0
GASTROINTESTINAL		
Nausea	15	8
Diarrhea	12	11
Minor Gastrointestinal Upset	11	6
Anorexia	4	3
Flatulence	2	0
Vomiting	1	1
Gastrointestinal Bleeding	1	0
Burning Throat	1	0
Thirst	1	0
INTEGUMENTARY		
Rash	1	4
Pruritus	2	2
Dry Skin	2	0
Pigment Changes	0	3
Easy Bruising	3	0
Flushing	1	0
Night Sweats	0	1
Fingertip—Peeling Skin	1	0
Thinning Hair	1	1
BREAST CHANGES		
Tenderness	66	64
Enlargement		
Mild	60	54
Moderate	10	16
Marked	0	5
MISCELLANEOUS		
Lethargy Alone	4	3
Depression	0	2
Emotional Lability	2	0
Insomnia	3	0
Headache	1	1
Anxiety	1	0
Chest Pain	1	1
Hot Flashes	0	1
Pain in Eyes	0	1
Tearing of Eyes	1	1
Tinnitus	0	1
LABORATORY ABNORMALITIES		
Hematologic		
Leukopenia	4	2
Thrombopenia	1	2
Hepatic		
Bilirubin Alone	1	5
Bilirubin and LDH	0	1
Bilirubin and SGOT	2	1
Bilirubin, LDH and SGOT	2	0
LDH and/or SGOT	31	28
Miscellaneous		
Hypercalcemia—Transient	0	1

OVERDOSAGE

Although there has been no experience with overdosage to date, it is reasonable to expect that such episodes may produce pronounced manifestations of the known adverse reactions. In the event of overdosage, the gastric contents should be evacuated by gastric lavage and symptomatic therapy should be initiated. Hematologic and hepatic parameters should be monitored for at least 6 weeks after overdosage of Emcyt.

DOSAGE AND ADMINISTRATION

The recommended daily dose is 14 mg per kg of body weight (ie, one 140 mg capsule for each 10 kg or 22 lb of body weight), given in 3 or 4 divided doses. Most patients in studies in the United States have been treated at a dosage range of 10 to 16 mg per kg per day.

Patients should be instructed to take Emcyt at least 1 hour before or 2 hours after meals. Emcyt should be swallowed with water. Milk, milk products and calcium-rich foods or drugs (such as calcium-containing antacids) must not be taken simultaneously with Emcyt.

Patients should be treated for 30 to 90 days before the physician determines the possible benefits of continued therapy. Therapy should be continued as long as the favorable response lasts. Some patients have been maintained on therapy for more than 3 years at doses ranging from 10 to 16 mg per kg of body weight per day.

Procedures for proper handling and disposal of anticancer drugs should be considered. Several guidelines on this subject have been published.[1-7] There is no general agreement that all of the procedures recommended in the guidelines are necessary or appropriate.

HOW SUPPLIED

White opaque capsules, each containing estramustine phosphate sodium as the disodium salt monohydrate equivalent to 140 mg estramustine phosphate—bottle of 100 (NDC 0013-0132-02).

NOTE: Emcyt should be stored at 36° to 46°F (2° to 8°C). Federal law prohibits dispensing without prescription.

REFERENCES

1. Recommendations for the Safe Handling of Parenteral Antineoplastic Drugs. NIH Publication No. 83-2621. For sale by the Superintendent of Documents, U.S. Government Printing Office, Washington, DC, 20402.
2. AMA Council Report, Guidelines for Handling Parenteral Antineoplastics. *JAMA.* 1985; 253 (11):1590–1592.
3. National Study Commission on Cytotoxic Exposure-Recommendations for Handling Cytotoxic Agents. Available from Louis P. Jeffrey, Sc.D., Chairman, National Study Commission on Cytotoxic Exposure, Massachusetts College of Pharmacy and Allied Health Sciences, 179 Longwood Avenue, Boston, Massachusetts 02115.
4. Clinical Oncological Society of Australia. Guidelines and Recommendations for Safe Handling of Antineoplastic Agents. *Med J Australia.* 1983; 1:426–428.
5. Jones RB, et al. Safe Handling of Chemotherapeutic Agents: A Report from the Mount Sinai Medical Center. *CA-A Cancer Journal for Clinicians.* 1983; (Sept/Oct) 258–263.
6. American Society of Hospital Pharmacists Technical Assistance Bulletin on Handling Cytotoxic and Hazardous Drugs. *Am J Hosp Pharm.* 1990; 47:1033–1049.
7. OSHA Work-Practice Guidelines for Personnel Dealing with Cytotoxic (Antineoplastic) Drugs. *Am J Hosp Pharm.* 1986; 43:1193–1204.

Pharmacia

Manufactured by: Hoffmann-La Roche Inc.
Nutley, N.J. 07110
for: Pharmacia Inc.
Columbus, OH 43216

11-B-085-04

©1994, Pharmacia Inc. 108001094 Revised: October 1994
13-06-76701-1094
13-20-76701-1094

ESTRING™
(estradiol vaginal ring)   ℞

1. ESTROGENS HAVE BEEN REPORTED TO INCREASE THE RISK OF ENDOMETRIAL CARCINOMA IN POSTMENOPAUSAL WOMEN.

   Close clinical surveillance of all women taking estrogens is important. Adequate diagnostic measures, including endometrial sampling when indicated, should be undertaken to rule out malignancy in all cases of undiagnosed persistent or recurring abnormal vaginal bleeding. There is no evidence that "natural" estrogens are more or less hazardous than "synthetic" estrogens at equi-estrogenic doses.

2. ESTROGENS SHOULD NOT BE USED DURING PREGNANCY.

   There is no indication for estrogen therapy during pregnancy or during immediate postpartum period. Estrogens are ineffective for the prevention or treatment of threatened or habitual abortion. Estrogens are not indicated for the prevention of postpartum breast engorgement.

   Estrogen therapy during pregnancy is associated with an increased risk of congenital defects in the reproductive organs of the fetus, and possibly other birth de-

fects. Studies of women who received diethylstilbestrol (DES) during pregnancy have shown that female offspring have an increased risk of vaginal adenosis, squamous cell dysplasia of the uterine cervix, and clear cell vaginal cancer later in life; male offspring have an increased risk of urogenital abnormalities and possibly testicular cancer later in life. The 1985 DES Task Force concluded that the use of DES during pregnancy is associated with a subsequent increased risk of breast cancer in the mothers, although a casual relationship remains unproven and the observed level of excess risk is similar to that for a number of other breast cancer risk factors.

DESCRIPTION

ESTRING™ (estradiol vaginal ring) is a slightly opaque ring with a whitish core containing a drug reservoir of 2 mg estradiol. Estradiol, silicone polymers and barium sulfate are combined to form the ring. When placed in the vagina, ESTRING releases estradiol, approximately 7.5 μg/24 hours, in a consistent stable manner over 90 days. ESTRING has the following dimensions: outer diameter 55 mm; cross-sectional diameter 9 mm; core diameter 2 mm. One ESTRING should be inserted into the upper third of the vaginal vault, to be worn continuously for three months.

Estradiol is chemically described as estra-1,3,5(10)-triene-3,17β-diol. The molecular formula of estradiol is $C_{18}H_{24}O_2$ and the structural formula is:

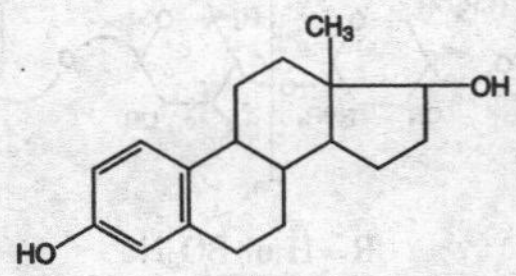

The molecular weight of estradiol is 272.39.

CLINICAL PHARMACOLOGY

Pharmacokinetics

ABSORPTION

Estrogens used in therapeutics are well absorbed through the skin, mucous membranes, and the gastrointestinal (GI) tract. The vaginal delivery of estrogens circumvents first-pass metabolism possibly reducing the induction of several other hepatic proteins.

In a Phase I study of 14 postmenopausal women, the insertion of ESTRING (estradiol vaginal ring) rapidly increased serum estradiol (E_2) levels attesting to the rapid absorption of estradiol via the vaginal mucosa. The time to attain peak serum estradiol levels (T_{max}) was 0.5 to 1 hour. Peak serum estradiol concentrations post-initial burst declined rapidly over the next 24 hours and were virtually indistinguishable from the baseline mean (range: 5 to 22 pg/mL). Serum levels of estradiol and estrone (E_1) over the following 12 weeks during which the ring was maintained in the vaginal vault remained relatively unchanged (see Table 1). The initial estradiol peak post-application of the second ring in the same women resulted in ~38% lower C_{max}, apparently due to reduced systemic absorption via the revitalized vaginal epithelium. The relative systemic exposure from the initial peak of ESTRING accounted for approximately 4% of the total estradiol exposure over the 12 week period.

The constant and stable release of estradiol from ESTRING was demonstrated in a Phase II study of 166–222 post-menopausal women who inserted up to four rings consecutively at three month intervals. Low dose systemic delivery of estradiol from ESTRING resulted in mean steady state serum estradiol estimates of 7.8, 7.0, 7.0, 8.1 pg/mL at weeks 12, 24, 36, and 48, respectively. Similar reproducibility is also seen in levels of estrone. Lower systemic exposure to estradiol and estrone is further supported by serum levels measured during a pivotal Phase III study.

In post-menopausal women, mean dose of estradiol systemically absorbed unchanged from ESTRING is ~8% [95% CI: 2.8–12.8%] of the daily amount released locally. Low systemic exposure to estradiol and estrone resulting from ESTRING should elicit lower estrogen-dependent effects.

DISTRIBUTION

Circulating, unbound estrogens are known to modulate pharmacological response. Estrogens circulate in blood bound to sex-hormone binding globulin (SHBG) and albumin. A dynamic equilibrium exists between the conjugated and the unconjugated forms of estradiol and estrone, which undergo rapid interconversion.

METABOLISM

Exogenously delivered or endogenously derived estrogens are primarily metabolized in the liver to estrone and estriol, which are also found in the systemic circulation. Estrogen metabolites are primarily excreted in the urine as glucuronides and sulphates. Of the several estrogen metabolites, urinary estrone and estrone sulphate (E_1S), post-ESTRING use, are in the normal post-menopausal range.

EXCRETION

Mean percent dose excreted in the 24-hour urine as estradiol, 4 and 12 weeks post-application of ESTRING in a Phase I study was 5 and 8%, respectively, of the daily released amount.

Drug-Drug Interactions

No formal *drug-drug* interactions studies have been done with ESTRING. It is anticipated that lower exposure to systemic estrogens may reduce the potential for drug interactions thus maintaining the benefit to risk ratio of concomitant drugs.

TABLE 1: PHARMACOKINETIC MEAN ESTIMATES FOLLOWING ESTRING APPLICATION

Estrogen	C_{max} (pg/mL)	$C_{ss\text{-}48\ hr}$ (pg/mL)	$C_{ss\text{-}4w}$ (pg/mL)	Css–12w (pg/mL)
Estradiol (E_2)	63.2[a]	11.2	9.5	8.0
Baseline-adjusted E_2[b]	55.6	3.6	2.0	0.4
Estrone (E_1)	66.3	52.5	43.8	47.0
Baseline-adjusted E_1	20.0	6.2	−2.4	0.8

[a] n=14 [b] Based on means

Pharmacodynamics

In-vivo, estrogens diffuse through cell membranes, distribute throughout the cell, bind to and activate the estrogen receptors, thereby eliciting their biological effects. Estrogen receptors have been identified in tissues of the reproductive tract, breast, pituitary, hypothalamus, liver and bone of women. ESTRING delivers estradiol constantly at a mean rate of ~7.5 μg/24 hours for a period of up to 90 days. Its use in post-menopausal patients in Phase I and II studies showed no apparent effects on systemic levels of hepatic protein SHBG, or FSH. Lowering of the pretreatment vaginal pH from a mean of 6.0 to a mean of 4.6 (as found in fertile women) over the 12 to 48 week treatment period, and improvements evident in the vaginal mucosal epithelium seen in all studies attest to the local dynamic effects of estrogens.

INDICATIONS AND USAGE

ESTRING (estradiol vaginal ring) is indicated for the treatment of urogenital symptoms associated with post-menopausal atrophy of the vagina (such as dryness, burning, pruritus and dyspareunia) and/or the lower urinary tract (urinary urgency and dysuria).

CLINICAL STUDIES

Two pivotal controlled studies have demonstrated the efficacy of ESTRING (estradiol vaginal ring) in the treatment of post-menopausal urogenital symptoms due to estrogen deficiency.

In a U.S. study where ESTRING was compared with conjugated estrogens vaginal cream, no difference in efficacy between the treatment groups was found with respect to improvement in the physician's global assessment of vaginal symptoms (83% and 82% of patients receiving ESTRING and cream, respectively) and in the patient's global assessment of vaginal symptoms (83% and 82% of patients receiving ESTRING and cream, respectively) after 12 weeks of treatment. In an Australian study, ESTRING was also compared with conjugated estrogens vaginal cream and no difference in the physician's assessment of improvement of vaginal mucosal atrophy (79% and 75% for ESTRING and cream, respectively) or in the patient's assessment of improvement in vaginal dryness (82% and 76% for ESTRING and cream, respectively) after 12 weeks of treatment.

In the U.S. study, symptoms of dysuria and urinary urgency improved in 74% and 65%, respectively, of patients receiving ESTRING as assessed by the patient. In the Australian study, symptoms of dysuria and urinary urgency improved in 90% and 71%, respectively, of patients receiving ESTRING as assessed by the patient.

In both studies, ESTRING and conjugated estrogens vaginal cream had a similar ability to reduce vaginal pH levels and to mature the vaginal mucosa (as measured cytologically using the maturation index and/or the maturation value) after 12 weeks of treatment. In supportive studies, ESTRING was also shown to have a similar significant treatment effect on the maturation of the urethral mucosa.

Endometrial overstimulation, as evaluated in non-hysterectomized patients participating in the U.S. study by the progestogen challenge test and pelvic sonogram, was reported for none of the 58 (0%) patients receiving ESTRING and 4 of the 35 patients (11%) receiving conjugated estrogens vaginal cream.

Of the U.S. women who completed 12 weeks of treatment, 95% rated product comfort for ESTRING as excellent or very good compared with 65% of patients receiving conjugated estrogens vaginal cream, 95% of ESTRING patients judged the product to be very easy or easy to use compared with 88% of cream patients, and 82% gave ESTRING an overall rating of excellent or very good compared with 58% for the cream.

CONTRAINDICATIONS

1. Estrogens should not be used in women with any of the following conditions:
   a. Known or suspected pregnancy (see BOXED WARNING).
   b. Undiagnosed abnormal genital bleeding.
   c. Known or suspected cancer of the breast.
   d. Known or suspected estrogen-dependent neoplasia.
2. ESTRING (estradiol vaginal ring) should not be used in patients hypersensitive to any of its ingredients.

WARNINGS

1. Breast cancer. While the majority of studies have not shown an increased risk of breast cancer in women who have ever used estrogen replacement therapy, some have reported a moderately increased risk (relative risks of 1.3 to 2.0) in those taking higher doses or those taking lower doses for prolonged periods of time, especially in excess of ten years. Other studies have not shown this relationship.
2. Other. Congenital lesions with malignant potential, gallbladder disease, cardiovascular disease, elevated blood pressure and hypercalcemia have been associated with systemic estrogen treatment.

PRECAUTIONS

A. General

1. **Use of Progestins.** It is common practice with systemic administration of estrogen to add progestin for ten or more days during a cycle to lower the incidence of endometrial proliferation or hyperplasia. From the available clinical data, it seems unlikely that ESTRING would have adverse effects on the endometrium. Furthermore, addition of progestins to a patient being treated with ESTRING is not expected to result in vaginal bleeding.
2. **Physical Examination.** A complete medical and family history should be taken prior to the initiation of any estrogen therapy. The pretreatment and periodic physical examinations should include special reference to blood pressure, breasts, abdomen, and pelvic organs and should include a Papanicolaou smear. As a general rule, estrogen should not be prescribed for longer than one year without reexamining the patient.
3. **Uterine Bleeding and Mastodynia.** Although uncommon with ESTRING, certain patients may develop undesirable manifestations of estrogenic stimulation, such as abnormal uterine bleeding and mastodynia.
4. **Liver Disease.** ESTRING should be used with caution in patients with impaired liver function.
5. **Location of ESTRING.** Some women have experienced moving or gliding of ESTRING within the vagina. Instances of ESTRING being expelled from the vagina in connection with moving the bowels, strain, or constipation have been reported. If this occurs, ESTRING can be rinsed in lukewarm water and reinserted into the vagina by the patient.
6. **Vaginal Irritation.** ESTRING may not be suitable for women with narrow, short, or stenosed vaginas. Narrow vagina, vaginal stenosis, prolapse, and vaginal infections are conditions that make the vagina more susceptible to ESTRING-caused irritation or ulceration. Women with signs or symptoms of vaginal irritation should alert their physician.
7. **Vaginal Infection.** Vaginal infection is generally more common in postmenopausal women due to the lack of the normal flora of fertile women, especially lactobacillus, and the subsequent higher pH. Vaginal infections should be treated with appropriate antimicrobial therapy before initiation of ESTRING. If a vaginal infection develops during use of ESTRING, then ESTRING should be removed and reinserted only after the infection has been appropriately treated.
8. **Other.** Hypercoagulability and hyperlipidemia have been reported in women on other types of estrogen replacement therapy but, these have not been seen with ESTRING patients.

   Fluid retention is another known risk factor with estrogen therapy and may be harmful to patients with asthma, epilepsy, migraine and cardiac or renal dysfunction. ESTRING treatment has not been associated with any indication of increase in body weight up to 48 weeks of treatment.

B. Information for the Patient. See text of Patient Package Insert which appears below.

C. Drug-Drug and Drug-Laboratory Interactions. It is recommended that ESTRING be removed during treatment with other vaginally administered preparations. Drug-drug and drug-laboratory interactions have been reported with estrogen administration overall, but were

Continued on next page

Information on these Pharmacia & Upjohn products is based on labeling in effect June 1, 1996. Further information concerning these and other Pharmacia & Upjohn products may be obtained by direct inquiry to Medical Information, Pharmacia & Upjohn, Kalamazoo, MI 49001.

Consult 1997 supplements and future editions for revisions

Pharmacia & Upjohn—Cont.

not observed in clinical trials with ESTRING. However, the possibility of the following interactions should be considered when treating patients with ESTRING.

1. Accelerated prothrombin time, partial thromboplastin time, and platelet aggregation time; increased platelet count; increased factors II, VII antigen, VIII antigen, VIII coagulant activity, IX, X, XII, VII-X complex, II-VII-X complex, and beta-thromboglobulin; decreased levels of anti-factor Xa and antithrombin III, decreased antithrombin III activity; increased levels of fibrinogen and fibrinogen activity; increased plasminogen antigen and activity.
2. Increased plasma HDL and HDL-2 subfraction concentrations, reduced LDL cholesterol concentration, increased triglycerides levels.

D. Carcinogenesis, Mutagenesis, and Impairment of Fertility. Long term continuous administration of natural and synthetic estrogens in certain animal species increases the frequency of carcinomas of the breast, uterus, cervix, vagina, and liver (see **CONTRAINDICATIONS and BOXED WARNING**).

E. Pregnancy Category X. Estrogens should not be used during pregnancy. (See **CONTRAINDICATIONS AND BOXED WARNING**).

F. Nursing Mothers. This product is not intended for nursing mothers. As a general principal, the administration of any drug to nursing mothers should be done only when clearly necessary since many drugs are excreted in human milk. In addition, estrogen administration to nursing mothers has been shown to decrease the quantity and quality of the milk.

ADVERSE REACTIONS

The biological safety of the silicone elastomer has been studied in various *in vitro* and *in vivo* test models. The results show that the silicone elastomer is non-toxic, non-pyrogenic, non-irritating, and non-sensitizing. Long-term implantation induced encapsulation equal to or less than the negative control (polyethylene) used in the USP test. No toxic reaction or tumor formation was observed with the silicone elastomer.

In general, ESTRING (estradiol vaginal ring) was well tolerated. In the two pivotal controlled studies, discontinuation of treatment due to an adverse event was required by 5.4% of patients receiving ESTRING and 3.9% of patients receiving conjugated estrogens vaginal cream. The most common reason for withdrawal from ESTRING treatment is due to an adverse event were vaginal discomfort and gastrointestinal symptoms.

The adverse events reported with a frequency of 3% or greater in the two pivotal controlled studies by patients receiving ESTRING or conjugated estrogens vaginal cream are listed in Table 2.

Table 2: Adverse Events Reported by 3% or More of Patients Receiving Either ESTRING or Conjugated Estrogens Vaginal Cream in Two Pivotal Controlled Studies

ADVERSE EVENT	Estring (n=257) %	Conjugated Estrogens Vaginal Cream (n=129) %
Musculoskeletal		
Back Pain	6	8
Arthritis	4	2
Arthralgia	3	5
Skeletal Pain	2	4
CNS/Peripheral Nervous System		
Headache	13	16
Psychiatric		
Insomnia	4	0
Gastrointestinal		
Abdominal Pain	4	2
Nausea	3	2
Respiratory		
Upper Respiratory Tract Infection	5	6
Sinusitis	4	3
Pharyngitis	1	3
Urinary		
Urinary Tract Infection	2	7
Female Reproductive		
Leukorrhea	7	3
Vaginitis	5	2
Vaginal Discomfort/Pain	5	5
Vaginal Hemorrhage	4	5
Asymptomatic Genital Bacterial Growth	4	6
Breast Pain	1	7
Resistance Mechanisms		
Genital Moniliasis	6	7
Body as a Whole		
Flu-Like Symptoms	3	2
Hot Flushes	2	3
Allergy	1	4
Miscellaneous		
Family Stress	2	3

Other adverse events (listed alphabetically) occurring at a frequency of 1 to 3% in the two pivotal controlled studies by patients receiving ESTRING include: anxiety, bronchitis, chest pain, cystitis, dermatitis, diarrhea, dyspepsia, dysuria, flatulence, gastritis, genital eruption, genital pruritus, hemorrhoids, leg edema, migraine, otitis media, skin hypertrophy, syncope, toothache, tooth disorder, urinary incontinence.

The following additional adverse events were reported at least once by patients receiving ESTRING in the worldwide clinical program, which includes controlled and uncontrolled studies. A causal relationship with ESTRING has not been established.

Body as a Whole: Allergic reaction
CNS/Peripheral Nervous System: dizziness
Gastrointestinal: enlarged abdomen, vomiting
Metabolic/Nutritional Disorders: weight decrease or increase
Psychiatric: depression, decreased libido, nervousness
Reproductive: breast engorgement, breast enlargement, intermenstrual bleeding, genital edema, vulval disorder
Skin/Appendages: pruritus, pruritus ani
Urinary: micturition frequency, urethral disorder
Vascular: thrombophlebitis
Vision: abnormal vision

OVERDOSAGE

Given the nature and design of ESTRING (estradiol vaginal ring), it is unlikely that overdosage will occur. However, should overdosage occur, it may manifest itself as nausea, vomiting, and/or vaginal bleeding. Serious ill effects have not been reported following acute ingestion of large doses of estrogen-containing oral contraceptives by young children.

DOSAGE AND ADMINISTRATION

One ESTRING (estradiol vaginal ring) is to be inserted as deeply as possible into the upper one-third of the vaginal vault. The ring is to remain in place continuously for three months, after which it is to be removed and, if appropriate, replaced by a new ring. The need to continue treatment should be assessed at 3 or 6 month intervals.

Should the ring be removed or fall out at any time during the 90-day treatment period, the ring should be rinsed in lukewarm water and re-inserted by the patient, or, if necessary, by a physician or nurse.

Retention of the ring for greater than 90-days does not represent overdosage but will result in progressively greater underdosage with the attendant risk of loss of efficacy and increasing risk of vaginal infections and/or erosions.

Instructions for Insertion

ESTRING (estradiol vaginal ring) insertion

The ring should be pressed into an oval and inserted into the upper third of the vaginal vault. The exact position is not critical. When ESTRING is in place, the patient should not feel anything. If the patient feels discomfort, ESTRING is probably not far enough inside. Gently push ESTRING further into the vagina.

ESTRING use

ESTRING should be left in place continuously for 90 days and then, if continuation of therapy is deemed appropriate, replaced by a new ESTRING. The patient should not feel ESTRING when it is in place and it should not interfere with sexual intercourse. Straining at defecation may make ESTRING move down in the lower part of the vagina. If so, it may be pushed up again with a finger. If ESTRING is expelled totally from the vagina, it should be rinsed in lukewarm water and reinserted by the patient (or doctor/nurse if necessary).

ESTRING removal

ESTRING may be removed by hooking a finger through the ring and pulling it out.

For patient instructions, see Information for Patients.

HOW SUPPLIED

Each ESTRING™ (estradiol vaginal ring) is individually packaged in a heat-sealed rectangular pouch consisting of three layers, from outside to inside: polyester, aluminum foil, and low density polyethylene, respectively. The pouch is provided with a tear-off notch on one side.

NDC 0013-2150-36 ESTRING (estradiol vaginal ring) 2 mg—available in single packs.

STORAGE—Store at controlled room temperature 15° to 30°C (59° to 86°F).

CAUTION: Federal law prohibits dispensing without prescription.

101000496
April 19, 1996

FRAGMIN® ℞

(dalteparin sodium injection)
For *Subcutaneous Use Only*

DESCRIPTION

FRAGMIN® (dalteparin sodium injection)$^{+}$, is a sterile, low molecular weight heparin for injection. Each syringe contains 2500 (16 mg dalteparin sodium) or 5000 (32 mg dalteparin sodium) anti-Factor Xa International units in 0.2 mL (with reference to the W.H.O. First International Low Molecular Weight Heparin Reference Standard). Each syringe also contains water for injection and sodium chloride, when required, to maintain physiologic ionic strength. The pH of the injection is 5.0 to 7.5. FRAGMIN is preservative free and intended for use only as a single dose injection.

Dalteparin sodium is produced through controlled nitrous acid depolymerization of sodium heparin from porcine intestinal mucosa followed by a chromatographic purification process. It is composed of strongly acidic sulphated polysaccharide chains (oligosaccharide, containing 2,5-anhydro-D-mannitol residues as end groups) with an average molecular weight of 5000 and about 90% of the material within the range 2000-9000. The molecular weight distribution is:

< 3000 daltons	3.0-15.0%
3000 to 8000 daltons	65.0-78.0%
> 8000 daltons	14.0-26.0%

Structural Formula

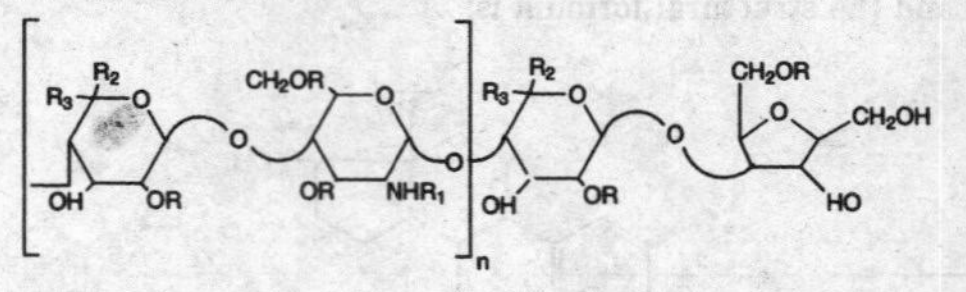

$R = H$ or SO_3Na
$R_1 = COCH_3$ or SO_3Na
$n = 3-20$ $R_2 = H$ $R_3 = COONa$
or
$R_2 = COONa$ $R_3 = H$

CLINICAL PHARMACOLOGY

Dalteparin is a low molecular weight heparin with antithrombotic properties. It acts by enhancing the inhibition of Factor Xa and thrombin by antithrombin. In man, dalteparin potentiates preferentially the inhibition of coagulation factor Xa, while only slightly affecting clotting time, e.g., activated partial thromboplastin time (APTT).

Pharmacodynamics:

Doses of FRAGMIN of up to 10,000 anti-Factor Xa IU administered subcutaneously as a single dose or two 5,000 IU doses 12 hours apart to healthy subjects do not produce a significant change in platelet aggregation, fibrinolysis, or global clotting tests such as prothrombin time (PT), thrombin time (TT) or APTT. Subcutaneous administration of FRAGMIN doses of 5,000 IU b.i.d. for seven consecutive days to patients undergoing abdominal surgery did not markedly affect APTT, Platelet Factor 4 (PF4), or lipoprotein lipase.

Pharmacokinetics:

Mean peak levels of plasma anti-Factor Xa activity following single subcutaneous doses of 2,500, 5,000 and 10,000 IU were 0.19 ± 0.04, 0.41 ± 0.07 and 0.82 ± 0.10 IU/mL, respectively, and were attained in about 4 hours in most subjects. Absolute bioavailability in healthy volunteers, measured as the anti-Factor Xa activity, was $87 \pm 6\%$. Increasing the dose from 2,500 to 10,000 IU resulted in an overall increase in anti-Factor Xa AUC that was greater than proportional by about one-third.

Peak anti - Factor Xa activity increased more or less linearly with dose over the same dose range. There appeared to be no appreciable accumulation of anti-Factor Xa activity with twice-daily dosing of 100 IU/kg subcutaneously for up to 7 days.

The volume of distribution for dalteparin anti-Factor Xa activity was 40 to 60 mL/kg. The mean plasma clearances of dalteparin anti-Factor Xa activity in normal volunteers following single intravenous bolus doses of 30 and 120 anti-Factor Xa IU/kg were 24.6 ± 5.4 and 15.6 ± 2.4 mL/ hr/kg, respectively. The corresponding mean disposition half-lives are 1.47 ± 0.3 and 2.5 ± 0.3 hr.

Following intravenous doses of 40 and 60 IU/kg, mean terminal half-lives were 2.1 ± 0.3 and 2.3 ± 0.4 hrs, respectively. Longer apparent terminal half-lives (3 to 5 hrs) are observed following subcutaneous dosing, possibly due to delayed absorption. In patients with chronic renal insufficiency requiring hemodialysis, the mean terminal half-life of anti-Factor Xa activity following a single intravenous dose of 5,000 IU FRAGMIN was 5.7 ± 2.0 hrs, i.e. considerably longer than values observed in healthy volunteers, therefore, greater accumulation can be expected in these patients.

Clinical Trials

FRAGMIN, administered once-daily beginning prior to surgery and continuing for 5 to 10 days after surgery, has been shown to prevent deep vein thrombosis (DVT) in patients at risk for thromboembolic complications (see INDICATIONS

and DOSAGE AND ADMINISTRATION). Data from two double-blind randomized controlled clinical trials performed in patients undergoing major abdominal surgery, summarized in the following tables, show that FRAGMIN 2500 IU was superior to placebo and similar to heparin in preventing DVT (see Tables 1 and 2).

Table 1
Abdominal Surgery

	Treatment Group	
	Fragmin	Placebo
Dosing Regimen	2500 IU qd	qd
Number of Patients Treated	102	102
Treatment Failures		
Total Thromboembolic Events (%)	4/91 (4.4)*	16/91 (17.6)
Proximal DVT (%)	0/91 (0)	5/91 (5.5)
Distal DVT (%)	4/91 (4.4)	11/91 (12.1)
PE (%)	0/91 (0)	2/91 (2.2)**

* P-value versus placebo =0.008
** Both patients also had DVT, 1 proximal and 1 distal

Table 2
Abdominal Surgery

	Treatment Group	
	Fragmin	Heparin
Dosing Regimen	2500 IU qd	5000 IU bid
Number of Patients Treated	195	196
Treatment Failures		
Total Thromboembolic Events (%)	7/178 (3.9)*	7/174 (4.0)
Proximal DVT (%)	3/178 (1.7)	4/174 (2.3)
Distal DVT (%)	3/178 (1.7)	3/174 (1.7)
PE (%)	1/178 (0.6)	0/174 (0)

* P-value versus heparin = 0.74

Data from a double-blind randomized controlled clinical trial show that FRAGMIN 5000 IU once daily is more effective than FRAGMIN 2500 IU once - daily in preventing DVT in patients undergoing abdominal surgery with malignancy (see Table 3).

Table 3
Abdominal Surgery Patients With Malignancy

	Intent to Treat	
	Fragmin	Fragmin
Dosing Regimen	2500 IU qd	5000 IU qd
Number of Patients treated	696	679
Treatment Failures		
Total Thromboembolic Events (%)	99/656 (15.1)*	60/645 (9.3)
Proximal DVT (%)	18/657 (2.7)	14/646 (2.2)
Distal DVT (%)	80/657 (12.2)	41/646 (6.3)
PE (%)		
Fatal	1/674 (0.1)	1/669 (0.1)
Non-fatal	2	4

* p=0.001

INDICATIONS AND USAGE

FRAGMIN is indicated for prophylaxis against deep vein thrombosis, which may lead to pulmonary embolism, in patients undergoing abdominal surgery who are at risk for thromboembolic complications.

Patients at risk include patients who are over 40 years of age, obese, undergoing surgery under general anesthesia lasting longer than 30 minutes or who have additional risk factors such as malignancy or a history of deep vein thrombosis or pulmonary embolism.

CONTRAINDICATIONS

FRAGMIN is contraindicated in patients with known hypersensitivity to the drug, active major bleeding, or thrombocytopenia associated with positive *in vitro* tests for anti-platelet antibody in the presence of FRAGMIN.

Patients with known hypersensitivity to heparin or pork products should not be treated with FRAGMIN.

WARNINGS

FRAGMIN is not intended for intramuscular administration.

FRAGMIN cannot be used interchangeably (unit for unit) with unfractionated heparin or other low molecular weight heparins.

FRAGMIN should be used with extreme caution in patients with history of heparin-induced thrombocytopenia.

Hemorrhage:
FRAGMIN, like other anticoagulants, should be used with extreme caution in patients who have an increased risk of hemorrhage, such as those with severe uncontrolled hypertension, bacterial endocarditis, congenital or acquired bleed-

	Fragmin vs. Heparin*				Fragmin vs. Placebo		Fragmin vs. Fragmin	
	Fragmin 2500 IU/ 24 hr	Heparin 10000 IU/ 24 hr	Fragmin 5000 IU/ 24 hr	Heparin 10000 IU/ 24 hr	Fragmin 2500 IU/ 24 hr	Placebo	Fragmin 2500 IU/ 24 hr	Fragmin 5000 IU/ 24 hr
Post-Operational Transfusions	5.7% (n=459)	7.9% (n=454)	15.9% (n=508)	12.7% (n=498)	7.7% (n=182)	7.1% (n=182)	8.7% (n=1025)	12.1% (n=1033)
Wound Hematoma	3.4% (n=467)	3.9% (n=467)	2.4% (n=508)	1.2% (n=498)	2.5% (n=79)	2.6% (n=77)	0.1% (n=1030)	0.4% (n=1039)
Reoperation due to Bleeding	0.5% (n=392)	0.8% (n=392)	0.8% (n=508)	0.4% (n=498)	1.3% (n=79)	1.3% (n=78)	0.2% (n=1030)	1.3% (n=1038)
Injection Site Hematoma	0.2% (n=466)	1.1% (n=464)	7.1% (n=506)	9.5% (n=493)	4.7% (n=172)	1.1% (n=174)	3.5% (n=1026)	5.5% (n=1035)

*FRAGMIN administered once-daily, heparin administered twice daily at a dose of 5000 IU.

ing disorders, active ulceration and angiodysplastic gastrointestinal disease, hemorrhagic stroke or shortly after brain, spinal or ophthalmological surgery.

As with other anticoagulants, bleeding can occur at any site during therapy with FRAGMIN. An unexpected drop in hematocrit or blood pressure should lead to a search for a bleeding site.

Thrombocytopenia:
Thrombocytopenia with platelet counts of $<50,000/mm^3$ and $<100,000/mm^3$ occurred in $<1\%$ and $<1\%$, respectively, of patients undergoing abdominal surgery.

Thrombocytopenia of any degree should be monitored closely. Heparin-induced thrombocytopenia can occur with the administration of FRAGMIN. The incidence of this complication is unknown at present.

PRECAUTIONS

General:
FRAGMIN should not be mixed with other injections or infusions unless specific compatibility data are available that support such mixing.

FRAGMIN should be used with caution in patients with bleeding diathesis, thrombocytopenia or platelet defects; severe liver or kidney insufficiency, hypertensive or diabetic retinopathy, and recent gastrointestinal bleeding.

If a thromboembolic event should occur despite dalteparin prophylaxis, FRAGMIN should be discontinued and appropriate therapy initiated.

Drug Interactions:
FRAGMIN should be used with care in patients receiving oral anticoagulants and/or platelet inhibitors because of increased risk of bleeding.

Laboratory Tests:
Periodic routine complete blood counts, including platelet count, and stool occult blood tests are recommended during the course of treatment with FRAGMIN. No special monitoring of blood clotting times (e.g., APTT) is needed.

Drug/Laboratory Test Interactions:
Elevations of Serum Transaminases:
Asymptomatic increases in transaminase levels (SGOT/AST and SGPT/ALT) greater than three times the upper of normal of the laboratory reference range have been reported in 1.7 and 4.3%, respectively, of patients during treatment with FRAGMIN. Similar significant increases in transaminase levels have also been observed in patients treated with heparin and other low molecular weight heparin. Such elevations are fully reversible and are rarely associated with increases in bilirubin. Since transaminase determinations are important in the differential diagnosis of myocardial infarction, liver disease and pulmonary emboli, elevations that might be caused by drugs like FRAGMIN should be interpreted with caution.

Carcinogenicity, Mutagenesis, Impairment of Fertility:
Dalteparin sodium has not been tested for its carcinogenic potential in long-term animal studies. It was not mutagenic in the in vitro Ames Test, mouse lymphoma cell forward mutation test and human lymphocyte chromosomal aberration test and in the *in vivo* mouse micronucleus test. Dalteparin sodium at subcutaneous doses up to 1,200 IU/kg (7080 IU/m^2) did not affect the fertility or reproductive performance of male and female rats.

Pregnancy: Pregnancy Category B.
Teratogenic Effects:
Reproduction studies with dalteparin sodium at intravenous doses up to 2400 IU/kg (14160 IU/m^2) in pregnant rats and 4800 IU/kg (40800 IU/m^2) in pregnant rabbits did not produce any evidence of impaired fertility or harm to the fetuses. There are, however, no adequate and well controlled studies in pregnant women. Because animal reproduction studies are not always predictive of human response, this drug should be used during pregnancy only if clearly needed.

Nursing Mothers:
It is not known whether dalteparin sodium is excreted in human milk.

Because many drugs are excreted in human milk, caution should be exercised when FRAGMIN is administered to a nursing mother.

Pediatric Use:
Safety and effectiveness in children has not been established.

ADVERSE REACTIONS

Hemorrhage:
The incidence of hemorrhagic complications during FRAGMIN treatment has been low. The most commonly reported side effect is hematoma at the injection site. The incidence of bleeding may increase with higher doses; however, in abdominal surgery patients with malignancy, no significant increase in bleeding was observed when comparing FRAGMIN 5000 IU to either FRAGMIN 2500 IU or low dose Heparin. In a study comparing FRAGMIN 5000 IU once daily to FRAGMIN 2500 IU once daily in patients undergoing surgery for malignancy, the incidence of bleeding events was 4.6% and 3.6%, respectively (n.s.). In a study comparing FRAGMIN 5000 IU once daily to heparin 5000 IU twice daily, the incidence of bleeding events was 3.2% and 2.7%, respectively (n.s.) in the malignancy subgroup.

The following table summarizes adverse bleeding events that occurred in clinical trials which studied FRAGMIN 2500 and 5000 IU administered once daily to abdominal surgery patients.

[See table on top of page.]

Thrombocytopenia:
During clinical trials with FRAGMIN in thromboprophylaxis, thrombocytopenia, platelet counts of $<50,000/mm^3$ and $<100,000/mm^3$ were reported in $<1\%$ and $<1\%$, respectively, of patients given FRAGMIN and $<1\%$ and 1% of patients given heparin.

Other:
Pain at injection site was seen in the following percentages of patients involved in clinical trials: 0% for FRAGMIN 2500 IU qd vs 0.4% for FRAGMIN 5000 IU bid; 4.5% for FRAGMIN 5000 IU qd vs 11.8% for heparin 5000 IU bid; 0% for FRAGMIN 2500 IU qd vs 0% for placebo and 1.1% for FRAGMIN 2500 IU qd vs 1.8% for FRAGMIN 5000 IU qd.

Allergic reactions (i.e., pruritus, rash, fever, injection site reaction, bulleous eruption) and skin necrosis have occurred rarely. A few cases of anaphylactoid reactions have been reported.

OVERDOSAGE

Symptoms/Treatment:
An excessive dosage of FRAGMIN may lead to hemorrhagic complications. These may generally be stopped by the slow intravenous injection of protamine sulfate (1% solution), at a dose of 1 mg protamine for every 100 anti-Xa IU of FRAGMIN given. A second infusion of 0.5 mg protamine sulfate per 100 anti-Xa IU of FRAGMIN may be administered if the APTT measured 2 to 4 hours after the first infusion remains prolonged. Even with these additional doses of protamine, the APTT may remain more prolonged than would usually be found following administration of conventional heparin. In all cases, the anti-Factor Xa activity is never completely neutralized (maximum about 60 to 75%).

Continued on next page

Information on these Pharmacia & Upjohn products is based on labeling in effect June 1, 1996. Further information concerning these and other Pharmacia & Upjohn products may be obtained by direct inquiry to Medical Information, Pharmacia & Upjohn, Kalamazoo, MI 49001.

Pharmacia & Upjohn—Cont.

Particular care should be taken to avoid overdosage with protamine sulfate. Administration of protamine sulfate can cause severe hypotensive and anaphylactoid reactions. Because fatal reactions, often resembling anaphylaxis, have been reported with protamine sulfate, it should be given only when resuscitation techniques and treatment of anaphylactic shock are readily available. For additional information, consult the labeling of Protamine Sulfate Injection, USP, products. A single subcutaneous dose of 100,000 IU/kg of FRAGMIN to mice caused a mortality of 8% (1/12) whereas 50,000 IU/kg was a non-lethal dose. The observed sign was hematoma at the site of injection.

DOSAGE AND ADMINISTRATION

In patients undergoing abdominal surgery with a risk of thromboembolic complications, 2500 IU should be administered subcutaneously only, each day, starting 1 to 2 hours prior to surgery and repeated once daily for 5 to 10 days postoperatively (refer to INDICATIONS).

In abdominal surgery associated with a high risk of thromboembolic complications, such as malignant disorder, 5000 IU should be administered subcutaneously only the evening before surgery and repeated once daily for 5 to 10 days postoperatively. Alternatively in patients with malignancy, the first 5000 IU dose can be administered as 2500 IU s.c. 1 to 2 hours prior to surgery with an additional 2500 IU s.c. dose 12 hours later and then 5000 IU once daily for 5 to 10 days.

Dosage adjustment and routine monitoring of coagulation parameters are not required if the dosage and administration recommendations specified above are followed.

Administration:

FRAGMIN is administered by subcutaneous injection. It must not be administered by intramuscular injection.

Subcutaneous injection technique: Patients should be sitting or lying down and FRAGMIN administered by deep subcutaneous injection. FRAGMIN may be injected in a U-shape area around the navel, the upper outer side of the thigh or the upper outer quadrangle of the buttock. The injection site should be varied daily. When the area around the navel or the thigh is used, using the thumb and forefinger, you must lift up a fold of skin while giving the injection. The entire length of the needle should be inserted at a 45 to 90 degree angle.

Parenteral drug products should be inspected visually for particulate matter and discoloration prior to administration, whenever solution and container permit.

HOW SUPPLIED

FRAGMIN® (dalteparin sodium injection) is available in packs of 10 single dose prefilled syringes in the following strength:

2500 anti-Factor Xa IU/0.2 mL
NDC 0013-2406-91
5000 anti-Factor Xa IU/0.2 mL
NDC 0013-2426-91

Each FRAGMIN prefilled syringe is affixed with a 27 gauge X $^1/_2$ inch needle.

Storage

Store at controlled room temperature 20° to 25° C (68° to 77°F) (see USP).

Caution: Federal law prohibits dispensing without prescription.

+ U.S. Patent 4,303,651

132010396 Revised March 20, 1996

GENOTROPIN™ ℞

[gen-ō" trō-pin]

(somatropin [rDNA origin] for injection)

DESCRIPTION

GENOTROPIN™ (somatropin [rDNA origin] for injection) is a polypeptide hormone of recombinant DNA origin. It has 191 amino acid residues and a molecular weight of 22,124 daltons. The amino acid sequence of the product is identical to that of human growth hormone of pituitary origin (somatropin). GENOTROPIN is synthesized in a strain of *Escherichia coli* that has been modified by the addition of the gene for human growth hormone. GENOTROPIN is a sterile white lyophilized powder intended for subcutaneous injection. GENOTROPIN, 1.5 mg is dispensed in a two-chamber cartridge. The front chamber contains recombinant somatropin 1.5 mg (approximately 4.5 IU), glycine 27.6 mg, sodium dihydrogen pho phate anhydrous 0.3 mg, disodium phosphate anhydrous 0.3 mg; the rear chamber contains 1.13mL water for injection. GENOTROPIN, 5.8 mg is dispensed in a two-chamber cartridge. The front chamber contains recombinant somatropin 5.8 mg (approximately 17.4 IU), glycine 2.2 mg, mannitol 1.8 mg, sodium dihydrogen phosphate anhydrous 0.32 mg and disodium phosphate anhydrous 0.31 mg; the rear chamber contains 0.3% m-Cresol (as a preservative) and mannitol 45 mg in 1.14 mL water for injection. GENOTROPIN is a highly purified preparation. The reconstituted recombinant somatropin solution has a concentration of either 1.3 mg/mL (approximately 4 IU/mL), for GENOTROPIN 1.5 mg, or 5 mg/mL (approximately 15 IU/mL), for GENOTROPIN 5.8 mg, an osmolality of approximately 300 mosm/kg, and a pH of approximately 6.7.

CLINICAL PHARMACOLOGY

GENOTROPIN stimulates linear growth in children with growth hormone deficiency. In vitro, preclinical and clinical tests have demonstrated that GENOTROPIN is therapeutically equivalent to somatropin and achieves similar pharmacokinetic profiles in normal adults. Treatment of growth hormone-deficient (GHD) children with GENOTROPIN produces increased growth rate and IGF-I (Insulin-like Growth Factor/Somatomedin-C) concentrations that are similar to those seen after therapy with somatropin.

In addition, the following actions have been demonstrated for GENOTROPIN and/or somatropin.

1. Tissue Growth
   A. Skeletal Growth: GENOTROPIN stimulates skeletal growth in children with GHD. The measurable increase in body length after administration of either GENOTROPIN or somatropin results from an effect on the epiphyseal plates of long bones. Concentrations of IGF-I, which may play a role in skeletal growth, are generally low in the serum of GHD children but tend to increase during treatment with GENOTROPIN. Elevations in mean serum alkaline phosphatase concentration are also seen.
   B. Cell Growth: It has been shown that there are fewer skeletal muscle cells in short-statured children who lack endogenous growth hormone as compared with normal children. Treatment with somatropin results in an increase in both the number and size of muscle cells.
2. Protein Metabolism
   Linear growth is facilitated in part by increased cellular protein synthesis. Nitrogen retention, as demonstrated by decreased urinary nitrogen excretion and serum urea nitrogen, follows the initiation of therapy with somatropin. Treatment with GENOTROPIN results in similar decreases.
3. Carbohydrate Metabolism
   Children with hypopituitarism sometimes experience fasting hypoglycemia that is improved by treatment with GENOTROPIN. Large doses of human growth hormone may impair glucose tolerance.
4. Lipid Metabolism
   In GHD patients, administration of somatropin has resulted in lipid mobilization, reduction in body fat stores, and increased plasma fatty acids.
5. Mineral Metabolism
   Retention of sodium, potassium, and phosphorus is induced by somatropin. Serum concentrations of inorganic phosphate are increased in patients with GHD after therapy with GENOTROPIN or somatropin. Serum calcium is not significantly altered by either GENOTROPIN or somatropin. Growth hormone could increase calciuria.

PHARMACOKINETICS

When compared to intravenous administration, approximately 80% of 1.5 mg GENOTROPIN was systemically available following subcutaneous (SC) injection in the thigh in a study using healthy male subjects.

In another study involving healthy male subjects following a SC injection dose of 0.033 mg/kg in the thigh, the extent of absorption (AUC) for 5mg/mL GENOTROPIN was 35% greater than that for 1.3 mg/mL GENOTROPIN. The mean (± standard deviation) peak (C_{max}) serum levels were 35.5 (± 14.5) ng/mL and 26.8 (± 14.2) ng/mL, respectively.

In a study involving children with growth hormone deficiency, 5 mg/mL GENOTROPIN following a SC injection dose of 0.033 mg/kg in the thigh, had a mean AUC that was 17% greater than 1.3 mg/mL GENOTROPIN. The mean C_{max} levels were 32.4 ng/mL and 25.2 ng/mL, respectively. Mean C_{max} levels were all achieved at approximately 3 to 4 hours and the apparent terminal half-life ($T_{1/2}$) is approximately 2 hours following SC injection.

INDICATION AND USAGE

GENOTROPIN is indicated for the long-term treatment of children who have growth failure due to an inadequate secretion of endogenous growth hormone. Other causes of short stature should be excluded.

CONTRAINDICATIONS

GENOTROPIN should not be used when there is any evidence of neoplastic activity. Intracranial lesions must be inactive and antitumor therapy complete prior to the institution of therapy. GENOTROPIN should be discontinued if there is evidence of tumor growth. Growth hormone should not be used in patients with fused epiphyses. Caution should be used if growth hormone is administered to children with diabetes mellitus.

WARNINGS

The 5.8 mg presentation of GENOTROPIN contains m-Cresol as a preservative. This product should not be used by patients with a known sensitivity to this preservative. The 1.5 mg presentation of GENOTROPIN is preservative-free. (See HOW SUPPLIED section).

PRECAUTIONS

General

Treatment with GENOTROPIN as with other growth hormone preparations, should be directed by physicians who are experienced in the diagnosis and management of patients with GHD.

Patients and caregivers who will administer GENOTROPIN in medically unsupervised situations should receive appropriate training and instruction on the proper use of GENOTROPIN from the physician or other suitably qualified health professional.

Patients with GHD secondary to an intracranial lesion should be examined frequently for progression or recurrence of the underlying disease process. Because human growth hormone may induce a state of insulin resistance, patients should be observed for evidence of glucose intolerance.

Concomitant glucocorticoid treatment may inhibit the growth promoting effect of human growth hormone. GHD patients with coexisting ACTH deficiency should have their glucocorticoid replacement dose carefully adjusted to avoid an inhibitory effect on growth. Hypothyroidism may develop during treatment with human growth hormone, and inadequate treatment of hypothyroidism may prevent an optimal response to human growth hormone. Therefore, GHD patients should have periodic thyroid function tests and be treated with thyroid hormone when indicated.

Patients with endocrine disorders, including GHD, have a higher incidence of slipped capital femoral epiphyses. Any child with the onset of a limp or complaints of hip or knee pain during growth hormone therapy should be evaluated.

Intracranial hypertension (IH) with papilledema, visual changes, headache, nausea and/or vomiting has been reported in a small number of patients treated with growth hormone products. Symptoms usually occurred within the first eight (8) weeks of the initiation of growth hormone therapy. In all reported cases, IH-associated signs and symptoms resolved after termination of therapy or a reduction of the growth hormone dose. Funduscopic examination of patients is recommended at the initiation, and periodically during the course of, growth hormone therapy.

Drug Interactions

Concomitant glucocorticoid treatment may inhibit the growth promoting effect of human growth hormone. GHD patients with coexisting ACTH deficiency should have their glucocorticoid replacement dose carefully adjusted to avoid an inhibitory effect on growth. See also PRECAUTIONS.

Carcinogenesis, Mutagenesis, Impairment of Fertility

Carcinogenicity studies have not been conducted with rhGH. No potential mutagenicity of rhGH was revealed in a battery of tests including the Ames test, induction of gene mutations in mammalian cells (L5178Y) in vitro and in intact bone marrow cells (rats). See **PREGNANCY** section below for effect on fertility.

Pregnancy: Pregnancy Category B

Reproduction studies carried out with GENOTROPIN at doses of 1, 3 and 10 IU/kg/day subcutaneously in the rat and 0.25, 1 and 4 IU/kg/day intramuscularly in the rabbit (highest doses approximately 24 times and 19 times the recommended human therapeutic levels, respectively) based on body surface area showed decreased maternal body weight gains but were not teratogenic. In rats dosed subcutaneously during gametogenesis and up to seven days of pregnancy, 10 IU/kg/day (approximately 24 times human dose) produced anestrus or extended estrus cycles in females and fewer and less motile sperm in males. When given to pregnant female rats (days 1–7 of gestation) at 10 IU/kg/day a very slight increase in fetal deaths was observed. At 3 IU/kg/day (approximately 7 times human dose) rats showed slightly extended estrus cycles whereas at 1 IU/kg/day no effects were noted. Peri- and post-natal studies in rats dosed with GENOTROPIN at doses of 1, 3 and 10 IU/kg/day produced growth promoting effects in the dams but not in the fetuses. Young rats at the highest dose showed increased weight gain during suckling but the effect was not apparent by 10 weeks of age. No adverse effects were observed on gestation, morphogenesis, parturition, lactation, post-natal development or reproductive capacity of the offsprings due to GENOTROPIN. There are, however, no adequate and well-controlled studies in pregnant woman. Because animal reproduction studies are not always predictive of human response, this drug should be used during pregnancy only if clearly needed.

Nursing Mothers

There have been no studies conducted with GENOTROPIN in nursing mothers. It is not known whether this drug is excreted in human milk. Because many drugs are excreted in human milk, caution should be exercised when GENOTROPIN is administered to a nursing woman.

ADVERSE REACTIONS

As with all protein drugs, a small number of patients may develop antibodies to the protein. Growth hormone antibody with binding lower than 2 mg/L has not been associated with growth attenuation. In some cases, when binding capacity is > 2mg/L, interference with growth response has been observed.

In 419 patients evaluated in clinical studies with GENOTROPIN, 244 had been treated previously with GENOTROPIN or other growth hormone preparations and 175 patients had received no previous growth hormone therapy. Antibodies to growth hormone (anti-hGH antibodies), were present in 6 previously treated patients at baseline. Three of the six became negative for anti-hGH antibodies during 6 to 12 months of treatment with GENOTROPIN. Of the remaining 413, eight (1.9%) developed detectable anti-hGH antibodies during GENOTROPIN treatment, none had an antibody binding capacity > 2 mg/L. There was no evidence that the growth response to GENOTROPIN was affected in these antibody positive patients.

GENOTROPIN preparations contain a small amount of periplasmic *Escherichia coli* peptides (PECP). Anti-PECP antibodies are found in a small number of patients treated with GENOTROPIN, but these appear to be of no clinical significance.

In clinical studies with GENOTROPIN, the following events were reported infrequently: injection site reactions, e.g., pain or burning associated with the injection, fibrosis, nodules, rash, inflammation, pigmentation, bleeding; lipoatrophy; headache; hematuria; hypothyroidism; mild hyperglycemia.

Leukemia has been reported in a small number of children who have been treated with growth hormone, including growth hormone of pituitary origin and recombinant somatropin. The relationship, if any, between leukemia and growth hormone therapy is uncertain.

OVERDOSAGE

The recommended subcutaneous dosage of GENOTROPIN is 0.16 to 0.24 mg/kg body weight/week given in 6 to 7 doses. There is little information on acute or chronic overdosage with GENOTROPIN. It is known that intravenously administered growth hormone has been shown to result in an acute decrease in plasma glucose. Subsequently, hyperglycemia was seen. It is thought that the same effect might occur on rare occasions with high dosage of GENOTROPIN administered subcutaneously. Long-term overdosage may result in signs and symptoms of acromegaly consistent with overproduction of human growth hormone.

DOSAGE AND ADMINISTRATION

GENOTROPIN dosage must be adjusted for the individual patient. Generally, a dose of 0.16 to 0.24 mg/kg body weight/week is recommended. The weekly GENOTROPIN dose should be divided into 6 to 7 **subcutaneous** injections. GENOTROPIN may be given in the thigh, buttocks or abdomen, the site of s.c. injections should be rotated daily in an attempt to prevent lipoatrophy.

GENOTROPIN must not be injected intravenously.

GENOTROPIN is supplied as a powder, filled in a two-chamber cartridge with the active substance in the front chamber and the diluent in the rear chamber. A reconstitution device is used to co-mix the diluent and the lyophilized powder. **Gently** tip the cartridge upside down a few times until the contents are completely dissolved. **Do not shake**; this may cause denaturation of the active ingredient. For more specific information see directions accompanying the reconstitution device.

All parenteral drug products should be inspected visually for particulate matter and discoloration prior to administration, whenever solution and container permit. If the solution is cloudy, the contents **MUST NOT** be injected.

After using the reconstitution device, **withdraw** the GENOTROPIN solution **using a** 0.5 mL or 1.0 mL **insulin syringe** with an attached needle.

Patients and caregivers who will administer GENOTROPIN in medically unsupervised situations should receive appropriate training and instruction on the proper use of GENOTROPIN from the physician or other suitably qualified health professional.

STABILITY AND STORAGE

GENOTROPIN should be stored under refrigeration 36° to 46°F (2°C to 8°C). (Do not freeze). Protect from light.

The GENOTROPIN 1.5 mg cartridge reconstituted with diluent (without preservative) may be stored under refrigeration for only up to 24 hours because it contains no antimicrobial agent. Use once only and discard any remaining solution.

The GENOTROPIN 5.8 mg cartridge is reconstituted with a diluent containing a preservative. Thus, after reconstitution, it may be stored under refrigeration for up to 14 days.

HOW SUPPLIED

GENOTROPIN (somatropin [rDNA origin] for injection) 1.5 mg, with a concentration of 1.3 mg/mL (approximately 4 IU/mL).

NDC 0013-2606-94 GENOTROPIN 1.5 mg Intra-Mix two-chamber cartridge (without preservative) preassembled in a reconstitution device and co-packaged with a pressure release needle, package of 5.

GENOTROPIN (somatropin [rDNA origin] for injection) 5.8 mg, with a concentration of 5 mg/mL (approximately 15 IU/mL).

NDC 0013-2616-94 GENOTROPIN 5.8 mg Intra-Mix two-chamber cartridge (with preservative) preassembled in a reconstitution device and co-packaged with a pressure release needle, package of 5.

NDC 0013-2616-81 GENOTROPIN 5.8 mg Intra-Mix two-chamber cartridge (with preservative) preassembled in a reconstitution device and co-packaged with a pressure release needle, package of 1.

NDC 0013-2626-94 GENOTROPIN 5.8 mg two-chamber cartridge (with preservative) for use with the GENOTROPIN Pen 5 injection device, and/or the GENOTROPIN Mixer reconstitution device, package of 5.

NDC 0013-2626-81 GENOTROPIN 5.8 mg two-chamber cartridge (with preservative) for use with the GENOTROPIN Pen 5 injection device, and/or the GENOTROPIN Mixer reconstitution device, package of 1.

Please see accompanying directions for use of the injection and/or reconstitution device.

Caution: Federal law prohibits dispensing without prescription.

121020496 April 4, 1996

Shown in Product Identification Guide, page 329

GLYNASE® PresTab® Tablets ℞

brand of micronized glyburide tablets
1.5, 3, and 6 mg

DESCRIPTION

GLYNASE PresTab Tablets contain micronized (smaller particle size) glyburide, which is an oral blood-glucose-lowering drug of the sulfonylurea class. Glyburide is a white, crystalline compound, formulated as GLYNASE PresTab Tablets of 1.5, 3, and 6 mg strengths for oral administration. Inactive ingredients: colloidal silicon dioxide, corn starch, lactose, magnesium stearate. In addition, the **3 mg** strength contains FD&C Blue No. 1 Aluminum Lake, and the **6 mg** tablet contains D&C Yellow No. 10 Aluminum Lake. The chemical name for glyburide is 1-[[p-[2-(5-chloro-o-anisamido)ethyl]phenyl]-sulfonyl]-3-cyclohexylurea and the molecular weight is 493.99. The structural formula is represented below:

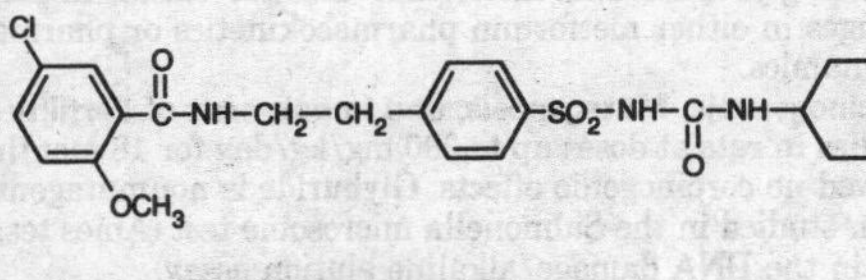

CLINICAL PHARMACOLOGY

Actions

Glyburide appears to lower the blood glucose acutely by stimulating the release of insulin from the pancreas, an effect dependent upon functioning beta cells in the pancreatic islets. The mechanism by which glyburide lowers blood glucose during long-term administration has not been clearly established. With chronic administration in Type II diabetic patients, the blood glucose lowering effect persists despite a gradual decline in the insulin secretory response to the drug. Extrapancreatic effects may be involved in the mechanism of action of oral sulfonylurea hypoglycemic drugs.

Some patients who are initially responsive to oral hypoglycemic drugs, including glyburide, may become unresponsive or poorly responsive over time. Alter natively, glyburide may be effective in some patients who have become unresponsive to one or more other sulfonylurea drugs.

In addition to its blood glucose lowering actions, glyburide produces a mild diuresis by enhancement of renal free water clearance. Disulfiram-like reactions have very rarely been reported in patients treated with glyburide.

Pharmacokinetics

Single dose studies with GLYNASE PresTab Tablets in normal subjects demonstrate significant absorption of glyburide within one hour, peak drug levels at about two to three hours, and low but detectable levels at twenty-four hours.

Bioavailability studies have demonstrated that GLYNASE PresTab Tablets 3 mg provide serum glyburide concentrations that are not bioequivalent to those from MICRONASE® Tablets 5 mg. Therefore, the patient should be retitrated.

In a single-dose bioavailability study (see Figure A) in which subjects received GLYNASE PresTab Tablets 3 mg and MICRONASE Tablets 5 mg with breakfast, the peak of the mean serum glyburide concentration-time curve was 97.2 ng/mL for GLYNASE PresTab Tablets 3 mg and 87.5 ng/mL for MICRONASE Tablets 5 mg. The mean of the individual maximum serum concentration values of glyburide (C_{max}) from GLYNASE PresTab Tablets 3 mg was 106 ng/mL and that from MICRONASE Tablets 5 mg was 104 ng/mL. The mean glyburide area under the serum concentration-time curve (AUC) for this study was 568 ng × hr/mL for GLYNASE PresTab Tablets 3 mg and 746 ng × hr/mL for MICRONASE Tablets 5 mg.

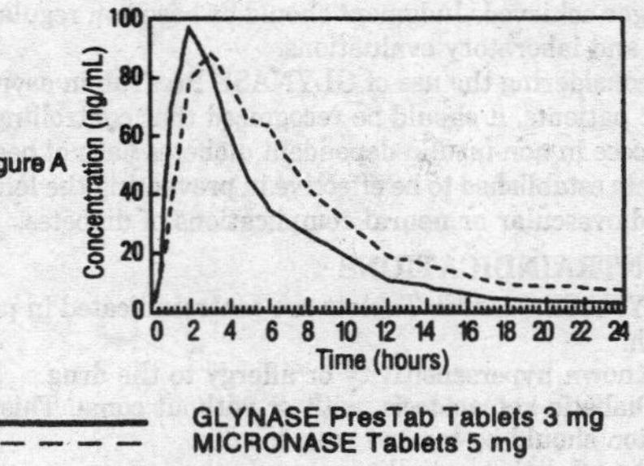

Mean serum levels of glyburide, as reflected by areas under the serum concentration-time curve, increase in proportion to corresponding increases in dose. Multiple dose studies with glyburide in diabetic patients demonstrate drug level concentration-time curves similar to single dose studies, indicating no buildup of drug in tissue depots.

The serum concentration of glyburide in normal subjects decreased with a half-life of about four hours.

In single dose studies in fasting normal subjects who were administered glyburide (MICRONASE Tablets) in doses ranging from 1.25 mg to 5 mg, the degree and duration of blood glucose lowering is proportional to the dose administered and to the area under the drug level concentration-time curve. The blood glucose lowering effect persists for 24 hours following single morning doses in nonfasting diabetic patients. Under conditions of repeated administration in diabetic patients, however, there is no reliable correlation between blood drug levels and fasting blood glucose levels. A one year study of diabetic patients treated with glyburide showed no reliable correlation between administered dose and serum drug level.

The major metabolite of glyburide is the 4-trans-hydroxy derivative. A second metabolite, the 3-cis-hydroxy derivative, also occurs. These metabolites probably contribute no significant hypoglycemic action in humans since they are only weakly active (1/400th and 1/40th as active, respectively, as glyburide) in rabbits.

Glyburide is excreted as metabolites in the bile and urine, approximately 50% by each route. This dual excretory pathway is qualitatively different from that of other sulfonylureas, which are excreted primarily in the urine.

Sulfonylurea drugs are extensively bound to serum proteins. Displacement from protein binding sites by other drugs may lead to enhanced hypoglycemic action. *In vitro*, the protein binding exhibited by glyburide is predominantly non-ionic, whereas that of other sulfonylureas (chlorpropamide, tolbutamide, tolazamide) is predominantly ionic. Acidic drugs such as phenylbutazone, warfarin, and salicylates displace the ionic-binding sulfonylureas from serum proteins to a far greater extent than the non-ionic binding glyburide. It has not been shown that this difference in protein binding will result in fewer drug-drug interactions with glyburide in clinical use.

INDICATIONS AND USAGE

GLYNASE PresTab Tablets are indicated as an adjunct to diet to lower the blood glucose in patients with non-insulin-dependent diabetes mellitus (Type II) whose hyperglycemia cannot be satisfactorily controlled by diet alone.

In initiating treatment for non-insulin-dependent diabetes, diet should be emphasized as the primary form of treatment. Caloric restriction and weight loss are essential in obese diabetic patient. Proper dietary management alone may be effective in controlling the blood glucose and symptoms of hyperglycemia. The importance of regular physical activity should also be stressed, and cardiovascular risk factors should be identified and corrective measures taken where possible. If this treatment program fails to reduce symptoms and/or blood glucose, the use of an oral sulfonylurea or insulin should be considered. Use of GLYNASE PresTab must be viewed by both the physician and patient as a treatment in addition to diet and not as a substitution or as a convenient mechanism for avoiding dietary restraint. Furthermore, loss of blood glucose control on diet alone may be transient, thus

Continued on next page

Information on these Pharmacia & Upjohn products is based on labeling in effect June 1, 1996. Further information concerning these and other Pharmacia & Upjohn products may be obtained by direct inquiry to Medical Information, Pharmacia & Upjohn, Kalamazoo, MI 49001.

Consult 1997 supplements and future editions for revisions

Pharmacia & Upjohn—Cont.

requiring only short-term administration of GLYNASE PresTab.

During maintenance programs, GLYNASE PresTab should be discontinued if satisfactory lowering of blood glucose is no longer achieved. Judgment should be based on regular clinical and laboratory evaluations.

In considering the use of GLYNASE PresTab in asymptomatic patients, it should be recognized that controlling blood glucose in non-insulin-dependent diabetes has not been definitely established to be effective in preventing the long-term cardiovascular or neural complications of diabetes.

CONTRAINDICATIONS

GLYNASE PresTab Tablets are contraindicated in patients with:

1. Known hypersensitivity or allergy to the drug.
2. Diabetic ketoacidosis, with or without coma. This condition should be treated with insulin.
3. Type I diabetes mellitus, as sole therapy.

SPECIAL WARNING ON INCREASED RISK OF CARDIOVASCULAR MORTALITY

The administration of oral hypoglycemic drugs has been reported to be associated with increased cardiovascular mortality as compared to treatment with diet alone or diet plus insulin. This warning is based on the study conducted by the University Group Diabetes Program (UGDP), a long-term prospective clinical trial designed to evaluate the effectiveness of glucose-lowering drugs in preventing or delaying vascular complications in patients with non-insulin-dependent diabetes. The study involved 823 patients who were randomly assigned to one of four treatment groups (Diabetes, 19 (Suppl. 2):747-830, 1970).

UGDP reported that patients treated for 5 to 8 years with diet plus a fixed dose of tolbutamide (1.5 grams per day) had a rate of cardiovascular mortality approximately $2^1/_2$ times that of patients treated with diet alone. A significant increase in total mortality was not observed, but the use of tolbutamide was discontinued based on the increase in cardiovascular mortality, thus limiting the opportunity for the study to show an increase in overall mortality. Despite controversy regarding the interpretation of these results, the findings of the UGDP study provide an adequate basis for this warning. The patient should be informed of the potential risks and advantages of GLYNASE PresTab and of alternative modes of therapy.

Although only one drug in the sulfonylurea class (tolbutamide) was included in this study, it is prudent from a safety standpoint to consider that this warning may also apply to other oral hypoglycemic drugs in this class, in view of their close similarities in mode of action and chemical structure.

PRECAUTIONS

Bioavailability studies have demonstrated that GLYNASE PresTab Tablets 3 mg provide serum glyburide concentrations that are not bioequivalent to those from MICRONASE Tablets 5 mg. Therefore, patients should be retitrated when transferred from MICRONASE or Diabeta or other oral hypoglycemic agents.

General

Hypoglycemia: All sulfonylureas are capable of producing severe hypoglycemia. Proper patient selection and dosage and instructions are important to avoid hypoglycemic episodes. Renal or hepatic insufficiency may cause elevated drug levels of glyburide and the latter may also diminish gluconeogenic capacity, both of which increase the risk of serious hypoglycemic reactions. Elderly, debilitated or malnourished patients, and those with adrenal or pituitary insufficiency, are particularly susceptible to the hypoglycemic action of glucose-lowering drugs. Hypoglycemia may be difficult to recognize in the elderly and in people who are taking beta-adrenergic blocking drugs. Hypoglycemia is more likely to occur when caloric intake is deficient, after severe or prolonged exercise, when alcohol is ingested, or when more than one glucose lowering drug is used. The risk of hypoglycemia may be increased with combination therapy.

Loss of Control of Blood Glucose: When a patient stabilized on any diabetic regimen is exposed to stress such as fever, trauma, infection or surgery, a loss of control may occur. At such times it may be necessary to discontinue GLYNASE PresTab and administer insulin.

The effectiveness of any hypoglycemic drug, including GLYNASE PresTab, in lowering blood glucose to a desired level decreases in many patients over a period of time which may be due to progression of the severity of diabetes or to diminished responsiveness to the drug. This phenomenon is known as secondary failure, to distinguish it from primary failure in which the drug is ineffective in an individual patient when GLYNASE PresTab is first given. Adequate adjustment of dose and adherence to diet should be assessed before classifying a patient as a secondary failure.

Information for Patients: Patients should be informed of the potential risks and advantages of GLYNASE PresTab and of alternative modes of therapy. They also should be informed about the importance of adherence to dietary instructions, of a regular exercise program, and of regular testing of urine and/or blood glucose.

The risks of hypoglycemia, its symptoms and treatment, and conditions that predispose to its development should be explained to patients and responsible family members. Primary and secondary failure also should be explained.

Laboratory Tests

Therapeutic response to GLYNASE PresTab Tablets should be monitored by frequent urine glucose tests and periodic blood glucose tests. Measurement of glycosylated hemoglobin levels may be helpful in some patients.

Drug Interactions

The hypoglycemic action of sulfonylureas may be potentiated by certain drugs including nonsteroidal anti-inflammatory agents and other drugs that are highly protein bound, salicylates, sulfonamides, chloramphenicol, probenecid, coumarins, monoamine oxidase inhibitors, and beta adrenergic blocking agents. When such drugs are administered to a patient receiving glyburide, the patient should be observed closely for hypoglycemia. When such drugs are withdrawn from a patient receiving glyburide, the patient should be observed closely for loss of control.

Certain drugs tend to produce hyperglycemia and may lead to loss control. These drugs include the thiazides and other diuretics, corticosteroids, phenothiazines, thyroid products, estrogens, oral contraceptives, phenytoin, nicotinic acid, sympathomimetics, calcium channel blocking drugs, and isoniazid. When such drugs are administered to a patient receiving glyburide, the patient should be closely observed for loss of control. When such drugs are withdrawn from a patient receiving glyburide, the patient should be observed closely for hypoglycemia.

A possible interaction between glyburide and ciprofloxacin, a fluoroquinolone antibiotic, has been reported, resulting in a potentiation of the hypoglycemic action of glyburide. The mechanism of action for this interaction is not known.

A potential interaction between oral miconazole and oral hypoglycemic agents leading to severe hypoglycemia has been reported. Whether this interaction also occurs with the intravenous, topical or vaginal preparations of miconazole is not known.

Metformin: In a single-dose interaction study in NIDDM subjects, decreases in glyburide AUC and C_{max} were observed, but were highly variable. The single-dose nature of this study and the lack of correlation between glyburide blood levels and pharmacodynamic effects, makes the clinical significance of this interaction uncertain. Coadministration of glyburide and metformin did not result in any changes in either metformin pharmacokinetics or pharmacodynamics.

Carcinogenesis, Mutagenesis, and Impairment of Fertility

Studies in rats at doses up to 300 mg/kg/day for 18 months showed no carcinogenic effects. Glyburide is nonmutagenic when studied in the Salmonella microsome test (Ames test) and in the DNA damage/alkaline elution assay.

No drug-related effects were noted in any of the criteria evaluated in the two-year oncogenicity study of glyburide in mice.

Pregnancy

Teratogenic Effects: Pregnancy Category B

Reproduction studies have been performed in rats and rabbits at doses up to 500 times the human dose and have revealed no evidence of impaired fertility or harm to the fetus due to glyburide. There are, however, no adequate and well controlled studies in pregnant women. Because animal reproduction studies are not always predictive of human response, this drug should be used during pregnancy only if clearly needed.

Because recent information suggests that abnormal blood glucose levels during pregnancy are associated with a higher incidence of congenital abnormalities, many experts recommend that insulin be used during pregnancy to maintain blood glucose as close to normal as possible.

Nonteratogenic Effects: Prolonged severe hypoglycemia (4 to 10 days) has been reported in neonates born to mothers who were receiving a sulfonylurea drug at the time of delivery. This has been reported more frequently with the use of agents with prolonged half-lives. If GLYNASE PresTab is used during pregnancy, it should be discontinued at least two weeks before the expected delivery date.

Nursing Mothers

Although it is not known whether glyburide is excreted in human milk, some sulfonylurea drugs are known to be excreted in human milk. Because the potential for hypoglycemia in nursing infants may exist, a decision should be made whether to discontinue nursing or to discontinue the drug, taking into account the importance of the drug to the mother. If the drug is discontinued, and if diet alone is inadequate for controlling blood glucose, insulin therapy should be considered.

Pediatric Use

Safety and effectiveness in children have not been established.

ADVERSE REACTIONS

Hypoglycemia: See PRECAUTIONS and OVERDOSAGE Sections.

Gastrointestinal Reactions: Cholestatic jaundice and hepatitis may occur rarely; GLYNASE PresTab Tablets should be discontinued if this occurs.

Liver function abnormalities, including isolated transaminase elevations, have been reported.

Gastrointestinal disturbances, eg, nausea, epigastric fullness, and heartburn are the most common reactions, having occurred in 1.8% of treated patients during clinical trials. They tend to be dose related and may disappear when dosage is reduced.

Dermatologic Reactions: Allergic skin reactions, eg, pruritus, erythema, urticaria, and morbilliform or maculopapular eruptions occurred in 1.5% of treated patients during clinical trials. These may be transient and may disappear despite continued use of glyburide. If skin reactions persist, the drug should be discontinued.

Porphyria cutanea tarda and photosensitivity reactions have been reported with sulfonylureas.

Hematologic Reactions: Leukopenia, agranulocytosis, thrombocytopenia, hemolytic anemia, aplastic anemia, and pancytopenia have been reported with sulfonylureas.

Metabolic Reactions: Hepatic porphyria and disulfiram-like reactions have been reported with sulfonylureas; however, hepatic porphyria has not been reported with glyburide and disulfiram-like reactions have been reported very rarely.

Cases of hyponatremia have been reported with glyburide and all other sulfonylureas, most often in patients who are on other medications or have medical conditions known to cause hyponatremia or increase release of antidiuretic hormone. The syndrome of inappropriate antidiuretic hormone (SIADH) secretion has been reported with certain other sulfonylureas, and it has been suggested that these sulfonylureas may augment the peripheral (antidiuretic) action of ADH and/or increase release of ADH.

Other Reactions: Changes in accommodation and/or blurred vision have been reported with glyburide and other sulfonylureas. These are thought to be related to fluctuation in glucose levels.

In addition to dermatologic reactions, allergic reactions such as angioedema, arthralgia, myalgia and vasculitis have been reported.

OVERDOSAGE

Overdosage of sulfonylureas, including glyburide, can produce hypoglycemia. Mild hypoglycemic symptoms, without loss of consciousness or neurological findings, should be treated aggressively with oral glucose and adjustments in drug dosage and/or meal patterns. Close monitoring should continue until the physician is assured that the patient is out of danger. Severe hypoglycemic reactions with coma, seizure, or other neurological impairment occur infrequently, but constitute medical emergencies requiring immediate hospitalization. If hypoglycemic coma is diagnosed or suspected, the patient should be given a rapid intravenous injection of concentrated (50%) glucose solution. This should be followed by a continuous infusion of a more dilute (10%) glucose solution at a rate which will maintain the blood glucose at a level above 100 mg/dL. Patients should be closely monitored for a minimum of 24 to 48 hours, since hypoglycemia may recur after apparent clinical recovery.

DOSAGE AND ADMINISTRATION

Patients should be retitrated when transferred from MICRONASE or Diabeta or other oral hypoglycemic agents.

There is no fixed dosage regimen for the management of diabetes mellitus with GLYNASE PresTab Tablets or any other hypoglycemic agent. In addition to the usual monitoring of urinary glucose, the patient's blood glucose must also be monitored periodically to determine the minimum effective dose for the patient; to detect primary failure, ie, inadequate lowering of blood glucose at the maximum recommended dose of medication; and to detect secondary failure, ie, loss of adequate blood glucose lowering response after an initial period of effectiveness. Glycosylated hemoglobin levels may also be of value in monitoring the patient's response to therapy.

Short-term administration of GLYNASE PresTab may be sufficient during periods of transient loss of control in patients usually controlled well on diet.

Usual Starting Dose

The suggested starting dose of GLYNASE PresTab is 1.5 to 3 mg daily, administered with breakfast or the first main meal. Those patients who may be more sensitive to hypoglycemic drugs should be started at 0.75 mg daily. (See PRECAUTIONS Section for patients at increased risk.) Failure to follow an appropriate dosage regimen may precipitate hypoglycemia. Patients who do not adhere to their prescribed dietary and drug regimen are more prone to exhibit unsatisfactory response to therapy.

Transfer From Other Hypoglycemic Therapy; Patients Receiving Other Oral Antidiabetic Therapy: Patients should be retitrated when transferred from MICRONASE or other

oral hypoglycemic agents. The initial daily dose should be 1.5 to 3 mg. When transferring patients from oral hypoglycemic agents other than chlorpropamide to GLYNASE PresTab, no transition period and no initial or priming dose are necessary. When transferring patients from chlorpropamide, particular care should be exercised during the first two weeks because the prolonged retention of chlorpropamide in the body and subsequent overlapping drug effects may provoke hypoglycemia.

Patients Receiving Insulin: Some Type II diabetic patients being treated with insulin may respond satisfactorily to GLYNASE PresTab. If the insulin dose is less than 20 units daily, substitution of GLYNASE PresTab 1.5 to 3 mg as a single daily dose may be tried. If the insulin dose is between 20 and 40 units daily, the patient may be placed directly on GLYNASE PresTab Tablets 3 mg daily as a single dose. If the insulin dose is more than 40 units daily, a transition period is required for conversion to GLYNASE PresTab. In these patients, insulin dosage is decreased by 50% and GLYNASE PresTab Tablets 3 mg daily is started. Please refer to Titration to Maintenance Dose for further explanation.

Titration to Maintenance Dose

The usual maintenance dose is in the range of 0.75 to 12 mg daily, which may be given as a single dose or in divided doses (See Dosage Interval Section). Dosage increases should be made in increments of no more than 1.5 mg at weekly intervals based upon the patient's blood glucose response.

No exact dosage relationship exists between GLYNASE PresTab and the other oral hypoglycemic agents, including MICRONASE or Diabeta. Although patients may be transferred from the maximum dose of other sulfonylureas, the maximum starting dose of 3 mg of GLYNASE PresTab Tablets should be observed. A maintenance dose of 3 mg of GLYNASE PresTab Tablets provides approximately the same degree of blood glucose control as 250 to 375 mg chlorpropamide, 250 to 375 mg tolazamide, 5 mg of glyburide (nonmicronized tablets), 500 to 750 mg acetohexamide, or 1000 to 1500 mg tolbutamide.

When transferring patients receiving more than 40 units of insulin daily, they may be started on a daily dose of GLYNASE PresTab Tablets 3 mg concomitantly with a 50% reduction in insulin dose. Progressive withdrawal of insulin and increase of GLYNASE PresTab in increments of 0.75 to 1.5 mg every 2 to 10 days is then carried out. During this conversion period when both insulin and GLYNASE PresTab are being used, hypoglycemia may rarely occur. During insulin withdrawal, patients should test their urine for glucose and acetone at least three times daily and report results to their physician. The appearance of persistent acetonuria with glycosuria indicates that the patient is a Type I diabetic who requires insulin therapy.

Maximum Dose

Daily doses of more than 12 mg are not recommended.

Dosage Interval

Once-a-day therapy is usually satisfactory. Some patients, particularly those receiving more than 6 mg daily, may have a more satisfactory response with twice-a-day dosage.

Specific Patient Populations

GLYNASE PresTab Tablets are not recommended for use in pregnancy or for use in children.

In elderly patients, debilitated or malnourished patients, and patients with impaired renal or hepatic function, the initial and maintenance dosing should be conservative to avoid hypoglycemic reactions. (See PRECAUTIONS Section.)

HOW SUPPLIED

GLYNASE PresTab Tablets are supplied as follows:

GLYNASE PresTab Tablets 1.5 mg

(white, ovoid, imprinted GLYNASE 1.5/PT Score PT, contour, scored)

Plastic Bottles of 100	NDC 0009-0341-01
Unit Dose Package of 100	NDC 0009-0341-02

GLYNASE PresTab Tablets 3 mg

(blue, ovoid, imprinted GLYNASE 3/PT Score PT, contour, scored)

Plastic Bottles of 100	NDC 0009-0352-01
Plastic Bottles of 500	NDC 0009-0352-03
Plastic Bottles of 1000	NDC 0009-0352-04
Unit Dose Package of 100	NDC 0009-0352-02

GLYNASE PresTab Tablets 6 mg

(yellow, ovoid, imprinted GLYNASE 6/PT Score PT, contour, scored)

Plastic Bottles of 100	NDC 0009-3449-01
Plastic Bottles of 500	NDC 0009-3449-03

The PresTab Tablet can be easily divided in half for a more flexible dosing regimen. Press gently on the score and the PresTab Tablet will split in even halves.

Caution: Federal law prohibits dispensing without prescription. Store at controlled room temperature 15° to 30° C (59° to 86° F). Dispensed in well closed containers with safety closures. Keep container tightly closed.

GLYNASE is a trademark of The Upjohn Company
PresTab is a trademark of The Upjohn Company
Diabeta is a trademark of
Hoechst-Roussel Pharmaceuticals, Inc.
Revised March 1996 814 930 007
691015

HALCION® Ⓒ℞

brand of triazolam tablets, USP

DESCRIPTION

HALCION Tablets contain triazolam, a triazolobenzodiazepine hypnotic agent.

Triazolam is a white crystalline powder, soluble in alcohol and poorly soluble in water. It has a molecular weight of 343.21.

The chemical name for triazolam is 8-chloro-6-(o-chlorophenyl)-1-methyl-4H-s-triazolo-[4,3-α][1,4] benzodiazepine.

The structural formula is represented below:

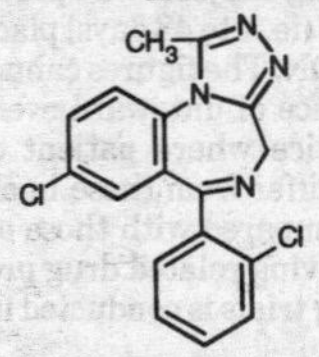

Each HALCION Tablet, for oral administration, contains 0.125 mg or 0.25 mg of triazolam. Inactive ingredients: **0.125 mg**-cellulose, corn starch, docusate sodium, lactose, magnesium stearate, silicon dioxide, sodium benzoate; **0.25 mg**-cellulose, corn starch, docusate sodium, FD&C Blue No. 2, lactose, magnesium stearate, silicon dioxide, sodium benzoate.

CLINICAL PHARMACOLOGY

Triazolam is a hypnotic with a short mean plasma half-life reported to be in the range of 1.5 to 5.5 hours. In normal subjects treated for 7 days with four times the recommended dosage, there was no evidence of altered systemic bioavailability, rate of elimination, or accumulation. Peak plasma levels are reached within 2 hours following oral administration. Following recommended doses of HALCION, triazolam peak plasma levels in the range of 1 to 6 ng/mL are seen. The plasma levels achieved are proportional to the dose given.

Triazolam and its metabolites, principally as conjugated glucuronides, which are presumably inactive, are excreted primarily in the urine. Only small amounts of unmetabolized triazolam appear in the urine. The two primary metabolites accounted for 79.9% of urinary excretion. Urinary excretion appeared to be biphasic in its time course.

HALCION Tablets 0.5 mg, in two separate studies, did not affect the prothrombin times or plasma warfarin levels in male volunteers administered sodium warfarin orally.

Extremely high concentrations of triazolam do not displace bilirubin bound to human serum albumin *in vitro*.

Triazolam ^{14}C was administered orally to pregnant mice. Drug-related material appeared uniformly distributed in the fetus with ^{14}C concentrations approximately the same as in the brain of the mother.

In sleep laboratory studies, HALCION Tablets significantly decreased sleep latency, increased the duration of sleep, and decreased the number of nocturnal awakenings. After 2 weeks of consecutive nightly administration, the drug's effect on total wake time is decreased, and the values recorded in the last third of the night approach baseline levels. On the first and/or second night after drug discontinuance (first or second post-drug night), total time asleep, percentage of time spent sleeping, and rapidity of falling asleep frequently were significantly less than on baseline (predrug) nights. This effect is often called "rebound" insomnia.

The type and duration of hypnotic effects and the profile of unwanted effects during administration of benzodiazepine drugs may be influenced by the biologic half-life of administered drug and any active metabolites formed. When half-lives are long, the drug or metabolites may accumulate during periods of nightly administration and be associated with impairments of cognitive and motor performance during waking hours; the possibility of interaction with other psychoactive drugs or alcohol will be enhanced. In contrast, if half-lives are short, the drug and metabolites will be cleared before the next dose is ingested, and carry-over effects related to excessive sedation or CNS depression should be minimal or absent. However, during nightly use for an extended period pharmacodynamic tolerance or adaptation to some effects of benzodiazepine hypnotics may develop. If the drug has a short half-life of elimination, it is possible that a relative deficiency of the drug or its active metabolites (ie, in relationship to the receptor site) may occur at some point in the interval between each night's use. This sequence of events may account for two clinical findings reported to occur after several weeks of nightly use of rapidly eliminated benzodiazepine hypnotics: 1) increased wakefulness during the last third of the night and 2) the appearance of increased daytime anxiety after 10 days of continuous treatment.

INDICATIONS AND USAGE

HALCION is indicated for the short-term treatment of insomnia (generally 7-10 days). Use for more than 2-3 weeks requires complete reevaluation of the patient (see WARNINGS).

Prescriptions for HALCION should be written for short-term use (7-10 days) and it should not be prescribed in quantities exceeding a 1-month supply.

CONTRAINDICATIONS

HALCION Tablets are contraindicated in patients with known hypersensitivity to this drug or other benzodiazepines.

Benzodiazepines may cause fetal damage when administered during pregnancy. An increased risk of congenital malformations associated with the use of diazepam and chlordiazepoxide during the first trimester of pregnancy has been suggested in several studies. Transplacental distribution has resulted in neonatal CNS depression following the ingestion of therapeutic doses of a benzodiazepine hypnotic during the last weeks of pregnancy.

HALCION is contraindicated in pregnant women. If there is a likelihood of the patient becoming pregnant while receiving HALCION, she should be warned of the potential risk to the fetus. Patients should be instructed to discontinue the drug prior to becoming pregnant. The possibility that a woman of childbearing potential may be pregnant at the time of institution of therapy should be considered.

WARNINGS

Sleep disturbance may be the presenting manifestation of a physical and/or psychiatric disorder. Consequently, a decision to initiate symptomatic treatment of insomnia should only be made after the patient has been carefully evaluated.

The failure of insomnia to remit after 7–10 days of treatment may indicate the presence of a primary psychiatric and/or medical illness.

Worsening of insomnia or the emergence of new abnormalities of thinking or behavior may be the consequence of an unrecognized psychiatric or physical disorder. These have also been reported to occur in association with the use of HALCION.

Because some of the adverse effects of HALCION appear to be dose related (see PRECAUTIONS and DOSAGE AND ADMINISTRATION), it is important to use the smallest possible effective dose. Elderly patients are especially susceptible to dose related adverse effects.

An increase in daytime anxiety has been reported for HALCION after as few as 10 days of continuous use. In some patients this may be a manifestation of interdose withdrawal (see CLINICAL PHARMACOLOGY). If increased daytime anxiety is observed during treatment, discontinuation of treatment may be advisable.

A variety of abnormal thinking and behavior changes have been reported to occur in association with the use of benzodiazepine hypnotics including HALCION. Some of these changes may be characterized by decreased inhibition, eg, aggressiveness and extroversion that seem excessive, similar to that seen with alcohol and other CNS depressants (eg, sedative/hypnotics). Other kinds of behavioral changes have also been reported, for example, bizarre behavior, agitation, hallucinations, depersonalization. In primarily depressed patients, the worsening of depression, including suicidal thinking, has been reported in association with the use of benzodiazepines.

It can rarely be determined with certainty whether a particular instance of the abnormal behaviors listed above is drug induced, spontaneous in origin, or a result of an underlying psychiatric or physical disorder. Nonetheless, the emergence of any new behavioral sign or symptom of concern requires careful and immediate evaluation.

Because of its depressant CNS effects, patients receiving triazolam should be cautioned against engaging in hazardous occupations requiring complete mental alertness such as operating machinery or driving a motor vehicle. For the same reason, patients should be cautioned about the concomitant ingestion of alcohol and other CNS depressant drugs during treatment with HALCION Tablets.

As with some, but not all benzodiazepines, anterograde amnesia of varying severity and paradoxical reactions have been reported following therapeutic doses of HALCION. Data from several sources suggest that anterograde amnesia may occur at a higher rate with HALCION than with other benzodiazepine hypnotics.

Continued on next page

Information on these Pharmacia & Upjohn products is based on labeling in effect June 1, 1996. Further information concerning these and other Pharmacia & Upjohn products may be obtained by direct inquiry to Medical Information, Pharmacia & Upjohn, Kalamazoo, MI 49001.

Pharmacia & Upjohn—Cont.

PRECAUTIONS

General: In elderly and/or debilitated patients it is recommended that treatment with HALCION Tablets be initiated at 0.125 mg to decrease the possibility of development of oversedation, dizziness, or impaired coordination.

Some side effects reported in association with the use of HALCION appear to be dose related. These include drowsiness, dizziness, light-headedness, and amnesia.

The relationship between dose and what may be more serious behavioral phenomena is less certain. Specifically, some evidence, based on spontaneous marketing reports, suggests that confusion, bizarre or abnormal behavior, agitation, and hallucinations may also be dose related, but this evidence is inconclusive. In accordance with good medical practice it is recommended that therapy be initiated at the lowest effective dose (see DOSAGE AND ADMINISTRATION).

Cases of "traveler's amnesia" have been reported by individuals who have taken HALCION to induce sleep while traveling, such as during an airplane flight. In some of these cases, insufficient time was allowed for the sleep period prior to awakening and before beginning activity. Also, the concomitant use of alcohol may have been a factor in some cases.

Caution should be exercised if HALCION is prescribed to patients with signs or symptoms of depression that could be intensified by hypnotic drugs. Suicidal tendencies may be present in such patients and protective measures may be required. Intentional overdosage is more common in these patients, and the least amount of drug that is feasible should be available to the patient at any one time.

The usual precautions should be observed in patients with impaired renal or hepatic function, chronic pulmonary insufficiency, and sleep apnea. In patients with compromised respiratory function, respiratory depression and apnea have been reported infrequently.

Information for patients: The text of a patient package insert is printed at the end of this insert. To assure safe and effective use of HALCION, the information and instructions provided in this patient package insert should be discussed with patients.

Laboratory tests: Laboratory tests are not ordinarily required in otherwise healthy patients.

Drug interactions: Both pharmacodynamic and pharmacokinetic interactions have been reported with benzodiazepines. In particular, triazolam produces additive CNS depressant effects when co-administered with other psychotropic medications, anticonvulsants, antihistamines, ethanol, and other drugs which themselves produce CNS depression.

Pharmacokinetic interactions can occur when triazolam is administered along with drugs that interfere with its metabolism. Specific examples, documented with evidence from controlled trials, show that the co-administration of either cimetidine or erythromycin with triazolam causes an approximate doubling of the elimination half-life and plasma levels of triazolam. Consequently, consideration of dose reduction may be appropriate in patients treated concomitantly with either cimetidine or erythromycin and triazolam.

Carcinogenesis, mutagenesis, impairment of fertility: No evidence of carcinogenic potential was observed in mice during a 24-month study with HALCION in doses up to 4,000 times the human dose.

Pregnancy:

1. Teratogenic effects: Pregnancy category X (see CONTRAINDICATIONS).

2. Non-teratogenic effects: It is to be considered that the child born of a mother who is on benzodiazepines may be at some risk for withdrawal symptoms from the drug, during the postnatal period. Also, neonatal flaccidity has been reported in an infant born of a mother who had been receiving benzodiazepines.

Nursing mothers: Human studies have not been performed; however, studies in rats have indicated that HALCION and its metabolites are secreted in milk. Therefore, administration of HALCION to nursing mothers is not recommended.

Pediatric use: Safety and efficacy of HALCION in children below the age of 18 have not been established.

ADVERSE REACTIONS

During placebo-controlled clinical studies in which 1,003 patients received HALCION Tablets, the most troublesome side effects were extensions of the pharmacologic activity of triazolam, eg, drowsiness, dizziness, or light-headedness.

The figures cited below are estimates of untoward clinical event incidence among subjects who participated in the relatively short duration (ie, 1 to 42 days) placebo-controlled clinical trials of HALCION. The figures cannot be used to predict precisely the incidence of untoward events in the course of usual medical practice where patient characteristics and other factors often differ from those in clinical trials. These figures cannot be compared with those obtained from other clinical studies involving related drug products and placebo, as each group of drug trials is conducted under a different set of conditions.

Comparison of the cited figures, however, can provide the prescriber with some basis for estimating the relative contributions of drug and nondrug factors to the untoward event incidence rate in the population studied. Even this use must be approached cautiously, as a drug may relieve a symptom in one patient while inducing it in others. (For example, an anticholinergic, anxiolytic drug may relieve dry mouth [a sign of anxiety] in some subjects but induce it [an untoward event] in others.)

	HALCION	PLACEBO
Number of Patients	1003	997
% Patients Reporting		
Central Nervous System		
Drowsiness	14.0	6.4
Headache	9.7	8.4
Dizziness	7.8	3.1
Nervousness	5.2	4.5
Light-headedness	4.9	0.9
Coordination disorders/ataxia	4.6	0.8
Gastrointestinal		
Nausea/vomiting	4.6	3.7

In addition to the relatively common (ie, 1% or greater) untoward events enumerated above, the following adverse events have been reported less frequently (ie, 0.9% to 0.5%): euphoria, tachycardia, tiredness, confusional states/memory impairment, cramps/pain, depression, visual disturbances.

Rare (ie, less than 0.5%) adverse reactions included constipation, taste alterations, diarrhea, dry mouth, dermatitis/allergy, dreaming/nightmares, insomnia, paresthesia, tinnitus, dysesthesia, weakness, congestion, death from hepatic failure in a patient also receiving diuretic drugs.

In addition to these untoward events for which estimates of incidence are available, the following adverse events have been reported in association with the use of HALCION and other benzodiazepines: amnestic symptoms (anterograde amnesia with appropriate or inappropriate behavior), confusional states (disorientation, derealization, depersonalization, and/or clouding of consciousness), dystonia, anorexia, fatigue, sedation, slurred speech, jaundice, pruritus, dysarthria, changes in libido, menstrual irregularities, incontinence, and urinary retention. Other factors may contribute to some of these reactions, eg, concomitant intake of alcohol or other drugs, sleep deprivation, an abnormal premorbid state, etc.

Other events reported include: paradoxical reactions such as stimulation, mania, an agitational state (restlessness, irritability, and excitation), increased muscle spasticity, sleep disturbances, hallucinations, delusions, aggressiveness, falling, somnambulism, syncope, inappropriate behavior and other adverse behavioral effects. Should these occur, use of the drug should be discontinued.

The following events have also been reported: chest pain, burning tongue/glossitis/stomatitis.

Laboratory analyses were performed on all patients participating in the clinical program for HALCION. The following incidences of abnormalities were observed in patients receiving HALCION and the corresponding placebo group. None of these changes were considered to be of physiological significance.

[See table on bottom of page.]

When treatment with HALCION is protracted, periodic blood counts, urinalysis, and blood chemistry analyses are advisable.

Minor changes in EEG patterns, usually low-voltage fast activity, have been observed in patients during therapy with HALCION and are of no known significance.

DRUG ABUSE AND DEPENDENCE

Controlled Substance: Triazolam is a controlled substance under the Controlled Substance Act, and HALCION Tablets have been assigned to Schedule IV.

Abuse, Dependence and Withdrawal: Withdrawal symptoms, similar in character to those noted with barbiturates and alcohol (convulsions, tremor, abdominal and muscle cramps, vomiting, sweating, dysphoria, perceptual disturbances and insomnia), have occurred following abrupt discontinuance of benzodiazepines, including HALCION. The more severe symptoms are usually associated with higher dosages and longer usage, although patients at therapeutic dosages given for as few as 1-2 weeks can also have withdrawal symptoms and in some patients there may be withdrawal symptoms (daytime anxiety, agitation) between nightly doses (see CLINICAL PHARMACOLOGY). Consequently, abrupt discontinuation should be avoided and a gradual dosage tapering schedule is recommended in any patient taking more than the lowest dose for more than a few weeks. The recommendation for tapering is particularly important in any patient with a history of seizure.

The risk of dependence is increased in patients with a history of alcoholism, drug abuse, or in patients with marked personality disorders. Such dependence-prone individuals should be under careful surveillance when receiving HALCION. As with all hypnotics, repeat prescriptions should be limited to those who are under medical supervision.

OVERDOSAGE

Because of the potency of triazolam, some manifestations of overdosage may occur at 2 mg, four times the maximum recommended therapeutic dose (0.5 mg).

Manifestations of overdosage with HALCION Tablets include somnolence, confusion, impaired coordination, slurred speech, and ultimately, coma. Respiratory depression and apnea have been reported with overdosages of HALCION. Seizures have occasionally been reported after overdosages.

Death has been reported in association with overdoses of triazolam by itself, as it has with other benzodiazepines. In addition, fatalities have been reported in patients who have overdosed with a combination of a single benzodiazepine, including triazolam, and alcohol; benzodiazepine and alcohol levels seen in some of these cases have been lower than those usually associated with reports of fatality with either substance alone.

As in all cases of drug overdosage, respiration, pulse, and blood pressure should be monitored and supported by general measures when necessary. Immediate gastric lavage should be performed. An adequate airway should be maintained. Intravenous fluids may be administered.

Flumazenil, a specific benzodiazepine receptor antagonist, is indicated for the complete or partial reversal of the sedative effects of benzodiazepines and may be used in situations when an overdose with a benzodiazepine is known or suspected. Prior to the administration of flumazenil, necessary measures should be instituted to secure airway, ventilation and intravenous access. Flumazenil is intended as an adjunct to, not as a substitute for, proper management of benzodiazepine overdose. Patients treated with flumazenil should be monitored for re-sedation, respiratory depression, and other residual benzodiazepine effects for an appropriate period after treatment. The prescriber should be aware of a risk of seizure in association with flumazenil treatment, particularly in long-term benzodiazepine users and in cyclic antidepressant overdose. The complete flumazenil package insert including CONTRAINDICATIONS, WARNINGS and PRECAUTIONS should be consulted prior to use.

	HALCION		PLACEBO	
Number of Patients	380		361	
% of Patients Reporting:	Low	High	Low	High
Hematology				
Hematocrit	*	*	*	*
Hemoglobin	*	*	*	*
Total WBC count	1.7	2.1	*	1.3
Neutrophil count	1.5	1.5	3.3	1.0
Lymphocyte count	2.3	4.0	3.1	3.8
Monocyte count	3.6	*	4.4	1.5
Eosinophil count	10.2	3.2	9.8	3.4
Basophil count	1.7	2.1	*	1.8
Urinalysis				
Albumin	—	1.1	—	*
Sugar	—	*	—	*
RBC/HPF	—	2.9	—	2.9
WBC/HPF	—	11.7	—	7.9
Blood chemistry				
Creatinine	2.4	1.9	3.6	1.5
Bilirubin	*	1.5	1.0	*
SGOT	*	5.3	*	4.5
Alkaline phosphatase	*	2.2	*	2.6

*Less than 1%

Experiments in animals have indicated that cardiopulmonary collapse can occur with massive intravenous doses of triazolam. This could be reversed with posi tive mechanical respiration and the intravenous infusion of norepinephrine bitartrate or metaraminol bitartrate. Hemodialysis and forced diuresis are probably of little value. As with the management of intentional overdosage with any drug, the physician should bear in mind that multiple agents may have been ingested by the patient.

The oral LD_{50} in mice is greater than 1,000 mg/kg and in rats is greater than 5,000 mg/kg.

DOSAGE AND ADMINISTRATION

It is important to individualize the dosage of HALCION Tablets for maximum beneficial effect and to help avoid significant adverse effects.

The recommended dose for most adults is 0.25 mg before retiring. A dose of 0.125 mg may be found to be sufficient for some patients (eg, low body weight). A dose of 0.5 mg should be used only for exceptional patients who do not respond adequately to a trial of a lower dose since the risk of several adverse reactions increases with the size of the dose administered. A dose of 0.5 mg should not be exceeded.

In geriatric and/or debilitated patients the recommended dosage range is 0.125 mg to 0.25 mg. Therapy should be initiated at 0.125 mg in this group and the 0.25 mg dose should be used only for exceptional patients who do not respond to a trial of the lower dose. A dose of 0.25 mg should not be exceeded in these patients.

As with all medications, the lowest effective dose should be used.

HOW SUPPLIED

HALCION Tablets are available in the following strengths and package sizes:

0.125 mg (white, elliptical, imprinted HALCION 0.125):

Unit of Use (10's) Reverse numbered	NDC 0009-0010-06
Unit Dose (100)	NDC 0009-0010-32
Bottles of 10	NDC 0009-0010-37
Bottles of 500	NDC 0009-0010-11

0.25 mg (powder blue, elliptical, scored, imprinted HALCION 0.25):

Unit of Use (10's) Reverse numbered	NDC 0009-0017-11
Unit Dose (100)	NDC 0009-0017-55
Bottles of 10	NDC 0009-0017-58
Bottles of 500	NDC 0009-0017-02

Store at controlled room temperature 15° to 30° C (59° to 86° F).

Caution: Federal law prohibits dispensing without prescription.

US Patent No. 3,987,052

The text of the patient insert for HALCION is set forth below.

PATIENT INFORMATION

INTRODUCTION

HALCION is intended to help you sleep. It is one of several benzodiazepine sleeping pills that have generally similar properties. Anyone who is considering using one of these medications should be aware of both their benefits and several important risks and limitations, including diminishing effectiveness with continued use and the possible development of dependence (addiction) and possibly mental changes particularly when the drugs are used for more than a few days to a week. This patient information statement is intended to provide you with knowledge about this class of medications in general and about HALCION in particular that will be useful to guide you in the safe use of this product, BUT IT SHOULD NOT REPLACE A DISCUSSION BETWEEN YOU AND YOUR PHYSICIAN ABOUT THE RISKS AND BENEFITS OF HALCION.

This leaflet will focus on the beneficial and adverse effects of all members of this class of medications, as well as some specific information about HALCION. There are some differences among these products, and your physician may wish to discuss any specific advantages and disadvantages of particular members of this drug class with you.

EFFECTIVENESS OF BENZODIAZEPINE SLEEPING PILLS

Benzodiazepine sleeping pills are effective medications and are relatively free of serious problems when they are used for short-term management of sleep problems (insomnia). Insomnia is not always the same. It may be reflected in difficulty in falling asleep, frequent awakening during the night, and/or early morning awakening. Insomnia is often transient in nature, responding to brief treatment with sleeping pills. Use for more than a short while requires discussion with your physician about the risks and benefits of prolonged use.

SIDE EFFECTS

Common Side Effects

The most common side effects of benzodiazepine sleeping pills are related to the ability of the medications to make you sleepy; drowsiness, dizziness, lightheadedness, and difficulty with coordination. Users must be cautious about engaging in hazardous activities requiring complete mental alertness, eg, operating machinery or driving a motor vehicle. Do not take alcohol while using HALCION. Benzodiazepine sleeping pills should not be used with other medications or substances that may cause drowsiness, without discussing said use with your physician.

How sleepy you are the day after you use one of these sleep medications depends on your individual response and on how quickly the product is eliminated from your body. The larger the dose, the more likely an individual will experience next day residual effects such as drowsiness. For this reason, it is important to use the lowest effective dose for each individual patient. Benzodiazepines that are eliminated rapidly, eg, HALCION, tend to cause less next day drowsiness but may cause more withdrawal problems the day after use (see below).

Special Concerns

Memory Problems

All benzodiazepine sleeping pills can cause a special type of amnesia (memory loss) in which a person may not recall events occurring during some period of time, usually several hours, after taking a drug. This is ordinarily not a problem, because the person taking a sleeping pill intends to be asleep during this vulnerable period of time. It can be a problem when the drugs are taken to induce sleep while traveling, such as during an airplane flight, because the person may awake before the effect of the drug is gone. This has been called "traveler's amnesia". HALCION is more likely than other members of the class to cause this problem.

Tolerance/Withdrawal Phenomena

Some loss of effectiveness or adaptation to the sleep inducing effects of these medications may develop after nightly use for more than a few weeks and there may be a degree of dependence that develops. For the benzodiazepine sleeping pills that are eliminated quickly from the body, a relative deficiency of the drug may occur at some point in the interval between each night's use. This can lead to (1) increased wakefulness during the last third of the night, and (2) the appearance of increased signs of daytime anxiety or nervousness. These two events have been reported in particular for HALCION.

There can be more severe 'withdrawal' effects when a benzodiazepine sleeping pill is stopped. Such effects can occur after discontinuing these drugs following use for only a week or two, but may be more common and more severe after longer periods of continuous use. One type of withdrawal phenomenon is the occurrence of what is known as 'rebound insomnia'. That is, on the first few nights after the drug is stopped, insomnia is actually worse than before the sleeping pill was given. Other withdrawal phenomena following abrupt stopping of benzodiazepine sleeping pills range from mild unpleasant feelings to a major withdrawal syndrome which may include abdominal and muscle cramps, vomiting, sweating, tremor, and rarely, convulsions. These more severe withdrawal phenomena are uncommon.

Dependence/Abuse Phenomena

All benzodiazepine sleeping pills can cause dependence (addiction), especially when used regularly for more than a few weeks or at higher doses. Some people develop a need to continue taking these drugs, either at the prescribed dose or at increasing doses, not so much for continued therapeutic effect, but rather, to avoid withdrawal phenomena and/or to achieve nontherapeutic effects. Individuals who have been dependent on alcohol or other drugs may be at particular risk of becoming dependent on drugs in this class, but all people appear to be at some risk. This possibility must be considered before extending the use of these drugs for more than a few weeks.

Mental and Behavioral Changes

A variety of abnormal thinking and behavior changes have been reported to occur in association with the use of benzodiazepine sleeping pills. Some of these changes are like the release of inhibition seen in association with alcohol, eg, aggressiveness and extroversion that seem out of character. Others, however, can be more unusual and more extreme, such as confusion, bizarre behavior, agitation, hallucinations, depersonalization, and worsening of depression, including suicidal thinking. It is rarely clear whether such events are induced by the drug being taken, are caused by some underlying illness or are simply spontaneous happenings. In fact, worsened insomnia may in some cases be associated with illnesses that were present before the medication was used. In any event, the most important fact is to understand that regardless of the cause, users of these medications should promptly report any mental or behavioral changes to their doctor.

Effects on Pregnancy

Certain benzodiazepines have been linked to birth defects when administered during the early months of pregnancy. In addition, the administration of benzodiazepines during the last weeks of pregnancy has been associated with sedation of the fetus. Consequently, the use of this drug should be avoided at any time during pregnancy.

SAFE USE OF BENZODIAZEPINE SLEEPING PILLS

To assure the safe and effective use of HALCION, you should adhere to the following cautions:

1. HALCION is a prescription medication and, therefore, should be used only as directed by your doctor. Follow your doctor's advice about how to take it, when to take it, and how long to take it. As with other prescription medication, HALCION should be taken only by the individual for whom it is prescribed.
2. Do not extend your use of HALCION beyond 7-10 days without first consulting your physician.
3. If you develop any unusual and disturbing thoughts or behavior during treatment with HALCION, you should discuss such problems with your physician.
4. Inform your physician about any alcohol consumption and medicine you are taking now, including drugs you may buy without a prescription. Do not use alcohol while taking HALCION.
5. Do not take HALCION in circumstances where a full night's sleep and elimination of the drug from the body are not possible before you would again need to be active and functional, eg, an overnight flight of less than 7-8 hours, because amnestic episodes have been reported in such situations.
6. Do not increase the prescribed dose except on the advice of your physician.
7. Until you experience how this medication affects you, do not drive a car or operate potentially dangerous machinery, etc.
8. Be aware that you may experience an increase in sleep difficulties (rebound insomnia) on the first night or two after discontinuing HALCION.
9. Inform your physician if you are planning to become pregnant, if you are pregnant, or if you become pregnant while you are taking this medicine. The use of HALCION should be avoided at any time during pregnancy.

Revised July 1993 812 110 525
691157

Shown in Product Identification Guide, page 329

HALOTESTIN® Ⓒ℞

brand of fluoxymesterone tablets, USP

DESCRIPTION

HALOTESTIN Tablets contain fluoxymesterone, an androgenic hormone.

Fluoxymesterone is a white or nearly white, odorless, crystalline powder, melting at or about 240° C, with some decomposition. It is practically insoluble in water, sparingly soluble in alcohol, and slightly soluble in chloroform.

The chemical name for fluoxymesterone is androst-4-en-3-one, 9-fluoro-11,17-dihydroxy-17-methyl-, (11β,17β)-. The molecular formula is $C_{20}H_{29}FO_3$ and the molecular weight 336.45.

The structural formula is represented below:

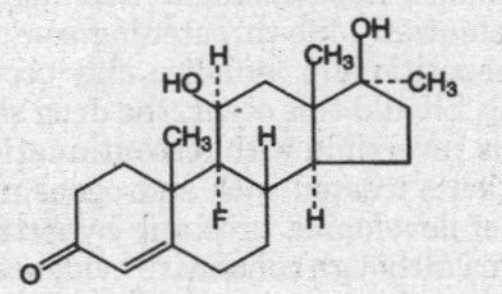

Each HALOTESTIN tablet, for oral administration, contains 2 mg, 5 mg or 10 mg fluoxymesterone. Inactive ingredients: calcium stearate, corn starch, FD&C Yellow no. 5, lactose, sorbic acid, sucrose, tragacanth. In addition, the **2 mg** tablet contains FD&C Yellow No. 6 and the **5 mg** and **10 mg** contain FD&C Blue No. 2.

CLINICAL PHARMACOLOGY

Endogenous androgens are responsible for normal growth and development of the male sex organs and for maintenance of secondary sex characteristics. These effects include growth and maturation of the prostate, seminal vesicles, penis, and scrotum; development of male hair distribution, such as beard, pubic, chest, and axillary hair; laryngeal enlargement, vocal cord thickening, and alterations in body musculature and fat distribution. Drugs in this class also cause retention of nitrogen, sodium, potassium, and phosphorus, and decreased urinary excretion of calcium. Androgens have been reported to increase protein anabolism and decrease protein catabolism. Nitrogen balance is improved only when there is sufficient intake of calories and protein.

Continued on next page

Information on these Pharmacia & Upjohn products is based on labeling in effect June 1, 1996. Further information concerning these and other Pharmacia & Upjohn products may be obtained by direct inquiry to Medical Information, Pharmacia & Upjohn, Kalamazoo, MI 49001.

Pharmacia & Upjohn—Cont.

Androgens are responsible for the growth spurt of adolescence and for eventual termination of linear growth, brought about by fusion of the epiphyseal growth centers. In children, exogenous androgens accelerate linear growth rates, but may cause disproportionate advancement in bone maturation. Use over long periods may result in fusion of the epiphyseal growth centers and termination of the growth process. Androgens have been reported to stimulate production of red blood cells by enhancing production of erythropoietic stimulation factor.
During exogenous administration of androgens, endogenous testosterone release is inhibited through feedback inhibition of pituitary luteinizing hormone (LH). At large doses of exogenous androgens, spermatogenesis may also be suppressed through feedback inhibition of pituitary follicle stimulating hormone (FSH).
Inactivation of testosterone occurs primarily in the liver.
The half-life of fluoxymesterone after oral administration is approximately 9.2 hours.

INDICATIONS AND USAGE

In the male—HALOTESTIN Tablets are indicated for:
1. Replacement therapy in conditions associated with symptoms of deficiency or absence of endogenous testosterone.
   a. Primary hypogonadism (congenital or acquired)—testicular failure due to cryptorchidism, bilateral torsion, orchitis, vanishing testis syndrome; or orchidectomy.
   b. Hypogonadotropic hypogonadism (congenital or acquired)—diopathic gonadotropin or LHRH deficiency, or pituitary-hypothalamic injury from tumors, trauma, or radiation.
2. Delayed puberty, provided it has been definitely established as such, and is not just a familial trait.

In the female—HALOTESTIN Tablets are indicated for palliation of androgen-responsive recurrent mammary cancer in women who are more than one year but less than five years postmenopausal, or who have been proven to have a hormone-dependent tumor as shown by previous beneficial response to castration.

CONTRAINDICATIONS

1. Known hypersensitivity to the drug
2. Males with carcinoma of the breast
3. Males with known or suspected carcinoma of the prostate gland
4. Women known or suspected to be pregnant
5. Patients with serious cardiac, hepatic or renal disease

WARNINGS

Hypercalcemia may occur in immobilized patients and in patients with breast cancer. If this occurs, the drug should be discontinued.
Prolonged use of high doses of androgens (principally the 17-α alkyl-androgens) has been associated with development of hepatic adenomas, hepatocellular carcinoma, and peliosis hepatis-all potentially life-threatening complications.
Cholestatic hepatitis and jaundice may occur with 17-α-alkyl-androgens. Should this occur, the drug should be discontinued. This is reversible with discontinuation of the drug.
Geriatric patients treated with androgens may be at an increased risk of developing prostatic hypertrophy and prostatic carcinoma although conclusive evidence to support this concept is lacking.
Edema, with or without congestive heart failure, may be a serious complication in patients with pre-existing cardiac, renal or hepatic disease.
Gynecomastia may develop and occasionally persists in patients being treated for hypogonadism.
Androgen therapy should be used cautiously in males with delayed puberty. Androgens can accelerate bone maturation without producing compensatory gain in linear growth. The effect on bone maturation should be monitored by assessing bone age of the wrist and hand every six months.
This drug has not been shown to be safe and effective for the enhancement of athletic performance. Because of the potential risk of serious adverse health effects, this drug should not be used for such purpose.

PRECAUTIONS

General
Women should be observed for signs of virilization which is usual following androgen use at high doses. Discontinuation of drug therapy at the time of evidence of mild virilism is necessary to prevent irreversible virilization. A decision may be made by the patient and the physician that some virilization will be tolerated during treatment for breast carcinoma.
Patients with benign prostatic hypertrophy may develop acute urethral obstruction. Priapism or excessive sexual stimulation may develop. Oligospermia may occur after prolonged administration or excessive dosage. If any of these effects appear, the androgen should be stopped and if restarted, a lower dosage should be utilized.
This product contains FD&C Yellow No. 5 (tartrazine) which may cause allergic-type reactions (including bronchial asthma) in certain susceptible individuals. Although the overall incidence of FD&C Yellow No. 5 (tartrazine) sensitivity in the general population is low, it is frequently seen in patients who also have aspirin hypersensitivity.

Information for patients
Patients should be instructed to report any of the following: nausea, vomiting, changes in skin color, and ankle swelling.
Males should be instructed to report too frequent or persistent erections of the penis and females any hoarseness, acne, changes in menstrual periods or increase in facial hair.

Laboratory tests
Women with disseminated breast carcinoma should have frequent determination of urine and serum calcium levels during the course of androgen therapy (See WARNINGS).
Because of the hepatotoxicity associated with the use of 17-alpha-alkylated androgens, liver function tests should be obtained periodically.
Periodic (every six months) X-ray examinations of bone age should be made during treatment of prepubertal males to determine the rate of bone maturation and the effects of androgen therapy on the epiphyseal centers.
Hemoglobin and hematocrit levels (to detect polycythemia) should be checked periodically in patients receiving long-term androgen administration.
Serum cholesterol may increase during androgen therapy.

Drug interactions
Androgens may increase sensitivity to oral anticoagulants. Dosage of the anticoagulant may require reduction in order to maintain satisfactory therapeutic hypoprothrombinemia.
Concurrent administration of oxyphenbutazone and androgens may result in elevated serum levels of oxyphenbutazone.
In diabetic patients, the metabolic effects of androgens may decrease blood glucose and, therefore, insulin requirements.

Drug/Laboratory test interferences
Androgens may decrease levels of thyroxine-binding globulin, resulting in decreased total T4 serum levels and increased resin uptake of T3 and T4. Free thyroid hormone levels remain unchanged, however, and there is no clinical evidence of thyroid dysfunction.

Carcinogenesis, mutagenesis, impairment of fertility
Animal data: Testosterone has been tested by subcutaneous injection and implantation in mice and rats. The implant induced cervical-uterine tumors in mice, which metastasized in some cases. There is suggestive evidence that injection of testosterone into some strains of female mice increases their susceptibility to hepatoma. Testosterone is also known to increase the number of tumors and decrease the degree of differentiation of chemically-induced carcinomas of the liver in rats.
Human data: There are rare reports of hepatocellular carcinoma in patients receiving long-term therapy with androgens in high doses. Withdrawal of the drugs did not lead to regression of the tumors in all cases.
Geriatric patients treated with androgens may be at an increased risk of developing prostatic hypertrophy and prostatic carcinoma although conclusive evidence to support this concept is lacking.
This compound has not been tested for mutagenic potential. However, as noted above, carcinogenic effects have been attributed to treatment with androgenic hormones. The potential carcinogenic effects likely occur through a hormonal mechanism rather than by a direct chemical interaction mechanism.
Impairment of fertility was not tested directly in animal species. However, as noted below under Adverse Reactions, oligospermia in males and amenorrhea in females are potential adverse effects of treatment with HALOTESTIN Tablets. There fore, impairment of fertility is a possible outcome of treatment with HALOTESTIN.

Pregnancy
Teratogenic effects: Pregnancy Category X. (See CONTRAINDICATIONS.)

Nursing mothers
HALOTESTIN is not recommended for use in nursing mothers.

Pediatric use
Androgen therapy should be used very cautiously in children and only by specialists aware of the adverse effects on bone maturation. Skeletal maturation must be monitored every six months by an X-ray of the hand and wrist (See WARNINGS).

ADVERSE REACTIONS

Endocrine and urogenital
Female: the most common side effects of androgen therapy are amenorrhea and other menstrual irregularities; inhibition of gonadotropin secretion; and virilization, including deepening of the voice and clitoral enlargement. The latter usually is not reversible after androgens are discontinued. When administered to a pregnant woman, androgens can cause virilization of external genitalia of the female fetus.
Male: Gynecomastia, and excessive frequency and duration of penile erections. Oligospermia may occur at high dosage.
Skin and appendages
Hirsutism, male pattern of baldness, seborrhea, and acne.
Fluid and electrolyte disturbances
Retention of sodium, chloride, water, potassium, calcium, and inorganic phosphates.
Gastrointestinal
Nausea, cholestatic jaundice, alterations in liver function tests, rarely hepatocellular neoplasms and peliosis hepatis (See WARNINGS).
Hematologic
Suppression of clotting factors II, V, VII, and X, bleeding in patients on concomitant anticoagulant therapy, and polycythemia.
Nervous system
Increased or decreased libido, headache, anxiety, depression, and generalized paresthesia.
Allergic
Hypersensitivity, including skin manifestations and anaphylactoid reactions.

DRUG ABUSE AND DEPENDENCE

Controlled Substance Class: Fluoxymesterone is a controlled substance under the Anabolic Steroids Control Act, and HALOTESTIN Tablets has been assigned to Schedule III.

OVERDOSAGE

There have been no reports of acute overdosage with the androgens.

DOSAGE AND ADMINISTRATION

The dosage will vary depending upon the individual, the condition being treated, and its severity. The total daily oral dose may be administered singly or in divided (three or four) doses.
Male hypogonadism: For complete replacement in the hypogonadal male, a daily dose of 5 to 20 mg will suffice in the majority of patients. It is usually preferable to begin treatment with full therapeutic doses which are later adjusted to individual requirements. Priapism is indicative of excessive dosage and is indication for temporary withdrawal of the drug.
Delayed puberty: Dosage should be carefully titrated utilizing a low dose, appropriate skeletal monitoring, and by limiting the duration of therapy to four to six months.
Inoperable carcinoma of the breast in the female: The recommended total daily dose for palliative therapy in advanced inoperable carcinoma of the breast is 10 to 40 mg. Because of its short action, fluoxymesterone should be administered to patients in divided, rather than single, daily doses to ensure more stable blood levels. In general, it appears necessary to continue therapy for at least one month for a satisfactory subjective response, and for two to three months for an objective response.

HOW SUPPLIED

HALOTESTIN Tablets, round and scored, are available in the following strengths and colors:

2 mg (peach)	
Bottles of 100	NDC 0009-0014-01
5 mg (light green)	
Bottles of 100	NDC 0009-0019-06
10 mg (green)	
Bottles of 30	NDC 0009-0036-03
Bottles of 100	NDC 0009-0036-04

Store at controlled room temperature 15°-30° C (59°-86° F).
Caution: Federal law prohibits dispensing without prescription.
Revised June 1991 810 804 304
691015

Shown in Product Identification Guide, page 329

IDAMYCIN® ℞

[eye-dă-mī-sĭn]
(IDARUBICIN HYDROCHLORIDE FOR INJECTION, USP)
FOR INTRAVENOUS USE ONLY

WARNINGS

1. IDAMYCIN should be given slowly into a freely flowing intravenous infusion. It must never be given intramuscularly or subcutaneously. Severe local tissue necrosis can occur if there is extravasation during administration.
2. As is the case with other anthracyclines the use of IDAMYCIN can cause myocardial toxicity leading to congestive heart failure. Cardiac toxicity is more common in patients who have received prior anthracyclines or who have pre-existing cardiac disease.
3. As is usual with antileukemic agents, severe myelosuppression occurs when IDAMYCIN is used at effective therapeutic doses.
4. It is recommended that IDAMYCIN be administered only under the supervision of a physician who is expe-

rienced in leukemia chemotherapy and in facilities with laboratory and supportive resources adequate to monitor drug tolerance and protect and maintain a patient compromised by drug toxicity. The physician and institution must be capable of responding rapidly and completely to severe hemorrhagic conditions and/or overwhelming infection.

5. Dosage should be reduced in patients with impaired hepatic or renal function. (See DOSAGE AND ADMINISTRATION).

DESCRIPTION

IDAMYCIN® (Idarubicin Hydrochloride for Injection, USP) is a sterile, synthetic antineoplastic anthracycline for intravenous use. Chemically, idarubicin hydrochloride is 5, 12-Naphthacenedione, 9-acetyl-7-[(3-amino-2,3,6-trideoxy-α-L-*lyxo*-hexopyranosyl)oxy]-7,8,9,10-tetrahydro - 6,9,11 -trihydroxy-hydrochloride, (7S-*cis*). The structural formula is as follows:

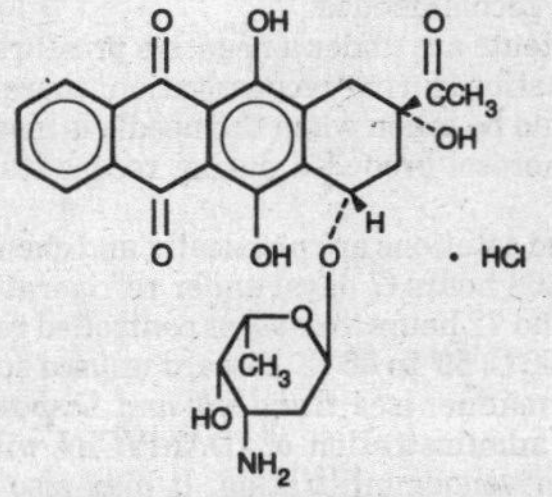

$C_{26}H_{27}NO_9 \cdot HCl$ M.W. 533.96

IDAMYCIN, a sterile parenteral, is available in 5 mg, 10 mg and 20 mg single use only vials.

Each 5 mg vial contains 5 mg Idarubicin Hydrochloride, USP and 50 mg of Lactose NF (hydrous) as an orange-red, lyophilized powder.

Each 10 mg vial contains 10 mg Idarubicin Hydrochloride, USP and 100 mg of Lactose NF (hydrous) as an orange-red, lyophilized powder.

Each 20 mg vial contains 20 mg Idarubicin Hydrochloride, USP and 200 mg of Lactose NF (hydrous) as an orange-red, lyophilized powder.

CLINICAL PHARMACOLOGY

IDAMYCIN is a DNA-intercalating analog of daunorubicin which has an inhibitory effect on nucleic acid synthesis and interacts with the enzyme topoisomerase II. The absence of a methoxy group at position 4 of the anthracycline structure gives the compound a high lipophilicity which results in an increased rate of cellular uptake compared with other anthracyclines.

Pharmacokinetic studies have been performed in adult leukemia patients with normal renal and hepatic function following intravenous administration of 10 to 12 mg/m² of IDAMYCIN daily for 3 to 4 days, as a single agent or combined with cytarabine (Ara-C). The plasma concentrations of IDAMYCIN are best described by a two or three compartment open model. The disposition profile shows a rapid distributive phase with a very high volume of distribution presumably reflecting extensive tissue binding. The plasma clearance is twice the expected hepatic plasma flow indicating extensive extrahepatic metabolism. The drug is eliminated predominately by biliary and to a lesser extent by renal excretion, mostly in the form of the primary metabolite, 13-dihydroidarubicin (idarubicinol).

The elimination rate of IDAMYCIN from plasma is slow with an estimated mean terminal half-life of 22 hours (range: 4 to 46 hours) when used as a single agent and 20 hours (range: 7 to 38 hours) when used in combination with cytarabine. The elimination of idarubicinol is considerably slower than that of the parent drug with an estimated mean terminal half-life that exceeds 45 hours; hence its plasma levels are sustained for a period greater than 8 days. As idarubicinol has cytotoxic activity it presumably contributes to the effects of IDAMYCIN.

The extent of drug and metabolite accumulation predicted in leukemia patients for Day 2 and 3 of dosing, based on the mean plasma levels and half-life obtained after the first dose, is 1.7- and 2.3-fold, respectively, and suggests no change in kinetics following a daily x 3 regimen.

The pharmacokinetics of IDAMYCIN have not been evaluated in leukemia patients with hepatic impairment. It is expected that in patients with moderate or severe hepatic dysfunction, the metabolism of IDAMYCIN may be impaired and lead to higher systemic drug levels.

Studies of cellular (nucleated blood and bone marrow cells) drug concentrations in leukemia patients have shown that peak cellular idarubicin concentrations are reached a few minutes after injection. Idarubicin and idarubicinol concentrations in nucleated blood and bone marrow cells are more than a hundred times the plasma concentrations. Idarubicin disappearance rates in plasma and cells were comparable with a terminal half-life of about 15 hours. The terminal half-life of idarubicinol in cells was about 72 hours.

Protein binding was studied *in vitro* by equilibrium dialysis at concentrations of idarubicin and idarubicinol similar to the maximum plasma level obtained in the pharmacokinetic studies. The percentages of idarubicin and idarubicinol bound to human plasma proteins averaged 97% and 94%, respectively. The binding is concentration independent.

IDAMYCIN studies in pediatric leukemia patients, at doses of 4.2 to 13.3 mg/m²/day x 3, suggest dose independent kinetics. There is no difference between the half-lives of the drug following daily x 3 or weekly x 3 administration.

Cerebrospinal fluid (CSF) levels of idarubicin and its active metabolite, idarubicinol, were measured in pediatric leukemia patients treated intravenously. Idarubicin was detected in 2 of 21 CSF samples (0.14 and 1.57 ng/mL), while idarubicinol was detected in 20 of these 21 CSF samples obtained 18 to 30 hours after dosing (mean = 0.51 ng/mL, range 0.22 to 1.05 ng/mL). The clinical relevance of these findings is currently being evaluated.

CLINICAL STUDIES

Four prospective randomized studies, three U.S. and one Italian, have been conducted to compare the efficacy and safety of idarubicin (IDR) to that of daunorubicin (DNR), each in combination with cytarabine (Ara-C) as induction therapy in previously untreated adult patients with acute myeloid leukemia (AML). These data are summarized in the following table and demonstrate significantly greater complete remission rates for the IDR regimen in two of the three U.S. studies and significantly longer overall survival for the IDR regimen in two of the three U.S. studies.

[See table above.]

	Induction[a] Regimen Dose in mg/m²-Daily × 3 Days		Complete Remission Rate, All Pts Randomized		Median Survival (Days) All Pts Randomized	
	IDR	DNR	IDR	DNR	IDR	DNR
U.S. (IND Studies)						
1. MSKCC* (Age ≤ 60 years)	12[b]	50[b]	51/65+ (78%)	38/65 (58%)	508+	435
2. SEG** (Age ≥ 15 years)	12[c]	45[c]	76/111+ (69%)	65/119 (55%)	328	277
3. U.S. Multicenter (Age ≥ 18 years)	13[c]	45[c]	68/101 (67%)	66/113 (58%)	393+	281
Foreign (non-IND study)						
GIMEMA*** (Age ≥ 55 years)	12[c]	45[c]	49/124 (40%)	49/125 (39%)	87	169

* Memorial Sloan Kettering Cancer Center
** Southeastern Cancer Study Group
*** Gruppo Italiano Malattie Ematologiche Maligne dell' Adulto
+ Overall $p < 0.05$, unadjusted for prognostic factors or multiple endpoints.
[a] Patients who had persistent leukemia after the first induction course received a second course.
[b] Ara-C 25 mg/m² bolus IV followed by 200 mg/m² daily × 5 days by continuous infusion.
[c] Ara-C 100 mg/m² daily × 7 days by continuous infusion.

There is no consensus regarding optional regimens to be used for consolidation; however, the following consolidation regimens were used in U.S. controlled trials. Patients received the same anthracycline for consolidation as was used for induction.

Studies 1 and 3 utilized 2 courses of consolidation therapy consisting of idarubicin 12 or 13 mg/m² daily for 2 days, respectively (or DNR 50 or 45 mg/m² daily for 2 days), and Ara-C, either 25 mg/m² by IV bolus followed by 200 mg/m² daily by continuous infusion for 4 days (Study 1), or 100 mg/m² daily for 5 days by continuous infusion (Study 3). A rest period of 4 to 6 weeks is recommended prior to initiation of consolidation and between the courses. Hematologic recovery is mandatory prior to initiation of each consolidation course.

Study 2 utilized 3 consolidation courses, administered at intervals of 21 days or upon hematologic recovery. Each course consisted of idarubicin 15 mg/m² IV for 1 dose (or DNR 50 mg/m² IV for 1 dose), Ara-C 100 mg/m² every 12 hours for 10 doses and 6-thioguanine 100 mg/m² po for 10 doses. If severe myelosuppression occurred, subsequent courses were given with 25% reduction in the doses of all drugs. In addition, this study included 4 courses of maintenance therapy (2 days of the same anthracycline as was used in induction and 5 days of Ara-C).

Toxicities and duration of aplasia were similar during induction on the 2 arms in the U.S. studies except for an increase in mucositis on the IDR arm in one study. During consolidation, duration of aplasia on the IDR arm was longer in all three studies and mucositis was more frequent in two studies. During consolidation, transfusion requirements were higher on the IDR arm in the two studies in which they were tabulated, and patients on the IDR arm in Study 3 spent more days on IV antibiotics (Study 3 used a higher dose of IDAMYCIN).

The benefit of consolidation and maintenance therapy in prolonging the duration of remission and survival is not proven.

Intensive maintenance with IDAMYCIN is not recommended in view of the considerable toxicity (including deaths in remission) experienced by patients during the maintenance phase of Study 2.

A higher induction death rate was noted in patients on the IDR arm in the Italian trial. Since this was not noted in patients of similar age in the U.S. trials, one may speculate that it was due to a difference in the level of supportive care.

INDICATIONS AND USAGE

IDAMYCIN in combination with other approved antileukemic drugs is indicated for the treatment of acute myeloid leukemia (AML) in adults. This includes French-American-British (FAB) classifications M1 through M7.

WARNINGS

IDAMYCIN is intended for administration under the supervision of a physician who is experienced in leukemia chemotherapy.

IDAMYCIN is a potent bone marrow suppressant. IDAMYCIN should not be given to patients with pre-existing bone marrow suppression induced by previous drug therapy or radiotherapy unless the benefit warrants the risk.

Severe myelosuppression will occur in all patients given a therapeutic dose of this agent for induction, consolidation or maintenance. Careful hematologic monitoring is required. Deaths due to infection and/or bleeding have been reported during the period of severe myelosuppression. Facilities with laboratory and supportive resources adequate to monitor drug tolerability and protect and maintain a patient compromised by drug toxicity should be available. It must be possible to treat rapidly and completely a severe hemorrhagic condition and/or a severe infection.

Pre-existing heart disease and previous therapy with anthracyclines at high cumulative doses or other potentially cardiotoxic agents are co-factors for increased risk of idarubicin-induced cardiac toxicity and the benefit to risk ratio of idarubicin therapy in such patients should be weighed before starting treatment with IDAMYCIN.

Myocardial toxicity as manifested by potentially fatal congestive heart failure, acute life-threatening arrhythmias or other cardiomyopathies may occur following therapy with IDAMYCIN. Appropriate therapeutic measures for the management of congestive heart failure and/or arrhythmias are indicated.

Cardiac function should be carefully monitored during treatment in order to minimize the risk of cardiac toxicity of the type described for other anthracycline compounds. The risk of such myocardial toxicity may be higher following concomitant or previous radiation to the mediastinal-pericardial area or in patients with anemia, bone marrow depression, infections, leukemic pericarditis and/or myocarditis. While there are no reliable means for predicting congestive heart failure, cardiomyopathy induced by anthracyclines is usually associated with a decrease of the left ventricular ejection fraction (LVEF) from pretreatment baseline values.

Since hepatic and/or renal function impairment can affect the disposition of IDAMYCIN, liver and kidney function should be evaluated with conventional clinical laboratory tests (using serum bilirubin and serum creatinine as indicators) prior to and during treatment. In a number of Phase III clinical trials, treatment was not given if bilirubin and/or creatinine serum levels exceeded 2 mg%. However, in one

Continued on next page

Information on these Pharmacia & Upjohn products is based on labeling in effect June 1, 1996. Further information concerning these and other Pharmacia & Upjohn products may be obtained by direct inquiry to Medical Information, Pharmacia & Upjohn, Kalamazoo, MI 49001.

Consult 1997 supplements and future editions for revisions

Pharmacia & Upjohn—Cont.

Phase III trial, patients with bilirubin levels between 2.6 and 5 mg% received the anthracycline with a 50% reduction in dose. Dose reduction of IDAMYCIN should be considered if the bilirubin and/or creatinine levels are above the normal range. (See DOSAGE AND ADMINISTRATION).

Pregnancy Category D - Idarubicin was embryotoxic and teratogenic in the rat at a dose of 1.2 mg/m^2/day or one tenth the human dose, which was nontoxic to dams. Idarubicin was embryotoxic but not teratogenic in the rabbit even at a dose of 2.4 mg/m^2/day or two tenths the human dose, which was toxic to dams. There is no conclusive information about idarubicin adversely affecting human fertility or causing teratogenesis.

There are no adequate and well-controlled studies in pregnant women. If IDAMYCIN is to be used during pregnancy, or if the patient becomes pregnant during therapy, the patient should be apprised of the potential hazard to the fetus. Women of childbearing potential should be advised to avoid pregnancy.

PRECAUTIONS

General

Therapy with IDAMYCIN requires close observation of the patient and careful laboratory monitoring. Hyperuricemia secondary to rapid lysis of leukemic cells may be induced. Appropriate measures must be taken to prevent hyperuricemia and to control any systemic infection before beginning therapy.

Extravasation of IDAMYCIN can cause severe local tissue necrosis. Extravasation may occur with or without an accompanying stinging or burning sensation even if blood returns well on aspiration of the infusion needle. If signs or symptoms of extravasation occur the injection or infusion should be terminated immediately and restarted in another vein. (See DOSAGE AND ADMINISTRATION).

Laboratory Tests

Frequent complete blood counts and monitoring of hepatic and renal function tests are recommended.

Carcinogenesis, Mutagenesis, Impairment of Fertility

Formal long-term carcinogenicity studies have not been conducted with IDAMYCIN. IDAMYCIN and related compounds have been shown to have mutagenic and carcinogenic properties when tested in experimental models (including bacterial systems, mammalian cells in culture and female Sprague-Dawley rats).

In male dogs given 1.8 mg/m^2 /day or more idarubicin (3 times/week for 13 weeks), testicular atrophy was observed with inhibition of spermiogenesis and sperm maturation, and few or no mature sperm. Effects were not readily reversible after an eight week recovery period.

Pregnancy Category D

(See WARNINGS).

Nursing Mothers

It is not known whether this drug is excreted in human milk. Because many drugs are excreted in human milk and because of the potential for serious adverse reactions in nursing infants from idarubicin, mothers should discontinue nursing prior to taking this drug.

Pediatric Use

Safety and effectiveness in children have not been established.

ADVERSE REACTIONS

Approximately 550 patients with AML have received IDAMYCIN in combination with Ara-C in controlled clinical trials worldwide. In addition, over 550 patients with acute leukemia have been treated in uncontrolled trials utilizing IDAMYCIN as a single agent or in combination. The table below lists the adverse experiences reported in U.S. Study 2 (see CLINICAL STUDIES) and is representative of the experiences in other studies. These adverse experiences constitute all reported or observed experiences, including those not considered to be drug related. Patients undergoing induction therapy for AML are seriously ill due to their disease, are receiving multiple transfusions, and concomitant medications including potentially toxic antibiotics and antifungal agents. The contribution of the study drug to the adverse experience profile is difficult to establish.

Induction Phase	Percentage of Patients	
	IDR	DNR
Adverse Experiences	(N=110)	(N=118)
Infection	95%	97%
Nausea & Vomiting	82%	80%
Hair Loss	77%	72%
Abdominal Cramps/ Diarrhea	73%	68%
Hemorrhage	63%	65%
Mucositis	50%	55%
Dermatologic	46%	40%
Mental Status	41%	34%
Pulmonary-Clinical	39%	39%
Fever (not elsewhere classified)	26%	28%
Headache	20%	24%
Cardiac-Clinical	16%	24%
Neurologic-Peripheral Nerves	7%	9%
Pulmonary Allergy	2%	4%
Seizure	4%	5%
Cerebellar	4%	4%

The duration of aplasia and incidence of mucositis were greater on the IDR arm than the DNR arm, especially during consolidation in some U.S. controlled trials (see CLINICAL STUDIES).

The following information reflects experience based on U.S. controlled clinical trials.

Myelosuppression

Severe myelosuppression is the major toxicity associated with IDAMYCIN therapy, but this effect of the drug is required in order to eradicate the leukemic clone. During the period of myelosuppression, patients are at risk of developing infection and bleeding which may be life-threatening or fatal.

Gastrointestinal

Nausea and/or vomiting, mucositis, abdominal pain and diarrhea were reported frequently, but were severe (equivalent to WHO Grade 4) in less than 5% of patients. Severe enterocolitis with perforation has been reported rarely. The risk of perforation may be increased by instrumental intervention. The possibility of perforation should be considered in patients who develop severe abdominal pain and appropriate steps for diagnosis and management should be taken.

Dermatologic

Alopecia was reported frequently and dermatologic reactions including generalized rash, urticaria and a bullous erythrodermatous rash of the palms and soles have occurred. The dermatologic reactions were usually attributed to concomitant antibiotic therapy. Local reactions including hives at the injection site have been reported.

Hepatic and Renal

Changes in hepatic and renal function tests have been observed. These changes were usually transient and occurred in the setting of sepsis and while patients were receiving potentially hepatotoxic and nephrotoxic antibiotics and antifungal agents. Severe changes in renal function (equivalent to WHO Grade 4) occurred in no more than 1% of patients, while severe changes in hepatic function (equivalent to WHO Grade 4) occurred in less than 5% of patients.

Cardiac

Congestive heart failure (frequently attributed to fluid overload), serious arrhythmias including atrial fibrillation, chest pain, myocardial infarction and asymptomatic declines in LVEF have been reported in patients undergoing induction therapy for AML. Myocardial insufficiency and arrhythmias were usually reversible and occurred in the setting of sepsis, anemia and aggressive intravenous fluid administration. The events were reported more frequently in patients over age 60 years and in those with pre-existing cardiac disease.

OVERDOSAGE

There is no known antidote to IDAMYCIN. Two cases of fatal overdosage in patients receiving therapy for AML have been reported. The doses were 135 mg/m^2 over 3 days and 45 mg/m^2 of idarubicin and 90 mg/m^2 of daunorubicin over a three day period.

It is anticipated that overdosage with idarubicin will result in severe and prolonged myelosuppression and possibly in increased severity of gastrointestinal toxicity. Adequate supportive care including platelet transfusions, antibiotics and symptomatic treatment of mucositis is required. The effect of acute overdose on cardiac function is not fully known, but severe arrhythmia occurred in 1 of the 2 patients exposed. It is anticipated that very high doses of idarubicin may cause acute cardiac toxicity and may be associated with a higher incidence of delayed cardiac failure.

Disposition studies with idarubicin in patients undergoing dialysis have not been carried out. The profound multicompartment behavior, extensive extravascular distribution and tissue binding, coupled with the low unbound fraction available in the plasma pool make it unlikely that therapeutic efficacy or toxicity would be altered by conventional peritoneal or hemodialysis.

DOSAGE AND ADMINISTRATION (See WARNINGS).

For induction therapy in adult patients with AML the following dose schedule is recommended:

IDAMYCIN 12 mg/m^2 daily for 3 days by slow (10 to 15 min) intravenous injection in combination with Ara-C. The Ara-C may be given as 100 mg/m^2 daily by continuous infusion for 7 days or as Ara-C 25 mg/m^2 intravenous bolus followed by Ara-C 200 mg/m^2 daily for 5 days continuous infusion. In patients with unequivocal evidence of leukemia after the first induction course, a second course may be administered. Administration of the second course should be delayed in patients who experience severe mucositis, until recovery from this toxicity has occurred, and a dose reduction of 25% is recommended. In patients with hepatic and/or renal impairment, a dose reduction of IDAMYCIN should be considered. IDAMYCIN should not be administered if the bilirubin level exceeds 5 mg%. (See WARNINGS).

The benefit of consolidation in prolonging the duration of remissions and survival is not proven. There is no consensus regarding optional regimens to be used for consolidation. (See CLINICAL STUDIES for doses used in U.S. Clinical studies).

Preparation of Solution

Caution in handling of the powder and preparation of the solution must be exercised as skin reactions associated with IDAMYCIN may occur. Skin accidently exposed to IDAMYCIN should be washed thoroughly with soap and water and if the eyes are involved, standard irrigation techniques should be used immediately. The use of goggles, gloves, and protective gowns is recommended during preparation and administration of the drug.

IDAMYCIN 5 mg, 10 mg and 20 mg vials should be reconstituted with 5 mL, 10 mL and 20 mL, respectively, of Sodium Chloride Injection USP (0.9%) to give a final concentration of 1 mg/mL of idarubicin hydrochloride. Bacteriostatic diluents are not recommended.

The vial contents are under a negative pressure to minimize aerosol formation during reconstitution; therefore, particular care should be taken when the needle is inserted. Inhalation of any aerosol produced during reconstitution must be avoided.

Reconstituted solutions are physically and chemically stable for at least 168 hours (7 days) under refrigeration (2° to 8°C, 36° to 46°F) and 72 hours (3 days) at controlled room temperature, (15° to 30°C, 59° to 86°F). Discard unused solutions in an appropriate manner (see *Handling and Disposal*).

Care in the administration of IDAMYCIN will reduce the chance of perivenous infiltration. It may also decrease the chance of local reactions such as urticaria and erythematous streaking. During intravenous administration of IDAMYCIN extravasation may occur with or without an accompanying stinging or burning sensation even if blood returns well on aspiration of the infusion needle. If any signs or symptoms of extravasation have occurred, the injection or infusion should be immediately terminated and restarted in another vein. If it is known or suspected that subcutaneous extravasation has occurred it is recommended that intermittent ice packs (1/2 hour immediately, then 1/2 hour 4 times per day for 3 days) be placed over the area of extravasation and that the affected extremity be elevated. Because of the progressive nature of extravasation reactions, the area of injection should be frequently examined and plastic surgery consultation obtained early if there is any sign of a local reaction such as pain, erythema, edema or vesication. If ulceration begins or there is severe persistent pain at the site of extravasation, early wide excision of the involved area should be considered.[1]

IDAMYCIN should be administered slowly (over 10 to 15 minutes) into the tubing of a freely running intravenous infusion of Sodium Chloride Injection USP (0.9%) or 5% Dextrose Injection USP. The tubing should be attached to a Butterfly needle or other suitable device and inserted preferably into a large vein.

Incompatibility

Unless specific compatibility data are available, IDAMYCIN should not be mixed with other drugs. Precipitation occurs with heparin. Prolonged contact with any solution of an alkaline pH will result in degradation of the drug.

Parenteral drug products should be inspected visually for particulate matter and discoloration prior to administration whenever solution and containers permit.

Handling and Disposal - Procedures for handling and disposal of anticancer drugs should be considered. Several guidelines on this subject have been published.[2-8] There is no general agreement that all of the procedures recommended in the guidelines are necessary or appropriate.

HOW SUPPLIED

IDAMYCIN (Idarubicin Hydrochloride for Injection, USP)

NDC 0013-2506-94	5 mg single dose vial. Available in 5 vial packs.
NDC 0013-2516-86	10 mg single dose vial. Available in single vials.
NDC 0013-2526-86	20 mg single dose vial. Available in single vials.

Store at controlled room temperature, 15° to 30°C (59° to 86°F), and protect from light.

CAUTION: Federal law prohibits dispensing without prescription.

Manufactured by:
PHARMACIA S.p.A.
MILAN, ITALY

REFERENCES

1. Rudolph R, Larson DL: Etiology and Treatment of Chemotherapeutic Agent Extravasation Injuries: A Review. J Clin Oncol 5: 1116-1126, 1987.
2. Recommendations for the Safe Handling of Parenteral Antineoplastic Drugs. NIH Publication No. 83-2621. For sale by the Superintendent of Documents, US Government Printing Office, Washington, DC 20402.

3. AMA Council Report, Guidelines for Handling Parenteral Antineoplastics, JAMA. 1985; 253 (11): 1590-1592.
4. National Study Commission on Cytotoxic Exposure-Recommendations for Handling Cytotoxic Agents. Available from Louis P. Jeffrey, Sc.D., Chairman, National Study Commission on Cytotoxic Exposure, Massachusetts College of Pharmacy and Allied Health Sciences, 179 Longwood Avenue, Boston, Massachusetts 02115.
5. Clinical Oncological Society of Australia. Guidelines and Recommendations for Safe Handling of Antineoplastic Agents. Med J Australia. 1983; 1:426-428.
6. Jones RB, et al: Safe Handling of Chemotherapeutic Agents: A Report from the Mount Sinai Medical Center. CA-A Cancer Journal for Clinicians. 1983; (Sept/Oct) 258-263.
7. American Society of Hospital Pharmacists Technical Assistance Bulletin on Handling Cytotoxic and Hazardous Drugs. Am J Hosp Pharm. 1990; 47:1033-1049.
8. OSHA Work-Practice Guidelines for Personnel Dealing with Cytotoxic (Antineoplastic) Drugs. Am J Hosp Pharm. 1986; 43:1193-1204.

052010496 Revised April 25, 1996

KAO LECTROLYTE™ OTC

Electrolyte Replenisher

DESCRIPTION

INGREDIENTS: Dextrose, Sodium Citrate, Potassium Chloride, Sodium Chloride, Aspartame*, Artificial Grape Flavor and FD&C Red #40 and FD&C Blue #1.

*Phenylketonurics: Contains Phenylalanine.

Each packet of Kao Lectrolyte provides: Sodium, 12 mEq; Potassium, 5 mEq; Chloride, 10 mEq; Citrate, 7 mEq; Dextrose, 5 grams; and Calories, 22.

Kao Lectrolyte comes Unflavored or in two great-tasting flavors—Grape and Bubble Gum—that children actually like, to make it easier for you to give them the electrolytes they need.

INDICATIONS AND USAGE

Replaces fluid and minerals lost during diarrhea and vomiting.

DOSAGE AND ADMINISTRATION

DIRECTIONS FOR PREPARATION:

Carefully measure and pour 8 fluid ounces (1 cup) of any safe drinking water (use cold water for best tasts) into clean container.

Important: Do not use less than 8 fluid ounces.

Add entire contents of one packet. Stir or shake well until powder is dissolved. Pour into bottle or cup. Use immediately or cover and store any prepared solution in refrigerator and use within 48 hours.

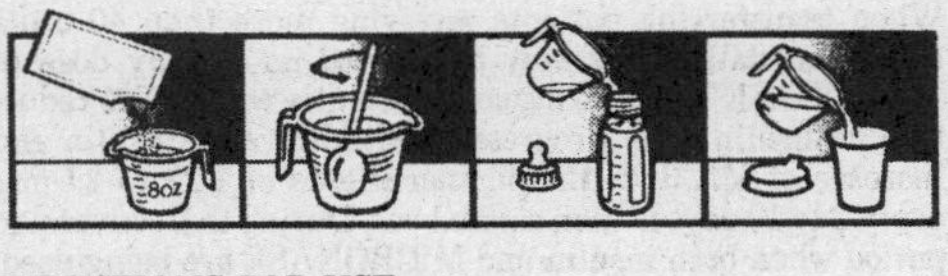

DIRECTIONS FOR USE:

For Children under 2 years of age, consult your physician before feeding Kao Lectrolyte.

For Children 2 years of age and older, provide 8 oz of Kao Lectrolyte every 3 to 4 hours. Discard any unused solution left in bottle or cup after feeding. Your child should be given from 1 to 2 quarts (4–8 packets) per day while the diarrhea continues. If there is vomiting or fever, or if diarrhea continues beyond 24 hours, consult your physician.

Kao Lectrolyte has been specially formulated to replace fluids and minerals lost in diarrhea and vomiting, in accordance with pediatric guidelines.

Contents per Liter	Kao Lectrolyte	Pediatric Guidelines
Sodium	50 mEq	40 mEq–60 mEq
Potassium	20 mEq	20 mEq
Carbohydrates	111 mEq	110–140 mEq
Citrate (Base)	30 mEq	20 mEq–30 mEq

HOW SUPPLIED

Four 6.5 gram (0.22 oz) Packets.

DO NOT USE IF CARTON IS OPENED OR IF FOIL PACKET IS TORN OR BROKEN.

Store unopened packets at controlled room temperature 20° to 25°C (68° to 77°F).

Marketed by: Pharmacia & Upjohn, Kalamazoo, MI 49001

Shown in Product Identification Guide, page 329

MICRONASE® ℞

[mīk-run-aze]

brand of glyburide tablets (1.25, 2.5, and 5 mg)

DESCRIPTION

MICRONASE Tablets contain glyburide, which is an oral blood-glucose-lowering drug of the sulfonylurea class. Glyburide is a white, crystalline compound, formulated as MICRONASE Tablets of 1.25, 2.5, and 5 mg strengths for oral administration. Inactive ingredients: colloidal silicon dioxide, dibasic calcium phosphate, magnesium stearate, microcrystalline cellulose, sodium alginate, talc. In addition, the **2.5 mg** contains aluminum oxide and FD&C Red No. 40 and the **5 mg** contains aluminum oxide and FD&C Blue No. 1. The chemical name for glyburide is 1-[[p-[2-(5-chloro-o-anisamido)-ethyl]phenyl]-sulfonyl]-3-cyclohexylurea and the molecular weight is 493.99. The structural formula is represented below.

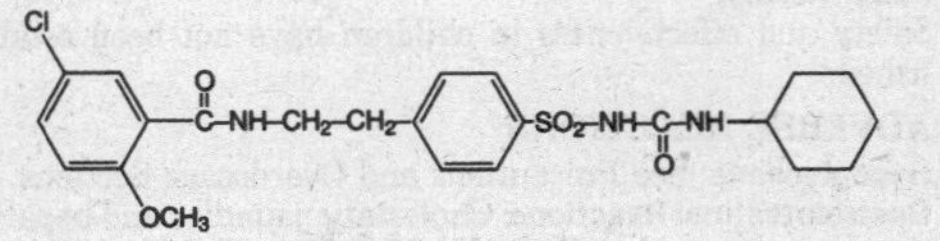

CLINICAL PHARMACOLOGY

Actions

Glyburide appears to lower the blood glucose acutely by stimulating the release of insulin from the pancreas, an effect dependent upon functioning beta cells in the pancreatic islets. The mechanism by which glyburide lowers blood glucose during long-term administration has not been clearly established. With chronic administration in Type II diabetic patients, the blood glucose lowering effect persists despite a gradual decline in the insulin secretory response to the drug. Extrapancreatic effects may be involved in the mechanism of action of oral sulfonyl urea hypoglycemic drugs.

Some patients who are initially responsive to oral hypoglycemic drugs, including MICRONASE, may become unresponsive or poorly responsive over time. Alternatively, MICRONASE Tablets may be effective in some patients who have become unresponsive to one or more other sulfonylurea drugs.

In addition to its blood glucose lowering actions, glyburide produces a mild diuresis by enhancement of renal free water clearance. Disulfiram-like reactions have very rarely been reported in patients treated with MICRONASE Tablets.

Pharmacokinetics

Single dose studies with MICRONASE Tablets in normal subjects demonstrate significant absorption of glyburide within one hour, peak drug levels at about four hours, and low but detectable levels at twenty-four hours. Mean serum levels of glyburide, as reflected by areas under the serum concentration-time curve, increase in proportion to corresponding increases in dose. Multiple dose studies with MICRONASE in diabetic patients demonstrate drug level concentration-time curves similar to single dose studies, indicating no buildup of drug in tissue depots. The decrease of glyburide in the serum of normal healthy individuals is biphasic; the terminal half-life is about 10 hours. In single dose studies in fasting normal subjects, the degree and duration of blood glucose lowering is proportional to the dose administered and to the area under the drug level concentration-time curve. The blood glucose lowering effect persists for 24 hours following single morning doses in nonfasting diabetic patients. Under conditions of repeated administration in diabetic patients, however, there is no reliable correlation between blood drug levels and fasting blood glucose levels. A one year study of diabetic patients treated with MICRONASE showed no reliable correlation between administered dose and serum drug level.

The major metabolite of glyburide is the 4-trans-hydroxy derivative. A second metabolite, the 3-cis-hydroxy derivative, also occurs. These metabolites probably contribute no significant hypoglycemic action in humans since they are only weakly active (1/400th and 1/40th as active, respectively, as glyburide) in rabbits.

Glyburide is excreted as metabolites in the bile and urine, approximately 50% by each route. This dual excretory pathway is qualitatively different from that of other sulfonylureas, which are excreted primarily in the urine.

Sulfonylurea drugs are extensively bound to serum proteins. Displacement from protein binding sites by other drugs may lead to enhanced hypoglycemic action. *In vitro*, the protein binding exhibited by glyburide is predominantly non-ionic, whereas that of other sulfonylureas (chlorpropamide, tolbutamide, tolazamide) is predominantly ionic. Acidic drugs such as phenylbutazone, warfarin, and salicylates displace the ionic-binding sulfonylureas from serum proteins to a far greater extent than the non-ionic binding glyburide. It has not been shown that this difference in protein binding will result in fewer drug-drug interactions with MICRONASE Tablets in clinical use.

INDICATIONS AND USAGE

MICRONASE Tablets are indicated as an adjunct to diet to lower the blood glucose in patients with non-insulin-dependent diabetes mellitus (Type II) whose hyperglycemia cannot be satisfactorily controlled by diet alone.

In initiating treatment for non-insulin-dependent diabetes, diet should be emphasized as the primary form of treatment. Caloric restriction and weight loss are essential in the obese diabetic patient. Proper dietary management alone may be effective in controlling the blood glucose and symptoms of hyperglycemia. The importance of regular physical activity should also be stressed, and cardiovascular risk factors should be identified and corrective measures taken where possible. If this treatment program fails to reduce symptoms and/or blood glucose, the use of an oral sulfonylurea or insulin should be considered. Use of MICRONASE must be viewed by both the physician and patient as a treatment in addition to diet and not as a substitution or as a convenient mechanism for avoiding dietary restraint. Furthermore, loss of blood glucose control on diet alone may be transient, thus requiring only short-term administration of MICRONASE.

During maintenance programs, MICRONASE should be discontinued if satisfactory lowering of blood glucose is no longer achieved. Judgment should be based on regular clinical and laboratory evaluations.

In considering the use of MICRONASE in asymptomatic patients, it should be recognized that controlling blood glucose in non-insulin-dependent diabetes has not been definitely established to be effective in preventing the long-term cardiovascular or neural complications of diabetes.

CONTRAINDICATIONS

MICRONASE Tablets are contraindicated in patients with:

1. Known hypersensitivity or allergy to the drug.
2. Diabetic ketoacidosis, with or without coma. This condition should be treated with insulin.
3. Type I diabetes mellitus, as sole therapy.

SPECIAL WARNING ON INCREASED RISK OF CARDIOVASCULAR MORTALITY

The administration of oral hypoglycemic drugs has been reported to be associated with increased cardiovascular mortality as compared to treatment with diet alone or diet plus insulin. This warning is based on the study conducted by the University Group Diabetes Program (UGDP), a long-term prospective clinical trial designed to evaluate the effectiveness of glucose-lowering drugs in preventing or delaying vascular complications in patients with non-insulin-dependent diabetes. The study involved 823 patients who were randomly assigned to one of four treatment groups (*Diabetes*, 19 (Suppl. 2):747-830, 1970).

UGDP reported that patients treated for 5 to 8 years with diet plus a fixed dose of tolbutamide (1.5 grams per day) had a rate of cardiovascular mortality approximately 2 1/2 times that of patients treated with diet alone. A significant increase in total mortality was not observed, but the use of tolbutamide was discontinued based on the increase in cardiovascular mortality, thus limiting the opportunity for the study to show an increase in overall mortality. Despite controversy regarding the interpretation of these results, the findings of the UGDP study provide an adequate basis for this warning. The patient should be informed of the potential risks and advantages of MICRONASE and of alternative modes of therapy.

Although only one drug in the sulfonylurea class (tolbutamide) was included in this study, it is prudent from a safety standpoint to consider that this warning may also apply to other oral hypoglycemic drugs in this class, in view of their close similarities in mode of action and chemical structure.

PRECAUTIONS

General

Hypoglycemia: All sulfonylureas are capable of producing severe hypoglycemia. Proper patient selection and dosage and instructions are important to avoid hypoglycemic episodes. Renal or hepatic insufficiency may cause elevated drug levels of glyburide and the latter may also diminish gluconeogenic capacity, both of which increase the risk of serious hypoglycemic reactions. Elderly, debilitated or malnourished patients, and those with adrenal or pituitary insufficiency, are particularly susceptible to the hypoglycemic action of glucose-lowering drugs.

Continued on next page

Information on these Pharmacia & Upjohn products is based on labeling in effect June 1, 1996. Further information concerning these and other Pharmacia & Upjohn products may be obtained by direct inquiry to Medical Information, Pharmacia & Upjohn, Kalamazoo, MI 49001.

Pharmacia & Upjohn—Cont.

Hypoglycemia may be difficult to recognize in the elderly and in people who are taking beta-adrenergic blocking drugs. Hypoglycemia is more likely to occur when caloric intake is deficient, after severe or prolonged exercise, when alcohol is ingested, or when more than one glucose lowering drug is used. The risk of hypoglycemia may be increased with combination therapy.

Loss of Control of Blood Glucose: When a patient stabilized on any diabetic regimen is exposed to stress such as fever, trauma, infection or surgery, a loss of control may occur. At such times it may be necessary to discontinue MICRONASE and administer insulin.

The effectiveness of any hypoglycemic drug, including MICRONASE, in lowering blood glucose to a desired level decreases in many patients over a period of time which may be due to progression of the severity of diabetes or to diminished responsiveness to the drug. This phenomenon is known as secondary failure, to distinguish it from primary failure in which the drug is ineffective in an individual patient when MICRONASE is first given. Adequate adjustment of dose and adherence to diet should be assessed before classifying a patient as a secondary failure.

Information for Patients: Patients should be informed of the potential risks and advantages of MICRONASE and of alternative modes of therapy. They also should be informed about the importance of adherence to dietary instructions, of a regular exercise program, and of regular testing of urine and/or blood glucose.

The risks of hypoglycemia, its symptoms and treatment, and conditions that predispose to its development should be explained to patients and responsible family members. Primary and secondary failure also should be explained.

Laboratory Tests

Therapeutic response to MICRONASE Tablets should be monitored by frequent urine glucose tests and periodic blood glucose tests. Measure ment of glycosylated hemoglobin levels may be helpful in some patients.

Drug Interactions

The hypoglycemic action of sulfonylureas may be potentiated by certain drugs including nonsteroidal anti-inflammatory agents and other drugs that are highly protein bound, salicylates, sulfonamides, chloramphenicol, probenecid, coumarins, monoamine oxidase inhibitors, and beta adrenergic blocking agents. When such drugs are administered to a patient receiving MICRONASE, the patient should be observed closely for hypoglycemia. When such drugs are withdrawn from a patient receiving MICRONASE, the patient should be observed closely for loss of control.

Certain drugs tend to produce hyperglycemia and may lead to loss of control. These drugs include the thiazides and other diuretics, corticosteroids, phenothiazines, thyroid products, estrogens, oral contraceptives, phenytoin, nicotinic acid, sympathomimetics, calcium channel blocking drugs, and isoniazid. When such drugs are administered to a patient receiving MICRONASE, the patient should be closely observed for loss of control. When such drugs are withdrawn from a patient receiving MICRONASE, the patient should be observed closely for hypoglycemia.

A possible interaction between glyburide and ciprofloxacin, a fluoroquinolone antibiotic, has been reported, resulting in a potentiation of the hypoglycemic action of glyburide. The mechanism for this interaction is not known.

A potential interaction between oral miconazole and oral hypoglycemic agents leading to severe hypoglycemia has been reported. Whether this interaction also occurs with the intravenous, topical or vaginal preparations of miconazole is not known.

Metformin: In a single-dose interaction study in NIDDM subjects, decreases in glyburide AUC and C_{max} were observed, but were highly variable. The single-dose nature of this study and the lack of correlation between glyburide blood levels and pharmacodynamic effects, makes the clinical significance of this interaction uncertain. Coadministration of glyburide and metformin did not result in any changes in either metformin pharmacokinetics or pharmacodynamics.

Carcinogenesis, Mutagenesis, and Impairment of Fertility

Studies in rats at doses up to 300 mg/kg/day for 18 months showed no carcinogenic effects. Glyburide is nonmutagenic when studied in the Salmonella microsome test (Ames test) and in the DNA damage/alkaline elution assay. No drug related effects were noted in any of the criteria evaluated in the two year oncogenicity study of glyburide in mice.

Pregnancy

Teratogenic Effects: Pregnancy Category B

Reproduction studies have been performed in rats and rabbits at doses up to 500 times the human dose and have revealed no evidence of impaired fertility or harm to the fetus due to glyburide. There are, however, no adequate and well controlled studies in pregnant women. Because animal reproduction studies are not always predictive of human response, this drug should be used during pregnancy only if clearly needed.

Because recent information suggests that abnormal blood glucose levels during pregnancy are associated with a higher incidence of congenital abnormalities, many experts recommend that insulin be used during pregnancy to maintain blood glucose as close to normal as possible.

Nonteratogenic Effects: Prolonged severe hypoglycemia (4 to 10 days) has been reported in neonates born to mothers who were receiving a sulfonylurea drug at the time of delivery. This has been reported more frequently with the use of agents with prolonged half-lives. If MICRONASE is used during pregnancy, it should be discontinued at least two weeks before the expected delivery date.

Nursing Mothers

Although it is not known whether glyburide is excreted in human milk, some sulfonylurea drugs are known to be excreted in human milk. Because the potential for hypoglycemia in nursing infants may exist, a decision should be made whether to discontinue nursing or to discontinue the drug, taking into account the importance of the drug to the mother. If the drug is discontinued, and if diet alone is inadequate for controlling blood glucose, insulin therapy should be considered.

Pediatric Use

Safety and effectiveness in children have not been established.

ADVERSE REACTIONS

Hypoglycemia: See Precautions and Overdosage Sections.

Gastrointestinal Reactions: Cholestatic jaundice and hepatitis may occur rarely; MICRONASE Tablets should be discontinued if this occurs.

Liver function abnormalities, including isolated transaminase elevations, have been reported.

Gastrointestinal disturbances, *eg*, nausea, epigastric fullness, and heartburn are the most common reactions, having occurred in 1.8% of treated patients during clinical trials. They tend to be dose related and may disappear when dosage is reduced.

Dermatologic Reactions: Allergic skin reactions, *eg*, pruritus, erythema, urticaria, and morbilliform or maculopapular eruptions occurred in 1.5% of treated patients during clinical trials. These may be transient and may disappear despite continued use of MICRONASE; if skin reactions persist, the drug should be discontinued.

Porphyria cutanea tarda and photosensitivity reactions have been reported with sulfonylureas.

Hematologic Reactions: Leukopenia, agranulocytosis, thrombocytopenia, hemolytic anemia, aplastic anemia, and pancytopenia have been reported with sulfonylureas.

Metabolic Reactions: Hepatic porphyria and disulfiram-like reactions have been reported with sulfonylureas; however, hepatic porphyria has not been reported with MICRONASE and disulfiram-like reactions have been reported very rarely.

Cases of hyponatremia have been reported with glyburide and all other sulfonylureas, most often in patients who are on other medications or have medical conditions known to cause hyponatremia or increase release of antidiuretic hormone. The syndrome of inappropriate antidiuretic hormone (SIADH) secretion has been reported with certain other sulfonylureas, and it has been suggested that these sulfonylureas may augment the peripheral (antidiuretic) action of ADH and/or increase release of ADH.

Other Reactions: Changes in accommodation and/or blurred vision have been reported with glyburide and other sulfonylureas. These are thought to be related to fluctuation in glucose levels.

In addition to dermatologic reactions, allergic reactions such as angioedema, arthralgia, myalgia and vasculitis have been reported.

OVERDOSAGE

Overdosage of sulfonylureas, including MICRONASE Tablets, can produce hypoglycemia. Mild hypoglycemic symptoms, without loss of consciousness or neurological findings, should be treated aggressively with oral glucose and adjustments in drug dosage and/or meal patterns. Close monitoring should continue until the physician is assured that the patient is out of danger. Severe hypoglycemic reactions with coma, seizure, or other neurological impairment occur infrequently, but constitute medical emergencies requiring immediate hospitalization. If hypoglycemic coma is diagnosed or suspected, the patient should be given a rapid intravenous injection of concentrated (50%) glucose solution. This should be followed by a continuous infusion of a more dilute (10%) glucose solution at a rate which will maintain the blood glucose at a level above 100 mg/dL. Patients should be closely monitored for a minimum of 24 to 48 hours, since hypoglycemia may recur after apparent clinical recovery.

DOSAGE AND ADMINISTRATION

There is no fixed dosage regimen for the management of diabetes mellitus with MICRONASE Tablets or any other hypoglycemic agent. In addition to the usual monitoring of urinary glucose, the patient's blood glucose must also be monitored periodically to determine the minimum effective dose for the patient; to detect primary failure, *ie*, inadequate lowering of blood glucose at the maximum recommended dose of medication; and to detect secondary failure, *ie*, loss of adequate blood glucose lowering response after an initial period of effectiveness. Glycosylated hemoglobin levels may also be of value in monitoring the patient's response to therapy.

Short-term administration of MICRONASE may be sufficient during periods of transient loss of control in patients usually controlled well on diet.

Usual Starting Dose

The usual starting dose of MICRONASE Tablets is 2.5 to 5 mg daily, administered with breakfast or the first main meal. Those patients who may be more sensitive to hypoglycemic drugs should be started at 1.25 mg daily. (See PRECAUTIONS Section for patients at increased risk.) Failure to follow an appropriate dosage regimen may precipitate hypoglycemia. Patients who do not adhere to their prescribed dietary and drug regimen are more prone to exhibit unsatisfactory response to therapy.

Transfer From Other Hypoglycemic Therapy Patients Receiving Other Oral Antidiabetic Therapy: Transfer of patients from other oral antidiabetic regimens to MICRONASE should be done conservatively and the initial daily dose should be 2.5 to 5 mg. When transferring patients from oral hypoglycemic agents other than chlorpropamide to MICRONASE, no transition period and no initial or priming dose are necessary. When transferring patients from chlorpropamide, particular care should be exercised during the first two weeks because the prolonged retention of chlorpropamide in the body and subsequent overlapping drug effects may provoke hypoglycemia.

Patients Receiving Insulin: Some Type II diabetic patients being treated with insulin may respond satisfactorily to MICRONASE. If the insulin dose is less than 20 units daily, substitution of MICRONASE Tablets 2.5 to 5 mg as a single daily dose may be tried. If the insulin dose is between 20 and 40 units daily, the patient may be placed directly on MICRONASE Tablets 5 mg daily as a single dose. If the insulin dose is more than 40 units daily, a transition period is required for conversion to MICRONASE. In these patients, insulin dosage is decreased by 50% and MICRONASE Tablets 5 mg daily is started. Please refer to Titration to Maintenance Dose for further explanation.

Titration to Maintenance Dose

The usual maintenance dose is in the range of 1.25 to 20 mg daily, which may be given as a single dose or in divided doses (See Dosage Interval Section). Dosage increases should be made in increments of no more than 2.5 mg at weekly intervals based upon the patient's blood glucose response.

No exact dosage relationship exists between MICRONASE and the other oral hypoglycemic agents. Although patients may be transferred from the maximum dose of other sulfonylureas, the maximum starting dose of 5 mg of MICRONASE Tablets should be observed. A maintenance dose of 5 mg of MICRONASE Tablets provides approximately the same degree of blood glucose control as 250 to 375 mg chlorpropamide, 250 to 375 mg tolazamide, 500 to 750 mg acetohexamide, or 1000 to 1500 mg tolbutamide.

When transferring patients receiving more than 40 units of insulin daily, they may be started on a daily dose of MICRONASE Tablets 5 mg concomitantly with a 50% reduction in insulin dose. Progressive withdrawal of insulin and increase of MICRONASE in increments of 1.25 to 2.5 mg every 2 to 10 days is then carried out. During this conversion period when both insulin and MICRONASE are being used, hypoglycemia may rarely occur. During insulin withdrawal, patients should test their urine for glucose and acetone at least three times daily and report results to their physician. The appearance of persistent acetonuria with glycosuria indicates that the patient is a Type I diabetic who requires insulin therapy.

Maximum Dose

Daily doses of more than 20 mg are not recommended.

Dosage Interval

Once-a-day therapy is usually satisfactory. Some patients, particularly those receiving more than 10 mg daily, may have a more satisfactory response with twice-a-day dosage.

Specific Patient Populations

MICRONASE is not recommended for use in pregnancy or for use in children.

In elderly patients, debilitated or malnourished patients, and patients with impaired renal or hepatic function, the initial and maintenance dosing should be conservative to avoid hypoglycemic reactions. (See PRECAUTIONS Section.)

HOW SUPPLIED

MICRONASE Tablets are supplied as follows:

MICRONASE Tablets 1.25 mg (White, Round, Scored, imprinted MICRONASE 1.25)

Bottles of 100	NDC 0009-0131-01

MICRONASE Tablets 2.5 mg (Dark Pink, Round, Scored, imprinted MICRONASE 2.5)

Bottles of 100	NDC 0009-0141-01
Bottles of 500	NDC 0009-0141-11
Bottles of 1000	NDC 0009-0141-03
Unit Dose Pkg of 100	NDC 0009-0141-02

MICRONASE Tablets 5 mg (Blue, Round, Scored imprinted MICRONASE 5)

Bottles of 30	NDC 0009-0171-11
Bottles of 60	NDC 0009-0171-12
Bottles of 100	NDC 0009-0171-05
Bottles of 500	NDC 0009-0171-06
Bottles of 1000	NDC 0009-0171-07
Unit Dose Pkg of 100	NDC 0009-0171-03

Caution: Federal law prohibits dispensing without prescription. Store at controlled room temperature 15° to 30° C (59° to 86° F). Dispensed in well closed containers with safety closures. Keep container tightly closed.

Revised November 1995 811 985 419
691015

MYCOBUTIN® ℞
(Rifabutin Capsules, USP)

DESCRIPTION
MYCOBUTIN® is the brand name for the antimycobacterial agent rifabutin. It is a semisynthetic ansamycin antibiotic derived from rifamycin S. MYCOBUTIN capsules for oral administration contain 150 mg of Rifabutin, USP per capsule, along with the inactive ingredients microcrystalline cellulose, magnesium stearate, red iron oxide, silica gel, sodium lauryl sulfate, titanium dioxide, and edible white ink.
The chemical name for rifabutin is 1′,4-didehydro-1-deoxy-1,4-dihydro-5′-(2-methylpropyl)-1-oxorifamycin XIV (Chemical Abstracts Service, 9th Collective Index) or (9*S*, 12*E*, 14*S*, 15*R*, 16*S*, 17*R*, 18*R*, 19*R*, 20*S*, 21*S*, 22*E*, 24*Z*)-6,16,18,20-tetrahydroxy -1′- isobutyl -14- methoxy -7,9,15,17,19,21,25 -heptamethyl-spiro [9,4-(epoxypentadeca[1, 11, 13]trienimino)-2*H*-furo[2′,3′:7,8]naphth[1,2-*d*]imidazole-2,4′-piperidine]-5,10,26-(3*H*,9*H*)-trione-16-acetate. Rifabutin has a molecular formula of $C_{46}H_{62}N_4O_{11}$, a molecular weight of 847.02 and the following structure:

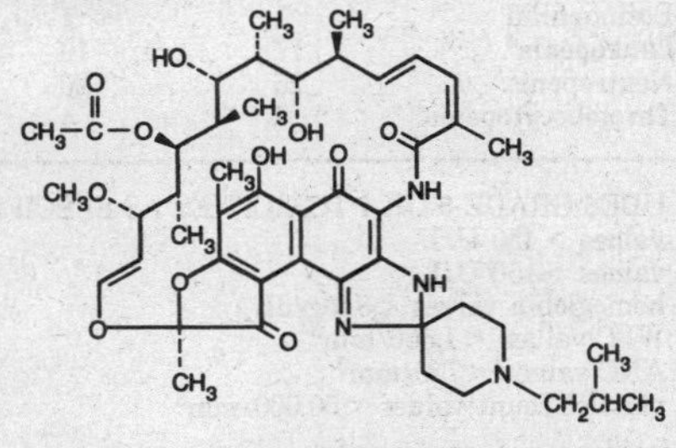

Rifabutin is a red-violet powder soluble in chloroform and methanol, sparingly soluble in ethanol, and very slightly soluble in water (0.19 mg/mL). Its log P value (the base 10 logarithm of the partition coefficient between n-octanol and water) is 3.2 (n-octanol/water).

CLINICAL PHARMACOLOGY
Pharmacokinetics
Following a single oral dose of 300 mg to nine healthy adult volunteers, MYCOBUTIN was readily absorbed from the gastrointestinal tract with mean (±SD) peak plasma levels (C_{max}) of 375 (±267) ng/mL (range: 141 to 1033 ng/mL) attained in 3.3 (±0.9) hours (T_{max} range: 2 to 4 hours). Plasma concentrations post -C_{max} declined in an apparent biphasic manner. Kinetic dose-proportionality has been established over the 300 to 600 mg dose range in nine healthy adult volunteers (crossover design) and in 16 early symptomatic human immunodeficiency virus (HIV)-positive patients over a 300 to 900 mg dose range. Rifabutin was slowly eliminated from plasma in seven healthy adult volunteers, presumably because of *distribution-limited elimination*, with a mean terminal half-life of 45 (±17) hours (range: 16 to 69 hours). Although the systemic levels of rifabutin following multiple dosing decreased by 38%, its terminal half-life remained unchanged. Rifabutin, due to its high lipophilicity, demonstrates a high propensity for distribution and intracellular tissue uptake. Estimates of apparent steady-state distribution volume (9.3 ± 1.5 L/kg) in five HIV-positive patients, following I.V. dosing, exceed total body water by approximately 15-fold. Substantially higher intracellular tissue levels than those seen in plasma have been observed in both rat and man. The lung to plasma concentration ratio, obtained at 12 hours, was found to be approximately 6.5 in four surgical patients administered an oral dose. Mean rifabutin steady-state trough levels ($C_{p,min}^{ss}$; 24-hour post-dose) ranged from 50 to 65 ng/mL in HIV-positive patients and in healthy adult volunteers. About 85% of the drug is bound in a concentration-independent manner to plasma proteins over a concentration range of 0.05 to 1 μg/mL. Binding does not appear to be influenced by renal or hepatic dysfunction.
Mean systemic clearance (CL_s/F) in healthy adult volunteers following a single oral dose was 0.69 (±0.32) L/hr/kg (range: 0.46 to 1.34 L/hr/kg). Renal and biliary clearance of unchanged drug each contribute approximately 5% to CL_s/F. About 30% of the dose is excreted in the feces. A mass-balance study in three healthy adult volunteers with ^{14}C-labeled drug has shown that 53% of the oral dose was excreted in the urine, primarily as metabolites. Of the five metabolites that have been identified, 25-O-desacetyl and 31-hydroxy are the most predominant, and show a plasma metabolite:parent area under the curve ratio of 0.10 and 0.07, respectively. The former has an activity equal to the parent drug and contributes up to 10% to the total antimicrobial activity.
Absolute bioavailability assessed in five HIV-positive patients, who received both oral and I.V. doses, averaged 20%. Total recovery of radioactivity in the urine indicates that at least 53% of the orally administered rifabutin dose is absorbed from the G.I. tract. The bioavailability of rifabutin from the capsule dosage form, relative to a solution, was 85% in 12 healthy adult volunteers. High-fat meals slow the rate without influencing the extent of absorption from the capsule dosage form. The overall pharmacokinetics of MYCOBUTIN are modified only slightly by alterations in hepatic function or age. MYCOBUTIN steady-state kinetics in early symptomatic HIV-positive patients are similar to healthy volunteers. Compared to healthy volunteers, steady-state kinetics of MYCOBUTIN are more variable in elderly patients (>70 years) and in symptomatic HIV-positive patients. Somewhat reduced drug distribution and faster elimination of rifabutin in patients with compromised renal function may result in decreased drug concentrations. The clinical implications of this are unknown.
No rifabutin disposition information is currently available in children or adolescents under 18 years of age.
Microbiology
Mechanism of Action
Rifabutin inhibits DNA-dependent RNA polymerase in susceptible strains of *Escherichia coli* and *Bacillus subtilis* but not in mammalian cells. In resistant strains of *E. coli*, rifabutin, like rifampin, did not inhibit this enzyme. It is not known whether rifabutin inhibits DNA-dependent RNA polymerase in *Mycobacterium avium* or in M. *intracellulare* which comprise *M. avium* complex (MAC).
Susceptibility Testing
In vitro susceptibility testing methods and diagnostic products used for determining minimum inhibitory concentration (MIC) values against *M. avium* complex (MAC) organisms have not been standardized. Breakpoints to determine whether clinical isolates of MAC and other mycobacterial species are susceptible or resistant to rifabutin have not been established.
In Vitro Studies
Rifabutin has demonstrated *in vitro* activity against *M. avium* complex (MAC) organisms isolated from both HIV-positive and HIV-negative people. While gene probe techniques may be used to identify these two organisms, many reported studies did not distinguish between these two species. The vast majority of isolates from MAC-infected, HIV-positive people are *M. avium*, whereas in HIV-negative people, about 40% of the MAC isolates are *M. intracellulare*.
Various *in vitro* methodologies employing broth or solid media, with and without polysorbate 80 (Tween 80), have been used to determine rifabutin MIC values for mycobacterial species. In general, MIC values determined in broth are several fold lower than that observed with methods employing solid media. Utilization of Tween 80 in these assays has been shown to further lower MIC values. However, MIC values were substantially higher for egg based compared to agar based solid media.
Rifabutin activity against 211 MAC isolates from HIV-positive people was evaluated *in vitro* utilizing a radiometric broth and an agar dilution method. Results showed that 78% and 82% of these isolates had MIC_{99} values of ≤0.25μg/mL and ≤1.0μg/mL, respectively, when evaluated by these two methods. Rifabutin was also shown to be active against phagocytized, *M avium* complex in a mouse macrophage cell culture model.
Rifabutin has *in vitro* activity against many strains of *Mycobacterium tuberculosis*. In one study, utilizing the radiometric broth method, each of 17 and 20 rifampin-naive clinical isolates tested from the United States and Taiwan, respectively, were shown to be susceptible to rifabutin concentrations of ≤0.125μg/mL.
Cross-resistance between rifampin and rifabutin is commonly observed with *M. tuberculosis* and *M. avium* complex isolates. Isolates of *M. tuberculosis* resistant to rifampin are likely to be resistant to rifabutin. Rifampicin and rifabutin MIC_{99} values against 523 isolates of *M. avium* complex were determined utilizing the agar dilution method (Ref. Heifets, Leonid B. and Iseman, Michael D. 1985. Determination of *in vitro* susceptibility of Mycobacteria to Ansamycin. Am. Rev. Respir. Dis. 132 (3):710-711).
[See table above.]

SUSCEPTIBILITY OF *M. AVIUM* COMPLEX STRAINS TO RIFAMPIN AND RIFABUTIN

		% of Strains Susceptible/Resistant to Different Concentrations of Rifabutin (μg/mL)			
Susceptibility to Rifampin (μg/mL)	Number of Strains	Susceptible to 0.5	Resistant to 0.5 only	Resistant to 1.0	Resistant to 2.0
Susceptible to 1.0	30	100.0	0.0	0.0	0.0
Resistant to 1.0 only	163	88.3	11.7	0.0	0.0
Resistant to 5.0	105	38.0	57.1	2.9	2.0
Resistant to 10.0	225	20.0	50.2	19.6	10.2
TOTAL	523	49.5	36.7	9.0	4.8

Rifabutin *in vitro* MIC_{99} values of ≤0.5 μg/mL, determined by the agar dilution method, for *M. kansasii*, *M. gordonae* and *M. marinum* have been reported; however, the clinical significance of these results is unknown.

INDICATIONS AND USAGE
MYCOBUTIN is indicated for the prevention of disseminated *Mycobacterium avium* complex (MAC) disease in patients with advanced HIV infection.
Clinical Studies
Two randomized, double-blind clinical trials (study 023 and study 027) compared MYCOBUTIN (300 mg/day) to placebo in patients with CDC-defined AIDS and CD4 counts ≤ 200 cells/μL. These studies accrued patients from 2/90 through 2/92. Study 023 enrolled 590 patients, with a median CD4 cell count at study entry of 42 cells/μL (mean 61). Study 027 enrolled 556 patients, with a median CD4 cell count at study entry of 40 cells/μL (mean 58).
Endpoints included the following:
(1) MAC bacteremia, defined as at least one blood culture positive for *M. avium* complex bacteria.
(2) Clinically significant disseminated MAC disease, defined as MAC bacteremia accompanied by signs or symptoms of serious MAC infection, including one or more of the following: fever, night sweats, rigors, weight loss, worsening anemia, and/or elevations in alkaline phosphatase.
(3) Survival

MAC bacteremia
Participants who received MYCOBUTIN were one-third to one-half as likely to develop MAC bacteremia as were participants who received placebo. These results were statistically significant (study 023: p<0.001; study 027: p = 0.002).
In study 023, the one-year cumulative incidence of MAC bacteremia, on an intent to treat basis, was 9% for patients randomized to MYCOBUTIN and 22% for patients randomized to placebo. In study 027, these rates were 13% and 28% for MYCOBUTIN-treated and placebo-treated patients, respectively.
Most cases of MAC bacteremia (approximately 90% in these studies) occurred among participants whose CD4 count at study entry was ≤ 100 cells/μL. The median and mean CD4 counts at onset of MAC bacteremia were 13 cells/μL and 24 cells/μL, respectively. These studies did not investigate the optimal time to begin MAC prophylaxis.
Clinically significant disseminated MAC disease
In association with the decreased incidence of bacteremia, patients on MYCOBUTIN showed reductions in the signs

Continued on next page

Information on these Pharmacia & Upjohn products is based on labeling in effect June 1, 1996. Further information concerning these and other Pharmacia & Upjohn products may be obtained by direct inquiry to Medical Information, Pharmacia & Upjohn, Kalamazoo, MI 49001.

Pharmacia & Upjohn—Cont.

and symptoms of disseminated MAC disease, including fever, night sweats, weight loss, fatigue, abdominal pain, anemia, and hepatic dysfunction.

Survival

The one year survival rates in study 023 were 77% for the MYCOBUTIN group and 77% for the placebo group. In study 027, the one year survival rates were 77% for the MYCOBUTIN group and 70% for the placebo group. These differences were not statistically significant.

CONTRAINDICATIONS

Rifabutin is contraindicated in patients who have had clinically significant hypersensitivity to this drug, or to any other rifamycins.

WARNINGS

MYCOBUTIN prophylaxis must not be administered to patients with active tuberculosis. Tuberculosis in HIV-positive patients is common and may present with atypical or extrapulmonary findings. Patients are likely to have a nonreactive purified protein derivative (PPD) despite active disease. In addition to chest X-ray and sputum culture, the following studies may be useful in the diagnosis of tuberculosis in the HIV-positive patient: blood culture, urine culture, or biopsy of a suspicious lymph node.

Patients who develop complaints consistent with active tuberculosis while on MYCOBUTIN prophylaxis should be evaluated immediately, so that those with active disease may be given an effective combination regimen of anti-tuberculosis medications. Administration of single-agent MYCOBUTIN to patients with active tuberculosis is likely to lead to the development of tuberculosis that is resistant both to MYCOBUTIN and to rifampin.

There is no evidence that MYCOBUTIN is effective prophylaxis against *M. tuberculosis*. Patients requiring prophylaxis against both *M. tuberculosis* and *Mycobacterium avium* complex may be given isoniazid and MYCOBUTIN concurrently.

PRECAUTIONS

Because MYCOBUTIN may be associated with neutropenia, and more rarely thrombocytopenia, physicians should consider obtaining hematologic studies periodically in patients receiving MYCOBUTIN prophylaxis.

Information for Patients

Patients should be advised of the signs and symptoms of both MAC and tuberculosis, and should be instructed to consult their physicians if they develop new complaints consistent with either of these diseases. In addition, since MYCOBUTIN may rarely be associated with myositis and uveitis, patients should be advised to notify their physicians if they develop signs or symptoms suggesting either of these disorders.

Urine, feces, saliva, sputum, perspiration, tears, and skin may be colored brown-orange with rifabutin and some of its metabolites. Soft contact lenses may be permanently stained. Patients to be treated with MYCOBUTIN should be made aware of these possibilities.

Drug Interactions

In 10 healthy adult volunteers and 8 HIV-positive patients, steady-state plasma levels of zidovudine (ZDV), an antiretroviral agent which is metabolized mainly through glucuronidation, were decreased after repeated MYCOBUTIN dosing; the mean decrease in C_{max} and AUC was decreased by 48% and 32%, respectively. *In vitro* studies have demonstrated that MYCOBUTIN does not affect the inhibition of HIV by ZDV.

Steady-state kinetics in 12 HIV-positive patients show that both the rate and extent of systemic availability of didanosine (ddI), was not altered after repeated dosing of MYCOBUTIN.

MYCOBUTIN has liver enzyme-inducing properties. The related drug rifampin is known to reduce the activity of a number of other drugs, including dapsone, narcotics (including methadone), anticoagulants, corticosteroids, cyclosporine, cardiac glycoside preparations, quinidine, oral contraceptives, oral hypoglycemic agents (sulfonylureas), and analgesics. Rifampin has also been reported to decrease the effects of concurrently administered ketoconazole, barbiturates, diazepam, verapamil, beta-adrenergic blockers, clofibrate, progestins, disopyramide, mexiletine, theophylline, chloramphenicol, and anticonvulsants. Because of the structural similarity of rifabutin and rifampin, MYCOBUTIN may be expected to have some effect on these drugs as well. However, unlike rifampin, MYCOBUTIN appears not to affect the acetylation of isoniazid. When rifabutin was compared with rifampin in a study with 8 healthy normal volunteers, rifabutin appeared to be a less potent enzyme inducer than rifampin. The significance of this finding for clinical drug interactions is not known. Dosage adjustment of drugs listed above may be necessary if they are given concurrently with MYCOBUTIN. Patients using oral contraceptives should consider changing to nonhormonal methods of birth control.

Carcinogenesis, Mutagenesis, Impairment of Fertility:

Long term carcinogenicity studies were conducted with rifabutin in mice and in rats. Rifabutin was not carcinogenic in mice at doses up to 180 mg/kg/day, or approximately 36 times the recommended human daily dose. Rifabutin was not carcinogenic in the rat at doses up to 60 mg/kg/day, about 12 times the recommended human dose.

Rifabutin was not mutagenic in the bacterial mutation assay (Ames Test) using both rifabutin-susceptible and resistant strains. Rifabutin was not mutagenic in *Schizosaccharomyces pombe P_1* and was not genotoxic in V-79 Chinese hamster cells, human lymphocytes *in vitro*, or mouse bone marrow cells *in vivo*.

Fertility was impaired in male rats given 160 mg/kg (32 times the recommended human daily dose).

Pregnancy:

Pregnancy Category B: Reproduction studies have been carried out in rats and rabbits given rifabutin using dose levels up to 200 mg/kg (40 times the recommended human daily dose). No teratogenicity was observed in either species. In rats, given 200 mg/kg/day, there was a decrease in fetal viability. In rats, at 40 mg/kg/day (8 times the recommended human daily dose), rifabutin caused an increase in fetal skeletal variants. In rabbits, at 80 mg/kg/day (16 times the recommended human daily dose), rifabutin caused maternotoxicity and increase in fetal skeletal anomalies. There are no adequate and well-controlled studies in pregnant women. Because animal reproduction studies are not always predictive of human response, rifabutin should be used in pregnant women only if the potential benefit justifies the potential risk to the fetus.

Nursing Mothers:

It is not known whether rifabutin is excreted in human milk. Because many drugs are excreted in human milk and because of the potential for serious adverse reactions in nursing infants, a decision should be made whether to discontinue nursing or discontinue the drug, taking into account the importance of the drug to the mother.

Pediatric Use:

Safety and effectiveness of rifabutin for prophylaxis of MAC in children have not been established. Limited safety data are available from treatment use in 22 HIV-positive children with MAC who received MYCOBUTIN in combination with at least two other antimycobacterials for periods from 1 to 183 weeks. Mean doses (mg/kg) for these children were: 18.5 (range 15.0 to 25.0) for infants one year of age; 8.6 (range 4.4 to 18.8) for children 2 to 10 years of age; and 4.0 (range 2.8 to 5.4) for adolescents 14 to 16 years of age. There is no evidence that doses greater than 5 mg/kg daily are useful. Adverse experiences were similar to those observed in the adult population, and included leukopenia, neutropenia and rash. Doses of MYCOBUTIN may be administered mixed with foods such as applesauce.

ADVERSE REACTIONS

MYCOBUTIN was generally well tolerated in the controlled clinical trials. Discontinuation of therapy due to an adverse event was required in 16% of patients receiving MYCOBUTIN compared to 8% of patients receiving placebo in these trials. Primary reasons for discontinuation of MYCOBUTIN were rash (4% of treated patients), gastrointestinal intolerance (3%), and neutropenia (2%).

The following table enumerates adverse experiences that occurred at a frequency of 1% or greater, among the patients treated with MYCOBUTIN in studies 023 and 027.

CLINICAL ADVERSE EXPERIENCES REPORTED IN ≥ 1% OF PATIENTS TREATED WITH MYCOBUTIN

ADVERSE EVENT	MYCOBUTIN (n=566) %	PLACEBO (n=580) %
BODY AS A WHOLE		
Abdominal Pain	4	3
Asthenia	1	1
Chest Pain	1	1
Fever	2	1
Headache	3	5
Pain	1	2
DIGESTIVE SYSTEM		
Anorexia	2	2
Diarrhea	3	3
Dyspepsia	3	1
Eructation	3	1
Flatulence	2	1
Nausea	6	5
Nausea and Vomiting	3	2
Vomiting	1	1
MUSCULOSKELETAL SYSTEM		
Myalgia	2	1
NERVOUS SYSTEM		
Insomnia	1	1
SKIN AND APPENDAGES		
Rash	11	8
SPECIAL SENSES		
Taste Perversion	3	1
UROGENITAL SYSTEM		
Discolored Urine	30	6

CLINICAL ADVERSE EVENTS REPORTED IN <1% OF PATIENTS WHO RECEIVED MYCOBUTIN

Considering data from the 023 and 027 pivotal trials, and from other clinical studies, MYCOBUTIN appears to be a likely cause of the following adverse events which occurred in less than 1% of treated patients: flu-like syndrome, hepatitis, hemolysis, arthralgia, myositis, chest pressure or pain with dyspnea, and skin discoloration.

The following adverse events have occurred in more than one patient receiving MYCOBUTIN, but an etiologic role has not been established: seizure, paresthesia, aphasia, confusion, and non-specific T wave changes on electrocardiogram.

When MYCOBUTIN was administered at doses from 1050 mg/day to 2400 mg/day, generalized arthralgia and uveitis were reported. These adverse experiences abated when MYCOBUTIN was discontinued.

The following table enumerates the changes in laboratory values that were considered as laboratory abnormalities in studies 023 and 027.

PERCENTAGE OF PATIENTS WITH LABORATORY ABNORMALITIES

LABORATORY ABNORMALITIES	MYCOBUTIN (n=566) %	PLACEBO (n=580) %
Chemistry:		
Increased Alkaline Phosphatase[1]	<1	3
Increased SGOT[2]	7	12
Increased SGPT[2]	9	11
Hematology:		
Anemia[3]	6	7
Eosinophilia	1	1
Leukopenia[4]	17	16
Neutropenia[5]	25	20
Thrombocytopenia[6]	5	4

INCLUDES GRADE 3 OR 4 TOXICITIES AS SPECIFIED:

1 all values >450 U/L

2 all values >150 U/L

3 all hemoglobin values <8.0 g/dL

4 all WBC values <1,500/mm^3

5 all ANC values <750/mm^3

6 all platelet count values <50,000/mm^3

The incidence of neutropenia in patients treated with MYCOBUTIN was significantly greater than in patients treated with placebo ($p = 0.03$). Although thrombocytopenia was not significantly more common among MYCOBUTIN treated patients in these trials, MYCOBUTIN has been clearly linked to thrombocytopenia in rare cases. One patient in study 023 developed thrombotic thrombocytopenic purpura, which was attributed to MYCOBUTIN.

Uveitis is rare when MYCOBUTIN is used as a single agent at 300 mg/day for prophylaxis of MAC in HIV-infected persons, even with the concomitant use of fluconazole and/or macrolide antibiotics. However, if higher doses of MYCOBUTIN are administered in combination with these agents, the incidence of uveitis is higher.

Patients who developed uveitis had mild to severe symptoms that resolved after treatment with corticosteroids and/or mydriatic eye drops; in some severe cases, however, resolution of symptoms occurred after several weeks.

When uveitis occurs, temporary discontinuance of MYCOBUTIN and ophthalmologic evaluation are recommended. In most mild cases, MYCOBUTIN may be restarted; however if signs or symptoms recur, use of MYCOBUTIN should be discontinued (Morbidity and Mortality Weekly Report, September 9, 1994).

ANIMAL TOXICOLOGY

Liver abnormalities, (increased bilirubin and liver weight), occurred in all species tested, in rats at doses 5 times, in monkeys at doses 8 times, and in mice at doses 6 times the recommended human daily dose. Testicular atrophy occurred in baboons at doses 4 times the recommended human dose, and in rats at doses 40 times the recommended human daily dose.

OVERDOSAGE

No information is available on accidental overdosage in humans.

Treatment

While there is no experience in the treatment of overdose with MYCOBUTIN, clinical experience with rifamycins suggest that gastric lavage to evacuate gastric contents (within a few hours of overdose), followed by instillation of an activated charcoal slurry into the stomach, may help absorb any remaining drug from the gastrointestinal tract.

Rifabutin is 85% protein bound and distributed extensively into tissues (Vss:8 to 9 L/kg). It is not primarily excreted via the urinary route (less than 10% as unchanged drug), therefore, neither hemodialysis nor forced diuresis is expected to enhance the systemic elimination of unchanged rifabutin from the body in a patient with MYCOBUTIN overdose.

DOSAGE AND ADMINISTRATION

It is recommended that 300 mg of MYCOBUTIN be administered once daily. For those patients with propensity to nausea, vomiting, or other gastrointestinal upset, administration of MYCOBUTIN at doses of 150 mg twice daily taken with food may be useful.

HOW SUPPLIED

MYCOBUTIN® (Rifabutin Capsules, USP) is supplied as hard gelatin capsules having an opaque red-brown cap and body, imprinted with MYCOBUTIN/PHARMACIA in white ink, each containing 150 mg of Rifabutin, USP.
MYCOBUTIN is available as follows:
NDC 0013-5301-17 Bottles of 100 capsules
Keep tightly closed and dispense in a tight container as defined in the USP. Store at controlled room temperature, 15° to 30°C (59° to 86°F).
CAUTION: Federal law prohibits dispensing without prescription.
Manufactured by:
PHARMACIA S.p.A.
ASCOLI PICENO, ITALY
057000496 Revised April 1, 1996
Shown in Product Identification Guide, page 329

OGEN® ℞
brand of estropipate tablets, USP

WARNINGS:

1. ESTROGENS HAVE BEEN REPORTED TO INCREASE THE RISK OF ENDOMETRIAL CARCINOMA IN POST-MENOPAUSAL WOMEN.

Close clinical surveillance of all women taking estrogens is important. Adequate diagnostic measures, including endometrial sampling when indicated, should be undertaken to rule out malignancy in all cases of undiagnosed persistent or recurring abnormal vaginal bleeding. There is no evidence that "natural" estrogens are more or less hazardous than "synthetic" estrogens at equi estrogenic doses.

2. ESTROGENS SHOULD NOT BE USED DURING PREGNANCY.

There is no indication for estrogen therapy during pregnancy or during the immediate postpartum period. Estrogens are ineffective for the prevention or treatment of threatened, or habitual abortion. Estrogens are not indicated for the prevention of postpartum breast engorgement.
Estrogen therapy during pregnancy is associated with an increased risk of congenital defects in the reproductive organs of the fetus, and possibly other birth defects. Studies of women who received diethylstilbestrol (DES) during pregnancy have shown that female offspring have an increased risk of vaginal adenosis, squamous cell dysplasia of the uterine cervix, and clear cell vaginal cancer later in life; male offspring have an increased risk of urogenital abnormalities and possibly testicular cancer later in life. The 1985 DES Task Force concluded that use of DES during pregnancy is associated with a subsequent increased risk of breast cancer in the mothers, although a causal relationship remains unproven and the observed level of excess risk is similar to that for a number of other breast cancer risk factors.

DESCRIPTION

OGEN (estropipate tablets), (formerly piperazine estrone sulfate), is a natural estrogenic substance prepared from purified crystalline estrone, solubilized as the sulfate and stabilized with piperazine. It is appreciably soluble in water and has almost no odor or taste - properties which are ideally suited for oral administration. The amount of piperazine in OGEN is not sufficient to exert a pharmacological action. Its addition ensures solubility, stability, and uniform potency of the estrone sulfate. Chemically estropipate, molecular weight: 436.56, is represented by estra-1,3,5(10)-trien-17-one,3-(sulfooxy)-, compound with piperazine (1:1). The structural formula may be represented as follows:

[See chemical structure at top of next column.]

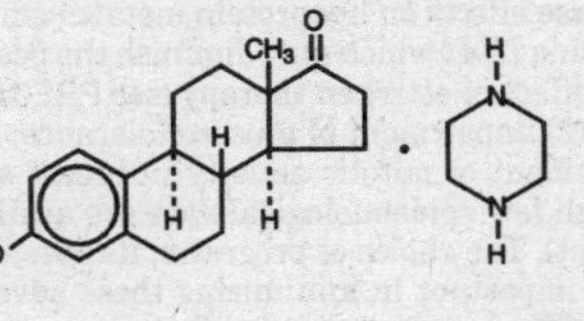

OGEN is available as tablets for oral administration containing either 0.75 mg (OGEN .625), 1.5 mg (OGEN 1.25), or 3 mg (OGEN 2.5) estropipate (Calculated as sodium estrone sulfate 0.625 mg, 1.25 mg, and 2.5 mg, respectively).

Inactive Ingredients

Each tablet contains: Colloidal silicon dioxide, dibasic potassium phosphate, hydrogenated vegetable oil wax, hydroxy propyl cellulose, lactose, magnesium stearate, microcrystalline cellulose, sodium starch glycolate and tromethamine.
OGEN .625 also contains: D&C Yellow No. 10 and FD&C Yellow No. 6.
OGEN 1.25 also contains: FD&C Yellow No. 6.
OGEN 2.5 also contains: FD&C Blue No. 2.

CLINICAL PHARMACOLOGY

Estrogen drug products act by regulating the transcription of a limited number of genes. Estrogens diffuse through cell membranes, distribute themselves throughout the cell, and bind to and activate the nuclear estrogen receptor, a DNA-binding protein which is found in estrogen-responsive tissues. The activated estrogen receptor binds to specific DNA sequences, or hormone-response elements, which enhance the transcription of adjacent genes and in turn lead to the observed effects. Estrogen receptors have been identified in tissues of the reproductive tract, breast, pituitary, hypothalamus, liver, and bone of women.
Estrogens are important in the development and maintenance of the female reproductive system and secondary sex characteristics. By a direct action, they cause growth and development of the uterus, Fallopian tubes, and vagina. With other hormones, such as pituitary hormones and progesterone, they cause enlargement of the breasts through promotion of ductal growth, stromal development, and the accretion of fat. Estrogens are intricately involved with other hormones, especially progesterone, in the processes of the ovulatory menstrual cycle and pregnancy, and affect the release of pituitary gonadotropins. They also contribute to the shaping of the skeleton, maintenance of tone and elasticity of urogenital structures, changes in the epiphyses of the long bones that allow for the pubertal growth spurt and its termination, and pigmentation of the nipples and genitals.
Estrogens occur naturally in several forms. The primary source of estrogen in normally cycling adult women is the ovarian follicle, which secretes 70 to 500 micrograms of estradiol daily, depending on the phase of the menstrual cycle. This is converted primarily to estrone, which circulates in roughly equal proportion to estradiol, and to small amounts of estriol. After menopause, most endogenous estrogen is produced by conversion of androstenedione, secreted by the adrenal cortex, to estrone by peripheral tissues. Thus, estrone—especially in its sulfate ester form—is the most abundant circulating estrogen in postmenopausal women. Although circulating estrogens exist in a dynamic equilibrium of metabolic interconversions, estradiol is the principal intracellular human estrogen and is substantially more potent than estrone or estriol at the receptor.
Estrogens used in therapy are well absorbed through the skin, mucous membranes, and gastrointestinal tract. When applied for a local action, absorption is usually sufficient to cause systemic effects. When conjugated with aryl and alkyl groups for parenteral administration, the rate of absorption of oily preparations is slowed with a prolonged duration of action, such that a single intramuscular injection of estradiol valerate or estradiol cypionate is absorbed over several weeks.
Administered estrogens and their esters are handled within the body essentially the same as the endogenous hormones. Metabolic conversion of estrogens occurs primarily in the liver (first pass effect), but also at local target tissue sites. Complex metabolic processes result in a dynamic equilibrium of circulating conjugated and unconjugated estrogenic forms which are continually interconverted, especially between estrone and estradiol and between esterified and unesterified forms. Although naturally-occurring estrogens circulate in the blood largely bound to sex hormone-binding globulin and albumin, only unbound estrogens enter target tissue cells. A significant proportion of the circulating estrogen exists as sulfate conjugates, especially estrone sulfate, which serves as a circulating reservoir for the formation of more active estrogenic species. A certain proportion of the estrogen is excreted into the bile and then reabsorbed from the intestine. During this enterohepatic recirculation, estrogens are desulfated and resulfated and undergo degradation through conversion to less active estrogens (estriol and other estrogens), oxidation to nonestrogenic substances (catecholestrogens, which interact with catecholamine metabolism, especially in the central nervous system), and conjugation with glucuronic acids (which are then rapidly excreted in the urine).
When given orally, naturally-occurring estrogens and their esters are extensively metabolized (first pass effect) and circulate primarily as estrone sulfate, with smaller amounts of other conjugated and unconjugated estrogenic species. This results in limited oral potency. By contrast, synthetic estrogens, such as ethinyl estradiol and the nonsteroidal estrogens, are degraded very slowly in the liver and other tissues, which results in their high intrinsic potency. Estrogen drug products administered by non-oral routes are not subject to first-pass metabolism, but also undergo significant hepatic uptake, metabolism, and enterohepatic recycling.

INDICATIONS AND USAGE

Estrogen drug products are indicated in the:
1. Treatment of moderate to severe vasomotor symptoms associated with the menopause. There is no adequate evidence that estrogens are effective for nervous symptoms or depression which might occur during menopause and they should not be used to treat these conditions.
2. Treatment of vulval and vaginal atrophy.
3. Treatment of hypoestrogenism due to hypogonadism, castration or primary ovarian failure.
4. Prevention of osteoporosis.

Since estrogen administration is associated with risk, selection of patients should ideally be based on prospective identification of risk factors for developing osteoporosis. Unfortunately, there is no certain way to identify those women who will develop osteoporotic fractures. Most prospective studies of efficacy for this indication have been carried out in white menopausal women, without stratification by other risk factors, and tend to show a universally salutary effect on bone. Thus, patient selection must be individualized based on the balance of risks and benefits. A more favorable risk/benefit ratio exists in a hysterectomized woman because she has no risk of endometrial cancer (see BOXED WARNINGS).
Estrogen replacement therapy reduces bone resorption and retards or halts postmenopausal bone loss. Case-control studies have shown an approximately 60 percent reduction in hip and wrist fractures in women whose estrogen replacement was begun within a few years of menopause. Studies also suggest that estrogen reduces the rate of vertebral fractures. Even when started as late as 6 years after menopause, estrogen prevents further loss of bone mass for as long as the treatment is continued. The results of a double-blind, placebo-controlled two-year study have shown that treatment with one tablet of OGEN .625 daily for 25 days (of a 31-day cycle per month) prevents vertebral bone mass loss in postmenopausal women. When estrogen therapy is discontinued, bone mass declines at a rate comparable to the immediate postmenopausal period. There is no evidence that estrogen replacement therapy restores bone mass to premenopausal levels.
At skeletal maturity there are sex and race differences in both the total amount of bone present and its density, in favor of men and blacks. Thus, women are at higher risk than men because they start with less bone mass and, for several years following natural or induced menopause, the rate of bone mass decline is accelerated. White and Asian women are at higher risk than black women.
Early menopause is one of the strongest predictors for the development of osteoporosis. In addition, other factors affecting the skeleton which are associated with osteoporosis include genetic factors (small build, family history), endocrine factors (nulliparity, thyrotoxicosis, hyperparathyroidism, Cushing's syndrome, hyperprolactinemia, Type I diabetes), lifestyle (cigarette smoking, alcohol abuse, sedentary exercise habits) and nutrition (below average body weight, dietary calcium intake).
The mainstays of prevention and management of osteoporosis are estrogen, an adequate lifetime calcium intake, and exercise. Postmenopausal women absorb dietary calcium less efficiently than premenopausal women and require an average of 1500 mg/day of elemental calcium to remain in neutral calcium balance. By comparison, premenopausal women require about 1000 mg/day and the average calcium intake in the USA is 400-600 mg/day. Therefore, when not contraindicated, calcium supplementation may be helpful.
Weight-bearing exercise and nutrition may be important adjuncts to the prevention and management of osteoporosis. Immobilization and prolonged bed rest produce rapid bone

Continued on next page

Information on these Pharmacia & Upjohn products is based on labeling in effect June 1, 1996. Further information concerning these and other Pharmacia & Upjohn products may be obtained by direct inquiry to Medical Information, Pharmacia & Upjohn, Kalamazoo, MI 49001.

Pharmacia & Upjohn—Cont.

loss, while weight-bearing exercise has been shown both to reduce bone loss and to increase bone mass. The optimal type and amount of physical activity that would prevent osteoporosis have not been established, however in two studies an hour of walking and running exercises twice or three times weekly significantly increased lumbar spine bone mass.

CONTRAINDICATIONS

Estrogens should not be used in individuals with any of the following conditions:
1. Known or suspected pregnancy (see BOXED WARNINGS). Estrogens may cause fetal harm when administered to a pregnant woman.
2. Undiagnosed abnormal genital bleeding.
3. Known or suspected cancer of the breast except in appropriately selected patients being treated for metastatic disease.
4. Known or suspected estrogen-dependent neoplasia.
5. Active thrombophlebitis or thromboembolic disorders.

WARNINGS

1. *Induction of malignant neoplasms.*
Endometrial cancer. The reported endometrial cancer risk among unopposed estrogen users is about 2-12-fold greater than in nonusers, and appears dependent on duration of treatment and on estrogen dose. Most studies show no significant increased risk associated with use of estrogens for less than one year. The greatest risk appears associated with prolonged use - with increased risks of 15-24-fold for five to ten years or more. In three studies, persistence of risk was demonstrated for 8 to over 15 years after cessation of estrogen treatment. In one study a significant decrease in the incidence of endometrial cancer occurred six months after estrogen withdrawal. Concurrent progestin therapy may offset this risk but the overall health impact in postmenopausal women is not known (see PRECAUTIONS).
Breast Cancer. While the majority of studies have not shown an increased risk of breast cancer in women who have ever used estrogen replacement therapy, some have reported a moderately increased risk (relative risks of 1.3-2.0) in those taking higher doses or those taking lower doses for prolonged periods of time, especially in excess of 10 years. Other studies have not shown this relationship.
Congenital lesions with malignant potential. Estrogen therapy during pregnancy is associated with an increased risk of fetal congenital reproductive tract disorders, and possibly other birth defects. Studies of women who received DES during pregnancy have shown that female offspring have an increased risk of vaginal adenosis, squamous cell dysplasia of the uterine cervix, and clear cell vaginal cancer later in life; male offspring have an increased risk of urogenital abnormalities and possibly testicular cancer later in life. Although some of these changes are benign, others are precursors of malignancy.
2. *Gallbladder disease.* Two studies have reported a 2- to 4-fold increase in the risk of gallbladder disease requiring surgery in women receiving postmenopausal estrogens.
3. *Cardiovascular disease.* Large doses of estrogen (5 mg conjugated estrogens per day), comparable to those used to treat cancer of the prostate and breast, have been shown in a large prospective clinical trial in men to increase the risks of nonfatal myocardial infarction, pulmonary embolism, and thrombophlebitis. These risks cannot necessarily be extrapolated from men to women. However, to avoid the theoretical cardiovascular risk to women caused by high estrogen doses, the dose for estrogen replacement therapy should not exceed the lowest effective dose.
4. *Elevated blood pressure.* Occasional blood pressure increases during estrogen replacement therapy have been attributed to idiosyncratic reactions to estrogens. More often, blood pressure has remained the same or has dropped. One study showed that postmenopausal estrogen users have higher blood pressure than nonusers. Two other studies showed slightly lower blood pressure among estrogen users compared to nonusers. Postmenopausal estrogen use does not increase the risk of stroke. Nonetheless, blood pressure should be monitored at regular intervals with estrogen use.
5. *Hypercalcemia.* Administration of estrogens may lead to severe hypercalcemia in patients with breast cancer and bone metastases. If this occurs, the drug should be stopped and appropriate measures taken to reduce the serum calcium level.

PRECAUTIONS

A. General
1. Addition of a progestin. Studies of the addition of a progestin for seven or more days of a cycle of estrogen administration have reported a lowered incidence of endometrial hyperplasia which would otherwise be induced by estrogen treatment. Morphological and biochemical studies of endometrium suggest that 10 to 14 days of progestin are needed to provide maximal maturation of the endometrium and to eliminate any hyperplastic changes. There are possible additional risks which may be associated with the inclusion of progestins in estrogen replacement regimens. These include: (1) adverse effects on lipoprotein metabolism (lowering HDL and raising LDL) which may diminish the possible cardioprotective effect of estrogen therapy (see PRECAUTIONS, D.4., below); (2) impairment of glucose tolerance; and (3) possible enhancement of mitotic activity in breast epithelial tissue (although few epidemiological data are available to address this point). The choice of progestin, its dose, and its regimen may be important in minimizing these adverse effects, but these issues remain to be clarified.
2. Physical examination. A complete medical and family history should be taken prior to the initiation of any estrogen therapy. The pretreatment and periodic physical examinations should include special reference to blood pressure, breasts, abdomen, and pelvic organs, and should include a Papanicolaou smear. As a general rule, estrogen should not be prescribed for longer than one year without reexamining the patient.
3. Hypercoagulability. Some studies have shown that women taking estrogen replacement therapy have hypercoagulability, primarily related to decreased antithrombin activity. This effect appears dose- and duration-dependent and is less pronounced than that associated with oral contraceptive use. Also, postmenopausal women tend to have increased coagulation parameters at baseline compared to premenopausal women. There is some suggestion that low dose postmenopausal mestranol may increase the risk of thromboembolism, although the majority of studies (of primarily conjugated estrogen users) report no such increase. There is insufficient information on hypercoagulability in women who have had previous thrombo embolic disease.
4. Familial hyperlipoproteinemia. Estrogen therapy may be associated with massive elevations of plasma triglycerides leading to pancreatitis and other complications in patients with familial defects of lipoprotein metabolism.
5. Fluid retention. Because estrogens may cause some degree of fluid retention, conditions which might be exacerbated by this factor, such as asthma, epilepsy, migraine, and cardiac or renal dysfunction, require careful observation.
6. Uterine bleeding and mastodynia. Certain patients may develop undesirable manifestations of estrogenic stimulation, such as abnormal uterine bleeding and mastodynia.
7. Impaired liver function. Estrogen may be poorly metabolized in patients with impaired liver function and should be administered with caution.
B. Information for the Patient. See text of Patient Package Insert below.
C. Laboratory Tests. Estrogen administration should generally be guided by clinical response at the smallest dose, rather than laboratory monitoring, for relief of symptoms for those indications in which symptoms are observable. For prevention and treatment of osteoporosis, however, see DOSAGE AND ADMINISTRATION section.
D. Drug/Laboratory Test Interactions.
1. Accelerated prothrombin time, partial thromboplastin time, and platelet aggregation time; increased platelet count; increased factors II, VII antigen, VIII antigen, VIII coagulant activity, IX, X, XII, VII-X complex, II-VII-X complex, and beta-thromboglobulin; decreased levels of antifactor Xa and antithrombin III, decreased antithrombin III activity; increased levels of fibrinogen and fibrinogen activity; increased plasminogen antigen and activity.
2. Increased thyroid-binding globulin (TBG) leading to increased circulating total thyroid hormone, as measured by protein-bound iodine (PBI), T4 levels (by column or by radioimmunoassay) or T3 levels by radioimmunoassay. T3 resin uptake is decreased, reflecting the elevated TBG. Free T4 and free T3 concentrations are unaltered.
3. Other binding proteins may be elevated in serum, i.e., corticosteroid binding globulin (CBG), sex hormone-binding globulin (SHBG), leading to increased circulating corticosteroids and sex steroids respectively. Free or biologically active hormone concentrations are unchanged. Other plasma proteins may be increased (angiotensinogen/renin substrate, alpha-1-antitrypsin, ceruloplasmin).
4. Increased plasma HDL and HDL-2 subfraction concentrations, reduced LDL cholesterol concentration, increased triglycerides levels.
5. Impaired glucose tolerance.
6. Reduced response to metyrapone test.
7. Reduced serum folate concentration.
E. Carcinogenesis, Mutagenesis, and Impairment of Fertility. Long term continuous administration of natural and synthetic estrogens in certain animal species increases the frequency of carcinomas of the breast, uterus, cervix, vagina, testis, and liver. See "CONTRAINDICATIONS" and "WARNINGS" sections.
F. Pregnancy Category X. Estrogens should not be used during pregnancy. See "CONTRAINDICATIONS" and BOXED WARNINGS.
G. Nursing Mothers. As a general principle, the administration of any drug to nursing mothers should be done only when clearly necessary since many drugs are excreted in human milk. In addition, estrogen administration to nursing mothers has been shown to decrease the quantity and quality of the milk.

ADVERSE REACTIONS

The following additional adverse reactions have been reported with estrogen therapy (see WARNINGS regarding induction of neoplasia, adverse effects on the fetus, increased incidence of gallbladder disease, cardiovascular disease, elevated blood pressure, and hypercalcemia).
1. *Genitourinary system.*
Changes in vaginal bleeding pattern and abnormal withdrawal bleeding or flow; breakthrough bleeding, spotting. Increase in size of uterine leiomyomata. Vaginal candidiasis. Change in amount of cervical secretion.
2. *Breast.*
Tenderness, enlargement.
3. *Gastrointestinal.*
Nausea, vomiting.
Abdominal cramps, bloating.
Cholestatic jaundice.
Increased incidence of gallbladder disease.
4. *Skin.*
Chloasma or melasma that may persist when drug is discontinued.
Erythema multiforme.
Erythema nodosum.
Hemorrhagic eruption.
Loss of scalp hair.
Hirsutism.
5. *Eyes.*
Steepening of corneal curvature.
Intolerance to contact lenses.
6. *Central Nervous System.*
Headache, migraine, dizziness.
Mental depression.
Chorea.
7. *Miscellaneous.*
Increase or decrease in weight.
Reduced carbohydrate tolerance.
Aggravation of porphyria.
Edema.
Changes in libido.

OVERDOSAGE

Serious ill effects have not been reported following acute ingestion of large doses of estrogen-containing oral contraceptives by young children. Overdosage of estrogen may cause nausea and vomiting, and withdrawal bleeding may occur in females.

DOSAGE AND ADMINISTRATION

1. For treatment of moderate to severe vasomotor symptoms, vulval and vaginal atrophy associated with the menopause, the lowest dose and regimen that will control symptoms should be chosen and medication should be discontinued as promptly as possible.
Attempts to discontinue or taper medication should be made at 3-month to 6-month intervals.
Usual dosage ranges:
Vasomotor symptoms—One OGEN .625 (0.75 mg estropipate) tablet to two OGEN 2.5 (3 mg estropipate) tablets per day. The lowest dose that will control symptoms should be chosen. If the patient has not menstruated within the last two months or more, cyclic administration is started arbitrarily. If the patient is menstruating, cyclic administration is started on day 5 of bleeding.
Vulval and vaginal atrophy—One OGEN .625 (0.75 mg estropipate) tablet to two OGEN 2.5 (3 mg estropipate) tablets daily, depending upon the tissue response of the individual patient. The lowest dose that will control symptoms should be chosen. Administer cyclically.
2. For treatment of female hypoestrogenism due to hypogonadism, castration, or primary ovarian failure.
Usual dosage ranges:
Female hypogonadism—A daily dose of one OGEN 1.25 (1.5 mg estropipate) tablet to three OGEN 2.5 (3 mg estropipate) tablets may be given for the first three weeks of a theoretical cycle, followed by a rest period of eight to ten days. The lowest dose that will control symptoms should be chosen. If bleeding does not occur by the end of this period, the same dosage schedule is repeated. The number of courses of estrogen therapy necessary to produce bleeding may vary depending on the responsiveness of the endometrium. If satisfactory withdrawal bleeding does not occur, an oral progestogen may be given in addition to estrogen during the third week of the cycle.
Female castration or primary ovarian failure—A daily dose of one OGEN 1.25 (1.5 mg estropipate) tablet to three OGEN 2.5 (3 mg estropipate) tablets may be given for the first three weeks of a theoretical cycle, followed by a rest period of eight to ten days. Adjust dosage upward or downward according to severity of symptoms and response of the patient. For maintenance, adjust dosage to lowest level that will provide effective control.
Treated patients with an intact uterus should be monitored closely for signs of endometrial cancer and appropriate diagnostic measures should be taken to rule out malignancy in the event of persistent or recurring abnormal vaginal bleeding.

3. For prevention of osteoporosis. A daily dose of one OGEN .625 (0.75 mg estropipate) tablet for 25 days of a 31-day cycle per month.

HOW SUPPLIED

OGEN (estropipate tablets, USP) is supplied as OGEN .625 (0.75 mg estropipate; calculated as sodium estrone sulfate 0.625 mg), yellow, scored tablets, imprinted U 3772, NDC 0009-3772-01; OGEN 1.25 (1.5 mg estropipate; calculated as sodium estrone sulfate 1.25 mg), peach-colored, scored tablets, imprinted U 3773, NDC 0009-3773-01; and OGEN 2.5 (3 mg estropipate; calculated as sodium estrone sulfate 2.5 mg), blue, scored tablets, imprinted U 3774, NDC 0009-3774-01. Tablets of all three dosage levels are standardized to provide uniform estrone activity and are scored to provide dosage flexibility. All tablet sizes of OGEN are available in bottles of 100.

Recommended storage: Store below 77°F (25°C).

PATIENT INFORMATION
WHAT YOU SHOULD KNOW ABOUT ESTROGENS

OGEN® ℞
brand of estropipate tablets, USP

INTRODUCTION

This leaflet describes when and how to use estrogens, and the risks and benefits of estrogen treatment.

Estrogens have important benefits but also some risks. You must decide, with your doctor, whether the risks to you of estrogen use are acceptable because of their benefits. If you use estrogens, check with your doctor to be sure you are using the lowest possible dose that works, and that you don't use them longer than necessary. How long you need to use estrogens will depend on the reason for use.

WARNINGS

ESTROGENS INCREASE THE RISK OF CANCER OF THE UTERUS IN WOMEN WHO HAVE HAD THEIR MENOPAUSE ("CHANGE OF LIFE").

If you use any estrogen-containing drug, it is important to visit your doctor regularly and report any unusual vaginal bleeding right away. Vaginal bleeding after menopause may be a warning sign of uterine cancer. Your doctor should evaluate any unusual vaginal bleeding to find out the cause.

ESTROGENS SHOULD NOT BE USED DURING PREGNANCY.

Estrogens do not prevent miscarriage (spontaneous abortion) and are not needed in the days following childbirth. If you take estrogens during pregnancy, your unborn child has a greater than usual chance of having birth defects. The risk of developing these defects is small, but clearly larger than the risk in children whose mothers did not take estrogens during pregnancy. These birth defects may affect the baby's urinary system and sex organs. Daughters born to mothers who took DES (an estrogen drug) have a higher than usual chance of developing cancer of the vagina or cervix when they become teenagers or young adults. Sons may have a higher than usual chance of developing cancer of the testicles when they become teenagers or young adults.

USES OF ESTROGEN

(Not every estrogen drug is approved for every use listed in this section. If you want to know which of these possible uses are approved for the medicine prescribed for you, ask your doctor or pharmacist to show you the professional labeling. You can also look up the specific estrogen product in a book called the "Physicians' Desk Reference", which is available in many book stores and public libraries. Generic drugs carry virtually the same labeling information as their brand name versions.)

+ To reduce moderate or severe menopausal symptoms.
Estrogens are hormones made by the ovaries of normal women. Between ages 45 and 55, the ovaries normally stop making estrogens. This leads to a drop in body estrogen levels which causes the "change of life" or menopause (the end of monthly menstrual periods). If both ovaries are removed during an operation before natural menopause takes place, the sudden drop in estrogen levels causes "surgical menopause".

When the estrogen levels begin dropping, some women develop very uncomfortable symptoms, such as feelings of warmth in the face, neck, and chest, or sudden intense episodes of heat and sweating ("hot flashes" or "hot flushes"). Using estrogen drugs can help the body adjust to lower estrogen levels and reduce these symptoms. Most women have only mild menopausal symptoms or none at all and do not need to use estrogen drugs for these symptoms. Others may need to take estrogens for a few months while their bodies adjust to lower estrogen levels. The majority of women do not need estrogen replacement for longer than six months for these symptoms.

+ To treat vulval and vaginal atrophy (itching, burning, dryness in or around the vagina, difficulty or burning on urination) associated with menopause.

+ To treat certain conditions in which a young woman's ovaries do not produce enough estrogen naturally.

+ To treat certain types of abnormal vaginal bleeding due to hormonal imbalance when your doctor has found no serious cause of the bleeding.

+ To treat certain cancers in special situations, in men and women.

+ To prevent thinning of bones.
Osteoporosis is a thinning of the bones that makes them weaker and allows them to break more easily. The bones of the spine, wrists and hips break most often in osteoporosis. Both men and women start to lose bone mass after about age 40, but women lose bone mass faster after the menopause. Using estrogens after the menopause slows down bone thinning and may prevent bones from breaking. Lifelong adequate calcium intake, either in the diet (such as dairy products) or by calcium supplements (to reach a total daily intake of 1000 milligrams per day before menopause or 1500 milligrams per day after menopause), may help to prevent osteoporosis. Regular weight-bearing exercise (like walking and running for an hour, two or three times a week) may also help to prevent osteoporosis. Before you change your calcium intake or exercise habits, it is important to discuss these lifestyle changes with your doctor to find out if they are safe for you.

Since estrogen use has some risks, only women who are likely to develop osteoporosis should use estrogens for prevention. Women who are likely to develop osteoporosis often have the following characteristics: white or Asian race, slim, cigarette smokers, and a family history of osteoporosis in a mother, sister, or aunt. Women who have relatively early menopause, often because their ovaries were removed during an operation ("surgical menopause"), are more likely to develop osteoporosis than women whose menopause happens at the average age.

WHO SHOULD NOT USE ESTROGENS

Estrogens should not be used:

+ During pregnancy (see BOXED WARNINGS).
If you think you may be pregnant, do not use any form of estrogen-containing drug. Using estrogens while you are pregnant may cause your unborn child to have birth defects. Estrogens do not prevent miscarriage.

+ If you have unusual vaginal bleeding which has not been evaluated by your doctor (see BOXED WARNINGS).
Unusual vaginal bleeding can be a warning sign of cancer of the uterus, especially if it happens after menopause. Your doctor must find out the cause of the bleeding so that he or she can recommend the proper treatment. Taking estrogens without visiting your doctor can cause you serious harm if your vaginal bleeding is caused by cancer of the uterus.

+ If you have had cancer.
Since estrogens increase the risk of certain types of cancer, you should not use estrogens if you have ever had cancer of the breast or uterus, unless your doctor recommends that the drug may help in the cancer treatment. (For certain patients with breast or prostate cancer, estrogens may help.)

+ If you have any circulation problems.
Estrogen drugs should not be used except in unusually special situations in which your doctor judges that you need estrogen therapy so much that the risks are acceptable. Men and women with abnormal blood clotting conditions should avoid estrogen use (see **DANGERS OF ESTROGENS**, below).

+ When they do not work.
During menopause, some women develop nervous symptoms or depression. Estrogens do not relieve these symptoms. You may have heard that taking estrogens for years after menopause will keep your skin soft and supple and keep you feeling young. There is no evidence for these claims and such long-term estrogen use may have serious risks.

+ After childbirth or when breastfeeding a baby.
Estrogens should not be used to try to stop the breasts from filling with milk after a baby is born. Such treatment may increase the risk of developing blood clots (see **DANGERS OF ESTROGENS**, below).

If you are breastfeeding, you should avoid using any drugs because many drugs pass through to the baby in the milk. While nursing a baby, you should take drugs only on the advice of your health care provider.

DANGERS OF ESTROGENS

+ Cancer of the uterus.
Your risk of developing cancer of the uterus gets higher the longer you use estrogens and the larger doses you use. One study showed that after women stop taking estrogens, this higher cancer risk quickly returns to the usual level of risk (as if you had never used estrogen therapy). Three other studies showed that the cancer risk stayed high for 8 to more than 15 years after stopping estrogen treatment. **Because of this risk, IT IS IMPORTANT TO TAKE THE LOWEST DOSE THAT WORKS AND TO TAKE IT ONLY AS LONG AS YOU NEED IT.**

Using progestin therapy together with estrogen therapy may reduce the higher risk of uterine cancer related to estrogen use (but see **OTHER INFORMATION**, below).

If you have had your uterus removed (total hysterectomy), there is no danger of developing cancer of the uterus.

+ Cancer of the breast.
Most studies have not shown a higher risk of breast cancer in women who have ever used estrogens. However, some studies have reported that breast cancer developed more often (up to twice the usual rate) in women who used estrogens for long periods of time (especially more than 10 years), or who used higher doses for shorter time periods.

Regular breast examinations by a health professional and monthly self-examination are recommended for all women.

+ Gallbladder disease.
Women who use estrogens after menopause are more likely to develop gallbladder disease needing surgery than women who do not use estrogens.

+ Abnormal blood clotting.
Taking estrogens may cause changes in your blood clotting system. These changes allow the blood to clot more easily, possibly allowing clots to form in your bloodstream. If blood clots do form in your bloodstream, they can cut off the blood supply to vital organs, causing serious problems. These problems may include a stroke (by cutting off blood to the brain), a heart attack (by cutting off blood to the heart), a pulmonary embolus (by cutting off blood to the lungs), or other problems. Any of these conditions may cause death or serious long term disability. How ever, most studies of low dose estrogen usage by women do not show an increased risk of these complications.

SIDE EFFECTS

In addition to the risks listed above, the following side effects have been reported with estrogen use:

Nausea and vomiting.

Breast tenderness or enlargement.

Enlargement of benign tumors ("fibroids") of the uterus.

Retention of excess fluid. This may make some conditions worsen, such as asthma, epilepsy, migraine, heart disease, or kidney disease.

A spotty darkening of the skin, particularly on the face.

REDUCING RISK OF ESTROGEN USE

If you use estrogens, you can reduce your risks by doing these things:

+ See your doctor regularly. While you are using estrogens, it is important to visit your doctor at least once a year for a check-up. If you develop vaginal bleeding while taking estrogens, you may need further evaluation. If members of your family have had breast cancer or if you have ever had breast lumps or an abnormal mammogram (breast x-ray), you may need to have more frequent breast examinations.

+ Reassess your need for estrogens. You and your doctor should reevaluate whether or not you still need estrogens at least every six months.

+ Be alert for signs of trouble. If any of these warning signals (or any other unusual symptoms) happen while you are using estrogens, call your doctor immediately:

Abnormal bleeding from the vagina (possible uterine cancer).

Pains in the calves or chest, sudden shortness of breath, or coughing blood (possible clot in the legs, heart, or lungs).

Severe headache or vomiting, dizziness, faintness, changes in vision or speech, weakness or numbness of an arm or leg (possible clot in the brain or eye).

Breast lumps (possible breast cancer; ask your doctor or health professional to show you how to examine your breasts monthly).

Yellowing of the skin or eyes (possible liver problem).

Pain, swelling, or tenderness in the abdomen (possible gallbladder problem).

OTHER INFORMATION

Some doctors may choose to prescribe a progestin, a different hormonal drug, for you to take together with your estrogen treatment. Progestins lower your risk of developing endometrial hyperplasia (a possible pre-cancerous condition of the uterus) while using estrogens. Taking estrogens and progestins together may also protect you from the higher risk of uterine cancer, but this has not been clearly established. Combined use of progestin and estrogen treatment may have additional risks, however. The possible risks include unhealthy effects on blood fats (especially a lowering of HDL cholesterol, the "good" blood fat which protects against heart disease risk), unhealthy effects on blood sugar (which might worsen a diabetic condition), and a possible further increase in the breast cancer risk which may be associated

Continued on next page

Information on these Pharmacia & Upjohn products is based on labeling in effect June 1, 1996. Further information concerning these and other Pharmacia & Upjohn products may be obtained by direct inquiry to Medical Information, Pharmacia & Upjohn, Kalamazoo, MI 49001.

Pharmacia & Upjohn—Cont.

with long-term estrogen use. The type of progestin drug used and its dosage schedule may be important in minimizing these effects.

Your doctor has prescribed this drug for you and you alone. Do not give the drug to anyone else.

If you will be taking calcium supplements as part of the treatment to help prevent osteoporosis, check with your doctor about how much to take.

Keep this and all drugs out of the reach of children. In case of overdose, call your doctor, hospital or poison control center immediately.

This leaflet provides a summary of the most important information about estrogens. If you want more information, ask your doctor or pharmacist to show you the professional labeling. The professional labeling is also published in a book called the "Physicians' Desk Reference", which is available in book stores and public libraries. Generic drugs carry virtually the same labeling information as their brand name versions.

HOW SUPPLIED

OGEN (estropipate tablets, USP) is supplied as: OGEN .625 (0.75 mg estropipate), yellow tablets; OGEN 1.25 (1.5 mg estropipate), peach-colored tablets; OGEN 2.5 (3 mg estropipate), blue tablets.

By Abbott Laboratories
North Chicago, IL 60064, USA
Revised March 1994 816 035 002

Shown in Product Identification Guide, page 329

OGEN® ℞
brand of estropipate vaginal cream, USP

WARNING:

1. ESTROGENS HAVE BEEN REPORTED TO INCREASE THE RISK OF ENDOMETRIAL CARCINOMA IN POSTMENOPAUSAL WOMEN.

Close clinical surveillance of all women taking estrogens is important. Adequate diagnostic measures, including endometrial sampling when indicated, should be undertaken to rule out malignancy in all cases of undiagnosed persistent or recurring abnormal vaginal bleeding. There is no evidence that "natural" estrogens are more or less hazardous than "synthetic" estrogens at equi-estrogenic doses.

2. ESTROGENS SHOULD NOT BE USED DURING PREGNANCY.

There is no indication for estrogen therapy during pregnancy or during the immediate postpartum period. Estrogens are ineffective for the prevention or treatment of threatened, or habitual abortion. Estrogens are not indicated for the prevention of postpartum breast engorgement.

Estrogen therapy during pregnancy is associated with an increased risk of congenital defects in the reproductive organs of the fetus, and possibly other birth defects. Studies of women who received diethylstilbestrol (DES) during pregnancy have shown that female offspring have an increased risk of vaginal adenosis, squamous cell dysplasia of the uterine cervix, and clear cell vaginal cancer later in life; male offspring have an increased risk of urogenital abnormalities and possibly testicular cancer later in life. The 1985 DES Task Force concluded that use of DES during pregnancy is associated with a subsequent increased risk of breast cancer in the mothers, although a causal relationship remains unproven and the observed level of excess risk is similar to that for a number of other breast cancer risk factors.

DESCRIPTION

OGEN (estropipate), (formerly piperazine estrone sulfate), is a natural estrogenic substance prepared from purified crystalline estrone, solubilized as the sulfate and stabilized with piperazine. It is appreciably soluble in water and has almost no odor or taste. The amount of piperazine in OGEN is not sufficient to exert a pharmacological action. Its addition ensures solubility, stability, and uniform potency of the estrone sulfate. Chemically estropipate, molecular weight: 436.56, is represented by estra-1,3,5(10)-trien-17-one,3-(sulfooxy)-, compound with piperazine (1:1). The structural formula may be represented as follows:

[See chemical structure at top of next column.]

Each gram of OGEN Vaginal Cream contains 1.5 mg estropipate in a base composed of the following ingredients: glycerin, mineral oil, glyceryl monostearate, polyethylene glycol ether complex of higher fatty alcohols, cetyl alcohol, anhydrous lanolin, sodium biphosphate, cis-N-(3-chloroallyl) hex-

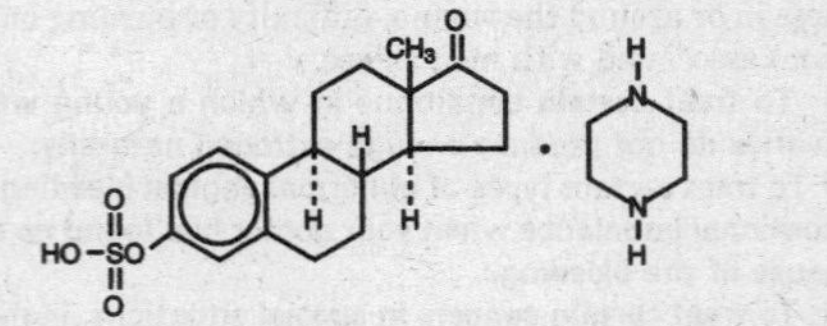

aminium chloride, propylparaben, methylparaben, piperazine hexahydrate, citric acid and water.

CLINICAL PHARMACOLOGY

Estrogen drug products act by regulating the transcription of a limited number of genes. Estrogens diffuse through cell membranes, distribute themselves throughout the cell, and bind to and activate the nuclear estrogen receptor, a DNA-binding protein which is found in estrogen-responsive tissues. The activated estrogen receptor binds to specific DNA sequences, or hormone-response elements, which enhance the transcription of adjacent genes and in turn lead to the observed effects. Estrogen receptors have been identified in tissues of the reproductive tract, breast, pituitary, hypothalamus, liver, and bone of women.

Estrogens are important in the development and maintenance of the female reproductive system and secondary sex characteristics. By a direct action, they cause growth and development of the uterus, Fallopian tubes, and vagina. With other hormones, such as pituitary hormones and progesterone, they cause enlargement of the breasts through promotion of ductal growth, stromal development, and the accretion of fat. Estrogens are intricately involved with other hormones, especially progesterone, in the processes of the ovulatory menstrual cycle and pregnancy, and affect the release of pituitary gonadotropins. They also contribute to the shaping of the skeleton, maintenance of tone and elasticity of urogenital structures, changes in the epiphyses of the long bones that allow for the pubertal growth spurt and its termination, and pigmentation of the nipples and genitals.

Estrogens occur naturally in several forms. The primary source of estrogen in normally cycling adult women is the ovarian follicle, which secretes 70 to 500 micrograms of estradiol daily, depending on the phase of the menstrual cycle. This is converted primarily to estrone, which circulates in roughly equal proportion to estradiol, and to small amounts of estriol. After menopause, most endogenous estrogen is produced by conversion of androstenedione, secreted by the adrenal cortex, to estrone by peripheral tissues. Thus, estrone — especially in its sulfate ester form — is the most abundant circulating estrogen in postmenopausal women. Although circulating estrogens exist in a dynamic equilibrium of metabolic interconversions, estradiol is the principal intracellular human estrogen and is substantially more potent than estrone or estriol at the receptor.

Estrogens used in therapy are well absorbed through the skin, mucous membranes, and gastrointestinal tract. When applied for a local action, absorption is usually sufficient to cause systemic effects. When conjugated with aryl and alkyl groups for parenteral administration, the rate of absorption of oily preparations is slowed with a prolonged duration of action, such that a single intramuscular injection of estradiol valerate or estradiol cypionate is absorbed over several weeks.

Administered estrogens and their esters are handled within the body essentially the same as the endogenous hormones. Metabolic conversion of estrogens occurs primarily in the liver (first pass effect), but also at local target tissue sites. Complex metabolic processes result in a dynamic equilibrium of circulating conjugated and unconjugated estrogenic forms which are continually interconverted, especially between estrone and estradiol and between esterified and unesterified forms. Although naturally-occurring estrogens circulate in the blood largely bound to sex hormone-binding globulin and albumin, only unbound estrogens enter target tissue cells. A significant proportion of the circulating estrogen exists as sulfate conjugates, especially estrone sulfate, which serves as a circulating reservoir for the formation of more active estrogenic species. A certain proportion of the estrogen is excreted into the bile and then reabsorbed from the intestine. During this enterohepatic recirculation, estrogens are desulfated and resulfated and undergo degradation through conversion to less active estrogens (estriol and other estrogens), oxidation to nonestrogenic substances (catecholestrogens, which interact with catecholamine metabolism, especially in the central nervous system), and conjugation with glucuronic acids (which are then rapidly excreted in the urine).

When given orally, naturally-occurring estrogens and their esters are extensively metabolized (first pass effect) and circulate primarily as estrone sulfate, with smaller amounts of other conjugated and unconjugated estrogenic species. This results in limited oral potency. By contrast, synthetic estrogens, such as ethinyl estradiol and the nonsteroidal estrogens, are degraded very slowly in the liver and other tissues, which results in their high intrinsic potency. Estrogen drug products administered by non-oral routes are not subject to first-pass metabolism, but also undergo significant hepatic uptake, metabolism, and enterohepatic recycling.

INDICATIONS AND USAGE

OGEN Vaginal Cream is indicated for the treatment of vulval and vaginal atrophy.

CONTRAINDICATIONS

Estrogens should not be used in individuals with any of the following conditions:

1. Known or suspected pregnancy (see boxed **WARNING**). Estrogens may cause fetal harm when administered to a pregnant woman.
2. Undiagnosed abnormal genital bleeding.
3. Known or suspected cancer of the breast except in appropriately selected patients being treated for metastatic disease.
4. Known or suspected estrogen-dependent neoplasia.
5. Active thrombophlebitis or thromboembolic disorders.

OGEN Vaginal Cream (estropipate) is contraindicated in patients hypersensitive to its ingredients.

WARNINGS

1. Induction of malignant neoplasms.

Endometrial cancer. The reported endometrial cancer risk among unopposed estrogen users is about 2 to 12 fold greater than in non-users, and appears dependent on duration of treatment and on estrogen dose. Most studies show no significant increased risk associated with use of estrogens for less than one year. The greatest risk appears associated with prolonged use — with increased risks of 15 to 24-fold for five to ten years or more. In three studies, persistence of risk was demonstrated for 8 to over 15 years after cessation of estrogen treatment. In one study a significant decrease in the incidence of endometrial cancer occurred six months after estrogen withdrawal. Concurrent progestin therapy may offset this risk but the overall health impact in postmenopausal women is not known (see **PRECAUTIONS**).

Breast Cancer. While the majority of studies have not shown an increased risk of breast cancer in women who have ever used estrogen replacement therapy, some have reported a moderately increased risk (relative risks of 1.3-2.0) in those taking higher doses or those taking lower doses for prolonged periods of time, especially in excess of 10 years. Other studies have not shown this relationship.

Congenital lesions with malignant potential. Estrogen therapy during pregnancy is associated with an increased risk of fetal congenital reproductive tract disorders, and possibly other birth defects. Studies of women who received DES during pregnancy have shown that female offspring have an increased risk of vaginal adenosis, squamous cell dysplasia of the uterine cervix, and clear cell vaginal cancer later in life; male offspring have an increased risk of urogenital abnormalities and possibly testicular cancer later in life. Although some of these changes are benign, others are precursors of malignancy.

2. Gallbladder disease. Two studies have reported a 2- to 4-fold increase in the risk of gallbladder disease requiring surgery in women receiving postmenopausal estrogens.

3. Cardiovascular disease. Large doses of estrogen (5 mg conjugated estrogens per day), comparable to those used to treat cancer of the prostate and breast, have been shown in a large prospective clinical trial in men to increase the risks of nonfatal myocardial infarction, pulmonary embolism, and thrombophlebitis. These risks cannot necessarily be extrapolated from men to women. However, to avoid the theoretical cardiovascular risk to women caused by high estrogen doses, the dose for estrogen replacement therapy should not exceed the lowest effective dose.

4. Elevated blood pressure. Occasional blood pressure increases during estrogen replacement therapy have been attributed to idiosyncratic reactions to estrogens. More often, blood pressure has remained the same or has dropped. One study showed that postmenopausal estrogen users have higher blood pressure than nonusers. Two other studies showed slightly lower blood pressure among estrogen users compared to nonusers. Postmenopausal estrogen use does not increase the risk of stroke. Nonetheless, blood pressure should be monitored at regular intervals with estrogen use.

5. Hypercalcemia. Administration of estrogens may lead to severe hypercalcemia in patients with breast cancer and bone metastases. If this occurs, the drug should be stopped and appropriate measures taken to reduce the serum calcium level.

PRECAUTIONS

A. General

1. Addition of a progestin. Studies of the addition of a progestin for seven or more days of a cycle of estrogen administration have reported a lowered incidence of endometrial hyperplasia which would otherwise be induced by estrogen treatment. Morphological and biochemical studies of endometrium suggest that 10 to 14 days of progestin are needed to provide maximal maturation of the endometrium and to eliminate any hyperplastic changes. There are possible addi-

tional risks which may be associated with the inclusion of progestins in estrogen replacement regimens. These include: (1) adverse effects on lipoprotein metabolism (lowering HDL and raising LDL) which may diminish the possible cardioprotective effect of estrogen therapy (see **PRECAUTIONS**, D.4., below); (2) impairment of glucose tolerance; and (3) possible enhancement of mitotic activity in breast epithelial tissue (although few epidemiological data are available to address this point). The choice of progestin, its dose, and its regimen may be important in minimizing these adverse effects, but these issues remain to be clarified.

2. Physical examination. A complete medical and family history should be taken prior to the initiation of any estrogen therapy. The pretreatment and periodic physical examinations should include special reference to blood pressure, breasts, abdomen, and pelvic organs, and should include a Papanicolaou smear. As a general rule, estrogen should not be prescribed for longer than one year without reexamining the patient.

3. Hypercoagulability. Some studies have shown that women taking estrogen replacement therapy have hypercoagulability, primarily related to decreased antithrombin activity. This effect appears dose- and duration-dependent and is less pronounced than that associated with oral contraceptive use. Also, postmenopausal women tend to have increased coagulation parameters at baseline compared to premenopausal women. There is some suggestion that low dose postmenopausal mestranol may increase the risk of thromboembolism, although the majority of studies (of primarily conjugated estrogens users) report no such increase. There is insufficient information on hypercoagulability in women who have had previous thromboembolic disease.

4. Familial hyperlipoproteinemia. Estrogen therapy may be associated with massive elevations of plasma triglycerides leading to pancreatitis and other complications in patients with familial defects of lipoprotein metabolism.

5. Fluid retention. Because estrogens may cause some degree of fluid retention, conditions which might be exacerbated by this factor, such as asthma, epilepsy, migraine, and cardiac or renal dysfunction, require careful observation.

6. Uterine bleeding and mastodynia. Certain patients may develop undesirable manifestations of estrogenic stimulation, such as abnormal uterine bleeding and mastodynia.

7. Impaired liver function. Estrogen may be poorly metabolized in patients with impaired liver function and should be administered with caution.

B. *Information for the Patient.* See text of Patient Package Insert that appears after **HOW SUPPLIED** section.

C. *Laboratory Tests.* Estrogen administration should generally be guided by clinical response at the smallest dose, rather than laboratory monitoring, for relief of symptoms for those indications in which symptoms are observable.

D. *Drug/Laboratory Test Interactions.*
1. Accelerated prothrombin time, partial thromboplastin time, and platelet aggregation time; increased platelet count; increased factors II, VII antigen, VIII antigen, VIII coagulant activity, IX, X, XII, VII—X complex, II—VII—X complex, and beta-thromboglobulin; decreased levels of anti-factor Xa and antithrombin III, decreased antithrombin III activity; increased levels of fibrinogen and fibrinogen activity; increased plasminogen antigen and activity.
2. Increased thyroid-binding globulin (TBG) leading to increased circulating total thyroid hormone, as measured by protein-bound iodine (PBI), T4 levels (by column or by radioimmunoassay) or T3 levels by radioimmunoassay. T3 resin uptake is decreased, reflecting the elevated TBG. Free T4 and free T3 concentrations are unaltered.
3. Other binding proteins may be elevated in serum, i.e., corticosteroid binding globulin (CBG), sex hormone-binding globulin (SHBG), leading to increased circulating corticosteroids and sex steroids respectively. Free or biologically active hormone concentrations are unchanged. Other plasma proteins may be increased (angiotensinogen/renin substrate, alpha-l-antitrypsin, ceruloplasmin).
4. Increased plasma HDL and HDL-2 subfraction concentrations, reduced LDL cholesterol concentration, increased triglycerides levels.
5. Impaired glucose tolerance.
6. Reduced response to metyrapone test.
7. Reduced serum folate concentration.

E. *Carcinogenesis, Mutagenesis, and Impairment of Fertility.* Long-term continuous administration of natural and synthetic estrogens in certain animal species increases the frequency of carcinomas of the breast, uterus, cervix, vagina, testis, and liver. See **CONTRAINDICATIONS** and **WARNINGS** sections.

F. *Pregnancy Category X.* Estrogens should not be used during pregnancy. See **CONTRAINDICATIONS** and boxed **WARNING.**

G. *Nursing Mothers* As a general principle, the administration of any drug to nursing mothers should be done only when clearly necessary since many drugs are excreted in human milk. In addition, estrogen administration to nursing mothers has been shown to decrease the quantity and quality of the milk.

ADVERSE REACTIONS

Hypersensitivity reactions, systemic effects such as breast tenderness, and rarely, withdrawal bleeding, have occurred with the use of topical estrogens. Local irritation (especially when prior inflammation is present) has occurred at initiation of therapy.

The following additional adverse reactions have been reported with estrogen therapy (see **WARNINGS** regarding induction of neoplasia, adverse effects on the fetus, increased incidence of gallbladder disease, cardiovascular disease, elevated blood pressure, and hypercalcemia).

1. *Genitourinary system.*
   Changes in vaginal bleeding pattern and abnormal withdrawal bleeding or flow; breakthrough bleeding, spotting.
   Increase in size of uterine leiomyomata.
   Vaginal candidiasis.
   Change in amount of cervical secretion.
2. *Breasts.*
   Tenderness, enlargement.
3. *Gastrointestinal.*
   Nausea, vomiting.
   Abdominal cramps, bloating.
   Cholestatic jaundice.
   Increased incidence of gallbladder disease.
4. *Skin.*
   Chloasma or melasma which may persist when drug is discontinued.
   Erythema multiforme.
   Erythema nodosum.
   Hemorrhagic eruption.
   Loss of scalp hair.
   Hirsutism.
5. *Eyes.*
   Steepening of corneal curvature.
   Intolerance to contact lenses.
6. *Central Nervous System.*
   Headache, migraine, dizziness.
   Mental depression.
   Chorea.
7. *Miscellaneous.*
   Increase or decrease in weight.
   Reduced carbohydrate tolerance.
   Aggravation of porphyria.
   Edema.
   Changes in libido.

OVERDOSAGE

Serious ill effects have not been reported following acute ingestion of large doses of estrogen-containing oral contraceptives by young children. Overdosage of estrogen may cause nausea and vomiting, and withdrawal bleeding may occur in females.

DOSAGE AND ADMINISTRATION

1. For treatment of vulval and vaginal atrophy associated with the menopause, the lowest dose and regimen that will control symptoms should be chosen and medication should be discontinued as promptly as possible.

Attempts to discontinue or taper medication should be made at 3-month to 6-month intervals.

Usual dosage range: Intravaginally, 2 to 4 grams of OGEN Vaginal Cream daily, depending upon the severity of the condition.

The following instructions for use are intended for the patient and are printed on the carton label for OGEN Vaginal Cream (estropipate).
1. Remove cap from tube.
2. Make sure plunger of applicator is all the way into the barrel.
3. Screw nozzle end of applicator onto the tube.
4. Squeeze tube to force sufficient cream into applicator so that number on plunger indicating prescribed dose is level with top of barrel.
5. Unscrew applicator from tube and replace cap on tube.
6. To deliver medication, insert end of applicator into vagina and push plunger all the way down.

Between uses, pull plunger out of barrel and wash applicator in warm, soapy water. DO NOT PUT APPLICATOR IN HOT OR BOILING WATER.

HOW SUPPLIED

OGEN (estropipate vaginal cream, USP), 1.5 mg estropipate per gram, is available in packages containing a $1^{1}/_{2}$ oz (42.5 g) tube with one plastic applicator calibrated at 1, 2, 3, and 4 g levels, (NDC 0009-3776-01).

RECOMMENDED STORAGE: Store below 86° F (30° C).

INFORMATION FOR PATIENTS

OGEN®   ℞

brand of estropipate vaginal cream, USP

INTRODUCTION

This leaflet describes when and how to use estrogens, and the risks and benefits of estrogen treatment.

Estrogens have important benefits but also some risks. You must decide, with your doctor, whether the risks to you of estrogen use are acceptable because of their benefits. If you use estrogens, check with your doctor to be sure you are us-

ing the lowest possible dose that works, and that you don't use them longer than necessary. How long you need to use estrogens will depend on the reason for use.

WARNINGS

ESTROGENS INCREASE THE RISK OF CANCER OF THE UTERUS IN WOMEN WHO HAVE HAD THEIR MENOPAUSE ("CHANGE OF LIFE").

If you use any estrogen-containing drug, it is important to visit your doctor regularly and report any unusual vaginal bleeding right away. Vaginal bleeding after menopause may be a warning sign of uterine cancer. Your doctor should evaluate any unusual vaginal bleeding to find out the cause.

ESTROGENS SHOULD NOT BE USED DURING PREGNANCY.

Estrogens do not prevent miscarriage (spontaneous abortion) and are not needed in the days following childbirth. If you take estrogens during pregnancy, your unborn child has a greater than usual chance of having birth defects. The risk of developing these defects is small, but clearly larger than the risk in children whose mothers did not take estrogens during pregnancy. These birth defects may affect the baby's urinary system and sex organs. Daughters born to mothers who took DES (an estrogen drug) have a higher than usual chance of developing cancer of the vagina or cervix when they become teenagers or young adults. Sons may have a higher than usual chance of developing cancer of the testicles when they become teenagers or young adults.

USES OF ESTROGEN

(Not every estrogen drug is approved for every use listed in this section. If you want to know which of these possible uses are approved for the medicine prescribed for you, ask your doctor or pharmacist to show you the professional labeling. You can also look up the specific estrogen product in a book called the "Physicians' Desk Reference," which is available in many book stores and public libraries. Generic drugs carry virtually the same labeling information as their brand name versions.)

+ To reduce moderate or severe menopausal symptoms. Estrogens are hormones made by the ovaries of normal women. Between ages 45 and 55, the ovaries normally stop making estrogens. This leads to a drop in body estrogen levels which causes the "change of life" or menopause (the end of monthly menstrual periods). If both ovaries are removed during an operation before natural menopause takes place, the sudden drop in estrogen levels causes "surgical menopause."

When the estrogen levels begin dropping, some women develop very uncomfortable symptoms, such as feelings of warmth in the face, neck, and chest, or sudden intense episodes of heat and sweating ("hot flashes" or "hot flushes"). Using estrogen drugs can help the body adjust to lower estrogen levels and reduce these symptoms. Most women have only mild menopausal symptoms or none at all and do not need to use estrogen drugs for these symptoms. Others may need to take estrogens for a few months while their bodies adjust to lower estrogen levels. The majority of women do not need estrogen replacement for longer than six months for these symptoms.

+ To treat vulval and vaginal atrophy (itching, burning, dryness in or around the vagina, difficulty or burning on urination) associated with menopause.

+ To treat certain conditions in which a young woman's ovaries do not produce enough estrogen naturally.

+ To treat certain types of abnormal vaginal bleeding due to hormonal imbalance when your doctor has found no serious cause of the bleeding.

+ To treat certain cancers in special situations, in men and women.

+ To prevent thinning of bones. Osteoporosis is a thinning of the bones that makes them weaker and allows them to break more easily. The bones of the spine, wrists and hips break most often in osteoporosis. Both men and women start to lose bone mass after about age 40, but women lose bone mass faster after the menopause. Using estrogens after the menopause slows down bone thinning and may prevent bones from breaking. Lifelong adequate calcium intake, either in the diet (such as dairy products) or by calcium supplements (to reach a total daily intake of 1000 milligrams per day before menopause or 1500 milligrams per day after menopause), may help to prevent osteoporosis. Regular weight-bearing exercise (like walking and running for an hour, two or three times a week) may also help to prevent osteoporosis.

Continued on next page

Information on these Pharmacia & Upjohn products is based on labeling in effect June 1, 1996. Further information concerning these and other Pharmacia & Upjohn products may be obtained by direct inquiry to Medical Information, Pharmacia & Upjohn, Kalamazoo, MI 49001.

Pharmacia & Upjohn—Cont.

Before you change your calcium intake or exercise habits, it is important to discuss these lifestyle changes with your doctor to find out if they are safe for you.
Since estrogen use has some risks, only women who are likely to develop osteoporosis should use estrogens for prevention. Women who are likely to develop osteoporosis often have the following characteristics: white or Asian race, slim, cigarette smokers, and a family history of osteoporosis in a mother, sister, or aunt. Women who have relatively early menopause, often because their ovaries were removed during an operation ("surgical menopause"), are more likely to develop osteoporosis than women whose menopause happens at the average age.

WHO SHOULD NOT USE ESTROGENS

Estrogens should not be used:
+ During pregnancy (see boxed **WARNING**). If you think you may be pregnant, do not use any form of estrogen-containing drug. Using estrogens while you are pregnant may cause your unborn child to have birth defects. Estrogens do not prevent miscarriage.
+ If you have unusual vaginal bleeding which has not been evaluated by your doctor (see boxed **WARNING**). Unusual vaginal bleeding can be a warning sign of cancer of the uterus, especially if it happens after menopause. Your doctor must find out the cause of the bleeding so that he or she can recommend the proper treatment. Taking estrogens without visiting your doctor can cause you serious harm if your vaginal bleeding is caused by cancer of the uterus.
+ If you have had cancer. Since estrogens increase the risk of certain types of cancer, you should not use estrogens if you have ever had cancer of the breast or uterus, unless your doctor recommends that the drug may help in the cancer treatment. (For certain patients with breast or prostate cancer, estrogens may help.)
+ If you have any circulation problems. Estrogen drugs should not be used except in unusually special situations in which your doctor judges that you need estrogen therapy so much that the risks are acceptable. Men and women with abnormal blood clotting conditions should avoid estrogen use (see **DANGERS OF ESTROGENS**, below).
+ When they do not work. During menopause, some women develop nervous symptoms or depression. Estrogens do not relieve these symptoms. You may have heard that taking estrogens for years after menopause will keep your skin soft and supple and keep you feeling young. There is no evidence for these claims and such long-term estrogen use may have serious risks.
+ After childbirth or when breastfeeding a baby. Estrogens should not be used to try to stop the breasts from filling with milk after a baby is born. Such treatment may increase the risk of developing blood clots (see Dangers of Estrogens, below).
If you are breastfeeding, you should avoid using any drugs because many drugs pass through to the baby in the milk. While nursing a baby, you should take drugs only on the advice of your health care provider.

DANGERS OF ESTROGENS

+ Cancer of the uterus. Your risk of developing cancer of the uterus gets higher the longer you use estrogens and the larger doses you use. One study showed that after women stop taking estrogens, this higher cancer risk quickly returns to the usual level of risk (as if you had never used estrogen therapy). Three other studies showed that the cancer risk stayed high for 8 to more than 15 years after stopping estrogen treatment. Because of this risk, **IT IS IMPORTANT TO TAKE THE LOWEST DOSE THAT WORKS AND TO TAKE IT ONLY AS LONG AS YOU NEED IT.**
Using progestin therapy together with estrogen therapy may reduce the higher risk of uterine cancer related to estrogen use (but see **OTHER INFORMATION**, below).
If you have had your uterus removed (total hysterectomy), there is no danger of developing cancer of the uterus.
+ Cancer of the breast. Most studies have not shown a higher risk of breast cancer in women who have ever used estrogens.
However, some studies have reported that breast cancer developed more often (up to twice the usual rate) in women who used estrogens for long periods of time (especially more than 10 years), or who used higher doses for shorter time periods.
Regular breast examinations by a health professional and monthly self-examination are recommended for all women.
+ Gallbladder disease. Women who use estrogens after menopause are more likely to develop gallbladder disease needing surgery than women who do not use estrogens.
+ Abnormal blood clotting. Taking estrogens may cause changes in your blood clotting system. These changes allow the blood to clot more easily, possibly allowing clots to form in your bloodstream. If blood clots do form in your bloodstream, they can cut off the blood supply to vital organs, causing serious problems. These problems may include a stroke (by cutting off blood to the brain), a heart attack (by cutting off blood to the heart), a pulmonary embolus (by cutting off blood to the lungs), or other problems. Any of these conditions may cause death or serious long-term disability. However, most studies of low dose estrogen usage by women do not show an increased risk of these complications.

SIDE EFFECTS

In addition to the risks listed above, the following side effects have been reported with estrogen use:
Nausea and vomiting.
Breast tenderness or enlargement.
Enlargement of benign tumors ("fibroids") of the uterus.
Retention of excess fluid. This may make some conditions worsen, such as asthma, epilepsy, migraine, heart disease, or kidney disease.
A spotty darkening of the skin, particularly on the face.

REDUCING RISK OF ESTROGEN USE

If you use estrogens, you can reduce your risks by doing these things:
+ See your doctor regularly. While you are using estrogens, it is important to visit your doctor at least once a year for a check-up. If you develop vaginal bleeding while taking estrogens, you may need further evaluation. If members of your family have had breast cancer or if you have ever had breast lumps or an abnormal mammogram (breast X-ray), you may need to have more frequent breast examinations.
+ Reassess your need for estrogens. You and your doctor should reevaluate whether or not you still need estrogens at least every six months.
+ Be alert for signs of trouble. If any of these warning signals (or any other unusual symptoms) happen while you are using estrogens, call your doctor immediately:
Abnormal bleeding from the vagina (possible uterine cancer).
Pains in the calves or chest, sudden shortness of breath, or coughing blood (possible clot in the legs, heart, or lungs).
Severe headache or vomiting, dizziness, faintness, changes in vision or speech, weakness or numbness of an arm or leg (possible clot in the brain or eye)
Breast lumps (possible breast cancer; ask your doctor or health professional to show you how to examine your breasts monthly).
Yellowing of the skin or eyes (possible liver problem).
Pain, swelling, or tenderness in the abdomen (possible gallbladder problem).

OTHER INFORMATION

Some doctors may choose to prescribe a progestin, a different hormonal drug, for you to take together with your estrogen treatment. Progestins lower your risk of developing endometrial hyperplasia (a possible pre-cancerous condition of the uterus) while using estrogens. Taking estrogens and progestins together may also protect you from the higher risk of uterine cancer, but this has not been clearly established. Combined use of progestin and estrogen treatment may have additional risks, however. The possible risks include unhealthy effects on blood fats (especially a lowering of HDL cholesterol, the "good" blood fat which protects against heart disease risk), unhealthy effects on blood sugar (which might worsen a diabetic condition), and a possible further increase in the breast cancer risk which may be associated with long-term estrogen use. The type of progestin drug used and its dosage schedule may be important in minimizing these effects.
Your doctor has prescribed this drug for you and you alone. Do not give the drug to anyone else.
If you will be taking calcium supplements as part of the treatment to help prevent osteoporosis, check with your doctor about how much to take.
Keep this and all drugs out of the reach of children. In case of overdose, call your doctor, hospital or poison control center immediately.
This leaflet provides a summary of the most important information about estrogens. If you want more information, ask your doctor or pharmacist to show you the professional labeling. The professional labeling is also published in a book called the "Physicians' Desk Reference," which is available in book stores and public libraries. Generic drugs carry virtually the same labeling information as their brand name versions.

HOW SUPPLIED

OGEN (estropipate vaginal cream, USP), 1.5 mg estropipate per gram, is available in packages containing a $1^1/_2$ oz (42.5 g) tube with one plastic applicator calibrated at 1, 2, 3, and 4 g levels, (NDC 0009-3776-01).
RECOMMENDED STORAGE: Store below 86° F (30° C).
Manufactured for
The Upjohn Company,
Kalamazoo, MI 49001, USA
By
Abbott Laboratories,
North Chicago, IL 60064, USA
Revised January 1995
03-4508-R2 (No. 2467) 816 007 002

Shown in Product Identification Guide, page 329

PREPIDIL® Gel ℞
brand of dinoprostone cervical gel
For Endocervical Use

DESCRIPTION

PREPIDIL Gel contains dinoprostone as the naturally occurring form of prostaglandin E_2 (PGE_2) and is designated chemically as (5Z, 11α, 13E, 15S) - 11,15 - Dihydroxy-9-oxo-prosta-5, 13-dien-1-oic acid. The molecular formula is $C_{20}H_{32}O_5$ and the molecular weight is 352.5. Dinoprostone occurs as a white to off-white crystalline powder with a melting point within the range of 65° to 69°C. It is soluble in ethanol, in 25% ethanol in water, and in water to the extent of 130 mg/100 mL. The active constituent of PREPIDIL Gel is dinoprostone 0.5 mg/3 g (2.5 mL gel); other constituents are colloidal silicon dioxide NF (240 mg/3 g) and triacetin USP (2760 mg/3 g).
The structural formula is represented below:

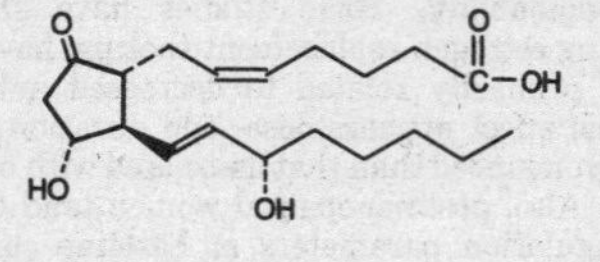

CLINICAL PHARMACOLOGY

PREPIDIL Gel (dinoprostone) administered endocervically may stimulate the myometrium of the gravid uterus to contract in a manner similar to contractions seen in the term uterus during labor. Whether or not this action results from a direct effect of dinoprostone on the myometrium has not been determined. Dinoprostone is also capable of stimulating smooth muscle of the gastrointestinal tract in humans. This activity may be responsible for the vomiting and/or diarrhea that is occasionally seen when dinoprostone is used for preinduction cervical ripening.
In laboratory animals, and also in humans, large doses of dinoprostone can lower blood pressure, probably as a result of its effect on smooth muscle of the vascular system. With the doses of dinoprostone used for cervical ripening this effect has not been seen. In laboratory animals, and also in humans, dinoprostone can elevate body temperature; however, with the dosing used for cervical ripening this effect has not been seen.
In addition to an oxytocic effect, there is evidence suggesting that this agent has a local cervical effect in initiating softening, effacement, and dilation. These changes, referred to as cervical ripening, occur spontaneously as the normal pregnancy progresses toward term and allow evacuation of uterine contents by decreasing cervical resistance at the same time that myometrial activity increases. While not completely understood, biochemical changes within the cervix during natural cervical ripening are similar to those following PGE_2-induced ripening. Further, it has been shown that these changes can take place independent of myometrial activity; however, it is quite likely that PGE_2 administered endocervically produces effacement and softening by combined contraction-inducing and cervical-ripening properties.
There is evidence to suggest that the changes that take place within the cervix are due to collagen degradation resulting from collagenase secretion as a response, at least in part, to PGE_2.
Using an unvalidated assay, the following information was determined. When PREPIDIL Gel was administered endocervically to women undergoing preinduction ripening, results from measurement of plasma levels of the metabolite 13,14-dihydro-15-keto-PGE_2 (DHK-PGE_2) showed that PGE_2 was relatively rapidly absorbed and the T_{max} was 0.5 to 0.75 hours. Plasma mean C_{max} for gel-treated subjects was 433 ± 51 pg/mL versus 137 ± 24 pg/mL for untreated controls. In those subjects in which a clinical response was observed, mean C_{max} was 484 ± 57 pg/mL versus 213 ± 69 pg/mL in nonresponders and 219 ± 92 pg/mL in control subjects who had positive clinical progression toward normal labor. These elevated levels in gel-treated subjects appear to be largely a result of absorption of PGE_2 from the gel rather than from endogenous sources.
PGE_2 is completely metabolized in humans. PGE_2 is extensively metabolized in the lungs, and the resulting metabolites are further metabolized in the liver and kidney. The major route of elimination of the products of PGE_2 metabolism is the kidneys.

INDICATIONS AND USAGE

PREPIDIL Gel is indicated for ripening an unfavorable cervix in pregnant women at or near term with a medical or obstetrical need for labor induction.

CONTRAINDICATIONS

Endocervically administered PREPIDIL Gel is not recommended for the following:
a. Patients in whom oxytocic drugs are generally contraindicated or where prolonged contractions of the uterus are considered inappropriate, such as:

- cases with a history of cesarean section or major uterine surgery
- cases in which cephalopelvic disproportion is present
- cases in which there is a history of difficult labor and/or traumatic delivery
- grand multiparae with six or more previous term pregnancies cases with non-vertex presentation
- cases with hyperactive or hypertonic uterine patterns
- cases of fetal distress where delivery is not imminent
- in obstetric emergencies where the benefit-to-risk ratio for either the fetus or the mother favors surgical intervention

b. Patients with hypersensitivity to prostaglandins or constituents of the gel.

c. Patients with placenta previa or unexplained vaginal bleeding during this pregnancy.

d. Patients for whom vaginal delivery is not indicated, such as vasa previa or active herpes genitalia.

WARNINGS
FOR HOSPITAL USE ONLY
Dinoprostone, as with other potent oxytocic agents, should be used only with strict adherence to recommended dosages. Dinoprostone should be administered by physicians in a hospital that can provide immediate intensive care and acute surgical facilities.

PRECAUTIONS
1. General Precautions:
During use, uterine activity, fetal status, and character of the cervix (dilation and effacement) should be carefully monitored either by auscultation or electronic fetal monitoring to detect possible evidence of undesired responses, eg, hypertonus, sustained uterine contractility, or fetal distress. In cases where there is a history of hypertonic uterine contractility or tetanic uterine contractions, it is recommended that uterine activity and the state of the fetus should be continuously monitored. The possibility of uterine rupture should be borne in mind when high-tone myometrial contractions are sustained. Feto-pelvic relationships should be carefully evaluated before use of PREPIDIL Gel (see CONTRAINDICATIONS).
Caution should be exercised in administration of PREPIDIL Gel in patients with:
- asthma or history of asthma
- glaucoma or raised intraocular pressure

Caution should be taken so as not to administer PREPIDIL Gel above the level of the internal os. Careful vaginal examination will reveal the degree of effacement which will regulate the size of the shielded endocervical catheter to be used. That is, the 20 mm endocervical catheter should be used if no effacement is present, and the 10 mm catheter should be used if the cervix is 50% effaced. Placement of PREPIDIL Gel into the extra-amniotic space has been associated with uterine hyperstimulation.
As PREPIDIL Gel is extensively metabolized in the lung, liver, and kidney, and the major route of elimination is the kidney, PREPIDIL Gel should be used with caution in patients with renal and hepatic dysfunction.

2. Patients With Ruptured Membranes:
Caution should be exercised in the administration of PREPIDIL Gel in patients with ruptured membranes. The safety of use of PREPIDIL Gel in these patients has not been determined.

3. Drug Interactions:
PREPIDIL Gel may augment the activity of other oxytocic agents and their concomitant use is not recommended. For the sequential use of oxytocin following PREPIDIL Gel administration, a dosing interval of 6–12 hours is recommended.

4. Carcinogenesis, Mutagenesis, Impairment of Fertility:
Carcinogenic bioassay studies have not been conducted in animals with PREPIDIL Gel due to the limited indications for use and short duration of administration. No evidence of mutagenicity was observed in the Micronucleus Test or Ames Assay.

5. Pregnancy, Teratogenic Effects:
PREGNANCY CATEGORY C
Prostaglandin E_2 produced an increase in skeletal anomalies in rats and rabbits. No effect would be expected clinically, when used as indicated, since PREPIDIL Gel is administered after the period of organogenesis. PREPIDIL Gel has been shown to be embryotoxic in rats and rabbits, and any dose that produces sustained increased uterine tone could put the embryo or fetus at risk. See statements under General Precautions.

ADVERSE REACTIONS
PREPIDIL Gel is generally well-tolerated. In controlled trials, in which 1731 women were entered, the following events were reported at an occurrence of ≥1%:
[See table above.]
In addition, in other trials amnionitis and intrauterine fetal sepsis have been associated with extra-amniotic intrauterine administration of PGE_2. Uterine rupture has been reported in association with the use of PREPIDIL Gel intracervically. Additional events reported in the literature, associated by

Adverse Reaction	PGE₂ (N=884) N	(%)	Control* (N=847) N	(%)
Maternal				
Uterine contractile abnormality	58	(6.6)	34	(4.0)
Any gastrointestinal effect	50	(5.7)	22	(2.6)
Back pain	27	(3.1)	0	(0)
Warm feeling in vagina	13	(1.5)	0	(0)
Fever	12	(1.4)	10	(1.2)
Fetal				
Any fetal heart rate abnormality	150	(17.0)	123	(14.5)
Bradycardia	36	(4.1)	26	(3.1)
Deceleration				
Late	25	(2.8)	18	(2.1)
Variable	38	(4.3)	29	(3.4)
Unspecified	19	(2.1)	19	(2.2)

* placebo gel or no treatment

the authors with the use of PREPIDIL Gel, included premature rupture of membranes, fetal depression (1 min Apgar < 7), and fetal acidosis (umbilical artery pH < 7.15).

DRUG ABUSE AND DEPENDENCE
No drug abuse or drug dependence has been seen with the use of PREPIDIL Gel.

OVERDOSAGE
Overdosage with PREPIDIL Gel may be expressed by uterine hypercontractility and uterine hypertonus. Because of the transient nature of PGE_2-induced myometrial hyperstimulation, nonspecific, conservative management was found to be effective in the vast majority of the cases; ie, maternal position change and administration of oxygen to the mother. β-adrenergic drugs may be used as a treatment of hyperstimulation following the administration of PGE_2 for cervical ripening.

DOSAGE AND ADMINISTRATION
NOTE: USE CAUTION IN HANDLING THIS PRODUCT TO PREVENT CONTACT WITH SKIN. WASH HANDS THOROUGHLY WITH SOAP AND WATER AFTER ADMINISTRATION.
PREPIDIL Gel should be brought to room temperature (59° to 86°F; 15° to 30°C) just prior to administration. Do not force the warming process by using a water bath or other source of external heat (eg, microwave oven).
To prepare the product for use, remove the peel-off seal from the end of the syringe. Then remove the protective end cap (to serve as plunger extension) and insert the protective end cap into the plunger stopper assembly in the barrel of syringe. Choose the appropriate length shielded catheter (10 mm or 20 mm) and aseptically remove the sterile shielded catheter from the package. Careful vaginal examination will reveal the degree of effacement which will regulate the size of the shielded endocervical catheter to be used. That is, the 20 mm endocervical catheter should be used if no effacement is present, and the 10 mm catheter should be used if the cervix is 50% effaced. Firmly attach the catheter hub to the syringe tip as evidenced by a distinct click. Fill the catheter with sterile gel by pushing the plunger assembly to expel air from the catheter prior to administration to the patient. Proper assembly of the dosing apparatus is shown below.

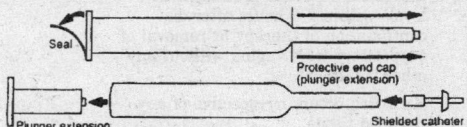

To properly administer the product, the patient should be in a dorsal position with the cervix visualized using a speculum. Using sterile technique, introduce the gel with the catheter provided into the cervical canal just below the level of the internal os. Administer the contents of the syringe by gentle expulsion and then remove the catheter. The gel is easily extrudable from the syringe. Use the contents of one syringe for one patient only. No attempt should be made to administer the small amount of gel remaining in the catheter. The syringe, catheter, and any unused package contents should be discarded after use. Following administration of PREPIDIL Gel, the patient should remain in the supine position for at least 15–30 minutes to minimize leakage from the cervical canal. If the desired response is obtained from PREPIDIL Gel, the recommended interval before giving intravenous oxytocin is 6–12 hours. If there is no cervical/uterine response to the initial dose of PREPIDIL Gel, repeat dosing may be given. The recommended repeat dose is 0.5 mg dinoprostone with a dosing interval of 6 hours. The need for additional dosing and the interval must be determined by the attending physician based on the course of clinical events. The maximum recommended cumulative dose for a 24-hour period is 1.5 mg of dinoprostone (7.5 mL PREPIDIL Gel).

HOW SUPPLIED
PREPIDIL Gel is available as a sterile semitranslucent viscous preparation for endocervical application: 0.5 mg PGE_2 per 3.0 g (2.5 mL) in syringe. In addition, each package contains two shielded catheters (10 mm and 20 mm tip) enclosed in sterile envelopes. The contents are not guaranteed sterile if envelopes are not intact.
Each 3-gram syringe applicator contains:
dinoprostone, 0.5 mg; colloidal silicon dioxide, 240 mg; triacetin, 2760 mg.
3 gram syringe   NDC 0009-3359-01
5 × 3 gram syringes   NDC 0009-3359-02
PREPIDIL Gel has a shelf life of 24 months when stored under continuous refrigeration (36° to 46°F; 2° to 8°C).
Caution: Federal law prohibits dispensing without prescription.
Manufactured by N.V. Upjohn S.A.,
Puurs-Belgium for
The Upjohn Company
Kalamazoo, MI 49001, USA
Revised January 1995

815 040 004
5R2685/1

PROSTIN E2®   ℞
brand of dinoprostone vaginal suppository

DESCRIPTION
PROSTIN E2 Vaginal Suppository, an oxytocic, contains dinoprostone as the naturally occurring prostaglandin E2 (PGE2).
Its chemical name is (5Z,11α,13E,15S)-11,15-Dihydroxy-9-oxo-prosta-5,13-dien-1-oic acid and the structural formula is represented below:

The molecular formula is $C_{20}H_{32}O_5$. The molecular weight of dinoprostone is 352.5. Dinoprostone occurs as a white crystalline powder. It has a melting point within the range of 64° to 71° C. Dinoprostone is soluble in ethanol and in 25% ethanol in water. It is soluble in water to the extent of 130 mg/100 mL.
Each suppository contains 20 mg of dinoprostone in a mixture of glycerides of fatty acids.

CLINICAL PHARMACOLOGY
PROSTIN E2 Vaginal Suppository administered intravaginally stimulates the myometrium of the gravid uterus to contract in a manner that is similar to the contractions seen in the term uterus during labor. Whether or not this action results from a direct effect of dinoprostone on the myometrium has not been determined with certainty at this time. Nonetheless, the myometrial contractions induced by the vaginal administration of dinoprostone are sufficient to produce evacuation of the products of conception from the uterus in the majority of cases.
Dinoprostone is also capable of stimulating the smooth muscle of the gastrointestinal tract of man. This activity may be responsible for the vomiting and/or diarrhea that is not uncommon when dinoprostone is used to terminate pregnancy.

Continued on next page

Information on these Pharmacia & Upjohn products is based on labeling in effect June 1, 1996. Further information concerning these and other Pharmacia & Upjohn products may be obtained by direct inquiry to Medical Information, Pharmacia & Upjohn, Kalamazoo, MI 49001.

Pharmacia & Upjohn—Cont.

In laboratory animals, and also in man, large doses of dinoprostone can lower blood pressure, probably as a consequence of its effect on the smooth muscle of the vascular system. With the doses of dinoprostone used for terminating pregnancy this effect has not been clinically significant. In laboratory animals, and also in man, dinoprostone can elevate body temperature. With the clinical doses of dinoprostone used for the termination of pregnancy some patients do exhibit temperature increases.

INDICATIONS AND USAGE

1. PROSTIN E2 Vaginal Suppository is indicated for the termination of pregnancy from the 12th through the 20th gestational week as calculated from the first day of the last normal menstrual period.
2. PROSTIN E2 is also indicated for evacuation of the uterine contents in the management of missed abortion or intrauterine fetal death up to 28 weeks of gestational age as calculated from the first day of the last normal menstrual period.
3. PROSTIN E2 is indicated in the management of nonmetastatic gestational trophoblastic disease (benign hydatidiform mole).

CONTRAINDICATIONS

1. Hypersensitivity to dinoprostone
2. Acute pelvic inflammatory disease
3. Patients with active cardiac, pulmonary, renal, or hepatic disease

---

WARNINGS

Dinoprostone, as with other potent oxytocic agents, should be used only with strict adherence to recommended dosages. Dinoprostone should be used by medically trained personnel in a hospital which can provide immediate intensive care and acute surgical facilities.

Dinoprostone does not appear to directly affect the fetoplacental unit. Therefore, the possibility does exist that the previable fetus aborted by dinoprostone could exhibit transient life signs. Dinoprostone is not indicated if the fetus in utero has reached the stage of viability. Dinoprostone should not be considered a feticidal agent.

Evidence from animal studies has suggested that certain prostaglandins may have some teratogenic potential. Therefore, any failed pregnancy termination with dinoprostone should be completed by some other means.

PROSTIN E2 Vaginal Suppository should not be used for extemporaneous preparation of any other dosage form.

Neither the PROSTIN E2 Vaginal Suppository, as dispensed nor any extemporaneous formulation made from the PROSTIN E2 Vaginal Suppository should be used for cervical ripening or other indication in the patient with term pregnancy.

PRECAUTIONS

1. General precautions

Animal studies lasting several weeks at high doses have shown that prostaglandins of the E and F series can induce proliferation of bone. Such effects have also been noted in newborn infants who have received prostaglandin E1 during prolonged treatment. There is no evidence that short term administration of PROSTIN E2 Vaginal Suppository can cause similar bone effects.

As in spontaneous abortion, where the process is sometimes incomplete, abortion induced by PROSTIN E2 may sometimes be incomplete. In such cases, other measures should be taken to assure complete abortion.

In patients with a history of asthma, hypo- or hypertension, cardiovascular disease, renal disease, hepatic disease, anemia, jaundice, diabetes or history of epilepsy, dinoprostone should be used with caution.

Dinoprostone administered by the vaginal route should be used with caution in the presence of cervicitis, infected endocervical lesions, or acute vaginitis.

As with any oxytocic agent, dinoprostone should be used with caution in patients with compromised (scarred) uteri.

Dinoprostone vaginal therapy is associated with transient pyrexia that may be due to its effect on hypothalamic thermoregulation. In the patients studied, temperature elevations in excess of 2° F (1.1° C) were observed in approximately one-half of the patients on the recommended dosage regimen. In all cases, temperature returned to normal on discontinuation of therapy. Differentiation of post-abortion endometritis from drug-induced temperature elevations is difficult, but with increasing clinical exposure and experience with PGE2 vaginal therapy the distinctions become more obviously apparent and are summarized below:
[See table below.]

2. Laboratory tests

When a pregnancy diagnosed as missed abortion is electively interrupted with intravaginal administration of dinoprostone, confirmation of intrauterine fetal death should be obtained in respect to a *negative pregnancy test* for chorionic gonadotropic activity (U.C.G. test or equivalent). When a pregnancy with late fetal intrauterine death is interrupted with intravaginal administration of dinoprostone, confirmation of intrauterine fetal death should be obtained prior to treatment.

3. Drug interactions

PROSTIN E2 may augment the activity of other oxytocic drugs. Concomitant use with other oxytocic agents is not recommended.

4. Carcinogenesis, mutagenesis, impairment of fertility

Carcinogenic bioassay studies have not been conducted in animals with PROSTIN E2 due to the limited indications for use and short duration of administration. No evidence of mutagenicity was observed in the Micronucleus Test or Ames Assay.

5. Pregnancy: Teratogenic Effects: Pregnancy Category C

Animal studies do not indicate that PROSTIN E2 is teratogenic, however, it has been shown to be embryotoxic in rats and rabbits and any dose which produces increased uterine tone could put the embryo or fetus at risk. See WARNINGS section.

ADVERSE REACTIONS

The most frequent adverse reactions observed with the use of dinoprostone for abortion are related to its contractile effect on smooth muscle.

In the patients studied, approximately two-thirds experienced vomiting, one-half temperature elevations, two-fifths diarrhea, one-third some nausea, one-tenth headache, and one-tenth shivering and chills.

In addition, approximately one-tenth of the patients studied exhibited transient diastolic blood pressure decreases of greater than 20 mmHg.

Two cases of myocardial infarction following the use of dinoprostone have been reported in patients with a history of cardiovascular disease.

It is not known whether these events were related to the administration of dinoprostone.

Adverse effects in decreasing order of their frequency, observed with the use of dinoprostone, not all of which are clearly drug related include:

Vomiting	Nocturnal leg cramps
Diarrhea	Uterine rupture
Nausea	Breast tenderness
Fever	Blurred vision
Headache	Coughing
Chills or shivering	Rash
Backache	Myalgia
Joint inflammation or pain new or exacerbated	Stiff neck Dehydration
Flushing or hot flashes	Tremor
Dizziness	Paresthesia
Arthralgia	Hearing impairment
Vaginal pain	Urine retention
Chest pain	Pharyngitis
Dyspnea	Laryngitis
Endometritis	Diaphoresis
Syncope or fainting sensation	Eye pain Wheezing
Vaginitis or vulvitis	Cardiac arrhythmia
Weakness	Skin discoloration
Muscular cramp or pain	Vaginismus
Tightness in chest	Tension

DOSAGE AND ADMINISTRATION

STORE IN A FREEZER NOT ABOVE −20° C (−4° F) BUT BRING TO ROOM TEMPERATURE JUST PRIOR TO USE. REMOVE FOIL BEFORE USE.

A suppository containing 20 mg of dinoprostone should be inserted high into the vagina. The patient should remain in the supine position for ten minutes following insertion. Additional intravaginal administration of each subsequent suppository should be at 3- to 5-hour intervals until abortion occurs. Within the above recommended intervals administration time should be determined by abortifacient progress, uterine contractility response, and by patient tolerance. Continuous administration of the drug for more than 2 days is not recommended.

HOW SUPPLIED

STORE IN A FREEZER NOT ABOVE −20° C (−4° F).

PROSTIN E2 Vaginal Suppositories are available in containers of one suppository each. Each suppository contains 20 mg of dinoprostone in a mixture of glycerides of fatty acids.

Caution: Federal law prohibits dispensing without prescription.

REVISED JUNE 1992

810 994 211
691693

Endometritis pyrexia	PGE2 induced pyrexia
1. **Time of onset:** Typically, on third post-abortional day (38° C or higher).	Within 15–45 minutes of suppository administration.
2. **Duration:** Untreated pyrexia and infection continue and may give rise to other infective pelvic pathology.	Elevations revert to pretreatment levels within 2–6 hours after discontinuation of therapy or removal of suppository from vagina without any other treatment.
3. **Retention:** Products of conception are often retained in the cervical os or uterine cavity.	Elevation occurs irrespective of any retained tissue.
4. **Histology:** Endometrium shows evidence of inflammatory lymphocytic infiltration with areas of necrotic hemorrhagic tissue.	Although the endometrial stroma may be edematous and vascular, there is relative absence of inflammatory reaction. Normal uterine involution not tender.
5. **The uterus:** Often remains boggy and soft with tenderness over the fundus, and pain on moving the cervix, on bimanual examination.	
6. **Discharge:** Often associated foul-smelling lochia and leukorrhea.	Lochia normal.

7. **Cervical culture**
The culture of pathological organisms from the cervix or uterine cavity after abortion does not, of itself, warrant the diagnosis of septic abortion in the absence of clinical evidence of sepsis. It is not uncommon to culture pathogens from cases of recent abortion *not* clinically infected. Persistent positive culture with clear clinical signs of infection are significant in the differential diagnosis.

8. **Blood count**
Leukocytosis and differential white cell counts are not of major clinical importance in distinguishing between the two conditions, since total WBC's may be increased as a result of infection and transient leukocytosis may also be drug induced.

In the absence of clinical or bacteriological evidence of intrauterine infection, supportive therapy for drug induced fevers includes the forcing of fluids. As all PGE2-induced fevers have been found to be transient or self-limiting, it is doubtful if any simple empirical measures for temperature reduction are indicated.

PROVERA®
brand of medroxyprogesterone acetate tablets, USP

℞

WARNING

THE USE OF PROVERA (MEDROXYPROGESTERONE ACETATE) DURING THE FIRST FOUR MONTHS OF PREGNANCY IS NOT RECOMMENDED.

Progestational agents have been used beginning with the first trimester of pregnancy in an attempt to prevent habitual abortion. There is no adequate evidence that such use is effective when such drugs are given during the first four months of pregnancy. Furthermore, in the vast majority of women, the cause of abortion is a defective ovum, which progestational agents could not be expected to influence. In addition, the use of progestational agents, with their uterine-relaxant properties, in patients with fertilized defective ova may cause a delay in spontaneous abortion. Therefore, the use of such drugs during the first four months of pregnancy is not recommended.

Several reports suggest an association between intra-uterine exposure to progestational drugs in the first trimester of pregnancy and genital abnormalities in male and female fetuses. The risk of hypospadias, 5 to 8 per 1,000 male births in the general population, may be approximately doubled with exposure to these drugs. There are insufficient data to quantify the risk to exposed female fetuses, but insofar as some of these drugs induce mild virilization of the external genitalia of the female fetus, and because of the increased association of hypospadias in the male fetus, it is prudent to avoid the use of these drugs during the first trimester of pregnancy.

If the patient is exposed to PROVERA Tablets (medroxyprogesterone acetate) during the first four months of pregnancy or if she becomes pregnant while taking this drug, she should be apprised of the potential risks to the fetus.

DESCRIPTION

PROVERA Tablets contain medroxyprogesterone acetate, which is a derivative of progesterone. It is a white to off-white, odorless crystalline powder, stable in air, melting between 200 and 210° C. It is freely soluble in chloroform, soluble in acetone and in dioxane, sparingly soluble in alcohol and in methanol, slightly soluble in ether, and insoluble in water.

The chemical name for medroxyprogesterone acetate is Pregn-4-ene-3,20-dione, 17-(acetyloxy)-6-methyl-, (6α)-. The structural formula is:

Each PROVERA tablet for oral administration contains 2.5 mg, 5 mg or 10 mg of medroxyprogesterone acetate. Inactive ingredients: calcium stearate, corn starch, lactose, mineral oil, sorbic acid, sucrose, talc. The 2.5 mg tablet contains FD&C Yellow no. 6.

ACTIONS

Medroxyprogesterone acetate, administered orally or parenterally in the recommended doses to women with adequate endogenous estrogen, transforms proliferative into secretory endometrium. Androgenic and anabolic effects have been noted, but the drug is apparently devoid of significant estrogenic activity. While parenterally administered medroxyprogesterone acetate inhibits gonadotropin production, which in turn prevents follicular maturation and ovulation, available data indicate that this does not occur when the usually recommended oral dosage is given as single daily doses.

INDICATIONS AND USAGE

Secondary amenorrhea; abnormal uterine bleeding due to hormonal imbalance in the absence of organic pathology, such as fibroids or uterine cancer.

CONTRAINDICATIONS

1. Thrombophlebitis, thromboembolic disorders, cerebral apoplexy or patients with a past history of these conditions.
2. Liver dysfunction or disease.
3. Known or suspected malignancy of breast or genital organs.
4. Undiagnosed vaginal bleeding.
5. Missed abortion.
6. As a diagnostic test for pregnancy.
7. Known sensitivity to PROVERA Tablets.

WARNINGS

1. The physician should be alert to the earliest manifestations of thrombotic disorders (thrombophlebitis, cerebrovascular disorders, pulmonary embolism, and retinal thrombosis). Should any of these occur or be suspected, the drug should be discontinued immediately.
2. Beagle dogs treated with medroxyprogesterone acetate developed mammary nodules some of which were malignant. Although nodules occasionally appeared in control animals, they were intermittent in nature, whereas the nodules in the drug-treated animals were larger, more numerous, persistent, and there were some breast malignancies with metastases. Their significance with respect to humans has not been established.
3. Discontinue medication pending examination if there is sudden partial or complete loss of vision, or if there is a sudden onset of proptosis, diplopia or migraine. If examination

reveals papilledema or retinal vascular lesions, medication should be withdrawn.
4. Detectable amounts of progestin have been identified in the milk of mothers receiving the drug. The effect of this on the nursing infant has not been determined.
5. Usage in pregnancy is not recommended (See WARNING Box).
6. Retrospective studies of morbidity and mortality in Great Britain and studies of morbidity in the United States have shown a statistically significant association between thrombophlebitis, pulmonary embolism, and cerebral thrombosis and embolism and the use of oral contraceptives.[1-4] The estimate of the relative risk of thromboembolism in the study by Vessey and Doll[3] was about sevenfold, while Sartwell and associates[4] in the United States found a relative risk of 4.4, meaning that the users are several times as likely to undergo thromboembolic disease without evident cause as nonusers. The American study also indicated that the risk did not persist after discontinuation of administration, and that it was not enhanced by long continued administration. The American study was not designed to evaluate a difference between products.

PRECAUTIONS

1. The pretreatment physical examination should include special reference to breast and pelvic organs, as well as Papanicolaou smear.
2. Because progestogens may cause some degree of fluid retention, conditions which might be influenced by this factor, such as epilepsy, migraine, asthma, cardiac or renal dysfunction, require careful observation.
3. In cases of breakthrough bleeding, as in all cases of irregular bleeding per vaginum, nonfunctional causes should be borne in mind. In cases of undiagnosed vaginal bleeding, adequate diagnostic measures are indicated.
4. Patients who have a history of psychic depression should be carefully observed and the drug discontinued if the depression recurs to a serious degree.
5. Any possible influence of prolonged progestin therapy on pituitary, ovarian, adrenal, hepatic or uterine functions awaits further study.
6. A decrease in glucose tolerance has been observed in a small percentage of patients on estrogen-progestin combination drugs. The mechanism of this decrease is obscure. For this reason, diabetic patients should be carefully observed while receiving progestin therapy.
7. The age of the patient constitutes no absolute limiting factor although treatment with progestins may mask the onset of the climacteric.
8. The pathologist should be advised of progestin therapy when relevant specimens are submitted.
9. Because of the occasional occurrence of thrombotic disorders, (thrombophlebitis, pulmonary embolism, retinal thrombosis, and cerebrovascular disorders) in patients taking estrogen-progestin combinations and since the mechanism is obscure, the physician should be alert to the earliest manifestation of these disorders.
10. Studies of the addition of a progestin product to an estrogen replacement regimen for seven or more days of a cycle of estrogen administration have reported a lowered incidence of endometrial hyperplasia. Morphological and biochemical studies of endometrium suggest that 10–13 days of a progestin are needed to provide maximal maturation of the endometrium and to eliminate any hyperplastic changes. Whether this will provide protection from endometrial carcinoma has not been clearly established. There are possible additional risks which may be associated with the inclusion of progestin in estrogen replacement regimen. The potential risks include adverse effects on carbohydrate and lipid metabolism. The dosage used may be important in minimizing these adverse effects.
11. Aminoglutethimide administered concomitantly with PROVERA may significantly depress the bioavailability of PROVERA.

Carcinogenesis, Mutagenesis, Impairment of Fertility.
Long-term intramuscular administration of PROVERA has been shown to produce mammary tumors in beagle dogs (see WARNINGS). There was no evidence of a carcinogenic effect associated with the oral administration of PROVERA to rats and mice. Medroxyprogesterone acetate was not mutagenic in a battery of in vitro or in vivo genetic toxicity assays. Medroxyprogesterone acetate at high doses is an antifertility drug and high doses would be expected to impair fertility until the cessation of treatment.

Information for the Patient
See Patient Information at end of insert.

ADVERSE REACTIONS

Pregnancy—(See WARNING Box for possible adverse effects on the fetus).
Breast—Breast tenderness or galactorrhea has been reported rarely.
Skin—Sensitivity reactions consisting of urticaria, pruritus, edema and generalized rash have occurred in an occasional

patient. Acne, alopecia and hirsutism have been reported in a few cases.
Thromboembolic Phenomena—Thromboembolic phenomena including thrombophlebitis and pulmonary embolism have been reported.
The following adverse reactions have been observed in women taking progestins including PROVERA Tablets:
breakthrough bleeding
spotting
change in menstrual flow
amenorrhea
edema
change in weight (increase or decrease)
changes in cervical erosion and cervical secretions
cholestatic jaundice
anaphylactoid reactions and anaphylaxis
rash (allergic) with and without pruritus
mental depression
pyrexia
insomnia
nausea
somnolence
A statistically significant association has been demonstrated between use of estrogen-progestin combination drugs and the following serious adverse reactions: thrombophlebitis; pulmonary embolism and cerebral thrombosis and embolism. For this reason patients on progestin therapy should be carefully observed.
Although available evidence is suggestive of an association, such a relationship has been neither confirmed nor refuted for the following serious adverse reactions:
neuro-ocular lesions, eg, retinal thrombosis and optic neuritis.
The following adverse reactions have been observed in patients receiving estrogen-progestin combination drugs:
rise in blood pressure in susceptible individuals
premenstrual-like syndrome
changes in libido
changes in appetite
cystitis-like syndrome
headache
nervousness
fatigue
backache
hirsutism
loss of scalp hair
erythema multiforme
erythema nodosum
hemorrhagic eruption
itching
dizziness
In view of these observations, patients on progestin therapy should be carefully observed.
The following laboratory results may be altered by the use of estrogen-progestin combination drugs:
Increased sulfobromophthalein retention and other hepatic function tests.
Coagulation tests: increase in prothrombin factors VII, VIII, IX and X.
Metyrapone test.
Pregnanediol determination.
Thyroid function: increase in PBI, and butanol extractable protein bound iodine and decrease in T3 uptake values.

DOSAGE AND ADMINISTRATION

Secondary Amenorrhea—PROVERA Tablets may be given in dosages of 5 to 10 mg daily for from 5 to 10 days. A dose for inducing an optimum secretory transformation of an endometrium that has been adequately primed with either endogenous or exogenous estrogen is 10 mg of PROVERA daily for 10 days. In cases of secondary amenorrhea, therapy may be started at any time. Progestin withdrawal bleeding usually occurs within three to seven days after discontinuing PROVERA therapy.
Abnormal Uterine Bleeding Due to Hormonal Imbalance in the Absence of Organic Pathology—Beginning on the calculated 16th or 21st day of the menstrual cycle, 5 to 10 mg of medroxyprogesterone acetate may be given daily for from 5 to 10 days. To produce an optimum secretory transformation of an endometrium that has been adequately primed with either endogenous or exogenous estrogen, 10 mg of medroxyprogesterone acetate daily for 10 days beginning on the 16th day of the cycle is suggested. Progestin withdrawal bleeding usually occurs within three to seven days after discontinuing therapy with PROVERA. Patients with a past history of recurrent episodes of abnormal uterine bleeding may benefit from planned menstrual cycling with PROVERA.

Continued on next page

Information on these Pharmacia & Upjohn products is based on labeling in effect June 1, 1996. Further information concerning these and other Pharmacia & Upjohn products may be obtained by direct inquiry to Medical Information, Pharmacia & Upjohn, Kalamazoo, MI 49001.

Pharmacia & Upjohn—Cont.

HOW SUPPLIED

PROVERA Tablets are available in the following strengths and package sizes:

2.5 mg (scored, round, orange)

Bottles of 30	NDC 0009-0064-06
Bottles of 100	NDC 0009-0064-04

5 mg (scored, hexagonal, white)

Bottles of 30	NDC 0009-0286-32
Bottles of 100	NDC 0009-0286-03

10 mg (scored, round, white)

Bottles of 30	NDC 0009-0050-09
Bottles of 100	NDC 0009-0050-02
Bottles of 500	NDC 0009-0050-11
DOSEPAK™ Unit of Use (10)	NDC 0009-0050-12

Store at controlled room temperature 15°–30°C (59°–86°F).

REFERENCES

1. Royal College of General Practitioners: Oral contraception and thromboembolic disease. J Coll Gen Pract **13**:267–279, 1967.
2. Inman WHW, Vessey MP: Investigation of deaths from pulmonary, coronary, and cerebral thrombosis and embolism in women of child-bearing age. Br Med J **2**:193–199, 1968.
3. Vessey MP, Doll R: Investigation of relation between use of oral contraceptives and thromboembolic disease. A further report. Br Med J **2**:651–657, 1969.
4. Sartwell PE, Masi AT, Arthes FG, et al: Thromboembolism and oral contraceptives: An epidemiological case-control study. Am J Epidemiol **90**:365–380, 1969.

The text of the patient insert for progesterone and progesterone-like drugs is set forth below.

PATIENT INFORMATION

PROVERA Tablets contain medroxyprogesterone acetate a progesterone. The information below is that which the U.S. Food and Drug Administration requires be provided for all patients taking progesterones. The information below relates only to the risk to the unborn child associated with use of progesterone during pregnancy. For further information on the use, side effects and other risks associated with this product, ask your doctor.

WARNING FOR WOMEN

Progesterone or progesterone-like drugs have been used to prevent miscarriage in the first few months of pregnancy. No adequate evidence is available to show that they are effective for this purpose. Furthermore, most cases of early miscarriage are due to causes which could not be helped by these drugs.

There is an increased risk of minor birth defects in children whose mothers take this drug during the first 4 months of pregnancy. Several reports suggest an association between mothers who take these drugs in the first trimester of pregnancy and genital abnormalities in male and female babies. The risk to the male baby is the possibility of being born with a condition in which the opening of the penis is on the underside rather than the tip of the penis (hypospadias). Hypospadias occurs in about 5 to 8 per 1,000 male births and is about doubled with exposure to these drugs. There is not enough information to quantify the risk to exposed female fetuses, but enlargement of the clitoris and fusion of the labia may occur, although rarely.

Therefore, since drugs of this type may induce mild masculinization of the external genitalia of the female fetus, as well as hypospadias in the male fetus, it is wise to avoid using the drug during the first trimester of pregnancy.

These drugs have been used as a test for pregnancy but such use is no longer considered safe because of possible damage to a developing baby. Also, more rapid methods for testing for pregnancy are now available.

If you take PROVERA and later find you were pregnant when you took it, be sure to discuss this with your doctor as soon as possible.

Caution: Federal law prohibits dispensing without prescription.

Revised January 1992 812 584 409

691015

Shown in Product Identification Guide, page 329

VANTIN® ℞

Tablets and Oral Suspension
Brand of cefpodoxime proxetil tablets
and cefpodoxime proxetil for oral suspension
For Oral Use Only

DESCRIPTION

Cefpodoxime proxetil is an orally administered, extended spectrum, semi-synthetic antibiotic of the cephalosporin class. The chemical name is (RS)-1-(isopropoxycarbonyloxy)ethyl (+)-(6R,7R)-7-[2-(2-amino-4-thiazolyl)-2-{(Z)-methoxyimino}acetamido]-3-methoxymethyl-8-oxo-5-thia-1-azabicyclo[4.2.0]oct-2-ene-2-carboxylate. Its empirical formula is $C_{21}H_{27}N_5O_9S_2$ and its structural formula is represented below:

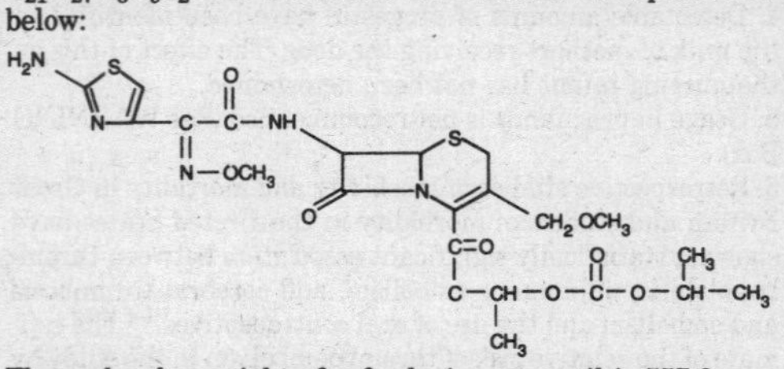

The molecular weight of cefpodoxime proxetil is 557,6.

Cefpodoxime proxetil is a prodrug; its active metabolite is cefpodoxime. All doses of cefpodoxime proxetil in this insert are expressed in terms of the active cefpodoxime moiety. The drug is supplied both as film-coated tablets and as flavored granules for oral suspension.

VANTIN Tablets contain cefpodoxime proxetil equivalent to 100 mg or 200 mg of cefpodoxime activity and the following inactive ingredients: carboxymethylcellulose calcium, carnauba wax, FD&C Yellow No. 6, hydroxypropylcellulose, hydroxypropylmethylcellulose, lactose hydrous, magnesium stearate, propylene glycol, sodium lauryl sulfate and titanium dioxide. In addition, the 100 mg film-coated tablets contain D&C Yellow No. 10 and the 200 mg film-coated tablets contain FD&C Red No. 40.

Each 5 mL of VANTIN for Oral Suspension contains cefpodoxime proxetil equivalent to 50 mg or 100 mg of cefpodoxime activity after constitution and the following inactive ingredients: artificial flavorings, butylated hydroxy anisole (BHA), carboxymethylcellulose sodium, carrageenan, citric acid, colloidal silicon dioxide, croscarmellose sodium, hydroxypropylcellulose, lactose, lactose hydrous, maltodextrin, microcrystalline cellulose, natural flavorings, propylene glycol alginate, sodium citrate hydrous, sodium benzoate, starch, sucrose, and vegetable oil.

CLINICAL PHARMACOLOGY

Absorption and Excretion:

Cefpodoxime proxetil is a prodrug that is absorbed from the gastrointestinal tract and de-esterified to its active metabolite, cefpodoxime. Following oral administration of 100 mg of cefpodoxime proxetil to fasting subjects, approximately 50% of the administered cefpodoxime dose was absorbed systemically. Over the recommended dosing range (100 to 400 mg), approximately 29 to 33% of the administered cefpodoxime dose was excreted unchanged in the urine in 12 hours. There is minimal metabolism of cefpodoxime *in vivo*.

Effects of food:

The extent of absorption (mean AUC) and the mean peak plasma concentration increased when film-coated tablets were administered with food. Following a 200 mg tablet dose taken with food, the AUC was 21 to 33% higher than under fasting conditions, and the peak plasma concentration averaged 3.1 mcg/mL in fed subjects versus 2.6 mcg/mL in fasted subjects. Time to peak concentration was not significantly different between fed and fasted subjects.

When a 200 mg dose of the suspension was taken with food, the extent of absorption (mean AUC) and mean peak plasma concentration in fed subjects were not significantly different from fasted subjects, but the rate of absorption was slower with food (48% increase in T_{max}).

Pharmacokinetics of Cefpodoxime Proxetil Film-coated Tablets:

Over the recommended dosing range, (100 to 400 mg), the rate and extent of cefpodoxime absorption exhibited dose-dependency; dose-normalized C_{max} and AUC decreased by up to 32% with increasing dose. Over the recommended dosing range, the T_{max} was approximately 2 to 3 hours and the $T_{1/2}$ ranged from 2.09 to 2.84 hours. Mean C_{max} was 1.4 mcg/mL for the 100 mg dose, 2.3 mcg/mL for the 200 mg dose, and 3.9 mcg/mL for the 400 mg dose. In patients with normal renal function, neither accumulation nor significant changes in other pharmacokinetic parameters were noted following multiple oral doses of up to 400 mg Q 12 hours.

CEFPODOXIME PLASMA LEVELS (mcg/mL)
IN FASTED ADULTS
AFTER FILM-COATED TABLET ADMINISTRATION
(Single Dose)

Dose (cefpodoxime equivalents)	Time after oral ingestion 1hr	2hr	3hr	4hr	6hr	8hr	12hr
100 mg	0.98	1.4	1.3	1.0	0.59	0.29	0.08
200 mg	1.5	2.2	2.2	1.8	1.2	0.62	0.18
400 mg	2.2	3.7	3.8	3.3	2.3	1.3	0.38

Pharmacokinetics of Cefpodoxime Proxetil Suspension:

In adult subjects, a 100 mg dose of oral suspension produced an average peak cefpodoxime concentration of approximately 1.5 mcg/mL (range: 1.1 to 2.1 mcg/mL), which is equivalent to that reported following administration of the 100 mg tablet. Time to peak plasma concentration and area under the plasma concentration-time curve (AUC) for the oral suspension were also equivalent to those produced with film-coated tablets in adults following a 100 mg oral dose. The pharmacokinetics of cefpodoxime were investigated in 18 patients aged 4 to 17 years. Each patient received a single, oral, 5 mg/kg dose of cefpodoxime oral suspension. Plasma and urine samples were collected for 12 hours after dosing. The plasma levels reported from this study are as follows:

CEFPODOXIME PLASMA LEVELS (mcg/mL)
IN FASTED PATIENTS
(4 to 17 YEARS OF AGE)
AFTER SUSPENSION ADMINISTRATION

Dose (cefpodoxime equivalents)	Time after oral ingestion 1hr	2hr	3hr	4hr	6hr	8hr	12hr
5 mg/kg[1]	1.6	2.4	2.3	1.9	0.96	0.41	0.091

[1] Dose did not exceed 200 mg.

Distribution:

Protein binding of cefpodoxime ranges from 22 to 33% in serum and from 21 to 29% in plasma.

Skin Blister:

Following multiple-dose administration every 12 hours for 5 days of 200 mg or 400 mg cefpodoxime proxetil, the mean maximum cefpodoxime concentration in skin blister fluid averaged 1.6 and 2.8 mcg/mL, respectively. Skin blister fluid cefpodoxime levels at 12 hours after dosing averaged 0.2 and 0.4 mcg/mL for the 200 mg and 400 mg multiple-dose regimens, respectively.

Tonsil Tissue:

Following a single, oral 100 mg cefpodoxime proxetil film-coated tablet, the mean maximum cefpodoxime concentration in tonsil tissue averaged 0.24 mcg/g at 4 hours post-dosing and 0.09 mcg/g at 7 hours post-dosing. Equilibrium was achieved between plasma and tonsil tissue within 4 hours of dosing. No detection of cefpodoxime in tonsillar tissue was reported 12 hours after dosing. These results demonstrated that concentrations of cefpodoxime exceeded the MIC_{90} of *S. pyogenes* for at least 7 hours after dosing of 100 mg of cefpodoxime proxetil.

Lung Tissue:

Following a single, oral 200 mg cefpodoxime proxetil film-coated tablet, the mean maximum cefpodoxime concentration in lung tissue averaged 0.63 mcg/g at 3 hours post-dosing, 0.52 mcg/g at 6 hours post-dosing, and 0.19 mcg/g at 12 hours post-dosing. The results of this study indicated that cefpodoxime penetrated into lung tissue and produced sustained drug concentrations for at least 12 hours after dosing at levels that exceeded the MIC_{90} for *S. pneumoniae* and *H. influenzae*.

CSF:

Adequate data on CSF levels of cefpodoxime are not available.

Effects of decreased renal function:

Elimination of cefpodoxime is reduced in patients with moderate to severe renal impairment (<50 mL/min creatinine clearance). (See PRECAUTIONS and DOSAGE AND ADMINISTRATION.) In subjects with mild impairment of renal function (50 to 80 mL/min creatinine clearance), the average plasma half-life of cefpodoxime was 3.5 hours. In subjects with moderate (30 to 49 mL/min creatinine clearance) or severe renal impairment (5 to 29 mL/min creatinine clearance), the half-life increased to 5.9 and 9.8 hours, respectively. Approximately 23% of the administered dose was cleared from the body during a standard 3-hour hemodialysis procedure.

Effect of hepatic impairment (cirrhosis):

Absorption was somewhat diminished and elimination unchanged in patients with cirrhosis. The mean cefpodoxime $T_{1/2}$ and renal clearance in cirrhotic patients were similar to those derived in studies of healthy subjects. Ascites did not appear to affect values in cirrhotic subjects. No dosage adjustment is recommended in this patient population.

Pharmacokinetics in Elderly Subjects:

Elderly subjects do not require dosage adjustments unless they have diminished renal function. (See PRECAUTIONS.) In healthy geriatric subjects, cefpodoxime half-life in plasma averaged 4.2 hours (vs 3.3 in younger subjects) and urinary recovery averaged 21% after a 400 mg dose was administered every 12 hours. Other pharmacokinetic parameters (C_{max}, AUC, and T_{max}) were unchanged relative to those observed in healthy young subjects.

Microbiology:

Cefpodoxime is active *in vitro* against a wide range of gram-positive and gram-negative bacteria. Cefpodoxime is highly stable in the presence of beta-lactamase enzymes. As a result, many organisms resistant to penicillins and some cephalosporins, due to the presence of beta-lactamases, may be susceptible to cefpodoxime.

The bactericidal activity of cefpodoxime results from its inhibition of cell wall synthesis. Cefpodoxime is usually active against the following organisms *in vitro* and in clinical infections. (See INDICATIONS AND USAGE.)

Gram-positive aerobes:

Staphylococcus aureus (including penicillinase-producing strains)

NOTE: Cefpodoxime is inactive against methicillin-resistant staphylococci.

Staphylococcus saprophyticus
Streptococcus pneumoniae
Streptococcus pyogenes
Gram-negative aerobes:
Escherichia coli
Haemophilus influenzae (including β-lactamase-producing strains)
Klebsiella pneumoniae
Moraxella (Branhamella) catarrhalis
Neisseria gonorrhoeae (including penicillinase-producing strains)
Proteus mirabilis
The following *in vitro* data are available; however, their clinical significance is unknown.

Cefpodoxime exhibits *in vitro* minimum inhibitory concentrations of 2.0 mcg/mL or less against most strains of the following organisms. The safety and effectiveness of cefpodoxime proxetil in treating infections due to these organisms have not been established in adequate and well-controlled trials.

Gram-positive aerobes:
Streptococcus agalactiae
Streptococcus spp. (Groups C, F, G)
NOTE: Cefpodoxime is inactive against most strains of *Enterococcus.*

Gram-negative aerobes:
Citrobacter diversus
Haemophilus parainfluenzae
Klebsiella oxytoca
Proteus vulgaris
Providencia rettgeri
NOTE: Cefpodoxime is inactive against most strains of *Pseudomonas* and *Enterobacter.*

Anaerobes
Peptostreptococcus magnus

SUSCEPTIBILITY TESTING

Diffusion Techniques: Quantitative methods that require measurement of zone diameters give the most precise estimate of the susceptibility of bacteria to antimicrobial agents. One such standardized procedure[1] recommended for use with the 10 mcg cefpodoxime disk is the National Committee for Clinical Laboratory Standards (NCCLS) approved procedure.

Interpretation involves correlation of the diameters obtained in the disk test with the minimum inhibitory concentration (MIC) for cefpodoxime.

Reports from the laboratory giving results of the standardized single disk susceptibility test using a 10 mcg cefpodoxime disk should be interpreted according to the following criteria:

Zone diameter (mm)	Interpretation
≥ 21	(S) Susceptible
18–20	(I) Intermediate
≤ 17	(R) Resistant

A report of "Susceptible" indicates that the pathogen is likely to be inhibited by generally achievable blood levels. A report of "Intermediate" indicates that the result should be considered equivocal, and, if the organism is not fully susceptible to alternative, clinically feasible drugs, the test should be repeated. This category implies clinical applicability in body sites where the drug is physiologically concentrated or in situations where high dosage of drug can be used. This category provides a buffer zone that prevents small uncontrolled technical factors from causing major discrepancies in interpretation. A report of "Resistant" indicates that achievable concentrations of the antibiotic are unlikely to be inhibitory and other therapy should be selected.

Standardized procedures require the use of laboratory control organisms. The 10 mcg disk should give the following zone diameters:

Organism	Zone diameter (mm)
Escherichia coli ATCC 25922	23–28
Staphylococcus aureus ATCC 25923	19–25

Cephalosporin "class disks" should not be used to test for susceptibility to cefpodoxime.

Dilution Technique: Use a standardized dilution method[2] (broth, agar, microdilution) or equivalent with cefpodoxime susceptibility powder. The MIC values should be interpreted according to the following criteria:

MIC (mcg/mL)	Interpretation
≤ 2	(S) Susceptible
4	(I) Intermediate
≥ 8	(R) Resistant

As with standard diffusion methods, dilution procedures require the use of laboratory control organisms. Standard cefpodoxime susceptibility powder should give the following MIC values:

Organism	MIC range (mcg/mL)
Escherichia coli ATCC 25922	0.25–1
Staphylococcus aureus ATCC 29213	1–8

NOTE: Susceptibility testing by dilution methods requires the use of cefpodoxime susceptibility powder. Cefpodoxime proxetil granules for oral use should NOT be used for *in vitro* susceptibility tests.

INDICATIONS AND USAGE

Cefpodoxime proxetil is indicated for the treatment of patients with mild to moderate infections caused by susceptible strains of the designated microorganisms in the conditions listed below. Recommended dosages, durations of therapy, and applicable patient populations vary among these infections. Please see DOSAGE AND ADMINISTRATION for specific recommendations.

LOWER RESPIRATORY TRACT
Community-acquired pneumonia caused by *S. pneumoniae* or *H. influenzae* (including beta-lactamase-producing strains). Acute bacterial exacerbation of chronic bronchitis caused by *S. pneumoniae, H. influenzae* (non-beta-lactamase- producing strains only), or *M. catarrhalis.* Data are insufficient at this time to establish efficacy in patients with acute bacterial exacerbations of chronic bronchitis caused by beta-lactamase-producing strains of *H. influenzae.*

SEXUALLY TRANSMITTED DISEASES
Acute, uncomplicated urethral and cervical gonorrhea caused by Neisseria gonorrhoeae (including penicillinase-producing strains)
Acute, uncomplicated ano-rectal infections in women due to Neisseria gonorrhoeae (including penicillinase-producing strains).
NOTE: The efficacy of cefpodoxime in treating male patients with rectal infections caused by *N. gonorrhoeae* has not been established. Data do not support the use of cefpodoxime proxetil in the treatment of pharyngeal infections due to *N. gonorrhoeae* in men or women.

SKIN AND SKIN STRUCTURES
Uncomplicated skin and skin structure infections caused by *Staphylococcus aureus* (including penicillinase-producing strains) or *Streptococcus pyogenes.* Abscesses should be surgically drained as clinically indicated.
NOTE: In clinical trials, successful treatment of uncomplicated skin and skin structure infections was dose-related. The effective therapeutic dose for skin infections was higher than those used in other recommended indications. (See DOSAGE AND ADMINISTRATION.)

UPPER RESPIRATORY TRACT
Acute otitis media caused by *Streptococcus pneumoniae, Haemophilus influenzae* (including β-lactamase-producing strains), or *Moraxella (Branhamella) catarrhalis.*
Pharyngitis and/or tonsillitis caused by *Streptococcus pyogenes.*
NOTE: Only penicillin by the intramuscular route of administration has been shown to be effective in the prophylaxis of rheumatic fever. Cefpodoxime proxetil is generally effective in the eradication of streptococci from the oropharynx. However, data establishing the efficacy of cefpodoxime proxetil for the prophylaxis of subsequent rheumatic fever are not available.

URINARY TRACT
Uncomplicated urinary tract infections (cystitis) caused by *Escherichia coli, Klebsiella pneumoniae, Proteus mirabilis,* or *Staphylococcus saprophyticus.*
NOTE: In considering the use of cefpodoxime proxetil in the treatment of cystitis, cefpodoxime proxetil's lower bacterial eradication rates should be weighed against the increased eradication rates and different safety profiles of some other classes of approved agents. (See CLINICAL STUDIES section.)

Appropriate specimens for bacteriological examination should be obtained in order to isolate and identify causative organisms and to determine their susceptibility to cefpodoxime. Therapy may be instituted while awaiting the results of these studies. Once these results become available, antimicrobial therapy should be adjusted accordingly.

CONTRAINDICATIONS

Cefpodoxime proxetil is contraindicated in patients with a known allergy to cefpodoxime or to the cephalosporin group of antibiotics.

WARNINGS

BEFORE THERAPY WITH CEFPODOXIME PROXETIL IS INSTITUTED, CAREFUL INQUIRY SHOULD BE MADE TO DETERMINE WHETHER THE PATIENT HAS HAD PREVIOUS HYPERSENSITIVITY REACTIONS TO CEFPODOXIME, OTHER CEPHALOSPORINS, PENICILLINS, OR OTHER DRUGS. IF CEFPODOXIME IS TO BE ADMINISTERED TO PENICILLIN-SENSITIVE PATIENTS, CAUTION SHOULD BE EXERCISED BECAUSE CROSS HYPERSENSITIVITY AMONG BETA-LACTAM ANTIBIOTICS HAS BEEN CLEARLY DOCUMENTED AND MAY OCCUR IN UP TO 10% OF PATIENTS WITH A HISTORY OF PENICILLIN ALLERGY. IF AN ALLERGIC REACTION TO CEFPODOXIME PROXETIL OCCURS, DISCONTINUE THE DRUG. SERIOUS ACUTE HYPERSENSITIVITY REACTIONS MAY REQUIRE TREATMENT WITH EPINEPHRINE AND OTHER EMERGENCY MEASURES, INCLUDING OXYGEN, INTRAVENOUS FLUIDS, INTRAVENOUS ANTIHISTAMINE, AND AIRWAY MANAGEMENT, AS CLINICALLY INDICATED. PSEUDOMEMBRANOUS COLITIS HAS BEEN REPORTED WITH NEARLY ALL ANTIBACTERIAL AGENTS, INCLUDING CEFPODOXIME, AND MAY RANGE IN SEVERITY FROM MILD TO LIFE-THREATENING. THEREFORE, IT IS IMPORTANT TO CONSIDER THIS DIAGNOSIS IN PATIENTS WHO PRESENT WITH DIARRHEA SUBSEQUENT TO THE ADMINISTRATION OF ANTIBACTERIAL AGENTS.

Extreme caution should be observed when using this product in patients at increased risk for antibiotic-induced, pseudomembranous colitis because of exposure to institutional settings, such as nursing homes or hospitals with endemic *C. difficile.*

Treatment with broad-spectrum antibiotics, including cefpodoxime proxetil, alters the normal flora of the colon and may permit overgrowth of clostridia. Studies indicate a toxin produced by *Clostridium difficile* is the primary cause of "antibiotic-associated colitis".

After the diagnosis of pseudomembranous colitis has been established, therapeutic measures should be initiated. Mild cases of pseudomembranous colitis usually respond to drug discontinuation alone. In moderate to severe cases, consideration should be given to management with fluids and electrolytes, protein supplementation, and treatment with an oral antibacterial drug effective against *C. difficile.*

A concerted effort to monitor for *C. difficile* in cefpodoxime treated patients with diarrhea was undertaken because of an increased incidence of diarrhea associated with *C. difficile* in early trials in normal subjects. *C. difficile* organisms or toxin was reported in 10% of the cefpodoxime-treated adult patients with diarrhea; however, no specific diagnosis of pseudomembranous colitis was made in these patients.

In post-marketing experience outside the United States, reports of pseudomembranous colitis associated with the use of cefpodoxime proxetil have been received.

PRECAUTIONS

General
In patients with transient or persistent reduction in urinary output due to renal insufficiency, the total daily dose of cefpodoxime proxetil should be reduced because high and prolonged serum antibiotic concentrations can occur in such individuals following usual doses. Cefpodoxime, like other cephalosporins, should be administered with caution to patients receiving concurrent treatment with potent diuretics. (See DOSAGE AND ADMINISTRATION).

As with other antibiotics, prolonged use of cefpodoxime proxetil may result in overgrowth of non-susceptible organisms. Repeated evaluation of the patient's condition is essential. If superinfection occurs during therapy, appropriate measures should be taken.

Drug Interactions
Antacids: Concomitant administration of high doses of antacids (sodium bicarbonate and aluminum hydroxide) or H_2 blockers reduces peak plasma levels by 24% to 42% and the extent of absorption by 27% to 32%, respectively. The rate of absorption is not altered by these concomitant medications. Oral anti-cholinergics (e.g., propantheline) delay peak plasma levels (47% increase in T_{max}), but do not affect the extent of absorption (AUC).

Probenecid: As with other beta-lactam antibiotics, renal excretion of cefpodoxime was inhibited by probenecid and resulted in an approximately 31% increase in AUC and 20% increase in peak cefpodoxime plasma levels.

Nephrotoxic drugs: Although nephrotoxicity has not been noted when cefpodoxime proxetil was given alone, close monitoring of renal function is advised when cefpodoxime proxetil is administered concomitantly with compounds of known nephrotoxic potential.

Drug/Laboratory Test Interactions
Cephalosporins, including cefpodoxime proxetil, are known to occasionally induce a positive direct Coombs' test.

Carcinogenesis, Mutagenesis, Impairment of Fertility
Long-term animal carcinogenesis studies of cefpodoxime proxetil have not been performed. Mutagenesis studies of cefpodoxime, including the Ames test both with and without metabolic activation, the chromosome aberration test, the unscheduled DNA synthesis assay, mitotic recombination and gene conversion, the forward gene mutation assay and the *in vivo* micronucleus test, were all negative. No untoward effects on fertility or reproduction were noted when 100 mg/kg/day or less (2 times the human dose based on mg/m²) was administered orally to rats.

Continued on next page

Information on these Pharmacia & Upjohn products is based on labeling in effect June 1, 1996. Further information concerning these and other Pharmacia & Upjohn products may be obtained by direct inquiry to Medical Information, Pharmacia & Upjohn, Kalamazoo, MI 49001.

Pharmacia & Upjohn—Cont.

Pregnancy—Teratogenic Effects:
Pregnancy Category B
Cefpodoxime proxetil was neither teratogenic nor embryocidal when administered to rats during organogenesis at doses up to 100 mg/kg/day (2 times the human dose based on mg/m^2) or to rabbits at doses up to 30 mg/kg/day (1-2 times the human dose based on mg/m^2).
There are, however, no adequate and well-controlled studies of cefpodoxime proxetil use in pregnant women. Because animal reproduction studies are not always predictive of human response, this drug should be used during pregnancy only if clearly needed.

Labor and Delivery:
Cefpodoxime proxetil has not been studied for use during labor and delivery. Treatment should only be given if clearly needed.

Nursing Mothers:
Cefpodoxime is excreted in human milk. In a study of 3 lactating women, levels of cefpodoxime in human milk were 0%, 2% and 6% of concomitant serum levels at 4 hours following a 200 mg oral dose of cefpodoxime proxetil. At 6 hours post-dosing, levels were 0%, 9% and 16% of concomitant serum levels. Because of the potential for serious reactions in nursing infants, a decision should be made whether to discontinue nursing or to discontinue the drug, taking into account the importance of the drug to the mother.

Pediatric Use
Safety and efficacy in infants less than 5 months of age have not been established.

Geriatric Use
Of the 3338 patients in multiple-dose clinical studies of cefpodoxime proxetil film-coated tablets, 521 (16%) were 65 and over, while 214 (6%) were 75 and over. No overall differences in effectiveness or safety were observed between the elderly and younger patients. In healthy geriatric subjects with normal renal function, cefpodoxime half-life in plasma averaged 4.2 hours and urinary recovery averaged 21% after a 400 mg dose was given every 12 hours for 15 days. Other pharmacokinetic parameters were unchanged relative to those observed in healthy younger subjects.
Dose adjustment in elderly patients with normal renal function is not necessary.

ADVERSE REACTIONS

Clinical Trials:

Film-coated Tablets (Multiple dose):
In clinical trials using multiple doses of cefpodoxime proxetil film-coated tablets, 3338 patients were treated with the recommended dosages of cefpodoxime (100 to 400 mg Q 12 hours). There were no deaths or permanent disabilities thought related to drug toxicity. Eighty-one (2.4%) patients discontinued medication due to adverse events thought possibly- or probably-related to drug toxicity. Sixty-six (66%) of the 100 patients who discontinued therapy (whether thought related to drug therapy or not) did so because of gastrointestinal disturbances, usually diarrhea. The percentage of cefpodoxime proxetil-treated patients who discontinued study drug because of adverse events was significantly greater at a dose of 800 mg daily than at a dose of 400 mg daily or at a dose of 200 mg daily. Adverse events thought possibly- or probably-related to cefpodoxime in multiple dose clinical trials (N=3338 cefpodoxime-treated patients) were:

Incidence greater than 1%:

Diarrhea	7.2%

Diarrhea or loose stools were dose related: decreasing from 10.6% of patients receiving 800 mg per day to 5.9% for those receiving 200 mg per day. Of patients with diarrhea, 10% had *C. difficile* organism or toxin in the stool. (See **WARNINGS**.)

Nausea	3.8%
Vaginal Fungal Infections	3.1%
Abdominal Pain	1.6%
Rash	1.4%
Headache	1.1%
Vomiting	1.1%

Incidence less than 1%:
Cardiovascular: Chest pain, hypotension.
Dermatologic: Fungal skin infection, skin scaling/peeling.
Endocrine: Menstrual irregularity.
Genital: Pruritus.
Gastrointestinal: Flatulence, decreased salivation, candidiasis, pseudomembranous colitis.
Hypersensitivity: Anaphylactic shock.
Metabolic: Decreased appetite.
Miscellaneous: Malaise, fever.
Central Nervous System: Dizziness, fatigue, anxiety, insomnia, flushing, nightmares, weakness.
Respiratory: Cough, epistaxis.
Special Senses: Taste alteration, eye itching, tinnitus.

Granules for Oral Suspension (Multiple dose):
In clinical trials using multiple doses of cefpodoxime proxetil granules for oral suspension, pediatric patients (90% of whom were less than 12 years of age) were treated with the recommended dosages of cefpodoxime (10 mg/kg/day divided Q 12 hours to a maximum equivalent adult dose). There were no deaths or permanent disabilities in any of the patients in these studies. Seven patients (<1%) discontinued medication due to adverse events thought possibly- or probably-related to drug toxicity. Primarily, these discontinuations were for gastrointestinal disturbances, usually diarrhea or diaper area rashes.
Adverse events thought possibly- or probably-related to cefpodoxime granules for oral suspension in multiple dose clinical trials (N=758 cefpodoxime-treated patients) were:

Incidence greater than 1%:

Diarrhea	7.0%

The incidence of diarrhea ranged from 17.8% in infants and toddlers to 4.1% in 2 to 12 year olds to 6.0% in adolescents.

Diaper Rash	3.5%
Other skin rashes	1.8%
Vomiting	1.7%

Incidence less than 1%:
Central Nervous System: Headache, irritability.
Dermatologic: Exacerbation of acne.
Genital: Pruritus or vaginitis.
Gastrointestinal: Nausea, abdominal pain, candidiasis.
Metabolic: Decreased appetite.
Miscellaneous: Fever.

Film-coated tablets (Single dose):
In clinical trials using a single dose of cefpodoxime proxetil film-coated tablets, 509 patients were treated with the recommended dosage of cefpodoxime (200 mg). There were no deaths or permanent disabilities thought related to drug toxicity in these studies.
Adverse events thought possibly- or probably-related to cefpodoxime in single dose clinical trials conducted in the United States were:

Incidence greater than 1%:

Nausea	1.4%
Diarrhea	1.2%

Incidence less than 1%:
Central Nervous System: Dizziness, headache, syncope.
Dermatologic: Rash.
Genital: Vaginitis.
Gastrointestinal: Abdominal pain.
Psychiatric: Anxiety.

Laboratory Changes (Adult patients):
Significant laboratory changes that have been reported in adult patients in clinical trials of cefpodoxime proxetil, without regard to drug relationship, were:
Hepatic: Transient increases in AST (SGOT), ALT (SGPT), GGT, alkaline phosphatase, bilirubin, and LDH.
Hematologic: Eosinophilia, leukocytosis, lymphocytosis, granulocytosis, basophilia, monocytosis, thrombocytosis, decreased hemoglobin, leukopenia, neutropenia, lymphocytopenia, thrombocytopenia, positive Coombs' test, and prolonged PT, and PTT.
Serum Chemistry: Increases in glucose, decreases in glucose, decreases in serum albumin, decreases in serum total protein.
Renal: Increases in BUN and creatinine.
Most of these abnormalities were transient and not clinically significant.

Laboratory Changes (Pediatric patients):
Significant laboratory changes that have been reported in pediatric patients in clinical trials of cefpodoxime proxetil, without regard to drug relationship, were:
Hematologic: Eosinophilia, decreased hemoglobin, decreased hematocrit.
Hepatic: Transiently increased ALT (SGPT)
Most of these abnormalities were transient and not clinically significant.

Post-marketing Experience:
The following serious adverse experiences have been reported: allergic reactions including Stevens-Johnson syndrome, toxic epidermal necrolysis, erythema multiforme and serum sickness-like reactions, pseudomembranous colitis, bloody diarrhea with abdominal pain, ulcerative colitis, rectorrhagia with hypotension, anaphylactic shock, acute liver injury, *in utero* exposure with miscarriage, purpuric nephritis, pulmonary infiltrate with eosinophilia, and eyelid dermatitis.
One death was attributed to pseudomembranous colitis and disseminated intravascular coagulation.

Cephalosporin Class Labeling:
In addition to the adverse reactions listed above which have been observed in patients treated with cefpodoxime proxetil, the following adverse reactions and altered laboratory tests have been reported for cephalosporin class antibiotics:
Adverse Reactions and Abnormal Laboratory Tests: Renal dysfunction, toxic nephropathy, hepatic dysfunction including cholestasis, aplastic anemia, hemolytic anemia, hemorrhage; agranulocytosis; and pancytopenia. Several cephalosporins have been implicated in triggering seizures, particularly in patients with renal impairment when the dosage was not reduced. (See **DOSAGE AND ADMINISTRATION** and **OVERDOSAGE**.) If seizures associated with drug therapy occur, the drug should be discontinued. Anticonvulsant therapy can be given if clinically indicated.

OVERDOSAGE

In acute rodent toxicity studies, a single 5 g/kg oral dose produced no adverse effects.
Information on overdosage in humans is not available. In the event of serious toxic reaction from overdosage, hemodialysis or peritoneal dialysis may aid in the removal of cefpodoxime from the body, particularly if renal function is compromised.
The toxic symptoms following an overdose of β-lactam antibiotics may include nausea, vomiting, epigastric distress, and diarrhea.

DOSAGE AND ADMINISTRATION

(See **INDICATIONS and USAGE** for indicated pathogens.)
FILM-COATED TABLETS:
VANTIN Tablets should be administered orally with food to enhance absorption. (See **CLINICAL PHARMACOLOGY**.)
The recommended dosages, durations of treatment, and applicable patient population are as described in the following chart: [See table below.]

Adults (age 13 years and older):

Type of Infection	Total Daily Dose	Dose Frequency	Duration
Acute community-acquired pneumonia	400 mg	200 mg Q 12 hours	14 days
Acute bacterial exacerbations of chronic bronchitis	400 mg	200 mg Q 12 hours	10 days
Uncomplicated gonorrhea (men and women) and rectal gonococcal infections (women)	200 mg	single dose	
Skin and skin structure	800 mg	400 mg Q 12 hours	7 to 14 days
Pharyngitis and/or tonsillitis	200 mg	100 mg Q 12 hours	10 days
Uncomplicated urinary tract infection	200 mg	100 mg Q 12 hours	7 days

GRANULES FOR ORAL SUSPENSION:
VANTIN for Oral Suspension may be given without regard to food. The recommended dosages, durations of treatment, and applicable patient populations are as described in the following chart:
[See first table at top of next page.]

Patients with Renal Dysfunction:
For patients with severe renal impairment (<30 mL/min creatinine clearance), the dosing intervals should be increased to Q 24 hours. In patients maintained on hemodialysis, the dose frequency should be 3 times/week after hemodialysis.
When only the serum creatinine level is available, the following formula (based on sex, weight, and age of the patient) may be used to estimate creatinine clearance (mL/min). For this estimate to be valid, the serum creatinine level should represent a steady state of renal function.

Males: (mL/min) $\frac{\text{Weight (kg)} \times (140\text{–age})}{72 \times \text{serum creatinine (mg/100 mL)}}$

Females: (mL/min) 0.85 × above value

Patients with Cirrhosis:
Cefpodoxime pharmacokinetics in cirrhotic patients (with or without ascites) are similar to those in healthy subjects. Dose adjustment is not necessary in this population.

Preparation of Suspension:
[See second table at top of next page.]
After mixing, the suspension should be stored in a refrigerator, 2° to 8°C (36° to 46°F). Shake well before using. Keep container tightly closed. The mixture may be used for 14 days. Discard unused portion after 14 days.

HOW SUPPLIED

VANTIN Tablets are available in the following strengths (cefpodoxime equivalent), colors, and sizes: 100 mg, (light orange, elliptical, debossed with U3617)

Bottles of 20	NDC 0009-3617-01
Bottles of 100	NDC 0009-3617-02
Unit dose packs of 100	NDC 0009-3617-03

200 mg, (coral red, elliptical, debossed with U3618)

Bottles of 20	NDC 0009-3618-01
Bottles of 100	NDC 0009-3618-02
Unit dose packs of 100	NDC 0009-3618-03

Adults (age 13 years and older):

Type of Infection	Total Daily Dose	Dose Frequency	Duration
Acute community-acquired pneumonia	400 mg	200 mg Q 12 hours	14 days
Uncomplicated gonorrhea (men and women) and rectal gonococcal infections (women)	200 mg	single dose	
Skin and skin structure	800 mg	400 mg Q 12 hours	7 to 14 days
Pharyngitis and/or tonsillitis	200 mg	100 mg Q 12 hours	10 days
Uncomplicated urinary tract infection	200 mg	100 mg Q 12 hours	7 days

Children (age 5 months through 12 years):

Type of Infection	Total Daily Dose	Dose Frequency	Duration
Acute otitis media	10 mg/kg/day (Max 400 mg/day)	10 mg/kg/ Q 24 h (Max 400 mg/dose) or 5 mg/kg Q 12 h (Max 200 mg/dose)	10 days
Pharyngitis and/or tonsillitis	10 mg/kg/day divided Q 12 hr (Max 200 mg/day)	5 mg/kg/Q 12 h (Max 100 mg/dose)	10 days

Constitution Directions For Oral Suspension

Bottle Size	Final Concentration	Directions
100 mL	50 mg per 5 mL	Suspend in a total of 58 mL of water. Method: First, tap the bottle to loosen granules. Then add the water in two portions, shaking well after each aliquot of water.
100 mL	100 mg per 5 mL	Suspend in a total of 57 mL of water. Method: First, tap the bottle to loosen granules. Then add the water in two portions, shaking well after each aliquot of water.

Store tablets between 15° and 30°C (59° to 86°F). Replace cap securely after each opening. Protect unit dose packs from excessive moisture.

VANTIN for Oral Suspension is available in the following strengths (cefpodoxime equivalents when constituted according to directions), flavor, and size:
50 mg/5 mL, lemon creme flavor in 100 mL bottles NDC 0009-3531-01
100 mg/5 mL, lemon creme flavor in 100 mL bottles NDC 0009-3615-01
Store unsuspended granules between 15° and 30°C (59° to 86°F).
Directions for mixing are included on the label. After mixing, suspension should be stored in a refrigerator, 2° to 8°C (36° to 46°F). Shake well before using. Keep container tightly closed. The mixture may be used for 14 days. Discard unused portion after 14 days.

REFERENCES

1. National Committee for Clinical Laboratory Standards, Approved Standard: Performance Standards for Antimicrobial Disk Susceptibility Tests, 4th Edition, Vol. 10(7):M2-A4, Villanova, PA, April, 1990.
2. National Committee for Clinical Laboratory Standards, Approved Standard: Methods for Dilution Antimicrobial Susceptibility Tests for Bacteria That Grow Aerobically, 2nd Edition, Vol. 10(8):M7-A2, Villanova, PA, April, 1990.

CLINICAL TRIALS:

Cystitis
In two double-blind, 2:1 randomized, comparative trials performed in adults in the United States, cefpodoxime proxetil was compared to other beta-lactam antibiotics. In these studies, the following bacterial eradication rates were obtained at 5 to 9 days after therapy:

Pathogen	Cefpodoxime	Comparators
E. coli	200/243 (82%)	99/123 (80%)
Other pathogens	34/42 (81%)	23/28 (82%)
K. pneumoniae		
P. mirabilis		
S. saprophyticus		
TOTAL	234/285 (82%)	122/151 (81%)

In these studies, clinical cure rates and bacterial eradication rates for cefpodoxime proxetil were comparable to the comparator agents; however, the clinical cure rates and bacteriologic eradication rates were lower than those observed with some other classes of approved agents for cystitis.

Acute Otitis Media Studies
In controlled studies of acute otitis media performed in the United States, where significant rates of β-lactamase-producing organisms were found, cefpodoxime proxetil was compared to other oral antibiotics. In these studies, using very strict evaluability criteria and microbiologic and clinical response criteria at the 15-to-28 day post-therapy follow-up, the following presumptive bacterial eradication/clinical cure outcomes (ie, clinical success) were obtained.

Pathogen	cefpodoxime proxetil 5 mg/kg Q12h × 10 d	comparator
H. influenzae	25/46 (54%)	18/36 (50%)
M. catarrhalis	20/42 (48%)	8/22 (36%)
S. pneumoniae	39/74 (53%)	19/37 (51%)

Pathogen	cefpodoxime proxetil 10 mg/kg Q24h × 10 d	comparator
H. influenzae	36/56 (64%)	12/21 (57%)
M. catarrhalis	14/18 (78%)	8/12 (67%)
S. pneumoniae	56/89 (63%)	21/38 (55%)

Caution: Federal law prohibits dispensing without prescription.
U.S. Patent Nos. 4,486,425; 4,409,215.
Licensed from Sankyo Company, Ltd., Japan and manufactured by Upjohn S.A., Puurs-Belgium for The Upjohn Company Kalamazoo, Michigan 49001, USA
Revised October 1995   815 267 009

Shown in Product Identification Guide, page 329

XANAX®   © ℞
brand of alprazolam tablets, USP

DESCRIPTION

XANAX Tablets contain alprazolam which is a triazolo analog of the 1,4 benzodiazepine class of central nervous system-active compounds.
The chemical name of alprazolam is 8-Chloro-1-methyl-6-phenyl-4H-s-triazolo [4,3-α] [1,4] benzodiazepine.
The structural formula is represented below:

Alprazolam is a white crystalline powder, which is soluble in methanol or ethanol but which has no appreciable solubility in water at physiological pH.
Each XANAX Tablet, for oral administration, contains 0.25, 0.5, 1 or 2 mg of alprazolam.
XANAX Tablets, 2 mg, are multi-scored and may be divided as shown below:

Complete 2 mg Tablet

Two 1 mg segments

Four 0.5 mg segments

Inactive ingredients: Cellulose, corn starch, docusate sodium, lactose, magnesium stearate, silicon dioxide and sodium benzoate. In addition, the 0.5 mg tablet contains FD&C Yellow No. 6 and the 1 mg tablet contains FD&C Blue No. 2.

CLINICAL PHARMACOLOGY

CNS agents of the 1,4 benzodiazepine class presumably exert their effects by binding at stereo specific receptors at several sites within the central nervous system. Their exact mechanism of action is unknown. Clinically, all benzodiazepines cause a dose-related central nervous system depressant activity varying from mild impairment of task performance to hypnosis.

Following oral administration, alprazolam is readily absorbed. Peak concentrations in the plasma occur in one to two hours following administration. Plasma levels are proportionate to the dose given; over the dose range of 0.5 to 3.0 mg, peak levels of 8.0 to 37 ng/mL were observed. Using a specific assay methodology, the mean plasma elimination half-life of alprazolam has been found to be about 11.2 hours (range: 6.3-26.9 hours) in healthy adults.

The predominant metabolites are α-hydroxy-alprazolam and a benzophenone derived from alprazolam. The biological activity of α-hydroxy-alprazolam is approximately one-half that of alprazolam. The benzophenone metabolite is essentially inactive. Plasma levels of these metabolites are extremely low, thus precluding precise pharmacokinetic description. However, their half-lives appear to be of the same order of magnitude as that of alprazolam. Alprazolam and its metabolites are excreted primarily in the urine.

The ability of alprazolam to induce human hepatic enzyme systems has not yet been determined. However, this is not a property of benzodiazepines in general. Further, alprazolam did not affect the prothrombin or plasma warfarin levels in male volunteers administered sodium warfarin orally.

In vitro, alprazolam is bound (80 percent) to human serum protein.

Changes in the absorption, distribution, metabolism and excretion of benzodiazepines have been reported in a variety of disease states including alcoholism, impaired hepatic function and impaired renal function. Changes have also been demonstrated in geriatric patients. A mean half-life of alprazolam of 16.3 hours has been observed in healthy elderly subjects (range: 9.0-26.9 hours, n=16) compared to 11.0 hours (range: 6.3-15.8 hours, n=16) in healthy adult subjects. In patients with alcoholic liver disease the half-life of alprazolam ranged between 5.8 and 65.3 hours (mean: 19.7 hours, n=17) as compared to between 6.3 and 26.9 hours (mean=11.4 hours, n=17) in healthy subjects. In an obese group of subjects the half-life of alprazolam ranged between 9.9 and 40.4 hours (mean=21.8 hours, n=12) as compared to between 6.3 and 15.8 hours (mean=10.6 hours, n=12) in healthy subjects.

Because of its similarity to other benzodiazepines, it is assumed that alprazolam undergoes transplacental passage and that it is excreted in human milk.

INDICATIONS AND USAGE

XANAX Tablets (alprazolam) are indicated for the management of anxiety disorder (a condition corresponding most closely to the APA Diagnostic and Statistical Manual [DSM-III-R] diagnosis of generalized anxiety disorder) or the short-term relief of symptoms of anxiety. Anxiety or tension associated with the stress of everyday life usually does not require treatment with an anxiolytic.

Generalized anxiety disorder is characterized by unrealistic or excessive anxiety and worry (apprehensive expectation) about two or more life circumstances, for a period of six months or longer, during which the person has been bothered more days than not by these concerns. At least 6 of the following 18 symptoms are often present in these patients: Motor Tension (trembling, twitching, or feeling shaky; muscle tension, aches, or soreness; restlessness; easy fatigability); Autonomic Hyperactivity (shortness of breath or smothering sensations; palpitations or accelerated heart rate; sweating, or cold clammy hands; dry mouth; dizziness or light-headedness; nausea, diarrhea, or other abdominal distress; flushes or chills; frequent urination; trouble swallowing or 'lump in throat'); Vigilance and Scanning (feeling keyed up or on edge; exaggerated startle response; difficulty concentrating or 'mind going blank' because of anxiety; trouble falling or staying asleep; irritability). These symptoms must not be secondary to another psychiatric disorder or caused by some organic factor.

Anxiety associated with depression is responsive to XANAX. XANAX is also indicated for the treatment of panic disorder, with or without agoraphobia.

Continued on next page

Information on these Pharmacia & Upjohn products is based on labeling in effect June 1, 1996. Further information concerning these and other Pharmacia & Upjohn products may be obtained by direct inquiry to Medical Information, Pharmacia & Upjohn, Kalamazoo, MI 49001.

Pharmacia & Upjohn—Cont.

Studies supporting this claim were conducted in patients whose diagnoses corresponded closely to the DSM-III-R criteria for panic disorder (see CLINICAL STUDIES).

Panic disorder is an illness characterized by recurrent panic attacks. The panic attacks, at least initially, are unexpected. Later in the course of this disturbance certain situations, eg, driving a car or being in a crowded place, may become associated with having a panic attack. These panic attacks are not triggered by situations in which the person is the focus of others' attention (as in social phobia). The diagnosis requires four such attacks within a four week period, or one or more attacks followed by at least a month of persistent fear of having another attack. The panic attacks must be characterized by at least four of the following symptoms: dyspnea or smothering sensations; dizziness, unsteady feelings, or faintness; palpitations or tachycardia; trembling or shaking; sweating; choking; nausea or abdominal distress; depersonalization or derealization; paresthesias; hot flashes or chills; chest pain or discomfort; fear of dying; fear of going crazy or of doing something uncontrolled. At least some of the panic attack symptoms must develop suddenly, and the panic attack symptoms must not be attributable to some known organic factors. Panic disorder is frequently associated with some symptoms of agoraphobia.

Demonstrations of the effectiveness of XANAX by systematic clinical study are limited to four months duration for anxiety disorder and four to ten weeks duration for panic disorder; however, patients with panic disorder have been treated on an open basis for up to eight months without apparent loss of benefit. The physician should periodically reassess the usefulness of the drug for the individual patient.

CONTRAINDICATIONS

XANAX Tablets are contraindicated in patients with known sensitivity to this drug or other benzodiazepines. XANAX may be used in patients with open angle glaucoma who are receiving appropriate therapy, but is contraindicated in patients with acute narrow angle glaucoma.

XANAX is contraindicated with ketoconazole and itraconazole, since these medications significantly impair the oxidative metabolism mediated by cytochrome P450 3A (CYP 3A) (see WARNINGS and PRECAUTIONS-Drug Interactions).

WARNINGS

Dependence and withdrawal reactions, including seizures:

Certain adverse clinical events, some life-threatening, are a direct consequence of physical dependence to XANAX. These include a spectrum of withdrawal symptoms; the most important is seizure (see DRUG ABUSE AND DEPENDENCE). Even after relatively short-term use at the doses recommended for the treatment of transient anxiety and anxiety disorder (ie, 0.75 to 4.0 mg per day), there is some risk of dependence. Post-marketing surveillance data suggest that the risk of dependence and its severity appear to be greater in patients treated with relatively high doses (above 4 mg per day) and for long periods (more than 8-12 weeks).

The importance of dose and the risks of XANAX as a treatment for panic disorder:

Because the management of panic disorder often requires the use of average daily doses of XANAX above 4 mg, the risk of dependence among panic disorder patients may be higher than that among those treated for less severe anxiety. Experience in randomized placebo-controlled discontinuation studies of patients with panic disorder showed a high rate of rebound and withdrawal symptoms in patients treated with XANAX compared to placebo treated patients.

Relapse or return of illness was defined as a return of symptoms characteristic of panic disorder (primarily panic attacks) to levels approximately equal to those seen at baseline before active treatment was initiated. Rebound refers to a return of symptoms of panic disorder to a level substantially greater in frequency, or more severe in intensity than seen at baseline. Withdrawal symptoms were identified as those which were generally not characteristic of panic disorder and which occurred for the first time more frequently during discontinuation than at baseline.

In a controlled clinical trial in which 63 patients were randomized to XANAX and where withdrawal symptoms were specifically sought, the following were identified as symptoms of withdrawal: heightened sensory perception, impaired concentration, dysosmia, clouded sensorium, paresthesias, muscle cramps, muscle twitch, diarrhea, blurred vision, appetite decrease and weight loss. Other symptoms, such as anxiety and insomnia, were frequently seen during discontinuation, but it could not be determined if they were due to return of illness, rebound or withdrawal.

In a larger database comprised of both controlled and uncontrolled studies in which 641 patients received XANAX, discontinuation-emergent symptoms which occurred at a rate of over 5% in patients treated with XANAX and at a greater rate than the placebo treated group were as follows:

[See table below.]

From the studies cited, it has not been determined whether these symptoms are clearly related to the dose and duration of therapy with XANAX in patients with panic disorder.

In two controlled trials of six to eight weeks duration where the ability of patients to discontinue medication was measured, 71%-93% of XANAX treated patients tapered completely off therapy compared to 89%-96% of placebo treated patients. The ability of patients to completely discontinue therapy with XANAX after long-term therapy has not been reliably determined.

Seizures attributable to XANAX were seen after drug discontinuance or dose reduction in 8 of 1980 patients with panic disorder or in patients participating in clinical trials where XANAX doses of greater than 4 mg daily for over 3 months were permitted. Five of these cases clearly occurred during abrupt dose reduction, or discontinuation from daily doses of 2 to 10 mg. Three cases occurred in situations where there was not a clear relationship to abrupt dose reduction or discontinuation. In one instance, seizure occurred after discontinuation from a single dose of 1 mg after tapering at a rate of 1 mg every three days from 6 mg daily. In two other instances, the relationship to taper is indeterminate; in both of these cases the patients had been receiving doses of 3 mg daily prior to seizure. The duration of use in the above 8 cases ranged from 4 to 22 weeks. There have been occasional voluntary reports of patients developing seizures while apparently tapering gradually from XANAX. The risk of seizure seems to be greatest 24-72 hours after discontinuation (see DOSAGE AND ADMINISTRATION for recommended tapering and discontinuation schedule).

Status epilepticus and its treatment:

The medical event voluntary reporting system shows that withdrawal seizures have been reported in association with the discontinuation of XANAX. In most cases, only a single seizure was reported; however, multiple seizures and status epilepticus were reported as well. Ordinarily, the treatment of status epilepticus of any etiology involves use of intravenous benzodiazepines plus phenytoin or barbiturates, maintenance of a patent airway and adequate hydration. For additional details regarding therapy, consultation with an appropriate specialist may be considered.

Interdose Symptoms:

Early morning anxiety and emergence of anxiety symptoms between doses of XANAX have been reported in patients with panic disorder taking prescribed maintenance doses of XANAX. These symptoms may reflect the development of tolerance or a time interval between doses which is longer than the duration of clinical action of the administered dose. In either case, it is presumed that the prescribed dose is not sufficient to maintain plasma levels above those needed to prevent relapse, rebound or withdrawal symptoms over the entire course of the interdosing interval. In these situations, it is recommended that the same total daily dose be given divided as more frequent administrations (see DOSAGE AND ADMINISTRATION).

Risk of dose reduction:

Withdrawal reactions may occur when dosage reduction occurs for any reason. This includes purposeful tapering, but also inadvertent reduction of dose (eg, the patient forgets, the patient is admitted to a hospital, etc.). Therefore, the dosage of XANAX should be reduced or discontinued gradually (see DOSAGE AND ADMINISTRATION).

XANAX Tablets are not of value in the treatment of psychotic patients and should not be employed in lieu of appropriate treatment for psychosis. Because of its CNS depressant effects, patients receiving XANAX should be cautioned against engaging in hazardous occupations or activities requiring complete mental alertness such as operating machinery or driving a motor vehicle. For the same reason, patients should be cautioned about the simultaneous ingestion of alcohol and other CNS depressant drugs during treatment with XANAX.

Benzodiazepines can potentially cause fetal harm when administered to pregnant women. If XANAX is used during pregnancy, or if the patient becomes pregnant while taking this drug, the patient should be apprised of the potential hazard to the fetus. Because of experience with other members of the benzodiazepine class, XANAX is assumed to be capable of causing an increased risk of congenital abnormalities when administered to a pregnant woman during the first trimester. Because use of these drugs is rarely a matter of urgency, their use during the first trimester should almost always be avoided. The possibility that a woman of childbearing potential may be pregnant at the time of institution of therapy should be considered. Patients should be advised that if they become pregnant during therapy or intend to become pregnant they should communicate with their physicians about the desirability of discontinuing the drug.

Alprazolam interaction with drugs that inhibit metabolism via cytochrome P450 3A:

The initial step in alprazolam metabolism is hydroxylation catalyzed by cyto chrome P450 3A (CYP 3A). Drugs that inhibit this metabolic pathway may have a profound effect on the clearance of alprazolam. Consequently, alprazolam should be avoided in patients receiving very potent inhibitors of CYP 3A. With drugs inhibiting CYP 3A to a lesser but still significant degree, alprazolam should be used only with caution and consideration of appropriate dosage reduction. For some drugs, an interaction with alprazolam has been quantified with clinical data; for other drugs, interactions are predicted from *in vitro* data and/or experience with similar drugs in the same pharmacologic class.

The following are examples of drugs known to inhibit the metabolism of alprazolam and/or related benzodiazepines, presumably through inhibition of CYP 3A.

Potent CYP 3A inhibitors:

Azole antifungal agents—Although *in vivo* interaction data with alprazolam are not available, ketoconazole and itraconazole are potent CYP 3A inhibitors and the coadministration of alprazolam with them is not recommended. Other azole-type antifungal agents should also be considered potent CYP 3A inhibitors and the coadministration of alprazolam with them is not recommended (see CONTRAINDICATIONS).

Drugs demonstrated to be CYP 3A inhibitors on the basis of clinical studies involving alprazolam (caution and consideration of appropriate alprazolam dose reduction are recommended during coadministration with the following drugs):

Nefazodone—Coadministration of nefazodone increased alprazolam concentration two-fold.

Fluvoxamine—Coadministration of fluvoxamine approx imately doubled the maximum plasma concentration of alprazolam, decreased clearance by 49%, increased half-life by 71%, and decreased measured psychomotor performance.

Cimetidine—Coadministration of cimetidine increased the maximum plasma concentration of alprazolam by 86%, decreased clearance by 42%, and increased half-life by 16%.

Other drugs possibly affecting alprazolam metabolism:

Other drugs possibly affecting alprazolam metabolism by inhibition of CYP 3A are discussed in the PRECAUTIONS section (see PRECAUTIONS-Drug Interactions).

PRECAUTIONS

General: If XANAX Tablets are to be combined with other psychotropic agents or anticonvulsant drugs, careful consideration should be given to the pharmacology of the agents to be employed, particularly with compounds which might potentiate the action of benzodiazepines (see DRUG INTERACTIONS).

As with other psychotropic medications, the usual precautions with respect to administration of the drug and size of the prescription are indicated for severely depressed patients or those in whom there is reason to expect concealed suicidal ideation or plans.

DISCONTINUATION-EMERGENT SYMPTOM INCIDENCE

Percentage of 641 XANAX-Treated Panic Disorder Patients Reporting Events

Body System/Event	
Neurologic	
Insomnia	29.5
Light-headedness	19.3
Abnormal involuntary movement	17.3
Headache	17.0
Muscular twitching	6.9
Impaired coordination	6.6
Muscle tone disorders	5.9
Weakness	5.8
Psychiatric	
Anxiety	19.2
Fatigue and Tiredness	18.4
Irritability	10.5
Cognitive disorder	10.3
Memory impairment	5.5
Depression	5.1
Confusional state	5.0
Gastrointestinal	
Nausea/Vomiting	16.5
Diarrhea	13.6
Decreased salivation	10.6
Metabolic-Nutritional	
Weight loss	13.3
Decreased appetite	12.8
Dermatological	
Sweating	14.4
Cardiovascular	
Tachycardia	12.2
Special Senses	
Blurred vision	10.0

It is recommended that the dosage be limited to the smallest effective dose to preclude the development of ataxia or oversedation which may be a particular problem in elderly or debilitated patients. (See DOSAGE AND ADMINISTRATION.) The usual precautions in treating patients with impaired renal, hepatic or pulmonary function should be observed. There have been rare reports of death in patients with severe pulmonary disease shortly after the initiation of treatment with XANAX. A decreased systemic alprazolam elimination rate (eg, increased plasma half-life) has been observed in both alcoholic liver disease patients and obese patients receiving XANAX (see CLINICAL PHARMACOLOGY).

Episodes of hypomania and mania have been reported in association with the use of XANAX in patients with depression.

Alprazolam has a weak uricosuric effect. Although other medications with weak uricosuric effect have been reported to cause acute renal failure, there have been no reported instances of acute renal failure attributable to therapy with XANAX.

Information for Patients:

For all users of XANAX:

To assure safe and effective use of benzodiazepines, all patients prescribed XANAX should be provided with the following guidance. In addition, panic disorder patients, for whom higher doses are typically prescribed, should be advised about the risks associated with the use of higher doses.

1. Inform your physician about any alcohol consumption and medicine you are taking now, including medication you may buy without a prescription. Alcohol should generally not be used during treatment with benzodiazepines.
2. Not recommended for use in pregnancy. Therefore, inform your physician if you are pregnant, if you are planning to have a child, or if you become pregnant while you are taking this medication.
3. Inform your physician if you are nursing.
4. Until you experience how this medication affects you, do not drive a car or operate potentially dangerous machinery, etc.
5. Do not increase the dose even if you think the medication does not work anymore without consulting your physician. Benzodiazepines, even when used as recommended, may produce emotional and/or physical dependence.
6. Do not stop taking this medication abruptly or decrease the dose without consulting your physician, since withdrawal symptoms can occur.

Additional advice for panic disorder patients:

The use of XANAX at the high doses (above 4 mg per day), often necessary to treat panic disorder, is accompanied by risks that you need to carefully consider. When used at high doses for long intervals, which may or may not be required for your treatment, XANAX has the potential to cause severe emotional and physical dependence in some patients and these patients may find it exceedingly difficult to terminate treatment. In two controlled trials of six to eight weeks duration where the ability of patients to discontinue medication was measured, 7 to 29% of XANAX treated patients did not completely taper off therapy. The ability of patients to completely discontinue therapy with XANAX after long-term therapy has not been reliably determined. In all cases, it is important that your physician help you discontinue this medication in a careful and safe manner to avoid overly extended use of XANAX.

In addition, the extended use at high doses appears to increase the incidence and severity of withdrawal reactions when XANAX is discontinued. These are generally minor but seizure can occur, especially if you reduce the dose too rapidly or discontinue the medication abruptly. Seizure can be life-threatening.

Laboratory Tests: Laboratory tests are not ordinarily required in otherwise healthy patients.

Drug Interactions: The benzodiazepines, including alprazolam, produce additive CNS depressant effects when coadministered with other psychotropic medications, anticonvulsants, antihistaminics, ethanol and other drugs which themselves produce CNS depression.

The steady state plasma concentrations of imipramine and desipramine have been reported to be increased an average of 31% and 20%, respectively, by the concomitant administration of XANAX Tablets in doses up to 4 mg/day. The clinical significance of these changes is unknown.

Drugs that inhibit alprazolam metabolism via cytochrome P450 3A: The initial step in alprazolam metabolism is hydroxylation catalyzed by cytochrome P450 3A (CYP 3A). Drugs which inhibit this metabolic pathway may have a profound effect on the clearance of alprazolam (see CONTRAINDICATIONS and WARNINGS for additional drugs of this type).

Drugs demonstrated to be CYP 3A inhibitors of possible clinical significance on the basis of clinical studies involving alprazolam (caution is recommended during coadministration with alprazolam):

Fluoxetine—Coadministration of fluoxetine with alprazolam increased the maximum plasma concentration of alprazolam by 46%, decreased clearance by 21%, increased half-life by 17%, and decreased measured psychomotor performance.

Propoxyphene—Coadministration of propoxyphene decreased the maximum plasma concentration of alprazolam by 6%, decreased clearance by 38%, and increased half-life by 58%.

Oral Contraceptives—Coadministration of oral contraceptives increased the maximum plasma concentration of alprazolam by 18%, decreased clearance by 22%, and increased half-life by 29%.

Drugs and other substances demonstrated to be CYP 3A inhibitors on the basis of clinical studies involving benzodiazepines metabolized similarly to alprazolam or on the basis of in vitro studies with alprazolam or other benzodiazepines (caution is recommended during coadministration with alprazolam):

Available data from clinical studies of benzodiazepines other than alprazolam suggest a possible drug interaction with alprazolam for the following: diltiazem, isoniazid, macrolide antibiotics such as erythromycin and clarithromycin, and grapefruit juice. Data from *in vitro* studies of alprazolam suggest a possible drug interaction with alprazolam for the following: sertraline and paroxetine. Data from *in vitro* studies of benzodiazepines other than alprazolam suggest a possible drug interaction for the following: ergotamine, cyclo sporine, amiodarone, nicardipine, and nifedipine. Caution is recommended during the coadministration of any of these with alprazolam (see WARNINGS).

Drug/Laboratory Test Interactions: Although interactions between benzodiazepines and commonly employed clinical laboratory tests have occasionally been reported, there is no consistent pattern for a specific drug or specific test.

Carcinogenesis, Mutagenesis, Impairment of Fertility: No evidence of carcinogenic potential was observed during 2-year bioassay studies of alprazolam in rats at doses up to 30 mg/kg/day (150 times the maximum recommended daily human dose of 10 mg/day) and in mice at doses up to 10 mg/kg/day (50 times the maximum recommended daily human dose).

Alprazolam was not mutagenic in the rat micronucleus test at doses up to 100 mg/kg, which is 500 times the maximum recommended daily human dose of 10 mg/day. Alprazolam also was not mutagenic *in vitro* in the DNA Damage/Alkaline Elution Assay or the Ames Assay.

Alprazolam produced no impairment of fertility in rats at doses up to 5 mg/kg/day, which is 25 times the maximum recommended daily human dose of 10 mg/day.

Pregnancy: Teratogenic Effects: Pregnancy Category D: (See WARNINGS Section).

Nonteratogenic Effects: It should be considered that the child born of a mother who is receiving benzodiazepines may be at some risk for withdrawal symptoms from the drug during the postnatal period. Also, neonatal flaccidity and respiratory problems have been reported in children born of mothers who have been receiving benzodiazepines.

Labor and Delivery: XANAX has no established use in labor or delivery.

Nursing Mothers: Benzodiazepines are known to be excreted in human milk. It should be assumed that alprazolam is as well. Chronic administration of diazepam to nursing mothers has been reported to cause their infants to become lethargic and to lose weight. As a general rule, nursing should not be undertaken by mothers who must use XANAX.

Pediatric Use: Safety and effectiveness of XANAX in individuals below 18 years of age have not been established.

ADVERSE REACTIONS

Side effects to XANAX Tablets, if they occur, are generally observed at the beginning of therapy and usually disappear upon continued medication. In the usual patient, the most frequent side effects are likely to be an extension of the pharmacological activity of alprazolam, eg, drowsiness or lightheadedness.

The data cited in the two tables below are estimates of untoward clinical event incidence among patients who participated under the following clinical conditions: relatively short duration (ie, four weeks) placebo-controlled clinical studies with dosages up to 4 mg/day of XANAX (for the management of anxiety disorders or for the short-term relief of the symptoms of anxiety) and short-term (up to ten weeks) placebo-controlled clinical studies with dosages up to 10 mg/day of XANAX in patients with panic disorder, with or without agoraphobia.

These data cannot be used to predict precisely the incidence of untoward events in the course of usual medical practice where patient characteristics, and other factors often differ from those in clinical trials. These figures cannot be compared with those obtained from other clinical studies involving related drug products and placebo as each group of drug trials are conducted under a different set of conditions.

Comparison of the cited figures, however, can provide the prescriber with some basis for estimating the relative contributions of drug and non-drug factors to the untoward event incidence in the population studied. Even this use must be approached cautiously, as a drug may relieve a symptom in one patient but induce it in others. (For example, an anxiolytic drug may relieve dry mouth [a symptom of anxiety] in some subjects but induce it [an untoward event] in others.) Additionally, for anxiety disorders the cited figures can provide the prescriber with an indication as to the frequency with which physician intervention (eg, increased surveillance, decreased dosage or discontinuation of drug therapy) may be necessary because of the untoward clinical event. [See table at bottom of next page.]

In addition to the relatively common (ie, greater than 1%) untoward events enumerated in the table above, the following adverse events have been reported in association with the use of benzodiazepines: dystonia, irritability, concentration difficulties, anorexia, transient amnesia or memory impairment, loss of coordination, fatigue, seizures, sedation, slurred speech, jaundice, musculoskeletal weakness, pruritus, diplopia, dysarthria, changes in libido, menstrual irregularities, incontinence and urinary retention.

PANIC DISORDER

	Treatment-Emergent Symptom Incidence*	
	XANAX	PLACEBO
Number of Patients	1388	1231
% of Patients Reporting:		
Central Nervous System		
Drowsiness	76.8	42.7
Fatigue and Tiredness	48.6	42.3
Impaired Coordination	40.1	17.9
Irritability	33.1	30.1
Memory Impairment	33.1	22.1
Light-headedness/Dizziness	29.8	36.9
Insomnia	29.4	41.8
Headache	29.2	35.6
Cognitive Disorder	28.8	20.5
Dysarthria	23.3	6.3
Anxiety	16.6	24.9
Abnormal Involuntary Movement	14.8	21.0
Decreased Libido	14.4	8.0
Depression	13.8	14.0
Confusional State	10.4	8.2
Muscular Twitching	7.9	11.8
Increased Libido	7.7	4.1
Change in Libido (Not Specified)	7.1	5.6
Weakness	7.1	8.4
Muscle Tone Disorders	6.3	7.5
Syncope	3.8	4.8
Akathisia	3.0	4.3
Agitation	2.9	2.6
Disinhibition	2.7	1.5
Paresthesia	2.4	3.2
Talkativeness	2.2	1.0
Vasomotor Disturbances	2.0	2.6
Derealization	1.9	1.2
Dream Abnormalities	1.8	1.5
Fear	1.4	1.0
Feeling Warm	1.3	0.5
Gastrointestinal		
Decreased Salivation	32.8	34.2
Constipation	26.2	15.4
Nausea/Vomiting	22.0	31.8
Diarrhea	20.6	22.8
Abdominal Distress	18.3	21.5
Increased Salivation	5.6	4.4
Cardio-Respiratory		
Nasal Congestion	17.4	16.5
Tachycardia	15.4	26.8
Chest Pain	10.6	18.1
Hyperventilation	9.7	14.5
Upper Respiratory Infection	4.3	3.7
Sensory		
Blurred Vision	21.0	21.4
Tinnitus	6.6	10.4
Musculoskeletal		
Muscular Cramps	2.4	2.4
Muscle Stiffness	2.2	3.3
Cutaneous		
Sweating	15.1	23.5
Rash	10.8	8.1
Other		
Increased Appetite	32.7	22.8
Decreased Appetite	27.8	24.1
Weight Gain	27.2	17.9
Weight Loss	22.6	16.5
Micturition Difficulties	12.2	8.6
Menstrual Disorders	10.4	8.7
Sexual Dysfunction	7.4	3.7

Continued on next page

Information on these Pharmacia & Upjohn products is based on labeling in effect June 1, 1996. Further information concerning these and other Pharmacia & Upjohn products may be obtained by direct inquiry to Medical Information, Pharmacia & Upjohn, Kalamazoo, MI 49001.

Pharmacia & Upjohn—Cont.

Edema	4.9	5.6
Incontinence	1.5	0.6
Infection	1.3	1.7

Events reported by 1% or more of XANAX patients are included.

In addition to the relatively common (ie, greater than 1%) untoward events enumerated in the table above, the following adverse events have been reported in association with the use of XANAX: seizures, hallucinations, depersonalization, taste alterations, diplopia, elevated bilirubin, elevated hepatic enzymes, and jaundice.

There have also been reports of withdrawal seizures upon rapid decrease or abrupt discontinuation of XANAX Tablets (see WARNINGS).

To discontinue treatment in patients taking XANAX, the dosage should be reduced slowly in keeping with good medical practice. It is suggested that the daily dosage of XANAX be decreased by no more than 0.5 mg every three days (see DOSAGE AND ADMINISTRATION). Some patients may require an even slower dosage reduction.

Panic disorder has been associated with primary and secondary major depressive disorders and increased reports of suicide among untreated patients. Therefore, the same precaution must be exercised when using the higher doses of XANAX in treating patients with panic disorders as is exercised with the use of any psychotropic drug in treating depressed patients or those in whom there is reason to expect concealed suicidal ideation or plans.

As with all benzodiazepines, paradoxical reactions such as stimulation, increased muscle spasticity, sleep disturbances, hallucinations and other adverse behavioral effects such as agitation, rage, irritability, and aggressive or hostile behavior have been reported rarely. In many of the spontaneous case reports of adverse behavioral effects, patients were receiving other CNS drugs concomitantly and/or were described as having underlying psychiatric conditions. Should any of the above events occur, alprazolam should be discontinued. Isolated published reports involving small numbers of patients have suggested that patients who have borderline personality disorder, a prior history of violent or aggressive behavior, or alcohol or substance abuse may be at risk for such events. Instances of irritability, hostility, and intrusive thoughts have been reported during discontinuation of alprazolam in patients with posttraumatic stress disorder.

Laboratory analyses were performed on patients participating in the clinical program for XANAX. The following incidences of abnormalities shown below were observed in patients receiving XANAX and in patients in the corresponding placebo group. Few of these abnormalities were considered to be of physiological significance.

	XANAX		PLACEBO	
	Low	High	Low	High
Hematology				
Hematocrit	*	*	*	*
Hemoglobin	*	*	*	*
Total WBC Count	1.4	2.3	1.0	2.0
Neutrophil Count	2.3	3.0	4.2	1.7
Lymphocyte Count	5.5	7.4	5.4	9.5
Monocyte Count	5.3	2.8	6.4	*
Eosinophil Count	3.2	9.5	3.3	7.2
Basophil Count	*	*	*	*
Urinalysis				
Albumin	—	*	—	*
Sugar	—	*	—	*
RBC/HPF	—	3.4	—	5.0
WBC/HPF	—	25.7	—	25.9
Blood Chemistry				
Creatinine	2.2	1.9	3.5	1.0
Bilirubin	*	1.6	*	*
SGOT	*	3.2	1.0	1.8
Alkaline Phosphatase	*	1.7	*	1.8

Less than 1%

When treatment with XANAX is protracted, periodic blood counts, urinalysis and blood chemistry analyses are advisable.

Minor changes in EEG patterns, usually low-voltage fast activity have been observed in patients during therapy with XANAX and are of no known significance. Post Introduction Reports: Various adverse drug reactions have been reported in association with the use of XANAX since market introduction. The majority of these reactions were reported through the medical event voluntary reporting system. Because of the spontaneous nature of the reporting of medical events and the lack of controls, a causal relationship to the use of XANAX cannot be readily determined. Reported events include: liver enzyme elevations, gynecomastia and galactorrhea.

DRUG ABUSE AND DEPENDENCE

Physical and Psychological Dependence: Withdrawal symptoms similar in character to those noted with sedative/hypnotics and alcohol have occurred following discontinuance of benzodiazepines, including XANAX. The symptoms can range from mild dysphoria and insomnia to a major syndrome that may include abdominal and muscle cramps, vomiting, sweating, tremors and convulsions. Distinguishing between withdrawal emergent signs and symptoms and the recurrence of illness is often difficult in patients undergoing dose reduction. The long term strategy for treatment of these phenomena will vary with their cause and the therapeutic goal. When necessary, immediate management of withdrawal symptoms requires re-institution of treatment at doses of XANAX sufficient to suppress symptoms. There have been reports of failure of other benzodiazepines to fully suppress these withdrawal symptoms. These failures have been attributed to incomplete cross-tolerance but may also reflect the use of an inadequate dosing regimen of the substituted benzodiazepine or the effects of concomitant medications.

While it is difficult to distinguish withdrawal and recurrence for certain patients, the time course and the nature of the symptoms may be helpful. A withdrawal syndrome typically includes the occurrence of new symptoms, tends to appear toward the end of taper or shortly after discontinuation, and will decrease with time. In recurring panic disorder, symptoms similar to those observed before treatment may recur either early or late, and they will persist.

While the severity and incidence of withdrawal phenomena appear to be related to dose and duration of treatment, withdrawal symptoms, including seizures, have been reported after only brief therapy with XANAX at doses within the recommended range for the treatment of anxiety (eg, 0.75 to 4 mg/day). Signs and symptoms of withdrawal are often more prominent after rapid decrease of dosage or abrupt discontinuance. The risk of withdrawal seizures may be increased at doses above 4 mg/day (see WARNINGS).

Patients, especially individuals with a history of seizures or epilepsy, should not be abruptly discontinued from any CNS depressant agent, including XANAX. It is recommended that all patients on XANAX who require a dosage reduction be gradually tapered under close supervision (see WARNINGS and DOSAGE AND ADMINISTRATION).

Psychological dependence is a risk with all benzodiazepines, including XANAX. The risk of psychological dependence may also be increased at higher doses and with longer term use, and this risk is further increased in patients with a history of alcohol or drug abuse. Some patients have experienced considerable difficulty in tapering and discontinuing from XANAX, especially those receiving higher doses for extended periods. Addiction-prone individuals should be under careful surveillance when receiving XANAX. As with all anxiolytics, repeat prescriptions should be limited to those who are under medical supervision.

Controlled Substance Class: Alprazolam is a controlled substance under the Controlled Substance Act by the Drug Enforce ment Ad ministration and XANAX Tablets have been assigned to Schedule IV.

OVERDOSAGE

Manifestations of alprazolam overdosage include somnolence, confusion, impaired coordination, diminished reflexes and coma. Death has been reported in association with overdoses of alprazolam by itself, as it has with other benzodiazepines. In addition, fatalities have been reported in patients who have overdosed with a combination of a single benzodiazepine, including alprazolam, and alcohol; alcohol levels seen in some of these patients have been lower than those usually associated with alcohol-induced fatality.

The acute oral LD_{50} in rats is 331-2171 mg/kg. Other experiments in animals have indicated that cardiopulmonary collapse can occur following massive intravenous doses of alprazolam (over 195 mg/kg; 975 times the maximum recommended daily human dose of 10 mg/day). Animals could be resuscitated with positive mechanical ventilation and the intravenous infusion of norepinephrine bitartrate.

Animal experiments have suggested that forced diuresis or hemodialysis are probably of little value in treating overdosage.

General Treatment of Overdose: Overdosage reports with XANAX Tablets are limited. As in all cases of drug overdosage, respiration, pulse rate, and blood pressure should be monitored. General supportive measures should be employed, along with immediate gastric lavage. Intravenous fluids should be administered and an adequate airway maintained. If hypotension occurs, it may be combated by the use of vasopressors. Dialysis is of limited value. As with the management of intentional overdosing with any drug, it should be borne in mind that multiple agents may have been ingested.

Flumazenil, a specific benzodiazepine receptor antagonist, is indicated for the complete or partial reversal of the sedative effects of benzodiazepines and may be used in situations when an overdose with a benzodiazepine is known or suspected. Prior to the administration of flumazenil, necessary measures should be instituted to secure airway, ventilation and intravenous access. Flumazenil is intended as an adjunct to, not as a substitute for, proper management of benzodiazepine overdose. Patients treated with flumazenil should be monitored for re-sedation, respiratory depression, and other residual benzodiazepine effects for an appropriate period after treatment. The prescriber should be aware of a risk of seizure in association with flumazenil treatment, particularly in long-term benzodiazepine users and in cyclic antidepressant overdose. The complete flumazenil package

	ANXIETY DISORDERS		
	Treatment-Emergent Symptom Incidence†		Incidence of Intervention Because of Symptom
	XANAX	**PLACEBO**	**XANAX**
Number of Patients	565	505	565
% of Patients Reporting:			
Central Nervous System			
Drowsiness	41.0	21.6	15.1
Light-headedness	20.8	19.3	1.2
Depression	13.9	18.1	2.4
Headache	12.9	19.6	1.1
Confusion	9.9	10.0	0.9
Insomnia	8.9	18.4	1.3
Nervousness	4.1	10.3	1.1
Syncope	3.1	4.0	
Dizziness	1.8	0.8	2.5
Akathisia	1.6	1.2	
Tiredness/Sleepiness	*	*	1.8
Gastrointestinal			
Dry Mouth	14.7	13.3	0.7
Constipation	10.4	11.4	0.9
Diarrhea	10.1	10.3	1.2
Nausea/Vomiting	9.6	12.8	1.7
Increased Salivation	4.2	2.4	
Cardiovascular			
Tachycardia/Palpitations	7.7	15.6	0.4
Hypotension	4.7	2.2	
Sensory			
Blurred Vision	6.2	6.2	0.4
Musculoskeletal			
Rigidity	4.2	5.3	
Tremor	4.0	8.8	0.4
Cutaneous			
Dermatitis/Allergy	3.8	3.1	0.6
Other			
Nasal Congestion	7.3	9.3	
Weight Gain	2.7	2.7	*
Weight Loss	2.3	3.0	*

* None reported
† Events reported by 1% or more of XANAX patients are included.

insert including CONTRAINDICATIONS, WARNINGS and PRECAUTIONS should be consulted prior to use.

DOSAGE AND ADMINISTRATION

Dosage should be individualized for maximum beneficial effect. While the usual daily dosages given below will meet the needs of most patients, there will be some who require higher doses. In such cases, dosage should be increased cautiously to avoid adverse effects.

Anxiety disorders and transient symptoms of anxiety:
Treatment for patients with anxiety should be initiated with a dose of 0.25 to 0.5 mg given three times daily. The dose may be increased to achieve a maximum therapeutic effect, at intervals of 3 to 4 days, to a maximum daily dose of 4 mg, given in divided doses. The lowest possible effective dose should be employed and the need for continued treatment reassessed frequently. The risk of dependence may increase with dose and duration of treatment.
In elderly patients, in patients with advanced liver disease or in patients with debilitating disease, the usual starting dose is 0.25 mg, given two or three times daily. This may be gradually increased if needed and tolerated. The elderly may be especially sensitive to the effects of benzodiazepines.
If side effects occur at the recommended starting dose, the dose may be lowered.
In all patients, dosage should be reduced gradually when discontinuing therapy or when decreasing the daily dosage. Although there are no systematically collected data to support a specific discontinuation schedule, it is suggested that the daily dosage be decreased by no more than 0.5 mg every three days. Some patients may require an even slower dosage reduction.

Panic disorder:
The successful treatment of many panic disorder patients has required the use of XANAX at doses greater than 4 mg daily. In controlled trials conducted to establish the efficacy of XANAX in panic disorder, doses in the range of 1 to 10 mg daily were used. The mean dosage employed was approximately 5 to 6 mg daily. Among the approximately 1700 patients participating in the panic disorder development program, about 300 received maximum XANAX dosages of greater than 7 mg/day, including approximately 100 patients who received maximum dosages of greater than 9 mg/day. Occasional patients required as much as 10 mg a day to achieve a successful response.
However, in the absence of systematic studies evaluating the dose response relationship, the dosing regimen for the administration of XANAX to patients with panic disorder must be based on generic principles. Generally, therapy should be initiated at a low dose to minimize the risk of adverse responses in patients especially sensitive to the drug. Thereafter, the dose can be increased at intervals equal to at least 5 times the elimination half-life (about 11 hours in young patients, about 16 hours in elderly patients). Longer titration intervals should probably be used because the maximum therapeutic response may not occur until after the plasma levels achieve steady state. Dose should be advanced until an acceptable therapeutic response (ie, a substantial reduction in or total elimination of panic attacks) is achieved, intolerance occurs, or the maximum recommended dose is attained. Because of the danger of withdrawal, abrupt discontinuation of treatment should be avoided. (See WARNINGS, PRECAUTIONS, DRUG ABUSE AND DEPENDENCE).

The following regimen is one that follows the principles outlined above:
Treatment may be initiated with a dose of 0.5 mg three times daily. Depending on the response, the dose may be increased at intervals of 3 to 4 days in increments of no more than 1 mg per day. Slower titration to the higher dose levels may be advisable to allow full expression of the pharmacodynamic effect of XANAX. To lessen the possibility of interdose symptoms, the times of administration should be distributed as evenly as possible throughout the waking hours, that is, on a three or four times per day schedule.
The necessary duration of treatment for panic disorder patients responding to XANAX is unknown. After a period of extended freedom from attacks, a carefully supervised tapered discontinuation may be attempted, but there is evidence that this may often be difficult to accomplish without recurrence of symptoms and/or the manifestation of withdrawal phenomena.
In any case, reduction of dose must be undertaken under close supervision and must be gradual. If significant withdrawal symptoms develop, the previous dosing schedule should be reinstituted and, only after stabilization, should a less rapid schedule of discontinuation be attempted. Although no experimental studies have been conducted to assess the comparative benefits of various discontinuation regimens, a possible approach is to reduce the dose by no more than 0.5 mg every three days, with the understanding that some patients may require an even more gradual discontinuation. Some patients may prove resistant to all discontinuation regimens.

HOW SUPPLIED

XANAX Tablets are available as follows:

0.25 mg (white, oval, scored, imprinted XANAX 0.25)

Bottles of 100	NDC 0009-0029-01
Reverse Numbered Unit Dose (100)	NDC 0009-0029-46
Bottles of 500	NDC 0009-0029-02
Bottles of 1000	NDC 0009-0029-14

0.5 mg (peach, oval, scored, imprinted XANAX 0.5)

Bottles of 100	NDC 0009-0055-01
Reverse Numbered Unit Dose (100)	NDC 0009-0055-46
Bottles of 500	NDC 0009-0055-03
Bottles of 1000	NDC 0009-0055-15

1 mg (blue, oval, scored, imprinted XANAX 1.0)

Bottles of 100	NDC 0009-0090-01
Reverse Numbered Unit Dose (100)	NDC 0009-0090-46
Bottles of 500	NDC 0009-0090-04
Bottles of 1000	NDC 0009-0090-13

2 mg (white, oblong, multi-scored, imprinted XANAX 2)

Bottles of 100	NDC 0009-0094-01
Bottles of 500	NDC 0009-0094-03

Store at controlled room temperature 15° to 30° C (59° to 86° F).

Caution: Federal law prohibits dispensing without prescription.

ANIMAL STUDIES

When rats were treated with alprazolam at 3, 10, and 30 mg/kg/day (15 to 150 times the maximum recommended human dose) orally for 2 years, a tendency for a dose related increase in the number of cataracts was observed in females and a tendency for a dose related increase in corneal vascularization was observed in males. These lesions did not appear until after 11 months of treatment.

CLINICAL STUDIES

Anxiety Disorders:
XANAX Tablets were compared to placebo in double blind clinical studies (doses up to 4 mg/day) in patients with a diagnosis of anxiety or anxiety with associated depressive symptomatology. XANAX was significantly better than placebo at each of the evaluation periods of these four week studies as judged by the following psychometric instruments: Physician's Global Impressions, Hamilton Anxiety Rating Scale, Target Symptoms, Patient's Global Impressions and Self-Rating Symptom Scale.

Panic Disorder:
Support for the effectiveness of XANAX in the treatment of panic disorder came from three short-term, placebo-controlled studies (up to 10 weeks) in patients with diagnoses closely corresponding to DSM-III-R criteria for panic disorder.
The average dose of XANAX was 5-6 mg/day in two of the studies, and the doses of XANAX were fixed at 2 and 6 mg/day in the third study. In all three studies, XANAX was superior to placebo on a variable defined as "the number of patients with zero panic attacks" (range, 37-83% met this criterion), as well as on a global improvement score. In two of the three studies, XANAX was superior to placebo on a variable defined as "change from baseline on the number of panic attacks per week" (range, 3.3-5.2), and also on a phobia rating scale. A subgroup of patients who were improved on XANAX during short-term treatment in one of these trials was continued on an open basis up to eight months, without apparent loss of benefit.

Revised February 1996 811 557 824
691439

Shown in Product Identification Guide, page 329

ZANOSAR® ℞

brand of streptozocin sterile powder

WARNING

ZANOSAR Sterile Powder should be administered under the supervision of a physician experienced in the use of cancer chemotherapeutic agents.
A patient need not be hospitalized but should have access to a facility with laboratory and supportive resources sufficient to monitor drug tolerance and to protect and maintain a patient compromised by drug toxicity. Renal toxicity is dose-related and cumulative and may be severe or fatal. Other major toxicities are nausea and vomiting which may be severe and at times treatment-limiting. In addition, liver dysfunction, diarrhea, and hematological changes have been observed in some patients. Streptozocin is mutagenic. When administered parenterally, it has been found to be tumorigenic or carcinogenic in some rodents.
The physician must judge the possible benefit to his patient against the known toxic effects of this drug in considering the advisability of therapy with ZANOSAR. He should be familiar with the following text before making his judgment and beginning treatment.

DESCRIPTION

Each vial of ZANOSAR Sterile Powder contains 1 g of the active ingredient streptozocin 2-deoxy-2-[[(methylnitrosoamino)carbonyl]amino]-α(and β)-D-glucopyranose and 220 mg citric acid anhydrous. ZANOSAR is available as a sterile, pale yellow, freeze-dried preparation for intravenous administration. The pH was adjusted with sodium hydroxide. When reconstituted as directed, the pH of the solution will be between 3.5 and 4.5. Streptozocin is a synthetic antineoplastic agent that is chemically related to other nitrosoureas used in cancer chemotherapy. Streptozocin is an ivory-colored crystalline powder with a molecular weight of 265.2. It is very soluble in water or physiological saline and is soluble in alcohol. The structural formula is represented below:

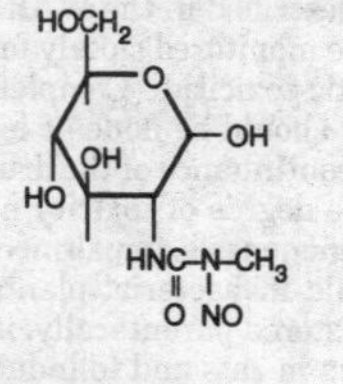

CLINICAL PHARMACOLOGY

Streptozocin inhibits DNA synthesis in bacterial and mammalian cells. In bacterial cells, a specific interaction with cytosine moieties leads to degradation of DNA. The biochemical mechanism leading to mammalian cell death has not been definitely established; streptozocin inhibits cell proliferation at a considerably lower level than that needed to inhibit precursor incorporation into DNA or to inhibit several of the enzymes involved in DNA synthesis. Although streptozocin inhibits the progression of cells into mitosis, no specific phase of the cell cycle is particularly sensitive to its lethal effects.
Streptozocin is active in the L1210 leukemic mouse over a fairly wide range of parenteral dosage schedules. In experiments in many animal species, streptozocin induced a diabetes that resembles human hyperglycemic nonketotic diabetes mellitus. This phenomenon, which has been extensively studied, appears to be mediated through a lowering of beta cell nicotinamide adenine dinucleotide (NAD) and consequent histopathologic alteration of pancreatic islet beta cells.
The metabolism and the chemical dissociation of streptozocin that occurs under physiologic conditions has not been extensively studied. When administered intravenously to a variety of experimental animals, streptozocin disappears from the blood very rapidly. In all species tested, it was found to concentrate in the liver and kidney. As much as 20% of the drug (or metabolites containing an N-nitrosourea group) is metabolized and/or excreted by the kidney. Metabolic products have not yet been identified.

INDICATIONS AND USAGE

ZANOSAR Sterile Powder is indicated in the treatment of metastatic islet cell carcinoma of the pancreas. Responses have been obtained with both functional and nonfunctional carcinomas. Because of its inherent renal toxicity, therapy with this drug should be limited to patients with symptomatic or progressive metastatic disease.

WARNINGS

Renal Toxicity

Many patients treated with ZANOSAR Sterile Powder have experienced renal toxicity, as evidenced by azotemia, anuria hypophosphatemia, glycosuria and renal tubular acidosis. **Such toxicity is dose-related and cumulative and may be severe or fatal.** Renal function must be monitored before and after each course of therapy. Serial urinalysis, blood urea nitrogen, plasma creatinine, serum electrolytes and creatinine clearance should be obtained prior to, at least weekly during, and for four weeks after drug administration. Serial urinalysis is particularly important for the early detection of proteinuria and should be quantitated with a 24 hour collection when proteinuria is detected. Mild proteinuria is one of the first signs of renal toxicity and may herald further deterioration of renal function. Reduction of the dose of ZANOSAR or discontinuation of treatment is suggested in the presence of significant renal toxicity.

Continued on next page

Information on these Pharmacia & Upjohn products is based on labeling in effect June 1, 1996. Further information concerning these and other Pharmacia & Upjohn products may be obtained by direct inquiry to Medical Information, Pharmacia & Upjohn, Kalamazoo, MI 49001.

Pharmacia & Upjohn—Cont.

Use of ZANOSAR in patients with preexisting renal disease requires a judgment by the physician of potential benefit as opposed to the known risk of serious renal damage.
This drug should not be used in combination with or concomitantly with other potential nephrotoxins.
When exposed dermally, some rats developed benign tumors at the site of application of streptozocin. Consequently, streptozocin may pose a carcinogenic hazard following topical exposure if not properly handled (see DOSAGE AND ADMINISTRATION).
See additional warnings at the beginning of this insert.

PRECAUTIONS

Laboratory Tests: Patients who are treated with ZANOSAR Sterile Powder must be monitored closely, particularly for evidence of renal, hepatic, and hematopoietic toxicity. Renal function tests are described in the WARNINGS section. Patients should also be monitored closely for evidence of hematopoietic and hepatic toxicities. Complete blood counts and liver function tests should be done at least weekly. Dosage adjustments or discontinuance of the drug may be indicated, depending upon the degree of toxicity noted.

Mutagenesis, Carcinogenesis, Impairment of Fertility: Streptozocin is mutagenic in bacteria, plants, and mammalian cells. When administered parenterally, it has been shown to induce renal tumors in rats and to induce liver tumors and other tumors in hamsters. Stomach and pancreatic tumors were observed in rats treated orally with streptozocin. Streptozocin has also been shown to be carcinogenic in mice.
Streptozocin adversely affected fertility when administered to male and female rats.

Pregnancy Category C: Reproduction studies revealed that streptozocin is teratogenic in the rat and has abortifacient effects in rabbits. When administered intravenously to pregnant monkeys, it appears rapidly in the fetal circulation. There are no studies in pregnant women. ZANOSAR should be used during pregnancy only if the potential benefit justifies the potential risk to the fetus.

Nursing Mothers: It is not known whether streptozocin is excreted in human milk. Because many drugs are excreted in human milk and because of the potential for serious adverse reactions in nursing infants, nursing should be discontinued in patients receiving ZANOSAR.

ADVERSE REACTIONS

Renal: See WARNINGS.

Gastrointestinal: Most patients treated with ZANOSAR Sterile Powder have experienced severe nausea and vomiting, occasionally requiring discontinuation of drug therapy. Some patients experienced diarrhea. A number of patients have experienced hepatic toxicity, as characterized by elevated liver enzyme (SGOT and LDH) levels and hypoalbuminemia.

Hematological: Hematological toxicity has been rare, most often involving mild decreases in hematocrit values. However, **fatal hematological toxicity with substantial reductions in leukocyte and platelet count** has been observed.

Metabolic: Mild to moderate abnormalities of glucose tolerance have been noted in some patients treated with ZANOSAR. These have generally been reversible, but insulin shock with hypoglycemia has been observed.

Genitourinary: Two cases of nephrogenic diabetes insipidus following therapy with ZANOSAR have been reported. One had spontaneous recovery and the second responded to indomethacin.

OVERDOSAGE

No specific antidote for ZANOSAR is known.

DOSAGE AND ADMINISTRATION

ZANOSAR Sterile Powder should be administered intravenously. It is not active orally. Although it has been administered intra-arterially, this is not recommended pending further evaluation of the possibility that adverse renal effects may be evoked more rapidly by this route of administration. Two different dosage schedules have been employed successfully with ZANOSAR.

Daily Schedule—The recommended dose for daily intravenous administration is 500 mg/m^2 of body surface area for five consecutive days every six weeks until maximum benefit or until treatment- limiting toxicity is observed. Dose escalation on this schedule is not recommended.

Weekly Schedule—The recommended initial dose for weekly intravenous administration is 1000 mg/m^2 of body surface area at weekly intervals for the first two courses (weeks). In subsequent courses, drug doses may be escalated in patients who have not achieved a therapeutic response and who have not experienced significant toxicity with the previous course of treatment. However, A SINGLE DOSE OF 1500 mg/m^2 BODY SURFACE AREA SHOULD NOT BE EXCEEDED as a greater dose may cause azotemia. When administered on this schedule, the median time to onset of response is about 17 days and the median time to maximum response is about 35 days. The median **total** dose to onset of response is about 2000 mg/m^2 body surface area and the median **total** dose to maximum response is about 4000 mg/m^2 body surface area.
The ideal duration of maintenance therapy with ZANOSAR has not yet been clearly established for either of the above schedules.
For patients with functional tumors, serial monitoring of fasting insulin levels allows a determination of biochemical response to therapy. For patients with either functional or nonfunctional tumors, response to therapy can be determined by measurable reductions of tumor size (reduction of organomegaly, masses, or lymph nodes).
Reconstitute ZANOSAR with 9.5 mL of Dextrose Injection USP, or 0.9% Sodium Chloride Injection USP. The resulting pale-gold solution will contain 100 mg of streptozocin and 22 mg of citric acid per mL. Where more dilute infusion solutions are desirable, further dilution in the above vehicles is recommended. The total storage time for streptozocin after it has been placed in solution should not exceed 12 hours. This product contains no preservatives and is not intended as a multiple-dose vial.
Caution in the handling and preparation of the powder and solution should be exercised, and the use of gloves is recommended. If ZANOSAR Sterile Powder or a solution prepared from ZANOSAR contacts the skin or mucosae, immediately wash the affected area with soap and water.
Procedures for proper handling and disposal of anticancer drugs should be considered. Several guidelines on this subject have been published.[4–9] There is no general agreement that all of the procedures recommended in the guidelines are necessary or appropriate.

HOW SUPPLIED

ZANOSAR Sterile Powder is supplied in 1 gram vials (NDC 0009-0844-01). Unopened vials of ZANOSAR should be stored at refrigeration temperatures (2° to 8° C) and protected from light (preferably stored in carton).

REFERENCES

1. Broder LE and Carter SK: *Ann Int Med*, 79:101-118, 1972.
2. Schein PS, O'Connell MJ, Blom J, Hubbard S, Magrath IT, Bergevin P, Wiernik PH, Ziegler TL, and DeVita VT: *Cancer*, 34:993-1000, 1974.
3. Moertel CG, *et al*: *Cancer Chemother Rep*, 55:303-307, 1972.
4. Recommendations for the Safe Handling of Parenteral Antineoplastic Drugs. NIH Publication No. 83-2621. For sale by the Superintendent of Documents, US Government Printing Office, Washington, DC 20402.
5. AMA Council Report. Guidelines for Handling Parenteral Antineoplastics. JAMA, March 15, 1985.
6. National Study Commission on Cytotoxic Exposure-Recommendations for Handling Cytotoxic Agents. Available from Louis P. Jeffrey, ScD, Director of Pharmacy Services, Rhode Island Hospital, 593 Eddy Street, Providence, Rhode Island 02902.
7. Clinical Oncological Society of Australia: Guidelines and recommendations for safe handling of antineoplastic agents. *Med J Australia* 1:426-428, 1983.
8. Jones RB, et al, Safe handling of chemotherapeutic agents: A report from the Mount Sinai Medical Center CA-A Cancer Journal for Clinicians Sept./Oct., 1983, pp. 258-263.
9. American Society of Hospital Pharmacists Technical assistance bulletin on handling cytotoxic drugs in hospitals. *AmJ Hosp Pharm* 42:131-137, 1985.

Caution: Federal law prohibits dispensing without prescription.

Revised July 1994 812 350 106
691272

ZINECARD® ℞

[zĭn "ă card ']
(dexrazoxane for injection)

DESCRIPTION

ZINECARD® (dexrazoxane for injection) is a sterile, pyrogen-free lyophilizate intended for intravenous administration. It is a cardioprotective agent for use in conjunction with doxorubicin.
Chemically, dexrazoxane is (S)-4,4'-(1-methyl-1,2-ethanediyl)bis-2,6-piperazinedione. The structural formula is as follows:

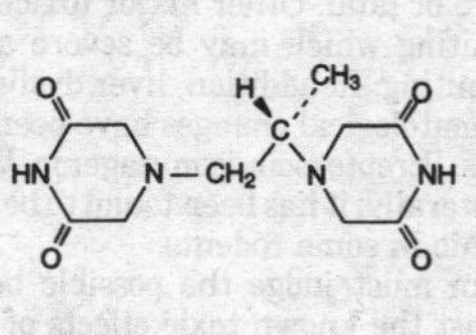

$C_{11}H_{16}N_4O_4$ M.W. 268.28

Dexrazoxane, a potent intracellular chelating agent is a derivative of EDTA. Dexrazoxane is a whitish crystalline powder which melts at 191° to 197°C. It is sparingly soluble in water and 0.1 N HCl, slightly soluble in ethanol and methanol and practically insoluble in nonpolar organic solvents. The pK_a is 2.1. Dexrazoxane has an octanol/water partition coefficient of 0.025 and degrades rapidly above a pH of 7.0.
ZINECARD is available in 250 mg and 500 mg single use only vials.
Each 250 mg vial contains dexrazoxane hydrochloride equivalent to 250 mg dexrazoxane. Hydrochloric Acid, NF is added for pH adjustment. When reconstituted as directed with the 25 mL vial of 0.167 Molar (M/6) Sodium Lactate Injection, USP diluent provided, each mL contains: 10 mg dexrazoxane. The pH of the resultant solution is 3.5 to 5.5.
Each 500 mg vial contains dexrazoxane hydrochloride equivalent to 500 mg dexrazoxane. Hydrochloric Acid, NF is added for pH adjustment. When reconstituted as directed with the 50 mL vial of 0.167 Molar (M/6) Sodium Lactate Injection, USP diluent provided, each mL contains: 10 mg dexrazoxane. The pH of the resultant solution is 3.5 to 5.5.

CLINICAL PHARMACOLOGY

Mechanism of Action: The mechanism by which ZINECARD exerts its cardioprotective activity is not fully understood. Dexrazoxane is a cyclic derivative of EDTA that readily penetrates cell membranes. Results of laboratory studies suggest that dexrazoxane is converted intracellularly to a ring-opened chelating agent that interferes with iron-mediated free radical generation thought to be responsible, in part, for anthracycline-induced cardiomyopathy.

Pharmacokinetics: The pharmacokinetics of dexrazoxane have been studied in advanced cancer patients with normal renal and hepatic function. Generally, the pharmacokinetics of dexrazoxane can be adequately described by a two-compartment open model with first-order elimination. Dexrazoxane has been administered as a 15 minute infusion over a dose-range of 60 to 900 mg/m^2 with 60 mg/m^2 of doxorubicin, and at a fixed dose of 500 mg/m^2 with 50 mg/m^2 doxorubicin. The disposition kinetics of dexrazoxane are dose-independent, as shown by linear relationship between the area under plasma concentration-time curves and administered doses ranging from 60 to 900 mg/m^2. The mean peak plasma concentration of dexrazoxane was 36.5 μg/mL at the end of the 15 minute infusion of a 500 mg/m^2 dose of Zinecard administered 15 to 30 minutes prior to the 50 mg/m^2 doxorubicin dose. The important pharmacokinetic parameters of dexrazoxane are summarized in the following table.
[See table on top of next page.]
Following a rapid distributive phase (∼.2 to 0.3 hours), dexrazoxane reaches post-distributive equilibrium within two to four hours. The estimated steady-state volume of distribution of dexrazoxane suggests its distribution primarily in the total body water (25 L/m^2). The mean systemic clearance and steady-state volume of distribution of dexrazoxane in two Asian female patients at 500 mg/m^2 dexrazoxane along with 50 mg/m^2 doxorubicin were 15.15 $L/h/m^2$ and 36.27 L/m^2, respectively, but their elimination half-life and renal clearance of dexrazoxane were similar to those of the ten Caucasian patients from the same study. Qualitative metabolism studies with Zinecard have confirmed the presence of unchanged drug, a diacid-diamide cleavage product, and two monoacid-monoamide ring products in the urine of animals and man. The metabolite levels were not measured in the pharmacokinetic studies.
Urinary excretion plays an important role in the elimination of dexrazoxane. Forty-two percent of the 500 mg/m^2 dose of Zinecard was excreted in the urine.

Protein Binding: *In vitro* studies have shown that Zinecard is not bound to plasma proteins.

Special Populations: The pharmacokinetics of Zinecard have not been evaluated in pediatric populations nor in hepatic or renal insufficiency patients.

Drug Interactions: There was no significant change in the pharmacokinetics of doxorubicin (50 mg/m^2) and its predominant metabolite, doxorubicinol, in the presence of dexrazoxane (500 mg/m^2) in a crossover study in cancer patients.

Clinical Studies: The ability of ZINECARD to prevent/reduce the incidence and severity of doxorubicin-induced cardiomyopathy was demonstrated in three prospectively randomized placebo-controlled studies. In these studies, patients were treated with a doxorubicin-containing regimen and either ZINECARD or placebo starting with the first course of chemotherapy. There was no restriction on the cumulative dose of doxorubicin. Cardiac function was assessed by measurement of the left ventricular ejection fraction (LVEF), utilizing resting multigated nuclear medicine (MUGA) scans, and by clinical evaluations. Patients receiving ZINECARD had significantly smaller mean decreases from baseline in LVEF and lower incidences of congestive heart failure than the control group. The difference in decline from baseline in LVEF was evident beginning with a cumulative doxorubicin dose of 150 mg/m^2 and reached statistical significance in patients who received ≥ 400 mg/m^2 of doxorubicin. In addition to evaluating the effect of ZINECARD on cardiac

SUMMARY OF MEAN (%CV[a]) DEXRAZOXANE PHARMACOKINETIC PARAMETERS AT A DOSAGE RATIO OF 10:1 OF ZINECARD: DOXORUBICIN

Dose Doxorubicin (mg/m²)	Dose Zinecard (mg/m²)	Number of Subjects	Elimination Half-Life (h)	Plasma Clearance (L/h/m²)	Renal Clearance (L/h/m²)	[b]Volume of Distribution (L/m²)
50	500	10	2.5 (16)	7.88 (18)	3.35 (36)	22.4 (22)
60	600	5	2.1 (29)	6.25 (31)	—	22.0 (55)

[a] Coefficient of variation
[b] Steady-state volume of distribution

function, the studies also assessed the effect of the addition of ZINECARD on the antitumor efficacy of the chemotherapy regimens. In one study (the largest of three breast cancer studies) patients with advanced breast cancer receiving fluorouracil, doxorubicin and cyclophosphamide (FAC) with ZINECARD had a lower response rate (48% vs 63%; p=0.007) and a shorter time to progression than patients who received FAC + placebo, although the survival of patients who did or did not receive ZINECARD with FAC was similar.

Two of the randomized breast cancer studies evaluating the efficacy and safety of FAC with either ZINECARD or placebo were amended to allow patients on the placebo arm who had attained a cumulative dose of doxorubicin of 300 mg/m² (six courses of FAC) to receive FAC with open-label ZINECARD for each subsequent course. This change in design allowed examination of whether there was a cardioprotective effect of Zinecard even when it was started after substantial exposure to doxorubicin.

Retrospective historical analyses were then performed to compare the likelihood of heart failure in patients to whom ZINECARD was added to the FAC regimen after they had received six (6) courses of FAC (and who then continued treatment with FAC therapy) with the heart failure rate in patients who had received six (6) courses of FAC and continued to receive this regimen without added ZINECARD. These analyses showed that the risk of experiencing a cardiac event (see Table 1 for definition) at a given cumulative dose of doxorubicin above 300 mg/m² was substantially greater in the 99 patients who did *not* receive ZINECARD beginning with their seventh course of FAC than in the 102 patients who did receive Zinecard (See Figure 1).

Table 1
The development of cardiac events is shown by:
1. Development of congestive heart failure, defined as having two or more of the following:
   a. Cardiomegaly by X-ray
   b. Basilar Rales
   c. S₃ Gallop
   d. Paroxysmal nocturnal dyspnea and/or orthopnea and/or significant dyspnea on exertion.
2. Decline from baseline in LVEF by ≥ 10% and ≥ below the lower limit of normal for the institution.
3. Decline in LVEF by ≥ 20% from baseline value.
4. Decline in LVEF to ≥ 5% below lower limit of normal for the institution.

Figure 1 displays the risk of developing congestive heart failure by cumulative dose of doxorubicin in patients who received ZINECARD starting with their seventh course of FAC compared to patients who did not. Patients unprotected by ZINECARD had a 13 times greater risk of developing congestive heart failure. Overall, 3% of patients treated with ZINECARD developed CHF compared with 22% of patients not receiving ZINECARD.

Figure 1
DOX Dose at Congestive Heart Failure (CHF)
FAC vs. FAC/Zinecard Patients
Patients Receiving At Least Seven Courses of Treatment

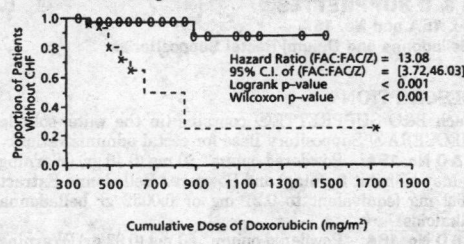

Because of its cardioprotective effect, ZINECARD permitted a greater percentage of patients to be treated with extended doxorubicin therapy. Figure 2 shows the number of patients still on treatment at increasing cumulative doses.

Figure 2
Cumulative Number of Patients On Treatment
FAC vs. FAC/Zinecard Patients
Patients Receiving at Least Seven Courses of Treatment

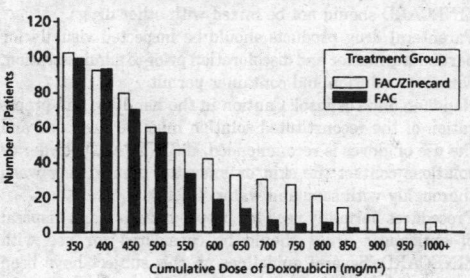

In addition to evaluating the cardioprotective efficacy of ZINECARD in this setting, the time to tumor progression and survival of these two groups of patients were also compared. There was a similar time to progression in the two groups and survival was at least as long for the group of patients that received ZINECARD starting with their seventh course, i.e., starting after a cumulative dose of doxorubicin of 300 mg/m². These time to progression and survival data should be interpreted with caution, however, because they are based on comparisons of groups entered sequentially in the studies and are not comparisons of prospectively randomized patients.

INDICATIONS AND USAGE
ZINECARD is indicated for reducing the incidence and severity of cardiomyopathy associated with doxorubicin administration in women with metastatic breast cancer who have received a cumulative doxorubicin dose of 300 mg/m² and who, in their physician's opinion, would benefit from continuing therapy with doxorubicin. It is not recommended for use with the initiation of doxorubicin therapy (see WARNINGS).

CONTRAINDICATIONS
ZINECARD should not be used with chemotherapy regimens that do not contain an anthracycline.

WARNINGS
ZINECARD may add to the myelosuppression caused by chemotherapeutic agents.
There is some evidence that the use of dexrazoxane concurrently with the initiation of fluorouracil, doxorubicin and cyclophosphamide (FAC) therapy interferes with the antitumor efficacy of the regimen, and this use is not recommended. In the largest of three breast cancer trials, patients who received dexrazoxane starting with their first cycle of FAC therapy had a lower response rate (48% vs 63%; p=0.007) and shorter time to progression than patients who did not receive dexrazoxane (see Clinical Studies section of CLINICAL PHARMACOLOGY). Therefore, ZINECARD should only be used in those patients who have received a cumulative doxorubicin dose of 300 mg/m² and are continuing with doxorubicin therapy.
Although clinical studies have shown that patients receiving FAC with ZINECARD may receive a higher cumulative dose of doxorubicin before experiencing cardiac toxicity than patients receiving FAC without ZINECARD, the use of ZINECARD in patients who have already received a cumulative dose of doxorubicin of 300 mg/m² without ZINECARD, does not eliminate the potential for anthracycline induced cardiac toxicity. Therefore, cardiac function should be carefully monitored.
Secondary malignancies (primarily acute myeloid leukemia) have been reported in patients treated chronically with oral razoxane. Razoxane is the racemic mixture, of which dexrazoxane is the S(+)-enantiomer. In these patients, the total cumulative dose of razoxane ranged from 26 to 480 grams and the duration of treatment was from 42 to 319 weeks. One case of T-cell lymphoma, a case of B-cell lymphoma and six to eight cases of cutaneous basal cell or squamous cell carcinoma have also been reported in patients treated with razoxane.

PRECAUTIONS
General
Doxorubicin should not be given prior to the intravenous injection of ZINECARD. ZINECARD should be given by slow I.V. push or rapid drip intravenous infusion from a bag. Doxorubicin should be given within 30 minutes after beginning the infusion with ZINECARD. (See DOSAGE AND ADMINISTRATION.)
As ZINECARD will always be used with cytotoxic drugs, patients should be monitored closely. While the myelosuppressive effects of ZINECARD at the recommended dose are mild, additive effects upon the myelosuppressive activity of chemotherapeutic agents may occur.
Laboratory tests
As ZINECARD may add to the myelosuppressive effects of cytotoxic drugs, frequent complete blood counts are recommended. (See ADVERSE REACTIONS).
Drug Interactions
ZINECARD does not influence the pharmacokinetics of doxorubicin.
Carcinogenesis, Mutagenesis, Impairment of Fertility (see WARNINGS section for information on human carcinogenicity) – No long-term carcinogenicity studies have been carried out with dexrazoxane in animals. Dexrazoxane was not mutagenic in the Ames test but was found to be clastogenic to human lymphocytes *in vitro* and to mouse bone marrow erythrocytes *in vivo* (micronucleus test).
The possible adverse effects of Zinecard on the fertility of humans and experimental animals, male or female, have not been adequately studied. Testicular atrophy was seen with dexrazoxane administration at doses as low as 30 mg/kg weekly for 6 weeks in rats (1/3 the human dose on a mg/m² basis) and as low as 20 mg/kg weekly for 13 weeks in dogs (approximately equal to the human dose on a mg/m² basis).
Pregnancy – *Pregnancy Category C* – Dexrazoxane was maternotoxic at doses of 2 mg/kg (1/40 the human dose on a mg/m² basis) and embryotoxic and teratogenic at 8 mg/kg (approximately 1/10 the human dose on a mg/m² basis) when given daily to pregnant rats during the period of organogenesis. Teratogenic effects in the rat included imperforate anus, microphthalmia, and anophthalmia. In offspring allowed to develop to maturity, fertility was impaired in the male and female rats treated in utero during organogenesis at 8 mg/kg. In rabbits, doses of 5 mg/kg (approximately 1/10 the human dose on a mg/m² basis) daily during the period of organogenesis were maternotoxic and dosages of 20 mg/kg (1/2 the human dose on a mg/m² basis) were embryotoxic and teratogenic. Teratogenic effects in the rabbit included several skeletal malformations such as short tail, rib and thoracic malformations, and soft tissue variations including subcutaneous, eye and cardiac hemorrhagic areas, as well as agenesis of the gallbladder and of the intermediate lobe of the lung. There are no adequate and well-controlled studies in pregnant women. ZINECARD should be used during pregnancy only if the potential benefit justifies the potential risk to the fetus.
Nursing Mothers – It is not known whether dexrazoxane is excreted in human milk. Because many drugs are excreted in human milk and because of the potential for serious adverse reactions in nursing infants exposed to dexrazoxane, mothers should be advised to discontinue nursing during dexrazoxane therapy.
Pediatric Use – Safety and effectiveness of dexrazoxane in children have not been established.

ADVERSE REACTIONS
ZINECARD at a dose of 500 mg/m² has been administered in combination with FAC in randomized, placebo-controlled, double-blind studies to patients with metastatic breast cancer. The dose of doxorubicin was 50 mg/m² in each of the trials. Courses were repeated every three weeks, provided recovery from toxicity had occurred. Table 2 below lists the incidence of adverse experiences for patients receiving FAC with either ZINECARD or placebo in the breast cancer studies. Adverse experiences occurring during courses 1 through 6 are displayed for patients receiving ZINECARD or placebo with FAC beginning with their first course of therapy (column 1 & 3, respectively). Adverse experiences occurring at course 7 and beyond for patients who received placebo with FAC during the first six courses and who then received either ZINECARD or placebo with FAC are also displayed (column 2 & 4, respectively).
[See Table 2 at bottom of next page.]
The adverse experiences listed above are likely attributable to the FAC regimen with the exception of pain on injection that was observed mainly on the ZINECARD arm.

Continued on next page

Information on these Pharmacia & Upjohn products is based on labeling in effect June 1, 1996. Further information concerning these and other Pharmacia & Upjohn products may be obtained by direct inquiry to Medical Information, Pharmacia & Upjohn, Kalamazoo, MI 49001.

Pharmacia & Upjohn—Cont.

Myelosuppression
Patients receiving FAC with ZINECARD experienced more severe leucopenia, granulocytopenia and thrombocytopenia at nadir than patients receiving FAC without ZINECARD, but recovery counts were similar for the two groups of patients.

Hepatic and Renal
Some patients receiving FAC + ZINECARD or FAC + placebo experienced marked abnormalities in hepatic or renal function tests, but the frequency and severity of abnormalities in bilirubin, alkaline phosphatase, BUN, and creatinine were similar for patients receiving FAC with or without ZINECARD.

OVERDOSAGE
There have been no instances of drug overdose in the clinical studies sponsored by either Pharmacia Inc. or the National Cancer Institute. The maximum dose administered during the cardioprotective trials was 1000 mg/m^2 every three weeks.

Disposition studies with ZINECARD have not been conducted in cancer patients undergoing dialysis, but retention of a significant dose fraction (> 0.4) of the unchanged drug in the plasma pool, minimal tissue partitioning or binding, and availability of greater than 90% of the systemic drug levels in the unbound form suggest that it could be removed using conventional peritoneal or hemodialysis.

There is no known antidote for dexrazoxane. Instances of suspected overdose should be managed with good supportive care until resolution of myelosuppression and related conditions is complete. Management of overdose should include treatment of infections, fluid regulation, and maintenance of nutritional requirements.

DOSAGE AND ADMINISTRATION
The recommended dosage ratio of ZINECARD:DOX is 10:1 (eg, 500 mg/m^2 ZINECARD:50 mg/m^2 DOX). ZINECARD must be reconstituted with 0.167 Molar (M/6) Sodium Lactate Injection, USP, to give a concentration of 10 mg ZINECARD for each mL of sodium lactate. The reconstituted solution should be given by slow I.V. push or rapid drip intravenous infusion from a bag. After completing the infusion of ZINECARD, and prior to a total elapsed time of 30 minutes (from the beginning of the ZINECARD infusion), the intravenous injection of doxorubicin should be given.

Reconstituted ZINECARD, when transferred to an empty infusion bag, is stable for 6 hours from the time of reconstitution when stored at controlled room temperature, 15° to 30°C (59° to 86°F) or under refrigeration, 2° to 8°C (36° to 46°F). DISCARD UNUSED SOLUTIONS.

The reconstituted ZINECARD solution may be diluted with either 0.9% Sodium Chloride Injection, USP or 5.0% Dextrose Injection, USP to a concentration range of 1.3 to 5.0 mg/mL in intravenous infusion bags. The resultant solutions are stable for 6 hours when stored at controlled room temperature, 15° to 30°C (59° to 86°F) or under refrigeration, 2° to 8°C (36° to 46°F). DISCARD UNUSED SOLUTIONS.

Incompatibility
ZINECARD should not be mixed with other drugs.

Parenteral drug products should be inspected visually for particulate matter and discoloration prior to administration, whenever solution and container permit.

Handling and Disposal: Caution in the handling and preparation of the reconstituted solution must be exercised and the use of gloves is recommended. If ZINECARD powder or solutions contact the skin or mucosae, immediately wash thoroughly with soap and water.

Procedures normally used for proper handling and disposal of anticancer drugs should be considered for use with ZINECARD. Several guidelines on this subject have been published.[1-7] There is no general agreement that all of the procedures recommended in the guidelines are necessary or appropriate.

HOW SUPPLIED
ZINECARD® (dexrazoxane for injection) is available in the following strengths as sterile, pyrogen-free lyophilizates.

NDC 0013-8715-62 250 mg single dose vial with a red flip-top seal, packaged in single vial packs.
(This package also contains a 25 mL vial of 0.167 Molar (M/6) Sodium Lactate Injection, USP.)

NDC 0013-8725-89 500 mg single dose vial with a blue flip-top seal, packaged in single vial packs.
(This package also contains a 50 mL vial of 0.167 Molar (M/6) Sodium Lactate Injection, USP.)
Store at controlled room temperature, 15° to 30°C (59° to 86°F). Reconstituted solutions of ZINECARD are stable for 6 hours at controlled room temperature or under refrigeration, 2° to 8°C (36° to 46°F). DISCARD UNUSED SOLUTIONS.

CAUTION: Federal law prohibits dispensing without prescription.

REFERENCES
1. Recommendations for the Safe Handling of Parenteral Antineoplastic Drugs. NIH Publication No. 83-2621. For sale by the Superintendent of Documents, U.S. Government Printing Office, Washington, DC 20402.
2. AMA Council Report. Guidelines for Handling Parenteral Antineoplastics JAMA. 1985 March 15.
3. National Study Commission on Cytotoxic Exposure-Recommendations for Handling Cytotoxic Agents. Available from Louis P. Jeffrey, Sc.D., Chairman, National Study Commission on Cytotoxic Exposure, Massachusetts College of Pharmacy and Allied Health Sciences, 179 Longwood Avenue, Boston, Massachusetts 02115.
4. Clinical Oncological Society of Australia. Guidelines and Recommendations for Safe Handling of Antineoplastic Agents. Med J Australia. 1983; 1:426–428.
5. Jones RB. et al. Safe handling of Chemotherapeutic Agents: A report from the Mount Sinai Medical Center. CA – A Cancer Journal for Clinicians. 1983; (Sept/Oct) 258–263.
6. American Society of Hospital Pharmacists Technical Assistance Bulletin on Handling Cytotoxic and Hazardous Drugs. Am J Hosp Pharm. 1990; 47:1033–1049.
7. OSHA Work-Practice Guidelines for Personnel Dealing with Cytotoxic (Antineoplastic) Drugs. Am J Hosp Pharm. 1986; 43:1193–1204.
770000496 April 1, 1996

PolyMedica Pharmaceuticals (U.S.A.), Inc.
11 STATE STREET
WOBURN, MA 01801

For Medical Information Contact:
In Emergencies:
Peter Etzel or Arthur Siciliano
(617) 933-2020
FAX: (617) 933-7992

ANESTACON® ℞
(lidocaine hydrochloride jelly, USP) 2%

DESCRIPTION
Each mL contains: Active: Lidocaine Hydrochloride 20 mg/ml (2%). Vehicle: Hydroxypropyl Methylcellulose 10 mg (1%). Preservative: Benzalkonium Chloride 0.1 mg (0.01%). Inactive: Sodium Chloride, Hydrochloric Acid and/or Sodium Hydroxide (to adjust pH to 6.0-7.0), Purified Water. The resulting mixture maximizes contact with mucosa and provides lubrication for instrumentation.

DM-00

HOW SUPPLIED
In 15 ml. unit-dose and 240 ml. disposable containers for SINGLE PATIENT USE.

B & O SUPPRETTES® Ⓒ ℞
No. 15A and No. 16A
(Belladonna and Opium) Rectal Suppositories

DESCRIPTION
Each B&O SUPPRETTE® contains (in the water-soluble NEOCERA® Suppository Base for rectal administration):
B&O No. 15A: Powdered opium* 30 mg (0.46 gr) (Warning —May be habit forming) and Powdered Belladonna Extract 16.2 mg (equivalent to 0.21 mg or 0.0032 gr belladonna alkaloids).
B&O No. 16A: Powdered opium* 60 mg (0.92 gr) (Warning —May be habit forming) and Powdered Belladonna Extract 16.2 mg (equivalent to 0.21 mg or 0.0032 gr belladonna alkaloids).
Store at room temperature. DO NOT REFRIGERATE.

HOW SUPPLIED
In strip packaged units of 12.

TABLE 2

PERCENTAGE (%) OF BREAST CANCER PATIENTS WITH ADVERSE EXPERIENCE

ADVERSE EXPERIENCE	FAC + ZINECARD		FAC + PLACEBO	
	Courses 1–6 N=413	Courses ≥ 7 N=102	Courses 1–6 N=458	Course ≥ 7 N=99
Alopecia	94	100	97	98
Nausea	77	51	84	60
Vomiting	59	42	72	49
Fatigue/Malaise	61	48	58	55
Anorexia	42	27	47	38
Stomatitis	34	26	41	28
Fever	34	22	29	18
Infection	23	19	18	21
Diarrhea	21	14	24	7
Pain on Injection	12	13	3	0
Sepsis	17	12	14	9
Neurotoxicity	17	10	13	5
Streaking/Erythema	5	4	4	2
Phlebitis	6	3	3	5
Esophagitis	6	3	7	4
Dysphagia	8	0	10	5
Hemorrhage	2	3	2	1
Extravasation	1	3	1	2
Urticaria	2	2	2	0
Recall Skin Reaction	1	1	2	0

CYSTOSPAZ® ℞
(hyoscyamine) Tablets
CYSTOSPAZ-M® ℞
(hyoscyamine sulfate) Timed-Release Capsules

DESCRIPTION
CYSTOSPAZ® is a pale blue uncoated compressed tablet for oral administration. It contains the parasympatholytic agent hyoscyamine as the free base. Each tablet contains: hyoscyamine 0.15 mg.
CYSTOSPAZ-M® is a light blue timed-release capsule containing hyoscyamine sulfate 0.375 mg.

CLINICAL PHARMACOLOGY
Through its parasympatholytic action, hyoscyamine relaxes smooth muscle spasm resulting from parasympathetic stimulation. It inhibits gastrointestinal propulsive motility and decreases gastric acid secretion. It also controls excessive pharyngeal, tracheal and bronchial secretions. It is the λ-isomer of atropine and therefore exhibits the same clinical effects as atropine. It is, however, approximately twice as active peripherally as atropine, since the latter is the racemic (dλ) form of hyoscyamine and d-hyoscyamine possesses only a very weak anti-cholinergic action. Since only one-half the atropine dose is required for λ-hyoscyamine, it has only one-half the unwanted central effects of atropine.[1]

INDICATIONS AND USAGE
In the management of disorders of the lower urinary tract associated with hypermotility. Although specific therapy is often required to remove the underlying cause of spasm, CYSTOSPAZ Tablets and CYSTOSPAZ-M Capsules are offered as antispasmodic agent dosage forms which may be combined with other forms of therapy where indicated. CYSTOSPAZ Tablets and CYSTOSPAZ-M capsules are effective as adjunctive therapy in the treatment of peptic ulcer and irritable bowel syndrome (irritable colon, spastic colon, mucous colitis), acute entercolitis and other functional gastrointestinal disorders.
CYSTOSPAZ Tablets and CYSTOSPAZ-M Capsules can also be used to control gastric secretion, visceral spasm and hypermotility in cystitis, pylorospasm and associated abdominal cramps. May be used in functional intestinal disorders to reduce symptoms such as those seen in mild dysenteries and diverticulitis. They are indicated (along with appropriate analgesics) in symptomatic relief of biliary and renal colic.

CONTRAINDICATIONS
Glaucoma, obstructive uropathy (for example, bladder neck obstruction due to prostatic hypertrophy); obstructive disease of the gastrointestinal tract (as in achalasia, pyloroduodenal stenosis); paralytic ileus, intestinal atony of elderly or debilitated patients; unstable cardiovascular status in acute hemorrhage; severe ulcerative colitis; toxic megacolon complicating ulcerative colitis; myasthenia gravis. Hypersensitivity to any of the ingredients.

WARNINGS
In the presence of high environmental temperature, heat prostration can occur with drug use (fever and heat stroke due to decreased sweating). Diarrhea may be an early symptom of incomplete intestinal obstruction, especially in patients with ileostomy or colostomy. In this instance, treatment with this drug would be inappropriate and possibly harmful. Like other anticholinergic agents, these products may produce drowsiness or blurred vision. In this event, the patient should be warned not to engage in activities requiring mental alertness such as operating a motor vehicle or other machinery or to perform hazardous work while taking this drug.

PRECAUTIONS
General: Use with caution in patients with autonomic neuropathy, hyperthyroidism, coronary heart disease, congestive heart failure, cardiac arrhythmias, and hypertension. Investigate any tachycardia before giving any anticholinergic drug since they may increase the heart rate. Use with caution in patients with hiatal hernia associated with reflux esophagitis.
Information for Patients: CYSTOSPAZ Tablets and CYSTOSPAZ-M Capsules may cause drowsiness, dizziness or blurred vision; patients should observe caution before driving, using machinery or performing other tasks requiring mental alertness. Use of CYSTOSPAZ Tablets or CYSTOSPAZ-M Capsules may decrease sweating resulting in heat prostration, fever or heat stroke; febrile patients or those who may be exposed to elevated environmental temperatures should use caution.

DRUG INTERACTIONS
Additive adverse effects resulting from cholinergic blockade may occur when CYSTOSPAZ® Tablets or CYSTOSPAZ-M Capsules are administered concomitantly with other antimuscarinics, amanatadine, haloperidol, phenothiazines, monoamine oxidase (MAO) inhibitors, tricyclic antidepressants or some antihistamines. Antacids may interfere with the absorption of CYSTOSPAZ Tablets or CYSTOSPAZ-M

Capsules; take CYSTOSPAZ Tablets or CYSTOSPAZ-M Capsules before meals and antacids after meals.
Carcinogenesis, Mutagenesis, Impairment Of Fertility: No long term studies in animals have been performed to determine the carcinogenic, mutagenic or impairment of fertility potential of CYSTOSPAZ Tablets or CYSTOSPAZ-M Capsules.
Pregnancy Category C—Animal reproduction studies have not been conducted with CYSTOSPAZ Tablets or CYSTOSPAZ-M Capsules. It is also not known whether CYSTOSPAZ Tablets or CYSTOSPAZ-M Capsules can cause fetal harm when administered to a pregnant woman or can affect reproduction capacity. CYSTOSPAZ Tablets or CYSTOSPAZ-M Capsules should be taken by a pregnant woman only if clearly needed.
Nursing Mothers—Hyoscyamine is excreted in human milk. Caution should be exercised when CYSTOSPAZ Tablets or CYSTOSPAZ-M Capsules are administered to a nursing woman.

ADVERSE REACTIONS
Adverse reactions may include dryness of the mouth; urinary hesitancy and retention; blurred vision; tachycardia; palpitations; mydriasis; cycloplegia; increased ocular tension; headache; nervousness; drowsiness; weakness; suppression of lactation; allergic reactions or drug idiosyncrasies; urticaria and other dermal manifestations; and decreased sweating. **Note:** Slight dryness of the mouth is an indication that parasympathetic blockage is effective.

DRUG ABUSE AND DEPENDENCE
A dependence on the use of CYSTOSPAZ Tablets or CYSTOSPAZ-M Capsules has not been reported and due to the nature of their ingredients, abuse of CYSTOSPAZ Tablets or CYSTOSPAZ-M Capsules is not expected.

OVERDOSAGE
Symptoms of overdosage include severe dryness of the mouth, nose, throat, and hot dry flushed skin, hyperpyrexia (especially in children), difficulty or inability to swallow, difficult speech, dilated pupils until iris almost disappears, restlessness and garrulity indicating an irritability of the brain, marked tremors, convulsions, respiratory failure, death.[1] In adults, symptoms of overdosage may begin in the range of ingestion of 0.6 to 1 mg with doses exceeding 1–2 mg eliciting more profound toxicity. Measures to be taken are immediate lavage of the stomach and injection of physostigmine 0.5 to 2 mg intravenously and repeated as necessary up to a total of 5 mg. Fever may be treated symptomatically (tepid water sponge baths, hypothermic blanket). Excitement to a degree which demands attention may be managed with sodium thiopental 2% solution given slowly intravenously or chloral hydrate (100–200 ml. of a 2% solution) by rectal infusion.

DOSAGE AND ADMINISTRATION
Adults: CYSTOSPAZ Tablets—One or two tablets four times daily or fewer if needed. CYSTOSPAZ-M Capsules—One capsule every twelve hours.
Children (12 and under): Reduce dosage in proportion to age and weight.

HOW SUPPLIED
CYSTOSPAZ Tablets— Bottles of 100 light blue tablets. Tablets are imprinted with a "W 2225". CYSTOSPAZ-M Capsules—Bottles of 100 light blue timed-release capsules. Capsules are identified with "W 2260" printed in black.

URISED® ℞

DESCRIPTION
URISED® is a blue, round, coated tablet for oral administration. It is a combination of antiseptics (Methenamine, Methylene Blue, Phenyl Salicylate, Benzoic Acid) and parasympatholytics (Atropine Sulfate, Hyoscyamine).
Each tablet contains: Methenamine 40.8 mg, Phenyl Salicylate 18.1 mg, Methylene Blue 5.4 mg, Benzoic Acid 4.5 mg, Atropine Sulfate 0.03 mg and Hyoscyamine (as the sulfate) 0.03 mg.

CLINICAL PHARMACOLOGY
Methenamine itself does not have antiseptic, irritant, or toxic properties in the urine. Methenamine, in an acid urine (pH 6 or below), hydrolyzes into formaldehyde within the urinary tract providing mild antiseptic activity. When given as directed and the daily urine volume is 1000 to 1500 mL, a daily dose of 2 grams will yield a urinary concentration of 18–60 mcg/mL of free formaldehyde in the urine. This is more than the minimal inhibitory dose of formaldehyde which must be available for most urinary tract pathogens. Methenamine is readily absorbed from the gastrointestinal tract and is rapidly excreted almost entirely in the urine. Methylene Blue and Benzoic Acid are mild but effective antiseptics which contribute to the antiseptic properties of Methenamine. Phenyl Salicylate is a mild analgesic and antipy-

retic with weak antiseptic activity. All of these compounds are readily absorbed from the gastrointestinal tract and excreted in the urine. Through parasympatholytic action, atropine and hyoscyamine relax smooth muscle spasms resulting from parasympathetic stimulation.

INDICATIONS AND USAGE
URISED is indicated for the relief of discomfort of the lower urinary tract caused by hypermotility resulting from inflammation or diagnostic procedures and in the treatment of cystitis, urethritis, and trigonitis when caused by organisms which maintain or produce an acid urine and are susceptible to formaldehyde.

CONTRAINDICATIONS
Glaucoma, urinary bladder neck obstruction, pyloric or duodenal obstruction, or cardiospasm. Hypersensitivity to any of the ingredients.

WARNINGS
Do not exceed recommended dose. Methenamine may combine with sulfonamides in the urine to give mutual antagonism and should not be used with sulfonamides.

PRECAUTIONS
Administer with caution to persons with known idiosyncrasy to atropine-like compounds and to patients suffering from cardiac disease. Bacteriological studies of the urine may be helpful in following the patient response. Methylene Blue interferes with the analysis for some urinary components such as free formaldehyde. Drugs and/or foods which produce an alkaline urine should be restricted.[3]
Patient should be advised that the urine may become blue to blue-green and the feces may be discolored as a result of excretion of Methylene Blue. Methenamine preparations should not be given to patients taking sulfonamides since insoluble precipitates may form with formaldehyde in the urine. No known long-term animal studies have been performed to evaluate carcinogenic potential. The precautions related to drug interaction, diagnostic interference, medical problems and side effects to use of belladonna alkaloids, should be observed.
Pregnancy Category C. Animal reproduction studies have not been conducted with URISED® tablets. It is also not known whether URISED tablets can cause fetal harm when administered to a pregnant woman or can affect reproduction capacity. URISED tablets should be given to a pregnant woman only if clearly needed.
Nursing Mothers: It is not known whether this drug is excreted in human milk. Because many drugs are excreted in human milk, caution should be exercised when URISED tablets are administered to a nursing woman.
Prolonged Use: There have been no studies to establish the safety of prolonged use in humans.

ADVERSE REACTIONS
Prolonged use may result in a generalized skin rash, pronounced dryness of the mouth, flushing, difficulty in initiating micturition, rapid pulse, dizziness or blurring of vision. If any of these reactions occurs, discontinue use immediately. Acute urinary retention may be precipitated in prostatic hypertrophy. See "OVERDOSAGE."

DRUG ABUSE AND DEPENDENCE
A dependence on the use of URISED has not been reported and due to the nature of its ingredients, abuse of URISED is not expected.

OVERDOSAGE
By exceeding the recommended dosage of URISED, symptomology related to the overdose of its individual active ingredients may be expected as follows:
Atropine Sulfate, Hyoscyamine: Symptoms associated with an overdosage of URISED will most probably be manifested in the symptoms related to overdosage of the alkaloids Atropine Sulfate and Hyoscyamine. Such symptoms as dryness of mucous membranes; dilatation of pupils; hot, dry, flushed skin; hyperpyrexia; tachycardia; palpitations; elevated blood pressure; coma; circulatory collapse and death from respiratory failure can occur due to overdosage of these alkaloids.
Methenamine: If large amounts of the drug (2–8 gm daily) are used over extended periods (3–4 weeks), bladder and gastrointestinal irritation, painful and frequent micturition, albuminuria and gross hematuria may be expected.
Methylene Blue: Symptoms of Methylene Blue overdosage associated with the overdosage of URISED are not expected to be discernible from those associated with the other active ingredients in URISED.
Benzoic Acid: Symptoms of Benzoic Acid overdosage associated with the overdosage of URISED are not expected to be discernible from those associated with the other active ingredients in URISED.
Phenyl Salicylate: Symptoms of Phenyl Salicylate overdosage include burning pain in throat and mouth, white necrotic lesions in the mouth, abdominal pain, vomiting, bloody diarrhea, pallor, sweating, weakness, headache, dizziness and tinnitus. The symptoms, however, are not expected to be

Continued on next page

PolyMedica Pharmaceuticals—Cont.

discernible from those associated with the other active ingredients in URISED.

DOSAGE AND ADMINISTRATION

Adults: Two tablets four times daily. See "PRECAUTIONS."
Usual pediatric dosage: Children up to 6 years of age—Use is not recommended. Children 6 years of age and older—Dosage must be individualized by physician.

HOW SUPPLIED

Bottles of 100 and 500 tablets. Tablets are imprinted with a "W 2183".

Pratt Pharmaceuticals Division
see Pfizer Inc

Procter & Gamble
P.O. BOX 5516
CINCINNATI, OH 45201

Direct Inquiries to:
Charles Lambert
(800) 358-8707

For Medical Emergencies:
Call Collect: (513) 558-4422

ALEVE®   OTC
[ə lēv´]
Naproxen Sodium Tablets, USP
Pain Reliever/Fever Reducer

ALLERGY WARNING

Do not take this product if you have had either hives or a severe allergic reaction after taking any pain reliever. Even though this product may not contain the same ingredient, ALEVE could cause similar reactions in patients allergic to other pain relieving drugs.

ALCOHOL WARNING

If you generally consume 3 or more alcohol-containing drinks per day, you should consult your doctor for advice on when and how you should take ALEVE and other pain relievers.

ACTIVE INGREDIENT

Each [tablet] [caplet] contains naproxen sodium 220 mg (naproxen 200 mg and sodium 20 mg).

INACTIVE INGREDIENTS

Magnesium Stearate, Microcrystalline Cellulose, Povidone, Talc, Opadry YS-1-4215.

INDICATIONS

For the temporary relief of minor aches and pains associated with the common cold, headache, toothache, muscular aches, backache, for the minor pain of arthritis, for the pain of menstrual cramps and for the reduction of fever.

DOSAGE AND ADMINISTRATION

<u>Adults:</u> Take 1 [tablet] [caplet] every 8 to 12 hours while symptoms persist. With experience, some people may find that an initial dose of 2 [tablets] [caplets] followed by 1 [tablet] [caplet] 12 hours later, if necessary, will give better relief. *Do not exceed 3 [tablets] [caplets] in 24 hours unless directed to do so by a doctor.* The smallest effective dose should be used. A full glass of water or other liquid is recommended with each dose.
<u>Adults over age 65:</u> Do not take more than 1 [tablet] [caplet] every 12 hours, unless directed to do so by a doctor.
<u>Children under age 12:</u> Do not give this product to children under 12, except under the advice and supervision of a doctor.

GENERAL WARNINGS

Do not take ALEVE for more than 10 days for pain, or for more than 3 days for fever, unless directed by a doctor. Consult a doctor if:
* your pain or fever persists or gets worse
* the painful area is red or swollen
* you take any other drugs on a regular basis
* you have had serious side effects from any pain reliever
* you have any new or unusual symptoms
* more than mild heartburn, upset stomach, or stomach pain occurs with use of this product or if even mild symptoms persist

Although naproxen sodium is indicated for the same conditions as aspirin, ibuprofen and acetaminophen, it should not be taken with them or other naproxen-containing products

except under a doctor's direction. As with any drug, if you are pregnant or nursing a baby, seek the advice of a health professional before using this product. IT IS ESPECIALLY IMPORTANT NOT TO USE NAPROXEN SODIUM DURING THE LAST 3 MONTHS OF PREGNANCY UNLESS SPECIFICALLY DIRECTED TO DO SO BY A DOCTOR BECAUSE IT MAY CAUSE PROBLEMS IN THE UNBORN CHILD OR COMPLICATIONS DURING DELIVERY.
Keep this and all drugs out of the reach of children. In case of accidental overdose, seek professional assistance or contact a poison control center immediately.
If you have questions, comments or problems, call 1-800-395-0689 to report them.

HOW SUPPLIED

Light blue round tablets or oval-shaped caplets debossed with "ALEVE". Child-resistant "Safety SquEASE" bottles of 24, 50, 100, and 150 (200 available in caplets) tablets or caplets, with fold-out back label containing important information on the 24 and 50 count bottles.

STORAGE

Store at room temperature. Avoid excessive heat (104°F or 40°C).

CHILDREN'S   OTC
VICKS® CHLORASEPTIC®
SORE THROAT LOZENGES
Benzocaine/Oral Anesthetic

(See PDR For Nonprescription Drugs.)

CHILDREN'S VICKS® CHLORASEPTIC®   OTC
SORE THROAT SPRAY
Phenol/Oral
Anesthetic/Antiseptic

(See PDR For Nonprescription Drugs.)

CHILDREN'S VICKS® DAYQUIL®   OTC
ALLERGY RELIEF
Nasal Decongestant/Antihistamine

(See PDR For Nonprescription Drugs.)

CHILDREN'S VICKS® NYQUIL®   OTC
COLD/COUGH RELIEF
Antihistamine/Nasal Decongestant/Cough Suppressant

(See PDR For Nonprescription Drugs.)

FEMSTAT® 3   OTC
(butoconazole nitrate)
2% vaginal cream
Antifungal

ACTIVE INGREDIENTS: Butoconazole Nitrate (2%).
INACTIVE INGREDIENTS: Cetyl Alcohol, Glyceryl Stearate (and) PEG-100 Stearate, Methylparaben and Propylparaben (preservatives), Mineral Oil, Polysorbate 60, Propylene Glycol, Sorbitan Monostearate, Stearyl Alcohol and Water (purified).
Femstat® 3 is the first 3-day medicine available without a prescription for the treatment of vaginal yeast (Candida) infections.
Femstat 3 is clinically proven to cure most yeast infections with only 3 days of treatment.
IF THIS IS THE FIRST TIME YOU HAVE HAD VAGINAL ITCH AND DISCOMFORT, CONSULT YOUR DOCTOR. IF YOU HAVE HAD A DOCTOR DIAGNOSE A VAGINAL YEAST INFECTION BEFORE AND HAVE THE SAME SYMPTOMS NOW, USE FEMSTAT 3 AS DIRECTED FOR 3 CONSECUTIVE DAYS.
Directions For Use:
Disposable Cardboard Applicator
IMPORTANT: In order to help ensure proper dosage, please familiarize yourself with the disposable applicator before using the product. To do this, pull the ends of the disposable applicator apart until you see an arrow pointing to the "full" line as described in step 3. Push the disposable applicator back together.
1. Open the tube of cream.
* Remove the cap from the tube.
* Turn the cap upside down.
* Using the point on the cap, puncture the protective seal on the tube.

2. Attach white end of disposable applicator over opening of tube of cream and push until secure.
3. Slowly squeeze the tube of cream until you see the "full" line on the disposable applicator appear.
4. Remove disposable applicator from tube of cream and use immediately.
5. Insert the disposable applicator into the vagina.
* Lie down with your knees bent to insert.
* Hold the applicator with your thumb and forefinger.
* Beginning with the white end, gently insert the applicator into the vagina.
* Insert as far as the applicator will go comfortably.
6. To dispense the cream, slowly push the blue end of the applicator in as far as it will go.
7. Remove the cardboard applicator and throw it away.
* Some cream may be left in the applicator, but if you pushed the blue end of the applicator until it stopped, you will be getting the proper dosage.
* Do not flush the disposable applicator in toilet.
8. Repeat steps #2 through #7 for the next two days, preferably at bedtime.
DO NOT USE TAMPONS.
Pre-Filled Applicator
1. Tear open the foil wrapper and remove one Femstat 3 prefilled applicator. The Femstat 3 applicator has a special tip on the end. Do not remove tip; do not use if tip has been removed. Do not warm applicator before using.
2. While holding the applicator firmly, pull the ring back to fully extend the plunger.
3. Hold the applicator by the outer cylinder with the thumb and forefinger. Lie down with your knees bent to insert the applicator into the vagina as far as it will go comfortably.
4. Push the plunger to release the cream. Remove the applicator and throw it away. Some cream may be left in the applicator, but if you pushed the plunger until it stopped, you are getting the proper dosage.
5. Repeat this procedure for the next two days, preferably at bedtime.
DO NOT USE TAMPONS.

WARNINGS:
* Do not use if you have abdominal pain, fever, or foul-smelling discharge. Contact your doctor immediately.
* If your infection isn't gone in three days, you may have a condition other than a yeast infection or you may need to use more medication. Consult your doctor. If your symptoms return within two months or if you think you have been exposed to the human immunodeficiency virus (HIV) that causes AIDS, consult your doctor immediately. Recurring infections may be a sign of pregnancy or a serious condition, such as AIDS or diabetes.
* Do not use this product if you are pregnant or think you may be pregnant, have diabetes, a positive HIV test or AIDS. Consult Your Doctor.
* Do not rely on condoms or diaphragms to prevent sexually transmitted diseases or pregnancy while using this product. This product may damage condoms and diaphragms and may cause them to fail. Use another method of birth control to prevent pregnancy while using this product.
* Do not use tampons while using this medicine.
* Do not use in girls under 12 years of age.
* Keep this and all drugs out of the reach of children.
* For vaginal use only. Do not use in eyes or take by mouth. In case of accidental ingestion, seek professional assistance or contact a Poison Control Center immediately.
* If your doctor has previously told you that you are sensitive or allergic to any Femstat product, do not use Femstat 3 without talking to your doctor first.

Do not use if overwrap is torn or missing. In addition, the tube opening should be sealed. **Do not use if seal has a hole in it or if the seal can not be seen.**
CONTENTS: Disposable Cardboard Applicator: One 20g (0.67 oz) tube of vaginal cream and 3 disposable applicators.
Pre-Filled Applicator: Three disposable applicators pre-filled to deliver 5 g vaginal cream (butoconazole nitrate 2%).
Avoid excessive heat above 30°C (86°F) and avoid freezing.
© 1996 P-S HPC
CONTENTS MADE IN CANADA
Distributed by Procter & Gamble
Cincinnati, OH 45202
If You Have Questions Or Comments.
If you have questions or comments about Femstat 3, please call toll-free, 1-800-353-3343. If you have questions about your infection, please call your doctor.

HEAD & SHOULDERS®   OTC
DANDRUFF SHAMPOO

(See PDR For Nonprescription Drugs.)

HEAD & SHOULDERS® DANDRUFF SHAMPOO DRY SCALP   OTC

(See PDR For Nonprescription Drugs.)

HEAD & SHOULDERS® INTENSIVE TREATMENT DANDRUFF AND SEBORRHEIC DERMATITIS SHAMPOO   OTC

(See PDR For Nonprescription Drugs.)

METAMUCIL®   OTC
[met uh-mū sil]
(psyllium husk fiber)

DESCRIPTION

Metamucil contains a bulk forming natural therapeutic fiber for restoring and maintaining regularity as recommended by a physician. It contains psyllium husk, a highly efficient fiber from the plant Plantago ovata. Metamucil contains no chemical stimulants and does not disrupt normal bowel function. Each dose contains approximately 3.4 grams of psyllium. Inactive ingredients, sodium, potassium, calories, carbohydrate, fat and phenylalanine content are shown in Table 1 for all forms and flavors. Phenylketonurics should be aware that phenylalanine is present in Metamucil products that contain aspartame. Metamucil Sugar-Free Regular Flavor contains no sugar and no artificial sweeteners.

Metamucil in powdered forms is gluten-free. Wafers contain gluten: Apple Crisp contains 0.7g/dose, Cinnamon Spice contains 0.5g/dose.

ACTIONS

The active ingredient in Metamucil is psyllium, a natural fiber which promotes elimination due to its bulking effect in the colon. This bulking effect is due to both the water-holding capacity of undigested fiber and the increased bacterial mass following partial fiber digestion. These actions result in enlargement of the lumen of the colon, and softer stool, thereby decreasing intraluminal pressure and straining, and speeding colonic transit in constipated patients.

INDICATIONS

Metamucil is indicated in the management of chronic constipation, irritable bowel syndrome, as adjunctive therapy in the constipation of diverticular disease, the bowel management of patients with hemorrhoids, for constipation associated with convalescence and senility and for occasional constipation during pregnancy when under the care of a physician. Pregnancy: Category B.

CONTRAINDICATIONS

Intestinal obstruction, fecal impaction. Known allergy to any component.

WARNINGS

Patients are advised they should not use the product without consulting a doctor when abdominal pain, nausea, or vomiting are present or if they have noticed a sudden change in bowel habits that persists over a period of two weeks, or rectal bleeding. Patients are advised to consult a physician if constipation persists for longer than one week, as this may be a sign of a serious medical condition. PATIENTS ARE CAUTIONED THAT TAKING THIS PRODUCT WITHOUT ADEQUATE FLUID MAY CAUSE IT TO SWELL AND BLOCK THE THROAT OR ESOPHAGUS AND MAY CAUSE CHOKING. THEY SHOULD NOT TAKE THE PRODUCT IF THEY HAVE DIFFICULTY IN SWALLOWING. IF THEY EX- PERIENCE CHEST PAIN, VOMITING, OR DIFFICULTY IN SWALLOWING OR BREATHING AFTER TAKING THIS PRODUCT, THEY ARE ADVISED TO SEEK IMMEDIATE MEDICAL ATTENTION. Psyllium products may cause allergic reaction in people sensitive to inhaled or ingested psyllium. Keep this and all medications out of the reach of children.

PRECAUTION

Notice to Health Care Professionals: To minimize the potential for allergic reaction, health care professionals who frequently dispense powdered psyllium products should avoid inhaling airborne dust while dispensing these products. Handling and Dispensing: To minimize generating airborne dust, spoon product from the canister into a glass according to label directions.

DOSAGE AND ADMINISTRATION

The usual adult dosage is 1 rounded teaspoonful or 1 rounded tablespoonful depending on product form. Generally the sugar-free products are dosed by the teaspoonful, sucrose-containing products by the tablespoonful. Some forms are available in packets. The appropriate dose should be mixed with 8 oz. of liquid (e.g., cool water, fruit juice, milk) following the labeled instructions. Metamucil wafers should be consumed with 8 oz. of liquid. THE PRODUCT (CHILD OR ADULT DOSE) SHOULD BE TAKEN WITH AT LEAST 8 OZ (A FULL GLASS) OF WATER OR OTHER FLUID. TAKING THIS PRODUCT WITHOUT ENOUGH LIQUID MAY CAUSE CHOKING (SEE WARNINGS). Metamucil can be taken orally one to three times a day, depending on the need and response. It may require continued use for 2 to 3 days to provide optimal benefit. Generally produces effect in 12–72 hours. For children (6 to 12 years old), use $1/_2$ the adult dose in/with 8 oz. of liquid, 1 to 3 times daily. Children under 6 consult a doctor.

TABLE 1

Forms/ Flavors	Inactive Ingredients	Sodium mg/Dose	Potassium mg/Dose	Phenylalanine mg/Dose	Dosage 1–3 Times Daily. Each Dose Contains 3.4 g Psyllium Husk Fiber	How Supplied
Smooth Texture Orange Flavor **METAMUCIL** Powder	Citric acid, D&C Yellow No. 10, FD&C Yellow No. 6, Flavoring, Sucrose	<5	30	—	1 rounded tablespoonful 12 g	Canisters: 20.3, 30.4 and 48 ozs. (Doses: 48, 72 and 114); Cartons: 30 and 100 single-dose packets (OTC)
Smooth Texture Sugar-Free Orange Flavor **METAMUCIL** Powder	Aspartame, Citric acid, D&C Yellow No. 10, FD&C Yellow No. 6, Flavoring, Maltodextrin	<5	30	25	1 rounded teaspoonful 5.8 g	Canisters: 10, 15, 23.3 ozs. and 36.8 ozs. (Doses: 48, 72, 114 and 180); Cartons: 30 single-dose packets (OTC), 100 single-dose packets (Institutional)
Smooth Texture Sugar-Free Regular Flavor **METAMUCIL** Powder	Citric Acid (less than 1%), Magnesium sulfate*, Maltodextrin	<5	30	—	1 rounded teaspoonful 5.8 g	Canisters: 10, 15 and 23.3 ozs. (Doses: 48, 72 and 114)
Original Texture Regular Flavor **METAMUCIL** Powder	Dextrose	<5	30	—	1 rounded teaspoonful 7 g	Canisters: 13, 19 and 29 ozs. (Doses: 48, 72 and 114)
Original Texture Orange Flavor **METAMUCIL** Powder	Citric acid, FD&C Yellow No. 6, Flavoring, Sucrose	<5	35	—	1 rounded tablespoonful 11 g	Canisters: 19, 29 and 44.2 ozs. (Doses: 48, 72 and 114)
Apple Crisp **METAMUCIL** Wafers	Ascorbic acid, Brown sugar, Cinnamon, Corn oil, Flavors, Fructose, Lecithin, Modified food starch, Molasses, Oat hull fiber, Sodium bicarbonate, Sucrose, Water, Wheat flour	20	50	—	2 wafers 25 g	Cartons: 12 doses; 24 doses
Cinnamon Spice **METAMUCIL** Wafers	Ascorbic acid, Cinnamon, Corn oil, Flavors, Fructose, Lecithin, Modified food starch, Molasses, Nutmeg, Oat hull fiber, Oats, Sodium bicarbonate, Sucrose, Water, Wheat flour	15	45	—	2 wafers 25 g	Cartons: 12 doses; 24 doses

* Metamucil Sugar-Free Regular Flavor contains 26 mg of magnesium per dose.

Continued on next page

Procter & Gamble—Cont.

NEW USERS: (Label statement)
Your doctor can recommend the right dosage of Metamucil to best meet your needs. In general, start by taking one dose each day. Gradually increase to three doses per day, if needed or recommended by your doctor. If minor gas or bloating occurs when you increase doses, try slightly reducing the amount you are taking.

HOW SUPPLIED
Powder: canisters (OTC) and cartons of single-dose packets (OTC and Institutional). Wafers: cartons of single-dose packets (OTC). (See Table 1).
[See Table 1 on bottom of preceding page.]

OIL OF OLAY®—Daily UV Protectant OTC
SPF 15 Beauty Fluid—Regular &
Fragrance Free
Procter & Gamble

(See PDR For Nonprescription Drugs.)

OIL OF OLAY®—Daily UV Protectant OTC
SPF 15 Moisture Replenishing
Cream—Regular & Fragrance Free
Procter & Gamble

(See PDR For Nonprescription Drugs.)

PEDIATRIC VICKS® 44d OTC
COUGH & HEAD CONGESTION RELIEF
Cough Suppressant/Nasal Decongestant

(See PDR For Nonprescription Drugs.)

PEDIATRIC VICKS® 44e OTC
CHEST COUGH & CHEST CONGESTION RELIEF
Cough Suppressant/Expectorant

(See PDR For Nonprescription Drugs.)

PEDIATRIC VICKS® 44m OTC
COUGH & COLD RELIEF
Cough Suppressant/Nasal
Decongestant/Antihistamine

(See PDR For Nonprescription Drugs.)

PEPTO-BISMOL® OTC
ORIGINAL LIQUID,
ORIGINAL AND CHERRY TABLETS
AND EASY-TO-SWALLOW CAPLETS
For upset stomach, indigestion, diarrhea, heartburn and nausea.

Multi-symptom Pepto-Bismol contains bismuth subsalicylate and is the only leading OTC stomach remedy clinically proven effective for both upper and lower GI symptoms. Pepto-Bismol is in more households than any other stomach remedy, making it a convenient recommendation with a name your patients will know. It has been clinically proven in double-blind placebo-controlled trials for relief of upset stomach symptoms and diarrhea.

DESCRIPTION
Each tablespoon (15 ml) of Pepto-Bismol Liquid contains 262 mg bismuth subsalicylate. Each tablespoonful of liquid contains a total of 130 mg non-aspirin salicylate. Pepto-Bismol liquid contains no sugar and is very low in sodium (less than 3 mg/tablespoonful). Inactive ingredients: benzoic acid, D&C Red No. 22, D&C Red No. 28, flavor, magnesium aluminum silicate, methylcellulose, saccharin sodium, salicylic acid, sodium salicylate, sorbic acid and water.
Each Pepto-Bismol Tablet contains 262 mg bismuth subsalicylate. Each tablet contains a total of 102 mg non-aspirin salicylate (99 mg non-aspirin salicylate for Cherry). Pepto-Bismol tablets contain no sugar and are very low in sodium (less than 2 mg/tablet). Inactive ingredients: adipic acid (in Cherry only), calcium carbonate, D&C Red No. 27, FD&C Red No. 40 (in Cherry only), flavors, magnesium stearate, mannitol, povidone, saccharin sodium and talc.
Each Pepto-Bismol Caplet contains 262 mg bismuth subsalicylate. Each caplet contains a total of 99 mg non-aspirin salicylate. Caplets contain no sugar and are low in sodium (less than 2 mg/caplet). Inactive ingredients include: calcium carbonate, D&C Red No. 27, magnesium stearate, mannitol, microcrystalline cellulose, polysorbate 80, povidone, silicon dioxide, and sodium starch glycolate.

INDICATIONS
Pepto-Bismol controls diarrhea within 24 hours, relieving associated abdominal cramps; soothes heartburn and indigestion without constipating; and relieves nausea and upset stomach.

ACTIONS
For upset stomach symptoms (i.e., indigestion, heartburn, nausea and fullness caused by over-indulgence), the active ingredient is believed to work via a topical effect on the stomach mucosa. For diarrhea, it is believed to work by several mechanisms in the gastrointestinal tract, including: 1) normalizing fluid movement via an antisecretory mechanism, 2) binding bacterial toxins and 3) antimicrobial activity.

WARNINGS
Children and teenagers who have or are recovering from chicken pox or flu should not use this medicine to treat nausea or vomiting. If nausea or vomiting is present, patients are advised to consult a doctor because this could be an early sign of Reye syndrome, a rare but serious illness.
This product contains non-aspirin salicylates. If taken with aspirin and ringing in the ears occurs, discontinue use. This product does not contain aspirin, but should not be administered to those patients who have a known allergy to aspirin or non-aspirin salicylates as an adverse reaction may occur. Caution is advised in the administration to patients taking medication for anticoagulation, diabetes and gout.
If diarrhea is accompanied by a high fever or continues more than 2 days, patients are advised to consult a physician. As with any drug, caution is advised in the administration to pregnant or nursing women.
Keep all medicine out of the reach of children.
Note: This medication may cause a temporary and harmless darkening of the tongue and/or stool. Stool darkening should not be confused with melena.

OVERDOSAGE
In case of overdose, patients are advised to contact a physician or Poison Control Center. Emesis induced by ipecac syrup is indicated in large ingestions provided ipecac can be administered within one hour of ingestion. Activated charcoal should be administered after gastric emptying. Patients should be evaluated for signs and symptoms of salicylate toxicity.

DOSAGE AND ADMINISTRATION
Liquid: Shake well before using.
Adults—   2 tablespoonsful
(1 dose cup, 30 ml)
Children (according to age)—
9–12 yrs.   1 tablespoonful
($^1/_2$ dose cup, 15 ml)
6–9 yrs.   2 teaspoonsful
($^1/_3$ dose cup, 10 ml)
3–6 yrs.   1 teaspoonful
($^1/_6$ dose cup, 5 ml)

Repeat dosage every $^1/_2$ to 1 hour, if needed, to a maximum of 8 doses in a 24-hour period. Drink plenty of clear fluids to help prevent dehydration which may accompany diarrhea. For children under 3 years of age, consult a physician.

Tablets:
Adults—Two tablets
Children (according to age)—
9–12 yrs.   1 tablet
6–9 yrs. $^2/_3$ tablet
3–6 yrs. $^1/_3$ tablet

Chew or dissolve in mouth. Repeat every $^1/_2$ to 1 hour as needed, to a maximum of 8 doses in a 24-hour period. Drink plenty of clear fluids to help prevent dehydration, which may accompany diarrhea. For children under 3 years of age, consult a physician.

Caplets:
Adults—Two caplets
Children (according to age)—
9–12 yrs.   1 caplet
6–9 yrs. $^2/_3$ caplet
3–6 yrs. $^1/_3$ caplet

Swallow caplet(s) with water, do not chew. Repeat every $^1/_2$ to 1 hour as needed, to a maximum of 8 doses in a 24-hour period. Drink plenty of clear fluids to help prevent dehydration, which may accompany diarrhea. For children under 3 years of age, consult a physician.

HOW SUPPLIED
Pepto-Bismol Liquid is available in: 4, 8, 12, 16 and 20 FL OZ bottles. Pepto-Bismol Tablets are pink, round, chewable tablets imprinted with a debossed triangle and "Pepto-Bismol" on one side. Tablets are available in: boxes of 30 and 48 (Original only). Caplets are available in bottles of 24 and 40. Caplets are imprinted with "Pepto-Bismol" on one side.

PEPTO-BISMOL® OTC
MAXIMUM STRENGTH LIQUID
For upset stomach, indigestion, diarrhea, heartburn and nausea.

Multi-symptom Pepto-Bismol contains bismuth subsalicylate and is the only leading OTC stomach remedy clinically proven effective for both upper and lower GI symptoms. Pepto-Bismol is in more households than any other stomach remedy, making it a convenient recommendation with a name your patients will know. It has been clinically-proven in double-blind placebo-controlled trials for relief of upset stomach symptoms and diarrhea.

DESCRIPTION
Each tablespoonful (15 ml) of Maximum Strength Pepto-Bismol Liquid contains 525 mg bismuth subsalicylate (236 mg non-aspirin salicylate). Maximum Strength Pepto-Bismol Liquid contains no sugar and is low in sodium (less than 3 mg/tablespoonful). Inactive ingredients include: benzoic acid, D&C Red No. 22, D&C Red No. 28, flavor, magnesium aluminum silicate, methylcellulose, saccharin sodium, salicylic acid, sodium salicylate, sorbic acid and water.

INDICATIONS
Maximum Strength Pepto-Bismol soothes upset stomach and indigestion without constipating; controls diarrhea within 24 hours, relieving associated abdominal cramps; and relieves heartburn and nausea.

ACTIONS
For upset stomach symptoms (i.e. indigestion, heartburn, nausea and fullness caused by over-indulgence), the active ingredient is believed to work via a topical effect on the stomach mucosa. For diarrhea, it is believed to work by several mechanisms in the gastrointestinal tract, including: 1) normalizing fluid movement via an antisecretory mechanism, 2) binding bacterial toxins, and 3) antimicrobial activity.

WARNINGS
Children and teenagers who have or are recovering from chicken pox or flu should not use this medicine to treat nausea or vomiting. If nausea or vomiting is present, patients are advised to consult a doctor because this could be an early sign of Reye syndrome, a rare but serious illness.
This product contains non-aspirin salicylates. If taken with aspirin and ringing in the ears occurs, discontinue use. This product does not contain aspirin, but should not be administered to those patients who have a known allergy to aspirin or other non-aspirin salicylates as an adverse reaction may occur. Caution is advised in the administration to patients taking medication for anticoagulation, diabetes and gout.
If diarrhea is accompanied by a high fever or continues more than 2 days, patients are advised to consult a physician. As with any drug, caution is advised in the administration to pregnant or nursing women.
Keep all medicine out of the reach of children.
Note: This medication may cause a temporary and harmless darkening of the tongue and/or stool. Stool darkening should not be confused with melena.

OVERDOSAGE
In case of overdose, patients are advised to contact a physician or Poison Control Center. Emesis induced by ipecac syrup is indicated in large ingestions provided ipecac can be administered within one hour of ingestion. Activated charcoal should be administered after gastric emptying. Patients should be evaluated for signs and symptoms of salicylate toxicity.

DOSAGE AND ADMINISTRATION
Shake well before using.
Adults—   2 tablespoonsful
(1 dose cup, 30 ml)
Children (according to age)—
9–12 yrs.   1 tablespoonful
($^1/_2$ dose cup, 15 ml)
6–9 yrs.   2 teaspoonsful
($^1/_3$ dose cup, 10 ml)
3–6 yrs.   1 teaspoonful
($^1/_6$ dose cup, 5 ml)

Repeat dosage every hour, if needed, to a maximum of 4 doses in a 24-hour period. Drink plenty of clear fluids to help prevent dehydration, which may accompany diarrhea.

HOW SUPPLIED
Maximum Strength Pepto-Bismol is available in: 4, 8, and 12 FL OZ bottles.

PEPTO DIARRHEA CONTROL® OTC
Loperamide Hydrochloride
Caplets

DESCRIPTION

Each caplet of Pepto Diarrhea Control contains 2 mg of Loperamide Hydrochloride and is scored and colored white.

ACTIONS

Pepto Diarrhea Control contains a clinically proven antidiarrheal medication, Loperamide Hydrochloride, that works in many cases with just one dose. Loperamide Hydrochloride acts by slowing intestinal motility and by affecting water and electrolyte movement through the bowel.

INDICATION

Pepto Diarrhea Control controls the symptoms of diarrhea.

DIRECTIONS

Drink plenty of clear fluids to help prevent dehydration, which may accompany diarrhea.

USUAL DOSAGE

Adults and children 12 years of age and older: Two caplets after first loose bowel movement followed by one caplet after each subsequent loose bowel movement but no more than four caplets a day for no more than two days.
Children 9–11 years old (60–95 lbs.): One caplet after first loose bowel movement, followed by one-half caplet after each subsequent loose bowel movement, but no more than three caplets a day for no more than two days.
Children 6–8 years old (48–59 lbs.): One caplet after first loose bowel movement, followed by one-half caplet after each subsequent loose bowel movement, but no more than two caplets a day for no more than two days.
Under 6 years old (up to 47 lbs.): Consult a physician. Not intended for children under 6 years old.

WARNINGS

DO NOT USE FOR MORE THAN TWO DAYS UNLESS DIRECTED BY A PHYSICIAN. Do not use if diarrhea is accompanied by high fever (greater than 101°F), or if blood is present in the stool, or if you have had a rash or other allergic reaction to Loperamide Hydrochloride. If you are taking antibiotics or have a history of liver disease, consult a physician before using this product. As with any drug, caution is advised in the administration to pregnant and nursing women. Keep this and all drugs out of the reach of children. In case of accidental overdose, seek professional assistance or contact a poison control center immediately.

OVERDOSAGE

Overdosage of Loperamide Hydrochloride in humans may result in constipation, CNS depression and nausea. A slurry of activated charcoal administered promptly after ingestion of Loperamide Hydrochloride can reduce the amount of drug which is absorbed. If vomiting occurs spontaneously upon ingestion, a slurry of 100 grams of activated charcoal may be administered orally as soon as fluids can be retained. If vomiting has not occurred, and CNS depression is evident, gastric lavage should be performed followed by administration of 100 grams of the activated charcoal slurry through the gastric tube. In the event of overdosage, patients should be monitored for signs of CNS depression for at least 24 hours. Children may be more sensitive to central nervous system effects than adults. If CNS depression is observed, naloxone may be administered. If responsive to naloxone, vital signs must be monitored carefully for recurrence of symptoms of drug overdose for at least 24 hours after the last dose of naloxone.

INACTIVE INGREDIENTS

Corn starch, lactose, magnesium stearate, microcrystalline cellulose.

HOW SUPPLIED

White scored caplets in 6's and 12's blister packaging which is tamper-evident and child-resistant. Caplets are imprinted with "Pepto DC" on one side, "2" and "MG" separated by score mark on other side.

PERCOGESIC® OTC
[*pĕr 'kō-gē-sĭk*]
Aspirin-free analgesic tablets
Pain Reliever/Fever Reducer

(See PDR For Nonprescription Drugs.)

PERIDEX® ℞
[*per-i-dex*]
(chlorhexidine gluconate)
Oral Rinse

PRODUCT OVERVIEW

KEY FACTS

Peridex is an antimicrobial oral rinse containing 0.12% chlorhexidine gluconate. Peridex has been shown to achieve significant reductions in gingivitis as characterized by gingival inflammation and associated bleeding which can complicate certain dental procedures. Approximately 30% of the active ingredient is retained in the oral cavity following a single rinsing. This retained active is slowly released into the oral fluids.

MAJOR USES

Peridex has proved to be clinically effective for use between dental visits as part of a professional program for the treatment of gingivitis as characterized by gingival bleeding and inflammation. Therapy should be initiated directly following an oral prophylaxis. Patients using Peridex should be reevaluated and given a thorough prophylaxis at intervals no longer than six months. Recommended use is a 30-second rinse of ½ fluid ounce (marked in cap) twice daily.

SAFETY INFORMATION

The most common side effects associated with chlorhexidine oral rinses are (1) an increase in staining of teeth and other oral surfaces on certain individuals, (2) an increase in supragingival calculus formation, and (3) an alteration in taste perception. Not all patients will experience a visually significant increase in tooth staining. Staining can be removed from most tooth surfaces by a conventional professional prophylaxis.

PRESCRIBING INFORMATION

PERIDEX® ℞
(chlorhexidine gluconate)
Oral Rinse

DESCRIPTION

Peridex is an oral rinse containing 0.12% chlorhexidine gluconate (1,1′ -hexamethylene bis [5-(p-chlorophenyl) biguanide] di-D-gluconate) in a base containing water, 11.6% alcohol, glycerin, PEG-40 sorbitan diisostearate, flavor, sodium saccharin, and FD&C Blue No. 1. Peridex is a near-neutral solution (pH range 5–7). Chlorhexidine gluconate is a salt of chlorhexidine and gluconic acid. Its chemical structure is:

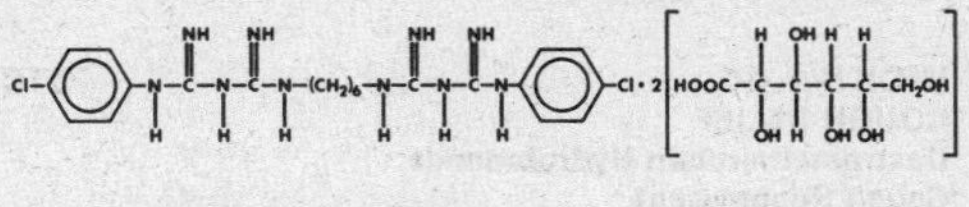

CLINICAL PHARMACOLOGY

Peridex provides microbicidal activity during oral rinsing. The clinical significance of Peridex's antimicrobial activities is not clear. Microbiological sampling of plaque has shown a general reduction of counts of certain assayed bacteria, both aerobic and anaerobic, ranging from 54–97% through six months' use.
Use of Peridex in a six-month clinical study did not result in any significant changes in bacterial resistance, overgrowth of potentially opportunistic organisms or other adverse changes in the oral microbial ecosystem. Three months after Peridex use was discontinued, the number of bacteria in plaque had returned to baseline levels and resistance of plaque bacteria to chlorhexidine gluconate was equal to that at baseline.

PHARMACOKINETICS

Pharmacokinetic studies with Peridex indicate approximately 30% of the active ingredient, chlorhexidine gluconate, is retained in the oral cavity following rinsing. This retained drug is slowly released into the oral fluids. Studies conducted on human subjects and animals demonstrate chlorhexidine gluconate is poorly absorbed from the gastrointestinal tract. The mean plasma level of chlorhexidine gluconate reached a peak of 0.206 μg/g in humans 30 minutes after they ingested a 300-mg dose of the drug. Detectable levels of chlorhexidine gluconate were not present in the plasma of these subjects 12 hours after the compound was administered. Excretion of chlorhexidine gluconate occurred primarily through the feces (∼90%). Less than 1% of the chlorhexidine gluconate ingested by these subjects was excreted in the urine.

INDICATION

Peridex is indicated for use between dental visits as part of a professional program for the treatment of gingivitis as characterized by redness and swelling of the gingivae, including gingival bleeding upon probing. Peridex has not been tested among patients with acute necrotizing ulcerative gingivitis (ANUG). For patients having coexisting gingivitis and periodontitis, see PRECAUTIONS.

CONTRAINDICATIONS

Peridex should not be used by persons who are known to be hypersensitive to chlorhexidine gluconate.

WARNINGS

The effect of Peridex on periodontitis has not been determined. An increase in supragingival calculus was noted in clinical testing in Peridex users compared with control users. It is not known if Peridex use results in an increase in subgingival calculus. Calculus deposits should be removed by a dental prophylaxis at intervals no greater than six months. Rare hypersensitivity and generalized allergic reactions have also been reported. Peridex should not be used by persons who have a sensitivity to it or its components.

PRECAUTIONS

GENERAL:

1. For patients having coexisting gingivitis and periodontitis, the presence or absence of gingival inflammation following treatment with Peridex should not be used as a major indicator of underlying periodontitis.
2. Peridex can cause staining of oral surfaces, such as tooth surfaces, restorations, and the dorsum of the tongue. Not all patients will experience a visually significant increase in toothstaining. In clinical testing, 56% of Peridex users exhibited a measurable increase in facial anterior stain, compared to 35% of control users after six months; 15% of Peridex users developed what was judged to be heavy stain, compared to 1% of control users after six months. Stain will be more pronounced in patients who have heavier accumulations of unremoved plaque.
   Stain resulting from use of Peridex does not adversely affect health of the gingivae or other oral tissues. Stain can be removed from most tooth surfaces by conventional professional prophylactic techniques. Additional time may be required to complete the prophylaxis.
   Discretion should be used when prescribing to patients with anterior facial restorations with rough surfaces or margins. If natural stain cannot be removed from these surfaces by a dental prophylaxis, patients should be excluded from Peridex treatment if permanent discoloration is unacceptable. Stain in these areas may be difficult to remove by dental prophylaxis and on rare occasions may necessitate replacement of these restorations.
3. Some patients may experience an alteration in taste perception while undergoing treatment with Peridex. Most patients accommodate to this effect with continued use of Peridex. No instances of permanent taste alteration due to Peridex have been reported.

USAGE IN PREGNANCY: Pregnancy Category B. Reproduction and fertility studies with chlorhexidine gluconate have been conducted. No evidence of impaired fertility was observed in rats at doses up to 100 mg/kg/day, and no evidence of harm to the fetus was observed in rats and rabbits at doses up to 300 mg/kg/day and 40 mg/kg/day, respectively. These doses are approximately 100, 300, and 40 times that which would result from a person's ingesting 30 ml (2 capfuls) of Peridex per day. Since controlled studies in pregnant women have not been conducted, the benefits of the drug in pregnant women should be weighed against possible risk to the fetus.

NURSING MOTHERS: It is not known whether this drug is excreted in human milk. Because many drugs are excreted in human milk, caution should be exercised when Peridex is administered to a nursing woman.
In parturition and lactation studies with rats, no evidence of impaired parturition or of toxic effects to suckling pups was observed when chlorhexidine gluconate was administered to dams at doses that were over 100 times greater than that which would result from a person's ingesting 30 ml (2 capfuls) of Peridex per day.

PEDIATRIC USE: Clinical effectiveness and safety of Peridex have not been established in children under the age of 18.

CARCINOGENESIS, MUTAGENESIS: In a drinking water study in rats, carcinogenesis was not observed. The highest dose of chlorhexidine gluconate used in this study, 38 mg/kg/day, is at least 500 times the amount that would be ingested from the recommended daily dose of Peridex.
In two mammalian *in vivo* mutagenic studies with chlorhexidine gluconate, mutagenesis was not observed. The highest dose of chlorhexidine gluconate used in a mouse dominant lethal assay was 1000 mg/kg/day and in a hamster cytogenetics test was 250 mg/kg/day, i.e., > 3200 times the amount that would be ingested from the recommended daily dose of Peridex.

ADVERSE REACTIONS

The most common side effects associated with chlorhexidine gluconate oral rinses are (1) an increase in staining of teeth and other oral surfaces, (2) an increase in calculus formation, and (3) an alteration in taste perception; see WARNINGS and PRECAUTIONS. No serious systemic adverse reactions

Continued on next page

Procter & Gamble—Cont.

associated with use of Peridex were observed in clinical testing.

Minor irritation and superficial desquamation of the oral mucosa have been noted in patients using Peridex, particularly among children.

Although there have been no reports of parotitis (inflammation or swelling of salivary glands) among Peridex users in controlled clinical studies, transient parotitis has been reported in research studies with chlorhexidine-containing mouthrinses.

OVERDOSAGE

Ingestion of 1 or 2 ounces of Peridex by a small child (~10 kg body weight) might result in gastric distress, including nausea, or signs of alcohol intoxication. Medical attention should be sought if more than 4 ounces of Peridex is ingested by a small child or if signs of alcohol intoxication develop.

DOSAGE AND ADMINISTRATION

Peridex therapy should be initiated directly following a dental prophylaxis. Patients using Peridex should be reevaluated and given a thorough prophylaxis at intervals no longer than six months.

Recommended use is twice daily oral rinsing for 30 seconds, morning and evening after toothbrushing. Usual dosage is ½ fl. oz. (marked in cap) of undiluted Peridex. Peridex is not intended for ingestion and should be expectorated after rinsing.

HOW SUPPLIED

Peridex is supplied as a blue liquid in dispenser packs of three 1-pint amber plastic bottles with child-resistant dispensing closures. Store above freezing (32°F).
NDC 37000-007- 01
Military-6505-01-253-8138

ORIGINAL VICKS® COUGH DROPS   OTC
Menthol Cough Suppressant/Oral Anesthetic
Cherry & Menthol Flavors

(See PDR For Nonprescription Drugs.)

VICKS® CHLORASEPTIC®   OTC
COUGH & THROAT DROPS
Menthol Cough Suppressant/Oral
Anesthetic
Cherry, Menthol & Honey Lemon Flavors

(See PDR For Nonprescription Drugs.)

VICKS® CHLORASEPTIC®   OTC
GARGLE & MOUTH RINSE
Phenol/oral anesthetic/antiseptic
Menthol Flavor

VICKS® CHLORASEPTIC ®   OTC
SORE THROAT SPRAY
Phenol/oral anesthetic/antiseptic
Cherry and Menthol Flavors

(See PDR For Nonprescription Drugs.)

VICKS® CHLORASEPTIC® SORE   OTC
THROAT LOZENGES
Cherry and Menthol Flavors
Menthol/Benzocaine
Oral Anesthetic

(See PDR For Nonprescription Drugs.)

VICKS® COUGH DROPS   OTC
Menthol Cough Suppressant/Oral
Anesthetic
Cherry & Menthol Flavors

(See PDR For Nonprescription Drugs.)

VICKS® DAYQUIL® ALLERGY RELIEF   OTC
12 HOUR EXTENDED RELEASE
Nasal Decongestant/Antihistamine

(See PDR For Nonprescription Drugs.)

VICKS® DAYQUIL® ALLERGY   OTC
RELIEF 4 HOUR
Nasal Decongestant/Antihistamine

(See PDR For Nonprescription Drugs.)

VICKS® DAYQUIL®   OTC
VICKS® DAYQUIL® LIQUICAPS   OTC
MULTI-SYMPTOM COLD/FLU RELIEF
Nasal Decongestant/Expectorant/
Pain Reliever/Cough Suppressant/
Fever Reducer

(See PDR For Nonprescription Drugs.)

VICKS® DAYQUIL®   OTC
SINUS PRESSURE & CONGESTION RELIEF
Nasal Decongestant/Expectorant

(See PDR For Nonprescription Drugs.)

VICKS® DAYQUIL®   OTC
SINUS PRESSURE & PAIN RELIEF
WITH IBUPROFEN
Nasal Decongestant/Pain Reliever

(See PDR For Nonprescription Drugs.)

VICKS® 44 LIQUICAPS®   OTC
COUGH, COLD & FLU RELIEF
Cough Suppressant/Nasal Decongestant/Antihistamine/
Pain Reliever-Fever Reducer

(See PDR For Nonprescription Drugs.)

VICKS® 44 LIQUICAPS® NON-DROWSY   OTC
COUGH & COLD RELIEF
Cough Suppressant/Nasal Decongestant

(See PDR For Nonprescription Drugs.)

VICKS® 44   OTC
COUGH RELIEF
Dextromethorphan Hydrobromide
Cough Suppressant

(See PDR For Nonprescription Drugs.)

VICKS® 44D   OTC
COUGH & HEAD CONGESTION RELIEF
Cough Suppressant/Nasal Decongestant

(See PDR For Nonprescription Drugs.)

VICKS® 44E   OTC
CHEST COUGH & CHEST CONGESTION RELIEF
Cough Suppressant/Expectorant

(See PDR For Nonprescription Drugs.)

VICKS® 44M   OTC
COUGH, COLD & FLU RELIEF
Cough Suppressant/Nasal
Decongestant/Antihistamine/
Pain Reliever-Fever Reducer

(See PDR For Nonprescription Drugs.)

VICKS® NYQUIL HOT THERAPY®   OTC
VICKS® NYQUIL® LIQUID
VICKS® NYQUIL LIQUICAPS®
[nī quil]
Multi-Symptom Cold/Flu Relief
Antihistamine/Cough Suppressant/
Pain Reliever/Nasal Decongestant/
Fever Reducer

(See PDR For Nonprescription Drugs.)

VICKS® SINEX®   OTC
[sī'něx]
NASAL SPRAY AND
ULTRA FINE MIST FOR SINUS RELIEF
Phenylephrine HCl Decongestant

(See PDR For Nonprescription Drugs.)

VICKS® SINEX® 12 HOUR   OTC
[sī'něx]
NASAL SPRAY AND ULTRA FINE MIST
FOR SINUS RELIEF
Oxymetazoline HCl Nasal Decongestant

(See PDR For Nonprescription Drugs.)

VICKS® VAPOR INHALER   OTC
l-Desoxyephedrine/Nasal
Decongestant

(See PDR For Nonprescription Drugs.)

VICKS® VAPORUB®   OTC
(cream) (ointment)
[vā'pō-rub]
Nasal Decongestant/Cough
Suppresssant/Topical Analgesic

(See PDR For Nonprescription Drugs.)

VICKS® VAPOSTEAM®   OTC
[vā'pō"stēm]
Liquid Medication for
Hot Steam Vaporizers.
Nasal Decongestant/Cough
Suppressant

(See PDR For Nonprescription Drugs.)

EDUCATIONAL MATERIAL

Procter & Gamble offers to health care professionals a variety of journal reprints and patient education materials on:
- pain management (Aleve)
- fiber therapy and related bowel disorders (Metamucil),
- H. pylori research and healthy traveling advice (Pepto-Bismol),
- caffeine reduction (Folgers), and
- pharmacy practice issues (Pharmacy Digest newsletter).

Additionally, selected professional samples of Procter & Gamble Health Care and Skin Care products are available to targeted health care specialists.

For these materials, please call 1-800/358-8707, or write:
Charles Lambert
Manager, Scientific Communications
The Procter & Gamble Company
Two Procter & Gamble Plaza
Cincinnati, OH 45201

Procter & Gamble Pharmaceuticals, Inc.
SHARON WOODS TECHNICAL CENTER
11520 REED HARTMAN HIGHWAY
CINCINNATI, OH 45241

Direct Inquiries to:
Customer Service
(800) 448-4878

For Medical Information Contact:
Medical Communications
(800) 836-0658
Fax: (800) 438-0138
or write
Procter & Gamble Pharmaceuticals
Medical Communications Department
11450 Grooms Road
Cincinnati, OH 45242-1434

In Emergencies:
Medical Communications
(800) 836-0658

Information on these Procter & Gamble Pharmaceuticals products is based on labeling in effect June 3, 1996. Further information on these and other Procter & Gamble Pharmaceuticals products may be obtained by direct inquiry to Procter & Gamble Pharmaceuticals, Medical Communications Department, 11370 Reed Hartman Highway, Cincinnati, OH 45241-2422, or phone 800-836-0658/FAX 800-438-0138.

ASACOL® ℞

[*āce 'ah-kol*]
(mesalamine)
Delayed-Release Tablets

DESCRIPTION

Each **Asacol** delayed-release tablet for oral administration contains 400 mg of mesalamine, an anti-inflammatory drug. The **Asacol** delayed-release tablets are coated with acrylic based resin, Eudragit S (methacrylic acid copolymer B, NF), which dissolves at pH 7 or greater, releasing mesalamine in the terminal ileum and beyond for topical anti-inflammatory action in the colon. Mesalamine has the chemical name 5-amino-2-hydroxybenzoic acid; its structural formula is:

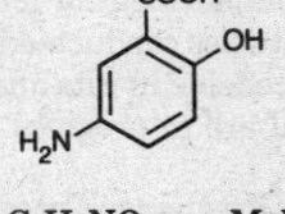

Molecular Formula: $C_7H_7NO_3$ Molecular Weight: 153.1

Inactive Ingredients: Each tablet contains colloidal silicon dioxide, dibutyl phthalate, edible black ink, iron oxide red, iron oxide yellow, lactose, magnesium stearate, methacrylic acid copolymer B (Eudragit S), polyethylene glycol, povidone, sodium starch glycolate, and talc.

CLINICAL PHARMACOLOGY

Mesalamine is thought to be the major therapeutically active part of the sulfasalazine molecule in the treatment of ulcerative colitis. Sulfasalazine is converted to equimolar amounts of sulfapyridine and mesalamine by bacterial action in the colon. The usual oral dose of sulfasalazine for active ulcerative colitis is 3 to 4 grams daily in divided doses, which provides 1.2 to 1.6 grams of mesalamine to the colon.

The mechanism of action of mesalamine (and sulfasalazine) is unknown, but appears to be topical rather than systemic. Mucosal production of arachidonic acid (AA) metabolites, both through the cyclooxygenase pathways, *i.e.*, prostanoids, and through the lipoxygenase pathways, *i.e.*, leukotrienes (LTs) and hydroxyeicosatetraenoic acids (HETEs), is increased in patients with chronic inflammatory bowel disease, and it is possible that mesalamine diminishes inflammation by blocking cyclooxygenase and inhibiting prostaglandin (PG) production in the colon.

Pharmacokinetics: **Asacol** tablets are coated with an acrylic-based resin that delays release of mesalamine until it reaches the terminal ileum and beyond. This has been demonstrated in human studies conducted with radiological and serum markers. Approximately 28% of the mesalamine in **Asacol** tablets is absorbed after oral ingestion, leaving the remainder available for topical action and excretion in the feces. Absorption of mesalamine is similar in fasted and fed subjects. The absorbed mesalamine is rapidly acetylated in the gut mucosal wall and by the liver. It is excreted mainly by the kidney as N-acetyl-5-amino-salicylic acid.

Mesalamine from orally administered **Asacol** tablets appears to be more extensively absorbed than the mesalamine released from sulfasalazine. Maximum plasma levels of mesalamine and N-acetyl-5-aminosalicylic acid following multiple **Asacol** doses are about 1.5 to 2 times higher than those following an equivalent dose of mesalamine in the form of sulfasalazine. Combined mesalamine and N-acetyl-5-aminosalicylic acid AUC's and urine drug dose recoveries following multiple doses of **Asacol** tablets are about 1.3 to 1.5 times higher than those following an equivalent dose of mesalamine in the form of sulfasalazine.

The t_{max} for mesalamine and its metabolite, N-acetyl-5-aminosalicylic acid, is usually delayed, reflecting the delayed release, and ranges from 4 to 12 hours. The half-lives of elimination ($t1/2_{elm}$) for mesalamine and N-acetyl-5-aminosalicylic acid are usually about 12 hours, but are variable, ranging from 2 to 15 hours. There is a large intersubject variability in the plasma concentrations of mesalamine and N-acetyl-5-aminosalicylic acid and in their elimination half-lives following administration of **Asacol** tablets.

Clinical Studies: Two placebo-controlled studies have demonstrated the efficacy of **Asacol** tablets in patients with mildly to moderately active ulcerative colitis. In one randomized, double-blind, multicenter trial of 158 patients, **Asacol** doses of 1.6 g/day and 2.4 g/day were compared to placebo. At the dose of 2.4 g/day, **Asacol** tablets reduced the disease activity, with 21 of 43 (49%) **Asacol** patients showing improvement in sigmoidoscopic appearance of the bowel compared to 12 of 44 (27%) placebo patients (p=0.048). In addition, significantly more patients in the **Asacol** 2.4 g/day group showed improvement in rectal bleeding and stool frequency. The 1.6 g/day dose did not produce consistent evidence of effectiveness.

In a second randomized, double-blind, placebo-controlled clinical trial of 6 weeks duration in 87 ulcerative colitis patients, **Asacol** tablets, at a dose of 4.8 g/day, gave sigmoidoscopic improvement in 28 of 38 (74%) patients compared to 10 of 38 (26%) placebo patients ($p < 0.001$). Also, more patients in the **Asacol** 4.8 g/day group showed improvement in overall symptoms.

The effect of **Asacol** (mesalamine) on sulfasalazine-induced impairment of male fertility was examined in an open-label study. Nine patients (age < 40 years) with chronic ulcerative colitis in clinical remission on sulfasalazine 2–3 g/day were crossed over to an equivalent **Asacol** dose (0.8–1.2 g/day) for 3 months. Improvement in sperm count ($p < 0.02$) and morphology ($p < 0.02$) occurred in all cases. Improvement in sperm motility ($p < 0.001$) occurred in 8 of the 9 patients.

INDICATIONS AND USAGE

Asacol tablets are indicated for the treatment of mildly to moderately active ulcerative colitis.

CONTRAINDICATIONS

Asacol tablets are contraindicated in patients with hypersensitivity to salicylates or to any of the components of the **Asacol** tablet.

PRECAUTIONS

General: Patients with pyloric stenosis may have prolonged gastric retention of **Asacol** tablets which could delay release of mesalamine in the colon.

Exacerbation of the symptoms of colitis, thought to have been caused by mesalamine or sulfasalazine has been reported in 3% of patients in controlled clinical trials. This acute reaction, characterized by cramping, abdominal pain, bloody diarrhea, and occasionally by fever, headache, malaise, pruritus, rash, and conjunctivitis, has been reported after the initiation of **Asacol** tablets as well as other mesalamine products. Symptoms usually abate when **Asacol** tablets are discontinued.

Some patients who have experienced a hypersensitivity reaction to sulfasalazine may have a similar reaction to **Asacol** tablets or to other compounds which contain or are converted to mesalamine.

Renal: Renal impairment, including minimal change nephropathy, and acute and chronic interstitial nephritis, has been reported in patients taking **Asacol** tablets as well as in patients taking other mesalamine products. In animal studies (rats, dogs), the kidney is the principal target organ for toxicity. At doses of approximately 750-1000 mg/kg [15-20 times the administered recommended human dose (based on a 50 kg person) on a mg/kg basis and 3-4 times on a mg/m^2 basis], mesalamine causes renal papillary necrosis. **Therefore, caution should be exercised when using Asacol (mesalamine) or other compounds converted to mesalamine or its metabolites in patients with known renal dysfunction or history of renal disease. It is recommended that all patients have an evaluation of renal function prior to initiation of Asacol tablets and periodically while on Asacol therapy.**

Information for Patients: Patients should be instructed to swallow the **Asacol** tablets whole, taking care not to break the outer coating. The outer coating is designed to remain intact to protect the active ingredient and thus ensure mesalamine availability for action in the colon. In 2–3% of patients in clinical studies, intact or partially intact tablets have been reported in the stool. If this occurs repeatedly, patients should contact their physician.

Drug Interactions: There are no known drug interactions.

Carcinogenesis, Mutagenesis, Impairment of Fertility: Long-term studies in animals have not been performed to evaluate the carcinogenicity potential of mesalamine. Mesalamine was not mutagenic in fluctuation assay in *K. pneumoniae* and Ames assay in *S. typhimurium*. Mesalamine, at oral doses up to 480 mg/kg/day, had no adverse effect on fertility or reproductive performance of male and female rats. The oligospermia and infertility in men associated with sulfasalazine have not been reported with **Asacol** delayed-release tablets.

Pregnancy: Teratogenic Effects:
Pregnancy Category B: Reproduction studies in rats and rabbits at oral doses up to 480 mg/kg/day have revealed no evidence of teratogenic effects or fetal toxicity due to mesalamine. There are, however, no adequate and well-controlled studies in pregnant women. Because animal reproduction studies are not always predictive of human response, this drug should be used during pregnancy only if clearly needed.

Nursing Mothers: Low concentrations of mesalamine and higher concentrations of its N-acetyl metabolite have been detected in human breast milk. While the clinical significance of this has not been determined, caution should be exercised when mesalamine is administered to a nursing woman.

Pediatric Use: Safety and effectiveness of **Asacol** tablets in pediatric patients have not been established.

ADVERSE REACTIONS

Asacol tablets have been evaluated in about 1830 inflammatory bowel disease patients (most patients with ulcerative colitis) in controlled and open-label studies. Adverse events seen in clinical trials with **Asacol** tablets have generally been mild and reversible. In two short-term (6 weeks) placebo-controlled clinical studies involving 245 patients, 155 of whom were randomized to **Asacol** tablets, five (3.2%) of the **Asacol** patients discontinued **Asacol** therapy because of adverse events as compared to two (2.2%) of the placebo patients. Adverse reactions leading to withdrawal from **Asacol** tablets included (each in one patient): diarrhea and colitis flare; dizziness, nausea, joint pain, and headache; rash, lethargy and constipation; dry mouth, malaise, lower back discomfort, mild disorientation, mild indigestion and cramping; headache, nausea, malaise, aching, vomiting, muscle cramps, a stuffy head, plugged ears, and fever.

Adverse events occurring at a frequency of 2% or greater in the two short-term, double-blind, placebo-controlled trials mentioned above are listed in Table 1 below. Overall, the incidence of adverse events seen with **Asacol** tablets was similar to placebo.

Table 1

Frequency (%) of Common Adverse Events Reported in Ulcerative Colitis Patients Treated with **Asacol** Tablets or Placebo in Double-Blind Controlled Studies

	Percent of Patients with Adverse Events	
Event	Placebo (n=87)	Asacol tablets (n=152)
Headache	36	35
Abdominal pain	14	18
Eructation	15	16
Pain	8	14
Nausea	15	13
Pharyngitis	9	11
Dizziness	8	8
Asthenia	15	7
Diarrhea	9	7
Back pain	5	7
Fever	8	6
Rash	3	6
Dyspepsia	1	6
Rhinitis	5	5
Arthralgia	3	5
Vomiting	2	5
Constipation	1	5
Hypertonia	3	5
Flatulence	7	3
Flu syndrome	2	3
Chills	2	3
Colitis exacerbation	0	3
Chest pain	2	3
Peripheral edema	2	3
Myalgia	1	3
Pruritius	0	3
Sweating	1	3
Dysmenorrhea	3	3

Of these adverse events, only rash showed a consistently higher frequency with increasing **Asacol** dose in these studies. In uncontrolled data, fever, flu syndrome, and headache also seemed dose-related.

In addition, the following adverse reactions were seen in 1–2% of the patients in the controlled studies: malaise, arthritis, increased cough, acne, and conjunctivitis.

Over 1800 patients have been treated with **Asacol** tablets in clinical studies. In addition to the adverse events listed above, the following adverse events also have been reported in controlled clinical studies, open-label studies, or foreign marketing experience. The relationship of the reported events to **Asacol** administration is unclear in many cases. Some complaints, including anorexia, joint pains, pyoderma gangrenosum, oral ulcers, and anemia could be part of the clinical presentation of inflammatory bowel disease.

Body as a Whole: Weakness, neck pain, abdominal enlargement, facial edema, edema.

Cardiovascular: Pericarditis (rare), myocarditis (rare), vasodilation, migraine.

Digestive: Anorexia, hepatitis (rare), pancreatitis, gastroenteritis, gastritis, increased appetite, cholecystitis, dry mouth, oral ulcers, perforated peptic ulcer (rare), bloody diarrhea, tenesmus.

Hematologic: Agranulocytosis (rare), aplastic anemia (rare), thrombocytopenia, eosinophilia, leukopenia, anemia, lymphadenopathy.

Musculoskeletal: Gout.

Nervous: Anxiety, insomnia, depression, somnolence, emotional lability, hyperesthesia, vertigo, nervousness, confusion, paresthesia, tremor, peripheral neuropathy (rare), transverse myelitis (rare), Guillain-Barré syndrome (rare).

Continued on next page

Procter & Gamble Pharm.—Cont.

Respiratory/Pulmonary: Sinusitis, eosinophilic pneumonia, interstitial pneumonitis, asthma exacerbation.
Skin: Alopecia, psoriasis (rare), pyoderma gangrenosum (rare), dry skin, erythema nodosum, urticaria.
Special Senses: Ear pain, eye pain, taste perversion, blurred vision, tinnitus.
Urogenital: Interstitial nephritis (See also Renal subsection in PRECAUTIONS), minimal change nephropathy (See also Renal subsection in PRECAUTIONS), dysuria, urinary urgency, hematuria, epididymitis, menorrhagia.
Laboratory Abnormalities: Elevated AST (SGOT) or ALT (SGPT), elevated alkaline phosphatase, elevated serum creatinine and BUN.
Hepatitis has been reported to occur rarely with **Asacol** tablets. More commonly, asymptomatic elevations of liver enzymes have occurred which usually resolve during continued use or with discontinuation of the drug.

DRUG ABUSE AND DEPENDENCY
Abuse: None reported.
Dependency: Drug dependence has not been reported with chronic administration of mesalamine.

OVERDOSAGE
One case of overdosage has been reported. A 3-year-old male ingested 2 grams of **Asacol** tablets. He was treated with ipecac and activated charcoal. No adverse events occurred. Oral doses of mesalamine in mice and rats of 5000 mg/kg and 4595 mg/kg, respectively, cause significant lethality.

DOSAGE AND ADMINISTRATION
The usual dosage in adults is two 400-mg tablets to be taken three times a day for a total daily dose of 2.4 grams for a duration of 6 weeks.

HOW SUPPLIED
Asacol tablets are available as red-brown, capsule-shaped tablets containing 400 mg mesalamine and imprinted "Asacol NE" in black.
NDC 0149-0752-02 Bottle of 100
Store at controlled room temperature (59°–86°F or 15°–30°C).
CAUTION: Federal law prohibits dispensing without prescription.
Procter & Gamble Pharmaceuticals
Cincinnati, Ohio 45202
under license from Tillotts Pharma AG,
the registered trademark owner.
Made in Germany
D-64331 Weiterstadt
REVISED APRIL 1996 75200-P7
Shown in Product Identification Guide, page 329

BRONTEX® Ⓒ℞
[brŏn -tex]
codeine phosphate/guaifenesin tablets

DESCRIPTION
Each **Brontex** tablet contains
codeine phosphate .... 10 mg
Warning—May be habit forming
guaifenesin .... 300 mg
Codeine phosphate is an opiate antitussive having the chemical name 7,8-didehydro-4,5α-epoxy-3-methoxy-17-methylmorphinan-6α-ol Phosphate (1:1) salt hemihydrate, with the following structure:

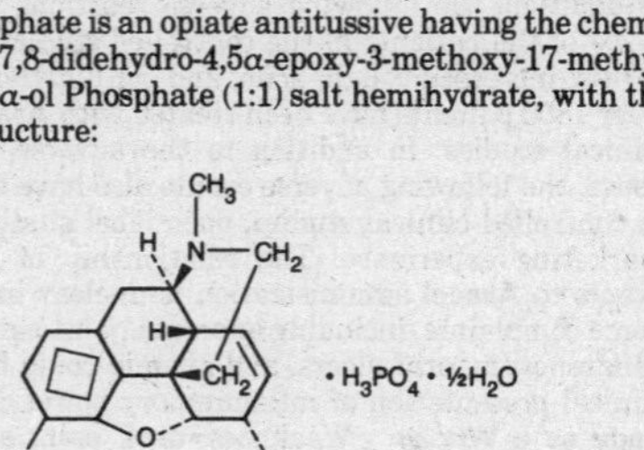

Guaifenesin is an expectorant having the chemical name, 1,2-propanediol, 3-(2-methoxyphenoxy)-, with the following stucture:

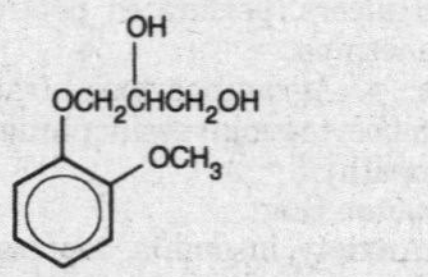

Inactive Ingredients: Compressible sugar, crospovidone, dioctyl sodium sulfosuccinate, FD&C Red No. 40 aluminum lake, FD&C Yellow No. 6 aluminum lake, hydroxypropyl cellulose, hydroxypropyl methylcellulose, magnesium stearate, microcrystalline cellulose, polyethylene glycol, silicon dioxide, sodium citrate, stearic acid, and titanium dioxide.

CLINICAL PHARMACOLOGY
Narcotic analgesics and antitussives, including codeine, exert their primary effect on the central nervous system and gastrointestinal tract. Codeine is an opiate agonist and is similar in structure and pharmacology to morphine. However, it is better absorbed orally, is less constipating, and produces less of an increase in biliary pressure than morphine. At therapeutic doses codeine produces less respiratory depression and has a lower risk of dependence and abuse than morphine.
Codeine suppresses the cough reflex by a direct effect on the cough center in the medulla and appears to exert a drying effect on respiratory tract mucosa and to increase viscosity of bronchial secretions.
Following oral administration, peak antitussive effect usually occurs within 1-2 hours and may persist for 4-6 hours. It is metabolized by the liver. Codeine undergoes O-demethylation, N-demethylation and partial conjugation with glucuronic acid and is excreted in the urine as norcodeine and morphine in the free and conjugated forms. Negligible amounts of codeine and its metabolites are found in the feces. Codeine crosses the placental barrier.
The analgesic effects of codeine are due to its central action; however, the precise sites and mechanisms of action have not been determined.
Guaifenesin promotes lower respiratory tract drainage by thinning bronchial secretions, increasing sputum volume, thereby facilitating removal of mucus.
This combination of the antitussive activity of codeine and the expectorant action of guaifenesin results in coughs becoming more productive and less frequent.

INDICATIONS AND USAGE
Temporarily relieves cough due to minor throat and bronchial irritation as may occur with a cold, or inhaled irritants. Helps loosen phlegm (mucus) and thin bronchial secretions to rid the bronchial passageways of bothersome mucus.

CONTRAINDICATIONS
Brontex tablets are contraindicated in patients with known hypersensitivity to any of its ingredients. **Brontex** tablets are contraindicated for use in patients with asthma.

WARNINGS
Codeine is not recommended for use in pediatric patients under 2 years of age. Pediatric patients under 2 years may be more susceptible to the respiratory depressant effects of codeine, including respiratory arrest, coma, and death.

PRECAUTIONS
General: Codeine should be used with extreme caution in patients with severe CNS depression, respiratory depression, or those prone to respiratory depression, acute alcoholism, chronic pulmonary disease and those with substantially decreased respiratory reserve. Codeine should be administered with caution in patients with acute abdominal conditions, convulsive disorders, significant hepatic or renal impairment, fever, hypothyroidism, Addison's disease, ulcerative colitis, prostatic hypertrophy, in patients with recent gastrointestinal or urinary tract surgery, and in the very young or elderly or debilitated patients.
Administration of codeine may be accompanied by histamine release and should be used with caution in pediatric patients with atopy.
Dosage of codeine should not be increased if cough fails to respond; an unresponsive cough should be reevaluated in 5 days or sooner for possible underlying pathology, such as foreign body or lower respiratory tract disease.
Codeine may cause or aggravate constipation.
Hypotensive Effects: Codeine may produce hypotension in ambulatory patients.
Head Injury and Increased Intracranial Pressure: The risk of respiratory depression and elevation of cerebrospinal fluid pressure is increased by opiate agonists, including codeine, in the presence of head injury, intracranial lesions, or a preexisting increase in intracranial pressure. They also may produce adverse reactions such as sedation and pupillary changes which may obscure the clinical course of patients with head injuries.
Respiratory Conditions with Productive Cough or Chronic Respiratory Disease: The risks and benefits of opiate agonists or cough suppressants, including codeine, should be carefully considered in illness associated with productive cough or in chronic respiratory disease where interference with ability to clear the tracheobronchial tree of secretions would have a deleterious effect on the patient's respiratory function.
Information for Patients: **Brontex** tablets may cause marked drowsiness or may impair the mental and/or physical abilities required for the performance of potentially hazardous tasks, such as driving a vehicle or operating machinery. Ambulatory patients should be told to avoid engaging in such activities until it is known that they do not become drowsy or dizzy from **Brontex** tablets. Pediatric patients should be supervised to avoid potential harm in bike riding or in other hazardous activities.
The concomitant use of alcohol or other central nervous system depressants, including opiate agonists, sedatives, hypnotics, and tranquilizers, may have an additive effect and should be avoided or their dosage reduced.
Codeine, like other opiate agonists, may produce orthostatic hypotension in some ambulatory patients. Patients should be cautioned accordingly.
Drug Interactions: Caution should be used when taking this product with CNS depressants including
alcohol, sedatives, tranquilizers and drugs used for depression, especially monoamine oxidase inhibitors (MAOIs). These combinations may cause greater sedation than is caused by the products used alone.
Drug/Laboratory Test Interactions: Guaifenesin has been reported to interfere with clinical laboratory determinations of urinary 5-hydroxyindoleacetic acid (5-HIAA) and urinary vanillylmandelic acid (VMA).
Because opiate agonists may increase biliary tract pressure, with resultant increases in plasma amylase or lipase levels, determination of these enzyme levels may be unreliable for 24 hours after an opiate agonist has been given.
Carcinogenesis, Mutagenesis, Impairment of Fertility: Studies with **Brontex** tablets in animals to evaluate carcinogenic, mutagenic, or impairment of fertility potential have not been conducted. Studies conducted by the National Toxicology Program with codeine in rats and mice to evaluate its carcinogenic potential are in progress.
Pregnancy:
Teratogenic Effects: Pregnancy Category C. Animal reproduction studies have not been conducted with **Brontex** tablets. It is also not known whether **Brontex** tablets can cause fetal harm when administered to a pregnant woman or can affect reproduction capacity. **Brontex** tablets should be given to a pregnant woman only if clearly needed.
Studies with codeine in hamsters and mice to evaluate its developmental toxicity potential have been reported by the National Toxicology Program. Codeine produced a decrease in mean fetal weight in both hamsters and mice, but did not produce structural malformations.
Nonteratogenic Effects: Dependence has been reported in newborns whose mothers took opiates regularly during pregnancy. Signs of withdrawal include irritability, excessive crying, tremors, hyperreflexia, fever, vomiting, and diarrhea. These signs usually disappear during the first few days of life.
Labor and Delivery: Use should be avoided during labor and delivery. Opiates cross the placental barrier. The closer to delivery and the larger the dose used, the greater the possibility of respiratory depression in the newborn. If the mother received opiates during labor, the newborn should be closely observed for signs of respiratory depression. Resuscitation, and in severe cases, naloxone may be required. Codeine may also prolong labor.
Nursing Mothers: Codeine is excreted in breast milk in amounts that are probably insignificant when given at usual therapeutic dose. It is not known whether guaifenesin is excreted in breast milk. Caution should be exercised when **Brontex** tablets are administered to a nursing mother.
The possibility of clinically important amounts of codeine being excreted in breast milk in individuals abusing codeine should be considered.
Pediatric Use: **Brontex** tablets are not recommended for use in pediatric patients below the age of 12 years.

ADVERSE REACTIONS
Nervous System: CNS depression, particularly respiratory depression, light-headedness, dizziness, sedation, euphoria, dysphoria, headache, transient hallucination, disorientation, visual disturbances, and convulsions.
Cardiovascular: Tachycardia, bradycardia, palpitation, faintness, syncope, orthostatic hypotension (common to opiate agonists), and circulatory depression.
Gastrointestinal: Nausea, vomiting, stomach pain, constipation, and biliary tract spasm. Patients with chronic ulcerative colitis may experience increased colonic motility; in patients with acute ulcerative colitis, toxic dilation has been reported.
Genitourinary: Oliguria and urinary retention; antidiuretic effect has been reported (common to opiate agonists).
Allergic: Infrequent pruritus, urticaria, angioneurotic edema, laryngeal edema, and rare anaphylactic reaction.
Other: Flushing of the face, sweating, and weakness.

DRUG ABUSE AND DEPENDENCE
Brontex tablets are a Schedule III Controlled Substance.
Codeine is known to be subject to abuse; however, the abuse potential of oral codeine is lower than that of most other opiate agonists because of its lower potency at therapeutic doses. However, codeine must be administered only under close supervision to patients with a history of drug abuse or dependence.
Psychological dependence, physical dependence, and tolerance are known to occur with codeine.

OVERDOSAGE

Signs and Symptoms: Serious overdose with codeine is characterized by respiratory depression (a decrease in respiratory rate and/or tidal volume, Cheyne-Stokes respiration, cyanosis), extreme somnolence progressing to stupor or coma, miosis (mydriasis may occur in terminal necrosis or hypoxia), skeletal muscle flaccidity, cold and clammy skin, and sometimes bradycardia and hypotension. In severe overdosage, apnea, circulatory collapse, cardiac arrest and death may occur.

Treatment: The treatment of overdosage should provide symptomatic and supportive care. Primary attention should be given to the reestablishment of adequate respiratory exchange through provision of a patent airway and the institution of assisted or controlled ventilation as necessary. The narcotic antagonist naloxone is a specific antidote against respiratory depression resulting from overdosage or unusual sensitivity to opiate agonists, including codeine. Therefore, an appropriate dose of naloxone hydrochloride (see package insert) may be administered, preferably by the intravenous route, and simultaneously with efforts at respiratory resuscitation. Since the duration of action of codeine may exceed that of the antagonist, the patient should be kept under continued surveillance and repeated doses of the antagonist should be administered as needed to maintain adequate respiration.

An antagonist should not be administered in the absence of clinically significant respiratory or cardiovascular depression. Oxygen, intravenous fluids, vasopressors and other supportive measures should be employed as indicated.

If the amount ingested is considered dangerous or excessive, induce vomiting with ipecac syrup unless the patient is convulsing, comatose, or has lost the gag reflex, in which case perform gastric lavage using a large-bore tube. If indicated, follow with activated charcoal and a saline cathartic.

DOSAGE AND ADMINISTRATION

Adults and pediatric patients 12 years of age and older: 1 tablet every 4 hours not to exceed 6 tablets in 24 hours.

Brontex tablets are not recommended for pediatric patients under 12 years of age.

HOW SUPPLIED

Brontex tablets are available as a red, capsule-shaped tablet, embossed **"BRONTEX"**.

NDC 0149-0440-01 bottle of 100

Store at controlled room temperature (59°–86°F or 15°–30°C).

CAUTION: Federal law prohibits dispensing without prescription.

Procter & Gamble Pharmaceuticals
Cincinnati, Ohio 45202
REVISED MAY 1995 44000–P2

Shown in Product Identification Guide, page 329

DANTRIUM® capsules ℞
[dan 'trē-um]
(dantrolene sodium)

> **Dantrium** (dantrolene sodium) has a potential for hepatotoxicity, and should not be used in conditions other than those recommended. Symptomatic hepatitis (fatal and non-fatal) has been reported at various dose levels of the drug. The incidence reported in patients taking up to 400 mg/day is much lower than in those taking doses of 800 mg or more per day. Even sporadic short courses of these higher dose levels within a treatment regimen markedly increased the risk of serious hepatic injury. Liver dysfunction as evidenced by blood chemical abnormalities alone (liver enzyme elevations) has been observed in patients exposed to **Dantrium** for varying periods of time. Overt hepatitis has occurred at varying intervals after initiation of therapy, but has been most frequently observed between the third and twelfth month of therapy. The risk of hepatic injury appears to be greater in females, in patients over 35 years of age, and in patients taking other medication(s) in addition to **Dantrium** (dantrolene sodium). **Dantrium** should be used only in conjunction with appropriate monitoring of hepatic function including frequent determination of SGOT or SGPT. If no observable benefit is derived from the administration of **Dantrium** after a total of 45 days, therapy should be discontinued. The lowest possible effective dose for the individual patient should be prescribed.

DESCRIPTION

The chemical formula of **Dantrium** (dantrolene sodium) is hydrated 1-[[[5-(4-nitrophenyl)-2-furanyl]methylene]amino]-2, 4-imidazolidinedione sodium salt. It is an orange powder, slightly soluble in water, but due to its slightly acidic nature the solubility increases somewhat in alkaline solution. The anhydrous salt has a molecular weight of 336. The hydrated salt contains approximately 15% water (3-1/2 moles) and has a molecular weight of 399. The structural formula for the hydrated salt is:

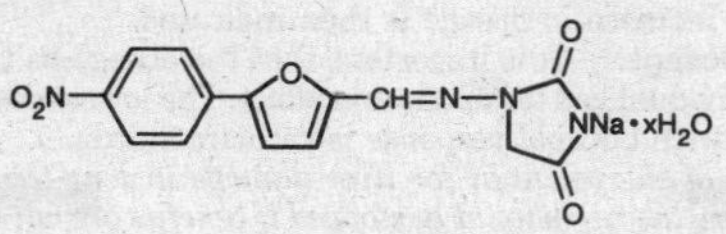

Dantrium is supplied in capsules of 25 mg, 50 mg, and 100 mg.

Inactive Ingredients: Each capsule contains edible black ink, FD&C Yellow No. 6, gelatin, lactose, magnesium stearate, starch, synthetic iron oxide red, synthetic iron oxide yellow, talc, and titanium dioxide.

CLINICAL PHARMACOLOGY

In isolated nerve-muscle preparation, **Dantrium** has been shown to produce relaxation by affecting the contractile response of the skeletal muscle at a site beyond the myoneural junction, directly on the muscle itself. In skeletal muscle, **Dantrium** dissociates the excitation-contraction coupling, probably by interfering with the release of Ca^{++} from the sarcoplasmic reticulum. This effect appears to be more pronounced in fast muscle fibers as compared to slow ones, but generally affects both. A central nervous system effect occurs, with drowsiness, dizziness, and generalized weakness occasionally present. Although **Dantrium** does not appear to directly affect the CNS, the extent of its indirect effect is unknown. The absorption of **Dantrium** after oral administration in humans is incomplete and slow but consistent, and dose-related blood levels are obtained. The duration and intensity of skeletal muscle relaxation is related to the dosage and blood levels. The mean biologic half-life of **Dantrium** in adults is 8.7 hours after a 100-mg dose. Specific metabolic pathways in the degradation and elimination of **Dantrium** in human subjects have been established. Metabolic patterns are similar in adults and pediatric patients. In addition to the parent compound, dantrolene, which is found in measurable amounts in blood and urine, the major metabolites noted in body fluids are the 5-hydroxy analog and the acetamido analog. Since **Dantrium** is probably metabolized by hepatic microsomal enzymes, enhancement of its metabolism by other drugs is possible. However, neither phenobarbital nor diazepam appears to affect **Dantrium** metabolism.

Clinical experience in the management of fulminant human malignant hyperthermia, as well as experiments conducted in malignant hyperthermia susceptible swine, have revealed that the administration of intravenous dantrolene, combined with indicated supportive measures, is effective in reversing the hypermetabolic process of malignant hyperthermia. Known differences between human and swine malignant hyperthermia are minor. The prophylactic administration of oral or intravenous dantrolene to malignant hyperthermia susceptible swine will attenuate or prevent the development of signs of malignant hyperthermia in a manner dependent upon the dosage of dantrolene administered and the intensity of the malignant hyperthermia triggering stimulus. Limited clinical experience with the administration of oral dantrolene to patients judged malignant hyperthermia susceptible, when combined with clinical experience in the use of intravenous dantrolene for the treatment of malignant hyperthermia and data derived from the above cited animal model experiments, suggests that oral dantrolene will also attenuate or prevent the development of signs of human malignant hyperthermia, provided that currently accepted practices in the management of such patients are adhered to (see INDICATIONS AND USAGE); intravenous dantrolene should also be available for use should the signs of malignant hyperthermia appear.

INDICATIONS AND USAGE

In Chronic Spasticity:

Dantrium is indicated in controlling the manifestations of clinical spasticity resulting from upper motor neuron disorders (*e.g.*, spinal cord injury, stroke, cerebral palsy, or multiple sclerosis). It is of particular benefit to the patient whose functional rehabilitation has been retarded by the sequelae of spasticity. Such patients must have presumably reversible spasticity where relief of spasticity will aid in restoring residual function. **Dantrium** is not indicated in the treatment of skeletal muscle spasm resulting from rheumatic disorders.

If improvement occurs, it will ordinarily occur within the dosage titration (see DOSAGE AND ADMINISTRATION), and will be manifested by a decrease in the severity of spasticity and the ability to resume a daily function not quite attainable without **Dantrium**.

Occasionally, subtle but meaningful improvement in spasticity may occur with **Dantrium** therapy. In such instances, information regarding improvement should be solicited from the patient and those who are in constant daily contact and attendance with him. Brief withdrawal of **Dantrium** for a period of 2 to 4 days will frequently demonstrate exacerbation of the manifestations of spasticity and may serve to confirm a clinical impression.

A decision to continue the administration of **Dantrium** on a long-term basis is justified if introduction of the drug into the patient's regimen:

- produces a significant reduction in painful and/or disabling spasticity such as clonus, or
- permits a significant reduction in the intensity and/or degree of nursing care required, or
- rids the patient of any annoying manifestation of spasticity considered important by the patient himself.

In Malignant Hyperthermia:

Oral **Dantrium** is also indicated preoperatively to prevent or attenuate the development of signs of malignant hyperthermia in known, or strongly suspect, malignant hyperthermia susceptible patients who require anesthesia and/or surgery. Currently accepted clinical practices in the management of such patients must still be adhered to (careful monitoring for early signs of malignant hyperthermia, minimizing exposure to triggering mechanisms and prompt use of intravenous dantrolene sodium and indicated supportive measures should signs of malignant hyperthermia appear); see also the package insert for **Dantrium®** (dantrolene sodium) **Intravenous.**

Oral **Dantrium** should be administered following a malignant hyperthermic crisis to prevent recurrence of the signs of malignant hyperthermia.

CONTRAINDICATIONS

Active hepatic disease, such as hepatitis and cirrhosis, is a contraindication for use of **Dantrium. Dantrium** is contraindicated where spasticity is utilized to sustain upright posture and balance in locomotion or whenever spasticity is utilized to obtain or maintain increased function.

WARNINGS

It is important to recognize that fatal and non-fatal liver disorders of an idiosyncratic or hypersensitivity type may occur with **Dantrium** therapy.

At the start of **Dantrium** therapy, it is desirable to do liver function studies (SGOT, SGPT, alkaline phosphatase, total bilirubin) for a baseline or to establish whether there is preexisting liver disease. If baseline liver abnormalities exist and are confirmed, there is a clear possibility that the potential for **Dantrium** hepatotoxicity could be enhanced, although such a possibility has not yet been established.

Liver function studies (*e.g.*, SGOT or SGPT) should be performed at appropriate intervals during **Dantrium** therapy. If such studies reveal abnormal values, therapy should generally be discontinued. Only where benefits of the drug have been of major importance to the patient, should reinitiation or continuation of therapy be considered. Some patients have revealed a return to normal laboratory values in the face of continued therapy while others have not.

If symptoms compatible with hepatitis, accompanied by abnormalities in liver function tests or jaundice appear, **Dantrium** should be discontinued. If caused by **Dantrium** and detected early, the abnormalities in liver function characteristically have reverted to normal when the drug was discontinued.

Dantrium therapy has been reinstituted in a few patients who have developed clinical and/or laboratory evidence of hepatocellular injury. If such reinstitution of therapy is done, it should be attempted only in patients who clearly need **Dantrium** and only after previous symptoms and laboratory abnormalities have cleared. The patient should be hospitalized and the drug should be restarted in very small and gradually increasing doses. Laboratory monitoring should be frequent and the drug should be withdrawn immediately if there is any indication of recurrent liver involvement. Some patients have reacted with unmistakable signs of liver abnormality upon administration of a challenge dose, while others have not.

Dantrium should be used with particular caution in females and in patients over 35 years of age in view of apparent greater likelihood of drug-induced, potentially fatal, hepatocellular disease in these groups.

Long-term safety of **Dantrium** in humans has not been established. Chronic studies in rats, dogs, and monkeys at dosages greater than 30 mg/kg/day showed growth or weight depression and signs of hepatopathy and possible occlusion nephropathy, all of which were reversible upon cessation of treatment. Sprague-Dawley female rats fed dantrolene sodium for 18 months at dosage levels of 15, 30, and 60 mg/kg/day showed an increased incidence of benign and malignant mammary tumors compared with concurrent controls and, at the highest dosage, an increase in the incidence of hepatic lymphangiomas and hepatic angiosarcomas. These effects were not seen in 2-1/2-year studies in Sprague-Dawley or Fischer 344 rats or in 2-year studies in mice of the HaM/ICR strain. Carcinogenicity in humans cannot be fully excluded, so that this possible risk of chronic administration must be weighed against the benefits of the drug (*i.e.*, after a brief trial) for the individual patient.

Continued on next page

Procter & Gamble Pharm.—Cont.

USAGE IN PREGNANCY

The safety of **Dantrium** for use in women who are or who may become pregnant has not been established. **Dantrium** should not be used in nursing mothers.

Usage in Pediatric Patients: The long-term safety of **Dantrium** in pediatric patients under the age of 5 years has not been established. Because of the possibility that adverse effects of the drug could become apparent only after many years, a benefit-risk consideration of the long-term use of **Dantrium** is particularly important in pediatric patients.

Drug Interactions: While a definite drug interaction with estrogen therapy has not yet been established, caution should be observed if the two drugs are to be given concomitantly. Hepatotoxicity has occurred more often in women over 35 years of age receiving concomitant estrogen therapy.

There are very rare reports of cardiovascular collapse in patients treated simultaneously with verapamil and dantrolene sodium. The combination of therapeutic doses of intravenous dantrolene sodium and verapamil in halothane/α-chloralose anesthetized swine has resulted in ventricular fibrillation and cardiovascular collapse in association with marked hyperkalemia. Until the relevance of these findings to humans is established, the combination of dantrolene sodium and verapamil is not recommended during the management of malignant hyperthermia.

PRECAUTIONS

Dantrium should be used with caution in patients with impaired pulmonary function, particularly those with obstructive pulmonary disease, and in patients with severely impaired cardiac function due to myocardial disease. It should be used with caution in patients with a history of previous liver disease or dysfunction (see WARNINGS).

Patients should be cautioned against driving a motor vehicle or participating in hazardous occupations while taking **Dantrium**. Caution should be exercised in the concomitant administration of tranquilizing agents.

Dantrium might possibly evoke a photosensitivity reaction; patients should be cautioned about exposure to sunlight while taking it.

ADVERSE REACTIONS

The most frequently occurring side effects of **Dantrium** have been drowsiness, dizziness, weakness, general malaise, fatigue, and diarrhea. These are generally transient, occurring early in treatment, and can often be obviated by beginning with a low dose and increasing dosage gradually until an optimal regimen is established. Diarrhea may be severe and may necessitate temporary withdrawal of **Dantrium** therapy. If diarrhea recurs upon readministration of **Dantrium**, therapy should probably be withdrawn permanently.

Other less frequent side effects, listed according to system, are:

Gastrointestinal: Constipation, GI bleeding, anorexia, swallowing difficulty, gastric irritation, abdominal cramps, nausea and/or vomiting.

Hepatobiliary: Hepatitis (see WARNINGS).

Neurologic: Speech disturbance, seizure, headache, lightheadedness, visual disturbance, diplopia, alteration of taste, insomnia.

Cardiovascular: Tachycardia, erratic blood pressure, phlebitis, heart failure.

Hematologic: Aplastic anemia, leukopenia, lymphocytic lymphoma.

Psychiatric: Mental depression, mental confusion, increased nervousness.

Urogenital: Increased urinary frequency, crystalluria, hematuria, difficult erection, urinary incontinence and/or nocturia, difficult urination and/or urinary retention.

Integumentary: Abnormal hair growth, acne-like rash, pruritus, urticaria, eczematoid eruption, sweating.

Musculoskeletal: Myalgia, backache.

Respiratory: Feeling of suffocation.

Special Senses: Excessive tearing.

Hypersensitivity: Pleural effusion with pericarditis, anaphylaxis.

Other: Chills and fever.

The published literature has included some reports of **Dantrium** use in patients with Neuroleptic Malignant Syndrome (NMS). **Dantrium** capsules are not indicated for the treatment of NMS and patients may expire despite treatment with **Dantrium** capsules.

DOSAGE AND ADMINISTRATION

For Use in Chronic Spasticity:

Prior to the administration of **Dantrium**, consideration should be given to the potential response to treatment. A decrease in spasticity sufficient to allow a daily function not otherwise attainable should be the therapeutic goal of treatment with **Dantrium**. Refer to INDICATIONS AND USAGE section for description of response to be anticipated.

It is important to establish a therapeutic goal (regain and maintain a specific function such as therapeutic exercise program, utilization of braces, transfer maneuvers, etc.) before beginning **Dantrium** therapy. Dosage should be increased until the maximum performance compatible with the dysfunction due to underlying disease is achieved. No further increase in dosage is then indicated.

Usual Dosage: It is important that the dosage be titrated and individualized for maximum effect. The lowest dose compatible with optimal response is recommended.

In view of the potential for liver damage in long-term **Dantrium** *use, therapy should be stopped if benefits are not evident within 45 days.*

Adults: Begin therapy with 25 mg once daily; increase to 25 mg two, three, or four times daily and then by increments of 25 mg up to as high as 100 mg two, three, or four times daily if necessary. As most patients will respond to a dose of 400 mg/day or less, rarely should doses higher than 400 mg/day be used (see Box Warning).

Each dosage level should be maintained for four to seven days to determine the patient's response. The dose should not be increased beyond, and may even have to be reduced to, the amount at which the patient received maximal benefit without adverse effects.

Pediatric Patients: A similar approach should be utilized starting with 0.5 mg/kg of body weight twice daily; this is increased to 0.5 mg/kg three or four times daily and then by increments of 0.5 mg/kg up to as high as 3 mg/kg two, three, or four times daily, if necessary. Doses higher than 100 mg four times daily should not be used in pediatric patients.

For Malignant Hyperthermia:

Preoperatively: Administer 4 to 8 mg/kg/day of oral **Dantrium** in 3 or 4 divided doses for one or two days prior to surgery, with the last dose being given approximately 3 to 4 hours before scheduled surgery with a minimum of water.

This dosage will usually be associated with skeletal muscle weakness and sedation (sleepiness or drowsiness); adjustment can usually be made within the recommended dosage range to avoid incapacitation or excessive gastrointestinal irritation (including nausea and/or vomiting).

Post Crisis Follow-up:

Oral **Dantrium** should also be administered following a malignant hyperthermia crisis, in doses of 4 to 8 mg/kg per day in four divided doses, for a one to three day period to prevent recurrence of the manifestations of malignant hyperthermia.

OVERDOSAGE

For acute overdosage, general supportive measures should be employed along with immediate gastric lavage.

Intravenous fluids should be administered in fairly large quantities to avert the possibility of crystalluria. An adequate airway should be maintained and artificial resuscitation equipment should be at hand. Electrocardi ographic monitoring should be instituted, and the patient carefully observed. To date, no experience has been reported with dialysis and its value in **Dantrium** overdosage is not known.

HOW SUPPLIED

Dantrium (dantrolene sodium) is available in:

25-mg opaque, orange and tan capsules:

NDC 0149-0030-05	bottle of 100
NDC 0149-0030-66	bottle of 500
NDC 0149-0030-77	hospital unit-dose strips in boxes of 100

50-mg opaque, orange and tan capsules:

NDC 0149-0031-05	bottle of 100

100-mg opaque, orange and tan capsules:

NDC 0149-0033-05	bottle of 100
NDC 0149-0033-77	hospital unit-dose strips in boxes of 100

Avoid excessive heat (over 104°F or 40°C).

Address medical inquiries to Procter & Gamble Pharmaceuticals, Medical Communications Dept., 11450 Grooms Rd, Cincinnati, OH 45242.

CAUTION: Federal law prohibits dispensing without prescription.

Procter & Gamble Pharmaceuticals
Cincinnati, Ohio 45202
REVISED JANUARY 1996 03001-U6

DANTRIUM® Intravenous ℞

[dan' trēum]
(dantrolene sodium for injection)

DESCRIPTION

Dantrium Intravenous is a sterile, non-pyrogenic, lyophilized formulation of dantrolene sodium for injection. **Dantrium Intravenous** is supplied in 70 mL vials containing 20 mg dantrolene sodium, 3000 mg mannitol, and sufficient sodium hydroxide to yield a pH of approximately 9.5 when reconstituted with 60 mL sterile water for injection USP (without a bacteriostatic agent).

Dantrium is classified as a direct-acting skeletal muscle relaxant. Chemically, **Dantrium** is hydrated 1-[[[5-(4-nitrophenyl)-2-furanyl]methylene]amino]-2,4-imidazolidinedione sodium salt. The structural formula for the hydrated salt is:

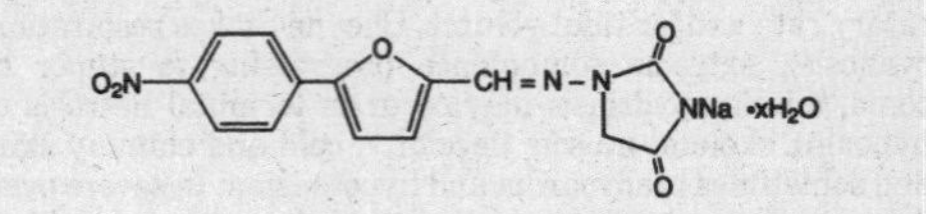

The hydrated salt contains approximately 15% water ($3\text{-}^{1}/_{2}$ moles) and has a molecular weight of 399. The anhydrous salt (dantrolene) has a molecular weight of 336.

CLINICAL PHARMACOLOGY

In isolated nerve-muscle preparation, **Dantrium** produces skeletal muscle relaxation by directly affecting the contractile response of the muscle at a site beyond the myoneural junction. In skeletal muscle, **Dantrium** dissociates excitation-contraction coupling, probably by interfering with the release of Ca++ from the sarcoplasmic reticulum. The administration of intravenous **Dantrium** to human volunteers is associated with loss of grip strength and weakness in the legs, as well as subjective CNS complaints (see also PRECAUTIONS, Information for Patients). Information concerning the passage of **Dantrium** across the blood-brain barrier is not available.

In the anesthetic-induced malignant hyperthermia (MH) syndrome, evidence points to an intrinsic abnormality of skeletal muscle tissue. In affected humans, it has been postulated that "triggering agents" (*e.g.*, general anesthetics and depolarizing neuromuscular blocking agents) produce a change within the cell which results in an elevated myoplasmic calcium. This elevated myoplasmic calcium activates acute cellular catabolic processes that cascade to the MH crisis.

It is hypothesized that addition of **Dantrium** to the "triggered" malignant hyperthermic muscle cell reestablishes a normal level of ionized calcium in the myoplasm. Inhibition of calcium release from the sarcoplasmic reticulum by **Dantrium** reestablishes the myoplasmic calcium equilibrium, increasing the percentage of bound calcium. In this way, physiologic, metabolic, and biochemical changes associated with the MH crisis may be reversed or attenuated. Experimental results in malignant hyperthermia susceptible (MHS) swine show that prophylactic administration of intravenous or oral dantrolene prevents or attenuates the development of vital sign and blood gas changes characteristic of malignant hyperthermia (MH) in a dose related manner. The efficacy of intravenous dantrolene in the treatment of human and porcine MH crisis, when considered along with prophylactic experiments in MHS swine, lends support to prophylactic use of oral or intravenous dantrolene in MHS humans. When prophylactic intravenous dantrolene is administered as directed, whole blood concentrations remain at a near steady state level for 3 or more hours after the infusion is completed. Clinical experience has shown that early vital sign and/or blood gas changes characteristic of MH may appear during or after anesthesia and surgery despite the prophylactic use of dantrolene and adherence to currently accepted patient management practices. These signs are compatible with attenuated MH and respond to the administration of additional i.v. dantrolene (see DOSAGE AND ADMINISTRATION). The administration of the recommended prophylactic dose of intravenous dantrolene to healthy volunteers was not associated with clinically significant cardiorespiratory changes.

Specific metabolic pathways for the degradation and elimination of **Dantrium** in humans have been established. Dantrolene is found in measurable amounts in blood and urine. Its major metabolites in body fluids are 5-hydroxy dantrolene and an acetylamino metabolite of dantrolene. Another metabolite with an unknown structure appears related to the latter. **Dantrium** may also undergo hydrolysis and subsequent oxidation forming nitrophenylfuroic acid.

The mean biologic half-life of **Dantrium** after intravenous administration is variable, between 4 to 8 hours under most experimental conditions. Based on assays of whole blood and plasma, slightly greater amounts of dantrolene are associated with red blood cells than with the plasma fraction of blood. Significant amounts of dantrolene are bound to plasma proteins, mostly albumin, and this binding is readily reversible.

Dantrium Intravenous (dantrolene sodium for injection)

Cardiopulmonary depression has not been observed in MHS swine following the administration of up to 7.5 mg/kg i.v. dantrolene. This is twice the amount needed to maximally diminish twitch response to single supramaximal peripheral nerve stimulation (95% inhibition). A transient, inconsistent, depressant effect on gastrointestinal smooth muscles has been observed at high doses.

INDICATIONS AND USAGE

Dantrium Intravenous is indicated, along with appropriate supportive measures, for the management of the fulminant hypermetabolism of skeletal muscle characteristic of MH

crises in patients of all ages. **Dantrium Intravenous** should be administered by continuous rapid intravenous push as soon as the MH reaction is recognized (*i.e.*, tachycardia, tachypnea, central venous desaturation, hypercarbia, metabolic acidosis, skeletal muscle rigidity, increased utilization of anesthesia circuit carbon dioxide absorber, cyanosis and mottling of the skin, and, in many cases, fever).

Dantrium Intravenous is also indicated preoperatively, and sometimes postoperatively, to prevent or attenuate the development of clinical and laboratory signs of malignant hyperthermia in individuals judged to be malignant hyperthermia susceptible.

CONTRAINDICATIONS

None.

WARNINGS

*The use of **Dantrium Intravenous** in the management of MH crisis is not a substitute for previously known supportive measures. These measures must be individualized, but it will usually be necessary to discontinue the suspect triggering agents, attend to increased oxygen requirements, manage the metabolic acidosis, institute cooling when necessary, monitor urinary output, and monitor for electrolyte imbalance.*

Since the effect of disease state and other drugs on the consequences of **Dantrium** related skeletal muscle weakness, including possible respiratory depression, cannot be predicted, patients who receive i.v. **Dantrium** preoperatively should have vital signs monitored.

If patients judged malignant hyperthermia susceptible are administered intravenous or oral **Dantrium** preoperatively, anesthetic preparation must still follow a standard MHS regimen, including the avoidance of known triggering agents. Monitoring for early clinical and metabolic signs of MH is indicated because attenuation of MH, rather than prevention, is possible. These signs usually call for the administration of additional i.v. dantrolene.

PRECAUTIONS

General: Care must be taken to prevent extravasation of **Dantrium** solution into the surrounding tissues due to the high pH of the intravenous formulation.

When mannitol is used for prevention or treatment of late renal complications of MH, the 3 g of mannitol needed to dissolve each 20 mg vial of i.v. **Dantrium** should be taken into consideration.

Information for Patients: Based upon data in human volunteers, it will sometimes be appropriate to tell patients who receive **Dantrium Intravenous** that decrease in grip strength and weakness of leg muscles, especially walking down stairs, can be expected postoperatively. In addition, symptoms such as "light-headedness" may be noted. Since some of these symptoms may persist for up to 48 hours, patients must not operate an automobile or engage in other hazardous activity during this time. Caution is also indicated at meals on the day of administration because difficulty swallowing and choking has been reported.

Drug Interactions: Dantrium is metabolized by the liver, and it is theoretically possible that its metabolism may be enhanced by drugs known to induce hepatic microsomal enzymes. However, neither phenobarbital nor diazepam appears to affect **Dantrium** metabolism. Binding to plasma protein is not significantly altered by diazepam, diphenylhydantoin, or phenylbutazone. Binding to plasma proteins is reduced by warfarin and clofibrate and increased by tolbutamide.

The combination of therapeutic doses of intravenous dantrolene sodium and verapamil in halothane/α-chloralose anesthetized swine has resulted in ventricular fibrillation and cardiovascular collapse in association with marked hyperkalemia. It is recommended that the combination of intravenous dantrolene sodium and calcium channel blockers, such as verapamil, not be used together during the management of malignant hyperthermia crisis until the relevance of these findings to humans is established.

Carcinogenesis, Mutagenesis, and Impairment of Fertility: Studies of **Dantrium** in animals to evaluate mutagenic potential and the effect on fertility have not been conducted. Sprague-Dawley female rats fed **Dantrium** for 18 months at dosage levels of 15, 30, and 60 mg/kg/day showed an increased incidence of benign and malignant mammary tumors compared with concurrent controls. At the highest dosage, there was an increase in the incidence of hepatic lymphangiomas and hepatic angiosarcomas. These effects were not seen in 30-month studies in Sprague-Dawley or Fischer-344 rats or in 24-month studies in mice of the HaM/ICR strain. Although the possibility that the drug may be carcinogenic in humans cannot be fully excluded, the risks associated with administration of **Dantrium Intravenous** in a life-threatening crisis would appear to be minimal.

Usage in Pregnancy: Pregnancy Category C: **Dantrium** has been shown to be embryocidal in the rabbit and has been shown to decrease pup survival in the rat when given at doses seven times the human oral dose. There are no adequate and well-controlled studies in pregnant women. **Dantrium Intravenous** should be used during pregnancy only if the potential benefit justifies the potential risk to the fetus.

Labor and Delivery: In one uncontrolled study, 100 mg per day of prophylactic oral **Dantrium** was administered to term pregnant patients awaiting labor and delivery. Dantrolene readily crossed the placenta, with maternal and fetal whole blood levels approximately equal at delivery; neonatal levels then fell approximately 50% per day for 2 days before declining sharply. No neonatal respiratory and neuromuscular side effects were detected at low dose. More data, at higher doses, are needed before more definitive conclusions can be made.

ADVERSE REACTIONS

There have been occasional reports of death following MH crisis even when treated with intravenous dantrolene; incidence figures are not available (the pre-dantrolene mortality of MH crisis was approximately 50%). Most of these deaths can be accounted for by late recognition, delayed treatment, inadequate dosage, lack of supportive therapy, intercurrent disease and/or the development of delayed complications such as renal failure or disseminated intravascular coagulopathy. In some cases there are insufficient data to completely rule out therapeutic failure of dantrolene.

There are rare reports of fatality in MH crisis, despite initial satisfactory response to i.v. dantrolene, which involve patients who could not be weaned from dantrolene after initial treatment.

The following adverse reactions are in approximate order of severity:

There are rare reports of pulmonary edema developing during the treatment of MH crisis in which the diluent volume and mannitol needed to deliver i.v. dantrolene possibly contributed.

There have been reports of thrombophlebitis following administration of intravenous dantrolene; actual incidence figures are not available.

There have been rare reports of urticaria and erythema possibly associated with the administration of i.v. **Dantrium**. There has been one case of anaphylaxis.

None of the serious reactions occasionally reported with long-term oral **Dantrium** use, such as hepatitis, seizures, and pleural effusion with pericarditis, have been reasonably associated with short-term **Dantrium Intravenous** therapy.

The following events have been reported in patients receiving oral dantrolene: aplastic anemia, leukopenia, lymphocytic lymphoma, and heart failure. (See package insert for **Dantrium** (dantrolene sodium) **Capsules** for a complete listing of adverse reactions.)

The published literature has included some reports of **Dantrium** use in patients with Neuroleptic Malignant Syndrome (NMS).

Dantrium Intravenous is not indicated for the treatment of NMS and patients may expire despite treatment with **Dantrium Intravenous.**

OVERDOSAGE

Because **Dantrium Intravenous** must be administered at a low concentration in a large volume of fluid, acute toxicity of **Dantrium** could not be assessed in animals. In 14-day (subacute) studies, the intravenous formulation of **Dantrium** was relatively non-toxic to rats at doses of 10 mg/kg/day and 20 mg/kg/day. While 10 mg/kg/day in dogs for 14 days evoked little toxicity, 20 mg/kg/day for 14 days caused hepatic changes of questionable biologic significance.

No data are available to define the symptomatology of an overdose of **Dantrium Intravenous.** If an overdose is suspected, treatment is symptomatic and supportive. There is no known antidote.

DOSAGE AND ADMINISTRATION

As soon as the MH reaction is recognized, all anesthetic agents should be discontinued; the administration of 100% oxygen is recommended. **Dantrium Intravenous** should be administered by continuous rapid intravenous push beginning at a minimum dose of 1 mg/kg, and continuing until symptoms subside or the maximum cumulative dose of 10 mg/kg has been reached.

If the physiologic and metabolic abnormalities reappear, the regimen may be repeated. It is important to note that administration of **Dantrium Intravenous** should be continuous until symptoms subside. The effective dose to reverse the crisis is directly dependent upon the individual's degree of susceptibility to MH, the amount and time of exposure to the triggering agent, and the time elapsed between onset of the crisis and initiation of treatment.

Pediatric Dose: Experience to date indicates that the dose of **Dantrium Intravenous** for pediatric patients is the same as for adults.

Preoperatively: Dantrium Intravenous and/or **Dantrium Capsules** may be administered preoperatively to patients judged MH susceptible as part of the overall patient management to prevent or attenuate the development of clinical and laboratory signs of MH.

Dantrium Intravenous: The recommended prophylactic dose of **Dantrium Intravenous** is 2.5 mg/kg, starting approximately 1-1/4 hours before anticipated anesthesia and infused over approximately 1 hour. This dose should prevent or attenuate the development of clinical and laboratory signs of MH provided that the usual precautions, such as avoidance of established MH triggering agents, are followed.

Additional **Dantrium Intravenous** may be indicated during anesthesia and surgery because of the appearance of early clinical and/or blood gas signs of MH or because of prolonged surgery (see also CLINICAL PHARMACOLOGY, WARNINGS, and PRECAUTIONS). Additional doses must be individualized.

Oral administration of Dantrium Capsules: Administer 4 to 8 mg/kg/day of oral **Dantrium** in 3 or 4 divided doses for one or two days prior to surgery, with the last dose being given with a minimum of water approximately 3 to 4 hours before scheduled surgery. Adjustment can usually be made within the recommended dosage range to avoid incapacitation (weakness, drowsiness, etc.) or excessive gastrointestinal irritation (nausea and/or vomiting). See also the package insert for **Dantrium Capsules.**

Post Crisis Follow-up: Dantrium Capsules, 4 to 8 mg/kg/day, in four divided doses should be administered for one to three days following a malignant hyperthermia crisis to prevent recurrence of the manifestations of malignant hyperthermia.

Intravenous **Dantrium** may be used postoperatively to prevent or attenuate the recurrence of signs of MH when oral **Dantrium** administration is not practical. The i.v. dose of **Dantrium** in the postoperative period must be individualized, starting with 1 mg/kg or more as the clinical situation dictates.

PREPARATION

Each vial of **Dantrium Intravenous** should be reconstituted by adding 60 mL of *sterile water for injection USP (without a bacteriostatic agent), and the vial shaken until the solution is clear.* 5% Dextrose Injection USP, 0.9% Sodium Chloride Injection USP, and other acidic solutions are not compatible with **Dantrium Intravenous** and should not be used. The contents of the vial must be *protected from direct light* and *used within 6 hours* after reconstitution. Store reconstituted solutions at controlled room temperature (59°F to 86°F or 15°C to 30°C).

Reconstituted **Dantrium Intravenous** should *not* be transferred to large glass bottles for prophylactic infusion due to precipitate formation observed with the use of some glass bottles as reservoirs.

For prophylactic infusion, the required number of individual vials of **Dantrium Intravenous** should be reconstituted as outlined above. The contents of individual vials are then transferred to a larger volume sterile intravenous plastic bag. Stability data on file at Procter & Gamble Pharmaceuticals indicate commercially available sterile plastic bags are acceptable drug delivery devices. However, it is recommended that the prepared infusion be inspected carefully for cloudiness and/or precipitation prior to dispensing and administration. Such solutions should not be used. While stable for 6 hours, it is recommended that the infusion be prepared immediately prior to the anticipated dosage administration time.

Parenteral drug products should be inspected visually for particulate matter and discoloration prior to administration.

HOW SUPPLIED

Dantrium Intravenous (**NDC** 0149-0734-02) is available in vials containing a sterile lyophilized mixture of 20 mg dantrolene sodium, 3000 mg mannitol, and sufficient sodium hydroxide to yield a pH of approximately 9.5 when reconstituted with 60 mL sterile water for injection USP (without a bacteriostatic agent).

Store unreconstituted product at controlled room temperature (59°F to 86°F or 15°C to 30°C) and avoid prolonged exposure to light.

Address medical inquiries to Procter & Gamble Pharmaceuticals, Medical Communications Department, 11450 Grooms Rd, Cincinnati, Ohio 45242-1434.

CAUTION: Federal law prohibits dispensing without prescription.

Procter & Gamble Pharmaceuticals
Cincinnati, Ohio 45202
REVISED JANUARY 1996 73402–P1

DIDRONEL® ℞

[dī′drō-nel]
(etidronate disodium)

DESCRIPTION

Didronel tablets contain either 200 mg or 400 mg of etidronate disodium, the disodium salt of (1-hydroxyethylidene) diphosphonic acid, for oral administration. This compound, also known as EHDP, regulates bone metabolism. It is a

Continued on next page

Procter & Gamble Pharm.—Cont.

white powder, highly soluble in water, with a molecular weight of 250 and the following structural formula:

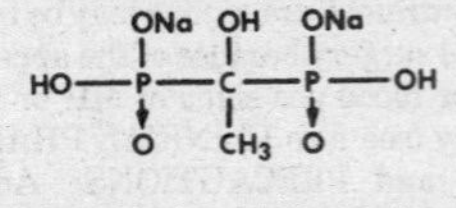

Inactive Ingredients: Each tablet contains magnesium stearate, microcrystalline cellulose, and starch.

CLINICAL PHARMACOLOGY

Didronel acts primarily on bone. It can inhibit the formation, growth, and dissolution of hydroxyapatite crystals and their amorphous precursors by chemisorption to calcium phosphate surfaces. Inhibition of crystal resorption occurs at lower doses than are required to inhibit crystal growth. Both effects increase as the dose increases.

Didronel is not metabolized. The amount of drug absorbed after an oral dose is approximately 3%. In normal subjects, plasma half-life ($t^1/_2$) of etidronate, based on non-compartmental pharmacokinetics is 1 to 6 hours. Within 24 hours, approximately half the absorbed dose is excreted in urine; the remainder is distributed to bone compartments from which it is slowly eliminated. Animal studies have yielded bone clearance estimates up to 165 days. In humans, the residence time on bone may vary due to such factors as specific metabolic condition and bone type. Unabsorbed drug is excreted intact in the feces. Preclinical studies indicate etidronate disodium does not cross the blood-brain barrier.

Didronel therapy does not adversely affect serum levels of parathyroid hormone or calcium.

Paget's Disease: Paget's disease of bone (osteitis deformans) is an idiopathic, progressive disease characterized by abnormal and accelerated bone metabolism in one or more bones. Signs and symptoms may include bone pain and/or deformity, neurologic disorders, elevated cardiac output and other vascular disorders, and increased serum alkaline phosphatase and/or urinary hydroxyproline levels. Bone fractures are common in patients with Paget's disease.

Didronel slows accelerated bone turnover (resorption and accretion) in pagetic lesions and, to a lesser extent, in normal bone. This has been demonstrated histologically, scintigraphically, biochemically, and through calcium kinetic and balance studies. Reduced bone turnover is often accompanied by symptomatic improvement, including reduced bone pain. Also, the incidence of pagetic fractures may be reduced, and elevated cardiac output and other vascular disorders may be improved by **Didronel** therapy.

Heterotopic Ossification: Heterotopic ossification, also referred to as myositis ossificans (circumscripta, progressiva or traumatica), ectopic calcification, periarticular ossification, or paraosteoarthropathy, is characterized by metaplastic osteogenesis. It usually presents with signs of localized inflammation or pain, elevated skin temperature, and redness. When tissues near joints are involved, functional loss may also be present.

Heterotopic ossification may occur for no known reason as in myositis ossificans progressiva or may follow a wide variety of surgical, occupational, and sports trauma (eg, hip arthroplasty, spinal cord injury, head injury, burns, and severe thigh bruises). Heterotopic ossification has also been observed in non-traumatic conditions (eg, infections of the central nervous system, peripheral neuropathy, tetanus, biliary cirrhosis, Peyronie's disease, as well as in association with a variety of benign and malignant neoplasms).

Clinical trials have demonstrated the efficacy of **Didronel** in heterotopic ossification following total hip replacement, or due to spinal cord injury.

—*Heterotopic ossification complicating total hip replacement* typically develops radiographically 3 to 8 weeks postoperatively in the pericapsular area of the affected hip joint. The overall incidence is about 50%; about one-third of these cases are clinically significant.

—*Heterotopic ossification due to spinal cord injury* typically develops radiographically 1 to 4 months after injury. It occurs below the level of injury, usually at major joints. The overall incidence is about 40%; about one-half of these cases are clinically significant.

Didronel chemisorbs to calcium hydroxyapatite crystals and their amorphous precursors, blocking the aggregation, growth, and mineralization of these crystals. This is thought to be the mechanism by which **Didronel** prevents or retards heterotopic ossification. There is no evidence **Didronel** affects mature heterotopic bone.

INDICATIONS AND USAGE

Didronel is indicated for the treatment of symptomatic Paget's disease of bone and in the prevention and treatment of heterotopic ossification following total hip replacement or due to spinal cord injury. **Didronel** is not approved for the treatment of osteoporosis.

Paget's Disease: **Didronel** is indicated for the treatment of symptomatic Paget's disease of bone. **Didronel** therapy usually arrests or significantly impedes the disease process as evidenced by:

—Symptomatic relief, including decreased pain and/or increased mobility (experienced by 3 out of 5 patients).
—Reductions in serum alkaline phosphatase and urinary hydroxy-proline levels (30% or more in 4 out of 5 patients).
—Histomorphometry showing reduced numbers of osteoclasts and osteoblasts, and more lamellar bone formation.
—Bone scans showing reduced radionuclide uptake at pagetic lesions.

In addition, reductions in pagetically elevated cardiac output and skin temperature have been observed in some patients.

In many patients, the disease process will be suppressed for a period of at least 1 year following cessation of therapy. The upper limit of this period has not been determined.

The effects of the **Didronel** treatment in patients with asymptomatic Paget's disease have not been studied. However, **Didronel** treatment of such patients may be warranted if extensive involvement threatens irreversible neurologic damage, major joints, or major weight-bearing bones.

Heterotopic Ossification: **Didronel** is indicated in the prevention and treatment of heterotopic ossification following total hip replacement or due to spinal cord injury.

Didronel reduces the incidence of clinically important heterotopic bone by about two-thirds. Among those patients who form heterotopic bone, **Didronel** retards the progression of immature lesions and reduces the severity by at least half. Follow-up data (at least 9 months posttherapy) suggest these benefits persist.

In total hip replacement patients, **Didronel** does not promote loosening of the prosthesis or impede trochanteric reattachment.

In spinal cord injury patients, **Didronel** does not inhibit fracture healing or stabilization of the spine.

CONTRAINDICATIONS

Didronel tablets are contraindicated in patients with known hypersensitivity to etidronate disodium or in patients with clinically overt osteomalacia.

WARNINGS

Paget's Disease: In Paget's patients the response to therapy may be of slow onset and continue for months after **Didronel** therapy is discontinued. Dosage should not be increased prematurely. A 90-day drug-free interval should be provided between courses of therapy.

Heterotopic Ossification: No specific warnings.

PRECAUTIONS

General: Patients should maintain an adequate nutritional status, particularly an adequate intake of calcium and vitamin D.

Therapy has been withheld from some patients with enterocolitis since diarrhea may be experienced, particularly at higher doses.

Didronel is not metabolized and is excreted intact via the kidney. Hyperphosphatemia may occur at doses of 10 to 20 mg/kg/day, apparently as a result of drug-related increases in tubular reabsorption of phosphate. Serum phosphate levels generally return to normal 2 to 4 weeks posttherapy. There is no experience to specifically guide treatment in patients with impaired renal function. **Didronel** dosage should be reduced when reductions in glomerular filtration rates are present. Patients with renal impairment should be closely monitored. In approximately 10% of patients in clinical trials of **Didronel® I. V. Infusion** (etidronate disodium) for hypercalcemia of malignancy, occasional, mild-to-moderate abnormalities in renal function (increases of >0.5 mg/dl serum creatinine) were observed during or immediately after treatment.

Didronel suppresses bone turnover, and may retard mineralization of osteoid laid down during the bone accretion process. These effects are dose and time dependent. Osteoid, which may accumulate noticeably at doses of 10 to 20 mg/kg/day, mineralizes normally posttherapy. In patients with fractures, especially of long bones, it may be advisable to delay or interrupt treatment until callus is evident.

Paget's Disease: In Paget's patients, treatment regimens exceeding the recommended (see DOSAGE AND ADMINISTRATION) daily maximum dose of 20 mg/kg or continuous administration of medication for periods greater than 6 months may be associated with osteomalacia and an increased risk of fracture.

Long bones predominantly affected by lytic lesions, particularly in those patients unresponsive to **Didronel** therapy, may be especially prone to fracture. Patients with predominantly lytic lesions should be monitored radiographically and biochemically to permit termination of **Didronel** in those patients unresponsive to treatment.

Drug Interactions: There have been isolated reports of patients experiencing increases in their prothrombin times when etidronate was added to warfarin therapy. The majority of these reports concerned variable elevations in prothrombin times without clinically significant sequelae. Although the relevance of these reports and any mechanism of coagulation alterations is unclear, patients on warfarin should have their prothrombin time monitored.

Carcinogenesis: Long-term studies in rats have indicated that **Didronel** is not carcinogenic.

Pregnancy: Teratogenic Effects: Pregnancy Category C. In teratology and developmental toxicity studies conducted in rats and rabbits treated with dosages of up to 100 mg/kg (5 to 20 times the clinical dose), no adverse or teratogenic effects have been observed in the offspring. Etidronate disodium has been shown to cause skeletal abnormalities in rats when given at oral dose levels of 300 mg/kg (15 to 60 times the human dose). Other effects on the offspring (including decreased live births) are at dosages that cause significant toxicity in the parent generation and are 25 to 200 times the human dose. The skeletal effects are thought to be the result of the pharmacological effects of the drug on bone.

There are no adequate and well-controlled studies in pregnant women, **Didronel** (etidronate disodium) should be used during pregnancy only if the potential benefit justifies the potential risk to the fetus.

Nursing Mothers: It is not known whether this drug is excreted in human milk. Because many drugs are excreted in human milk, caustion should be exercised when **Didronel** is administered to a nursing woman.

Pediatric Use: Safety and effectiveness in pediatric patients have not been established. Pediatric patients have been treated with **Didronel**, at doses recommended for adults, to prevent heterotopic ossifications or soft tissue calcifications. A rachitic syndrome has been reported infrequently at doses of 10 mg/kg/day and more for prolonged periods approaching or exceeding a year. The epiphyseal radiologic changes associated with retarded mineralization of new osteoid and cartilage, and occasional symptoms reported, have been reversible when medication is discontinued.

ADVERSE REACTIONS

The incidence of gastrointestinal complaints (diarrhea, nausea) is the same for **Didronel** at 5 mg/kg/day as for placebo, about 1 patient in 15. At 10 to 20 mg/kg/day the incidence may increase to 2 or 3 in 10. These complaints are often alleviated by dividing the total daily dose.

Paget's Disease: In Paget's patients, increased or recurrent bone pain at pagetic sites, and/or the onset of pain at previously asymptomatic sites has been reported. At 5 mg/kg/day about 1 patient in 10 (versus 1 in 15 in the placebo group) report these phenomena. At higher doses the incidence rises to about 2 in 10. When therapy continues, pain resolves in some patients but persists in others.

Heterotopic Ossification: No specific adverse reactions.

Worldwide Postmarketing Experience: The worldwide postmarketing experience for etidronate disodium reflects its use in the following approved indications: Paget's disease, heterotopic ossification, and hypercalcemia of malignancy. It also reflects the use of etidronate disodium for osteoporosis where approved in countries outside the US. Other adverse events that have been reported and were thought to be possibly related to etidronate disodium include the following: alopecia; arthropathies, including arthralgia and arthritis; bone fracture; esophagitis; glossitis; hypersensitivity reactions, including angioedema, follicular eruption, macular rash, maculopapular rash, pruritus, a single case of Stevens-Johnson syndrome, and urticaria; osteomalacia; neuropsychiatric events, including amnesia, confusion, depression, and hallucination; and paresthesias.

In patients receiving etidronate disodium, there have been rare reports of agranulocytosis, pancytopenia, and a report of leukopenia with recurrence on rechallenge. In addition, there have been rare reports of exacerbation of asthma. Exacerbation of existing peptic ulcer disease has been reported in a few patients. In one patient, perforation also occurred.

OVERDOSAGE

Clinical experience with acute **Didronel** overdosage is extremely limited. Decreases in serum calcium following substantial overdosage may be expected in some patients. Signs and symptoms of hypocalcemia also may occur in some of these patients. Some patients may develop vomiting. In one event, an 18-year-old female who ingested an estimated single dose of 4000 to 6000 mg (67 to 100 mg/kg) of **Didronel** was reported to be mildly hypocalcemic (7.52 mg/dl) and experienced paresthesia of the fingers. Hypocalcemia resolved 6 hours after lavage and treatment with intravenous calcium gluconate. A 92-year-old female who accidentally received 1600 mg of etidronate disodium per day for 3.5 days experienced marked diarrhea and required treatment for electrolyte imbalance. Orally administered etidronate disodium may cause hematologic abnormalities in some patients (see ADVERSE REACTIONS).

Etidronate disodium suppresses bone turnover and may retard mineralization of osteoid laid down during the bone accretion process. These effects are dose and time dependent. Osteoid which may accumulate noticeably at doses of 10 to 20 mg/kg/day of chronic, continuous dosing mineralizes normally posttherapy.

Prolonged continuous treatment (chronic overdosage) has been reported to cause nephrotic syndrome and fracture.

Gastric lavage may remove unabsorbed drug. Standard procedures for treating hypocalcemia, including the administration of Ca^{++} intravenously, would be expected to restore physiologic amounts of ionized calcium and relieve signs and symptoms of hypocalcemia. Such treatment has been effective.

DOSAGE AND ADMINISTRATION

Didronel should be taken as a single, oral dose. However, should gastrointestinal discomfort occur, the dose may be divided. To maximize absorption, patients should avoid taking the following items within two hours of dosing:

—Food, especially food high in calcium, such as milk or milk products.
—Vitamins with mineral supplements or antacids which are high in metals such as calcium, iron, magnesium, or aluminum.

***Paget's Disease:* Initial Treatment Regimens:** 5 to 10 mg/kg/day, not to exceed 6 months, or 11 to 20 mg/kg/day, not to exceed 3 months.

The recommended initial dose is 5 mg/kg/day for a period not to exceed 6 months. Doses above 10 mg/kg/day should be reserved for when 1) lower doses are ineffective or 2) there is an overriding need to suppress rapid bone turnover (especially when irreversible neurologic damage is possible) or reduce elevated cardiac output. Doses in excess of 20 mg/kg/day are not recommended.

Retreatment Guidelines: Retreatment should be initiated only after 1) a **Didronel**-free period of at least 90 days and 2) there is biochemical, symptomatic or other evidence of active disease process. It is advisable to monitor patients every 3 to 6 months although some patients may go drug free for extended periods. Retreatment regimens are the same as for initial treatment. For most patients the original dose will be adequate for retreatment. If not, consideration should be given to increasing the dose within the recommended guidelines.

Heterotopic Ossification: The following treatment regimens have been shown to be effective:

—Total Hip Replacement Patients: 20 mg/kg/day for 1 month before and 3 months after surgery (4 months total).
—Spinal Cord Injured Patients: 20 mg/kg/day for 2 weeks followed by 10 mg/kg/day for 10 weeks (12 weeks total). **Didronel** therapy should begin as soon as medically feasible following the injury, preferably prior to evidence of heterotopic ossification.

Retreatment has not been studied.

HOW SUPPLIED

Didronel is available as 200-mg, white, rectangular tablets with "P & G" on one face and "402" on the other.

NDC 0149-0405-60 bottle of 60

400-mg, white, scored, capsule-shaped tablets with "N E" on one face and "406" on the other.

NDC 0149-0406-60 bottle of 60

Avoid excessive heat (over 104°F or 40°C).

CAUTION: Federal law prohibits dispensing without prescription.

Procter & Gamble Pharmaceuticals
Cincinnati, Ohio 45202
REVISED APRIL 1996 40560-P7

Shown in Product Identification Guide, page 329

HELIDAC™ Therapy ℞

(bismuth subsalicylate/metronidazole/tetracycline hydrochlride)

THESE PRODUCTS ARE INTENDED ONLY FOR USE AS DESCRIBED. The individual products contained in this package should not be used alone or in combination for other purposes. The information described in this labeling concerns only the use of these products as indicated in this combination package. For information on use of the individual components when dispensed as individual medications outside this combined use for treating *Helicobacter pylori,* please see the package inserts for each individual product.

WARNING

Metronidazole has been shown to be carcinogenic in mice and rats. (See **PRECAUTIONS.**) Unnecessary use of the drug should be avoided. Its use should be reserved for the conditions described in the **INDICATIONS AND USAGE** section below.

DESCRIPTION

HELIDAC Therapy consists of 112 bismuth subsalicylate 262.4-mg chewable tablets, 56 metronidazole 250-mg tablets, USP, and 56 tetracycline hydrochloride 500-mg capsules, USP for oral administration.

Bismuth subsalicylate chewable tablets: Each pink round tablet contains 262.4 mg bismuth subsalicylate (102 mg salicylate) for oral administration.

Bismuth subsalicylate is a fine, white, odorless, and tasteless powder that is stable and non-hygroscopic. It is a highly insoluble salt of trivalent bismuth and salicylic acid.

Bismuth subsalicylate is 2-Hydroxybenzoic acid bismuth (3+) salt with the following structural formula:

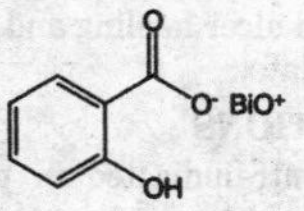

Molecular weight: 362.11

Inactive Ingredients: Each bismuth subsalicylate chewable tablet contains calcium carbonate, D&C Red No. 27 aluminum lake, flavor, magnesium stearate, mannitol, povidone, saccharin sodium, and talc.

Metronidazole tablets, USP: Each white round tablet contains 250 mg metronidazole. Metronidazole is 2-Methyl-5-nitroimidazole-1-ethanol, with the following structural formula:

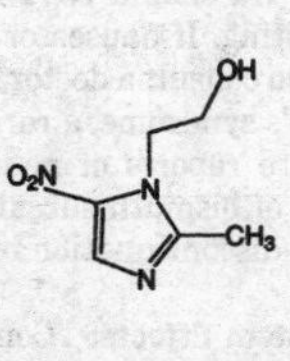

Molecular weight: 171.16

Inactive Ingredients: Each metronidazole tablet contains lactose monohydrate, magnesium stearate, microcrystalline cellulose, povidone, sodium starch glycolate, and stearic acid.

Tetracycline hydrochloride capsules, USP: Each pink and white capsule contains 500 mg tetracycline hydrochloride, causing it to appear pale orange and white in color when filled. Tetracycline is a yellow, odorless, crystalline powder. Tetracycline is stable in air but exposure to strong sunlight causes it to darken. Its potency is affected in solutions of pH below 2 and is rapidly destroyed by alkali hydroxide solutions. Tetracycline is very slightly soluble in water, freely soluble in dilute acid and in alkali hydroxide solutions, sparingly soluble in alcohol, and practically insoluble in chloroform and ether.

Tetracycline hydrochloride is (4S,4aS,5aS,6S,12aS)-4 (Dimethylamino) 1,4,4a,5,5a,6,11,12a-octahydro-3,6,10,12,12a-pentahydroxy-6-methyl-1,11-dioxo-2-naphthacenecarboxamide monohydrochloride, with the following structural formula:

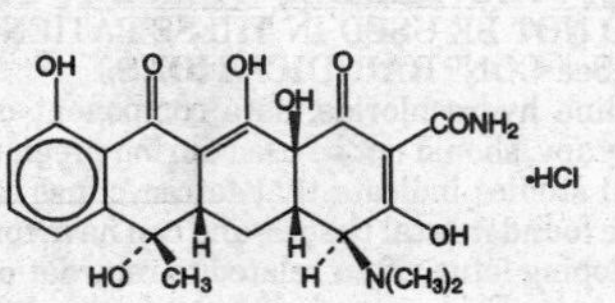

Molecular weight: 480.90

Inactive Ingredients: Each tetracycline hydrochloride capsule contains colloidal silicon dioxide, white ink, FD&C Red No. 40, gelatin, pregelatinized starch, stearic acid, and titanium dioxide.

CLINICAL PHARMACOLOGY

Pharmacokinetics: Pharmacokinetics for the HELIDAC Therapy components (bismuth subsalicylate chewable tablets, metronidazole tablets, and tetracycline hydrochloride capsules) when coadministered has not been studied. There is no information about the gastric mucosal concentrations of bismuth, metronidazole, and tetracycline after administration of these agents concomitantly or in combination with an acid suppressive agent. The systemic pharmacokinetic information presented below is based on studies in which each product was administered alone.

Bismuth Subsalicylate: Upon oral administration, bismuth subsalicylate is almost completely hydrolyzed in the gastrointestinal tract to bismuth and salicylic acid. Thus, the pharmacokinetics of bismuth subsalicylate following oral administration can be described by the individual pharmacokinetics of bismuth and salicylic acid.

Bismuth: Less than 1% of bismuth from oral doses of bismuth subsalicylate is absorbed from the gastrointestinal tract into the systemic circulation. Absorbed bismuth is distributed throughout the body. Bismuth is highly bound to plasma proteins (>90%). Bismuth has multiple disposition half-lives with an intermediate half-life of 5 to 11 days and a terminal half-life of 21 to 72 days. Elimination of bismuth is primarily through urinary and biliary routes with a renal clearance of 50 ± 18 mL/min. The mean trough blood bismuth concentration after 2 weeks oral administration of 787 mg bismuth subsalicylate (3 chewable tablets) four times daily under fasted condition was 5.1 ± 3.1 ng/mL. In another study, the mean trough blood bismuth concentration after 2 weeks oral administration of 525 mg bismuth subsalicylate (as PEPTO-BISMOL® liquid suspension) four times daily was 5 ng/mL with the highest value being 32 ng/mL.

Salicylic Acid: More than 80% of the salicylic acid is absorbed from oral doses of bismuth subsalicylate chewable tablets. Salicylic acid is about 90% plasma protein bound. The volume of distribution is about 170 mL/kg of body weight. Salicylic acid is extensively metabolized and about 10% is excreted unchanged in the urine. The metabolic clearance of salicylic acid is saturable; accordingly, nonlinear pharmacokinetics is observed at bismuth subsalicylate doses above 525 mg. Salicylic acid metabolic clearance is lower in females than in males. The terminal half-life of salicylic acid upon a single oral dose of 525 mg bismuth subsalicylate is between 2 to 5 hours. After a single oral dose of 525 mg bismuth subsalicylate (2 chewable tablets), the mean peak plasma salicylic acid concentration was 13.1 ± 3.4 μg/mL under fasted condition. The mean steady-state serum total salicylate concentration after 2 weeks oral administration of 525 mg bismuth subsalicylate (as PEPTO-BISMOL liquid suspension) four times daily was 24 μg/mL with the highest value being 70 μg/mL.

Metronidazole: Following oral administration, metronidazole is well absorbed, with peak plasma concentrations occurring between 1 and 2 hours after administration. Plasma concentrations of metronidazole are proportional to the administered dose, with oral administration of 250 mg producing a peak plasma concentration of 6 μg/mL. Studies reveal no significant bioavailability differences between males and females; however because of weight differences, the resulting plasma levels in males are generally lower.

Metronidazole is the major component appearing in the plasma, with lesser quantities of the 2-hydroxymethyl metabolite also being present. Less than 20% of the circulating metronidazole is bound to plasma proteins. Metronidazole also appears in cerebrospinal fluid, saliva, and breast milk in concentrations similar to those found in plasma.

The average elimination half-life in normal volunteers is 8 hours. The major route of elimination of metronidazole and its metabolites is via the urine (60% to 80% of the dose), with fecal excretion accounting for 6% to 15% of the dose. The metabolites that appear in the urine result primarily from side-chain oxidation [1-(β-hydroxyethyl)-2-hydroxymethyl-5-nitroimidazole and 2-methyl-5-nitroimidazole-1-yl-acetic acid] and glucuronide conjugation, with unchanged metronidazole accounting for approximately 20% of the total. Renal clearance of metronidazole is approximately 10 mL/min/1.73 m^2.

Decreased renal function does not alter the single-dose pharmacokinetics of metronidazole. In patients with decreased liver function plasma clearance of metronidazole is decreased.

Tetracycline Hydrochloride: Tetracyclines are readily absorbed and are bound to plasma proteins in varying degrees. They are concentrated by the liver in the bile and excreted in the urine and feces at high concentrations in a biologically active form.

The relative contribution of systemic versus local antimicrobial activity against *H. pylori* for agents used in eradication therapy has not been established.

Microbiology: Bismuth subsalicylate, metronidazole, and tetracycline individually have demonstrated *in vitro* activity against most susceptible strains of *Helicobacter pylori.*

Helicobacter: *Helicobacter pylori:* Metronidazole resistance has been increasing in the U.S. and mostly occurs in patients previously treated with metronidazole. Some *H. pylori* strains isolated from patients treated with bismuth, metronidazole, and tetracycline demonstrate an increase in metronidazole MIC's, indicating decreasing susceptibility and increasing resistance.

In the clinical studies, pretreatment and emerging resistance were not assessed for bismuth subsalicylate, metronidazole, or tetracycline, because susceptibility testing was not performed. No adequate data were collected during the clinical studies to indicate that bismuth subsalicylate can either decrease or increase metronidazole resistance.

It is recommended that all patients not eradicated of *H. pylori* following bismuth subsalicylate, metronidazole, and tetracycline treatment be considered to have *H. pylori* resistant to metronidazole. Patients who fail therapy should not be retreated with a regimen containing metronidazole.

In vitro* Activity of Bismuth Subsalicylate, Metronidazole, and Tetracycline Hydrochloride against *Helicobacter pylori: Bismuth subsalicylate, metronidazole, and tetracycline individually have demonstrated *in vitro* activity against most susceptible strains of *Helicobacter pylori* isolated from patients with duodenal ulcers.

In vitro susceptibility testing methods (broth microdilution, agar dilution, E-test, and disk diffusion) and diagnostic products currently available for determining minimum inhibi-

Continued on next page

Procter & Gamble Pharm.—Cont.

tory concentrations (MIC's) and zone sizes have not been standardized, validated, or approved for testing *H. pylori*. MIC values and zone sizes will vary depending on the susceptibility testing methodology employed, media, growth additives, inoculum concentration tested, growth phase, incubation atmosphere, and time.

INDICATIONS AND USAGE

The components of the HELIDAC Therapy (bismuth subsalicylate, metronidazole, and tetracycline hydrochloride), in combination with an H_2 antagonist are indicated for the treatment of patients with an active duodenal ulcer associated with *Helicobacter pylori* infection. The eradication of *H. pylori* has been demonstrated to reduce the risk of duodenal ulcer recurrence. Appropriate doses of H_2 antagonists for the treatment of active duodenal ulcers should be prescribed for ulcer healing. (See DOSAGE AND ADMINISTRATION.)
It is recommended that all patients not eradicated of *Helicobacter pylori* following HELIDAC Therapy plus an H_2 antagonist should be considered to have *Helicobacter pylori* resistant to metronidazole. Patients who fail therapy should not be retreated with a regimen containing metronidazole. (See Microbiology subsection.)

CLINICAL STUDIES

Investigators in the U.S. (Graham et al., 1991, 1992, and Cutler et al., 1993) and Germany (Labenz et al., 1993) studied the effect of therapy on the eradication of *H. pylori* using bismuth subsalicylate, metronidazole, and tetracycline hydrochloride. The patient population in these studies consisted predominantly of duodenal ulcer patients with active disease. In addition to bismuth subsalicylate, metronidazole, tetracycline hydrochloride triple therapy, most patients were also prescribed antisecretory therapy at doses recommended for ulcer healing, with the majority receiving ranitidine. The primary efficacy variable used in these studies to determine effectiveness of therapy was *H. pylori* eradication, or cure of infection. Use of cure of infection as a surrogate for reduced ulcer recurrence is based on an extensive review of the literature (Hopkins RJ, Girardi LS, Turney EA. The relationship between *H. pylori* eradication and reduced duodenal and gastric ulcer recurrence: A review. Gastroenterol 1996; 110:1244-52). Eradication rates are derived from results of the randomized, controlled study of Graham et al. and the uncontrolled, nonrandomized study of Cutler et al. *H. pylori* eradication was defined as no positive test (culture, histology, rapid urease, or C^{13} breath test) at least 4 weeks following the end of treatment. In the analysis performed, dropouts and patients with missing *H. pylori* tests post-treatment were excluded. HELIDAC Therapy (bismuth subsalicylate, metronidazole, and tetracycline hydrochloride) was effective in eradicating *H. pylori*.

Helicobacter pylori Eradication Rates in Patients with Duodenal Ulcer

Investigator	Eradication Rate in Duodenal Ulcer Patients[†]	95% Confidence Intervals
Graham[1,2]	77% (n=39)	61%–89%
Cutler[3]	82% (n=51)	70%–92%

[†]Evaluable patients were defined as having a confirmed duodenal ulcer within 2 years prior to treatment and having taken 14 days of bismuth subsalicylate, metronidazole, and tetracycline (range 11 to 17 days). Eradication was defined as no evidence of *H. pylori* infection by culture, histology, rapid urease test and/or urea breath test from at least 4 weeks post-treatment up to 1 year post-treatment.
Graham et al. 1992 (2) studied long-term outcome in patients treated for active duodenal ulcer by frequently monitoring for ulcer recurrence for up to 1 year after therapy. This study compared patients who received bismuth subsalicylate (BSS), metronidazole (MTZ), and tetracycline hydrochloride (TCN) for 2 weeks with ranitidine to those who received ranitidine alone. The ulcer recurrence rates at 6 months and 1 year, regardless of post-treatment eradication status, are summarized below for patients who were *H. pylori* positive at baseline.

Ulcer Recurrence at 6 Months and 1 Year[†]

Ulcer Recurrence Rates	All Patients	*H. pylori* Negative Patients Post-Treatment
6 Months Post-Treatment		
BSS/MTZ/TCN		
+Ranitidine	4% (1/25)	6% (1/18)
Ranitidine	85% (17/20)	100% (1/1)
1 Year Post-Treatment		
BSS/MTZ/TCN		
+Ranitidine	9% (2/22)	13% (2/16)
Ranitidine	95% (18/19)	100% (1/1)

[†]Includes all patients randomized to therapy who were *H. pylori* positive at baseline (by culture, histology, and/or urea breath test) who had ulcer healing and 24 or 48 weeks of endoscopic follow-up data.

CONTRAINDICATIONS

This therapy is contraindicated in pregnant or nursing women, pediatric patients, in patients with renal or hepatic impairment, and in those with known hypersensitivity to bismuth subsalicylate, metronidazole or other nitroimidazole derivatives, or any of the tetracyclines. (See WARNINGS and PRECAUTIONS.) This product does not contain aspirin but should not be administered to those patients who have a known allergy to aspirin or salicylates.

WARNINGS

Bismuth Subsalicylate

Children and teenagers who have or who are recovering from chicken pox or flu should NOT use this medicine to treat nausea or vomiting. If nausea or vomiting is present, patients are advised to consult a doctor because this could be an early sign of Reye's syndrome, a rare but serious illness. There have been rare reports of neurotoxicity associated with excessive doses of bismuth subsalicylate. Effects have been reversible with discontinuation of therapy.

Metronidazole

Central Nervous System Effects: Convulsive seizures and peripheral neuropathy, the latter characterized mainly by numbness or paresthesia of an extremity, have been reported in patients treated with metronidazole. The prevalence and severity of the neuropathy are directly related to the cumulative dose and duration of therapy, being most prevalent in patients taking high doses for prolonged treatment periods. The appearance of abnormal neurologic signs demands the prompt discontinuation of metronidazole therapy. Metronidazole should be administered with caution to patients with central nervous system diseases.

Tetracycline

THE USE OF DRUGS OF THE TETRACYCLINE CLASS DURING TOOTH DEVELOPMENT (LAST HALF OF PREGNANCY, INFANCY, AND CHILDHOOD TO THE AGE OF 8 YEARS) MAY CAUSE PERMANENT DISCOLORATION OF THE TEETH (YELLOW-GRAY-BROWN). This adverse reaction is more common during long-term use of the drugs but has been observed following repeated short-term courses. Enamel hypoplasia has also been reported. TETRACYCLINE HYDROCHLORIDE, AS A COMPONENT OF THE HELIDAC THERAPY, THEREFORE, SHOULD NOT BE USED IN THESE PATIENT POPULATIONS. (See CONTRAINDICATIONS.)
Tetracycline hydrochloride, as a component of the HELIDAC Therapy, should not be used during pregnancy. Results of animal studies indicate that tetracyclines cross the placenta, are found in fetal tissues, and can have toxic effects on the developing fetus (often related to retardation of skeletal development). Evidence of embryotoxicity has also been noted in animals treated early in pregnancy. If this drug is used during pregnancy or if the patient becomes pregnant while taking this drug, the patient should be apprised of the potential hazard to the fetus.
Photosensitivity manifested by an exaggerated sunburn reaction has been observed in some individuals taking tetracyclines. Patients apt to be exposed to direct sunlight or ultraviolet light should be advised that this reaction can occur with tetracycline drugs. Treatment should be discontinued at the first evidence of skin erythema.
The antianabolic action of the tetracyclines may cause an increase in blood urea nitrogen (BUN). While this is not a problem in those with normal renal function, in patients with significantly impaired renal function, higher serum levels of tetracycline may lead to azotemia, hyperphosphatemia, and acidosis.

PRECAUTIONS

General:

Bismuth Subsalicylate

Bismuth subsalicylate may cause a temporary and harmless darkening of the tongue and/or black stool. Stool darkening should not be confused with melena.

Metronidazole

Patients with severe hepatic disease metabolize metronidazole slowly, with resultant accumulation of metronidazole and its metabolites in the plasma. (See CONTRAINDICATIONS.) Metronidazole is a nitroimidazole and should be used with care in patients with evidence of, or history of, blood dyscrasia. A mild leukopenia has been observed; however, no persistent hematologic abnormalities attributable to metronidazole have been observed.
Known or previously unrecognized candidiasis may present more prominent symptoms during therapy with metronidazole and requires treatment with a candicidal agent.

Tetracycline

As with other antibiotics, use of tetracycline hydrochloride may result in overgrowth of nonsusceptible organisms, including fungi. If superinfection occurs, tetracycline should be discontinued and appropriate therapy should be instituted.
Pseudotumor cerebri (benign intracranial hypertension) in adults has been associated with the use of tetracyclines. The usual clinical manifestations are headache and blurred vision. While this condition and related symptoms usually resolve soon after discontinuation of the tetracycline, the possibility for permanent sequelae exists.
Information for Patients: Each dose includes 4 pills: 2 pink round chewable tablets (bismuth subsalicylate), 1 white round tablet (metronidazole), and 1 orange and white capsule (tetracycline hydrochloride). Each dose (all 4 pills) should be taken 4 times a day, at mealtimes and bedtime. Patients should be instructed to chew and swallow the pink round tablets (bismuth subsalicylate tablets) and to swallow the white round tablet (metronidazole tablet) and the pale orange and white capsule (tetracycline hydrochloride capsule) whole with a full glass of water (8 ounces). Concomitantly prescribed H_2 antagonist therapy should be taken as directed.
Administration of adequate amounts of fluid, particularly with the bedtime dose of tetracycline hydrochloride, is recommended to reduce the risk of esophageal irritation and ulceration. (See ADVERSE REACTIONS.)
Missed doses can be made up by continuing the normal dosing schedule until the medication is gone. Patients should not take double doses. (If more than 4 doses are missed, the prescriber should be contacted.)
This treatment regimen includes salicylates. If taken with aspirin and ringing in the ears occurs, the prescriber should be consulted concerning discontinuation of the aspirin therapy until the HELIDAC Therapy is completed.
Concurrent use of tetracyclines may render oral contraceptives less effective. Patients should be advised to use a different or additional form of contraception. Breakthrough bleeding has been reported. Women who become pregnant while taking components of the HELIDAC Therapy should be advised to notify their prescriber immediately. (See CONTRAINDICATIONS and WARNINGS.)
Alcoholic beverages should be avoided while taking metronidazole and for at least 1 day afterward. (See DRUG INTERACTIONS.)
Patients taking tetracycline hydrochloride should be cautioned to avoid exposure to sun or sun lamps. (See WARNINGS.)
Bismuth subsalicylate may cause temporary and harmless darkening of the tongue and/or black stool. Stool darkening should not be confused with melena (blood in the stool).
Drug Interactions: Individual components of the HELIDAC Therapy have a potential interaction with anticoagulants. Tetracycline has been shown to depress plasma prothrombin activity. Metronidazole has been reported to potentiate the anticoagulant effect of warfarin and other oral coumarin anticoagulants, resulting in a prolongation of prothrombin time. Salicylates may cause an increased risk of bleeding when administered with anticoagulant therapy. Therefore, monitoring anticoagulant therapy with appropriate adjustment of the anticoagulant dosage may be warranted if concurrent therapy is instituted.
Caution is advised in the administration of bismuth subsalicylate to patients taking medication for diabetes (possible enhanced hypoglycemic effect when given with salicylates) or patients taking aspirin, probenecid, or sulfinpyrazone.
Absorption of tetracyclines is impaired by antacids containing aluminum, calcium, or magnesium; preparations containing iron, zinc, or sodium bicarbonate; or milk or dairy products.
There is an anticipated reduction in tetracycline systemic absorption due to an interaction with bismuth and/or calcium carbonate, an excipient of bismuth subsalicylate tablets. The clinical significance of this is unknown as the relative contribution of systemic versus local antimicrobial activity against *H. pylori* for these agents has not been established.
Since bacteriostatic drugs, such as the tetracycline class of antibiotics, may interfere with the bactericidal action of penicillin, it is not advisable to administer these drugs concomitantly.
The concurrent use of tetracycline and methoxyflurane has been reported to result in fatal renal toxicity.
Concurrent use of tetracycline may render oral contraceptives less effective. Patients should be advised to use a different or additional form of contraception. Breakthrough bleeding has been reported. Women who become pregnant while on the HELIDAC Therapy should be advised to notify their prescriber immediately.
The simultaneous administration of drugs that decrease microsomal liver enzyme activity, such as cimetidine, may prolong the half-life and decrease plasma clearance of metronidazole.
The simultaneous administration of drugs that induce microsomal liver enzymes, such as phenytoin or phenobarbital,

may accelerate the elimination of metronidazole, resulting in reduced plasma levels; impaired clearance of phenytoin has also been reported.

In patients stabilized on relatively high doses of lithium, short-term metronidazole therapy has been associated with elevation of serum lithium and, in a few cases, signs of lithium toxicity. Serum lithium and serum creatinine should be obtained several days after beginning metronidazole to detect any increase that may precede clinical symptoms of lithium intoxication.

Alcoholic beverages should not be consumed during metronidazole therapy and for at least 1 day afterward because abdominal cramps, nausea, vomiting, headaches, and flushing may occur.

Psychotic reactions have been reported in alcoholic patients who are using metronidazole and disulfiram concurrently. Metronidazole should not be given to patients who have taken disulfiram within the last 2 weeks.

Drug/Laboratory Test Interactions: Bismuth absorbs x-rays and may interfere with x-ray diagnostic procedures of the gastrointestinal tract.

Bismuth subsalicylate may cause a temporary and harmless darkening of the stool. However, this does not interfere with standard tests for occult blood.

Metronidazole may interfere with certain types of determinations of serum chemistry values, such as aspartate aminotransferase (AST, SGOT), alanine aminotranferase (ALT, SGPT), lactate dehydrogenase (LDH), triglycerides, and hexokinase glucose. Values of zero may be observed. All of the assays in which interference has been reported involve enzymatic coupling of the assay to oxidation-reduction of nicotine adenine dinucleotide ($NAD^+ \rightleftarrows NADH$). Interference is due to the similarity in absorbance peaks of NADH (340 nm) and metronidazole (322 nm) at pH 7.

Carcinogenesis, Mutagenesis, Impairment of Fertility: Metronidazole has shown evidence of carcinogenic activity in a number of studies involving chronic, oral administration in mice and rats. Prominent among the effects in the mouse was an increased incidence of pulmonary tumorigenesis. This has been observed in all six reported studies in that species, including one study in which the animals were dosed on an intermittent schedule (administration during every fourth week only). At very high dose levels, 500 mg/kg/day, (approximately two times the recommended maximum human dose based on mg/m^2), there was a statistically significant increase in the incidence of malignant liver tumors in male mice. Also, the published results of one of the mouse studies indicate an increase in the incidence of malignant lymphomas as well as pulmonary neoplasms associated with lifetime feeding of the drug. All these effects are statistically significant. Long-term, oral-dosing studies in the rat showed statistically significant increases in the incidence of various neoplasms, particularly in mammary and hepatic tumors, among female rats administered metronidazole over those noted in the concurrent female control groups. Two lifetime tumorigenicity studies in hamsters have been performed and reported to be negative.

There has been no evidence of carcinogenicity for tetracycline hydrochloride in studies conducted with rats and mice. Some related antibiotics (oxytetracycline, minocycline) have shown evidence of oncogenic activity in rats.

No long-term toxicity studies have been conducted with bismuth subsalicylate.

No long-term studies have been performed to evaluate the effect of the combined use of bismuth subsalicylate, metronidazole, and tetracycline on carcinogenesis, mutagenesis, or impairment of fertility.

Although metronidazole has shown mutagenic activity in a number of *in vitro* assay systems, studies in mammals (*in vivo*) have failed to demonstrate a potential for genetic damage.

In two *in vitro* mammalian cell assay systems (L51784y mouse lymphoma and Chinese hamster lung cells), there was evidence of mutagenicity by tetracycline hydrochloride at concentrations of 60 and 10 μg/mL, respectively.

Bismuth did not show mutagenic potential in the NTP salmonella plate assay.

No reproductive toxicity studies have been conducted with bismuth subsalicylate.

Tetracycline hydrochloride had no effect on fertility when administered in the diet to male and female rats at a daily intake of 25 times the human dose.

Metronidazole, at doses up to 400 mg/kg/day (approximately 3.5 times the recommended maximum human dose based on mg/m^2) for 28 days, failed to produce any adverse effects on fertility and testicular function in male rats.

Pregnancy: Teratogenic Effects. Pregnancy Category D: Category D is based on the pregnancy category for tetracycline hydrochloride. (See **CONTRAINDICATIONS** and **WARNINGS, Tetracycline** subsection.)

Non-teratogenic Effects: (See **WARNINGS.**)

Pregnant women with renal disease may be more prone to develop tetracycline-associated liver failure.

Labor and Delivery: The effect of this therapy on labor and delivery is unknown.

Nursing Mothers: Metronidazole and tetracycline are both secreted into human milk. Because of the potential for tumorigenicity shown for metronidazole in mouse and rat studies, and because of the potential for serious adverse reactions in nursing infants from tetracyclines, a decision should be made whether to discontinue nursing or to discontinue therapy, taking into account the importance of the therapy to the mother. Metronidazole is secreted in human milk in concentrations similar to those found in plasma. (See **CONTRAINDICATIONS.**)

Pediatric Use: Safety and effectiveness in pediatric patients infected with *H. pylori* have not been established. (See **CONTRAINDICATIONS** and **WARNINGS.**)

Geriatric Use: Elderly patients may suffer from asymptomatic renal and hepatic dysfunction. Care should be taken when administering this therapy to this patient population.

ADVERSE REACTIONS

The most common adverse reactions (≥1%) reported in clinical trials when all three components of this therapy were given concomitantly are listed in the table below. The majority of the adverse reactions were related to the gastrointestinal tract, were reversible, and infrequently led to discontinuation of therapy.

Incidence of Adverse Reactions Reported in Clinical Trials (≥ 1.0%)†

	BSS/MTZ/TCN‡ n=197	Ranitidine n=73
Adverse Reactions	**% Pts**	**% Pts**
Nausea	10.2%	1.4%
Diarrhea	5.1%	0%
Abdominal Pain	3.0%	0%
Melena	2.5%	0%
Anal Discomfort	1.5%	0%
Anorexia	1.5%	0%
Dizziness	1.5%	0%
Paresthesia	1.5%	0%
Vomiting	1.5%	0%
Asthenia	1.0%	0%
Constipation	1.0%	0%
Insomnia	1.0%	0%
Pain	1.0%	0%
Upper Respiratory Infection	1.0%	0%

† Includes reactions reported at ≥1.0% in patients taking BSS/MTZ/TCN

‡Most patients were on concomitant acid suppression therapy

The additional adverse reactions (<1%) reported in clinical trials when all three components of this therapy were given concomitantly are listed below and divided by body system:

Gastrointestinal: dry mouth, dyspepsia, dysphagia, flatulence, gastrointestinal hemorrhage, glossitis, stomatitis

Skin: photosensitivity reaction (see **WARNINGS**), rash

Cardiovascular: hypertension, myocardial infarction

CNS: nervousness

Musculoskeletal: rheumatoid arthritis

Other: malaise, syncope

The following adverse reactions from the labeling for bismuth subsalicylate are provided for information.

Gastrointestinal: black stools

Mouth: temporary and harmless darkening of the tongue

The following adverse reactions from the labeling for metronidazole are provided for information.

Gastrointestinal: The most common adverse reactions reported have been referable to the gastrointestinal tract, particularly nausea reported by about 12% of patients, sometimes accompanied by headache, anorexia, and occasionally vomiting; diarrhea, epigastric distress, and abdominal cramping. Constipation has also been reported.

Mouth: A sharp, unpleasant metallic taste is not unusual. Furry tongue, glossitis, stomatitis have occurred; these may be associated with a sudden overgrowth of *Candida* which may occur during therapy.

Blood: Reversible neutropenia (leukopenia); rarely, reversible thrombocytopenia.

Cardiovascular: Flattening of the T-wave may be seen in electrocardiographic tracings.

CNS: Convulsive seizures, peripheral neuropathy, dizziness, vertigo, incoordination, ataxia, confusion, irritability, depression, weakness, and insomnia. Two serious adverse reactions reported in patients treated with metronidazole have been convulsive seizures and peripheral neuropathy, the latter characterized mainly by numbness or paresthesia of an extremity. Since persistent peripheral neuropathy has been reported in some patients receiving prolonged administration of metronidazole, patients should be specifically warned about these reactions and should be told to stop the drug and report immediately to their physicians if any neurologic symptoms occur.

Hypersensitivity: urticaria, erythematous rash, flushing, nasal congestion, dryness of mouth (or vagina or vulva), and fever

Renal: Dysuria, cystitis, polyuria, incontinence, and a sense of pelvic pressure. Instances of darkened urine have been reported by approximately one patient in 100,000. Although the pigment which is probably responsible for this phenomenon has not been positively identified, it is almost certainly a metabolite of metronidazole and seems to have no clinical significance.

Other: Proliferation of *Candida* in the vagina, dyspareunia, decrease of libido, proctitis, and fleeting joint pains sometimes resembling "serum sickness." If patients receiving metronidazole drink alcoholic beverages, they may experience abdominal distress, nausea, vomiting, flushing, or headache. A modification of the taste of alcoholic beverages has also been reported. Crohn's disease patients are known to have an increased incidence of gastrointestinal and certain extraintestinal cancers. There have been some reports in the medical literature of breast and colon cancer in Crohn's disease patients who have been treated with metronidazole at high doses for extended periods of time. A cause and effect relationship has not been established. Rare cases of pancreatitis, which abated on withdrawal of the drug, have been reported.

The following adverse reactions from the labeling for tetracycline hydrochloride are provided for information.

Gastrointestinal: Anorexia, nausea, epigastric distress, vomiting, diarrhea, glossitis, black hairy tongue, dysphagia, enterocolitis, and inflammatory lesions (with monilial overgrowth) in the anogenital region. Rare instances of esophagitis and esophageal ulceration have been reported in patients taking the tetracycline-class antibiotics in capsule and tablet form. Most of the patients who experienced esophageal irritation took the medication immediately before going to bed. (See **DOSAGE AND ADMINISTRATION.**)

Liver: Hepatotoxicity and liver failure have been observed in patients receiving large doses of tetracycline and in tetracycline-treated patients with renal impairment. Increases in liver enzymes and hepatic toxicity have been reported rarely.

Teeth: Permanent discoloration of teeth may be caused during tooth development. Enamel hypoplasia has also been reported. (See **WARNINGS.**)

Blood: hemolytic anemia, thrombocytopenia, thrombocytopenic purpura, neutropenia, and eosinophilia

CNS: Pseudotumor cerebri (benign intracranial hypertension) in adults and bulging fontanels in infants. (See **PRECAUTIONS: Tetracycline** subsection.) Dizziness, tinnitus, and visual disturbances have been reported. Myasthenic syndrome has been reported rarely.

Hypersensitivity: urticaria, angioneurotic edema, anaphylaxis, anaphylactoid purpura, pericarditis, exacerbation of systemic lupus erythematosus and serum sickness-like reactions, as fever, rash, and arthralgia

Renal: Rise in BUN has been reported and is apparently dose related. (See **WARNINGS.**)

Skin: Maculopapular and erythematous rashes have been reported. Exfoliative dermatitis has been rarely reported. Photosensitivity (see **WARNINGS**), onycholysis, and discoloration of the nails have been reported rarely.

Other: When given over prolonged periods, tetracyclines have been reported to produce brown-black microscopic discoloration of thyroid glands. No abnormalities of thyroid function studies are known to occur.

OVERDOSAGE

In case of an overdose, patients should contact a physician, poison control center, or emergency room. If all three components of this therapy are involved in an overdose, acute treatment should focus on the salicylate intoxication. There is neither a pharmacologic basis nor data suggesting an increased toxicity of the combination compared to individual components.

Bismuth Subsalicylate: The main concern of an acute bismuth subsalicylate (BSS) overdose focuses on the salicylate burden and not on bismuth, since less than 1% of the bismuth is normally absorbed. Each 262.4-mg tablet of BSS contains an amount of salicylate comparable to approximately 130 mg aspirin. Acute ingestion of less than 150 mg/kg of aspirin (i.e., less than one tablet of bismuth subsalicylate per kilogram of body weight) is not expected to lead to toxicity. Mild to moderate toxicity may result from the ingestion of 150 to 300 mg/kg, while severe toxicity may occur from ingestions over 300 mg/kg. Salicylate intoxication is well described in the literature and presents a complex clinical picture. Multiple respiratory and metabolic effects result in fluid, electrolyte, glucose, and acid-base disturbances. Initial symptoms of salicylate toxicity include hyperpnea, nausea, vomiting, tinnitus, hyperpyrexia, lethargy, tachycardia, and confusion. In severe cases, these symptoms may progress to severe hyperpnea, convulsions, pulmonary or cerebral edema, respiratory failure, cardiovascular collapse, coma, and death.

Continued on next page

Procter & Gamble Pharm.—Cont.

Treatment: There is no specific antidote for salicylate poisoning. If there are no contraindications, vomiting should be induced as soon as possible with syrup of ipecac, or gastric lavage should be instituted, provided that no more than one hour has elapsed since ingestion. Activated charcoal and a cathartic may be administered as primary decontamination therapy in those cases where greater than one hour has elapsed since ingestion, or to further decontaminate the gastrointestinal tract in those who have already received ipecac or gastric lavage. Plasma salicylate levels may be useful; a common nomogram can be used to help predict the severity of intoxication. Supportive and symptomatic treatment should be provided, with emphasis on correcting fluid, electrolyte, blood glucose, and acid-base disturbances. (Note: An acidotic blood pH increases the un-ionized salicylate form, allowing more to reach the central nervous system.) Elimination may be enhanced by urinary alkalinization, hemodialysis, or hemoperfusion. Since hemodialysis aids in correcting acid-base disturbances, this method may be preferred over hemoperfusion.

Metronidazole: Single oral doses of metronidazole, up to 19.5 g in adults, have been reported without resultant serious toxicity in suicide attempts and accidental overdoses. Symptoms reported include nausea, vomiting, and ataxia. Neurotoxic effects, including seizures and peripheral neuropathy, have been reported after 5 to 7 days of doses of 6 to 10.4 g every other day.

Treatment: There is no specific antidote for metronidazole overdose. Management of the patient should consist of symptomatic and supportive therapy. Metronidazole is dialyzable.

Tetracycline: The acute toxicity of tetracycline in overdose is not well established in the literature. Therapeutic and overdose quantities of tetracycline can cause gastrointestinal symptoms such as nausea, vomiting, and diarrhea.

Treatment: There is no specific antidote for tetracycline overdose. Management of the patient should consist of symptomatic and supportive therapy. Tetracycline is not dialyzable.

DOSAGE AND ADMINISTRATION

Adults: The recommended dosages are: bismuth subsalicylate, 525 mg (two 262.4 mg-chewable tablets), metronidazole, 250 mg (one 250-mg tablet), and tetracycline hydrochloride, 500 mg (one 500-mg capsule) taken four times daily (q.i.d.) for 14 days plus an H_2 antagonist approved for the treatment of acute duodenal ulcer. Patients should be instructed to take the medicines at meals and at bedtime. The bismuth subsalicylate tablets should be chewed and swallowed. The metronidazole tablet and tetracycline hydrochloride capsule should be swallowed whole with a full glass of water (8 ounces). Concomitantly prescribed H_2 antagonist therapy should be taken as directed.

Ingestion of adequate amounts of fluid, particularly with the bedtime dose of tetracycline hydrochloride, is recommended to reduce the risk of esophageal irritation and ulceration. (See **ADVERSE REACTIONS**.)

Missed doses can be made up by continuing the normal dosing schedule until the medication is gone. Patients should not take double doses. If more than 4 doses are missed, the prescriber should be contacted.

HOW SUPPLIED

The HELIDAC Therapy is supplied in a carton containing patient instructions, patient reminders, and 14 blister cards, each card containing the following daily dosage:

- 8 bismuth subsalicylate 262.4-mg chewable tablets, each pink round tablet engraved "PG 11"
- 4 metronidazole 250–mg tablets, each white round tablet engraved "PG" on the upper half and "10" on the lower half of the tablet
- 4 tetracycline hydrochloride 500-mg capsules, each pale orange and white capsule printed "PG 12" in white ink

NDC 0149-0495-01 carton containing 14 days of therapy

Store at controlled room temperature 20°-25°C (68°-77°F) [See USP].

REFERENCES

1. Graham DY, Lew GM, Evans DG, Evans DJ Jr, Klein PD. Effect of triple therapy (antibiotics plus bismuth) on duodenal ulcer healing. Ann Intern Med 1991; 115:266-69.

2. Graham DY, Lew GM, Klein PD, Evans DG, Evans DJ Jr, Saeed ZA, Malaty HM. Effect of treatment of *Helicobacter pylori* infection on the long-term recurrence of gastric or duodenal ulcer. Ann Int Med 1992; 116:705-08.

3. Cutler AF, Schubert TT. Long-term *Helicobacter pylori* recurrence after successful eradication with triple therapy. Am J Gastroenterol 1993; 88:1359-61.

CAUTION: Federal law prohibits dispensing without prescription.

Sold Under U.S. Patent No. 5,256,684

PEPTO-BISMOL is the registered trademark of The Procter & Gamble Company.

Bismuth subsalicylate tablets are manufactured by Procter & Gamble Pharmaceuticals. Metronidazole 250-mg tablets, USP and tetracycline hydrochloride 500-mg capsules, USP are manufactured by Zenith Laboratories, Inc., Northvale, New Jersey 07647

Procter & Gamble Pharmaceuticals
Cincinnati, Ohio 45202
AUGUST 1996 49501–P2

MACROBID® ℞

[mak'ró bid]

(nitrofurantoin monohydrate/macrocrystals)
Capsules

DESCRIPTION

Nitrofurantoin is an antibacterial agent specific for urinary tract infections. The **Macrobid**® brand of nitrofurantoin is a hard gelatin capsule shell containing the equivalent of 100 mg of nitrofurantoin in the form of 25 mg of nitrofurantoin macrocrystals and 75 mg of nitrofurantoin monohydrate.

The chemical name of nitrofurantoin macrocrystals is 1-[[[5-nitro-2-furanyl]methylene]amino]-2,4-imidazolidinedione.

The chemical structure is the following:

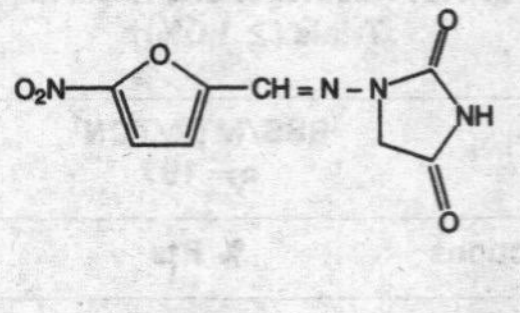

Molecular Weight: 238.16

The chemical name of nitrofurantoin monohydrate is 1-[[[5-nitro-2-furanyl]methylene]amino]-2,4-imidazolidinedione monohydrate. The chemical structure is the following:

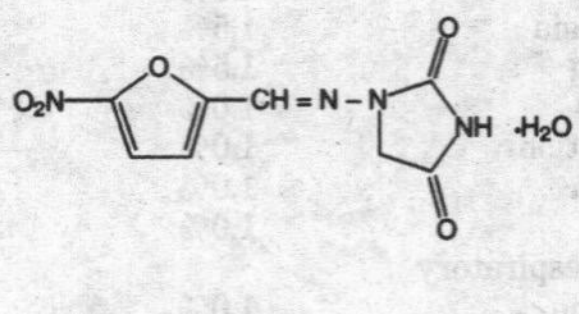

Molecular Weight: 256.17

Inactive Ingredients: Each capsule contains carbomer 934P, corn starch, compressible sugar, D&C Yellow No. 10, edible gray ink, FD&C Blue No. 1, FD&C Red No. 40, gelatin, lactose, magnesium stearate, povidone, talc, and titanium dioxide.

CLINICAL PHARMACOLOGY

Each **Macrobid** capsule contains two forms of nitrofurantoin. Twenty-five percent is macrocrystalline nitrofurantoin, which has slower dissolution and absorption than nitrofurantoin monohydrate. The remaining 75% is nitrofurantoin monohydrate contained in a powder blend which, upon exposure to gastric and intestinal fluids, forms a gel matrix that releases nitrofurantoin over time. Based on urinary pharmacokinetic data, the extent and rate of urinary excretion of nitrofurantoin from the 100-mg **Macrobid** capsule are similar to those of the 50-mg or 100-mg **Macrodantin**® (nitrofurantoin macrocrystals) capsule. Approximately 20–25% of a single dose of nitrofurantoin is recovered from the urine unchanged over 24 hours.

Plasma nitrofurantoin concentrations after a single oral dose of the 100-mg **Macrobid** capsule are low, with peak levels usually less than 1 mcg/mL. Nitrofurantoin is highly soluble in urine, to which it may impart a brown color. When **Macrobid** is administered with food, the bioavailability of nitrofurantoin is increased by approximately 40%.

Microbiology: Nitrofurantoin is bactericidal in urine at therapeutic doses. The mechanism of the antimicrobial action of nitrofurantoin is unusual among antibacterials. Nitrofurantoin is reduced by bacterial flavoproteins to reactive intermediates which inactivate or alter bacterial ribosomal proteins and other macromolecules. As a result of such inactivations, the vital biochemical processes of protein synthesis, aerobic energy metabolism, DNA synthesis, RNA synthesis, and cell wall synthesis are inhibited. The broad-based nature of this mode of action may explain the lack of acquired bacterial resistance to nitrofurantoin, as the necessary multiple and simultaneous mutations of the target macromolecules would likely be lethal to the bacteria. Development of resistance to nitrofurantoin has not been a significant problem since its introduction in 1953. Cross-resistance with antibiotics and sulfonamides has not been observed, and transferable resistance is, at most, a very rare phenomenon.

Nitrofurantoin, in the form of **Macrobid**, has been shown to be active against most strains of the following bacteria both *in vitro* and in clinical infections: (See **INDICATIONS AND USAGE**.)

Gram-Positive Aerobes
Staphylococcus saprophyticus
Gram-Negative Aerobes
Escherichia coli

Nitrofurantoin also demonstrates *in vitro* activity against the following microorganisms, although the clinical significance of these data with respect to treatment with **Macrobid** is unknown:

Gram-Positive Aerobes
Coagulase-negative staphylococci (including *Staphylococcus epidermidis*)
Enterococcus faecalis
Staphylococcus aureus
Streptococcus agalactiae
Group D streptococci
Viridans group streptococci
Gram-Negative Aerobes
Citrobacter amalonaticus
Citrobacter diversus
Citrobacter freundii
Klebsiella oxytoca
Klebsiella ozaenae

Nitrofurantoin is not active against most strains of *Proteus* species or *Serratia* species. It has no activity against *Pseudomonas* species.

Antagonism has been demonstrated *in vitro* between nitrofurantoin and quinolone antimicrobials. The clinical significance of this finding is unknown.

Susceptibility Tests:

Diffusion Techniques:

Quantitative methods that require measurement of zone diameters give the most precise estimate of the susceptibility of bacteria to antimicrobial agents. One such standard procedure,[1] which has been recommended for use with disks to test susceptibility of organisms to nitrofurantoin, uses the 300-mcg nitrofurantoin disk. Interpretation involves the correlation of the diameter obtained in the disk test with the minimum inhibitory concentration (MIC) for nitrofurantoin.

Reports from the laboratory giving results of the standard single-disk susceptibility test with a 300-mcg nitrofurantoin disk should be interpreted according to the following criteria:

Zone Diameter (mm)	Interpretation
≥17	Susceptible
15–16	Intermediate
≤14	Resistant

A report of "susceptible" indicates that the pathogen is likely to be inhibited by generally achievable urinary levels. A report of "intermediate" indicates that the result be considered equivocal and, if the organism is not fully susceptible to alternative clinically feasible drugs, the test should be repeated. This category provides a buffer zone which prevents small uncontrolled technical factors from causing major discrepancies in interpretations. A report of "resistant" indicates that achievable concentrations are unlikely to be inhibitory, and other therapy should be selected.

Standardized procedures require the use of laboratory control organisms. The 300-mcg nitrofurantoin disk should give the following zone diameters:

Organism	Zone Diameter (mm)
E. coli ATCC 25922	20–25
S. aureus ATCC 25923	18–22

Dilution Techniques:

Use a standardized dilution method[2] (broth, agar, microdilution) or equivalent with nitrofurantoin powder. The MIC values obtained should be interpreted according to the following criteria:

MIC (mcg/mL)	Interpretation
≤32	Susceptible
64	Intermediate
≥128	Resistant

As with standard diffusion techniques, dilution methods require the use of laboratory control organisms. Standard nitrofurantoin powder should provide the following MIC values:

Organism	MIC (mcg/mL)
E. coli ATCC 25922	4–16
S. aureus ATCC 29213	8–32
E. faecalis ATCC 29212	4–16

INDICATIONS AND USAGE

Macrobid is indicated only for the treatment of acute uncomplicated urinary tract infections (acute cystitis) caused by susceptible strains of *Escherichia coli* or *Staphylococcus saprophyticus.*

Nitrofurantoin is not indicated for the treatment of pyelonephritis or perinephric abscesses.

Nitrofurantoins lack the broader tissue distribution of other therapeutic agents approved for urinary tract infections. Consequently, many patients who are treated with **Macrobid** are predisposed to persistence or reappearance of bacteriu-

ria. (See CLINICAL STUDIES.) Urine specimens for culture and susceptibility testing should be obtained before and after completion of therapy. If persistence or reappearance of bacteriuria occurs after treatment with **Macrobid**, other therapeutic agents with broader tissue distribution should be selected. In considering the use of **Macrobid**, lower eradication rates should be balanced against the increased potential for systemic toxicity and for the development of antimicrobial resistance when agents with broader tissue distribution are utilized.

CONTRAINDICATIONS

Anuria, oliguria, or significant impairment of renal function (creatinine clearance under 60 mL per minute or clinically significant elevated serum creatinine) are contraindications. Treatment of this type of patient carries an increased risk of toxicity because of impaired excretion of the drug.

Because of the possibility of hemolytic anemia due to immature erythrocyte enzyme systems (glutathione instability), the drug is contraindicated in pregnant patients at term (38-42 weeks gestation), during labor and delivery, or when the onset of labor is imminent. For the same reason, the drug is contraindicated in neonates under one month of age.

Macrobid is also contraindicated in those patients with known hypersensitivity to nitrofurantoin.

WARNINGS

ACUTE, SUBACUTE, OR CHRONIC PULMONARY REACTIONS HAVE BEEN OBSERVED IN PATIENTS TREATED WITH NITROFURANTOIN. IF THESE REACTIONS OCCUR, **MACROBID** SHOULD BE DISCONTINUED AND APPROPRIATE MEASURES TAKEN. REPORTS HAVE CITED PULMONARY REACTIONS AS A CONTRIBUTING CAUSE OF DEATH.

CHRONIC PULMONARY REACTIONS (DIFFUSE INTERSTITIAL PNEUMONITIS OR PULMONARY FIBROSIS, OR BOTH) CAN DEVELOP INSIDIOUSLY. THESE REACTIONS OCCUR RARELY AND GENERALLY IN PATIENTS RECEIVING THERAPY FOR SIX MONTHS OR LONGER. CLOSE MONITORING OF THE PULMONARY CONDITION OF PATIENTS RECEIVING LONG-TERM THERAPY IS WARRANTED AND REQUIRES THAT THE BENEFITS OF THERAPY BE WEIGHED AGAINST POTENTIAL RISKS. (SEE RESPIRATORY REACTIONS.)

Hepatic reactions, including hepatitis, cholestatic jaundice, chronic active hepatitis, and hepatic necrosis, occur rarely. Fatalities have been reported. The onset of chronic active hepatitis may be insidious, and patients should be monitored periodically for changes in biochemical tests that would indicate liver injury. If hepatitis occurs, the drug should be withdrawn immediately and appropriate measures should be taken.

Peripheral neuropathy, which may become severe or irreversible, has occurred. Fatalities have been reported. Conditions such as renal impairment (creatinine clearance under 60 mL per minute or clinically significant elevated serum creatinine), anemia, diabetes mellitus, electrolyte imbalance, vitamin B deficiency, and debilitating disease may enhance the occurrence of peripheral neuropathy. Patients receiving long-term therapy should be monitored periodically for changes in renal function.

Optic neuritis has been reported rarely in postmarketing experience with nitrofurantoin formulations.

Cases of hemolytic anemia of the primaquine-sensitivity type have been induced by nitrofurantoin. Hemolysis appears to be linked to a glucose-6-phosphate dehydrogenase deficiency in the red blood cells of the affected patients. This deficiency is found in 10 percent of Blacks and a small percentage of ethnic groups of Mediterranean and Near-Eastern origin. Hemolysis is an indication for discontinuing **Macrobid**; hemolysis ceases when the drug is withdrawn.

Pseudomembranous colitis has been reported with nearly all antibacterial agents, including nitrofurantoin, and may range from mild to life threatening. Therefore, it is important to consider this diagnosis in patients with diarrhea subsequent to the administration of antibacterial agents.

Treatment with antibacterial agents alters the normal flora of the colon and may permit overgrowth of clostridia. Studies indicate that a toxin produced by *Clostridium difficile* is one primary cause of antibiotic-associated colitis.

After the diagnosis of pseudomembranous colitis has been established, appropriate therapeutic measures should be initiated. Mild cases of pseudomembranous colitis usually respond to drug discontinuation alone. In moderate to severe cases, consideration should be given to management with fluids and electrolytes, protein supplementation, and treatment with an antibacterial drug clinically effective against *Clostridium difficile* colitis.

PRECAUTIONS

Information for Patients: Patients should be advised to take **Macrobid** with food (ideally breakfast and dinner) to further enhance tolerance and improve drug absorption. Patients should be instructed to complete the full course of therapy; however, they should be advised to contact their physician if any unusual symptoms occur during therapy.

Patients should be advised not to use antacid preparations containing magnesium trisilicate while taking **Macrobid**.

Drug Interactions: Antacids containing magnesium trisilicate, when administered concomitantly with nitrofurantoin, reduce both the rate and extent of absorption. The mechanism for this interaction probably is adsorption of nitrofurantoin onto the surface of magnesium trisilicate.

Uricosuric drugs, such as probenecid and sulfinpyrazone, can inhibit renal tubular secretion of nitrofurantoin. The resulting increase in nitrofurantoin serum levels may increase toxicity, and the decreased urinary levels could lessen its efficacy as a urinary tract antibacterial.

Drug/Laboratory Test Interactions: As a result of the presence of nitrofurantoin, a false-positive reaction for glucose in the urine may occur. This has been observed with Benedict's and Fehling's solutions but not with the glucose enzymatic test.

Carcinogenesis, Mutagenesis, Impairment of Fertility: Nitrofurantoin was not carcinogenic when fed to female Holtzman rats for 44.5 weeks or to female Sprague-Dawley rats for 75 weeks. Two chronic rodent bioassays utilizing male and female Sprague-Dawley rats and two chronic bioassays in Swiss mice and in BDF_1 mice revealed no evidence of carcinogenicity.

Nitrofurantoin presented evidence of carcinogenic activity in female $B6C3F_1$ mice as shown by increased incidences of tubular adenomas, benign mixed tumors, and granulosa cell tumors of the ovary. In male F344/N rats, there were increased incidences of uncommon kidney tubular cell neoplasms, osteosarcomas of the bone, and neoplasms of the subcutaneous tissue. In one study involving subcutaneous administration of 75 mg/kg nitrofurantoin to pregnant female mice, lung papillary adenomas of unknown significance were observed in the F1 generation.

Nitrofurantoin has been shown to induce point mutations in certain strains of *Salmonella typhimurium* and forward mutations in L5178Y mouse lymphoma cells. Nitrofurantoin induced increased numbers of sister chromatid exchanges and chromosomal aberrations in Chinese hamster ovary cells but not in human cells in culture. Results of the sex-linked recessive lethal assay in Drosophila were negative after administration of nitrofurantoin by feeding or by injection. Nitrofurantoin did not induce heritable mutation in the rodent models examined.

The significance of the carcinogenicity and mutagenicity findings relative to the therapeutic use of nitrofurantoin in humans is unknown.

The administration of high doses of nitrofurantoin to rats causes temporary spermatogenic arrest; this is reversible on discontinuing the drug. Doses of 10 mg/kg/day or greater in healthy human males may, in certain unpredictable instances, produce a slight to moderate spermatogenic arrest with a decrease in sperm count.

Pregnancy:

Teratogenic effects: Pregnancy Category B. Several reproduction studies have been performed in rabbits and rats at doses up to six times the human dose and have revealed no evidence of impaired fertility or harm to the fetus due to nitrofurantoin. In a single published study conducted in mice at 68 times the human dose (based on mg/kg administered to the dam), growth retardation and a low incidence of minor and common malformations were observed. However, at 25 times the human dose, fetal malformations were not observed; the relevance of these findings to humans is uncertain. There are, however, no adequate and well-controlled studies in pregnant women. Because animal reproduction studies are not always predictive of human response, this drug should be used during pregnancy only if clearly needed.

Non-teratogenic effects: Nitrofurantoin has been shown in one published transplacental carcinogenicity study to induce lung papillary adenomas in the F1 generation mice at doses 19 times the human dose on a mg/kg basis. The relationship of this finding to potential human carcinogenesis is presently unknown. Because of the uncertainty regarding the human implications of these animal data, this drug should be used during pregnancy only if clearly needed.

Labor and Delivery: See CONTRAINDICATIONS.

Nursing Mothers: Nitrofurantoin has been detected in human breast milk in trace amounts. Because of the potential for serious adverse reactions from nitrofurantoin in nursing infants under one month of age, a decision should be made whether to discontinue nursing or to discontinue the drug, taking into account the importance of the drug to the mother. (See CONTRAINDICATIONS.)

Pediatric Use: **Macrobid** is contraindicated in infants below the age of one month. (See CONTRAINDICATIONS.) Safety and effectiveness in pediatric patients below the age of twelve years have not been established.

ADVERSE REACTIONS

In clinical trials of **Macrobid**, the most frequent clinical adverse events that were reported as possibly or probably drug-related were nausea (8%), headache (6%), and flatulence (1.5%). Additional clinical adverse events reported as possibly or probably drug-related occurred in less than 1% of patients studied and are listed below within each body system in order of decreasing frequency:

Gastrointestinal: Diarrhea, dyspepsia, abdominal pain, constipation, emesis

Neurologic: Dizziness, drowsiness, amblyopia

Respiratory: Acute pulmonary hypersensitivity reaction (see **WARNINGS**)

Allergic: Pruritus, urticaria

Dermatologic: Alopecia

Miscellaneous: Fever, chills, malaise

The following additional clinical adverse events have been reported with the use of nitrofurantoin:

Gastrointestinal: Sialadenitis, pancreatitis. There have been sporadic reports of pseudomembranous colitis with the use of nitrofurantoin. The onset of pseudomembranous colitis symptoms may occur during or after antimicrobial treatment. (See **WARNINGS**.)

Neurologic: Peripheral neuropathy, which may become severe or irreversible, has occurred. Fatalities have been reported. Conditions such as renal impairment (creatinine clearance under 60 mL per minute or clinically significant elevated serum creatinine), anemia, diabetes mellitus, electrolyte imbalance, vitamin B deficiency, and debilitating diseases may increase the possibility of peripheral neuropathy. (See **WARNINGS**.)

Asthenia, vertigo, and nystagmus also have been reported with the use of nitrofurantoin.

Benign intracranial hypertension (pseudotumor cerebri), confusion, depression, optic neuritis, and psychotic reactions have been reported rarely. Bulging fontanels, as a sign of benign intracranial hypertension in infants, have been reported rarely.

Respiratory:

CHRONIC, SUBACUTE, OR ACUTE PULMONARY HYPERSENSITIVITY REACTIONS MAY OCCUR WITH THE USE OF NITROFURANTOIN.

CHRONIC PULMONARY REACTIONS GENERALLY OCCUR IN PATIENTS WHO HAVE RECEIVED CONTINUOUS TREATMENT FOR SIX MONTHS OR LONGER. MALAISE, DYSPNEA ON EXERTION, COUGH, AND ALTERED PULMONARY FUNCTION ARE COMMON MANIFESTATIONS WHICH CAN OCCUR INSIDIOUSLY. RADIOLOGIC AND HISTOLOGIC FINDINGS OF DIFFUSE INTERSTITIAL PNEUMONITIS OR FIBROSIS, OR BOTH, ARE ALSO COMMON MANIFESTATIONS OF THE CHRONIC PULMONARY REACTION. FEVER IS RARELY PROMINENT.

THE SEVERITY OF CHRONIC PULMONARY REACTIONS AND THEIR DEGREE OF RESOLUTION APPEAR TO BE RELATED TO THE DURATION OF THERAPY AFTER THE FIRST CLINICAL SIGNS APPEAR. PULMONARY FUNCTION MAY BE IMPAIRED PERMANENTLY, EVEN AFTER CESSATION OF THERAPY. THE RISK IS GREATER WHEN CHRONIC PULMONARY REACTIONS ARE NOT RECOGNIZED EARLY.

In subacute pulmonary reactions, fever and eosinophilia occur less often than in the acute form. Upon cessation of therapy, recovery may require several months. If the symptoms are not recognized as being drug-related and nitrofurantoin therapy is not stopped, the symptoms may become more severe.

Acute pulmonary reactions are commonly manifested by fever, chills, cough, chest pain, dyspnea, pulmonary infiltration with consolidation or pleural effusion on x-ray, and eosinophilia. Acute reactions usually occur within the first week of treatment and are reversible with cessation of therapy. Resolution often is dramatic. (See **WARNINGS**.)

Changes in EKG (eg, non-specific ST/T wave changes, bundle branch block) have been reported in association with pulmonary reactions.

Cyanosis has been reported rarely.

Hepatic: Hepatic reactions, including hepatitis, cholestatic jaundice, chronic active hepatitis, and hepatic necrosis, occur rarely. (See **WARNINGS**.)

Allergic: Lupus-like syndrome associated with pulmonary reaction to nitrofurantoin has been reported. Also, angioedema; maculopapular, erythematous, or eczematous eruptions; anaphylaxis; arthralgia; myalgia; drug fever; and chills have been reported.

Dermatologic: Exfoliative dermatitis and erythema multiforme (including Stevens-Johnson syndrome) have been reported rarely.

Hematologic: Cyanosis secondary to methemoglobinemia has been reported rarely.

Miscellaneous: As with other antimicrobial agents, superinfections caused by resistant organisms, eg, *Pseudomonas* species or *Candida* species, can occur.

In clinical trials of **Macrobid**, the most frequent laboratory adverse events (1-5%), without regard to drug relationship, were as follows: eosinophilia, increased AST (SGOT), increased ALT (SGPT), decreased hemoglobin, increased serum phosphorus. The following laboratory adverse events also have been reported with the use of nitrofurantoin: glucose-6-phosphate dehydrogenase deficiency anemia (see

Continued on next page

Procter & Gamble Pharm.—Cont.

WARNINGS), agranulocytosis, leukopenia, granulocytopenia, hemolytic anemia, thrombocytopenia, megaloblastic anemia. In most cases, these hematologic abnormalities resolved following cessation of therapy. Aplastic anemia has been reported rarely.

OVERDOSAGE

Occasional incidents of acute overdosage of nitrofurantoin have not resulted in any specific symptoms other than vomiting. Induction of emesis is recommended. There is no specific antidote, but a high fluid intake should be maintained to promote urinary excretion of the drug. Nitrofurantoin is dialyzable.

DOSAGE AND ADMINISTRATION

Macrobid capsules should be taken with food.

Adults and Pediatric patients Over 12 Years: One 100-mg capsule every 12 hours for seven days.

HOW SUPPLIED

Macrobid is available as 100-mg opaque black and yellow capsules imprinted "Macrobid" on the black portion and "Norwich Eaton" on the yellow portion.

NDC 0149-0710-01 bottle of 100

Store at controlled room temperature (59° to 86°F or 15° to 30°C).

CAUTION: Federal law prohibits dispensing without prescription.

REFERENCES

1. National Committee for Clinical Laboratory Standards. Performance Standards for Antimicrobial Disk Susceptibility Tests—Fourth Edition. Approved Standard NCCLS Document M2-A4, Vol. 10, No. 7, NCCLS, Villanova, PA, 1990.
2. National Committee for Clinical Laboratory Standards. Methods for Dilution Antimicrobial Susceptibility Tests for Bacteria that Grow Aerobically—Second Edition. Approved Standard NCCLS Document M7-A2, Vol. 10, No. 8, NCCLS, Villanova, PA, 1990.

CLINICAL STUDIES

Controlled clinical trials comparing **Macrobid** 100 mg p.o. q12h and **Macrodantin** 50 mg p.o. q6h in the treatment of acute uncomplicated urinary tract infections demonstrated approximately 75% microbiologic eradication of susceptible pathogens in each treatment group.

Procter & Gamble Pharmaceuticals
Cincinnati, Ohio 45202
REVISED JULY 1996 71001-P8

Shown in Product Identification Guide, page 329

MACRODANTIN® ℞

[mak" rō-dan' tin]
(nitrofurantoin macrocrystals)

DESCRIPTION

Macrodantin (nitrofurantoin macrocrystals) is a synthetic chemical of controlled crystal size. It is a stable, yellow, crystalline compound. **Macrodantin** is an antibacterial agent for specific urinary tract infections. It is available in 25-mg, 50-mg, and 100-mg capsules for oral administration.

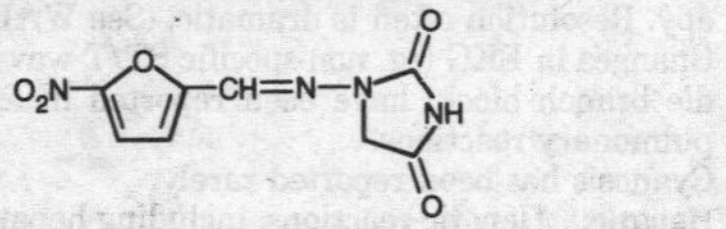

1-[[(5-NITRO-2-FURANYL)METHYLENE]AMINO]-2, 4-IMIDAZOLIDINEDIONE

Inactive Ingredients: Each capsule contains edible black ink, gelatin, lactose, starch, talc, titanium dioxide, and may contain FD&C Yellow No.6 and D&C Yellow No.10.

CLINICAL PHARMACOLOGY

Macrodantin is a larger crystal form of **Furadantin®** (nitrofurantoin). The absorption of **Macrodantin** is slower and its excretion somewhat less when compared to **Furadantin**. Blood concentrations at therapeutic dosage are usually low. It is highly soluble in urine, to which it may impart a brown color.

Following a dose regimen of 100 mg q.i.d. for 7 days, average urinary drug recoveries (0-24 hours) on day 1 and day 7 were 37.9% and 35.0%.

Unlike many drugs, the presence of food or agents delaying gastric emptying can increase the bioavailability of **Macrodantin**, presumably by allowing better dissolution in gastric juices.

Microbiology: Nitrofurantoin is bactericidal in urine at therapeutic doses. The mechanism of the antimicrobial action of nitrofurantoin is unusual among antibacterials. Nitrofurantoin is reduced by bacterial flavoproteins to reactive intermediates which inactivate or alter bacterial ribosomal proteins and other macromolecules. As a result of such inactivations, the vital biochemical processes of protein synthesis, aerobic energy metabolism, DNA synthesis, RNA synthesis, and cell wall synthesis are inhibited. The broad-based nature of this mode of action may explain the lack of acquired bacterial resistance to nitrofurantoin, as the necessary multiple and simultaneous mutations of the target macromolecules would likely be lethal to the bacteria. Development of resistance to nitrofurantoin has not been a significant problem since its introduction in 1953. Cross-resistance with antibiotics and sulfonamides has not been observed, and transferable resistance is, at most, a very rare phenomenon.

Nitrofurantoin, in the form of **Macrodantin**, has been shown to be active against most strains of the following bacteria both *in vitro* and in clinical infections: (See INDICATIONS AND USAGE.)

Gram-Positive Aerobes
Staphylococcus aureus
Enterococci (*e.g., Enterococcus faecalis*)

Gram-Negative Aerobes
Escherichia coli

NOTE: Some strains of *Enterobacter* species and *Klebsiella* species are resistant to nitrofurantoin.

Nitrofurantoin also demonstrates *in vitro* activity against the following microorganisms, although the clinical significance of these data with respect to treatment with **Macrodantin** is unknown:

Gram-Positive Aerobes
Coagulase-negative staphylococci
(including *Staphylococcus epidermidis* and *Staphylococcus saprophyticus*)
Streptococcus agalactiae
Group D streptococci
Viridans group streptococci

Gram-Negative Aerobes
Citrobacter amalonaticus
Citrobacter diversus
Citrobacter freundii
Klebsiella oxytoca
Klebsiella ozaenae

Nitrofurantoin is not active against most strains of *Proteus* species or *Serratia* species. It has no activity against *Pseudomonas* species.

Antagonism has been demonstrated *in vitro* between nitrofurantoin and quinolone antimicrobial agents. The clinical significance of this finding is unknown.

Susceptibility Tests:

Diffusion Techniques:

Quantitative methods that require measurement of zone diameters give the most precise estimate of the susceptibility of bacteria to antimicrobial agents. One such standard procedure,[1] which has been recommended for use with disks to test susceptibility of organisms to nitrofurantoin, uses the 300-mcg nitrofurantoin disk. Interpretation involves the correlation of the diameter obtained in the disk test with the minimum inhibitory concentration (MIC) for nitrofurantoin.

Reports from the laboratory giving results of the standard single-disk susceptibility test with a 300-mcg nitrofurantoin disk should be interpreted according to the following criteria:

Zone Diameter (mm)	Interpretation
≥17	Susceptible
15-16	Intermediate
≤14	Resistant

A report of "susceptible" indicates that the pathogen is likely to be inhibited by generally achievable urinary levels. A report of "intermediate" indicates that the result be considered equivocal and, if the organism is not fully susceptible to alternative clinically feasible drugs, the test should be repeated. This category provides a buffer zone which prevents small uncontrolled technical factors from causing major discrepancies in interpretations. A report of "resistant" indicates that achievable concentrations are unlikely to be inhibitory, and other therapy should be selected.

Standardized procedures require the use of laboratory control organisms. The 300-mcg nitrofurantoin disk should give the following zone diameters:

Organism	Zone Diameter (mm)
E. coli ATCC 25922	20-25
S. aureus ATCC 25923	18-22

Dilution Techniques:

Use a standardized dilution method[2] (broth, agar, microdilution) or equivalent with nitrofurantoin powder. The MIC values obtained should be interpreted according to the following criteria:

MIC (mcg/mL)	Interpretation
≤32	Susceptible
64	Intermediate
≥128	Resistant

As with standard diffusion techniques, dilution methods require the use of laboratory control organisms. Standard nitrofurantoin powder should provide the following MIC values:

Organism	MIC (mcg/mL)
E. coli ATCC 25922	4-16
S. aureus ATCC 29213	8-32
E. faecalis ATCC 29212	4-16

INDICATIONS AND USAGE

Macrodantin is specifically indicated for the treatment of urinary tract infections when due to susceptible strains of *Escherichia coli*, enterococci, *Staphylococcus aureus*, and certain susceptible strains of *Klebsiella* and *Enterobacter* species.

Nitrofurantoin is not indicated for the treatment of pyelonephritis or perinephric abscesses.

Nitrofurantoins lack the broader tissue distribution of other therapeutic agents approved for urinary tract infections. Consequently, many patients who are treated with **Macrodantin** are predisposed to persistence or reappearance of bacteriuria. Urine specimens for culture and susceptibility testing should be obtained before and after completion of therapy. If persistence or reappearance of bacteriuria occurs after treatment with **Macrodantin**, other therapeutic agents with broader tissue distribution should be selected. In considering the use of **Macrodantin**, lower eradication rates should be balanced against the increased potential for systemic toxicity and for the development of antimicrobial resistance when agents with broader tissue distribution are utilized.

CONTRAINDICATIONS

Anuria, oliguria, or significant impairment of renal function (creatinine clearance under 60 mL per minute or clinically significant elevated serum creatinine) are contraindications. Treatment of this type of patient carries an increased risk of toxicity because of impaired excretion of the drug.

Because of the possibility of hemolytic anemia due to immature erythrocyte enzyme systems (glutathione instability), the drug is contraindicated in pregnant patients at term (38-42 weeks gestation), during labor and delivery, or when the onset of labor is imminent. For the same reason, the drug is contraindicated in neonates under one month of age.

Macrodantin is also contraindicated in those patients with known hypersensitivity to nitrofurantoin.

WARNINGS

ACUTE, SUBACUTE, OR CHRONIC PULMONARY REACTIONS HAVE BEEN OBSERVED IN PATIENTS TREATED WITH NITROFURANTOIN. IF THESE REACTIONS OCCUR, MACRODANTIN SHOULD BE DISCONTINUED AND APPROPRIATE MEASURES TAKEN. REPORTS HAVE CITED PULMONARY REACTIONS AS A CONTRIBUTING CAUSE OF DEATH.

CHRONIC PULMONARY REACTIONS (DIFFUSE INTERSTITIAL PNEUMONITIS OR PULMONARY FIBROSIS, OR BOTH) CAN DEVELOP INSIDIOUSLY. THESE REACTIONS OCCUR RARELY AND GENERALLY IN PATIENTS RECEIVING THERAPY FOR SIX MONTHS OR LONGER. CLOSE MONITORING OF THE PULMONARY CONDITION OF PATIENTS RECEIVING LONG-TERM THERAPY IS WARRANTED AND REQUIRES THAT THE BENEFITS OF THERAPY BE WEIGHED AGAINST POTENTIAL RISKS. (SEE RESPIRATORY REACTIONS.)

Hepatic reactions, including hepatitis, cholestatic jaundice, chronic active hepatitis, and hepatic necrosis, occur rarely. Fatalities have been reported. The onset of chronic active hepatitis may be insidious, and patients should be monitored periodically for changes in biochemical tests that would indicate liver injury. If hepatitis occurs, the drug should be withdrawn immediately and appropriate measures should be taken.

Peripheral neuropathy, which may become severe or irreversible, has occurred. Fatalities have been reported. Conditions such as renal impairment (creatinine clearance under 60 mL per minute or clinically significant elevated serum creatinine), anemia, diabetes mellitus, electrolyte imbalance, vitamin B deficiency, and debilitating disease may enhance the occurrence of peripheral neuropathy. Patients receiving long-term therapy should be monitored periodically for changes in renal function.

Optic neuritis has been reported rarely in postmarketing experience with nitrofurantoin formulations.

Cases of hemolytic anemia of the primaquine-sensitivity type have been induced by nitrofurantoin. Hemolysis appears to be linked to a glucose-6-phosphate dehydrogenase deficiency in the red blood cells of the affected patients. This deficiency is found in 10 percent of Blacks and a small percentage of ethnic groups of Mediterranean and Near-Eastern origin. Hemolysis is an indication for discontinuing **Macrodantin**; hemolysis ceases when the drug is withdrawn.

Pseudomembranous colitis has been reported with nearly all antibacterial agents, including nitrofurantoin, and may range from mild to life threatening. Therefore, it is important to consider this diagnosis in patients with diarrhea subsequent to the administration of antibacterial agents.

Treatment with antibacterial agents alters the normal flora of the colon and may permit overgrowth of clostridia. Studies

indicate that a toxin produced by *Clostridium difficile* is one primary cause of antibiotic-associated colitis.

After the diagnosis of pseudomembranous colitis has been established, appropriate therapeutic measures should be initiated. Mild cases of pseudomembranous colitis usually respond to drug discontinuation alone. In moderate to severe cases, consideration should be given to management with fluids and electrolytes, protein supplementation, and treatment with an antibacterial drug clinically effective against *Clostridium difficile* colitis.

PRECAUTIONS

Information for Patients: Patients should be advised to take **Macrodantin** with food to further enhance tolerance and improve drug absorption. Patients should be instructed to complete the full course of therapy; however, they should be advised to contact their physician if any unusual symptoms occur during therapy.

Many patients who cannot tolerate microcrystalline nitrofurantoin are able to take **Macrodantin** without nausea.

Patients should be advised not to use antacid preparations containing magnesium trisilicate while taking **Macrodantin**.

Drug Interactions: Antacids containing magnesium trisilicate, when administered concomitantly with nitrofurantoin, reduce both the rate and extent of absorption. The mechanism for this interaction probably is adsorption of nitrofurantoin onto the surface of magnesium trisilicate.

Uricosuric drugs, such as probenecid and sulfinpyrazone, can inhibit renal tubular secretion of nitrofurantoin. The resulting increase in nitrofurantoin serum levels may increase toxicity, and the decreased urinary levels could lessen its efficacy as a urinary tract antibacterial.

Drug/Laboratory Test Interactions: As a result of the presence of nitrofurantoin, a false-positive reaction for glucose in the urine may occur. This has been observed with Benedict's and Fehling's solutions but not with the glucose enzymatic test.

Carcinogenesis, Mutagenesis, Impairment of Fertility: Nitrofurantoin was not carcinogenic when fed to female Holtzman rats for 44.5 weeks or to female Sprague-Dawley rats for 75 weeks. Two chronic rodent bioassays utilizing male and female Sprague-Dawley rats and two chronic bioassays in Swiss mice and in BDF_1 mice revealed no evidence of carcinogenicity.

Nitrofurantoin presented evidence of carcinogenic activity in female $B6C3F_1$ mice as shown by increased incidences of tubular adenomas, benign mixed tumors, and granulosa cell tumors of the ovary. In male F344/N rats, there were increased incidences of uncommon kidney tubular cell neoplasms, osteosarcomas of the bone, and neoplasms of the subcutaneous tissue. In one study involving subcutaneous administration of 75 mg/kg nitrofurantoin to pregnant female mice, lung papillary adenomas of unknown significance were observed in the F1 generation.

Nitrofurantoin has been shown to induce point mutations in certain strains of *Salmonella typhimurium* and forward mutations in L5178Y mouse lymphoma cells. Nitrofurantoin induced increased numbers of sister chromatid exchanges and chromosomal aberrations in Chinese hamster ovary cells but not in human cells in culture. Results of the sex-linked recessive lethal assay in Drosophila were negative after administration of nitrofurantoin by feeding or by injection. Nitrofurantoin did not induce heritable mutation in the rodent models examined.

The significance of the carcinogenicity and mutagenicity findings relative to the therapeutic use of nitrofurantoin in humans is unknown.

The administration of high doses of nitrofurantoin to rats causes temporary spermatogenic arrest; this is reversible on discontinuing the drug. Doses of 10 mg/kg/day or greater in healthy human males may, in certain unpredictable instances, produce a slight to moderate spermatogenic arrest with a decrease in sperm count.

Pregnancy:

Teratogenic effects: Pregnancy Category B. Several reproduction studies have been performed in rabbits and rats at doses up to six times the human dose and have revealed no evidence of impaired fertility or harm to the fetus due to nitrofurantoin. In a single published study conducted in mice at 68 times the human dose (based on mg/kg administered to the dam), growth retardation and a low incidence of minor and common malformations were observed. However, at 25 times the human dose, fetal malformations were not observed; the relevance of these findings to humans is uncertain. There are, however, no adequate and well-controlled studies in pregnant women. Because animal reproduction studies are not always predictive of human response, this drug should be used during pregnancy only if clearly needed.

Non-teratogenic effects: Nitrofurantoin has been shown in one published transplacental carcinogenicity study to induce lung papillary adenomas in the F1 generation mice at doses 19 times the human dose on a mg/kg basis. The relationship of this finding to potential human carcinogenesis is presently unknown. Because of the uncertainty regarding the human implications of these animal data, this drug should be used during pregnancy only if clearly needed.

Labor and Delivery: See CONTRAINDICATIONS.

Nursing Mothers: Nitrofurantoin has been detected in human breast milk in trace amounts. Because of the potential for serious adverse reactions from nitrofurantoin in nursing infants under one month of age, a decision should be made whether to discontinue nursing or to discontinue the drug, taking into account the importance of the drug to the mother. (See CONTRAINDICATIONS.)

Pediatric Use: Macrodantin is contraindicated in infants below the age of one month. (See CONTRAINDICATIONS.)

ADVERSE REACTIONS

Respiratory:

CHRONIC, SUBACUTE, OR ACUTE PULMONARY HYPERSENSITIVITY REACTIONS MAY OCCUR.

CHRONIC PULMONARY REACTIONS OCCUR GENERALLY IN PATIENTS WHO HAVE RECEIVED CONTINUOUS TREATMENT FOR SIX MONTHS OR LONGER. MALAISE, DYSPNEA ON EXERTION, COUGH, AND ALTERED PULMONARY FUNCTION ARE COMMON MANIFESTATIONS WHICH CAN OCCUR INSIDIOUSLY. RADIOLOGIC AND HISTOLOGIC FINDINGS OF DIFFUSE INTERSTITIAL PNEUMONITIS OR FIBROSIS, OR BOTH, ARE ALSO COMMON MANIFESTATIONS OF THE CHRONIC PULMONARY REACTION. FEVER IS RARELY PROMINENT.

THE SEVERITY OF CHRONIC PULMONARY REACTIONS AND THEIR DEGREE OF RESOLUTION APPEAR TO BE RELATED TO THE DURATION OF THERAPY AFTER THE FIRST CLINICAL SIGNS APPEAR. PULMONARY FUNCTION MAY BE IMPAIRED PERMANENTLY, EVEN AFTER CESSATION OF THERAPY. THE RISK IS GREATER WHEN CHRONIC PULMONARY REACTIONS ARE NOT RECOGNIZED EARLY.

In subacute pulmonary reactions, fever and eosinophilia occur less often than in the acute form. Upon cessation of therapy, recovery may require several months. If the symptoms are not recognized as being drug-related and nitrofurantoin therapy is not stopped, the symptoms may become more severe.

Acute pulmonary reactions are commonly manifested by fever, chills, cough, chest pain, dyspnea, pulmonary infiltration with consolidation or pleural effusion on x-ray, and eosinophilia. Acute reactions usually occur within the first week of treatment and are reversible with cessation of therapy. Resolution often is dramatic. (See **WARNINGS**.)

Changes in EKG (eg, non-specific ST/T wave changes, bundle branch block) have been reported in association with pulmonary reactions.

Cyanosis has been reported rarely.

Hepatic: Hepatic reactions, including hepatitis, cholestatic jaundice, chronic active hepatitis, and hepatic necrosis, occur rarely. (See **WARNINGS**.)

Neurologic: Peripheral neuropathy, which may become severe or irreversible, has occurred. Fatalities have been reported. Conditions such as renal impairment (creatinine clearance under 60 mL per minute or clinically significant elevated serum creatinine), anemia, diabetes mellitus, electrolyte imbalance, vitamin B deficiency, and debilitating diseases may increase the possibility of peripheral neuropathy. (See **WARNINGS**.)

Asthenia, vertigo, and nystagmus also have been reported with the use of nitrofurantoin.

Benign intracranial hypertension (pseudotumor cerebri), confusion, depression, optic neuritis, and psychotic reactions have been reported rarely. Bulging fontanels, as a sign of benign intracranial hypertension in infants, have been reported rarely.

Dermatologic: Exfoliative dermatitis and erythema multiforme (including Stevens-Johnson syndrome) have been reported rarely. Transient alopecia also has been reported.

Allergic: A lupus-like syndrome associated with pulmonary reactions to nitrofurantoin has been reported. Also, angioedema; maculopapular, erythematous, or eczematous eruptions; pruritus; urticaria; anaphylaxis; arthralgia; myalgia; drug fever; and chills have been reported.

Gastrointestinal: Nausea, emesis, and anorexia occur most often. Abdominal pain and diarrhea are less common gastrointestinal reactions. These dose-related reactions can be minimized by reduction of dosage. Sialadenitis and pancreatitis have been reported. There have been sporadic reports of pseudomembranous colitis with the use of nitrofurantoin. The onset of pseudomembranous colitis symptoms may occur during or after antimicrobial treatment. (See **WARNINGS**.)

Hematologic: Cyanosis secondary to methemoglobinemia has been reported rarely.

Miscellaneous: As with other antimicrobial agents, superinfections caused by resistant organisms, eg, *Pseudomonas* species or *Candida* species, can occur.

Laboratory Adverse Events: The following laboratory adverse events have been reported with the use of nitrofurantoin: increased AST (SGOT), increased ALT (SGPT), decreased hemoglobin, increased serum phosphorus, eosinophilia, glucose-6-phosphate dehydrogenase deficiency anemia (see **WARNINGS**), agranulocytosis, leukopenia, granulocytopenia, hemolytic anemia, thrombocytopenia, megaloblastic anemia. In most cases, these hematologic abnormalities resolved following cessation of therapy. Aplastic anemia has been reported rarely.

OVERDOSAGE

Occasional incidents of acute overdosage of **Macrodantin** have not resulted in any specific symptoms other than vomiting. Induction of emesis is recommended. There is no specific antidote, but a high fluid intake should be maintained to promote urinary excretion of the drug. It is dialyzable.

DOSAGE AND ADMINISTRATION

Macrodantin should be given with food to improve drug absorption and, in some patients, tolerance.

Adults: 50-100 mg four times a day – the lower dosage level is recommended for uncomplicated urinary tract infections.

Pediatric patients: 5-7 mg/kg of body weight per 24 hours, given in four divided doses (contraindicated under one month of age).

Therapy should be continued for one week or for at least 3 days after sterility of the urine is obtained. Continued infection indicates the need for reevaluation.

For long-term suppressive therapy in adults, a reduction of dosage to 50-100 mg at bedtime may be adequate. For long-term suppressive therapy in pediatric patients, doses as low as 1 mg/kg per 24 hours, given in a single dose or in two divided doses, may be adequate. **SEE WARNINGS SECTION REGARDING RISKS ASSOCIATED WITH LONG-TERM THERAPY.**

HOW SUPPLIED

Macrodantin is available as follows:

25-mg opaque, white capsule imprinted with one black line encircling the capsule and coded "MACRODANTIN 25 mg" and "0149-0007".*

NDC 0149-0007-05 bottle of 100

50-mg opaque, yellow and white capsule imprinted with two black lines encircling the capsule and coded "MACRODANTIN 50 mg" and "0149-0008".*

NDC 0149-0008-05 bottle of 100
NDC 0149-0008-66 bottle of 500
NDC 0149-0008-67 bottle of 1000
NDC 0149-0008-77 hospital unit-dose strips in box of 100

100-mg opaque, yellow capsule imprinted with three black lines encircling the capsule and coded "MACRODANTIN 100 mg" and "0149-0009".*

NDC 0149-0009-05 bottle of 100
NDC 0149-0009-66 bottle of 500
NDC 0149-0009-67 bottle of 1000
NDC 0149-0009-77 hospital unit-dose strips in box of 100

*Capsule design, registered trademark of Procter & Gamble Pharmaceuticals.

CAUTION: Federal law prohibits dispensing without prescription.

REFERENCES

1. National Committee for Clinical Laboratory Standards. Performance Standards for Antimicrobial Disk Susceptibility Tests - Fourth Edition. Approved Standard NCCLS Document M2-A4, Vol. 10, No. 7, NCCLS, Villanova, PA, 1990.
2. National Committee for Clinical Laboratory Standards. Methods for Dilution Antimicrobial Susceptibility Tests for Bacteria that Grow Aerobically - Second Edition. Approved Standard NCCLS Document M7-A2, Vol. 10, No. 8, NCCLS, Villanova, PA, 1990.

Procter & Gamble Pharmaceuticals
Cincinnati, Ohio 45202
REVISED JULY 1996 00700–U6

Shown in Product Identification Guide, page 329

EDUCATIONAL MATERIAL

Procter & Gamble Pharmaceuticals offers a wide range of educational services to the medical profession. Please write to Manager, Professional Meetings & Conventions, Procter & Gamble Pharmaceuticals, Sharon Woods Technical Center, 11520 Reed Hartman Highway, Cincinnati, OH 45241 for further information.

- **Sponsorship of Educational Seminars**
- **Patient Education Booklets**
- **Resident/Fellow Conferences**
- **Newsletters**

The Purdue Frederick Company
100 CONNECTICUT AVENUE
NORWALK, CT 06850-3590

For Medical Information Contact:
Generally:
Medical Department
(203) 853-0123

OxyContin™ 10 mg Tablets
OxyContin™ 20 mg Tablets
OxyContin™ 40 mg Tablets
see listing under Purdue Pharma L.P., page 2163

OxyIR™ Capsules—see listing under Purdue Pharma L.P., page 2167.

ALFERON® N INJECTION ℞
Interferon alfa-n3
(Human Leukocyte Derived)

DESCRIPTION

Alferon® N Injection [Interferon alfa-n3 (Human Leukocyte Derived)] is a sterile aqueous formulation of purified, natural, human interferon alpha proteins for use by injection. Alferon® N Injection consists of interferon alpha proteins comprising approximately 166 amino acids ranging in molecular weights from 16,000 to 27,000 daltons. The specific activity of Interferon alfa-n3 is approximately equal to, or greater than, 2×10^8 IU/mg of protein.

Alferon® N Injection is manufactured from pooled units of human leukocytes which have been induced by incomplete infection with an avian virus (Sendai virus) to produce Interferon alfa-n3. The manufacturing process includes immunoaffinity chromatography with a murine monoclonal antibody, acidification (pH 2) for 5 days at 4°C, and gel filtration chromatography.

Since Alferon® N Injection is manufactured using source leukocytes, human, donor screening is performed to minimize the risk that the leukocytes could contain infectious agents. In addition, the manufacturing process contains steps which have been shown to inactivate viruses, and there has been no evidence of infection transmission to recipients in clinical trials. The laboratory and clinical data obtained support the conclusion that Alferon® N Injection is equivalent to other products derived from human blood or plasma which are free of risk of transmission of infectious agents, such as immunoglobulin and albumin.

The Alferon® N Injection manufacturing process was evaluated for quantitative removal or inactivation of model pathogenic viruses. The viruses were deliberately added to the leukocytes in amounts far exceeding those present in contaminated blood, i.e., $\geq 10^9$ infectious units per milliliter. The manufacturing process yielded a cumulative reduction of $\geq 10^{14}$ of infectious HIV-1, i.e., $\geq 10^{6.5}$ removal by acid inactivation and $\geq 10^{7.9}$ removal by the purification process. In the validation studies, there was 10^8 reduction in the titer of hepatitis B virus as determined by HBsAg assay, and a 10^9 reduction in the infectious titer of herpes simplex virus-1 (HSV-1). Cultivation of Alferon® N Injection Purified Drug Concentrate with human indicator cells, i.e., MRC-5 cells, peripheral blood leukocytes in the presence of Cyclosporin A, and fetal cord blood cells, did not detect the presence of infectious viruses.

As part of a validation study, Alferon® N Injection [Interferon alfa-n3 (Human Leukocyte Derived)] was examined for the presence of the following viruses; Sendai virus (SV), HIV-1, HTLV-I, HBV, HSV-1, CMV, and EBV. Alferon® N Injection contained no detectable quantities of these viruses. In addition other studies, i.e., Polymerase Chain Reaction (PCR) and Dot Blot Hybridization (DBH), have shown no detectable genetic material from these viruses in Alferon® N Injection. The sensitivity of the PCR was 10 copies for HIV-1 (env gene probe) and 10 copies for HBV (S/P gene probe). The sensitivity of the DBH was 1 pg for EBV, < 10 pg for CMV, < 10 pg for HSV-1, and < 2 pg for SV. Furthermore, sera from 105 patients treated with Alferon® N Injection (95 with condylomata acuminata and 10 with cancer) were tested for antibody HIV-1 and HIV p24 antigen. There was no evidence to suggest transmission of HIV-1 by Alferon® N Injection. Sera from 135 patients with condylomata, acuminata treated with Alferon® N Injection were tested to determine abnormal SGOT laboratory values. There was no evidence to suggest transmission of hepatitis by Alferon® N Injection based on both SGOT results and patient data collected during clinical trials.

Alferon® N Injection has been extensively purified using immunoaffinity chromatography with a murine monoclonal antibody, acidification (pH 2) for 5 days at 4°C, and gel filtration chromatography. Alferon® N Injection has been subjected to the acid treatment for five days during its manufacture in order to reduce the risk of viral transmission. Subsequent analyses of the Alferon® N Injection Purified Drug Concentrate confirm the absence of detectable infectious or non-infectious viral particles.

The leukocyte nutrient medium contains the antibotic neomycin sulfate at a concentration of 35 mg/L; however, neomycin sulfate is not detectable in the final product, i.e., < 0.64 μg/ml.

Murine immunoglobulin (IgG) is detected in the Alferon® N Injection Purified Drug Concentrate at levels below 0.15% of the Interferon alfa-n3 protein. This equates to levels less than 8 ng of murine IgG per million IU Interferon alfa-n3 (range of 0.9 to 5.6 ng typically found).

Alferon® N Injection [Interferon alfa-n3 (Human Leukocyte Derived)] is available in an injectable solution containing 5 million IU Alferon® N Injection per vial for intralesional injection. The solution is clear and colorless. Each milliliter (ml) contains five million IU of Interferon alfa-n3 in phosphate buffered saline (8.0 mg sodium chloride, 1.74 mg sodium phosphate dibasic, 0.20 mg potassium phosphate monobasic, and 0.20 mg potassium chloride) containing 3.3 mg phenol as a preservative and 1 mg Albumin (Human) as a stabilizer.

CLINICAL PHARMACOLOGY

General Interferons are naturally occuring proteins with both antiviral and antiproliferative properties. They are produced and secreted in response to viral infections and to a variety of other synthetic and biological inducers. Three major families of interferons have been identified: alpha, beta, and gamma. The interferon alpha family contains at least 15 different molecular species. Their molecular weights range from 16,000 to 27,000 daltons.

Interferons bind to specific membrane receptors on cell surfaces. Interferon alfa-n3 has been shown to bind to the same receptors as Interferon alfa-2b. The receptors have a high degree of selectivity for the binding of human but not mouse interferon. This correlates with the high species specificity found in laboratory studies.

Binding of interferon to membrane receptors initiates a series of events including induction of protein synthesis. These actions are followed by a variety of cellular responses, including inhibition of virus replication and suppression of cell proliferation. Immunomodulation, including enhancement of phagocytosis by macrophages, augmentation of the cytotoxicity of lymphocytes and enhancement of human leukocyte antigen expression occurs in response to exposure to interferons. One or more of these activities may contribute to the therapeutic effect of interferon.

Pharmacokinetics In a study of intralesional use of Alferon® N Injection [Interferon alfa-n3 (Human Leukocyte Derived)] for the treatment of condylomata acuminata, plasma concentrations of interferon were below the detection limit of the assay, i.e., ≤ 3 IU/ml. Minor systemic effects (e.g., myalgias, fever, and headaches) were noted, indicating that some of the injected interferon entered the systemic circulation (See ADVERSE REACTIONS).

Condylomata Acuminata Condylomata acuminata (venereal or genital warts) are associated with infections of human papilloma virus (HPV), especially HPV type-6 and possibly type-11. Given the antiviral and antiproliferative activities of interferons and the viral etiology of condylomata, a placebo-controlled clinical trial was conducted to evaluate the safety and efficacy of intralesional injection of Alferon® N Injection in the treatment of condylomata acuminata.

In a multicenter randomized double-blind, placebo-controlled clinical trial, intralesional administration of Alferon® N Injection was an effective treatment for condylomata acuminata.[1–4] One hundred fifty-six patients were evaluable for efficacy (81 Alferon® N Injection patients and 75 placebo patients). Patients had a mean of five warts (range was 2-14) and all warts were treated. Patients were injected intralesionally with a mean of 225,000 IU of Alferon® N Injection per wart 2 times a week for up to 8 weeks. Overall, 80% ($^{65}/_{81}$) of patients treated with Alferon® N Injection had a complete or partial resolution of warts compared with 44% ($^{33}/_{75}$) of placebo-treated patients ($p < 0.001$). Alferon® N Injection was significantly more effective than placebo in producing a complete resolution of warts ($p < 0.001$), as shown by the following table:

[See Table 1 below.]

Of the patients who had a complete resolution of warts, approximately half ($^{21}/_{44}$) the patients had complete resolution of warts by the end of treatment, and half ($^{23}/_{44}$) had complete resolution of warts during the three months after the cessation of treatment. Patients with complete resolution of warts were followed for a median of 48 weeks. Overall, 76% ($^{31}/_{41}$) of Alferon® N Injection [Interferon alfa-n3 (Human Leukocyte Derived)]-treated patients who achieved complete resolution of warts remained clear of all treated lesions during follow-up, while 79% ($^{11}/_{14}$) of the placebo-treated patients remained clear of all treated lesions during follow-up.

A total of 762 evaluable warts were injected in this trial. Of the 407 Alferon® N Injection-treated warts, 73% ($^{297}/_{407}$) completely resolved, as compared to 35% ($^{125}/_{355}$) of the placebo-treated warts ($p < 0.0001$). Alferon® N Injection was effective in treating lesions of all sizes, and there was no difference in resolution for perianal, penile, or vulvar lesions.

There was no difference in resolution for patients who had received prior treatment of their warts and for those who had not. Among patients with recalcitrant warts (i.e., warts that were refractory to previous treatment or recurring), 82% ($^{58}/_{71}$) of the evaluable patients had complete or partial resolution of warts due to intralesional administration of Alferon® N Injection as compared to 43% ($^{29}/_{67}$) of placebo patients ($p < 0.001$). Fifty-four percent ($^{38}/_{71}$) of the evaluable Alferon® N Injection patients had complete resolution of warts as compared to 18% ($^{12}/_{67}$) of placebo patients ($p < 0.001$). Patients with primary occurrence of genital warts (i.e., no prior treatment of warts) had a similar resolution rate compared to the patients with recalcitrant warts: 70% ($^{7}/_{10}$) had complete or partial resolution of warts due to Alferon® N Injection treatment and 60% ($^{6}/_{10}$) had complete resolution of warts, as compared to 50% ($^{4}/_{8}$) of placebo recipients who had complete or partial resolution of warts and 38% ($^{3}/_{8}$) who had complete resolution. Overall, 83% ($^{5}/_{6}$) of Alferon® N Injection [Interferon alfa-n3 (Human Leukocyte Derived)]-treated patients with primary occurrence, who achieved complete resolution of warts, remained clear of all treated lesions during a median follow-up of 52 weeks. Because the number of patients with primary occurrence of warts was small (10 Alferon® N Injection recipients and 8 placebo recipients), the difference between Alferon® N Injection and placebo treatment was not statistically significant. However, when the resolution of primary warts was examined, 75% ($^{33}/_{44}$) of the Alferon® N Injection-treated primary warts resolved completely as compared to 39% ($^{11}/_{28}$) of the placebo-treated primary warts ($p = 0.003$).

In an open clinical trial using a once a week treatment schedule for up to 16 weeks, 28 patients were evaluable for efficacy. Eighty-nine percent ($^{25}/_{28}$) of patients had a complete or partial resolution of warts following treatment with Alferon® N Injection. The condylomata acuminata resolved completely in 46% ($^{13}/_{28}$) of the patients. Of the 154 warts treated, 77% ($^{118}/_{154}$) resolved completely.

After injections of Alferon® N Injection, side effects were minor and transient. After 4 weeks of treatment, the frequency of adverse reactions was similar in Alferon® N Injection and placebo treatment groups. The most frequent side effects were myalgias, fever, and headache (See ADVERSE REACTIONS).

Antigenicity

1. Alferon® N Injection
   One hundred and five (105) patients treated with Alferon® N Injection during clinical trials were tested for the presence of anti-interferon antibodies using three different antibody assays: Immunoradiometric Assay (IRMA), Enzyme Linked Immunosorbent Assay (ELISA), and neutralization by the Cytopathic Effect Assay (CPE). To date, no antibodies to Interferon alfa-n3 have been detected in any of the patients.
2. Mouse Proteins
   No hypersensitivity reactions to the components in Alferon® N Injection [Interferon alfa-n3 (Human Leukocyte Derived)] have been observed. Alferon® N Injection uses a murine monoclonal antibody in one of the purification procedures. A possibility exists that patients treated with Alferon® N Injection may develop hypersensitivity to the mouse proteins. However, none of the patients receiving Alferon® N Injection during clinical trials developed antibodies or hypersensitivity to mouse proteins (See CONTRAINDICATIONS).

Table 1

Degree of Resolution as Measured By Total Wart Volume per Patient

	Percent of Patients with:			
	Complete Resolution	Partial Resolution (≥50% resolution)	Minor Resolution (<50% resolution)	Progression/ No change
Alferon® (n = 81)	54%	26%	15%	5%
Placebo (n = 75)	20%	24%	13%	43%

3. Egg Protein

The initial stage in the manufacture of Alferon® N Injection uses Sendai virus which was grown in chicken eggs as the specific Interferon alfa-n3 inducer. Although no egg protein (ovalbumin) has been detected in the initial stage of interferon manufacture using an ELISA (sensitivity of 16 ng/ml), a possibility exists that patients treated with Alferon® N Injection may develop hypersensitivity to egg protein (See CONTRAINDICATIONS).

INDICATIONS AND USAGE

Alferon® N Injection is indicated for the intralesional treatment of refractory or recurring external condylomata acuminata in patients 18 years of age or older (See DOSAGE AND ADMINISTRATION).

The physician should select patients for treatment with Alferon® N Injection after consideration of a number of factors: the locations and sizes of the lesions, past treatment and response thereto, and the patient's ability to comply with the treatment regimen. Alferon® N Injection is particularly useful for patients who have not responded satisfactorily to other treatment modalities, e.g., podophyllin resin, surgery, laser or cryotherapy.

There have been no studies with this product in adolescents. This product is not recommended for use in patients less than 18 years of age.

CONTRAINDICATIONS

Alferon® N Injection is contraindicated in patients with known hypersensitivity to human interferon alpha or any component of the product. The product also is contraindicated in patients who have anaphylactic sensitivity to mouse immunoglobulin (IgG), egg protein or neomycin.

WARNINGS

Because of the fever and other "flu-like" symptoms associated with Alferon® N Injection [Interferon alfa-n3 (Human Leukocyte Derived)] (See ADVERSE REACTIONS), it should be used cautiously in patients with debilitating medical conditions such as cardiovascular disease (e.g., unstable angina and uncontrolled congestive heart failure), severe pulmonary disease (e.g., chronic obstructive pulmonary disease), or diabetes mellitus with ketoacidosis. Alferon® N Injection should be used cautiously in patients with coagulation disorders (e.g., thrombophlebitis, pulmonary embolism and hemophilia), severe myelosuppression, or seizure disorders. Acute, serious hypersensitivity reactions (e.g., urticaria, angioedema, bronchoconstriction, and anaphylaxis) have not been observed in patients receiving Alferon® N Injection. However, if such reactions develop, drug administration should be discontinued immediately and appropriate medical therapy should be instituted.

PRECAUTIONS

General Patients being treated with Alferon® N Injection should be informed of the benefits and risks associated with the treatment. Because the manufacturing process, strength, and type of interferon (e.g., natural, human leukocyte interferon versus single-subspecies recombinant interferon) may vary for different interferon formulations, changing brands may require a change in dosage. Therefore, physicians are cautioned not to change from one interferon product to another without considering these factors.

Information for Patients Patients should be informed of the early signs of hypersensitivity reactions including hives, generalized urticaria, tightness of the chest, wheezing, hypotension, and anaphylaxis, and should be advised to contact their physician if these symptoms occur.

Patients being treated with Alferon® N Injection should be informed of benefits and risks associated with treatment. Patients should be cautioned not to change brands of interferon without medical consultation, as a change in dosage may occur.

Carcinogenesis, Mutagenesis, Impairment of Fertility Studies with Alferon® N Injection [Interferon alfa-n3 (Human Leukocyte Derived)] have not been performed to determine carcinogenicity, mutagenicity, or the effect on fertility. In studies with adult females, interferon alpha has been shown to affect the menstrual cycle and decrease serum estradiol and progesterone levels[5].

Alferon® N Injection should be used with caution in fertile men. Fertile women should be cautioned to use effective contraception while being treated with Alferon® N Injection. Changes in the menstrual cycle and abortions have been reported to occur in non-human primates given extremely high doses of recombinant interferon alpha[6]. In these studies, Macaca mulatta (rhesus monkeys) were given interferon daily by intramuscular injection. When given at daily intramuscular doses 326 times the average intralesional dose of Alferon® N Injection (120 times the maximum recommended dose), this recombinant interferon formulation produced menstrual cycle changes in the monkeys.

In human clinical trials with Alferon® N Injection, menstrual cycle data were reported by 51 patients (36 Alferon® N Injection and 15 placebo). There was no significant difference between Alferon® N Injection and placebo treatment groups with regard to menstrual cycle changes.

PREGNANCY Pregnancy Category C Animal reproduction studies have not been conducted with Alferon® N Injection. It is also not known whether Alferon® N Injection can cause fetal harm when administered to a pregnant woman or can affect reproductive capacity. Alferon® N Injection should be given to a pregnant woman only if clearly needed. Changes in the menstrual cycle and abortions have been reported to occur in non-human primates given extremely high doses of recombinant interferon alpha. In these studies, Macaca mulatta (rhesus monkeys) were given interferon daily by intramuscular injection. Abortifacient effects were noted when the recombinant interferon alpha was given daily during early to mid-gestation at intramuscular doses of 978 times the average intralesional dose of Alferon® N Injection [Interferon alfa-n3 (Human Leukocyte Derived)] (360 times the maximum recommended dose).

Nursing Mothers It is not known whether Alferon® N Injection is excreted in human milk. Studies in mice have shown that mouse interferons are excreted in milk[7]. Because many drugs are excreted in human milk and because of the potential for serious adverse reactions in nursing infants, a decision should be made whether to discontinue nursing or to not initiate drug treatment, taking into account the importance of the drug to the mother and the potential risk to the infant.

Pediatric Use Safety and effectiveness have not been established in patients below the age of 18 years.

ADVERSE REACTIONS

Adverse reactions were evaluated in 202 patients with condylomata acuminata receiving Alferon® N Injection by intralesional administration and in 31 patients with cancer receiving Alferon® N Injection by systemic administration. In the double-blind efficacy trial for the treatment of condylomata acuminata, 104 patients were treated with doses of Alferon® N Injection of 0.05 million to 2.5 million IU per treatment session (average dose = 0.92 million IU per treatment session) by intralesional injection. In open trials, an additional 98 patients received a dose range of 0.05 to 4.6 million IU of Alferon® N Injection per treatment session (average dose = 1.12 million IU per treatment session). Patients with cancer were given doses of Alferon® N Injection of 3 million, 9 million, or 15 million IU per day for ten days by intramuscular injection.

Adverse Reactions in Patients with Condylomata Acuminata A total of 104 patients with condylomata acuminata was treated with Alferon® N Injection during the double-blind clinical trial. Adverse reactions were reported to be likely, unlikely, or not known to be related to Alferon® N Injection. Adverse reactions consisted primarily of "flu-like" symptoms (myalgias, fever, and/or headache) which were in most cases mild or moderate, and transient, and did not interfere with treatment.

The "flu-like" adverse reactions, consisting of fever myalgias, and/or headache, occurred primarily after the first treatment session and were reported by 30% of the patients. The frequency of "flu-like" adverse reactions abated with repeated dosing of Alferon® N Injection [Interferon alfa-n3 (Human Leukocyte Derived)] so that the incidences due to Alferon® N Injection and placebo were similar after three to four weeks of treatment (after six to eight treatment sessions). "Flu-like" symptoms were relieved by administration of acetaminophen.

Adverse reactions were reported at least once during the course of treatment in the following percentages of patients in each treatment group:

Table 2
Percent of Patients with Adverse Reactions

Adverse Reactions:	Alferon® (n = 104)	Placebo (n = 85)
Autonomic Nervous System		
Sweating	2%	1%
Vasovagal Reaction	2%	0%
Body as a Whole		
Fever	40%	19%
Chills	14%	2%
Fatigue	14%	6%
Malaise	9%	9%
Skin		
Generalized Pruritis	2%	0%
Central & Peripheral Nervous System		
Dizziness	9%	4%
Insomnia	2%	1%
Gastrointestinal System		
Nausea	4%	7%
Vomiting	3%	0%
Dyspepsia/Heartburn	3%	1%
Diarrhea	2%	2%
Musculoskeletal System		
Arthralgia	5%	1%
Back Pain	4%	1%
Myalgias	45%	15%
Headache	31%	15%
Psychiatric Disorders		
Depression	2%	1%
Nasopharyngeal		
Nose/sinus drainage	2%	2%

Most of the systemic adverse reactions were mild or moderate. Severe systemic adverse reactions were reported by 18% of Alferon® N Injection [Interferon alfa-n3 (Human Leukocyte Derived)]-treated patients and 13% of placebo-treated patients (not a statistically significant difference). Most of the severe systemic adverse reactions reported were "flu-like". Other severe systemic adverse reactions included back pain, insomnia, and sensitivity to allergens. Those adverse reactions which were reported by 1% of patients treated with Alferon® N Injection in the double-blind trial include: left groin lymph node swelling, tongue hyperaesthesia, thirst, tingling of legs/feet, hot sensation on bottom of feet, strange taste in mouth, increased salivation, heat intolerance, visual disturbances, pharyngitis, sensitivity to allergens, muscle cramps, nose bleed, throat tightness, and papular rash on neck. Additional adverse reactions which were reported by 1% of patients treated with placebo include: pharyngitis, oral pain, penile discharge, cold, knuckle stiffness, herpes outbreak, cough, disorientation, and weight/appetite loss.

Additional adverse reactions which occurred only in open clinical trials of intralesional use of Alferon® N Injection for treatment of condylomata acuminata were herpes labialis, hot flashes, nervousness, decrease in concentration, dysuria, photosensitivity, and swollen lymph nodes. These reactions occurred in 1% of the patients. One patient with a history of epilepsy, who was not taking anticonvulsant medication, had a grand mal seizure while being treated with Alferon® N Injection; this seizure was judged to be unrelated to Alferon® N Injection administration.

Application Site Disorders The frequency of application site disorders (such as itching and pain) for patients treated with Alferon® N Injection was significantly less than that reported with placebo (12% versus 26%). No severe application site disorders were reported by patients treated with Alferon® N Injection, while 7% of placebo-treated patients reported severe disorders.

Labortory Test Values Abnormalities were seen with statistically equivalent frequencies in both the Alferon® N Injection and placebo groups. None of the laboratory abnormalities were considered clinically significant. The abnormalities in the Alferon® N Injection [Interferon alfa-n3 (Human Leukocyte Derived)]-treated patients consisted primarily of decreased WBC (11%). Decreases also occurred in 4% of the placebo patients (not a statistically significant difference). The abnormalities in Alferon® N Injection-treated patients involved increases of only one WHO grade.

Adverse Reactions in Patients with Cancer Thirty-one patients with cancer were treated with a maximum of ten intramuscular injections of Alferon® N Injection in doses of 3 million IU, 9 million IU, or 15 million IU per treatment session. The occurrence of adverse reactions was judged to be unrelated to the dose of Alferon® N Injection. The following adverse reactions were reported at least once (the percentage of patients experiencing the reaction is indicated in parentheses): chills (87%), fever (81%), anorexia (68%), malaise (65%), nausea (48%), vomiting (29%), myalgias (16%), arthralgia (10%), chest pains (10%), soreness at injection site (10%), sleepiness (10%), headache (10%), diarrhea (6%), fatigue (6%), low blood pressure (6%), sore mouth/stomatitis (6%), and blurred vision (6%). Those adverse reactions which were each reported by only one patient treated with Alferon® N Injection include: stiff shoulders, face flushed, edema, dry mouth, mucositis, coughing, numbness, numbness in hands, numbness in fingers, pain on ocular rotation, shakes/shivers, ringing in ears, cramps, constipation, muscle soreness, confusion, light-headedness, depression, upset stomach, and sweating. The following adverse

Continued on next page

Purdue Frederick—Cont.

reactions were reported as severe by at least one patient (the percentage of patients experiencing the reaction is indicated in parentheses): fever (55%), malaise (54%), anorexia (45%), chills (45%), nausea (16%), myalgias (13%), vomiting (10%), fatigue (6%), low blood pressure (6%), chest pains (6%), sore mouth/stomatitis (6%), headache (3%), diarrhea (3%), sleepiness (3%), arthralgia (3%), blurred vision (3%), stiff shoulders (3%), numbness (3%), pain on ocular rotation (3%), muscle soreness (3%), confusion (3%), light-headedness (3%), depression (3%), and sweating (3%).

The number and percentage of patients with cancer who experienced a significant abnormal laboratory test value (values that changed from WHO Grades 0, 1, or 2 at baseline to WHO Grades 3 or 4 during or after treatment) at least once during the trials are shown in the following table:

Table 3
Abnormal Laboratory Test Values

	Cancer (n = 31)
Hemoglobin Level	2 (7%)
White Blood Cell Count	1 (3%)
Platelet Count	1 (3%)
GGT	1 (6%)
SGOT	1 (3%)
Alkaline Phosphatase	2 (8%)
Total Bilirubin	1 (4%)

DOSAGE AND ADMINISTRATION

The recommended dose of Alferon® N Injection [Interferon alfa-n3 (Human Leukocyte Derived)] for the treatment of condylomata acuminata is 0.05 ml (250,000 IU) per wart. Alferon® N Injection should be administered twice weekly for up to 8 weeks. The maximum recommended dose per treatment session is 0.5 ml (2.5 million IU). Alferon® N Injection should be injected into the base of each wart, preferably using a 30 gauge needle. For large warts, Alferon® N Injection may be injected at several points around the periphery of the wart, using a total dose of 0.05 ml per wart. The minimum effective dose of Alferon® N Injection for the treatment of condylomata acuminata has not been established. Moderate to severe adverse experiences may require modification of the dosage regimen or, in some cases, termination of therapy with Alferon® N Injection.

Genital warts usually begin to disappear after several weeks of treatment with Alferon® N Injection. Treatment should continue for a maximum of 8 weeks. In clinical trials with Alferon® N Injection, many patients who had partial resolution of warts during treatment experienced further resolution of their warts after cessation of treatment. Of the patients who had complete resolution of warts due to treatment, half the patients had complete resolution of warts by the end of the treatment and half had complete resolution of warts during the 3 months after cessation of treatment. Thus, it is recommended that no further therapy (Alferon® N Injection or conventional therapy) be administered for 3 months after the initial 8-week course of treatment unless the warts enlarge or new warts appear. Studies to determine the safety and efficacy of a second course of treatment with Alferon® N Injection [Interferon alfa-n3 (Human Leukocyte Derived)] have not been conducted.

Parenteral drug products should be inspected visually for particulate matter and discoloration prior to administration, whenever solution and container permit.

HOW SUPPLIED

Injectable Solution: 5 Million IU Alferon® N Injection per vial. Each vial contains 1 ml of Alferon® N Injection. Each ml of Alferon® N Injection contains 5 million IU of Interferon alfa-n3, 3.3 mg of phenol, and 1 mg of Albumin (Human) in a pH 7.4 phosphate buffered saline solution (8.0 mg/ml sodium chloride, 1.74 mg/ml sodium phosphate dibasic, 0.20 mg/ml potassium phosphate monobasic, and 0.20 mg/ml potassium chloride). One vial per box. (NDC 0034-1019-01).

STORAGE

Alferon® N Injection should be stored at 2° to 8°C (36° to 46°F). Do not freeze. Do not shake.
CAUTION: FEDERAL (U.S.A.) LAW PROHIBITS DISPENSING WITHOUT PRESCRIPTION.

REFERENCES

1. Friedman-Kien, AE, Eron, LJ, Conant, M, et al., *JAMA*, *259*: 533–538, 1988.
2. Kirby, P. (editorial comment), *JAMA*, *259*: 570–572, 1988.
3. Friedman-Kien, AE, Plasse, TF, et al., *Papilloma Viruses: Molecular and Clinical Aspects* [Howley, PM, Broker, TR (eds)], New York, Alan R. Liss, Inc., 1986, pp. 217–233.
4. Geffen, JR, Klein, RJ, Friedman-Kien, AE, *J Infect. Dis.*, *150*: 612–615, 1984.
5. Kauppila, A, et al., *Int. J. Cancer*, *29*: 291–294, 1982.
6. Trown, PW, et al., *Cancer*, *57* (Suppl):1648–1656, 1986.
7. Schafer, TW, et al., *Science*, *176*: 1326–1327, 1972.

Manufactured by:
Interferon Sciences, Inc.
783 Jersey Avenue
New Brunswick, NJ 08901
U.S. Lic. No. 930
Distributed by:
The Purdue Frederick Company
100 Connecticut Avenue
Norwalk, CT 06850-3590
01-B-01   8/90   B3126

BETADINE® FIRST AID CREAM   OTC
[bā'tăh-dĭn"]
(povidone-iodine, 5%)

ACTION AND USES

BETADINE First Aid Cream is a topical antiseptic containing 5% povidone-iodine (PVP-I) in an oil-in-water emulsion. It is virtually nonirritating, nonstinging and nonburning when applied to open cuts, burns or scrapes. It kills most bacteria and other pathogens virtually on contact. It enhances healing of minor wounds and has a very broad spectrum of microbicidal activity.
BETADINE First Aid Cream is easy to apply and remove. It is preservative-free.

ADMINISTRATION

Apply directly to affected area as needed. May be bandaged.

WARNINGS

For External Use Only. In case of deep or puncture wounds or serious burns, consult physician. If redness, irritation, swelling or pain persists or increases, or if infection occurs, discontinue use and consult physician. Keep out of reach of children.

SUPPLIED

½ oz. plastic tube, with an applicator tip for easy and economical application.
Copyright 1991, 1996. The Purdue Frederick Company

BETADINE®   OTC
BRAND First Aid Antibiotics + Moisturizer Ointment
[Bā'tăh-dĭn"]
Each gram contains: Polymyxin B Sulfate (10,000 IU) and Bacitracin Zinc (500 IU) in a cholesterolized ointment base.

ACTION AND USES

BETADINE Brand First Aid Antibiotics + Moisturizer Ointment is a topical antibiotic in a cholesterolized ointment base. It is formulated to help heal and prevent infection in minor cuts, scrapes and burns.

ADVANTAGES

Its unique formula of two broad-spectrum antibiotics plus moisturizer fights infection while helping to heal damaged skin.

ADMINISTRATION

Clean affected area. Apply small amount (an amount equal to the surface area of the tip of the finger) on the area 1 to 3 times daily. May be covered with a sterile bandage.

WARNINGS

For External Use Only. Do not use in the eyes or apply over large areas of the body. In case of deep or puncture wounds, animal bites, or serious burns, consult a physician. Stop use and consult a physician if the condition persists or gets worse. Do not use longer than 1 week unless directed by a physician. Keep this and all medications out of the reach of children. In case of accidental ingestion, seek professional assistance or contact a Poison Control Center immediately.

SUPPLIED

½ oz. & 1 oz. plastic tubes, with an applicator-tip for easy and economical application.
Copyright 1996, The Purdue Frederick Company

BETADINE® MEDICATED GEL   OTC
[bā'tăh-dĭn"]
(povidone-iodine, 10%)

ACTION AND USES

BETADINE Medicated Gel provides prompt, soothing, symptomatic relief of minor vaginal irritation, itching and soreness associated with vaginitis due to *Candida albicans*, *Trichomonas vaginalis*, and *Gardnerella vaginalis*. Offers relief from annoying vaginal symptoms and odor.

ADVANTAGES

Its gel formulation is convenient for evening application to irritated vaginal tissue. It is gentle and virtually nonirritating to delicate vaginal tissue. It is nongreasy and nonsticky. Its active ingredient—the broad-spectrum microbicide povidone-iodine—significantly and rapidly reduces the aerobic and anaerobic bacterial count.

DIRECTIONS FOR USE

Insert one applicatorful of BETADINE Medicated Gel. A sanitary napkin should be worn. When external irritation is present, it may be applied manually to the affected area. Treatment should be continued for seven days.

WARNINGS

Do not use during pregnancy or while nursing except with the approval of your physician. If symptoms persist after seven days of treatment, or redness, swelling or pain develops, discontinue use and consult physician. Women with iodine sensitivity should not use this product. Keep out of reach of children.

HOW SUPPLIED

18 g tubes (approximately 1 use) and 3 oz. tubes (approximately 14 uses), each packaged with a convenient, easy-to-use vaginal applicator.
Copyright 1991, 1996. The Purdue Frederick Company

BETADINE® MEDICATED DOUCHE   OTC
CONCENTRATE
[bā'tăh-dĭn"]
(povidone-iodine, 10%)

A pleasantly scented solution, BETADINE Medicated Douche is indicated for the prompt symptomatic relief of minor vaginal irritation, itching and soreness. May be used as a cleansing douche.

ADVANTAGES

Low surface tension, with uniform wetting action to assist penetration into vaginal crypts and crevices. Microbicidal activity is retained in the presence of moderate quantities of blood, pus, mucosal secretions and soap and water. Virtually nonirritating to vaginal mucosa. Will not stain skin or natural fabrics.

DIRECTIONS FOR USE

Professional Labeling
Suggested Regimen For Therapeutic Use: In the office, swab the cervix and vulvovaginal area with BETADINE Solution. Prescribe BETADINE Medicated Douche: Two tablespoonfuls of BETADINE Douche Concentrate or two ½ fl. oz. packets to a quart of lukewarm water once daily for five days. If further therapy is warranted, douching should be continued through the next cycle. The patient may be instructed to return for an office visit following two weeks of therapy.
Directions For Deodorizing and Cleansing Douche: Two (2) tablespoonfuls of BETADINE Douche Concentrate to a quart of lukewarm water once or twice per week.
Directions for prompt symptomatic relief of minor vaginal irritation and itching: Fill 2 capfuls (2 tablespoonfuls) with douche. Mix with a quart of lukewarm water. Repeat procedure each day and use once daily for five days. Continue use for the full five days, even if symptoms are relieved earlier.

WARNINGS

Douching does not prevent pregnancy. Do not use during pregnancy or while nursing except with the approval of your physician. If symptoms persist after five days of use, or redness, swelling or pain develops, discontinue use and consult a physician. As a cleansing and deodorizing douche, do not use more often than twice weekly. Women with iodine sensitivity should not use this product. Douching is reported to be associated with Pelvic Inflammatory Disease, a serious infection of the reproductive system. Keep out of reach of children.

HOW SUPPLIED

1 oz. and 8 oz. plastic bottles. Disposable ½ oz. (1 tablespoonful) packets. Also available: BETADINE Medicated Douche Kit 8 oz. (approximately 20 uses), BETADINE Medicated Disposable Douche (single- and twin-pack) and BETADINE Pre-Mixed Medicated Disposable Douche, which requires no measuring or mixing (single- and twin-pack).
Copyright 1991, 1996. The Purdue Frederick Company
Norwalk, CT 06850-3590

BETADINE® OINTMENT OTC
[bā'tăh-dīn"]
(povidone-iodine, 10%)

ACTION
Betadine ointment, in a water-soluble base, is a topical microbicide active against organisms commonly encountered in skin and wound infections.

INDICATIONS
Therapeutically, It may be used as an adjunct to systemic therapy where indicated; for primary or secondary topical infections, infected surgical incisions, infected decubitus or stasis ulcers, pyodermas, secondarily infected dermatoses, and infected traumatic lesions.
Prophylactically: It may be used to prevent microbial contamination in burns, incisions and other topical lesions; for degerming skin in hyperalimentation and catheter care. Its use for abrasions, minor cuts and wounds may prevent the development of infections and permit wound healing.

ADMINISTRATION
Apply directly to affected area as needed. Nonocclusion allows air to reach the wound. May be bandaged.

WARNINGS
For External Use Only. In case of deep or puncture wounds or serious burns, consult physician. If redness, irritation, swelling or pain persists or increases, or if infection occurs, discontinue use and consult physician. Keep out of reach of children.

SUPPLIED
1/32 oz. and 1/8 oz. packettes; 1 oz. tubes; 16 oz. (1 lb.).
Copyright 1991, 1996. The Purdue Frederick Company

BETADINE® SKIN CLEANSER OTC
[bā'tăh-dīn"]
(povidone-iodine, 7.5%)

BETADINE Skin Cleanser, a sudsing, antiseptic bactericidal, virucidal liquid cleanser, forms a rich, golden lather.

INDICATIONS
Aids in degerming the skin of patients with common pathogens, including *Staphylococcus aureus*. To help prevent the recurrence of acute inflammatory skin infections caused by iodine-susceptible pyogenic bacteria. In pyodermas, as a topical adjunct to systemic antimicrobial therapy. Aids in removal of foreign material such as dirt and debris.

DIRECTIONS FOR USE
Wet the skin, apply a sufficient amount to work up a rich golden lather. Allow lather to remain about 3 minutes. Then rinse thoroughly with water. Repeat 2–3 times a day or as directed by physician.

WARNINGS
For External Use Only. In case of deep or puncture wounds or serious burns, consult physician. If redness, irritation, swelling or pain persists or increases, or if infection occurs, discontinue use and consult physician. Keep out of reach of children.

HOW SUPPLIED
1 fl. oz. and 4 fl. oz. plastic bottles.

NOTE
Blue stains on starched linen will wash off with soap and water.
Copyright 1991, 1996. The Purdue Frederick Company

BETADINE® SOLUTION OTC
[bā'tăh-dīn"]
(povidone-iodine, 10%)
Topical Antiseptic Bactericide/Virucide

INDICATIONS
For preoperative prepping of operative site, including the vagina, and as a general topical bactericide/virucide for: disinfection of wounds; emergency treatment of lacerations and abrasions; second- and third-degree burns; as a prophylactic anti-infective agent in hospital and office procedures, including postoperative application to incisions to help prevent infection; oral moniliasis (thrush); bacterial and mycotic skin infections; decubitus and stasis ulcers; as a preoperative swab in the mouth and throat.

ADMINISTRATION
Apply full strength as often as needed as a paint, spray, or wet soak. May be bandaged.

WARNINGS
For External Use Only. In preoperative prepping, avoid "pooling" beneath the patient. Prolonged exposure to wet solution may cause irritation or rarely, severe skin reactions.

In rare instance of local irritation or sensitivity, discontinue use. Do not heat prior to application.

HOW SUPPLIED
1/2 oz., 4 oz., 8 oz., 16 oz. (1 pt.), 32 oz. (1 qt.) and 1 gal. plastic bottles and 1 oz. packettes.

ALSO AVAILABLE
BETADINE® Solution Swab Aid® Pads for degerming small areas of skin or mucous membranes prior to injections, aspirations, catheterization and surgery; boxes of 100 packettes. Also: disposable BETADINE® Solution Swabsticks, in packettes of 1's and 3's. BETADINE® Aerosol Spray in 3 oz. bottles.
Copyright 1991, 1996. The Purdue Frederick Company

BETADINE® SURGICAL SCRUB OTC
[bā'tăh-dīn"]
(povidone-iodine, 7.5%)
Topical Antiseptic Bactericide/Virucide

INDICATIONS
A broad-spectrum antiseptic, bactericidal, virucidal sudsing skin cleanser for pre- and postoperative scrubbing or washing by hospital operating room personnel; for preoperative use on patients; and general use as an antiseptic microbicide in physician's office. Forms rich, golden lather.

DIRECTIONS FOR USE
A.   For Preoperative Washing by Operating Personnel
1.   Wet hands and forearms with water. Pour about 5 cc. (1 teaspoonful) of BETADINE Surgical Scrub on the palm of the hand and spread over both hands and forearms. Without adding more water, rub the Scrub thoroughly over all areas for about five minutes. Use a brush if desired. Clean thoroughly under fingernails. Add a little water and develop copious suds. Rinse thoroughly under running water.
2.   Complete the wash by scrubbing with another 5 cc. of BETADINE Surgical Scrub in the same way.

B.   For Preoperative Use on Patients
After the skin area is shaved, wet it with water. Apply BETADINE Surgical Scrub (1 cc. is sufficient to cover an area of 20-30 square inches), develop lather and scrub thoroughly for about five minutes. Rinse off by aid of sterile gauze saturated with water. The area may then be painted with BETADINE Solution or sprayed with BETADINE Aerosol Spray and allowed to dry.

C.   For Use in the Physician's Office
Use for washing whenever a germicidal soap is required. For maximum degerming of the hands proceed as under (A). To prepare the patient's skin proceed as under (B).
Note: Blue stains on starched linen will wash off with soap and water.

WARNINGS
For External Use Only. Do not heat prior to application. In rare instances of local irritation or sensitivity, discontinue use. Keep out of reach of children.

SUPPLIED
16 oz. (1 pint) plastic bottle with and without pump, 32 oz. (1 quart) and 1 gal. plastic bottles, and 1/2 oz. packettes.
Copyright 1991, 1996. The Purdue Frederick Company
Norwalk, CT 06850-3590

BETADINE® MEDICATED VAGINAL SUPPOSITORIES OTC
[bā'tăh-dīn"]
(povidone-iodine, 10%)

ACTION AND USES
Provides prompt symptomatic relief of minor vaginal irritation, itching and soreness. Its active ingredient—the broad-spectrum microbicide povidone-iodine—significantly and rapidly reduces the aerobic and anaerobic microbial count. Offers soothing relief from annoying vaginal symptoms and odor.

ADVANTAGES
Each measured-dose suppository is convenient for application to irritated vaginal tissue in the evening or at night. The suppositories are gentle and virtually nonirritating to delicate vaginal tissue. Nonstaining to skin and natural fabrics, color can be washed off with soap and water.

DIRECTIONS FOR USE
1. Unwrap a suppository and gently insert its smaller end into the applicator. 2. Lie down, insert the applicator high into the vagina, then push plunger to release the suppository. Wear a sanitary napkin. 3. To clean, push plunger out of tube, wash both parts in hot water, then replace plunger. 4. Continue treatment for seven days.

WARNINGS
Do not use during pregnancy or while nursing except with the approval of your physician. If symptoms persist after seven days of treatment, or redness, swelling or pain develops, discontinue use and consult your physician. Women with iodine sensitivity should not use this product. Keep out of reach of children.

HOW SUPPLIED
7 Suppositories packaged with a convenient, easy-to-use applicator and patient instruction booklet.
Copyright 1991, 1996. The Purdue Frederick Company

BETASEPT® Surgical Scrub 4% OTC
[bā'tăh-sĕp-t"]
(chlorhexidine gluconate)

ACTION AND USES
BETASEPT Surgical Scrub (chlorhexidine gluconate) is an antiseptic/antimicrobial skin cleanser for hand scrubbing or washing by operating room personnel, for hand-washing by medical personnel, for pre-operative skin preparation, and for skin wound and general skin cleansing.
BETASEPT Surgical Scrub provides rapid bactericidal action and has a persistent antimicrobial effect against a wide range of microorganisms.

ADVANTAGES
BETASEPT Surgical Scrub is uniquely kind to hands, helping to reduce drying and roughness—a feature that encourages hospital personnel to follow correct hand-washing procedures.
BETASEPT Surgical Scrub is formulated in a highly viscous base which can help reduce waste and per-use cost during prepping and hand-washing. No unnecessary pink tint has been added.

DIRECTIONS FOR USE
Surgical Hand Scrub:
Wet hands and forearms with water. Scrub for 3 minutes with about 5 mL of BETASEPT Surgical Scrub and a wet brush, paying particular attention to the nails, cuticles and interdigital spaces. A separate nail cleaner may be used. Rinse thoroughly. Wash for an additional 3 minutes with 5 mL of BETASEPT Surgical Scrub and rinse under running water. Dry thoroughly.
Personnel Hand Wash:
Wet hands with water. Dispense about 5 mL of BETASEPT Surgical Scrub into cupped hands and wash in a vigorous manner for 15 seconds. Rinse and dry thoroughly.
Pre-Operative Skin Preparation:
Apply BETASEPT Surgical Scrub liberally to surgical site and swab for at least 2 minutes. Dry with a sterile towel. Repeat procedure for an additional 2 minutes and again dry with a sterile towel.
Skin Wound and General Skin Cleansing:
Wounds which involve more than the superficial layers of the skin should not be routinely treated with BETASEPT Surgical Scrub. BETASEPT Surgical Scrub should not be used for repeated general skin cleansing of large body areas except in those patients whose underlying condition makes it necessary to reduce the bacterial population of the skin. To use, thoroughly rinse the area to be cleansed with water. Apply the minimum amount of BETASEPT Surgical Scrub necessary to cover the skin or wound area and wash gently. Rinse again thoroughly.

WARNINGS
FOR EXTERNAL USE ONLY. KEEP OUT OF EYES, EARS AND MOUTH. BETASEPT SURGICAL SCRUB SHOULD NOT BE USED AS A PRE-OPERATIVE SKIN PREPARATION OF THE FACE OR HEAD. MISUSE OF PRODUCTS CONTAINING CHLORHEXIDINE GLUCONATE HAS BEEN REPORTED TO CAUSE SERIOUS AND PERMANENT EYE INJURY WHEN IT HAS BEEN PERMITTED TO ENTER AND REMAIN IN THE EYE DURING SURGICAL PROCEDURES. IF BETASEPT SURGICAL SCRUB SHOULD CONTACT THESE AREAS, RINSE OUT PROMPTLY AND THOROUGHLY WITH WATER.
Avoid contact with meninges. Betasept Surgical Scrub should not be used by persons who have sensitivity to it or its components. Chlorhexidine gluconate has been reported to cause deafness when instilled in the middle ear through perforated ear drums. Irritation, sensitization and generalized allergic reactions have been reported with chlorhexidine-containing products, especially in the genital areas. If adverse reactions occur, discontinue use immediately and if severe, contact a physician. Keep this and all drugs out of the reach of children. In case of accidental ingestion, seek professional assistance or contact a Poison Control Center immediately.
Avoid excessive heat (above 104°F).

Continued on next page

Purdue Frederick—Cont.

HOW SUPPLIED

BETASEPT Surgical Scrub 4% is packaged in 1 gallon, 32 oz., 32 oz. with pump, 16 oz., 8 oz., and 4 oz. plastic bottles.

Copyright 1993, 1996, The Purdue Frederick Company, Norwalk, CT 06850-3590

CARDIOQUIN® ℞

(quinidine polygalacturonate)
tablets

DESCRIPTION

Quinidine is an antimalarial schizonticide and an antiarrhythmic agent with class 1a activity; it is the d-isomer of quinine, and its molecular weight is 324.43. Quinidine polygalacturonate is a polymer of quinidine and galacturonic acid; its structural formula is

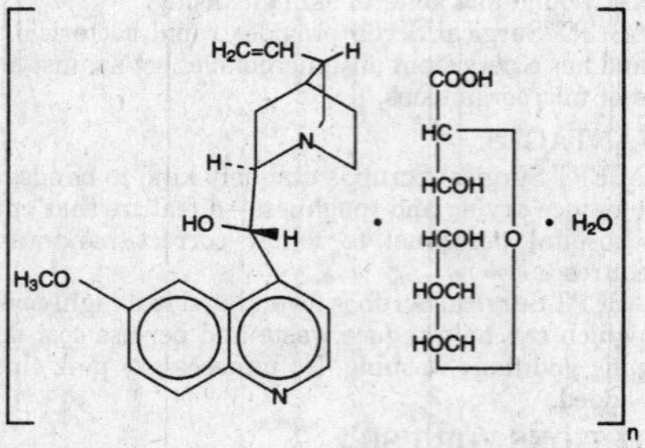

and its empirical formula is $(C_{20}H_{24}N_2O_2{\bullet}C_6H_{10}O_7{\bullet}H_2O)_n$. The molecular weight of the monomer is 536.58, of which 60.46% is quinidine base. Quinidine polygalacturonate is a creamy white, amorphous powder, sparingly soluble in water but freely soluble in hot 40% ethanol. Each CARDIOQUIN tablet contains 275 mg of quinidine polygalacturonate (166 mg of quinidine base); the inactive ingredients include corn starch, lactose, magnesium stearate, povidone, and talc.

CLINICAL PHARMACOLOGY

Pharmacokinetics and Metabolism The absolute bioavailability of orally-administered CARDIOQUIN is about 70%, but this varies widely (45–100%) between patients. The less-than-complete bioavailability is the result of first-pass metabolism in the liver. Peak serum levels generally appear about 2 hours after dosing; absorption is delayed, but not changed in extent, when the drug is taken with food.

The **volume of distribution** of quinidine is 2–3 L/kg in healthy young adults, but this may be reduced to as little as 0.5 L/kg in patients with congestive heart failure, or increased to 3–5 L/kg in patients with cirrhosis of the liver. At concentrations of 2–5 mg/L (6.5–16.2 μmol/L), the fraction of quinidine bound to plasma proteins (mainly to α_1-acid glycoprotein and to albumin) is 80–88% in adults and older children, but it is lower in pregnant women, and in infants and neonates it may be as low as 50–70%. Because α_1-acid glycoprotein levels are increased in response to stress, serum levels of total quinidine may be greatly increased in settings such as acute myocardial infarction, even though the serum content of unbound (active) drug may remain normal. Protein binding is also increased in chronic renal failure, but binding abruptly descends toward or below normal when heparin is administered for hemodialysis.

Quinidine **clearance** typically proceeds at 3–5 mL/min/kg in adults, but clearance in children may be twice or three times as rapid. The elimination half-life is about 6–8 hours in adults and 3–4 hours in children. Quinidine clearance is unaffected by hepatic cirrhosis, so the increased volume of distribution seen in cirrhosis leads to a proportionate increase in the elimination half-life.

Most quinidine is eliminated hepatically via the action of cytochrome P450IIIA4; there are several different hydroxylated metabolites, and some of these have antiarrhythmic activity.

The most important of quinidine's metabolites is 3-hydroxyquinidine (3HQ), serum levels of which can approach those of quinidine in patients receiving conventional doses of CARDIOQUIN. The volume of distribution of 3HQ appears to be larger than that of quinidine, and the elimination half-life of 3HQ is about 12 hours.

As measured by antiarrhythmic effects in animals, by QT_c prolongation in human volunteers, or by various *in vitro* techniques, 3HQ has at least half the antiarrhythmic activity of the parent compound, so it may be responsible for a substantial fraction of the effect of CARDIOQUIN in chronic use.

When the urine pH is less than 7, about 20% of administered quinidine appears unchanged in the urine, but this fraction drops to as little as 5% when the urine is more alkaline. Renal clearance involves both glomerular filtration and active tubular secretion, moderated by (pH-dependent) tubular reabsorption. The net renal clearance is about 1 mL/min/kg in healthy adults.

When renal function is taken into account, quinidine clearance is apparently independent of patient age.

Assays of serum quinidine levels are widely available, but the results of modern assays may not be consistent with results cited in the older medical literature. The serum levels of quinidine cited in this package insert are those derived from specific assays, using either benzene extraction or (preferably) reverse-phase high-pressure liquid chromatography. In matched samples, older assays might unpredictably have given results that were as much as two or three times higher. A typical "therapeutic" concentration range is 2–6 mg/L (6.2–18.5 μmol/L).

Mechanisms of action In patients with malaria, quinidine acts primarily as an intra-erythrocytic schizonticide, with little effect upon sporozoites or upon pre-erythrocytic parasites. Quinidine is gametocidal to *Plasmodium vivax* and *P. malariae*, but not to *P. falciparum*.

In cardiac muscle and in Purkinje fibers, quinidine depresses the rapid inward depolarizing sodium current, thereby slowing phase-0 depolarization and reducing the amplitude of the action potential without affecting the resting potential. In normal Purkinje fibers, it reduces the slope of phase-4 depolarization, shifting the threshold voltage upward toward zero. The result is slowed conduction and reduced automaticity in all parts of the heart, with increase of the effective refractory period relative to the duration of the action potential in the atria, ventricles, and Purkinje tissues. Quinidine also raises the fibrillation thresholds of the atria and ventricles, and it raises the ventricular defibrillation threshold as well. Quinidine's actions fall into class 1a in the Vaughn-Williams classification.

By slowing conduction and prolonging the effective refractory period, quinidine can interrupt or prevent reentrant arrhythmias and arrhythmias due to increased automaticity, including atrial flutter, atrial fibrillation, and paroxysmal supraventricular tachycardia.

In patients with the sick sinus syndrome, quinidine can cause marked sinus node depression and bradycardia. In most patients, however, quinidine is associated with an increase in sinus rate.

Quinidine prolongs the QT interval in a dose-related fashion. This may lead to increased ventricular automaticity and polymorphic ventricular tachycardias, including *torsades de pointes* (see **Warnings**).

In addition, quinidine has anticholinergic activity, it has negative inotropic activity, and it acts peripherally as an α-adrenergic antagonist (that is, as a vasodilator).

Clinical effects

Maintenance of sinus rhythm after conversion from atrial fibrillation: In six trials (published between 1970 and 1984) with a total of 808 patients, quinidine (418 patients) was compared to nontreatment (258 patients) or placebo (132 patients) for the maintenance of sinus rhythm after cardioversion from chronic atrial fibrillation. Quinidine was consistently more efficacious in maintaining sinus rhythm, but a meta-analysis found that mortality in the quinidine-exposed patients (2.9%) was significantly greater than mortality in the patients who had not been treated with active drug (0.8%). Suppression of atrial fibrillation with quinidine has theoretical patient benefits (*e.g.,* improved exercise tolerance; reduction in hospitalization for cardioversion; lack of arrhythmia-related palpitations, dyspnea, and chest pain; reduced incidence of systemic embolism and/or stroke), but these benefits have never been demonstrated in clinical trials. Some of these benefits (*e.g.,* reduction in stroke incidence) may be achievable by other means (anticoagulation).

By slowing the rate of atrial flutter/fibrillation, quinidine can decrease the degree of atrioventricular block and cause an increase, sometimes marked, in the rate at which supraventricular impulses are successfully conducted by the atrioventricular node, with a resultant paradoxical increase in ventricular rate (see **Warnings**).

Non-life-threatening ventricular arrhythmias: In studies of patients with a variety of ventricular arrhythmias (mainly frequent ventricular premature beats and non-sustained ventricular tachycardia), quinidine (total N=502) has been compared to flecainide (N=141), mexiletine (N=246), propafenone (N=53), and tocainide (N=67). In each of these studies, the mortality in the quinidine group was numerically greater than the mortality in the comparator group. When the studies were combined in a meta-analysis, quinidine was associated with a statistically significant threefold relative risk of death.

At therapeutic doses, quinidine's only consistent effect upon the surface electrocardiogram is an increase in the QT interval. This prolongation can be monitored as a guide to safety, and it may provide better guidance than serum drug levels (see **Warnings**).

INDICATIONS AND USAGE

Conversion of atrial fibrillation/flutter: In patients with symptomatic atrial fibrillation/flutter whose symptoms are not adequately controlled by measures that reduce the rate of ventricular response, CARDIOQUIN is indicated as a means of restoring normal sinus rhythm. If this use of CARDIOQUIN does not restore sinus rhythm within a reasonable time (see **Dosage and Administration**), then CARDIOQUIN should be discontinued.

Reduction of frequency of relapse into atrial fibrillation/flutter: Chronic therapy with CARDIOQUIN is indicated for some patients at high risk of symptomatic atrial fibrillation/flutter, generally patients who have had previous episodes of atrial fibrillation/flutter that were so frequent and poorly tolerated as to outweigh, in the judgment of the physician and the patient, the risks of prophylactic therapy with CARDIOQUIN. The increased risk of death should specifically be considered. CARDIOQUIN should be used only after alternative measures (*e.g.,* use of other drugs to control the ventricular rate) have been found to be inadequate.

In patients with histories of frequent symptomatic episodes of atrial fibrillation/flutter, the goal of therapy should be an increase in the average time between episodes. In most patients, the tachyarrhythmia *will recur* during therapy, and a single recurrence should not be interpreted as therapeutic failure.

Suppression of ventricular arrhythmias: CARDIOQUIN is also indicated for the suppression of recurrent documented ventricular arrhythmias, such as sustained ventricular tachycardia, that in the judgment of the physician are life-threatening. Because of the proarrhythmic effects of quinidine, its use with ventricular arrhythmias of lesser severity is generally not recommended, and treatment of patients with asymptomatic ventricular premature contractions should be avoided. Where possible, therapy should be guided by the results of programmed electrical stimulation and/or Holter monitoring with exercise.

Antiarrhythmic drugs (including CARDIOQUIN) have not been shown to enhance survival in patients with ventricular arrhythmias.

CONTRAINDICATIONS

Quinidine is contraindicated in patients who are known to be allergic to it, or who have developed thrombocytopenic purpura during prior therapy with quinidine or quinine.

In the absence of a functioning artificial pacemaker, quinidine is also contraindicated in any patient whose cardiac rhythm is dependent upon a junctional or idioventricular pacemaker, including patients in complete atrioventricular block.

Quinidine is also contraindicated in patients who, like those with myasthenia gravis, might be adversely affected by an anticholinergic agent.

WARNINGS

Mortality:

> **In many trials of antiarrhythmic therapy for non-life-threatening arrhythmias, active antiarrhythmic therapy has resulted in increased mortality; the risk of active therapy is probably greatest in patients with structural heart disease.**
>
> **In the case of quinidine used to prevent or defer recurrence of atrial flutter/fibrillation, the best available data come from a meta-analysis described under** Clinical Pharmacology/Clinical Effects **above. In the patients studied in the trials there analyzed, the mortality associated with the use of quinidine was more than three times as great as the mortality associated with the use of placebo.**
>
> **Another meta-analysis, also described under** Clinical Pharmacology/Clinical Effects, **showed that in patients with various non-life-threatening ventricular arrhythmias, the mortality associated with the use of quinidine was consistently greater than that associated with the use of any of a variety of alternative antiarrhythmics.**

Proarrhythmic effects: Like many other drugs (including all other class 1a antiarrhythmics), quinidine prolongs the QT_c interval, and this can lead to *torsades de pointes*, a life-threatening ventricular arrhythmia (see **Overdosage**). The risk of *torsades* is increased by any of: bradycardia, hypokalemia, hypomagnesemia, and high serum levels of quinidine, but it may appear in the absence of any of these risk factors. The best predictor of this arrhythmia appears to be the length of the QT_c interval, and quinidine should be used with extreme care in patients who have preexisting long-QT syndromes, who have histories of *torsades de pointes* of any cause, or who have previously responded to quinidine (or other drugs that prolong ventricular repolarization) with marked lengthening of the QT_c interval. Estimation of the incidence of *torsades* in patients with therapeutic levels of quinidine is not possible from the available data.

Other ventricular arrhythmias that have been reported with quinidine include frequent extrasystoles, ventricular tachycardia, ventricular flutter, and ventricular fibrillation.

Paradoxical increase in ventricular rate in atrial flutter/fibrillation: When quinidine is administered to patients with atrial flutter/fibrillation, the desired pharmacologic reversion to sinus rhythm may (rarely) be preceded by a slowing of the atrial rate with a consequent increase in the rate of beats conducted to the ventricles. The resulting ventricular rate may be very high (greater than 200 beats per minute) and poorly tolerated. This hazard may be decreased if partial atrioventricular block is achieved prior to initiation of quinidine therapy, using conduction-reducing drugs such as digitalis, verapamil, diltiazem, or a β-receptor blocking agent.

Exacerbated bradycardia in sick sinus syndrome: In patients with the sick sinus syndrome, quinidine has been associated with marked sinus node depression and bradycardia.

Pharmacokinetic considerations: Renal or hepatic dysfunction causes the elimination of quinidine to be slowed, while congestive heart failure causes a reduction in quinidine's apparent volume of distribution. Any of these conditions can lead to quinidine toxicity if dosage is not appropriately reduced. In addition, interactions with coadministered drugs can alter the serum concentration and activity of quinidine, leading either to toxicity or to lack of efficacy if the dose of quinidine is not appropriately modified (see **Precautions/Drug Interactions**).

Vagolysis: Because quinidine opposes the atrial and A-V nodal effects of vagal stimulation, physical or pharmacological vagal maneuvers undertaken to terminate paroxysmal supraventricular tachycardia may be ineffective in patients receiving quinidine.

PRECAUTIONS

Heart block: In patients without implanted pacemakers who are at high risk of complete atrioventricular block (e.g., those with digitalis intoxication, second-degree atrioventricular block, or severe intraventricular conduction defects), quinidine should be used only with caution.

Drug Interactions

Altered pharmacokinetics of quinidine: Drugs that alkalinize the urine (**carbonic-anhydrase inhibitors, sodium bicarbonate, thiazide diuretics**) reduce renal elimination of quinidine.

By pharmacokinetic mechanisms that are not well understood, quinidine levels are increased by coadministration of **amiodarone** or **cimetidine**. Very rarely, and again by mechanisms not understood, quinidine levels are decreased by coadministration of **nifedipine**.

Hepatic elimination of quinidine may be accelerated by coadministration of drugs (**phenobarbital, phenytoin, rifampin**) that induce production of cytochrome P450IIIA4.

Perhaps because of competition for the P450IIIA4 metabolic pathway, quinidine levels rise when **ketoconazole** is coadministered.

Coadministration of propranolol usually does not affect quinidine pharmacokinetics, but in some studies the β-blocker appeared to cause increases in the peak serum levels of quinidine, decreases in quinidine's volume of distribution, and decreases in total quinidine clearance. The effects (if any) of coadministration of other β-blockers on quinidine pharmacokinetics have not been adequately studied.

Hepatic clearance of quinidine is significantly reduced during coadministration of **verapamil**, with corresponding increases in serum levels and half-life.

Altered pharmacokinetics of other drugs: Quinidine slows the elimination of **digoxin** and simultaneously reduces digoxin's apparent volume of distribution. As a result, serum digoxin levels may be as much as doubled. When quinidine and digoxin are coadministered, digoxin doses usually need to be reduced. Serum levels of **digitoxin** are also raised when quinidine is coadministered, although the effect appears to be smaller.

By a mechanism that is not understood, quinidine potentiates the anticoagulatory action of **warfarin**, and the anticoagulant dosage may need to be reduced.

Cytochrome P450IID6 is an enzyme critical to the metabolism of many drugs, notably including **mexiletine**, some phenothiazines, and most polycyclic antidepressants. Constitutional deficiency of cytochrome P450IID6 is found in less than 1% of Orientals, in about 2% of American blacks, and in some 8% of American whites.

Testing with debrisoquine is sometimes used to distinguish the P450IID6-deficient "poor metabolizers" from the majority-phenotype "extensive metabolizers."

When drugs whose metabolism is P450IID6-dependent are given to poor metabolizers, the serum levels achieved are higher, sometimes much higher, than the serum levels achieved when identical doses are given to extensive metabolizers. To obtain similar clinical benefit without toxicity, doses given to poor metabolizers may need to be greatly reduced. In the cases of prodrugs whose actions are actually mediated by P450IID6-produced metabolites (for example, **codeine and hydrocodone**, whose analgesic and antitussive effects appear to be mediated by morphine and hydromor-

phone, respectively), it may not be possible to achieve the desired clinical benefits in poor metabolizers.

Quinidine is not metabolized by cytochrome P450IID6, but therapeutic serum levels of quinidine inhibit the action of cytochrome P450IID6, effectively converting extensive metabolizers into poor metabolizers. Caution must be exercised whenever quinidine is prescribed together with drugs metabolized by cytochrome P450IID6.

Perhaps by competing for pathways of renal clearance, coadministration of quinidine causes an increase in serum levels of **procainamide**.

Serum levels of **haloperidol** are increased when quinidine is coadministered.

Presumably because both drugs are metabolized by cytochrome P450IIIA4, coadministration of quinidine causes variable slowing of the metabolism of **nifedipine**. Interactions with other dihydropyridine calcium-channel blockers have not been reported, but these agents (including **felodipine, nicardipine, and nimodipine**) are all dependent upon P450IIIA4 for metabolism, so similar interactions with quinidine should be anticipated.

Altered pharmacodynamics of other drugs: Quinidine's anticholinergic, vasodilating, and negative inotropic actions may be additive to those of other drugs with these effects, and antagonistic to those of drugs with cholinergic, vasoconstricting, and positive inotropic effects. For example, when quinidine and **verapamil** are coadministered in doses that are each well tolerated as monotherapy, hypotension attributable to additive peripheral α-blockade is sometimes reported.

Quinidine potentiates the actions of depolarizing (succinylcholine, decamethonium) and nondepolarizing (d-tubocurarine, pancuronium) **neuromuscular blocking agents**. These phenomena are not well understood, but they are observed in animal models as well as in humans. In addition, in vitro addition of quinidine to the serum of pregnant women reduces the activity of pseudo-cholinesterase, an enzyme that is essential to the metabolism of succinylcholine.

Non-interaction of quinidine with other drugs: Quinidine has no clinically significant effect on the pharmacokinetics of **diltiazem, flecainide, mephenytoin, metoprolol, propafenone, propranolol, quinine, timolol,** or **tocainide**. Conversely, the pharmacokinetics of quinidine are not significantly affected by **caffeine, ciprofloxacin, digoxin, diltiazem, felodipine, omeprazole,** or **quinine**. Quinidine's pharmacokinetics are also unaffected by cigarette smoking.

Information for patients: Before prescribing CARDIOQUIN as prophylaxis against recurrence of atrial fibrillation, the physician should inform the patient of the risks and benefits to be expected (see **Clinical Pharmacology**). Discussion should include the facts:

- that the goal of therapy will be a reduction (probably not to zero) in the frequency of episodes of atrial fibrillation; and
- that reduced frequency of fibrillatory episodes may be expected, if achieved, to bring symptomatic benefits; but
- that no data are available to show that reduced frequency of fibrillatory episodes will reduce the risks of irreversible harm through stroke or death; and in fact
- that such data as are available suggest that treatment with CARDIOQUIN is likely to increase the patient's risk of death.

Carcinogenesis, mutagenesis, impairment of fertility Animal studies to evaluate quinidine's carcinogenic or mutagenic potential have not been performed. Similarly, there are no animal data as to quinidine's potential to impair fertility.

Pregnancy

Pregnancy Category C. Animal reproductive studies have not been conducted with quinidine. There are no adequate and well-controlled studies in pregnant women. Quinidine should be given to a pregnant woman only if clearly needed. In one neonate whose mother had received quinidine throughout her pregnancy, the serum level of quinidine was equal to that of the mother, with no apparent ill effect. The level of quinidine in amniotic fluid was about three times higher than that found in serum.

Labor and delivery Quinine is known to be oxytocic in humans, but there are no adequate data as to quinidine's effects (if any) on human labor and delivery.

Nursing mothers Quinidine is present in human milk at levels slightly lower than those in maternal serum; a human infant ingesting such milk should (scaling directly by weight) be expected to develop serum quinidine levels at least an order of magnitude lower than those of the mother. On the other hand, the pharmacokinetics and pharmacodynamics of quinidine in human infants have not been adequately studied, and neonates' reduced protein binding of quinidine may increase their risk of toxicity at low total serum levels. Administration of quinidine should (if possible) be avoided in lactating women who continue to nurse.

Geriatric use

Safety and efficacy of quinidine in elderly patients has not been systematically studied.

Pediatric use

In antimalarial trials, quinidine was as safe and effective in pediatric patients as in adults. Notwithstanding the known

pharmacokinetic differences between children and adults (see **Pharmacokinetics and Metabolism**), children in these trials received the same doses (on a mg/kg basis) as adults. Safety and effectiveness of antiarrhythmic use in children have not been established.

ADVERSE REACTIONS

Quinidine preparations have been used for many years, but there are only sparse data from which to estimate the incidence of various adverse reactions. The adverse reactions most frequently reported have consistently been gastrointestinal, including diarrhea, nausea, vomiting, and heartburn/esophagitis. In one study of 245 adult outpatients who received quinidine to suppress premature ventricular contractions, the incidences of reported adverse experiences were as shown in the table below. The most serious quinidine-associated adverse reactions are described above under **Warnings**.

Adverse Experiences in a 245-Patient PVC Trial	Incidence	(%)
diarrhea	85	(35)
"upper gastrointestinal distress"	55	(22)
lightheadedness	37	(15)
headache	18	(7)
fatigue	17	(7)
palpitations	16	(7)
angina-like pain	14	(6)
weakness	13	(5)
rash	11	(5)
visual problems	8	(3)
change in sleep habits	7	(3)
tremor	6	(2)
nervousness	5	(2)
discoordination	3	(1)

Vomiting and diarrhea can occur as isolated reactions to therapeutic levels of quinidine, but they may also be the first signs of **cinchonism**, a syndrome that may also include tinnitus, reversible high-frequency hearing loss, deafness, vertigo, blurred vision, diplopia, photophobia, headache, confusion, and delirium. Cinchonism is most often a sign of chronic quinidine toxicity, but it may appear in sensitive patients after a single moderate dose.

A few cases of **hepatotoxicity**, including granulomatous hepatitis, have been reported in patients receiving quinidine. All of these have appeared during the first few weeks of therapy, and most (not all) have remitted once quinidine was withdrawn.

Autoimmune and inflammatory syndromes associated with quinidine therapy have included fever, urticaria, flushing, exfoliative rash, bronchospasm, psoriaform rash, pruritus and lymphadenopathy, hemolytic anemia, vasculitis, thrombocytopenic purpura, uveitis, angioedema, agranulocytosis, the sicca syndrome, arthralgia, myalgia, elevation in serum levels of skeletal-muscle enzymes, a disorder resembling systemic lupus erythematosus, and pneumonitis.

Convulsions, apprehension, and ataxia have been reported, but it is not clear that these were not simply the results of hypotension and consequent cerebral hypoperfusion. There are many reports of syncope. Acute psychotic reactions have been reported to follow the first dose of quinidine, but these reactions appear to be extremely rare.

Other adverse reactions occasionally reported include depression, mydriasis, disturbed color perception, night blindness, scotomata, optic neuritis, visual field loss, photosensitivity, and abnormalities of pigmentation.

OVERDOSAGE

Overdoses with various oral formulations of quinidine have been well described. Death has been described after a 5-gram ingestion by a toddler, while an adolescent was reported to survive after ingesting 8 grams of quinidine.

The most important ill effects of acute quinidine overdoses are ventricular arrhythmias and hypotension. Other signs and symptoms of overdose may include vomiting, diarrhea, tinnitus, high frequency hearing loss, vertigo, blurred vision, diplopia, photophobia, headache, confusion, and delirium.

Arrhythmias: Serum quinidine levels can be conveniently assayed and monitored, but the electrocardiographic QT_c interval is a better predictor of quinidine-induced ventricular arrhythmias.

The necessary treatment of hemodynamically unstable polymorphic ventricular tachycardia (including torsades de pointes) is withdrawal of treatment with quinidine and either immediate cardioversion or, if a cardiac pacemaker is in place or immediately available, immediate overdrive pacing. After pacing or cardioversion, further treatment must be guided by the length of the QT_c interval.

Quinidine-associated ventricular tachyarrhythmias with normal underlying QT_c intervals have not been adequately studied. Because of the theoretical possibility of QT-prolonging effects that might be additive to those of quinidine, other

Continued on next page

Purdue Frederick—Cont.

antiarrhythmics with Class I (disopyramide, procainamide) or Class III activities should (if possible) be avoided. Similarly, although the use of bretylium in quinidine overdose has not been reported, it is reasonable to expect that the α-blocking properties of bretylium might be additive to those of quinidine, resulting in problematic hypotension.
If the post-cardioversion QT_c interval is prolonged, then the pre-cardioversion polymorphic ventricular tachyarrhythmia was (by definition) *torsades de pointes*. In this case, lidocaine and bretylium are unlikely to be of value, and other Class I antiarrhythmics (disopyramide, procainamide) are likely to exacerbate the situation. Factors contributing to QT_c prolongation (especially hypokalemia and hypomagnesemia) should be sought out and (if possible) aggressively corrected. Prevention of recurrent *torsades* may require sustained overdrive pacing or the cautious administration of isoproterenol (30–150 ng/kg/min).
Hypotension: Quinidine-induced hypotension that is not due to an arrhythmia is likely to be a consequence of quinidine-related α-blockade and vasorelaxation. Simple repletion of central volume (Trendelenburg positioning, saline infusion) may be sufficient therapy; other interventions reported to have been beneficial in this setting are those that increase peripheral vascular resistance, including α-agonist catecholamines (norepinephrine, metaraminol) and the Military Anti-Shock Trousers.
Treatment: To obtain up-to-date information about the treatment of overdose, a good resource is your certified Regional Poison Control Center. Telephone numbers of certified poison control centers are listed in the *Physicians' Desk Reference (PDR)*. In managing overdose, consider the possibilities of multiple-drug overdoses, drug-drug interactions, and unusual drug kinetics in your patient.
Accelerated removal: Adequate studies of orally administered activated charcoal in human overdoses of quinidine have not been reported, but there are animal data showing significant enhancement of systemic elimination following this intervention, and there is at least one human case report in which the elimination half-life of quinidine in the serum was apparently shortened by repeated gastric lavage. Activated charcoal should be avoided if an ileus is present; the conventional dose is 1 gram/kg, administered every 2–6 hours as a slurry with 8 mL/kg of tap water.
Although renal elimination of quinidine might theoretically be accelerated by maneuvers to acidify the urine, such maneuvers are potentially hazardous and of no demonstrated benefit.
Quinidine is not usefully removed from the circulation by dialysis.
Following quinidine overdose, drugs that delay elimination of quinidine (cimetidine, carbonic-anhydrase inhibitors, thiazide diuretics) should be withdrawn unless absolutely required.

DOSAGE AND ADMINISTRATION

The dosage of quinidine varies considerably depending upon the general condition and the cardiovascular state of the patient.
Conversion of atrial fibrillation/flutter to sinus rhythm Especially in patients with known structural heart disease or other risk factors for toxicity, initiation or dose-adjustment of treatment with CARDIOQUIN should generally be performed in a setting where facilities and personnel for monitoring and resuscitation are continuously available. Patients with symptomatic atrial fibrillation/flutter should be treated with CARDIOQUIN only after ventricular rate control (*e.g.*, with digitalis or β-blockers) has failed to provide satisfactory control of symptoms.
Adequate trials have not identified an optimal regimen of CARDIOQUIN for conversion of atrial fibrillation/flutter to sinus rhythm. In one reported regimen, the patient first receives two tablets (550 mg; 333 mg of quinidine base) of CARDIOQUIN every six hours. If this regimen has not resulted in conversion after 4 or 5 doses, then the dose is cautiously increased. If, at any point during administration, the QRS complex widens to 130% of its pre-treatment duration; the QT_c interval widens to 130% of its pre-treatment duration and is then longer than 500 ms; P waves disappear; or the patient develops significant tachycardia, symptomatic bradycardia, or hypotension, then CARDIOQUIN is discontinued and other means of conversion (e.g., direct-current cardioversion) are considered.
Reduction of frequency of relapse into atrial fibrillation/flutter
In a patient with a history of frequent symptomatic episodes of atrial fibrillation/flutter, the goal of therapy with CARDIOQUIN should be an increase in the average time between episodes. In most patients, the tachyarrhythmia *will recur* during therapy with CARDIOQUIN, and a single recurrence should not be interpreted as therapeutic failure.
Especially in patients with known structural heart disease or other risk factors for toxicity, initiation or dose-adjustment of treatment with CARDIOQUIN should generally be performed in a setting where facilities and personnel for monitoring and resuscitation are continuously available. Monitoring should be continued for two or three days after initiation of the regimen on which the patient will be discharged.
Therapy with CARDIOQUIN should begin with one tablet (275 mg; 166 mg of quinidine base) every six to eight hours. If this regimen is well tolerated, if the serum quinidine level is still well within the laboratory's therapeutic range, and if the average time between arrhythmic episodes has not been satisfactorily increased, then the dose may be cautiously raised. The total daily dosage should be reduced if the QRS complex widens to 130% of its pre-treatment duration; the QT_c interval widens to 130% of its pre-treatment duration and is longer than 500 ms: P waves disappear; or the patient develops significant tachycardia, symptomatic bradycardia, or hypotension.
Suppression of ventricular arrhythmias
Dosing regimens for the use of quinidine polygalacturonate in suppressing life-threatening ventricular arrhythmias have not been adequately studied. Described regimens have generally been similar to the regimen described just above for the prophylaxis of symptomatic atrial fibrillation/flutter. Where possible, therapy should be guided by the results of programmed electrical stimulation and/or Holter monitoring with exercise.

HOW SUPPLIED

CARDIOQUIN is supplied as 275-mg, white, round, scored, uncoated tablets embossed **PF** on one side and **C275** on the other. The tablets are available in opaque white plastic bottles containing 100 tablets (**NDC** #0034-5470-80) and 500 tablets (**NDC** #0034-5470-90).
Store tablets at controlled room temperature (15–30°C; 59–86°F).
CAUTION: Federal (USA) law prohibits dispensing without prescription.
The Purdue Frederick Company
Norwalk, CT 06850-3590
Copyright© 1990, 1995
The Purdue Frederick Company
August 2, 1995 O8038

CERUMENEX® EARDROPS ℞

[*sĕ-rū 'mĕn-ĕx"*]
(triethanolamine polypeptide oleate-condensate)

DESCRIPTION

CERUMENEX Eardrops contain Triethanolamine Polypeptide Oleate-Condensate (10%). Inactive Ingredients: Chlorobutanol 0.5%, Propylene Glycol and Water. Triethanolamine Polypeptide Oleate is a hygroscopic-miscible solution with low surface tension and optimal viscosity of 50–90 cps. It also has a slightly acid pH range (5.0–6.0) to approximate the surface of a normal ear canal.

CLINICAL PHARMACOLOGY

CERUMENEX Eardrops emulsify and disperse excess or impacted earwax. The triethanolamine polypeptide oleate, a surfactant, in a hygroscopic vehicle lyses cerumen to facilitate removal by subsequent water irrigation.

INDICATIONS AND USAGE

For removal of impacted cerumen prior to ear examination, otologic therapy and/or audiometry.

CONTRAINDICATIONS

Perforated tympanic membrane or otitis media is considered a contraindication to the use of this medication in the external ear canal.
A history of hypersensitivity to CERUMENEX Eardrops or to any of its components is also a contraindication to the use of this medication.

WARNINGS

Discontinue promptly if sensitization or irritation occurs.

PRECAUTIONS

General
It is recommended that the following precautions be observed in prescribing and administration of this agent:
1. Extreme caution is indicated in patients with demonstrable dermatologic idiosyncrasies or with history of allergic reactions in general.
2. Exposure of the ear canal to the CERUMENEX Eardrops should be limited to 15–30 minutes.
3. When administering CERUMENEX Eardrops, care must be taken to avoid undue exposure of the skin outside the ear during the instillation and the flushing out of the medication. If the medication comes in contact with the skin, the area should be washed with soap and water. Use of proper technique (see Dosage and Administration) will help avoid such undue exposure.
4. CERUMENEX Eardrops should be used only with caution in external otitis.

Information for Patients
1. Patients should be cautioned to avoid placing the applicator tip into the ear canal.
2. Patients should be cautioned to gently flush the ear with lukewarm water.
3. Patients should be warned to use CERUMENEX Eardrops in ears only. Surrounding skin should be promptly rinsed of any excess drops.
4. Patients should be instructed not to leave CERUMENEX Eardrops in the ear for longer than 30 minutes. A second application may be made, if needed, but more frequent use must be indicated by the physician.
5. Patients must be instructed not to exceed the time of exposure, nor to use the medication more frequently than directed by the physician.
6. Patients should be advised to discontinue the use of the medication in case of a possible reaction and to consult their physician promptly.

Carcinogenesis, Mutagenesis, Impairment of Fertility
Long-term animal studies have not been performed to evaluate the carcinogenic potential or the effect on fertility of CERUMENEX Eardrops.
Pregnancy
Teratogenic Effects: Pregnancy Category C. Animal reproduction studies have not yet been conducted with CERUMENEX Eardrops. It is also not known whether CERUMENEX Eardrops can cause fetal harm when administered to a pregnant woman or can affect reproduction capacity. CERUMENEX Eardrops should be given to a pregnant woman only if clearly needed.
Nursing Mothers
It is not known whether this drug is excreted in human milk. Because many drugs are excreted in human milk, caution should be exercised when CERUMENEX Eardrops are administered to a nursing mother.
Pediatric Use
Safety and effectiveness in children have not been established.

ADVERSE REACTIONS

Clinical Reactions of Possible Allergic Origin
Localized dermatitis reactions were reported in about 1% of 2,700 patients treated, ranging from a very mild erythema and pruritus of the external canal to a severe eczematoid reaction involving the external ear and periauricular tissue, generally with duration of 2–10 days. Other reactions which have been reported in connection with the use of CERUMENEX Eardrops include allergic contact dermatitis, skin ulcerations, burning and pain at the application site and skin rash.

DOSAGE AND ADMINISTRATION

1. Fill ear canal with CERUMENEX Eardrops with the patient's head tilted at a 45° angle.
2. Insert cotton plug and allow to remain 15–30 minutes.
3. Then gently flush with lukewarm water, using a soft rubber syringe (avoid excessive pressure). Exposure of skin outside the ear to the drug should be avoided. The procedure may be repeated if the first application fails to clear the impaction.

CAUTION: Federal Law Prohibits Dispensing Without a Prescription.
FOR EXTERNAL USE IN THE EAR ONLY

HOW SUPPLIED

CERUMENEX Eardrops (triethanolamine polypeptide oleate-condensate) are supplied in 6 ml (NDC 0034-5490-06) and 12 ml (NDC 0034-5490-12) bottles with a cellophane wrapped dropper.
Store at Controlled Room Temperature 15–30°C (59–86°F).
Copyright 1991, The Purdue Frederick Company
Norwalk, CT 06850-3590
May 15, 1991 L8037

DHCplus® CAPSULES Ⓒ III

DESCRIPTION

Each light aqua and bluish-green capsule contains:
Dihydrocodeine Bitartrate 16 mg
(Warning—May be habit forming.)

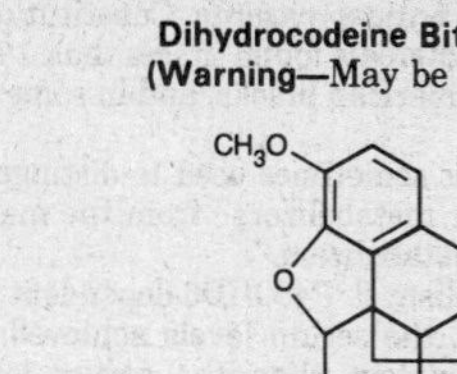

$C_{18}H_{23}NO_3 \cdot C_4H_6O_6$ 451.46
6-hydroxy-3-methoxy-N-methyl-4,5-epoxy-morphinan Bitartrate

[See chemical structure at top of next column.]

Acetaminophen 356.4 mg

HO—⬡—NHCOCH₃

$C_8H_9NO_2$ 151.16
N-(4-Hydroxyphenyl)acetamide

Caffeine 30 mg

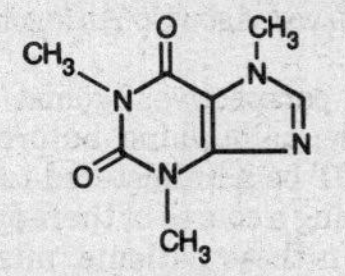

$C_8H_{10}N_4O_2$ (anhydrous) 194.19
3,7-Dihydro-1,3,7-trimethyl-1H-purine-2,6-dione

DHCplus® Capsules also contain the following inactive ingredients: Croscarmellose sodium, FD&C Blue No. 1, FD&C Green No. 3, Gelatin, Silicon dioxide, Syloid 244 FP, Sodium lauryl sulfate, Corn starch, Titanium dioxide and Zinc stearate.

CLINICAL PHARMACOLOGY

DHCplus® Capsules contain dihydrocodeine which is a semi-synthetic narcotic analgesic related to codeine, with multiple actions qualitatively similar to those of codeine; the most prominent of these involve the central nervous system and organs with smooth muscle components. The principal action of therapeutic value is analgesia.
DHCplus® Capsules also contain acetaminophen, a non-opiate, non-salicylate analgesic, and antipyretic.
DHCplus® Capsules contain caffeine as an analgesic adjuvant. Caffeine is also a CNS and cardiovascular stimulant.

INDICATIONS AND USAGE

DHCplus® Capsules are indicated for the relief of moderate to moderately severe pain.

CONTRAINDICATIONS

Hypersensitivity to dihydrocodeine, codeine, acetaminophen, caffeine, or the other components noted above.

WARNINGS

Dihydrocodeine may impair the mental and/or physical abilities required for the performance of potentially hazardous tasks such as driving a car or operating machinery.

PRECAUTIONS

General:
DHCplus® Capsules should be given with caution to certain patients such as the elderly or debilitated.
Acetaminophen is relatively non-toxic at therapeutic doses, but should be used with caution in patients with severe renal or hepatic disease.
Caffeine in high doses may produce CNS and cardiovascular stimulation and GI irritation.
Information for Patients:
Dihydrocodeine may impair the mental and/or physical abilities required for the performance of potentially hazardous tasks such as driving a car or operating machinery. The patient using DHCplus® Capsules should be cautioned accordingly.
Drug Interactions:
Dihydrocodeine
Patients receiving other narcotic analgesics, general anesthetics, tranquilizers, sedative-hypnotics, or other CNS depressants (including alcohol) concomitantly with DHCplus® Capsules may exhibit an additive CNS depression. When such combined therapy is contemplated, the dose of one or both agents should be reduced.
Caffeine
Caffeine may enhance the cardiac inotropic effects of beta-adrenergic stimulating agents. Co-administration of caffeine and disulfiram may lead to a substantial decrease in caffeine clearance. Caffeine may increase the metabolism of other drugs such as phenobarbital and aspirin. Caffeine accumulation may occur when products or foods containing caffeine are consumed concomitantly with quinolones such as ciprofloxacin.
Pregnancy:
Teratogenic Effects—Pregnancy Category C. Animal reproduction studies have not been conducted with DHCplus® Capsules. It is also not known whether DHCplus® Capsules can cause fetal harm when administered to pregnant women or can affect reproduction capacity in males and females. DHCplus® Capsules should be given to a pregnant woman only if clearly needed.
Nursing Mothers:
Because of the potential for serious adverse reactions in nursing infants from DHCplus® Capsules, a decision should be made whether to discontinue nursing or to discontinue the drug, taking into account the importance of the drug to the mother.
Pediatric Use:
Safety and effectiveness in children have not been established.

ADVERSE REACTIONS

The most frequently observed reactions include light-headedness, dizziness, drowsiness, sedation, nausea, vomiting, constipation, pruritus, and skin reactions.

DRUG ABUSE AND DEPENDENCE

DHCplus® Capsules are subject to the provisions of the Controlled Substance Act, and has been placed in Schedule III. Dihydrocodeine can produce drug dependence of the codeine type and therefore has the potential of being abused. Psychic dependence, physical dependence, and tolerance may develop upon repeated administration of dihydrocodeine, and it should be prescribed and administered with the same degree of caution appropriate to the use of other oral narcotic-containing medications.
Prolonged, high intake of caffeine may produce tolerance, and habituation. Physical signs of withdrawal, such as headaches, irritation, nervousness, anxiety, and dizziness, may occur upon abrupt discontinuation.

OVERDOSAGE

Following an acute overdosage with DHCplus® Capsules, toxicity may result from the dihydrocodeine, acetaminophen, or, less likely, caffeine component. An overdose is a potentially lethal polydrug overdose situation, and consultation with a regional poison control center is recommended. A listing of the poison control centers can be found in standard references such as the *Physicians' Desk Reference®*.
Signs and Symptoms and Laboratory Findings:
Toxicity from *dihydrocodeine* is typical of opiates and includes pinpoint pupils, respiratory depression, and loss of consciousness. Convulsions, cardiovascular collapse, and death may occur. With *acetaminophen*, dose-dependent hepatic necrosis is the most serious adverse effect. Renal tubular necrosis, hypoglycemic coma, thrombocytopenia may occur. Early symptoms of hepatotoxicity include nausea, vomiting, diaphoresis, and general malaise. Clinical and laboratory evidence of hepatic toxicity may not be apparent until 48 to 72 hours post-ingestion. In adults, hepatic toxicity has rarely been reported with acute overdoses of less than 10 grams or fatalities with less than 15 grams. Acute *caffeine* poisoning may cause insomnia, restlessness, tremor, delirium, tachycardia, extrasystoles, and seizures.
Because overdose information on DHCplus® Capsules is limited, it is unclear which of the signs and symptoms of toxicity would manifest in any particular overdose situation.
Treatment:
Immediate treatment includes support of cardiorespiratory function and measures to reduce drug absorption. Vomiting should be induced with syrup of ipecac, if the patient is alert and has adequate laryngeal reflexes. Oral activated charcoal should follow. The first dose should be accompanied by an appropriate cathartic. Gastric lavage may be necessary. Hypotension is usually hypovolemic and should be treated with fluids. Endotracheal intubation and artificial respiration may be necessary. Peritoneal or hemodialysis may be necessary. If hypoprothrombinemia occurs, Vitamin K should be administered.
The pure opioid antagonist, naloxone, is a specific antidote against repiratory depression which results from opioid overdose. Naloxone hydrochloride (usually 0.4 to 2.0 mg) should be administered intravenously; however, because its duration of action is relatively short, the patient must be carefully monitored until spontaneous respiration is reliably re-established. Re-administration may be necessary. Naloxone should not be given in the absence of clinically significant respiratory or circulatory depression secondary to opioid overdose.
In adults and adolescents, regardless of the quantity of acetaminophen reported to have been ingested, administer acetylcysteine immediately if 24 hours or less have elapsed from the reported time since ingestion. Do not await the plasma concentration determination of acetaminophen before administering acetylcysteine. Serum liver enzyme levels should be quantitated. Therapy in children involves a similar treatment scheme; however, a regional Poison Control Center should be contacted.
No specific antidote is available for caffeine. In addition to the supportive measures above, administration of demulcents such as aluminum hydroxide gel may diminish GI irritation. Seizures may be treated with intravenous diazepam or a barbiturate.

DOSAGE AND ADMINISTRATION

The usual adult dose is two (2) DHCplus® Capsules orally every four (4) hours. Dosage should be adjusted according to the severity of the pain and the response of the patient. No more than twelve (12) capsules should be taken in a 24-hour period.

HOW SUPPLIED

DHCplus® (Dihydrocodeine Bitartrate, Acetaminophen, and Caffeine) Capsules are available in light aqua and bluish-green capsules imprinted with PURDUE on the capsule top containing Dihydrocodeine Bitartrate 16 mg (**Warning**—May be habit forming.), Acetaminophen 356.4 mg, Caffeine 30 mg. Supplied in bottles of 100 capsules (NDC 0034-8000-80).
Store at controlled room temperature, 15°–30°C (59°–86°F). Protect from moisture.
Dispense in a tight, light-resistant container as defined in the U.S.P.

CAUTION

Federal law prohibits dispensing without prescription.
DIST.: The Purdue Frederick Company
Norwalk, CT 06850-3590
Copyright© 1993, 1995, The Purdue Frederick Company
June 20, 1995   E3888
Shown in Product Identification Guide, page 329

MS CONTIN® 15 mg Tablets ⓒ
MS CONTIN® 30 mg Tablets ⓒ
MS CONTIN® 60 mg Tablets ⓒ
MS CONTIN® 100 mg Tablets ⓒ

MS CONTIN® 200 mg Tablets*
(For use in opioid tolerant patients only.) ⓒ

[em es "kŏn "těn]
Morphine Sulfate Controlled-Release
WARNING: May be habit forming.

DESCRIPTION

Chemically, morphine sulfate is 7,8-didehydro-4,5α-epoxy-17- methylmorphinan-3,6 α-diol sulfate (2:1) (salt) pentahydrate and has the following structural formula:

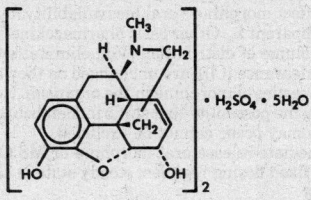

Each MS CONTIN 15 mg Controlled-Release Tablet contains: 15 mg Morphine sulfate U.S.P. Inactive ingredients: Cetostearyl alcohol, FD&C Blue No. 2, Hydroxyethyl cellulose, Hydroxypropyl methylcellulose, Lactose, Magnesium stearate, Talc, Titanium dioxide and other ingredients.
Each MS CONTIN 30 mg Controlled-Release Tablet contains: 30 mg Morphine sulfate U.S.P. Inactive ingredients: Cetostearyl alcohol, D&C Red No. 7, FD&C Blue No. 1, Hydroxyethyl cellulose, Hydroxypropyl methylcellulose, Lactose, Magnesium stearate, Talc, Titanium dioxide and other ingredients.
Each MS CONTIN 60 mg Controlled-Release Tablet contains: 60 mg Morphine sulfate U.S.P. Inactive ingredients: Cetostearyl alcohol, D&C Red No. 30, D&C Yellow No. 10, Hydroxyethyl cellulose, Hydroxypropyl methylcellulose, Lactose, Magnesium stearate, Talc, Titanium dioxide and other ingredients.
Each MS CONTIN 100 mg Controlled-Release Tablet contains: 100 mg Morphine sulfate U.S.P. Inactive ingredients: Cetostearyl alcohol, Hydroxyethyl cellulose, Hydroxypropyl methylcellulose, Magnesium stearate, Synthetic black iron oxide, Talc, Titanium dioxide and other ingredients.
MS CONTIN 200 mg Tablets*
(For use in opioid tolerant patients only.)
Each MS CONTIN 200 mg Controlled-Release Tablet* contains: 200 mg Morphine sulfate U.S.P. Inactive ingredients: Cetostearyl alcohol, D&C Yellow No. 10, FD&C Blue No. 1, Hydroxyethyl cellulose, Hydroxypropyl cellulose, Hydroxypropyl methylcellulose, Magnesium stearate, Polyethylene glycol, Talc, Titanium dioxide.
***FOR USE IN OPIOID TOLERANT PATIENTS ONLY.**

CLINICAL PHARMACOLOGY

Metabolism and Pharmacokinetics
MS CONTIN is a controlled-release tablet containing morphine sulfate. Following oral administration of a given dose of morphine, the amount ultimately absorbed is essentially the same whether the source is MS CONTIN or a conventional formulation. Morphine is released from MS CONTIN somewhat more slowly than from conventional oral preparations. Because of pre-systemic elimination (i.e., metabolism in the gut wall and liver) only about 40% of the administered dose reaches the central compartment.
Once absorbed, morphine is distributed to skeletal muscle, kidneys, liver, intestinal tract, lungs, spleen and brain. Morphine also crosses the placental membranes and has been found in breast milk.
Although a small fraction (less than 5%) of morphine is demethylated, for all practical purposes, virtually all morphine is converted to glucuronide metabolites; among these,

Continued on next page

Purdue Frederick—Cont.

morphine-3-glucuronide is present in the highest plasma concentration following oral administration.

The glucuronide system has a very high capacity and is not easily saturated even in disease. Therefore, rate of delivery of morphine to the gut and liver should not influence the total and, probably, the relative quantities of the various metabolites formed. Moreover, even if rate affected the relative amounts of each metabolite formed, it should be unimportant clinically because morphine's metabolites are ordinarily inactive.

The following pharmacokinetic parameters show considerable inter-subject variation but are representative of average values reported in the literature. The volume of distribution (Vd) for morphine is 4 liters per kilogram, and its terminal elimination half-life is normally 2 to 4 hours. Following the administration of conventional oral morphine products, approximately fifty percent of the morphine that will reach the central compartment intact reaches it within 30 minutes. Following the administration of an equal amount of MS CONTIN to normal volunteers, however, this extent of absorption occurs, on average, after 1.5 hours.

The possible effect of food upon the systemic bioavailability of MS CONTIN has not been systematically evaluated for all strengths. Data from at least one study suggests that concurrent administration of MS CONTIN with a fatty meal may cause a slight decrease in peak plasma concentration.

Variation in the physical/mechanical properties of a formulation of an oral morphine drug product can affect both its absolute bioavailability and its absorption rate constant (k_a). The formulation employed in MS CONTIN has not been shown to affect morphine's oral bioavailability, but does decrease its apparent k_a. Other basic pharmacokinetic parameters (e.g., volume of distribution [Vd], elimination rate constant [k_e], clearance [Cl]), are unchanged as they are fundamental properties of morphine in the organism. However, in chronic use, the possibility that shifts in metabolite to parent drug ratios may occur cannot be excluded.

When immediate-release oral morphine or MS CONTIN is given on a fixed dosing regimen, steady state is achieved in about a day.

For a given dose and dosing interval, the AUC and average blood concentration of morphine at steady state (Css) will be independent of the specific type of oral formulation administered so long as the formulations have the same absolute bioavailability. The absorption rate of a formulation will, however, affect the maximum (Cmax) and minimum (Cmin) blood levels and the times of their occurrence.

PHARMACODYNAMICS

The effects described below are common to all morphine-containing products.

Central Nervous System

The principal actions of therapeutic value of morphine are analgesia and sedation (i.e., sleepiness and anxiolysis).

The precise mechanism of the analgesic action is unknown. However, specific CNS opiate receptors and endogenous compounds with morphine-like activity have been identified throughout the brain and spinal cord and are likely to play a role in the expression of analgesic effects.

Morphine produces respiratory depression by direct action on brain stem respiratory centers. The mechanism of respiratory depression involves a reduction in the responsiveness of the brain stem respiratory centers to increases in carbon dioxide tension, and to electrical stimulation.

Morphine depresses the cough reflex by direct effect on the cough center in the medulla. Antitussive effects may occur with doses lower than those usually required for analgesia. Morphine causes miosis, even in total darkness. Pinpoint pupils are a sign of narcotic overdose but are not pathognomonic (e.g., pontine lesions of hemorrhagic or ischemic origins may produce similar findings). Marked mydriasis rather than miosis may be seen with worsening hypoxia.

Gastrointestinal Tract and Other Smooth Muscle

Gastric, biliary and pancreatic secretions are decreased by morphine. Morphine causes a reduction in motility associated with an increase in tone in the antrum of the stomach and duodenum. Digestion of food in the small intestine is delayed and propulsive contractions are decreased. Propulsive peristaltic waves in the colon are decreased, while tone is increased to the point of spasm. The end result is constipation. Morphine can cause a marked increase in biliary tract pressure as a result of spasm of sphincter of Oddi.

Cardiovascular System

Morphine produces peripheral vasodilation which may result in orthostatic hypotension. Release of histamine can occur and may contribute to narcotic-induced hypotension. Manifestations of histamine release and/or peripheral vasodilation may include pruritus, flushing, red eyes and sweating.

Plasma Level- Analgesia Relationships

In any particular patient, both analgesic effects and plasma morphine concentrations are related to the morphine dose. In non-tolerant individuals, plasma morphine concentra-

tion-efficacy relationships have been demonstrated and suggest that opiate receptors occupy effector compartments, leading to a lag-time, or hysteresis, between rapid changes in plasma morphine concentrations and effects of such changes. The most direct and predictable concentration-effect relationships can, therefore, be expected at distribution equilibrium and/or steady state conditions. In general, the minimum effective analgesic concentration in the plasma of non tolerant patients ranges from approximately 5 to 20ng/ml.

While plasma morphine-efficacy relationships can be demonstrated in non-tolerant individuals, they are influenced by a wide variety of factors and are not generally useful as a guide to the clinical use of morphine. The effective dose in opioid-tolerant patients may be 10–50 times as great (or greater) than the appropriate dose for opioid-naive individuals. Dosages of morphine should be chosen and must be titrated on the bases of clinical evaluation of the patient and the balance between therapeutic and adverse effects.

For any fixed dose and dosing interval, MS CONTIN will have at steady state, a lower Cmax and a higher Cmin than conventional morphine. This is a potential advantage; a reduced fluctuation in morphine concentration during the dosing interval should keep morphine blood levels more centered within the theoretical "therapeutic window." (Fluctuation for a dosing interval is defined as [Cmax-Cmin]/[Css-average].) On the other hand, the degree of fluctuation in serum morphine concentration might conceivably affect other phenomena. For example, reduced fluctuations in blood morphine concentrations might influence the rate of tolerance induction.

The elimination of morphine occurs primarily as renal excretion of 3-morphine glucuronide. A small amount of the glucuronide conjugate is excreted in the bile, and there is some minor enterohepatic recycling. Because morphine is primarily metabolized to inactive metabolites, the effects of renal disease on morphine's elimination are not likely to be pronounced. However, as with any drug, caution should be taken to guard against unanticipated accumulation if renal and/or hepatic function is seriously impaired.

INDICATIONS AND USAGE

MS CONTIN is a controlled-release oral morphine formulation indicated for the relief of moderate to severe pain. It is intended for use in patients who require repeated dosing with potent opioid analgesics over periods of more than a few days.

The MS CONTIN 200 mg Tablet strength is a high dose, controlled-release, oral morphine formulation indicated for the relief of pain in opioid tolerant patients only.

CONTRAINDICATIONS

MS CONTIN is contraindicated in patients with known hypersensitivity to the drug, in patients with respiratory depression in the absence of resuscitative equipment, and in patients with acute or severe bronchial asthma.

MS CONTIN is contraindicated in any patient who has or is suspected of having a paralytic ileus.

WARNINGS

(See also: CLINICAL PHARMACOLOGY)

Impaired Respiration

Respiratory depression is the chief hazard of all morphine preparations. Respiratory depression occurs most frequently in the elderly and debilitated patients, as well as in those suffering from conditions accompanied by hypoxia or hypercapnia when even moderate therapeutic doses may dangerously decrease pulmonary ventilation.

Morphine should be used with extreme caution in patients with chronic obstructive pulmonary disease or cor pulmonale, and in patients having a substantially decreased respiratory reserve, hypoxia, hypercapnia, or preexisting respiratory depression. In such patients, even usual therapeutic doses of morphine may decrease respiratory drive while simultaneously increasing airway resistance to the point of apnea.

Head Injury and Increased Intracranial Pressure

The respiratory depressant effects of morphine with carbon dioxide retention and secondary elevation of cerebrospinal fluid pressure may be markedly exaggerated in the presence of head injury, other intracranial lesions, or preexisting increase in intracranial pressure. Morphine produces effects which may obscure neurologic signs of further increases in pressure in patients with head injuries.

Hypotensive Effect

MS CONTIN, like all opioid analgesics, may cause severe hypotension in an individual whose ability to maintain his blood pressure has already been compromised by a depleted blood volume, or a concurrent administration of drugs such as phenothiazines or general anesthetics. (See also: PRECAUTIONS: Drug Interactions.) MS CONTIN may produce orthostatic hypotension in ambulatory patients.

MS CONTIN, like all opioid analgesics, should be administered with caution to patients in circulatory shock, since vasodilation produced by the drug may further reduce cardiac output and blood pressure.

Interactions with other CNS Depressants

MS CONTIN, like all opioid analgesics, should be used with great caution and in reduced dosage in patients who are concurrently receiving other central nervous system depressants including sedatives or hypnotics, general anesthetics, phenothiazines, other tranquilizers and alcohol because respiratory depression, hypotension and profound sedation or coma may result.

Interactions with Mixed Agonist/Antagonist Opioid Analgesics

From a theoretical perspective, agonist/antagonist analgesics (i.e., pentazocine, nalbuphine, butorphanol and buprenorphine) should NOT be administered to a patient who has received or is receiving a course of therapy with a pure opioid agonist analgesic. In these patients, mixed agonist/antagonist analgesics may reduce the analgesic effect or may precipitate withdrawal symptoms.

Drug Dependence

Morphine can produce drug dependence and has a potential for being abused. Tolerance as well as psychological and physical dependence may develop upon repeated administration. Physical dependence, however, is not of paramount importance in the management of terminally ill patients or any patients in severe pain. Abrupt cessation or a sudden reduction in dose after prolonged use may result in withdrawal symptoms. After prolonged exposure to opioid analgesics, if withdrawal is necessary, it must be undertaken gradually. (See DRUG ABUSE AND DEPENDENCE.)

Infants born to mothers physically dependent on opioid analgesics may also be physically dependent and exhibit respiratory depression and withdrawal symptoms. (See DRUG ABUSE AND DEPENDENCE.)

PRECAUTIONS

(See also: CLINICAL PHARMACOLOGY)

Special precautions regarding MS CONTIN 200 mg Tablets
MS CONTIN 200 mg Tablets are for use only in opioid tolerant patients requiring daily morphine equivalent dosages of 400 mg or more. Care should be taken in its prescription and patients should be instructed against use by individuals other than the patient for whom it was prescribed, as this may have severe medical consequences for that individual.

General

MS CONTIN is intended for use in patients who require more than several days continuous treatment with a potent opioid analgesic. The controlled-release nature of the formulation allows it to be administered on a more convenient schedule than conventional immediate-release oral morphine products. (See CLINICAL PHARMACOLOGY: "Metabolism and Pharmacokinetics".) However, MS CONTIN does not release morphine continuously over the course of a dosing interval. The administration of single doses of MS CONTIN on a q12 hour dosing schedule will result in higher peak and lower trough plasma levels than those that occur when an identical daily dose of morphine is administered using conventional oral formulations on a q4h regimen. The clinical significance of greater fluctuations in morphine plasma level has not been systematically evaluated. (See DOSAGE AND ADMINISTRATION)

As with any potent opioid, it is critical to adjust the dosing regimen for each patient individually, taking into account the patient's prior analgesic treatment experience. Although it is clearly impossible to enumerate every consideration that is important to the selection of the initial dose and dosing interval of MS CONTIN, attention should be given to 1) the daily dose, potency, and characteristics of the opioid the patient has been taking previously (e.g., whether it is a pure agonist or mixed agonist/antagonist), 2) the reliability of the relative potency estimate used to calculate the dose of morphine needed [N.B. potency estimates may vary with the route of administration], 3) the degree of opioid tolerance, if any, and 4) the general condition and medical status of the patient.

Selection of patients for treatment with MS CONTIN should be governed by the same principles that apply to the use of morphine or other potent opioid analgesics. Specifically, the increased risks associated with its use in the following populations should be considered: the elderly or debilitated and those with severe impairment of hepatic, pulmonary or renal function; myxedema or hypothyroidism; adrenocortical insufficiency (e.g., Addison's Disease); CNS depression or coma; toxic psychosis; prostatic hypertrophy or urethral stricture; acute alcoholism; delirium tremens; kyphoscoliosis; or inability to swallow.

The administration of morphine, like all opioid analgesics, may obscure the diagnosis or clinical course in patients with acute abdominal conditions.

Morphine may aggravate preexisting convulsions in patients with convulsive disorders. Morphine should be used with caution in patients about to undergo surgery of the biliary tract since it may cause spasm of the sphincter of Oddi. Similarly, morphine should be used with caution in patients with acute pancreatitis secondary to biliary tract disease.

Information for Patients

If clinically advisable, patients receiving MS CONTIN should be given the following instructions by the physician:

1. Appropriate pain management requires changes in the dose to maintain best pain control. Patients should be advised of the need to contact their physician if pain control is inadequate, but not to change the dose of MS CONTIN without consulting their physician.
2. Morphine may impair mental and/or physical ability required for the performance of potentially hazardous tasks (e.g., driving, operating machinery). Patients started on MS CONTIN or whose dose has been changed should refrain from dangerous activity until it is established that they are not adversely affected.
3. Morphine should not be taken with alcohol or other CNS depressants (sleep aids, tranquilizers) because additive effects including CNS depression may occur. A physician should be consulted if other prescription medications are currently being used or are prescribed for future use.
4. For women of childbearing potential who become or are planning to become pregnant, a physician should be consulted regarding analgesics and other drug use.
5. Upon completion of therapy, it may be appropriate to taper the morphine dose, rather than abruptly discontinue it.
6. While psychological dependence ("addiction") to morphine used in the treatment of pain is very rare, morphine is one of a class of drugs known to be abused and should be handled accordingly.
7. The MS CONTIN 200 mg Tablet is for use only in opioid tolerant patients requiring daily morphine equivalent dosages of 400 mg or more. Special care must be taken to avoid accidental ingestion or the use by individuals (including children) other than the patient for whom it was originally prescribed, as such unsupervised use may have severe, even fatal, consequences.

Drug Interactions (See WARNINGS)

The concomitant use of other central nervous system depressants including sedatives or hypnotics, general anesthetics, phenothiazines, tranquilizers and alcohol may produce additive depressant effects. Respiratory depression, hypotension and profound sedation or coma may occur. When such combined therapy is contemplated, the dose of one or both agents should be reduced. Opioid analgesics, including MS CONTIN, may enhance the neuromuscular blocking action of skeletal muscle relaxants and produce an increased degree of respiratory depression.

Carcinogenicity/Mutagenicity/Impairment of Fertility

Studies of morphine sulfate in animals to evaluate the drug's carcinogenic and mutagenic potential or the effect on fertility have not been conducted.

Pregnancy

Teratogenic effects—CATEGORY C: Adequate animal studies on reproduction have not been performed to determine whether morphine affects fertility in males or females. There are no well-controlled studies in women, but marketing experience does not include any evidence of adverse effects on the fetus following routine (short-term) clinical use of morphine sulfate products. Although there is no clearly defined risk, such experience cannot exclude the possibility of infrequent or subtle damage to the human fetus.

MS CONTIN should be used in pregnant women only when clearly needed. (See also: PRECAUTIONS: Labor and Delivery, and DRUG ABUSE AND DEPENDENCE.)

Nonteratogenic effects: Infants born from mothers who have been taking morphine chronically may exhibit withdrawal symptoms.

Labor and Delivery

MS CONTIN is not recommended for use in women during and immediately prior to labor. Occasionally, opioid analgesics may prolong labor through actions which temporarily reduce the strength, duration and frequency of uterine contractions. However, this effect is not consistent and may be offset by an increased rate of cervical dilatation which tends to shorten labor.

Neonates whose mothers received opioid analgesics during labor should be observed closely for signs of respiratory depression. A specific narcotic antagonist, naloxone, should be available for reversal of narcotic-induced respiratory depression in the neonate.

Nursing Mothers

Low levels of *morphine* have been detected in the breast milk. Withdrawal symptoms can occur in breast-feeding infants when maternal administration of morphine sulfate is stopped. Ordinarily, nursing should not be undertaken while a patient is receiving MS CONTIN since morphine may be excreted in the milk.

Pediatric Use

Use of MS CONTIN has not been evaluated systematically in children.

ADVERSE REACTIONS

The adverse reactions caused by morphine are essentially those observed with other opioid analgesics. They include the following major hazards: respiratory depression, apnea, and to a lesser degree, circulatory depression; respiratory arrest, shock and cardiac arrest.

Most Frequently Observed

Constipation, lightheadedness, dizziness, sedation, nausea, vomiting, sweating, dysphoria and euphoria.

Some of these effects seem to be more prominent in ambulatory patients and in those not experiencing severe pain. Some adverse reactions in ambulatory patients may be alleviated if the patient lies down.

Less Frequently Observed Reactions

Central Nervous System: Weakness, headache, agitation, tremor, uncoordinated muscle movements, seizure, alterations of mood (nervousness, apprehension, depression, floating feelings), dreams, muscle rigidity, transient hallucinations and disorientation, visual disturbances, insomnia and increased intracranial pressure.

Gastrointestinal: Dry mouth, constipation, biliary tract spasm, laryngospasm, anorexia, diarrhea, cramps and taste alterations.

Cardiovascular: Flushing of the face, chills, tachycardia, bradycardia, palpitation, faintness, syncope, hypotension and hypertension.

Genitourinary: Urine retention or hesitance, reduced libido and/or potency.

Dermatologic: Pruritus, urticaria, other skin rashes, edema and diaphoresis.

Other: Antidiuretic effect, paresthesia, muscle tremor, blurred vision, nystagmus, diplopia and miosis.

DRUG ABUSE AND DEPENDENCE

Opioid analgesics may cause psychological and physical dependence (see WARNINGS). Physical dependence results in withdrawal symptoms in patients who abruptly discontinue the drug or may be precipitated through the administration of drugs with narcotic antagonist activity, e.g., naloxone or mixed agonist/antagonist analgesics (pentazocine, etc.; See also OVERDOSAGE). Physical dependence usually does not occur to a clinically significant degree until after several weeks of continued narcotic usage. Tolerance, in which increasingly large doses are required in order to produce the same degree of analgesia, is initially manifested by a shortened duration of analgesic effect, and, subsequently, by decreases in the intensity of analgesia.

In chronic pain patients, and in narcotic-tolerant cancer patients, the administration of MS CONTIN should be guided by the degree of tolerance manifested. Physical dependence, per se, is not ordinarily a concern when one is dealing with opioid-tolerant patients whose pain and suffering is associated with an irreversible illness.

If MS CONTIN is abruptly discontinued, a moderate to severe abstinence syndrome may occur. The opioid agonist abstinence syndrome is characterized by some or all of the following: restlessness, lacrimation, rhinorrhea, yawning, perspiration, gooseflesh, restless sleep or "yen" and mydriasis during the first 24 hours. These symptoms often increase in severity and over the next 72 hours may be accompanied by increasing irritability, anxiety, weakness, twitching and spasms of muscles; kicking movements; severe backache, abdominal and leg pains; abdominal and muscle cramps; hot and cold flashes, insomnia; nausea, anorexia, vomiting, intestinal spasm, diarrhea; coryza and repetitive sneezing; increase in body temperature, blood pressure, respiratory rate and heart rate. Because of excessive loss of fluids through sweating, vomiting and diarrhea, there is usually marked weight loss, dehydration, ketosis, and disturbances in acid-base balance. Cardiovascular collapse can occur. Without treatment most observable symptoms disappear in 5–14 days; however, there appears to be a phase of secondary or chronic abstinence which may last for 2–6 months characterized by insomnia, irritability, and muscular aches.

If treatment of physical dependence of patients on MS CONTIN is necessary, the patient may be detoxified by gradual reduction of the dosage. Gastrointestinal disturbances or dehydration should be treated accordingly.

OVERDOSAGE

Acute overdosage with morphine is manifested by respiratory depression, somnolence progressing to stupor or coma, skeletal muscle flaccidity, cold and clammy skin, constricted pupils, and, sometimes, bradycardia and hypotension.

In the treatment of overdosage, primary attention should be given to the re-establishment of a patent airway and institution of assisted or controlled ventilation. The pure opioid antagonist, naloxone, is a specific antidote against respiratory depression which results from opioid overdose. Naloxone (usually 0.4 to 2.0 mg) should be administered intravenously; however, because its duration of action is relatively short, the patient must be carefully monitored until spontaneous respiration is reliably re-established. If the response to naloxone is suboptimal or not sustained, additional naloxone may be re-administered, as needed, or given by continuous infusion to maintain alertness and respiratory function; however, there is no information available about the cumulative dose of naloxone that may be safely administered.

Naloxone should not be administered in the absence of clinically significant respiratory or circulatory depression secondary to morphine overdose. Naloxone should be administered cautiously to persons who are known, or suspected to be physically dependent on MS CONTIN. In such cases, an abrupt or complete reversal of narcotic effects may precipitate an acute abstinence syndrome.

Note: In an individual physically dependent on opioids, administration of the usual dose of the antagonist will precipitate an acute withdrawal syndrome. The severity of the withdrawal syndrome produced will depend on the degree of physical dependence and the dose of the antagonist administered. Use of a narcotic antagonist in such a person should be avoided. If necessary to treat serious respiratory depression in the physically dependent patient, the antagonist should be administered with care and by titration with smaller than usual doses of the antagonist.

Supportive measures (including oxygen, vasopressors) should be employed in the management of circulatory shock and pulmonary edema accompanying overdose as indicated. Cardiac arrest or arrhythmias may require cardiac massage or defibrillation.

DOSAGE AND ADMINISTRATION

(See also: CLINICAL PHARMACOLOGY, WARNINGS AND PRECAUTIONS sections)

MS CONTIN TABLETS ARE TO BE TAKEN WHOLE, AND ARE NOT TO BE BROKEN, CHEWED OR CRUSHED. TAKING BROKEN, CHEWED OR CRUSHED MS CONTIN TABLETS COULD LEAD TO THE RAPID RELEASE AND ABSORPTION OF A POTENTIALLY TOXIC DOSE OF MORPHINE.

MS CONTIN is intended for use in patients who require more than several days continuous treatment with a potent opioid analgesic. The controlled-release nature of the formulation allows it to be administered on a more convenient schedule than conventional immediate-release oral morphine products. (See CLINICAL PHARMACOLOGY: "Metabolism and Pharmacokinetics".) However, MS CONTIN does not release morphine continuously over the course of a dosing interval. The administration of single doses of MS CONTIN on a q12h dosing schedule will result in higher peak and lower trough plasma levels than those that occur when an identical daily dose of morphine is administered using conventional oral formulations on a q4h regimen. The clinical significance of greater fluctuations in morphine plasma level has not been systematically evaluated.

As with any potent opioid drug product, it is critical to adjust the dosing regimen for each patient individually, taking into account the patient's prior analgesic treatment experience. Although it is clearly impossible to enumerate every consideration that is important to the selection of initial dose and dosing interval of MS CONTIN, attention should be given to 1) the daily dose, potency and precise characteristics of the opioid the patient has been taking previously (e.g., whether it is a pure agonist or mixed agonist/antagonist), 2) the reliability of the relative potency estimate used to calculate the dose of morphine needed [N.B. potency estimates may vary with the route of administration], 3) the degree of opioid tolerance, if any, and 4) the general condition and medical status of the patient.

The following dosing recommendations, therefore, can only be considered suggested approaches to what is actually a series of clinical decisions in the management of the pain of an individual patient.

Conversion from Conventional Oral Morphine to MS CONTIN

A patient's daily morphine requirement is established using immediate-release oral morphine (dosing every 4 to 6 hours). The patient is then converted to MS CONTIN in either of two ways: 1) by administering one-half of the patient's 24-hour requirement as MS CONTIN on an every 12-hour schedule; or, 2) by administering one-third of the patient's daily requirement as MS CONTIN on an every eight hour schedule. With either method, dose and dosing interval is then adjusted as needed (see discussion below). The 15 mg tablet should be used for initial conversion for patients whose total daily requirement is expected to be less than 60 mg. The 30 mg tablet strength is recommended for patients with a daily morphine requirement of 60 to 120 mg. When the total daily dose is expected to be greater than 120 mg, the appropriate combination of tablet strengths should be employed.

Conversion from Parenteral Morphine or Other Opioids (Parenteral or Oral) to MS CONTIN

MS CONTIN can be administered as the initial oral morphine drug product; in this case, however, particular care must be exercised in the conversion process. Because of uncertainty about, and intersubject variation in, relative estimates of opioid potency and cross tolerance, initial dosing regimens should be conservative; that is, an underestimation of the 24-hour oral morphine requirement is preferred to an overestimate. To this end, initial individual doses of MS CONTIN should be estimated conservatively. In patients whose daily morphine requirements are expected to be less than or equal to 120 mg per day, the 30 mg tablet strength is recommended for the initial titration period. Once a stable dose regimen is reached, the patient can be converted to the

Continued on next page

Purdue Frederick—Cont.

60 mg or 100 mg tablet strength, or appropriate combination of tablet strengths, if desired.
Estimates of the relative potency of opioids are only approximate and are influenced by route of administration, individual patient differences, and possibly, by an individual's medical condition. Consequently, it is difficult to recommend any fixed rule for converting a patient to MS CONTIN directly. The following general points should be considered, however.

1. *Parenteral to oral morphine ratio:* Estimates of the oral to parenteral potency of morphine vary. Some authorities suggest that a dose of oral morphine only three times the daily parenteral morphine requirement may be sufficient in chronic use settings.
2. *Other parenteral or oral opioids to oral morphine:* Because there is lack of systemic evidence bearing on these types of analgesic substitutions, specific recommendations are not possible.

Physicians are advised to refer to published relative potency data, keeping in mind that such ratios are only approximate. In general, it is safer to underestimate the daily dose of MS CONTIN required and rely upon ad hoc supplementation to deal with inadequate analgesia. (See discussion which follows.)
Use of MS CONTIN as the first opioid analgesic
There has been no systematic evaluation of MS CONTIN as an initial opioid analgesic in the management of pain. Because it may be more difficult to titrate a patient using a controlled-release morphine, it is ordinarily advisable to begin treatment using an immediate-release formulation.
Considerations in the Adjustment of Dosing Regimens
Whatever the approach, if signs of excessive opioid effects are observed early in a dosing interval, the next dose should be reduced. If this adjustment leads to inadequate analgesia, that is, "breakthrough" pain occurs late in the dosing interval, the dosing interval may be shortened. Alternatively, a supplemental dose of a short-acting analgesic may be given. As experience is gained, adjustments can be made to obtain an appropriate balance between pain relief, opioid side effects, and the convenience of the dosing schedule.
In adjusting dosing requirements, it is recommended that the dosing interval never be extended beyond 12 hours because the administration of very large single doses may lead to acute overdose. (N.B. MS CONTIN is a controlled-release formulation; it does not release morphine continuously over the dosing interval.)
For patients with low daily morphine requirements, the 15 mg tablet should be used.
Special Instructions for MS CONTIN 200 mg Tablets
(For use in opioid tolerant patients only.)
The MS CONTIN 200 mg tablet is for use only in opioid tolerant patients requiring daily morphine equivalent dosages of 400 mg or more. It is recommended that this strength be reserved for patients that have already been titrated to a stable analgesic regimen using lower strengths of MS CONTIN or other opioid.
Conversion from MS CONTIN to parenteral opioids:
When converting a patient from MS CONTIN to parenteral opioids, it is best to assume that the parenteral to oral potency is high. NOTE THAT THIS IS THE CONVERSE OF THE STRATEGY USED WHEN THE DIRECTION OF CONVERSION IS FROM THE PARENTERAL TO ORAL FORMULATIONS. IN BOTH CASES, HOWEVER, THE AIM IS TO ESTIMATE THE NEW DOSE CONSERVATIVELY. For example, to estimate the required 24-hour dose of morphine for IM use, one could employ a conversion of 1 mg of morphine IM for every 6 mg of morphine as MS CONTIN. Of course, the IM 24-hour dose would have to be divided by six and administered on a q4h regimen. This approach is recommended because it is least likely to cause overdose.
Safety and Handling
MS CONTIN TABLETS ARE TO BE TAKEN WHOLE, AND ARE NOT TO BE BROKEN, CHEWED, OR CRUSHED. TAKING BROKEN, CHEWED, OR CRUSHED MS CONTIN TABLETS COULD LEAD TO THE RAPID RELEASE AND ABSORPTION OF A POTENTIALLY TOXIC DOSE OF MORPHINE.
The MS CONTIN 200 mg Tablet strength is for use only in opioid tolerant patients requiring daily morphine equivalent dosages of 400 mg or more. This strength is potentially toxic if accidentally ingested and patients and their families should be instructed to take special care to avoid accidental or intentional ingestion by individuals other than those for whom the medication was originally prescribed.

HOW SUPPLIED

NDC 0034-0514-10: MS CONTIN (morphine sulfate controlled-release tablets) 15 mg are supplied in opaque plastic bottles containing 100 tablets.
NDC 0034-0514-90: MS CONTIN (morphine sulfate controlled-release tablets) 15 mg are supplied in opaque plastic bottles containing 500 tablets.
NDC 0034-0514-25: MS CONTIN (morphine sulfate controlled-release tablets) 15 mg are supplied in unit dose packaging with 25 individually numbered tablets per card; one card per tuck end carton.
NDC 0034-0515-50: MS CONTIN (morphine sulfate controlled-release tablets) 30 mg are supplied in opaque plastic bottles containing 50 tablets.
NDC 0034-0515-10: MS CONTIN (morphine sulfate controlled-release tablets) 30 mg are supplied in opaque plastic bottles containing 100 tablets.
NDC 0034-0515-45: MS CONTIN (morphine sulfate controlled-release tablets) 30 mg are supplied in opaque plastic bottles containing 250 tablets.
NDC 0034-0515-90: MS CONTIN (morphine sulfate controlled-release tablets) 30 mg are supplied in opaque plastic bottles containing 500 tablets.
NDC 0034-0515-25: MS CONTIN (morphine sulfate controlled-release tablets) 30 mg are supplied in unit dose packaging with 25 individually numbered tablets per card; one card per tuck end carton.
NDC 0034-0516-10: MS CONTIN (morphine sulfate controlled-release tablets) 60 mg are supplied in opaque plastic bottles containing 100 tablets.
NDC 0034-0516-90: MS CONTIN (morphine sulfate controlled-release tablets) 60 mg are supplied in opaque plastic bottles containing 500 tablets.
NDC 0034-0516-25: MS CONTIN (morphine sulfate controlled-release tablets) 60 mg are supplied in unit dose packaging with 25 individually numbered tablets per card; one card per tuck end carton.
NDC 0034-0517-10: MS CONTIN (morphine sulfate controlled-release tablets) 100 mg are supplied in opaque plastic bottles containing 100 tablets.
NDC 0034-0517-90: MS CONTIN (morphine sulfate controlled-release tablets) 100 mg are supplied in opaque plastic bottles containing 500 tablets.
NDC 0034-0517-25: MS CONTIN (morphine sulfate controlled-release tablets) 100 mg are supplied in unit dose packaging with 25 individually numbered tablets per card; one card per tuck end carton.
NDC 0034-0513-10: MS CONTIN (morphine sulfate controlled-release tablets) 200 mg are supplied in opaque plastic bottles containing 100 tablets.
NDC 0034-0513-25: MS CONTIN (morphine sulfate controlled-release tablets) 200 mg are supplied in unit dose packaging with 25 individually numbered tablets per card; one card per tuck end carton.
15 mg: Each round, blue-colored tablet bears the symbol PF on one side and M15 on the other side.
30 mg: Each round, lavender-colored tablet bears the symbol PF on one side and M30 on the other side.
60 mg: Each round, orange-colored tablet bears the symbol PF on one side and M60 on the other side.
100 mg: Each round, gray-colored tablet bears the symbol PF on one side and 100 on the other side.
200 mg: Each capsule-shaped, green-colored tablet bears the symbol PF on one side and 200 on the other side.
Store tablets at controlled room temperature 15°–30°C (59°–86°F).
Dispense in tight, light-resistant container.

CAUTION

DEA Order Form Required.
Federal law prohibits dispensing without prescription.
THE PURDUE FREDERICK COMPANY
Norwalk, CT 06850-3590
Copyright © 1987, 1991, 1993, 1994, The Purdue Frederick Company
U.S. Patent Numbers 4235870 and 4366310
January 28, 1994 **G3220**
Shown in Product Identification Guide, page 329

MSIR® Oral Solution Ⓒ
[em 'es ī"ahr]
(morphine sulfate)
MSIR® Oral Solution Concentrate Ⓒ
(morphine sulfate)
MSIR® Immediate-Release Oral Tablets Ⓒ
(morphine sulfate)
MSIR® Immediate-Release Oral Capsules Ⓒ
(morphine sulfate)
WARNING: May be habit forming

DESCRIPTION

Chemically, morphine sulfate is 7,8 didehydro-4,5-α-epoxy-17-methylmorphinan-3,6 α-diol sulfate (2:1) (salt) pentahydrate and has the following structural formula:
[See chemical structure at top of next column.]
MSIR Oral Solution
Each 5 mL of MSIR Oral Solution contains:
Morphine Sulfate .... 10 or 20 mg
Inactive Ingredients: Edetate disodium, FD&C Red. No. 40, Glycerin, Invert Sugar, Sodium benzoate, Sodium chloride, Sucrose, Artificial & Natural Flavors, and other ingredients.

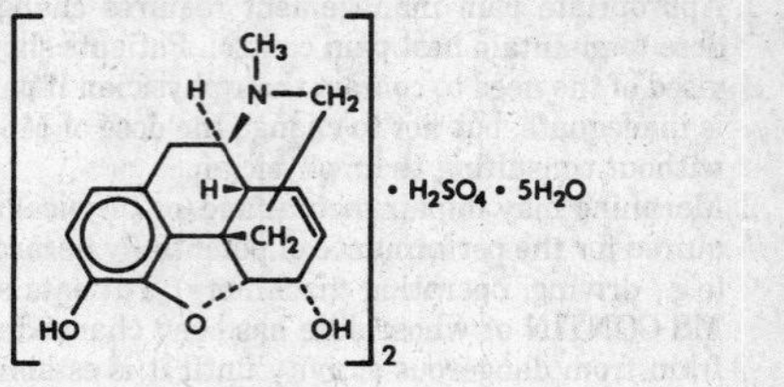

MSIR Oral Solution Concentrate
Each 1 mL of MSIR Oral Solution Concentrate contains:
Morphine Sulfate .... 20 mg
Inactive Ingredients: Edetate disodium, Sodium benzoate, and other ingredients.
MSIR Tablets
Each MSIR Tablet for oral administration contains:
Morphine Sulfate .... 15 or 30 mg
Inactive Ingredients: Corn starch, Lactose, Magnesium stearate, and Talc.
MSIR Capsules
Each MSIR Capsule for oral administration contains:
Morphine Sulfate .... 15 or 30 mg
Inactive Ingredients: FD&C Blue No. 1, FD&C Blue No. 2, FD&C Red No. 40, FD&C Yellow No. 6, Gelatin, Hydroxypropyl methylcellulose, Lactose, Polyethylene glycol, Polysorbate 80, Polyvinylpyrrolidone, Starch, Sucrose, Titanium dioxide, and other ingredients. In addition, the 30 mg capsule contains Black iron oxide and D&C Red No. 28.

WARNING: May be habit forming

CLINICAL PHARMACOLOGY

Metabolism and Pharmacokinetics
MSIR Solutions, Tablets and Capsules containing morphine sulfate are for oral administration and are conventional immediate release products. Only about 40% of the administered dose reaches the central compartment because of presystemic elimination (i.e., metabolism in the gut wall and liver).
Once absorbed, morphine is distributed to skeletal muscle, kidneys, liver, intestinal tract, lungs, spleen and brain. Morphine also crosses the placental membranes and has been found in breast milk.
Although a small fraction (less than 5%) of morphine is demethylated, for all practical purposes, virtually all morphine is converted to glucuronide metabolites; among these, morphine-3-glucuronide is present in the highest plasma concentration following oral administration.
The glucuronide system has a very high capacity and is not easily saturated even in disease. Therefore, rate of delivery of morphine to the gut and liver should not influence the total and, probably, the relative quantities of the various metabolites formed. Moreover, even if rate affected the relative amounts of each metabolite formed, it should be unimportant clinically because morphine's metabolites are ordinarily inactive.
The following pharmacokinetic parameters show considerable intersubject variation but are representative of average values reported in the literature. The volume of distribution (Vd) for morphine is 4 liters per kilogram, and its terminal elimination half-life is approximately 2 to 4 hours. Following the administration of conventional oral morphine products, approximately fifty percent of the morphine that will reach the central compartment intact, reaches it within 30 minutes.
Variation in the physical/mechanical properties of a formulation of an oral morphine drug product can affect both its absolute bioavailability and its absorption rate constant (k_a). The basic pharmacokinetic parameters (e.g., volume of distribution [Vd], elimination rate constant [k_e], clearance [Cl]) are fundamental properties of morphine in the organism. However, in chronic use, the possibility that shifts in metabolite to parent drug ratios may occur cannot be excluded.
When immediate-release oral morphine is given on a fixed dosing regimen, steady state is achieved in about a day.
For a given dose and dosing interval, the AUC and average blood concentration of morphine at steady state (Css) will be independent of the specific type of oral formulation administered so long as the formulations have the same absolute bioavailability. The absorption rate of a formulation will, however, affect the maximum (Cmax) and minimum (Cmin) blood levels and the times of their occurrence.
While there is no predictable relationship between morphine blood levels and analgesic response, effective analgesia will not occur below some minimum blood level in a given patient. The minimum effective blood level for analgesia will vary among patients, especially among patients who have been previously treated with potent mu (μ) agonist opioids. Similarly, there is no predictable relationship between blood morphine concentration and untoward clinical responses; again, however, higher concentrations are more likely to be toxic than lower ones.
The elimination of morphine occurs primarily as renal excretion of 3-morphine glucuronide. A small amount of the

glucuronide conjugate is excreted in the bile, and there is some minor enterohepatic recycling.

The elimination half-life of morphine is reported to vary between 2 and 4 hours. Thus, steady-state is probably achieved on most regimens within a day. Because morphine is primarily metabolized to inactive metabolites, the effects of renal disease on morphine's elimination are not likely to be pronounced. However, as with any drug, caution should be taken to guard against unanticipated accumulation if renal and/or hepatic function is seriously impaired.

Individual differences in the metabolism of morphine suggest that MSIR Oral Solutions, Tablets and Capsules be dosed conservatively according to the dosing initiation and titration recommendations in the Dosage and Administration section.

PHARMACODYNAMICS

The effects described below are common to all morphine-containing products.

Central Nervous System

The principal actions of therapeutic value of morphine are analgesia and sedation (i.e., sleepiness and anxiolysis).

The precise mechanism of analgesic action is unknown. However, specific CNS opiate receptors and endogenous compounds with morphine-like activity have been identified throughout the brain and spinal cord and are likely to play a role in the expression of analgesic effects.

Morphine produces respiratory depression by direct action on brain stem respiratory centers. The mechanism of respiratory depression involves a reduction in the responsiveness of the brain stem respiratory centers to increases in carbon dioxide tension, and to electrical stimulation.

Morphine depresses the cough reflex by direct effect on the cough center in the medulla. Antitussive effects may occur with doses lower than those usually required for analgesia. Morphine causes miosis, even in total darkness. Pinpoint pupils are a sign of narcotic overdose but are not pathognomonic (e.g., pontine lesions of hemorrhagic or ischemic origins may produce similar findings). Marked mydriasis rather than miosis may be seen with worsening hypoxia.

Gastrointestinal Tract and Other Smooth Muscle

Gastric, biliary and pancreatic secretions are decreased by morphine. Morphine causes a reduction in motility associated with an increase in tone in the antrum of the stomach and duodenum. Digestion of food in the small intestine is delayed and propulsive contractions are decreased. In addition, propulsive peristaltic waves in the colon are decreased, while tone is increased to the point of spasm. The end result is constipation. Morphine can cause a marked increase in biliary tract pressure as a result of spasm of the sphincter of Oddi.

Cardiovascular System

Morphine produces peripheral vasodilation which may result in orthostatic hypotension. Release of histamine can occur and may contribute to narcotic-induced hypotension. Manifestations of histamine release and/or peripheral vasodilation may include pruritus, flushing, red eyes and sweating.

INDICATIONS AND USAGE

MSIR Oral Solutions, Tablets and Capsules are indicated for the relief of moderate to severe pain.

CONTRAINDICATIONS

MSIR Oral Solutions, Tablets and Capsules are contraindicated in patients with known hypersensitivity to the drug, in patients with respiratory depression in the absence of resuscitative equipment, and in patients with acute or severe bronchial asthma.

MSIR Oral Solutions, Tablets and Capsules are contraindicated in any patient who has or is suspected of having a paralytic ileus.

WARNINGS (See also: CLINICAL PHARMACOLOGY)

Impaired Respiration

Respiratory depression is the chief hazard of all morphine preparations. Respiratory depression occurs most frequently in elderly and debilitated patients, and those suffering from conditions accompanied by hypoxia or hypercapnia when even moderate therapeutic doses may dangerously decrease pulmonary ventilation.

Morphine should be used with extreme caution in patients with chronic obstructive pulmonary disease or cor pulmonale, and in patients having a substantially decreased respiratory reserve, hypoxia, hypercapnia, or preexisting respiratory depression. In such patients, even usual therapeutic doses of morphine may decrease respiratory drive while simultaneously increasing airway resistance to the point of apnea.

Head Injury and Increased Intracranial Pressure

The respiratory depressant effects of morphine with carbon dioxide retention and secondary elevation of cerebrospinal fluid pressure may be markedly exaggerated in the presence of head injury, other intracranial lesions, or preexisting increase in intracranial pressure. Morphine produces effects which may obscure neurologic signs of further increase in pressure in patients with head injuries.

Hypotensive Effects

MSIR Oral Solutions, Tablets and Capsules, like all opioid analgesics, may cause severe hypotension in an individual whose ability to maintain his blood pressure has already been compromised by a depleted blood volume, or a concurrent administration of drugs such as phenothiazines, or general anesthetics. (See also: PRECAUTIONS: Drug Interactions.) MSIR Oral Solutions, Tablets and Capsules may produce orthostatic hypotension in ambulatory patients.

MSIR Oral Solutions, Tablets and Capsules, like all opioid analgesics, should be administered with caution to patients in circulatory shock, since vasodilation produced by the drug may further reduce cardiac output and blood pressure.

Interactions with Other CNS Depressants

MSIR Oral Solutions, Tablets and Capsules, like all opioid analgesics, should be used with great caution and in reduced dosage in patients who are concurrently receiving other central nervous system depressants including sedatives or hypnotics, general anesthetics, phenothiazines, other tranquilizers and alcohol, because respiratory depression, hypotension and profound sedation or coma may result.

Interactions with Mixed Agonist/Antagonist Opioid Analgesics

From a theoretical perspective, agonist/antagonist analgesics (i.e., pentazocine, nalbuphine, butorphanol and buprenorphine) should NOT be administered to a patient who has received or is receiving a course of therapy with a pure agonist opioid analgesic. In these patients, mixed agonist-antagonist analgesics may reduce the analgesic effect or may precipitate withdrawal symptoms.

Drug Dependence

Morphine can produce drug dependence and has a potential for being abused. Tolerance and psychological and physical dependence may develop upon repeated administration. Physical dependence, however, is not of paramount importance in the management of terminally ill patients or any patient in severe pain. Abrupt cessation or a sudden reduction in dose after prolonged use may result in withdrawal symptoms. After prolonged exposure to opioid analgesics, if withdrawal is necessary, it must be undertaken gradually. (See DRUG ABUSE AND DEPENDENCE.)

Infants born to mothers physically dependent on opioid analgesics may also be physically dependent and exhibit respiratory depression and withdrawal symptoms. (See DRUG ABUSE AND DEPENDENCE.)

PRECAUTIONS (See also: CLINICAL PHARMACOLOGY)

General

MSIR Oral Solutions, Tablets and Capsules are intended for use in patients who require a potent opioid analgesic for relief of moderate to severe pain.

Selection of patients for treatment with MSIR Oral Solutions, Tablets and Capsules should be governed by the same principles that apply to the use of morphine and other potent opioid analgesics. Specifically, the increased risks associated with its use in the following populations should be considered: the elderly or debilitated and those with severe impairment of hepatic, pulmonary or renal function; myxedema or hypothyroidism; adrenocortical insufficiency (e.g., Addison's Disease); CNS depression or coma; toxic psychoses; prostatic hypertrophy or urethral stricture; acute alcoholism; delirium tremens; kyphoscoliosis or inability to swallow.

The administration of morphine, like all opioid analgesics, may obscure the diagnosis or clinical course in patients with acute abdominal conditions.

Morphine may aggravate preexisting convulsions in patients with convulsive disorders.

Morphine should be used with caution in patients about to undergo surgery of the biliary tract, since it may cause spasm of the sphincter of Oddi. Similarly, morphine should be used with caution in patients with acute pancreatitis secondary to biliary tract disease.

Information for Patients

If clinically advisable, patients receiving MSIR Oral Solutions, Tablets and Capsules should be given the following instructions by the physician.

1. Morphine may produce physical and/or psychological dependence. For this reason, the dose of the drug should not be adjusted without consulting a physician.
2. Morphine may impair mental and/or physical ability required for the performance of potentially hazardous tasks (e.g., driving, operating machinery).
3. Morphine should not be taken with alcohol or other CNS depressants (sleep aids, tranquilizers) because additive effects including CNS depression may occur. A physician should be consulted if other prescription medications are currently being used or are prescribed for future use.
4. For women of childbearing potential who become or are planning to become pregnant, a physician should be consulted regarding analgesics and other drug use.

Drug Interactions (See also WARNINGS)

The concomitant use of other central nervous system depressants including sedatives or hypnotics, general anesthetics, phenothiazines, tranquilizers and alcohol may produce additive depressant effects. Respiratory depression, hypotension and profound sedation or coma may occur. When such combined therapy is contemplated, the dose of one or both agents should be reduced. Opioid analgesics, including MSIR Oral Solutions, Tablets and Capsules, may enhance the neuromuscular blocking action of skeletal muscle relaxants and produce an increased degree of respiratory depression.

Carcinogenicity/Mutagenicity/Impairment of Fertility

Studies of morphine sulfate in animals to evaluate the drug's carcinogenic and mutagenic potential or the effect on fertility have not been conducted.

Pregnancy

Teratogenic effects—CATEGORY C: Adequate animal studies on reproduction have not been performed to determine whether morphine affects fertility in males or females. There are no well-controlled studies in women, but marketing experience does not include any evidence of adverse effects on the fetus following routine (short-term) clinical use of morphine sulfate products. Although there is no clearly defined risk, such experience cannot exclude the possibility of infrequent or subtle damage to the human fetus. MSIR Oral Solutions, Tablets and Capsules should be used in pregnant women only when clearly needed. (See also: PRECAUTIONS: Labor and Delivery, and DRUG ABUSE AND DEPENDENCE.)

Nonteratogenic effects: Infants born from mothers who have been taking morphine chronically may exhibit withdrawal symptoms.

Labor and Delivery

MSIR Oral Solutions, Tablets and Capsules are not recommended for use in women during and immediately prior to labor. Occasionally, opioid analgesics may prolong labor through actions which temporarily reduce the strength, duration and frequency of uterine contractions. However, this effect is not consistent and may be offset by an increased rate of cervical dilatation which tends to shorten labor.

Neonates whose mothers received opioid analgesics during labor should be observed closely for signs of respiratory depression. A specific narcotic antagonist, naloxone, should be available for reversal of narcotic-induced respiratory depression in the neonate.

Nursing Mothers

Low levels of morphine have been detected in human milk. Withdrawal symptoms can occur in breast-feeding infants when maternal administration of morphine sulfate is stopped. Nursing should not be undertaken while a patient is receiving MSIR Oral Solutions, Tablets and Capsules since morphine may be excreted in the milk.

Pediatric Use

MSIR Oral Solutions, Tablets and Capsules have not been evaluated systematically in children.

ADVERSE REACTIONS

The adverse reactions caused by morphine are essentially the same as those observed with other opioid analgesics. They include the following major hazards: respiratory depression, apnea, and to a lesser degree, circulatory depression; respiratory arrest, shock, and cardiac arrest.

Most Frequently Observed

Constipation, lightheadedness, dizziness, sedation, nausea, vomiting, sweating, dysphoria and euphoria.

Some of these effects seem to be more prominent in ambulatory patients and in those not experiencing severe pain. Some adverse reactions in ambulatory patients may be alleviated if the patient lies down.

Less Frequently Observed Reactions

Central Nervous System: Weakness, headache, agitation, tremor, uncoordinated muscle movements, seizure, alterations of mood (nervousness, apprehension, depression, floating feelings), dreams, muscle rigidity, transient hallucinations and disorientation, visual disturbances, insomnia and increased intracranial pressure.

Gastrointestinal: Dry mouth, biliary tract spasm, laryngospasm, anorexia, diarrhea, cramps and taste alterations.

Cardiovascular: Flushing of the face, chills, tachycardia, bradycardia, palpitation, faintness, syncope, hypotension and hypertension.

Genitourinary: Urinary retention or hesitance, reduced libido, and/or potency.

Dermatologic: Pruritus, urticaria, other skin rashes, edema and diaphoresis.

Other: Antidiuretic effect, paresthesia, muscle tremor, blurred vision, nystagmus, diplopia and miosis.

DRUG ABUSE AND DEPENDENCE

Opioid analgesics may cause psychological and physical dependence. (See WARNINGS.) Physical dependence results in withdrawal symptoms in patients who abruptly discontinue the drug or may be precipitated through the administration of drugs with narcotic antagonist activity, e.g., naloxone or mixed agonist/antagonist analgesics (pentazocine, etc.: see also OVERDOSE). Physical dependence usually does not occur to a clinically significant degree until after several weeks of continued narcotic usage. Tolerance, in which increasingly large doses are required in order to produce the

Continued on next page

Purdue Frederick—Cont.

same degree of analgesia, is initially manifested by a shortened duration of analgesic effect, and, subsequently, by decreases in the intensity of analgesia.

In chronic-pain patients and in narcotic-tolerant cancer patients, the administration of MSIR Oral Solutions, Tablets and Capsules should be guided by the degree of tolerance manifested. Physical dependence, per se, is not ordinarily a concern when one is dealing with opioid-tolerant patients whose pain and suffering is associated with an irreversible illness.

If MSIR Oral Solutions, Tablets and Capsules are abruptly discontinued, a moderate to severe abstinence syndrome may occur. The opioid agonist abstinence syndrome is characterized by some or all of the following: restlessness, lacrimation, rhinorrhea, yawning, perspiration, cutis anserina, restless sleep known as the "yen" and mydriasis during the first 24 hours. These symptoms often increase in severity and over the next 72 hours may be accompanied by increasing irritability, anxiety, weakness, twitching and spasms of muscles; kicking movements; severe backache, abdominal and leg pains; abdominal and muscle cramps; hot and cold flashes; insomnia; nausea, anorexia, vomiting, intestinal spasm, diarrhea; coryza and repetitive sneezing; and increase in body temperature, blood pressure, respiratory rate and heart rate. Because of excessive loss of fluids through sweating, vomiting and diarrhea, there is usually marked weight loss, dehydration, ketosis, and disturbances in acid-base balance. Cardiovascular collapse can occur. Without treatment, most observable symptoms disappear in 5-14 days; however, there appears to be a phase of secondary or chronic abstinence which may last for 2–6 months, characterized by insomnia, irritability, and muscular aches.

If treatment of physical dependence on MSIR Oral Solutions, Tablets and Capsules is necessary, the patient may be detoxified by gradual reduction of the dosage. Gastrointestinal disturbances or dehydration should be treated accordingly.

OVERDOSE

Acute overdosage with morphine is manifested by respiratory depression, somnolence progressing to stupor or coma, skeletal muscle flaccidity, cold and clammy skin, constricted pupils, and, sometimes, bradycardia and hypotension.

In the treatment of overdosage, primary attention should be given to the re-establishment of a patent airway and institution of assisted or controlled ventilation. The pure opioid antagonist, naloxone, is a specific antidote against respiratory depression which results from opioid overdose. Naloxone (usually 0.4 to 2.0 mg) should be administered intravenously; however, because its duration of action is relatively short, the patient must be carefully monitored until spontaneous respiration is reliably reestablished. If the response to naloxone is suboptimal or not sustained, additional naloxone may be re-administered, as needed, or given by continuous infusion to maintain alertness and respiratory function; however, there is no information available about the cumulative dose of naloxone that may be safely administered. Naloxone should not be administered in the absence of clinically significant respiratory or circulatory depression secondary to morphine overdose. Naloxone should be administered cautiously to persons who are known or suspected to be physically dependent on morphine. In such cases, an abrupt or complete reversal of narcotic effects may precipitate an acute abstinence syndrome.

Note: In an individual physically dependent on opioids, administration of the usual dose of the antagonist will precipitate an acute withdrawal syndrome. The severity of the withdrawal syndrome produced will depend on the degree of physical dependence and the dose of the antagonist administered. Use of a narcotic antagonist in such a person should be avoided. If necessary to treat serious respiratory depression in the physically dependent patient the antagonist should be administered with extreme care and by titration with smaller than usual doses of the antagonist.

Supportive measures (including oxygen, vasopressors) should be employed in the management of circulatory shock and pulmonary edema accompanying overdose as indicated. Cardiac arrest or arrhythmias may require cardiac massage or defibrillation.

DOSAGE AND ADMINISTRATION: (See also: CLINICAL PHARMACOLOGY, WARNINGS AND PRECAUTIONS sections)

Dosage of morphine is a patient-dependent variable, which must be individualized according to patient metabolism, age and disease state and also response to morphine. Each patient should be maintained at the lowest dosage level that will produce acceptable analgesia. As the patient's well-being improves after successful relief of moderate to severe pain, periodic reduction of dosage and/or extension of dosing interval should be attempted to minimize exposure to morphine.

Usual Adult Oral Dose: 5 to 30 mg every four (4) hours or as directed by physician, administered either as MSIR Oral Solutions, MSIR Oral Tablets or MSIR Oral Capsules. For control of pain in terminal illness, it is recommended that the appropriate dose of MSIR Oral Solutions, MSIR Oral Tablets or MSIR Oral Capsules be given on a regularly scheduled basis every four hours at the minimum dose to achieve acceptable analgesia. If converting a patient from another narcotic to morphine sulfate on the basis of standard equivalence tables, a 1 to 3 ratio of parenteral to oral morphine equivalence is suggested. This ratio is conservative and may underestimate the amount of morphine required. If this is the case, the dose of MSIR Oral Solutions, MSIR Oral Tablets or MSIR Oral Capsules should be gradually increased to achieve acceptable analgesia and tolerable side effects.

Sprinkling Contents of Capsule on Food or Liquids: MSIR Oral Capsules may be carefully opened and the entire beaded contents added to a small amount of cool, soft food, such as applesauce or pudding, or a liquid, such as water or orange juice. The bead-food mixture should be swallowed immediately and not stored for future use.

HOW SUPPLIED

MSIR (morphine sulfate) Oral Solution:
(pleasantly flavored)
10 mg per 5 mL.
NDC 0034-0521-02: high density polyethylene plastic bottle of 120 mL with child-resistant closure.
20 mg per 5 mL.
NDC 0034-0522-02: high density polyethylene plastic bottle of 120 mL with child-resistant closure.

MSIR (morphine sulfate) Oral Solution Concentrate:
(unflavored)
20 mg per 1 mL.
NDC 0034-0523-01: high density polyethylene plastic, child-resistant closure bottle with child-resistant dropper in 30 mL size.
NDC 0034-0523-02: high density polyethylene plastic, child-resistant closure bottle with child-resistant dropper in 120 mL size.
Discard opened bottle of Oral Solution after 90 days. Protect from light.

MSIR (morphine sulfate) Tablets:
15 mg round, white scored tablets
NDC 0034-0518-10: opaque plastic bottle containing 100 tablets. Each tablet bears the symbol *PF* on the scored side and *MI 15* on the other side.
30 mg capsule-shaped, white scored tablets
NDC 0034-0519-10: opaque plastic bottle containing 100 tablets. Each tablet bears the symbol *PF* on the scored side and *MI 30* on the other side.
MSIR (morphine sulfate) Capsules:
15 mg capsules, white opaque capsule body with blue cap
NDC 0034-1025-15: opaque plastic bottle containing 50 capsules. Each capsule bears the symbols "*PF MSIR 15* " and "*THIS END UP.*"
30 mg capsules, gray opaque capsule body with lavender cap
NDC 0034-1026-30: opaque plastic bottle containing 50 capsules. Each capsule bears the symbols "*PF MSIR 30* " and "*THIS END UP.*"
Store MSIR Oral Solutions, Tablets and Capsules at controlled room temperature 15°to 30°C (59°– 86°F).
CAUTION:
DEA Order Form Required.
Federal law prohibits dispensing without prescription.
THE PURDUE FREDERICK COMPANY
Norwalk, CT 06850-3590
Copyright© 1985, 1990, 1991, 1992, 1993, 1994, 1995
The Purdue Frederick Company
January 30, 1995   G3154
Shown in Product Identification Guide, pages 329 and 330

SENOKOT® CHILDREN'S SYRUP   OTC
[sĕn 'ŏ-kŏt]
(extract of senna concentrate)*

ACTION AND USES
To relieve functional constipation in children from two to under 12 years of age, Senokot Children's Syrup generally produces bowel movement in 6 to 12 hours. Taken at bedtime, it works gently overnight.

DESCRIPTION
Each teaspoon of Senokot Children's Syrup contains 8.8 mg sennosides. Active Ingredient: Extract of Senna Concentrate. Inactive Ingredients: Methylparaben, Potassium sorbate, Propylparaben, Sucrose, Water, Natural and artificial chocolate flavor, and other ingredients.
Formulated without alcohol, Senokot Children's Syrup has an appealing chocolaty flavor. It may be given with ice cream or stirred into milk. Its natural active ingredient is concentrated, making it effective with smaller doses than other children's laxatives.

ADMINISTRATION AND DOSAGE
Recommended Dosage (or as directed by a doctor):
Take preferably at bedtime.

AGE	STARTING	MAXIMUM
6 to under 12 years of age	1-1½ tsp. once/day	1½ tsp. twice/day
2 to under 6 years of age	½-¾ tsp. once/day	¾ tsp. twice/day
Under 2 years	Consult a physician	

SENOKOT Children's Syrup is packaged with a free measuring cup to help assure accurate dosing.

WARNINGS
Do not use laxative products when abdominal pain, nausea, or vomiting are present unless directed by a doctor. If there has been a sudden change in the child's bowel movements that persists over a period of 2 weeks, consult a doctor before using a laxative. Laxative products should not be used for a period longer than 1 week unless directed by a doctor. Rectal bleeding or failure to have a bowel movement after use of a laxative may indicate a serious condition. Discontinue use and consult a doctor. As with any drug, if the user is pregnant or nursing a baby, seek the advice of a health professional before taking this product. In case of accidental overdose, seek professional assistance or contact a Poison Control Center immediately. Keep out of children's reach.

HOW SUPPLIED
2.5 fl. oz. plastic bottles; packaged with measuring cup.
Copyright 1996, The Purdue Frederick Company, Norwalk, CT 06850-3590

SENOKOT® TABLETS/GRANULES   OTC
[sen 'o-kot]

SenokotXTRA® Tablets   OTC
(standardized senna concentrate)

SENOKOT-S® Tablets   OTC
(standardized senna concentrate and docusate sodium)
Natural Laxative/Stool Softener Combination

INDICATIONS
SENOKOT Tablets/Granules and Double-Strength SenokotXTRA Tablets contain a natural vegetable derivative, standardized for uniform action. Each Double-Strength SenokotXTRA Tablet contains twice the active ingredient in one SENOKOT Tablet; patients may take one Double-Strength SenokotXTRA Tablet instead of two SENOKOT Tablets.

Senokot Laxatives provide a virtually colon-specific action which is gentle, effective and predictable, generally producing bowel movement in 6 to 12 hours. SENOKOT has been found to be effective even in many previously intractable cases of functional constipation. SENOKOT preparations may aid in rehabilitation of the constipated patient by facilitating regular elimination. At proper dosage levels, SENOKOT preparations are virtually free of adverse reactions (such as loose stools or abdominal discomfort) and enjoy high patient acceptance. Numerous and extensive clinical studies show their high degree of effectiveness in several types of functional constipation: geriatric and postpartum, drug-induced, pediatric, as well as in functional constipation concurrent with heart disease or anorectal surgery.

SENOKOT-S Tablets are designed to relieve both aspects of functional constipation—bowel inertia and hard, dry stools. They provide a natural neuroperistaltic stimulant combined with a classic stool softener, standardized senna concentrate gently stimulates the colon while docusate sodium softens the stool for smoother and easier evacuation. This coordinated dual action of the two ingredients results in colon-specific, predictable laxative effect, generally producing bowel movement in 6 to 12 hours. Flexibility of dosage permits fine adjustment to individual requirements. SENOKOT-S Tablets are highly suitable for relief of postsurgical and postpartum constipation, and effectively counteract drug-induced constipation.

DESCRIPTION
SENOKOT Tablets: Each tablet contains 8.6 mg sennosides.
Active Ingredient: Standardized Senna Concentrate.
Inactive Ingredients: Corn starch, Glycerin, Lactose, Magnesium Stearate, Talc and other ingredients.
SENOKOT Granules: (cocoa-flavored): Each teaspoonful contains 15 mg sennosides.
Active Ingredient: Standardized Senna Concentrate.
Inactive Ingredients: Cocoa, Malt extract, Sodium lauryl sulfate, Sucrose, Vanillin and other ingredients.
SenokotXTRA Tablets: Each tablet contains 17 mg sennosides.
Active Ingredient: Standardized Senna Concentrate.
Inactive Ingredients: Corn Starch, Glycerin, Lactose, Magnesium stearate, Talc and other ingredients.

SENOKOT-S Tablets: Each tablet contains 8.6 mg sennosides and 50 mg of docusate sodium. Active Ingredients: Docusate Sodium and Standardized Senna Concentrate. Inactive Ingredients: Cellulosic polymers, Corn starch, FD&C Yellow No. 10, FD&C Yellow No. 6 (Sunset Yellow), Guar Gum, Lactose, Polyethylene glycol, Talc, Titanium dioxide, and other ingredients.

RECOMMENDED DOSAGE

(or as directed by a doctor): Take preferably at bedtime. For older, debilitated, and OB/GYN patients, the physician may consider prescribing $1/2$ the initial dose. Senokot Tablets and Granules are available for children under 6 years of age. For children under 2 years of age, consult a doctor.

SENOKOT Tablets and SENOKOT-S Tablets:

Recommended Dosage (or as directed by a doctor): Take preferably at bedtime.

AGE	STARTING	MAXIMUM
Adults and children 12 years of age and over	2 tablets once a day	4 tablets twice a day
6 to under 12 years of age	1 tablet once a day	2 tablets twice a day
2 to under 6 years of age	$1/2$ tablet once a day	1 tablet twice a day
Under 2 years	Consult a physician.	

Double-Strength SenokotXTRA Tablets:

Recommended Dosage (or as directed by a doctor): Take preferably at bedtime.

AGE	STARTING	MAXIMUM
Adults and children 12 years of age and over	1 tablet once a day	2 tablets twice a day
6 to under 12 years of age	$1/2$ tablet once a day	1 tablet twice a day

SENOKOT Granules

(May be eaten plain, mixed with liquids such as milk to make a delicious drink, or sprinkled on foods.):

AGE	STARTING	MAXIMUM
Adults and children 12 years of age and over	1 teaspoon once a day	2 teaspoons twice a day
6 to under 12 years of age	$1/2$ teaspoon once a day	1 teaspoon twice a day
2 to under 6 years of age	$1/4$ teaspoon once a day	$1/2$ teaspoon twice a day
Under 2 years	Consult a physician.	

WARNINGS

Do not use laxative products when abdominal pain, nausea or vomiting are present unless directed by a doctor. If you have noticed a sudden change in bowel movements that persists over a period of 2 weeks, consult a doctor before using a laxative. Laxative products should not be used for a period longer than 1 week unless directed by a doctor. Rectal bleeding or failure to have a bowel movement after use of a laxative may indicate a serious condition. Discontinue use and consult your doctor. As with any drug, if you are pregnant or nursing a baby, seek the advice of a health professional before using this product. In case of accidental overdose, seek professional assistance or contact a Poison Control Center immediately. Keep out of children's reach.

HOW SUPPLIED

Tablets: Boxes of 10 and 20; bottles of 50, 100 and 1000. Unit Strip Packs in boxes of 100 tablets: each tablet individually sealed. Double-Strength SenokotXTRA Tablets: Boxes of 12 and 36.
Senokot-S Tablets are supplied in packages of 10, bottles of 30, 60, and 1000 tablets, and Unit Strip Boxes of 100 tablets.
Granules: 2, 6, and 12 oz. plastic containers.

ALSO AVAILABLE

SENOKOT Syrup (extract of senna concentrate) in bottles of 2 and 8 fl. oz. Each teaspoon of SENOKOT Syrup contains 8.8 mg sennosides.
Active Ingredient: Extract of Senna Concentrate.
Inactive Ingredients: Alcohol 7% by volume, Methyl paraben, Potassium sorbate, Propylparaben, Sodium lauryl sulfate, Sucrose, Water, Natural and artificial flavors and other ingredients.
Copyright 1991, 1996. The Purdue Frederick Company

TRILISATE® TABLETS/LIQUID

[tril'i-sāt"]
(choline magnesium trisalicylate)
500 mg, 750 mg, or 1000 mg salicylate content

℞

DESCRIPTION

TRILISATE Tablets/Liquid are nonsteroidal, anti-inflammatory preparations containing choline magnesium trisalicylate which is freely soluble in water. The absolute structure of choline magnesium trisalicylate is not known at this time. Choline magnesium trisalicylate has a molecular formula of $C_{26}H_{29}O_{10}NMg$, a molecular weight of 539.8, and it may be represented in the solid form as:

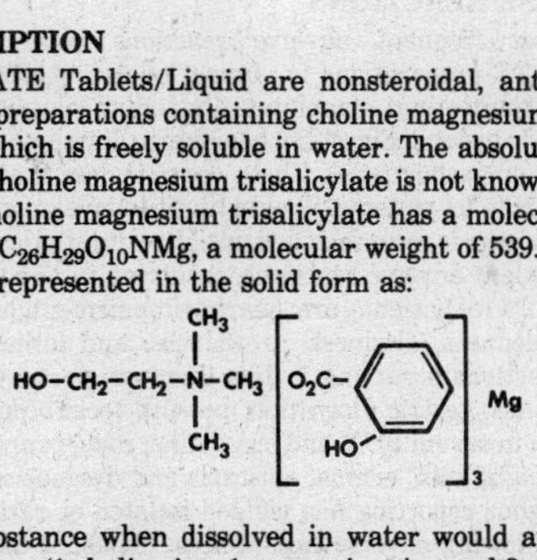

$$HO-CH_2-CH_2-N^{CH_3}_{CH_3}-CH_3 \left[O_2C-\bigcirc-HO \right]_3 Mg$$

This substance when dissolved in water would appear to form 5 ions (1 choline ion, 1 magnesium ion and 3 salicylate ions) which may be represented as:

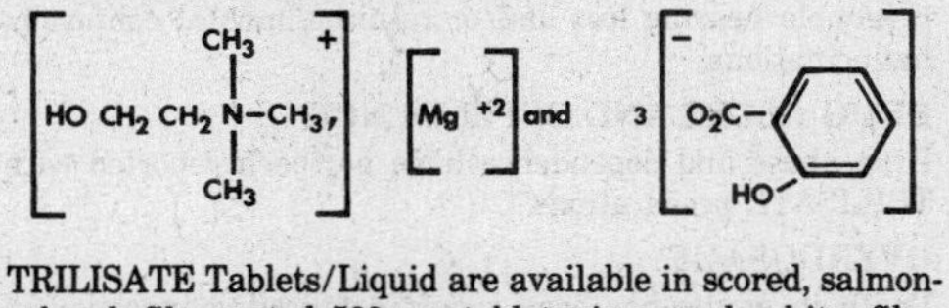

$$\left[HO\ CH_2\ CH_2\ N^{CH_3}_{CH_3}-CH_3 \right]^+ \left[Mg \right]^{+2} and\ 3 \left[O_2C-\bigcirc-HO \right]^-$$

TRILISATE Tablets/Liquid are available in scored, salmon-colored, film-coated 500 mg tablets; in scored, white, film-coated 750 mg tablets, and in scored, red, film-coated 1000 mg tablets. TRILISATE Liquid is a cherry cordial-flavored liquid providing 500 mg salicylate content per teaspoonful (5 ml) for oral administration.
Each 500 mg tablet contains 293 mg of choline salicylate combined with 362 mg of magnesium salicylate to provide 500 mg salicylate content. Each 750 mg tablet contains 440 mg of choline salicylate combined with 544 mg of magnesium salicylate to provide 750 mg salicylate content. Each 1000 mg tablet contains 587 mg of choline salicylate combined with 725 mg magnesium salicylate to provide 1000 mg salicylate content. TRILISATE Liquid contains 293 mg of choline salicylate combined with 362 mg of magnesium salicylate to provide 500 mg salicylate per teaspoonful (5 ml) in a clear amber, cherry cordial-flavored vehicle.
Inactive Ingredients: Each 500 mg tablet contains Carboxymethylcellulose sodium, Edetate disodium, FD&C Yellow No. 6, Polyethylene glycol, Polysorbate 20, Polysorbate 80, Stearic acid, Talc, and other ingredients.
Each 750 mg tablet contains Carboxymethylcellulose sodium, Edetate disodium, Hydroxypropyl methylcellulose, Polyethylene glycol, Polysorbate 20, Stearic acid, Talc, Titanium dioxide, and other ingredients.
Each 1000 mg tablet contains Carboxymethylcellulose sodium, Edetate disodium, FD&C Red No. 40, FD&C Yellow No. 6, FD&C Blue No. 2, Hydroxypropyl methylcellulose, Polyethylene glycol, Polysorbate 20, Polysorbate 80, Stearic acid, Talc, Titanium dioxide and other ingredients.
Each teaspoonful (5 ml) of Liquid contains: Caramel, Carboxymethylcellulose sodium, Edetate disodium, FD&C Yellow No. 6, Glycerin, High fructose corn syrup, Potassium sorbate, Water, and Artificial Flavors.

CLINICAL PHARMACOLOGY

TRILISATE Tablets/Liquid contain salicylate with anti-inflammatory, analgesic and antipyretic action. On ingestion of TRILISATE Tablets/Liquid, the salicylate moiety is absorbed rapidly and reaches peak blood levels within an average of one to two hours after single doses of the tablets or liquid. The primary route of excretion is renal: the excretion products are chiefly the glycine and glucuronide conjugates. At higher serum salicylate concentrations, the glycine conjugation pathway becomes rapidly saturated. Thus, the slower glucuronide conjugation pathway becomes the rate limiting step for salicylate excretion. In addition, salicylate excreted in the bile as glucuronide conjugate may be reabsorbed. These factors account for the prolongation of salicylate half-life and the nonlinear increase in plasma salicylate level as the salicylate dose is increased. The serum concentration of salicylate is increased by conditions that decrease glomerular filtration rate or proximal tubular secretion.
The bioequivalence of TRILISATE Liquid and Tablets 500 mg/750 mg/1000 mg has been established. With the tablets, a steady-state condition is usually reached after 4 to 5 doses, and the half-life of elimination, on repeated administration of tablets, is 9 to 17 hours. This permits a maintenance dosage schedule of once or twice daily. Unlike aspirin and certain other non-steroidal anti-inflammatory agents, such as arylpropionic acid derivatives and arylacetic acid derivatives, choline magnesium trisalicylate, at therapeutic

dosage levels, does not affect platelet aggregation, as shown by in-vitro and in-vivo studies.

INDICATIONS AND USAGE

Osteoarthritis, Rheumatoid Arthritis and Acute Painful Shoulder: Salicylates are considered the base therapy of choice in the arthritides; and TRILISATE preparations are indicated for the relief of the signs and symptoms of rheumatoid arthritis, osteoarthritis and other arthritides. TRILISATE Tablets or Liquid are indicated in the long-term management of these diseases and especially in the acute flare of rheumatoid arthritis. TRILISATE Tablets or Liquid are also indicated for the treatment of acute painful shoulder.
TRILISATE preparations are effective and generally well tolerated, and are logical choices whenever salicylate treatment is indicated. They are particularly suitable when a once-a-day or b.i.d. dosage regimen is important to patient compliance; when gastrointestinal intolerance to aspirin is encountered; when gastrointestinal microbleeding or hematologic effects of aspirin are considered a patient hazard; and when interference (or the risk of interference) with normal platelet function by aspirin or by propionic acid derivatives is considered to be clinically undesirable. Use of TRILISATE Liquid is appropriate when a liquid dosage form is preferred, as in the elderly patient.
The efficacy of TRILISATE preparations has not been studied in those patients who are designated by the American Rheumatism Association as belonging in Functional Class IV (incapacitated, largely or wholly bedridden or confined to a wheelchair, with little or no self-care). Analgesic and Antipyretic Action: TRILISATE Tablets/Liquid are also indicated for the relief of mild to moderate pain and for antipyresis.
Pediatric Use: In children, TRILISATE preparations are indicated for conditions requiring anti-inflammatory or analgesic action—such as juvenile rheumatoid arthritis and other appropriate conditions. In a four-week open label pilot study of patients with juvenile rheumatoid arthritis, children from 6 to 16 years of age previously on aspirin received weight adjusted doses (50–60 mg/kg) of TRILISATE 500 mg tablets on a divided b.i.d. schedule with subsequent dose titration to achieve therapeutic serum salicylate levels. Eighty-three percent (83%) of the patients rated the therapeutic effect of TRILISATE as good or excellent. Tinnitus, was reported by one patient and elevated SGOT levels at Week 1, which decreased during the trial, were detected in two patients. (See WARNINGS section).

CONTRAINDICATIONS

Patients who are hypersensitive to non-acetylated salicylates should not take TRILISATE Tablets or Liquid.

WARNINGS

Reye Syndrome is a rare but serious disease which may develop in children and teenagers who have chicken pox, influenza, or flu symptoms. While the cause of Reye Syndrome is unknown, some studies suggest a possible association between the development of Reye Syndrome and the use of medicines containing acetylated salicylates or aspirin. TRILISATE Tablets and Liquid are a combination of choline salicylate and magnesium salicylate which are nonacetylated salicylates, and there have been no reported cases associating TRILISATE with Reye Syndrome. Nevertheless, TRILISATE, as a salicylate-containing product, is not recommended for use in children and teenagers with chicken pox, influenza or flu symptoms.

PRECAUTIONS

General Precautions: As with other salicylates and nonsteroidal anti-inflammatory drugs, TRILISATE preparations should be used with caution in patients with acute or chronic renal insufficiency, with acute or chronic hepatic dysfunction, or with gastritis or peptic ulcer disease.
Although reports exist of cross reactivity, including bronchospasm, with the use of non-acetylated salicylate products in aspirin-sensitive patients, TRILISATE preparations were found to be well tolerated with regard to pulmonary function and respiratory symptoms when these parameters were monitored in a group of documented aspirin-sensitive asthmatics dosed with TRILISATE in both controlled and open label studies.[1]
Concurrent use of other salicylate-containing products and TRILISATE preparations can lead to an increase in plasma salicylate concentration and may result in potentially toxic salicylate levels.
Laboratory Tests: Plasma salicylate levels can be periodically assessed during treatment with TRILISATE preparations to determine whether a therapeutically effective anti-inflammatory concentration of 15 to 30 mg/100 ml (150–300 micrograms/ml) is being maintained. Manifestations of systemic salicylate intoxication are usually not seen until the concentration exceeds 30 mg/100 ml. However, such tests rarely differentiate between the active free and inactive protein bound salicylate components. Since protein binding

Continued on next page

Purdue Frederick—Cont.

of salicylate is affected by age, nutritional status, competitive binding of other drugs, and underlying disease (e.g. rheumatoid arthritis), plasma salicylate level determinations may not always accurately reflect efficacious or toxic levels of active free salicylate. Acidification of the urine can significantly diminish the renal clearance of salicylate and increase plasma salicylate concentrations.

Drug Interactions: Foods and drugs that alter urine pH may affect renal clearance of salicylate and plasma salicylate concentrations. Raising urine pH, as with chronic antacid use, can enhance renal salicylate clearance and diminish plasma salicylate concentration; urine acidification can decrease urinary salicylate excretion and increase plasma levels.

When salicylate drug products are concurrently dosed with other plasma protein bound drug products, adverse effects may result. Although TRILISATE preparations are a rational choice for anti-inflammatory and analgesic therapy in patients on oral anticoagulants due to their demonstrated lack of effect in vivo and in vitro on platelet aggregation, bleeding time, platelet count, prothrombin time, and serum thromboxane B2 generation[1-7], the potential exists for increased levels of unbound warfarin with their concurrent use. Prothrombin time should be closely monitored and warfarin dose appropriately adjusted when therapy with TRILISATE preparations is initiated. The effect of TRILISATE on blood prothrombin levels has not been established. Salicylates may increase the therapeutic as well as toxic effects of methotrexate, particularly when administered in chemotherapeutic doses, by inhibition of renal methotrexate excretion and by displacement of plasma protein bound methotrexate. Caution should be exercised in administering TRILISATE to rheumatoid arthritis patients on methotrexate. When sulfonylurea oral hypoglycemic agents are co-administered with salicylates, the hypoglycemic effect may be enhanced via increased insulin secretion or by displacement of sulfonylurea agents from binding sites. Insulin-treated diabetics on high doses of salicylates should also be closely monitored for a similar hypoglycemic response. Other drugs with which salicylate competes for protein binding sites, and whose plasma concentration or free fraction may be altered by concurrent salicylate administration, include the following: phenytoin, valproic acid, and carbonic anhydrase inhibitors.

The efficacy of uricosuric agents may be decreased when administered with salicylate products. Although low doses of salicylate (1 to 2 grams per day) have been reported to decrease urate excretion and elevate plasma urate concentrations, intermediate doses (2 to 3 grams per day) usually do not alter urate excretion. Larger salicylate doses (over 5 grams per day) can induce uricosuria and lower plasma urate levels.

Corticosteroids can reduce plasma salicylate levels by increasing renal elimination and perhaps by also stimulating hepatic metabolism of salicylates. By monitoring plasma salicylate levels, salicylate dosage may be titrated to accommodate changes in corticosteroid dose or to avoid salicylate toxicity during corticosteroid taper.

Drug/Laboratory Test Interactions: Free T4 values may be increased in patients on salicylate drug products due to competitive plasma protein binding; a concurrent decrease in total plasma T4 may be observed. Thyroid function is not affected.

Carcinogenesis: No long-term animal studies have been performed with TRILISATE to evaluate its carcinogenic potential.

Use in Pregnancy: Pregnancy Category C. Animal reproduction studies have not been conducted with TRILISATE preparations. It is also not known whether TRILISATE can cause fetal harm when administered to a pregnant woman or can affect reproduction capacity. TRILISATE should be given to a pregnant woman only if clearly needed. Because of the known effects of other salicylate drug products on the fetal cardiovascular system (closure of ductus arteriosus), use during late pregnancy should be avoided.

Labor and Delivery: The effects of TRILISATE on labor and delivery in pregnant women are unknown. Since prolonged gestation and prolonged labor due to prostaglandin inhibition have been reported with the use of other salicylate products, the use of TRILISATE preparations near term is not recommended. Other salicylate products have also been associated with alterations in maternal and neonatal hemostasis mechanisms and with perinatal mortality.

Nursing Mothers: Salicylate is excreted in human milk. Peak milk salicylate levels are delayed, occurring as long as 9 to 12 hours post dose, and the milk:plasma ratio has been reported to be as high as 0.34. Because of the potential for significant salicylate absorption by the nursing infant, caution should be exercised when TRILISATE is administered to a nursing woman.

Geriatric Use: The elderly may be prone to more side effects from salicylates than younger patients due to an age-related decline in renal clearance and/or increased use of concomitant medication. The elderly are more likely than younger patients to be taking a number of medications, some of which may affect the plasma protein binding of salicylate and thus increase the amount of free salicylate.

ADVERSE REACTIONS

The most frequent adverse reactions observed with TRILISATE preparations in clinical trials[7-12] are tinnitus and gastrointestinal complaints (including nausea, vomiting, gastric upset, indigestion, heartburn, diarrhea, constipation and epigastric pain). These occur in less than twenty percent (20%) of patients. Should tinnitus develop, reduction of daily dosage is recommended until the tinnitus is resolved. Less frequent adverse reactions, occurring in less than two percent (2%) of patients, are: hearing impairment, headache, lightheadedness, dizziness, drowsiness, and lethargy. Adverse reactions occurring in less than one percent (1%) of patients are: gastric ulceration, positive fecal occult blood, elevation in serum BUN and creatinine, rash, pruritus, anorexia, weight gain, edema, epistaxis and dysgeusia.

Spontaneous reporting has yielded isolated or rare reports of the following adverse experiences: duodenal ulceration, elevated hepatic transaminases, hepatitis, esophagitis, asthma, erythema multiforme, urticaria, ecchymoses, irreversible hearing loss and/or tinnitus, mental confusion, hallucinations.

DRUG ABUSE AND DEPENDENCE

Drug abuse and dependence have not been reported with TRILISATE preparations.

OVERDOSAGE

Death in adults has been reported following ingestion of doses from 10 to 30 grams of salicylate; however, larger doses have been taken without resulting fatality.

Symptoms: Salicylate intoxication, known as salicylism, may occur with large doses or extended therapy. Common symptoms of salicylism include headache, dizziness, tinnitus, hearing impairment, confusion, drowsiness, sweating, vomiting, diarrhea, and hyperventilation. A more severe degree of salicylate intoxication can lead to CNS disturbances, alteration in electrolyte balance, respiratory and metabolic acidosis, hyperthermia, and dehydration.

Treatment: Reduction of further absorption of salicylate from the gastrointestinal tract can be achieved via emesis, gastric lavage, use of activated charcoal, or a combination of the above. Appropriate I.V. fluids should be administered to correct dehydration, electrolyte imbalance, and acidosis and to maintain adequate renal function. To accelerate salicylate excretion, forced diuresis with alkalinizing solution is recommended. In extreme cases, peritoneal dialysis or hemodialysis should be considered for effective salicylate removal.

DOSAGE AND ADMINISTRATION

ADULTS: In rheumatoid arthritis, osteoarthritis, the more severe arthritides, and acute painful shoulder, the recommended starting dosage is 1500 mg given b.i.d. Some patients may be treated with 3000 mg given once per day (h.s.) In the elderly patient, a daily dosage of 2250 mg given as 750 mg t.i.d. may be efficacious and well tolerated. Dosage should be adjusted in accordance with the patient's response. In patients with renal dysfunction, monitor salicylate levels and adjust dose accordingly.

ELDERLY: In the elderly patients, a daily dosage of 2250 mg given as 750 mg t.i.d. may be efficacious and well tolerated. Dosage should be adjusted in accordance with the patient's response. In patients with renal dysfunction, monitor salicylate levels and adjust dose accordingly.

For mild to moderate pain or for antipyresis, the usual dosage is 2000 mg to 3000 mg daily in divided doses (b.i.d.). Based on patient response or salicylate blood levels, dosage may be adjusted to achieve optimum therapeutic effect. Salicylate blood levels should be in the range of 15 to 30 mg/100 ml for anti-inflammatory effect and 5 to 15 mg/100 ml for analgesia and antipyresis.

Each 500 mg tablet or teaspoonful is equivalent in salicylate content to 10 gr of aspirin; each 750 mg tablet, to 15 gr of aspirin; and each 1000 mg tablet, to 20 gr of aspirin.

If the physician prefers, the recommended daily dosage may be administered on a t.i.d. schedule.

As with other therapeutic agents, individual dosage adjustment is advisable, and a number of patients may require higher or lower dosages than those recommended. Certain patients require 2 to 3 weeks of therapy for optimal effect.

CHILDREN: Usual daily dose for children for anti-inflammatory or analgesic action:

TRILISATE 500 mg Tablets/Liquid and TRILISATE 750 mg and 1000 mg Tablets, 50 mg/kg/day.

Weight (kg)	Total daily dose
12–13	500 mg
14–17	750 mg
18–22	1000 mg
23–27	1250 mg
28–32	1500 mg
33–37	1750 mg

Total daily doses should be administered in divided doses (b.i.d.). Doses of TRILISATE preparations are calculated as the total daily dose of 50 mg/kg/day for children of 37 kg body weight or less and 2250 mg/day for heavier children. TRILISATE Liquid is available for greater convenience in treating younger patients and those adult patients unable to swallow a solid dosage form.

CAUTION

Federal law prohibits dispensing without a prescription.

HOW SUPPLIED

NDC 0034-0500-80: TRILISATE 500 mg Tablets (scored, salmon-colored, film-coated) supplied in bottles of 100 tablets.

NDC 0034-0500-50: TRILISATE 500 mg Tablets (scored, salmon-colored, film-coated) supplied in bottles of 500 tablets.

NDC 0034-0500-10: TRILISATE 500 mg Tablets (scored, salmon-colored, film-coated) supplied in unit dose packaging with 10 tablets per card. Ten cards are packed in each carton; 10 cartons are packed in each shipper.

NDC 0034-0505-80: TRILISATE 750 mg Tablets (scored, white, film-coated) in bottles of 100 tablets.

NDC 0034-0505-50: TRILISATE 750 mg Tablets (scored, white, film-coated) in bottles of 500 tablets.

NDC 0034-0505-10: TRILISATE 750 mg Tablets (scored, white, film-coated) supplied in unit dose packaging with 10 tablets per card. Ten cards are packed in each carton; 10 cartons are packed in each shipper.

NDC 0034-0510-80: TRILISATE 1000 mg Tablets (scored, red, film-coated) in bottles of 100 tablets.

NDC 0034-0520-80: TRILISATE Liquid in bottles of 8 fl. oz. (237 ml).

Store at controlled room temperature 59° to 86°F (15° to 30°C).

REFERENCES

1. Szczeklik, A et al; Choline magnesium trisalicylate in patients with aspirin-induced asthma; *Eur Respir J;* 3:535–539, 1990.
2. Zucker, MB and Rothwell KB; Differential influences of salicylate compounds on platelet aggregation and serotonin release; *Current Therapeutic Research;* 23(2), Feb 1987.
3. Stuart, JJ and Pisko, EJ; Choline magnesium trisalicylate does not impair platelet aggregation; *Pharmatherapeutica;* 2(8):547, 1981.
4. Danesh, BJZ, Saniabadi, AR, Russell, RI et al; Therapeutic potential of choline magnesium trisalicylate as an alternative to aspirin for patients with bleeding tendencies; *Scottish Medical Journal;* 32:167–168, 1987.
5. Danesh, BJZ, McLaren, M. Russell, RI et al; Does nonacetylated salicylate inhibit thromboxane biosynthesis in human platelets? *Scottish Medical Journal;* 33: 315–316, 1988.
6. Danesh, BJZ, McLaren, M, Russell, RI et al; Comparison of the effect of aspirin and choline magnesium trisalicylate on thromboxane biosynthesis in human platelets: role of the acetyl moiety; *Haemostasis;* 19:169–173, 1989.
7. Data on file. Medical Department. The Purdue Frederick Company, 1989.
8. Blechman, WJ, and Lechner, BL; Clinical comparative evaluation of choline magnesium trisalicylate and acetylsalicylic acid in rheumatoid arthritis; *Rheumatology and Rehabilitation;* 18:119–124, 1979.
9. McLaughlin, G; Choline magnesium trisalicylate vs. naproxen in rheumatoid arthritis; *Current Therapeutic Research;* 32(4):579–585, 1982.
10. Ehrlich, GE; Miller, SB; and Zeiders, RS; Choline magnesium trisalicylate vs. ibuprofen in rheumatoid arthritis; *Rheumatology and Rehabilitation;* 19:30–41, 1980.
11. Goldenberg, A; Rudnicki, RD, and Koonce, ML; Clinical comparison of efficacy and safety of choline magnesium trisalicylate and indomethacin in treating osteoarthritis; *Current Therapeutic Research;* 24(3):245–260, 1978.
12. Guerin, BK and Burnstein, SL; Conservative therapy of acute painful shoulder; *Orthopedic Review;* XI(7):29–37, 1982.

The Purdue Frederick Company, Norwalk, CT 06850-3590

Copyright © 1982, 1991, 1995, The Purdue Frederick Company

U.S. Patent Number 4067974

December 7, 1995   R145

Shown in Product Identification Guide, page 330

UNIPHYL® ℞

[ū´nĭ-fĭl]

400 mg and 600 mg Tablets
(theophylline)
UNICONTIN® Controlled-Release System

DESCRIPTION

Uniphyl® (theophylline, anhydrous) Tablets in a controlled-release system allows a 24-hour dosing interval for appropriate patients.

Theophylline is structurally classified as a methylxanthine. It occurs as a white, odorless, crystalline powder with a bitter taste. Anhydrous theophylline has the chemical name 1H-Purine-2,6-dione,3,7-dihydro-1,3-dimethyl-, and is represented by the following structural formula:

The molecular formula of anhydrous theophylline is $C_7H_8N_4O_2$ with a molecular weight of 180.17.

Each controlled-release tablet for oral administration, contains 400 or 600 mg of anhydrous theophylline per tablet.

Inactive Ingredients: Cetostearyl alcohol, Hydroxymethyl cellulose, Magnesium stearate, Povidone and Talc.

CLINICAL PHARMACOLOGY

Mechanism of Action: Theophylline has two distinct actions in the airways of patients with reversible obstruction; smooth muscle relaxation (i.e., bronchodilation) and suppression of the response of the airways to stimuli (i.e., non-bronchodilator prophylactic effects). While the mechanisms of action of theophylline are not known with certainty, studies in animals suggest that bronchodilatation is mediated by the inhibition of two isozymes of phosphodiesterase (PDE III and, to a lesser extent, PDE IV) while non-bronchodilator prophylactic actions are probably mediated through one or more different molecular mechanisms, that do not involve inhibition of PDE III or antagonism of adenosine receptors. Some of the adverse effects associated with theophylline appear to be mediated by inhibition of PDE III (e.g., hypotension, tachycardia, headache, and emesis) and adenosine receptor antagonism (e.g., alterations in cerebral blood flow). Theophylline increases the force of contraction of diaphragmatic muscles. This action appears to be due to enhancement of calcium uptake through an adenosine-mediated channel.

Serum Concentration-Effect Relationship: Bronchodilation occurs over the serum theophylline concentration range of 5–20 mcg/mL. Clinically important improvement in symptom control has been found in most studies to require peak serum theophylline concentrations >10 mcg/mL, but patients with mild disease may benefit from lower concentrations. At serum theophylline concentrations >20 mcg/mL, both the frequency and severity of adverse reactions increase. In general, maintaining peak serum theophylline concentrations between 10 and 15 mcg/mL will achieve most of the drug's potential therapeutic benefit while minimizing the risk of serious adverse events.

Pharmacokinetics:

Overview Theophylline is rapidly and completely absorbed after oral administration in solution or immediate-release solid oral dosage form. Theophylline does not undergo any appreciable pre-systemic elimination, distributes freely into fat-free tissues and is extensively metabolized in the liver. The pharmacokinetics of theophylline vary widely among similar patients and cannot be predicted by age, sex, body weight or other demographic characteristics. In addition, certain concurrent illnesses and alterations in normal physiology (see Table I) and co-administration of other drugs (see Table II) can significantly alter the pharmacokinetic characteristics of theophylline. Within-subject variability in metabolism has also been reported in some studies, especially in acutely ill patients. It is, therefore, recommended that serum theophylline concentrations be measured frequently in acutely ill patients (e.g., at 24-hr intervals) and periodically in patients receiving long-term therapy, e.g., at 6–12 month intervals. More frequent measurements should be made in the presence of any condition that may significantly alter theophylline clearance (see PRECAUTIONS, Laboratory tests).

[See table 1 above.]

Absorption Uniphyl® administered in the fed state is completely absorbed after oral administration.

In a single-dose crossover study, two 400 mg Uniphyl® Tablets were administered to 19 normal volunteers in the morning or evening immediately following the same standardized meal (769 calories consisting of 97 grams carbohydrates, 33 grams protein and 27 grams fat). There was no evidence of dose dumping nor were there any significant differences in

Table I. Mean and range of total body clearance and half-life of theophylline related to age and altered physiological states.¶

Population Characteristics	Total body clearance* mean (range)‡ (mL/kg/min)	Half-life mean (range)‡ (hr)
Age		
Premature neonates		
postnatal age 3–15 days	0.29 (0.09–0.49)	30 (17–43)
postnatal age 25–57 days	0.64 (0.04–1.2)	20 (9.4–30.6)
Term infants		
postnatal age 1–2 days	NR†	25.7 (25–26.5)
postnatal age 3–30 weeks	NR†	11 (6–29)
Children		
1–4 years	1.7 (0.5–2.9)	3.4 (1.2–5.6)
4–12 years	1.6 (0.8–2.4)	NR†
13–15 years	0.9 (0.48–1.3)	NR†
6–17 years	1.4 (0.2–2.6)	3.7 (1.5–5.9)
Adults (16–60 years)		
otherwise healthy		
non-smoking asthmatics	0.65 (0.27–1.03)	8.7 (6.1–12.8)
Elderly (>60 years)		
non-smokers with normal cardiac, liver, and renal function	0.41 (0.21–0.61)	9.8 (1.6–18)
Concurrent illness or altered physiological state		
Acute pulmonary edema	0.33** (0.07–2.45)	19** (3.1–82)
COPD->60 years, stable		
non-smoker >1 year	0.54 (0.44–0.64)	11 (9.4–12.6)
COPD with cor pulmonale	0.48 (0.08–0.88)	NR†
Cystic fibrosis (14–28 years)	1.25 (0.31–2.2)	6.0 (1.8–10.2)
Fever associated with acute viral respiratory illness (children 9–15 years)	NR†	7.0 (1.0–13)
Liver disease		
cirrhosis	0.31** (0.1–0.7)	32** (10–56)
acute hepatitis	0.35 (0.25–0.45)	19.2 (16.6–21.8)
cholestasis	0.65 (0.25–1.45)	14.4 (5.7–31.8)
Pregnancy		
1st trimester	NR†	8.5 (3.1–13.9)
2nd trimester	NR†	8.8 (3.8–13.8)
3rd trimester	NR†	13.0 (8.4–17.6)
Sepsis with multi-organ failure	0.47 (0.19–1.9)	18.8 (6.3–24.1)
Thyroid disease		
hypothyroid	0.38 (0.13–0.57)	11.6 (8.2–25)
hyperthyroid	0.8 (0.68–0.97)	4.5 (3.7–5.6)

¶ For various North American patient populations from literature reports. Different rates of elimination and consequent dosage requirements have been observed among other peoples.

* Clearance represents the volume of blood completely cleared of theophylline by the liver in one minute. Values listed were generally determined at serum theophylline concentrations <20 mcg/mL; clearance may decrease and half-life may increase at higher serum concentrations due to non-linear pharmacokinetics.

‡ Reported range or estimated range (mean ± 2 SD) where actual range not reported.

† NR = not reported or not reported in a comparable format.

**Median

Note: In addition to the factors listed above, theophylline clearance is increased and half-life decreased by low carbohydrate/high protein diets, parenteral nutrition, and daily consumption of charcoal-broiled beef. A high carbohydrate/low protein diet can decrease the clearance and prolong the half-life of theophylline.

pharmacokinetic parameters attributable to time of drug administration. On the morning arm, the pharmacokinetic parameters were AUC=241.9±83.0 mcg hr/mL, Cmax=9.3±2.0 mcg/mL, Tmax=12.8±4.2 hours. On the evening arm, the pharmacokinetic parameters were AUC=219.7±83.0 mcg hr/mL, Cmax=9.2±2.0 mcg/mL, Tmax=12.5±4.2 hours.

A study in which Uniphyl® 400 mg tablets were administered to 17 fed adult asthmatics produced similar theophylline level-time curves when administered in the morning or evening. Serum levels were generally higher in the evening regimen but there were no statistically significant differences between the two regimens.

	MORNING	EVENING
AUC (0–24 hrs) (mcg hr/mL)	236.0±76.7	256.0±80.4
Cmax (mcg/mL)	14.5±4.1	16.3±4.5
Cmin (mcg/mL)	5.5±2.9	5.0±2.5
Tmax (hours)	8.1±3.7	10.1±4.1

A single-dose study in 15 normal fasting male volunteers whose theophylline inherent mean elimination half-life was verified by a liquid theophylline product to be 6.9±2.5 (S.D.) hours were administered two or three 400 mg Uniphyl® Tablets. The relative bioavailability of Uniphyl® given in the fasting state in comparison to an immediate-release product was 59%. Peak serum theophylline levels occurred at 6.9±5.2 (S.D.) hours, with a normalized (to 800 mg) peak level being 6.2±2.1 (S.D.) mcg/mL. The apparent elimination half-life for the 400 mg Uniphyl® Tablets was 17.2±5.8 (S.D.) hours. Steady-state pharmacokinetics were determined in a study in 12 fasted patients with chronic reversible obstructive pulmonary disease. All were dosed with two 400 mg Uniphyl®

Tablets given once daily in the morning and a reference controlled-release BID product administered as two 200 mg tablets given 12 hours apart. The pharmacokinetic parameters obtained for Uniphyl® Tablets given at doses of 800 mg once daily in the morning were virtually identical to the corresponding parameters for the reference drug when given as 400 mg BID. In particular, the AUC, Cmax and Cmin values obtained in this study were as follows:

	Uniphyl® Tablets 800 mg Q24h±S.D.	Reference Drug 400 mg Q12h±S.D.
AUC, (0–24 hours), mcg hr/mL	288.9±21.5	283.5±38.4
Cmax, mcg/mL	15.7±2.8	15.2±2.1
Cmin, mcg/mL	7.9±1.6	7.8±1.7
Cmax-Cmin diff.	7.7±1.5	7.4±1.5

Single-dose studies in which subjects were fasted for twelve (12) hours prior to and an additional four (4) hours following dosing, demonstrated reduced bioavailability as compared to dosing with food. One single-dose study in 20 normal volunteers dosed with two (2) 400 mg tablets in the morning, compared dosing under these fasting conditions with dosing immediately prior to a standardized breakfast (769 calories, consisting of 97 grams carbohydrates, 33 grams protein and 27 grams fat). Under fed conditions, the pharmacokinetic parameters were: AUC=231.7±92.4 mcg hr/mL, Cmax=8.4±2.6 mcg/mL, Tmax=17.3±6.7 hours. Under fasting conditions, these parameters were

Continued on next page

Purdue Frederick—Cont.

AUC=141.2±6.53 mcg hr/mL, Cmax=5.5±1.5 mcg/mL, Tmax=6.5±2.1 hours.

Another single-dose study in 21 normal male volunteers, dosed in the evening, compared fasting to a standardized high calorie, high fat meal (870–1,020 calories, consisting of 33 grams protein, 55–75 grams fat, 58 grams carbohydrates). In the fasting arm subjects received one Uniphyl® 400 mg Tablet at 8 p.m. after an eight hour fast followed by a further four hour fast. In the fed arm, subjects were again dosed with one 400 mg Uniphyl® Tablet, but at 8 p.m. immediately after the high fat content standardized meal cited above. The pharmacokinetic parameters (normalized to 800 mg) fed were AUC=221.8±40.9 mcg hr/mL, Cmax=10.9±1.7 mcg/mL, Tmax=11.8±2.2 hours. In the fasting arm, the pharmacokinetic parameters (normalized to 800 mg) were AUC=146.4±40.9 mcg hr/mL, Cmax=6.7±1.7 mcg/mL, Tmax=7.3±2.2 hours.

Thus, administration of single Uniphyl® doses to healthy normal volunteers, under prolonged fasted conditions (at least 10 hour overnight fast before dosing followed by an additional four (4) hour fast after dosing) results in decreased bioavailability. However, there was no failure of this delivery system leading to a sudden and unexpected release of a large quantity of theophylline with Uniphyl® Tablets even when they are administered with a high fat, high calorie meal.

Similar studies were conducted with the 600 mg Uniphyl® Tablet. A single-dose study in 24 subjects with an established theophylline clearance of ≤ 4 L/hr, compared the pharmacokinetic evaluation of one 600 mg Uniphyl® Tablet and one and one-half 400 mg Uniphyl® Tablets under fed (using a standard high fat diet) and fasted conditions. The results of this 4-way randomized crossover study demonstrate the bioequivalence of the 400 mg and 600 mg Uniphyl® Tablets. Under fed conditions, the pharmacokinetic results for the one and one-half 400 mg Tablets were AUC=214.64±55.88 mcg hr/mL, Cmax=10.58±2.21 mcg/mL and Tmax=9.00±2.64 hours, and for the 600 mg Tablet were AUC=207.85±48.9 mcg hr/mL, Cmax=10.39±1.91 mcg/mL and Tmax=9.58 ±1.86 hours. Under fasted conditions the pharmacokinetic results for the one and one-half 400 mg Tablets were AUC=191.85±51.1 mcg hr/mL, Cmax=7.37±1.83 mcg/mL and Tmax=8.08±4.39 hours, and for the 600 mg Tablet were AUC=199.39±70.27 mcg hr/mL, Cmax=7.66±2.09 mcg/mL and Tmax=9.67±4.89 hours.

In this study the mean fed/fasted ratios for the one and one-half 400 mg Tablets and the 600 mg Tablet were about 112% and 104%, respectively.

In another study, the bioavailability of the 600 mg Uniphyl® Tablet was examined with morning and evening administration. This single-dose, crossover study in 22 healthy males was conducted under fed (standard high fat diet) conditions. The results demonstrated no clinically significant difference in the bioavailability of the 600 mg Uniphyl® Tablet administered in the morning or in the evening. The results were: AUC=233.6±45.1 mcg hr/mL, Cmax=10.6±1.3 mcg/mL and Tmax=12.5±3.2 hours with morning dosing; AUC=209.8±46.2 mcg hr/mL, Cmax=9.7±1.4 mcg/mL and Tmax=13.7±3.3 hours with evening dosing. The PM/AM ratio was 89.3%.

The absorption characteristics of Uniphyl® Tablets (theophylline, anhydrous) have been extensively studied. A steady-state crossover bioavailability study in 22 normal males compared two Uniphyl® 400 mg Tablets administered q24h at 8 a.m. immediately after breakfast with a reference controlled-release theophylline product administered BID in fed subjects at 8 a.m. immediately after breakfast and 8 p.m. immediately after dinner (769 calories, consisting of 97 grams carbohydrates, 33 grams protein and 27 grams fat). The pharmacokinetic parameters for Uniphyl® 400 mg Tablets under these steady-state conditions were AUC=203.3±87.1 mcg hr/mL, Cmax=12.1±3.8 mcg/mL, Cmin=4.50±3.6, Tmax=8.8±4.6 hours. For the reference BID product, the pharmacokinetic parameters were AUC=219.2±88.4 mcg hr/mL, Cmax=11.0±4.1 mcg/mL, Cmin=7.28±3.5, Tmax=6.9±3.4 hours. The mean percent fluctuation [(Cmax-Cmin/Cmin) × 100] = 169% for the once-daily regimen and 51% for the reference product BID regimen.

The bioavailability of the 600 mg Uniphyl® tablet was further evaluated in a multiple dose, steady-state study in 26 healthy males comparing the 600 mg Tablet to one and one-half 400 mg Uniphyl® tablets. All subjects had previously established theophylline clearances of ≤ 4L/hr and were dosed once-daily for 6 days under fed conditions. The results showed no clinically significant difference between the 600 mg and one and one-half 400 mg Uniphyl® tablet regimens. Steady-state results were:

	600 MG TABLET FED	600 MG (ONE + ONE-HALF 400 MG TABLETS) FED
AUC 0–24hrs (mcg hr/mL)	209.77±51.04	212.32±56.29
Cmax (mcg/mL)	12.91±2.46	13.17±3.11
Cmin (mcg/mL)	5.52±1.79	5.39±1.95
Tmax (hours)	8.62±3.21	7.23±2.35
Percent Fluctuation	183.73±54.02	179.72±28.86

The bioavailability ratio for the 600/400 mg tablets was 98.8%. Thus, under all study conditions the 600 mg tablet is bioequivalent to one and one-half 400 mg tablets.

Studies demonstrate that as long as subjects were either consistently fed or consistently fasted, there is similar bioavailability with once-daily administration of Uniphyl® tablets whether dosed in the morning or evening.

Distribution Once theophylline enters the systemic circulation, about 40% is bound to plasma protein, primarily albumin. Unbound theophylline distributes throughout body water, but distributes poorly into body fat. The apparent volume of distribution of theophylline is approximately 0.45 L/kg (range 0.3–0.7 L/kg) based on ideal body weight. Theophylline passes freely across the placenta, into breast milk and into the cerebrospinal fluid (CSF). Saliva theophylline concentrations approximate unbound serum concentrations, but are not reliable for routine or therapeutic monitoring unless special techniques are used. An increase in the volume of distribution of theophylline, primarily due to reduction in plasma protein binding, occurs in premature neonates, patients with hepatic cirrhosis, uncorrected acidemia, the elderly and in women during the third trimester of pregnancy. In such cases, the patient may show signs of toxicity at total (bound + unbound) serum concentrations of theophylline in the therapeutic range (10–20 mcg/mL) due to elevated concentrations of the pharmacologically active unbound drug. Similarly, a patient with decreased theophylline binding may have a sub-therapeutic total drug concentration while the pharmacologically active unbound concentration is in the therapeutic range. If only total serum theophylline concentration is measured, this may lead to an unnecessary and potentially dangerous dose increase. In patients with reduced protein binding, measurement of unbound serum theophylline concentration provides a more reliable means of dosage adjustment than measurement of total serum theophylline concentration. Generally, concentrations of unbound theophylline should be maintained in the range of 6–12 mcg/mL

Metabolism Following oral dosing, theophylline does not undergo any measurable first-pass elimination. In adults and children beyond one year of age, approximately 90% of the dose is metabolized in the liver. Biotransformation takes place through demethylation to 1-methylxanthine and 3-methylxanthine and hydroxylation to 1,3-dimethyluric acid. 1-methylxanthine is further hydroxylated, by xanthine oxidase, to 1-methyluric acid. About 6% of a theophylline dose is N-methylated to caffeine. Theophylline demethylation to 3-methylxanthine is catalyzed by cytochrome P-450 1A2, while cytochromes P-450 2E1 and P-450 3A3 catalyze the hydroxylation to 1,3-dimethyluric acid. Demethylation to 1-methylxanthine appears to be catalyzed either by cytochrome P-450 1A2 or a closely related cytochrome. In neonates, the N-demethylation pathway is absent while the function of the hydroxylation pathway is markedly deficient. The activity of these pathways slowly increases to maximal levels by one year of age.

Caffeine and 3-methylxanthine are the only theophylline metabolites with pharmacologic activity. 3-methylxanthine has approximately one tenth the pharmacologic activity of theophylline and serum concentrations in adults with normal renal function are <1 mcg/mL. In patients with end-stage renal disease, 3-methylxanthine may accumulate to concentrations that approximate the unmetabolized theophylline concentration. Caffeine concentrations are usually undetectable in adults regardless of renal function. In neonates, caffeine may accumulate to concentrations that approximate the unmetabolized theophylline concentration and thus, exert a pharmacologic effect.

Both the N-demethylation and hydroxylation pathways of theophylline biotransformation are capacity-limited. Due to the wide intersubject variability of the rate of theophylline metabolism, non-linearity of elimination may begin in some patients at serum theophylline concentrations <10 mcg/mL. Since this non-linearity results in more than proportional changes in serum theophylline concentrations with changes in dose, it is advisable to make increases or decreases in dose in small increments in order to achieve desired changes in serum theophylline concentrations (see DOSAGE AND ADMINISTRATION, Table VI). Accurate prediction of dose-dependency of theophylline metabolism in patients *a priori* is not possible, but patients with very high initial clearance rates (i.e., low steady-state serum theophylline concentrations at above average doses) have the greatest likelihood of experiencing large changes in serum theophylline concentration in response to dosage changes.

Excretion In neonates, approximately 50% of the theophylline dose is excreted unchanged in the urine. Beyond the first three months of life, approximately 10% of the theophylline dose is excreted unchanged in the urine. The remainder is excreted in the urine mainly as 1,3-dimethyluric acid (35–40%), 1-methyluric acid (20–25%) and 3-methylxanthine (15–20%). Since little theophylline is excreted unchanged in the urine and since active metabolites of theophylline (i.e., caffeine, 3-methylxanthine) do not accumulate to clinically significant levels even in the face of end-stage renal disease, no dosage adjustment for renal insufficiency is necessary in adults and children > 3 months of age. In contrast, the large fraction of the theophylline dose excreted in the urine as unchanged theophylline and caffeine in neonates requires careful attention to dose reduction and frequent monitoring of serum theophylline concentrations in neonates with reduced renal function (See WARNINGS).

Serum Concentrations at Steady State After multiple doses of theophylline, steady state is reached in 30–65 hours (average 40 hours) in adults. At steady state, on a dosage regimen with 24-hour intervals, the expected mean trough concentration is approximately 50% of the mean peak concentration, assuming a mean theophylline half-life of 8 hours. The difference between peak and trough concentrations is larger in patients with more rapid theophylline clearance. In these patients administration of Uniphyl® may be required more frequently (every 12 hours).

Special Populations (See Table I for mean clearance and half-life values)

Geriatric The clearance of theophylline is decreased by an average of 30% in healthy elderly adults (> 60 yrs) compared to healthy young adults. Careful attention to dose reduction and frequent monitoring of serum theophylline concentrations are required in elderly patients (see WARNINGS).

Pediatrics The clearance of theophylline is very low in neonates (see WARNINGS). Theophylline clearance reaches maximal values by one year of age, remains relatively constant until about 9 years of age and then slowly decreases by approximately 50% to adult values at about age 16. Renal excretion of unchanged theophylline in neonates amounts to about 50% of the dose, compared to about 10% in children older than three months and in adults. Careful attention to dosage selection and monitoring of serum theophylline concentrations are required in pediatric patients (see WARNINGS and DOSAGE AND ADMINISTRATION).

Gender Gender differences in theophylline clearance are relatively small and unlikely to be of clinical significance. Significant reduction in theophylline clearance, however, has been reported in women on the 20th day of the menstrual cycle and during the third trimester of pregnancy.

Race Pharmacokinetic differences in theophylline clearance due to race have not been studied.

Renal insufficiency Only a small fraction, e.g., about 10%, of the administered theophylline dose is excreted unchanged in the urine of children greater than three months of age and adults. Since little theophylline is excreted unchanged in the urine and since active metabolites of theophylline (i.e., caffeine, 3-methylxanthine) do not accumulate to clinically significant levels even in the face of end-stage renal disease, no dosage adjustment for renal insufficiency is necessary in adults and children > 3 months of age. In contrast, approximately 50% of the administered theophylline dose is excreted unchanged in the urine in neonates. Careful attention to dose reduction and frequent monitoring of serum theophylline concentrations are required in neonates with decreased renal function (see WARNINGS).

Hepatic Insufficiency Theophylline clearance is decreased by 50% or more in patients with hepatic insufficiency (e.g., cirrhosis, acute hepatitis, cholestasis). Careful attention to dose reduction and frequent monitoring of serum theophylline concentrations are required in patients with reduced hepatic function (see WARNINGS).

Congestive Heart Failure (CHF) Theophylline clearance is decreased by 50% or more in patients with CHF. The extent of reduction in theophylline clearance in patients with CHF appears to be directly correlated to the severity of the cardiac disease. Since theophylline clearance is independent of liver blood flow, the reduction in clearance appears to be due to impaired hepatocyte function rather than reduced perfusion. Careful attention to dose reduction and frequent monitoring of serum theophylline concentrations are required in patients with CHF (see WARNINGS).

Smokers Tobacco and marijuana smoking appears to increase the clearance of theophylline by induction of metabolic pathways. Theophylline clearance has been shown to increase by approximately 50% in young adult tobacco smokers and by approximately 80% in elderly tobacco smokers compared to non-smoking subjects. Passive smoke exposure has also been shown to increase theophylline clearance by up to 50%. Abstinence from tobacco smoking for one week causes a reduction of approximately 40% in theophylline clearance. Careful attention to dose reduction and frequent monitoring of serum theophylline concentrations are required in patients who stop smoking (see WARNINGS). Use

of nicotine gum has been shown to have no effect on theophylline clearance.

Fever Fever, regardless of its underlying cause, can decrease the clearance of theophylline. The magnitude and duration of the fever appear to be directly correlated to the degree of decrease of theophylline clearance. Precise data are lacking, but a temperature of 39°C (102°F) for at least 24 hours is probably required to produce a clinically significant increase in serum theophylline concentrations. Children with rapid rates of theophylline clearance (i.e., those who require a dose that is substantially larger than average [e.g., > 22 mg/kg/day] to achieve a therapeutic peak serum theophylline concentration when afebrile) may be at greater risk of toxic effects from decreased clearance during sustained fever. Careful attention to dose reduction and frequent monitoring of serum theophylline concentrations are required in patients with sustained fever (see WARNINGS).

Miscellaneous Other factors associated with decreased theophylline clearance include the third trimester of pregnancy, sepsis with multiple organ failure, and hypothyroidism. Careful attention to dose reduction and frequent monitoring of serum theophylline concentrations are required in patients with any of these conditions (see WARNINGS). Other factors associated with increased theophylline clearance include hyperthyroidism and cystic fibrosis.

Clinical Studies: In patients with chronic asthma, including patients with severe asthma requiring inhaled corticosteroids or alternate-day oral corticosteroids, many clinical studies have shown that theophylline decreases the frequency and severity of symptoms, including nocturnal exacerbations, and decreases the "as needed" use of inhaled beta-2 agonists. Theophylline has also been shown to reduce the need for short courses of daily oral prednisone to relieve exacerbations of airway obstruction that are unresponsive to bronchodilators in asthmatics.

In patients with chronic obstructive pulmonary disease (COPD), clinical studies have shown that theophylline decreases dyspnea, air trapping, the work of breathing, and improves contractility of diaphragmatic muscles with little or no improvement in pulmonary function measurements.

INDICATIONS AND USAGE

Theophylline is indicated for the treatment of the symptoms and reversible airflow obstruction associated with chronic asthma and other chronic lung diseases, e.g., emphysema and chronic bronchitis.

CONTRAINDICATIONS

Uniphyl® is contraindicated in patients with a history of hypersensitivity to theophylline or other components in the product.

WARNINGS

Concurrent Illness: Theophylline should be used with extreme caution in patients with the following clinical conditions due to the increased risk of exacerbation of the concurrent condition.

Active peptic ulcer disease
Seizure disorders
Cardiac arrhythmias (not including bradyarrhythmias)

Conditions That Reduce Theophylline Clearance: There are several readily identifiable causes of reduced theophylline clearance. ***If the total daily dose is not appropriately reduced in the presence of these risk factors, severe and potentially fatal theophylline toxicity can occur.*** Careful consideration must be given to the benefits and risks of theophylline use and the need for more intensive monitoring of serum theophylline concentrations in patients with the following risk factors:

Age

Neonates (term and premature)
Children < 1 year
Elderly (> 60 years)

Concurrent Diseases

Acute pulmonary edema
Congestive heart failure
Cor-pulmonale
Fever; ≥ 102° for 24 hours or more; or lesser temperature elevations for longer periods
Hypothyroidism
Liver disease, cirrhosis, acute hepatitis
Reduced renal function in infants < 3 months of age
Sepsis with multi-organ failure
Shock

Cessation of Smoking

Drug Interactions

Adding a drug that inhibits theophylline metabolism (e.g., cimetidine, erythromycin, tacrine) or stopping a concurrently administered drug that enhances theophylline metabolism (e.g., carbamazepine, rifampin). (See PRECAUTIONS, Drug Interactions, Table II).

When Signs or Symptoms of Theophylline Toxicity Are Present:

Whenever a patient receiving theophylline develops nausea or vomiting, particularly repetitive vomiting, or other signs or symptoms consistent with theophylline toxicity (even if another cause may be suspected), additional doses of theophylline should be withheld and a serum theophylline concentration measured immediately. Patients should be instructed not to continue any dosage that causes adverse effects and to withhold subsequent doses until the symptoms have resolved, at which time the clinician may instruct the patient to resume the drug at a lower dosage (see DOSAGE AND ADMINISTRATION, Dosing Guidelines, Table VI).

Dosage Increases: Increases in the dose of theophylline should not be made in response to an acute exacerbation of symptoms of chronic lung disease since theophylline provides little added benefit to inhaled $beta_2$-selective agonists and systemically administered corticosteroids in this circumstance and increases the risk of adverse effects. A peak steady-state serum theophylline concentration should be measured before increasing the dose in response to persistent chronic symptoms to ascertain whether an increase in dose is safe. Before increasing the theophylline dose on the basis of a low serum concentration, the clinician should consider whether the blood sample was obtained at an appropriate time in relationship to the dose and whether the patient has adhered to the prescribed regimen (see PRECAUTIONS, Laboratory Tests).

As the rate of theophylline clearance may be dose-dependent (i.e., steady-state serum concentrations may increase disproportionately to the increase in dose), an increase in dose based upon a sub-therapeutic serum concentration measurement should be conservative. In general, limiting dose increases to about 25% of the previous total daily dose will reduce the risk of unintended excessive increases in serum theophylline concentration (see DOSAGE AND ADMINISTRATION, Table VI).

PRECAUTIONS

General: Careful consideration of the various interacting drugs and physiologic conditions that can alter theophylline clearance and require dosage adjustment should occur prior to initiation of theophylline therapy, prior to increases in theophylline dose, and during follow up (see WARNINGS). The dose of theophylline selected for initiation of therapy should be low and, ***if tolerated,*** increased slowly over a period of a week or longer with the final dose guided by monitoring serum theophylline concentrations and the patient's clinical response (see DOSAGE AND ADMINISTRATION, Table V).

Monitoring Serum Theophylline Concentrations: Serum theophylline concentration measurements are readily available and should be used to determine whether the dosage is appropriate. Specifically, the serum theophylline concentration should be measured as follows:

1. When initiating therapy to guide final dosage adjustment after titration.
2. Before making a dose increase to determine whether the serum concentration is sub-therapeutic in a patient who continues to be symptomatic.
3. Whenever signs or symptoms of theophylline toxicity are present.
4. Whenever there is a new illness, worsening of a chronic illness or a change in the patient's treatment regimen that may alter theophylline clearance (e.g., fever > 102°F sustained for ≥ 24 hours, hepatitis, or drugs listed in Table II are added or discontinued).

To guide a dose increase, the blood sample should be obtained at the time of the expected peak serum theophylline concentration; 12 hours after an evening dose or 9 hours after a morning dose at steady-state. For most patients, steady-state will be reached after 3 days of dosing when no doses have been missed, no extra doses have been added, and none of the doses have been taken at unequal intervals. A trough concentration (i.e., at the end of the dosing interval) provides no additional useful information and may lead to an inappropriate dose increase since the peak serum theophylline concentration can be two or more times greater than the trough concentration with an immediate-release formulation. If the serum sample is drawn more than 12 hours after the evening dose, or more than 9 hours after a morning dose, the results must be interpreted with caution since the concentration may not be reflective of the peak concentration. In contrast, when signs or symptoms of theophylline toxicity are present, a serum sample should be obtained as soon as possible, analyzed immediately, and the result reported to the clinician without delay. In patients in whom decreased serum protein binding is suspected (e.g., cirrhosis, women during the third trimester of pregnancy), the concentration of unbound theophylline should be measured and the dosage adjusted to achieve an unbound concentration of 6–12 mcg/mL.

Saliva concentrations of theophylline cannot be used reliably to adjust dosage without special techniques.

Effects on Laboratory Tests: As a result of its pharmacological effects, theophylline at serum concentrations within the 10–20 mcg/mL range modestly increases plasma glucose (from a mean of 88 mg% to 98 mg%), uric acid (from a mean of 4 mg/dl to 6 mg/dl), free fatty acids (from a mean of 451 μEq/l to 800 μEq/l, total cholesterol (from a mean of 140 vs 160 mg/dl), HDL (from a mean of 36 to 50 mg/dl), HDL/LDL ratio (from a mean of 0.5 to 0.7), and urinary free cortisol excretion (from a mean of 44 to 63 mcg/24 hr). Theophylline at serum concentrations within the 10–20 mcg/mL range may also transiently decrease serum concentrations of triiodothyronine (144 before, 131 after one week and 142 ng/dL after 4 weeks of theophylline). The clinical importance of these changes should be weighed against the potential therapeutic benefit of theophylline in individual patients.

Information for Patients: The patient (or parent/care giver) should be instructed to seek medical advice whenever nausea, vomiting, persistent headache, insomnia or rapid heart beat occurs during treatment with theophylline, even if another cause is suspected. The patient should be instructed to contact their clinician if they develop a new illness, especially if accompanied by a persistent fever, if they experience worsening of a chronic illness, if they start or stop smoking cigarettes or marijuana, or if another clinician adds a new medication or discontinues a previously prescribed medication. Patients should be instructed to inform all clinicians involved in their care that they are taking theophylline, especially when a medication is being added or deleted from their treatment. Patients should be instructed to not alter the dose, timing of the dose, or frequency of administration without first consulting their clinician. If a dose is missed, the patient should be instructed to take the next dose at the usually scheduled time and to not attempt to make up for the missed dose.

Uniphyl® tablets can be taken once a day in the morning or evening. It is recommended that Uniphyl® be taken with meals. Patients should be advised that if they choose to take Uniphyl® with food it should be taken consistently with food and if they take it in a fasted condition it should routinely be taken fasted. It is important that the product whenever dosed be dosed consistently with or without food.

Uniphyl® tablets are not to be chewed or crushed. The scored tablet may be split. Patients receiving Uniphyl® tablets may pass an intact matrix tablet in the stool or via colostomy. These matrix tablets usually contain little or no residual theophylline.

Drug Interactions: Theophylline interacts with a wide variety of drugs. The interaction may be pharmacodynamic, i.e., alterations in the therapeutic response to theophylline or another drug or occurrence of adverse effects without a change in serum theophylline concentration. More frequently, however, the interaction is pharmacokinetic, i.e., the rate of theophylline clearance is altered by another drug resulting in increased or decreased serum theophylline concentrations. Theophylline only rarely alters the pharmacokinetics of other drugs.

The drugs listed in Table II have the potential to produce clinically significant pharmacodynamic or pharmacokinetic interactions with theophylline. The information in the "Effect" column of Table II assumes that the interacting drug is being added to a steady-state theophylline regimen. If theophylline is being initiated in a patient who is already taking a drug that inhibits theophylline clearance (e.g., cimetidine, erythromycin), the dose of theophylline required to achieve a therapeutic serum theophylline concentration will be smaller. Conversely, if theophylline is being initiated in a patient who is already taking a drug that enhances theophylline clearance (e.g., rifampin), the dose of theophylline required to achieve a therapeutic serum theophylline concentration will be larger. Discontinuation of a concomitant drug that increases theophylline clearance will result in accumulation of theophylline to potentially toxic levels, unless the theophylline dose is appropriately reduced. Discontinuation of a concomitant drug that inhibits theophylline clearance will result in decreased serum theophylline concentrations, unless the theophylline dose is appropriately increased.

The drugs listed in Table III have either been documented not to interact with theophylline or do not produce a clinically significant interaction (i.e., < 15% change in theophylline clearance).

The listing of drugs in Tables II and III are current as of February 9, 1995. New interactions are continuously being reported for theophylline, especially with new chemical entities. **The clinician should not assume that a drug does not interact with theophylline if it is not listed in Table II.** Before addition of a newly available drug in a patient receiving theophylline, the package insert of the new drug and/or the medical literature should be consulted to determine if an interaction between the new drug and theophylline has been reported.

[See Table II on next page.]

Table III. Drugs that have been documented not to interact with theophylline or drugs that produce no clinically significant interaction with theophylline.*

albuterol, systemic and inhaled	mebendazole
amoxicillin	medroxyprogesterone
ampicillin, with or without sulbactam	methylprednisolone
atenolol	metronidazole
azithromycin	metoprolol
caffeine, dietary ingestion	nadolol
	nifedipine
	nizatidine

Continued on next page

Purdue Frederick—Cont.

cefaclor	norfloxacin
co-trimoxazole (trimethoprim and sulfamethoxazole)	ofloxacin
	omeprazole
diltiazem	prednisone, prednisolone
dirithromycin	ranitidine
enflurane	rifabutin
famotidine	roxithromycin
felodipine	sorbitol (purgative doses
finasteride	do not inhibit
hydrocortisone	theophylline
isoflurane	absorption)
isoniazid	sucralfate
isradipine	terbutaline, systemic
influenza vaccine	terfenadine
ketoconazole	tetracycline
lomefloxacin	tocainide

* Refer to PRECAUTIONS, Drug Interactions for information regarding table.

Drug-Food Interactions: The bioavailability of Uniphyl® tablets (theophylline, anhydrous) has been studied with co-administration of food. In three single-dose studies, subjects given Uniphyl® 400 mg or 600 mg tablets with a standardized high-fat meal were compared to fasted conditions. Under fed conditions, the peak plasma concentration and bioavailability were increased; however, a precipitous increase in the rate and extent of absorption was not evident (See **Pharmacokinetics-Absorption**). The increased peak and extent of absorption under fed conditions suggests that dosing should be ideally administered consistently either with or without food.

The Effect of Other Drugs on Theophylline Serum Concentration Measurements: Most serum theophylline assays in clinical use are immunoassays which are specific for theophylline. Other xanthines such as caffeine, dyphylline, and pentoxifylline are not detected by these assays. Some drugs (e.g., cefazolin, cephalothin), however, may interfere with certain HPLC techniques. Caffeine and xanthine metabolites in neonates or patients with renal dysfunction may cause the reading from some dry reagent office methods to be higher than the actual serum theophylline concentration.

Carcinogenesis, Mutagenesis, and Impairment of Fertility: Long term carcinogenicity studies have been carried out in mice (oral doses 30–150 mg/kg) and rats (oral doses 5–75 mg/kg). Results are pending.

Theophylline has been studied in Ames salmonella, in vivo and in vitro cytogenetics, micronucleus and Chinese hamster ovary test systems and has not been shown to be genotoxic. In a 14 week continuous breeding study, theophylline, administered to mating pairs of B6C3F$_1$ mice at oral doses of 120, 270 and 500 mg/kg (approximately 1.0–3.0 times the human dose on a mg/m^2 basis) impaired fertility, as evidenced by decreases in the number of live pups per litter, decreases in the mean number of litters per fertile pair, and increases in the gestation period at the high dose as well as decreases in the proportion of pups born alive at the mid and high dose. In 13 week toxicity studies, theophylline was administered to F344 rats and B6C3F$_1$ mice at oral doses of 40–300 mg/kg (approximately 2.0 times the human dose on a mg/m^2 basis). At the high dose, systemic toxicity was observed in both species including decreases in testicular weight.

Pregnancy: CATEGORY C: There are no adequate and well controlled studies in pregnant women. Additionally, there are no teratogenicity studies in non-rodents (e.g., rabbits). Theophylline was not shown to be teratogenic in CD-1 mice at oral doses up to 400 mg/kg, approximately 2.0 times the human dose on a mg/m^2 basis or in CD-1 rats at oral doses up to 260 mg/kg, approximately 3.0 times the recommended human dose on a mg/m^2 basis. At a dose of 220 mg/kg, embryotoxicity was observed in rats in the absence of maternal toxicity.

Nursing Mothers: Theophylline is excreted into breast milk and may cause irritability or other signs of mild toxicity in nursing human infants. The concentration of theophylline in breast milk is about equivalent to the maternal serum concentration. An infant ingesting a liter of breast milk containing 10–20 mcg/mL of theophylline per day is likely to receive 10–20 mg of theophylline per day. Serious adverse effects in the infant are unlikely unless the mother has toxic serum theophylline concentrations.

Pediatric Use: Theophylline is safe and effective for the approved indications in pediatric patients. The maintenance dose of theophylline must be selected with caution in pediatric patients since the rate of theophylline clearance is highly variable across the pediatric age range (see CLINICAL PHARMACOLOGY, Table I, WARNINGS, and DOSAGE AND ADMINISTRATION, Table V).

Geriatric Use: Elderly patients are at significantly greater risk of experiencing serious toxicity from theophylline than younger patients due to pharmacokinetic and pharmacody-

Table II. Clinically significant drug interactions with theophylline*.

Drug	Type of Interaction	Effect**
Adenosine	Theophylline blocks adenosine receptors.	Higher doses of adenosine may be required to achieve desired effect.
Alcohol	A single large dose of alcohol (3 mL/kg of whiskey) decreases theophylline clearance for up to 24 hours.	30% increase
Allopurinol	Decreases theophylline clearance at allopurinol doses ≥ 600 mg/day.	25% increase
Aminoglutethimide	Increases theophylline clearance by induction of microsomal enzyme activity.	25% decrease
Carbamazepine	Similar to aminoglutethimide.	30% decrease
Cimetidine	Decreases theophylline clearance by inhibiting cytochrome P450 1A2.	70% increase
Ciprofloxacin	Similar to cimetidine.	40% increase
Clarithromycin	Similar to erythromycin.	25% increase
Diazepam	Benzodiazepines increase CNS concentrations of adenosine, a potent CNS depressant, while theophylline blocks adenosine receptors.	Larger diazepam doses may be required to produce desired level of sedation. Discontinuation of theophylline without reduction of diazepam dose may result in respiratory depression.
Disulfiram	Decreases theophylline clearance by inhibiting hydroxylation and demethylation.	50% increase
Enoxacin	Similar to cimetidine.	300% increase
Ephedrine	Synergistic CNS effects	Increased frequency of nausea, nervousness, and insomnia.
Erythromycin	Erythromycin metabolite decreases theophylline clearance by inhibiting cytochrome P450 3A3.	35% increase. Erythromycin steady-state serum concentrations decrease by a similar amount.
Estrogen	Estrogen containing oral contraceptives decrease theophylline clearance in a dose-dependent fashion. The effect of progesterone on theophylline clearance is unknown.	30% increase
Flurazepam	Similar to diazepam.	Similar to diazepam
Fluvoxamine	Similar to cimetidine.	Similar to cimetidine
Halothane	Halothane sensitizes the myocardium to catecholamines, theophylline increases release of endogenous catecholamines.	Increased risk of ventricular arrhythmias.
Interferon, human recombinant alpha-A	Decreases theophylline clearance.	100% increase
Isoproterenol (IV)	Increases theophylline clearance.	20% decrease
Ketamine	Pharmacologic	May lower theophylline seizure threshold.
Lithium	Theophylline increases renal lithium clearance.	Lithium dose required to achieve a therapeutic serum concentration increased an average of 60%.
Lorazepam	Similar to diazepam.	Similar to diazepam.
Methotrexate (MTX)	Decreases theophylline clearance.	20% increase after low dose MTX, higher dose MTX may have a greater effect.
Mexiletine	Similar to disulfiram.	80% increase
Midazolam	Similar to diazepam.	Similar to diazepam.
Moricizine	Increases theophylline clearance.	25% decrease
Pancuronium	Theophylline may antagonize non-depolarizing neuromuscular blocking effects; possibly due to phosphodiesterase inhibition.	Larger dose of pancuronium may be required to achieve neuromuscular blockade.
Pentoxifylline	Decreases theophylline clearance.	30% increase
Phenobarbital (PB)	Similar to aminoglutethimide.	25% decrease after two weeks of concurrent PB.
Phenytoin	Phenytoin increases theophylline clearance by increasing microsomal enzyme activity. Theophylline decreases phenytoin absorption.	Serum theophylline and phenytoin concentrations decrease about 40%.
Propafenone	Decreases theophylline clearance and pharmacologic interaction.	40% increase. Beta-2 blocking effect may decrease efficacy of theophylline.
Propranolol	Similar to cimetidine and pharmacologic interaction.	100% increase. Beta-2 blocking effect may decrease efficacy of theophylline.
Rifampin	Increases theophylline clearance by increasing cytochrome P450 1A2 and 3A3 activity.	20–40% decrease
Sulfinpyrazone	Increases theophylline clearance by increasing demethylation and hydroxylation. Decreases renal clearance of theophylline.	20% decrease
Tacrine	Similar to cimetidine, also increases renal clearance of theophylline.	90% increase
Thiabendazole	Decreases theophylline clearance.	190% increase
Ticlopidine	Decreases theophylline clearance.	60% increase
Troleandomycin	Similar to erythromycin.	33–100% increase depending on troleandomycin dose.
Verapamil	Similar to disulfiram.	20% increase

* Refer to PRECAUTIONS, Drug Interactions for further information regarding table.
** Average effect on steady-state theophylline concentration or other clinical effect for pharmacologic interactions. Individual patients may experience larger changes in serum theophylline concentration than the value listed.

namic changes associated with aging. Theophylline clearance is reduced in patients greater than 60 years of age, resulting in increased serum theophylline concentrations in response to a given theophylline dose. Protein binding may be decreased in the elderly resulting in a larger proportion of the total serum theophylline concentration in the pharmacologically active unbound form. For these reasons, the maximum daily dose of theophylline in patients greater than 60 years of age ordinarily should not exceed 400 mg/day unless the patient continues to be symptomatic and the peak steady-state serum theophylline concentration is <10 mcg/mL (see DOSAGE AND ADMINISTRATION). Theophylline doses greater than 400 mg/d should be prescribed with caution in elderly patients.

ADVERSE REACTIONS

Adverse reactions associated with theophylline are generally mild when peak serum theophylline concentrations are <20 mcg/mL and mainly consist of transient caffeine-like adverse effects such as nausea, vomiting, headache, and insomnia. When peak serum theophylline concentrations exceed 20 mcg/mL, however, theophylline produces a wide range of adverse reactions including persistent vomiting, cardiac arrhythmias, and intractable seizures which can be lethal (see OVERDOSAGE). The transient caffeine-like adverse reactions occur in about 50% of patients when theophylline therapy is initiated at doses higher than recommended initial doses (e.g., >300 mg/day in adults and >12 mg/kg/day in children beyond >1 year of age). During the initiation of theophylline therapy, caffeine-like adverse effects may transiently alter patient behavior, especially in school age children, but this response rarely persists. Initiation of theophylline therapy at a low dose with subsequent slow titration to a predetermined age-related maximum dose will significantly reduce the frequency of these transient adverse effects (see DOSAGE AND ADMINISTRATION, Table V). In a small percentage of patients (<3% of children and <10% of adults) the caffeine-like adverse effects persist during maintenance therapy, even at peak serum theophylline concentrations within the therapeutic range (i.e., 10–20 mcg/mL). Dosage reduction may alleviate the caffeine-like adverse effects in these patients, however, persistent adverse effects should result in a reevaluation of the need for continued theophylline therapy and the potential therapeutic benefit of alternative treatment.

Other adverse reactions that have been reported at serum theophylline concentrations <20 mcg/mL include diarrhea, irritability, restlessness, fine skeletal muscle tremors, and transient diuresis. In patients with hypoxia secondary to COPD, multifocal atrial tachycardia and flutter have been reported at serum theophylline concentrations ≥15 mcg/mL. There have been a few isolated reports of seizures at serum theophylline concentrations <20 mcg/mL in patients with an underlying neurological disease or in elderly patients. The occurrence of seizures in elderly patients with serum theophylline concentrations <20 mcg/mL may be secondary to decreased protein binding resulting in a larger proportion of the total serum theophylline concentration in the pharmacologically active unbound form. The clinical characteristics of the seizures reported in patients with serum theophylline concentrations <20 mcg/mL have generally been milder than seizures associated with excessive serum theophylline concentrations resulting from an overdose (i.e. they have generally been transient, often stopped without anticonvulsant therapy, and did not result in neurological residua).

Table IV. Manifestations of theophylline toxicity.*

	Percentage of patients reported with sign or symptom			
	Acute Overdose (Large Single Ingestion)		Chronic Overdosage (Multiple Excessive Doses)	
Sign/Symptom	Study 1 (n=157)	Study 2 (n=14)	Study 1 (n=92)	Study 2 (n=102)
Asymptomatic	NR**	0	NR**	6
Gastrointestinal				
Vomiting	73	93	30	61
Abdominal Pain	NR**	21	NR**	12
Diarrhea	NR**	0	NR**	14
Hematemesis	NR**	0	NR**	2
Metabolic/Other				
Hypokalemia	85	79	44	43
Hyperglycemia	98	NR**	18	NR**
Acid/base disturbance	34	21	9	5
Rhabdomyolysis	NR**	7	NR**	0
Cardiovascular				
Sinus tachycardia	100	86	100	62
Other supraventricular tachycardias	2	21	12	14
Ventricular premature beats	3	21	10	19
Atrial fibrillation or flutter	1	NR**	12	NR**
Multifocal atrial tachycardia	0	NR**	2	NR**
Ventricular arrhythmias with hemodynamic instability	7	14	40	0
Hypotension/shock	NR**	21	NR**	8
Neurologic				
Nervousness	NR**	64	NR**	21
Tremors	38	29	16	14
Disorientation	NR**	7	NR**	11
Seizures	5	14	14	5
Death	3	21	10	4

* These data are derived from two studies in patients with serum theophylline concentrations >30 mcg/mL. In the first study (Study #1—Shanon, *Ann Intern Med* 1993; 119:1161–67), data were prospectively collected from 249 consecutive cases of theophylline toxicity referred to a regional poison center for consultation. In the second study (Study #2—Sessler, *Am J Med* 1990;88:567–76), data were retrospectively collected from 116 cases with serum theophylline concentrations >30 mcg/mL among 6000 blood samples obtained for measurement of serum theophylline concentrations in three emergency departments. Differences in the incidence of manifestations of theophylline toxicity between the two studies may reflect sample selection as a result of study design (e.g., in Study #1, 48% of the patients had acute intoxications versus only 10% in Study #2) and different methods of reporting results.

**NR=Not reported in a comparable manner.

OVERDOSAGE

General: The chronicity and pattern of theophylline overdosage significantly influences clinical manifestations of toxicity, management and outcome. There are two common presentations: (1) *acute overdose,* i.e., ingestion of a single large excessive dose (>10 mg/kg), as occurs in the context of an attempted suicide or isolated medication error, and (2) *chronic overdosage,* i.e., ingestion of repeated doses that are excessive for the patient's rate of theophylline clearance. The most common causes of chronic theophylline overdosage include patient or care giver error in dosing, clinician prescribing of an excessive dose or a normal dose in the presence of factors known to decrease the rate of theophylline clearance, and increasing the dose in response to an exacerbation of symptoms without first measuring the serum theophylline concentration to determine whether a dose increase is safe.

Severe toxicity from theophylline overdose is a relatively rare event. In one health maintenance organization, the frequency of hospital admissions for chronic overdosage of theophylline was about 1 per 1000 person-years exposure. In another study, among 6000 blood samples obtained for measurement of serum theophylline concentration, for any reason, from patients treated in an emergency department, 7% were in the 20–30 mcg/mL range and 3% were >30 mcg/mL. Approximately two-thirds of the patients with serum theophylline concentrations in the 20–30 mcg/mL range had one or more manifestations of toxicity while >90% of patients with serum theophylline concentrations >30 mcg/mL were clinically intoxicated. Similarly, in other reports, serious toxicity from theophylline is seen principally at serum concentrations >30 mcg/mL.

Several studies have described the clinical manifestations of theophylline overdose and attempted to determine the factors that predict life-threatening toxicity. In general, patients who experience an acute overdose are less likely to experience seizures than patients who have experienced a chronic overdosage, unless the peak serum theophylline concentration is >100 mcg/mL. After a chronic overdosage, generalized seizures, life-threatening cardiac arrhythmias, and death may occur at serum theophylline concentrations >30 mcg/mL. The severity of toxicity after chronic overdosage is more strongly correlated with the patient's age than the peak serum theophylline concentration; patients >60 years are at the greatest risk for severe toxicity and mortality after a chronic overdosage. Pre-existing or concurrent disease may also significantly increase the susceptibility of a patient to a particular toxic manifestation, e.g., patients with neurologic disorders have an increased risk of seizures and patients with cardiac disease have an increased risk of cardiac arrhythmias for a given serum theophylline concentration compared to patients without the underlying disease.

The frequency of various reported manifestations of theophylline overdose according to the mode of overdose are listed in Table IV.

Other manifestations of theophylline toxicity include increases in serum calcium, creatine kinase, myoglobin and leukocyte count, decreases in serum phosphate and magnesium, acute myocardial infarction, and urinary retention in men with obstructive uropathy.

Seizures associated with serum theophylline concentrations >30 mcg/mL are often resistant to anticonvulsant therapy and may result in irreversible brain injury if not rapidly controlled. Death from theophylline toxicity is most often secondary to cardiorespiratory arrest and/or hypoxic encephalopathy following prolonged generalized seizures or intractable cardiac arrhythmias causing hemodynamic compromise.

Overdose Management: General Recommendations for Patients with Symptoms of Theophylline Overdose or Serum Theophylline Concentrations >30 mcg/mL (Note: Serum theophylline concentrations may continue to increase after presentation of the patient for medical care.)

1. While simultaneously instituting treatment, contact a regional poison center to obtain updated information and advice on individualizing the recommendations that follow.
2. Institute supportive care, including establishment of intravenous access, maintenance of the airway, and electrocardiographic monitoring.
3. Treatment of seizures Because of the high morbidity and mortality associated with theophylline-induced seizures, treatment should be rapid and aggressive. Anticonvulsant therapy should be initiated with an intravenous benzodiazepine, e.g., diazepam, in increments of 0.1–0.2 mg/kg every 1–3 minutes until seizures are terminated. Repetitive seizures should be treated with a loading dose of phenobarbital (20 mg/kg infused over 30–60 minutes). Case reports of theophylline overdose in humans and animal studies suggest that phenytoin is ineffective in terminating theophylline-induced seizures. The doses of benzodiazepines and phenobarbital required to terminate theophylline-induced seizures are close to the doses that may cause severe respiratory depression or respiratory arrest; the clinician should therefore be prepared to provide assisted ventilation. Elderly patients and patients with COPD may be more susceptible to the respiratory depressant effects of anticonvulsants. Barbiturate-induced coma or administration of general anesthesia may be required to terminate repetitive seizures or status epilepticus. General anesthesia should be used with caution in patients with theophylline overdose because fluorinated volatile anesthetics may sensitize the myocardium to endogenous catecholamines released by theophylline. Enflurane appears less likely to be associated with this effect than halothane and may, therefore, be safer. Neuromuscular blocking agents alone should not be used to terminate seizures since they abolish the musculoskeletal manifestations without terminating seizure activity in the brain.
4. Anticipate Need for Anticonvulsants in patients with theophylline overdose who are at high risk for theophylline-induced seizures, e.g., patients with acute overdoses and serum theophylline concentrations >100 mcg/mL or chronic overdosage in patients >60 years of age with serum theophylline concentrations >30 mcg/mL, the need for anticonvulsant therapy should be anticipated. A benzodiazepine such as diazepam should be drawn into a syringe and kept at the patient's bedside and medical personnel qualified to treat seizures should be immediately available. In selected patients at high risk for theophylline-induced seizures, consideration should be given to the administration of prophylactic anticonvulsant therapy. Situations where prophylactic anticonvulsant therapy should be considered in high risk patients include anticipated delays in instituting methods for extracorporeal removal of theophylline (e.g., transfer of a high risk patient from one health care facility to another for extracorporeal removal) and clinical circumstances that significantly interfere with efforts to enhance theophylline clearance (e.g., a neonate where dialysis may not be technically feasible or a patient with vomiting unresponsive to antiemetics who is unable to tolerate multiple-dose oral activated charcoal). In animal studies, prophylactic administration of phenobarbital, but not phenytoin, has been shown to delay the onset of theophylline-induced generalized seizures and to increase the dose of theophylline required to induce seizures (i.e., markedly increases the LD_{50}). Although there are no controlled studies in humans, a loading dose of intravenous phenobarbital (20 mg/kg infused over 60 minutes) may delay or prevent life-threatening seizures in high risk patients while efforts to enhance theophylline clearance are continued. Phenobarbital may cause respiratory depression, particularly in elderly patients and patients with COPD.
5. Treatment of cardiac arrhythmias Sinus tachycardia and simple ventricular premature beats are not harbingers of life-threatening arrhythmias, they do not require treatment in the absence of hemodynamic compromise, and they resolve with declining serum theophylline concentra-

Continued on next page

Purdue Frederick—Cont.

tions. Other arrhythmias, especially those associated with hemodynamic compromise, should be treated with antiarrhythmic therapy appropriate for the type of arrhythmia.

6. Gastrointestinal decontamination Oral activated charcoal (0.5 g/kg up to 20 g and repeat at least once 1–2 hours after the first dose) is extremely effective in blocking the absorption of theophylline throughout the gastrointestinal tract, even when administered several hours after ingestion. If the patient is vomiting, the charcoal should be administered through a nasogastric tube or after administration of an antiemetic. Phenothiazine antiemetics such as prochlorperazine or perphenazine should be avoided since they can lower the seizure threshold and frequently cause dystonic reactions. A single dose of sorbitol may be used to promote stooling to facilitate removal of theophylline bound to charcoal from the gastrointestinal tract. Sorbitol, however, should be dosed with caution since it is a potent purgative which can cause profound fluid and electrolyte abnormalities, particularly after multiple doses. Commercially available fixed combinations of liquid charcoal and sorbitol should be avoided in young children and after the first dose in adolescents and adults since they do not allow for individualization of charcoal and sorbitol dosing. Ipecac syrup should be avoided in theophylline overdoses. Although ipecac induces emesis, it does not reduce the absorption of theophylline unless administered within 5 minutes of ingestion and even then is less effective than oral activated charcoal. Moreover, ipecac induced emesis may persist for several hours after a single dose and significantly decrease the retention and the effectiveness of oral activated charcoal.

7. Serum Theophylline Concentration Monitoring The serum theophylline concentration should be measured immediately upon presentation, 2–4 hours later, and then at sufficient intervals, e.g., every 4 hours, to guide treatment decisions and to assess the effectiveness of therapy. Serum theophylline concentrations may continue to increase after presentation of the patient for medical care as a result of continued absorption of theophylline from the gastrointestinal tract. Serial monitoring of serum theophylline serum concentrations should be continued until it is clear that the concentration is no longer rising and has returned to non-toxic levels.

8. General Monitoring Procedures Electrocardiographic monitoring should be initiated on presentation and continued until the serum theophylline level has returned to a non-toxic level. Serum electrolytes and glucose should be measured on presentation and at appropriate intervals indicated by clinical circumstances. Fluid and electrolyte abnormalities should be promptly corrected. **Monitoring and treatment should be continued until the serum concentration decreases below 20 mcg/mL.**

9. Enhance clearance of theophylline Multiple-dose oral activated charcoal (e.g., 0.5 mg/kg up to 20 g, every two hours) increases the clearance of theophylline at least twofold by adsorption of theophylline secreted into gastrointestinal fluids. Charcoal must be retained in, and pass through, the gastrointestinal tract to be effective; emesis should therefore be controlled by administration of appropriate antiemetics. Alternatively, the charcoal can be administered continuously through a nasogastric tube in conjunction with appropriate antiemetics. A single dose of sorbitol may be administered with the activated charcoal to promote stooling to facilitate clearance of the adsorbed theophylline from the gastrointestinal tract. Sorbitol alone does not enhance clearance of theophylline and should be dosed with caution to prevent excessive stooling which can result in severe fluid and electrolyte imbalances. Commercially available fixed combinations of liquid charcoal and sorbitol should be avoided in young children and after the first dose in adolescents and adults since they do not allow for individualization of charcoal and sorbitol dosing. In patients with intractable vomiting, extracorporeal methods of theophylline removal should be instituted (see OVERDOSAGE, Extracorporeal Removal).

Specific Recommendations:

Acute Overdose

A. Serum Concentration > 20 < 30 mcg/mL
1. Administer a single dose of oral activated charcoal.
2. Monitor the patient and obtain a serum theophylline concentration in 2–4 hours to insure that the concentration is not increasing.

B. Serum Concentration > 30 < 100 mcg/mL
1. Administer multiple dose oral activated charcoal and measures to control emesis.
2. Monitor the patient and obtain serial theophylline concentrations every 2–4 hours to gauge the effectiveness of therapy and to guide further treatment decisions.
3. Institute extracorporeal removal if emesis, seizures, or cardiac arrhythmias cannot be adequately controlled (see OVERDOSAGE, Extracorporeal Removal).

C. Serum Concentration > 100 mcg/mL
1. Consider prophylactic anticonvulsant therapy.
2. Administer multiple-dose oral activated charcoal and measures to control emesis.
3. Consider extracorporeal removal, even if the patient has not experienced a seizure (see OVERDOSAGE, Extracorporeal Removal).
4. Monitor the patient and obtain serial theophylline concentrations every 2–4 hours to gauge the effectiveness of therapy and to guide further treatment decisions.

Chronic Overdosage

A. Serum Concentration > 20 < 30 mcg/mL (with manifestations of theophylline toxicity)
1. Administer a single dose of oral activated charcoal.
2. Monitor the patient and obtain a serum theophylline concentration in 2–4 hours to insure that the concentration is not increasing.

B. Serum Concentration > 30 mcg/mL in patients < 60 years of age
1. Administer multiple-dose oral activated charcoal and measures to control emesis.
2. Monitor the patient and obtain serial theophylline concentrations every 2–4 hours to gauge the effectiveness of therapy and to guide further treatment decisions.
3. Institute extracorporeal removal if emesis, seizures, or cardiac arrhythmias cannot be adequately controlled (see OVERDOSAGE, Extracorporeal Removal).

C. Serum Concentration > 30 mcg/mL in patients ≥ 60 years of age
1. Consider prophylactic anticonvulsant therapy.
2. Administer multiple-dose oral activated charcoal and measures to control emesis.
3. Consider extracorporeal removal even if the patient has not experienced a seizure (see OVERDOSAGE, Extracorporeal Removal).
4. Monitor the patient and obtain serial theophylline concentrations every 2–4 hours to gauge the effectiveness of therapy and to guide further treatment decisions.

Extracorporeal Removal: Increasing the rate of theophylline clearance by extracorporeal methods may rapidly decrease serum concentrations, but the risks of the procedure must be weighed against the potential benefit. Charcoal hemoperfusion is the most effective method of extracorporeal removal, increasing theophylline clearance up to six fold, but serious complications, including hypotension, hypocalcemia, platelet consumption and bleeding diatheses may occur. Hemodialysis is about as efficient as multiple-dose oral activated charcoal and has a lower risk of serious complications than charcoal hemoperfusion. Hemodialysis should be considered as an alternative when charcoal hemoperfusion is not feasible and multiple-dose oral charcoal is ineffective because of intractable emesis. Serum theophylline concentrations may rebound 5–10 mcg/mL after discontinuation of charcoal hemoperfusion or hemodialysis due to redistribution of theophylline from the tissue compartment. Peritoneal dialysis is ineffective for theophylline removal; exchange transfusions in neonates have been minimally effective.

DOSAGE AND ADMINISTRATION

Uniphyl® 400 or 600 mg Tablets can be taken once a day in the morning or evening. It is recommended that Uniphyl be taken with meals. Patients should be advised that if they choose to take Uniphyl® with food it should be taken consistently with food and if they take it in a fasted condition it should routinely be taken fasted. It is important that the product whenever dosed be dosed consistently with or without food.

Uniphyl® Tablets are not to be chewed or crushed. The scored tablet may be split. Infrequently, patients receiving Uniphyl® 400 or 600 mg Tablets may pass an intact matrix tablet in the stool or via colostomy. These matrix tablets usually contain little or no residual theophylline.

Stabilized patients, 12 years of age or older, who are taking an immediate-release or controlled-release theophylline product may be transferred to once-daily administration of 400 mg or 600 mg Uniphyl® Tablets on a mg-for-mg basis. It must be recognized that the peak and trough serum theophylline levels produced by the once-daily dosing may vary from those produced by the previous product and/or regimen.

General Considerations: The steady-state peak serum theophylline concentration is a function of the dose, the dosing interval, and the rate of theophylline absorption and clearance in the individual patient. Because of marked individual differences in the rate of theophylline clearance, the dose required to achieve a peak serum theophylline concentration in the 10–20 mcg/mL range varies fourfold among otherwise similar patients in the absence of factors known to alter theophylline clearance (e.g., 400–1600 mg/day in adults < 60 years old and 10–36 mg/kg/day in children 1–9 years old). For a given population there is no single theophylline dose that will provide both safe and effective serum concentrations for all patients. Administration of the median theophylline dose required to achieve a therapeutic serum theophylline concentration in a given population may result in

either sub-therapeutic or potentially toxic serum theophylline concentrations in individual patients. For example, at a dose of 900 mg/d in adults < 60 years or 22 mg/kg/d in children 1–9 years, the steady-state peak serum theophylline concentration will be < 10 mcg/mL in about 30% of patients, 10–20 mcg/mL in about 50% and 20–30 mcg/mL in about 20% of patients. **The dose of theophylline must be individualized on the basis of peak serum theophylline concentration measurements in order to achieve a dose that will provide maximum potential benefit with minimal risk of adverse effects.**

Transient caffeine-like adverse effects and excessive serum concentrations in slow metabolizers can be avoided in most patients by starting with a sufficiently low dose and slowly increasing the dose, if judged to be clinically indicated, in small increments (See Table V). Dose increases should only be made if the previous dosage is well tolerated and at intervals of no less than 3 days to allow serum theophylline concentrations to reach the new steady-state. Dosage adjustment should be guided by serum theophylline concentration measurement (see PRECAUTIONS, Laboratory Tests and DOSAGE AND ADMINISTRATION, Table VI). Health care providers should instruct patients and care givers to discontinue any dosage that causes adverse effects, to withhold the medication until these symptoms are gone and to then resume therapy at a lower, previously tolerated dosage (see WARNINGS).

If the patient's symptoms are well controlled, there are no apparent adverse effects, and no intervening factors that might alter dosage requirements (see WARNINGS and PRECAUTIONS), serum theophylline concentrations should be monitored at 6 month intervals for rapidly growing children and at yearly intervals for all others. In acutely ill patients, serum theophylline concentrations should be monitored at frequent intervals, e.g., every 24 hours.

Theophylline distributes poorly into body fat, therefore, mg/kg dose should be calculated on the basis of ideal body weight.

Table V contains theophylline dosing titration schema recommended for patients in various age groups and clinical circumstances. Table VI contains recommendations for theophylline dosage adjustment based upon serum theophylline concentrations. **Application of these general dosing recommendations to individual patients must take into account the unique clinical characteristics of each patient. In general, these recommendations should serve as the upper limit for dosage adjustments in order to decrease the risk of potentially serious adverse events associated with unexpected large increases in serum theophylline concentration.**

Table V. Dosing initiation and titration (as anhydrous theophylline).*

A. Children (12–15 years) and adults (16–60 years) without risk factors for impaired clearance.

Titration Step	Children < 45 kg	Children > 45 kg and adults
1. Starting Dosage	12–14 mg/kg/day up to a maximum of 300 mg/day admin. QD*	300–400 mg/day† admin. QD*
2. After 3 days, if tolerated, increase dose to:	16 mg/kg/day up to a maximum of 400 mg/day admin. QD*	400–600 mg/day† admin. QD*
3. After 3 more days, if tolerated and if needed increase dose to:	20 mg/kg/day up to a maximum of 600 mg/day admin. QD*	As with all theophylline products, doses greater than 600 mg should be titrated according to blood level (See Table VI)

†If caffeine-like adverse effects occur, then consideration should be given to a lower dose and titrating the dose more slowly (see ADVERSE REACTIONS).

B. Patients With Risk Factors For Impaired Clearance, The Elderly (> 60 Years), And Those In Whom It Is Not Feasible To Monitor Serum Theophylline Concentrations:
In children 12–15 years of age, the theophylline dose should not exceed 16 mg/kg/day up to a maximum of 400 mg/day in the presence of risk factors for reduced theophylline clearance (see WARNINGS) or if it is not feasible to monitor serum theophylline concentrations.

In adolescents ≥ 16 years and adults, including the elderly, the theophylline dose should not exceed 400 mg/day in the presence of risk factors for reduced theophylline clearance (see WARNINGS) or if it is not feasible to monitor serum theophylline concentrations.

*Patients with more rapid metabolism clinically identified by higher than average dose requirements, should receive a smaller dose more frequently (every 12 hours) to prevent breakthrough symptoms resulting from low trough concentrations before the next dose.

Table VI. Dosage adjustment guided by serum theophylline concentration.

Peak Serum Concentration	Dosage Adjustment
<9.9 mcg/mL	If symptoms are not controlled and current dosage is tolerated, increase dose about 25%. Recheck serum concentration after three days for further dosage adjustment.
10–14.9 mcg/mL	If symptoms are controlled and current dosage is tolerated, maintain dose and recheck serum concentration at 6–12 month intervals.¶ If symptoms are not controlled and current dosage is tolerated consider adding additional medication(s) to treatment regimen.
15–19.9 mcg/mL	Consider 10% decrease in dose to provide greater margin of safety even if current dosage is tolerated.¶
20–24.9 mcg/mL	Decrease dose by 25% even if no adverse effects are present. Recheck serum concentration after 3 days to guide further dosage adjustment.
25–30 mcg/mL	Skip next dose and decrease subsequent doses at least 25% even if no adverse effects are present. Recheck serum concentration after 3 days to guide further dosage adjustment. If symptomatic, consider whether overdose treatment is indicated (see recommendations for chronic overdosage).
>30 mcg/mL	Treat overdose as indicated (see recommendations for chronic overdosage). If theophylline is subsequently resumed, decrease dose by at least 50% and recheck serum concentration after 3 days to guide further dosage adjustment.

¶ Dose reduction and/or serum theophylline concentration measurement is indicated whenever adverse effects are present, physiologic abnormalities that can reduce theophylline clearance occur (e.g., sustained fever), or a drug that interacts with theophylline is added or discontinued (see WARNINGS).

HOW SUPPLIED

Uniphyl® (theophylline, anhydrous) 400 mg Controlled-Release Tablets are supplied in white-opaque plastic bottles containing 100 tablets (NDC 0034-7004-80) or 500 tablets (NDC 0034-7004-70).

Each round, white, scored 400 mg tablet bears the symbol PF on one side and is marked U400 on the other side.

Uniphyl® (theophylline, anhydrous) 600 mg Controlled-Release Tablets are supplied in white-opaque plastic bottles containing 100 tablets (NDC 0034-7006-80).

Each rectangular, concave, white 600 mg scored tablet bears the symbol PF on one side and is marked U600 on the other side.

Store at controlled room temperature 15°–30°C (59°–86°F).

Dispense in tight, light-resistant container.

CAUTION: Federal law prohibits dispensing without prescription.

The Purdue Frederick Company
Norwalk, CT 06850-3590

Copyright © 1996 The Purdue Frederick Company
U.S. Patent Numbers 4,235,870 and 4,366,310
June 12, 1996   R1374

Shown in Product Identification Guide, page 330

Purdue Pharma L.P.
100 CONNECTICUT AVENUE
NORWALK, CT 06850-3590

DHCplus® Capsules—see listing under The Purdue Frederick Company, page 2148.

MS Contin® Tablets—see listing under The Purdue Frederick Company, page 2149.

MSIR® Capsules—see listing under The Purdue Frederick Company, page 2152.

MSIR® Tablets—see listing under The Purdue Frederick Company, page 2152.

MSIR® Liquid—see listing under The Purdue Frederick Company, page 2152.

OXYCONTIN™   Ⓒ Ⴥ
(OXYCODONE HCL CONTROLLED-RELEASE) TABLETS
Warning-May be habit forming.
10mg 20mg 40mg

DESCRIPTION
OxyContin™ (oxycodone hydrochloride controlled-release) tablets are an opioid analgesic supplied in 10 mg, 20 mg, and 40 mg tablet strengths for oral administration. The tablet strengths describe the amount of oxycodone per tablet as the hydrochloride salt. The structural formula for oxycodone hydrochloride is as follows:

$C_{18}H_{21}NO_4 \bullet HCl$ MW 351.83

The chemical formula is 4, 5-epoxy-14-hydroxy-3-methoxy-17-methylmorphinan-6-one hydrochloride.

Oxycodone is a white, odorless crystalline powder derived from the opium alkaloid, thebaine. Oxycodone hydrochloride dissolves in water (1 g in 6 to 7 mL). It is slightly soluble in alcohol (octanol water partition coefficient 0.7). The tablets contain the following inactive ingredients: ammonio methacrylate copolymer, hydroxypropyl methylcellulose, lactose, magnesium stearate, povidone, red iron oxide (20 mg strength tablet only), stearyl alcohol, talc, titanium dioxide, triacetin, yellow iron oxide (40 mg strength tablet only), and other ingredients.

CLINICAL PHARMACOLOGY
Central Nervous System
Oxycodone is a pure agonist opioid whose principal therapeutic action is analgesia. Other therapeutic effects of oxycodone include anxiolysis, euphoria and feelings of relaxation. Like all pure opioid agonists, there is no ceiling effect to analgesia, such as is seen with partial agonists or non-opioid analgesics.

The precise mechanism of the analgesic action is unknown. However, specific CNS opioid receptors for endogenous compounds with opioid-like activity have been identified throughout the brain and spinal cord and play a role in the analgesic effects of this drug.

Oxycodone produces respiratory depression by direct action on brain stem respiratory centers. The respiratory depression involves both a reduction in the responsiveness of the brain stem respiratory centers to increases in carbon dioxide tension and to electrical stimulation.

Oxycodone depresses the cough reflex by direct effect on the cough center in the medulla. Antitussive effects may occur with doses lower than those usually required for analgesia. Oxycodone causes miosis, even in total darkness. Pinpoint pupils are a sign of opioid overdose but are not pathognomonic. Marked mydriasis rather than miosis may be seen due to hypoxia in overdose situations.

Gastrointestinal Tract and Other Smooth Muscle
Oxycodone causes a reduction in motility associated with an increase in smooth muscle tone in the antrum of the stomach and duodenum. Digestion of food in the small intestine is delayed and propulsive contractions are decreased. Propulsive peristaltic waves in the colon are decreased, while tone may be increased to the point of spasm resulting in constipation. Other opioid-induced effects may include a reduction in gastric, biliary and pancreatic secretions, spasm of sphincter of Oddi, and transient elevations in serum amylase.

Cardiovascular System
Oxycodone may produce release of histamine with or without associated peripheral vasodilation. Manifestations of histamine release and/or peripheral vasodilation may include pruritus, flushing, red eyes, sweating, and/or orthostatic hypotension.

Concentration—Efficacy Relationships (Pharmacodynamics)
Studies in normal volunteers and patients reveal predictable relationships between oxycodone dosage and plasma oxycodone concentrations, as well as between concentration and certain expected opioid effects. In normal volunteers these include pupillary constriction, sedation and overall "drug effect" and in patients, analgesia and feelings of "relaxation." In non-tolerant patients, analgesia is not usually seen at a plasma oxycodone concentration of less than 5–10 ng/mL.

As with all opioids, the minimum effective plasma concentration for analgesia will vary widely among patients, especially among patients who have been previously treated with potent agonist opioids. As a result, patients need to be treated with individualized titration of dosage to the desired effect. The minimum effective analgesic concentration of oxycodone for any individual patient may increase with re-

peated dosing due to an increase in pain and/or the development of tolerance.

Concentration—Adverse Experience Relationships
OxyContin™ tablets are associated with typical opioid-related adverse experiences similar to those seen with immediate-release oxycodone and all opioids. There is a general relationship between increasing oxycodone plasma concentration and increasing frequency of dose-related opioid adverse experiences such as nausea, vomiting, CNS effects and respiratory depression. In opioid-tolerant patients, the situation is altered by the development of tolerance to opioid-related side effects, and the relationship is poorly understood.

As with all opioids, the dose must be individualized (see DOSAGE AND ADMINISTRATION), because the effective analgesic dose for some patients will be too high to be tolerated by other patients.

PHARMACOKINETICS AND METABOLISM
The activity of OxyContin™ (oxycodone hydrochloride controlled-release) tablets is primarily due to the parent drug oxycodone. OxyContin tablets are designed to provide controlled delivery of oxycodone over 12 hours. Oxycodone is well absorbed from OxyContin tablets with an oral bioavailability of from 60% to 87%. The relative oral bioavailability of OxyContin to immediate-release oral dosage forms is 100%. Upon repeated dosing in normal volunteers, steady-state levels were achieved within 24–36 hours of dosing. Dose proportionality has been established for the 10 mg, 20 mg and 40 mg tablet strengths for both peak plasma levels (C_{max}) and extent of absorption (AUC). Oxycodone is extensively metabolized and eliminated primarily in the urine as both conjugated and unconjugated metabolites. The apparent elimination half-life of oxycodone following the administration of OxyContin was 4.5 hours compared to 3.2 hours for immediate-release oxycodone.

Absorption
About 60% to 87% of an oral dose of oxycodone reaches the central compartment in comparison to a parenteral dose. This high oral bioavailability is due to low pre-systemic and/or first-pass metabolism. In normal volunteers the $t^1/_2$ of absorption is 0.4 hours for immediate-release oral oxycodone. In contrast, OxyContin tablets exhibit a biphasic absorption pattern with two apparent absorption half-times of 0.6 and 6.9 hours, which describes the initial release of oxycodone from the tablet followed by a prolonged release.

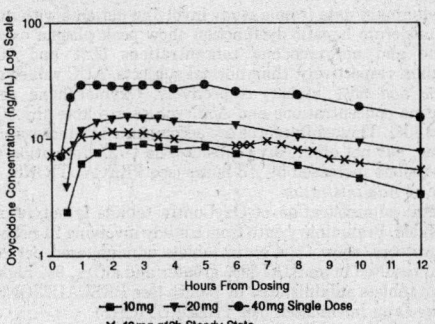

Plasma Oxycodone By Time

- ■ 10mg   ▼ 20mg   ● 40mg Single Dose
- ✕ 10mg q12h Steady-State

Dose proportionality has been established for the 10 mg, 20 mg and 40 mg tablet strengths for both peak plasma concentrations (C_{max}) and extent of absorption (AUC) (see Table 1 below). Given the short half-life of elimination of oxycodone from OxyContin, steady-state plasma concentrations of oxycodone are achieved within 24–36 hours of initiation of dosing with OxyContin tablets. In a study comparing 10 mg of OxyContin every 12 hours to 5 mg of immediate-release oxycodone every 6 hours the two treatments were found to be equivalent for AUC and C_{max}, and similar for C_{min} (trough) concentrations. There was less fluctuation in plasma concentrations for the OxyContin tablets than for the immediate-release formulation.

[See Table 1 at bottom of next page.]

Food Effects
In contrast to immediate-release formulations, food has no significant effect on the absorption of oxycodone from OxyContin. Oxycodone release from OxyContin tablets is pH independent.

Distribution
Following intravenous administration, the volume of distribution (Vss) for oxycodone was 2.6L/kg. Oxycodone binding to plasma protein at 37C° and a pH of 7.4 was about 45%. Once absorbed, oxycodone is distributed to skeletal muscle, liver, intestinal tract, lungs, spleen and brain. Oxycodone has been found in breast milk (see PRECAUTIONS).

Metabolism
Oxycodone hydrochloride is extensively metabolized to noroxycodone, oxymorphone, and their glucuronides. The

Continued on next page

Purdue Pharma L.P.—Cont.

major circulating metabolite is noroxycodone with an AUC ratio of 0.6 relative to that of oxycodone. Noroxycodone is reported to be a considerably weaker analgesic than oxycodone. Oxymorphone, although possessing analgesic activity, is present in the plasma only in low concentrations. The correlation between oxymorphone concentrations and opioid effects was much less than that seen with oxycodone plasma concentrations. The analgesic activity profile of other metabolites is not known at present.

The formation of oxymorphone, but not noroxycodone, is mediated by CYP2D6 and as such its formation can, in theory, be affected by other drugs (see Drug-Drug Interactions).

Excretion
Oxycodone and its metabolites are excreted primarily via the kidney. The amounts measured in the urine have been reported as follows: free oxycodone up to 19%; conjugated oxycodone up to 50%; free oxymorphone 0%; conjugated oxymorphone ≤ 14%; both free and conjugated noroxycodone have been found in the urine but not quantified. The total plasma clearance was 0.8 L/min for adults.
Special Populations
Elderly
The plasma concentrations of oxycodone are only nominally affected by age, being 15% greater in elderly as compared to young subjects. There were no differences in adverse event reporting between young and elderly subjects.
Gender
Female subjects have, on average, plasma oxycodone concentrations up to 25% higher than males on a body weight adjusted basis. The reason for this difference is unknown.
Renal Impairment
Preliminary data from a study involving patients with mild to severe renal dysfunction (creatinine clearance < 60 mL/min) show peak plasma oxycodone and noroxycodone concentrations 50% and 20% higher, respectively and AUC values for oxycodone, noroxycodone and oxymorphone 60%, 50% and 40% higher than normal subjects, respectively. This is accompanied by an increase in sedation but not by differences in respiratory rate, pupillary constriction, or several other measures of drug effect. There was an increase in $t^1/_2$ of elimination for oxycodone of only 1 hour (see PRECAUTIONS).
Hepatic Impairment
Preliminary data from a study involving patients with mild to moderate hepatic dysfunction show peak plasma oxycodone and noroxycodone concentrations 50% and 20% higher, respectively, than normal subjects. AUC values are 95% and 65% higher, respectively. Oxymorphone peak plasma concentrations and AUC values are lower by 30% and 40%. These differences are accompanied by increases in some, but not other, drug effects. The $t^1/_2$ elimination for oxycodone increased by 2.3 hours (see PRECAUTIONS).
Rectal Administration
Rectal administration of OxyContin tablets is not recommended. Preliminary data from a study involving 21 normal volunteers, show OxyContin tablets administered per rectum resulted in an AUC 39% greater and a C_{max} 9% higher than tablets administered by mouth (see PRECAUTIONS).
Drug-Drug Interactions (see PRECAUTIONS)
Oxycodone is metabolized in part via CYP2D6 to oxymorphone which represents less than 15% of the total administered dose. This route of elimination can be blocked by a variety of drugs (e.g., certain cardiovascular drugs and anti-depressants). Patients receiving such drugs concomitantly with OxyContin do not appear to present different therapeutic profiles than other patients.

CLINICAL TRIALS

OxyContin™ (oxycodone hydrochloride controlled-release) tablets were evaluated in studies involving 713 patients with either cancer or non-cancer pain. All patients receiving OxyContin were dosed q12h. Efficacy comparable to other forms of oral oxycodone was demonstrated in clinical studies using pharmacokinetic, pharmacodynamic and efficacy outcomes. The outcome of these trials indicated: (1) a positive relationship between dose and plasma oxycodone concentration, (2) a positive relationship between plasma oxycodone concentration and analgesia, and (3) an observed peak to trough variation in plasma concentration with OxyContin lying within the observed range established with qid dosing of immediate-release oxycodone in clinical populations at the same total daily dose.

In clinical trials, OxyContin tablets were substituted for a wide variety of analgesics, including acetaminophen (APAP), aspirin (ASA), other non-steroidal anti-inflammatory drugs (NSAIDs), opioid combination products and single-entity opioids, primarily morphine. In cancer patients receiving adequate opioid therapy at baseline, pain intensity scores and acceptability of therapy remained unchanged by transfer to OxyContin. For non-cancer pain patients who had moderate to severe pain at baseline on prn opioid therapy, pain control and acceptability of therapy improved with the introduction of fixed-interval therapy with OxyContin.
Use in Cancer Pain
OxyContin was studied in three double-blind, controlled clinical trials involving 341 cancer patients and several open-label trials with therapy durations of over 10 months.
Two, double-blind, controlled clinical studies indicated that OxyContin dosed q12h produced analgesic efficacy equivalent to immediate-release oxycodone dosed qid at the same total daily dose. Peak and trough plasma concentrations attained were similar to those attained with immediate-release oxycodone at equivalent total daily doses. With titration to analgesic effect and proper use of rescue medication, nearly every patient achieved adequate pain control with OxyContin.
In the third study, a double-blind, active-controlled, crossover trial, OxyContin dosed q12h was shown to be equivalent in efficacy and safety to immediate-release oxycodone dosed qid at the same total daily dose. Patients were able to be titrated to an acceptable analgesic effect with either OxyContin or immediate-release oxycodone with both treatments providing stable pain control within 2 days in most patients.
In patients with cancer pain, the total daily OxyContin doses tested ranged from 20 mg to 640 mg per day. The average total daily dose was approximately 105 mg per day.
Studies in Non-Cancer Pain
A double-blind, placebo-controlled, fixed-dose, parallel group study was conducted in 133 patients with moderate to severe osteoarthritis pain, who were judged as having inadequate pain control with prn opioids and maximal non-steroidal anti-inflammatory therapy. In this study, 20 mg OxyContin q12h significantly decreased pain and improved quality of life, mood and sleep, relative to placebo. Both dose-concentration and concentration-effect relationships were noted with a minimum effective plasma oxycodone concentration of approximately 5–10 ng/mL.
In a double-blind, active-controlled, crossover study involving 57 patients with low-back pain inadequately controlled with prn opioids and non-opioid therapy, OxyContin administered q12h provided analgesia equivalent to immediate-release oxycodone administered qid. Patients could be titrated to an acceptable analgesic effect with either OxyContin or immediate-release forms of oxycodone.
Single-Dose Comparison with Standard Therapy
A single-dose, double-blind, placebo-controlled, post-operative study of 182 patients was conducted utilizing graded doses of OxyContin (10, 20 and 30 mg). Twenty and 30 mg of OxyContin gave equivalent peak analgesic effect compared to two oxycodone 5 mg / acetaminophen 325 mg tablets and to 15 mg immediate-release oxycodone, while the 10 mg dose of OxyContin was intermediate between both the immediate-release and combination products and placebo. The onset of

analgesic action with OxyContin occurred within 1 hour in most patients following oral administration.
OxyContin is not recommended pre-operatively (preemptive analgesia) or for the management of pain in the immediate post-operative period (the first 12 to 24 hours following surgery) because the safety or appropriateness of fixed-dose, long-acting opioids in this setting has not been established.
Other Clinical Trials
In open-label trials involving approximately 200 patients with cancer-related and non-cancer pain, dosed according to the package insert recommendations, appropriate analgesic effectiveness was noted without regard to age, gender, race, or disease state. There were no unusual drug interactions observed in patients receiving a wide range of medications common in these populations.
For opioid-naive patients, the average total daily dose of OxyContin was approximately 40 mg per day. There was no evidence of oxycodone and metabolite accumulation during 8 months of therapy. For cancer pain patients the average total daily dose was 105 mg (range 20 to 720 mg) per day. There was a significant decrease in acute opioid-related side effects, except for constipation, during the first several weeks of therapy. Development of significant tolerance to analgesia was uncommon.

INDICATIONS AND USAGE

OxyContin™ tablets are a controlled-release oral formulation of oxycodone hydrochloride indicated for the management of moderate to severe pain where use of an opioid analgesic is appropriate for more than a few days. (See: CLINICAL PHARMACOLOGY; CLINICAL TRIALS).

CONTRAINDICATIONS

OxyContin™ is contraindicated in patients with known hypersensitivity to oxycodone, or in any situation where opioids are contraindicated. This includes patients with significant respiratory depression (in unmonitored settings or the absence of resuscitative equipment), and patients with acute or severe bronchial asthma or hypercarbia. OxyContin is contraindicated in any patient who has or is suspected of having paralytic ileus.

WARNINGS

OxyContin™ (oxycodone hydrochloride controlled-release) TABLETS ARE TO BE SWALLOWED WHOLE, AND ARE NOT TO BE BROKEN, CHEWED OR CRUSHED. TAKING BROKEN, CHEWED OR CRUSHED OxyContin TABLETS COULD LEAD TO THE RAPID RELEASE AND ABSORPTION OF A POTENTIALLY TOXIC DOSE OF OXYCODONE.
Respiratory Depression
Respiratory depression is the chief hazard from all opioid agonist preparations. Respiratory depression occurs most frequently in elderly or debilitated patients, usually following large initial doses in non-tolerant patients, or when opioids are given in conjunction with other agents that depress respiration.
Oxycodone should be used with extreme caution in patients with significant chronic obstructive pulmonary disease or cor pulmonale, and in patients having a substantially decreased respiratory reserve, hypoxia, hypercapnia, or preexisting respiratory depression. In such patients, even usual therapeutic doses of oxycodone may decrease respiratory drive to the point of apnea. In these patients alternative non-opioid analgesics should be considered, and opioids should be employed only under careful medical supervision at the lowest effective dose.
Head Injury
The respiratory depressant effects of opioids include carbon dioxide retention and secondary elevation of cerebrospinal fluid pressure, and may be markedly exaggerated in the presence of head injury, intracranial lesions, or other sources of preexisting increased intracranial pressure. Oxycodone produces effects on pupillary response and consciousness which may obscure neurologic signs of further increases in intracranial pressure in patients with head injuries.
Hypotensive Effect
OxyContin™, like all opioid analgesics, may cause severe hypotension in an individual whose ability to maintain blood pressure has been compromised by a depleted blood volume, or after concurrent administration with drugs such as phenothiazines or other agents which compromise vasomotor tone. OxyContin may produce orthostatic hypotension in ambulatory patients. OxyContin, like all opioid analgesics, should be administered with caution to patients in circulatory shock, since vasodilation produced by the drug may further reduce cardiac output and blood pressure.

PRECAUTIONS

General
OxyContin™ (oxycodone hydrochloride controlled-release) tablets are intended for use in patients who require oral pain therapy with an opioid agonist of more than a few days duration. As with any opioid analgesic, it is critical to adjust the

Table 1
Mean [% coefficient variation]

Regimen/Dosage Form	AUC (ng·hr/mL)†	C_{max} (ng/mL)	T_{max} (hrs)	Trough Conc. (ng/mL)
Single Dose				
10 mg OxyContin	100.7 [26.6]	10.6 [20.1]	2.7 [44.1]	n.a.
20 mg OxyContin	207.5 [35.9]	21.4 [36.6]	3.2 [57.9]	n.a.
40 mg OxyContin	423.1 [33.3]	39.3 [34.0]	3.1 [77.4]	n.a.
Multiple Dose				
10 mg OxyContin Tablets q12h	103.6 [38.6]	15.1 [31.0]	3.2 [69.5]	7.2 [48.1]
5 mg immediate-release q6h	99.0 [36.2]	15.5 [28.8]	1.6 [49.7]	7.4 [50.9]

† for single-dose AUC=AUC_{0-inf}; for multiple-dose AUC=AUC_{0-T}

dosing regimen individually for each patient (see DOSAGE AND ADMINISTRATION).

Selection of patients for treatment with OxyContin should be governed by the same principles that apply to the use of similar controlled-release opioid analgesics (see INDICATIONS AND USAGE). Opioid analgesics given on a fixed-dosage schedule have a narrow therapeutic index in certain patient populations, especially when combined with other drugs, and should be reserved for cases where the benefits of opioid analgesia outweigh the known risks of respiratory depression, altered mental state, and postural hypotension. Physicians should individualize treatment in every case, using non-opioid analgesics, prn opioids and/or combination products, and chronic opioid therapy with drugs such as OxyContin in a progressive plan of pain management such as outlined by the World Health Organization, the Agency for Health Care Policy and Research, and the American Pain Society.

Use of OxyContin is associated with increased potential risks and should be used only with caution in the following conditions: acute alcoholism; adrenocortical insufficiency (e.g., Addison's disease); CNS depression or coma; delirium tremens; debilitated patients; kyphoscoliosis associated with respiratory depression; myxedema or hypothyroidism; prostatic hypertrophy or urethral stricture; severe impairment of hepatic, pulmonary or renal function; and toxic psychosis. The administration of oxycodone, like all opioid analgesics, may obscure the diagnosis or clinical course in patients with acute abdominal conditions. Oxycodone may aggravate convulsions in patients with convulsive disorders, and all opioids may induce or aggravate seizures in some clinical settings.

Interactions with other CNS Depressants

OxyContin, like all opioid analgesics, should be used with caution and started in a reduced dosage ($^1/_3$ to $^1/_2$ of the usual dosage) in patients who are concurrently receiving other central nervous system depressants including sedatives or hypnotics, general anesthetics, phenothiazines, other tranquilizers and alcohol. Interactive effects resulting in respiratory depression, hypotension, profound sedation or coma may result if these drugs are taken in combination with the usual doses of OxyContin.

Interactions with Mixed Agonist/Antagonist Opioid Analgesics

Agonist/antagonist analgesics (i.e., pentazocine, nalbuphine, butorphanol and buprenorphine) should be administered with caution to a patient who has received or is receiving a course of therapy with a pure opioid agonist analgesic such as oxycodone. In this situation, mixed agonist/antagonist analgesics may reduce the analgesic effect of oxycodone and/or may precipitate withdrawal symptoms in these patients.

Ambulatory Surgery

OxyContin is not recommended pre-operatively (preemptive analgesia) or for the management of pain in the immediate post-operative period (the first 12 to 24 hours following surgery) for patients not previously taking the drug, because its safety in this setting has not been established.

Patients who are already receiving OxyContin tablets as part of ongoing analgesic therapy may be safely continued on the drug if appropriate dosage adjustments are made considering the procedure, other drugs given and the temporary changes in physiology caused by the surgical intervention (see PRECAUTIONS: Drug-Drug Interactions, and DOSAGE AND ADMINISTRATION).

Use in Pancreatic/Biliary Tract Disease

Oxycodone may cause spasm of the sphincter of Oddi and should be used with caution in patients with biliary tract disease, including acute pancreatitis. Opioids like oxycodone may cause increases in the serum amylase level.

Tolerance and Physical Dependence

Tolerance is the need for increasing doses of opioids to maintain a defined effect such as analgesia (in the absence of disease progression or other external factors). Physical dependence is the occurrence of withdrawal symptoms after abrupt discontinuation of a drug or upon administration of an antagonist. Physical dependence and tolerance are not unusual during chronic opioid therapy.

Significant tolerance should not occur in most of the patients treated with the lowest doses of oxycodone. It should be expected, however, that a fraction of cancer patients will develop some degree of tolerance and require progressively higher dosages of OxyContin to maintain pain control during chronic treatment. Regardless of whether this occurs as a result of increased pain secondary to disease progression or pharmacological tolerance, dosages can usually be increased safely by adjusting the patient's dose to maintain an acceptable balance between pain relief and side effects. The dosage should be selected according to the patient's individual analgesic response and ability to tolerate side effects. Tolerance to the analgesic effect of opioids is usually paralleled by tolerance to side effects, except for constipation.

Physical dependence results in withdrawal symptoms in patients who abruptly discontinue the drug or may be precipitated through the administration of drugs with opioid antagonist activity (see OVERDOSAGE). If OxyContin is abruptly discontinued in a physically dependent patient, an abstinence syndrome may occur. This is characterized by some or all of the following: restlessness, lacrimation, rhinorrhea, yawning, perspiration, chills, myalgia and mydriasis. Other symptoms also may develop, including: irritability, anxiety, backache, joint pain, weakness, abdominal cramps, insomnia, nausea, anorexia, vomiting, diarrhea, or increased blood pressure, respiratory rate or heart rate.

If signs and symptoms of withdrawal occur, patients should be treated by reinstitution of opioid therapy followed by a gradual, tapered dose reduction of OxyContin combined with symptomatic support (see DOSAGE AND ADMINISTRATION: Cessation of Therapy).

Information for Patients/Caregivers

If clinically advisable, patients receiving OxyContin (oxycodone hydrochloride controlled-release) tablets or their caregivers should be given the following information by the physician, nurse, pharmacist or caregiver:

1. Patients should be advised that OxyContin tablets were designed to work properly only if swallowed whole. They may release all their contents at once if broken, chewed or crushed, resulting in a risk of overdose.
2. Patients should be advised to report episodes of breakthrough pain and adverse experiences occurring during therapy. Individualization of dosage is essential to make optimal use of this medication.
3. Patients should be advised not to adjust the dose of OxyContin without consulting the prescribing professional.
4. Patients should be advised that OxyContin may impair mental and/or physical ability required for the performance of potentially hazardous tasks (e.g., driving, operating heavy machinery).
5. Patients should not combine OxyContin with alcohol or other central nervous system depressants (sleep aids, tranquilizers) except by the orders of the prescribing physician, because additive effects may occur.
6. Women of childbearing potential who become, or are planning to become, pregnant should be advised to consult their physician regarding the effects of analgesics and other drug use during pregnancy on themselves and their unborn child.
7. Patients should be advised that OxyContin is a potential drug of abuse. They should protect it from theft, and it should never be given to anyone other than the individual for whom it was prescribed.
8. Patients should be advised that they may pass empty matrix "ghosts" (tablets) via colostomy or in the stool, and that this is of no concern since the active medication has already been absorbed.
9. Patients should be advised that if they have been receiving treatment with OxyContin for more than a few weeks and cessation of therapy is indicated, it may be appropriate to taper the OxyContin dose, rather than abruptly discontinue it, due to the risk of precipitating withdrawal symptoms. Their physician can provide a dose schedule to accomplish a gradual discontinuation of the medication.

Laboratory Monitoring

Due to the broad range of plasma concentrations seen in clinical populations, the varying degrees of pain, and the development of tolerance, plasma oxycodone measurements are usually not helpful in clinical management. Plasma concentrations of the active drug substance may be of value in selected, unusual or complex cases.

Interactions with Alcohol and Drugs of Abuse

Oxycodone may be expected to have additive effects when used in conjunction with alcohol, other opioids or illicit drugs which cause central nervous system depression.

Use in Drug and Alcohol Addiction

OxyContin is an opioid with no approved use in the management of addictive disorders. Its proper usage in individuals with drug or alcohol dependence, either active or in remission, is for the management of pain requiring opioid analgesia.

Drug-Drug Interactions

Opioid analgesics, including OxyContin, may enhance the neuromuscular blocking action of skeletal muscle relaxants and produce an increased degree of respiratory depression. Oxycodone is metabolized in part to oxymorphone via CYP2D6. While this pathway may be blocked by a variety of drugs (e.g., certain cardiovascular drugs and antidepressants), such blockade has not yet been shown to be of clinical significance with this agent. Clinicians should be aware of this possible interaction, however.

Use with CNS Depressants

OxyContin, like all opioid analgesics, should be started at $^1/_3$ to $^1/_2$ of the usual dosage in patients who are concurrently receiving other central nervous system depressants including sedatives or hypnotics, general anesthetics, phenothiazines, centrally acting anti-emetics, tranquilizers and alcohol because respiratory depression, hypotension and profound sedation or coma may result. No specific interaction between oxycodone and monoamine oxidase inhibitors has been observed, but caution in the use of any opioid in patients taking this class of drugs is appropriate.

Mutagenicity

Studies of oxycodone in animals to evaluate its carcinogenic and mutagenic potential have not been conducted owing to the length of clinical experience with the drug substance.

Pregnancy

Teratogenic Effects—Category B: Reproduction studies have been performed in rats and rabbits by oral administration at doses up to 8 mg/kg (48 mg/m^2) and 125 mg/kg (1375 mg/m^2), respectively. These doses are 4 and 60 times a human dose of 120 mg/day (74 mg/m^2), based on mg/kg of a 60 kg adult (0.7 and 19 times this human dose based upon mg/m^2). The results did not reveal evidence of harm to the fetus due to oxycodone. There are, however, no adequate and well-controlled studies in pregnant women. Because animal reproduction studies are not always predictive of human response, this drug should be used during pregnancy only if clearly needed.

Nonteratogenic Effects—Neonates whose mothers have been taking oxycodone chronically may exhibit respiratory depression and/or withdrawal symptoms, either at birth and/or in the nursery.

Labor and Delivery

OxyContin is not recommended for use in women during and immediately prior to labor and delivery because oral opioids may cause respiratory depression in the newborn.

Nursing Mothers

Low concentrations of oxycodone have been detected in breast milk. Withdrawal symptoms can occur in breast-feeding infants when maternal administration of an opioid analgesic is stopped. Ordinarily, nursing should not be undertaken while a patient is receiving OxyContin since oxycodone may be excreted in the milk.

Pediatric Use

Safety and effectiveness in pediatric patients below the age of 18 have not been established with this dosage form of oxycodone. However, oxycodone has been used extensively in the pediatric population in other dosage forms, as have the excipients used in this formulation. No specific increased risk is expected from the use of this form of oxycodone in pediatric patients old enough to safely take tablets if dosing is adjusted for the patient's weight (see DOSAGE AND ADMINISTRATION). It must be remembered that OxyContin tablets cannot be crushed or divided for administration.

Geriatric Use

In controlled pharmacokinetic studies in elderly subjects (greater than 65 years) the clearance of oxycodone appeared to be slightly reduced. Compared to young adults, the plasma concentrations of oxycodone were increased approximately 15%. In clinical trials with appropriate initiation of therapy and dose titration, no untoward or unexpected side effects were seen based on age, and the usual doses and dosing intervals are appropriate for the geriatric patient. As with all opioids, the starting dose should be reduced to $^1/_3$ to $^1/_2$ of the usual dosage in debilitated, non-tolerant patients.

Hepatic Impairment

A study of OxyContin in patients with hepatic impairment indicates greater plasma concentrations than those with normal function. The initiation of therapy at $^1/_3$ to $^1/_2$ the usual doses and careful dose titration is warranted.

Renal Impairment

In patients with renal impairment, as evidenced by decreased creatinine clearance (< 60 mL/min.), the concentrations of oxycodone in the plasma are approximately 50% higher than in subjects with normal renal function. Dose initiation should follow a conservative approach. Dosages should be adjusted according to the clinical situation.

Gender Differences

In pharmacokinetic studies, opioid-naive females demonstrate up to 25% higher average plasma concentrations and greater frequency of typical opioid adverse events than males, even after adjustment for body weight. The clinical relevance of a difference of this magnitude is low for a drug intended for chronic usage at individualized dosages, and there was no male/female difference detected for efficacy or adverse events in clinical trials.

Rectal Administration

OxyContin Tablets are not recommended for administration per rectum. A study in normal volunteers showed a significantly greater AUC and higher C$_{max}$ during this route of administration (see PHARMACOKINETICS AND METABOLISM).

ADVERSE REACTIONS

Serious adverse reactions which may be associated with OxyContin™ (oxycodone hydrochloride controlled-release) tablet therapy in clinical use are those observed with other opioid analgesics, including: respiratory depression, apnea, respiratory arrest, and (to an even lesser degree) circulatory depression, hypotension or shock (see OVERDOSE). The non-serious adverse events seen on initiation of therapy with OxyContin are typical opioid side effects. These events are dose-dependent, and their frequency depends upon the dose, the clinical setting, the patient's level of opioid tolerance, and host factors specific to the individual. They should

Continued on next page

Purdue Pharma L.P.—Cont.

be expected and managed as a part of opioid analgesia. The most frequent (>5%) include constipation, nausea, somnolence, dizziness, vomiting, pruritus, headache, dry mouth, sweating and asthenia.

In many cases the frequency of these events during initiation of therapy may be minimized by careful individualization of starting dosage, slow titration, and the avoidance of large swings in the plasma concentrations of the opioid. Many of these adverse events will cease or decrease in intensity as OxyContin therapy is continued and some degree of tolerance is developed.

In clinical trials comparing OxyContin with immediate-release oxycodone and placebo, the most common adverse events (>5%) reported by patients (pts) at least once during therapy were:

Table 2

	OxyContin n=227 #pts (%)		Immediate-Release n=225 #pts (%)		Placebo n=45 #pts (%)	
Constipation	52	(23)	58	(26)	3	(7)
Nausea	52	(23)	60	(27)	5	(11)
Somnolence	52	(23)	55	(24)	2	(4)
Dizziness	29	(13)	35	(16)	4	(9)
Pruritus	29	(13)	28	(12)	1	(2)
Vomiting	27	(12)	31	(14)	3	(7)
Headache	17	(7)	19	(8)	3	(7)
Dry Mouth	13	(6)	15	(7)	1	(2)
Asthenia	13	(6)	16	(7)	—	—
Sweating	12	(5)	13	(6)	1	(2)

The following adverse experiences were reported in OxyContin treated patients with an incidence between 1% and 5%. In descending order of frequency they were anorexia, nervousness, insomnia, fever, confusion, diarrhea, abdominal pain, dyspepsia, rash, anxiety, euphoria, dyspnea, postural hypotension, chills, twitching, gastritis, abnormal dreams, thought abnormalities, and hiccups.

The following adverse reactions occurred in less than 1% of patients involved in clinical trials:

General: accidental injury, chest pain, facial edema, malaise, neck pain, pain

Cardiovascular: migraine, syncope, vasodilation, ST depression

Digestive: dysphagia, eructation, flatulence, gastrointestinal disorder, increased appetite, nausea and vomiting, stomatitis

Hemic and Lymphatic: lymphadenopathy

Metabolic and Nutritional: dehydration, edema, hyponatremia, peripheral edema, syndrome of inappropriate antidiuretic hormone secretion, thirst

Nervous: abnormal gait, agitation, amnesia, depersonalization, depression, emotional lability, hallucination, hyperkinesia, hypesthesia, hypotonia, malaise, paresthesia, seizures, speech disorder, stupor, tinnitus, tremor, vertigo, withdrawal syndrome with or without seizures

Respiratory: cough increased, pharyngitis, voice alteration

Skin: dry skin, exfoliative dermatitis

Special Senses: abnormal vision, taste perversion

Urogenital: dysuria, hematuria, impotence, polyuria, urinary retention, urination impaired

DRUG ABUSE AND DEPENDENCE

(Addiction)

OxyContin™ is a mu-agonist opioid with an abuse liability similar to morphine and is a Schedule II controlled substance. Oxycodone products are common targets for both drug abusers and drug addicts. Delayed absorption, as provided by OxyContin tablets, is believed to reduce the abuse liability of a drug.

Drug addiction (drug dependence, psychological dependence) is characterized by a preoccupation with the procurement, hoarding, and abuse of drugs for non-medicinal purposes. Drug dependence is treatable, utilizing a multi-disciplinary approach, but relapse is common. Iatrogenic "addiction" to opioids legitimately used in the management of pain is very rare. "Drug seeking" behavior is very common to addicts. Tolerance and physical dependence in pain patients are *not* signs of psychological dependence. Preoccupation with achieving adequate pain relief can be appropriate behavior in a patient with poor pain control. Most chronic pain patients limit their intake of opioids to achieve a balance between the benefits of the drug and dose-limiting side effects. Physicians should be aware that psychological dependence may not be accompanied by concurrent tolerance and symptoms of physical dependence in all addicts. In addition, abuse of opioids can occur in the absence of true psychological dependence and is characterized by misuse for non-medical purposes, often in combination with other psychoactive substances.

OxyContin consists of a dual-polymer matrix, intended for oral use only. Parenteral venous injection of the tablet con-

stituents, especially talc, can be expected to result in local tissue necrosis and pulmonary granulomas.

OVERDOSAGE

Acute overdosage with oxycodone can be manifested by respiratory depression, somnolence progressing to stupor or coma, skeletal muscle flaccidity, cold and clammy skin, constricted pupils, bradycardia, hypotension, and death.

In the treatment of oxycodone overdosage, primary attention should be given to the re-establishment of a patent airway and institution of assisted or controlled ventilation. Supportive measures (including oxygen and vasopressors) should be employed in the management of circulatory shock and pulmonary edema accompanying overdose as indicated. Cardiac arrest or arrhythmias may require cardiac massage or defibrillation.

The pure opioid antagonists such as naloxone or nalmefene are specific antidotes against respiratory depression from opioid overdose. Opioid antagonists should not be administered in the absence of clinically significant respiratory or circulatory depression secondary to oxycodone overdose. They should be administered cautiously to persons who are known, or suspected to be, physically dependent on any opioid agonist including OxyContin™. In such cases, an abrupt or complete reversal of opioid effects may precipitate an acute abstinence syndrome. The severity of the withdrawal syndrome produced will depend on the degree of physical dependence and the dose of the antagonist administered. Please see the prescribing information for the specific opioid antagonist for details of their proper use.

DOSAGE AND ADMINISTRATION

General Principles

OxyContin™ (oxycodone hydrochloride controlled-release) TABLETS ARE TO BE SWALLOWED WHOLE, AND ARE NOT TO BE BROKEN, CHEWED OR CRUSHED. TAKING BROKEN, CHEWED OR CRUSHED OxyContin TABLETS COULD LEAD TO THE RAPID RELEASE AND ABSORPTION OF A POTENTIALLY TOXIC DOSE OF OXYCODONE.

In treating pain it is vital to assess the patient regularly and systematically. Therapy should also be regularly reviewed and adjusted based upon the patient's own reports of pain and side effects and the health professional's clinical judgment.

OxyContin is intended for the management of moderate to severe pain in patients who require treatment with an oral opioid analgesic for more than a few days. The controlled-release nature of the formulation allows it to be effectively administered every 12 hours. (See CLINICAL PHARMACOLOGY; PHARMACOKINETICS AND METABOLISM.) While symmetric (same dose AM and PM), around-the-clock, q12h dosing is appropriate for the majority of patients, some patients may benefit from asymmetric (different dose given in AM than in PM) dosing, tailored to their pain pattern. It is usually appropriate to treat a patient with only one opioid for around-the-clock therapy.

Initiation of Therapy

It is critical to initiate the dosing regimen for each patient individually, taking into account the patient's prior opioid and non-opioid analgesic treatment. Attention should be given to:

(1) the general condition and medical status of the patient

(2) the daily dose, potency and kind of the analgesic(s) the patient has been taking

(3) the reliability of the conversion estimate used to calculate the dose of oxycodone

(4) the patient's opioid exposure and opioid tolerance (if any)

(5) the balance between pain control and adverse experiences Care should be taken to use low initial doses of OxyContin in patients who are not already opioid tolerant, especially those who are receiving concurrent treatment with muscle relaxants, sedatives, or other CNS active medications (see PRECAUTIONS: Drug-Drug Interactions).

Patients Not Already Taking Opioids (opioid naive)

Clinical trials have shown that patients may initiate analgesic therapy with OxyContin. A reasonable starting dose for most patients who are opioid naive is 10 mg q12h. If a non-opioid analgesic [aspirin (ASA), acetaminophen (APAP) or a non-steroidal anti-inflammatory (NSAID)] is being provided, it may be continued. If the current non-opioid is discontinued, early upward dose titration may be necessary.

Conversion from Fixed-Ratio Opioid/APAP, ASA, or NSAID Combination Drugs

Patients who are taking 1 to 5 tablets/capsules/caplets per day of a regular strength fixed-combination opioid/non-opioid should be started on 10 to 20 mg OxyContin q12h. For patients taking 6 to 9 tablets/capsules/ caplets, a starting dose of 20 to 30 mg q12h is suggested. For those taking 10 to 12 tablets, caplets or capsules a day, 30 to 40 mg q12h should be considered. The non-opioid may be continued as a separate drug. Alternatively, a different non-opioid analgesic may be selected. If the decision is made to discontinue the non-opioid analgesic, consideration should be given to early upward titration.

Patients Currently on Opioid Therapy

If a patient has been receiving opioid-containing medications prior to OxyContin therapy, the total daily (24-hour) dose of the other opioids should be determined.

1. Using standard conversion ratio estimates (see Table 3 below), multiply the mg/day of the previous opioids by the appropriate multiplication factors to obtain the equivalent total daily dose of oral oxycodone.
2. Divide this 24-hour oxycodone dose in half to obtain the twice a day (q12h) dose of OxyContin.
3. Round down to a dose which is appropriate for the tablet strengths available (10, 20, and 40 mg tablets).
4. Discontinue all other around-the-clock opioid drugs when OxyContin therapy is initiated.

No fixed conversion ratio is likely to be satisfactory in all patients, especially patients receiving large opioid doses. The recommended doses shown in Table 3 are only a starting point, and close observation and frequent titration are indicated until patients are stable on the new therapy.

Table 3

Multiplication Factors for Converting the Daily Dose of Prior Opioids to the Daily Dose of Oral Oxycodone*

(Mg/Day Prior Opioid × Factor=Mg/Day Oral Oxycodone)

	Oral Prior Opioid	Parenteral Prior Opioid
Oxycodone	1	—
Codeine	0.15	—
Fentanyl TTS	SEE BELOW	SEE BELOW
Hydrocodone	0.9	—
Hydromorphone	4	20
Levorphanol	7.5	15
Meperidine	0.1	0.4
Methadone	1.5	3
Morphine	0.5	3

* To be used only for conversion to oral oxycodone. For patients receiving high-dose parenteral opioids, a more conservative conversion is warranted. For example, for high-dose parenteral morphine, use 1.5 instead of 3 as a multiplication factor.

In all cases, supplemental analgesia (see below) should be made available in the form of immediate-release oral oxycodone or another suitable short-acting analgesic.

OxyContin can be safely used concomitantly with usual doses of non-opioid analgesics and analgesic adjuvants, provided care is taken to select a proper initial dose (see PRECAUTIONS).

Conversion from Transdermal Fentanyl to OxyContin

Eighteen hours following the removal of the transdermal fentanyl patch, OxyContin treatment can be initiated. Although there has been no systematic assessment of such conversion, a conservative oxycodone dose, approximately 10 mg q12h of OxyContin, should be initially substituted for each 25 µg/hr fentanyl transdermal patch. The patient should be followed closely for early titration as there is very limited clinical experience with this conversion.

Managing Expected Opioid Adverse Experiences

Most patients receiving opioids, especially those who are opioid naive, will experience side effects. Frequently the side effects from OxyContin are transient, but may require evaluation and management. Adverse events such as constipation should be anticipated and treated aggressively and prophylactically with a stimulant laxative and/or stool softener. Patients do not usually become tolerant to the constipating effects of opioids.

Other opioid-related side effects such as sedation and nausea are usually self-limited and often do not persist beyond the first few days. If nausea persists and is unacceptable to the patient, treatment with anti-emetics or other modalities may relieve these symptoms and should be considered.

Patients receiving OxyContin may pass an intact matrix "ghost" in the stool or via colostomy. These ghosts contain little or no residual oxycodone and are of no clinical consequence.

Individualization of Dosage

Once therapy is initiated, pain relief and other opioid effects should be frequently assessed. Patients should be titrated to adequate effect (generally mild or no pain with the regular use of no more than two doses of supplemental analgesia per 24 hours). Rescue medication should be available (see: Supplemental Analgesia). Because steady-state plasma concentrations are approximated within 24 to 36 hours, dosage adjustment may be carried out every 1 to 2 days. It is most appropriate to increase the q12h dose, not the dosing frequency. There is no clinical information on dosing intervals shorter than q12h. As a guideline, except for the increase from 10 mg to 20 mg q12h, the total daily oxycodone dose usually can be increased by 25% to 50% of the current dose at each increase.

If signs of excessive opioid-related adverse experiences are observed, the next dose may be reduced. If this adjustment leads to inadequate analgesia, a supplemental dose of immediate-release oxycodone may be given. Alternatively, non-opioid analgesic adjuvants may be employed. Dose adjust-

ments should be made to obtain an appropriate balance between pain relief and opioid-related adverse experiences.

If significant adverse events occur before the therapeutic goal of mild or no pain is achieved, the events should be treated aggressively. Once adverse events are under control, upward titration should continue to an acceptable level of pain control.

During periods of changing analgesic requirements, including initial titration, frequent contact is recommended between physician, other members of the health-care team, the patient and the caregiver/family.

Supplemental Analgesia

Most cancer patients given around-the-clock therapy with controlled-release opioids will need to have immediate-release medication available for "rescue" from breakthrough pain or to prevent pain that occurs predictably during certain patient activities (incident pain).

Rescue medication can be immediate-release oxycodone, either alone or in combination with acetaminophen, aspirin or other NSAIDs as a supplemental analgesic. The supplemental analgesic should be prescribed at $^1/_4$ to $^1/_3$ of the 12-hour OxyContin dose as shown in Table 4. The rescue medication is dosed as needed for breakthrough pain and administered one hour before anticipated incident pain. If more than two doses of rescue medication are needed within 24 hours, the dose of OxyContin should be titrated upward. Caregivers and patients using prn rescue analgesia in combination with around-the-clock opioids should be advised to report incidents of breakthrough pain to the physician managing the patient's analgesia (see Information for Patients/Caregivers).

Table 4

Table of Appropriate Supplemental Analgesia

OxyContin q12h Dose (mg)	prn Rescue Dose immediate-release oxycodone (mg)
10 (1×10 mg)	5
20 (2×10 mg)	5
30 (3×10 mg)	10
40 (2×20 mg)	10
60 (3×20 mg)	15
80 (2×40 mg)	20
120 (3×40 mg)	30

Maintenance of Therapy

The intent of the titration period is to establish a patient-specific q12h dose that will maintain adequate analgesia with acceptable side effects for as long as pain relief is necessary. Should pain recur then the dose can be incrementally increased to re-establish pain control. The method of therapy adjustment outlined above should be employed to re-establish pain control.

During chronic therapy, especially for non-cancer pain syndromes, the continued need for around-the-clock opioid therapy should be reassessed periodically (e.g., every 6 to 12 months) as appropriate.

Cessation of Therapy

When the patient no longer requires therapy with OxyContin tablets, patients receiving doses of 20–60 mg/day can usually have the therapy stopped abruptly without incident. However, higher doses should be tapered over several days to prevent signs and symptoms of withdrawal in the physically dependent patient. The daily dose should be reduced by approximately 50% for the first two days and then reduced by 25% every two days thereafter until the total dose reaches the dose recommended for opioid naive patients (10 or 20 mg q12h). Therapy can then be discontinued.

If signs of withdrawal appear, tapering should be stopped. The dose should be slightly increased until the signs and symptoms of opioid withdrawal disappear. Tapering should then begin again but with longer periods of time between each dose reduction.

Conversion from OxyContin to Parenteral Opioids

To avoid overdose, conservative dose conversion ratios should be followed. Initiate treatment with about 50% of the estimated equianalgesic daily dose of parenteral opioid divided into suitable individual doses based on the appropriate dosing interval, and titrate based upon the patient's response.

SAFETY AND HANDLING

OxyContin™ (oxycodone hydrochloride controlled-release) tablets are solid dosage forms that pose no known health risk to health-care providers beyond that of any controlled substance. As with all such drugs, care should be taken to prevent diversion or abuse by proper handling.

HOW SUPPLIED

OxyContin™ (oxycodone hydrochloride controlled-release) 10 mg tablets are round, unscored, white-colored, convex tablets bearing the symbol OC on one side and 10 on the other. They are supplied as follows:

NDC 59011-100-10: child-resistant closure, opaque plastic bottles of 100

NDC 59011-100-25: unit dose packaging with 25 individually numbered tablets per card; one card per tuck end carton

OxyContin (oxycodone hydrochloride controlled-release) 20 mg tablets are round, unscored, pink-colored, convex tablets bearing the symbol OC on one side and 20 on the other. They are supplied as follows:

NDC 59011-103-10: child-resistant closure, opaque plastic bottles of 100

NDC 59011-103-25: unit dose packaging with 25 individually numbered tablets per card; one card per tuck end carton

OxyContin (oxycodone hydrochloride controlled-release) 40 mg tablets are round, unscored, yellow-colored, convex tablets bearing the symbol OC on one side and 40 on the other. They are supplied as follows:

NDC 59011-105-10: child-resistant closure, opaque plastic bottles of 100

NDC 59011-105-25: unit dose packaging with 25 individually numbered tablets per card; one card per tuck end carton

Store tablets at controlled room temperature 15–30°C (59–86°F).

Dispense in tight, light-resistant container.

CAUTION

DEA Order Form Required.

Federal law prohibits dispensing without prescription.

Manufactured by The PF Laboratories, Inc.
Totowa, N.J. 07512
Distributed by Purdue Pharma L.P.
Norwalk, CT 06850-3590
Copyright© 1995, 1996 Purdue Pharma L.P.
U.S. Patent Numbers 4,861,598; 4,970,075; 5,266,331; 5,508,042.
February 13, 1996
C4909 00P010

Shown in Product Identification Guide, page 330

OxyIR™ Ⓒ℞
(oxycodone hydrochloride immediate-release) capsules

DESCRIPTION

Each capsule contains:
oxycodone hydrochloride .... 5 mg.
(WARNING: May be habit forming)

Oxycodone is 14-hydroxydihydrocodeinone, a white odorless crystalline powder which is derived from the opium alkaloid, thebaine, and may be represented by the following structural formula:

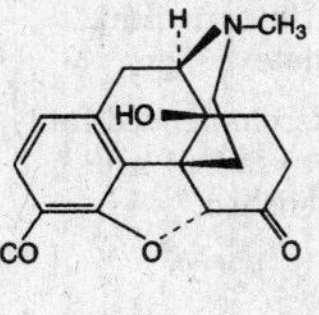

ACTIONS

The analgesic ingredient, oxycodone, is a semisynthetic narcotic with multiple actions qualitatively similar to those of morphine; the most prominent of these involve the central nervous system and organs composed of smooth muscle. The principal actions of therapeutic value of oxycodone are analgesia and sedation.

Oxycodone is similar to codeine and methadone in that it retains at least one half of its analgesic activity when administered orally.

INDICATIONS

For the relief of moderate to moderately severe pain.

CONTRAINDICATIONS

Hypersensitivity to oxycodone.

WARNINGS

Drug Dependence: Oxycodone can produce drug dependence of the morphine type, and therefore, has the potential for being abused. Psychic dependence, physical dependence and tolerance may develop upon repeated adminstration of this drug, and it should be prescribed and administered with the same degree of caution appropriate to the use of other oral narcotic-containing medications. Like other narcotic-containing medications, this drug is subject to the Federal Controlled Substances Act.

Usage in Ambulatory Patients: Oxycodone may impair the mental and/or physical abilities required for the performance of potential hazardous tasks such as driving a car or operating machinery. The patient using this drug should be cautioned accordingly.

Interaction with Other Central Nervous System Depressants: Patients receiving other narcotic analgesics, general anesthetics, phenothiazines, other tranquilizers, sedative-hypnotics or other CNS depressants (including alcohol) concomitantly with oxycodone hydrochloride may exhibit an additive CNS depression. When such combined therapy is contemplated, the dose of one or both agents should be reduced.

Usage in Pregnancy: Safe use in pregnancy has not been established relative to possible adverse effects on fetal development. Therefore, this drug should not be used in pregnant women unless, in the judgment of the physician, the potential benefits outweigh the possible hazards.

Usage in Children: This drug should not be administered to children.

PRECAUTIONS

Head injury and Increased Intracranial Pressure: The respiratory depressant effects of narcotics and their capacity to elevate cerebrospinal fluid pressure may be markedly exaggerated in the presence of head injury, other intracranial lesions or a pre-existing increase in intracranial pressure. Furthermore, narcotics produce adverse reactions which may obscure the clinical course of patients with head injuries.

Acute Abdominal Conditions: The administration of this drug or other narcotics may obscure the diagnosis or clinical course in patients with acute abdominal conditions.

Specal Risk Patients: This drug should be given with caution to certain patients such as the elderly, or debilitated, and those with severe impairment of hepatic or renal function, hypothyroidism, Addison's disease and prostatic hypertrophy or urethral stricture.

DRUG INTERACTIONS

The CNS depressant effects of oxycodone hydrochloride may be additive with that of other CNS depressants. See WARNINGS.

ADVERSE REACTIONS

The most frequently observed reactions include light-headedness, dizziness, sedation, nausea and vomiting. These effects seem to be more prominent in ambulatory than in nonambulatory patients, and some of these adverse reactions may be alleviated if the patient lies down.

Other adverse reactions include euphoria, dysphoria, constipation, skin rash and pruritus.

MANAGEMENT OF OVERDOSAGE

Signs and Symptoms: Serious overdose of oxycodone hydrochloride is characterized by respiratory depression (a decrease in respiratory rate and/or tidal volume, Cheyne-Stokes respiration, cyanosis), extreme somnolence progressing to stupor or coma, skeletal muscle flaccidity, cold and clammy skin, and sometimes bradycardia and hypotension. In severe overdosage, apnea, circulatory collapse, cardiac arrest and death may occur.

Treatment: Primary attention should be given to the reestablishment of adequate respiratory exchange through provision of a patent airway and the institution of assisted or controlled ventilation. The narcotic antagonist naloxone is a specific antidote against respiratory depression which may result from overdosage or unusual sensitivity to narcotics, including oxycodone. Therefore, an appropriate dose of naloxone (usual initial adult dose: 0.4 mg) should be administered, preferably by the intravenous route, simultaneously with efforts at respiratory resuscitation. Since the duration of action of oxycodone may exceed that of the antagonist, the patient should be kept under continued surveillance and repeated doses of the antagonist should be adminstered as needed to maintain adequate respiration. An antagonist should not be administered in the absence of clinically significant respiratory or cardiovascular depression.

Oxygen, intravenous fluids, vasopressors and other supportive measures should be employed as indicated.

Gastric emptying may be useful in removing unabsorbed drug.

DOSAGE AND ADMINISTRATION

Dosage should be adjusted to the severity of the pain and the response of the patient. It may occasionally be necessary to exceed the usual dosage recommended below in cases of more severe pain or in those patients who have become tolerant to the analgesic effects of narcotics. This drug is given orally. The usual adult dosage is one 5 mg capsule every 6 hours as needed for pain.

HOW SUPPLIED

5 mg capsules, Cap: Beige Imprinted with O-IR; Body: Orange Imprinted with PF5mg.

NDC 59011-201-10:
Bottle of 100 Capsules

DEA Order Form Required.

Caution: Federal law prohibits dispensing without prescription.

Manufactured by:
The P.F. Laboratories, Inc.
Totowa, NJ 07512
Distributed by:
Purdue Pharma L.P.
Norwalk, CT 06850-3590
Copyright © 1995
February 2, 1995
A4597

Shown in Product Identification Guide, page 330

R&D Laboratories, Inc.
4640 ADMIRALTY WAY, SUITE 710
MARINA DEL REY, CA 90292

Direct Inquiries to:
Rhoda Makoff, PhD
(310) 305-8053
(800) 338-9066
FAX (310) 305-8103

For Medical Emergencies:
Dwight Makoff, M.D.
(310) 652-9162

AMIN–AID® INSTANT DRINK   OTC
Essential Amino Acid and Calorie Supplement

DESCRIPTION
Amin-Aid® is recommended for dietary management of patients with nutritional deficiencies resulting from acute or chronic renal failure.

HOW SUPPLIED
Amin-Aid® Instant Drink is packaged 12 packages per carton, 2 cartons per case (24 packages per case).

Flavor	NDC No.
Orange	54391-6100-24
Lemon-Lime	54391-6105-24
Strawberry	54391-6103-24
Berry	54391-6104-24

Manufactured by McGaw, Inc. For R & D Laboratories, Inc.

CALCI–CHEW®   OTC

1.25 gm USP grade calcium carbonate chewable tablets—500 mg elemental calcium. Packaged as three separate flavors—cherry, lemon, orange.

DESCRIPTION
Tablets supplying 1.25 gm USP grade calcium carbonate. Contains no dyes and no sodium.

INDICATIONS
For use as calcium supplementation and in the treatment of hypocalcemia.

DOSAGE
For hypocalcemia, use as necessary to restore calcium to normal levels. For patients with impaired calcium absorption or on a calcium restricted diet, give under a physician's guidance.

HOW SUPPLIED
Plastic bottles of 100 tablets.

FLAVOR	NDC No.
CHERRY	54391-0025-2
LEMON	54391-0225-2
ORANGE	54391-0325-2

CALCI–MIX®   OTC

1.25 gm USP grade calcium carbonate powdered in pull apart capsules. Contains 500 mg of elemental calcium. Can be swallowed or pulled apart and sprinkled on food or in drink.

DESCRIPTION
Gelatin capsules containing 1.25 gm USP grade calcium carbonate. Contains no sodium and no dyes.

INDICATIONS
For use as calcium supplementation and in the treatment of hypocalcemia.

DOSAGE
For hypocalcemia, use as necessary to restore calcium to normal levels. For patients with impaired calcium absorption or on a calcium restricted diet, give under a physician's guidance.

SUPPLIED
Plastic bottles of 100 capsules. NDC 54391-0027-3.

---

d-BIOTIN   OTC

10 mg. d-Biotin in capsules for Biotin replacement. Supplied in plastic bottles of 60 capsules.
NDC 54391-0003-9

DIABEVITE®   OTC
[dī'ă-bə-vīt]
Antioxidant-Rich Vitamin and Mineral Supplement

DESCRIPTION
An antioxidant-rich vitamin/mineral supplement designed to provide nutritional support for the diabetic patient with a restricted or poor diet. Suitable for both insulin dependent and non-insulin dependent diabetics with normal renal function. Diabetic patients with impaired renal function should use Nephro-Vite® RX. Consult a physician. Contains no added sugar, starch, or preservatives.

INGREDIENTS PER TABLET

EACH TABLET PROVIDES:			%USRDA*
Vitamin A (Acetate)	625	IU	12%
Vitamin A (Beta Carotene)	625	IU	12%
Vitamin B1 (Thiamine Mononitrate)	1.5	mg	100%
Vitamin B2 (Riboflavin)	1.7	mg	100%
Niacinamide	20	mg	100%
Vitamin B6 (Pyridoxine HCl)	2	mg	100%
Vitamin B12 (Cyanocobalamin)	6	mcg	100%
Vitamin C (Ascorbic Acid)	250	mg	417%
Vitamin D2 (Ergocalciferol)	100	IU	25%
Vitamin E (d-Alpha Tocopheryl Succinate)	100	IU	333%
Folic Acid	800	mcg	200%
Biotin	300	mcg	100%
Pantothenic Acid (d-Calcium Pantothenate)	10	mg	100%
Chromium (ChromeMate® GTF) [InterHealth]	200	mcg	**
Copper (Gluconate)	2	mg	100%
Magnesium (Oxide)	100	mg	25%
Selenium (Proteinate)	25	mcg	**
Zinc (Opti-Zinc™) [InterHealth]	15	mg	100%
Manganese (Gluconate)	2.5	mg	**

*Percentage U.S. Recommended Daily Allowance for adults and children over 4 years of age.
**USRDA not established.

DOSAGE
One tablet daily.

HOW SUPPLIED
White, film coated tablet in plastic bottles of 60. Store tightly in a cool, dry place.
NDC #54391-3010-09

L-CARNITINE   OTC

250 mg capsules.
Plastic bottles of 60 capsules
NDC 54391-0050-9

MAG-CARB™   OTC
[măg-kărb]
A Nutritional Supplement

DESCRIPTION
A 250 mg magnesium carbonate supplement packaged in a gel capsule, delivering 70 mg of elemental magnesium. Used as a general supplement and especially suitable for the transplant recipient on cyclosporin therapy who is at risk for magnesium deficiency.

INGREDIENTS
Magnesium carbonate, magnesium stearate, cellulose, and gelatin.

DOSAGE
As needed or prescribed.

HOW SUPPLIED
Clear gelatin capsules in plastic bottles of 100. Store tightly in a cool, dry place.
NDC #54391-0031-03

NEPHRO–CALCI®   OTC

1.5 gm USP grade calcium carbonate tablets—600 mg elemental calcium.

DESCRIPTION
Tablets supplying 1.5 gm of (USP grade) calcium carbonate. Contains no dyes.

INDICATIONS
For use as calcium supplementation and in the treatment of hypocalcemia.

DOSAGE
For hypocalcemia, use as necessary to restore calcium to normal levels. For patients with impaired calcium absorption and patients on a calcium restricted diet give under a physician's guidance.

SUPPLIED
Plastic bottles of 100 tablets. NDC 54391-0026-3.

NEPHRO–DERM®   OTC

Non-steroidal skin cream for the relief of uremic itching. Nephro-Derm® contains Eucerin®*, camphor, and menthol as its active ingredients and is formulated to help relieve general and uremic itching. This product is supplied in 4 oz jars.
NDC 54391-2000-4

*®Beiersdorf, Inc., Norwalk, CT

NEPHRO–FER®   OTC

Ferrous fumarate preparation for oral iron supplementation.

DESCRIPTION
Each tablet supplies 350 mg of ferrous fumarate—115 mg of elemental iron. Contains no dyes.

INDICATIONS
Patients taking EPO requiring oral iron supplementation—particularly patients who experience gastric problems with ferrous sulfate. Appropriate for any iron supplementation. (See Nephro-Fer® Rx for side effects.)

DOSAGE
One to three tablets daily as required, under the supervision of a physician.

SUPPLIED
Brown oval tablets marked RD13.
Plastic bottles of 100 tablets. NDC 54391-0013-9.

NEPHRO-FER® Rx   ℞
Iron Supplement With Folic Acid

Oral iron supplement. For any patient needing iron supplementation for documented iron deficiency. Suitable for certain patients undergoing therapy with erythropoietin.

DESCRIPTION
Each tablet contains 324 mg ferrous fumarate—106.9 mg elemental iron—and 1 mg folic acid. Product does not contain any coloring agents/dyes. Ferrous fumarate may be better tolerated than ferrous sulfate in some patients.

INDICATIONS
Renal failure patients and patients who have documented iron deficiency. Patients undergoing erythropoietin therapy who risk iron deficiency.

DOSAGE
One to three tablets daily between meals as required to correct iron deficiency.

SIDE EFFECTS
Transient bloating, flatulence, constipation, and diarrhea. Ingestion of greater than 400 mg per day of elemental iron can result in nausea and vomiting.

PRECAUTION
Folic acid can mask the symptoms of anemia.

SUPPLIED
Brown, oval tablets marked RD33.
Plastic bottles of 120 tablets. NDC 54391-1313-6.
For use under medical supervision.

NEPHRAMINE® ℞

5.4% Essential Amino Acid Injection

DESCRIPTION

5.4% NephrAmine® (Essential Amino Acid Injection) is a sterile, nonpyrogenic solution containing crystalline essential amino acids plus histidine. Each 250 mL unit provides Rose's recommended daily intake of essential amino acids plus 625 mg of histidine, considered essential for uremics. The total nitrogen content of a 250 mL unit is approximately 1.6 grams (10 g of protein equivalent) in 14 grams of amino acids. All amino acids designated USP are the "L" isomer.

Each 100 mL contains:

Histidine USP*	0.25 g
Isoleucine USP	0.56 g
Leucine USP	0.88 g
Lysine	0.64 g
(added as Lysine Acetate USP	0.90 g)
Methionine USP	0.88 g
Phenylalanine USP	0.88 g
Threonine USP	0.40 g
Tryptophan USP	0.20 g
Valine USP	0.64 g
Cysteine	<0.014 g
(as Cysteine HCl·H_2O USP	<0.020 g)
Sodium Bisulfite (as an antioxidant)	<0.05 g
Water for Injection USP	qs

pH adjusted with Sodium Hydroxide NF as required
pH: 6.5 (6.0–7.0): Calculated Osmolarity: 435 mOsmol/liter
Total Nitrogen: Approx. 0.65 g/100 mL
Concentration of Electrolytes (mEq/liter): Sodium 5 Chloride <3, Acetate Approx. 44

* Histidine is considered an essential amino acid in uremic patients

[1] Rose WC: The sequence of events leading to the establishment of the amino acid needs of man **Am J Public Health: 1968: 58(11)**: 2020–2027

CLINICAL PHARMACOLOGY

NephrAmine® provides an intravenously compatible mixture of essential amino acids which, when infused with hypertonic dextrose as a source of calories, plus electrolytes, minerals, and vitamins provides in a small volume of fluid all ingredients (with the exception of essential fatty acids) needed for total parenteral nutrition in patients with renal disease.

Infusion of NephrAmine® and hypertonic dextrose provides essential amino acids and calories for protein synthesis to promote improved cellular metabolic balance. Infusion of these components can decrease the rate of rise of blood urea nitrogen (bun) and minimize deterioration of serum potassium, magnesium and phosphorus balance in patients with impaired renal function. The extent to which essential amino acids and calories promote incorporation of waste urea nitrogen into newly synthesized amino acids in man, as it does in experimental animals, is, so far, not established.

The accelerated decrease in serum creatinine levels seen in patients with limited extra-renal complications suggests that treatment with NephrAmine® and hypertonic dextrose leads to earlier return of renal function in patients with potentially reversible acute renal failure. By providing nutritional support and promoting biochemical improvement as well as earlier return of renal function, NephrAmine® and hypertonic dextrose decrease morbidity associated with acute renal failure.

It is thought that acetate from lysine acetate, under the condition of parenteral nutrition, does not impact net acid-base balance when renal and respiratory functions are normal. Clinical evidence seems to support this thinking; however, confirmatory experimental evidence is not available.

The amounts of sodium and chloride present are not of clinical significance.

INDICATIONS AND USAGE

5.4% NephrAmine® (Essential Amino Acid Injection) is indicated for adult and pediatric use, in conjunction with other measures, to provide nutritional support for uremic patients, particularly when oral nutrition is infeasible or impractical. See ***Special Precautions in Pediatric Patients*** for additional information.

CONTRAINDICATIONS

NephrAmine® is contraindicated in patients with severe, uncorrected electrolyte and acid-base imbalance, hyperammonemia, decreased (subcritical) circulating blood volume, inborn errors of amino acid metabolism, or hypersensitivity to one or more amino acids present in the solution.

WARNINGS

This product contains sodium bisulfite, a sulfite that may cause allergic-type reactions including anaphylactic symptoms and life-threatening or less severe asthmatic episodes in certain susceptible people. The overall prevalence of sulfite sensitivity in the general population is unknown and probably low. Sulfite sensitivity is seen more frequently in asthmatic than in nonasthmatic people.

Safe and effective use of central venous nutrition requires a knowledge of nutrition as well as clinical expertise in recognition and treatment of the complications which can occur. **Frequent clinical evaluation and laboratory determinations are necessary for proper monitoring of central venous nutrition.** Studies should include blood sugar, serum proteins, kidney and liver function tests, electrolytes, hemogram, carbon dioxide combining power, serum osmolarity, blood cultures, blood ammonia levels, and circulating blood volume.

NephrAmine® does not replace dialysis and conventional supportive therapy in patients with renal failure.

Administration of NephrAmine® to children or low birthweight infants, especially in high doses, may result in hyperammononemia.

Clinically significant hypokalemia, hypophosphatemia, or hypomagnesemia may occur as a result of therapy with NephrAmine® and hypertonic dextrose and replacement therapy may become necessary.

Administration of nitrogen in any form to patients with marked hepatic insufficiency or hepatic coma may result in plasma amino acid imbalances, hyperammonemia, or central nervous system deterioration. NephrAmine® should, therefore, be used with caution in such patients.

The intravenous administration of these solutions can cause fluid and/or solute overload resulting in dilution of serum electrolyte concentrations, overhydration, congested states or pulmonary edema. The risk of dilutional states is inversely proportional to the solute concentration of the solution infused. The risk of solute overload causing congested states with peripheral and pulmonary edema is directly proportional to the concentration of the solution.

Conservative doses of amino acids should be given, dictated by the nutritional status of the patient.

PRECAUTIONS

General

Clinical evaluation and periodic laboratory determinations are necessary to monitor changes in fluid balance, electrolyte concentrations, and acid-base balance during prolonged parenteral therapy or whenever the condition of the patient warrants such evaluation. Significant deviations from normal concentrations may require the use of additional electrolyte supplements.

In order to promote urea nitrogen reutilization in patients with renal failure, it is essential to provide adequate calories with minimal amounts of the essential amino acids, and to severely restrict the intake of nonessential nitrogen. Hypertonic dextrose solutions are a convenient and metabolically effective source of concentrated calories.

Fluid balance must be carefully monitored in patients with renal failure and care should be taken to avoid circulatory overload, particularly in association with cardiac insufficiency.

In patients with myocardial infarct, infusion of amino acids should always be accompanied by dextrose, since in anoxia, free fatty acids cannot be utilized by the myocardium, and energy must be produced anaerobically from glycogen or glucose.

Strongly hypertonic nutrient solutions should be administered through an indwelling intravenous catheter with the tip located in the superior vena cava.

Special care must be taken when giving hypertonic dextrose to glucose-intolerant patients such as diabetic or prediabetic and uremic patients; especially when the latter are receiving peritoneal dialysis. To prevent severe hyperglycemia in such patients, insulin may be required.

Administration of glucose at a rate exceeding the patient's utilization may lead to hyperglycemia, coma, and death.

Administration of amino acids without carbohydrates may result in the accumulation of ketone bodies in the blood. Correction of this ketonemia may be achieved by the administration of carbohydrates. Abrupt cessation of hypertonic dextrose infusion may result in rebound hypoglycemia.

When 5.4% NephrAmine® (Essential Amino Acid Injection) is subjected to changes in temperature, there is a chance that some transient crystallization of amino acids may occur. Thorough shaking of the bottle for about one minute should redissolve the amino acids. If the amino acids do not completely redissolve, the bottle must be rejected.

To minimize the risk of possible incompatibilities arising from mixing this solution with other additives that may be prescribed, the final infusate should be inspected for cloudiness or precipitation immediately after mixing, prior to administration, and periodically during administration.

Use only if solution is clear and vacuum is present.

Usage in Pregnancy

Pregnancy Category C. Animal reproduction studies have not been conducted with 5.4% NephrAmine® (Essential Amino Acid Injection). It is also not known whether NephrAmine® can cause fetal harm when administered to a pregnant woman or can affect reproduction capacity. NephrAmine® should be given to a pregnant woman only if clearly needed.

Special Precautions for Central Venous Nutrition

Administration by central venous catheter should be used only by those familiar with this technique and its complications.

Central venous nutrition may be associated with complications which can be prevented or minimized by careful attention to all aspects of the procedure including solution preparation, administration, and patient monitoring. **It is essential that a carefully prepared protocol, based on current medical practices, be followed, preferably by an experienced team.**

SEE PACKAGE INSERT FOR ADDITIONAL INFORMATION ON CENTRAL VENOUS ADMINISTRATION.

Special Precautions in Patients with Renal Insufficiency

Frequent laboratory studies are necessary in patients with renal insufficiency due to underlying metabolic abnormalities. Hyperglycemia, a frequent complication, may not be reflected by glycosuria in renal failure. Blood glucose, therefore, must be determined frequently, often every six hours to guide dosage of dextrose and insulin if required.

Serum concentrations of potassium, phosphorus, and magnesium may dramatically decline with successful treatment, individually or together; these substances should be supplemented as required. Special care must be taken to avoid hypokalemia in digitalized patients, or those with cardiac arrhythmias.

Special Precautions in Pediatric Patients

5.4% NephrAmine® (Essential Amino Acid Injection) should be used with special caution in pediatric patients, especially low birth-weight infants, due to limited clinical experience.

Laboratory and clinical monitoring of pediatric patients, especially when nutritionally depleted, must be extensive and frequent. Initial total daily dose should be low, and increased slowly. Dosage of NephrAmine® above one gram of essential amino acids per kilogram body weight per day is not recommended.

Frequent monitoring of blood glucose is required in low birth-weight or septic infants as infusion of hypertonic dextrose carries a greater risk of hyperglycemia in such patients.

The absence of arginine in NephrAmine® may accentuate the risk of hyperammonemia in infants.

ADVERSE REACTIONS

See **WARNINGS** and ***Special Precautions for Central Venous Nutrition.***

Reactions which may occur because of the solution or the technique of administration include febrile response, infection at the site of injection, venous thrombosis, and hypervolemia.

Symptoms may result from an excess or deficit of one or more of the ions present in the solution infused, therefore, frequent monitoring of electrolyte levels is essential.

Infrequent instances of hyperammonemia have been reported following administration of essential amino acid solutions to patients with massive gastrointestinal hemorrhage, nonuremic infants and children or following administration of higher than recommended doses to adult or pediatric patients. Serum ammonia levels and clinical symptoms may subside when the infusions are discontinued.

Phosphorus deficiency may lead to impaired tissue oxygenation and acute hemolytic anemia. Relative to calcium, excessive phosphorus intake can precipitate hypocalcemia with cramps, tetany and muscular hyperexcitability.

If an adverse reaction does occur, discontinue the infusion, evaluate the patient, institute appropriate therapeutic countermeasures and save the remainder of the fluid for examination if deemed necessary.

OVERDOSAGE

In the event of a fluid or solute overload during parenteral therapy, reevaluate the patient's condition, and institute appropriate corrective treatment.

DOSAGE AND ADMINISTRATION

The objective of nutritional management of renal decompensation is the provision of sufficient amino acid and caloric suppport for protein synthesis without greatly exceeding the renal capacity to excrete metabolic wastes.

Three grams of nitrogen per day provided as essential amino acids with adequate calories produce nitrogen equilibrium in many stable patients with chronic uremia. Although nitrogen requirements may be higher in stressed or acutely uremic patients, or those on dialysis, provision of additional nitrogen may not be possible due to fluid intake limits or glucose intolerance.

The usual methods of determining individual patient requirements for amino acids such as nitrogen balance or daily body weight are difficult to perform or interpret in the uremic patient. Therefore, dosage is guided by the patient's fluid intake limits and glucose and nitrogen tolerances, as well as metabolic and clinical response. Rate of rise of blood urea nitrogen generally diminishes with infusion of essential

Continued on next page

R&D Laboratories—Cont.

amino acids. However, excessive intake of dietary protein or increased protein catabolism may alter this response.

Adults: Generally, 250 to 500 mL of 5.4% NephrAmine® (Essential Amino Acid Injection), containing approximately 1.6 to 3.2 grams of nitrogen (in 13.4 to 26.8 grams of essential amino acids), are given daily. Adequate calories should be provided simultaneously. Each 250 mL of NephrAmine® is typically mixed aseptically with 500 mL of 70% dextrose to yield a solution of 1.8% NephrAmine® in 47% dextrose. This mixture provides a calorie-to-nitrogen ratio of 744.1.

Children: Initial total daily dose should be low and increased slowly. Dosage of NephrAmine above one gram of essential amino acids per kg of body weight per day is not recommended. See *Special Precautions in Pediatric Patients* for additional information.

Fat emulsion coadministration should be considered when prolonged (more than 5 days) parenteral nutrition is required in order to prevent essential fatty acid deficiency (E.F.A.D.). Serum lipids should be monitored for evidence of E.F.A.D. in patients maintained on fat free TPN.

Electrolyte supplementation may be required. Undiluted NephrAmine® contains 5 mEq/liter of sodium. Elevated serum potassium, phosphorus, and magnesium levels generally decrease during treatment with NephrAmine®. Although these effects are beneficial, especially in acute renal failure, in some instances the reduction may be so great that supplementation of these electrolytes is required, especially in the presence of cardiac arrhythmias or digitalis toxicity. During periods of anuria or oliguria, electrolyte supplementation should be done with caution, even if serum levels are in the low normal range.

Compatibility of electrolyte additives to the 5.4% NephrAmine® (Essential Amino Acid Injection)/hypertonic dextrose mixture must be considered, and potentially incompatible ions such as calcium and phosphate may be added to alternate infusion bottles to avoid precipitation. In patients with hyperchloremic or other metabolic acidosis, sodium and potassium may be added as acetate or lactate salts to provide bicarbonate precursor. The electrolyte content of NephrAmine® must be considered when calculating daily electrolyte intake. Serum electrolytes, including magnesium and phosphorus, should be monitored frequently.

If a patient's nutritional intake is primarily parenteral, water soluble vitamins should also be provided.

Hypertonic mixtures of essential amino acids and dextrose may be safely administered by continuous infusion through a central venous catheter with the tip located in the superior vena cava. Initial infusion rates should be slow, generally 20–30 mL/hour. Increases by increments of 10 mL/hour each 24 hours are recommended to a maximum of 60–100 mL/hour. If administration rate should fall behind schedule, no attempt to "catch up" to planned intake should be made. Administration rate is governed by the patient's nitrogen, fluid, and glucose tolerance. Uremic patients are frequently glucose intolerant, especially in association with peritoneal dialysis, and may require the administration of exogenous insulin to prevent hyperglycemia. Blood glucose levels must be determined frequently. To prevent rebound hypoglycemia, a solution containing 5% dextrose should be administered when hypertonic dextrose infusions are abruptly discontinued.

Parenteral drug products should be inspected visually for particulate matter and discoloration prior to administration, whenever solution and container permit.

Care must be taken to avoid incompatible admixtures. Consult with pharmacist.

HOW SUPPLIED

5.4% NephrAmine® (Essential Amino Acid Injection) is supplied sterile and nonpyrogenic in glass containers packaged 12 per case.

NDC No.: 54391-1909-20   Size: 250 mL

Exposure of pharmaceutical products to heat should be minimized. Avoid excessive heat. Protect from freezing. It is recommended that the product be stored at room temperature (25°C); however, brief exposure up to 40°C does not adversely affect the product. Protect from light until use.

Manufactured By McGaw, Inc. For R&D Laboratories, Inc. For Medical Emergencies:
McGaw Stat Line
(800) 854-6851

NEPHRO–VITE®Rx
Vitamin Formulation For Renal Patients

DESCRIPTION

The process of dialysis causes vitamin losses necessitating the regular replacement of the water soluble vitamins. It is important not to over supplement some vitamins. Vitamin A should not be supplemented and vitamin C supplementation

should be limited to 60 mg per day to avoid the risk of increased oxalate formation.

Each tablet provides:

	Nephro-Vite®Rx	Nephro-Vite®
Vitamin C	60 mg	60 mg
Vitamin B$_1$	1.5 mg	1.5 mg
Vitamin B$_2$	1.7 mg	1.7 mg
Niacinamide	20 mg	20 mg
Vitamin B$_6$	10 mg	10 mg
Vitamin B$_{12}$	6 mcg	6 mcg
Folic Acid	1 mg	.8 mg
Pantothenic Acid	10 mg	10 mg
Biotin	300 mcg	300 mcg

INDICATIONS

Dialysis patients; Azotemic patients not on dialysis who eat poorly.

PRECAUTION

See Folic Acid Precaution under Nephro-Vite® +Fe

DOSAGE

One tablet daily.

SUPPLIED

Film coated, round yellow tablets, marked RD 12.
Plastic bottles of 100. NDC 54391-1002-1.
For use under medical supervision.

NEPHRO–VITE®   OTC
Vitamin Formulation For Renal Patients

Renal vitamin replacement formulation—see table under Nephro-Vite® Rx for description. Same dosage as Nephro-Vite® Rx.
Film coated, round yellow tablets marked RD 02.
Supplied in plastic bottles of 100. NDC 54391-0002-1.

NEPHRO-VITE® +Fe   ℞
Vitamin Formulation For Renal Patients With Iron

COMPOSITION

Same as Nephro-Vite® Rx with the addition of 304 mg of ferrous fumarate—100 mg of elemental iron.

INDICATIONS

For any patient needing vitamin and iron supplementation for documented iron deficiency. Suitable for pre-dialysis and end stage renal disease patients.

PRECAUTION

Folic acid may partially correct the hematological damage due to vitamin B$_{12}$ deficiency of pernicious anemia while the associated neurological damage progresses.

ADVERSE REACTIONS

Allergic sensitization has been reported following administration of folic acid. Iron sensitivity to low doses of iron has been reported and high doses result in iron toxicity. Transient bloating, flatulence, constipation and diarrhea. Ingestion of greater than 400 mg/day of iron can result in nausea and vomiting.

DOSAGE

One tablet daily between meals or as prescribed by a physician.

HOW SUPPLIED

Film coated, oval tablets marked RD23 in plastic bottles of 120 tablets.
NDC 54391-2213-6
For use under medical supervision.

REGAIN® MEDICAL NUTRITION BAR   OTC
[rē·gain]

DESCRIPTION

An effective oral nutrition supplement formulated for the malnourished renal failure patient. High nutritional value with no increase in fluid intake. Lower in sodium, potassium, phosphorus, and magnesium. Low in dextrose and sucrose.

DOSAGE

One bar daily or as prescribed by a medical professional.

HOW SUPPLIED

3 oz. bar; packaged in cases of 24, available in 3 flavors (vanilla, strawberry, malt) each with cocoa coating. Store in a cool place, 24°C (75°F) or less.
NDC: 54391-0240-05 vanilla; 54391-0140-05 malt; 54391-0040-05 strawberry

---

Reckitt & Colman Pharmaceuticals Inc.
1909 HUGUENOT ROAD
RICHMOND, VA 23235

Direct Inquiries to:
Professional Services
(804) 379-1090
FAX: (804) 379-1215

For Medical Information Contact:
In Emergencies
Medical Department
(804) 379-1090
FAX: (804) 379-1215

BUPRENEX®   © ℞
[būp´rĕn-ex]
(buprenorphine hydrochloride)
INJECTABLE

DESCRIPTION

Buprenex (buprenorphine hydrochloride) is a narcotic under the Controlled Substances Act due to its chemical derivation from thebaine. Chemically, it is 17-(cyclopropylmethyl)-α-(1,1-dimethylethyl)-4, 5-epoxy-18, 19-dihydro-3-hydroxy-6-methoxy-α-methyl-6, 14-ethenomorphinan-7-methanol, hydrochloride [5α, 7α(S)]. Buprenorphine hydrochloride is a white powder, weakly acidic and with limited solubility in water. Buprenex is a clear, sterile, injectable agonist-antagonist analgesic intended for intravenous or intramuscular administration. Each ml of Buprenex contains 0.324 mg buprenorphine hydrochloride (equivalent to 0.3 mg buprenorphine), 50 mg anhydrous dextrose, water for injection and HCl to adjust pH. Buprenorphine hydrochloride has the molecular formula, $C_{29}H_{41}NO_4 \cdot HCl$, and the following structure:

Molecular weight: 504.09

CLINICAL PHARMACOLOGY

Buprenex is a parenteral opioid analgesic with 0.3 mg Buprenex being approximately equivalent to 10 mg morphine sulfate in analgesic and respiratory depressant effects in adults. Pharmacological effects occur as soon as 15 minutes after intramuscular injection and persist for 6 hours or longer. Peak pharmacologic effects usually are observed at 1 hour. When used intravenously, the times to onset and peak effect are shortened.

The limits of sensitivity of available analytical methodology precluded demonstration of bioequivalence between intramuscular and intravenous routes of administration. In postoperative adults, pharmacokinetic studies have shown elimination half-lives ranging from 1.2–7.2 hours (mean 2.2 hours) after intravenous administration of 0.3 mg of buprenorphine. A single, ten-patient, pharmacokinetic study of doses of 3 μg/kg in children (age 5-7 years) showed a high inter-patient variability, but suggests that the clearance of the drug may be higher in children than in adults. This is supported by at least one repeat-dose study in postoperative pain that showed an optimal inter-dose interval of 4–5 hours in pediatric patients as opposed to the recommended 6–8 hours in adults.

Buprenorphine, in common with morphine and other phenolic opioid analgesics, is metabolized by the liver and its clearance is related to hepatic blood flow. Studies in patients anesthetized with 0.5% halothane have shown that this anesthetic decreases hepatic blood flow by about 30%.

Mechanism of Analgesic Action: Buprenex exerts its analgesic effect via high affinity binding to μ subclass opiate receptors in the central nervous system. Although Buprenex may be classified as a partial agonist, under the conditions of recommended use it behaves very much like classical μ agonists such as morphine. One unusual property of Buprenex observed in *in vitro* studies is its very slow rate of dissociation from its receptor. This could account for its longer duration of action than morphine, the unpredictability of its reversal

by opioid antagonists, and its low level of manifest physical dependence.

Narcotic Antagonist Activity: Buprenorphine demonstrates narcotic antagonist activity and has been shown to be equipotent with naloxone as an antagonist of morphine in the mouse tail flick test.

Cardiovascular Effects: Buprenex may cause a decrease or, rarely, an increase in pulse rate and blood pressure in some patients.

Effects on Respiration: Under usual conditions of use in adults, both Buprenex and morphine show similar dose-related respiratory depressant effects. At adult therapeutic doses, Buprenex (0.3 mg buprenorphine) can decrease respiratory rate in an equivalent manner to an equianalgesic dose of morphine (10 mg). (See WARNINGS.)

INDICATIONS AND USAGE

Buprenex is indicated for the relief of moderate to severe pain.

CONTRAINDICATIONS

Buprenex should not be administered to patients who have been shown to be hypersensitive to the drug.

WARNINGS

Impaired Respiration: As with other potent opioids, clinically significant respiratory depression may occur within the recommended dose range in patients receiving therapeutic doses of buprenorphine. Buprenex should be used with caution in patients with compromised respiratory function (e.g., chronic obstructive pulmonary disease, cor pulmonale, decreased respiratory reserve, hypoxia, hypercapnia, or preexisting respiratory depression). Particular caution is advised if Buprenex is administered to patients taking or recently receiving drugs with CNS/respiratory depressant effects. In patients with the physical and/or pharmacological risk factors above, the dose should be reduced by approximately one-half.

NALOXONE MAY NOT BE EFFECTIVE IN REVERSING THE RESPIRATORY DEPRESSION PRODUCED BY BUPRENEX. THEREFORE, AS WITH OTHER POTENT OPIOIDS, THE PRIMARY MANAGEMENT OF OVERDOSE SHOULD BE THE REESTABLISHMENT OF ADEQUATE VENTILATION WITH MECHANICAL ASSISTANCE OF RESPIRATION, IF REQUIRED.

Interaction with Other Central Nervous System Depressants: Patients receiving Buprenex in the presence of other narcotic analgesics, general anesthetics, antihistamines, benzodiazepines, phenothiazines, other tranquilizers, sedative/hypnotics or other CNS depressants (including alcohol) may exhibit increased CNS depression. When such combined therapy is contemplated, it is particularly important that the dose of one or both agents be reduced.

Head Injury and Increased Intracranial Pressure: Buprenex, like other potent analgesics, may itself elevate cerebrospinal fluid pressure and should be used with caution in head injury, intracranial lesions and other circumstances where cerebrospinal pressure may be increased. Buprenex can produce miosis and changes in the level of consciousness which may interfere with patient evaluation.

Use in Ambulatory Patients: Buprenex may impair the mental or physical abilities required for the performance of potentially dangerous tasks such as driving a car or operating machinery. Therefore, Buprenex should be administered with caution to ambulatory patients who should be warned to avoid such hazards.

Use in Narcotic-Dependent Patients: Because of the narcotic antagonist activity of Buprenex, use in the physically dependent individual may result in withdrawal effects.

PRECAUTIONS

General: Buprenex should be administered with caution in the elderly, debilitated patients, in children and those with severe impairment of hepatic, pulmonary, or renal function; myxedema or hypothyroidism; adrenal cortical insufficiency (e.g., Addison's disease); CNS depression or coma; toxic psychoses; prostatic hypertrophy or urethral stricture; acute alcoholism, delirium tremens; or kyphoscoliosis.

Because Buprenex is metabolized by the liver, the activity of Buprenex may be increased and/or extended in those individuals with impaired hepatic function or those receiving other agents known to decrease hepatic clearance.

Buprenex has been shown to increase intracholedochal pressure to a similar degree as other opioid analgesics, and thus should be administered with caution to patients with dysfunction of the biliary tract.

Information for Patients: The effects of Buprenex, particularly drowsiness, may be potentiated by other centrally acting agents such as alcohol or benzodiazepines. It is particularly important that in these circumstances patients must not drive or operate machinery. Buprenex has some pharmacologic effects similar to morphine which in susceptible patients may lead to self-administration of the drug when pain no longer exists. Patients must not exceed the dosage of Buprenex prescribed by their physician. Patients should be urged to consult their physician if other prescription medica-

tions are currently being used or are prescribed for future use.

Drug Interactions: Drug interactions common to other potent opioid analgesics also may occur with Buprenex. Particular care should be taken when Buprenex is used in combination with central nervous system depressant drugs (see WARNINGS). Although specific information is not presently available, caution should be exercised when Buprenex is used in combination with MAO inhibitors. There have been reports of respiratory and cardiovascular collapse in patients who received therapeutic doses of diazepam and Buprenex. A suspected interaction between Buprenex and phenprocoumon resulting in purpura has been reported.

Carcinogenesis, Mutagenesis, Impairment of Fertility: The effects of Buprenex on fertility and gestation indices were investigated in rats by the subcutaneous and intramuscular routes at doses 10 to 1,000 times the proposed human doses. Dystocia was noted in dams treated with 1,000 times the human dose. No effects on fertility or gestation were noted in these Segment 1 studies.

Pregnancy: Pregnancy Category C. Reproduction studies have been performed in the rat at doses which ranged from 10 to 1,000 times the proposed human dose by the subcutaneous and intramuscular routes and 160 times the proposed human dose by the intravenous route. By the intramuscular route, Buprenex produced mild but statistically significant (p < 0.05) post-implantation losses and early fetal deaths at 10 and 100 but not 1,000 times the proposed human dose. No fetal malformations were noted in rats at any dose when Buprenex was administered by subcutaneous, intramuscular, or intravenous routes. In rabbits, intramuscularly administered Buprenex produced a dose-related trend for extra rib formation which attained statistical significance (p < 0.01) at 1,000 times the proposed human dose. By the intravenous route, doses in rats of 40 and 160 times the proposed human dose of Buprenex caused a slight increase in post-implantation losses that may have been treatment-related. No major fetal malformations were noted in drug treated groups when administered by intramuscular or intravenous routes.

There are no adequate and well-controlled studies in pregnant women. Buprenex should be used during pregnancy only if the potential benefit justifies the potential risk to the fetus.

Labor and Delivery: The safety of Buprenex given during labor and delivery has not been established.

Nursing Mothers: An apparent lack of milk production during general reproduction studies with Buprenex in rats caused decreased viability and lactation indices. It is unknown at this time whether or not Buprenex is excreted in human milk. Despite the lack of specific knowledge on this issue, it is reasonable to assume that Buprenex will enter human milk and caution should be exercised in the use of Buprenex when it is administered to nursing mothers.

Pediatric Use: The safety and effectiveness of Buprenex have been established for children between 2 and 12 years of age. Use of Buprenex in children is supported by evidence from adequate and well controlled trials of Buprenex in adults, with additional data from studies of 960 children ranging in age from 9 months to 18 years of age. Data is available from a pharmacokinetic study, several controlled clinical trials, and several large post-marketing studies and case series. The available information provides reasonable evidence that Buprenex may be used safely in children ranging from 2–12 years of age, and that it is of similar effectiveness in children as in adults.

ADVERSE REACTIONS

The most frequent side effect in clinical studies involving 1,133 patients was sedation which occurred in approximately two-thirds of the patients. Although sedated, these patients could easily be aroused to an alert state.

Other less frequent adverse reactions occurring in 5–10% of the patients were:

Nausea	Dizziness/Vertigo

Occurring in 1–5% of the patients:

Sweating	Headache
Hypotension	Nausea/Vomiting
Vomiting	Hypoventilation
Miosis	

The following adverse reactions were reported to have occurred in less than 1% of the patients:

CNS Effect: confusion, blurred vision, euphoria, weakness/fatigue, dry mouth, nervousness, depression, slurred speech, paresthesia.

Cardiovascular: hypertension, tachycardia, bradycardia.

Gastrointestinal: constipation.

Respiratory: dyspnea, cyanosis.

Dermatological: pruritus.

Ophthalmological: diplopia, visual abnormalities.

Miscellaneous: injection site reaction, urinary retention, dreaming, flushing/warmth, chills/cold, tinnitus, conjunctivitis, Wenckebach block, and psychosis.

Other effects observed infrequently include malaise, hallucinations, depersonalization, coma, dyspepsia, flatulence, apnea, rash, amblyopia, tremor, and pallor.

The following reactions have been reported to occur rarely: loss of appetite, dysphoria/agitation, diarrhea, urticaria, and convulsions/lack of muscle coordination.

In the United Kingdom, buprenorphine hydrochloride was made available under monitored release regulation during the first year of sale, and yielded data from 1,736 physicians on 9,123 patients (17,120 administrations). Data on 240 children under the age of 18 years were included in this monitored release program. No important new adverse effects attributable to buprenorphine hydrochloride were observed.

DRUG ABUSE AND DEPENDENCE

Buprenorphine hydrochloride is a partial agonist of the morphine type: i.e., it has certain opioid properties which may lead to psychic dependence of the morphine type due to an opiate-like euphoric component of the drug. Direct dependence studies have shown little physical dependence upon withdrawal of the drug. However, caution should be used in prescribing to individuals who are known to be drug abusers or ex-narcotic addicts. The drug may not substitute in acutely dependent narcotic addicts due to its antagonist component and may induce withdrawal symptoms.

OVERDOSAGE

Manifestations: Clinical experience with Buprenex overdosage has been insufficient to define the signs of this condition at this time. Although the antagonist activity of buprenorphine may become manifest at doses somewhat above the recommended therapeutic range, doses in the recommended therapeutic range may produce clinically significant respiratory depression in certain circumstances. (See WARNINGS.)

Treatment: The respiratory and cardiac status of the patients should be monitored carefully. Primary attention should be given to the reestablishment of adequate respiratory exchange through provision of a patent airway and institution of assisted or controlled ventilation. Oxygen, intravenous fluids, vasopressors, and other supportive measures should be employed as indicated. Doxapram, a respiratory stimulant, may be used. NALOXONE MAY NOT BE EFFECTIVE IN REVERSING THE RESPIRATORY DEPRESSION PRODUCED BY BUPRENEX. THEREFORE, AS WITH OTHER POTENT OPIOIDS, THE PRIMARY MANAGEMENT OF OVERDOSE SHOULD BE THE REESTABLISHMENT OF ADEQUATE VENTILATION WITH MECHANICAL ASSISTANCE OF RESPIRATION, IF REQUIRED.

DOSAGE AND ADMINISTRATION

Adults: The usual dosage for persons 13 years of age and over is 1 ml Buprenex (0.3 mg buprenorphine) given by deep intramuscular or slow (over at least 2 minutes) intravenous injection at up to 6-hour intervals, as needed. Repeat once (up to 0.3 mg) if required, 30 to 60 minutes after initial dosage, giving consideration to previous dose pharmacokinetics, and thereafter only as needed. In high-risk patients (e.g., elderly, debilitated, presence of respiratory disease, etc.) and/or in patients where other CNS depressants are present, such as in the immediate postoperative period, the dose should be reduced by approximately one-half. Extra caution should be exercised with the intravenous route of administration, particularly with the initial dose.

Occasionally, it may be necessary to administer single doses of up to 0.6 mg to adults depending on the severity of the pain and the response of the patient. This dose should only be given I.M. and only to adult patients who are not in a high risk category (see WARNINGS and PRECAUTIONS). At this time, there are insufficient data to recommend single doses greater than 0.6 mg for long-term use.

Children: Buprenex has been used in children 2–12 years of age at doses between 2–6 micrograms/kg of body weight given every 4–6 hours. There is insufficient experience to recommend a dose in infants below the age of two years, single doses greater than 6 micrograms/kg of body weight, or the use of a repeat or second dose at 30–60 minutes (such as is used in adults). Since there is some evidence that not all children clear buprenorphine faster than adults, fixed interval or "round-the-clock" dosing should not be undertaken until the proper inter-dose interval has been established by clinical observation of the child. Physicians should recognize that, as with adults, some pediatric patients may not need to be remedicated for 6–8 hours.

Safety and Handling: Buprenex is supplied in sealed ampuls and poses no known environmental risk to health care providers. Accidental dermal exposure should be treated by removal of any contaminated clothing and rinsing the affected area with water.

Buprenex is a potent narcotic, and like all drugs of this class has been associated with abuse and dependence among health care providers. To control the risk of diversion, it is recommended that measures appropriate to the health care setting be taken to provide rigid accounting, control of wastage, and restriction of access.

Parenteral drug products should be inspected visually for particulate matter and discoloration prior to administration, whenever solution and container permit.

Continued on next page

Reckitt & Colman—Cont.

HOW SUPPLIED
Buprenex (buprenorphine hydrochloride) is supplied in clear glass snap-ampuls of 1 ml (0.3 mg buprenorphine).
NDC 12496-0757-1
Avoid excessive heat (over 104°F or 40°C). Protect from prolonged exposure to light.

CAUTION
Federal law prohibits dispensing without prescription.
Manufactured by:
Reckitt & Colman Products,
Hull, England HU8 7DS.

Distributed by:
Reckitt & Colman Pharmaceuticals Inc.,
Richmond, VA 23235.
Buprenex® is a trademark of Reckitt & Colman (Overseas) Limited.
REVISED JANUARY 1993

912801

Shown in Product Identification Guide, page 330

Reed & Carnrick
DIVISION OF BLOCK DRUG COMPANY, INC
257 CORNELISON AVENUE
JERSEY CITY, NJ 07302

The following products previously marketed by Reed & Carnrick are now marketed by Schwarz Pharma.

Actinex Cream
Colyte & Colyte Flavored
Cortifoam
Dilatrate-SR
Epifoam
Ethamolin
Levatol
Proctocream-HC 2.5%
Proctofoam-HC
Proctofoam-NS (Non-Steroid)
Trichotine Liquid, Vaginal Douche
Trichotine Powder, Vaginal Douche

Reedco, Inc.
ROAD # 3, KM 76.9
HCO4 BOX 4013
HUMACAO, PUERTO RICO 00791-9502

Direct Inquiries to:
Block Drug Company, Inc.
Consumer Affairs
(201) 434-3000, Ext. 1308
FAX: (201) 434-5739

For Medical Information Contact:
In Emergencies:
Block Drug Company, Inc.
Consumer Affairs
(800) 365-6500, Ext. 1308
FAX: (201) 434-5739

KWELL® Cream and Lotion ℞
(lindane) 1%

DESCRIPTION
KWELL Cream and Lotion (lindane) 1% are an ectoparasiticide and ovicide effective against Sarcoptes scabiei (scabies). The inactive ingredients of Kwell Cream are stearic acid, glycerin, lanolin, 2-amino-2-methyl-1-propanol, perfume and purified water, forming a pleasantly water dispersible cream. In addition to the active ingredient, lindane, Kwell Lotion contains glyceryl monostearate, cetyl alcohol, stearic acid, trolamine, 2-amino-2-methyl-1-propanol, methyl p-hydroxybenzoate, butyl p-hydroxybenzoate, carrageenan, perfume and purified water to form a non-greasy lotion. Lindane, which is the highly purified gamma isomer of 1, 2, 3, 4, 5, 6, hexachlorocyclohexane, has the following chemical structure:

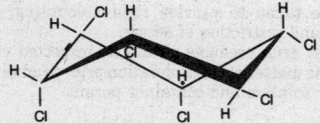

CLINICAL PHARMACOLOGY
KWELL exerts its parasiticidal action by being directly absorbed in the parasites and their ova. Feldmann and Maibach[1] reported approximately 10% absorption of a lindane acetone solution applied to the forearm and left in place for 24 hours. Dale, et al[2] reported a blood level of 290 ng/ml associated with convulsions following the accidental ingestion of a lindane-containing product. Ginsburg[3] found a mean peak blood level of 28 ng/ml 6 hours after total body application of KWELL to scabietic infants and children. The half-life was determined to be 18 hours.

INDICATIONS AND USAGE
KWELL is indicated for the treatment of patients infested with Sarcoptes scabiei (scabies).

CONTRAINDICATIONS
KWELL is contraindicated for premature neonates because their skin may be more permeable and their liver enzymes may not be sufficiently developed. It is also contraindicated for patients with Norwegian (crusted) scabies due to possible increased absorption. It is also contraindicated for patients with known seizure disorders and for individuals with a known sensitivity to the product or any of its components.

WARNINGS
LINDANE PENETRATES HUMAN SKIN AND HAS THE POTENTIAL FOR CNS TOXICITY (SEE CLINICAL PHARMACOLOGY SECTION). KWELL SHOULD BE USED ACCORDING TO RECOMMENDED DOSAGE (SEE DIRECTIONS FOR USE) ESPECIALLY ON INFANTS, PREGNANT WOMEN AND NURSING MOTHERS. ANIMAL STUDIES INDICATE THAT POTENTIAL TOXIC EFFECTS OF TOPICALLY APPLIED LINDANE ARE GREATER IN THE YOUNG. SEIZURES AND, IN RARE INSTANCES, DEATHS HAVE BEEN REPORTED AFTER EXCESS DOSAGE, OVER-EXPOSURE, FREQUENT REAPPLICATIONS, AND ACCIDENTAL AND INTENTIONAL INGESTION OF LINDANE. THESE INSTANCES OF PATIENT MISUSE HAVE BEEN ASSOCIATED WITH LACK OF PATIENT UNDERSTANDING OF DIRECTIONS OF USE, PRESCRIBING OR DISPENSING EXCESSIVE QUANTITIES, AND IMPROPER REAPPLICATIONS. IN EXCEEDINGLY RARE CASES SEIZURES HAVE BEEN REPORTED WHEN USED ACCORDING TO DIRECTIONS. NO RESIDUAL EFFECTS OF KWELL TREATMENT HAVE BEEN DEMONSTRATED; THEREFORE, THIS PRODUCT SHOULD NOT BE USED TO WARD OFF A POSSIBLE INFESTATION.
If accidental ingestion occurs prompt gastric lavage is indicated. Because oils may enhance absorption, saline rather than oily cathartics should be used. Central nervous excitation can be controlled by the administration of pentobarbital, phenobarbital or diazepam.

PRECAUTIONS
General
Care should be taken to avoid contact with the eyes. If such contact occurs, eyes should be immediately flushed with water. If irritation or sensitization occurs, the patient should be advised to consult a physician.
Geriatric
Dosage may have to be reduced due to the possibility of increased absorption through elderly skin.
Information to Patients
Patients must be instructed on the proper use of the medication, especially as to amount applied and duration of use. Patient Directions for Use must accompany the product.

LABORATORY TESTS
No laboratory tests are needed for the proper use of this medication.

DRUG INTERACTIONS
Oils may enhance absorption; therefore, simultaneous use of creams, ointments or oils should be avoided.

CARCINOGENESIS
Although no studies have been conducted with KWELL, numerous long term feeding studies have been conducted in mice and rats to evaluate the carcinogenic potential of the technical grade of hexachlorocyclohexane (BHC) as well as the alpha, beta, gamma (lindane) and delta isomers. Both oral and topical applications have been evaluated. Nagasaki, et al[4] Goto, et al[5] and Hanada, et al[6] found varying amounts of benign and malignant hepatomas associated with BHC and the alpha, delta and epsilon isomers. None reported a carcinogenic potential for lindane. Tumors were found only in the animals which had received the alpha isomer. Weisse and Herbst[7] also evaluated the carcinogenic potential of lindane in mice but could find no evidence of lindane carcinogenicity. The National Cancer Institute[8] also found no evidence of carcinogenicity.
Thorpe and Walker[9] compared beta BHC with lindane, dieldrin, DDT and hexabarbital in mice. Despite the unusually high incidence of tumors in the control group, they concluded that 600 ppm of lindane was associated with a significant increase of hepatoma and thus considerd it a tumorigen.

Orr[10] and Kashyap, et al[11] evaluated the carcinogenic potential in mice of topically applied BHC. In neither study was there any evidence of a tumorigenic or carcinogenic potential associated with topical application of BHC.
Mutagenicity tests have been used as predictive information about the carcinogenicity of various chemical compounds. Numerous types of mutagenicity tests have been performed with lindane. The results of these tests do not indicate that lindane is mutagenic.

PREGNANCY
Teratogenic Effects
Pregnancy category B: Reproduction, including multigeneration, studies have been performed in mice, rats, rabbits, pigs and dogs at doses up to 10 times the human dose and have revealed no evidence of impaired fertility or harm to the fetus due to orally administered lindane. There are, however, no adequate and well controlled studies in pregnant women. Because animal reproduction studies are not always predictive of human responses, the recommended dosage should not be exceeded on pregnant women. They should be treated no more than twice during a pregnancy.

NURSING MOTHERS
Lindane is secreted in human milk in low concentrations. Studies conducted in the United States as well as in Europe and South America found levels of lindane in human milk ranging from 0 to 113 ppb as the result of ingestion of foods which had been treated with lindane. There appeared to be no difference in concentrations between country and urban dwellers. Although the levels of lindane found in blood after topical application with KWELL make is unlikely that amounts of lindane sufficient to cause serious adverse reactions will be excreted in the milk of nursing mothers who have used KWELL, an alternate method of feeding may be used for 4 days if there is any concern.

PEDIATRIC USE
Refer to the Contraindications and Warnings sections.

ADVERSE REACTIONS
Lindane has been reported to cause central nervous stimulation ranging from dizziness to convulsions. Cases of convulsions have been reported in connection with KWELL therapy. However, these incidents were almost always associated with accidental oral ingestion or misuse of the product. In exceedingly rare cases, seizures have been reported when used according to directions. Eczematous eruptions due to irritation from this product have also been reported. Incidence of these adverse reactions is relatively infrequent, occurring in less than 1 in 100,000 patients.

DRUG ABUSE AND DEPENDENCE
KWELL is not subject to abuse, nor is there any dependence on the drug.

OVERDOSAGE
Overdosage or oral ingestion of KWELL can cause central nervous system excitation and, if taken in sufficient quantities, convulsions may occur.
If accidental ingestion occurs, prompt gastric lavage should be instituted. However, since oils favor absorption, saline cathartics for intestinal evacuation should be given rather than oil laxatives. If central nervous system manifestations occur, they can be antagonized by the administration of pentobartital, phenobartital or diazepam.

DOSAGE AND ADMINISTRATION
CAUTION: USE ONLY AS DIRECTED. DO NOT EXCEED RECOMMENDED DOSAGE.
No residual effects of KWELL treatment have been demonstrated, therefore, this product should not be used to ward off a possible infestation. However, sexual contacts should be treated simultaneously.
NOTE: PLEASE READ CAREFULLY.
DIRECTIONS FOR USE:
WARNING:
THIS PRODUCT CAN BE POISONOUS IF MISUSED. CHILDREN MUST NOT BE ALLOWED TO APPLY THIS DRUG WITHOUT DIRECT ADULT SUPERVISION. USE THE CREAM OR LOTION FOR SCABIES ONLY. APPLY ONLY ONCE. USE ONLY ENOUGH TO COVER THE BODY IN A THIN LAYER. 1 OUNCE (HALF OF A 2 OUNCE CONTAINER) SHOULD BE ALL THAT IS NEEDED FOR CHILDREN UNDER 6 YEARS OF AGE; 1 TO 2 OUNCES FOR OLDER CHILDREN AND ADULTS. DO NOT LEAVE ON FOR MORE THAN 12 HOURS. DO NOT INGEST. KEEP AWAY FROM MOUTH AND EYES. COVER INFANT'S HANDS AND FEET DURING TREATMENT TO PREVENT SUCKING OR LICKING OF CREAM OR LOTION. DO NOT USE IF OPEN WOUNDS, CUTS OR SORES ARE PRESENT, UNLESS DIRECTED BY YOUR PHYSICIAN.
(LOTION: SHAKE WELL)
1. APPLY THIS PREPARATION TO DRY SKIN IN A THIN LAYER AND RUB IN THOROUGHLY.
2. TRIM NAILS AND APPLY UNDER NAILS WITH TOOTHBRUSH (THROW AWAY TOOTHBRUSH AFTER USE).

3. IF A WARM BATH IS TAKEN BEFORE APPLICATION ALLOW THE SKIN TO DRY AND COOL COMPLETELY BEFORE APPLYING THE MEDICATION.
4. A TOTAL BODY APPLICATION SHOULD BE MADE FROM THE NECK DOWN, INCLUDING SOLES OF FEET, UNLESS OTHERWISE DIRECTED BY YOUR PHYSICIAN.
5. THE CREAM OR LOTION SHOULD BE LEFT ON FOR 8 TO 12 HOURS (USUALLY OVERNIGHT) AND THEN REMOVED BY THOROUGH WASHING (BATH OR SHOWER).
6. AVOID UNNECESSARY CONTACT WITH YOUR SKIN IF YOU ARE APPLYING TO ANOTHER PERSON. IF TREATING MORE THAN ONE PERSON, PERSON APPLYING THE CREAM OR LOTION (ESPECIALLY PREGNANT OR NURSING WOMEN) SHOULD WEAR RUBBER GLOVES.
7. ALL RECENTLY WORN CLOTHING, UNDERWEAR AND PAJAMAS, AND USED SHEETS, PILLOW CASES, AND TOWELS SHOULD BE WASHED IN VERY HOT WATER OR DRY-CLEANED.

AFTER ONE APPLICATION, ITCHING WILL CONTINUE FOR SEVERAL WEEKS. THIS IS NORMAL AND DOES NOT REQUIRE REAPPLICATION.

IF YOU HAVE ANY QUESTIONS OR CONCERNS ABOUT YOUR CONDITION OR USE OF THE CREAM OR LOTION, CONTACT YOUR PHYSICIAN.

CAUTION: Federal law prohibits dispensing without prescription.

HOW SUPPLIED

KWELL Cream in tubes of 60 grams.
KWELL Lotion in bottles of patient-size 2 fl. oz. (59 ml), pharmacy-size only 16 fl. oz. (473 ml) and pharmacy-size only 1 gallon (3.8 liters).

REFERENCES

1. Feldmann, R. J. and Maibach, H.I., *Toxicol. Appl. Pharmacol.* 28:126, 1974
2. Dale, W.E., Curley, A. and Cueto, C., *Life Sci.* 5:47, 1966
3. Ginsburg, C.M., et al., *J. Pediat.* 91:998, 1977
4. Nagasaki, T., Tomii, S., Mega, T., Marugami, M. and Ito, N., *Gann* (Cancer) 63:393, 1972
5. Goto, M., Hattori, M., Miyagawa, T. and Enomoto, M., *Chemosphere* 6:279, 1972
6. Hanada, M., Yatani, C. and Miyaji, T., *Gann* 64:511, 1973
7. Weisse, I. and Herbst, M., *Toxicol.* 7:233, 1977
8. Technical Report Series, NCI-CG-TR-14, *HEW PUBLICATIONS,* No. (NIH) 77-814
9. Thorpe, E. and Walker, A.I.T., *Food Cosm. Toxicol.* 11:433, 1973
10. Orr, J.W., *Nature* 162:189, 1948
11. Kashyap, S.K. et al., *J. Environ. Sci. Health* 14:305, 1979

Revised May 1994
Manufactured by Reedco, Inc., Humacao, P.R. 00791
a subsidiary of Block Drug Company, Inc.

KWELL® Shampoo ℞
(lindane) 1%
(hexachlorocyclohexane)

DESCRIPTION

KWELL Shampoo (lindane) 1% is an ectoparasiticide and ovicide effective against Pediculosis capitis (head lice), Pediculosis pubis (crab lice) and their ova. In addition to the active ingredient, lindane, it contains trolamine lauryl sulfate, polysorbate 60, acetone and purified water to form a cosmetically pleasant shampoo. Lindane, which is the highly purified gamma isomer of 1, 2, 3, 4, 5, 6, hexachlorocyclohexane, has the following chemical structure:

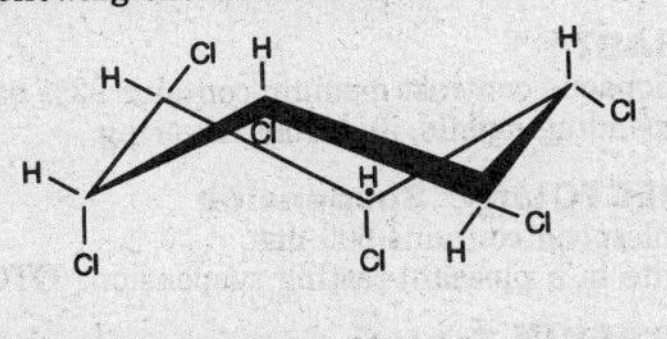

CLINICAL PHARMACOLOGY

KWELL Shampoo exerts its parasiticidal action by being directly absorbed into the parasites and their ova. Dale et al[1] reported a blood level of 290 ng/ml associated with convulsions following the accidental ingestion of a lindane containing product. Analysis of blood taken from subjects before and after the use of KWELL Shampoo showed a mean peak blood level of only 3 ng/ml which appeared at six hours and disappeared at eight hours after the shampoo was applied.[2]

INDICATIONS AND USAGE

Because post-treatment pruritus is common and may lead to misuse, KWELL lindane shampoo is indicated only for the treatment of patients with pediculosis capitis (head lice) and pediculosis pubis (crab lice) who have either failed to respond to adequate doses, or are intolerant of, other approved therapies. Reinfestation should be considered carefully before attributing the posttreatment presence of ectoparasites to a failure of response to adequate doses of other approved therapies.

CONTRAINDICATIONS

KWELL Shampoo is contraindicated for premature neonates because their skin may be more permeable than full term infants and their liver enzymes may not be sufficiently developed. It is also contraindicated for patients with known seizure disorders and for individuals with a known sensitivity to the product or any of its components.

WARNINGS

LINDANE PENETRATES HUMAN SKIN AND HAS THE POTENTIAL FOR CNS TOXICITY (SEE CLINICAL PHARMACOLOGY SECTION). KWELL SHAMPOO SHOULD BE USED ACCORDING TO RECOMMENDED DOSAGE (SEE DIRECTIONS FOR USE) ESPECIALLY ON INFANTS, PREGNANT WOMEN AND NURSING MOTHERS. ANIMAL STUDIES INDICATE THAT POTENTIAL TOXIC EFFECTS OF TOPICALLY APPLIED LINDANE ARE GREATER IN THE YOUNG. SEIZURES, AND, IN RARE INSTANCES, DEATHS HAVE BEEN REPORTED AFTER EXCESS DOSAGE, OVER-EXPOSURE, FREQUENT REAPPLICATIONS, AND ACCIDENTAL AND INTENTIONAL INGESTION OF LINDANE. THESE INSTANCES OF PATIENT MISUSE HAVE BEEN ASSOCIATED WITH LACK OF PATIENT UNDERSTANDING OF DIRECTIONS FOR USE, PRESCRIBING OR DISPENSING EXCESSIVE QUANTITIES, AND IMPROPER REAPPLICATIONS. IN EXCEEDINGLY RARE CASES SEIZURES HAVE BEEN REPORTED WHEN USED ACCORDING TO DIRECTIONS. NO RESIDUAL EFFECTS OF KWELL TREATMENT HAVE BEEN DEMONSTRATED; THEREFORE, THIS PRODUCT SHOULD NOT BE USED TO WARD OFF A POSSIBLE INFESTATION.

If accidental ingestion occurs prompt gastric lavage is indicated. Because oils may enhance absorption, saline rather than oily cathartics should be used. Central nervous excitation can be controlled by the administration of pentobarbital, phenobarbital or diazepam.

PRECAUTIONS

General
Care should be taken to avoid contact with the eyes. If such contact occurs, eyes should be immediately flushed with water. If irritation or sensitization occurs, the patient should be advised to consult a physician.

Information to Patients
Patients must be instructed on the proper use of this medication, especially as to amount applied and duration of use. Directions for use must accompany the product.

LABORATORY TESTS

No laboratory tests are needed for the proper use of this medication.

DRUG INTERACTIONS

Oils may enhance absorption, therefore, avoid using oil treatments, or oil based hair dressings or conditioners immediately before and after applying KWELL Shampoo.

CARCINOGENESIS

Although no studies have been conducted with KWELL Shampoo, numerous long term feeding studies have been conducted in mice and rats to evaluate the carcinogenic potential of the technical grade of hexachlorocyclohexane (BHC) as well as the alpha, beta, gamma (lindane) and delta isomers. Both oral and topical applications have been evaluated. Nagasaki,[3] Goto[4] and Hanada[5] found varying amounts of benign and malignant hepatomas associated with BHC and the alpha, delta and epsilon isomers. None reported a carcinogenic potential for lindane. Tumors were found only in the animals which had received the alpha isomer. Weisse and Herbst[6] also evaluated the carcinogenic potential of lindane in mice but could find no evidence of lindane carcinogenicity. The National Cancer Institute[7] had also found no evidence of carcinogenicity.

Thorpe and Walker[8] compared beta BHC with lindane, dieldrin, DDT and hexabarbital in mice. Despite the unusually high incidence of tumors in the control group, they concluded that 600 ppm of lindane was associated with a significant increase in the incidence of hepatoma and thus, considered it a tumorigen.

Orr[9] and Kashyap, et al[10] evaluated the carcinogenic potential in mice of topically applied BHC. In neither study was there any evidence of a tumorigenic or carcinogenic potential associated with the topical application of BHC.

Mutagenicity tests have been used as predictive information about the carginogenicity of various chemical compounds. Numerous types of mutagenicity tests have been performed with lindane. The results of these tests do not indicate that lindane is mutagenic.

PREGNANCY

Teratogenic Effects
Pregnancy category B: Reproduction, including multigeneration, studies have been performed in mice, rats, rabbits, pigs and dogs at doses up to 10 times the human dose and have revealed no evidence of impaired fertility or harm to the fetus due to orally administered lindane. There are, however, no adequate and well controlled studies in pregnant women. Because animal reproduction studies are not always predictive of human response, the recommended dosage should not be exceeded on pregnant women. They should be treated no more than twice during a pregnancy.

NURSING MOTHERS

Lindane is secreted in human milk in low concentrations. Studies conducted in the United States as well as in Europe and South America found levels of lindane in human milk ranging from 0 to 113 ppb as the result of ingestion of foods which had been treated with lindane. There appeared to be no difference in concentrations between country and urban dwellers. Although the levels of lindane found in blood after topical application with KWELL Shampoo make it unlikely that amounts of lindane sufficient to cause serious adverse reactions will be excreted in the milk of nursing mothers who have used KWELL Shampoo, an alternate method of feeding may be used for 4 days if there is any concern.

PEDIATRIC USE

Refer to the Contraindications and Warnings sections.

ADVERSE REACTIONS

Lindane has been reported to cause central nervous stimulation ranging from dizziness to convulsions. Cases of convulsions have been reported in connection with KWELL Shampoo therapy. However, these incidents were almost always associated with accidental oral ingestion or misuse of the product. In exceedingly rare cases, seizures have been reported when used according to directions. Eczematous eruptions due to irritation from this product have also been reported. Incidence of these adverse reactions is relatively infrequent, occurring in less than 1 in 100,000 patients.

DRUG ABUSE AND DEPENDENCE

KWELL Shampoo is not subject to abuse nor is there any dependence on the drug.

OVERDOSAGE

Overdosage or oral ingestion of KWELL Shampoo can cause central nervous system excitation and, if taken in sufficient quantities, convulsions may occur.

If accidental ingestion occurs, prompt gastric lavage should be instituted. However, since oils favor absorption, saline cathartics for ingestinal evacuation should be given rather than oil laxatives. If central nervous system manifestations occur, they can be antagonized by the administration of pentobarbital, phenobarbital or diazepam.

DOSAGE AND ADMINISTRATION

CAUTION: USE ONLY AS DIRECTED. DO NOT EXCEED RECOMMENDED DOSAGE.

No residual effects of KWELL Shampoo treatment have been demonstrated, therefore, this product should not be used to ward off a possible infestation. However, sexual contacts should be treated simultaneously.

NOTE: PLEASE READ CAREFULLY.

DIRECTIONS FOR USE:

NOTE: PLEASE SEE NEW INDICATIONS AND USAGE BEFORE PROVIDING DIRECTIONS

WARNING:

THIS PRODUCT CAN BE POISONOUS IF MISUSED. CHILDREN MUST NOT BE ALLOWED TO APPLY THIS DRUG WITHOUT DIRECT ADULT SUPERVISION. USE SHAMPOO FOR HEAD AND PUBIC LICE ONLY. DO NOT USE FOR SCABIES. USE ONLY IN AMOUNTS DIRECTED BELOW. IN NO CASE SHOULD MORE THAN 2 OUNCES BE USED BY ONE PERSON IN ONE APPLICATION. DO NOT INGEST. KEEP AWAY FROM MOUTH AND EYES. DO NOT USE IF OPEN WOUNDS, CUTS OR SORES ARE PRESENT ON SCALP OR GROIN, UNLESS DIRECTED BY YOUR PHYSICIAN.

AVOID USING OIL TREATMENTS, OIL BASED HAIR DRESSINGS OR CONDITIONERS IMMEDIATELY BEFORE AND AFTER APPLYING KWELL SHAMPOO.

(SHAKE WELL)

1. BEFORE APPLYING KWELL SHAMPOO, USE REGULAR SHAMPOO (WITHOUT CONDITIONERS), RINSE AND COMPLETELY DRY HAIR.
2. USE 1 OUNCE (HALF OF A 2 OUNCE BOTTLE) FOR SHORT HAIR; 1.5 OUNCES (THREE-QUARTERS OF A 2 OUNCE BOTTLE) FOR MEDIUM LENGTH HAIR; AND FULL 2 OUNCE BOTTLE FOR LONG HAIR.
3. APPLY SHAMPOO DIRECTLY TO DRY HAIR WITHOUT ADDING WATER. WORK THOROUGHLY INTO THE HAIR AND ALLOW TO REMAIN IN PLACE FOR 4 MINUTES ONLY.
4. AFTER 4 MINUTES, ADD SMALL QUANTITIES OF WATER TO HAIR UNTIL A GOOD LATHER FORMS.
5. IMMEDIATELY RINSE ALL LATHER AWAY. AVOID UNNECESSARY CONTACT OF LATHER WITH OTHER BODY SURFACES.
6. TOWEL BRISKLY AND REMOVE NITS WITH NIT COMB OR TWEEZERS.

Continued on next page

Reedco—Cont.

7. AVOID UNNECESSARY CONTACT WITH YOUR SKIN IF YOU ARE APPLYING SHAMPOO TO ANOTHER PERSON. IF TREATING MORE THAN ONE PERSON, PERSON APPLYING SHAMPOO (ESPECIALLY PREGNANT AND/OR NURSING WOMEN) SHOULD WEAR RUBBER GLOVES.

RE-TREATMENT IS USUALLY NOT NECESSARY, BUT PRESENCE OF LIVING LICE IN HAIR 7 DAYS AFTER TREATMENT INDICATES THAT RE-TREATMENT MAY BE NECESSARY. DO NOT RETREAT WITHOUT THE ADVICE OF A PHYSICIAN.

CAUTION: Federal law prohibits dispensing without prescription.

HOW SUPPLIED
KWELL Shampoo in bottles of patient-size 2 fl. oz. (59 ml), and pharmacy-size only 16 fl. oz. (473 ml).

REFERENCES
1. Dale, W.E., Curly A. and Cueto, C., *Life Sci* 5:47, 1966.
2. Data on File at Reed & Carnrick.
3. Nagasaki, T., Tomii, S., Mega, T., Marugami, M. and Ito, N., *Gann* (Cancer) 63:393, 1972.
4. Goto, M., Hattori, M., Miyagawa, T. and Enomoto, M., *Chemosphere* 6:279, 1972.
5. Hanada, M., Yatani, C., Miyaji, T., *Gann* 64:511, 1973.
6. Weisse, I. and Herbst, M., *Toxicol* 7:233, 1977.
7. Technical Report Series, NCI-CG-TR-14, *HEW PUBLICATIONS*, No. (NIH) 77-814.
8. Thorpe, E. and Walker, A.I.T., *Food Cosme. Toxicol.* 11:433, 1973.
9. Orr, J.W., *Nature* 162:189, 1948.
10. Kashyap, S.K. et al., *J. Environ. Sci. Health* 14:305, 1979.
Revised March 1992
Manufactured by Reedco, Inc., Humacao, P.R. 00791 a subsidiary of Block Drug Company, Inc.

4030120010

Respa Pharmaceuticals, Inc.
P.O. BOX 88222
CAROL STREAM, IL 60188

Direct Inquiries to:
(630) 462-9986
FAX: (630) 462-9934

RESPA-DM TABLETS
DYE FREE

Each tablet contain 30 mg Dextromethorphan and 600 mg Guaifenesin
DOSAGE
12 yr. and older 1 or 2 tab. B.I.D. 6 to 12 1 tab. B.I.D.

RESPA-GF TABLETS
DYE FREE

Each tablet contain 600 mg Guaifenesin
DOSAGE
12 yr. and older 1 or 2 tab. B.I.D. 6 to 12 1 tab. B.I.D.

RESPA-1ST TABLETS
DYE FREE

Each tab. contain 60 mg Pseudoephedrine and 600 mg Guaifenesin
DOSAGE
12 yr. and older 1 or 2 tab. B.I.D. 6 to 12 1 tab. B.I.D.

RESPAHIST CAPSULES ℞
DYE FREE

Each capsule contain 6 mg Brompheniramine and 60 mg Pseudoephedrine
DOSAGE
12 yr. and older 1 or 2 capsules B.I.D. 6 to 12 1 Capsule B.I.D.

RESPA-A.R.M. Tablets ℞
DYE FREE

Each tablet contains: 25 mg Phenylephrine HCL, 50 mg Phenylpropanolamine HCL, 8 mg Chlorpheniramine MAL, Belladonna Alkaloids (Hyoscyamine Sulfate, Atropine Sulfate and Scopolamine Hydrobromide)
DOSAGE
Adults and Children over 12 years of age 1 tab B.I.D.

Rexar Pharmacal
A division Of Richwood Pharmaceutical Company Inc.
396 ROCKAWAY AVENUE
VALLEY STREAM, NY 11581

See Richwood Pharmaceutical Co.

Rhône-Poulenc Rorer Pharmaceuticals Inc.
500 ARCOLA ROAD
COLLEGEVILLE, PA 19426-0107

Direct Inquiries to:
QUALITY ASSURANCE QUESTIONS:
John Chiles, Manager, Quality Control
(610) 454-3130
REGULATORY AFFAIRS QUESTIONS:
Ron Panner, Director, Regulatory Affairs
(610) 454-3026
For Medical Information Contact:
PRODUCT INFORMATION/ADVERSE DRUG EXPERIENCES/EMERGENCIES:
Medical Information and Education
1-800-340-7502
(610) 454-8110

Following is a list of Rhône-Poulenc Rorer Pharmaceuticals Inc. products. Full prescribing information is provided on the following pages for those products indicated by an asterisk. For further information, please call Rhône-Poulenc Rorer Medical Information and Education at 1-800-340-7502 or (610) 454-8110.

H.P. ACTHAR® GEL ℞
40 USP Units/mL and 80 USP Units/mL
Repository corticotropin injection available in strengths of 40 USP Units or 80 USP Units per mL.

*AZMACORT® Oral Inhaler ℞
Each metered-dose inhaler contains 60 mg triamcinolone acetonide. Each oral inhaler unit delivers 240 actuations of approximately 100 mcg of triamcinolone acetonide.
Pictured in Product Identification Guide, page 330

BAROTRAST® ℞
This radiopaque contrast medium contains 92.5% barium sulfate, suspending agents, and sodium saccharin.

*CALCIMAR® Injection, Synthetic ℞
Each 2-mL vial contains 400 I.U. (200 I.U. per mL) calcitonin-salmon as a sterile solution for subcutaneous or intramuscular injection.

CALEL-D ® Tablets
Each tablet provides 500 mg of elemental Calcium (50% of U.S. RDA) from calcium carbonate and 200 I.U. of Vitamin D₃ (Cholecalciferol) (50% of U.S. RDA).

*DDAVP® Injection ℞
Each mL of sterile, aqueous solution for injection provides 4.0 mcg desmopressin acetate.
Pictured in Product Identification Guide, page 330

*DDAVP® Injection 15 μg/mL ℞
Each mL of sterile, aqueous solution for injection provides 15 μg desmopressin acetate.
Pictured in Product Identification Guide, page 330

*DDAVP® Nasal Spray 5 mL ℞
*DDAVP® Rhinal Tube 2.5 mL ℞
Each mL of aqueous solution for intranasal use provides 0.1 mg desmopressin acetate.
Pictured in Product Identification Guide, page 330

*DDAVP™ Tablets ℞
Each tablet contains either 0.1 or 0.2 mg desmopressin acetate.
Pictured in Product Identification Guide, page 330

DEMI-REGROTON® Tablets ℞
See Regroton® Tablets.

DIALUME® Capsules ℞
Each capsule contains aluminum hydroxide (calcium aluminum basic carbonate) powder 500 mg (aluminum content equivalent to 383 mg Al(OH)₃); sodium content not more than 1.2 mg, magnesium content not more than 1.0 mg, calcium content not more than 40 mg.

*DILACOR XR® Extended-release Capsules ℞
Each capsule contains multiple units of diltiazem HCl 60 mg in a Geomatrix™ controlled-release system, resulting in 120-mg, 180-mg, and 240-mg dosage strengths.
Pictured in Product Identification Guide, page 330

ESOPHOTRAST® Cream ℞
This radiopaque contrast medium contains 560 mg per gm (100% w/v) barium sulfate, suspending agent, and fruit flavoring.

HYGROTON® Tablets ℞
25 mg, 50 mg, and 100 mg
Each tablet contains 25 mg, 50 mg, or 100 mg chlorthalidone, USP.

*INTAL® Inhaler ℞
Each metered-dose aerosol unit delivers at least 112 (8.1 g canister) or at least 200 (14.2 g canister) inhalations containing 800 mcg cromolyn sodium. Product of Fisons Corporation, a Rhône-Poulenc Rorer Company.
Pictured in Product Identification Guide, page 330

*INTAL® Nebulizer Solution ℞
Each 2-mL ampule contains 20 mg cromolyn sodium inhalation solution, USP, in purified water. Product of Fisons Corporation, a Rhône-Poulenc Rorer Company.
Pictured in Product Identification Guide, page 330

*LOVENOX® Injection ℞
Each prefilled syringe contains 30 mg of enoxaparin sodium in 0.3 mL of Water for Injection.
Pictured in Product Identification Guide, page 330

LOZOL® Tablets ℞
Each tablet contains 1.25 mg or 2.5 mg indapamide.

*NASACORT® AQ Nasal Spray ℞
Metered-dose pump spray unit delivers 120 actuations of 55 mcg aqueous triamcinolone acetonide.
Pictured in Product Identification Guide, page 330

*NASACORT® Nasal Inhaler ℞
This metered-dose aerosol unit delivers 100 actuations of 55 mcg of triamcinolone acetonide.
Pictured in Product Identification Guide, page 330

*NASALCROM® Nasal Solution ℞
Each unit delivers at least 100 (13-mL bottle) or at least 200 (26-mL bottle) metered sprays containing 5.2 mg cromolyn sodium nasal solution, USP. Product of Fisons Corporation, a Rhône-Poulenc Rorer Company.

NICOBID® Tempules® ℞
125 mg, 250 mg, and 500 mg
Each timed-release capsule contains 125 mg, 250 mg, or 500 mg of niacin (nicotinic acid).

NICOLAR® Tablets ℞
Each tablet contains 500 mg of niacin (nicotinic acid).

*NITROLINGUAL® SPRAY ℞
A 200-dose metered sublingual aerosol delivering 0.4 mg of nitroglycerin per actuation.
Pictured in Product Identification Guide, page 330

*ONCASPAR® ℞
Each 5-mL vial contains pegaspargase 750 IU/mL in a clear, colorless, phosphate buffered saline solution.
Pictured in Product Identification Guide, page 330

ORATRAST® ℞
This radiopaque contrast medium contains 92% barium sulfate, suspending agents, and lime flavoring.

PAREPECTOLIN® Suspension
Each tablespoon contains 600 mg attapulgite in a pleasant-tasting suspension. (OTC)

*PENETREX™ Tablets ℞
Each 200-mg and 400-mg film-coated tablet contains enoxacin sesquihydrate equivalent to 200 mg and 400 mg of anhydrous enoxacin, respectively.
Pictured in Product Identification Guide, page 330

REGROTON® Tablets ℞
DEMI-REGROTON® Tablets ℞
Each Regroton tablet provides 50 mg chlorthalidone, USP, and 0.25 mg reserpine, USP.
Each Demi-Regroton tablet provides 25 mg chlorthalidone, USP, and 0.125 mg reserpine, USP.

*RILUTEK® Tablets ℞
Each film-coated tablet contains 50 mg riluzole.
Pictured in Product Identification Guide, page 330

***SLO-BID™ Gyrocaps®** ℞
50 mg, 75 mg, 100 mg, 125 mg, 200 mg, and 300 mg
Each extended-release capsule contains theophylline, anhydrous, USP.
Pictured in Product Identification Guide, page 330

SLO-PHYLLIN® Tablets ℞
100 mg and 200 mg
Each tablet contains 100 mg or 200 mg theophylline, anhydrous, USP.

SLO-PHYLLIN® Syrup ℞
Each 15 mL contains 80 mg theophylline, anhydrous, USP.

SLO-PHYLLIN® GG Capsules, Syrup ℞
Each capsule or 15 mL of syrup contains 150 mg of theophylline, anhydrous, and 90 mg of guaifenesin.

***TAXOTERE® for Injection Concentrate** ℞
Single-dose vials contain either Taxotere (docetaxel) 80 mg Concentrate for Infusion or Taxotere (docetaxel) 20 mg Concentrate for Infusion with accompanying diluent. Taxotere Concentrate for Infusion contains polysorbate 80.
Pictured in Product Identification Guide, page 331

***TILADE® Inhaler** ℞
Metered-dose aerosol unit delivers at least 104 metered inhalations of 1.75 mg nedocromil sodium from the mouthpiece. Product of Fisons Corporation, a Rhône-Poulenc Rorer Company.
Pictured in Product Identification Guide, page 330

TUSSAR® DM Syrup
Each 5 mL contains 15 mg dextromethorphan hydrobromide, USP; 2 mg chlorpheniramine maleate, USP; and 30 mg psuedoephedrine HCl, USP.

TUSSAR®-2 Syrup Ⓒ
Each 5 mL contains 10 mg codeine phosphate, USP; 30 mg pseudoephedrine HCl, USP; 100 mg guaifenesin, USP; and 2.5% alcohol.
(Warning: May be habit-forming.)

TUSSAR® SF Syrup Ⓒ
(Sugar Free)
Formulation identical to Tussar–2, except Tussar SF contains saccharin-sorbitol base for patients who must limit sugar intake. Alcohol content 2.5%.
(Warning: May be habit-forming.)

*** Please see full prescribing information on the following pages.**

AZMACORT® ℞
[*ăz ′ma-kort*]
(triamcinolone acetonide)
Oral Inhaler

FOR ORAL INHALATION ONLY

PRODUCT OVERVIEW

KEY FACTS

Azmacort® is an anti-inflammatory steroid in a metered-dose aerosol unit containing at least 240 actuations. Each actuation releases approximately 200 mcg triamcinolone acetonide, of which approximately 100 mcg are delivered from the unit. **Azmacort** provides effective local steroid activity with minimal systemic effect. Triamcinolone acetonide is a very potent derivative of triamcinolone.

MAJOR USES

Azmacort® Oral Inhaler is indicated only for patients who require chronic treatment with corticosteroids for the control of symptoms of bronchial asthma. **Azmacort®** Oral Inhaler is not to be regarded as a bronchodilator and is not indicated for rapid relief of bronchospasm.

SAFETY INFORMATION

Azmacort® Oral Inhaler is contraindicated in the primary treatment of status asthmaticus or other acute episodes of asthma requiring intensive measures. Particular care is needed in patients transferred from systemically active corticosteroids to **Azmacort®** inhaler because deaths due to adrenal insufficiency have occurred in asthmatic patients during and after such a transfer. Patients who are on immunosuppressant doses of corticosteroids should be warned to avoid exposure to chickenpox or measles and, if exposed, to obtain medical advice.

PRESCRIBING INFORMATION

AZMACORT® ℞
[*ăz ′ma-kort*]
(triamcinolone acetonide)
Oral Inhaler

For Oral Inhalation Only
Shake Well Before Using

DESCRIPTION

Triamcinolone acetonide, USP, the active ingredient in **Azmacort®** Oral Inhaler, is a glucocorticosteroid with a molecular weight of 434.5 and with the chemical designation 9-Fluoro-11β, 16α, 17, 21-tetrahydroxypregna-1, 4-diene-3, 20-dione cyclic 16, 17-acetal with acetone. ($C_{24}H_{31}FO_6$).

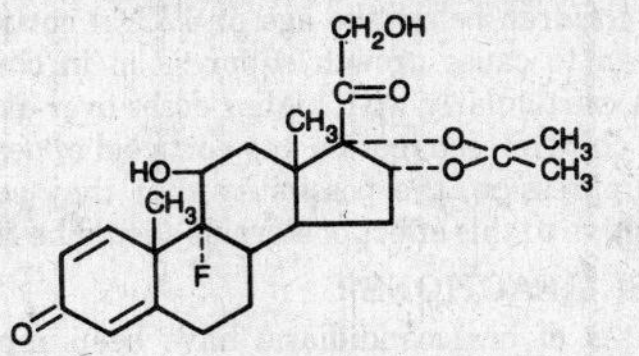

Azmacort Oral Inhaler is a metered-dose aerosol unit containing a microcrystalline suspension of triamcinolone acetonide in the propellant dichlorodifluoromethane and dehydrated alcohol USP 1% w/w. Each canister contains 60 mg triamcinolone acetonide. Each actuation releases approximately 200 mcg triamcinolone acetonide, of which approximately 100 mcg are delivered from the unit (*in-vitro* testing). There are at least 240 actuations in one **Azmacort** aerosol canister. After 240 actuations, the amount delivered per actuation may not be consistent and the unit should be discarded.

CLINICAL PHARMACOLOGY

The precise mechanism of the action of the inhaled drug is unknown. However, use of the inhaler makes it possible to provide effective local steroid activity with minimal systemic effect.
Triamcinolone acetonide is a more potent derivative of triamcinolone. Although triamcinolone itself is approximately one to two times as potent as prednisone in animal models of inflammation, triamcinolone acetonide is approximately 8 times more potent than prednisone.
Pharmacokinetic studies with radiolabeled triamcinolone acetonide have been carried out by the oral route and intravenous route in several species. The pharmacokinetic behavior of the triamcinolone acetonide was similar in all species within each route of administration. The major portion of the dose was eliminated in the feces irrespective of route of administration with only one species (rabbit) showing significant urinary excretion of radioactivity.
The results of studies in which triamcinolone acetonide was administered as an aerosol showed rapid disappearance of radioactivity from the lungs comparable to that observed following oral administration with peak blood levels occurring in one to two hours. Virtually no radioactivity was present in the lung and trachea 24 hours after dosing.
Based upon intravenous dosing of triamcinolone acetonide phosphate ester, the half-life of triamcinolone acetonide was reported to be 88 minutes. The volume of distribution (Vd) reported was 99.5 L (SD $\pm$ 27.5) and clearance was 45.2 L/hour (SD $\pm$ 9.1) for triamcinolone acetonide. The plasma half-life of corticoids does not correlate well with the biologic half-life.
Three metabolites of triamcinolone acetonide have been identified. They are 6β-hydroxytriamcinolone acetonide, 21-carboxytriamcinolone acetonide and 21-carboxy-6β-hydroxytriamcinolone acetonide. All three metabolites are expected to be substantially less active than the parent compound due to (a) the dependence of anti-inflammatory activity on the presence of a 21-hydroxyl group, (b) the decreased activity observed upon 6-hydroxylation, and (c) the markedly increased water solubility favoring rapid elimination. There appeared to be some quantitative differences in the metabolites among species. No differences were detected in metabolic pattern as a function of route of administration.

INDICATIONS

Azmacort Oral Inhaler is indicated only for patients who require chronic treatment with corticosteroids for the control of the symptoms of bronchial asthma. Such patients would include those already receiving systemic corticosteroids and selected patients who are inadequately controlled on a non-steroid regimen and in whom steroid therapy has been withheld because of concern over potential adverse effects.
Azmacort Oral Inhaler is *NOT* indicated:
1. For relief of asthma which can be controlled by bronchodilators and other non-steroid medications.
2. In patients who require systemic corticosteroid treatment infrequently.
3. In the treatment of non-asthmatic bronchitis.

CONTRAINDICATIONS

Azmacort Oral Inhaler is contraindicated in the primary treatment of status asthmaticus or other acute episodes of asthma where intensive measures are required.
Hypersensitivity to any of the ingredients of this preparation contraindicates its use.

WARNINGS

Particular care is needed in patients who are transferred from systemically active corticosteroids to **Azmacort** Oral Inhaler because deaths due to adrenal insufficiency have occurred in asthmatic patients during and after transfer from systemic corticosteroids to aerosolized steroids in recommended doses. After withdrawal from systemic corticosteroids, a number of months is usually required for recovery of hypothalamic-pituitary-adrenal (HPA) function. For some patients who have received large doses of oral steroids for long periods of time before therapy with **Azmacort** Oral Inhaler is initiated, recovery may be delayed for one year or longer. During this period of HPA suppression, patients may exhibit signs and symptoms of adrenal insufficiency when exposed to trauma, surgery or infections, particularly gastroenteritis or other conditions with acute electrolyte loss. Although **Azmacort** Oral Inhaler may provide control of asthmatic symptoms during these episodes, in recommended doses it supplies only normal physiological amounts of corticosteroid systemically and does NOT provide the increased systemic steroid which is necessary for coping with these emergencies.
During periods of stress or a severe asthmatic attack, patients who have been recently withdrawn from systemic corticosteroids should be instructed to resume systemic steroids (in large doses) immediately and to contact their physician for further instruction. These patients should also be instructed to carry a warning card indicating that they may need supplementary systemic steroids during periods of stress or a severe asthma attack.

Localized infections with *Candida albicans* have occurred infrequently in the mouth and pharynx. These areas should be examined by the treating physician at each patient visit. The percentage of positive mouth and throat cultures for *Candida albicans* did not change during a year of continuous therapy. The incidence of clinically apparent infection is low (2.5%). These infections may disappear spontaneously or may require treatment with appropriate antifungal therapy or discontinuance of treatment with **Azmacort** Oral Inhaler.
Children who are on immunosuppressant drugs are more susceptible to infections than healthy children. Chickenpox and measles, for example, can have a more serious or even fatal course in children on immunosuppressant doses of corticosteroids. In such children, or in adults who have not had these diseases, particular care should be taken to avoid exposure. If exposed, therapy with varicella zoster immune globulin (VZIG) or pooled intravenous immunoglobulin (IVIG), as appropriate, may be indicated. If chickenpox develops, treatment with antiviral agents may be considered.
Azmacort Oral Inhaler is not to be regarded as a bronchodilator and is not indicated for rapid relief of bronchospasm.
Patients should be instructed to contact their physician immediately when episodes of asthma which are not responsive to bronchodilators occur during the course of treatment with **Azmacort** Oral Inhaler. During such episodes, patients may require therapy with systemic corticosteroids.
There is no evidence that control of asthma can be achieved by the administration of **Azmacort** Oral Inhaler in amounts greater than the recommended doses, which appear to be the therapeutic equivalent of approximately 10 mg/day of oral prednisone.
The use of **Azmacort** Oral Inhaler with alternate-day systemic prednisone could increase the likelihood of HPA suppression compared to a therapeutic dose of either one alone. Therefore, **Azmacort** Oral Inhaler should be used with caution in patients already receiving alternate-day prednisone treatment for any disease.
Transfer of patients from systemic steroid therapy to **Azmacort** Oral Inhaler may unmask allergic conditions previously suppressed by the systemic steroid therapy, *e.g.,* rhinitis, conjunctivitis, and eczema.

PRECAUTIONS

During withdrawal from oral steroids, some patients may experience symptoms of systemically active steroid withdrawal, *e.g.,* joint and/or muscular pain, lassitude and depression, despite maintenance or even improvement of respiratory function (see DOSAGE AND ADMINISTRATION for details). Although steroid withdrawal effects are usually transient and not severe, severe and even fatal exacerbation of asthma can occur if the previous daily oral corticosteroid requirement had significantly exceeded 10 mg/day of prednisone or equivalent.
In responsive patients, inhaled corticosteroids will often permit control of asthmatic symptoms with less suppression of HPA function than therapeutically equivalent oral doses of prednisone. Since triamcinolone acetonide is absorbed into the circulation and can be systemically active, the beneficial effects of **Azmacort** Oral Inhaler in minimizing or preventing HPA dysfunction may be expected only when recommended dosages are not exceeded.
Suppression of HPA function has been reported in volunteers who received 4000 mcg daily of triamcinolone acetonide. In addition, suppression of HPA function has been

Continued on next page

Rhône-Poulenc Rorer—Cont.

reported in some patients who have received recommended doses for as little as 6 to 12 weeks. Since the response of HPA function to inhaled corticosteroids is highly individualized, the physician should consider this information when treating patients.

Because of the possibility of systemic absorption of inhaled corticosteroids, patients treated with these drugs should be observed carefully for any evidence of systemic corticosteroid effects including suppression of growth in children. Particular care should be taken in observing patients postoperatively or during periods of stress for evidence of a decrease in adrenal function.

The long-term effects of triamcinolone acetonide inhaler in human subjects are not completely known, although patients have received **Azmacort** Oral Inhaler on a continuous basis for periods of two years or longer. While there has been no clinical evidence of adverse experiences, the local effects of the agent on developmental or immunologic processes in the mouth, pharynx, trachea and lung are also unknown.

Azmacort Oral Inhaler should be used with caution, if at all, in patients with active or quiescent tuberculous infections of the respiratory tract or in patients with untreated fungal, bacterial, or systemic viral infections or ocular herpes simplex. The potential effects of long-term administration of **Azmacort** Oral Inhaler on lung or other tissues are unknown. However, pulmonary infiltrates with eosinophilia have occurred in patients receiving other inhaled corticosteroids.

When used at excessive doses, systemic corticosteroid effects such as hypercorticism and adrenal suppression may appear. If such changes occur, **Azmacort** Oral Inhaler should be discontinued slowly, consistent with accepted procedures for discontinuing oral steroid therapy.

Information for Patients: Patients who are on immunosuppressant doses of corticosteroids should be warned to avoid exposure to chickenpox or measles and, if exposed, to obtain medical advice.

Carcinogenesis, Mutagenesis: No evidence of treatment-related carcinogenicity was demonstrated after two years of once daily oral administration of triamcinolone acetonide at a maximum daily dose of 1.0 mcg/kg/day (6.1 mcg/m^2/day) in male or female rats and 3.0 mcg/kg/day (12.9 mcg/m^2/day) in male or female mice.

Impairment of Fertility: Male and female rats which were administered oral triamcinolone acetonide at doses as high as 15 mcg/kg/day (110 mcg/m^2/day, as calculated on a surface area basis) exhibited no evidence of impaired fertility. The maximum human dose, for comparison, is 22.9 mcg/kg/day (889 mcg/m^2/day). However, a few female rats which received maternally toxic doses of 8 or 15 mcg/kg/day (60 mcg/m^2/day or 110 mcg/m^2/day, respectively, as calculated on a surface area basis) exhibited dystocia and prolonged delivery. Developmental toxicity, which included increases in fetal resorptions and stillbirths and decreases in pup body weight and survival, also occurred at the maternally toxic doses (2.5–15.0 mcg/kg/day or 20–110 mcg/m^2/day, as calculated on a surface area basis). Reproductive performance of female rats and effects on fetuses and offspring were comparable between groups that received placebo and non-toxic or marginally toxic doses (0.5 and 1.0 mcg/kg/day or 3.8 mcg/m^2/day and 7.0 mcg/m^2/day).

Pregnancy: Pregnancy Category C. Like other corticoids, triamcinolone acetonide has been shown to be teratogenic in rats and rabbits. Teratogenic effects, which occurred in both species at 0.02, 0.04 and 0.08 mg/kg/day (approximately 135, 270 and 540 mcg/m^2/day in the rat and 320, 640 and 1280 mcg/m^2/day in the rabbit, as calculated on a surface area basis), included a low incidence of cleft palate and/or internal hydrocephaly and axial skeletal defects. Teratogenic effects, including CNS and cranial malformations, have also been observed in non-human primates at 0.5 mg/kg/day (approximately 6.7 mg/m^2/day). Administration of aerosol by inhalation to pregnant rats and rabbits produced embryotoxic and fetotoxic effects which were comparable to those produced by administration by other routes. There are no adequate and well-controlled studies in pregnant women. Triamcinolone acetonide should be used during pregnancy only if the potential benefit justifies the potential risk to the fetus.

Experience with oral corticoids since their introduction in pharmacologic as opposed to physiologic doses suggests that rodents are more prone to teratogenic effects from corticoids than humans. In addition, because there is a natural increase in glucocorticoid production during pregnancy, most women will require a lower exogenous steroid dose and many will not need corticoid treatment during pregnancy.

Nonteratogenic Effects: Hypoadrenalism may occur in infants born of mothers receiving corticosteroids during pregnancy. Such infants should be carefully observed.

Nursing Mothers: It is not known whether triamcinolone acetonide is excreted in human milk. Because other corticosteroids are excreted in human milk, caution should be exercised when **Azmacort** Oral Inhaler is administered to nursing women.

Pediatric Use: Safety and effectiveness have not been established in children below the age of 6. Oral corticoids have been shown to cause growth suppression in children and teenagers, particularly with higher doses over extended periods. If a child or teenager on any corticoid appears to have growth suppression, the possibility that they are particularly sensitive to this effect of steroids should be considered.

ADVERSE REACTIONS

A few cases of oral candidiasis have been reported (see WARNINGS). In addition, some patients receiving **Azmacort** Oral Inhaler have experienced hoarseness, dry throat, irritated throat and dry mouth. Increased wheezing and cough have been reported infrequently as has facial edema. These adverse effects have generally been mild and transient.

DOSAGE AND ADMINISTRATION

All patients should be instructed that the **Azmacort** Oral Inhaler must be used on a regular daily basis rather than *prn*. Reliable dosage delivery cannot be assured after 240 actuations and patients should be cautioned against longer use of individual canisters.

Good oral hygiene including rinsing of the mouth after inhalation is recommended.

Adults: The usual dosage is two inhalations (approximately 200 mcg) given three to four times a day. The maximal daily intake should not exceed 16 inhalations (1600 mcg) in adults. Higher initial doses (12 to 16 inhalations per day) may be advisable in patients with more severe asthma, the dosage then being adjusted downward according to the response of the patient. In some patients maintenance can be accomplished when the total daily dose is given on a twice a day schedule.

Children 6 to 12 years of age: The usual dosage is one or two inhalations (100 to 200 mcg) given three to four times a day according to the response of the patient. The maximal daily intake should not exceed 12 inhalations (1200 mcg) in children 6 to 12 years of age. Insufficient clinical data exist with respect to the administration of **Azmacort** Oral Inhaler in children below the age of 6. The long-term effects of inhaled steroids on growth are still under evaluation.

Patients receiving bronchodilators by inhalation should be advised to use the bronchodilator before **Azmacort** Oral Inhaler in order to enhance penetration of triamcinolone acetonide into the bronchial tree. After use of an aerosol bronchodilator, several minutes should elapse before use of the **Azmacort** Oral Inhaler to reduce the potential toxicity from the inhaled fluorocarbon propellants in the two aerosols.

Different considerations must be given to the following groups of patients in order to obtain the full therapeutic benefit of **Azmacort** Oral Inhaler:

Patients not receiving systemic steroids: The use of **Azmacort** Oral Inhaler is straightforward in patients who are inadequately controlled with non-steroid medications but in whom systemic steroid therapy has been withheld because of concern over potential adverse reactions. In patients who respond to **Azmacort**, an improvement in pulmonary function is usually apparent within one to two weeks after the start of **Azmacort** Oral Inhaler.

Patients receiving systemic steroids: In those patients dependent on systemic steroids, transfer to **Azmacort** Oral Inhaler and subsequent management may be more difficult because recovery from impaired adrenal function is usually slow. Such suppression has been known to last for up to 12 months or longer. Clinical studies, however, have demonstrated that **Azmacort** Oral Inhaler may be effective in the management of these asthmatic patients and may permit replacement or significant reduction in the dosage of systemic corticosteroids.

The patient's asthma should be reasonably stable before treatment with **Azmacort** Oral Inhaler is started. Initially, the inhaler should be used concurrently with the patient's usual maintenance dose of systemic steroid. After approximately one week, gradual withdrawal of the systemic steroid is started by reducing the dose. The next reduction is made after an interval of one or two weeks, depending on the response of the patient. Generally, these decrements should not exceed 2.5 mg of prednisone or its equivalent. A slow rate of withdrawal cannot be overemphasized. During withdrawal, some patients may experience symptoms of systemically active steroid withdrawal, *e.g.*, joint and/or muscular pain, lassitude and depression, despite maintenance or even improvement of respiratory function. Such patients should be encouraged to continue with the inhaler but should be watched carefully for objective signs of adrenal insufficiency, such as hypotension and weight loss. If evidence of adrenal insufficiency occurs, the systemic steroid dose should be boosted temporarily and thereafter further withdrawal should continue more slowly. No clinical studies have been conducted evaluating **Azmacort** with alternate day prednisone regimens. However, based on the results of such a study with another inhaled corticosteroid, inhaled corticosteroids generally are not recommended for chronic use with alternate day prednisone regimens (see WARNINGS).

During periods of stress or a severe asthma attack, transfer patients will require supplementary treatment with systemic steroids. Exacerbations of asthma which occur during the course of treatment with **Azmacort** Oral Inhaler should be treated with a short course of systemic steroid which is gradually tapered as these symptoms subside. There is no evidence that control of asthma can be achieved by administration of **Azmacort** Oral Inhaler in amounts greater than the recommended doses.

Directions for Use: An illustrated leaflet of patient instructions for proper use accompanies each package of **Azmacort** Oral Inhaler.

HOW SUPPLIED

Azmacort Oral Inhaler contains 60 mg triamcinolone acetonide in a 20 gram package which delivers at least 240 actuations. It is supplied with an oral adapter and patient's leaflet of instructions: box of one. NDC 0075-0060-37

CONTENTS UNDER PRESSURE: Do not puncture. Do not use or store near heat or open flame. Exposure to temperatures above 120°F may cause bursting. Never throw container into fire or incinerator. Keep out of reach of children.

STORE AT ROOM TEMPERATURE.

Note: The indented statement below is required by the Federal government's Clean Air Act for all products containing or manufactured with chlorofluorocarbons (CFCs):

> WARNING: Contains CFC-12, a substance which harms public health and environment by destroying ozone in the upper atmosphere.

A notice similar to the above WARNING has been placed in the "Information For The Patient" portion of this package insert pursuant to EPA regulations.

CAUTION

Federal (U.S.A.) law prohibits dispensing without prescription.

Military and Veterans Administration: 20 gram inhaler (NSN 6505-01-206-9233).

Rev. 11/95 IN-6337

Marketed by

RHÔNE-POULENC RORER PHARMACEUTICALS INC.

Collegeville, PA, U.S.A. 19426-0107

Shown in Product Identification Guide, page 330

CALCIMAR® ℞

[kal 'sĭ-mar]

(calcitonin-salmon)

INJECTION, SYNTHETIC

PRODUCT OVERVIEW

KEY FACTS

CALCIMAR® Injection, Synthetic is a synthetic polypeptide of 32 amino acids in the same linear sequence found in calcitonin of salmon origin. It is provided as a sterile solution in 2 mL vials containing 400 I.U. (200 I.U. per mL) for subcutaneous or intramuscular injection.

MAJOR USES

CALCIMAR® Injection, Synthetic is indicated for the relief of bone pain and other symptoms of Paget's disease, for the treatment of hypercalcemia, and for the treatment of postmenopausal osteoporosis (PMO) to prevent the progressive loss of bone mass. Adequate calcium and Vitamin D intake in conjunction with CALCIMAR is essential to prevent the progressive loss of bone mass in PMO.

SAFETY INFORMATION

Skin testing should be considered prior to treatment with calcitonin because of its protein nature. Careful instruction in sterile injection technique should be given to the patient and to other persons who may administer CALCIMAR.

PRESCRIBING INFORMATION

CALCIMAR® ℞

[kal 'sĭ-mar]

(calcitonin-salmon)

INJECTION, SYNTHETIC

DESCRIPTION

Calcitonin is a polypeptide hormone secreted by the parafollicular cells of the thyroid gland in mammals and by the ultimobranchial gland of birds and fish.

CALCIMAR® (calcitonin-salmon) Injection, Synthetic is a synthetic polypeptide of 32 amino acids in the same linear sequence that is found in calcitonin of salmon origin. This is shown by the following graphic formula:

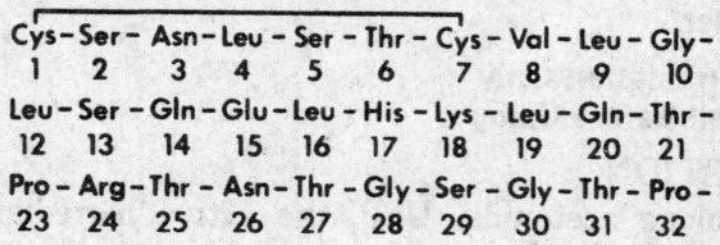
Cys-Ser-Asn-Leu-Ser-Thr-Cys-Val-Leu-Gly-Lys-
1 2 3 4 5 6 7 8 9 10 11
Leu-Ser-Gln-Glu-Leu-His-Lys-Leu-Gln-Thr-Tyr-
12 13 14 15 16 17 18 19 20 21 22
Pro-Arg-Thr-Asn-Thr-Gly-Ser-Gly-Thr-Pro-NH2
23 24 25 26 27 28 29 30 31 32

It is provided in sterile solution for subcutaneous or intramuscular injection. Each milliliter contains 200 I.U. (MRC) of calcitonin-salmon, 5 mg phenol (as preservative), with sodium chloride, sodium acetate, acetic acid, and sodium hydroxide to adjust tonicity and pH.

The activity of CALCIMAR is stated in International Units (equal to MRC or Medical Research Council units) based on bio-assay in comparison with the International Reference Preparation of Calcitonin, Salmon for Bioassay, distributed by the National Institute for Biological Standards and Control, Holly Hill, London.

CLINICAL PHARMACOLOGY

Calcitonin acts primarily on bone, but direct renal effects and actions on the gastrointestinal tract are also recognized. Calcitonin-salmon appears to have actions essentially identical to calcitonins of mammalian origin, but its potency per mg is greater and it has a longer duration of action. The actions of calcitonin on bone and its role in normal human bone physiology are still incompletely understood.

Bone —Single injections of calcitonin cause a marked transient inhibition of the ongoing bone resorptive process. With prolonged use, there is a persistent, smaller decrease in the rate of bone resorption. Histologically this is associated with a decreased number of osteoclasts and an apparent decrease in their resorptive activity. Decreased osteocytic resorption may also be involved. There is some evidence that initially bone formation may be augmented by calcitonin through increased osteoblastic activity. However, calcitonin will probably not induce a long-term increase in bone formation. Animal studies indicate that endogenous calcitonin, primarily through its action on bone, participates with parathyroid hormone in the homeostatic regulation of blood calcium. Thus, high blood calcium levels cause increased secretion of calcitonin which, in turn, inhibits bone resorption. This reduces the transfer of calcium from bone to blood and tends to return blood calcium to the normal level. The importance of this process in humans has not been determined. In normal adults, who have a relatively low rate of bone resorption, the administration of exogenous calcitonin results in only a slight decrease in serum calcium. In normal children and in patients with generalized Paget's disease, bone resorption is more rapid and decreases in serum calcium are more pronounced in response to calcitonin.

Paget's Disease of Bone (osteitis deformans)— Paget's disease is a disorder of uncertain etiology characterized by abnormal and accelerated bone formation and resorption in one or more bones. In most patients only small areas of bone are involved and the disease is not symptomatic. In a small fraction of patients, however, the abnormal bone may lead to bone pain and bone deformity, cranial and spinal nerve entrapment, or spinal cord compression. The increased vascularity of the abnormal bone may lead to high output congestive heart failure.

Active Paget's disease involving a large mass of bone may increase the urinary hydroxyproline excretion (reflecting breakdown of collagen-containing bone matrix) and serum alkaline phosphatase (reflecting increased bone formation). Calcitonin-salmon, presumably by an initial blocking effect on bone resorption, causes a decreased rate of bone turnover with a resultant fall in the serum alkaline phosphatase and urinary hydroxyproline excretion in approximately $^2/_3$ of patients treated. These biochemical changes appear to correspond to changes toward more normal bone, as evidenced by a small number of documented examples of: 1) radiologic regression of Pagetic lesions, 2) improvement of impaired auditory nerve and other neurologic function, 3) decreases (measured) in abnormally elevated cardiac output. These improvements occur extremely rarely, if ever, spontaneously (elevated cardiac output may disappear over a period of years when the disease slowly enters a sclerotic phase; in the cases treated with calcitonin, however, the decreases were seen in less than one year).

Some patients with Paget's disease who have good biochemical and/or symptomatic responses initially, later relapse. Suggested explanations have included the formation of neutralizing antibodies and the development of secondary hyperparathyroidism, but neither suggestion appears to explain adequately the majority of relapses.

Although the parathyroid hormone levels do appear to rise transiently during each hypocalcemic response to calcitonin, most investigators have been unable to demonstrate persistent hypersecretion of parathyroid hormone in patients treated chronically with calcitonin.

Circulating antibodies to calcitonin after 2–18 months' treatment have been reported in about half of the patients with Paget's disease in whom antibody studies were done, but calcitonin treatment remained effective in many of these cases. Occasionally patients with high antibody titers are found. These patients usually will have suffered a biochemical relapse of Paget's disease and are unresponsive to the acute hypocalcemic effects of calcitonin.

Hypercalcemia —In clinical trials, CALCIMAR has been shown to lower the elevated serum calcium of patients with carcinoma (with or without demonstrated metastases), multiple myeloma or primary hyperparathyroidism (lesser response). Patients with higher values for serum calcium tend to show greater reduction during CALCIMAR therapy. The decrease in calcium occurs about 2 hours after the first injection and lasts for about 6-8 hours. CALCIMAR given every 12 hours maintained a calcium lowering effect for about 5-8 days, the time period evaluated for most patients during the clinical studies. The average reduction of 8-hour post-injection serum calcium during this period was about 9 percent.

Kidney —Calcitonin increases the excretion of filtered phosphate, calcium, and sodium by decreasing their tubular reabsorption. In some patients the inhibition of bone resorption by calcitonin is of such magnitude that the consequent reduction of filtered calcium load more than compensates for the decrease in tubular reabsorption of calcium. The result in these patients is a decrease rather than an increase in urinary calcium.

Transient increases in sodium and water excretion may occur after the initial injection of calcitonin. In most patients these changes return to pre-treatment levels with continued therapy.

Gastrointestinal tract —Increasing evidence indicates that calcitonin has significant actions on the gastrointestinal tract. Short-term administration results in marked transient decreases in the volume and acidity of gastric juice and in the volume and the trypsin and amylase content of pancreatic juice. Whether these effects continue to be elicited after each injection of calcitonin during chronic therapy has not been investigated.

Metabolism —The metabolism of calcitonin-salmon has not yet been studied clinically. Information from animal studies with calcitonin-salmon and from clinical studies with calcitonins of porcine and human origin suggest that calcitonin-salmon is rapidly metabolized by conversion to smaller inactive fragments, primarily in the kidneys, but also in the blood and peripheral tissues. A small amount of unchanged hormone and its inactive metabolites are excreted in the urine.

It appears that calcitonin-salmon cannot cross the placental barrier and its passage to the cerebrospinal fluid or to breast milk has not been determined.

INDICATIONS AND USAGE

CALCIMAR is indicated for the treatment of symptomatic Paget's disease of bone, the treatment of hypercalcemia, and the treatment of postmenopausal osteoporosis.

Paget 's Disease —At the present time effectiveness has been demonstrated principally in patients with moderate to severe disease characterized by polyostotic involvement with elevated serum alkaline phosphatase and urinary hydroxyproline excretion.

In these patients, the biochemical abnormalities were substantially improved (more than 30% reduction) in about $^2/_3$ of patients studied, and bone pain was improved in a similar fraction. A small number of documented instances of reversal of neurologic deficits has occurred, including improvement in the basilar compression syndrome, and improvement of spinal cord and spinal nerve lesions. At present there is too little experience to predict the likelihood of improvement of any given neurologic lesion. Hearing loss, the most common neurologic lesion of Paget's disease, is improved infrequently (4 of 29 patients studied audiometrically).

Patients with increased cardiac output due to extensive Paget's disease have had measured decreases in cardiac output while receiving calcitonin. The number of treated patients in this category is still too small to predict how likely such a result will be.

The large majority of patients with localized, especially monostotic disease do not develop symptoms and most patients with mild symptoms can be managed with analgesics. There is no evidence that the prophylactic use of calcitonin is beneficial in asymptomatic patients, although treatment may be considered in exceptional circumstances in which there is extensive involvement of the skull or spinal cord with the possibility of irreversible neurologic damage. In these instances treatment would be based on the demonstrated effect of calcitonin on Pagetic bone, rather than on clinical studies in the patient population in question.

Hypercalcemia —CALCIMAR is indicated for early treatment of hypercalcemic emergencies, along with other appropriate agents, when a rapid decrease in serum calcium is required, until more specific treatment of the underlying disease can be accomplished. It may also be added to existing therapeutic regimens for hypercalcemia such as intravenous fluids and furosemide, oral phosphate or corticosteroids, or other agents.

Postmenopausal Osteoporosis —CALCIMAR is indicated for the treatment of postmenopausal osteoporosis in conjunction with adequate calcium and vitamin D intake to prevent the progressive loss of bone mass. No evidence currently exists to indicate whether or not CALCIMAR decreases the risk of vertebral crush fractures or spinal deformity. A recent controlled study, which was discontinued prior to completion because of questions regarding its design and implementation, failed to demonstrate any benefit of CALCIMAR on fracture rate. No adequate controlled trials have examined the effect of calcitonin-salmon injection on vertebral bone mineral density beyond one year of treatment. Two controlled studies with CALCIMAR have shown an increase in total body calcium at one year, followed by a trend to decreasing total body calcium (still above baseline) at two years. It has been suggested that those postmenopausal patients having increased rates of bone turnover may be more likely to respond to antiresorptive agents such as CALCIMAR.

CONTRAINDICATIONS

Clinical allergy to synthetic calcitonin-salmon.

WARNINGS

Allergic Reactions

Because calcitonin is protein in nature, the possibility of a systemic allergic reaction exists. Administration of calcitonin-salmon has been reported in a few cases to cause serious allergic-type reactions (*e.g.* bronchospasms, swelling of the tongue or throat, and anaphylactic shock), and in one case, death due to anaphylaxis. The usual provisions should be made for the emergency treatment of such a reaction should it occur. Allergic reactions should be differentiated from generalized flushing and hypotension.

Skin testing should be considered prior to treatment with calcitonin, particularly for patients with suspected sensitivity to calcitonin. The following procedure is suggested: Prepare a dilution at 10 I.U. per mL by withdrawing $^1/_{20}$ mL (0.05 mL) in a tuberculin syringe and filling it to 1.0 mL with Sodium Chloride Injection, USP. Mix well, discard 0.9 mL and inject intracutaneously 0.1 mL (approximately 1 I.U.) on the inner aspect of the forearm. Observe the injection site 15 minutes after injection. The appearance of more than mild erythema or wheal constitutes a positive response.

General

The incidence of osteogenic sarcoma is known to be increased in Paget's disease. Pagetic lesions, with or without therapy, may appear by X-ray to progress markedly, possibly with some loss of definition of periosteal margins. Such lesions should be evaluated carefully to differentiate these from osteogenic sarcoma.

PRECAUTIONS

1. General

The administration of calcitonin possibly could lead to hypocalcemic tetany. Provisions for parenteral calcium administration should be available during the first several administrations of calcitonin.

2. Laboratory Tests

Periodic examinations of urine sediment of patients on chronic therapy are recommended.

Coarse granular casts and casts containing renal tubular epithelial cells were reported in young adult volunteers at bed rest who were given calcitonin-salmon to study the effect on immobilization osteoporosis. There was no other evidence of renal abnormality and the urine sediment became normal after calcitonin was stopped. Urine sediment abnormalities have not been reported by other investigators.

3. Instructions for the patient

Careful instruction in sterile injection technique should be given to the patient, and to other persons who may administer CALCIMAR.

4. Carcinogenesis, Mutagenesis, and Impairment of Fertility

An increased incidence of pituitary adenomas has been observed in one-year toxicity studies in Sprague-Dawley rats administered calcitonin-salmon at dosages of 20 and 80 I.U./kg/day and in Fisher 344 rats given 80 I.U./kg/day. The relevance of these findings to humans is unknown. Calcitonin-salmon was not mutagenic in tests using *Salmonella typhimurium*, *Escherichia coli*, and Chinese Hamster V79 cells.

5. Pregnancy: Teratogenic effects. Category C.

Calcitonin-salmon has been shown to cause a decrease in fetal birth weights in rabbits when given in doses 14–56 times the dose recommended for human use. Since calcitonin does not cross the placental barrier, this finding may be due to metabolic effect of calcitonin on the pregnant animal. There are no adequate and well-controlled studies in pregnant women. CALCIMAR should be used during pregnancy only if the potential benefit justifies the potential risk to the fetus.

6. Nursing Mothers

It is not known whether this drug is excreted in human milk. As a general rule, nursing should not be undertaken while a patient is on this drug since many drugs are excreted in human milk. Calcitonin has been shown to inhibit lactation in animals.

7. Pediatric Use

Disorders of bone in children referred to as juvenile Paget's disease have been reported rarely. The relationship of these disorders to adult Paget's disease has not been established and experience with the use of calcitonin in these disorders is very limited. There are no adequate data to support the use of CALCIMAR in children.

Continued on next page

Rhône-Poulenc Rorer—Cont.

ADVERSE REACTIONS

Gastrointestinal System—Nausea with or without vomiting has been noted in about 10% of patients treated with calcitonin. It is most evident when treatment is first initiated and tends to decrease or disappear with continued administration.

Dermatologic/Hypersensitivity—Local inflammatory reactions at the site of subcutaneous or intramuscular injection have been reported in about 10% of patients. Flushing of face or hands occurred in about 2% to 5% of patients. Skin rashes have been reported occasionally. Administration of calcitonin-salmon has been reported in a few cases to cause serious allergic-type reactions (*e.g.* bronchospasms, swelling of the tongue or throat, and anaphylactic shock), and in one case, death due to anaphylaxis. (SEE WARNINGS.)

OVERDOSAGE

A dose of 1000 I.U. subcutaneously may produce nausea and vomiting as the only adverse effects. Doses of 32 units per kg per day for one or two days demonstrate no other adverse effects.

Data on chronic high dose administration are insufficient to judge toxicity.

DOSAGE AND ADMINISTRATION

Paget's Disease— The recommended starting dose of calcitonin in Paget's disease is 100 I.U. (0.5 mL) per day administered subcutaneously (preferred for outpatient self-administration) or intramuscularly. Drug effect should be monitored by periodic measurement of serum alkaline phosphatase and 24-hour urinary hydroxyproline (if available) and evaluation of symptoms. A decrease toward normal of the biochemical abnormalities is usually seen, if it is going to occur, within the first few months. Bone pain may also decrease during that time. Improvement of neurologic lesions, when it occurs, requires a longer period of treatment, often more than one year.

In many patients doses of 50 I.U. (0.25 mL) per day or every other day are sufficient to maintain biochemical and clinical improvement. At the present time, however, there are insufficient data to determine whether this reduced dose will have the same effect as the higher dose on forming more normal bone structure. It appears preferable, therefore, to maintain the higher dose in any patient with serious deformity or neurological involvement.

In any patient with a good response initially who later relapses, either clinically or biochemically, the possibility of antibody formation should be explored. The patient may be tested for antibodies by an appropriate specialized test or evaluated for the possibility of antibody formation by critical clinical evaluation.

Patient compliance should also be assessed in the event of relapse.

In patients who relapse, whether because of antibodies or for unexplained reasons, a dosage increase beyond 100 I.U. per day does not usually appear to elicit an improved response.

Hypercalcemia—The recommended starting dose of CALCIMAR in hypercalcemia is 4 I.U./kg body weight every 12 hours by subcutaneous or intramuscular injection. If the response to this dose is not satisfactory after one or two days, the dose may be increased to 8 I.U./kg every 12 hours. If the response remains unsatisfactory after two more days, the dose may be further increased to a maximum of 8 I.U./kg every 6 hours.

Postmenopausal Osteoporosis—The recommended dose of calcitonin is 100 I.U. per day administered subcutaneously or intramuscularly. Patients should also receive supplemental calcium such as calcium carbonate 1.5 g daily and an adequate vitamin D intake (400 units daily). An adequate diet is also essential.

The minimum effective dose of CALCIMAR for the prevention of vertebral bone mineral density loss has not been established. Data from a single one-year placebo-controlled study with calcitonin-salmon injection suggested that 100 I.U. every other day might be effective in preserving vertebral bone mineral density. Baseline and interval monitoring of biochemical markers of bone resorption/turnover (*e.g.*, fasting A.M., urine hydroxyproline to creatinine ratio) and of bone mineral density may be useful in achieving the minimum effective dose.

If the volume of CALCIMAR to be injected exceeds 2 mL, intramuscular injection is preferable and multiple sites of injection should be used.

Parenteral drug products should be inspected visually for particulate matter and discoloration prior to administration whenever solution and container permit.

HOW SUPPLIED

CALCIMAR is available as a sterile solution in 2 mL vials containing 200 I.U. per mL (NDC 0075-1306-01).

Store in refrigerator, 2°–8°C (36°–46°F).

Military: NSN 6505-01-079-2635.

CAUTION: FEDERAL (U.S.A.) LAW PROHIBITS DISPENSING WITHOUT PRESCRIPTION. 20109

Rev. 10/92 IN-4001H

RHÔNE-POULENC RORER PHARMACEUTICALS INC.
Collegeville, PA, U.S.A. 19426-0107

DDAVP® Injection ℞
(desmopressin acetate)

DESCRIPTION

DDAVP® Injection (desmopressin acetate) is a synthetic analogue of the natural pituitary hormone 8-arginine vasopressin (ADH), an antidiuretic hormone affecting renal water conservation. It is chemically defined as follows:

Mol. Wt. 1183.32

Empirical Formula: $C_{46}H_{64}N_{14}O_{12}S_2 \cdot C_2H_4O_2 \cdot 3H_2O$

$$\overset{\text{O}}{\overset{\|}{\text{SCH}_2\text{CH}_2\text{C}}}\text{-Tyr-Phe-Gln-Asn-Cys-Pro-D-Arg-Gly-NH}_2\cdot$$

1 2 3 4 5 6 7 8 9

$$CH_3COOH \cdot 3H_2O$$

1-(3-mercaptopropionic acid)-8-D-arginine vasopressin monoacetate (salt) trihydrate

DDAVP Injection is provided as a sterile, aqueous solution for injection.

Each mL provides:	Desmopressin acetate	4.0 mcg
	Sodium chloride	9.0 mg
	Hydrochloric acid to adjust pH to 4	

The 10 mL vial contains chlorobutanol as a preservative (5.0 mg/mL).

CLINICAL PHARMACOLOGY

DDAVP Injection contains as active substance, 1-(3-mercaptopropionic acid)-8-D-arginine vasopressin, a synthetic analogue of the natural hormone arginine vasopressin. One mL (4 mcg) of DDAVP (desmopressin acetate) solution has an antidiuretic activity of about 16 IU; 1 mcg of DDAVP is equivalent to 4 IU.

DDAVP has been shown to be more potent than arginine vasopressin in increasing plasma levels of factor VIII activity in patients with hemophilia and von Willebrand's disease Type I.

Dose-response studies were performed in healthy persons, using doses of 0.1 to 0.4 mcg/kg body weight, infused over a 10-minute period. Maximal dose response occurred at 0.3 to 0.4 mcg/kg. The response to DDAVP of factor VIII activity and plasminogen activator is dose-related, with maximal plasma levels of 300 to 400 percent of initial concentrations obtained after infusion of 0.4 mcg/kg body weight. The increase is rapid and evident within 30 minutes, reaching a maximum at a point ranging from 90 minutes to two hours. The factor VIII related antigen and ristocetin cofactor activity were also increased to a smaller degree, but still are dose-dependent.

1. The biphasic half-lives of DDAVP were 7.8 and 75.5 minutes for the fast and slow phases, respectively, compared with 2.5 and 14.5 minutes for lysine vasopressin, another form of the hormone. As a result, DDAVP (desmopressin acetate) provides a prompt onset of antidiuretic action with a long duration after each administration.
2. The change in structure of arginine vasopressin to DDAVP has resulted in a decreased vasopressor action and decreased actions on visceral smooth muscle relative to the enhanced antidiuretic activity, so that clinically effective antidiuretic doses are usually below threshold levels for effects on vascular or visceral smooth muscle.
3. When administered by injection, DDAVP has an antidiuretic effect about ten times that of an equivalent dose administered intranasally.
4. The bioavailability of the subcutaneous route of administration was determined qualitatively using urine output data. The exact fraction of drug absorbed by that route of administration has not been quantitatively determined.
5. The percentage increase of factor VIII levels in patients with mild hemophilia A and von Willebrand's disease was not significantly different from that observed in normal healthy individuals when treated with 0.3 mcg/kg of DDAVP infused over 10 minutes.
6. Plasminogen activator activity increases rapidly after DDAVP infusion, but there has been no clinically significant fibrinolysis in patients treated with DDAVP.
7. The effect of repeated DDAVP administration when doses were given every 12 to 24 hours has generally shown a gradual diminution of the factor VIII activity increase noted with a single dose. The initial response is reproducible in any particular patient if there are 2 or 3 days between administrations.

INDICATIONS AND USAGE

Hemophilia A

DDAVP Injection is indicated for patients with hemophilia A with factor VIII coagulant activity levels greater than 5%.

DDAVP will often maintain hemostasis in patients with hemophilia A during surgical procedures and postoperatively when administered 30 minutes prior to scheduled procedure.

DDAVP will also stop bleeding in hemophilia A patients with episodes of spontaneous or trauma-induced injuries such as hemarthroses, intramuscular hematomas or mucosal bleeding.

DDAVP is not indicated for the treatment of hemophilia A with factor VIII coagulant activity levels equal to or less than 5%, or for the treatment of hemophilia B, or in patients who have factor VIII antibodies.

In certain clinical situations, it may be justified to try DDAVP in patients with factor VIII levels between 2%–5%; however, these patients should be carefully monitored.

von Willebrand's Disease (Type I)

DDAVP Injection is indicated for patients with mild to moderate classic von Willebrand's disease (Type I) with factor VIII levels greater than 5%. DDAVP will often maintain hemostasis in patients with mild to moderate von Willebrand's disease during surgical procedures and postoperatively when administered 30 minutes prior to the scheduled procedure.

DDAVP will usually stop bleeding in mild to moderate von Willebrand's patients with episodes of spontaneous or trauma-induced injuries such as hemarthroses, intramuscular hematomas or mucosal bleeding.

Those von Willebrand's disease patients who are least likely to respond are those with severe homozygous von Willebrand's disease with factor VIII coagulant activity and factor VIII von Willebrand factor antigen levels less than 1%. Other patients may respond in a variable fashion depending on the type of molecular defect they have. Bleeding time and factor VIII coagulant activity, ristocetin cofactor activity, and von Willebrand factor antigen should be checked during administration of DDAVP to ensure that adequate levels are being achieved.

DDAVP is not indicated for the treatment of severe classic von Willebrand's disease (Type I) and when there is evidence of an abnormal molecular form of factor VIII antigen. See WARNING.

Diabetes Insipidus

DDAVP Injection is indicated as antidiuretic replacement therapy in the management of central (cranial) diabetes insipidus and for the management of the temporary polyuria and polydipsia following head trauma or surgery in the pituitary region. DDAVP is ineffective for the treatment of nephrogenic diabetes insipidus.

DDAVP is also available as an intranasal preparation. However, this means of delivery can be compromised by a variety of factors that can make nasal insufflation ineffective or inappropriate. These include poor intranasal absorption, nasal congestion and blockage, nasal discharge, atrophy of nasal mucosa, and severe atrophic rhinitis. Intranasal delivery may be inappropriate where there is an impaired level of consciousness. In addition, cranial surgical procedures, such as transsphenoidal hypophysectomy, create situations where an alternative route of administration is needed as in cases of nasal packing or recovery from surgery.

CONTRAINDICATION

DDAVP Injection is contraindicated in individuals with known hypersensitivity to desmopressin acetate or any of the components of **DDAVP Injection.**

WARNINGS

Patients who do not have need of antidiuretic hormone for its antidiuretic effect, in particular those who are young or elderly, should be cautioned to ingest only enough fluid to satisfy thirst, in order to decrease the potential occurrence of water intoxication and hyponatremia.

Fluid intake should be adjusted downward, particularly in very young and elderly patients, in order to decrease the potential occurrence of water intoxication and hyponatremia.

Particular attention should be paid to the possibility of the rare occurrence of an extreme decrease in plasma osmolality that may result in seizures which could lead to coma.

DDAVP should not be used to treat patients with Type IIB von Willebrand's disease since platelet aggregation may be induced.

PRECAUTIONS

GENERAL: For injection use only.

DDAVP Injection (desmopressin acetate) has infrequently produced changes in blood pressure causing either a slight elevation in blood pressure or a transient fall in blood pressure and a compensatory increase in heart rate. The drug should be used with caution in patients with coronary artery insufficiency and/or hypertensive cardiovascular disease.

DDAVP Injection should be used with caution in patients with conditions associated with fluid and electrolyte imbal-

ance, such as cystic fibrosis, because these patients are prone to hyponatremia.
There have been rare reports of thrombotic events following **DDAVP Injection** in patients predisposed to thrombus formation. No causality has been determined, however, the drug should be used with caution in these patients.
Severe allergic reactions have been reported rarely. Fatal anaphylaxis has been reported in one patient who received intravenous DDAVP (desmopressin acetate). It is not known whether antibodies to **DDAVP Injection** (desmopressin acetate) are produced after repeated injections.

Hemophilia A
Laboratory tests for assessing patient status include levels of factor VIII coagulant, factor VIII antigen and factor VIII ristocetin cofactor (von Willebrand factor) as well as activated partial thromboplastin time. Factor VIII coagulant activity should be determined before giving DDAVP for hemostasis. If factor VIII coagulant activity is present at less than 5% of normal, DDAVP should not be relied on.

von Willebrand's Disease
Laboratory tests for assessing patient status include levels of factor VIII coagulant activity, factor VIII ristocetin cofactor activity, and factor VIII von Willebrand factor antigen. The skin bleeding time may be helpful in following these patients.

Diabetes Insipidus
Laboratory tests for monitoring the patient include urine volume and osmolality. In some cases, plasma osmolality may be required.

DRUG INTERACTIONS: Although the pressor activity of DDAVP is very low compared with the antidiuretic activity, use of doses as large as 0.3 mcg/kg of DDAVP with other pressor agents should be done only with careful patient monitoring.
DDAVP has been used with epsilon aminocaproic acid without adverse effects.

CARCINOGENICITY, MUTAGENICITY, IMPAIRMENT OF FERTILITY: There have been no long-term studies in animals to assess the carcinogenic, mutagenic, or impairment of fertility potential of DDAVP (desmopressin acetate).

PREGNANCY CATEGORY B: Reproduction studies performed in rats and rabbits by the subcutaneous route at doses up to 10μg/kg/day have revealed no evidence of harm to the fetus due to desmopressin acetate. This dose is equivalent to 10 times (for Factor VIII stimulation) or 38 times (for diabetes insipidus) the systemic human dose based on mg/M^2 surface area.
There are no adequate and well-controlled studies in pregnant women. Several publications of desmopressin acetate's use in the management of diabetes insipidus during pregnancy are available; these include a few anecdotal reports of congenital anomalies and low birth weight babies. However, no causal connection between these events and desmopressin acetate has been established. A 15-year, Swedish epidemiologic study of the use of desmopressin acetate in pregnant women with diabetes insipidus found the rate of birth defects to be no greater than that in the general population. As opposed to preparations containing natural hormones, desmopressin acetate in antidiuretic doses has no uterotonic action and the physician will have to weigh the therapeutic advantages against the possible risks in each case.

NURSING MOTHERS: There have been no controlled studies in nursing mothers. A single study in postpartum women demonstrated a marked change in plasma, but little if any change in assayable DDAVP in breast milk following an intranasal dose of 10 mcg. It is not known whether this drug is excreted in human milk. Because many drugs are excreted in human milk, caution should be exercised when DDAVP is administered to a nursing woman.

PEDIATRIC USE: Use in infants and children will require careful fluid intake restriction to prevent possible hyponatremia and water intoxication. ***DDAVP Injection** should not be used in infants younger than three months* in the treatment of hemophilia A or von Willebrand's disease; safety and effectiveness in children under 12 years of age with diabetes insipidus have not been established.

ADVERSE REACTIONS

Infrequently, DDAVP has produced transient headache, nausea, mild abdominal cramps and vulval pain. These symptoms disappeared with reduction in dosage. Occasionally, injection of DDAVP has produced local erythema, swelling or burning pain. Occasional facial flushing has been reported with the administration of DDAVP. **DDAVP Injection** has infrequently produced changes in blood pressure causing either a slight elevation or a transient fall and a compensatory increase in heart rate. Severe allergic reactions including anaphylaxis have been reported rarely with **DDAVP Injection** (desmopressin acetate).
See WARNING for the possibility of water intoxication and hyponatremia.
There have been rare reports of thrombotic events (acute cerebrovascular thrombosis, acute myocardial infarction) following **DDAVP Injection** in patients predisposed to thrombus formation.

OVERDOSAGE

See ADVERSE REACTIONS above. In case of overdosage, the dosage should be reduced, frequency of administration decreased, or the drug withdrawn according to the severity of the condition.
There is no known specific antidote for desmopressin acetate or **DDAVP Injection.**
An oral LD_{50} has not been established. An intravenous dose of 2 mg/kg in mice demonstrated no effect.

DOSAGE AND ADMINISTRATION

Hemophilia A and von Willebrand's Disease (Type I)
DDAVP Injection is administered as an intravenous infusion at a dose of 0.3 mcg DDAVP/kg body weight diluted in sterile physiological saline and infused slowly over 15 to 30 minutes. In adults and children weighing more than 10 kg, 50 mL of diluent is used; in children weighing 10 kg or less, 10 mL of diluent is used. Blood pressure and pulse should be monitored during infusion. If **DDAVP Injection** is used preoperatively, it should be administered 30 minutes prior to the scheduled procedure.
The necessity for repeat administration of DDAVP or use of any blood products for hemostasis should be determined by laboratory response as well as the clinical condition of the patient. The tendency toward tachyphylaxis (lessening of response) with repeated administration given more frequently than every 48 hours should be considered in treating each patient.

Diabetes Insipidus
This formulation is administered subcutaneously or by direct intravenous injection. **DDAVP Injection** (desmopressin acetate) dosage must be determined for each patient and adjusted according to the pattern of response. Response should be estimated by two parameters: adequate duration of sleep and adequate, not excessive, water turnover.
The usual dosage range in adults is 0.5 mL (2.0 mcg) to 1 mL (4.0 mcg) daily, administered intravenously or subcutaneously, usually in two divided doses. The morning and evening doses should be separately adjusted for an adequate diurnal rhythm of water turnover. For patients who have been controlled on intranasal DDAVP and who must be switched to the injection form, either because of poor intranasal absorption or because of the need for surgery, the comparable antidiuretic dose of the injection is about one-tenth the intranasal dose.
Parenteral drug products should be inspected visually for particulate matter and discoloration prior to administration whenever solution and container permit.

HOW SUPPLIED

DDAVP Injection (desmopressin acetate) is available as a sterile solution in cartons of ten 1 mL single-dose ampules (NDC 0075-2451-01) and in 10 mL multiple-dose vials (NDC 0075-2451-53), each containing 4.0 mcg DDAVP per mL.
KEEP REFRIGERATED AT 2°–8°C (36°–46°F).
Caution: Federal (U.S.A.) law prohibits dispensing without prescription.
Military: 4 mcg/mL—10 × 1 mL (NSN 6505-01-224-7450).
Rev. 3/95 IN-4708H
Manufactured for
RHÔNE-POULENC RORER PHARMACEUTICALS INC.
Collegeville, PA, U.S.A. 19426-0107
By Ferring Pharmaceuticals, Malmö, Sweden
Shown in Product Identification Guide, page 330

DDAVP® ℞
(desmopressin acetate)
Injection 15 μg/mL

PRODUCT OVERVIEW

KEY FACTS

DDAVP® Injection 15 μg/mL (desmopressin acetate) is a synthetic analogue of the natural pituitary hormone 8-arginine vasopressin (ADH), an antidiuretic hormone affecting renal water conservation. DDAVP Injection 15 μg/mL is provided as a sterile, aqueous solution for injection. The ampules contain either 1 mL (15 μg) or 2 mL (30 μg).

MAJOR USES

Hemophilia A: DDAVP Injection 15 μg/mL is indicated for patients with hemophilia A with factor VIII coagulant activity levels greater than 5%.
von Willebrand's Disease (Type I): DDAVP Injection 15 μg/mL is indicated for patients with mild to moderate classic von Willebrand's disease (Type I) with factor VIII levels greater than 5%.

SAFETY INFORMATION

DDAVP Injection 15 μg/mL is contraindicated in individuals with known hypersensitivity to desmopressin acetate or to any of the components of **DDAVP Injection 15 μg/mL.**

WARNINGS

Patients who do not have need of antidiuretic hormone for its antidiuretic effect, in particular those who are young or elderly, should be cautioned to ingest only enough fluid to satisfy thirst, in order to decrease the potential occurrence of water intoxication and hyponatremia.
Fluid intake should be adjusted downward, particularly in very young and elderly patients, in order to decrease the potential occurrence of water intoxication and hyponatremia.
Particular attention should be paid to the possibility of the rare occurrence of an extreme decrease in plasma osmolality that may result in seizures which could lead to coma.
DDAVP should not be used to treat patients with Type IIB von Willebrand's disease since platelet aggregation may be induced.
DDAVP Injection 15 μg/mL should be used with caution in patients with conditions associated with fluid and electrolyte imbalance, such as cystic fibrosis, because these patients are prone to hyponatremia.
For injection use only.

DDAVP® ℞
(desmopressin acetate)
Injection 15 μg/mL

DESCRIPTION

DDAVP® (desmopressin acetate) is a synthetic analogue of the natural pituitary hormone 8-arginine vasopressin (ADH), an antidiuretic hormone affecting renal water conservation. It is chemically defined as follows:
Mol. Wt. 1183.32
Empirical Formula: $C_{46}H_{64}N_{14}O_{12}S_2 \cdot C_2H_4O_2 \cdot 3H_2O$

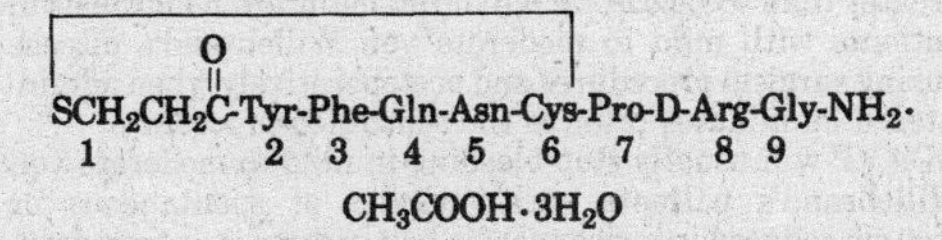

O
SCH2CH2C-Tyr-Phe-Gln-Asn-Cys-Pro-D-Arg-Gly-NH2·
1 2 3 4 5 6 7 8 9
CH3COOH·3H2O

1-(3-mercaptopropionic acid)-8-D-arginine vasopressin monoacetate (salt) trihydrate
DDAVP (desmopressin acetate) Injection 15 μg/mL is provided as a sterile, aqueous solution for injection.
Each mL provides:

Desmopressin acetate	15.0 μg
Sodium chloride	9.0 mg

Hydrochloric acid to adjust pH to 4
The ampules contain either 1 mL (15 μg) or 2 mL (30 μg).

CLINICAL PHARMACOLOGY

DDAVP Injection 15 μg/mL contains as active substance, 1-(3-mercaptopropionic acid)-8-D-arginine vasopressin, a synthetic analogue of the natural hormone arginine vasopressin. One mL (15 μg) of DDAVP (desmopressin acetate) solution has an antidiuretic activity of about 60 IU; 1 μg of DDAVP is equivalent to 4 IU.
DDAVP has been shown to be more potent than arginine vasopressin in increasing plasma levels of factor VIII activity in patients with hemophilia and von Willebrand's disease Type I.
Dose-response studies were performed in healthy persons, using doses of 0.1 to 0.4 μg/kg body weight, infused over a 10-minute period. Maximal dose response occurred at 0.3 to 0.4 μg/kg. The response to DDAVP of factor VIII activity and plasminogen activator is dose-related, with maximal plasma levels of 300 to 400 percent of initial concentrations obtained after infusion of 0.4 μg/kg body weight. The increase is rapid and evident within 30 minutes, reaching a maximum at a point ranging from 90 minutes to two hours. The factor VIII related antigen and ristocetin cofactor activity were also increased to a smaller degree, but still are dose-dependent.

1. The biphasic half-lives of DDAVP were 7.8 and 75.5 minutes for the fast and slow phases, respectively, compared with 2.5 and 14.5 minutes for lysine vasopressin, another form of the hormone. As a result, DDAVP (desmopressin acetate) provides a prompt onset of antidiuretic action with a long duration after each administration.
2. The change in structure of arginine vasopressin to DDAVP has resulted in a decreased vasopressor action and decreased actions on visceral smooth muscle relative to the enhanced antidiuretic activity, so that clinically effective antidiuretic doses are usually below threshold levels for effects on vascular or visceral smooth muscle.
3. When administered by injection, DDAVP has an antidiuretic effect about ten times that of an equivalent dose administered intranasally.
4. The percentage increase of factor VIII levels in patients with mild hemophilia A and von Willebrand's disease was not significantly different from that observed in normal healthy individuals when treated with 0.3 μg/kg of DDAVP infused over 10 minutes.

Continued on next page

Rhône-Poulenc Rorer–Cont.

5. Plasminogen activator activity increases rapidly after DDAVP infusion, but there has been no clinically significant fibrinolysis in patients treated with DDAVP.
6. The effect of repeated DDAVP administration when doses were given every 12 to 24 hours has generally shown a gradual diminution of the factor VIII activity increase noted with a single dose. The initial response is reproducible in any particular patient if there are 2 or 3 days between administrations.

INDICATIONS AND USAGE

Hemophilia A: DDAVP Injection 15 μg/mL is indicated for patients with hemophilia A with factor VIII coagulant activity levels greater than 5%.

DDAVP will often maintain hemostasis in patients with hemophilia A during surgical procedures and postoperatively when administered 30 minutes prior to scheduled procedure.

DDAVP will also stop bleeding in hemophilia A patients with episodes of spontaneous or trauma-induced injuries such as hemarthroses, intramuscular hematomas or mucosal bleeding.

DDAVP is not indicated for the treatment of hemophilia A with factor VIII coagulant activity levels equal to or less than 5%, or for the treatment of hemophilia B, or in patients who have factor VIII antibodies.

In certain clinical situations, it may be justified to try DDAVP in patients with factor VIII levels between 2%–5%; however, these patients should be carefully monitored.

von Willebrand's Disease (Type I): DDAVP Injection 15 μg/mL is indicated for patients with mild to moderate classic von Willebrand's disease (Type I) with factor VIII levels greater than 5%. DDAVP will often maintain hemostasis in patients with mild to moderate von Willebrand's disease during surgical procedures and postoperatively when administered 30 minutes prior to the scheduled procedure.

DDAVP will usually stop bleeding in mild to moderate von Willebrand's patients with episodes of spontaneous or trauma-induced injuries such as hemarthroses, intramuscular hematomas or mucosal bleeding.

Those von Willebrand's disease patients who are least likely to respond are those with severe homozygous von Willebrand's disease with factor VIII coagulant activity and factor VIII von Willebrand factor antigen levels less than 1%. Other patients may respond in a variable fashion depending on the type of molecular defect they have. Bleeding time and factor VIII coagulant activity, ristocetin cofactor activity, and von Willebrand factor antigen should be checked during administration of DDAVP to ensure that adequate levels are being achieved.

DDAVP is not indicated for the treatment of severe classic von Willebrand's disease (Type I) and when there is evidence of an abnormal molecular form of factor VIII antigen. See WARNING.

CONTRAINDICATIONS

DDAVP Injection 15 μg/mL is contraindicated in individuals with known hypersensitivity to desmopressin acetate or to any of the components of **DDAVP Injection 15 μg/mL**.

WARNINGS

Patients who do not have need of antidiuretic hormone for its antidiuretic effect, in particular those who are young or elderly, should be cautioned to ingest only enough fluid to satisfy thirst, in order to decrease the potential occurrence of water intoxication and hyponatremia.

Fluid intake should be adjusted downward, particularly in very young and elderly patients, in order to decrease the potential occurrence of water intoxication and hyponatremia.

Particular attention should be paid to the possibility of the rare occurrence of an extreme decrease in plasma osmolality that may result in seizures which could lead to coma.

DDAVP should not be used to treat patients with Type IIB von Willebrand's disease since platelet aggregation may be induced.

PRECAUTIONS

General: For injection use only.

DDAVP (desmopressin acetate) **Injection 15 μg/mL** has infrequently produced changes in blood pressure causing either a slight elevation in blood pressure or a transient fall in blood pressure and a compensatory increase in heart rate. The drug should be used with caution in patients with coronary artery insufficiency and/or hypertensive cardiovascular disease.

DDAVP Injection 15 μg/mL should be used with caution in patients with conditions associated with fluid and electrolyte imbalance, such as cystic fibrosis, because these patients are prone to hyponatremia.

There have been rare reports of thrombotic events following **DDAVP Injection 15 μg/mL** in patients predisposed to thrombus formation. No causality has been determined, however, the drug should be used with caution in these patients.

Severe allergic reactions have been reported rarely. Fatal anaphylaxis has been reported in one patient who received intravenous DDAVP (desmopressin acetate). It is not known whether antibodies to **DDAVP Injection 15 μg/mL** are produced after repeated injections.

Hemophilia A: Laboratory tests for assessing patient status include levels of factor VIII coagulant, factor VIII antigen and factor VIII ristocetin cofactor (von Willebrand factor) as well as activated partial thromboplastin time. Factor VIII coagulant activity should be determined before giving DDAVP for hemostasis. If factor VIII coagulant activity is present at less than 5% of normal, DDAVP should not be relied on.

von Willebrand's Disease: Laboratory tests for assessing patient status include levels of factor VIII coagulant activity, factor VIII ristocetin cofactor activity, and factor VIII von Willebrand factor antigen. The skin bleeding time may be helpful in following these patients.

Drug Interactions: Although the pressor activity of DDAVP is very low compared with the antidiuretic activity, use of doses as large as 0.3 μg/kg of DDAVP with other pressor agents should be done only with careful patient monitoring.

DDAVP has been used with epsilon aminocaproic acid without adverse effects.

Carcinogenicity, Mutagenicity, Impairment of Fertility: There have been no long-term studies in animals to assess the carcinogenic, mutagenic, or impairment of fertility potential of DDAVP (desmopressin acetate).

Pregnancy Category B: Reproduction studies performed in rats and rabbits by the subcutaneous route at doses up to 10 μg/kg/day have revealed no evidence of harm to the fetus due to desmopressin acetate. This dose is equivalent to 10 times the systemic human dose for Factor VIII stimulation based on mg/M^2 surface area.

There are no adequate and well-controlled studies in pregnant women. Several publications of desmopressin acetate's use in the management of diabetes insipidus during pregnancy are available; these include a few anecdotal reports of congenital anomalies and low birth weight babies. However, no causal connection between these events and desmopressin acetate has been established. A 15-year, Swedish epidemiologic study of the use of desmopressin acetate in pregnant women with diabetes insipidus found the rate of birth defects to be no greater than that in the general population. As opposed to preparations containing natural hormones, desmopressin acetate in antidiuretic doses has no uterotonic action and the physician will have to weigh the therapeutic advantages against the possible risks in each case.

Nursing Mothers: There have been no controlled studies in nursing mothers. A single study in postpartum women demonstrated a marked change in plasma, but little if any change in assayable DDAVP in breast milk following an intranasal dose of 10 μg. It is not known whether this drug is excreted in human milk. Because many drugs are excreted in human milk, caution should be exercised when DDAVP is administered to a nursing woman.

Pediatric Use: Use in infants and children will require careful fluid intake restriction to prevent possible hyponatremia and water intoxication. ***DDAVP Injection 15 μg/mL** should not be used in infants less than three months of age* in the treatment of hemophilia A or von Willebrand's disease.

ADVERSE REACTIONS

Infrequently, DDAVP has produced transient headache, nausea, mild abdominal cramps and vulval pain. These symptoms disappeared with reduction in dosage. Occasionally, injection of DDAVP has produced local erythema, swelling or burning pain. Occasional facial flushing has been reported with the administration of DDAVP. Intravenous administration of DDAVP Injection has infrequently produced changes in blood pressure causing either a slight elevation or a transient fall and a compensatory increase in heart rate. Severe allergic reactions including anaphylaxis have been reported rarely with intravenous administration of DDAVP Injection (desmopressin acetate).

See WARNING for the possibility of water intoxication and hyponatremia.

There have been rare reports of thrombotic events (acute cerebrovascular thrombosis, acute myocardial infarction) following intravenous administration of DDAVP Injection in patients predisposed to thrombus formation.

OVERDOSAGE

See ADVERSE REACTIONS above. In case of overdosage, the dosage should be reduced, frequency of administration decreased, or the drug withdrawn according to the severity of the condition.

There is no known specific antidote for desmopressin acetate or DDAVP Injection.

An oral LD_{50} has not been established. An intravenous dose of 2 mg/kg in mice demonstrated no effect.

DOSAGE AND ADMINISTRATION

Hemophilia A and von Willebrand's Disease (Type I): DDAVP Injection 15 μg/mL is administered as an intravenous infusion at a dose of 0.3 μg DDAVP/kg body weight diluted in sterile physiological saline and infused slowly over 15 to 30 minutes. In adults and children weighing more than 10 kg, 50 mL of diluent is recommended; in children weighing 10 kg or less, 10 mL of diluent is recommended. Blood pressure and pulse should be monitored during infusion. If **DDAVP Injection 15 μg/mL** is used preoperatively, it should be administered 30 minutes prior to the scheduled procedure.

The necessity for repeat administration of DDAVP or use of any blood products for hemostasis should be determined by laboratory response as well as the clinical condition of the patient. The tendency toward tachyphylaxis (lessening of response) with repeated administration given more frequently than every 48 hours should be considered in treating each patient.

Parenteral drug products should be inspected visually for particulate matter and discoloration prior to administration whenever solution and container permit.

HOW SUPPLIED

DDAVP (desmopressin acetate) **Injection 15 μg/mL** is available as a sterile solution in cartons of five 1 mL ampules (NDC 0075-0945-01) and five 2 mL ampules (NDC 0075-0945-02). Each vial is marked with two red rings and contains 15 μg desmopressin acetate per mL.

KEEP REFRIGERATED AT 2°–8°C (36°–46°F).

Caution: Federal (U.S.A.) law prohibits dispensing without prescription.

Manufactured for
RHÔNE-POULENC RORER PHARMACEUTICALS INC.
COLLEGEVILLE, PA 19426
By Ferring Pharmaceuticals, Malmö, Sweden
Rev. 5/95 IN-6531

Shown in Product Identification Guide, page 330

DDAVP® Nasal Spray ℞
(desmopressin acetate)
DDAVP® Rhinal Tube ℞
(desmopressin acetate)

COMBINED PRODUCT OVERVIEW

KEY FACTS

DDAVP® (desmopressin acetate) is a synthetic analogue of the natural pituitary hormone 8-arginine vasopressin (ADH), an antidiuretic hormone affecting renal water conservation. DDAVP Nasal Spray and DDAVP Rhinal Tube are each provided as an aqueous solution for intranasal use only.

MAJOR USES

DDAVP is indicated for the management of primary nocturnal enuresis. It may be used alone or adjunctive to behavioral conditioning or other nonpharmacological intervention. It has been shown to be effective in some cases that are refractory to conventional therapies.

DDAVP is also indicated as antidiuretic replacement therapy in the management of central cranial diabetes insipidus and for management of the temporary polyuria and polydipsia following head trauma or surgery in the pituitary region. DDAVP is not effective for the treatment of nephrogenic diabetes insipidus.

SAFETY INFORMATION

Patients who do not have need of antidiuretic hormone for its antidiuretic effect (i.e. those who are young or elderly) should be cautioned to ingest only enough fluid to satisfy thirst in order to decrease the potential occurrence of water intoxication and hyponatremia.

DDAVP® Nasal Spray ℞
(desmopressin acetate)
DDAVP® Rhinal Tube ℞
(desmopressin acetate)
COMBINED PRESCRIBING INFORMATION

DESCRIPTION

DDAVP® (desmopressin acetate) is a synthetic analogue of the natural pituitary hormone 8-arginine vasopressin (ADH), an antidiuretic hormone affecting renal water conservation. It is chemically defined as follows:

Mol. wt. 1183.32

Empirical formula: $C_{46}H_{64}N_{14}O_{12}S_2 \cdot C_2H_4O_2 \cdot 3H_2O$

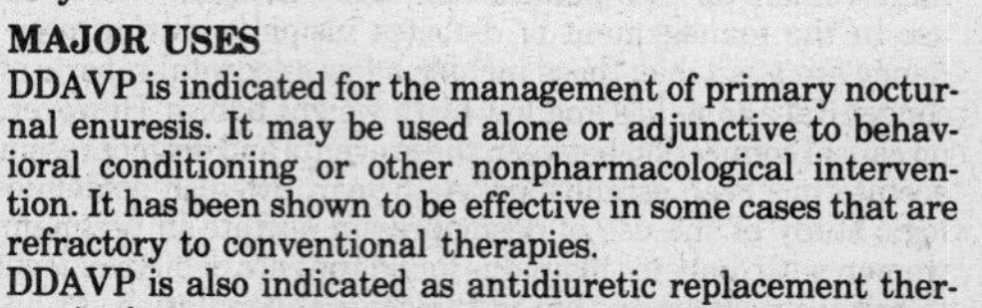
O
SCH2CH2C-Tyr-Phe-Gln-Asn-Cys-Pro-D-Arg-Gly-NH2·
1 2 3 4 5 6 7 8 9
CH3COOH·3H2O

1-(3-mercaptopropionic acid)-8-D-arginine vasopressin monoacetate (salt) trihydrate

DDAVP Nasal Spray (desmopressin acetate) and DDAVP Rhinal Tube (desmopressin acetate) are each provided as an aqueous solution for intranasal use.

Each mL contains:

Desmopressin acetate	0.1 mg
Chlorobutanol	5.0 mg
Sodium Chloride	9.0 mg

Hydrochloric acid to adjust pH to approximately 4
The DDAVP Nasal Spray compression pump delivers 0.1 mL (10 mcg) of DDAVP per spray.

CLINICAL PHARMACOLOGY

DDAVP contains as active substance 1-(3-mercaptopropionic acid)-8-D-arginine vasopressin, which is a synthetic analogue of the natural hormone arginine vasopressin. One mL (0.1 mg) of intranasal DDAVP has an antidiuretic activity of about 400 IU; 10 mcg of desmopressin acetate is equivalent to 40 IU.

1. The biphasic half-lives for intranasal DDAVP were 7.8 and 75.5 minutes for the fast and slow phases, compared with 2.5 and 14.5 minutes for lysine vasopressin, another form of the hormone used in this condition. As a result, intranasal DDAVP provides a prompt onset of antidiuretic action with a long duration after each administration.
2. The change in structure of arginine vasopressin to DDAVP has resulted in a decreased vasopressor action and decreased actions on visceral smooth muscle relative to the enhanced antidiuretic activity, so that clinically effective antidiuretic doses are usually below threshold levels for effects on vascular or visceral smooth muscle.
3. DDAVP administered intranasally has an antidiuretic effect about one-tenth that of an equivalent dose administered by injection.

INDICATIONS AND USAGE

Primary Nocturnal Enuresis: DDAVP Nasal Spray and DDAVP Rhinal Tube are indicated for the management of primary nocturnal enuresis. It may be used alone or adjunctive to behavioral conditioning or other non-pharmacological intervention. It has been shown to be effective in some cases that are refractory to conventional therapies.

Central Cranial Diabetes Insipidus: DDAVP Nasal Spray and DDAVP Rhinal Tube are indicated as antidiuretic replacement therapy in the management of central cranial diabetes insipidus and for management of the temporary polyuria and polydipsia following head trauma or surgery in the pituitary region. It is ineffective for the treatment of nephrogenic diabetes insipidus.

The use of DDAVP Nasal Spray or DDAVP Rhinal Tube in patients with an established diagnosis will result in a reduction in urinary output with increase in urine osmolality and a decrease in plasma osmolality. This will allow the resumption of a more normal life-style with a decrease in urinary frequency and nocturia.

There are reports of an occasional change in response with time, usually greater than 6 months. Some patients may show a decreased responsiveness, others a shortened duration of effect. There is no evidence this effect is due to the development of binding antibodies but may be due to a local inactivation of the peptide.

Patients are selected for therapy by establishing the diagnosis by means of the water deprivation test, the hypertonic saline infusion test, and/or the response to antidiuretic hormone. Continued response to intranasal DDAVP can be monitored by urine volume and osmolality.

DDAVP is also available as a solution for injection when the intranasal route may be compromised. These situations include nasal congestion and blockage, nasal discharge, atrophy of nasal mucosa, and severe atrophic rhinitis. Intranasal delivery may also be inappropriate where there is an impaired level of consciousness. In addition, cranial surgical procedures, such as transsphenoidal hypophysectomy create situations where an alternative route of administration is needed as in cases of nasal packing or recovery from surgery.

CONTRAINDICATIONS

DDAVP Nasal Spray and DDAVP Rhinal Tube are contraindicated in individuals with known hypersensitivity to desmopressin acetate or to any of the components of DDAVP Nasal Spray or DDAVP Rhinal Tube.

WARNINGS

1. For intranasal use only.
2. In very young and elderly patients in particular, fluid intake should be adjusted downward in order to decrease the potential occurrence of water intoxication and hyponatremia. Particular attention should be paid to the possibility of the rare occurrence of an extreme decrease in plasma osmolality that may result in seizures which could lead to coma.

PRECAUTIONS

General: Intranasal DDAVP at high dosage has infrequently produced a slight elevation of blood pressure, which disappeared with a reduction in dosage. The drug should be used with caution in patients with coronary artery insufficiency and/or hypertensive cardiovascular disease because of possible rise in blood pressure.

DDAVP should be used with caution in patients with conditions associated with fluid and electrolyte imbalance, such as cystic fibrosis, because these patients are prone to hyponatremia.

Rare severe allergic reactions have been reported with DDAVP. Anaphylaxis has been reported with intravenous administration of DDAVP Injection, but not with DDAVP intranasal.

Central Cranial Diabetes Insipidus: Since DDAVP is used intranasally, changes in the nasal mucosa such as scarring, edema, or other disease may cause erratic, unreliable absorption in which case intranasal DDAVP should not be used. For such situations, DDAVP Injection should be considered.

Primary Nocturnal Enuresis: If changes in the nasal mucosa have occurred, unreliable absorption may result. DDAVP intranasal solution should be discontinued until the nasal problems resolve.

Information for Patients: Patients should be informed that the DDAVP Nasal Spray bottle accurately delivers 50 doses of 10 mcg each. Any solution remaining after 50 doses should be discarded since the amount delivered thereafter may be substantially less than 10 mcg of drug. No attempt should be made to transfer remaining solution to another bottle. Patients should be instructed to read accompanying directions on use of the spray pump carefully before use.

Laboratory Tests: Laboratory tests for following the patient with central cranial diabetes insipidus or post-surgical or head trauma-related polyuria and polydipsia include urine volume and osmolality. In some cases plasma osmolality measurements may be required. For the healthy patient with primary nocturnal enuresis, serum electrolytes should be checked at least once if therapy is continued beyond 7 days.

Drug Interactions: Although the pressor activity of DDAVP is very low compared to the antidiuretic activity, use of large doses of intranasal DDAVP with other pressor agents should only be done with careful patient monitoring.

Carcinogenesis, Mutagenesis, Impairment of Fertility: There have been no long-term studies in animals to assess the carcinogenic, mutagenic, or impairment of fertility potential of DDAVP (desmopressin acetate).

Pregnancy—Category B: Reproduction studies performed in rats and rabbits by the subcutaneous route at doses up to 10 mcg/kg/day have revealed no evidence of harm to the fetus due to desmopressin acetate. This dose is equivalent to 10 times (for Factor VIII stimulation) or 38 times (for diabetes insipidus) the systemic human dose based on mg/M^2 surface area.

There are no adequate and well-controlled studies in pregnant women. Several publications of desmopressin acetate's use in the management of diabetes insipidus during pregnancy are available; these include a few anecdotal reports of congenital anomalies and low birth weight babies. However, no causal connection between these events and desmopressin acetate has been established. A 15-year, Swedish epidemiologic study of the use of desmopressin acetate in pregnant women with diabetes insipidus found the rate of birth defects to be no greater than that in the general population. As opposed to preparations containing natural hormones, desmopressin acetate in antidiuretic doses has no uterotonic action and the physician will have to weigh the therapeutic advantages against the possible risks in each case.

Nursing Mothers: There have been no controlled studies in nursing mothers. A single study in postpartum women demonstrated a marked change in plasma, but little if any change in assayable DDAVP® in breast milk following an intranasal dose of 10 mcg. It is not known whether this drug is excreted in human milk. Because many drugs are excreted in human milk, caution should be exercised when DDAVP is administered to a nursing woman.

Pediatric Use:

Primary Nocturnal Enuresis: DDAVP Nasal Spray and DDAVP Rhinal Tube have been used in childhood nocturnal enuresis. Short-term (4–8 weeks) DDAVP intranasal administration has been shown to be safe and modestly effective in children aged 6 years or older with severe childhood nocturnal enuresis. Adequately controlled studies with intranasal DDAVP in primary nocturnal enuresis have not been conducted beyond 4–8 weeks. The dose should be individually adjusted to achieve the best results.

Central Cranial Diabetes Insipidus: DDAVP Nasal Spray and DDAVP Rhinal Tube have been used in children with diabetes insipidus. Use in infants and children will require careful fluid intake restriction to prevent possible hyponatremia and water intoxication. The dose must be individually adjusted to the patient with attention in the very young to the danger of an extreme decrease in plasma osmolality with resulting convulsions. Dose should start at 0.05 mL or less.

Since the spray cannot deliver less than 0.1 mL (10 mcg), smaller doses should be administered using the rhinal tube delivery system. Do not use the nasal spray in pediatric patients requiring less than 0.1 mL (10 mcg) per dose.

There are reports of an occasional change in response with time, usually greater than 6 months. Some patients may show a decreased responsiveness, others a shortened duration of effect. There is no evidence this effect is due to the development of binding antibodies but may be due to a local inactivation of the peptide.

ADVERSE REACTIONS

Infrequently, high dosages of intranasal DDAVP have produced transient headache and nausea. Nasal congestion, rhinitis and flushing have also been reported occasionally along with mild abdominal cramps. These symptoms disappeared with reduction in dosage. Nosebleed, sore throat, cough and upper respiratory infections have also been reported.

The following table lists the percent of patients having adverse experiences without regard to relationship to study drug from the pooled pivotal study data for nocturnal enuresis.

ADVERSE REACTION	PLACEBO (N=59) %	DDAVP 20 mcg (N=60) %	DDAVP 40 mcg (N=61) %
BODY AS A WHOLE			
Abdominal Pain	0	2	2
Asthenia	0	0	2
Chills	0	0	2
Headache	0	2	5
Throat Pain	2	0	0
NERVOUS SYSTEM			
Depression	2	0	0
Dizziness	0	0	3
RESPIRATORY SYSTEM			
Epistaxis	2	3	0
Nostril Pain	0	2	0
Respiratory Infection	2	0	0
Rhinitis	2	8	3
CARDIOVASCULAR SYSTEM			
Vasodilation	2	0	0
DIGESTIVE SYSTEM			
Gastrointestinal Disorder	0	2	0
Nausea	0	0	2
SKIN & APPENDAGES			
Leg Rash	2	0	0
Rash	2	0	0
SPECIAL SENSES			
Conjunctivitis	0	2	0
Edema Eyes	0	2	0
Lachrymation Disorder	0	0	2

See WARNING for the possibility of water intoxication and hyponatremia.

OVERDOSAGE

See ADVERSE REACTIONS above. In case of overdosage, the dose should be reduced, frequency of administration decreased, or the drug withdrawn according to the severity of the condition. There is no known specific antidote for desmopressin acetate or DDAVP.

An oral LD_{50} has not been established. An intravenous dose of 2 mg/kg in mice demonstrated no effect.

DOSAGE AND ADMINISTRATION

Primary Nocturnal Enuresis: Dosage should be adjusted according to the individual. The recommended initial dose for those 6 years of age and older is 20 mcg or 0.2 mL solution intranasally at bedtime. Adjustment up to 40 mcg is suggested if the patient does not respond. Some patients may respond to 10 mcg and adjustment to that lower dose may be done if the patient has shown a response to 20 mcg. It is recommended that one-half of the dose be administered per nostril. Adequately controlled studies with intranasal DDAVP in primary nocturnal enuresis have not been conducted beyond 4–8 weeks.

Central Cranial Diabetes Insipidus: DDAVP Nasal Spray and DDAVP Rhinal Tube dosage must be determined for each individual patient and adjusted according to the diurnal pattern of response. Response should be estimated by two parameters: adequate duration of sleep and adequate, not excessive, water turnover. Patients with nasal congestion and blockage have often responded well to intranasal DDAVP. The nasal spray pump can only deliver doses of 0.1 mL (10 mcg) or multiples of 0.1 mL. If doses other than these are required, the rhinal tube delivery system may be used. DDAVP Rhinal Tube is administered into the nose through a soft, flexible plastic rhinal tube that has four graduation marks on it that measure 0.2, 0.15, 0.1, and 0.05 mL. The usual dosage range in adults is 0.1 to 0.4 mL daily, either as a single dose or divided into two or three doses. Most adults require 0.2 mL daily in two divided doses. The morning and evening doses should be separately adjusted for an adequate diurnal rhythm of water turnover. For children aged 3 months to 12 years, the usual dosage range is 0.05 to 0.3 mL daily, either as a single dose or divided into two doses. About $^1/_4$ to $^1/_3$ of patients can be controlled by a single daily dose of DDAVP administered intranasally.

Continued on next page

Rhône-Poulenc Rorer–Cont.

HOW SUPPLIED

DDAVP Nasal Spray is available as a 5 mL bottle with spray pump delivering 50 doses of 10 mcg (NDC 0075-2450-02).
KEEP REFRIGERATED AT 2°–8°C (36°–46°F). When traveling, product will maintain stability for up to 3 weeks when stored at room temperature, 22°C (72°F).
DDAVP Rhinal Tube is available in a 2.5 mL vial packaged with two rhinal tube applicators per carton (NDC 0075-2450-01).
KEEP REFRIGERATED AT 2°–8°C (36°–46°F). When traveling, closed bottles will maintain stability for 3 weeks when stored at room temperature, 22°C (72°F).
Military: DDAVP Rhinal Tube, 1 × 2.5 mL (NSN 6505-01-145-6338). DDAVP Nasal Spray, 1 × 5.0 mL (NSN 6505-01-320-5579).

CAUTION

Federal (U.S.A.) law prohibits dispensing without prescription.
Rev. 3/95 IN-0368E
Rev. 3/95 IN-0369F
Manufactured for:
RHÔNE-POULENC RORER PHARMACEUTICALS INC.
Collegeville, PA, U.S.A. 19426-0107
By: Ferring Pharmaceuticals, Malmö, Sweden
Shown in Product Identification Guide, page 330

DDAVP™ Tablets ℞
(desmopressin acetate)

DESCRIPTION

DDAVP™ (desmopressin acetate) is a synthetic analogue of the natural pituitary hormone 8-arginine vasopressin (ADH), an antidiuretic hormone affecting renal water conservation. DDAVP™ Tablets contain either 0.1 or 0.2 mg desmopressin acetate. Inactive ingredients include: lactose, potato starch, magnesium stearate and povidone. It is chemically defined as follows:
Mol. Wt. 1183.34
Empirical Formula: $C_{46}H_{64}N_{14}O_{12}S_2 \cdot C_2H_4O_2 \cdot 3H_2O$

SCH_2CH_2CO-Tyr-Phe-Gln-Asn-Cys-Pro-D-Arg-Gly-NH_2 • CH_3COOH • $3H_2O$
1 2 3 4 5 6 7 8 9

1-(3-mercaptopropionic acid)-8-D-arginine vasopressin monoacetate (salt) trihydrate
Route of Administration: Oral

CLINICAL PHARMACOLOGY

DDAVP Tablets contain as active substance, desmopressin acetate, a synthetic analogue of the natural hormone arginine vasopressin.
Dose response studies in patients with diabetes insipidus have demonstrated that oral doses of 0.025 mg to 0.4 mg produced clinically significant antidiuretic effects. In most patients, doses of 0.1 mg to 0.2 mg produced optimal antidiuretic effects lasting up to eight hours. With doses of 0.4 mg, antidiuretic effects were observed for up to 12 hours; measurements beyond 12 hours were not recorded. Increasing oral doses produced dose dependent increases in the plasma levels of DDAVP.
The plasma half-life of DDAVP followed a monoexponential time course with $t^{1}/_{2}$ values of $1^{1}/_{2}$ to $2^{1}/_{2}$ hours which was independent of dose.
The bioavailability of DDAVP oral tablets is about 5% compared to intranasal DDAVP, and about 0.15% compared to intravenous DDAVP. The time to reach maximum plasma DDAVP levels ranged from 0.9 to 1.5 hours following oral or intranasal administration, respectively. Following administration of DDAVP Tablets, the onset of antidiuretic effect occurs at around 1 hour, and it reaches a maximum at about 4 to 7 hours based on the measurement of increased urine osmolality.
The use of DDAVP Tablets in patients with an established diagnosis will result in a reduction in urinary output with an accompanying increase in urine osmolality. These effects usually will allow resumption of a more normal life style when there is a decrease in urinary frequency and nocturia.
There are reports of an occasional change in response to the intranasal formulations of DDAVP (DDAVP Nasal Spray and DDAVP Rhinal Tube). Usually, the change occurs over a period of time greater than six months. This change may be due to decreased responsiveness, or to shortened duration of effect. There is no evidence that this effect is due to the development of binding antibodies, but may be due to a local inactivation of the peptide. No lessening of effect has been seen in the 46 patients who were treated with DDAVP Tablets for 12 to 44 months and no serum antibodies to desmopressin were detected.
The change in structure of arginine vasopressin to desmopressin acetate resulted in less vasopressor activity and decreased action on visceral smooth muscle relative to enhanced antidiuretic activity. Consequently, clinically effective antidiuretic doses are usually below the threshold for effects on vascular or visceral smooth muscle. In the four long-term studies of DDAVP Tablets, no increases in blood pressure in 46 patients receiving DDAVP Tablets for periods up to 12 to 44 months were reported.
In one study, the pharmacodynamic characteristics of DDAVP Tablets and intranasal formulation were compared during an 8-hour dosing interval at steady state. The doses administered to 36 hydrated (water loaded) healthy male adult volunteers every 8 hours were 0.1, 0.2, 0.4 mg orally and 0.01 mg intranasally by rhinal tube. The results are shown in the following table:

Mean Changes from Baseline (SE) in Pharmacodynamic parameters in Normal Healthy Adult Volunteers

Treatment	Total Urine Volume in mL	Maximum Urine Osmolality in mOsm/kg
0.1 mg PO q8h	−3689.3 (149.6)	514.8 (21.9)
0.2 mg PO q8h	−4429.9 (149.6)	686.3 (21.9)
0.4 mg PO q8h	−4998.8 (149.6)	769.3 (21.9)
0.01 mg IN q8h	−4844.9 (149.6)	754.1 (21.9)

With respect to the mean values of total urine volume decrease and maximum urine osmolality increase from baseline, the 90% confidence limits estimated that the 0.4 mg and 0.2 mg oral dose produced between 95% and 110% and 84% to 99% of pharmacodynamic activity, respectively, when compared to the 0.01 mg intranasal dose.
While both the 0.2 mg and 0.4 mg oral doses are considered pharmacodynamically similar to the 0.01 mg intranasal dose, the pharmacodynamic data on an inter-subject basis was highly variable and, therefore, individual dosing is recommended.
In another study in diabetes insipidus patients, the pharmacodynamic characteristics of DDAVP Tablet and intranasal formulations were compared over a 12-hour period. Ten fluid-controlled patients under age 18 were administered tablet doses of 0.2 mg and 0.4 mg, and intranasal doses of 10 μg and 20 μg.

Mean Peak Pharmacodynamic parameters in Pediatric and Adolescent Diabetes Insipidus Patients (± std)

Treatment	Urine Volume in mL/min.	Maximum Urine Osmolality in mOsm/kg
10 μg IN	0.3 (± 0.15)	717.0 (± 224.63)
20 μg IN	0.3 (± 0.25)	761.8 (± 298.82)
0.2 mg PO	0.3 (± 0.12)	678.3 (± 147.91)
0.4 mg PO	0.2 (± 0.15)	787.2 (± 73.34)

All four dose formulations (10 μg IN, 20 μg IN, 0.20 mg PO and 0.40 mg PO) have a similar, pronounced pharmacodynamic effect on urine volume and urine osmolality. At two hours after study drug administration, mean urine volume was 4 mL/min and urine osmolality was >500 mOsm/kg. Mean plasma osmolality remained relatively constant over the time course recorded (0 to 12 hours). A statistical separation from baseline did not occur at any dose or time point. In these patients, the 0.2 mg tablets and the 10 μg intranasal spray exhibited similar pharmacodynamic profiles as did the 0.4 mg tablets and the 20 μg intranasal spray formulation. In another study of adult diabetes insipidus patients previously controlled on DDAVP intranasal spray, after one week of self-titration from spray to tablets, patients' diuresis was controlled with 0.1 mg DDAVP Tablets t.i.d.

INDICATIONS AND USAGE

Central Cranial Diabetes Insipidus: DDAVP Tablets are indicated as antidiuretic replacement therapy in the management of central (cranial) diabetes insipidus and for the management of the temporary polyuria and polydipsia following head trauma or surgery in the pituitary region. DDAVP is ineffective for the treatment of nephrogenic diabetes insipidus.
Patients are selected for therapy by establishing the diagnosis by means of the water deprivation test, the hypertonic saline infusion test, and/or response to antidiuretic hormone. Continued response to DDAVP can be monitored by urine volume and osmolality.

CONTRAINDICATION

DDAVP Tablets are contraindicated in individuals with known hypersensitivity to desmopressin acetate or to any of the components of DDAVP Tablets.

WARNINGS

In very young and elderly patients, in particular, fluid intake should be adjusted downward to decrease the potential occurrence of water intoxication and hyponatremia. Particular attention should be paid to the possibility of the rare occurrence of an extreme decrease in plasma osmolality that may result in seizures which could lead to coma.

PRECAUTIONS

General: Intranasal formulations of DDAVP at high doses and DDAVP Injection have infrequently produced a slight elevation of blood pressure which disappears with a reduction of dosage. Although this effect has not been observed when single oral doses up to 0.6 mg have been administered, the drug should be used with caution in patients with coronary artery insufficiency and/or hypertensive cardiovascular disease, because of a possible rise in blood pressure.
DDAVP should be used with caution in patients with conditions associated with fluid and electrolyte imbalance, such as cystic fibrosis, because these patients are prone to hyponatremia.
Rare severe allergic reactions have been reported with DDAVP. Anaphylaxis has been reported with intravenous administration of DDAVP Injection, but not with DDAVP Tablets.
Laboratory Tests: Laboratory tests for monitoring the patient with central cranial diabetes insipidus or post-surgical or head trauma-related polyuria and polydipsia include urine volume and osmolality. In some cases, measurements of plasma osmolality may be necessary.
Drug Interactions: Although the pressor activity of DDAVP is very low compared to its antidiuretic activity, large doses of DDAVP Tablets should be used with other pressor agents only with careful patient monitoring.
Carcinogenicity, Mutagenicity, Impairment of Fertility: There have been no long-term studies in animals to assess the carcinogenic, mutagenic or impairment of fertility potential of DDAVP (desmopressin acetate).
Pregnancy—Category B: Fertility studies have not been done. Teratology studies in rats and rabbits at doses from 0.05 to 10 μg/kg/day (approximately 0.1 times the maximum systemic human exposure in rats and up to 38 times the maximum systemic human exposure in rabbits based on surface area, mg/m²) revealed no harm to the fetus due to DDAVP (desmopressin acetate). There are, however, no adequate and well-controlled studies in pregnant women. Because animal studies are not always predictive of human response, this drug should be used during pregnancy only if clearly needed.
Several publications of desmopressin acetate's use in the management of diabetes insipidus during pregnancy are available; these include a few anecdotal reports of congenital anomalies and low birth weight babies. However, no causal connection between these events and desmopressin acetate has been established. A 15-year, Swedish epidemiologic study of the use of desmopressin acetate in pregnant women with diabetes insipidus found the rate of birth defects to be no greater than that in the general population. However, the statistical power of this study is low. As opposed to preparations containing natural hormones, desmopressin acetate in antidiuretic doses has no uterotonic action and the physician will have to weigh the possible therapeutic advantages against the possible risks in each case.
Nursing Mothers: There have been no controlled studies in nursing mothers. A single study in postpartum women demonstrated a marked change in plasma, but little if any change in assayable DDAVP in breast milk following an intranasal dose of 10 μg.
It is not known whether the drug is excreted in human milk. Because many drugs are excreted in human milk, caution should be exercised when DDAVP is administered to nursing mothers.
Pediatric Use:
Central Cranial Diabetes Insipidus: DDAVP™ Tablets have been used safely in children, age 4 years and older, with diabetes insipidus for periods up to 44 months. In younger children the dose must be individually adjusted in order to prevent an excessive decrease in plasma osmolality leading to hyponatremia and possible convulsions; dosing should start at 0.05 mg ($^{1}/_{2}$ of the 0.1 mg tablet). Use of DDAVP Tablets in children requires careful fluid intake restrictions to prevent possible hyponatremia and water intoxication.

ADVERSE REACTIONS

Infrequently, large doses of the intranasal formulations of DDAVP and DDAVP Injection have produced transient headache, nausea, flushing and mild abdominal cramps. These symptoms have disappeared with reduction in dosage. In long-term clinical studies in which patients with diabetes insipidus were followed for periods up to 12 to 44 months of DDAVP Tablet therapy, transient increases in SGOT, no higher than 1.5 times the upper limit of normal were expected. Elevated SGOT returned to the normal range despite continued use of DDAVP Tablets.
See WARNINGS for the possibility of water intoxication and hyponatremia.

OVERDOSAGE

See ADVERSE REACTIONS above. In case of overdose, the dose should be reduced, frequency of administration decreased, or the drug withdrawn according to the severity of the condition. There is no known specific antidote for DDAVP.

An oral LD_{50} has not been established. Oral doses up to 0.2 mg/kg/day have been administered to dogs and rats for 6 months without any significant drug-related toxicities reported. An intravenous dose of 2 mg/kg in mice demonstrated no effect.

DOSAGE AND ADMINISTRATION

Central Cranial Diabetes Insipidus: The dosage of DDAVP Tablets must be determined for each individual patient and adjusted according to the diurnal pattern of response. Response should be estimated by two parameters: adequate duration of sleep and adequate, not excessive, water turnover. Patients previously on intranasal DDAVP therapy should begin tablet therapy twelve hours after the last intranasal dose. During the initial dose titration period, patients should be observed closely and appropriate safety parameters measured to assure adequate response. Patients should be monitored at regular intervals during the course of DDAVP Tablet therapy to assure adequate antidiuretic response. Modifications in dosage regimen should be implemented as necessary to assure adequate water turnover.

Adults and children: It is recommended that patients be started on doses of 0.05 mg ($^1/_2$ of the 0.1 mg tablet) two times a day and individually adjusted to their optimum therapeutic dose. Most patients in clinical trials found that the optimal dosage range is 0.1 mg to 0.8 mg daily, administered in divided doses. Each dose should be separately adjusted for an adequate diurnal rhythm of water turnover. Total daily dosage should be increased or decreased in the range of 0.1 mg to 1.2 mg divided t.i.d. or b.i.d. as needed to obtain adequate antidiuresis. See PEDIATRIC USE section for special considerations when administering desmopressin acetate to pediatric diabetes insipidus patients.

HOW SUPPLIED

Strength	Size	NDC 0075-	Color	Markings
0.1 mg	Bottle of 100	0016-00	White	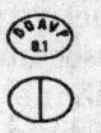 (DDAVP 0.1)
				⊖
0.2 mg	Bottle of 100	0026-00	White	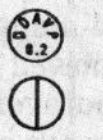 (DDAVP 0.2)
				⊖

Store at controlled room temperature between 15° to 30°C (59° to 86°F). Avoid exposure to excessive heat or light.
Caution: Federal (U.S.A.) law prohibits dispensing without prescription.
Manufactured for
RHÔNE-POULENC RORER PHARMACEUTICALS INC.
COLLEGEVILLE, PA 19426
By
Ferring Pharmaceuticals, Malmö, Sweden
Rev. 3/96
IN-5547A
413951

Shown in Product Identification Guide, page 330

DILACOR XR® ℞
[dil'a-kor]
(diltiazem HCl)
Extended-release Capsules

PRODUCT OVERVIEW
KEY FACTS
Dilacor XR capsules contain multiple units of diltiazem HCl Extended-release 60 mg, resulting in 120 mg, 180 mg or 240 mg dosage strengths.
Dilacor XR capsules contain a degradable controlled-release tablet formulation designed to release diltiazem over a 24-hour period. Geomatrix™, a registered trademark of Jago Research AG, Zollikon, Switzerland, is a patented controlled-release system incorporated in the tablets.

MAJOR USES
Dilacor XR is indicated for the treatment of hypertension. Diltiazem hydrochloride may be used alone or in combination with other antihypertensive medications, such as diuretics.
Dilacor XR is indicated for the management of chronic stable angina.
Dosage: Hypertension. Dosages must be adjusted to each patient's needs, starting with 180 or 240 mg once-daily. Based on the antihypertensive effect, the dose may be adjusted as needed. Individual patients, particularly ≥ 60 years of age, may respond to a lower dose of 120 mg. The usual dosage range studied in clinical trials was 180 to 480 mg once daily. Although current clinical experience with the 540 mg dose is limited, the dose may be increased to 540 mg with little or no increased risk of adverse reactions.

Dosage: Angina. Dosages for the treatment of angina should be adjusted to each patient's needs, starting with a dose of 120 mg once daily, which may be titrated to doses of up to 480 mg once daily. When necessary, titration may be carried out over a 7 to 14 day period.

SAFETY INFORMATION
Diltiazem hydrochloride is contraindicated in: (1) patients with sick sinus syndrome except in the presence of a functioning ventricular pacemaker; (2) patients with second or third degree AV block except in the presence of a functioning ventricular pacemaker; (3) patients with hypotension (less than 90 mmHg systolic); (4) patients who have demonstrated hypersensitivity to the drug; and (5) patients with acute myocardial infarction and pulmonary congestion as documented by X-ray on admission.

PRESCRIBING INFORMATION

DILACOR XR® ℞
(diltiazem HCl)
Extended-release Capsules

DESCRIPTION
Dilacor XR® (diltiazem hydrochloride) is a calcium ion influx inhibitor (slow channel blocker or calcium antagonist). Chemically, diltiazem hydrochloride is 1,5-Benzothiazepin-4(5H)one,3-(acetyloxy)-5-[2-(dimethylamino) ethyl]-2,3-dihydro-2-(4-methoxyphenyl)-, monohydrochloride, (+)-cis-. Its molecular formula is $C_{22}H_{26}N_2O_4S \cdot HCl$ and its molecular weight is 450.98. Its structural formula is as follows:

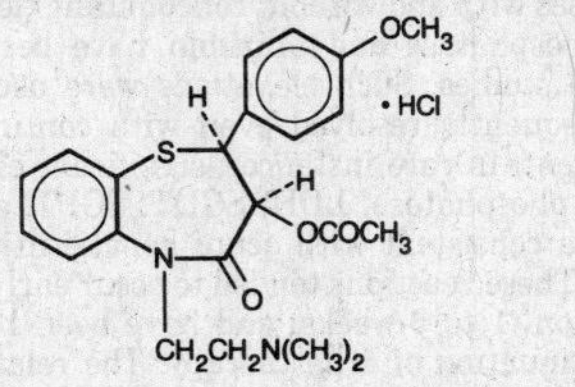

Diltiazem hydrochloride is a white to off-white crystalline powder with a bitter taste. It is soluble in water, methanol and chloroform.
Dilacor XR capsules contain multiple units of diltiazem HCl Extended-release 60 mg, resulting in 120 mg, 180 mg or 240 mg dosage strengths.
Inactive Ingredients: Dilacor XR capsules also contain mannitol, ethyl cellulose, hydroxypropyl methylcellulose, hydrogenated castor oil, ferric oxides, silicon dioxide, magnesium stearate, gelatin, D&C Yellow No. 10, FD&C Red No. 40, D&C Red No. 28, and titanium dioxide. The 120 mg dosage form contains pregelatinized starch.
For oral administration.

CLINICAL PHARMACOLOGY
The therapeutic benefits of diltiazem hydrochloride are believed to be related to its ability to inhibit the influx of calcium ions during membrane depolarization of cardiac and vascular smooth muscle.
Mechanisms of Action. Hypertension. Dilacor XR produces its antihypertensive effect primarily by relaxation of vascular smooth muscle with a resultant decrease in peripheral vascular resistance. The magnitude of blood pressure reduction is related to the degree of hypertension; thus hypertensive individuals experience an antihypertensive effect, whereas there is only a modest fall in blood pressure in normotensives.
Angina. Diltiazem HCl has been shown to produce increases in exercise tolerance, probably due to its ability to reduce myocardial oxygen demand. This is accomplished via reductions in heart rate and systemic blood pressure at submaximal and maximal work loads.
Diltiazem has been shown to be a potent dilator of coronary arteries, both epicardial and subendocardial. Spontaneous and ergonovine-induced coronary artery spasm are inhibited by diltiazem.
In animal models, diltiazem interferes with the slow inward (depolarizing) current in excitable tissue. It causes excitation-contraction uncoupling in various myocardial tissues without changes in the configuration of the action potential. Diltiazem produces relaxation of coronary vascular smooth muscle and dilation of both large and small coronary arteries at drug levels which cause little or no negative inotropic effect. The resultant increases in coronary blood flow (epicardial and subendocardial) occur in ischemic and nonischemic models and are accompanied by dose-dependent decreases in systemic blood pressure and decreases in peripheral resistance.
Hemodynamic and Electrophysiologic Effects. Like other calcium antagonists, diltiazem decreases sinoatrial and atrioventricular conduction in isolated tissues and has a negative inotropic effect in isolated preparations. In the intact animal, prolongation of the AH interval can be seen at higher doses.
In man, diltiazem prevents spontaneous and ergonovine-provoked coronary artery spasm. It causes a decrease in peripheral vascular resistance and a modest fall in blood pressure in normotensive individuals. In exercise tolerance studies in patients with ischemic heart disease, diltiazem reduces the double product (HR × SBP) for any given work load. Studies to date, primarily in patients with good ventricular function, have not revealed evidence of a negative inotropic effect. Cardiac output, ejection fraction and left ventricular end diastolic pressure have not been affected. Such data have no predictive value with respect to effects in patients with poor ventricular function. Increased heart failure has, however, been reported in occasional patients with pre-existing impairment of ventricular function. There are as yet few data on the interaction of diltiazem and beta-blockers in patients with poor ventricular function. Resting heart rate is usually slightly reduced by diltiazem.
Dilacor XR produces antihypertensive effects both in the supine and standing positions. Postural hypotension is infrequently noted upon suddenly assuming an upright position. Diltiazem decreases vascular resistance, increases cardiac output (by increasing stroke volume), and produces a slight decrease or no change in heart rate. No reflex tachycardia is associated with the chronic antihypertensive effects.
During dynamic exercise, increases in diastolic pressure are inhibited while maximum achievable systolic pressure is usually reduced. Heart rate at maximum exercise does not change or is slightly reduced.
Diltiazem antagonizes the renal and peripheral effects of angiotensin II. No increased activity of the renin-angiotensin-aldosterone axis has been observed. Chronic therapy with diltiazem produces no change or an increase in plasma catecholamines. Hypertensive animal models respond to diltiazem with reductions in blood pressure and increased urinary output and natriuresis without a change in the urinary sodium/potassium ratio. In man, transient natriuresis and kaliuresis have been reported, but only in high intravenous doses of 0.5 mg/kg of body weight.
Diltiazem-associated prolongation of the AH interval is not more pronounced in patients with first-degree heart block. In patients with sick sinus syndrome, diltiazem significantly prolongs sinus cycle length (up to 50% in some cases). Intravenous diltiazem in doses of 20 mg prolongs AH conduction time and AV node functional and effective refractory periods approximately 20%.
In two short-term, double-blind, placebo-controlled studies, 303 hypertensive patients were treated with once-daily Dilacor XR in doses of up to 540 mg. There were no instances of greater than first-degree atrioventricular block, and the maximum increase in the PR interval was .08 seconds. No patients were prematurely discontinued from the medication due to symptoms related to prolongation of the PR interval.
Pharmacodynamics. In one short-term, double-blind, placebo-controlled study, Dilacor XR 120, 240, 360 and 480 mg/day demonstrated a dose-related antihypertensive response among patients with mild to moderate hypertension. Statistically significant decreases in trough mean supine diastolic blood pressure were seen through four weeks of treatment: 120 mg/day (−5.1 mmHg); 240 mg/day (−6.9 mmHg); 360 mg/day (−6.9 mmHg); and 480 mg/day (−10.6 mmHg). Statistically significant decreases in trough mean supine systolic blood pressure were also seen through four weeks of treatment: 120 mg/day (−2.6 mmHg); 240 mg/day (−6.5 mmHg); 360 mg/day (−4.8 mmHg); and 480 mg/day (−10.6 mmHg). The proportion of evaluable patients exhibiting a therapeutic response (supine diastolic blood pressure <90 mmHg or decrease >10 mmHg) was greater as the dose increased: 31%, 42%, 48% and 69% with the 120, 240, 360 and 480 mg/day diltiazem groups, respectively. Similar findings were observed for standing systolic and diastolic blood pressures. The trough (24 hours after a dose) antihypertensive effect of Dilacor XR retained more than one-half of the response seen at peak (3–6 hours after administration).
Significant reductions of mean supine blood pressure (at trough) in patients with mild to moderate hypertension were also seen in a short-term, double-blind, dose-escalation, placebo-controlled study after 2 weeks of once-daily Dilacor XR 180 mg/day (diastolic: −6.1 mmHg; systolic: −4.7 mmHg) and again, 2 weeks after escalation to 360 mg/day (diastolic: −9.3 mmHg; systolic: −7.2 mmHg). However, a further increase in dose to 540 mg/day for 2 weeks provided only a minimal further increase in the antihypertensive effect (diastolic: −10.2 mmHg; systolic: −6.7 mmHg).
Dilacor XR, given at 120 mg, 240 mg, and 480 mg/day, in a randomized, multicenter, double-blind, placebo-controlled, parallel group, dose-ranging study, in 189 patients with chronic angina, demonstrated a dose-related increase in exercise time by Exercise Tolerance Test (ETT) and a reduction in rates of anginal attacks (based on individual patients diaries). The improvement in total exercise time (using the Bruce protocol), measured at trough exercise periods, for placebo, 120 mg, 240 mg, and 480 mg, was 20, 37, 49, and 56 seconds, respectively.

Continued on next page

Rhône-Poulenc Rorer—Cont.

Pharmacokinetics and Metabolism. Diltiazem is well-absorbed from the gastrointestinal tract, and is subject to an extensive first-pass effect. When given as an immediate release oral formulation, the absolute bioavailability (compared to intravenous administration) of diltiazem is approximately 40%. Diltiazem undergoes extensive hepatic metabolism in which 2% to 4% of the unchanged drug appears in the urine. Total radioactivity measurement following short IV administration in healthy volunteers suggests the presence of other unidentified metabolites which attain higher concentrations than those of diltiazem and are more slowly eliminated; half-life of total radioactivity is about 20 hours compared to 2 to 5 hours for diltiazem. *In-vitro* binding studies show diltiazem HCl is 70% to 80% bound to plasma proteins. Competitive *in-vitro* ligand binding studies have also shown diltiazem HCl binding is not altered by therapeutic concentrations of digoxin, HCTZ, phenylbutazone, propranolol, salicylic acid, or warfarin. The plasma elimination half-life of diltiazem is approximately 3.0 to 4.5 hours. Desacetyl-diltiazem, the major metabolite of diltiazem, which is also present in the plasma at concentrations of 10% to 20% of the parent drug, is approximately 25% to 50% as potent a coronary vasodilator as diltiazem. Therapeutic blood levels of diltiazem hydrochloride appear to be in the range of 40-200 ng/mL. There is a departure from linearity when dose strengths are increased; the half-life is slightly increased with dose.

A study that compared patients with normal hepatic function to patients with cirrhosis found an increase in half-life and a 69% increase in bioavailability in the hepatically impaired patients. A single study in patients with severely impaired renal function showed no difference in the pharmacokinetic profile of diltiazem compared to patients with normal renal function.

Dilacor XR capsules contain a degradable controlled-release tablet formulation designed to release diltiazem over a 24-hour period. Geomatrix™, a registered trademark of Jago Research AG, Zollikon, Switzerland, is a patented controlled-release system incorporated in the tablets. Controlled absorption of diltiazem begins within 1 hour, with maximum plasma concentrations being achieved 4 to 6 hours after administration. The apparent steady-state half-life of diltiazem following once-daily administration of Dilacor XR capsules ranges from 5 to 10 hours. This prolongation of half-life is attributed to continued absorption of diltiazem rather than to alterations in its elimination.

Neither the absolute bioavailability of Dilacor XR capsules nor its relative bioavailability compared to immediate release products has been definitively determined. No information is currently available as to the relative bioavailability of Dilacor XR capsules compared to other approved controlled-release diltiazem products.

As the dose of Dilacor XR capsules is increased from a daily dose of 120 mg to 240 mg, there is an increase in the AUC of 2.3 fold. When the dose is increased from 240 mg to 360 mg, AUC increases 1.6 fold and when increased from 240 mg to 480 mg, AUC increases 2.4 fold.

In-vivo release of diltiazem occurs throughout the gastrointestinal tract, with controlled release still occurring for up to 24 hours after administration, as determined by radio-labelled methods. As the once-daily dose of Dilacor XR was increased, departures from linearity were noted. There were disproportionate increases in area under the curve for doses from 120 mg to 480 mg.

The presence of food did not affect the ability of Dilacor XR to maintain a continuous release of drug for up to 24 hours after administration. Simultaneous administration of Dilacor XR with a high-fat breakfast had a modest effect on diltiazem bioavailability with AUC increasing by 13% and C_{max} by 37%.

INDICATIONS AND USAGE

Dilacor XR is indicated for the treatment of hypertension. Diltiazem hydrochloride may be used alone or in combination with other antihypertensive medications, such as diuretics.

Dilacor XR is indicated for the management of chronic stable angina.

CONTRAINDICATIONS

Diltiazem hydrochloride is contraindicated in: (1) patients with sick sinus syndrome except in the presence of a functioning ventricular pacemaker; (2) patients with second or third degree AV block except in the presence of a functioning ventricular pacemaker; (3) patients with hypotension (less than 90 mmHg systolic); (4) patients who have demonstrated hypersensitivity to the drug; and (5) patients with acute myocardial infarction and pulmonary congestion as documented by X-ray on admission.

WARNINGS

1. Cardiac Conduction. Diltiazem hydrochloride prolongs AV node refractory periods without significantly prolonging sinus node recovery time, except in patients with sick sinus syndrome. This effect may rarely result in abnormally slow heart rates (particularly in patients with sick sinus syndrome) or second, or third degree AV block (22 of 10,119 patients, or 0.2%); 41% of these 22 patients were receiving concomitant β-adrenoceptor antagonists versus 17% of the total group. Concomitant use of diltiazem with beta-blockers or digitalis may result in additive effects on cardiac conduction. A patient with Prinzmetal's angina developed periods of asystole (2 to 5 seconds) after a single 60 mg dose of diltiazem.

2. Congestive Heart Failure. Although diltiazem has a negative inotropic effect in isolated animal tissue preparations, hemodynamic studies in humans with normal ventricular function have not shown a reduction in cardiac index nor consistent negative effects on contractility (dp/dt). An acute study of oral diltiazem in patients with impaired ventricular function (ejection fraction of 24% ± 6%) showed improvement in indices of ventricular function without significant decrease in contractile function (dp/dt). Worsening of congestive heart failure has been reported in patients with preexisting impairment of ventricular function. Experience with the use of diltiazem hydrochloride in combination with beta-blockers in patients with impaired ventricular function is limited. Caution should be exercised when using this combination.

3. Hypotension. Decreases in blood pressure associated with diltiazem hydrochloride therapy may occasionally result in symptomatic hypotension.

4. Acute Hepatic Injury. Mild elevations of serum transaminases with and without concomitant elevation in alkaline phosphatase and bilirubin have been observed in clinical studies. Such elevations were usually transient and frequently resolved even with continued diltiazem treatment. In rare instances, significant elevations in alkaline phosphatase, LDH, SGOT, SGPT, and other phenomena consistent with acute hepatic injury have been noted. These reactions tended to occur early after therapy initiation (1 to 6 weeks) and have been reversible upon discontinuation of drug therapy. The relationship to diltiazem is uncertain in some cases, but probable in some others (see PRECAUTIONS).

PRECAUTIONS

General. Diltiazem hydrochloride is extensively metabolized by the liver and is excreted by the kidneys and in bile. As with any drug given over prolonged periods, laboratory parameters should be monitored at regular intervals. The drug should be used with caution in patients with impaired renal or hepatic function. In subacute and chronic dog and rat studies designed to produce toxicity, high doses of diltiazem were associated with hepatic damage. In special subacute hepatic studies, oral doses of 125 mg/kg and higher in rats were associated with histological changes in the liver which were reversible when the drug was discontinued. In dogs, doses of 20 mg/kg were also associated with hepatic changes; however, these changes were reversible with continued dosing.

Dermatological events (see ADVERSE REACTIONS) may be transient and may disappear despite continued use of diltiazem hydrochloride. However, skin eruptions progressing to erythema multiforme and/or exfoliative dermatitis have also been infrequently reported. Should a dermatologic reaction persist, the drug should be discontinued.

Although Dilacor XR utilizes a slowly disintegrating matrix, caution should still be used in patients with preexisting severe gastrointestinal narrowing (pathologic or iatrogenic). There have been no reports of obstructive symptoms in patients with known strictures in association with the ingestion of Dilacor XR.

Information for Patients. Dilacor XR capsules should be taken on an empty stomach. Patients should be cautioned that the Dilacor XR capsules should not be opened, chewed or crushed, and should be swallowed whole.

Drug Interaction. Due to the potential for additive effects, caution and careful titration are warranted in patients receiving diltiazem hydrochloride concomitantly with any agents known to affect cardiac contractility and/or conduction (see WARNINGS). Pharmacologic studies indicate that there may be additive effects in prolonging AV conduction when using beta-blockers or digitalis concomitantly with diltiazem hydrochloride (see WARNINGS). As with all drugs, care should be exercised when treating patients with multiple medications. Diltiazem hydrochloride undergoes biotransformation by cytochrome P-450 mixed function oxidase. Co-administration of diltiazem hydrochloride with other agents which follow the same route of biotransformation may result in the competitive inhibition of metabolism. Especially in patients with renal and/or hepatic impairment, dosages of similarly metabolized drugs, particularly those of low therapeutic ratio such as cyclosporin, may require adjustment when starting or stopping concomitantly administered diltiazem hydrochloride to maintain optimum therapeutic blood levels. Concomitant administration of diltiazem with carbamazepine has been reported to result in elevated plasma levels of carbamazepine, resulting in toxicity in some cases.

Beta-Blockers: Controlled and uncontrolled domestic studies suggest that concomitant use of diltiazem hydrochloride and beta-blockers is usually well-tolerated, but available data are not sufficient to predict the effects of concomitant treatment in patients with left ventricular dysfunction or cardiac conduction abnormalities. Administration of diltiazem hydrochloride concomitantly with propranolol in five normal volunteers resulted in increased propranolol levels in all subjects and the bioavailability of propranolol was increased approximately 50%. If combination therapy is initiated or withdrawn in conjunction with propranolol, an adjustment in the propranolol dose may be warranted (see WARNINGS).

Cimetidine: A study in six healthy volunteers has shown a significant increase in peak diltiazem plasma levels (58%) and area-under-the-curve (53%) after a 1-week course of cimetidine at 1,200 mg per day and diltiazem 60 mg per day. Ranitidine produced smaller, nonsignificant increases. The effect may be mediated by cimetidine's known inhibition of hepatic cytochrome P-450, the enzyme system responsible for the first-pass metabolism of diltiazem. Patients currently receiving diltiazem therapy should be carefully monitored for a change in pharmacological effect when initiating and discontinuing therapy with cimetidine. An adjustment in the diltiazem dose may be warranted.

Digitalis: Administration of diltiazem hydrochloride with digoxin in 24 healthy male subjects increased plasma digoxin concentrations approximately 20%. Another investigator found no increase in digoxin levels in 12 patients with coronary artery disease. Since there have been conflicting results regarding the effect of digoxin levels, it is recommended that digoxin levels be monitored when initiating, adjusting, and discontinuing diltiazem hydrochloride therapy to avoid possible over- or under-digitalization (see WARNINGS).

Anesthetics: The depression of cardiac contractility, conductivity, and automaticity as well as the vascular dilation associated with anesthetics may be potentiated by calcium channel blockers. When used concomitantly, anesthetics and calcium channel blockers should be titrated carefully.

Carcinogenesis, Mutagenesis, Impairment of Fertility. A 24-month study in rats and an 18-month study in mice showed no evidence of carcinogenicity. There was also no mutagenic response *in-vitro* or *in-vivo* in mammalian cell assays or *in-vitro* in bacteria. No evidence of impaired fertility was observed in male or female rats at oral doses of up to 100 mg/kg/day.

Pregnancy. Category C. Reproduction studies have been conducted in mice, rats and rabbits. Administration of doses ranging from 4 to 6 times (depending on species) the upper limit of the optimum dosage range in clinical trials (480 mg q.d. or 8 mg/kg q.d. for a 60 kg patient) has resulted in embryo and fetal lethality. These studies have revealed, in one species or another, a propensity to cause abnormalities of the skeleton, heart, retina and tongue. Also observed were reductions in early individual pup weights and pup survival, prolonged delivery and increased incidence of stillbirths. There are no well-controlled studies in pregnant women; therefore, use diltiazem hydrochloride in pregnant women only if the potential benefit justifies the potential risk to the fetus.

Nursing Mothers. Diltiazem is excreted in human milk. One report suggests that concentrations in breast milk may approximate serum levels. If use of diltiazem hydrochloride is deemed essential, an alternative method of infant feeding should be instituted.

Pediatric Use. Safety and effectiveness in children have not been established.

ADVERSE REACTIONS

Serious adverse reactions to diltiazem hydrochloride have been rare in studies with other formulations, as well as with Dilacor XR®. It should be recognized, however, that patients with impaired ventricular function and cardiac conduction abnormalities have usually been excluded from these studies.

Hypertension: The most common adverse events (frequency ≥1%) in placebo-controlled, clinical hypertension studies with Dilacor XR using daily doses up to 540 mg, are listed in the table below with placebo-treated patients included for comparison.

MOST COMMON ADVERSE EVENTS IN
DOUBLE-BLIND, PLACEBO-CONTROLLED
HYPERTENSION TRIALS

Adverse Events (COSTART Term)	Dilacor XR®* n=303 # pts (%)	Placebo n=87 # pts (%)
rhinitis	29 (9.6)	7 (8.0)
headache	27 (8.9)	12 (13.8)
pharyngitis	17 (5.6)	4 (4.6)
constipation	11 (3.6)	2 (2.3)
cough increase	9 (3.0)	2 (2.3)
flu syndrome	7 (2.3)	1 (1.1)
edema, peripheral	7 (2.3)	0 (0.0)

myalgia	7 (2.3)	0 (0.0)
diarrhea	6 (2.0)	0 (0.0)
vomiting	6 (2.0)	0 (0.0)
sinusitis	6 (2.0)	1 (1.1)
asthenia	5 (1.7)	0 (0.0)
pain, back	5 (1.7)	2 (2.3)
nausea	5 (1.7)	1 (1.1)
dyspepsia	4 (1.3)	0 (0.0)
vasodilatation	4 (1.3)	0 (0.0)
injury, accident	4 (1.3)	0 (0.0)
pain, abdominal	3 (1.0)	0 (0.0)
arthrosis	3 (1.0)	0 (0.0)
insomnia	3 (1.0)	0 (0.0)
dyspnea	3 (1.0)	0 (0.0)
rash	3 (1.0)	1 (1.1)
tinnitus	3 (1.0)	0 (0.0)

* Adverse events occurring in 1% or more of patients receiving Dilacor XR.

Angina: The most common adverse events (frequency ≥1%) in a placebo-controlled, short-term (2 week) clinical angina study with Dilacor XR are listed in the table below with placebo-treated patients included for comparison. In this trial, following a placebo phase, patients were randomly assigned to once-daily doses of either 120, 240 or 480 mg of Dilacor XR.

MOST COMMON ADVERSE EVENTS IN A DOUBLE-BLIND, PLACEBO-CONTROLLED SHORT-TERM, ANGINA TRIAL

Adverse Events (COSTART Term)	Dilacor XR®* n=139 # pts (%)	Placebo n=50 # pts (%)
asthenia	5 (3.6)	2 (4.0)
headache	4 (2.9)	3 (6.0)
pain, back	4 (2.9)	1 (2.0)
rhinitis	4 (2.9)	1 (2.0)
constipation	3 (2.2)	1 (2.0)
nausea	3 (2.2)	0 (0.0)
edema, peripheral	3 (2.2)	1 (2.0)
dizziness	3 (2.2)	0 (0.0)
cough, increased	3 (2.2)	0 (0.0)
bradycardia	2 (1.4)	0 (0.0)
fibrillation, atrial	2 (1.4)	0 (0.0)
arthralgia	2 (1.4)	0 (0.0)
dream, abnormal	2 (1.4)	0 (0.0)
dyspnea	2 (1.4)	0 (0.0)
pharyngitis	2 (1.4)	1 (2.0)

* Adverse events occurring in 1% or more of patients receiving Dilacor XR.

Infrequent Adverse Events. The following additional events (COSTART Terms), listed by body system, were reported infrequently (less than 1%) in all subjects, hypertensive (n=425) or angina (n=318) patients who received Dilacor XR, or with other formulations of diltiazem.

Hypertension. Cardiovascular: First-degree AV block, arrhythmia, postural hypotension, tachycardia, pallor, palpitations, phlebitis, ECG abnormality, ST elevation.
Nervous System: Vertigo, hypertonia, paresthesia, dizziness, somnolence.
Digestive System: Dry mouth, anorexia, tooth disorder, eructation.
Skin and Appendages: Sweating, urticaria, skin hypertrophy (nevus).
Respiratory System: Epistaxis, bronchitis, respiratory disorder.
Urogenital System: Cystitis, kidney calculus, impotence, dysmenorrhea, vaginitis, prostate disease.
Metabolic and Nutritional Disorders: Gout, edema.
Musculoskeletal System: Arthralgia, bursitis, bone pain.
Hemic and Lymphatic System: Lymphadenopathy.
Body as a Whole: Pain, unevaluable reaction, neck pain, neck rigidity, fever, chest pain, malaise.
Special Senses: Amblyopia (blurred vision), ear pain.
Angina. Cardiovascular: Palpitations, AV block, sinus bradycardia, bigeminal extrasystole, angina pectoris, hypertension, hypotension, myocardial infarct, myocardial ischemia, syncope, vasodilatation, ventricular extrasystole.
Nervous System: Abnormal thinking, neuropathy, paresthesia.
Digestive System: Diarrhea, dyspepsia, vomiting, colitis, flatulence, GI hemorrhage, stomach ulcers.
Skin and Appendages: Contact dermatitis, pruritus, sweating.
Respiratory System: Respiratory distress.
Urogenital System: Kidney failure, pyelonephritis, urinary tract infection.
Metabolic and Nutritional Disorders: Weight increase.
Musculoskeletal System: Myalgia.
Body as a Whole: Chest pain, accidental injury, infection.
Special Senses: Eye hemorrhage, ophthalmitis, otitis media, taste perversion, tinnitus.

Strength	Size	NDC 0075-	Color	Markings
120 mg	Bottles of 100	0250-00	gold cap white body	DilacorXR 120 mg
	Bottles of 1000	0250-99		
180 mg	Bottles of 100	0251-00	orange cap white body	DilacorXR 180 mg
	Unit Dose 100	0251-62		
	Bottles of 1000	0251-99		
240 mg	Bottles of 100	0252-00	brown cap white body	DilacorXR 240 mg
	Unit Dose 100	0252-62		
	Bottles of 1000	0252-99		

There have been post-marketing reports of Stevens-Johnson syndrome and toxic epidermal necrolysis associated with the use of diltiazem hydrochloride.

OVERDOSAGE OR EXAGGERATED RESPONSE

Overdosage experience with oral diltiazem hydrochloride has been limited. The administration of ipecac to induce vomiting and activated charcoal to reduce drug absorption have been advocated as initial means of intervention. In addition to gastric lavage, the following measures should also be considered:

Bradycardia: Administer atropine (0.60 mg to 1.0 mg). If there is no response to vagal blockade, administer isoproterenol cautiously.
High-Degree AV Block: Treat as for bradycardia above. Fixed high-degree AV block should be treated with cardiac pacing.
Cardiac Failure: Administer inotropic agents (dopamine or dobutamine) and diuretics.
Hypotension: Vasopressors (e.g. dopamine, or levarterenol bitartrate).

Actual treatment and dosage should depend on the severity of the clinical situation as well as the judgment and experience of the treating physician.

Due to extensive metabolism, plasma concentrations after a standard dose of diltiazem can vary over tenfold, which significantly limits their value in evaluating cases of overdosage.

Charcoal hemoperfusion has been used successfully as an adjunct therapy to hasten drug elimination. Overdoses with as much as 10.8 gm of oral diltiazem have been successfully treated using appropriate supportive care.

DOSAGE AND ADMINISTRATION

Hypertensive or anginal patients who are treated with other formulations of diltiazem can safely be switched to Dilacor XR capsules at the nearest equivalent total daily dose. Subsequent titration to higher or lower doses may, however, be necessary and should be initiated as clinically indicated.

Studies have shown a slight increase in the rate of absorption of Dilacor XR, when ingested with a high-fat breakfast; therefore, administration in the morning on an empty stomach is recommended.

Patients should be cautioned that the Dilacor XR capsules should not be opened, chewed or crushed and should be swallowed whole.

Dosage: Hypertension. Dosages must be adjusted to each patient's needs, starting with 180 mg or 240 mg once-daily. Based on the antihypertensive effect, the dose may be adjusted as needed. Individual patients, particularly ≥ 60 years of age, may respond to a lower dose of 120 mg. The usual dosage range studied in clinical trials was 180 mg to 480 mg once daily. Although current clinical experience with the 540 mg dose is limited, the dose may be increased to 540 mg with little or no increased risk of adverse reactions. Doses should not exceed 540 mg once-daily.

While a dose of Dilacor XR given once-daily may produce an antihypertensive effect similar to the same total daily dose given in divided doses, individual dose adjustment may be needed.

Dosage: Angina. Dosages for the treatment of angina should be adjusted to each patient's needs, starting with a dose of 120 mg once-daily, which may be titrated to doses of up to 480 mg once-daily. When necessary, titration may be carried out over a 7 to 14 day period.

Concomitant Use with Other Cardiovascular Agents.
1. **Sublingual Nitroglycerin** may be taken as required to abort acute anginal attacks during diltiazem hydrochloride therapy.
2. **Prophylactic Nitrate Therapy**—Diltiazem hydrochloride may be safely co-administered with short- and long-acting nitrates.

3. **Beta-blockers.** (See WARNINGS and PRECAUTIONS.)
4. **Antihypertensives**—Diltiazem hydrochloride has an additive antihypertensive effect when used with other antihypertensive agents. Therefore, the dosage of diltiazem hydrochloride or the concomitant antihypertensives may need to be adjusted when adding one to the other.

HOW SUPPLIED
[See table above.]

	National Stock Number	
Strength	Size	NSN
120 mg	Bottles of 100	6505-01-365-8942
	Bottles of 1000	6505-01-393-7440
180 mg	Bottles of 100	6505-01-355-3602
	Bottles of 1000	6505-01-393-7319
240 mg	Bottles of 100	6505-01-355-3601
	Bottles of 1000	6505-01-393-7437

STORE AT CONTROLLED ROOM TEMPERATURE, 15°–30°C (59°–86°F).
CAUTION: FEDERAL (U.S.A.) LAW PROHIBITS DISPENSING WITHOUT PRESCRIPTION.
Rev. 2/96   IN-5887
RHÔNE-POULENC RORER PHARMACEUTICALS INC.
Collegeville, PA, U.S.A. 19426-0107
Shown in Product Identification Guide, page 330

INTAL® Inhaler   ℞
[in'tăl]
(cromolyn sodium inhalation aerosol)

DESCRIPTION

The active ingredient of INTAL Inhaler is cromolyn sodium, USP. It is an inhaled anti-inflammatory agent for the preventive management of asthma. Cromolyn sodium is disodium 5,5'-[(2-hydroxytrimethylene)dioxy]bis[4-oxo-4H-1-benzopyran-2-carboxylate]. The empirical formula is $C_{23}H_{14}Na_2O_{11}$; the molecular weight is 512.34. Cromolyn sodium is water soluble, odorless, white, hydrated crystalline powder. It is tasteless at first, but leaves a slightly bitter aftertaste.

The molecular structure of cromolyn sodium is:

INTAL Inhaler (cromolyn sodium inhalation aerosol) is a metered dose aerosol unit for oral inhalation containing micronized cromolyn sodium, sorbitan trioleate with dichlorotetrafluoroethane and dichlorodifluoromethane as propellants. Each actuation delivers approximately 800 mcg cromolyn sodium through the mouthpiece to the patient. Each 8.1 g canister delivers at least 112 metered inhalations (56 doses); each 14.2 g canister delivers at least 200 metered inhalations (100 doses).

CLINICAL PHARMACOLOGY

In vitro and *in vivo* animal studies have shown that cromolyn sodium inhibits sensitized mast cell degranulation which occurs after exposure to specific antigens. Cromolyn sodium acts by inhibiting the release of mediators from mast cells. Studies show that cromolyn sodium indirectly blocks calcium ions from entering the mast cell, thereby preventing mediator release.

Continued on next page

Rhône-Poulenc Rorer–Cont.

Cromolyn sodium inhibits both the immediate and non-immediate bronchoconstrictive reactions to inhaled antigen. Cromolyn sodium also attenuates bronchospasm caused by exercise, toluene diisocyanate, aspirin, cold air, sulfur dioxide, and environmental pollutants, at least in some patients. Cromolyn sodium has no intrinsic bronchodilator or antihistamine activity.

After administration of cromolyn sodium capsules by inhalation, approximately 8% of the total dose administered is absorbed and rapidly excreted unchanged, approximately equally divided between urine and bile. The remainder of the dose is either exhaled or deposited in the oropharynx, swallowed, and excreted via the alimentary tract.

INDICATIONS AND USAGE

INTAL Inhaler is a prophylactic agent indicated in the management of patients with bronchial asthma.

In patients whose symptoms are sufficiently frequent to require a continuous program of medication, INTAL Inhaler is given by inhalation on a regular daily basis (see Dosage and Administration). The effect of INTAL Inhaler is usually evident after several weeks of treatment, although some patients show an almost immediate response.

If improvement occurs, it will ordinarily occur within the first 4 weeks of administration as manifested by a decrease in the severity of clinical symptoms of asthma, or in the need for concomitant therapy, or both.

In patients who develop acute bronchoconstriction in response to exposure to exercise, toluene diisocyanate, environmental pollutants, known antigens, etc., INTAL Inhaler should be used shortly before exposure to the precipitating factor, i.e., within 10–15 minutes but not more than 60 minutes (see Dosage and Administration). INTAL Inhaler may be effective in relieving bronchospasm in some, but not all, patients with exercise induced bronchospasm.

CONTRAINDICATIONS

INTAL Inhaler is contraindicated in those patients who have shown hypersensitivity to cromolyn sodium or other ingredients in this preparation.

WARNINGS

INTAL Inhaler has no role in the treatment of an acute attack of asthma, especially status asthmaticus. Severe anaphylactic reactions can occur after cromolyn sodium administration. The recommended dosage should be decreased in patients with decreased renal or hepatic function. INTAL Inhaler should be discontinued if the patient develops eosinophilic pneumonia (or pulmonary infiltrates with eosinophilia). Because of the propellants in this preparation, it should be used with caution in patients with coronary artery disease or a history of cardiac arrhythmias.

PRECAUTIONS

General: In view of the biliary and renal routes of excretion for cromolyn sodium, consideration should be given to decreasing the dosage or discontinuing the administration of the drug in patients with impaired renal or hepatic function.

Occasionally, patients may experience cough and/or bronchospasm following cromolyn sodium inhalation. At times, patients who develop bronchospasm may not be able to continue administration despite prior bronchodilator administration. Rarely, very severe bronchospasm has been encountered.

Carcinogenesis, Mutagenesis, Impairment of Fertility: Long term studies in mice (12 months intraperitoneal treatment followed by 6 months observation), hamsters (12 months intraperitoneal treatment followed by 12 months observation), and rats (18 months subcutaneous treatment) showed no neoplastic effect of cromolyn sodium.

No evidence of chromosomal damage or cytotoxicity was obtained in various mutagenesis studies.

No evidence of impaired fertility was shown in laboratory animal reproduction studies.

Pregnancy: Pregnancy Category B. Reproduction studies with cromolyn sodium administered parenterally to pregnant mice, rats, and rabbits in doses up to 338 times the human clinical dose produced no evidence of fetal malformations. Adverse fetal effects (increased resorptions and decreased fetal weight) were noted only at the very high parenteral doses that produced maternal toxicity. There are, however, no adequate and well-controlled studies in pregnant women. Because animal reproduction studies are not always predictive of human response, this drug should be used during pregnancy only if clearly needed.

Drug Interaction During Pregnancy: Cromolyn sodium and isoproterenol were studied following subcutaneous injections in pregnant mice. Cromolyn sodium alone in doses of 60 to 540 mg/kg (38 to 338 times the human dose) did not cause significant increases in resorptions or major malformations. Isoproterenol alone at a dose of 2.7 mg/kg (90 times the human dose) increased both resorptions and malformations. The addition of cromolyn sodium (338 times the human dose) to isoproterenol (90 times the human dose) appears to have increased the incidence of both resorptions and malformations.

Nursing Mothers: It is not known whether this drug is excreted in human milk, therefore, caution should be exercised when INTAL Inhaler is administered to a nursing woman and the attending physician must make a benefit/risk assessment in regard to its use in this situation.

Pediatric Use: Safety and effectiveness in pediatric patients below the age of 5 years have not been established. For young pediatric patients unable to utilize the Inhaler, INTAL Nebulizer Solution (cromolyn sodium inhalation solution, USP) is recommended. Because of the possibility that adverse effects of this drug could become apparent only after many years, a benefit/risk consideration of the long-term use of INTAL Inhaler is particularly important in pediatric patients.

ADVERSE REACTIONS

In controlled clinical studies of INTAL Inhaler, the most frequently reported adverse reactions attributed to cromolyn sodium treatment were:

Throat irritation or dryness
Bad taste
Cough
Wheeze
Nausea

The most frequently reported adverse reactions attributed to other forms of cromolyn sodium (on the basis of reoccurrence following readministration) involve the respiratory tract and are: bronchospasm [sometimes severe, associated with a precipitous fall in pulmonary function (FEV_1)], cough, laryngeal edema (rare), nasal congestion (sometimes severe), pharyngeal irritation, and wheezing.

Adverse reactions which occur infrequently and are associated with administration of the drug are: anaphylaxis, angioedema, dizziness, dysuria and urinary frequency, joint swelling and pain, lacrimation, nausea and headache, rash, swollen parotid gland, urticaria, pulmonary infiltrates with eosinophilia, substernal burning, and myopathy.

The following adverse reactions have been reported as rare events and it is unclear whether they are attributable to the drug: anemia, exfoliative dermatitis, hemoptysis, hoarseness, myalgia, nephrosis, periarteritic vasculitis, pericarditis, peripheral neuritis, photodermatitis, sneezing, drowsiness, nasal itching, nasal bleeding, nasal burning, serum sickness, stomachache, polymyositis, vertigo, and liver disease.

OVERDOSAGE

No action other than medical observation should be necessary.

DOSAGE AND ADMINISTRATION

For management of bronchial asthma in adults and pediatric patients (5 years of age and over) who are able to use the Inhaler, the usual starting dosage is two metered inhalations four times daily at regular intervals. This dose should not be exceeded. Not all patients will respond to the recommended dose and there is evidence to suggest, at least in younger patients, that a lower dose may provide efficacy.

Patients with chronic asthma should be advised that the effect of INTAL Inhaler therapy is dependent upon its administration at regular intervals, as directed. INTAL Inhaler should be introduced into the patient's therapeutic regimen when the acute episode has been controlled, the airway has been cleared, and the patient is able to inhale adequately.

For the prevention of acute bronchospasm which follows exercise, exposure to cold dry air or environmental agents, the usual dose is two metered inhalations shortly, i.e., 10–15 minutes but not more than 60 minutes, before exposure to the precipitating factor.

INTAL Inhaler Therapy in Relation to Other Treatments for Asthma: Non-steroidal agents: INTAL Inhaler should be *added* to the patient's existing treatment regimen (e.g., bronchodilators). When a clinical response to INTAL Inhaler is evident, usually within two to four weeks, and if the asthma is under good control, an attempt may be made to decrease concomitant medication usage gradually.

If concomitant medications are eliminated or required on no more than a prn basis, the frequency of administration of INTAL Inhaler may be titrated downward to the lowest level consistent with the desired effect. The usual decrease is from two metered inhalations four times daily to three times daily to twice daily. It is important that the dosage be reduced gradually to avoid exacerbation of asthma. It is emphasized that in patients whose dosage has been titrated to fewer than four inhalations per day, an increase in the dosage of INTAL Inhaler and the introduction of, or increase in, symptomatic medications may be needed if the patient's clinical condition deteriorates.

Corticosteroids: In patients chronically receiving corticosteroids for the management of bronchial asthma, the dosage should be maintained following the introduction of INTAL Inhaler. If the patient improves, an attempt to decrease corticosteroids should be made. Even if the corticosteroid-dependent patient fails to show symptomatic improvement following INTAL Inhaler administration, the potential to reduce corticosteroids may nonetheless be present. Thus, gradual tapering of corticosteroid dosage may be attempted. It is important that the dose be reduced slowly, maintaining close supervision of the patient to avoid an exacerbation of asthma.

It should be borne in mind that prolonged corticosteroid therapy frequently causes an impairment in the activity of the hypothalamic-pituitary-adrenal axis and a reduction in the size of the adrenal cortex. A potentially critical degree of impairment or insufficiency may persist asymptomatically for some time even after gradual discontinuation of adrenocortical steroids. Therefore, if a patient is subjected to significant stress, such as a severe asthmatic attack, surgery, trauma, or severe illness while being treated or within one year (occasionally up to two years) after corticosteroid treatment has been terminated, consideration should be given to reinstituting corticosteroid therapy. When respiratory function is impaired, as may occur in severe exacerbation of asthma, a temporary increase in the amount of corticosteroids may be required to regain control of the patient's asthma.

It is particularly important that great care be exercised if for any reason cromolyn sodium is withdrawn in cases where its use has permitted a reduction in the maintenance dose of corticosteroids. In such cases, continued close supervision of the patient is essential since there may be sudden reappearance of severe manifestations of asthma which will require immediate therapy and possible reintroduction of corticosteroids.

HOW SUPPLIED

INTAL Inhaler, 8.1 g or 14.2 g canister, box of one. Supplied with mouthpiece and patient instructions.

NDC 0585-0675-01	14.2 g canister
NDC 0585-0675-02	8.1 g canister

Store between 15°–30°C (59°–86°F). Contents under pressure. Do not puncture, incinerate, or place near sources of heat. Keep out of the reach of children.

Note: The indented statement below is required by the Federal government's Clean Air Act for all products containing or manufactured with chlorofluorocarbons (CFC's).

> WARNING: Contains CFC-12 and CFC-114, substances which harm public health and environment by destroying ozone in the upper atmosphere.

A notice similar to the above WARNING has been placed in the "Patient Instructions for Use" portion of this package circular pursuant to EPA regulations.

CAUTION: Federal law prohibits dispensing without prescription.

Marketed by:
FISONS Pharmaceuticals
Fisons Corporation
Rochester, NY 14623 U.S.A.
Made in England
Manufactured by:
Health Care Specialties Division
3M Health Care Limited
Loughborough, England LE11 1EP
INTAL, FISONS, and the blue and white colors applied to the Inhaler are Registered Trademarks of Fisons plc. Rev. 10/95 RFO43E

Shown in Product Identification Guide page 330

INTAL® Nebulizer Solution ℞
(cromolyn sodium inhalation solution, USP)
For Inhalation Use Only—Not for Injection

DESCRIPTION

The active ingredient of INTAL Nebulizer Solution is cromolyn sodium, USP. It is an inhaled anti-inflammatory agent for the preventive management of asthma. Cromolyn sodium is the disodium salt of 1,3 bis (2-carboxychromon-5-yloxy)-2-hydroxypropane. The empirical formula is $C_{23}H_{14}Na_2O_{11}$; the molecular weight is 512.34. Cromolyn sodium is a water soluble, odorless, white, hydrated crystalline powder. It is tasteless at first, but leaves a slightly bitter aftertaste. INTAL Nebulizer Solution is clear, colorless, sterile, and has a target pH of 5.5.

The molecular structure is:

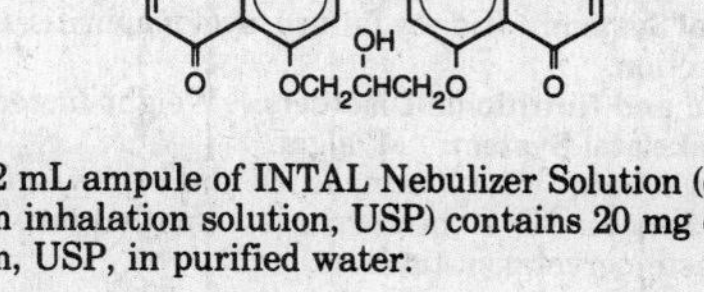

Each 2 mL ampule of INTAL Nebulizer Solution (cromolyn sodium inhalation solution, USP) contains 20 mg cromolyn sodium, USP, in purified water.

CLINICAL PHARMACOLOGY

In vitro and *in vivo* animal studies have shown that cromolyn sodium inhibits sensitized mast cell degranulation which occurs after exposure to specific antigens. Cromolyn sodium acts by inhibiting the release of mediators from mast cells. Studies show that cromolyn sodium indirectly blocks calcium ions from entering the mast cell, thereby preventing mediator release.

Cromolyn sodium inhibits both the immediate and nonimmediate bronchoconstrictive reactions to inhaled antigen. Cromolyn sodium also attenuates bronchospasm caused by exercise, toluene diisocyanate, aspirin, cold air, sulfur dioxide, and environmental pollutants.

Cromolyn sodium has no intrinsic bronchodilator or antihistamine activity.

After administration by inhalation, approximately 8% of the total cromolyn sodium dose administered is absorbed and rapidly excreted unchanged, approximately equally divided between urine and bile. The remainder of the dose is either exhaled or deposited in the oropharynx, swallowed and excreted via the alimentary tract.

INDICATIONS AND USAGE

INTAL is a prophylactic agent indicated in the management of patients with bronchial asthma.

In patients whose symptoms are sufficiently frequent to require a continuous program of medication, INTAL is given by inhalation on a regular daily basis (see **DOSAGE AND ADMINISTRATION**). The effect of INTAL is usually evident after several weeks of treatment, although some patients show an almost immediate response.

In patients who develop acute bronchoconstriction in response to exposure to exercise, toluene diisocyanate, environmental pollutants, etc., INTAL should be given shortly before exposure to the precipitating factor (see **DOSAGE AND ADMINISTRATION**).

CONTRAINDICATIONS

INTAL is contraindicated in those patients who have shown hypersensitivity to cromolyn sodium.

WARNINGS

INTAL has no role in the treatment of status asthmaticus.

PRECAUTIONS

General: Occasionally, patients may experience cough and/or bronchospasm following INTAL inhalation. At times, patients who develop bronchospasm may not be able to continue INTAL administration despite prior bronchodilator administration. Rarely, very severe bronchospasm has been encountered.

Symptoms of asthma may recur if INTAL is reduced below the recommended dosage or discontinued.

Information for Patients: INTAL is to be taken as directed by the physician. Because it is preventive medication, it may take up to four weeks before the patient experiences maximum benefit.

INTAL Nebulizer Solution should be used in a power-driven nebulizer with an adequate airflow rate equipped with a suitable face mask or mouthpiece.

For additional information, see the accompanying leaflet entitled "Living a Full Life with Asthma."

Carcinogenesis, Mutagenesis, and Impairment of Fertility: Long term studies in mice (12 months intraperitoneal treatment followed by 6 months observation), hamsters (12 months intraperitoneal treatment followed by 12 months observation), and rats (18 months subcutaneous treatment) showed no neoplastic effect of cromolyn sodium.

No evidence of chromosomal damage or cytotoxicity was obtained in various mutagenesis studies.

No evidence of impaired fertility was shown in laboratory animal reproduction studies.

Pregnancy: Pregnancy Category B. Reproduction studies with cromolyn sodium administered parenterally to pregnant mice, rats, and rabbits in doses up to 338 times the human clinical dose produced no evidence of fetal malformations. Adverse fetal effects (increased resorptions and decreased fetal weight) were noted only at the very high parenteral doses that produced maternal toxicity. There are, however, no adequate and well-controlled studies in pregnant women. Because animal reproduction studies are not always predictive of human response, this drug should be used during pregnancy only if clearly needed.

Drug Interaction During Pregnancy: Cromolyn sodium and isoproterenol were studied following subcutaneous injections in pregnant mice. Cromolyn sodium alone in doses of 60 to 540 mg/kg (38 to 338 times the human dose) did not cause significant increases in resorptions or major malformations. Isoproterenol alone at a dose of 2.7 mg/kg (90 times the human dose) increased both resorptions and malformations. The addition of cromolyn sodium (338 times the human dose) to isoproterenol (90 times the human dose) appears to have increased the incidence of both resorptions and malformations.

Nursing Mothers: It is not known whether this drug is excreted in human milk. Because many drugs are excreted in human milk, caution should be exercised when INTAL is administered to a nursing woman.

Pediatric Use: Safety and effectiveness in children below the age of 2 years have not been established.

ADVERSE REACTIONS

Clinical experience with the use of INTAL suggests that adverse reactions are rare events. The following adverse reactions have been associated with INTAL Nebulizer Solution: cough, nasal congestion, nausea, sneezing, and wheezing. Other reactions have been reported in clinical trials; however, a causal relationship could not be established: drowsiness, nasal itching, nose bleed, nose burning, serum sickness, and stomachache.

In addition, adverse reactions have been reported with INTAL Capsules (cromolyn sodium for inhalation, USP). The most common side effects are associated with inhalation of the powder and include transient cough (1 in 5 patients) and mild wheezing (1 in 25 patients). These effects rarely require treatment or discontinuation of the drug.

Information on the incidence of adverse reactions to INTAL Capsules has been derived from U.S. postmarketing surveillance experience. The following adverse reactions attributed to INTAL, based upon recurrence following readministration, have been reported in less than 1 in 10,000 patients: laryngeal edema, swollen parotid gland, angioedema, bronchospasm, joint swelling and pain, dizziness, dysuria and urinary frequency, nausea, cough, wheezing, headache, nasal congestion, rash, urticaria, and lacrimation.

Other adverse reactions have been reported in less than 1 in 100,000 patients, and it is unclear whether these are attributable to the drug: anaphylaxis, nephrosis, periarteritic vasculitis, pericarditis, peripheral neuritis, pulmonary infiltrates with eosinophilia, polymyositis, exfoliative dermatitis, hemoptysis, anemia, myalgia, hoarseness, photodermatitis, and vertigo.

OVERDOSAGE

There is no clinical syndrome associated with an overdosage of cromolyn sodium. Acute toxicity testing in a wide variety of species has demonstrated an extremely low order of toxicity for cromolyn sodium, regardless of whether administration was parenteral, oral or by inhalation. Parenteral administration in mice, rats, guinea pigs, hamsters, and rabbits demonstrated an LD_{50} in the region of 4000 mg/kg. Intravenous administration in monkeys also indicated a similar order of toxicity. The highest dose administered by the oral route in rats and mice was 8000 mg/kg, and at this dose level no deaths occurred. By inhalation, even in long term studies, it proved impossible to achieve toxic dose levels of cromolyn sodium in a range of mammalian species.

DOSAGE AND ADMINISTRATION

For management of bronchial asthma in adults and children (two years of age and over), the usual starting dosage is the contents of one ampule administered by nebulization four times a day at regular intervals.

Patients with chronic asthma should be advised that the effect of INTAL therapy is dependent upon its administration at regular intervals, as directed. INTAL should be introduced into the patient's therapeutic regimen when the acute episode has been controlled, the airway has been cleared and the patient is able to inhale adequately.

For the prevention of acute bronchospasm which follows exercise or exposure to cold dry air, environmental agents (e.g., animal danders, toluene diisocyanate, pollutants), etc., the usual dose is the contents of one ampule administered by nebulization shortly before exposure to the precipitating factor.

It should be emphasized to the patient that the drug is poorly absorbed when swallowed and is not effective by this route of administration.

INTAL Therapy in Relation to Other Treatments for Asthma: Non-steroidal agents

INTAL should be *added* to the patient's existing treatment regimen (e.g., bronchodilators). When a clinical response to INTAL is evident, usually within two to four weeks, and if the asthma is under good control, an attempt may be made to decrease concomitant medication usage gradually.

If concomitant medications are eliminated or required on no more than a prn basis, the frequency of administration of INTAL may be titrated downward to the lowest level consistent with the desired effect. The usual decrease is from four to three ampules per day. It is important that the dosage be reduced gradually to avoid exacerbation of asthma. It is emphasized that in patients whose dosage has been titrated to fewer than four ampules per day, an increase in the dose of INTAL and the introduction of, or increase in, symptomatic medications may be needed if the patient's clinical condition deteriorates.

Corticosteroids

In patients chronically receiving corticosteroids for the management of bronchial asthma, the dosage should be maintained following the introduction of INTAL. If the patient improves, an attempt to decrease corticosteroids should be made. Even if the corticosteroid-dependent patient fails to show symptomatic improvement following INTAL administration, the potential to reduce corticosteroids may nonetheless be present. Thus, gradual tapering of corticosteroid dosage may be attempted. It is important that the dose be reduced slowly, maintaining close supervision of the patient to avoid an exacerbation of asthma.

It should be borne in mind that prolonged corticosteroid therapy frequently causes an impairment in the activity of the hypothalamic-pituitary-adrenal axis and a reduction in the size of the adrenal cortex. A potentially critical degree of impairment or insufficiency may persist asymptomatically for some time even after gradual discontinuation of adrenocortical steroids. Therefore, if a patient is subjected to significant stress, such as a severe asthmatic attack, surgery, trauma or severe illness while being treated or within one year (occasionally up to two years) after corticosteroid treatment has been terminated, consideration should be given to reinstituting corticosteroid therapy. When respiratory function is impaired, as may occur in severe exacerbation of asthma, a temporary increase in the amount of corticosteroids may be required to regain control of the patient's asthma.

It is particularly important that great care be exercised if, for any reason, INTAL is withdrawn in cases where its use has permitted a reduction in the maintenance dose of corticosteroids. It such cases, continued close supervision of the patient is essential since there may be sudden reappearance of severe manifestations of asthma which will require immediate therapy and possible reintroduction of corticosteroids.

HOW SUPPLIED

INTAL Nebulizer Solution is a colorless solution supplied in a low density polyethylene plastic unit dose ampule with 12 ampules per foil pouch. Each 2 mL ampule contains 20 mg cromolyn sodium, USP, in purified water.

NDC 0585-0673-02	60 ampules × 2 mL
NDC 0585-0673-03	120 ampules × 2 mL

INTAL Nebulizer Solution should be stored between 15°–30°C (59°–86°F) and protected from light. Do not use if it contains a precipitate or becomes discolored. Keep out of the reach of children.

Store ampules in foil pouch until ready for use.

CAUTION: Federal law prohibits dispensing without prescription.

Marketed by:
FISONS Pharmaceuticals
Fisons Corporation
Rochester, NY 14623 U.S.A.
Manufactured by:
Automatic Liquid Packaging, Inc.
Woodstock, IL 60098
INTAL and FISONS are registered trademarks
of Fisons plc.   Rev. 4/94
©1994, Fisons Corporation   RF078B

Shown in Product Identification Guide, page 330

PRESCRIBING INFORMATION

LOVENOX®   ℞
(enoxaparin sodium) Injection

DESCRIPTION

Enoxaparin sodium is a sterile, low molecular weight heparin for injection. Each syringe contains 30 mg enoxaparin sodium in 0.3 mL Water for Injection. The approximate anti-Factor Xa activity per syringe is 3000 IU (with reference to the W.H.O. First International Low Molecular Weight Heparin Reference Standard). Nitrogen is used in the headspace to inhibit oxidation. The pH of the injection is 5.5–7.5. The solution is preservative-free and intended for use only as a single-dose injection.

Enoxaparin is obtained by alkaline degradation of heparin benzyl ester derived from porcine intestinal mucosa. Its structure is characterized by a 2-O-sulfo-4-enepyranosuronic acid group at the non-reducing end and a 2-N,6-O-disulfo-D-glucosamine at the reducing end of the chain. The substance is the sodium salt. The average molecular weight is about 4500. The molecular weight distribution is:

< 2000 daltons	≤20%
2000 to 8000 daltons	≥68%
> 8000 daltons	≤15%

STRUCTURAL FORMULA
[See chemical structure at top of next column.]

CLINICAL PHARMACOLOGY

Enoxaparin is a low molecular weight heparin which has antithrombotic properties. In man enoxaparin is characterized by a higher ratio of anti-Factor Xa to anti-Factor IIa activity (3.35 ± 0.89) than unfractionated heparin ($1.22 \pm$

Continued on next page

Rhône-Poulenc Rorer–Cont.

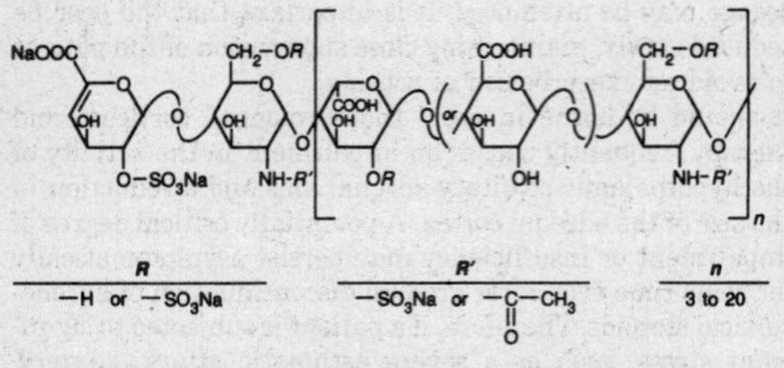

0.13). Following the administration of a single subcutaneous dose of up to 90 mg of enoxaparin to healthy subjects, no appreciable change was observed in fibrinogen level and other parameters of fibrinolysis. At the recommended doses, single injections of enoxaparin do not significantly influence platelet aggregation or affect global clotting tests (*i.e.* prothrombin time [PT] or activated partial thromboplastin time [APTT]).

Pharmacodynamics

Maximum anti-Factor Xa and antithrombin (anti-Factor IIa) activities occur 3 to 5 hours after subcutaneous injection of enoxaparin. Mean peak anti-Factor Xa activity was 0.16 IU/mL (1.58 µg/mL) and 0.38 IU/mL (3.83 µg/mL) after the 20 mg and the 40 mg clinically tested doses, respectively. Mean absolute bioavailability of enoxaparin based on anti-Factor Xa activity is 92% in healthy volunteers. The volume of distribution of anti-Factor Xa activity is about 6 L. Following i.v. dosing, the total body clearance of enoxaparin is 25 mL/min. Elimination half-life based on anti-Factor Xa activity was about 4.5 hours after subcutaneous administration. Following a 40 mg dose significant anti-Factor Xa activity persists in plasma for about 12 hours. There appears to be no appreciable increase in anti-Factor Xa activity after dosing for 3 days in young healthy subjects. Clearance and C_{max} derived from anti-Factor Xa values following single and multiple s.c. dosing in elderly subjects and subjects with renal failure were close to those observed in normal subjects. An increase of 25% in the area under anti-Factor Xa activity versus time curve was observed following once daily dosing in healthy elderly subjects for 10 days. The kinetics of anti-Factor Xa activity in anuric patients undergoing dialysis are similar to those in historical control normal subjects following i.v. dosing.

The decline of anti-Factor Xa activity with time was parallel to the decay curve of plasma total radioactivity (^{99m}Tc) in healthy volunteers. Following intravenous dosing of enoxaparin labeled with the gamma-emitter, ^{99m}Tc, 40% of radioactivity and 8–20% of anti-Factor Xa activity were recovered in urine in 24 hours.

CLINICAL TRIALS

Lovenox has been shown to prevent postoperative deep vein thrombosis (DVT) following hip or knee replacement surgery.

In a double-blind study, Lovenox 30 mg q12h sc was compared to placebo in hip replacement patients. Treatment was initiated within 12–24 hours post-surgery and was continued for 10–14 days post-operatively.

Treatment Group	Treatment Group: Lovenox	Placebo
Dosing Regimen	30 mg q12h n (%)	q12h n (%)
All Treated Patients	50 (100%)	50 (100%)
Treatment Failures		
Total DVT (%)	5 (10%)*	23 (46%)
Proximal DVT (%)	1 (2%)**	11 (22%)

* p value versus placebo = 0.0002
** p value versus placebo = 0.0134

A double-blind, multicenter study compared three dosing regimens of Lovenox in hip replacement patients. Treatment was initiated within two days post-surgery and was continued for 7–11 days post-operatively.

[See table below.]

There was no significant difference between the 30 mg BID and 40 mg QD regimens.

In a double-blind study with 99 patients undergoing knee replacement surgery, Lovenox 30 mg q12h sc was compared to placebo. Treatment was initiated within 12–24 hours post-operatively and was continued up to 15 days post-operatively. The incidence of post-operative proximal and total deep vein thrombosis was significantly lower for enoxaparin compared to placebo.

Treatment Group	Treatment Group: Lovenox	Placebo
Dosing Regimen	30 mg q12h n (%)	q12h n (%)
All Knee Replacement Patients	47 (100%)	52 (100%)
Treatment Failures		
Total DVT (%)	5 (11%)* (95% CI: 1–21%)	32 (62%) (95% CI: 47–76%)
Proximal DVT (%)	0 (0%)** (95% Upper CL: 5%)	7 (13%) (95% CI: 3–24%)

* p value versus placebo = 0.0001
CI = Confidence Interval
** p value versus placebo = 0.013
CL = Confidence Limit

Additionally, in an open-label, parallel group, randomized clinical study in patients undergoing elective knee replacement surgery, Lovenox 30 mg q12h sc was compared to unfractionated heparin 5000 U q8h sc. Treatment was initiated post-operatively and continued up to 14 days. The incidence of deep vein thrombosis was significantly lower for enoxaparin compared to heparin.

Dose	Treatment Group: Lovenox 10 mg QD	30 mg q12h	40 mg QD
	n (%)	n (%)	n (%)
All Treated Patients	161 (100%)	208 (100%)	199 (100%)
Treatment Failures			
Total DVT (%)	40 (25%)	22 (11%)*	27 (14%)**
Proximal DVT (%)	17 (11%)	8 (4%)	9 (5%)

* p value versus Lovenox 10 mg QD = 0.0008
** p value versus Lovenox 10 mg QD = 0.0168

INDICATIONS AND USAGE

Lovenox Injection is indicated for the prevention of deep vein thrombosis, which may lead to pulmonary embolism, following hip or knee replacement surgery.

CONTRAINDICATIONS

Lovenox Injection is contraindicated in patients with active major bleeding, in patients with thrombocytopenia associated with a positive *in vitro* test for anti-platelet antibody in the presence of enoxaparin sodium, or in patients with hypersensitivity to enoxaparin sodium.

Patients with known hypersensitivity to heparin or pork products should not be treated with Lovenox Injection.

WARNINGS

Lovenox Injection is not intended for intramuscular administration.

Lovenox cannot be used interchangeably (unit for unit) with unfractionated heparin or other low molecular weight heparins as they differ in their manufacturing process, molecular weight distribution, anti-Xa and anti-IIa activities, units and dosage. Special attention and compliance with the instructions for use specific to each proprietary medicinal product is therefore required.

Lovenox should be used with extreme caution in patients with a history of heparin-induced thrombocytopenia.

Hemorrhage:

Lovenox Injection, like other anticoagulants, should be used with extreme caution in conditions with increased risk of hemorrhage, such as bacterial endocarditis, congenital or acquired bleeding disorders, active ulcerative and angiodysplastic gastrointestinal disease, hemorrhagic stroke, or shortly after brain, spinal or ophthalmological surgery, or in patients treated concomitantly with platelet inhibitors.

Bleeding can occur at any site during therapy with enoxaparin. An unexplained fall in hematocrit or blood pressure should lead to a search for a bleeding site.

Neuraxial Anesthesia and Post-operative Indwelling Epidural Catheter Use:

Spinal/Epidural Anesthesia: As with other anticoagulants, there have been rare cases of neuraxial hematomas reported with the concurrent use of enoxaparin and spinal/epidural anesthesia resulting in long-term or permanent paralysis. The risk of these rare events may be higher with the use of post-operative indwelling epidural catheters.

Thrombocytopenia:

Thrombocytopenia can occur with the administration of Lovenox. Moderate thrombocytopenia (platelet counts between 100,000/mm^3 and 50,000/mm^3) occurred at a rate of 1.9% in patients given Lovenox, 2.0% in patients given heparin, and 1.7% in patients given placebo following hip or knee replacement surgery in clinical trials.

Platelet counts less than 50,000/mm^3 occurred at a rate of 0.1% in patients given Lovenox, 0.5% in patients given heparin, and 0% in patients given placebo in the same trials.

Thrombocytopenia of any degree should be monitored closely. If the platelet count falls below 100,000/mm^3, enoxaparin should be discontinued. Rare cases of thrombocytopenia with thrombosis have also been observed in clinical practice. The rate of incidence of this complication in usual medical practice is unknown at present.

PRECAUTIONS

General:

Lovenox Injection should not be mixed with other injections or infusions. Lovenox Injection should be used with care in patients with a bleeding diathesis, uncontrolled arterial hypertension or a history of recent gastrointestinal ulceration and hemorrhage. Elderly patients and patients with renal insufficiency may show delayed elimination of enoxaparin. Enoxaparin should be used with care in these patients.

If thromboembolic events occur despite enoxaparin prophylaxis, Lovenox should be discontinued and appropriate therapy initiated.

Laboratory Tests:

Periodic complete blood counts, including platelet count, and stool occult blood tests are recommended during the course of treatment with Lovenox Injection.

Drug Interactions:

It is recommended that agents which affect hemostasis be discontinued prior to Lovenox therapy as they may enhance the risk of hemorrhage. These agents include medications such as: oral anticoagulants, and/or platelet inhibitors including acetylsalicylic acid, salicylates, NSAIDs (including ketorolac tromethamine), dipyridamole, or sulfinpyrazone. If co-administration cannot be avoided and their use is essential, conduct close clinical and laboratory monitoring (see Laboratory Tests, PRECAUTIONS).

Drug/Laboratory Test Interactions:

Elevations of Serum Transaminases

Asymptomatic increases in aspartate (AST [SGOT]) and alanine (ALT [SGPT]) aminotransferase levels greater than three times the upper limit of normal of the laboratory reference range have been reported in 2 of 10 normal subjects and in up to 4% of patients during treatment with Lovenox® Injection. Similar significant increases in aminotransferase levels have also been observed in patients and normal volunteers treated with heparin and other low molecular weight heparins. Such elevations are fully reversible and are rarely associated with increases in bilirubin. Since aminotransferase determinations are important in the differential diagnosis of myocardial infarction, liver disease and pulmonary emboli, elevations that might be caused by drugs like Lovenox should be interpreted with caution.

Carcinogenesis, Mutagenesis, Impairment of Fertility:

No long-term studies in animals have been performed to evaluate carcinogenic potential of enoxaparin. Enoxaparin was not mutagenic in *in vitro* tests, including the Ames test, mouse lymphoma cell forward mutation test, and human lymphocyte chromosomal aberration test and the *in vivo* rat bone marrow chromosomal aberration test. Enoxaparin was found to have no effect on fertility or reproductive performance of male and female rats at subcutaneous doses up to 20 mg/kg/day or 141 mg/m^2/day. The maximum received human dose in clinical trials was 1.5 mg/kg/day or 48.4 mg/m^2/day.

Pregnancy: Teratogenic Effects

Pregnancy category B: Teratology studies have been conducted in rats and rabbits at subcutaneous doses of enoxaparin up to 30 mg/kg/day or 211 mg/m^2/day and 410 mg/m^2/day, respectively. The maximum received human dose in clinical trials was 1.5 mg/kg/day or 48.4 mg/m^2/day. There was no evidence of teratogenic effects or fetotoxicity due to enoxaparin. There are, however, no adequate and well-controlled studies in pregnant women. Because animal reproduction studies are not always predictive of human response, this drug should be used during pregnancy only if clearly needed.

Non-teratogenic Effects

There have been a few spontaneous post-marketing reports of fetal death while using enoxaparin; none of the cases have been definitively associated with the use of the drug. In one case, placental hemorrhage and detachment were found in association with the fetal death. If enoxaparin is used during pregnancy, or if the patient becomes pregnant while taking this drug, the patient should be apprised of the potential hazard to the fetus.

Nursing Mothers:

It is not known whether this drug is excreted in human milk. Because many drugs are excreted in human milk, caution should be exercised when enoxaparin is administered to nursing women.

Pediatric Use:

Safety and effectiveness of enoxaparin in pediatric patients has not been established.

ADVERSE REACTIONS

Hemorrhage:

The incidence of hemorrhagic complications during Lovenox Injection treatment has been low.

Adverse Events Occurring at ≥2% Incidence in Enoxaparin Treated Patients*

	Enoxaparin 30 mg q12h n = 1080		Heparin 15000 U/24h n = 766		Placebo n = 115	
Adverse Event	**Severe**	**Total**	**Severe**	**Total**	**Severe**	**Total**
Fever	<1%	5%	<1%	4%	0%	3%
Hemorrhage	<1%	4%	1%	4%	0%	3%
Nausea	<1%	3%	<1%	2%	0%	2%
Hypochromic anemia	<1%	2%	2%	5%	<1%	7%
Edema	<1%	2%	<1%	2%	0%	2%
Peripheral edema	<1%	3%	<1%	4%	0%	3%

*(Excluding Unrelated Adverse Events)

The following rates of major bleeding events have been reported during clinical trials with Lovenox Injection and heparin and placebo in patients undergoing hip or knee replacement surgery.

Major Bleeding Episodes*

	Enoxaparin 30 mg q12h	Heparin 15000 U/24h	Placebo
Hip Replacement	n = 786	n = 541	n =50
Surgery	31 [4%]	32 [6%]	2 [4%]
Knee Replacement	n = 294	n = 225	n = 65
Surgery	3 [1%]	3 [1%]	2 [3%]

*Bleeding complications were considered major if accompanied by a significant clinical event or if hemoglobin decreased by ≥2 g/dL or transfusion of 2 or more units of blood products was required.

Thrombocytopenia:
During clinical trials with Lovenox Injection, moderate thrombocytopenia, defined as a platelet count between 100,000/mm^3 and 50,000/mm^3, occurred at a rate of 1.9% in patients given Lovenox, 2.0% in patients given heparin, and 1.7% in patients given placebo following hip or knee replacement surgery.
Platelet counts less than 50,000/mm^3 occurred at a rate of 0.1% in patients given Lovenox, 0.5% in patients given heparin, and 0% in patients given placebo in the same trials. Rare cases of thrombocytopenia with thrombosis have also been observed in clinical practice (see WARNINGS).

Local Irritation:
Mild local irritation, pain, hematoma and erythema may follow subcutaneous injection of Lovenox Injection.

Other:
Other adverse effects that were thought to be possibly or probably related to treatment with Lovenox Injection, heparin or placebo in clinical trials with patients undergoing hip or knee replacement surgery, and that occurred at a rate of at least 2% in the enoxaparin group, are shown below.
[See table at top of page.]

Ongoing Safety Surveillance
There have been rare reports of neuraxial hematoma formation with concurrent use of enoxaparin and spinal/epidural anesthesia, and post-operative indwelling catheters. These events resulted in varying degrees of neurologic injuries including long-term or permanent paralysis.
Other reports include: skin necrosis at the injection site, inflammatory nodules at the injection site, purpura, systemic allergic reactions, and thrombocythemia.

OVERDOSAGE:

SYMPTOMS/TREATMENT:
Accidental overdosage following administration of Lovenox Injection may lead to hemorrhagic complications. This may be largely neutralized by the slow intravenous injection of protamine sulfate (1% solution). The dose of protamine sulfate should be equal to the dose of Lovenox Injection injected: 1 mg protamine sulfate should be administered to neutralize 1 mg Lovenox Injection. A second infusion of 0.5 mg protamine sulfate per 1 mg of Lovenox Injection may be administered if the APTT measured 2 to 4 hours after the first infusion remains prolonged. However, even with higher doses of protamine, the APTT may remain more prolonged than under normal conditions found following administration of conventional heparin. In all cases, the anti-Factor Xa activity is never completely neutralized (maximum about 60%). Particular care should be taken to avoid overdosage with protamine sulfate. Administration of protamine sulfate can cause severe hypotensive and anaphylactoid reactions. Because fatal reactions, often resembling anaphylaxis, have been reported with protamine sulfate, it should be given only when resuscitation techniques and treatment of anaphylactic shock are readily available. For additional information consult the labeling of Protamine Sulfate Injection, USP, products.
A single subcutaneous dose of 46.4 mg/kg enoxaparin was lethal to rats. The symptoms of acute toxicity were ataxia, decreased motility, dyspnea, cyanosis and coma.

DOSAGE AND ADMINISTRATION

Adult Dosage:
In patients undergoing hip or knee replacement surgery, the recommended dose of Lovenox Injection is 30 mg twice daily administered by subcutaneous injection with the initial dose given within 12–24 hours post-operatively provided hemostasis has been established. Treatment should be continued throughout the period of post-operative care until the risk of deep vein thrombosis has diminished. Up to 14 days administration has been well tolerated in controlled clinical trials. The average duration of administration is 7 to 10 days.
All patients should be screened prior to prophylactic administration of Lovenox to rule out a bleeding disorder. There is usually no need for daily monitoring of the effect of Lovenox in patients with normal presurgical coagulation parameters.

Administration:
Lovenox Injection is administered by subcutaneous injection. It must not be administered by intramuscular injection.
Subcutaneous injection technique: Patients should be lying down and Lovenox Injection administered by deep subcutaneous injection. To avoid the loss of drug, do not expel the air bubble from the syringe before the injection. Administration should be alternated between the left and right anterolateral and left and right posterolateral abdominal wall. The whole length of the needle should be introduced into a skin fold held between the thumb and forefinger; the skin fold should be held throughout the injection. To minimize bruising, do not rub the injection site after completion of the injection.
Enoxaparin injection is a clear colorless to pale-yellow sterile solution and as with other parenteral drug products should be inspected visually for particulate matter and discoloration prior to administration.

HOW SUPPLIED

Lovenox Injection is available in packs of 10 prefilled syringes, NDC 0075-0624-30. Each Lovenox (enoxaparin sodium) prefilled syringe is affixed with a 27 gauge × $^1/_2$ inch needle. Lovenox contains 30 mg enoxaparin sodium in 0.3 mL of Water for Injection. Lovenox has an anti-Factor Xa activity of approximately 3000 IU (with reference to the W.H.O. First International Low Molecular Weight Heparin Reference Standard).
Lovenox Injection should be stored at or below 25°C. Do not freeze.
Caution: Federal (U.S.A.) law prohibits dispensing without prescription.
National Stock Number: 10 × 3 mL/syringe (NSN 6505-01-377-1444).
Made in France.
Rev. 8/96 IN-1107L
RHÔNE-POULENC RORER PHARMACEUTICALS INC.
COLLEGEVILLE, PA 19426
Shown in Product Identification Guide, page 330

NASACORT® ℞

[na'za · cort]
(triamcinolone acetonide)
Nasal Inhaler
For Intranasal Use Only
Shake Well Before Using

DESCRIPTION

Triamcinolone acetonide, USP, the active ingredient in **Nasacort**® Nasal Inhaler, is a glucocorticosteroid with a molecular weight of 434.5 and with the chemical designation 9-Fluoro-11β,16α,17, 21-tetrahydroxypregna-1, 4-diene-3, 20-dione cyclic 16,17-acetal with acetone. ($C_{24}H_{31}FO_6$).

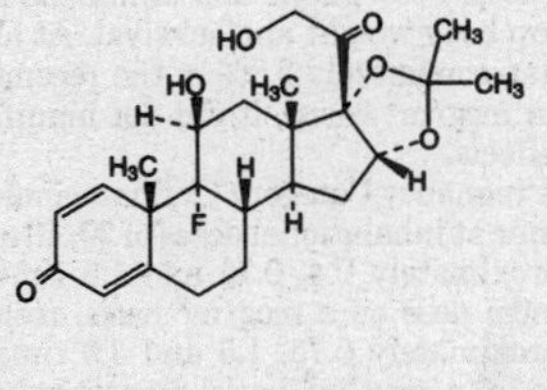

Nasacort Nasal Inhaler is a metered-dose aerosol unit containing a microcrystalline suspension of triamcinolone acetonide in dichlorodifluoromethane and dehydrated alcohol USP 0.7% w/w. Each canister contains 15 mg triamcinolone acetonide. Each actuation delivers 55 mcg triamcinolone acetonide from the nasal actuator to the patient (estimated from *in vitro* testing). There are at least 100 actuations in one **Nasacort** Nasal Inhaler canister. **After 100 actuations, the amount delivered per actuation may not be consistent and the unit should be discarded.** Patients are provided with a check-off card to track usage as part of the Information for Patients tear-off sheet.

CLINICAL PHARMACOLOGY

Triamcinolone acetonide is a more potent derivative of triamcinolone. Although triamcinolone itself is approximately one to two times as potent as prednisone in animal models of inflammation, triamcinolone acetonide is approximately 8 times more potent than prednisone.
Although the precise mechanism of corticosteroid antiallergic action is unknown, corticosteroids are very effective. However, they do not have an immediate effect on allergic signs and symptoms. When allergic symptoms are very severe, local treatment with recommended doses (microgram) of any available topical corticosteroids are not as effective as treatment with larger doses (milligram) of oral or parenteral formulations. When corticosteroids are prematurely discontinued, symptoms may not recur for several days.
Based upon intravenous dosing of triamcinolone acetonide phosphate ester, the half-life of triamcinolone acetonide was reported to be 88 minutes. The volume of distribution (Vd) reported was 99.5 L (SD ± 27.5) and clearance was 45.2 L/hour (SD ± 9.1) for triamcinolone acetonide. The plasma half-life of corticosteroids does not correlate well with the biologic half-life.
When administered intranasally to man at 440 mcg/day dose, the peak plasma concentration was <1 ng/mL and occurred on average at 3.4 hours (range 0.5 to 8.0 hours) post-dosing. The apparent half-life was 4.0 hours (range 1.0 to 7.0 hours); however, this value probably reflects lingering absorption. Intranasal doses below 440 mcg/day gave sparse data and did not allow for the calculation of meaningful pharmacokinetic parameters.
In animal studies using rats and dogs, three metabolites of triamcinolone acetonide have been identified. They are 6β-hydroxytriamcinolone acetonide, 21-carboxytriamcinolone acetonide and 21-carboxy-6β-hydroxytriamcinolone acetonide. All three metabolites are expected to be substantially less active than the parent compound due to (a) the dependence of anti-inflammatory activity on the presence of a 21-hydroxyl group, (b) the decreased activity observed upon 6-hydroxylation, and (c) the markedly increased water solubility favoring rapid elimination. There appeared to be some quantitative differences in the metabolites among species. No differences were detected in metabolic pattern as a function of route of administration.

CLINICAL TRIALS

In double-blind, parallel, placebo-controlled clinical trials of seasonal and perennial allergic rhinitis, in adults and adolescents in fixed total daily doses of 110, 220 and 440 mcg per day, the responses to aerosolized triamcinolone acetonide demonstrated a statistically significant improvement over placebo. In open label trials where the doses were sometimes adjusted according to patients' signs and symptoms, the daily doses and regimens varied. The most commonly used dose was 110 mcg per day.
Nasacort Nasal Inhaler, at a dose of 220 mcg once daily, has also been studied in two double-blind, placebo-controlled trials of two and four weeks duration in children ages 6 through 11 years with seasonal and perennial allergic rhinitis. These trials included 162 males and 91 females. **Nasacort** administered at a fixed dose of 220 mcg once daily resulted in consistent and statistically significant reductions of allergic rhinitis symptoms over vehicle placebo.
In attempting to determine if systemic absorption played a role in the response to **Nasacort**, a clinical study comparing intranasal and depot intramuscular triamcinolone acetonide was conducted. The doses used were based on bioavailability studies of each formulation. The final doses of **Nasacort** 440 mcg once a day and Kenalog®-40, 4 mg intramuscularly once a week, were chosen to deliver comparable total amounts of weekly triamcinolone acetonide. However, the weekly injection yielded sustained plasma levels throughout the dosing interval while the daily **Nasacort** application resulted in daily peak and trough concentrations, the mean of which was 3.5 times below the Kenalog plasma levels.
Both topical **Nasacort** and intramuscular Kenalog-40 were clinically effective. In addition, in some studies there was evidence of improvement of eye symptoms. This suggests that **Nasacort**, at least to some degree is acting by a systemic mechanism.
In order to evaluate the effects of systemic absorption on the Hypothalamic-Pituitary-Adrenal (HPA) axis, **Nasacort** administered to adults in doses of 440 mcg once a day was compared to placebo and 42 days of a single morning dose of prednisone 10 mg. Adrenal response to a six-hour cosyntropin

Continued on next page

Rhône-Poulenc Rorer–Cont.

stimulation test suggests that intranasal **Nasacort** 440 mcg/day for six weeks did not measurably affect adrenal activity. Conversely, oral prednisone at 10 mg/day significantly reduced the response to ACTH.

No evidence of adrenal axis suppression was observed in 26 pediatric patients exposed for 6 weeks to systemic levels of triamcinolone acetonide higher than the systemic levels observed following administration of the maximum recommended dose of **Nasacort** Nasal Inhaler.

INDIVIDUALIZATION OF DOSAGE

Individual patients will experience a variable time to onset and degree of symptom relief when using **Nasacort**. It is recommended that dosing be started at 220 mcg once a day and the effect be assessed in four to seven days.

Adults and Children 12 years of age and older: Some relief can be expected in approximately two-thirds of patients within four to seven days. If greater effect is desired an increase of dose to 440 mcg once a day can be tried. If adequate relief has not been obtained by the third week of **Nasacort** treatment, alternate forms of treatment should be considered.

A dose-response between 110 mcg/day (one spray/nostril/day) and 440 mcg/day (four sprays/nostril/day) is not clearly discernible. In general, in the clinical trials the highest dose tended to provide relief sooner. This suggests an alternative approach to starting therapy with **Nasacort**, *e.g.*, starting treatment with 440 mcg (four sprays/nostril/day) and then, depending on the patient's response, decreasing the dose by one spray per day every four to seven days. Although **Nasacort** may be used at 220 mcg/day or 440 mcg/day divided into two or four times a day, the degree of relief does not seem to be significantly different compared to once-a-day dosing. As with other nasal corticosteroids, the vehicle used to deliver the corticosteroid, may cause symptoms that are difficult to distinguish from the patient's rhinitis symptoms. Thus, depending upon the balance between these vehicle side effects and the benefits of treatment, in determining the optimal dose for the relief of symptoms, individual patients may need to have a trial of high and low doses.

Children 6 through 11 years of age: In children 6 through 11 years of age, it is recommended that dosing be started at 220 mcg given as two sprays (55 mcg/spray) in each nostril once a day. In clinical trials, significant relief of rhinitis symptoms in children was observed as early as the fourth day of treatment and generally, it took one to two weeks to achieve maximum benefit. If adequate relief has not been obtained by the third week of **Nasacort** treatment, alternate forms of treatment should be considered.

In general, it is always desirable to titrate an individual patient to the minimum effective dose to reduce the possibility of side effects. In clinical trials, after symptoms have been brought under control at the recommended starting doses, reducing the daily dose to 110 mcg (one spray in each nostril once per day) has been shown to be effective in controlling symptoms in approximately one-half of adult patients being treated long-term for allergic rhinitis. (See **PRECAUTIONS, WARNINGS, Information for Patients** and **ADVERSE REACTIONS** sections).

INDICATIONS AND USAGE

Nasacort Nasal Inhaler is indicated for the nasal treatment of seasonal and perennial allergic rhinitis symptoms in adults and children 6 years of age and older.

CONTRAINDICATIONS

Hypersensitivity to any of the ingredients of this preparation contraindicates its use.

WARNINGS

The replacement of a systemic corticosteroid with a topical corticoid can be accompanied by signs of adrenal insufficiency and, in addition, some patients may experience symptoms of withdrawal, *e.g.*, joint and/or muscular pain, lassitude and depression. Patients previously treated for prolonged periods with systemic corticosteroids and transferred to topical corticoids should be carefully monitored for acute adrenal insufficiency in response to stress. In those patients who have asthma or other clinical conditions requiring long-term systemic corticosteroid treatment, too rapid a decrease in systemic corticosteroids may cause a severe exacerbation of their symptoms.

Children who are on immunosuppressant drugs are more susceptible to infections than healthy children. Chickenpox and measles, for example, can have a more serious or even fatal course in children on immunosuppressant doses of corticosteroids. In such children, or in adults who have not had these diseases, particular care should be taken to avoid exposure. If exposed, therapy with varicella-zoster immune globulin (VZIG) or pooled intravenous immunoglobulin (IVIG), as appropriate, may be indicated. If chickenpox develops, treatment with antiviral agents may be considered.

The use of **Nasacort** Nasal Inhaler with alternate-day systemic prednisone could increase the likelihood of hypothalamic-pituitary-adrenal (HPA) suppression compared to a therapeutic dose of either one alone. Therefore, **Nasacort** Nasal Inhaler should be used with caution in patients already receiving alternate-day prednisone treatment for any disease.

PRECAUTIONS

General: In clinical studies with triamcinolone acetonide administered intranasally, the development of localized infections of the nose and pharynx with *Candida albicans* has rarely occurred. When such an infection develops, it may require treatment with appropriate local therapy and discontinuance of treatment with **Nasacort** Nasal Inhaler.

Triamcinolone acetonide administered intranasally has been shown to be absorbed into the systemic circulation in humans. Patients with active rhinitis showed absorption similar to that found in normal volunteers. **Nasacort** at 440 mcg/day for 42 days did not measurably affect adrenal response to a six hour cosyntropin test. In the same study, prednisone 10 mg/day significantly reduced adrenal response to ACTH over the same period (see **CLINICAL TRIALS** section).

Nasacort Nasal Inhaler should be used with caution, if at all, in patients with active or quiescent tuberculous infections of the respiratory tract or in patients with untreated fungal, bacterial, or systemic viral infections or ocular herpes simplex.

Because of the inhibitory effect of corticosteroids on wound healing in patients who have experienced recent nasal septal ulcers, nasal surgery or trauma, a corticosteroid should be used with caution until healing has occurred. As with other nasally inhaled corticosteroids, nasal septal perforations have been reported in rare instances.

When used at excessive doses, systemic corticosteroid effects such as hypercorticism and adrenal suppression may appear. If such changes occur, **Nasacort** Nasal Inhaler should be discontinued slowly, consistent with accepted procedures for discontinuing oral steroid therapy.

Information for Patients: Patients being treated with **Nasacort** Nasal Inhaler should receive the following information and instructions.

Patients who are on immunosuppressant doses of corticosteroids should be warned to avoid exposure to chickenpox or measles and, if exposed, to obtain medical advice.

Patients should use **Nasacort** Nasal Inhaler at regular intervals since its effectiveness depends on its regular use. A decrease in symptoms may occur as soon as 12 hours after starting steroid therapy and generally can be expected to occur within a few days of initiating therapy in allergic rhinitis. The patient should take the medication as directed and should not exceed the prescribed dosage. The patient should contact the physician if symptoms do not improve after three weeks, or if the condition worsens. Nasal irritation and/or burning or stinging after use of the spray occur only rarely with this product. The patient should contact the physician if they occur.

For the proper use of this unit and to attain maximum improvement, the patient should read and follow the accompanying patient instructions carefully. Spraying triamcinolone acetonide directly onto the nasal septum should be avoided. Because the amount dispensed per puff may not be consistent, it is important to shake the canister well. Also, the canister should be discarded after 100 actuations.

Carcinogenesis, Mutagenesis: No evidence of treatment-related carcinogenicity was demonstrated after 2 years of once daily gavage administration of triamcinolone acetonide at doses of 0.05, 0.2 and 1.0 mcg/kg (approximately 0.1, 0.4 and 1.8% of the recommended clinical dose on a mcg/m^2 basis) in the rat and 0.1, 0.6 and 3.0 mcg/kg (approximately 0.1, 0.6 and 3.0% of the recommended clinical dose on a mcg/m^2 basis) in the mouse.

Mutagenesis studies with triamcinolone acetonide have not been conducted.

Impairment of Fertility: No evidence of impaired fertility was demonstrated when oral doses up to 15 mcg/kg (approximately 28% of the recommended clinical dose on a mcg/m^2 basis) were administered to female and male rats. However, triamcinolone acetonide at oral doses of 8.0 mcg/kg (approximately 15.0% of the recommended clinical dose on a mcg/m^2 basis) caused dystocia and prolonged delivery and at oral doses of 5.0 mcg/kg (approximately 9.0% of the recommended clinical dose on a mcg/m^2 basis) and above produced increases in fetal resorptions and stillbirths as well as decreases in pup body weight and survival. At an oral dose of 1.0 mcg/kg (approximately 2.0% of the recommended clinical dose on a mcg/m^2 basis), it did not manifest the above mentioned effects.

Pregnancy: Pregnancy Category C. Triamcinolone acetonide was teratogenic at inhalational doses of 20, 40 and 80 mcg/kg in rats (approximately 0.4, 0.75 and 1.5 times the recommended clinical dose on a mcg/m^2 basis, respectively) and rabbits (approximately 0.75, 1.5 and 3.0 times the recommended dose on a mcg/m^2 basis, respectively). Triamcinolone acetonide was also teratogenic at an inhalational dose of 500 mcg/kg in monkeys (approximately 18 times the recommended clinical dose on a mcg/m^2 basis). Dose-related teratogenic effects in rats and rabbits included cleft palate, internal hydrocephaly, and axial skeletal defects. Teratogenic effects observed in the monkey were CNS and cranial malformations. There are no adequate and well-controlled studies in pregnant women. Triamcinolone acetonide should be used during pregnancy only if the potential benefits justify the potential risk to the fetus.

Experience with oral corticoids since their introduction in pharmacologic as opposed to physiologic doses suggests that rodents are more prone to teratogenic effects from corticoids than humans. In addition, because there is a natural increase in glucocorticoid production during pregnancy, most women will require a lower exogenous steroid dose and many will not need corticoid treatment during pregnancy.

Nonteratogenic Effects: Hypoadrenalism may occur in infants born of mothers receiving corticosteroids during pregnancy. Such infants should be carefully observed.

Nursing Mothers: It is not known whether triamcinolone acetonide is excreted in human milk. Because other corticosteroids are excreted in human milk, caution should be exercised when **Nasacort** Nasal Inhaler is administered to nursing women.

Pediatric Use: Safety and effectiveness have not been established in children below the age of 6. Oral corticosteroids have been shown to cause growth suppression in children and teenagers, particularly with higher doses over extended periods. If a child or teenager on any corticosteroid appears to have growth suppression, the possibility that they are particularly sensitive to this effect of steroids should be considered.

ADVERSE REACTIONS

Adults and Children 12 years of age and older: In controlled and uncontrolled studies, 1257 adult and adolescent patients received treatment with intranasal triamcinolone acetonide. Adverse reactions are based on the 567 patients who received a product similar to the marketed **Nasacort** canister.

These patients were treated for an average of 48 days (range 1 to 117 days). The 145 patients enrolled in uncontrolled studies received treatment from 1 to 820 days (average 332 days). The most prevalent adverse experience was headache, being reported by approximately 18% of the patients who received **Nasacort**. Nasal irritation was reported by 2.8% of the patients receiving **Nasacort**. Other nasopharyngeal side effects were reported by fewer than 5% of the patients who received **Nasacort** and included: dry mucous membranes, naso-sinus congestion, throat discomfort, sneezing, and epistaxis. The complaints do not usually interfere with treatment and in the controlled and uncontrolled studies approximately 1% of patients have discontinued because of these nasal adverse effects. In the event of accidental overdose, an increased potential for these adverse experiences may be expected, but systemic adverse experiences are unlikely (see **OVERDOSAGE** section).

Children 6 through 11 years of age: Adverse event data in children 6 through 11 years of age are derived from two controlled clinical trials of two and four weeks duration. In these trials, 127 patients received fixed doses of 220 mcg/day of triamcinolone acetonide for an average of 22 days (range 8 to 33 days).

Adverse events occurring at an incidence of 3% or greater and more common among children treated with 220 mcg triamcinolone acetonide daily than vehicle placebo were:

Adverse Events	220 mcg of triamcinolone acetonide daily (n=127)	Vehicle placebo (n=322)
Epistaxis	11.0%	9.3%
Cough	9.4%	9.3%
Fever	7.9%	5.6%
Nausea	6.3%	3.1%
Throat discomfort	5.5%	5.3%
Otitis	4.7%	3.7%
Dyspepsia	4.7%	2.2%

Adverse events occurring at a rate of 3% or greater that were more common in the placebo group were upper respiratory tract infection, headache and concurrent infection.

Only 1.6% of patients discontinued due to adverse experiences. No patient discontinued due to a serious adverse event related to **Nasacort** therapy.

Though not observed in controlled clinical trials of **Nasacort** Nasal Inhaler in children, cases of nasal septum perforation among pediatric users have been reported in post-marketing surveillance of this product.

DOSAGE AND ADMINISTRATION

A decrease in symptoms may occur as soon as 12 hours after starting steroid therapy and generally can be expected to occur within a few days of initiating therapy in allergic rhinitis.

If improvement is not evident after 2 to 3 weeks, the patient should be re-evaluated. (See **INDIVIDUALIZATION OF DOSAGE** section).

Adults and Children 12 years of age and older: The recommended starting dose of **Nasacort** Nasal Inhaler is 220 mcg

per day given as two sprays (55 mcg/spray) in each nostril once a day. If needed, the dose may be increased to 440 mcg per day (55 mcg/spray) either as once-a-day dosage or divided up to four times a day, i.e., twice a day (two sprays/nostril), or four times a day (one spray/nostril). After the desired effect is obtained, some patients may be maintained on a dose of as little as one spray (55 mcg) in each nostril once a day (total daily dose 110 mcg per day).

Children 6 through 11 years of age: The recommended starting dose of **Nasacort** Nasal Inhaler is 220 mcg per day given as two sprays (55 mcg/spray) in each nostril once a day. Once the maximal effect has been achieved, it is always desirable to titrate the patient to the minimum effective dose. **Nasacort** Nasal Inhaler is not recommended for children below 6 years of age since adequate numbers of patients have not been studied in this age group.

Directions for Use: Illustrated Patient's Instructions for use accompany each package of **Nasacort** Nasal Inhaler.

OVERDOSAGE

Acute overdosage with this dosage form is unlikely. The acute topical application of the entire 15 mg of the canister would most likely cause nasal irritation and headache. It would be unlikely to see acute systemic adverse effects even if the entire 15 mg of triamcinolone acetonide was administered intranasally all at once.

HOW SUPPLIED

Nasacort Nasal Inhaler is supplied as an aerosol canister which will provide 100 metered dose actuations. Each actuation delivers 55 mcg triamcinolone acetonide through the nasal actuator. The **Nasacort** Nasal Inhaler canister and accompanying nasal actuator are designed to be used together. The **Nasacort** Nasal Inhaler canister should not be used with other nasal actuators and the supplied nasal actuator should not be used with other products' canisters. **Nasacort** Nasal Inhaler is supplied with a white plastic nasal actuator and patient instructions. Net weight of the canister contents is 10 grams.
NDC 0075-1505-43.

CONTENTS UNDER PRESSURE

Avoid spraying in eyes.
Do not puncture. Do not use or store near heat or open flame. Exposure to temperatures above 120°F may cause bursting. Never throw container into fire or incinerator. Keep out of reach of children. Store at controlled room temperature, 15°–30°C (59°–86°F).
Note: The indented statement below is required by the Federal government's Clean Air Act for all products containing or manufactured with chlorofluorocarbons (CFC's):

> WARNING: Contains CFC-12, a substance which harms public health and the environment by destroying ozone in the upper atmosphere.

A notice similar to the above WARNING has been placed in the "Information For The Patient" portion of this package insert under the Environmental Protection Agency's (EPA's) regulations. The patient's warning states that the patient should consult his or her physician if there are questions about alternatives.
Caution: Federal (U.S.A.) law prohibits dispensing without prescription.
U.S. Pat. No. 4,767,612
Rev. 5/96
IN-0479H
Military and Veterans Administration: 1 × 10 gm (NSN 6505-01-345-2880).
Marketed by
RHÔNE-POULENC RORER PHARMACEUTICALS INC.
500 ARCOLA ROAD
COLLEGEVILLE, PA 19426
Shown in Product Identification Guide, page 330

NASACORT® AQ ℞
[na′za · cort]
(triamcinolone acetonide)
Nasal Spray
For intranasal use only.
Shake Well Before Using

DESCRIPTION

Triamcinolone acetonide, USP, the active ingredient in **Nasacort® AQ** Nasal Spray, is a corticosteroid with a molecular weight of 434.51 and with the chemical designation 9-Fluoro- 11β,16α,17,21-tetrahydroxypregna- 1,4-diene-3,20-dione cyclic 16,17-acetal with acetone ($C_{24}H_{31}FO_6$).
[See chemical structure at top of next column.]
Nasacort AQ Nasal Spray is an unscented, thixotropic, water-based metered-dose pump spray formulation unit containing a microcrystalline suspension of triamcinolone acetonide in an aqueous medium. Microcrystalline cellulose, carboxymethylcellulose sodium, polysorbate 80, dextrose, benzalkonium chloride, and edetate disodium are contained in this aqueous medium; hydrochloric acid or sodium hydrox-

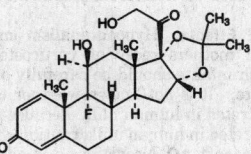

ide may be added to adjust the pH to a target of 5.0 within a range of 4.5 and 6.0.
Each bottle contains 9.075 mg triamcinolone acetonide. Each actuation delivers 55 mcg triamcinolone acetonide from the nasal actuator to the patient (estimated from *in vitro* testing) after an initial priming of 5 sprays. It will remain adequately primed for 2 weeks. If the product is not used for more than 2 weeks, then it can be adequately reprimed with one spray. There are at least 120 actuations in one **Nasacort AQ** Nasal Spray bottle. **After 120 actuations, the amount of triamcinolone acetonide delivered per actuation may not be consistent and the unit should be discarded.**
In the Information for Patients tear-off sheet, patients are provided with a check-off form to track usage.

CLINICAL PHARMACOLOGY

Triamcinolone acetonide is a more potent derivative of triamcinolone. Although triamcinolone itself is approximately one to two times as potent as prednisone in animal models of inflammation, triamcinolone acetonide is approximately 8 times more potent than prednisone.
Although the precise mechanism of corticosteroid antiallergic action is unknown, corticosteroids are very effective. However, when allergic symptoms are very severe, local treatment with recommended doses (microgram) of any available topical corticosteroid are not as effective as treatment with larger doses (milligram) of oral or parenteral formulations.
With **Nasacort AQ,** an improvement in some patient symptoms may be seen within the first day of treatment, and generally, it takes one week of treatment to reach maximum benefit. Similarly when corticosteroids are prematurely discontinued symptoms may not recur for several days.
Based upon intravenous dosing of triamcinolone acetonide phosphate ester, the half-life of triamcinolone acetonide was reported to be 88 minutes. The volume of distribution (Vd) reported was 99.5 L (SD ± 27.5) and clearance was 45.2 L/hour (SD ± 9.1) for triamcinolone acetonide. The plasma half-life of corticosteroids does not correlate well with the biologic half-life.
Pharmacokinetic characterization of the **Nasacort AQ** Nasal Spray formulation was determined in both normal subjects and in patients with allergic rhinitis. Single dose intranasal administration of 220 mcg of **Nasacort AQ** Nasal Spray in normal subjects and patients demonstrated minimal absorption of triamcinolone acetonide. The mean peak plasma concentration was approximately 0.5 ng/mL (range: 0.1 to 1.0 ng/mL) and occurred at 1.5 hours post dose. The mean plasma drug concentration was less than 0.06 ng/mL at 12 hours, and below the assay detection limit at 24 hours. The average terminal half-life was 3.1 hours. The range of mean $AUC_{0-\infty}$ values was 1.4 ng·hr/mL to 4.7 ng·hr/mL between doses of 110 mcg to 440 mcg in both patients and healthy volunteers. Dose proportionality was demonstrated in both normal subjects and in allergic rhinitis patients following single intranasal doses of 110 mcg or 220 mcg **Nasacort AQ** Nasal Spray. The C_{max} and AUC of the 440 mcg dose increased less than proportionally when compared to 110 and 220 mcg doses.
In animal studies using rats and dogs, three metabolites of triamcinolone acetonide have been identified. They are 6β-hydroxytriamcinolone acetonide, 21-carboxytriamcinolone acetonide and 21-carboxy-6β-hydroxytriamcinolone acetonide. All three metabolites are expected to be substantially less active than the parent compound due to (a) the dependence of anti-inflammatory activity on the presence of a 21-hydroxyl group, (b) the decreased activity observed upon 6-hydroxylation, and (c) the markedly increased water solubility favoring rapid elimination. There appeared to be some quantitative differences in the metabolites among species. No differences were detected in metabolic pattern as a function of route of administration.
In order to determine if systemic absorption plays a role in **Nasacort AQ's** treatment of allergic rhinitis symptoms, a two week double-blind, placebo-controlled clinical study was conducted comparing **Nasacort AQ,** orally ingested triamcinolone acetonide, and placebo in 297 patients with seasonal allergic rhinitis. The study demonstrated that the therapeutic efficacy of **Nasacort AQ** Nasal Spray can be attributed to the topical effects of triamcinolone acetonide.
In order to evaluate the effects of systemic absorption on the Hypothalamic-Pituitary-Adrenal (HPA) axis, a clinical study was performed comparing 220 mcg or 440 mcg

Nasacort AQ per day, or 10 mg prednisone per day with placebo for 42 days. Adrenal response to a six-hour cosyntropin stimulation test showed that **Nasacort AQ** administered at doses of 220 mcg and 440 mcg had no statistically significant effect on HPA activity versus placebo. Conversely, oral prednisone at 10 mg/day significantly reduced the response to ACTH.

CLINICAL TRIALS

The safety and efficacy of **Nasacort AQ** Nasal Spray has been evaluated in 10 double-blind, placebo-controlled clinical trials of two to four weeks duration in adults and children 12 years and older with seasonal or perennial allergic rhinitis. The number of patients treated with **Nasacort AQ** Nasal Spray in these studies was 1266; of these patients, 675 were males and 591 were females.
Overall, the results of these clinical trials showed that **Nasacort AQ** Nasal Spray 220 mcg once daily (2 sprays in each nostril) when compared to placebo provides statistically significant relief of nasal symptoms including sneezing, stuffiness, discharge, and itching.

INDIVIDUALIZATION OF DOSAGE

It is recommended that dosing be started at 220 mcg as 2 sprays in each nostril once daily for adults and children 12 years and older.
An improvement in some patient symptoms may be seen within the first day of treatment, and generally, it takes one week of treatment to reach maximum benefit. Initial assessment for response should be made during this time frame and periodically until the patient's symptoms are stabilized. If adequate relief of symptoms has not been obtained after 3 weeks of treatment, **Nasacort AQ** Nasal Spray should be discontinued.
It is always desirable to titrate an individual patient to the minimum effective dose to reduce the possibility of side effects. Therefore, when the maximum benefit has been achieved and symptoms have been controlled, reducing the dose to 110 mcg (one spray in each nostril once per day) has been shown to be effective in maintaining control of the allergic rhinitis symptoms in patients who were initially controlled at 220 mcg/day. (See PRECAUTIONS, WARNINGS, Information for Patients, and ADVERSE REACTIONS sections.)

INDICATIONS AND USAGE

Nasacort AQ Nasal Spray is indicated for the treatment of seasonal and perennial allergic rhinitis symptoms.

CONTRAINDICATIONS

Hypersensitivity to any of the ingredients of this preparation contraindicates its use.

WARNINGS

The replacement of a systemic corticosteroid with a topical corticosteroid can be accompanied by signs of adrenal insufficiency and, in addition, some patients may experience symptoms of withdrawal; e.g., joint and/or muscular pain, lassitude and depression. Patients previously treated for prolonged periods with systemic corticosteroids and transferred to topical corticosteroids should be carefully monitored for acute adrenal insufficiency in response to stress. In those patients who have asthma or other clinical conditions requiring long-term systemic corticosteroid treatment, too rapid a decrease in systemic corticosteroids may cause a severe exacerbation of their symptoms.
Children who are on immunosuppressant drugs are more susceptible to infections than healthy children. Chickenpox and measles, for example, can have a more serious or even fatal course in children on immunosuppressant doses of corticosteroids. In such children, or in adults who have not had these diseases, particular care should be taken to avoid exposure. If exposed, therapy with varicella-zoster immune globulin (VZIG) or pooled intravenous immunoglobulin (IVIG), as appropriate, may be indicated. If chickenpox develops, treatment with antiviral agents may be considered.
The use of **Nasacort AQ** Nasal Spray with alternate day systemic prednisone could increase the likelihood of hypothalamic-pituitary-adrenal (HPA) suppression compared to a therapeutic dose of either one alone. Therefore, **Nasacort AQ** Nasal Spray should be used with caution in patients already receiving alternate-day prednisone treatment for any disease.

PRECAUTIONS

General: In clinical studies with triamcinolone acetonide nasal spray, the development of localized infections of the nose and pharynx with *Candida albicans* has rarely occurred. When such an infection develops it may require treatment with appropriate local or systemic therapy and discontinuance of treatment with **Nasacort AQ** Nasal Spray. Triamcinolone acetonide aqueous administered intranasally has been shown to be minimally absorbed into the systemic circulation in humans. Patients with active rhinitis showed absorption similar to that found in normal volunteers. Daily doses of 220 mcg or 440 mcg **Nasacort AQ** Nasal Spray, 10

Continued on next page

Rhône-Poulenc Rorer–Cont.

mg prednisone each was compared to placebo. Adrenal response to a six-hour cosyntropin test showed that **Nasacort AQ** Nasal Spray in doses of 220 or 440 mcg/day for six weeks had no statistically significant effect on adrenal activity. In the same study prednisone 10 mg/day significantly reduced adrenal response to synthetic ACTH over the same period.

Nasacort AQ Nasal Spray should be used with caution, if at all, in patients with active or quiescent tuberculous infections of the respiratory tract or in patients with untreated fungal, bacterial, or systemic viral infections or ocular herpes simplex.

Because of the inhibitory effect of corticosteroids, in patients who have experienced recent nasal septal ulcers, nasal surgery or trauma, a corticosteroid should be used with caution until healing has occurred. As with other nasally inhaled corticosteroids, nasal septal perforations have been reported in rare instances.

When used at excessive doses, systemic corticosteroid effects such as hypercorticism and adrenal suppression may appear. If such changes occur, **Nasacort® AQ** Nasal Spray should be discontinued slowly, consistent with accepted procedures for discontinuing oral steroid therapy.

Information for Patients: Patients being treated with **Nasacort AQ** Nasal Spray should receive the following information and instructions. Patients who are on immunosuppressant doses of corticosteroids should be warned to avoid exposure to chickenpox or measles and, if exposed, to obtain medical advice.

Patients should use **Nasacort AQ** Nasal Spray at regular intervals since its effectiveness depends on its regular use. (See **DOSAGE AND ADMINISTRATION** section.)

An improvement in some patient symptoms may be seen within the first day of treatment, and generally, it takes one week of treatment to reach maximum benefit. Initial assessment for response should be made during this time frame and periodically until the patient's symptoms are stabilized.

The patient should take the medication as directed and should not exceed the prescribed dosage. The patient should contact the physician if symptoms do not improve after three weeks, or if the condition worsens. For the proper use of this unit and to attain maximum improvement, the patient should read and follow the accompanying patient instructions carefully.

It is important to shake the bottle well before each use. **Also, the bottle should be discarded after 120 actuations since the amount of triamcinolone acetonide delivered thereafter per actuation may be substantially less than 55 mcg of drug.** Do not transfer any remaining suspension to another bottle.

Carcinogenesis, Mutagenesis: No evidence of treatment-related carcinogenicity was demonstrated after two years of once daily gavage of triamcinolone acetonide at doses of 0.05, 0.2 and 1.0 mcg/kg (approximately 0.2, 0.7 and 4.0% of the recommended clinical dose on a mcg/m^2 basis) in the rat and 0.1, 0.6 and 3.0 mcg/kg (approximately 0.2, 1.0 and 6.0% of the recommended clinical dose on a mcg/m^2 basis) in the mouse.

Mutagenesis studies with triamcinolone acetonide have not been carried out.

Impairment of Fertility: No evidence of impaired fertility was manifested when oral doses of up to 15.0 mcg/kg (55.0% of the recommended clinical dose on a mcg/m^2 basis) were administered to female and male rats. However, triamcinolone acetonide at oral doses of 8.0 mcg/kg (approximately 30.0% of the recommended clinical dose on a mcg/m^2 basis) caused dystocia and prolonged delivery and at oral doses of 5.0 mcg/kg (approximately 20.0% of the recommended clinical dose on a mcg/m^2 basis) and above caused increases in fetal resorptions and stillbirths and decreases in pup body weight and survival. At a lower dose of 1.0 mcg/kg (approximately 4.0% of the recommended clinical dose on a mcg/m^2 basis), it did not induce the aforementioned effects.

Pregnancy: Pregnancy Category C. Triamcinolone acetonide has been shown to be teratogenic at inhalational doses of 20, 40 and 80 mcg/kg in rats (approximately 0.75, 1.5 and 3.0 times the recommended clinical dose on a mcg/m^2 basis, respectively), in rabbits at the same doses (approximately 1.5, 3.0 and 6.0 times the recommended clinical dose on a mcg/m^2 basis, respectively) and in monkeys, at an inhalational dose of 500 mcg/kg (approximately 37.0 times the recommended clinical dose on a mcg/m^2 basis). Dose-related teratogenic effects in rats and rabbits included cleft palate and/or internal hydrocephaly and axial skeletal defects whereas the effects observed in the monkey were CNS and/or cranial malformations. There are no adequate and well-controlled studies in pregnant women. Triamcinolone acetonide should be used in pregnancy only if the potential benefit justifies the potential risk to the fetus.

Since their introduction, experience with oral corticosteroids in pharmacologic as opposed to physiologic doses suggests that rodents are more prone to teratogenic effects from corticosteroids than humans. In addition, because there is a natural increase in glucocorticoid production during pregnancy, most women will require a lower exogenous steroid dose and many will not need corticosteroid treatment during pregnancy.

Nonteratogenic Effects: Hypoadrenalism may occur in infants born of mothers receiving corticosteroids during pregnancy. Such infants should be carefully observed.

Nursing Mothers: It is not known whether triamcinolone acetonide is excreted in human milk. Because other corticosteroids are excreted in human milk, caution should be exercised when **Nasacort AQ** Nasal Spray is administered to nursing women.

Pediatric Use: Safety and effectiveness have not been established in children below the age of 12. Oral corticosteroids have been shown to cause growth suppression in children and teenagers, particularly with higher doses over extended periods. If a child or teenager on any corticosteroid appears to have growth suppression, the possibility that they are particularly sensitive to this effect of steroids should be considered.

ADVERSE REACTIONS

In placebo-controlled, double-blind and open-label clinical studies, 1483 patients received treatment with triamcinolone acetonide aqueous nasal spray. These patients were treated for an average duration of 50.7 days. In the controlled trials (2-5 weeks duration) from which the following adverse reaction data is derived, 1394 patients were treated with **Nasacort AQ** Nasal Spray for an average of 18.7 days. In the long-term, open-label study, 172 patients received treatment for an average duration of 286 days.

Adverse events occurring at an incidence of 2% or greater and more common among patients treated with 220 mcg triamcinolone acetonide daily than placebo were:

Adverse Events	Triamcinolone acetonide 220 mcg (N=857) %	Placebo (N=962) %
Increase in cough	2.1	1.5
Epistaxis	2.7	0.8
Pharyngitis	5.1	3.6

Also, those adverse events occurring at an incidence of 2% or greater and more common among patients treated with placebo than 220 mcg triamcinolone acetonide daily were: headache and rhinitis.

Nasal septum perforation was reported in one patient although relationship to **Nasacort AQ** Nasal Spray has not been established.

In the event of accidental overdose, an increased potential for these adverse experiences may be expected, but systemic adverse experiences are unlikely. (See **OVERDOSAGE** section.)

DOSAGE AND ADMINISTRATION

An improvement in some patient symptoms may be seen within the first day of treatment, and generally, it takes one week of treatment to reach maximum benefit. If adequate relief of symptoms has not been obtained after 3 weeks of treatment, **Nasacort AQ** Nasal Spray should be discontinued. (See **INDIVIDUALIZATION OF DOSAGE** section.)

Adults and children 12 years of age and older: The recommended starting dose is 220 mcg as two sprays in each nostril once daily.

It is always desirable to titrate an individual patient to the minimum effective dose to reduce the possibility of side effects. Therefore, when the maximum benefit has been achieved and symptoms have been controlled, reducing the dose to 110 mcg has been shown to be effective in maintaining control of the allergic rhinitis symptoms in patients who were initially controlled at 220 mcg/day.

Directions For Use: Illustrated Patient's Instructions for use accompany each package of **Nasacort AQ** Nasal Spray.

OVERDOSAGE

Like any other nasally administered corticosteroid, acute overdosing is unlikely in view of the total amount of active ingredient present. In the event that the entire contents of the bottle were administered all at once, via either oral or nasal application, clinically significant systemic adverse events would most likely not result. The patient may experience some gastrointestinal upset.

HOW SUPPLIED

Nasacort AQ Nasal Spray is a nonchlorofluorocarbon (CFC) containing metered-dose pump spray which will provide 120 actuations. Net weight of the bottle contents is 16.5 grams. It is supplied in a high-density polyethylene container with a metered-dose pump unit, nasal adapter, and patient instructions.

NDC 0075-1506-16.

Caution: Federal (U.S.A.) law prohibits dispensing without prescription. Keep out of reach of children.

Store at controlled room temperature, 15° - 30°C (59° - 86°F).

Rev. 5/96

IN-6361

Manufactured by
RHÔNE-POULENC RORER PHARMACEUTICALS INC.
500 ARCOLA ROAD
COLLEGEVILLE, PA 19426

Shown in Product Identification Guide, page 330

NASALCROM® NASAL SOLUTION ℞

[*nāz 'ŭl-krōm* ″]

(cromolyn sodium nasal solution, USP)

DESCRIPTION

Each mL of NASALCROM Nasal Solution (cromolyn sodium nasal solution, USP) contains 40 mg cromolyn sodium in purified water with 0.01% benzalkonium chloride to preserve and 0.01% EDTA (edetate disodium) to stabilize the solution. NASALCROM possesses a natural pH of 4.5–6.5 and negligible titratable acidity.

Chemically, cromolyn sodium is disodium 5,5'-[(2-hydroxytrimethylene) dioxy] bis [4-oxo-4*H*-1-benzopyran-2-carboxylate]. The empirical formula is $C_{23}H_{14}Na_2O_{11}$; the molecular weight is 512.34. Cromolyn sodium is a water soluble, odorless, white, hydrated crystalline powder. It is tasteless at first, but leaves a slightly bitter aftertaste.

The molecular structure is:

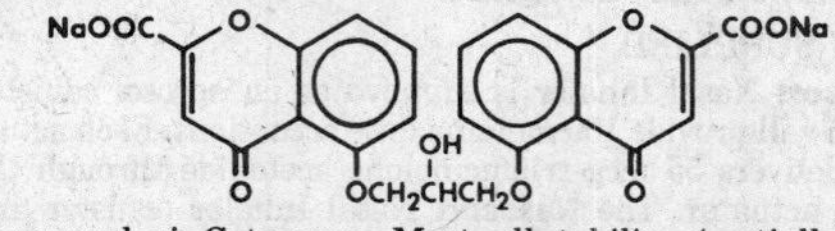

Pharmacologic Category: Mast cell stabilizer/ antiallergic.

Therapeutic Category: Antiallergic.

After priming the delivery system for NASALCROM, each actuation of the unit delivers a metered spray containing 5.2 mg of cromolyn sodium. The contents of one bottle delivers at least 100 sprays (13 mL bottle) or 200 sprays (26 mL bottle).

CLINICAL PHARMACOLOGY

In vitro and *in vivo* animal studies have shown that cromolyn sodium inhibits the degranulation of sensitized mast cells which occurs after exposure to specific antigens. Cromolyn sodium inhibits the release of histamine and SRS-A (the slow-reacting substance of anaphylaxis). Rhinitis induced by the inhalation of specific antigens can be inhibited to varying degrees by pretreatment with NASALCROM.

Another activity demonstrated *in vitro* is the capacity of cromolyn sodium to inhibit the degranulation of non-sensitized rat mast cells by phospholipase A and the subsequent release of chemical mediators. An additional *in vitro* study showed that cromolyn sodium did not inhibit the enzymatic activity of released phospholipase A on its specific substrate.

Cromolyn sodium has no intrinsic bronchodilator or antihistamine activity.

Cromolyn sodium is poorly absorbed from the gastrointestinal tract. After instillation of NASALCROM, less than 7% of the total dose administered is absorbed and is rapidly excreted unchanged in the bile and urine. The remainder of the dose is expelled from the nose, or swallowed and excreted via the alimentary tract.

INDICATIONS

NASALCROM is indicated for the prevention and treatment of the symptoms of allergic rhinitis.

CONTRAINDICATIONS

NASALCROM is contraindicated in those patients who have shown hypersensitivity to any of the ingredients.

PRECAUTIONS

General: Some patients may experience transient nasal stinging and/or sneezing immediately following instillation of NASALCROM. Except in rare occurrences, these experiences have not caused discontinuation of therapy.

In view of the biliary and renal routes of excretion for cromolyn sodium, consideration should be given to decreasing the dosage or discontinuing the administration of the drug in patients with impaired renal or hepatic function.

Carcinogenesis, Mutagenesis, and Impairment of Fertility: Long term studies in mice (12 months intraperitoneal treatment followed by 6 months observation), hamsters (12 months intraperitoneal treatment followed by 12 months observation), and rats (18 months subcutaneous treatment) showed no neoplastic effect of cromolyn sodium.

No evidence of chromosomal damage or cytotoxicity was obtained in various mutagenesis studies.

No evidence of impaired fertility was shown in laboratory animal reproduction studies.

Pregnancy: Pregnancy Category B. Reproduction studies with cromolyn sodium administered parenterally to pregnant mice, rats, and rabbits in doses up to 338 times the human clinical dose produced no evidence of fetal malformations. Adverse fetal effects (increased resorptions and decreased fetal weight) were noted only at the very high parenteral doses that produced maternal toxicity. There are, however, no adequate and well-controlled studies in pregnant women. Because animal reproduction studies are not always

predictive of human response, this drug should be used during pregnancy only if clearly needed.

Drug Interaction During Pregnancy: Cromolyn sodium and isoproterenol were studied following subcutaneous injections in pregnant mice. Cromolyn sodium alone in doses of 60 to 540 mg/kg (38 to 338 times the human dose) did not cause significant increases in resorptions or major malformations. Isoproterenol alone at a dose of 2.7 mg/kg (90 times the human dose) increased both resorptions and malformations. The addition of cromolyn sodium (338 times the human dose) to isoproterenol (90 times the human dose) appears to have increased the incidence of both resorptions and malformations.

Nursing Mothers: It is not known whether this drug is excreted in human milk. Because many drugs are excreted in human milk, caution should be exercised when NASALCROM is administered to a nursing woman.

Pediatric Use: Safety and effectiveness in pediatric patients below the age of 6 years have not been established.

ADVERSE REACTIONS

The most frequent adverse reactions occurring in the 430 patients included in the clinical trials with NASALCROM were sneezing (1 in 10 patients), nasal stinging (1 in 20), nasal burning (1 in 25), and nasal irritation (1 in 40). Headaches and bad taste were reported in about 1 in 50 patients. Epistaxis, postnasal drip, and rash were reported in less than one percent of the patients. One patient in the clinical trials developed anaphylaxis.

Adverse reactions which have occurred in the use of other cromolyn sodium formulations for inhalation include angioedema, joint pain and swelling, urticaria, cough, and wheezing. Other reactions reported rarely are serum sickness, periarteritic vasculitis, polymyositis, pericarditis, photodermatitis, exfoliative dermatitis, peripheral neuritis, and nephrosis.

DOSAGE AND ADMINISTRATION

The dose for adults and children 6 years and older is **one spray in each nostril** 3–4 times daily at regular intervals. If needed, this dose may be increased to one spray to each nostril 6 times daily. The patient should be instructed to clear the nasal passages before administering the spray and should inhale through the nose during administration.

In the management of seasonal (pollenotic) rhinitis, and for prevention of rhinitis caused by exposure to other types of specific inhalant allergens, treatment with NASALCROM will be more effective if started prior to expected contact with the offending allergen. Treatment should be continued throughout the period of exposure, i.e., until the pollen season is over or until exposure to the offending allergen is terminated.

In the management of perennial allergic rhinitis, the effects of treatment with NASALCROM may become apparent only after two to four weeks of treatment. The concomitant use of antihistamines and/or nasal decongestants may be necessary during the initial phase of treatment, but the need for this type of medication should diminish and may be eliminated when the full benefit of NASALCROM is achieved.

HOW SUPPLIED

NASALCROM is available in bottles of 13 mL and 26 mL. Each fully assembled unit consists of a pump unit and actuator with cover in position on the bottle of nasal solution. The amount of cromolyn sodium in each bottle is: 13 mL—520 mg (40 mg/mL); 26 mL—1040 mg (40 mg/mL).

NDC 0585-0671-03   13 mL bottle
(fully assembled unit)
NDC 0585-0671-04   26 mL bottle
(fully assembled unit)

NASALCROM should be stored between 15°–30°C (59°–86°F). Protect from light.

CAUTION: Federal law prohibits dispensing without prescription.

FISONS Pharmaceuticals
Fisons Corporation
Rochester, NY 14623 U.S.A.
Made in France
NASALCROM, NASALMATIC and FISONS are
Registered Trademarks of Fisons plc.
© 1995, Fisons Corporation.   Rev. 12/95
RF037F

NITROLINGUAL® SPRAY   ℞
(nitroglycerin lingual aerosol)
0.4 mg/metered dose

PRODUCT OVERVIEW

KEY FACTS

Nitrolingual® Spray is a metered dose aerosol containing 200 doses of nitroglycerin. Each metered dose of Nitrolingual Spray delivers 0.4 mg of nitroglycerin per actuation. Nitrolingual Spray offers guaranteed potency for 4 years from date of manufacture.

MAJOR USES

Nitrolingual® Spray is indicated for acute relief of an attack or prophylaxis of angina pectoris due to coronary artery disease.

SAFETY INFORMATION

Nitrolingual® Spray is contraindicated in patients who have shown purported hypersensitivity or idiosyncrasy to it or other nitrates or nitrites.
NOTE: THE SPRAY SHOULD NOT BE INHALED.

PRESCRIBING INFORMATION

NITROLINGUAL® SPRAY   ℞
(nitroglycerin lingual aerosol)
0.4 mg/metered dose

DESCRIPTION

Nitroglycerin, an organic nitrate, is a vasodilator which has effects on both arteries and veins. The chemical name for nitroglycerin is 1,2,3-propanetriol trinitrate ($C_3H_5N_3O_9$). The compound has a molecular weight of 227.09. The chemical structure is:

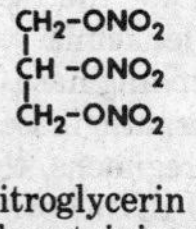

$$CH_2-ONO_2$$
$$CH-ONO_2$$
$$CH_2-ONO_2$$

Nitrolingual® Spray (nitroglycerin lingual aerosol 0.4 mg) is a metered dose aerosol containing nitroglycerin in propellants (dichlorodifluoromethane and dichlorotetrafluoroethane). Each metered dose of Nitrolingual Spray delivers 0.4 mg of nitroglycerin per spray emission. This product delivers nitroglycerin in the form of spray droplets onto or under the tongue. Inactive ingredients: caprylic/capric/diglyceryl succinate, ether, flavors.

CLINICAL PHARMACOLOGY

The principal pharmacological action of nitroglycerin is relaxation of vascular smooth muscle, producing a vasodilator effect on both peripheral arteries and veins with more prominent effects on the latter. Dilation of the post-capillary vessels, including large veins, promotes peripheral pooling of blood and decreases venous return to the heart, thereby reducing left ventricular end-diastolic pressure (pre-load). Arteriolar relaxation reduces systemic vascular resistance and arterial pressure (after-load).

The mechanism by which nitroglycerin relieves angina pectoris is not fully understood. Myocardial oxygen consumption or demand (as measured by the pressure-rate product, tension-time index, and stroke-work index) is decreased by both the arterial and venous effects of nitroglycerin and presumably, a more favorable supply-demand ratio is achieved. While the large epicardial coronary arteries are also dilated by nitroglycerin, the extent to which this action contributes to relief of exertional angina is unclear.

Nitroglycerin is rapidly metabolized *in vivo*, with a liver reductase enzyme having primary importance in the formation of glycerol nitrate metabolites and inorganic nitrate. Two active major metabolites, 1,2- and 1,3-dinitroglycerols, the products of hydrolysis, although less potent as vasodilators, have longer plasma half-lives than the parent compound. The dinitrates are further metabolized to mononitrates (considered biologically inactive with respect to cardiovascular effects) and ultimately glycerol and carbon dioxide.

Therapeutic doses of nitroglycerin may reduce systolic, diastolic, and mean arterial blood pressure. Effective coronary perfusion pressure is usually maintained, but can be compromised if blood pressure falls excessively or increased heart rate decreases diastolic filling time.

Elevated central venous and pulmonary capillary wedge pressures, pulmonary vascular resistance and systemic vascular resistance are also reduced by nitroglycerin therapy. Heart rate is usually slightly increased, presumably a reflex response to the fall in blood pressure. Cardiac index may be increased, decreased, or unchanged. Patients with elevated left ventricular filling pressure and systemic vascular resistance values in conjunction with a depressed cardiac index are likely to experience an improvement in cardiac index. On the other hand, when filling pressures and cardiac index are normal, cardiac index may be slightly reduced.

A pharmacokinetic study in 13 healthy men showed no statistically significant differences between the mean values for maximum plasma concentration and time to achieve maximum plasma level with equal doses (0.8 mg) of Nitrolingual Spray and sublingual nitroglycerin tablets. Peak plasma concentration after 0.8 mg of Nitrolingual occurred within 4 minutes and the apparent plasma half-life was approximately 5 minutes. In a randomized, double-blind study in patients with exertional angina pectoris dose-related increases in exercise tolerance were seen following doses of 0.2, 0.4, and 0.8 mg delivered by metered spray.

INDICATIONS AND USAGE

Nitrolingual Spray is indicated for acute relief of an attack or prophylaxis of angina pectoris due to coronary artery disease.

CONTRAINDICATIONS

Nitrolingual Spray is contraindicated in patients who have shown purported hypersensitivity or idiosyncrasy to it or other nitrates or nitrites.

WARNINGS

The use of any form of nitroglycerin during the early days of acute myocardial infarction requires particular attention to hemodynamic monitoring and clinical status.

PRECAUTIONS

(General)—Severe hypotension, particularly with upright posture, may occur even with small doses of nitroglycerin. The drug, therefore, should be used with caution in subjects who may have volume depletion from diuretic therapy or in patients who have low systolic blood pressure (e.g., below 90 mm Hg). Paradoxical bradycardia and increased angina pectoris may accompany nitroglycerin-induced hypotension.

Nitrate therapy may aggravate the angina caused by hypertrophic cardiomyopathy.

Tolerance to this drug and cross-tolerance to other nitrates and nitrites may occur. Tolerance to the vascular and antianginal effects of nitrates has been demonstrated in clinical trials, experience through occupational exposure, and in isolated tissue experiments in the laboratory.

In industrial workers continuously exposed to nitroglycerin, tolerance clearly occurs. Moreover, physical dependence also occurs since chest pain, acute myocardial infarction, and even sudden death have occurred during temporary withdrawal of nitroglycerin from the workers. In various clinical trials in angina patients, there are reports of anginal attacks being more easily provoked and of rebound in the hemodynamic effects soon after nitrate withdrawal. The relative importance of these observations to the routine, clinical use of nitroglycerin is not known.

DRUG INTERACTIONS: Alcohol may enhance sensitivity to the hypotensive effects of nitrates. Nitroglycerin acts directly on vascular muscle. Therefore, any other agents that depend on vascular smooth muscle as the final common path can be expected to have decreased or increased effect depending upon the agent.

Marked symptomatic orthostatic hypotension has been reported when calcium channel blockers and oral controlled-release nitroglycerin were used in combination. Dose adjustments of either class of agents may be necessary.

CARCINOGENESIS, MUTAGENESIS, IMPAIRMENT OF FERTILITY: Animal carcinogenesis studies with sublingual nitroglycerin have not been performed.

Rats receiving up to 434 mg/kg/day of dietary nitroglycerin for 2 years developed dose-related fibrotic and neoplastic changes in liver, including carcinomas, and interstitial cell tumors in testes. At high dose, the incidences of hepatocellular carcinomas in both sexes were 52% vs. 0% in controls, and incidences of testicular tumors were 52% vs. 8% in controls. Incidences of pituitary adenomas and female mammary tumors normally seen in aged rats were significantly reduced, consistent with treatment-related decrease in food intake and body weight; increased life span was also seen in the high dose females. Lifetime dietary administration of up to 1058 mg/kg/day of nitroglycerin was not tumorigenic in mice.

Nitroglycerin was weakly mutagenic in Ames tests performed in two different laboratories. Nevertheless, there was no evidence of mutagenicity in an *in vivo* dominant lethal assay with male rats treated with doses up to about 363 mg/kg/day, p.o., or in *in vitro* cytogenic tests in rat and dog tissues.

In a three-generation reproduction study, rats received dietary nitroglycerin at doses up to about 434 mg/kg/day for six months prior to mating of the F_0 generation with treatment continuing through successive F_1 and F_2 generations. The high dose was associated with decreased feed intake and body weight gain in both sexes at all matings. No specific effect on the fertility of the F_0 generation was seen. Infertility noted in subsequent generations, however, was attributed to increased interstitial cell tissue and aspermatogenesis in the high-dose males. In this three-generation study there was no clear evidence of teratogenicity.

PREGNANCY: Pregnancy Category C – Animal teratology studies have not been conducted with nitroglycerin spray. Teratology studies in rats and rabbits, however, were conducted with topically applied nitroglycerin ointment at doses up to 80 mg/kg/day and 240 mg/kg/day, respectively. No toxic effects on dams or fetuses were seen at any dose tested. There are no adequate and well-controlled studies in pregnant women. Nitroglycerin should be given to pregnant women only if clearly needed.

NURSING MOTHERS: It is not known whether nitroglycerin is excreted in human milk. Because many drugs are excreted in human milk, caution should be exercised when Nitrolingual Spray is administered to a nursing woman.

PEDIATRIC USE: The safety and effectiveness of nitroglycerin in children have not been established.

Continued on next page

Rhône-Poulenc Rorer—Cont.

ADVERSE REACTIONS

Adverse reaction to Nitrolingual Spray, particularly headache and hypotension, is generally dose-related. In clinical trials at various doses of nitroglycerin, the following adverse effects have been observed:

Headache, which may be severe and persistent, is the most commonly reported side effect of nitroglycerin with an incidence on the order of about 50% in some studies. Cutaneous vasodilation with flushing may occur. Transient episodes of dizziness and weakness, as well as other signs of cerebral ischemia associated with postural hypotension, may occasionally develop. An occasional individual may exhibit marked sensitivity to the hypotensive effects of nitrates and severe responses (nausea, vomiting, weakness, restlessness, pallor, perspiration, and collapse) may occur even with therapeutic doses. Drug rash and/or exfoliative dermatitis have been reported in patients receiving nitrate therapy. Nausea and vomiting appear to be uncommon.

OVERDOSAGE

Signs and Symptoms:

Nitrate overdosage may result in: severe hypotension, persistent throbbing headache, vertigo, palpitation, visual disturbance, flushing and perspiring skin (later becoming cold and cyanotic), nausea and vomiting (possibly with colic and even bloody diarrhea), syncope (especially in the upright posture), methemoglobinemia with cyanosis and anorexia, initial hypernea, dyspnea and slow breathing, slow pulse (dicrotic and intermittent), heart block, increased intracranial pressure with cerebral symptoms of confusion and moderate fever, paralysis and coma followed by clonic convulsions, and possibly death due to circulatory collapse.

Treatment of Overdosage:

Keep the patient recumbent in a shock position and comfortably warm. Gastric lavage may be of use if the medication has only recently been swallowed. Passive movement of the extremities may aid venous return. Administer oxygen and artificial ventilation, if necessary. If methemoglobinemia is present, administration of methylene blue (1% solution), 1–2 mg per kilogram of body weight intravenously, may be required.

Methemoglobinemia:

Case reports of clinically significant methemoglobinemia are rare at conventional doses of organic nitrates. The formation of methemoglobin is dose-related and in the case of genetic abnormalities of hemoglobin that favor methemoglobin formation, even conventional doses of organic nitrates could produce harmful concentrations of methemoglobin.

WARNING

Epinephrine is ineffective in reversing the severe hypotensive events associated with overdosage. It and related compounds are contraindicated in this situation.

DOSAGE AND ADMINISTRATION

At the onset of an attack, one or two metered doses should be sprayed onto or under the tongue. No more than three metered doses are recommended within a 15-minute period. If the chest pain persists, prompt medical attention is recommended. Nitrolingual Spray may be used prophylactically five to ten minutes prior to engaging in activities which might precipitate an acute attack.

During application the patient should rest, ideally in the sitting position. The canister should be held vertically with the valve head uppermost and the spray orifice as close to the mouth as possible. The dose should preferably be sprayed onto the tongue by pressing the button firmly and the mouth should be closed immediately after each dose. THE SPRAY SHOULD NOT BE INHALED. Patients should be instructed to familiarize themselves with the position of the spray orifice, which can be identified by the finger rest on top of the valve, in order to facilitate orientation for administration at night.

HOW SUPPLIED

Nitrolingual Spray, 14.49 g (Net Contents) containing 200 metered doses, box of one. (NDC 0075-0850-84)

Note: The indented statement below is required by the Federal government's Clean Air Act for all products containing or manufactured with chlorofluorocarbons (CFCs):

WARNING: Contains CFC-11 and CFC-12, substances which harm public health and environment by destroying ozone in the upper atmosphere.

A notice similar to the above WARNING has been placed in the "Information For The Patient" portion of this package insert pursuant to EPA regulations.

STORE AT ROOM TEMPERATURE. Do not expose to temperatures exceeding 50°C (122°F).

CAUTION

Federal (U.S.A.) law prohibits dispensing without prescription.

Military and Veterans Administration: 0.4 mg–14.49 gm (NSN 6505-01-246-3781).

Rev. 3/94   IN-2997K
Manufactured by:
G. Pohl-Boskamp GmbH & Co.
D-25551 Hohenlockstedt
Germany
Distributed by:
RHÔNE-POULENC RORER PHARMACEUTICALS INC.
Collegeville, PA, U.S.A. 19426-0107
Shown in Product Identification Guide, page 330

ONCASPAR®   ℞

[ən '-cə-spər]
(pegaspargase)

PRODUCT OVERVIEW

KEY FACTS

ONCASPAR® (pegaspargase) is a modified version of the enzyme L-asparaginase. It is an oncolytic agent used in combination chemotherapy for the treatment of patients with acute lymphoblastic leukemia who are hypersensitive to native forms of L-asparaginase. Oncaspar was clinically researched as PEG-L-asparaginase. As a component of selected multiple agent regimens, the recommended dose of **ONCASPAR®** is 2,500 IU/m² every 14 days by either the intramuscular or intravenous route of administration. When a remission is obtained, appropriate maintenance therapy may be instituted. **ONCASPAR®** may be used as part of a maintenance regimen.

MAJOR USES

ONCASPAR® is indicated for patients with acute lymphoblastic leukemia who require L-asparaginase in their treatment regimen, but have developed hypersensitivity to the native forms of L-asparaginase. **ONCASPAR®**, like native L-asparaginase, is generally used in combination with other chemotherapeutic agents, such as vincristine, methotrexate, cytarabine, daunorubicin, and doxorubicin.[1,5] Use of **ONCASPAR®** as a single agent should only be undertaken when multi-agent chemotherapy is judged to be inappropriate for the patient.

SAFETY INFORMATION

ONCASPAR® is contraindicated in patients with pancreatitis or a history of pancreatitis. **ONCASPAR®** is contraindicated in patients who have had significant hemorrhagic events associated with prior L-asparaginase therapy. **ONCASPAR®** is also contraindicated in patients who have had previous serious allergic reactions, such as generalized urticaria, bronchospasm, laryngeal edema, hypotension, or other unacceptable adverse reactions to **ONCASPAR®**.

PRESCRIBING INFORMATION

ONCASPAR®   ℞

[ən '-cə-spər]
(pegaspargase)

DESCRIPTION

ONCASPAR®, the ENZON trademark for pegaspargase, is a modified version of the enzyme L-asparaginase. It is an oncolytic agent used in combination chemotherapy for the treatment of patients with acute lymphoblastic leukemia who are hypersensitive to native forms of L-asparaginase (as described in **CLINICAL PHARMACOLOGY**).

The generic name for **ONCASPAR®** is **pegaspargase**. The chemical name is monomethoxypolyethylene glycol succinimidyl L-asparaginase. L-asparaginase is modified by covalently conjugating units of monomethoxypolyethylene glycol (PEG), molecular weight of 5,000, to the enzyme, forming the active ingredient PEG-L-asparaginase. The L-asparaginase (L-asparagine amidohydrolase, type EC-2, EC 3.5.1.1) used in the manufacture of **ONCASPAR®** is derived from *Escherichia coli*. ENZON purchases the enzyme L-asparaginase in bulk from Merck, Sharp and Dohme, Division of Merck & Co., Inc., West Point, PA 19486, U.S. License Number 2. Merck & Co., Inc. supplies bulk L-asparaginase as a licensed intermediate for further manufacture by ENZON into PEG-L-asparaginase. Merck & Co., Inc. can only assume responsibility for the bulk intermediate supplied to ENZON. **ONCASPAR®** is supplied as an isotonic sterile solution in phosphate buffered saline, pH 7.3, for intramuscular or intravenous administration only. The solution is clear, colorless and contains no preservatives. It is supplied in 5 mL single-dose vials.

ONCASPAR® activity is expressed in International Units (IU) according to the recommendation of the International Union of Biochemistry. One IU of L-asparaginase is defined as that amount of enzyme required to generate 1 μmol of ammonia per minute at pH 7.3 and 37°C.

Each milliliter of **ONCASPAR®** contains:

PEG-L-asparaginase	750 IU ± 20%
Monobasic sodium phosphate, USP	1.20 mg ± 5%
Dibasic sodium phosphate, USP	5.58 mg ± 5%
Sodium chloride, USP	8.50 mg ± 5%
Water for injection, USP	qs to 1.0 mL

The specific activity of **ONCASPAR®** is at least 85 IU per milligram protein.

CLINICAL PHARMACOLOGY

Leukemic cells are unable to synthesize asparagine due to a lack of asparagine synthetase and are dependent on an exogenous source of asparagine for survival. Rapid depletion of asparagine which results from treatment with the enzyme L-asparaginase, kills the leukemic cells. Normal cells, however, are less affected by the rapid depletion due to their ability to synthesize asparagine. This is an approach to therapy based on a specific metabolic defect in some leukemic cells which do not produce asparagine synthetase.[1]

In a study in predominately L-asparaginase naive adult patients with leukemia and lymphoma, initial plasma levels of L-asparaginase following intravenous administration were determined. Plasma half-life did not appear to be influenced by dose levels, and it could not be correlated with age, sex, surface area, renal or hepatic function, diagnosis or extent of disease. Apparent volume of distribution was equal to estimated plasma volume. L-asparaginase was measurable for at least 15 days following the initial treatment with **ONCASPAR®**. The enzyme could not be detected in the urine.[2]

In a study of newly diagnosed pediatric patients with acute lymphoblastic leukemia (ALL) who received either a single intramuscular injection of **ONCASPAR®** (2,500 IU/m²), *E. coli* L-asparaginase (25,000 IU/m²), or *Erwinia* L-asparaginase (25,000 IU/m²), the plasma half-lives for the three forms of L-asparaginase were:[3]

PLASMA HALF-LIVES OF THREE FORMS OF L-ASPARAGINASE

Treatment Group	No. of Patients	Mean (Days)	Standard Deviation
ONCASPAR®	10	5.73	3.24
E. coli L-asparaginase	17	1.24	0.17
Erwinia L-asparaginase	10	0.65	0.13

In this same study of newly diagnosed pediatric ALL patients, the *in vivo* early leukemic cell kill after a single intramuscular injection of native *E. coli* L-asparaginase (25,000 IU/m²), *Erwinia* L-asparaginase (25,000 IU/m²), and **ONCASPAR®** (2,500 IU/m²) during a five day "investigational window" was studied.[4] Bone marrow aspirates were taken before and five days after a single dose of one of the three different forms of L-asparaginase. Rhodamine-123 (RH-123), a selectively incorporated fluorescent mitochondrial dye, was used in an *in vitro* assay on the bone marrow aspirates to ascertain cell viability. The percent reduction of viable lymphoblasts at day five for each group is presented in the following table:[4]

RHODAMINE-123 (*IN VIVO* CELL KILL)

Treatment Group	No. of Patients	Percent Reduction of Viable Lymphoblasts At Day 5 Mean ± S.D.
ONCASPAR®	21	55.7 ± 10.2
E. coli L-asparaginase	28	57.8 ± 10.1
Erwinia L-asparaginase	19	57.9 ± 13.8

In three pharmacokinetic studies, 37 relapsed ALL patients received **ONCASPAR®** at 2,500 IU/m² every two weeks. The plasma half-life of **ONCASPAR®** was 3.24 ± 1.83 days in nine patients who were previously hypersensitive to native L-asparaginase and 5.69 ± 3.25 days in 28 non-hypersensitive patients. The area under the curve was 9.50 ± 3.95 IU/mL/day in the previously hypersensitive patients, and 9.83 ± 5.94 IU/mL/day in the non-hypersensitive patients.

Hypersensitivity Reactions

Hypersensitivity reactions to *E. coli* L-asparaginase have been reported in the literature in 3% to 73% of patients.[1] Patients in **ONCASPAR®** clinical studies were considered to be previously hypersensitive if they experienced a systemic rash, urticaria, bronchospasm, laryngeal edema, or hypotension following administration of any form of native L-asparaginase. Patients were also considered to be previously hypersensitive if they experienced local erythema, urticaria, or swelling, greater than two centimeters, for at least ten minutes following administration of any form of native L-asparaginase. The National Cancer Institute Common Toxicity Criteria (CTC) were used to classify the severity of the hypersensitivity reactions. These are: grade 1 — transient rash (mild); grade 2 — mild bronchospasm (moderate); grade 3 — moderate bronchospasm and/or serum sickness (severe); grade 4 — hypotension and/or anaphylaxis (life-threatening). Additionally, most transient local urticaria were considered grade 2 hypersensitivity reactions, while most sustained urticaria distant from the injection site were considered grade 3 hypersensitivity reactions. In general, the moderate to life-threatening hypersensitivity reactions

were considered dose-limiting; that is, they required L-asparaginase treatment to be discontinued.

In separate studies, **ONCASPAR®** was administered intravenously to 48 patients and intramuscularly to 126 patients. The incidence of hypersensitivity reactions when **ONCASPAR®** was administered intramuscularly was 30% in patients who were previously hypersensitive to native L-asparaginase and 11% in non-hypersensitive patients (p-value of 0.007). The incidence of hypersensitivity reactions when **ONCASPAR®** was administered intravenously was 60% in patients who were previously hypersensitive to native L-asparaginase and 12% in non-hypersensitive patients. Since only five previously hypersensitive patients received **ONCASPAR®** intravenously, no meaningful analysis of the incidence of hypersensitivity reactions was possible between either the previously hypersensitive and non-hypersensitive patients, or between the intravenous and intramuscular routes of administration.

The overall incidence of hypersensitivity reactions in 174 patients who received **ONCASPAR®** in five clinical studies is shown in the table below:

INCIDENCE OF ONCASPAR® HYPERSENSITIVITY REACTIONS

		CTC GRADE OF HYPERSENSITIVITY REACTION				
PATIENT STATUS	**N**	**1**	**2**	**3**	**4**	**TOTAL**
Previously Hypersensitive Patients	62	7	8	4	1	20 (32%)
Non-Hypersensitive Patients	112	5	4	1	1	11 (10%)
Total Patients	174	12	12	5	2	31 (18%)

The probability of a previously hypersensitive or non-hypersensitive patient completing 8 doses of **ONCASPAR®** therapy without developing a dose-limiting hypersensitivity reaction was 77% and 95%, respectively.

All of the 62 hypersensitive patients treated with **ONCASPAR®** in five clinical studies had previous hypersensitivity reactions to one or more of the native forms of L-asparaginase. Of the 35 patients who had previous hypersensitivity reactions to *E. coli* L-asparaginase only, 5 (14%) had **ONCASPAR®** dose-limiting hypersensitivity reactions. Of the 27 patients who had hypersensitivity reactions to both *E. coli* and *Erwinia* L-asparaginase, 7 (26%) had **ONCASPAR®** dose-limiting hypersensitivity reactions. The overall incidence of dose-limiting hypersensitivity reactions in 174 patients treated with **ONCASPAR®** was 9% (19% in 62 hypersensitive and 3% in 112 non-hypersensitive patients). Of the total of 9% dose-limiting hypersensitivity reactions, 1% were anaphylactic (CTC grade 4) and the other 8% were ≤ CTC grade 3.

Clinical Activity

ONCASPAR® was evaluated as part of combination therapy in four open label studies comprising 42 multiply-relapsed, previously hypersensitive acute leukemia patients [39 (93%) with ALL] at a dose of 2,000 or 2,500 IU/m^2 administered intramuscularly or intravenously every 14 days during induction combination chemotherapy. The reinduction response rate was 50% (36% complete remissions and 14% partial remissions), with a 95% confidence interval of 35% to 65%. This response rate is comparable to that reported in the literature for relapsed patients treated with native L-asparaginase as part of combination chemotherapy.[1]

ONCASPAR® was also shown to have some activity as a single agent in multiply-relapsed hypersensitive ALL patients, the majority of whom were pediatric. Treatment with **ONCASPAR®** resulted in three responses (one complete remission and two partial remissions) in nine previously hypersensitive patients who would not have been able to receive any further L-asparaginase treatment.

ONCASPAR® was also studied in non-hypersensitive, relapsed ALL patients who were randomized to receive two doses of **ONCASPAR®** at 2,500 IU/m^2 every 14 days or twelve doses of *E. coli* L-asparaginase at 10,000 IU/m^2 three times a week during a 28 day induction combination chemotherapy regimen (which included vincristine and prednisone). Although the enrollment in this study was too small to be conclusive, the data showed that for 20 patients there was no significant difference between the overall response rates of 60% and 50%, respectively, or the complete remission rates of 50% and 50%, respectively.

ONCASPAR® was administered during maintenance therapy regimens to 33 previously hypersensitive patients. The average number of doses received during maintenance therapy was 5.8 (range of 1 to 24) and the average duration of maintenance therapy was 126 (range of 1 to 513) days for this patient population.

INDICATIONS AND USAGE

ONCASPAR® is indicated for patients with acute lymphoblastic leukemia who require L-asparaginase in their treatment regimen, but have developed hypersensitivity to the native forms of L-asparaginase **(SEE CLINICAL PHARMACOLOGY)**. **ONCASPAR®**, like native L-asparaginase, is generally used in combination with other chemotherapeutic agents, such as vincristine, methotrexate, cytarabine, daunorubicin, and doxorubicin.[1,5] Use of **ONCASPAR®** as a single agent should only be undertaken when multi-agent chemotherapy is judged to be inappropriate for the patient.

CONTRAINDICATIONS

ONCASPAR® is contraindicated in patients with pancreatitis or a history of pancreatitis. **ONCASPAR®** is contraindicated in patients who have had significant hemorrhagic events associated with prior L-asparaginase therapy. **ONCASPAR®** is also contraindicated in patients who have had previous serious allergic reactions, such as generalized urticaria, bronchospasm, laryngeal edema, hypotension, or other unacceptable adverse reactions to **ONCASPAR®**.

WARNINGS

It is recommended that **ONCASPAR®** be given under the supervision of an individual who is qualified by training and experience to administer cancer chemotherapeutic agents. Especially in patients with known hypersensitivity to the other forms of L-asparaginase, hypersensitivity reactions to **ONCASPAR®**, including life-threatening anaphylaxis, may occur during therapy. As a routine precaution, patients should be kept under observation for one hour with resuscitation equipment and other agents necessary to treat anaphylaxis (epinephrine, oxygen, intravenous steroids, etc.) available.

PRECAUTIONS

General

This drug may be a contact irritant, and the solution must be handled and administered with care. Gloves are recommended. Inhalation of vapors and contact with skin or mucous membranes, especially those of the eyes, must be avoided. In case of contact, wash with copious amounts of water for at least 15 minutes. Anaphylactic reactions require the immediate use of epinephrine, oxygen, intravenous steroids, and antihistamines. Patients taking **ONCASPAR®** are at higher than usual risk for bleeding problems, especially with simultaneous use of other drugs that have anticoagulant properties, such as aspirin, and non-steroidal anti-inflammatories **(SEE DRUG INTERACTIONS)**. **ONCASPAR®** may have immunosuppressive activity. Therefore, it is possible that use of the drug in patients may predispose the patient to infection. Severe hepatic and central nervous system toxicity following multi-agent chemotherapy that includes **ONCASPAR®** may occur. Caution appears warranted when treating patients with **ONCASPAR®** given in combination with hepatotoxic agents, particularly when liver dysfunction is present.

Patients undergoing **ONCASPAR®** therapy must be carefully monitored and the therapeutic regimen adjusted according to response and toxicity. Physicians using a given treatment regimen incorporating **ONCASPAR®** should be thoroughly familiar with its benefits and risks.

Information For Patients

Patients should be informed of the possibility of hypersensitivity reactions, including immediate anaphylaxis, to **ONCASPAR®**. Patients taking **ONCASPAR®** are at higher than usual risk for bleeding problems. Patients should be instructed that the simultaneous use of **ONCASPAR®** with other drugs that may increase the risk of bleeding should be avoided **(SEE DRUG INTERACTIONS)**. **ONCASPAR®** may affect the ability of the liver to function normally in some patients. Therapy with **ONCASPAR®** may increase the toxicity of other medications **(SEE DRUG INTERACTIONS)**. **ONCASPAR®** may have immunosuppressive activity. Therefore, it is possible that use of the drug in patients may predispose the patient to infection. Patients should notify their physicians of any adverse reactions that occur.

Laboratory Tests

A fall in circulating lymphoblasts is often noted after initiating therapy. This may be accompanied by a marked rise in serum uric acid. As a guide to the effects of therapy, the patient's peripheral blood count and bone marrow should be monitored.

Frequent serum amylase determinations should be obtained to detect early evidence of pancreatitis **(SEE CONTRAINDICATIONS)**. Blood sugar should be monitored during therapy with **ONCASPAR®** because hyperglycemia may occur. When using **ONCASPAR®** in conjunction with hepatotoxic chemotherapy, patients should be monitored for liver dysfunction.

ONCASPAR® may affect a number of plasma proteins; therefore, monitoring of fibrinogen, PT, and PTT may be indicated.

Drug Interactions

Unfavorable interactions of L-asparaginase with some antitumor agents have been demonstrated.[1] It is recommended, therefore, that **ONCASPAR®** be used in combination regimens only by physicians familiar with the benefits and risks of a given regimen. Depletion of serum proteins by **ONCASPAR®** may increase the toxicity of other drugs which are protein bound. Additionally, during the period of its inhibition of protein synthesis and cell replication, **ONCASPAR®** may interfere with the action of drugs such as methotrexate, which require cell replication for their lethal effects. **ONCASPAR®** may interfere with the enzymatic detoxification of other drugs, particularly in the liver. Physicians using a given treatment regimen should be thoroughly familiar with its benefits and risks.

Imbalances in coagulation factors have been noted with the use of **ONCASPAR®** predisposing to bleeding and/or thrombosis. Caution should be used when administering any concurrent anticoagulant therapy, such as coumadin, heparin, dipyridamole, aspirin, or non-steroidal anti-inflammatories.

Carcinogenesis, Mutagenesis, Impairment of Fertility

Long-term carcinogenic studies in animals have not been performed with **ONCASPAR®** nor have studies been performed on impairment of fertility. **ONCASPAR®** did not exhibit a mutagenic effect when tested against *Salmonella typhimurium* strains in the Ames assay.

Pregnancy

Pregnancy Category C. Animal reproduction studies have not been conducted with **ONCASPAR®**. It is also not known whether **ONCASPAR®** can cause fetal harm when administered to a pregnant woman or can affect reproduction capacity. **ONCASPAR®** should be given to a pregnant woman only if clearly needed.

Nursing Mothers

It is not known whether **ONCASPAR®** is excreted in human milk. Because many drugs are excreted in human milk and because of the potential for serious adverse reactions due to **ONCASPAR®** in nursing infants, a decision should be made to discontinue nursing or discontinue the drug, taking into account the importance of the drug to the mother.

ONCASPAR® ADVERSE REACTIONS

Adverse reactions have been reported in adults and pediatric patients. Overall, the adult patients treated with **ONCASPAR®** had a somewhat higher incidence of known L-asparaginase toxicities, except for hypersensitivity reactions, than the pediatric patients treated with **ONCASPAR®**.

Excluding hypersensitivity reactions, the most frequently occurring known L-asparaginase related toxicities and adverse experiences reported for the 174 patients in clinical studies were chemical hepatotoxicities and coagulopathies, the majority of which did not result in any significant clinical events. The incidence of significant clinical events included clinical pancreatitis (1%), hyperglycemia requiring insulin therapy (3%), and thrombosis (4%).

The following adverse reactions related to **ONCASPAR®** were reported for 174 patients in five clinical studies.

The adverse reactions reported most frequently (greater than 5%) were allergic reactions (which may have included rash, erythema, edema, pain, fever, chills, urticaria, dyspnea, or bronchospasm), SGPT increase, nausea and/or vomiting, fever and malaise.

The adverse reactions reported occasionally (greater than 1% but less than 5%) were anaphylactic reactions, dyspnea, injection site hypersensitivity, lip edema, rash, urticaria, abdominal pain, chills, pain in the extremities, hypotension, tachycardia, thrombosis, anorexia, diarrhea, jaundice, abnormal liver function test, decreased anticoagulant effect, disseminated intravascular coagulation, decreased fibrinogen, hemolytic anemia, leukopenia, pancytopenia, thrombocytopenia, increased thromboplastin, injection site pain, injection site reaction, bilirubinemia, hyperglycemia, hyperuricemia, hypoglycemia, hypoproteinemia, peripheral edema, increased SGOT, arthralgia, myalgia, convulsion, headache, night sweats, and paresthesia.

The adverse reactions reported rarely (less than 1%) were bronchospasm, petechial rash, face edema, lesional edema, sepsis, septic shock, chest pain, endocarditis, hypertension, constipation, flatulence, gastrointestinal pain, hepatomegaly, increased appetite, liver fatty deposits, coagulation disorder, increased coagulation time, decreased platelet count, purpura, increased amylase, edema, excessive thirst, hyperammonemia, hyponatremia, weight loss, bone pain, joint disorder, confusion, dizziness, emotional lability, somnolence, increased cough, epistaxis, upper respiratory infection, erythema simplex, pruritus, hematuria, increased urinary frequency, and abnormal kidney function.

The following **ONCASPAR®** related adverse reactions have been observed in patients with hematologic malignancies, primarily acute lymphoblastic leukemia (approximately 75%), non-Hodgkins lymphoma (approximately 13%), acute myelogenous leukemia (approximately 3%), and a variety of solid tumors (approximately 9%):

HYPERSENSITIVITY REACTIONS: a variety of hypersensitivity reactions have occurred. These reactions may be acute or delayed, and include acute anaphylaxis, bronchospasm, dyspnea, urticaria, arthralgia, erythema, induration, edema, pain, tenderness, hives, swelling, lip edema, chills, fever, and skin rashes **(SEE WARNINGS AND CONTRAINDICATIONS)**.

Continued on next page

Rhône-Poulenc Rorer–Cont.

PANCREATIC FUNCTION: pancreatitis, sometimes fulminant and fatal, has occurred. Increased serum amylase and lipase have also occurred.
LIVER FUNCTION: a variety of liver function abnormalities have been observed, including elevations of SGOT, SGPT, and bilirubin (direct and indirect). Jaundice, ascites, and hypoalbuminemia, which may be associated with peripheral edema, have been observed. These abnormalities usually are reversible on discontinuance of therapy, and some reversal may occur during the course of therapy. Fatty changes in the liver and liver failure have occurred.
HEMATOLOGIC: hypofibrinogenemia, prolonged prothrombin times, prolonged partial thromboplastin times, and decreased antithrombin III have been observed. Superficial and deep venous thrombosis, sagittal sinus thrombosis, venous catheter thrombosis, and atrial thrombosis have occurred. Leukopenia, agranulocytosis, pancytopenia, thrombocytopenia, disseminated intravascular coagulation, severe hemolytic anemia, and anemia have been observed. Clinical hemorrhage, which may be fatal; easy bruisability, and ecchymosis have also been observed.
METABOLIC: mild to severe hyperglycemia has been observed in low incidence, and usually responds to discontinuation of **ONCASPAR®** and the judicious use of intravenous fluid and insulin. Hypoglycemia, increased thirst and hyponatremia, uric acid nephropathy, hyperuricemia, hypoproteinemia, and peripheral edema have also been observed. Hypoalbuminemia, proteinuria, weight loss, and metabolic acidosis have occurred. Therapy with **ONCASPAR®** is associated with an increase in blood ammonia during the conversion of L-asparagine to aspartic acid by the enzyme.
NEUROLOGIC: status epilepticus and temporal lobe seizures, somnolence, coma, malaise, mental status changes, dizziness, emotional lability, headache, lip numbness, finger paresthesia, mood changes, night sweats, and a Parkinson-like syndrome have occurred. Mild to severe confusion, disorientation, and paresthesia have also occurred. These side effects usually have reversed spontaneously after treatment was stopped.
RENAL: increased BUN, increased creatinine, increased urinary frequency, hematuria due to thrombopenia, severe hemorrhagic cystitis, renal dysfunction, and renal failure have been observed.
CARDIOVASCULAR: chest pain, subacute bacterial endocarditis, hypertension, severe hypotension, and tachycardia have occurred.
DIGESTIVE: anorexia, constipation, decreased appetite, diarrhea, indigestion, flatulence, gas, gastrointestinal pain, mucositis, hepatomegaly, elevated gamma-glutamyltranspeptidase, increased appetite, mouth tenderness, severe colitis, and nausea and/or vomiting have been observed.
MUSCULOSKELETAL: diffuse and local musculoskeletal pain, arthralgia, joint stiffness, and cramps have occurred.
RESPIRATORY: cough, epistaxis, severe bronchospasm, and upper respiratory infection have been observed.
SKIN/APPENDAGES: itching, alopecia, fever blister, purpura, hand whiteness and fungal changes, nail whiteness and ridging, erythema simplex, jaundice, and petechial rash have occurred.
GENERAL: localized edema, injection site reactions (including pain, swelling, or redness), malaise, infection, sepsis, fatigue, and septic shock may occur.

OVERDOSAGE

Three patients received 10,000 IU/m^2 of **ONCASPAR®** as an intravenous infusion. One patient experienced a slight increase in liver enzymes. A second patient developed a rash ten minutes after the start of the infusion, which was controlled with the administration of an antihistamine and by slowing down the infusion rate. A third patient did not experience any adverse reactions.

DOSAGE AND ADMINISTRATION

As a component of selected multiple agent regimens, the recommended dose of **ONCASPAR®** is 2,500 IU/m^2 every 14 days by either the intramuscular or intravenous route of administration.
The preferred route of administration, however, is the intramuscular route because of the lower incidence of hepatotoxicity, coagulopathy, and gastrointestinal and renal disorders compared to the intravenous route of administration.
The safety and effectiveness of **ONCASPAR®** have been established in patients with known previous hypersensitivity to L-asparaginase whose ages ranged from 1 to 21 years old. The recommended dose of **ONCASPAR®** for children with a body surface area ≥ 0.6 m^2 is 2,500 IU/m^2 administered every 14 days. The recommended dose of **ONCASPAR®** for children with a body surface area <0.6 m^2 is 82.5 IU/kg administered every 14 days.
Do not administer ONCASPAR® if there is any indication that the drug has been frozen. Although there may not be an apparent change in the appearance of the drug, ONCASPAR®'s activity is destroyed after freezing.
When administering **ONCASPAR®** intramuscularly, the volume at a single injection site should be limited to 2 mL. If the volume to be administered is greater than 2 mL, multiple injection sites should be used.
When administered intravenously, **ONCASPAR®** should be given over a period of 1 to 2 hours in 100 mL of sodium chloride or dextrose injection 5%, through an infusion that is already running.
Anaphylactic reactions require the immediate use of antihistamines, epinephrine, oxygen, and intravenous steroids.
Use of **ONCASPAR®** as the sole induction agent should be undertaken only in an unusual situation when a combined regimen, which uses other chemotherapeutic agents such as vincristine, methotrexate, cytarabine, daunorubicin, or doxorubicin, is inappropriate because of toxicity or other specific patient-related factors, or in patients refractory to other therapy. When **ONCASPAR®** is to be used as the sole induction agent, the recommended dosage regimen is also 2,500 IU/m^2 every 14 days.
When a remission is obtained, appropriate maintenance therapy may be instituted. **ONCASPAR®** may be used as part of a maintenance regimen.
Parenteral drug products should be inspected visually for particulate matter, cloudiness or discoloration prior to administration, whenever solution and container permit.

HOW SUPPLIED

Dosage Form
ONCASPAR®: Use only one dose per vial; do not re-enter the vial. Discard unused portions. Do not save unused drug for later administration.
Sterile solution for injection in ready to use single-use vials. Preservative free.
Quantity per Individual Container
5 mL per vial containing 750 IU/mL **ONCASPAR®** in a clear, colorless, phosphate buffered saline solution, pH 7.3. Each vial contains 3,750 IU of **ONCASPAR®**.
Handling and Storage
Avoid excessive agitation. DO NOT SHAKE.
Keep refrigerated at +2°C to +8°C (36°F to 46°F).
Do not use if cloudy or if precipitate is present.
Do not use if stored at room temperature for more than 48 hours.
DO NOT FREEZE. Do not use product if it is known to have been frozen. Freezing destroys activity, which cannot be detected visually.
NDC 0075-0640-05
U.S. Patent 4,179,337 and pat. pending

40 Kingsbridge Road
Piscataway, NJ 08854-3998 USA

01/21/94

REFERENCES

1. Capizzi, RL and Holcenberg, JS. Asparaginase. In: Holland and Frei (eds). *Cancer Med* third edition, Lea and Febiger, Phila. PA, 1993.
2. Ho, DH, et al. Clinical pharmacology of polyethylene glycol-L-asparaginase. *Drug Metab Dispos* 14 (3): 349–352, 1986.
3. Asselin, BL, et al. Comparative Pharmacokinetic Studies of Three L-asparaginase Preparations. *J Clin Oncology* (11): 1780–1786, 1993.
4. Data on File at ENZON.
5. Clavell, LA, et al. Four-agent induction and intensive asparaginase therapy for treatment of childhood acute lymphoblastic leukemia. *N Engl J Med* 315 (11): 657–663, 1986.

IN-1724
PN 200-040 Rev. 2/94
Mfg. by: Enzon, Inc.
Piscataway, NJ 08854 USA
License No. 1171
Dist. by: Rhône-Poulenc Rorer Pharmaceuticals Inc.
Collegeville, PA 19426-0107 U.S.A.
Shown in Product Identification Guide, page 330

PENETREX™ ℞
(enoxacin) Tablets

DESCRIPTION

Penetrex™ (enoxacin) is a broad-spectrum azafluoroquinolone antibacterial agent for oral administration. Enoxacin is 1-ethyl-6-fluoro-1,4-dihydro-4-oxo-7-(1-piperazinyl)-1,8-naphthyridine-3-carboxylic acid sesquihydrate. The chemical structure of enoxacin is:

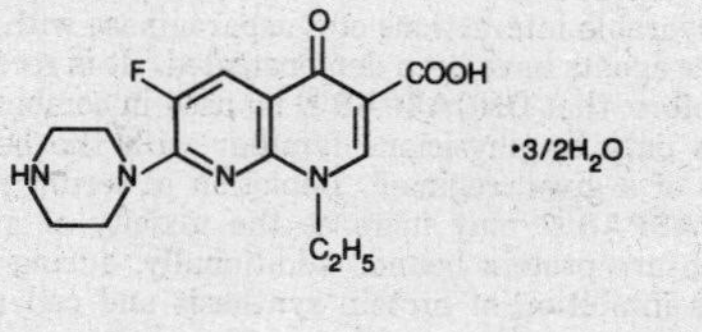

Its empirical formula is $C_{15}H_{17}N_4O_3F \cdot 1^1/_2\ H_2O$, and its molecular weight is 320.32 (anhydrous). Enoxacin is an ivory-to-slightly yellow powder. In dilute aqueous solution, it is unstable in strong sunlight.
Penetrex is available in 200 mg and 400 mg film-coated tablets. Each "200" and "400" Penetrex tablet contains enoxacin sesquihydrate equivalent to 200 mg and 400 mg of anhydrous enoxacin, respectively. Each Penetrex 200 mg and 400 mg tablet contains the following inactive ingredients: cellulose microcrystalline NF, colloidal silicon dioxide NF, croscarmellose sodium NF, FD&C Blue No. 2 aluminum lake, hydroxypropyl cellulose NF, hydroxypropyl methylcellulose, magnesium stearate USP, polyethylene glycol, simethicone, sorbic acid, stearate emulsifiers, and titanium dioxide.

CLINICAL PHARMACOLOGY

Following oral administration to healthy subjects, peak plasma enoxacin concentrations were achieved within 1 to 3 hours. Absolute oral bioavailability of enoxacin is approximately 90%. Maximum plasma concentrations of enoxacin average 0.93 μg/mL and 2.0 μg/mL after single 200 mg and 400 mg doses, respectively. Enoxacin plasma half-life is 3 to 6 hours. Enoxacin is excreted primarily via the kidney. After a single dose, greater than 40% was recovered in urine by 48 hours as unchanged drug. In elderly patients, the mean peak enoxacin plasma concentration was 50% higher than that in young adult volunteers receiving comparable single doses of enoxacin. This appears to correspond to age-associated reduction of renal function in the elderly population. Five metabolites of enoxacin have been identified in human urine and account for 15% to 20% of the administered dose.
Enoxacin diffuses into cervix, fallopian tube, and myometrium at levels approximately 1–2 times those achieved in plasma, and into kidney and prostate at levels approximately 2–4 times those achieved in plasma. Studies have not been conducted to assess the penetration of enoxacin into human cerebrospinal fluid.
Enoxacin is approximately 40% bound to plasma proteins in healthy subjects and is approximately 14% bound to plasma proteins in patients with impaired renal function.
The effect of food on the absorption of enoxacin from the tablet formulation has not been studied.
Some isozymes of the cytochrome P-450 hepatic microsomal enzyme system are inhibited by enoxacin. This inhibition results in significant drug/drug interactions with theophylline and caffeine. Enoxacin interferes with the metabolism of theophylline, resulting in a dose-related decrease in theophylline clearance. Elevated serum theophylline concentrations may increase the risk of theophylline-related adverse reactions. (See **PRECAUTIONS: Drug Interactions.**)
Clearance of enoxacin is reduced in patients with impaired renal function (creatinine clearance ≤ 30 mL/min/1.73 m^2), and dosage adjustment is necessary. (See **DOSAGE AND ADMINISTRATION.**)

MICROBIOLOGY

Enoxacin is an inhibitor of the bacterial enzyme DNA gyrase and is a bactericidal agent. Enoxacin may be active against pathogens resistant to drugs that act by different mechanisms.
Enoxacin has been shown to be active against most strains of the following organisms both *in vitro* and in clinical infections: (See **INDICATIONS AND USAGE.**)
Gram-positive aerobes: *Staphylococcus epidermidis, Staphylococcus saprophyticus.*
Gram-negative aerobes: *Enterobacter cloacae, Escherichia coli, Klebsiella pneumoniae, Neisseria gonorrhoeae, Proteus mirabilis, Pseudomonas aeruginosa.*
The following *in vitro* data are available but their clinical significance is unknown.
In addition, enoxacin exhibits *in vitro* minimum inhibitory concentrations (MICs) of 2.0 μg/mL or less against most strains of the following organisms; however, the safety and effectiveness of enoxacin in treating clinical infections due to these organisms have not been established in adequate and well-controlled trials.
Gram-negative aerobes: *Aeromonas hydrophila, Citrobacter diversus, Citrobacter freundii, Citrobacter koseri, Enterobacter aerogenes, Haemophilus ducreyi, Klebsiella oxytoca, Klebsiella ozaenae, Morganella morganii, Proteus vulgaris, Providencia stuartii, Providencia alcalifaciens, Serratia marcescens, Serratia proteomaculans* (formerly *S. liquefaciens*).
Many strains of *Streptococcus* species and anaerobes are usually resistant to enoxacin.
The activity of enoxacin against *Treponema pallidum* has not been evaluated; however, other quinolones are not active against *T. pallidum.* (See **WARNINGS.**)
Cross-resistance with other quinolones has been demonstrated.
The addition of human serum has no effect on the *in vitro* MIC values; however, enoxacin activity is decreased in acidic (pH 5.5) environments.

Susceptibility Testing
Diffusion Techniques: Quantitative methods that require measurement of zone diameters give the most precise estimate of susceptibility of bacteria to antimicrobial agents.

One such standardized procedure[1] that has been recommended for use with disks to test susceptibility of organisms to enoxacin uses the 10-µg enoxacin disk.

Interpretation involves the correlation of the diameter obtained in the disk test with the minimum inhibitory concentration (MIC) for enoxacin.

Reports from the laboratory giving results of the standard single-disk susceptibility test with a 10-µg enoxacin disk should be interpreted according to the following criteria:

Zone Diameter (mm)	Interpretation
≥ 18	(S) Susceptible
15–17	(MS) Moderately susceptible
≤ 14	(R) Resistant

A report of "Susceptible" indicates that the pathogen is likely to be inhibited by generally achievable blood concentrations. A report of "Moderately susceptible" suggests that the organism would be susceptible if high dosage is used or if the infection is confined to tissues or fluids in which high antimicrobial levels are attained. A report of "Resistant" indicates that achievable drug concentrations are unlikely to be inhibitory, and other therapy should be selected.

Standardized susceptibility test procedures require the use of laboratory control organisms. The 10-µg enoxacin disk should give the following zone diameters:

Organism	Zone Diameter (mm)
Escherichia coli (ATCC 25922)	28–36
Neisseria gonorrhoeae (ATCC 49226)	43–51
Pseudomonas aeruginosa (ATCC 27853)	22–28
Staphylococcus aureus (ATCC 25923)	22–28

Other quinolone antibacterial disks should not be substituted when performing susceptibility tests for enoxacin because of spectrum differences. The 10-µg enoxacin disk should be used for all *in vitro* testing of isolates for enoxacin susceptibility using diffusion techniques.

Dilution Techniques: Use a standardized dilution method[2] (broth, agar, or microdilution) or equivalent with enoxacin powder. The MIC values obtained should be interpreted according to the following criteria:

MIC (µg/mL)	Interpretation
≤ 2	(S) Susceptible
4	(MS) Moderately susceptible
≥ 8	(R) Resistant

As with standard diffusion methods, dilution procedures require the use of laboratory control organisms. Standard enoxacin powder should give the following MIC values:

Organism	MIC (µg/mL)
Enterococcus faecalis (ATCC 29212)	2–16
Escherichia coli (ATCC 25922)	0.06–0.25
Neisseria gonorrhoeae (ATCC 49226)	0.015–0.06
Pseudomonas aeruginosa (ATCC 27853)	2–8
Staphylococcus aureus (ATCC 29213)	0.5–2

INDICATIONS AND USAGE

Penetrex™ (enoxacin) is indicated for the treatment of adults (≥ 18 years of age) with the following infections caused by susceptible strains of the designated microorganisms:

Sexually Transmitted Diseases (See **WARNINGS.**) Uncomplicated urethral or cervical gonorrhea due to *Neisseria gonorrhoeae.*

Urinary Tract: Uncomplicated urinary tract infections (cystitis) due to *Escherichia coli, Staphylococcus epidermidis**, or *Staphylococcus saprophyticus**.

Complicated urinary tract infections due to *Escherichia coli, Klebsiella pneumoniae, Proteus mirabilis, Pseudomonas aeruginosa, Staphylococcus epidermidis*, or *Enterobacter cloacae**.

*Efficacy for this organism in this organ system at the recommended dose was studied in fewer than ten infections. The dosage regimens for complicated and uncomplicated urinary tract infections are different. (See **DOSAGE AND ADMINISTRATION.**)

Penicillinase production should have no effect on enoxacin activity.

Appropriate culture and susceptibility tests should be performed before treatment in order to isolate and identify organisms causing the infection and to determine their susceptibility to enoxacin. Therapy with enoxacin may be initiated while awaiting the results of these studies; therapy should be adjusted if necessary once the results are known. Culture and susceptibility testing performed periodically during therapy will provide information not only on the therapeutic effect of the antimicrobial agent but also on the possible emergence of bacterial resistance.

CONTRAINDICATIONS

Penetrex is contraindicated in persons with a history of hypersensitivity, tendinitis, or tendon rupture associated with the use of enoxacin or any member of the quinolone group of antimicrobial agents.

WARNINGS

THE SAFETY AND EFFECTIVENESS OF ENOXACIN IN CHILDREN, ADOLESCENTS (UNDER THE AGE OF 18 YEARS), PREGNANT WOMEN, AND LACTATING WOMEN HAVE NOT BEEN ESTABLISHED. (See PRECAUTIONS: Pregnancy, Nursing Mothers, and Pediatric Use.) Enoxacin has been shown to cause arthropathy in immature rats and dogs when given in oral doses approximately 1.5 and 3.8 times, respectively, the highest human clinical dose based on a mg/m² basis after a four-week dosage regimen. Gross and histopathological examination of the weight-bearing joints of the dogs revealed lesions of the cartilage. Other quinolones also produce erosions of cartilage of weight-bearing joints and other signs of arthropathy in immature animals of various species. (See **ANIMAL PHARMACOLOGY.**)

Convulsions and abnormal electroencephalograms have been reported in some patients receiving enoxacin. Increased intracranial pressure, and toxic psychoses have been reported in patients receiving drugs in this class. Quinolones may also cause central nervous system stimulation which may lead to: tremors, restlessness/agitation, nervousness/anxiety, lightheadedness, confusion, hallucinations, paranoia, depression, nightmares, insomnia, and, rarely, suicidal thoughts or acts. These reactions may occur following the first dose. If these reactions occur in patients receiving enoxacin, the drug should be discontinued and appropriate measures instituted. As with all quinolones, enoxacin should be used with caution in patients with known or suspected CNS disorder that may predispose to seizures or lower the seizure threshold (e.g., severe cerebral arteriosclerosis, epilepsy) or in the presence of other risk factors that may predispose to seizures or lower the seizure threshold (e.g., certain drug therapy, renal dysfunction). (See **PRECAUTIONS: General, Information for Patients, Drug Interactions and ADVERSE REACTIONS.**)

Enoxacin is a potent inhibitor of the hepatic microsomal enzyme system, resulting in significant drug/drug interactions with theophylline and caffeine. (See **PRECAUTIONS: Drug Interactions.**)

Serious and occasionally fatal hypersensitivity (anaphylactoid or anaphylactic) reactions, some following the first dose, have been reported in patients receiving quinolone therapy. Some reactions were accompanied by cardiovascular collapse, loss of consciousness, tingling, pharyngeal or facial edema, dyspnea, urticaria, or itching. Only a few patients had a history of previous hypersensitivity reactions. Serious hypersensitivity reactions have also been reported following treatment with enoxacin. If an allergic reaction to enoxacin occurs, discontinue the drug. Serious acute hypersensitivity reactions may require immediate treatment with epinephrine. Oxygen, intravenous fluids, antihistamines, corticosteroids, pressor amines, and airway management, including intubation, should be administered as indicated.

Pseudomembranous colitis has been reported with nearly all antibacterial agents, including enoxacin, and may range in severity from mild to life-threatening. Therefore, it is important to consider this diagnosis in patients who present with diarrhea subsequent to the administration of antibacterial agents.

Treatment with broad-spectrum antibacterial agents alters the normal flora of the colon and may permit overgrowth of clostridia. Studies indicate that a toxin produced by *Clostridium difficile* is a primary cause of "antibiotic-associated colitis."

After the diagnosis of pseudomembranous colitis has been established, therapeutic measures should be initiated.

Mild cases of pseudomembranous colitis usually respond to discontinuation of the drug alone. In moderate to severe cases, consideration should be given to management with fluids and electrolytes, protein supplementation, and treatment with an antibacterial drug clinically effective against *C. difficile* colitis.

Ruptures of the shoulder, hand and Achilles tendons that required surgical repair or resulted in prolonged disability have been reported with fluoroquinolone antimicrobials. Enoxacin should be discontinued if the patient experiences pain, inflammation or rupture of a tendon. Patients should rest and refrain from exercise until the diagnosis of tendinitis or tendon rupture has been confidently excluded. Tendon rupture can occur at anytime during or after therapy with enoxacin.

Enoxacin has not been shown to be effective in the treatment of syphilis. Antimicrobial agents used in high doses for short periods of time to treat gonorrhea may mask or delay the symptoms of incubating syphilis. All patients with gonorrhea should have a serologic test for syphilis at the time of diagnosis. Patients treated with enoxacin should have a follow-up serologic test for syphilis after 3 months.

PRECAUTIONS

General: Alteration of the dosage regimen is necessary for patients with impaired renal function (creatinine clearance ≤ 30 mL/min/1.73 m²). (See **DOSAGE AND ADMINISTRATION.**)

As with other quinolones, enoxacin should be used with caution in patients with a known or suspected CNS disorder that may predispose to seizures or lower the seizure threshold (e.g., severe cerebral arteriosclerosis, epilepsy) or in the presence of other risk factors that may predispose to seizures or lower the seizure threshold (e.g., certain drug therapy, renal dysfunction). (See **WARNINGS and Drug Interactions**).

Moderate-to-severe phototoxicity reactions have been observed in patients exposed to direct sunlight while receiving enoxacin or some other drugs in this class. Excessive sunlight should be avoided. Therapy should be discontinued if phototoxicity occurs.

Ophthalmologic abnormalities, including cataracts and multiple punctate lenticular opacities, have been noted in patients undergoing treatment with enoxacin, as well as with some other quinolones, but have also been observed in patients receiving placebo in comparative trials. In clinical trials using multiple-dose therapy, ophthalmic tissue levels of enoxacin and other quinolones were significantly higher than respective plasma concentrations. The causal relationship, if any, of quinolones to lenticular abnormalities has not been established.

Decreased spermatogenesis and subsequent decreased fertility were noted in rats and dogs treated with doses of enoxacin that produced plasma levels in the animals three times higher than those produced in humans at the recommended therapeutic dosage. The potential for enoxacin to affect spermatogenesis in male patients is unknown.

Information for Patients:
Patients should be advised:

- not to take magnesium-, aluminum-, or calcium-containing antacids, bismuth subsalicylate, products containing iron, or multivitamins containing zinc for 8 hours prior to enoxacin or for 2 hours after enoxacin administration (see **PRECAUTIONS: Drug Interactions**);
- to drink fluids liberally;
- to avoid consumption of caffeine-containing products (certain drugs, coffee, tea, chocolate, certain carbonated beverages) during enoxacin therapy (see **PRECAUTIONS: Drug Interactions**);
- that convulsions have been reported in patients taking quinolones, including enoxacin, and to notify their physicians before taking this drug if there is a history of this condition;
- that enoxacin may cause dizziness and lightheadedness and, therefore, patients should know how they react to enoxacin before they operate an automobile or machinery or engage in activities requiring mental alertness and coordination;
- to discontinue treatment and inform their physician if they experience pain, inflammation, or rupture of a tendon, and to rest and refrain from exercise until the diagnosis of tendinitis or tendon rupture has been confidently excluded;
- that enoxacin may be associated with hypersensitivity reaction, even following the first dose, and to discontinue the drug at the first sign of a skin rash or other allergic reaction;
- to avoid undue exposure to excessive sunlight while receiving enoxacin and to discontinue therapy if phototoxicity occurs.

Drug Interactions
Bismuth: Bismuth subsalicylate, given concomitantly with enoxacin or 60 minutes following enoxacin administration, decreased enoxacin bioavailability by approximately 25%. Thus, concomitant administration of enoxacin and bismuth subsalicylate should be avoided.

Caffeine: Enoxacin is a potent inhibitor of the cytochrome P-450 isozymes responsible for the metabolism of methylxanthines. In a multiple-dose study, enoxacin caused a dose-related increase in the mean elimination half-life of caffeine, thereby decreasing the clearance of caffeine by up to 80% and leading to a five-fold increase in the AUC and the half-life of caffeine. Trough plasma enoxacin levels were also 20% higher when caffeine and enoxacin were administered concomitantly. Caffeine-related adverse effects have occurred in patients consuming caffeine while on therapy with enoxacin. (See **WARNINGS.**)

Cyclosporine: Elevated serum levels of cyclosporine have been reported with concomitant use of cyclosporine with other members of the quinolone class.

Digoxin: Enoxacin may raise serum digoxin levels in some individuals. If signs and symptoms suggestive of digoxin toxicity occur when enoxacin and digoxin are given concomitantly, physicians are advised to obtain serum digoxin levels and adjust digoxin doses appropriately.

Non-steroidal anti-inflammatory agents: Seizures have been reported in patients taking enoxacin concomitantly with the

Continued on next page

Rhône-Poulenc Rorer —Cont.

nonsteroidal anti-inflammatory drug fenbufen. Animal studies also suggest an increased potential for seizures when these two drugs are given concomitantly. Fenbufen is not approved in the United States at this time.

Sucralfate and antacids: Quinolones form chelates with metal cations. Therefore, administration of quinolones with antacids containing calcium, magnesium, or aluminum; with sucralfate; with divalent or trivalent cations such as iron; or with multivitamins containing zinc may substantially interfere with drug absorption and result in insufficient plasma and tissue quinolone concentrations. Antacids containing aluminum hydroxide and magnesium hydroxide reduce the oral absorption of enoxacin by 75%. The oral bioavailability of enoxacin is reduced by 60% with coadministration of ranitidine. These agents should not be taken for 8 hours before or for 2 hours after enoxacin administration.

Theophylline: Enoxacin is a potent inhibitor of the cytochrome P-450 isozymes responsible for the metabolism of methylxanthines. Enoxacin interferes with the metabolism of theophylline resulting in a 42% to 74% dose-related decrease in theophylline clearance and a subsequent 260% to 350% increase in serum theophylline levels. Theophylline-related adverse effects have occurred in patients when theophylline and enoxacin were coadministered. (See **WARNINGS.**)

Warfarin: Quinolones, including enoxacin, decrease the clearance of R-warfarin, the less active isomer of racemic warfarin. Enoxacin does not affect the clearance of the active S-isomer, and changes in clotting time have not been observed when enoxacin and warfarin were coadministered. Nevertheless, the prothrombin time or other suitable coagulation test should be monitored when warfarin or its derivatives and enoxacin are given concomitantly.

Carcinogenesis, Mutagenesis, Impairment of Fertility: Long-term studies in animals to determine the carcinogenic potential of enoxacin have not been conducted.

Genetic toxicology tests included *in vitro* mutagenicity and cytogenetic assays and *in vivo* cytogenetic and micronucleus tests. Enoxacin did not induce point mutations in bacterial cells or mitotic gene conversion in yeast cells, with or without metabolic activation. Enoxacin did not induce sister chromatid exchanges or structural chromosomal aberrations in mammalian cells *in vitro,* with or without metabolic activation. In addition, enoxacin did not induce chromosomal aberrations in mice.

There was a minimal, dose-related, statistically significant increase in micronuclei at high doses in mice. The significance of these findings, in the absence of effects in other test systems, is not established.

Enoxacin produced no consistent effects on fertility and reproductive parameters in female rats given oral doses of enoxacin at levels up to 1000 mg/kg. Decreased spermatogenesis and subsequent impaired fertility was noted in male rats given oral doses of 1000 mg/kg. This dose is approximately 13-fold greater than the highest human clinical daily oral dose of 16 mg/kg, assuming a 50 kg person and based on a mg/m^2 basis.

Pregnancy: *Teratogenic effects.* Pregnancy Category C. Studies with enoxacin given orally to mice and rats have shown no evidence of teratogenic potential. The intravenous infusion of enoxacin into pregnant rabbits at doses of 10 to 50 mg/kg caused dose-related maternal toxicity (venous irritation, body weight loss, and reduced food intake) and, at 50 mg/kg, fetal toxicity (increased post-implantation loss and stunted fetuses).

At 50 mg/kg, the incidence of fetal malformations was significantly increased in the presence of overt maternal and fetal toxicity. There are no adequate and well-controlled studies in pregnant women. Enoxacin should be used during pregnancy only if the potential benefit justifies the potential risk to the fetus. (See **WARNINGS.**)

Nursing Mothers: It is not known whether enoxacin is excreted in human milk. Enoxacin is excreted in the milk of lactating rats. Because drugs of this class are excreted in human milk and because of the potential for serious adverse reactions from enoxacin in nursing infants, a decision should be made whether to discontinue nursing or to discontinue the drug, taking into account the importance of the drug to the mother.

Pediatric Use: Safety and effectiveness in children and adolescents below the age of 18 years have not been established. Enoxacin causes arthropathy in juvenile animals. (See **WARNINGS** and **ANIMAL PHARMACOLOGY.**)

Geriatric Use: In multiple-dose clinical trials of enoxacin, elderly patients (≥ 65 years of age) experienced significantly more overall adverse events than patients under 65 years of age. However, the incidence of drug-related adverse reactions was comparable between age groups.

ADVERSE REACTIONS

Single-Dose Studies

During clinical trials, approximately 9% of patients treated with a single dose of 400 mg of enoxacin for uncomplicated urethral or endocervical gonorrhea reported adverse events. The most frequently reported events in single-dose trials, without regard to drug relationship, were nausea and vomiting (2%). Events that occurred in less than 1% of patients are listed below.

CENTRAL NERVOUS SYSTEM: headache, dizziness, somnolence; GASTROINTESTINAL: abdominal pain; GYNECOLOGIC: vaginal moniliasis; SKIN/HYPERSENSITIVITY: rash; LABORATORY ABNORMALITIES: increased AST (SGOT), decreased hemoglobin, decreased hematocrit, eosinophilia, leukocytosis, leukopenia, thrombocytosis, increased urinary protein, increased alkaline phosphatase, increased ALT (SGPT), increased bilirubin, hyperkalemia.

Multiple-Dose Studies

The incidence of adverse events reported by patients in multiple-dose clinical trials, without regard to drug relationship, was 23%. The incidence of drug-related adverse reactions in multiple-dose clinical trials was 16%. Among patients receiving multiple-dose therapy, enoxacin was discontinued because of an adverse event in 3.8% of patients.

The following events were considered likely to be drug-related in patients receiving multiple doses of enoxacin in clinical trials: nausea and/or vomiting 6%, dizziness 2%, headache 1%, abdominal pain 1%, diarrhea 1%, dyspepsia 1%.

The most frequently reported events in all multiple-dose clinical trials, without regard to drug relationship, were as follows: nausea and/or vomiting 8%, dizziness and/or vertigo 3%, headache 2%, diarrhea 2%, abdominal pain 2%, insomnia 1%, dyspepsia 1%, rash 1%, nervousness and/or anxiety 1%, unusual taste 1%, pruritus 1%.

Additional events that occurred in less than 1% of patients but > 0.1% of patients are listed below.

BODY AS A WHOLE: asthenia, fatigue, fever, malaise, back pain, chest pain, edema, chills; GASTROINTESTINAL: flatulence, constipation, dry mouth/throat, stomatitis, anorexia, gastritis, bloody stools; CENTRAL NERVOUS SYSTEM: somnolence, tremor, convulsions, paresthesia, confusion, agitation, depression, syncope, myoclonus, depersonalization, hypertonia; SKIN/HYPERSENSITIVITY: photosensitivity reaction, urticaria, hyperhidrosis, mycotic infection, erythema multiforme, toxic epidermal necrolysis, Stevens-Johnson syndrome; SPECIAL SENSES: tinnitus, conjunctivitis, visual disturbances including amblyopia; MUSCULOSKELETAL: myalgia, arthralgia; CARDIOVASCULAR: palpitations, tachycardia, vasodilation; RESPIRATORY: dyspnea, cough, epistaxis; HEMIC AND LYMPHATIC: purpura; UROGENITAL: vaginal moniliasis, vaginitis, urinary incontinence, renal failure.

The following adverse events occurred in less than 0.1% of patients in multiple-dose clinical trials but were considered significant: pseudomembranous colitis, hyperkinesia, amnesia, ataxia, hypotonia, psychosis, emotional lability, hallucination, schizophrenic reaction.

LABORATORY CHANGES: The following laboratory abnormalities appeared in ≥ 1.0% of patients receiving multiple doses of enoxacin: elevated AST (SGOT), elevated ALT (SGPT). It is not known whether these abnormalities were caused by the drug or the underlying conditions.

Worldwide Post-Marketing Experience

The most frequent spontaneously-reported adverse events in the worldwide post-marketing experience with multiple- and single-dose enoxacin use have been rashes, seizures/convulsions, and photosensitivity reactions; however, there is no evidence that the incidences of these events were larger than those observed in the clinical trials population.

Quinolone-class adverse reactions: Although not reported in completed clinical studies with enoxacin, a variety of adverse events have been reported with other quinolones.

Clinical adverse events include: erythema nodosum, hepatic necrosis, possible exacerbation of myasthenia gravis, nystagmus, intestinal perforation, hyperpigmentation, interstitial nephritis, polyuria, urinary retention, renal calculi, cardiopulmonary arrest, cerebral thrombosis, and laryngeal or pulmonary edema.

Laboratory adverse events include: agranulocytosis, elevation of serum triglycerides and/or serum cholesterol, prolongation of the prothrombin time, candiduria, and crystalluria.

OVERDOSAGE

In the event of acute overdosage, the stomach should be emptied by inducing vomiting or by gastric lavage and the patient carefully observed and given supportive treatment. Enoxacin is poorly removed (< 5% over 4 hours) by hemodialysis.

DOSAGE AND ADMINISTRATION

Penetrex™ (enoxacin) should be taken at least one hour before or at least two hours after a meal.

See **INDICATIONS AND USAGE** for information on appropriate pathogens and patient populations.

Sexually Transmitted Diseases

Uncomplicated urethral or cervical gonorrhea: 400 mg single dose

Urinary Tract Infections

Uncomplicated urinary tract infections: 200 mg q12h for 7 days

Complicated urinary tract infections: 400 mg q12h for 14 days

Dosage Adjustment for Renal Impairment: Dosage should be adjusted in patients with a creatinine clearance value of 30 $mL/min/1.73\ m^2$ or less. After a normal initial dose, the dosing interval should be adjusted as follows:

Creatinine Clearance	Dosage Adjustment	Dosage Interval
> 30 $mL/min/1.73\ m^2$	None	12 hours
≤ 30 $mL/min/1.73\ m^2$	1/2 recommended dose	12 hours

When only the serum creatinine is known, the following formula may be used to estimate creatinine clearance.

Men:

$$\text{creatinine clearance (mL/min)} = \frac{\text{Weight (kg)} \times (140 - \text{age})}{72 \times \text{serum creatinine (mg/dL)}}$$

Women: 0.85 × the value calculated for men.

The serum creatinine should represent a steady state of renal function.

Dosage adjustment is not necessary in elderly patients with normal renal function, but dose should be adjusted according to the previous guidelines in elderly patients with compromised renal function.

HOW SUPPLIED

[See table below.]

Store at controlled room temperature, 15° to 30°C (59° to 86°F).

ANIMAL PHARMACOLOGY

Enoxacin and other members of the quinolone class have been shown to cause arthropathy in immature animals of most species tested. (See **WARNINGS.**)

REFERENCES

1. National Committee for Clinical Laboratory Standards, Performance Standards for Antimicrobial Disk Susceptibility Tests—Fourth Edition. Approved Standard NCCLS Document M2-A4, Vol. 10, No. 7, NCCLS, Villanova, PA, 1990.
2. National Committee for Clinical Laboratory Standards, Methods for Dilution Antimicrobial Susceptibility Tests for Bacteria that Grow Aerobically—Second Edition. Approved Standard NCCLS Document M7-A2, Vol. 10, No. 8, NCCLS, Villanova, PA, 1990.

Caution: Federal (U.S.A.) law prohibits dispensing without a prescription.

Rev. 8/96 IN-5391A

Distributed by

RHÔNE-POULENC RORER PHARMACEUTICALS INC.

Collegeville, PA, U.S.A. 19426-0107

Shown in Product Identification Guide, page 330

Strength	Size	NDC 0075-	Color	Markings
200 mg	Bottles of 50	5100-50	light blue	5100
400 mg	Bottles of 50	5140-50	dark blue	5140

RILUTEK® ℞

(riluzole) Tablets

[rĭl-ū-tĕk]

DESCRIPTION

RILUTEK® (riluzole) is a member of the benzothiazole class. Chemically, riluzole is 2-amino-6-(trifluoromethoxy) benzothiazole. Its molecular formula is $C_8H_5F_3N_2OS$ and its molecular weight is 234.2. Its structural formula is as follows:

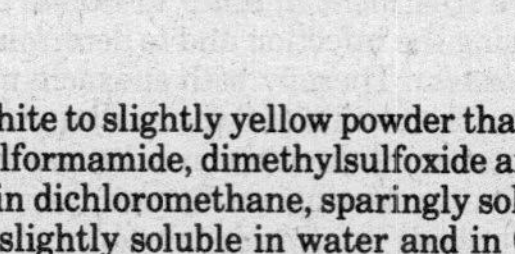

Riluzole is a white to slightly yellow powder that is very soluble in dimethylformamide, dimethylsulfoxide and methanol, freely soluble in dichloromethane, sparingly soluble in 0.1 N HCl and very slightly soluble in water and in 0.1 N NaOH. RILUTEK is available as a capsule-shaped, white, film-coated tablet for oral administration containing 50 mg of

riluzole. Each tablet is engraved with "RPR 202" on one side.
Inactive Ingredients: Core: anhydrous dibasic calcium phosphate, USP; microcrystalline cellulose, NF; anhydrous colloidal silica, NF; magnesium stearate, NF; croscarmellose sodium, NF. **Film coating:** hydroxypropyl methylcellulose, USP; polyethylene glycol 6000; titanium dioxide, USP.

CLINICAL PHARMACOLOGY

Mechanism of Action

The etiology and pathogenesis of amyotrophic lateral sclerosis (ALS) are not known, although a number of hypotheses have been advanced. One hypothesis is that motor neurons, made vulnerable through either genetic predisposition or environmental factors, are injured by glutamate. In some cases of familial ALS the enzyme superoxide dismutase has been found to be defective.

The mode of action of RILUTEK is unknown. Its pharmacological properties include the following, some of which may be related to its effect: 1) an inhibitory effect on glutamate release, 2) inactivation of voltage-dependent sodium channels, and 3) ability to interfere with intracellular events that follow transmitter binding at excitatory amino acid receptors.

Riluzole has also been shown, in a single study, to delay median time to death in a transgenic mouse model of ALS. These mice express human superoxide dismutase bearing one of the mutations found in one of the familial forms of human ALS.

It is also neuroprotective in various *in vivo* experimental models of neuronal injury involving excitotoxic mechanisms. In *in vitro* tests, riluzole protected cultured rat motor neurons from the excitotoxic effects of glutamic acid and prevented the death of cortical neurons induced by anoxia.

Due to its blockade of glutamatergic neurotransmission, riluzole also exhibits myorelaxant and sedative properties in animal models at doses of 30 mg/kg (about 20 times the recommended human daily dose) and anticonvulsant properties at a dose of 2.5 mg/kg (about 2 times the recommended human daily dose).

Pharmacokinetics

Riluzole is well-absorbed (approximately 90%), with average absolute oral bioavailability of about 60% (CV = 30%). Pharmacokinetics are linear over a dose range of 25–100 mg given every 12 hours. A high fat meal decreases absorption, reducing AUC by about 20% and peak blood levels by about 45%. The mean elimination half-life of riluzole is 12 hours (CV = 35%) after repeated doses. With multiple-dose administration, riluzole accumulates in plasma by about 2 fold and steady-state is reached in less than 5 days. Riluzole is 96% bound to plasma proteins, mainly to albumin and lipoproteins over the clinical concentration range.

The 50 mg market tablet was equivalent, with respect to AUC, to the tablet used in the dose ranging clinical trials, while the C_{max} was approximately 30% higher. Both tablets have been used in clinical trials. However, if doses greater than those recommended are given, it is likely that higher plasma levels will be achieved, the safety of which has not been established (see DOSAGE AND ADMINISTRATION).

Metabolism and Elimination

Riluzole is extensively metabolized to six major and a number of minor metabolites, not all of which have been identified. Some metabolites appear pharmacologically active in *in vitro* assays. The metabolism of riluzole is mostly hepatic and consists of cytochrome P450-dependent hydroxylation and glucuronidation.

There is marked inter-individual variability in the clearance of riluzole, probably attributable to variability of CYP 1A2 activity, the principal isozyme involved in N-hydroxylation. *In vitro* studies using liver microsomes show that hydroxylation of the primary amine group producing N-hydroxyriluzole is the main metabolic pathway in human, monkey, dog and rabbit. In humans, cytochrome P450 1A2 is the principal isozyme involved in N-hydroxylation. *In vitro* studies predict that CYP 2D6, CYP 2C19, CYP 3A4 and CYP 2E1 are unlikely to contribute significantly to riluzole metabolism in humans. Whereas direct glucuroconjugation of riluzole (involving the glucurotransferase isoform UGT-HP4) is very slow in human liver microsomes, N-hydroxyriluzole is readily conjugated at the hydroxylamine group resulting in the formation of O- (>90%) and N-glucuronides.

Following a single 150 mg dose of ^{14}C-riluzole to 6 healthy males, 90% and 5% of the radioactivity was recovered in the urine and feces respectively over a period of 7 days. Glucuronides accounted for more than 85% of the metabolites in urine. Only 2% of a riluzole dose was recovered in the urine as unchanged drug.

Special Populations

The pharmacokinetics of riluzole have not been studied in renally and hepatically impaired subjects, nor is there information about the effects of smoking, age and gender on the pharmacokinetics of riluzole but certain differences in population subsets should be anticipated (see PRECAUTIONS).

Hepatic and Renal Disease: Since riluzole is extensively metabolized and subsequently excreted in the urine, it is likely that functional hepatic and renal impairment will reduce the clearance of riluzole and its metabolites and give higher plasma levels (see PRECAUTIONS and WARNINGS).

Age: Age-related decreased renal function would be expected to give higher plasma levels of riluzole and metabolites. However, in controlled clinical trials, in which approximately 30% of patients were over 65, there were no differences in adverse events between younger and older patients (see PRECAUTIONS).

Gender: CYP 1A2 activity has been reported to be lower in women than in men. Therefore, a gender effect on riluzole kinetics may be expected in women, resulting in higher blood concentrations of riluzole and its metabolites (see PRECAUTIONS). No gender effect on favorable or adverse effects of riluzole was seen in controlled trials, however.

Smoking: Cigarette smoking is known to induce CYP 1A2. Patients who smoke cigarettes would be expected to eliminate riluzole faster. There is no information, however, on the effect of, or need for, dosage adjustment in these patients.

Race: Clearance of riluzole in Japanese subjects native to Japan was found to be 50% lower as compared to Caucasians after normalizing for body weight. Although it is not clear if this difference is due to genetic or environmental factors (*e.g.*, smoking, alcohol, coffee, and dietary preferences), it is possible that Japanese subjects may possess a lower capacity (oxidative and/or conjugative) for metabolizing riluzole. There are no studies, however, of lower doses in Japanese subjects (see PRECAUTIONS).

Clinical Trials

The efficacy of RILUTEK as a treatment of ALS was established in two adequate and well-controlled trials in which the time to tracheostomy or death was longer for patients randomized to RILUTEK than for those randomized to placebo.

These studies admitted patients with either familial or sporadic ALS, a disease duration of less than 5 years, and a baseline forced vital capacity greater than or equal to 60%.

In one study, performed in France and Belgium, 155 ALS patients were followed for at least 13 months (maximum duration 18 months) after being randomized to either 100 mg/day (given 50 mg BID) of RILUTEK or placebo.

Figure 1, which follows, displays the survival curves for time to death or tracheostomy. The vertical axis represents the proportion of individuals alive without tracheostomy at various times following treatment initiation (horizontal axis). Although these survival curves were not statistically significantly different when evaluated by the analysis specified in the study protocol (Logrank test p = 0.12), the difference was found to be significant by another appropriate analysis (Wilcoxon test p = 0.05). As seen, the study showed an early increase in survival in patients given riluzole. Among the patients in whom treatment failed during the study (tracheostomy or death) there was a difference between the treatment groups in median survival of approximately 90 days. There was no statistically significant difference in mortality at the end of the study.

Figure 1: Kaplan-Meier Survival Curves

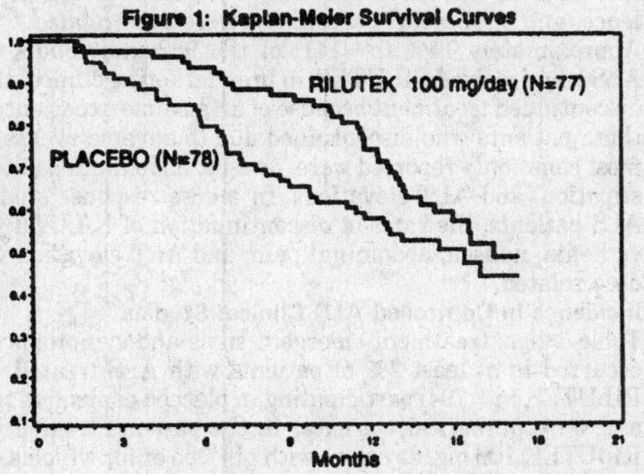

In the second study, performed in both Europe and North America, 959 ALS patients were followed for at least 1 year (North American centers) and up to 18 months (European centers) after being randomized to either 50, 100, 200 mg/day of RILUTEK or placebo.

Figure 2, which follows, displays the survival curves for time to death or tracheostomy for patients randomized to either 100 mg/day of RILUTEK or placebo. Although these survival curves were not statistically significantly different when evaluated by the analysis specified in the study protocol (Logrank test p = 0.076), the difference was found to be significant by another appropriate analysis (Wilcoxon test p = 0.05). Not displayed in Figure 2 are the results of 50 mg/day of RILUTEK which could not be statistically distinguished from placebo and the results of 200 mg/day which are essentially identical to 100 mg/day. As seen, the study showed an early increase in survival in patients given riluzole. Among the patients in whom treatment failed during the study (tracheostomy or death) there was a difference between the treatment groups in median survival of approximately 60 days. There was no statistically significant difference in mortality at the end of the study.

[See Figure at top of next column.]

Figure 2: Kaplan-Meier Survival Curves

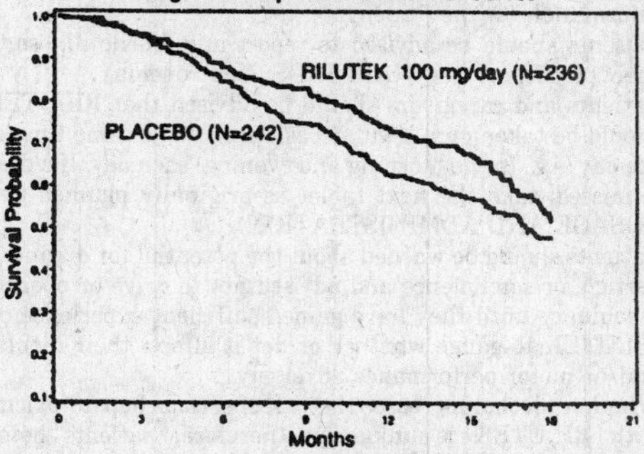

Although riluzole improved early survival in both studies, measures of muscle strength and neurological function did not show a benefit.

INDICATIONS AND USAGE

RILUTEK is indicated for the treatment of patients with amyotrophic lateral sclerosis (ALS). Riluzole extends survival and/or time to tracheostomy.

CONTRAINDICATIONS

RILUTEK is contraindicated in patients who have a history of severe hypersensitivity reactions to riluzole or any of the tablet components.

WARNINGS

Liver Injury/Monitoring Liver Chemistries

RILUTEK should be prescribed with care in patients with current evidence or history of abnormal liver function indicated by significant abnormalities in serum transaminase (ALT/SGPT; AST/SGOT), bilirubin, and/or gamma-glutamate transferase (GGT) levels (see PRECAUTIONS and DOSAGE AND ADMINISTRATION SECTIONS). Baseline elevations of several LFTs (especially elevated bilirubin) should preclude the use of RILUTEK.

RILUTEK, even in patients without a prior history of liver disease, causes serum aminotransferase elevations. Experience in almost 800 ALS patients indicates that about 50% of riluzole-treated patients will experience at least one ALT/SGPT level above the upper limit of normal, about 8% will have elevations > 3 × ULN, and about 2% of patients will have elevations > 5 × ULN. A single non-ALS patient with epilepsy treated with concomitant carbamazepine and phenobarbital experienced marked, rapid elevations of liver enzymes with jaundice (ALT 26 × ULN, AST 17 × ULN, and bilirubin 11 × ULN) four months after starting RILUTEK; these returned to normal 7 weeks after treatment discontinuation.

Maximum increases in serum ALT usually occurred within 3 months after the start of riluzole therapy and were usually transient when < 5 times ULN. In trials, if ALT levels were <5 times ULN, treatment continued and ALT levels usually returned to below 2 times ULN within 2 to 6 months. Treatment in studies was discontinued, however, if ALT levels exceeded 5 × ULN, so that there is no experience with continued treatment of ALS patients once ALT values exceed 5 times ULN (see PRECAUTIONS: Laboratory Tests). There were rare instances of jaundice.

Liver chemistries should be monitored (see PRECAUTIONS).

Neutropenia

Among approximately 4000 patients given riluzole for ALS, there were three cases of marked neutropenia (absolute neutrophil count less than 500/mm^3), all seen within the first 2 months of riluzole treatment. In one case, neutrophil counts rose on continued treatment. In a second case, counts rose after therapy was stopped. A third case was more complex, with marked anemia as well as neutropenia and the etiology of both is uncertain. Patients should be warned to report any febrile illness to their physicians. The report of a febrile illness should prompt treating physicians to check white blood cell counts.

PRECAUTIONS

Use in Patients with Concomitant Disease

RILUTEK should be used with caution in patients with concomitant liver and/or renal insufficiency (see WARNINGS, CLINICAL PHARMACOLOGY). In particular, in cases of RILUTEK-induced hepatic injury manifested by elevated liver enzymes, the effect of the hepatic injury on RILUTEK metabolism is unknown.

Special Populations

Riluzole should be used with caution in elderly patients whose hepatic or renal functions may be compromised due to age. Also, females and Japanese patients may possess a lower metabolic capacity to eliminate riluzole compared to males and Caucasian subjects, respectively (see CLINICAL PHARMACOLOGY: Special Populations).

Continued on next page

Rhône-Poulenc Rorer–Cont.

Information for the Patient

Patients should be advised to report any febrile illness to their physicians (see WARNINGS: Neutropenia).

Patients and caregivers should be advised that RILUTEK should be taken on a regular basis and at the same time of the day (*e.g.,* in the morning and evening) each day. If a dose is missed, take the next tablet as originally planned (see DOSAGE AND ADMINISTRATION).

Patients should be warned about the potential for dizziness, vertigo, or somnolence and advised not to drive or operate machinery until they have gained sufficient experience on RILUTEK to gauge whether or not it affects their mental and/or motor performance adversely.

Whether alcohol increases the risk of serious hepatotoxicity with RILUTEK is unknown; therefore, patients being treated with RILUTEK should be discouraged from drinking excessive amounts of alcohol.

Patients should also be made aware that RILUTEK should be stored at temperatures between 20°-25°C (68°-77°F) and protected from bright light.

RILUTEK must be kept out of the reach of children.

Laboratory Tests

It is recommended that serum aminotransferases including ALT levels be measured before and during riluzole therapy. Serum ALT levels should be evaluated every month during the first 3 months of treatment, every 3 months during the remainder of the first year, and periodically thereafter. Serum ALT levels should be evaluated more frequently in patients who develop elevations (see WARNINGS).

As noted in the WARNINGS Section, there is no experience with continued treatment of patients once ALT exceeds 5 × ULN. If a decision is made to continue to treat these patients, frequent monitoring (at least weekly) of complete liver function is recommended. Treatment should be discontinued if ALT exceeds 10 × ULN or if clinical jaundice develops. Because there is no experience with rechallenge of patients who have had RILUTEK discontinued for ALT > 5 × ULN, no recommendations about restarting RILUTEK can be made.

In the two controlled trials in patients with ALS, the frequency with which values for hemoglobin, hematocrit, and erythrocyte counts fell below the lower limit of normal was greater in RILUTEK-treated patients than in placebo-treated patients; however, these changes were mild and transient. The proportions of patients observed with abnormally low values for these parameters showed a dose-response relationship. Only one patient was discontinued from treatment because of severe anemia. The significance of this finding is unknown.

Drug Interactions

There have been no clinical studies designed to evaluate the interaction of riluzole with other drugs.

As with all drugs, the potential for interaction by a variety of mechanisms is a possibility.

Hepatotoxic Drugs: The clinical trials in ALS excluded patients on concomitant medications which were potentially hepatotoxic, (*e.g.,* allopurinol, methyldopa, sulfasalazine). Accordingly, there is no information about the safety of administering RILUTEK in conjunction with such medications. If the practitioner chooses to prescribe such a combination, caution should be exercised.

Drugs Highly Bound To Plasma Proteins: Riluzole is highly bound (96%) to plasma proteins, binding mainly to serum albumin and to lipoproteins. The effect of riluzole (up to 5 mcg/mL) on warfarin (5 mcg/mL) binding did not show any displacement of warfarin. Conversely, riluzole binding was unaffected by the addition of warfarin, digoxin, imipramine and quinine at high therapeutic concentrations.

Effect of Other Drugs On Riluzole Metabolism: *In vitro* studies using human liver microsomal preparations suggest that CYP 1A2 is the principal isozyme involved in the initial oxidative metabolism of riluzole and, therefore, potential interactions may occur when riluzole is given concurrently with agents that affect CYP 1A2 activity. Potential inhibitors of CYP 1A2 (*e.g.,* caffeine, phenacetin, theophylline, amitriptyline, and quinolones) could decrease the rate of riluzole elimination, while inducers of CYP 1A2 (*e.g.,* cigarette smoke, charcoal-broiled food, rifampicin, and omeprazole) could increase the rate of riluzole elemination.

Effect of Riluzole On the Metabolism of Other Drugs: CYP 1A2 is the principal isoenzyme involved in the initial oxidative metabolism of riluzole; potential interactions may occur when riluzole is given concurrently with other agents which are also metabolized primarily by CYP 1A2 (*e.g.,* theophylline, caffeine and tacrine). Currently, it is not known whether riluzole has any potential for enzyme induction in humans.

Drug Laboratory Test Interactions: None known

Carcinogenesis, Mutagenesis, Impairment of Fertility

Long-term studies to determine the carcinogenic potential of riluzole have not yet been completed.

The genotoxic potential of riluzole was evaluated in the bacterial mutagenicity (Ames) test, the mouse lymphoma mutation assay in L5178Y cells, the *in vitro* chromosomal aberration assay in human lymphocytes and the *in vivo* rat cytogenetic assay and *in vivo* mouse micronucleus assay in bone marrow. There was no evidence of mutagenic or clastogenic potential in the Ames test, the mouse lymphoma assay, or the *in vivo* assays in the mouse and rat. There was an equivocal clastogenic response in the *in vitro* lymphocyte chromosomal aberration assay.

Riluzole impaired fertility when administered to male and female rats prior to and during mating at an oral dose of 15 mg/kg or 1.5 times the maximum daily dose on a mg/m^2 basis (see PRECAUTIONS: "Pregnancy" for effects on fertility).

Pregnancy

Pregnancy category C:

Oral administration of riluzole to pregnant animals during the period of organogenesis caused embryotoxicity in rats and rabbits at doses of 27 mg/kg and 60 mg/kg, respectively, or 2.6 and 11.5 times, respectively, the recommended maximum human daily dose on a mg/m^2 basis. Evidence of maternal toxicity was also observed at these doses.

When administered to rats prior to and during mating (males and females) and throughout gestation and lactation (females), riluzole produced adverse effects on pregnancy (decreased implantations, increased intrauterine death) and offspring viability and growth at an oral dose of 15 mg/kg or 1.5 times the maximum daily dose on a mg/m^2 basis.

There are no adequate and well-controlled studies in pregnant women. Riluzole should be used during pregnancy only if the potential benefit justifies the potential risk to the fetus.

Nursing Women

In rat studies, ^{14}C-riluzole was detected in maternal milk. It is not known whether riluzole is excreted in human breast milk. Because many drugs are excreted in human milk, and because the potential for serious adverse reactions in nursing infants from RILUTEK® is unknown, women should be advised not to breast-feed during treatment with RILUTEK.

Use in the Elderly

Age-related compromised renal and hepatic function may cause a decrease in clearance of riluzole (see CLINICAL PHARMACOLOGY: Special Populations). In controlled clinical trials, about 30% of patients were over 65. There were no differences in adverse effects between younger and older patients.

Pediatric Use

The safety and the effectiveness of RILUTEK in pediatric patients have not been established.

ADVERSE REACTIONS

The most commonly observed AEs associated with the use of RILUTEK more frequently than placebo treated patients, were: asthenia, nausea, dizziness, decreased lung function, diarrhea, abdominal pain, pneumonia, vomiting, vertigo, circumoral paresthesia, anorexia, and somnolence. Asthenia, nausea, dizziness, diarrhea, anorexia, vertigo, somnolence, and circumoral paresthesia were dose related.

Approximately 14% (n=141) of the 982 individuals with ALS who received RILUTEK in pre-marketing clinical trials discontinued treatment because of an adverse experience. Of those patients who discontinued due to adverse events, the most commonly reported were: nausea, abdominal pain, constipation, and ALT elevations. In a dose response study in ALS patients, the rates of discontinuation of RILUTEK for asthenia, nausea, abdominal pain, and ALT elevation were dose related.

Incidence in Controlled ALS Clinical Studies

Table 1 lists treatment-emergent signs and symptoms that occurred in at least 2% of patients with ALS treated with RILUTEK (n=794) participating in placebo-controlled trials and were numerically greater in the patients treated with RILUTEK 100 mg/day than with placebo or for which a dose response relationship is suggested.

The prescriber should be aware that these figures cannot be used to predict the frequency of adverse experiences in the course of usual medical practice where patient characteristics and other factors may differ from those prevailing during clinical studies. Inspection of these frequencies, however, does provide the prescriber with one basis to estimate the relative contribution of drug and non-drug factors to the AE incidences in the population studied.

Table 1
Adverse Events Occurring in Placebo-Controlled Clinical Trials

Percentage of patients reporting events*

Body System/ Adverse Event*	Riluzole 50 mg/day (N=237)	Riluzole 100 mg/day (N=313)	Riluzole 200 mg/day (N=244)	Placebo (N=320)
Body as a Whole				
Asthenia	14.8	19.2	20.1	12.2
Headache	8.0	7.3	7.0	6.6
Abdominal pain	6.8	5.1	7.8	3.8
Back pain	1.7	3.2	4.1	2.5
Aggravation reaction	0.4	1.3	2.0	0.9
Malaise	0.4	0.6	1.2	0.0
Digestive				
Nausea	12.2	16.3	20.5	10.6
Vomiting	4.2	4.2	4.5	1.6
Dyspepsia	2.5	3.8	6.1	5.0
Anorexia	3.8	3.2	8.6	3.8
Diarrhea	5.5	2.9	9.0	3.1
Flatulence	2.5	2.6	2.0	1.9
Stomatitis	0.8	1.0	1.2	0.0
Tooth disorder	0.0	1.0	1.2	0.3
Oral Moniliasis	0.4	0.6	1.2	0.3
Nervous				
Hypertonia	5.9	6.1	5.3	5.9
Depression	4.2	4.5	6.1	5.0
Dizziness	5.1	3.8	12.7	2.5
Dry mouth	3.0	3.5	2.0	3.4
Insomnia	2.1	3.5	2.9	3.4
Somnolence	0.8	1.9	4.1	1.3
Vertigo	2.5	1.9	4.5	0.9
Circumoral paresthesia	1.3	1.6	3.3	0.0
Skin and Appendages				
Pruritus	3.8	3.8	2.5	3.1
Eczema	0.8	1.6	1.6	0.6
Alopecia	0.0	1.0	1.2	0.6
Exfoliative dermatitis	0.0	0.6	1.2	0.0
Respiratory				
Decreased lung function	13.1	10.2	16.0	9.4
Rhinitis	8.9	6.4	7.8	6.3
Increased cough	2.1	2.6	3.7	1.6
Sinusitis	0.4	1.0	1.6	0.9
Cardiovascular				
Hypertension	6.8	5.1	3.3	4.1
Tachycardia	1.3	2.6	2.0	1.3
Phlebitis	0.4	1.0	0.8	0.3
Palpitation	0.4	0.6	1.2	0.9
Postural hypotension	0.8	0.0	1.6	0.6
Metabolic and Nutritional Disorders				
Weight loss	4.6	4.8	3.7	4.7
Peripheral edema	4.2	2.9	3.3	2.2
Musculoskeletal System				
Arthralgia	5.1	3.5	1.6	3.4
Urogenital System				
Urinary tract infection	2.5	2.6	4.5	2.2
Dysuria	0.0	1.0	1.2	0.3

Other Adverse Events Observed

Other events which occurred in more than 2% of patients treated with RILUTEK 100 mg/day but equally or more frequently in the placebo group included: accidental injury, apnea, bronchitis, constipation, death, dysphagia, dyspnea, flu syndrome, heart arrest, increased sputum, pneumonia, and respiratory disorder.

The overall adverse event profile for RILUTEK was similar between females and males, and was independent of age. Because the largest non-white racial subgroup was only 2% of patients exposed to RILUTEK (18/794) in placebo-controlled trials, there are insufficient data to support a statement regarding the distribution of adverse experience reports by race. In ALS studies, dizziness did occur more commonly in females (11%) than in males (4%). There was not a difference between females and males in the rates of discontinuation of RILUTEK for individual adverse experiences.

Other Adverse Events Observed During All Clinical Trials

RILUTEK has been administered to 1713 individuals during all clinical trials, some of which were placebo-controlled. During these trials, all adverse events were recorded by the clinical investigators using terminology of their own choosing. To provide a meaningful estimate of the proportion of individuals having adverse events, similar types of events were grouped into a smaller number of standardized categories using modified COSTART dictionary terminology. The frequencies presented represent the proportion of the 1713 individuals exposed to RILUTEK who experienced an event of the type cited on at least one occasion while receiving RILUTEK. All reported events are included except those already listed in the previous table, those too general to be informative, and those not reasonably associated with the use of the drug.

Events are further classified within body system categories and enumerated in order of decreasing frequency using the following definitions: *frequent* adverse events are defined as

those occurring in at least 1/100 patients; *infrequent* adverse events are those occurring in 1/100 to 1/1000 patients; *rare* adverse events are those occurring in fewer than 1/1000 patients.

*** = AE frequency ≤ to placebo**

Body as a Whole: *Frequent:* Hostility*. *Infrequent:* Abscess*, sepsis*, photosensitivity reaction*, cellulitis, face edema*, hernia, peritonitis, attempted suicide, injection site reaction, chills*, flu syndrome, intentional injury, enlarged abdomen, neoplasm. *Rare:* Acrodynia, hypothermia, moniliasis*, rheumatoid arthritis.

Digestive System: *Infrequent:* Increased appetite, intestinal obstruction*, fecal impaction, gastrointestinal hemorrhage, gastrointestinal ulceration, gastritis*, fecal incontinence, jaundice, hepatitis, glossitis, gum hemorrhage*, pancreatitis, tenesmus, esophageal stenosis. *Rare:* Cheilitis*, cholecystitis, hematemesis, melena*, biliary pain, proctitis, pseudomembranous enterocolitis, enlarged salivary gland, tongue discoloration, tooth caries.

Nervous System: *Frequent:* Agitation*, tremor. *Infrequent:* Hallucinations, personality disorder*, abnormal thinking*, coma, paranoid reaction*, manic reaction, ataxia, extrapyramidal syndrome, hypokinesia, urinary retention, emotional lability, delusions, apathy, hypesthesia, incoordination, confusion*, convulsion, leg cramps, amnesia, dysarthria, increased libido, stupor, subdural hematoma, abnormal gait, delirium, depersonalization, facial paralysis, hemiplegia, decreased libido, myoclonus. *Rare:* Abnormal dreams, acute brain syndrome, CNS depression, dementia, cerebral embolism, euphoria*, hypotonia, ileus*, peripheral neuritis, psychosis*, psychotic depression, schizophrenic reaction, trismus, wristdrop.

Skin and Appendages: *Infrequent:* Skin ulceration, urticaria, psoriasis, seborrhea*, skin disorder, fungal dermatitis*. *Rare:* Angioedema, contact dermatitis, erythema multiforme, furunculosis*, skin moniliasis, skin granuloma, skin nodule.

Respiratory System: *Infrequent:* Hiccup, pleural disorder*, asthma, epistaxis, hemoptysis, yawn, hyperventilation*, lung edema*, hypoventilation*, lung carcinoma, hypoxia, laryngitis, pleural effusion, pneumothorax*, respiratory moniliasis, stridor.

Cardiovascular System: *Infrequent:* Syncope*, hypotension, heart failure, migraine, peripheral vascular disease, angina pectoris*, myocardial infarction*, ventricular extrasystoles, cerebral hemorrhage, atrial fibrillation*, bundle branch block, congestive heart failure, pericarditis, lower extremity embolus, myocardial ischemia*, shock*. *Rare:* Bradycardia, cerebral ischemia, hemorrhage, mesenteric artery occlusion, subarachnoid hemorrhage, supraventricular tachycardia*, thrombosis, ventricular fibrillation, ventricular tachycardia.

Metabolic and Nutritional Disorders: *Infrequent:* Gout*, respiratory acidosis, edema, thirst*, hypokalemia, hyponatremia, weight gain*. *Rare:* Generalized edema, hypercalcemia, hypercholesteremia.

Endocrine System: *Infrequent:* Diabetes mellitus, thyroid neoplasia. *Rare:* Diabetes insipidus, parathyroid disorder.

Hemic and Lymphatic System: *Infrequent:* Anemia*, leukocytosis, leukopenia, ecchymosis. *Rare:* Neutropenia, aplastic anemia, cyanosis, hypochromic anemia, iron deficiency anemia, lymphadenopathy, petechiae*, purpura.

Musculoskeletal System: *Infrequent:* Arthrosis, myasthenia*, bone neoplasm. *Rare:* Bone necrosis, osteoporosis, tetany.

Special Senses: *Infrequent:* Amblyopia, ophthalmitis. *Rare:* Blepharitis, cataract, deafness, diplopia*, ear pain, glaucoma, hyperacusis, photophobia, taste loss, vestibular disorder.

Urogenital System: *Infrequent:* Urinary urgency, urine abnormality, urinary incontinence, kidney calculus, hematuria, impotence, prostate carcinoma, kidney pain, metrorrhagia, priapism. *Rare:* Amenorrhea, breast abscess, breast pain, nephritis*, nocturia, pyelonephritis, enlarged uterine fibroids, uterine hemorrhage, vaginal moniliasis.

Laboratory Tests: *Infrequent:* Increased gamma glutamyl transferase, abnormal liver function/tests, increased alkaline phosphatase, positive direct Coombs test, increased gamma globulins. *Rare:* increased lactic dehydrogenase.

OVERDOSAGE

There have been no reports of overdose with RILUTEK. No specific antidote or information on treatment of overdosage with RILUTEK is available. In the event of overdose, RILUTEK therapy should be discontinued immediately. Treatment should be supportive and directed toward alleviating symptoms.

The estimated oral median lethal dose is 94 mg/kg and 39 mg/kg for male mice and rats, respectively.

DOSAGE AND ADMINISTRATION

The recommended dose for RILUTEK is 50 mg every 12 hours. No increased benefit can be expected from higher daily doses, but adverse events are increased.

RILUTEK tablets should be taken at least an hour before, or two hours after, a meal to avoid a food-related decrease in bioavailability.

Special Populations

Patients with Impaired Renal or Hepatic Function: Studies have not yet been completed in these populations (see WARNINGS, PRECAUTIONS, CLINICAL PHARMACOLOGY).

HOW SUPPLIED

RILUTEK 50 mg tablets are white, film-coated, capsule-shaped and engraved with "RPR 202" on one side. RILUTEK is supplied in bottles of 60 tablets, NDC 0075-7700-60. These bottles are designed with a special dispensing flip cap to aid dispensing with minimum effort.

STORE AT CONTROLLED ROOM TEMPERATURE 20°–25°C (68°–77°F) AND PROTECT FROM BRIGHT LIGHT. KEEP OUT OF THE REACH OF CHILDREN.

Caution: Federal law prohibits dispensing without prescription.

Manufactured in Ireland

RHÔNE-POULENC RORER PHARMACEUTICALS INC.
COLLEGEVILLE, PA 19426
IN-5336A Rev. 1/96

Shown in Product Identification Guide, page 330

SLO-BID™ ℞
[*slō 'bid"*]
(Theophylline, Extended-release Capsules, USP)
50 mg, 75 mg, 100 mg, 125 mg, 200 mg, and 300 mg Gyrocaps®

PRODUCT OVERVIEW

KEY FACTS

Slo-bid™ Gyrocaps® contain theophylline, anhydrous in the form of long-acting beads within a dye-free hard gelatin capsule for oral administration (intact or sprinkled). Theophylline is a bronchodilator and is a member of the xanthine class of chemical compounds.

MAJOR USES

Slo-bid™ is indicated for relief and/or prevention of symptoms of asthma and reversible bronchospasm associated with chronic bronchitis and emphysema.

SAFETY INFORMATION

Slo-bid™ is contraindicated in persons who have shown hypersensitivity to any of the components of this product. It is not intended for patients experiencing an acute episode of bronchospasm. Such patients require *rapid* relief of symptoms and should be treated with an immediate-release or intravenous theophylline preparation. Status asthmaticus should be considered a medical emergency. Adverse reactions are usually due to overdose.

PRESCRIBING INFORMATION

SLO-BID™ ℞
[*slō 'bid"*]
(Theophylline, Extended-release Capsules, USP)
50 mg, 75 mg, 100 mg, 125 mg, 200 mg, and 300 mg Gyrocaps®

DESCRIPTION

Slo-bid™ Gyrocaps® contain 50 mg, 75 mg, 100 mg, 125 mg, 200 mg, or 300 mg theophylline, anhydrous in the form of long-acting beads within a dye-free hard gelatin capsule and are intended for oral administration. Theophylline is a bronchodilator structurally classified as a xanthine derivative. Slo-bid Gyrocaps can be administered with a 12-hour dosing interval for a majority of patients and a 24-hour dosing interval for selected patients (see DOSAGE AND ADMINISTRATION section for description of appropriate patient population).

Theophylline is 1*H*-Purine-2, 6-dione,3, 7-dihydro-1,3-dimethyl represented by the following structural formula:

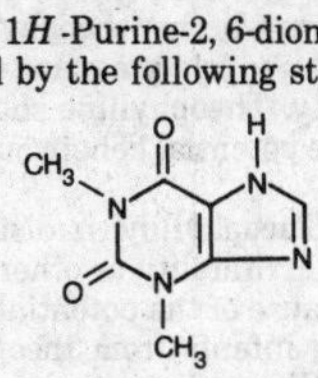

Theophylline is a white, odorless, crystalline powder having a bitter taste.

CLINICAL PHARMACOLOGY

Theophylline directly relaxes the smooth muscle of the bronchial airways and pulmonary blood vessels, thus acting as a bronchodilator and smooth muscle relaxant. It has also been demonstrated that aminophylline has a potent effect on diaphragmatic contractility in normal persons and may then be capable of reducing fatigability and thereby improve contractility in patients with chronic obstructive airways disease. The exact mode of action remains unsettled. Although theophylline does cause inhibition of phosphodiesterase with a resultant increase in intracellular cyclic AMP, other agents similarly inhibit the enzyme producing a rise of cyclic AMP but are unassociated with any demonstrable bronchodilation. Other mechanisms proposed include an effect on translocation of intracellular calcium; prostaglandin antagonism; stimulation of catecholamines endogenously; inhibition of cyclic guanosine monophosphate metabolism and adenosine receptor antagonism. None of these mechanisms has been proved, however.

In vitro, theophylline has been shown to act synergistically with beta agonists, and there are now available data that do demonstrate an additive effect *in vivo* with combined use.

Pharmacokinetics:

The half-life of theophylline is influenced by a number of known variables. It may be prolonged in chronic alcoholics, particularly those with liver disease (cirrhosis or alcoholic liver disease), in patients with congestive heart failure and in those patients taking certain other drugs (See PRECAUTIONS, Drug Interactions).

Newborns and neonates have extremely slow clearance rates compared to older infants and children, i.e., those over one year. Older children have rapid clearance rates while most nonsmoking adults have clearance rates between these two extremes. In premature neonates the decreased clearance is related to oxidative pathways that have yet to be established.

Theophylline Elimination Characteristics
Half-life (in hours)

	Range	Mean
Children	1–9	3.7
Adults	3–15	7.7

In cigarette smokers (1–2 packs/day) the mean half-life is 4–5 hours, much shorter than in nonsmokers. The increase in clearance associated with smoking is presumably due to stimulation of the hepatic metabolic pathway by components of cigarette smoke. The duration of this effect after cessation of smoking is unknown but may require 6 months to 2 years before the rate approaches that of the nonsmoker.

In a single-dose bioavailability study in 18 normal subjects, 300 mg extended-release Slo-bid Gyrocaps produced mean peak serum concentrations of 3.5 ± 0.7 μg/mL at a mean time of 7.8 ± 1.8 hours after dosing. Subjects fasted overnight before dosing and four hours after the dose. When compared to a syrup dosage form, relative bioavailability of Slo-bid Gyrocaps was about 91%. At steady state in a multiple-dose bioavailability study in 18 normal subjects with q12h dosing (600–1000 mg/day), the mean peak-trough variation was 3.5 ± 0.9 μg/mL. The mean C_{max} and C_{min} were 12.9 ± 3.0 and 9.4 ± 2.5 μg/mL, respectively. The mean percent fluctuation $[((C_{max} - C_{min})/C_{min}) \times 100]$ was 40 ± 15%. Subjects fasted 12 hours before the dose and 4 hours after the dose was administered on the days that the blood samples were drawn. A multiple-dose bioequivalence study with 15 asthmatic children, ages 9–16, comparing Slo-bid Gyrocaps administered as intact capsules and as the beaded contents sprinkled on applesauce with b.i.d. dosing (150–600 mg/dose) indicated no significant differences in maximum and minimum theophylline concentrations, time to achieve peak concentration, and peak-trough differences. The bioavailability as measured by comparing area under the curves ($AUC_{0-12\ hours}$ granules/$AUC_{0-12\ hours}$ capsules) was 0.990 ± 0.214.

Taking Slo-bid immediately after a high-fat content meal may result in a decrease in the rate of absorption (lower C_{max} and later T_{max}) but with no significant difference in the extent of absorption (see PRECAUTIONS, Drug-Food Interactions). In a single-dose bioavailability study, 24 normal adult nonsmoking subjects were given 900 mg extended-release Slo-bid Gyrocaps with food and under fasting conditions. Results (mean ± S.D.) showed:

	Food	Fasting
$AUC\ 0 \rightarrow \infty$ (μg-hr/mL)	260.5±60.6	280.5±68.7
C_{max} (μg/mL)	10.57±2.00	12.49±2.15
T_{max} (hr)	9.8±2.1	7.0±1.4

Steady-state pharmacokinetics were determined in 26 normal male volunteers (with theophylline clearance rates less than or equal to 5.0 L/hr and/or a theophylline elimination half-life of 6 to 12 hours) who received 900 mg of theophylline per day for five days. Twenty-six were dosed with three 300 mg extended-release Slo-bid Gyrocaps administered 24 hours apart immediately after the consumption of breakfast, and seventeen were dosed with one 300 mg, one 100 mg, and one 50 mg Slo-bid Gyrocap administered 12 hours apart (immediately after consuming breakfast and two hours after the consumption of dinner).

The pharmacokinetic parameters obtained for the extended-release Slo-bid Gyrocaps given as 900 mg once daily in the morning after a high-fat content breakfast were essentially the same as those parameters obtained after Slo-bid Gyrocaps administered in the widely-acceptable, approved manner of twice-daily. In particular, the area-under-the-curve

Continued on next page

Rhône-Poulenc Rorer—Cont.

values were 238 ± 27 (S.D.) and 251 ± 29 μg-hr/mL for the products administered q24h and q12h, respectively. Mean C_{max} values of 13.2 ± 2.0 μg/mL and 12.2 ± 2.2 μg/mL and C_{min} values of 5.9 ± 1.0 μg/mL and 8.6 ± 1.1 μg/mL were obtained after q24h and q12h administration, respectively. The mean percent fluctuation $[((C_{max}-C_{min})/C_{min}) \times 100]$ was 140 ± 66% (S.D.) and 40 ± 15% (S.D.) when Slo-bid was given once- or twice-daily, respectively.

INDICATIONS AND USAGE

For relief and/or prevention of symptoms from asthma and reversible bronchospasm associated with chronic bronchitis and emphysema.

CONTRAINDICATIONS

Slo-bid is contraindicated in individuals who have shown hypersensitivity to any of the components of this product or to xanthine derivatives. It is also contraindicated in patients with active peptic ulcer disease and in individuals with underlying seizure disorders (unless receiving appropriate anticonvulsant medication).

WARNINGS

Serum levels above 20 μg/mL are rarely found after appropriate administration of the recommended doses. However, in individuals in whom theophylline plasma clearance is reduced *for any reason,* even conventional doses may result in increased serum levels and potential toxicity. Reduced theophylline clearance has been documented in the following readily identifiable groups: 1) patients with impaired renal or liver function; 2) patients over 55 years of age, particularly males and those with chronic lung disease; 3) those with cardiac failure from any cause; 4) patients with sustained high fever; 5) neonates and infants under 1 year of age; and 6) those patients taking certain drugs (see PRECAUTIONS, Drug Interactions). Frequently, such patients have markedly prolonged theophylline serum levels following discontinuation of the drug.

Decreased clearance of theophylline may be associated with either influenza immunization or active influenza, and with other viral infections.

It is important to consider reduction of dosage and measurement of serum theophylline levels in the above individuals.

Serious side effects such as ventricular arrhythmias, convulsions or even death may appear as the first sign of toxicity without any previous warning. Less serious signs of theophylline toxicity (i.e., nausea and restlessness) may occur frequently when initiating therapy but are usually transient; when such signs are persistent during maintenance therapy, they are often associated with serum concentrations above 20 μg/mL. Stated differently, *serious toxicity is not reliably preceded by less severe side effects.* A serum concentration measurement is the only reliable method of identifying a potential for life-threatening toxicity.

Many patients who require theophylline exhibit tachycardia due to their underlying disease process, so the cause/effect relationship to elevated serum theophylline concentrations may not be appreciated.

Theophylline products may cause or worsen arrhythmias and any significant change in rate and/or rhythm warrants monitoring and further investigation.

Studies in laboratory animals (minipigs, rodents and dogs) recorded the occurrence of cardiac arrhythmias and sudden death (with histologic evidence of myocardial necrosis) when beta agonists and methylxanthines were administered concurrently. The significance of these findings when applied to humans is currently unknown.

PRECAUTIONS

General: On the average, theophylline half-life is shorter in cigarette and marijuana smokers than in nonsmokers, but smokers can have half-lives as long as nonsmokers. Theophylline should not be administered concurrently with other xanthine preparations. Use with caution in patients with hypoxemia, hypertension or with a history of peptic ulcer. Theophylline may occasionally act as a local irritant to the GI tract, although GI symptoms are more commonly centrally mediated and associated with serum drug concentrations over 20 μg/mL.

Xanthines can potentiate hypokalemia resulting from $beta_2$ agonist therapy, steroids, diuretics, other xanthines and hypoxia. Particular caution is advised in severe asthma. It is recommended that serum potassium levels be monitored in such situations.

Information for Patients:

The physician should reinforce the importance of taking only the prescribed dose at the prescribed time intervals. The patient should alert the physician if symptoms occur repeatedly, especially near the end of a dosing interval. When prescribing administration by the sprinkle method, details of the proper technique should be explained to the patient.

Laboratory Test: Serum levels should be monitored periodically to determine the theophylline levels associated with observed clinical response and to identify the potential for toxicity. For such measurements, the serum sample should be obtained at the time of peak concentration, approximately 5–9 hours after the morning dose. It is important that the patient has not missed or taken additional doses during the previous 48 hours and that dosing intervals have been reasonably equally spaced.

DOSE ADJUSTMENT BASED ON SERUM THEOPHYLLINE MEASUREMENTS WHEN THESE INSTRUCTIONS HAVE NOT BEEN FOLLOWED MAY RESULT IN RECOMMENDATIONS THAT PRESENT RISK OF TOXICITY TO THE PATIENT.

Drug Interactions:

Drug-Drug: Toxic synergism with ephedrine has been documented and may occur with some other sympathomimetic bronchodilators. In addition, the following drug interactions have been demonstrated:

Drug	Effect
Theophylline with:	
Allopurinol (high dose)	Increased serum theophylline levels
Cimetidine	Increased serum theophylline levels
Ciprofloxacin	Increased serum theophylline levels
Erythromycin, Troleandomycin	Increased serum theophylline levels
Lithium carbonate	Increased renal excretion of lithium
Oral contraceptives	Increased serum theophylline levels
Propranolol	Increased serum theophylline levels
Phenytoin	Decreased theophylline and phenytoin serum levels
Rifampin	Decreased serum theophylline levels

Drug-Food: Taking Slo-bid immediately after a high-fat content meal such as 8 ounces whole milk, 2 fried eggs, 2 strips bacon, one bran muffin with butter, 2 ounces hash brown potatoes (about 789 calories, including approximately 49 g of fat) may result in a decrease in the rate of absorption, but with no significant difference in the extent of absorption (see CLINICAL PHARMACOLOGY, Pharmacokinetics). The influence of the type and amount of other foods, as well as the time interval between drug and food, has not been studied.

Drug/Laboratory Test Interactions: Currently available analytic methods, including high-pressure liquid chromatography and immunoassay techniques, for measuring serum theophylline levels are specific. Metabolites and other drugs generally do not affect the results. Other new analytic methods are also now in use. The physician should be aware of the laboratory method used and whether other drugs will interfere with the assay for theophylline.

Carcinogenesis, Mutagenesis, Impairment of Fertility: Long-term carcinogenicity studies have not been performed with theophylline.

Chromosome-breaking activity was detected in human cell cultures at concentrations of theophylline up to 50 times the therapeutic serum concentrations in humans. Theophylline was not mutagenic in the dominant lethal assay in male mice given theophylline intraperitoneally in doses up to 30 times the maximum daily human oral dose.

Studies to determine the effect on fertility have not been performed with theophylline.

Pregnancy: Pregnancy Category C—Reproduction studies performed in mice and rats at oral doses from 7 to 17 times the human dose (maximum human dose for adults assumed to be 13 mg/kg/day) have indicated that theophylline may cause malformations, but these effects only occurred at or near doses that were toxic to the maternal animals. There are no adequate and well-controlled studies in pregnant women. It is not known whether theophylline can cause fetal harm when administered to a pregnant woman or can affect reproduction capacity. Theophylline should be used during pregnancy only if the potential benefit justifies the potential risk to the fetus.

Nursing Mothers: Theophylline is distributed into breast milk and may cause irritability or other signs of toxicity in nursing infants. Because of the potential for serious adverse reactions in nursing infants from theophylline, a decision should be made whether to discontinue nursing or to discontinue the drug, taking into account the importance of the drug to the mother.

Pediatric Use: Safety and effectiveness of Slo-bid Gyrocaps administered:

1. Every 24 hours in children under 12 years of age, have not been established.
2. Every 12 hours in children under 6 years of age, have not been established.

ADVERSE REACTIONS

The following adverse reactions have been observed, but there has not been enough systematic collection of data to support an estimate of their frequency. The most consistent adverse reactions are usually due to overdosage.

Gastrointestinal: nausea, vomiting, epigastric pain, hematemesis, diarrhea.

Central Nervous System: headaches, irritability, restlessness, insomnia, reflex hyperexcitability, muscle twitching, clonic and tonic generalized convulsions.

Cardiovascular: palpitation, tachycardia, extrasystoles, flushing, hypotension, circulatory failure, ventricular arrhythmias.

Respiratory: tachypnea.

Renal: potentiation of diuresis.

Other: alopecia, hyperglycemia, inappropriate ADH syndrome, rash.

OVERDOSAGE

Management: It is suggested that the management principles (consistent with the clinical status of the patient when first seen) outlined below be instituted and that simultaneous contact with a Regional Poison Control Center be established. In this way both updated information and individualization regarding therapy may be provided.

1. When potential oral overdose is established and seizure has not occurred:
   a) If patient is alert and seen soon after ingestion, induction of emesis may be of value. Gastric lavage has been demonstrated to be of no value in influencing outcome in patients who present more than 1 hour after ingestion.
   b) Administer a cathartic. Sorbitol solution is reported to be of value.
   c) Administer repeated doses of activated charcoal and monitor theophylline serum levels.
   d) Prophylactic administration of phenobarbital has been shown to increase the seizure threshold in laboratory animals, and administration of this drug may be of value.
   e) Monitor serum potassium.
2. If patient presents with a seizure:
   a) Establish an airway.
   b) Administer oxygen.
   c) Treat the seizure with intravenous diazepam 0.1 to 0.3 mg/kg up to 10 mg. If seizures cannot be controlled, the use of general anesthesia should be considered.
   d) Monitor vital signs, maintain blood pressure and provide adequate hydration.
3. Postseizure Coma:
   a) Maintain airway and oxygenation.
   b) If a result of oral medication, follow above recommendations to prevent absorption of drug, but intubation and lavage will have to be performed instead of inducing emesis and the cathartic and charcoal will need to be introduced via a large-bore gastric lavage tube.
   c) Continue to provide full supportive care and adequate hydration until the drug is metabolized. In general, drug metabolism is sufficiently rapid so as not to warrant dialysis. If repeated oral activated charcoal is ineffective (as noted by stable or rising serum levels), charcoal hemoperfusion may be indicated.

DOSAGE AND ADMINISTRATION

Taking Slo-bid immediately after a high-fat-content meal may alter its rate of absorption (see CLINICAL PHARMACOLOGY and PRECAUTIONS, Drug-Food Interactions). However, the differences are usually small and Slo-bid may normally be administered without regard to meals.

Effective use of theophylline (i.e., the concentration of drug in the serum associated with optimal benefit and minimal risk of toxicity) is considered to occur when the theophylline concentration is maintained from 10 to 20 μg/mL. The early studies from which these levels were derived were carried out in patients immediately or shortly after recovery from acute exacerbations of their disease (some hospitalized with status asthmaticus).

Although the 20 μg/mL level remains appropriate as a critical value (above which toxicity is more likely to occur) for safety purposes, additional data are now available that indicate that the serum theophylline concentrations required to produce maximum physiologic benefit may, in fact, fluctuate with the degree of bronchospasm present and are variable. Therefore, the physician should individualize the range appropriate to the patient's requirements, based on both symptomatic response and improvement in pulmonary function.

It should be stressed that serum theophylline concentrations maintained at the upper level of the 10 to 20 μg/mL range may be associated with potential toxicity when factors known to reduce theophylline clearance are operative. (See WARNINGS.)

If it is not possible to obtain serum level determinations, restriction of the daily dose (in otherwise healthy adults) to not greater than 13 mg/kg/day, to a maximum of 900 mg, in divided doses will result in relatively few patients exceeding serum levels of 20 μg/mL and the resultant greater risk of toxicity.

Caution should be exercised for younger children who cannot complain of minor side effects. Older adults, those with cor

pulmonale, congestive heart failure, and/or liver disease may have unusually low dosage requirements and thus may experience toxicity at the maximal dosage recommended below.

Theophylline does not distribute into fatty tissue. Dosage should be calculated on the basis of lean (ideal) body weight where mg/kg doses are presented.

Frequency of Dosing: When immediate-release products with rapid absorption are used, dosing to maintain serum levels generally requires administration every 6 hours. This is particularly true in children, but dosing intervals up to 8 hours may be satisfactory in adults since they eliminate the drug at a slower rate. Some children, and adults requiring higher than average doses (those having rapid rates of clearance, e.g., half-lives of under 6 hours) may benefit and be more effectively controlled during chronic therapy when given products with extended-release characteristics since these provide longer dosing intervals and/or less fluctuation in serum concentration between dosing. Those extended-release products which provide flexibility in dosage through formulations of varying strengths are also helpful in controlling serum levels. Dosage guidelines are approximations only and the wide range of theophylline clearance between individuals (particularly those with concomitant disease) make indiscriminate usage hazardous.

Dosage Guidelines:

I. Acute Symptoms

NOTE: Status asthmaticus should be considered a medical emergency and is defined as that degree of bronchospasm that is not rapidly responsive to usual doses of conventional bronchodilators. Optimal therapy for such patients frequently requires both *additional medication* parenterally administered, and *close monitoring*, preferably in an intensive care setting.

Slo-bid is not intended for patients experiencing an acute episode of bronchospasm (associated with asthma, chronic bronchitis, or emphysema). Such patients require *rapid* relief of symptoms and should be treated with an immediate-release or intravenous theophylline preparation (or other bronchodilators) and not with extended-release products.

II. Chronic Therapy

A. Initiating Therapy with an Immediate-Release Product

It is recommended that the appropriate dosage be established using an immediate-release preparation. A dosage form that allows small incremental doses is desirable for initiating therapy. A liquid preparation should be considered for children to permit easier and more accurate dosage adjustment. Slow clinical titration is generally preferred to help assure acceptance and safety of the medication and to allow the patient to develop tolerance to transient caffeine-like side effects. Then, if the total 24-hour dose can be given by use of the available strengths of this product, the patient can usually be switched to Slo-bid, giving one third of the daily dose at 8-hour intervals or one half the daily dose at 12-hour intervals. Patients who metabolize theophylline rapidly, such as the young, smokers, and some nonsmoking adults are the most likely candidates for dosing at 8-hour intervals. Such patients can generally be identified as having trough serum concentrations lower than desired or repeatedly exhibiting symptoms near the end of a dosing interval.

		Dose per 8 hours	Dose per 12 hours
Age 6–under 9 years	24 mg/kg/day	8.0 mg/kg	12.0 mg/kg
Age 9–under 12 years	20 mg/kg/day	6.7 mg/kg	10.0 mg/kg
Age 12–under 16 years	18 mg/kg/day	6.0 mg/kg	9.0 mg/kg
Age over 16 years	13 mg/kg/day	4.3 mg/kg	6.5 mg/kg
	OR 900 mg		
	(WHICHEVER IS LESS)		

B. Initiating Therapy with Slo-bid Gyrocaps

Alternatively, therapy can be initiated with Slo-bid Gyrocaps since they are available in dosage strengths that permit titration and adjustments of dosage (in adults and older children). Children weighing less than 25 kg should have their daily dosage requirements established with Slo-Phyllin® 80 mg Syrup to permit small dosage increments.

Initial Dose: 16 mg/kg/24 hours or 400 mg/24 hours (whichever is less) of anhydrous theophylline in 2 or 3 divided doses at 8- or 12-hour intervals.

Increasing Dose: The above dosage may be increased in approximately 25-percent increments at 3-day intervals so long as the drug is tolerated. Following each adjustment, if the clinical response is satisfactory and serum levels can be measured, then such measurements should be obtained as directed under section IV (below). If serum levels cannot be obtained, then that dosage level should be maintained. Dosage increases may be made in this manner until the maximum dose indicated in section III (below) is reached.

It is important that no patient be maintained on any dosage that is not tolerated. When instructing patients to increase dosage according to the schedule above, they should be told not to take a subsequent dose if apparent side effects occur and to resume therapy at a lower dose once adverse effects have disappeared.

C. Sprinkling Contents on Food

Slo-bid Gyrocaps may be administered by carefully opening the capsule and sprinkling the beaded contents on a spoonful of soft food such as applesauce or pudding; the soft food should be swallowed immediately without chewing and followed with a glass of cool water or juice to ensure complete swallowing of the beads. It is recommended that the food used should not be hot and should be soft enough to be swallowed without chewing. Any bead/food mixture should be used immediately and not stored for future use. SUBDIVIDING THE CONTENTS OF A CAPSULE IS NOT RECOMMENDED.

D. Once-Daily Dosing

The slow absorption rate of this preparation may allow once-daily administration in adult nonsmokers with appropriate total body clearance and other patients with low dosage requirements. Once-daily dosing should be considered only after the patient has been gradually and satisfactorily titrated to therapeutic levels with q12h dosing. Once-daily dosing should be based on twice the q12h dose and should be initiated at the end of the last q12h dosing interval. The trough concentration (C_{min}) obtained following conversion to once-daily dosing may be lower (especially in high clearance patients) and the peak concentration (C_{max}) may be higher (especially in low clearance patients) than that obtained with q12h dosing. If symptoms recur, or signs of toxicity appear during the once-daily dosing interval, dosing on the q12h basis should be reinstituted.

It is essential that serum theophylline concentrations be monitored before and after transfer to once-daily dosing. Food and posture, along with changes associated with circadian rhythm, may influence the rate of absorption and/or clearance rates of theophylline from extended-release dosage forms administered at night. The exact relationship of these and other factors to nighttime serum concentrations and the clinical significance of such findings require additional study. Therefore, it is not recommended that Slo-bid, when used as a once-a-day product, be administered at night.

III. Maximum Dose of Theophylline Where the Serum Concentration is Not Measured:

WARNING: DO NOT ATTEMPT TO MAINTAIN ANY DOSE THAT IS NOT TOLERATED.

Not to exceed the following:
[See table above.]

IV. Measurement of Serum Theophylline Concentrations During Chronic Therapy

If the above maximum doses are to be maintained or exceeded, serum theophylline measurement is essential (See PRECAUTIONS, Laboratory Tests for guidance).

V. Final Adjustment of Dosage

Dosage adjustment after serum theophylline measurement

If serum theophylline is:		Directions:
Within desired range		Maintain dosage if tolerated.
Too high	20 to 25 µg/mL	Decrease doses by about 10% and recheck serum level after 3 days.
	25 to 30 µg/mL	Skip next dose and decrease subsequent doses by about 25%. Recheck serum level after 3 days.
	Over 30 µg/mL	Skip next 2 doses and decrease subsequent doses by 50%. Recheck serum level after 3 days.
Too low		Increase dosage by 25% at 3-day intervals until either the desired serum concentration and/or clinical response is achieved. The total daily dose may need to be administered at more frequent intervals if symptoms occur repeatedly at the end of a dosing interval.

The serum concentration may be rechecked at appropriate intervals, but at least at the end of any adjustment period. When the patient's condition is otherwise clinically stable and none of the recognized factors which alter elimination are present, measurement of serum levels need be repeated only every 6 to 12 months.

STORAGE CONDITIONS

Store at room temperature. Protect from excessive heat, light and moisture.

CAUTION

Federal (U.S.A.) law prohibits dispensing without prescription. Keep this and all medications out of the reach of children.

HOW SUPPLIED

[See table at left.]

Military: 50 mg—100s (NSN 6505-01-172-2852), 50 mg—10 x 10s (NSN 6505-01-324-6969), 75 mg—100s (NSN 6505-01-289-2007), 75 mg—10 x 10s (NSN 6505-01-324-6971), 100 mg—100s (NSN 6505-01-166-9018), 100 mg—1000s (NSN 6505-01-180-3221), 100 mg—10 x 10s (NSN 6505-01-324-6970), 125 mg—100s (NSN 6505-01-289-2006), 125 mg—10 x 10s (NSN 6505-01-324-6972), 200 mg—100s (NSN 6505-01-166-8989), 200 mg—1000s (NSN 6505-01-173-1906), 300 mg—100s (NSN 6505-01-164-8736), 300 mg—1000s (NSN 6505-01-172-1054), 300 mg—10 x 10s (NSN 6505-01-164-8737).

RHÔNE-POULENC RORER PHARMACEUTICALS INC.
Collegeville, PA, U.S.A. 19426-0107
Rev. 1/96   IN-0221E
Shown in Product Identification Guide, page 330

Strength	Size	NDC 0075-	Color	Markings
50 mg	Bottles of 100	0057-00	Opaque white capsule	50 printed in red
	Unit Dose 100	0057-62		
75 mg	Bottles of 100	1075-00	Opaque white capsule	75 printed in red
	Unit Dose 100	1075-62		
100 mg	Bottles of 100	0100-00	Opaque white capsule	100 printed in red
	Bottles of 1000	0100-99		
	Unit Dose 100	0100-62		
125 mg	Bottles of 100	1125-00	Opaque white capsule	125 print in red
	Unit Dose 100	1125-62		
200 mg	Bottles of 100	0200-00	Opaque white capsule	200 printed in red
	Bottles of 1000	0200-99		
	Unit Dose 100	0200-62		
300 mg	Bottles of 100	0300-00	Opaque white capsule	300 printed in red
	Bottles of 1000	0300-99		
	Unit Dose 100	0300-62		

Continued on next page

Rhône-Poulenc Rorer—Cont.

TAXOTERE® ℞
[tax-ō-tēr]
(docetaxel)
for Injection Concentrate

Caution: Federal law prohibits dispensing without prescription.

WARNING

TAXOTERE® (docetaxel) for Injection Concentrate should be administered under the supervision of a qualified physician experienced in the use of antineoplastic agents. Appropriate management of complications is possible only when adequate diagnostic and treatment facilities are readily available.

The incidence of treatment-related mortality associated with TAXOTERE® therapy is increased in patients with abnormal liver function and in patients receiving higher doses (see **WARNINGS**).

TAXOTERE® should generally not be given to patients with bilirubin > upper limit of normal (ULN), or to patients with SGOT and/or SGPT > 1.5 x ULN concomitant with alkaline phosphatase > 2.5 x ULN. Patients with elevations of bilirubin or abnormalities of transaminase concurrent with alkaline phosphatase are at increased risk for the development of grade 4 neutropenia, febrile neutropenia, infections, severe thrombocytopenia, severe stomatitis, severe skin toxicity, and toxic death. Patients with isolated elevations of transaminase > 1.5 x ULN also had a higher rate of febrile neutropenia grade 4 but did not have an increased incidence of toxic death. Bilirubin, SGOT or SGPT, and alkaline phosphatase values should be obtained prior to each cycle of TAXOTERE® therapy and reviewed by the treating physician.

TAXOTERE® therapy should not be given to patients with neutrophil counts of < 1500 cells/mm³. In order to monitor the occurrence of neutropenia, which may be severe and result in infection, frequent blood cell counts should be performed on all patients receiving TAXOTERE®.

Severe hypersensitivity reactions characterized by hypotension and/or bronchospasm, or generalized rash/erythema occurred in 0.9% of patients who received the recommended dexamethasone premedication. Hypersensitivity reactions requiring discontinuation of the TAXOTERE® infusion were reported in five patients who did not receive premedication. These reactions resolved after discontinuation of the infusion and the administration of appropriate therapy. TAXOTERE® must not be given to patients who have a history of severe hypersensitivity reactions to TAXOTERE® or to other drugs formulated with polysorbate 80.

Severe fluid retention occurred in 6% of patients despite use of a 5-day dexamethasone premedication regimen. It was characterized by one or more of the following events: poorly tolerated peripheral edema, generalized edema, pleural effusion requiring urgent drainage, dyspnea at rest, cardiac tamponade, or pronounced abdominal distention (due to ascites).

DESCRIPTION

Docetaxel is an antineoplastic agent belonging to the taxoid family. It is prepared by semisynthesis beginning with a precursor extracted from the renewable needle biomass of yew plants. The chemical name for docetaxel is (2R,3S)-N-carboxy-3-phenylisoserine,N-tert-butyl ester,13-ester with 5β-20-epoxy-1,2α,4,7β,10β,13α-hexahydroxytax-11-en-9-one 4-acetate 2-benzoate, trihydrate. Docetaxel has the following structural formula:

Docetaxel is a white to almost-white powder with an empirical formula of $C_{43}H_{53}NO_{14} \cdot 3H_2O$, and a molecular weight of 861.9. It is highly lipophilic and practically insoluble in water. TAXOTERE® (docetaxel) for Injection Concentrate is a clear yellow to brownish-yellow viscous solution. TAXOTERE® is sterile, non-pyrogenic, and is available in single-dose vials containing 20 mg (0.5 mL) or 80 mg (2.0 mL) docetaxel (anhydrous). Each mL contains 40 mg docetaxel (anhydrous) and 1040 mg polysorbate 80.

TAXOTERE® for Injection Concentrate requires dilution prior to use. A sterile, non-pyrogenic, single-dose diluent is supplied for that purpose. The diluent for TAXOTERE® contains 13% ethanol in Water for Injection, and is supplied in 1.5 mL (to be used with 20 mg TAXOTERE® for Injection Concentrate) and 6.0 mL (to be used with 80 mg TAXOTERE® for Injection Concentrate) vials.

CLINICAL PHARMACOLOGY

Docetaxel is an antineoplastic agent that acts by disrupting the microtubular network in cells that is essential for mitotic and interphase cellular functions. Docetaxel binds to free tubulin and promotes the assembly of tubulin into stable microtubules while simultaneously inhibiting their disassembly. This leads to the production of microtubule bundles without normal function and to the stabilization of microtubules, which results in the inhibition of mitosis in cells. Docetaxel's binding to microtubules does not alter the number of protofilaments in the bound microtubules, a feature which differs from most spindle poisons currently in clinical use.

HUMAN PHARMACOKINETICS

The pharmacokinetics of docetaxel have been evaluated in cancer patients after administration of 20 – 115 mg/m² in phase I studies. The area under the curve (AUC) was dose proportional following doses of 70 – 115 mg/m² with infusion times of one to two hours. Docetaxel's pharmacokinetic profile is consistent with a three-compartment pharmacokinetic model, with half-lives for the α, β, and γ phases of 4 min, 36 min, and 11.1 hr, respectively. The initial rapid decline represents distribution to the peripheral compartments and the late (terminal) phase is due, in part, to a relatively slow efflux of docetaxel from the peripheral compartment. Mean values for total body clearance and steady state volume of distribution were 21 L/h/m² and 113 L, respectively. Mean total body clearance for Japanese patients dosed at the range of 10-90 mg/m² was similar to that of European/American populations dosed at 100 mg/m², suggesting no significant difference in the elimination of docetaxel in the two populations.

A study of ¹⁴C-docetaxel was conducted in three cancer patients. Docetaxel was eliminated in both the urine and feces following oxidative metabolism of the tert–butyl ester group, but fecal excretion was the main elimination route. Within seven days, urinary and fecal excretion accounted for approximately 6% and 75% of the administered radioactivity, respectively. About 80% of the radioactivity recovered in feces is excreted during the first 48 hours as one major and 3 minor metabolites with very small amounts (less than 8%) of unchanged drug. Based on in vitro studies, isoenzymes of the cytochrome P4503A (CYP 3A) subfamily appear to be involved in docetaxel metabolism.

A population pharmacokinetic analysis was carried out after TAXOTERE® treatment of 535 patients dosed at 100 mg/m². Pharmacokinetic parameters estimated by this analysis were very close to those estimated from phase I studies. The pharmacokinetics of docetaxel were not influenced by age or gender and docetaxel total body clearance was not modified by pretreatment with dexamethasone. In patients with clinical chemistry data suggestive of mild to moderate liver function impairment (SGOT and/or SGPT > 1.5 times the upper limit of normal (ULN) concomitant with alkaline phosphatase > 2.5 times ULN), total body clearance was lowered by an average of 27%, resulting in a 38% increase in systemic exposure (AUC). This average, however, includes a substantial range and there is, at present, no measurement that would allow recommendation for dose adjustment in such patients. Patients with combined abnormalities of transaminase and alkaline phosphatase should, in general, not be treated with TAXOTERE®.

In vitro studies showed that docetaxel is about 94% protein bound, mainly to α_1–acid glycoprotein, albumin, and lipoproteins. In three cancer patients, the in vitro binding to plasma proteins was found to be approximately 97%. Dexamethasone does not affect the protein binding of docetaxel.

CLINICAL STUDIES

The efficacy and safety of TAXOTERE® has been evaluated in advanced breast carcinoma patients in independent clinical studies at doses of 100, 75, and 60 mg/m².

Safety and Efficacy at 100 mg/m²: The safety and efficacy of TAXOTERE® have been evaluated in three phase II studies which were conducted in a total of 134 patients with anthracycline-resistant, locally advanced or metastatic breast carcinoma. Anthracycline resistance was defined as progressive disease on anthracyclines for advanced disease or relapse on anthracycline adjuvant therapy. In these studies, TAXOTERE® was administered at a 100 mg/m² dose given as a one-hour infusion every 3 weeks.

The overall response rate (ORR) considering all patients (intent-to-treat) was 41% and the complete response (CR) was 2%. The median survival time was 43 weeks. In the evaluable patients (see table), the ORR was 47% and the CR was 2.8%. Overall response rates (ORR), duration of response, and time to progression are shown in the following table:

Efficacy Of TAXOTERE® In Anthracycline-Resistant Breast Cancer Patients Treated At 100 mg/m²

		(95% C.I.)
Overall Response Rates		
Intent-to-Treat Patients (n=134)	41%	(33–49)
Evaluable Patients (n=106)*	47%	(38–57)
Response Rate in Patients		
with Visceral Involvement		
Intent-to-Treat Patients (n=95)	37%	
Evaluable Patients (n=76)*	43%	
Median Response Duration**	6 months	(2.1–17.5)
Median Time to Progression**	4 months	(0.2–17.5)
Median Survival**	10 months	(0.2–24.6+)
1 Year Survival**	43%	

* Evaluable patients include those meeting the study eligibility requirements and having received at least two cycles of TAXOTERE® unless disease progression occurred earlier.

** Intent-to-treat population

For the 134 anthracycline-resistant breast cancer patients who received TAXOTERE®, 127 had normal LFTs (see table for definition) at baseline, and 7 had elevated LFTs at baseline. Patients with elevated LFTs at baseline had an increased incidence of thrombocytopenia, infection, febrile neutropenia, and death considered at least possibly treatment related. The following table shows the incidence of important hematologic adverse events during the study:

[See table at left.]

Hematologic Adverse Events In Anthracycline-Resistant Breast Cancer Patients Treated At 100 mg/m² With Normal Or Elevated Baseline Liver Function Tests

Adverse Event		Normal LFTs* at Baseline n=127 %	Elevated LFTs** at Baseline n=7 %
Neutropenia			
Any	<2000 cells/mm³	99.2	100
Grade 4	<500 cells/mm³	94.5	100
Thrombocytopenia			
Any	<100,000 cells/mm³	11.8	71.4
Grade 4	<20,000 cells/mm³	0	14.3
Anemia	<11 g/dL	98.4	85.7
Infection***			
Any		25.2	71.4
Grade 3 and 4		7.1	57.1
Febrile Neutropenia****			
By Patient		22.0	42.9
By Course		4.0	14.3
Septic Death		0.8	14.3
Non-Septic Death		0	14.3

*   Normal LFTs: Transaminases ≤1.5 times ULN or alkaline phosphatase ≤2.5 times ULN or isolated elevations of transaminases or alkaline phosphatase up to 5 times ULN.

**   Elevated LFTs: SGOT and/or SGPT >1.5 times ULN concurrent with alkaline phosphatase >2.5 times ULN.

*** Incidence of infection requiring hospitalization and/or intravenous antibiotics was 13.4% (n=17) among the 127 patients with normal LFTs at baseline. There were two patients with grade 2, one with grade 3, and fourteen with grade 4 neutropenia.

**** Febrile Neutropenia: ANC grade 4 with fever >38° C with IV antibiotics and/or hospitalization.

The following table shows important non-hematologic adverse events for the anthracycline-resistant breast cancer patients with normal and elevated LFTs at baseline:

Non-Hematologic Adverse Events In Anthracycline-Resistant Breast Cancer Patients Treated At 100 mg/m^2 With Normal Or Elevated Baseline Liver Function Tests

Adverse Event	Normal LFTs* at Baseline n=127 %	Elevated LFTs** at Baseline n=7 %
Acute Hypersensitivity Reaction		
Regardless of Premedication		
Any	11.8	0
Severe	0	0
Fluid Retention***		
Regardless of Type of Premedication		
Any	56.7	57.1
Severe	9.4	14.3
With Recommended Premedication	n=29	n=3
Any	41.4	66.6
Severe	3.4	33.3
Neurosensory		
Any	66.1	42.9
Severe	7.1	0
Myalgia	35.4	57.1
Cutaneous		
Any	62.2	57.1
Severe	10.2	14.3
Asthenia		
Any	80.3	42.9
Severe	22.8	28.6
Stomatitis		
Any	55.9	71.4
Severe	8.7	57.1

* Normal LFTs: Transaminases ≤1.5 times ULN or alkaline phosphatase ≤2.5 times ULN or isolated elevations of transaminases or alkaline phosphatase up to 5 times ULN.

** Elevated Liver Function: SGOT and/or SGPT >1.5 times ULN concurrent with alkaline phosphatase >2.5 times ULN.

*** Fluid Retention includes (by COSTART): edema (peripheral, localized, generalized, lymphedema, pulmonary edema, and edema otherwise not specified) and effusion (pleural, pericardial, and ascites).

Safety at 75 mg/m^2: TAXOTERE® at a dose of 75 mg/m^2 every 3 weeks has been evaluated in two phase II studies in 55 previously untreated patients with normal liver function and locally advanced or metastatic breast carcinoma. The following table shows the important hematologic adverse events in these studies:

Hematologic Adverse Events In 55 Breast Cancer Patients Treated With 75 mg/m^2

Adverse Event		%
Neutropenia		
Any	<2000 cells/mm^3	98.1
Grade 4	<500 cells/mm^3	80.0
Thrombocytopenia		
Any	<100,000 cells/mm^3	5.5
Grade 4	<20,000 cells/mm^3	0
Anemia	<11 g/dL	89.1
Infection		
Any		21.8
Grade 3 and 4		0
Febrile Neutropenia*		
By Patient		1.8
Septic Death		0
Non-Septic Death		0

* Febrile Neutropenia: ANC grade 4 with fever >38°C with IV antibiotics and/or hospitalization.

The following table shows the important non-hematologic adverse events at 75 mg/m^2:

Non-Hematologic Adverse Events In 55 Breast Cancer Patients Treated With 75 mg/m^2

Adverse Event	%
Acute Hypersensitivity Reaction*	
Any	29.1
Severe	1.8
Fluid Retention**	
Any	69.1
Severe	10.9
Neurosensory	
Any	38.2
Severe	1.8
Myalgia	
Any	12.7
Severe	1.8

Cutaneous	
Any	47.3
Severe	1.8
Asthenia	
Any	63.6
Severe	7.3
Stomatitis	
Any	30.9
Severe	3.6

* Regardless of premedication
** Without recommended premedication

Safety and Efficacy at 60 mg/m^2: The safety and efficacy of TAXOTERE® have been evaluated in three phase II Japanese studies in 174 patients (3 patients had elevated LFTs) who had received prior chemotherapy for locally advanced or metastatic breast carcinoma; 26 patients had progression of disease as best response to prior anthracycline treatment. In the 26 patients who had progression of disease as best response to prior anthracycline treatment, the ORR was 34.6% (95% C.I.: 17.2 – 55.7) and the CR was 3.8%. The median duration of response was 4 months.

The following table shows important hematologic adverse events for the Japanese breast cancer trials:

Hematologic Adverse Events In 174 Breast Cancer Patients Treated With 60 mg/m^2 Who Had Received Prior Chemotherapy In Trials Conducted In Japan

Adverse Event		%
Neutropenia		
Any	<2000 cells/mm^3	95.4
Grade 4	<500 cells/mm^3	74.9
Thrombocytopenia		
Any	<100,000 cells/mm^3	14.4
Grade 4	<20,000 cells/mm^3	1.1
Anemia	<11 g/dL	64.9
Infection		
Any		1.1
Grade 3 and 4		0
Febrile Neutropenia*		
By Patient		0
Septic Death		1.1
Non-Septic Death		0

* Febrile Neutropenia: ANC grade 3/4 concomitant with fever >38.1° C.

The following table shows important non-hematologic adverse events for the Japanese breast cancer trials; the incidence of severe non-hematologic toxicity in patients dosed at 60 mg/m^2 is negligible:

Non-Hematologic Adverse Events In 174 Breast Cancer Patients Treated With 60 mg/m^2 Who Had Received Prior Chemotherapy In Trials Conducted In Japan

Adverse Event	%
Acute Hypersensitivity Reaction	
Any	0.6
Severe	0
Fluid Retention*	
Any	12.6
Severe	0
Neurosensory	
Any	19.5
Severe	0
Cutaneous	
Any	30.5
Severe	0
Myalgia	
Any	3.4
Severe	0
Asthenia	
Any	65.5
Severe	0
Stomatitis	
Any	19.0
Severe	0.6

* without premedication

INDICATIONS AND USAGE

TAXOTERE® (docetaxel) for Injection Concentrate is indicated for the treatment of patients with locally advanced or metastatic breast cancer who have progressed during anthracycline-based therapy or have relapsed during anthracycline-based adjuvant therapy.

CONTRAINDICATIONS

TAXOTERE® is contraindicated in patients who have a history of severe hypersensitivity reactions to docetaxel or to other drugs formulated with polysorbate 80.

TAXOTERE® should not be used in patients with neutrophil counts of < 1500 cells/mm^3.

WARNINGS

TAXOTERE® (docetaxel) for Injection Concentrate should be administered under the supervision of a qualified physi-

cian experienced in the use of antineoplastic agents. Appropriate management of complications is possible only when adequate diagnostic and treatment facilities are readily available.

Toxic Deaths: TAXOTERE® administered at 100 mg/m^2 was associated with deaths considered possibly or probably related to treatment in 2.4% (34/1435) of patients with normal liver function and in 11% (6/55) of patients with abnormal liver function (SGOT and/or SGPT > 1.5 times ULN together with AP > 2.5 times ULN). Among patients dosed at 60 mg/m^2, mortality related to treatment occurred in 0.6% (3/481) of patients with normal liver function, and in 3 of 7 patients with abnormal liver function. Approximately half of these deaths occurred during the first cycle. Sepsis accounted for the majority of the deaths.

Premedication Regimen: Although the optimal premedication regimen is not defined, all patients should be premedicated with oral corticosteroids such as dexamethasone 16 mg per day (e.g., 8 mg BID) for 5 days starting 1 day prior to TAXOTERE® to reduce the severity of fluid retention and hypersensitivity reactions (see **DOSAGE AND ADMINISTRATION** section).

Hypersensitivity Reactions: Patients should be observed closely for hypersensitivity reactions, especially during the first and second infusions. Severe hypersensitivity reactions characterized by hypotension and/or bronchospasm, or generalized rash/erythema occurred in 0.9% of patients who received the recommended premedication. Hypersensitivity reactions requiring discontinuation of the TAXOTERE® infusion were reported in 5 out of 1260 patients who did not receive premedication. Patients with a history of severe hypersensitivity reactions should not be rechallenged with TAXOTERE®.

Hematologic Effects: Neutropenia (less than 2000 neutrophils/mm^3) occurs in virtually all patients given 60–100 mg/m^2 of TAXOTERE® and grade 4 neutropenia (less than 500 cells/mm^3) occurs in nearly all patients given 100 mg/m^2 and 75–80% of patients given 60–75 mg/m^2. Frequent monitoring of blood counts is, therefore, essential so that dose can be adjusted. TAXOTERE® should not be administered to patients with neutrophils < 1500 cells/mm^3. Febrile neutropenia occurred in about 12% of patients given 100 mg/m^2 but was very uncommon in patients given 60–75 mg/m^2. Hematologic responses, febrile reactions and infections, and rates of septic death for different regimens are dose related and are described in CLINICAL STUDIES. Three breast cancer patients with severe liver impairment (bilirubin > 1.7 times ULN) developed fatal gastrointestinal bleeding associated with severe drug-induced thrombocytopenia.

Hepatic Impairment: (see **BOXED WARNING**).

Fluid Retention: (see **BOXED WARNING**).

Pregnancy: TAXOTERE® can cause fetal harm when administered to pregnant women. Studies in both rats and rabbits at doses equal to or greater than 0.3 and 0.03 mg/kg/day, respectively (about 1/50 and 1/300 the daily maximum recommended human dose on a mg/m^2 basis), administered during the period of organogenesis, have shown that TAXOTERE® is embryotoxic and fetotoxic (characterized by intrauterine mortality, increased resorption, reduced fetal weight, and fetal ossification delay). The doses indicated above also caused maternal toxicity.

There are no adequate and well-controlled studies in pregnant women using TAXOTERE®. If TAXOTERE® is used during pregnancy, or if the patient becomes pregnant while receiving this drug, the patient should be apprised of the potential hazard to the fetus or potential risk for loss of the pregnancy. Women of childbearing potential should be advised to avoid becoming pregnant during therapy with TAXOTERE®.

PRECAUTIONS

General: Responding patients may not experience an improvement in performance status on therapy and may experience worsening. The relationship between changes in performance status, response to therapy and treatment-related side effects has not been established.

Hematologic Effects: In order to monitor the occurrence of myelotoxicity, it is recommended that frequent peripheral blood cell counts be performed on all patients receiving TAXOTERE®. Patients should not be retreated with subsequent cycles of TAXOTERE® until neutrophils recover to a level > 1500 cells/mm^3 and platelets recover to a level > 100,000 cells/mm^3.

A 25% reduction in the dose of TAXOTERE® is recommended during subsequent cycles following severe neutropenia (< 500 cells/mm^3) lasting 7 days or more, febrile neutropenia, or a grade 4 infection in a TAXOTERE® cycle (see **DOSAGE AND ADMINISTRATION** section).

Hypersensitivity Reactions: Hypersensitivity reactions may occur within a few minutes following initiation of a TAXOTERE® infusion. If minor reactions such as flushing or localized skin reactions occur, interruption of therapy is not required. More severe reactions, however, require the

Continued on next page

Rhône-Poulenc Rorer—Cont.

immediate discontinuation of TAXOTERE® and aggressive therapy. All patients should be premedicated with an oral corticosteroid prior to the initiation of the infusion of TAXOTERE® (see WARNINGS: Premedication Regimen).

Cutaneous: Localized erythema of the extremities with edema followed by desquamation has been observed. In case of severe skin toxicity, an adjustment in dosage is recommended (see DOSAGE AND ADMINISTRATION section). The discontinuation rate due to skin toxicity was 1.7%.

Fluid Retention: Severe fluid retention has been reported following TAXOTERE® therapy (see BOXED WARNING and ADVERSE REACTIONS). Patients should be premedicated with oral corticosteroids prior to each TAXOTERE® administration to reduce the incidence and severity of fluid retention (see DOSAGE AND ADMINISTRATION section). Patients with pre-existing effusions should be closely monitored from the first dose for the possible exacerbation of the effusions.

In patients who received the recommended premedication, moderate fluid retention occurred in 17.4% with severe fluid retention in 6% and a 1.7% discontinuation rate. Fluid retention was completely, but sometimes slowly, reversible following discontinuation of TAXOTERE® (median of 29 weeks). The median cumulative dose to onset of moderate or severe fluid retention was 705 mg/m^2 in patients receiving premedication. Patients developing peripheral edema may be treated with standard measures, e.g., salt restriction, oral diuretic(s).

Neurologic: Severe neurosensory symptoms (paresthesia, dysesthesia, pain) were observed among 7% of 134 patients with anthracycline-resistant breast cancer. When these occur, dosage must be adjusted. If symptoms persist, treatment should be discontinued (see DOSAGE AND ADMINISTRATION section). Patients who experienced neurotoxicity in clinical trials and for whom follow-up information on the complete resolution of the event was available had spontaneous reversal of symptoms within a median of 9 weeks from onset (range: 0 to 106 weeks) and only about 3.8% of patients required discontinuation due to neurotoxicity. Peripheral motor neuropathy mainly manifested as distal extremity weakness occurred in 13.4% (7.1% severe) of the 127 anthracycline-resistant breast cancer patients with normal LFTs. No neuromotor toxicity was reported in the 7 patients with elevated LFTs.

Asthenia: Severe asthenia has been reported in 11.1% of the patients but has led to treatment discontinuation in only 2.6% of the patients. Severe asthenia was reported in 23% of 134 patients with anthracycline-resistant breast cancer and 5.5% of the 786 cycles received. Symptoms of fatigue and weakness may last a few days up to several weeks and may be associated with deterioration of performance status in patients with progressive disease.

Drug Interactions: There have been no formal clinical studies to evaluate the drug interactions of TAXOTERE® with other medications. In vitro studies have shown that the metabolism of docetaxel may be modified by the concomitant administration of compounds that induce, inhibit or are metabolized by cytochrome P450 3A4, such as cyclosporine, terfenadine, ketoconazole, erythromycin, and troleandomycin. Caution should be exercised with these drugs when treating patients receiving TAXOTERE® as there is a potential for a significant interaction.

Carcinogenicity, Mutagenicity, Impairment of Fertility: No studies have been conducted to assess the carcinogenic potential of TAXOTERE®. TAXOTERE® has been shown to be clastogenic in the in vitro chromosome aberration test in CHO-K$_1$ cells and in the in vivo micronucleus test in the mouse, but it did not induce mutagenicity in the Ames test, or the CHO/HGPRT gene mutation assays. TAXOTERE® produced no impairment of fertility in rats when administered in multiple i.v. doses of up to 0.3 mg/kg (about 1/50 the recommended human dose on a mg/m^2 basis), but decreased testicular weights were reported. This correlates with findings of a 10–cycle toxicity study (dosing once every 21 days for 6 months) in rats and dogs in which testicular atrophy or degeneration was observed at i.v. doses of 5 mg/kg in rats and 0.375 mg/kg in dogs (about 1/3 and 1/15 the recommended human dose on a mg/m^2 basis, respectively). An increased frequency of dosing in rats produced similar effects at lower dose levels.

Pregnancy: Pregnancy Category D (see WARNINGS section).

Nursing Mothers: It is not known whether TAXOTERE® is excreted in human milk. Because many drugs are excreted in human milk, and because of the potential for serious adverse reactions in nursing infants from TAXOTERE®, mothers should discontinue nursing prior to taking the drug.

Pediatric Use: The safety and effectiveness of TAXOTERE® in pediatric patients have not been established.

ADVERSE REACTIONS

There were 1495 patients enrolled in 37 clinical trials conducted in North America and Europe (624 breast carcinoma patients and 866 patients with other tumor types) who received TAXOTERE® at an initial dose of 100 mg/m^2 every 3 weeks. Five patients were not evaluable for toxicity since they discontinued TAXOTERE® treatment due to acute hypersensitivity reactions with the first infusion. At least 95% of these patients did not receive hematopoietic support. The following table lists adverse reactions that occurred in at least 5% of 1435 patients with normal liver function tests at baseline (Normal LFTs: Transaminases ≤ 1.5 times ULN or alkaline phosphatase ≤ 2.5 times ULN or isolated elevations of transaminases or alkaline phosphatase up to 5 times ULN) as well as all deaths and adverse reactions in patients with abnormal liver function tests. These reactions were considered possibly or probably related to TAXOTERE®. The safety profile is generally similar in patients receiving TAXOTERE® for the treatment of breast carcinoma or for other tumor types.

[See table at left.]

Hematologic: Bone marrow suppression was the major dose-limiting toxicity of TAXOTERE®. Neutropenia is reversible and not cumulative. The median day to nadir was 8 days, while the median duration of severe neutropenia (<500 cells/mm^3) was 7 days. Among patients with normal liver function treated with TAXOTERE®, severe neutropenia occurred in 76% and lasted for more than 7 days in 4.3% of cycles. Anemia was reported in 89.5% of patients, with severe cases being reported in 8.4% of the patients (see WARNINGS section).

Febrile neutropenia (<500 cells/mm^3 with fever >38°C with IV antibiotics and/or hospitalization) occurred in 11.8% of the patients with normal liver function (3% of the cycles). Infectious episodes occurred in 21.7% of the patients (6.2% of the cycles) and were fatal in 1.6% of those treated with TAXOTERE® (1.4% in breast cancer patients).

Thrombocytopenia (<100,000 cells/mm^3) occurred in 7.5% of the patients with normal liver function. Bleeding episodes were reported in 2.3% of the patients. A fatal gastrointestinal hemorrhage associated with thrombocytopenia was reported in one patient. Three breast cancer patients with severe liver impairment (bilirubin > 1.7 times ULN) developed fatal gastrointestinal bleeding associated with severe drug-induced thrombocytopenia.

Hypersensitivity Reactions: Hypersensitivity reactions requiring discontinuation of the TAXOTERE® infusion were reported in 5 patients of 1260 who did not receive premedication. Severe hypersensitivity reactions characterized by hypotension and/or bronchospasm, or generalized rash/erythema have been observed in only 0.9% of patients with normal liver function receiving the recommended premedication regimen and none of these patients had to discontinue therapy.

Minor events, including flushing, rash with or without pruritus, chest tightness, back pain, dyspnea, drug fever, or chills, have been reported and resolved after discontinuing the infusion and appropriate therapy (see WARNINGS section).

Fluid Retention (see BOXED WARNING): Events such as edema and weight gain and, less frequently, pleural effusion, pericardial effusion or ascites have been described. Among 229 patients with normal liver function receiving the recommended pretreatment, severe fluid retention was observed in 6%, causing treatment discontinuation in 1.7%. When it occurs, peripheral edema usually starts at the lower extremi-

Summary Of Adverse Events In Patients Receiving TAXOTERE® At 100 mg/m²

Adverse Event		Normal LFTs* at Baseline n=1435 %	Elevated LFTs** at Baseline n=55 %
Hematologic			
Neutropenia	<2000 cells/mm³	96.3	96.0
	<500 cells/mm³	76.0	86.0
Leukopenia	<4000 cells/mm³	96.5	98.1
	<1000 cells/mm³	31.0	44.2
Thrombocytopenia	<100,000 cells/mm³	7.5	27.3
Anemia	<11 g/dL	89.5	92.7
	<8 g/dL	8.4	30.9
Febrile Neutropenia		11.8	26.4
Septic Death		1.8	3.6
Non-Septic Death		0.6	7.3
Infections			
Any		21.7	32.7
Severe		5.6	16.4
Fever in absence of Infection			
Any		30.2	50.9
Severe		1.7	9.1
Hypersensitivity Reactions			
with recommended premedication		n=229	n=6
Any		15.7	0
Severe		0.9	0
Fluid Retention			
with recommended premedication		n=229	n=6
Any		48.5	66.7
Severe		5.2	33.3
Neurosensory			
Any		53.7	41.8
Severe		3.9	0
Neuromotor (principally distal extremity weakness)			
Any		13.4	5.5
Severe		3.7	1.8
Cutaneous			
Any		58.5	61.8
Severe		5.6	10.9
Nail Changes			
Any		28.2	18.2
Severe		2.6	4.6
Gastrointestinal			
Nausea		40.4	40.0
Diarrhea		40.4	32.7
Vomiting		24.0	25.5
Alopecia		80.0	61.8
Asthenia			
Any		61.5	54.5
Severe		11.1	23.6
Stomatitis			
Any		42.3	47.3
Severe		5.3	14.5
Myalgia			
Any		19.4	18.2
Severe		1.4	1.9
Arthralgia		8.6	7.3
Infusion Site Reactions		5.6	3.6

* Normal LFTs: Transaminases ≤1.5 times ULN or alkaline phosphatase ≤2.5 times ULN or isolated elevations of transaminases or alkaline phosphatase up to 5 times ULN.

** Elevated LFTs: SGOT and/or SGPT >1.5 times ULN concurrent with alkaline phosphatase >2.5 times ULN.

ties and may become generalized with a median weight gain of 2 kg. Fluid retention is cumulative in incidence and severity. The median cumulative dose to onset of moderate or severe fluid retention was 705 mg/m^2. Fluid retention was completely reversible, resolving a median of 29 weeks (range: 0 to 42+ weeks) from the last TAXOTERE® infusion.

Cutaneous: Reversible cutaneous reactions characterized by a rash including localized eruptions, mainly on the feet and/or hands, but also on the arms, face or thorax, usually associated with pruritus, have been observed. Eruptions generally occurred within one week after TAXOTERE® infusion, recovered before the next infusion and were not disabling. Severe symptoms, such as eruptions followed by desquamation, occurred in 5.6% of the patients and rarely led to interruption or discontinuation of TAXOTERE® treatment. Alopecia occurred in 80% of patients, and it was severe in 61.8% of patients.

Severe nail disorders occurred in 2.6% of the patients. These reactions were characterized by hypo- or hyperpigmentation, and occasionally by onycholysis (in 0.8% of patients) and pain.

Neurologic: Neurosensory symptoms characterized by paresthesia, dysesthesia or pain (including burning sensation) have been reported in patients receiving TAXOTERE®. Severe reactions were observed in 3.9%.

Neuromotor events characterized mainly by weakness have been reported and were severe in 3.7% of the patients.

Gastrointestinal: Gastrointestinal reactions (nausea, and/or vomiting, and/or diarrhea) were generally mild to moderate and severe reactions occurred in 8.2% of the patients. Stomatitis was reported in 42.3% of patients receiving TAXOTERE®. Severe reactions were observed in 5.3% of patients.

Cardiovascular: Hypotension occurred in 3.6% of the patients; 3.4% required treatment. Clinically meaningful events such as heart failure, sinus tachycardia, atrial flutter, dysrhythmia, unstable angina, pulmonary edema, and hypertension occurred rarely.

Infusion Site Reactions: Infusion site reactions were generally mild and consisted of hyperpigmentation, inflammation, redness or dryness of the skin, phlebitis, extravasation, or swelling of the vein.

Hepatic: In patients with normal LFTs at baseline, bilirubin values greater than the ULN occurred in 8.9% of patients. Increases in SGOT or SGPT > 1.5 times the ULN, or alkaline phosphatase > 2.5 times ULN, were observed in 18.1% and 7.6% of patients, respectively. During the study, increases in SGOT and/or SGPT > 1.5 times ULN concomitant with alkaline phosphatase > 2.5 times ULN occurred in 4.5% of patients with normal LFTs at baseline. (Whether these changes were related to the drug or underlying disease has not been established.)

Ongoing Evaluation: The following serious adverse events of uncertain relationship to TAXOTERE® have been reported:

- Body as a whole: abdominal pain, diffuse pain, chest pain
- Cardiovascular: atrial fibrillation, deep vein thrombosis, ECG abnormalities, thrombophlebitis, pulmonary embolism, syncope, tachycardia
- Digestive: constipation, duodenal ulcer, esophagitis, gastrointestinal hemorrhage, intestinal obstruction, ileus
- Nervous: confusion
- Respiratory: dyspnea, acute pulmonary edema, acute respiratory distress syndrome
- Urogenital: renal insufficiency

OVERDOSAGE

There is no known antidote for TAXOTERE® overdosage. In case of overdosage, the patient should be kept in a specialized unit where vital functions can be closely monitored. Anticipated complications of overdosage include: bone marrow suppression, peripheral neurotoxicity, and mucositis.

There were two reports of overdose. One patient received 150 mg/m^2 and the other received 200 mg/m^2 as one-hour infusions. Both patients experienced severe neutropenia, mild asthenia, cutaneous reactions, and mild paresthesia, and recovered without incident.

In mice, lethality was observed following single i.v. doses that were ≥ 154 mg/kg (about 4.5 times the recommended human dose on a mg/m^2 basis); neurotoxicity associated with paralysis, non-extension of hind limbs and myelin degeneration was observed in mice at 48 mg/kg (about 1.5 times the recommended human dose on a mg/m^2 basis). In male and female rats, lethality was observed at a dose of 20 mg/kg, (comparable to the recommended human dose on a mg/m^2 basis) and was associated with abnormal mitosis and necrosis of multiple organs.

DOSAGE AND ADMINISTRATION

For treatment of patients with locally advanced or metastatic carcinoma of the breast after progression during anthracycline-based therapy for metastatic disease or relapse during anthracycline-based adjuvant therapy, the recommended dose of TAXOTERE® is 60–100 mg/m^2 administered intravenously over 1 hour every three weeks.

Premedication Regimen: All patients should be premedicated with oral corticosteroids such as dexamethasone 16 mg per day (*e.g.*, 8 mg BID) for 5 days starting 1 day prior to TAXOTERE® administration in order to reduce the incidence and severity of fluid retention as well as the severity of hypersensitivity reactions (see **WARNINGS** and **PRECAUTIONS** sections).

Dosage Adjustments During Treatment: Patients who are dosed initially at 100 mg/m^2 and who experience either febrile neutropenia, neutrophils < 500 cells/mm^3 for more than one week, severe or cumulative cutaneous reactions, or severe peripheral neuropathy during TAXOTERE® therapy should have the dosage adjusted from 100 mg/m^2 to 75 mg/m^2. If the patient continues to experience these reactions, the dosage should either be decreased from 75 mg/m^2 to 55 mg/m^2 or the treatment should be discontinued. Conversely, patients who are dosed initially at 60 mg/m^2 and who do not experience febrile neutropenia, neutrophils < 500 cells/mm^3 for more than one week, severe or cumulative cutaneous reactions, or severe peripheral neuropathy during TAXOTERE® therapy may tolerate higher doses.

Special Populations:

Hepatic Impairment: Patients with bilirubin > ULN should generally not receive TAXOTERE®. Also, patients with SGOT and/or SGPT > 1.5 x ULN concomitant with alkaline phosphatase > 2.5 x ULN should generally not receive TAXOTERE®.

Children: The safety and effectiveness of docetaxel in pediatric patients below the age of 16 years have not been established.

Elderly: No dosage adjustments are required for use in elderly.

PREPARATION AND ADMINISTRATION PRECAUTIONS

TAXOTERE® is a cytotoxic anticancer drug and, as with other potentially toxic compounds, caution should be exercised when handling and preparing TAXOTERE® solutions. The use of gloves is recommended. Please refer to **Handling and Disposal** section.

If TAXOTERE® concentrate, premix solution, or infusion solution should come into contact with the skin, immediately and thoroughly wash with soap and water. If TAXOTERE® concentrate, premix solution, or infusion solution should come into contact with mucosa, immediately and thoroughly wash with water.

TAXOTERE® for Injection Concentrate requires dilution prior to administration. Please follow the preparation instructions provided below. Note: Both the TAXOTERE® for Injection Concentrate and the diluent vials contain an overfill.

A. Preparation of the Premix Solution

1. Remove the appropriate number of vials of TAXOTERE® for Injection Concentrate and diluent from the refrigerator. Allow the vials to stand at room temperature for approximately 5 minutes.
2. Aseptically withdraw the entire contents of the diluent vial into a syringe and transfer it to the vial of TAXOTERE® for Injection Concentrate.
   Information regarding fill volumes is listed below:

Strength	Vial Content	Diluent Vial
TAXOTERE® 20 mg	23.6 mg/0.59 mL	1.83 mL
TAXOTERE® 80 mg	94.4 mg/2.36 mL	7.33 mL

   This will assure a final premix concentration of 10 mg docetaxel/mL.
3. Gently rotate each premix solution vial for approximately 15 seconds to assure full mixture of the concentrate and diluent.
4. The TAXOTERE® premix solution (10 mg docetaxel/mL) should be clear; however, there may be some foam on top of the solution due to the polysorbate 80. Allow the premix solution to stand for a few minutes to allow any foam to dissipate. It is not required that all foam dissipate prior to continuing the preparation process.

B. Preparation of the Infusion Solution

1. Aseptically withdraw the required amount of TAXOTERE® premix solution (10 mg docetaxel/mL) with a calibrated syringe and inject the required volume of premix solution into a 250 mL infusion bag or bottle of either 0.9% Sodium Chloride solution or 5% Dextrose solution to produce a final concentration of 0.3 to 0.9 mg/mL.
   If a dose greater than 240 mg of TAXOTERE® is required, use a larger volume of the infusion vehicle so that a concentration of 0.9 mg/mL TAXOTERE® is not exceeded.
2. Thoroughly mix the infusion by manual rotation.
3. As with all parenteral products, TAXOTERE® should be inspected visually for particulate matter or discoloration prior to administration whenever the solution and container permit. If the TAXOTERE® for Injection premix solution or infusion solution is not clear or appears to have precipitation, the solution should be discarded.

TAXOTERE® infusion solution should be administered intravenously as a one-hour infusion under ambient room temperature and lighting conditions.

Contact of the undiluted concentrate with plasticized PVC equipment or devices used to prepare solutions for infusion is not recommended. In order to minimize patient exposure to the plasticizer DEHP (di-2-ethylexyl phthalate), which may be leached from PVC infusion bags or sets, diluted TAXOTERE® solution should be stored in bottles (glass, polypropylene) or plastic bags (polypropylene, polyolefin) and administered through polyethylene-lined administration sets.

Stability: Unopened vials of TAXOTERE® are stable until the expiration date indicated on the package when stored refrigerated, 2° to 8°C (36° to 46°F), and protected from bright light. Freezing does not adversely affect the product.

HOW SUPPLIED

TAXOTERE® for Injection Concentrate is supplied in a single-dose vial as a sterile, pyrogen-free, non-aqueous, viscous solution with an accompanying sterile, non-pyrogenic, diluent (13% ethanol in Water for Injection) vial. The following strengths are available:

TAXOTERE® 80 mg (NDC 0075-8001-80)

TAXOTERE® (docetaxel) 80 mg Concentrate for Infusion: 80 mg docetaxel in 2 mL polysorbate 80 (Fill: 94.4 mg docetaxel in 2.36 mL polysorbate 80) and diluent for TAXOTERE® 80 mg. 13% (w/w) ethanol in Water for Injection (Fill: 7.33 mL). Both items are in a blister pack in one carton.

TAXOTERE® 20 mg (NDC 0075-8001-20)

TAXOTERE® (docetaxel) 20 mg Concentrate for Infusion: 20 mg docetaxel in 0.5 mL polysorbate 80 (Fill: 23.6 mg docetaxel in 0.59 mL polysorbate 80) and diluent for TAXOTERE® 20 mg. 13% (w/w) ethanol in Water for Injection (Fill: 1.83 mL). Both items are in a blister pack in one carton.

Storage: Store refrigerated, 2° to 8°C (36° to 46°F). Retain in the original package to protect from bright light.

TAXOTERE® premix solution (10 mg TAXOTERE®/mL) and fully prepared TAXOTERE® infusion solution (in either 0.9% Sodium Chloride solution or 5% Dextrose solution) should be used as soon as possible after preparation. However, the premix solution is stable for 8 hours either at room temperature, 15° to 25°C (59° to 77°F), or stored refrigerated, 2° to 8°C (36° to 46°F).

Handling and Disposal: Procedures for proper handling and disposal of anticancer drugs should be considered. Several guidelines on this subject have been published[1–4]. There is no general agreement that all of the procedures recommended in the guidelines are necessary or appropriate.

REFERENCES

1. OSHA Work-Practice Guidelines for Personnel Dealing with Cytotoxic (Antineoplastic) Drugs. *Am J Hosp Pharm.* 1986; 43(5): 1193–1204.
2. American Society of Hospital Pharmacists Technical Assistance Bulletin on Handling Cytotoxic and Hazardous Drugs. *Am J Hosp Pharm.* 1990; 47(95): 1033–1049.
3. AMA Council Report. Guidelines for Handling Parenteral Antineoplastics. *JAMA.* 1985; 253(11): 1590–1592.
4. Oncology Nursing Society Clinical Practice Committee. Cancer Chemotherapy Guidelines. Module II–Recommendations of Nursing Practice in the Acute Care Setting. *ONS.* 1988; 2–14.

RHÔNE-POULENC RORER PHARMACEUTICALS INC.
COLLEGEVILLE, PA 19426

For drug information and reimbursement assistance, call 1-800-996-ONCO (6626).

Shown in Product Identification Guide, page 331

TILADE® INHALER ℞
[*tī lādĕ*]
(nedocromil sodium inhalation aerosol)

DESCRIPTION

TILADE (nedocromil sodium) is an inhaled anti-inflammatory agent for the preventive management of asthma. Nedocromil sodium is a pyranoquinoline with the chemical name 4H-Pyrano[3,2-g]quinoline-2,8-dicarboxylic acid, 9-ethyl-6,9-dihydro-4, 6-dioxo-10-propyl-, disodium salt, and it has a molecular weight of 415.3. The empirical formula is $C_{19}H_{15}NNa_2O_7$. Nedocromil sodium, a yellow powder, is soluble in water.

Continued on next page

Rhône-Poulenc Rorer—Cont.

The molecular structure of nedocromil sodium is:

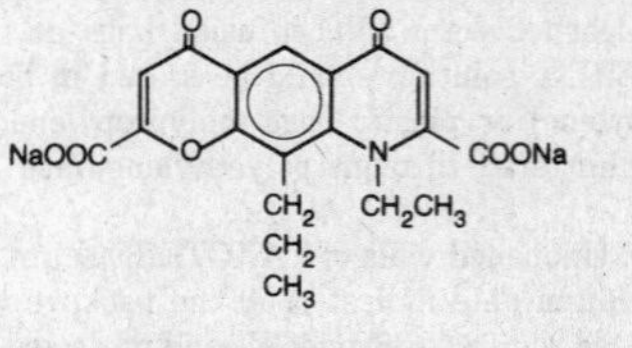

Chemical Class: Pyranoquinoline

TILADE Inhaler (nedocromil sodium inhalation aerosol) is a pressurized metered-dose aerosol suspension for oral inhalation containing micronized nedocromil sodium, sorbitan trioleate with dichlorotetrafluoroethane and dichlorodifluoromethane as propellants. Each actuation delivers from the mouthpiece 1.75 mg nedocromil sodium. Each 16.2 g canister provides at least 104 metered inhalations.

CLINICAL PHARMACOLOGY

Cellular and Animal Studies: Nedocromil sodium has been shown to inhibit the *in vitro* activation of, and mediator release from, a variety of inflammatory cell types associated with asthma, including eosinophils, neutrophils, macrophages, mast cells, monocytes, and platelets. *In vitro* studies on cells obtained by bronchoalveolar lavage from antigen-sensitized macaque monkeys show that nedocromil sodium inhibits the release of mediators including histamine, leukotriene C_4 and prostaglandin D_2. Similar studies with human bronchoalveolar cells showed inhibition of histamine release from mast cells and beta-glucuronidase release from macrophages.

Nedocromil sodium has been tested in experimental models of asthma using allergic animals and shown to inhibit the development of early and late bronchoconstriction responses to inhaled antigen. The development of airway hyper-responsiveness to nonspecific bronchoconstrictors was also inhibited. Nedocromil sodium reduced antigen-induced increases in airway microvasculature leakage when administered intravenously in a model system.

Clinical Studies: Nedocromil sodium has been shown to inhibit acutely the bronchoconstrictor response to several kinds of challenge. Pretreatment with single doses of nedocromil sodium inhibited the bronchoconstriction caused by sulfur dioxide, inhaled neurokinin A, various antigens, exercise, cold air, fog, and adenosine monophosphate.

Nedocromil sodium has no intrinsic bronchodilator, antihistamine, or glucocorticoid activity.

Nedocromil sodium, when delivered by inhalation at the recommended dose, has no known therapeutic systemic activity.

Pharmacokinetics and Bioavailability: Systemic bioavailability of nedocromil sodium administered as an inhaled aerosol is low. In a single dose study involving 20 healthy subjects who were administered a 3.5 mg dose of nedocromil sodium (2 actuations of 1.75 mg each), the mean AUC was 5.0 ng × hr/mL and the mean Cmax was 1.6 ng/mL attained about 28 minutes after dosing. The mean half life was 3.3 hours. Urinary excretion over 12 hours averaged 3.4% of the administered dose, of which approximately 75% was excreted in the first six hours of dosing.

In a multiple dose study, six healthy volunteers (3 males and 3 females) received a 3.5 mg single dose followed by 3.5 mg four times a day for seven consecutive days. Accumulation of the drug was not observed. Following single and multiple dose inhalations, urinary excretion of nedocromil accounted for 5.6% and 12% of the drug administered, respectively. After intravenous administration, urinary excretion of nedocromil was approximately 70%. The absolute bioavailability of nedocromil was thus 8% (5.6/70) for single and 17% (12/70) for multiple inhaled doses.

Similarly, in a multiple dose study of 12 asthmatic patients, each given a 3.5 mg single dose followed by 3.5 mg four times a day for one month, both single dose and multiple dose inhalation gave a mean high plasma concentration of 2.8 ng/mL between 5 and 90 minutes, mean AUC of 5.6 ng × hr/mL, and a mean terminal half life of 1.5 hours. The mean 24-hour urinary excretion after either single or multiple dose administration represented approximately 5% of the administered dose.

Studies involving very high oral doses of nedocromil (600 mg single dose, and subsequently 200 mg three times a day for seven days), showed an absolute bioavailability of less than 2%. In a radiolabeled (^{14}C) nedocromil study involving two healthy males, urinary excretion accounted for 64% of the dose, fecal excretion for 36%.

Protein binding—Nedocromil is approximately 89% protein bound to human plasma over a concentration range of 0.5 to 50 μg/mL. This binding is reversible.

Metabolism—Nedocromil is not metabolized after IV administration and is excreted unchanged.

CLINICAL STUDIES

The worldwide clinical trial experience with TILADE comprises 5352 patients. Studies have been conducted both at twice daily and at four times daily dosage regimens. Evidence from these studies indicates that the four times daily regimen has been more effective than the twice daily regimen. A lower dose (two or three times daily) can be considered in patients under good control on the four times daily regimen (see DOSAGE AND ADMINISTRATION).

1. TILADE vs. Placebo: The effectiveness of TILADE given four times daily was examined in a 14 week double-blind, placebo-controlled, parallel group trial in five centers in 120 patients (60/treatment). To be eligible for entry, the asthmatic patients had to be controlled using only sustained-release theophylline (SRT) and beta-agonists. Two weeks after the test therapies were begun the SRT was discontinued and four weeks after that oral beta-agonists were stopped. Beta-agonist metered dose inhalers could still be used after 6 weeks. Efficacy was assessed by symptom scores recorded on diary cards completed on a daily basis by the patients. Each morning the patient recorded nighttime asthma on a 0–2 scale, (0=slept well, no asthma; 1=woke once because of asthma; 2=woke more than once because of asthma). Before bedtime the patients recorded daytime asthma and cough on a 0–5 scale (0=no symptoms of asthma/cough today; 5=asthma/cough symptoms were noticed most of the day and caused a lot of trouble). At the end of the treatment phase, patients and clinicians were asked for their opinions on the effectiveness of the treatment based on a five point scale (1=very effective; 5=made condition worse). The results of these evaluations are shown in Table 1; TILADE was significantly superior to placebo for all measurements.

TABLE 1

Variable	Time Period	TILADE Mean	Placebo Mean
Daytime Asthma[1]	Weeks 7–14	1.26	2.08
Nighttime Asthma[2]	Weeks 7–14	0.67	0.96
Cough[1]	Weeks 7–14	0.68	1.49
Patient's Opinion[2]	Week 14	2.27	3.55
Clinician's Opinion[2]	Week 14	2.13	3.48
FEV_1[2] (liters)	Week 2	2.69	2.18
FEV_1[2] (liters)	Week 6	2.65	2.15
FEV_1[2] (liters)	Week 10	2.55	2.15
FEV_1[2] (liters)	Week 14	2.59	2.10

1: TILADE significantly better than Placebo, $p < 0.05$
2: TILADE significantly better than Placebo, $p < 0.01$

The FEV_1 percentage change relative to baseline is shown in Figure 1; these also favored TILADE over placebo throughout the study, with an effect seen first at the two week measurement.

FIGURE 1

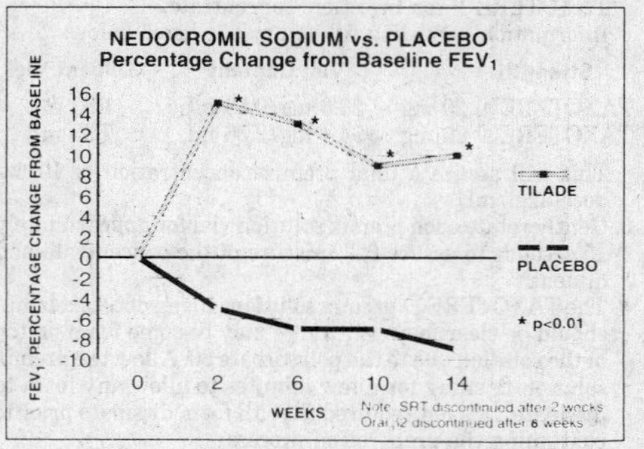

This study shows that TILADE improves symptom control and pulmonary function when it is added to a prn inhaled beta-adrenergic bronchodilator regimen and that a beneficial effect could be detected within two weeks.

2. TILADE vs. Cromolyn Sodium vs. Placebo: The effectiveness of TILADE was compared to cromolyn sodium and placebo in an eight week, double-blind, parallel group, 12 center trial during which medication was given four times daily. Three hundred and six patients were randomized to treatment (103/TILADE; 104/cromolyn sodium; 99/placebo). All patients were SRT dependent and this drug was stopped prior to starting the test treatment. Efficacy was assessed on the basis of diary card symptom scores and FEV_1. The diary scores were the same as used in the 14 week study except that nighttime symptoms were recorded on a 0–3 scale. The primary efficacy variable was a summary symptom score derived by averaging the scores for daytime asthma, nighttime asthma and cough. The results of the study are shown in Table 2.

[See table 2 below.]

This study corroborates the findings of the 14 week study, showing that TILADE is effective in the management of symptoms and pulmonary function in primarily atopic mild to moderate asthmatics. Both active treatments were statistically significantly better than placebo for the primary efficacy variable (summary symptom score); TILADE and cromolyn sodium were not significantly different for this parameter. A statistically significant difference favoring cromolyn sodium was, however, seen for nighttime asthma and FEV_1.

In laboratory studies, pretreatment with TILADE before an anticipated challenge can prevent the bronchoconstriction associated with sulfur dioxide, cold air, fog, exercise, allergen challenge, adenosine monophospate, and neurokinin A. Controlled studies have not been carried out to assess the clinical significance of these findings.

In allergic asthmatics who are well controlled on cromolyn sodium, there is no evidence that the substitution of TILADE for cromolyn sodium would confer additional benefit to the patient. Efficacy with one agent is not known to be predictive of efficacy with the other.

The presently available data on the relative efficacy of TILADE and cromolyn sodium are inconclusive.

INDICATIONS AND USAGE

TILADE Inhaler is indicated for maintenance therapy in the management of patients with mild to moderate bronchial asthma. TILADE is not indicated for the reversal of acute bronchospasm.

CONTRAINDICATIONS

TILADE Inhaler is contraindicated in those patients who have shown hypersensitivity to nedocromil sodium or other ingredients in this preparation.

WARNINGS

TILADE Inhaler is not a bronchodilator and, therefore, should not be used for the reversal of acute bronchospasm, particularly status asthmaticus. TILADE should ordinarily be continued during acute exacerbations, unless the patient becomes intolerant to the use of inhaled dosage forms.

As with other inhaled asthma medications, paradoxical bronchospasm, which can be life-threatening, has been reported rarely in postmarketing experience. If it occurs, discontinue treatment with TILADE immediately and institute alternative therapy.

PRECAUTIONS

General: If systemic or inhaled steroid therapy is at all reduced, patients must be monitored carefully. TILADE has not been shown to be able to substitute for the total dose of steroids.

Information for Patients: TILADE must be taken regularly to achieve benefit, even during symptom-free periods. Because the therapeutic effect depends upon topical application to the lungs, it is essential that patients be properly instructed in the correct method of use (see Patient Instruction leaflet). An illustrated leaflet for the patient is included in each TILADE Inhaler pack.

Drug Interactions: TILADE has been co-administered with other anti-asthma therapies including inhaled and oral bronchodilators and inhaled corticosteroids. There are no known adverse drug interactions.

TABLE 2

Variable	Time Period	TILADE Mean	Placebo Mean	Cromolyn Sodium Mean
Summary Score[1]	Weeks 3–8	1.30	1.76	1.13
Daytime Asthma[1]	Weeks 3–8	1.59	2.05	1.41
Nighttime Asthma[2]	Weeks 3–8	0.91	1.23	0.77
Cough[3]	Weeks 3–8	1.11	1.58	0.93
FEV_1[2]	Weeks 3–8	2.46	2.23	2.56
Patient's Opinion[1]	Week 8	2.54	3.39	2.22
Clinician's Opinion[1]	Week 8	2.60	3.43	2.39

1: TILADE significantly better than Placebo, $p < 0.001$
2: TILADE significantly better than Placebo, $p < 0.01$, cromolyn sodium significantly better than TILADE, $p < 0.05$
3: TILADE significantly better than Placebo, $p < 0.05$

Carcinogenesis, Mutagenesis, Impairment of Fertility: A two-year inhalation chronic/carcinogenicity study of nedocromil sodium in Wistar rats showed no carcinogenic potential. The maximum achievable daily dose of 24 mg/kg corresponded to 86 times the maximum human daily aerosol dose of 0.28 mg/kg (based on eight actuations of 1.75 mg to a 50 kg person). Assuming 5% systemic absorption in man, and comparing calculated exposure to measured exposure in rats, systemic exposure in rats in this study was about 40 times human exposure. A 21-month oral dietary carcinogenicity study of nedocromil sodium performed in B6C3F1 mice with daily doses up to 180 mg/kg showed no carcinogenic potential. Systemic exposure in the mouse, calculated as above for the rats, was about six times that in humans, or about 20 times that in humans based on free drug concentrations in plasma. The exposure of the GI tract in top dose animals corresponded to 643 times the human daily dose since, in man, most of an inhaled dose is subsequently swallowed. Nedocromil sodium showed no mutagenic potential in the Ames Salmonella/microsome plate assay, mitotic gene conversion in *S. cerevisiae*, mouse lymphoma forward mutation and mouse micronucleus assays.

Reproduction and fertility studies in mice and rats showed no effects on male or female fertility at subcutaneous doses of 100 mg/kg/day.

Pregnancy: Pregnancy Category B. Reproduction studies performed in mice, rats and rabbits using subcutaneous doses of 100 mg/kg/day, revealed no evidence of impaired fertility or harm to the fetus due to nedocromil sodium. There are, however, no adequate and well-controlled studies in pregnant women. Because animal reproduction studies are not always predictive of human response, this drug should be used during pregnancy only if clearly needed.

Nursing Mothers: It is not known whether this drug is excreted in human milk. Because many drugs are excreted in human milk, caution should be exercised when TILADE is administered to a nursing woman.

Pediatric Use: Safety and effectiveness in children below the age of 12 years have not been established.

ADVERSE REACTIONS

TILADE is generally well tolerated. Adverse event information was derived from 5352 patients receiving TILADE in controlled and open-label clinical trials of 2–52 weeks in duration. A total of 3538 patients received two inhalations four times a day. An additional 1814 patients received two inhalations twice daily or some other dose regimen. Seventy-three percent of patients were exposed to study drug for eight weeks or longer.

Of the 3538 patients who received two inhalations of TILADE four times a day, 2042 were in placebo-controlled trials and of these 7% withdrew from the trials due to adverse events, compared to 6% of the 1875 patients who received placebo.

The reasons for withdrawal were generally similar in the TILADE and placebo-treated groups, except that patients withdrew due to bad taste statistically more frequently on TILADE than on placebo. Headache reported as severe or very severe was experienced by 1.2 percent of TILADE patients and 0.9 percent of placebo patients, some with nausea and ill feeling.

The events reported with a frequency of 1% or greater across all placebo-controlled studies are displayed below for all patients who received TILADE or placebo at two inhalations four times daily.

[See table above.]

Other adverse events present at less than the 1% level of occurrence, but that might be related to TILADE administration, include rash, arthritis, tremor and a sensation of warmth.

Elevations of SGPT were noted in 3.3% of patients on nedocromil sodium vs. 1.7% on placebo. The average elevation over placebo was 10 I.U. with only two patients increasing by more than 100 I.U. and none becoming ill. The clinical significance of these elevations is unclear.

Rare cases of paradoxical bronchospasm (see WARNINGS) have been reported from postmarketing experience. Isolated cases of pneumonitis with eosinophilia (PIE syndrome) and anaphylaxis have also been reported in which a relationship to drug is undetermined.

OVERDOSAGE

There is no experience to date with overdose of TILADE in humans. Animal studies by several routes of administration (inhalation, oral, intravenous, subcutaneous) have demonstrated little potential for significant toxicity in humans from inhalation of high doses of nedocromil sodium. Head shaking/tremor and salivation were observed in beagle dogs following daily inhalation doses of 5 mg/kg and transient hypotension was detected following daily subcutaneous doses of 8 mg/kg. In addition, clonic convulsions were observed in dogs following daily inhalation doses of 20 mg/kg plus subcutaneous doses of 20 mg/kg giving peak plasma levels of 7.6 µg/mL, some three orders of magnitude greater than peak plasma levels (2.5 ng/mL) of the human daily dose. Specific tests designed to evaluate CNS activity demon-

strated no effects due to nedocromil sodium, and nedocromil sodium does not pass the blood brain barrier. Therefore, overdosage is unlikely to result in clinical manifestations requiring more than observation and discontinuation of the drug where appropriate.

DOSAGE AND ADMINISTRATION

The recommended dosage for symptomatic adults and children (12 years of age and over) is two inhalations four times a day at regular intervals to provide 14 mg of TILADE per day. Maintenance therapy should be initiated at the same dose. In patients under good control on four times daily dosing (i.e., patients whose only medication need is occasional [not more than twice a week] inhaled or oral beta-agonists, and who have no serious exacerbations with respiratory infections) a lower dose can be tried. If use of lower doses is attempted, TILADE should first be reduced to a three times daily regimen (10.5 mg of TILADE per day) then, after several weeks on continued good control, to twice a day (7 mg of TILADE per day).

TILADE Inhaler should be added to the patient's existing treatment regimen (e.g., bronchodilators). When a clinical response to TILADE Inhaler is evident and if the asthma is under good control, an attempt may be made to decrease concomitant medication usage gradually.

Proper inhalational technique is essential (see Patient Instruction leaflet).

Patients should be advised that the optimal effect of TILADE therapy depends upon its administration at regular intervals, even during symptom-free periods.

HOW SUPPLIED

TILADE Inhaler is available in 16.2 g canisters providing at least 104 metered inhalations. Available in single and double canister packs. Each pack is supplied with patient instructions and white plastic mouthpiece(s), one per canister, bearing the TILADE logo.

NDC 0585-0685-02   One 16.2 g Canister (104 Metered Inhalations)

NDC 0585-0685-04   Two 16.2 g Canisters (2 × 104 Metered Inhalations)

Store between 2°–30°C (36°–86°F). Do not freeze. Contents under pressure. Do not puncture, incinerate, place near sources of heat or use with other mouthpieces. Keep out of the reach of children.

Note: the indented statement below is required by the Federal government's Clean Air Act for all products containing or manufactured with chlorofluorocarbons (CFC's).

> WARNING: Contains CFC-12 and CFC-114, substances which harm public health and environment by destroying ozone in the upper atmosphere.

A notice similar to the above WARNING has been placed in the "Patient Instructions for Use" portion of this package circular pursuant to EPA regulations.

CAUTION: Federal law prohibits dispensing without prescription.

ADVERSE EVENT (AE)	% Experiencing AE		% Withdrawing	
	Tilade (n=2042)	Placebo (n=1875)	Tilade	Placebo
Special Senses				
Unpleasant Taste*	12.6%	3.6%	2.1%	0.4%
Respiratory System Disorders				
Coughing	7.0	7.2	1.4	1.4
Pharyngitis	5.7	5.0	0.6	0.5
Rhinitis*	4.6	3.0	0.1	0.1
Upper Respiratory Tract Infection*	3.9	2.4	0.1	0.1
Sputum Increased	1.7	1.4	0.1	0.2
Bronchitis	1.2	1.3	0.1	0.1
Dyspnea	2.8	3.8	0.9	1.3
Bronchospasm**	5.4	8.2	1.5	2.3
Gastro-Intestinal Tract				
Nausea*	4.0	2.1	1.3	0.7
Vomiting*	1.7	0.9	0.2	0.4
Dyspepsia*	1.3	0.6	0.1	0.1
Mouth Dry	1.0	0.9	0.1	0.2
Diarrhea	0.9	0.9	0.1	0.0
Abdominal Pain*	1.2	0.5	0.2	0.1
Central and Peripheral Nervous System				
Dizziness	0.9	1.2	0.1	0.2
Dysphonia	1.0	0.6	0.1	0.1
Body as a Whole				
Headache	6.0	4.7	0.5	0.3
Chest Pain	4.0	3.9	0.9	0.6
Fatigue	1.1	0.7	0.2	0.1
Resistance Mechanism Disorders				
Infection Viral	2.4	3.4	0.1	0.1

Table includes data from double-bind group comparative studies at four times per day dosing.
* Statistically significant (p ≤ 0.05) higher frequency of events on TILADE.
** Statistically significant (p ≤ 0.05) higher frequency of events on Placebo.

FISONS Pharmaceuticals
Fisons Corporation
Rochester, NY 14623 U.S.A.
Made in England
TILADE and FISONS are Registered
Trademarks of Fisons plc.   Rev. 10/94
©1994, Fisons Corporation   RF302E

Shown in Product Identification Guide, page 330

Richwood Pharmaceutical Company Inc.
7900 TANNER'S GATE DRIVE, SUITE 200 FLORENCE, KENTUCKY 41042

Direct Inquiries to:
(606) 282-2100
FAX: (606) 282-2103

ACUPRIN 81™ Adult Low Dose Aspirin.   OTC
Contains 81 mg of enteric coated aspirin.

81 mg 120's NDC 58521-081-01
81 mg 500's NDC 58521-081-05

ADDERALL® TABLETS   C Ⅱ ℞

> AMPHETAMINES HAVE A HIGH POTENTIAL FOR ABUSE. ADMINISTRATION OF AMPHETAMINES FOR PROLONGED PERIODS OF TIME MAY LEAD TO DRUG DEPENDENCE AND MUST BE AVOIDED. PARTICULAR ATTENTION SHOULD BE PAID TO THE POSSIBILITY OF SUBJECTS OBTAINING AMPHETAMINES FOR NON-THERAPEUTIC USE OR DISTRIBUTION TO OTHERS, AND THE DRUGS SHOULD BE PRESCRIBED OR DISPENSED SPARINGLY.

DESCRIPTION

A single entity amphetamine product combining the neutral sulfate salts of dextroamphetamine and amphetamine, with the dextro isomer of amphetamine saccharate and d, l-amphetamine aspartate.

EACH TABLET CONTAINS:	10 mg	.20 mg
Dextroamphetamine Saccharate	2.5 mg	.5 mg
Amphetamine Aspartate	2.5 mg	.5 mg
Dextroamphetamine Sulfate USP	2.5 mg	.5 mg
Amphetamine Sulfate USP	2.5 mg	.5 mg
Total amphetamine base equivalence	6.3 mg	.12.6 mg

Continued on next page

Richwood Pharmaceutical—Cont.

Inactive Ingredients: sucrose, lactose, corn starch, acacia and magnesium stearate.

Colors: ADDERALL 10 mg contains FD & C Blue #1
ADDERALL 20 mg contains FD & C Yellow #6 as a color additive

CLINICAL PHARMACOLOGY

Amphetamines are non-catecholamine sympathomimetic amines with CNS stimulant activity. Peripheral actions include elevation of systolic and diastolic blood pressures and weak bronchodilator and respiratory stimulant action.

There is neither specific evidence which clearly establishes the mechanism whereby amphetamine produces mental and behavioral effects in children, nor conclusive evidence regarding how these effects relate to the condition of the central nervous system.

INDICATIONS

Attention Deficit Disorder with Hyperactivity: Adderall is indicated as an integral part of a total treatment program which typically includes other remedial measures (psychological, educational, social) for a stabilizing effect in children with behavioral syndrome characterized by the following group of developmentally inappropriate symptoms: moderate to severe distractibility, short attention span, hyperactivity, emotional lability, and impulsivity. The diagnosis of this syndrome should not be made with finality when these symptoms are only of comparatively recent origin. Nonlocalizing (soft) neurological signs, learning disability and abnormal EEG may or may not be present, and a diagnosis of central nervous system dysfunction may or may not be warranted.

In Narcolepsy

CONTRAINDICATIONS

Advanced arteriosclerosis, symptomatic cardiovascular disease, moderate to severe hypertension, hyperthyroidism, known hypersensitivity or idiosyncrasy to the sympathomimetic amines, glaucoma.

Agitated states.

Patients with a history of drug abuse.

During or within 14 days following the administration of monoamine oxidase inhibitors (hypertensive crises may result).

WARNINGS

When tolerance to the "anorectic" effect develops, the recommended dose should not be exceeded in an attempt to increase the effect; rather, the drug should be discontinued. Clinical experience suggests that in psychotic children, administration of amphetamine may exacerbate symptoms of behavior disturbance and thought disorder. Data are inadequate to determine whether chronic administration of amphetamine may be associated with growth inhibition; therefore, growth should be monitored during treatment.

Usage in Nursing Mothers: Amphetamines are excreted in human milk. Mothers taking amphetamines should be advised to refrain from nursing.

PRECAUTIONS

General: Caution is to be exercised in prescribing amphetamines for patients with even mild hypertension.

The least amount feasible should be prescribed or dispensed at one time in order to minimize the possibility of overdosage.

Information for Patients: Amphetamines may impair the ability of the patient to engage in potentially hazardous activities such as operating machinery or vehicles; the patient should therefore be cautioned accordingly.

Drug Interactions: *Acidifying agents*—Gastrointestinal acidifying agents (guanethidine, reserpine, glutamic acid HCl, ascorbic acid, fruit juices, etc.) lower absorption of amphetamines.

Urinary acidifying agents—(ammonium chloride, sodium acid phosphate, etc.) Increase the concentration of the ionized species of the amphetamine molecule, thereby increasing urinary excretion. Both groups of agents lower blood levels and efficacy of amphetamines.

Adrenergic blockers—Adrenergic blockers are inhibited by amphetamines.

Alkalinizing agents—Gastrointestinal alkalinizing agents (sodium bicarbonate, etc.) increase absorption of amphetamines. Urinary alkalinizing agents (acetazolamide, some thiazides) increase the concentration of the non-ionized species of the amphetamine molecule, thereby decreasing urinary excretion. Both groups of agents increase blood levels and therefore potentiate the actions of amphetamines.

Antidepressants, tricyclic—Amphetamines may enhance the activity of tricyclic or sympathomimetic agents; d-amphetamine with desipramine or protriptyline and possibly other tricyclics cause striking and sustained increases in the concentration of d-amphetamine in the brain; cardiovascular effects can be potentiated.

MAO inhibitors—MAOI antidepressants, as well as a metabolite of furazolidone, slow amphetamine metabolism. This slowing potentiates amphetamines, increasing their effect on the release of norepinephrine and other monoamines from adrenergic nerve endings; this can cause headaches and other signs of hypertensive crisis. A variety of neurological toxic effects and malignant hyperpyrexia can occur, sometimes with fatal results.

Antihistamines—Amphetamines may counteract the sedative effect of antihistamines.

Antihypertensives—Amphetamines may antagonize the hypotensive effects of antihypertensives.

Chlorpromazine—Chlorpromazine blocks dopamine and norepinephrine reuptake, thus inhibiting the central stimulant effects of amphetamines, and can be used to treat amphetamine poisoning.

Ethosuximide—Amphetamines may delay intestinal absorption of ethosuximide.

Haloperidol—Haloperidol blocks dopamine and norepinephrine reuptake, thus inhibiting the central stimulant effects of amphetamines.

Lithium carbonate—The antiobesity and stimulatory effects of amphetamines may be inhibited by lithium carbonate.

Meperidine—Amphetamines potentiate the analgesic effect of meperidine.

Methenamine therapy—Urinary excretion of amphetamines is increased, and efficacy is reduced, by acidifying agents used in methenamine therapy.

Norepinephrine—Amphetamines enhance the adrenergic effect of norepinephrine.

Phenobarbital—Amphetamines may delay intestinal absorption of phenobarbital; co-administration of phenobarbital may produce a synergistic anticonvulsant action.

Phenytoin—Amphetamines may delay intestinal absorption of phenytoin; co-administration of phenytoin may produce a synergistic anticonvulsant action.

Propoxyphene—In cases of propoxyphene overdosage, amphetamine CNS stimulation is potentiated and fatal convulsions can occur.

Veratrum alkaloids—Amphetamines inhibit the hypotensive effect of veratrum alkaloids.

Drug/Laboratory Test Interactions:

- Amphetamines can cause a significant elevation in plasma corticosteroid levels. This increase is greatest in the evening.
- Amphetamines may interfere with urinary steroid determinations.

Carcinogenesis/Mutagenesis: Mutagenicity studies and long-term studies in animals to determine the carcinogenic potential of Amphetamine, have not been performed.

Pregnancy—Teratogenic Effects: Pregnancy Category C. Amphetamine has been shown to have embryotoxic and teratogenic effects when administered to A/Jax mice and C57BL mice in doses approximately 41 times the maximum human dose. Embryotoxic effects were not seen in New Zealand white rabbits given the drug in doses 7 times the human dose nor in rats given 12.5 times the maximum human dose. While there are no adequate and well-controlled studies in pregnant women, there has been one report of severe congenital bony deformity, tracheoesophageal fistula, and anal atresia (vater association) in a baby born to a woman who took dextroamphetamine sulfate with lovastatin during the first trimester of pregnancy. Amphetamines should be used during pregnancy only if the potential benefit justifies the potential risk to the fetus.

Nonteratogenic Effects: Infants born to mothers dependent on amphetamines have an increased risk of premature delivery and low birth weight. Also, these infants may experience symptoms of withdrawal as demonstrated by dysphoria, including agitation, and significant lassitude.

Pediatric Use: Long-term effects of amphetamines in children have not been well established. Amphetamines are not recommended for use in children under 3 years of age with Attention Deficit Disorder with Hyperactivity described under INDICATIONS AND USAGE.

Amphetamines have been reported to exacerbate motor and phonic tics and Tourette's syndrome. Therefore, clinical evaluation for tics and Tourette's syndrome in children and their families should precede use of stimulant medications.

Drug treatment is not indicated in all cases of Attention Deficit Disorder with Hyperactivity and should be considered only in light of the complete history and evaluation of the child. The decision to prescribe amphetamines should depend on the physician's assessment of the chronicity and severity of the child's symptoms and their appropriateness for his/her age. Prescription should not depend solely on the presence of one or more of the behavioral characteristics. When these symptoms are associated with acute stress reactions, treatment with amphetamines is usually not indicated.

ADVERSE REACTIONS

Cardiovascular: Palpitations, tachycardia, elevation of blood pressure. There have been isolated reports of cardiomyopathy associated with chronic amphetamine use.

Central Nervous System: Psychotic episodes at recommended doses (rare), overstimulation, restlessness, dizziness, insomnia, euphoria, dyskinesia, dysphoria, tremor, headache, exacerbation of motor and phonic tics and Tourette's syndrome.

Gastrointestinal: Dryness of the mouth, unpleasant taste, diarrhea, constipation, other gastrointestinal disturbances. Anorexia and weight loss may occur as undesirable effects when amphetamines are used for other than the anorectic effect.

Allergic: Urticaria.

Endocrine: Impotence, changes in libido.

DRUG ABUSE AND DEPENDENCE

Dextroamphetamine sulfate is a Schedule II controlled substance.

Amphetamines have been extensively abused. Tolerance, extreme psychological dependence, and severe social disability have occurred. There are reports of patients who have increased the dosage to many times that recommended. Abrupt cessation following prolonged high dosage administration results in extreme fatigue and mental depression; changes are also noted on the sleep EEG. Manifestations of chronic intoxication with amphetamines include severe dermatoses, marked insomnia, irritability, hyperactivity, and personality changes. The most severe manifestation of chronic intoxication is psychosis, often clinically indistinguishable from schizophrenia. This is rare with oral amphetamines.

OVERDOSAGE

Individual patient response to amphetamines varies widely. While toxic symptoms occasionally occur as an idiosyncrasy at doses as low as 2 mg, they are rare with doses of less than 15 mg; 30 mg can produce severe reactions, yet doses of 400 to 500 mg are not necessarily fatal.

In rats, the oral LD50 of dextroamphetamine sulfate is 96.8 mg/kg.

Symptoms: Manifestations of acute overdosage with amphetamines include restlessness, tremor, hyperreflexia, rapid respiration, confusion, assaultiveness, hallucinations, panic states, hyperpyrexia and rhabdomolysis.

Fatigue and depression usually follow the central stimulation.

Cardiovascular effects include arrhythmias, hypertension or hypotension and circulatory collapse.

Gastrointestinal symptoms include nausea, vomiting, diarrhea, and abdominal cramps. Fatal poisoning is usually preceded by convulsions and coma.

Treatment: Consult with a Certified Poison Control Center for up to date guidance and advice. Management of acute amphetamine intoxication is largely symptomatic and includes gastric lavage, administration of activated charcoal, administration of a cathartic and sedation. Experience with hemodialysis or peritoneal dialysis is inadequate to permit recommendation in this regard. Acidification of the urine increases amphetamine excretion, but is believed to increase risk of acute renal failure if myoglobinuria is present. If acute, severe hypertension complicates amphetamine overdosage, administration of intravenous phentolamine (Regitine®, CIBA) has been suggested. However, a gradual drop in blood pressure will usually result when sufficient sedation has been achieved. Chlorpromazine antagonizes the central stimulant effects of amphetamines and can be used to treat amphetamine intoxication.

DOSAGE AND ADMINISTRATION

Regardless of indication, amphetamines should be administered at the lowest effective dosage and dosage should be individually adjusted. Late evening doses should be avoided because of the resulting insomnia.

Attention Deficit Disorder with Hyperactivity: Not recommended for children under 3 years of age. In children from 3 to 5 years of age, start with 2.5 mg daily; daily dosage may be raised in increments of 2.5 mg at weekly intervals until optimal response is obtained.

In children 6 years of age and older, start with 5 mg once or twice daily; daily dosage may be raised in increments of 5 mg at weekly intervals until optimal response is obtained. Only in rare cases will it be necessary to exceed a total of 40 mg per day. Give first dose on awakening; additional doses (1 or 2) at intervals of 4 to 6 hours.

Where possible, drug administration should be interrupted occasionally to determine if there is a recurrence of behavioral symptoms sufficient to require continued therapy.

Narcolepsy: Usual dose 5 mg to 60 mg per day in divided doses, depending on the individual patient response.

Narcolepsy seldom occurs in children under 12 years of age; however, when it does, dextroamphetamine sulfate, may be used. The suggested initial dose for patients aged 6–12 is 5 mg daily; daily dose may be raised in increments of 5 mg at weekly intervals until optimal response is obtained. In patients 12 years of age and older, start with 10 mg daily; daily dosage may be raised in increments of 10 mg at weekly intervals until optimal response is obtained. If bothersome adverse reactions appear (e.g., insomnia or anorexia), dosage should be reduced. Give first dose on awakening; additional doses (1 or 2) at intervals of 4 to 6 hours.

HOW SUPPLIED

ADDERALL® 10 mg: Blue double-scored tablet, debossed "AD" on one side and "10" on the other side (NDC 58521-032-01)
ADDERALL® 20 mg: Orange double-scored tablet, debossed "AD" on one side and "20" on the other side (NDC 58521-033-01)
In bottles of 100 tablets.
Dispense in a tight, light-resistant container as defined in the U.S.P.
Store at controlled room temperature 15°-30°C (59°-86°F).
CAUTION: Federal law prohibits dispensing without prescription.
Richwood Pharmaceutical Company Inc.
Florence, KY 41042

MG #10185 Revised: May 1996

Shown in Product Identification Guide, page 331

BELLATAL™ ℞

DESCRIPTION

Each scored, white, compressed, oral tablet contains:

Phenobarbital USP	16.2 mg
Warning: May be habit forming.	
From:	
Hyoscyamine Sulfate USP	0.1037 mg
Atropine Sulfate USP	0.0194 mg
Scopolamine Hydrobromide USP	0.0065 mg

HOW SUPPLIED

Scored, white, compressed oral tablets debossed.
0478/5477
Bottle of 100 NDC 58521-162-01
Dispense in a tight container as defined in the USP.
RICHWOOD PHARMACEUTICAL COMPANY INC.
FLORENCE, KY 41042

MG#10179

DEXTROSTAT™ Ⓒ ℞

Dextroamphetamine Sulfate Tablets, USP

WARNING

AMPHETAMINES HAVE A HIGH POTENTIAL FOR ABUSE, ADMINISTRATION OF AMPHETAMINES FOR PROLONGED PERIODS OF TIME MAY LEAD TO DRUG DEPENDENCE AND MUST BE AVOIDED. PARTICULAR ATTENTION SHOULD BE PAID TO THE POSSIBILITY OF SUBJECTS OBTAINING AMPHETAMINES FOR NONTHERAPEUTIC USE OR DISTRIBUTION TO OTHERS, AND THE DRUGS SHOULD BE PRESCRIBED OR DISPENSED SPARINGLY.

DESCRIPTION

DextroStat™ (dextroamphetamine sulfate) is the dextro isomer of the compound *d,l*-amphetamine sulfate, a sympathomimetic amine of the amphetamine group. Chemically, dextroamphetamine is *d*-alpha-methylphenethlamine, and is present in all forms of DextroStat™ as the neutral sulfate. It has a chemical formula of $(C_9H_{13}N)_2 \cdot H_2SO_4$ and a molecular weight of 368.50.
Structural Formula:

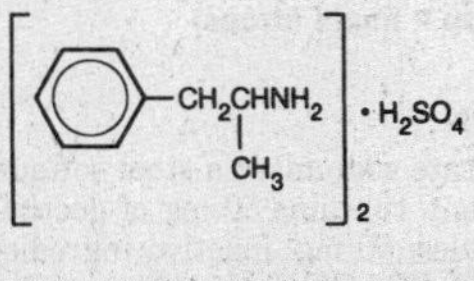

Each round, yellow, scored tablet contains dextroamphetamine sulfate USP; and is debossed as follows: 5 mg—debossed "RP" on one side and "51" on the other side; 10 mg—debossed "RP" on one side and "52" on the other side. Inactive ingredients consist of acacia, corn starch, lactose monohydrate, magnesium stearate, sucrose, 10 mg tablet contains sodium starch glycolate, 5 mg and 10 mg tablets contain FD&C Yellow #5 (tartrazine).

CLINICAL PHARMACOLOGY

Amphetamines are non-catecholamine, sympathomimetic amines with CNS stimulant activity. Peripheral actions include elevations of systolic and diastolic blood pressures and weak bronchodilator and respiratory stimulant action.
There is neither specific evidence which clearly establishes the mechanism whereby amphetamines produce mental and behavioral effects in children, nor conclusive evidence regarding how these effects relate to the condition of the central nervous system.

Pharmacokinetics
The single ingestion of two 5 mg tablets by healthy volunteers produced an average peak dextroamphetamine blood level of 29.2 ng/mL at 2 hours post-administration. The average half-life was 10.25 hours. The average urinary recovery was 45% in 48 hours.

INDICATIONS AND USAGE

DextroStat™ (dextroamphetamine sulfate is indicated:

1. **In Narcolepsy.**
2. **In Attention Deficit Disorder with Hyperactivity,** as an integral part of a total treatment program which typically includes other remedial measures (psychological, educational, social) for a stabilizing effect in children with a behavioral syndrome characterized by the following group of developmentally inappropriate symptoms: moderate to severe distractibility, short attention span, hyperactivity, emotional lability, and impulsivity, The diagnosis of this syndrome should not be made with finality when these symptoms are only of comparatively recent origin. Nonlocalizing (soft) neurological signs, learning disability and abnormal EEG may or may not be present, and a diagnosis of central nervous system dysfunction may or may not be warranted.

CONTRAINDICATIONS

Advanced arteriosclerosis, symptomatic cardiovascular disease, moderate to severe hypertension, hyperthyroidism, known hypersensitivity or idiosyncrasy to the sympathomimetic amines, glaucoma.
Agitated states.
Patients with a history of drug abuse.
During or within 14 days following the administration of monoamine oxidase inhibitors (hypertensive crises may result).

PRECAUTIONS

General: Caution is to be exercised in prescribing amphetmaines for patients with even mild hypertension.
The least amount feasible should be prescribd or dispensed at one time in order to minimize the possibility of overdosage.
These products contain FD&C Yellow No. 5 (tartrazine), which may cause allergic-type reactions (including bronchial asthma) in certain susceptible individuals. Although the overall incidence of FD&C Yellow No. 5 (tartrazine) sensitivity in the general population is low, it is frequently seen in patients who also have aspirin hypersensitivity.
Information for Patients: Amphetamines may impair the ability of the patient to engage in potentially hazardous activities such as operating machinery or vehicles; the patient should therefore be cautioned accordingly.
Drug Interactions
Acidifying agents—Gastrointestinal acidifying agents (guanethidine, reserpine, glutaminc acid HCl, ascorbic acid, fruit juices, etc.) lower absorption of amphetamines. Urinary acidifying agents (ammonium chloride, sodium acid phosphate, etc.) increase the concentration of the ionized species of the amphetamine molecule, thereby increasing urinary excretion. Both groups of agents lower blood levels and efficacy of amphetamines.
Adrenergic blockers—Adrenergic blockers are inhibited by amphetamines.
Alkalinizing agents—Gastrointestinal alkalinizing agents (sodium bicarbonate, etc.) increase absorption of amphetamines. Urinary alkalinizing agents (acetazolamide, some thiazides) increase the concentration of the non-ionized species of the amphetamine molecule, thereby decreasing urinary excretion. Both groups of agents increase blood levels and therefore potentiate the actions of amphetamines.
Antidepressants, tricyclic—Amphetamines may enhance the activity of tricyclic or sympathomimetic agents; *d*-amphetamine with desipramine or protriptyline and possibly other tricyclics cause striking and sustained increases in the concentration of *d*-amphetamine in the brain; cardiovascular effects can be potentiated.
MAO inhibitors—MAOI antidepressants, as well as a metabolite of furazolidone, slow amphetamine metabolism. This slowing potentiates amphetamines, increasing their effect on the release of norepinephrine and other monoamines from adrenergic nerve endings; this can cause headaches and other signs of hypertensive crisis. A variety of neurological toxic effects and malignant hyperpyrexia can occur, sometimes with fatal results.
Antihistamines—Amphetamines may counteract the sedative effect of amphetamines.
Antihypertensives—Amphetamines may antagonize the hypotensive effects of antihypertensives.
Chlorpromazine—Chlorpromazine blocks dopamine and norepinephrine reuptake, thus inhibiting the central stimulant effects of amphetamines, and can be used to treat amphetamine poisoning.
Ethosuximide—Amphetamines may delay intestinal absorption of ethosuximide.
Haloperidol—Haloperidol blocks dopamine and norepinephrine reuptake, thus inhibiting the central stimulant effects of amphetamines.
Meperidine—Amphetamines potentiate the analgesic effect of meperidine.
Methenamine therapy—Urinary excretion of amphetamines is increased, and efficacy is reduced, by acidifying agents used in methenamine therapy.
Norepinephrine—Amphetamines enhance the adrenergic effect of norepinephrine.
Phenobarbital—Amphetamines may delay intestinal absorption of phenobarbital; co-administration of phenobarbital may produce a synergistic anticonvulsant action.
Phenytoin-Amphetamines may delay intestinal absorption of phenytoin; co-administration of phenytoin may produce a synergistic anticonvulsant action.
Propoxyphene—In cases of propoxyphene overdosage, amphetamine CNS stimulation is potentiated and fatal convulsions can occur.
Veratrum alkaloids—Amphetamines inhibit the hypotensive effect of veratrum alkaloids.
Drug/Laboratory Test
Interactions

- Amphetamines can cause a significant elevation in plasma corticosteroid levels. This increase is greatest in the evening.
- Amphetamines may interfere with urinary steroid determinations.

Carcinogenesis/Mutagenesis: Mutagenicity studies and long-term studies in animals to determine the carcinogenic potential of DextroStat™ (dextroamphetamine sulfate) have not been performed.
Pregnancy-Teratogenic Effects: Pregnancy Category C. Amphetamine has been shown to have embryotoxic and teratogenic effects when administered to A/Jax mice and C57BL mice in doses approximately 41 times the maximum human dose. Embryotoxic effects were not seen in New Zealand white rabbits given the drug in doses 7 times the human dose nor in rats given 12.5 times the maximum human dose. While there are no adequate and well-controlled studies in pregnant women, there has been one report of severe congenital bony deformity, tracheoesophageal fistula, and anal atresia (Vater association) in a baby born to a woman who took dextroamphetamine sulfate with lovastatin during the first trimester of pregnancy. Amphetamines should be used during pregnancy only if the potential benefit justifies the potential risk to the fetus.
Nonteratogenic Effects: Infants born to mothers dependent on amphetamines have an increased risk of premature delivery and low birth weight. Also, these infants may experience symptoms of withdrawal as demonstrated by dysphoria, including agitation, and significant lassitude.
Nursing Mothers: Amphetamines are excreted in human milk. Mothers taking amphetamines should be advised to refrain from nursing.
Pediatric Use: Long-term effects of amphetamines in pediatric patients have not been well established.
Amphetamines are not recommended for use in children under 3 years of age with Attention Deficit Disorder with Hyperactivity described under INDICATIONS AND USAGE.
Clinical experience suggests that in psychotic pediatric patients, administration of amphetamines may exacerbate symptoms of behavior disturbance and thought disorder.
Amphetamines have been reported to exacerbate motor and phonic tics and Tourette's syndrome. Therefore, clinical evaluation for tics and Tourette's syndrome in pediatric patients and their families should precede use of stimulant medications.
Data are inadequate to determine whether chronic administration of amphetamines may be associated with growth inhibition; therefore, growth should be monitored during treatment.
Drug treatment is not indicated in all cases of Attention Deficit Disorder with Hyperactivity and should be considered only in light of the complete history and evaluation of the pediatric patient. The decision to prescribe amphetamines should depend on the physician's assessment of the chronicity and severity of the pediatric patient's symptoms and their appropriateness for his/her age.
Prescription should not depend solely on the presence of one or more of the behavioral characteristics.
When these symptoms are associated with acute stress reactions, treatment with amphetamines is usually not indicated.

ADVERSE REACTIONS

Cardiovascular: Palpitations, tachycardia, elevation of blood pressure. There have been isolated reports of cardioimyopathy associated with chronic amphetamine use.
Central Nervous System:
Psychotic episodes at recommended doses (rare), overstimulation, restlessness, dizziness, insomnia, euphoria, dyskinesia, dysphoria, tremor, headache, exacerbation of motor and phonic tics and Tourette's syndrome.

Continued on next page

Richwood Pharmaceutical—Cont.

Gastrointestinal: Dryness of the mouth, unpleasant taste, diarrhea, constipation, other gastrointestinal disturbances. Anorexia and weight loss may occur as undesirable effects.
Allergic: Urticaria.
Endocrine: Impotence, changes in libido.

DRUG ABUSE AND DEPENDENCE

Dextroamphetamine sulfate is a Schedule II controlled substance.

Amphetamines have been extensively abused. Tolerance, extreme psychological dependence and severe social disability have occurred. There are reports of patients who have increased the dosage to many times that recommended. Abrupt cessation following prolonged high dosage administration results in extreme fatigue and mental depression; changes are also noted on the sleep EEG.

Manifestation of chronic intoxication with amphetamines include severe dermatoses, marked insomnia, irritability, hyperactivity and personality changes. The most severe manifestation of chronic intoxication is psychosis, often clinically indistinguishable from schizophrenia. This is rare with oral amphetamines.

OVERDOSAGE

Individual patient response to amphetamines varies widely. While toxic symptoms occasionally occur as an idiosyncrasy at doses as low as 2 mg, they are rare with doses of less than 15 mg; 30 mg can produce severe reactions, yet doses of 400 to 500 mg are not necessarily fatal.

In rats, the oral LD_{50} of dextroamphetamine sulfate is 96.8 mg/kg.

Manifestations of acute overdosage with amphetamines include restlessness, tremor, hyperreflexia, rhabdomyolysis, rapid respiration, hyperpyrexia, confusion, assultiveness, hallucinations, panic states.

Fatigue and depression usually follow the central stimulation.

Cardiovascular effects include arrhythmias, hypertension or hypotension and circulatory collapse. Gastrointestinal symptoms include nausea, vomiting, diarrhea and abdominal cramps. Fatal poisoning is usually preceded by convulsions and coma.

TREATMENT—Management of acute amphetamine intoxication is largely symptomatic and includes gastric lavage and sedation with a barbiturate. Experience with hemodialysis or peritoneal dialysis is inadequate to permit recommendation in this regard. Acidification of the urine increases amphetamine excretion. If acute, severe hypertension complicates amphetamine overdosage, administration of intravenous phentolamine (Regitine®, CIBA) has been suggested. However, a gradual drop in blood pressure will usually result when sufficient sedation has been achieved.

Chlorpromazine antagonizes the central stimulant effects of amphetamines and can be used to treat amphetamine intoxication.

DOSAGE AND ADMINISTRATION

Amphetamines should be administered at the lowest effective dosage and dosage should be individually adjusted. Late evening doses should be avoided because of the resulting insomnia.

Narcolepsy: Usual dose 5 to 60 mg per day in divided doses, depending on the individual patient response.

Narcolepsy seldom occurs in children under 12 years of age; however, when it does, DextroStat™ (dextroamphetamine sulfate) may be used. The suggested initial dose for patients aged 6 to 12 is 5 mg daily; daily dose may be raised in increments of 5 mg at weekly intervals until optimal response is obtained. In patients 12 years of age and older, start with 10 mg daily; daily dosage may be raised in increments of 10 mg at weekly intervals until optimal response is obtained. If bothersome adverse reactions appear (e.g., insomnia or anorexia), disage should be reduced. Give first dose on awakening; additional doses (1 or 2) at intervals of 4 to 6 hours.

Attention Deficit Disorder with Hyperactivity: Not recommended for children under 3 years of age.

In children from 3 to 5 years of age, start with 2.5 mg daily; daily dosage may be raised in increments of 2.5 mg at weekly intervals until optimal response is obtained.

In children 6 years of age and older, start with 5 mg once or twice daily; daily dosage may be raised in increments of 5 mg at weekly intervals until optimal response is obtained. Only in rare cases will it be necessary to exceed a total of 40 mg per day.

Give first dose on awakening; additional doses (1 or 2) at intervals of 4 to 6 hours.

When possible, drug administration should be interrupted occasionally to determine if there is a recurrence of behavioral symptoms sufficient to require continued therapy.

HOW SUPPLIED

DextroStat™, (dextroamphetamine sulfate) Tablets are available as follows:

5 mg Yellow, Round, Scored Tablet debossed "RP" on one side and "51" on the other side.

NDC #: 58521-451-01 for 100s
       58521-451-05 for 500s
       58521-451-10 for 1000s

10 mg Yellow, Round, Double-Scored Tablet debossed "RP" on one side and "52" on the other side.

NDC #: 58521-452-01 for 100s
       58521-452-05 for 500s

Dispense in a tight container as defined in the USP. Store at controlled room temperature 15°–30°C (59°–86°F).
DEA Order Form Required.
Richwood Pharmaceutical Company Inc.
Florence, KY 41042
MG #9245   Rev 7/96
Shown in Product Identification Guide, page 331

DOSAFLEX®   OTC
Senna Liquid Concentrate
Stimulant Laxative
Pleasant tasting syrup

INDICATIONS

For the relief of occasional constipation or irregularity. This product generally produces bowel movement in 6 to 12 hours.
RECOMMENDED DOSE (preferably at bedtime)
CHILDREN: 5–15 years: 1 to 2 teaspoonfuls (maximum 2 tsp. twice in a day): 1–5 years: $^{1}/_{2}$ to 1 teaspoonful (maximum 1 tsp. twice in a day): 1 month to 1 year: $^{1}/_{4}$ to $^{1}/_{2}$ teaspoonful (maximum $^{1}/_{2}$ tsp. twice in a day). **ADULTS:** 2 to 3 teaspoonfuls (maximum 3 tsp. twice in a day). See important dosage information on side. Alcohol 7% by volume. **Diabetic Patients Note:** Consult your physician concerning the sugar content of DOSAFLEX™ Liquid (approximately 3.5 grams per teaspoonful).

HOW SUPPLIED

237 mL (8 oz) Bottle
NDC # 58521-086-80

MS/L™   Ⓒ Ⓡ
MORPHINE SULFATE
IMMEDIATE RELEASE ORAL SOLUTION
(WARNING: May be habit forming)

DESCRIPTION

Each 5 mL of Morphine Sulfate Oral Solution contains:
Morphine Sulfate USP .... 10 mg

HOW SUPPLIED

Morphine Sulfate Immediate Release Oral Solution (Unflavored)
10 mg per 5 mL
NDC 58521-110-50: Bottles of 500 mL

MS/L CONCENTRATE™   Ⓒ Ⓡ
MORPHINE SULFATE IMMEDIATE RELEASE
CONCENTRATED ORAL SOLUTION
(WARNING: May be habit forming)

DESCRIPTION

Each 5mL of Morphine Sulfate immediate release concentrated oral solution contains:
Morphine Sulfate USP .... 100 mg

HOW SUPPLIED

Morphine Sulfate Immediate Release Concentrated Oral Solution
20 mg per mL
NDC 58521-120-58: Bottles of 120 mL with calibrated dropper.

MS/S™   Ⓒ Ⓡ
Rectal Morphine Sulfate Suppositories
(WARNING—May be habit forming)

DESCRIPTION

Suppositories contain 5, 10, 20, or 30 mg of morphine sulfate.

HOW SUPPLIED

MS/S Suppositories are individually sealed in unit dose packets of 12 suppositories per carton.

5 mg Pink carton	NDC 58521-005-12
10 mg Light blue carton	NDC 58521-010-12
20 mg Light green carton	NDC 58521-020-12
30 mg Purple carton	NDC 58521-030-12

OBY-CAP™   Ⓒ Ⓡ
PHENTERMINE HYDROCHLORIDE CAPSULES USP

DESCRIPTION

Phentermine hydrochloride is a white, odorless, hygroscopic, crystalline powder which is soluble in water and lower alcohols; slightly soluble in chloroform and insoluble in ether. OBY-CAP (Phentermine Hydrochloride Capsules, USP), for oral administration, contains 30 mg of phentermine hydrochloride (equivalent to 24 mg of phentermine base). Inactive Ingredients: Lactose, Starch and Talc.

HOW SUPPLIED

OBY-CAP 30 mg is available as Hard Gelatin Yellow Capsules #3 Imprinted RPC-69.
Bottle of 100 NDC 58521-333-01
Store at controlled room temperature 15°-30°C (59°-86°F).
Dispense in a tight container as defined in the USP.

Roberts Pharmaceutical Corp.
4 INDUSTRIAL WAY WEST
EATONTOWN, NJ 07724

Direct Inquiries to:
Customer Service
(908) 389-1182
(800) 828-2088
FAX: (908) 389-1014

For Medical Information Contact:
(800) 992-9306

CHERACOL®   Ⓒ
Expectorant
Cough Suppressant

DESCRIPTION

Cheracol cough syrup is an antitussive and expectorant formula for the temporary relief of coughs. Calms the cough control center and relieves coughing due to minor throat and bronchial irritation associated with a cold or inhaled irritants. Helps loosen phlegm and drain bronchial tubes to make coughs more productive. Each teaspoonful (5 mL) contains the following:
ACTIVE INGREDIENTS:
Codeine Phosphate .... 10 mg
(Warning—May be habit forming)
Guaifenesin .... 100 mg
Alcohol 4.75%

INACTIVE INGREDIENTS: benzoic acid, flavors, fragrances, fructose, glycerin, propylene glycol, FD&C Red No. 40, sodium chloride, sucrose, and purified water.

HOW SUPPLIED

2 FL OZ bottles (NDC 54092-402-60)
4 FL OZ bottles (NDC 54092-402-04)
16 FL OZ bottles (NDC 54092-402-16)
Store at controlled room temperature: 15°–30°C (59°–86°F).

COLACE®   OTC
[kōlās]
docusate sodium,
capsules ● syrup ● liquid (drops)

DESCRIPTION

Colace® (docusate sodium) is a stool softener.
Active Ingredient: contains 50 mg of docusate sodium.
Colace® Capsules, 50 mg, inactive ingredients: citric acid, D&C Red No. 33, FD&C Red No. 40, nonporcine gelatin, edible ink, polyethylene glycol, propylene glycol, and purified water.
Active Ingredient: contains 100 mg of docusate sodium.
Colace® Capsules, 100 mg, inactive ingredients: citric acid, D&C Red No. 33, FD&C Red No. 40, FD&C Yellow No. 6, nonporcine gelatin, edible ink, polyethylene glycol, propylene glycol, titanium dioxide, and purified water.
Active Ingredient: each mL contains 10 mg of docusate sodium.
Colace® Liquid, 1%, inactive ingredients: citric acid, D&C Red No. 33, methylparaben, poloxamer, polyethylene glycol, propylene glycol, propylparaben, sodium citrate, vanillin, and purified water.
Active Ingredient: each 5 mL contains 20 mg of docusate sodium.
Colace® Syrup, 20 mg/5 mL, inactive ingredients: alcohol (not more than 1%), citric acid, D&C Red No. 33, FD&C Red No. 40, flavor (natural), menthol, methylparaben, pepper-

mint oil, poloxamer, polyethylene glycol, propylparaben, sodium citrate, sucrose, and purified water.

ACTIONS AND USES

Colace®, a surface-active agent, helps to keep stools soft for easy, natural passage and is not a laxative, thus, not habit forming. Useful in constipation due to hard stools, in painful anorectal conditions, in cardiac and other conditions in which maximum ease of passage is desirable to avoid difficult or painful defecation, and when peristaltic stimulants are contraindicated.

Note: When peristaltic stimulation is needed due to inadequate bowel motility, see Peri-Colace® (laxative and stool softener).

CONTRAINDICATIONS

There are no known contraindications to Colace®.

WARNING

As with any drug, pregnant or nursing women should seek the advice of a health professional before using this product.

SIDE EFFECTS

The incidence of side effects—none of a serious nature—is exceedingly small. Bitter taste, throat irritation, and nausea (primarily associated with the use of the syrup and liquid) are the main side effects reported. Rash has occurred.

ADMINISTRATION AND DOSAGE

Orally—Suggested daily Dosage: *Adults and older children:* 50 to 200 mg *Children 6 to 12:* 40 to 120 mg *Children 3 to 6:* 20 to 60 mg. *Infants and children under 3:* 10 to 40 mg. The higher doses are recommended for initial therapy. Dosage should be adjusted to individual response. The effect on stools is usually apparent 1 to 3 days after the first dose. Colace® liquid or syrup must be given in a 6 oz. to 8 oz. glass of milk or fruit juice or in infant's formula to prevent throat irritation. *In enemas*—Add 5 to 10 mL Colace® liquid) to a retention or flushing enema.

HOW SUPPLIED

Colace® capsules, 50 mg
  NDC 54092-052-30 Bottles of 30
  NDC 54092-052-60 Bottles of 60
  NDC 54092-052-52 Cartons of 100
    single unit packs
Colace® capsules, 100 mg
  NDC 54092-053-30 Bottles of 30
  NDC 54092-053-60 Bottles of 60
  NDC 54092-053-02 Bottles of 250
  NDC 54092-053-10 Bottles of 1000
  NDC 54092-053-52 Cartons of 100
    single unit packs
Note: Colace® capsules should be stored at controlled room temperature (59°–86°F or 15°–30°C)
Colace® liquid, 1% solution; 10 mg/mL (with calibrated dropper)
  NDC 54092-414-16 Bottles of 16 fl oz
  NDC 54092-414-30 Bottles of 30 mL
Colace® syrup, 20 mg/5-mL teaspoon; contains not more than 1% alcohol
  NDC 54092-415-08 Bottles of 8 fl oz
  NDC 54092-415-16 Bottles of 16 fl oz
Manufactured for:
Roberts Laboratories Inc., a subsidiary of
ROBERTS PHARMACEUTICAL CORPORATION
Eatontown, NJ 07724 USA

COLACE®-T   OTC
[*kō lās*]
docusate sodium, capsules, 50 mg
Stool Softener Travel Size

> COLACE® a laxative for the prevention of dry, hard stools. By drawing water into the stool, COLACE® makes passage easier and more comfortable.

DESCRIPTION

Active Ingredient: Each capsule contains 50 mg of docusate sodium.
Inactive Ingredients: Citric acid, D&C Red No. 33, FD&C Red No. 40, non-porcine gelatin, edible ink, polyethylene glycol, propylene glycol, and purified water.
Usual Daily Dose: Adults and Children 12 years and older: 1 to 6 capsules; **Children 6 to 12 years old:** 1 to 3 capsules. The highest dose should be taken until the first bowel movement; thereafter, a lower dose should be taken for maintenance. The effect of COLACE® on the stools may not be apparent until 1 to 3 days after the first oral dose.

WARNING

As with any drug, pregnant or nursing women should seek the advice of a health professional before using this product.

Keep this and all medication out of the reach of children. Store at or below 30°C (86°F). Protect from freezing.

HOW SUPPLIED

10 CAPSULES
Manufactured for Roberts Laboratories Inc., a subsidiary of
ROBERTS PHARMACEUTICAL CORP., Eatontown, NJ 07724, USA
by R.P. Scherer, St. Petersburg, FL 33716
Copyright© 1996 Roberts Laboratories Inc., Made in USA
052 1104 001   1/96
*Among stool softeners

COLACE®-T   OTC
[*kō lās*]
docusate sodium capsules, 100 mg
Stool Softener Travel Size

> COLACE® a laxative for the prevention of dry, hard stools. By drawing water into the stool, COLACE® makes passage easier and more comfortable.

DESCRIPTION

Active Ingredient: Each capsule contains 100 mg of docusate sodium.
Inactive Ingredients: Citric acid, D&C Red No. 33, FD&C Red No. 40, FD&C Yellow No. 6, non-porcine gelatin, edible ink, polyethylene glycol, propylene glycol, titanium dioxide, and purified water.
Usual Daily Dose: Adults and Children 12 years and older: 1 to 3 capsules; **Children 6 to 12 years old:** 1 capsule. The highest dose should be taken until the first bowel movement; thereafter, a lower dose should be taken for maintenance. The effect of COLACE® on the stools may not be apparent until 1 to 3 days after the first oral dose.

WARNING

As with any drug, pregnant or nursing women should seek the advice of a health professional before using this product.
Keep this and all medication out of the reach of children. Store at or below 30°C (86°F). Protect from freezing.

HOW SUPPLIED

10 CAPSULES
Manufactured for Roberts Laboratories Inc., a subsidiary of
ROBERTS PHARMACEUTICAL CORP., Eatontown, NJ 07724, USA
by R.P. Scherer, St. Petersburg, FL 33716
Copyright© 1996 Roberts Laboratories Inc., Made in USA
053 1104 001   1/96
*Among stool softeners

COLACE MICROENEMA   OTC
[*kō lās*]
(docusate sodium)
(for rectal use only)

DESCRIPTION

Active ingredient: Each 5 mL contains 200 mg of docusate sodium.
Inactive ingredients: Citric acid, sodium benzoate, hydroxypropyl methylcellulose, apricot kernel oil PEG-8 esters. PEG-6 and PEG-32 and glycol stearate, glycerin 96%, and purified water.
Indications: For relief of occasional constipation (irregularity).
Directions for use: Adults and children 3 years of age and older: Express a drop of the mixture to lubricate the tip if necessary. Slowly insert the full length (half length for children 3 to 12 years old) of the nozzle into the rectum. Squeeze out the entire contents of the tube. Remove the nozzle completely before releasing grip on the tube, otherwise the contents may flow back into the tube.
Do not use in children under 3 years of age, except under the advise of a physician.
This product generally produces bowel movement in 2 to 15 minutes.

WARNINGS

Do not use laxative products when abdominal pain, nausea, or vomiting are present, unless directed by a doctor. If you have noticed a sudden change in bowel habits that persists over a period of 2 weeks, consult a doctor before using a laxative. Laxative products should not be used for a period longer than 1 week unless directed by a doctor. Rectal bleeding or failure to have a bowel movement after use of a laxative may indicate a serious condition. Discontinue use and consult your doctor.
Keep this and all medication out of the reach of children. Store from 15°C to 30°C.

HOW SUPPLIED

200 mg
3 × 5 mL Microenemas
NDC 54092-491-70
Manufactured for
Roberts Laboratories Inc., a subsidiary of
ROBERTS PHARMACEUTICAL CORP.
Eatontown, NJ 07724, USA
Copyright© 1995 Roberts Laboratories Inc.
491 7004 001   10/95

COMHIST® LA   ℞
[*kŏm 'hist*]
COMHIST®   ℞
(chlorpheniramine maleate/
phenyltoloxamine citrate/phenylephrine hydrochloride)

ACTIVE INGREDIENTS

Each **Comhist®** yellow scored tablet for oral administration contains
chlorpheniramine maleate .... 2 mg
phenyltoloxamine citrate .... 25 mg
phenylephrine hydrochloride .... 10 mg

ACTIVE INGREDIENTS

Each **COMHIST® LA** yellow and clear extended-release capsule for oral administration contains:
chlorpheniramine maleate .... 4 mg
phenyltoloxamine citrate .... 50 mg
phenylephrine hydrochloride .... 20 mg
in a special base to provide a prolonged therapeutic effect. This product contains ingredients of the following therapeutic classes: antihistamine and decongestant.
Chlorpheniramine maleate is an antihistamine having the chemical name S/B: 2-pyridinepropanamine, γ-(4-chlorophenyl)-N,N-dimethyl (Z)-2-butenedioate(1:1) with the following structure:

Phenyltoloxamine citrate is an antihistamine having the chemical name N,N-dimethyl-2-(α-phenyl-o-tolyloxy) ethylamine dihydrogen citrate with the following structure:

Phenylephrine hydrochloride is a decongestant having the chemical name 3-hydroxy-α[(methylamino)methyl]benzenemethanol hydrochloride with the following structure:

INACTIVE INGREDIENTS

Each COMHIST® tablet contains compressible sugar, magnesium stearate, microcrystalline cellulose, and D&C Yellow No. 10.
Each COMHIST® LA capsule contains dicalcium phosphate anhydrous, pharmaceutical glaze, sucrose, cornstarch, talc, titanium dioxide, gelatin, D&C Yellow No. 10, and FD&C Yellow No. 6.

HOW SUPPLIED

COMHIST® LA is available as a yellow and clear capsule imprinted "ROBERTS" and "COMHIST-LA 065".
NDC 54092-065-01 Bottle of 100
Store from 15° to 30°C (59° to 86°F)
Dispense in a tight container.
COMHIST® is available as a round, yellow, scored tablet debossed "COMHIST" on the smooth side and "RPC" and "066" on the scored side.
NDC 54092-066-01   Bottle of 100
Store from 15° to 30°C (59° to 86°F)

CAUTION

United States law prohibits dispensing without prescription.
Manufactured for
Roberts Laboratories Inc.
a subsidiary of
Roberts Pharmaceutical Corporation
Eatontown, New Jersey 07724 USA

                                        COMLA-X7

Continued on next page

Roberts—Cont.

DOPAR® ℞
(levodopa)

Toward reducing the high incidence of adverse reactions, it is necessary to individualize the therapy and to gradually increase the dosage to the desired therapeutic level.

DESCRIPTION

Chemically, levodopa is 3-hydroxy-L-tyrosine. It is a colorless, crystalline compound, slightly soluble in water and insoluble in alcohol, with a molecular weight of 197.2 and the following structural formula:

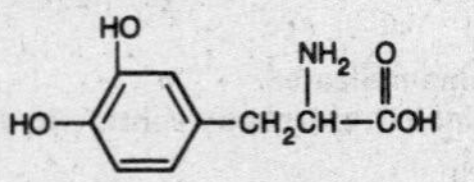

HOW SUPPLIED

Dopar® is available as follows:
100 mg: opaque, green capsule imprinted "Roberts 060" and "Dopar 100mg"
NDC 54092-060-01 bottle of 100.
250 mg: opaque green and white capsule imprinted "Roberts 061" and "Dopar 250mg"
NDC 54092-061-01 bottle of 100
500 mg: opaque green capsule imprinted "Roberts 062" and "Dopar 500mg"
NDC 54092-062-01 bottle of 100
Manufactured for:
Roberts Laboratories Inc.
a wholly owned subsidiary of
Roberts Pharmaceutical Corporation
Eatontown, New Jersey 07724 USA

ELTROXIN™ ℞
(Levothyroxine Sodium Tablets USP)

For Oral Administration

INGREDIENTS

Active: Levothyroxine Sodium USP,
Inactive: Lactose, corn starch, acacia powder, magnesium stearate, purified water, also contains the following colors (by strength):

Strength (mcg)	Color(s)
25	FD&C Yellow #6 Aluminum Lake.
50	none.
75	FD&C Blue #2, FD&C Red #40.
88	D&C Yellow #10, FD&C Yellow #6, FD&C Blue #1.
100	FD&C Yellow #6 Aluminum Lake.
112	FD&C Red #40 Aluminum Lake, FD&C Yellow #6 Aluminum Lake.
125	FD&C Yellow #6, FD&C Red #40, FD&C Blue #1.
137	FD&C Yellow #6 Aluminum Lake, FD&C Red #40 Aluminum Lake.
150	FD&C Blue #2 Aluminum Lake.
175	FD&C Red #40 Aluminum Lake, FD&C Blue #2 Aluminum Lake.
200	FD&C Red #3.
300	D&C Yellow #10 Aluminum Lake, FD&C Blue #1 Aluminum Lake.

DESCRIPTION

ELTROXIN™ (Levothyroxine Sodium Tablets USP) contain synthetic crystalline L-3,3′,5,5′-tretraoidothyronine sodium salt [levothyroxine (T_4) sodium]. Synthetic T_4 is similar to that produced in the human thyroid gland. T_4 contains four iodine atoms and is formed by the coupling of two molecules of diiodotyrsine (DIT).
Levothyroxine (T_4) Sodium has an empirical formula of $C_{15}H_{10}I_4NNaO_4xH_2O$, molecular weight of 798.86 (anhydrous), and structural formula as shown:

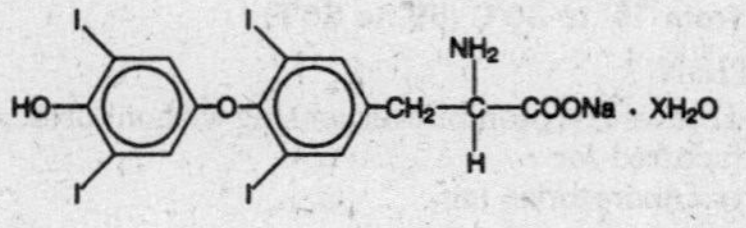

CLINICAL PHARMACOLOGY

The steps in the synthesis of thyroid hormones are controlled by thyrotropin (Thyroid Stimulating Hormone, TSH) secreted by the anterior pituitary. This hormone's secretion is in turn controlled by a feedback mechanism effected by the thyroid hormones themselves and by thyrotropin releasing hormone (TRH), a tripeptide of hypothalamic origin. Endogenous thyroid hormone secretion is suppressed when exogenous thyroid hormones are administered to euthyroid individuals in excess of the normal gland's secretion.
The mechanisms by which thyroid hormones exert their physiologic action are not well understood. These hormones enhance oxygen consumption by most tissues of the body and increase the basal metabolic rate and the metabolism of carbohydrates, lipids, and proteins. Thus they exert a profound influence on every organ system in the body and are of particular importance in the development of the central nervous system.
The normal thyroid gland contains approximately 200 mcg of levothyroxine (T_4) per gram of gland and 15 mcg of triiodothyronine (T_3) per gram. The ratio of these two hormones in the circulation does not represent the ratio in the thyroid gland, since about 80 percent of peripheral triiodothyronine comes from monodeiodination of levothyroxine at the 5 position (outer ring). Peripheral monodeiodination of levothyroxine at the 5 position (inner ring) results in the formation of reverse triiodothyronine (rT_3), which is calorigenically inactive. These facts would seem to advocate levothyroxine as the treatment of choice for the hypothyroid patient and to militate against the administration of hormone combinations which, while normalizing thyroxine levels, may produce triiodothyronine levels in the thyrotoxic range.
Triiodothyronine (T_3) levels is low in the fetus and newborn, in old age, in chronic caloric-deprivation, hepatic cirrhosis, renal failure, surgical stress, and chronic illnesses representing what has been called the "low triiodothyronine syndrome".

PHARMACOKINETICS

Animal studies have shown that T_4 is only partially absorbed from the gastrointestinal tract. The degree of absorption is dependent on the vehicle used for its administration and by the character of the intestinal contents, the intestinal flora, including plasma protein, soluble dietary factors, all of which bind thyroid hormone and thereby make it unavailable for diffusion.
Depending on other factors, absorption has varied from 48 to 79 percent of the administered dose. Fasting increases absorption. Malabsorption syndromes, as well as dietary factors, (children's soybean formula, concomitant use of anionic exchange resins such as cholestyramine) cause excessive fecal loss.
More than 99 percent of circulating hormones are bound to serum proteins, including thyroxine-binding globuline (TMG), thyroxine-binding prealbumin (TBPA), and albumin (TBa), whose capacities and affinities vary for the hormones. The higher affinity of levothyroxine (T_4) for both TBG and TBPA as compared to triiodothyronine (T_3) partially explains the higher serum levels and longer half-life of the former hormone. Both protein-bound hormones exist in equilibrium with minute amounts of free hormones, the latter accounting for the metabolic activity.
Deiodination of levothyroxine (T_4) occurs at a number of sites, including liver, kidney, and other tissues. The conjugated hormone, in the form of glucoronide or sulfate, is found in the bile and gut where it may complete an enterohepatic circulation. 85 percent of levothyroxine (T_4) metabolized daily is deiodinated.

INDICATIONS AND USAGE

Levothyroxine Sodium Tablets USP are indicated:

1. As replacement or supplemental therapy in patients with hypothyroidism of any etiology, except transient hypothyroidism during the recovery phase of subacute thyroiditis. This category includes cretinism, myxedema, and ordinary hypothyroidism in patients of any age (children, adults, the elderly), or state (including pregnancy); primary hypothyroidism resulting from functional deficiency, primary atrophy, partial or total absence of thyroid gland, or the effects of surgery, radiation, or drugs, with or without the presence of goiter; and secondary (pituitary) or tertiary (hypothalamic) hypothyroidism) (see CONTRAINDICATIONS and PRECAUTIONS).
2. As a pituitary TSH suppressant, in the treatment or prevention of various types of euthyroid goiters, including thyroid nodules, subacute or chronic lymphocytic thyroiditis (Hashimoto's), multinodular goiter, and in the management of thyroid cancer.
3. As a diagnostic agent in suppression tests to aid in the diagnosis of suspected mild hyperthyroidism or thyroid gland autonomy.

WARNINGS:
Drugs with thyroid hormone activity, alone or together with other therapeutic agents, have been used for the treatment of obesity. In euthyroid patients, doses within the range of daily hormonal requirements are ineffective for weight reduction. Larger doses may produce serious or even life threatening manifestations of toxicity, particularly when given in association with sympathomimetic amines such as those used for their anorectic effects.

CONTRAINDICATIONS

Thyroid hormone preparations are generally contraindicated in patients with diagnosed but as yet uncorrected adrenal cortical insufficiency, untreated thyrotoxicosis, and apparent hypersensitivity to any of their active or extraneous constituents. There is no well documented evidence from the literature, however, of true allergic or idiosyncratic reactions to thyroid hormone.
The use of thyroid hormones in the therapy of obesity, alone or combined with other drugs is unjustified and has been shown to be ineffective. Neither is their use justified for the treatment of male or female infertility unless this condition is accompanied by hypothyroidism.

PRECAUTIONS

General: Thyroid hormones should be used with great caution in a number of circumstances where the integrity of the cardiovascular system, particularly the coronary arteries, is suspected. These include patients with angina pectoris or the elderly, who have a greater likelihood of occult cardiac disease. In these patients, therapy should be initiated with low doses, i.e., 25–50 mcg levothyroxine (T_4). When, in such patients, a euthyroid state can only be reached at the expense of an aggravation of the cardiovascular disease, thyroid hormone dosage should be reduced.
Thyroid hormone therapy in patients with concomitant diabetes mellitus or insipidus or adrenal cortical insufficiency aggravates the intensity of their symptoms. Appropriate adjustments of the various therapeutic measures directed at these concomitant endocrine diseases are required, the therapy of myxedema coma may require simultaneous administration of glucocorticoids (see DOSAGE AND ADMINISTRATION).
Hypothyroidism decreases and hyperthyroidism increases the sensitivity to oral anticoagulants. Prothrombin time should be closely monitored in thyroid treated patients on oral anticoagulants and dosage of the latter agents adjusted on the basis of frequent prothrombin time determinations.
In infants, excessive doses of thyroid hormone preparations may produce craniosynostosis.
Information for Patient: Patients on thyroid hormone preparations and parents of children on thyroid therapy should be informed that:

1. Replacement therapy is to be taken essentially for life, with the exception of cases of transient hypothyroidism, usually associated with thyroiditis, and in those patients receiving a therapeutic trial of the drug.
2. They should immediately report during the course of therapy any signs or symptoms of thyroid hormone toxicity, e.g., chest pain, increased pulse rate, palpitations, excessive sweating, heat intolerance, nervousness, or any other unusual event.
3. In case of concomitant diabetes mellitus, the daily dosage of antidiabetic medication may need readjustment as thyroid hormone replacement is achieved. If thyroid medication is stopped, a downward readjustment of the dosage of insulin or oral hypoglycemic agent may be necessary to avoid hypoglycemia. At all times, close monitoring of blood or urinary glucose levels is mandatory in such patients.
4. In case of concomitant oral anticoagulant therapy, the prothrombin time should be measured frequently to determine if the dosage of oral anticoagulants is to be readjusted.
5. Partial loss of hair may be experienced by children in the first few months of thyroid therapy, but this is usually a transient phenomenon and later recovery is usually the rule.

Laboratory Tests: Treatment of patients with thyroid hormones requires the periodic assessment of thyroid status by means of appropriate laboratory tests, by full clinical evaluation, or both. The TSH suppression test can be used to test the effectiveness of the thyroid preparation bearing in mind the relative insensitivity of the infant pituitary to the negative feedback effect of thyroid hormones. Serum T_4 levels can be used to test the effectiveness of levothyroxine sodium. When the total serum T_4 is low but TSH is normal, a test specific to assess unbound (free) T_4 levels is warranted. Specific measurements of T_4 and T_3 by competitive protein binding or radioimmunoassay are not influenced by blood levels of organic or inorganic iodine and have essentially replaced older tests of thyroid hormone measurements, i.e., PBI, BEI, and T_4 by column.
Drug Interactions: *Oral Anticoagulants*—Thyroid hormones appear to increase catabolism of vitamin K-dependent clotting factors. If oral anticoagulants are also being given, compensatory increases in clotting factor synthesis are impaired. Patients stabilized on oral anticoagulants who are found to require thyroid replacement therapy should be watched very closely when therapy is started. If a patient is

truly hypothyroid, it is likely that a reduction in anticoagulant dosage will be required. No special precautions appear to be necessary when oral anticoagulant therapy is begun in a patient already stabilized on maintenance thyroid replacement therapy.

Insulin or Oral Hypoglycemics—Initiating thyroid replacement therapy may cause increases in insulin or oral hypoglycemic requirements. The effects seen are poorly understood and depend upon a variety of factors such as dose and type of thyroid preparations and endocrine status of the patient. Patients receiving insulin or oral hypoglycemics should be closely watched during initiation of thyroid replacement therapy.

Cholestyramine—Cholestyramine binds both T_4 and T_3 in the intestine, thus impairing absorption of these thyroid hormones. *In vitro* studies indicate that the binding is not easily reversed. Therefore, four to five hours should elapse between administration of cholestyramine or similar resins and thyroid hormones.

Estrogen, Oral Contraceptives—Estrogens tend to increase serum thyroxine-binding globulin (TBG). In a patient with a nonfunctioning thyroid gland who is receiving thyroid replacement therapy, free levothyroxine may be decreased when estrogens are started thus increasing thyroid requirements. However, if the patient's thyroid gland has sufficient function, the decreased free thyroxine will result in a compensatory increase in thyroxine output by the thyroid. Therefore, patients without a functioning thyroid gland who are on thyroid replacement therapy may need to increase their thyroid dose if estrogens or estrogen-containing oral contraceptives are given.

Drug/Laboratory Test Interactions: The following drugs or moieties are known to interfere with some laboratory tests performed in patients on thyroid hormone therapy: Androgens, corticosteroids, estrogens, oral contraceptives containing estrogens, iodine-containing preparations, and the numerous preparations containing salicylates.

1. Changes in TBG concentration should be taken into consideration in the interpretation of T_4 and T_3 values. Pregnancy, estrogens, and estrogen-containing oral contraceptives increase TBG concentrations. TBG may also be increased during infectious hepatitis. Decreases in TBG concentrations are observed in nephrosis, acromegaly, and after androgen or corticosteroid therapy. Familial hyper- or hypo-thyroxine-binding-globulinemias have been described. The incidence of TBG deficiency approximates 1 in 9000. The binding of thyroxine by TBPA is inhibited by salicylates; in such cases, the unbound (free) hormone should be measured. Alternatively, an indirect measure of free thyroxine, such as the Free Thyroxine Index (FTI) may be used.

2. Medicinal or dietary iodine interferes with all *in vivo* tests of radioiodine uptake, producing low uptakes which may not be reflective of a true decrease in hormone synthesis.

3. The persistence of clinical and laboratory evidence of hypothyroidism in spite of adequate dosage replacement indicates either poor patient compliance, poor absorption, or inactivity of the preparation. Intracellular resistance to thyroid hormone is quite rare, and is suggested by clinical signs and symptoms of hypothyroidism in the presence of high serum T_4 levels.

Carcinogenesis, Mutagenesis, and Impairment of Fertility: A reportedly apparent association between prolonged thyroid therapy and breast cancer has not been confirmed and patients on thyroid therapy for established indications should not discontinue therapy. No confirmatory long-term studies in animals have been performed to evaluate carcinogenic potential, mutagenicity, or impairment of fertility in either males or females.

Pregnancy-Category A: Thyroid hormones do not readily cross the placental barrier. The clinical experience to date does not indicate any adverse effect on fetuses when thyroid hormones are administered to pregnant women. On the basis of current knowledge, thyroid replacement therapy to hypothyroid women should not be discontinued during pregnancy.

Nursing Mothers: Minimal amounts of thyroid hormones are excreted in human milk. Thyroid is not associated with serious adverse reactions and does not have known tumorigenic potential. Caution should be exercised when thyroid is administered to a nursing woman, adequate replacement doses of levothyroxine are generally needed to maintain normal lactation.

Pediatric Use: Pregnant mothers provide little or no thyroid hormone to the fetus. The incidence of congenital hypothyroidism is relatively high (1 in 4,000) and the hypothyroid fetus would not derive any benefit from the small amounts of hormone crossing the placental barrier. Routine determinations of serum T_4 and/or TSH are strongly advised in neonates in view of the deleterious effects of thyroid deficiency on growth and development.

Treatment should be initiated immediately upon diagnosis, and maintained for life, unless transient hypothyroidism is suspected, in which case, therapy may be interrupted for 2 to 8 weeks after the age of 3 years to reassess the condition.

Cessation of therapy is justified in patients who have maintained a normal TSH during those 2 to 8 weeks.

ADVERSE REACTIONS

Adverse reactions other than those indicative of hyperthyroidism because of therapeutic overdosage, either initially or during maintenance periods, are rare (see OVERDOSAGE).

OVERDOSAGE

Signs and Symptoms: Excessive doses of thyroid medicine result in hypermetabolic state resembling, in every respect, the condition of endogenous origin. The condition may be self-induced.

Treatment of Overdosage: Dosage should be reduced or therapy temporarily discontinued if signs and symptoms of overdosage appear. Treatment may be reinstated at a lower dosage. In normal individuals, normal hypothalamic-pituitary-thyroid axis function is restored in 6 to 8 weeks after thyroid suppression.

Treatment of acute massive thyroid hormone overdosage is aimed at reducing gastrointestinal absorption of the drugs and counter-acting central and peripheral effects, mainly those of increased sympathetic activity. Vomiting may be induced initially if further gastrointestinal absorption can reasonably be prevented and barring contraindications such as coma, convulsions, or loss of the gagging reflex. Treatment is symptomatic and supportive. Oxygen may be administered and ventilation maintained. Cardiac glycosides may be indicated if congestive heart failure develops. Measures to control fever, hypoglycemia, or fluid loss should be instituted if needed. Antiadrenergic agents, particularly propranolol, have been used advantageously in the treatment of increased sympathetic activity. Propranolol may be administered intravenously at a dosage of 1 to 3 mg over a 10 minute period or orally, 80 to 160 mg/day, especially when no contraindications exist for its use. Other adjunctive measures may include administration of cholestyramine to interfere with thyroxine absorption, and glucocorticoids to inhibit conversion of T_4 to T_3.

DOSAGE AND ADMINISTRATION

The dosage and rate of administration of Levothyroxine Sodium Tablets USP is determined by the indication and must in every case be individualized according to patient response and laboratory findings.

Hypothyroidism: Therapy is usually instituted using low doses, with increments which depend on the cardiovascular status of the patient. The usual starting dose is 50 mcg with increments of 25 mcg every 2 to 3 weeks. A lower starting dosage, 25 mcg/day or less, is recommended in patients with long standing hypothyroidism, particularly if cardiovascular impairment is suspected, in which case extreme caution is recommended. The appearance of angina is an indication for a reduction in dosage. Most patients require not more than 200 mcg/day. Failure to respond to doses of 300 mcg suggests lack of compliance or malabsorption. Adequate therapy usually results in normal TSH and T_4 levels after 2 to 3 weeks of the maintenance dose.

Readjustment of thyroid hormone dosage should be made within the first four weeks of therapy, after proper clinical and laboratory evaluations.

Myxedema Coma: Myxedema coma is usually precipitated in the hypothyroid patient by intercurrent illness or drugs such as sedatives and anesthetics and should be considered a medical emergency. Therapy should be directed at the correction of electrolyte disturbances and possible infection besides the administration of thyroid hormones. Corticosteroids should be administered routinely. T_4 may be administered via a nasogastric tube but the preferred route of administration is intravenous. Levothyroxine sodium (T_4) is given at a starting dose of 400 mcg (100 mcg/mL) given rapidly, and is usually well tolerated, even in the elderly. In the presence of concomitant heart disease, the sudden administration of such large doses of L-thyroxine intravenously is clearly not without its cardiovascular risks. Under such circumstances, intravenous therapy should not be undertaken without weighing the alternative risks of the myxedema coma and the cardiovascular disease. Clinical judgement in this situation may dictate smaller intravenous doses. The initial dose is followed by daily supplements of 100 to 200 mcg given intravenously. Normal T_4 levels are achieved in 24 hours followed in 3 days by three-fold evaluation of T3. Continued daily administration of lesser amounts parenterally should be maintained until the patient is fully capable of accepting a daily oral dose. A daily maintenance dose of 50–100 mcg parenterally should suffice to maintain the euthyroid state, once established. Oral therapy would be resumed as soon as the clinical situation has been stabilized and the patient is able to take oral medication.

TSH Suppression in Thyroid Cancer, Nodules, and Euthyroid Goiters: Exogenous thyroid hormone may produce regression of metastases from follicular and papillary carcinoma of the thyroid and is used as ancillary therapy of these conditions following surgery or radioactive iodine. Medullary carcinoma of the thyroid is usually unresponsive to this therapy. TSH should be suppressed to low or undetectable levels. Therefore, larger amounts of thyroid hormone than those

used for replacement therapy are frequently required. This therapy is also used in treating nontoxic solitary nodules and multinodule goiters, and to prevent thyroid enlargement in chronic (Hashimoto's) thyroiditis.

Thyroid Suppression Therapy: Administration of thyroid hormone in doses higher than those produced physiologically by the gland results in suppression of the production of endogenous hormone. This is the basis for the thyroid suppression test and is used as an aid in the diagnosis of patients with signs of mild hyperthyroidism in whom base line laboratory tests appear normal, or to demonstrate thyroid gland autonomy in patients with Graves' ophthalmopathy. ^{131}I uptake is determined before and after the administration of the exogenous hormone. A fifty percent or greater suppression of uptake indicates a normal thyroid-pituitary axis and thus rules out thyroid gland autonomy.

For adults, the average suppressive dose of levothyroxine (T_4) is 2.6 mcg/kg of body weight per day given for 7 to 10 days. These doses usually yield normal serum T_4 and T_3 levels and lack of responses to TSH.

Levothyroxine sodium should be administered cautiously to patients in whom there is a strong suspicion of thyroid gland autonomy, in view of the fact that the exogenous hormone effects will be additive to the endogenous source.

Pediatric Dosage: Pediatric dosage should follow the recommendations summarized in Table 1. In infants with congenital hypothyroidism, therapy with full doses should be instituted as soon as the diagnosis has been made. Levothyroxine Sodium Tablets may be given to infants and children who cannot swallow intact tablets by crushing the proper dose tablet and suspending the freshly crushed tablet in a small amount of water or formula. The suspension can be given by spoon or dropper. DO NOT STORE THE SUSPENSION FOR ANY PERIOD OF TIME. The crushed tablet may also be sprinkled over a small amount of food, such as cooked cereal or applesauce.

Table 1
Recommended Pediatric Dosage For Congenital Hypothroidism*

Levothyroxine Sodium Tablets USP		
Age	Dose per day	Daily dose per kg of body weight
0–6 mos	25–50 mcg	8–10 mcg
6–12 mos	50–75 mcg	6–8 mcg
1–5 yrs	75–100 mcg	5–6 mcg
6–12 yrs	100–150 mcg	4–5 mcg

* To be adjusted on the basis of clinical response and laboratory tests (see Laboratory Tests)

HOW SUPPLIED

ELTROXIN™ (Levothyroxine Sodium Tablets USP): round tablets. Scored on one side and debossed with the potency (mcg). ELTROXIN™ is available in bottles of 100 in strengths of 25 mcg, 50 mcg, 75 mcg, 88 mcg, 100 mcg, 112 mcg, 125 mcg, 137 mcg, 150 mcg, 175 mcg, 200 mcg, 300 mcg, and in bottles of 500 in the strength of 100 mcg.

Store from 15°–25°C (59°–77°F).

Caution: Federal law prohibits dispensing without a prescription.

Manufactured for Roberts Laboratories Inc., a subsidiary of **ROBERTS PHARMACEUTICAL CORPORATION,** Eatontown, NJ 07724, USA
by **GLAXO WELLCOME INC.,** Toronto, Ontario, Canada M8Z 5S6
™A Trademark of Glaxo Group Ltd.: licensed use.

EMINASE®   ℞
[*em-in-āz*]
brand of ANISTREPLASE

DESCRIPTION

Eminase® (anistreplase) is the p-anisoylated derivative of the Lys-Plasminogen-Streptokinase activator complex prepared *in vitro* by acylating human plasma-derived, purified, heat-treated, Lys-Plasminogen and purified Streptokinase from group C β-hemolytic streptococci. *Eminase*® has a molecular weight of about 131,000. Each vial of *Eminase*® is supplied as a sterile, lyophilized, white to off-white powder containing 30 units of Anistreplase, < 3 mg dimethylsulfoxide, < 0.2 mg sodium hydroxide and the following buffers and stabilizers: 150 μg p-amidinophenyl-p'-anisate (acylating agent), 100 mg mannitol, 46 mg L-lysine, 30 mg Albumin (Human), < 2 mg glycerol, and 1.3 mg ε-aminocaproic acid. *Eminase*® is intended only for intravenous (I.V.) injection after reconstitution with **Sterile Water for Injection,** USP. The preparation contains no preservatives and is intended to be used as a single dose. Potency is expressed in units of Anistreplase by using a reference standard which is specific for

Continued on next page

Roberts—Cont.

Eminase ® and is not comparable with units used for other fibrinolytics.

The Lys-Plasminogen and the Streptokinase used in the manufacture of *Eminase* ® are prepared under U.S. license by Oesterreichisches Institut fuer Haemoderivate GmbH and Behringwerke AG, respectively, under shared manufacturing arrangements.

CLINICAL PHARMACOLOGY

Eminase ® is an inactive derivative of a fibrinolytic enzyme with the catalytic center of the activator complex temporarily blocked by an anisoyl group. The anisoyl group does not decrease the high fibrin-binding ability of the complex. *Eminase* ® is made *in vitro* from Lys-Plasminogen and Streptokinase. *Eminase* ® differs from the complex initially formed *in vivo* upon administration of Streptokinase; the latter complex contains predominately glu-plasminogen. Activation of *Eminase* ® occurs with release of the anisoyl group by deacylation, a non-enzymatic first-order process with a half-life *in vitro* in human blood of about 2 hours. In solution, deacylation of *Eminase* ® starts immediately and the enzymatically active Lys-Plasminogen-Streptokinase activator complex is progressively formed. The production of plasmin from plasminogen by deacylated *Eminase* ® can take place in the bloodstream or within the thrombus; the latter process is catalytically more efficient but both may contribute to thrombolysis. The half-life of fibrinolytic activity of the circulating *Eminase* ® is 70 to 120 minutes (mean 94 minutes). A number of controlled clinical studies have been performed with *Eminase* ® to demonstrate benefit. Heparin anticoagulation was administered to all patients routinely following (about 4 to 6 hours) dosing with *Eminase* ®.

Randomized, controlled studies have demonstrated that *Eminase* ® reduces mortality when administered within 6 hours of the onset of the symptoms of acute myocardial infarction (AMI). The benefit of mortality reduction occurs acutely and is maintained for at least 1 year.

In a study of 1258 patients (AIMS trial), mortality at 30 days postinfarction was decreased (47.2%, p = 0.0001) in patients receiving *Eminase* ® as compared with placebo. At 1 year, the reduction in mortality was maintained (38%, p = 0.001). The incidence of heart failure was less in patients treated with *Eminase* ® (17.9%) compared with patients who received placebo (23.3%).[1,2] Similar mortality results were obtained from a smaller, randomized, controlled trial.[1,3]

In a double-blind, randomized trial of *Eminase* ® compared with heparin bolus, left ventricular function was improved and infarction size reduced. There was significantly (p < 0.01, two sample t-test) higher left ventricular ejection fraction (LVEF) for the *Eminase* ® treatment group (53%) compared with the heparin treatment group (47.5%) when measured 4 days after treatment (intent-to-treat analysis). This difference was maintained when patients were reexamined by radionuclide ventriculography at day 19, even when patients who experienced successful angioplasty were excluded from the analysis (p = 0.04). About 3 weeks after treatment, mean infarct size was 24% lower in the patients treated with *Eminase* ® compared with those treated with heparin (n = 188, p = 0.02).[1,4] Similarly, if those patients who experienced successful angioplasty were excluded from the analysis, the mean infarct size in patients treated with *Eminase* ® was significantly less than that of heparin-treated patients (p < 0.01).

In randomized, comparative studies reperfusion rates of between 50% and 68% have been reported in patients receiving *Eminase* ® within 6 hours of symptom onset. However, for maximum rates of reperfusion, treatment should be initiated as soon as possible after onset of symptoms.

In two studies,[1,5,6] *Eminase* ® and intracoronary (IC) Streptokinase were compared in patients with angiographically proven coronary artery occlusion. Reperfusion occurred about 45 minutes after the start of therapy for both treatment groups. When therapy was initiated within 4 hours of onset of AMI symptoms reperfusion rates of 59% (n = 87) and 68% (n = 41) were observed for *Eminase* ® compared with 59% (n = 85) and 70% (n = 43) for IC Streptokinase. Of those patients who had coronary artery reperfusion, angiographically demonstrated reocclusion occurred within 24 hours in 3% to 4% of those treated with *Eminase* ® and in 7% to 12% of those treated with Streptokinase.[1,5,6]

In a well-controlled, randomized study, a patency rate of 72% was obtained with *Eminase* ® compared with 53% for I.V. Streptokinase. Patency for the 107 patients was determined by posttreatment angiography.[1,7]

Eminase ® was also found to have a favorable risk/benefit profile in elderly patients (> 65 years, n = 940) who participated in clinical trials. Use of *Eminase* ® in patients over 75 years old has not been adequately studied.

INDICATIONS AND USAGE

Eminase ® is indicated for use in the management of acute myocardial infarction (AMI) in adults, for the lysis of thrombi obstructing coronary arteries, the reduction of infarct size, the improvement of ventricular function following AMI, and the reduction of mortality associated with AMI. Treatment should be initiated as soon as possible after the onset of AMI symptoms (see CLINICAL PHARMACOLOGY).

CONTRAINDICATIONS

Because thrombolytic therapy increases the risk of bleeding, *Eminase* ® is contraindicated in the following situations:
- active internal bleeding
- history of cerebrovascular accident
- recent (within 2 months) intracranial or intraspinal surgery or trauma (see WARNINGS)
- intracranial neoplasm, arteriovenous malformation, or aneurysm
- known bleeding diathesis
- severe, uncontrolled hypertension

Eminase ® should not be administered to patients having experienced severe allergic reactions to either this product or Streptokinase.

WARNINGS

Bleeding: (See ADVERSE REACTIONS) The most common complication associated with *Eminase* ® therapy is bleeding. The types of bleeding associated with thrombolytic therapy can be divided into two broad categories:
1. Internal bleeding involving the gastrointestinal tract, genitourinary tract, retroperitoneal, ocular, or intracranial sites.
2. Superficial or surface bleeding, observed mainly at invaded or disturbed sites (e.g., venous cutdowns, arterial punctures, sites of recent surgical intervention).

The concomitant use of heparin anticoagulation may contribute to the bleeding. Some of the hemorrhagic episodes occurred 1 or more days after the effects of *Eminase* ® had dissipated, but while heparin therapy was continuing.

As fibrin is lysed during *Eminase* ® therapy, bleeding from recent puncture sites may occur. Therefore, thrombolytic therapy requires careful attention to all potential bleeding sites (including catheter insertion sites, arterial and venous puncture sites, cutdown sites, and needle puncture sites). Intramuscular injections and nonessential handling of the patient should be avoided during treatment with *Eminase* ®. Venipunctures should be performed carefully and only as required.

Should an arterial puncture be necessary following administration of *Eminase* ®, it is preferable to use an upper-extremity vessel that is accessible to manual compression. A pressure dressing should be applied, and the puncture site should be checked frequently for evidence of bleeding.

Each patient being considered for therapy with *Eminase* ® should be carefully evaluated and anticipated benefits should be weighed against potential risks associated with therapy.

In the following conditions, the risks of *Eminase* ® therapy may be increased and should be weighed against the anticipated benefits:
- recent (within 10 days) major surgery (e.g., coronary artery bypass graft, obstetrical delivery, organ biopsy, previous puncture of noncompressible vessels)
- cerebrovascular disease
- recent gastrointestinal or genitourinary bleeding (within 10 days)
- recent trauma (within 10 days) including cardiopulmonary resuscitation
- hypertension: systolic BP ≥ 180 mmHg and/or diastolic BP ≥ 110 mmHg
- high likelihood of left heart thrombus (e.g., mitral stenosis with atrial fibrillation)
- subacute bacterial endocarditis
- acute pericarditis
- hemostatic defects including those secondary to severe hepatic or renal disease
- pregnancy
- age > 75 years (Use of *Eminase* ® in patients over 75 years old has not been adequately studied.)
- diabetic hemorrhagic retinopathy or other hemorrhagic ophthalmic conditions
- septic thrombophlebitis or occluded AV cannula at seriously infected site
- patients currently receiving oral anticoagulants (e.g., warfarin sodium)
- any other condition in which bleeding constitutes a significant hazard or would be particularly difficult to manage because of its location

Arrhythmias: Coronary thrombolysis may result in arrhythmias associated with reperfusion. These arrhythmias (such as sinus bradycardia, accelerated idioventricular rhythm, ventricular premature depolarizations, ventricular tachycardia, ventricular fibrillation) are not different from those often seen in the ordinary course of acute myocardial infarction and may be managed with standard antiarrhythmic measures. It is recommended that antiarrhythmic therapy for bradycardia and/or ventricular irritability be available when injections of *Eminase* ® are administered.

Hypotension: Hypotension, sometimes severe, not secondary to bleeding or anaphylaxis, has occasionally been observed soon after intravenous *Eminase* ® administration. Patients should be monitored closely and, should symptomatic or alarming hypotension occur, appropriate symptomatic treatment should be administered.

PRECAUTIONS

General: Standard management of myocardial infarction should be implemented concomitantly with *Eminase* ® treatment. Invasive procedures should be minimized (see WARNINGS). Anaphylactoid reactions have rarely been reported in patients who received *Eminase* ®. Accordingly, adequate treatment provisions such as epinephrine should be available for immediate use.

Readministration: Because of the increased likelihood of resistance due to antistreptokinase antibody, Eminase ® (anistreplase) may not be as effective if administered more than 5 days after prior *Eminase* ® or Streptokinase therapy, particularly between 5 days and 12 months. Increased antistreptokinase antibody levels after *Eminase* ® or Streptokinase may also increase the risk of allergic reactions following readministration.

Repeated administration of *Eminase* ® within 1 week of the initial dose has occurred in a small number of patients treated for AMI and non-AMI conditions. The incidence of hematomas/bruising was somewhat greater in those patients who received repeat doses of *Eminase* ® but otherwise the adverse event profile was similar to those who received 1 dose.

Laboratory Tests: Intravenous administration of *Eminase*® will cause marked decreases in plasminogen and fibrinogen and increases in thrombin time (TT), activated partial thromboplastin time (APTT), and prothrombin time (PT).

Results of coagulation tests and/or measures of fibrinolytic activity performed during *Eminase* ® therapy may be unreliable unless specific precautions are taken to prevent *in vitro* artifacts. *Eminase* ® when present in blood in pharmacologic concentrations, remains active under *in vitro* conditions. This can lead to degradation of fibrinogen in blood samples removed for analysis. Collection of blood samples in the presence of aprotinin (2000 to 3000 KIU/mL) can, to some extent, mitigate this phenomenon.

Drug Interactions: The interaction of *Eminase* ® (anistreplase) with other cardioactive drugs has not been studied. In addition to bleeding associated with heparin and vitamin K antagonists, drugs that alter platelet function (such as aspirin and dipyridamole) may increase the risk of bleeding if administered prior to *Eminase* ® therapy.

Use of Anticoagulants: *Eminase* ® alone or in combination with antiplatelet agents and anticoagulants may cause bleeding complications. Therefore, careful monitoring is advised, especially at arterial puncture sites. In clinical studies, a majority of patients treated received anticoagulant therapy postdosing with *Eminase* ® during their hospital stay and a minority received heparin pretreatment with *Eminase*®. The use of antiplatelet agents increased the incidence of bleeding events similarly in patients treated with *Eminase* ® or nonthrombolytic therapy. There was no evidence of a synergistic effect of combined *Eminase* ® and antiplatelet agents on bleeding events. In addition, there was no difference in the incidence of hemorrhagic CVAs in *Eminase* ®-treated patients who did or did not receive aspirin.

Carcinogenesis, Mutagenesis, Impairment of Fertility: Long-term studies in animals have not been performed to evaluate the carcinogenic potential or the effect on fertility. Studies to determine mutagenicity and chromosomal aberration assays in human lymphocytes were negative at all concentrations tested.

Pregnancy (Category C): Animal reproduction studies have not been conducted with *Eminase* ®. It is also not known whether *Eminase* ® can cause fetal harm when administered to a pregnant woman or can affect reproduction capacity. *Eminase* ® should be given to a pregnant woman only if clearly needed.

Nursing Mothers: It is not known whether *Eminase* ® is excreted in human milk. Because many drugs are excreted in human milk, the physician should decide whether the patient should discontinue nursing or not receive *Eminase*®.

Pediatric Use: Safety and effectiveness of Eminase® (anistreplase) in children have not been established.

ADVERSE REACTIONS

Bleeding: The incidence of bleeding (major or minor) varied widely from study to study and may depend on the use of arterial catheterization and other invasive procedures, patient population, and/or concomitant therapy. The overall incidence of bleeding in patients treated with *Eminase* ® in clinical trials (n = 5275) was 14.6%, with nonpuncture-site bleeding occurring in 10.2%, and puncture-site bleeding occurring in 5.7%, of these patients. Bleeding at the puncture site occurred more frequently in clinical trials in which the patients underwent immediate coronary catheterization

(13.3%, n = 637) compared with those who did not (3.0%, n = 2023). The incidence of presumed intracranial bleeding within 7 days postdosing with *Eminase* ® was 0.57% (n = 5275); 0.34% etiology confirmed hemorrhagic; 0.23% etiology not confirmed) compared to 0.16% (n = 1249) after non-thrombolytic therapy.

In the AIMS trial the overall incidence of bleeding in patients treated with *Eminase* ® was 14.8% compared with 3.8% for placebo. The incidence of specific bleeding events was:

Type of Bleeding	EMINASE® (n=500)	Placebo (n=501)
Puncture site	4.6%	<1%
Nonpuncture site hematoma	2.8%	<1%
Hematuria/Genitourinary	2.4%	<1%
Hemoptysis	2.2%	<1%
Gastrointestinal hemorrhage	2.0%	1.4%
Intracranial	1.0%	<1%
Gum/Mouth hemorrhage	1.0%	0
Epistaxis	<1%	<1%
Anemia	<1%	<1%
Eye hemorrhage	<1%	<1%
Hemorrhage (unspecified)	<1%	0

In this study there was no difference between *Eminase* ® and placebo in the incidence of major bleeding events. Should serious bleeding (not controlled by local pressure) occur in a critical location (intracranial, gastrointestinal, retroperitoneal, pericardial), any concomitant heparin should be terminated immediately and the administration of protamine to reverse heparinization should be considered. If necessary, the bleeding tendency can be reversed with appropriate replacement therapy.

Minor bleeding can be anticipated mainly at invaded or disturbed sites. If such bleeding occurs, local measures should be taken to control the bleeding (**see WARNINGS**).

Cardiovascular: The most frequently reported adverse experiences in *Eminase* ® clinical trials (n = 5275) were arrhythmia/conduction disorders which were reported in 38% of patients treated with *Eminase* ® and 46% of non-thrombolytic control patients. Hypotension occurred in 10.4% of patients treated with *Eminase* ® compared to 7.9% for patients who received nonthrombolytic treatment (**see WARNINGS**).

Allergic-type Reactions: Anaphylactic and anaphylactoid reactions have been observed rarely (0.2%) in patients treated with *Eminase* ® and are similar in incidence to Streptokinase (0.1% anaphylactic shock in 1 study). These included symptoms such as bronchospasm or angioedema. Other milder or delayed effects such as urticaria, itching, flushing, rashes and eosinophilia have been occasionally observed. A delayed purpuric rash appearing 1 to 2 weeks after treatment has been reported in 0.3% of patients. The rash may also be associated with arthralgia, ankle edema, gastrointestinal symptoms, mild hematuria, mild proteinuria and vasculitis. This syndrome was self-limiting and without long-term sequelae.

Risk of Viral Transmission: Six batches of *Eminase* ® (five different batches of Lys-Plasminogen) were used in clinical trials designed specifically to monitor possible hepatitis non-A, non-B transmission. No case of hepatitis was diagnosed in patients receiving *Eminase*®. Lys-Plasminogen is derived from human plasma obtained from FDA approved sources and tested for absence of viral contamination, including human immunodeficiency virus type-1 (HIV-1) and hepatitis B surface antigen. The manufacturing process includes a vapor-heat treatment step for inactivation of viruses. The entire manufacturing process has also been validated to yield a cumulative reduction of $\geq 10^{21}$ fold HIV-1 infectious particles, i.e., $\geq 10^6$ infectious particles removed by vapor-heat treatment and a cumulative total of $\geq 10^{15}$ infectious particles removed by the various steps in the purification process.

Causal Relationship Unknown: Since the following experiences may also be associated with AMI or other therapy, the causal relationship to *Eminase* ® administration is unknown. The following adverse experiences were infrequently (<10%) reported in clinical trials: **Body as a Whole**—chills, fever, headache, shock; **Cardiovascular**—cardiac rupture, chest pain, emboli; **Dermatology**—purpura, sweating; **Gastrointestinal**—nausea and/or vomiting; **Hemic and Lymphatic**—thrombocytopenia; **Metabolic and Nutritional**—elevated transaminase levels; **Musculoskeletal**—arthralgia; **Nervous**—agitation, dizziness, paresthesia, tremor, vertigo; **Respiratory**—dyspnea, lung edema. The following adverse experiences were rarely (less than one in a thousand) reported with use of commercially distributed *Eminase*®: **Nervous**—Guillain Barré syndrome; **Respiratory**—adult respiratory distress syndrome.

DOSAGE AND ADMINISTRATION

Administer *Eminase* ® as soon as possible after the onset of symptoms. The recommended dose is 30 units of *Eminase* ® administered only by intravenous injection over 2 to 5 minutes into an intravenous line or vein.

Reconstitution:
1. Slowly add 5 mL of Sterile Water for Injection, USP, by directing the stream of fluid against the side of the vial.
2. Gently roll the vial, mixing the dry powder and fluid. Do not shake. Try to minimize foaming.
3. The reconstituted preparation is a colorless to pale yellow transparent solution. Before administration, the product should be visually inspected for particulate matter and discoloration.
4. Withdraw the entire contents of the vial.
5. The reconstituted solution should not be further diluted before administration or added to any infusion fluids. No other medications should be added to the vial or syringe containing *Eminase*®.
6. If *Eminase* ® is not administered within 30 minutes of reconstitution, it should be discarded.

HOW SUPPLIED

Eminase ® is supplied as a sterile, lyophilized powder in 30-unit vials. NDC 54092-543-30.

Storage: Store lyophilized *Eminase* ® between 2° and 8°C (36° to 46°F).

Do not use beyond the expiration date printed on the vial.

REFERENCES

1. Data on File. SmithKline Beecham Pharmaceuticals, Philadelphia.
2. AIMS Trial Study Group. Effect of intravenous APSAC on mortality after acute myocardial infarction: preliminary report of a placebo-controlled clinical trial. Lancet 1988; 1:545–9.
3. Meinertz T, Kasper W, Schumacher M, Just H for the APSAC multicenter trial group. The German multicenter trial of anisoylated plasminogen streptokinase activator complex versus heparin for acute myocardial infarction. Am J Cardiol 1988; 62:347–51.
4. Bassand JP, Machecourt J, Cassagnes J, et al. Multicenter trial of intravenous anisoylated plasminogen streptokinase activator complex (APSAC) in acute myocardial infarction: effects on infarct size and left ventricular function. J Am Coll Cardiol 1989; 13:988–97.
5. Anderson JL, Rothbard RL, Hackworthy RA, et al. Multicenter reperfusion trial of intravenous anisoylated plasminogen streptokinase activator complex (APSAC) in acute myocardial infarction: controlled comparison with intracoronary streptokinase. J Am Coll Cardiol 1988; 11:1153–63.
6. Bonnier HJRM, Visser RF, Klomps HC, Hoffmann HJML and the Dutch Invasive Reperfusion Study Group. Comparison of intravenous anisoylated plasminogen streptokinase activator complex and intracoronary streptokinase in acute myocardial infarction. Am J Cardiol 1988; 62:25–30.
7. Brochier ML, Quilliet L, Kulbertus H, et al. Intravenous anisoylated plasminogen streptokinase activator complex versus intravenous streptokinase in evolving myocardial infarction: preliminary data from a randomized multicentre study. Drugs 1987; 33(Suppl 3):140–5.

Manufactured by:
SmithKline Beecham Pharma GmbH
Munich, Germany

U.S. License No. 1097

Distributed by:
Roberts Laboratories Inc.
a subsidiary of
ROBERTS PHARMACEUTICAL CORP.
Eatontown, NJ 07724, USA

Veterans Administration/Military/PHS—Vial, 30 mL, 6505-01-314-7922. EM:L3

Shown in Product Identification Guide, page 331

ENTUSS™-D Tablets
ENTUSS™-D Jr. Liquid
ENTUSS™-D Liquid
Decongestant
Expectorant
Cough Suppressant

DESCRIPTION

Entuss™-D liquid, Entuss™-D Jr. liquid, and Entuss™-D tablets are an antitussive, decongestant and expectorant formula for the temporary relief of dry nonproductive cough and nasal congestion associated with the common cold, or respiratory allergies.

ENTUSS™-D Tablets

Each white capsule-shaped tablet contains the following
ACTIVE INGREDIENTS:
Hydrocodone Bitartrate .... 5 mg
(Warning–May be habit forming)
Pseudoephedrine Hydrochloride .... 30 mg
Guaifenesin .... 300 mg
INACTIVE INGREDIENTS: corn starch, gelatin, lactose, magnesium stearate and talc.

HOW SUPPLIED

A white bisected capsule-shaped tablet, embossed on the bisected side with "RPC" and "142". Bottles of 100 tablets (NDC 54092-142-01).

ENTUSS™-D Jr. Liquid

is a red tropical fruit punch flavored liquid for oral administration. Each teaspoonful (5 mL) contains the following
ACTIVE INGREDIENTS:
Hydrocodone Bitartrate .... 2.5 mg
(Warning–May be habit forming)
Pseudoephedrine Hydrochloride .... 30 mg
Guaifenesin .... 100 mg
Alcohol .... 5%.
INACTIVE INGREDIENTS: citric acid anhydrous, ethyl maltol, liquid glucose, methylparaben, propylene glycol, propylparaben, purified water, saccharin sodium, sodium hydroxide, sorbitol solution, and sucrose with FD&C Red No. 40 and natural and artificial flavor. May also contain other ingredients.

HOW SUPPLIED

4 FL OZ bottle (NDC 54092-439-04)
16 FL OZ bottle (NDC 54092-439-16)

ENTUSS™ Liquid is a clear, colorless, sweet-tasting syrup for oral administration which is Sugar-Free, Alcohol-Free, Dye-Free and Corn-Free. Each teaspoonful (5 mL) contains the following
ACTIVE INGREDIENTS:
Hydrocodone Bitartrate .... 5 mg
(Warning–May be habit forming)
Pseudoephedrine Hydrochloride .... 30 mg
Potassium Guaiacolsulfonate .... 300 mg
INACTIVE INGREDIENTS: benzoic acid, citric acid, flavor, propylene glycol, purified water, saccharin sodium and sorbitol.

HOW SUPPLIED

16 FL OZ bottles (NDC 54092-438-16)

ENTUSS™ Tablets
Expectorant
Cough Suppressant

DESCRIPTION

Entuss™ is an antitussive and expectorant formula for the temporary relief of dry, non-productive cough due to colds, or allergies. Each tablet contains the following
ACTIVE INGREDIENTS:
Hydrocodone Bitartrate .... 5 mg
(Warning–May be habit forming)
Guaifenesin .... 300 mg
INACTIVE INGREDIENTS: lactose, starch, gelatin, FD&C Yellow No. 6, magnesium stearate and talc.
HOW SUPPLIED: Bottles of 100 (NDC 54092-141-01)-Light orange scored tablets imprinted "RPC" and "141".

ENTUSS™ Expectorant
Cough Suppressant

DESCRIPTION

Entuss™ is an antitussive and expectorant formula for the temporary relief of cough associated with the common cold or bronchial irritants. A light amber color, apricot sweet-tasting syrup for oral administration which is Alcohol-Free, Corn-Free, Tartrazine-Free and Sugar-Free. Each teaspoonful (5 mL) contains the following
ACTIVE INGREDIENTS:
Hydrocodone Bitartrate .... 5 mg
(Warning–May be habit forming)
Potassium Guaiacolsulfonate .... 300 mg
INACTIVE INGREDIENTS: sorbitol, propylene glycol, saccharin sodium, benzoic acid, citric acid, flavor and FD&C Yellow No. 6.

HOW SUPPLIED

4 FL OZ bottle (NDC 54092-437-04)
16 FL OZ bottle (NDC 54092-437-16)

Store all Entuss products in tight, light-resistant containers, as defined in the USP, at controlled room temperature: 15°–30°C (59°–86°F). Dispense in child-resistant containers.
CAUTION: Federal law prohibits dispensing without a prescription.

ETHMOZINE®
(moricizine hydrochloride)
TABLETS

℞

DESCRIPTION

ETHMOZINE® (moricizine hydrochloride) is an orally active antiarrhythmic drug available for administration in tablets containing 200 mg, 250 mg and 300 mg of moricizine hydrochloride. The chemical name of moricizine hydrochloride is 10-(3-morpholinopropionyl) phenothiazine-2-carbamic acid ethyl ester hydrochloride and the structural formula is represented as follows:
[See chemical structure at top of next column.]

Continued on next page

Roberts—Cont.

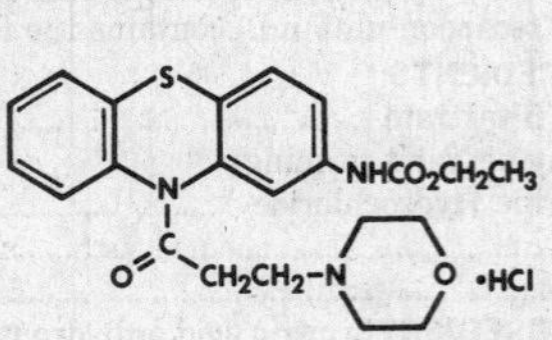

MW=464

Moricizine hydrochloride is a white to tan crystalline powder, freely soluble in water and has a pKa of 6.4 (weak acid). ETHMOZINE® tablets contain: lactose, microcrystalline cellulose, sodium starch glycolate, magnesium stearate, and dyes (FD&C Blue 1, D&C Yellow 10 and FD&C Yellow 6 [200 mg tablet]; FD&C Yellow 6 and FD&C Red 40 [250 mg tablet]; FD&C Blue 1 [300 mg tablet]).

CLINICAL PHARMACOLOGY

Mechanism of Action

ETHMOZINE® is a Class I antiarrhythmic agent with potent local anesthetic activity and myocardial membrane stabilizing effects. ETHMOZINE® reduces the fast inward current carried by sodium ions.

In isolated dog Purkinje fibers, ETHMOZINE® shortens Phase II and III repolarization, resulting in a decreased action potential duration and effective refractory period. A dose-related decrease in the maximum rate of Phase 0 depolarization (V_{max}) occurs without effect on maximum diastolic potential or action potential amplitude. The sinus node and atrial tissue of the dog are not affected.

Electrophysiology

Electrophysiology studies in patients with ventricular tachycardia have shown that ETHMOZINE®, at daily doses of 750 mg and 900 mg, prolongs atrioventricular conduction. Both AV nodal conduction time (AH interval) and His-Purkinje conduction time (HV interval) are prolonged by 10–13% and 21–26%, respectively. The PR interval is prolonged by 16–20% and the QRS by 7–18%. Prolongations of 2–5% in the corrected QT interval result from widening of the QRS interval, but there is shortening of the JT interval, indicating an absence of significant effect on ventricular repolarization. Intra-atrial conduction or atrial effective refractory periods are not consistently affected. In patients without sinus node dysfunction, ETHMOZINE® has minimal effects on sinus cycle length and sinus node recovery time. These effects may be significant in patients with sinus node dysfunction (see PRECAUTIONS: Electrocardiographic Changes/Conduction Abnormalities).

Hemodynamics

In patients with impaired left ventricular function, ETHMOZINE® has minimal effects on measurements of cardiac performance such as cardiac index, stroke volume index, pulmonary capillary wedge pressure, systemic or pulmonary vascular resistance or ejection fraction, either at rest or during exercise. ETHMOZINE® is associated with a small, but consistent increase in resting blood pressure and heart rate. Exercise tolerence in patients with ventricular arrhythmias is unaffected. In patients with a history of congestive heart failure or angina pectoris, exercise duration and rate-pressure product at maximal exercise are unchanged during ETHMOZINE® administration. Nonetheless, in some cases worsened heart failure in patients with severe underlying heart disease has been attributed to ETHMOZINE®.

Other Pharmacologic Effects

Although ETHMOZINE® is chemically related to the neuroleptic phenothiazines, it has no demonstrated central or peripheral dopaminergic activity in animals. Moreover, in patients on chronic ETHMOZINE®, serum prolactin levels did not increase.

Pharmacokinetics/Pharmacodynamics

The antiarrhythmic and electrophysiologic effects of ETHMOZINE® are not related in time course or intensity to plasma moricizine concentrations or to the concentrations of any identified metabolite, all of which have short (2–3 hours) half-lives. Following single doses of ETHMOZINE®, there is a prompt prolongation of the PR interval, which becomes normal within 2 hours, consistent with the rapid fall of plasma moricizine. JT interval shortening, however, peaks at about 6 hours and persists for at least 10 hours. Although an effect on VPD rates is seen within 2 hours after dosing, the full effect is seen after 10–14 hours and persists in full, when therapy is terminated, for more than 10 hours, after which the effect decays slowly, and is still substantial at 24 hours. This suggests either an unidentified, active, long half-life metabolite or a structural or functional "deep compartment" with slow entry from, and release to, the plasma. The following description of parent compound pharmacokinetics is therefore of uncertain relevance to clinical actions.

Following oral administration, ETHMOZINE® undergoes significant first-pass metabolism resulting in an absolute bioavailability of approximately 38%. Peak plasma concentrations of ETHMOZINE® are usually reached within 0.5–2 hours. Administration 30 minutes after a meal delays the rate of absorption, resulting in lower peak plasma concentrations, but the extent of absorption is not altered. ETHMOZINE® plasma levels are proportional to dose over the recommended therapeutic dose range.

The apparent volume of distribution after oral administration is very large (≥300L) and is not significantly related to body weight. ETHMOZINE® is approximately 95% bound to human plasma proteins. This binding interaction is independent of ETHMOZINE® plasma concentration.

ETHMOZINE® undergoes extensive biotransformation. Less than 1% of orally administered ETHMOZINE® is excreted unchanged in the urine. There are at least 26 metabolites, but no single metabolite has been found to represent as much as 1% of the administered dose, and as stated above, antiarrhythmic response has relatively slow onset and offset. Two metabolites are pharmacologically active in at least one animal model: moricizine sulfoxide and phenothiazine-2-carbamic acid ethyl ester sulfoxide. Each of these metabolites represents a small percentage of the administered dose (<0.6%), is present in lower concentrations in the plasma than the parent drug, and has a plasma elimination half-life of approximately three hours.

ETHMOZINE® has been shown to induce its own metabolism. Average ETHMOZINE® plasma concentrations in patients decrease with multiple dosing. This decrease in plasma levels of parent drug does not appear to affect clinical outcome for patients receiving chronic ETHMOZINE® therapy.

The plasma half-life of ETHMOZINE® is 1.5–3.5 hours (most values about 2 hours) following single or multiple oral doses in patients with ventricular ectopy. Approximately 56% of the administered dose is execreted in the feces and 39% is excreted in the urine. Some ETHMOZINE® is also recycled through enterohepatic circulation.

CLINICAL ACTIONS

ETHMOZINE® at daily doses of 600–900 mg produces a dose- related reduction in the occurrence of frequent ventricular premature depolarizations (VPDs) and reduces the incidence of nonsustained and sustained ventricular tachycardia (VT). In controlled clinical trials, ETHMOZINE® has been shown to have antiarrhythmic activity that is generally similar to that of disopyramide, propranolol, and quinidine at the doses studied. In controlled and compassionate use programmed electrical stimulation studies (PES), ETHMOZINE® prevented the induction of sustained ventricular tachycardia in approximately 25% (19/75) of patients. In a post-marketing randomized comparative PES study, ETHMOZINE® had a response rate of approximately 12% (7/59). Activity of ETHMOZINE® is maintained during long-term use.

ETHMOZINE® is effective in treating ventricular arrhythmias in patients with and without organic heart disease. ETHMOZINE® may be effective in patients in whom other antiarrhythmic agents are ineffective, not tolerated and/or contraindicated.

Arrhythmia exacerbation or "rebound" is not noted following discontinuation of ETHMOZINE® therapy.

INDICATIONS AND USAGE

ETHMOZINE® is indicated for the treatment of documented ventricular arrhythmias, such as sustained ventricular tachycardia, that, in the judgement of the physician are life- threatening. Because of the proarrhythmic effects of ETHMOZINE®, its use with lesser arrhythmias is generally not recommended. Treatment of patients with asymptomatic ventricular premature contractions should be avoided.

Initiation of ETHMOZINE® treatment, as with other antiarrhythmic agents used to treat life-threatening arrhythmias, should be carried out in the hospital.

Antiarrhythmic drugs have not been shown to enhance survival in patients with ventricular arrhythmias.

CONTRAINDICATIONS

ETHMOZINE® (moricizine hydrochloride) is contraindicated in patients with pre-existing second- or third-degree AV block and in patients with right bundle branch block when associated with left hemiblock (bifascicular block) unless a pacemaker is present. ETHMOZINE® is also contraindicated in the presence of cardiogenic shock or known hypersensitivity to the drug.

WARNINGS

Mortality

ETHMOZINE® was one of three antiarrhythmic drugs included in the National Heart Lung and Blood Institute's Cardiac Arrhythmia Suppression Trial (CAST), a long-term multi-center, randomized, double-blind study in patients with asymptomatic non-life-threatening ventricular arrhythmias who had a myocardial infarction more than 6 days, but less than 2 years, previously. An excessive mortality or nonfatal cardiac arrest rate was seen in patients treated with both of the other agents included in the trial, which led to discontinuation of those 2 arms of the trial. The average duration of treatment with these agents was 10 months. The ETHMOZINE® and placebo arms of the trial were continued in the NHLBI sponsored CAST II. In this randomized, double-blind trial, patients with asymptomatic, non-life-threatening arrhythmias who had had a myocardial infarction within 4 to 90 days and left ventricular ejection fraction ≤0.40 prior to enrollment were evaluated. The average duration of treatment with ETHMOZINE® in this study was 18 months. The study was discontinued because there was no possibility of demonstrating a benefit toward improved survival with ETHMOZINE® and because of an evolving adverse trend after long-term treatment.

The applicability of the CAST results to other populations (e.g. those without recent myocardial infarction) is uncertain. Considering the known proarrhythmic properties of ETHMOZINE® and the lack of evidence of improved survival for any antiarrhythmic drug in patients without life-threatening arrhythmias, the use of ETHMOZINE®, as well as other antiarrhythmic agents, should be reserved for patients with structural heart disease.

Proarrhythmia

Like other antiarrhythmic drugs, ETHMOZINE® can provoke new rhythm disturbances or make existing arrhythmias worse. These proarrhythmic effects can range from an increase in the frequency of VPDs to the development of new or more severe ventricular tachycardia, e.g., tachycardia that is more sustained or more resistant to conversion to sinus rhythm, with potentially fatal consequences. It is often not possible to distinguish a proarrhythmic effect from the patient's underlying rhythm disorder, so that the occurrence rates given below must be considered approximations. Note also that drug-induced arrhythmias can generally be identified only when they occur early after starting the drug and when the rhythm can be identified, usually because the patient is being monitored. It is clear from the NIH sponsored CAST (Cardiac Arrhythmia Suppression Trial) that some antiarrhythmic drugs can cause increased sudden death mortality, presumably due to new arrhythmias or asystole that do not appear early after treatment but that represent a sustained increased risk.

Domestic pre-marketing trials included 1072 patients given ETHMOZINE®; 397 had baseline lethal arrhythmias (sustained VT or VF and non-sustained VT with hemodynamic symptoms) and 576 had potentially lethal arrhythmias (increased VPDs or NSVT in patients with known structural heart disease, active ischemia, congestive heart failure or an LVEF<40% and/or CI<2.0 l/min/m²). In this population there were 40 (3.7%) identified proarrhythmic events, 26 (2.5%) of which were serious, either fatal (6), new hemodynamically significant sustained VT or VF (4), new sustained VT that was not hemodynamically significant (11) or sustained VT that became syncopal/presyncopal when it had not been before (5). Proarrhythmic effects described as incessant ventricular tachycardia were observed in the post-marketing PES study and in post-marketing adverse event reports.

In general, serious proarrhythmic effects in the domestic pre-marketing trials were equally common in patients with more and less severe arrhythmias, 2.5% in the patients with baseline lethal arrhythmias vs. 2.8% in patients with potentially lethal arrhythmias, although the patients with serious effects were more likely to have a history of sustained VT (38% vs. 23%). In the post-marketing comparative PES study, patients treated with ETHMOZINE® (250–300 mg TID) had a proarrhythmia rate of 14% (8/59).

Five of the six fatal proarrhythmic events were in patients with baseline lethal arrhythmias; four had prior cardiac arrests. Rates and severity of proarrhythmic events were similar in patients given 600–900 mg of ETHMOZINE® per day and those given higher doses. Patients with proarrhythmic events were more likely than the overall population to have coronary artery disease (85% vs. 67%), history of acute myocardial infarction (75% vs. 53%), congestive heart failure (60% vs. 43%), and cardiomegaly (55% vs. 33%). All of the six proarrhythmic deaths were in patients with coronary artery disease; 5/6 each had documented acute myocardial infarction, congestive heart failure, and cardiomegaly.

Electrolyte Disturbances

Hypokalemia, hyperkalemia, or hypomagnesemia may alter the effects of Class I antiarrhythmic drugs. Electrolyte imbalances should be corrected before administration of ETHMOZINE®.

Sick Sinus Syndrome

ETHMOZINE® should be used only with extreme caution in patients with sick sinus syndrome, as it may cause sinus bradycardia, sinus pause or sinus arrest.

PRECAUTIONS

General:

Electrocardiographic Changes/Conduction Abnormalities

ETHMOZINE® slows AV nodal and intraventricular conduction, producing dose-related increases in the PR and QRS intervals. In clinical trials, the average increase in the PR interval was 12% and the QRS interval was 14%. Although

the QTC interval is increased, this is wholly because of QRS prolongation; the JT interval is shortened, indicating the absence of significant slowing of ventricular repolarization. The degree of lengthening of PR and QRS intervals does not predict efficacy.

In controlled clinical trials and in open studies, the overall incidence of delayed ventricular conduction, including new bundle branch block pattern, was approximately 9.4%. In patients without baseline conduction abnormalities, the frequency of second-degree AV block was 0.2% and third-degree AV block did not occur. In patients with baseline conduction abnormalities, the frequencies of second-degree AV block and third-degree AV block were 0.9% and 1.4%, respectively.

ETHMOZINE® therapy was discontinued in 1.6% of patients due to electrocardiographic changes (0.6% due to sinus pause or asystole, 0.2% to AV block, 0.2% to junctional rhythm, 0.4% to intraventricular conduction delay, and 0.2% to wide QRS and/or PR interval).

In patients with pre-existing conduction abnormalities, ETHMOZINE® therapy should be initiated cautiously. If second- or third-degree AV block occurs, ETHMOZINE® therapy should be discontinued unless a ventricular pacemaker is in place. When changing the dose of ETHMOZINE® or adding concomitant medications which may also affect cardiac conduction, patients should be monitored electrocardiographically.

Hepatic Impairment

Patients with significant liver dysfunction have reduced plasma clearance and an increased half-life of ETHMOZINE®. Although the precise relationship of ETHMOZINE® levels to effect is not clear, patients with hepatic disease should be treated with lower doses and closely monitored for excessive pharmacological effects, including effects on ECG intervals, before dosage adjustment. Patients with severe liver disease should be administered ETHMOZINE® with particular care, if at all (See DOSAGE AND ADMINISTRATION).

Renal Impairment

Plasma levels of intact ETHMOZINE® are unchanged in hemodialysis patients, but a significant portion (39%) of ETHMOZINE® is metabolized and excreted in the urine. Although no identified active metabolite is known to increase in people with renal failure, metabolites of unrecognized importance could be affected. For this reason, ETHMOZINE® should be administered cautiously in patients with impaired renal function. Patients with significant renal dysfunction should be started on lower doses and monitored for excessive pharmacologic effects, including ECG intervals, before dosage adjustment (See DOSAGE AND ADMINISTRATION).

Congestive Heart Failure

Most patients with congestive heart failure have tolerated the recommended ETHMOZINE® daily doses without unusual toxicity or change in effect. Pharmacokinetic differences between ETHMOZINE® patients with and without congestive heart failure were not apparent (See Hepatic Impairment above). In some cases, worsened heart failure has been attributed to ETHMOZINE®. Patients with pre-existing heart failure should be monitored carefully when ETHMOZINE® is initiated.

Effects on Pacemaker Threshold

The effect of ETHMOZINE® on the sensing and pacing thresholds of artificial pacemakers has not been sufficiently studied. In such patients, pacing parameters must be monitored, if ETHMOZINE® is used.

Drug Interactions

No significant changes in serum digoxin levels or pharmacokinetics have been observed in patients or healthy subjects receiving concomitant ETHMOZINE® therapy. Concomitant use was associated with additive prolongation of the PR interval, but not with a significant increase in the rate of second- or third-degree AV block.

Concomitant administration of cimetidine resulted in a decrease in ETHMOZINE® clearance of 49% and a 1.4 fold increase in plasma levels in healthy subjects. During clinical trials, no significant changes in the efficacy or tolerance of ETHMOZINE® have been observed in patients receiving concomitant cimetidine therapy. Patients on cimetidine should have ETHMOZINE® therapy initiated at relatively low doses, not more than 600 mg/day. Patients should be monitored when concomitant cimetidine therapy is instituted or discontinued or when the ETHMOZINE® dose is changed.

Concomitant administration of beta blocker therapy did not reveal significant changes in overall electrocardiographic intervals in patients. In one controlled study, ETHMOZINE® (moricizine hydrochloride) and propranolol administered concomitantly produced a small additive increase in the PR interval.

Theophylline clearance and plasma half-life were significantly affected by multiple dose ETHMOZINE® administration when both conventional and sustained release theophylline were given to healthy subjects (clearance increased 44–66% and plasma half-life decreased 19–33%). Plasma theophylline levels should be monitored when concomitant ETHMOZINE® is initiated or discontinued.

Because of possible additive pharmocologic effects, caution is indicated when ETHMOZINE® is used with any drug that affects cardiac electrophysiology. Uncontrolled experience in patients indicates no serious adverse interaction during the concomitant use of ETHMOZINE® and diuretics, vasodilators, antihypertensive drugs, calcium channel blockers, beta-blockers, angiotensin-converting enzyme inhibitors, or warfarin. Plasma warfarin levels, warfarin pharmacokinetics, and prothrombin times were unaffected during multiple dose ETHMOZINE® administration to young, healthy, male subjects in a controlled study. However, there are isolated reports of the need to either increase or decrease warfarin doses after initiation of ETHMOZINE®. Some patients who were taking warfarin with a stable prothrombin time experienced excessive prolongation of the prothrombin time following the initiation of ETHMOZINE®. In some cases, liver enzymes also were elevated. Bleeding or bruising may occur. When ETHMOZINE® is started or stopped in a patient stabilized on warfarin, more frequent prothrombin time monitoring is advisable.

Results from *in vitro* studies do not suggest alterations in ETHMOZINE plasma protein binding in the presence of other highly plasma protein bound drugs.

CARCINOGENESIS, MUTAGENESIS, IMPAIRMENT OF FERTILITY

In a 24-month mouse study in which ETHMOZINE® was administered in the feed at concentrations calculated to provide doses ranging up to 320 mg/kg/day, ovarian tubular adenomas and granulosa cell tumors were limited in occurrence to ETHMOZINE® treated animals. Although the findings were of borderline statistical significance, or not statistically significant, historical control data indicate that both of these tumors are uncommon in the strain of mouse studied.

In a 24-month study in which ETHMOZINE® was administered by gavage to rats at doses of 25, 50 and 100 mg/kg/day, Zymbal's Gland Carcinoma was observed in one mid-dose and two high-dose males. This tumor appears to be uncommon in the strain of rat studied. Rats of both sexes showed a dose-related increase in hepatocellular cholangioma (also described as bile ductile cystadenoma or cystic hyperplasia) along with fatty metamorphosis, possibly due to disruption of hepatic choline utilization for phospholipid biosynthesis. The rat is known to be uniquely sensitive to alteration in choline metabolism.

ETHMOZINE® was not mutagenic when assayed for genotoxicity in *in vitro* bacterial (Ames test) and mammalian (Chinese hamster ovary/hypoxanthine-guanine phosphoribosyl transferase and sister chromatid exchange) cell systems or in *in vivo* mammalian systems (rat bone cytogenicity and mouse micronucleus).

A general reproduction and fertility study was conducted in rats at dose levels up to 6.7 times the maximum recommended human dose of 900 mg/day (based upon 50 kg human body weight) and revealed no evidence of impaired male or female fertility.

Pregnancy—Teratogenic Effects:

Pregnancy Category B

Teratology studies have been performed with ETHMOZINE® in rats and in rabbits at doses up to 6.7 and 4.7 times the maximum recommended human daily dose, respectively, and have revealed no evidence of harm to the fetus. There are, however, no adequate and well-controlled studies in pregnant women. Because animal reproduction studies are not always predictive of human response, ETHMOZINE® should be used during pregnancy only if clearly needed.

Pregnancy—Nonteratogenic Effects:

In a study in which rats were dosed with ETHMOZINE® prior to mating, during mating and throughout gestation and lactation, dose levels 3.4 and 6.7 times the maximum recommended human daily dose produced a dose-related decrease in pup and maternal weight gain, possibly related to a larger litter size. In a study in which dosing was begun on Day 15 of gestation, ETHMOZINE®, at a level 6.7 times the maximum recommended human daily dose, produced a retardation in maternal weight gain but no effect on pup growth.

Nursing Mothers

ETHMOZINE® is secreted in the milk of laboratory animals and has been reported to be present in human milk. Because of the potential for serious adverse reactions in nursing infants from ETHMOZINE®, a decision should be made whether to discontinue the drug, taking into account the importance of the drug to the mother.

Pediatric Use

The safety and effectiveness of ETHMOZINE® in children less than 18 years of age have not been established.

ADVERSE REACTIONS

The most serious adverse reaction reported for ETHMOZINE® is proarrhythmia (see WARNINGS). This occurred in 3.7% of 1072 patients with ventricular arrhythmias who received a wide range of doses under a variety of circumstances.

In addition to discontinuations because of proarrhythmias, in controlled clinical trials and in open studies, adverse reactions led to discontinuation of ETHMOZINE® in 7% of 1105 patients with ventricular and supraventricular arrhythmias, including 3.2% due to nausea, 1.6% due to ECG abnormalities (principally conduction defects, sinus pause, junctional rhythm, or AV block), 1% due to congestive heart failure and 0.3–0.4% due to dizziness, anxiety, drug fever, urinary retention, blurred vision, gastrointestinal upset, rash, and laboratory abnormalities.

The most frequently occurring adverse reactions in the 1072 patients (including all adverse experiences whether or not considered ETHMOZINE®-related by the investigator) were dizziness (15.1%), nausea (9.6%), headache (8.0%), fatigue (5.9%), palpitations (5.8%) and dyspnea (5.7%). Dizziness appears to be related to the size of each dose. In a comparison of 900 mg/day given at 450 mg b.i.d. or 300 mg t.i.d., more than 20% of patients experienced dizziness on the b.i.d. regimen vs. 12% on the t.i.d. regimen.

Adverse reactions reported by less than 5%, but in 2% or greater of the patients were: sustained ventricular tachycardia, hypesthesias, abdominal pain, dyspepsia, vomiting, sweating, cardiac chest pain, asthenia, nervousness, paresthesias, congestive heart failure, musculoskeletal pain, diarrhea, dry mouth, cardiac death, sleep disorders and blurred vision.

Adverse reactions infrequently reported (in less than 2% of the patients) were:

Cardiovascular—hypotension, hypertension, syncope, supraventricular arrhythmias (including atrial fibrillation/flutter), cardiac arrest, bradycardia, pulmonary embolism, myocardial infarction, vasodilation, cerebrovascular events, thrombophlebitis;

Nervous System—tremor, anxiety, depression, euphoria, confusion, somnolence, agitation, seizure, coma, abnormal gait, hallucinations, nystagmus, diplopia, speech disorder, akathisia, loss of memory, ataxia, abnormal coordination, dyskinesia, vertigo, tinnitus;

Genitourinary—urinary retention or frequency, dysuria, urinary incontinence, kidney pain, impotence, decreased libido;

Respiratory—hyperventilation, apnea, asthma, pharyngitis, cough, sinusitus;

Gastrointestinal—anorexia, bitter taste, dysphagia, flatulence, ileus;

Other—drug fever, hypothermia, temperature intolerence, eye pain, rash, pruritus, dry skin, urticaria, swelling of the lips and tongue, periorbital edema.

During ETHMOZINE® therapy, two patients developed thrombocytopenia that may have been drug-related. Clinically significant elevations in liver function tests (bilirubin, serum transaminases) and jaundice consistent with hepatitis were rarely reported. Although a cause and effect relationship has not been established, caution is advised in patients who develop unexplained signs of hepatic dysfunction, and consideration should be given to discontinuing therapy.

Three patients developed rechallenge-confirmed drug fever, with one patient experiencing an elevation above 103°F (to 105°F. with rigors). Fevers occurred at about 2 weeks in 2 cases, and after 21 weeks in the third. Fevers resolved within 48 hours of discontinuation of moricizine.

Adverse reactions were generally similar in patients over 65 (n=375) and under 65 (n=697), although discontinuation of therapy for reasons other than proarrhythmia was more common in older patients (13.9% vs. 7.7%). Overall mortality was greater in older patients (9.3% vs. 3.9%), but those were not deaths attributed to treatment and the older patients had more serious underlying heart disease.

The following table compares the most common (occurrence in more than 2% of the patients) non-cardiac adverse reactions (i.e., drug-related or of unknown relationship) in controlled clinical trials during the first one to two weeks of therapy with ETHMOZINE®, quinidine, placebo, disopyramide, or propranolol in patients with ventricular arrhythmias.

[See table at top of next page.]

OVERDOSAGE

Deaths have occurred after accidental or intentional overdosages of 2,250 and 10,000 mg of ETHMOZINE® (moricizine hydrochloride), respectively.

Signs, Symptoms and Laboratory Findings Associated with an Overdosage of Drug

Overdosage with ETHMOZINE® may produce emesis, lethargy, coma, syncope, hypotension, conduction disturbances, exacerbation of congestive heart failure, myocardial infarction, sinus arrest, arrhythmias (including junctional bradycardia, ventricular tachycardia, ventricular fibrillation and asystole), and respiratory failure.

Lethal Dose in Animals

Oral doses of ETHMOZINE® of about 200 mg/kg in dogs, 250 mg/kg in monkeys, 420 mg/kg in mice and 905 mg/kg in rats were lethal to about one-half of the animals exposed.

Continued on next page

Roberts—Cont.

INCIDENCE (%) OF THE MOST COMMON ADVERSE REACTIONS (THERAPY DURATION = 1–14 DAYS)

Adverse Reactions	>2% Moricizine No.	%	>2% Placebo No.	%	>2% Quinidine No.	%	>5% Disopyramide No.	%	>5% Propranolol No.	%
Total No. of Patients	1072		618		110		31		24	
Dizziness	121	11.3	33	5.3	8	7.3	—		2	8.3
Nausea	74	6.9	18	2.9	7	6.4	3	9.7	—	
Headache	62	5.8	27	4.4	—		—		4	16.7
Pain	41	3.8	31	5.0	6	5.5	2	6.5	—	
Dyspnea	41	3.8	22	3.6	—		—		—	
Hypesthesia	40	3.7	—		3	2.7	—		—	
Fatigue	33	3.1	16	2.6	6	5.5	2	6.5	3	12.5
Vomiting	22	2.1	—		—		—		—	
Dry Mouth	—		—		—		11	35.5	—	
Nervousness	—		—		—		3	9.7	—	
Blurred vision	—		—		3	2.7	2	6.5	3	12.5
Diarrhea	—		—		25	22.7	—		—	
Constipation	—		—		—		2	6.5	—	
Somnolence	—		—		—		—		2	8.3
Urinary Retention	—		—		—		4	12.9	—	

Death was usually preceded by tremors, convulsions and respiratory depression.

Recommended General Treatment Procedures

A specific antidote for ETHMOZINE® has not been identified. In the event of overdosage, treatment should be supportive. Patients should be hospitalized and monitored for cardiac, respiratory and CNS changes. Advanced life support systems, including an intracardiac pacing catheter, should be provided where necessary. Acute overdosage should be treated with appropriate gastric evacuation, and with special care to avoid aspiration. Accidental introduction of ETHMOZINE® into the lungs of monkeys resulted in rapid arrhythmic death.

DOSAGE AND ADMINISTRATION

The dosage of ETHMOZINE® must be individualized on the basis of antiarrhythmic response and tolerance. Clinical, cardiac rhythm monitoring, electrocardiogram intervals, exercise testing, and/or programmed electrical stimulation testing may be used to guide antiarrhythmic response and dosage adjustment. In general, the patients will be at high risk and should be hospitalized for the initiation of therapy (see INDICATIONS AND USAGE).

The usual adult dosage is between 600 and 900 mg per day, given every 8 hours in three equally divided doses. Within this range, the dosage can be adjusted as tolerated, in increments of 150 mg/day at 3-day intervals, until the desired effect is obtained. Patients with life-threatening arrhythmias who exhibit a beneficial response as judged by objective criteria (Holter monitoring, programmed electrical stimulation, exercise testing, etc.) can be maintained on chronic ETHMOZINE® therapy. As the antiarrhythmic effect of ETHMOZINE® persists for more than 12 hours, some patients whose arrhythmias are well-controlled on a Q8H regimen may be given the same total daily dose in a Q12H regimen to increase convenience and help assure compliance. When higher doses are used, patients may experience more dizziness and nausea on the Q12 hour regimen.

Patients with Hepatic Impairment

Patients with hepatic disease should be started at 600 mg/day or lower and monitored closely, including measurement of ECG intervals, before dosage adjustment.

Patients with Renal Impairment

Patients with significant renal dysfunction should be started at 600mg/day or lower and monitored closely, including measurement of ECG intervals, before dosage adjustment.

Transfer to ETHMOZINE®

Recommendations for transferring patients from another antiarrhythmic to ETHMOZINE® can be given based on theoretical considerations. Previous antiarrhythmic therapy should be withdrawn for 1–2 plasma half-lives before starting ETHMOZINE® at the recommended dosages. In patients in whom withdrawal of a previous antiarrhythmic is likely to produce life-threatening arrhythmias, hospitalization is recommended.

Transferred From	Start ETHMOZINE®
Quinidine, Disopyramide	6–12 hours after last dose
Procainamide	3–6 hours after last dose
Encainide, Propafenone, Tocainide, or Mexiletine	8–12 hours after last dose
Flecainide	12–24 hours after last dose

HOW SUPPLIED

ETHMOZINE® (moricizine hydrochloride) is available as oval, convex, film-coated tablets as follows:

200 mg (light green): Bottles of 100 (NDC 54092-046-01) Hospital Unit Dose Carton of 100 (NDC 54092-046-52)

250 mg (light orange): Bottles of 100 (NDC 54092-047-01) Hospital Unit Dose Carton of 100 (NDC 54092-047-52)

300 mg (light blue): Bottles of 100 (NDC 54092-048-01) Hospital Unit Dose Carton of 100 (NDC 54092-048-52)

Store from 15°–30°C (59°–86°F) in a tightly-closed, light resistant container. Protect from light.

Manufactured for:
Roberts Laboratories Inc.
a wholly owned subsidiary of
Roberts Pharmaceutical Corporation
Eatontown, New Jersey 07724
US Patent 3,864,487

Shown in Product Identification Guide, page 331

FURACIN® topical cream ℞
[fewr' a-sin]
(nitrofurazone)

FURACIN® soluble dressing ℞
[fewr' a-sin]
(nitrofurazone)

DESCRIPTION

Chemically, Furacin is nitrofurazone, 2-[(5-nitro-2- furanyl)-methylene]hydrazinecarboxamide, with the following structure:

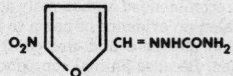

O_2N ... $CH = NNHCONH_2$

Furacin soluble dressing is a preparation containing 0.2% nitrofurazone in Solubase® (a water-soluble base of polyethylene glycols 3350, 900, and 300).
Furacin Soluble Dressing is an antibacterial agent for topical use.
Furacin topical cream is a preparation containing 0.2% Furacin in a water-miscible base consisting of glycerin, cetyl alcohol, mineral oil, an ethoxylated fatty alcohol, methylparaben, propylparaben, and purified water.
Furacin Topical Cream is an antibacterial agent for topical use.

CLINICAL PHARMACOLOGY

Furacin nitrofurazone soluble dressing and topical cream are a nitrofuran that is bactericidal for most pathogens commonly causing surface infections, including *Staphylococcus aureus*, *Streptococcus*, *Escherichia coli*, *Clostridium perfringens*, *Aerobacter aerogenes*, and *Proteus*.
Furacin soluble dressing and topical cream inhibits a number of bacterial enzymes, especially those involved in the aerobic and anaerobic degradation of glucose and pyruvate. The activity appears to involve the pyruvate dehydrogenase system as well as citrate synthetase, malate dehydrogenase, glutathione reductase, and pyruvate decarboxylase. Glutathione reductase inhibition may be caused by control of pentose phosphate metabolism. Although Furacin soluble dressing and topical cream inhibits a variety of enzymes, it is not considered to be a general enzyme inactivator since many enzymes are not inhibited by this compound.

INDICATIONS AND USAGE

Furacin soluble dressing and topical cream are a topical antibacterial agent indicated for adjunctive therapy of patients with second- and third-degree burns when bacterial resistance to other agents is a real or potential problem.
It is also indicated in skin grafting where bacterial contamination may cause graft rejection and/or donor site infection particularly in hospitals with historical resistant-bacteria epidemics.
There is no known evidence of effectiveness of this product in the treatment of minor burns or surface bacterial infections involving wounds, cutaneous ulcers, or the various pyodermas.

CONTRAINDICATIONS

Known sensitization to any of the components of this preparation is a contraindication for use.

WARNINGS

None

PRECAUTIONS

General: Use of topical antimicrobials occasionally allows overgrowth of nonsusceptible organisms including fungi. If this occurs, or if irritation, sensitization or superinfection develops, treatment with Furacin Soluble Dressing should be discontinued and appropriate therapy instituted.
General: Use of Furacin topical cream occasionally allows overgrowth of nonsusceptible organisms including fungi and *Pseudomonas*. If this occurs, or if irritation, sensitization or superinfection develops, treatment with Furacin topical cream should be discontinued and appropriate therapy instituted.
Carcinogenesis, Mutagenesis, and Impairment of Fertility: Nitrofurazone has been shown to produce mammary tumors when fed at high doses to female Sprague-Dawley rats. The relevance of this to topical use in humans is unknown. *Dietary* dosage levels of 60 and 30 mg/kg/day shortened the onset time of the typical mammary gland tumors associated with older female rats. These tumors exhibited the same histological characteristics seen in the spontaneously occurring tumors, and were seen only in the female animals. No mammary tumors were seen in rats treated with nitrofurazone orally in the diet for 1 year at levels of approximately 11 mg/kg/day. Spermatogenic arrest was noted in the male rats in dietary dosage levels of 30 mg/kg/day and above, after one year on test.
Pregnancy: Pregnancy Category C: Nitrofurazone has been shown to have an embryocidal effect in rabbits when given in oral doses thirty times the human dose. There are no adequate and well controlled studies in pregnant women. Furacin soluble dressing and Furacin topical cream should be used during pregnancy only if the potential benefit justifies the potential risk to the fetus.
Nursing mothers: It is not known whether this drug is excreted in human milk. Because many drugs are excreted in human milk and because of the potential for tumorigenicity shown for nitrofurazone in animal studies, a decision should be made whether to discontinue nursing or to discontinue the drug, taking into account the importance of the drug to the mother.
Pediatric use: Safety and effectiveness in children have not been established.

ADVERSE REACTIONS

Instances of clinical skin reactions have been reported for patients treated with Furacin formulations. Symptoms appear as varying degrees of contact dermatitides such as rash, pruritus, and local edema. Although the exact incidence such reactions is difficult to determine, historically, a survey of world literature and clinical data indicates an overall incidence of approximately 1%. Allergic reactions to Furacin soluble dressing and Furacin topical cream should be treated symptomatically.

DOSAGE AND ADMINISTRATION

Apply Furacin soluble dressing directly to the lesion with a spatula, or first place on gauze. Impregnated gauze may be used. Reapply depending on the preferred dressing technique. Flushing the dressing with sterile saline facilitates its removal.
Apply Furacin topical cream directly to the lesion, or first place on gauze. Reapply once daily or every few days, depending on the usual dressing technique.

PREPARATION OF IMPREGNATED GAUZE

Sterile gauze strips are placed in a tray and covered with Furacin Soluble Dressing. Repeat the procedure, adding several layers of gauze for each layer of Furacin Soluble Dressing. Sprinkling a little sterile water on each layer of dressing will minimize any color change from autoclaving. Cover the tray very loosely and autoclave at 121°C for 30 minutes at 15 to 20 pounds pressure. To impregnate bandage rolls, place some Furacin Soluble Dressing in the bottom of a glass jar. Stand rolls on end. Place more Furacin Soluble Dressing on top. Cover top of jar with aluminum foil. Autoclave at 121°C for 45 minutes to 20 pounds pressure. Do not

store impregnated bandage rolls for more than 24 hours. Autoclaving more than once is not recommended.

ANIMAL TOXICOLOGY

The oral administration of nitrofurazone for 7 days to rats at extremely high dosage levels of 240 mg/kg/day produced severe hepatorenal lesions whereas only renal changes were seen when the dosage level was reduced to 60 mg/kg/day for 60 days. Dogs treated orally with nitrofurazone for 400 days at levels of 11 mg/kg/day showed no toxic effects related to drug treatment. The single intravenous administration in dogs of 20, 35, or 75 mg/kg nitrofurazone produced clinical signs of lacrimation, salivation, emesis, diarrhea, excitation, weakness, ataxia, and weight loss, whereas 100 mg/kg/day produced convulsions and death. There was no evidence of toxicosis in rhesus monkeys treated with doses of nitrofurazone as high as 58 mg/kg/day for 10 weeks and 23 mg/kg/day for 63 weeks. The peroral LD 50 of nitrofurazone in mice and rats is 747 and 590 mg/kg/respectively. For bacterial sensitivity tests: **Furacin** Sensi-Discs are available from BBL, Division of BioQuest or BBL Microbiology Systems, Becton Dickinson and Co.

HOW SUPPLIED

Furacin soluble dressing is available in:
NDC 54092-310-28 tube of 28 grams
NDC 54092-310-56 tube of 56 grams
NDC 54092-310-16 jar of 454 grams
Furacin topical cream is available in:
NDC 54092-311-28 tube of 28 grams
Storage: Avoid exposure to direct sunlight, strong fluorescent lighting, alkaline materials, and excessive heat (over 104°F or 40°C).

CAUTION

Federal law prohibits dispensing without prescription.
Manufactured for
Roberts Laboratories Inc.,
a subsidiary of
ROBERTS PHARMACEUTICAL CORPORATION
Eatontown, New Jersey 07724 USA
by Procter & Gamble Pharmaceuticals
Norwich, NY 13815

FUROXONE® ℞
[*fewr-ox 'ōne*]
(furazolidone)
Tablets and Liquid

DESCRIPTION

Furoxone (furazolidone) is one of the synthetic antimicrobial nitrofurans. It is a stable, yellow, crystalline compound with the following structure:

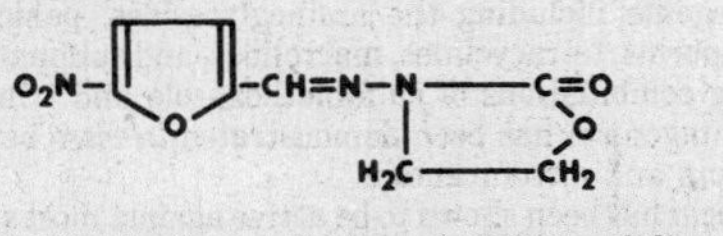

3-(5-nitrofurfurylideneamino)-2-oxazolidinone

Inactive Ingredients: Furoxone tablets contain calcium pyrophosphate, FD&C Blue #2, magnesium stearate, starch, and sucrose. Furoxone liquid contains carboxymethylcellulose sodium, flavors, glycerin, magnesium aluminum silicate, methylparaben, propylparaben, purified water, and saccharin sodium.

ACTION

Furoxone has a broad antibacterial spectrum covering the majority of gastrointestinal tract pathogens including *E. coli*, staphylococci, *Salmonella, Shigella, Proteus, Aerobacter aerogenes, Vibrio cholerae*[9,10,11] and *Giardia lamblia*.[5,6] Its bactericidal activity is based upon its interference with several bacterial enzyme systems; this antimicrobial action minimizes the development of resistant organisms. It neither significantly alters the normal bowel flora nor results in fungal overgrowth. The brown color found in the urine with adequate dosage is of no clinical significance.

INDICATIONS

Indicated in the specific and symptomatic treatment of bacterial or protozoal diarrhea and enteritis caused by susceptible organisms. Furoxone products are well tolerated, have a very low incidence of adverse reactions.

CONTRAINDICATIONS

1. To obviate an Antabuse® (disulfiram)-like reaction which may occur in some patients, the ingestion of alcohol should be avoided during or within four days after Furoxone therapy (see ADVERSE REACTIONS).
2. IN GENERAL MAOI DRUGS, TYRAMINE-CONTAINING FOODS AND INDIRECTLY-ACTING SYMPATHOMIMETIC AMINES ARE CONTRAINDICATED OR SHOULD BE USED WITH CAUTION IN PATIENTS RECEIVING FUROXONE (SEE PRECAUTIONS).
3. INFANTS UNDER 1 MONTH SHOULD NOT RECEIVE FUROXONE (SEE ADVERSE REACTIONS AND DOSAGE FOR CHILDREN).[4] THE FUROXONE CONCENTRATION IN THE BREAST MILK OF LACTATING WOMEN HAS NOT BEEN DETERMINED. THEREFORE THE SAFETY IN THIS CIRCUMSTANCE HAS NOT BEEN ESTABLISHED.
4. Prior sensitivity to Furoxone is a contraindication.

WARNINGS

(See CONTRAINDICATIONS listed above.)
Use In Pregnancy: The safety of Furoxone during the childbearing age has not been established; as with any potent antibacterial, Furoxone must be administered with caution during the childbearing age. However, animal breeding studies have revealed no evidence of teratogenicity following the administration of Furoxone for long periods of time and at doses far in excess of those recommended for the human. There have been no clinical reports regarding this possible adverse effect on the fetus or the newborn infant.

PRECAUTIONS

Monoamine Oxidase Inhibition:[7] Effective inhibition of monoamine oxidase by furazolidone has been demonstrated experimentally in man by the enhancement of tyramine and amphetamine sensitivity and by the directly measured monoamine oxidase inhibition.
A period of five days of furazolidone administration in the recommended doses in these patients was required to give an enhancement of the tyramine and amphetamine sensitivities by two to threefold. Administration of furazolidone in the recommended dose of 400 mg/day for a period of five days should not subject the adult patient to an undue hazard of hypertensive crisis due to monoamine oxidase inhibition. Hypertensive crises have never been reported even after the peroral administration of larger doses and/or for doses given over longer periods of time. Controlled studies reveal no signs or symptoms of hypertensive crisis even after the peroral administration of Furoxone in doses of 400 mg/day in excess of 48 consecutive months.[8]
If administered in doses larger than recommended or in excess of five days, the indications must be weighed against the possible hazards of hypertensive crisis related to the accumulation of monoamine oxidase inhibition. If indications are sufficient, the patients should be informed of drugs and foods which predispose to hypertensive crises:

(A) Other known MAOI drugs; however, when indicated they should be prescribed with caution and at a reduced dosage.
(B) Tyramine-containing foods such as broad beans, yeast extracts, strong unpasteurized cheeses, beer, wine, pickled herring, chicken livers, and fermented products are contraindicated.
(C) Indirectly-acting sympathomimetic amines such as those found in nasal decongestants (phenylephrine, ephedrine) and anorectics (amphetamines) are contraindicated.
(D) Likewise, sedatives, antihistamines, tranquilizers, and narcotics should be used in reduced dosages and with caution.

Orthostatic hypotension and hypoglycemia may occur.
Carcinogenesis, Mutagenesis, Impairment of Fertility: Furazolidone has shown evidence of tumorigenic activity in several studies involving chronic, high-dose oral administration to rodents. Promotion of the development of mammary neoplasia has been demonstrated in rats of two strains. Prominent among the findings in mice was that furazolidone caused significant increases in malignant lung tumors. The relevance of these animal findings, particularly in relationship to short-term therapy in humans, is not established.

ADVERSE REACTIONS

A few hypersensitivity reactions to Furoxone have been reported including a fall in blood pressure, urticaria, fever, arthralgia, and a vesicular morbilliform rash. These reactions subsided following withdrawal of the drug.
Nausea, emesis, headache, or malaise occur occasionally and may be minimized or eliminated by reduction in dosage or withdrawal of the drug.
Rarely, individuals receiving Furoxone have exhibited an Antabuse® (disulfiram)-like reaction to alcohol characterized by flushing, slight temperature elevation, dyspnea, and in some instances, a sense of constriction within the chest. All symptomatology disappeared within 24 hours with no lasting ill effects. During nine years of clinical use and approximately 3.5 million courses of therapy (in the U.S.A. alone) in the published literature and documented case reports 43 cases have been reported—of which 14 were produced under experimental conditions with planned doses of the compound in excess of those recommended.
Three of these experienced a fall in blood pressure necessitating active therapy. Indications are that levarterenol (Levophed®) may be used to combat such hypotensive episodes since human studies show that this drug is not potentiated in patients treated with Furoxone. (Indirectly acting pressor agents should be avoided.) The ingestion of alcohol in any form should be avoided during Furoxone therapy and for four days thereafter to prevent this reaction.
Furoxone may cause mild reversible intravascular hemolysis in certain ethnic groups of Mediterranean and Near-Eastern origin, and Negroes.[1,3] This is due to an intrinsic defect of red blood cell metabolism in a small percentage of these ethnic groups, making them unusually susceptible to hemolysis by numerous compounds.[2] It is necessary to observe such patients closely while receiving Furoxone and to discontinue its use if there is any indication of hemolysis.
Should not be administered to infants under 1 month of age because of the possibility of producing a hemolytic anemia due to immature enzyme systems (glutathione instability) in the early neonatal period.[4]
Colitis, proctitis, anal pruritus, staphylococcic enteritis and renal or hepatic toxicity have not been a significant problem with Furoxone.

DOSAGE AND ADMINISTRATION

FUROXONE TABLETS, 100 mg each, are green and scored to facilitate adjustment of dosage.
Average Adult Dosage: One 100 mg tablet four times daily.
Average Dosage for Children: Those 5 years of age or older should receive 25 to 50 mg ($\frac{1}{4}$ to $\frac{1}{2}$ tablet) four times daily. The tablet dosage may be crushed and given in a spoonful of corn syrup.
FUROXONE LIQUID composition: each 15 ml tablespoonful contains Furoxone 50 mg per 15 ml (3.33 mg per ml) in a light-yellow aqueous vehicle. Suitable flavoring, suspending and preservative agents complete the formulation. (See Inactive Ingredients.) It is stable in storage. Prior to administering Furoxone Liquid shake the bottle vigorously. It should be dispensed in amber bottles.
Average Adult Dosage: Two tablespoonfuls four times daily.
Average Dosage for Children:
5 years or older—$\frac{1}{2}$ to 1 tablespoonful four times daily (7.5–15.0 ml)
1 to 4 years old—1 to $1\frac{1}{2}$ teaspoonfuls four times daily (5.0–7.5 ml)
1 month to 1 year—$\frac{1}{2}$ to 1 teaspoonful four times daily (2.5–5.0 ml)
This dosage is based on an average dose of 5 mg of Furoxone per Kg (2.3 mg per lb) of body weight given in four equally divided doses during 24 hours. The maximal dose of 8.8 mg of Furoxone per Kg (4 mg per lb) of body weight per 24 hours should probably not be exceeded because of the possibility of producing nausea or emesis. If these are severe, the dosage should be reduced.
The average case of diarrhea treated with Furoxone will respond within 2 to 5 days of therapy. Occasional patients may require a longer term of therapy. If satisfactory clinical response is not obtained within 7 days it indicates that the pathogen is refractory to Furoxone and the drug should be discontinued. Adjunctive therapy with other antibacterial agents or bismuth salts is not contraindicated. (N.B. Refer to WARNINGS.)
In order to administer furazolidone in doses larger than recommended or in excess of five days the indications must be weighed against the possible hazards of hypertensive crisis related to the accumulation of monoamine oxidase inhibition. If indications are sufficient, the patient should be informed of drugs and foods which predispose to hypertensive crises. (See PRECAUTIONS.)

HOW SUPPLIED

Furoxone Tablets, 100mg each, coded "Roberts 130", are supplied in amber bottles containing 20 tablets NDC 54092-130-20 and 100 tablets NDC 54092-130-01. (Should be dispensed in amber bottles.)
Furoxone Liquid is supplied in amber bottles containing 60 ml NDC 54092-430-60 and 473 ml NDC 54092-430-16. (Should be dispensed in amber bottles.)

REFERENCES

1 Kellermeyer, R.S., Tarlov, A.R., Schrier, S.L., and Alving, A.S.J. Lab. Clin. Med. 52:827–828 (Nov) 1958.
2 Tarlov et al. Arch. Int. Med. 109:209–234, 1962.
3 Kellermeyer et al. J.A.M.A. 180: No. 5, 388–394, 1962.
4 Zinkham, Pediatrics 23:18–32, 1959; Gross & Hurwitz, Pediatrics 22:453, 1958.
5 Fallas Vargas, M Un Nuevo Tratamiento para la Giardiasis (A New Treatment for Giardiasis). Rev. Med. Costa Rica 19:269–284 (July) 1962.
6 Webster, B. H. Furazolidone in the Treatment of Giardiasis. Amer. J. Dig. Diseases 5:618–622 (July) 1960.
7 Oates, J.A., Pettinger, W.A. Inhibition of Monoamine Oxidase by Furazolidone in Man. Data on file: Office of the Medical Director, Roberts Pharmaceutical Corp. Available upon request.
8 Kirsner, Joseph B., M.D., Ph.D. Data on file: Office of the Medical Director, Roberts Pharmaceutical Corp. Available upon request.
9 Neogy, K.N., et al. Furazolidone in Cholera, Journ. Indian Med. Assoc. 48:137, 1967.
10 Chaudhuri, R.N. et al. Furazolidone in Cholera. Lancet 2:909 (Oct 30) 1965.

Continued on next page

Roberts—Cont.

11 Curlin, G. Comparison of Antibiotic Regimens in Cholera. Abstracts of papers, Epidemiological Intelligence Service Conference, Atlanta, Ga., April 11–14, 1967, p. 11.

FUROXONE (FURAZOLIDONE) SENSI-DISCS for laboratory determination of bacterial sensitivity are available from BBL, division of BioQuest.

CAUTION

Federal law prohibits dispensing without prescription.
Store at controlled room temperature: 15°–30°C (59°–86°F). Do not refrigerate.
Manufactured for
Roberts Laboratories Inc.
a subsidiary of
Roberts Pharmaceutical Corporation
Eatontown, New Jersey 07724 USA

NORETHIN™ 1/50M-21 ℞
NORETHIN™ 1/50M-28 ℞
(Norethindrone and Mestranol Tablets USP)

NORETHIN™ 1/35E-21 ℞
NORETHIN™ 1/35E-28 ℞
(Norethindrone and Ethinyl Estradiol Tablets USP)

DESCRIPTION

Norethin™ 1/35E-21 and Norethin™ 1/35-28. Each white tablet contains 1 mg of norethindrone and 35 mcg of ethinyl estradiol, and the inactive ingredients include calcium acetate, calcium phosphate, corn starch, hydrogenated castor oil, and povidone. Each blue tablet in the Norethin 1/35E-28 package is a placebo containing no active ingredients, and the inactive ingredients include calcium sulfate, corn starch, FD&C Blue No. 1 Lake, magnesium stearate, and sucrose.
Norethin™ 1/50M-21 and Norethin™ 1/50M-28. Each white tablet contains 1 mg of norethindrone and 50 mcg of mestranol, and the inactive ingredients include calcium acetate, calcium phosphate, corn starch, hydrogenated castor oil, and povidone. Each blue tablet in the Norethin 1/50M-28 package is a placebo containing no active ingredients, and the inactive ingredients include calcium sulfate, corn starch, FD&C Blue No. 1 Lake, magnesium stearate, and sucrose.
The chemical name for norethindrone is 17-hydroxy-19-nor-17α-preg-4-en-20-yn-3-one, for ethinyl estradiol it is 19-nor-17α-pregna-1,3,5(10)-trien-20-yne-3,17-diol, and for mestranol it is 3-methoxy-19-nor-17α-pregna-1,3,5(10)-trien-20-yn-17-ol. the structural formulas are as follows:

norethindrone

mestranol

ethinyl estradiol

HOW SUPPLIED

Norethin™ 1/35E:
Each white Norethin 1/35E tablet is round in shape, with a debossed RPC and 071 on one side and 1/35 on the other side, and contains 1 mg of norethindrone and 35 mcg of ethinyl estradiol.
Norethin™ 1/35E-21 (NDC 54092-087-21) is packaged in cartons of six compact tablet dispensers of 21 tablets each.
Norethin™ 1/35E-28 (NDC 54092-071-28) is packaged in cartons of six compact tablet dispensers. Each dispenser contains 21 white tablets and 7 blue placebo tablets. (Placebo tablets have a debossed ROBERTS on one side and "P"on the other side.)

Norethin™ 1/50M:
Each white Norethin 1/50M tablet is round in shape, with a debossed UPC and 072 on one side and 1/50 on the other side, and contains 1 mg of norethindrone and 50 mcg of mestranol.
Norethin™ 1/50M-211 (NDC 54092-088-21) is packaged in cartons of six compact tablet dispensers of 21 tablets each.
Norethin™ 1/50M-28 (NDC 54092-072-28) is packaged in cartons of six compact tablet dispensers. Each dispenser contains 21 white tablets and 7 blue placebo tablets. (Placebo tablets have debossed ROBERTS on one side and a "P"on the other side.)
Caution: Federal law prohibits dispensing without prescription.
Manufactured for
Roberts Laboratories Inc., a subsidy of
ROBERTS PHARMACEUTICAL CORP.
Eatontown, NJ 07724, USA
by Searle & Co.
San Juan, Puerto Rico 00936

NOROXIN® Tablets ℞
(Norfloxacin), U.S.P.

DESCRIPTION

NOROXIN+ (Norfloxacin) is a synthetic, broad-spectrum antibacterial agent for oral administration. Norfloxacin, a fluoroquinolone, is 1-ethyl-6-fluoro-1,4-dihydro-4-oxo-7-(1-piperazinyl)-3-quinolinecarboxylic acid. Its empirical formula is $C_{16}H_{18}FN_3O_3$ and the structural formula is:

Norfloxacin is a white to pale yellow crystalline powder with a molecular weight of 319.34 and a melting point of about 221℃. It is freely soluble in glacial acetic acid, and very slightly soluble in ethanol, methanol and water.
NOROXIN is available in 400-mg tablets. Each tablet contains the following inactive ingredients: cellulose, croscarmellose sodium, hydroxypropyl cellulose, hydroxypropyl methylcellulose, iron oxide, magnesium stearate, and titanium dioxide.
Norfloxacin, a fluoroquinolone, differs from non-fluorinated quinolones by having a fluorine atom at the 6 position and a piperazine moiety at the 7 position.

+ Registered trademark of MERCK & CO., INC.

CLINICAL PHARMACOLOGY

In fasting healthy volunteers, at least 30–40% of an oral dose of NOROXIN is absorbed. Absorption is rapid following single doses of 200 mg, 400 mg and 800 mg. At the respective doses, mean peak serum and plasma concentrations of 0.8, 1.5 and 2.4 µg/mL are attained approximately one hour after dosing. The presence of food may decrease absorption. The effective half-life of norfloxacin in serum and plasma is 3–4 hours. Steady-state concentrations of norfloxacin will be attained within two days of dosing.
In healthy older volunteers (65–75 years of age with normal renal function for their age), norfloxacin is eliminated more slowly because of their slightly decreased renal function. Drug absorption appears unaffected. However, the effective half-life of norfloxacin in these elderly subjects is 4 hours.
The disposition of norfloxacin in patients with creatinine clearance rates greater than 30 mL/min/1.73m² is similar to that in healthy volunteers. In patients with creatinine clearance rates equal to or less than 30 mL/min/1.73m², the renal elimination of norfloxacin decreases so that the effective serum half-life is 6.5 hours. In these patients, alteration of dosage is necessary (see DOSAGE AND ADMINISTRATION). Drug absorption appears unaffected by decreasing renal function.
Norfloxacin is eliminated through metabolism, biliary excretion, and renal excretion. After a single 400-mg dose of NOROXIN, mean antimicrobial activities equivalent to 278, 773, and 82 µg of norfloxacin/g of feces were obtained at 12, 24, and 48 hours, respectively. Renal excretion occurs by both glomerular filtration and tubular secretion as evidenced by the high rate of renal clearance (approximately 275 mL/min). Within 24 hours of drug administration, 26 to 32% of the administered dose is recovered in the urine as norfloxacin with an additional 5–8% being recovered in the urine as six active metabolites of lesser antimicrobial potency. Only a small percentage (less than 1%) of the dose is recovered thereafter. Fecal recovery accounts for another 30% of the administered dose.
Two to three hours after a single 400-mg dose, urinary concentrations of 200 µg/mL or more are attained in the urine. In healthy volunteers, mean urinary concentrations of norfloxacin remain above 30 µg/mL for at least 12 hours following a 400-mg dose. The urinary pH may affect the solubility of norfloxacin. Norfloxacin is least soluble at urinary pH of 7.5 with greater solubility occurring at pHs above and below this value. The serum protein binding of norfloxacin is between 10 and 15%.
The following are mean concentrations of norfloxacin in various fluids and tissues measured 1 to 4 hours post-dose after two 400-mg doses, unless otherwise indicated:

Renal Parenchyma	7.3 µg/g
Prostate	2.5 µg/g
Seminal Fluid	2.7 µg/mL
Testicle	1.6 µg/g
Uterus/Cervix	3.0 µg/g
Vagina	4.3 µg/g
Fallopian Tube	1.9 µg/g
Bile	6.9 µg/mL (after two 200-mg doses)

Microbiology
Norfloxacin has *in vitro* activity against a broad range of gram-positive and gram-negative aerobic bacteria. The fluorine atom at the 6 position provides increased potency against gram-negative organisms, and the piperazine moiety at the 7 position is responsible for anti-pseudomonal activity. Norfloxacin inhibits bacterial deoxyribonucleic acid synthesis and is bactericidal. At the molecular level, three specific events are attributed to norfloxacin in *E. coli* cells:
1) inhibition of the ATP-dependent DNA supercoiling reaction catalyzed by DNA gyrase,
2) inhibition of the relaxation of supercoiled DNA,
3) promotion of double-stranded DNA breakage.
Resistance to norfloxacin due to spontaneous mutation *in vitro* is a rare occurrence (range: 10^{-9} to 10^{-12} cells). Resistant organisms have emerged during therapy with norfloxacin in less than 1% of patients treated. Organisms in which development of resistance is greatest are the following:
Pseudomonas aeruginosa
Klebsiella pneumoniae
Acinetobacter species
Enterococcus species
For this reason, when there is a lack of satisfactory clinical response, repeat culture and susceptibility testing should be done. Nalidixic acid-resistant organisms are generally susceptible to norfloxacin *in vitro*; however, these organisms may have higher MICs to norfloxacin than nalidixic acid-susceptible strains. There is generally no cross-resistance between norfloxacin and other classes of antibacterial agents. Therefore, norfloxacin may demonstrate activity against indicated organisms resistant to some other antimicrobial agents including the aminoglycosides, penicillins, cephalosporins, tetracyclines, macrolides, and sulfonamides, including combinations of sulfamethoxazole and trimethoprim. Antagonism has been demonstrated *in vitro* between norfloxacin and nitrofurantoin.
Norfloxacin has been shown to be active against most strains of the following organisms both *in vitro* and in clinical infections (see INDICATIONS AND USAGE):
Gram-positive aerobes:
Enterococcus faecalis
Staphylococcus aureus
Staphylococcus epidermidis
Staphylococcus saprophyticus
Streptococcus agalactiae
Gram-negative aerobes:
Citrobacter freundii
Enterobacter aerogenes
Enterobacter cloacae
Escherichia coli
Klebsiella pneumoniae
Neisseria gonorrhoeae
Proteus mirabilis
Proteus vulgaris
Pseudomonas aeruginosa
Serratia marcescens
Norfloxacin has been shown to be active *in vitro* against most strains of the following organisms; however, the clinical significance of these data is unknown.
Gram-positive aerobes:
Bacillus cereus
Gram-negative aerobes:
Acinetobacter calcoaceticus
Aeromonas species
Alcaligenes species
Campylobacter species
Citrobacter diversus
Edwardsiella tarda
Flavobacterium species
Hafnia alvei
Klebsiella oxytoca
Klebsiella rhinoscleromatis
Morganella morganii

Providencia alcalifaciens
Providencia rettgeri
Providencia stuartii
Salmonella species
Shigella species
Vibrio cholerae
Vibrio parahemolyticus
Yersinia enterocolitica

Other:
Ureaplasma urealyticum

NOROXIN is not generally active against obligate anaerobes.

Norfloxacin has not been shown to be active against *Treponema pallidum.* (See WARNINGS.)

Susceptibility Tests

Diffusion Techniques: Quantitative methods that require measurement of zone diameters give the most precise estimate of the susceptibility of bacteria to antimicrobial agents. One such procedure is the National Committee for Clinical Laboratory Standards (NCCLS) approved procedure (M2-A4–Performance Standards for Antimicrobial Disk Susceptibility Tests 1990). This method has been recommended for use with the 10-μg norfloxacin disk to test susceptibility to norfloxacin. Interpretation involves correlation of the diameters obtained in the disk test with minimum inhibitory concentration (MIC) for norfloxacin. Reports from the laboratory giving results of the standard single-disk susceptibility test with a 10-μg norfloxacin disk should be interpreted according to the following criteria **(these criteria apply to isolates from urinary tract or prostatic infections):**

Zone diameter (mm)	Interpretation
≥17	(S) Susceptible
13–16	(I) Intermediate
≤12	(R) Resistant

A report of "Susceptible" indicates that the pathogen is likely to be inhibited by generally achievable urine/prostatic tissue levels. A report of "Intermediate" indicates that the test results be considered equivocal or indeterminate. A report of "Resistant" indicates that achievable concentrations of the antibiotic are unlikely to be inhibitory and other therapy should be selected.

Standardized procedures require the use of laboratory control organisms. The 10-μg norfloxacin disk should give the following zone diameter:

Organism	Zone diameter (mm)
E. coli ATCC 25922	28–35
P. aeruginosa ATCC 27853	22–29
S. aureus ATCC 25923	17–28

Other quinolone antibacterial disks should not be substituted when performing susceptibility tests for norfloxacin because of spectrum differences with norfloxacin. The 10-μg norfloxacin disk should be used for all *in vitro* testing of isolates using diffusion techniques.

Dilution Techniques: Broth and agar dilution methods, such as those recommended by the NCCLS (M7-A2—Methods for Dilution Antimicrobial Susceptibility Tests for Bacteria that Grow Aerobically 1990), may be used to determine the minimum inhibitory concentration (MIC) of norfloxacin. MIC test results should be interpreted according to the following criteria **(these criteria apply to isolates from urinary tract or prostatic infections):**

MIC (μg/mL)	Interpretation
≤4	(S) Susceptible
8	(I) Intermediate
≥16	(R) Resistant

As with standard diffusion methods, dilution procedures require the use of laboratory control organisms. Standard norfloxacin powder should give the following MIC values:

Organism	MIC range (μg/mL)
E. coli ATCC 25922	0.03–0.12
E. faecalis ATCC 29212	2.0–8.0
P. aeruginosa ATCC 27853	1.0–4.0
S. aureus ATCC 29213	0.05–2.0

INDICATIONS AND USAGE

NOROXIN is indicated for the treatment of adults with the following infections caused by susceptible strains of the designated microorganisms:

Urinary tract infections:
Uncomplicated urinary tract infections (including cystitis) due to *Enterococcus faecalis, Escherichia coli, Klebsiella pneumoniae, Proteus mirabilis, Pseudomonas aeruginosa, Staphylococcus epidermidis, Staphylococcus saprophyticus, Citrobacter freundii*, Enterobacter aerogenes*, Enterobacter cloacae*, Proteus vulgaris*, Staphylococcus aureus**, or *Streptococcus agalactiae**.

Complicated urinary tract infections due to *Enterococcus faecalis, Escherichia coli, Klebsiella pneumoniae, Proteus mirabilis, Pseudomonas aeruginosa*, or *Serratia marcescens**.

Sexually transmitted diseases (See WARNINGS.):
Uncomplicated urethral and cervical gonorrhea due to *Neisseria gonorrhoeae.*

Prostatitis:
Prostatitis due to *Escherichia coli.*

(See DOSAGE AND ADMINISTRATION for appropriate dosing instructions.)

Penicillinase production should have no effect on norfloxacin activity.

Appropriate culture and susceptibility tests should be performed before treatment in order to isolate and identify organisms causing the infection and to determine their susceptibility to norfloxacin. Therapy with norfloxacin may be initiated before results of these tests are known; once results become available, appropriate therapy should be given. Repeat culture and susceptibility testing performed periodically during therapy will provide information not only on the therapeutic effect of the antimicrobial agents but also on the possible emergence of bacterial resistance.

* Efficacy for this organism in this organ system was studied in fewer than 10 infections.

CONTRAINDICATIONS

NOROXIN (norfloxacin) is contraindicated in persons with a history of hypersensitivity, tendinitis, or tendon rupture associated with the use of norfloxacin or any member of the quinolone group of antimicrobial agents.

WARNINGS

THE SAFETY AND EFFICACY OF ORAL NORFLOXACIN IN CHILDREN, ADOLESCENTS (UNDER THE AGE OF 18), PREGNANT WOMEN, AND NURSING MOTHERS HAVE NOT BEEN ESTABLISHED. (See PRECAUTIONS–*Pregnancy, Nursing Mothers* and *Pediatric Use.*) The oral administration of single doses of norfloxacin, 6 times** the recommended human clinical dose (on a mg/kg basis), caused lameness in immature dogs. Histologic examination of the weight-bearing joints of these dogs revealed permanent lesions of the cartilage. Other quinolones also produced erosions of the cartilage in weight-bearing joints and other signs of arthropathy in immature animals of various species. (See ANIMAL PHARMACOLOGY.)

Convulsions have been reported in patients receiving norfloxacin. Convulsions, increased intracranial pressure, and toxic psychoses have been reported in patients receiving drugs in this class. Quinolones may also cause central nervous system (CNS) stimulation which may lead to tremors, restlessness, lightheadedness, confusion, and hallucinations. If these reactions occur in patients receiving norfloxacin, the drug should be discontinued and appropriate measures instituted.

The effects of norfloxacin on brain function or on the electrical activity of the brain have not been tested. Therefore, until more information becomes available, norfloxacin, like all other quinolones, should be used with caution in patients with known or suspected CNS disorders, such as severe cerebral arteriosclerosis, epilepsy, and other factors which predispose to seizures. (See ADVERSE REACTIONS.)

Serious and occasionally fatal hypersensitivity (anaphylactoid or anaphylactic) reactions, some following the first dose, have been reported in patients receiving quinolone therapy. Some reactions were accompanied by cardiovascular collapse, loss of consciousness, tingling, pharyngeal or facial edema, dyspnea, urticaria and itching. Only a few patients had a history of hypersensitivity reactions. If an allergic reaction to norfloxacin occurs, discontinue the drug. Serious acute hypersensitivity reactions may require immediate emergency treatment with epinephrine. Oxygen, intravenous fluids, antihistamines, corticosteroids, pressor amines, and airway management, including intubation, should be administered as indicated.

Pseudomembranous colitis has been reported with nearly all antibacterial agents, including norfloxacin, and may range in severity from mild to life-threatening. Therefore, it is important to consider this diagnosis in patients who present with diarrhea subsequent to the administration of antibacterial agents.

Treatment with antibacterial agents alters the normal flora of the colon and may permit overgrowth of clostridia. Studies indicate that a toxin produced by *Clostridium difficile* is one primary cause of "antibiotic-associated colitis".

After the diagnosis of pseudomembranous colitis has been established, therapeutic measures should be initiated. Mild cases of pseudomembranous colitis usually respond to drug discontinuation alone. In moderate to severe cases, consideration should be given to management with fluids and electrolytes, protein supplementation, and treatment with an antibacterial drug clinically effective against *C. difficile* colitis.

Ruptures of the shoulder, hand, and Achilles tendons that required surgical repair or resulted in prolonged disability have been reported with norfloxacin. Norfloxacin should be discontinued if the patient experiences pain, inflammation, or rupture of a tendon. Patients should rest and refrain from exercise until the diagnosis of tendinitis or tendon rupture has been confidently excluded. Tendon rupture can occur at any time during or after therapy with norfloxacin.

Norfloxacin has not been shown to be effective in the treatment of syphilis. Antimicrobial agents used in high doses for short periods of time to treat gonorrhea may mask or delay the symptoms of incubating syphilis. All patients with gonorrhea should have a serologic test for syphilis at the time of diagnosis. Patients treated with norfloxacin should have a follow-up serologic test for syphilis after three months.

Transient hearing loss (rare), tinnitus, diplopia

Other adverse events reported with quinolones include: agranulocytosis, albuminuria, candiduria, crystalluria, cylindruria, dysphagia, elevation of blood glucose, elevation of serum cholesterol, elevation of serum potassium, elevation of serum triglycerides, hematuria, hepatic necrosis, symptomatric hypoglycemia, nystagmus, postural hypotension, prolongation of prothrombin time, and vaginal candidiasis.

**Based on a patient weight of 50 kg.

PRECAUTIONS

General:

Needle-shaped crystals were found in the urine of some volunteers who received either placebo, 800 mg norfloxacin, or 1600 mg norfloxacin (at or twice the recommended daily dose, respectively) while participating in a double-blind, crossover study comparing single doses of norfloxacin with placebo. While crystalluria is not expected to occur under usual conditions with a dosage regimen of 400 mg b.i.d., as a precaution, the daily recommended dosage should not be exceeded and the patient should drink sufficient fluids to ensure a proper state of hydration and adequate urinary output.

Alteration in dosage regimen is necessary for patients with impaired renal function (see DOSAGE AND ADMINISTRATION).

Moderate to severe phototoxicity reactions have been observed in patients who are exposed to excessive sunlight while receiving some members of this drug class. Excessive sunlight should be avoided. Therapy should be discontinued if phototoxicity occurs.

Rarely, hemolytic reactions have been reported in patients with latent or actual defects in glucose-6-phosphate dehydrogenase activity who take quinolone antibacterial agents, including norfloxacin. (See ADVERSE REACTIONS.)

Information for Patients

Patients should be advised:

—to drink fluids liberally.

—that norfloxacin should be taken at least one hour before or at least two hours after a meal or milk ingestion.

—that multivitamins or other products containing iron or zinc, or antacids should not be taken within the two-hour period before or within the two-hour period after taking norfloxacin. (See *Drug Interactions.*)

—that norfloxacin can cause dizziness and lightheadedness and, therefore, patients should know how they react to norfloxacin before they operate an automobile or machinery or engage in activities requiring mental alertness and coordination.

—to discontinue treatment and inform their physician if they experience pain, inflammation, or rupture of a tendon, and to rest and refrain from exercise until the diagnosis of tendinitis or tendon rupture has been confidently excluded.

—that norfloxacin may be associated with hypersensitivity reactions, even following the first dose, and to discontinue the drug at the first sign of a skin rash or other allergic reaction.

—to avoid undue exposure to excessive sunlight while receiving norfloxacin and to discontinue therapy if phototoxicity occurs.

—that some quinolones may increase the effects of theophylline and/or caffeine. (See *Drug Interactions.*)

Laboratory Tests

As with any potent antibacterial agent, periodic assessment of organ system functions, including renal, hepatic, and hematopoietic, is advisable during prolonged therapy.

Drug Interactions

Elevated plasma levels of theophylline have been reported with concomitant quinolone use. There have been reports of theophylline-related side effects in patients on concomitant therapy with norfloxacin and theophylline. Therefore, monitoring of theophylline plasma levels should be considered and dosage of theophylline adjusted as required.

Elevated serum levels of cyclosporine have been reported with concomitant use of cyclosporine with norfloxacin. Therefore cyclosporine serum levels should be monitored and appropriate cyclosporine dosage adjustments made when these drugs are used concomitantly.

Quinolones, including norfloxacin, may enhance the effects of the oral anticoagulant warfarin or its derivatives. When these products are administered concomitantly, prothrombin time or other suitable coagulation tests should be closely monitored.

Continued on next page

Roberts—Cont.

Diminished urinary excretion of norfloxacin has been reported during the concomitant administration of probenecid and norfloxacin.

The concomitant use of nitrofurantoin is not recommended since nitrofurantoin may antagonize the antibacterial effect of NOROXIN in the urinary tract.

Multivitamins, or other products containing iron or zinc, antacids or sucralfate should not be administered concomitantly with, or within 2 hours of, the administration of norfloxacin, because they may interfere with absorption resulting in lower serum and urine levels of norfloxacin.

Some quinolones have also been shown to interfere with the metabolism of caffeine. This may lead to reduced clearance of caffeine and a prolongation of its plasma half-life.

Carcinogenesis, Mutagenesis, Impairment of Fertility
No increase in neoplastic changes was observed with norfloxacin as compared to controls in a study in rats, lasting up to 96 weeks at doses 8–9 times** the usual human dose (on a mg/kg basis).

Norfloxacin was tested for mutagenic activity in a number of *in vivo* and *in vitro* tests. Norfloxacin had no mutagenic effect in the dominant lethal test in mice and did not cause chromosomal aberrations in hamsters or rats at doses 30–60 times** the usual human dose (on a mg/kg basis). Norfloxacin had no mutagenic activity *in vitro* in the Ames microbial mutagen test, Chinese hamster fibroblasts and V-79 mammalian cell assay. Although norfloxacin was weakly positive in the Rec-assay for DNA repair, all other mutagenic assays were negative including a more sensitive test (V-79).

Norfloxacin did not adversely affect the fertility of male and female mice at oral doses up to 30 times** the usual human dose (on a mg/kg basis).

Pregnancy
Teratogenic Effects. Pregnancy Category C. Norfloxacin has been shown to produce embryonic loss in monkeys when given in doses 10 times** the maximum daily total human dose (on a mg/kg basis). At this dose, peak plasma levels obtained in monkeys were approximately 2 times those obtained in humans. There has been no evidence of a teratogenic effect in any of the animal species tested (rat, rabbit, mouse, monkey) at 6–50 times** the maximum daily human dose (on a mg/kg basis). There are, however, no adequate and well controlled studies in pregnant women. Norfloxacin should be used during pregnancy only if the potential benefit justifies the potential risk to the fetus.

Nursing Mothers
It is not known whether norfloxacin is excreted in human milk.

When a 200-mg dose of NOROXIN was administered to nursing mothers, norfloxacin was not detected in human milk. However, because the dose studied was low, because other drugs in this class are secreted in human milk, and because of the potential for serious adverse reactions from norfloxacin in nursing infants, a decision should be made to discontinue nursing or to discontinue the drug, taking into account the importance of the drug to the mother.

Pediatric Use
The safety and effectiveness of oral norfloxacin in children and adolescents below the age of 18 years have not been established. Norfloxacin causes arthropathy in juvenile animals of several animal species. (See WARNINGS and ANIMAL PHARMACOLOGY.)

**Based on a patient weight of 50 kg.

ADVERSE REACTIONS

Single-Dose Studies
In clinical trials involving 82 healthy subjects and 228 patients with gonorrhea, treated with a single dose of norfloxacin, 6.5% reported drug-related adverse experiences. However, the following incidence figures were calculated without reference to drug relationship.

The most common adverse experiences (> 1.0%) were: dizziness (2.6%), nausea (2.6%), headache (2.0%), and abdominal cramping (1.6%).

Additional reactions (0.3%–1.0%) were: anorexia, diarrhea, hyperhidrosis, asthenia, anal/rectal pain, constipation, dyspepsia, flatulence, tingling of the fingers, and vomiting.

Laboratory adverse changes considered drug-related were reported in 4.5% of patients/subjects. These laboratory changes were: increased AST (SGOT) (1.6%), decreased WBC (1.3%), decreased platelet count (1.0%), increased urine protein (1.0%), decreased hematocrit and hemoglobin (0.6%), and increased eosinophils (0.6%).

Multiple-Dose Studies
In clinical trials involving 52 healthy subjects and 1980 patients with urinary tract infections or prostatitis, treated with multiple doses of norfloxacin, 3.6% reported drug-related adverse experiences. However, the incidence figures below were calculated without reference to drug relationship.

The most common adverse experiences (> 1.0%) were: nausea (4.2%), headache (2.8%), dizziness (1.7%), and asthenia (1.3%).

Additional reactions (0.3%–1.0%) were: abdominal pain, back pain, constipation, diarrhea, dry mouth, dyspepsia/heartburn, fever, flatulence, hyperhidrosis, loose stools, pruritus, rash, somnolence, and vomiting.

Less frequent reactions (0.1%–0.2%) included: abdominal swelling, allergies, anorexia, anxiety, bitter taste, blurred vision, bursitis, chest pain, chills, depression, dysmenorrhea, edema, erythema, foot or hand swelling, insomnia, mouth ulcer, myocardial infarction, palpitation, pruritus ani, renal colic, sleep disturbances, and urticaria.

Abnormal laboratory values observed in these patients/subjects were: eosinophilia (1.5%), elevation of ALT (SGPT) (1.4%), decreased WBC and/or neutrophil count (1.4%), elevation of AST (SGOT) (1.4%), and increased alkaline phosphatase (1.1%). Those occurring less frequently included increased BUN, increased LDH, increased serum creatinine, decreased hematocrit, and glycosuria.

Post Marketing
The most frequently reported adverse reaction in post-marketing experience is rash.

CNS effects characterized as generalized seizures and myoclonus have been reported with NOROXIN®. A causal relationship to NOROXIN® has not been established (see WARNINGS). Visual disturbances have been reported with drugs in this class.

The following additional adverse reactions have been reported since the drug was marketed:

Hypersensitivity Reactions
Hypersensitivity reactions have been reported including anaphylactoid reactions, angioedema, dyspnea, vasculitis, urticaria, arthritis, arthralgia and myalgia (see WARNINGS).

Skin
Toxic epidermal necrolysis, Stevens-Johnson syndrome and erythema multiforme, exfoliative dermatitis, photosensitivity

Gastrointestinal
Pseudomembranous colitis, hepatitis, jaundice including cholestatic jaundice, pancreatitis (rare), stomatitis. The onset of pseudomembranous colitis symptoms may occur during or after antibacterial treatment. (See WARNINGS.)

Renal
Interstitial nephritis, renal failure

Nervous System/Psychiatric
Peripheral neuropathy, Guillain-Barré syndrome, ataxia, paresthesia; psychic disturbances including psychotic reactions and confusion

Musculoskeletal
Tendinitis, tendon rupture, possible exacerbation of myasthenia gravis

Hematologic
Neutropenia, leukopenia, hemolytic anemia, sometimes associated with glucose-6-phosphate dehydrogenase deficiency; thrombocytopenia

Special Senses
Transient hearing loss (rare), tinnitus, diplopia

Other adverse events reported with quinolones include: agranulocytosis, albuminuria, candiduria, crystalluria, cylindruria, dysphagia, elevation of blood glucose, elevation of serum cholesterol, elevation of serum potassium, elevation of serum triglycerides, hematuria, hepatic necrosis, symptomatic hypoglycemia, nystagmus, postural hypotension, prolongation of prothrombin time, and vaginal candidiasis.

OVERDOSAGE

No significant lethality was observed in male and female mice and rats at single oral doses up to 4 g/kg.

In the event of acute overdosage, the stomach should be emptied by inducing vomiting or by gastric lavage, and the patient carefully observed and given symptomatic and supportive treatment. Adequate hydration must be maintained.

DOSAGE AND ADMINISTRATION

Tablets NOROXIN should be taken at least one hour before or at least two hours after a meal or milk ingestion. Tablets NOROXIN should be taken with a glass of water. Patients receiving NOROXIN should be well hydrated (see PRECAUTIONS).

Normal Renal Function
The recommended daily dose of NOROXIN is as described in the following chart:
[See table below.]

Renal Impairment
NOROXIN may be used for the treatment of urinary tract infections in patients with renal insufficiency. In patients with a creatinine clearance rate of 30 mL/min/1.73m^2 or less, the recommended dosage is one 400-mg tablet once daily for the duration given above. At this dosage, the urinary concentration exceeds the MICs for most urinary pathogens susceptible to norfloxacin, even when the creatinine clearance is less than 10 mL/min/1.73m^2.

When only the serum creatinine level is available, the following formula (based on sex, weight, and age of the patient) may be used to convert this value into creatinine clearance. The serum creatinine should represent a steady state of renal function.

Males: $\dfrac{(\text{weight in kg}) \times (140 - \text{age})}{(72) \times \text{serum creatinine (mg/100 mL)}}$

Females: $(0.85) \times (\text{above value})$

Elderly
Elderly patients being treated for urinary tract infections who have a creatinine clearance of greater than 30 mL/min/1.73m^2 should receive the dosages recommended under

Normal Renal Function.
Elderly patients being treated for urinary tract infections who have a creatinine clearance of 30 mL/min/1.73m^2 or less should receive 400 mg once daily as recommended under *Renal Impairment.*

HOW SUPPLIED

Tablets NOROXIN 400 mg are dark pink, oval shaped, film-coated tablets, coded MSD 705 on one side and NOROXIN on the other. They are supplied as follows:
NDC 54092-097-01 bottles of 100.

Storage
Tablets NOROXIN should be stored in a tightly-closed container. Avoid storage at temperatures above 40°C (104°F).

ANIMAL PHARMACOLOGY

Norfloxacin and related drugs have been shown to cause arthropathy in immature animals of most species tested (see WARNINGS).

Crystalluria has occurred in laboratory animals tested with norfloxacin. In dogs, needle-shaped drug crystals were seen in the urine at doses of 50 mg/kg/day. In rats, crystals were reported following doses of 200 mg/kg/day.

Embryo lethality and slight maternotoxicity (vomiting and anorexia) were observed in cynomolgus monkeys at doses of 150 mg/kg/day or higher.

Ocular toxicity, seen with some related drugs, was not observed in any norfloxacin-treated animals.

Manufactured by:
Merck & Co., Inc.
West Point, PA 19486, USA

Infection	Description	Unit Dose	Frequency	Duration	Daily Dose
Urinary Tract	Uncomplicated UTI's (crystitis) due to *E. coli, K. pneumoniae,* or *P. mirabilis*	400 mg	q12h	3 days	800 mg
	Uncomplicated UTI's due to other indicated organisms	400 mg	q12h	7–10 days	800 mg
	Complicated UTI's	400 mg	q12h	10–21 days	800 mg
Sexually Transmitted Diseases	Uncomplicated Gonorrhea	800 mg	single dose	1 day	800 mg
Prostatitis	Acute or Chronic	400 mg	q12h	28 days	800 mg

Distributed by:
Roberts Laboratories, Inc. a subsidiary of
Roberts Pharmaceutical Corp.
Eatontown, NJ 07724, USA
Shown in Product Identification Guide, page 331

NUCOFED® Syrup and Capsules ℞
NUCOFED® EXPECTORANT Syrup
NUCOFED® PEDIATRIC EXPECTORANT Syrup

NUCOFED® Syrup and Capsules
DESCRIPTION
ACTIVE INGREDIENTS
Nucofed® Syrup and Nucofed® Capsules are antitussive-decongestants containing in each 5ml (teaspoonful) and each capsule: Codeine Phosphate, 20 mg (Warning: May Be Habit Forming) Pseudoephedrine Hydrochloride, 60mg. Codeine Phosphate and Pseudoephedrine Hydrochloride are represented by the following chemical names and structural formulas:

Codeine Phosphate

7,8-Didehydro-4,5α-epoxy-3-methoxy-17-methylmorphinan-6α-ol phosphate (1:1) salt hemihydrate

Pseudoephedrine HCl

[S-(R*.R*)]-α-[1-(Methylamino)ethyl]benzene methanol hydrochloride
INACTIVE INGREDIENTS
SYRUP: citric acid, flavorings, glycerin, propylene glycol, sodium benzoate, sorbitol, sucrose, (2.25 gm/5mL), D&C Yellow No. 10, and FD&C Blue No. 1.
Capsules: starch, lactose, magnesium stearate, FD&C Yellow No. 6, FD&C Blue No. 1, and D&C Yellow No. 10.

NUCOFED® EXPECTORANT Syrup
DESCRIPTION
Nucofed® Expectorant is an antitussive-decongestant-expectorant syrup for oral administration containing in each 5 ml (teaspoonful): codeine phosphate, 20mg (Warning: May Be Habit Forming): pseudoephedrine HCl, 60mg: guaifenesin, 200mg; alcohol, 12.5%.
The structural formulas and chemical names for codeine phosphate and pseudoephedrine hydrochloride are shown above. The structural formula and chemical name for guaifenesin is shown below.

Guaifenesin

3-(O-Methoxyphenoxy)-1,2-propanediol
INACTIVE INGREDIENTS
D&C Yellow 10, FD&C Red 40, flavoring, glycerin, saccharin sodium, sodium chloride, and sucrose.

NUCOFED® PEDIATRIC EXPECTORANT Syrup
DESCRIPTION
Nucofed® Pediatric Expectorant is an antitussive-decongestant-expectorant syrup for oral administration containing in each 5 ml (teaspoonful): codeine phosphate, 10mg (Warning: May Be Habit Forming): pseudoephedrine HCl, 30mg: guaifenesin, 100mg; alcohol, 6%.
INACTIVE INGREDIENTS
edetate disodium, FD&C Red 40, flavorings, glycerin, potassium sorbate, saccharin sodium, sodium chloride, and sucrose.

NUCOFED® Syrup and Capsules
Codeine Phosphate. Codeine causes suppression of the cough reflex by a direct effect on the cough center in the medulla and appears to exert a drying effect on respiratory tract mucosa and to increase viscosity of bronchial secretions.
Codeine is well absorbed from the gastrointestinal tract. Following oral administration, peak antitussive effects usually can be expected to occur within 1–2 hours and may persist for a period of four hours. Codeine is metabolized in the liver. The drug undergoes O-demethylation, N-demethyla-

tion, and partial conjugation with glucuronic acid, and is excreted mainly in the urine as norcodeine and morphine in the free and conjugated forms.
Codeine appears in breast milk of nursing mothers, and has been reported to cross the placental barrier.
Pseudoephedrine Hydrochloride. Pseudoephedrine is a physiologically active stereoisomer of ephedrine, which acts directly on *alpha-*, and, to a lesser degree, *beta-*adrenergic receptors. The *alpha-*adrenergic effects are believed to result from the reduced production of cyclic adenosine-3′, 5′ monophosphate (cyclic -AMP) by inhibition of the enzyme adenyl cyclase, whereas *beta-*adrenergic effects appear to be caused by the stimulation of adenyl cyclase activity.
Pseudoephedrine acts directly on *alpha-*adrenergic receptors in the respiratory tract mucosa producing vasoconstriction that results in shrinkage of swollen nasal mucous membranes, reduction of tissue hyperemia, edema, and nasal congestion, and an increase in nasal airway patency. Drainage of sinus secretions is increased and obstructed eustachian ostia may be opened. Relaxation of bronchial smooth muscle by stimulation of $beta_2$ adrenergic receptors may also occur. Following oral administration, significant bronchodilation has not been demonstrated consistently.
Nasal decongestion usually occurs within 30 minutes and persists for 4–6 hours after oral administration of 60 mg of pseudoephedrine hydrochloride.
Although specific information is not available, pseudoephedrine is presumed to cross the placenta and to enter cerebrospinal fluid. It is incompletely metabolized in the liver by N-demethylation to an inactive metabolite. Both are excreted in the urine with 55%–75% of a dose being unchanged.
Nucofed® Expectorant Syrup, and Nucofed® Pediatric Expectorant Syrup.
Guaifenesin. Guaifenesin, by increasing respiratory tract fluid, reduces the viscosity of tenacious secretions and acts as an expectorant. Guaifenesin is excreted in the urine mainly as glucuronates and sulfonates.

INDICATIONS AND USAGE
NUCOFED® Syrup and Capsules
NUCOFED® EXPECTORANT Syrup
NUCOFED® PEDIATRIC EXPECTORANT Syrup
NUCOFED is indicated for symptomatic relief when both coughing and congestion are associated with upper respiratory infections and related conditions such as common cold, bronchitis, influenza, and sinusitis.

CONTRAINDICATIONS
Hypersensitivity to any of the product's ingredients.

WARNINGS
Persons with a high fever; persistent cough, such as occurs with smoking, asthma, emphysema; cough accompanied by excessive phlegm (mucus); persons with chronic pulmonary disease; shortness of breath; or children taking other drugs should not take this product. May cause or aggravate constipation.
Do not exceed recommended dosage because at higher doses nervousness, dizziness, or sleeplessness may occur.
If symptoms do not improve within 7 days, consult a physician before continuing use.

PRECAUTIONS
General. Inasmuch as the active ingredients of **Nucofed®** **Syrup and Capsules** consist of **Codeine Phosphate and Pseudoephedrine Hydrochloride, and Nucofed® Expectorant and Nucofed® Pediatric Expectorant Syrups** consist of Codeine Phosphate, Pseudoephedrine Hydrochloride and Guaifenesin, this medication should be used with caution in the presence of the following:
● Cardiovascular disease (of any etiology)
● Diabetes mellitus; closed-angle glaucoma
● Hypertension (of any severity)
● Abnormal thyroid function
● Prostatic hypertrophy
● Addison's disease
● Chronic ulcerative colitis
● History of drug abuse or dependence
● Chronic respiratory disease or impairment
● Functional impairment of the liver or kidney
Information for Patients: Patients taking **NUCOFED®** products should be cautioned not to drive or do jobs requiring alertness, to get up slowly from a lying or sitting position and to lie down if nausea occurs.
Drug Interactions Prescribe with caution to patients taking any of the following:
● Beta adrenergic blockers—may increase the press effect of pseudoephedrine.
● Digitalis glycosides—may increase the possibility of cardiac arrhythmias.
● Antihypertensive agents including Veratrum alkaloids—hypotensive effects may be decreased.
● Monoamine oxidase (MAO) inhibitors—may potentiate the pressor effect of Pseudoephedrine and may result in a hypertensive crisis.

● Sympathomimetics—may have increased effects, or may increase the effects of pseudoephedrine, thereby increasing the potential for side effects.
● Tricyclic antidepressants—may antagonize the effects of pseudoephrine and may increase the effects of the antidepressants or codeine.
● CNS depressants
● Alcohol
● General anesthetics
● Anticholinergics—may result in paralytic ileus.
Drug Interaction Precaution: Persons taking a prescription monoamine oxidase inhibitor (MAOI), should not use this product before 2 weeks after stopping the MAOI drug.
Laboratory Test Interactions
● Codeine may cause an elevation in serum amylase levels, due to the spasm-producing potential of narcotic analgesics on the sphincter of Oddi.
Nucofed® Expectorant Syrup and Nucofed® Pediatric Expectorant Syrup
● Guaifenesin is known to interfere with the colorimetric determination of 5-hydroxyindole-acetic acid (5-HIAA) and vanilmandelic acid (VMA).
Pregnancy: Category C
Animal reproduction studies have not been conducted with codeine, pseudoephedrine and guaifenesin. Thus, it is not known whether these compounds can cause fetal harm when administered to pregnant women or whether they affect reproductive capacity. Accordingly, NUCOFED products should be given to pregnant women only if clearly needed.
Nursing Mothers
Codeine and Pseudoephedrine are excreted in breast milk; therefore, caution should be exercised when this medication is administered to nursing mother.
Pediatric Use
Do not give Nucofed® Syrup, Nucofed® Expectorant or Nucofed® Pediatric Expectorant to children under two years of age or Nucofed Capsules to children under 12 years of age.

ADVERSE REACTIONS
Based on the composition of Nucofed® Syrup and Capsules, Nucofed® Expectorant and Nucofed® Pediatric Expectorant, the following side effects may occur: nervousness, restlessness, sleeplessness, drowsiness, difficult or painful urination, dizziness or lightheadedness, headache, nausea, and vomiting, constipation, trembling, troubled breathing, increase in sweating, unusual paleness, weakness, and changes in heart rate.

DRUG ABUSE AND DEPENDENCE
NUCOFED® Syrup and Capsules and NUCOFED® Expectorant Syrup is placed in Schedule III of the Controlled Substances Act.
NUCOFED® Pediatric Expectorant Syrup is placed in Schedule V of the Controlled Substances Act.

OVERDOSAGE
Nucofed® Syrup and Capsules contain codeine phosphate and pseudoephedrine hydrochloride; Nucofed® Expectorant Syrup and Nucofed Pediatric Expectorant Syrup contain codeine phosphate, pseudoephedrine hydrochloride and guaifenesin. Overdosage as a result of these products should be treated based upon the symptomatology of the patient as it relates to the individual ingredient. Treatment of acute overdosage would probably be based upon treating the patient for codeine toxicity which may be manifested as:
● Gradual drowsiness, dizziness, heaviness of the head, weariness, diminution of sensibility, and loss of sensation.
● Nausea and vomiting.
● A transient excitement stage, characterized by extreme restlessness, delirium, and rarely epileptiform convulsions, is sometimes seen.
● Bilateral miosis progressing to pinpoint pupils which do not react to light or accommodation. The pupils may dilate during terminal asphyxia.
● Itching of the skin and nose, sometimes with skin rashes and urticaria.
● Coma, with muscular relaxation and depressed or absent superficial and deep reflexes. A Babinski toe sign may appear.
● Marked slowing of the respiratory rate with inadequate pulmonary ventilation and consequent cyanosis. Breathing becomes stertorous and irregular (Cheyne-Stokes or Biot).
● The pulse is slow and the blood pressure gradually falls to shock levels. Urine formation ceases or is reduced to a very slow rate.
NUCOFED® Syrup and Capsules and NUCOFED® Expectorant Syrup
The lethal dose of codeine for an adult is about 0.5–1.0 g. Treat as a narcotic overdose.
NUCOFED® Pediatric Expectorant Syrup
The lethal dose of codeine for an adult is about 0.5–1.0 g. Reliable information regarding the lethal dose in children is not available. Treatment is as recommended for narcotics.

Continued on next page

Consult 1997 supplements and future editions for revisions

Roberts—Cont.

DOSAGE AND ADMINISTRATION

NUCOFED® Syrup and Capsules
Recommended Dosage: CAPSULE
Adults: 1 capsule every 6 hours, not to exceed 4 capsules in 24 hours. Not recommended for children under 12 years of age.
Recommended Dosage: SYRUP
Adults and children 12 years of age and older: 1 teaspoonful every 4-6 hours, not to exceed 6 teaspoonfuls (120 mg of codeine) in 24 hours.
Children 6 to under 12 years: ½ teaspoonful every 4-6 hours, not to exceed 3 teaspoonfuls (60 mg of codeine) in 24 hours.
2 to under 6 years: ¼ teaspoonful every 6 hours, not to exceed 1 teaspoonful in 24 hours.
NUCOFED® Expectorant Syrup
Recommended Dosage:
Adults and children 12 years of age and over: 1 teaspoonful every 6 hours, not to exceed 4 teaspoonfuls in 24 hours.
Children: 6 to under 12 years: ½ teaspoonful every 6 hours, not to exceed 2 teaspoonfuls in 24 hours.
2 to under 6 years: ¼ teaspoonful every 6 hours, not to exceed 1 teaspoonful in 24 hours. A special measuring device should be used to give an accurate dose of this product to children under 6 years of age. Giving a higher dose than recommended could result in serious side effects.
NUCOFED® Pediatric Expectorant Syrup
Recommended Dosage:
Adults and Children 12 years of age and over: 2 teaspoonfuls every 6 hours, not to exceed 8 teaspoonfuls in 24 hours.
Children: 6 to under 12 years: 1 teaspoonful every 6 hours, not to exceed 4 teaspoonfuls in 24 hours.
2 to under 6 years: ½ teaspoonful every 6 hours, not to exceed 2 teaspoonfuls in 24 hours.
DO NOT Give these products to children under 2 years old, unless under the advice and supervision of a physician.

HOW SUPPLIED

NUCOFED® Syrup and Capsules
Nucofed Syrup, Green, Mint Flavored
NDC 54092-403-16   Pints
Nucofed Capsules, Green Top, Clear Bottom
NDC 54092-005-60   Bottles of 60
NUCOFED® Expectorant Syrup
Red, Wintergreen Flavored Syrup
NDC 54092-404-16   Pints
NUCOFED® Pediatric Expectorant Syrup
Red, Strawberry Flavored Syrup
NDC 54092-405-16   Pints
Store at or below 25°C (77°F), keep from freezing.

CAUTION

Federal law prohibits dispensing without prescription.
Manufactured for
Roberts Laboratories Inc.
a wholly owned subsidiary of
ROBERTS PHARMACEUTICAL CORPORATION
Eatontown, NJ 07724

PERI-COLACE® capsules • syrup   OTC
(casanthranol and docusate sodium)

DESCRIPTION

Peri-Colace® is a combination of the mild stimulant laxative casanthranol, and the stool-softener Colace® (docusate sodium). Each capsule contains 30 mg of casanthranol and 100 mg of Colace®; the syrup contains 30 mg of casanthranol and 60 mg of Colace® per 15-mL tablespoon (10 mg of casanthranol and 20 mg of Colace® per 5-mL teaspoon) and 10% alcohol.
Peri-Colace® Capsules contain the following inactive ingredients: D&C Red No. 33, FD&C Red No. 40, non-porcine gelatin, edible ink, polyethylene glycol, propylene glycol, titanium dioxide, and purified water.
Peri-Colace® Syrup contains the following inactive ingredients: alcohol (10% v/v), citric acid, flavors, methyl salicylate, methylparaben, poloxamer, polyethylene glycol, propylparaben, sodium citrate, sorbitol solution, sucrose, and purified water.

ACTION AND USES

Peri-Colace® provides gentle peristaltic stimulation and helps to keep stools soft for easier passage. Bowel movement is induced gently—usually overnight or in 8 to 12 hours. Nausea, griping, abnormally loose stools, and constipation rebound are minimized. Useful in management of chronic or temporary constipation.
Note: To prevent hard stools when laxative stimulation is not needed or undesirable, see Colace® (stool softener).

WARNINGS

Do not use when abdominal pain, nausea, or vomiting is present. Frequent or prolonged use of this preparation may result in dependence on laxatives.
As with any drug, pregnant or nursing women should seek the advice of a health professional before using this product.

SIDE EFFECTS

The incidence of side effects—none of a serious nature—is exceedingly small. Nausea, abdominal cramping or discomfort, diarrhea, and rash are the main side effects reported.

ADMINISTRATION AND DOSAGE

Adults —1 or 2 capsules, or 1 or 2 tablespoons syrup at bedtime, or as indicated. In severe cases, dosage may be increased to 2 capsules or 2 tablespoons twice daily, or 3 capsules at bedtime. *Children* —1 to 3 teaspoons of syrup at bedtime, or as indicated. Peri-Colace® syrup must be given in a 6 oz. to 8 oz. glass of milk or fruit juice or in infant's formula to prevent throat irritation.

OVERDOSAGE

In addition to symptomatic treatment, gastric lavage, if timely, is recommended in cases of large overdosage.

HOW SUPPLIED

Peri-Colace® Capsules
  NDC 54092-054-30 Bottles of 30
  NDC 54092-054-60 Bottles of 60
  NDC 54092-054-02 Bottles of 250
  NDC 54092-054-10 Bottles of 1000
  NDC 54092-054-52 Cartons of 100 single unit packs
Note: Peri-Colace® capsules should be stored at controlled room temperatures (59°–86°F or 15°–30°C).
Peri-Colace® Syrup
  NDC 54092-418-08 Bottles of 8 fl oz
  NDC 54092-418-16 Bottles of 16 fl oz
Peri-Colace®-T
  NDC 54092-054-11 Blister Pack of 10
Manufactured for:
Roberts Laboratories Inc., a subsidiary of
ROBERTS PHARMACEUTICAL CORPORATION
Eatontown, NJ 07724 USA

PRO-BANTHINE® Tablets   ℞
[prō-ban 'thīne]
(propantheline bromide)

DESCRIPTION

Pro-Banthine® (probantheline bromide) oral tablets contain 15 mg or $7^{1}/_{2}$ mg of the anticholinergic propantheline bromide, (2-hydroxyethyl)diisopropylmethylammonium bromide xanthene-9-carboxylate.
The structural formula of probantheline bromide® is

Propantheline bromide is very soluble in water, alcohol, and chloroform, but it is practically insoluble in ether and in benzene. Its molecular weight is 448.40.
Inactive ingredients: include calcium carbonate, corn starch, edible ink, flavor, lactose, magnesium carbonate, magnesium stearate, sucrose, talc, titanium dioxide, and waxes. The 15-mg tablet also contains red oxide and yellow oxide as coloring agents.

CLINICAL PHARMACOLOGY

Probantheline bromide® inhibits gastrointestinal motility and diminishes gastric acid secretion. The drug also inhibits the action of acetylcholine at the postganglionic nerve endings of the parasympathetic nervous system.
Propantheline bromide is extensively metabolized in man primarily by hydrolysis to the inactive compounds xanthene-9-carboxylic acid and (2-hydroxyethyl) diisopropylmethylammonium bromide. After a single 30-mg oral dose given as two 15-mg tablets, the mean peak plasma concentration of propantheline was 21 ng/ml at 1 hour in 6 healthy subjects. The plasma elimination half-life of propantheline is about 1.6 hours. Approximately 70% of the dose is excreted in the urine, mostly as metabolites. The urinary excretion of propantheline is about 3% after oral tablet administration.

INDICATIONS AND USAGE

Pro-Banthine® (propantheline bromide) tablets are effective as adjunctive therapy in the treatment of peptic ulcer.

CONTRAINDICATIONS

Propantheline bromide is contraindicated in patients with:
1. Glaucoma, since mydriasis is to be avoided.
2. Obstructive disease of the gastrointestinal tract (pyloroduodenal stenosis, achalasia, paralytic ileus, etc).
3. Obstructive uropathy (e.g., bladder-neck obstruction due to prostatic hypertrophy).
4. Intestinal atony of elderly or debilitated patients.
5. Severe ulcerative colitis or toxic megacolon complicating ulcerative colitis.
6. Unstable cardiovascular adjustment in acute hemorrhage.
7. Myasthenia gravis.

WARNINGS

In the presence of a high environmental temperature, heat prostration (fever and heat stroke due to decreased sweating) can occur with the use of Pro-Banthine®.
Diarrhea may be an early symptom of incomplete intestinal obstruction, especially in patients with ileostomy or colostomy. In this instance treatment with propantheline bromide would be inappropriate and possibly harmful.
With overdosage, a curare-like action may occur (ie, neuromuscular blockade leading to muscular weakness and possible paralysis).
Propantheline bromide may cause increased heart rate and, therefore, should be used with caution in patients with heart disease.

PRECAUTIONS

General: Propantheline bromide should be used with caution in the elderly and in all patients with autonomic neuropathy, hepatic or renal disease, hyperthyroidism, coronary heart disease, congestive heart failure, cardiac tachyarrhythmias, hypertension, or hiatal hernia associated with reflux esophagitis, since anticholinergics may aggravate this condition.
In patients with ulcerative colitis, large doses of propantheline bromide may suppress intestinal motility to the point of producing paralytic ileus and, for this reason, may precipitate or aggravate toxic megacolon, a serious complication of the disease.
Information for patients: Propantheline bromide may produce drowsiness or blurred vision. The patient should be cautioned regarding activities requiring mental alertness, such as operating a motor vehicle or other machinery or performing hazardous work, while taking this drug.
Drug interactions: Anticholinergics may delay absorption of other medication given concomitantly.
Excessive cholinergic blockade may occur if propantheline bromide is given concomitantly with belladonna alkaloids, synthetic or semisynthetic anticholinergic agents, narcotic analgesics such as meperidine, Type 1 antiarrhythmic drugs (e.g., disopyramide, procainamide, or quinidine), antihistamines, phenothiazines, tricyclic antidepressants, or other psychoactive drugs. Propantheline bromide may also potentiate the sedative effect of phenothiazines. Increased intraocular pressure may result from concurrent administration of anticholinergics and corticosteroids.
Concurrent use of propantheline bromide with slow-dissolving tablets of digoxin may cause increased serum digoxin levels. This interaction can be avoided by using only those digoxin tablets that rapidly dissolve by USP standards.
Carcinogenesis, mutagenesis, impairment of fertility: No long-term fertility, carcinogenicity, or mutagenesis studies have been done with propantheline bromide.
Pregnancy: Pregnancy Category C. Animal reproduction studies have not been conducted with propantheline bromide. It is also not known whether propantheline bromide can cause fetal harm when administered to a pregnant woman or can affect reproduction capacity. Propantheline bromide should be given to a pregnant woman only if clearly needed.
Nursing mothers: It is not known whether this drug is excreted in human milk. Because many drugs are excreted in human milk, caution should be exercised when propantheline bromide is administered to a nursing woman. Suppression of lactation may occur with anticholinergic drugs.
Pediatric use: Safety and effectiveness in children have not been established.

ADVERSE REACTIONS

Varying degrees of drying of salivary secretions may occur as well as decreased sweating. Ophthalmic side effects include blurred vision, mydriasis, cycloplegia, and increased ocular tension. Other reported adverse reactions include urinary hesitancy and retention, tachycardia, palpitations, loss of the sense of taste, headache, nervousness, mental confusion, drowsiness, weakness, dizziness, insomnia, nausea, vomiting, constipation, bloated feeling, impotence, suppression of lactation, and allergic reactions or drug idiosyncrasies, including anaphylaxis, urticaria, and other dermal manifestations.

OVERDOSAGE

The symptoms of overdosage with propantheline bromide progress from an intensification of the usual side effects to

CNS disturbances (from restlessness and excitement to psychotic behavior), circulatory changes (flushing, fall in blood pressure, circulatory failure), respiratory failure, paralysis, and coma.
Measures to be taken are (1) immediate induction of emesis or lavage of the stomach, (2) injection of physostigmine 0.5 to 2 mg intravenously, repeated as necessary up to a total of 5 mg, and (3) monitoring of vital signs and managing as necessary.
Fever may be treated symptomatically (cooling blanket or alcohol sponging). Excitement of a degree which demands attention may be managed with thiopental sodium 2% solution given slowly intravenously, or diazepam, 5 to 10 mg intravenously or 10 mg intramuscularly. In the event of progression of the curare-like effect to paralysis of the respiratory muscles, mechanical respiration should be instituted and maintained until effective respiratory action returns.
The oral LD_{50} of propantheline bromide is 780 mg/kg in the mouse and 370 mg/kg in the rat.

DOSAGE AND ADMINISTRATION

The usual initial adult dosage of **Pro-Banthīne®** tablets is 15 mg taken 30 minutes before each meal (3 times daily), and 30 mg at bedtime (a total of 75 mg daily). Subsequent dosage adjustment should be made according to the patient's individual response and tolerance. The administration of one $7^1/_2$-mg tablet 30 minutes before each meal (3 times daily) is convenient for patients with mild manifestations, for geriatric patients, and for those of small stature.

HOW SUPPLIED

Pro-Banthīne® 15-mg tablets are round, peach colored, sugar coated, with RPC imprinted on one side and 074 on the other side. Bottles of 100 NDC 54092-074-01, and bottles of 500 NDC 54092-074-05, cartons containing 100 unit-dose, individually blister-sealed tablets NDC 54092-074-52.
Pro-Banthīne® $7^1/_2$-mg tablets are round, white, sugar coated, with RPC imprinted on one side and 073 on the other side; bottles of 100. NDC 54092-073-01
Store below 25°C (77°F).
Caution: United States law prohibits dispensing without prescription.
Manufactured for
Roberts Laboratories Inc., a subsidiary of
ROBERTS PHARMACEUTICAL CORPORATION
Eatontown, New Jersey 07724, USA
by Searle & Co.
San Juan, Puerto Rico 00936

QUIBRON® ℞
[*kwĭ'bron*]
(theophylline-guaifenesin)

QUIBRON®-300 ℞
(theophylline-guaifenesin)

QUIBRON®-T ℞
(theophylline Tablets, USP)
ACCUDOSE™ Tablets
IMMEDIATE RELEASE BRONCHODILATOR

QUIBRON®-T/SR ℞
(theophylline anhydrous)
ACCUDOSE™ Tablets
SUSTAINED-RELEASE BRONCHODILATOR

DESCRIPTION

QUIBRON®-T TABLETS
ACCUDOSE™Tablets
IMMEDIATE-RELEASE BRONCHODILATOR
Theophylline is a bronchodilator structurally classified as a xanthine derivative. It occurs as a white, odorless, crystalline powder having a bitter taste. Theophylline anhydrous has the chemical name, 1 H-purine-2,6-dione,3,7-dihydro-1,3-dimethyl-, and is represented by the following structural formula:

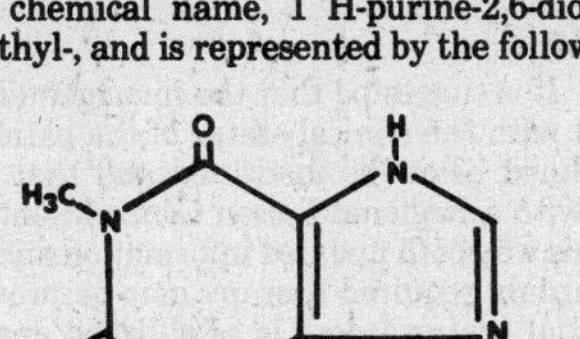

QUIBRON®-T tablets provide 300 mg of anhydrous theophylline as an oral bronchodilator in an immediate release formulation combined with the convenience of the unique **ACCUDOSE** tablet design. With functional trisects and bisects, QUIBRON®-T tablets can be conveniently and accurately divided into 100, 150, and 200 mg segments to provide a variety of dosing increments, as required.

QUIBRON®-T tablets	
One-third tablet	= 100 mg
One-half tablet	= 150 mg
Two-thirds tablet	= 200 mg
One tablet	= 300 mg

Inactive Ingredients: microcrystalline cellulose, yellow ferric oxide, hydroxypropyl methylcellulose 2910, lactose, magnesium stearate, colloidal silicon dioxide, and sodium starch glycolate.

QUIBRON® AND QUIBRON®-300
Guaifenesin is an expectorant classified as a guaiacol compound. It occurs as a white to slightly yellow crystalline powder with a bitter, aromatic taste. Guaifenesin has the chemical name, 3-(o-Methoxyphenoxy)-1,2-propanediol, and is represented by the following structural formula:

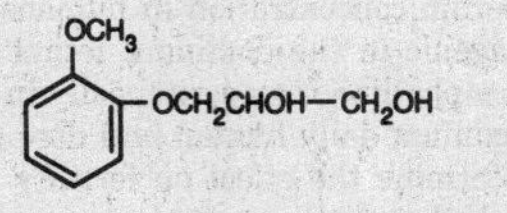

QUIBRON® is available as soft gelatin capsules intended for oral administration, containing 150 mg of theophylline anhydrous and 90 mg of guaifenesin. QUIBRON®-300 is available as soft gelatin capsules intended for oral administration, containing 300 mg of theophylline anhydrous and 180 mg of guaifenesin. These products contain the following inactive ingredients: D&C Yellow No. 10, non-porcine gelatin, glycerin, edible ink, polyethylene glycol, and titanium dioxide.

QUIBRON®-T/SR **ACCUDOSE Tablets**
SUSTAINED-RELEASE BRONCHODILATOR
QUIBRON®-T/SR tablets provide 300 mg of anhydrous theophylline as an oral bronchodilator in a sustained release formulation combined with the convenience of the unique divided tablet design. With functional trisects and bisects, QUIBRON®-T/SR tablets can be conveniently and accurately divided into 100-, 150-, and 200-mg segments to provide a variety of dosing increments, as required.

QUIBRON®-T/SR tablets	
One-third tablet	= 100 mg
One-half tablet	= 150 mg
Two-thirds tablet	= 200 mg
One tablet	= 300 mg

Inactive Ingredient: microcrystalline cellulose.

CLINICAL PHARMACOLOGY

QUIBRON®, QUIBRON®-300, QUIBRON®-T
Theophylline
Mode of Action
Theophylline directly relaxes the smooth muscle of the bronchial airways and pulmonary blood vessels, thus acting mainly as a bronchodilator and smooth muscle relaxant. It has also been demonstrated that aminophylline has a potent effect on diaphragmatic contractility in normal persons and may then be capable of reducing fatigability and thereby improve contractility in patients with chronic obstructive airways disease. The exact mode of action remains unsettled. Although theophylline does cause inhibition of phosphodiesterase with a resultant increase in intracellular cyclic AMP, other agents similarly inhibit the enzyme producing a rise of cyclic AMP, but are unassociated with any demonstrable bronchodilation. Other mechanisms proposed include an effect on translocation of intracellular calcium; prostaglandin antagonism; endogenous stimulation of catecholamines; inhibition of cyclic guanosine monophosphate metabolism and adenosine receptor antagonism. None of these mechanisms has been proven, however.
In vitro, theophylline has been shown to act synergistically with Beta-agonists and there are now available data which do demonstrate an additive effect *in vivo* with combined use.
Pharmacokinetics
The half-life of theophylline is influenced by a number of known variables. It may be prolonged in chronic alcoholics, particularly those with liver disease (cirrhosis or alcoholic liver disease), in patients with congestive heart failure, and in those patients taking certain other drugs (see PRECAUTIONS, Drug Interactions). Neonates have extremely slow clearance rates compared to older infants and children, e.g., those over 1 year. Older children have rapid clearance rates while most nonsmoking adults have clearance rates between these two extremes. In premature neonates the decreased clearance is related to oxidative pathways that have yet to be established.

Theophylline Elimination Characteristics

	Half-Life (in hours)	
	Range	Mean
Children	1–9	3.7
Adults	3–15	7.7

In cigarette smokers (1 to 2 packs/day) the mean half-life is 4 to 5 hours, much shorter than in nonsmokers. The increase in clearance associated with smoking is presumably due to stimulation of the hepatic metabolic pathway by components of cigarette smoke. The duration of this effect after cessation of smoking is unknown but may require 6 months to 2 years before the rate approaches that of the nonsmoker.

QUIBRON® AND QUIBRON®-300
Guaifenesin
Mode of Action
Guaifenesin increases respiratory tract secretions, possibly by stimulating the goblet cells.
Pharmacokinetics
Guaifenesin appears to be well absorbed, but its pharmacokinetics have not been well studied.
QUIBRON®-T/SR
Pharmacokinetics
The half-life of theophylline is influenced by a number of known variables. It may be prolonged in chronic alcoholics, particularly those with liver disease (cirrhosis or alcoholic liver disease), in patients with congestive heart failure, and in those patients taking certain other drugs (see PRECAUTIONS, Drug Interactions).
Neonates have extremely slow clearance rates compared to older infants and children, e.g., those over 1 year. Older children have rapid clearance rates, while most nonsmoking adults have clearance rates between these two extremes. In premature neonates, the decreased clearance is related to oxidative pathways that have yet to be established.

Theophylline Elimination Characteristics

	Half-life (in hours)	
	Range	**Mean**
Children	1–9	3.7
Adults	3–15	7.7

In cigarette smokers (1 to 2 packs/day) the mean half-life is 4 to 5 hours, much shorter than in nonsmokers. The increase in clearance associated with smoking is presumably due to stimulation of the hepatic metabolic pathway by components of cigarette smoke. The duration of this effect after cessation of smoking is unknown but may require 6 months to 2 years before the rate approaches that of the nonsmoker.
In a single-dose study of QUIBRON®-T/SR (theophylline, anhydrous), a 300-mg dose in 12 fasted normal male subjects gave a mean peak plasma level of 5.26 ± 1.04 μg/mL at 6.25 ± 1.10 (S.D.) hours.
In a multi-dose, steady of 16 adult patients with a mean age of 39.0 years, the patients were dose-titrated to a therapeutically effective level without toxicity. Doses were administered once every 12 hours and ranged from 7.8 mg/kg/24 hours to 18.6 mg/kg/24 hours with a mean dose of 10.0 ± 2.8 (S.D.) mg/kg/24 hours. No food-fasting conditions were imposed in the study. A mean C_{max} of 13.9 ± 3.2 (S.D.) μg/mL, a mean C_{min} of 7.7 ± 2.0 (S.D.) μg/mL, and a mean percent fluctuation $[(C_{max} - C_{min})/C_{min} \times 100]$ of 87.1 ± 49.6 (S.D.) resulted from the study.
In a multi-dose, steady state study of 15 patients with a mean age of 14.4 years, the patients were dose-titrated to a therapeutically effective level without toxicity. Doses were administered once every 12 hours and ranged from 9.1 mg/kg/24 hours to 22.6 mg/kg/24 hours with a mean dose of 13.3 ± 3.9 (S.D.) mg/kg/24 hours. No food-fasting conditions were imposed in the study. A mean C_{max} of 13.8 ± 3.9 (S.D.) μg/mL, a mean C_{min} of 8.0 ± 2.5 (S.D.) μg/mL, and a mean percent fluctuation $[(C_{max} - C_{min})/C_{min} \times 100]$ of 85.4 ± 57.7 (S.D.) resulted from the study.
In a multiple-dose bioavailability study in 16 normal volunteers, when tested against an immediate-release reference tablet, QUIBRON®-T/SR was found to be 98% bioavailable.

INDICATIONS AND USAGE

QUIBRON®Capsules, QUIBRON®-300 Capsules, QUIBRON®-T tablets, and QUIBRON®-T/SR tablets are indicated for relief and/or prevention of symptoms from asthma and reversible bronchospasm associated with chronic bronchitis and emphysema.

CONTRAINDICATIONS

QUIBRON®Capsules, QUIBRON®-300 Capsules, QUIBRON®-T tablets, and QUIBRON®-T/SR tablets are contraindicated in individuals who have shown hypersensitivity to their components. They are also contraindicated in patients with active peptic ulcer disease, and in individuals with underlying seizure disorders (unless receiving appropriate anticonvulsant medication).

WARNINGS

Excessive doses may be associated with toxicity, although increasing the dose of theophylline may enhance response. The likelihood of serious toxicity increases significantly when the serum theophylline concentration exceeds 20 μg/mL. Therefore, determination of serum theophylline levels is recommended to assure maximal benefit without excessive risk.
Serum levels above 20 μg/mL are rarely found after appropriate administration of the recommended doses. However, in individuals in whom theophylline plasma clearance is reduced **for any reason,** even conventional doses may result in increased serum levels and potential toxicity. Reduced theophylline clearance has been documented in the following readily identifiable groups: 1) patients with impaired

Continued on next page

Roberts—Cont.

liver function; 2) patients over 55 years of age, particularly males and those with chronic lung disease; 3) those with cardiac failure from any cause; 4) patients with sustained high fever; 5) neonates and infants under 1 year of age; and 6) those patients taking certain drugs (see PRECAUTIONS, Drug Interactions). Frequently, such patients have markedly prolonged theophylline serum levels following discontinuation of the drug. Reduction of dosage and laboratory monitoring is especially appropriate in the above individuals.

Serious side effects such as ventricular arrhythmias, convulsions or even death may appear as the first sign of toxicity without any previous warning. Less serious signs of theophylline toxicity (ie, nausea and restlessness) may occur frequently when initiating therapy, but are usually transient; when such signs are persistent during maintenance therapy, they are often associated with serum concentrations above 20 μg/mL. Stated differently: *serious toxicity is not reliably preceded by less severe side effects*. A serum concentration measurement is the only reliable method of predicting potentially life-threatening toxicity.

Many patients who require theophylline exhibit tachycardia due to their underlying disease process, so that the cause/effect relationship to elevated serum theophylline concentrations may not be appreciated. Theophylline products may cause or worsen arrhythmias and any significant change in rate and/or rhythm warrants monitoring and further investigation.

Studies in laboratory animals (minipigs, rodents, and dogs) recorded the occurrence of cardiac arrhythmias and sudden death (with histologic evidence of myocardial necrosis) when β-agonists and methylxanthines were administered concurrently. The significance of these findings when applied to humans is currently unknown.

PRECAUTIONS

QUIBRON®, QUIBRON®-300, AND QUIBRON®-T
General

On the average, theophylline half-life is shorter in cigarette and marijuana smokers than in nonsmokers, but smokers can have half-lives as long as nonsmokers. Theophylline should not be administered concurrently with other xanthines. Use with caution in patients with hypoxemia, hypertension, or those with history of peptic ulcer. Theophylline may occasionally act as a local irritant to G.I. tract although gastrointestinal symptoms are more commonly centrally mediated and associated with serum drug concentrations over 20 μg/mL.

Information for Patients

The importance of taking only the prescribed dose and time interval between doses should be reinforced.

Laboratory Tests

Serum levels should be monitored periodically to determine the theophylline level associated with observed clinical response and as the method of predicting toxicity. For such measurements, the serum sample should be obtained at the time of peak concentration, 1 to 2 hours after administration for immediate release products. It is important that the patient will not have missed or taken additional doses during the previous 48 hours and that dosing intervals will have been reasonably equally spaced. DOSAGE ADJUSTMENT BASED ON SERUM THEOPHYLLINE MEASUREMENTS WHEN THESE INSTRUCTIONS HAVE NOT BEEN FOLLOWED MAY RESULT IN RECOMMENDATIONS THAT PRESENT RISK OF TOXICITY TO THE PATIENT.

Drug Interactions

Toxic synergism with ephedrine has been documented and may occur with other sympathomimetic bronchodilators. In addition, the following drug interactions have been demonstrated:

Theophylline with:	
Allopurinol (high dose)	Increased serum theophylline levels
Cimetidine	Increased serum theophylline levels
Ciprofloxacin	Increased serum theophylline levels
Erythromycin, Troleandomycin	Increased serum theophylline levels
Lithium Carbonate	Increased renal excretion of lithium
Oral Contraceptives	Increased serum theophylline levels
Phenytoin	Decreased theophylline and phenytoin serum levels
Propranolol	Increased serum theophylline levels
Rifampin	Decreased serum theophylline levels

Drug-Laboratory Test Interactions

Currently available analytical methods, including high pressure liquid chromatography and immunoassay techniques, for measuring serum theophylline levels are specific. Metabolites and other drugs generally do not affect the results. Other new analytic methods are also now in use. The physician should be aware of the laboratory method used and whether other drugs will interfere with the assay for theophylline.

Carcinogenesis, Mutagenesis, and Impairment of Fertility

Long-term carcinogenicity studies have not been performed with theophylline.

Chromosome-breaking activity was detected in human cell cultures at concentrations of theophylline up to 50 times the therapeutic serum concentration in humans. Theophylline was not mutagenic in the dominant lethal assay in male mice given theophylline intraperitoneally in doses up to 30 times the maximum daily human oral dose.

Studies to determine the effect on fertility have not been performed with theophylline.

Pregnancy

Category C—Animal reproduction studies have not been conducted with theophylline. It is also not known whether theophylline can cause fetal harm when administered to a pregnant woman or can affect reproduction capacity. Xanthines should be given to a pregnant woman only if clearly needed.

Nursing Mothers

Theophylline is distributed into breast milk and may cause irritability or other signs of toxicity in nursing infants. Because of the potential for serious adverse reactions in nursing infants from theophylline, a decision should be made whether to discontinue nursing or to discontinue the drug, taking into account the importance of the drug to the mother.

Pediatric Use

Safety and effectiveness of QUIBRON®, QUIBRON®-300, QUIBRON®-T, and QUIBRON®-T/SR in children under 6 years of age have not been established.

Safety and effectiveness of theophylline immediate-release products in children under 1 year of age have not been established. Because of the potential difficulty of drug administration (eg, tablet swallowability) and the inability to provide small and precise incremental doses, it is recommended that a liquid theophylline preparation be used for children under 6 years of age.

QUIBRON®T/SR

PRECAUTIONS

General

On the average, theophylline half-life is shorter in cigarette and marijuana smokers than in nonsmokers, but smokers can have half-lives as long as nonsmokers. Theophylline should not be administered concurrently with other xanthines. Use with caution in patients with hypoxemia, hypertension, or those with a history of peptic ulcer. Theophylline may occasionally act as a local irritant to the GI tract, although gastrointestinal symptoms are more commonly centrally mediated and associated with serum drug concentrations over 20 μg/mL.

Information for Patients

QUIBRON®-T/SR Tablets should not be chewed or crushed. The importance of taking only the prescribed dose and time interval between doses should be reinforced.

The patient should alert the physician if symptoms occur repeatedly, especially near the end of a dosing interval.

Drug Interactions

Toxic synergism with ephedrine has been documented and may occur with other sympathomimetic bronchodilators. In addition, the folowing drug interactions have been demonstrated:

Theophylline with:	
Allopurinol (high dose)	Increased serum theophylline levels
Cimetidine	Increased serum theophylline levels
Ciprofloxacin	Increased serum theophylline levels
Erythromycin, Troleandomycin	Increased serum theophylline levels
Litium carbonate	Increased rnal excretion of lithium
Oral contraceptives	Increased serum theophylline levels
Phenytoin	Decreased theophylline and phenytoin serum levels
Propranolol	Increased serum theophylline levels
Rifampin	Decreased serum theophylline levels

Drug-Food Interactions

QUIBRON®-T/SR has not been adequately studied to determine whether its bioavailability is altered when it is given with food.

Available data suggests that drug administration at the time of food ingestion may influence the absorption characteristics of some or all theophylline controlled-release products, resulting in serum values different from those found after administration in the fasting state.

A drug-food effect, if any, would likely have its greatest clinical significance when high theophylline serum levels are being maintained and/or when large single doses (> 13 mg/kg or 900 mg) of a controlled-release theophylliine product are given. The influence of type and amount of food on performance of controlled-release theophylline products is under study at this time.

Drug-Laboratory Test Interactions

Currently available analytical methods, including high-pressure liquid chromatography and immunoassay techniques, for measuring serum theophylline levels are specific. Metabolites and other drugs generally do not affect the results. Other new analytic methods are also now in use. The physician should be aware of the laboratory method used and whether other drugs will interfere with the assay for theophylline.

Carcinogenesis, Mutagenesis, and Impairment of Fertility

Long-term carcinogenicity studies have not been performed with theophylline.

Chromosome-breaking activity was detected in human cell cultures at concentrations of theophylline up to 50 times the therapeutic serum concentration in humans. Theophylline was not mutagenic in the dominant lethal assay i male mice given theophylline intraperitoneally in doses up to 30 times the maximum daily human oral dose.

Studies to determine the effect on fertility have not been performed with theophylline.

Pregnancy

Category C —Animal reproduction studies have not been conducted with theophylline. It is also not known whether theophylline can cause fetal harm when administered to a pregnant woman or whether it affects reproductive capacity. Xanthines should be given to a pregnant woman only if clearly needed.

Nursing Mothers

Theophylline is distributed into breast milk and may cause irritability or other signs of toxicity in nursing infants. Because of the potential for serious adverse reactions in nursing infants, a decision should be made whether to discontinue nursing or to discontinue the drug, taking into account the importance of the drug to the mother.

Pediatric Use

Safety and effectiveness of sustained-release theophylline in children under 6 years of age have not been established. Because of the potential difficulty of drug administration (e.g., tablet swallowability) and the inability to provide small and precise incremental doses, it is recommended that a liquid theophylline preparation be used for children under 6 years of age.

ADVERSE REACTIONS

QUIBRON®, QUIBRON®-300, QUIBRON®-T, and QUIBRON®-T/SR

The following adverse reactions have been observed, but there has not been enough systematic collection of data to support an estimate of their frequency. The most consistent adverse reactions are usually due to overdosage.

1. *Gastrointestinal:* nausea, vomiting, epigastric pain, hematemesis, diarrhea.
2. *Central nervous system:* headaches, irritability, restlessness, insomnia, reflex hyperexcitability, muscle twitching, clonic and tonic generalized convulsions.
3. *Cardiovascular:* palpitation, tachycardia, extrasystoles, flushing, hypotension, circulatory failure, ventricular arrhythmias.
4. *Respiratory:* tachypnea.
5. *Renal:* potentiation of diuresis.
6. *Others:* alopecia, hyperglycemia, inappropriate ADH syndrome, rash.

OVERDOSAGE

Management: It is suggested that the management principles (consistent with the clinical status of the patient when first seen) outlined below be instituted and that simultaneous contact with a Regional Poison Control Center be established. In this way both updated information and individualization regarding required therapy may be provided.

1. When potential oral overdose is established and seizure has not occurred:
   a) If patient is alert and seen within the early hours after ingestion, induction of emesis may be of value. Gastric lavage has been demonstrated to be of no value in influencing outcome in patients who present more than 1 hour after ingestion.
   b) Administer a cathartic. Sorbitol solution is reported to be of value. This is particularly important if a sustained release preparation has been taken.
   c) Administer repeated doses of activated charcoal and monitor theophylline serum levels. Monitor vital signs, maintain blood pressure, and provide adequate hydration.
   d) Prophylactic administration of phenobarbital has been shown to increase the seizure threshold in laboratory

animals, and administration of this drug can be considered.

2. If patient presents with a seizure:
   a) Establish an airway.
   b) Administer oxygen.
   c) Treat the seizure with intravenous diazepam, 0.1 to 0.3 mg/kg, up to 10 mg. If seizures cannot be controlled, the use of general anesthesia should be considered.
   d) Monitor vital signs, maintain blood pressure, and provide adequate hydration.
3. If postseizure coma is present:
   a) Maintain airway and oxygenation.
   b) If a result of oral medication, follow above recommendations to prevent absorption of the drug, but intubation and lavage will have to be performed instead of inducing emesis, and the cathartic and charcoal will need to be introduced via a large bore gastric lavage tube.
   c) Continue to provide full supportive care and adequate hydration until the drug is metabolized. In general, drug metabolism is sufficiently rapid so as not to warrant dialysis. If repeated oral activated charcoal is ineffective (as noted by stable or rising serum levels) charcoal hemoperfusion may be indicated.

DOSAGE AND ADMINISTRATION

QUIBRON®-T/SR (theophylline, anhydrous), has not been adequately studied for its bioavailability when administered with food (see PRECAUTIONS, Drug-Food Interactions).

QUIBRON, QUIBRON-300, QUIBRON-T, and QUIBRON®-T/SR

Effective use of theophylline (ie, the concentration of drug in the serum associated with optimal benefit and minimal risk of toxicity) is considered to occur when the theophylline concentration is maintained from 10 to 20 μg/mL. The early studies from which these levels were derived were carried out in patients immediately or shortly after recovery from acute exacerbations of their disease (some hospitalized with status asthmaticus).

Although the 20 μg/mL level remains appropriate as a critical value (above which toxicity is more likely to occur) for safety purposes, additional data are now available which indicate that the serum theophylline concentrations required to produce maximum physiologic benefit may, in fact, fluctuate with the degree of bronchospasm present and are variable. Therefore, the physician should individualize the range appropriate to the patient's requirements, based on both symptomatic response and improvement in pulmonary function. It should be stressed that serum theophylline concentrations maintained at the upper level of the 10- to 20-μg/mL range may be associated with potential toxicity when factors known to reduce theophylline clearance are operative. (See WARNINGS).

If it is not possible to obtain serum level determinations, restriction of the daily dose (in otherwise healthy adults) to not greater than 13 mg/kg/day, to a maximum of 900 mg, in divided doses will result in relatively few patients exceeding serum levels of 20 μg/mL and, therefore, no greater risk of toxicity.

Caution should be exercised for younger children who cannot complain of minor side effects. Older adults, those with cor pulmonale, congestive heart failure, and/or liver disease may have unusually low dosage requirements and thus may experience toxicity at the maximal dosage recommended below.

Theophylline does not distribute into fatty tissue. Dosage should be calculated on the basis of lean (ideal) body weight where mg/kg doses are presented.

Frequency of Dosing: When immediate-release products with rapid absorption are used, dosing to maintain serum levels generally requires administration every 6 hours. This is particularly true in children, but dosing intervals up to 8 hours may be satisfactory in adults since they eliminate the drug at a slower rate. Some children, and adults requiring higher-than-average doses (those having rapid rates of clearance, e.g., half-lives of under 6 hours), may benefit and be more effectively controlled during chronic therapy when given products with sustained-release characteristics since these provide longer dosing intervals and/or less fluctuation in serum concentration between dosing. Dosage guidelines are approximations only and the wide range of theophylline clearance between individuals (particularly those with concomitant disease) makes indiscriminate usage hazardous.

Dosage Guidelines

I. Acute symptoms of bronchospasm requiring rapid attainment of theophylline serum levels for bronchodilation. QUIBRON®-T/SR is not intended for use in status asthmaticus or with patients experiencing an acute episode of bronchospasm (associated with asthma, chronic bronchitis, or emphysema). Such patients require ***rapid*** relief of symptoms and should be treated with an immediate-release or intravenous theophylline preparation (or other bronchodilators) and not with controlled-release products.

NOTE: Status asthmaticus should be considered a medical emergency and is defined as that degree of bronchospasm which is not rapidly responsive to usual doses of conventional bronchodilators. Optimal therapy for such patients frequently requires both ***additional medication,*** parenterally administered, and ***close monitoring,*** preferably in an intensive care setting.

If serum theophylline Is:		Directions:
Within desired range		Maintain dosage if tolerated.
Too high	20 to 25μg/mL	Decrease dosage by about 10% and recheck serum levels after 3 days.
	25 to 30μg/mL	Skip the next dose and decrease subsequent doses by about 25%. Recheck serum level after 3 days.
	Over 30μg/mL	Skip next 2 doses and decrease subsequent doses by 50%. Recheck serum level after 3 days.
Too low		Increase dosage by 25% at 3-day intervals until either the desired serum concentration and/or clinical response is achieved. The total daily dose may need to be administered at more frequent intervals if symptoms occur repeatedly at the end of a dosing interval.

II. Chronic Therapy

A. Initiating Therapy with an Immediate-Release Product. It is recommended that the appropriate dosage be established using an immediate-release preparation. A dosage form that allows small incremental doses is desirable for initiation therapy. A liquid preparation should be considered for children to permit easier and more accurate dosage adjustment. Slow clinical titration is generally preferred to help assure acceptance and safety of the medication and to allow the patient to develop tolerance in transient caffeine-like side effects. Then, if the total 24-hour dose can be given by use of the available strengths of this product, the patient can usually be switched to QUIBRON®-T/SR (theophylline, anhydrous), giving one-third of the daily dose at 8-hour intervals or one-half the daily dose at 12-hour intervals. Patients who metabolize theophylline rapidly, such as the young, smokers, and some nonsmoking adults are the most likely candidates for dosing at 8-hour intervals. Such patients can generally be identified as having trough serum concentrations lower than desired or repeatedly exhibiting symptoms near the end of a dosing interval.

B. Initiating Therapy with QUIBRON®-T/SR

Alternatively, therapy can be initiated with QUIBRON®-T/SR ACCUDOSE™ Tablets, since they are designed to be divided into segments which provide a variety of dosing increments that permit titration and adjustments of dosage (in adults and older children). Children weighing less than 25 kg should have their daily dosage requirements established with a liquid theophylline preparation to permit small dosage increments.

Initial Dose: 16 mg/kg/24 hours or 400 mg/24 hours (whichever is less) of QUIBRON®-T/SR in divided doses at 8- or 12-hour intervals.

Increasing Dose: The above dosage may be increased in approximately 25% increments at 3-day intervals, so long as the drug is tolerated; until clinical response is satisfactory or the maximum dose as indicated in Section III (below) is reached. The serum concentration should be checked at these intervals, but at a minimum, should be determined at the end of this adjustment period.

It is important that no patient be maintained on any dosage that is not tolerated. When instructing patients to increase dosage according to the schedule above, they should be told not to take a subsequent dose if apparent side effects occur and to resume therapy at a lower dose once adverse effects have disappeared.

III. Maximum Dose of Theophylline Where the Serum Concentration is not Measured:

WARNING: DO NOT ATTEMPT TO MAINTAIN ANY DOSE THAT IS NOT TOLERATED.

Not to exceed the following: (or 900 mg, whichever is less)

Age 6* to under 9 years	24 mg/kg/day
Age 9 to under 12 years	20 mg/kg/day
Age 12 to under 16 years	18 mg/kg/day
Age 16 years and older	13 mg/kg/day

*1 for QUIBRON®-T

IV. Measurement of Serum Theophylline Concentrations During Chronic Therapy:

If the above maximum doses are to be maintained or exceeded, serum theophylline measurement is essential. (See PRECAUTIONS, Laboratory Tests, for guidance.)

V. Final Adjustment of Dosage:

Dosage adjustment after serum theophylline measurement.

[See table on top of page.]

The serum concentration should be rechecked at appropriate intervals, but at least at the end of the adjustment period. When the patient's condition is otherwise clinically stable and none of the recognized factors which alter elimination are present, measurement of serum levels needs to be repeated only every 6 to 12 months.

DOSAGE OF THEOPHYLLINE TO PROVIDE mg ANHYDROUS THEOPHYLLINE/kg BODY WEIGHT*/DOSE

Body Weight*		Approximate Dose in mg		
Lbs	kg	3 mg/kg	4 mg/kg	5 mg/kg
40	18	54	72	90
60	27	81	108	135
70	32	96	128	160
80	36	108	144	180
90	41	123	164	205
100	45	135	180	225
120	55	165	220	275
140	64	192		320
160	73	219		365
180	82	246		410
200	91	273		455
220	100	300		500

* For obese patients, use lean (e.g., ideal) body weight.

HOW SUPPLIED

QUIBRON® Capsules: One piece, opaque yellow, soft gelatin capsules printed "Roberts" and "067" containing 150 mg anhydrous theophylline and 90 mg guaifenesin.

NDC 54092-067-01 Bottles of 100
NDC 54092-067-10 Bottls of 1000
NDC 54092-067-52 Unit Dose 100's

QUIBRON®-300 Capsules: One piece, half opaque white/half opaque yellow, soft gelatin capsules with the "Roberts" and "068" containing 300 mg anhydrous theophylline and 180 mg guaifenesin.

NDC m54092-068-01 Bottles of 100

Store from 15°-25°C (59°-77°F). Dispense in a tight container as defined in the USP

QUIBRON®-T Tablets: Ivory in the **ACCUDOSE™** Tablet design p;rinted "RP" and "069" debossed on one side, containing 300 mg anhydrous theophylline.

NDC 54092-069-01 Bottles of 100

Store from 15°-25°C (59°-77°F).

QUIBRON®-T/SR Tablets: White in the "**ACCUDOSE**"™ Tablet design with debossed "RP" and "070" on one side containing 300 mg anhydrous theophylline.

NDC 54092-070-01 Bottles of 100
NDC 54092-070-05 Bottles of 500

Patent Nos. 4,465,660; 4,547,358; 4,215,104

Store from 15°-25°C (59°-77°F).

CAUTION: Federal law prohibits dispensing without a prescription.

Manufactured for
Roberts Laboratories Inc.,
a subsidiary of
ROBERTS PHARMACEUTICAL CORPORATION
Eatontown, NJ 07724 USA

SALURON® ℞
(Hydroflumethiazide)
SALURON Tablets—for oral administration

DESCRIPTION

Saluron® is a potent oral diuretic-antihypertensive agent of low toxicity. Each tablet contains the following

ACTIVE INGREDIENT

Hydroflumethiazide .... 50 mg

INACTIVE INGREDIENTS

cellulose microcrystalline, lactose, magnesium stearate, silicon dioxide collidal and sodium starch glycolate.

HOW SUPPLIED

Saluron® tablets, scored, 50 mg, in bottles of 100 (NDC 54092-055-01).

Store from 15°-25°C (59°-77°F).

Dispense in a tight, light-resistant container as defined in the USP.

CAUTION: Federal law prohibits dispensing without a prescription.

Continued on next page

Roberts—Cont.

SALUTENSIN®
SALUTENSIN-DEMI® ℞
(Hydroflumethiazide, Reserpine)
SALUTENSIN Tablets—for oral administration
Antihypertensive

> **Warning**
> This fixed combination drug is not indicated for initial therapy of hypertension. Hypertension requires therapy titrated to the individual patient. If the fixed combination represents the dosage so determined, its use may be more convenient in patient management. The treatment of hypertension is not static, but must be reevaluated as conditions in each patient warrant.

DESCRIPTION

Salutensin® and Salutensin-Demi® tablets for oral administration combine two antihypertensive agents: hydroflumethiazide and reserpine, and is indicated for hypertension. Each Salutensin® tablet contains the following

ACTIVE INGREDIENTS:

Saluron® (hydroflumethiazide) .... 50 mg
Reserpine .... 0.125 mg.

Each Salutensin-Demi® tablet contains the following

ACTIVE INGREDIENTS

Saluron® (hydroflumethiazide) .... 25 mg
Reserpine .... 0.125 mg

INACTIVE INGREDIENTS

Salutensin® Tablets: D&C Yellow No. 10 Lake, FD&C Blue No. 1 Lake 12%, lactose, magnesium stearate, povidone, starch, and sucrose.
Salutensin-Demi® Tablets: D&C Red No. 30 Lake, D&C Yellow No. 10 Lake, lactose, magnesium stearate, povidone, starch, and sucrose.

HOW SUPPLIED

Salutensin® tablets are round, green, and contain 50 mg of Saluron® (hydroflumethiazide) and 0.125 mg of reserpine. Bottles of 100 (NDC 54092-056-01) and bottles of 1000 (NDC 54092-056-10).
Salutensin-Demi Tablets are round, pale yellow, and contain 25 mg of Saluron® (hydroflumethiazide) and 0.125 mg of reserpine. Bottles of 100 (NDC 54092-057-01).
Store below 30°C (86°F).
Dispense in a tight, light-resistant container as defined in the USP.
CAUTION: Federal law prohibits dispensing without a prescription.

SUPPRELIN® (histrelin acetate) INJECTION ℞

DESCRIPTION

SUPPRELIN® (histrelin acetate) Injection contains a synthetic nonapeptide agonist of the naturally occurring gonadotropin releasing hormone (GnRH or LHRH). The analog possesses a greater potency than the natural sequence hormone. The amino acid sequence and chemical name of histrelin acetate is:
5-oxo-L-prolyl-L-histidyl-L-tryptophyl-L-seryl-L-tyrosyl-N^{t}-benzyl-D-histidyl-L-leucyl-L-arginyl-N-ethyl-L-prolinamide acetate (salt) [$C_{66}H_{86}N_{18}O_{12}$·(1.7–2.8 moles) CH_3COOH. (0.6–7.0 moles) H_20].
The molecular weight of the peptide base is 1323.52.

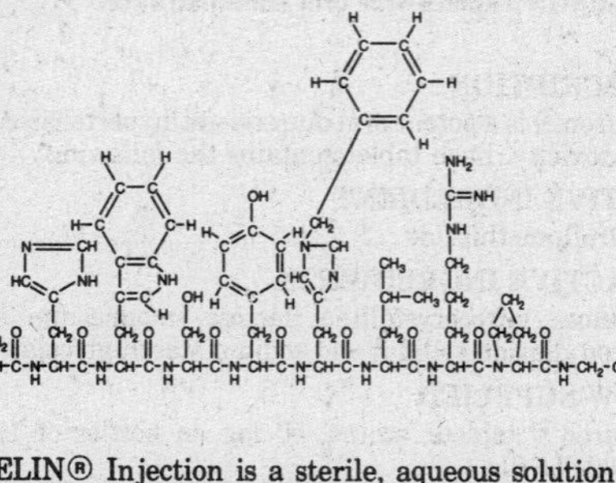

SUPPRELIN® Injection is a sterile, aqueous solution for subcutaneous administration available in single-use vials of 0.6 mL. It contains histrelin equivalent to either 200 mcg/mL, 500 mcg/mL, or 1000 mcg/mL peptide base with 0.9% sodium chloride and 10% mannitol. The pH of the 200 mcg/mL solution is 4.5–6.5 and the pH of the 500 mcg/mL and 1000 mcg/mL solutions is 4.5–6.0. All solutions are unbuffered, hypertonic and contain no preservative.

CLINICAL PHARMACOLOGY

SUPPRELIN® Injection, a GnRH agonist, is a potent inhibitor of gonadotropin secretion when administered daily in therapeutic doses. Both animal and human studies indicate that following an initial stimulatory phase, chronic, subcutaneous administration of histrelin acetate desensitizes responsiveness of the pituitary gonadotropin which, in turn, causes a reduction in ovarian and testicular steroidogenesis.
Although animal studies have shown that *acute* administration of SUPPRELIN® (histrelin acetate) Injection results in stimulation of the reproductive system, *chronic* SUPPRELIN® Injection administration in the rat delays sexual development, inhibits estrous cyclicity and pregnancy, reduces reproductive organ weight and inhibits ovarian and testicular steroidogenesis in a reversible fashion. In the rabbit, chronic administration of SUPPRELIN® Injection resulted in decreased reproductive organ weights.
In human studies, chronic administration of SUPPRELIN® Injection controls the secretion of pituitary gonadotropins resulting in decreased sex steroid levels and in the regression of secondary sexual characteristics in children with precocious puberty. In girls, menses cease, serum estradiol levels are decreased to prepubertal levels, linear growth velocities decrease, skeletal maturation is slowed, and adult height predictions increase. In boys, testicular steroidogenesis is inhibited and testicular volume is reduced.
Continuous SUPPRELIN® Injection administration to patients with central precocious puberty can be monitored by standard GnRH testing and by serial determinations of sex steroid levels. The decreases in LH, FSH, and sex steroid levels are evident within three months of the initiation of therapy. These effects have been demonstrated in the 10 female patients who were studied for periods up to eighteen months. The metabolism, distribution, and excretion of SUPPRELIN® Injection in humans have not been determined.

INDICATIONS AND USAGE

SUPPRELIN® Injection is indicated for the control of the biochemical and clinical manifestations of central precocious puberty.
Selection of Patients

1. Only patients with centrally mediated precocious puberty (either idiopathic or neurogenic and occurring before age 8 years in girls or 9.5 years in boys) should receive SUPPRELIN® Injection treatment.
2. Before treatment with SUPPRELIN® (histrelin acetate) Injection is instituted, a thorough physical and endocrinologic evaluation should be performed. This should include:
   a. Height and weight as baseline for serial monitoring.
   b. Hand and wrist x-ray for bone age determination, to document advanced skeletal age and as baseline for serially monitoring predicted height.
   c. Total sex steriod level (estradiol or testosterone).
   d. Adrenal steroid level, to exclude congenital adrenal hyperplasia.
   e. Beta-Human Chorionic Gonadotropin level, to rule out a chorionic gonadotropin-secreting tumor.
   f. GnRH stimulation test, to demonstrate activation of the Hypothalamic-Pituitary-Gonadal (HPG) axis.
   g. Pelvic/adrenal/testicular ultrasound, to rule out a steroid-secreting tumor and to document gonadal size for serial monitoring.
   h. Computerized tomography of the head, to rule out previously undiagnosed intracranial tumor.
3. Patients must be able to maintain compliance with a *daily* regimen of injections.

CONTRAINDICATIONS

SUPPRELIN® Injection should not be administered to patients known to be hypersensitive to any of its components.
SUPPRELIN® Injection is contraindicated in women who are or may become pregnant while receiving the drug and in nursing mothers. There was increased fetal size and mortality in rats and increased fetal mortality in rabbits but not in mice after SUPPRELIN® Injection administration. Other responses to SUPPRELIN® Injection included dystocia, a greater incidence of unilateral hydroureter, and incomplete ossification in rat fetuses in all treated groups. When administered to rabbits on days 6–18 of pregnancy at doses of 20 to 80 mcg/kg/day (2 to 8 times the human dose), SUPPRELIN® Injection produced early termination of pregnancy and increased fetal death. In rats administered SUPPRELIN® Injection on days 7–20 of pregnancy at doses of 1 to 15 mcg/kg/day (0.1 to 1.5 times the human dose) there was an increase in fetal resorptions. In mice treated on days 6–15 of pregnancy at 10 to 100 times the human dose Supprelin® Injection had no adverse effects. The effects on fetal mortality are expected consequences of the alterations in hormonal levels brought about by the drug. If this drug is inadvertently used during pregnancy or in the rare event that a patient becomes pregnant while taking this drug, she should be apprised of the potential hazard to the fetus.
It is not known if this drug is excreted in human milk, but because many drugs are excreted in human milk and because of the potential for serious adverse reactions in nursing infants from SUPPRELIN® Injection, the drug should not be given to nursing mothers.

WARNINGS

Non-compliance with drug regimen or inadequate dosing may result in inadequate control of the pubertal process. The consequences of poor control include the return of pubertal signs such as menses, breast development, and testicular growth. The long-term consequences of inadequate control of gonadal steroid secretion are unknown, but may include a further compromise of adult stature.
Serious hypersensitivity reactions (angioedema, urticaria) have been reported following SUPPRELIN® (histrelin acetate) Injection administration. Clinical manifestations may include: cardiovascular collapse, hypotension, tachycardia, loss of consciousness, angioedema, bronchospasm, dyspnea, urticaria, flushing and pruritus. If any allergic reaction occurs, therapy with SUPPRELIN® should be discontinued. Serious acute hypersensitivity reactions may require emergency medical treatment.

PRECAUTIONS

General: Studies in rats and monkeys have indicated that all of the known biochemical and antifertility effects of SUPPRELIN® Injection are reversible. Because animal studies are not always predictive of human response, and because children who have received SUPPRELIN® Injection have not been followed sufficiently long to ensure reactivation of the HPG axis following long-term therapy, this drug should be used only when the benefits to the patient outweigh the potential risks. In addition, the patient (and/or guardian) should be advised that hypogonadism may result if the HPG axis fails to reactivate after the drug is discontinued.
Information to patient: Prior to SUPPRELIN® Injection therapy, patients and their families should be informed of the importance of complying with the schedule of single, daily injections, given at approximately the same time each day. If injections are not given daily, the pubertal process may be reactivated. SUPPRELIN® Injection contains no preservative. Patients should be informed that vials are to be used once and any unused solution is to be discarded. Medication should be allowed to reach room temperature before injecting. Daily injections should be rotated through different body sites (upper arms, thighs, abdomen).
Patients should be made aware of the required monitoring of their condition and of the potential risks of therapy. Within the first month of therapy, girls being treated with SUPPRELIN® (histrelin acetate) Injection may experience a light menstrual flow. This menstrual flow is common and likely is related to the lower estrogen levels brought about by treatment, and the withdrawal of estrogen support from the endometrium.
Irritation, redness, or swelling at the injection sites may occur. If these reactions are severe, or do not go away, the patient's doctor should be notified.
The patients and their families should be advised to discontinue the drug and seek medical attention at the first sign of skin rash, urticaria, rapid heartbeat, difficulty in swallowing and breathing, or any swelling which may suggest angioedema (See Warnings and Adverse Reactions).
Clinical Evaluations/Laboratory Tests: An initial pelvic ultrasound should be performed to exclude other conditions before treating with SUPPRELIN® Injection. The patient should be monitored carefully after 3 months and every 6 to 12 months thereafter by serial clinical evaluations, repeated height measurements, bone age determinations (yearly), and serial GnRH testing to document that gonadotropin responsiveness of the pituitary remains prepubertal while on therapy. During the initial agonistic phase of treatment, the patient may demonstrate transient increases in breast tissue, moodiness, vaginal secretions, or testicular volume. After this initial agonistic phase (usually one to three weeks), control of the biochemical and physical manifestations of puberty should remain as long as chronic therapy is in effect. Treatment should be discontinued when the onset of puberty is desired. Following the discontinuation of SUPPRELIN® Injection treatment, the onset of normal puberty should be documented. In addition, patients should be monitored to assess menstrual cyclicity, reproductive function, and ultimate adult height.
Carcinogenesis, Mutagenesis, and Impairment of Fertility: Carcinogenicity studies were conducted in rats for 2 years at doses of 5, 25 or 150 mcg/kg/day (up to 15 times the human dose) and in mice for 18 months at doses of 20, 200, or 2000 mcg/kg/day (up to 200 times the human dose). As seen with other GnRH agonists, SUPPRELIN® (histrelin acetate) Injection administration was associated with an increase in tumors of hormonally responsive tissues. There was a significant increase in pituitary adenomas in rats. There was an increase in pancreatic islet-cell adenomas in treated female rats and a non-dose-related increase in testicular Leydig-cell tumors (highest incidence in the low-dose group). In mice, there was a significant increase in mammary-gland adenocarcinomas in all treated females. In addition, there were increases in stomach papillomas in male rats given high

doses, and an increase in histiocytic sarcomas in female mice at the highest dose.

Mutagenicity studies have not been performed. Fertility studies have been conducted in rats and monkeys given subcutaneous daily doses of SUPPRELIN® Injection up to 180 mcg/kg for 6 months and full reversibility of fertility suppression was demonstrated. The development and reproductive performance of offspring from parents treated with SUPPRELIN® Injection has not been investigated.

Pregnancy, Teratogenic effects: Pregnancy Category X. See "CONTRAINDICATIONS" section.

Nursing Mothers: See "CONTRAINDICATIONS" section.

Pediatric Use: Safety and effectiveness in children below the age of two years have not been established.

ADVERSE REACTIONS

At least one adverse experience was reported for 139 of the 183 (76%) children in clinical studies of central precocious puberty. Three of the 183 children (2%) stopped therapy due to a hypersensitivity reaction.

Adverse experience considered related or probably related to drug therapy included:

skin reactions at the medication site (redness, swelling, and itching)	45%
vaginal bleeding (usually only one episode within 1 to 3 weeks of starting therapy lasting several days)	22%
urticaria	4%
purpura	2%
convulsions (increased frequency)	2%
visual disturbances	2%
hot flashes/flushes	2%
edema (other than at medication site)	2%
mood changes	2%
erythema (other than at medication site)	1%
conduct disorder	1%

Other adverse experiences considered possibly related to drug therapy and reported in at least 1% of patients are as follows:

Cardiovascular: (1–3%)—palpitations, tachycardia, epistaxis, hypertension, migraine headache, pallor.
Endocrine: (6%)—leukorrhea; (1%)—goiter, hyperlipidemia, anemia, breast edema, breast pain, breast discharge, glycosuria
Gastrointestinal: (3–10%)—gastrointestinal pain, abdominal pain, nausea, vomiting, diarrhea; (1–3%)—GI cramps, GI distress, constipation, decreased appetite, and increased thirst
Miscellaneous: (14%)—pyrexia; (6%)—extremity pain; (1–3%)—fatigue, chills, malaise, neck, chest or trunk pain, viral infection
Musculoskeletal: (4%)—arthralgia; (1%)—pain, hypotonia
Nervous System: (22%)—headache; 1–3%)—somnolence, lethergy, dizziness impared consciousness, syncope, tremor, hyperkinesia, nervousness, anxiety, depression
Respiratory: (3–10%)—cough, pharyngitis; (1–3%)—hyperventilation, upper respiratory infection
Skin: (7%)—rash; (1–3%—pruritus, dyschromia, keratoderma, alopecia, sweating
Special Senses: (1–3%)—abnormal pupillary function, otalgia, hearing loss, polyopia, photophobia
Urogenital: (1–3%)—irritation or odor or pruritus or infections of the female genitalia, polyuria, dysuria, urinary frequency, incontinence, hematuria, nocturia

Acute generalized (angioedema, urticaria) hypersensitivity reactions have been reported (See: Warnings and Precautions).

Other Patients

SUPPRELIN® (histrelin acetate) injection has been studied in other patients for various indications (N=196). Adverse experiences occurring in 2% or more of the study population are:

Cardiovascular: (35%)—vasodilation; (3%)—edema, migraine headache, hypertension
Endocrine: (12%)—vaginal dryness; (3–10%)—metrorrhagia, breast pain, breast edema; (2–3%)—leukorrhea, breast discharge, decreased breast size, tenderness of female genitalia
Gastrointestinal: (3–10%)—nausea, GI pain, flatulence, decreased appetitie, dyspepsia; (2–3%)—vomiting, constipation, diarrhea, GI cramps, gastritis
Miscellaneous: (12%)—abdominal pain; (3–10%)—pain in trunk, body, or extremities, fatigue, pyrexia, weight gain, chest pain, viral infection; (2–3%)—chills, malaise, head/face pain, neck pain, purpura
Musculoskeletal: (3–10%)—arthralgia, joint stiffness, muscle cramps (2–3%)—muscle stiffness, myalgia
Nervous System: (22%)—headache; (3–10%)—mood changes, nervousness, dizziness, depression, libido changes, insomnia, anxiety; (2–3%)—paresthesia, cognitive changes, syncope
Respiratory: (3–10%)—upper respiratory infection, pharyngitis, respiratory congestion; (2–3%)—cough, asthma, breathing disorder, rhinorrhea, bronchitis, sinusitis
Skin: (12%)—skin reaction at the medication site; (3–10%)—acne, rash, sweating; (2–3%)—keratoderma, pruritus, pain
Special Senses: (6%)—visual disturbances; (2–3%)—ear congestion, otalgia
Urogenital: (3–10%)—pain of female genitalia, vaginitis, dysmenorrhea; (2–3%)—dyspareunia, dysuria, hypertrophy of female genitalia, pruritus of external female genitalia

Urticaria which was reported by less than 2% of the population, may be clinically significant.

DRUG ABUSE AND DEPENDENCE

No instances of drug abuse or dependence have been reported.

OVERDOSAGE

SUPPRELIN® (histrelin acetate) injection of up to 200 mcg/kg (rats, rabbits), or 2000 mcg/kg (mice) resulted in no systemic toxicity. This represents 20 to 200 times the maximal recommended human dose of 10 mcg/kg/day.

DOSAGE AND ADMINISTRATION

The dose of SUPPRELIN® Injection that is recommended for the treatment of central precocious puberty is 10 mcg/kg of body weight administered as a single, daily subcutaneous injection. If prepubertal levels of sex steroids and/or a prepubertal gonadotropin response to GnRH testing are not achieved within the first 3 months of treatment, the patient should be reevaluated. Doses greater than 10 mcg/kg/day have not been evaluated in clinical trials. The injection site should be varied daily.

NOTE: Parenteral drug products should be inspected visually for discoloration and particulate matter before use. SUPPRELIN® Injection contains no preservative. Vials are to be used once. Any unused solution is to be discarded.

HOW SUPPLIED

SUPPRELIN® Injection is supplied in a 30-day kit of single-use vials that deliver 0.6 mL of a sterile, preservative-free solution. Each kit contains 30 vials of the same strength of SUPPRELIN® Injection expressed as mcg of peptide base 30 syringes with needles, prescribing information and patient information.

NDC#	SUPPRELIN® Injection Strength (mcg peptide base)	SUPPRELIN® Injection per Vial (0.6 mL)
54092-637-75	200 mcg/mL	120 mcg
54092-638-75	500 mcg/mL	300 mcg
54092-639-75	1000 mcg/mL	600 mcg

Store refrigerated at 2–8°C (36–46°F) and protect from light. Remove vial from packaging only at time of use. Allow vial to reach room temperature before injecting contents. Discard unused portion of the vial after administration.

CAUTION

U.S. law prohibits dispensing without prescription.
U.S. patent No. 4,244,946.
Manufactured for
Roberts Laboratories Inc.
a subsidiary of
ROBERTS PHARMACEUTICAL CORPORATION
Eatontown, New Jersey 07724 USA
by Schering-Plough Products Inc.
Manati, Puerto Rico

17727702

Shown in Product Identification Guide, page 331

TIGAN® ℞
[*tī'găn*]
brand of trimethobenzamide hydrochloride
CAPSULES
SUPPOSITORIES
INJECTABLE

DESCRIPTION

Chemically, trimethobenzamide HCl is N-[p-[2-(dimethylamino) -ethoxy] benzyl]-3,4,5-trimethoxybenzamide hydrochloride. It has a molecular weight of 424.93 and the following structural formula:

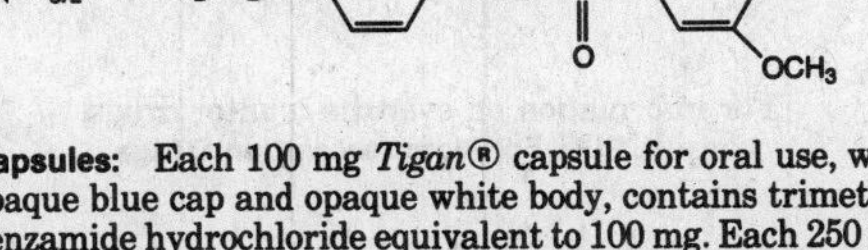
• HCl
OCH3
(CH3)2N—CH2CH2O
CH2NHC
O
OCH3
OCH3

Capsules: Each 100 mg *Tigan®* capsule for oral use, with opaque blue cap and opaque white body, contains trimethobenzamide hydrochloride equivalent to 100 mg. Each 250 mg *Tigan®* capsule for oral use, with opaque blue cap and body, contains trimethobenzamide hydrochloride equivalent to 250 mg. Both caps and bodies of the 100 and 250 mg capsules are imprinted with TIGAN® 100 mg and TIGAN® 250 mg, respectively.

Inactive Ingredients: FD&C Blue No. 1, FD&C Red No. 3, lactose, magnesium stearate, starch and titanium dioxide.

Suppositories (200 mg): Each suppository contains 200 mg trimethobenzamide hydrochloride and 2% benzocaine in a base compounded with polysorbate 80, white beeswax and propylene glycol monostearate.

Suppositories, Pediatric (100 mg): Each suppository contains 100 mg trimethobenzamide hydrochloride and 2% benzocaine in a base compounded with polysorbate 80, white beeswax and propylene glycol monostearate.

Ampuls: Each 2 mL ampul contains 200 mg trimethobenzamide hydrochloride compounded with 0.2% parabens (methyl and propyl) as preservatives, 1 mg sodium citrate and 0.4 mg citric acid as buffers and pH adjusted to approximately 5.0 with sodium hydroxide.

Multi-Dose Vials: Each mL contains 100 mg trimethobenzamide hydrochloride compounded with 0.45% phenol as preservative, 0.5 mg sodium citrate and 0.2 mg citric acid as buffers and pH adjusted to approximately 5.0 with sodium hydroxide.

Thera-Ject® (Disposable Syringes): Each 2 mL contains 200 mg trimethobenzamide hydrochloride compounded with 0.45% phenol as preservative, 1 mg sodium citrate and 0.4 mg citric acid as buffers, 0.2 mg disodium edetate as stabilizer and pH adjusted to approximately 5.0 with sodium hydroxide.

ACTIONS

The mechanism of action of *Tigan®* as determined in animals is obscure, but may be the chemoreceptor trigger zone (CTZ), an area in the medulla oblongata through which emetic impulses are conveyed to the vomiting center; direct impulses to the vomiting center apparently are not similarly inhibited. In dogs pretreated with trimethobenzamide HCl, the emetic response to apomorphine is inhibited, while little or no protection is afforded against emesis induced by intragastric copper sulfate.

INDICATIONS

Tigan® is indicated for the control of nausea and vomiting.

CONTRAINDICATIONS

The injectable form of *Tigan®* in children, the suppositories in premature or newborn infants, and use in patients with known hypersensitivity to trimethobenzamide are contraindicated. Since the suppositories contain benzocaine they should not be used in patients known to be sensitive to this or similar local anesthetics.

WARNINGS

Caution should be exercised when administering *Tigan®* to children for the treatment of vomiting. Antiemetics are not recommended for treatment of uncomplicated vomiting in children and their use should be limited to prolonged vomiting of known etiology. There are three principal reasons for caution:

1. There has been some suspicion that centrally acting antiemetics may contribute, in combination with viral illnesses (a possible cause of vomiting in children), to development of Reye's syndrome, a potentially fatal acute childhood encephalopathy with visceral fatty degeneration, especially involving the liver. Although there is no confirmation of this suspicion, caution is nevertheless recommended.
2. The extrapyramidal symptoms which can occur secondary to *Tigan®* may be confused with the central nervous system signs of an undiagnosed primary disease responsible for the vomiting, e.g., Reye's syndrome or other encephalopathy.
3. It has been suspected that drugs with hepatotoxic potential, such as *Tigan®*, may unfavorably alter the course of Reye's syndrome. Such drugs should therefore be avoided in children whose signs and symptoms (vomiting) could represent Reye's syndrome. It should also be noted that salicylates and acetaminophen are hepatotoxic at large doses. Although it is not known that at usual doses they would represent a hazard in patients with the underlying hepatic disorder of Reye's syndrome, these drugs, too, should be avoided in children whose signs and symptoms could represent Reye's syndrome, unless alternative methods of controlling fever are not successful.

Tigan® may produce drowsiness. Patients should not operate motor vehicles or other dangerous machinery until their individual responses have been determined. Reye's syndrome has been associated with the use of *Tigan®* and other drugs, including antiemetics, although their contribution, if any, to the cause and course of the disease has not been established. This syndrome is characterized by an abrupt onset shortly following a nonspecific febrile illness, with persistent, severe vomiting, lethargy, irrational behavior, progressive encephalopathy leading to coma, convulsions and death.

Continued on next page

Roberts—Cont.

Usage in Pregnancy: Trimethobenzamide hydrochloride was studied in reproduction experiments in rats and rabbits and no teratogenicity was suggested. The only effects observed were an increased percentage of embryonic resorptions or stillborn pups in rats administered 20 mg and 100 mg/kg and increased resorptions in rabbits receiving 100 mg/kg. In each study these adverse effects were attributed to one or two dams. The relevance to humans is not known. Since there is no adequate experience in pregnant or lactating women who have received this drug, safety in pregnancy or in nursing mothers has not been established.

Usage with Alcohol: Concomitant use of alcohol with *Tigan®* may result in an adverse drug interaction.

PRECAUTIONS

During the course of acute febrile illness, encephalitides, gastroenteritis, dehydration and electrolyte imbalance, especially in children and the elderly or debilitated, CNS reactions such as opisthotonos, convulsions, coma and extrapyramidal symptoms have been reported with and without use of *Tigan®* (trimethobenzamide hydrochloride) or other antiemetic agents. In such disorders caution should be exercised in administering *Tigan,®* particularly to patients who have recently received other CNS-acting agents (phenothiazines, barbiturates, belladonna derivatives). It is recommended that severe emesis should not be treated with an antiemetic drug alone; where possible the cause of vomiting should be established. Primary emphasis should be directed toward the restoration of body fluids and electrolyte balance, the relief of fever and relief of the causative disease process. Overhydration should be avoided since it may result in cerebral edema.

The antiemetic effects of *Tigan®* may render diagnosis more difficult in such conditions as appendicitis and obscure signs of toxicity due to overdosage of other drugs.

ADVERSE REACTIONS

There have been reports of hypersensitivity reactions and Parkinson-like symptoms. There have been instances of hypotension reported following parenteral administration to surgical patients. There have been reports of blood dyscrasias, blurring of vision, coma, convulsions, depression of mood, diarrhea, disorientation, dizziness, drowsiness, headache, jaundice, muscle cramps and opisthotonos. If these occur, the administration of the drug should be discontinued. Allergic-type skin reactions have been observed; therefore, the drug should be discontinued at the first sign of sensitization. While these symptoms will usually disappear spontaneously, symptomatic treatment may be indicated in some cases.

DOSAGE AND ADMINISTRATION

(See WARNINGS and PRECAUTIONS.)
Dosage should be adjusted according to the indication for therapy, severity of symptoms and the response of the patient.
CAPSULES, 250 mg and 100 mg
Usual Adult Dosage
One 250 mg capsule t.i.d. or q.i.d.
Usual Children's Dosage
30 to 90 lbs: One or two 100 mg capsules t.i.d. or q.i.d.
SUPPOSITORIES, 200 mg (not to be used in premature or newborn infants)
Usual Adult Dosage
One suppository (200 mg) t.i.d. or q.i.d.
Usual Children's Dosage
Under 30 lbs: One-half suppository (100 mg) t.i.d. or q.i.d.
30 to 90 lbs: One-half to one suppository (100 to 200 mg) t.i.d. or q.i.d.
SUPPOSITORIES, PEDIATRIC, 100 mg (not to be used in premature or newborn infants)
Usual Children's Dosage
Under 30 lbs: One suppository (100 mg) t.i.d. or q.i.d.
30 to 90 lbs: One to two suppositories (100 to 200 mg) t.i.d. or q.i.d.
INJECTABLE, 100 mg/mL (not for use in children)
Usual Adult Dosage
2 mL (200 mg) t.i.d. or q.i.d. intramuscularly.
NOTE: The injectable form is intended for intramuscular administration only; it is not recommended for intravenous use.
Intramuscular administration may cause pain, stinging, burning, redness and swelling at the site of injection. Such effects may be minimized by deep injection into the upper outer quadrant of the gluteal region, and by avoiding the escape of solution along the route.

CAUTION

Federal law prohibits dispensing without prescription.

STORAGE

Store *Tigan®* from 15° to 30°C (59° to 86°F).

HOW SUPPLIED

Capsules, 100 mg trimethobenzamide hydrochloride each, bottles of 100; 250 mg trimethobenzamide hydrochloride each, bottles of 100 and 500
NDC 54092-186-01 100 mg 100's
NDC 54092-187-01 250 mg 100's
NDC 54092-187-05 250 mg 500's
Suppositories, Pediatric, 100 mg, boxes of 10
Suppositories, 200 mg, boxes of 10 and 50
NDC 54092-503-10 100 mg (box of 10)
NDC 54092-504-10 200 mg (box of 10)
NDC 54092-504-50 200 mg (box of 50)
Ampuls, 2 mL, boxes of 10
NDC 54092-540-02 100 mg/mL in 2 mL ampul
Multi-Dose Vials, 20 mL
NDC 54092-541-20 100 mg/mL in 20 mL Multi-Dose Vials
Thera-Ject® (Disposable Syringes), 2 mL, boxes of 25
NDC 54092-542-02 100 mg/mL in 2 mL Thera-Ject® Disposable Syringes
Manufactured for
Roberts Laboratories Inc.,
a subsidiary of
ROBERTS PHARMACEUTICAL CORP.
Eatontown, NJ 07724, USA
Veterans Administration/Military/PHS—Capsules, 250 mg, 100's. 6505-01-333-7733; 250 mg, 500's, 6505-00-965-2319; Suppositories, 100 mg, 10's, 6505-01-153-3395; 200 mg, 10's, 6505-01-234-4444; 200 mg, 50's, 6505-00-890-1819; Vials, 100 mg/mL, 2 mL, 1's, 6505-00-949-1410; 100 mg/mL, 20 mL, 1's, 6505-00-951-4759; Thera-Ject®, 2 mL, 1's, 6505-01-048-0827.
TN: L1
Shown in Product Identification Guide, page 331

TOPICYCLINE®

(tetracycline hydrochloride)
for Topical Solution

DESCRIPTION

TOPICYCLINE® is a topical antibiotic preparation containing 2.2 mg. of tetracyline hydrochloride per ml as the active ingredient, as well as 4-epitetracycline hydrochloride and sodium bisulfite in an aqueous base of 40% ethanol, citric acid and n-decyl methyl sulfoxide. Tetracycline is 4-(dimethylamino)-1,4,4a,5,5a,6,11,12a-octahydro-3,6,10,12,12a-pentahydroxy-6-methyl-1,11-dioxo-2-naphthacenecarboxamide, the structural formula of which is
Tetracycline Structure

HOW SUPPLIED

TOPICYCLINE® is supplied in a single carton containing a powder and a liquid which must be combined prior to using. Complete instructions for mixing are provided on the carton. Once combined, the TOPICYCLINE bottle contains 70 ml of medication. This constitutes about an eight-week supply for treating the face and neck, or about a four-week supply for treating the face, neck and additional acne involved areas. Differences in individual usage habits will result in variation from these averages.
NDC 54092-315-70, 70 ml as dispensed.
TOPICYCLINE® should be kept at controlled room temperature 59°F–86°F (15°C-30°C) or below.
Manufactured for
Roberts Laboratories, Inc.
a subsidiary of
ROBERTS PHARMACEUTICAL CORPORATION
Eatontown, New Jersey 07724
Shown in Product Identification Guide, page 331

For information on over-the-counter drugs, consult **PDR For Nonprescription Drugs**

A. H. Robins Company
1407 CUMMINGS DRIVE
RICHMOND, VA 23220

Direct General Inquiries to:
(610) 688-4400

For Emergency Medical Information Contact:
Day: (800) 934-5556 8:30 AM to 4:30 PM (Eastern Standard Time), Weekdays only
Night: (610) 688-4400 (Emergencies only; non-emergencies should wait until the next day)
For Medical/Pharmacy Inquiries on Marketed Products Call:
Medical Affairs, (800) 934-5556 8:30 AM to 4:30 PM (Eastern Standard Time), Weekdays only

DIMETANE®-DC   ℂ ℞
[di'mĕ-tāne]
COUGH SYRUP
SUGAR-FREE

DESCRIPTION

Dimetane-DC Cough Syrup is a light bluish-pink syrup with a raspberry flavor.
Each 5 mL (1 teaspoonful) contains:
Brompheniramine Maleate, USP...................................... 2.0 mg
Phenylpropanolamine
    Hydrochloride, USP.. 12.5 mg
Codeine Phosphate, USP... 10.0 mg
    (Warning: May be habit forming)
        Alcohol 0.95 percent
In a palatable aromatic vehicle.
Inactive Ingredients: Citric Acid, FD&C Blue 1, FD&C Red 40, Flavors, Glycerin, Sodium Benzoate, Sorbitol, Water. Antihistamine/Nasal Decongestant/Antitussive syrup for oral administration.

CLINICAL PHARMACOLOGY

Brompheniramine maleate is a histamine antagonist, specifically an H_1-receptor-blocking agent belonging to the alkylamine class of antihistamines. Antihistamines appear to compete with histamine for receptor sites on effector cells. Brompheniramine also has anticholinergic (drying) and sedative effects. Among the antihistaminic effects, it antagonizes the allergic response (vasodilatation, increased vascular permeability, increased mucus secretion) of nasal tissue. Brompheniramine is well absorbed from the gastrointestinal tract, with peak plasma concentration after a single oral dose of 4 mg reached in 5 hours; urinary excretion is the major route of elimination, mostly as products of biodegradation; the liver is assumed to be the main site of metabolic transformation.
Phenylpropanolamine hydrochloride is a sympathomimetic drug which is readily absorbed from the gastrointestinal tract and produces nasal vasoconstriction (decongestion). Phenylpropanolamine stimulates both α and β-adrenergic receptors, similar to ephedrine. Part of its peripheral action is indirect and is due to the displacement of norepinephrine from storage sites, but it also has direct effect on the adrenergic receptors.
Codeine is an opiate analgesic and antitussive. Codeine calms the cough control center.

INDICATIONS AND USAGE

For relief of coughs and upper respiratory symptoms, including nasal congestion, associated with allergy or the common cold.

CONTRAINDICATIONS

Hypersensitivity to any of the ingredients. Do not use in the newborn, in premature infants, in nursing mothers, in patients with severe hypertension or severe coronary artery disease, or in those receiving monoamine oxidase (MAO) inhibitors.
Antihistamines should not be used to treat lower respiratory tract conditions including asthma.

WARNINGS

Especially in infants and small children, antihistamines in overdosage may cause hallucinations, convulsions, death. Codeine may cause or aggravate constipation.
Antihistamines may diminish mental alertness. In the young child, they may produce excitation.

PRECAUTIONS

General: Because of its antihistamine component, Dimetane-DC Cough Syrup should be used with caution in patients with a history of bronchial asthma, narrow angle glaucoma, gastrointestinal obstruction, or urinary bladder neck obstruction. Because of its sympathomimetic component, Dimetane-DC Cough Syrup should be used with caution in patients with diabetes, hypertension, heart disease, or thyroid disease.

Information for Patients: Patients should be warned about engaging in activities requiring mental alertness, such as driving a car or operating dangerous machinery.

Drug Interactions: Antihistamines have additive effects with alcohol and other CNS depressants (hypnotics, sedatives, tranquilizers, antianxiety agents, etc.). MAO inhibitors prolong and intensify the anticholinergic (drying) effects of antihistamines. MAO inhibitors may enhance the effect of phenylpropanolamine. Sympathomimetics may reduce the effects of antihypertensive drugs.

Carcinogenesis, Mutagenesis: Long-term studies in animals to evaluate carcinogenic and mutagenic potential have not been performed.

Pregnancy Category C: Animal reproduction studies have not been conducted with Dimetane-DC Cough Syrup. It is also not known whether Dimetane-DC Cough Syrup can cause fetal harm when administered to a pregnant woman or can affect reproduction capacity. Dimetane-DC Cough Syrup should be given to a pregnant woman only if clearly needed. Reproduction studies of brompheniramine maleate (one of the components of the Dimetane formulations) in rats and mice at doses up to 16 times the maximum human dose have revealed no evidence of impaired fertility or harm to the fetus.

Nursing Mothers: Because of the higher risk of intolerance of antihistamines in small infants generally, and in newborns and prematures in particular, and the fact that codeine appears in human milk, Dimetane-DC Cough Syrup is contraindicated in nursing mothers.

ADVERSE REACTIONS

The most frequent adverse reactions to Dimetane-DC Cough Syrup are: sedation; dryness of mouth, nose and throat; thickening of bronchial secretions; dizziness. Other adverse reactions may include:

Dermatologic: Urticaria, drug rash, photosensitivity, pruritus.

Cardiovascular System: Hypotension, hypertension, cardiac arrhythmias.

CNS: Disturbed coordination, tremor, irritability, insomnia, visual disturbances, weakness, nervousness, convulsions, headache, euphoria, and dysphoria.

G. U. System: Urinary frequency, difficult urination.

G. I. System: Epigastric discomfort, anorexia, nausea, vomiting, diarrhea, constipation.

Respiratory System: Tightness of chest and wheezing, shortness of breath. At higher doses, codeine has most of the disadvantages of morphine including respiratory depression.

Hematologic System: Hemolytic anemia, thrombocytopenia, agranulocytosis.

DRUG ABUSE AND DEPENDENCE

Codeine can produce drug dependence of the morphine type, and therefore has the potential for being abused. Psychic dependence, physical dependence and tolerance may develop upon repeated administration of this drug, and it should be prescribed and administered with the same degree of caution appropriate to the use of other oral narcotic medications. Dimetane-DC Cough Syrup is subject to the Federal Controlled Substances Act (Schedule V).

OVERDOSAGE

Signs and Symptoms: Serious overdose with codeine is characterized by respiratory depression, extreme somnolence progressing to stupor or coma. In severe overdosage, apnea, circulatory collapse, cardiac arrest and death may occur. The central nervous system effects from overdosage of brompheniramine may vary from depression to stimulation. Anticholinergic effects may also occur. Overdosage of phenylpropanolamine may be associated with tachycardia, hypertension and cardiac arrhythmias.

Toxic Doses: Doses of 800 mg or more of codeine have caused partial loss of consciousness, delirium, restlessness, excitement, tremors, convulsions and collapse; or respiratory paralysis with such sequelae as mydriasis, marked vasodilatation, and finally death. A $2^1/_2$-year-old child survived a dose of 300–900 mg of brompheniramine; the lethal dose of phenylpropanolamine is in the range of 50 mg/kg.

Treatment: Respiratory depression should be treated promptly. Oxygen, intravenous fluids, vasopressors and other supportive measures should be employed as indicated. If necessary, reestablishment of adequate respiratory exchange through provision of a patent airway and the institution of assisted or controlled ventilation must be provided. The narcotic antagonist, naloxone, is a specific antidote to codeine-induced respiratory depression, and should be administered by the intravenous route if appropriate (see package insert for naloxone). Since the duration of action of codeine may exceed that of the antagonist, the patient should be kept under constant surveillance.

Gastric emptying may be useful in removing unabsorbed drug, either by inducing emesis or lavage; precautions against aspiration must be taken. Stimulants or depressants should be used cautiously and only when specifically indicated. If marked excitement is present, one of the short-acting barbiturates or chloral hydrate may be used.

DOSAGE AND ADMINISTRATION

Adults and children 12 years of age and over: 2 teaspoonfuls every 4 hours. Children 6 to under 12 years: 1 teaspoonful every 4 hours. Children 2 to under 6 years: $^1/_2$ teaspoonful every 4 hours. Use of codeine-containing preparations is not recommended for children under 2 years of age.

Do not exceed 6 doses during a 24-hour period.

HOW SUPPLIED

Dimetane-DC Cough Syrup is a light bluish-pink syrup containing in each 5 mL (1 teaspoonful): brompheniramine maleate 2 mg, phenylpropanolamine HCl 12.5 mg, and codeine phosphate 10 mg; available in pints (NDC 0031-1833-25).

Store at controlled room temperature, between 15°C and 30°C (59°F and 86°F).

Dispense in tight, light-resistant container.

DIMETANE®–DX ℞

[di 'mĕ-tāne]

COUGH SYRUP

SUGAR-FREE

DESCRIPTION

Dimetane-DX Cough Syrup is a light-red syrup with a butterscotch flavor.

Each 5 mL (1 teaspoonful) contains:

Brompheniramine Maleate, USP	2 mg
Pseudoephedrine Hydrochloride, USP	30 mg
Dextromethorphan Hydrobromide, USP	10 mg
Alcohol 0.95 percent	

In a palatable, aromatic vehicle.

Inactive Ingredients: Citric Acid, FD&C Red 40, FD&C Yellow 6, Flavors, Glycerin, Saccharin Sodium, Sodium Benzoate, Sorbitol, Water.

Antihistamine/Nasal Decongestant/Antitussive syrup for oral administration.

CLINICAL PHARMACOLOGY

Brompheniramine maleate is a histamine antagonist, specifically an H_1-receptor-blocking agent belonging to the alkylamine class of antihistamines. Antihistamines appear to compete with histamine for receptor sites on effector cells. Brompheniramine also has anticholinergic (drying) and sedative effects. Among the antihistaminic effects, it antagonizes the allergic response (vasodilatation, increased vascular permeability, increased mucus secretion) of nasal tissue. Brompheniramine is well absorbed from the gastrointestinal tract, with peak plasma concentration after single, oral dose of 4 mg reached in 5 hours; urinary excretion is the major route of elimination, mostly as products of biodegradation; the liver is assumed to be the main site of metabolic transformation.

Pseudoephedrine acts on sympathetic nerve endings and also on smooth muscle, making it useful as a nasal decongestant. The nasal decongestant effect is mediated by the action of pseudoephedrine on α-sympathetic receptors, producing vasoconstriction of the dilated nasal arterioles. Following oral administration, effects are noted within 30 minutes with peak activity occurring at approximately one hour.

Dextromethorphan acts centrally to elevate the threshold for coughing. It has no analgesic or addictive properties. The onset of antitussive action occurs in 15 to 30 minutes after administration and is of long duration.

INDICATIONS AND USAGE

For relief of coughs and upper respiratory symptoms, including nasal congestion, associated with allergy or the common cold.

CONTRAINDICATIONS

Hypersensitivity to any of the ingredients. Do not use in the newborn, in premature infants, in nursing mothers, in patients with severe hypertension or severe coronary artery disease, or in those receiving monoamine oxidase (MAO) inhibitors.

Antihistamines should not be used to treat lower respiratory tract conditions including asthma.

WARNINGS

Especially in infants and small children, antihistamines in overdosage may cause hallucinations, convulsions, and death.

Antihistamines may diminish mental alertness. In the young child, they may produce excitation.

PRECAUTIONS

General: Because of its antihistamine component, Dimetane-DX Cough Syrup should be used with caution in patients with a history of bronchial asthma, narrow angle glaucoma, gastrointestinal obstruction, or urinary bladder neck obstruction. Because of its sympathomimetic component, Dimetane-DX Cough Syrup should be used with caution in patients with diabetes, hypertension, heart disease, or thyroid disease.

Information for Patients: Patients should be warned about engaging in activities requiring mental alertness, such as driving a car or operating dangerous machinery.

Drug Interactions: Antihistamines have additive effects with alcohol and other CNS depressants (hypnotics, sedatives, tranquilizers, antianxiety agents, etc.). MAO inhibitors prolong and intensify the anticholinergic (drying) effects of antihistamines. MAO inhibitors may enhance the effect of pseudoephedrine. Sympathomimetics may reduce the effects of antihypertensive drugs.

Carcinogenesis, Mutagenesis, Impairment of Fertility

Animal studies of Dimetane-DX Cough Syrup to assess the carcinogenic and mutagenic potential or the effect on fertility have not been performed.

Pregnancy

Teratogenic Effects—Pregnancy Category C

Animal reproduction studies have not been conducted with Dimetane-DX Cough Syrup. It is also not known whether Dimetane-DX Cough Syrup can cause fetal harm when administered to a pregnant woman or can affect reproduction capacity. Dimetane-DX Cough Syrup should be given to a pregnant woman only if clearly needed.

Reproduction studies of brompheniramine maleate (a component of Dimetane-DX Cough Syrup) in rats and mice at doses up to 16 times the maximum human dose have revealed no evidence of impaired fertility or harm to the fetus.

Nursing Mothers: Because of the higher risk of intolerance of antihistamines in small infants generally, and in newborns and prematures in particular, Dimetane-DX Cough Syrup is contraindicated in nursing mothers.

ADVERSE REACTIONS

The most frequent adverse reactions to Dimetane-DX Cough Syrup are: sedation; dryness of mouth, nose and throat; thickening of bronchial secretions; dizziness. Other adverse reactions may include:

Dermatologic: Urticaria, drug rash, photosensitivity, pruritus.

Cardiovascular System: Hypotension, hypertension, cardiac arrhythmias, palpitation.

CNS: Disturbed coordination, tremor, irritability, insomnia, visual disturbances, weakness, nervousness, convulsions, headache, euphoria, and dysphoria.

G. U. System: Urinary frequency, difficult urination.

G. I. System: Epigastric discomfort, anorexia, nausea, vomiting, diarrhea, constipation.

Respiratory System: Tightness of chest and wheezing, shortness of breath.

Hematologic System: Hemolytic anemia, thrombocytopenia, agranulocytosis.

OVERDOSAGE

Signs and Symptoms: Central nervous system effects from overdosage of brompheniramine may vary from depression to stimulation, especially in children. Anticholinergic effects may be noted. Toxic doses of pseudoephedrine may result in CNS stimulation, tachycardia, hypertension, and cardiac arrhythmias; signs of CNS depression may occasionally be seen. Dextromethorphan in toxic doses will cause drowsiness, ataxia, nystagmus, opisthotonos, and convulsive seizures.

Toxic Doses: Data suggest that individuals may respond in an unexpected manner to apparently small amounts of a particular drug. A 2½-year-old child survived the ingestion of 21 mg/kg of dextromethorphan exhibiting only ataxia, drowsiness, and fever, but seizures have been reported in 2 children following the ingestion of 13–17 mg/kg. Another 2½-year-old child survived a dose of 300–900 mg of brompheniramine. The toxic dose of pseudoephedrine should be less than that of ephedrine, which is estimated to be 50 mg/kg.

Treatment: Induce emesis if patient is alert and is seen prior to 6 hours following ingestion. Precautions against aspiration must be taken, especially in infants and small children. Gastric lavage may be carried out, although in some instances tracheostomy may be necessary prior to lavage. Naloxone hydrochloride 0.005 mg/kg intravenously may be of value in reversing the CNS depression that may occur from an overdose of dextromethorphan. CNS stimulants may counter CNS depression. Should CNS hyperactivity or convulsive seizures occur, intravenous short-acting barbiturates may be indicated. Hypertensive responses and/or tachycardia should be treated appropriately. Oxygen, intravenous fluids, and other supportive measures should be employed as indicated.

DOSAGE AND ADMINISTRATION

Adults and children 12 years of age and over: 2 teaspoonfuls every 4 hours. Children 6 to under 12 years: 1 teaspoonful every 4 hours. Children 2 to under 6 years: ½ teaspoonful every 4 hours. Children 6 months to under 2 years: Dosage to be established by physician.

Do not exceed 6 doses during a 24-hour period.

Continued on next page

A. H. Robins—Cont.

HOW SUPPLIED

Dimetane-DX Cough Syrup is a light-red syrup containing in each 5 mL (1 teaspoonful) brompheniramine maleate 2 mg, pseudoephedrine hydrochloride 30 mg and dextromethorphan hydrobromide 10 mg, available in pints (NDC 0031-1836-25) and gallons (NDC 0031-1836-29).

Store at controlled room temperature, between 15°C and 30°C (59°F and 86°F).

Dispense in tight, light-resistant container.

DONNATAL® TABLETS ℞
DONNATAL® CAPSULES ℞
DONNATAL® ELIXIR ℞

[don 'nă-tal]

DESCRIPTION

Each Donnatal tablet, capsule or 5 mL (teaspoonful) of elixir (23% alcohol) contains:

Phenobarbital, USP	16.2 mg
(Warning: May be habit forming)	
Hyoscyamine Sulfate, USP	0.1037 mg
Atropine Sulfate, USP	0.0194 mg
Scopolamine Hydrobromide, USP	0.0065 mg

INACTIVE INGREDIENTS:

Tablets: Dibasic Calcium Phosphate, Magnesium Stearate, Microcrystalline Cellulose, Silicon Dioxide, Sodium Starch Glycolate, Stearic Acid, Sucrose. May contain Corn Starch, Dextrose, or Invert Sugar.

Capsules: Corn Starch, Edible Ink, D&C Yellow 10 and FD&C Green 3 or FD&C Blue 1 and FD&C Yellow 6, FD&C Blue 2 Aluminum Lake, Gelatin, Lactose, Sucrose. May contain FD&C Red 40 and Yellow 6 Aluminum Lakes.

Elixir: D&C Yellow 10, FD&C Blue 1, FD&C Yellow 6, Flavors, Glucose, Saccharin Sodium, Water.

ACTIONS

This drug combination provides natural belladonna alkaloids in a specific, fixed ratio combined with phenobarbital to provide peripheral anticholinergic/antispasmodic action and mild sedation.

INDICATIONS

Based on a review of this drug by the National Academy of Sciences—National Research Council and/or other information, FDA has classified the following indications as "possibly" effective:

For use as adjunctive therapy in the treatment of irritable bowel syndrome (irritable colon, spastic colon, mucous colitis) and acute enterocolitis.

May also be useful as adjunctive therapy in the treatment of duodenal ulcer. IT HAS NOT BEEN SHOWN CONCLUSIVELY WHETHER ANTICHOLINERGIC/ANTISPASMODIC DRUGS AID IN THE HEALING OF A DUODENAL ULCER, DECREASE THE RATE OF RECURRENCES OR PREVENT COMPLICATIONS.

CONTRAINDICATIONS

Glaucoma, obstructive uropathy (for example, bladder neck obstruction due to prostatic hypertrophy); obstructive disease of the gastrointestinal tract (as in achalasia, pyloroduodenal stenosis, etc.); paralytic ileus, intestinal atony of the elderly or debilitated patient; unstable cardiovascular status in acute hemorrhage; severe ulcerative colitis especially if complicated by toxic megacolon; myasthenia gravis; hiatal hernia associated with reflux esophagitis.

Donnatal is contraindicated in patients with known hypersensitivity to any of the ingredients. Phenobarbital is contraindicated in acute intermittent porphyria and in those patients in whom phenobarbital produces restlessness and/or excitement.

WARNINGS

In the presence of a high environmental temperature, heat prostration can occur with belladonna alkaloids (fever and heatstroke due to decreased sweating).

Diarrhea may be an early symptom of incomplete intestinal obstruction, especially in patients with ileostomy or colostomy. In this instance treatment with this drug would be inappropriate and possibly harmful.

Donnatal may produce drowsiness or blurred vision. The patient should be warned, should these occur, not to engage in activities requiring mental alertness, such as operating a motor vehicle or other machinery, and not to perform hazardous work.

Phenobarbital may decrease the effect of anticoagulants, and necessitate larger doses of the anticoagulant for optimal effect. When the phenobarbital is discontinued, the dose of the anticoagulant may have to be decreased.

Phenobarbital may be habit forming and should not be administered to individuals known to be addiction prone or to those with a history of physical and/or psychological dependence upon drugs.

Since barbiturates are metabolized in the liver, they should be used with caution and initial doses should be small in patients with hepatic dysfunction.

PRECAUTIONS

Use with caution in patients with: autonomic neuropathy, hepatic or renal disease, hyperthyroidism, coronary heart disease, congestive heart failure, cardiac arrhythmias, tachycardia, and hypertension.

Belladonna alkaloids may produce a delay in gastric emptying (antral stasis) which would complicate the management of gastric ulcer.

Theoretically, with overdosage, a curare-like action may occur.

CARCINOGENESIS, MUTAGENESIS. Long-term studies in animals have not been performed to evaluate carcinogenic potential.

PREGNANCY CATEGORY C. Animal reproduction studies have not been conducted with Donnatal. It is not known whether Donnatal can cause fetal harm when administered to a pregnant woman or can affect reproduction capacity. Donnatal should be given to a pregnant woman only if clearly needed.

NURSING MOTHERS. It is not known whether this drug is excreted in human milk. Because many drugs are excreted in human milk, caution should be exercised when Donnatal is administered to a nursing mother.

ADVERSE REACTIONS

Adverse reactions may include xerostomia; urinary hesitancy and retention; blurred vision; tachycardia; palpitation; mydriasis; cycloplegia; increased ocular tension; loss of taste sense; headache; nervousness; drowsiness; weakness; dizziness; insomnia; nausea; vomiting; impotence; suppression of lactation; constipation; bloated feeling; musculoskeletal pain; severe allergic reaction or drug idiosyncrasies, including anaphylaxis, urticaria and other dermal manifestations; and decreased sweating. Elderly patients may react with symptoms of excitement, agitation, drowsiness, and other untoward manifestations to even small doses of the drug.

Phenobarbital may produce excitement in some patients, rather than a sedative effect. In patients habituated to barbiturates, abrupt withdrawal may produce delirium or convulsions.

DOSAGE AND ADMINISTRATION

The dosage of Donnatal should be adjusted to the needs of the individual patient to assure symptomatic control with a minimum of adverse effects.

Donnatal Tablets or Capsules. Adults: One or two Donnatal tablets or capsules three or four times a day according to condition and severity of symptoms.

Donnatal Elixir. Adults: One or two teaspoonfuls of elixir three or four times a day according to conditions and severity of symptoms.

Children (Elixir)—may be dosed every 4 or 6 hours.:

Body Weight	Starting Dosage q4h	Starting Dosage q6h
10 lb (4.5 kg)	0.5 mL	0.75 mL
20 lb (9.1 kg)	1.0 mL	1.5 mL
30 lb (13.6 kg)	1.5 mL	2.0 mL
50 lb (22.7 kg)	1/2 tsp	3/4 tsp
75 lb (34.0 kg)	3/4 tsp	1 tsp
100 lb (45.4 kg)	1 tsp	1 1/2 tsp

OVERDOSAGE

The signs and symptoms of overdose are headache, nausea, vomiting, blurred vision, dilated pupils, hot and dry skin, dizziness, dryness of the mouth, difficulty in swallowing, CNS stimulation. Treatment should consist of gastric lavage, emetics, and activated charcoal. If indicated, parenteral cholinergic agents such as physostigmine or bethanechol chloride, should be added.

HOW SUPPLIED

Donnatal® Tablets. White, compressed, scored and embossed "R"; in bottles of 100 (NDC 0031-4250-63), 1000 (NDC 0031-4250-74) and Dis-Co® Unit Dose Packs of 100 (NDC 0031-4250-64).

Donnatal® Capsules. Green and white, monogrammed "AHR" and "4207"; in bottles of 100 (NDC 0031-4207-63).

Donnatal® Elixir. Green, citrus flavored, in 4 fl. oz. (NDC 0031-4221-12), pints (NDC 0031-4221-25), gallons (NDC 0031-4221-29) and 5 mL Dis-Co® Unit Dose Packs (4 × 25s) (NDC 0031-4221-13).

Store at controlled room temperature, between 20°C and 25°C (68°F and 77°F).

Dispense in tight, light-resistant container.

Shown in Product Identification Guide, page 331

DONNATAL EXTENTABS® ℞

[don 'nă-tal ĕks "tĕn 'tabs]

DESCRIPTION

Each Donnatal Extentabs tablet contains:

Phenobarbital, USP (¾ gr)	48.6 mg
(Warning: May be habit forming)	
Hyoscyamine Sulfate, USP	0.3111 mg
Atropine Sulfate, USP	0.0582 mg
Scopolamine Hydrobromide, USP	0.0195 mg

Each Donnatal Extentabs tablet contains the equivalent of three Donnatal tablets. Extentabs are designed to release the ingredients gradually to provide effects for up to twelve (12) hours.

Inactive Ingredients: Acacia, Acetylated Monoglycerides, Calcium Sulfate, Carnauba Wax, D&C Yellow 10, Edible Ink, FD&C Blue 1, FD&C Blue 2 Aluminum Lake, FD&C Yellow 6, Gelatin, Guar Gum, Magnesium Stearate, Polysorbates, Shellac, Sodium Phosphate, Sucrose, Titanium Dioxide, Wheat Flour, White Wax and other ingredients, one of which is a corn derivative. May include FD&C Red 40 and Yellow 6 Aluminum Lakes.

ACTIONS

This drug combination provides natural belladonna alkaloids in a specific, fixed ratio combined with phenobarbital to provide peripheral anticholinergic/antispasmodic action and mild sedation.

INDICATIONS

Based on a review of this drug by the National Academy of Sciences—National Research Council and/or other information, FDA has classified the following indications as "possibly" effective:

For use as adjunctive therapy in the treatment of irritable bowel syndrome (irritable colon, spastic colon, mucous colitis) and acute enterocolitis.

May also be useful as adjunctive therapy in the treatment of duodenal ulcer. IT HAS NOT BEEN SHOWN CONCLUSIVELY WHETHER ANTICHOLINERGIC/ANTISPASMODIC DRUGS AID IN THE HEALING OF A DUODENAL ULCER, DECREASE THE RATE OF RECURRENCES OR PREVENT COMPLICATIONS.

CONTRAINDICATIONS

Glaucoma, obstructive uropathy (for example, bladder neck obstruction due to prostatic hypertrophy); obstructive disease of the gastrointestinal tract (as in achalasia, pyloroduodenal stenosis, etc.); paralytic ileus, intestinal atony of the elderly or debilitated patient; unstable cardiovascular status in acute hemorrhage; severe ulcerative colitis especially if complicated by toxic megacolon; myasthenia gravis, hiatal hernia associated with reflux esophagitis.

Donnatal is contraindicated in patients with known hypersensitivity to any of the ingredients. Phenobarbital is contraindicated in acute intermittent porphyria and in those patients in whom phenobarbital produces restlessness and/or excitement.

WARNINGS

In the presence of a high environmental temperature, heat prostration can occur with belladonna alkaloids (fever and heatstroke due to decreased sweating).

Diarrhea may be an early symptom of incomplete intestinal obstruction, especially in patients with ileostomy or colostomy. In this instance treatment with this drug would be inappropriate and possibly harmful.

Donnatal may produce drowsiness or blurred vision. The patient should be warned, should these occur, not to engage in activities requiring mental alertness, such as operating a motor vehicle or other machinery, and not to perform hazardous work.

Phenobarbital may decrease the effect of anticoagulants and necessitate larger doses of the anticoagulant for optimal effect. When the phenobarbital is discontinued, the dose of the anticoagulant may have to be decreased.

Phenobarbital may be habit forming and should not be administered to individuals known to be addiction prone or to those with a history of physical and/or psychological dependence upon drugs.

Since barbiturates are metabolized in the liver, they should be used with caution and initial doses should be small in patients with hepatic dysfunction.

PRECAUTIONS

Use with caution in patients with: autonomic neuropathy, hepatic or renal disease, hyperthyroidism, coronary heart disease, congestive heart failure, cardiac arrhythmias, tachycardia, and hypertension.

Belladonna alkaloids may produce a delay in gastric emptying (antral stasis) which would complicate the management of gastric ulcer.

Theoretically, with overdosage, a curare-like action may occur.

Carcinogenesis, mutagenesis. Long-term studies in animals have not been performed to evaluate carcinogenic potential.

Pregnancy Category C. Animal reproduction studies have not been conducted with Donnatal. It is not known whether Donnatal can cause fetal harm when administered to a pregnant woman or can affect reproduction capacity. Donnatal should be given to a pregnant woman only if clearly needed.

Nursing mothers. It is not known whether this drug is excreted in human milk. Because many drugs are excreted in human milk, caution should be exercised when Donnatal is administered to a nursing mother.

ADVERSE REACTIONS

Adverse reactions may include xerostomia; urinary hesitancy and retention; blurred vision; tachycardia; palpitation; mydriasis; cycloplegia; increased ocular tension; loss of taste sense; headache; nervousness; drowsiness; weakness; dizziness; insomnia; nausea; vomiting; impotence; suppression of lactation; constipation; bloated feeling; musculoskeletal pain; severe allergic reaction or drug idiosyncrasies, including anaphylaxis, urticaria and other dermal manifestations; and decreased sweating. Elderly patients may react with symptoms of excitement, agitation, drowsiness, and other untoward manifestations to even small doses of the drug.

Phenobarbital may produce excitement in some patients, rather than a sedative effect. In patients habituated to barbiturates, abrupt withdrawal may produce delirium or convulsions.

DOSAGE AND ADMINISTRATION

The dosage of Donnatal Extentabs should be adjusted to the needs of the individual patient to assure symptomatic control with a minimum of adverse reactions. The usual dose is one tablet every twelve (12) hours. If indicated, one tablet every eight (8) hours may be given.

OVERDOSAGE

The signs and symptoms of overdose are headache, nausea, vomiting, blurred vision, dilated pupils; hot and dry skin, dizziness, dryness of the mouth, difficulty in swallowing, CNS stimulation. Treatment should consist of gastric lavage, emetics, and activated charcoal. If indicated, parenteral cholinergic agents such as physostigmine or bethanechol chloride should be added.

HOW SUPPLIED

Pale green, coated tablets, monogrammed AHR and Donnatal Extentab in bottles of 100 (NDC 0031-4235-63) and 500 (NDC 0031-4235-70); and Dis-Co® Unit Dose Packs of 100 (NDC 0031-4235-64).

Store at controlled room temperature, between 15°C and 30°C (59°F and 86°F).

Dispense in well-closed, light-resistant container.

Shown in Product Identification Guide, page 331

DONNAZYME® Tablets ℞

[*don 'nā " zīm*]

Pancreatic Enzyme Replacement

DESCRIPTION

Donnazyme tablets are available for oral administration.

Each tablet contains:

Pancreatin, USP equivalent .... 500 mg

which provides not less than the following enzymatic activity—

Lipase	1,000 USP Units
Protease	12,500 USP Units
Amylase	12,500 USP Units

Inactive Ingredients: Acacia, Acetylated Monoglycerides, Calcium Sulfate, Carnauba Wax, Cellulose Acetate Phthalate, Corn Starch, D&C Yellow 10 Aluminum Lake, Diethyl Phthalate, Edible Ink, FD&C Blue 1 Aluminum Lake, FD&C Yellow 6 Aluminum Lake, Gelatin, Methylparaben, Microcrystalline Cellulose, Polysorbates, Povidone, Propylparaben, Shellac, Sodium Benzoate, Stearic Acid, Sucrose, Titanium Dioxide, Wheat Flour, White Wax. May contain Docusate Sodium.

CLINICAL PHARMACOLOGY

The outer layer of Donnazyme tablets is gastric-soluble. The core of the tablet contains pancreatin. It is designed to disintegrate in the alkaline medium of the duodenum where it releases the active enzyme components of pancreatin (trypsin, amylase and lipase). Trypsin breaks down larger protein fractions into peptides; amylase converts starch into maltose; lipase splits fat into fatty acids and glycerin.

INDICATIONS AND USAGE

Donnazyme is indicated for the treatment of exocrine pancreatic insufficiency.

CONTRAINDICATIONS

Donnazyme is contraindicated in patients with known hypersensitivity to the drug.

WARNINGS

Do not take this product if you are allergic to pork.

Do not take this product unless directed by a physician.

Do not exceed the labeled dose unless directed by a physician.

Do not chew tablets.

Swallow tablets quickly to lessen potential for mouth irritation.

PRECAUTIONS

Carcinogenesis, mutagenesis: Long-term studies in animals have not been performed to evaluate carcinogenic potential.

Pregnancy Category C. Animal reproduction studies have not been conducted with Donnazyme. It is not known whether Donnazyme can cause fetal harm when administered to a pregnant woman or can affect reproduction capacity. Donnazyme should be given to a pregnant woman only if clearly needed.

Nursing mothers: It is not known whether this drug is excreted in human milk. Because many drugs are excreted in human milk, caution should be exercised when Donnazyme is administered to a nursing mother.

Pediatric Use: Safety and effectiveness in children have not been established.

ADVERSE REACTIONS

Skin rash is the most frequently reported adverse reaction to Donnazyme and appears to be associated with hypersensitivity to pork protein in the pancreatin. At high doses, a laxative effect may occur.

OVERDOSAGE

Excessive dosage may produce a laxative effect. Systemic toxicity does not occur.

DOSAGE AND ADMINISTRATION

Two tablets with each meal and 2 tablets taken with food eaten between meals or as directed by a physician. Donnazyme tablets should be swallowed whole and not crushed or chewed.

HOW SUPPLIED

Kelly green tablets in bottles of 100 (NDC 0031-4650-63).

Store at controlled room temperature, between 15°C and 30°C (59°F and 86°F). Dispense in tight container.

Shown in Product Identification Guide, page 331

DOPRAM® INJECTABLE ℞

[*do 'pram*]

brand of Doxapram Hydrochloride Injection, USP

DESCRIPTION

Dopram Injectable (Doxapram Hydrochloride Injection, USP) is a clear, colorless, sterile, non-pyrogenic, aqueous solution with pH 3.5—5.0, for intravenous administration.

Each 1 mL contains:

Doxapram Hydrochloride, USP	20 mg
Benzyl Alcohol, NF (as preservative)	0.9%
Water for Injection, USP	q.s.

Due to its benzyl alcohol content, Dopram Injectable should not be used in newborns.

Dopram Injectable is a respiratory stimulant.

Doxapram hydrochloride is a white to off-white, crystalline powder, sparingly soluble in water, alcohol and chloroform. It has the following chemical name:

1-ethyl-4-[2-(4-morpholinyl)ethyl]-3,3-diphenyl-2-pyrrolidinone monohydrochloride, monohydrate.

CLINICAL PHARMACOLOGY

Doxapram hydrochloride produces respiratory stimulation mediated through the peripheral carotid chemoreceptors. As the dosage level is increased, the central respiratory centers in the medulla are stimulated with progressive stimulation of other parts of the brain and spinal cord.

The onset of respiratory stimulation following the recommended single intravenous injection of doxapram hydrochloride usually occurs in 20–40 seconds with peak effect at 1–2 minutes. The duration of effect may vary from 5–12 minutes.

The respiratory stimulant action is manifested by an increase in tidal volume associated with a slight increase in respiratory rate.

A pressor response may result following doxapram administration. Provided there is no impairment of cardiac function, the pressor effect is more marked in hypovolemic than in normovolemic states. The pressor response is due to the improved cardiac output rather than peripheral vasoconstriction. Following doxapram administration an increased release of catecholamines has been noted.

Although opiate induced respiratory depression is antagonized by doxapram, the analgesic effect is not affected.

INDICATIONS

1. ***Postanesthesia.***
   a. When the possibility of airway obstruction and/or hypoxia have been eliminated, doxapram may be used to stimulate respiration in patients with drug-induced postanesthesia respiratory depression or apnea other than that due to muscle relaxant drugs.
   b. To pharmacologically stimulate deep breathing in the so-called "stir-up" regimen in the postoperative patient. (Simultaneous administration of oxygen is desirable.)
2. ***Drug-induced central nervous system depression.***
   Exercising care to prevent vomiting and aspiration, doxapram may be used to stimulate respiration, hasten arousal, and to encourage the return of laryngopharyngeal reflexes in patients with mild to moderate respiratory and CNS depression due to drug overdosage.
3. ***Chronic pulmonary disease associated with acute hypercapnia.***
   Doxapram is indicated as a temporary measure in hospitalized patients with acute respiratory insufficiency superimposed on chronic obstructive pulmonary disease. Its use should be for a short period of time (approximately 2 hours) as an aid in the prevention of elevation of arterial CO_2 tension during the administration of oxygen. It should not be used in conjuction with mechanical ventilation.

CONTRAINDICATIONS

Due to its benzyl alcohol content, Dopram Injectable should not be used in newborns.

Doxapram should not be used in patients with epilepsy or other convulsive disorders.

Doxapram is contraindicated in patients with mechanical disorders of ventilation such as mechanical obstruction, muscle paresis, flail chest, pneumothorax, acute bronchial asthma, pulmonary fibrosis or other conditions resulting in restriction of chest wall, muscles of respiration or alveolar expansion.

Doxapram is contraindicated in patients with evidence of head injury or cerebral vascular accident and in those with significant cardiovascular impairment, severe hypertension, or known hypersensitivity to the drug.

WARNINGS

1. ***In postanesthetic use.***
   a. Doxapram is neither an antagonist to muscle relaxant drugs nor a specific narcotic antagonist. Adequacy of airway and oxygenation must be assured prior to doxapram administration.
   b. Doxapram should be administered with great care and only under careful supervision to patients with hypermetabolic states such as hyperthyroidism or pheochromocytoma.
   c. Since narcosis may recur after stimulation with doxapram, care should be taken to maintain close observation until the patient has been fully alert for ½ to 1 hour.
2. ***In drug-induced CNS and respiratory depression.***
   Doxapram alone may not stimulate adequate spontaneous breathing or provide sufficient arousal in patients who are ***severely*** depressed either due to respiratory failure or to CNS depressant drugs, but should be used as an adjunct to established supportive measures and resuscitative techniques.
3. ***In chronic obstructive pulmonary disease.***
   a. Because of the associated increased work of breathing, do not increase the rate of infusion of doxapram in severely ill patients in an attempt to lower pCO_2.
   b. Doxapram should not be used in conjunction with mechanical ventilation.

PRECAUTIONS

1. ***General.***
   a. An adequate airway is essential.
   b. Recommended dosages of doxapram should be employed and maximum total dosages should not be exceeded. In order to avoid side effects, it is advisable to use the minimum effective dosage.
   c. Monitoring of the blood pressure and deep tendon reflexes is recommended to prevent overdosage.
   d. Vascular extravasation or use of a single injection site over an extended period should be avoided since either may lead to thrombophlebitis or local skin irritation.
   e. Rapid infusion may result in hemolysis.
   f. Lowered pCO_2 induced by hyperventilation produces cerebral vasoconstriction and slowing of the cerebral circulation. This should be taken into consideration on an individual basis.
   g. Intravenous short-acting barbiturates, oxygen and resuscitative equipment should be readily available to manage overdosage manifested by excessive central nervous system stimulation. Slow administration of the drug, and careful observation of the patient during administration and for some time subsequently are advisable. These precautions are to assure that the protective reflexes have been restored and to prevent possible post-hyperventilation hypoventilation.
   h. Doxapram should be administered cautiously to patients receiving sympathomimetic or monoamine oxi-

Continued on next page

A. H. Robins—Cont.

dase inhibiting drugs, since an additive pressor effect may occur.

i. Blood pressure increases are generally modest but significant increases have been noted in some patients. Because of this doxapram is not recommended for use in severe hypertension (see Contraindications).

j. If sudden hypotension or dyspnea develops, doxapram should be stopped.

2. *In postanesthetic use.*

a. The same consideration to pre-existing disease states should be exercised as in non-anesthetized individuals. See Contraindications and Warnings covering use in hypertension, asthma, disturbances of respiratory mechanics including airway obstruction, CNS disorders including increased cerebrospinal fluid pressure, convulsive disorders, acute agitation, and profound metabolic disorders.

b. See Drug Interactions.

3. *In chronic obstructive pulmonary disease.*

a. Arrhythmias seen in some patients in acute respiratory failure secondary to chronic obstructive pulmonary disease are probably the result of hypoxia. Doxapram should be used with caution in these patients.

b. Arterial blood gases should be drawn prior to the initiation of doxapram infusion and oxygen administration, then at least every ½ hour. Doxapram administration does not diminish the need for careful monitoring of the patient or the need for supplemental oxygen in patients with acute respiratory failure. Doxapram should be stopped if the arterial blood gases deteriorate, and mechanical ventilation initiated.

Drug Interactions: Administration of doxapram to patients who are receiving sympathomimetic or monoamine oxidase inhibiting drugs may result in an additive pressor effect. (See Precautions.)

In patients who have received muscle relaxants, doxapram may temporarily mask the residual effects of muscle relaxant drugs.

In patients who have received anesthetics known to sensitize the myocardium to catecholamines, such as halothane, cyclopropane and enflurane, initiation of doxapram therapy should be delayed for at least 10 minutes following discontinuance of anesthesia, since an increase in epinephrine release has been noted with doxapram.

Carcinogenesis, mutagenesis, impairment of fertility. No carcinogenic or mutagenic studies have been performed using doxapram. Doxapram did not adversely affect the breeding performance of rats.

Pregnancy Category B. Reproduction studies have been performed in rats at doses up to 1.6 times the human dose and have revealed no evidence of impaired fertility or harm to the fetus due to doxapram. There are, however, no adequate and well-controlled studies in pregnant women. Since the animals in the reproduction studies were dosed by the IM and oral routes and animal reproduction studies, in general, are not always predictive of human response, this drug should be used during pregnancy only if clearly needed.

Nursing mothers. It is not known whether this drug is excreted in human milk. Because many drugs are excreted in human milk, caution should be exercised when doxapram hydrochloride is administered to a nursing mother.

Pediatric use. The use of the preservative benzyl alcohol in the newborn has been associated with metabolic, CNS, respiratory, circulatory, and renal dysfunction. Safety and effectiveness in children below the age of 12 years have not been established.

ADVERSE REACTIONS

The following adverse reactions have been reported:

1. *Central and autonomic nervous systems.*

Pyrexia, flushing, sweating; pruritus and paresthesia, such as a feeling of warmth, burning, or hot sensation, especially in the area of genitalia and perineum; apprehension, disorientation, pupillary dilatation, headache, dizziness, hyperactivity, involuntary movements, muscle spasticity, increased deep tendon reflexes, clonus, bilateral Babinski, and convulsions.

2. *Respiratory.*

Dyspnea, cough, tachypnea, laryngospasm, bronchospasm, hiccough, and rebound hypoventilation.

3. *Cardiovascular.*

Phlebitis, variations in heart rate, lowered T-waves, arrhythmias, chest pain, tightness in chest. A mild to moderate increase in blood pressure is commonly noted and may be of concern in patients with severe cardiovascular diseases.

4. *Gastrointestinal.*

Nausea, vomiting, diarrhea, desire to defecate.

5. *Genitourinary.*

Stimulation of urinary bladder with spontaneous voiding; urinary retention.

6. *Laboratory determinations.*

A decrease in hemoglobin, hematocrit, or red blood cell count has been observed in postoperative patients. In the presence of pre-existing leukopenia, a further decrease in WBC has been observed following anesthesia and treatment with doxapram hydrochloride. Elevation of BUN and albuminuria have also been observed. As some of the patients cited above had received multiple drugs concomitantly, a cause and effect relationship could not be determined.

OVERDOSAGE

Signs and Symptoms. Symptoms of overdosage are extensions of the pharmacologic effects of the drug. Excessive pressor effect, tachycardia, skeletal muscle hyperactivity, and enhanced deep tendon reflexes may be early signs of overdosage. Therefore, the blood pressure, pulse rate and deep tendon reflexes should be evaluated periodically and the dosage or infusion rate adjusted accordingly.

Convulsive seizures are unlikely at recommended dosages. In unanesthetized animals, the convulsant dose is 70 times greater than the respiratory stimulant dose. Intravenous LD_{50} values in the mouse and rat were approximately 75 mg/kg and in the cat and dog were 40–80 mg/kg.

Except for management of chronic obstructive pulmonary disease associated with acute hypercapnia, the maximum recommended dosage is 3 GRAMS/24 HOURS. (See Dosage and Administration.)

Management. There is no specific antidote for doxapram. Management should be symptomatic. Short-acting intravenous barbiturates, oxygen and resuscitative equipment should be used as needed for supportive treatment.

There is no evidence that doxapram is dialyzable; further, the half-life of doxapram makes it unlikely that dialysis would be appropriate in managing overdose with this drug.

DOSAGE AND ADMINISTRATION

1. Doxapram hydrochloride is compatible with 5% and 10% dextrose in water or normal saline. ADMIXTURE OF DOXAPRAM WITH ALKALINE SOLUTIONS SUCH AS 2.5% THIOPENTAL SODIUM, BICARBONATE, OR AMINOPHYLLINE WILL RESULT IN PRECIPITATION OR GAS FORMATION.

2. *In postanesthetic use.*

a. By i.v. injection (see Table I. Dosage for postanesthetic use—I.V.) Slow administration of the drug and careful observation of the patient during administration and for some time subsequently are advisable. [See table I below.]

b. By infusion. The solution is prepared by adding 250 mg of doxapram (12.5 mL) to 250 mL of dextrose or saline solution. The infusion is initiated at a rate of approximately 5 mg/minute until a satisfactory respiratory response is observed, and maintained at a rate of 1–3 mg/minute. The rate of infusion should be adjusted to sustain the desired level of respiratory stimulation with a minimum of side effects. The recommended total dosage by infusion is 4 mg/kg (2.0 mg/lb), or approximately 300 mg for the average adult.

3. *In the management of drug-induced CNS depression.*

(See Table II. Dosage for drug-induced CNS depression.) [See table II above.]

METHOD ONE

Using Single and/or Repeat Single I.V. *Injections.*

a. Give priming dose of 1.0 mg/lb (2.0 mg/kg) body weight and repeat in 5 minutes.

b. Repeat same dose q1–2h until patient wakens. Watch for relapse into unconsciousness or development of respiratory depression, since Dopram does not affect the metabolism of CNS-depressant drugs.

c. If relapse occurs, resume injections q1–2h until arousal is sustained, or total maximum daily dose (3 grams) is given. Allow patients to sleep until 24 hours have elapsed from first injection of Dopram, using assisted or automatic respiration if necessary.

d. Repeat procedure the following day until patient breathes spontaneously and sustains desired level of consciousness, or until maximum dosage (3 grams) is given.

e. Repetitive doses should be administered only to patients who have shown response to the initial dose.

f. Failure to respond appropriately indicates the need for neurologic evaluation for a possible central nervous system source of sustained coma.

METHOD TWO

By Intermittent I.V. *Infusion.*

a. Give priming dose as in Method One.

b. If patient wakens, watch for relapse; if no response, continue general supportive treatment for 1–2 hours and repeat Dopram. If some respiratory stimulation occurs, prepare I.V. infusion by adding 250 mg of Dopram (12.5 mL) to 250 mL of saline or dextrose solution. Deliver at rate of 1–3 mg/min (60–180 mL/hr) according to size of patient and depth of coma. Discontinue Dopram if patient begins to waken or at end of 2 hours.

c. Continue supportive treatment for ½ to 2 hours and repeat Step b.

d. Do not exceed 3 grams/day.

4. *Chronic obstructive pulmonary disease associated with acute hypercapnia.*

a. One vial of doxapram (400 mg) should be mixed with 180 mL of dextrose or saline solution (concentration of 2.0 mg/mL). The infusion should be started at 1–2 mg/minute (½–1 mL/minute); if indicated, increase to a maximum of 3 mg/minute. Arterial blood gases should be determined prior to the onset of doxapram's administration and at least every half hour during the two hours of infusion to insure against the insidious development of CO_2-RETENTION AND ACIDOSIS. Alteration of oxygen concentration or flow rate may necessitate adjustment in the rate of doxapram infusion.

b. Predictable blood gas patterns are more readily established with a continuous infusion of doxapram. If the blood gases show evidence of deterioration, the infusion of doxapram should be discontinued.

c. ADDITIONAL INFUSIONS BEYOND THE SINGLE MAXIMUM TWO HOUR ADMINISTRATION PERIOD ARE NOT RECOMMENDED.

Table II. Dopram Injectable Dosage for drug-induced CNS depression.

Level of Depression	METHOD ONE Priming dose single/repeat i.v. injection		METHOD TWO Rate of intermittent i.v. infusion	
	mg/kg	mg/lb	mg/kg/hr	mg/lb/hr
Mild*	1.0	0.5	1.0–2.0	0.5–1.0
Moderate†	2.0	1.0	2.0–3.0	1.0–1.5

*Mild Depression
Class 0: Asleep, but can be aroused and can answer questions.
Class 1: Comatose, will withdraw from painful stimuli, reflexes intact.
†Moderate Depression
Class 2: Comatose, will not withdraw from painful stimuli, reflexes intact.
Class 3: Comatose, reflexes absent, no depression of circulation or respiration.

Table I. Dopram Injectable Dosage for postanesthetic use—I.V.

I.V. Administration	Recommended dosage		Maximum dose per single injection		Maximum total dose	
	mg/kg	mg/lb	mg/kg	mg/lb	mg/kg	mg/lb
Single Injection	0.5–1.0	0.25–0.5	1.5	0.70	1.5	0.70
Repeat Injections (5 min. intervals)	0.5–1.0	0.25–0.5	1.5	0.70	2.0	1.0
Infusion	0.5–1.0	0.25–0.5	—	—	4.0	2.0

Parenteral drug products should be inspected visually for particulate matter and discoloration prior to administration, whenever solution and container permit.

HOW SUPPLIED

Dopram Injectable (doxapram hydrochloride injection) is available in 20 mL multiple dose vials containing 20 mg of doxapram hydrochloride per mL. with benzyl alcohol 0.9% as the preservative (NDC 0031-4849-83).

Store at Controlled Room Temperature, Between 15°C and 30°C (59°F and 86°F).

Manufactured for A. H. Robins Company, Richmond, Virginia 23220 by Elkins-Sinn, Inc., Cherry Hill, New Jersey 08003-4099.

MICRO–K EXTENCAPS® ℞
[mi'cro" K ĕks"tĕn'caps]
MICRO–K 10 EXTENCAPS® ℞
(Potassium Chloride Extended-Release Capsules, USP)

DESCRIPTION

Micro-K Extencaps are pale orange, hard gelatin capsules, each containing 600 mg of dispersible, small crystalline particles of potassium chloride (equivalent to 8 mEq K), monogrammed Micro-K and AHR/5720.

Micro-K 10 Extencaps are pale orange and opaque white, hard gelatin capsules, each containing 750 mg of dispersible, small crystalline particles of potassium chloride (equivalent to 10 mEq K) monogrammed Micro-K 10 and AHR/5730.

Each particle of potassium chloride (KCl) is microencapsulated with a polymeric coating which allows for the controlled release of potassium and chloride ions over an eight- to ten-hour period. The dispersibility of the microcapsules and the controlled release of ions are intended to minimize the likelihood of high localized concentrations of potassium chloride and resultant mucosal ulceration within the gastrointestinal tract.

The polymeric coating forming the microcapsules functions as a water-permeable membrane. Fluids pass through the membrane and gradually dissolve the potassium chloride within the microcapsules. The resulting potassium chloride solution slowly diffuses outward through the membrane.

Inactive Ingredients: Edible Ink, Ethylcellulose, FD&C Blue 2 Aluminum Lake, FD&C Yellow 6, Gelatin, Magnesium Stearate, Sodium Lauryl Sulfate, Titanium Dioxide. May contain FD&C Red 40 and Yellow 6 Aluminum Lakes.

ACTIONS

Potassium ion is the principal intracellular cation of most body tissues. Potassium ions participate in a number of essential physiological processes, including the maintenance of intracellular tonicity, the transmission of nerve impulses, the contraction of cardiac, skeletal, and smooth muscle and the maintenance of normal renal function.

Potassium depletion may occur whenever the rate of potassium loss through renal excretion and/or loss from the gastrointestinal tract exceeds the rate of potassium intake. Such depletion usually develops slowly as a consequence of prolonged therapy with oral diuretics, primary or secondary hyperaldosteronism, diabetic ketoacidosis, severe diarrhea, or inadequate replacement of potassium in patients on prolonged parenteral nutrition. Potassium depletion due to these causes is usually accompanied by a concomitant deficiency of chloride and is manifested by hypokalemia and metabolic alkalosis. Potassium depletion may produce weakness, fatigue, disturbances of cardiac rhythm (primarily ectopic beats), prominent U-waves in the electrocardiogram, and in advanced cases, flaccid paralysis and/or impaired ability to concentrate urine.

Potassium depletion associated with metabolic alkalosis is managed by correcting the fundamental causes of the deficiency whenever possible and administering supplemental potassium chloride, in the form of high potassium food or potassium chloride solution, capsules or tablets. In rare circumstances (e.g., patients with renal tubular acidosis) potassium depletion may be associated with metabolic acidosis and hyperchloremia. In such patients potassium replacement should be accomplished with potassium salts other than the chloride, such as potassium bicarbonate, potassium citrate, or potassium acetate.

INDICATIONS

BECAUSE OF REPORTS OF INTESTINAL AND GASTRIC ULCERATION AND BLEEDING WITH SLOW-RELEASE POTASSIUM CHLORIDE PREPARATIONS, THESE DRUGS SHOULD BE RESERVED FOR THOSE PATIENTS WHO CANNOT TOLERATE OR REFUSE TO TAKE LIQUID OR EFFERVESCENT POTASSIUM PREPARATIONS OR FOR PATIENTS IN WHOM THERE IS A PROBLEM OF COMPLIANCE WITH THESE PREPARATIONS.

1. For therapeutic use in patients with hypokalemia with or without metabolic alkalosis; in digitalis intoxication and in patients with hypokalemic familial periodic paralysis.
2. For prevention of potassium depletion when the dietary intake of potassium is inadequate in the following conditions: patients receiving digitalis and diuretics for congestive heart failure; hepatic cirrhosis with ascites; states of aldosterone excess with normal renal function; potassium-losing nephropathy, and certain diarrheal states.
3. The use of potassium salts in patients receiving diuretics for uncomplicated essential hypertension is often unnecessary when such patients have a normal dietary pattern. Serum potassium should be checked periodically, however, and, if hypokalemia occurs, dietary supplementation with potassium-containing foods may be adequate to control milder cases. In more severe cases, supplementation with potassium salts may be indicated.

CONTRAINDICATIONS

Potassium supplements are contraindicated in patients with hyperkalemia since a further increase in serum potassium concentration in such patients can produce cardiac arrest. Hyperkalemia may complicate any of the following conditions: chronic renal failure, systemic acidosis such as diabetic acidosis, acute dehydration, extensive tissue breakdown as in severe burns, adrenal insufficiency, or the administration of a potassium-sparing diuretic (e.g., spironolactone, triamterene, amiloride) (see OVERDOSAGE).

Controlled release formulations of potassium chloride have produced esophageal ulceration in certain cardiac patients with esophageal compression due to an enlarged left atrium. Potassium supplementation, when indicated in such patients, should be given as a liquid preparation.

All solid oral dosage forms of potassium chloride are contraindicated in any patient in whom there is structural, pathological (e.g., diabetic gastroparesis) or pharmacologic (use of anticholinergic agents or other agents with anticholinergic properties at sufficient doses to exert anticholinergic effects) cause for arrest or delay in capsule passage through the gastrointestinal tract.

WARNINGS

Hyperkalemia. In patients with impaired mechanisms for excreting potassium, the administration of potassium salts can produce hyperkalemia and cardiac arrest. This occurs most commonly in patients given potassium by the intravenous route but may also occur in patients given potassium orally. Potentially fatal hyperkalemia can develop rapidly and be asymptomatic.

The use of potassium salts in patients with chronic renal disease, or any other condition which impairs potassium excretion, requires particularly careful monitoring of the serum potassium concentration and appropriate dosage adjustments.

Interaction with Potassium-Sparing Diuretics. Hypokalemia should not be treated by the concomitant administration of potassium salts and a potassium-sparing diuretic (e.g., spironolactone or triamterene), since the simultaneous administration of these agents can produce severe hyperkalemia.

Interaction with Angiotensin Converting Enzyme Inhibitors. Angiotensin converting enzyme (ACE) inhibitors (e.g., captopril, enalapril) will produce some potassium retention by inhibiting aldosterone production. Potassium supplements should be given to patients receiving ACE inhibitors only with close monitoring.

Gastrointestinal lesions. Potassium chloride tablets have produced stenotic and/or ulcerative lesions of the small bowel and deaths, in addition to upper gastrointestinal bleeding. These lesions are caused by a high localized concentration of potassium ion in the region of a rapidly dissolving tablet which injures the bowel wall and thereby produces obstruction, hemorrhage, or perforation.

Micro-K Extencaps contain microcapsules which disperse upon dissolution of the hard gelatin capsule. The microcapsules are formulated to provide a controlled release of potassium chloride. The dispersibility of the microcapsules and the controlled release of ions from the microcapsules are intended to minimize the possibility of a high local concentration near the gastrointestinal mucosa and the ability of the KCl to cause stenosis or ulceration. Other means of accomplishing this (e.g., incorporation of KCl into a wax matrix) have reduced the frequency of such lesions to less than one per 100,000 patient years (compared to 40–50 per 100,000 patient years with enteric-coated KCl), but have not eliminated them. The frequency of GI lesions with Micro-K Extencaps is, at present, unknown. Micro-K Extencaps should be discontinued immediately and the possibility of bowel obstruction or perforation considered if severe vomiting, abdominal pain, distention, or gastrointestinal bleeding occurs.

Metabolic Acidosis. Hypokalemia in patients with metabolic *acidosis* should be treated with an alkalinizing potassium salt such as potassium bicarbonate, potassium citrate, or potassium acetate.

PRECAUTIONS

General: The diagnosis of potassium depletion is ordinarily made by demonstrating hypokalemia in a patient with a clinical history suggesting some cause for potassium depletion. In interpreting the serum potassium level, the physician should bear in mind that acute alkalosis per se can produce hypokalemia in the absence of a deficit in total body potassium, while acute acidosis per se can increase the serum potassium concentration into the normal range even in the presence of a reduced total body potassium. The treatment of potassium depletion, particularly in the presence of cardiac disease, renal disease, or acidosis, requires careful attention to acid-base balance and appropriate monitoring of serum electrolytes, the electrocardiogram, and the clinical status of the patient.

Information for Patients:

Physicians should consider reminding the patient of the following:

To take each dose with meals and with water or other suitable liquid.

To take this medicine following the frequency and amount prescribed by the physician. This is especially important if the patient is also taking diuretics and/or digitalis preparations.

To check with the physician if there is trouble swallowing capsules or if the capsules seem to stick in the throat.

To check with the physician at once if tarry stools or other evidence of gastrointestinal bleeding is noticed.

To take each dose without crushing, chewing, or sucking the capsule.

Laboratory Tests:

Regular serum potassium determinations are recommended, especially in patients with renal insufficiency or diabetic nephropathy.

When blood is drawn for analysis of plasma potassium it is important to recognize that artifactual elevations can occur after improper venipuncture technique or as a result of *in vitro* hemolysis of the sample.

Drug Interactions:

Potassium-sparing diuretic, angiotensin converting enzyme inhibitors: see WARNINGS.

Carcinogenesis, Mutagenesis, Impairment of Fertility: Carcinogenicity, mutagenicity and fertility studies in animals have not been performed. Potassium is a normal dietary constituent.

Pregnancy Category C:

Animal reproduction studies have not been conducted with Micro-K. It is unlikely that potassium supplementation that does not lead to hyperkalemia would have an adverse effect on the fetus or would affect reproductive capacity.

Nursing Mothers:

The normal potassium ion content of human milk is about 13 mEq per liter. Since oral potassium becomes part of the body potassium pool, so long as body potassium is not excessive, the contribution of potassium chloride supplementation should have little or no effect on the level in human milk.

Pediatric Use:

Safety and effectiveness in children have not been established.

ADVERSE REACTIONS

One of the most severe adverse effects is hyperkalemia (see CONTRAINDICATIONS, WARNINGS, AND OVERDOSAGE).

Gastrointestinal bleeding and ulceration have been reported in patients treated with Micro-K Extencaps (see WARNINGS).

In addition to gastrointestinal bleeding and ulceration, perforation and obstruction have been reported in patients treated with other solid KCl dosage forms, and may occur with Micro-K Extencaps.

The most common adverse reactions to the oral potassium salts are nausea, vomiting, abdominal pain/discomfort, and diarrhea. These symptoms are due to irritation of the gastrointestinal tract and are best managed by taking the dose with meals, or reducing the amount taken at one time.

OVERDOSAGE

The administration of oral potassium salts to persons with normal excretory mechanisms for potassium rarely causes serious hyperkalemia. However, if excretory mechanisms are impaired or if potassium is administered too rapidly intravenously, potentially fatal hyperkalemia can result (see Contraindications and Warnings). It is important to recognize that hyperkalemia is usually asymptomatic and may be manifested only by an increased serum potassium concentration and characteristic electrocardiogram changes (peaking of T-waves, loss of P-wave, depression of S-T segment, and prolongation of the QT interval). Late manifestations include muscle paralysis and cardiovascular collapse from cardiac arrest.

Treatment measures for hyperkalemia include the following: (1) elimination of foods and medications containing potassium and of potassium-sparing diuretics; (2) intravenous administration of 300 to 500 ml/hr of 10% dextrose solution containing 10–20 units of insulin per 1,000 ml; (3) correction of acidosis, if present, with intravenous sodium bicarbonate; (4) use of exchange resins, hemodialysis, or peritoneal dialysis.

In treating hyperkalemia, it should be recalled that in patients who have been stabilized on digitalis, too rapid a lowering of the serum potassium concentration can produce digitalis toxicity.

Continued on next page

A. H. Robins—Cont.

DOSAGE AND ADMINISTRATION

The usual dietary intake of potassium by the average adult is 40 to 80 mEq per day. Potassium depletion sufficient to cause hypokalemia usually requires the loss of 200 or more mEq of potassium from the total body store.

Dosage must be adjusted to the individual needs of each patient, but typically is around 20 mEq per day for the prevention of hypokalemia and 40 to 100 mEq per day for the treatment of potassium depletion.

	For Prevention	For Treatment
Micro-K Extencaps (8 mEq K)	2 or 3 Extencaps/day (16–24 mEq K)	5 to 12 Extencaps/day (40–96 mEq K)
Micro-K 10 Extencaps (10 mEq K)	2 Extencaps/day (20 mEq K)	4 to 10 Extencaps/day (40–100 mEq K)

If more than 2 Extencaps are prescribed per day, the total daily dosage should be divided into two or more separate doses. Those patients having difficulty swallowing the capsules may be advised to sprinkle the contents onto a spoonful of soft food to facilitate ingestion.

HOW SUPPLIED

Micro-K Extencaps® are pale orange capsules monogrammed Micro-K and AHR/5720, each containing 600 mg microencapsulated potassium chloride (equivalent to 8 mEq K) in bottles of 100 (NDC 0031-5720-63), 500 (NDC 0031-5720-70) and Dis-Co® unit dose packs of 100 (NDC 0031-5720-64).

Micro-K 10 Extencaps® are pale orange and opaque white capsules monogrammed Micro-K 10 and AHR/5730, each containing 750 mg microencapsulated potassium chloride (equivalent to 10 mEq K) in bottles of 100 (NDC 0031-5730-63), 100 Unit-of-Use (NDC 0031-5730-68), bottles of 500 (NDC 0031-5730-70), and Dis-Co® unit dose packs of 100 (NDC 0031-5730-64).

Store at controlled room temperature, between 15°C and 30°C (59°F and 86°F). Dispense in tight container.

CAUTION: Federal law prohibits dispensing without a prescription.

Animal Toxicology: The ulcerogenic potential of microencapsulated KCl was studied in anesthetized cats by direct applications on exteriorized gastric mucosa. The microcapsules of KCl were found to be non-ulcerogenic and significantly less irritating than wax-matrix tablets and 20% solution of KCl.

In groups of monkeys (up to 8 monkeys per group) receiving different formulations of potassium chloride at equivalent daily dosage (2400 mg KCl) for four and one-half days, Micro-K Extencaps showed no tendency to cause intestinal ulceration (similar to liquid KCl and a wax-matrix preparation but in contrast to an enteric-coated KCl tablet) and minimal gastric irritation (less than a wax-matrix preparation).

Shown in Product Identification Guide, page 331

MICRO-K® LS ℞

[mi 'cro "k]

brand of Potassium Chloride
Extended-Release Formulation
for Liquid Suspension

DESCRIPTION

Micro-K LS is an oral dosage form of microencapsulated potassium chloride. Each packet contains 1.5 g of potassium chloride, USP equivalent to 20 mEq of potassium. Micro-K LS is comprised of specially formulated granules. After reconstitution with 2–6 fl oz of water and 1 minute of stirring, the suspension is odorless and tasteless.

Each crystal of potassium chloride (KCl) is microencapsulated with an insoluble polymeric coating which functions as a semipermeable membrane; it allows for the controlled release of potassium and chloride ions over an eight–ten hour period. The controlled release of K^+ ions by the microcapsular membrane is intended to reduce the likelihood of a high localized concentration of potassium chloride at any point on the mucosa of the gastrointestinal tract. Fluids pass through the membrane and gradually dissolve the potassium chloride within the microcapsules. The resulting potassium chloride solution slowly diffuses outward through the membrane.

Micro-K LS is an electrolyte replenisher. The chemical name of the active ingredient is potassium chloride and the structural formula is KCl. Potassium Chloride, USP occurs as a white, granular powder or as colorless crystals. It is odorless and has a saline taste. Its solutions are neutral to litmus. It is freely soluble in water and insoluble in alcohol.

Inactive Ingredients: Docusate Sodium, Ethylcellulose, Povidone, Silicon Dioxide, Sucrose, and another ingredient.

CLINICAL PHARMACOLOGY

The potassium ion is the principal intracellular cation of most body tissues. Potassium ions participate in a number of essential physiological processes including the maintenance of intracellular tonicity, the transmission of nerve impulses, the contraction of cardiac, skeletal, and smooth muscle, and the maintenance of normal renal function.

The intracellular concentration of potassium is approximately 150 to 160 mEq per liter. The normal adult plasma concentration is 3.5 to 5 mEq per liter. An active ion transport system maintains this gradient across the plasma membrane.

Potassium is a normal dietary constituent and under steady-state conditions the amount of potassium absorbed from the gastrointestinal tract is equal to the amount excreted in the urine. The usual dietary intake of potassium is 50 to 100 mEq per day.

Potassium depletion will occur whenever the rate of potassium loss through renal excretion and/or loss from the gastrointestinal tract exceeds the rate of potassium intake. Such depletion usually develops as a consequence of therapy with diuretics, primary or secondary hyperaldosteronism, diabetic ketoacidosis, or inadequate replacement of potassium in patients on prolonged parenteral nutrition. Depletion can develop rapidly with severe diarrhea, especially if associated with vomiting. Potassium depletion due to these causes is usually accompanied by a concomitant loss of chloride and is manifested by hypokalemia and metabolic alkalosis. Potassium depletion may produce weakness, fatigue, disturbances of cardiac rhythm (primarily ectopic beats), prominent U-waves in the electrocardiogram, and, in advanced cases, flaccid paralysis and/or impaired ability to concentrate urine.

If potassium depletion associated with metabolic alkalosis cannot be managed by correcting the fundamental cause of the deficiency, e.g., where the patient requires long-term diuretic therapy, supplemental potassium in the form of high potassium food or potassium chloride may be able to restore normal potassium levels.

In rare circumstances (e.g., patients with renal tubular acidosis) potassium depletion may be associated with metabolic acidosis and hyperchloremia. In such patients potassium replacement should be accomplished with potassium salts other than the chloride, such as potassium bicarbonate, potassium citrate, potassium acetate, or potassium gluconate.

INDICATIONS AND USAGE

BECAUSE OF REPORTS OF INTESTINAL AND GASTRIC ULCERATION AND BLEEDING WITH CONTROLLED RELEASE POTASSIUM CHLORIDE PREPARATIONS, THESE DRUGS SHOULD BE RESERVED FOR THOSE PATIENTS WHO CANNOT TOLERATE OR REFUSE TO TAKE IMMEDIATE RELEASE LIQUIDS/EFFERVESCENT POTASSIUM PREPARATIONS OR FOR PATIENTS IN WHOM THERE IS A PROBLEM OF COMPLIANCE WITH THESE PREPARATIONS.

1. For the treatment of patients with hypokalemia, with or without metabolic alkalosis; in digitalis intoxication; and in patients with hypokalemic familial periodic paralysis. If hypokalemia is the result of diuretic therapy, consideration should be given to the use of a lower dose of diuretic, which may be sufficient without leading to hypokalemia.
2. For the prevention of hypokalemia in patients who would be at particular risk if hypokalemia were to develop, e.g., digitalized patients or patients with significant cardiac arrhythmias, hepatic cirrhosis with ascites, states of aldosterone excess with normal renal function, potassium losing nephropathy, and certain diarrheal states.

The use of potassium salts in patients receiving diuretics for uncomplicated essential hypertension is often unnecessary when such patients have a normal dietary pattern and when low doses of the diuretic are used. Serum potassium should be checked periodically, however, and if hypokalemia occurs, dietary supplementation with potassium-containing foods may be adequate to control milder cases. In more severe cases, and if dose adjustment of the diuretic is ineffective or unwarranted, supplementation with potassium salts may be indicated.

CONTRAINDICATIONS

Potassium supplements are contraindicated in patients with hyperkalemia since a further increase in serum potassium concentration in such patients can produce cardiac arrest. Hyperkalemia may complicate any of the following conditions: chronic renal failure, systemic acidosis such as diabetic acidosis, acute dehydration, extensive tissue breakdown as in severe burns, adrenal insufficiency, or the administration of a potassium-sparing diuretic (e.g., spironolactone, triamterene, amiloride) (see OVERDOSAGE).

Controlled release formulations of potassium chloride have produced esophageal ulceration in certain cardiac patients with esophageal compression due to an enlarged left atrium. Potassium supplementation, when indicated in such patients, should be given as an immediate release liquid preparation.

All solid oral dosage forms of potassium chloride are contraindicated in any patient in whom there is structural, pathological (e.g., diabetic gastroparesis) or pharmacologic (use of anticholinergic agents or other agents with anticholinergic properties at sufficient doses to exert anticholinergic effects) cause for arrest or delay in tablet or capsule-passage through the gastrointestinal tract.

WARNINGS

Hyperkalemia (see OVERDOSAGE). In patients with impaired mechanisms for excreting potassium, the administration of potassium salts can produce hyperkalemia and cardiac arrest. This occurs most commonly in patients given potassium by the intravenous route but may also occur in patients given potassium orally. Potentially fatal hyperkalemia can develop rapidly and be asymptomatic. The use of potassium salts in patients with chronic renal disease, or any other condition which impairs potassium excretion, requires particularly careful monitoring of the serum potassium concentration and appropriate dosage adjustment.

Interaction with Potassium-Sparing Diuretics. Hypokalemia should not be treated by the concomitant administration of potassium salts and a potassium-sparing diuretic (e.g., spironolactone, triamterene or amiloride) since the simultaneous administration of these agents can produce severe hyperkalemia.

Interaction with Angiotensin Converting Enzyme Inhibitors. Angiotensin converting enzyme (ACE) inhibitors (e.g., captopril, enalapril) will produce some potassium retention by inhibiting aldosterone production. Potassium supplements should be given to patients receiving ACE inhibitors only with close monitoring.

Gastrointestinal Lesions. Solid oral dosage forms of potassium chloride can produce ulcerative and/or stenotic lesions of the gastrointestinal tract. Based on spontaneous adverse reaction reports, enteric coated preparations of potassium chloride are associated with an increased frequency of small bowel lesions (40–50 per 100,000 patient years) compared to sustained release wax matrix formulations (less than one per 100,000 patient years). Because of the lack of extensive marketing experience with microencapsulated products, a comparison between such products and wax matrix or enteric coated products is not available. Micro-K LS is administered as a liquid suspension of microencapsulated potassium chloride formulated to provide a controlled rate of release of potassium chloride and thus to minimize the possibility of a high local concentration of potassium near the gastrointestinal wall.

Prospective trials have been conducted in normal human volunteers in which the upper gastrointestinal tract was evaluated by endoscopic inspection before and after one week of solid oral potassium chloride therapy. The ability of this model to predict events occurring in usual clinical practice is unknown. Trials which approximated usual clinical practice did not reveal any clear differences between the wax matrix and microencapsulated dosage forms. In contrast, there was a higher incidence of gastric and duodenal lesions in subjects receiving a high dose of a wax matrix controlled release formulation under conditions which did not resemble usual or recommended clinical practice (i.e., 96 mEq per day in divided doses of potassium chloride administered to fasted patients, in the presence of an anticholinergic drug to delay gastric emptying). The upper gastrointestinal lesions observed by endoscopy were asymptomatic and were not accompanied by evidence of bleeding (hemoccult testing). The relevance of these findings to the usual conditions (i.e., non-fasting, no anticholinergic agent, smaller doses) under which controlled release potassium chloride products are used is uncertain; epidemiologic studies have not identified an elevated risk, compared to microencapsulated products, for upper gastrointestinal lesions in patients receiving wax matrix formulations. Micro-K LS should be discontinued immediately and the possibility of ulceration, obstruction or perforation considered if severe vomiting, abdominal pain, distention, or gastrointestinal bleeding occurs.

Diarrhea or Dehydration. Micro-K LS contains, as a dispersing agent, docusate sodium, which also increases stool water and is used as a stool softener. Clinical studies with Micro-K LS indicate that minor changes in stool consistency may be common, although usually are well-tolerated. However, rarely patients may experience diarrhea or cramping abdominal pain. Patients with severe or chronic diarrhea or who are dehydrated ordinarily should not be prescribed Micro-K LS.

Metabolic Acidosis. Hypokalemia in patients with metabolic acidosis should be treated with an alkalinizing potassium salt such as potassium bicarbonate, potassium citrate, potassium acetate, or potassium gluconate.

PRECAUTIONS

General: The diagnosis of potassium depletion is ordinarily made by demonstrating hypokalemia in a patient with a clinical history suggesting some cause for potassium depletion. In interpreting the serum potassium level, the physician should bear in mind that acute alkalosis *per se* can produce hypokalemia in the absence of a deficit in total body potassium while acute acidosis *per se* can increase the serum potassium concentration into the normal range even in the presence of a reduced total body potassium. The treatment of potassium depletion, particularly in the presence of cardiac

disease, renal disease, or acidosis requires careful attention to acid-base balance and appropriate monitoring of serum electrolytes, the electrocardiogram, and the clinical status of the patient.

Information for Patients: Physicians should consider reminding the patient of the following:

To take each dose with meals mixed in water or other suitable liquid.

To take this medicine following the frequency and amount prescribed by the physician. This is especially important if the patient is also taking diuretics and/or digitalis preparations.

To inform patients that this product contains as a dispersing agent the stool softener, docusate sodium, which may change stool consistency, or rarely produce diarrhea or cramps.

To check with the physician at once if tarry stools or other evidence of gastrointestinal bleeding is noticed.

Laboratory Tests: Regular serum potassium determinations are recommended, especially in patients with renal insufficiency or diabetic nephropathy.

When blood is drawn for analysis of plasma potassium, it is important to recognize that artifactual elevations can occur after improper venipuncture technique or as a result of *in vitro* hemolysis of the sample.

Drug Interactions: Potassium-sparing diuretics, angiotensin converting enzyme inhibitors: see WARNINGS.

Carcinogenesis, Mutagenesis, Impairment of Fertility: Carcinogenicity, mutagenicity, and fertility studies in animals have not been performed. Potassium is a normal dietary constituent.

Pregnancy Category C. Animal reproduction studies have not been conducted with Micro-K LS. It is unlikely that potassium supplementation that does not lead to hyperkalemia would have an adverse effect on the fetus or would affect reproductive capacity.

Nursing Mothers: The normal potassium ion content of human milk is about 13 mEq per liter. Since oral potassium becomes part of the body potassium pool, so long as body potassium is not excessive, the contribution of potassium chloride supplementation should have little or no effect on the level in human milk.

Pediatric Use: Safety and effectiveness in children have not been established.

ADVERSE REACTIONS

One of the most severe adverse effects is hyperkalemia (see CONTRAINDICATIONS, WARNINGS, AND OVERDOSAGE).

Gastrointestinal bleeding and ulceration have been reported in patients treated with microencapsulated KCl (see WARNINGS).

In addition to bleeding and ulceration, perforation and obstruction have been reported in patients treated with solid KCl dosage forms, and may occur with Micro-K LS.

The most common adverse reactions to the oral potassium salts are nausea, vomiting, flatulence, abdominal pain/discomfort, and diarrhea. These symptoms are due to irritation of the gastrointestinal tract and are best managed by taking the dose with meals, or reducing the amount taken at one time.

Skin rash has been reported rarely with potassium preparations.

In a controlled clinical study Micro-K LS was associated with an increased frequency of gastrointestinal intolerance (e.g., diarrhea, loose stools, abdominal pain, etc.) compared to equal doses (100 mEq/day) of Micro-K Extencaps (see WARNINGS, Diarrhea or Dehydration). This finding was attributed to an inactive ingredient used in the Micro-K LS formulation that is not present in the Micro-K Extencaps formulation.

OVERDOSAGE

The administration of oral potassium salts to persons with normal excretory mechanisms for potassium rarely causes serious hyperkalemia. However, if excretory mechanisms are impaired, or if potassium is administered too rapidly intravenously, potentially fatal hyperkalemia can result (see CONTRAINDICATIONS and WARNINGS). It is important to recognize that hyperkalemia is usually asymptomatic and may be manifested only by an increased serum potassium concentration (6.5–8.0 mEq/L) and characteristic electrocardiographic changes (peaking of T-waves, loss of P-wave, depression of S-T segment, and prolongation of the QT interval). Late manifestations include muscle paralysis and cardiovascular collapse from cardiac arrest (9–12 mEq/L).

Treatment measures for hyperkalemia include the following:

1. Elimination of foods and medications containing potassium and of any agents with potassium-sparing properties;
2. Intravenous administration of 300 to 500 mL/hr of 10% dextrose solution containing 10–20 units of crystalline insulin per 1,000 mL;
3. Correction of acidosis, if present, with intravenous sodium bicarbonate;
4. Use of exchange resins, hemodialysis, or peritoneal dialysis.

In treating hyperkalemia, it should be recalled that in patients who have been stabilized on digitalis, too rapid a lowering of the serum potassium concentration can produce digitalis toxicity.

DOSAGE AND ADMINISTRATION

The usual dietary potassium intake by the average adult is 50 to 100 mEq per day. Potassium depletion sufficient to cause hypokalemia usually requires the loss of 200 or more mEq of potassium from the total body store.

Dosage must be adjusted to the individual needs of each patient. The dose for the prevention of hypokalemia is typically in the range of 20 mEq per day. Doses of 40–100 mEq per day or more are used for the treatment of potassium depletion. Dosage should be divided if more than 20 mEq per day are given such that no more than 20 mEq is given in a single dose.

Usual Adult dose—One Micro-K LS 20 mEq packet 1 to 5 times daily, depending on the requirements of the patient. This product must be suspended in a liquid, preferably water, or sprinkled on food prior to ingestion.

Suspension in Water: Pour contents of packet slowly into approximately 2–6 fluid ounces (¼–¾ glassful) of water. Stir thoroughly for approximately 1 minute until slightly thickened, then drink. The entire contents of the packet must be used immediately and not stored for future use. Any microcapsule/water mixture should be used immediately and not stored for future use.

Suspension in Liquids other than Water: Studies conducted using orange juice, tomato juice, apple juice and milk as the suspending liquid have shown that the quantity of fluid used to suspend one Micro-K LS packet MUST be limited to ***2 fluid ounces (¼ glassful)***. The use of volumes greater than 2 fluid ounces substantially reduces the dose of potassium chloride delivered. If a liquid other than water is used to suspend Micro-K LS then the contents of the packet should be slowly poured into ***2 fluid ounces (¼ glassful)*** of liquid. Stir thoroughly for approximately 1 minute, then drink. The entire contents of the packet must be used immediately and not stored for future use. Any microcapsule/liquid mixture should be used immediately and not stored for future use.

Sprinkling Contents on Food: Micro-K LS may be given on soft food that may be swallowed easily without chewing, such as applesauce or pudding. After sprinkling the contents of the packet on the food, it should be swallowed immediately without chewing and followed with a glass of cool water, milk, or juice to ensure complete swallowing of all the microcapsules. Do not store microcapsule/food mixture for future use.

HOW SUPPLIED

Micro-K LS containing 1.5 g microencapsulated potassium chloride (equivalent to 20 mEq K) per packet in cartons of 30 (NDC 0031-5760-56) and 100 packets (NDC 0031-5760-63).

Store at controlled room temperature, between 15°C and 30°C (59°F and 86°F).

CAUTION: Federal law prohibits dispensing without prescription.

PHENAPHEN® WITH CODEINE NO. 3 Ⓒ℞
PHENAPHEN® WITH CODEINE NO. 4 Ⓒ℞

[fen 'ah-fen"]

(Acetaminophen and Codeine Phosphate Capsules)

DESCRIPTION

Each Phenaphen® with Codeine No. 3 capsule contains:

Acetaminophen, USP .... 325 mg
Codeine Phosphate, USP .... 30 mg
(Warning: May be habit forming)

Inactive Ingredients: D&C Yellow 10, Edible Ink, FD&C Blue 1, (FD&C Green 3 *and* Red 40), FD&C Yellow 6, Gelatin, Magnesium Stearate, Sodium Starch Glycolate, Stearic Acid.

Each Phenaphen® with Codeine No. 4 capsule contains:

Acetaminophen, USP .... 325 mg
Codeine Phosphate, USP .... 60 mg
(Warning: May be habit forming)

Inactive Ingredients: Corn Starch, D&C Yellow 10, Edible Ink, FD&C Green 3 or Blue 1, FD&C Yellow 6, Gelatin, Lactose, Magnesium Stearate, Sodium Starch Glycolate, Stearic Acid.

Acetaminophen, 4′-hydroxyacetanilide, is a non-opiate, nonsalicylate analgesic and antipyretic which occurs as a white, odorless, crystalline powder, possessing a slightly bitter taste.

Codeine is an alkaloid, obtained from opium or prepared from morphine by methylation. Codeine phosphate occurs as fine, white, needle-shaped crystals, or white, crystalline powder. It is affected by light. Its chemical name is: 7,8-didehydro-4, 5α-epoxy-3-methoxy-17-methylmorphinan-6α-ol phosphate (1:1) (salt) hemihydrate.

HOW SUPPLIED

Phenaphen with Codeine No. 3, black and green capsules in bottles of 100 (NDC 0031-6257-63) and 500 (NDC 0031-6257-70).

Phenaphen with Codeine No. 4, green and white capsules in bottles of 100 (NDC 0031-6274-63).

Store at controlled room temperature, between 15°C and 30°C (59°F and 86°F).

Dispense capsules in tight, light-resistant container.

For prescribing information write to Professional Service, Wyeth-Ayerst Laboratories, P.O. Box 8299, Philadelphia, PA 19101, or contact your local Wyeth-Ayerst representative.

PONDIMIN® TABLETS Ⓒ℞

[pŏn 'dĭ-min]

brand of Fenfluramine Hydrochloride Tablets—20 mg

DESCRIPTION

Pondimin® (fenfluramine hydrochloride) is an anorectic drug for oral administration. Immediate release tablets containing 20 mg fenfluramine hydrochloride are orange, scored, compressed tablets engraved "AHR" and "6447". The inactive ingredients are corn starch, FD&C Yellow 6, magnesium stearate, microcrystalline cellulose, silicon dioxide, sodium lauryl sulfate. Pondimin has the chemical name, N- ethyl -α- methyl -3- (trifluoromethyl) benzeneethanamine hydrochloride.

CLINICAL PHARMACOLOGY

Fenfluramine is a sympathomimetic amine, the pharmacologic activity of which differs somewhat from that of the prototype drugs of this class used in obesity, the amphetamines, in appearing to produce more central nervous system depression than stimulation.

The mechanism of action of Pondimin is unclear but may be related to brain levels (or turnover rates) of serotonin or to increased glucose utilization. The antiappetite effects of Pondimin are suppressed by serotonin-blocking drugs and by drugs that lower brain levels of the amine. Furthermore, decreased serotonin levels produced by selective brain lesions suppress the action of Pondimin.

In a study of 20 normal males, fenfluramine increased glucose utilization, resulting in decreased blood glucose levels. Experimental work in animals suggested that increased glucose utilization activated the satiety center and decreased the activity of the feeding center. Perhaps by this mechanism Pondimin inhibits appetite. The relationship between glucose utilization and serotonin has not been clarified.

Fenfluramine is well-absorbed from the gastrointestinal tract, and a maximal anorectic effect is generally seen after 2 to 4 hours. In man, fenfluramine is de-ethylated to norfenfluramine which is subsequently oxidized to m-trifluoromethyl benzoic acid and excreted as the glycine conjugate, m-trifluoromethylhippuric acid. Other compounds found in the urine include unchanged fenfluramine and norfenfluramine.

The rate of excretion of fenfluramine is pH dependent, with much smaller amounts appearing in an alkaline than in an acid urine.

The half-life of fenfluramine is said to be about 20 hours, compared with 5 hours for amphetamines; however, if urinary excretion is rapid and the pH maintained in the acidic range (below pH 5), half-life can be reduced to 11 hours. Fenfluramine and norfenfluramine reach steady state concentrations in plasma within 3 to 4 days following chronic dosage.

The greatest weight loss is seen in those patients who maintain the highest levels of Pondimin. A 2-to-3-kg weight loss over 6 weeks is associated with a plasma level of 0.1 mcg/mL (or 10 mcg/100 mL).

Fenfluramine is widely distributed in almost all body tissues. It is soluble in lipids and crosses the blood-brain barrier. Fenfluramine crosses the placenta readily in monkeys.

INDICATIONS AND USAGE

Pondimin is indicated in the management of exogenous obesity as a short-term (a few weeks) adjunct in a regimen of weight reduction based on caloric restriction.

Drugs of this class used in obesity are commonly known as "anorectics" or "anorexigenics." It has not been established, however, that the action of such drugs in treating obesity is primarily one of appetite suppression. Other central nervous system actions or metabolic effects may be involved.

Adult obese subjects instructed in dietary management and treated with "anorectic" drugs, lose more weight on the average than those treated with placebo and diet, as determined in relatively short-term trials.

The average magnitude of increased weight loss of drug-treated patients over placebo-treated is only a fraction of a pound a week. The rate of weight loss is greatest in the first weeks of therapy for both drug and placebo subjects and

Continued on next page

A. H. Robins—Cont.

tends to decrease in succeeding weeks. The possible origins of the increased weight loss due to the various drug effects are not established. The average amount of weight loss associated with the use of an "anorectic" drug varies from trial to trial, and the increased weight loss appears to be related in part to variables other than the drug prescribed such as the physician-investigator, the population treated and the diet prescribed. Studies do not permit conclusions as to the relative importance of the drug and non-drug factors on weight loss.

The natural history of obesity is measured in years, whereas the studies cited are restricted to a few weeks duration; thus, the total impact of drug-induced weight loss over that of diet alone must be considered clinically limited.

CONTRAINDICATIONS

Fenfluramine is contraindicated in patients with glaucoma or with hypersensitivity to fenfluramine or other sympathomimetic amines. Do not administer fenfluramine during or within 14 days following the administration of monoamine oxidase inhibitors, since hypertensive crises may result. Patients with a history of drug abuse should not receive this drug.

Do not administer fenfluramine to patients with alcoholism since psychiatric symptoms (paranoia, depression, psychosis) have been reported in a few such patients who had been administered this drug.

Fenfluramine should also generally be avoided in patients with psychotic illness. There have been reports of schizophrenic patients who have become agitated, delusional, and assaultive.

A fatal cardiac arrest has been reported shortly after the induction of anesthesia in a patient who had been taking fenfluramine prior to surgery. Fenfluramine may have a catecholamine-depleting effect when administered for prolonged periods of time; therefore, potent anesthetic agents should be administered with caution to patients taking fenfluramine. If general anesthesia cannot be avoided, full cardiac monitoring and facilities for instant resuscitative measures are a minimum necessity.

WARNINGS

Primary Pulmonary Hypertension
A 2-year, international (5 country), case-control (epidemiological) study identified 95 primary pulmonary hypertension (PPH) cases; 20 of these had been exposed to anorexigens in the past, and 9 of the 20 had been exposed to anorexigens for longer than three months. In this study, the use of anorexigens for longer than 3 months was associated with an increase in the risk of developing PPH (odds ratio=9.1, 95% confidence interval=2.6–31.5). This increased risk of PPH was concentrated in persons who had used the drugs within the preceding year; there was no significant increase in risk for persons who had taken the drugs more than 1 year ago or for persons who had used these agents for 3 months or less. In the general population, the yearly occurrence of PPH is estimated to be about 1–2 cases per 1,000,000 persons. Therefore, the case-control study indicated an estimated risk associated with the long-term use of anorexigen drugs of about 18 cases per million persons exposed per year. According to the case-control study, obesity itself (body mass index ≥ 30 kg/m²) was also associated with an increase of about two-fold in the risk of developing PPH.

PPH is a serious condition; the 4-year survival rate has been reported to be 55%.

The initial symptom of pulmonary hypertension is generally dyspnea. Other initial symptoms include: angina pectoris, syncope, or lower extremity edema. *Patients should be advised to report immediately any deterioration in exercise tolerance. Treatment should be discontinued in patients who develop new, unexplained symptoms of dyspnea, angina pectoris, syncope, or lower extremity edema. These patients should be evaluated for the etiology of these symptoms and the possible presence of pulmonary hypertension.* (See also Precautions— GENERAL.)

When tolerance to the "anorectic" effect develops, the maximum recommended dose should not be exceeded in an attempt to increase the effect; rather, the drug should be discontinued.

PRECAUTIONS

GENERAL
Fenfluramine differs in its pharmacological profile from other "anorectic" drugs with which the prescribing practitioner may be familiar. Correspondingly, there are possible adverse effects not associated with other "anorectics"; such effects include those of diarrhea, sedation, and depression. The possibility of these effects should be weighed against the possible advantage of decreased central nervous system stimulation and/or abuse potential.

There have been cases of pulmonary hypertension reported coincident with fenfluramine use. Most of these cases involved women between the ages of 29 and 68, some of whom were receiving concomitant treatment with other medica-

tions (including other appetite suppressants). In the majority of these cases, symptoms of pulmonary hypertension developed in current users of fenfluramine or in patients who had used it within the past 12 months. Most patients required hospitalization, with treatment including diuretics, calcium antagonists, vasodilatory agents, β-adrenergic blockers, and anticoagulants. In some cases, patients required heart-lung transplants. Death due to cardiac or hemodynamic/respiratory complications has occurred. Patients taking fenfluramine should be advised to report immediately any deterioration in exercise tolerance. (See also **Warnings—***Primary Pulmonary Hypertension.*)

Use only with caution in hypertension, with monitoring of blood pressure, since evidence is insufficient to rule out a possible adverse effect on blood pressure in some hypertensive patients. The drug is not recommended in severely hypertensive patients. The drug is not recommended for patients with symptomatic cardiovascular disease including arrhythmias.

Caution should be exercised in prescribing fenfluramine for patients with a history of mental depression. Further depression of mood may become evident while the patient is on fenfluramine or following withdrawal of fenfluramine. Symptoms of depression occurring immediately following abrupt withdrawal can be readily controlled by reinstituting Pondimin®, followed by a gradual tapering off of the daily dose.

INFORMATION FOR PATIENTS

Fenfluramine may impair the ability of the patient to engage in potentially hazardous activities such as operating machinery or driving a motor vehicle (see "**Adverse Reactions**"); the patient should be cautioned accordingly. The patient should also be advised to avoid alcoholic beverages while taking Pondimin.

DRUG INTERACTIONS

Fenfluramine may increase slightly the effect of antihypertensive drugs, e.g., guanethidine, methyldopa, reserpine. Other CNS depressant drugs should be used with caution in patients taking fenfluramine, since the effects may be additive.

There are no adequate and well-controlled studies in pregnant women. Pondimin should be used during pregnancy only if the potential benefit justifies the potential risk to the fetus.

CARCINOGENESIS, MUTAGENESIS

No carcinogenic studies or mutagenic studies have been undertaken with this drug.

PREGNANCY CATEGORY C

Pondimin was shown to produce a questionable embryotoxic effect in rats and a reduced conception rate when given in a dose of 20 times the human dose. However, additional reproduction studies in rats, rabbits, mice, and monkeys at doses up to, respectively, 5 times, 20 times, 1 time, and 5 times the human dose yielded negative results.

LABOR AND DELIVERY

The effect of fenfluramine during labor or delivery on the mother and the fetus is unknown. The effect on later growth, development, and functional maturation of the child is unknown.

NURSING MOTHERS

It is not known whether this drug is excreted in human milk. Because many drugs are excreted in human milk, caution should be exercised when fenfluramine is administered to a nursing mother.

PEDIATRIC USE

Safety and effectiveness in children below the age of 12 years have not been established.

ADVERSE REACTIONS

The most common adverse reactions of fenfluramine are drowsiness, diarrhea, and dry mouth. Less frequent adverse reactions reported in association with fenfluramine are:
Autonomic–Sweating; chills; blurred vision.
Cardiovascular–Pulmonary hypertension (see **Warnings** and **Precautions**); palpitation; hypotension; hypertension; fainting.
Central Nervous System–Dizziness; confusion; incoordination; headache; elevated mood; depression; anxiety, nervousness or tension; insomnia; weakness or fatigue; increased or decreased libido; agitation, dysarthria.
Gastrointestinal–Constipation; abdominal pain; nausea.
Genitourinary–Dysuria; urinary frequency.
Miscellaneous–Eye irritation; myalgia; fever; chest pain; bad taste.
Respiratory–Pulmonary hypertension (see **Warnings** and **Precautions**).
Skin–Alopecia; rash; urticaria; burning sensation.

DRUG ABUSE AND DEPENDENCE

Pondimin (fenfluramine hydrochloride) is a controlled substance in Schedule IV. Fenfluramine is related chemically to the amphetamines, although it differs somewhat pharmacologically. The amphetamines and related stimulant drugs have been extensively abused and can produce tolerance and severe psychological dependence, as well as other adverse organic and mental changes. In this regard, there has been a report of abuse of fenfluramine by subjects with a history of

abuse of other drugs. Abuse of 80 to 400 milligrams of the drug has been reported to be associated with euphoria, derealization, and perceptual changes. Fenfluramine did not produce signs of dependence in animals and appears to produce sedation more often than CNS stimulation at therapeutic doses. Its abuse potential appears qualitatively different from that of amphetamines. The possibility that fenfluramine may induce dependence should be kept in mind when evaluating the desirability of including the drug in the weight reduction programs of individual patients.

OVERDOSAGE

SIGNS AND SYMPTOMS
Only limited data have been reported concerning clinical effects and management of overdosage of fenfluramine. Agitation and drowsiness, confusion, flushing, tremor (or shivering), fever, sweating, abdominal pain, hyperventilation, and dilated non-reactive pupils seem frequent in fenfluramine overdosage. Reflexes may be either exaggerated or depressed and some patients may have rotary nystagmus. Tachycardia may be present, but blood pressure may be normal or only slightly elevated. Convulsions, coma, and ventricular extrasystoles, culminating in ventricular fibrillation, and cardiac arrest, may occur at higher dosages.

HUMAN TOXICITY
Less than 5 mg/kg are toxic to humans. Five-ten mg/kg may produce coma and convulsions. Reported single overdoses have ranged from 300 to 2000 mg; the lowest reported fatal dose was a few hundred mg in a small child, and the highest reported nonfatal dose was 1800 mg in an adult. Most deaths were apparently due to respiratory failure and cardiac arrest.

Toxic effects will appear within 30 to 60 minutes and may progress rapidly to potentially fatal complications in 90 to 240 minutes. Symptoms may persist for extended periods depending upon the dose ingested.

MANAGEMENT
After overdosage, only a small percentage of the drug is excreted in the urine. Forced acid diuresis has been recommended only in extreme cases in which the patient survives the early hours of intoxication but fails to show decisive improvement from other measures. Hemodialysis and peritoneal dialysis are of theoretical advantage but have not been used clinically.

Reportedly the treatment of fenfluramine intoxication should include:
• *Gastric lavage* (but not drug-induced emesis because the patient may become unconscious at a very early stage.)
• In the event that gastric lavage is not feasible due to trismus, consult an anesthesiologist for endotracheal intubation after administration of muscle relaxants; only then should gastric evacuation be tried.
• Administration of activated charcoal after emesis or lavage may reduce absorption of drug.
• *Monitoring of vital functions*. If necessary, mechanical respiration, defibrillation, or "cardioversion" should be instituted.
• *Drug therapy*. Diazepam or phenobarbital for convulsions or muscular hyperactivity. In the presence of extreme tachycardia: propranolol; in the presence of ventricular extrasystoles: lidocaine; in the presence of hyperpyrexia: chlorpromazine.

Since fenfluramine has been shown to have a slight lowering effect on blood sugar in some patients, the theoretical possibility of hypoglycemia should be borne in mind although this effect has not been reported in cases of clinical overdosage.

DOSAGE AND ADMINISTRATION

The usual dose is one 20 mg tablet three times daily before meals. Depending on the degree of effectiveness and side effects, the dosage may be increased at weekly intervals by one tablet (20 mg) daily until a maximum dosage of two tablets three times daily is attained. Total dosage of fenfluramine should not exceed 120 mg per day.

HOW SUPPLIED

Pondimin® is available in 20 mg orange, scored, compressed tablets monogrammed "AHR" and "6447", in bottles of 100 (NDC 0031-6447-63) and 500 (NDC 0031-6447-70).

Store at controlled room temperature, between 20°C and 25°C (68°F and 77°F).
Dispense in well-closed container.
Shown in Product Identification Guide, page 331

QUINIDEX EXTENTABS® Tablets ℞
[kwĭn´ĭ˝deks ĕks˝tĕn´tabs]
(quinidine sulfate extended-release tablets, USP)

DESCRIPTION

Quinidine is an antimalarial schizonticide and an antiarrhythmic agent with Class Ia activity; it is the d-isomer of quinine, and its molecular weight is 324.43. Quinidine sulfate is the sulfate salt of quinidine; its chemical name is cinchonan-9-ol, 6'-methoxy-, (9S)-, sulfate(2:1) dihydrate; its structural formula is

[See structure at top of next column.]

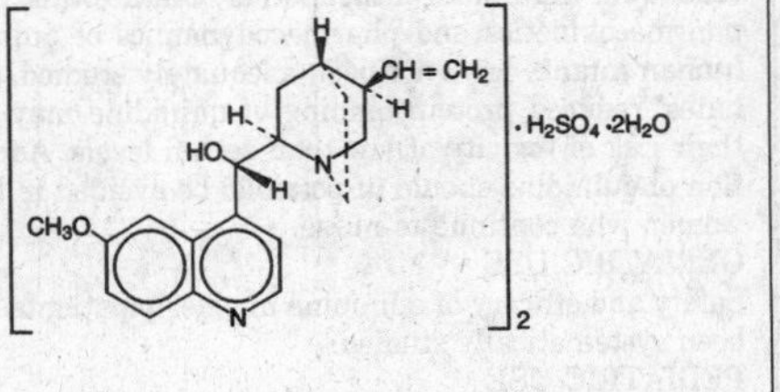

its empirical formula is $(C_{20}H_{24}N_2O_2)_2 \cdot H_2SO_4 \cdot 2H_2O$; and its molecular weight is 782.95, of which 82.9% is quinidine base.

Each Quinidex Extentabs® tablet contains 300 mg of quinidine sulfate (249 mg of quinidine base) in a formulation to provide extended release; the inactive ingredients are acacia, acetylated monoglycerides, calcium sulfate, carnauba wax, edible ink, FD&C Blue 2, gelatin, guar gum, magnesium oxide, magnesium stearate, polysorbates, shellac, sucrose, titanium dioxide, white wax, and other ingredients, one of which is a corn derivative. Tablets may also contain FD&C Red 40 and FD&C Yellow 6 Aluminum Lakes.

CLINICAL PHARMACOLOGY

PHARMACOKINETICS

The absolute bioavailability of quinidine from Quinidex is about 70%, but this varies widely (45–100%) between patients. The less-than-complete bioavailability is the result of first-pass metabolism in the liver. Peak serum levels generally appear about 6 hours after dosing.

Although the effect of food upon Quinidex absorption has not been studied, peak serum quinidine levels obtained from immediate-release quinidine sulfate are known to be delayed by nearly an hour (without change in total absorption) when these products are taken with food.

The **volume of distribution** of quinidine is 2 to 3 L/kg in healthy young adults, but this may be reduced to as little as 0.5 L/kg in patients with congestive heart failure, or increased to 3 to 5 L/kg in patients with cirrhosis of the liver.

At concentrations of 2 to 5 mg/L (6.5 to 16.2 μmol/L), the fraction of quinidine bound to plasma proteins (mainly to α_1-acid glycoprotein and to albumin) is 80 to 88% in adults and older children, but it is lower in pregnant women, and in infants and neonates it may be as low as 50 to 70%. Because α_1-acid glycoprotein levels are increased in response to stress, serum levels of total quinidine may be greatly increased in settings such as acute myocardial infarction, even though the serum content of unbound (active) drug may remain normal. Protein binding is also increased in chronic renal failure, but binding abruptly descends toward or below normal when heparin is administered for hemodialysis.

Quinidine **clearance** typically proceeds at 3 to 5 mL/min/kg in adults, but clearance in children may be twice or three times as rapid. The elimination half-life is 6 to 8 hours in adults and 3 to 4 hours in children. Quinidine clearance is unaffected by hepatic cirrhosis, so the increased volume of distribution seen in cirrhosis leads to a proportionate increase in the elimination half-life.

Most quinidine is eliminated hepatically via the action of cytochrome $P_{450}IIIA_4$; there are several different hydroxylated metabolites, and some of these have antiarrhythmic activity.

The most important of quinidine's metabolites is 3-hydroxyquinidine (3HQ), serum levels of which can approach those of quinidine in patients receiving conventional doses of Quinidex. The volume of distribution of 3HQ appears to be larger than that of quinidine, and the elimination half-life of 3HQ is about 12 hours.

As measured by antiarrhythmic effects in animals, by QT_c prolongation in human volunteers, or by various *in vitro* techniques, 3HQ has at least half the antiarrhythmic activity of the parent compound, so it may be responsible for a substantial fraction of the effect of Quinidex in chronic use.

When the urine pH is less than 7, about 20% of administered quinidine appears unchanged in the urine, but this fraction drops to as little as 5% when the urine is more alkaline. Renal clearance involves both glomerular filtration and active tubular secretion, moderated by (pH-dependent) tubular reabsorption. The new renal clearance is about 1 mL/min/kg in healthy adults.

When renal function is taken into account, quinidine clearance is apparently independent of patient age.

Assays of serum quinidine levels are widely available, but the results of modern assays may not be consistent with results cited in the older medical literature. The serum levels of quinidine cited in this package insert are those derived from specific assays, using either benzene extraction or (preferably) reverse-phase high-pressure liquid chromatography. In matched samples, older assays might unpredictably have given results that were as much as two or three times higher. A typical "therapeutic" concentration range is 2 to 6 mg/L (6.2 to 18.5 μmol/L).

MECHANISMS OF ACTION

In patients with malaria, quinidine acts primarily as an intra-erythrocytic schizonticide, with little effect upon sporozites or upon pre-erythrocytic parasites. Quinidine is gametocidal to *Plasmodium vivax* and *P. malariae*, but not to *P. falciparum*.

In cardiac muscle and in Purkinje fibers, quinidine depresses the rapid inward depolarizing sodium current, thereby slowing phase-0 depolarization and reducing the amplitude of the action potential without affecting the resting potential. In normal Purkinje fibers, it reduces the slope of phase-4 depolarization, shifting the threshold voltage upward toward zero. The result is slow conduction and reduced automaticity in all parts of the heart, with increase of the effective refractory period relative to the duration of the action potential in the atria, ventricles, and Purkinje tissues. Quinidine also raises the fibrillation thresholds of the atria and ventricles, and it raises the ventricular *de*fibrillation threshold as well. Quinidine's actions fall into Class la in the Vaughan-Williams classification.

By slowing conduction and prolonging the effective refractory period, quinidine can interrupt or prevent reentrant arrhythmias and arrhythmias due to increased automaticity, including atrial flutter, atrial fibrillation, and paroxysmal supraventricular tachycardia.

In patients with the sick sinus syndrome, quinidine can cause marked sinus node depression and bradycardia. In most patients, however, use of quinidine is associated with an increase in the sinus rate.

Quinidine prolongs the QT interval in a dose-related fashion. This may lead to increased ventricular automaticity and polymorphic ventricular tachycardias, including *torsades de pointes* (see **WARNINGS**).

In addition, quinidine has anticholinergic activity, it has negative inotropic activity, and it acts peripherally as an α-adrenergic antagonist (that is, as a vasodilator).

CLINICAL EFFECTS

Maintenance of sinus rhythm after conversion from atrial fibrillation: In six clinical trials (published between 1970 and 1984) with a total of 808 patients, quinidine (418 patients) was compared to nontreatment (258 patients) or placebo (132 patients) for the maintenance of sinus rhythm after cardioversion from chronic atrial fibrillation. Quinidine was consistently more efficacious in maintaining sinus rhythm, but a meta-analysis found that mortality in the quinidine-exposed patients (2.9%) was significantly greater than mortality in the patients who had not been treated with active drug (0.8%). Suppression of atrial fibrillation with quinidine has theoretical patient benefits (e.g., improved exercise tolerance; reduction in hospitalization for cadioversion; lack of arrhythmia-related palpitations, dyspnea, and chest pain; reduced incidence of systemic embolism and/or stroke), but these benefits have never been demonstrated in clinical trials. Some of these benefits (e.g., reduction in stroke incidence) may be achievable by other means (anticoagulation).

By slowing the rate of atrial flutter/fibrillation, quinidine can decrease the degree of atrioventricular block and cause an increase, sometimes marked, in the rate at which supraventricular impulses are successfully conducted by the atrioventricular node, with a resultant paradoxical increase in ventricular rate (see **WARNINGS**).

Non-life-threatening ventricular arrhythmias: In studies of patients with a variety of ventricular arrhythmias (mainly frequent ventricular premature beats and non-sustained ventricular tachycardia), quinidine (total N=502) has been compared to flecainide (N=141), mexiletine (N=246), propafenone (N=53), and tocainide (N=67). In each of these studies, the mortality in the quinidine group was numerically greater than the mortality in the comparator group. When the studies were combined in a meta-analysis, quinidine was associated with a statistically significant threefold relative risk of death.

At therapeutic doses, quinidine's only consistent effect upon the surface electrocardiogram is an increase in the QT interval. This prolongation can be monitored as a guide to safety, and it may provide better guidance than serum drug levels (see **WARNINGS**).

INDICATIONS AND USAGE

CONVERSION OF ATRIAL FIBRILLATION/FLUTTER

In patients with symptomatic atrial fibrillation/flutter whose symptoms are not adequately controlled by measures that reduce the rate of ventricular response, Quinidex is indicated as a means of restoring normal sinus rhythm. If this use of Quinidex does not restore sinus rhythm within a reasonable time (see **DOSAGE AND ADMINISTRATION**), then Quinidex should be discontinued.

REDUCTION OF FREQUENCY OF RELAPSE INTO ATRIAL FIBRILLATION/FLUTTER

Chronic therapy with Quinidex is indicated for some patients at high risk of symptomatic atrial fibrillation/flutter; generally patients who have had previous episodes of atrial fibrillation/flutter that were so frequent and poorly tolerated as to outweigh, in the judgment of the physician and the patient, the risks of prophylactic therapy with Quinidex. The increased risk of death should specifically be considered. Quinidex should be used only after alternative measures (e.g., use of other drugs to control ventricular rate) have been found to be inadequate.

In patients with histories of frequent symptomatic episodes of atrial fibrillation/flutter, the goal of therapy should be an increase in the average time between episodes. In most patients, the tachyarrhythmia *will recur* during therapy, and a single recurrence should not be interpreted as therapeutic failure.

SUPPRESSION OF VENTRICULAR ARRHYTHMIAS

Quinidex is also indicated for the suppression of recurrent documented ventricular arrhythmias, such as sustained ventricular tachycardia, that in the judgment of the physician are life-threatening. Because of the proarrhythmic effects of quinidine, its use with ventricular arrhythmias of lesser severity is generally not recommended, and treatment of patients with asymptomatic ventricular premature contractions should be avoided. Where possible, therapy should be guided by the results of programmed electrical stimulation and/or Holter monitoring with exercise.

Antiarrhythmic drugs (including Quinidex) have not been shown to enhance survival in patients with ventricular arrhythmias.

CONTRAINDICATIONS

Quinidine is contraindicated in patients who are known to be allergic to it, or who have developed thrombocytopenic purpura during prior therapy with quinidine or quinine.

In the absence of a functioning artificial pacemaker, quinidine is also contraindicated in any patient whose cardiac rhythm is dependent upon a junctional or idioventricular pacemaker, including patients in complete atrioventricular block.

Quinidine is also contraindicated in patients who, like those will myasthenia gravis, might be adversely affected by an anticholinergic agent.

WARNINGS

MORTALITY

In many trials of antiarrhythmic therapy for non-life-threatening arrhythmias, active antiarrhythmic therapy has resulted in increased mortality; the risk of active therapy is probably greatest in patients with structural heart disease.

In the case of quinidine used to prevent or defer recurrence of atrial flutter/fibrillation, the best available data come from a meta-analysis described under Clinical Pharmacology—CLINICAL EFFECTS above. In the patients studied in the trials there analyzed, the mortality associated with the use of quinidine was more than three times as great as the mortality associated with the use of placebo.

Another meta-analysis, also described under Clinical Pharmacology—CLINICAL EFFECTS, showed that in patients with various non-life-threatening ventricular arrhythmias, the mortality associated with the use of quinidine was consistently greater than that associated with the use of any of a variety of alternative antiarrhythmics.

PROARRHYTHMIC EFFECTS

Like many other drugs (including all other Class la antiarrhythmics), quinidine prolongs the QT_c interval, and this can lead to *torsades de pointes*, a life-threatening ventricular arrhythmia (see **OVERDOSAGE**). The risk of *torsades* is increased by bradycardia, hypokalemia, hypomagnesemia, or high serum levels of quinidine, but it may appear in the absence of any of these risk factors. The best predictor of this arrhythmia appears to be the length of the QT_c interval, and quinidine should be used with extreme care in patients who have preexisting long-QT syndromes, who have histories of *torsades de pointes* of any cause, or who have previously responded to quinidine (or other drugs that prolong ventricular repolarization) with marked lengthening of the QT_c interval. Estimation of the incidence of *torsades* in patients with therapeutic levels of quinidine is not possible from the available data.

Other ventricular arrhythmias that have been reported with quinidine include frequent extrasystoles, ventricular tachycardia, ventricular flutter, and ventricular fibrillation.

PARADOXICAL INCREASE IN VENTRICULAR RATE IN ATRIAL FLUTTER/FIBRILLATION

When quinidine is administered to patients with atrial flutter/fibrillation the desired pharmacologic reversion to sinus rhythm may (rarely) be preceded by a showing of the atrial rate with a consequent increase in the rate of beats conducted to the ventricles. The resulting ventricular rate may be very high (greater than 200 beats per minute) and poorly

Continued on next page

A. H. Robins—Cont.

tolerated. This hazard may be decreased if partial atrioventricular block is achieved prior to initiation of quinidine therapy, using conduction-reducing drugs such as digitalis, verapamil, diltiazem, or a β-receptor blocking agent.

EXACERBATED BRADYCARDIA IN SICK SINUS SYNDROME

In patients with the sick sinus syndrome, quinidine has been associated with marked sinus node depression and bradycardia.

PHARMACOKINETIC CONSIDERATIONS

Renal or hepatic dysfunction causes the elimination of quinidine to be slowed, while congestive heart failure causes a reduction in quinidine's apparent volume of distribution. Any of these conditions can lead to quinidine toxicity if dosage is not appropriately reduced. In addition, interactions with coadministered drugs can alter the serum concentration and activity of quinidine, leading either to toxicity or to lack of efficacy if the dose of quinidine is not appropriately modified. (See **PRECAUTIONS**—DRUG INTERACTIONS.)

VAGOLYSIS

Because quinidine opposes the atrial and A-V nodal effects of vagal stimulation, physical or pharmacological vagal maneuvers undertaken to terminate paroxysmal supraventricular tachycardia may be ineffective in patients receiving quinidine.

PRECAUTIONS

GENERAL

All the precautions applying to regular quinidine therapy apply to this product. Hypersensitivity or anaphylactoid reactions to quinidine, although rare, should be considered, especially during the first weeks of therapy. Hospitalization for close clinical observation, electrocardiographic monitoring, and determination of serum quinidine levels are indicated when large doses of quinidine are used or with patients who present an increased risk.

LABORATORY TESTS

Periodic blood counts and liver and kidney function tests should be performed during long-term therapy; the drug should be discontinued if blood dyscrasias or evidence of hepatic or renal dysfunction occurs.

HEART BLOCK

In patients without implanted pacemakers who are at high risk of complete atrioventricular block (e.g., those with digitalis intoxication, second-degree atrioventricular block, or severe intraventricular conduction defects), quinidine should be used only with caution.

DRUG INTERACTIONS

Altered pharmacokinetics of quinidine: Drugs that alkalinize the urine (**carbonic-anhydrase inhibitors, sodium bicarbonate, thiazide diuretics**) reduce renal elimination of quinidine.

By pharmacokinetic mechanisms that are not well understood, quinidine levels are increased by coadministration of **amiodarone** or **cimetidine.** Very rarely, and again by mechanisms not understood, quinidine levels are decreased by coadministration of **nifedipine.**

Hepatic elimination of quinidine may be accelerated by coadministration of drugs (**phenobarbital, phenytoin, rifampin**) that induce production of cytochrome $P_{450}IIIA_4$.

Perhaps because of competition for the $P_{450}IIIA_4$ metabolic pathway, quinidine levels rise when **ketaconazole** is coadministered.

Coadministration of **propranolol** usually does not affect quinidine pharmacokinetics, but in some studies the β-blocker appeared to cause increases in the peak serum levels of quinidine, decreases in quinidine's volume of distribution, and decreases in total quinidine clearance. The effects (if any) of coadministration of **other β-blockers** on quinidine pharmacokinetics have not been adequately studied.

Hepatic clearance of quinidine is significantly reduced during coadministration of **verapamil**, with corresponding increases in serum levels and half-life.

Altered pharmacokinetics of other drugs: Quinidine slows the elimination of **digoxin** and simultaneously reduces digoxin's apparent volume of distribution. As a result, serum digoxin levels may be as much as doubled. When quinidine and digoxin are coadministered, digoxin doses usually need to be reduced. Serum levels of **digitoxin** are also raised when quinidine is coadministered, although the effect appears to be smaller.

By a mechanism that is not understood, quinidine potentiates the anticoagulatory action of **warfarin**, and the anticoagulant dosage may need to be reduced.

Cytochrome $P_{450}IID_6$ is an enzyme critical to the metabolism of many drugs, notably including **mexiletine**, some **phenothiazines**, and most **polycyclic antidepressants**. Constitutional deficiency of cytochrome $P_{450}IID_6$ is found in less than 1% of Orientals, in about 2% of American blacks, and in about 8% of American whites. Testing with debrisoquine is sometimes used to distinguish the $P_{450}IID_6$-deficient "poor metabolizers" from the majority-phenotype "extensive metabolizers."

When drugs whose metabolism is $P_{450}IID_6$-dependent are given to poor metabolizers, the serum levels achieved are higher, sometimes much higher, than the serum levels achieved when identical doses are given to extensive metabolizers. To obtain similar clinical benefit without toxicity, doses given to poor metabolizers may need to be greatly reduced. In the cases of prodrugs whose actions are actually mediated by $P_{450}IID_6$-produced metabolites (for example, **codeine** and **hydrocodone**, whose analgesic and antitussive effects appear to be mediated by morphine and hydromorphone, respectively), it may not be possible to achieve the desired clinical benefits in poor metabolizers.

Quinidine is not metabolized by cytochrome $P_{450}IID_6$, but therapeutic serum levels of quinidine inhibit the action of cytochrome $P_{450}IID_6$, effectively converting extensive metabolizers into poor metabolizers. Caution must be exercised whenever quinidine is prescribed together with drugs metabolized by cytochrome $P_{450}IID_6$.

Perhaps by competing for pathways of renal clearance, coadministration of quinidine causes an increase in serum levels of **procainamide.**

Serum levels of **haloperidol** are increased when quinidine is coadministered.

Presumably because both drugs are metabolized by cytochrome $P_{450}IIIA_4$, coadministration of quinidine causes variable slowing of the metabolism of **nifedipine**. Interactions with other dihydropyridine calcium-channel blockers have not been reported, but these agents (including **felodipine, nicardipine,** and **nimodipine**) are all dependent upon $P_{450}IIIA_4$ for metabolism, so similar interactions with quinidine should be anticipated.

Altered pharmacodynamics of other drugs: Quinidine's anticholinergic, vasodilating, and negative inotropic actions may be additive to those of other drugs with these effects, and antagonistic to those of drugs with cholinergic, vasoconstricting, and positive inotropic effects. For example, when quinidine and **verapamil** are coadministered in doses that are each well tolerated as monotherapy, hypotension attributable to additive peripheral α-blockade is sometimes reported.

Quinidine potentiates the actions of depolarizing (succinylcholine, decamethonium) and nondepolarizing (d-tubocurarine, pancuronium) **neuromuscular blocking agents**. These phenomena are not well understood, but they are observed in animals models as well as in humans. In addition, *in vitro* addition of quinidine to the serum of pregnant women reduces the activity of pseudocholinesterase, an enzyme that is essential to the metabolism of succinylcholine.

Non-interactions of quinidine with other drugs: Quinidine has no clinically significant effect on the pharmacokinetics of **diltiazem, flecainide, mephenytoin, metoprolol, propafenone, propranolol, quinine, timolol,** or **tocainide.**

Conversely, the pharmacokinetics of quinidine are not significantly affected by **caffeine, ciprofloxacin, digoxin, diltiazem, felodipine, omeprazole,** or **quinine**. Quinidine's pharmacokinetics are also unaffected by cigarette smoking.

INFORMATION FOR PATIENTS

Before prescribing Quinidex Extentabs® as prophylaxis against recurrence of atrial fibrillation, the physician should inform the patient of the risks and benefits to be expected (see **CLINICAL PHARMACOLOGY**).

Discussion should include the facts

- that the goal of therapy will be a reduction (probably not to zero) in the frequency of episodes of atrial fibrillation; and
- that reduced frequency of fibrillatory episodes may be expected, if achieved, to bring symptomatic benefit; but
- that no data are available to show that reduced frequency of fibrillatory episodes will reduce the risks of irreversible harm through stroke or death; and in fact
- that such data as are available suggest that treatment with Quinidex is likely to increase the patient's risk of death.

CARCINOGENESIS, MUTAGENESIS, IMPAIRMENT OF FERTILITY

Animal studies to evaluate quinidine's carcinogenic or mutagenic potential have not been performed. Similarly, there are no animal data as to quinidine's potential to impair fertility.

PREGNANCY

Pregnancy Category C: Animal reproductive studies have not been conducted with quinidine. There are no adequate and well-controlled studies in pregnant women. Quinidine should be given to a pregnant woman only if clearly needed.

In one neonate whose mother had received quinidine throughout her pregnancy, the serum level of quinidine was equal to that of the mother, with no apparent ill effect. The level of quinidine in amniotic fluid was about three times higher than that found in serum.

LABOR AND DELIVERY

Quinine is said to be oxytocic in humans, but there are no adequate data as to quinidine's effects (if any) on human labor and delivery.

NURSING MOTHERS

Quinidine is present in human milk at levels slightly lower than those in maternal serum; a human infant ingesting such milk should (scaling directly by weight) be expected to develop serum quinidine levels at least an order of magnitude lower than those of the mother. On the other hand, the pharmacokinetics and pharmacodynamics of quinidine in human infants have not been adequately studied, and neonates' reduced protein binding of quinidine may increase their risk of toxicity at low total serum levels. Administration of quinidine should (if possible) be avoided in lactating women who continue to nurse.

GERIATRIC USE

Safety and efficacy of quinidine in elderly patients have not been systematically studied.

PEDIATRIC USE

In antimalarial trials, quinidine was as safe and effective in pediatric patients as in adults. Notwithstanding the known pharmacokinetic differences between the pediatric population and adults (see **CLINICAL PHARMACOLOGY**—PHARMACOKINETICS), pediatric patients in these trials received the same doses (on a mg/kg basis) as adults.

Safety and effectiveness of the antiarrhythmic use of quinidine in pediatric patients have not been established in well-controlled clinical trials.

ADVERSE REACTIONS

Quinidine preparations have been used for many years, but there are only sparse data from which to estimate the incidence of various adverse reactions. The adverse reactions most frequently reported have consistently been gastrointestinal, including diarrhea, nausea, vomiting, and heartburn/esophagitis. In one study of 245 adult outpatients who received quinidine to suppress premature ventricular contractions, the incidences of reported adverse experiences were as shown in the table below. The most serious quinidine-associated adverse reactions are described above under **WARNINGS**.

Adverse Experiences in a 245-Patient PVC Trial

	Incidence (%)
diarrhea	85 (35)
"upper gastrointestinal distress"	55 (22)
light-headedness	37 (15)
headache	18 (7)
fatigue	17 (7)
palpitations	16 (7)
angina-like pain	14 (6)
weakness	13 (5)
rash	11 (5)
visual problems	8 (3)
change in sleep habits	7 (3)
tremor	6 (2)
nervousness	5 (2)
discoordination	3 (1)

Vomiting and diarrhea can occur as isolated reactions to therapeutic levels of quinidine, but they also may be the first signs of **cinchonism**, a syndrome that also may include tinnitus, reversible high-frequency hearing loss, deafness, vertigo, blurred vision, diplopia, photophobia, headache, confusion, and delirium. Cinchonism is most often a sign of chronic quinidine toxicity, but it may appear in sensitive patients after a single moderate dose.

A few cases of **hepatotoxicity**, including granulomatous hepatitis, have been reported in patients receiving quinidine. All of these have appeared during the first few weeks of therapy, and most (not all) have remitted once quinidine was withdrawn.

Autoimmune and inflammatory syndromes associated with quinidine therapy have included pneumonitis, fever, urticaria, flushing, exfoliative rash, bronchospasm, psoriasiform rash, pruritus and lymphadenopathy, hemolytic anemia, vasculitis, thrombocytopenic purpura, uveitis, angioedema, agranulocytosis, the sicca syndrome, arthralgia, myalgia, elevation in serum levels of skeletal-muscle enzymes, and a disorder resembling systemic lupus erythematosus.

Convulsions, apprehension, and ataxia have been reported, but it is not clear that these were not simply the results of hypotension and consequent cerebral hypoperfusion. There are many reports of syncope. Acute psychotic reactions have been reported to follow the first dose of quinidine, but these reactions appear to be extremely rare.

Other adverse reactions occasionally reported include depression, mydriasis, disturbed color perception, night blindness, scotomata, optic neuritis, visual field loss, photosensitivity, and abnormalities of pigmentation.

OVERDOSAGE

Overdoses with various oral formulations of quinidine have been well described. Death has been described after a 5-gram ingestion by a toddler, while an adolescent was reported to survive after ingesting 8 grams of quinidine.

The most important ill effects of acute quinidine overdoses are ventricular arrhythmias and hypotension. Other signs and symptoms of overdose may include vomiting, diarrhea, tinnitus, high-frequency hearing loss, vertigo, blurred vision, diplopia, photophobia, headache, confusion, and delirium.

ARRHYTHMIAS

Serum quinidine levels can be conveniently assayed and monitored, but the electrocardiographic QT_c interval is a

better predictor of quinidine-induced ventricular arrhythmias.

The necessary treatment of hemodynamically unstable polymorphic ventricular tachycardia (including *torsades de pointes*) is withdrawal of treatment with quinidine and either immediate cardioversion or, if a cardiac pacemaker is in place or immediately available, immediate overdrive pacing. After pacing or cardioversion, further management must be guided by the length of the QT_c interval.

Quinidine-associated ventricular tachyarrhythmias with normal underlying QT_c intervals have not been adequately studied. Because of the theoretical possibility of QT-prolonging effects that might be additive to those of quinidine, other antiarrhythmics with Class I (disopyramide, procainamide) or Class III activities should (if possible) be avoided. Similarly, although the use of bretylium in quinidine overdose has not been reported, it is reasonable to expect that the α-blocking properties of bretylium might be additive to those of quinidine, resulting in problematic hypotension.

If the post-cardioversion QT_c interval is prolonged, then the pre-cardioversion polymorphic ventricular tachyarrhythmia was (by definition) *torsades de pointes*. In this case, lidocaine and bretylium are unlikely to be of value, and other Class I antiarrhythmics (disopyramide, procainamide) are likely to exacerbate the situation. Factors contributing to QT_c prolongation (especially hypokalemia and hypomagnesemia) should be sought out and (if possible) aggressively corrected. Prevention of recurrent *torsades* may require sustained overdrive pacing or the cautious administration of isoproterenol (30 to 150 ng/kg/min).

HYPOTENSION

Quinidine-induced hypotension that is not due to an arrhythmia is likely to be a consequence of quinidine-related α-blockade and vasorelaxation. Simple repletion of central volume (Trendelenburg positioning, saline infusion) may be sufficient therapy; other interventions reported to have been beneficial in this setting are those that increase peripheral vascular resistance, including α-agonist catecholamines (norepinephrine, metaraminol) and the Military Anti-Shock Trousers.

TREATMENT

Adequate studies of orally-administered activated charcoal in human overdoses of quinidine have not been reported, but there are animal data showing significant enhancement of systemic elimination following this intervention, and there is at least one human case report in which the elimination half-life of quinidine in the serum was apparently shortened by repeated gastric lavage. Activated charcoal should be avoided if an ileus is present; the conventional dose is 1 gram/kg, administered every 2 to 6 hours as a slurry with 8 mL/kg of tap water. Although renal elimination of quinidine might theoretically be accelerated by maneuvers to acidify the urine, such maneuvers are potentially hazardous and of no demonstrated benefit.

Quinidine is not usefully removed from the circulation by dialysis. Following quinidine overdose, drugs that delay elimination of quinidine (cimetidine, carbonic-anhydrase inhibitors, thiazide diuretics) should be withdrawn unless absolutely required.

In managing overdose, consider the possibilities of multiple-drug overdoses, drug-drug interactions, and unusual drug kinetics in your patient.

DOSAGE AND ADMINISTRATION

CONVERSION OF ATRIAL FIBRILLATION/FLUTTER TO SINUS RHYTHM

Especially in patients with known structural heart disease or other risk factors for toxicity, initiation or dose-adjustment of treatment with Quinidex should generally be performed in a setting where facilities and personnel for monitoring and resuscitation are continuously available.

Patients with symptomatic atrial fibrillation/flutter should be treated with Quinidex only after ventricular rate control (e.g., with digitalis or β-blockers) has failed to provide satisfactory control of symptoms. Adequate trials have not identified an optimal regimen of Quinidex for conversion of atrial fibrillation/flutter to sinus rhythm. Therapy with Quinidex should begin with one tablet (300 mg; 249 mg of quinidine base) every 8 to 12 hours. If this regimen is well tolerated, if the serum quinidine level is still well within the laboratory's therapeutic range, and if this regimen has not resulted in conversion, then the dose may be cautiously raised. If, at any point during administration, the QRS complex widens to 130% of its pre-treatment duration; the QT_c interval widens to 130% of its pre-treatment duration and is then longer than 500 ms; P waves disappear; or the patient develops significant tachycardia, symptomatic bradycardia, or hypotension, then Quinidex is discontinued, and other means of conversion (e.g., direct-current cardioversion) are considered.

REDUCTION OF FREQUENCY OF RELAPSE INTO ATRIAL FIBRILLATION/FLUTTER

In a patient with a history of frequent symptomatic episodes of atrial fibrillation/flutter, the goal of therapy with Quinidex should be an increase in the average time between episodes. In most patients, the tachyarrhythmia *will recur* during therapy with Quinidex, and a single recurrence should not be interpreted as therapeutic failure.

Especially in patients with known structural heart disease or other risk factors for toxicity, initiation or dose-adjustment of treatment with Quinidex should generally be performed in a setting where facilities and personnel for monitoring and resuscitation are continously available.

Monitoring should be continued for two or three days after initiation of the regimen on which the patient will be discharged.

Therapy with Quinidex should begin with one tablet (300 mg; 249 mg of quinidine base) every eight to twelve hours. If this regimen is well tolerated, if the serum quinidine level is still well within the laboratory's therapeutic range, and if the average time between arrhythmic episodes has not been satisfactorily increased, then the dose may be cautiously raised. The total daily dosage should be reduced if the QRS complex interval widens to 130% of its pre-treatment duration; the QT_c interval widens to 130% of its pre-treatment duration and is then longer than 500 ms; P waves disappear; or the patient develops significant tachycardia, symptomatic bradycardia, or hypotension.

SUPPRESSION OF VENTRICULAR ARRHYTHMIAS

Dosing regimens for the use of quinidine sulfate in suppressing life-threatening ventricular arrhythmias have not been adequately studied.

Described regimens have generally been similar to the regimen described just above for the prophylaxis of symptomatic atrial fibrillation/flutter. Where possible, therapy should be guided by the results of programmed electrical stimulation and/or Holter monitoring with exercise.

HOW SUPPLIED

Quinidex Extentabs® Tablets (quinine sulfate extended-release tablets, USP) are 300 mg, white, sugar-coated, round tablets marked with "QUINIDEX" and "AHR". The tablets are available in bottles and in DIS-CO® unit-dose packages as follows:

bottle of 100	NDC 0031-6649-63
bottle of 250	NDC 0031-6649-67
unit-dose pack of 100	NDC 0031-6649-64

Store tablets at controlled room temperature, 20°–25°C (68°–77°F).

Dispense in well-closed, light-resistant container.

Caution: Federal law prohibits dispensing without prescription.

Shown in Product Identification Guide, page 331

REGLAN® Tablets ℞

[*rĕg'lan*]

(Metoclopramide Tablets, USP)

REGLAN® Syrup

(Metoclopramide Oral Solution, USP)

REGLAN® Injectable

(Metoclopramide Injection, USP)

DESCRIPTION

For oral administration, Reglan Tablets (Metoclopramide Tablets, USP) 10 mg are white. scored, capsule-shaped tablets engraved Reglan on one side and AHR 10 on the opposite side.

Each tablet contains:

Metoclopramide base 10 mg
(as the monohydrochloride monohydrate)

INACTIVE INGREDIENTS: Magnesium Stearate, Mannitol, Microcrystalline Cellulose, Stearic Acid.

Reglan Tablets (Metoclopramide Tablets, USP) 5 mg are green, elliptical-shaped tablets engraved Reglan 5 on one side and AHR on the opposite side.

Each tablet contains:

Metoclopramide base 5 mg
(as the monohydrochloride monohydrate)

INACTIVE INGREDIENTS: Corn Starch, D&C Yellow 10 Lake, FD&C Blue 1 Aluminum Lake, Lactose, Microcrystalline Cellulose, Silicon Dioxide, Stearic Acid.

Reglan Syrup (Metoclopramide Oral Solution, USP) is an orange-colored, palatable, aromatic, sugar-free liquid.

Each 5 mL (1 teaspoonful) contains:

Metoclopramide base 5 mg
(as the monohydrochloride monohydrate)

INACTIVE INGREDIENTS: Citric Acid, FD&C Yellow 6, Flavors, Glycerin, Methylparaben, Propylparaben, Sorbitol, Water.

For parenteral administration, Reglan Injectable (Metoclopramide Injection, USP) is a clear, colorless, sterile solution with a pH of 4.5–6.5 for intravenous or intramuscular administration.

CONTAINS NO PRESERVATIVE.

2 mL and 10 mL single dose vials/ampuls; 30 mL single dose vial

Each 1 mL contains:

Metoclopramide base 5 mg
(as the monohydrochloride monohydrate)

Sodium Chloride, USP 8.5 mg, Water for Injection, USP q.s. pH adjusted, when necessary, with hydrochloric acid and/or sodium hydroxide.

Metoclopramide hydrochloride is a white crystalline, odorless substance, freely soluble in water. Chemically, it is 4-amino-5-chloro-N-[2-(diethylamino)ethyl]-2-methoxy benzamide monohydrochloride monohydrate. Molecular weight: 354.3.

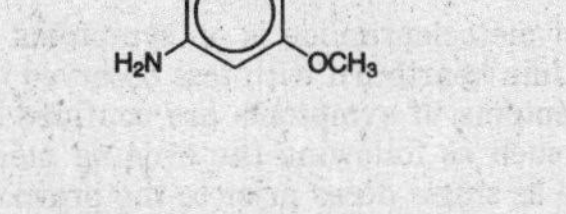

CLINICAL PHARMACOLOGY

Metoclopramide stimulates motility of the upper gastrointestinal tract without stimulating gastric, biliary, or pancreatic secretions. Its mode of action is unclear. It seems to sensitize tissues to the action of acetylcholine. The effect of metoclopramide on motility is not dependent on intact vagal innervation, but it can be abolished by anticholinergic drugs. Metoclopramide increases the tone and amplitude of gastric (especially antral) contractions, relaxes the pyloric sphincter and the duodenal bulb, and increases peristalsis of the duodenum and jejunum resulting in accelerated gastric emptying and intestinal transit. It increases the resting tone of the lower esophageal sphincter. It has little, if any effect on the motility of the colon or gallbladder.

In patients with gastroesophageal reflux and low LESP (lower esophageal sphincter pressure), single oral doses of metoclopramide produce dose-related increases in LESP. Effects begin at about 5 mg and increase through 20 mg (the largest dose tested). The increase in LESP from a 5 mg dose lasts about 45 minutes and that of 20 mg lasts between 2 and 3 hours. Increased rate of stomach emptying has been observed with single oral doses of 10 mg.

The antiemetic properties of metoclopramide appear to be a result of its antagonism of central and peripheral dopamine receptors. Dopamine produces nausea and vomiting by stimulation of the medullary chemoreceptor trigger zone (CTZ), and metoclopramide blocks stimulation of the CTZ by agents like l-dopa or apomorphine which are known to increase dopamine levels or to possess dopamine-like effects. Metoclopramide also abolishes the slowing of gastric emptying caused by apomorphine.

Like the phenothiazines and related drugs, which are also dopamine antagonists, metoclopramide produces sedation and may produce extrapyramidal reactions, although these are comparatively rare (see **Warnings**). Metoclopramide inhibits the central and peripheral effects of apomorphine, induces release of prolactin and causes a transient increase in circulating aldosterone levels, which may be associated with transient fluid retention.

The onset of pharmacological action of metoclopramide is 1 to 3 minutes following an intravenous dose, 10 to 15 minutes following intramuscular administration, and 30 to 60 minutes following an oral dose; pharmacological effects persist for 1 to 2 hours.

PHARMACOKINETICS: Metoclopramide is rapidly and well absorbed. Relative to an intravenous dose of 20 mg, the absolute oral bioavailability of metoclopramide is 80% ± 15.5% as demonstrated in a crossover study of 18 subjects. Peak plasma concentrations occur at about 1–2 hr after a single oral dose. Similar time to peak is observed after individual doses at steady state.

In a single dose study of 12 subjects the area under the drug concentration-time curve increases linearly with doses from 20 to 100 mg. Peak concentrations increase linearly with dose; time to peak concentrations remains the same; whole body clearance is unchanged; and the elimination rate remains the same. The average elimination half-life in individuals with normal renal function is 5–6 hr. Linear kinetic processes adequately describe the absorption and elimination of metoclopramide.

Approximately 85% of the radioactivity of an orally administered dose appears in the urine within 72 hr. Of the 85% eliminated in the urine, about half is present as free or conjugated metoclopramide.

The drug is not extensively bound to plasma proteins (about 30%). The whole body volume of distribution is high (about 3.5 L/kg) which suggests extensive distribution of drug to the tissues.

Renal impairment affects the clearance of metoclopramide. In a study with patients with varying degrees of renal impairment, a reduction in creatinine clearance was correlated with a reduction in plasma clearance, renal clearance, nonrenal clearance, and increase in elimination half-life. The kinetics of metoclopramide in the presence of renal impairment remained linear however. The reduction in clearance

Continued on next page

A. H. Robins—Cont.

as a result of renal impairment suggests that adjustment downward of maintenance dosage should be done to avoid drug cumulation.

INDICATIONS AND USAGE

SYMPTOMATIC GASTROESOPHAGEAL REFLUX: Reglan Tablets and Syrup are indicated as short-term (4 to 12 weeks) therapy for adults with symptomatic, documented gastroesophageal reflux who fail to respond to conventional therapy.

The principal effect of metoclopramide is on symptoms of postprandial and daytime heartburn with less observed effect on nocturnal symptoms. If symptoms are confined to particular situations, such as following the evening meal, use of metoclopramide as single doses prior to the provocative situation should be considered, rather than using the drug throughout the day. Healing of esophageal ulcers and erosions has been endoscopically demonstrated at the end of a 12-week trial using doses of 15 mg q.i.d. As there is no documented correlation between symptoms and healing of esophageal lesions, patients with documented lesions should be monitored endoscopically.

DIABETIC GASTROPARESIS (DIABETIC GASTRIC STASIS). Reglan (Metoclopramide Hydrochloride, USP) is indicated for the relief of symptoms associated with acute and recurrent diabetic gastric stasis. The usual manifestations of delayed gastric emptying (e.g., nausea, vomiting, heartburn, persistent fullness after meals and anorexia) appear to respond to Reglan within different time intervals. Significant relief of nausea occurs early and continues to improve over a three-week period. Relief of vomiting and anorexia may precede the relief of abdominal fullness by one week or more.

THE PREVENTION OF NAUSEA AND VOMITING ASSOCIATED WITH EMETOGENIC CANCER CHEMOTHERAPY. Reglan Injectable is indicated for the prophylaxis of vomiting associated with emetogenic cancer chemotherapy.

THE PREVENTION OF POSTOPERATIVE NAUSEA AND VOMITING. Reglan Injectable is indicated for the prophylaxis of postoperative nausea and vomiting in those circumstances where nasogastric suction is undesirable.

SMALL BOWEL INTUBATION. Reglan Injectable may be used to facilitate small bowel intubation in adults and children in whom the tube does not pass the pylorus with conventional maneuvers.

RADIOLOGICAL EXAMINATION. Reglan Injectable may be used to stimulate gastric emptying and intestinal transit of barium in cases where delayed emptying interferes with radiological examination of the stomach and/or small intestine.

CONTRAINDICATIONS

Metoclopramide should not be used whenever stimulation of gastrointestinal motility might be dangerous, e.g., in the presence of gastrointestinal hemorrhage, mechanical obstruction, or perforation.

Metoclopramide is contraindicated in patients with pheochromocytoma because the drug may cause a hypertensive crisis, probably due to release of catecholamines from the tumor. Such hypertensive crises may be controlled by phentolamine.

Metoclopramide is contraindicated in patients with known sensitivity or intolerance to the drug.

Metoclopramide should not be used in epileptics or patients receiving other drugs which are likely to cause extrapyramidal reactions, since the frequency and severity of seizures or extrapyramidal reactions may be increased.

WARNINGS

Mental depression has occurred in patients with and without prior history of depression. Symptoms have ranged from mild to severe and have included suicidal ideation and suicide. Metoclopramide should be given to patients with a prior history of depression only if the expected benefits outweigh the potential risks.

Extrapyramidal symptoms, manifested primarily as acute dystonic reactions, occur in approximately 1 in 500 patients treated with the usual adult dosages of 30–40 mg/day of metoclopramide. These usually are seen during the first 24–48 hours of treatment with metoclopramide, occur more frequently in children and young adults, and are even more frequent at the higher doses used in prophylaxis of vomiting due to cancer chemotherapy. These symptoms may include involuntary movements of limbs and facial grimacing, torticollis, oculogyric crisis, rhythmic protrusion of tongue, bulbar type of speech, trismus, or dystonic reactions resembling tetanus. Rarely, dystonic reactions may present as stridor and dyspnea, possibly due to laryngospasm. If these symptoms should occur, inject 50 mg Benadryl® (diphenhydramine hydrochloride) intramuscularly, and they usually will subside. Cogentin® (benztropine mesylate), 1 to 2 mg intramuscularly, may also be used to reverse these reactions.

Parkinsonian-like symptoms have occurred, more commonly within the first 6 months after beginning treatment with metoclopramide, but occasionally after longer periods. These symptoms generally subside within 2–3 months following discontinuance of metoclopramide. Patients with preexisting Parkinson's disease should be given metoclopramide cautiously, if at all, since such patients may experience exacerbation of parkinsonian symptoms when taking metoclopramide.

TARDIVE DYSKINESIA: Tardive dyskinesia, a syndrome consisting of potentially irreversible, involuntary, dyskinetic movements may develop in patients treated with metoclopramide. Although the prevalence of the syndrome appears to be highest among the elderly, especially elderly women, it is impossible to predict which patients are likely to develop the syndrome. Both the risk of developing the syndrome and the likelihood that it will become irreversible are believed to increase with the duration of treatment and the total cumulative dose.

Less commonly, the syndrome can develop after relatively brief treatment periods at low doses; in these cases, symptoms appear more likely to be reversible.

There is no known treatment for established cases of tardive dyskinesia although the syndrome may remit, partially or completely, within several weeks-to-months after metoclopramide is withdrawn. Metoclopramide itself, however, may suppress (or partially suppress) the signs of tardive dyskinesia, thereby masking the underlying disease process. The effect of this symptomatic suppression upon the long-term course of the syndrome is unknown. Therefore, the use of metoclopramide for the symptomatic control of tardive dyskenesia is not recommended.

PRECAUTIONS

GENERAL. In one study in hypertensive patients, intravenously administered metoclopramide was shown to release catecholamines; hence, caution should be exercised when metoclopramide is used in patients with hypertension.

Intravenous injections of undiluted metoclopramide should be made slowly allowing 1 to 2 minutes for 10 mg since a transient but intense feeling of anxiety and restlessness, followed by drowsiness, may occur with rapid administration.

Intravenous administration of Reglan Injectable diluted in a parenteral solution should be made slowly over a period of not less than 15 minutes.

Giving a promotility drug such as metoclopramide theoretically could put increased pressure on suture lines following a gut anastomosis or closure. Although adverse events related to this possibility have not been reported to date, the possibility should be considered and weighed when deciding whether to use metoclopramide or nasogastric suction in the prevention of postoperative nausea and vomiting.

INFORMATION FOR PATIENTS: Metoclopramide may impair the mental and/or physical abilities required for the performance of hazardous tasks such as operating machinery or driving a motor vehicle. The ambulatory patient should be cautioned accordingly.

DRUG INTERACTIONS. The effects of metoclopramide on gastrointestinal motility are antagonized by anticholinergic drugs and narcotic analgesics. Additive sedative effects can occur when metoclopramide is given with alcohol, sedatives, hypnotics, narcotics or tranquilizers.

The finding that metoclopramide releases catecholamines in patients with essential hypertension suggests that it should be used cautiously, if at all, in patients receiving monoamine oxidase inhibitors.

Absorption of drugs from the stomach may be diminished (e.g., digoxin) by metoclopramide, whereas the rate and/or extent of absorption of drugs from the small bowel may be increased (e.g., acetaminophen, tetracycline, levodopa, ethanol, cyclosporine).

Gastroparesis (gastric stasis) may be responsible for poor diabetic control in some patients. Exogenously administered insulin may begin to act before food has left the stomach and lead to hypoglycemia. Because the action of metoclopramide will influence the delivery of food to the intestines and thus the rate of absorption, insulin dosage or timing of dosage may require adjustment.

CARCINOGENESIS, MUTAGENESIS, IMPAIRMENT OF FERTILITY: A 77-week study was conducted in rats with oral doses up to about 40 times the maximum recommended human daily dose. Metoclopramide elevates prolactin levels and the elevation persists during chronic administration. Tissue culture experiments indicate that approximately one-third of human breast cancers are prolactin-dependent *in vitro*, a factor of potential importance if the prescription of metoclopramide is contemplated in a patient with previously detected breast cancer. Although disturbances such as galactorrhea, amenorrhea, gynecomastia, and impotence have been reported with prolactin-elevating drugs, the clinical significance of elevated serum prolactin levels is unknown for most patients. An increase in mammary neoplasms has been found in rodents after chronic administration of prolactin-stimulating neuroleptic drugs and metoclopramide. Neither clinical studies nor epidemiologic studies conducted to date, however, have shown an association between chronic administration of these drugs and mammary tumorigenesis; the available evidence is too limited to be conclusive at this time.

An Ames mutagenicity test performed on metoclopramide was negative.

PREGNANCY CATEGORY B. Reproduction studies Performed in rats, mice, and rabbits by the I.V., I.M., S.C. and oral routes at maximum levels ranging from 12 to 250 times the human dose have demonstrated no impairment of fertility or significant harm to the fetus due to metoclopramide. There are, however, no adequate and well-controlled studies in pregnant women. Because animal reproduction studies are not always predictive of human response, this drug should be used during pregnancy only if clearly needed.

NURSING MOTHERS. Metoclopramide is excreted in human milk. Caution should be exercised when metoclopramide is administered to a nursing mother.

PEDIATRIC USE. There are insufficient data to support efficacy or make dosage recommendations for metoclopramide in patients less than 18 years of age except as stated to facilitate small bowel intubation (see **Overdosage** and **Dosage and Administration**).

ADVERSE REACTIONS

In general, the incidence of adverse reactions correlates with the dose and duration of metoclopramide administration. The following reactions have been reported, although in most instances, data do not permit an estimate of frequency:

CNS EFFECTS. Restlessness, drowsiness, fatigue and lassitude occur in approximately 10% of patients receiving the most commonly prescribed dosage of 10 mg q.i.d. (see **Precautions**). Insomnia, headache, confusion, dizziness or mental depression with suicidal ideation (see **Warnings**) occur less frequently. In cancer chemotherapy patients being treated with 1–2 mg/kg per dose, incidence of drowsiness is about 70%. There are isolated reports of convulsive seizures without clearcut relationship to metoclopramide. Rarely, hallucinations have been reported.

EXTRAPYRAMIDAL REACTIONS (EPS). Acute dystonic reactions, the most common type of EPS associated with metoclopramide, occur in approximately 0.2% of patients (1 in 500) treated with 30 to 40 mg of metoclopramide per day. In cancer chemotherapy patients receiving 1–2 mg/kg per dose, the incidence is 2% in patients over the ages of 30–35, and 25% or higher in children and young adults who have not had prophylactic administration of diphenhydramine. Symptoms include involuntary movements of limbs, facial grimacing, torticollis, oculogyric crisis, rhythmic protrusion of tongue, bulbar type of speech, trismus, opisthotonus (tetanus-like reactions) and rarely, stridor and dyspnea, possibly due to laryngospasm; ordinarily these symptoms are readily reversed by diphenhydramine (see **Warnings**).

Parkinsonian-like symptoms may include bradykinesia, tremor, cogwheel rigidity, mask-like facies (see **Warnings**). Tardive dyskinesia most frequently is characterized by involuntary movements of the tongue, face, mouth or jaw, and sometimes by involuntary movements of the trunk and/or extremities; movements may be choreoathetotic in appearance (see **Warnings**).

Motor restlessness (akathisia) may consist of feelings of anxiety, agitation, jitteriness, and insomnia, as well as inability to sit still, pacing, foot-tapping. These symptoms may disappear spontaneously or respond to a reduction in dosage.

ENDOCRINE DISTURBANCES. Galactorrhea, amenorrhea, gynecomastia, impotence secondary to hyperprolactinemia (see **Precautions**). Fluid retention secondary to transient elevation of aldosterone (see **Clinical Pharmacology**).

CARDIOVASCULAR. Hypotension, hypertension supraventricular tachycardia, and bradycardia (see **Contraindications** and **Precautions**).

GASTROINTESTINAL. Nausea and bowel disturbances, primarily diarrhea.

HEPATIC. Rarely, cases of hepatotoxicity, characterized by such findings as jaundice and altered liver function tests, when metoclopramide was administered with other drugs with known hepatotoxic potential.

RENAL. Urinary frequency and incontinence.

HEMATOLOGIC. A few cases of neutropenia, leukopenia, or agranulocytosis, generally without clearcut relationship to metoclopramide. Methemoglobinemia, especially with overdosage in neonates (see **Overdosage**).

ALLERGIC REACTIONS. A few cases of rash, urticaria, or bronchospasm, especially in patients with a history of asthma. Rarely, angioneurotic edema, including glossal or laryngeal edema.

MISCELLANEOUS. Visual disturbances. Porphyria. Rare occurrences of neuroleptic malignant syndrome (NMS) have been reported. This potentially fatal syndrome is comprised of the symptom complex of hyperthermia, altered consciousness, muscular rigidity and autonomic dysfunction. Transient flushing of the face and upper body, without alterations in vital signs, following high doses intravenously.

OVERDOSAGE

Symptoms of overdosage may include drowsiness, disorientation and extrapyramidal reactions. Anticholinergic or antiparkinson drugs or antihistamines with anticholinergic

properties may be helpful in controlling the extrapyramidal reactions. Symptoms are self-limiting and usually disappear within 24 hours.
Hemodialysis removes relatively little metoclopramide, probably because of the small amount of the drug in blood relative to tissues. Similarly, continuous ambulatory peritoneal dialysis does not remove significant amounts of drug. It is unlikely that dosage would need to be adjusted to compensate for losses through dialysis. Dialysis is not likely to be an effective method of drug removal in overdose situations.
Unintentional overdose due to misadministration has been reported in patients between the age of 2 months and 7 years with the use of Reglan syrup. While there was no consistent pattern to the reports associated with these overdoses, events included seizures, extrapyramidal reactions, and lethargy.
Methemoglobinemia has occurred in premature and full-term neonates who were given overdoses of metoclopramide (1–4 mg/kg/day orally, intramuscularly or intravenously for 1–3 or more days). Methemoglobinemia has not been reported in neonates treated with 0.5 mg/kg/day in divided doses. Methemoglobinemia can be reversed by the intravenous administration of methylene blue.

DOSAGE AND ADMINISTRATION

FOR THE RELIEF OF SYMPTOMATIC GASTROESOPHAGEAL REFLUX: Administer from 10 mg to 15 mg Reglan (Metoclopramide Hydrochloride, USP) orally up to q.i.d. 30 minutes before each meal and at bedtime, depending upon symptoms being treated and clinical response (see **Clinical Pharmacology** and **Indications and Usage**). If symptoms occur only intermittently or at specific times of the day, use of metoclopramide in single doses up to 20 mg prior to the provoking situation may be preferred rather than continuous treatment. Occasionally, patients (such as elderly patients) who are more sensitive to the therapeutic or adverse effects of metoclopramide will require only 5 mg per dose.
Experience with esophageal erosions and ulcerations is limited, but healing has thus far been documented in one controlled trial using q.i.d. therapy at 15 mg/dose, and this regimen should be used when lesions are present, so long as it is tolerated (see **Adverse Reactions**). Because of the poor correlation between symptoms and endoscopic appearance of the esophagus, therapy directed at esophageal lesions is best guided by endoscopic evaluation.
Therapy longer than 12 weeks has not been evaluated and cannot be recommended.
FOR THE RELIEF OF SYMPTOMS ASSOCIATED WITH DIABETIC GASTROPARESIS (DIABETIC GASTRIC STASIS): Administer 10 mg of metoclopramide 30 minutes before each meal and at bedtime for two to eight weeks, depending upon response and the likelihood of continued well-being upon drug discontinuation.
The initial route of administration should be determined by the severity of the presenting symptoms. If only the earliest manifestations of diabetic gastric stasis are present, oral administration of Reglan may be initiated. However, if severe symptoms are present, therapy should begin with Reglan Injectable (I.M. or I.V.). Doses of 10 mg may be administered slowly by the intravenous route over a 1- to 2-minute period.
Administration of Reglan Injectable (Metoclopramide Injection, USP) up to 10 days may be required before symptoms subside, at which time oral administration may be instituted. Since diabetic gastric stasis is frequently recurrent, Reglan therapy should be reinstituted at the earliest manifestation.
FOR THE PREVENTION OF NAUSEA AND VOMITING ASSOCIATED WITH EMETOGENIC CANCER CHEMOTHERAPY: For doses in excess of 10 mg, Reglan Injectable should be diluted in 50 mL of a parenteral solution.
The preferred parenteral solution is Sodium Chloride Injection (normal saline), which when combined with Reglan Injectable, can be stored frozen for up to 4 weeks. Reglan Injectable is degraded when admixed and frozen with Dextrose-5% in Water. Reglan Injectable diluted in Sodium Chloride Injection, Dextrose-5% in Water, Dextrose-5% in 0.45% Sodium Chloride, Ringer's Injection or Lactated Ringer's Injection may be stored up to 48 hours (without freezing) after preparation if protected from light. All dilutions may be stored unprotected from light under normal light conditions up to 24 hours after preparation.
Intravenous infusions should be made slowly over a period of not less than 15 minutes, 30 minutes before beginning cancer chemotherapy and repeated every 2 hours for two doses, then every 3 hours for three doses.
The initial two doses should be 2 mg/kg if highly emetogenic drugs such as cisplatin or dacarbazine are used alone or in combination. For less emetogenic regimens, 1 mg/kg per dose may be adequate.
If extrapyramidal symptoms should occur, inject 50 mg Benadryl® (diphenhydramine hydrochloride) intramuscularly, and EPS usually will subside.
FOR THE PREVENTION OF POSTOPERATIVE NAUSEA AND VOMITING: Reglan Injectable should be given intramuscularly near the end of surgery. The usual adult dose is 10 mg; however, doses of 20 mg may be used.
TO FACILITATE SMALL BOWEL INTUBATION: If the tube has not passed the pylorus with conventional maneuvers in 10 minutes, a single dose (undiluted) may be administered slowly by the intravenous route over a 1- to 2-minute period.
The recommended single dose is: Adults—10 mg metoclopramide base. Pediatric patients (6–14 years of age)—2.5 to 5 mg metoclopramide base; (under 6 years of age)—0.1 mg/kg metoclopramide base.
TO AID IN RADIOLOGICAL EXAMINATIONS: In patients where delayed gastric emptying interferes with radiological examination of the stomach and/or small intestine, a single dose may be administered slowly by the intravenous route over a 1- to 2-minute period.
For dosage, see intubation, above.
Use in Patients with Renal or Hepatic Impairment: Since metoclopramide is excreted principally through the kidneys, in those patients whose creatinine clearance is below 40 mL/min, therapy should be initiated at approximately one-half the recommended dosage. Depending upon clinical efficacy and safety considerations, the dosage may be increased or decreased as appropriate.
See **Overdosage** section for information regarding dialysis.
Metoclopramide undergoes minimal hepatic metabolism, except for simple conjugation. Its safe use has been described in patients with advanced liver disease whose renal function was normal.
NOTE: Parenteral drug products should be inspected visually for particulate matter and discoloration prior to administration, whenever solution and container permit.
Admixture Compatibilities. Reglan Injectable (Metoclopramide Injection, USP) is compatible for mixing and injection with the following dosage forms to the extent indicated below:
PHYSICALLY AND CHEMICALLY COMPATIBLE UP TO 48 HOURS. Cimetidine Hydrochloride (SK&F), Mannitol, USP (Abbott), Potassium Acetate, USP (Invenex), Potassium Chloride, USP (ESI), Potassium Phosphate, USP (Invenex).
PHYSICALLY COMPATIBLE UP TO 48 HOURS. Ascorbic Acid, USP (Abbott), Benztropine Mesylate, USP (MS&D), Cytarabine, USP (Upjohn), Dexamethasone Sodium Phosphate, USP (ESI, MS&D), Diphenhydramine Hydrochloride, USP (Parke-Davis), Doxorubicin Hydrochloride, USP (Adria), Heparin Sodium, USP (ESI), Hydrocortisone Sodium Phosphate (MS&D), Lidocaine Hydrochloride, USP (ESI), Magnesium Sulfate, USP (ESI), Multi-Vitamin Infusion (must be refrigerated-USV), Vitamin B Complex with Ascorbic Acid (Roche).
PHYSICALLY COMPATIBLE UP TO 24 HOURS *(Do not use if precipitation occurs).* Aminophylline, USP (ESI), Clindamycin Phosphate, USP (Upjohn), Cyclophosphamide, USP (Mead-Johnson), Insulin, USP (Lilly), Methylprednisolone Sodium Succinate, USP (ESI).
CONDITIONALLY COMPATIBLE *(Use within one hour after mixing or may be infused directly into the same running IV line).* Ampicillin Sodium, USP (Bristol), Calcium Gluconate, USP (ESI), Cisplatin (Bristol), Erythromycin Lactobionate, USP (Abbott), Methotrexate Sodium, USP (Lederle), Penicillin G Potassium, USP (Squibb), Tetracycline Hydrochloride, USP (Lederle).
INCOMPATIBLE *(Do Not Mix).* Cephalothin Sodium, USP (Lilly), Chloramphenicol Sodium, USP (Parke-Davis), Sodium Bicarbonate, USP (Abbott).

HOW SUPPLIED

Each white, capsule-shaped, scored Reglan® Tablet contains 10 mg metoclopramide base (as the monohydrochloride monohydrate). Available in bottles of 100 (NDC 0031-6701-63), and 500 tablets (NDC 0031-6701-70) and Dis-Co® Unit Dose Packs of 100 tablets (NDC 0031-6701-64).
Each green, elliptical-shaped Reglan® Tablet contains 5 mg metoclopramide base (as the monohydrochloride monohydrate). Available in bottles of 100 (NDC 0031-6705-63) and Dis-Co® Unit Dose Packs of 100 tablets (NDC 0031-6705-64). Dispense tablets in tight, light-resistant container.
Reglan® Syrup, 5 mg metoclopramide base (as the monohydrochloride monohydrate) per 5 mL, available in pints (NDC 0031-6706-25). Dispense syrup in tight, light-resistant container.
Preservative-free:
Reglan® Injectable, 5 mg metoclopramide base (as the monohydrochloride monohydrate) per mL; available in 2 mL single dose vials in cartons of 25 (NDC 0031-6709-72), 10 mL single dose vials in cartons of 25 (NDC 0031-6709-78); and 30 mL single dose vials in cartons of 25 (NDC 0031-6709-24); 2 mL ampuls in cartons of 5 (NDC 0031-6709-90) and 25 (NDC 0031-6709-95).
[See table above.]

Container	Total Contents #	Concentration #	Administration
2 mL single dose vial/ampul	10 mg	5 mg/mL	FOR IV or IM ADMINISTRATION
10 mL single dose vial/ampul	50 mg	5 mg/mL	FOR IV INFUSION ONLY; DILUTE BEFORE USING
30 mL single dose vial	150 mg	5 mg/mL	FOR IV INFUSION ONLY; DILUTE BEFORE USING

Metoclopramide base (as the monohydrochloride monohydrate)

Store vials and ampuls in carton until used. Do not store open single dose vials or ampuls for later use, as they contain no preservative.
Dilutions may be stored unprotected from light under normal light conditions up to 24 hours after preparation.
TABLETS, SYRUP AND INJECTABLE SHOULD BE STORED AT CONTROLLED ROOM TEMPERATURE BETWEEN 20°C and 25°C (68°F and 77°F).
Reglan Injectable is manufactured for Pharmaceutical Division, A. H. Robins Company, Richmond, Virginia 23220 by Elkins-Sinn, Inc., Cherry Hill, NJ 08003.

Tablets Shown in Product Identification Guide, page 331
Injectable Shown in Identification Guide, page 331

ROBAXIN® INJECTABLE ℞
[ro″baks′in]
brand of Methocarbamol Injection, USP

DESCRIPTION

Methocarbamol has the following structural formula:

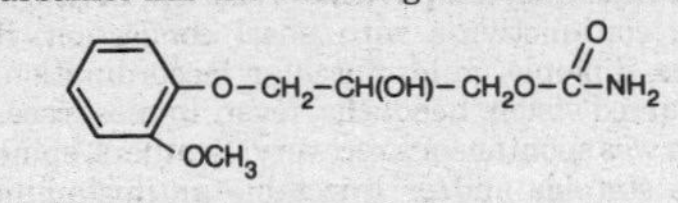

3-(2-methoxyphenoxy)-1,2-propanediol
1-carbamate, or methocarbamol

Robaxin Injectable is a parenteral dosage form.
Each mL contains:
Methocarbamol, USP **100 mg**; Polyethylene Glycol 300, NF 0.5 mL; Water for Injection, USP q.s. pH adjusted, when necessary, with hydrochloric acid and/or sodium hydroxide.
AFTER MIXING WITH I.V. INFUSION FLUIDS, **DO NOT REFRIGERATE.**

ACTIONS

The mechanism of action of methocarbamol in humans has not been established, but may be due to general central nervous system depression. It has no direct action on the contractile mechanism of striated muscle, the motor end plate or the nerve fiber.

INDICATIONS

The injectable form of methocarbamol is indicated as an adjunct to rest, physical therapy, and other measures for the relief of discomfort associated with acute, painful musculoskeletal conditions. The mode of action of this drug has not been clearly identified, but may be related to its sedative properties. Methocarbamol does not directly relax tense skeletal muscles in man.

CONTRAINDICATIONS

Robaxin Injectable should not be administered to patients with known or suspected renal pathology. This caution is necessary because of the presence of polyethylene glycol 300 in the vehicle.
A much larger amount of polyethylene glycol 300 than is present in recommended doses of Robaxin Injectable is known to have increased pre-existing acidosis and urea retention in patients with renal impairment. Although the amount present in this preparation is well within the limits of safety, caution dictates this contraindication.
Robaxin Injectable is contraindicated in patients hypersensitive to any of the ingredients.

WARNINGS

Since methocarbamol may possess a general central nervous system depressant effect, patients receiving Robaxin Inject-

Continued on next page

A. H. Robins—Cont.

able (methocarbamol injection) should be cautioned about combined effects with alcohol and other CNS depressants.
Safe use of Robaxin Injectable has not been established with regard to possible adverse effects upon fetal development. Therefore, Robaxin Injectable should not be used in women who are or may become pregnant and particularly during early pregnancy unless in the judgment of the physician the potential benefits outweigh the possible hazards.

PRECAUTIONS

As with other agents administered either intravenously or intramuscularly, careful supervision of dose and rate of injection should be observed. Rate of injection should not exceed 3 mL per minute—i.e., one 10 mL vial in approximately three minutes. Since Robaxin Injectable is hypertonic, vascular extravasation must be avoided. A recumbent position will reduce the likelihood of side reactions.
Blood aspirated into the syringe does not mix with the hypertonic solution. This phenomenon occurs with many other intravenous preparations. The blood may be safely injected with the methocarbamol, or the injection may be stopped when the plunger reaches the blood, whichever the physician prefers.
The total dosage should not exceed 30 mL (three vials) a day for more than three consecutive days except in the treatment of tetanus.
Caution should be observed in using the injectable form in suspected or known epileptic patients.
Safety and effectiveness in children below the age of 12 years have not been established except in tetanus. See special directions for use in tetanus.
It is not known whether this drug is secreted in human milk. As a general rule, nursing should not be undertaken while a patient is on a drug since many drugs are excreted in human milk.
Methocarbamol may cause a color interference in certain screening tests for 5-hydroxyindoleacetic acid (5-HIAA) and vanillylmandelic acid (VMA).

ADVERSE REACTIONS

Dizziness, lightheadedness, drowsiness, vertigo, fainting, syncope, hypotension, gastrointestinal upset, metallic taste, thrombophlebitis, sloughing at the site of injection, pain at the site of injection, anaphylactic reaction, urticaria, pruritus, rash, conjunctivitis with nasal congestion, flushing, nystagmus, diplopia, mild muscular incoordination, bradycardia, blurred vision, headache, fever. In most cases of syncope there was spontaneous recovery. In others, epinephrine, injectable steroids and/or injectable antihistamines were employed to hasten recovery. Certain of these complaints may have been due to any overly rapid rate of intravenous injection.
The onset of convulsive seizures during intravenous administration has been reported, including instances in known epileptics. The psychic trauma of the procedure may have been a contributing factor. Although several observers have reported success in terminating epileptiform seizures with Robaxin Injectable, its administration to patients with epilepsy is not recommended.

DOSAGE AND ADMINISTRATION

For Intravenous and Intramuscular Use Only. Total adult dosage should not exceed 30 mL (3 vials) a day for more than 3 consecutive days except in the treatment of tetanus. A like course may be repeated after a lapse of 48 hours if the condition persists. Dosage and frequency of injection should be based on the severity of the condition being treated and therapeutic response noted.
For the relief of symptoms of moderate degree, 10 mL (one vial) may be adequate. Ordinarily this injection need not be repeated, as the administration of the oral form will usually sustain the relief initiated by the injection. For the severest cases or in postoperative conditions in which oral administration is not feasible, 20 to 30 mL (two to three vials) may be required.
Directions for Intravenous Use. Robaxin Injectable may be administered undiluted directly into the vein at a ***maximum rate of three mL per minute.*** It may also be added to an intravenous drip of Sodium Chloride Injection (Sterile Isotonic Sodium Chloride Solution for Parenteral Use) or five per cent Dextrose Injection (Sterile 5 per cent Dextrose Solution); one vial given as a single dose should not be diluted to more than 250 mL for I. V. infusion. Care should be exercised to avoid vascular extravasation of this hypertonic solution which may result in thrombophlebitis. It is preferable that the patient be in a recumbent position during and for at least 10 to 15 minutes following the injection.
Directions for Intramuscular Use. When the intramuscular route is indicated, not more than five mL (one-half vial) should be injected into each gluteal region. The injections may be repeated at eight hour intervals, if necessary. When satisfactory relief of symptoms is achieved, it can usually be maintained with tablets.
Not Recommended for Subcutaneous Administration.
Special Directions for Use in Tetanus: There is clinical evidence which suggests that methocarbamol may have a beneficial effect in the control of the neuromuscular manifestations of tetanus. It does not, however, replace the usual procedure of debridement, tetanus antitoxin, penicillin, tracheotomy, attention to fluid balance, and supportive care. Robaxin Injectable should be added to the regimen as soon as possible.
For adults: Inject one or two vials directly into the tubing of a previously inserted indwelling needle. An additional 10 mL or 20 mL may be added to the infusion bottle so that a total of up to 30 mL (three vials) is given as the initial dose (note Precautions). This procedure should be repeated every six hours until conditions allow for the insertion of a nasogastric tube. Crushed Robaxin (methocarbamol) tablets suspended in water or saline may then be given through this tube. Total daily oral doses up to 24 grams may be required as judged by patient response.
For children: A minimum initial dose of 15 mg/kg is recommended. This dosage may be repeated every six hours as indicated. The maintenance dosage may be given by injection into the tubing or by I.V. infusion with an appropriate quantity of fluid. See directions for I.V. use.

HOW SUPPLIED

Robaxin Injectable—10 mL single dose vials in packages of 5 (NDC 0031-7409-87) and 25 (NDC 0031-7409-94).
Manufactured for A. H. ROBINS CO., by ELKINS-SINN, INC.

Shown in Product Identification Guide, page 331

ROBAXIN® ℞
[*ro"baks'ĭn*]
brand of Methocarbamol Tablets, USP
500 mg per tablet

ROBAXIN®-750 ℞
brand of Methocarbamol Tablets, USP
750 mg per tablet

DESCRIPTION

Inactive Ingredients: ROBAXIN—Corn Starch, FD&C Yellow 6 Aluminum Lake, Hydroxypropyl Cellulose, Hydroxypropyl Methylcellulose, Magnesium Stearate, Polysorbate 20, Povidone, Propylene Glycol, Saccharin Sodium, Sodium Lauryl Sulfate, Sodium Starch Glycolate, Stearic Acid, Titanium Dioxide.
ROBAXIN-750—Corn Starch, D&C Yellow 10 Aluminum Lake, FD&C Yellow 6 Aluminum Lake, Hydroxypropyl Cellulose, Hydroxypropyl Methylcellulose, Magnesium Stearate, Polysorbate 20, Povidone, Propylene Glycol, Saccharin Sodium, Sodium Lauryl Sulfate, Sodium Starch Glycolate, Stearic Acid, Titanium Dioxide.
Methocarbamol has the following structural formula:

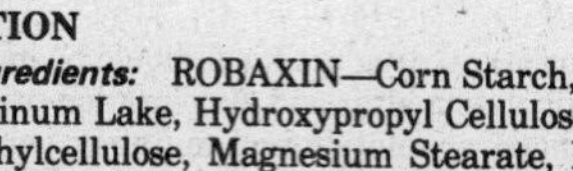

3-(2-methoxyphenoxy)-1,2-propanediol
1-carbamate, or methocarbamol

ACTIONS

The mechanism of action of methocarbamol in humans has not been established, but may be due to general central nervous system depression. It has no direct action on the contractile mechanism of striated muscle, the motor end plate or the nerve fiber.

INDICATIONS

Robaxin (methocarbamol) is indicated as an adjunct to rest, physical therapy, and other measures for the relief of discomforts associated with acute, painful musculoskeletal conditions. The mode of action of this drug has not been clearly identified, but may be related to its sedative properties. Methocarbamol does not directly relax tense skeletal muscles in man.

CONTRAINDICATIONS

Robaxin is contraindicated in patients hypersensitive to any of the ingredients.

WARNINGS

Since methocarbamol may possess a general central nervous system depressant effect, patients receiving Robaxin/Robaxin-750 (methocarbamol tablets) should be cautioned about combined effects with alcohol and other CNS depressants.
Safe use of methocarbamol has not been established with regard to possible adverse effects upon fetal development. Therefore, methocarbamol tablets should not be used in women who are or may become pregnant and particularly during early pregnancy unless in the judgment of the physician the potential benefits outweigh the possible hazards.

PRECAUTIONS

Safety and effectiveness in children below the age of 12 years have not been established.
It is not known whether this drug is secreted in human milk. As a general rule, nursing should not be undertaken while a patient is on a drug since many drugs are excreted in human milk.
Methocarbamol may cause a color interference in certain screening tests for 5-hydroxyindoleacetic acid (5-HIAA) and vanilmandelic acid (VMA).

ADVERSE REACTIONS

Lightheadedness, dizziness, drowsiness, nausea, allergic manifestations such as urticaria, pruritus, rash, conjunctivitis with nasal congestion, blurred vision, headache, fever.

DOSAGE AND ADMINISTRATION

Robaxin (methocarbamol), 500 mg—Adults: initial dosage, 3 tablets q.i.d.; maintenance dosage, 2 tablets q.i.d.
Robaxin-750 (methocarbamol), 750 mg— Adults: initial dosage, 2 tablets q.i.d.; maintenance dosage, 1 tablet q.4h. or 2 tablets t.i.d.
Six grams a day are recommended for the first 48 to 72 hours of treatment. (For severe conditions 8 grams a day may be administered.) Thereafter, the dosage can usually be reduced to approximately 4 grams a day.

HOW SUPPLIED

Robaxin—light orange, round, film-coated tablets monogrammed Robaxin and AHR in bottles of 100 (NDC 0031-7429-63), and 500 (NDC 0031-7429-70).
Robaxin-750—orange, capsule-shaped, film-coated tablets monogrammed Robaxin-750 and AHR in bottles of 100 (NDC 0031-7449-63), 500 (NDC 0031-7449-70), and Dis-Co® unit dose packs of 100 (NDC 0031-7449-64).
Store at Controlled Room Temperature, between 15°C and 30°C (59°F and 86°F).
Dispense in tight container.
Also available in the injectable form, 1 g methocarbamol in each 10 ml vial (NDC 0031-7409).

Shown in Product Identification Guide, page 331

ROBAXISAL® TABLETS ℞
[*ro"baks'ĭ-sal"*]

DESCRIPTION

For oral administration, Robaxisal is available as a pink and white laminated tablet containing:

Methocarbamol, USP	400 mg
Aspirin, USP	325 mg

Inactive Ingredients: Corn Starch, FD&C Red 3, Magnesium Stearate, Povidone, Sodium Lauryl Sulfate, Sodium Starch Glycolate, Stearic Acid.
Methocarbamol has the following structural formula and chemical name:

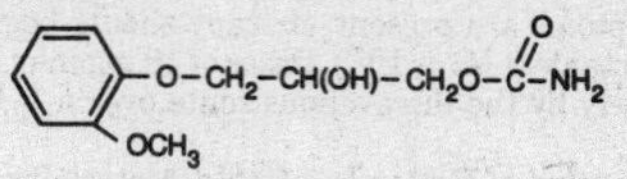

3-(2-Methoxyphenoxy)-1,2-propanediol
1-Carbamate

ACTIONS

Robaxisal provides a double approach to the management of discomforts associated with musculoskeletal disorders.
Methocarbamol. The mechanism of action of methocarbamol in humans has not been established, but may be due to general central nervous system depression. It has no direct action on the contractile mechanism of striated muscle, the motor end plate or the nerve fiber.
Aspirin. Aspirin is a mild analgesic with anti-inflammatory and antipyretic activity.

INDICATIONS

Robaxisal is indicated as an adjunct to rest, physical therapy, and other measures for the relief of discomfort associated with acute, painful musculoskeletal conditions. The mode of action of methocarbamol has not been clearly identified but may be related to its sedative properties. Methocarbamol does not directly relax tense skeletal muscles in man.

CONTRAINDICATIONS

Hypersensitivity to methocarbamol or aspirin.

WARNINGS

Since methocarbamol may possess a general central nervous system depressant effect, patients receiving Robaxisal should be cautioned about combined effects with alcohol and other CNS depressants.

PRECAUTIONS

Products containing aspirin should be administered with caution to patients with gastritis or peptic ulceration, or those receiving hypoprothrombinemic anticoagulants.

Methocarbamol may cause a color interference in certain screening tests for 5-hydroxyindoleacetic acid (5-HIAA) and vanilmandelic acid (VMA).

Pregnancy. Safe use of Robaxisal has not been established with regard to possible adverse effects upon fetal development. Therefore, Robaxisal should not be used in women who are or may become pregnant and particularly during early pregnancy unless in the judgment of the physician the potential benefits outweigh the possible hazards.

Nursing Mothers. It is not known whether methocarbamol is secreted in human milk; however, aspirin does appear in human milk in moderate amounts. It can produce a bleeding tendency either by interfering with the function of the infant's platelets or by decreasing the amount of prothrombin in the blood. The risk is minimal if the mother takes the aspirin just after nursing and if the infant has an adequate store of vitamin K. As a general rule, nursing should not be undertaken while a patient is on a drug.

Pediatric Use. Safety and effectiveness in children 12 years of age and below have not been established.

Use in Activities Requiring Mental Alertness. Robaxisal may rarely cause drowsiness. Until the patient's response has been determined, he should be cautioned against the operation of motor vehicles or dangerous machinery.

ADVERSE REACTIONS

The most frequent adverse reaction to methocarbamol is dizziness or lightheadedness and nausea. This occurs in about one in 20–25 patients. Less frequent reactions are drowsiness, blurred vision, headache, fever, allergic manifestations such as urticaria, pruritus, and rash.

Adverse reactions that have been associated with the use of aspirin include: nausea and other gastrointestinal discomfort, gastritis, gastric erosion, vomiting, constipation, diarrhea, angio-edema, asthma, rash, pruritus, urticaria.

Gastrointestinal discomfort may be minimized by taking Robaxisal with food.

DOSAGE AND ADMINISTRATION

Adults and children over 12 years of age: Two tablets four times daily. Three tablets four times daily may be used in severe conditions for one to three days in patients who are able to tolerate salicylates. These dosage recommendations provide respectively 3.2 and 4.8 grams of methocarbamol per day.

OVERDOSAGE

Toxicity due to overdosage of methocarbamol is unlikely; however, acute overdosage of aspirin may cause symptoms of salicylate intoxication.

Treatment of Overdosage. Supportive therapy for 24 hours, as methocarbamol is excreted within that time. If salicylate intoxication occurs, especially in children, the hyperpnea may be controlled with sodium bicarbonate. Judicious use of 5% CO_2 with 95% O_2 may be of benefit. Abnormal electrolyte patterns should be corrected with appropriate fluid therapy.

HOW SUPPLIED

Robaxisal® is supplied as pink and white laminated, compressed tablets in bottles of 100 (NDC 0031-7469-63), and 500 (NDC 0031-7469-70).

Store at controlled room temperature, between 15°C and 30°C (59°F and 86°F).

Dispense in well-closed container.

Shown in Product Identification Guide, page 331

ROBINUL® TABLETS ℞

[ro 'bĭ-nul]

ROBINUL® FORTE TABLETS ℞

brand of Glycopyrrolate Tablets, USP

DESCRIPTION

Robinul and Robinul Forte tablets contain the synthetic anticholinergic, glycopyrrolate. Glycopyrrolate is a quaternary ammonium compound with the following chemical name: 3-[(cyclopentylhydroxyphenylacetyl)oxy]-1,1-dimethylpyrrolidinium bromide.

Robinul tablets are scored, compressed white tablets engraved AHR. Each tablet contains:

Glycopyrrolate, USP .... 1 mg

Robinul Forte tablets are scored, compressed white tablets engraved $\frac{AHR}{2}$.

Each tablet contains:

Glycopyrrolate, USP .... 2 mg

Inactive Ingredients: Dibasic Calcium Phosphate, Lactose, Magnesium Stearate, Povidone, Sodium Starch Glycolate.

ACTIONS

Glycopyrrolate, like other anticholinergic (antimuscarinic) agents, inhibits the action of acetylcholine on structures innervated by postganglionic cholinergic nerves and on smooth muscles that respond to acetylcholine but lack cholinergic innervation. These peripheral cholinergic receptors are present in the autonomic effector cells of smooth muscle, cardiac muscle, the sino-atrial node, the atrioventricular node, exocrine glands, and, to a limited degree, in the autonomic ganglia. Thus, it diminishes the volume and free acidity of gastric secretions and controls excessive pharyngeal, tracheal, and bronchial secretions.

Glycopyrrolate antagonizes muscarinic symptoms (e.g., bronchorrhea, bronchospasm, bradycardia, and intestinal hypermotility) induced by cholinergic drugs such as the anticholinesterases.

The highly polar quaternary ammonium group of glycopyrrolate limits its passage across lipid membranes, such as the blood-brain barrier, in contrast to atropine sulfate and scopolamine hydrobromide, which are non-polar tertiary amines which penetrate lipid barriers easily.

INDICATIONS

For use as adjunctive therapy in the treatment of peptic ulcer.

CONTRAINDICATIONS

Glaucoma; obstructive uropathy (for example, bladder neck obstruction due to prostatic hypertrophy); obstructive disease of the gastrointestinal tract (as in achalasia, pyloroduodenal stenosis, etc.); paralytic ileus; intestinal atony of the elderly or debilitated patient; unstable cardiovascular status in acute hemorrhage; severe ulcerative colitis; toxic megacolon complicating ulcerative colitis; myasthenia gravis. Robinul (glycopyrrolate) tablets are contraindicated in those patients with a hypersensitivity to glycopyrrolate.

WARNINGS

In the presence of a high environmental temperature, heat prostration (fever and heat stroke due to decreased sweating) can occur with use of Robinul.

Diarrhea may be an early symptom of incomplete intestinal obstruction, especially in patients with ileostomy or colostomy. In this instance treatment with this drug would be inappropriate and possibly harmful.

Robinul (glycopyrrolate) may produce drowsiness or blurred vision. In this event, the patient should be warned not to engage in activities requiring mental alertness such as operating a motor vehicle or other machinery, or performing hazardous work while taking this drug.

Theoretically, with overdosage, a curare-like action may occur, i.e., neuromuscular blockade leading to muscular weakness and possible paralysis.

Pregnancy. The safety of this drug during pregnancy has not been established. The use of any drug during pregnancy requires that the potential benefits of the drug be weighed against possible hazards to mother and child. Reproduction studies in rats revealed no teratogenic effects from glycopyrrolate; however, the potent anticholinergic action of this agent resulted in diminished rates of conception and of survival at weaning, in a dose-related manner. Other studies in dogs suggest that this may be due to diminished seminal secretion which is evident at high doses of glycopyrrolate. Information on possible adverse effects in the pregnant female is limited to uncontrolled data derived from marketing experience. Such experience has revealed no reports of teratogenic or other fetus-damaging potential. No controlled studies to establish the safety of the drug in pregnancy have been performed.

Nursing mothers. It is not known whether this drug is secreted in human milk. As a general rule, nursing should not be undertaken while a patient is on a drug since many drugs are excreted in human milk.

Pediatric Use. Since there is no adequate experience in children who have received this drug, safety and efficacy in children have not been established.

PRECAUTIONS

Use Robinul with caution in the elderly and in all patients with:

- Autonomic neuropathy.
- Hepatic or renal disease.
- Ulcerative colitis—large doses may suppress intestinal motility to the point of producing a paralytic ileus and for this reason may precipitate or aggravate "toxic megacolon," a serious complication of the disease.
- Hyperthyroidism, coronary heart disease, congestive heart failure, cardiac tachyarrhythmias, tachycardia, hypertension and prostatic hypertrophy.
- Hiatal hernia associated with reflux esophagitis, since anticholinergic drugs may aggravate this condition.

ADVERSE REACTIONS

Anticholinergics produce certain effects, most of which are extensions of their fundamental pharmacological actions. Adverse reactions to anticholinergics in general may include xerostomia; decreased sweating; urinary hesitancy and retention; blurred vision; tachycardia; palpitations; dilatation of the pupil; cycloplegia; increased ocular tension; loss of taste; headaches; nervousness; mental confusion; drowsiness; weakness; dizziness; insomnia; nausea; vomiting; constipation; bloated feeling; impotence; suppression of lactation; severe allergic reaction or drug idiosyncrasies including anaphylaxis, urticaria and other dermal manifestations.

Robinul (glycopyrrolate) is chemically a quaternary ammonium compound; hence, its passage across lipid membranes, such as the blood-brain barrier, is limited in contrast to atropine sulfate and scopolamine hydrobromide. For this reason the occurrence of CNS related side effects is lower, in comparison to their incidence following administration of anticholinergics which are chemically tertiary amines that can cross this barrier readily.

OVERDOSAGE

The symptoms of overdosage of glycopyrrolate are peripheral in nature rather than central.

1. To guard against further absorption of the drug—use gastric lavage, cathartics and/or enemas.
2. To combat peripheral anticholinergic effects (residual mydriasis, dry mouth, etc.)—utilize a quaternary ammonium anticholinesterase, such as neostigmine methylsulfate.
3. To combat hypotension—use pressor amines (norepinephrine, metaraminol) i.v.; and supportive care.
4. To combat respiratory depression—administer oxygen; utilize a respiratory stimulant such as Dopram® i.v.; artificial respiration.

DOSAGE AND ADMINISTRATION

The dosage of Robinul or Robinul Forte should be adjusted to the needs of the individual patient to assure symptomatic control with a minimum of adverse reactions. The presently recommended maximum daily dosage of glycopyrrolate is 8 mg.

Robinul (glycopyrrolate, 1 mg) tablets. The recommended initial dosage of Robinul for adults is one tablet three times daily (in the morning, early afternoon, and at bedtime). Some patients may require two tablets at bedtime to assure overnight control of symptoms. For maintenance, a dosage of one tablet twice a day is frequently adequate.

Robinul Forte (glycopyrrolate, 2 mg) tablets. The recommended dosage of Robinul Forte for adults is one tablet two or three times daily at equally spaced intervals.

Robinul tablets are not recommended for use in children under the age of 12 years.

DRUG INTERACTIONS

There are no known drug interactions.

HOW SUPPLIED

Robinul (glycopyrrolate, 1 mg) tablets in bottles of 100 (NDC 0031-7824-63).

Robinul Forte (glycopyrrolate, 2 mg) tablets in bottles of 100 (NDC 0031-7840-63).

Shown in Product Identification Guide, page 331

ROBINUL® INJECTABLE ℞

[ro 'bĭ-nul]

brand of Glycopyrrolate Injection, USP

DESCRIPTION

Robinul (glycopyrrolate) is a synthetic anticholinergic agent. Each 1 mL contains:

Glycopyrrolate, USP .... 0.2 mg

Water for Injection, USP .... q.s.

Benzyl Alcohol, NF (preservative) 0.9%

pH adjusted, when necessary, with hydrochloric acid and/or sodium hydroxide.

For Intramuscular or Intravenous administration.

Glycopyrrolate is a quaternary ammonium compound with the following chemical name:

3[(cyclopentylhydroxyphenylacetyl)oxy]-1,1-dimethyl pyrrolidinium bromide.

Unlike atropine, glycopyrrolate is completely ionized at physiological pH values.

Robinul Injectable is a clear, colorless, sterile liquid; pH 2.0–3.0.

CLINICAL PHARMACOLOGY

Glycopyrrolate, like other anticholinergic (antimuscarinic) agents, inhibits the action of acetylcholine on structures innervated by postganglionic cholinergic nerves and on smooth muscles that respond to acetylcholine but lack cholinergic innervation. These peripheral cholinergic receptors are present in the autonomic effector cells of smooth muscle, cardiac muscle, the sinoatrial node, the atrioventricular node, exocrine glands, and, to a limited degree, in the autonomic ganglia. Thus, it diminishes the volume and free acidity of gastric secretions and controls excessive pharyngeal, tracheal, and bronchial secretions.

Glycopyrrolate antagonizes muscarinic symptoms (e.g., bronchorrhea, bronchospasm, bradycardia, and intestinal hypermotility) induced by cholinergic drugs such as the anticholinesterases.

The highly polar quaternary ammonium group of glycopyrrolate limits its passage across lipid membranes, such as the blood-brain barrier, in contrast to atropine sulfate and scopolamine hydrobromide, which are non-polar tertiary amines which penetrate lipid barriers easily.

Continued on next page

A. H. Robins—Cont.

Peak effects occur approximately 30 to 45 minutes after intramuscular administration. The vagal blocking effects persist for 2 to 3 hours and the antisialagogue effects persist up to 7 hours, periods longer than for atropine. With intravenous injection, the onset of action is generally evident within one minute.

INDICATIONS AND USAGE

In Anesthesia: Robinul (glycopyrrolate) Injectable is indicated for use as a preoperative antimuscarinic to reduce salivary, tracheobronchial, and pharyngeal secretions; to reduce the volume and free acidity of gastric secretions; and, to block cardiac vagal inhibitory reflexes during induction of anesthesia and intubation. When indicated, Robinul Injectable may be used intraoperatively to counteract drug-induced or vagal traction reflexes with the associated arrhythmias. Glycopyrrolate protects against the peripheral muscarinic effects (e.g., bradycardia and excessive secretions) of cholinergic agents such as neostigmine and pyridostigmine given to reverse the neuromuscular blockade due to nondepolarizing muscle relaxants.

In Peptic Ulcer: For use in adults as adjunctive therapy for the treatment of peptic ulcer when rapid anticholinergic effect is desired or when oral medication is not tolerated.

CONTRAINDICATIONS

Known hypersensitivity to glycopyrrolate.
Due to its benzyl alcohol content, Robinul Injectable should not be used in newborns (children less than 1 month of age).
In addition, in the management of *peptic ulcer* patients, because of the longer duration of therapy, Robinul Injectable may be contraindicated in patients with concurrent glaucoma; obstructive uropathy (for example, bladder neck obstruction due to prostatic hypertrophy); obstructive disease of the gastrointestinal tract (as in achalasia, pyloroduodenal stenosis, etc.); paralytic ileus, intestinal atony of the elderly or debilitated patient; unstable cardiovascular status in acute hemorrhage; severe ulcerative colitis; toxic megacolon complicating ulcerative colitis; myasthenia gravis.

WARNINGS

This drug should be used with great caution, if at all, in patients with glaucoma or asthma.
In the ambulatory patient. Robinul (glycopyrrolate) may produce drowsiness or blurred vision. The patient should be cautioned regarding activities requiring mental alertness such as operating a motor vehicle or other machinery or performing hazardous work while taking this drug.
In addition, in the presence of a high environmental temperature, heat prostration (fever and heat stroke due to decreased sweating) can occur with use of Robinul (glycopyrrolate).
Diarrhea may be an early symptom of incomplete intestinal obstruction, especially in patients with ileostomy or colostomy. In this instance treatment with Robinul (glycopyrrolate) would be inappropriate and possibly harmful.

PRECAUTIONS

General.
Investigate any tachycardia before giving glycopyrrolate since an increase in the heart rate may occur.
Use with caution in patients with: coronary artery disease; congestive heart failure; cardiac arrhythmias; hypertension; hyperthyroidism.
In managing ulcer patients, use Robinul with caution in the elderly and in all patients with autonomic neuropathy, hepatic or renal disease, ulcerative colitis or hiatal hernia, since anticholinergic drugs may aggravate these conditions. With overdosage, a curare-like action may occur.
Drug Interactions. The intravenous administration of any anticholinergic in the presence of cyclopropane anesthesia can result in ventricular arrhythmias; therefore, caution should be observed if Robinul (glycopyrrolate) Injectable is used during cyclopropane anesthesia. If the drug is given in small incremental doses of 0.1 mg or less, the likelihood of producing ventricular arrhythmias is reduced.
Carcinogenesis, mutagenesis, impairment of fertility. Long-term studies in animals have not been performed to evaluate carcinogenic potential. In the teratology studies, diminished rates of conception and of survival at weaning were observed in rats, in a dose-related manner. Studies in dogs suggest that this may be due to diminished seminal secretion which is evident at high doses of glycopyrrolate.
Pregnancy Category B. Reproduction studies have been performed in rats and rabbits up to 1000 times the human dose and have revealed no teratogenic effects from glycopyrrolate. There are, however, no adequate and well-controlled studies in pregnant women. Because animal reproduction studies are not always predictive of human response, this drug should be used during pregnancy only if clearly needed.
Nursing Mothers. It is not known whether this drug is excreted in human milk. Because many drugs are excreted in human milk, caution should be exercised when Robinul is administered to a nursing woman.

Pediatric Use. Safety and effectiveness in children below the age of 12 years have not been established for the management of peptic ulcer.

ADVERSE REACTIONS

Anticholinergics produce certain effects, most of which are extensions of their pharmacologic actions. Adverse reactions to anticholinergics in general may include dry mouth; urinary hesitancy and retention; blurred vision due to mydriasis; increased ocular tension; tachycardia; palpitation; decreased sweating; loss of taste; headache; nervousness; drowsiness; weakness; dizziness; insomnia; nausea; vomiting; impotence; suppression of lactation; constipation; bloated feeling; severe allergic reaction or drug idiosyncrasies including anaphylaxis; urticaria and other dermal manifestations; some degree of mental confusion and/or excitement, especially in elderly persons.
Robinul is chemically a quaternary ammonium compound; hence, its passage across lipid membranes, such as the blood-brain barrier is limited in contrast to atropine sulfate and scopolamine hydrobromide. For this reason the occurrence of CNS related side effects is lower, in comparison to their incidence following administration of anticholinergics which are chemically tertiary amines that can cross this barrier readily.

OVERDOSAGE

To combat peripheral anticholinergic effects, a quaternary ammonium anticholinesterase such as neostigmine methylsulfate (which does not cross the blood-brain barrier) may be given intravenously in increments of 0.25 mg in adults. This dosage may be repeated every five to ten minutes until anticholinergic overactivity is reversed or up to a maximum of 2.5 mg. Proportionately smaller doses should be used in children. Indication for repetitive doses of neostigmine should be based on close monitoring of the decrease in heart rate and the return of bowel sounds.
In the unlikely event that CNS symptoms (excitement, restlessness, convulsions, psychotic behavior) occur, physostigmine (which does cross the blood-brain barrier) should be used. Physostigmine 0.5 to 2 mg should be slowly administered intravenously and repeated as necessary up to a total of 5 mg in adults. Proportionately smaller doses should be used in children.
Fever should be treated symptomatically. In the event of a curare-like effect on respiratory muscles, artificial respiration should be instituted and maintained until effective respiratory action returns.

DOSAGE AND ADMINISTRATION

Robinul (glycopyrrolate) Injectable may be administered intramuscularly, or intravenously, without dilution, in the following indications:
Adults: *Preanesthetic Medication.* The recommended dose of Robinul (glycopyrrolate) Injectable is 0.002 mg (0.01 mL) per pound of body weight by intramuscular injection, given 30 to 60 minutes prior to the anticipated time of induction of anesthesia or at the time the preanesthetic narcotic and/or sedative are administered.
Intraoperative Medication. Robinul (glycopyrrolate) Injectable may be used during surgery to counteract drug induced or vagal traction reflexes with the associated arrhythmias (e.g., bradycardia). It should be administered intravenously as single doses of 0.1 mg (0.5 mL) and repeated, as needed, at intervals of 2–3 minutes. The usual attempts should be made to determine the etiology of the arrhythmia, and the surgical or anesthetic manipulations necessary to correct parasympathetic imbalance should be performed.
Reversal of Neuromuscular Blockade. The recommended dose of Robinul (glycopyrrolate) Injectable is 0.2 mg (1.0 mL) for each 1.0 mg of neostigmine or 5.0 mg of pyridostigmine. In order to minimize the appearance of cardiac side effects, the drugs may be administered simultaneously by intravenous injection and may be mixed in the same syringe.
Children: (Read Contraindications). *Preanesthetic Medication.* The recommended dose of Robinul (glycopyrrolate) Injectable in children 1 month to 12 years of age is 0.002 mg (0.01 mL) per pound of body weight intramuscularly, given 30 to 60 minutes prior to the anticipated time of induction of anesthesia or at the time the preanesthetic narcotic and/or sedative are administered.
Children 1 month to 2 years of age may require up to 0.004 mg (0.02 mL) per pound of body weight.
Intraoperative Medication. Because of the long duration of action of Robinul (glycopyrrolate) if used as preanesthetic medication, additional Robinul (glycopyrrolate) Injectable for anticholinergic effect intraoperatively is rarely needed; in the event it is required the recommended pediatric dose is 0.002 mg (0.01 mL) per pound of body weight intravenously, not to exceed 0.1 mg (0.5 mL) in a single dose which may be repeated, as needed, at intervals of 2–3 minutes. The usual attempts should be made to determine the etiology of the arrhythmia, and the surgical or anesthetic manipulations necessary to correct parasympathetic imbalance should be performed.
Reversal of Neuromuscular Blockade. The recommended pediatric dose of Robinul (glycopyrrolate) Injectable is

0.2 mg (1.0 mL) for each 1.0 mg of neostigmine or 5.0 mg of pyridostigmine. In order to minimize the appearance of cardiac side effects, the drugs may be administered simultaneously by intravenous injection and may be mixed in the same syringe.
Adults: *Peptic Ulcer.* The usual recommended dose of Robinul Injectable is 0.1 mg (0.5 mL) administered at 4-hour intervals, 3 or 4 times daily intravenously or intramuscularly. Where more profound effect is required, 0.2 mg (1.0 mL) may be given. Some patients may need only a single dose, and frequency of administration should be dictated by patient response up to a maximum of four times daily.
Robinul Injectable is not recommended for peptic ulcers in children under 12 years of age. (See Precautions.)
NOTE: Parenteral drug products should be inspected visually for particulate matter and discoloration prior to administration whenever solution and container permit.
Admixture Compatibilities. Robinul (glycopyrrolate) Injectable is compatible for mixing and injection with the following injectable dosage forms: 5% and 10% glucose in water or saline; atropine sulfate, USP; Antilirium® (physostigmine salicylate); Benadryl® (diphenhydramine HCl); codeine phosphate, USP; Emete-Con® (benzquinamide HCl); hydromorphone HCl, USP; Inapsine® (droperidol); Innovar® (droperidol and fentanyl citrate); Largon® (propiomazine HCl); Levo-Dromoran® (levorphanol tartrate); lidocaine, USP; Mepergan® (meperidine and promethazine HCls); meperidine HCl, USP; Mestinon® /Regonol® (pyridostigmine bromide); morphine sulfate, USP; Nisentil® (alphaprodine HCl); Nubain® (nalbuphine HCl); Numorphan® (oxymorphone HCl); Pantopon® (opium alkaloids HCls); procaine HCl, USP; promethazine HCl, USP; Prostigmin® (neostigmine methylsulfate, USP); scopolamine HBr, USP; Sparine® (promazine HCl); Stadol® (butorphanol tartrate); Sublimaze® (fentanyl citrate); Talwin® (pentazocine lactate); Tigan® (trimethobenzamide HCl); Vesprin® (triflupromazine HCl); and Vistaril® (hydroxyzine HCl). Robinul Injectable may be administered via the tubing of a running infusion of physiological saline or lactated Ringer's solution.
Since the stability of glycopyrrolate is questionable above a pH of 6.0, do *not* combine Robinul Injectable in the same syringe with Brevital® (methohexital Na); Chloromycetin® (chloramphenicol Na succinate); Dramamine® (dimenhydrinate); Nembutal® (pentobarbital Na); Pentothal® (thiopental Na); Seconal® (secobarbital Na); sodium bicarbonate (Abbott); or Valium® (diazepam). A gas will evolve or a precipitate may form. Mixing with Decadron® (dexamethasone Na phosphate) or a buffered solution of lactated Ringer's solution will result in a pH higher than 6.0. Mixing chlorpromazine HCl, USP, or Compazine® (prochlorperazine) with other agents in a syringe is not recommended by the manufacturer, although the mixture with Robinul Injectable is physically compatible.

HOW SUPPLIED

Robinul (glycopyrrolate) Injectable, 0.2 mg/mL, is available in 1 mL single dose vials packaged in 25's (NDC 0031-7890-11), 2 mL single dose vials packaged in 25's (NDC 0031-7890-95), 5 mL multiple dose vials packaged individually (NDC 0031-7890-93) and in 25's (NDC 0031-7890-06), and 20 mL (NDC 0031-7890-83) multiple dose vials.
Store at controlled room temperature, between 15°C and 30°C (59°F and 86°F).
Manufactured for Pharmaceutical Division, A. H. Robins Company, by Elkins-Sinn, Inc.
Shown in Product Identification Guide, page 331

ROBITUSSIN A–C®   ℂ
[ro "bĭ-tuss 'ĭn]
Expectorant
Cough Suppressant
Sugar-Free

Robitussin and Codeine
Each 5 mL (1 teaspoonful) contains:
Guaifenesin, USP .... 100 mg
Codeine Phosphate, USP .... 10 mg
  (Warning: May be habit forming)
Alcohol 3.5 percent
In a palatable, aromatic syrup
Inactive Ingredients: Caramel, Citric Acid, FD&C Red 40, Flavors, Glycerin, Saccharin Sodium, Sodium Benzoate, Sorbitol, Water.

ACTIONS

Robitussin A-C combines the expectorant, guaifenesin, with the cough suppressant, codeine. Guaifenesin enhances the output of lower respiratory tract fluid. The enhanced flow of less viscid secretions promotes and facilitates the removal of mucus. Codeine is a centrally acting agent which elevates the threshold for cough.
As a result, dry, unproductive coughs become more productive and less frequent.

Under Federal law, Robitussin A-C is available without a prescription. Certain state laws may differ. The container label contains the following indications, warnings and drug interaction precaution statements and directions:

INDICATIONS

Temporarily controls cough due to minor throat and bronchial irritation as may occur with the common cold or inhaled irritants. Helps loosen phlegm (mucus) and thin bronchial secretions to make coughs more productive.

WARNINGS

A persistent cough may be a sign of a serious condition. If cough persists for more than 1 week, tends to recur, or is accompanied by fever, rash, or persistent headache, consult a doctor. Do not take this product for persistent or chronic cough such as occurs with smoking, asthma, chronic bronchitis, emphysema, or if cough is accompanied by excessive phlegm (mucus) unless directed by a doctor. Adults and children who have a chronic pulmonary disease or shortness of breath, or children who are taking other drugs, should not take this product unless directed by a doctor. May cause or aggravate constipation. As with any drug, if you are pregnant or nursing a baby, seek the advice of a health professional before using this product.

PROFESSIONAL NOTE: Guaifenesin has been shown to produce a color interference with certain clinical laboratory determinations of 5-hydroxyindoleacetic acid (5-HIAA) and vanillylmandelic acid (VMA).

DRUG INTERACTION PRECAUTION

Caution should be used when taking this product with sedatives, tranquilizers and drugs used for depression, especially monoamine oxidase inhibitors (MAOIs). These combinations may cause greater sedation (drowsiness) than is caused by the products used alone.

DIRECTIONS

Take orally as stated below or use as directed by a doctor. Adults and children 12 years of age and over: 2 teaspoonfuls every 4 hours, not to exceed 12 teaspoonfuls in a 24-hour period; children 6 to under 12 years: 1 teaspoonful every 4 hours, not to exceed 6 teaspoonfuls in a 24-hour period; children under 6 years: consult a doctor. A special measuring device should be used to give an accurate dose of this product to children under 6 years of age. Giving a higher dose than recommended by a doctor could result in serious side effects for a child. Use of codeine-containing preparations is not recommended for children under 2 years of age. Do not exceed recommended dosage.

HOW SUPPLIED

Bottles of 4 fl. oz. (NDC 0031-8674-12), pints (NDC 0031-8674-25), and gallons (NDC 0031-8674-29).

ROBITUSSIN® –DAC

[ro"bĭ-tuss'ĭn]
Expectorant
Nasal Decongestant
Cough-Suppressant
Sugar-Free

Each 5 mL (1 teaspoonful) contains:
Guaifenesin, USP ....100 mg
Pseudoephedrine
 Hydrochloride, USP ....30 mg
Codeine Phosphate, USP ....10 mg
 (Warning: May be habit forming)
In a palatable, aromatic syrup
Alcohol 1.9 percent
Inactive Ingredients: Caramel, Citric Acid, FD&C Red 40, Flavors, Glycerin, Saccharin Sodium, Sodium Benzoate, Sorbitol, Water.

ACTIONS

Robitussin-DAC combines the expectorant, guaifenesin, the nasal decongestant, pseudoephedrine, and the cough suppressant, codeine. Guaifenesin enhances the output of lower respiratory tract fluid. The enhanced flow of less viscid secretions promotes and facilitates the removal of mucus. Codeine is a centrally acting agent which elevates the threshold for cough. As a result, dry, unproductive coughs become more productive and less frequent. The nasal decongestant, pseudoephedrine, reduces the swelling of nasal passages.

Under Federal law, Robitussin-DAC is available without a prescription. Certain state laws may differ. The container label contains the following indications, warnings and drug interaction precaution statements and directions:

INDICATIONS

Temporarily relieves nasal congestion and controls cough due to minor throat and bronchial irritation as may occur with the common cold or inhaled irritants. Temporarily restores freer breathing through the nose. Helps loosen phlegm (mucus) and thin bronchial secretions to make coughs more productive.

WARNINGS

A persistent cough may be a sign of a serious condition. If cough persists for more than 1 week, tends to recur, or is accompanied by fever, rash, or persistent headache, consult a doctor. Do not take this product for persistent or chronic cough such as occurs with smoking, asthma, chronic bronchitis, emphysema, or if cough is accompanied by excessive phlegm (mucus) unless directed by a doctor. Adults and children who have a chronic pulmonary disease or shortness of breath, or children who are taking other drugs, should not take this product unless directed by a doctor. Do not take this product if you have high blood pressure, heart disease, diabetes or thyroid disease, except under the advice and supervision of a doctor. Do not exceed recommended dosage because at higher doses nervousness, dizziness or sleeplessness may occur. May cause or aggravate constipation. As with any drug, if you are pregnant or nursing a baby, seek the advice of a health professional before using this product.

PROFESSIONAL NOTE: Guaifenesin has been shown to produce a color interference with certain clinical laboratory determinations of 5-hydroxyindoleacetic acid (5-HIAA) and vanillylmandelic acid (VMA).

DRUG INTERACTION PRECAUTION

Do not take this product if you are presently taking a prescription drug for high blood pressure or depression, especially monoamine oxidase inhibitors (MAOIs), without first consulting your doctor.

DIRECTIONS

Take orally as stated below or use as directed by a doctor. Adults and children 12 years of age and over: 2 teaspoonfuls every 4 hours, not to exceed 8 teaspoonfuls in a 24-hour period; children 6 to under 12 years: 1 teaspoonful every 4 hours, not to exceed 4 teaspoonfuls in a 24-hour period; children under 6 years: consult a doctor. A special measuring device should be used to give an accurate dose of this product to children under 6 years of age. Giving a higher dose than recommended by a doctor could result in serious side effects for a child. Use of codeine-containing preparations is not recommended for children under 2 years of age. Do not exceed recommended dosage.

HOW SUPPLIED

Bottles of 4 fl. oz. (NDC 0031-8680-12) and one pint (NDC 0031-8680-25).

TENEX®   ℞

[ten'ex]
(Guanfacine Hydrochloride)
1 mg Tablets
2 mg Tablets

DESCRIPTION

Tenex (guanfacine hydrochloride) is a centrally acting antihypertensive with α_2-adrenoceptor agonist properties in tablet form for oral administration.

The chemical name of Tenex (guanfacine hydrochloride) is N-amidino-2-(2,6-dichlorophenyl) acetamide hydrochloride and its molecular weight is 282.56.

Guanfacine hydrochloride is a white to off-white powder; sparingly soluble in water and alcohol and slightly soluble in acetone. The tablets contain the following inactive ingredients:

1 mg—FD&C Red 40 aluminum lake, Lactose, Microcrystalline cellulose, Povidone, Stearic Acid.

2 mg—D&C Yellow 10 aluminum lake, Lactose, Microcrystalline cellulose, Povidone, Stearic Acid.

CLINICAL PHARMACOLOGY

Tenex (guanfacine hydrochloride) is an orally active antihypertensive agent whose principal mechanism of action appears to be stimulation of central α_2-adrenergic receptors. By stimulating these receptors, guanfacine reduces sympathetic nerve impulses from the vasomotor center to the heart and blood vessels. This results in a decrease in peripheral vascular resistance and a reduction in heart rate.

The dose-response relationship for blood pressure and adverse effects of guanfacine given once a day as monotherapy has been evaluated in patients with mild to moderate hypertension. In this study patients were randomized to placebo or to 0.5 mg, 1 mg, 2 mg, 3 mg, or 5 mg of Tenex. Results are shown in the following table. A useful effect was not observed overall until doses of 2 mg were reached, although responses in white patients were seen at 1 mg; 24 hour effectiveness of 1 mg to 3 mg doses was documented using 24 hour ambulatory monitoring. While the 5 mg dose added an increment of effectiveness, it caused an unacceptable increase in adverse reactions.

[See first table below.]

Controlled clinical trials in patients with mild to moderate hypertension who were receiving a thiazide-type diuretic have defined the dose-response relationship for blood pressure response and adverse reactions of guanfacine given at bedtime and have shown that the blood pressure response to guanfacine can persist for 24 hours after a single dose. In the 12-week, placebo-controlled dose-response study, patients were randomized to placebo or to doses of 0.5, 1, 2, and 3 mg of guanfacine, in addition to 25 mg chlorthalidone, each given at bedtime. The observed mean changes from baseline, tabulated below, indicate the similarity of response for placebo and the 0.5 mg dose. Doses of 1, 2, and 3 mg resulted in decreased blood pressure in the sitting position with no real differences among the three doses. In the standing position there was some increase in response with dose.

[See second table below.]

While most of the effectiveness of guanfacine in combination (and as monotherapy in white patients) was present at 1 mg, adverse reactions at this dose were not clearly distinguishable from those associated with placebo. Adverse reactions were clearly present at 2 and 3 mg (see Adverse Reactions).

In a second 12-week, placebo-controlled study of 1, 2 or 3 mg of Tenex (guanfacine hydrochloride) administered with 25 mg of chlorthalidone once daily, a significant decrease in blood pressure was maintained for a full 24 hours after dosing. While there was no significant difference between the 12 and 24 hour blood pressure readings, the fall in blood pressure at 24 hours was numerically smaller, suggesting possible escape of blood pressure in some patients and the need for individualization of therapy.

In a double-blind, randomized trial, either guanfacine or clonidine was given at recommended doses with 25 mg chlorthalidone for 24 weeks and then abruptly discontinued. Results showed equal degrees of blood pressure reduction with the two drugs and there was no tendency for blood pressures to increase despite maintenance of the same daily dose of the two drugs. Signs and symptoms of rebound phenomena were infrequent upon discontinuation of either drug. Abrupt withdrawal of clonidine produced a rapid return of diastolic and especially, systolic blood pressure to approximately pretreatment levels, with occasional values significantly greater than baseline, whereas guanfacine withdrawal produced a more gradual increase to pre-treatment levels, but also with occasional values significantly greater than baseline.

Mean Changes (mm Hg) from Baseline in Seated Systolic and Diastolic Blood Pressure for Patients Completing 4 to 8 Weeks of Treatment with Guanfacine Monotherapy

Mean Change S/D* Seated	n = (range)	Placebo	0.5 mg	1 mg	2 mg	3 mg	5 mg
White Patients	11–30	–1/–5	–6/–8	–8/–9	–12/–11	–15/–12	–18/–16
Black Patients	8–28	–3/–5	0/–2	–3/–5	–7/–7	–8/–9	–19/–15

* S/D = Systolic/diastolic blood pressure.

Mean Decreases (mm Hg) in Seated and Standing Blood Pressure for Patients Treated with Guanfacine in Combination with Chlorthalidone

Mean Change	n =	Placebo 63	0.5 mg 63	1 mg 64	2 mg 58	3 mg 59
S/D* Seated		–5/–7	–5/–6	–14/–13	–12/–13	–16/–13
S/D* Standing		–3/–5	–5/–4	–11/–9	–9/–10	–15/–12

* S/D = Systolic/diastolic blood pressure

Continued on next page

A. H. Robins—Cont.

Pharmacodynamics: Hemodynamic studies in man showed that the decrease in blood pressure observed after single-dose or long-term oral treatment with guanfacine was accompanied by a significant decrease in peripheral resistance and a slight reduction in heart rate (5 beats/min). Cardiac output under conditions of rest or exercise was not altered by guanfacine.

Tenex (guanfacine hydrochloride) lowered elevated plasma renin activity and plasma catecholamine levels in hypertensive patients, but this does not correlate with individual blood-pressure responses.

Growth hormone secretion was stimulated with single oral doses of 2 and 4 mg of guanfacine. Long-term use of Tenex had no effect on growth hormone levels.

Guanfacine had no effect on plasma aldosterone. A slight but insignificant decrease in plasma volume occurred after one month of guanfacine therapy. There were no changes in mean body weight or electrolytes.

Pharmacokinetics: Relative to an intravenous dose of 3 mg, the absolute oral bioavailability of guanfacine is about 80%. Peak plasma concentrations occur from 1 to 4 hours with an average of 2.6 hours after single oral doses or at steady state. The area under the concentration-time curve (AUC) increases linearly with the dose.

In individuals with normal renal function, the average elimination half-life is approximately 17 hr (range 10–30 hr). Younger patients tend to have shorter elimination half-lives (13–14 hr) while older patients tend to have half-lives at the upper end of the range. Steady state blood levels were attained within 4 days in most subjects.

In individuals with normal renal function, guanfacine and its metabolites are excreted primarily in the urine. Approximately 50% (40–75%) of the dose is eliminated in the urine as unchanged drug; the remainder is eliminated mostly as conjugates of metabolites produced by oxidative metabolism of the aromatic ring.

The guanfacine-to-creatinine clearance ratio is greater than 1.0, which would suggest that tubular secretion of drug occurs.

The drug is approximately 70% bound to plasma proteins, independent of drug concentration.

The whole body volume of distribution is high (a mean of 6.3 L/kg), which suggests a high distribution of drug to the tissues.

The clearance of guanfacine in patients with varying degrees of renal insufficiency is reduced, but plasma levels of drug are only slightly increased compared to patients with normal renal function. When prescribing for patients with renal impairment, the low end of the dosing range should be used. Patients on dialysis also can be given usual doses of guanfacine hydrochloride as the drug is poorly dialyzed.

INDICATIONS AND USAGE

Tenex (guanfacine hydrochloride) is indicated in the management of hypertension. Tenex may be given alone or in combination with other antihypertensive agents, especially thiazide-type diuretics.

CONTRAINDICATIONS

Tenex is contraindicated in patients with known hypersensitivity to guanfacine hydrochloride.

PRECAUTIONS

General. Like other antihypertensive agents, Tenex (guanfacine hydrochloride) should be used with caution in patients with severe coronary insufficiency, recent myocardial infarction, cerebrovascular disease or chronic renal or hepatic failure.

Sedation. Tenex, like other orally active central α-2-adrenergic agonists, causes sedation or drowsiness, especially when beginning therapy. These symptoms are dose-related (see Adverse Reactions). When Tenex is used with other centrally active depressants (such as phenothiazines, barbiturates, or benzodiazepines), the potential for additive sedative effects should be considered.

Rebound. Abrupt cessation of therapy with orally active central α-2 adrenergic agonists may be associated with increases (from depressed on-therapy levels) in plasma and urinary catecholamines, symptoms of "nervousness and anxiety" and, less commonly, increases in blood pressure to levels significantly greater than those prior to therapy.

Information for Patients. Patients who receive Tenex should be advised to exercise caution when operating dangerous machinery or driving motor vehicles until it is determined that they do not become drowsy or dizzy from the medication. Patients should be warned that their tolerance for alcohol and other CNS depressants may be diminished. Patients should be advised not to discontinue therapy abruptly.

Laboratory Tests. In clinical trials, no clinically relevant laboratory test abnormalities were identified as causally related to drug during short-term treatment with Tenex (guanfacine hydrochloride).

Adverse Reaction	Placebo n=59	0.5 mg n=60	1 mg n=61	2 mg n=60	3 mg n=59
Dry Mouth	0%	10%	10%	42%	54%
Somnolence	8%	5%	10%	13%	39%
Asthenia	0%	2%	3%	7%	3%
Dizziness	8%	12%	2%	8%	15%
Headache	8%	13%	7%	5%	3%
Impotence	0%	0%	0%	7%	3%
Constipation	0%	2%	0%	5%	15%
Fatigue	2%	2%	5%	8%	10%

Adverse Reaction	Placebo n=73	0.5 mg n=72	1 mg n=72	2 mg n=72	3 mg n=72
Dry Mouth	5 (7%)	4 (5%)	6 (8%)	8 (11%)	20 (28%)
Somnolence	1 (1%)	3 (4%)	0 (0%)	1 (1%)	10 (14%)
Asthenia	0 (0%)	2 (3%)	0 (0%)	2 (2%)	7 (10%)
Dizziness	2 (2%)	1 (1%)	3 (4%)	6 (8%)	3 (4%)
Headache	3 (4%)	4 (3%)	3 (4%)	1 (1%)	2 (2%)
Impotence	1 (1%)	1 (0%)	0 (0%)	1 (1%)	3 (4%)
Constipation	0 (0%)	0 (0%)	0 (0%)	1 (1%)	1 (1%)
Fatigue	3 (3%)	2 (3%)	2 (3%)	5 (6%)	3 (4%)

Drug Interactions. The potential for increased sedation when Tenex is given with other CNS-depressant drugs should be appreciated.

The administration of guanfacine concomitantly with a known microsomal enzyme inducer (phenobarbital or phenytoin) to two patients with renal impairment reportedly resulted in significant reductions in elimination half-life and plasma concentration. In such cases, therefore, more frequent dosing may be required to achieve or maintain the desired hypotensive response. Further, if guanfacine is to be discontinued in such patients, careful tapering of the dosage may be necessary in order to avoid rebound phenomena (see *Rebound* above).

Anticoagulants. Ten patients who were stabilized on oral anticoagulants were given guanfacine, 1–2 mg/day, for 4 weeks. No changes were observed in the degree of anticoagulation.

In several well-controlled studies, guanfacine was administered together with diuretics with no drug interactions reported. In the long-term safety studies, Tenex was given concomitantly with many drugs without evidence of any interactions. The principal drugs given (number of patients in parentheses) were: cardiac glycosides (115), sedatives and hypnotics (103), coronary vasodilators (52), oral hypoglycemics (45), cough and cold preparations (45), NSAIDs (38), antihyperlipidemics (29), antigout drugs (24), oral contraceptives (18), bronchodilators (13), insulin (10), and beta blockers (10).

Drug/Laboratory Test Interactions. No laboratory test abnormalities related to the use of Tenex (guanfacine hydrochloride) have been identified.

Carcinogenesis, Mutagenesis, Impairment of Fertility. No carcinogenic effect was observed in studies of 78 weeks in mice at doses more than 150 times the maximum recommended human dose and 102 weeks in rats at doses more than 100 times the maximum recommended human dose. In a variety of test models, guanfacine was not mutagenic.

No adverse effects were observed in fertility studies in male and female rats.

Pregnancy Category B. Administration of guanfacine to rats at 70 times the maximum recommended human dose and to rabbits at 20 times the maximum recommended human dose resulted in no evidence of harm to the fetus. Higher doses (100 and 200 times the maximum recommended human dose in rabbits and rats respectively) were associated with reduced fetal survival and maternal toxicity. Rat experiments have shown that guanfacine crosses the placenta.

There are, however, no adequate and well-controlled studies in pregnant women. Because animal reproduction studies are not always predictive of human response, this drug should be used during pregnancy only if clearly needed.

Labor and Delivery. Tenex (guanfacine hydrochloride) is not recommended in the treatment of acute hypertension associated with toxemia of pregnancy. There is no information available on the effects of guanfacine on the course of labor and delivery.

Nursing Mothers. It is not known whether Tenex (guanfacine hydrochloride) is excreted in human milk. Because many drugs are excreted in human milk, caution should be exercised when Tenex is administered to a nursing woman. Experiments with rats have shown that guanfacine is excreted in the milk.

Pediatric Use. Safety and effectiveness in children under 12 years of age have not been demonstrated. Therefore, the use of Tenex in this age group is not recommended.

ADVERSE REACTIONS

Adverse reactions noted with Tenex (guanfacine hydrochloride) are similar to those of other drugs of the central α-2 adrenoreceptor agonist class: dry mouth, sedation (somnolence), weakness (asthenia), dizziness, constipation, and impotence. While the reactions are common, most are mild and tend to disappear on continued dosing.

Skin rash with exfoliation has been reported in a few cases; although clear cause and effect relationships to Tenex could not be established, should a rash occur, Tenex should be discontinued and the patient monitored appropriately.

In the dose-response monotherapy study described under Clinical Pharmacology, the frequency of the most commonly observed adverse reactions showed a dose relationship from 0.5 to 3 mg as follows:

[See first table above.]

The percent of patients who dropped out because of adverse reactions are shown below for each dosage group.

	Placebo	0.5 mg	1 mg	2 mg	3 mg
Percent dropouts	0%	2.0%	5.0%	13%	32%

The most common reasons for dropouts among patients who received guanfacine were dry mouth, somnolence, dizziness, fatigue, weakness, and constipation.

In the 12-week, placebo-controlled, dose-response study of guanfacine administered with 25 mg chlorthalidone at bedtime, the frequency of the most commonly observed adverse reactions showed a clear dose relationship from 0.5 to 3 mg as follows:

[See second table at top of page.]

There were 41 premature terminations because of adverse reactions in this study. The percent of patients who dropped out and the dose at which the dropout occurred were as follows:

Dose:	Placebo	0.5 mg	1 mg	2 mg	3 mg
Percent dropouts	6.9%	4.2%	3.2%	6.9%	8.3%

Reasons for dropouts among patients who received guanfacine were: somnolence, headache, weakness, dry mouth, dizziness, impotence, insomnia, constipation, syncope, urinary incontinence, conjunctivitis, paresthesia, and dermatitis.

In a second 12-week placebo-controlled combination therapy study in which the dose could be adjusted upward to 3 mg per day in 1-mg increments at 3-week intervals, i.e., a setting more similar to ordinary clinical use, the most commonly recorded reactions were: dry mouth, 47%; constipation, 16%; fatigue, 12%; somnolence, 10%; asthenia, 6%; dizziness, 6%; headache, 4%; and insomnia, 4%.

Reasons for dropouts among patients who received guanfacine were: somnolence, dry mouth, dizziness, impotence, constipation, confusion, depression, and palpitations.

In the clonidine/guanfacine comparison described in Clinical Pharmacology, the most common adverse reactions noted were as follows:

Adverse Reactions	Guanfacine (n = 279)	Clonidine (n = 278)
Dry mouth	30%	37%
Somnolence	21%	35%
Dizziness	11%	8%
Constipation	10%	5%
Fatigue	9%	8%
Headache	4%	4%
Insomnia	4%	3%

Adverse reactions occurring in 3% or less of patients in the three controlled trials of Tenex with a diuretic were:

Cardiovascular— bradycardia, palpitations, substernal pain

Gastrointestinal— abdominal pain, diarrhea, dyspepsia, dysphagia, nausea

CNS— amnesia, confusion, depression, insomnia, libido decrease

ENT disorders— rhinitis, taste perversion, tinnitus

Eye disorders— conjunctivitis, iritis, vision disturbance

Musculoskeletal— leg cramps, hypokinesia

Respiratory— dyspnea

Dermatologic— dermatitis, pruritus, purpura, sweating

Urogenital— testicular disorder, urinary incontinence

Other— malaise, paresthesia, paresis

Adverse reaction reports tend to decrease over time. In an open-label trial of one year's duration, 580 hypertensive subjects were given guanfacine, titrated to achieve goal blood pressure, alone (51%), with diuretic (38%), with beta blocker (3%), with diuretic plus beta blocker (6%), or with diuretic plus vasodilator (2%). The mean daily dose of guanfacine reached was 4.7 mg.

Adverse Reaction	Incidence of adverse reactions at any time during the study	Incidence of adverse reactions at the end of one year
	n=580	n=580
Dry mouth	60%	15%
Drowsiness	33%	6%
Dizziness	15%	1%
Constipation	14%	3%
Weakness	5%	1%
Headache	4%	0.2%
Insomnia	5%	0%

There were 52 (8.9%) dropouts due to adverse effects in this 1-year trial. The causes were: dry mouth (n = 20), weakness (n = 12), constipation (n = 7), somnolence (n = 3), nausea (n = 3), orthostatic hypotension (n = 2), insomnia (n = 1), rash (n = 1), nightmares (n = 1), headache (n = 1), and depression (n = 1).

Postmarketing Experience. An open-label postmarketing study involving 21,718 patients was conducted to assess the safety of Tenex (guanfacine hydrochloride) 1 mg/day given at bedtime for 28 days. Tenex was administered with or without other antihypertensive agents. Adverse events reported in the postmarketing study at an incidence greater than 1% included dry mouth, dizziness, somnolence, fatigue, headache and nausea. The most commonly reported adverse events in this study were the same as those observed in controlled clinical trials.

Less frequent, possibly Tenex-related events observed in the postmarketing study and/or reported spontaneously include:

BODY AS A WHOLE: asthenia, chest pain, edema, malaise, tremor

CARDIOVASCULAR: bradycardia, palpitations, syncope, tachycardia

CENTRAL NERVOUS SYSTEM: paresthesias, vertigo

EYE DISORDERS; blurred vision

GASTROINTESTINAL SYSTEM: abdominal pain, constipation, diarrhea, dyspepsia

LIVER AND BILIARY SYSTEM: abnormal liver function tests

MUSCULO-SKELETAL SYSTEM: arthralgia, leg cramps, leg pain, myalgia

PSYCHIATRIC: agitation, anxiety, confusion, depression, insomnia, nervousness

REPRODUCTIVE SYSTEM, MALE: impotence

RESPIRATORY SYSTEM: dyspnea

SKIN AND APPENDAGES: alopecia, dermatitis, exfoliative dermatitis, pruritus, rash

SPECIAL SENSES: alterations in taste

URINARY SYSTEM: nocturia, urinary frequency

Rare, serious disorders with no definitive cause and effect relationship to Tenex have been reported spontaneously and/or in the postmarketing study. These events include acute renal failure, cardiac fibrillation, cerebrovascular accident, congestive heart failure, heart block, and myocardial infarction.

Drug Abuse and Dependence: No reported abuse or dependence has been associated with the administration of Tenex (guanfacine hydrochloride).

OVERDOSAGE

Signs and Symptoms. Drowsiness, lethargy, bradycardia and hypotension have been observed following overdose with guanfacine.

A 25-year-old female intentionally ingested 60 mg. She presented with severe drowsiness and bradycardia of 45 beats/minute. Gastric lavage was performed and an infusion of isoproterenol (0.8 mg in 12 hours) was administered. She recovered quickly and without sequelae.

A 28-year-old female who ingested 30–40 mg developed only lethargy, was treated with activated charcoal and a cathartic, was monitored for 24 hours, and was discharged in good health.

A 2-year-old male weighing 12 kg, who ingested up to 4 mg of guanfacine, developed lethargy. Gastric lavage (followed by activated charcoal and sorbitol slurry via NG tube) removed some tablet fragments within 2 hours after ingestion, and vital signs were normal. During 24-hour observation in ICU, systolic pressure was 58 and heart rate 70 at 16 hours post-ingestion. No intervention was required, and the child was discharged fully recovered the next day.

Treatment of Overdosage. Gastric lavage and supportive therapy as appropriate. Guanfacine is not dializable in clinically significant amounts (2.4%).

DOSAGE AND ADMINISTRATION

The recommended initial dose of Tenex (guanfacine hydrochloride) when given alone or in combination with another antihypertensive drug is 1 mg daily given at bedtime to minimize somnolence. If after 3 to 4 weeks of therapy, 1 mg does not give a satisfactory result, a dose of 2 mg may be given, although most of the effect of Tenex is seen at 1 mg (see Clinical Pharmacology). Higher daily doses have been used, but adverse reactions increase significantly with doses above 3 mg/day.

The frequency of rebound hypertension is low, but it can occur. When rebound occurs, it does so after 2–4 days, which is delayed compared with clonidine hydrochloride. This is consistent with the longer half-life of guanfacine. In most cases, after abrupt withdrawal of guanfacine, blood pressure returns to pretreatment levels slowly (within 2–4 days) without ill effects.

HOW SUPPLIED

Tenex is available in 2 tablet strengths of guanfacine (as the hydrochloride salt) as follows:

1 mg—light pink, diamond-shaped tablet embossed with a 1 and engraved AHR on one side and engraved TENEX on the other side in bottles of 100 (NDC 0031-8901-63) and 500 (NDC 0031-8901-70) and Dis-Co® Unit Dose Packs of 100 (NDC 0031-8901-64).

2 mg—yellow, diamond-shaped tablet, one side engraved TENEX, other side engraved 2 with AHR below it in bottles of 100 (NDC 0031-8903-63).

Store at controlled room temperature, between 20°C and 25°C (68°F and 77°F). Dispense in tight, light-resistant container.

Shown in Product Identification Guide, page 331

VIOKASE® ℞

[vi´o-kās]

(Pancrelipase, USP)

Tablets

Powder

DESCRIPTION

Viokase (Pancrelipase, USP) is a pancreatic enzyme concentrate of porcine origin containing standardized lipase, protease, and amylase as well as other pancreatic enzymes. Viokase is available in tablet and powder dosage form for oral administration.

The enzyme potencies of the tablets and powder are:

	Each Tablet	Each 0.7g powder (¼ teaspoonful)
Lipase, USP Units	8,000	16,800
Protease, USP Units	30,000	70,000
Amylase, USP Units	30,000	70,000

Inactive Ingredients:

TABLETS—Lactose, Magnesium Stearate, Sodium Chloride, Stearic Acid.

POWDER—Lactose, Sodium Chloride.

CLINICAL PHARMACOLOGY

The natural digestive enzymes in Viokase hydrolyze fats into fatty acids and glycerol, split protein into amino acids, and convert carbohydrates to dextrins and short chain sugars. Under conditions of the USP test method (in vitro) Viokase has the following total digestive capacity:

	Each Tablet	Each 0.7g powder
Dietary Fat, grams	28	59
Dietary Protein, grams	30	70
Dietary Starch, grams	30	70

Viokase Tablets are not enteric coated.

The digestive capacity of a pancreatic enzyme concentrate depends on the amount that passes through the stomach unchanged and is available at the site of action in the small intestine.

INDICATIONS

Viokase (Pancrelipase, USP) is indicated as a digestive aid in the treatment of exocrine pancreatic insufficiency as associated with but not limited to cystic fibrosis, chronic pancreatitis, pancreatectomy, or obstruction of the pancreas ducts.

CONTRAINDICATIONS

Do not use in patients hypersensitive to pork protein.

PRECAUTIONS

General: Individuals previously sensitized to trypsin, pancreatin or pancrelipase may have allergic manifestations.

Information for patients: Viokase should not be held in the mouth as the proteolytic action may cause irritation of the mucosa.

Avoid inhalation of the powder when administering Viokase.

Carcinogenesis, Mutagenesis, Impairment of Fertility: Long-term studies in animals have not been performed to evaluate carcinogenic potential.

Pregnancy Category C. Animal reproduction studies have not been conducted with Viokase. It is also not known whether Viokase can cause fetal harm when administered to a pregnant woman or can affect reproduction capacity. Viokase should be given to a pregnant woman only if clearly needed.

Nursing Mothers: It is not known whether this drug is excreted in human milk. Because many drugs are excreted in human milk, caution should be exercised when Viokase is administered to a nursing mother.

ADVERSE REACTIONS

The dust or finely powdered pancreatic enzyme concentrate is irritating to the nasal mucosa and the respiratory tract. It has been documented that inhalation of the airborne powder can precipitate an asthma attack. The literature also contains several references to asthma due to inhalation in patients sensitized to pancreatic enzyme concentrates. Extremely high doses of exogenous pancreatic enzymes have been associated with hyperuricemia and hyperuricosuria. Overdosage of pancreatic enzyme concentrate may cause diarrhea or transient intestinal upset.

OVERDOSAGE

Acute toxicity determinations in animals have not been possible since the maximum dose that could be given orally produced no toxic reaction. In chronic feeding tests, rats developed swollen salivary glands. This is believed due to the proteolytic activity and the mucosal irritation caused by tissue digestion.

No acute toxic reactions have been reported.

DOSAGE AND ADMINISTRATION

Powder: Dosage for patients with cystic fibrosis—¼ teaspoonful (0.7 grams) with meals.

Tablets: Dosage for patients with cystic fibrosis or chronic pancreatitis—1 to 3 tablets with meals or as directed by physician. As a digestive aid in patients with pancreatectomy or obstruction of pancreatic ducts—1 to 2 tablets taken at 2-hour intervals or as directed by physician.

HOW SUPPLIED

Tablets—Tan, round, compressed tablets engraved Viokase/AHR on one side and 9111 on the other side in bottles of 100 (NDC 0031-9111-63) and 500 (NDC 0031-9111-70).

Powder—Tan powder in bottles of 4 oz. (113.5 grams) (NDC 0031-9115-12) and 8 oz. (227 grams) (NDC 0031-9115-25).

Store in tightly closed container in a dry place at a temperature not exceeding 25°C (77°F).

Dispense tablets and powder in tight container, preferably with a desiccant.

CLINICAL STUDIES

The effectiveness of Viokase as a digestive aid in the treatment of patients with exocrine pancreatic insufficiency has been documented in the literature as follows:

1. Regan, PT, Malagelada J-R, DiMagno EP, Glanzman SL, Go VLW: Comparative effects of antacids, cimetidine and enteric coating on the therapeutic response to oral enzymes in severe pancreatic insufficiency. N. Engl. J. Med. 297:854-8, 1977.

2. Graham DY: Enzyme replacement therapy of exocrine pancreatic insufficiency in man. N. Engl. J. Med. 296:1314-7, 1977.

Shown in Product Identification Guide, page 331

For EMERGENCY telephone numbers, consult the **Manufacturers Index.**

Roche Pharmaceuticals

Roche Laboratories Inc.
340 Kingsland Street
Nutley, NJ 07110-1199

For Medical Information:
Routine Inquires:
Write: Professional Product Information Department
Call: (800) 526-6367
In Emergencies:
(800) 526-6367
(24-hour service)
Adverse Drug Experiences:
(800) 526-6367

ACCUTANE® ℞
[*acc 'u-tane*]
(isotretinoin)
CAPSULES

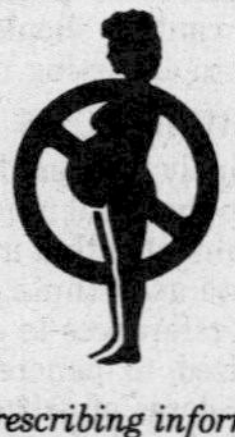

Avoid Pregnancy

The folllowing text is complete prescribing information based on official labeling in effect June 1996.

CONTRAINDICATION AND WARNING: Accutane must not be used by females who are pregnant or who may become pregnant while undergoing treatment. Although not every fetus exposed to Accutane has resulted in a deformed child, there is an extremely high risk that a deformed infant can result if pregnancy occurs while taking Accutane in any amount even for short periods of time. Potentially any fetus exposed during pregnancy can be affected. Presently, there is no accurate means of determining after Accutane exposure which fetus has been affected and which fetus has not been affected.

Accutane is contraindicated in women of childbearing potential unless the patient meets all of the following conditions:

- **has severe disfiguring nodular acne that is recalcitrant to standard therapies (see INDICATIONS AND USAGE section for definition)**
- **is reliable in understanding and carrying out instructions**
- **is capable of complying with the mandatory contraceptive measures**
- **has received both oral and written warnings of the hazards of taking Accutane during pregnancy and exposing a fetus to the drug**
- **has received both oral and written warnings of the risk of possible contraception failure and of the need to use two reliable forms of contraception simultaneously, unless abstinence is the chosen method, or the patient has undergone a hysterectomy and has acknowledged in writing her understanding of these warnings and of the need for using dual contraceptive methods**
- **has had a negative serum or urine pregnancy test with a sensitivity of at least 50 mIU/mL within 1 week prior to beginning therapy**
- **will begin therapy only on the second or third day of the next normal menstrual period**

It is recommended that a prescription for Accutane should not be issued by the physician until a report of a negative pregnancy test has been obtained and the patient has begun her menstrual period. It is also recommended that pregnancy testing and contraception counseling be repeated on a monthly basis. To encourage compliance with this recommendation, the physician should prescribe no more than a 1 month supply of the drug.

Major human fetal abnormalities related to Accutane administration have been documented: CNS abnormalities (including cerebral abnormalities, cerebellar malformation, hydrocephalus, microcephaly, cranial nerve deficit); skull abnormality; external ear abnormalities (including anotia, micropinna, small or absent external auditory canals); eye abnormalities (including microphthalmia); cardiovascular abnormalities; facial dysmorphia; cleft palate; thymus gland abnormality; parathyroid hormone deficiency. In some cases death has occurred with certain of the abnormalities previously noted. Cases of IQ scores less than 85 with or without obvious CNS abnormalities have also been reported. There is an increased risk of spontaneous abortion. In addition, premature births have been reported.

Effective contraception must be used for at least 1 month before beginning Accutane therapy, during therapy and for 1 month following discontinuation of therapy even where there has been a history of infertility, unless due to hysterectomy. It is recommended that two reliable forms of contraception be used simultaneously unless abstinence is the chosen method.

If pregnancy does occur during treatment, the physician and patient should discuss the desirability of continuing the pregnancy.

Accutane should be prescribed only by physicians who have special competence in the diagnosis and treatment of severe recalcitrant nodular acne, are experienced in the use of systemic retinoids and understand the risk of teratogenicity if Accutane is used during pregnancy.

DESCRIPTION

Accutane (isotretinoin), a retinoid which inhibits sebaceous gland function and keratinization, is available in 10-mg, 20-mg and 40-mg soft gelatin capsules for oral administration. Each capsule also contains beeswax, butylated hydroxyanisole, edetate disodium, hydrogenated soybean oil flakes, hydrogenated vegetable oil and soybean oil. Gelatin capsules contain glycerin and parabens (methyl and propyl), with the following dye systems: 10 mg—iron oxide (red) and titanium dioxide; 20 mg—FD&C Red No. 3, FD&C Blue No. 1 and titanium dioxide; 40 mg—FD&C Yellow No. 6, D&C Yellow No. 10 and titanium dioxide.

Chemically, isotretinoin is 13-*cis* -retinoic acid and is related to both retinoic acid and retinol (vitamin A). It is a yellow-orange to orange crystalline powder with a molecular weight of 300.44.

CLINICAL PHARMACOLOGY

The exact mechanism of action of Accutane is unknown.

Nodular Acne: Clinical improvement in nodular acne patients occurs in association with a reduction in sebum secretion. The decrease in sebum secretion is temporary and is related to the dose and duration of treatment with Accutane, and reflects a reduction in sebaceous gland size and an inhibition of sebaceous gland differentiation.[1]

Clinical Pharmacokinetics: The pharmacokinetic profile of isotretinoin is predictable and can be described using linear pharmacokinetic theory.

After oral administration of 80 mg (two 40-mg capsules), peak blood concentrations ranged from 167 to 459 ng/mL (mean 256 ng/mL) and mean time to peak was 3.2 hours in normal volunteers, while in acne patients peak concentrations ranged from 98 to 535 ng/mL (mean 262 ng/mL) with a mean time to peak of 2.9 hours. The drug is 99.9% bound in human plasma almost exclusively to albumin. The terminal elimination half-life of isotretinoin ranged from 10 to 20 hours in volunteers and patients. Following an 80-mg liquid suspension oral dose of ^{14}C-isotretinoin, ^{14}C-activity in blood declined with a half-life of 90 hours. Relatively equal amounts of radioactivity were recovered in the urine and feces with 65% to 83% of the dose recovered.

The major identified metabolite in blood is 4-*oxo* -isotretinoin. The mean elimination half-life of this metabolite is 25 hours (range 17–50 hours). Tretinoin and 4-*oxo* -tretinoin were also observed. After two 40-mg capsules of isotretinoin, maximum concentrations of the metabolite of 87 to 399 ng/mL occurred at 6 to 20 hours. The blood concentration of the major metabolite generally exceeded that of isotretinoin after 6 hours.

When taken with food or milk, the oral absorption of isotretinoin is increased.

The mean $\pm$ SD minimum steady-state blood concentration of isotretinoin was 160 $\pm$ 19 ng/mL in 10 patients receiving 40-mg bid doses. After single and multiple doses, the mean ratio of areas under the blood concentration:time curves of 4-*oxo*-isotretinoin to isotretinoin was 3 to 3.5.

Tissue Distribution in Animals: Tissue distribution of ^{14}C-isotretinoin in rats after oral dosing revealed high concentrations of radioactivity in many tissues after 15 minutes, with a maximum in 1 hour, and declining to nondetectable levels by 24 hours in most tissues. After 7 days, however, low levels of radioactivity were detected in the liver, ureter, adrenal, ovary and lacrimal gland.

INDICATIONS AND USAGE

Severe recalcitrant nodular acne: Accutane is indicated for the treatment of severe recalcitrant nodular acne. Nodules are inflammatory lesions with a diameter of 5 mm or greater. The nodules may become suppurative or hemorrhagic. "Severe," by definition,[2] means "many" as opposed to "few or several" nodules. Because of significant adverse effects associated with its use, Accutane should be reserved for patients with severe nodular acne who are unresponsive to conventional therapy, including systemic antibiotics.

A single course of therapy has been shown to result in complete and prolonged remission of disease in many patients.[1,3,4] If a second course of therapy is needed, it should not be initiated until at least 8 weeks after completion of the first course, because experience has shown that patients may continue to improve while off Accutane.

CONTRAINDICATIONS

Pregnancy: Category X. See boxed CONTRAINDICATION and WARNING.

Accutane should not be given to patients who are sensitive to parabens, which are used as preservatives in the gelatin capsule.

WARNINGS

Pseudotumor Cerebri: **Accutane use has been associated with a number of cases of pseudotumor cerebri (benign intracranial hypertension). Early signs and symptoms of pseudotumor cerebri include papilledema, headache, nausea and vomiting, and visual disturbances. Patients with these symptoms should be screened for papilledema and, if present, they should be told to discontinue Accutane immediately and be referred to a neurologist for further diagnosis and care.**

Decreased Night Vision: A number of cases of decreased night vision have occurred during Accutane therapy. Because the onset in some patients was sudden, patients should be advised of this potential problem and warned to be cautious when driving or operating any vehicle at night. Visual problems should be carefully monitored.

Corneal Opacities: Corneal opacities have occurred in patients receiving Accutane for acne and more frequently when higher drug dosages were used in patients with disorders of keratinization. All Accutane patients experiencing visual difficulties should discontinue the drug and have an ophthalmological examination. The corneal opacities that have been observed in patients treated with Accutane have either completely resolved or were resolving at follow-up 6 to 7 weeks after discontinuation of the drug. See ADVERSE REACTIONS.

Inflammatory Bowel Disease: Accutane has been temporally associated with inflammatory bowel disease (including regional ileitis) in patients without a prior history of intestinal disorders. Patients experiencing abdominal pain, rectal bleeding or severe diarrhea should discontinue Accutane immediately.

Lipids: Blood lipid determinations should be performed before Accutane is given and then at intervals until the lipid response to Accutane is established, which usually occurs within 4 weeks. See PRECAUTIONS.

Approximately 25% of patients receiving Accutane experienced an elevation in plasma triglycerides. Approximately 15% developed a decrease in high density lipoproteins and about 7% showed an increase in cholesterol levels. These effects on triglycerides, HDL and cholesterol were reversible upon cessation of Accutane therapy.

Patients with increased tendency to develop hypertriglyceridemia include those with diabetes mellitus, obesity, increased alcohol intake and familial history.

The cardiovascular consequences of hypertriglyceridemia are not well understood, but may increase the patient's risk status. In addition, acute pancreatitis, sometimes associated with elevation of serum triglycerides in excess of 800 mg/dL, has been reported. Therefore, every attempt should be made to control significant triglyceride elevation.

Some patients have been able to reverse triglyceride elevation by reduction in weight, restriction of dietary fat and alcohol, and reduction in dose while continuing Accutane.[5]

An obese male patient with Darier's disease developed elevated triglycerides and subsequent eruptive xanthomas.[6]

Hyperostosis: In clinical trials of disorders of keratinization with a mean dose of 2.24 mg/kg/day, a high prevalence of skeletal hyperostosis was noted. Two children showed x-ray findings suggestive of premature closure of the epiphysis. Additionally, skeletal hyperostosis was noted in 6 of 8 patients in a prospective study of disorders of keratinization.[7] Minimal skeletal hyperostosis has also been observed by x-rays in prospective studies of nodular acne patients treated with a single course of therapy at recommended doses.

Hepatotoxicity: Several cases of clinical hepatitis have been noted which are considered to be possibly or probably related to Accutane therapy. Additionally, mild to moderate elevations of liver enzymes have been observed in approximately 15% of individuals treated during clinical trials, some of which normalized with dosage reduction or continued administration of the drug. If normalization does not readily occur or if hepatitis is suspected during treatment with Accutane, the drug should be discontinued and the etiology further investigated.

Animal Studies: In rats given 32 or 8 mg/kg/day of isotretinoin for 18 months or longer, the incidences of focal calcification, fibrosis and inflammation of the myocardium, calcification of coronary, pulmonary and mesenteric arteries and metastatic calcification of the gastric mucosa were

greater than in control rats of similar age. Focal endocardial and myocardial calcifications associated with calcification of the coronary arteries were observed in two dogs after approximately 6 to 7 months of treatment with isotretinoin at a dosage of 60 to 120 mg/kg/day.
In dogs given isotretinoin chronically at a dosage of 60 mg/kg/day, corneal ulcers and corneal opacities were encountered at a higher incidence than in control dogs. In general, these ocular changes tended to revert toward normal when treatment with isotretinoin was stopped, but did not completely clear during the observation period.
In rats given isotretinoin at a dosage of 32 mg/kg/day for approximately 15 weeks, long bone fracture has been observed.

PRECAUTIONS

Information for Patients: **Females of childbearing potential should be instructed that they must not be pregnant when Accutane therapy is initiated, and that they should use effective contraception while taking Accutane and for 1 month after Accutane has been stopped. They should also sign a consent form prior to beginning Accutane therapy. See boxed CONTRAINDICATION AND WARNING.**
Because of the relationship of Accutane to vitamin A, patients should be advised against taking vitamin supplements containing vitamin A to avoid additive toxic effects.
Patients should be informed that transient exacerbation of acne has been seen, generally during the initial period of therapy.
Patients should be informed that they may experience decreased tolerance to contact lenses during and after therapy.
It is recommended that patients not donate blood during therapy and for 1 month following discontinuance of the drug.
Laboratory Tests: The incidence of hypertriglyceridemia is 1 patient in 4 on Accutane therapy. Pretreatment and follow-up blood lipids should be obtained under fasting conditions. After consumption of alcohol at least 36 hours should elapse before these determinations are made. It is recommended that these tests be performed at weekly or biweekly intervals until the lipid response to Accutane is established.
Since elevations of liver enzymes have been observed during clinical trials, pretreatment and follow-up liver function tests should be performed at weekly or biweekly intervals until the response to Accutane has been established.
Certain patients receiving Accutane have experienced problems in the control of their blood sugar. In addition, new cases of diabetes have been diagnosed during Accutane therapy, although no causal relationship has been established.
Some patients undergoing vigorous physical activity while on Accutane therapy have experienced elevated CPK levels; however, the clinical significance is unknown.
Carcinogenesis, Mutagenesis and Impairment of Fertility: In Fischer 344 rats given oral isotretinoin at dosages of 8 or 32 mg/kg/day for greater than 18 months, there was an increased incidence of pheochromocytoma; the incidence of adrenal medullary hyperplasia was also increased at the higher dosage. The relatively high level of spontaneous pheochromocytomas occurring in the Fischer 344 rat makes it a poor model for study of this tumor. The increase in adrenal medullary proliferative lesions following chronic treatment with relatively high dosages of oral isotretinoin may be an accentuation of a genetic predisposition in the Fischer 344 rat; therefore, the relevance of this tumor to the human population is uncertain. In addition, decreased incidences of liver adenomas, liver angiomas and leukemia were noted at the dose levels of 8 and 32 mg/kg/day.
The Ames test was conducted with isotretinoin in two laboratories. The results of the tests in one laboratory were negative while in the second laboratory a weakly positive response (less than 1.6 × background) was noted in *S. typhimurium* TA100 when the assay was conducted with metabolic activation. No dose-response effect was seen and all other strains were negative. Additionally, other tests designed to assess genotoxicity (Chinese hamster cell assay, mouse micronucleus test, *S. cerevisiae* D7 assay, in vitro clastogenesis assay with human-derived lymphocytes and unscheduled DNA synthesis assay) were all negative.
No adverse effects on gonadal function, fertility, conception rate, gestation or parturition were observed in rats at oral doses of isotretinoin of 2, 8 or 32 mg/kg/day.
In dogs, testicular atrophy was noted after treatment with oral isotretinoin for approximately 30 weeks at dosages of 20 or 60 mg/kg/day. In general, there was microscopic evidence for appreciable depression of spermatogenesis but some sperm were observed in all testes examined and in no instance were completely atrophic tubules seen. In studies of 66 men, 30 of whom were patients with nodular acne under treatment with oral isotretinoin, no significant changes were noted in the count or motility of spermatozoa in the ejaculate. In a study of 50 men (ages 17 to 32 years) receiving Accutane (isotretinoin) therapy for nodular acne, no significant effects were seen on ejaculate volume, sperm count, total sperm motility, morphology or seminal plasma fructose.
Pregnancy: **Category X. See boxed CONTRAINDICATION AND WARNING.**
Nursing Mothers: It is not known whether this drug is excreted in human milk. Because of the potential for adverse effects, nursing mothers should not receive Accutane.

ADVERSE REACTIONS

Clinical: Many of the side effects and adverse reactions seen or expected in patients receiving Accutane are similar to those described in patients taking high doses of vitamin A.
The percentages of adverse reactions listed below reflect the total experience in Accutane studies, including investigational studies of disorders of keratinization, with the exception of those pertaining to dry skin and mucous membranes. These latter reflect the experience only in patients with nodular acne because reactions relating to dryness are more commonly recognized as adverse reactions in this disease.
Included in this category are dry skin, skin fragility, pruritus, epistaxis, dry nose and dry mouth, which may be seen in up to 80% of nodular acne patients.
The most frequent adverse reaction to Accutane is cheilitis, which occurs in over 90% of patients. A less frequent reaction was conjunctivitis (about 2 patients in 5).
Skeletal hyperostosis has been observed on x-rays of patients treated with Accutane. See WARNINGS. Other types of bone abnormalities have also been reported; however, no causal relationship has been established.
Approximately 16% of patients treated with Accutane developed musculoskeletal symptoms (including arthralgia) during treatment. In general, these were mild to moderate and have occasionally required discontinuation of drug. Less frequently, transient pain in the chest has also been reported. These symptoms generally cleared rapidly after discontinuation of Accutane but in rare cases have persisted.
Less than 1 patient in 10 experienced rash (including erythema, seborrhea and eczema); thinning of hair, which in rare cases has persisted.
Approximately 1 patient in 20 experienced peeling of palms and soles, skin infections, nonspecific urogenital findings, nonspecific gastrointestinal symptoms, fatigue, headache and increased susceptibility to sunburn.
Accutane has been associated with a number of cases of pseudotumor cerebri, some of which involved concomitant use of tetracyclines. See WARNINGS.
The following CNS reactions have been reported and may bear no relationship to therapy—seizures, emotional instability, dizziness, nervousness, drowsiness, malaise, weakness, insomnia, lethargy and paresthesias.
Depression has been reported in some patients on Accutane therapy. In some of these patients, this has subsided with discontinuation of therapy and recurred with reinstitution of therapy.
The following reactions have been reported in less than 1% of patients and may bear no relationship to therapy—changes in skin pigment (hypo- and hyperpigmentation), flushing, urticaria, bruising, disseminated herpes simplex, edema, hair problems (other than thinning), hirsutism, respiratory infections, weight loss, erythema nodosum, paronychia, nail dystrophy, bleeding and inflammation of the gums, abnormal menses, optic neuritis, photophobia, eye lid inflammation, arthritis, anemia, palpitation, tachycardia, lymphadenopathy, sweating, tinnitus and voice alteration.
Reports of acne fulminaris and vasculitis, including Wegener's granulomatosis, have been received, but no causal relationship to Accutane therapy has been established.
In Accutane studies to date, of 72 patients who had normal pretreatment ophthalmological examinations, 5 developed corneal opacities while on Accutane (all 5 patients had a disorder of keratinization). Corneal opacities have also been reported in nodular acne patients treated with Accutane. See WARNINGS. Dry eyes and decrease in night vision have been reported and in rare instances have persisted. See WARNINGS. Cataracts, Keratitis and visual disturbances have also been reported.
Accutane has been temporally associated with inflammatory bowel disease. See WARNINGS.
Delayed wound healing has been reported. As may be seen with healing inflammatory acne lesions, an occasional exaggerated healing response, manifested by exuberant granulation tissue with crusting, has been reported in patients receiving therapy with Accutane. Pyogenic granuloma has also been diagnosed in a number of cases.
Laboratory: Accutane therapy induces change in serum lipids in a significant number of treated subjects. Approximately 25% of patients had elevation of plasma triglycerides. Five out of 135 patients treated for nodular acne and 32 out of 298 total subjects treated for all diagnoses showed an elevation of triglycerides above 500 mg percent. About 16% of patients showed a mild to moderate decrease in serum high density lipoprotein (HDL) levels while receiving treatment with Accutane and about 7% of patients experienced minimal elevations of serum cholesterol during treatment. Abnormalities of serum triglycerides, HDL and cholesterol were reversible upon cessation of Accutane therapy.
Approximately 40% of patients receiving Accutane developed elevated sedimentation rates, often from elevated baseline values.
From 1 in 10 to 1 in 5 patients showed decreases in red blood cell parameters and white blood cell counts, elevated platelet counts, white cells in the urine, increased alkaline phosphatase, SGOT, SGPT, GGTP or LDH. See WARNINGS: Hepatotoxicity.
Less than 1 in 10 patients showed proteinuria, microscopic or gross hematuria, elevated fasting blood sugar, elevated CPK, hyperuricemia or thrombocytopenia.
Dose Relationship and Duration: Cheilitis and hypertriglyceridemia are usually dose-related.
Most adverse reactions were reversible when therapy was discontinued; however, some have persisted after cessation of therapy. (See WARNINGS and ADVERSE REACTIONS.)
Overdosage: The oral LD_{50} of isotretinoin is greater than 4000 mg/kg in rats and mice and is approximately 1960 mg/kg in rabbits. Overdose has been associated with vomiting, facial flushing, cheilosis, abdominal pain, headache, dizziness and ataxia. All symptoms quickly resolved without apparent residual effects.

DOSAGE AND ADMINISTRATION

The recommended dosage range for Accutane is 0.5 to 2 mg/kg given in 2 divided doses daily for 15 to 20 weeks. In studies comparing 0.1, 0.5 and 1 mg/kg/day,[8] it was found that all doses provided initial clearing of disease but there was a greater need for retreatment with the lower dose(s).
It is recommended that for most patients the initial dose of Accutane be 0.5 to 1 mg/kg/day. Patients whose disease is very severe or is primarily manifested on the body may require up to the maximum recommended dose, 2 mg/kg/day. During treatment, the dose may be adjusted according to response of the disease and/or the appearance of clinical side effects—some of which may be dose-related.
If the total nodule count has been reduced by more than 70% prior to completing 15 to 20 weeks of treatment, the drug may be discontinued. After a period of 2 months or more off therapy, and if warranted by persistent or recurring severe nodular acne, a second course of therapy may be initiated.
Contraceptive measures must be followed for any subsequent course of therapy.
Accutane should be administered with food.

ACCUTANE DOSING BY BODY WEIGHT

Body Weight		Total Mg/Day		
kilograms	pounds	0.5 mg/kg	1 mg/kg	2 mg/kg
40	88	20	40	80
50	110	25	50	100
60	132	30	60	120
70	154	35	70	140
80	176	40	80	160
90	198	45	90	180
100	220	50	100	200

HOW SUPPLIED

Soft gelatin capsules, 10 mg (light pink), imprinted ACCUTANE 10 ROCHE. Boxes of 100 containing 10 Prescription Paks of 10 capsules (NDC 0004-0155-49).
Soft gelatin capsules, 20 mg (maroon), imprinted ACCUTANE 20 ROCHE. Boxes of 100 containing 10 Prescription Paks of 10 capsules (NDC 0004-0169-49).
Soft gelatin capsules, 40 mg (yellow), imprinted ACCUTANE 40 ROCHE. Boxes of 100 containing 10 Prescription Paks of 10 capsules (NDC 0004-0156-49).
Store at 59° to 86°F; 15° to 30°C. Protect from light.

REFERENCES

1. Peck GL, Olsen TG, Yoder FW, Strauss JS, Downing DT, Pandya M, Butkus D, Arnaud-Battandier J: Prolonged remissions of cystic and conglobate acne with 13-*cis* -retinoic acid. *N Engl J Med 300*:329–333, 1979. 2. Pochi PE, Shalita AR, Strauss JS, Webster SB: Report of the consensus conference on acne classification. *J Am Acad Dermatol 24*:495–500, 1991. 3. Farrell LN, Strauss JS, Stranieri AM: The treatment of severe cystic acne with 13-*cis* -retinoic acid. Evaluation of sebum production and the clinical response in a multiple-dose trial. *J Am Acad Dermatol 3*:602–611, 1980. 4. Jones H, Blanc D, Cunliffe WJ: 13-*cis* -retinoic acid and acne. *Lancet 2*:1048–1049, 1980. 5. Katz RA, Jorgensen H, Nigra TP: Elevation of serum triglyceride levels from oral isotretinoin in disorders of keratinization. *Arch Dermatol 116*:1369–1372, 1980. 6. Dicken CH, Connolly SM: Eruptive xanthomas associated with isotretinoin (13-*cis* -retinoic acid). *Arch Dermatol 116*: 951–952, 1980. 7. Ellis CN, Madison KC, Pennes DR, Martel W, Voorhees JJ: Isotretinoin therapy is associated with early skeletal radiographic changes. *J Am Acad Dermatol 10*:1024–1029, 1984. 8. Strauss JS, Rapini RP, Shalita AR, Konecky E, Pochi PE, Comite H, Exner JH: Isotretinoin

Continued on next page

Roche Laboratories—Cont.

therapy for acne: Results of a multicenter dose-response study. *J Am Acad Dermatol 10:*490–496, 1984.

PATIENT INFORMATION/CONSENT

Accutane must not be used by females who are pregnant or who may become pregnant while undergoing treatment.

IMPORTANT INFORMATION AND WARNING: Accutane can cause severe birth defects if it is taken when a female is pregnant. There is an extremely high risk that you will have a severely deformed baby if:

- you are pregnant when you start taking Accutane,
- you become pregnant while you are taking Accutane,
- you do not wait 1 month after you stop taking Accutane before becoming pregnant.

It is recommended that you and your doctor schedule an appointment every month to repeat the pregnancy test and check your body's response to Accutane. For your health and well-being, be sure to keep your appointments as scheduled.

THE CONSENT

My treatment with Accutane has been personally explained to me by Dr. ______________.

The following points of information, among others, have been specifically discussed and made clear:

1. I, ________________________________,
(Patient's Name)
understand that Accutane is a very powerful medicine used to treat severe nodular acne that did not get better with other treatments including oral antibiotics.
INITIALS: ________
2. I understand that I must not take Accutane if I am pregnant or may become pregnant during treatment.
INITIALS: ________
3. I understand that severe birth defects have occurred in babies of females who took Accutane during pregnancy. I have been warned by my doctor that there is an extremely high risk of severe damage to my unborn baby if I am pregnant or become pregnant while taking Accutane.
INITIALS: ________
4. I have been told by my doctor that effective birth control (contraception) must be used for at least 1 month before starting Accutane, all during Accutane therapy and for 1 month after Accutane treatment has stopped. My doctor has told me that I must either abstain from sexual intercourse or use two reliable kinds of birth control at the same time. I have also been told that any method of birth control can fail. I must use two forms of reliable birth control simultaneously even if I think I cannot become pregnant, unless I abstain from sexual intercourse or have had a hysterectomy.
INITIALS: ________
5. I know that I must have a blood or urine test done by my doctor that shows I am not pregnant within 1 week before starting Accutane, and I understand that I must wait until the second or third day of my next normal menstrual period before starting Accutane.
INITIALS: ________
6. My doctor has told me that I can participate in the "Patient Referral" program for an initial free pregnancy test and birth control counseling session by a consulting physician.
INITIALS: ________
7. I also know that I must immediately stop taking Accutane if I become pregnant while taking the drug and immediately contact my doctor to discuss the desirability of continuing the pregnancy. I also know that I must immediately contact my doctor if I become pregnant during the month after stopping Accutane.
INITIALS: ________
8. I have carefully read the Accutane patient brochure, "Important information concerning your treatment with Accutane," given to me by my doctor. I understand all of its contents and have talked over any questions I have with my doctor. INITIALS: ________
9. I am not now pregnant, nor do I plan to become pregnant for 1 month after I have completely finished taking Accutane. INITIALS: ________
10. My doctor has told me that I can participate in a survey concerning Accutane use in females by completing an additional form. INITIALS: ________

I now authorize Dr. ______________ to begin my treatment with Accutane.

____
Patient, Parent or Guardian — Date

____
Address

____

____
Telephone Number

I have fully explained to the patient, ____________, the nature and purpose of the treatment described above and the risks to females of childbearing potential. I have asked the patient if she has any questions regarding her treatment with Accutane and have answered those questions to the best of my ability.

____
Physician — Date

Revised: February 1995

Shown in Product Identification Guide, page 331

ANCOBON® ℞

[an 'co-bon]

brand of flucytosine

CAPSULES

The following text is complete prescribing information based on official labeling in effect June 1996.

> **WARNING**
>
> **Use with extreme caution in patients with impaired renal function. Close monitoring of hematologic, renal and hepatic status of all patients is essential. These instructions should be thoroughly reviewed before administration of Ancobon.**

DESCRIPTION

Ancobon (flucytosine), an antifungal agent, is available as 250-mg and 500-mg capsules for oral administration. Each capsule also contains corn starch, lactose and talc. Gelatin capsule shells contain parabens (butyl, methyl, propyl) and sodium propionate, with the following dye systems: 250-mg capsules—black iron oxide, FD&C Blue No. 1, FD&C Yellow No. 6, D&C Yellow No. 10 and titanium dioxide; 500-mg capsules—black iron oxide and titanium dioxide. Chemically, flucytosine is 5-fluorocytosine, a fluorinated pyrimidine which is related to fluorouracil and floxuridine. It is a white to off-white crystalline powder with a molecular weight of 129.09.

CLINICAL PHARMACOLOGY

Flucytosine is rapidly and virtually completely absorbed following oral administration. Bioavailability estimated by comparing the area under the curve of serum concentrations after oral and intravenous administration showed 78% to 89% absorption of the oral dose. Peak blood concentrations of 30 to 40 mcg/mL were reached within 2 hours of administration of a 2-gm oral dose to normal subjects. The mean blood concentrations were approximately 70 to 80 mcg/mL 1 to 2 hours after a dose in patients with normal renal function who received a 6-week regimen of flucytosine (150 mg/kg/day given in divided doses every 6 hours) in combination with amphotericin B. The half-life in the majority of normal subjects ranged between 2.4 and 4.8 hours. Flucytosine is excreted via the kidneys by means of glomerular filtration without significant tubular reabsorption. More than 90% of the total radioactivity after oral administration was recovered in the urine as intact drug. Approximately 1% of the dose is present in the urine as the α-fluoro-β-ureido-propionic acid metabolite. A small portion of the dose is excreted in the feces.

The half-life of flucytosine is prolonged in patients with renal insufficiency; the average half-life in nephrectomized or anuric patients was 85 hours (range: 29.9 to 250 hours). A linear correlation was found between the elimination rate constant of flucytosine and creatinine clearance.

In vitro studies have shown that 2.9% to 4% of flucytosine is protein-bound over the range of therapeutic concentrations found in the blood. Flucytosine readily penetrates the blood-brain barrier, achieving clinically significant concentrations in cerebrospinal fluid. Studies in pregnant rats have shown that flucytosine injected intraperitoneally crosses the placental barrier (see PRECAUTIONS).

Microbiology

Flucytosine has in vitro and in vivo activity against Candida and Cryptococcus. Although the exact mode of action is unknown, it has been proposed that flucytosine acts directly on fungal organisms by competitive inhibition of purine and pyrimidine uptake and indirectly by intracellular metabolism to 5-fluorouracil. Flucytosine enters the fungal cell via cytosine permease; thus, flucytosine is metabolized to 5-fluorouracil within fungal organisms. The 5-fluorouracil is extensively incorporated into fungal RNA and inhibits synthesis of both DNA and RNA. The result is unbalanced growth and death of the fungal organism. Antifungal synergism between Ancobon and polyene antibiotics, particularly amphotericin B, has been reported.

Actions

Flucytosine has in vitro and in vivo activity against Candida and Cryptococcus. The exact mode of action against these fungi is not known. Ancobon is not metabolized significantly when given orally to man.

Susceptibility

Cryptococcus: Most strains initially isolated from clinical material have shown flucytosine minimal inhibitory concentrations (MIC's) ranging from .46 to 7.8 mcg/mL. Any isolate with an MIC greater than 12.5 mcg/mL is considered resistant. In vitro resistance has developed in originally susceptible strains during therapy. It is recommended that clinical cultures for susceptibility testing be taken initially and at weekly intervals during therapy. The initial culture should be reserved as a reference in susceptibility testing of subsequent isolates.

Candida: As high as 40% to 50% of the pretreatment clinical isolates of Candida have been reported to be resistant to flucytosine. It is recommended that susceptibility studies be performed as early as possible and be repeated during therapy. An MIC value greater than 100 mcg/mL is considered resistant.

Interference with in vitro activity of flucytosine occurs in complex or semisynthetic media. In order to rely upon the recommended in vitro interpretations of susceptibility, it is essential that the broth medium and the testing procedure used be that described by Shadomy.[1]

INDICATIONS AND USAGE

Ancobon is indicated only in the treatment of serious infections caused by susceptible strains of Candida and/or Cryptococcus. *Candida:* Septicemia, endocarditis and urinary system infections have been effectively treated with flucytosine. Limited trials in pulmonary infections justify the use of flucytosine. *Cryptococcus:* Meningitis and pulmonary infections have been treated effectively. Studies in septicemias and urinary tract infections are limited, but good responses have been reported.

CONTRAINDICATIONS

Ancobon should not be used in patients with a known hypersensitivity to the drug.

WARNINGS

Ancobon must be given with extreme caution to patients with impaired renal function. Since Ancobon is excreted primarily by the kidneys, renal impairment may lead to accumulation of the drug. Ancobon blood concentrations should be monitored to determine the adequacy of renal excretion in such patients.[1] Dosage adjustments should be made in patients with renal insufficiency to prevent progressive accumulation of active drug.

Ancobon must be given with extreme caution to patients with bone marrow depression. Patients may be more prone to depression of bone marrow function if they: 1) have a hematologic disease, 2) are being treated with radiation or drugs which depress bone marrow, or 3) have a history of treatment with such drugs or radiation. Frequent monitoring of hepatic function and of the hematopoietic system is indicated during therapy.

PRECAUTIONS

General: Before therapy with Ancobon is instituted, electrolytes (because of hypokalemia) and the hematologic and renal status of the patient should be determined (see WARNINGS). Close monitoring of the patient during therapy is essential.

Laboratory Tests: Since renal impairment can cause progressive accumulation of the drug, blood concentrations and kidney function should be monitored during therapy. Hematologic status (leucocyte and thrombocyte count) and liver function (alkaline phosphatase, SGOT and SGPT) should be determined at frequent intervals during treatment as indicated.

Drug Interactions: Cytosine arabinoside, a cytostatic agent, has been reported to inactivate the antifungal activity of Ancobon by competitive inhibition. Drugs which impair glomerular filtration may prolong the biological half-life of flucytosine. Antifungal synergism between Ancobon and polyene antibiotics, particularly amphotericin B, has been reported.

Drug/Laboratory Test Interactions: Measurement of serum creatinine levels should be determined by the Jaffe method, since Ancobon does not interfere with the determination of creatinine values by this method, as it does when the dry-slide enzymatic method with the Kodak Ektachem analyzer is used.

Carcinogenesis, Mutagenesis, Impairment of Fertility: Ancobon has not undergone adequate animal testing to evaluate carcinogenic potential. The mutagenic potential of Ancobon was evaluated in Ames-type studies with five different mutants of *S. typhimurium* and no mutagenicity was detected in the presence or absence of activating enzymes. Ancobon was nonmutagenic in three different repair assay systems.

There have been no adequate trials in animals on the effects of Ancobon on fertility or reproductive performance. The fertility and reproductive performance of the offspring (F_1 generation) of mice treated with 100, 200 or 400 mg/kg/day of flucytosine on days 7 to 13 of gestation was studied; the *in utero* treatment had no adverse effect on the fertility or reproductive performance of the offspring.

Pregnancy: Teratogenic Effects. Pregnancy Category C. Ancobon has been shown to be teratogenic in the rat and mouse at doses of 40 mg/kg/day (ie, 0.27 times the maximum recommended human dose). There are no adequate and well-controlled studies in pregnant women. Ancobon should be used during pregnancy only if the potential benefit justifies the potential risk to the fetus.

The teratogenicity of Ancobon is apparently species-related. Although there is confirmation of rat teratogenicity in the published literature, three studies in the mouse and studies in the rabbit and monkey have failed to reveal a teratogenic liability.

Nursing Mothers: It is not known whether this drug is excreted in human milk. Because many drugs are excreted in human milk and because of the potential for serious adverse reactions in nursing infants from Ancobon, a decision should be made whether to discontinue nursing or to discontinue the drug, taking into account the importance of the drug to the mother.

Pediatric Use: Safety and effectiveness in children have not been established.

ADVERSE REACTIONS

The adverse reactions which have occurred during treatment with Ancobon are grouped according to organ system affected.

Cardiovascular: Cardiac arrest.

Respiratory: Respiratory arrest, chest pain, dyspnea.

Dermatologic: Rash, pruritus, urticaria, photosensitivity.

Gastrointestinal: Nausea, emesis, abdominal pain, diarrhea, anorexia, dry mouth, duodenal ulcer, gastrointestinal hemorrhage, hepatic dysfunction, jaundice, ulcerative colitis, bilirubin elevation.

Genitourinary: Azotemia, creatinine and BUN elevation, crystalluria, renal failure.

Hematologic: Anemia, agranulocytosis, aplastic anemia, eosinophilia, leukopenia, pancytopenia, thrombocytopenia.

Neurologic: Ataxia, hearing loss, headache, paresthesia, parkinsonism, peripheral neuropathy, pyrexia, vertigo, sedation.

Psychiatric: Confusion, hallucinations, psychosis.

Miscellaneous: Fatigue, hypoglycemia, hypokalemia, weakness.

OVERDOSAGE

There is no experience with intentional overdosage. It is reasonable to expect that overdosage may produce pronounced manifestations of the known clinical adverse reactions. Prolonged serum concentrations in excess of 100 mcg/mL may be associated with an increased incidence of toxicity, especially gastrointestinal (diarrhea, nausea, vomiting), hematologic (leukopenia, thrombocytopenia) and hepatic (hepatitis).

In the management of overdosage, prompt gastric lavage or the use of an emetic is recommended. Adequate fluid intake should be maintained, by the intravenous route if necessary, since Ancobon is excreted unchanged via the renal tract. The hematologic parameters should be monitored frequently; liver and kidney function should be carefully monitored. Should any abnormalities appear in any of these parameters, appropriate therapeutic measures should be instituted. Since hemodialysis has been shown to rapidly reduce serum concentrations in anuric patients, this method may be considered in the management of overdosage.

DOSAGE AND ADMINISTRATION

The usual dosage of Ancobon is 50 to 150 mg/kg/day administered in divided doses at 6-hour intervals. Nausea or vomiting may be reduced or avoided if the capsules are given a few at a time over a 15-minute period. If the BUN or the serum creatinine is elevated, or if there are other signs of renal impairment, the initial dose should be at the lower level (see WARNINGS).

HOW SUPPLIED

Capsules, 250 mg (gray and green), imprinted ANCOBON® 250 ROCHE; bottles of 100 (NDC 0004-0077-01). *Capsules,* 500 mg (gray and white), imprinted ANCOBON® 500 ROCHE, bottles of 100 (NDC 0004-0079-01).

REFERENCE

1. Shadomy S: *Appl Microbiol.* June 1969, 17: 871–877.

Revised: June 1994

Shown in Product Identification Guide, page 331

BACTRIM™ ℞

[bac'trim]

brand of trimethoprim and sulfamethoxazole

IV INFUSION

The following text is complete prescribing information based on official labeling in effect June 1996.

DESCRIPTION

Bactrim (trimethoprim and sulfamethoxazole) IV Infusion, a sterile solution for intravenous infusion only, is a synthetic antibacterial combination product. Each 5 mL contains 80 mg trimethoprim (16 mg/mL) and 400 mg sulfamethoxazole (80 mg/mL) compounded with 40% propylene glycol, 10% ethyl alcohol and 0.3% diethanolamine; 1% benzyl alcohol and 0.1% sodium metabisulfite added as preservatives, water for injection, and pH adjusted to approximately 10 with sodium hydroxide.

Trimethoprim is 2,4-diamino-5-(3,4,5-trimethoxybenzyl)pyrimidine. It is a white to light yellow, odorless, bitter compound with a molecular weight of 290.3.

Sulfamethoxazole is N^1-(5-methyl-3-isoxazolyl)sulfanilamide. It is an almost white, odorless, tasteless compound with a molecular weight of 253.28.

CLINICAL PHARMACOLOGY

Following a 1-hour intravenous infusion of a single dose of 160 mg trimethoprim and 800 mg sulfamethoxazole to 11 patients whose weight ranged from 105 lbs to 165 lbs (mean, 143 lbs), the peak plasma concentrations of trimethoprim and sulfamethoxazole were 3.4 ± 0.3 μg/mL and 46.3 ± 2.7 μg/mL, respectively. Following repeated intravenous administration of the same dose at 8-hour intervals, the mean plasma concentrations just prior to and immediately after each infusion at steady state were 5.6 ± 0.6 μg/mL and 8.8 ± 0.9 μg/mL for trimethoprim and 70.6 ± 7.3 μg/mL and 105.6 ± 10.9 μg/mL for sulfamethoxazole. The mean plasma half-life was 11.3 ± 0.7 hours for trimethoprim and 12.8 ± 1.8 hours for sulfamethoxazole. All of these 11 patients had normal renal function, and their ages ranged from 17 to 78 years (median, 60 years).[1]

Pharmacokinetic studies in children and adults suggest an age-dependent half-life of trimethoprim, as indicated in the following table.[2]

Age (years)	No. of Patients	Mean TMP Half-life (hours)
<1	2	7.67
1–10	9	5.49
10–20	5	8.19
20–63	6	12.82

Patients with severely impaired renal function exhibit an increase in the half-lives of both components, requiring dosage regimen adjustment (See DOSAGE AND ADMINISTRATION section).

Both trimethoprim and sulfamethoxazole exist in the blood as unbound, protein-bound and metabolized forms; sulfamethaxazole also exists as the conjugated form. The metabolism of sulfamethoxazole occurs predominately by N_4-acetylation, although the glucuronide conjugate has been identified. The principal metabolites of trimethoprim are the 1- and 3-oxides and the 3′- and 4′-hydroxy derivatives. The free forms of trimethoprim and sulfamethoxazole are considered to be the therapeutically active forms. Approximately 44% of trimethoprim and 70% of sulfamethoxazole are bound to plasma proteins. The presence of 10 mg percent sulfamethoxazole in plasma decreases the protein binding of trimethoprim by an insignificant degree; trimethoprim does not influence the protein binding of sulfamethoxazole.

Excretion of trimethoprim and sulfamethoxazole is primarily by the kidneys through both glomerular filtration and tubular secretion. Urine concentrations of both trimethoprim and sulfamethoxazole are considerably higher than are the concentrations in the blood. The percent of dose excreted in urine over a 12-hour period following the intravenous administration of the first dose of 240 mg of trimethoprim and 1200 mg of sulfamethoxazole on day 1 ranged from 17% to 42.4% as free trimethoprim; 7% to 12.7% as free sulfamethoxazole; and 36.7% to 56% as total (free plus the N_4-acetylated metabolite) sulfamethoxazole. When administered together as Bactrim, neither trimethoprim nor sulfamethoxazole affects the urinary excretion pattern of the other. Both trimethoprim and sulfamethoxazole distribute to sputum and vaginal fluid; trimethoprim also distributes to bronchial secretions, and both pass the placental barrier and are excreted in breast milk.

Microbiology: Sulfamethoxazole inhibits bacterial synthesis of dihydrofolic acid by competing with *para*-aminobenzoic acid (PABA). Trimethoprim blocks the production of tetrahydrofolic acid from dihydrofolic acid by binding to and reversibly inhibiting the required enzyme, dihydrofolate reductase. Thus, Bactrim blocks two consecutive steps in the biosynthesis of nucleic acids and proteins essential to many bacteria.

In vitro studies have shown that bacterial resistance develops more slowly with Bactrim than with either trimethoprim or sulfamethoxazole alone.

In vitro serial dilution tests have shown that the spectrum of antibacterial activity of Bactrim includes common bacterial pathogens with the exception of *Pseudomonas aeruginosa.* The following organisms are usually susceptible: *Escherichia coli, Klebsiella* species, *Enterobacter* species, *Morganella morganii, Proteus mirabilis,* indole-positive *Proteus* species including *Proteus vulgaris, Haemophilus influenzae* (including ampicillin-resistant strains), *Streptococcus pneumoniae, Shigella flexneri* and *Shigella sonnei.* It should be noted, however, that there are little clinical data on the use of Bactrim IV Infusion in serious systemic infections due to *Haemophilus influenzae* and *Streptococcus pneumoniae.*

[See table above.]

REPRESENTATIVE MINIMUM INHIBITORY CONCENTRATION VALUES FOR BACTRIM-SUSCEPTIBLE ORGANISMS (MIC—μg/mL)

Bacteria	TMP alone	SMX alone	TMP/SMX (1:20) TMP	TMP/SMX (1:20) SMX
Escherichia coli	0.05–1.5	1.0–245	0.05–0.5	0.95–9.5
Proteus species (indole positive)	0.5– 5.0	7.35–300	0.05–1.5	0.95– 28.5
Morganella morganii	0.5–5.0	7.35–300	0.05–1.5	0.95–28.5
Proteus mirabilis	0.5–1.5	7.35–30	0.05–0.15	0.95–2.85
Klebsiella species	0.15–5.0	2.45–245	0.05–1.5	0.95–28.5
Enterobacter species	0.15–5.0	2.45–245	0.05–1.5	0.95–28.5
Haemophilus influenzae	0.15–1.5	2.85–95	0.015–0.15	0.285–2.85
Streptococcus pneumoniae	0.15–1.5	7.35–24.5	0.05–0.15	0.95–2.85
*Shigella flexneri**	<0.01–0.04	<0.16–>320	<0.002–0.03	0.04–0.625
*Shigella sonnei**	0.02– 0.08	0.625–>320	0.004–0.06	0.08– 1.25

TMP = trimethoprim   SMX = sulfamethoxazole

*Rudoy RC, Nelson JD, Haltalin KC. *Antimicrob Agents Chemother.* May 1974;5:439–443.

The recommended quantitative disc susceptibility method may be used for estimating the susceptibility of bacteria to Bactrim.[3,4] With this procedure, a report from the laboratory of "Susceptible to trimethoprim and sulfamethoxazole" indicates that the infection is likely to respond to therapy with Bactrim. If the infection is confined to the urine, a report of "Intermediate susceptibility to trimethoprim and sulfamethoxazole" also indicates that the infection is likely to respond. A report of "Resistant to trimethoprim and sulfamethoxazole" indicates that the infection is unlikely to respond to therapy with Bactrim.

INDICATIONS AND USAGE

Pneumocystis Carinii Pneumonia: Bactrim IV Infusion is indicated in the treatment of *Pneumocystis carinii* pneumonia in children and adults.

Shigellosis: Bactrim IV Infusion is indicated in the treatment of enteritis caused by susceptible strains of *Shigella flexneri* and *Shigella sonnei* in children and adults.

Urinary Tract Infections: Bactrim IV Infusion is indicated in the treatment of severe or complicated urinary tract infections due to susceptible strains of *Escherichia coli, Klebsiella* species, *Enterobacter* species, *Morganella morganii* and *Proteus* species when oral administration of Bactrim is not feasible and when the organism is not susceptible to single-agent antibacterials effective in the urinary tract.

Although appropriate culture and susceptibility studies should be performed, therapy may be started while awaiting the results of these studies.

CONTRAINDICATIONS

Bactrim is contraindicated in patients with a known hypersensitivity to trimethoprim or sulfonamides and in patients with documented megaloblastic anemia due to folate deficiency. Bactrim is also contraindicated in pregnant patients and nursing mothers, because sulfonamides pass the placenta and are excreted in the milk and may cause kernicterus. Bactrim is contraindicated in infants less than 2 months of age.

WARNINGS

FATALITIES ASSOCIATED WITH THE ADMINISTRATION OF SULFONAMIDES, ALTHOUGH RARE, HAVE OCCURRED DUE TO SEVERE REACTIONS, INCLUDING STEVENS-JOHNSON SYNDROME, TOXIC EPIDERMAL NECROLYSIS, FULMINANT HEPATIC NECROSIS, AGRANULOCYTOSIS, APLASTIC ANEMIA AND OTHER BLOOD DYSCRASIAS.

Continued on next page

Roche Laboratories—Cont.

BACTRIM SHOULD BE DISCONTINUED AT THE FIRST APPEARANCE OF SKIN RASH OR ANY SIGN OF ADVERSE REACTION. Clinical signs, such as rash, sore throat, fever, arthralgia, cough, shortness of breath, pallor, purpura or jaundice may be early indications of serious reactions. In rare instances a skin rash may be followed by more severe reactions, such as Stevens-Johnson syndrome, toxic epidermal necrolysis, hepatic necrosis or serious blood disorder. Complete blood counts should be done frequently in patients receiving sulfonamides.

BACTRIM SHOULD NOT BE USED IN THE TREATMENT OF STREPTOCOCCAL PHARYNGITIS. Clinical studies have documented that patients with group A β-hemolytic streptococcal tonsillopharyngitis have a greater incidence of bacteriologic failure when treated with Bactrim than do those patients treated with penicillin, as evidenced by failure to eradicate this organism from the tonsillopharyngeal area.

Bactrim IV Infusion contains sodium metabisulfite, a sulfite that may cause allergic-type reactions, including anaphylactic symptoms and life-threatening or less severe asthmatic episodes in certain susceptible people. The overall prevalence of sulfite sensitivity in the general population is unknown and probably low. Sulfite sensitivity is seen more frequently in asthmatic than in nonasthmatic people.

PRECAUTIONS

General: Bactrim should be given with caution to patients with impaired renal or hepatic function, to those with possible folate deficiency (eg, the elderly, chronic alcoholics, patients receiving anticonvulsant therapy, patients with malabsorption syndrome, and patients in malnutrition states) and to those with severe allergies or bronchial asthma. In glucose-6-phosphate dehydrogenase deficient individuals, hemolysis may occur. This reaction is frequently dose-related.

Local irritation and inflammation due to extravascular infiltration of the infusion have been observed with Bactrim IV Infusion. If these occur the infusion should be discontinued and restarted at another site.

Use in the Elderly: There may be an increased risk of severe adverse reactions in elderly patients, particularly when complicating conditions exist, eg, impaired kidney and/or liver function, or concomitant use of other drugs. Severe skin reactions, generalized bone marrow suppression (see WARNINGS and ADVERSE REACTIONS sections) or a specific decrease in platelets (with or without purpura) are the most frequently reported severe adverse reactions in elderly patients. In those concurrently receiving certain diuretics, primarily thiazides, an increased incidence of thrombocytopenia with purpura has been reported. Appropriate dosage adjustments should be made for patients with impaired kidney function (see DOSAGE AND ADMINISTRATION section).

Use in the Treatment of Pneumocystis Carinii Pneumonia in Patients with Acquired Immunodeficiency Syndrome (AIDS): AIDS patients may not tolerate or respond to Bactrim in the same manner as non-AIDS patients. The incidence of side effects, particularly rash, fever, leukopenia, and elevated aminotransferase (transaminase) values, with Bactrim therapy in AIDS patients who are being treated for *Pneumocystis carinii* pneumonia has been reported to be greatly increased compared with the incidence normally associated with the use of Bactrim in non-AIDS patients.

Laboratory Tests: Appropriate culture and susceptibility studies should be performed before and throughout treatment. Complete blood counts should be done frequently in patients receiving Bactrim; if a significant reduction in the count of any formed blood element is noted, Bactrim should be discontinued. Urinalyses with careful microscopic examination and renal function tests should be performed during therapy, particularly for those patients with impaired renal function.

Drug Interactions: In elderly patients concurrently receiving certain diuretics, primarily thiazides, an increased incidence of thrombocytopenia with purpura has been reported.

It has been reported that Bactrim may prolong the prothrombin time in patients who are receiving the anticoagulant warfarin. This interaction should be kept in mind when Bactrim is given to patients already on anticoagulant therapy, and the coagulation time should be reassessed.

Bactrim may inhibit the hepatic metabolism of phenytoin. Bactrim, given at a common clinical dosage, increased the phenytoin half-life by 39% and decreased the phenytoin metabolic clearance rate by 27%. When administering these drugs concurrently, one should be alert for possible excessive phenytoin effect.

Sulfonamides can also displace methotrexate from plasma protein binding sites, thus increasing free methotrexate concentrations.

Drug/Laboratory Test Interactions: Bactrim, specifically the trimethoprim component, can interfere with a serum methotrexate assay as determined by the competitive binding protein technique (CBPA) when a bacterial dihydrofolate reductase is used as the binding protein. No interference occurs, however, if methotrexate is measured by a radioimmunoassay (RIA).

The presence of trimethoprim and sulfamethoxazole may also interfere with the Jaffé alkaline picrate reaction assay for creatinine, resulting in overestimations of about 10% in the range of normal values.

Carcinogenesis, Mutagenesis, Impairment of Fertility:

Carcinogenesis: Long-term studies in animals to evaluate carcinogenic potential have not been conducted with Bactrim IV Infusion.

Mutagenesis: Bacterial mutagenic studies have not been performed with sulfamethoxazole and trimethoprim in combination. Trimethoprim was demonstrated to be nonmutagenic in the Ames assay. No chromosomal damage was observed in human leukocytes cultured in vitro with sulfamethoxazole and trimethoprim alone or in combination; the concentrations used exceeded blood levels of these compounds following therapy with Bactrim. Observations of leukocytes obtained from patients treated with Bactrim revealed no chromosomal abnormalities.

Impairment of Fertility: Bactrim IV Infusion has not been studied in animals for evidence of impairment of fertility. However, studies in rats at oral dosages as high as 70 mg/kg trimethoprim plus 350 mg/kg sulfamethoxazole daily showed no adverse effects on fertility or general reproductive performance.

Pregnancy: Teratogenic Effects: Pregnancy Category C. In rats, oral doses of 533 mg/kg sulfamethoxazole or 200 mg/kg trimethoprim produced teratological effects manifested mainly as cleft palates.

The highest dose which did not cause cleft palates in rats was 512 mg/kg sulfamethoxazole or 192 mg/kg trimethoprim when administered separately. In two studies in rats, no teratology was observed when 512 mg/kg of sulfamethoxazole was used in combination with 128 mg/kg of trimethoprim. In one study, however, cleft palates were observed in one litter out of 9 when 355 mg/kg of sulfamethoxazole was used in combination with 88 mg/kg of trimethoprim.

In some rabbit studies, an overall increase in fetal loss (dead and resorbed and malformed conceptuses) was associated with doses of trimethoprim six times the human therapeutic dose.

While there are no large, well-controlled studies on the use of trimethoprim and sulfamethoxazole in pregnant women, Brumfitt and Pursell,[5] in a retrospective study, reported the outcome of 186 pregnancies during which the mother received either placebo or oral trimethoprim and sulfamethoxazole. The incidence of congenital abnormalities was 4.5% (3 of 66) in those who received placebo and 3.3% (4 of 120) in those receiving trimethoprim and sulfamethoxazole. There were no abnormalities in the 10 children whose mothers received the drug during the first trimester. In a separate survey, Brumfitt and Pursell also found no congenital abnormalities in 35 children whose mothers had received oral trimethoprim and sulfamethoxazole at the time of conception or shortly thereafter.

Because trimethoprim and sulfamethoxazole may interfere with folic acid metabolism, Bactrim IV Infusion should be used during pregnancy only if the potential benefit justifies the potential risk to the fetus.

Nonteratogenic Effects: See CONTRAINDICATIONS section.

Nursing Mothers: See CONTRAINDICATIONS section.

Pediatric Use: Bactrim IV Infusion is not recommended for infants younger than two months of age (see CONTRAINDICATIONS section).

ADVERSE REACTIONS

The most common adverse effects are gastrointestinal disturbances (nausea, vomiting, anorexia) and allergic skin reactions (such as rash and urticaria). **FATALITIES ASSOCIATED WITH THE ADMINISTRATION OF SULFONAMIDES, ALTHOUGH RARE, HAVE OCCURRED DUE TO SEVERE REACTIONS, INCLUDING STEVENS-JOHNSON SYNDROME, TOXIC EPIDERMAL NECROLYSIS, FULMINANT HEPATIC NECROSIS, AGRANULOCYTOSIS, APLASTIC ANEMIA AND OTHER BLOOD DYSCRASIAS (SEE WARNINGS SECTION).** Local reaction, pain and slight irritation on IV administration are infrequent. Thrombophlebitis has rarely been observed.

Hematologic: Agranulocytosis, aplastic anemia, thrombocytopenia, leukopenia, neutropenia, hemolytic anemia, megaloblastic anemia, hypoprothrombinemia, methemoglobinemia, eosinophilia.

Allergic Reactions: Stevens-Johnson syndrome, toxic epidermal necrolysis, anaphylaxis, allergic myocarditis, erythema multiforme, exfoliative dermatitis, angioedema, drug fever, chills, Henoch-Schoenlein purpura, serum sickness-like syndrome, generalized allergic reactions, generalized skin eruptions, conjunctival and scleral injection, photosensitivity, pruritus, urticaria and rash. In addition, periarteritis nodosa and systemic lupus erythematosus have been reported.

Gastrointestinal: Hepatitis (including cholestatic jaundice and hepatic necrosis), elevation of serum transaminase and bilirubin, pseudomembraneous enterocolitis, pancreatitis, stomatitis, glossitis, nausea, emesis, abdominal pain, diarrhea, anorexia.

Genitourinary: Renal failure, interstitial nephritis, BUN and serum creatinine elevation, toxic nephrosis with oliguria and anuria, and crystalluria.

Neurologic: Aseptic meningitis, convulsions, peripheral neuritis, ataxia, vertigo, tinnitus, headache.

Psychiatric: Hallucinations, depression, apathy, nervousness.

Endocrine: The sulfonamides bear certain chemical similarities to some goitrogens, diuretics (acetazolamide and the thiazides) and oral hypoglycemic agents. Cross-sensitivity may exist with these agents. Diuresis and hypoglycemia have occurred rarely in patients receiving sulfonamides.

Musculoskeletal: Arthralgia and myalgia.

Respiratory: Pulmonary infiltrates.

Miscellaneous: Weakness, fatigue, insomnia.

OVERDOSAGE

Acute: Since there has been no extensive experience in humans with single doses of Bactrim IV Infusion in excess of 25 mL (400 mg trimethoprim and 2000 mg sulfamethoxazole), the maximum tolerated dose in humans is unknown. Signs and symptoms of overdosage reported with sulfonamides include anorexia, colic, nausea, vomiting, dizziness, headache, drowsiness and unconsciousness. Pyrexia, hematuria and crystalluria may be noted. Blood dyscrasias and jaundice are potential late manifestations of overdosage.

Signs of acute overdosage with trimethoprim include nausea, vomiting, dizziness, headache, mental depression, confusion and bone marrow depression.

General principles of treatment include the administration of intraveneous fluids if urine output is low and renal function is normal. Acidification of the urine will increase renal elimination of trimethoprim. The patient should be monitored with blood counts and appropriate blood chemistries, including electrolytes. If a significant blood dyscrasia or jaundice occurs, specific therapy should be instituted for these complications. Peritoneal dialysis is not effective and hemodialysis is only moderately effective in eliminating trimethoprim and sulfamethoxazole.

Chronic: Use of Bactrim IV Infusion at high doses and/or for extended periods of time may cause bone marrow depression manifested as thrombocytopenia, leukopenia and/or megaloblastic anemia. If signs of bone marrow depression occur, the patient should be given leucovorin 5 to 15 mg daily until normal hematopoiesis is restored.

Animal Toxicity: The LD_{50} of Bactrim IV Infusion in mice is 700 mg/kg or 7.3 mL/kg; in rats and rabbits the LD_{50} is > 500 mg/kg or > 5.2 mL/kg. The vehicle produced the same LD_{50} in each of these species as the active drug.

The signs and symptoms noted in mice, rats and rabbits with Bactrim IV Infusion or its vehicle at the high IV doses used in acute toxicity studies included ataxia, decreased motor activity, loss of righting reflex, tremors or convulsions, and/or respiratory depression.

DOSAGE AND ADMINISTRATION

CONTRAINDICATED IN INFANTS LESS THAN 2 MONTHS OF AGE. CAUTION—BACTRIM IV INFUSION MUST BE DILUTED IN 5% DEXTROSE IN WATER SOLUTION PRIOR TO ADMINISTRATION. DO NOT MIX BACTRIM IV INFUSION WITH OTHER DRUGS OR SOLUTIONS. RAPID INFUSION OR BOLUS INJECTION MUST BE AVOIDED.

Dosage:

CHILDREN AND ADULTS:

Pneumocystis Carinii Pneumonia: Total daily dose is 15 to 20 mg/kg (based on the trimethoprim component) given in 3 or 4 equally divided doses every 6 to 8 hours for up to 14 days. One investigator noted that a total daily dose of 10 to 15 mg/kg was sufficient in 10 adult patients with normal renal function.[6]

Severe Urinary Tract Infections and Shigellosis: Total daily dose is 8 to 10 mg/kg (based on the trimethoprim component) given in 2 or 4 equally divided doses every 6, 8 or 12 hours for up to 14 days for severe urinary tract infections and 5 days for shigellosis. The maximum recommended daily dose is 60 mL per day.

For Patients with Impaired Renal Function: When renal function is impaired, a reduced dosage should be employed using the following table:

Creatinine Clearance (mL/min)	Recommended Dosage Regimen
Above 30	Usual standard regimen
15–30	1/2 the usual regimen
Below 15	Use not recommended

Method of Preparation: Bactrim IV Infusion must be diluted. EACH 5 ML SHOULD BE ADDED TO 125 ML OF 5% DEXTROSE IN WATER. After diluting with 5% dextrose in water the solution should not be refrigerated and should be

REPRESENTATIVE MINIMUM INHIBITORY CONCENTRATION VALUES FOR BACTRIM-SUSCEPTIBLE ORGANISMS
(MIC—μg/mL)

Bacteria	TMP alone	SMX alone	TMP/SMX (1:20) TMP	TMP/SMX (1:20) SMX
Escherichia coli	0.05–1.5	1.0– 245	0.05– 0.5	0.95–9.5
Escherichia coli (enterotoxigenic strains)	0.015– 0.15	0.285– > 950	0.005–0.15	0.095– 2.85
Proteus species (indole positive)	0.5– 5.0	7.35–300	0.05–1.5	0.95– 28.5
Morganella morganii	0.5–5.0	7.35– 300	0.05– 1.5	0.95–28.5
Proteus mirabilis	0.5–1.5	7.35– 30	0.05– 0.15	0.95–2.85
Klebsiella species	0.15–5.0	2.45– 245	0.05– 1.5	0.95–28.5
Enterobacter species	0.15–5.0	2.45– 245	0.05– 1.5	0.95–28.5
Haemophilus influenzae	0.15–1.5	2.85– 95	0.015– 0.15	0.285–2.85
Streptococcus pneumoniae	0.15–1.5	7.35– 24.5	0.05– 0.15	0.95–2.85
*Shigella flexneri**	< 0.01–0.04	< 0.16– > 320	< 0.002– 0.03	0.04–0.625
*Shigella sonnei**	0.02–0.08	0.625– > 320	0.004–0.06	0.08–1.25

TMP = trimethoprim SMX = sulfamethoxazole
*Rudoy RC, Nelson JD, Haltalin KC. *Antimicrob Agents Chemother.* May 1974;5:439–443.

used within 6 hours. If a dilution of 5 mL per 100 mL of 5% dextrose in water is desired, it should be used within 4 hours. If upon visual inspection there is cloudiness or evidence of crystallization after mixing, the solution should be discarded and a fresh solution prepared.

Multidose Vials: After initial entry into the vial, the remaining contents must be used within 48 hours.

The following infusion systems have been tested and found satisfactory: unit-dose glass containers; unit-dose polyvinyl chloride and polyolefin containers. No other systems have been tested and therefore no others can be recommended.

Dilution: EACH 5 ML OF BACTRIM IV INFUSION SHOULD BE ADDED TO 125 ML OF 5% DEXTROSE IN WATER.

Note: In those instances where fluid restriction is desirable, each 5 mL may be added to 75 mL of 5% dextrose in water. Under these circumstances the solution should be mixed just prior to use and should be administered within 2 hours. If upon visual inspection there is cloudiness or evidence of crystallization after mixing, the solution should be discarded and a fresh solution prepared.

DO NOT MIX BACTRIM IV INFUSION–5% DEXTROSE IN WATER WITH DRUGS OR SOLUTIONS IN THE SAME CONTAINER.

Administration: The solution should be given by intravenous infusion over a period of 60 to 90 minutes. Rapid infusion or bolus injection must be avoided. Bactrim IV Infusion should not be given intramuscularly.

HOW SUPPLIED

10-mL *Vials,* containing 160 mg trimethoprim (16 mg/mL) and 800 mg sulfamethoxazole (80 mg/mL) for infusion with 5% dextrose in water. Boxes of 10 (NDC 0004-1955-01).

30-mL *Multidose Vials,* each 5 mL containing 80 mg trimethoprim (16 mg/mL) and 400 mg sulfamethoxazole (80 mg/mL) for infusion with 5% dextrose in water. Boxes of 1 (NDC 0004-1958-01).

STORE AT ROOM TEMPERATURE (15°–30°C or 59°–86°F). DO NOT REFRIGERATE.

Bactrim is also available as *DS (double strength) Tablets* (white, notched, capsule shaped), containing 160 mg trimethoprim and 800 mg sulfamethoxazole—bottles of 100 (NDC 0004-0117-01), 250 (NDC 0004-0117-04) and 500 (NDC 0004-0117-14). Imprint on tablets: (front) BACTRIM-DS; (back) ROCHE.

Tablets (light green, scored, capsule shaped), containing 80 mg trimethoprim and 400 mg sulfamethoxazole—bottles of 100 (NDC 0004-0050-01). Imprint on tablets: (front) BACTRIM; (back) ROCHE.

Pediatric Suspension (pink, cherry flavored), containing 40 mg trimethoprim and 200 mg sulfamethoxazole per teaspoonful (5 mL)—bottles of 16 oz (1 pint) (NDC 0004-1033-28).

REFERENCES

1. Grose WE, Bodey GP, Loo TL. Clinical Pharmacology of Intravenously Administered Trimethoprim-Sulfamethoxazole. *Antimicrob Agents Chemother.* Mar 1979;15:447-451. 2. Siber GR, Gorham C, Durbin W, Lesko L, Levin MJ. Pharmacology of Intravenous Trimethoprim-Sulfamethoxazole in Children and Adults. *Current Chemotherapy and Infectious Diseases.* American Society for Microbiology, Washington, D.C., 1980, Vol. 1, pp. 691-692. 3. Bauer AW, Kirby WMM, Sherris JC, Turck M. Antibiotic Susceptibility Testing by a Standardized Single Disk Method. *Am J Clin Pathol.* Apr 1966;45:493-496. 4. National Committee for Clinical Laboratory Standards. *Performance Standards for Antimicrobial Disc Susceptibility Test.* 771 East Lancaster Avenue, Villanova, Pennsylvania 19085: Approved Standard ASM-2. 5. Brumfitt W, Pursell R. Trimethoprim/Sulfamethoxazole in the Treatment of Bacteriuria in Women. *J Infect Dis.* Nov 1973;128 (Suppl):S657-S663. 6. Winston DJ, Lau WK, Gale RP, Young LS. Trimethoprim-Sulfamethoxazole for the Treatment of *Pneumocystis carinii* pneumonia. *Ann Intern Med.* June 1980;92:762-769.

Revised: March 1994.

BACTRIM™ ℞

[*bac'trim*]
brand of trimethoprim and sulfamethoxazole
DS (double strength) Tablets,
Tablets
and
Pediatric Suspension

The following text is complete prescribing information based on official labeling in effect June 1996.

DESCRIPTION

Bactrim (trimethoprim and sulfamethoxazole) is a synthetic antibacterial combination product available in DS (double strength) tablets, tablets and pediatric suspension for oral administration. Each DS tablet contains 160 mg trimethoprim and 800 mg sulfamethoxazole plus magnesium stearate, pregelatinized starch and sodium starch glycolate. Each tablet contains 80 mg trimethoprim and 400 mg sulfamethoxazole plus magnesium stearate, pregelatinized starch, sodium starch glycolate, FD&C Blue No. 1 lake, FD&C Yellow No. 6 lake and D&C Yellow No. 10 lake. Each teaspoonful (5 mL) of the pediatric suspension contains 40 mg trimethoprim and 200 mg sulfamethoxazole in a vehicle containing 0.3 percent alcohol, edetate disodium, glycerin, microcrystalline cellulose, parabens (methyl and propyl), polysorbate 80, saccharin sodium, simethicone, sorbitol, sucrose, FD&C Yellow No. 6, FD&C Red No. 40, flavors and water.

Trimethoprim is 2,4-diamino-5-(3,4,5-trimethoxybenzyl) pyrimidine. It is a white to light yellow, odorless, bitter compound with a molecular weight of 290.3.

Sulfamethoxazole is N^1-(5-methyl-3-isoxazolyl)sulfanilamide. It is almost white, odorless, tasteless compound with a molecular weight of 253.28.

CLINICAL PHARMACOLOGY

Bactrim is rapidly absorbed following oral administration. Both sulfamethoxazole and trimethoprim exist in the blood as unbound, protein-bound and metabolized forms; sulfamethoxazole also exists as the conjugated form. The metabolism of sulfamethoxazole occurs predominately by N_4-acetylation, although the glucuronide conjugate has been identified. The principal metabolites of trimethoprim are the 1- and 3-oxides and the 3′- and 4′- hydroxy derivatives. The free forms of sulfamethoxazole and trimethoprim are considered to be the therapeutically active forms. Approximately 44% of trimethoprim and 70% of sulfamethoxazole are bound to plasma proteins. The presence of 10 mg percent sulfamethoxazole in plasma decreases the protein binding of trimethoprim by an insignificant degree; trimethoprim does not influence the protein binding of sulfamethoxazole.

Peak blood levels for the individual components occur 1 to 4 hours after oral administration. The mean serum half-lives of sulfamethoxazole and trimethoprim are 10 and 8 to 10 hours, respectively. However, patients with severely impaired renal function exhibit an increase in the half-lives of both components, requiring dosage regimen adjustment (see DOSAGE AND ADMINISTRATION section). Detectable amounts of trimethoprim and sulfamethoxazole are present in the blood 24 hours after drug administration. During administration of 160 mg trimethoprim and 800 mg sulfamethoxazole bid, the mean steady-state plasma concentration of trimethoprim was 1.72 μg/mL. The steady-state mean plasma levels of free and total sulfamethoxazole were 57.4 μg/mL and 68.0 μg/mL, respectively. These steady-state levels were achieved after three days of drug administration.[1]

Excretion of sulfamethoxazole and trimethoprim is primarily by the kidneys through both glomerular filtration and tubular secretion. Urine concentrations of both sulfamethoxazole and trimethoprim are considerably higher than are the concentrations in the blood. The average percentage of the dose recovered in urine from 0 to 72 hours after a single oral dose of Bactrim is 84.5% for total sulfonamide and 66.8% for free trimethoprim. Thirty percent of the total sulfonamide is excreted as free sulfamethoxazole, with the remaining as N_4-acetylated metabolite.[2] When administered together as Bactrim, neither sulfamethoxazole nor trimethoprim affects the urinary excretion pattern of the other.

Both trimethoprim and sulfamethoxazole distribute to sputum, vaginal fluid and middle ear fluid; trimethoprim also distributes to bronchial secretion, and both pass the placental barrier and are excreted in breast milk.

Microbiology: Sulfamethoxazole inhibits bacterial synthesis of dihydrofolic acid by competing with *para*-aminobenzoic acid (PABA). Trimethoprim blocks the production of tetrahydrofolic acid from dihydrofolic acid by binding to and reversibly inhibiting the required enzyme, dihydrofolate reductase. Thus, Bactrim blocks two consecutive steps in the biosynthesis of nucleic acids and proteins essential to many bacteria.

In vitro studies have shown that bacterial resistance develops more slowly with Bactrim than with either trimethoprim or sulfamethoxazole alone.

In vitro serial dilution tests have shown that the spectrum of antibacterial activity of Bactrim includes the common urinary tract pathogens with the exception of *Pseudomonas aeruginosa.* The following organisms are usually susceptible: *Escherichia coli, Klebsiella* species, *Enterobacter* species, *Morganella morganii, Proteus mirabilis,* and indole-positive *Proteus* species including *Proteus vulgaris.* The usual spectrum of antimicrobial activity of Bactrim includes the following bacterial pathogens isolated from middle ear exudate and from bronchial secretions: *Haemophilus influenzae,* including ampicillin-resistant strains, and *Streptococcus pneumoniae. Shigella flexneri* and *Shigella sonnei* are usually susceptible. The usual spectrum also includes enterotoxigenic strains of *Escherichia coli* (ETEC) causing bacterial gastroenteritis.

[See table above.]

The recommended quantitative disc susceptibility method may be used for estimating the susceptibility of bacteria to Bactrim.[3,4] With this procedure, a report from the laboratory of "Susceptible to trimethoprim and sulfamethoxazole" indicates that the infection is likely to respond to therapy with Bactrim. If the infection is confined to the urine, a report of "Intermediate susceptibility to trimethoprim and sulfamethoxazole" also indicates that the infection is likely to respond. A report of "Resistant to trimethoprim and sulfamethoxazole" indicates that the infection is unlikely to respond to therapy with Bactrim.

INDICATIONS AND USAGE

Urinary Tract Infections: For the treatment of urinary tract infections due to susceptible strains of the following organisms: *Escherichia coli, Klebsiella* species, *Enterobacter* species, *Morganella morganii, Proteus mirabilis* and *Proteus vulgaris.* It is recommended that initial episodes of uncomplicated urinary tract infections be treated with a single effective antibacterial agent rather than the combination.

Acute Otitis Media: For the treatment of acute otitis media in children due to susceptible strains of *Streptococcus pneumoniae* or *Haemophilus influenzae* when in the judgment of the physician Bactrim offers some advantage over the use of other antimicrobial agents. To date, there are limited data on the safety of repeated use of Bactrim in children under two years of age. Bactrim is not indicated for prophylactic or prolonged administration in otitis media at any age.

Acute Exacerbations of Chronic Bronchitis in Adults: For the treatment of acute exacerbations of chronic bronchitis due to susceptible strains of *Streptococcus pneumoniae* or *Haemophilus influenzae* when in the judgment of the physician Bactrim offers some advantage over the use of a single antimicrobial agent.

Shigellosis: For the treatment of enteritis caused by susceptible strains of *Shigella flexneri* and *Shigella sonnei* when antibacterial therapy is indicated.

Pneumocystis Carinii Pneumonia: For the treatment of documented *Pneumocystis carinii* pneumonia. For prophylaxis against *Pneumocystis carinii* pneumonia in individuals who are immunosuppressed and considered to be at an increased risk of developing *Pneumocystis carinii* pneumonia.

Travelers' Diarrhea in Adults: For the treatment of travelers' diarrhea due to susceptible strains of enterotoxigenic *E. coli.*

CONTRAINDICATIONS

Bactrim is contraindicated in patients with a known hypersensitivity to trimethoprim or sulfonamides and in patients

Continued on next page

Roche Laboratories—Cont.

with documented megaloblastic anemia due to folate deficiency. Bactrim is also contraindicated in pregnant patients and nursing mothers, because sulfonamides pass the placenta and are excreted in the milk and may cause kernicterus. Bactrim is contraindicated in infants less than 2 months of age.

WARNINGS: FATALITIES ASSOCIATED WITH THE ADMINISTRATION OF SULFONAMIDES, ALTHOUGH RARE, HAVE OCCURRED DUE TO SEVERE REACTIONS, INCLUDING STEVENS-JOHNSON SYNDROME, TOXIC EPIDERMAL NECROLYSIS, FULMINANT HEPATIC NECROSIS, AGRANULOCYTOSIS, APLASTIC ANEMIA AND OTHER BLOOD DYSCRASIAS.

BACTRIM SHOULD BE DISCONTINUED AT THE FIRST APPEARANCE OF SKIN RASH OR ANY SIGN OF ADVERSE REACTION. Clinical signs, such as rash, sore throat, fever, arthralgia, cough, shortness of breath, pallor, purpura or jaundice may be early indications of serious reactions. In rare instances a skin rash may be followed by more severe reactions, such as Stevens-Johnson syndrome, toxic epidermal necrolysis, hepatic necrosis or serious blood disorder. Complete blood counts should be done frequently in patients receiving sulfonamides.

BACTRIM SHOULD NOT BE USED IN THE TREATMENT OF STREPTOCOCCAL PHARYNGITIS. Clinical studies have documented that patients with group A β-hemolytic streptococcal tonsillopharyngitis have a greater incidence of bacteriologic failure when treated with Bactrim than do those patients treated with penicillin, as evidenced by failure to eradicate this organism from the tonsillopharyngeal area.

PRECAUTIONS

General: Bactrim should be given with caution to patients with impaired renal or hepatic function, to those with possible folate deficiency (eg, the elderly, chronic alcoholics, patients receiving anticonvulsant therapy, patients with malabsorption syndrome, and patients in malnutrition states) and to those with severe allergies or bronchial asthma. In glucose-6-phosphate dehydrogenase deficient individuals, hemolysis may occur. This reaction is frequently dose-related.

Use in the Elderly: There may be an increased risk of severe adverse reactions in elderly patients, particularly when complicating conditions exist, eg, impaired kidney and/or liver function, or concomitant use of other drugs. Severe skin reactions, generalized bone marrow suppression (see WARNINGS and ADVERSE REACTIONS sections) or a specific decrease in platelets (with or without purpura) are the most frequently reported severe adverse reactions in elderly patients. In those concurrently receiving certain diuretics, primarily thiazides, an increased incidence of thrombocytopenia with purpura has been reported. Appropriate dosage adjustments should be made for patients with impaired kidney function (see DOSAGE AND ADMINISTRATION section).

Use in the Treatment of and Prophylaxis for Pneumocystis Carinii Pneumonia in Patients with Acquired Immunodeficiency Syndrome (AIDS): AIDS patients may not tolerate or respond to Bactrim in the same manner as non-AIDS patients. The incidence of side effects, particularly rash, fever, leukopenia and elevated aminotransferase (transaminase) values, with Bactrim therapy in AIDS patients who are being treated for *Pneumocystis carinii* pneumonia has been reported to be greatly increased compared with the incidence normally associated with the use of Bactrim in non-AIDS patients. Adverse effects are generally less severe in patients receiving Bactrim for prophylaxis. A history of mild intolerance to Bactrim in AIDS patients does not appear to predict intolerance of subsequent secondary prophylaxis.[5] However, if a patient develops skin rash or any sign of adverse reaction, therapy with Bactrim should be reevaluated (see WARNINGS).

Information for Patients: Patients should be instructed to maintain an adequate fluid intake in order to prevent crystalluria and stone formation.

Laboratory Tests: Complete blood counts should be done frequently in patients receiving Bactrim; if a significant reduction in the count of any formed blood element is noted, Bactrim should be discontinued. Urinalyses with careful microscopic examination and renal function tests should be performed during therapy, particularly for those patients with impaired renal function.

Drug Interactions: In elderly patients concurrently receiving certain diuretics, primarily thiazides, an increased incidence of thrombocytopenia with purpura has been reported. It has been reported that Bactrim may prolong the prothrombin time in patients who are receiving the anticoagulant warfarin. This interaction should be kept in mind when Bactrim is given to patients already on anticoagulant therapy, and the coagulation time should be reassessed. Bactrim may inhibit the hepatic metabolism of phenytoin. Bactrim, given at a common clinical dosage, increased the phenytoin half-life by 39% and decreased the phenytoin metabolic clearance rate by 27%. When administering these drugs concurrently, one should be alert for possible excessive phenytoin effect.

Sulfonamides can also displace methotrexate from plasma protein binding sites, thus increasing free methotrexate concentrations.

Drug/Laboratory Test Interactions: Bactrim, specifically the trimethoprim component, can interfere with a serum methotrexate assay as determined by the competitive binding protein technique (CBPA) when a bacterial dihydrofolate reductase is used as the binding protein. No interference occurs, however, if methotrexate is measured by a radioimmunoassay (RIA).

The presence of trimethoprim and sulfamethoxazole may also interfere with the Jaffé alkaline picrate reaction assay for creatinine, resulting in overestimations of about 10% in the range of normal values.

Carcinogenesis, Mutagenesis, Impairment of Fertility:

Carcinogenesis: Long-term studies in animals to evaluate carcinogenic potential have not been conducted with Bactrim.

Mutagenesis: Bacterial mutagenic studies have not been performed with sulfamethoxazole and trimethoprim in combination. Trimethoprim was demonstrated to be nonmutagenic in the Ames assay. No chromosomal damage was observed in human leukocytes in vitro with sulfamethoxazole and trimethoprim alone or in combination; the concentrations used exceeded blood levels of these compounds following therapy with Bactrim. Observations of leukocytes obtained from patients treated with Bactrim revealed no chromosomal abnormalities.

Impairment of Fertility: No adverse effects on fertility or general reproductive performance were observed in rats given oral dosages as high as 70 mg/kg/day trimethoprim plus 350 mg/kg/day sulfamethoxazole.

Pregnancy: Teratogenic Effects: Pregnancy Category C. In rats, oral doses of 533 mg/kg sulfamethoxazole or 200 mg/kg trimethoprim produced teratologic effects manifested mainly as cleft palates.

The highest dose which did not cause cleft palates in rats was 512 mg/kg sulfamethoxazole or 192 mg/kg trimethoprim when administered separately. In two studies in rats, no teratology was observed when 512 mg/kg of sulfamethoxazole was used in combination with 128 mg/kg of trimethoprim. In one study, however, cleft palates were observed in one litter out of 9 when 355 mg/kg of sulfamethoxazole was used in combination with 88 mg/kg of trimethoprim.

In some rabbit studies, an overall increase in fetal loss (dead and resorbed and malformed conceptuses) was associated with doses of trimethoprim 6 times the human therapeutic dose.

While there are no large, well-controlled studies on the use of trimethoprim and sulfamethoxazole in pregnant women, Brumfitt and Pursell,[6] in a retrospective study, reported the outcome of 186 pregnancies during which the mother received either placebo or trimethoprim and sulfamethoxazole. The incidence of congenital abnormalities was 4.5% (3 of 66) in those who received placebo and 3.3% (4 of 120) in those receiving trimethoprim and sulfamethoxazole. There were no abnormalities in the 10 children whose mothers received the drug during the first trimester. In a separate survey, Brumfitt and Pursell also found no congenital abnormalities in 35 children whose mothers had received oral trimethoprim and sulfamethoxazole at the time of conception or shortly thereafter.

Because trimethoprim and sulfamethoxazole may interfere with folic acid metabolism, Bactrim should be used during pregnancy only if the potential benefit justifies the potential risk to the fetus.

Nonteratogenic Effects: See CONTRAINDICATIONS section.

Nursing Mothers: See CONTRAINDICATIONS section.

Pediatric Use: Bactrim is not recommended for infants younger than 2 months of age (see INDICATIONS and CONTRAINDICATIONS sections).

ADVERSE REACTIONS

The most common adverse effects are gastrointestinal disturbances (nausea, vomiting, anorexia) and allergic skin reactions (such as rash and urticaria). **FATALITIES ASSOCIATED WITH THE ADMINISTRATION OF SULFONAMIDES, ALTHOUGH RARE, HAVE OCCURRED DUE TO SEVERE REACTIONS, INCLUDING STEVENS-JOHNSON SYNDROME, TOXIC EPIDERMAL NECROLYSIS, FULMINANT HEPATIC NECROSIS, AGRANULOCYTOSIS, APLASTIC ANEMIA AND OTHER BLOOD DYSCRASIAS (SEE WARNINGS SECTION).**

Hematologic: Agranulocytosis, aplastic anemia, thrombocytopenia, leukopenia, neutropenia, hemolytic anemia, megaloblastic anemia, hypoprothrombinemia, methemoglobinemia, eosinophilia.

Allergic Reactions: Stevens-Johnson syndrome, toxic epidermal necrolysis, anaphylaxis, allergic myocarditis, erythema multiforme, exfoliative dermatitis, angioedema, drug fever, chills, Henoch-Schoenlein purpura, serum sickness-like syndrome, generalized allergic reactions, generalized skin eruptions, photosensitivity, conjunctival and scleral injection, pruritus, urticaria and rash. In addition, periarteritis nodosa and systemic lupus erythematosus have been reported.

Gastrointestinal: Hepatitis (including cholestatic jaundice and hepatic necrosis), elevation of serum transaminase and bilirubin, pseudomembranous enterocolitis, pancreatitis, stomatitis, glossitis, nausea, emesis, abdominal pain, diarrhea, anorexia.

Genitourinary: Renal failure, interstitial nephritis, BUN and serum creatinine elevation, toxic nephrosis with oliguria and anuria, and crystalluria.

Neurologic: Aseptic meningitis, convulsions, peripheral neuritis, ataxia, vertigo, tinnitus, headache.

Psychiatric: Hallucinations, depression, apathy, nervousness.

Endocrine: The sulfonamides bear certain chemical similarities to some goitrogens, diuretics (acetazolamide and the thiazides) and oral hypoglycemic agents. Cross-sensitivity may exist with these agents. Diuresis and hypoglycemia have occurred rarely in patients receiving sulfonamides.

Musculoskeletal: Arthralgia and myalgia.

Respiratory: Pulmonary infiltrates.

Miscellaneous: Weakness, fatigue, insomnia.

OVERDOSAGE

Acute: The amount of a single dose of Bactrim that is either associated with symptoms of overdosage or is likely to be life-threatening has not been reported. Signs and symptoms of overdosage reported with sulfonamides include anorexia, colic, nausea, vomiting, dizziness, headache, drowsiness and unconsciousness. Pyrexia, hematuria and crystalluria may be noted. Blood dyscrasias and jaundice are potential late manifestations of overdosage.

Signs of acute overdosage with trimethoprim include nausea, vomiting, dizziness, headache, mental depression, confusion and bone marrow depression.

General principles of treatment include the institution of gastric lavage or emesis, forcing oral fluids, and the administration of intravenous fluids if urine output is low and renal function is normal. Acidification of the urine will increase renal elimination of trimethoprim. The patient should be monitored with blood counts and appropriate blood chemistries, including electrolytes. If a significant blood dyscrasia or jaundice occurs, specific therapy should be instituted for these complications. Peritoneal dialysis is not effective and hemodialysis is only moderately effective in eliminating trimethoprim and sulfamethoxazole.

Chronic: Use of Bactrim at high doses and/or for extended periods of time may cause bone marrow depression manifested as thrombocytopenia, leukopenia and/or megaloblastic anemia. If signs of bone marrow depression occur, the patient should be given leucovorin 5 to 15 mg daily until normal hematopoiesis is restored.

DOSAGE AND ADMINISTRATION

Not recommended for use in infants less than 2 months of age.

Urinary Tract Infections and Shigellosis in Adults and Children, and Acute Otitis Media in Children:

Adults: The usual adult dosage in the treatment of urinary tract infections is 1 Bactrim DS (double strength) tablet, 2 Bactrim tablets or 4 teaspoonfuls (20 mL) of Bactrim Pediatric Suspension every 12 hours for 10 to 14 days. An identical daily dosage is used for 5 days in the treatment of shigellosis.

Children: The recommended dose for children with urinary tract infections or acute otitis media is 8 mg/kg trimethoprim and 40 mg/kg sulfamethoxazole per 24 hours, given in two divided doses every 12 hours for 10 days. An identical daily dosage is used for 5 days in the treatment of shigellosis. The following table is a guideline for the attainment of this dosage:

Children 2 months of age or older:

Weight		Dose—every 12 hours	
lb	kg	Teaspoonfuls	Tablets
22	10	1 (5 mL)	—
44	20	2 (10 mL)	1
66	30	3 (15 mL)	1$^1/_2$
88	40	4 (20 mL)	2 or 1 DS tablet

For Patients with Impaired Renal Function: When renal function is impaired, a reduced dosage should be employed using the following table:

Creatinine Clearance (mL/min)	Recommended Dosage Regimen
Above 30	Usual standard regimen
15–30	$^1/_2$ the usual regimen
Below 15	Use not recommended

Acute Exacerbations of Chronic Bronchitis in Adults:
The usual adult dosage in the treatment of acute exacerbations of chronic bronchitis is 1 Bactrim DS (double strength)

tablet, 2 Bactrim tablets or 4 teaspoonfuls (20 mL) of Bactrim Pediatric Suspension every 12 hours for 14 days.

Pneumocystis Carinii Pneumonia:

Treatment: Adults and Children:

The recommended dosage for patients with documented *Pneumocystis carinii* pneumonia is 15 to 20 mg/kg trimethoprim and 75 to 100 mg/kg sulfamethoxazole per 24 hours given in equally divided doses every 6 hours for 14 to 21 days.[7] The following table is a guideline for the upper limit of this dosage.

Weight		Dose—every 6 hours	
lb	kg	Teaspoonfuls	Tablets
18	8	1 (5 mL)	—
35	16	2 (10 mL)	1
53	24	3 (15 mL)	$1^1/_2$
70	32	4 (20 mL)	2 or 1 DS tablet
88	40	5 (25 mL)	$2^1/_2$
106	48	6 (30 mL)	3 or $1^1/_2$ DS tablets
141	64	8 (40 mL)	4 or 2 DS tablets
176	80	10 (50 mL)	5 or $2^1/_2$ DS Tablets

For the lower limit dose (15 mg/kg trimethoprim and 75 mg/kg sulfamethoxazole per 24 hours) administer 75% of the dose in the above table.

Prophylaxis:

Adults:

The recommended dosage for prophylaxis in adults is 1 Bactrim DS (double strength) tablet daily.[8]

Children:

For children, the recommended dose is 150 mg/m²/day trimethoprim with 750 mg/m²/day sulfamethoxazole given orally in equally divided doses twice a day, on 3 consecutive days per week. The total daily dose should not exceed 320 mg trimethoprim and 1600 mg sulfamethoxazole.[9] The following table is a guideline for the attainment of this dosage in children:

Body Surface Area	Dose—every 12 hours	
(m²)	Teaspoonfuls	Tablets
0.26	$^1/_2$ (2.5 mL)	—
0.53	1 (5 mL)	$^1/_2$
1.06	2 (10 mL)	1

Travelers' Diarrhea in Adults:

For the treatment of travelers' diarrhea, the usual adult dosage is 1 Bactrim DS (double strength) tablet; 2 Bactrim tablets or 4 teaspoonfuls (20 mL) of Pediatric Suspension every 12 hours for 5 days.

HOW SUPPLIED

DS (double strength) Tablets (white, notched, capsule shaped), containing 160 mg trimethoprim and 800 mg sulfamethoxazole—bottles of 100 (NDC 0004-0117-01), 250 (NDC 0004-0117-04) and 500 (NDC 0004-0117-14). Imprint on tablets: (front) BACTRIM-DS; (back) ROCHE.

Tablets (light green, scored, capsule shaped), containing 80 mg trimethoprim and 400 mg sulfamethoxazole—bottles of 100 (NDC 0004-0050-01). Imprint on tablets: (front) BACTRIM; (back) ROCHE.

Pediatric Suspension (pink, cherry flavored), containing 40 mg trimethoprim and 200 mg sulfamethoxazole per teaspoonful (5 mL)—bottles of 16 oz (1 pint) (NDC 0004-1033-28). TABLETS SHOULD BE STORED AT 15°–30°C (59°–86°F) IN A DRY PLACE AND PROTECTED FROM LIGHT. SUSPENSION SHOULD BE STORED AT 15°–30°C (59°–86°F) AND PROTECTED FROM LIGHT.

REFERENCES

1. Kremers P, Duvivier J, Heusghem C. Pharmacokinetic Studies of Co-Trimoxazole in Man after Single and Repeated Doses. *J Clin Pharmacol.* Feb-Mar 1974; 14:112–117. 2. Kaplan SA, et al. Pharmacokinetic Profile of Trimethoprim-Sulfamethoxazole in Man. *J Infect Dis.* Nov 1973; 128 (Suppl): S547–S555. 3. *Federal Register.* 1972; 37:20527–20529, 4. Bauer AW, Kirby WMM, Sherris JC, Turck M. Antibiotic Susceptibility Testing by a Standardized Single Disk Method. *Am J Clin Path.* Apr 1966; 45:493–496. 5. Hardy DW, et al. A controlled trial of trimethoprim-sulfamethoxazole or aerosolized pentamidine for secondary prophylaxis of *Pneumocystis carinii* pneumonia in patients with the acquired immunodeficiency syndrome. *N Engl J Med.* 1992; 327: 1842–1848. 6. Brumfitt W, Pursell R. Trimethoprim/Sulfamethoxazole in the Treatment of Bacteriuria in Women. *J Infect Dis.* Nov 1973; 128 (Suppl): S657–S663. 7. Masur H. Prevention and treatment of *Pneumocystis* pneumonia. *N Engl J Med.* 1992;327:1853–1880. 8. Recommendations for prophylaxis against *Pneumocystis carinii* pneumonia for adults and adolescents infected with human immunodeficiency virus. *MMWR,* 1992; 41(RR-4):1–11. 9. CDC Guidelines for prophylaxis against *Pneumocystis carinii* pneumonia for children infected with human immunodeficiency virus. *MMWR.* 1991;40(RR-2);1–13.

Revised: January 1994

Shown in Product Identification Guide, page 331

		U.S. RDA— Adults and children 4 or more years of age	U.S. RDA— Pregnant or lactating women
	Quantity		
Vitamin C (ascorbic acid)	500 mg	60 mg	60 mg
Vitamin B₁ (as thiamine mononitrate)	15 mg	1.5 mg	1.7 mg
Vitamin B₂ (riboflavin)	15 mg	1.7 mg	2 mg
Niacin (as niacinamide)	100 mg	20 mg	20 mg
Vitamin B₆ (as pyridoxine HCl)	4 mg	2 mg	2.5 mg
Pantothenic acid	18 mg	10 mg	10 mg
(as calcium *d*-pantothenate)			
Folic acid	0.5 mg	0.4 mg	0.8 mg
Vitamin B₁₂ (cyanocobalamin)	5 mcg	6 mcg	8 mcg

BEROCCA®   ℞

[*ber-o'ka*]

TABLETS

(See accompanying table).

The following text is complete prescribing information based on official labeling in effect June 1996.

[See table above.]

Each tablet also contains povidone, hydrogenated vegetable oil, magnesium oxide, magnesium stearate, carnauba wax, hydroxypropyl methylcellulose, polyethylene glycol, polysorbate 80, and peppermint flavor with the following colorants: D&C yellow #10 Aluminum Lake (AL), titanium dioxide, FD&C Blue #2AL, and FD&C Red #40 AL.

DESCRIPTION

Berocca is a prescription-only oral multivitamin tablet specially formulated for prophylactic or therapeutic nutritional supplementation in conditions requiring water-soluble vitamins.

Berocca tablets supply *therapeutic* levels of ascorbic acid, vitamins B₁, B₂, B₆, niacin and pantothenic acid and a *supplemental* level of vitamin B₁₂. Berocca tablets also supply a supplemental level of folic acid for pregnant or lactating women and a therapeutic level for adults and children four or more years of age.

CLINICAL PHARMACOLOGY

Vitamins are essential for normal metabolic functions including hematopoiesis. The B-complex vitamins are necessary for the conversion of carbohydrate, protein and fat into tissue and energy.

Ascorbic acid (C) is involved in collagen formation and tissue repair.

The water-soluble vitamins (B-complex and C) are not significantly stored by the body; excess quantities are excreted in the urine. They must be replenished regularly through diet or other means to maintain essential tissue levels. Thus, these vitamins are rapidly depleted in conditions interfering with their intake or absorption.

INDICATIONS AND USAGE

Berocca is indicated for supportive nutritional supplementation in conditions in which water-soluble vitamins are required prophylactically or therapeutically. These include:

Conditions causing depletion, or reduced absorption or bioavailability of water-soluble vitamins—

Gastrointestinal disorders, chronic alcoholism, febrile illnesses, prolonged or wasting diseases, hyperthyroidism or poorly-controlled diabetes.

Conditions resulting in increased needs for water-soluble vitamins—

Pregnancy, severe burns, recovery from surgery.

CONTRAINDICATIONS

Berocca is contraindicated in patients known to be hypersensitive to any of its components.

WARNINGS

Berocca is not intended for treatment of pernicious anemia or other megaloblastic anemias where vitamin B₁₂ is deficient. Neurologic involvement may develop or progress, despite temporary remission of anemia, in patients with vitamin B₁₂ deficiency who receive supplemental folic acid and who are inadequately treated with B₁₂.

PRECAUTIONS

General: Certain conditions listed above may require additional nutritional supplementation. During pregnancy, for instance, supplementation with fat-soluble vitamins and minerals may be required according to the dietary habits of the individual. Berocca is not intended for treatment of severe specific deficiencies.

Information for the Patient: Because toxic reactions have been reported with injudicious use of certain vitamins, urge patients to follow your specific instructions regarding dosage

---

regimen. As with any medication, advise patients to keep Berocca out of reach of children.

Drug and Treatment Interactions: As little as 5 mg pyridoxine daily can decrease the efficacy of levodopa in the treatment of parkinsonism. Therefore, Berocca is not recommended for patients undergoing such therapy.

ADVERSE REACTIONS

Adverse reactions have been reported with specific vitamins, but generally at levels substantially higher than those in Berocca. However, allergic and idiosyncratic reactions are possible at lower levels.

DOSAGE AND ADMINISTRATION

Usual adult dosage: one tablet daily.

Berocca is available on prescription only.

HOW SUPPLIED

Light green, capsule-shaped tablets—bottles of 100 (NDC 0004-0020-01).

Engraved on tablets: BEROCCA
                              ROCHE

Revised: November 1993

Shown in Product Identification Guide, page 331

BEROCCA® PLUS   ℞

[*ber-o'ka*]

TABLETS

The following text is complete prescribing information based on official labeling in effect June 1996.

(See accompanying table.)

[See table at top of next page.]

DESCRIPTION

Berocca Plus is a prescription-only oral multivitamin/mineral tablet specially formulated for prophylactic or therapeutic nutritional supplementation in physiologically stressful conditions.

Berocca Plus supplies: *therapeutic* levels of water-soluble vitamins (ascorbic acid and all B-complex vitamins except biotin); *supplemental* levels of biotin, fat-soluble vitamins (A and E) and minerals (iron, chromium, manganese, copper and zinc); plus magnesium.

CLINICAL PHARMACOLOGY

Vitamins and minerals are essential for normal metabolic functions including hematopoiesis. The B-complex vitamins are necessary for the conversion of carbohydrate, protein and fat into tissue and energy. Ascorbic acid is involved in tissue repair and collagen formation. Vitamin A is necessary for proper functioning of the retina; it appears to be essential to the integrity of epithelial cells. Vitamin E is an antioxidant which preserves essential cellular constituents. Magnesium is a structural component of body tissues; iron, chromium, manganese, copper and zinc serve as catalysts in enzyme systems which perform vital cellular functions.

Water-soluble vitamins (B-complex and C) are not significantly stored by the body and must be replaced continually to maintain essential tissue levels; excess quantities are excreted in urine. These vitamins are rapidly depleted in conditions interfering with their intake or absorption. Berocca Plus supplies therapeutic levels of vitamin C and all B-complex vitamins (except biotin).

Fat-soluble vitamins and several trace minerals, however, can accumulate in the body and do not need replacement as frequently. Therefore, Berocca Plus supplies more conservative levels of vitamins A and E and various essential minerals.

Specifically, Berocca Plus contains an adequate level of vitamin B₆ (25 mg) to normalize the tryptophan metabolism disturbance which has been associated with the use of estrogenic oral contraceptives or other estrogen therapy. It provides zinc (22.5 mg) which facilitates wound healing, the level of folic acid (0.8 mg) recommended during pregnancy,

Continued on next page

Roche Laboratories—Cont.

Each Berocca® Plus tablet contains:	Quantity	U.S. RDA—Adults and children 4 or more years of age	U.S. RDA—Pregnant or lactating women
Fat-Soluble Vitamins			
Vitamin A (as vitamin A acetate)	5000 IU	5000 IU	8000 IU
Vitamin E (as *dl*-alpha tocopheryl acetate)	30 IU	30 IU	30 IU
Water-Soluble Vitamins			
Vitamin C (ascorbic acid)	500 mg	60 mg	60 mg
Vitamin B_1 (as thiamine mononitrate)	20 mg	1.5 mg	1.7 mg
Vitamin B_2 (riboflavin)	20 mg	1.7 mg	2 mg
Niacin (as niacinamide)	100 mg	20 mg	20 mg
Vitamin B_6 (as pyridoxine HCl)	25 mg	2 mg	2.5 mg
Biotin	0.15 mg	0.30 mg	0.30 mg
Pantothenic acid (as calcium pantothenate)	25 mg	10 mg	10 mg
Folic acid	0.8 mg	0.4 mg	0.8 mg
Vitamin B_{12} (cyanocobalamin)	50 mcg	6 mcg	8 mcg
Minerals			
Iron (as ferrous fumarate)	27 mg	18 mg	18 mg
Chromium (as chromium nitrate)	0.1 mg	0.05–0.2 mg*	
Magnesium (as magnesium oxide)	50 mg	400 mg	450 mg
Manganese (as manganese dioxide)	5 mg	2.5–5 mg*	
Copper (as cupric oxide)	3 mg	2 mg	2 mg
Zinc (as zinc oxide)	22.5 mg	15 mg	15 mg

Each tablet also contains carnauba wax, ethylcellulose, ethyl vanillin, hydroxypropyl methylcellulose, magnesium stearate, povidone, silicon dioxide, stearic acid, triacetin and flavor with the following dyes: yellow iron oxide and titanium dioxide.
*Not established. Estimated by NAS/NRC as safe and adequate daily dietary intake for adults.

and ascorbic acid (500 mg) which has been demonstrated to improve the absorption of inorganic iron.

INDICATIONS

Berocca Plus is indicated for prophylactic or therapeutic nutritional supplementation in physiologically stressful conditions. These include:

Conditions causing depletion, or reduced absorption or bioavailability of essential vitamins and minerals—
Inadequate intake due to highly restricted or unbalanced diets such as those frequently associated with anorexic conditions and other states of severe malnutrition.
Gastrointestinal disorders, chronic alcoholism, chronic or acute infections (especially those involving febrile illness), prolonged or wasting disease, congestive heart failure, hyperthyroidism, poorly controlled diabetes or other physiologic stress.
Also, patients on estrogenic oral contraceptives or other estrogen therapy, antibacterials which affect intestinal microflora, or other interfering drugs.

Certain conditions resulting from severe B-vitamin or ascorbic acid deficiency—
Cheilosis, gingivitis, stomatitis and certain other classic water-soluble vitamin deficiency syndromes.

Conditions resulting in increased needs for essential vitamins and minerals—
Recovery from surgery or trauma involving severe burns, fractures or other extensive tissue damage.
Also, pregnant women and those with heavy menstrual bleeding.

CONTRAINDICATIONS

Berocca Plus is contraindicated in patients hypersensitive to any of its components.

WARNINGS

Not intended for treatment of pernicious anemia or other megaloblastic anemias where vitamin B_{12} is deficient. Neurologic involvement may develop or progress, despite temporary remission of anemia, in patients with vitamin B_{12} deficiency who receive supplemental folic acid and who are inadequately treated with B_{12}.

PRECAUTIONS

General: Certain conditions listed above may require additional nutritional supplementation. During pregnancy, for instance, supplementation with vitamin D and calcium may be required according to the dietary habits of the individual. Berocca Plus is not intended for treatment of severe specific deficiencies.
Information for the Patient: Because toxic reactions have been reported with injudicious use of certain vitamins and minerals, urge patients to follow your specific instructions regarding dosage regimen. Advise patients to keep Berocca Plus out of reach of children.
Drug and Treatment Interactions: As little as 5 mg pyridoxine daily can decrease the efficacy of levodopa in the treatment of parkinsonism. Therefore, Berocca Plus is not recommended for patients undergoing such therapy.

ADVERSE REACTIONS

Adverse reactions have been reported with specific vitamins and minerals, but generally at levels substantially higher than those in Berocca Plus. However, allergic and idiosyncratic reactions are possible at lower levels. Iron, even at the usual recommended levels, has been associated with gastrointestinal intolerance in some patients.

DOSAGE AND ADMINISTRATION

Usual adult dosage: 1 tablet daily. Not recommended for children. *Berocca Plus is available on prescription only.*

HOW SUPPLIED

Golden yellow, capsule-shaped tablets—bottles of 100.
Imprint on tablets: (front) BEROCCA PLUS; (back) ROCHE.
Revised: November 1985

Shown in Product Identification Guide, page 331

BUMEX® ℞
[*bu'mex*]
brand of bumetanide
TABLETS
INJECTION

The following text is complete prescribing information based on official labeling in effect June 1996.

> **WARNING**
> Bumex (bumetanide) is a potent diuretic which, if given in excessive amounts, can lead to a profound diuresis with water and electrolyte depletion. Therefore, careful medical supervision is required, and dose and dosage schedule have to be adjusted to the individual patient's needs. (See DOSAGE AND ADMINISTRATION.)

DESCRIPTION

Bumex® (bumetanide) is a loop diuretic, available as scored tablets, 0.5 mg (light green), 1 mg (yellow) and 2 mg (peach) for oral administration; each tablet also contains lactose, magnesium stearate, microcrystalline cellulose, corn starch and talc, with the following dye systems: 0.5 mg—D&C Yellow No. 10 and FD&C Blue No. 1; 1 mg—D&C Yellow No. 10; 2 mg—red iron oxide. Also as 2-mL ampuls, 2-mL vials, 4-mL vials and 10-mL vials (0.25 mg/mL) for intravenous or intramuscular injection as a sterile solution, each 2 mL of which contains 0.5 mg (0.25 mg/mL) bumetanide compounded with 0.85% sodium chloride and 0.4% ammonium acetate as buffers; 0.01% edetate disodium; 1% benzyl alcohol as preservative, and pH adjusted to approximately 7 with sodium hydroxide.
Chemically, bumetanide is 3-(butylamino)-4-phenoxy-5-sulfamoylbenzoic acid. It is a practically white powder having a calculated molecular weight of 364.41.

CLINICAL PHARMACOLOGY

Bumex is a loop diuretic with a rapid onset and short duration of action. Pharmacological and clinical studies have shown that 1 mg Bumex has a diuretic potency equivalent to approximately 40 mg furosemide. The major site of Bumex action is the ascending limb of the loop of Henle.
The mode of action has been determined through various clearance studies in both humans and experimental animals. Bumex inhibits sodium reabsorption in the ascending limb of the loop of Henle, as shown by marked reduction of free-water clearance (C_{H_2O}) during hydration and tubular free-water reabsorption ($T^{C}H_2O$) during hydropenia. Reabsorption of chloride in the ascending limb is also blocked by Bumex, and Bumex is somewhat more chloruretic than natriuretic.
Potassium excretion is also increased by Bumex, in a dose-related fashion.
Bumex may have an additional action in the proximal tubule. Since phosphate reabsorption takes place largely in the proximal tubule, phosphaturia during Bumex-induced diuresis is indicative of this additional action. This is further supported by the reduction in the renal clearance of Bumex by probenecid, associated with diminution in the natriuretic response. This proximal tubular activity does not seem to be related to an inhibition of carbonic anhydrase. Bumex does not appear to have a noticeable action on the distal tubule.
Bumex decreases uric acid excretion and increases serum uric acid. Following oral administration of Bumex the onset of diuresis occurs in 30 to 60 minutes. Peak activity is reached between 1 and 2 hours. At usual doses (1 to 2 mg) diuresis is largely complete within 4 hours; with higher doses, the diuretic action lasts for 4 to 6 hours. Diuresis starts within minutes following an intravenous injection and reaches maximum levels within 15 to 30 minutes.
Several pharmacokinetic studies have shown that Bumex, administered orally or parenterally, is eliminated rapidly in humans, with a half-life of between 1 and $1^1/_2$ hours. Plasma protein-binding is in the range of 94% to 96%.
Oral administration of carbon-14 labeled Bumex to human volunteers revealed that 81% of the administered radioactivity was excreted in the urine, 45% of it as unchanged drug. Urinary and biliary metabolites identified in this study were formed by oxidation of the N-butyl side chain. Biliary excretion of Bumex amounted to only 2% of the administered dose.

INDICATIONS AND USAGE

Bumex is indicated for the treatment of edema associated with congestive heart failure, hepatic and renal disease, including the nephrotic syndrome.
Almost equal diuretic response occurs after oral and parenteral administration of Bumex. Therefore, if impaired gastrointestinal absorption is suspected or oral administration is not practical, Bumex should be given by the intramuscular or intravenous route.
Successful treatment with Bumex following instances of allergic reactions to furosemide suggests a lack of cross-sensitivity.

CONTRAINDICATIONS

Bumex is contraindicated in anuria. Although Bumex can be used to induce diuresis in renal insufficiency, any marked increase in blood urea nitrogen or creatinine, or the development of oliguria during therapy of patients with progressive renal disease, is an indication for discontinuation of treatment with Bumex. Bumex is also contraindicated in patients in hepatic coma or in states of severe electrolyte depletion until the condition is improved or corrected. Bumex is contraindicated in patients hypersensitive to this drug.

WARNINGS

1. Volume and electrolyte depletion. The dose of Bumex should be adjusted to the patient's need. Excessive doses or too frequent administration can lead to profound water loss, electrolyte depletion, dehydration, reduction in blood volume and circulatory collapse with the possibility of vascular thrombosis and embolism, particularly in elderly patients.
2. Hypokalemia. Hypokalemia can occur as a consequence of Bumex administration. Prevention of hypokalemia requires particular attention in the following conditions: patients receiving digitalis and diuretics for congestive heart failure, hepatic cirrhosis and ascites, states of aldosterone excess with normal renal function, potassium-losing nephropathy, certain diarrheal states, or other states where hypokalemia is thought to represent particular added risks to the patient, ie, history of ventricular arrhythmias.
In patients with hepatic cirrhosis and ascites, sudden alterations of electrolyte balance may precipitate hepatic encephalopathy and coma. Treatment in such patients is best initiated in the hospital with small doses and careful monitoring of the patient's clinical status and electrolyte balance. Supplemental potassium and/or spironolactone may prevent hypokalemia and metabolic alkalosis in these patients.
3. Ototoxicity. In cats, dogs and guinea pigs, Bumex has been shown to produce ototoxicity. In these test animals Bumex was 5 to 6 times more potent than furosemide and, since the diuretic potency of Bumex is about 40 to 60 times furosemide, it is anticipated that blood levels necessary to produce ototoxicity will rarely be achieved. The potential exists, however, and must be considered a risk of intravenous therapy, especially at high doses, repeated frequently in the face of renal excretory function impairment. Potentiation of aminoglycoside ototoxicity has not been tested for Bumex. Like other members of this class of diuretics, Bumex probably shares this risk.
4. Allergy to sulfonamides. Patients allergic to sulfonamides may show hypersensitivity to Bumex.

5. Thrombocytopenia. Since there have been rare spontaneous reports of thrombocytopenia from postmarketing experience, patients should be observed regularly for possible occurrence of thrombocytopenia.

PRECAUTIONS

General: Serum potassium should be measured periodically and potassium supplements or potassium-sparing diuretics added if necessary. Periodic determinations of other electrolytes are advised in patients treated with high doses or for prolonged periods, particularly in those on low salt diets. Hyperuricemia may occur; it has been asymptomatic in cases reported to date. Reversible elevations of the BUN and creatinine may also occur, especially in association with dehydration and particularly in patients with renal insufficiency. Bumex may increase urinary calcium excretion with resultant hypocalcemia.

Diuretics have been shown to increase the urinary excretion of magnesium; this may result in hypomagnesemia.

Laboratory Tests: Studies in normal subjects receiving Bumex revealed no adverse effects on glucose tolerance, plasma insulin, glucagon and growth hormone levels, but the possibility of an effect on glucose metabolism exists. Periodic determinations of blood sugar should be done, particularly in patients with diabetes or suspected latent diabetes.

Patients under treatment should be observed regularly for possible occurrence of blood dyscrasias, liver damage or idiosyncratic reactions, which have been reported occasionally in foreign marketing experience. The relationship of these occurrences to Bumex use is not certain.

Drug Interactions:
1. Drugs with ototoxic potential (see WARNINGS): Especially in the presence of impaired renal function, the use of parenterally administered Bumex in patients to whom aminoglycoside antibiotics are also being given should be avoided, except in life-threatening conditions.
2. Drugs with nephrotoxic potential: There has been no experience on the concurrent use of Bumex with drugs known to have a nephrotoxic potential. Therefore, the simultaneous administration of these drugs should be avoided.
3. Lithium: Lithium should generally not be given with diuretics (such as Bumex) because they reduce its renal clearance and add a high risk of lithium toxicity.
4. Probenecid: Pretreatment with probenecid reduces both the natriuresis and hyperreninemia produced by Bumex. This antagonistic effect of probenecid on Bumex natriuresis is not due to a direct action on sodium excretion but is probably secondary to its inhibitory effect on renal tubular secretion of bumetanide. Thus, probenecid should not be administered concurrently with Bumex.
5. Indomethacin: Indomethacin blunts the increases in urine volume and sodium excretion seen during Bumex treatment and inhibits the bumetanide-induced increase in plasma renin activity. Concurrent therapy with Bumex is thus not recommended.
6. Antihypertensives: Bumex may potentiate the effect of various antihypertensive drugs, necessitating a reduction in the dosage of these drugs.
7. Digoxin: Interaction studies in humans have shown no effect on digoxin blood levels.
8. Anticoagulants: Interaction studies in humans have shown Bumex to have no effect on warfarin metabolism or on plasma prothrombin activity.

Carcinogenesis, Mutagenesis, Impairment of Fertility: Bumex was devoid of mutagenic activity in various strains of *Salmonella typhimurium* when tested in the presence or absence of an in vitro metabolic activation system. An 18-month study showed an increase in mammary adenomas of questionable significance in female rats receiving oral doses of 60 mg/kg/day (2000 times a 2-mg human dose). A repeat study at the same doses failed to duplicate this finding.

Reproduction studies were performed to evaluate general reproductive performance and fertility in rats at oral dose levels of 10, 30, 60 or 100 mg/kg/day. The pregnancy rate was slightly decreased in the treated animals; however, the differences were small and not statistically significant.

Pregnancy: Teratogenic Effects: Pregnancy Category C. Bumex is neither teratogenic nor embryocidal in mice when given in doses up to 3400 times the maximum human therapeutic dose.

Bumex has been shown to be nonteratogenic, but it has a slight embryocidal effect in rats when given in doses of 3400 times the maximum human therapeutic dose and in rabbits at doses of 3.4 times the maximum human therapeutic dose. In one study, moderate growth retardation and increased incidence of delayed ossification of sternebrae were observed in rats at oral doses of 100 mg/kg/day, 3400 times the maximum human therapeutic dose. These effects were associated with maternal weight reductions noted during dosing. No such adverse effects were observed at 30 mg/kg/day (1000 times the maximum human therapeutic dose). No fetotoxicity was observed at 1000 to 2000 times the human therapeutic dose.

In rabbits, a dose-related decrease in litter size and an increase in resorption rate were noted at oral doses of 0.1 and 0.3 mg/kg/day (3.4 and 10 times the maximum human thera-

peutic dose). A slightly increased incidence of delayed ossification of sternebrae occurred at 0.3 mg/kg/day; however, no such adverse effects were observed at the dose of 0.03 mg/kg/day. The sensitivity of the rabbit to Bumex parallels the marked pharmacologic and toxicologic effects of the drug in this species.

Bumex was not teratogenic in the hamster at an oral dose of 0.5 mg/kg/day (17 times the maximum human therapeutic dose). Bumex was not teratogenic when given intravenously to mice and rats at doses up to 140 times the maximum human therapeutic dose.

There are no adequate and well-controlled studies in pregnant women. A small investigational experience in the United States and marketing experience in other countries to date have not indicated any evidence of adverse effects on the fetus, but these data do not rule out the possibility of harmful effects. Bumex should be given to a pregnant woman only if the potential benefit justifies the potential risk to the fetus.

Nursing Mothers: It is not known whether this drug is excreted in human milk. As a general rule, nursing should not be undertaken while the patient is on Bumex since it may be excreted in human milk.

Pediatric Use: Safety and effectiveness in children below the age of 18 have not been established.

ADVERSE REACTIONS

The most frequent clinical adverse reactions considered probably or possibly related to Bumex are muscle cramps (seen in 1.1% of treated patients), dizziness (1.1%), hypotension (0.8%), headache (0.6%), nausea (0.6%), and encephalopathy (in patients with preexisting liver disease) (0.6%). One or more of these adverse reactions have been reported in approximately 4.1% of Bumex-treated patients.

Less frequent clinical adverse reactions to Bumex are impaired hearing (0.5%), pruritus (0.4%), electrocardiogram changes (0.4%), weakness (0.2%), hives (0.2%), abdominal pain (0.2%), arthritic pain (0.2%), musculoskeletal pain (0.2%), rash (0.2%) and vomiting (0.2%). One or more of these adverse reactions have been reported in approximately 2.9% of Bumex-treated patients.

Other clinical adverse reactions, which have each occurred in approximately 0.1% of patients, are vertigo, chest pain, ear discomfort, fatigue, dehydration, sweating, hyperventilation, dry mouth, upset stomach, renal failure, asterixis, itching, nipple tenderness, diarrhea, premature ejaculation and difficulty maintaining an erection.

Laboratory abnormalities reported have included hyperuricemia (in 18.4% of patients tested), hypochloremia (14.9%), hypokalemia (14.7%), azotemia (10.6%), hyponatremia (9.2%), increased serum creatinine (7.4%), hyperglycemia (6.6%), and variations in phosphorus (4.5%), CO_2 content (4.3%), bicarbonate (3.1%) and calcium (2.4%). Although manifestations of the pharmacologic action of Bumex, these conditions may become more pronounced by intensive therapy.

Also reported have been thrombocytopenia (0.2%) and deviations in hemoglobin (0.8%), prothrombin time (0.8%), hematocrit (0.6%), WBC (0.3%) and differential counts (0.1%). There have been rare spontaneous reports of thrombocytopenia from postmarketing experience.

Diuresis induced by Bumex may also rarely be accompanied by changes in LDH (1.0%), total serum bilirubin (0.8%), serum proteins (0.7%), SGOT (0.6%), SGPT (0.5%), alkaline phosphatase (0.4%), cholesterol (0.4%) and creatinine clearance (0.3%). Increases in urinary glucose (0.7%) and urinary protein (0.3%) have also been seen.

OVERDOSAGE

Overdosage can lead to acute profound water loss, volume and electrolyte depletion, dehydration, reduction of blood volume and circulatory collapse with a possibility of vascular thrombosis and embolism. Electrolyte depletion may be manifested by weakness, dizziness, mental confusion, anorexia, lethargy, vomiting and cramps. Treatment consists of replacement of fluid and electrolyte losses by careful monitoring of the urine and electrolyte output and serum electrolyte levels.

DOSAGE AND ADMINISTRATION

Dosage should be individualized with careful monitoring of patient response.

Oral Administration: The usual total daily dosage of Bumex is 0.5 to 2 mg and in most patients is given as a single dose.

If the diuretic response to an initial dose of Bumex is not adequate, in view of its rapid onset and short duration of action, a second or third dose may be given at 4- to 5-hour intervals up to a maximum daily dose of 10 mg. An intermittent dose schedule, whereby Bumex is given on alternate days or for 3 to 4 days with rest periods of 1 to 2 days in between, is recommended as the safest and most effective method for the continued control of edema. In patients with hepatic failure, the dosage should be kept to a minimum, and if necessary, dosage increased very carefully.

Because cross-sensitivity with furosemide has rarely been observed, Bumex can be substituted at approximately a

1:40 ratio of Bumex to furosemide in patients allergic to furosemide.

Parenteral Administration: Bumex may be administered parenterally (IV or IM) to patients in whom gastrointestinal absorption may be impaired or in whom oral administration is not practical.

Parenteral treatment should be terminated and oral treatment instituted as soon as possible.

The usual initial dose is 0.5 to 1 mg intravenously or intramuscularly. Intravenous administration should be given over a period of 1 to 2 minutes. If the response to an initial dose is deemed insufficient, a second or third dose may be given at intervals of 2 to 3 hours, but should not exceed a daily dosage of 10 mg.

Miscibility and Parenteral Solutions: The compatibility tests of Bumex injection (0.25 mg/mL, 2-mL ampuls) with 5% dextrose in water, 0.9% sodium chloride, and lactated Ringer's solution in both glass and plasticized PVC (Viaflex) containers have shown no significant absorption effect with either containers, nor a measurable loss of potency due to degradation of the drug. However, solutions should be freshly prepared and used within 24 hours.

Parenteral drug products should be inspected visually for particulate matter and discoloration prior to administration whenever solution and container permit.

HOW SUPPLIED

Tablets, 0.5 mg (light green), bottles of 100 (NDC 0004-0125-01) and 500 (NDC 0004-0125-14) and 5000 (NDC 0004-0125-11); Tel-E-Dose® packages of 100 (NDC 0004-0125-49). 1 mg (yellow), bottles of 100 (NDC 0004-0121-01), 500 (NDC 0004-0121-14) and 5000 (NDC 0004-0121-11); Tel-E-Dose® packages of 100 (NDC 0004-0121-49). 2 mg (peach), bottles of 100 (NDC 0004-0162-01) and 5000 (NDC 0004-0162-11); Tel-E-Dose® packages of 100 (NDC 0004-0162-07).

Imprint on tablets: 0.5 mg—ROCHE BUMEX 0.5; 1 mg—ROCHE BUMEX 1; 2 mg—ROCHE BUMEX 2.

Ampuls (0.25 mg/mL), 2 mL, boxes of 10 (NDC 0004-1944-06). *Vials* (0.25 mg/mL), 2 mL, boxes of 10 (NDC 0004-1968-01); 4 mL, boxes of 10 (NDC 0004-1969-01); 10 mL, boxes of 10 (NDC 0004-1970-01).

Store all tablets, vials and ampuls at 59° to 86° F.
Revised: September 1993
Shown in Product Identification Guide, page 331

CARDENE® ℞
[kar 'deen]
**(nicardipine hydrochloride)
Capsules**

DESCRIPTION

CARDENE capsules for oral administration each contain 20 mg or 30 mg of nicardipine hydrochloride. CARDENE is a calcium ion influx inhibitor (slow channel blocker or calcium channel blocker).

Nicardipine hydrochloride is a dihydropyridine structure with the IUPAC (International Union of Pure and Applied Chemistry) chemical name 2-(benzyl-methyl amino)ethyl methyl 1,4-dihydro-2,6-dimethyl-4-(*m*-nitrophenyl)-3,5-pyridinedicarboxylate monohydrochloride.

Nicardipine hydrochloride is a greenish-yellow, odorless, crystalline powder that melts at about 169°C. It is freely soluble in chloroform, methanol and glacial acetic acid, sparingly soluble in anhydrous ethanol, slightly soluble in n-butanol, water, 0.01 M potassium dihydrogen phosphate, acetone and dioxane, very slightly soluble in ethyl acetate, and practically insoluble in benzene, ether and hexane. It has a molecular weight of 515.99.

CARDENE is available in hard gelatin capsules containing 20 mg or 30 mg nicardipine hydrochloride with magnesium stearate and pregelatinized starch as the inactive ingredients. The 20 mg strength is provided in opaque white-white capsules with a brilliant blue band, while the 30 mg capsules are opaque light blue-powder blue with a brilliant blue band. The colorants used in the 20 mg capsules are titanium dioxide, D&C Red No. 7 Calcium Lake and FD&C Blue No. 1 and the 30 mg capsules use titanium dioxide, FD&C Blue No. 1, D&C Yellow No. 10 Aluminum Lake, D&C Red No. 7 Calcium Lake and FD&C Blue No. 2.

CLINICAL PHARMACOLOGY

Mechanism of Action: CARDENE is a calcium entry blocker (slow channel blocker or calcium ion antagonist) that inhibits the transmembrane influx of calcium ions into cardiac muscle and smooth muscle without changing serum calcium concentrations. The contractile processes of cardiac muscle and vascular smooth muscle are dependent upon the movement of extracellular calcium ions into these cells through specific ion channels. The effects of CARDENE are more selective to vascular smooth muscle than cardiac muscle. In animal models, CARDENE produces relaxation of

Continued on next page

Roche Laboratories—Cont.

coronary vascular smooth muscle at drug levels that cause little or no negative inotropic effect.

Pharmacokinetics and Metabolism: CARDENE is completely absorbed following oral doses administered as capsules. Plasma levels are detectable as early as 20 minutes following an oral dose and maximal plasma levels are observed within 30 minutes to 2 hours (mean T_{max} = 1 hour). While CARDENE is completely absorbed, it is subject to saturable first pass metabolism and the systemic bioavailability is about 35% following a 30 mg oral dose at steady state.

When CARDENE was administered 1 or 3 hours after a high fat meal, the mean C_{max} and mean AUC were lower (20% to 30%) than when CARDENE was given to fasting subjects. These decreases in plasma levels observed following a meal may be significant, but the clinical trials establishing the efficacy and safety of CARDENE were done in patients without regard to the timing of meals. Thus the results of these trials reflect the effects of meal-induced variability.

The pharmacokinetics of CARDENE are nonlinear due to saturable hepatic first pass metabolism. Following oral administration, increasing doses result in a disproportionate increase in plasma levels. Steady-state C_{max} values following 20, 30 and 40 mg doses every 8 hours averaged 36, 88 and 133 ng/mL, respectively. Hence, increasing the dose from 20 to 30 mg every 8 hours more than doubled C_{max} and increasing the dose from 20 to 40 mg every 8 hours increased C_{max} more than threefold. A similar disproportionate increase in AUC with dose was observed. Considerable inter-subject variability in plasma levels was also observed.

Post-absorption kinetics of CARDENE are also non-linear, although there is a reproducible terminal plasma half-life that averaged 8.6 hours following 30 and 40 mg doses at steady state (tid). The terminal half-life represents the elimination of less than 5% of the absorbed drug (measured by plasma concentrations). Elimination over the first 8 hours after dosing is much faster with a half-life of 2 to 4 hours. Steady-state plasma levels are achieved after 2 to 3 days of tid dosing (every 8 hours) and are twofold higher than after a single dose.

CARDENE is highly protein bound (>95%) in human plasma over a wide concentration range.

CARDENE is metabolized extensively by the liver; less than 1% of intact drug is detected in the urine. Following a radioactive oral dose in solution, 60% of the radioactivity was recovered in the urine and 35% in feces. Most of the dose (over 90%) was recovered within 48 hours of dosing. CARDENE does not induce its own metabolism and does not induce hepatic microsomal enzymes.

The steady-state pharmacokinetics of CARDENE in elderly hypertensive patients (≥65 years) are similar to those obtained in young normal adults. After 1 week of CARDENE dosing at 20 mg three times a day, the C_{max}, T_{max}, AUC, terminal plasma half-life and the extent of protein binding of CARDENE observed in healthy elderly hypertensive patients did not differ significantly from those observed in young normal volunteers.

CARDENE plasma levels were higher in patients with mild renal impairment (baseline serum creatinine concentration ranged from 1.2 to 5.5 mg/dL) than in normal subjects. After 30 mg CARDENE tid at steady state, C_{max} and AUC were approximately twofold higher in these patients.

Because CARDENE is extensively metabolized by the liver, the plasma levels of the drug are influenced by changes in hepatic function. CARDENE plasma levels were higher in patients with severe liver disease (hepatic cirrhosis confirmed by liver biopsy or presence of endoscopically-confirmed esophageal varices) than in normal subjects. After 20 mg CARDENE bid at steady state, C_{max} and AUC were 1.8 and fourfold higher, and the terminal half-life was prolonged to 19 hours in these patients.

Hemodynamics: In man, CARDENE produces a significant decrease in systemic vascular resistance. The degree of vasodilation and the resultant hypotensive effects are more prominent in hypertensive patients. In hypertensive patients, nicardipine reduces the blood pressure at rest and during isometric and dynamic exercise. In normotensive patients, a small decrease of about 9 mm Hg in systolic and 7 mm Hg in diastolic blood pressure may accompany this fall in peripheral resistance. An increase in heart rate may occur in response to the vasodilation and decrease in blood pressure, and in a few patients this heart rate increase may be pronounced. In clinical studies mean heart rate at time of peak plasma levels was usually increased by 5 to 10 beats per minute compared to placebo, with the greater increases at higher doses, while there was no difference from placebo at the end of the dosing interval. Hemodynamic studies following intravenous dosing in patients with coronary artery disease and normal or moderately abnormal left ventricular function have shown significant increases in ejection fraction and cardiac output with no significant change, or a small decrease, in left ventricular end-diastolic pressure (LVEDP). Although there is evidence that CARDENE increases coronary blood flow, there is no evidence that this property plays any role in its effectiveness in stable angina. In patients with coronary artery disease, intracoronary administration of nicardipine caused no direct myocardial depression. CARDENE does, however, have a negative inotropic effect in some patients with severe left ventricular dysfunction and could, in patients with very impaired function, lead to worsened failure.

"Coronary Steal," the detrimental redistribution of coronary blood flow in patients with coronary artery disease (diversion of blood from underperfused areas toward better perfused areas), has not been observed during nicardipine treatment. On the contrary, nicardipine has been shown to improve systolic shortening in normal and hypokinetic segments of myocardial muscle, and radio-nuclide angiography has confirmed that wall motion remained improved during an increase in oxygen demand. Nonetheless, occasional patients have developed increased angina upon receiving nicardipine. Whether this represents steal in those patients, or is the result of increased heart rate and decreased diastolic pressure, is not clear.

In patients with coronary artery disease nicardipine improves L.V. diastolic distensibility during the early filling phase, probably due to a faster rate of myocardial relaxation in previously underperfused areas. There is little or no effect on normal myocardium, suggesting the improvement is mainly by indirect mechanisms such as afterload reduction, and reduced ischemia. Nicardipine has no negative effect on myocardial relaxation at therapeutic doses. The clinical consequences of these properties are as yet undemonstrated.

Electrophysiologic Effects: In general, no detrimental effects on the cardiac conduction system were seen with the use of CARDENE.

CARDENE increased the heart rate when given intravenously during acute electrophysiologic studies and prolonged the corrected QT interval to a minor degree. The sinus node recovery times and SA conduction times were not affected by the drug. The PA, AH and HV intervals* and the functional and effective refractory periods of the atrium were not prolonged by CARDENE, and the relative and effective refractory periods of the His-Purkinje system were slightly shortened after intravenous CARDENE.

*PA = conduction time from high to low right atrium, AH = conduction time from low right atrium to His bundle deflection or AV nodal conduction time,
HV = conduction time through the His bundle and the bundle branch-Purkinje system.

Renal Function: There is a transient increase in electrolyte excretion, including sodium. CARDENE does not cause generalized fluid retention, as measured by weight changes, although 7% to 8% of the patients experience pedal edema.

Effects in Angina Pectoris: In controlled clinical trials of up to 12 weeks duration in patients with chronic stable angina, CARDENE increased exercise tolerance and reduced nitroglycerin consumption and the frequency of anginal attacks. The antianginal efficacy of CARDENE (20 to 40 mg) has been demonstrated in four placebo-controlled studies involving 258 patients with chronic stable angina. In exercise tolerance testing, CARDENE significantly increased time to angina, total exercise duration and time to 1 mm ST segment depression. Included among these four studies was a dose-definition study in which dose-related improvements in exercise tolerance at 1 and 4 hours postdosing and reduced frequency of anginal attacks were seen at doses of 10, 20 and 30 mg tid. Effectiveness at 10 mg tid was, however, marginal. In a fifth placebo-controlled study, the antianginal efficacy of CARDENE was demonstrated at 8 hours postdose (trough). The sustained efficacy of CARDENE has been demonstrated over long-term dosing. Blood pressure fell in patients with angina by about 10/8 mm Hg at peak blood levels and was little different from placebo at trough blood levels.

Effects in Hypertension: CARDENE produced dose-related decreases in both systolic and diastolic blood pressure in clinical trials. The antihypertensive efficacy of CARDENE administered three times daily has been demonstrated in three placebo-controlled studies involving 517 patients with mild to moderate hypertension. The blood pressure responses in the three studies were statistically significant from placebo at peak (1 hour postdosing) and trough (8 hours postdosing) although it is apparent that well over half of the antihypertensive effect is lost by the end of the dosing interval. The results from placebo controlled studies of CARDENE given three times daily are shown in the following table:
[See table below.]

SYSTOLIC BP (mm Hg)

Dose	Number of Patients	Mean Peak Response	Mean Trough Response	Trough/Peak
20 mg	50	−10.3	−4.9	48%
	52	−17.6	−7.9	45%
30 mg	45	−14.5	−7.2	50%
	44	−14.6	−7.5	51%
40 mg	50	−16.3	−9.5	58%
	38	−15.9	−6.0	38%

DIASTOLIC BP (mm Hg)

Dose	Number of Patients	Mean Peak Response	Mean Trough Response	Trough/Peak
20 mg	50	−10.6	−4.6	43%
	52	− 9.0	−2.9	32%
30 mg	45	−12.8	−4.9	38%
	44	−14.2	−4.3	30%
40 mg	50	−15.4	−5.9	38%
	38	−14.8	−3.7	25%

The responses are shown as differences from the concurrent placebo control group. The large changes between peak and trough effects were not accompanied by observed side effects at peak response times. In a study using 24 hour intra-arterial blood pressure monitoring, the circadian variation in blood pressure remained unaltered, but the systolic and diastolic blood pressures were reduced throughout the whole 24 hours.

When added to beta-blocker therapy, CARDENE further lowers both systolic and diastolic blood pressure.

INDICATIONS AND USAGE

I. Stable Angina: CARDENE is indicated for the management of patients with chronic stable angina (effort-associated angina). CARDENE may be used alone or in combination with beta-blockers.

II. Hypertension: CARDENE is indicated for the treatment of hypertension. CARDENE may be used alone or in combination with other antihypertensive drugs. In administering nicardipine it is important to be aware of the relatively large peak to trough differences in blood pressure effect. (See DOSAGE AND ADMINISTRATION.)

CONTRAINDICATIONS

CARDENE is contraindicated in patients with hypersensitivity to the drug.

Because part of the effect of CARDENE is secondary to reduced afterload, the drug is also contraindicated in patients with advanced aortic stenosis. Reduction of diastolic pressure in these patients may worsen rather than improve myocardial oxygen balance.

WARNINGS

Increased Angina: About 7% of patients in short-term placebo-controlled angina trials have developed increased frequency, duration or severity of angina on starting CARDENE or at the time of dosage increases, compared with 4% of patients on placebo. Comparisons with beta-blockers also show a greater frequency of increased angina, 4% vs 1%. The mechanism of this effect has not been established. (See ADVERSE REACTIONS.)

Use in Patients with Congestive Heart Failure: Although preliminary hemodynamic studies in patients with congestive heart failure have shown that CARDENE reduced afterload without impairing myocardial contractility, it has a negative inotropic effect in vitro and in some patients. Caution should be exercised when using the drug in congestive heart failure patients, particularly in combination with a beta-blocker.

Beta-Blocker Withdrawal: CARDENE is not a beta-blocker and therefore gives no protection against the dangers of abrupt beta-blocker withdrawal; any such withdrawal should be by gradual reduction of the dose of beta-blocker, preferably over 8 to 10 days.

PRECAUTIONS

General: *Blood Pressure:* Because CARDENE decreases peripheral resistance, careful monitoring of blood pressure during the initial administration and titration of CARDENE is suggested. CARDENE, like other calcium channel blockers, may occasionally produce symptomatic hypotension. Caution is advised to avoid systemic hypotension when administering the drug to patients who have sustained an acute cerebral infarction or hemorrhage. Because of prominent effects at the time of peak blood levels, initial titration should be performed with measurements of blood pressure at peak effect (1 to 2 hours after dosing) and just before the next dose.

Use in Patients with Impaired Hepatic Function: Since the liver is the major site of biotransformation and since CARDENE is subject to first pass metabolism, the drug should be used with caution in patients having impaired liver function or reduced hepatic blood flow. Patients with severe liver disease developed elevated blood levels (fourfold increase in AUC) and prolonged half-life (19 hours) of CARDENE. (See DOSAGE AND ADMINISTRATION.)

Use in Patients with Impaired Renal Function: When CARDENE 20 mg or 30 mg tid was given to hypertensive patients with mild renal impairment, mean plasma concentrations, AUC and C_{max} were approximately twofold higher in renally impaired patients than in healthy controls. Doses

in these patients must be adjusted. (See CLINICAL PHARMACOLOGY and DOSAGE AND ADMINISTRATION.)

Drug Interactions: *Beta-Blockers:* In controlled clinical studies, adrenergic beta-receptor blockers have been frequently administered concomitantly with CARDENE. The combination is well tolerated.

Cimetidine: Cimetidine increases CARDENE plasma levels. Patients receiving the two drugs concomitantly should be carefully monitored.

Digoxin: Some calcium blockers may increase the concentration of digitalis preparations in the blood. CARDENE usually does not alter the plasma levels of digoxin; however, serum digoxin levels should be evaluated after concomitant therapy with CARDENE is initiated.

Maalox: Coadministration of Maalox TC had no effect on CARDENE absorption.

Fentanyl Anesthesia: Severe hypotension has been reported during fentanyl anesthesia with concomitant use of a beta-blocker and a calcium channel blocker. Even though such interactions were not seen during clinical studies with CARDENE, an increased volume of circulating fluids might be required if such an interaction were to occur.

Cyclosporine: Concomitant administration of nicardipine and cyclosporine results in elevated plasma cyclosporine levels. Plasma concentrations of cyclosporine should therefore be closely monitored, and its dosage reduced accordingly, in patients treated with nicardipine.

When therapeutic concentrations of *furosemide, propranolol, dipyridamole, warfarin, quinidine* or *naproxen* were added to human plasma (in vitro), the plasma protein binding of CARDENE was not altered.

Carcinogenesis, Mutagenesis, Impairment of Fertility: Rats treated with nicardipine in the diet (at concentrations calculated to provide daily dosage levels of 5, 15 or 45 mg/kg/day) for 2 years showed a dose-dependent increase in thyroid hyperplasia and neoplasia (follicular adenoma/carcinoma). One and 3 month studies in the rat have suggested that these results are linked to a nicardipine-induced reduction in plasma thyroxine (T_4) levels with a consequent increase in plasma levels of thyroid stimulating hormone (TSH). Chronic elevation of TSH is known to cause hyperstimulation of the thyroid. In rats on an iodine deficient diet, nicardipine administration for 1 month was associated with thyroid hyperplasia that was prevented by T_4 supplementation. Mice treated with nicardipine in the diet (at concentrations calculated to provide daily dosage levels of up to 100 mg/kg/day) for up to 18 months showed no evidence of neoplasia of any tissue and no evidence of thyroid changes. There was no evidence of thyroid pathology in dogs treated with up to 25 mg nicardipine/kg/day for 1 year and no evidence of effects of nicardipine on thyroid function (plasma T_4 and TSH) in man. There was no evidence of a mutagenic potential of nicardipine in a battery of genotoxicity tests conducted on microbial indicator organisms, in micronucleus tests in mice and hamsters, or in a sister chromatid exchange study in hamsters. No impairment of fertility was seen in male or female rats administered nicardipine at oral doses as high as 100 mg/kg/day (50 times the 40 mg tid maximum recommended antianginal or antihypertensive dose in man, assuming a patient weight of 60 kg).

Pregnancy: Pregnancy Category C. Nicardipine was embryocidal when administered orally to pregnant Japanese White rabbits, during organogenesis, at 150 mg/kg/day (a dose associated with marked body weight gain suppression in the treated doe) but not at 50 mg/kg/day (25 times the maximum recommended antianginal or antihypertensive dose in man). No adverse effects on the fetus were observed when New Zealand albino rabbits were treated, during organogenesis, with up to 100 mg nicardipine/kg/day (a dose associated with significant mortality in the treated doe). In pregnant rats administered nicardipine orally at up to 100 mg/kg/day (50 times the maximum recommended human dose) there was no evidence of embryolethality or teratogenicity. However, dystocia, reduced birth weights, reduced neonatal survival, and reduced neonatal weight gain were noted. There are no adequate and well-controlled studies in pregnant women. CARDENE should be used during pregnancy only if the potential benefit justifies the potential risk to the fetus.

Nursing Mothers: Studies in rats have shown significant concentrations of CARDENE in maternal milk following oral administration. For this reason it is recommended that women who wish to breast-feed should not take this drug.

Pediatric Use: Safety and efficacy in patients under the age of 18 have not been established.

Use in the Elderly: Pharmacokinetic parameters did not differ between elderly hypertensive patients (≥65 years) and healthy controls after 1 week of CARDENE treatment at 20 mg tid. Plasma CARDENE concentrations in elderly hypertensive patients were similar to plasma concentrations in healthy young adult subjects when CARDENE was administered at doses of 10, 20 and 30 mg tid, suggesting that the pharmacokinetics of CARDENE are similar in young and elderly hypertensive patients. No significant differences in responses to CARDENE have been observed in elderly patients and the general adult population of patients who participated in clinical studies.

ADVERSE REACTIONS

In multiple-dose US and foreign controlled short-term (up to 3 months) studies 1910 patients received CARDENE alone or in combination with other drugs. In these studies adverse events were reported spontaneously; adverse experiences were generally not serious but occasionally required dosage adjustment and about 10% of patients left the studies prematurely because of them. Peak responses were not observed to be associated with adverse effects during clinical trials, but physicians should be aware that adverse effects associated with decreases in blood pressure (tachycardia, hypotension, etc.) could occur around the time of the peak effect. Most adverse effects were expected consequences of the vasodilator effects of CARDENE.

Angina: The incidence rates of adverse effects in anginal patients were derived from multicenter, controlled clinical trials. Following are the rates of adverse effects for CARDENE (n=520) and placebo (n=310), respectively, that occurred in 0.4% of patients or more. These represent events considered probably drug-related by the investigator (except for certain cardiovascular events that were recorded in a different category). Where the frequency of adverse effects for CARDENE and placebo is similar, causal relationship is uncertain. The only dose-related effects were pedal edema and increased angina.

Percent of Patients with Adverse Effects in Controlled Studies (Incidence of discontinuations shown in parentheses)

Adverse Experience	CARDENE (n=520)	PLACEBO (n=310)
Pedal Edema	7.1 (0)	0.3 (0)
Dizziness	6.9 (1.2)	0.6 (0)
Headache	6.4 (0.6)	2.6 (0)
Asthenia	5.8 (0.4)	2.6 (0)
Flushing	5.6 (0.4)	1.0 (0)
Increased Angina	5.6 (3.5)	4.2 (1.9)
Palpitations	3.3 (0.4)	0.0 (0)
Nausea	1.9 (0)	0.3 (0)
Dyspepsia	1.5 (0.6)	0.6 (0.3)
Dry Mouth	1.4 (0)	0.3 (0)
Somnolence	1.4 (0)	1.0 (0)
Rash	1.2 (0.2)	0.3 (0)
Tachycardia	1.2 (0.2)	0.6 (0)
Myalgia	1.0 (0)	0.0 (0)
Other Edema	1.0 (0)	0.0 (0)
Paresthesia	1.0 (0.2)	0.3 (0)
Sustained Tachycardia	0.8 (0.6)	0.0 (0)
Syncope	0.8 (0.2)	0.0 (0)
Constipation	0.6 (0.2)	0.6 (0)
Dyspnea	0.6 (0)	0.0 (0)
Abnormal ECG	0.6 (0.6)	0.0 (0)
Malaise	0.6 (0)	0.0 (0)
Nervousness	0.6 (0)	0.3 (0)
Tremor	0.6 (0)	0.0 (0)

In addition, adverse events were observed that are not readily distinguishable from the natural history of the atherosclerotic vascular disease in these patients. Adverse events in this category each occurred in <0.4% of patients receiving CARDENE and included myocardial infarction, atrial fibrillation, exertional hypotension, pericarditis, heart block, cerebral ischemia, and ventricular tachycardia. It is possible that some of these events were drug-related.

Hypertension: The incidence rates of adverse effects in hypertensive patients were derived from multicenter, controlled clinical trials. Following are the rates of adverse effects for CARDENE (n=1390) and placebo (n=211), respectively, that occurred in 0.4% of patients or more. These represent events considered probably drug-related by the investigator. Where the frequency of adverse effects for CARDENE and placebo is similar, causal relationship is uncertain. The only dose-related effect was pedal edema.

Percent of Patients with Adverse Effects in Controlled Studies (Incidence of discontinuations shown in parentheses)

Adverse Experience	CARDENE (n=1390)	PLACEBO (n=211)
Flushing	9.7 (2.1)	2.8 (0)
Headache	8.2 (2.6)	4.7 (0)
Pedal Edema	8.0 (1.8)	0.9 (0)
Asthenia	4.2 (1.7)	0.5 (0)
Palpitations	4.1 (1.0)	0.0 (0)
Dizziness	4.0 (1.8)	0.0 (0)
Tachycardia	3.4 (1.2)	0.5 (0)
Nausea	2.2 (0.9)	0.9 (0)
Somnolence	1.1 (0.1)	0.0 (0)
Dyspepsia	0.8 (0.3)	0.5 (0)
Insomnia	0.6 (0.1)	0.0 (0)
Malaise	0.6 (0.1)	0.0 (0)
Other Edema	0.6 (0.3)	1.4 (0)
Abnormal Dreams	0.4 (0)	0.0 (0)
Dry Mouth	0.4 (0.1)	0.0 (0)
Nocturia	0.4 (0)	0.0 (0)
Rash	0.4 (0.4)	0.0 (0)
Vomiting	0.4 (0.4)	0.0 (0)

Rare Events: The following rare adverse events have been reported in clinical trials or the literature:

Body as a Whole: infection, allergic reaction

Cardiovascular: hypotension, postural hypotension, atypical chest pain, peripheral vascular disorder, ventricular extrasystoles, ventricular tachycardia

Digestive: sore throat, abnormal liver chemistries

Musculoskeletal: arthralgia

Nervous: hot flashes, vertigo, hyperkinesia, impotence, depression, confusion, anxiety

Respiratory: rhinitis, sinusitis

Special Senses: tinnitus, abnormal vision, blurred vision

Urogenital: increased urinary frequency

OVERDOSAGE

Overdosage with a 600 mg single dose (15 to 30 times normal clinical dose) has been reported. Marked hypotension (blood pressure unobtainable) and bradycardia (heart rate 20 bpm in normal sinus rhythm) occurred, along with drowsiness, confusion and slurred speech. Supportive treatment with a vasopressor resulted in gradual improvement with normal vital signs approximately 9 hours posttreatment.

Based on results obtained in laboratory animals, overdosage may cause systemic hypotension, bradycardia (following initial tachycardia) and progressive atrioventricular conduction block. Reversible hepatic function abnormalities and sporadic focal hepatic necrosis were noted in some animal species receiving very large doses of nicardipine.

For treatment of overdose standard measures (for example, evacuation of gastric contents, elevation of extremities, attention to circulating fluid volume and urine output) including monitoring of cardiac and respiratory functions should be implemented. The patient should be positioned so as to avoid cerebral anoxia. Frequent blood pressure determinations are essential. Vasopressors are clinically indicated for patients exhibiting profound hypotension. Intravenous calcium gluconate may help reverse the effects of calcium entry blockade.

DOSAGE AND ADMINISTRATION

Angina: The dose should be individually titrated for each patient beginning with 20 mg three times daily. Doses in the range of 20 to 40 mg three times a day have been shown to be effective. At least 3 days should be allowed before increasing the CARDENE dose to ensure achievement of steady state plasma drug concentrations.

Concomitant Use With Other Antianginal Agents:

1. Sublingual NTG may be taken as required to abort acute anginal attacks during CARDENE therapy.
2. Prophylactic Nitrate Therapy: CARDENE may be safely coadministered with short- and long-acting nitrates.
3. Beta-blockers: CARDENE may be safely coadministered with beta-blockers. (See *Drug Interactions.*)

Hypertension: The dose of CARDENE should be individually adjusted according to the blood pressure response beginning with 20 mg three times daily. The effective doses in clinical trials have ranged from 20 mg to 40 mg three times daily. The maximum blood pressure lowering effect occurs approximately 1 to 2 hours after dosing. **To assess the adequacy of blood pressure response, the blood pressure should be measured at trough (8 hours after dosing). Because of the prominent peak effects of nicardipine, blood pressure should be measured 1 to 2 hours after dosing, particularly during initiation of therapy.** (See PRECAUTIONS: Blood Pressure, INDICATIONS and CLINICAL PHARMACOLOGY—Peak/Trough Effects in Hypertension.) At least 3 days should be allowed before increasing the CARDENE dose to ensure achievement of steady state plasma drug concentrations.

Concomitant Use With Other Antihypertensive Agents:

1. Diuretics: CARDENE may be safely coadministered with thiazide diuretics.
2. Beta-blockers: CARDENE may be safely coadministered with beta-blockers. (See *Drug Interactions.*)

Special Patient Populations: *Renal Insufficiency:* Although there is no evidence that CARDENE impairs renal function, careful dose titration beginning with 20 mg tid is advised. (See PRECAUTIONS.)

Hepatic Insufficiency: CARDENE should be administered cautiously in patients with severely impaired hepatic function. A suggested starting dose of 20 mg twice a day is advised with individual titration based on clinical findings maintaining the twice a day schedule. (See PRECAUTIONS.)

Congestive Heart Failure: Caution is advised when titrating CARDENE dosage in patients with congestive heart failure. (See WARNINGS.)

HOW SUPPLIED

CARDENE® 20 mg capsules are available in opaque white-white hard gelatin capsules with a brilliant blue band and printed CARDENE 20 mg on the cap and ROCHE on the

Continued on next page

Roche Laboratories—Cont.

capsule body. These are supplied in bottles of 100 (NDC 0033-2437-42) and bottles of 500 (NDC 0033-2437-62).
CARDENE® 30 mg capsules are available in opaque light blue-powder blue hard gelatin capsules with a brilliant blue band and printed CARDENE 30 mg on the cap and ROCHE on the capsule body. These are supplied in bottles of 100 (NDC 0033-2438-42) and bottles of 500 (NDC 0033-2438-62). Store bottles at 15° to 30°C (59° to 86° F) and dispense in light resistant containers.
Revised: August 1995

Shown in Product Identification Guide, page 331

CARDENE® SR
(nicardipine hydrochloride)
Sustained Release Capsules

℞

DESCRIPTION

CARDENE® SR is a sustained release formulation of CARDENE®. CARDENE SR capsules for oral administration each contain 30 mg, 45 mg or 60 mg of nicardipine hydrochloride. Nicardipine hydrochloride is a calcium ion influx inhibitor (slow channel blocker or calcium entry blocker).
Nicardipine hydrochloride is a dihydropyridine derivative with the IUPAC (International Union of Pure and Applied Chemistry) chemical name (±)-2-(benzyl-methyl amino) ethyl methyl 1,4-dihydro-2,6-dimethyl-4-(m-nitrophenyl)-3, 5-pyridinedicarboxylate monohydrochloride.
Nicardipine hydrochloride is a greenish-yellow, odorless, crystalline powder that melts at about 169°C. It is freely soluble in chloroform, methanol and glacial acetic acid, sparingly soluble in anhydrous ethanol, slightly soluble in n-butanol, water, 0.01 M potassium dihydrogen phosphate, acetone and dioxane, very slightly soluble in ethyl acetate, and practically insoluble in benzene, ether and hexane. It has a molecular weight of 515.99.
CARDENE SR is available in hard gelatin capsules containing 30 mg, 45 mg or 60 mg nicardipine hydrochloride. All strengths contain a two component capsule fill. A powder component containing 25% of total nicardipine hydrochloride dose contains pregelatinized starch and magnesium stearate as inactive ingredients. A spherical granule component containing 75% of total nicardipine hydrochloride dose also contains microcrystalline cellulose, starch, lactose and methacrylic acid copolymer Type C as inactive ingredients. The colorants used in the 30 mg capsules are titanium dioxide, FD&C Red No. 40 and Red Iron Oxide, and the colorants used in the 45 mg and 60 mg capsules are titanium dioxide and FD&C Blue No. 2.

CLINICAL PHARMACOLOGY

Mechanism of Action: Nicardipine is a calcium entry blocker (slow channel blocker or calcium ion antagonist) that inhibits the transmembrane influx of calcium ions into cardiac muscle and smooth muscle without changing serum calcium concentrations. The contractile processes of cardiac muscle and vascular smooth muscle are dependent upon the movement of extracellular calcium ions into these cells through specific ion channels. The effects of nicardipine are more selective to vascular smooth muscle than cardiac muscle. In animal models, nicardipine produces relaxation of coronary vascular smooth muscle at drug levels that cause little or no negative inotropic effect.
Pharmacokinetics and Metabolism: Nicardipine is completely absorbed following oral doses administered as capsules, and the systemic bioavailability is about 35% following a 30 mg oral dose at steady state. The pharmacokinetics of nicardipine are nonlinear due to saturable hepatic first-pass metabolism.
Following oral administration of CARDENE SR, plasma levels are detectable as early as 20 minutes and maximal plasma levels are achieved as a broad peak generally between 1 and 4 hours. The average terminal plasma half-life of nicardipine is 8.6 hours. Following oral administration increasing doses result in disproportionate increases in plasma levels. Steady-state C_{max} values following 30, 45 and 60 mg doses every 12 hours averaged 13.4, 34.0 and 58.4 ng/mL, respectively. Hence, increasing the dose twofold increases maximum plasma levels four- to fivefold. A similar disproportionate increase is observed with AUC. In comparison with equivalent daily doses of CARDENE capsules, CARDENE SR shows a significant reduction in C_{max}. CARDENE SR also has somewhat lower bioavailability than CARDENE except at the highest dose. Minimum plasma levels produced by equivalent daily doses are similar. CARDENE SR thus exhibits significantly reduced fluctuation in plasma levels in comparison to CARDENE capsules.
When CARDENE SR was administered with a high fat breakfast, mean C_{max} was 45% lower, AUC was 25% lower and trough levels were 75% higher than when CARDENE SR was given in the fasting state. Thus, taking CARDENE SR with the meal reduced the fluctuation in plasma levels.

Clinical trials establishing the safety and efficacy of CARDENE SR were carried out in patients without regard to the timing of meals.
Nicardipine is highly protein bound (>95%) in human plasma over a wide concentration range.
Nicardipine is metabolized extensively by the liver; less than 1% of intact drug is detected in the urine. Following a radioactive oral dose in solution, 60% of the radioactivity was recovered in the urine and 35% in feces. Most of the dose (over 90%) was recovered within 48 hours of dosing. Nicardipine does not induce its own metabolism and does not induce hepatic microsomal enzymes.
The pharmacokinetics of CARDENE SR in elderly hypertensive patients (mean age 70 years) were compared to those in younger hypertensive patients (mean age 44 years). After a single dose and after 1 week of dosing with CARDENE SR there were no significant differences in C_{max}, T_{max}, AUC or clearance between the young and elderly patients. In both groups of patients, steady-state plasma levels were significantly higher than following a single dose. In the elderly patients, a disproportional increase in plasma levels with dose was observed similar to that observed in normal subjects.
Nicardipine plasma levels following administration of CARDENE SR in hypertensive patients with moderate renal impairment (creatinine clearance 10 to 55 mL/min) were significantly higher following a single oral dose and at steady state than in hypertensive patients with mildly impaired renal function (creatinine clearance >55 mL/min). After 45 mg CARDENE SR bid at steady state, C_{max} and AUC were two- to threefold higher in the patients with moderate renal impairment. Plasma levels in patients with mildly impaired renal function were similar to those in normal subjects.
In patients with severe renal impairment undergoing routine hemodialysis, plasma levels following a single dose of CARDENE SR were not significantly different from those patients with mildly impaired renal function.
Because nicardipine is extensively metabolized by the liver, the plasma levels of the drug are influenced by changes in hepatic function. Following administration of CARDENE capsules, nicardipine plasma levels were higher in patients with severe liver disease (hepatic cirrhosis confirmed by liver biopsy or presence of endoscopically-confirmed esophageal varices) than in normal subjects. After 20 mg CARDENE bid at steady state, C_{max} and AUC were 1.8 and fourfold higher, and the terminal half-life was prolonged to 19 hours in these patients. CARDENE SR has not been studied in patients with severe liver disease.
Hemodynamics: In man, nicardipine produces a significant decrease in systemic vascular resistance. The degree of vasodilation and the resultant hypotensive effects are more prominent in hypertensive patients. In hypertensive patients, nicardipine reduces the blood pressure at rest and during isometric and dynamic exercise. In normotensive patients, a small decrease of about 9 mm Hg in systolic and 7 mm Hg in diastolic blood pressure may accompany this fall in peripheral resistance. An increase in heart rate may occur in response to the vasodilation and decrease in blood pressure, and in a few patients this heart rate increase may be pronounced. In clinical studies mean heart rate at time of peak plasma levels was usually increased by 5 to 10 beats per minute compared to placebo, with the greater increases at higher doses, while there was no difference from placebo at the end of the dosing interval. Hemodynamic studies following intravenous dosing in patients with coronary artery disease and normal or moderately abnormal left ventricular function have shown significant increases in ejection fraction and cardiac output with no significant change, or a small decrease, in left ventricular end-diastolic pressure (LVEDP). Although there is evidence that nicardipine increases coronary blood flow, there is no evidence that this property plays any role in its effectiveness in stable angina. In patients with coronary artery disease, intracoronary administration of nicardipine caused no direct myocardial depression. CARDENE does, however, have a negative inotropic effect in some patients with severe left ventricular dysfunction and could, in patients with very impaired function, lead to worsened failure.
"Coronary Steal," the detrimental redistribution of coronary blood flow in patients with coronary artery disease (diversion of blood from underperfused areas toward better perfused areas), has not been observed during nicardipine treatment. On the contrary, nicardipine has been shown to improve systolic shortening in normal and hypokinetic segments of myocardial muscle, and radionuclide angiography has confirmed that wall motion remained improved during an increase in oxygen demand. Nonetheless, occasional patients have developed increased angina upon receiving nicardipine. Whether this represents steal in those patients, or is the result of increased heart rate and decreased diastolic pressure, is not clear.
In patients with coronary artery disease nicardipine improves L.V. diastolic distensibility during the early filling phase, probably due to a faster rate of myocardial relaxation in previously underperfused areas. There is little or no effect on normal myocardium, suggesting the improvement is

mainly by indirect mechanisms such as afterload reduction and reduced ischemia. Nicardipine has no negative effect on myocardial relaxation at therapeutic doses. The clinical consequences of these properties are as yet undemonstrated.
Electrophysiologic Effects: In general, no detrimental effects on the cardiac conduction system were seen with the use of CARDENE.
Nicardipine increased the heart rate when given intravenously during acute electrophysiologic studies and prolonged the corrected QT interval to a minor degree. The sinus node recovery times and SA conduction times were not affected by the drug. The PA, AH and HV intervals* and the functional and effective refractory periods of the atrium were not prolonged by nicardipine and the relative and effective refractory periods of the His-Purkinje system were slightly shortened after intravenous nicardipine.
*PA=conduction time from high to low right atrium, AH= conduction time from low right atrium to His bundle deflection or AV nodal conduction time, HV=conduction time through the His bundle and the bundle branch-Purkinje system.
Renal Function: There is a transient increase in electrolyte excretion, including sodium. CARDENE does not cause generalized fluid retention, as measured by weight changes.
Effects in Hypertension: CARDENE SR produced decreases in both systolic and diastolic blood pressure throughout the dosing interval in clinical trials. The antihypertensive efficacy of CARDENE SR administered twice daily has been demonstrated using in-clinic blood pressure measures in placebo-controlled trials involving patients with mild to moderate hypertension and in trials using 12 or 24 hour ambulatory blood pressure monitoring.

INDICATIONS AND USAGE

CARDENE SR is indicated for the treatment of hypertension. CARDENE SR may be used alone or in combination with other antihypertensive drugs.

CONTRAINDICATIONS

CARDENE is contraindicated in patients with hypersensitivity to the drug.
Because part of the effect of CARDENE is secondary to reduced afterload, the drug is also contraindicated in patients with advanced aortic stenosis. Reduction of diastolic pressure by any means in these patients may worsen rather than improve myocardial oxygen balance.

WARNINGS

Increased Angina in Patients with Angina: In short-term placebo-controlled angina trials with CARDENE (an immediate release oral dosage form of nicardipine), about 7% of patients on CARDENE (compared with 4% of patients on placebo) have developed increased frequency, duration or severity of angina. Comparisons with beta-blockers also show a greater frequency of increased angina, 4% vs 1%. The mechanism of this effect has not been established.
Use in Patients with Congestive Heart Failure: Although preliminary hemodynamic studies in patients with congestive heart failure have shown that CARDENE reduced afterload without impairing myocardial contractility, it has a negative inotropic effect in vitro and in some patients. Caution should be exercised when using the drug in congestive heart failure patients, particularly in combination with a beta-blocker.
Beta-Blocker Withdrawal: CARDENE is not a beta-blocker and therefore gives no protection against the dangers of abrupt beta-blocker withdrawal; any such withdrawal should be by gradual reduction of the dose of beta-blocker, preferably over 8 to 10 days.

PRECAUTIONS

General: Blood Pressure: Because CARDENE decreases peripheral resistance, careful monitoring of blood pressure during the initial administration and titration of CARDENE is suggested. CARDENE, like other calcium channel blockers, may occasionally produce symptomatic hypotension. Caution is advised to avoid systemic hypotension when administering the drug to patients who have sustained an acute cerebral infarction or hemorrhage.
Use in Patients with Impaired Hepatic Function: Since the liver is the major site of biotransformation and since CARDENE is subject to first-pass metabolism, CARDENE should be used with caution in patients having impaired liver function or reduced hepatic blood flow. Patients with severe liver disease developed elevated blood levels (fourfold increase in AUC) and prolonged half-life (19 hours) of CARDENE.
Use in Patients with Impaired Renal Function: When CARDENE SR 45 mg bid was given to hypertensive patients with moderate renal impairment, mean AUC and C_{max} values were approximately two- to threefold higher than in patients with mild renal impairment. Doses in these patients must be adjusted. Mean AUC and C_{max} values were similar in patients with mildly impaired renal function and normal volunteers. (See CLINICAL PHARMACOLOGY and DOSAGE AND ADMINISTRATION.)
Drug Interactions: Beta-Blockers: In controlled clinical studies, adrenergic beta-receptor blockers have been frequently

administered concomitantly with CARDENE. The combination is well tolerated.

Cimetidine: Cimetidine increases CARDENE plasma levels. Patients receiving the two drugs concomitantly should be carefully monitored.

Digoxin: Some calcium blockers may increase the concentration of digitalis preparations in the blood. CARDENE usually does not alter the plasma levels of digoxin; however, serum digoxin levels should be evaluated after concomitant therapy with CARDENE is initiated.

Fentanyl Anesthesia: Severe hypotension has been reported during fentanyl anesthesia with concomitant use of a beta-blocker and a calcium channel blocker. Even though such interactions were not seen during clinical studies with CARDENE, an increased volume of circulating fluids might be required if such an interaction were to occur.

Cyclosporine: Concomitant administration of nicardipine and cyclosporine results in elevated plasma cyclosporine levels. Plasma concentrations of cyclosporine should therefore be closely monitored, and its dosage reduced accordingly, in patients treated with nicardipine.

When therapeutic concentrations of *furosemide, propranolol, dipyridamole, warfarin, quinidine* or *naproxen* were added to human plasma (in vitro), the plasma protein binding of CARDENE was not altered.

Carcinogenesis, Mutagenesis, Impairment of Fertility: Rats treated with nicardipine in the diet (at concentrations calculated to provide daily dosage levels of 5, 15 or 45 mg/kg/day) for 2 years showed a dose-dependent increase in thyroid hyperplasia and neoplasia (follicular adenoma/carcinoma). One and 3 month studies in the rat have suggested that these results are linked to a nicardipine-induced reduction in plasma thyroxine (T_4) levels with a consequent increase in plasma levels of thyroid stimulating hormone (TSH). Chronic elevation of TSH is known to cause hyperstimulation of the thyroid. In rats on an iodine deficient diet, nicardipine administration for 1 month was associated with thyroid hyperplasia that was prevented by T_4 supplementation. Mice treated with nicardipine in the diet (at concentrations calculated to provide daily dosage levels of up to 100 mg/kg/day) for up to 18 months showed no evidence of neoplasia of any tissue and no evidence of thyroid changes. There was no evidence of thyroid pathology in dogs treated with up to 25 mg nicardipine/kg/day for 1 year and no evidence of effects of nicardipine on thyroid function (plasma T_4 and TSH) in man.

There was no evidence of a mutagenic potential of nicardipine in a battery of genotoxicity tests conducted on microbial indicator organisms, in micronucleus tests in mice and hamsters, or in a sister chromatid exchange study in hamsters.

No impairment of fertility was seen in male or female rats administered nicardipine at oral doses as high as 100 mg/kg/day (50 times the maximum recommended daily dose in man, assuming a patient weight of 60 kg).

Pregnancy: Pregnancy Category C. Nicardipine was embryocidal when administered orally to pregnant Japanese White rabbits, during organogenesis, at 150 mg/kg/day (a dose associated with marked body weight gain suppression in the treated doe) but not at 50 mg/kg/day (25 times the maximum recommended dose in man). No adverse effects on the fetus were observed when New Zealand albino rabbits were treated, during organogenesis, with up to 100 mg nicardipine/kg/day (a dose associated with significant mortality in the treated doe). In pregnant rats administered nicardipine orally at up to 100 mg/kg/day (50 times the maximum recommended human dose) there was no evidence of embryolethality or teratogenicity. However, dystocia, reduced birth weights, reduced neonatal survival and reduced neonatal weight gain were noted. There are no adequate and well-controlled studies in pregnant women. CARDENE SR should be used during pregnancy only if the potential benefit justifies the potential risk to the fetus.

Nursing Mothers: Studies in rats have shown significant concentrations of nicardipine in maternal milk following oral administration. For this reason it is recommended that women who wish to breastfeed should not take this drug.

Pediatric Use: Safety and efficacy in patients under the age of 18 have not been established.

Use in the Elderly: Pharmacokinetic parameters did not differ significantly between elderly hypertensive patients (mean age: 70 years) and younger hypertensive patients (mean age: 44 years) after 1 week of treatment with CARDENE SR. No significant differences in response to CARDENE have been observed in elderly patients and the general adult population of patients who have participated in studies.

ADVERSE EVENTS

In multiple-dose US and foreign controlled studies, 667 patients received CARDENE SR. In these studies adverse events were elicited by nondirected and in some cases directed questioning; adverse events were generally not serious and about 9% of patients withdrew prematurely from the studies because of them.

Hypertension: The incidence rates of adverse events in hypertensive patients were derived from placebo-controlled clinical trials. Following are the rates of adverse events for CARDENE SR (n=322) and placebo (n=140), respectively, that occurred in 0.6% of patients or more on CARDENE SR. These represent events considered probably drug related by the investigator. Where the frequency of adverse events for CARDENE SR and placebo is similar, causal relationship is uncertain. The only dose-related effect was pedal edema.

Percentage of Patients with Probably Drug Related Adverse Events in Placebo-Controlled Studies

Adverse Event	CARDENE SR (n=322)	Placebo (n=140)
Headache	6.2	7.1
Pedal Edema	5.9	1.4
Vasodilatation	4.7	1.4
Palpitation	2.8	1.4
Nausea	1.9	0.7
Dizziness	1.6	0.7
Asthenia	0.9	0.7
Postural Hypotension	0.9	0
Increased Urinary Frequency	0.6	0
Pain	0.6	0
Rash	0.6	0
Sweating Increased	0.6	0
Vomiting	0.6	0

Incidence (%) of Discontinuations Due to Any Adverse Event in Placebo-Controlled Studies

Adverse Event	CARDENE SR (n=322)	Placebo (n=140)
Headache	2.5	1.4
Palpitation	2.2	0.7
Dizziness	1.9	0.7
Asthenia	1.9	0
Pedal Edema	1.2	0
Nausea	1.2	0
Rash	0.9	0.7
Diarrhea	0.9	0
Tachycardia	0.9	0
Blurred Vision	0.6	0
Chest Pain	0.6	0
Face Edema	0.6	0
Myocardial Infarct	0.6	0
Vasodilatation	0.6	0
Vomiting	0.6	0

Uncontrolled experience in over 300 patients with hypertension treated for up to 27.5 months with CARDENE SR has shown no unexpected adverse events or increase in incidence of adverse events compared to the controlled clinical trials.

Rare Events: The following rare adverse events have been reported in clinical trials or the literature:

Body as a Whole: infection, allergic reaction

Cardiovascular: hypotension, atypical chest pain, peripheral vascular disorder, ventricular extrasystoles, ventricular tachycardia, angina pectoris

Digestive: sore throat, abnormal liver chemistries

Musculoskeletal: arthralgia

Nervous: hot flashes, vertigo, hyperkinesia, impotence, depression, confusion, anxiety

Respiratory: rhinitis, sinusitis

Special Senses: tinnitus, abnormal vision, blurred vision

Angina: Data are available from only 91 patients with chronic stable angina pectoris who received CARDENE SR 30 to 60 mg administered twice daily in open-label clinical trials. Fifty-eight of these patients were treated for at least 30 days. The four most frequently reported adverse events thought by the investigators to be probably related to the use of CARDENE SR were vasodilatation (5.5%), pedal edema (4.4%), asthenia (4.4%) and dizziness (3.3%).

OVERDOSAGE

Three overdosages with CARDENE or CARDENE SR have been reported. Two occurred in adults, 1 of whom ingested 600 mg of CARDENE and the other 2160 mg of CARDENE SR. Symptoms included marked hypotension, bradycardia, palpitations, flushing, drowsiness, confusion and slurred speech. All symptoms resolved without sequelae. The third overdosage occurred in a 1-year-old child who ingested half of the powder in a 30 mg CARDENE capsule. The child remained asymptomatic.

Based on results obtained in laboratory animals, overdosage may cause systemic hypotension, bradycardia (following initial tachycardia) and progressive atrioventricular conduction block. Reversible hepatic function abnormalities and sporadic focal hepatic necrosis were noted in some animal species receiving very large doses of nicardipine.

For treatment of overdose standard measures (for example, evacuation of gastric contents, elevation of extremities, attention to circulating fluid volume and urine output) including monitoring of cardiac and respiratory functions should be implemented. The patient should be positioned so as to avoid cerebral anoxia. Frequent blood pressure determinations are essential. Vasopressors are clinically indicated for patients exhibiting profound hypotension. Intravenous calcium gluconate may help reverse the effects of calcium entry blockade.

DOSAGE AND ADMINISTRATION

The dose of CARDENE SR should be individually adjusted according to the blood pressure response beginning with 30 mg two times daily. The effective doses in clinical trials have ranged from 30 mg to 60 mg two times daily. The maximum blood pressure lowering effect at steady state is sustained from 2 hours until 6 hours after dosing.

When initiating therapy or upon increasing dose, blood pressure should be measured 2 to 4 hours after the first dose or dose increase, as well as at the end of a dosing interval.

The total daily dose of immediate release nicardipine (CARDENE) may not be a useful guide to judging the effective dose of CARDENE SR. Patients currently receiving immediate release nicardipine may be titrated with CARDENE SR starting at their current total daily dose of immediate release nicardipine and then reexamined to assess the adequacy of blood pressure control.

Concomitant Use with Other Antihypertensive Agents:

1. Diuretics: CARDENE may be safely coadministered with thiazide diuretics.
2. Beta-Blockers: CARDENE may be safely coadministered with beta-blockers. (See *Drug Interactions.*)

Special Patient Populations: *Renal Insufficiency:* Although there is no evidence that CARDENE SR impairs renal function, careful dose titration beginning with 30 mg CARDENE SR bid is advised. (See PRECAUTIONS.)

Hepatic Insufficiency: CARDENE SR has not been studied in patients with severe liver impairment. (See PRECAUTIONS.)

Congestive Heart Failure: Caution is advised when titrating CARDENE SR dosage in patients with congestive heart failure. (See WARNINGS.)

HOW SUPPLIED

CARDENE® SR 30 mg capsules are available in opaque pink-pink hard gelatin capsules. The capsule cap is printed with CARDENE SR 30 mg and the capsule body is printed with ROCHE. These are supplied in bottles of 60 (NDC 0004-0180-22) and bottles of 200 (NDC 0004-0180-91).

CARDENE® SR 45 mg capsules are available in opaque powder blue-powder blue hard gelatin capsules. The capsule cap is printed with CARDENE SR 45 mg and the capsule body is printed with ROCHE. These are supplied in bottles of 60 (NDC 0004-0181-22) and bottles of 200 (NDC 0004-0181-91).

CARDENE® SR 60 mg capsules are available in opaque light blue-white hard gelatin capsules. The capsule cap is printed with CARDENE SR 60 mg and the capsule body is printed with ROCHE. These are supplied in bottles of 60 (NDC 0004-0182-22) and bottles of 200 (NDC 0004-0182-91).

Store bottles at 15° to 30°C (59° to 86°F) and dispense in light-resistant containers, such as the manufacturer's original container.

Revised: February 1996

Shown in Product Identification Guide, page 332

CELLCEPT® ℞

[Sel'sep]

(mycophenolate mofetil capsules)

The following text is complete prescribing information based on official labeling in effect June 1996.

WARNING

Increased susceptibility to infection and the possible development of lymphoma may result from immunosuppression. Only physicians experienced in immunosuppressive therapy and management of renal transplant patients should use CellCept®. Patients receiving the drug should be managed in facilities equipped and staffed with adequate laboratory and supportive medical resources. The physician responsible for maintenance therapy should have complete information requisite for the follow-up of the patient.

DESCRIPTION

CellCept (mycophenolate mofetil) is the 2-morpholinoethyl ester of mycophenolic acid (MPA), an immunosuppressive agent.

The chemical name for mycophenolate mofetil is 2-morpholinoethyl (E)-6-(1,3-dihydro-4-hydroxy-6-methoxy-7-methyl-3-oxo-5-isobenzofuranyl)-4-methyl-4-hexenoate. It has an empirical formula of $C_{23}H_{31}NO_7$, and a molecular weight of 433.50.

Continued on next page

Roche Laboratories—Cont.

CellCept is available for oral administration as capsules containing 250 mg of mycophenolate mofetil. Inactive ingredients include croscarmellose sodium, magnesium stearate, povidone (K-90) and pregelatinized starch. The capsule shells contain black iron oxide, FD&C blue #2, gelatin, red iron oxide, silicon dioxide, sodium lauryl sulfate, titanium dioxide, and yellow iron oxide.

Mycophenolate mofetil is a white to off-white crystalline powder. It is slightly soluble in water (43 μg/mL at pH 7.4); the solubility increases in acidic medium (4.27 mg/mL at pH 3.6). It is freely soluble in acetone, soluble in methanol, and sparingly soluble in ethanol. The apparent partition coefficient in 1-octanol/water (pH 7.4) buffer solution is 238. The pKa values for mycophenolate mofetil are 5.6 for the morpholino group and 8.5 for the phenolic group.

CLINICAL PHARMACOLOGY

Mechanism of Action

Mycophenolate mofetil has been demonstrated in experimental animal models to prolong the survival of allogeneic transplants (kidney, heart, liver, intestine, limb, small bowel, pancreatic islets, and bone marrow). Mycophenolate mofetil has also been shown to reverse ongoing acute rejection in the canine renal and rat cardiac allograft models. Mycophenolate mofetil also inhibited proliferative arteriopathy in experimental models of aortic and heart allografts in rats, as well as in primate cardiac xenografts. Mycophenolate mofetil was used alone or in combination with other immunosuppressive agents in these studies. Mycophenolate mofetil has been demonstrated to inhibit immunologically-mediated inflammatory responses in animal models and to inhibit tumor development and prolong survival in murine tumor transplant models.

Mycophenolate mofetil is rapidly absorbed following oral administration and hydrolyzed to form MPA, which is the active metabolite. MPA is a potent, selective, uncompetitive and reversible inhibitor of inosine monophosphate dehydrogenase (IMPDH), and therefore inhibits the *de novo* pathway of guanosine nucleotide synthesis without incorporation into DNA. Because T- and B-lymphocytes are critically dependent for their proliferation on *de novo* synthesis of purines whereas other cell types can utilize salvage pathways, MPA has potent cytostatic effects on lymphocytes. MPA inhibits proliferative responses of T- and B-lymphocytes to both mitogenic and allospecific stimulation. Addition of guanosine or deoxyguanosine reverses the cytostatic effects of MPA on lymphocytes. MPA also suppresses antibody formation by B-lymphocytes. MPA prevents the glycosylation of lymphocyte and monocyte glycoproteins that are involved in intercellular adhesion to endothelial cells and may inhibit recruitment of leukocytes into sites of inflammation and graft rejection. Mycophenolate mofetil did not inhibit early events in the activation of human peripheral blood mononuclear cells, such as the production of interleukin-1 (IL-1) and interleukin-2 (IL-2), but did block the coupling of these events to DNA synthesis and proliferation.

Pharmacokinetics

Following oral administration, mycophenolate mofetil undergoes rapid and extensive absorption and complete presystemic metabolism to MPA, the active metabolite. MPA is metabolized to form the phenolic glucuronide of MPA (MPAG) which is not pharmacologically active. Mycophenolate mofetil is not measurable systemically in plasma following oral administration.

Absorption: In 12 healthy volunteers, the mean absolute bioavailability of oral mycophenolate mofetil relative to IV mycophenolate mofetil (based on MPA AUC) was 94%. The area under the plasma-concentration time curve (AUC) for MPA appears to increase in a dose-proportional fashion in renal transplant patients receiving multiple doses of mycophenolate mofetil up to a daily dose of 3 g (see table below on pharmacokinetic parameters in renal transplant patients). Immediately post-transplant (<40 days), mean AUC and Cmax are approximately 50% lower in renal transplant patients than that observed in healthy volunteers or in stable renal transplant patients.

Food (27 g fat, 650 calories) had no effect on the extent of absorption (MPA AUC) of mycophenolate mofetil when administered at doses of 1.5 g b.i.d. to renal transplant patients. However, MPA Cmax was decreased by 40% in the presence of food. (See DOSAGE AND ADMINISTRATION.)

Distribution: The mean ($\pm$SD) apparent volume of distribution of MPA in twelve healthy volunteers is approximately 3.6 ($\pm$1.5) and 4.0 ($\pm$1.2) L/kg following IV and oral administration, respectively. MPA, at clinically relevant concentrations, is 97% bound to plasma albumin. MPAG is 82% bound to plasma albumin at MPAG concentration ranges that are normally seen in stable renal transplant patients; however, at higher MPAG concentrations (observed in patients with renal impairment or delayed graft function), the binding of MPA may be reduced as a result of

competition between MPAG and MPA for protein binding. Mean blood to plasma ratio of radioactivity concentrations was approximately 0.6 indicating that MPA and MPAG do not extensively distribute into the cellular fractions of blood.

In vitro studies to evaluate the effect of other agents on the binding of MPA to human serum albumin (HSA) or plasma proteins showed that salicylate (at 25 mg/dL with HSA) and MPAG (at $\geq$ 460 μg/mL with plasma proteins) increased the free fraction of MPA. At concentrations that exceeded what is encountered clinically, cyclosporine, digoxin, naproxen, prednisone, propranolol, tacrolimus, theophylline, tolbutamide, and warfarin did not increase the free fraction of MPA. MPA at concentrations as high as 100 μg/mL had little effect on the binding of warfarin, digoxin or propranolol, but decreased the binding of theophylline from 53% to 45% and phenytoin from 90% to 87%.

Metabolism: Mycophenolate mofetil undergoes complete presystemic metabolism to MPA, the active metabolite. MPA is metabolized principally by glucuronyl transferase to form the phenolic glucuronide of MPA (MPAG) which is not pharmacologically active. The following metabolites of the 2-hydroxyethylmorpholino moiety are also recovered in the urine following oral administration of mycophenolate mofetil to healthy subjects: N-(2-carboxymethyl)-morpholine, N-(2-hydroxyethyl)-morpholine, and the N-oxide of N-(2-hydroxyethyl)-morpholine.

Secondary peaks in the plasma MPA concentration-time profile are usually observed 6-12 hours post-dose. The coadministration of cholestyramine (4 g t.i.d.) resulted in approximately a 40% decrease in the MPA AUC (largely as a consequence of lower concentrations in the terminal portion of the profile). These observations suggest that enterohepatic recirculation contributes to MPA plasma concentrations.

Increased plasma concentrations of mycophenolate mofetil metabolites (MPA 50% increase and MPAG about 3–6 fold increase) are observed in patients with renal insufficiency. (See CLINICAL PHARMACOLOGY: Special Populations.)

Excretion: Negligible amount of drug is excreted as MPA (<1% of dose) in the urine. Orally administered radiolabeled mycophenolate mofetil resulted in complete recovery of the administered dose; with 93% of the administered dose recovered in the urine and 6% recovered in feces. Most (about 87%) of the administered dose is excreted in the urine as MPAG. MPA and MPAG are usually not removed by hemodialysis. However, at high MPAG plasma concentrations (>100 μg/mL), small amounts of MPAG are removed.

Mean ($\pm$SD) apparent half-life and plasma clearance of MPA are 17.9 ($\pm$6.5) hours and 193 ($\pm$48) mL/min following oral administration and 16.6 ($\pm$5.8) hours and 177 ($\pm$31) mL/min following IV administration, respectively.

Pharmacokinetics in Healthy Volunteers and Renal Transplant Patients: Shown below are the mean ($\pm$SD) pharmacokinetic parameters for MPA following the administration of oral mycophenolate mofetil given as single doses to healthy volunteers and multiple doses to renal transplant patients. As noted below, MPA AUC and Cmax in early transplant patients (<40 days post-transplant) are approximately 50% lower as compared to healthy volunteers or to stable renal transplant patients.

[See first table above.]

Special Populations

Shown below are the mean ($\pm$SD) pharmacokinetic parameters for MPA following the administration of oral mycophenolate mofetil given as single doses to subjects with renal and hepatic impairment.

[See second table above.]

PHARMACOKINETIC PARAMETERS FOR MPA
[mean ($\pm$SD)]
FOLLOWING ADMINISTRATION OF MYCOPHENOLATE MOFETIL TO HEALTHY VOLUNTEERS (SINGLE DOSE) AND RENAL TRANSPLANT PATIENTS (MULTIPLE DOSES)

Healthy Volunteers (no. of subjects)	Dose	Tmax (h)	Cmax (μg/mL)	Total AUC (μg·h/mL)
(n=129) *(n=117)	1 g	0.80 ($\pm$0.36)	24.5 ($\pm$9.5)	63.9* ($\pm$16.2)
Time After Renal Transplantation (no. of patients)	**Dose**	**Tmax (h)**	**Cmax (μg/mL)**	**Interdosing Interval AUC$_{0-12}$ (μg·h/mL)**
Early (<40 days) (n=25)	1 g b.i.d.	1.31 ($\pm$0.76)	8.16 ($\pm$4.50)	27.3 ($\pm$10.9)
Early (<40 days) (n=27)	1.5 g b.i.d.	1.21 ($\pm$0.81)	13.5 ($\pm$8.18)	38.4 ($\pm$15.4)
Late (>3 months) (n=23)	1.5 g b.i.d.	0.90 ($\pm$0.24)	24.1 ($\pm$12.1)	65.3 ($\pm$35.4)

PHARMACOKINETIC PARAMETERS FOR MPA
[mean ($\pm$SD)]
FOLLOWING SINGLE DOSES OF MYCOPHENOLATE MOFETIL IN CHRONIC RENAL AND HEPATIC IMPAIRMENT

Renal Impairment (no. of patients)	Dose	Tmax (h)	Cmax (μg/mL)	AUC$_{0-96}$ (μg·h/mL)
Healthy Volunteers GFR >80 mL/min/1.73m^2 (n=6)	1 g	0.75 ($\pm$0.27)	25.3 ($\pm$7.99)	45.0 ($\pm$22.6)
Mild Renal Impairment GFR 50-80 mL/min/1.73m^2 (n=6)	1 g	0.75 ($\pm$0.27)	26.0 ($\pm$3.82)	59.9 ($\pm$12.9)
Moderate Renal Impairment GFR 25-49 mL/min/1.73m^2 (n=6)	1 g	0.75 ($\pm$0.27)	19.0 ($\pm$13.2)	52.9 ($\pm$25.5)
Severe Renal Impairment GFR <25 mL/min/1.73m^2 (n=7)	1 g	1.00 ($\pm$0.41)	16.3 ($\pm$10.8)	78.6 ($\pm$46.4)
Hepatic Impairment (no. of patients)	**Dose**	**Tmax (h)**	**Cmax (μg/mL)**	**AUC$_{0-48}$ (μg·h/mL)**
Healthy Volunteers (n=6)	1 g	0.63 ($\pm$0.14)	24.3 ($\pm$5.73)	29.0 ($\pm$5.78)
Alcoholic cirrhosis (n=18)	1 g	0.85 ($\pm$0.58)	22.4 ($\pm$10.1)	29.8 ($\pm$10.7)

Renal Insufficiency: In a single-dose study (6 volunteers per group), plasma MPA AUCs observed in volunteers with severe chronic renal impairment [glomerular filtration rate (GFR) < 25 mL/min/1.73 m^2] were about 75% higher relative to those observed in healthy volunteers (GFR > 80 mL/min/1.73 m^2). In addition, the single dose plasma MPAG AUC was 3–6 fold higher in volunteers with severe renal impairment than in volunteers with mild renal impairment or healthy volunteers, consistent with the known renal elimination of MPAG. Multiple dosing of mycophenolate mofetil in patients with severe chronic renal impairment has not been studied. No data are available on the safety of long-term exposure to this level of MPAG. (See PRECAUTIONS: General and DOSAGE AND ADMINISTRATION.)

In patients with delayed graft function post-transplant, mean MPA AUC$_{0-12}$ was comparable to that seen in post-transplant patients without delayed graft function. Mean plasma MPAG AUC$_{0-12}$ was 2–3 fold higher than in post-transplant patients without delayed graft function. (See PRECAUTIONS: General and DOSAGE AND ADMINISTRATION.)

The pharmacokinetics of mycophenolate mofetil are not altered by hemodialysis. Hemodialysis usually does not remove MPA or MPAG. At high concentrations of MPAG (> 100 μg/mL), hemodialysis removes only small amounts of MPAG.

Hepatic Insufficiency: In a single dose (1 g) study of 18 volunteers with alcoholic cirrhosis and 6 healthy volunteers, hepatic MPA glucuronidation processes appeared to be relatively unaffected by hepatic parenchymal disease when pharmacokinetic parameters of healthy volunteers and alcoholic cirrhosis patients within this study were compared. However, it should be noted that for unexplained reasons, the healthy volunteers in this study had about a 50% lower AUC as compared to healthy volunteers in other studies, thus making comparisons between volunteers with alcoholic cirrhosis and healthy volunteers difficult. Effects of hepatic disease on this process probably depend on the particular disease. Hepatic disease with other etiologies may show a different effect.

Pediatrics: Very limited pharmacokinetic data are available for pediatric renal transplant recipients. Data on these patients collected on day 21 post-transplant are presented in the table below: [See first table above.]

Gender: Data obtained from several studies were pooled to look at any gender related differences in the pharmacokinetics of MPA (data were adjusted to 1 g dose). Mean ($\pm$SD) MPA AUC$_{0-12}$ for males (n=79) was 32.0 ($\pm$14.5) and for females (n=41) was 36.5 ($\pm$18.8) μg·h/mL while mean ($\pm$SD) MPA Cmax was 9.96 ($\pm$6.19) in the males and 10.6 ($\pm$5.64) μg/mL in the females. These differences are not of clinical significance.

Clinical Studies

The safety and efficacy of CellCept in combination with corticosteroids and cyclosporine for the prevention of organ rejection following allogeneic renal transplants were assessed in three randomized, double-blind, multicenter trials.

These studies compared two dose levels of CellCept (1.0 g b.i.d. and 1.5 g b.i.d.) with azathioprine (2 studies) or placebo (1 study) when administered in combination with cyclosporine (Sandimmune®) and corticosteroids to prevent acute rejection episodes. One study also included antithymocyte globulin (ATGAM®) induction therapy. The three studies are described by geographic location of the investigational sites. One study was conducted in the USA at 14 sites, one study was conducted in Europe at 20 sites, and one study was conducted in Europe, Canada, and Australia at a total of 21 sites.

The primary efficacy endpoint was the proportion of patients in each treatment group who experienced treatment failure within the first six months after transplantation (defined as biopsy-proven acute rejection on treatment or the occurrence of death, graft loss or early termination from the study for any reason without prior biopsy-proven rejection). Cell-Cept, when administered with antithymocyte globulin (ATGAM®) induction (one study) and with cyclosporine and corticosteroids (all three studies), was compared to the following three therapeutic regimens: (1) antithymocyte globulin (ATGAM®) induction/azathioprine/cyclosporine/corticosteroids, (2) azathioprine/cyclosporine/corticosteroids, and (3) cyclosporine/corticosteroids.

CellCept, in combination with corticosteroids and cyclosporine reduced (statistically significant at the < 0.05 level) the incidence of treatment failure within the first 6 months following transplantation. The following tables summarize the results of these studies. These tables show (1) the proportion of patients experiencing treatment failure, (2) the proportion of patients who experienced biopsy-proven acute rejection on treatment, and (3) early termination, for any reason other than graft loss or death, without a prior biopsy-proven rejection episode. Patients who prematurely discontinued treatment were followed for the occurrence of death or graft loss, and the cumulative incidence of graft loss and patient death are summarized separately. Patients who prematurely discontinued treatment were not followed for the occurrence

of acute rejection after termination. More patients discontinued receiving CellCept (without prior biopsy-proven rejection, death or graft loss) than discontinued in the control groups, with the highest rate in the CellCept 3 g/day group. Therefore, the acute rejection rates may be underestimates, particularly in the CellCept 3 g/day group.
[See second table above.]
[See third table above.]
[See fourth table above.]
Cumulative incidence of twelve-month graft loss and patient death are presented below. No advantage of CellCept with respect to graft loss and patient death was established. Numerically, patients receiving CellCept 2 g/day and 3 g/day experienced a better outcome than controls in all three studies; patients receiving CellCept 2 g/day experienced a better outcome than CellCept 3 g/day in two of the three studies. Patients in all treatment groups who terminated treatment early were found to have a poor outcome with respect to graft loss and patient death at one year.
[See table at top of next page.]

INDICATIONS AND USAGE

CellCept is indicated by the prophylaxis of organ rejection in patients receiving allogeneic renal transplants. CellCept should be used concomitantly with cyclosporine and corticosteroids.

CONTRAINDICATIONS

Allergic reactions to CellCept have been observed; therefore, CellCept is contraindicated in patients with a hypersensitivity to mycophenolate mofetil, mycophenolic acid or any component of the drug product.

WARNINGS

(See boxed WARNING.)
Patients receiving immunosuppressive regimens involving combinations of drugs, including CellCept, as part of an immunosuppressive regimen are at increased risk of developing lymphomas and other malignancies, particularly of the skin. The risk appears to be related to the intensity and duration of immunosuppression rather than to the use of any specific agent. Oversuppression of the immune system can also increase susceptibility to infection. CellCept has been administered in combination with the following agents in clinical trials: antithymocyte globulin (ATGAM®), OKT3 (Orthoclone OKT®3), cyclosporine (Sandimmune®), and

Continued on next page

PHARMACOKINETIC PARAMETERS FOR MPA
[mean $\pm$ (SD)]
FOLLOWING MULTIPLE ORAL DOSES OF MYCOPHENOLATE MOFETIL IN PEDIATRIC RENAL TRANSPLANT PATIENTS

Age Range	Dose	Tmax (h)	Cmax (μg/mL)	AUC$_{0-12}$ (μg·h/mL)
≥ 3 mo to < 6 yr (Mean = 2.75) (n=4)	15 mg/kg b.i.d.	1.25 ($\pm$0.87)	3.70 ($\pm$2.08)	13.6 ($\pm$8.69)
≥ 6 yr to < 12 yr (Mean = 9.0) (n=4)	15 mg/kg b.i.d.	0.50 ($\pm$0.00)	13.5 ($\pm$4.48)	23.4 ($\pm$2.84)
≥ 12 yr to 18 yr (Mean = 15.6) (n=5)	15 mg/kg b.i.d.	0.50 ($\pm$0.00)	13.2 ($\pm$6.86)	30.0 ($\pm$8.34)
≥ 12 yr to 18 yr (Mean = 14.0) (n=7)	23 mg/kg b.i.d.	1.14 ($\pm$0.80)	10.6 ($\pm$9.59)	28.3 ($\pm$12.8)

Incidence of Treatment Failure
(Biopsy-Proven Rejection or Early Termination for Any Reason)

USA Study (n=499 patients)	CellCept 2 g/day (n=167 patients)	CellCept 3 g/day (n=166 patients)	Azathioprine 1–2 mg/kg/day (n=166 patients)
All treatment failures	31.1%	31.3%	47.6%
Early termination without prior acute rejection*	9.6%	12.7%	6.0%
Biopsy-proven rejection episode on treatment	19.8%	17.5%	38.0%

Europe/Canada/ Australia Study (n=503 patients)	CellCept 2 g/day (n=173 patients)	CellCept 3 g/day (n=164 patients)	Azathioprine 100–150 mg/day (n=166 patients)
All treatment failures	38.2%	34.8%	50.0%
Early termination without prior acute rejection*	13.9%	15.2%	10.2%
Biopsy-proven rejection episode on treatment	19.7%	15.9%	35.5%

Europe Study (n=491 patients)	CellCept 2 g/day (n=165 patients)	CellCept 3 g/day (n=160 patients)	Placebo (n=166 patients)
All treatment failures	30.3%	38.8%	56.0%
Early termination without prior acute rejection*	11.5%	22.5%	7.2%
Biopsy-proven rejection episode on treatment	17.0%	13.8%	46.4%

* Does not include death and graft loss as reason for early termination.

Roche Laboratories—Cont.

corticosteroids. The efficacy and safety of the use of CellCept in combination with other immunosuppressive agents have not been determined.

Lymphoproliferative disease or lymphoma developed in patients receiving CellCept with other immunosuppressive agents in approximately 1% of patients in the controlled studies of prevention of rejection. (See ADVERSE REACTIONS.)

Adverse effects on fetal development (including malformations) occurred when pregnant rats and rabbits were dosed during organogenesis. These responses occurred at doses lower than those associated with maternal toxicity, and at doses below the recommended clinical dose. There are no adequate and well-controlled studies in pregnant women. However, as CellCept has been shown to have teratogenic effects in animals, it may cause fetal harm when administered to a pregnant woman. Therefore, CellCept should not be used in pregnant women unless the potential benefit justifies the potential risk to the fetus.

Women of childbearing potential should have a negative serum or urine pregnancy test with a sensitivity of at least 50 mIU/mL within 1 week prior to beginning therapy. It is recommended that CellCept therapy should not be initiated by the physician until a report of a negative pregnancy test has been obtained.

Effective contraception must be used before beginning CellCept therapy, during therapy, and for 6 weeks following discontinuation of therapy, even where there has been a history of infertility, unless due to hysterectomy. Two reliable forms of contraception must be used simultaneously unless abstinence is the chosen method. If pregnancy does occur during treatment, the physician and patient should discuss the desirability of continuing the pregnancy. (See PRECAUTIONS: Pregnancy and Information for Patients.)

In the three controlled studies for prevention of rejection, similar rates of fatal infections/sepsis (<2%) occurred in patients while receiving CellCept or control therapy in combination with other immunosuppressive agents. (See ADVERSE REACTIONS.)

Up to 2.0% of patients receiving CellCept for prevention of rejection developed severe neutropenia [absolute neutrophil count (ANC) $<0.5 \times 10^3/\mu L$]. (See ADVERSE REACTIONS.) Patients receiving CellCept should be monitored for neutropenia. (See PRECAUTIONS: Laboratory Tests.) The development of neutropenia may be related to CellCept itself, concomitant medications, viral infections, or some combination of these causes. If neutropenia develops (ANC $<1.3 \times 10^3/\mu L$), dosing with CellCept should be interrupted or the dose reduced, appropriate diagnostic tests performed, and the patient managed appropriately. (See DOSAGE AND ADMINISTRATION.) Neutropenia has been observed most frequently in the period from 31 to 180 days post-transplant in patients treated for prevention of rejection.

PRECAUTIONS

General

Gastrointestinal tract hemorrhage has been observed in approximately 3% of patients treated with CellCept. Gastrointestinal tract perforations have rarely been observed. Most patients receiving CellCept were also receiving other drugs known to be associated with those complications. Patients with active peptic ulcer disease were excluded from enrollment in studies with mycophenolate mofetil. Because CellCept has been associated with an increased incidence of digestive system adverse events, including infrequent cases of gastrointestinal tract ulceration, hemorrhage, and perforation, CellCept should be administered with caution in patients with active serious digestive system disease.

Subjects with severe chronic renal impairment (GFR <25 mL/min/1.73 m^2) who have received single doses of CellCept showed higher plasma MPA and MPAG AUCs relative to subjects with lesser degrees of renal impairment or normal healthy volunteers. No data are available on the safety of long-term exposure to these levels of MPAG. Doses of CellCept greater than 1 g administered twice a day should be avoided and they should be carefully observed. (See CLINICAL PHARMACOLOGY: Pharmacokinetics and DOSAGE AND ADMINISTRATION.)

In patients with delayed graft function post-transplant, mean MPA AUC_{0-12} was comparable, but MPAG AUC_{0-12} was 2–3 fold higher, compared to that seen in post-transplant patients without delayed graft function. In the three controlled studies of prevention of rejection, there were 298 of 1,483 patients (20%) with delayed graft function. Although patients with delayed graft function have a higher incidence of certain adverse events (anemia, thrombocytopenia, hyperkalemia) than patients without delayed graft function, these events were not more frequent in patients receiving CellCept than azathioprine or placebo. No dose adjustment is recommended for these patients, however, they should be carefully observed. (See CLINICAL PHARMACOLOGY: Pharmacokinetics and DOSAGE AND ADMINISTRATION.)

Cumulative Incidence of Combined Graft Loss and Patient Death at 12 Months

Study	CellCept 2 g/day	CellCept 3 g/day	Control (Azathioprine or Placebo)
USA	8.5%	11.5%	12.2%
Europe/ Canada/ Australia	11.7%	11.0%	13.6%
Europe	8.5%	10.0%	11.5%

It is recommended that CellCept not be administered concomitantly with azathioprine because such concomitant administration has not been studied clinically.

In view of the significant reduction in the AUC of MPA by cholestyramine, caution should be used in the concomitant administration of CellCept with drugs that interfere with enterohepatic recirculation because of the potential to reduce the efficacy of CellCept. (See PRECAUTIONS: Drug Interactions.)

Information for Patients

Patients should be informed of the need for repeated appropriate laboratory tests while they are receiving CellCept. Patients should be given complete dosage instructions and informed of the increased risk of lymphoproliferative disease and certain other malignancies. Women of childbearing potential should be instructed of the potential risks during pregnancy, and that they should use effective contraception before beginning CellCept therapy, during therapy and for 6 weeks after CellCept has been stopped. (See WARNINGS and PRECAUTIONS: Pregnancy.)

Laboratory Tests

Complete blood counts should be performed weekly during the first month, twice monthly for the second and third months of treatment, then monthly through the first year. (See WARNINGS, ADVERSE REACTIONS, and DOSAGE AND ADMINISTRATION.)

Drug Interactions

Drug interaction studies with mycophenolate mofetil have been conducted with acyclovir, antacids, cholestyramine, cyclosporine, ganciclovir, oral contraceptives, and trimethoprim/sulfamethoxazole. Drug interaction studies have not been conducted with other drugs that may be commonly administered to renal transplant patients. CellCept has not been administered concomitantly with azathioprine.

acyclovir: Coadministration of mycophenolate mofetil (1 g) and acyclovir (800 mg) to twelve healthy volunteers resulted in no significant change in MPA AUC and Cmax. However, MPAG and acyclovir plasma AUCs were increased 10.6% and 21.9%, respectively. Because MPAG plasma concentrations are increased in the presence of renal impairment, as are acyclovir concentrations, the potential exists for the two drugs to compete for tubular secretion further increasing the concentrations of both drugs.

antacids with magnesium and aluminum hydroxides: Absorption of a single-dose of mycophenolate mofetil (2.0 g) was decreased when administered to ten rheumatoid arthritis patients also taking Maalox® TC (10 mL q.i.d.). The Cmax and AUC_{0-24} for MPA were 33% and 17% lower, respectively, than when mycophenolate mofetil was administered alone after fasting conditions. CellCept may be administered to patients who are also taking antacids containing magnesium and aluminum hydroxides; however, it is recommended that CellCept and the antacid not be administered simultaneously.

cholestyramine: Following single-dose administration of 1.5 g mycophenolate mofetil to twelve healthy volunteers pretreated with 4 g t.i.d. of cholestyramine for 4 days, MPA AUC decreased approximately 40%. This decrease is consistent with interruption of enterohepatic recirculation which may be due to binding of recirculating MPAG with cholestyramine in the intestine. CellCept is not recommended to be given with cholestyramine or other agents that may interfere with enterohepatic recirculation.

cyclosporine: Cyclosporine (Sandimmune®) pharmacokinetics (at doses of 275 to 415 mg/day) were unaffected by single and multiple doses of 1.5 g b.i.d. of mycophenolate mofetil in ten stable renal transplant patients. The mean (±SD) AUC_{0-12} and Cmax of cyclosporine after 14 days of multiple doses of mycophenolate mofetil were 3290 (±822) ng·h/mL and 753 (±161) ng/mL, respectively, compared to 3245 (±1088) ng·h/mL and 700 (±246) ng/mL, respectively, one week before administration of mycophenolate mofetil. The effect of cyclosporine on mycophenolate mofetil pharmacokinetics could not be evaluated in this study, however, plasma concentrations of MPA were similar to that for healthy volunteers.

ganciclovir: Following single-dose administration to twelve stable renal transplant patients, no pharmacokinetic inteeraction was observed between mycophenolate mofetil (1.5 g) and IV ganciclovir (5 mg/kg). Mean (±SD) ganciclovir AUC and Cmax (n=10) were 54.3 (±19.0) μg·h/mL and 11.5 (±1.8) μg/mL, respectively after coadministration of the two drugs, compared to 51.0 (±17.0) μg·h/mL and 10.6 (±2.0) μg/mL, respectively after administration of IV ganciclovir alone. The mean (±SD) AUC and Cmax of MPA (n=12) after coadministration were 80.9 (±21.6) μg·h/mL and 27.8 (±13.9) μg/mL, respectively compared to values of 80.3 (±16.4) μg·h/mL and 30.9 (±11.2) μg/mL, respectively after administration of mycophenolate mofetil alone. Because MPAG plasma concentrations are increased in the presence of renal impairment, as are ganciclovir concentrations, the potential exists for the two drugs to compete for tubular secretion and thus further increases in concentrations of both drugs may occur.

oral contraceptives: Following single-dose administration to fifteen healthy women, no pharmacokinetic interaction was observed between mycophenolate mofetil (1.0 g) and two tablets of Ortho-Novum® 7/7/7 (1 mg norethindrone [NET] and 35 μg estradiol ethinyl [EE]). This single-dose study suggests the lack of a gross pharmacokinetic interaction, but cannot exclude the possibility of changes in the pharmacokinetics of the oral contraceptive under long term dosing conditions with CellCept which might adversely affect the efficacy of the oral contraceptive.

trimethoprim/sulfamethoxazole: Following single dose administration of mycophenolate mofetil (1.5 g) to twelve healthy male volunteers on day 8 of a 10 day course of Bactrim® DS (trimethoprim 160 mg/sulfamethoxazole 800 mg) administered b.i.d., no effect on the bioavailability of MPA was observed. The mean (±SD) AUC and Cmax of MPA after concomitant administration were 75.2 (±19.8) μg·h/mL and 34.0 (±6.6) μg/mL, respectively compared to 79.2 (±27.9) and 34.2 (±10.7), respectively after administration of mycophenolate mofetil alone.

other interactions: The measured value for renal clearance of MPAG indicates removal occurs by renal tubular secretion as well as glomerular filtration. Consistent with this, coadministration of probenecid, a known inhibitor of tubular secretion, with mycophenolate mofetil in monkeys results in a 3-fold increase in plasma MPAG AUC and a 2-fold increase in plasma MPA AUC. Thus, other drugs known to undergo renal tubular secretion may compete with MPAG and thereby raise plasma concentrations of MPAG or the other drug undergoing tubular secretion.

Drugs that alter the gastrointestinal flora may interact with mycophenolate mofetil by disrupting enterohepatic recirculation. Interference of MPAG hydrolysis may lead to less MPA available for absorption.

Carcinogenesis, Mutagenesis, Impairment of Fertility

In a 104-week oral carcinogenicity study in mice, mycophenolate mofetil in daily doses up to 180 mg/kg was not tumorigenic. The highest dose tested was 0.5 times the recommended clinical dose (2 g/day) when corrected for differences in body surface area (BSA). In a 104-week oral carcinogenicity study in rats, mycophenolate mofetil in daily doses up to 15 mg/kg was not tumorigenic. The highest dose was 0.08 times the recommended clinical dose when corrected for BSA. While these animal doses were lower than those given to patients, they were maximal in those species and were considered adequate to evaluate the potential for human risk. (See WARNINGS.)

Mycophenolate mofetil was not genotoxic, with or without metabolic activation, in several assays: the bacterial mutation assay, the yeast mitotic gene conversion assay, the mouse micronucleus aberration assay, or the Chinese hamster ovary cell (CHO) chromosomal aberration assay.

Mycophenolate mofetil had no effect on fertility of male rats at oral doses up to 20 mg/kg/day. This dose represents 0.1 times the recommended clinical dose when corrected for BSA. In a female fertility and reproduction study conducted in rats, oral doses of 4.5 mg/kg/day caused malformations (principally of the head and eyes) in the first generation offspring in the absence of maternal toxicity. This dose was 0.02 times the recommended clinical dose when corrected for BSA. No effects on fertility or reproductive parameters were evident in the dams or in the subsequent generation.

Pregnancy: Category C

In teratology studies in rats and rabbits, fetal resorptions and malformations occurred in rats at 6 mg/kg/day and in rabbits at 90 mg/kg/day, in the absence of maternal toxicity. These levels are equivalent to 0.03–0.92 times the recom-

mended clinical dose on a BSA basis. In a female fertility and reproduction study conducted in rats, oral doses of 4.5 mg/kg/day caused malformations (principally of the head and eyes) in the first generation offspring in the absence of maternal toxicity. This dose was 0.02 times the recommended clinical dose when corrected by BSA.

There are no adequate and well-controlled studies in pregnant women. CellCept should not be used in pregnant women unless the potential benefit justifies the potential risk to the fetus. Effective contraception must be used before beginning CellCept therapy, during therapy and for 6 weeks after CellCept has been stopped. (See WARNINGS, PRECAUTIONS: Information for Patients.)

Nursing Mothers
Studies in rats treated with mycophenolate mofetil have shown mycophenolic acid to be excreted in milk. It is not known whether this drug is excreted in human milk. Because many drugs are excreted in human milk and because of the potential for serious adverse reactions in nursing infants from mycophenolate mofetil, a decision should be made whether to discontinue nursing or to discontinue the drug, taking into account the importance of the drug to the mother.

Pediatric Patients
Safety and effectiveness in pediatric patients have not been established. Very limited pharmacokinetic data are available in pediatric patients. (See CLINICAL PHARMACOLOGY: Pharmacokinetics.)

ADVERSE REACTIONS
The principal adverse reactions associated with the administration of CellCept include diarrhea, leukopenia, sepsis and vomiting, and there is evidence of a higher frequency of certain types of infections.

The incidence of adverse events for CellCept was determined in three randomized comparative double-blind trials in prevention of rejection in renal transplant patients. Because of the lower overall reporting of events in the European placebo-controlled, prevention of rejection study, these data were not combined with the other two active-controlled prevention trials, but are instead presented separately.

Safety data are summarized below for all patients in the double-blind prevention studies while receiving treatment; approximately 53% of these patients have been treated for more than 1 year. Adverse events that were reported in ≥10% of patients in either CellCept treatment group are presented below for the two active-controlled studies combined (USA and Europe/Canada/Australia) and for the one European placebo-controlled study. Opportunistic infections are summarized separately.
[See table at right.]

The above data demonstrate that in three controlled trials for prevention of rejection, patients receiving 2 g per day of CellCept had an overall better safety profile than did patients receiving 3 g per day of CellCept. Sepsis, which was generally CMV viremia, was slightly more common in patients treated with CellCept, with an incidence of 18–22%, compared to 16% in patients receiving azathioprine and 14% in patients receiving placebo. In the digestive system, diarrhea was most clearly increased in patients receiving CellCept, with an incidence of up to 36%, compared to 21% for patients receiving azathioprine and 14% for patients receiving placebo.

The incidence of malignancies among the 1,483 patients enrolled in controlled trials for the prevention of rejection who were followed for ≥1 year was similar to the incidence reported in the literature for renal allograft recipients. There was a slight increase in the incidence of lymphoproliferative disease in the CellCept treatment groups compared to the placebo and azathioprine groups. (See WARNINGS.) The following table summarizes the incidence of malignancies observed in the prevention of rejection trials.
[See first table at top of next page.]

Up to 2.0% of patients receiving CellCept for prevention of rejection have developed severe neutropenia [absolute neutrophil count (ANC) <0.5 × 10³/μL]. (See WARNINGS, PRECAUTIONS: Laboratory Tests, and DOSAGE AND ADMINISTRATION.)

The following tables show the incidence of opportunistic infections that occurred in the transplant population in the prevention of rejection trials:
[See second table at top of next page.]

In the three controlled studies for prevention of rejection, similar rates of fatal infections/sepsis (<2%) occurred in patients while receiving CellCept or control therapy in combination with other immunosuppressive agents. (See WARNINGS.)

The following adverse events, not mentioned in any of the tables above, were reported with ≥3% incidence in patients treated with CellCept: BODY AS A WHOLE: abdomen enlarged, accidental injury, chills and fever, cyst, face edema, flu syndrome, hemorrhage, hernia, malaise, pelvic pain; HEMIC AND LYMPHATIC: ecchymosis, polycythemia; UROGENITAL: albuminuria, dysuria, hydronephrosis, impotence, pain, pyelonephritis, urinary frequency, urinary tract disorder; CARDIOVASCULAR: angina pectoris, atrial

Adverse Events in Prevention of Renal Allograft Rejection
USA Study Combined with Europe/Canada/Australia Study

	CellCept 2 g/day (n=336)	CellCept 3 g/day (n=330)	Azathioprine 1–2 mg/kg/day or 100–150 mg/day (n=326)
Body as a Whole			
Pain	33.0%	31.2%	32.2%
Abdominal pain	24.7	27.6	23.0
Fever	21.4	23.3	23.3
Headache	21.1	16.1	21.2
Infection	18.2	20.9	19.9
Sepsis	17.6	19.7	15.6
Asthenia	13.7	16.1	19.9
Chest pain	13.4	13.3	14.7
Back pain	11.6	12.1	14.1
Hemic and Lymphatic			
Anemia	25.6	25.8	23.6
Leukopenia	23.2	34.5	24.8
Thrombocytopenia	10.1	8.2	13.2
Hypochromic anemia	7.4	11.5	9.2
Leukocytosis	7.1	10.9	7.4
Urogenital			
Urinary tract infection	37.2	37.0	33.7
Hematuria	14.0	12.1	11.3
Kidney tubular necrosis	6.3	10.0	5.8
Cardiovascular			
Hypertension	32.4	28.2	32.2
Metabolic and Nutritional			
Peripheral edema	28.6	27.0	28.2
Hypercholesteremia	12.8	8.5	11.3
Hypophosphatemia	12.5	15.8	11.7
Edema	12.2	11.8	13.5
Hypokalemia	10.1	10.0	8.3
Hyperkalemia	8.9	10.3	16.9
Hyperglycemia	8.6	12.4	15.0
Digestive			
Diarrhea	31.0	36.1	20.9
Constipation	22.9	18.5	22.4
Nausea	19.9	23.6	24.5
Dyspepsia	17.6	13.6	13.8
Vomiting	12.5	13.6	9.2
Nausea and vomiting	10.4	9.7	10.7
Oral moniliasis	10.1	12.1	11.3
Respiratory			
Infection	22.0	23.9	19.6
Dyspnea	15.5	17.3	16.6
Cough increased	15.5	13.3	15.0
Pharyngitis	9.5	11.2	8.0
Skin and Appendages			
Acne	10.1	9.7	6.4
Rash	7.7	6.4	10.4
Nervous System			
Tremor	11.0	11.8	12.3
Insomnia	8.9	11.8	10.4
Dizziness	5.7	11.2	11.0

Europe Study

	CellCept 2 g/day (n=165)	CellCept 3 g/day (n=160)	Placebo (n=166)
Body as a Whole			
Sepsis	21.8%	17.5%	13.9%
Infection	12.7	15.6	13.3
Abdominal pain	12.1	11.9	11.4
Hemic and Lymphatic			
Leukopenia	11.5	16.3	4.2
Urogenital			
Urinary tract infection	45.5	44.4	37.3
Urinary tract disorder	6.7	10.6	4.2
Cardiovascular			
Hypertension	17.6	16.9	19.3
Digestive			
Diarrhea	16.4	18.8	13.9
Respiratory			
Infection	15.8	13.1	9.0
Bronchitis	8.5	11.9	8.4
Penumonia	3.6	10.6	10.8

fibrillation, cardiovascular disorder, hypotension, palpitation, peripheral vascular disorder, postural hypotension, tachycardia, thrombosis, vasodilatation; METABOLIC AND NUTRITIONAL: acidosis, alkaline phosphatase increased, creatinine increased, dehydration, gamma glutamyl transpeptidase increased, hypercalcemia, hyperlipemia, hyperuricemia, hypervolemia, hypocalcemia, hypoglycemia, hypoproteinemia, lactic dehydrogenase increased, SGOT increased, SGPT increased, weight gain; DIGESTIVE: anorexia, esophagitis, flatulence, gastritis, gastroenteritis, gas-

trointestinal hemorrhage, gastrointestinal moniliasis, gingivitis, gum hyperplasia, hepatitis, ileus, infection, liver function tests abnormal, mouth ulceration, rectal disorder; RESPIRATORY: asthma, lung disorder, lung edema, pleural effusion, rhinitis, sinusitis; SKIN AND APPENDAGES: alopecia, fungal dermatitis, hirsutism, pruritis, skin benign neoplasm, skin disorder, skin hypertrophy, skin ulcer, sweating; NERVOUS: anxiety, depression, hypertonia, paresthe-

Continued on next page

Roche Laboratories—Cont.

Malignancies Observed in Prevention of Renal Rejection Trials

	CellCept 2 g/day	CellCept 3 g/day	Placebo	Azathioprine 1–2 mg/kg/day or 100–150 mg/day
	(n=501)	(n=490)	(n=166)	(n=326)
Lymphoma/lympho-proliferative disease	0.6%	1.0%	0.0%	0.3%
Non-melanoma skin carcinoma	4.0	1.6	0.0	2.4
Other malignancy	0.8	1.4	1.8	1.8

Opportunistic Infections in Prevention of Renal Rejection Trials
USA Study Combined with Europe/Canada/Australia Study

	CellCept 2 g/day	CellCept 3 g/day	Azathioprine 1–2 mg/kg/day or 100-150 mg/day
	(n=336)	(n=330)	(n=326)
Herpes simplex	16.7%	20.0%	19.0%
CMV			
viremia/syndrome	13.4	12.4	13.8
tissue invasive disease	8.3	11.5	6.1
Herpes zoster	6.0	7.6	5.8
Candida			
fungemia/disseminated	0.6	0.6	0.3
tissue invasive	0.6	0.6	0.3
Aspergillus/Mucor invasive disease	0.3	0.9	0.3
Pneumocystis carinii	0.3	0.0	1.2

Europe Study

	CellCept 2 g/day	CellCept 3 g/day	Placebo
	(n=165)	(n=160)	(n=166)
Herpes simplex	15.2%	12.5%	6.0%
CMV			
viremia/syndrome	15.2	15.0	13.3
tissue invasive disease	3.6	7.5	2.4
Herpes zoster	6.7	6.9	2.4
Candida			
fungemia/disseminated	0.0	0.6	0.0
tissue invasive	0.0	0.6	0.0
Pneumocystis carinii	0.0	0.0	2.4

sia, somnolence; ENDOCRINE: diabetes mellitus, parathyroid disorder; MUSCULO-SKELETAL: arthralgia, joint disorder, leg cramps, myalgia, myasthenia; SPECIAL SENSES: amblyopia, cataract (not specified), conjunctivitis.

OVERDOSAGE

There has been no reported experience of overdosage of mycophenolate mofetil in humans. The highest dose administered to renal transplant patients have been 4 g per day. In limited experience with cardiac and hepatic transplant patients, the highest doses used were 4 g or 5 g per day. At doses of 4 g or 5 g per day, there appears to be a higher rate, compared to the use of 3 g per day or less, of gastrointestinal intolerance (nausea, vomiting, and/or diarrhea), and occasional hematologic abnormalities, principally neutropenia, leading to a need to reduce or discontinue dosing.

In acute oral toxicity studies, no deaths occurred in adult mice at doses up to 4000 mg/kg or in adult monkeys at doses up to 1000 mg/kg; these were the highest doses of mycophenolate mofetil tested in these species. These doses represent 11 times the recommended clinical dose when corrected for BSA. In adult rats, deaths occurred after single oral doses of 500 mg/kg of mycophenolate mofetil. The dose represents approximately 3 times the recommended clinical dose when corrected for BSA.

MPA and MPAG are usually not removed by hemodialysis. However, at high MPAG plasma concentrations (>100 μg/mL), small amounts of MPAG are removed. By increasing excretion of the drug, MPA can be removed by bile acid sequestrants, such as cholestyramine.

DOSAGE AND ADMINISTRATION

The initial dose of CellCept should be given within 72 hours following transplantation. A dose of 1.0 g administered twice a day (daily dose of 2 g) is recommended for use in combination with corticosteroids and cyclosporine in renal transplant patients. Although a dose of 1.5 g administered twice daily (daily dose of 3 g) was used in clinical trials and was shown to be safe and effective, no efficacy advantage could be established. Patients receiving 2 g per day of CellCept demonstrated an overall better safety profile than did patients receiving 3 g per day of CellCept. Food had no effect on MPA AUC, but has been shown to decrease MPA Cmax by 40%. It

is recommended that CellCept be administered on an empty stomach.

Dosage Adjustments
In patients with severe chronic renal impairment (GFR <25 mL/min/1.73m²) outside of the immediate post-transplant period, doses of CellCept greater than 1 g administered twice a day should be avoided. These patients should also be carefully observed. No dose adjustments are needed in patients experiencing delayed graft function post-operatively. (See CLINICAL PHARMACOLOGY: Pharmacokinetics and PRECAUTIONS: General.)

If neutropenia develops (ANC <1.3 × 10³/μL), dosing with CellCept should be interrupted or the doses reduced, appropriate diagnostic tests performed, and the patient managed appropriately. (See WARNINGS, ADVERSE REACTIONS, and PRECAUTIONS: Laboratory Tests.)

HANDLING AND DISPOSAL

Because mycophenolate mofetil has demonstrated teratogenic effects in rats and rabbits, CellCept capsules should not be opened or crushed. Avoid inhalation or direct contact with skin or mucous membranes of the powder contained in CellCept capsules. If such contact occurs, wash thoroughly with soap and water; rinse eyes with plain water.

HOW SUPPLIED

CellCept capsules are blue/brown, two-piece hard gelatin capsules, printed in black with "CellCept 250" on the blue cap and "Roche" on the brown body. Supplied in the following presentations:

NDC Number	Size
NDC 0004-0259-01	Bottle of 100
NDC 0004-0259-43	Bottle of 500

STORAGE

Store at 15° to 30°C (59° to 86°F).

CAUTION:

Federal (USA) law prohibits dispensing without a prescription.
Manufactured by Syntex Puerto Rico, Inc., Humacao, Puerto Rico 00791 for Roche Laboratories.

June 1995

Shown in Product Identification Guide, page 331

CYTOVENE®-IV ℞
(ganciclovir sodium for injection)

CYTOVENE® ℞
(ganciclovir capsules)

> THE CLINICAL TOXICITY OF CYTOVENE AND CYTOVENE-IV INCLUDES GRANULOCYTOPENIA, ANEMIA AND THROMBOCYTOPENIA. IN ANIMAL STUDIES GANCICLOVIR WAS CARCINOGENIC, TERATOGENIC AND CAUSED ASPERMATOGENESIS. CYTOVENE-IV IS INDICATED FOR USE *ONLY* IN THE TREATMENT OF CYTOMEGALOVIRUS (CMV) RETINITIS IN IMMUNOCOMPROMISED PATIENTS AND FOR THE PREVENTION OF CMV DISEASE IN TRANSPLANT PATIENTS AT RISK FOR CMV DISEASE. CYTOVENE CAPSULES ARE INDICATED *ONLY* FOR PREVENTION OF CMV DISEASE IN PATIENTS WITH ADVANCED HIV INFECTION AT RISK FOR CMV DISEASE, AND FOR MAINTENANCE TREATMENT OF CMV RETINITIS IN IMMUNOCOMPROMISED PATIENTS (see INDICATIONS AND USAGE section). BECAUSE CYTOVENE CAPSULES ARE ASSOCIATED WITH A RISK OF MORE RAPID RATE OF CMV RETINITIS PROGRESSION, THEY SHOULD BE USED AS MAINTENANCE TREATMENT ONLY IN THOSE PATIENTS FOR WHOM THIS RISK IS BALANCED BY THE BENEFIT ASSOCIATED WITH AVOIDING DAILY INTRAVENOUS INFUSIONS.

DESCRIPTION

Ganciclovir is a synthetic guanine derivative active against cytomegalovirus (CMV). CYTOVENE-IV and CYTOVENE are the brand names for ganciclovir sodium for injection and ganciclovir capsules, respectively.

CYTOVENE-IV is available as sterile lyophilized powder in strength of 500 mg per vial for intravenous administration only. Each vial of CYTOVENE-IV contains the equivalent of 500 mg ganciclovir as the sodium salt (46 mg sodium). Reconstitution with 10 mL of Sterile Water for Injection, USP, yields a solution with pH 11 and a ganciclovir concentration of approximately 50 mg/mL. Further dilution in an appropriate intravenous solution must be performed before infusion (see DOSAGE AND ADMINISTRATION section).

CYTOVENE is available as 250 mg capsules. Each capsule contains 250 mg ganciclovir and inactive ingredients croscarmellose sodium, magnesium stearate and povidone. The hard gelatin shell consists of gelatin, titanium dioxide, yellow iron oxide and FD&C Blue No. 2.

Ganciclovir is a white to off-white crystalline powder with a molecular formula of $C_9H_{13}N_5O_4$ and a molecular weight of 255.23. The chemical name for ganciclovir is 9-[[2-hydroxy-1-(hydroxymethyl)ethoxy]methyl]guanine. Ganciclovir is a polar hydrophilic compound with a solubility of 2.6 mg/mL in water at 25°C and an n-octanol/water partition coefficient of 0.022. The pK_as for ganciclovir are 2.2 and 9.4

Ganciclovir, when formulated as monosodium salt in the IV dosage form, is a white to off-white lyophilized powder with a molecular formula of $C_9H_{12}N_5NaO_4$, and molecular weight of 277.22. The chemical name for ganciclovir sodium is 9-[[2-hydroxy-1-(hydroxymethyl)ethoxy]methyl]guanine, monosodium salt. The lyophilized powder has an aqueous solubility of greater than 50 mg/mL at 25°C. At physiological pH, ganciclovir sodium exists as the un-ionized form with a solubility of approximately 6 mg/mL at 37°C.

All doses in this insert are specified in terms of ganciclovir.

CLINICAL PHARMACOLOGY

Virology
Mechanism of Action: Ganciclovir is an acyclic nucleoside analogue of 2'-deoxyguanosine that inhibits replication of herpes viruses both in vitro and in vivo. Sensitive human viruses include cytomegalovirus (CMV), herpes simplex virus-1 and -2, herpesvirus type 6, Epstein-Barr virus, varicella zoster virus and hepatitis B virus.[1-4] Clinical studies have been limited to assessment of efficacy in patients with CMV infection.

Ganciclovir must be converted to the corresponding triphosphate in order to exert its antiviral activity. In herpes simplex virus-infected cells, the initial conversion to the monophosphate is catalyzed by a viral thymidine kinase.[5] In contrast, in CMV-infected cells a protein kinase homologue, encoded by the CMV gene UL97, may be responsible for the initial phosphorylation of ganciclovir.[6,7] Cellular kinases, in CMV-infected cells, subsequently phosphorylate ganciclovir monophosphate to the diphosphate and active triphosphate moieties.[8,9] It has been shown that the levels of ganciclovir-triphosphate are as much as 100-fold greater in CMV-in-

fected cells than in uninfected cells, indicating a preferential phosphorylation of ganciclovir in virus-infected cells.[9] Ganciclovir triphosphate, once formed, appears quite stable and persists for days in the CMV-infected cell.[9] The antiviral activity of ganciclovir-triphosphate is believed to be the result of inhibition of viral DNA synthesis by two known modes: (1) competitive inhibition of viral DNA polymerases; (2) direct incorporation into viral DNA, resulting in eventual termination of viral DNA elongation. The cellular DNA polymerase alpha is also inhibited, but at a higher concentration than required for inhibition of viral DNA polymerase.

Antiviral Activity: The median concentration of ganciclovir that effectively inhibits the replication of either laboratory strains or clinical isolates of CMV (ED_{50}) has ranged from 0.02 to 3.48 μg/mL. The relationship of in vitro sensitivity of CMV to ganciclovir and clinical response has not been established. Ganciclovir inhibits mammalian cell proliferation in vitro at higher concentrations: IC_{50} values range from 30 to 725 μg/mL[4,10] with the exception of bone marrow-derived colony-forming cells that are more sensitive with IC_{50} values ranging from 0.028 to 0.7 μg/mL.[4,11]

Clinical Antiviral Effect of CYTOVENE-IV and CYTOVENE Capsules

CYTOVENE-IV: Of 314 immunocompromised patients enrolled in an open-label study of the treatment of life- or sight-threatening CMV disease with CYTOVENE-IV solution, 121 patients were identified who had a positive culture for CMV within 7 days prior to treatment and had sequential viral cultures after treatment with CYTOVENE-IV.[12] Post-treatment virologic response was defined as conversion to culture negativity, or a greater than 100-fold decrease in CMV infectious units, as shown in the following table:

Virologic Response

Culture Source	No. Patients Cultured	No. (%) Patients Responding	Median Days to Response
Urine	107	93 (87)	8
Blood	41	34 (83)	8
Throat	21	19 (90)	7
Semen	6	6 (100)	15

The antiviral activity of CYTOVENE-IV solution was demonstrated in two separate placebo-controlled studies for the prevention of CMV disease in transplant recipients. One hundred forty-nine heart allograft recipients who were either CMV seropositive or had received seropositive heart allografts were randomized to treatment with CYTOVENE-IV solution (5 mg/kg bid for 14 days followed by 6 mg/kg qd for 5 days/week for an additional 14 days) or placebo.[13] Seventy-two CMV culture-positive allogeneic bone marrow[14] transplant recipients were randomized to treatment with CYTOVENE-IV solution (5 mg/kg bid for 7 days followed by 5 mg/kg qd) or placebo until day 100 post-transplant. CYTOVENE-IV suppressed CMV shedding in heart allograft and bone marrow allograft recipients. The antiviral effect of CYTOVENE-IV solution in these patients is summarized in the following table:

[See first table on top of next page.]

CYTOVENE Capsules: The antiviral activity of CYTOVENE capsules was confirmed in two randomized, controlled trials comparing CYTOVENE-IV solution with CYTOVENE capsules for the maintenance treatment of CMV retinitis in patients with AIDS. Serial cultures of urine were obtained, and cultures of semen, biopsy specimens, blood, and other sources also were obtained when available. Only a small proportion of patients remained culture-positive during maintenance therapy with either CYTOVENE-IV solution or CYTOVENE capsules. There were no statistically significant differences in the rates of positive cultures between the treatment groups. The antiviral effect of CYTOVENE capsules in the patients in the two studies is summarized in the following table:

[See second table on top of next page.]

A placebo-controlled study of CYTOVENE capsules (1000 mg every 8 hours) for prevention of CMV disease in individuals with advanced HIV infection (ICM 1654) evaluated antiviral activity as measured by CMV isolation in culture. The majority of cultures tested were from urine. At baseline, 40% (176/436) and 44% (92/210) of ganciclovir and placebo recipients, respectively, had positive cultures, either in urine or blood. After 2 months on study treatment, 10% of ganciclovir recipients had positive cultures, compared with 44% of placebo recipients. The weighted mean monthly prevalence of positive cultures for study months 2 to 20 was 11.2% and 46.0% for ganciclovir and placebo recipients, respectively.

Viral Resistance: The current working definition of CMV resistance to ganciclovir in in vitro assays is $IC_{50} > 3.0$ μg/mL (12.0 μM). CMV resistance to ganciclovir has been observed in individuals with AIDS and CMV retinitis who have never received ganciclovir therapy. In a controlled study of oral ganciclovir for prevention of CMV disease in HIV+ individuals, cultures were available for 437 individuals who had received treatment for at least 90 days. Of these, 132 had at least one positive culture. Eighteen of these isolates have been tested for reduced sensitivity, and one was found to be resistant to ganciclovir. This resistant isolate was associated with subsequent treatment failure for retinitis. Viral resistance has also been observed in patients receiving prolonged treatment for CMV retinitis with CYTOVENE-IV.[15-19]
The possibility of viral resistance should be considered in patients who show poor clinical response or experience persistent viral excretion during therapy. The principal mechanism of resistance to ganciclovir in CMV is the decreased ability to form the active triphosphate moiety; resistant viruses have been described that contain mutations in the UL97 gene of CMV that controls phosphorylation of ganciclovir.[6,7,20-24] Mutations in the viral DNA polymerase have also been reported to confer viral resistance to ganciclovir.[23,24]

Pharmacokinetics

BECAUSE THE MAJOR ELIMINATION PATHWAY FOR GANCICLOVIR IS RENAL, DOSAGE REDUCTIONS ACCORDING TO CREATININE CLEARANCE ARE REQUIRED FOR CYTOVENE-IV AND SHOULD BE CONSIDERED FOR CYTOVENE CAPSULES. FOR DOSING INSTRUCTIONS IN PATIENTS WITH RENAL IMPAIRMENT, REFER TO THE SECTION ON DOSAGE AND ADMINISTRATION.

Absorption: The absolute bioavailability of oral ganciclovir under fasting conditions was approximately 5% (n=6) and following food was 6% to 9% (n=32). When ganciclovir was administered orally with food at a total daily dose of 3 g/day (500 mg q3h, 6 times daily and 1000 mg tid), the steady-state absorption as measured by area under the serum concentration vs time curve (AUC) over 24 hours and maximum serum concentrations (C_{max}) were similar following both regimens with an AUC_{0-24} of 15.9±4.2 (mean±SD) and 15.4±4.3 μg·hr/mL and C_{max} of 1.02±0.24 and 1.18±0.36 μg/mL, respectively (n=16).
At the end of a 1-hour intravenous infusion of 5 mg/kg ganciclovir, total AUC ranged between 22.1±3.2 (n=16) and 26.8±6.1 μg·hr/mL (n=16) and C_{max} ranged between 8.27±1.02 (n=16) and 9.0±1.4 μg/mL (n=16).
Food Effects: When CYTOVENE capsules were given with a meal containing 602 calories and 46.5% fat at a dose of 1000 mg every 8 hours to 20 HIV-positive subjects, the steady-state AUC increased by 22±22% (range: −6% to 68%) and there was a significant prolongation of time to peak serum concentrations (T_{max}) from 1.8±0.8 to 3.0±0.6 hours and a higher C_{max} (0.85±0.25 vs 0.96±0.27 μg/mL) (n=20).

Distribution: The steady-state volume of distribution of ganciclovir after intravenous administration was 0.74±0.15 L/kg (n=98). For CYTOVENE capsules, no correlation was observed between AUC and reciprocal weight (range: 55 to 128 kg); oral dosing according to weight is not required. Cerebrospinal fluid concentrations obtained 0.25 and 5.67 hours postdose in 3 patients who received 2.5 mg/kg ganciclovir intravenously q8h or q12h ranged from 0.31 to 0.68 μg/mL[25] representing 24% to 70% of the respective plasma concentrations. Binding to plasma proteins was 1% to 2% over ganciclovir concentrations of 0.5 and 51 μg/mL.

Metabolism: Following oral administration of a single 1000 mg dose of ^{14}C-labelled ganciclovir, 86±3% of the administered dose was recovered in the feces and 5±1% was recovered in the urine (n=4). No metabolite accounted for more than 1% to 2% of the radioactivity recovered in urine or feces.

Elimination: When administered intravenously, ganciclovir exhibits linear pharmacokinetics over the range of 1.6 to 5.0 mg/kg and when administered orally, it exhibits linear kinetics up to a total daily dose of 4 g/day. Renal excretion of unchanged drug by glomerular filtration and active tubular secretion is the major route of elimination of ganciclovir. In patients with normal renal function, 91.3±5.0% (n=4) of intravenously administered ganciclovir was recovered unmetabolized in the urine. Systemic clearance of intravenously administered ganciclovir was 3.52±0.80 mL/min/kg (n=98) while renal clearance was 3.20±0.80 mL/min/kg (n=47), accounting for 91±11% of the systemic clearance (n=47). After oral administration of ganciclovir, steady state is achieved within 24 hours. Renal clearance following oral administration was 3.1±1.2 mL/min/kg (n=22). Half-life was 3.5±0.9 hours (n=98) following IV administration and 4.8±0.9 (n=39) following oral administration.

Special Populations

Renal Impairment: The pharmacokinetics following intravenous administration of CYTOVENE-IV solution were evaluated in 10 immunocompromised patients with renal impairment who received doses ranging from 1.25 to 5.0 mg/kg.

CrCl (mL/min)	n	Dose	Clearance (mL/min) Mean±SD	Half-life (hours) Mean±SD
50–79	4	3.2 - 5 mg/kg	128±63	4.6±1.4
25–49	3	3 - 5 mg/kg	57±8	4.4±0.4
<25	3	1.25 - 5 mg/kg	30±13	10.7±5.7

The pharmacokinetics following oral administration of CYTOVENE capsules were evaluated in 8 solid organ transplant recipients; dose was modified according to estimated creatinine clearance:

CrCl (mL/min)	n	Dose	AUC_{0-24}* (μg·hr/mL) Mean±SD	Half-life (hours)
50–69	4	1000 mg q8h	49.1±12.2	NC‡
25–49	1	1000 mg qd	27.4	18.2
10–24	1	500 mg qd	10.7	15.7
<10	2	500 mg tiw†	25.6±5.9	NC‡

* Estimated or actual
† Three times weekly, after hemodialysis
‡ Not Calculated since half-life exceeded sampling interval

Hemodialysis reduces plasma concentrations of ganciclovir by about 50% after both intravenous and oral administration.
Race and Gender: The effects of race and gender were studied in subjects receiving a dose regimen of 1000 mg every 8 hours. Although the numbers of blacks (16%) and Hispanics (20%) were small, there appeared to be a trend towards a lower steady-state C_{max} and AUC_{0-8} in these subpopulations as compared to Caucasians. No definitive conclusions regarding gender differences could be made because of the small number of females (12%); however, no differences between males and females were observed.
Pediatrics: Ganciclovir pharmacokinetics were studied in 27 neonates, aged 2 to 49 days. At an intravenous dose of 4 mg/kg (n=14) or 6 mg/kg (n=13), the pharmacokinetic parameters were, respectively, C_{max} of 5.5±1.6 and 7.0±1.6 μg/mL, systemic clearance of 3.14±1.75 and 3.56±1.27 mL/min/kg, and $t_{1/2}$ of 2.4 hours (harmonic mean) for both.[26]

Ganciclovir pharmacokinetics were also studied in 10 children, aged 9 months to 12 years. The pharmacokinetic characteristics of ganciclovir were the same after single and multiple (q12h) intravenous doses (5 mg/kg). The steady state volume of distribution was 0.64 ± 0.22 L/kg, C_{max} was 7.9 ± 3.9 μg/mL, systemic clearance was 4.7 ± 2.2 mL/min/kg, and $t_{1/2}$ was 2.4 ± 0.7 hours. The pharmacokinetics of intravenous ganciclovir in neonates and children are similar to those observed in adults.
Elderly: No studies have been conducted in adults older than 65 years of age.

INDICATIONS AND USAGE

CYTOVENE-IV is indicated for the treatment of CMV retinitis in immunocompromised patients, including patients with acquired immunodeficiency syndrome (AIDS). CYTOVENE-IV is also indicated for the prevention of CMV disease in transplant recipients at risk for CMV disease (see CLINICAL TRIALS section below).
CYTOVENE capsules are indicated for the prevention of CMV disease in individuals with advanced HIV infection at risk for developing CMV disease. CYTOVENE capsules are also indicated as an alternative to the intravenous formulation for maintenance treatment of CMV retinitis in immunocompromised patients, including patients with AIDS, in whom retinitis is stable following appropriate induction therapy and for whom the risk of more rapid progression is balanced by the benefit associated with avoiding daily IV infusions (see CLINICAL TRIALS section below).
SAFETY AND EFFICACY OF **CYTOVENE-IV** AND **CYTOVENE** HAVE NOT BEEN ESTABLISHED FOR CONGENITAL OR NEONATAL CMV DISEASE; NOR FOR THE TREATMENT OF ESTABLISHED CMV DISEASE OTHER THAN RETINITIS; NOR FOR USE IN NON-IMMUNOCOMPROMISED INDIVIDUALS. THE SAFETY AND EFFICACY OF **CYTOVENE** CAPSULES HAVE NOT BEEN ESTABLISHED FOR TREATING ANY MANIFESTATION OF CMV DISEASE OTHER THAN MAINTENANCE TREATMENT OF CMV RETINITIS.

Clinical Trials:

1. Treatment of CMV Retinitis

The diagnosis of CMV retinitis should be made by indirect ophthalmoscopy. Other conditions in the differential diagnosis of CMV retinitis include candidiasis, toxoplasmosis, histoplasmosis, retinal scars and cotton wool spots, any of which may produce a retinal appearance similar to CMV. For this reason it is essential that the diagnosis of CMV be established by an ophthalmologist familiar with the retinal presentation of these conditions. The diagnosis of CMV retinitis may be supported by culture of CMV from urine, blood, throat or other sites, but a negative CMV culture does not rule out CMV retinitis.

Continued on next page

Roche Laboratories—Cont.

Studies with CYTOVENE-IV: In a retrospective, non-randomized, single-center analysis of 41 patients with AIDS and CMV retinitis diagnosed by ophthalmologic examination between August 1983 and April 1988, treatment with CYTOVENE-IV solution resulted in a significant delay in mean (median) time to first retinitis progression compared to untreated controls [105 (71) days from diagnosis versus 35 (29) days from diagnosis].[27] Patients in this series received induction treatment of CYTOVENE-IV 5 mg/kg bid for 14 to 21 days followed by maintenance treatment with either 5 mg/kg once daily, 7 days per week or 6 mg/kg once daily, 5 days per week (see DOSAGE AND ADMINISTRATION section).

In a controlled, randomized, study conducted between February 1989 and December 1990,[28] immediate treatment with CYTOVENE-IV was compared to delayed treatment in 42 patients with AIDS and peripheral CMV retinitis; 35 of 42 patients (13 in the immediate-treatment group and 22 in the delayed-treatment group) were included in the analysis of time to retinitis progression. Based on masked assessment of fundus photographs, the mean [95% Cl] and median [95% Cl] times to progression of retinitis were 66 days [39, 94] and 50 days [40, 84], respectively, in the immediate-treatment group compared to 19 days [11, 27] and 13.5 days [8, 18], respectively, in the delayed-treatment group.

[See table at top of next page.]

ICM 1653: In this randomized, open-label, parallel group trial, conducted between March 1991 and November 1992, patients with AIDS and newly diagnosed CMV retinitis received a 3-week induction course of CYTOVENE-IV solution, 5 mg/kg bid for 14 days followed by 5 mg/kg once daily for 1 additional week.[29] Following the 21-day intravenous induction course, patients with stable CMV retinitis were randomized to receive 20 weeks of maintenance treatment with either CYTOVENE-IV solution, 5 mg/kg once daily, or CYTOVENE capsules, 500 mg 6 times daily (3000 mg/day). The study showed that the mean [95% Cl] and median [95% Cl] times to progression of CMV retinitis, as assessed by masked reading of fundus photographs, were 57 days [44, 70] and 29 days [28, 43], respectively, for patients on oral therapy compared to 62 days [50, 73] and 49 days [29, 61], respectively, for patients on intravenous therapy. The difference [95% Cl] in the mean time to progression between the oral and intravenous therapies (oral–IV) was −5 days [−22, 12]. See Figure 1 for comparison of the proportion of patients remaining free of progression over time.

ICM 1774: In this three-arm, randomized, open-label, parallel group trial, conducted between June 1991 and August 1993, patients with AIDS and stable CMV retinitis following from 4 weeks to 4 months of treatment with CYTOVENE-IV solution were randomized to receive maintenance treatment with CYTOVENE-IV solution, 5 mg/kg once daily, CYTOVENE capsules, 500 mg 6 times daily, or CYTOVENE capsules, 1000 mg tid for 20 weeks. The study showed that the mean [95% Cl] and median [95% Cl] times to progression of CMV retinitis, as assessed by masked reading of fundus photographs, were 54 days [48, 60] and 42 days [31, 54], respectively, for patients on oral therapy compared to 66 days [56, 76] and 54 days [41, 69], respectively, for patients on intravenous therapy. The difference [95% Cl] in the mean time to progression between the oral and intravenous therapies (oral–IV) was −12 days [−24, 0]. See Figure 2 for comparison of the proportion of patients remaining free of progression over time.

AVI 034: In this randomized, open-label, parallel group trial, conducted between June 1991 and February 1993, patients with AIDS and newly diagnosed (81%) or previously treated (19%) CMV retinitis who had tolerated 10 to 21 days of induction treatment with CYTOVENE-IV, 5 mg/kg twice daily, were randomized to receive 20 weeks of maintenance treatment with either CYTOVENE capsules, 500 mg 6 times daily or CYTOVENE-IV solution, 5 mg/kg/day.[30] The mean [95% Cl] and median [95% Cl] times to progression of CMV retinitis, as assessed by masked reading of fundus photographs, were 51 days [44, 57] and 41 days [31, 45], respectively, for patients on oral therapy compared to 62 days [52, 72] and 60 days [42, 83], respectively, for patients on intravenous therapy. The difference [95% Cl] in the mean time to progression between the oral and intravenous therapies (oral–IV) was −11 days [−24, 1]. See Figure 3 for comparison of the proportion of patients remaining free of progression over time.

Other CMV retinitis outcomes as assessed by masked reading of fundus photographs in the three studies, and visual acuity data, are presented in the following table. Because of low event rates among these endpoints, these studies are underpowered to rule out significant differences in these endpoints.

[See second table on top of next page.]

	Patients with Positive CMV Cultures			
	Heart Allograft		**Bone Marrow Allograft**	
Time	CYTOVENE-IV	Placebo	CYTOVENE-IV	Placebo
Pre-Treatment	1/67 (2%)	5/64 (8%)	37/37 (100%)	35/35 (100%)
Week 2	2/75 (3%)	11/67 (16%)	2/31 (6%)	19/28 (68%)
Week 4	3/66 (5%)	28/66 (43%)	0/24 (0%)	16/20 (80%)

Patients with Positive CMV Cultures in Two Controlled Clinical Trials

	Patients With Newly Diagnosed CMV Retinitis*		Patients With Stable, Previously Treated CMV Retinitis†	
	CYTOVENE-IV Solution	CYTOVENE Capsules	CYTOVENE-IV Solution	CYTOVENE Capsules‡
At Start of Maintenance	5/37 (13.5%)	9/37 (24.3%)	2/66 (3.0%)	5/137 (3.6%)
Anytime During Maintenance	3/48 (6.3%)	4/44 (9.1%)	1/45 (2.2%)	7/99 (7.1%)

* Study ICM 1653. 3 weeks of treatment with IV ganciclovir before start of maintenance
† Study ICM 1774. 4 weeks to 4 months treatment with IV ganciclovir before start of maintenance
‡ Data from 6 times daily and 3 times daily regimens pooled

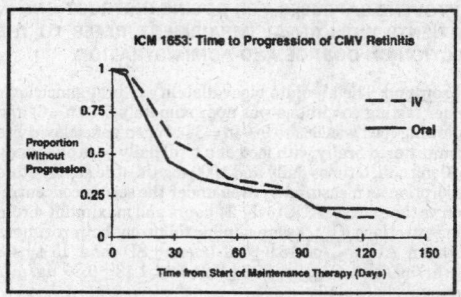

Figure 1 - ICM 1653

ICM 1653: Time to Progression of CMV Retinitis

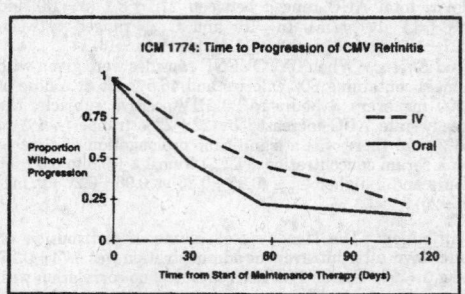

Figure 2 - ICM 1774

ICM 1774: Time to Progression of CMV Retinitis

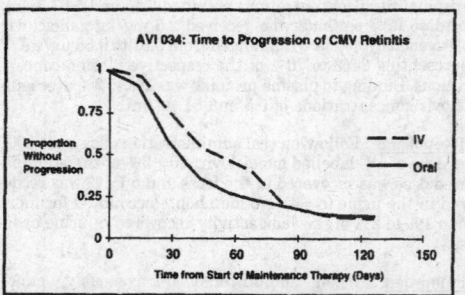

Figure 3 - AVI 034

AVI 034: Time to Progression of CMV Retinitis

2. Prevention of CMV Disease in Subjects with AIDS

ICM 1654: In a double-blind study conducted between November 1992 and July 1994, 725 subjects with AIDS, who were CMV seropositive and/or culture positive, were randomized to receive CYTOVENE capsules, 1000 mg, every 8 hours, or placebo. The study population had a median age of 38 years (range: 21 to 69); were 99% male; were 82% Caucasian, 10% Hispanic, 7% African-American and 1% Asian; and had a median CD_4 count of 21 (range: 0 to 100). The mean observation time was 351 days (range: 5 to 621). As shown in the following table, significantly more placebo recipients developed CMV disease.

Incidence of CMV Disease at 6, 12 and 18 Months after Enrollment (Kaplan-Meier Estimates)

	Incidence (Number Still at Risk) CMV Disease			
	Ganciclovir		Placebo	
6 months	8%	(397)	11%	(190)
12 months	14%	(225)	26%	(92)
18 months	20%	(27)	39%	(9)

3. Prevention of CMV Disease in Transplant Recipients

CYTOVENE-IV was evaluated in three randomized, controlled trials of prevention of CMV disease in organ transplant recipients.

ICM 1496: In a randomized, double-blind, placebo-controlled study of 149 heart transplant recipients[13] at risk for CMV infection (CMV seropositive or a seronegative recipient of an organ from a CMV seropositive donor), there was a statistically significant reduction in the overall incidence of CMV disease in patients treated with CYTOVENE-IV. Immediately post-transplant, patients received CYTOVENE-IV solution 5 mg/kg bid for 14 days followed by 6 mg/kg qd for 5 days/week for an additional 14 days. Twelve of the 76 (16%) patients treated with CYTOVENE-IV versus 31 of the 73 (43%) placebo-treated patients developed CMV disease during the 120-day post-transplant observation period. No significant differences in hematologic toxicities were seen between the two treatment groups (refer to table in ADVERSE EVENTS section).

ICM 1689: In a randomized, double-blind, placebo-controlled study of 72 bone marrow transplant recipients[14] with asymptomatic CMV infection (CMV positive culture of urine, throat or blood) there was a statistically significant reduction in the incidence of CMV disease in patients treated with CYTOVENE-IV solution following successful hematopoietic engraftment. Patients with virologic evidence of CMV infection received CYTOVENE-IV 5 mg/kg bid for 7 days followed by 5 mg/kg qd through day 100 post-transplant. One of the 37 (3%) patients treated with CYTOVENE-IV versus 15 of the 35 (43%) placebo-treated patients developed CMV disease during the study. At 6 months post-transplant, there continued to be a statistically significant reduction in the incidence of CMV disease in patients treated with CYTOVENE-IV. Six of 37 (16%) patients treated with CYTOVENE-IV versus 15 of the 35 (43%) placebo-treated patients developed disease through 6 months post-transplant. The overall rate of survival was statistically significantly higher in the group treated with CYTOVENE-IV, both at day 100 and day 180 post-transplant. Although the differences in hematologic toxicities were not statistically significant, the incidence of neutropenia was higher in the group treated with CYTOVENE-IV (refer to table in ADVERSE EVENTS section).

ICM 1570: A second, randomized, unblinded study evaluated 40 allogeneic bone marrow transplant recipients at risk for CMV disease.[31] Patients underwent bronchoscopy and bronchoalveolar lavage (BAL) on day 35 post-transplant. Patients with histologic, immunologic or virologic evidence of CMV infection in the lung were then randomized to observation or treatment with CYTOVENE-IV solution (5 mg/kg bid for 14 days followed by 5 mg/kg qd 5 days/week until day 120). Four of 20 (20%) patients treated with CYTOVENE-IV and 14 of 20 (70%) control patients developed interstitial pneumonia. The incidence of CMV disease was significantly lower in the group treated with CYTOVENE-IV, consistent with the results observed in ICM 1689.

CONTRAINDICATIONS
CYTOVENE and CYTOVENE-IV are contraindicated in patients with hypersensitivity to ganciclovir or acyclovir.

WARNINGS
Hematologic: CYTOVENE-IV and CYTOVENE should not be administered if the absolute neutrophil count is less than 500 cells/µL or the platelet count is less than 25,000 cells/µL. Granulocytopenia (neutropenia), anemia and thrombocytopenia have been observed in patients treated with CYTOVENE-IV and CYTOVENE. The frequency and severity of these events vary widely in different patient populations (see ADVERSE EVENTS section).

CYTOVENE-IV and CYTOVENE should, therefore, be used with caution in patients with pre-existing cytopenias or with a history of cytopenic reactions to other drugs, chemicals or irradiation. Granulocytopenia usually occurs during the first or second week of treatment but may occur at any time during treatment. Cell counts usually begin to recover within 3 to 7 days of discontinuing drug. Colony-stimulating factors have been shown to increase neutrophil and white blood cell counts in patients receiving CYTOVENE-IV solution for treatment of CMV retinitis.[32-33]

Impairment of Fertility: Animal data indicate that administration of ganciclovir causes inhibition of spermatogenesis and subsequent infertility. These effects were reversible at lower doses and irreversible at higher doses (see Carcinogenesis, Mutagenesis and Impairment of Fertility in PRECAUTIONS section). Although data in humans have not been obtained regarding this effect, it is considered probable that ganciclovir at the recommended doses causes temporary or permanent inhibition of spermatogenesis. Animal data also indicate that suppression of fertility in females may occur.

Teratogenesis: Because of the mutagenic and teratogenic potential of ganciclovir, women of childbearing potential should be advised to use effective contraception during treatment. Similarly, men should be advised to practice barrier contraception during and for at least 90 days following treatment with CYTOVENE-IV or CYTOVENE (see Pregnancy: Category C).

PRECAUTIONS

General
In clinical studies with CYTOVENE-IV, the maximum single dose administered was 6 mg/kg by intravenous infusion over 1 hour. Larger doses have resulted in increased toxicity. It is likely that more rapid infusions would also result in increased toxicity (see OVERDOSAGE section). Administration of CYTOVENE-IV solution should be accompanied by adequate hydration.

Initially, reconstituted solutions of CYTOVENE-IV have a high pH (pH 11). Despite further dilution in intravenous fluids, phlebitis and/or pain may occur at the site of intravenous infusion. Care must be taken to infuse solutions containing CYTOVENE-IV only into veins with adequate blood flow to permit rapid dilution and distribution (see DOSAGE AND ADMINISTRATION section).

Since ganciclovir is excreted by the kidneys, normal clearance depends on adequate renal function. IF RENAL FUNCTION IS IMPAIRED, DOSAGE ADJUSTMENTS ARE REQUIRED. FOR CYTOVENE-IV AND SHOULD BE CONSIDERED FOR CYTOVENE CAPSULES. Such adjustments should be based on measured or estimated creatinine clearance values. (see DOSAGE AND ADMINISTRATION section).

Information for Patients
All patients should be informed that the major toxicities of ganciclovir are granulocytopenia (neutropenia), anemia and thrombocytopenia and that dose modifications may be required, including discontinuation. The importance of close monitoring of blood counts while on therapy should be emphasized. Patients should be informed that ganciclovir has been associated with elevations in serum creatinine.

Patients should be instructed to take CYTOVENE capsules with food to maximize bioavailability.

Patients should be advised that ganciclovir has caused decreased sperm production in animals and may cause infertility in humans. Women of childbearing potential should be advised that ganciclovir causes birth defects in animals and should not be used during pregnancy. Women of childbearing potential should be advised to use effective contraception during treatment with CYTOVENE-IV or CYTOVENE. Similarly, men should be advised to practice barrier contraception during and for at least 90 days following treatment with CYTOVENE-IV or CYTOVENE.

Patients should be advised that ganciclovir causes tumors in animals. Although there is no information from human studies, ganciclovir should be considered a potential carcinogen.

All HIV+ Patients: These patients may be receiving zidovudine (Retrovir). Patients should be counseled that treatment with both ganciclovir and zidovudine simultaneously may not be tolerated by some patients and may result in severe granulocytopenia (neutropenia). Patients with AIDS may be receiving didanosine (Videx). Patients should be counseled that concomitant treatment with both ganciclovir and didanosine can cause didanosine serum concentrations to be significantly increased.

HIV+Patients with CMV Retinitis: Ganciclovir is not a cure for CMV retinitis, and immunocompromised patients may continue to experience progression of retinitis during or following treatment. Patients should be advised to have ophthalmologic follow-up examinations at a minimum of every 4 to 6 weeks while being treated with CYTOVENE-IV or CYTOVENE. Some patients will require more frequent follow-up.

Transplant Recipients: Transplant recipients should be counseled regarding the high frequency of impaired renal function in transplant recipients who received CYTOVENE-

Studies Comparing CYTOVENE Capsules to CYTOVENE-IV:

Population Characteristics in Studies ICM 1653, ICM 1774 and AVI 034

		ICM 1653 (n=121)	ICM 1774 (n=225)	AVI 034 (n=159)
Median age (years)		38	37	39
Range		24–62	22–56	23–62
Sex	Males	116 (96%)	222 (99%)	148 (93%)
	Females	5 (4%)	3 (1%)	10 (6%)
Ethnicity	Asian	3 (3%)	5 (2%)	7 (4%)
	Black	11 (9%)	9 (4%)	3 (2%)
	Caucasian	98 (81%)	186 (83%)	140 (88%)
	Other	9 (7%)	25 (11%)	8 (5%)
Median CD$_4$ Count		9.5	7.0	10.0
Range		0–141	0–80	0–320
Mean (SD) Observation Time (days)		107.9 (43.0)	97.6 (42.5)	80.9 (47.0)

Other Ophthalmologic Endpoints Assessed Using Fundus Photographs and Changes in Snellen Visual Acuity During Maintenance Treatment of CMV Retinitis with CYTOVENE Capsules, 3 g/day, versus CYTOVENE-IV Solution, 5 mg/kg/day, in Three Controlled Clinical Trials

	Study ICM 1653 IV	Study ICM 1653 Oral	Study ICM 1774 IV	Study ICM 1774 Oral	Study AVI 034 IV	Study AVI 034 Oral
Subjects Developing Bilateral Retinitis*	3/34 (9%)	9/42 (21%)	7/52 (13%)	17/89 (19%)	6/31 (19%)	7/70 (10%)
95% Confidence Interval	[0%, 18%]	[9%, 34%]	[4%, 22%]	[11%, 27%]	[5%, 33%]	[3%, 17%]
Oral-IV Difference	13%		6%		−9%	
95% Confidence Interval	[−3%, +28%]		[−7%, +18%]		[−25%, +6%]	
Subjects with Progression Into Zone 1*	3/52 (6%)	6/56 (11%)	7/59 (12%)	20/127 (16%)	1/33 (3%)	1/86 (1%)
95% Confidence Interval	[0%, 12%]	[3%, 18%]	[4%, 20%]	[9%, 22%]	[0%, 9%]	[0%, 3%]
Oral-IV Difference	5%		4%		−2%	
95% Confidence Interval	[−5%, +15%]		[−7%, +14%]		[−8%, +4%]	
Subjects with Deterioration of Visual Acuity	14/57 (25%)	12/60 (20%)	11/69 (16%)	28/150 (19%)	5/44 (11%)	18/110 (16%)
95% Confidence Interval	[13%, 36%]	[10%, 30%]	[7%, 25%]	[12%, 25%]	[2%, 21%]	[9%, 23%]
Oral-IV Difference	−5%		3%		5%	
95% Confidence Interval	[−20%, +11%]		[−8%, +13%]		[−7%, +17%]	

* The rates of development of bilateral CMV retinitis and of progression into Zone 1 in studies 1774 and 034 may be underestimated when assessed by photography because photographic assessment was discontinued at the time of funduscopically-determined progression, which may have occurred earlier.

IV solution in controlled clinical trials, particularly in patients receiving concomitant administration of nephrotoxic agents such as cyclosporine and amphotericin B. Although the specific mechanism of this toxicity, which in most cases was reversible, has not been determined, the higher rate of renal impairment in patients receiving CYTOVENE-IV solution compared with those who received placebo in the same trials may indicate that CYTOVENE-IV played a significant role.

Laboratory Testing
Due to the frequency of neutropenia, anemia and thrombocytopenia in patients receiving CYTOVENE-IV and CYTOVENE (see ADVERSE EVENTS section), it is recommended that complete blood counts and platelet counts be performed frequently, especially in patients in whom ganciclovir or other nucleoside analogues have previously resulted in leukopenia or in whom neutrophil counts are less than 1000 cells/µL at the beginning of treatment. Increased serum creatinine levels have been observed in trials evaluating both CYTOVENE-IV and CYTOVENE. Patients should have serum creatinine or creatinine clearance values monitored carefully to allow for dosage adjustments in renally impaired patients (see DOSAGE AND ADMINISTRATION section).

Drug Interactions
Didanosine: At an oral dose of 1000 mg of CYTOVENE every 8 hours and didanosine, 200 mg every 12 hours, the steady-state didanosine AUC$_{0-12}$ increased $111\pm114\%$ (range: 10% to 493%) when didanosine was administered either 2 hours prior to or concurrent with administration of CYTOVENE (n=12 patients, 23 observations). A decrease in steady-state ganciclovir AUC of $21\pm17\%$ (range: −44% to 5%) was observed when didanosine was administered 2 hours prior to administration of CYTOVENE, but ganciclovir AUC was not affected by the presence of didanosine when the two drugs were administered simultaneously (n=12). There were no significant changes in renal clearance for either drug.

When the standard intravenous ganciclovir induction dose (5 mg/kg infused over 1 hour every 12 hours) was coadminis-

Continued on next page

Roche Laboratories—Cont.

tered with didanosine at a dose of 200 mg orally every 12 hours, the steady-state didanosine AUC_{0-12} increased 70 ± 40% (range: 3% to 121%, n=11) and C_{max} increased 49 ± 48% (range: 28% to 125%). In a separate study, when the standard intravenous ganciclovir maintenance dose (5 mg/kg infused over 1 hour every 24 hours) was coadministered with didanosine at a dose of 200 mg orally every 12 hours, didanosine AUC_{0-12} increased 50 ± 26% (range 22% to 110%, n=11) and C_{max} increased 36 ± 36% (range: −27% to 94%) over the first didanosine dosing interval. Didanosine plasma concentrations (AUC_{12-24}) were unchanged during the dosing intervals when ganciclovir was not coadministered. Ganciclovir pharmacokinetics were not affected by didanosine. In neither study were there significant changes in the renal clearance of either drug.

Zidovudine: At an oral dose of 1000 mg of CYTOVENE every 8 hours, mean steady-state ganciclovir AUC_{0-8} decreased 17±25% (range: −52% to 23%) in the presence of zidovudine, 100 mg every 4 hours (n=12). Steady-state zidovudine AUC_{0-4} increased 19±27% (range: −11% to 74%) in the presence of ganciclovir.

Since both zidovudine and ganciclovir have the potential to cause neutropenia and anemia, some patients may not tolerate concomitant therapy with these drugs at full dosage.

Probenecid: At an oral dose of 1000 mg of CYTOVENE every 8 hours (n=10), ganciclovir AUC_{0-8} increased 53±91% (range: −14% to 299%) in the presence of probenecid, 500 mg every 6 hours. Renal clearance of ganciclovir decreased 22±20% (range: −54% to −4%), which is consistent with an interaction involving competition for renal tubular secretion.

Imipenem-cilastatin: Generalized seizures have been reported in patients who received ganciclovir and imipenem-cilastatin. These drugs should not be used concomitantly unless the potential benefits outweigh the risks.

Other Medications: It is possible that drugs that inhibit replication of rapidly dividing cell populations such as bone marrow, spermatogonia and germinal layers of skin and gastrointestinal mucosa may have additive toxicity when administered concomitantly with ganciclovir. Therefore, drugs such as dapsone, pentamidine, flucytosine, vincristine, vinblastine, adriamycin, amphotericin B, trimethoprim/sulfamethoxazole combinations or other nucleoside analogues, should be considered for concomitant use with ganciclovir only if the potential benefits are judged to outweigh the risks.

No formal drug interaction studies of CYTOVENE-IV or CYTOVENE and drugs commonly used in transplant recipients have been conducted. Increases in serum creatinine were observed in patients treated with CYTOVENE-IV plus either cyclosporine or amphotericin B, drugs with known potential for nephrotoxicity (see ADVERSE EVENTS section). In a retrospective analysis of 93 liver allograft recipients receiving ganciclovir (5mg/kg infused over 1 hour every 12 hours) and oral cyclosporine (at therapeutic doses), there was no evidence of an effect on cyclosporine whole blood concentrations.

Carcinogenesis, Mutagenesis*

Ganciclovir was carcinogenic in the mouse at oral doses of 20 and 1000 mg/kg/day (approximately 0.1x and 1.4x, respectively, the mean drug exposure in humans following the recommended intravenous dose of 5 mg/kg, based on area under the plasma concentration curve [AUC] comparisons). At the dose of 1000 mg/kg/day there was a significant increase in the incidence of tumors of the preputial gland in males, forestomach (nonglandular mucosa) in males and females, and reproductive tissues (ovaries, uterus, mammary gland, clitoral gland and vagina) and liver in females. At the dose of 20 mg/kg/day, a slightly increased incidence of tumors was noted in the preputial and harderian glands in males, forestomach in males and females, and liver in females. No carcinogenic effect was observed in mice administered ganciclovir at 1 mg/kg/day (estimated as 0.01x the human dose based on AUC comparison). Except for histiocytic sarcoma of the liver, ganciclovir-induced tumors were generally of epithelial or vascular origin. Although the preputial and clitoral glands, forestomach and harderian glands of mice do not have human counterparts, ganciclovir should be considered a potential carcinogen in humans.

Ganciclovir increased mutations in mouse lymphoma cells and DNA damage in human lymphocytes in vitro at concentrations between 50 to 500 and 250 to 2000 μg/mL, respectively. In the mouse micronucleus assay, ganciclovir was clastogenic at doses of 150 and 500 mg/kg (IV) (2.8 to 10x human exposure based on AUC) but not 50 mg/kg (exposure approximately comparable to the human based on AUC). Ganciclovir was not mutagenic in the Ames Salmonella assay at concentrations of 500 to 5000 μg/mL.

Impairment of Fertility*

Ganciclovir caused decreased mating behavior, decreased fertility, and an increased incidence of embryolethality in female mice following intravenous doses of 90 mg/kg/day (approximately 1.7x the mean drug exposure in humans following the dose of 5 mg/kg, based on AUC comparisons). Ganciclovir caused decreased fertility in male mice and hypospermatogenesis in mice and dogs following daily oral or intravenous administration of doses ranging from 0.2 to 10 mg/kg. Systemic drug exposure (AUC) at the lowest dose showing toxicity in each species ranged from 0.03 to 0.1x the AUC of the recommended human intravenous dose.

Pregnancy: Category C*

Ganciclovir has been shown to be embryotoxic in rabbits and mice following intravenous administration and teratogenic in rabbits. Fetal resorptions were present in at least 85% of rabbits and mice administered 60 mg/kg/day and 108 mg/kg/day (2x the human exposure based on AUC comparisons), respectively. Effects observed in rabbits included: fetal growth retardation, embryolethality, teratogenicity and/or maternal toxicity. Teratogenic changes included cleft palate, anophthalmia/microphthalmia, aplastic organs (kidney and pancreas), hydrocephaly and brachygnathia. In mice, effects observed were maternal/fetal toxicity and embryolethality.

Daily intravenous doses of 90 mg/kg administered to female mice prior to mating, during gestation, and during lactation caused hypoplasia of the testes and seminal vesicles in the month-old male offspring, as well as pathologic changes in the nonglandular region of the stomach (see Carcinogenesis, Mutagenesis subsection). The drug exposure in mice as estimated by the AUC was approximately 1.7x the human AUC.

Ganciclovir may be teratogenic or embryotoxic at dose levels recommended for human use. There are no adequate and well-controlled studies in pregnant women. CYTOVENE-IV or CYTOVENE should be used during pregnancy only if the potential benefits justify the potential risk to the fetus.

***Footnote:** All dose comparisons presented in the Carcinogenesis, Mutagenesis, Impairment of Fertility and Pregnancy subsections are based on the human AUC following administration of a single 5 mg/kg intravenous infusion of CYTOVENE-IV as used during the maintenance phase of treatment. Compared with the single 5 mg/kg intravenous infusion, human exposure is doubled during the intravenous induction phase (5 mg/kg bid) and approximately halved during maintenance treatment with CYTOVENE capsules (1000 mg tid). The cross-species dose comparisons should be divided by 2 for intravenous induction treatment with CYTOVENE-IV and multiplied by 2 for CYTOVENE capsules.

Nursing Mothers

It is not known whether ganciclovir is excreted in human milk. However, many drugs are excreted in human milk and, because carcinogenic and teratogenic effects occurred in animals treated with ganciclovir, the possibility of serious adverse reactions from ganciclovir in nursing infants is considered likely (see Pregnancy: Category C section). Mothers should be instructed to discontinue nursing if they are receiving CYTOVENE-IV or CYTOVENE. The minimum interval before nursing can safely be resumed after the last dose of CYTOVENE-IV or CYTOVENE is unknown.

Pediatric Use

SAFETY AND EFFICACY OF CYTOVENE-IV AND CYTOVENE IN CHILDREN HAVE NOT BEEN ESTABLISHED. THE USE OF CYTOVENE-IV OR CYTOVENE IN CHILDREN WARRANTS EXTREME CAUTION DUE TO THE PROBABILITY OF LONG-TERM CARCINOGENICITY AND REPRODUCTIVE TOXICITY. ADMINISTRATION TO CHILDREN SHOULD BE UNDERTAKEN ONLY AFTER CAREFUL EVALUATION AND ONLY IF THE POTENTIAL BENEFITS OF TREATMENT OUTWEIGH THE RISKS.

The spectrum of adverse events reported in 120 immunocompromised pediatric clinical trial participants with serious CMV infections receiving CYTOVENE-IV solution were similar to those reported in adults. Granulocytopenia (17%) and thrombocytopenia (10%) were the most common adverse events reported.

Sixteen children (8 months to 15 years of age) with life- or sight-threatening CMV infections were evaluated in an open-label CYTOVENE-IV solution pharmacokinetics study. Adverse events reported for more than 1 child were as follows: hypokalemia (4/16, 25%), abnormal kidney function (3/16, 19%), sepsis (3/16, 19%), thrombocytopenia (3/16, 19%), leukopenia (2/16, 13%), coagulation disorder (2/16, 13%), hypertension (2/16, 13%), pneumonia (2/16, 13%), and immune system disorder (2/16, 13%).

There has been very limited clinical experience using CYTOVENE-IV for the treatment of CMV retinitis in patients under the age of 12 years. Two children (ages 9 and 5 years) showed improvement or stabilization of retinitis for 23 and 9 months, respectively. These children received induction treatment with 2.5 mg/kg tid followed by maintenance therapy with 6 to 6.5 mg/kg once per day, 5 to 7 days per week. When retinitis progressed during once-daily maintenance therapy, both children were treated with the 5 mg/kg bid regimen. Two other children (ages 2.5 and 4 years) who received similar induction regimens showed only partial or no response to treatment. Another child, a 6-year-old with T-cell dysfunction, showed stabilization of retinitis for 3 months while receiving continuous infusions of CYTOVENE-IV at doses of 2 to 5 mg/kg/24 hours. Continuous infusion treatment was discontinued due to granulocytopenia.

Eleven of the 72 patients in the placebo-controlled trial in bone marrow transplant recipients were children, ranging from 3 to 10 years of age (5 treated with CYTOVENE-IV and 6 with placebo). Five of the pediatric patients treated with CYTOVENE-IV received 5 mg/kg intravenously bid for up to 7 days; 4 patients went on to receive 5 mg/kg qd up to day 100 post-transplant. Results were similar to those observed in adult transplant recipients treated with CYTOVENE-IV. Two of the 6 placebo-treated pediatric patients developed CMV pneumonia, versus none of the 5 patients treated with CYTOVENE-IV. The spectrum of adverse events in the pediatric group was similar to that observed in the adult patients.

CYTOVENE capsules have not been studied in children under age 13.

Use in Patients with Renal Impairment

CYTOVENE-IV and CYTOVENE should be used with caution in patients with impaired renal function because the half-life and plasma/serum concentrations of ganciclovir will be increased due to reduced renal clearance (see DOSAGE AND ADMINISTRATION and ADVERSE EVENTS: Renal Toxicity sections).

Hemodialysis has been shown to reduce plasma levels of ganciclovir by approximately 50%.

Use in Elderly Patients

The pharmacokinetic profiles of CYTOVENE-IV and CYTOVENE in elderly patients have not been established. Since elderly individuals frequently have a reduced glomerular filtration rate, particular attention should be paid to assessing renal function before and during administration of CYTOVENE-IV or CYTOVENE (see DOSAGE AND ADMINISTRATION section).

ADVERSE EVENTS

Adverse events that occurred during clinical trials of CYTOVENE-IV solution and CYTOVENE capsules are summarized below, according to the participating study subject population.

Subjects with AIDS: Three controlled, randomized, phase 3 trials comparing CYTOVENE-IV and CYTOVENE capsules for maintenance treatment of CMV retinitis have been completed. During these trials, CYTOVENE-IV or CYTOVENE capsules were prematurely discontinued in 9% of subjects because of adverse events, new or worsening intercurrent illnesses, or laboratory abnormalities. In a placebo-controlled, randomized, phase 3 trial of CYTOVENE capsules for prevention of CMV disease in AIDS, treatment was prematurely discontinued because of adverse events, new or worsening intercurrent illness, or laboratory abnormalities in 19.5% of subjects treated with CYTOVENE capsules and 16% of subjects receiving placebo. Laboratory data and adverse events reported during the conduct of these controlled trials are summarized below.

Laboratory Data:

[See table at top of next page.]

Overall, in the treatment studies, subjects treated with CYTOVENE-IV solution experienced lower minimum ANCs and hemoglobin levels, consistent with more neutropenia and anemia, compared with those who received CYTOVENE capsules (p=0.024 for neutropenia; p=0.027 for anemia). In the prevention study, subjects treated with CYTOVENE capsules also experienced lower minimum ANCs compared with those who received placebo ($p < 0.001$).

For the majority of subjects in the treatment studies, maximum serum creatinine levels were < 1.5 mg/dL and no difference was noted between CYTOVENE-IV solution and CYTOVENE capsules for the occurrence of renal impairment. Serum creatinine elevations ≥ 2.5 mg/dL occurred in < 2% of all subjects, and no significant differences were noted in the time from the start of maintenance to the occurrence of elevations in serum creatinine values. In the prevention study, 20% of subjects treated with CYTOVENE capsules had maximum serum creatinine levels of 1.5 mg/dL or greater, compared to 13% on placebo (p=0.013). Of subjects in ganciclovir and placebo treatment groups, 24% and 20%, respectively, experienced creatinine elevations more than 25% over baseline levels.

Adverse Events: The following table shows selected adverse events reported in 5% or more of the subjects in three controlled clinical trials during treatment with either CYTOVENE-IV solution (5 mg/kg/day) or CYTOVENE capsules (3000 mg/day), and in one controlled clinical trial in which CYTOVENE capsules (3000 mg/day) were compared to placebo for the prevention of CMV disease.

[See second table on top of next page.]

Retinal Detachment: Retinal detachment has been observed in subjects with CMV retinitis both before and after initiation of therapy with ganciclovir. Its relationship to therapy with ganciclovir is unknown. Retinal detachment occurred in 11% of patients treated with CYTOVENE-IV solution and in 8% of patients treated with CYTOVENE capsules. Patients with CMV retinitis should have frequent

ophthalmologic evaluations to monitor the status of their retinitis and to detect any other retinal pathology.

Transplant Recipients: There have been three controlled clinical trials of CYTOVENE-IV solution for the prevention of CMV disease in transplant recipients.[13,14,31] Laboratory data and adverse events reported during these trials are summarized below.

Laboratory Data:

The following table shows the frequency of granulocytopenia (neutropenia) and thrombocytopenia observed:

[See table at top of next page.]

The following table shows the frequency of elevated serum creatinine values in these controlled clinical trials:

[See second table at top of next page.]

In a placebo-controlled clinical trial conducted in heart allograft recipients (ICM 1496), more patients receiving CYTOVENE-IV solution had elevation of serum creatinine to values exceeding 2.5 mg/dL than patients receiving placebo (18% vs 4%, respectively). These increases in serum creatinine, up to 5.5 mg/dL in 1 patient, were transient and occurred primarily during the first week of treatment with CYTOVENE-IV solution. In a randomized, open-label study of CYTOVENE-IV solution in bone marrow allograft recipients (ICM 1570), more patients treated with CYTOVENE-IV solution experienced serum creatinine values exceeding 1.5 mg/dL than patients who were not treated (70% vs 35%, respectively). These elevations in serum creatinine, up to 3.2 mg/dL in 1 patient, were transient and occurred intermittently throughout the 3-month study. Most patients in these studies also received cyclosporine. In a second study in bone marrow transplant patients that was placebo-controlled (ICM 1689), no differences in elevations of serum creatinine were seen between the patients receiving CYTOVENE-IV solution and those receiving placebo. The mechanism of impairment of renal function is not known. However, careful monitoring of renal function during therapy with CYTOVENE-IV solution is essential, especially for those patients receiving concomitant agents that may cause nephrotoxicity.

General: Other adverse events that were thought to be "probably" or "possibly" related to CYTOVENE-IV solution or CYTOVENE capsules in clinical studies in either subjects with AIDS or transplant recipients are listed below. These events all occurred with a frequency of 1% or less unless otherwise noted.

Body as a Whole: abdomen enlarged, abscess, asthenia (6%), back pain, cellulitis, chest pain, chills and fever, drug level increased (ganciclovir), edema, face edema, headache (4%), injection site abscess, injection site edema, injection site hemorrhage, injection site inflammation (2%), injection site pain, injection site phlebitis, laboratory test abnormality, malaise, pain (2%), photosensitivity reaction, neck pain, neck rigidity.

Digestive System: abnormal liver function test (2%), aphthous stomatitis, constipation, dyspepsia (4%), dysphagia, eructation, esophagitis, fecal incontinence, gastritis, gastrointestinal hemorrhage, hepatitis, jaundice, melena, mouth ulceration, nausea and vomiting (2%), pancreatitis, tongue disorder

Hemic and Lymphatic System: eosinophilia, hypochromic anemia, marrow depression, pancytopenia, splenomegaly

Respiratory System: cough increased, dyspnea, pharyngitis

Nervous System: abnormal dreams, abnormal gait, agitation, amnesia, anxiety, ataxia, coma, confusion, depression, dizziness, dry mouth (2%), emotional lability, euphoria, hypertonia, hyperkinesia, hypesthesia, insomnia (2%), libido decreased, manic reaction, myoclonus, nervousness, psychosis, seizures, somnolence, thinking abnormal, tremor, trismus. (Overall, probably or possibly related neurologic system events occurred in approximately 5% of patients).

Skin and Appendages: acne, alopecia, dry skin, fixed eruption, maculopapular rash, skin discoloration, urticaria, vesiculobullous rash

Special Senses: abnormal vision, amblyopia, blindness, conjunctivitis, deafness, ear pain, eye pain, glaucoma, photophobia, taste perversion, tinnitus

Metabolic and Nutritional Disorders: alkaline phosphatase increased, creatinine increased, creatine phosphokinase increased, decreased blood sugar, hyperglycemia, hypokalemia, increased blood urea nitrogen (BUN), lactic dehydrogenase increased, SGOT increased, SGPT increased, weight loss (2%)

Cardiovascular System: arrhythmia, deep thrombophlebitis, hypertension, hypotension, migraine, phlebitis (2%), vasodilatation

Urogenital System: breast pain, creatinine clearance decreased, hematuria, impotence, kidney failure, kidney function abnormal, urinary frequency, urinary tract infection

Musculoskeletal System: arthralgia, bone pain, leg cramps, myalgia, myasthenia

Selected Laboratory Abnormalities in Trials for Treatment of CMV Retinitis and Prevention of CMV Disease

Treatment	CMV Retinitis Treatment* CYTOVENE Capsules[†] 3000 mg/day	CYTOVENE-IV[‡] 5 mg/kg/day	CMV Disease Prevention [§] CYTOVENE Capsules" 3000 mg/day	Placebo [¶]
Subjects, number	320	175	478	234
Neutropenia:				
<500 ANC/μL	18%	25%	10%	6%
500–<749	17%	14%	16%	7%
750–<1000	19%	26%	22%	16%
Anemia:				
Hemoglobin:				
<6.5 g/dL	2%	5%	1%	<1%
6.5–<8.0	10%	16%	5%	3%
8.0–<9.5	25%	26%	15%	16%
Maximum Serum Creatinine:				
≥2.5 mg/dL	1%	2%	1%	2%
≥1.5–<2.5	12%	14%	19%	11%

* Pooled data from Treatment Studies, ICM 1653, Study ICM 1774, and Study AVI 034.
† Mean time on therapy = 91 days, including allowed reinduction treatment periods
‡ Mean time on therapy = 103 days, including allowed reinduction treatment periods
§ Data from Prevention Study, ICM 1654
" Mean time on ganciclovir = 269 days
¶ Mean time on placebo = 240 days
(See discussion of clinical trials under INDICATIONS AND USAGE section.)

Selected Adverse Events Reported in ≥5% of Subjects in Three Randomized Phase 3 Studies Comparing CYTOVENE Capsules to CYTOVENE-IV Solution for Maintenance Treatment of CMV Retinitis and in One Phase 3 Randomized Study Comparing Cytovene Capsules to Placebo for Prevention of CMV Disease

Body System	Adverse Event	Maintenance Treatment Studies Capsules (n=326)	IV (n=179)	Prevention Study Capsules (n=478)	Placebo (n=234)
Body as a Whole	Fever	38%	48%	35%	33%
	Abdominal Pain	17%	19%	21%	21%
	Infection	9%	13%	8%	4%
	Chills	7%	10%	7%	4%
	Sepsis	4%	15%	3%	2%
Digestive System	Diarrhea	41%	44%	48%	42%
	Nausea	26%	25%	30%	33%
	Anorexia	15%	14%	19%	16%
	Vomiting	13%	13%	14%	11%
	Flatulence	6%	3%	9%	11%
Hemic and Lymphatic System	Leukopenia	29%	41%	17%	9%
	Anemia	19%	25%	9%	7%
	Thrombocytopenia	6%	6%	3%	1%
Respiratory System	Pneumonia	6%	8%	7%	7%
Nervous System	Neuropathy	8%	9%	21%	15%
	Paresthesia	6%	10%	6%	6%
Other	Rash	15%	10%	23%	26%
	Sweating	11%	12%	14%	12%
	Pruritis	6%	5%	10%	9%
	Vitreous Disorder	6%	4%	1%	1%
Catheter Related*	Total Catheter Events	6%	22%	—	—
	Catheter Infection	4%	9%	—	—
	Catheter Sepsis	1%	8%	—	—

*Some of these events also appear under other body systems.

The following adverse events reported in patients receiving ganciclovir may be potentially fatal: pancreatitis, sepsis and multiple organ failure.

Adverse Events Reported During Postmarketing Experience with CYTOVENE-IV

Listed below are adverse events reported spontaneously since the marketing introduction of CYTOVENE-IV that have not been included previously based on experience during clinical trials. These events have been reported infrequently, and data are insufficient to estimate an incidence at which they have occurred or to establish a relationship to ganciclovir use. These events may have occurred as part of an underlying disease process and do not necessarily represent the type, severity or prevalence of adverse events occurring in clinical practice. These voluntary reports include: acidosis, allergic reaction, anaphylactic reaction, arthritis, bronchospasm, cardiac arrest, cardiac conduction abnormality, cataracts, cholestasis, congenital anomaly, dry eyes, dysesthesia, dysphasia, elevated triglyceride levels, encephalopathy, exfoliative dermatitis, extrapyramidal reaction, facial palsy, hallucinations, hemolytic anemia, hepatic failure, hepatitis, hyponatremia, inappropriate serum ADH, infertility, intestinal ulceration, intracranial hypertension, irritability, loss of memory, loss of sense of smell, myelopathy, perforated intestine, peripheral ischemia, pulmonary fibrosis, rhabdomyolysis, Stevens-Johnson syndrome, stroke, testicular hypotrophy, Torsades de Pointes, vasculitis, ventricular tachycardia.

OVERDOSAGE

CYTOVENE-IV: Overdosage with CYTOVENE-IV has been reported in 17 patients (13 adults and 4 children under 2 years of age). Five patients experienced no adverse events following overdosage at the following doses: 7 doses of 11 mg/kg over a 3-day period (adult), single dose of 3500 mg (adult), single dose of 500 mg (72.5 mg/kg) followed by 48 hours of peritoneal dialysis (4-month-old), single dose of approximately 60 mg/kg followed by exchange transfusion (18-month-old), 2 doses of 500 mg instead of 31 mg (21-month-old).

Irreversible pancytopenia developed in 1 adult with AIDS and CMV colitis after receiving 3000 mg of CYTOVENE-IV solution on each of 2 consecutive days. He experienced wors-

Continued on next page

Roche Laboratories—Cont.

ening GI symptoms and acute renal failure that required short-term dialysis. Pancytopenia developed and persisted until his death from a malignancy several months later. Other adverse events reported following overdosage included: persistent bone marrow suppression (1 adult with neutropenia and thrombocytopenia after a single dose of 6000 mg), reversible neutropenia or granulocytopenia (4 adults, overdoses ranging from 8 mg/kg daily for 4 days to a single dose of 25 mg/kg), hepatitis (1 adult receiving 10 mg/kg daily, and one 2 kg infant after a single 40 mg dose), renal toxicity (1 adult with transient worsening of hematuria after a single 500 mg dose, and 1 adult with elevated creatinine (5.2 mg/dL) after a single 5000 to 7000 mg dose), and seizure (1 adult with known seizure disorder after 3 days of 9 mg/kg). In addition, 1 adult received 0.4 mL (instead of 0.1 mL) CYTOVENE-IV solution by intravitreal injection, and experienced temporary loss of vision and central retinal artery occlusion secondary to increased intraocular pressure related to the injected fluid volume.

CYTOVENE Capsules: There have been no reports of overdosage with CYTOVENE capsules. Doses as high as 6000 mg/day, given either as 1000 mg 6 times daily or as 2000 mg tid, did not result in overt toxicity other than transient neutropenia. Daily doses of more than 6000 mg have not been studied.

Since ganciclovir is dialyzable, dialysis may be useful in reducing serum concentrations. Adequate hydration should be maintained. The use of hematopoietic growth factors should be considered.

DOSAGE AND ADMINISTRATION

CAUTION—DO NOT ADMINISTER CYTOVENE-IV SOLUTION BY RAPID OR BOLUS INTRAVENOUS INJECTION. THE TOXICITY OF CYTOVENE-IV MAY BE INCREASED AS A RESULT OF EXCESSIVE PLASMA LEVELS.

CAUTION—INTRAMUSCULAR OR SUBCUTANEOUS INJECTION OF RECONSTITUTED CYTOVENE-IV SOLUTION MAY RESULT IN SEVERE TISSUE IRRITATION DUE TO HIGH pH (11).

Dosage

THE RECOMMENDED DOSE FOR CYTOVENE-IV SOLUTION AND CYTOVENE CAPSULES SHOULD NOT BE EXCEEDED. THE RECOMMENDED INFUSION RATE FOR CYTOVENE-IV SOLUTION SHOULD NOT BE EXCEEDED.

For Treatment of CMV Retinitis for Patients with Normal Renal Function:

1. Induction Treatment

The recommended initial dose for patients with normal renal function is 5 mg/kg (given intravenously at a constant rate over 1 hour) every 12 hours for 14 to 21 days. CYTOVENE capsules should not be used for induction treatment.

2. Maintenance Treatment

CYTOVENE-IV: Following induction treatment, the recommended maintenance dose of CYTOVENE-IV solution is 5 mg/kg given as a constant-rate intravenous infusion over 1 hour once daily, 7 days per week or 6 mg/kg once daily, 5 days per week.

CYTOVENE Capsules: Following induction treatment, the recommended maintenance dose of CYTOVENE capsules is 1000 mg tid with food. Alternatively, the dosing regimen of 500 mg 6 times daily every 3 hours with food, during waking hours, may be used.

For patients who experience progression of CMV retinitis while receiving maintenance treatment with either formulation of ganciclovir, reinduction treatment is recommended.

For the Prevention of CMV Disease in Patients with Advanced HIV Infection and Normal Renal Function

CYTOVENE Capsules: The recommended prophylactic dose of CYTOVENE capsules is 1000 mg tid with food.

For the Prevention of CMV Disease in Transplant Recipients with Normal Renal Function

The recommended initial dose of CYTOVEVE-IV solution for patients with normal renal function is 5 mg/kg (given intravenously at a constant rate over 1 hour) every 12 hours for 7 to 14 days, followed by 5 mg/kg once daily, 7 days per week or 6 mg/kg once daily, 5 days per week.

The duration of treatment with CYTOVENE-IV solution in transplant recipients is dependent upon the duration and degree of immunosuppression. In controlled clinical trials in bone marrow allograft recipients, treatment was continued until day 100 to 120 post-transplantation. CMV disease occurred in several patients who discontinued treatment with CYTOVENE-IV solution prematurely. In heart allograft recipients, the onset of newly diagnosed CMV disease occurred after treatment with CYTOVENE-IV was stopped at day 28 post-transplant, suggesting that continued dosing may be necessary to prevent late occurrence of CMV disease

Controlled Trials—Transplant Recipients

	Heart Allograft*		Bone Marrow Allograft†	
	CYTOVENE-IV (n=76)	Placebo (n=73)	CYTOVENE-IV (n=57)	Control (n=55)
Neutropenia				
Minimum ANC <500/μL	4%	3%	12%	6%
Minimum ANC 500–1000/μL	3%	8%	29%	17%
TOTAL ANC ≤1000/μL	7%	11%	41%	23%
Thrombocytopenia				
Platelet count <25,000/μL	3%	1%	32%	28%
Platelet count 25,000–50,000/μL	5%	3%	25%	37%
TOTAL Platelet ≤50,000/μL	8%	4%	57%	65%

* Study ICM 1496. Mean duration of treatment=28 days
† Study ICM 1570 and ICM 1689. Mean duration of treatment=45 days
(See discussion of clinical trials under INDICATIONS AND USAGE section.)

Controlled Trials—Transplant Recipients

	Heart Allograft ICM 1496		Bone Marrow Allograft			
			ICM 1570		ICM 1689	
Maximum Serum Creatinine Levels	CYTOVENE-IV (n=76)	Placebo (n=73)	CYTOVENE-IV (n=20)	Control (n=20)	CYTOVENE-IV (n=37)	Placebo (n=35)
Serum Creatinine ≥2.5 mg/dL	18%	4%	20%	0%	0%	0%
Serum Creatinine ≥1.5 – <2.5 mg/dL	58%	69%	50%	35%	43%	44%

in this patient population (see INDICATIONS AND USAGE section for a more detailed discussion).

Renal Impairment

CYTOVENE-IV: For patients with impairment of renal function, refer to the table below for recommended doses of CYTOVENE-IV solution and adjust the dosing interval as indicated:

[See table at top of next page.]

Dosing for patients undergoing hemodialysis should not exceed 1.25 mg/kg 3 times per week, following each hemodialysis session. CYTOVENE-IV should be given shortly after completion of the hemodialysis session, since hemodialysis has been shown to reduce plasma levels by approximately 50%.

CYTOVENE Capsules: In patients with renal impairment, the dose of CYTOVENE capsules should be modified as shown below:

Creatinine Clearance* mL/min	CYTOVENE Capsule Doses
≥70	1000 mg tid or 500 mg q3h, 6x/day
50–69	1500 mg qd or 500 mg tid
25–49	1000 mg qd or 500 mg bid
10–24	500 mg qd
<10	500 mg 3 times per week, following hemodialysis

* Creatinine clearance can be related to serum creatinine by the following formulae:

$$\text{Creatinine clearance for males} = \frac{(140 - \text{age [yrs]}) (\text{body wt [kg]})}{(72) (\text{serum creatinine [mg/dL]})}$$

$$\text{Creatinine clearance for females} = 0.85 \times \text{male value}$$

Patient Monitoring

Due to the frequency of granulocytopenia and thrombocytopenia in patients receiving ganciclovir (see ADVERSE EVENTS section), it is recommended that complete blood counts and platelet counts be performed frequently, especially in patients in whom ganciclovir or other nucleoside analogues have previously resulted in cytopenia, or in whom neutrophil counts are less than 1000 cells/μL at the beginning of treatment. Patients should have serum creatinine or creatinine clearance values followed carefully to allow for dosage adjustments in renally impaired patients (see DOSAGE AND ADMINISTRATION section).

Reduction of Dose

Dosage reductions in renally impaired patients are required for CYTOVENE-IV and should be considered for CYTO-

VENE capsules (see Renal Impairment section). Dosage reductions should also be considered for those with neutropenia, anemia and/or thrombocytopenia (see ADVERSE EVENTS section). Ganciclovir should not be administered in patients with severe neutropenia (ANC less than 500/μL) or severe thrombocytopenia (platelets less than 25,000/μL).

Method of Preparation of CYTOVENE-IV Solution

Each 10 mL clear glass vial contains ganciclovir sodium equivalent to 500 mg of ganciclovir and 46 mg of sodium. The contents of the vial should be prepared for administration in the following manner:

1. Reconstituted Solution:

a. Reconstitute lyophilized CYTOVENE-IV by injecting 10 mL of Sterile Water for Injection, USP, into the vial. DO NOT USE BACTERIOSTATIC WATER FOR INJECTION CONTAINING PARABENS. IT IS INCOMPATIBLE WITH CYTOVENE-IV AND MAY CAUSE PRECIPITATION.

b. Shake the vial to dissolve the drug.

c. Visually inspect the reconstituted solution for particulate matter and discoloration prior to proceeding with infusion solution. Discard the vial if particulate matter or discoloration is observed.

d. Reconstituted solution in the vial is stable at room temperature for 12 hours. It should not be refrigerated.

2. Infusion Solution:

Based on patient weight, the appropriate volume of the reconstituted solution (ganciclovir concentration 50 mg/mL) should be removed from the vial and added to an acceptable (see below) infusion fluid (typically 100 mL) for delivery over the course of 1 hour. Infusion concentrations greater than 10 mg/mL are not recommended. The following infusion fluids have been determined to be chemically and physically compatible with CYTOVENE-IV solution: 0.9% Sodium Chloride, 5% Dextrose, Ringer's Injection, and Lactated Ringer's Injection, USP.

CYTOVENE-IV, when reconstituted with sterile water for injection, further diluted with 0.9% sodium chloride injection, and stored refrigerated at 5°C in polyvinyl chloride (PVC) bags, remains physically and chemically sterile for 14 days

However, because CYTOVENE-IV is reconstituted with non-bacteriostatic sterile water, it is recommended that the infusion solution be used within 24 hours of dilution to reduce the risk of bacterial contamination. The infusion solution should be refrigerated. Freezing is not recommended.

Handling and Disposal

Caution should be exercised in the handling and preparation of solutions of CYTOVENE-IV and in the handling of CYTOVENE capsules. Solutions of CYTOVENE-IV are alkaline (pH 11). Avoid direct contact with the skin or mucous membranes of the powder contained in CYTOVENE capsules or of CYTOVENE-IV solutions. If such contact occurs, wash thoroughly with soap and water; rinse eyes thoroughly

Creatinine Clearance* (mL/min)	CYTOVENE-IV Induction Dose (mg/kg)	Dosing Interval (hours)	CYTOVENE-IV Maintenance Dose (mg/kg)	Dosing Interval (hours)
≥70	5.0	12	5.0	24
50–69	2.5	12	2.5	24
25–49	2.5	24	1.25	24
10–24	1.25	24	0.625	24
<10	1.25	3 times per week, following hemodialysis	0.625	3 times per week, following hemodialysis

* Creatinine clearance can be related to serum creatinine by the formulae given below.

with plain water. CYTOVENE capsules should not be opened or crushed.

Because ganciclovir shares some of the properties of antitumor agents (ie, carcinogenicity and mutagenicity), consideration should be given to handling and disposal according to guidelines issued for antineoplastic drugs. Several guidelines on this subject have been published.[34–39]

There is no general agreement that all of the procedures recommended in the guidelines are necessary or appropriate.

HOW SUPPLIED

CYTOVENE®-IV (ganciclovir sodium for injection) is supplied in 10 mL sterile vials, each containing ganciclovir sodium equivalent to 500 mg of ganciclovir, in cartons of 25 (NDC 0004-6940-03).

Store vials at temperatures below 40°C (104°F).

CYTOVENE® (ganciclovir capsules) 250 mg are two-pieced, size No. 1, opaque green hard gelatin capsules with ROCHE and CYTOVENE 250 imprinted on the capsules in dark blue ink and with two blue lines partially encircling the capsule body. Each capsule contains 250 mg of ganciclovir as a white to off-white powder. CYTOVENE capsules are supplied as follows: Bottles of 180 capsules (NDC 0004-0269-48)

Store at 15°–30°C (59°–86°F).

REFERENCES

1. Agut H, Huraux J-M, Collandre H, Montagnier L. Susceptibility of human herpesvirus 6 to acyclovir and ganciclovir. Lancet. 1989; 2: 626. Letter. **2.** Russler SK, Tapper MA, Carrigan DR. Susceptibility of human herpesvirus 6 to acyclovir and ganciclovir. Lancet. 1989; 2:382. Letter. **3.** Locarnini S, Guo K, Lucas R, Gust I. Inhibition of HBV DNA replication by ganciclovir in patients with AIDS. Lancet. 1989; 2:1225–1226. Letter. **4.** Faulds D, Heel RC. Ganciclovir: a review of its antiviral activity, pharmacokinetic properties and therapeutic efficacy in cytomegalovirus infections. Drugs. 1990; 39:597–638. **5.** Field AK, Biron KK. The end of innocence revisited: resistance of herpesviruses to antiviral drugs. Clin Microbiology Rev. 1994; 7:1–13. **6.** Littler E, Stuart AD, Chee MS. Human cytomegalovirus UL97 open reading frame encodes a protein that phosphorylates the antiviral nucleoside analogue ganciclovir. Nature. 1992; 358:160–162. **7.** Sullivan V, Talarico CL, Stanat SC, Davis M, Coen DM, Biron KK. A protein kinase homologue controls phosphorylation of ganciclovir in human cytomegalovirus-infected cells. [Published erratum appears in Nature 1992; 359:85] Nature. 1992; 358:162–164. **8.** Smee DF. Interaction of 9-(1,3-dihydroxy-2-propoxymethyl)guanine with cytosol and mitochondrial deoxyguanosine kinases: possible role in anticytomegalovirus activity. Mol Cell Biochem. 1985; 69:75–81. **9.** Biron KK, Stanat SC, Sorrell JB, Fyfe JA, Keller PM, Lambe CU, Nelson DJ. Metabolic activation of the nucleoside analog 9-{[2-hydroxy-1-(hydroxymethyl)ethoxy]methyl}guanine in human diploid fibroblasts infected with human cytomegalovirus. Proc Natl Acad Sci (USA). 1985; 82:2473–2477. **10.** Freitas VR, Smee DF, Chernow M, Boehme R, Matthews TR. Activity of 9-(1,3-dihydroxy-2-propoxymethyl)guanine compared with that of acyclovir against human, monkey, and rodent cytomegaloviruses. Antimicrob Agents Chemother. 1985; 28:240–245. **11.** Sommadossi J-P, Carlisle R. Toxicity of 3'-azido-3'-deoxythymidine and 9-(1,3-dihydroxy-2-propoxymethyl)guanine for normal human hematopoietic progenitor cells in vitro. Antimicrob Agents Chemother. 1987; 31:452–454. **12.** Buhles WC, Mastre BJ, Tinker AJ, Strand V, Koretz SH, the Syntex Collaborative Ganciclovir Treatment Study Group. Ganciclovir treatment of life- or sight-threatening cytomegalovirus infection: experience in 314 immunocompromised patients. Rev Infect Dis. 1988; 10:495–506. **13.** Merigan TC, Renlund DG, Keay S, et al. A controlled trial of ganciclovir to prevent cytomegalovirus disease after heart transplantation. New Engl J Med. 1992; 326:1182–1186. **14.** Goodrich JM, Mori M, Gleaves CA, et al. Early treatment with ganciclovir to prevent cytomegalovirus disease after allogeneic bone marrow transplantation. New Engl J Med. 1991; 325:1601–1607. **15.** Erice A, Chou S, Biron KK, Stanat SC, Balfour HH Jr, Jordan MC. Progressive disease due to ganciclovir-resistant cytomegalovirus in immunocompromised patients. New Eng J Med. 1989; 320:289–293. **16.** Drew WL, Miner RC, Busch DF, et al. Prevalence of resistance in patients receiving ganciclovir for serious cytomegalovirus infection. J Infect Dis. 1991; 163:716–719. **17.** Jacobson MA, Drew WL, Feinberg J, O'Donnell JJ, Whitmore PV, Miner RD, Parenti D. Foscarnet therapy for ganciclovir-resistant cytomegalovirus retinitis in patients with AIDS. J Infect Dis. 1991; 163:1348–1351. **18.** Pepin J-M, Simon F, Dussault A, Collin G, Dazza M-C., Brun-Vezinet F. Rapid determination of human cytomegalovirus susceptibility to ganciclovir directly from clinical specimen primocultures. J Clin Microbiol. 1992; 30:2917–2920. **19.** Tseng LF. Rapid and simple antiviral sensitivity testing of cytomegalovirus (CMV). In: Abstract Book of the 92nd General Meeting of the American Society for Microbiology; May 26–30, 1992; New Orleans, LA. Abstract. **20.** Biron KK, Fyfe JA, Stanat SC, Leslie LK, Sorrell JB, Lambe CU, Coen DM. A human cytomegalovirus mutant resistant to the nucleoside analog 9-{[2-hydroxy-1-(hydroxymethyl)ethoxy]methyl}guanine (BW B759U) induces reduced levels of BW B759U triphosphate. Proc Natl Acad Sci (USA). 1986; 83:8769–8773. **21.** Stanat SC, Reardon JE, Erice A, Jordan MC, Drew WL, Biron KK. Ganciclovir-resistant cytomegalovirus clinical isolates: mode of resistance to ganciclovir. Antimicrob Agents Chemother. 1991; 35:2191–2197. **22.** Lurain NS, Spafford LE, Thompson KD. Mutation in the UL97 open reading frame of human cytomegalovirus strains resistant to ganciclovir. J. Virol. 1994; 68:4427–4431. **23.** Sullivan V, Biron KK, Talarico C, Stanat SC, Davis M, Pozzi L, Coen DM. A point mutation in the human cytomegalovirus DNA polymerase gene confers resistance to ganciclovir and phosphonylmethoxyalkyl derivatives. Antimicrob Agents Chemother. 1993; 37:19–25. **24.** Lurain NS, Thompson KD, Holmes EW, Sullivan Read G. Point mutations in the DNA polymerase gene of human cytomegalovirus strains resistant to ganciclovir. J Virol. 1992; 66:7146–7152. **25.** Fletcher C, Sawchuk R, Chinnock B, deMiranda P, Balfour HH Jr. Human pharmacokinetics of the antiviral drug DHPG. Clin Pharmacol Ther. 1986; 40:281–286. **26.** Trang JM, Kidd L, Gruber W, Storch G, Demmler G, Jacobs R, Dankner W, Starr S, Pass R, Stagno S, Alford C, Soong S-J, Whitley RJ, Sommadossi J-P. Linear single-dose pharmacokinetics of ganciclovir in newborns with congenital cytomegalovirus infections. Clin Pharmacol Ther. 1993; 53:15–21. **27.** Jabs DA, Enger C, Bartlett JG. Cytomegalovirus retinitis and acquired immunodeficiency syndrome. Arch Ophthalmol. 1989;107:75–80. **28.** Spector, SA, Weingeis T, Pollard R, et al. A randomized, controlled study of intravenous ganciclovir therapy for cytomegalovirus peripheral retinitis in patients with AIDS. J Inf Dis. 1993; 168:557–563. **29.** Drew, WL, Ives, D, Lalezari JP, et al. Oral ganciclovir as maintenance treatment for cytomegalovirus retinitis in patients with AIDS. New Engl J Med. 1995; 333:615–620. **30.** The Oral Ganciclovir European and Australian Cooperative Study Group. Intravenous versus oral ganciclovir: European/Australian comparative study of efficacy and safety in the prevention of cytomegalovirus retinitis recurrence in patients with AIDS. AIDS. 1995; 9:471–477. **31.** Schmidt GM, Horak DA, Niland JC, Duncan SR, Forman SJ, Zaia JA. The City of Hope-Stanford-Syntex CMV Study Group. A randomized, controlled trial of prophylactic ganciclovir for cytomegalovirus pulmonary infection in recipients of allogeneic bone marrow transplants. New Engl J Med. 1991; 15:1005–1011. **32.** Hardy WD. Combined ganciclovir and recombinant human granulocyte-macrophage colony-stimulating factor in the treatment of cytomegalovirus retinitis in AIDS patients. J Acquir Immune Defic Syndr. 1991; 4:S22–S28. **33.** Jacobson MA, Stanley HD, Heard SE. Ganciclovir with recombinant methionyl human granulocyte colony-stimulating factor for treatment of cytomegalovirus disease in AIDS patients. AIDS. 1992; 6:515–517. **34.** Recommendations for the Safe Handling of Cytotoxic Drugs. Washington, DC: Superintendent of Documents; 1992. US Government Printing Office publication NIH 92-2621. **35.** Council on Scientific Affairs: Guidelines for Handling Parenteral Antineoplastics. JAMA. 1985; 253:1590–1592. **36.** Recommendations for Handling Cytotoxic Agents, September 1987. National Study Commission of Cytotoxic Exposure. Available from: Louis P. Jeffrey, Sc. D., President Emeritus, Massachusetts College of Pharmacy and Allied Health Sciences, Boston, MA. **37.** Guidelines and recommendations for safe handling of antineoplastic agents. Med J Aust. 1983; (April 30):426–428. **38.** Jones RB, Frank R, Mass T. Safe handling of chemotherapeutic agents: a report from the Mount Sinai Medical Center, CA. Cancer J Clin. 1983; 33:258–263. **39.** American Society of Hospital Pharmacists technical assistance bulletin on handling cytotoxic and hazardous drugs. Am J Hosp Pharm. 1990; 47:1033–1049.

CYTOVENE-IV for intravenous infusion manufactured by Warner-Lambert Company, Morris Plains, NJ 07950 and CYTOVENE Capsules for oral administration manufactured by Syntex Puerto Rico, Inc., Humacao, Puerto Rico 00791

Revised: August 1996

Shown in Product Identification Guide, page 332

EC-NAPROSYN™ ℞

[nă' pro-sin]

(naproxen) Delayed-Release Tablets

NAPROSYN® ℞

(naproxen) Tablets

ANAPROX®/ANAPROX® DS ℞

[an' ă-prox]

(naproxen sodium) Tablets

NAPROSYN® ℞

(naproxen) Suspension

DESCRIPTION

Naproxen is a member of the arylacetic acid group of nonsteroidal anti-inflammatory drugs. The chemical names for naproxen and naproxen sodium are (S)-6-methoxy-α-methyl-2-naphthaleneacetic acid and (S)-6-methoxy-α-methyl-2-naphthaleneacetic acid, sodium salt, respectively.

Naproxen is an odorless, white to off-white crystalline substance. It is lipid-soluble, practically insoluble in water at low pH and freely soluble in water at high pH. The octanol/water partition coefficient of naproxen at pH 7.4 is 1.6 to 1.8. Naproxen sodium is a white to creamy white, crystalline solid, freely soluble in water at neutral pH.

NAPROSYN (naproxen) Tablets contain 250 mg, 375 mg or 500 mg of naproxen and croscarmellose sodium, iron oxides, povidone and magnesium stearate.

EC-NAPROSYN (naproxen) Delayed-Release Tablets are enteric-coated tablets containing 375 mg or 500 mg of naproxen and croscarmellose sodium, povidone and magnesium stearate. The enteric coating dispersion contains methacrylic acid copolymer, talc, triethyl citrate, sodium hydroxide and purified water. The dispersion may also contain simethicone emulsion. The dissolution of this enteric-coated naproxen tablet is pH dependent with rapid dissolution above pH 6. There is no dissolution below pH 4.

Each ANAPROX 275 mg and ANAPROX DS 550 mg tablet contains naproxen sodium, the active ingredient, with magnesium stearate, microcrystalline cellulose, povidone and talc. The coating suspension for the ANAPROX 275 mg tablet may contain hydroxypropyl methylcellulose 2910, Opaspray K-1-4210A, polyethylene glycol 8000 or Opadry YS-1-4215. The coating suspension for the ANAPROX DS 550 mg tablet may contain hydroxypropyl methylcellulose 2910, Opaspray K-1-4227, polyethylene glycol 8000 or Opadry YS-1-4216.

NAPROSYN (naproxen) Suspension for oral administration contains 125 mg/5 mL of naproxen in a vehicle containing sucrose, magnesium aluminum silicate, sorbitol solution and sodium chloride (30 mg/5 mL, 1.5 mEq), methylparaben, fumaric acid, FD&C Yellow #6, imitation pineapple flavor, imitation orange flavor and purified water. The pH of the suspension ranges from 2.2 to 3.7.

CLINICAL PHARMACOLOGY

Naproxen is a nonsteroidal anti-inflammatory drug (NSAID) with analgesic and antipyretic properties. The sodium salt of naproxen has been developed as a more rapidly absorbed formulation of naproxen for use as an analgesic. The naproxen anion inhibits prostaglandin synthesis but beyond this its mode of action is unknown.

Pharmacokinetics: Naproxen itself is rapidly and completely absorbed from the gastrointestinal tract with an in vivo bioavailability of 95%. The different dosage forms of NAPROSYN are bioequivalent in terms of extent of absorption (AUC) and peak concentration (C_{max}); however, the products do differ in their pattern of absorption. These differences between naproxen products are related to both the chemical form of naproxen used and its formulation. Even with the observed differences in pattern of absorption, the elimination half-life of naproxen is unchanged across products ranging from 12 to 17 hours. Steady-state levels of naproxen are reached in 4 to 5 days and the degree of naproxen accumulation is consistent with this half-life. This suggests that the differences in pattern of release play only a negligible role in the attainment of steady-state plasma levels.

Continued on next page

Roche Laboratories—Cont.

Absorption
Immediate Release: After administration of NAPROSYN tablets, peak plasma levels are attained in 2 to 4 hours. After oral administration of ANAPROX, peak plasma levels are attained in 1 to 2 hours. The difference in rates between the two products is due to the increased aqueous solubility of the sodium salt of naproxen used in ANAPROX. Peak plasma levels of naproxen given as NAPROSYN Suspension are attained in 1 to 4 hours.

Delayed Release: EC-NAPROSYN is designed with a pH-sensitive coating to provide a barrier to disintegration in the acidic environment of the stomach and to lose integrity in the more neutral environment of the small intestine. The enteric polymer coating selected for EC-NAPROSYN dissolves above pH 6. When EC-NAPROSYN was given to fasted subjects, peak plasma levels were attained about 4 to 6 hours following the first dose (range 2 to 12 hours). An in vivo study in man using radiolabeled EC-NAPROSYN tablets demonstrated that EC-NAPROSYN dissolves primarily in the small intestine rather than the stomach, so the absorption of the drug is delayed until the stomach is emptied. When EC-NAPROSYN and NAPROSYN were given to fasted subjects ($n=24$) in a crossover study following 1 week of dosing, differences in time to peak plasma levels (T_{max}) were observed, but there were no differences in total absorption as measured by C_{max} and AUC:

	EC-NAPROSYN* 500 mg bid	NAPROSYN* 500 mg bid
C_{max} (µg/mL)	94.9 (18%)	97.4 (13%)
T_{max} (hours)	4 (39%)	1.9 (61%)
AUC_{0-12hr} (µg-hr/mL)	845 (20%)	767 (15%)

* Mean value (coefficient of variation)

Antacid Effects: When EC-NAPROSYN was given as a single dose with antacid (54 mEq buffering capacity), the peak plasma levels of naproxen were unchanged, but the time to peak was reduced (mean T_{max} fasted 5.6 hours, mean T_{max} with antacid 5 hours), although not significantly.

Food Effects: When EC-NAPROSYN was given as a single dose with food, peak plasma levels in most subjects were achieved in about 12 hours (range 4 to 24 hours). Residence time in the small intestine until disintegration was independent of food intake. The presence of food prolonged the time the tablets remained in the stomach, time to first detectable serum naproxen levels, and time to maximal naproxen levels (T_{max}), but did not affect peak naproxen levels (C_{max}).

Distribution
Naproxen has a volume of distribution of 0.16 L/kg. At therapeutic levels naproxen is greater than 99% albumin-bound. At doses of naproxen greater than 500 mg/day there is less than proportional increase in plasma levels due to an increase in clearance caused by saturation of plasma protein binding at higher doses (average trough C_{ss} 36.5, 49.2 and 56.4 mg/L with 500, 1000 and 1500 mg daily doses of naproxen). However, the concentration of unbound naproxen continues to increase proportionally to dose.

Metabolism
Naproxen is extensively metabolized to 6-0-desmethyl naproxen and both parent and metabolites do not induce metabolizing enzymes.

Elimination
The clearance of naproxen is 0.13 mL/min/kg. Approximately 95% of the naproxen from any dose is excreted in the urine, primarily as naproxen (less than 1%), 6-0-desmethyl naproxen (less than 1%) or their conjugates (66% to 92%). The plasma half-life of the naproxen anion in humans ranges from 12 to 17 hours. The corresponding half-lives of both naproxen's metabolites and conjugates are shorter than 12 hours and their rates of excretion have been found to coincide closely with the rate of naproxen disappearance from the plasma. In patients with renal failure metabolites may accumulate.

Special Populations
Children: In children of 5 to 16 years of age with arthritis, plasma naproxen levels following a 5 mg/kg single dose of naproxen suspension (see DOSAGE AND ADMINISTRATION) were found to be similar to those found in normal adults following a 500 mg dose. The terminal half-life appears to be similar in children and adults. Pharmacokinetic studies of naproxen were not performed in children of less than 5 years of age. EC-NAPROSYN has not been studied in subjects under the age of 18.

Renal Insufficiency: Naproxen pharmacokinetics has not been determined in subjects with renal insufficiency. Given that naproxen, its metabolites, and conjugates are primarily excreted by the kidney, the potential exists for naproxen metabolites to accumulate in the presence of renal insufficiency.

CLINICAL STUDIES

General Information: Naproxen has been studied in patients with rheumatoid arthritis, osteoarthritis, juvenile arthritis, ankylosing spondylitis, tendinitis and bursitis, and acute gout. Improvement in patients treated for rheumatoid arthritis was demonstrated by a reduction in joint swelling, a reduction in duration of morning stiffness, a reduction in disease activity as assessed by both the investigator and patient, and by increased mobility as demonstrated by a reduction in walking time. Generally, response to naproxen has not been found to be dependent on age, sex, severity or duration of rheumatoid arthritis.

In patients with osteoarthritis, the therapeutic action of naproxen has been shown by a reduction in joint pain or tenderness, an increase in range of motion in knee joints, increased mobility as demonstrated by a reduction in walking time, and improvement in capacity to perform activities of daily living impaired by the disease.

In a clinical trial comparing standard formulations of naproxen 375 mg bid (750 mg a day) versus 750 mg bid (1500 mg/day), 9 patients in the 750 mg group terminated prematurely because of adverse events. Nineteen patients in the 1500 mg group terminated prematurely because of adverse events. Most of these adverse events were gastrointestinal events.

In clinical studies in patients with rheumatoid arthritis, osteoarthritis and juvenile arthritis, naproxen has been shown to be comparable to aspirin and indomethacin in controlling the aforementioned measures of disease activity, but the frequency and severity of the milder gastrointestinal adverse effects (nausea, dyspepsia, heartburn) and nervous system adverse effects (tinnitus, dizziness, lightheadedness) were less in naproxen-treated patients than in those treated with aspirin or indomethacin.

In patients with ankylosing spondylitis, naproxen has been shown to decrease night pain, morning stiffness and pain at rest. In double-blind studies the drug was shown to be as effective as aspirin, but with fewer side effects.

In patients with acute gout, a favorable response to naproxen was shown by significant clearing of inflammatory changes (eg, decrease in swelling, heat) within 24 to 48 hours, as well as by relief of pain and tenderness.

Naproxen has been studied in patients with mild to moderate pain secondary to postoperative, orthopedic, postpartum episiotomy and uterine contraction pain and dysmenorrhea. Onset of pain relief can begin within 1 hour in patients taking naproxen and within 30 minutes in patients taking naproxen sodium. Analgesic effect was shown by such measures as reduction of pain intensity scores, increase in pain relief scores, decrease in numbers of patients requiring additional analgesic medication, and delay in time to remedication. The analgesic effect has been found to last for up to 12 hours.

Naproxen may be used safely in combination with gold salts and/or corticosteroids; however, in controlled clinical trials, when added to the regimen of patients receiving corticosteroids, it did not appear to cause greater improvement over that seen with corticosteroids alone. Whether naproxen has a "steroid-sparing" effect has not been adequately studied. When added to the regimen of patients receiving gold salts, naproxen did result in greater improvement. Its use in combination with salicylates is not recommended because there is evidence that aspirin increases the rate of excretion of naproxen and data are inadequate to demonstrate that naproxen and aspirin produce greater improvement over that achieved with aspirin alone. In addition, as with other NSAIDs the combination may result in higher frequency of adverse events than demonstrated for either product alone. In ^{51}Cr blood loss and gastroscopy studies with normal volunteers, daily administration of 1000 mg of naproxen as 1000 mg of NAPROSYN® (naproxen) or 1100 mg of ANAPROX® (naproxen sodium) has been demonstrated to cause statistically significantly less gastric bleeding and erosion than 3250 mg of aspirin.

Three 6-week, double-blind multicenter studies with EC-NAPROSYN™ (naproxen) (375 or 500 mg bid, $n=385$) and NAPROSYN (375 or 500 mg bid, $n=279$) were conducted comparing EC-NAPROSYN with NAPROSYN including 355 rheumatoid arthritis and osteoarthritis patients who had a recent history of NSAID-related GI symptoms. These studies indicated that EC-NAPROSYN and NAPROSYN showed no significant differences in efficacy or safety and had similar prevalence of minor GI complaints. Individual patients, however, may find one formulation preferable to the other.

Five hundred and fifty-three patients received EC-NAPROSYN during long-term open label trials (mean length of treatment was 159 days). The rates for clinically-diagnosed peptic ulcers and GI bleeds were similar to what has been historically reported for long-term NSAID use.

INDIVIDUALIZATION OF DOSAGE

Although NAPROSYN, NAPROSYN Suspension, EC-NAPROSYN, ANAPROX and ANAPROX DS all circulate in the plasma as naproxen, they have pharmacokinetic differences that may affect onset of action. Onset of pain relief can begin within 30 minutes in patients taking naproxen sodium and within 1 hour in patients taking naproxen. Because EC-NAPROSYN dissolves in the small intestine rather than in the stomach, the absorption of the drug is delayed compared to the other naproxen formulations (see CLINICAL PHARMACOLOGY).

The recommended strategy for initiating therapy is to choose a formulation and a starting dose likely to be effective for the patient and then adjust the dosage based on observation of benefit and/or adverse events. A lower dose should be considered in patients with renal or hepatic impairment or in elderly patients (see PRECAUTIONS).

Analgesia/Dysmenorrhea/Bursitis and Tendinitis:
Because the sodium salt of naproxen is more rapidly absorbed, ANAPROX/ANAPROX DS is recommended for the management of acute painful conditions when prompt onset of pain relief is desired. The recommended starting dose is 550 mg followed by 550 mg every 12 hours or 275 mg every 6 to 8 hours, as required. The initial total daily dose should not exceed 1375 mg of naproxen sodium. Thereafter, the total daily dose should not exceed 1100 mg of naproxen sodium. NAPROSYN may also be used for treatment of acute pain and dysmenorrhea. EC-NAPROSYN is not recommended for initial treatment of acute pain because absorption of naproxen is delayed compared to other naproxen-containing products (see CLINICAL PHARMACOLOGY and INDICATIONS AND USAGE).

Acute Gout: The recommended starting dose is 750 mg of NAPROSYN followed by 250 mg every 8 hours until the attack has subsided. ANAPROX may also be used at a starting dose of 825 mg followed by 275 mg every 8 hours as needed. EC-NAPROSYN is not recommended because of the delay in absorption (see CLINICAL PHARMACOLOGY).

Osteoarthritis/Rheumatoid Arthritis/Ankylosing Spondylitis: The recommended dose of naproxen is NAPROSYN or NAPROSYN Suspension 250 mg, 375 mg or 500 mg taken twice daily (morning and evening) or EC-NAPROSYN 375 mg or 500 mg taken twice daily. Naproxen sodium may also be used (see DOSAGE AND ADMINISTRATION).

During long-term administration the dose of naproxen may be adjusted up or down depending on the clinical response of the patient. A lower daily dose may suffice for long-term administration. In patients who tolerate lower doses well, the dose may be increased to 1500 mg per day when a higher level of anti-inflammatory/analgesic activity is required. When treating patients with naproxen 1500 mg/day (as NAPROSYN or 1650 mg of ANAPROX), the physician should observe sufficient increased clinical benefit to offset the potential increased risk. The morning and evening doses do not have to be equal in size and administration of the drug more frequently than twice daily does not generally make a difference in response (see CLINICAL PHARMACOLOGY).

Juvenile Arthritis: The use of NAPROSYN Suspension allows for more flexible dose titration. In children, doses of 5 mg/kg/day produced plasma levels of naproxen similar to those seen in adults taking 500 mg of naproxen (see CLINICAL PHARMACOLOGY).

The recommended total daily dose is approximately 10 mg/kg given in 2 divided doses (ie, 5 mg/kg given twice a day) (see DOSAGE AND ADMINISTRATION).

INDICATIONS AND USAGE

Naproxen as NAPROSYN, EC-NAPROSYN, ANAPROX, ANAPROX DS or NAPROSYN Suspension are indicated for the treatment of rheumatoid arthritis, osteoarthritis, ankylosing spondylitis and juvenile arthritis.

Naproxen as NAPROSYN Suspension is recommended for juvenile rheumatoid arthritis in order to obtain the maximum dosage flexibility based on the child's weight.

Naproxen as NAPROSYN, ANAPROX, ANAPROX DS and NAPROSYN Suspension are also indicated for the treatment of tendinitis, bursitis, acute gout, and for the management of pain and primary dysmennorhea. EC-NAPROSYN is not recommended for initial treatment of acute pain because the absorption of naproxen is delayed compared to absorption from other naproxen-containing products (see CLINICAL PHARMACOLOGY and DOSAGE AND ADMINISTRATION).

CONTRAINDICATIONS

All naproxen products are contraindicated in patients who have had allergic reactions to prescription as well as to over-the-counter products containing naproxen. It is also contraindicated in patients in whom aspirin or other nonsteroidal anti-inflammatory/analgesic drugs induce the syndrome of asthma, rhinitis and nasal polyps. Both types of reactions have the potential of being fatal. Anaphylactoid reactions to naproxen, whether of the true allergic type or the pharmacologic idiosyncratic (eg, aspirin hypersensitivity syndrome) type, usually but not always occur in patients with a known history of such reactions. Therefore, careful questioning of patients for such things as asthma, nasal polyps, urticaria and hypotension associated with nonsteroidal anti-inflammatory drugs before starting therapy is important. In addition, if such symptoms occur during therapy, treatment should be discontinued.

WARNINGS

Risk of GI Ulceration, Bleeding and Perforation with NSAID Therapy:
Serious gastrointestinal toxicity such as bleeding, ulceration and perforation can occur at any time, with or without warning symptoms, in patients treated chronically with NSAID therapy. Although minor upper gastrointestinal problems, such as dyspepsia, are common, usually developing early in therapy, physicians should remain alert for ulceration and bleeding in patients treated chronically with NSAIDs even in the absence of previous GI tract symptoms. In patients observed in clinical trials of several months to 2 years' duration, symptomatic upper GI ulcers, gross bleeding or perforation appear to occur in approximately 1% of patients treated for 3 to 6 months and in about 2% to 4% of patients treated for 1 year.

Physicians should inform patients about the signs and/or symptoms of serious GI toxicity and what steps to take if they occur.

Studies to date with all naproxen products have not identified any subset of patients not at risk of developing peptic ulceration and bleeding or any differences between different naproxen products in their propensity to cause peptic ulceration and bleeding. Except for a prior history of serious GI events and other risk factors known to be associated with peptic ulcer disease, such as alcoholism, smoking, etc., no risk factors (eg, age, sex) have been associated with increased risk. Elderly or debilitated patients seem to tolerate ulceration or bleeding less well than other individuals and most spontaneous reports of fatal GI events are in this population. Studies to date are inconclusive concerning the relative risk of various NSAIDs in causing such reactions. High doses of any NSAID probably carry a greater risk of these reactions, although controlled clinical trials showing this do not exist in most cases. In considering the use of relatively large doses (within the recommended dosage range), sufficient benefit should be anticipated to offset the potential increased risk of GI toxicity.

PRECAUTIONS

General: NAPROXEN-CONTAINING PRODUCTS SUCH AS NAPROSYN, EC-NAPROSYN, ANAPROX, ANAPROX DS, NAPROSYN SUSPENSION, ALEVE®, AND OTHER NAPROXEN PRODUCTS SHOULD NOT BE USED CONCOMITANTLY SINCE THEY ALL CIRCULATE IN THE PLASMA AS THE NAPROXEN ANION.

If the steroid dose is reduced or eliminated during therapy, the steroid dosage should be reduced slowly and the patients should be observed closely for any evidence of adverse effects, including adrenal insufficiency and exacerbation of symptoms of arthritis.

Patients with initial hemoglobin values of 10 grams or less who are to receive long-term therapy should have hemoglobin values determined periodically.

The antipyretic and anti-inflammatory activities of the drug may reduce fever and inflammation, thus diminishing their utility as diagnostic signs in detecting complications of presumed noninfectious, noninflammatory painful conditions. Because of adverse eye findings in animal studies with drugs of this class, it is recommended that ophthalmic studies be carried out if any change or disturbance in vision occurs.

Renal Effects: As with other nonsteroidal anti-inflammatory drugs, long-term administration of naproxen to animals has resulted in renal papillary necrosis and other abnormal renal pathology. In humans, there have been reports of acute interstitial nephritis, hematuria, proteinuria and occasionally nephrotic syndrome associated with naproxen-containing products and other NSAIDs since they have been marketed.

A second form of renal toxicity has been seen in patients taking naproxen as well as other nonsteroidal anti-inflammatory drugs. In patients with prerenal conditions leading to a reduction in renal blood flow or blood volume, where the renal prostaglandins have a supportive role in the maintenance of renal perfusion, administration of a nonsteroidal anti-inflammatory drug may cause a dose-dependent reduction in prostaglandin formation and precipitate overt renal decompensation. Patients at greatest risk of this reaction are those with impaired renal function, heart failure, liver dysfunction, those taking diuretics and the elderly. Discontinuation of nonsteroidal anti-inflammatory therapy is typically followed by recovery to the pretreatment state.

Naproxen and its metabolites are eliminated primarily by the kidneys; therefore, the drug should be used with caution in patients with significantly impaired renal function, and the monitoring of serum creatinine and/or creatinine clearance is advised in these patients. Caution should be used if the drug is given to patients with creatinine clearance of less than 20 mL/minute because accumulation of naproxen metabolites has been seen in such patients.

Chronic alcoholic liver disease and probably other diseases with decreased or abnormal plasma proteins (albumin) reduce the total plasma concentration of naproxen, but the plasma concentration of unbound naproxen is increased. Caution is advised when high doses are required and some

adjustment of dosage may be required in these patients. It is prudent to use the lowest effective dose.

Studies indicate that although total plasma concentration of naproxen is unchanged, the unbound plasma fraction of naproxen is increased in the elderly. Caution is advised when high doses are required and some adjustment of dosage may be required in elderly patients. As with other drugs used in the elderly, it is prudent to use the lowest effective dose.

Hepatic Function: As with other nonsteroidal anti-inflammatory drugs, borderline elevations of one or more liver tests may occur in up to 15% of patients. These abnormalities may progress, may remain essentially unchanged, or may be transient with continued therapy. The SGPT (ALT) test is probably the most sensitive indicator of liver dysfunction. Meaningful (3 times the upper limit of normal) elevations of SGPT or SGOT (AST) occurred in controlled clinical trials in less than 1% of patients. A patient with symptoms and/or signs suggesting liver dysfunction or in whom an abnormal liver test has occurred, should be evaluated for evidence of the development of more severe hepatic reaction while on therapy with naproxen. Severe hepatic reactions, including jaundice and cases of fatal hepatitis, have been reported with naproxen as with other nonsteroidal anti-inflammatory drugs. Although such reactions are rare, if abnormal liver tests persist or worsen, if clinical signs and symptoms consistent with liver disease develop, or if systemic manifestations occur (eg, eosinophilia, rash, etc.), naproxen should be discontinued.

Fluid Retention and Edema: Peripheral edema has been observed in some patients receiving naproxen. Since each ANAPROX or ANAPROX DS tablet contains 25 mg or 50 mg of sodium (about 1 mEq per each 250 mg of naproxen), and each teaspoonful of NAPROSYN Suspension contains 39 mg (about 1.5 mEq per each 125 mg of naproxen) of sodium, this should be considered in patients whose overall intake of sodium must be severely restricted. For these reasons, ANAPROX, ANAPROX DS and NAPROSYN Suspension should be used with caution in patients with fluid retention, hypertension or heart failure.

Information for Patients: Naproxen, in NAPROSYN, EC-NAPROSYN, ANAPROX, ANAPROX DS and NAPROSYN Suspension, like other drugs of this class, is not free of side effects. The side effects of these formulations of naproxen can cause discomfort and, rarely, there are more serious side effects, such as gastrointestinal bleeding, which may result in hospitalization and even fatal outcomes.

NSAIDs (Nonsteroidal Anti-Inflammatory Drugs) are often essential agents in the management of arthritis and have a major role in the treatment of pain, but they also may be commonly employed for conditions which are less serious. Physicians may wish to discuss with their patients the potential risks (see WARNINGS, PRECAUTIONS and ADVERSE REACTIONS) and likely benefits of naproxen treatment particularly when it is used for less serious conditions where treatment without NSAIDs may represent an acceptable alternative to both the patient and physician.

Caution should be exercised by patients whose activities require alertness if they experience drowsiness, dizziness, vertigo or depression during therapy with naproxen.

Laboratory Tests: Because serious GI tract ulceration and bleeding can occur without warning symptoms, physicians should follow patients chronically treated with naproxen for signs and symptoms of ulceration and bleeding and should inform them of the importance of this follow-up and what they should do if certain signs and symptoms do appear (see WARNINGS, **Risk of GI Ulcerations, Bleeding and Perforation with NSAID Therapy**).

Drug Interactions: The use of NSAIDs in patients who are receiving ACE inhibitors may potentiate renal disease states (see PRECAUTIONS, *Renal Effects*).

In vitro studies have shown that naproxen anion, because of its affinity for protein, may displace from their binding sites other drugs which are also albumin-bound (see CLINICAL PHARMACOLOGY, **Pharmacokinetics**).

Theoretically, the naproxen anion itself could likewise be displaced. Short-term controlled studies failed to show that taking the drug significantly affects prothrombin times when administered to individuals on coumarin-type anticoagulants. Caution is advised nonetheless, since interactions have been seen with other nonsteroidal agents of this class. Similarly, patients receiving the drug and a hydantoin, sulfonamide or sulfonylurea should be observed for signs of toxicity to these drugs (see CLINICAL STUDIES, *General Information*).

Concomitant administration of naproxen and aspirin is not recommended because naproxen is displaced from its binding sites during the concomitant administration of aspirin, resulting in lower plasma concentrations and peak plasma levels.

The natriuretic effect of furosemide has been reported to be inhibited by some drugs of this class. Inhibition of renal lithium clearance leading to increases in plasma lithium concentrations has also been reported. Naproxen and other nonsteroidal anti-inflammatory drugs can reduce the antihypertensive effect of propranolol and other beta-blockers.

Probenecid given concurrently increases naproxen anion plasma levels and extends its plasma half-life significantly. Caution should be used if naproxen is administered concomitantly with methotrexate. Naproxen, naproxen sodium and other nonsteroidal anti-inflammatory drugs have been reported to reduce the tubular secretion of methotrexate in an animal model, possibly increasing the toxicity of methotrexate.

Due to the gastric pH elevating effects of H2-blockers, sucralfate and intensive antacid therapy, concomitant administration of EC-NAPROSYN is not recommended.

Drug/Laboratory Test Interactions: Naproxen may decrease platelet aggregation and prolong bleeding time. This effect should be kept in mind when bleeding times are determined.

The administration of naproxen may result in increased urinary values for 17-ketogenic steroids because of an interaction between the drug and/or its metabolites with m-dinitrobenzene used in this assay. Although 17-hydroxy-corticosteroid measurements (Porter-Silber test) do not appear to be artifactually altered, it is suggested that therapy with naproxen be temporarily discontinued 72 hours before adrenal function tests are performed if the Porter-Silber test is to be used.

Naproxen may interfere with some urinary assays of 5-hydroxy indoleacetic acid (5HIAA).

Carcinogenesis: A 2-year study was performed in rats to evaluate the carcinogenic potential of naproxen at rat doses of 8, 16 and 24 mg/kg/day (50, 100 and 150 mg/m^2). The maximum dose used was 0.28 times the systemic exposure to humans at the recommended dose. No evidence of tumorigenicity was found.

Pregnancy: Teratogenic Effects: Pregnancy Category B. Reproduction studies have been performed in rats at 20 mg/kg/day (125 mg/m^2/day, 0.23 times the human systemic exposure), rabbits at 20 mg/kg/day (220 mg/m^2/day, 0.27 times the human systemic exposure), and mice at 170 mg/kg/day (510 mg/m^2/day, 0.28 times the human systemic exposure) with no evidence of impaired fertility or harm to the fetus due to the drug. There are no adequate and well-controlled studies in pregnant women. Because animal reproduction studies are not always predictive of human response, naproxen should not be used during pregnancy unless clearly needed.

Nonteratogenic Effects: There is some evidence to suggest that when inhibitors of prostaglandin synthesis are used to delay preterm labor there is an increased risk of neonatal complications such as necrotizing enterocolitis, patent ductus arteriosus, intracranial hemorrhage. Naproxen treatment given in late pregnancy to delay parturition has been associated with persistent pulmonary hypertension, renal dysfunction and abnormal prostaglandin E levels in preterm infants. Because of the known effect of drugs of this class on the human fetal cardiovascular system (closure of ductus arteriosus), use during third trimester should be avoided.

Nursing Mothers: The naproxen anion has been found in the milk of lactating women at a concentration of approximately 1% of that found in plasma. Because of the possible adverse effects of prostaglandin-inhibiting drugs on neonates, use in nursing mothers should be avoided.

Pediatric Use: Safety and effectiveness in children below the age of 2 years have not been established. Pediatric dosing recommendations for juvenile arthritis are based on well-controlled studies (see DOSAGE AND ADMINISTRATION). There are no adequate effectiveness or dose-response data for other pediatric conditions, but the experience in juvenile arthritis and other use experience have established that single doses of 2.5 to 5 mg/kg (as naproxen suspension, see DOSAGE AND ADMINISTRATION), with total daily dose not exceeding 15 mg/kg/day, are well tolerated in children over 2 years of age.

ADVERSE REACTIONS

The following adverse reactions are divided into three parts based on frequency and whether or not the possibility exists of a causal relationship between naproxen and these adverse events. In those reactions listed as "Probable Causal Relationship" there is at least 1 case for each adverse reaction where there is evidence to suggest that there is a causal relationship between drug usage and the reported event.

Adverse reactions reported in controlled clinical trials in 960 patients treated for rheumatoid arthritis or osteoarthritis are treated below. In general, reactions in patients treated chronically were reported 2 to 10 times more frequently than they were in short-term studies in the 962 patients treated for mild to moderate pain or for dysmenorrhea. The most frequent complaints reported related to the gastrointestinal tract.

A clinical study found gastrointestinal reactions to be more frequent and more severe in rheumatoid arthritis patients taking daily doses of 1500 mg naproxen compared to those taking 750 mg naproxen (see CLINICAL PHARMACOLOGY).

Continued on next page

Roche Laboratories—Cont.

In controlled clinical trials with about 80 children and in well-monitored, open-label studies with about 400 children with juvenile arthritis treated with naproxen, the incidence of rash and prolonged bleeding times were increased, the incidence of gastrointestinal and central nervous system reactions were about the same, and the incidence of other reactions were lower in children than in adults.

The following adverse reactions are divided into three parts based on frequency and causal relationship. Incidence greater than 1% (Probable Causal Relationship):

Gastrointestinal: constipation*, heartburn*, abdominal pain*, nausea*, dyspepsia, diarrhea, stomatitis.

Central Nervous System: headache*, dizziness*, drowsiness*, lightheadedness, vertigo.

Dermatologic: itching (pruritus)*, skin eruptions*, ecchymoses*, sweating, purpura.

Special Senses: tinnitus*, hearing disturbances, visual disturbances.

Cardiovascular: edema*, dyspnea*, palpitations.

General: thirst.

*Incidence of reported reaction between 3% and 9%. Those reactions occurring in less than 3% of the patients are unmarked. Incidence less than 1% (Probable Causal Relationship):

The following adverse reactions were reported less frequently than 1% during controlled clinical trials and through voluntary reports since marketing. Those reactions observed through voluntary reporting since marketing are italicized.

Gastrointestinal: *abnormal liver function tests, colitis*, gastrointestinal bleeding and/or *perforation, hematemesis*, jaundice, pancreatitis, melena, vomiting.

Renal: *glomerular nephritis, hematuria, hyperkalemia, interstitial nephritis, nephrotic syndrome, renal disease, renal failure, renal papillary necrosis.*

Hematologic: agranulocytosis, *eosinophilia, granulocytopenia, leukopenia*, thrombocytopenia.

Central Nervous System: *depression, dream abnormalities*, inability to concentrate, *insomnia, malaise, myalgia, muscle weakness.*

Dermatologic: *alopecia, photosensitive dermatitis, urticaria*, skin rashes, *photosensitivity reactions resembling porphyria cutanea tarda, epidermolysis bullosa.*

Special Senses: *hearing impairment.*

Cardiovascular: *congestive heart failure.*

Respiratory: *eosinophilic pneumonitis.*

General: *anaphylactoid reactions, angioneurotic edema, menstrual disorders, pyrexia (chills and fever).*

Incidence less than 1% (Causal Relationship Unknown):

These observations are being listed to serve as alerting information to the physician.

Hematologic: *aplastic anemia, hemolytic anemia.*

Central Nervous System: *aseptic meningitis, cognitive dysfunction.*

Dermatologic: *epidermal necrolysis, erythema multiforme, Stevens-Johnson syndrome.*

Gastrointestinal: *nonpeptic gastrointestinal ulceration, ulcerative stomatitis.*

Cardiovascular: *vasculitis.*

General: *hyperglycemia, hypoglycemia.*

OVERDOSAGE

Significant naproxen overdosage may be characterized by drowsiness, heartburn, indigestion, nausea or vomiting. Because naproxen sodium may be rapidly absorbed, high and early blood levels should be anticipated. A few patients have experienced seizures, but it is not clear whether or not these were drug-related. It is not known what dose of the drug would be life threatening. The oral LD_{50} of the drug is 543 mg/kg in rats, 1234 mg/kg in mice, 4110 mg/kg in hamsters, and greater than 1000 mg/kg in dogs.

Should a patient ingest a large number of tablets or a large volume of suspension, accidentally or purposefully, the stomach may be emptied and usual supportive measures employed. In animals 0.5 g/kg of activated charcoal was effective in reducing plasma levels of naproxen. Hemodialysis does not decrease the plasma concentration of naproxen because of the high degree of its protein binding.

DOSAGE AND ADMINISTRATION

Rheumatoid Arthritis, Osteoarthritis, and Ankylosing Spondylitis

[See table at bottom of page.]

To maintain the integrity of the enteric coating, the EC-NAPROSYN tablet should not be broken, crushed or chewed during ingestion.

During long-term administration, the dose of naproxen may be adjusted up or down depending on the clinical response of the patient. A lower daily dose may suffice for long-term administration. The morning and evening doses do not have to be equal in size and the administration of the drug more frequently than twice daily is not necessary.

In patients who tolerate lower doses well, the dose may be increased to naproxen 1500 mg per day for limited periods when a higher level of anti-inflammatory/analgesic activity is required. When treating such patients with naproxen 1500 mg/day, the physician should observe sufficient increased clinical benefits to offset the potential increased risk (see CLINICAL PHARMACOLOGY and INDIVIDUALIZATION OF DOSAGE).

Juvenile Arthritis: The recommended total daily dose of naproxen is approximately 10 mg/kg given in 2 divided doses (ie, 5 mg/kg given twice a day). A measuring cup marked in $^1/_2$ teaspoon and 2.5 milliliter increments is provided with the NAPROSYN Suspension. The following table may be used as a guide for dosing of NAPROSYN Suspension:

Child's Weight	Dose	Administered as
13 kg (29 lb)	62.5 mg bid	2.5 mL (1/2 tsp) twice daily
25 kg (55 lb)	125 mg bid	5.0 mL (1 tsp) twice daily
38 kg (84 lb)	187.5 mg bid	7.5 mL (1 1/2 tsp) twice daily

Management of Pain, Primary Dysmenorrhea and Acute Tendinitis and Bursitis: The recommended starting dose is 550 mg of naproxen sodium as ANAPROX/ANAPROX DS followed by 550 mg every 12 hours or 275 mg every 6 to 8 hours as required. The initial total daily dose should not exceed 1375 mg of naproxen sodium. Thereafter, the total daily dose should not exceed 1100 mg of naproxen sodium. NAPROSYN may also be used but EC-NAPROSYN is not recommended for initial treatment of acute pain because absorption of naproxen is delayed compared to other naproxen containing products (see CLINICAL PHARMACOLOGY, INDICATIONS AND USAGE, and INDIVIDUALIZATION OF DOSAGE).

Acute Gout: The recommended starting dose is 750 mg of NAPROSYN followed by 250 mg every 8 hours until the attack has subsided. ANAPROX may also be used at a starting dose of 825 mg followed by 275 mg every 8 hours. EC-NAPROSYN is not recommended because of the delay in absorption (see CLINICAL PHARMACOLOGY).

HOW SUPPLIED

NAPROSYN Tablets: 250 mg: yellow, round-shaped, biconvex, debossed with "NAPROSYN" on one side and "250" on the other. Packaged in light-resistant bottles of 100 and 500.

100's (bottle): NDC 18393-272-42; 500's (bottle): NDC 18393-272-62.

375 mg: peach, capsule-shaped, debossed with "NAPROSYN" on one side and "375" on the other. Packaged in light-resistant bottles of 100 and 500.

100's (bottle): NDC 18393-273-42; 500's (bottle): NDC 18393-273-62.

500 mg: yellow, capsule-shaped, debossed with "NAPROSYN" on one side and "500" on the other. Packaged in light-resistant bottles of 100 and 500.

100's (bottle): NDC 18393-277-42; 500's (bottle): NDC 18393-277-62.

Store at 15° to 30°C (59° to 86°F) in well-closed containers; dispense in light-resistant containers.

NAPROSYN Suspension: 125 mg/5 mL (contains 39 mg sodium, about 1.5 mEq/teaspoon): Available in 1 pint (474 mL) light-resistant bottles (NDC 18393-278-20). Measuring cups are provided so that one can be dispensed with each prescription.

Store at 15° to 30°C (59° to 86°F); avoid excessive heat, above 40°C (104°F). Dispense in light-resistant container.

NAPROSYN	250 mg or 375 mg or 500 mg	twice daily twice daily twice daily
ANAPROX	275 mg (naproxen 250 mg with 25 mg sodium)	twice daily
ANAPROX DS	550 mg (naproxen 500 mg with 50 mg sodium)	twice daily
NAPROSYN Suspension	250 mg (10 mL/2 tsp) or 375 mg (15 mL/3 tsp) or 500 mg (20 mL/4 tsp)	twice daily twice daily twice daily
EC-NAPROSYN	375 mg or 500 mg	twice daily twice daily

EC-NAPROSYN Delayed-Release Tablets: 375 mg: white, capsule shaped, imprinted with "EC-NAPROSYN" on one side and "375" on the other, in light-resistant bottles of 100.

100's (bottle): NDC 18393-255-42.

500 mg: white, capsule-shaped, imprinted with "EC-NAPROSYN" on one side and "500" on the other, in light-resistant bottles of 100.

100's (bottle): NDC 18393-256-42.

Store at 15° to 30°C (59° to 86°F) in well-closed containers; dispense in light-resistant containers.

ANAPROX Tablets: Naproxen sodium 275 mg: light blue, oval-shaped, film-coated, debossed with "ROCHE" on one side and "ANAPROX" on the other. Packaged in bottles of 100 and 500.

100's (bottle): NDC 18393-274-42; 500's (bottle): NDC 18393-274-62.

Store at 15° to 30°C (59° to 86°F) in well-closed containers.

ANAPROX DS Tablets: Naproxen sodium 550 mg: dark blue, capsule-shaped, film-coated, debossed with "ROCHE" on one side and "ANAPROX DS" on the other. Packaged in bottles of 100 and 500.

100's (bottle): NDC 18393-276-42; 500's (bottle): NDC 18393-276-62.

Store at 15° to 30°C (59° to 86°F) in well-closed containers.

Manufactured by Syntex Puerto Rico, Inc.
Humacao, PR 00791
Revised: September 1995

Shown in Product Identification Guide, page 332

EFUDEX ® ℞

[ef'u-dex]
brand of fluorouracil
TOPICAL SOLUTIONS AND CREAM

The following text is complete prescribing information based on official labeling in effect June 1996.

DESCRIPTION

Efudex Solutions and Cream are topical preparations containing the fluorinated pyrimidine 5-fluorouracil, an antineoplastic antimetabolite.

Efudex Solution consists of 2% or 5% fluorouracil on a weight/weight basis, compounded with propylene glycol, tris(hydroxymethyl)aminomethane, hydroxypropyl cellulose, parabens (methyl and propyl) and disodium edetate.

Efudex Cream contains 5% fluorouracil in a vanishing cream base consisting of white petrolatum, stearyl alcohol, propylene glycol, polysorbate 60 and parabens (methyl and propyl).

Chemically, fluorouracil is 5-fluoro-2,4(1*H*,3*H*)-pyrimidinedione. It is a white to practically white, crystalline powder which is sparingly soluble in water and slightly soluble in alcohol. One gram of fluorouracil is soluble in 100 mL of propylene glycol. The molecular weight of 5-fluorouracil is 130.08.

CLINICAL PHARMACOLOGY

There is evidence that the metabolism of fluorouracil in the anabolic pathway blocks the methylation reaction of deoxyuridylic acid to thymidylic acid. In this manner fluorouracil interferes with the synthesis of deoxyribonucleic acid (DNA) and to a lesser extent inhibits the formation of ribonucleic acid (RNA). Since DNA and RNA are essential for cell division and growth, the effect of fluorouracil may be to create a thymine deficiency which provokes unbalanced growth and death of the cell. The effects of DNA and RNA deprivation are most marked on those cells which grow more rapidly and take up fluorouracil at a more rapid rate. The catabolic metabolism of fluorouracil results in degradation products (eg, CO_2, urea, α-fluoro-β-alanine) which are inactive.

Systemic absorption studies of topically applied fluorouracil have been performed on patients with actinic keratoses using tracer amounts of ^{14}C-labeled fluorouracil added to a 5% preparation. All patients had been receiving nonlabeled fluorouracil until the peak of the inflammatory reaction occurred (2 to 3 weeks), ensuring that the time of maximum absorption was used for measurement. One gram of labeled preparation was applied to the entire face and neck and left in place for 12 hours. Urine samples were collected. At the end of 3 days, the total recovery ranged between 0.48% and 0.94% with an average of 0.76%, indicating that approximately 5.98% of the topical dose was absorbed systemically. If applied twice daily, this would indicate systemic absorption of topical fluorouracil to be in the range of 5 to 6 mg per daily dose of 100 mg. In an additional study negligible amounts of labeled material were found in plasma, urine and expired CO_2 after 3 days of treatment with topically applied ^{14}C-labeled fluorouracil.

INDICATIONS AND USAGE

Efudex is recommended for the topical treatment of multiple actinic or solar keratoses. In the 5% strength it is also useful in the treatment of superficial basal cell carcinomas when conventional methods are impractical, such as with multiple

lesions or difficult treatment sites. Safety and efficacy in other indications have not been established.

The diagnosis should be established prior to treatment, since this method has not been proven effective in other types of basal cell carcinomas. With isolated, easily accessible basal cell carcinomas, surgery is preferred since success with such lesions is almost 100%. The success rate with Efudex Cream and Solution is approximately 93%, based on 113 lesions in 54 patients. Twenty-five lesions treated with the solution produced 1 failure and 88 lesions treated with the cream produced 7 failures.

CONTRAINDICATIONS

Efudex may cause fetal harm when administered to a pregnant woman.

There are no adequate and well-controlled studies in pregnant women with either the topical or the parenteral forms of fluorouracil. One birth defect (cleft lip and palate) has been reported in the newborn of a patient using Efudex as recommended. One birth defect (ventricular septal defect) and cases of miscarriage have been reported when Efudex was applied to mucous membrane areas. Multiple birth defects have been reported in a fetus of a patient treated with intravenous fluorouracil.

Animal reproduction studies have not been conducted with Efudex. Fluorouracil administered parenterally has been shown to be teratogenic in mice, rats, and hamsters when given at doses equivalent to the usual human intravenous dose; however, the amount of fluorouracil absorbed systematically after topical administration to actinic keratoses is minimal (see CLINICAL PHARMACOLOGY). Fluorouracil exhibited maximum teratogenicity when given to mice as single intraperitoneal injections of 10 to 40 mg/kg on Day 10 or 12 of gestation. Similarly, intraperitoneal doses of 12 to 37 mg/kg given to rats between Days 9 and 12 of gestation and intramuscular doses of 3 to 9 mg/kg given to hamsters between Days 8 and 11 of gestation were teratogenic and/or embryotoxic (ie, resulted in increased resorptions of embryolethality). In monkeys, divided doses of 40 mg/kg given between Days 20 and 24 of gestation were not teratogenic. Doses higher than 40 mg/kg resulted in abortion.

Efudex is contraindicated in women who are or may become pregnant during therapy. If this drug is used during pregnancy, or if the patient becomes pregnant while using this drug, the patient should be apprised of the potential hazard to the fetus.

Efudex is also contraindicated in patients with known hypersensitivity to any of its components.

WARNINGS

Application to mucous membranes should be avoided due to the possibility of local inflammation and ulceration. Additionally, cases of miscarriage and a birth defect (ventricular septal defect) have been reported when Efudex was applied to mucous membrane areas during pregnancy.

Occlusion of the skin with resultant hydration has been shown to increase precutaneous penetration of several topical preparations. If any occlusive dressing is used in treatment of basal cell carcinoma, there may be an increase in the severity of inflammatory reactions in the adjacent normal skin. A porous gauze dressing may be applied for cosmetic reasons without increase in reaction.

Exposure to ultraviolet rays should be minimized during and immediately following treatment with Efudex because the intensity of the reaction may be increased.

PRECAUTIONS

General: There is a possibility of increased absorption through ulcerated or inflamed skin.

Information for Patients: Patients should be forewarned that the reaction in the treated areas may be unsightly during therapy and, usually, for several weeks following cessation of therapy. Patients should be instructed to avoid exposure to ultraviolet rays during and immediately following treatment with Efudex because the intensity of the reaction may be increased. If Efudex is applied with the fingers, the hands should be washed immediately afterward. Efudex should not be applied on the eyelids or directly into the eyes, nose or mouth because irritation may occur.

Laboratory Tests: Solar keratoses which do not respond should be biopsied to confirm the diagnosis. Follow-up biopsies should be performed as indicated in the management of superficial basal cell carcinoma.

Carcinogenesis, Mutagenesis, Impairment of Fertility: Adequate long-term studies in animals to evaluate carcinogenic potential have not been conducted with fluorouracil. Studies with the active ingredient of Efudex, 5-fluorouracil, have shown positive effects in in vitro tests for mutagenicity and on impairment of fertility.

5-Fluorouracil was positive in three in vitro cell neoplastic transformation assays. In the C3H/10T^1/$_2$ clone 8 mouse embryo cell system, the resulting morphologically transformed cells formed tumors when inoculated into immunosuppressed syngeneic mice.

While no evidence for mutagenic activity was observed in the Ames test (3 studies), fluorouracil has been shown to be mutagenic in the survival count rec-assay with *Bacillus subtilis*

and in the Drosophilia wing-hair spot test. Fluorouracil produced petite mutations in *Saccharomyces cerevisiae* and was positive in the micronucleus test (bone marrow cells of male mice).

Fluorouracil was clastogenic in vitro (ie, chromatid gaps, breaks and exchanges) in Chinese hamster fibroblasts at concentrations of 1.0 and 2.0 μg/mL and has been shown to increase sister chromatid exchange in vitro in human lymphocytes. In addition, 5-fluorouracil has been reported to produce an increase in numerical and structural chromosome aberrations in peripheral lymphocytes of patients treated with this product.

Doses of 125 to 250 mg/kg, administered intraperitoneally, have been shown to induce chromosomal aberrations and changes in chromosome organization of spermatogonia in rats. Spermatogonial differentiation was also inhibited by fluorouracil, resulting in transient infertility. However, in studies with a strain of mouse which is sensitive to the induction of sperm head abnormalities after exposure to a range of chemical mutagens and carcinogens, fluorouracil was inactive at oral doses of 5 to 80 mg/kg/day. In female rats, fluorouracil administered intraperitoneally at doses of 25 and 50 mg/kg during the preovulatory phase of oogenesis significantly reduced the incidence of fertile matings, delayed the development of preimplantation and postimplantation embryos, increased the incidence of preimplantation lethality and induced chromosomal anomalies in these embryos. Single dose intravenous and intraperitoneal injections of 5-fluorouracil have been reported to kill differentiated spermatogonia and spermatocytes (at 500 mg/kg) and to produce abnormalities in spermatids (at 50 mg/kg) in mice.

Pregnancy: **Teratogenic Effects: Pregnancy Category X:** See CONTRAINDICATIONS section.

Nursing Mothers: It is not known whether Efudex is excreted in human milk. Because there is some systemic absorption of fluorouracil after topical administration (see CLINICAL PHARMACOLOGY), because many drugs are excreted in human milk, and because of the potential for serious adverse reactions in nursing infants, a decision should be made whether to discontinue nursing or to discontinue use of the drug, taking into account the importance of the drug to the mother.

Pediatric Use: Safety and effectiveness in children have not been established.

ADVERSE REACTIONS

The most frequent adverse reactions to Efudex occur locally and are often related to an extension of the pharmacological activity of the drug. These include burning, crusting, allergic contact dermatitis erosions, erythema, hyperpigmentation, irritation, pain, photosensitivity, pruritus, scarring rash, soreness and ulceration. Ulcerations, other local reactions, cases of miscarriage and a birth defect (ventricular septal defect) have been reported when Efudex was applied to mucous membrane areas. Leukocytosis is the most frequent hematological side effect.

Although a causal relationship is remote, other adverse reactions which have been reported infrequently are:

Central Nervous System: Emotional upset, insomnia, irritability.

Gastrointestinal: Medicinal taste, stomatitis.

Hematological: Eosinophilia, thrombocytopenia, toxic granulation.

Integumentary: Alopecia, blistering, bullous pemphigoid, discomfort, ichthyosis, scaling, suppuration, swelling, telangiectasia, tenderness, urticaria, skin rash.

Special Senses: Conjunctival reaction, corneal reaction, lacrimation, nasal irritation.

Miscellaneous: Herpes simplex.

OVERDOSAGE

There have been no reports of overdosage with Efudex. The oral LD$_{50}$ for the 5% topical cream was 234 mg/kg in rats and 39 mg/kg in dogs. These doses represented 11.7 and 1.95 mg/kg of fluorouracil, respectively. Studies with a 5% topical solution yielded an oral LD$_{50}$ of 214 mg/kg in rats and 28.5 mg/kg in dogs, corresponding to 10.7 and 1.43 mg/kg of fluorouracil, respectively. The topical application of the 5% cream to rats yielded an LD$_{50}$ of greater than 500 mg/kg.

DOSAGE AND ADMINISTRATION

When Efudex is applied to a lesion, a response occurs with the following sequence: erythema, usually followed by vesiculation, desquamation, erosion and reepithelialization.

Efudex should be applied preferably with a nonmetal applicator or suitable glove. If Efudex is applied with the fingers, the hands should be washed immediately afterward.

Actinic or Solar Keratosis: Apply cream or solution twice daily in an amount sufficient to cover the lesions. Medication should be continued until the inflammatory response reaches the erosion stage, at which time use of the drug should be terminated. The usual duration to therapy is from 2 to 4 weeks. Complete healing of the lesions may not be evident for 1 to 2 months following cessation of Efudex therapy.

Superficial Basal Cell Carcinomas: **Only the 5% strength is recommended.** Apply cream or solution twice daily in an amount sufficient to cover the lesions. Treatment should be

continued for at least 3 to 6 weeks. Therapy may be required for as long as 10 to 12 weeks before the lesions are obliterated. As in any neoplastic condition, the patient should be followed for a reasonable period of time to determine if a cure has been obtained.

HOW SUPPLIED

Efudex Solution is available in 10-mL drop dispensers containing either 2% (NDC 0004-1704-06) or 5% (NDC 0004-1705-06) fluorouracil on a weight/weight basis compounded with propylene glycol, tris(hydroxymethyl)aminomethane, hydroxypropyl cellulose, parabens (methyl and propyl) and disodium edetate.

Efudex Cream is available in 25-gm tubes containing 5% fluorouracil (NDC 0004-1506-03) in a vanishing cream base consisting of white petrolatum, stearyl alcohol, propylene glycol, polysorbate 60 and parabens (methyl and propyl). Store in tight containers at room temperature (59° to 86°F; 15° to 30°C).

Revised May 1995

FANSIDAR® ℞
[fan 'sid-ar]
brand of sulfadoxine and pyrimethamine
TABLETS

The following text is complete prescribing information based on official labeling in effect June 1996.

> **WARNING: FATALITIES ASSOCIATED WITH THE ADMINISTRATION OF FANSIDAR HAVE OCCURRED DUE TO SEVERE REACTIONS, INCLUDING STEVENS-JOHNSON SYNDROME AND TOXIC EPIDERMAL NECROLYSIS. FANSIDAR PROPHYLAXIS SHOULD BE DISCONTINUED AT THE FIRST APPEARANCE OF SKIN RASH, IF A SIGNIFICANT REDUCTION IN THE COUNT OF ANY FORMED BLOOD ELEMENTS IS NOTED, OR UPON THE OCCURRENCE OF ACTIVE BACTERIAL OR FUNGAL INFECTIONS.**

DESCRIPTION

Fansidar is an antimalarial agent, each tablet containing 500 mg N^1-(5,6-dimethoxy-4-pyrimidinyl) sulfanilamide (sulfadoxine) and 25 mg 2,4-diamino-5-(p-chlorophenyl)-6-ethylpyrimidine (pyrimethamine). Each tablet also contains corn starch, gelatin, lactose, magnesium stearate and talc.

CLINICAL PHARMACOLOGY

Fansidar is an antimalarial agent which acts by reciprocal potentiation of its two components, achieved by a sequential blockade of two enzymes involved in the biosynthesis of folinic acid within the parasites. Fansidar is effective against certain strains of *Plasmodium falciparum* that are resistant to chloroquine.

Both the sulfadoxine and the pyrimethamine of Fansidar are absorbed orally and are excreted mainly by the kidney. Following a single tablet administration, sulfadoxine peak plasma concentrations of 51 to 76 mcg/mL were achieved in 2.5 to 6 hours and the pyrimethamine peak plasma concentrations of 0.13 to 0.4 mcg/mL were achieved in 1.5 to 8 hours. The apparent half-life of elimination of sulfadoxine ranged from 100 to 231 hours with a mean of 169 hours, whereas pyrimethamine half-lives ranged from 54 to 148 hours with a mean of 111 hours. Both drugs appear in breast milk of nursing mothers.

INDICATIONS AND USAGE

Fansidar is indicated for the treatment of *P. falciparum* malaria for those patients in whom chloroquine resistance is suspected. Malaria prophylaxis with Fansidar is indicated for travelers to areas where chloroquine-resistant *P. falciparum* malaria is endemic. However, strains of *P. falciparum* may be encountered which have developed resistance to Fansidar.

CONTRAINDICATIONS

Prophylactic (repeated) use of Fansidar is contraindicated in patients with severe renal insufficiency, marked liver parenchymal damage or blood dyscrasias. Hypersensitivity to pyrimethamine or sulfonamides. Patients with documented megaloblastic anemia due to folate deficiency. Infants less than 2 months of age. Pregnancy at term and during the nursing period because sulfonamides pass the placenta and are excreted in the milk and may cause kernicterus.

WARNINGS

> **FATALITIES ASSOCIATED WITH THE ADMINISTRATION OF FANSIDAR HAVE OCCURRED DUE TO SEVERE REACTIONS, INCLUDING STEVENS-JOHNSON SYNDROME AND TOXIC EPIDERMAL NECROLYSIS. FANSIDAR PROPHYLAXIS SHOULD BE DISCONTIN-**

Continued on next page

Roche Laboratories—Cont.

UED AT THE FIRST APPEARANCE OF SKIN RASH, IF A SIGNIFICANT REDUCTION IN THE COUNT OF ANY FORMED BLOOD ELEMENTS IS NOTED, OR UPON THE OCCURRENCE OF ACTIVE BACTERIAL OR FUNGAL INFECTIONS.

Fatalities associated with the administration of sulfonamides, although rare, have occurred due to severe reactions, including fulminant hepatic necrosis, agranulocytosis, aplastic anemia and other blood dyscrasias. Fansidar prophylactic regimen has been reported to cause leukopenia during a treatment of 2 months or longer. This leukopenia is generally mild and reversible.

PRECAUTIONS

1. *General:* Fansidar should be given with caution to patients with impaired renal or hepatic function, to those with possible folate deficiency and to those with severe allergy or bronchial asthma. As with some sulfonamide drugs, in glucose-6-phosphate dehydrogenase-deficient individuals, hemolysis may occur. Urinalysis with microscopic examination and renal function tests should be performed during therapy of those patients who have impaired renal function.

2. *Information for the Patient:* Patients should be warned that at the first appearance of a skin rash, they should stop use of Fansidar and seek medical attention immediately. Adequate fluid intake must be maintained in order to prevent crystalluria and stone formation.

Patients should also be warned that the appearance of sore throat, fever, arthralgia, cough, shortness of breath, pallor, purpura, jaundice or glossitis may be early indications of serious disorders which require prophylactic treatment to be stopped and medical treatment to be sought.

Females should be cautioned against becoming pregnant and should not breast feed their infants during Fansidar therapy or prophylactic treatment.

Patients should be warned to keep Fansidar out of reach of children.

3. *Laboratory Tests:* Periodic blood counts and analysis of urine for crystalluria are desirable during prolonged prophylaxis.

4. *Drug Interactions:* There have been reports which may indicate an increase in incidence and severity of adverse reactions when chloroquine is used with Fansidar as compared to the use of Fansidar alone. Fansidar is compatible with quinine and with antibiotics. However, antifolic drugs such as sulfonamides or trimethoprim-sulfamethoxazole combinations should not be used while the patient is receiving Fansidar for antimalarial prophylaxis. Fansidar has not been reported to interfere with antidiabetic agents.

If signs of folic acid deficiency develop, Fansidar should be discontinued. Folinic acid (leucovorin) may be administered in doses of 5 mg to 15 mg intramuscularly daily, for 3 days or longer, for depressed platelet or white blood cell counts in patients with drug-induced folic acid deficiency when recovery is too slow.

5. *Carcinogenesis, Mutagenesis, Impairment of Fertility:* Pyrimethamine was not found carcinogenic in female mice or in male and female rats. The carcinogenic potential of pyrimethamine in male mice could not be assessed from the study because of markedly reduced life-span. Pyrimethamine was found to be mutagenic in laboratory animals and also in human bone marrow following 3 or 4 consecutive daily doses totaling 200 mg to 300 mg. Pyrimethamine was not found mutagenic in the Ames test. Testicular changes have been observed in rats treated with 105 mg/kg/day of Fansidar and with 15 mg/kg/day of pyrimethamine alone. Fertility of male rats and the ability of male or female rats to mate were not adversely affected at dosages of up to 210 mg/kg/day of Fansidar. The pregnancy rate of female rats was not affected following their treatment with 10.5 mg/kg/day, but was significantly reduced at dosages of 31.5 mg/kg/day or higher, a dosage approximately 30 times the weekly human prophylactic dose or higher.

6. *Pregnancy:* Teratogenic Effects: Pregnancy Category C. Fansidar has been shown to be teratogenic in rats when given in weekly doses approximately 12 times the weekly human prophylactic dose. Teratology studies with pyrimethamine plus sulfadoxine (1:20) in rats showed the minimum oral teratogenic dose to be approximately 0.9 mg/kg pyrimethamine plus 18 mg/kg sulfadoxine. In rabbits, no teratogenic effects were noted at oral doses as high as 20 mg/kg pyrimethamine plus 400 mg/kg sulfadoxine.

There are no adequate and well-controlled studies in pregnant women. However, due to the teratogenic effect shown in animals and because pyrimethamine plus sulfadoxine may interfere with folic acid metabolism, Fansidar therapy should be used during pregnancy only if the potential benefit justifies the potential risk to the fetus. Women of childbearing potential who are traveling to areas where malaria is endemic should be warned against becoming pregnant.

Nonteratogenic Effects: See "CONTRAINDICATIONS" section.

7. *Nursing Mothers:* See "CONTRAINDICATIONS" section.

8. *Pediatric Use:* Fansidar should not be given to infants less than 2 months of age because of inadequate development of the glucuronide-forming enzyme system.

ADVERSE REACTIONS

For completeness, all major reactions to sulfonamides and to pyrimethamine are included below, even though they may not have been reported with Fansidar. See WARNINGS and PRECAUTIONS (*Information for the Patient*) sections.

Blood Dyscrasias: Agranulocytosis, aplastic anemia, megaloblastic anemia, thrombopenia, leukopenia, hemolytic anemia, purpura, hypoprothrombinemia, methemoglobinemia and eosinophilia.

Allergic Reactions: Erythema multiforme, Stevens-Johnson syndrome, generalized skin eruptions, toxic epidermal necrolysis, urticaria, serum sickness, pruritus, exfoliative dermatitis, anaphylactoid reactions, periorbital edema, conjunctival and scleral injection, photosensitization, arthralgia and allergic myocarditis.

Gastrointestinal Reactions: Glossitis, stomatitis, nausea, emesis, abdominal pains, hepatitis, hepatocellular necrosis, diarrhea and pancreatitis.

C.N.S. Reactions: Headache, peripheral neuritis, mental depression, convulsions, ataxia, hallucinations, tinnitus, vertigo, insomnia, apathy, fatigue, muscle weakness and nervousness.

Respiratory Reactions: Pulmonary infiltrates.

Miscellaneous Reactions: Drug fever, chills, and toxic nephrosis with oliguria and anuria. Periarteritis nodosa and L. E. phenomenon have occurred.

The sulfonamides bear certain chemical similarities to some goitrogens, diuretics (acetazolamide and the thiazides) and oral hypoglycemic agents. Diuresis and hypoglycemia have occurred rarely in patients receiving sulfonamides. Cross-sensitivity may exist with these agents. Rats appear to be especially susceptible to the goitrogenic effects of sulfonamides, and long-term administration has produced thyroid malignancies in the species.

OVERDOSAGE

Acute intoxication may be manifested by anorexia, vomiting and central nervous system stimulation (including convulsions), followed by megaloblastic anemia, leukopenia, thrombocytopenia, glossitis and crystalluria. In acute intoxication, emesis and gastric lavage followed by purges may be of benefit. The patient should be adequately hydrated to prevent renal damage. The renal and hematopoietic systems should be monitored for at least one month after an overdosage. If the patient is having convulsions, the use of a parenteral barbiturate is indicated. For depressed platelet or white blood cell counts, folinic acid (leucovorin) should be administered in a dosage of 5 mg to 15 mg intramuscularly daily for 3 days or longer.

DOSAGE AND ADMINISTRATION

(See INDICATIONS AND USAGE section):

(a) *Treatment of Acute Attack of Malaria*

A single dose of the following number of Fansidar Tablets is used in sequence with quinine or alone:

Adults	2 to 3 tablets
9 to 14 years	2 tablets
4 to 8 years	1 tablet
Under 4 years	1/2 tablet

(b) *Malaria Prophylaxis*

The first dose of Fansidar should be taken 1 or 2 days before departure to an endemic area; administration should be continued during the stay and for 4 to 6 weeks after return.

	Once Weekly	Once Every Two Weeks
Adults	1 tablet	2 tablets
9 to 14 years	3/4 tablet	1 1/2 tablets
4 to 8 years	1/2 tablet	1 tablet
Under 4 years	1/4 tablet	1/2 tablet

HOW SUPPLIED

Scored tablets, containing 500 mg sulfadoxine and 25 mg pyrimethamine—Tel-E-Dose® packages of 25 (NDC-0004-0161-03). Imprint on tablets: FANSIDAR ROCHE

Revised: October 1993

Shown in Product Identification Guide, page 332

FLUOROURACIL ℞

[flu "ro-u 'ra-sil]

INJECTION

The following text is complete prescribing information based on official labeling in effect June 1996.

WARNING

It is recommended that FLUOROURACIL be given only by or under the supervision of a qualified physician who is experienced in cancer chemotherapy and who is well versed in the use of potent antimetabolites. Because of the possibility of severe toxic reactions, it is recommended that patients be hospitalized at least during the initial course of therapy.

DESCRIPTION

FLUOROURACIL INJECTION, an antineoplastic antimetabolite, is a sterile, nonpyrogenic injectable solution for intravenous administration. Each 10-mL contains 500 mg fluorouracil; pH is adjusted to approximately 9.2 with sodium hydroxide.

Chemically, fluorouracil, a fluorinated pyrimidine, is 5-fluoro-2,4 (*1H,3H*)-pyrimidinedione. It is a white to practically white crystalline powder which is sparingly soluble in water. The molecular weight of fluorouracil is 130.08.

CLINICAL PHARMACOLOGY

There is evidence that the metabolism of fluorouracil in the anabolic pathway blocks the methylation reaction of deoxyuridylic acid to thymidylic acid. In this manner, fluorouracil interferes with the synthesis of deoxyribonucleic acid (DNA) and to a lesser extent inhibits the formation of ribonucleic acid (RNA). Since DNA and RNA are essential for cell division and growth, the effect of fluorouracil may be to create a thymine deficiency which provokes unbalanced growth and death of the cell. The effects of DNA and RNA deprivation are most marked on those cells which grow more rapidly and which take up fluorouracil at a more rapid rate.

Following intravenous injection, fluorouracil distributes into tumors, intestinal mucosa, bone marrow, liver and other tissues throughout the body. In spite of its limited lipid solubility, fluorouracil diffuses readily across the blood-brain barrier and distributes into cerebrospinal fluid and brain tissue.

Seven percent to 20% of the parent drug is excreted unchanged in the urine in 6 hours; of this over 90% is excreted in the first hour. The remaining percentage of the administered dose is metabolized, primarily in the liver. The catabolic metabolism of fluorouracil results in degradation products (eg, CO_2, urea and α-fluoro-β-alanine) which are inactive. The inactive metabolites are excreted in the urine over the next 3 to 4 hours. When fluorouracil is labeled in the six carbon position, thus preventing the ^{14}C metabolism to CO_2, approximately 90% of the total radioactivity is excreted in the urine. When fluorouracil is labeled in the two carbon position approximately 90% of the total radioactivity is excreted in expired CO_2. Ninety percent of the dose is accounted for during the first 24 hours following intravenous administration.

Following intravenous administration of fluorouracil, the mean half-life of elimination from plasma is approximately 16 minutes, with a range of 8 to 20 minutes, and is dose dependent. No intact drug can be detected in the plasma 3 hours after an intravenous injection.

INDICATIONS AND USAGE

Fluorouracil is effective in the palliative management of carcinoma of the colon, rectum, breast, stomach and pancreas.

CONTRAINDICATIONS

Fluorouracil therapy is contraindicated for patients in a poor nutritional state, those with depressed bone marrow function, those with potentially serious infections or those with a known hypersensitivity to Fluorouracil.

WARNINGS

THE DAILY DOSE OF FLUOROURACIL IS NOT TO EXCEED 800 MG. IT IS RECOMMENDED THAT PATIENTS BE HOSPITALIZED DURING THEIR FIRST COURSE OF TREATMENT.

Fluorouracil should be used with extreme caution in poor risk patients with a history of high-dose pelvic irradiation or previous use of alkylating agents, those who have a widespread involvement of bone marrow by metastatic tumors or those with impaired hepatic or renal function.

Rarely, unexpected, severe toxicity (eg, stomatitis, diarrhea, neutropenia and neurotoxicity) associated with 5-FU has been attributed to deficiency of dipyrimidine dehydrogenase activity.[1] A few patients have been rechallenged with 5-FU and despite 5-FU dose lowering, toxicity recurred and progressed with worse morbidity. Absence of this catabolic enzyme appears to result in prolonged clearance of 5-FU.

Pregnancy: Teratogenic Effects: Pregnancy Category D. Fluorouracil may cause fetal harm when administered to a pregnant woman. Fluorouracil has been shown to be teratogenic in laboratory animals. Fluorouracil exhibited maximum teratogenicity when given to mice as single intraperitoneal injections of 10 to 40 mg/kg on day 10 or 12 of gestation. Similarly, intraperitoneal doses of 12 to 37 mg/kg given to rats between days 9 and 12 of gestation and intramuscular

doses of 3 to 9 mg given to hamsters between days 8 and 11 of gestation were teratogenic. Malformations included cleft palates, skeletal defects and deformed appendages, paws and tails. The dosages which were teratogenic in animals are 1 to 3 times the maximum recommended human therapeutic dose. In monkeys, divided doses of 40 mg/kg given between days 20 and 24 of gestation were not teratogenic.

There are no adequate and well-controlled studies with Fluorouracil in pregnant women. While there is no evidence of teratogenicity in humans due to Fluorouracil, it should be kept in mind that other drugs which inhibit DNA synthesis (eg, methotrexate and aminopterin) have been reported to be teratogenic in humans. Women of childbearing potential should be advised to avoid becoming pregnant. If the drug is used during pregnancy, or if the patient becomes pregnant while taking the drug, the patient should be told of the potential hazard to the fetus. Fluorouracil should be used during pregnancy only if the potential benefit justifies the potential risk to the fetus.

Combination Therapy: Any form of therapy which adds to the stress of the patient, interferes with nutrition or depresses bone marrow function will increase the toxicity of Fluorouracil.

Rarely, unexpected, severe toxicity (eg, stomatitis, diarrhea, neutropenia and neurotoxicity) associated with 5-FU has been attributed to deficiency of dipyrimidine dehydrogenase activity.[1] A few patients have been rechallenged with 5-FU and despite 5-FU dose lowering, toxicity recurred and progressed with worse morbidity. Absence of this catabolic enzyme appears to result in prolonged clearance of 5-FU.

PRECAUTIONS

General: Fluorouracil is a highly toxic drug with a narrow margin of safety. Therefore, patients should be carefully supervised, since therapeutic response is unlikely to occur without some evidence of toxicity. Severe hematological toxicity, gastrointestinal hemorrhage and even death may result from the use of Fluorouracil despite meticulous selection of patients and careful adjustment of dosage. Although severe toxicity is more likely in poor risk patients, fatalities may be encountered occasionally even in patients in relatively good condition.

Therapy is to be discontinued promptly whenever one of the following signs of toxicity appears:

Stomatitis or esophagopharyngitis, at the first visible sign.

Leukopenia (WBC under 3500) or a rapidly falling white blood count.

Vomiting, intractable.

Diarrhea, frequent bowel movements or watery stools.

Gastrointestinal ulceration and bleeding.

Thrombocytopenia (platelets under 100,000).

Hemorrhage from any site.

The administration of 5-fluorouracil has been associated with the occurrence of palmar-plantar erythrodysesthesia syndrome, also known as hand-foot syndrome. This syndrome has been characterized as a tingling sensation of hands and feet which may progress over the next few days to pain when holding objects or walking. The palms and soles become symmetrically swollen and erythematous with tenderness of the distal phalanges, possibly accompanied by desquamation. Interruption of therapy is followed by gradual resolution over 5 to 7 days. Although pyridoxine has been reported to ameliorate the palmar-plantar erythrodysesthesia syndrome, its safety and effectiveness have not been established.

Information for Patients: Patients should be informed of expected toxic effects, particularly oral manifestations. Patients should be alerted to the possibility of alopecia as a result of therapy and should be informed that it is usually a transient effect.

Laboratory Tests: White blood counts with differential are recommended before each dose.

Drug Interactions: Leucovorin calcium may enhance the toxicity of fluorouracil.

Also see WARNINGS section.

Carcinogenesis, Mutagenesis, Impairment of Fertility: Carcinogenesis: Long-term studies in animals to evaluate the carcinogenic potential of fluorouracil have not been conducted. However, there was no evidence of carcinogenicity in small groups of rats given fluorouracil orally at doses of 0.01, 0.3, 1 or 3 mg per rat 5 days per week for 52 weeks, followed by a 6-month observation period. Also, in other studies, 33 mg/kg of flourouracil was administered intravenously to male rats once a week for 52 weeks followed by observation for the remainder of their lifetimes with no evidence of carcinogenicity. Female mice were given 1 mg of fluorouracil intravenously once a week for 16 weeks with no effect on the incidence of lung adenomas. On the basis of the available data, no evaluation can be made of the carcinogenic risk of fluorouracil to humans.

Mutagenesis: Oncogenic transformation of fibroblasts from mouse embryo has been induced in vitro by fluorouracil, but the relationship between oncogenicity and mutagenicity is not clear. Fluorouracil has been shown to be mutagenic to several strains of *Salmonella typhimurium*, including TA 1535, TA 1537 and TA 1538, and to *Saccharomyces cerevisiae*,

although no evidence of mutagenicity was found with *Salmonella typhimurium* strains TA 92, TA 98 and TA 100. In addition, a positive effect was observed in the micronucleus test on bone marrow cells of the mouse, and fluorouracil at very high concentrations produced chromosomal breaks in hamster fibroblasts in vitro.

Impairment of Fertility: Fluorouracil has not been adequately studied in animals to permit an evaluation of its effects on fertility and general reproductive performance. However, doses of 125 or 250 mg/kg, administered intraperitoneally, have been shown to induce chromosomal aberrations and changes in chromosomal organization of spermatogonia in rats. Spermatogonial differentiation was also inhibited by fluorouracil, resulting in transient infertility. However, in studies with a strain of mouse which is sensitive to the induction of sperm head abnormalities after exposure to a range of chemical mutagens and carcinogens, fluorouracil did not produce any abnormalities at oral doses of up to 80 mg/kg/day. In female rats, fluorouracil, administered intraperitoneally at weekly doses of 25 or 50 mg/kg for 3 weeks during the pre-ovulatory phases of oogenesis, significantly reduced the incidence of fertile matings, delayed the development of pre- and post-implantation embryos, increased the incidence of pre-implantation lethality and induced chromosomal anomalies in these embryos. In a limited study in rabbits, a single 25 mg/kg dose of fluorouracil or 5 daily doses of 5 mg/kg had no effect on ovulation, appeared not to affect implantation and had only a limited effect in producing zygote destruction. Compounds such as fluorouracil, which interfere with DNA, RNA and protein synthesis, might be expected to have adverse effects on gametogenesis.

Pregnancy: Pregnancy Category D. See WARNINGS section.

Nonteratogenic Effects: Fluorouracil has not been studied in animals for its effects on peri- and postnatal development. However, fluorouracil has been shown to cross the placenta and enter into fetal circulation in the rat. Administration of fluorouracil has resulted in increased resorptions and embryolethality in rats. In monkeys, maternal doses higher than 40 mg/kg resulted in abortion of all embryos exposed to fluorouracil. Compounds which inhibit DNA, RNA and protein synthesis might be expected to have adverse effects on peri- and postnatal development.

Nursing Mothers: It is not known whether fluorouracil is excreted in human milk. Because fluorouracil inhibits DNA, RNA and protein synthesis, mothers should not nurse while receiving this drug.

Pediatric Use: Safety and effectiveness in children have not been established.

ADVERSE REACTIONS

Stomatitis and esophagopharyngitis (which may lead to sloughing and ulceration), diarrhea, anorexia, nausea and emesis are commonly seen during therapy.

Leukopenia usually follows every course of adequate therapy with Fluorouracil. The lowest white blood cell counts are commonly observed between the 9th and 14th days after the first course of treatment, although uncommonly the maximal depression may be delayed for as long as 20 days. By the 30th day the count has usually returned to the normal range. Alopecia and dermatitis may be seen in a substantial number of cases. The dermatitis most often seen is a pruritic maculopapular rash usually appearing on the extremities and less frequently on the trunk. It is generally reversible and usually responsive to symptomatic treatment.

Other adverse reactions are:

Hematologic: pancytopenia, thrombocytopenia, agranulocytosis, anemia.

Cardiovascular: myocardial ischemia, angina.

Gastrointestinal: gastrointestinal ulceration and bleeding.

Allergic Reactions: anaphylaxis and generalized allergic reactions.

Neurologic: acute cerebellar syndrome (which may persist following discontinuance of treatment), nystagmus, headache.

Dermatologic: dry skin; fissuring; photosensitivity, as manifested by erythema or increased pigmentation of the skin; vein pigmentation, palmar-plantar erythrodysesthesia syndrome, as manifested by tingling of the hands and feet followed by pain, erythema and swelling.

Ophthalmic: lacrimal duct stenosis, visual changes, lacrimation, photophobia.

Psychiatric: disorientation, confusion, euphoria.

Miscellaneous: thrombophlebitis, epistaxis, nail changes (including loss of nails).

OVERDOSAGE

The possibility of overdosage with Fluorouracil is unlikely in view of the mode of administration. Nevertheless, the anticipated manifestations would be nausea, vomiting, diarrhea, gastrointestinal ulceration and bleeding, bone marrow depression (including thrombocytopenia, leukopenia and agranulocytosis). No specific antidotal therapy exists. Patients who have been exposed to an overdose of Fluorouracil should be monitored hematologically for at least four weeks.

Should abnormalities appear, appropriate therapy should be utilized.

The acute intravenous toxicity of fluorouracil is as follows:

Species	LD$_{50}$ (mg/kg±S.E.)
Mouse	340±17
Rat	165±26
Rabbit	27±5.1
Dog	31.5±3.8

DOSAGE AND ADMINISTRATION

General Instructions: Fluorouracil Injection should be administered only intravenously, using care to avoid extravasation. No dilution is required.

All dosages are based on the patient's actual weight. However, the estimated lean body mass (dry weight) is used if the patient is obese or if there has been a spurious weight gain due to edema, ascites or other forms of abnormal fluid retention.

It is recommended that prior to treatment each patient be carefully evaluated in order to estimate as accurately as possible the optimum initial dosage of Fluorouracil.

Dosage: 12 mg/kg are given intravenously once daily for 4 successive days. The daily dose should not exceed 800 mg. *If no toxicity is observed,* 6 mg/kg are given on the 6th, 8th, 10th and 12th days *unless toxicity occurs.* No therapy is given on the 5th, 7th, 9th or 11th days. *Therapy is to be discontinued at the end of the 12th day, even if no toxicity has become apparent.* (See WARNINGS and PRECAUTIONS sections.)

Poor risk patients or those who are not in an adequate nutritional state (see CONTRAINDICATIONS and WARNINGS sections) should receive 6 mg/kg/day for 3 days. *If no toxicity is observed,* 3 mg/kg may be given on the 5th, 7th and 9th days *unless toxicity occurs.* No therapy is given on the 4th, 6th or 8th days. The daily dose should not exceed 400 mg.

A sequence of injections on either schedule constitutes a "course of therapy."

Maintenance Therapy: In instances where toxicity has not been a problem, it is recommended that therapy be continued using either of the following schedules:

1. Repeat dosage of first course every 30 days after the last day of the previous course of treatment.

2. When toxic signs resulting from the initial course of therapy have subsided, administer a maintenance dosage of 10 to 15 mg/kg/week as a single dose. Do not exceed 1 gm per week.

The patient's reaction to the previous course of therapy should be taken into account in determining the amount of the drug to be used, and the dosage should be adjusted accordingly. Some patients have received from 9 to 45 courses of treatment during periods which ranged from 12 to 60 months.

Procedures for proper handling and disposal of anticancer drugs should be considered. Several guidelines on this subject have been published.[2-7] There is no general agreement that all of the procedures recommended in the guidelines are necessary or appropriate.

Note: Parenteral drug products should be inspected visually for particulate matter and discoloration prior to administration, whenever solution and container permit. Although the Fluorouracil solution may discolor slightly during storage, the potency and safety are not adversely affected. If a precipitate occurs due to exposure to low temperatures, resolubilize by heating to 140°F and shaking vigorously; allow to cool to body temperature before using.

HOW SUPPLIED

For intravenous use—10-mL single-use vials, boxes of 10 (NDC 0004-1977-01). Each 10 mL contains 500 mg fluorouracil in a colorless to faint yellow aqueous solution, with pH adjusted to approximately 9.2 with sodium hydroxide.

Store at room temperature (59° to 86°F; 15° to 30°C). Protect from light.

REFERENCES

1. Harris BE, Carpenter JT, Diasio RB: Severe 5-Fluorouracil Toxicity Secondary to Dihydropyrimidine Dehydrogenase Deficiency. A potentially more common pharmacogenetic syndrome. *Cancer.* August 1, 1991; 68:499–501.

2. Recommendations for the safe handling of parenteral antineoplastic drugs. Washington, DC, U.S. Government Printing Office (NIH Publication No. 83-2621).

3. AMA Council Report. Guidelines for handling parenteral antineoplastics. *JAMA.* Mar 15, 1985; 253:1590–1592.

4. National Study Commission on Cytotoxic Exposure: Recommendations for handling cytotoxic agents. Available from Louis P. Jeffrey, ScD, Director of Pharmacy Services, Rhode Island Hospital, 593 Eddy Street, Providence, Rhode Island 02902.

5. Clinical Oncological Society of Australia: Guidelines and recommendations for safe handling of antineoplastic agents. *Med J Aust.* Apr 30, 1983; 1:426–428.

6. Jones RB, Frank R. Mass T: Safe handling of chemotherapeutic agents: a report from the Mount Sinai Medical Center. *CA.* Sept–Oct 1983; 33:258–263.

Continued on next page

Roche Laboratories—Cont.

7. ASHP technical assistance bulletin on handling cytotoxic drugs in hospitals. *Am J Hosp Pharm.* Jan 1985; 42:131–137.

Revised: August 1994

STERILE ℞
FUDR
[*ef-u-dee-are*]
brand of floxuridine

The following text is complete prescribing information based on official labeling in effect June 1996.

> **WARNING**
> It is recommended that FUDR be given only by or under the supervision of a qualified physician who is experienced in cancer chemotherapy and intra-arterial drug therapy and is well versed in the use of potent antimetabolites.
> Because of the possibility of severe toxic reactions, all patients should be hospitalized for initiation of the first course of therapy.

DESCRIPTION

Sterile FUDR (floxuridine), an antineoplastic antimetabolite, is available as a sterile, nonpyrogenic, lyophilized powder for reconstitution. Each vial contains 500 mg of floxuridine which is to be reconstituted with 5 mL of sterile water for injection. An appropriate amount of reconstituted solution is then diluted with a parenteral solution for intra-arterial infusion (see DOSAGE AND ADMINISTRATION section).

Floxuridine is a fluorinated pyrimidine. Chemically, floxuridine is 2′-deoxy-5-fluorouridine with an empirical formula of $C_9H_{11}FN_2O_5$. It is a white to off-white odorless solid which is freely soluble in water.

The 2% aqueous solution has a pH of between 4.0 to 5.5. The molecular weight of floxuridine is 246.19.

CLINICAL PHARMACOLOGY

When FUDR is given by rapid intra-arterial injection it is apparently rapidly catabolized to 5-fluorouracil. Thus, rapid injection of FUDR produces the same toxic and antimetabolic effects as does 5-fluorouracil. The primary effect is to interfere with the synthesis of deoxyribonucleic acid (DNA) and to a lesser extent inhibit the formation of ribonucleic acid (RNA). However, when FUDR is given by continuous intra-arterial infusion its direct anabolism to FUDR-monophosphate is enhanced, thus increasing the inhibition of DNA.

Floxuridine is metabolized in the liver. The drug is excreted intact and as urea, fluorouracil, α-fluoro-β-ureidopropionic acid, dihydrofluorouracil, α-fluoro-β-guanidopropionic acid and α-fluoro-β-alanine in the urine; it is also expired as respiratory carbon dioxide. Pharmacokinetic data on intra-arterial infusion of FUDR are not available.

INDICATIONS AND USAGE

FUDR is effective in the palliative management of gastrointestinal adenocarcinoma metastatic to the liver, when given by continuous regional intra-arterial infusion in carefully selected patients who are considered incurable by surgery or other means. Patients with known disease extending beyond an area capable of infusion via a single artery should, except in unusual circumstances, be considered for systemic therapy with other chemotherapeutic agents.

CONTRAINDICATIONS

FUDR therapy is contraindicated for patients in a poor nutritional state, those with depressed bone marrow function or those with potentially serious infections.

WARNINGS

BECAUSE OF THE POSSIBILITY OF SEVERE TOXIC REACTIONS, ALL PATIENTS SHOULD BE HOSPITALIZED FOR THE FIRST COURSE OF THERAPY.

FUDR should be used with extreme caution in poor risk patients with impaired hepatic or renal function or a history of high-dose pelvic irradiation or previous use of alkylating agents. The drug is not intended as an adjuvant to surgery.

FUDR may cause fetal harm when administered to a pregnant woman. It has been shown to be teratogenic in the chick embryo, mouse (at doses of 2.5 to 100 mg/kg) and rat (at doses of 75 to 150 mg/kg). Malformations included cleft palates; skeletal defects; and deformed appendages, paws and tails. The dosages which were teratogenic in animals are 4.2 to 125 times the recommended human therapeutic dose.

There are no adequate and well-controlled studies with FUDR in pregnant women. If this drug is used during pregnancy or if the patient becomes pregnant while taking (receiving) this drug, the patient should be apprised of the potential hazard to the fetus. Women of childbearing potential should be advised to avoid becoming pregnant.

Combination Therapy: Any form of therapy which adds to the stress of the patient, interferes with nutrition or depresses bone marrow function will increase the toxicity of FUDR.

PRECAUTIONS

General: Sterile FUDR is a highly toxic drug with a narrow margin of safety. Therefore, patients should be carefully supervised since therapeutic response is unlikely to occur without some evidence of toxicity. Severe hematological toxicity, gastrointestinal hemorrhage and even death may result from the use of FUDR despite meticulous selection of patients and careful adjustment of dosage. Although severe toxicity is more likely in poor risk patients, fatalities may be encountered occasionally even in patients in relatively good condition.

Therapy is to be discontinued promptly whenever one of the following signs of toxicity appears:
Myocardial ischemia
Stomatitis or esophagopharyngitis, at the first visible sign
Leukopenia (WBC under 3500) or a rapidly falling white blood count
Vomiting, intractable
Diarrhea, frequent bowel movements or watery stools
Gastrointestinal ulceration and bleeding
Thrombocytopenia (platelets under 100,000)
Hemorrhage from any site

Information For Patients: Patients should be informed of expected toxic effects, particularly oral manifestations. Patients should be alerted to the possibility of alopecia as a result of therapy and should be informed that it is usually a transient effect.

Laboratory Tests: Careful monitoring of the white blood count and platelet count is recommended.

Drug Interactions: See WARNINGS section.

Carcinogenesis, Mutagenesis, Impairment Of Fertility:
Carcinogenesis: Long-term studies in animals to evaluate the carcinogenic potential of floxuridine have not been conducted. On the basis of the available data, no evaluation can be made of the carcinogenic risk of FUDR to humans.

Mutagenesis: Oncogenic transformation of fibroblasts from mouse embryo has been induced in vitro by FUDR, but the relationship between oncogenicity and mutagenicity is not clear. Floxuridine has also been shown to be mutagenic in human leukocytes in vitro and in the *Drosophila* test system. In addition, 5-fluorouracil, to which floxuridine is catabolized when given by intra-arterial injection, has been shown to be mutagenic in in vitro tests.

Impairment Of Fertility: The effects of floxuridine on fertility and general reproductive performance have not been studied in animals. However, because floxuridine is catabolized to 5-fluorouracil, it should be noted that 5-fluorouracil has been shown to induce chromosomal aberrations and changes in chromosome organization of spermatogonia in rats at doses of 125 or 250 mg/kg, administered intraperitoneally.

Spermatogonial differentiation was also inhibited by fluorouracil, resulting in transient infertility. In female rats, fluorouracil, administered intraperitoneally at doses of 25 or 50 mg/kg during the preovulatory phase of oogenesis, significantly reduced the incidence of fertile matings, delayed the development of pre- and post-implantation embryos, increased the incidence of preimplantation lethality and induced chromosomal anomalies in these embryos. Compounds such as FUDR, which interfere with DNA, RNA and protein synthesis, might be expected to have adverse effects on gametogenesis.

Pregnancy: Teratogenic Effects: Pregnancy category D. See WARNINGS section. Floxuridine has been shown to be teratogenic in the chick embryo, mouse (at doses of 2.5 to 100 mg/kg) and rat (at doses of 75 to 150 mg/kg). Malformations included cleft palates, skeletal defects and deformed appendages, paws and tails. The dosages which were teratogenic in animals are 4.2 to 125 times the recommended human therapeutic dose.

There are no adequate and well-controlled studies with FUDR in pregnant women. While there is no evidence of teratogenicity in humans due to FUDR, it should be kept in mind that other drugs which inhibit DNA synthesis (eg, methotrexate and aminopterin) have been reported to be teratogenic in humans. FUDR should be used during pregnancy only if the potential benefit justifies the potential risk to the fetus.

Nonteratogenic Effects: Floxuridine has not been studied in animals for its effects on peri- and postnatal development. However, compounds which inhibit DNA, RNA and protein synthesis might be expected to have adverse effects on peri- and postnatal development.

Nursing Mothers: It is not known whether FUDR is excreted in human milk. Because FUDR inhibits DNA and RNA synthesis, mothers should not nurse while receiving this drug.

Pediatric Use: Safety and effectiveness in children have not been established.

ADVERSE REACTIONS

Adverse reactions to the arterial infusion of FUDR are generally related to the procedural complications of regional arterial infusion.

The more common adverse reactions to the drug are nausea, vomiting, diarrhea, enteritis, stomatitis and localized erythema. The more common laboratory abnormalities are anemia, leukopenia, thrombocytopenia and elevations of alkaline phosphatase, serum transaminase, serum bilirubin and lactic dehydrogenase.

Other adverse reactions are:

Gastrointestinal: duodenal ulcer, duodenitis, gastritis, bleeding, gastroenteritis, glossitis, pharyngitis, anorexia, cramps, abdominal pain; possible intra- and extrahepatic biliary sclerosis, as well as acalculous cholecystitis.

Dermatologic: alopecia, dermatitis, nonspecific skin toxicity, rash.

Cardiovascular: myocardial ischemia.

Miscellaneous Clinical Reactions: fever, lethargy, malaise, weakness.

Laboratory Abnormalities: BSP, prothrombin, total proteins, sedimentation rate and thrombopenia.

Procedural Complications of Regional Arterial Infusion: arterial aneurysm; arterial ischemia; arterial thrombosis; embolism; fibromyositis; thrombophlebitis; hepatic necrosis; abscesses; infection at catheter site; bleeding at catheter site; catheter blocked, displaced or leaking.

The following adverse reactions have not been reported with FUDR but have been noted following the administration of 5-fluorouracil. While the possibility of these occurring following FUDR therapy is remote because of its regional administration, one should be alert for these reactions following the administration of FUDR because of the pharmacological similarity of these two drugs: pancytopenia, agranulocytosis, myocardial ischemia, angina, anaphylaxis, generalized allergic reactions, acute cerebellar syndrome, nystagmus, headache, dry skin, fissuring, photosensitivity, pruritic maculopapular rash, increased pigmentation of the skin, vein pigmentation, lacrimal duct stenosis, visual changes, lacrimation, photophobia, disorientation, confusion, euphoria, epistaxis and nail changes, including loss of nails.

OVERDOSAGE

The possibility of overdosage with FUDR is unlikely in view of the mode of administration. Nevertheless, the anticipated manifestations would be nausea, vomiting, diarrhea, gastrointestinal ulceration and bleeding, bone marrow depression (including thrombocytopenia, leukopenia and agranulocytosis). No specific antidotal therapy exists. Patients who have been exposed to an overdosage of FUDR should be monitored hematologically for at least 4 weeks. Should abnormalities appear, appropriate therapy should be utilized.

The acute intravenous toxicity of floxuridine is as follows:

Species	LD_{50} (mg/kg ± S.E.)
Mouse	880 ± 51
Rat	670 ± 73
Rabbit	94 ± 19.6
Dog	157 ± 46

DOSAGE AND ADMINISTRATION

Each vial must be reconstituted with 5 mL of sterile water for injection to yield a solution containing approximately 100 mg of floxuridine/mL. The calculated daily dose(s) of the drug is then diluted with 5% dextrose or 0.9% sodium chloride injection to a volume appropriate for the infusion apparatus to be used. The administration of FUDR is best achieved with the use of an appropriate pump to overcome pressure in large arteries and to ensure a uniform rate of infusion.

Parenteral drug products should be inspected visually for particulate matter and discoloration prior to administration whenever solution and container permit.

The recommended therapeutic dosage schedule of FUDR by continuous arterial infusion is 0.1 to 0.6 mg/kg/day. The higher dosage ranges (0.4 to 0.6 mg) are usually employed for hepatic artery infusion because the liver metabolizes the drug, thus reducing the potential for systemic toxicity. Therapy can be given until adverse reactions appear. (See PRECAUTIONS section.) When these side effects have subsided, therapy may be resumed. The patient should be maintained on therapy as long as response to FUDR continues.

Procedures for proper handling and disposal of anticancer drugs should be considered. Several guidelines on this subject have been published.[1–6] There is no general agreement that all of the procedures recommended in the guidelines are necessary or appropriate.

HOW SUPPLIED

500 mg Sterile FUDR (floxuridine) powder in a 5-mL vial (NDC 0004-1935-08). This is to be reconstituted with 5 mL sterile water for injection.

The sterile powder should be stored at 59° to 86°F (15° to 30°C). Reconstituted vials should be stored under refrigeration (36° to 46°F, 2° to 8°C) for not more than 2 weeks.

REFERENCES

1. Recommendations for the safe handling of parenteral antineoplastic drugs. Washington, DC, US Government Printing Office NIH publication 83-2621.
2. AMA Council Report. Guidelines for handling parenteral antineoplastics. *JAMA*. Mar 15, 1985, 253:1590–1592,
3. National Study Commission on Cytotoxic Exposure: Recommendations for handling cytotoxic agents. Available from Louis P. Jeffrey, ScD, Director of Pharmacy Services, Rhode Island Hospital, 593 Eddy Street, Providence, Rhode Island 02902.
4. Clinical Oncological Society of Australia: Guidelines and recommendations for safe handling of antineoplastic agents. *Med J Aust*. Apr 30, 1983, 1:426–428.
5. Jones RB, Frank R, Mass T: Safe handling of chemotherapeutic agents: a report from the Mount Sinai Medical Center. *CA* Sept–Oct, 1983, 33:258–263.
6. ASHP technical assistance bulletin on handling cytotoxic drugs in hospitals. *Am J Hosp Pharm*. Jan, 1985, 42:131–137.

Revised: July 1994

GANTANOL® ℞

[gan 'tan-ol]
brand of sulfamethoxazole
TABLETS

The following text is complete prescribing information based on official labeling in effect June 1996.

DESCRIPTION

Gantanol® (sulfamethoxazole) is an intermediate-dosage antibacterial sulfonamide available in tablets. Each tablet contains 0.5 gm sulfamethoxazole plus corn starch, polyvinyl acetate, polyvinyl alcohol, magnesium stearate, FD&C Blue No. 1 Lake, FD&C Yellow No. 6 Lake and D&C Yellow No. 10 Lake.

Sulfamethoxazole is N^1-(5-methyl-3-isoxazolyl)sulfanilamide. It is an almost white, odorless, tasteless compound with a molecular weight of 253.28.

CLINICAL PHARMACOLOGY

Sulfamethoxazole is rapidly absorbed following oral administration. It exists in the blood as unbound, protein-bound, metabolized and conjugated forms. The metabolism of sulfamethoxazole occurs predominately by N_4-acetylation, although the glucuronide conjugate has been identified. The free form is considered to be the therapeutically active form. Approximately 70% of sulfamethoxazole is bound to plasma proteins; of the unbound portion, 80% to 90% is in the nonacetylated form.

Following a single 1-gm oral dose in 12 volunteer male subjects, the mean peak plasma concentration of 38 mcg/mL of intact sulfamethoxazole was achieved by 2 hours. The mean half-life of sulfamethoxazole is approximately 10 hours. However, patients with severely impaired renal function, as shown by a creatinine clearance of less than 30 mL/minute, exhibit an increase of the half-life of sulfamethoxazole, requiring dosage regimen adjustment.

Sulfamethoxazole is excreted primarily by the kidneys chiefly through glomerular filtration but also through tubular secretion. Urine concentrations of sulfamethoxazole are considerably higher than are the concentrations in blood. Eighty percent to 100% of the dose is excreted in the urine as total sulfamethoxazole, of which 30% is intact drug with the remaining as the N_4-acetylated metabolite.

Sulfamethoxazole diffuses into cerebrospinal fluid, with peak concentrations occurring at 8 hours and reaching approximately 14% of simultaneous plasma concentrations. The drug has also been shown to distribute to aqueous humor, vaginal fluid and middle ear fluid; it also passes the placental barrier and is excreted in breast milk.

Microbiology: The systemic sulfonamides are bacteriostatic agents and the spectrum of activity is similar for all. Sulfonamides inhibit bacterial synthesis of dihydrofolic acid by competing with *para*-aminobenzoic acid (PABA). Resistant strains are capable of utilizing folic acid precursors or preformed folic acid.

INDICATIONS AND USAGE

Acute, recurrent or chronic urinary tract infections (primarily pyelonephritis, pyelitis and cystitis) due to susceptible organisms (usually *E. coli, Klebsiella-Enterobacter,* staphylococcus, *Proteus mirabilis* and, less frequently, *Proteus vulgaris*) in the absence of obstructive uropathy or foreign bodies.

Meningococcal meningitis prophylaxis when sulfonamide-sensitive group A strains are known to prevail in family groups or larger closed populations. (The prophylactic usefulness of sulfonamides when group B or C infections are prevalent has not been proven and in closed population groups may be harmful.)

Acute otitis media due to *Haemophilus influenzae* when used concomitantly with adequate doses of penicillin.

Trachoma. Inclusion conjunctivitis. Nocardiosis. Chancroid.

Toxoplasmosis as adjunctive therapy with pyrimethamine.

Malaria due to chloroquine-resistant strains of *Plasmodium falciparum,* when used as adjunctive therapy.

Important Note: In vitro sulfonamide susceptibility tests are not always reliable. The test must be carefully coordinated with bacteriologic and clinical response. When the patient is already taking sulfonamides, follow-up cultures should have aminobenzoic acid added to the culture media.

Currently, the increasing frequency of resistant organisms is a limitation of the usefulness of antibacterial agents including the sulfonamides, especially in the treatment of chronic and recurrent urinary tract infections.

Wide variation in blood concentrations may result with identical doses. Blood concentrations should be measured in patients receiving sulfonamides for serious infections. Free sulfonamide blood concentrations of 5 to 15 mg/100 mL may be considered therapeutically effective for most infections, with blood concentrations of 12 to 15 mg/100 mL optimal for serious infections; 20 mg/100 mL should be the maximum total sulfonamide concentration, since adverse reactions occur more frequently above this concentration.

CONTRAINDICATIONS

Hypersensitivity to sulfonamides. Infants less than 2 months of age (except in the treatment of congenital toxoplasmosis as adjunctive therapy with pyrimethamine). Pregnancy at term and during the nursing period because sulfonamides pass the placenta and are excreted in the milk and may cause kernicterus.

WARNINGS

The sulfonamides should not be used for the treatment of group A beta-hemolytic streptococcal infections. In an established infection, they will not eradicate the streptococcus, and therefore will not prevent sequelae such as rheumatic fever and glomerulonephritis.

Deaths associated with the administration of sulfonamides have been reported from hypersensitivity reactions, hepatocellular necrosis, agranulocytosis, aplastic anemia and other blood dyscrasias.

The presence of clinical signs such as sore throat, fever, arthralgia, cough, shortness of breath, pallor, purpura or jaundice may be early indications of serious reactions, including serious blood disorders.

PRECAUTIONS

General: Sulfonamides should be given with caution to patients with impaired renal or hepatic function and to those with severe allergy or bronchial asthma. In glucose-6-phosphate dehydrogenase-deficient individuals, hemolysis may occur. This reaction is frequently dose-related.

Information for Patients: Patients should be instructed to maintain an adequate fluid intake in order to prevent crystalluria and stone formation.

Laboratory Tests: Complete blood counts should be done frequently in patients receiving sulfonamides. If a significant reduction in the count of any formed blood element is noted, Gantanol should be discontinued. Urinalyses with careful microscopic examination and renal function tests should be performed during therapy, particularly for those patients with impaired renal function.

Drug Interactions: In elderly patients concurrently receiving certain diuretics, primarily thiazides, an increased incidence of thrombopenia with purpura has been reported.

It has been reported that sulfamethoxazole may prolong the prothrombin time in patients who are receiving the anticoagulant warfarin. This interaction should be kept in mind when Gantanol is given to patients already on anticoagulant therapy, and the coagulation time should be reassessed.

Sulfamethoxazole may inhibit the hepatic metabolism of phenytoin. At a 1.6 gm dose, sulfamethoxazole produced a slight but significant increase in the half-life of phenytoin but did not produce a corresponding decrease in the metabolic clearance rate. When administering these drugs concurrently, one should be alert for possible excessive phenytoin effect.

Sulfonamides can also displace methotrexate from plasma protein-binding sites, thus increasing free methotrexate concentrations.

The presence of sulfamethoxazole may interfere with the Jaffé alkaline picrate reaction assay for creatinine, resulting in overestimations of about 10% in the range of normal values.

Carcinogenesis, Mutagenesis, Impairment of Fertility: *Carcinogenesis:* Sulfamethoxazole has not been adequately tested in animals to permit an evaluation of its carcinogenic potential.

Mutagenesis: Bacterial mutagenic studies have not been performed with sulfamethoxazole. No chromosomal damage was observed in human leukocytes cultured in vitro with sulfamethoxazole; the concentrations used exceeded blood levels of sulfamethoxazole following therapy with Gantanol.

Impairment of Fertility: No adverse effects on fertility or general reproductive performance were observed in rats given sulfamethoxazole in oral dosages as high as 350 mg/kg/day.

Pregnancy: Teratogenic Effects: Pregnancy Category C. In rats, oral doses of 533 mg/kg of sulfamethoxazole produced teratologic effects manifested mainly as cleft palates. The highest dose which did not cause cleft palates in rats was 512 mg/kg of sulfamethoxazole. In rabbits, 150 to 350 mg/kg/day increased maternal mortality but had no deleterious effects on fetal development.

There are no adequate and well-controlled studies of Gantanol in pregnant women. Gantanol should be used during pregnancy only if the potential benefit justifies the potential risk to the fetus.

Nonteratogenic Effects: See CONTRAINDICATIONS section.

Nursing Mothers: See CONTRAINDICATIONS section.

Pediatric Use: Gantanol is not recommended in infants under 2 months of age, except in the treatment of congenital toxoplasmosis as adjunctive therapy with pyrimethamine. (See CONTRAINDICATIONS section.) At the present time there are insufficient clinical data on prolonged or recurrent therapy in chronic renal diseases of children under 6 years of age.

ADVERSE REACTIONS

Included in the listing that follows are adverse reactions that have not been reported with this specific drug; however, the pharmacologic similarities among the sulfonamides require that each of the reactions be considered with Gantanol administration.

Hematologic: Agranulocytosis, aplastic anemia, thrombocytopenia, leukopenia, hemolytic anemia, purpura, hypoprothrombinemia, methemoglobinemia, neutropenia, eosinophilia.

Allergic Reactions: Anaphylaxis, allergic myocarditis, serum sickness, conjunctival and scleral injection, generalized allergic reactions. In addition, periarteritis nodosa and systemic lupus erythematosus have been reported.

Dermatologic: Stevens-Johnson syndrome, epidermal necrolysis, erythema multiforme, exfoliative dermatitis, photosensitivity, pruritus, urticaria, rash, generalized skin eruptions.

Gastrointestinal: Hepatitis, hepatocellular necrosis, pseudomembranous enterocolitis, pancreatitis, stomatitis, glossitis, nausea, emesis, abdominal pain, diarrhea, anorexia.

Genitourinary: Creatinine elevation, toxic nephrosis with oliguria and anuria. The frequency of renal complications is considerably lower in patients receiving the more soluble sulfonamides.

Neurologic: Convulsions, peripheral neuritis, ataxia, vertigo, tinnitus, headache.

Psychiatric: Hallucinations, depression, apathy.

Endocrine: The sulfonamides bear certain chemical similarities to some goitrogens, diuretics (acetazolamide and the thiazides) and oral hypoglycemic agents. Cross-sensitivity may exist with these agents. Diuresis and hypoglycemia have occurred rarely in patients receiving sulfonamides.

Musculoskeletal: Arthralgia, myalgia.

Respiratory: Pulmonary infiltrates.

Miscellaneous: Edema (including periorbital), pyrexia, chills, weakness, fatigue, insomnia.

OVERDOSAGE

Acute: The amount of a single dose of sulfamethoxazole that is either associated with symptoms of overdosage or is likely to be life-threatening has not been reported. Signs and symptoms of overdosage reported with sulfonamides include anorexia, colic, nausea, vomiting, dizziness, headache, drowsiness and unconsciousness. Pyrexia, hematuria and crystalluria may be noted. Blood dyscrasias and jaundice are potential late manifestations of overdosage.

General principles of treatment include the institution of gastric lavage or emesis; forcing oral fluids; and the administration of intravenous fluids if urine output is low and renal function is normal. The patient should be monitored with blood counts and appropriate blood chemistries, including electrolytes. If a significant blood dyscrasia or jaundice occurs, specific therapy should be instituted for these complications. Peritoneal dialysis is not effective and hemodialysis is only moderately effective in eliminating sulfamethoxazole.

Chronic: Use of sulfamethoxazole at high doses and/or for extended periods of time may cause bone marrow depression manifested as thrombocytopenia, leukopenia and/or megaloblastic anemia. If signs of bone marrow depression occur, the patient should be given leucovorin 3 to 6 mg intramuscularly daily for 3 days, or as required to restore normal hematopoiesis.

ANIMAL TOXICITY

The oral LD_{50} of sulfamethoxazole is 2300 mg/kg in mice, 3000 mg/kg in rats and >2000 mg/kg in rabbits.

DOSAGE AND ADMINISTRATION

Systemic sulfonamides are contraindicated in infants under 2 months of age, except in the treatment of congenital toxoplasmosis as adjunctive therapy with pyrimethamine.

Continued on next page

Roche Laboratories—Cont.

The usual dosage schedules are as follows:

Infants (2 Months or Older) and Children	Initial Dose (50–60 mg/kg)	Dose Morning and Evening Daily Thereafter (25–30 mg/kg)
20 lbs	1 tablet (0.5 gm)	1/2 tablet (0.25 gm)
40 lbs	2 tablets (1 gm)	1 tablet (0.5 gm)
60 lbs	3 tablets (1.5 gm)	1 1/2 tablets (0.75 gm)
80 lbs	4 tablets (2 gm)	2 tablets (1 gm)

The maximum dose for children should not exceed 75 mg/kg/24 hours.

Adults		
Mild to Moderate Infections	4 tablets (2 gm)	2 tablets (1 gm)

Severe Infections: 4 tablets (2 gm) initially, followed by 2 tablets (1 gm) three times daily thereafter.

Patients with impaired renal function (creatinine clearance below 20 to 30 mL/min) require decreased dosage adjustment.

HOW SUPPLIED

Tablets (pale green, scored), containing 0.5 gm sulfamethoxazole—bottles of 100 (NDC 0004-0010-01); Tel-E-Dose® packages of 100 (NDC 0004-0010-49). Imprint on tablets: GANTANOL® ROCHE.

Revised: March 1994

Shown in Product Identification Guide, page 332

GANTRISIN® ℞

[*găn 'tris-in*]

brand of sulfisoxazole

TABLETS

GANTRISIN® ℞

brand of acetyl sulfisoxazole

PEDIATRIC SUSPENSION AND SYRUP

The following text is complete prescribing information based on official labeling in effect June 1996.

DESCRIPTION

Gantrisin (sulfisoxazole) is an antibacterial sulfonamide available in tablets, pediatric suspension and syrup for oral administration. Each tablet contains 0.5 gm sulfisoxazole with corn starch, gelatin, lactose and magnesium stearate. Each teaspoonful (5 mL) of the pediatric suspension contains the equivalent of approximately 0.5 gm sulfisoxazole in the form of acetyl sulfisoxazole in a vehicle containing 0.3% alcohol, carboxymethylcellulose (sodium), citric acid, methylcellulose, parabens (methyl and propyl), partial invert sugar, sodium citrate, sorbitan monolaurate, sucrose, flavors and water. Each teaspoonful (5 mL) of the syrup contains the equivalent of approximately 0.5 gm sulfisoxazole in the form of acetyl sulfisoxazole in a vehicle containing 0.9% alcohol, benzoic acid, carrageenan, citric acid, cocoa, sodium citrate, sorbitan monolaurate, sucrose, flavors and water.

Sulfisoxazole is N^1-(3,4-dimethyl-5-isoxazolyl)sulfanilamide. It is a white to slightly yellowish, odorless, slightly bitter, crystalline powder that is soluble in alcohol and very slightly soluble in water. Sulfisoxazole has a molecular weight of 267.30.

Acetyl sulfisoxazole, the tasteless form of sulfisoxazole, is N^1-acetyl sulfisoxazole and must be distinguished from N^4-acetyl sulfisoxazole, which is a metabolite of sulfisoxazole. Acetyl sulfisoxazole is a white or slightly yellow, crystalline powder that is slightly soluble in alcohol and practically insoluble in water. Acetyl sulfisoxazole has a molecular weight of 309.34.

CLINICAL PHARMACOLOGY

Following oral administration, sulfisoxazole is rapidly and completely absorbed; the small intestine is the major site of absorption, but some of the drug is absorbed from the stomach. Sulfonamides are present in the blood as free, conjugated (acetylated and possibly other forms) and protein-bound forms. The amount present as "free" drug is considered to be the therapeutically active form. Approximately 85% of a dose of sulfisoxazole is bound to plasma proteins, primarily to albumin; 65% to 72% of the unbound portion is in the nonacetylated form.

Maximum plasma concentrations of intact sulfisoxazole following a single 2-gm oral dose of sulfisoxazole to healthy adult volunteers ranged from 127 to 211 mcg/mL (mean, 169 mcg/mL) and the time of peak plasma concentration ranged from 1 to 4 hours (mean, 2.5 hours). The elimination half-life of sulfisoxazole ranged from 4.6 to 7.8 hours after oral administration. The elimination of sulfisoxazole has been shown to be slower in elderly subjects (63 to 75 years) with diminished renal function (creatinine clearance, 37 to 68 mL/min).[1] After multiple-dose oral administration of 500 mg q.i.d. to healthy volunteers, the average steady-state plasma concentrations of intact sulfisoxazole ranged from 49.9 to 88.8 mcg/mL (mean, 63.4 mcg/mL).[2]

Wide variation in blood levels may result following identical doses of a sulfonamide. Blood levels should be measured in patients receiving sulfonamides at the higher recommended doses or being treated for serious infections. Free sulfonamide blood levels of 50 to 150 mcg/mL may be considered therapeutically effective for most infections, with blood levels of 120 to 150 mcg/mL being optimal for serious infections. The maximum sulfonamide level should not exceed 200 mcg/mL, since adverse reactions occur more frequently above this concentration.

N^1-acetyl sulfisoxazole is metabolized to sulfisoxazole by digestive enzymes in the gastrointestinal tract and is absorbed as sulfisoxazole. This enzymatic splitting is presumed to be responsible for slower absorption and lower peak blood concentrations than are attained following administration of an equal oral dose of sulfisoxazole. With continued administration of acetyl sulfisoxazole, blood concentrations approximate those of sulfisoxazole. Following a single 4-gm dose of acetyl sulfisoxazole to healthy volunteers, maximum plasma concentrations of sulfisoxazole ranged from 122 to 282 mcg/mL (mean, 181 mcg/mL) for the pediatric suspension and from 101 to 202 mcg/mL (mean, 144 mcg/mL) for the syrup, and occurred between 2 and 6 hours postadministration. The half-lives of elimination from plasma ranged from 5.4 to 7.4 and from 5.9 to 8.5 hours, respectively.

Sulfisoxazole and its acetylated metabolites are excreted primarily by the kidneys through glomerular filtration. Concentrations of sulfisoxazole are considerably higher in the urine than in the blood. The mean urinary excretion recovery following oral administration of sulfisoxazole is 97% within 48 hours, of which 52% is intact drug, with the remaining as the N^4-acetylated metabolite. Following administration of acetyl sulfisoxazole syrup or suspension, approximately 58% is excreted in the urine as total drug within 72 hours.

Sulfisoxazole is distributed only in extracellular body fluid. It is excreted in human milk. It readily crosses the placental barrier and enters into fetal circulation and also crosses the blood-brain barrier. In healthy subjects, cerebrospinal fluid concentrations of sulfisoxazole vary; in patients with meningitis, however, concentrations of free drug in cerebrospinal fluid as high as 94 mcg/mL have been reported.

Microbiology: The sulfonamides are bacteriostatic agents and the spectrum of activity is similar for all. Sulfonamides inhibit bacterial synthesis of dihydrofolic acid by preventing the condensation of the pteridine with aminobenzoic acid through competitive inhibition of the enzyme dihydropteroate synthetase. Resistant strains have altered dihydropteroate synthetase with reduced affinity for sulfonamides or produce increased quantities of aminobenzoic acid.

Susceptibility Tests: *Diffusion Techniques:* Quantitative methods that require measurement of zone diameters give the most precise estimate of the susceptibility of bacteria to antimicrobial agents. One such standard procedure[3] which has been recommended for use with disks to test susceptibility of organisms to sulfisoxazole uses the 250- or 300-mcg sulfisoxazole disk. Interpretation involves the correlation of the diameter obtained in the disk test with the minimum inhibitory concentration (MIC) for sulfisoxazole.

Reports from the laboratory giving results of the standard single-disk susceptibility test with a 250- or 300-mcg sulfisoxazole disk should be interpreted according to the following criteria:

Zone Diameter (mm)	Interpretation
≥17	Susceptible
13–16	Moderately susceptible
≤12	Resistant

A report of "susceptible" indicates that the pathogen is likely to be inhibited by generally achievable blood levels. A report of "moderately susceptible" suggests that the organism would be susceptible if high dosage is used or if the infection is confined to tissues and fluids in which high antimicrobial levels are attained. A report of "resistant" indicates that achievable concentrations are unlikely to be inhibitory, and other therapy should be selected.

Standardized procedures require the use of laboratory control organisms. The 250- or 300-mcg sulfisoxazole disk should give the following zone diameters:

Organism	Zone Diameter (mm)
E. coli ATCC 25922	18–26 mm
S. aureus ATCC 25923	24–34 mm

Dilution Techniques: Use a standardized dilution method[4] (broth, agar, microdilution) or equivalent with sulfisoxazole powder. The MIC values obtained should be interpreted according to the following criteria:

MIC (mcg/mL)	Interpretation
≤256	Susceptible
≥512	Resistant

As with standard diffusion techniques, dilution methods require the use of laboratory control organisms. Dilutions of standard sulfisoxazole powder should provide the following MIC values:

Organism	MIC (mcg/mL)
S. aureus ATCC 29213	32–128
E. faecalis ATCC 29212	32–128
E. coli ATCC 25922	8–32

INDICATIONS AND USAGE

Acute, recurrent or chronic urinary tract infections (primarily pyelonephritis, pyelitis and cystitis) due to susceptible organisms (usually *Escherichia coli, Klebsiella-Enterobacter,* staphylococcus, *Proteus mirabilis* and, less frequently, *Proteus vulgaris*) in the absence of obstructive uropathy or foreign bodies.

Meningococcal meningitis where the organism has been demonstrated to be susceptible. *Haemophilus influenzae* meningitis as adjunctive therapy with parenteral streptomycin.

Meningococcal meningitis prophylaxis when sulfonamide-sensitive group A strains are known to prevail in family groups or larger closed populations. (The prophylactic usefulness of sulfonamides when group B or C infections are prevalent has not been proven and in closed population groups may be harmful.)

Acute otitis media due to *Haemophilus influenzae* when used concomitantly with adequate doses of penicillin or erythromycin (see appropriate labeling for prescribing information).

Trachoma. Inclusion conjunctivitis. Nocardiosis. Chancroid.

Toxoplasmosis as adjunctive therapy with pyrimethamine.

Malaria due to chloroquine-resistant strains of *Plasmodium falciparum,* when used as adjunctive therapy.

Currently, the increasing frequency of resistant organisms is a limitation of the usefulness of antibacterial agents including the sulfonamides, especially in the treatment of chronic and recurrent urinary tract infections.

Important Note: In vitro sulfonamide susceptibility tests are not always reliable. The test must be carefully coordinated with bacteriologic and clinical response. When the patient is already taking sulfonamides, follow-up cultures should have aminobenzoic acid added to the culture media.

CONTRAINDICATIONS

Gantrisin is contraindicated in the following patient populations: patients with a known hypersensitivity to sulfonamides; children younger than 2 months (except in the treatment of congenital toxoplasmosis as adjunctive therapy with pyrimethamine); pregnant women *at term;* and mothers nursing infants less than 2 months of age.

Use in pregnant women at term, in children less than 2 months of age and in mothers nursing infants less than 2 months of age is contraindicated because sulfonamides may promote kernicterus in the newborn by displacing bilirubin from plasma proteins.

WARNINGS

FATALITIES ASSOCIATED WITH THE ADMINISTRATION OF SULFONAMIDES, ALTHOUGH RARE, HAVE OCCURRED DUE TO SEVERE REACTIONS, INCLUDING STEVENS-JOHNSON SYNDROME, TOXIC EPIDERMAL NECROLYSIS, FULMINANT HEPATIC NECROSIS, AGRANULOCYTOSIS, APLASTIC ANEMIA AND OTHER BLOOD DYSCRASIAS.

SULFONAMIDES, INCLUDING SULFISOXAZOLE, SHOULD BE DISCONTINUED AT THE FIRST APPEARANCE OF SKIN RASH OR ANY SIGN OF AN ADVERSE REACTION. In rare instances, a skin rash may be followed by more severe reactions such as Stevens-Johnson syndrome, toxic epidermal necrolysis, hepatic necrosis and serious blood disorders. (See PRECAUTIONS.)

Clinical signs such as rash, sore throat, fever, arthralgia, pallor, purpura or jaundice may be early indications of serious reactions.

Cough, shortness of breath and pulmonary infiltrates are hypersensitivity reactions of the respiratory tract that have been reported in association with sulfonamide treatment.

The sulfonamides should not be used for the treatment of group A beta-hemolytic streptococcal infections. In an established infection, they will not eradicate the streptococcus and, therefore, will not prevent sequelae such as rheumatic fever.

Pseudomembranous colitis has been reported with nearly all antibacterial agents, including sulfisoxazole, and may range in severity from mild to life-threatening. Therefore, it is important to consider this diagnosis in patients who present with diarrhea subsequent to the administration of antibacterial agents.

Treatment with antibacterial agents alters the normal flora of the colon and may permit overgrowth of clostridia. Studies

indicate that toxin produced by *Clostridium difficile* is one primary cause of "antibiotic-associated colitis."

After the diagnosis of pseudomembranous colitis has been established, therapeutic measures should be initiated. Mild cases of pseudomembranous colitis usually respond to drug discontinuation alone. In moderate to severe cases, consideration should be given to management with fluids and electrolytes, protein supplementation, and treatment with an antibacterial drug clinically effective against *C. difficile* colitis.

PRECAUTIONS

General: Sulfonamides should be given with caution to patients with impaired renal or hepatic function and to those with severe allergy or bronchial asthma. In glucose-6-phosphate dehydrogenase-deficient individuals, hemolysis may occur; this reaction is frequently dose-related.

The frequency of resistant organisms limits the usefulness of antibacterial agents, including the sulfonamides, as sole therapy in the treatment of urinary tract infections. Since sulfonamides are bacteriostatic and not bactericidal, a complete course of therapy is needed to prevent immediate regrowth and the development of resistant uropathogens.

Information for Patients: Patients should maintain an adequate fluid intake to prevent crystalluria and stone formation.

Laboratory Tests: Complete blood counts should be done frequently in patients receiving sulfonamides. If a significant reduction in the count of any formed blood element is noted, sulfonamide therapy should be discontinued. Urinalyses with careful microscopic examination and renal function tests should be performed during therapy, particularly for those patients with impaired renal function. Blood levels should be measured in patients receiving a sulfonamide for serious infections. (See INDICATIONS AND USAGE.)

Drug Interactions: It has been reported that sulfisoxazole may prolong the prothrombin time in patients who are receiving anticoagulants, including warfarin. This interaction should be kept in mind when Gantrisin is given to patients already on anticoagulant therapy, and prothrombin time or other suitable coagulation test should be monitored.

It has been proposed that sulfisoxazole competes with thiopental for plasma protein binding. In one study involving 48 patients, intravenous sulfisoxazole resulted in a decrease in the amount of thiopental required for anesthesia and in a shortening of the awakening time. It is not known whether chronic oral doses of sulfisoxazole would have a similar effect. Until more is known about this interaction, physicians should be aware that patients receiving sulfisoxazole might require less thiopental for anesthesia.

Sulfonamides can displace methotrexate from plasma protein-binding sites, thus increasing free methotrexate concentrations. Studies in man have shown sulfisoxazole infusions to decrease plasma protein-bound methotrexate by one-fourth.

Sulfisoxazole can also potentiate the blood sugar lowering activity of sulfonylureas, as well as cause hypoglycemia by itself.

Carcinogenesis, Mutagenesis, Impairment of Fertility:

Carcinogenesis: Sulfisoxazole was not carcinogenic to mice in either sex when administered by gavage for 103 weeks at dosages up to approximately 18 times the highest recommended human daily dose or to rats at 4 times the highest recommended human daily dose. Rats appear to be especially susceptible to the goitrogenic effects of sulfonamides and long-term administration of sulfonamides has resulted in thyroid malignancies in this species.

Mutagenesis: There are no studies available that adequately evaluate the mutagenic potential of Gantrisin. Ames mutagenic assays have not been performed with sulfisoxazole. However, sulfisoxazole was not observed to be mutagenic in *E. coli* Sd-4-73 when tested in the absence of a metabolic activating system.

Impairment of Fertility: Gantrisin has not undergone adequate trials relating to impairment of fertility. In a reproduction study in rats given 7 times the highest recommended human dose per day of sulfisoxazole, no effects were observed regarding mating behavior, conception rate or fertility index (percent pregnant).

Pregnancy:

Teratogenic Effects: Pregnancy Category C. At dosages 7 times the highest recommended human daily dose, sulfisoxazole was not teratogenic in either rats or rabbits. However, in two other teratogenicity studies, cleft palates developed in both rats and mice, and skeletal defects were also observed in rats after administration of 9 times the highest recommended human daily dose of sulfisoxazole.

There are no adequate and well-controlled studies of Gantrisin in pregnant women. It is not known whether Gantrisin can cause fetal harm when administered to a pregnant woman prior to term or can affect reproduction capacity. Gantrisin should be used during pregnancy only if the potential benefit justifies the potential risk to the fetus.

Nonteratogenic Effects: Kernicterus may occur in the newborn as a result of treatment of a pregnant woman *at term* with sulfonamides. (See CONTRAINDICATIONS.)

Nursing Mothers: Gantrisin is excreted in human milk. Because of the potential for the development of kernicterus in neonates due to the displacement of bilirubin from plasma proteins by sulfisoxazole, a decision should be made whether to discontinue nursing or discontinue the drug taking into account the importance of the drug to the mother. (See CONTRAINDICATIONS.)

Pediatric Use: Gantrisin is not recommended for use in infants younger than 2 months of age except in the treatment of congenital toxoplasmosis as adjunctive therapy with pyrimethamine. (See CONTRAINDICATIONS.)

ADVERSE REACTIONS

The listing that follows includes adverse reactions both that have been reported with Gantrisin and some which have not been reported with this specific drug; however, the pharmacologic similarities among the sulfonamides require that each of the reactions be considered with the administration of any of the Gantrisin dosage forms.

Allergic/Dermatologic: Anaphylaxis, erythema multiforme (Stevens-Johnson syndrome), toxic epidermal necrolysis, exfoliative dermatitis, angioedema, arteritis and vasculitis, allergic myocarditis, serum sickness, rash, urticaria, pruritus, photosensitivity, and conjunctival and scleral injection, generalized allergic reactions and generalized skin eruptions. In addition, periarteritis nodosa and systemic lupus erythematosus have been reported. (See WARNINGS.)

Cardiovascular: Tachycardia, palpitations, syncope, cyanosis.

Endocrine: The sulfonamides bear certain chemical similarities to some goitrogens, diuretics (acetazolamide and thiazides) and oral hypoglycemia agents. Cross-sensitivity may exist with these agents. Development of goiter, diuresis and hypoglycemia have occurred rarely in patients receiving sulfonamides.

Gastrointestinal: Hepatitis, hepatocellular necrosis, jaundice, pseudomembranous colitis, nausea, emesis, anorexia, abdominal pain, diarrhea, gastrointestinal hemorrhage, melena, flatulence, glossitis, stomatitis, salivary gland enlargement, pancreatitis.

Onset of pseudomembranous colitis symptoms may occur during or after treatment with sulfisoxazole. (See WARNINGS.)

Sulfisoxazole has been reported to cause increased elevations of liver-associated enzymes in patients with hepatitis.

Genitourinary: Crystalluria, hematuria, BUN and creatinine elevations, nephritis and toxic nephrosis with oliguria and anuria. Acute renal failure and urinary retention have also been reported. The frequency of renal complications, commonly associated with some sulfonamides, is lower in patients receiving the more soluble sulfonamides such as sulfisoxazole.

Hematologic: Leukopenia, agranulocytosis, aplastic anemia, thrombocytopenia, purpura, hemolyticanemia, anemia, eosinophilia, clotting disorders including hypoprothombinemia, and hypofibrinogenemia, sulfhemoglobinemia, methemoglobinemia.

Musculoskeletal: Arthralgia, myalgia.

Neurologic: Headache, dizziness, peripheral neuritis, paresthesia, convulsions, tinnitus, vertigo, ataxia, intracranial hypertension.

Psychiatric: Psychosis, hallucination, disorientation, depression, anxiety, apathy.

Respiratory: Cough, shortness of breath, pulmonary infiltrates. (See WARNINGS.)

Vascular: Angioedema, arteritis, vasculitis.

Miscellaneous: Edema (including periorbital), pyrexia, drowsiness, weakness, fatigue, lassitude, rigors, flushing, hearing loss, insomnia, pneumonitis, chills.

OVERDOSAGE

The amount of a single dose of sulfisoxazole that is associated with symptoms of overdosage or is likely to be life-threatening has not been reported. Signs and symptoms of overdosage reported with sulfonamides include anorexia, colic, nausea, vomiting, dizziness, headache, drowsiness and unconsciousness. Pyrexia, hematuria and crystalluria may be noted. Blood dyscrasias and jaundice are potential late manifestations of overdosage.

General principles of treatment include the immediate discontinuation of the drug; institution of gastric lavage or emesis; forcing oral fluids; and the administration of intravenous fluids if urine output is low and renal function is normal. The patient should be monitored with blood counts and appropriate blood chemistries, including electrolytes. If the patient becomes cyanotic, the possibility of methemoglobinemia should be considered and, if present, the condition should be treated appropriately with intravenous 1% methylene blue. If a significant blood dyscrasia or jaundice occurs, specific therapy should be instituted for these complications.

Peritoneal dialysis is not effective and hemodialysis is only moderately effective in eliminating sulfonamides.

DOSAGE AND ADMINISTRATION

Systemic sulfonamides are contraindicated in infants under 2 months of age, except in the treatment of congenital toxoplasmosis as adjunctive therapy with pyrimethamine.

Usual Dose for Infants over 2 Months of Age and Children: Initial dose: One half of the 24-hour dose. Maintenance dose: 150 mg/kg/24 hours or 4 gm/M^2/24 hours—dose to be divided into 4 to 6 doses/24 hours. The maximum dose should not exceed 6 gm/24 hours.

Usual Adult Dose: Initial dose: 2 to 4 gm. Maintenance dose: 4 to 8 gm/24 hours, divided in 4 to 6 doses/24 hours.

HOW SUPPLIED

Tablets (white, scored), containing 0.5 gm sulfisoxazole—bottles of 100 (NDC 0004-0009-01) and 500 (NDC 0004-0009-14); Tel-E-Dose® packages of 100 (NDC 0004-0009-49). Imprint on tablets: ROCHE GANTRISIN®.

Pediatric Suspension (raspberry flavored), containing acetyl sulfisoxazole equivalent to approximately 0.5 gm sulfisoxazole per teaspoonful (5 mL)—bottles of 4 oz (NDC 0004-1003-30) and 16 oz (1 pint) (NDC 0004-1003-28).

Syrup (chocolate flavored), containing acetyl sulfisoxazole equivalent to approximately 0.5 gm sulfisoxazole per teaspoonful (5 mL)—bottles of 16 oz (1 pint) (NDC 0004-1004-28).

REFERENCES

1. Boisvert A, Barbeau G, Belanger PM. Pharmacokinetics of sulfisoxazole in young and elderly subjects. *Gerontology.* 1984;30:125–131.
2. Oie S, Gambertoglio JG, Fleckenstein L. Comparison of the disposition of total and unbound sulfisoxazole after single and multiple dosing. *J Pharmacokinet Biopharm.* 1982;10:157–172.
3. National Committee for Clinical Laboratory Standards. *Performance Standards for Antimicrobial Disk Susceptibility Tests.* 4th ed. Villanova, PA: April 1990. Approved Standard NCCLS Document M2-A4, Vol. 10, No. 7 NCCLS.
4. National Committee for Clinical Laboratory Standards. *Methods for Dilution Antimicrobial Susceptibility Tests for Bacteria that Grow Aerobically.* 2nd ed. Villanova, PA: April 1990. Approved Standard NCCLS Document M7-A2, Vol. 10, No. 8 NCCLS.

Revised: April 1993

HIVID® ℞

[*hiv′id*]

(zalcitabine)

TABLETS

WARNING

THE USE OF HIVID HAS BEEN ASSOCIATED WITH SIGNIFICANT CLINICAL ADVERSE REACTIONS, SOME OF WHICH ARE POTENTIALLY FATAL. HIVID CAN CAUSE SEVERE PERIPHERAL NEUROPATHY AND BECAUSE OF THIS SHOULD BE USED WITH EXTREME CAUTION IN PATIENTS WITH PREEXISTING NEUROPATHY. HIVID MAY ALSO RARELY CAUSE PANCREATITIS AND PATIENTS WHO DEVELOP ANY SYMPTOMS SUGGESTIVE OF PANCREATITIS WHILE USING HIVID SHOULD HAVE THERAPY SUSPENDED IMMEDIATELY UNTIL THIS DIAGNOSIS IS EXCLUDED.

RARE OCCURRENCES OF POTENTIALLY FATAL LACTIC ACIDOSIS IN THE ABSENCE OF HYPOXEMIA AND SEVERE HEPATOMEGALY WITH STEATOSIS HAVE BEEN REPORTED WITH THE USE OF NUCLEOSIDE ANALOGUES, INCLUDING ZIDOVUDINE AND HIVID. IN ADDITION, RARE CASES OF HEPATIC FAILURE AND DEATH CONSIDERED POSSIBLY RELATED TO UNDERLYING HEPATITIS B AND HIVID MONOTHERAPY HAVE BEEN REPORTED (SEE WARNINGS AND PRECAUTIONS).

DESCRIPTION

HIVID is the Hoffmann-La Roche brand of zalcitabine [formerly called 2′,3′-dideoxycytidine (ddC)], a synthetic pyrimidine nucleoside analogue active against the human immunodeficiency virus (HIV). HIVID is available as film-coated tablets for oral administration in strengths of 0.375 mg and 0.750 mg. Each tablet also contains the inactive ingredients lactose, microcrystalline cellulose, croscarmellose sodium, magnesium stearate, hydroxypropyl methylcellulose, polyethylene glycol and polysorbate 80 along with the following colorant system: 0.375 mg tablet—synthetic brown, black, red and yellow iron oxides, and titanium dioxide; 0.750 mg tablet—synthetic black iron oxide and titanium dioxide. The chemical name for zalcitabine is 4-amino-1-beta-D-2′,3′-dideoxyribofuranosyl-2-(1H)-pyrimidone or 2′,3′-dideoxycytidine with the molecular formula $C_9H_{13}N_3O_3$ and a molecular weight of 211.22.

Zalcitabine is a white to off-white crystalline powder with an aqueous solubility of 76.4 mg/mL at 25°C.

Continued on next page

Roche Laboratories—Cont.

MICROBIOLOGY

Mechanism of Action: Zalcitabine is a synthetic nucleoside analogue of the naturally occurring nucleoside deoxycytidine, in which the 3′-hydroxyl group is replaced by hydrogen. Within cells, zalcitabine is converted to the active metabolite, dideoxycytidine 5′-triphosphate (ddCTP), by the sequential action of cellular enzymes. Dideoxycytidine 5′-triphosphate inhibits the activity of the HIV-reverse transcriptase both by competing for utilization of the natural substrate, deoxycytidine 5′-triphosphate (dCTP), and by its incorporation into viral DNA. The lack of a 3′-OH group in the incorporated nucleoside analogue prevents the formation of the 5′ to 3′ phosphodiester linkage essential for DNA chain elongation and, therefore, the viral DNA growth is terminated. The active metabolite, ddCTP, is also an inhibitor of cellular DNA polymerase-beta and mitochondrial DNA polymerase-gamma and has been reported to be incorporated into the DNA of cells in culture.

In Vitro HIV Susceptibility: The in vitro anti-HIV activity of zalcitabine was assessed by infecting cell lines of lymphoblastic and monocytic origin and peripheral blood lymphocytes with laboratory and clinical isolates of HIV. The IC50 and IC95 values (50% and 95% inhibitory concentration) were in the range of 30 to 500 nM and 100 to 1000 nM, respectively (1 nM = 0.21 ng/mL). Zalcitabine showed antiviral activity in all acute infections; however, activity was substantially less in chronically infected cells. In drug combination studies with zidovudine (ZDV) or saquinavir, zalcitabine showed additive to synergistic activity in cell culture. The relationship between the in vitro susceptibility of HIV to reverse-transcriptase inhibitors and the inhibition of HIV replication in humans has not been established.

Drug Resistance: HIV isolates with a reduction in sensitivity to zalcitabine (ddC) have been isolated from a small number of patients treated with HIVID by 1 year of therapy. Genetic analysis of these isolates showed point mutations (Lys 65 Arg or Asn, Thr 69 Asp, Leu 74 Val, Val 75 Thr or Ala, Met 184 Val or Tyr 215 Cys) in the pol gene that encodes for the reverse transcriptase. Combination therapy with HIVID and ZDV does not appear to prevent the emergence of zidovudine-resistant isolates.

Cross-resistance: The potential for cross-resistance between HIV-reverse transcriptase inhibitors and HIV-protease inhibitors is low because of the different enzyme targets involved. The point mutation at position 69 appears to be specific to ddC in its selection and effect. Additionally, the point mutations at positions 65, 74, 75 and 184 are associated with resistance to didanosine (ddI), that at position 75 with resistance to stavudine (d4T), and those at positions 65 (Lys to Arg) and 184 (Met to Val) with resistance to lamivudine (3TC). HIV isolates with multidrug resistance to ZDV, ddI, ddC, d4T and 3TC were recovered from a small number of patients treated for 1 year with the combination of ZDV, ddI or ddC. The pattern of resistance mutations in the combination therapy was different (Ala 62 Val, Val 75 Ile, Phe 77 Leu, Phe 116 Tyr and Gln 151 Met) from monotherapy with mutation 151 being most significant for multidrug resistance.

CLINICAL PHARMACOLOGY

Pharmacokinetics: The pharmacokinetics of zalcitabine has been evaluated in studies in HIV-infected patients following 0.01 mg/kg, 0.03 mg/kg and 1.5 mg oral doses, and a 1.5 mg intravenous dose administered as a 1-hour infusion.

Absorption and Bioavailability in Adults: Following oral administration to HIV-infected patients, the mean absolute bioavailability of zalcitabine was >80% (30% CV, range 23% to 124%, n=19). The absorption rate of a 1.5 mg oral dose of zalcitabine (n=20) was reduced when administered with food. This resulted in a 39% decrease in mean maximum plasma concentrations (C_{max}) from 25.2 ng/mL (35% CV, range 11.6 to 37.5 ng/mL) to 15.5 ng/mL (24% CV, range 9.1 to 23.7 ng/mL), and a twofold increase in time to achieve maximum plasma concentrations from a mean of 0.8 hours under fasting conditions to 1.6 hours when the drug was given with food. The extent of absorption (as reflected by AUC) was decreased by 14%, from 72 ng·hr/mL (28% CV, range 43 to 119 ng·hr/mL) to 62 ng·hr/mL (23% CV, range 42 to 91 ng·hr/mL). The clinical relevance of these decreases is unknown. Absorption of zalcitabine does not appear to be reduced in patients with diarrhea not caused by an identified pathogen.

Distribution in Adults: The steady-state volume of distribution following intravenous administration of a 1.5 mg dose of zalcitabine averaged 0.534 (± 0.127) L/kg (24% CV, range 0.304 to 0.734 L/kg, n=20). Cerebrospinal fluid obtained from 9 patients at 2 to 3.5 hours following 0.06 mg/kg or 0.09 mg/kg intravenous infusion showed measurable concentrations of zalcitabine. The CSF:plasma concentration ratio ranged from 9% to 37% (mean 20%), demonstrating penetration of the drug through the blood-brain barrier. The clinical relevance of these ratios has not been evaluated.

Metabolism and Elimination in Adults: Zalcitabine is phosphorylated intracellularly to zalcitabine triphosphate, the active substrate for HIV-reverse transcriptase. Concentrations of zalcitabine triphosphate are too low for quantitation following administration of therapeutic doses to humans.

Zalcitabine does not undergo a significant degree of metabolism by the liver. The primary metabolite of zalcitabine that has been identified is dideoxyuridine (ddU), which accounts for less than 15% of an oral dose in both urine and feces (n=4). Approximately 10% of an orally administered radiolabeled dose of zalcitabine appears in the feces (n=10), comprised primarily of unchanged drug and ddU. Renal excretion of unchanged drug appears to be the primary route of elimination, accounting for approximately 80% of an intravenous dose and 60% of an orally administered dose within 24 hours after dosing (n=19). The mean elimination half-life is 2 hours and generally ranges from 1 to 3 hours in individual patients. Total clearance following an intravenous dose averaged 285 mL/min (29% CV, range 165 to 447 mL/min, n=20). Renal clearance averaged approximately 235 mL/min or about 80% of total clearance (30% CV, range 129 to 348 mL/min, n=20). Renal clearance exceeds glomerular filtration rate suggesting renal tubular secretion contributes to the elimination of zalcitabine by the kidneys.

In patients with impaired kidney function, prolonged elimination of zalcitabine may be expected. Preliminary results from 7 patients with renal impairment (estimated creatinine clearance <55 mL/min) indicate that the half-life was prolonged (up to 8.5 hours) in these patients compared to those with normal renal function. Maximum plasma concentrations were higher in some patients after a single dose (see PRECAUTIONS).

In patients with normal renal function, the pharmacokinetics of zalcitabine was not altered during 3 times daily multiple dosing (n=9). Accumulation of drug in plasma during this regimen was negligible. The drug was <4% bound to plasma proteins, indicating that drug interactions involving binding-site displacement are unlikely (see *Drug Interactions*).

Drug Interactions: *Zidovudine:* There was no significant pharmacokinetic interaction between zidovudine and zalcitabine when single doses of zalcitabine (1.5 mg) and zidovudine (200 mg) were coadministered to 12 HIV-positive patients.

Probenecid: Following administration of a single oral 1.5 mg dose of zalcitabine alone during probenecid treatment (500 mg at 8 and 2 hours before and 4 hours after zalcitabine dosing) to 12 HIV-positive patients, mean renal clearance decreased from 310 mL/min (28% CV) to 180 mL/min (22% CV) and AUC increased from 59 ng·hr/mL (27% CV) to 91 ng·hr/mL (22% CV), indicating an increase in exposure of approximately 50% to zalcitabine. Mean half-life of zalcitabine increased from 1.7 to 2.5 hours (see PRECAUTIONS).

Cimetidine: Administration of a single dose of 1.5 mg zalcitabine with a single dose of 800 mg cimetidine to 12 HIV-positive patients resulted in a decrease in renal clearance from 224 mL/min (27% CV) to 171 mL/min (39% CV) and an increase in AUC from 75 ng·hr/mL (29% CV) to 102 ng·hr/mL (35% CV) (see PRECAUTIONS) indicating an increase in exposure of approximately 36% to zalcitabine.

Maalox: Concomitant administration of Maalox TC (30 mL) with single dose of 1.5 mg zalcitabine to 12 HIV-positive patients resulted in a decrease in mean C_{max} from 25.2 ng/mL (28% CV) to 18.4 ng/mL (34% CV) and AUC from 75 ng·hr/mL (29% CV, n=10) to 58 ng·hr/mL (36% CV, n=10) indicating a decrease in bioavailability of approximately 25% to zalcitabine (see PRECAUTIONS).

Metoclopramide: Administration of a single dose of 1.5 mg zalcitabine with 20 mg metoclopramide (10 mg 1 hour before and 10 mg 4 hours after zalcitabine dose) to 12 HIV-positive patients resulted in a decrease in AUC from 69 ng·hr/mL (16% CV) to 62 ng·hr/mL (21% CV) indicating a decrease in bioavailability of approximately 10% (see PRECAUTIONS).

Loperamide: Administration of a single dose of 1.5 mg zalcitabine during loperamide treatment (4 mg 16 hours before zalcitabine, 2 mg at 10 and 4 hours before zalcitabine and 2 mg 2 hours after the zalcitabine dose) to 12 HIV-positive patients with diarrhea resulted in no significant pharmacokinetic interaction between zalcitabine and loperamide.

Pharmacokinetics in Children: For pharmacokinetic properties in children, see PRECAUTIONS: *Pediatric Use.* Limited pharmacokinetic data have been reported for 5 HIV-positive children using doses of 0.03 and 0.04 mg/kg HIVID administered orally every 6 hours.[1] The mean bioavailability of zalcitabine in these children was 54% and mean apparent systemic clearance was 150 mL/min/m^2. Due to the small number of subjects and different analytical techniques, it is difficult to make comparisons between pediatric and adult data.

INDICATIONS AND USAGE

Combination Therapy: HIVID in combination with zidovudine is indicated for the treatment of HIV infection in patients with limited prior exposure to zidovudine (<3 months). This indication is based on study results showing a reduction in the rate of disease progression (AIDS-defining events or death) in patients with limited prior antiretroviral therapy who were treated with the combination of HIVID and zidovudine (see *Description of Clinical Studies*). HIVID is also indicated in combination with protease inhibitors for the treatment of HIV based on studies showing greater changes in surrogate markers in regimens when HIVID was initiated concomitantly with a protease inhibitor.

HIVID Monotherapy: HIVID is indicated for the treatment of HIV infection in patients with advanced HIV disease who are intolerant to or who have disease progression while receiving alternative antiretroviral therapy (see *Description of Clinical Studies*).

The duration of clinical benefit from antiretroviral therapy may be limited. Alterations in antiretroviral therapy should be considered if disease progression occurs during treatment.

Description of Clinical Studies: *Combination Therapy:* The use of HIVID in combination with zidovudine is based on the clinical results from study ACTG 175. ACTG 175 was a randomized, double-blind, controlled trial that compared zidovudine 200 mg tid; didanosine 200 mg bid; zidovudine+didanosine; and zidovudine+HIVID 0.750 mg tid. A total of 2467 HIV-infected adults (mean baseline CD4 count = 352 cells/mm^3) with no prior AIDS-defining event enrolled with the following demographics: male (82%), Caucasian (70%), mean age of 35 years, asymptomatic HIV infection (81%) and prior antiretroviral use (57%, mean duration = 89.5 weeks). The overall mean duration of study treatment was 99 weeks. The incidence of AIDS-defining events or death is shown in the following table:

[See table at left.]

HIVID Monotherapy: The indication for HIVID use as monotherapy is based on the results of CPCRA 002, a randomized, multicenter, open-label study in which HIVID was compared to ddI as treatment for patients with advanced HIV infection (median CD4 cell count = 37 cells/mm^3) who were clinically intolerant to ZDV, or who had met criteria for having disease progression while receiving ZDV.[2] Patients in this study had a mean of 17.5 months of prior ZDV use. The median duration of treatment for both HIVID and ddI was 34 weeks. The results demonstrate that HIVID was at least as efficacious as ddI in terms of time to an AIDS-defining event or death, while for survival alone the results favored HIVID. However, most of the patients (66%) in either group had disease progression over the median 16 months of follow-up. Overall rates of study drug intolerance, discontinuation and adverse events were similar for the two groups, although the types of events were different.

A clinical study (N3300/ACTG 114) has demonstrated ZDV to be superior to HIVID as monotherapy for advanced HIV disease (CD4 cell count ≤200 cells/mm^3) in previously untreated patients.[3,4] The final analysis of this study indicated that 134 patients (42%) in the HIVID group with a median follow-up of 85 weeks and 120 patients (38%) in the ZDV

Table 1. First AIDS-defining Event or Death and Death Only by Study Arm and Antiretroviral Experience in ACTG 175

Antiretroviral Experience	Event	Treatment: zidovudine	zidovudine+ didanosine	zidovudine+ HIVID	didanosine
	n	619	613	615	620
Overall	AIDS/Death	96 (16%)	65 (11%)	76 (12%)	71 (11%)
	Death Only	54 (9%)	31 (5%)	40 (7%)	29 (5%)
	n	269	263	267	268
Naive	AIDS/Death	32 (12%)	20 (8%)	16 (6%)	23 (9%)
	Death Only	18 (7%)	11 (4%)	9 (3%)	11 (4%)
	n	350	350	348	352
Experienced	AIDS/Death	64 (18%)	45 (13%)	60 (17%)	48 (14%)
	Death Only	36 (10%)	20 (6%)	31 (9%)	18 (5%)

group with a median follow-up of 96 weeks died with a relative risk for mortality of ZDV to HIVID of 0.54.

CONTRAINDICATIONS

HIVID is contraindicated in patients with clinically significant hypersensitivity to zalcitabine or to any of the excipients contained in the tablets.

WARNINGS

SIGNIFICANT CLINICAL ADVERSE REACTIONS, SOME OF WHICH ARE POTENTIALLY FATAL, HAVE BEEN REPORTED WITH HIVID MONOTHERAPY AND WITH HIVID IN COMBINATION WITH ZIDOVUDINE. PATIENTS WITH DECREASED CD4 CELL COUNTS APPEAR TO HAVE AN INCREASED INCIDENCE OF ADVERSE EVENTS.

1. Peripheral Neuropathy:

THE MAJOR CLINICAL TOXICITY OF HIVID IS PERIPHERAL NEUROPATHY, WHICH MAY OCCUR IN UP TO 1/3 OF PATIENTS WITH ADVANCED DISEASE TREATED WITH HIVID. The incidence in patients with less-advanced disease is lower.

HIVID-related peripheral neuropathy is a sensorimotor neuropathy characterized initially by numbness and burning dysesthesia involving the distal extremities. These symptoms may be followed by sharp shooting pains or severe continuous burning pain if the drug is not withdrawn. The neuropathy may progress to severe pain requiring narcotic analgesics and is potentially irreversible. In some patients, symptoms of neuropathy may initially progress despite discontinuation of HIVID. With prompt discontinuation of HIVID, the neuropathy is usually slowly reversible.

There are no data regarding the use of HIVID in patients with preexisting peripheral neuropathy since these patients were excluded from clinical trials; therefore, HIVID should be used with extreme caution in these patients. Individuals with moderate or severe peripheral neuropathy, as evidenced by symptoms accompanied by objective findings, are advised to avoid HIVID.

HIVID should be stopped promptly when moderate discomfort from numbness, tingling, burning or pain of the extremities progresses, or any related symptoms occur that are accompanied by an objective finding.

2. Pancreatitis:

PANCREATITIS, WHICH HAS BEEN FATAL IN SOME CASES, HAS BEEN OBSERVED WITH THE ADMINISTRATION OF HIVID ALONE OR THE COMBINATION OF HIVID WITH ZIDOVUDINE. Pancreatitis is an uncommon complication of HIVID monotherapy or in combination with zidovudine, occurring in up to 1.1% of patients. The occurrence of asymptomatic elevated serum amylase of any etiology while on HIVID monotherapy was 1.6%.

Patients with a history of pancreatitis or known risk factors for the development of pancreatitis should be followed more closely while on HIVID therapy. Of 528 HIVID-treated patients enrolled in an expanded-access safety study (N3544), who had a history of prior pancreatitis or increased amylase, 28 (5.3%) developed pancreatitis and an additional 23 (4.4%) developed asymptomatic elevated serum amylase.

Treatment with HIVID monotherapy or HIVID in combination with zidovudine should be stopped immediately if clinical signs or symptoms (nausea, vomiting, abdominal pain) or if abnormalities in laboratory values (hyperamylasemia associated with dysglycemia, rising triglyceride level, decreasing serum calcium) suggestive of pancreatitis should occur. If clinical pancreatitis develops during HIVID administration, it is recommended that HIVID be permanently discontinued. Treatment with HIVID should also be interrupted if treatment with another drug known to cause pancreatitis (eg, intravenous pentamidine) is required (see *Drug Interactions*).

3. Hepatic Toxicity:

RARE OCCURRENCES OF POTENTIALLY FATAL LACTIC ACIDOSIS IN THE ABSENCE OF HYPOXEMIA AND SEVERE HEPATOMEGALY WITH STEATOSIS HAVE BEEN REPORTED WITH THE USE OF NUCLEOSIDE ANALOGUES, INCLUDING ZIDOVUDINE AND HIVID.[5,6] IN ADDITION, RARE CASES OF HEPATIC FAILURE AND DEATH CONSIDERED POSSIBLY RELATED TO UNDERLYING HEPATITIS B AND HIVID MONOTHERAPY HAVE BEEN REPORTED. Treatment with HIVID in patients with preexisting liver disease, liver enzyme abnormalities, a history of ethanol abuse or hepatitis should be approached with caution. HIVID should be interrupted or discontinued in the setting of deterioration of liver function tests, hepatic steatosis, progressive hepatomegaly or unexplained lactic acidosis. In clinical trials, drug interruption was recommended if liver function tests exceeded >5 times the upper limit of normal.

4. Other Serious Toxicities:

a) *Oral Ulcers:* Severe oral ulcers occurred in up to 3% of patients receiving HIVID in CPCRA 002 and ACTG 175; less severe oral ulcerations have occurred at higher frequencies in other clinical trials.

b) *Esophageal Ulcers:* Infrequent cases of esophageal ulcers have also been attributed to HIVID therapy. Interruption of HIVID should be considered in patients who develop esophageal ulcers that do not respond to specific treatment for opportunistic pathogens in order to assess a possible relationship to HIVID.

c) *Cardiomyopathy/Congestive Heart Failure:* Cardiomyopathy and congestive heart failure in patients with AIDS have been associated with the use of nucleoside analogues. Infrequent cases have been reported in patients receiving HIVID. Treatment with HIVID in patients with baseline cardiomyopathy or history of congestive heart failure should be approached with caution.

d) *Anaphylactoid Reaction:* An anaphylactoid reaction was reported in a patient receiving both HIVID and zidovudine. In addition, there have been several reports of urticaria without other signs of anaphylaxis.

PRECAUTIONS

General:

1. *Renal Impairment:* Patients with renal impairment (estimated creatinine clearance <55 mL/min) may be at a greater risk of toxicity from HIVID due to decreased drug clearance. Dosage adjustment is recommended in these patients (see DOSAGE AND ADMINISTRATION).
2. *Lymphoma:* High doses of zalcitabine, administered for 3 months to $B_6C_3F_1$ mice (resulting in plasma concentrations over 1000 times those seen in patients taking the recommended doses of HIVID) induced an increased incidence of thymic lymphoma.[7] Although the pathogenesis of the effect is uncertain, a predisposition to chemically induced thymic lymphoma and high rates of spontaneous lymphoreticular neoplasms have previously been noted in this strain of mice.[8]

The incidence of lymphomas was reviewed in 13 comparative studies conducted by Roche, the NIAID and the NCI, as well as 7 Roche expanded-access studies that included HIVID. In 1 study, ACTG 155, a statistically significant increased rate of lymphomas was seen in patients receiving HIVID or combination HIVID and zidovudine compared to zidovudine alone (rates of 0, 1.3 and 2.3 per 100 person years for zidovudine, HIVID, and combination HIVID and zidovudine, respectively; log rank p-value=0.01, pooling HIVID, and combination HIVID and zidovudine vs zidovudine, p-value=0.003). Based on review of the literature, the incidence of lymphomas in HIV-infected patients with advanced disease on zidovudine monotherapy would be expected to be approximately 1 to 2 per 100 person years of follow-up.

None of the other comparative studies evaluated showed a statistically significant difference in rates of lymphomas in patients receiving either HIVID monotherapy or combination HIVID and zidovudine. In a large, controlled clinical trial (ACTG 175) HIVID in combination with zidovudine was not associated with an increase in the incidence of lymphoma over that seen with zidovudine monotherapy (6 of 615 and 9 of 619, respectively).

Information for Patients: Patients should be informed that HIVID is not a cure for HIV infection and that they may continue to develop illnesses associated with advanced HIV infection including opportunistic infections. Since it is frequently difficult to determine whether symptoms are a result of drug effect or underlying disease manifestation, patients should be encouraged to report all changes in their condition to their physician. Patients should be informed that the use of HIVID or other antiretroviral drugs does not preclude the ongoing need to maintain practices designed to prevent transmission of HIV. Women of childbearing age should use effective contraception while using HIVID.

Patients should be instructed that the major toxicity of HIVID is peripheral neuropathy. Pancreatitis and hepatic toxicity are other serious and potentially life-threatening toxicities that have been reported in patients treated with HIVID monotherapy or in combination with zidovudine. Patients should be advised of the early symptoms of these conditions and instructed to promptly report them to their physician. Since the development of peripheral neuropathy appears to be dose-related to HIVID, patients should be advised to follow their physicians' instructions regarding the prescribed dose.

Laboratory Tests: Complete blood counts and clinical chemistry tests should be performed prior to initiating HIVID monotherapy or combination therapy with HIVID and zidovudine and at appropriate intervals thereafter. Baseline testing of serum amylase and triglyceride levels should be performed in individuals with a prior history of pancreatitis, increased amylase, those on parenteral nutrition or with a history of ethanol abuse.

Drug Interactions: The concomitant use of HIVID with drugs that have the potential to cause peripheral neuropathy should be avoided where possible. Drugs that have been associated with peripheral neuropathy include chloramphenicol, cisplatin, dapsone, disulfiram, ethionamide, glutethimide, gold, hydralazine, iodoquinol, isoniazid, metronidazole, nitrofurantoin, phenytoin, ribavirin and vincristine. Concomitant use of HIVID with didanosine is not recommended.

Treatment with HIVID should be interrupted when the use of a drug that has the potential to cause pancreatitis is required. Death due to fulminant pancreatitis possibly related to intravenous pentamidine and HIVID has been reported. If intravenous pentamidine is required to treat *Pneumocystis carinii* pneumonia, treatment with HIVID should be interrupted (see WARNINGS).

Drugs such as amphotericin, foscarnet and aminoglycosides may increase the risk of developing peripheral neuropathy or other HIVID-associated toxicities by interfering with the renal clearance of zalcitabine (thereby raising systemic exposure). Patients who require the use of one of these drugs with HIVID should have frequent clinical and laboratory monitoring with dosage adjustment for any significant change in renal function. Concomitant administration of probenecid or cimetidine decreases the elimination of zalcitabine, most likely by inhibition of renal tubular secretion of zalcitabine. Patients receiving these drugs in combination with zalcitabine should be monitored for signs of toxicity and the dose of zalcitabine reduced if warranted.

Absorption of zalcitabine is moderately reduced (approximately 25%) when coadministered with magnesium/aluminum containing antacid products. The clinical significance of this reduction is not known, hence zalcitabine is not recommended to be ingested simultaneously with magnesium/aluminum containing antacids. Bioavailability is mildly reduced (approximately 10%) when zalcitabine and metoclopramide are coadministered (see CLINICAL PHARMACOLOGY: *Drug Interactions*).

Carcinogenesis, Mutagenesis and Impairment of Fertility:

Carcinogenesis: Carcinogenicity studies in animals have not yet been completed.

Mutagenesis: There was no evidence of mutagenicity in Ames tests, Chinese Hamster lung cell tests and mouse lymphoma cell tests. An unscheduled DNA synthesis assay was performed in rat hepatocytes with no increases in DNA repair. An in vitro mammalian cell transformation assay was positive at doses of 500 mcg/mL and higher. Human peripheral blood lymphocytes were exposed to zalcitabine, with and without metabolic activation; at 1.5 mcg/mL and higher, dose-related increases in chromosomal aberration were seen. Oral doses of zalcitabine at 2500 and 4500 mg/kg were clastogenic in the mouse micronucleus assay.

Impairment of Fertility: Fertility and reproductive performance were assessed in rats at plasma concentrations up to 2142 times those achieved with the maximum recommended human dose (MRHD) based on AUC measurements. No adverse effects on rate of conception or general reproductive performance were observed. The highest dose was associated with embryolethality and evidence of teratogenicity. The next lower dose studied (plasma concentrations equivalent to 485 times the MRHD) was associated with a lower frequency of embryotoxicity but no teratogenicity. The fertility of F1 males was significantly reduced at a calculated dose of 2142 (but not 485) times the MRHD (based on AUC measurements) in a teratology study in which rat mothers were dosed on gestation days 7 to 15. No adverse effects were observed on the fertility of parents or F1 generation in the study of fertility and general reproductive performance or in the perinatal and postnatal reproduction study.

Pregnancy: Teratogenic Effects: Pregnancy Category C. Zalcitabine has been shown to be teratogenic in mice at calculated exposure levels of 1365 and 2730 times that of the MRHD (based on AUC measurements). In rats, zalcitabine was teratogenic at a calculated exposure level of 2142 times the MRHD but not at an exposure level of 485 times the MRHD. In a perinatal and postnatal study in the rat, a high incidence of hydrocephalus was observed in the F1 offspring derived from litters of dams treated with 1071 (but not 485) times the MRHD (based on AUC measurements). There are no adequate and well-controlled studies of zalcitabine in pregnant women. HIVID should be used during pregnancy only if the potential benefit justifies the potential risk to the fetus. Fertile women should not receive HIVID unless they are using effective contraception during therapy. If pregnancy occurs, physicians are encouraged to report such cases by calling (800) 526-6367.

Nonteratogenic Effects: Increased embryolethality was observed in pregnant mice at doses 2730 times the MRHD and in pregnant rats above 485 (but not 98) times the MRHD (based on AUC measurements). Average fetal body weight was significantly decreased in mice at doses of 1365 times the MRHD and in rats at 2142 times the MRHD (based on AUC measurements). In a perinatal and postnatal study, the learning and memory of a significant number of F1 offspring were impaired, and they tended to stay hyperactive for a longer period of time. These effects, observed at a calculated exposure level of 1071 (but not 485) times the MRHD (based on AUC measurements), were considered to result from extensive damage to or gross underdevelopment of the brain of these F1 offspring consistent with the finding of hydrocephalus.

Nursing Mothers: The US Public Health Service Centers for Disease Control and Prevention advises HIV-infected women not to breastfeed to avoid postnatal transmission of

Continued on next page

Roche Laboratories—Cont.

HIV to a child who may not yet be infected. It is not known whether zalcitabine is excreted in human milk.

Pediatric Use: Pharmacokinetics in Pediatric Patients: Limited pharmacokinetic data have been reported for 5 HIV-positive pediatric patients using doses of 0.03 and 0.04 mg/kg HIVID administered orally every 6 hours.[1] The mean bioavailability of zalcitabine in these pediatric patients was 54% and mean apparent systemic clearance was 150 mL/min/m^2. Due to the small number of subjects and different analytical techniques, it is difficult to make comparisons between pediatric and adult data.

Safety and effectiveness of HIVID in combination with zidovudine or as monotherapy in HIV-infected children younger than 13 years of age has not been established.

ADVERSE REACTIONS
(See WARNINGS.)

Tables 2 and 3 summarize the clinical adverse events and laboratory abnormalities, respectively, that occurred in ≥1% of patients in the comparative monotherapy trial (CPCRA 002) of HIVID vs didanosine (ddI), and the comparative combination trial (ACTG 175) of zidovudine (ZDV) monotherapy vs HIVID and zidovudine combination therapy, respectively. Other studies have found a higher or lower incidence of adverse experiences depending upon disease status, generally being lower in patients with less advanced disease.

[See Table 2 below.]
[See Table 3 above.]

Additional clinical adverse experiences associated with HIVID that occurred in <1% of patients in CPCRA 002 (at least possibly related, Grade 3 or higher), ACTG 175 (any relationship, Grade 3/4) or in other clinical studies are listed below by body system. Several of these events occurred in slightly higher rates in other studies. The incidence of adverse experiences varied in different studies, generally being lower in patients with less-advanced disease.

Body as a Whole: abnormal weight loss, asthenia, cachexia, chest tightness or pain, chills, cutaneous/allergic reaction, debilitation, difficulty moving, dry eyes/mouth, edema, facial pain or swelling, flank pain, flushing, increased sweating, lymphadenopathy, malaise, night sweats, pain, pelvic/groin pain, rigors.

Cardiovascular: abnormal cardiac movement, arrhythmia, atrial fibrillation, cardiac failure, cardiac dysrhythmias, cardiomyopathy, heart racing, hypertension, palpitation, subarachnoid hemorrhage, syncope, tachycardia, ventricular ectopy.

Endocrine/Metabolic: abnormal triglycerides, abnormal lipase, altered serum glucose, decreased bicarbonate, diabetes mellitus, glycosuria, gout, hot flushes, hypercalcemia, hyperkalemia, hyperlipemia, hypernatremia, hyperuricemia, hypocalcemia, hypoglycemia, hypokalemia, hypomagnesemia, hyponatremia, hypophosphatemia, increased nonprotein nitrogen.

Gastrointestinal: abdominal bloating or cramps, acute pancreatitis, anal/rectal pain, anorexia, bleeding gums, bloody or black stools, colitis, dental abscess, dry mouth, dyspepsia, dysphagia, enlarged abdomen, epigastric pain, eructation, esophageal pain, esophageal ulcers, esophagitis, flatulence, gagging with pills, gastritis, gastrointestinal hemorrhage, gingivitis, glossitis, gum disorder, heartburn, hemorrhagic pancreatitis, hemorrhoids, increased saliva, left quadrant pain, melena, mouth lesion, odynophagia, painful sore gums, painful swallowing, pancreatitis, rectal hemorrhage, rectal mass, rectal ulcers, salivary gland enlargement, sore tongue, sore throat, tongue disorder, tongue ulcer, toothache, unformed/loose stools, vomiting.

Hematologic: absolute neutrophil count alteration, anemia, epistaxis, decreased hematocrit, granulocytosis, hemoglobinemia, leukopenia, neutrophilia, platelet alteration, purpura, thrombus, unspecified hematologic toxicity, white blood cell alteration.

Hepatic: abnormal lactate dehydrogenase, bilirubinemia, cholecystitis, decreased alkaline phosphatase, hepatitis, hepatocellular damage, hepatomegaly, increased alkaline phosphatase.

Musculoskeletal: arthralgia, arthritis, arthropathy, arthrosis, back pain, backache, bone pains/aches, bursitis, cold extremities, extremity pain, joint inflammation, leg cramps, muscle aches, muscle weakness, muscle disorder, muscle stiffness, muscle cramps, myalgia, myopathy, myositis, neck pain, rib pain, stiff neck.

Neurological: abnormal coordination, aphasia, ataxia, Bell's palsy, confusion, decreased concentration, decreased neurological function, disequilibrium, dizziness, dysphonia, facial nerve palsy, focal motor seizures, grand mal seizure, hyperkinesia, hypertonia, hypokinesia, memory loss, migraine, neuralgia, neuritis, paralysis, seizures, speech disorder, status epilepticus, stupor, tremor, twitch, vertigo.

Psychological: acute psychotic disorder, acute stress reaction, agitation, amnesia, anxiety, confusion, decreased motivation, decreased sexual desire, depersonalization, emotional lability, euphoria, hallucination, impaired concentration, insomnia, manic reaction, mood swings, nervousness, paranoid state, somnolence, suicide attempt.

Respiratory: acute nasopharyngitis, chest congestion, coughing, cyanosis, difficulty breathing, dry nasal mucosa, dyspnea, flu-like symptoms, hemoptysis, nasal discharge, pharyngitis, rales/Rhonchi, respiratory distress, sinus congestion, sinus pain, sinusitis, wheezing.

Skin: acne, alopecia, bullous eruptions, carbuncle/furuncle, cellulitis, cold sore, dermatitis, dry skin, dry rash desquamation, erythematous rash, exfoliative dermatitis, finger inflammation, follicular rash, impetigo, infection, itchy rash, lip blisters/lesions, macular/papular rash, maculopapular rash, moniliasis, mucocutaneous/skin disorder, nail

Table 3. Percentage of Patients with Laboratory Abnormalities Protocol Grade 3/4

	CPCRA 002* ZDV Intolerant or Failure		ACTG 175 ZDV Naive/Experienced	
	HIVID 0.750 mg q8h	ddI 250 mg q12h	ZDV 200 mg q8h	HIVID+ZDV 0.750 mg q8h+200 mg q8h
	n=237	n=230	n=619	n=615
Laboratory Abnormality				
Anemia (<7.5 gm/dL)	8.4	7.4	1.8	3.1
Leukopenia (<1500 cells/mm^3)	13.1	9.6	N/A	N/A
Eosinophilia (>1000 cells/mm^3 or 25%)	2.5	1.7	N/A	N/A
Neutropenia (<750 cells/mm^3)	16.9	11.7	1.9	4.2
Thrombocytopenia (<50,000 cells/mm^3)	1.3	4.8	1.1	1.8
CPK Elevation* (>4 × ULN)	0.8	0.0	5.8	5.7
ALT (SGPT) (>5 × ULN)	N/A	N/A	3.6	5.0
AST (SGOT) (>5 × ULN)	7.6	5.7	2.9	4.1
Bilirubin (>2.5 × ULN)	0.8	0.9	0.5	1.0
GGT (>5 × ULN)	N/A	N/A	0.5	1.0
Amylase (>2 × ULN)	5.1	3.9	1.0	1.5
Hyperglycemia* (>250 mg/dL)	0.0	1.7	0.8	2.0

* Grade 3 or higher reported for CPCRA 002
N/A Not available

Table 2. Percentage of Patients with Clinical Adverse Experience ≥ Grade 3*,[†] in ≥ 1% of Patients Receiving HIVID

	CPCRA 002* ZDV Intolerant or Failure		ACTG 175[‡] ZDV Naive/Experienced	
	HIVID 0.750 mg q8h	ddI 250 mg q12h	ZDV 200 mg q8h	HIVID+ZDV 0.750 mg q8h+200 mg q8h
	n=237	n=230	n=619	n=615
Body System/Adverse Event				
Systemic				
Fatigue	3.8	2.6	2.7	2.3
Headache	2.1	1.3	2.4	2.6
Fever	1.7	0.4	2.7	2.9
Gastrointestinal				
Abdominal Pain	3.0	7.0	2.3	1.8
Oral Lesions/Stomatitis§	3.0	0.0	0.6	1.5
Vomiting/Nausea§	3.4	7.0	4.9	2.1
Diarrhea/Constipation§	2.5	17.4	2.9	1.0
Hepatic				
Abnormal Hepatic Function	8.9	7.0	"	"
Neurological				
Convulsions	1.3	2.2		
Peripheral Neuropathy¶	28.3	13.0	3.1	3.3
Skin				
Rash/Pruritus/Urticaria	3.4	3.9	1.8	1.6
Metabolic and Nutrition				
Pancreatitis	0.0	1.7	0.2	0.5
Psychological Depression	0.4	0.0	1.1	1.8
Musculoskeletal				
Painful/Swollen Joints	0.4	0.0	0.3	1.0

* Grade 2 Adverse Events possibly or probably related to treatment or unassessable were included if study drug dosage was changed or interrupted.
[†] Grade 3 severity: event causing marked limitation in activity, requiring medical care and possible hospitalization.
Grade 4 severity: completely disabling, unable to care for self, requiring active medical intervention, probable hospitalization or hospice care.
[‡] All relationships.
§ Adverse experiences were combined to form this category.
" See Table 3.
¶ CPCRA 002 included patients who were dose-adjusted for Grade 2 events; ACTG 175 required dose adjustment for Grade 2 peripheral neuropathy but recorded only Grade 3 events.

disorder, photosensitivity reaction, pruritic disorder, pruritus, skin disorder, skin lesions, skin fissure, skin ulcer, urticaria.

Special Senses: abnormal vision, blurred vision, burning eyes, decreased taste, decreased vision, ear pain/problem, ear blockage, eye abnormality, eye inflammation, eye itching, eye pain, eye irritation, eye redness, eye hemorrhage, fluid in ears, hearing loss, increased tears, loss of taste, mucopurulent conjunctivitis, parosmia, photophobia, smell dysfunction, taste perversion, tinnitus, unequal-sized pupils, xerophthalmia, yellow sclera.

Urogenital: abnormal renal function, acute renal failure, albuminuria, bladder pain, dysuria, frequent urination, genital lesion/ulcer, increased blood urea nitrogen, increased creatinine, micturition frequency, nocturia, painful penis sore, pain on urination, penile edema, polyuria, renal cyst, renal calculus, testicular swelling, toxic nephropathy, urinary retention, vaginal itch, vaginal ulcer, vaginal pain, vaginal/cervix disorder, vaginal discharge.

OVERDOSAGE

Acute Overdosage: Inadvertent pediatric overdoses have occurred with doses up to 1.5 mg/kg HIVID. The children had prompt gastric lavage and treatment with activated charcoal and had no sequelae. Mixed overdoses including HIVID and other drugs have led to drowsiness and vomiting (with HIVID or placebo, zidovudine and trimethoprim/sulfamethoxazole [TMP/SMX]), or increased GGT (with 18.75 mg HIVID with zidovudine and lormetazepam) or increased creatine phosphokinase (with HIVID or placebo, zidovudine, fluconazole, dapsone and wine). There is no experience with acute HIVID overdosage at higher doses and sequelae are unknown. There is no known antidote for HIVID overdosage. It is not known whether zalcitabine is dialyzable by peritoneal dialysis or hemodialysis.

Chronic Overdosage: In the early Phase 1 studies, all patients receiving zalcitabine at approximately 6 times the current total daily recommended dose experienced peripheral neuropathy by week 10. Eighty percent of patients who received approximately 2 times the current total daily recommended dose experienced peripheral neuropathy by week 12.

DOSAGE AND ADMINISTRATION

The recommended monotherapy regimen is one 0.750 mg tablet of HIVID orally every 8 hours (2.25 mg HIVID total daily dose). The recommended combination regimen is one 0.750 mg tablet of HIVID orally, administered concomitantly with 200 mg of zidovudine every 8 hours (2.25 mg HIVID total daily dose and 600 mg zidovudine total daily dose). Based on preliminary data, the recommended HIVID dosage reduction for patients with impaired renal function is: creatinine clearance 10 to 40 mL/min: 0.750 mg of HIVID q12h; creatinine clearance <10 mL/min: 0.750 mg of HIVID q24h.

Monitoring of Patients: Periodic complete blood counts and clinical chemistry tests should be performed. Serum amylase levels should be monitored in those individuals who have a history of elevated amylase, pancreatitis, ethanol abuse, who are on parenteral nutrition or who are otherwise at high risk of pancreatitis. Careful monitoring for signs or symptoms suggestive of peripheral neuropathy is recommended, particularly in individuals with a low CD4 cell count or who are at a greater risk of developing peripheral neuropathy while on therapy (see WARNINGS).

Dose Adjustment for Monotherapy with HIVID and in Combination Therapy with HIVID and Other Antiretroviral Agents: For toxicities that are likely to be associated with HIVID (eg, peripheral neuropathy, severe oral ulcers, pancreatitis, elevated liver function tests especially in patients with chronic Hepatitis B) HIVID should be interrupted or dose reduced. FOR SEVERE TOXICITIES OR THOSE PERSISTING AFTER DOSE REDUCTION, HIVID SHOULD BE INTERRUPTED. For recipients of combination therapy with HIVID and other antiretroviral agents, dose adjustments or interruption for each drug should be based on the known toxicity profile of the individual drugs. SEE INFORMATION FOR EACH DRUG USED IN COMBINATION FOR A DESCRIPTION OF KNOWN DRUG-ASSOCIATED ADVERSE REACTIONS.

Patients developing moderate discomfort with signs or symptoms of peripheral neuropathy should stop HIVID. HIVID-associated peripheral neuropathy may continue to worsen despite interruption of HIVID. HIVID should be reintroduced at 50% dose—0.375 mg q8h only if all findings related to peripheral neuropathy have improved to mild symptoms. HIVID should be permanently discontinued if patients experience severe discomfort related to peripheral neuropathy or moderate discomfort that progresses. If other moderate to severe clinical adverse reactions or laboratory abnormalities (such as increased liver function tests) occur, then HIVID and/or the other potential causative agent(s) should be interrupted until the adverse reaction abates. HIVID and/or the other potential causative agent(s) should then be carefully reintroduced at lower doses if appropriate. If adverse reactions recur at the reduced dose, therapy should be discontinued. The minimum effective dose of HIVID in combination with zidovudine for the treatment of adult patients with advanced HIV infection has not been established.

In patients with poor bone marrow reserve, particularly those patients with advanced symptomatic HIV disease, frequent monitoring of hematologic indices is recommended to detect serious anemia or granulocytopenia. Significant toxicities, such as anemia (hemoglobin of <7.5 gm/dL or reduction of >25% of baseline) and/or granulocytopenia (granulocyte count of <750 cells/mm^3 or reduction of >50% from baseline), may require a treatment interruption of HIVID and zidovudine until evidence of marrow recovery is observed. For less severe anemia or granulocytopenia, a reduction in daily dose of zidovudine in those patients receiving combination therapy may be adequate. In patients who experience hematologic toxicity, reduction in hemoglobin may occur as early as 2 to 4 weeks after initiation of therapy, and granulocytopenia usually occurs after 6 to 8 weeks of therapy. In patients who develop significant anemia, dose modification does not necessarily eliminate the need for transfusion. If marrow recovery occurs following dose modification, gradual increases in dose may be appropriate depending on hematologic indices and patient tolerance. For more details, refer to the complete product information for zidovudine.

HOW SUPPLIED

HIVID 0.375 mg tablets are oval, beige, film-coated tablets with "HIVID 0.375" imprinted on one side and "ROCHE" on the other side—bottles of 100 (NDC 0004-0220-01). HIVID 0.750 mg tablets are oval, gray, film-coated tablets with "HIVID 0.750" imprinted on one side and "ROCHE" on the other side—bottles of 100 (NDC 0004-0221-01).

The tablets should be stored in tightly closed bottles at 59° to 86°F (15° to 30°C).

REFERENCES

1. Pizzo PA, Butler K, Balis F, et al. Dideoxycytidine alone and in an alternating schedule with zidovudine in children with symptomatic human immunodeficiency virus infection. *J Pediatr.* 1990;117(5): 799–808.
2. Abrams DI, Goldman AI, Launer C, et al. A comparative trial of didanosine or zalcitabine after treatment with zidovudine in patients with human immunodeficiency virus infection. *N Engl J Med.* 1994;330(10): 657–662.
3. Follansbee S, Drew L, Olson R, et al. The efficacy of zalcitabine (ddC, HIVID) versus zidovudine (ZDV) as monotherapy in ZDV-naive patients with advanced HIV disease; a randomized, double-blind, comparative trial (ACTG 114; N3300). IXth International Conference on AIDS/IV STD World Congress, Berlin, Germany, June 7–11, 1993. Poster PO-B26-2113.
4. Remick S, Follansbee S, Olson R, et al. Safety and tolerance of zalcitabine (ddC, HIVID) in a double-blind comparative trial (ACTG 114; N3300). IXth International Conference on AIDS/IV STD World Congress, Berlin, Germany, June 7–11, 1993. Poster PO-B26-2115.
5. "Dear Doctor" letter, Burroughs Wellcome Co., June 1, 1993.
6. Food and Drug Administration Antiviral Drugs Advisory Committee Meeting, "Mitochondrial Damage Associated with Nucleoside Analogues," Rockville, Md, Sept 21, 1993.
7. Sanders VM, Elwell MR, Heath JE, et al. Induction of Thymic Lymphoma in Mice Administered the Dideoxynucleoside ddC. *Fundamental and Applied Toxicology.* 1995;27: 263–269.
8. Irons RD, Le AT, Som DB, et al. 2′3′-Dideoxycytidine-induced Thymic Lymphoma Correlates with Species-specific Suppression of a Subpopulation of Primitive Hematopoietic Progenitor Cells in Mouse but Not Rat or Human Bone Marrow. *J Clin Invest.* 1995;95: 2777–2782.

Revised: June 1996

Shown in Product Identification Guide, page 332

INVIRASE™ ℞

(saquinavir mesylate)
CAPSULES

> **WARNING**
> The indication for INVIRASE for the treatment of HIV infection is based on changes in surrogate markers. At present there are no results from controlled clinical trials evaluating the effect of regimens containing INVIRASE on survival or the clinical progression of HIV infection, such as the occurrence of opportunistic infections or malignancies.

DESCRIPTION

INVIRASE brand of saquinavir mesylate is an inhibitor of the human immunodeficiency virus (HIV) protease. INVIRASE is available as light brown and green, opaque hard gelatin capsules for oral administration in a 200-mg strength (as saquinavir free base). Each capsule also contains the inactive ingredients lactose, microcrystalline cellulose, povidone K30, sodium starch glycolate, talc and magnesium stearate. Each capsule shell contains gelatin and water with the following dye systems: red iron oxide, yellow iron oxide, black iron oxide, FD&C Blue #2 and titanium dioxide. The chemical name for saquinavir mesylate is N-tert-butyl-decahydro-2-[2(R)-hydroxy-4-phenyl-3(S)- [[N-(2-quinolylcarbonyl)-L-asparaginyl]amino]butyl]-(4aS,8aS)-isoquinoline-3 (S)-carboxamide methanesulfonate with a molecular formula $C_{38}H_{50}N_6O_5 \cdot CH_4O_3S$ and a molecular weight of 766.96. The molecular weight of the free base is 670.86. Saquinavir mesylate is a white to off-white, very fine powder with an aqueous solubility of 2.22 mg/mL at 25°C.

CLINICAL PHARMACOLOGY

Mechanism of Action: HIV protease cleaves viral polyprotein precursors to generate functional proteins in HIV-infected cells. The cleavage of viral polyprotein precursors is essential for maturation of infectious virus. Saquinavir mesylate, henceforth referred to as saquinavir, is a synthetic peptide-like substrate analogue that inhibits the activity of HIV protease and prevents the cleavage of viral polyproteins.

Microbiology: *Antiviral Activity In Vitro:* The in vitro antiviral activity of saquinavir was assessed in lymphoblastoid and monocytic cell lines and in peripheral blood lymphocytes. Saquinavir inhibited HIV activity in both acutely and chronically infected cells. IC50 values (50% inhibitory concentration) were in the range of 1 to 30 nM. In cell culture saquinavir demonstrated additive to synergistic effects against HIV in double and triple combination regimens with reverse transcriptase inhibitors zidovudine (ZDV), zalcitabine (ddC) and didanosine (ddI), without enhanced cytotoxicity.

Resistance: HIV isolates with reduced susceptibility to saquinavir have been selected in vitro. Genotypic analyses of these isolates showed substitution mutations in the HIV protease at amino acid positions 48 (Glycine to Valine) and 90 (Leucine to Methionine).

Phenotypic and genotypic changes in HIV isolates from patients treated with saquinavir were also monitored in Phase 1/2 clinical trials. Phenotypic changes were defined as a tenfold decrease in sensitivity from baseline. Two viral protease mutations (L90M and/or G48V, the former predominating) were found in virus from treated, but not untreated, patients. The incidence across studies of phenotypic and genotypic changes in the subsets of patients studied for a period of 16 to 74 weeks (median observation time approximately 1 year) is shown in Table 1. However, the clinical relevance of phenotypic and genotypic changes associated with saquinavir therapy has not been established.

[See Table 1 on top of next page.]

Cross-resistance to Other Antiretrovirals: The potential for HIV cross-resistance between protease inhibitors has not been fully explored. Therefore, it is unknown what effect saquinavir therapy will have on the activity of subsequent protease inhibitors. Cross-resistance between saquinavir and reverse transcriptase inhibitors is unlikely because of the different enzyme targets involved. ZDV-resistant HIV isolates have been shown to be sensitive to saquinavir in vitro.

Pharmacokinetics: The pharmacokinetic properties of saquinavir have been evaluated in healthy volunteers (n=351) and HIV-infected patients (n=270) after single and multiple oral doses of 25, 75, 200 and 600 mg tid and in healthy volunteers after intravenous doses of 6, 12, 36 or 72 mg (n=21).

Absorption and Bioavailability in Adults: Following multiple dosing (600 mg tid) in HIV-infected patients (n=29), the steady-state area under the plasma concentration versus time curve (AUC) was 2.5 times (95% CI 1.6 to 3.8) higher than that observed after a single dose. HIV-infected patients administered saquinavir 600 mg tid, with the instructions to take saquinavir after a meal or substantial snack, had AUC and maximum plasma concentration (Cmax) values which were about twice those observed in healthy volunteers receiving the same treatment regimen (Table 2).

Table 2. Mean (%CV) AUC and Cmax in Patients and Healthy Volunteers

	AUC_8 (dose interval) (ng·h/mL)	Cmax (ng/mL)
Healthy Volunteers (n=6)	359.0 (46)	90.39 (49)
Patients (n=113)	757.2 (84)	253.3 (99)

Absolute bioavailability averaged 4% (CV 73%, range: 1% to 9%) in 8 healthy volunteers who received a single 600 mg dose (3 × 200 mg) of saquinavir following a high fat break-

Continued on next page

Roche Laboratories—Cont.

fast (48 g protein, 60 g carbohydrate, 57 g fat; 1006 kcal). The low bioavailability is thought to be due to a combination of incomplete absorption and extensive first-pass metabolism.

Food Effect: The mean 24-hour AUC after a single 600 mg oral dose (6 × 100 mg) in healthy volunteers (n=6) was increased from 24 ng·h/mL (CV 33%), under fasting conditions, to 161 ng·h/mL (CV 35%) when saquinavir was given following a high fat breakfast (48 g protein, 60 g carbohydrate, 57 g fat; 1006 kcal). Saquinavir 24-hour AUC and Cmax (n=6) following the administration of a higher calorie meal (943 kcal, 54 g fat) were on average two times higher than after a lower calorie, lower fat meal (355 kcal, 8 g fat). The effect of food has been shown to persist for up to 2 hours.

Distribution in Adults: The mean steady-state volume of distribution following intravenous administration of a 12-mg dose of saquinavir (n=8) was 700 L (CV 39%), suggesting saquinavir partitions into tissues. Saquinavir was approximately 98% bound to plasma proteins over a concentration range of 15 to 700 ng/mL. In 2 patients receiving saquinavir 600 mg tid, cerebrospinal fluid concentrations were negligible when compared to concentrations from matching plasma samples.

Metabolism and Elimination in Adults: In vitro studies using human liver microsomes have shown that the metabolism of saquinavir is cytochrome P450 mediated with the specific isoenzyme, CYP3A4, responsible for more than 90% of the hepatic metabolism. Based on in vitro studies, saquinavir is rapidly metabolized to a range of mono- and di-hydroxylated inactive compounds. In a mass balance study using 600 mg ^{14}C-saquinavir (n=8), 88% and 1% of the orally administered radioactivity, was recovered in feces and urine, respectively, within 5 days of dosing. In an additional 4 subjects administered 10.5 mg ^{14}C-saquinavir intravenously, 81% and 3% of the intravenously administered radioactivity was recovered in feces and urine, respectively, within 5 days of dosing. In mass balance studies, 13% of circulating radioactivity in plasma was attributed to unchanged drug after oral administration and the remainder attributed to saquinavir metabolites. Following intravenous administration, 66% of circulating radioactivity was attributed to unchanged drug and the remainder attributed to saquinavir metabolites, suggesting that saquinavir undergoes extensive first-pass metabolism.

Systemic clearance of saquinavir was rapid, 1.14 L/h/kg (CV 12%) after intravenous doses of 6, 36 and 72 mg. The mean residence time of saquinavir was 7 hours (n=8).

Special Populations: Hepatic or Renal Impairment: Saquinavir pharmacokinetics in patients with hepatic or renal insufficiency has not been investigated (see PRECAUTIONS).

Gender, Race and Age: Pharmacokinetic data were available for 17 women in the Phase 1/2 studies. Pooled data did not reveal an apparent effect of gender on the pharmacokinetics of saquinavir.

The effect of race on the pharmacokinetics of saquinavir has not been evaluated, due to the small numbers of minorities for whom pharmacokinetic data were available.

Saquinavir pharmacokinetics has not been investigated in patients >65 years of age or in pediatric patients (<16 years).

Drug Interactions: HIVID and ZDV: Concomitant use of INVIRASE with HIVID® (zalcitabine, ddC) and ZDV has been studied (as triple combination) in adults. Pharmacokinetic data suggest that the absorption, metabolism and elimination of each of these drugs are unchanged when they are used together.

Ketoconazole: Concomitant administration of ketoconazole (200 mg qd) and saquinavir (600 mg tid) to 12 healthy volunteers resulted in steady-state saquinavir AUC and Cmax values which were three times those seen with saquinavir alone. No dose adjustment is required when the two drugs are coadministered at the doses studied. Ketoconazole pharmacokinetics was unaffected by coadministration with saquinavir.

Rifampin: Coadministration of rifampin (600 mg qd) and saquinavir (600 mg tid) to 12 healthy volunteers decreased the steady-state AUC and Cmax of saquinavir by approximately 80%.

Rifabutin: Preliminary data from 12 HIV-infected patients indicate that the steady-state AUC of saquinavir (600 mg tid) was decreased by 40% when saquinavir was coadministered with rifabutin (300 mg qd).

INDICATIONS AND USAGE

INVIRASE in combination with nucleoside analogues is indicated for the treatment of HIV infection when therapy is warranted (see *Description of Clinical Studies* below). This indication is based on changes in surrogate markers in patients who initiated INVIRASE concomitantly with other antiretroviral agents. There are no results available from clinical trials confirming the clinical benefit of combination therapy with INVIRASE on HIV disease progression or survival.

Description of Clinical Studies: The activity of INVIRASE in combination with HIVID and/or ZDV in HIV infection has been evaluated in three double-blind, randomized trials in a total of 810 patients with advanced HIV infection.

Table 1. Frequency of Genotypic and Phenotypic Changes in Selected Patients Treated with Saquinavir

	Genotypic*		Phenotypic†	
	24 Week	1 Year	24 Week	1 Year
Monotherapy	3/8 (38%)	15/33 (45%)	2/22 (9%)	5/11 (45%)
Combination Therapy	5/30 (17%)	16/52 (31%)	0/23 (0%)	11/29 (38%)

*Double mutation (G48V and L90M) has occurred in 2 of 33 patients receiving monotherapy. The double mutation has not occurred with combination therapy.

†Phenotypic changes have been defined as at least a tenfold change in sensitivity relative to baseline. In a few patients genotypic and phenotypic changes were unrelated.

Table 3. Summary of Mean Log_{10} Plasma RNA Results from Major INVIRASE Clinical Studies*

	V13330 (Italy) Naive patients			NV14255/ACTG229 (USA) ZDV-experienced			Surrogate Marker Analysis NV14256 (North America)		
	ZDV	SAQ†	ZDV+ SAQ†	ZDV+ ddC	ZDV+ SAQ†	ZDV+ddC +SAQ†	ddC	SAQ†	SAQ† +ddC
n Enrolled	17	19	20	100	99	98	145	159	147
Prior ZDV									
n	—	—	—	99	98	97	134	151	136
Median Duration (days)	—	—	—	659	713	647	614	459	442
Log_{10} Plasma RNA by PCR (copies/mL)									
n	17	19	20	100	97	96	114	124	119
Mean Baseline (n)	5.2 (13)	5.2 (15)	5.2 (15)	4.7 (100)	4.8 (97)	4.8 (96)	5.2 (114)	5.1 (124)	5.1 (119)
Mean Change from Baseline Week 16	-0.6	-0.2	-1.0	-0.3	0.0	-0.5	-0.4	-0.1	-0.6
Mean Change from Baseline Week 24	—	—	—	-0.2	0.0	-0.6	-0.4	-0.1	-0.5

*NOTE: THE CLINICAL SIGNIFICANCE OF CHANGES IN HIV VIRAL RNA DURING THERAPY IS UNKNOWN.

†Saquinavir (SAQ) at 600 mg tid

—Indicates not applicable

Advanced Patients without Prior ZDV Therapy: A dose-ranging study (Italy, V13330) conducted in 92 ZDV-naive patients (mean baseline CD_4=179) studied INVIRASE at doses of 75 mg, 200 mg and 600 mg tid in combination with ZDV 200 mg tid compared to INVIRASE 600 mg tid alone and ZDV alone.

In analyses of average CD_4 changes over 16 weeks, treatment with the combination of INVIRASE 600 mg tid + ZDV produced greater CD_4 cell increases than ZDV monotherapy (see Fig. 1). The CD_4 changes of ZDV in combination with doses of INVIRASE lower than 600 mg tid were no greater than that of ZDV alone.

Advanced Patients with Prior ZDV Therapy: In ACTG229/NV14255, 295 patients (mean baseline CD_4=165) with prolonged ZDV treatment (median 713 days) were randomized to receive either INVIRASE 600 mg tid + HIVID + ZDV (triple combination), INVIRASE 600 mg tid + ZDV or HIVID + ZDV. In analyses of average CD_4 changes over 24 weeks, the triple combination produced greater increases in CD_4 cell counts (see Fig. 2) compared to that of HIVID + ZDV. There were no significant differences in CD_4 changes among patients receiving INVIRASE + ZDV and HIVID + ZDV.

Study NV14256 (North America) is an ongoing, randomized, double-blind study comparing INVIRASE 600 mg tid + HIVID to HIVID monotherapy and INVIRASE monotherapy in patients with advanced HIV infection and at least 16 weeks of prior ZDV treatment. The study remains blinded with respect to clinical endpoints of disease progression; however, analyses of CD_4 changes over 16 weeks were conducted for a cohort of 423 patients. These analyses showed that the combination of INVIRASE + HIVID was associated with greater CD_4 increases than either HIVID or INVIRASE as monotherapy (see Fig. 3).

Comparisons of data across studies (NV14256 compared to ACTG229/NV14255) suggest that when INVIRASE was added to a regimen of prolonged prior zidovudine, there was little activity contributed by continuing ZDV.

HIV RNA: The clinical significance of changes in HIV-RNA measurements have not been established. Table 3 compares log RNA reductions at 16 and 24 weeks among INVIRASE combination treatment arms in three clinical trials. Monotherapy arms are included for reference. Overall, RNA reductions were greater in INVIRASE/nucleoside combination regimens compared to nucleoside monotherapy controls.

CONTRAINDICATIONS

INVIRASE is contraindicated in patients with clinically significant hypersensitivity to saquinavir or to any of the components contained in the capsule.

PRECAUTIONS

General: The safety profile of INVIRASE in children younger than 16 years has not been established.

If a serious or severe toxicity occurs during treatment with INVIRASE, INVIRASE should be interrupted until the etiology of the event is identified or the toxicity resolves. At that time, resumption of treatment with full dose INVIRASE may be considered. For nucleoside analogues used in combination with INVIRASE, physicians should refer to the complete product information for these drugs for dose adjustment recommendations and for information regarding drug-associated adverse reactions.

[See Table 3 above.]

[See Figures at top of next column.]

Caution should be exercised when administering INVIRASE to patients with hepatic insufficiency since patients with baseline liver function tests >5 times the upper limit of normal were not included in clinical studies.

Resistance/Cross-resistance: The potential for HIV cross-resistance between protease inhibitors has not been fully explored. Therefore, it is unknown what effect saquinavir therapy will have on the activity of subsequent protease inhibitors (see *Microbiology*).

Information for Patients: Patients should be informed that INVIRASE is not a cure for HIV infection and that they may continue to acquire illnesses associated with advanced HIV infection, including opportunistic infections. INVIRASE has not been shown to reduce the incidence or frequency of such illnesses, and patients should be advised to remain under the care of a physician while using INVIRASE.

Patients should be told that the long-term effects of INVIRASE are unknown at this time. They should be informed that INVIRASE therapy has not been shown to reduce the risk of transmitting HIV to others through sexual contact or blood contamination.

Patients should be advised that INVIRASE should be taken within 2 hours after a full meal (see *Pharmacokinetics*). When INVIRASE is taken without food, concentrations of saquinavir in the blood are substantially reduced and may result in no antiviral activity.

Laboratory Tests: No consistent alterations in standard laboratory tests have been associated with the use of INVIRASE. Clinical chemistry tests should be performed prior to initiating INVIRASE therapy and at appropriate intervals thereafter. For comprehensive information concerning laboratory test alterations associated with use of individual nucleoside analogues, physicians should refer to the complete product information for these drugs.

Drug Interactions: *Metabolic Enzyme Inducers:* INVIRASE should not be administered concomitantly with rifampin,

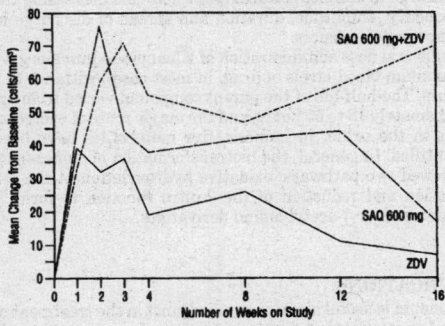

Fig. 1. Mean CD₄ Changes (cells/mm³) from Baseline in Study V13330 (Italy)

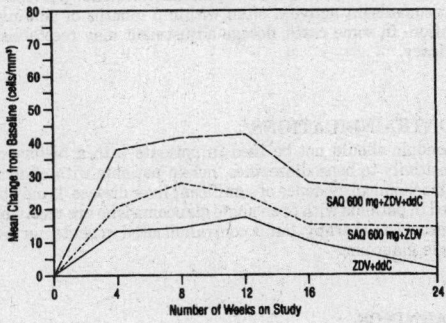

Fig. 2. Mean CD₄ Changes (cells/mm³) from Baseline in Study ACTG229/NV14255

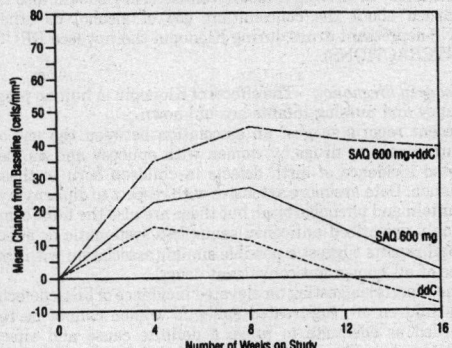

Fig. 3. Mean CD₄ Changes (cells/mm³) from Baseline in Study NV14256

Table 4. Percentage of Patients, by Study Arm, with Clinical Adverse Experiences Considered at Least Possibly Related to Study Drug or of Unknown Relationship and of Moderate, Severe or Life-threatening Intensity, Occurring in ≥ 2% of Patients in NV14255/ACTG229 and NV14256

ADVERSE EVENT	NV14255/ACTG229			NV14256		
	SAQ+ZDV n=99	SAQ+ddC+ZDV n=98	ddC+ZDV n=100	ddC n=145	SAQ n=159	SAQ+ddC n=147
GASTROINTESTINAL						
Diarrhea	3.0	1.0	—	1.4	3.8	3.4
Abdominal Discomfort	2.0	3.1	4.0	1.4	1.3	0.7
Nausea	—	3.1	3.0	0.7	1.9	0.7
Dyspepsia	1.0	1.0	2.0	2.1	—	0.7
Abdominal Pain	2.0	1.0	2.0	0.7	1.9	0.7
Mucosa Damage	—	—	4.0	1.4	—	0.7
Buccal Mucosa Ulceration	—	2.0	2.0	9.0	2.5	4.1
CENTRAL AND PERIPHERAL NERVOUS SYSTEM						
Headache	2.0	2.0	2.0	4.1	0.6	0.7
Paresthesia	2.0	3.1	4.0	0.7	1.0	1.0
Extremity Numbness	2.0	1.0	4.0	—	—	0.7
Dizziness	—	2.0	1.0	—	—	—
Peripheral Neuropathy	—	1.0	2.0	5.5	—	4.8
BODY AS A WHOLE						
Asthenia	6.1	9.2	10.0	0.7	1.3	0.7
Appetite Disturbances	—	1.0	2.0	—	—	—
SKIN AND APPENDAGES						
Rash	—	—	3.0	0.7	1.3	1.4
Pruritus	—	—	2.0	—	—	—
MUSCULOSKELETAL DISORDERS						
Musculoskeletal Pain	2.0	2.0	4.0	—	0.6	0.7
Myalgia	1.0	—	3.0	1.4	—	—

—Indicates no events reported

since rifampin decreases saquinavir concentrations by 80% (see *Pharmacokinetics*). Rifabutin also substantially reduces saquinavir plasma concentrations by 40%. Other drugs that induce CYP3A4 (eg, phenobarbital, phenytoin, dexamethasone, carbamazepine) may also reduce saquinavir plasma concentrations. If therapy with such drugs is warranted, physicians should consider using alternatives when a patient is taking INVIRASE.

Other Potential Interactions: Coadministration of terfenadine, astemizole or cisapride with drugs that are known to be potent inhibitors of the cytochrome P4503A pathway (ie, ketoconazole, itraconazole, etc.) may lead to elevated plasma concentrations of terfenadine, astemizole or cisapride which may in turn prolong QT intervals leading to rare cases of serious cardiovascular adverse events. Although INVIRASE is not a strong inhibitor of cytochrome P4503A, pharmacokinetic interaction studies with INVIRASE and terfenadine, astemizole or cisapride have not been conducted. Physicians should use alternatives to terfenadine, astemizole or cisapride when a patient is taking INVIRASE. Other compounds that are substrates of CYP3A4 (eg, calcium channel blockers, clindamycin, dapsone, quinidine, triazolam) may have elevated plasma concentrations when coadministered with INVIRASE; therefore, patients should be monitored for toxicities associated with such drugs.

Carcinogenesis, Mutagenesis and Impairment of Fertility:
Carcinogenesis: Carcinogenicity studies in rats and mice have not yet been completed.
Mutagenesis: Mutagenicity and genotoxicity studies, with and without metabolic activation where appropriate, have shown that saquinavir has no mutagenic activity in vitro in either bacterial (Ames test) or mammalian cells (Chinese

hamster lung V79/HPRT test). Saquinavir does not induce chromosomal damage in vivo in the mouse micronucleus assay or in vitro in human peripheral blood lymphocytes, and does not induce primary DNA damage in vitro in the unscheduled DNA synthesis test.
Impairment of Fertility: Fertility and reproductive performance were not affected in rats at plasma exposures (AUC values) up to five times those achieved in humans at the recommended dose.
Pregnancy: Teratogenic Effects: Category B. Reproduction studies conducted with saquinavir in rats have shown no embryotoxicity or teratogenicity at plasma exposures (AUC values) up to five times those achieved in humans at the recommended dose or in rabbits at plasma exposures four times those achieved at the recommended clinical dose. Studies in rats indicated that exposure to saquinavir from late pregnancy through lactation at plasma concentrations (AUC values) up to five times those achieved in humans at the recommended dose had no effect on the survival, growth and development of offspring to weaning. Because animal reproduction studies are not always predictive of human response, INVIRASE should be used during pregnancy after taking into account the importance of the drug to the mother. Presently, there are no reports of infants being born after women receiving INVIRASE in clinical trials became pregnant.
Nursing Mothers: The US Public Health Service Centers for Disease Control and Prevention advises HIV-infected women not to breastfeed to avoid postnatal transmission of HIV to a child who may not yet be infected. It is not known whether INVIRASE is excreted in human milk.
Pediatric Use: Safety and effectiveness of INVIRASE in HIV-infected children or adolescents younger than 16 years of age have not been established.

ADVERSE REACTIONS
(see PRECAUTIONS)
The safety of INVIRASE was studied in 688 patients who received the drug either alone or in combination with ZDV and/or HIVID (zalcitabine, ddC). The majority of adverse events were of mild intensity. The most frequently reported adverse events among patients receiving INVIRASE (excluding those toxicities known to be associated with ZDV and HIVID when used in combinations) were diarrhea, abdominal discomfort and nausea.
INVIRASE did not alter the pattern, frequency or severity of known major toxicities associated with the use of HIVID and/or ZDV. Physicians should refer to the complete product information for these drugs (or other antiretroviral agents as appropriate) for drug-associated adverse reactions to other nucleoside analogues.
In an open label protocol, NV15114, in which 33 patients received treatment with INVIRASE, ZDV and lamivudine for 4 to 16 weeks, no unexpected toxicities were reported.
Table 4 lists clinical adverse events that occurred in ≥2% of patients receiving INVIRASE 600 mg tid alone or in combi-

nation with ZDV and/or HIVID in two trials. Median duration of treatment in NV14255/ACTG229 (triple combination study) was 48 weeks; median duration of treatment among the surrogate analysis cohort analyzed for safety (n=451) in NV14256 was 42 weeks.
Rare occurrences of the following serious adverse experiences have been reported during clinical trials of INVIRASE and were considered at least possibly related to use of study drugs: confusion, ataxia and weakness; acute myeloblastic leukemia; hemolytic anemia; attempted suicide; Stevens-Johnson syndrome; seizures; severe cutaneous reaction associated with increased liver function tests; isolated elevation of transaminases; thrombophlebitis; headache; thrombocytopenia; exacerbation of chronic liver disease with Grade 4 elevated liver function tests; jaundice, ascites, and right and left upper quadrant abdominal pain; drug fever; pancreatitis leading to death; and nephrolithiasis. These events were reported from a database of >6000 patients. Over 100 patients on saquinavir therapy have been followed for >2 years.
[See Table 4 above.]
[See Table 5 on top of next page.]
Table 5 shows the percentage of patients with marked laboratory abnormalities in studies NV14255/ACTG229 and NV14256. Marked laboratory abnormalities are defined as a Grade 3 or 4 abnormality in a patient with a normal baseline value or a Grade 4 abnormality in a patient with a Grade 1 abnormality at baseline (ACTG Grading System).
Monotherapy and Combination Studies: Other clinical adverse experiences of any intensity, at least remotely related to INVIRASE, including those in <2% of patients on arms containing INVIRASE in studies NV14255/ACTG229 and NV14256, and those in smaller clinical trials, are listed below by body system.
Body as a Whole: Allergic reaction, chest pain, edema, fever, intoxication, parasites external, retrosternal pain, shivering, wasting syndrome, weight decrease
Cardiovascular: Cyanosis, heart murmur, heart valve disorder, hypertension, hypotension, syncope, vein distended
Endocrine/Metabolic: Dehydration, dry eye syndrome, hyperglycemia, weight increase, xerophthalmia
Gastrointestinal: Cheilitis, constipation, dysphagia, eructation, feces bloodstained, feces discolored, gastralgia, gastritis, gastrointestinal inflammation, gingivitis, glossitis, hemorrhage rectum, hemorrhoids, hepatomegaly, hepatosplenomegaly, melena, pain pelvic, painful defecation, pancreatitis, parotid disorder, salivary glands disorder, stomatitis, tooth disorder, vomiting
Hematologic: Anemia, microhemorrhages, pancytopenia, splenomegaly, thrombocytopenia
Musculoskeletal: Arthralgia, arthritis, back pain, cramps muscle, musculoskeletal disorders, stiffness, tissue changes, trauma

Continued on next page

Roche Laboratories—Cont.

Table 5. Percentage of Patients, by Treatment Group, with Marked Laboratory Abnormalities*
in NV14255/ACTG229 and NV14256

| | NV14255/ACTG229 | | | | NV14256 | |
	SAQ+ZDV n=99	SAQ+ZDV+ddC n=98	ZDV+ddC n=100	ddC n=145	SAQ n=159	SAQ+ddC n=147
BIOCHEMISTRY						
Calcium (high)	1	0	0	<1	0	0
Creatine Phosphokinase	10	12	7	6	4	7
Glucose (low)	0	0	0	4	5	4
Glucose (high)	0	0	0	0	<1	<1
Phosphorus	2	1	0	0	0	0
Potassium (high)	0	0	0	1	<1	<1
Potassium (low)	0	0	0	0	<1	0
Serum Amylase	2	1	1	<1	<1	2
SGOT (AST)	2	2	0	3	<1	<1
SGPT (ALT)	0	3	1	3	<1	<1
Total Bilirubin	1	0	0	0	<1	0
Uric Acid	0	0	1	Not assessed	Not assessed	Not assessed
HEMATOLOGY						
Neutrophils (low)	2	2	8	0	0	0
Hemoglobin (low)	0	0	1	0	<1	0
Platelets (low)	0	0	2	0	0	<1

* Marked Laboratory Abnormality defined as a shift from Grade 0 to at least Grade 3 or from Grade 1 to Grade 4 (ACTG Grading System)

Neurological: Ataxia, bowel movements frequent, confusion, convulsions, dysarthria, dysesthesia, heart rate disorder, hyperesthesia, hyperreflexia, hyporeflexia, mouth dry, numbness face, pain facial, paresis, poliomyelitis, progressive multifocal leukoencephalopathy, spasms, tremor

Psychological: Agitation, amnesia, anxiety, depression, dreaming excessive, euphoria, hallucination, insomnia, intellectual ability reduced, irritability, lethargy, libido disorder, overdose effect, psychic disorder, somnolence, speech disorder

Reproductive System: Prostate enlarged, vaginal discharge

Resistance Mechanism: Abscess, angina tonsillaris, candidiasis, hepatitis, herpes simplex, herpes zoster, infection bacterial, infection mycotic, infection staphylococcal, influenza, lymphadenopathy, tumor

Respiratory: Bronchitis, cough, dyspnea, epistaxis, hemoptysis, laryngitis, pharyngitis, pneumonia, respiratory disorder, rhinitis, sinusitis, upper respiratory tract infection

Skin and Appendages: Acne, dermatitis, dermatitis seborrheic, eczema, erythema, folliculitis, furunculosis, hair changes, hot flushes, photosensitivity reaction, pigment changes skin, rash maculopapular, skin disorder, skin nodule, skin ulceration, sweating increased, urticaria, verruca, xeroderma

Special Senses: Blepharitis, earache, ear pressure, eye irritation, hearing decreased, otitis, taste alteration, tinnitus, visual disturbance

Urinary System: Micturition disorder, urinary tract infection

OVERDOSAGE

No acute toxicities or sequelae were noted in 1 patient who ingested 8 grams of INVIRASE as a single dose. The patient was treated with induction of emesis within 2 to 4 hours after ingestion. In an exploratory Phase 2 study of oral dosing with INVIRASE at 7200 mg/day (1200 mg q4h), there were no serious toxicities reported through the first 25 weeks of treatment.

DOSAGE AND ADMINISTRATION

The recommended dose for INVIRASE in combination with a nucleoside analogue is three 200-mg capsules three times daily taken within 2 hours after a full meal.
Please refer to the complete prescribing information for each of the nucleoside analogues for the recommended dose of these agents.
INVIRASE should be used only in combination with an active antiretroviral nucleoside analogue regimen. Concomitant therapy should be based on a patient's prior drug exposure.

Monitoring of Patients: Clinical chemistry tests should be performed prior to initiating INVIRASE therapy and at appropriate intervals thereafter. For comprehensive patient monitoring recommendations for other nucleoside analogues, physicians should refer to the complete product information for these drugs.

Dose Adjustment for Combination Therapy with INVIRASE: For toxicities that may be associated with INVIRASE, the drug should be interrupted. INVIRASE at doses less than 600 mg tid are not recommended since lower doses have not shown antiviral activity. For recipients of combination therapy with INVIRASE and nucleoside analogues, dose adjustment of the nucleoside analogue should be based on the known toxicity profile of the individual drug. Physicians should refer to the complete product information for these drugs for comprehensive dose adjustment recommendations and drug-associated adverse reactions of nucleoside analogues.

HOW SUPPLIED

INVIRASE 200-mg capsules are light brown and green opaque capsules with ROCHE and 0245 imprinted on the capsule shell—bottles of 270 (NDC 0004-0245-15).
The capsules should be stored at 59° to 86°F (15° to 30°C) in tightly closed bottles.

Manufactured by F. Hoffmann-La Roche
& Co., Ltd., Basle, Switzerland or
Roche Laboratories Inc., Nutley, New Jersey
Revised: June 1996
Shown in Product Identification Guide, page 332

KLONOPIN®
[klon'o-pin]
(clonazepam)

℞

The following text is complete prescribing information based on official labeling in effect June 1996.

DESCRIPTION

Klonopin is available as scored tablets containing 0.5 mg, 1 mg or 2 mg clonazepam. Each tablet also contains lactose, magnesium stearate, microcrystalline cellulose and corn starch, with the following dye systems: 0.5 mg—FD&C Yellow No. 6; 1 mg—FD&C Blue No. 1 and FD&C Blue No. 2. Chemically, clonazepam is 5-(2-chlorophenyl)-1,3-dihydro-7-nitro-2H-1,4-benzodiazepin-2-one. It is a light yellow crystalline powder. It has a molecular weight of 315.7.

ACTIONS

In laboratory animals, Klonopin exhibits several pharmacologic properties which are characteristic of the benzodiazepine class of drugs. Convulsions produced in rodents by pentylenetetrazol or electrical stimulation are antagonized, as are convulsions produced by photic stimulation in susceptible baboons. A taming effect in aggressive primates, muscle

weakness and hypnosis are likewise produced by Klonopin. In humans it is capable of suppressing the spike and wave discharge in absence seizures (petit mal) and decreasing the frequency, amplitude, duration and spread of discharge in minor motor seizures.
Single oral dose administration of Klonopin to humans gave maximum blood levels of drug, in most cases, within 1 to 2 hours. The half-life of the parent compound varied from approximately 18 to 50 hours, and the major route of excretion was in the urine. In humans, five metabolites have been identified. In general, the biotransformation of clonazepam followed two pathways: oxidative hydroxylation at the C-3 position and reduction of the 7-nitro function to form 7-amino and/or 7-acetyl-amino derivatives.

INDICATIONS

Klonopin is useful alone or as an adjunct in the treatment of the Lennox-Gastaut syndrome (petit mal variant), akinetic and myoclonic seizures. In patients with absence seizures (petit mal) who have failed to respond to succinimides, Klonopin may be useful.
In some studies, up to 30% of patients have shown a loss of anticonvulsant activity, often within 3 months of administration. In some cases, dosage adjustment may reestablish efficacy.

CONTRAINDICATIONS

Klonopin should not be used in patients with a history of sensitivity to benzodiazepines, nor in patients with clinical or biochemical evidence of significant liver disease. It may be used in patients with open angle glaucoma who are receiving appropriate therapy, but is contraindicated in acute narrow angle glaucoma.

WARNINGS

Since Klonopin produces CNS depression, patients receiving this drug should be cautioned against engaging in hazardous occupations requiring mental alertness, such as operating machinery or driving a motor vehicle. They should also be warned about the concomitant use of alcohol or other CNS-depressant drugs during Klonopin therapy (see DRUG INTERACTIONS).

Usage in Pregnancy: The effects of Klonopin in human pregnancy and nursing infants are unknown.
Recent reports suggest an association between the use of anticonvulsant drugs by women with epilepsy and an elevated incidence of birth defects in children born to these women. Data are more extensive with respect to diphenylhydantoin and phenobarbital, but these are also the most commonly prescribed anticonvulsants; less systematic or anecdotal reports suggest a possible similar association with the use of all known anticonvulsant drugs.
The reports suggesting an elevated incidence of birth defects in children of drug-treated epileptic women cannot be regarded as adequate to prove a definite cause and effect relationship. There are intrinsic methodologic problems in obtaining adequate data on drug teratogenicity in humans; the possibility also exists that other factors, eg, genetic factors or the epileptic condition itself, may be more important than drug therapy in leading to birth defects. The great majority of mothers on anticonvulsant medication deliver normal infants. It is important to note that anticonvulsant drugs should not be discontinued in patients in whom the drug is administered to prevent seizures because of the strong possibility of precipitating status epilepticus with attendant hypoxia and threat to life. In individual cases where the severity and frequency of the seizure disorder are such that the removal of medication does not pose a serious threat to the patient, discontinuation of the drug may be considered prior to and during pregnancy, although it cannot be said with any confidence that even mild seizures do not pose some hazards to the developing embryo or fetus. These considerations should be weighed in treating or counseling epileptic women of childbearing potential.
Use of Klonopin in women of childbearing potential should be considered only when the clinical situation warrants the risk. Mothers receiving Klonopin should not breast-feed their infants.
In a two-generation reproduction study with Klonopin given orally to rats at 10 or 100 mg/kg/day, there was a decrease in the number of pregnancies and a decrease in the number of offspring surviving until weaning. When Klonopin was administered orally to pregnant rabbits at 0.2, 1, 5 or 10 mg/kg/day, a nondose-related incidence of cleft palates, open eyelids, fused sternebrae and limb defects was observed at the 0.2 and 5 mg/kg/day levels. Nearly all of the malformations were seen from one dam in each of the affected dosages.

Usage in Children: Because of the possibility that adverse effects on physical or mental development could become apparent only after many years, a benefit-risk consideration of the long-term use of Klonopin is important in pediatric patients.
Withdrawal symptoms of the barbiturate type have occurred after the discontinuation of benzodiazepines (see DRUG ABUSE AND DEPENDENCE section).

PRECAUTIONS
When used in patients in whom several different types of seizure disorders coexist, Klonopin may increase the incidence or precipitate the onset of generalized tonic-clonic seizures (grand mal). This may require the addition of appropriate anticonvulsants or an increase in their dosages. The concomitant use of valproic acid and clonazepam may produce absence status.
Periodic blood counts and liver function tests are advisable during long-term therapy with Klonopin.
The abrupt withdrawal of Klonopin, particularly in those patients on long-term, high-dose therapy, may precipitate status epilepticus. Therefore, when discontinuing Klonopin, gradual withdrawal is essential. While Klonopin is being gradually withdrawn, the simultaneous substitution of another anticonvulsant may be indicated. Metabolites of Klonopin are excreted by the kidneys; to avoid their excess accumulation, caution should be exercised in the administration of the drug to patients with impaired renal function.
Klonopin may produce an increase in salivation. This should be considered before giving the drug to patients who have difficulty handling secretions. Because of this and the possibility of respiratory depression, Klonopin should be used with caution in patients with chronic respiratory diseases.
Information for Patients: To assure the safe and effective use of benzodiazepines, patients should be informed that, since benzodiazepines may produce psychological and physical dependence, it is advisable that they consult with their physician before either increasing the dose or abruptly discontinuing this drug.

ADVERSE REACTIONS
The most frequently occurring side effects of Klonopin are referable to CNS depression. Experience to date has shown that drowsiness has occurred in approximately 50% of patients and ataxia in approximately 30%. In some cases, these may diminish with time; behavior problems have been noted in approximately 25% of patients. Others, listed by system, are:
Neurologic: Abnormal eye movements, aphonia, choreiform movements, coma, diplopia, dysarthria, dysdiadochokinesis, "glassy-eyed" appearance, headache, hemiparesis, hypotonia, nystagmus, respiratory depression, slurred speech, tremor, vertigo.
Psychiatric: Confusion, depression, amnesia, hallucinations, hysteria, increased libido, insomnia, psychosis, suicidal attempt (the behavior effects are more likely to occur in patients with a history of psychiatric disturbances).
Respiratory: Chest congestion, rhinorrhea, shortness of breath, hypersecretion in upper respiratory passages.
Cardiovascular: Palpitations.
Dermatologic: Hair loss, hirsutism, skin rash, ankle and facial edema.
Gastrointestinal: Anorexia, coated tongue, constipation, diarrhea, dry mouth, encopresis, gastritis, hepatomegaly, increased appetite, nausea, sore gums.
Genitourinary: Dysuria, enuresis, nocturia, urinary retention.
Musculoskeletal: Muscle weakness, pains.
Miscellaneous: Dehydration, general deterioration, fever, lymphadenopathy, weight loss or gain.
Hematopoietic: Anemia, leukopenia, thrombocytopenia, eosinophilia.
Hepatic: Transient elevations of serum transaminases and alkaline phosphatase.

DRUG ABUSE AND DEPENDENCE
Withdrawal symptoms, similar in character to those noted with barbiturates and alcohol (eg, convulsions, psychosis, hallucinations, behavioral disorder, tremor, abdominal and muscle cramps) have occurred following abrupt discontinuance of clonazepam. The more severe withdrawal symptoms have usually been limited to those patients who received excessive doses over an extended period of time. Generally milder withdrawal symptoms (eg, dysphoria and insomnia) have been reported following abrupt discontinuance of benzodiazepines taken continuously at therapeutic levels for several months. Consequently, after extended therapy, abrupt discontinuation should generally be avoided and a gradual dosage tapering schedule followed. Addiction-prone individuals (such as drug addicts or alcoholics) should be under careful surveillance when receiving clonazepam or other psychotropic agents because of the predisposition of such patients to habituation and dependence.

DRUG INTERACTIONS
The CNS-depressant action of the benzodiazepine class of drugs may be potentiated by alcohol, narcotics, barbiturates, nonbarbiturate hypnotics, antianxiety agents, the phenothiazines, thioxanthene and butyrophenone classes of antipsychotic agents, monoamine oxidase inhibitors and the tricyclic antidepressants, and by other anticonvulsant drugs.

OVERDOSAGE
Symptoms of Klonopin overdosage, like those produced by other CNS depressants, include somnolence, confusion, coma and diminished reflexes. Treatment includes monitoring of respiration, pulse and blood pressure, general supportive measures and immediate gastric lavage. Intravenous fluids should be administered and an adequate airway maintained. Hypotension may be combated by the use of levarterenol or metaraminol. Methylphenidate or caffeine and sodium benzoate may be given to combat CNS depression. Dialysis is of no known value.

DOSAGE AND ADMINISTRATION
Infants and Children: Klonopin is administered orally. In order to minimize drowsiness, the initial dose for infants and children (up to 10 years of age or 30 kg of body weight) should be between 0.01 and 0.03 mg/kg/day but not to exceed 0.05 mg/kg/day given in two or three divided doses. Dosage should be increased by no more than 0.25 to 0.5 mg every third day until a daily maintenance dose of 0.1 to 0.2 mg/kg of body weight has been reached unless seizures are controlled or side effects preclude further increase. Whenever possible, the daily dose should be divided into three equal doses. If doses are not equally divided, the largest dose should be given before retiring.
Adults: The initial dose for adults should not exceed 1.5 mg/day divided into three doses. Dosage may be increased in increments of 0.5 to 1 mg every 3 days until seizures are adequately controlled or until side effects preclude any further increase. Maintenance dosage must be individualized for each patient depending upon response. Maximum recommended daily dose is 20 mg.
The use of multiple anticonvulsants may result in an increase of depressant adverse effects. This should be considered before adding Klonopin to an existing anticonvulsant regimen.

HOW SUPPLIED
Scored tablets—0.5 mg, orange; 1 mg, blue; 2 mg, white—bottles of 100; Tel-E-Dose® packages of 100, available in boxes of four reverse-numbered cards of 25.
Manufactured by Roche Pharma, Inc., Manati, Puerto Rico 00674 or Roche Laboratories Inc., Nutley, New Jersey 07110
Revised: July 1991

Shown in Product Identification Guide, page 332

LARIAM® ℞
[lar-é-um]
brand of mefloquine hydrochloride
TABLETS

The following text is complete prescribing information based on official labeling in effect June 1996.

DESCRIPTION
Lariam (mefloquine hydrochloride) is an antimalarial agent available as 250-mg tablets of mefloquine hydrochloride (equivalent to 228.0 mg of the free base) for oral administration.

Mefloquine hydrochloride is a 4-quinolinemethanol derivative with the specific chemical name of (R*, S*)-(±)-α-2-piperidinyl-2,8-bis (trifluoromethyl)-4-quinolinemethanol hydrochloride. It is a 2-aryl substituted chemical structural analog of quinine. The drug is a white to almost white crystalline compound, slightly soluble in water.
Mefloquine hydrochloride has a calculated molecular weight of 414.78.
The inactive ingredients are ammonium-calcium alginate, corn starch, crospovidone, lactose, magnesium stearate, microcrystalline cellulose, poloxamer #331 and talc.

CLINICAL PHARMACOLOGY
Mefloquine is an antimalarial agent which acts as a blood schizonticide. Its exact mechanism of action is not known.
Pharmacokinetic studies of mefloquine in healthy male subjects showed that a significant lagtime occurred after drug administration, and the terminal elimination half-life varied widely (13 to 24 days) with a mean of about 3 weeks. Mefloquine is a mixture of enantiomeric molecules whose rates of release, absorption, transport, action, degradation and elimination may differ. A valid pharmacokinetic model may not exist in such a case.
Additional studies in European subjects showed slightly greater concentrations of drug for longer periods of time. The absorption half-life was 0.36 to 2 hours, and the terminal elimination half-life was 15 to 33 days. The primary metabolite was identified and its concentrations were found to surpass the concentrations of mefloquine.
Multiple-dose kinetic studies confirmed the long elimination half-lives previously observed. The mean metabolite to mefloquine ratio measured at steady-state was found to range between 2.3 and 8.6.
The total clearance of the drug, which is essentially all hepatic, is approximately 30 mL/min. The volume of distribution, approximately 20 L/kg, indicates extensive distribution. The drug is highly bound (98%) to plasma proteins and concentrated in blood erythrocytes, the target cells in malaria, at a relatively constant erythrocyte-to-plasma concentration ratio of about 2.
The pharmacokinetics of mefloquine in patients with compromised renal function and compromised hepatic function have not been studied.
In vitro and *in vivo* studies showed no hemolysis associated with glucose-6-phosphate dehydrogenase deficiency. (See ANIMAL TOXICOLOGY for additional information.)
Microbiology: Strains of *Plasmodium falciparum* resistant to mefloquine have been reported.

INDICATIONS AND USAGE
Treatment of Acute Malaria Infections: Lariam is indicated for the treatment of mild to moderate acute malaria caused by mefloquine-susceptible strains of *P. falciparum* (both chloroquine-susceptible and resistant strains) or by *Plasmodium vivax*. There are insufficient clinical data to document the effect of mefloquine in malaria caused by *P. ovale* or *P. malariae*.

Note: Patients with acute *P. vivax* malaria, treated with Lariam, are at high risk of relapse because Lariam does not eliminate exoerythrocytic (hepatic phase) parasites. To avoid relapse, after initial treatment of the acute infection with Lariam, patients should subsequently be treated with an 8-aminoquinoline (eg, primaquine).

Prevention of Malaria: Lariam is indicated for the prophylaxis of *P. falciparum* and *P. vivax* malaria infections, including prophylaxis of chloroquine-resistant strains of *P. falciparum*.

CONTRAINDICATIONS
Use of this drug is contraindicated in patients with a known hypersensitivity to mefloquine or related compounds (eg, quinine).

WARNINGS
In case of life-threatening, serious or overwhelming malaria infections due to *P. falciparum*, patients should be treated with an intravenous antimalarial drug. Following completion of intravenous treatment, Lariam may be given orally to complete the course of therapy.
Concomitant administration of Lariam and quinine, quinidine or drugs producing beta-adrenergic blockade may produce electrocardiographic abnormalities or cardiac arrest. Concomitant administration of Lariam and quinine or chloroquine may increase the risk of convulsions. Data on the use of halofantrine subsequent to administration of Lariam suggests a significant, potentially fatal, prolongation of the QTc interval of the ECG. Therefore, halofantrine should not be given simultaneously with or subsequent to Lariam. (see PRECAUTIONS: *Drug Interactions*.)

PRECAUTIONS
General: Caution should be exercised with regard to driving, piloting airplanes and operating machines, as dizziness, a disturbed sense of balance, neurological or psychiatric reactions have been reported during and following the use of Lariam. These effects may occur after therapy is discontin-

Continued on next page

Roche Laboratories—Cont.

ued due to the long half-life of the drug. During prophylactic use, if signs of unexplained anxiety, depression, restlessness or confusion are noticed, these may be considered prodromal to a more serious event. In these cases, the drug must be discontinued. Larium should be used with caution in patients with psychiatric disturbances because mefloquine use has been associated with emotional disturbances (see ADVERSE REACTIONS section).

This drug has not been administered for longer than 1 year. If the drug is to be administered for a prolonged period, periodic evaluations including liver function tests should be performed. Although retinal abnormalities seen in humans with long-term chloroquine use have not been observed with mefloquine use, long-term feeding of mefloquine to rats resulted in dose-related ocular lesions (retinal degeneration, retinal edema and lenticular opacity at 12.5 mg/kg/day and higher). (See ANIMAL TOXICOLOGY.) Therefore, periodic ophthalmic examinations are recommended.

Parenteral studies in animals show that mefloquine, a myocardial depressant, possesses 20% of the antifibrillatory action of quinidine and produces 50% of the increase in the PR interval reported with quinine. The effect of mefloquine on the compromised cardiovascular system has not been evaluated. However, transitory and clinically silent ECG alterations have been reported during the use of mefloquine. Alterations included sinus bradycardia, sinus arrhythmia, first degree AV-block, prolongation of the QTc interval and abnormal T waves (see also cardiovascular effects under PRECAUTIONS: *Drug Interactions* and ADVERSE REACTIONS). The benefits of Lariam therapy should be weighed against the possibility of adverse effects in patients with cardiac disease.

Laboratory Tests: Periodic evaluation of hepatic function should be performed during prolonged prophylaxis.

Drug Interactions: Drug-drug interactions with Lariam have not been explored in detail. There is one report of cardiopulmonary arrest, with full recovery, in a patient who was taking a beta blocker (propranolol), (see also WARNINGS and PRECAUTIONS: *General*). The effects of mefloquine on the compromised cardiovascular system have not been evaluated. The benefits of Lariam therapy should be weighed against the possibility of adverse effects in patients with cardiac disease.

Because of the danger of a potentially fatal prolongation of the QTc interval, halofantrine should not be given simultaneously with or subsequent to Lariam (see also WARNINGS).

Lariam should not be used concurrently with quinine or quinidine. If these drugs are to be used in the initial treatment of severe malaria, Lariam administration should be delayed at least 12 hours after the last dose.

Patients taking Lariam while taking valproic acid had loss of seizure control and lower than expected valproic acid blood levels. Therefore, patients concurrently taking antiseizure medication and Lariam should have the blood level of their antiseizure medication monitored and the dosage adjusted appropriately.

In clinical trials the concomitant administration of sulfadoxine and pyrimethamine did not alter the adverse reaction profile.

Carcinogenesis, Mutagenesis, Impairment of Fertility:
Carcinogenesis: The carcinogenic potential of mefloquine was studied in rats and mice in 2-year feeding studies at doses up to 30 mg/kg/day. No treatment-related increases in tumor of any type were noted.

Mutagenesis: The mutagenic potential of mefloquine was studied in a variety of assay systems including: Ames test, a host-mediated assay in mice, fluctuation tests and a mouse micronucleus assay. Several of these assays were performed with and without prior metabolic activation. In no instance was evidence obtained for the mutagenicity of mefloquine.

Impairment of Fertility: Fertility studies in rats at doses of 5, 20 and 50 mg/kg/day of mefloquine have demonstrated adverse effects on fertility in the male at the high dose of 50 mg/kg/day, and in the female at doses of 20 and 50 mg/kg/day. Histopathological lesions were noted in the epididymides from male rats at doses of 20 and 50 mg/kg/day. Administration of 250 mg/week of mefloquine (base) in adult males for 22 weeks failed to reveal any deleterious effects on human spermatozoa.

Pregnancy: Teratogenic Effects. Pregnancy Category C. Mefloquine has been demonstrated to be teratogenic in rats and mice at a dose of 100 mg/kg/day. In rabbits, a high dose of 160 mg/kg/day was embryotoxic and teratogenic, and a dose of 80 mg/kg/day was teratogenic but not embryotoxic. There are no adequate and well-controlled studies in pregnant women. Mefloquine should be used during pregnancy only if the potential benefit justifies the potential risk to the fetus. Women of childbearing potential who are traveling to areas where malaria is endemic should be warned against becoming pregnant.

Nursing Mothers: Mefloquine is excreted in human milk. Based on a study in a few subjects, low concentrations (3% to 4%) of mefloquine were excreted in human milk following a dose equivalent to 250 mg of the free base. Because of the potential for serious adverse reactions in nursing infants from mefloquine, a decision should be made whether to discontinue the drug, taking into account the importance of the drug to the mother.

Pediatric Use: Safety and effectiveness in children have not been established. Two studies of mefloquine in children living in endemic areas for *P. falciparum* were conducted. All children in these studies had at least a low level of parasitemia and 18% to 40% had significant parasitemia with or without mild malaria symptoms. When given 20 to 30 mg/kg of mefloquine as a single dose, all children with fever became afebrile, and 92% of those with significant parasitemia had a satisfactory response to treatment. While incomplete follow-up was obtained in these studies, nausea and vomiting occurred in approximately 10% and 20%, respectively, and dizziness was seen in approximately 40% of children.

ADVERSE REACTIONS

Clinical: At the doses used for treatment of acute malaria infections, the symptoms possibly attributable to drug administration cannot be distinguished from those symptoms usually attributable to the disease itself.

Among subjects who received mefloquine for prophylaxis of malaria, the most frequently observed adverse experience was vomiting (3%). Dizziness, syncope, extrasystoles and other complaints affecting less than 1% were also reported. Among subjects who received mefloquine for treatment, the most frequently observed adverse experiences included: dizziness, myalgia, nausea, fever, headache, vomiting, chills, diarrhea, skin rash, abdominal pain, fatigue, loss of appetite and tinnitus. Those side effects occurring in less than 1% included bradycardia, hair loss, emotional problems, pruritus, asthenia, transient emotional disturbances and telogen effluvium (loss of resting hair). Seizures have also been reported.

Two serious adverse reactions were cardiopulmonary arrest in one patient shortly after ingesting a single prophylactic dose of mefloquine while concomitantly using propranolol (see WARNINGS and PRECAUTIONS), and encephalopathy of unknown etiology during prophylactic mefloquine administration. The relationship of encephalopathy to drug administration could not be clearly established.

Post Marketing: Post-marketing surveillance indicates that the same adverse experiences are reported during prophylaxis, as well as acute treatment.

The following additional adverse reactions have been reported during post-marketing surveillance: vertigo, visual disturbances, central nervous system disturbances (eg, psychotic manifestations, hallucinations, confusion, anxiety and depression), insomnia, abnormal dreams, forgetfulness, motor and sensory neuropathy, hypertension, hypotension, flushing, tachycardia, palpitations, uticaria, Stevens-Johnson syndrome and erythema multiforma.

Laboratory: The most frequently observed laboratory alterations which could be possibly attributable to drug administration were decreased hematocrit, transient elevation of transaminases, leukopenia and thrombocytopenia. These alterations were observed in patients with acute malaria who received treatment doses of the drug and were attributed to the disease itself.

During prophylactic administration of mefloquine to indigenous populations in malaria-endemic areas, the following occasional alterations in laboratory values were observed: transient elevation of transaminases, leukocytosis or thrombocytopenia.

OVERDOSAGE

The following procedure is recommended in case of overdosage: Induce vomiting or perform gastric lavage, as appropriate. Monitor cardiac function and neurologic and psychiatric status for at least 24 hours. Provide symptomatic and intensive supportive treatment as required, particularly for cardiovascular disturbances. Treat vomiting or diarrhea with standard fluid therapy.

DOSAGE AND ADMINISTRATION (see INDICATIONS AND USAGE section):

(a) Treatment of mild to moderate malaria in adults caused by *P. vivax* or mefloquine-susceptible strains of *P. falciparum*—5 tablets (1250 mg) mefloquine hydrochloride to be given as a single oral dose. The drug should not be taken on an empty stomach and should be administered with at least 8 oz (240 mL) of water.

If a full treatment course has been administered without clinical cure, alternative treatment should be given. Similarly, if previous prophylaxis with mefloquine has failed, Larium should not be used for curative treatment.

Note: Patients with acute *P. vivax* malaria, treated with Lariam, are at high risk of relapse because Lariam does not eliminate exoerythrocytic (hepatic phase) parasites. To avoid relapse after initial treatment of the acute infection with Lariam, patients should subsequently be treated with an 8-aminoquinoline (eg, primaquine).

(b) Malaria prophylaxis—one 250 mg Lariam tablet once weekly.

Prophylactic drug administration should begin 1 week before departure to an endemic area. Subsequent weekly doses should always be taken on the same day of the week. To reduce the risk of malaria after leaving an endemic area, prophylaxis should be continued for 4 additional weeks. Tablets should not be taken on an empty stomach and should be administered with at least 8 oz (240 mL) of water.

HOW SUPPLIED

Lariam is available as scored, white, round tablets, containing 250 mg of mefloquine hydrochloride in Tel-E-Dose packages of 25 (NDC 0004-0172-02). Imprint on tablets: LARIAM 250 ROCHE.

Tablets should be stored at 15°–30°C (59°–86°F).

ANIMAL TOXICOLOGY

Ocular lesions were observed in rats fed mefloquine daily for 2 years. All surviving rats given 30 mg/kg/day had ocular lesions in both eyes characterized by retinal degeneration, opacity of the lens and retinal edema. Similar but less severe lesions were observed in 80% of female and 22% of male rats fed 12.5 mg/kg/day for 2 years. At doses of 5 mg/kg/day, only corneal lesions were observed. They occurred in 9% of rats studied.

Manufactured by
F. Hoffmann-La Roche & Co., Ltd.,
Basle, Switzerland
Revised: August 1994
Shown in Product Identification Guide, page 332

LARODOPA®   ℞
[lar"o-do'pa]
brand of levodopa

The following text is complete prescribing information based on official labeling in effect June 1, 1996.

> In order to reduce the high incidence of adverse reactions, it is necessary to individualize the therapy and to gradually increase the dosage to the desired therapeutic level.

DESCRIPTION

Larodopa is available as tablets containing 0.1 gm, 0.25 gm or 0.5 gm levodopa. Each tablet also contains corn starch, magnesium stearate, microcrystalline cellulose, povidone, talc and D&C Red No. 7 lake dye.

Chemically, levodopa is $(-)$-3-(3,4-dihydroxyphenyl)-*L*-alanine. It is a colorless, crystalline compound, slightly soluble in water and insoluble in alcohol, with a molecular weight of 197.2.

ACTIONS

Evidence indicates that the symptoms of Parkinson's disease are related to depletion of striatal dopamine. Since dopamine apparently does not cross the blood-brain barrier, its administration is ineffective in the treatment of Parkinson's disease. However, levodopa, the levorotatory isomer of dihydroxyphenylalanine (dopa) which is the metabolic precursor of dopamine, does cross the blood-brain barrier. Presumably it is converted into dopamine in the basal ganglia. This is generally thought to be the mechanism whereby oral levodopa acts in relieving the symptoms of Parkinson's disease.

The major urinary metabolites of levodopa in man appear to be dopamine and homovanillic acid (HVA). In 24-hour urine samples, HVA accounts for 13% to 42% of the ingested dose of levodopa.

INDICATIONS

Larodopa is indicated in the treatment of idiopathic Parkinson's disease (Paralysis Agitans), postencephalitic parkinsonism, symptomatic parkinsonism which may follow injury to the nervous system by carbon monoxide intoxication, and manganese intoxication. It is indicated in those elderly patients believed to develop parkinsonism in association with cerebral arteriosclerosis.

CONTRAINDICATIONS

Monoamine oxidase (MAO) inhibitors and Larodopa should not be given concomitantly and these inhibitors must be discontinued 2 weeks prior to initiating therapy with Larodopa. Larodopa is contraindicated in patients with known hypersensitivity to the drug and in narrow angle glaucoma.

Because levodopa may activate a malignant melanoma, it should not be used in patients with suspicious, undiagnosed skin lesions or a history of melanoma.

WARNINGS

Larodopa should be administered cautiously to patients with severe cardiovascular or pulmonary disease, bronchial asthma, renal, hepatic or endocrine disease.

Care should be exercised in administering Larodopa to patients with a history of myocardial infarction who have residual atrial, nodal or ventricular arrhythmias. If Larodopa is necessary in this type of patient, it should be used in a facility with a coronary care unit or an intensive care unit.
One must be on the alert for the possibility of upper gastrointestinal hemorrhage in those patients with a past history of active peptic ulcer disease.
All patients should be carefully observed for the development of depression with concomitant suicidal tendencies.
Psychotic patients should be treated with caution.
Pyridoxine hydrochloride (vitamin B_6) in oral doses of 10 to 25 mg rapidly reverses the toxic and therapeutic effects of Larodopa. This should be considered before recommending vitamin preparations containing pyridoxine hydrochloride (vitamin B_6).
Usage in Pregnancy: The safety of Larodopa in women who are or who may become pregnant has not been established; hence it should be given only when the potential benefits have been weighed against possible hazards to mother and child. Studies in rodents have shown that levodopa at dosages in excess of 200 mg/kg/day has an adverse effect on fetal and postnatal growth and viability.
Larodopa should not be used in nursing mothers.
Usage in Children: The safety of Larodopa under the age of 12 has not been established.

PRECAUTIONS

Periodic evaluations of hepatic, hematopoietic, cardiovascular and renal function are recommended during extended therapy in all patients.
Patients with chronic wide angle glaucoma may be treated cautiously with Larodopa, provided the intraocular pressure is well controlled and the patient monitored carefully for changes in intraocular pressure during therapy.
Postural hypotensive episodes have been reported as adverse reactions. Therefore, Larodopa should be administered to patients on antihypertensive drug cautiously (for patients receiving pargyline, see note on MAO inhibitors contraindications), and it may be necessary to adjust the dosage of the antihypertensive drugs.

ADVERSE REACTIONS

The most serious adverse reactions associated with the administration of Larodopa having frequent occurrences are: adventitious movements such as choreiform and/or dystonic movements. Other serious adverse reactions with a lower incidence are: cardiac irregularities and/or palpitations, orthostatic hypotensive episodes, bradykinetic episodes (the "on-off" phenomena), mental changes including paranoid ideation and psychotic episodes, depression with or without the development of suicidal tendencies, dementia, and urinary retention.
Rarely, gastrointestinal bleeding, development of duodenal ulcer, hypertension, phlebitis, hemolytic anemia, agranulocytosis, and convulsions have been observed. (The causal relationship between convulsions and Larodopa has not been established.)
Adverse reactions of a less serious nature having a relatively frequent occurrence are the following: anorexia, nausea and vomiting with or without abdominal pain and distress, dry mouth, dysphagia, sialorrhea, ataxia, increased hand tremor, headache, dizziness, numbness, weakness and faintness, bruxism, confusion, insomnia, nightmares, hallucinations and delusions, agitation and anxiety, malaise, fatigue and euphoria. Occurring with a lesser order of frequency are the following: muscle twitching and blepharospasm (which may be taken as an early sign of overdosage; consideration of dosage reduction may be made at this time), trismus, burning sensation of the tongue, bitter taste, diarrhea, constipation, flatulence, flushing, skin rash, increased sweating, bizarre breathing patterns, urinary incontinence, diplopia, blurred vision, dilated pupils, hot flashes, weight gain or loss, dark sweat and/or urine.
Rarely, oculogyric crises, sense of stimulation, hiccups, development of edema, loss of hair, hoarseness, priapism and activation of latent Horner's syndrome have been observed.
Elevations of blood urea nitrogen, SGOT, SGPT, LDH, bilirubin, alkaline phosphatase or protein-bound iodine have been reported; and the significance of this is not known. Occasional reductions in WBC, hemoglobin, and hematocrit have been noted.
Leukopenia has occurred and requires cessation, at least temporarily, of Larodopa administration. The Coombs' test has occasionally become positive during extended therapy.
Elevations of uric acid have been noted when colorimetric method was used but not when uricase method was used.

OVERDOSAGE

For acute overdosage general supportive measures should be employed, along with immediate gastric lavage. Intravenous fluids should be administered judiciously and an adequate airway maintained.
Electrocardiographic monitoring should be instituted and the patient carefully observed for the possible development of arrhythmias; if required, appropriate antiarrhythmic therapy should be given. Consideration should be given to the possibility of multiple drug ingestion by the patient. To date, no experience has been reported with dialysis; hence its value in Larodopa overdosage is not known. Although pyridoxine hydrochloride (vitamin B_6) has been reported to reverse the antiparkinson effects of Larodopa, its usefulness in the management of acute overdosage has not been established.

DOSAGE AND ADMINISTRATION

The optimal daily dose of Larodopa, ie, the dose producing maximal improvement with tolerated side effects, must be determined and *carefully titrated for each individual patient.*
The usual initial dosage is 0.5 to 1 gm daily, divided in two or more doses with food.
The total daily dosage is then increased gradually in increments not more than 0.75 gm every 3 to 7 days as tolerated.
The usual optimal therapeutic *dosage should not exceed 8 gm.*
The exceptional patient may carefully be given more than 8 gms as required. In some patients, a significant therapeutic response may not be obtained until 6 months of treatment.

In the event general anesthesia is required, Larodopa therapy may be continued as long as the patient is able to take fluids and medication by mouth. If therapy is temporarily interrupted, the usual daily dosage may be administered as soon as the patient is able to take oral medication. Whenever therapy has been interrupted for longer periods, dosage should again be adjusted gradually; however, in many cases the patient can be rapidly titrated to his previous therapeutic dosage.

HOW SUPPLIED

Tablets, pink, scored, each containing levodopa 0.1 gm (NDC 0004-0072-01), 0.25 gm (NDC 0004-0057-01) or 0.5 gm (NDC 0004-0056-01)—bottles of 100.
Revised: May 1991

Shown in Product Identification Guide, page 332

LEVO-DROMORAN® Ⓒ ℞
[lee″vo dro′mo-ran]
brand of
levorphanol tartrate
AMPULS, VIALS, TABLETS

WARNING: May be habit forming

DESCRIPTION

Levo-Dromoran (levorphanol tartrate) is a potent opioid analgesic with empirical formula $C_{17}H_{23}NO \cdot C_4H_6O_6 \cdot 2H_2O$ and molecular weight 443.5. Each mg of levorphanol tartrate is equivalent to 0.58 mg levorphanol base. Chemically levorphanol is levo-3-hydroxy-N-methylmorphinan. The USP nomenclature is 17-methylmorphinan 3-ol tartrate (1:1) (Salt) dihydrate. The material has 3 asymmetric carbon atoms.
Levorphanol tartrate is a white crystalline powder, soluble in water and ether but insoluble in chloroform.
Each 1-mL ampul contains 2 mg levorphanol tartrate, 1.8 mg methyl paraben preservative, 0.2 mg propyl paraben preservative, sodium hydroxide to adjust pH to approximately 4.3 and Water for Injection.
Each milliliter in the 10 mL vials contains 2 mg levorphanol tartrate, 4.5 mg phenol preservative, sodium hydroxide to adjust pH to approximately 4.3 and Water for Injection.
Each tablet contains 2 mg levorphanol tartrate, lactose, corn starch, stearic acid and talc.

CLINICAL PHARMACOLOGY

Pharmacodynamics: Levo-Dromoran is a potent synthetic opioid similar to morphine in its actions. Like other mu-agonist opioids it is believed to act at receptors in the periventricular and periaqueductal gray matter in both the brain and spinal cord to alter the transmission and perception of pain. Onset of analgesia and peak analgesic effect following administration of levorphanol are similar to morphine when administered at equianalgesic doses.
Levorphanol produces a degree of respiratory depression similar to that produced by morphine at equianalgesic doses, and like many mu-opioid drugs, levorphanol produces euphoria or has a positive effect on mood in many individuals. Two mg of intramuscular levorphanol tartrate depresses respiration to a degree approximately equivalent to that produced by 10 to 15 mg of intramuscular morphine in man. The hemodynamic changes after intravenous administration of levorphanol have not been studied in man but are expected to clinically resemble those seen after morphine.
As with other opioids, the blood levels required for analgesia are determined by the opioid tolerance of the patient and are likely to rise with chronic use. The rate of development of tolerance is highly variable and is determined by the dose, dosing interval, age, use of concomitant drugs and physical status of the patient. While blood levels of opioid drugs may be helpful in assessing individual cases, dosage is usually adjusted by careful clinical observation of the patient.
Pharmacokinetics: The pharmacokinetics of levorphanol have been studied in a limited number of cancer patients following intravenous (IV), intramuscular (IM) and oral (PO) administration. Following IV administration, plasma concentrations of levorphanol decline in a triexponential manner with a terminal half-life of approximately 11 to 16 hours and a clearance of 0.78 to 1.1 L/kg/hr. Based on terminal half-life, steady-state plasma concentrations should be achieved by the third day of dosing. Levorphanol is rapidly distributed (< 1 hr) and redistributed (1 to 2 hours) following IV administration and has a steady-state volume of distribution of 10 to 13 L/kg. In vitro studies of protein binding indicate that levorphanol is only 40% bound to plasma proteins.
No pharmacokinetic studies of the absorption of IM levorphanol are available, but clinical data suggests that absorption is rapid with onset of effects within 15 to 30 minutes of administration.
Levorphanol is well absorbed after PO administration with peak plasma concentrations occurring approximately 1 hour after dosing. The bioavailability of levorphanol tablets compared to IM or IV administration is not known.
Plasma concentrations of levorphanol following chronic administration in patients with cancer increased with the dose, but the analgesic effect was dependent on the degree of opioid tolerance of the patient. Expected steady-state plasma concentrations for a 6-hour dosing interval can reach 2 to 5 times those following a single dose, depending on the patient's individual clearance of the drug. Very high plasma concentrations of levorphanol can be reached in patients on chronic therapy due to the long half-life of the drug. One study in 11 patients using the drug for control of cancer pain reported plasma concentrations from 5 to 10 ng/mL after a single 2-mg dose up to 50 to 100 ng/mL after repeated oral doses of 20 to 50 mg/day.
Animal studies suggest that levorphanol is extensively metabolized in the liver and is eliminated as the glucuronide metabolite. This renally excreted inactive glucuronide metabolite accumulates with chronic dosing in plasma at concentrations that reach fivefold that of the parent compound.
The effects of age, gender, hepatic and renal disease on the pharmacokinetics of levorphanol are not known. As with all drugs of this class, patients at the extremes of age are expected to be more susceptible to adverse effects because of a greater pharmacodynamic sensitivity and probable increased variability in pharmacokinetics due to age or disease.

CLINICAL TRIALS

Clinical trials have been reported in the medical literature that investigated the use of Levo-Dromoran as a preoperative medication, as a postoperative analgesic and in the management of chronic pain due primarily to malignancy. In each of these clinical settings Levo-Dromoran has been shown to be an effective analgesic of the mu-opioid type and similar to morphine, meperidine or fentanyl.
A single 2 mg intramuscular dose of Levo-Dromoran was studied as a routine preoperative medication in 100 patients as part of a blinded 1500 patient trial of a number of synthetic opioids and was found to provide sedation similar to that observed with 100 mg meperidine or 10 mg of methadone.
Levo-Dromoran has been studied in chronic cancer patients. Dosages were individualized to each patient's level of opioid tolerance. In one study, starting doses of 2 mg twice a day often had to be advanced by 50% or more within a few weeks of starting therapy. A study of levorphanol indicates that the relative potency is approximately 4 to 8 times that of morphine, depending on the specific circumstances of use. In postoperative patients, intramuscular levorphanol was determined to be about 8 times as potent as intramuscular morphine, whereas in cancer patients with chronic pain, it was found to be only about 4 times as potent.

INDIVIDUALIZATION OF DOSAGE

Accepted medical practice dictates that the dose of any opioid analgesic be appropriate to the degree of pain to be relieved, the clinical setting, the physical condition of the patient, and the kind and dose of concurrent medication. This is especially important during recovery from anesthesia because of the residual CNS-depressant effects of anesthetic agents and the adverse effects of surgery on respiratory reserve. In consequence, the dose of Levo-Dromoran should be reduced under circumstances likely to increase the patient's sensitivity to the adverse effects of opioids. As there is substantial redistribution involved in the kinetics of levorphanol, the duration of effect of a single dose may vary and physicians must judge the need for a repeat dose based on the clinical response of the patient. Clinicians are advised to remember that while the long terminal half-life of levorphanol may reduce the need for postoperative analgesics, the administration of an excessive dose preoperatively may cause a delay in the return of spontaneous respirations or prolonged hypoventilation in the postoperative period. In addition, accumulation of the drug following excessive dos-

Continued on next page

Roche Laboratories—Cont.

age postoperatively may prolong or result in hypoventilation.

Levo-Dromoran has a long half-life similar to methadone or other slowly excreted opioids, rather than quickly excreted agents such as morphine or meperidine. Slowly excreted drugs may have some advantages in the management of chronic pain. Unfortunately, the duration of pain relief after a single dose of a slowly excreted opioid cannot always be predicted from pharmacokinetic principles, and the interdose interval may have to be adjusted to suit the patient's individual pharmacodynamic response.

Levo-Dromoran is 4 to 8 times as potent as morphine and has a longer half-life. Because there is incomplete cross-tolerance among opioids, when converting a patient from morphine to Levo-Dromoran, the total *daily* dose of oral Levo-Dromoran should begin at approximately $^1/_{15}$ to $^1/_{12}$ of the total *daily* dose of oral morphine that such patients had previously required and then the dose should be adjusted to the patient's clinical response. If a patient is to be placed on fixed-schedule dosing (round-the-clock) with this drug, care should be taken to allow adequate time after each dose change (approximately 72 hours) for the patient to reach a new steady-state before a subsequent dose adjustment to avoid excessive sedation due to drug accumulation.

INDICATIONS

Levo-Dromoran is indicated for the management of moderate to severe pain or as a preoperative medication where an opioid analgesic is appropriate.

CONTRAINDICATIONS

Levo-Dromoran is contraindicated in patients hypersensitive to levorphanol tartrate.

WARNINGS

Respiratory Depression: Levo-Dromoran, like morphine, may be expected to produce serious or potentially fatal respiratory depression if given in an excessive dose, too frequently, or if given in full dosage to compromised or vulnerable patients. This is because the doses required to produce analgesia in the general clinical population may cause serious respiratory depression in vulnerable patients. Safe usage of this potent opioid requires that the dose and dosage interval be individualized to each patient based on the severity of the pain, weight, age, diagnosis and physical status of the patient, and the kind and dose of concurrently administered medication.

The initial dose of Levo-Dromoran should be reduced by 50% or more when the drug is given to patients with any condition affecting respiratory reserve or in conjunction with other drugs affecting the respiratory center. Subsequent doses should then be individually titrated according to the patient's response. Respiratory depression produced by levorphanol tartrate can be reversed by naloxone, a specific antagonist (see OVERDOSAGE).

Preexisting Pulmonary Disease: Because Levo-Dromoran causes respiratory depression, it should be administered with caution to patients with impaired respiratory reserve or respiratory depression from some other cause (eg, from other medication, uremia, severe infection, obstructive respiratory conditions, restrictive respiratory diseases, intrapulmonary shunting or chronic bronchial asthma). As with other strong opioids, use of Levo-Dromoran in acute or severe bronchial asthma is not recommended (see *Respiratory Depression*).

Head Injury and Increased Intracranial Pressure: The respiratory depressant effects of Levo-Dromoran with carbon dioxide retention and secondary elevation of cerebral spinal fluid pressure may be markedly exaggerated in the presence of head injury, other intracranial lesions or pre-existing increase in intracranial pressure. Opioids, including Levo-Dromoran, produce effects that may obscure neurological signs of further increase in pressure in patients with head injuries. In addition, Levo-Dromoran may affect level of consciousness that may complicate neurological evaluation.

Cardiovascular Effects: The use of Levo-Dromoran in acute myocardial infarction or in cardiac patients with myocardial dysfunction or coronary insufficiency should be limited because the effects of levorphanol on the work of the heart are unknown.

Hypotensive Effect: The administration of Levo-Dromoran may result in severe hypotension in the postoperative patient or in any individual whose ability to maintain blood pressure has been compromised by a depleted blood volume or by administration of drugs, such as phenothiazines or general anesthetics. Opioids may produce orthostatic hypotension in ambulatory patients.

Use in Liver Disease: Levo-Dromoran should be administered with caution to patients with extensive liver disease who may be vulnerable to excessive sedation due to increased pharmacodynamic sensitivity or impaired metabolism of the drug.

Biliary Surgery: Levo-Dromoran has been shown to cause moderate to marked rises in pressure in the common bile duct when given in analgesic doses. It is not recommended for use in biliary surgery.

Use in Alcoholism or Drug Dependence: Levo-Dromoran has an abuse potential as great as morphine, and the prescription of this drug must always balance the prospective benefits against the risk of abuse and dependence. The use of levorphanol in patients with a history of alcohol or other drug dependence, either active or in remission, has not been specifically studied (see DRUG ABUSE AND DEPENDENCE).

PRECAUTIONS

General: As with other opioids, the administration of Levo-Dromoran may obscure the diagnosis or clinical course in patients with acute abdominal conditions. Levo-Dromoran should be administered with caution and the initial dose should be reduced in patients who are elderly or debilitated and in those patients with severe impairment of hepatic or renal function, hypothyroidism, Addison's disease, toxic psychosis, prostatic hypertrophy or urethral stricture, acute alcoholism, or delirium tremens.

Information for Patients: If Levo-Dromoran is administered to ambulatory patients, they should be cautioned against engaging in hazardous occupations requiring complete mental alertness such as operating machinery or driving a motor vehicle. They should also be warned that concurrent use of Levo-Dromoran with central nervous system depressants (eg, alcohol, sedatives, hypnotics, other opioids, barbiturates, tricyclic antidepressants, phenothiazines, tranquilizers, skeletal muscle relaxants and antihistamines) may result in additive central nervous system depressant effects. Patients should be made aware of the risk of orthostatic hypotension, dizziness and syncope in ambulatory patients taking Levo-Dromoran.

Drug Interactions: *Interactions with Other CNS Agents:* Concurrent use of Levo-Dromoran with all central nervous system depressants (eg, alcohol, sedatives, hypnotics, other opioids, general anesthetics, barbiturates, tricyclic antidepressants, phenothiazines, tranquilizers, skeletal muscle relaxants and antihistamines) may result in additive central nervous system depressant effects. Respiratory depression, hypotension, and profound sedation or coma may occur. When such combined therapy is contemplated, the dose of one or both agents should be reduced. Although no interaction between MAO inhibitors and Levo-Dromoran has been observed, it is not recommended for use with MAO inhibitors.

Most cases of serious or fatal adverse events involving Levo-Dromoran reported to the manufacturer or the FDA have involved either the administration of large initial doses or too frequent doses of the drug to nonopioid tolerant patients, or the simultaneous administration of levorphanol with other drugs affecting respiration (see INDIVIDUALIZATION OF DOSAGE and WARNINGS). The initial dose of levorphanol should be reduced by approximately 50% or more when it is given to patients along with another drug affecting respiration.

Interactions with Mixed Agonist/Antagonist Opioid Analgesics: Agonist/antagonist analgesics (eg, pentazocine, nalbuphine, butorphanol, dezocine and buprenorphine) should NOT be administered to a patient who has received or is receiving a course of therapy with a pure agonist opioid analgesic such as Levo-Dromoran. In opioid-dependent patients, mixed agonist/antagonist analgesics may precipitate withdrawal symptoms.

Use in Ambulatory Patients: Levo-Dromoran has been used in both inpatient and outpatient settings, but both physicians and patients must be aware of the risk of orthostatic hypotension, dizziness and syncope in ambulatory patients.

As with other opioids, the use of Levo-Dromoran may impair mental and/or physical abilities required for the performance of potentially hazardous tasks or for the exercise of normal good judgement and patients and staff should be advised accordingly.

Concurrent use of Levo-Dromoran with central nervous system depressants (eg, alcohol, sedatives, hypnotics, other opioids, barbiturates, tricyclic antidepressants, phenothiazines, tranquilizers, skeletal muscle relaxants and antihistamines) may result in additive central nervous system depressant effects.

Carcinogenesis, Mutagenesis, Impairment of Fertility: No information about the effects of Levo-Dromoran on carcinogenesis, mutagenesis, or fertility is available.

Pregnancy: Teratogenic Effects: Pregnancy Category C. Levo-Dromoran has been shown to be teratogenic in mice when given at a single oral dose of 25 mg/kg. The tested dose caused a near 50% mortality of the mouse embryos. There are no adequate and well-controlled studies in pregnant women. Levo-Dromoran should be used in pregnancy only if the potential benefit justifies the potential risk to the fetus.

Nonteratogenic Effects: Babies born to mothers who have been taking opioids regularly prior to delivery may be physically dependent.

A study in rabbits has demonstrated that at doses of 1.5 to 20 mg/kg, Levo-Dromoran administered intravenously crosses the placental barrier and depresses fetal respiration.

Labor and Delivery: The use of Levo-Dromoran in labor and delivery in humans has not been studied. However, as with other opioids, administration of Levo-Dromoran to the mother during labor and delivery may result in respiratory depression in the newborn. Therefore, its use during labor and delivery is not recommended.

Nursing Mothers: Studies of levorphanol concentrations in breast milk have not been performed. However, morphine, which is structurally similar to levorphanol, is excreted in human milk. Because of the potential for serious adverse reactions from Levo-Dromoran in nursing infants, a decision should be made whether to discontinue nursing or to discontinue the drug, taking into account the importance of the drug to the mother.

Pediatric Use: Levo-Dromoran is not recommended in children under the age of 18 years as the safety and efficacy of the drug in this population has not been established.

Geriatric Use: The initial dose of Levo-Dromoran should be reduced by 50% or more in the infirm elderly patient, even though there have been no reports of unexpected adverse events in older populations. All drugs of this class may be associated with a profound or prolonged effect in elderly patients for both pharmacokinetic and pharmacodynamic reasons and caution is indicated.

ADVERSE REACTIONS

In approximately 1400 patients treated with Levo-Dromoran in controlled clinical trials, the type and incidence of side effects were those expected of an opioid analgesic, and no unforeseen or unusual toxicity was reported.

Drugs of this type are expected to produce a cluster of typical opioid effects in addition to analgesia, consisting of nausea, vomiting, altered mood and mentation, pruritus, flushing, difficulties in urination, constipation and biliary spasm. The frequency and intensity of these effects appears to be dose related. Although listed as adverse events these are expected pharmacologic actions of these drugs and should be interpreted as such by the clinician.

The following adverse events have been reported with the use of Levo-Dromoran:

Body as a Whole: abdominal pain, dry mouth, sweating

Cardiovascular System: cardiac arrest, shock, hypotension, arrhythmias including bradycardia and tachycardia, palpitations, extra-systoles

Digestive System: nausea, vomiting, dyspepsia, biliary tract spasm

Nervous System: coma, suicide attempt, convulsions, depression, dizziness, confusion, lethargy, abnormal dreams, abnormal thinking, nervousness, drug withdrawal, hypokinesia, dyskinesia, hyperkinesia, CNS stimulation, personality disorder, amnesia, insomnia

Respiratory System: apnea, cyanosis, hypoventilation

Skin & Appendages: pruritus, urticaria, rash, injection site reaction

Special Senses: abnormal vision, pupillary disorder, diplopia

Urogenital System: kidney failure, urinary retention, difficulty urinating

DRUG ABUSE AND DEPENDENCE

Warning: May be Habit Forming

Levo-Dromoran is a Schedule II Controlled Substance. All drugs of this class (mu-opioids of the morphine type) are habit forming and should be stored, prescribed, used and disposed of accordingly. Psychological/physical dependence and tolerance may develop upon repeated administration of Levo-Dromoran.

Discontinuation of Levo-Dromoran after chronic use has been reported to result in withdrawal syndromes, and some reports of overuse and self-reported addiction have been received. Neither withdrawal nor withdrawal symptoms are usually expected in postoperative patients who used the drug for less than a week or in patients who are gradually tapered off the drug after longer use.

OVERDOSAGE

Most reports of overdosage known to the manufacturer and to the FDA involve three clinical situations. These are: 1. the use of larger than recommended doses or too frequent doses, 2. administration of the drug to children or small adults without any reduction in dosage, and 3. the use of the drug in ordinary dosage in patients compromised by concurrent illness.

As with all opioids, overdose can occur due to accidental or intentional misuse of this product, especially in infants and children who may gain access to the drug in the home. Based on its pharmacology, levorphanol overdosage would be expected to produce signs of respiratory depression, cardiovascular failure (especially in predisposed patients) and/or central nervous system depression. Serious overdosage with Levo-Dromoran is characterized by respiratory depression (a decrease in respiratory rate and/or tidal volume, periodic breathing, cyanosis), extreme somnolence progressing to stupor or coma, skeletal muscle flaccidity, cold and clammy skin, constricted pupils, and sometimes bradycardia and hypotension. In severe overdosage, apnea, circulatory collapse, cardiac arrest and death may occur.

Treatment: The specific treatment of suspected levorphanol tartrate overdosage is immediate establishment of an adequate airway and ventilation, followed (if necessary) by intravenous naloxone. The respiratory and cardiac status of the patient should be continuously monitored and appropriate supportive measures instituted, such as oxygen, intravenous fluids and/or vasopressors, if required. Physicians are reminded that the duration of levorphanol action far exceeds the duration of action of naloxone, and repeated dosing with naloxone may be required. Naloxone should be administered cautiously to persons known or suspected to be physically dependent on Levo-Dromoran. In such cases an abrupt and complete reversal of opioid effects may precipitate an acute abstinence syndrome. If necessary to administer naloxone to the physically dependent patient, the antagonist should be administered with extreme care and by titration with smaller than usual doses of the antagonist.

DOSAGE AND ADMINISTRATION

Intravenous: The usual recommended starting dose for IV administration is up to 1 mg, given in divided doses, by slow injection. This may be repeated in 3 to 6 hours as needed, provided the patient is assessed for signs of hypoventilation or excessive sedation. Dosage should be adjusted according to the severity of the pain; age, weight and physical status of the patient; the patient's underlying diseases; use of concomitant medications; and other factors (see INDIVIDUALIZATION OF DOSAGE, WARNINGS and PRECAUTIONS). Total *daily* doses or more than 4 to 8 mg IV in 24 hours are generally not recommended as starting doses in nonopioid tolerant patients; lower total *daily* doses may be appropriate.
Intramuscular or Subcutaneous: The usual recommended starting dose for IM or SC administration is 1 to 2 mg. This may be repeated in 6 to 8 hours as needed, provided the patient is assessed for signs of hypoventilation or excessive sedation. Dosage should be adjusted according to the severity of the pain; age, weight and physical status of the patient; the patient's underlying diseases; use of concomitant medications; and other factors (see INDIVIDUALIZATION OF DOSAGE, WARNINGS and PRECAUTIONS). Total *daily* doses of more than 3 to 8 mg IM in 24 hours are generally not recommended as starting doses in nonopioid tolerant patients; lower total *daily* doses may be appropriate.
Oral: The usual recommended starting dose for oral administration is 2 mg. This may be repeated in 6 to 8 hours as needed, provided the patient is assessed for signs of hypoventilation and excessive sedation. If necessary, the dose may be increased to up to 3 mg every 6 to 8 hours, after adequate evaluation of the patient's response. Higher doses may be appropriate in opioid tolerant patients. Dosage should be adjusted according to the severity of the pain; age, weight and physical status of the patient; the patient's underlying diseases; use of concomitant medications; and other factors (see INDIVIDUALIZATION OF DOSAGE, WARNINGS and PRECAUTIONS). Total oral *daily* doses of more than 6 to 12 mg in 24 hours are generally not recommended as starting doses in nonopioid tolerant patients; lower total *daily* doses may be appropriate.
Use in Chronic Pain: The dosage of Levo-Dromoran in patients with cancer or with other conditions for which chronic opioid therapy is indicated must be individualized (see INDIVIDUALIZATION OF DOSAGE). Levo-Dromoran is 4 to 8 times as potent as morphine and has a longer half-life. Because there is incomplete cross-tolerance among opioids, when converting a patient from morphine to Levo-Dromoran, the total *daily* dose of oral Levo-Dromoran should begin at approximately $^1/_{15}$ to $^1/_{12}$ of the total *daily* dose of oral morphine that such patients had previously required and then the dose should be adjusted to the patient's clinical response. If a patient is to be placed on fixed-schedule dosing (round-the-clock) with this drug, care should be taken to allow adequate time after each dose change (approximately 72 hours) for the patient to reach a new steady-state before a subsequent dose adjustment to avoid excessive sedation due to drug accumulation.
Use in The Perioperative Period: Levo-Dromoran has been used for analgesic action during premedication and the postoperative period. Factors to be considered in determining the dosage include age, body weight, physical status, underlying pathological condition, use of other drugs, type of anesthesia used, the surgical procedure involved and the severity of pain (see INDIVIDUALIZATION OF DOSAGE, WARNINGS and PRECAUTIONS).
Premedication: The preoperative medication dose of Levo-Dromoran should be individualized (see INDIVIDUALIZATION OF DOSAGE, WARNINGS and PRECAUTIONS). The usual dose for healthy young adults is 1 to 2 mg intramuscularly or subcutaneously, administered 60 to 90 minutes before surgery. Older or debilitated patients usually require less drug. Two mg of Levo-Dromoran is approximately equivalent to 10 to 15 mg of morphine or 100 mg of meperidine.
NOTE: Parenteral drug products should be inspected visually for particulate matter and discoloration prior to administration, whenever solution and container permit.
Pharmaceutical Incompatibilities of Levo-Dromoran: Levorphanol tartrate injection has been reported to be physically

incompatible with solutions containing aminophylline, ammonium chloride, amobarbital sodium, chlorothiazide sodium, heparin sodium, methicillin sodium, nitrofurantoin sodium, novobiocin sodium, pentobarbital sodium, perphenazine, phenobarbital sodium, phenytoin sodium, secobarbital sodium, sodium bicarbonate, sodium iodide, sulfadiazine sodium, sulfisoxazole diethanolamine and thiopental sodium.
Safety and Handling: Levo-Dromoran is packaged in sealed systems that have a low risk of accidental exposure to health care workers. Ordinary care should be taken to avoid aerosol generation while preparing a syringe for use. Significant absorption from accidental dermal exposure is unlikely, and spilled Levo-Dromoran should be washed from the skin by rinsing with cool water. As with all controlled substances, abuse by health care personnel is possible and the drug should be handled accordingly.

HOW SUPPLIED

Ampuls: 1 mL, 2 mg/mL levorphanol tartrate—boxes of 10 (NDC 0004-1910-06).
Multiple-Dose Vials: 10 mL, 2 mg/mL levorphanol tartrate—boxes of 1 (NDC 0004-1911-06).
Scored Oral Tablets: 2 mg levorphanol tartrate—bottles of 100 (NDC 0004-0044-01).
Storage: Tablets should be stored at 59° to 86°F (15° to 30°C). Dispense in tight containers as defined in USP/NF.
Parenteral dosage forms should be stored at 59° to 86° F (15° to 30°C).
WARNING: May be habit forming.
   DEA Order Form Required.
         Revised: January 1995
Shown in Product Identification Guide, page 332

LIDEX®   ℞
[*li'dex*]
(fluocinonide)
Cream 0.05%
Gel 0.05%
Ointment 0.05%
Topical Solution 0.05%

LIDEX-E®   ℞
(fluocinonide)
Cream 0.05%   ℞

SYNALAR®
[*sin'ă-lahr*]
(fluocinolone acetonide)
Cream 0.025%
Topical Solution 0.01%

DESCRIPTION

These preparations are all intended for topical administration.
LIDEX preparations have as their active component the corticosteroid fluocinonide, which is the 21-acetate ester of fluocinolone acetonide and has the chemical name pregna-1,4-diene-3,20-dione, 21-(acetyloxy)-6,9-difluoro-11-hydroxy-16,17-[(1-methylethylidene)bis(oxy)]-, (6α,11β, 16α)-.
LIDEX cream contains fluocinonide 0.5 mg/g in FAPG® cream, a specially formulated cream base consisting of citric acid, 1,2,6-hexanetriol, polyethylene glycol 8000, propylene glycol and stearyl alcohol. This white cream vehicle is greaseless, non-staining, anhydrous and completely water miscible. The base provides emollient and hydrophilic properties. In this formulation the active ingredient is totally in solution.
LIDEX gel contains fluocinonide 0.5 mg/g in a specially formulated gel base consisting of carbomer 940, edetate disodium, propyl gallate, propylene glycol, sodium hydroxide and/or hydrochloric acid (to adjust the pH), and water (purified). This clear, colorless thixotropic vehicle is greaseless, non-staining and completely water miscible. In this formulation the active ingredient is totally in solution.
LIDEX ointment contains fluocinonide 0.5 mg/g in a specially formulated ointment base consisting of glyceryl monostearate, white petrolatum, propylene carbonate, propylene glycol, and white wax. It provides the occlusive and emollient effects desirable in an ointment. In this formulation the active ingredient is totally in solution.
LIDEX topical solution contains fluocinonide 0.5 mg/mL in a solution of alcohol (35%), citric acid, diisopropyl adipate, and propylene glycol. In this formulation the active ingredient is totally in solution.
LIDEX-E cream contains fluocinonide 0.5 mg/g in a water-washable aqueous emollient base of cetyl alcohol, citric acid, mineral oil, polysorbate 60, propylene glycol, sorbitan monostearate, stearyl alcohol, and water (purified).
SYNALAR preparations have as their active component the corticosteroid fluocinolone acetonide, which has the chemical name pregna-1,4-diene-3,20-dione,6,9-difluoro-11,21-

dihydroxy-16,17-[(1-methylethylidene)bis(oxy)]-,(6α,11β, 16α)-.
SYNALAR cream contains fluocinolone acetonide 0.25 mg/g in a water-washable aqueous base of stearyl alcohol, propylene glycol, cetyl alcohol, polyoxyl 20 cetostearyl ether, mineral oil, white wax, simethicone, butylated hydroxytoluene, edetate disodium, citric acid, and purified water, with methylparaben and propylparaben as preservatives.
SYNALAR solution contains fluocinolone acetonide 0.1 mg/mL in a water-washable base of citric acid and propylene glycol.

CLINICAL PHARMACOLOGY

Topical corticosteroids share anti-inflammatory, antipruritic and vasoconstrictive actions.
The mechanism of anti-inflammatory activity of the topical corticosteroids is unclear. Various laboratory methods, including vasoconstrictor assays, are used to compare and predict potencies and/or clinical efficacies of the topical corticosteroids. There is some evidence to suggest that a recognizable correlation exists between vasoconstrictor potency and therapeutic efficacy in man.
Pharmacokinetics: The extent of percutaneous absorption of topical corticosteroids is determined by many factors including the vehicle, the integrity of the epidermal barrier, and the use of occlusive dressings. A significantly greater amount of fluocinonide is absorbed from the solution than from the cream or gel formulations.
Topical corticosteroids can be absorbed from normal intact skin. Inflammation and/or other disease processes in the skin increase percutaneous absorption. Occlusive dressings substantially increase the percutaneous absorption of topical corticosteroids. Thus, occlusive dressings may be a valuable therapeutic adjunct for treatment of resistant dermatoses. (See DOSAGE AND ADMINISTRATION.)
Once absorbed through the skin, topical corticosteroids are handled through pharmacokinetic pathways similar to systemically administered corticosteroids. Corticosteroids are bound to plasma proteins in varying degrees. Corticosteroids are metabolized primarily in the liver and are then excreted by the kidneys. Some of the topical corticosteroids and their metabolites are also excreted into the bile.

INDICATIONS AND USAGE

These products are indicated for the relief of the inflammatory and pruritic manifestations of corticosteroid-responsive dermatoses.

CONTRAINDICATIONS

Topical corticosteroids are contraindicated in those patients with a history of hypersensitivity to any of the components of the preparation.

PRECAUTIONS

General: Systemic absorption of topical corticosteroids has produced reversible hypothalamic-pituitary-adrenal (HPA) axis suppression, manifestations of Cushing's syndrome, hyperglycemia, and glucosuria in some patients. Conditions which augment systemic absorption include the application of the more potent steroids, use over large surface areas, prolonged use and the addition of occlusive dressings.
Therefore, patients receiving a large dose of a potent topical steroid applied to a large surface area or under an occlusive dressing should be evaluated periodically for evidence of HPA axis suppression by using the urinary free cortisol and ACTH stimulation tests. If HPA axis suppression is noted, an attempt should be made to withdraw the drug, to reduce the frequency of application, or to substitute a less potent steroid.
Recovery of HPA axis function is generally prompt and complete upon discontinuation of the drug. Infrequently, signs and symptoms of steroid withdrawal may occur, requiring supplemental systemic corticosteroids.
Pediatric patients may absorb proportionally larger amounts of topical corticosteroids and thus be more susceptible to systemic toxicity. (See PRECAUTIONS—Pediatric Use).
Not for ophthalmic use. Severe irritation is possible if fluocinonide solution contacts the eye. If that should occur, immediate flushing of the eye with a large volume of water is recommended.
If irritation develops, topical corticosteroids should be discontinued and appropriate therapy instituted.
As with any topical corticosteroid product, prolonged use may produce atrophy of the skin and subcutaneous tissues. When used on intertriginous or flexor areas, or on the face, this may occur even with short-term use.
In the presence of dermatological infections, the use of an appropriate antifungal or antibacterial agent should be instituted. If a favorable response does not occur promptly, the corticosteroid should be discontinued until the infection has been adequately controlled.
Information for the Patient: Patients using topical corticosteroids should receive the following information and instructions:

Continued on next page

Roche Laboratories—Cont.

1. This medication is to be used as directed by the physician. It is for external use only. Avoid contact with the eyes. If there is contact with the eyes and severe irritation occurs, immediately flush with a large volume of water.
2. Patients should be advised not to use this medication for any disorder other than for which it was prescribed.
3. The treated skin area should not be bandaged or otherwise covered or wrapped as to be occlusive unless directed by the physician.
4. Patients should report any signs of local adverse reactions especially under occlusive dressing.
5. Parents of pediatric patients should be advised not to use tight-fitting diapers or plastic pants on a child being treated in the diaper area, as these garments may constitute occlusive dressings.

Laboratory Tests: The following tests may be helpful in evaluating HPA axis suppression: Urinary free cortisol test and ACTH stimulation test.

Carcinogenesis, Mutagenesis, and Impairment of Fertility: Long-term animal studies have not been performed to evaluate the carcinogenic potential or the effect on fertility of topical corticosteroids.
Studies to determine mutagenicity with prednisolone and hydrocortisone have revealed negative results.

Pregnancy Category C: Corticosteroids are generally teratogenic in laboratory animals when administered systemically at relatively low dosage levels. The more potent corticosteroids have been shown to be teratogenic after dermal application in laboratory animals. There are no adequate and well-controlled studies in pregnant women on teratogenic effects from topically applied corticosteroids. Therefore, topical corticosteroids should be used during pregnancy only if the potential benefit justifies the potential risk to the fetus. Drugs of this class should not be used extensively on pregnant patients, in large amounts, or for prolonged periods of time.

Nursing Mothers: It is not known whether topical administration of corticosteroids could result in sufficient systemic absorption to produce detectable quantities in breast milk. Systemically administered corticosteroids are secreted into breast milk in quantities *not* likely to have a deleterious effect on the infant. Nevertheless, caution should be exercised when topical corticosteroids are administered to a nursing woman.

Pediatric Use: Pediatric patients may demonstrate greater susceptibility to topical corticosteroid-induced HPA axis suppression and Cushing's syndrome than mature patients because of a larger skin surface area to body weight ratio.
Parents of pediatric patients should be advised not to use tight-fitting diapers or plastic pants on a child being treated in the diaper area as these garments may constitute occlusive dressings.
Hypothalamic-pituitary-adrenal (HPA) axis suppression, Cushing's syndrome, and intracranial hypertension have been reported in children receiving topical corticosteroids. Manifestations of adrenal suppression in children include linear growth retardation, delayed weight gain, low plasma cortisol levels, and absence of response to ACTH stimulation. Manifestations of intracranial hypertension include bulging fontanelles, headaches, and bilateral papilledema.
Administration of topical corticosteroids to children should be limited to the least amount compatible with an effective therapeutic regimen. Chronic corticosteroid therapy may interfere with the growth and development of children.

ADVERSE REACTIONS

The following local adverse reactions are reported infrequently with topical corticosteroids, but may occur more frequently with the use of occlusive dressings. These reactions are listed in an approximate decreasing order of occurrence: burning, itching, irritation, dryness, folliculitis, hypertrichosis, acneiform eruptions, hypopigmentation, perioral dermatitis, allergic contact dermatitis, maceration of the skin, secondary infection, skin atrophy, striae, miliaria.

OVERDOSAGE

Topically applied corticosteroids can be absorbed in sufficient amounts to produce systemic effects (See PRECAUTIONS).

DOSAGE AND ADMINISTRATION

Topical corticosteroids are generally applied to the affected area as a thin film from two to four times daily depending on the severity of the condition. In hairy sites, the hair should be parted to allow direct contact with the lesion.
Occlusive dressings may be used for the management of psoriasis or recalcitrant conditions. Some plastic films may be flammable and due care should be exercised in their use. Similarly, caution should be employed when such films are used on children or left in their proximity, to avoid the possibility of accidental suffocation.
If an infection develops, the use of occlusive dressings should be discontinued and appropriate antimicrobial therapy instituted.

HOW SUPPLIED

Lidex Cream 0.05%—15 g Tube (NDC 0004-2511-04), 30 g Tube (0004-2511-23), 60 g Tube (NDC 0004-2511-22), 120 g Tube (NDC 0004-2511-51). Store at 59° to 86°F (15° to 30°C). Avoid excessive heat, above 104°F (40°C).
Lidex Gel 0.05%—15 g Tube (NDC 0004-2507-04), 30 g Tube (0004-2507-23), 60 g Tube (NDC 0004-2507-22). Store at 59° to 86°F (15° to 30°C).
Lidex Ointment 0.05%—15 g Tube (NDC 0004-2514-04), 30 g Tube (NDC 0004-2514-23), 60 g Tube (NDC 0004-2514-22), 120 g Tube (NDC 0004-2514-51). Store at 59° to 86°F (15° to 30°C). Avoid temperature above 86°F (30°C).
Lidex Topical Solution 0.05%—Plastic squeeze bottles: 20 cc (NDC 0004-2517-26), 60 cc (NDC 0004-2517-22). Store at 59° to 86°F (15° to 30°C). Avoid excessive heat, above 104°F (40°C).
Lidex-E Cream 0.05%—15 g Tube (NDC 0004-2513-04), 30 g Tube (NDC 0004-2513-23), 60 g Tube (NDC 0004-2513-22). Store at 59° to 86°F (15° to 30°C). Avoid excessive heat, above 104°F (40°C).
Synalar Cream 0.025%—15 g Tube (NDC 0004-2501-04), 60 g Tube (NDC 0004-2501-22). Store at 59° to 86°F (15° to 30°C). Avoid freezing and excessive heat, above 104°F (40°C).
Synalar Topical Solution 0.01%—20 cc (NDC 0004-2502-26), 60 cc (NDC 0004-2502-22). Store at 59° to 86°F (15° to 30°C). Avoid freezing.

Revised: August 1996

MATULANE® ℞

[*mat'u-lane*]
brand of procarbazine hydrochloride
CAPSULES

The following text is complete prescribing information based on official labeling in effect June 1996.

WARNING
It is recommended that MATULANE be given only by or under the supervision of a physician experienced in the use of potent antineoplastic drugs. Adequate clinical and laboratory facilities should be available to patients for proper monitoring of treatment.

DESCRIPTION

Matulane (procarbazine hydrochloride), a hydrazine derivative antineoplastic agent, is available as capsules containing the equivalent of 50 mg procarbazine as the hydrochloride. Each capsule also contains corn starch, mannitol and talc. Gelatin capsule shells contain parabens (methyl and propyl), potassium sorbate, titanium dioxide, FD&C Yellow No. 6 and D&C Yellow No. 10.
Chemically, procarbazine hydrochloride is *N*-isopropyl-α-(2-methylhydrazino)-*p*-toluamide monohydrochloride. It is a white to pale yellow crystalline powder which is soluble but unstable in water or aqueous solutions. The molecular weight of procarbazine hydrochloride is 257.76.

CLINICAL PHARMACOLOGY

The precise mode of cytotoxic action of procarbazine has not been clearly defined. There is evidence that the drug may act by inhibition of protein, RNA and DNA synthesis. Studies have suggested that procarbazine may inhibit transmethylation of methyl groups of methionine into t-RNA. The absence of functional t-RNA could cause the cessation of protein synthesis and consequently DNA and RNA synthesis. In addition, procarbazine may directly damage DNA. Hydrogen peroxide, formed during the auto-oxidation of the drug, may attack protein sulfhydryl groups contained in residual protein which is tightly bound to DNA.
Procarbazine is metabolized primarily in the liver and kidneys. The drug appears to be auto-oxidized to the azo derivative with the release of hydrogen peroxide. The azo derivative isomerizes to the hydrazone, and following hydrolysis splits into a benzylaldehyde derivative and methylhydrazine. The methylhydrazine is further degraded to CO_2 and CH_4 and possibly hydrazine, whereas the aldehyde is oxidized to *N*-isopropylterephthalamic acid, which is excreted in the urine.
Procarbazine is rapidly and completely absorbed. Following oral administration of 30 mg of ^{14}C-labeled procarbazine, maximum peak plasma radioactive concentrations were reached within 60 minutes.
After intravenous injection, the plasma half-life of procarbazine is approximately 10 minutes. Approximately 70% of the radioactivity is excreted in the urine as *N*-isopropylterephthalamic acid within 24 hours following both oral and intravenous administration of ^{14}C-labeled procarbazine.
Procarbazine crosses the blood-brain barrier and rapidly equilibrates between plasma and cerebrospinal fluid after oral administration.

INDICATIONS AND USAGE

Matulane is indicated for use in combination with other anticancer drugs for the treatment of Stage III and IV Hodgkin's disease. Matulane is used as part of the MOPP (nitrogen mustard, vincristine, procarbazine, prednisone) regimen.

CONTRAINDICATIONS

Matulane is contraindicated in patients with known hypersensitivity to the drug or inadequate marrow reserve as demonstrated by bone marrow aspiration. Due consideration of this possible state should be given to each patient who has leukopenia, thrombocytopenia or anemia.

WARNINGS

To minimize CNS depression and possible potentiation, barbiturates, antihistamines, narcotics, hypotensive agents or phenothiazines should be used with caution. Ethyl alcohol should not be used since there may be an Antabuse (disulfiram)-like reaction. Because Matulane exhibits some monoamine oxidase inhibitory activity, sympathomimetic drugs, tricyclic antidepressant drugs (eg, amitriptyline HCl, imipramine HCl) and other drugs and foods with known high tyramine content, such as wine, yogurt, ripe cheese and bananas, should be avoided. A further phenomenon of toxicity common to many hydrazine derivatives is hemolysis and the appearance of Heinz-Ehrlich inclusion bodies in erythrocytes.
Pregnancy: Teratogenic Effects: Pregnancy Category D. Procarbazine hydrochloride can cause fetal harm when administered to a pregnant woman. While there are no adequate and well-controlled studies with procarbazine hydrochloride in pregnant women, there are case reports of malformations in the offspring of women who were exposed to procarbazine hydrochloride in combination with other antineoplastic agents during pregnancy. Matulane should be used during pregnancy only if the potential benefit justifies the potential risk to the fetus. If this drug is used during pregnancy, or if the patient becomes pregnant while taking this drug, the patient should be apprised of the potential hazard to the fetus. Women of childbearing potential should be advised to avoid becoming pregnant. Procarbazine hydrochloride is teratogenic in the rat when given at doses approximately 4 to 13 times the maximum recommended human therapeutic dose of 6 mg/kg/day.
Nonteratogenic Effects: Procarbazine hydrochloride has not been adequately studied in animals for its effects on peri- and postnatal development. However, neurogenic tumors were noted in the offspring of rats given intravenous injections of 125 mg/kg of procarbazine hydrochloride on day 22 of gestation. Compounds which inhibit DNA, RNA and protein synthesis might be expected to have adverse effects on peri- and postnatal development.
Carcinogenesis, Mutagenesis and Impairment of Fertility: Carcinogenesis: The carcinogenicity of procarbazine hydrochloride in mice, rats and monkeys has been reported in a considerable number of studies. Instances of a second nonlymphoid malignancy, including acute myelocytic leukemia, have been reported in patients with Hodgkin's disease treated with procarbazine in combination with other chemotherapy and/or radiation. The International Agency for Research on Cancer (IARC) considers that there is "sufficient evidence" for the human carcinogenicity of procarbazine hydrochloride when it is given in intensive regimens which include other antineoplastic agents but that there is inadequate evidence of carcinogenicity in humans given procarbazine hydrochloride alone.
Mutagenesis: Procarbazine hydrochloride has been shown to be mutagenic in a variety of bacterial and mammalian test systems.
Impairment of Fertility: Azoospermia and antifertility effects associated with procarbazine hydrochloride administration in combination with other chemotherapeutic agents for treating Hodgkin's disease have been reported in human clinical studies. Since these patients received multicombination therapy, it is difficult to determine to what extent procarbazine hydrochloride alone was involved in the male germ-cell damage. The usual Segment 1 fertility/reproduction studies in laboratory animals have not been carried out with procarbazine hydrochloride. However, compounds which inhibit DNA, RNA and/or protein synthesis might be expected to have adverse effects on gametogenesis. Unscheduled DNA synthesis in the testis of rabbits and decreased fertility in male mice treated with procarbazine hydrochloride have been reported.

PRECAUTIONS

General: Undue toxicity may occur if Matulane is used in patients with impairment of renal and/or hepatic function. When appropriate, hospitalization for the initial course of treatment should be considered.
If radiation or a chemotherapeutic agent known to have marrow-depressant activity has been used, an interval of one month or longer without such therapy is recommended before starting treatment with Matulane. The length of this interval may also be determined by evidence of bone marrow recovery based on successive bone marrow studies.
Prompt cessation of therapy is recommended if any one of the following occurs:
Central nervous system signs or symptoms such as paresthesias, neuropathies or confusion.

Leukopenia (white blood count under 4000).

Thrombocytopenia (platelets under 100,000).

Hypersensitivity reaction.

Stomatitis—The first small ulceration or persistent spot soreness around the oral cavity is a signal for cessation of therapy.

Diarrhea—Frequent bowel movements or watery stools.

Hemorrhage or bleeding tendencies.

Bone marrow depression often occurs 2 to 8 weeks after the start of treatment. If leukopenia occurs, hospitalization of the patient may be needed for appropriate treatment to prevent systemic infection.

Information for Patients: Patients should be warned not to drink alcoholic beverages while on Matulane therapy since there may be an Antabuse (disulfiram)-like reaction. They should also be cautioned to avoid foods with known high tyramine content such as wine, yogurt, ripe cheese and bananas. Over-the-counter drug preparations which contain antihistamines or sympathomimetic drugs should also be avoided. Patients taking Matulane should also be warned against the use of prescription drugs without the knowledge and consent of their physician.

Laboratory Tests: Baseline laboratory data should be obtained prior to initiation of therapy. The hematologic status as indicated by hemoglobin, hematocrit, white blood count (WBC), differential, reticulocytes and platelets should be monitored closely—at least every 3 or 4 days.

Hepatic and renal evaluation are indicated prior to beginning therapy. Urinalysis, transaminase, alkaline phosphatase and blood urea nitrogen tests should be repeated at least weekly.

Drug Interactions: See WARNINGS section.

No cross-resistance with other chemotherapeutic agents, radiotherapy or steroids has been demonstrated.

Carcinogenesis, Mutagenesis and Impairment of Fertility: See WARNINGS section.

Pregnancy: Pregnancy Category D. See WARNINGS section.

Nursing Mothers: It is not known whether Matulane is excreted in human milk. Because of the potential for tumorigenicity shown for procarbazine hydrochloride in animal studies, mothers should not nurse while receiving this drug.

ADVERSE REACTIONS

Leukopenia, anemia and thrombopenia occur frequently. Nausea and vomiting are the most commonly reported side effects.

Other adverse reactions are:

Hematologic: Pancytopenia; eosinophilia; hemolytic anemia; bleeding tendencies such as petechiae, purpura, epistaxis and hemoptysis.

Gastrointestinal: Hepatic dysfunction, jaundice, stomatitis, hematemesis, melena, diarrhea, dysphagia, anorexia, abdominal pain, constipation, dry mouth.

Neurologic: Coma, convulsions, neuropathy, ataxia, paresthesia, nystagmus, diminished reflexes, falling, foot drop, headache, dizziness, unsteadiness.

Cardiovascular: Hypotension, tachycardia, syncope.

Ophthalmic: Retinal hemorrhage, papilledema, photophobia, diplopia, inability to focus.

Respiratory: Pneumonitis, pleural effusion, cough.

Dermatologic: Herpes, dermatitis, pruritus, alopecia, hyperpigmentation, rash, urticaria, flushing.

Allergic: Generalized allergic reactions.

Genitourinary: Hematuria, urinary frequency, nocturia.

Musculoskeletal: Pain, including myalgia and arthralgia; tremors.

Psychiatric: Hallucinations, depression, apprehension, nervousness, confusion, nightmares.

Endocrine: Gynecomastia in prepubertal and early pubertal boys.

Miscellaneous: Intercurrent infections, hearing loss, pyrexia, diaphoresis, lethargy, weakness, fatigue, edema, chills, insomnia, slurred speech, hoarseness, drowsiness.

Second nonlymphoid malignancies, including acute myelocytic leukemia and malignant myelosclerosis, and azoospermia have been reported in patients with Hodgkin's disease treated with procarbazine in combination with other chemotherapy and/or radiation.

OVERDOSAGE

The major manifestations of overdosage with Matulane would be anticipated to be nausea, vomiting, enteritis, diarrhea, hypotension, tremors, convulsions and coma. Treatment should consist of either the administration of an emetic or gastric lavage. General supportive measures such as intravenous fluids are advised. Since the major toxicity of procarbazine hydrochloride is hematologic and hepatic, patients should have frequent complete blood counts and liver function tests throughout their period of recovery and for a minimum of two weeks thereafter. Should abnormalities appear in any of these determinations, appropriate measures for correction and stabilization should be immediately undertaken.

The estimated mean lethal dose of procarbazine hydrochloride in laboratory animals varied from approximately 150 mg/kg in rabbits to 1300 mg/kg in mice.

DOSAGE AND ADMINISTRATION

The following doses are for administration of the drug as a single agent. When used in combination with other anticancer drugs, the Matulane dose should be appropriately reduced, eg, in the MOPP regimen, the Matulane dose is 100 mg/m^2 daily for 14 days. All dosages are based on the patient's actual weight. However, the estimated lean body mass (dry weight) is used if the patient is obese or if there has been a spurious weight gain due to edema, ascites or other forms of abnormal fluid retention.

Adults—To minimize the nausea and vomiting experienced by a high percentage of patients beginning Matulane therapy, single or divided doses of 2 to 4 mg/kg/day for the first week are recommended. Daily dosage should then be maintained at 4 to 6 mg/kg/day until maximum response is obtained or until the white blood count falls below 4000/cmm or the platelets fall below 100,000/cmm. When maximum response is obtained, the dose may be maintained at 1 to 2 mg/kg/day. Upon evidence of hematologic or other toxicity (see PRECAUTIONS section), the drug should be discontinued until there has been satisfactory recovery. After toxic side effects have subsided, therapy may then be resumed at the discretion of the physician, based on clinical evaluation and appropriate laboratory studies, at a dosage of 1 to 2 mg/kg/day.

Children—Very close clinical monitoring is mandatory. Undue toxicity, evidenced by tremors, coma and convulsions, has occurred in a few cases. Dosage, therefore, should be individualized. The following dosage schedule is provided as a guideline only.

Fifty (50) mg per square meter of body surface per day is recommended for the first week. Dosage should then be maintained at 100 mg per square meter of body surface per day until maximum response is obtained or until leukopenia or thrombocytopenia occurs. When maximum response is attained, the dose may be maintained at 50 mg per square meter of body surface per day. Upon evidence of hematologic or other toxicity (see PRECAUTIONS section), the drug should be discontinued until there has been satisfactory recovery, based on clinical evaluation and appropriate laboratory tests. After toxic side effects have subsided, therapy may then be resumed.

Procedures for proper handling and disposal of anticancer drugs should be considered. Several guidelines on this subject have been published.[1-6] There is no general agreement that all of the procedures recommended in the guidelines are necessary or appropriate.

HOW SUPPLIED

Capsules, ivory, containing the equivalent of 50 mg procarbazine as the hydrochloride; bottles of 100 (NDC 0004-0053-01). Imprint on capsules; MATULANE® ROCHE.

REFERENCES

1. Recommendations for the safe handling of parenteral antineoplastic drugs. Washington, DC, U.S. Government Printing Office (NIH Publication No. 83-2621).
2. AMA Council Report. Guidelines for handling parenteral antineoplastics. *JAMA* 253:1590–1592, Mar 15, 1985.
3. National Study Commission on Cytotoxic Exposure: Recommendations for handling cytotoxic agents. Available from Louis P. Jeffrey, ScD, Director of Pharmacy Services, Rhode Island Hospital, 593 Eddy Street, Providence, Rhode Island 02902.
4. Clinical Oncological Society of Australia: Guidelines and recommendations for safe handling of antineoplastic agents. *Med. J. Aust 1*:426–428, Apr 30, 1983.
5. Jones RB, Frank R, Mass T: Safe handling of chemotherapeutic agents: a report from the Mount Sinai Medical Center. *CA 33*:258–263, Sept–Oct 1983.
6. ASHP technical assistance bulletin on handling cytotoxic drugs in hospitals. *Am J Hosp Pharm 42*:131–137, Jan 1985.

Revised: November 1993

Shown in Product Identification Guide, page 332

NASALIDE®   ℞

[na′ză-lide]

(flunisolide)

Nasal Solution

0.025%

DESCRIPTION

NASALIDE® (flunisolide) nasal solution is intended for administration as a spray to the nasal mucosa. Flunisolide, the active component of NASALIDE nasal solution, is an anti-inflammatory steroid with the chemical name: 6α-fluoro-11β,16α,17,21-tetrahydroxypregna-1,4-diene-3,20-dione cyclic 16,17-acetal with acetone (USAN).

Flunisolide is a white to creamy white crystalline powder with a molecular weight of 434.49. It is soluble in acetone,

sparingly soluble in chloroform, slightly soluble in methanol, and practically insoluble in water. It has a melting point of about 245°C.

Each 25 mL spray bottle contains flunisolide 6.25 mg (0.25 mg/mL) in a solution of propylene glycol, polyethylene glycol 3350, citric acid, sodium citrate, butylated hydroxyanisole, edetate disodium, benzalkonium chloride and purified water, with NaOH and/or HCl added to adjust the pH to approximately 5.3. It contains no fluorocarbons.

After priming the delivery system for NASALIDE, each actuation of the unit delivers a metered droplet spray containing approximately 25 mcg of flunisolide. The size of the droplets produced by the unit is in excess of 8 microns to facilitate deposition on the nasal mucosa. The contents of one nasal spray bottle deliver at least 200 sprays.

CLINICAL PHARMACOLOGY

NASALIDE has demonstrated potent glucocorticoid and weak mineralocorticoid activity in classical animal test systems. As a glucocorticoid it is several hundred times more potent than the cortisol standard. Clinical studies with flunisolide have shown therapeutic activity on nasal mucous membranes with minimal evidence of systemic activity at the recommended doses.

A study in approximately 100 patients that compared the recommended dose of flunisolide nasal solution with an oral dose providing equivalent systemic amounts of flunisolide has shown that the clinical effectiveness of NASALIDE, when used topically as recommended, is due to its direct local effect and not to an indirect effect through systemic absorption.

Following administration of flunisolide to man, approximately half of the administered dose is recovered in the urine and half in the stool; 65% to 70% of the dose recovered in urine is the primary metabolite, which has undergone loss of the 6α fluorine and addition of a 6β hydroxy group. Flunisolide is well absorbed but is rapidly converted by the liver to the much less active primary metabolite and to glucuronate and/or sulfate conjugates. Because of first-pass liver metabolism, only 20% of the flunisolide reaches the systemic circulation when it is given orally whereas 50% of the flunisolide administered intranasally reaches the systemic circulation unmetabolized. The plasma half-life of flunisolide is 1 to 2 hours.

The effects of flunisolide on hypothalamic-pituitary-adrenal (HPA) axis function have been studied in adult volunteers. NASALIDE was administered intranasally as a spray in total doses over 7 times the recommended dose (2200 mcg, equivalent to 88 sprays/day) in 2 subjects for 4 days, about 3 times the recommended dose (800 mcg, equivalent to 32 sprays/day) in 4 subjects for 4 days, and over twice the recommended dose (700 mcg, equivalent to 28 sprays/day) in 6 subjects for 10 days. Early morning plasma cortisol concentrations and 24-hour urinary 17-ketogenic steroids were measured daily. There was evidence of decreased endogenous cortisol production at all three doses.

In controlled studies, NASALIDE was found to be effective in reducing symptoms of stuffy nose, runny nose and sneezing in most patients. These controlled clinical studies have been conducted in 488 adult patients at doses ranging from 8 to 16 sprays (200–400 mcg) per day and 127 children at doses ranging from 6 to 8 sprays (150 to 200 mcg) per day for periods as long as 3 months. In 170 patients who had cortisol levels evaluated at baseline and after 3 months or more of flunisolide treatment, there was no unequivocal flunisolide-related depression of plasma cortisol levels.

The mechanisms responsible for the anti-inflammatory action of corticosteroids and for the activity of the aerosolized drug on the nasal mucosa are unknown.

INDICATIONS

NASALIDE is indicated for the topical treatment of the symptoms of seasonal or perennial rhinitis when effectiveness of or tolerance to conventional treatment is unsatisfactory.

Clinical studies have shown that improvement is based on a local effect rather than systemic absorption and is usually apparent within a few days after starting NASALIDE. However, symptomatic relief may not occur in some patients for as long as 2 weeks. Although systemic effects are minimal at recommended doses, NASALIDE should not be continued beyond 3 weeks in the absence of significant symptomatic improvement.

NASALIDE should not be used in the presence of untreated localized infection involving nasal mucosa.

CONTRAINDICATIONS

Hypersensitivity to any of the ingredients.

WARNINGS

The replacement of a systemic corticosteroid with a topical corticoid can be accompanied by signs of adrenal insufficiency, and in addition some patients may experience symptoms of withdrawal, eg, joint and/or muscular pain, lassitude and depression. Patients previously treated for pro-

Continued on next page

Roche Laboratories—Cont.

longed periods with systemic corticosteroids and transferred to NASALIDE should be carefully monitored to avoid acute adrenal insufficiency in response to stress.

When transferred to NASALIDE, careful attention must be given to patients previously treated for prolonged periods with systemic corticosteroids. This is particularly important in those patients who have associated asthma or other clinical conditions, where too rapid a decrease in systemic corticosteroids may cause a severe exacerbation of their symptoms. The use of NASALIDE with alternate-day prednisone systemic treatment could increase the likelihood of HPA suppression compared to a therapeutic dose of either one alone. Therefore, NASALIDE treatment should be used with caution in patients already on alternate-day prednisone regimens for any disease.

Persons who are on drugs that suppress the immune system are more susceptible to infections than healthy individuals. Chicken pox and measles, for example, can have a more serious or even fatal course in nonimmune children or adults on corticosteroids. In such children or adults who have not had these diseases, particular care should be taken to avoid exposure. How the dose, route and duration of corticosteroid administration affects the risk of developing a disseminated infection is not known. The contribution of the underlying disease and/or prior corticosteroid treatment to the risk is also not known. If exposed to chicken pox, prophylaxis with varicella zoster immune globulin (VZIG) may be indicated. If exposed to measles, prophylaxis with pooled intramuscular immunoglobulin (IG) may be indicated. (See the respective package insert for complete VZIG and IG prescribing information.) If chicken pox develops, treatment with antiviral agents may be considered.

PRECAUTIONS

General: In clinical studies with flunisolide administered intranasally, the development of localized infections of the nose and pharynx with *Candida albicans* has occurred only rarely. When such an infection develops it may require treatment with appropriate local therapy or discontinuance of treatment with NASALIDE.

Flunisolide is absorbed into the circulation. Use of excessive doses of NASALIDE may suppress hypothalamic-pituitary-adrenal function.

Flunisolide should be used with caution, if at all in patients with active or quiescent tuberculosis infections of the respiratory tract or in untreated fungal, bacterial or systemic viral infections or ocular herpes simplex.

Because of the inhibitory effect of corticosteroids on wound healing, in patients who have experienced recent nasal septal ulcers, recurrent epistaxis, nasal surgery or trauma, a nasal corticosteroid should be used with caution until healing has occurred.

Although systemic effects have been minimal with recommended doses, this potential increases with excessive dosages. Therefore, larger than recommended doses should be avoided.

Information for Patients: Patients should use NASALIDE at regular intervals since its effectiveness depends on its regular use. The patient should take the medication as directed. It is not acutely effective and the prescribed dosage should not be increased. Instead, nasal vasoconstrictors or oral antihistamines may be needed until the effects of NASALIDE are fully manifested. One to 2 weeks may pass before full relief is obtained. The patient should contact the physician if symptoms do not improve, or if the condition worsens, or if sneezing or nasal irritation occurs.

Persons who are on immunosuppressant doses of corticosteroids should be warned to avoid exposure to chicken pox or measles. Patients should also be advised that if they are exposed, medical advice should be sought without delay.

For the proper use of this unit and to attain maximum improvement, the patient should read and follow the accompanying Patient Instructions carefully.

Carcinogenesis: Long-term studies were conducted in mice and rats using oral administration to evaluate the carcinogenic potential of the drug. There was an increase in the incidence of pulmonary adenomas in mice but not in rats.

Female rats receiving the highest oral dose had an increased incidence of mammary adenocarcinoma compared to control rats. An increased incidence of this tumor type has been reported for other corticosteroids.

Impairment of Fertility: Female rats receiving high doses of flunisolide (200 mcg/kg/day) showed some evidence of impaired fertility. Reproductive performance in the low (8 mcg/kg/day) and mid-dose (40 mcg/kg/day) groups was comparable to controls.

Pregnancy: Teratogenic Effects: Pregnancy Category C. As with other corticosteroids, flunisolide has been shown to be teratogenic in rabbits and rats at doses of 40 and 200 mcg/kg/day respectively. It was also fetotoxic in these animal reproductive studies. There are no adequate and well-controlled studies in pregnant women. Flunisolide should be

used during pregnancy only if the potential benefit justifies the potential risk to the fetus.

Nursing Mothers: It is not known whether this drug is excreted in human milk. Because other corticosteroids are excreted in human milk, caution should be exercised when flunisolide is administered to nursing women.

ADVERSE REACTIONS

Adverse reactions reported in controlled clinical trials and long-term open studies in 595 patients treated with NASALIDE are described below. Of these patients, 409 were treated for 3 months or longer, 323 for 6 months or longer, 259 for 1 year or longer and 91 for 2 years or longer.

In general, side effects elicited in the clinical studies have been primarily associated with the nasal mucous membranes. The most frequent complaints were those of mild transient nasal burning and stinging, which were reported in approximately 45% of the patients treated with NASALIDE in placebo-controlled and long-term studies. These complaints do not usually interfere with treatment; in only 3% of patients was it necessary to decrease dosage or stop treatment because of these symptoms. Approximately the same incidence of mild transient nasal burning and stinging was reported in patients on placebo as was reported in patients treated with NASALIDE in controlled studies, implying that these complaints may be related to the vehicle or the delivery system. The incidence of complaints of nasal burning and stinging decreased with increasing duration of treatment.

Other side effects reported at a frequency of 5% or less were: nasal congestion, sneezing, epistaxis and/or bloody mucus, nasal irritation, watery eyes, sore throat, nausea and/or vomiting and headaches. As with other nasally inhaled corticosteroids, nasal septal perforations have been reported in rare instances with the use of flunisolide nasal solutions. Temporary or permanent loss of the sense of smell and taste have also been reported with the use of flunisolide nasal solutions.

Systemic corticosteroid side effects were not reported during the controlled clinical trials. If recommended doses are exceeded, or if individuals are particularly sensitive, symptoms of hypercorticism, ie, Cushing's syndrome, could occur.

OVERDOSAGE

IV flunisolide in animals at doses up to 4 mg/kg showed no effect. One spray bottle contains 6.25 mg of NASALIDE; therefore acute overdosage is unlikely.

DOSAGE AND ADMINISTRATION

The therapeutic effects of corticosteroids, unlike those of decongestants, are not immediate. This should be explained to the patient in advance in order to ensure cooperation and continuation of treatment with the prescribed dosage regimen. Full therapeutic benefit requires regular use and is usually evident within a few days. However, a longer period of therapy may be required for some patients to achieve maximum benefit (up to 3 weeks). If no improvement is evident by that time, NASALIDE should not be continued. Patients with blocked nasal passages should be encouraged to use a decongestant just before NASALIDE administration to ensure adequate penetration of the spray. Patients should also be advised to clear their nasal passages of secretions prior to use.

Adults: The recommended starting dose of NASALIDE is 2 sprays (50 mcg) in each nostril 2 times a day (total dose 200 mcg/day). If needed, this dose may be increased to 2 sprays in each nostril 3 times a day (total dose 300 mcg/day).

Children 6 to 14 years: The recommended starting dose of NASALIDE is 1 spray (25 mcg) in each nostril 3 times a day or 2 sprays (50 mcg) in each nostril 2 times a day (total dose 150 to 200 mcg/day). NASALIDE is not recommended for use in children less than 6 years of age as safety and efficacy studies, including possible adverse effects on growth, have not been conducted.

Maximum total daily doses should not exceed 8 sprays in each nostril for adults (total dose 400 mcg/day) and 4 sprays in each nostril for children under 14 years of age (total dose 200 mcg/day). Since there is no evidence that exceeding the maximum recommended dosage is more effective and increased systemic absorption would occur, higher doses should be avoided.

After the desired clinical effect is obtained, the maintenance dose should be reduced to the smallest amount necessary to control the symptoms. Approximately 15% of patients with perennial rhinitis may be maintained on as little as 1 spray in each nostril per day.

HOW SUPPLIED

Each 25 mL NASALIDE nasal solution spray bottle (NDC 0004-2906-03) contains 6.25 mg (0.25 mg/mL) of flunisolide and is supplied in a nasal pump dispenser with dust cover and with a patient leaflet of instructions.
Store at 15°–30°C (59°–86°F).

Revised: August 1995

NASAREL™

℞

[Nā'ză ril]
(flunisolide)
Nasal Solution 0.025%

The following text is complete prescribing information based on official labeling in effect June 1996

DESCRIPTION

Flunisolide, the active component of NASAREL nasal solution, is an anti-inflammatory glucocorticosteroid with the chemical name: 6α-fluoro-11β,16α,17,21 tetrahydroxy-pregna-1,4-diene-3,20-dione cyclic 16, 17-acetal with acetone, hemihydrate.

Flunisolide is a white to creamy white crystalline powder with a molecular weight of 443.51. It is soluble in acetone, sparingly soluble in chloroform, slightly soluble in methanol, and practically insoluble in water. It has a melting point of about 245°C. The octanol:water partition coefficient is 2.17 at neutral pH.

NASAREL is a metered dose manual pump spray unit containing 0.025% w/w flunisolide in an aqueous medium containing benzalkonium chloride, butylated hydroxytoluene, citric acid, edetate disodium, polyethylene glycol 400, polysorbate 20, propylene glycol, sodium citrate dihydrate, sorbitol, and purified water. Sodium hydroxide and/or hydrochloric acid may be added to adjust the pH to approximately 5.2. It contains no fluorocarbons. Each 25 mL spray bottle contains 6.25 mg of flunisolide.

After initial priming (five to six actuations), each actuation of the pump spray unit delivers a metered spray containing approximately 25 mcg of flunisolide. The size of 99.5% of the droplets produced by the unit is greater than 8 microns. The contents of one nasal spray bottle deliver 200 sprays in addition to the priming sprays.

CLINICAL PHARMACOLOGY

General Pharmacology: Flunisolide nasal solution has demonstrated potent glucocorticoid and weak mineralocorticoid activity in classical animal test systems. As a glucocorticoid it was 180 times more potent than the cortisol standard in a rat anti-granuloma assay.

Pharmacokinetics: Flunisolide is well absorbed and is rapidly converted by the liver to the much less active primary metabolite and to glucuronide and sulfate conjugates. The primary metabolite results from the loss of the 6-alpha fluorine and addition of a 6-beta hydroxy group. Following administration of radiolabeled flunisolide to man, approximately half of the label is recovered in the urine and half in the stool. The primary metabolite accounts for 65–70% of the amount recovered in the urine. Due to first-pass liver metabolism, only 20% of an oral flunisolide dose reaches the systemic circulation unmetabolized as compared to 50% of an intranasal dose. The plasma half-life of flunisolide is 1–2 hours.

In a pharmacokinetic study comparing NASAREL with NASALIDE®, the original formulation, the two formulations were not bioequivalent. The total absorption of NASAREL was 25% less than that of NASALIDE, and the peak plasma concentration was 30% lower. The clinical significance of these differences is likely to be small, particularly since clinical efficacy is attributable to a local effect on the nasal mucosa. (see PHARMACODYNAMICS.)

Pharmacodynamics: A study in approximately 100 patients compared control of hay fever symptoms by the recommended dose of flunisolide as NASALIDE (200 mcg/day) with control by an oral dose of flunisolide providing equivalent plasma levels. The results demonstrated that the clinical effectiveness was due to the direct topical effect of flunisolide and not to an indirect effect through systemic absorption.

The effects of flunisolide on hypothalamic-pituitary-adrenal (HPA) axis function have been studied in adult volunteers. Flunisolide as NASALIDE, the original nasal formulation, was administered to 20 subjects intranasally in average total daily doses ranging from approximately 350 mcg to 2200 mcg (equivalent to about 14–88 sprays per day) for 4–10 days. Early morning plasma cortisol concentrations and 24-hour urinary 17-ketogenic steroids were measured daily. There was no consistent effect on endogenous cortisol production, although evidence of mild adrenal suppression was seen in some subjects.

Controlled studies evaluated adult patients receiving average total daily doses ranging from approximately 50 to 400 mcg (equivalent to about 2–16 sprays per day) of NASALIDE, the original flunisolide nasal solution, for periods as long as three months. Three hundred and thirty-nine patients from these studies were entered into a long-term open label study. Morning plasma cortisol levels were available for 182 patients at baseline, 129 after six months, and 36 after 12 months of continuous treatment with flunisolide. No effect of flunisolide on cortisol production was detected.

The mechanisms responsible for the anti-inflammatory action of corticosteroids and for their effect on the nasal mucosa are not completely understood.

CLINICAL TRIALS

The effectiveness of NASAREL was tested in 289 patients for up to 6 weeks at doses up to 300 mcg per day. NASAREL was shown to be effective in treating the symptoms of allergic rhinitis, including rhinorrhea, nasal congestion and sneezing.

A pivotal, 3-center trial involved 196 patients with seasonal allergic rhinitis randomized to NASALIDE, the vehicle of NASALIDE, NASAREL and the vehicle of NASAREL. Both active treatments were statistically significantly more effective than the vehicles. There was not statistically significant difference in efficacy between NASALIDE and NASAREL. The two formulations do differ in the nature and incidence of adverse complaints. There were more reports of nasal burning and stinging with NASALIDE and more problems related to taste, such as aftertaste, with NASAREL, owing to the differences in their respective vehicles. Some patients may prefer one formulation to the other.

INDIVIDUALIZATION OF DOSAGE

The therapeutic effects of corticosteroid nasal sprays, unlike those of decongestants, are not immediate. This should be explained to the patient in advance in order to ensure cooperation and continuation of treatment with the prescribed dosage regimen. Full therapeutic benefit requires regular use and is usually evident within a few days. A longer period of therapy may be required for some patients. However, NASAREL should not be continued beyond 3 weeks in the absence of significant symptomatic improvement (see PRECAUTIONS, WARNINGS, INFORMATION FOR PATIENTS and ADVERSE REACTIONS sections).

A starting dose of 2 sprays in each nostril twice daily is recommended. If greater control of symptoms is needed, the dose may be increased to 2 sprays in each nostril 3 times a day. For adults, maximum total daily doses should not exceed 8 sprays in each nostril per day (400 mcg/day).

After the desired clinical effect is obtained, the maintenance dose should be reduced to the smallest amount necessary to control the symptoms. Some patients with perennial rhinitis may be maintained on as little as one spray in each nostril per day. It is always desirable to titrate an individual patient to the minimum effective dose to reduce the possibility of side effects.

NASAREL and NASALIDE should not be considered to be identical. Physicians should consider the observed differences in the mean responses in terms of side effects (see ADVERSE REACTIONS) and flunisolide absorption (see PHARMACOKINETICS) in treating individual patients.

For children 6 to 14 years of age, the recommended starting dose of NASAREL is one spray (25 mcg) in each nostril 3 times a day (total dose 150 mcg/day) or 2 sprays (50 mcg) in each nostril 2 times a day (total dose 200 mcg/day). Maximum daily doses should not exceed 4 sprays in each nostril per day (total dose 200 mcg/day) as the safety and efficacy of higher doses have not been established. NASAREL is not recommended for use in children less than 6 years of age as the safety and efficacy have not been assessed in this age group.

INDICATIONS AND USAGE

NASAREL is indicated for the management of the symptoms of seasonal or perennial rhinitis.

CONTRAINDICATIONS

Hypersensitivity to any of the ingredients.
NASAREL should not be used in the presence of untreated localized infection involving the nasal mucosa.

WARNINGS

The replacement of a systemic corticosteroid with a topical corticoid can be accompanied by signs of adrenal insufficiency, and in addition some patients may experience symptoms of withdrawal, e.g., joint and/or muscular pain, lassitude and depression. Patients previously treated for prolonged periods with systemic corticosteroids and transferred to NASAREL should be carefully monitored to avoid acute adrenal insufficiency in response to stress.

Careful attention must also be given to patients who have associated asthma or other clinical conditions where too rapid a decrease in systemic corticosteroids may exacerbate their symptoms.

The use of NASAREL with systemic prednisone as alternate day therapy or with daily doses of less than 7.5 mg could increase the likelihood of hypothalamic-pituitary- adrenal axis suppression compared to a therapeutic dose of either one alone. Therefore, NASAREL treatment should be used with caution in patients already on prednisone regimens for any disease.

Persons who are on drugs which suppress the immune system are more susceptible to infections than healthy individuals. Chicken pox and measles, for example, can have a more serious or even fatal course in non-immune children or adults on corticosteroids. In such children or adults who have not had these diseases, particular care should be taken to avoid exposure. How the dose, route and duration of corticosteroid administration affects the risk of developing a disseminated infection is not known. The contribution of the underlying disease and/or prior corticosteroid treatment to the risk is also not known. If exposed to chicken pox, prophylaxis with varicella zoster immune globulin (VZIG) may be indicated. If exposed to measles, prophylaxis with pooled intramuscular immunoglobulin (IG) may be indicated. (See the respective package insert for complete. VZIG and IG prescribing information). If chicken pox develops, treatment with antiviral agents may be considered.

PRECAUTIONS

General: In clinical studies with flunisolide administered intranasally, the development of localized infections of the nose and pharynx with Candida albicans has occurred only rarely. When such an infection develops it may require treatment with appropriate local therapy or discontinuance of treatment with NASAREL.

Since there is no evidence that exceeding the maximum recommended dose of NASAREL is more effective, higher doses should be avoided.

Patients should be advised to clear their nasal passages of secretions prior to use. NASAREL should not be used in the presence of untreated local infection involving the nasal mucosa.

Flunisolide should be used with caution, if at all, in patients with active or quiescent tuberculosis infections, fungal, bacterial or systemic viral infections or ocular herpes simplex. As with other nasally inhaled corticosteroids, nasal septal perforations have been reported in rare instances with the use of flunisolide nasal solutions. Temporary or permanent loss of the sense of smell and taste have also been reported with the use of flunisolide nasal solutions.

Because of the inhibitory effect of corticosteroids on wound healing, a nasal corticosteroid should be used with caution in patients who have experienced recent nasal septal ulcers, recurrent epistaxis, nasal surgery or trauma, until healing has occurred.

Although systemic corticoid effects typical of Cushing's syndrome are minimal with recommended doses of topical steroids, this potential increases with excessive doses. If recommended doses are exceeded with long-term use, or if individuals are particularly sensitive, symptoms of hypercorticism could occur including suppression of hypothalamic-pituitary-adrenal function and/or retardation of growth in children or teenagers. Therefore, larger than recommended doses of NASAREL should be avoided.

Information for Patients: Patients should use NASAREL at regular intervals since its effectiveness depends on its regular use. Patients should take the medication as directed and should not exceed the prescribed dose. A decrease in symptoms can be expected to occur within a few days of initiating therapy in allergic rhinitis patients. Patients should contact their physician if the condition worsens, if sneezing or nasal irritation occurs, or if symptoms do not improve by three weeks.

Persons taking immunosuppressant doses of corticosteroids should be warned to avoid exposure to chicken pox or measles. Patients should also be advised that if they are exposed, medical advice should be sought without delay.

For the proper use of this unit and to attain maximum improvement, the patient should read and follow the accompanying Patient Instructions carefully.

Carcinogenesis: Long-term studies were conducted in mice and rats using oral administration to evaluate the carcinogenic potential of the drug. Flunisolide was administered to mice at doses of 5, 50 and 500 $\mu g/kg/day$ (15, 150, and 1500 $\mu g/\mu^2$ respectively) and to rats at doses of 0.5, 1, and 2.5 $\mu g/kg/day$ (3.0, 5.9, and 14.8 $\mu g/m^2$ respectively). There was an increase in the incidence of benign pulmonary adenomas in mice, but not in rats.

Female rats receiving the highest oral dose had an increased incidence of mammary adenocarcinoma compared to control rats. An increased incidence of this tumor type has been reported for other corticosteroids.

Impairment of Fertility: Female rats receiving high doses of flunisolide (200 $\mu g/kg/day$ or 1180 $\mu g/m^2$ body surface area) showed some evidence of impairment fertility. Reproductive performance in the low (8 $\mu g/kg/day$ or 47.2 $\mu g/m^2$) and mid-dose (40 $\mu g/kg/day$ or 236 $\mu g/m^2$) groups was comparable to controls.

Pregnancy: Teratogenic effects: Pregnancy Category C. As with other corticosteroids, flunisolide has been shown to be teratogenic in rabbits and rats at doses of 40 and 200 mcg/kg/day (480 $\mu g/m^2$ and 1180 $\mu g/m^2$) respectively. It was also fetotoxic in these animals reproductive studies. There are no adequate and well-controlled studies in pregnant women. Flunisolide should be used during pregnancy only if the potential benefit justifies the potential risk to the fetus.

Nursing Mothers: It is not known whether this drug is excreted in human milk. Because other corticosteroids are excreted in human milk, caution should be exercised when flunisolide is administered to nursing women.

ADVERSE REACTIONS

The adverse event rates listed below are based on symptoms spontaneously reported in multidose controlled clinical trials in comparing NASAREL and NASALIDE for treatment of allergic rhinitis. In patients receiving NASAREL the most common adverse events were transient aftertaste (17%) and transient nasal burning and stinging (13%). These symptoms did not usually interfere with treatment.

Adverse Event Rates for NASAREL:
Incidence Greater than 1% (probably causally related)
Respiratory: Nasal burning/stinging (13%), epistaxis*, nasal dryness, pharyngitis, cough increased
Gastrointestinal: Nausea
Special Senses: Aftertaste (17%)
Incidence 1% or Less (probably causally related)
Respiratory: Hoarseness
Special Senses: Abnormal sense of smell
Incidence 1% or less (causal relationship unknown)[1]
Respiratory: Sinusitis

Adverse Event Rates for NASALIDE:
Incidence Greater than 1% (probably causally related)
Respiratory: Nasal burning/stinging (44%), epistaxis*, nasal dryness*, pharyngitis*, cough increased
Gastrointestinal: Nausea
Special Senses: Aftertaste (8%)
Incidence 1% or Less (probably causally related)
Respiratory: Hoarseness, nasal ulcer
Incidence 1% or Less (causal relationship unknown)[1]
Respiratory: Sinusitis

*Incidence of reported reaction between 3% and 9%. Those reactions occurring in less than 3% of the patients are unmarked.

[1]Reactions occurred under circumstances where the causal relationship has not been clearly established; they are presented as alerting information for physicians.

OVERDOSAGE

In mice, rats and dogs, intravenous flunisolide at doses up to 4 mg/kg showed no effect. One spray bottle contains 6.25 mg of flunisolide; therefore acute overdosage is unlikely.

DOSAGE AND ADMINISTRATION

For adults, the recommended starting dose of NASAREL is two sprays (50 mcg) in each nostril 2 times a day (total dose 200 mcg/day): the effect should be assessed in 4 to 7 days (See INDIVIDUALIZATION OF DOSAGE section). Some relief can be expected in approximately two-thirds of patients within that time. This dose may be increased to 2 sprays in each nostril 3 times a day (total dose 300 mcg/day) if greater effect is needed. For adults, maximum total daily doses should not exceed 8 sprays in each nostril per day (400 mcg/day). After the desired clinical effect is obtained, the maintenance dose should be reduced to the smallest amount necessary to control the symptoms (See INDIVIDUALIZATION OF DOSAGE section).

For children 6 to 14 years of age, the recommended starting dose of NASAREL is one spray (25 mcg) in each nostril 3 times a day (total dose 150 mcg/day) or 2 sprays (50 mcg) in each nostril 2 times a day (total dose 200 mcg/day). For children 6 to 14 years of age, maximum daily doses should not exceed 4 sprays in each nostril per day (total dose 200 mcg/day) as the safety and efficacy of higher doses have not been established.

NASAREL is not recommended for use in children less than 6 years of age as safety and efficacy, including possible adverse effects on growth, have not been assessed in this age group.

NASAREL and NASALIDE should not be considered to be identical products. Physicians should consider the observed differences in the mean responses in terms of side effects (see ADVERSE REACTIONS) and flunisolide absorption (see PHARMACOKINETICS) in treating individual patients.

HOW SUPPLIED

Each 25 mL of NASAREL 0.025% nasal solution (6.25 mg flunisolide) is supplied in a spray bottle fitted with a meter pump, nasal adapter and a white protective cap (NDC # 0004-1708-09). The unit contains 200 metered sprays and comes with a patient instruction leaflet.

Store at 15°–30°C (59°–86°F).

April 1995

ROCALTROL®   ℞

[ro-cal'trol]
brand of calcitriol
CAPSULES

The following text is complete prescribing information based on official labeling in effect June 1996.

DESCRIPTION

Rocaltrol (calcitriol) is a synthetic vitamin D analog which is active in the regulation of the absorption of calcium from the gastrointestinal tract and its utilization in the body. It is available in capsules containing 0.25 mcg or 0.5 mcg calcitriol. Each capsule also contains butylated hydroxyanisole (BHA), butylated hydroxytoluene (BHT) and fractionated triglyceride of coconut oil. Gelatin capsule shells contain

Continued on next page

Roche Laboratories—Cont.

glycerin, parabens (methyl and propyl) and sorbitol, with the following dye systems: 0.25 mcg—FD&C Yellow No. 6 and titanium dioxide; 0.5 mcg—FD&C Red No. 3, FD&C Yellow No. 6 and titanium dioxide.

Calcitriol is a colorless, crystalline compound which occurs naturally in humans. It has a calculated molecular weight of 416.65 and is soluble in organic solvents but relatively insoluble in water. Chemically, calcitriol is 9,10-seco(5Z,7E)-5,7,10(19)-cholestatriene-1α, 3β, 25-triol.

The other names frequently used for calcitriol are 1α,25-dihydroxycholecalciferol, 1,25-dihydroxyvitamin D_3, 1,25-DHCC, 1,25$(OH)_2D_3$ and 1,25-diOHC.

CLINICAL PHARMACOLOGY

Man's natural supply of vitamin D depends mainly on exposure to the ultraviolet rays of the sun for conversion of 7-dehydrocholesterol in the skin to vitamin D_3 (cholecalciferol). Vitamin D_3 must be metabolically activated in the liver and the kidney before it is fully active as a regulator of calcium and phosphorus metabolism at target tissues. The initial transformation of vitamin D_3 is catalyzed by a vitamin D_3-25-hydroxylase enzyme (25-OHase) present in the liver, and the product of this reaction is 25-hydroxyvitamin D_3 [25-$(OH)D_3$]. Hydroxylation of 25-$(OH)D_3$ occurs in the mitochondria of kidney tissue, activated by the renal 25-hydroxyvitamin D_3-1 alpha-hydroxylase (alpha-OHase), to produce 1,25-$(OH)_2D_3$ (calcitriol), the active form of vitamin D_3. Several metabolites of calcitriol have been identified which include:

1α, 25, $(OH)_2$-24-oxo-D_3
1α, 23,25$(OH)_3$-24-oxo-D_3
1α, 24R,25$(OH)_3D_3$
1α, 25R$(OH)_2$-26-23S-lactone D_3
1α, 25S,26$(OH)_3D_3$
1α, 25$(OH)_2$-23-oxo-D_3
1α, 25R,26$(OH)_3$-23-oxo-D_3
1α, (OH)24,25,26,27-tetranor-COOH-D_3

The two known sites of action of calcitriol are intestine and bone. A calcitriol receptor-binding protein appears to exist in the mucosa of human intestine. Additional evidence suggests that calcitriol may also act on the kidney and the parathyroid glands. Calcitriol is the most active known form of vitamin D_3 in stimulating intestinal calcium transport. In acutely uremic rats calcitriol has been shown to stimulate intestinal calcium absorption. The kidneys of uremic patients cannot adequately synthesize calcitriol, the active hormone formed from precursor vitamin D. Resultant hypocalcemia and secondary hyperparathyroidism are a major cause of the metabolic bone disease of renal failure. However, other bone-toxic substances which accumulate in uremia (eg, aluminum) may also contribute.

The beneficial effect of Rocaltrol in renal osteodystrophy appears to result from correction of hypocalcemia and secondary hyperparathyroidism. It is uncertain whether Rocaltrol produces other independent beneficial effects.

Calcitriol is rapidly absorbed from the intestine. Peak serum concentrations (above basal values) were reached within 3 to 6 hours following oral administration of single doses of 0.25 to 1.0 mcg of Rocaltrol. The half-life of calcitriol elimination from serum was found to range from 3 to 6 hours. Following a single oral dose of 0.5 mcg, mean serum concentrations of calcitriol rose from a baseline value of 40.0 ± 4.4 (S.D.) pg/ml to 60.0 ± 4.4 pg/mL at 2 hours, and declined to 53.0 ± 6.9 at 4 hours, 50 ± 7.0 at 8 hours, 44 ± 4.6 at 12 hours and 41.5 ± 5.1 at 24 hours. The duration of pharmacologic activity of a single dose of calcitriol is about 3 to 5 days.

Calcitriol and other vitamin D metabolites are transported in blood, bound to specific plasma proteins. Enterohepatic recycling and biliary excretion of calcitriol occurs. Following intravenous administration of radiolabeled calcitriol in normal subjects, approximately 27% and 7% of the radioactivity appeared in the feces and urine, respectively, within 24 hours. When a 1-mcg oral dose of radiolabeled calcitriol was administered to normals, approximately 10% of the total radioactivity appeared in urine within 24 hours. Cumulative excretion of radioactivity on the sixth day following intravenous administration of radiolabeled calcitriol averaged 16% in urine and 49% in feces.

There is evidence that maternal calcitriol may enter the fetal circulation. Calcitriol may be excreted in human milk.

INDICATIONS AND USAGE

Rocaltrol is indicated in the management of hypocalcemia and the resultant metabolic bone disease in patients undergoing chronic renal dialysis. In these patients, Rocaltrol administration enhances calcium absorption, reduces serum alkaline phosphatase levels and may reduce elevated parathyroid hormone levels and the histological manifestations of osteitis fibrosa cystica and defective mineralization.

Rocaltrol is also indicated in the management of hypocalcemia and its clinical manifestations in patients with postsurgical hypoparathyroidism, idiopathic hypoparathyroidism, and pseudohypoparathyroidism.

CONTRAINDICATIONS

Rocaltrol should not be given to patients with hypercalcemia or evidence of vitamin D toxicity.

WARNINGS

Since Rocaltrol is the most potent metabolite of vitamin D available, pharmacologic doses of vitamin D and its derivatives should be withheld during Rocaltrol treatment to avoid possible additive effects and hypercalcemia.

Both appropriate oral phosphate-binders and a low phosphate diet should be used to control serum phosphate levels in patients undergoing dialysis.

Magnesium-containing antacids and Rocaltrol should not be used concomitantly in patients on chronic renal dialysis because such use may lead to the development of hypermagnesemia.

Overdosage of any form of vitamin D is dangerous (see also OVERDOSAGE). Progressive hypercalcemia due to overdosage of vitamin D and its metabolites may be so severe as to require emergency attention. Chronic hypercalcemia can lead to generalized vascular calcification, nephrocalcinosis and other soft-tissue calcification. **The serum calcium times phospate (Ca × P) product should not be allowed to exceed 70.** Radiographic evaluation of suspect anatomical regions may be useful in the early detection of this condition.

Studies in dogs and rats given calcitriol for up to 26 weeks have shown that small increases of calcitriol above endogenous levels can lead to abnormalities of calcium metabolism with the potential for calcification of many tissues in the body.

PRECAUTIONS

General: Excessive dosage of Rocaltrol induces hypercalcemia and in some instances hypercalciuria; therefore, early in treatment during dosage adjustment, serum calcium should be determined twice weekly. In dialysis patients, a fall in serum alkaline phosphatase levels usually antedates the appearance of hypercalcemia and may be an indication of impending hypercalcemia. Should hypercalcemia develop, the drug should be discontinued immediately. Rocaltrol should be given cautiously to patients on digitalis, because hypercalcemia in such patients may precipitate cardiac arrhythmias.

In patients with normal renal function, chronic hypercalcemia may be associated with an increase in serum creatinine. While this is usually reversible, it is important in such patients to pay careful attention to those factors which may lead to hypercalcemia. Rocaltrol therapy should always be started at the lowest possible dose and should not be increased without careful monitoring of the serum calcium. An estimate of daily dietary calcium intake should be made and the intake adjusted when indicated.

Patients with normal renal function taking Rocaltrol should avoid dehydration. Adequate fluid intake should be maintained.

Information for the Patient: The patient and his or her parents or spouse should be informed about compliance with dosage instructions, adherence to instructions about diet and calcium supplementation and avoidance of the use of unapproved nonprescription drugs. Patients should also be carefully informed about the symptoms of hypercalcemia (see ADVERSE REACTIONS section).

Laboratory Tests: For dialysis patients, serum calcium, phosphorus, magnesium and alkaline phosphatase should be determined periodically. For hypoparathyroid patients, serum calcium, phosphorus and 24-hour urinary calcium should be determined periodically.

Drug Interactions: Cholestyramine has been reported to reduce intestinal absorption of fat-soluble vitamins; as such it may impair intestinal absorption of Rocaltrol. (Also see WARNINGS and PRECAUTIONS [General] sections.)

Carcinogenesis, Mutagenesis, Impairment of Fertility: Long-term studies in animals have not been conducted to evaluate the carcinogenic potential of Rocaltrol. There was no evidence of mutagenicity as studied by the Ames method. No significant effects of Rocaltrol on fertility and/or general reproductive performances were reported.

Pregnancy: Teratogenic Effects: Pregnancy Category C. Rocaltrol has been found to be teratogenic in rabbits when given in doses 4 and 15 times the dose recommended for human use. All 15 fetuses in 3 litters at these doses showed external and skeletal abnormalities. However, none of the other 23 litters (156 fetuses) showed significant abnormalities compared with controls. Teratogenicity studies in rats showed no evidence of teratogenic potential. There are no adequate and well-controlled studies in pregnant women. Rocaltrol should be used during pregnancy only if the potential benefit justifies the potential risk to the fetus.

Nonteratogenic Effects: In the rabbit, dosages of 0.3 mcg/kg/day administered on days 7 to 18 of gestation resulted in 19% maternal mortality, a decrease in mean fetal body weight and a reduced number of newborn surviving to 24 hours. A study of peri- and postnatal development in rats resulted in hypercalcemia in the offspring of dams given Rocaltrol at doses of 0.08 or 0.3 mcg/ kg/day, hypercalcemia and hypophosphatemia in dams at doses of 0.08 or 0.3 mcg/

kg/day, and increased serum urea nitrogen in dams given Rocaltrol at a dose of 0.3 mcg/kg/day. In another study in rats, maternal weight gain was slightly reduced at a dose of 0.3 mcg/kg/day administered on days 7 to 15 of gestation. The offspring of a woman administered 17 to 36 mcg/day of Rocaltrol (17 to 144 times the recommended dose) during pregnancy manifested mild hypercalcemia in the first 2 days of life which returned to normal at day 3.

Nursing Mothers: Calcitriol may be excreted in human milk. Because many drugs are excreted in human milk and because of the potential for serious adverse reactions from Rocaltrol in nursing infants, a mother should not nurse while taking this drug.

Pediatric Use: Safety and efficacy of Rocaltrol in children undergoing dialysis have not been established.

ADVERSE REACTIONS

Since Rocaltrol is believed to be the active hormone which exerts vitamin D activity in the body, adverse effects are, in general, similar to those encountered with excessive vitamin D intake. The early and late signs and symptoms of vitamin D intoxication associated with hypercalcemia include:

Early: Weakness, headache, somnolence, nausea, vomiting, dry mouth, constipation, muscle pain, bone pain and metallic taste.

Late: Polyuria, polydipsia, anorexia, weight loss, nocturia, conjunctivitis (calcific), pancreatitis, photophobia, rhinorrhea, pruritus, hyperthermia, decreased libido, elevated BUN, albuminuria, hypercholesterolemia, elevated SGOT and SGPT, ectopic calcification, nephrocalcinosis, hypertension, cardiac arrhythmias and, rarely, overt psychosis.

In clinical studies on hypoparathyroidism and pseudohypoparathyroidism, hypercalcemia was noted on at least one occasion in about 1 in 3 patients and hypercalciuria in about 1 in 7. Elevated serum creatinine levels were observed in about 1 in 6 patients (approximately one half of whom had normal levels at baseline).

One case of erythema multiforme and one case of allergic reaction (swelling of lips and hives all over the body) were confirmed by rechallenge.

OVERDOSAGE

Administration of Rocaltrol to patients in excess of their daily requirements can cause hypercalcemia, hypercalciuria and hyperphosphatemia. High intake of calcium and phosphate concomitant with Rocaltrol may lead to similar abnormalities. High levels of calcium in the dialysate bath may contribute to the hypercalcemia.

Treatment of Hypercalcemia and Overdosage: General treatment of hypercalcemia (greater than 1 mg/dL above the upper limit of the normal range) consists of immediate discontinuation of Rocaltrol therapy, institution of a low calcium diet and withdrawal of calcium supplements. Serum calcium levels should be determined daily until normocalcemia ensues. Hypercalcemia frequently resolves in 2 to 7 days. When serum calcium levels have returned to within normal limits, Rocaltrol therapy may be reinstituted at a dose of 0.25 mcg/day less than prior therapy. Serum calcium levels should be obtained at least twice weekly after all dosage changes and subsequent dosage titration. In dialysis patients, persistent or markedly elevated serum calcium levels may be corrected by dialysis against a calcium-free dialysate.

Treatment of Accidental Overdosage of Rocaltrol: The treatment of acute accidental overdosage of Rocaltrol should consist of general supportive measures. If drug ingestion is discovered within a relatively short time, induction of emesis or gastric lavage may be of benefit in preventing further absorption. If the drug has passed through the stomach, the administration of mineral oil may promote its fecal elimination. Serial serum electrolyte determinations (especially calcium), rate of urinary calcium excretion and assessment of electrocardiographic abnormalities due to hypercalcemia should be obtained. Such monitoring is critical in patients receiving digitalis. Discontinuation of supplemental calcium and a low calcium diet are also indicated in accidental overdosage. Due to the relatively short duration of the pharmacological action of calcitriol, further measures are probably unnecessary. Should, however, persistent and markedly elevated serum calcium levels occur, there are a variety of therapeutic alternatives which may be considered, depending on the patient's underlying condition. These include the use of drugs such as phosphates and corticosteroids as well as measures to induce an appropriate forced diuresis. The use of peritoneal dialysis against a calcium-free dialysate has also been reported.

DOSAGE AND ADMINISTRATION

The optimal daily dose of Rocaltrol must be carefully determined for each patient.

The effectiveness of Rocaltrol therapy is predicated on the assumption that each patient is receiving an adequate daily intake of calcium. The U.S. RDA for calcium in adults is 800 to 1200 mg. To ensure that each patient receives an adequate daily intake of calcium, the physician should either prescribe a calcium supplement or instruct the patient in proper dietary measures.

Dialysis Patients: The recommended initial dose of Rocaltrol is 0.25 mcg/day. If a satisfactory response in the biochemical parameters and clinical manifestations of the disease state is not observed, dosage may be increased by 0.25 mcg/day at 4- to 8-week intervals. During this titration period, serum calcium levels should be obtained at least twice weekly, and if hypercalcemia is noted, the drug should be immediately discontinued until normocalcemia ensues. Patients with normal or only slightly reduced serum calcium levels may respond to Rocaltrol doses of 0.25 mcg every other day. Most patients undergoing hemodialysis respond to doses between 0.5 and 1 mcg/day.

Oral Rocaltrol may normalize plasma ionized calcium in some uremic patients, yet fail to suppress parathyroid hyperfunction. In these individuals with autonomous parathyroid hyperfunction, oral Rocaltrol may be useful to maintain normocalcemia, but has not been shown to be adequate treatment for hyperparathyroidism.

Hypoparathyroidism: The recommended initial dose of Rocaltrol is 0.25 mcg/day given in the morning. If a satisfactory response in the biochemical parameters and clinical manifestations of the disease is not observed, the dose may be increased at 2- to 4-week intervals. During the dosage titration period, serum calcium levels should be obtained at least twice weekly, and, if hypercalcemia is noted, Rocaltrol should be immediately discontinued until normocalcemia ensues. Careful consideration should also be given to lowering the dietary calcium intake.

Most adult patients and pediatric patients age 6 years and older have responded to dosages in the range of 0.5 to 2 mcg daily. Pediatric patients in the 1–5 year age group with hypoparathyroidism have usually been given 0.25 to 0.75 mcg daily. The number of treated patients with pseudohypoparathyroidism less than 6 years of age is too small to make dosage recommendations.

HOW SUPPLIED

0.25 mcg calcitriol in soft gelatin, light orange, oval capsules, imprinted ROCALTROL 0.25 ROCHE; bottles of 30 (NDC 0004-0143-23), and bottles of 100, (NDC 0004-0143-01).

0.5 mcg calcitriol in soft gelatin, dark orange, oblong capsules, imprinted ROCALTROL 0.5 ROCHE; bottles of 100, (NDC 0004-0144-01).

Rocaltrol should be protected from heat and light.

Revised: June 1996

Shown in Product Identification Guide, page 332

ROCEPHIN® ℞
[ro-sef'in]
(sterile ceftriaxone sodium)
STERILE VIALS

The following text is complete prescribing information based on official labeling in effect June 1996.

DESCRIPTION

Rocephin is a sterile, semisynthetic, broad-spectrum cephalosporin antibiotic for intravenous or intramuscular administration. Ceftriaxone sodium is (6R,7R)-7-[2-(2-Amino-4-thiazolyl)glyoxylamido] -8- oxo -3- [[(1,2,5,6-tetrahydro-2-methyl-5,6-dioxo-as-triazin-3-yl)thio]methyl]-5-thia-1-azabicyclo[4.2.0]oct-2-ene-2-carboxylic acid, 7^2-(Z)-(O-methyloxime), disodium salt, sesquaterhydrate.

The chemical formula of ceftriaxone sodium is $C_{18}H_{16}N_8Na_2O_7S_3 \cdot 3.5H_2O$. It has a calculated molecular weight of 661.59.

Rocephin is a white to yellowish-orange crystalline powder which is readily soluble in water, sparingly soluble in methanol and very slightly soluble in ethanol. The pH of a 1% aqueous solution is approximately 6.7. The color of Rocephin solutions ranges from light yellow to amber, depending on the length of storage, concentration and diluent used. Rocephin contains approximately 83 mg (3.6 mEq) of sodium per gram of ceftriaxone activity.

CLINICAL PHARMACOLOGY

Average plasma concentrations of ceftriaxone following a single 30-minute intravenous (IV) infusion of a 0.5, 1 or 2 gm dose and intramuscular (IM) administration of a single 0.5

TABLE 1
Ceftriaxone Plasma Concentrations After Single Dose Administration

Dose/Route	Average Plasma Concentrations (mcg/mL)								
	0.5 hr	1 hr	2 hr	4 hr	6 hr	8 hr	12 hr	16 hr	24 hr
0.5 gm IV*	82	59	48	37	29	23	15	10	5
0.5 gm IM 250 mg/mL	22	33	38	35	30	26	16	ND	5
0.5 gm IM 350 mg/mL	20	32	38	34	31	24	16	ND	5
1 gm IV*	151	111	88	67	53	43	28	18	9
1 gm IM	40	68	76	68	56	44	29	ND	ND
2 gm IV*	257	192	154	117	89	74	46	31	15

* I.V. doses were infused at a constant rate over 30 minutes.
† ND = Not determined.

(250 mg/mL or 350 mg/mL concentrations) or 1 gm dose in healthy subjects are presented in Table 1.
[See table above.]

Ceftriaxone was completely absorbed following IM administration with mean maximum plasma concentrations occurring between 2 and 3 hours postdosing. Multiple IV or IM doses ranging from 0.5 to 2 gm at 12- to 24-hour intervals resulted in 15% to 36% accumulation of ceftriaxone above single dose values.

Ceftriaxone concentrations in urine are high, as shown in Table 2.
[See table below.]

Thirty-three percent to 67% of a ceftriaxone dose was excreted in the urine as unchanged drug and the remainder was secreted in the bile and ultimately found in the feces as microbiologically inactive compounds. After a 1 gm IV dose, average concentrations of ceftriaxone, determined from 1 to 3 hours after dosing, were 581 mcg/mL in the gallbladder bile, 788 mcg/mL in the common duct bile, 898 mcg/mL in the cystic duct bile, 78.2 mcg/gm in the gallbladder wall and 62.1 mcg/mL in the concurrent plasma.

Over a 0.15 to 3 gm dose range in healthy adult subjects, the values of elimination half-life ranged from 5.8 to 8.7 hours; apparent volume of distribution from 5.78 to 13.5 L; plasma clearance from 0.58 to 1.45 L/hour; and renal clearance from 0.32 to 0.73 L/hour. Ceftriaxone is reversibly bound to human plasma proteins, and the binding decreased from a value of 95% bound at plasma concentrations of < 25 mcg/mL to a value of 85% bound at 300 mcg/mL.

The average values of maximum plasma concentration, elimination half-life, plasma clearance and volume of distribution after a 50 mg/kg IV dose and after a 75 mg/kg IV dose in pediatric patients suffering from bacterial meningitis are shown in Table 3. Ceftriaxone penetrated the inflamed meninges of infants and children; CSF concentrations after a 50 mg/kg IV dose and after a 75 mg/kg IV dose are also shown in Table 3.

TABLE 3
Average Pharmacokinetic Parameters of Ceftriaxone in Pediatric Patients with Meningitis

	50 mg/kg IV	75 mg/kg IV
Maximum Plasma Concentrations (mcg/mL)	216	275
Elimination Half-life (hr)	4.6	4.3
Plasma Clearance (mL/hr/kg)	49	60
Volume of Distribution (mL/kg)	338	373
CSF Concentration—inflamed meninges (mcg/mL)	5.6	6.4
Range (mcg/mL)	1.3-18.5	1.3-44
Time after dose (hr)	3.7 (± 1.6)	3.3 (± 1.4)

Compared to that in healthy adult subjects, the pharmacokinetics of ceftriaxone were only minimally altered in elderly subjects and in patients with renal impairment or hepatic dysfunction (Table 4); therefore, dosage adjustments are not necessary for these patients with ceftriaxone dosages up to 2

gm per day. Ceftriaxone was not removed to any significant extent from the plasma by hemodialysis. In 6 of 26 dialysis patients, the elimination rate of ceftriaxone was markedly reduced, suggesting that plasma concentrations of ceftriaxone should be monitored in these patients to determine if dosage adjustments are necessary.

[See table 4 at bottom of next page.]

Microbiology: The bactericidal activity of ceftriaxone results from inhibition of cell wall synthesis. Ceftriaxone has a high degree of stability in the presence of beta-lactamases, both penicillinases and cephalosporinases, of gram-negative and gram-positive bacteria. Ceftriaxone is usually active against the following microorganisms in vitro and in clinical infections (see INDICATIONS AND USAGE):

GRAM-NEGATIVE AEROBES:
Acinetobacter calcoaceticus
Enterobacter aerogenes
Enterobacter cloacae
Escherichia coli
Haemophilus influenzae (including ampicillin-resistant strains)
Haemophilus parainfluenzae
Klebsiella oxytoca
Klebsiella pneumoniae
Morganella morganii
Neisseria gonorrhoeae (including penicillinase- and nonpenicillinase-producing strains)
Neisseria meningitidis
Proteus mirabilis
Proteus vulgaris
Serratia marcescens
Ceftriaxone is also active against many strains of *Pseudomonas aeruginosa*.
NOTE: Many strains of the above organisms that are multiply resistant to other antibiotics; eg, penicillins, cephalosporins and aminoglycosides, are susceptible to ceftriaxone.
GRAM-POSITIVE AEROBES:
Staphylococcus aureus (including penicillinase-producing strains)
Staphylococcus epidermidis
Streptococcus pneumoniae
Streptococcus pyogenes
Viridans group streptococci
NOTE: Methicillin-resistant streptococci are resistant to cephalosporins, including ceftriaxone. Most strains of Group D streptococci and enterococci; eg, *Enterococcus (Streptococcus) faecalis*, are resistant.
ANAEROBES:
Bacteroides fragilis
Clostridium species
Peptostreptococcus species
NOTE: Most strains of *C. difficile* are resistant.
Ceftriaxone also demonstrates in vitro activity against most strains of the following microorganisms, although the clinical significance is unknown:
GRAM-NEGATIVE AEROBES:
Citrobacter diversus
Citrobacter freundii
Providencia species (including *Providencia rettgeri*)
Salmonella species (including *S. typhi*)
Shigella species
GRAM-POSITIVE AEROBES:
Streptococcus agalactiae
ANAEROBES:
Bacteroides bivius
Bacteroides melaninogenicus

Susceptibility Test: Diffusion Techniques: Quantitative methods that require the measurement of zone diameters give the most precise estimate of the susceptibility of bacteria to antimicrobial agents. One such standard procedure[1] which has been recommended for use with disks to test susceptibility of organisms to ceftriaxone uses a 30-mcg ceftriaxone disk. Interpretation involves the correlation of the diameters obtained in the disk test with the minimum inhibitory concentration (MIC) for ceftriaxone.

TABLE 2
Urinary Concentrations of Ceftriaxone After Single Dose Administration

Dose/Route	Average Urinary Concentrations (mcg/mL)					
	0-2 hr	2-4 hr	4-8 hr	8-12 hr	12-24 hr	24-48 hr
0.5 gm IV	526	366	142	87	70	15
0.5 gm IM	115	425	308	127	96	28
1 gm IV	995	855	293	147	132	32
1 gm IM	504	628	418	237	ND*	ND
2 gm IV	2692	1976	757	274	198	40

*ND = Not determined.

Continued on next page

Roche Laboratories—Cont.

Reports from the laboratory giving results of the standardized single disk susceptibility test using a 30-mcg ceftriaxone disk should be interpreted for ceftriaxone according to the following criteria:

Zone Diameter (mm)	Interpretation
≥ 18	(S) Susceptible
14-17	(MS) Moderately Susceptible
≤ 13	(R) Resistant

A report of "Susceptible" indicates that the pathogen is likely to be inhibited by generally achievable levels. A report of "Moderately Susceptible" suggests that the organism would be susceptible if high dosage (not to exceed 4 gm per day) is used or if the infection is confined to tissues and fluids in which high antimicrobial levels are attained. A report of "Resistant" indicates that achievable concentrations are unlikely to be inhibitory, and other therapy should be selected.

Standardized procedures require the use of laboratory control organisms. The 30-mcg ceftriaxone disk should give the following zone diameters:

Organism	Zone Diameter (mm)
Staphylococcus aureus ATCC® 25923	22-28
Escherichia coli ATCC® 25922	29-35
Pseudomonas aeruginosa ATCC® 27853	17-23

Dilution Techniques:
Use a standardized dilution method[2] (broth, agar, microdilution) or equivalent with ceftriaxone powder. The MIC values obtained should be interpreted according to the following criteria:

MIC (mcg/mL)	Interpretation
≤ 16	Susceptible
> 16-< 64	Moderately Susceptible
≥ 64	Resistant

As with standard diffusion techniques, dilution methods require the use of laboratory control organisms. Standard ceftriaxone powder should provide the following MIC values:

Organism	MIC (mcg/mL)
Staphylococcus aureus ATCC® 29213	1-8
Escherichia coli ATCC® 25922	0.03-0.12
Pseudomonas aeruginosa ATCC® 27853	8-32

INDICATIONS AND USAGE

Rocephin is indicated for the treatment of the following infections when caused by susceptible organisms:

LOWER RESPIRATORY TRACT INFECTIONS caused by Streptococcus pneumoniae, Staphylococcus aureus, Haemophilus influenzae, Haemophilus parainfluenzae, Klebsiella pneumoniae, Escherichia coli, Enterobacter aerogenes, Proteus mirabilis or Serratia marcescens.

SKIN AND SKIN STRUCTURE INFECTIONS caused by Staphylococcus aureus, Staphylococcus epidermidis, Streptococcus pyogenes, Viridans group streptococci, Escherichia coli, Enterobacter cloacae, Klebsiella oxytoca, Klebsiella pneumoniae, Proteus mirabilis, Morganella morganii*, Pseudomonas aeruginosa, Serratia marcescens, Acinetobacter calcoaceticus, Bacteroides fragilis* or Peptostreptococcus species.

URINARY TRACT INFECTIONS (complicated and uncomplicated) caused by Escherichia coli, Proteus mirabilis, Proteus vulgaris, Morganella morganii or Klebsiella pneumoniae.

UNCOMPLICATED GONORRHEA (cervical/urethral and rectal) caused by Neisseria gonorrhoeae, including both penicillinase- and nonpenicillinase-producing strains, and pharyngeal gonorrhea caused by nonpenicillinase-producing strains of Neisseria gonorrhoeae.

PELVIC INFLAMMATORY DISEASE caused by Neisseria gonorrhoeae. Rocephin, like other cephalosporins, has no activity against Chlamydia trachomatis. Therefore, when cephalosporins are used in the treatment of patients with pelvic inflammatory disease and C. trachomatis is one of the suspected pathogens, appropriate antichlamydial coverage should be added.

BACTERIAL SEPTICEMIA caused by Staphylococcus aureus, Streptococcus pneumoniae, Escherichia coli, Haemophilus influenzae or Klebsiella pneumoniae.

BONE AND JOINT INFECTIONS caused by Staphylococcus aureus, Streptococcus pneumoniae, Escherichia coli, Proteus mirabilis, Klebsiella pneumoniae or Enterobacter species.

INTRA-ABDOMINAL INFECTIONS caused by Escherichia coli, Klebsiella pneumoniae, Bacteroides fragilis, Clostridium species (Note: most strains of C. difficile are resistant) or Peptostreptococcus species.

MENINGITIS caused by Haemophilus influenzae, Neisseria meningitidis or Streptococcus pneumoniae. Rocephin has also been used successfully in a limited number of cases of meningitis and shunt infection caused by Staphylococcus epidermidis* and Escherichia coli.*

* Efficacy for this organism in this organ system was studied in fewer than ten infections.

SURGICAL PROPHYLAXIS: The preoperative administration of a single 1 gm dose of Rocephin may reduce the incidence of postoperative infections in patients undergoing surgical procedures classified as contaminated or potentially contaminated (eg, vaginal or abdominal hysterectomy or cholecystectomy for chronic calculous cholecystitis in high-risk patients, such as those over 70 years of age, with acute cholecystitis not requiring therapeutic antimicrobials, obstructive jaundice or common duct bile stones) and in surgical patients for whom infection at the operative site would present serious risk (eg, during coronary artery bypass surgery). Although Rocephin has been shown to have been as effective as cefazolin in the prevention of infection following coronary artery bypass surgery, no placebo-controlled trials have been conducted to evaluate any cephalosporin antibiotic in the prevention of infection following coronary artery bypass surgery.

When administered prior to surgical procedures for which it is indicated, a single 1 gm dose of Rocephin provides protection from most infections due to susceptible organisms throughout the course of the procedure.

Before instituting treatment with Rocephin, appropriate specimens should be obtained for isolation of the causative organism and for determination of its susceptibility to the drug. Therapy may be instituted prior to obtaining results of susceptibility testing.

CONTRAINDICATIONS

Rocephin is contraindicated in patients with known allergy to the cephalosporin class of antibiotics.

WARNINGS

BEFORE THERAPY WITH ROCEPHIN IS INSTITUTED, CAREFUL INQUIRY SHOULD BE MADE TO DETERMINE WHETHER THE PATIENT HAS HAD PREVIOUS HYPERSENSITIVITY REACTIONS TO CEPHALOSPORINS, PENICILLINS OR OTHER DRUGS. THIS PRODUCT SHOULD BE GIVEN CAUTIOUSLY TO PENICILLIN-SENSITIVE PATIENTS. ANTIBIOTICS SHOULD BE ADMINISTERED WITH CAUTION TO ANY PATIENT WHO HAS DEMONSTRATED SOME FORM OF ALLERGY, PARTICULARLY TO DRUGS. SERIOUS ACUTE HYPERSENSITIVITY REACTIONS MAY REQUIRE THE USE OF SUBCUTANEOUS EPINEPHRINE AND OTHER EMERGENCY MEASURES.

Pseudomembranous colitis has been reported with nearly all antibacterial agents, including ceftriaxone, and may range in severity from mild to life-threatening. Therefore, it is important to consider this diagnosis in patients who present with diarrhea subsequent to the administration of antibacterial agents.

Treatment with antibacterial agents alters the normal flora of the colon and may permit overgrowth of clostridia. Studies indicate that a toxin produced by Clostridium difficile is one primary cause of "antibiotic-associated colitis."

After the diagnosis of pseudomembranous colitis has been established, appropriate therapeutic measures should be initiated. Mild cases of pseudomembranous colitis usually respond to drug discontinuance alone. In moderate to severe cases, consideration should be given to management with fluids and electrolytes, protein supplementation and treatment with an oral antibacterial drug effective against C. difficile colitis.

PRECAUTIONS

General: Although transient elevations of BUN and serum creatinine have been observed, at the recommended dosages, the nephrotoxic potential of Rocephin is similar to that of other cephalosporins.

Ceftriaxone is excreted via both biliary and renal excretion (see CLINICAL PHARMACOLOGY). Therefore, patients with renal failure normally require no adjustment in dosage when usual doses of Rocephin are administered, but concentrations of drug in the serum should be monitored periodically. If evidence of accumulation exists, dosage should be decreased accordingly.

Dosage adjustments should not be necessary in patients with hepatic dysfunction; however, in patients with both hepatic dysfunction and significant renal disease, Rocephin dosage should not exceed 2 gm daily without close monitoring of serum concentrations.

Alterations in prothrombin times have occurred rarely in patients treated with Rocephin. Patients with impaired vitamin K synthesis or low vitamin K stores (eg, chronic hepatic disease and malnutrition) may require monitoring of prothrombin time during Rocephin treatment. Vitamin K administration (10 mg weekly) may be necessary if the prothrombin time is prolonged before or during therapy.

Prolonged use of Rocephin may result in overgrowth of non-susceptible organisms. Careful observation of the patient is essential. If superinfection occurs during therapy, appropriate measures should be taken.

Rocephin should be prescribed with caution in individuals with a history of gastrointestinal disease, especially colitis.

There have been reports of sonographic abnormalities in the gallbladder of patients treated with Rocephin; some of these patients also had symptoms of gallbladder disease. These abnormalities appear on sonography as an echo without acoustical shadowing suggesting sludge or as an echo with acoustical shadowing which may be misinterpreted as gallstones. The chemical nature of the sonographically detected material has been determined to be predominantly a ceftriaxone-calcium salt. The condition appears to be transient and reversible upon discontinuation of Rocephin and institution of conservative management. Therefore, Rocephin should be discontinued in patients who develop signs and symptoms suggestive of gallbladder disease and/or the sonographic findings described above.

Carcinogenesis, Mutagenesis, Impairment of Fertility:
Carcinogenesis: Considering the maximum duration of treatment and the class of the compound, carcinogenicity studies with ceftriaxone in animals have not been performed. The maximum duration of animal toxicity studies was 6 months.
Mutagenesis: Genetic toxicology tests included the Ames test, a micronucleus test and a test for chromosomal aberrations in human lymphocytes cultured in vitro with ceftriaxone. Ceftriaxone showed no potential for mutagenic activity in these studies.
Impairment of Fertility: Ceftriaxone produced no impairment of fertility when given intravenously to rats at daily doses up to 586 mg/kg/day, approximately 20 times the recommended clinical dose of 2 gm/day.
Pregnancy: Teratogenic Effects: Pregnancy Category B. Reproductive studies have been performed in mice and rats at doses up to 20 times the usual human dose and have no evidence of embryotoxicity, fetotoxicity or teratogenicity. In primates, no embryotoxicity or teratogenicity was demonstrated at a dose approximately 3 times the human dose. There are, however, no adequate and well-controlled studies in pregnant women. Because animal reproductive studies are not always predictive of human response, this drug should be used during pregnancy only if clearly needed. Nonteratogenic Effects: In rats, in the Segment I (fertility and general reproduction) and Segment III (perinatal and postnatal) studies with intravenously administered ceftriaxone, no adverse effects were noted on various reproductive parameters during gestation and lactation, including postnatal growth, functional behavior and reproductive ability of the offspring, at doses of 586 mg/kg/day or less.
Nursing Mothers: Low concentrations of ceftriaxone are excreted in human milk. Caution should be exercised when Rocephin is administered to a nursing woman.
Pediatric Use: Safety and effectiveness of Rocephin in neonates, infants and children have been established for the dosages described in the DOSAGE AND ADMINISTRATION section. In vitro studies have shown that ceftriaxone, like some other cephalosporins, can displace bilirubin from serum albumin. Rocephin should not be administered to hyperbilirubinemic neonates, especially prematures.

ADVERSE REACTIONS

Rocephin is generally well tolerated. In clinical trials, the following adverse reactions, which were considered to be related to Rocephin therapy or of uncertain etiology, were observed:

LOCAL REACTIONS—pain, induration and tenderness was 1% overall. Phlebitis was reported in < 1% after IV administration. The incidence of injection site reaction was 17% (3/

TABLE 4
Average Pharmacokinetic Parameters of Ceftriaxone in Humans

Subject Group	Elimination Half-Life (hr)	Plasma Clearance (L/hr)	Volume of Distribution (L)
Healthy Subjects	5.8-8.7	0.58-1.45	5.8-13.5
Elderly Subjects (mean age, 70.5 yr)	8.9	0.83	10.7
Patients with renal impairment			
Hemodialysis patients			
(0-5 mL/min)*	14.7	0.65	13.7
Severe (5-15 mL/min)	15.7	0.56	12.5
Moderate (16-30 mL/min)	11.4	0.72	11.8
Mild (31-60 mL/min)	12.4	0.70	13.3
Patients with liver disease	8.8	1.1	13.6

* Creatinine clearance.

Diluent	Concentration mg/mL	Storage Room Temp. (25°C)	Storage Refrigerated (4°C)
Sterile Water for Injection	100	3 days	10 days
	250, 350	24 hours	3 days
0.9% Sodium Chloride Solution	100	3 days	10 days
	250, 350	24 hours	3 days
5% Dextrose Solution	100	3 days	10 days
	250, 350	24 hours	3 days
Bacteriostatic Water + 0.9% Benzyl Alcohol	100	24 hours	10 days
	250, 350	24 hours	3 days
1% Lidocaine Solution (without epinephrine)	100	24 hours	10 days
	250, 350	24 hours	3 days

17) after IM administration of 350 mg/mL and 5% (1/20) after IM administration of 250 mg/mL.
HYPERSENSITIVITY—rash (1.7%). Less frequently reported (<1%) were pruritus, fever or chills.
HEMATOLOGIC—eosinophilia (6%), thrombocytosis (5.1%) and leukopenia (2.1%). Less frequently reported (<1%) were anemia, hemolytic anemia, neutropenia, lymphopenia, thrombocytopenia and prolongation of the prothrombin time.
GASTROINTESTINAL—diarrhea (2.7%). Less frequently reported (<1%) were nausea or vomiting, and dysgeusia. The onset of pseudomembranous colitis symptoms may occur during or after antibacterial treatment (see WARNINGS).
HEPATIC—elevations of SGOT (3.1%) or SGPT (3.3%). Less frequently reported (<1%) were elevations of alkaline phosphatase and bilirubin.
RENAL—elevations of the BUN (1.2%). Less frequently reported (<1%) were elevations of creatinine and the presence of casts in the urine.
CENTRAL NERVOUS SYSTEM—headache or dizziness were reported occasionally (<1%).
GENITOURINARY—moniliasis or vaginitis were reported occasionally (<1%).
MISCELLANEOUS—diaphoresis and flushing were reported occasionally (<1%).
Other rarely observed adverse reactions (<0.1%) include leukocytosis, lymphocytosis, monocytosis, basophilia, a decrease in the prothrombin time, jaundice, gallbladder sludge, glycosuria, hematuria, anaphylaxis, bronchospasm, serum sickness, abdominal pain, colitis, flatulence, dyspepsia, palpitations and epistaxis.

DOSAGE AND ADMINISTRATION

Rocephin may be administered intravenously or intramuscularly.
ADULTS: The usual adult daily dose is 1 to 2 grams given once a day (or in equally divided doses twice a day) depending on the type and severity of infection. The total daily dose should not exceed 4 grams.
If *C. trachomatis* is a suspected pathogen, appropriate antichlamydial coverage should be added, because ceftriaxone sodium has no activity against this organism.
For the treatment of uncomplicated gonococcal infections, a single intramuscular dose of 250 mg is recommended.
For preoperative use (surgical prophylaxis), a single dose of 1 gram administered intravenously 1/2 to 2 hours before surgery is recommended.
CHILDREN: For the treatment of skin and skin structure infections, the recommended total daily dose is 50 to 75 mg/kg given once a day (or in equally divided doses twice a day). The total daily dose should not exceed 2 grams.
For the treatment of serious miscellaneous infections other than meningitis, the recommended total daily dose is 50 to 75 mg/kg, given in divided doses every 12 hours. The total daily dose should not exceed 2 grams.
In the treatment of meningitis, it is recommended that the initial therapeutic dose be 100 mg/kg (not to exceed 4 grams). Thereafter, a total daily dose of 100 mg/kg/day (not to exceed 4 grams daily) is recommended. The daily dose may be administered once a day (or in equally divided doses every 12 hours). The usual duration of therapy is 7 to 14 days.
Generally, Rocephin therapy should be continued for at least 2 days after the signs and symptoms of infection have disappeared. The usual duration of therapy is 4 to 14 days; in complicated infections, longer therapy may be required.
When treating infections caused by *Streptococcus pyogenes*, therapy should be continued for at least 10 days.
No dosage adjustment is necessary for patients with impairment of renal or hepatic function; however, blood levels should be monitored in patients with severe renal impairment (eg, dialysis patients) and in patients with both renal and hepatic dysfunctions.
DIRECTIONS FOR USE: Intramuscular Administration: Reconstitute Rocephin powder with the appropriate diluent (see COMPATIBILITY-STABILITY section).
After reconstitution, each 1 mL of solution contains approximately 250 mg or 350 mg equivalent of ceftriaxone according to the amount of diluent indicated below. If required, more dilute solutions could be utilized. **A 350 mg/mL concentration is not recommended for the 250 mg vial since it may not be possible to withdraw the entire contents.** As with all intramuscular preparations, Rocephin should be injected well within the body of a relatively large muscle; aspiration helps to avoid unintentional injection into a blood vessel.

Vial Dosage Size	Amount of Diluent to be Added 250 mg/mL	350 mg/mL
250 mg	0.9 mL	—
500 mg	1.8 mL	1.0 mL
1 gm	3.6 mL	2.1 mL
2 gm	7.2 mL	4.2 mL

Intramuscular Convenience Kit: For the 500 mg vial, withdraw 1 mL of diluent, discard the remainder. Inject diluent into vial, shake vial thoroughly to form solution. Withdraw entire contents of vial into syringe to equal approximately 1.4 mL.
For 1 gm vial, withdraw entire contents of diluent (2.1 mL). Inject diluent into vial, shake vial thoroughly to form solution. Withdraw entire contents of vial into syringe to equal approximately 2.8 mL.
Intravenous Administration: Rocephin should be administered intravenously by infusion over a period of 30 minutes. Concentrations between 10 mg/mL and 40 mg/mL are recommended; however, lower concentrations may be used if desired. Reconstitute vials or "piggyback" bottles with an appropriate IV diluent (see COMPATIBILITY-STABILITY section).

Vial Dosage Size	Amount of Diluent to be Added
250 mg	2.4 mL
500 mg	4.8 mL
1 gm	9.6 mL
2 gm	19.2 mL

After reconstitution, each 1 mL of solution contains approximately 100 mg equivalent of ceftriaxone. Withdraw entire contents and dilute to the desired concentration with the appropriate IV diluent.

Piggyback Bottle Dosage Size	Amount of Diluent to be Added
1 gm	10 mL
2 gm	20 mL

After reconstitution, further dilute to 50 mL or 100 mL volumes with the appropriate IV diluent.
COMPATIBILITY AND STABILITY: Rocephin sterile powder should be stored at room temperature—77°F (25°C)—or below and protected from light. After reconstitution, protection from normal light is not necessary. The color of solutions ranges from light yellow to amber, depending on the length of storage, concentration and diluent used.
Rocephin *intramuscular* solutions remain stable (loss of potency less than 10%) for the following time periods: [See table at top of page.]
Rocephin *intravenous* solutions, at concentrations of 10, 20 and 40 mg/mL, remain stable (loss of potency less than 10%) for the following time periods stored in glass or PVC containers: [See table below.]
Similarly, Rocephin *intravenous* solutions, at concentrations of 100 mg/mL, remain stable in the IV piggyback glass containers for the above specified time periods.
The following *intravenous* Rocephin solutions are stable at room temperature (25°C) for 24 hours, at concentrations between 10 mg/mL and 40 mg/mL: Sodium Lactate (PVC container), 10% Invert Sugar (glass container), 5% Sodium Bicarbonate (glass container), Freamine III (glass container), Normosol-M in 5% Dextrose (glass and PVC containers), Ionosol-B in 5% Dextrose (glass container), 5% Mannitol (glass container), 10% Mannitol (glass container).
After the indicated stability time periods, unused portions of solutions should be discarded.

Diluent	Storage Room Temp. (25°C)	Storage Refrigerated (4°C)
Sterile Water	3 days	10 days
0.9% Sodium Chloride Solution	3 days	10 days
5% Dextrose Solution	3 days	10 days
10% Dextrose Solution	3 days	10 days
5% Dextrose + 0.9% Sodium Chloride Solution*	3 days	Incompatible
5% Dextrose + 0.45% Sodium Chloride Solution	3 days	Incompatible

*Data available for 10 to 40 mg/mL concentrations in this diluent in PVC containers only.

Rocephin reconstituted with 5% Dextrose or 0.9% Sodium Chloride solution at concentrations between 10 mg/mL and 40 mg/mL, and then stored in frozen state (−20°C) in PVC or polyolefin containers, remains stable for 26 weeks.
Frozen solutions should be thawed at room temperature before use. After thawing, unused portions should be discarded. **DO NOT REFREEZE.**
Rocephin solutions should *not* be physically mixed with or piggybacked into solutions containing other antimicrobial drugs or into diluent solutions other than those listed above, due to possible incompatibility.

ANIMAL PHARMACOLOGY

Concretions consisting of the precipitated calcium salt of ceftriaxone have been found in the gallbladder bile of dogs and baboons treated with ceftriaxone.
These appeared as a gritty sediment in dogs that received 100 mg/kg/day for 4 weeks. A similar phenomenon has been observed in baboons but only after a protracted dosing period (6 months) at higher dose levels (335 mg/kg/day or more). The likelihood of this occurrence in humans is considered to be low, since ceftriaxone has a greater plasma half-life in humans, the calcium salt of ceftriaxone is more soluble in human gallbladder bile and the calcium content of human gallbladder bile is relatively low.

HOW SUPPLIED

Rocephin is supplied as a sterile crystalline powder in glass vials and piggyback bottles. The following packages are available:
Vials containing 250 mg equivalent of ceftriaxone. Box of 1 (NDC 0004-1962-02) and box of 10 (NDC 0004-1962-01).
Vials containing 500 mg equivalent of ceftriaxone. Box of 1 (NDC 0004-1963-02) and box of 10 (NDC 0004-1963-01).
Vials containing 1 gm equivalent of ceftriaxone. Box of 1 (NDC 0004-1964-04) and box of 10 (NDC 0004-1964-01).
Piggyback bottles containing 1 gm equivalent of ceftriaxone. Box of 1 (NDC 0004-1964-02).
Vials containing 2 gm equivalent of ceftriaxone. Box of 10 (NDC 0004-1965-01).
Piggyback bottles containing 2 gm equivalent of ceftriaxone. Box of 1 (NDC 0004-1965-02).
Bulk pharmacy containers, containing 10 gm equivalent of ceftriaxone. Box of 1 (NDC 0004-1971-01). NOT FOR DIRECT ADMINISTRATION.
Rocephin is also supplied in an Intramuscular Convenience Kit, available in two strengths, consisting of a vial of ceftriaxone sodium as a sterile crystalline powder and a vial of Xylocaine®-MPF 1% (lidocaine HCl Injection, USP).
The following strengths are available:
Kit containing 1 vial of 500 mg equivalent of ceftriaxone, plus 1 vial of 2.1 mL Xylocaine (NDC 0004-1963-39).
Kit containing 1 vial of 1 gm equivalent of ceftriaxone, plus 1 vial of 2.1 mL Xylocaine (NDC 0004-1964-39).
Xylocaine®-MPF 1% (lidocaine HCl Injection, USP) is manufactured for Roche Laboratories Inc. by Astra USA, Inc., Westborough, MA 01581.
Rocephin is also supplied as a sterile crystalline powder in ADD-Vantage®* Vials as follows:
ADD-Vantage Vials containing 1 gm equivalent of ceftriaxone. Box of 10 (NDC 0004-1964-05).
ADD-Vantage Vials containing 2 gm equivalent of ceftriaxone. Box of 10 (NDC 0004-1965-05).
Rocephin (ceftriaxone sodium injection), also supplied premixed as a frozen, iso-osmotic, sterile, nonpyrogenic solution of ceftriaxone sodium in 50 mL single dose Galaxy®† containers (PL 2040 plastic), is manufactured for Roche Laboratories Inc., by Baxter Healthcare Corporation, Deerfield, Illinois 60015. The following strengths are available:
1 gm equivalent of ceftriaxone, iso-osmotic with approximately 1.9 gm Dextrose Hydrous, USP, added (NDC 0004-2002-78).
2 gm equivalent of ceftriaxone, iso-osmotic with approximately 1.2 gm Dextrose Hydrous, USP, added (NDC 0004-2003-78).
NOTE: Store Rocephin in the frozen state at or below −20°C/−4°F.

* Registered trademark of Abbott Laboratories, Inc.
† Registered trademark of Baxter International Inc.

Continued on next page

Roche Laboratories—Cont.

REFERENCES

1. National Committee for Clinical Standards, *Performance Standards for Antimicrobial Disk Susceptibility Tests.* 5th ed. Villanova, PA:1993. Approved Standard NCCLS Document M2-A5, Vol. 13, No. 7, NCCLS.
2. National Committee for Clinical Laboratory Standards, *Methods for Dilution Antimicrobial Susceptibility Tests for Bacteria That Grow Aerobically.* 3rd ed. Villanova, PA:1993. Approved Standard NCCLS Document M7-A3, Vol. 13, No. 25, NCCLS.

Revised: January 1996

ROFERON®-A ℞

[ro-fear'on]
(Interferon alfa-2a, recombinant)

DESCRIPTION

Roferon-A (Interferon alfa-2a, recombinant) is a sterile protein product for use by injection. Roferon-A is manufactured by recombinant DNA technology that employs a genetically engineered *E. coli* bacterium containing DNA that codes for the human protein. Interferon alfa-2a, recombinant is a highly purified protein containing 165 amino acids, and it has an approximate molecular weight of 19,000 daltons. The purification procedure includes affinity chromatography using a murine monoclonal antibody. Fermentation is carried out in a defined nutrient medium containing the antibiotic tetracycline hydrochloride, 5 mg/L. However, the presence of the antibiotic is not detectable in the final product. Roferon-A is supplied as an injectable solution or as a sterile powder for injection with its accompanying diluent.

Injectable Solution:

3 million IU (11.1 mcg/mL) Roferon-A per vial—The solution is colorless and each mL contains 3 million IU of Interferon alfa-2a, recombinant, 7.21 mg sodium chloride, 0.2 mg polysorbate 80, 10 mg benzyl alcohol as a preservative and 0.77 mg ammonium acetate.

9 million IU (33.3 mcg/0.9 mL) Roferon-A per vial—The solution is colorless and each 9 mL contains 9 million IU of Interferon alfa-2a, recombinant, 6.49 mg sodium chloride, 0.18 mg polysorbate 80, 9 mg benzyl alcohol as a preservative and 0.69 mg ammonium acetate.

18 million IU (66.7 mcg/3 mL) Roferon-A per vial—The solution is colorless and each mL contains 6 million IU of Interferon alfa-2a, recombinant, 7.21 mg sodium chloride, 0.2 mg polysorbate 80, 10 mg benzyl alcohol as a preservative and 0.77 mg ammonium acetate. Each 0.5 mL contains 3 million IU of Interferon alfa-2a, recombinant.

36 million IU (133.3 mcg/mL) Roferon-A per vial—The solution is colorless and each mL contains 36 million IU of Interferon alfa-2a, recombinant, 7.21 mg sodium chloride, 0.2 mg polysorbate 80, 10 mg benzyl alcohol as a preservative and 0.77 mg ammonium acetate. This dosage form should not be used for the treatment of hairy cell leukemia.

Based on the specific activity of 2.7×10^8 IU/mg protein, the corresponding quantities of Interferon alfa-2a, recombinant in the vials described above are approximately 3 million IU (11.1 mcg/mL), 6 million IU (22.2 mcg/mL), 9 million IU (33.3 mcg/0.9 mL), 18 million IU (66.7 mcg/3 mL) and 36 million IU (133.3 mcg/mL).

Sterile Powder for Injection:

18 million IU Roferon-A per vial—The powder is white to beige and when reconstituted with 3 mL of Diluent for Sterile Powder for Injection each 1 mL of reconstituted solution contains 6 million IU of Interferon alfa-2a, recombinant, 9 mg sodium chloride, 1.67 mg Albumin (Human) and 3.3 mg phenol as a preservative. Each 0.5 mL contains 3 million IU of Interferon alfa-2a, recombinant.

Diluent for Sterile Powder for Injection:

3 mL per vial—Each mL contains 6 mg sodium chloride and 3.3 mg phenol as a preservative.

The route of administration is subcutaneous or intramuscular.

CLINICAL PHARMACOLOGY

The mechanism by which Interferon alfa-2a, recombinant, or any other interferon, exerts antitumor activity is not clearly understood. However, it is believed that direct antiproliferative action against tumor cells and modulation of the host immune response play important roles in the antitumor activity.

The biological activities of Interferon alfa-2a, recombinant are species-restricted, ie, they are expressed in a very limited number of species other than humans. As a consequence, preclinical evaluation of Interferon alfa-2a, recombinant has involved in vitro experiments with human cells and some in vivo experiments.[1] Using human cells in culture, Interferon alfa-2a, recombinant has been shown to have antiproliferative and immunomodulatory activities that are very similar to those of the mixture of interferon alfa subtypes produced by human leukocytes. In vivo, Interferon alfa-2a, recombinant has been shown to inhibit the growth of several human tumors growing in immunocompromised (nude) mice. Because of its species-restricted activity, it has not been possible to demonstrate antitumor activity in immunologically intact syngeneic tumor model systems, where effects on the host immune system would be observable. However, such antitumor activity has been repeatedly demonstrated with, for example, mouse interferon-alfa in transplantable mouse tumor systems. The clinical significance of these findings is unknown.

The metabolism of Interferon alfa-2a, recombinant is consistent with that of alfa interferons in general. Alfa interferons are totally filtered through the glomeruli and undergo rapid proteolytic degradation during tubular reabsorption, rendering a negligible reappearance of intact alfa interferon in the systemic circulation. Small amounts of radiolabeled Interferon alfa-2a, recombinant appear in the urine of isolated rat kidneys, suggesting near complete reabsorption of Interferon alfa-2a, recombinant catabolites. Liver metabolism and subsequent biliary excretion are considered minor pathways of elimination for alfa interferons.

The serum concentrations of Interferon alfa-2a, recombinant reflected a large intersubject variation in both healthy volunteers and patients with disseminated cancer.

In healthy people, Interferon alfa-2a, recombinant exhibited an elimination half-life of 3.7 to 8.5 hours (mean 5.1 hours), volume of distribution at steady-state of 0.223 to 0.748 L/kg (mean 0.400 L/kg) and a total body clearance of 2.14 to 3.62 mL/min/kg (mean 2.79 mL/min/kg) after a 36 million IU (2.2×10^8 pg) intravenous infusion. After intramuscular and subcutaneous administrations of 36 million IU, peak serum concentrations ranged from 1500 to 2580 pg/mL (mean 2020 pg/mL) at a mean time to peak of 3.8 hours and from 1250 to 2320 pg/mL (mean 1730 pg/mL) at a mean time to peak of 7.3 hours, respectively. The apparent fraction of the dose absorbed after intramuscular injection was greater than 80%. The pharmacokinetics of Interferon alfa-2a, recombinant after single intramuscular doses to patients with disseminated cancer were similar to those found in healthy volunteers. Dose proportional increases in serum concentrations were observed after single doses up to 198 million IU. There were no changes in the distribution or elimination of Interferon alfa-2a, recombinant during twice daily (0.5 to 36 million IU), once daily (1 to 54 million IU), or three times weekly (1 to 136 million IU) dosing regimens up to 28 days of dosing. Multiple intramuscular doses of Interferon alfa-2a, recombinant resulted in an accumulation of two to four times the single dose serum concentrations. There is no pharmacokinetic information in patients with hairy cell leukemia, AIDS-related Kaposi's sarcoma and chronic myelogenous leukemia.

Serum neutralizing activity, determined by a highly sensitive enzyme immunoassay, and a neutralization bioassay, was detected in approximately 25% of all patients who received Roferon-A.[2] Antibodies to human leukocyte interferon may occur spontaneously in certain clinical conditions (cancer, systemic lupus erythematosus, herpes zoster) in patients who have never received exogenous interferon.[3] The significance of the appearance of serum neutralizing activity is not known.

CLINICAL STUDIES: Studies have shown that Roferon-A can produce clinically meaningful tumor regression or disease stabilization in patients with hairy cell leukemia or in patients with AIDS-related Kaposi's sarcoma.[4-6] In Ph-positive Chronic Myelogenous Leukemia, Roferon-A supplemented with intermittent chemotherapy has been shown to prolong overall survival and to delay disease progression compared to patients treated with chemotherapy alone.[7] In addition, Roferon-A has been shown to produce sustained complete cytogenetic responses in a small subset of patients with CML in chronic phase. The activity of Roferon-A in Ph-negative CML has not been determined.

EFFECTS ON HAIRY CELL LEUKEMIA: A multicenter US phase II study (N2752) enrolled 218 patients; 75 were evaluable for efficacy in a preliminary analysis; 218 patients were evaluable for safety. Patients were to receive a starting dose of Roferon-A up to 6 MIU/m2/day, for an induction period of 4 to 6 months. Responding patients were to receive 12 months maintenance therapy.

During the first 1 to 2 months of treatment of patients with hairy cell leukemia, significant depression of hematopoiesis was likely to occur. Subsequently, there was improvement in circulating blood cell counts. Of the 75 patients who were evaluable for efficacy following at least 16 weeks of therapy, 46 (61%) achieved complete or partial response. Twenty-one patients (28%) had a minor remission, eight (11%) remained stable, and none had worsening of disease. All patients who achieved either a complete or partial response had complete or partial normalization of all peripheral blood elements including hemoglobin level, white blood cell, neutrophil, monocyte and platelet counts with a concomitant decrease in peripheral blood and bone marrow hairy cells. Responding patients also exhibited a marked reduction in red blood cell and platelet transfusion requirements, a decrease in infectious episodes and improvement in performance status. The probability of survival for two years in patients receiving Roferon-A (94%) was statistically increased compared to a historical control group (75%).

EFFECTS ON AIDS-RELATED KAPOSI'S SARCOMA: In six studies with Roferon-A, doses of 3 to 54 million IU daily were evaluated for the treatment of AIDS-related Kaposi's sarcoma in more than 350 patients. Four dosage regimens of Roferon-A were evaluated for initial induction. Thirty-nine patients received 3 million IU daily; 99 patients received an escalating regimen of 3 million, 9 million and 18 million IU each daily for 3 days, followed by 36 million IU daily; 119 patients received 36 million IU daily; and 16 patients received doses greater than 36 million IU to a maximum of 54 million IU daily. An additional 91 patients received Roferon-A in combination with vinblastine. The best response rate associated with acceptable toxicity was observed when Roferon-A was administered as a single agent at a dose of 36 million IU daily. The escalating regimen of 3 to 36 million IU daily provided equivalent therapeutic benefit with some amelioration of acute toxicity in some patients. In AIDS-related Kaposi's sarcoma, lower doses were less effective in inducing tumor regression and doses higher than 36 million IU daily were associated with unacceptable toxicity. As summarized in Table 1, the likelihood of response to Roferon-A varied with the clinical manifestations of human immunodeficiency virus (HIV) infection. Patients with prior opportunistic infection or B symptoms are unlikely to respond to treatment with Roferon-A.

[See table 1 below.]

Patients who were otherwise asymptomatic, with no prior opportunistic infection and near-normal levels of CD_4 lymphocytes, experienced higher response rates. Responding patients with a baseline CD_4 lymphocyte count greater than 200 cells/mm^3 had a distinct survival advantage over both responding patients with a baseline CD_4 lymphocyte count of 200 cells/mm^3 or less and nonresponding patients regardless of their baseline CD_4 lymphocyte count. Median survival for responding patients with CD_4 lymphocyte counts of greater than 200 to 400 cells/mm^3 had not been reached but was greater than 32.7 months from the initiation of therapy. For responding patients with CD_4 lymphocyte counts of greater than 400 cells/mm^3, the median survival had not been reached but was greater than 29.5 months.

A classification system for staging AIDS-related Kaposi's sarcoma has been described based on location and extent of disease. In studies of Roferon-A, no difference was noted in response rates for patients with different stages of Kaposi's sarcoma. Likelihood of response was related to manifestations of HIV infection (baseline CD_4 lymphocyte count, prior opportunistic infection or B symptoms) and not to extent of tumor involvement. The median time to response was 2.7 months. The median duration of response for patients achieving a partial or complete response was 6.3 and 20.7 months, respectively. Complete and partial responses lasting in excess of three years have been observed. Therapy was discontinued because of progression of Kaposi's sarcoma, development of severe opportunistic infection or severe adverse effects. The median time to discontinuation of treatment was 12.5 months for responding patients and 2.3 months for patients who did not respond.

EFFECTS ON Ph-POSITIVE CHRONIC MYELOGENOUS LEUKEMIA (CML): Roferon-A was evaluated in two trials of patients with chronic phase CML. Study DM84-38 was a single center phase II study conducted at the MD Anderson Cancer Center, which enrolled 91 patients, 81% were previously treated, 82% were Ph positive, and 63% received

---

Table 1

Likelihood of Response to Roferon-A in Patients with
AIDS-Related Kaposi's Sarcoma

No. Pts.*	CD$_4$(T$_4$) Lymphocyte Count (cells/mm^3)	Objective Response Rate (%)		
		CR	PR	Total
83	0–200	3.6	3.6	7.2
51	201–400	15.7	11.8	27.5
33	>400	24.2	21.2	45.4

In the 28 patients evaluated who had prior opportunistic infection or B symptoms, the response rate was 3.6%.
* Patients had no prior opportunistic infection or B symptoms. B symptoms include night sweats, weight loss of greater than 10% of body weight or 15 lbs., or fever greater than 100°F without an identifiable source of infection.

Roferon-A within 1 year of diagnosis. Study MI400 was a multicenter randomized phase III study conducted in Italy by the Italian Cooperative Study Group on CML in 335 patients; 226 Roferon-A and 109 chemotherapy. Patients with Ph-positive, newly diagnosed or minimally treated CML were randomized (ratio 2:1) to either Roferon-A or conventional chemotherapy with either hydroxyurea or busulfan. In study DM84-38, patients started Roferon-A at 9 MIU/day, whereas in study MI400, it was progressively escalated from 3 to 9 MIU/day over the first month. In both trials, dose escalation for insufficient hematologic response, and dose attenuation or interruption for toxicity was permitted. No formal guidelines for dose attenuation were given in the chemotherapy arm of study MI400. In addition, in the Roferon-A arm, the MI400 protocol allowed the addition of intermittent single agent chemotherapy for insufficient hematologic response to Roferon-A alone. In this trial, 44% of the Roferon-A treated patients also received intermittent single agent chemotherapy at some time during the study.

The two studies were analyzed according to uniform response criteria. For hematologic response: complete response (WBC $< 9.10^9$/L, normalization of the differential with no immature forms in the peripheral blood, disappearance of splenomegaly), partial response ($> 50\%$ decrease from baseline of WBC to $< 20.10^9$/L). For cytogenetic response: complete response (0% Ph-positive metaphases), partial response (1% to 34% Ph-positive metaphases).

In study DM84-38, the median survival from initiation of Roferon-A was 47 months. In study MI400, the median survival for the patients on the interferon arm was 69 months, which was significantly better than the 55 months seen in the chemotherapy control group (48 patients in study MI400 proceeded to BMT and in study DM84-38, 15 patients proceeded to BMT). Roferon-A treatment significantly delayed disease progression to blastic phase as evidenced by a median time to disease progression of 69 months compared to 46 months with chemotherapy.

By multivariate analysis of prognostic factors associated with all 335 patients entered into the randomized study, treatment with Roferon-A (with or without intermittent additional chemotherapy; p = 0.006), Sokal index[8] (p = 0.006) and WBC (p = 0.023) were the three variables associated with an improved survival, independent of other baseline characteristics (Karnofsky performance status and hemoglobin being the other factors entered into the model).

In study MI400, overall hematologic responses, [complete responses (CR) and partial responses (PR)], were observed in approximately 60% of patients treated with Roferon-A (40% CR, 20% PR), compared to 70% with chemotherapy (30% CR, 40% PR). The median time to reach a complete hematologic response was 5 months in the Roferon-A arm and 4 months in the chemotherapy arm. The overall cytogenetic response rate (CR+PR), in patients receiving Roferon-A, was 10% and 12% in studies MI400 and DM84-38, respectively, according to the intent-to-treat principle. In contrast, only 2% of the patients in the chemotherapy arm of study MI400 achieved a cytogenetic response (with no complete responses). Cytogenetic responses were observed only in patients who had complete hematologic responses. In study DM84-38, hematologic and cytogenetic response rates were higher in the subset of patients treated with Roferon-A within 1 year of diagnosis (76% and 17%, respectively) compared to the subset initiating Roferon-A therapy more than 1 year from diagnosis (29% and 4%, respectively). In an exploratory analysis, patients who achieve a cytogenetic response live longer than those who did not.

Severe adverse events were observed in 66% and 31% of patients on study DM84-38 and MI400, respectively. Dose reduction and temporary cessation of therapy was required frequently. Permanent cessation of Roferon-A, due to intolerable side effects, was required in 15% and 23% of patients on studies DM84-38 and MI400, respectively (see ADVERSE REACTIONS).

Limited data are available on the use of Roferon-A in children with Ph-positive, adult-type CML. A published report on 15 children with CML suggest a safety profile similar to that seen in adult CML; clinical responses were also observed[9] (see DOSAGE AND ADMINISTRATION).

INDICATIONS AND USAGE

Roferon-A is indicated for the treatment of hairy cell leukemia and AIDS-related Kaposi's sarcoma in patients 18 years of age or older. In addition, it is indicated for chronic phase, Philadelphia chromosome (Ph) positive chronic myelogenous leukemia (CML) patients who are minimally pretreated (within 1 year of diagnosis).

FOR PATIENTS WITH AIDS-RELATED KAPOSI'S SARCOMA: Roferon-A is useful for the treatment of AIDS-related Kaposi's sarcoma in a select group of patients. In determining whether a patient should be treated, the physician should assess the likelihood of response based on the clinical manifestations of HIV infection, including prior opportunistic infections, presence of B symptoms, and CD_4 count, and the manifestations of Kaposi's sarcoma requiring treatment (see CLINICAL PHARMACOLOGY).

CONTRAINDICATIONS

Roferon-A is contraindicated in patients with known hypersensitivity to alfa interferon, mouse immunoglobulin or any component of the product. The injectable solutions contain benzyl alcohol and are contraindicated in any individual with a known allergy to that preservative.

WARNINGS

Roferon-A should be administered under the guidance of a qualified physician (see DOSAGE AND ADMINISTRATION). Appropriate management of the therapy and its complications is possible only when adequate diagnostic and treatment facilities are readily available.

DEPRESSION AND SUICIDAL BEHAVIOR INCLUDING SUICIDAL IDEATION, SUICIDAL ATTEMPTS AND SUICIDES HAVE BEEN REPORTED IN ASSOCIATION WITH TREATMENT WITH ALFA INTERFERONS, INCLUDING ROFERON-A. Patients to be treated with Roferon-A should be informed that depression and suicidal ideation may be side effects of treatment and should be advised to report these side effects immediately to the prescribing physician. Patients receiving Roferon-A therapy should receive close monitoring for the occurrence of depressive symptomatology. Cessation of treatment should be considered for patients experiencing depression. Although dose reduction or treatment cessation may lead to resolution of the depressive symptomatology, depression may persist and suicides have occurred after withdrawing therapy (see PRECAUTIONS and ADVERSE REACTIONS).

Roferon-A should not be used for the treatment of visceral AIDS-related Kaposi's sarcoma associated with rapidly progressive or life-threatening disease.

Roferon-A should be used with caution in patients with severe preexisting cardiac disease, severe renal or hepatic disease, seizure disorders and/or compromised central nervous system function.

Infrequently, severe or fatal gastrointestinal hemorrhage has been reported in association with alfa interferon therapy.

Because of the possibility of severe or even fatal adverse reactions, patients should be informed not only of the benefits of therapy but also of the risks involved.

Roferon-A should be administered with caution to patients with cardiac disease or with any history of cardiac illness. It is likely that acute, self-limited toxicities (ie, fever, chills) frequently associated with Roferon-A administration may exacerbate preexisting cardiac conditions. Rarely, myocardial infarction has occurred in patients receiving Roferon-A. Cases of cardiomyopathy have been observed on rare occasions in patients treated with alfa-interferons.

Caution should be exercised when administering Roferon-A to patients with myelosuppression or when Roferon-A is used in combination with other agents that are known to cause myelosuppression. Synergistic toxicity has been observed when Roferon-A is administered in combination with zidovudine (AZT).[10] The effects of Roferon-A when combined with other drugs used in the treatment of AIDS-related disease are not known.

Central nervous system adverse reactions have been reported in a number of patients. These reactions included decreased mental status, dizziness, impaired memory, agitation, manic behavior and psychotic reactions. More severe obtundation and coma have been rarely observed. Most of these abnormalities were mild and reversible within a few days to three weeks upon dose reduction or discontinuation of Roferon-A therapy. Careful periodic neuropsychiatric monitoring of all patients is recommended.

Leukopenia and elevation of hepatic enzymes occurred frequently but were rarely dose-limiting. Thrombocytopenia occurred less frequently. Proteinuria and increased cells in urinary sediment were also seen infrequently. Dose-limiting hepatic or renal toxicities were unusual. Infrequently, severe renal toxicities, sometimes requiring renal dialysis, have been reported with alfa interferon therapy alone or in combination with IL-2 (see PRECAUTIONS).

The injectable solutions contain benzyl alcohol and should not be used by patients with a known allergy to benzyl alcohol. Also, this product is not indicated for use in neonates or infants and should not be used by patients in that age group. There have been rare reports of death in neonates and infants associated with excessive exposure to benzyl alcohol. The amount of benzyl alcohol at which toxicity or adverse effects may occur in neonates or infants is not known (see CONTRAINDICATIONS and PRECAUTIONS: *Pediatric Use*).

PRECAUTIONS

General: In all instances where the use of Roferon-A is considered for chemotherapy, the physician must evaluate the need and usefulness of the drug against the risk of adverse reactions. Most adverse reactions are reversible if detected early. If severe reactions occur, the drug should be reduced in dosage or discontinued and appropriate corrective measures should be taken according to the clinical judgment of the physician. Reinstitution of Roferon-A therapy should be carried out with caution and with adequate consideration of

the further need for the drug and, alertness to possible recurrence of toxicity. The minimum effective doses of Roferon-A for treatment of hairy cell leukemia, AIDS-related Kaposi's sarcoma, and chronic myelogenous leukemia have not been established.

Variations in dosage and adverse reactions exist among different brands of Interferon. Therefore, do not use different brands of Interferon in a single treatment regimen.

Information for Patient: Patients should be cautioned not to change brands of Interferon without medical consultation, as a change in dosage may result. Patients should be informed regarding the potential benefits and risks attendant to the use of Roferon-A. If home use is determined to be desirable by the physician, instructions on appropriate use should be given, including review of the contents of the enclosed Patient Information Sheet. Patients should be well hydrated, especially during the initial stages of treatment. Patients should be thoroughly instructed in the importance of proper disposal procedures and cautioned against reusing syringes and needles. If home use is prescribed, a puncture resistant container for the disposal of used syringes and needles should be supplied to the patient. The full container should be disposed of according to directions provided by the physician.

Patients receiving high dose alfa-interferon should be cautioned against performing tasks that require complete mental alertness such as operating machinery or driving a motor vehicle. Patients to be treated with Roferon-A should be informed that depression and suicidal ideation may be side effects of treatment and should be advised to report these side effects immediately to the prescribing physician.

Laboratory Tests: Complete blood counts and clinical chemistry tests should be performed before initiation of Roferon-A therapy and at appropriate periods during therapy. Since responses of hairy cell leukemia, AIDS-related Kaposi's sarcoma, and chronic myelogenous leukemia are not generally observed for one to three months after initiation of treatment, very careful monitoring for severe depression of blood cell counts is warranted during the initial phase of treatment.

Those patients who have preexisting cardiac abnormalities and/or are in advanced stages of cancer should have electrocardiograms taken before and during the course of treatment.

Drug Interactions: Roferon-A, apparently through an unknown effect on certain microsomal enzyme systems, has been reported to reduce the clearance of theophylline.[11,12] The clinical relevance of this interaction is presently unknown. Interactions between Roferon-A and other drugs have not been fully evaluated. Caution should be exercised when administering Roferon-A in combination with other potentially myelosuppressive agents (see WARNINGS).

Other Drug Interactions: Alfa-Interferons may affect the oxidative metabolic process by reducing the activity of hepatic microsomal cytochrome enzymes in the P450 group. Although the clinical relevance is still unclear, this should be taken into account when prescribing concomitant therapy with drugs metabolized by this route. Reduced clearance of theophylline following the concomitant administration of alfa-interferons has been reported.

It has been observed that the neurotoxic, hematotoxic or cardiotoxic effects of previously or concurrently administered drugs may be increased by interferons. Interactions could occur following concurrent administration of centrally-acting drugs. Use of Roferon-A in conjunction with interleukin-2 may potentiate risks of renal failure.

Carcinogenesis, Mutagenesis, Impairment of Fertility:

Carcinogenesis: Roferon-A has not been tested for its carcinogenic potential.

Mutagenesis: A. Internal studies—Ames tests using six different tester strains, with and without metabolic activation, were performed with Roferon-A up to a concentration of 1920 µg/plate. There was no evidence of mutagenicity. Human lymphocyte cultures were treated in vitro with Roferon-A at noncytotoxic concentrations. No increase in the incidence of chromosomal damage was noted.

B. Published studies—There are no published studies on the mutagenic potential of Roferon-A. However, a number of studies on the genotoxicity of human leukocyte interferon have been reported.

A chromosomal defect following the addition of human leukocyte interferon to lymphocyte cultures from a patient suffering from a lymphoproliferative disorder has been reported.

In contrast, other studies have failed to detect chromosomal abnormalities following treatment of lymphocyte cultures from healthy volunteers with human leukocyte interferon. It has also been shown that human leukocyte interferon protects primary chick embryo fibroblasts from chromosomal aberrations produced by gamma rays.

Impairment of Fertility: Roferon-A has been studied for its effect on fertility in Macaca mulatta (rhesus monkeys). Nonpregnant rhesus females treated with Roferon-A at doses of 5

Continued on next page

Roche Laboratories—Cont.

and 25 million IU/kg/day have shown menstrual cycle irregularities, including prolonged or shortened menstrual periods and erratic bleeding; these cycles were considered to be anovulatory on the basis that reduced progesterone levels were noted and that expected increases in preovulatory estrogen and luteinizing hormones were not observed. These monkeys returned to a normal menstrual rhythm following discontinuation of treatment.

Pregnancy: Teratogenic Effects: Pregnancy Category C. Roferon-A has been shown to demonstrate a statistically significant increase in abortifacient activity in rhesus monkeys when given at approximately 20 to 500 times the human dose. A study in pregnant rhesus monkeys treated with 1, 5 or 25 million IU/kg/day of Roferon-A in their early to midfetal period (days 22 to 70 of gestation) has failed to demonstrate teratogenic activity for Roferon-A.

There are no adequate and well-controlled studies in pregnant women.

Nonteratogenic Effects: Dose-related abortifacient activity was observed in pregnant rhesus monkeys treated with 1, 5 or 25 million IU/kg/day of Roferon-A in their early to midfetal period (days 22 to 70 of gestation). A late-fetal period study (days 79 to 100 of gestation) is in progress and as yet there have been no reports of any increased rate of abortion.

Usage in Pregnancy: Safe use in human pregnancy has not been established. Therefore, Roferon-A should be used during pregnancy only if the potential benefit justifies the potential risk to the fetus. Information from primate studies showed dose-related menstrual irregularities and an increased incidence of spontaneous abortions. Decreases in serum estradiol and progesterone concentrations have been reported in women treated with human leukocyte interferon.[13] Therefore, fertile women should not receive Roferon-A unless they are using effective contraception during the therapy period.

Male fertility and teratologic evaluations have yielded no significant adverse effects to date.

Nursing Mothers: It is not known whether this drug is excreted in human milk. Because many drugs are excreted in human milk and because of the potential for serious adverse reactions in nursing infants from Roferon-A, a decision should be made whether to discontinue nursing or to discontinue the drug, taking into account the importance of the drug to the mother.

Pediatric Use: Use of Roferon-A in children with Ph-positive adult-type CML is supported by evidence from adequate and well-controlled studies of Roferon-A in adults with additional data from the literature on the use of alfa interferon in children with CML. A published report on 15 children with Ph-positive adult-type CML suggests a safety profile similar to that seen in adult CML; clinical responses were also observed[9] (see DOSAGE AND ADMINISTRATION).

The injectable solutions are not indicated for use in neonates or infants and should not be used by patients in that age group. There have been rare reports of death in neonates and infants associated with excessive exposure to benzyl alcohol. The amount of benzyl alcohol at which toxicity or adverse effects may occur in neonates or infants is not known.

ADVERSE REACTIONS

Depressive illness and suicidal behavior, including suicidal ideation and suicides, have been reported in association with the use of alfa interferon products. The incidence of reported depression has varied substantially among trials, possibly related to the underlying disease, dose, duration of therapy, and degree of monitoring, but has been reported to be 15% or higher (see WARNINGS).

FOR PATIENTS WITH HAIRY CELL LEUKEMIA:
Constitutional (100%): Fever (92%), fatigue (86%), headache (64%), chills (64%), weight loss (33%), dizziness (21%) and flu-like symptoms (16%).
Integumentary (79%): Skin rash (44%), diaphoresis (22%), partial alopecia (17%), dry skin (17%) and pruritus (13%).
Musculoskeletal (73%): Myalgia (71%), joint or bone pain (25%) and arthritis or polyarthritis (5%).
Gastrointestinal (69%): Anorexia (43%), nausea/vomiting (39%) and diarrhea (34%).
Head and neck (45%): Throat irritation (21%), rhinorrhea (12%) and sinusitis (11%).
Pulmonary (40%): Coughing (16%), dyspnea (12%) and pneumonia (11%).
Central nervous system (39%): Dizziness (21%), depression (16%), sleep disturbance (10%), decreased mental status (10%), anxiety (6%), lethargy (6%), visual disturbance (6%) and confusion (5%).
Cardiovascular (39%): Chest pain (11%), edema (11%) and hypertension (11%).
Pain (34%): Pain (24%) and pain in back (16%).
Peripheral nervous system (23%): Paresthesia (12%) and numbness (12%).
Rarely (<5%), central nervous system effects including gait disturbance, nervousness, syncope and vertigo, as well as cardiac adverse events including murmur, thrombophlebitis

and hypotension were reported. Adverse experiences that occurred rarely, and may have been related to underlying disease, included ecchymosis, epistaxis, bleeding gums and petechiae. Urticaria and inflammation at the site of injection were also rarely observed.

FOR PATIENTS WITH AIDS-RELATED KAPOSI'S SARCOMA:
Flu-like Symptoms—Fatigue (95%), fever (74%), myalgia (69%), headache (66%), chills (41%) and arthralgia (24%).
Gastrointestinal—Anorexia (65%), nausea (51%), diarrhea (42%), emesis (17%) and abdominal pain (15%).
Central and Peripheral Nervous System—Dizziness (40%), decreased mental status (17%), depression (16%), paresthesia (8%), confusion (8%), diaphoresis (7%), visual disturbances (5%), sleep disturbances (5%) and numbness (3%).
Pulmonary and Cardiovascular—Coughing (27%), dyspnea (11%), edema (9%), chest pain (4%) and hypotension (4%).
Skin—Partial alopecia (22%), rash (11%) and dry skin or pruritus (5%).
Other—Weight loss (25%), change in taste (25%), dryness or inflammation of the oropharynx (14%), night sweats (8%) and rhinorrhea (4%).
Occasionally (<3%) nervous system effects including anxiety, nervousness, emotional lability, vertigo and forgetfulness, as well as cardiac adverse events, including palpitations and arrhythmia, were reported. Other adverse experiences that occurred occasionally (<3%) and may have been related to underlying disease, included sinusitis, constipation, chest congestion, pneumonia, urticaria, and flatulence. Adverse experiences which occurred rarely (<1%) included ataxia, seizures, cyanosis, gastric distress, bronchospasm, pain at injection site, earache, eye irritation and rhinitis. Miscellaneous adverse experiences such as poor coordination, lethargy, muscle contractions, neuropathy, tremor, involuntary movement, syncope, aphasia, aphonia, dysarthria, amnesia, weakness and flushing of skin were observed in less than 0.5% of patients. Cases of cardiomyopathy have been observed on rare occasions in patients treated with alfa-interferons.

FOR PATIENTS WITH CHRONIC MYELOGENOUS LEUKEMIA:
For patients with chronic myelogenous leukemia, the percentage of adverse events, whether related to drug therapy or not, experienced by patients treated with rIFNα-2a is given below. Severe adverse events were observed in 66% and 31% of patients on study DM84-38 and MI400, respectively. Dose reduction and temporary cessation of therapy was required frequently. Permanent cessation of Roferon-A, due to intolerable side effects, was required in 15% and 23% of patients on studies DM84-38 and MI400, respectively.
Flu-like Symptoms—Fever (92%), asthenia or fatigue (88%), myalgia (68%), chills (63%), arthralgia/bone pain (47%) and headache (44%).
Gastrointestinal—Anorexia (48%), nausea/vomiting (37%) and diarrhea (37%).
Central and Peripheral Nervous System—Headache (44%), depression (28%), decreased mental status (16%), dizziness (11%), sleep disturbances (11%), paresthesia (8%), involuntary movements (7%) and visual disturbance (6%).
Pulmonary and Cardiovascular—Coughing (19%), dyspnea (8%) and dysrhythmia (7%).
Skin—Hair changes (including alopecia) (18%), skin rash (18%), sweating (15%), dry skin (7%) and pruritus (7%).
Uncommon adverse events (<4%) reported in clinical studies included chest pain, syncope, hypotension, impotence, alterations in taste or hearing, confusion, seizures, memory loss, disturbances of libido, bruising and coagulopathy. Miscellaneous adverse events that were rarely observed included Coombs' positive hemolytic anemia, aplastic anemia, hypothyroidism, cardiomyopathy, hypertriglyceridemia and bronchospasm.

IN OTHER INVESTIGATIONAL STUDIES OF ROFERON-A:
The following infrequent adverse events have been reported in one or more of the approved clinical indications as well as with the investigational use of Roferon-A (<5%): pancreatitis, colitis, gastrointestinal hemorrhage, stomatitis, thyroid dysfunction (including hypothyroidism and hyperthyroidism), diabetes (in some patients requiring insulin therapy), and pneumonitis (some cases responding to interferon cessation and corticosteroid therapy). In addition to the adverse experiences noted above, other adverse experiences that occurred included: abdominal fullness, hypermotility, hepatitis, gait disturbance, hallucinations, encephalopathy, psychomotor retardation, coma, stroke, transient ischemic attacks, dysphasia, sedation, apathy, irritability, hyperactivity, claustrophobia, loss of libido, congestive heart failure, myocardial infarction, Raynaud's phenomenon, hot flashes, tachypnea, ischemic retinopathy, excessive salivation and anaphylactic reactions. These adverse experiences occurred rarely (<1%).
The following events have been rarely observed (<3%) in some patients receiving Roferon-A: vasculitis, arthritis, hemolytic anemia and lupus erythematosus syndrome. The mechanism by which these events develop and their rela-

tionship to Roferon-A therapy are unclear. Similar events have been reported for other types of interferon.
ABNORMAL LABORATORY TEST VALUES: The percentage of patients with Hairy Cell Leukemia, with AIDS-related Kaposi's Sarcoma, and with Chronic Myelogenous Leukemia who experienced a severe or life-threatening abnormal laboratory test value at least once during their treatment with Roferon-A is shown in the following table:

SEVERE OR LIFE-THREATENING ABNORMAL LABORATORY TEST VALUES

	Hairy Cell Leukemia (n=218)	AIDS-related Kaposi's Sarcoma (n=241)	Chronic Myelogenous Leukemia‡ US study (n=91)	non-US study (n=219)
Leukopenia	45%*	49%	20%	3%
Neutropenia	68%*	52%	22%	0%
Thrombocytopenia	62%*	35%	27%	5%
Anemia (Hb)	31%*	27%	15%	4%
SGOT	9%	46%	5%	1%
Alk. Phosphatase	3%	11%	3%	1%
LDH	<1%	10%	NA	NA
Bilirubin	<1%	<1%	0%	0%
BUN	<1%	0%	0%	0%
Serum Creatinine	<1%	<1%	0%	0%
Proteinuria	10%†	<1%	NA	NA

* In the majority of patients, initial hematologic laboratory test values were abnormal due to their underlying disease.
† Ten percent of the patients experienced a proteinuria >1+ at least once.
‡ Patients enrolled in the two clinical studies receiving at least one dose of Roferon-A.
NA=Not Assessed

HAIRY CELL LEUKEMIA: Increases in serum phosphorus (≥1.6mmol/L) and serum uric acid (≥9.1mg/dL) were observed in 9% and 10% of patients, respectively. The increase in serum uric acid is likely to be related to the underlying disease. Decreases in serum calcium (≤1.9mmol/L) and serum phosphorus (≤0.9mmol/L) were seen in 28% and 22% of patients, respectively.
CHRONIC MYELOGENOUS LEUKEMIA: In the two clinical studies, a severe or life-threatening anemia was seen in up to 15% of patients. A severe or life-threatening leukopenia and thrombocytopenia were observed in up to 20% and 27% of patients, respectively. Changes were usually reversible when therapy was discontinued. One case of aplastic anemia and one case of Coombs' positive hemolytic anemia were seen in 310 patients treated with rIFNα-2a in clinical studies. Severe cytopenias led to discontinuation of therapy in 4% of all Roferon-A treated patients.
Transient increases in liver transaminases or alkaline phosphatase of any intensity were seen in up to 50% of patients during treatment with Roferon-A. Only 5% of patients had a severe or life-threatening increase in SGOT. In the clinical studies, such abnormalities required termination of therapy in less than 1% of patients.

DOSAGE AND ADMINISTRATION

The recommended dosages of Roferon-A differ for hairy cell leukemia, AIDS-related Kaposi's sarcoma and chronic myelogenous leukemia. See indication-specific dosages below.
Note: Parenteral drug products should be inspected visually for particulate matter and discoloration before administration, whenever solution and container permit.
HAIRY CELL LEUKEMIA: Prior to initiation of therapy, tests should be performed to quantitate peripheral blood hemoglobin, platelets, granulocytes and hairy cells and bone marrow hairy cells. These parameters should be monitored periodically (eg, monthly) during treatment to determine whether response to treatment has occurred. If a patient does not respond within 6 months, treatment should be discontinued. If a response to treatment does occur, treatment should be continued until no further improvement is observed and these laboratory parameters have been stable for about 3 months. Patients with hairy cell leukemia have been treated for up to 24 consecutive months. The optimal duration of treatment for this disease has not been determined. The induction dose of Roferon-A is 3 million IU daily for 16 to 24 weeks, administered as a subcutaneous or intramuscular injection. Subcutaneous administration is particularly suggested for, but not limited to, thrombocytopenic patients (platelet count <50,000) or for patients at risk for bleeding. The recommended maintenance dose is 3 million IU, three times per week. Dose reduction by one-half or withholding of individual doses may be needed when severe adverse reactions occur. The use of doses higher than 3 million IU is not recommended in hairy cell leukemia. The 36 million IU dosage form should not be used for the treatment of hairy cell leukemia.
AIDS-RELATED KAPOSI'S SARCOMA: Roferon-A is useful for the treatment of AIDS-related Kaposi's sarcoma in

a select group of patients. In determining whether a patient should be treated, the physician should assess the likelihood of response based on the clinical manifestations of HIV infection and the manifestations of Kaposi's sarcoma requiring treatment (see CLINICAL PHARMACOLOGY).

Indicator lesion measurements and total lesion count should be performed before initiation of therapy. These parameters should be monitored periodically (eg, monthly) during treatment to determine whether response to treatment or disease stabilization has occurred. When disease stabilization or a response to treatment occurs, treatment should continue until there is no further evidence of tumor or until discontinuation is required because of a severe opportunistic infection or adverse effects. The optimal duration of treatment for this disease has not been determined.

The recommended induction dose of Roferon-A is 36 million IU daily for 10 to 12 weeks, administered as an intramuscular or subcutaneous injection. Subcutaneous administration is particularly suggested for, but not limited to, patients who are thrombocytopenic (platelet count < 50,000) or who are at risk for bleeding. The recommended maintenance dose is 36 million IU, three times per week. If severe reactions occur, the dose should be modified (50% reduction) or therapy should be temporarily discontinued until the adverse reactions abate. An escalating schedule of 3 million IU, 9 million IU and 18 million IU each daily for 3 days followed by 36 million IU daily for the remainder of the 10- to 12-week induction period has also produced equivalent therapeutic benefit with some amelioration of the acute toxicity in some patients.

CHRONIC MYELOGENOUS LEUKEMIA: For patients with Ph-positive CML in chronic phase: Prior to initiation of therapy, a diagnosis of Philadelphia chromosome positive CML in chronic phase by the appropriate peripheral blood, bone marrow and other diagnostic testing should be made. Monitoring of hematologic parameters should be done regularly (eg, monthly). Since significant cytogenetic changes are not readily apparent until after hematologic response has occurred, and usually not until several months of therapy have elapsed, cytogenetic monitoring may be performed at less frequent intervals. Achievement of complete cytogenetic response has been observed up to 2 years following the start of Roferon-A treatment.

The recommended initial dose of Roferon-A is 9 million units daily administered as a subcutaneous or intramuscular injection. Based on clinical experience[3], short-term tolerance may be improved by gradually increasing the dose of Roferon-A over the first week of administration from 3 MIU daily for 3 days to 6 MIU daily for 3 days to the target dose of 9 MIU daily for the duration of the treatment period.

The optimal dose and duration of therapy have not yet been determined. Even though the median time to achieve a complete hematologic response was 5 months in study MI400, hematologic responses have been observed up to 18 months after treatment start. Treatment should be continued until disease progression. If severe side effects occur, a treatment interruption or a reduction in either the dose or the frequency of injections may be necessary to achieve the individual maximally tolerated dose (see PRECAUTIONS).

Limited data are available on the use of Roferon-A in children with CML. In one report of 15 children with Ph-positive, adult-type CML doses between 2.5 to 5 MIU/m^2/day given intramuscularly were tolerated.[9] In another study, severe adverse effects including deaths were noted in children with previously untreated, Ph-negative, juvenile CML, who received interferon doses of 30 MIU/m^2/day.[14]

HOW SUPPLIED

Single Use Injectable Solution:

3 million IU Roferon-A per vial— Each 1 mL contains 3 million IU of Interferon alfa-2a, recombinant, 7.21 mg sodium chloride, 0.2 mg polysorbate 80, 10 mg benzyl alcohol as a preservative and 0.77 mg ammonium acetate. Boxes of 1 (NDC 0004-2009-09).

9 million IU Roferon-A per vial—Each 0.9 mL contains 9 million IU of Interferon alfa-2a, recombinant, 6.49 mg sodium chloride, 0.18 mg polysorbate 80, 9 mg benzyl alcohol as a preservative and 0.69 mg ammonium acetate. For single dose administration, withdraw 0.9 mL using a 1 mL syringe. Also can be used as a multidose vial. Boxes of 1 (NDC 0004-2010-09).

36 million IU Roferon-A per vial —Each 1 mL contains 36 million IU of Interferon alfa-2a, recombinant, 7.21 mg sodium chloride, 0.2 mg polysorbate 80, 10 mg benzyl alcohol as a preservative and 0.77 mg ammonium acetate. This dosage form should not be used for the treatment of hairy cell leukemia. Boxes of 1 (NDC 0004-2012-09).

Multidose Injectable Solution:

9 million IU Roferon-A per vial —Each 0.3 mL contains 3 million IU of Interferon alfa-2a, recombinant, 2.16 mg sodium chloride, 0.06 mg polysorbate 80, 3 mg benzyl alcohol as a preservative and 0.23 mg ammonium acetate. Also can be used as a single use vial. Once the vial is entered, it must be used within 30 days. The 9 million IU multidose vial contains an average of 13 million IU of Interferon alfa-2a, recombinant in order to provide the delivery of three 0.3 mL doses, each containing 3 million IU of Roferon-A Interferon alfa-2a, recombinant for injection. Boxes of 1 (NDC 0004-2010-09).

18 million IU Roferon-A per vial—Each 1 mL contains 6 million IU of Interferon alfa-2a, recombinant, 7.21 mg sodium chloride, 0.2 mg polysorbate 80, 10 mg benzyl alcohol as a preservative and 0.77 mg ammonium acetate. Each 0.5 mL contains 3 million IU of Interferon alfa-2a, recombinant. Once the vial is entered, it must be used within 30 days. The 18 million IU multidose vial contains an average of 22.8 million IU of Interferon alfa-2a, recombinant in order to provide the delivery of six 0.5 mL doses, each containing 3 million IU of Roferon-A Interferon alfa-2a, recombinant for injection. Boxes of 1 (NDC 0004-2011-09).

Sterile Powder for Injection:

18 million IU Roferon-A per vial— Reconstitute with 3 mL diluent and swirl gently to dissolve. When reconstituted with accompanying Diluent for Roferon-A, each 1 mL of reconstituted solution contains 6 million IU Interferon alfa-2a, recombinant, 9 mg sodium chloride, 1.67 mg Albumin (Human) and 3.3 mg phenol as a preservative. Each 0.5 mL contains 3 million IU of Interferon alfa-2a, recombinant. Once the powder is reconstituted, it must be used within 30 days. Boxes of 1 (NDC 0004-1993-09).

Storage: The sterile powder and its accompanying diluent, the reconstituted solution and the injectable solution should be stored in the refrigerator at 36° to 46°F (2° to 8°C). Do *not* freeze or shake.

REFERENCES

1. Trown PW, et al. *Cancer.* 1986; 57 (suppl):1648-1656. 2. Itri LM, et al. *Cancer.* 1987; 59:668-674. 3. Jones GJ, Itri LM. *Cancer.* 1986; 57(suppl):1709-1715. 4. Foon KA, et al. *Blood.* 1984; 64(suppl 1):164a. 5. Quesada Jr, et al. *Cancer.* 1986; 57 (suppl):1678-1680. 6. Krown SE, et al. *N Eng J Med.* 1984; 308:1071-1076. 7. The Italian Cooperative Study Group on CML. *N Engl J Med.* 1994; 330:820-825. 8. Sokal JE et al. *Blood.* 1984; 63(4):789-799. 9. Dow LW, et al. *Cancer.* 1991; 68:1678-1684. 10. Krown SE, et al. *Proc Am Soc Clin Oncol.* 1988; 7:1. 11. Williams SJ, et al. *Lancet.* 1987; 2:939-941. 12. Jonkman JHG, et al. *Br J Clin Pharmacol.* 1989; 2(27):795-802. 13. Kauppila A, et al. *Int J Cancer.* 1982; 29:291-294. 14. Maybee D, et al. *Proc Annu Meet Am Soc Clin Oncol.* 1992; 11:A950.

Revised June 1996

ROMAZICON® ℞

[ro-măs 'ĕ-kŏn]

(flumazenil)

INJECTION

The following text is complete prescribing information based on official labeling in effect June 1996.

DESCRIPTION

ROMAZICON® (flumazenil) is a benzodiazepine receptor antagonist. Chemically, flumazenil is ethyl 8-fluoro-5,-6-dihydro-5-methyl-6-oxo-4H-imidazo [1,5-a](1,4) benzodiazepine-3-carboxylate. Flumazenil has an imidazobenzodiazepine structure and a calculated molecular weight of 303.3.

Flumazenil is a white to off-white crystalline compound with an octanol:buffer partition coefficient of 14 to 1 at pH 7.4. It is insoluble in water but slightly soluble in acidic aqueous solutions. ROMAZICON is available as a sterile parenteral dosage form for intravenous administration. Each mL contains 0.1 mg of flumazenil compounded with 1.8 mg of methylparaben, 0.2 mg of propylparaben, 0.9% sodium chloride, 0.01% edetate disodium, and 0.01% acetic acid; the pH is adjusted to approximately 4 with hydrochloric acid and/or, if necessary, sodium hydroxide.

CLINICAL PHARMACOLOGY

Flumazenil, an imidazobenzodiazepine derivative, antagonizes the actions of benzodiazepines on the central nervous system. Flumazenil competitively inhibits the activity at the benzodiazepine recognition site on the GABA/benzodiazepine receptor complex. Flumazenil is a weak partial agonist in some animal models of activity, but has little or no agonist activity in man. Flumazenil does not antagonize the central nervous system effects of drugs affecting GABA-ergic neurons by means other than the benzodiazepine receptor (including ethanol, barbiturates, or general anesthetics) and does not reverse the effects of opioids.

PHARMACODYNAMICS: Intravenous ROMAZICON has been shown to antagonize sedation, impairment of recall, psychomotor impairment and ventilatory depression produced by benzodiazepines in healthy human volunteers.

The duration and degree of reversal of benzodiazepine effects are related to the dose and plasma concentrations of flumazenil as shown in the following data from a study in normal volunteers.

[See Figure at top of next column.]

Generally, doses of approximately 0.1 to 0.2 mg (corresponding to peak plasma levels of 3 to 6 ng/mL) produce partial antagonism, whereas higher doses of 0.4 to 1 mg (peak

Magnitude and Duration of Reversal of Sedation as a Function of Flumazenil Dose*
Flumazenil doses of 0.2, 0.6 & 1 mg
(blood level in ng/mL)

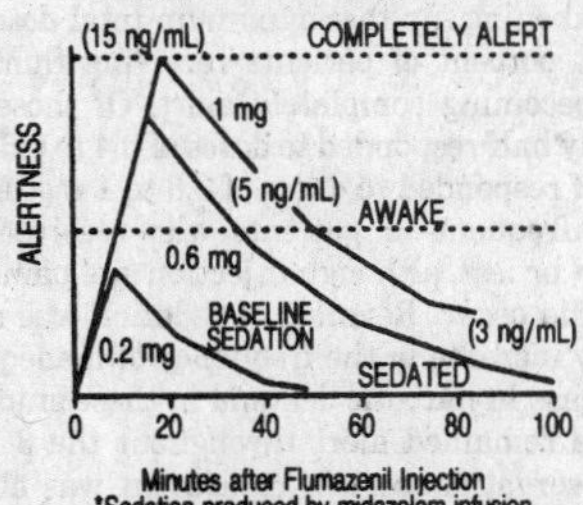

Minutes after Flumazenil Injection
*Sedation produced by midazolam infusion at a rate of 0.06–0.20 mg/kg/hr in healthy volunteers

plasma levels of 12 to 28 ng/mL) usually produce complete antagonism in patients who have received the usual sedating doses of benzodiazepines. The onset of reversal is usually evident within 1 to 2 minutes after the injection is completed. Eighty percent response will be reached within 3 minutes, with the peak effect occurring at 6 to 10 minutes. The duration and degree of reversal are related to the plasma concentration of the sedating benzodiazepine as well as the dose of ROMAZICON given.

In healthy volunteers, ROMAZICON did not alter intraocular pressure when given alone and reversed the decrease in intraocular pressure seen after administration of midazolam.

PHARMACOKINETICS: After IV administration, plasma concentrations of flumazenil follow a two compartment open pharmacokinetic model with an initial distribution half-life of 7 to 15 minutes and a terminal half-life of 41 to 79 minutes. Peak concentrations of flumazenil are proportional to dose, with an apparent initial volume of distribution of 0.5 L/kg. After redistribution the apparent volume of distribution (V_{ss}) ranges from 0.77 to 1.60L/kg. Protein binding is approximately 50% and the drug shows no preferential partitioning into red blood cells.

Flumazenil is a highly extracted drug. Clearance of flumazenil occurs primarily by hepatic metabolism and is dependent on hepatic blood flow. In pharmacokinetic studies of normal volunteers, total clearance ranges from 0.7 to 1.3 L/hr/kg, with less than 1% of the administered dose eliminated unchanged in the urine. The major metabolites of flumazenil identified in urine are the de-ethylated free acid and its glucuronide conjugate. In preclinical studies there was no evidence of pharmacologic activity exhibited by the de-ethylated free acid. Elimination of radiolabelled drug is essentially complete within 72 hours, with 90% to 95% of the radioactivity appearing in urine and 5% to 10% in the feces.

Pharmacokinetic Parameters Following a 5-minute infusion of a total of 1 mg of ROMAZICON Mean (Coefficient of variation, Range)

C_{max}(ng/mL)	24 (38%, 11–43)
AUC (ng · hr/mL)	15 (22%, 10–22)
V_{ss}(L/kg)	1 (24%, 0.8–1.6)
Cl (L/hr/kg)	1 (20%, 0.7–1.4)
Half-life (min)	54 (21%, 41–79)

The pharmacokinetics of flumazenil are not significantly affected by gender, age, renal failure (creatinine clearance < 10mL/min), or hemodialysis beginning 1 hour after drug administration. Mean total clearance is decreased to 40% to 60% of normal in patients with moderate liver dysfunction and to 25% of normal in patients with severe liver dysfunction compared with age-matched healthy subjects. This results in a prolongation of the half-life from 0.8 hours in healthy subjects to 1.3 hours in patients with moderate hepatic impairment and 2.4 hours in severely impaired patients. Ingestion of food during an intravenous infusion of the drug results in a 50% increase in clearance, most likely due to the increased hepatic blood flow that accompanies a meal. The pharmacokinetic profile of flumazenil is unaltered in the presence of benzodiazepine agonists and the kinetic profiles of those benzodiazepines are unaltered by flumazenil.

CLINICAL TRIALS

ROMAZICON has been administered to reverse the effects of benzodiazepines in conscious sedation, general anesthesia, and the management of suspected benzodiazepine overdose.

CONSCIOUS SEDATION: ROMAZICON was studied in four trials in 970 patients who received an average of 30 mg diazepam or 10 mg midazolam for sedation (with or without a narcotic) in conjunction with both inpatient and outpatient diagnostic or surgical procedures. ROMAZICON was effective in reversing the sedating and psychomotor effects of the benzodiazepine, however, amnesia was less completely and less consistently reversed. In these studies, ROMAZICON

Continued on next page

Roche Laboratories—Cont.

was administered as an initial dose of 0.4 mg I.V. (two doses of 0.2 mg) with additional 0.2 mg doses as needed to achieve complete awakening, up to a maximum total dose of 1 mg. Seventy-eight percent of patients receiving flumazenil responded by becoming completely alert. Of those patients, approximately half responded to doses of 0.4 to 0.6 mg, while the other half responded to doses of 0.8 to 1 mg. Adverse effects were infrequent in patients who received 1 mg of ROMAZICON or less, although injection site pain, agitation and anxiety did occur. Reversal of sedation was not associated with any increase in the frequency of inadequate analgesia or increase in narcotic demand in these studies. While most patients remained alert throughout the 3 hour post-procedure observation period, resedation was observed to occur in 3% to 9% of the patients, and was most common in patients who had received high doses of benzodiazepine. (See PRECAUTIONS.)

GENERAL ANESTHESIA: ROMAZICON was studied in four trials in 644 patients who received midazolam as an induction and/or maintenance agent in both balanced and inhalational anesthesia. Midazolam was generally administered in doses ranging from 5 to 80 mg, alone and/or in conjunction with muscle relaxants, nitrous oxide, regional or local anaesthetics, narcotics and/or inhalational anesthetics. Flumazenil was given as an initial dose of 0.2 mg IV, with additional 0.2 mg doses as needed to reach a complete response, up to a maximum total dose of 1 mg. These doses were effective in reversing sedation and restoring psychomotor function, but did not completely restore memory as tested by picture recall. ROMAZICON was not as effective in the reversal of sedation in patients who had received multiple anesthetic agents in addition to benzodiazepines.

Eighty-one percent of patients sedated with midazolam responded to flumazenil by becoming completely alert or just slightly drowsy. Of those patients, 36% responded to doses of 0.4 to 0.6 mg, while 64% responded to doses of 0.8 to 1 mg.

Resedation in patients who responded to ROMAZICON occurred in 10% to 15% of patients studied and was more common with larger doses of midazolam (> 20 mg), long procedures (> 60 minutes) and use of neuromuscular blocking agents. (See PRECAUTIONS.)

MANAGEMENT OF SUSPECTED BENZODIAZEPINE OVERDOSE: ROMAZICON was studied in two trials in 497 patients who were presumed to have taken an overdose of a benzodiazepine, either alone or in combination with a variety of other agents. In these trials, 299 patients were proven to have taken a benzodiazepine as part of the overdose, and 80% of the 148 who received ROMAZICON responded by an improvement in level of consciousness. Of the patients who responded to flumazenil, 75% responded to a total dose of 1 to 3 mg.

Reversal of sedation was associated with an increased frequency of symptoms of CNS excitation. Of the patients treated with flumazenil, 1% to 3% were treated for agitation or anxiety. Serious side effects were uncommon, but six seizures were observed in 446 patients treated with flumazenil in these studies. Four of these 6 patients had ingested a large dose of cyclic antidepressants, which increased the risk of seizures. (See WARNINGS.)

INDIVIDUALIZATION OF DOSAGE

GENERAL PRINCIPLES: The serious adverse effects of ROMAZICON are related to the reversal of benzodiazepine effects. Using more than the minimally effective dose of ROMAZICON is tolerated by most patients but may complicate the management of patients who are physically dependent on benzodiazepines or patients who are depending on benzodiazepines for therapeutic effect (such as suppression of seizures in cyclic antidepressant overdose).

In high-risk patients, it is important to administer the smallest amount of ROMAZICON that is effective. The 1-minute wait between individual doses in the dose-titration recommended for general clinical populations may be too short for high-risk patients. This is because it takes 6 to 10 minutes for any single dose of flumazenil to reach full effects. Practitioners should slow the rate of administration of ROMAZICON administered to high-risk patients as recommended below.

ANESTHESIA AND CONSCIOUS SEDATION: ROMAZICON is well tolerated at the recommended doses in individuals who have no tolerance to (or dependence on) benzodiazepines. The recommended dosages and titration rates in anesthesia and conscious sedation (0.2 to 1 mg given at 0.2 mg/min) are well tolerated in patients receiving the drug for reversal of a single benzodiazepine exposure in most clinical settings (see Adverse Events). The major risk will be resedation because the duration of effect of a long-acting (or large dose of a short-acting) benzodiazepine may exceed that of ROMAZICON. Resedation may be treated by giving a repeat dose at no less than 20-minute intervals. For repeat treatment, no more than 1 mg (at 0.2 mg/min doses) should be given at any one time and no more than 3 mg should be given in any one hour.

OVERDOSE PATIENTS: The risk of confusion, agitation, emotional lability and perceptual distortion with the doses recommended in patients with benzodiazepine overdose (3 to 5 mg administered as 0.5 mg/min) may be greater than that expected with lower doses and slower administration. The recommended doses represent a compromise between a desirable slow awakening and the need for prompt response and a persistent effect in the overdose situation. If circumstances permit, the physician may elect to use the 0.2 mg/minute titration rate to slowly awaken the patient over 5 to 10 minutes, which may help to reduce signs and symptoms on emergence.

ROMAZICON has no effect in cases where benzodiazepines are not responsible for sedation. Once doses of 3 to 5 mg have been reached without clinical response, additional ROMAZICON is likely to have no effect.

PATIENTS TOLERANT TO BENZODIAZEPINES: ROMAZICON may cause benzodiazepine withdrawal symptoms in individuals who have been taking benzodiazepines long enough to have some degree of tolerance. Patients who had been taking benzodiazepines prior to entry into the ROMAZICON trials who were given flumazenil in doses over 1 mg experienced withdrawal-like events 2 to 5 times more frequently than patients who received less than 1 mg.

In patients who may have tolerance to benzodiazepines, as indicated by clinical history or by the need for larger than usual doses of benzodiazepine, slower titration rates of 0.1 mg/min and lower total doses may help reduce the frequency of emergent confusion and agitation. In such cases special care must be taken to monitor the patients for resedation because of the lower doses of ROMAZICON used.

PATIENTS PHYSICALLY DEPENDENT ON BENZODIAZEPINES: ROMAZICON is known to precipitate withdrawal seizures in patients who are physically dependent on benzodiazepines, even if such dependence was established in a relatively few days of high dose sedation in Intensive Care Unit environments. The risk of either seizures or resedation in such cases is high and patients have experienced seizures before regaining consciousness. ROMAZICON should be used in such settings with extreme caution, since the use of flumazenil in this situation has not been studied and no information as to dose and rate of titration is available. ROMAZICON should be used in such patients only if the potential benefits of using the drug outweigh the risks of precipitated seizures. Physicians are directed to the scientific literature for the most current information in this area.

INDICATIONS AND USAGE

ROMAZICON is indicated for the complete or partial reversal of the sedative effects of benzodiazepines in cases where general anesthesia has been induced and/or maintained with benzodiazepines, where sedation has been produced with benzodiazepines for diagnostic and therapeutic procedures, and for the management of benzodiazepine overdose.

CONTRAINDICATIONS

ROMAZICON is contraindicated:

- in patients with a known hypersensitivity to flumazenil or to benzodiazepines.
- in patients who have been given a benzodiazepine for control of a potentially life-threatening condition (*e.g.* control of intracranial pressure or status epilepticus).
- in patients who are showing signs of serious cyclic antidepressant overdose. (See WARNINGS.)

WARNINGS

THE USE OF ROMAZICON HAS BEEN ASSOCIATED WITH THE OCCURRENCE OF SEIZURES.

THESE ARE MOST FREQUENT IN PATIENTS WHO HAVE BEEN ON BENZODIAZEPINES FOR LONG-TERM SEDATION OR IN OVERDOSE CASES WHERE PATIENTS ARE SHOWING SIGNS OF SERIOUS CYCLIC ANTIDEPRESSANT OVERDOSE.

PRACTITIONERS SHOULD INDIVIDUALIZE THE DOSAGE OF ROMAZICON AND BE PREPARED TO MANAGE SEIZURES.

Risk of Seizures: The reversal of benzodiazepine effects may be associated with the onset of seizures in certain high-risk populations. Possible risk factors for seizures include: concurrent major sedative-hypnotic drug withdrawal, recent therapy with repeated doses of parenteral benzodiazepines, myoclonic jerking or seizure activity prior to flumazenil administration in overdose cases, or concurrent cyclic anti-depressant poisoning.

ROMAZICON is not recommended in cases of serious cyclic antidepressant poisoning, as manifested by motor abnormalities (twitching, rigidity, focal seizure), dysrhythmia (wide QRS, ventricular dysrhythmia, heart block), anticholinergic signs (mydriasis, dry mucosa, hypo-peristalsis), and cardiovascular collapse at presentation. In such cases ROMAZICON should be withheld and the patient should be allowed to remain sedated (with ventilatory and circulatory support as needed) until the signs of antidepressant toxicity have subsided. Treatment with ROMAZICON has no known benefit to the seriously ill mixed-overdose patient other than reversing sedation and should not be used in cases where seizures (from any cause) are likely.

Most convulsions associated with flumazenil administration require treatment and have been successfully managed with benzodiazepines, phenytoin or barbiturates. Because of the presence of flumazenil, higher than usual doses of benzodiazepines may be required.

HYPOVENTILATION: Patients who have received ROMAZICON for the reversal of benzodiazepine effects (after conscious sedation or general anesthesia) should be monitored for resedation, respiratory depression, or other residual benzodiazepine effects for an appropriate period (up to 120 minutes) based on the dose and duration of effect of the benzodiazepine employed.

This is because ROMAZICON has not been established in patients as an effective treatment for hypoventilation due to benzodiazepine administration. In healthy male volunteers, ROMAZICON is capable of reversing benzodiazepine-induced depression of the ventilatory responses to hypercapnia and hypoxia after a benzodiazepine alone. However, such depression may recur because the ventilatory effects of typical doses of ROMAZICON (1 mg or less) may wear off before the effects of many benzodiazepines. The effects of ROMAZICON on ventilatory response following sedation with a benzodiazepine in combination with an opioid are inconsistent and have not been adequately studied. The availability of flumazenil does not diminish the need for prompt detection of hypoventilation and the ability to effectively intervene by establishing an airway and assisting ventilation.

Overdose cases should always be monitored for resedation until the patients are stable and resedation in unlikely.

PRECAUTIONS

RETURN OF SEDATION: ROMAZICON may be expected to improve the alertness of patients recovering from a procedure involving sedation or anesthesia with benzodiazepines, but should not be substituted for an adequate period of post-procedure monitoring. The availability of ROMAZICON does not reduce the risks associated with the use of large doses of benzodiazepines for sedation.

Patients should be monitored for resedation, respiratory depression (See WARNINGS), or other persistent or recurrent agonist effects for an adequate period of time after administration of ROMAZICON.

Resedation is least likely in cases where ROMAZICON is administered to reverse a low dose of a short-acting benzodiazepine (< 10 mg midazolam). It is most likely in cases where a large single or cumulative dose of a benzodiazepine has been given in the course of a long procedure along with neuromuscular blocking agents and multiple anesthetic agents.

Profound resedation was observed in 1% to 3% of patients in the clinical studies. In clinical situations where resedation must be prevented, physicians may wish to repeat the initial dose (up to 1 mg of ROMAZICON given at 0.2 mg/min) at 30 minutes and possibly again at 60 minutes. This dosage schedule, although not studied in clinical trials, was effective in preventing resedation in a pharmacologic study in normal volunteers.

USE IN THE ICU: ROMAZICON should be used with caution in the Intensive Care Unit because of the increased risk of unrecognized benzodiazepine dependence in such settings. ROMAZICON may produce convulsions in patients physically dependent on benzodiazepines. (See INDIVIDUALIZATION OF DOSAGE AND WARNINGS.)

Administration of ROMAZICON to diagnose benzodiazepine-induced sedation in the Intensive Care Unit is not recommended due to the risk of adverse events as described above. In addition, the prognostic significance of a patient's failure to respond to flumazenil in cases confounded by metabolic disorder, traumatic injury, drugs other than benzodiazepines, or any other reasons not associated with benzodiazepine receptor occupancy is not known.

USE IN OVERDOSE: ROMAZICON is intended as an adjunct to, not as a substitute for, proper management of airway, assisted breathing, circulatory access and support, internal decontamination by lavage and charcoal, and adequate clinical evaluation.

Necessary measures should be instituted to secure airway, ventilation and intravenous access prior to administering flumazenil. Upon arousal patients may attempt to withdraw endotracheal tubes and/or intravenous lines as the result of confusion and agitation following awakening.

HEAD INJURY: ROMAZICON should be used with caution in patients with head injury as it may be capable of precipitating convulsions or altering cerebral blood flow in patients receiving benzodiazepines. It should be used only by practitioners prepared to manage such complications should they occur.

USE WITH NEUROMUSCULAR BLOCKING AGENTS: ROMAZICON should not be used until the effects of neuromuscular blockade have been fully reversed.

USE IN PSYCHIATRIC PATIENTS: ROMAZICON has been reported to provoke panic attacks in patients with a history of panic disorder.

PAIN ON INJECTION: To minimize the likelihood of pain or inflammation at the injection site, ROMAZICON should be administered through a freely flowing intravenous infusion into a large vein. Local irritation may occur following extravasation into perivascular tissues.

USE IN RESPIRATORY DISEASE: The primary treatment of patients with serious lung disease who experience serious respiratory depression due to benzodiazepines should be appropriate ventilatory support (See PRECAUTIONS) rather than the administration of ROMAZICON. Flumazenil is capable of partially reversing benzodiazepine-induced alterations in ventilatory drive in healthy volunteers, but has not been shown to be clinically effective.

USE IN CARDIOVASCULAR DISEASE: ROMAZICON did not increase the work of the heart when used to reverse benzodiazepines in cardiac patients when given at a rate of 0.1 mg/min in total doses of less than 0.5 mg in studies reported in the clinical literature. Flumazenil alone had no significant effects on cardiovascular parameters when administered to patients with stable ischemic heart disease.

USE IN LIVER DISEASE: The clearance of ROMAZICON is reduced to 40% to 60% of normal in patients with mild to moderate hepatic disease and to 25% of normal in patients with severe hepatic dysfunction. (See PHARMACOKINETICS.) While the dose of flumazenil used for initial reversal of benzodiazepine effects is not affected, repeat doses of the drug in liver disease should be reduced in size or frequency.

USE IN DRUG AND ALCOHOL DEPENDENT PATIENTS: ROMAZICON should be used with caution in patients with alcoholism and other drug dependencies due to the increased frequency of benzodiazepine tolerance and dependence observed in these patient populations. ROMAZICON is not recommended either as a treatment for benzodiazepine dependence or for the management of protracted benzodiazepine abstinence syndromes, as such use has not been studied.

The administration of flumazenil can precipitate benzodiazepine withdrawal in animals and man. This has been seen in healthy volunteers treated with therapeutic doses of oral lorazepam for up to 2 weeks who exhibited effects such as hot flushes, agitation and tremor when treated with cumulative doses of up to 3 mg doses of flumazenil.

Similar adverse experiences suggestive of flumazenil precipitation of benzodiazepine withdrawal have occurred in some patients in clinical trials. Such patients had a short-lived syndrome characterized by dizziness, mild confusion, emotional lability, agitation (with signs and symptoms of anxiety), and mild sensory distortions. This response was dose-related, most common at doses above 1 mg, rarely required treatment other than reassurance and was usually short lived. When required (5 to 10 cases), these patients were successfully treated with usual doses of a barbiturate, a benzodiazepine, or other sedative drug.

Practitioners should assume that flumazenil administration may trigger dose-dependent withdrawal syndromes in patients with established physical dependence on benzodiazepines and may complicate the management of withdrawal syndromes for alcohol, barbiturates and cross-tolerant sedatives.

DRUG INTERACTIONS

Interaction with central nervous system depressants other than benzodiazepines has not been specifically studied; however, no deleterious interactions were seen when ROMAZICON was administered after narcotics, inhalational anesthetics, muscle relaxants and muscle relaxant antagonists administered in conjunction with sedation or anesthesia.

Particular caution is necessary when using ROMAZICON in cases of mixed drug overdosage since the toxic effects (such as convulsions and cardiac dysrhythmias) of other drugs taken in overdose (especially cyclic antidepressants) may emerge with the reversal of the benzodiazepine effect by flumazenil. (See WARNINGS.)

The pharmacokinetics of benzodiazepines are unaltered in the presence of flumazenil.

USE IN AMBULATORY PATIENTS: The effects of ROMAZICON may wear off before a long-acting benzodiazepine is completely cleared from the body. In general, if a patient shows no signs of sedation within 2 hours after a 1 mg dose of flumazenil, serious resedation at a later time is unlikely. An adequate period of observation must be provided for any patient in whom either long-acting benzodiazepines (such as diazepam) or large doses of short-acting benzodiazepines (such as >10 mg of midazolam) have been used. (See INDIVIDUALIZATION OF DOSAGE.)

Because of the increased risk of adverse reactions in patients who have been taking benzodiazepines on a regular basis, it is particularly important that physicians query carefully about benzodiazepine, alcohol and sedative use as part of the history prior to any procedure in which the use of ROMAZICON is planned. (See DRUG AND ALCOHOL DEPENDENT PATIENTS.)

INFORMATION FOR PATIENTS: ROMAZICON does not consistently reverse amnesia. Patients cannot be expected to remember information told to them in the post-procedure period and instructions given to patients should be reinforced in writing or given to a responsible family member. Physicians are advised to discuss with their patients, both before surgery and at discharge, that although the patient may feel alert at the time of discharge, the effects of the benzodiazepine may recur. As a result, the patient should be instructed, preferably in writing, that their memory and judgment may be impaired and specifically advised:

1. Not to engage in any activities requiring complete alertness, and not to operate hazardous machinery or a motor vehicle until at least 18 to 24 hours after discharge, and it is certain no residual sedative effects of the benzodiazepine remain.
2. Not to take any alcohol or non-prescription drugs for 18 to 24 hours after flumazenil administration or if the effects of the benzodiazepine persist.

LABORATORY TESTS: No specific laboratory tests are recommended to follow the patient's response or to identify possible adverse reactions.

DRUG/LABORATORY TEST INTERACTIONS: The possible interaction of flumazenil with commonly used laboratory tests has not been evaluated.

CARCINOGENESIS, MUTAGENESIS, IMPAIRMENT OF FERTILITY: Carcinogenesis: No studies in animals to evaluate the carcinogenic potential of flumazenil have been conducted.

Mutagenesis: No evidence for mutagenicity was noted in the Ames test using five different tester strains. Assays for mutagenic potential in *S. cerevisiae* D7 and in Chinese hamster cells were considered to be negative as were blastogenesis assays *in vitro* in peripheral human lymphocytes and *in vivo* in a mouse micronucleus assay. Flumazenil caused a slight increase in unscheduled DNA synthesis in rat hepatocyte culture at concentrations which were also cytotoxic; no increase in DNA repair was observed in male mouse germ cells in an *in vivo* DNA repair assay.

Impairment of fertility: A reproduction study in male and female rats did not show any impairment of fertility at oral dosages of 125 mg/kg/day. From the available data on the area under the curve (AUC) in animals and man the dose represented 120 × the human exposure from a maximum recommended intravenous dose of 5 mg.

PREGNANCY: CATEGORY C. There are no adequate and well-controlled studies of the use of flumazenil in pregnant women. Flumazenil should be used during pregnancy only if the potential benefit justifies the potential risk to the fetus.

Teratogenic Effects: Flumazenil has been studied for teratogenicity in rats and rabbits following oral treatments of up to 150 mg/kg/day. The treatments during the major organogenesis were on days 6 to 15 of gestation in the rat and days 6 to 18 of gestation in the rabbit. No teratogenic effects were observed in rats or rabbits at 150 mg/kg; the dose, based on the available data on the area under the plasma concentration-time curve (AUC) represented 120 × to 600 × the human exposure from a maximum recommended intravenous dose of 5 mg in humans. In rabbits, embryocidal effects (as evidenced by increased pre-implantation and post-implantation losses) were observed at 50 mg/kg or 200 × the human exposure from a maximum recommended intravenous dose of 5 mg. The no-effect dose of 15 mg/kg in rabbits represents 60 × the human exposure.

Nonteratogenic Effects: An animal reproduction study was conducted in rats at oral dosages of 5, 25 and 125 mg/kg/day of flumazenil. Pup survival was decreased during the lactating period, pup liver weight at weaning was increased for the high-dose group (125 mg/kg/day) and incisor eruption and ear opening in the offspring were delayed; the delay in ear opening was associated with a delay in the appearance of the auditory startle response. No treatment-related adverse effects were noted for the other dose groups. Based on the available data from AUC, the effect level (125 mg/kg), represents 120 × the human exposure from 5 mg, the maximum recommended intravenous dose in humans. The no-effect level represents 24 × the human exposure from an intravenous dose of 5 mg.

LABOR AND DELIVERY: The use of ROMAZICON to reverse the effects of benzodiazepines used during labor and delivery is not recommended because the effects of the drug in the newborn are unknown.

NURSING MOTHERS: Caution should be exercised when deciding to administer ROMAZICON to a nursing woman because it is not known whether flumazenil is excreted in human milk.

PEDIATRIC USE: ROMAZICON is not recommended for use in children (either for the reversal of sedation, the management of overdose or the resuscitation of the newborn), as no clinical studies have been performed to determine the risks, benefits and dosages to be used.

GERIATRIC USE: The pharmacokinetics of flumazenil have been studied in the elderly and are not significantly different from younger patients. Several studies of ROMAZICON in patients over the age of 65 and one study in patients over the age of 80 suggest that while the doses of benzodiazepine used to induce sedation should be reduced, ordinary doses of ROMAZICON may be used for reversal.

ADVERSE REACTIONS

SERIOUS ADVERSE REACTIONS: Deaths have occurred in patients who received ROMAZICON in a variety of clinical settings. The majority of deaths occurred in patients with serious underlying disease or in patients who had ingested large amounts of non-benzodiazepine drugs, (usually cyclic antidepressants) as part of an overdose.

Serious adverse events have occurred in all clinical settings, and convulsions are the most common serious adverse event reported. ROMAZICON administration has been associated with the onset of convulsions in patients who are relying on benzodiazepine effects to control seizures, are physically dependent on benzodiazepines, or who have ingested large doses of other drugs. (See WARNINGS.)

Two of the 446 patients who received ROMAZICON in controlled clinical trials for the management of a benzodiazepine overdosage had cardiac dysrhythmias (1 ventricular tachycardia, 1 junctional tachycardia).

ADVERSE EVENTS IN CLINICAL STUDIES: The following adverse reactions were considered to be related to ROMAZICON administration (both alone and for the reversal of benzodiazepine effects) and were reported in studies involving 1875 individuals who received flumazenil in controlled trials. Adverse events most frequently associated with flumazenil alone were limited to dizziness, injection site pain, increased sweating, headache and abnormal or blurred vision (3% to 9%).

BODY AS A WHOLE: Fatigue (asthenia, malaise), Headache, Injection Site Pain*, Injection Site Reaction (thrombophlebitis, skin abnormality, rash)

CARDIOVASCULAR SYSTEM: Cutaneous vasodilation (sweating, flushing, hot flushes)

DIGESTIVE SYSTEM: Nausea and Vomiting (11%)

NERVOUS SYSTEM: Agitation (anxiety, nervousness, dry mouth, tremor, palpitations, insomnia, dyspnea, hyperventilation)*, Dizziness (vertigo, ataxia) (10%), Emotional lability (crying abnormal, depersonalization, euphoria, increased tears, depression, dysphoria, paranoia).

SPECIAL SENSES: Abnormal Vision (visual field defect, diplopia), Paresthesia (sensation abnormal, hypoesthesia)

All adverse reactions occurred in 1% to 3% of cases unless otherwise marked.
*indicates reaction in 3% to 9% of cases.
Observed percentage reported if greater than 9%.

The following adverse events were observed infrequently (less than 1%) in the clinical studies, but were judged as probably related to ROMAZICON administration and/or reversal of benzodiazepine effects:

NERVOUS SYSTEM: Confusion (difficulty concentrating, delirium), Convulsions (See WARNINGS), Somnolence (stupor)

SPECIAL SENSES: Abnormal Hearing (transient hearing impairment, hyperacusis, tinnitus).

The following adverse events occurred with frequencies less than 1% in the clinical trials. Their relationship to ROMAZICON administration is unknown, but they are included as alerting information for the physician.

BODY AS A WHOLE: Rigors, shivering.

CARDIOVASCULAR: Arrythmia (atrial, nodal, ventricular extrasystoles), bradycardia, tachycardia, hypertension, chest pain.

DIGESTIVE SYSTEM: Hiccup.

NERVOUS SYSTEM: Speech disorder (dysphonia, thick tongue).

Not included in this list is operative site pain that occurred with the same frequency in patients receiving placebo as in patients receiving flumazenil for reversal of sedation following a surgical procedure.

DRUG ABUSE AND DEPENDENCE

ROMAZICON acts as a benzodiazepine antagonist, blocks the effects of benzodiazepines in animals and man, antagonizes benzodiazepine reinforcement in animal models, produces dysphoria in normal subjects, and has had no reported abuse in foreign marketing. Although ROMAZICON has a benzodiazepine-like structure it does not act as a benzodiazepine agonist in man and is not a controlled substance.

OVERDOSAGE

Large intravenous doses of ROMAZICON, when administered to healthy normal volunteers in the absence of a benzodiazepine agonist, produced no serious adverse reactions, severe signs or symptoms, or clinically significant laboratory test abnormalities. In clinical studies, most adverse reactions to flumazenil were an extension of the pharmacologic effects of the drug in reversing benzodiazepine effects.

Reversal with an excessively high dose of ROMAZICON may produce anxiety, agitation, increased muscle tone, hyperesthesia and possibly convulsions. Convulsions have been

Continued on next page

Roche Laboratories—Cont.

treated with barbiturates, benzodiazepines and phenytoin, generally with prompt resolution of the seizures. (See WARNINGS.)

DOSE AND ADMINISTRATION

ROMAZICON is recommended for intravenous use only. It is compatible with 5% dextrose in water, lactated Ringer's and normal saline solutions. If ROMAZICON is drawn into a syringe or mixed with any of these solutions, it should be discarded after 24 hours. For optimum sterility, ROMAZICON should remain in the vial until just before use. As with all parenteral drug products, ROMAZICON should be inspected visually for particulate matter and discoloration prior to administration, whenever solution and container permit.

To minimize the likelihood of pain at the injection site, ROMAZICON should be administered through a freely running intravenous infusion into a large vein.

REVERSAL OF CONSCIOUS SEDATION OR IN GENERAL ANESTHESIA: For the reversal of the sedative effects of benzodiazepines administered for conscious sedation or general anesthesia, the recommended initial dose of ROMAZICON is 0.2 mg (2 mL) administered intravenously over 15 seconds. If the desired level of consciousness is not obtained after waiting an additional 45 seconds, a further dose of 0.2 mg (2 mL) can be injected and repeated at 60-second intervals where necessary (up to a maximum of 4 additional times) to a maximum total dose of 1 mg (10 mL). The dose should be individualized based on the patient's response, with most patients responding to doses of 0.6 to 1 mg. (See INDIVIDUALIZATION OF DOSAGE.)

In the event of resedation, repeated doses may be administered at 20 minute intervals as needed. For repeat treatment, no more than 1 mg (given as 0.2 mg/min) should be administered at any one time, and no more than 3 mg should be given in any one hour.

It is recommended that ROMAZICON be administered as the series of small injections described (not as a single bolus injection) to allow the practitioner to control the reversal of sedation to the approximate endpoint desired and to minimize the possibility of adverse effects. (See INDIVIDUALIZATION OF DOSAGE.)

MANAGEMENT OF SUSPECTED BENZODIAZEPINE OVERDOSE: For initial management of a known or suspected benzodiazepine overdose, the recommended initial dose of ROMAZICON is 0.2 mg (2 mL) administered intravenously over 30 seconds. If the desired level of consciousness is not obtained after waiting 30 seconds, a further dose of 0.3 mg (3 mL) can be administered over another 30 seconds. Further doses of 0.5 mg (5 mL) can be administered over 30 seconds at 1-minute intervals up to a cumulative dose of 3 mg. Do not rush the administration of ROMAZICON. Patients should have a secure airway and intravenous access before administration of the drug and be awakened gradually. (See PRECAUTIONS.)

Most patients with benzodiazepine overdose will respond to a cumulative dose of 1–3 mg of ROMAZICON, and doses beyond 3 mg do not reliably produce additional effects. On rare occasions, patients with a partial response at 3 mg may require additional titration up to a total dose of 5 mg (administered slowly in the same manner).

If a patient has not responded 5 minutes after receiving a cumulative dose of 5 mg ROMAZICON, the major cause of sedation is likely not to be due to benzodiazepines, and additional ROMAZICON is likely to have no effect.

In the event of resedation, repeated doses may be given at 20-minute intervals if needed. For repeat treatment, no more than 1 mg (given as 0.5 mg/min) should be given at any one time and no more than 3 mg should be given in any one hour.

SAFETY AND HANDLING: ROMAZICON is supplied in sealed dosage forms and poses no known risk to the health care provider. Routine care should be taken to avoid aerosol generation when preparing syringes for injection, and spilled medication should be rinsed from the skin with cool water.

HOW SUPPLIED

5 mL multiple-use vials containing 0.1 mg/mL flumazenil: Boxes of 10 (NDC 0004-6911-06).

10 mL multiple-use vials containing 0.1 mg/mL flumazenil: Boxes of 10 (NDC 0004-6912-06).

Store at 59° to 86°F (15° to 30°C).

Revised: October 1994

SYNALAR®
(fluocinolone acetonide)
Cream 0.025%
Topical Solution 0.01%

Refer to entry under LIDEX® (fluocinonide) Cream 0.05%.

TEGISON® ℞
[*teg'is-on*]
etretinate
CAPSULES

The following text is complete prescribing information based on official labeling in effect June 1996.

CONTRAINDICATION

Tegison must not be used by females who are pregnant, who intend to become pregnant, or who are unreliable or may not use reliable contraception while undergoing treatment. The period of time during which pregnancy must be avoided after treatment is concluded has not been determined. Tegison blood levels of 0.5 to 12 ng/mL have been reported in 5 of 47 patients in the range of 2.1 to 2.9 years after treatment was concluded. The length of time necessary to wait after discontinuation of treatment to assure that no drug will be detectable in the blood has not been determined. The significance of undetectable blood levels relative to the risk of teratogenicity is unknown.

Major human fetal abnormalities related to Tegison administration have been reported, including meningomyelocoele, meningoencephalocoele, multiple synostoses, facial dysmorphia, syndactylies, absence of terminal phalanges, malformations of hip, ankle and forearm, low set ears, high palate, decreased cranial volume, and alterations of the skull and cervical vertebrae on x-ray.

Women of childbearing potential must not be given Tegison until pregnancy is excluded. It is strongly recommended that a pregnancy test be performed within 2 weeks prior to initiating Tegison therapy. Tegison therapy should start on the second or third day of the next normal menstrual period. An effective form of contraception must be used for at least 1 month before Tegison therapy, during therapy and following discontinuation of Tegison therapy for an indefinite period of time.

Females should be fully counseled on the serious risks to the fetus should they become pregnant while undergoing treatment or after discontinuation of therapy. If pregnancy does occur, the physician and patient should discuss the desirability of continuing the pregnancy.

DESCRIPTION

Tegison (etretinate), a retinoid, is available in 10-mg and 25-mg gelatin capsules for oral administration. Each capsule also contains corn starch, lactose and talc. Gelatin capsule shells contain parabens (methyl and propyl) and potassium sorbate, with the following dye systems: 10 mg—iron oxide (yellow, black and red); FD&C Blue No. 2 and titanium dioxide; 25 mg—iron oxide (yellow, black and red) and titanium dioxide.

Chemically, etretinate is ethyl (*all-E*)-9-(4-methoxy-2,3,6-trimethylphenyl)-3,7-dimethyl-2,4,6,8-nonatetraenoate and is related to both retinoic acid and retinol (vitamin A). It is a greenish-yellow to yellow powder with a calculated molecular weight of 354.5.

CLINICAL PHARMACOLOGY

The mechanism of action of Tegison is unknown.

Clinical: Improvement in psoriatic patients occurs in association with a decrease in scale, erythema and thickness of lesions, as well as histological evidence of normalization of epidermal differentiation, decreased stratum corneum thickness and decreased inflammation in the epidermis and dermis.

Pharmacokinetics: The pharmacokinetic profile of etretinate is predictable and is linear following single and multiple doses. Etretinate is extensively metabolized following oral dosing, with significant first-pass metabolism to the acid form, which also has the all-*trans* structure and is pharmacologically active. Subsequent metabolism results in the 13-*cis* acid form, chain-shortened breakdown products and conjugates that are ultimately excreted in the bile and urine.

After a 6-month course of therapy with doses ranging from 25 mg once daily to 25 mg four times daily, Cmax values ranged from 102 to 389 ng/mL and occurred at Tmax values of 2 to 6 hours. In one study the apparent terminal half-life after six months of therapy was approximately 120 days. In another study of 47 patients treated chronically with etretinate, 5 had detectable serum drug levels (in the range of 0.5 to 12 ng/mL) 2.1 to 2.9 years after therapy was discontinued. The long half-life appears to be due to storage of etretinate in adipose tissue.

Etretinate is more than 99% bound to plasma proteins, predominantly lipoproteins, whereas its active metabolite, the all-*trans* acid form, is predominantly bound to albumin. Concentrations of etretinate in blister fluid after 6 weeks of dosing were approximately one-tenth of those observed in plasma. Concentrations of etretinate and its all-*trans* acid metabolite in epidermal specimens obtained after 1 to 36 months of therapy were a function of location; subcutis > > serum > epidermis > dermis. Similarly, liver concentrations of etretinate in patients receiving therapy for 6 months were generally higher than concomitant plasma concentrations and tended to be higher in livers with a higher degree of fatty infiltration.

Studies in normal volunteers indicated that, when compared with the fasting state, the absorption of etretinate was increased by whole milk or a high-lipid diet.

INDICATIONS AND USAGE

Tegison is indicated for the treatment of severe recalcitrant psoriasis, including the erythrodermic and generalized pustular types. Because of significant adverse effects associated with its use, Tegison should be prescribed only by physicians knowledgeable in the systemic use of retinoids and reserved for patients with severe recalcitrant psoriasis who are unresponsive to or intolerant of standard therapies: topical tar plus UVB light; psoralens plus UVA light; systemic corticosteroids; and methotrexate.

The use of Tegison resulted in clinical improvement in the majority of patients treated. Complete clearing of the disease was observed after 4 to 9 months of therapy in 13% of all patients treated for severe psoriasis. This included complete clearing in 16% of patients with erythrodermic psoriasis and 37% of patients with generalized pustular psoriasis.

After discontinuation of Tegison the majority of patients experience some degree of relapse by the end of two months.

TABLE I
ADVERSE EVENTS FREQUENTLY REPORTED DURING CLINICAL TRIALS
PERCENT OF PATIENTS REPORTING

BODY SYSTEM	>75%	50%–75%	25%–50%	10%–25%
Mucocutaneous	Dry nose Chapped lips	Excessive thirst Sore mouth	Nosebleed	Cheilitis Sore tongue
Dermatologic	Loss of hair Palm/sole/ fingertip peeling	Dry skin Itching Rash Red scaly face Skin fragility	Bruising Sunburn	Nail disorder Skin peeling
Musculoskeletal	Hyperostosis*	Bone/joint pain	Muscle cramps	
Central Nervous		Fatigue	Headache	Fever
Special Senses		Irritation of eyes	Eyeball pain Eyelid abnormalities	Abnormalities of: —conjunctiva —cornea —lens —retina Conjunctivitis Decrease in visual acuity Double vision
Gastrointestinal			Abdominal pain Changes in appetite	Nausea

*In a retrospective study of 45 patients, 38 of whom received long-term etretinate therapy, 32 (84%) had radiographic evidence of hyperostosis. See WARNINGS.

After relapse, subsequent 4- to 9-month courses of Tegison therapy resulted in approximately the same clinical response as experienced during the initial course of therapy.

CONTRAINDICATIONS

Pregnancy: Category X. See boxed CONTRAINDICATION.

WARNINGS

Pseudotumor cerebri: Tegison and other retinoids have been associated with cases of pseudotumor cerebri (benign intracranial hypertension). Early signs and symptoms of pseudotumor cerebri include papilledema, headache, nausea and vomiting, and visual disturbances. Patients with these symptoms should be examined for papilledema and, if present, they should discontinue Tegison immediately and be referred for neurologic diagnosis and care.

Hepatotoxicity: Of the 652 patients treated in U.S. clinical trials, 10 had clinical or histologic hepatitis considered possibly or probably related to Tegison treatment. Liver function tests returned to normal in 8 of these patients after Tegison was discontinued; 1 patient had histologic changes resembling chronic active hepatitis 6 months off therapy, and 1 patient had no follow-up available. There have been 4 reports of hepatitis-related deaths worldwide; 2 of these patients had received etretinate for a month or less before presenting with hepatic symptoms. Elevations of AST (SGOT), ALT (SGPT) or LDH have occurred in 18%, 23% and 15%, respectively, of individuals treated with Tegison. Cases with pathology findings of hepatic fibrosis, necrosis and/or cirrhosis which may be related to Tegison therapy have been reported. If hepatotoxicity is suspected during treatment with Tegison, the drug should be discontinued and the etiology further investigated.

Ophthalmic effects: Corneal erosion, abrasion, irregularity and punctate staining have occurred in patients treated with Tegison, although these effects were absent or improved after therapy was stopped in those patients who had follow-up examinations. Corneal opacities have occurred in patients receiving isotretinoin; they had either completely resolved or were resolving at follow-up 6 to 7 weeks after discontinuation of the drug. Other ophthalmic effects that have occurred in Tegison patients include decreased visual acuity and blurring of vision, minimal posterior subcapsular cataract, iritis, blot retinal hemorrhage, scotoma and photophobia. A number of cases of decreased night vision have occurred during Tegison therapy. Because the onset in some patients was sudden, patients should be advised of this potential problem and warned to be cautious when driving or operating any vehicle at night. Any Tegison patient experiencing visual difficulties should discontinue the drug and have an ophthalmological examination.

Hyperostosis: There is a very high likelihood of the development of hyperostosis with Tegison therapy. In one clinical trial, 45 patients with a mean age of 40 years were retrospectively evaluated for evidence of hyperostosis. They had received etretinate at a mean dose of 0.8 mg/kg for a mean duration of 33 months at the time of x-ray. Eleven patients had psoriasis, while 34 patients had a disorder of keratinization. Of these, 38 patients who continued to receive etretinate at an average dose of 0.8 mg/kg/day for an average duration of 60 months, 32 (84%) had radiographic evidence of extraspinal tendon and ligament calcification. The most common sites of involvement were the ankles (76%), pelvis (53%) and knees (42%); spinal changes were uncommon. Involvement tended to be bilateral and multifocal. There were no bone or joint symptoms at the sites of radiographic abnormalities in 47% of the affected patients.

Lipids: Blood lipid determinations should be performed before Tegison is administered and then at intervals of 1 or 2 weeks until the lipid response to Tegison is established; this usually occurs within 4 to 8 weeks.

Approximately 45% of patients receiving Tegison during clinical trials experienced an elevation of plasma triglycerides. Approximately 37% developed a decrease in high density lipoproteins and about 16% showed an increase in cholesterol levels. These effects on triglycerides, HDL and cholesterol were reversible after cessation of Tegison therapy.

Patients with an increased tendency to develop hypertriglyceridemia include those with diabetes mellitus, obesity, increased alcohol intake or a familial history of these conditions.

Hypertriglyceridemia, hypercholesterolemia and lowered HDL may increase a patient's cardiovascular risk status. In addition, elevation of serum triglycerides in excess of 800 mg/dL has been associated with acute pancreatitis. Therefore, every attempt should be made to control significant elevations of triglycerides or cholesterol or significant decreases in HDL. Some patients have been able to reverse triglyceride and cholesterol elevations or HDL decrease by

reduction in weight or restriction of dietary fat and alcohol while continuing Tegison therapy.

Cardiovascular Effects: During clinical trials of 652 patients, 21 significant cardiovascular adverse incidents were reported, all in patients who had a strong history of cardiovascular risk. These incidents were not considered related to Tegison therapy except for two cases of myocardial infarction: 1 which was considered possibly related to Tegison therapy and 1 for which a relationship was not specified.

Animal Studies: In general, the signs of etretinate toxicity in rats, mice and dogs are dose-related with respect to incidence, onset and severity. In rodents, the most striking manifestations of this toxicity are bone fractures; no evidence of fractures was observed in a 1-year dog study. Other dose-related changes in some animals treated with etretinate in subchronic or chronic toxicity studies include alopecia, erythema, reductions in body weight and food consumption, stiffness, altered gait, hematologic changes, elevations in serum alkaline phosphatase and testicular atrophy with microscopic evidence of reduced spermatogenesis.

PRECAUTIONS

Information for Patients: Women of childbearing potential should be advised that they must not be pregnant when Tegison therapy is initiated, and that they should use an effective form of contraception for 1 month prior to Tegison therapy, while taking Tegison and after Tegison has been discontinued. Tegison has been found in the blood of some patients 2 to 3 years after the drug was discontinued. See boxed CONTRAINDICATION.

Because of the relationship of Tegison to vitamin A, patients should be advised against taking vitamin A supplements to avoid possible additive toxic effects.

TABLE II
LESS FREQUENT ADVERSE EVENTS REPORTED DURING CLINICAL TRIALS
(SOME OF WHICH MAY BEAR NO RELATIONSHIP TO THERAPY)
PERCENT OF PATIENTS REPORTING

BODY SYSTEM	1%–10%	<1%
Mucocutaneous	Dry eyes Mucous membrane abnormalities Dry mouth Gingival bleeding/inflammation	Decreased mucous secretion Rhinorrhea
Dermatologic	Hair abnormalities Bullous eruption Cold/clammy skin Onycholysis Paronychia Pyogenic granuloma Changes in perspiration	Abnormal skin odor Granulation tissue Healing impairment Herpes simplex Hirsutism Increased pore size Sensory skin changes Skin atrophy Skin fissures Skin infection Skin nodule Skin ulceration Urticaria
Musculoskeletal	Myalgia	Gout Hyperkinesia Hypertonia
Central Nervous System	Dizziness Lethargy Changes in sensation Pain Rigors	Abnormal thinking Amnesia Anxiety Depression Pseudotumor cerebri Emotional lability Faint feeling Flu-like symptoms
Special Senses	Abnormal lacrimation Abnormal vision Abnormalities of: —Extraocular musculature —Ocular tension —Pupil —Vitreous Earache Otitis externa	Change in equilibrium Ear drainage Ear infection Hearing change Night vision decrease Photophobia Visual change Scotoma
Gastrointestinal	Hepatitis	Constipation Diarrhea Melena Flatulence Weight loss Oral ulcers Taste perversion Tooth caries
Cardiovascular	Cardiovascular thrombotic or obstructive events Edema	Atrial fibrillation Chest pain Coagulation disorder Phlebitis Postural hypotension Syncope
Respiratory	Dyspnea	Coughing Increased sputum Dysphonia Pharyngitis
Renal		Kidney stones
Urogenital		Abnormal menses Atrophic vaginitis Dysuria Polyuria Urinary retention
Other	Malignant neoplasms	*Continued on next page*

Roche Laboratories—Cont.

Patients should be advised that transient exacerbation of psoriasis is commonly seen during the initial period of therapy.

Patients should be informed that they may experience decreased tolerance to contact lenses during and after therapy.

Laboratory Tests: See WARNINGS section. In clinical studies, the incidence of hypertriglyceridemia was 1 patient in 2, that of hypercholesterolemia 1 patient in 6, and that of decreased HDL 1 patient in 3 during Tegison therapy. Pretreatment and follow-up blood lipids should be obtained under fasting conditions. If alcohol has been consumed, at least 36 hours should elapse before these determinations are made. It is recommended that these tests be performed at weekly or biweekly intervals until the lipid response to Tegison is established.

Elevations of AST (SGOT), ALT (SGPT) or LDH have occurred in 18%, 23% and 15%, respectively, of individuals treated with Tegison. It is recommended that these tests be performed prior to initiation of Tegison therapy, at 1 to 2 week intervals for the first 1 to 2 months of therapy and thereafter at intervals of 1 to 3 months, depending on the response to Tegison administration.

Drug Interactions: Little information is available on drug interactions with Tegison; however, concomitant consumption of milk increases the absorption of etretinate. See *Pharmacokinetics* and DOSAGE AND ADMINISTRATION sections.

Carcinogenesis, Mutagenesis, Impairment of Fertility:
Carcinogenesis: In a 2-year study, male or female Sprague-Dawley rats given etretinate by dietary admixture at doses up to 3 mg/kg/day (two times the maximum recommended human therapeutic dose) had no increase in tumor incidence. In an 80-week study, Crl:CD-1 (lCR) BR mice were given etretinate by dietary admixture at doses of 1 to 5 mg/kg/day. An increased incidence of blood vessel tumors (hemangiomas and hemangiosarcomas in several different tissue sites) was noted in the high-dose male group (4 to 5 mg/kg/day) but not in the female group.

Mutagenesis: Etretinate was evaluated by the Ames test in a host-mediated assay, in the micronucleus test, and in a "treat and plate" test using the diploid yeast strain *S. cerevisiae* D7. Except for a weakly positive response in the Ames test using the tester strain TA 100, there was no evidence of genotoxicity. No differences in the rate of sister chromatid exchange (SCE) were noted in lymphocytes of patients before and after 4 weeks of treatment with therapeutic doses of etretinate.

Impairment of Fertility: In a study of fertility and general reproductive performance in rats, no etretinate-related effects were observed at doses up to 2.5 mg/kg/day. At a dose of 5 mg/kg/day (approximately three times the maximum recommended human therapeutic dose) the readiness of the treated animals to copulate was reduced but the pregnancy rate was unaffected. The number of viable young at birth and their postnatal weight gain and survival were adversely affected at the high dose. The pregnancy rate of the untreated first generation animals and postnatal weight gain of the untreated second generation animals were also reduced. No adverse effects on sperm production were noted in 12 psoriatic patients given 75 mg/day of etretinate for 1 month and 50 mg/day for an additional 2 months. However, testicular atrophy was noted in subchronic and chronic rat studies and in a chronic dog study, in some cases at doses approaching those recommended for use in humans. Decreased sperm counts were reported in a 13-week dog study at doses as low as 3 mg/kg/day (approximately twice the maximum recommended human dose). Spermatogenic arrest also was reported with chronic administration of the all-*trans* metabolite to dogs.

Pregnancy: Category X. See boxed CONTRAINDICATION. The following limited preliminary data must not be read or understood to diminish the serious risk of teratogenicity set forth in the boxed pregnancy CONTRAINDICATION.

Thirty women worldwide have been reported as having taken 1 or more doses of Tegison during pregnancy. In 29 cases in which information was available, there were a total of 10 congenital abnormalities. The occurrence of congenital abnormalities was 4 of 20 among delivered infants, 2 of 2 among spontaneously aborted fetuses, and 4 of 7 among induced abortions.

A further 38 women are reported to have become pregnant within 24 months after discontinuing Tegison therapy. Because congenital abnormalities have been reported in these pregnancies, it cannot be stated that there is a "safe" time to become pregnant after Tegison therapy. In 37 cases in which information was available, there were a total of 3 congenital abnormalities. The occurrence of congenital abnormalities was 2 of 29 among delivered infants, 0 of 1 among spontaneously aborted fetuses, and 1 of 5 among induced abortions. Two stillbirths with no apparent congenital abnormalities were attributed to other causes.

Nonteratogenic Effects: No adverse effects on various parameters of late gestation and lactation were observed in rats at doses of etretinate up to 4 mg/kg/day (approximately

three times the maximum human recommended dose). At doses of 8 mg/kg/day (approximately five times the maximum human recommended dose) of etretinate, the rate of stillbirths was increased and neonatal weight gain and survival rate were markedly reduced.

Nursing Mothers: Studies have shown that etretinate is excreted in the milk of lactating rats; however, it is not known whether this drug is excreted in human milk. Because of the potential for adverse effects, nursing mothers should not receive Tegison.

Pediatric Use: No clinical studies have been conducted in the U. S. using Tegison in children. Ossification of interosseous ligaments and tendons of the extremities has been reported. Two children showed x-ray changes suggestive of premature epiphyseal closure during treatment with Tegison. Skeletal hyperostosis has also been reported after treatment with isotretinoin. It is not known if any of these effects occur more commonly in children, but concern should be greater because of the growth process. Pretreatment x-rays for bone age including x-rays of the knees, followed by yearly monitoring, are advised. In addition, pain or limitation of motion should be evaluated with appropriate radiological examination. Because of the lack of data on the use of etretinate in children and the possibility of their being more sensitive to effects of the drug, this product should be used only when all alternative therapies have been exhausted.

ADVERSE EVENTS

Clinical: Hepatitis was observed in about 1.5% of patients treated with Tegison in clinical trials. Pathology findings of hepatic fibrosis, necrosis and/or cirrhosis have been reported. See WARNINGS section.

Tegison has been associated with pseudotumor cerebri. See WARNINGS section.

Hypervitaminosis A produces a wide spectrum of signs and symptoms of primarily the mucocutaneous, musculoskeletal, hepatic and central nervous systems. Nearly all of the clinical adverse events reported to date with Tegison administration resemble those of the hypervitaminosis A syndrome. Table I lists the adverse events frequently reported during clinical trials in which 652 patients were treated either for psoriasis (591 patients) or a disorder of keratinization (61 patients). Table II lists less frequently reported adverse events in these same patients. However the number of patients evaluated for each adverse event was not 652 in every case.

[See Table I on page 2314.]

[See Table II on preceding page.]

Laboratory: Tegison therapy induces change in serum lipids in a significant number of treated patients. Approximately 45% of patients experienced elevation in serum triglycerides, 37% a decrease in high density lipoproteins and 16% an increase in cholesterol levels.

Approximately 46% of patients had elevations of triglycerides above 250 mg/dL, 54% had decreases of HDL below 36 mg%, and 19% had elevations of cholesterol above 300 mg%. One case of eruptive xanthomas associated with triglyceride levels greater than 1000 mg% has been reported.

Elevations of AST (SGOT), ALT (SGPT) or LDH were experienced by 18%, 23% and 15%, respectively, of individuals treated with Tegison. In most of the patients, the elevations were slight to moderate and became normal either during therapy or after cessation of treatment. See WARNINGS section.

Table III lists the laboratory abnormalities reported during clinical trials. Data for patients who received intermittent courses of therapy for periods up to five years are included. Any instance of two consecutive values outside the range of normal, or an abnormal value with no follow-up during therapy, was considered to be possibly related to Tegison.

[See Table III above.]

OVERDOSAGE

There has been no experience with acute overdosage in humans.

The acute oral and intraperitoneal toxicities (LD_{50}) of etretinate capsules in mice and rats were greater than 4000 mg/kg. The acute oral toxicity (LD_{50}) of etretinate substance in 4% solution was 2300 mg/kg in mice and 1300 mg/kg in rats.

DOSAGE AND ADMINISTRATION

There is intersubject variation in the absorption and the rate of metabolism of Tegison. Individualization of dosage is required to achieve the maximal therapeutic response with a tolerable degree of side effects. Therapy with Tegison should generally be initiated at a dosage of 0.75 to 1 mg/kg of body weight/day taken in divided doses. A maximum dose of 1.5 mg/kg/day should not be exceeded. Erythrodermic psoriasis may respond to lower initial doses of 0.25 mg/kg/day increased by 0.25 mg/kg/day each week until optimal initial response is attained.

Maintenance doses of 0.5 to 0.75 mg/kg/day may be initiated after initial response, generally after 8 to 16 weeks of ther-

TABLE III
LABORATORY ABNORMALITIES REPORTED DURING CLINICAL TRIALS
PERCENT OF PATIENTS REPORTING

BODY SYSTEM	25%–50%	10%–25%	1%–10%
Hematologic	Increased: —MCHC (60%) —MCH —Reticulocytes —PTT —ESR	Decreased: —Hemoglobin/HCT —RBC —MCV Increased platelets Increased or decreased: —WBC and components —Prothrombin time	Decreased: —Platelets —MCH —MCHC —PTT Increased: —Hemoglobin/HCT —RBC
Urinary		WBC in urine	Proteinuria Glycosuria Microscopic hematuria Casts in urine Acetonuria Hemoglobinuria
Hepatic	Increased triglycerides	Increased: —AST (SGOT) —ALT (SGPT) —Alkaline phosphatase —GGTP —Globulin —Cholesterol	Increased bilirubin Increased or decreased: —Total protein —Albumin
Renal			Increased: —BUN —Creatinine
Electrolytes	Increased or decreased potassium	Increased or decreased: —Venous CO_2 —Sodium —Chloride	
Miscellaneous	Increased or decreased: —Calcium —Phosphorus	Increased or decreased FBS	Increased CPK

apy. In general, therapy should be terminated in patients whose lesions have sufficiently resolved. Relapses may be treated as outlined for initial therapy.

Tegison should be administered with food.

HOW SUPPLIED

Brown and green capsules, 10 mg, imprinted TEGISON 10 ROCHE; Prescription Paks of 30 (NDC 0004-0177-57). Brown and caramel capsules, 25 mg, imprinted TEGISON 25 ROCHE; Prescription Paks of 30 (NDC 0004-0179-57). STORE AT 59° TO 86°F (15° TO 30°C). PROTECT FROM LIGHT.

Revised: January 1994

Shown in Product Identification Guide, page 332

Tel-E-Ject® ℞

Available in the following product: VERSED® (midazolam HCl) disposable syringes, 10 mg.

Shown in Product Identification Guide, page 332

TICLID® Tablets ℞
[tye'klid]
(ticlopidine hydrochloride)

DESCRIPTION

TICLID (ticlopidine hydrochloride) is a platelet aggregation inhibitor. Chemically it is 5-[(2-chlorophenyl)methyl]-4,5,6,7-tetrahydrothieno [3,2-c] pyridine hydrochloride.

Ticlopidine hydrochloride is a white crystalline solid. It is freely soluble in water and self buffers to a pH of 3.6. It also dissolves freely in methanol, is sparingly soluble in methylene chloride and ethanol, slightly soluble in acetone and insoluble in a buffer solution of pH 6.3. It has a molecular weight of 300.25.

TICLID tablets for oral administration are provided as white, oval, film-coated, blue-imprinted tablets containing 250 mg of ticlopidine hydrochloride. Each tablet also contains citric acid, magnesium stearate, microcrystalline cellulose, povidone, starch and stearic acid as inactive ingredients. The white film coating contains hydroxypropylmethyl cellulose, polyethylene glycol and titanium dioxide. Each tablet is printed with blue ink, which includes FD&C Blue #1 aluminum lake as the colorant. The tablets are identified with TICLID on one side and 250 on the reverse side.

CLINICAL PHARMACOLOGY

Mechanism of Action: When taken orally, ticlopidine hydrochloride causes a time and dose-dependent inhibition of both platelet aggregation and release of platelet granule constituents, as well as a prolongation of bleeding time. The intact drug has no significant in vitro activity at the concentrations attained in vivo; and, although analysis of urine and plasma indicates at least twenty metabolites, no metabolite which accounts for the activity of ticlopidine has been isolated.

Ticlopidine hydrochloride, after oral ingestion, interferes with platelet membrane function by inhibiting ADP-induced platelet-fibrinogen binding and subsequent platelet-platelet interactions. The effect on platelet function is irreversible for the life of the platelet, as shown both by persistent inhibition of fibrinogen binding after washing platelets ex vivo and by inhibition of platelet aggregation after resuspension of platelets in buffered medium.

Pharmacokinetics and Metabolism: After oral administration of a single 250-mg dose, ticlopidine hydrochloride is rapidly absorbed with peak plasma levels occurring at approximately 2 hours after dosing and is extensively metabolized. Absorption is greater than 80%. Administration after meals results in a 20% increase in the AUC of ticlopidine.

Ticlopidine hydrochloride displays nonlinear pharmacokinetics and clearance decreases markedly on repeated dosing. In older volunteers the apparent half-life of ticlopidine after a single 250-mg dose is about 12.6 hours; with repeat dosing at 250 mg bid, the terminal elimination half-life rises to 4 to 5 days and steady-state levels of ticlopidine hydrochloride in plasma are obtained after approximately 14 to 21 days.

Ticlopidine hydrochloride binds reversibly (98%) to plasma proteins, mainly to serum albumin and lipoproteins. The binding to albumin and lipoproteins is nonsaturable over a wide concentration range. Ticlopidine also binds to alpha-1 acid glycoprotein. At concentrations attained with the recommended dose, only 15% or less ticlopidine in plasma is bound to this protein.

Ticlopidine hydrochloride is metabolized extensively by the liver; only trace amounts of intact drug are detected in the urine. Following an oral dose of radioactive ticlopidine hydrochloride administered in solution, 60% of the radioactivity is recovered in the urine and 23% in the feces. Approximately 1/3 of the dose excreted in the feces is intact ticlopidine hydrochloride, possibly excreted in the bile. Ticlopidine hydrochloride is a minor component in plasma (5%) after a

single dose, but at steady state is the major component (15%). Approximately 40% to 50% of the radioactive metabolites circulating in plasma are covalently bound to plasma proteins, probably by acylation.

Clearance of ticlopidine decreases with age. Steady-state trough values in elderly patients (mean age 70 years) are about twice those in young volunteer populations.

Hepatically Impaired Patients: The effect of decreased hepatic function on the pharmacokinetics of TICLID was studied in 17 patients with advanced cirrhosis. The average plasma concentration of ticlopidine in these subjects was slightly higher than that seen in older subjects in a separate trial (see CONTRAINDICATIONS).

Renally Impaired Patients: Patients with mildly (Ccr 50 to 80 mL/min) or moderately (Ccr 20 to 50 mL/min) impaired renal function were compared to normal subjects (Ccr 80 to 150 mL/min) in a study of the pharmacokinetic and platelet pharmacodynamic effects of TICLID (250 mg bid) for 11 days. Concentrations of unchanged TICLID were measured after a single 250-mg dose and after the final 250-mg dose on Day 11. AUC values of ticlopidine increased by 28 and 60% in mild and moderately impaired patients, respectively, and plasma clearance decreased by 37 and 52%, respectively; but there were no statistically significant differences in ADP-induced platelet aggregation. In this small study (26 patients), bleeding times showed significant prolongation only in the moderately impaired patients.

Pharmacodynamics: In healthy volunteers over the age of 50, substantial inhibition (over 50%) of ADP-induced platelet aggregation is detected within 4 days after administration of ticlopidine hydrochloride 250 mg bid, and maximum platelet aggregation inhibition (60% to 70%) is achieved after 8 to 11 days. Lower doses cause less, and more delayed, platelet aggregation inhibition, while doses above 250 mg bid give little additional effect on platelet aggregation but an increased rate of adverse effects. The dose of 250 mg bid is the only dose that has been evaluated in controlled clinical trials.

After discontinuation of ticlopidine hydrochloride, bleeding time and other platelet function tests return to normal within 2 weeks in the majority of patients.

At the recommended therapeutic dose (250 mg bid), ticlopidine hydrochloride has no known significant pharmacological actions in man other than inhibition of platelet function and prolongation of the bleeding time.

CLINICAL TRIALS

The effect of ticlopidine on the risk of stroke and cardiovascular events was studied in two multicenter, randomized, double-blind trials.

1. Study in Patients Experiencing Stroke Precursors: In a trial comparing ticlopidine and aspirin (The Ticlopidine Aspirin Stroke Study or TASS), 3069 patients (1987 men, 1082 women) who had experienced such stroke precursors as transient ischemic attack (TIA), transient monocular blindness (amaurosis fugax), reversible ischemic neurological deficit or minor stroke, were randomized to ticlopidine 250 mg bid or aspirin 650 mg bid. The study was designed to follow patients for at least 2 and up to 5 years.

Over the duration of the study, TICLID significantly reduced the risk of fatal and nonfatal stroke by 24% (p = .011) from 18.1 to 13.8 per 100 patients followed for 5 years, compared to aspirin. During the first year, when the risk of stroke is greatest, the reduction in risk of stroke (fatal and nonfatal) compared to aspirin was 48%; the reduction was similar in men and women.

TASS - Fatal or Nonfatal Stroke

2. Study in Patients Who Had a Completed Atherothrombotic Stroke: In a trial comparing ticlopidine with placebo (The Canadian American Ticlopidine Study or CATS) 1073 patients who had experienced a previous atherothrombotic stroke were treated with TICLID 250 mg bid or placebo for up to 3 years.

TICLID significantly reduced the overall risk of stroke by 24% (p = .017) from 24.6 to 18.6 per 100 patients followed for 3 years, compared to placebo. During the first year the reduction in risk of fatal and nonfatal stroke over placebo was 33%.

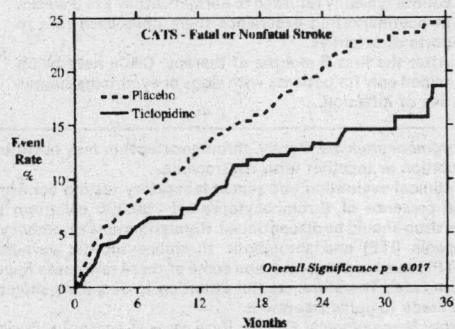

CATS - Fatal or Nonfatal Stroke

Overall Significance p = 0.017

INDICATIONS AND USAGE

TICLID is indicated to reduce the risk of thrombotic stroke (fatal or nonfatal) in patients who have experienced stroke precursors, and in patients who have had a completed thrombotic stroke.

Because TICLID is associated with a risk of neutropenia/agranulocytosis, which may be life-threatening (see WARNINGS), TICLID should be reserved for patients who are intolerant to aspirin therapy where indicated to prevent stroke.

CONTRAINDICATIONS

The use of TICLID is contraindicated in the following conditions:

- Hypersensitivity to the drug
- Presence of hematopoietic disorders such as neutropenia and thrombocytopenia
- Presence of a hemostatic disorder or active pathological bleeding (such as bleeding peptic ulcer or intracranial bleeding)
- Patients with severe liver impairment

WARNINGS

Neutropenia: Neutropenia defined in these studies as an ANC < 1200 neutrophils/mm³ occurred in 50 of 2048 (2.4%) stroke patients who received TICLID in clinical trials.

Severe Neutropenia (< 450 neutrophils/mm³):
Severe neutropenia and/or agranulocytosis occurred in 17 of the 2048 (0.8%) patients who received TICLID. When the drug was discontinued in these patients, the neutrophil counts returned to normal (> 1200 neutrophils/mm³) within 1 to 3 weeks.

Mild to Moderate Neutropenia (451 to 1200 neutrophils/mm³):
Mild to moderate neutropenia occurred in 33 of the 2048 (1.6%) patients who received TICLID. Eleven of the patients discontinued treatment and recovered within a few days. In the remaining 22 patients, the neutropenia was transient and did not require discontinuation of therapy.

The onset of severe neutropenia usually occurs 3 weeks to 3 months after the start of therapy. Nevertheless, in postmarketing experience there have been some reports of severe neutropenia beyond that time. The bone marrow typically showed a reduction in myeloid precursors. The onset of neutropenia may occur suddenly.

It is, therefore, essential that CBCs (including platelet count) and white cell differentials be performed every 2 weeks, starting at baseline before treatment is initiated to the end of the third month of therapy with TICLID, but more frequent monitoring is necessary for patients whose absolute neutrophil counts have been consistently declining or are 30% less than the baseline count. Because of the long plasma half-life of TICLID, it is recommended that any patient who discontinues TICLID for any reason within the first 90 days continue to have CBC (including platelet count) monitoring and white cell differential for at least another 2 weeks after discontinuation of therapy.

Neutropenia (an absolute neutrophil count [ANC] of less than 1200 neutrophils/mm³) is calculated as follows: ANC = WBC x % neutrophils. If clinical evaluation and repeat laboratory testing confirm the presence of neu-

Continued on next page

Roche Laboratories—Cont.

tropenia (<1200/mm³), the drug should be discontinued.

In clinical trials when therapy was discontinued immediately upon detection of neutropenia, the neutrophil counts typically returned to normal within 1 to 3 weeks. In postmarketing experience there have been rare reports of fatalities.

After the first 3 months of therapy, CBCs need be obtained only for patients with signs or symptoms suggestive of infection.

Thrombocytopenia: Rarely, thrombocytopenia may occur in isolation or together with neutropenia.

If clinical evaluation and repeat laboratory testing confirm the presence of thrombocytopenia (<80,000 cells/mm³), the drug should be discontinued. Rarely, immune thrombocytopenia (ITP) and thrombotic thrombocytopenic purpura (TTP) have been reported, and some of these rare cases have been fatal. Therefore, careful attention to diagnosis should be made to guide treatment.

Other Hematological Effects: Rare cases of agranulocytosis, pancytopenia or aplastic anemia have been reported in postmarketing experience, some of which have been fatal. All forms of hematological adverse reactions are potentially fatal.

Cholesterol Elevation: TICLID therapy causes increased serum cholesterol and triglycerides. Serum total cholesterol levels are increased 8% to 10% within 1 month of therapy and persist at that level. The ratios of the lipoprotein subfractions are unchanged.

Anticoagulant Drugs: The tolerance and safety of coadministration of TICLID with heparin, oral anticoagulants or fibrinolytic agents has not been established. If a patient is switched from an anticoagulant or fibrinolytic drug to TICLID, the former drug should be discontinued prior to TICLID administration.

PRECAUTIONS

General: TICLID should be used with caution in patients who may be at risk of increased bleeding from trauma, surgery or pathological conditions. If it is desired to eliminate the antiplatelet effects of TICLID prior to elective surgery, the drug should be discontinued 10 to 14 days prior to surgery. Several controlled clinical studies have found increased surgical blood loss in patients undergoing surgery during treatment with ticlopidine. In TASS and CATS it was recommended that patients have ticlopidine discontinued prior to elective surgery. Several hundred patients underwent surgery during the trials, and no excessive surgical bleeding was reported.

Prolonged bleeding time is normalized within 2 hours after administration of 20 mg methylprednisolone IV. Platelet transfusions may also be used to reverse the effect of TICLID on bleeding. Platelet transfusions are usually not indicated in patients with TTP on ticlopidine.

GI Bleeding: TICLID prolongs template bleeding time. The drug should be used with caution in patients who have lesions with a propensity to bleed (such as ulcers). Drugs that might induce such lesions should be used with caution in patients on TICLID (see CONTRAINDICATIONS).

Use in Hepatically Impaired Patients: Since ticlopidine is metabolized by the liver, dosing of TICLID or other drugs metabolized in the liver may require adjustment upon starting or stopping concomitant therapy. Because of limited experience in patients with severe hepatic disease, who may have bleeding diatheses, the use of TICLID is not recommended in this population (see CLINICAL PHARMACOLOGY and CONTRAINDICATIONS).

Use in Renally Impaired Patients: There is limited experience in patients with renal impairment. Decreased plasma clearance, increased AUC values and prolonged bleeding times can occur in renally impaired patients. In controlled clinical trials no unexpected problems have been encountered in patients having mild renal impairment, and there is no experience with dosage adjustment in patients with greater degrees of renal impairment. Nevertheless, for renally impaired patients, it may be necessary to reduce the dosage of ticlopidine or discontinue it altogether if hemorrhagic or hematopoietic problems are encountered (see CLINICAL PHARMACOLOGY).

Information for the Patient (See PPI): Patients should be told that a decrease in the number of white blood cells (neutropenia) can occur with TICLID, especially during the first 3 months of treatment and that, if neutropenia is severe, it could result in an increased risk of infection. They should be told it is critically important to obtain the scheduled blood tests to detect neutropenia. Patients should also be reminded to contact their physicians if they experience any indication of infection such as fever, chills and sore throat, all of which may be consequences of neutropenia.

All patients should be told that it may take them longer than usual to stop bleeding when they take TICLID and that they should report any unusual bleeding to their physician. Pa-

tients should tell physicians and dentists that they are taking TICLID before any surgery is scheduled and before any new drug is prescribed.

Patients should be told to report promptly side effects of TICLID such as severe or persistent diarrhea, skin rashes or subcutaneous bleeding or any signs of cholestasis, such as yellow skin or sclera, dark urine or light colored stools. Patients should be told to take TICLID with food or just after eating in order to minimize gastrointestinal discomfort.

Laboratory Tests: Liver Function: TICLID therapy has been associated with elevations of alkaline phosphatase and transaminases, which generally occurred within 1 to 4 months of therapy initiation. In controlled clinical trials the incidence of elevated alkaline phosphatase (greater than two times upper limit of normal) was 7.6% in ticlopidine patients, 6% in placebo patients and 2.5% in aspirin patients. The incidence of elevated AST (SGOT) (greater than two times upper limit of normal) was 3.1% in ticlopidine patients, 4% in placebo patients and 2.1% in aspirin patients. No progressive increases were observed in closely monitored clinical trials (eg, no transaminase greater than 10 times the upper limit of normal was seen), but most patients with these abnormalities had therapy discontinued. Occasionally patients had developed minor elevations in bilirubin.

Based on postmarketing and clinical trial experience, liver function testing, including SGPT and GGTP, should be considered whenever liver dysfunction is suspected, particularly during the first 4 months of treatment.

Drug Interactions: Therapeutic doses of TICLID caused a 30% increase in the plasma half-life of antipyrine and may cause analogous effects on similarly metabolized drugs. Therefore, the dose of drugs metabolized by hepatic microsomal enzymes with low therapeutic ratios or being given to patients with hepatic impairment may require adjustment to maintain optimal therapeutic blood levels when starting or stopping concomitant therapy with ticlopidine. Studies of specific drug interactions yielded the following results:

Aspirin and other NSAIDS: Ticlopidine potentiates the effect of aspirin or other NSAIDS on platelet aggregation. The safety of concomitant use of ticlopidine with aspirin or other NSAIDS has not been established. Aspirin did not modify the ticlopidine-mediated inhibition of ADP-induced platelet aggregation, but ticlopidine potentiated the effect of aspirin on collagen-induced platelet aggregation. Concomitant use of aspirin and ticlopidine is not recommended (see PRECAUTIONS—GI Bleeding).

Antacids: Administration of TICLID after antacids resulted in an 18% decrease in plasma levels of ticlopidine.

Cimetidine: Chronic administration of cimetidine reduced the clearance of a single dose of TICLID by 50%.

Digoxin: Coadministration of TICLID with digoxin resulted in a slight decrease (approximately 15%) in digoxin plasma levels. Little or no change in therapeutic efficacy of digoxin would be expected.

Theophylline: In normal volunteers, concomitant administration of TICLID resulted in a significant increase in the theophylline elimination half-life from 8.6 to 12.2 hours and a comparable reduction in total plasma clearance of theophylline.

Phenobarbital: In 6 normal volunteers, the inhibitory effects of TICLID on platelet aggregation were not altered by chronic administration of phenobarbital.

Phenytoin: In vitro studies demonstrated that ticlopidine does not alter the plasma protein binding of phenytoin. However, the protein binding interactions of ticlopidine and its metabolites have not been studied in vivo. Several cases of elevated phenytoin plasma levels with associated somnolence and lethargy have been reported following coadministration with TICLID. Caution should be exercised in coadministering this drug with TICLID, and it may be useful to remeasure phenytoin blood concentrations.

Propranolol: In vitro studies demonstrated that ticlopidine does not alter the plasma protein binding of propranolol. However, the protein binding interactions of ticlopidine and its metabolites have not been studied in vivo. Caution should be exercised in coadministering this drug with TICLID.

Other Concomitant Therapy: Although specific interaction studies were not performed, in clinical studies TICLID was used concomitantly with beta blockers, calcium channel blockers and diuretics without evidence of clinically significant adverse interactions (see PRECAUTIONS).

Food Interaction: The oral bioavailability of ticlopidine is increased by 20% when taken after a meal. Administration of TICLID with food is recommended to maximize gastrointestinal tolerance. In controlled trials TICLID was taken with meals.

Carcinogenesis, Mutagenesis and Impairment of Fertility: In a 2-year oral carcinogenicity study in rats, ticlopidine at daily doses of up to 100 mg/kg (610 mg/m²) was not tumorigenic. For a 70-kg person (1.73m² body surface area) the dose represents 14 times the recommended clinical dose on a mg/kg basis and two times the clinical dose on body surface area basis. In a 78-week oral carcinogenicity study in mice, ticlopidine at daily doses up to 275 mg/kg (1180 mg/m²) was not tumorigenic. The dose represents 40 times the recommended

clinical dose on a mg/kg basis and four times the clinical dose on body surface area basis.

Ticlopidine was not mutagenic in in vitro Ames test, rat hepatocyte DNA-repair assay and Chinese hamster fibroblast chromosomal aberration test and in in vivo mouse spermatozoid morphology test, Chinese hamster micronucleus test and Chinese hamster bone marrow cell sister chromatid exchange test. Ticlopidine was found to have no effect on fertility of male and female rats at oral doses up to 400 mg/kg/day.

Pregnancy: Teratogenic Effects: Pregnancy: Category B. Teratology studies have been conducted in mice (doses up to 200 mg/kg/day), rats (doses up to 400 mg/kg/day) and rabbits (doses up to 200 mg/kg/day). Doses of 400 mg/kg in rats, 200 mg/kg/day in mice and 100 mg/kg in rabbits produced maternal toxicity, as well as fetal toxicity, but there was no evidence of a teratogenic potential of ticlopidine. There are, however, no adequate and well-controlled studies in pregnant women. Because animal reproduction studies are not always predictive of a human response, this drug should be used during pregnancy only if clearly needed.

Nursing Mothers: Studies in rats have shown ticlopidine is excreted in the milk. It is not known whether this drug is excreted in human milk. Because many drugs are excreted in human milk and because of the potential for serious adverse reactions in nursing infants from ticlopidine, a decision should be made whether to discontinue nursing or to discontinue the drug, taking into account the importance of the drug to the mother.

Pediatric Use: Safety and efficacy in patients under the age of 18 have not been established.

Geriatric Use: Clearance of ticlopidine is somewhat lower in elderly patients and trough levels are increased. The major clinical trials with TICLID were conducted in an elderly population with an average age of 64 years. Of the total number of patients in the therapeutic trials, 45% of patients were over 65 years old and 12% were over 75 years old. No overall differences in effectiveness or safety were observed between these patients and younger patients, and other reported clinical experience has not identified differences in responses between the elderly and younger patients, but greater sensitivity of some older individuals cannot be ruled out.

ADVERSE REACTIONS:

Adverse reactions were relatively frequent with over 50% of patients reporting at least one. Most (30% to 40%) involved the gastrointestinal tract. Most adverse effects are mild, but 21% of patients discontinued therapy because of an adverse event, principally diarrhea, rash, nausea, vomiting, GI pain and neutropenia. Most adverse effects occur early in the course of treatment, but a new onset of adverse effects can occur after several months.

The incidence rates of adverse events listed in the following table were derived from multicenter, controlled clinical trials described above comparing TICLID, placebo and aspirin over study periods of up to 5.8 years. Adverse events considered by the investigator to be probably drug-related that occurred in at least 1% of patients treated with TICLID are shown in the following table:

Percent of Patients with Adverse Events in Controlled Studies

Event	TICLID (n=2048) Incidence	Aspirin (n=1527) Incidence	Placebo (n=536) Incidence
Any Events	60.0 (20.9)	53.2 (14.5)	34.3 (6.1)
Diarrhea	12.5 (6.3)	5.2 (1.8)	4.5 (1.7)
Nausea	7.0 (2.6)	6.2 (1.9)	1.7 (0.9)
Dyspepsia	7.0 (1.1)	9.0 (2.0)	0.9 (0.2)
Rash	5.1 (3.4)	1.5 (0.8)	0.6 (0.9)
GI Pain	3.7 (1.9)	5.6 (2.7)	1.3 (0.4)
Neutropenia	2.4 (1.3)	0.8 (0.1)	1.1 (0.4)
Purpura	2.2 (0.2)	1.6 (0.1)	0.0 (0.0)
Vomiting	1.9 (1.4)	1.4 (0.9)	0.9 (0.4)
Flatulence	1.5 (0.1)	1.4 (0.3)	0.0 (0.0)
Pruritus	1.3 (0.8)	0.3 (0.1)	0.0 (0.0)
Dizziness	1.1 (0.4)	0.5 (0.4)	0.0 (0.0)
Anorexia	1.0 (0.4)	0.5 (0.3)	0.0 (0.0)
Abnormal Liver Function Test	1.0 (0.7)	0.3 (0.3)	0.0 (0.0)

Incidence of discontinuation, regardless of relationship to therapy, is shown in parentheses.

Hematological: Neutropenia/thrombocytopenia (see WARNINGS), agranulocytosis, eosinophilia, pancytopenia, thrombocytosis and bone marrow depression have been reported.

Gastrointestinal: TICLID therapy has been associated with a variety of gastrointestinal complaints including diarrhea and nausea. The majority of cases are mild, but about 13% of patients discontinued therapy because of these. They usually occur within 3 months of initiation of therapy and typically are resolved within 1 to 2 weeks without discontinuation of therapy. If the effect is severe or persistent, therapy should be discontinued. In some cases of severe or bloody diarrhea, colitis was later diagnosed.

Hemorrhagic: TICLID has been associated with increased bleeding, spontaneous post-traumatic bleeding and perioperative bleeding including, but not limited to, gastrointestinal bleeding. It has also been associated with a number of bleeding complications such as ecchymosis, epistaxis, hematuria and conjunctival hemorrhage.

Intracerebral bleeding was rare in clinical trials with TICLID, with an incidence no greater than that seen with comparator agents (ticlopidine 0.5%, aspirin 0.6%, placebo 0.75%). It has also been reported postmarketing.

Rash: Ticlopidine has been associated with a maculopapular or urticarial rash (often with pruritus). Rash usually occurs within 3 months of initiation of therapy with a mean onset time of 11 days. If drug is discontinued, recovery occurs within several days. Many rashes do not recur on drug rechallenge. There have been rare reports of severe rashes, including Stevens-Johnson syndrome, erythema multiforme and exfoliative dermatitis.

Less Frequent Adverse Reactions (Probably Related): Clinical adverse experiences occurring in 0.5% to 1% of patients in the controlled trials include:

Digestive System: GI fullness
Skin and Appendages: urticaria
Nervous System: headache
Body as a Whole: asthenia, pain
Hemostatic System: epistaxis
Special Senses: tinnitus

In addition, rarer, relatively serious events have also been reported from postmarketing experience: Hemolytic anemia with reticulocytosis, aplastic anemia, immune thrombocytopenia, thrombotic thrombocytopenic purpura (TTP), hepatitis, hepatocellular jaundice, cholestatic jaundice, hepatic necrosis, peptic ulcer, renal failure, nephrotic syndrome, hyponatremia, vasculitis, sepsis, angioedema, allergic pneumonitis, systemic lupus (positive ANA), peripheral neuropathy, serum sickness, arthropathy and myositis.

OVERDOSAGE

One case of deliberate overdosage with TICLID has been reported by foreign postmarketing surveillance program. A 38-year-old male took a single 6000-mg dose of TICLID (equivalent to 24 standard 250-mg tablets). The only abnormalities reported were increased bleeding time and increased SGPT. No special therapy was instituted and the patient recovered without sequelae.

Single oral doses of ticlopidine at 1600 mg/kg and 500 mg/kg were lethal to rats and mice, respectively. Symptoms of acute toxicity were GI hemorrhage, convulsions, hypothermia, dyspnea, loss of equilibrium and abnormal gait.

DOSAGE AND ADMINISTRATION

The recommended dose of TICLID is 250 mg bid taken with food. Other doses have not been studied in controlled trials for these indications.

HOW SUPPLIED

TICLID is available in white, oval, film-coated 250-mg tablets, printed in blue with TICLID on one side and 250 on the other. They are provided in unit of use bottles of 30 tablets (NDC 0004-0018-23) and 60 tablets (NDC 0004-0018-22) and 500 tablets (NDC 0004-0018-14) or in cartons of 100 blister-packed tablets (NDC 0004-0018-81).

Store at 15° to 30°C (59° to 86°F).

IMPORTANT INFORMATION ABOUT TICLID
(ticlopidine HCl) Tablets

The information in this leaflet is intended to help you use TICLID safely. Please read the leaflet carefully. Although it does not contain all the detailed medical information that is provided to your doctor, it provides facts about TICLID that are important for you to know. If you still have questions after reading this sheet or if you have questions at any time during your treatment with TICLID, check with your doctor.

Special Warning for Users of TICLID/Necessary Blood Tests: Your doctor has prescribed TICLID tablets (250 mg) to help reduce your risk of having a stroke, either because you have had a stroke already (to decrease the chance of another one) or because a stroke is threatening.

TICLID is recommended only for patients who cannot take aspirin, which also can decrease the risk of stroke. This is because TICLID can, on occasion, cause a serious white blood cell abnormality. A small percentage of people who take TICLID (about 2.4%) develop a large fall in the number of their white cells (a condition called neutropenia) that can be life-threatening because it leaves them unable to fight infection. If neutropenia occurs, it typically does so during the first 3 months of treatment.

To make sure you don't develop this problem, your doctor will arrange for you to have your blood tested before you start taking TICLID and then every 2 weeks for the first 3 months you are on TICLID. If detected, neutropenia can almost always be reversed, but if left untreated, neutropenia can lead to fatal infection. It is therefore essential that you keep your appointments for the blood tests and that you call your doctor immediately if you have any sign of an infection, such as fever, chills or sore throat, because these can mean that you have neutropenia. If you stop taking TICLID for any

reason within the first 3 months, you will still need to have your blood tested for an additional 2 weeks after you have stopped taking TICLID.

Other Warnings and Precautions: A few people may develop jaundice while being treated with TICLID. The signs of jaundice are yellowing of the skin or the whites of the eyes or consistent darkening in the color of urine or lightening in the color of stools. **If these symptoms occur, contact your doctor immediately.**

TICLID should be used only as directed by your doctor. Do not give TICLID to anyone else. **Keep TICLID out of reach of children!**

Some people may have such side effects as diarrhea, skin rash, stomach or intestinal discomfort. If any of these problems are persistent, or if you are concerned about them, bring them to your doctor's attention.

It may take longer than usual to stop bleeding when taking TICLID. Tell your doctor if you have any more bleeding or bruising than usual, and be sure to let your doctor or dentist know that you are taking TICLID if you have emergency surgery. Also, tell your doctor well in advance of any planned surgery (including tooth extraction), because he or she may recommend that you stop taking TICLID temporarily.

How TICLID Works: A stroke occurs when a clot (or thrombus) forms in a blood vessel in the brain or forms in another part of the body and breaks off, then travels to the brain (an embolus). In both cases the blood supply to part of the brain is blocked and that part of the brain is damaged. TICLID works by making the blood less likely to clot, although not so much less that it causes you to become likely to bleed, unless you have a bleeding disorder or some injury (such as a bleeding ulcer of the stomach or intestine) that is especially likely to bleed.

Who Should Not Take TICLID? Contact your doctor immediately and do not take TICLID if:
● you have an allergic reaction to TICLID
● you have a blood disorder or a serious bleeding problem, such as a bleeding stomach ulcer
● you have severe liver disease or other liver problems
● you are pregnant or you are planning to become pregnant
● you are breastfeeding

Revised: August 1995
Shown in Product Identification Guide, page 332

TORADOL® IV/IM/ORAL ℞
[tō rah-dol]
(ketorolac tromethamine)

WARNING

TORADOL, a nonsteroidal anti-inflammatory drug (NSAID), is indicated for the short-term (up to 5 days) management of moderately severe acute pain that requires analgesia at the opioid level. It is NOT indicated for minor or chronic painful conditions. TORADOL is a potent NSAID analgesic, and its administration carries many risks. The resulting NSAID-related adverse events can be serious in certain patients for whom TORADOL is indicated, especially when the drug is used inappropriately. Increasing the dose of TORADOL beyond the label recommendations will not provide better efficacy but will result in increasing the risk of developing serious adverse events.

GASTROINTESTINAL EFFECTS
● TORADOL can cause peptic ulcers, gastrointestinal bleeding and/or perforation. Therefore, TORADOL is CONTRAINDICATED in patients with active peptic ulcer disease, in patients with recent gastrointestinal bleeding or perforation, and in patients with a history of peptic ulcer disease or gastrointestinal bleeding.

RENAL EFFECTS
● TORADOL is CONTRAINDICATED in patients with advanced renal impairment and in patients at risk for renal failure due to volume depletion (see WARNINGS).

RISK OF BLEEDING
● TORADOL inhibits platelet function and is, therefore, CONTRAINDICATED in patients with suspected or confirmed cerebrovascular bleeding, patients with hemorrhagic diathesis, incomplete hemostasis and those at high risk of bleeding (see WARNINGS and PRECAUTIONS).
● TORADOL is CONTRAINDICATED as prophylactic analgesic before any major surgery and is CONTRAINDICATED intraoperatively when hemostasis is critical because of the increased risk of bleeding.

HYPERSENSITIVITY
● Hypersensitivity reactions, ranging from bronchospasm to anaphylactic shock, have occurred and appropriate counteractive measures must be available when administering the first dose of TORADOL IV/IM (see CONTRAINDICATIONS and WARNINGS). TORADOL is CONTRAINDICATED in patients with previ-

ously demonstrated hypersensitivity to ketorolac tromethamine or allergic manifestations to aspirin or other nonsteroidal anti-inflammatory drugs (NSAIDs).

INTRATHECAL OR EPIDURAL ADMINISTRATION
● TORADOL is CONTRAINDICATED for intrathecal or epidural administration due to its alcohol content.

LABOR, DELIVERY AND NURSING
● The use of TORADOL in labor and delivery is CONTRAINDICATED because it may adversely affect fetal circulation and inhibit uterine contractions.
● The use of TORADOL is CONTRAINDICATED in nursing mothers because of the potential adverse effects of prostaglandin-inhibiting drugs on neonates.

CONCOMITANT USE WITH NSAIDs
● TORADOL is CONTRAINDICATED in patients currently receiving ASA or NSAIDs because of the cumulative risk of inducing serious NSAID-related side effects.

DOSAGE AND ADMINISTRATION
TORADOL^ORAL
● TORADOL^ORAL is indicated only as continuation therapy to TORADOL^IV/IM, and the combined duration of use of TORADOL^IV/IM and TORADOL^ORAL is not to exceed 5 days because of the increased risk of serious adverse events.
● The recommended total daily dose of TORADOL^ORAL (maximum 40 mg) is significantly lower than for TORADOL^IV/IM (maximum 120 mg) (see DOSAGE AND ADMINISTRATION and *Transition from TORADOL^IV/IM to TORADOL^ORAL*).

SPECIAL POPULATIONS
● Dosage should be adjusted for patients 65 years or older, for patients under 50 kg (110 lbs) of body weight (see DOSAGE AND ADMINISTRATION) and for patients with moderately elevated serum creatinine (see WARNINGS). Doses of TORADOL^IV/IM are not to exceed 60 mg (total dose per day) in these patients.

DESCRIPTION

TORADOL (ketorolac tromethamine) is a member of the pyrrolo-pyrrole group of nonsteroidal anti-inflammatory drugs (NSAIDs). The chemical name for ketorolac tromethamine is (±)-5-benzoyl-2,3-dihydro-1H-pyrrolizine-1-carboxylic acid, compound with 2-amino-2-(hydroxymethyl)-1,3-propanediol.

TORADOL is a racemic mixture of [−]S and [+]R ketorolac tromethamine. Ketorolac tromethamine may exist in three crystal forms. All forms are equally soluble in water. Ketorolac tromethamine has a pKa of 3.5 and an n-octanol/water partition coefficient of 0.26. The molecular weight of ketorolac tromethamine is 376.41.

TORADOL is available for intravenous (IV) or intramuscular (IM) administration as: 15 mg in 1 mL (1.5%) and 30 mg in 1 mL (3%) in sterile solution; 60 mg in 2 mL (3%) of ketorolac tromethamine in sterile solution is available for IM administration only. The solutions contain 10% (w/v) alcohol, USP, and 6.68 mg, 4.35 mg and 8.70 mg, respectively, of sodium chloride in sterile water. The pH is adjusted with sodium hydroxide or hydrochloric acid, and the solutions are packaged with nitrogen. The sterile solutions are clear and slightly yellow in color.

TORADOL^ORAL is available as round, white, film-coated, red-printed tablets. Each tablet contains 10 mg ketorolac tromethamine, the active ingredient, with added lactose, magnesium stearate and microcrystalline cellulose. The white film-coating contains hydroxypropyl methylcellulose, polyethylene glycol and titanium dioxide.

The tablets are printed with red ink that includes FD&C Red #40 Aluminum lake as the colorant. There is a large T printed on both sides of the tablet, as well as the word TORADOL on one side, and the word ROCHE on the other.

CLINICAL PHARMACOLOGY

Pharmacodynamics: Ketorolac tromethamine is a nonsteroidal anti-inflammatory drug (NSAID). Ketorolac tromethamine inhibits synthesis of prostaglandins and may be considered a peripherally acting analgesic. The biological activity of ketorolac tromethamine is associated with the S-form. Ketorolac tromethamine possesses no sedative or anxiolytic properties.

Pain relief was statistically different after TORADOL dosing from that of placebo at $1/2$ hour (the first time point at which it was measured) following the largest recommended doses of TORADOL and by 1 hour following the smallest recommended doses. The peak analgesic effect occurred within 2 to 3 hours and was not statistically significantly different over the recommended dosage range of TORADOL. The greatest difference between large and small doses of TORADOL by either route was in the duration of analgesia.

Pharmacokinetics: Ketorolac tromethamine is a racemic mixture of [−]S- and [+]R-enantiomeric forms, with the S-form having analgesic activity.

Continued on next page

Roche Laboratories—Cont.

Comparison of IV, IM and Oral Pharmacokinetics: The pharmacokinetics of ketorolac tromethamine, following IV, IM and oral doses of TORADOL, are compared in Table 1. The extent of bioavailability following administration of the ORAL and IM forms of TORADOL was equal to that following an IV bolus.

Linear Kinetics: Following administration of single ORAL, IM or IV doses of TORADOL in the recommended dosage ranges, the clearance of the racemate does not change. This implies that the pharmacokinetics of ketorolac tromethamine in humans, following single or multiple IM, IV or recommended oral doses of TORADOL, are linear. At the higher recommended doses, there is a proportional increase in the concentrations of free and bound racemate.

Binding and Distribution: The ketorolac tromethamine racemate has been shown to be highly protein bound (99%). Nevertheless, even plasma concentrations as high as 10 μg/mL will only occupy approximately 5% of the albumin binding sites. Thus, the unbound fraction for each enantiomer will be constant over the therapeutic range. A decrease in serum albumin, however, will result in increased free drug concentrations.

The mean apparent volume ($V\beta$) of ketorolac tromethamine following complete distribution was approximately 13 liters. This parameter was determined from single-dose data.

Metabolism: Ketorolac tromethamine is largely metabolized in the liver. The metabolic products are hydroxylated and conjugated forms of the parent drug. The products of metabolism, and some unchanged drug, are excreted in the urine.

Clearance and Excretion: A single-dose study with 10 mg TORADOL (n=9) demonstrated that the S-enantiomer is cleared approximately two times faster than the R-enantiomer and that the clearance was independent of the route of administration. This means that the ratio of S/R plasma concentrations decreases with time after each dose. There is little or no inversion of the R- to S- form in humans. The clearance of the racemate in normal subjects, elderly individuals and in hepatically and renally impaired patients is outlined in Table 2.

The half-life of the ketorolac tromethamine S-enantiomer was approximately 2.5 hours (SD ± 0.4) compared with 5 hours (SD ± 1.7) for the R-enantiomer. In other studies, the half-life for the racemate has been reported to lie within the range of 5 to 6 hours.

Accumulation: TORADOL administered as an IV bolus every 6 hours for 5 days to healthy subjects (n=13), showed no significant difference in C_{max} on Day 1 and Day 5. Trough levels averaged 0.29 μg/mL (SD ± 0.13) on Day 1 and 0.55 μg/mL (SD ± 0.23) on Day 6. Steady state was approached after the fourth dose.

Accumulation of ketorolac tromethamine has not been studied in special populations (elderly patients, renal failure patients or hepatic disease patients).

Effect of Food: Oral administration of TORADOL after a high-fat meal resulted in decreased peak and delayed time-to-peak concentrations of ketorolac tromethamine by about 1 hour. Antacids did not affect the extent of absorption.

Kinetics in Special Populations: Elderly Patients: Based on single-dose data only, the half-life of the ketorolac tromethamine racemate increased from 5 to 7 hours in the elderly (65 to 78 years) compared with young healthy volunteers (24 to 35 years) (see Table 2). There was little difference in the C_{max} for the two groups (elderly, 2.52 μg/mL ± 0.77; young, 2.99 μg/mL ± 1.03) (see PRECAUTIONS—*Use in the Elderly*).

Renally Impaired Patients: Based on single-dose data only, the mean half-life of ketorolac tromethamine in renally impaired patients is between 6 and 19 hours and is dependent on the extent of the impairment. There is poor correlation between creatinine clearance and total ketorolac tromethamine clearance in the elderly and populations with renal impairment (r=0.5).

In patients with renal disease, the AUC_∞ of each enantiomer increased by approximately 100% compared with healthy volunteers. The volume of distribution doubles for the S-enantiomer and increases by 1/5th for the R-enantiomer. The increase in volume of distribution of ketorolac tromethamine implies an increase in unbound fraction.

The AUC_∞-ratio of the ketorolac tromethamine enantiomers in healthy subjects and patients remained similar, indicating there was no selective excretion of either enantiomer in patients compared to healthy subjects (see WARNINGS—*Renal Effects*).

Hepatic Effects: There was no significant difference in estimates of half-life, AUC_∞ and C_{max} in 7 patients with liver disease compared to healthy volunteers (see PRECAUTIONS—*Hepatic Effects*).

Clinical Studies: The analgesic efficacy of intramuscularly, intravenously and orally administered TORADOL was in-

Table 1
Table of Approximate Average Pharmacokinetic Parameters (Mean ± SD)
Following Oral, Intramuscular and Intravenous Doses of TORADOL

Pharmacokinetic Parameters (units)	Oral*		Intramuscular†		Intravenous Bolus‡	
	10 mg	15 mg	30 mg	60 mg	15 mg	30 mg
Bioavailability (extent)			100%			
T_{max}^1 (min)	44 ± 34	33 ± 21§	44 ± 29	33 ± 21§	1.1 ± 0.7§	2.9 ± 1.8
C_{max}^2 (μg/mL) [single-dose]	0.87 ± 0.22	1.14 ± 0.32§	2.42 ± 0.68	4.55 ± 1.27§	2.47 ± 0.51§	4.65 ± 0.96
C_{max} (μg/mL) [steady state qid]	1.05 ± 0.26§	1.56 ± 0.44§	3.11 ± 0.87§	N/A"	3.09 ± 1.17§	6.85 ± 2.61
C_{min}^3 (μg/mL) [steady state qid]	0.29 ± 0.07§	0.47 ± 0.13§	0.93 ± 0.26§	N/A	0.61 ± 0.21§	1.04 ± 0.35
C_{avg}^4 (μg/mL) [steady state qid]	0.59 ± 0.20§	0.94 ± 0.29§	1.88 ± 0.59§	N/A	1.09 ± 0.30§	2.17 ± 0.59
$V\beta^5$ (L/kg)			——0.175 ± 0.039——		0.210 ± 0.044	

% Dose metabolized = <50   % Dose excreted in feces = 6

% Dose excreted in urine = 91   % Plasma protein binding = 99

* Derived from PO pharmacokinetic studies in 77 normal fasted volunteers
† Derived from IM pharmacokinetic studies in 54 normal volunteers
‡ Derived from IV pharmacokinetic studies in 24 normal volunteers

[1]Time-to-peak plasma concentration
[2]Peak plasma concentration
[3]Trough plasma concentration
[4]Average plasma concentration
[5]Volume of distribution

§Mean value was simulated from observed plasma concentration data and standard deviation was simulated from percent coefficient of variation for observed C_{max} and T_{max} data
"Not applicable because 60 mg is only recommended as a single dose

Table 2
The Influence of Age, Liver and Kidney Function, on the Clearance
and Terminal Half-life of TORADOL (IM[1] and ORAL[2])

Type of Subjects	Total Clearance [In L/h/kg][3]		Terminal Half-life [In hours]	
	IM Mean (range)	ORAL Mean (range)	IM Mean (range)	ORAL Mean (range)
Normal Subjects IM (n=54) mean age=32, range=18–60 Oral (n=77) mean age=32, range=20–60	0.023 (0.010–0.046)	0.025 (0.013–0.050)	5.3 (3.5–9.2)	5.3 (2.4–9.0)
Healthy Elderly Subjects IM (n=13), Oral (n=12) mean age=72, range=65–78	0.019 (0.013–0.034)	0.024 (0.018–0.034)	7.0 (4.7–8.6)	6.1 (4.3–7.6)
Patients with Hepatic Dysfunction IM and Oral (n=7) mean age=51, range 43–64	0.029 (0.013–0.066)	0.033 (0.019–0.051)	5.4 (2.2–6.9)	4.5 (1.6–7.6)
Patients with Renal Impairment IM (n=25), Oral (n=9) serum creatinine=1.9–5.0 mg/dL, mean age (IM)=54, range=35–71 mean age (Oral)=57, range=39–70	0.015 (0.005–0.043)	0.016 (0.007–0.052)	10.3 (5.9–19.2)	10.8 (3.4–18.9)
Renal Dialysis Patients IM and Oral (n=9) mean age=40, range 27–63	0.016 (0.003–0.036)	—	13.6 (8.0–39.1)	—

[1]Estimated from 30 mg single IM doses of ketorolac tromethamine
[2]Estimated from 10 mg single oral doses of ketorolac tromethamine
[3]Liters/hour/kilogram

IV Administration: In normal subjects (n=37), the total clearance of 30 mg IV-administered TORADOL was 0.030 (0.017–0.051) L/h/kg. The terminal half-life was 5.6 (4.0–7.9) hours.

vestigated in two postoperative pain models: general surgery (orthopedic, gynecologic and abdominal) and oral surgery (removal of impacted third molars). The studies were double-blind, single- and multiple-dose, parallel trial designs in patients with moderate to severe pain at baseline. TORADOL[IV/IM] was compared as follows: IM to meperidine or morphine administered intramuscularly and IV to morphine administered either directly IV or through a PCA (Patient-Controlled Analgesia) pump.

Short-Term Use (up to 5 days) Studies: In the comparisons of intramuscular administration during the first hour, the onset of analgesic action was similar for TORADOL and the narcotics, but the duration of analgesia was longer with TORADOL than with the opioid comparators meperidine or morphine.

[See Table 1 above.]
[See Table 2 above.]

In a multidose, postoperative (general surgery) double-blind trial of TORADOL[IM] 30 mg versus morphine 6 and 12 mg IM, each drug given on an as needed basis for up to 5 days, the overall analgesic effect of TORADOL[IM] 30 mg was between that of morphine 6 and 12 mg. The majority of patients

treated with either TORADOL or morphine were dosed for up to 3 days; a small percentage of patients received 5 days of dosing.

In clinical settings where perioperative morphine was allowed, TORADOL[IV] 30 mg, given once or twice as needed, provided analgesia comparable to morphine 4 mg IV once or twice as needed.

There was relatively limited experience with 5 consecutive days of TORADOL[IV] use in controlled clinical trials, as most patients were given the drug for 3 days or less. The adverse events seen with IV-administered TORADOL were similar to those observed with IM-administered TORADOL, as would be expected based on the similar pharmacokinetics and bioequivalence (AUC, clearance, plasma half-life) of IV and IM routes of TORADOL administration.

Clinical Studies with Concomitant Use of Opioids: Clinical studies in postoperative pain management have demonstrated that TORADOL[IV/IM], when used in combination with opioids, significantly reduced opioid consumption. This combination may be useful in the subpopulation of patients especially prone to opioid-related complications. TORADOL and narcotics should not be administered in the same syringe.

In a postoperative study, where all patients received morphine by a PCA device, patients treated with TORADOL^{IV} as fixed intermittent boluses (eg, 30 mg initial dose followed by 15 mg q3h), required significantly less morphine (26%) than the placebo group. Analgesia was significantly superior, at various postdosing pain assessment times, in the patients receiving TORADOL^{IV} plus PCA morphine as compared to patients receiving PCA-administered morphine alone.

Postmarketing Surveillance Study: A large postmarketing observational, nonrandomized study, involving approximately 10,000 patients receiving TORADOL, demonstrated that the risk of clinically serious gastrointestinal (GI) bleeding was dose-dependent (see Tables 3A and 3B). This was particularly true in elderly patients who received an average daily dose greater than 60 mg/day of TORADOL (Table 3A).

Table 3
Incidence of Clinically Serious GI Bleeding as Related to Age, Total Daily Dose, and History of GI Perforation, Ulcer, Bleeding (PUB) after up to 5 Days of Treatment with TORADOL$^{IV/IM}$

A. Patients without History of PUB

	Total Daily Dose of TORADOL$^{IV/IM}$			
Age of Patients	≤60 mg	>60 to 90 mg	>90 to 120 mg	>120 mg
<65 years of age	0.4%	0.4%	0.9%	4.6%
≥65 years of age	1.2%	2.8%	2.2%	7.7%

B. Patients with History of PUB

	Total Daily Dose of TORADOL$^{IV/IM}$			
Age of Patients	≤60 mg	>60 to 90 mg	>90 to 120 mg	>120 mg
<65 years of age	2.1%	4.6%	7.8%	15.4%
≥65 years of age	4.7%	3.7%	2.8%	25.0%

INDICATIONS AND USAGE

TORADOL is indicated for the short-term (≤5 days) management of moderately severe acute pain that requires analgesia at the opioid level, usually in a postoperative setting. Therapy should always be initiated with TORADOL$^{IV/IM}$, and TORADOL^{ORAL} is to be used only as continuation treatment, if necessary. Combined use of TORADOL$^{IV/IM}$ and TORADOL^{ORAL} is not to exceed 5 days of use because of the potential of increasing the frequency and severity of adverse reactions associated with the recommended doses (see WARNINGS, PRECAUTIONS, DOSAGE AND ADMINISTRATION and ADVERSE REACTIONS). Patients should be switched to alternative analgesics as soon as possible, but TORADOL therapy is not to exceed 5 days.

TORADOL$^{IV/IM}$ has been used concomitantly with morphine and meperidine and has shown an opioid-sparing effect. For breakthrough pain, it is recommended to supplement the lower end of the TORADOL$^{IV/IM}$ dosage range with low doses of narcotics prn, unless otherwise contraindicated. TORADOL$^{IV/IM}$ and narcotics should not be administered in the same syringe (see DOSAGE AND ADMINISTRATION—*Pharmaceutical Information for TORADOL$^{IV/IM}$*).

CONTRAINDICATIONS

(see also Boxed WARNING):

- TORADOL is CONTRAINDICATED in patients with active peptic ulcer disease, in patients with recent gastrointestinal bleeding or perforation and in patients with a history of peptic ulcer disease or gastrointestinal bleeding.
- TORADOL is CONTRAINDICATED in patients with advanced renal impairment or in patients at risk for renal failure due to volume depletion (see WARNINGS for correction of volume depletion).
- TORADOL is CONTRAINDICATED in labor and delivery because, through its prostaglandin synthesis inhibitory effect, it may adversely affect fetal circulation and inhibit uterine contractions, thus increasing the risk of uterine hemorrhage.
- The use of TORADOL is CONTRAINDICATED in nursing mothers because of the potential adverse effects of prostaglandin-inhibiting drugs on neonates.
- TORADOL is CONTRAINDICATED in patients with previously demonstrated hypersensitivity to ketorolac tromethamine, allergic manifestations to aspirin or other nonsteroidal anti-inflammatory drugs (NSAIDs).
- TORADOL is CONTRAINDICATED as prophylactic analgesic before any major surgery and is CONTRAINDICATED intraoperatively when hemostasis is critical because of the increased risk of bleeding.
- TORADOL inhibits platelet function and is, therefore, CONTRAINDICATED in patients with suspected or confirmed cerebrovascular bleeding, hemorrhagic diathesis, incomplete hemostasis and those at high risk of bleeding (see WARNINGS and PRECAUTIONS).
- TORADOL is CONTRAINDICATED in patients currently receiving ASA or NSAIDs because of the cumulative risks of inducing serious NSAID-related adverse events.
- TORADOL$^{IV/IM}$ is CONTRAINDICATED for neuraxial (epidural or intrathecal) administration due to its alcohol content.
- The concomitant use of TORADOL and probenecid is CONTRAINDICATED.

WARNINGS

(see also Boxed WARNING):

The combined use of TORADOL$^{IV/IM}$ and TORADOL^{ORAL} is not to exceed 5 days.

The most serious risks associated with TORADOL are:

- ***Gastrointestinal Ulcerations, Bleeding and Perforation:*** TORADOL is CONTRAINDICATED in patients with previously documented peptic ulcers and/or GI bleeding. Serious gastrointestinal toxicity, such as bleeding, ulceration and perforation, can occur at any time, with or without warning symptoms, in patients treated with TORADOL. Studies to date with NSAIDs have not identified any subset of patients not at risk of developing peptic ulceration and bleeding. Elderly or debilitated patients seem to tolerate ulceration or bleeding less well than other individuals, and most spontaneous reports of fatal GI events are in this population. Postmarketing experience with parenterally administered TORADOL suggests that there may be a greater risk of gastrointestinal ulcerations, bleeding and perforation in the elderly.
The incidence and severity of gastrointestinal complications increases with increasing dose of, and duration of treatment with, TORADOL. In a nonrandomized, in-hospital postmarketing surveillance study comparing parenteral TORADOL to parenteral opioids, higher rates of clinically serious GI bleeding were seen in patients <65 years of age who received an average total daily dose of more than 90 mg of TORADOL$^{IV/IM}$ per day (see CLINICAL PHARMACOLOGY—*Postmarketing Surveillance Study*).
The same study showed that elderly (≥65 years of age) and debilitated patients are more susceptible to gastrointestinal complications. A history of peptic ulcer disease was revealed as another risk factor that increases the possibility of developing serious gastrointestinal complications during TORADOL therapy (see Tables 3A and 3B).
- ***Impaired Renal Function: TORADOL should be used with caution in patients with impaired renal function or a history of kidney disease because it is a potent inhibitor of prostaglandin synthesis.*** Renal toxicity with TORADOL has been seen in patients with conditions leading to a reduction in blood volume and/or renal blood flow where renal prostaglandins have a supportive role in the maintenance of renal perfusion. In these patients administration of TORADOL may cause a dose-dependent reduction in renal prostaglandin formation and may precipitate acute renal failure. Patients at greatest risk of this reaction are those with impaired renal function, dehydration, heart failure, liver dysfunction, those taking diuretics and the elderly. Discontinuation of TORADOL therapy is usually followed by recovery to the pretreatment state.
Renal Effects: TORADOL and its metabolites are eliminated primarily by the kidneys, which, in patients with reduced creatinine clearance, will result in diminished clearance of the drug (see CLINICAL PHARMACOLOGY). Therefore, TORADOL should be used with caution in patients with impaired renal function (see DOSAGE AND ADMINISTRATION) and such patients should be followed closely. With the use of TORADOL, there have been reports of acute renal failure, nephritis and nephrotic syndrome.
Because patients with underlying renal insufficiency are at increased risk of developing acute renal failure, the risks and benefits should be assessed prior to giving TORADOL to these patients. Hence, in patients with moderately elevated serum creatinine, it is recommended that the daily dose of TORADOL$^{IV/IM}$ be reduced by half, not to exceed 60 mg/day. **TORADOL IS CONTRAINDICATED IN PATIENTS WITH SERUM CREATININE CONCENTRATIONS INDICATING ADVANCED RENAL IMPAIRMENT** (see CONTRAINDICATIONS).
Hypovolemia should be corrected before treatment with TORADOL is initiated.
- ***Fluid Retention and Edema:*** Fluid retention, edema, retention of NaCl, oliguria, elevations of serum urea nitrogen and creatinine have been reported in clinical trials with TORADOL. Therefore, TORADOL should be used only very cautiously in patients with cardiac decompensation, hypertension or similar conditions.
- ***Hemorrhage:*** Because prostaglandins play an important role in hemostasis and NSAIDs affect platelet aggregation as well, use of TORADOL in patients who have coagulation disorders should be undertaken very cautiously, and those patients should be carefully monitored. Patients on therapeutic doses of anticoagulants (eg, heparin or dicumarol derivatives) have an increased risk of bleeding complications if given TORADOL concurrently; therefore, physicians should administer such concomitant therapy only extremely cautiously. The concurrent use of TORADOL and prophylactic low-dose heparin (2500 to 5000 units q12h), warfarin and dextrans have not been studied extensively, but may also be associated with an increased risk of bleeding. Until data from such studies are available, physicians should carefully weigh the benefits against the risks and use such concomitant therapy in these patients only extremely cautiously. In patients who receive anticoagulants for any reason, there is an increased risk of intramuscular hematoma formation from administered TORADOL^{IM} (see PRECAUTIONS—*Drug Interactions*). Patients receiving therapy that affects hemostasis should be monitored closely.
In postmarketing experience, postoperative hematomas and other signs of wound bleeding have been reported in association with the perioperative use of TORADOL$^{IV/IM}$. Therefore, perioperative use of TORADOL should be avoided and postoperative use be undertaken with caution when hemostasis is critical (see WARNINGS and PRECAUTIONS).
- ***Anaphylactoid Reactions:*** Anaphylactoid reactions may occur in patients without a known previous exposure or hypersensitivity to aspirin, TORADOL or other NSAIDs, or in individuals with a history of angioedema, bronchospastic reactivity (eg, asthma) and nasal polyps. Anaphylactoid reactions, like anaphylaxis, may have a fatal outcome.

PRECAUTIONS

General:

- *Hepatic Effects: TORADOL should be used with caution in patients with impaired hepatic function or a history of liver disease.* Treatment with TORADOL may cause elevations of liver enzymes, and, in patients with pre-existing liver dysfunction, it may lead to the development of a more severe hepatic reaction. The administration of TORADOL should be discontinued in patients in whom an abnormal liver test has occurred as a result of TORADOL therapy.
- *Hematologic Effects:* TORADOL inhibits platelet aggregation and may prolong bleeding time; therefore, it is contraindicated as a preoperative medication, and caution should be used when hemostasis is critical. Unlike aspirin, the inhibition of platelet function by TORADOL disappears within 24 to 48 hours after the drug is discontinued. TORADOL does not appear to affect platelet count, prothrombin time (PT) or partial thromboplastin time (PTT). In controlled clinical studies, where TORADOL was administered intramuscularly or intravenously postoperatively, the incidence of clinically significant postoperative bleeding was 0.4% for TORADOL compared to 0.2% in the control groups receiving narcotic analgesics.

Information for Patients: TORADOL is a potent NSAID and may cause serious side effects such as gastrointestinal bleeding or kidney failure, which may result in hospitalization and even fatal outcome.

Physicians, when prescribing TORADOL, should inform their patients of the potential risks of TORADOL treatment (see Boxed WARNING, WARNINGS, PRECAUTIONS and ADVERSE REACTIONS sections). *Advise patients not to give TORADOL^{ORAL} to other family members and to discard any unused drug.*

Remember that the total duration of TORADOL therapy is not to exceed 5 days.

Drug Interactions: Ketorolac is highly bound to human plasma protein (mean 99.2%).

The in vitro binding of ***warfarin*** to plasma proteins is only slightly reduced by ketorolac tromethamine (99.5% control vs 99.3%) when ketorolac plasma concentrations reach 5 to 10 μg/mL. Ketorolac does not alter ***digoxin*** protein binding. In vitro studies indicate that, at therapeutic concentrations of ***salicylate*** (300 μg/mL), the binding of ketorolac was reduced from approximately 99.2% to 97.5%, representing a potential twofold increase in unbound ketorolac plasma levels. Therapeutic concentrations of ***digoxin, warfarin, ibuprofen, naproxen, piroxicam, acetaminophen, phenytoin*** and ***tolbutamide*** did not alter ketorolac tromethamine protein binding.

In a study involving 12 volunteers, TORADOL^{ORAL} was coadministered with a single dose of 25 mg ***warfarin***, causing no significant changes in pharmacokinetics or pharmacodynamics of warfarin. In another study, TORADOL$^{IV/IM}$ was given with two doses of 5000 U of ***heparin*** to 11 healthy volunteers, resulting in a mean template bleeding time of 6.4 minutes (3.2 to 11.4 min) compared to a mean of 6.0 minutes (3.4 to 7.5 min) for heparin alone and 5.1 minutes (3.5 to 8.5 min) for placebo. Although these results do not indicate a significant interaction between TORADOL and warfarin or heparin, the administration of TORADOL to patients taking anticoagulants should be done extremely cautiously, and patients should be closely monitored (see WARNINGS and PRECAUTIONS).

Continued on next page

Roche Laboratories—Cont.

TORADOL[IV/IM] reduced the diuretic response to *furosemide* in normovolemic healthy subjects by approximately 20% (mean sodium and urinary output decreased 17%).

Concomitant administration of TORADOL[ORAL] and *probenecid* resulted in decreased clearance of ketorolac and significant increases in ketorolac plasma levels (total AUC increased approximately threefold from 5.4 to 17.8 µg/h/mL) and terminal half-life increased approximately twofold from 6.6 to 15.1 hours. Therefore, concomitant use of TORADOL and probenecid is contraindicated.

Inhibition of renal *lithium* clearance, leading to an increase in plasma lithium concentration, has been reported with some prostaglandin synthesis-inhibiting drugs. The effect of TORADOL on plasma lithium has not been studied, but cases of increased lithium plasma levels during TORADOL therapy have been reported.

Concomitant administration of *methotrexate* and some NSAIDs has been reported to reduce the clearance of methotrexate, enhancing the toxicity of methotrexate. The effect of TORADOL on methotrexate clearance has not been studied. In postmarketing experience there have been reports of a possible interaction between TORADOL[IV/IM] and *non-depolarizing muscle relaxants* that resulted in apnea. The concurrent use of TORADOL with muscle relaxants has not been formally studied.

Concomitant use of *ACE inhibitors* may increase the risk of renal impairment, particularly in volume-depleted patients.

Sporadic cases of seizures have been reported during concomitant use of TORADOL and *antiepileptic drugs* (phenytoin, carbamazepine).

Hallucinations have been reported when TORADOL was used in patients taking *psychoactive drugs* (fluoxetine, thiothixene, alprazolam).

TORADOL[IV/IM] has been administered concurrently with *morphine* in several clinical trials of postoperative pain without evidence of adverse interactions. Do not mix TORADOL and morphine in the same syringe.

There is no evidence in animal or human studies that TORADOL induces or inhibits hepatic enzymes capable of metabolizing itself or other drugs.

Carcinogenesis, Mutagenesis and Impairment of Fertility: An 18-month study in mice with oral doses of ketorolac tromethamine at 2 mg/kg/day (0.9 times the human systemic exposure at the recommended IM or IV dose of 30 mg qid, based on area-under-the-plasma-concentration curve [AUC]), and a 24-month study in rats at 5 mg/kg/day (0.5 times the human AUC) showed no evidence of tumorigenicity.

Ketorolac tromethamine was not mutagenic in the Ames test, unscheduled DNA synthesis and repair, and in forward mutation assays. Ketorolac tromethamine did not cause chromosome breakage in the in vivo mouse micronucleus assay. At 1590 µg/mL and at higher concentrations, ketorolac tromethamine increased the incidence of chromosomal aberrations in Chinese hamster ovarian cells.

Impairment of fertility did not occur in male or female rats at oral doses of 9 mg/kg (0.9 times the human AUC) and 16 mg/kg (1.6 times the human AUC) of ketorolac tromethamine, respectively.

Pregnancy: Pregnancy Category C. Reproduction studies have been performed during organogenesis using daily oral doses of ketorolac tromethamine at 3.6 mg/kg (0.37 times the human AUC) in rabbits and at 10 mg/kg (1.0 times the human AUC) in rats. Results of these studies did not reveal evidence of teratogenicity to the fetus. Oral doses of ketorolac tromethamine at 1.5 mg/kg (0.14 times the human AUC), administered after gestation Day 17, caused dystocia and higher pup mortality in rats. There are no adequate and well-controlled studies of TORADOL in pregnant women. TORADOL should be used during pregnancy only if the potential benefit justifies the potential risk to the fetus.

Labor and Delivery: The use of TORADOL is contraindicated in labor and delivery because, through its prostaglandin synthesis inhibitory effect, it may adversely affect fetal circulation and inhibit uterine contractions, thus increasing the risk of uterine hemorrhage (see CONTRAINDICATIONS).

Lactation and Nursing: After a single administration of 10 mg of TORADOL[ORAL] to humans, the maximum milk concentration observed was 7.3 ng/mL, and the maximum milk-to-plasma ratio was 0.037. After 1 day of dosing (qid), the maximum milk concentration was 7.9 ng/mL, and the maximum milk-to-plasma ratio was 0.025. Because of the possible adverse effects of prostaglandin-inhibiting drugs on neonates, use in nursing mothers is contraindicated.

Pediatric Use: Safety and efficacy in children (less than 16 years of age) have not been established. Therefore, use of TORADOL in children is not recommended.

Use in the Elderly (≥ 65 years of age): Because ketorolac tromethamine may be cleared more slowly by the elderly (see CLINICAL PHARMACOLOGY) who are also more sensitive to the adverse effects of NSAIDs (see WAR-

NINGS—*Renal Effects*), extra caution and reduced dosages (see DOSAGE AND ADMINISTRATION) must be used when treating the elderly with TORADOL[IV/IM]. The lower end of the TORADOL[IV/IM] dosage range is recommended for patients over 65 years of age, and total daily dose is not to exceed 60 mg. The incidence and severity of gastrointestinal complications increases with increasing dose of, and duration of treatment with, TORADOL.

ADVERSE REACTIONS

Adverse reaction rates increase with higher doses of TORADOL. Practitioners should be alert for the severe complications of treatment with TORADOL, such as GI ulceration, bleeding and perforation, postoperative bleeding, acute renal failure, anaphylactic and anaphylactoid reactions and liver failure (see Boxed WARNING, WARNINGS, PRECAUTIONS and DOSAGE AND ADMINISTRATION). These NSAID-related complications can be serious in certain patients for whom TORADOL is indicated, especially when the drug is used inappropriately.

The Adverse Reactions Listed Below Were Reported In Clinical Trials As Probably Related To TORADOL:

● *Incidence Greater Than 1%*
Percentage of incidence in parentheses for those events reported in 3% or more patients.
Body as a Whole: edema (4%)
Cardiovascular: hypertension
Dermatologic: pruritus, rash
Gastrointestinal: nausea (12%), dyspepsia (12%), gastrointestinal pain (13%), diarrhea (7%), constipation, flatulence, gastrointestinal fullness, vomiting, stomatitis
Hemic and Lymphatic: purpura
Nervous System: headache (17%), drowsiness (6%), dizziness (7%), sweating
Injection-site pain was reported by 2% of patients in multidose studies.

● *Incidence 1% or Less*
Body as a Whole: weight gain, fever, infections, asthenia
Cardiovascular: palpitation, pallor, syncope
Dermatologic: urticaria
Gastrointestinal: gastritis, rectal bleeding, eructation, anorexia, increased appetite
Hemic and Lymphatic: epistaxis, anemia, eosinophilia
Nervous System: tremors, abnormal dreams, hallucinations, euphoria, extrapyramidal symptoms, vertigo, paresthesia, depression, insomnia, nervousness, excessive thirst, dry mouth, abnormal thinking, inability to concentrate, hyperkinesis, stupor
Respiratory: dyspnea, pulmonary edema, rhinitis, cough
Special Senses: abnormal taste, abnormal vision, blurred vision, tinnitus, hearing loss
Urogenital: hematuria, proteinuria, oliguria, urinary retention, polyuria, increased urinary frequency
The Following Adverse Events Were Reported From Postmarketing Experience:
Body as a Whole: hypersensitivity reactions such as anaphylaxis, anaphylactoid reaction, laryngeal edema, tongue edema (see Boxed WARNING, WARNINGS), myalgia
Cardiovascular: hypotension, flushing
Dermatologic: Lyell's syndrome, Stevens-Johnson syndrome, exfoliative dermatitis, maculopapular rash, urticaria
Gastrointestinal: peptic ulceration, GI hemorrhage, GI perforation (see Boxed WARNING, WARNINGS), melena, acute pancreatitis
Hemic and Lymphatic: postoperative wound hemorrhage (rarely requiring blood transfusion—see Boxed WARNING, WARNINGS and PRECAUTIONS), thrombocytopenia, leukopenia
Hepatic: hepatitis, liver failure, cholestatic jaundice
Nervous System: convulsions, psychosis, aseptic meningitis
Respiratory: asthma, bronchospasm
Urogenital: acute renal failure (see Boxed WARNING, WARNINGS), flank pain with or without hematuria and/or azotemia, nephritis, hyponatremia, hyperkalemia, hemolytic uremic syndrome

OVERDOSAGE

In controlled overdosage, daily doses of 360 mg of TORADOL[IV/IM] given for 5 days (three times the highest recommended dose), caused abdominal pain and peptic ulcers which healed after discontinuation of dosing. Metabolic acidosis has been reported following intentional overdosage. Dialysis does not significantly clear ketorolac tromethamine from the blood stream.

DOSAGE AND ADMINISTRATION

THE COMBINED DURATION OF USE OF TORADOL[IV/IM] AND TORADOL[ORAL] IS NOT TO EXCEED 5 DAYS.
THE USE OF TORADOL[ORAL] IS ONLY INDICATED AS CONTINUATION THERAPY TO TORADOL[IV/IM]
TORADOL[IV/IM]
TORADOL[IV/IM] may be used as a single or multiple dose on a regular or prn schedule for the management of moderately severe acute pain that requires analgesia at the opioid level, usually in a postoperative setting. Hypovolemia should be corrected prior to the administration of TORADOL (see WARNINGS—*Renal Effects*). Patients should be switched to

alternative analgesics as soon as possible, but TORADOL therapy is not to exceed 5 days.

When administering TORADOL[IV/IM], the IV bolus must be given over no less than 15 seconds. The IM administration should be given slowly and deeply into the muscle. The analgesic effect begins in ~30 minutes with maximum effect in 1 to 2 hours after dosing IV or IM. Duration of analgesic effect is usually 4 to 6 hours.

Single-Dose Treatment: The Following Regimen Should Be Limited To Single Administration Use Only
IM Dosing:
● *Patients < 65 years of age:* One dose of 60 mg.
● *Patients ≥ 65 years of age, renally impaired and/or less than 50 kg (110 lbs) of body weight:* One dose of 30 mg.
IV Dosing:
● *Patients < 65 years of age:* One dose of 30 mg.
● *Patients ≥ 65 years of age, renally impaired and/or less than 50 kg (110 lbs) of body weight:* One dose of 15 mg.
Multiple-Dose Treatment (IV or IM)
● *Patients < 65 years of age:* The recommended dose is 30 mg TORADOL[IV/IM] every 6 hours. The maximum daily dose should not exceed 120 mg.
● *For Patients ≥ 65 years of age, renally impaired patients (see WARNINGS) and patients less than 50 kg (110 lbs):* The recommended dose is 15 mg TORADOL[IV/IM] every 6 hours. The maximum daily dose for these populations should not exceed 60 mg.

For breakthrough pain do not increase the dose or the frequency of TORADOL. Consideration should be given to supplementing these regimens with low doses of opioids prn unless otherwise contraindicated.

Pharmaceutical Information for TORADOL[IV/IM]: Parenteral drug products should be inspected visually for particulate matter and discoloration prior to administration whenever solution and container permit.

TORADOL[IV/IM] should not be mixed in a small volume (eg, in a syringe) with morphine sulfate, meperidine hydrochloride, promethazine hydrochloride or hydroxyzine hydrochloride; this will result in precipitation of ketorolac from solution.

TORADOL[ORAL] is indicated ONLY as continuation therapy to TORADOL[IV/IM] for the management of moderately severe acute pain that requires analgesia at the opioid level (see also PRECAUTIONS—*Information for Patients*).

Transition from TORADOL[IV/IM] to TORADOL[ORAL]: The recommended TORADOL[ORAL] dose is as follows:
● *Patients < 65 years of age:* 2 tablets as a first oral dose for patients who received **60 mg IM single dose, 30 mg IV single dose or 30 mg multiple dose.** TORADOL[IV/IM] followed by 1 tablet TORADOL[ORAL] every 4 to 6 hours, not to exceed 40 mg/24 h of TORADOL[ORAL].
● *Patients ≥ 65 years of age, renally impaired and/or less than 50 kg (110 lbs) of body weight:* 1 tablet as a first oral dose for patients who received **30 mg IM single dose, 15 mg IV single dose or 15 mg multiple dose.** TORADOL[IV/IM] followed by 1 tablet TORADOL[ORAL] every 4 to 6 hours, not to exceed 40 mg/24 h of TORADOL[ORAL].

Shortening the recommended dosing intervals may result in increased frequency and severity of adverse reactions.

The maximum combined duration of use (parenteral and oral TORADOL) is limited to 5 days.

The TUBEX® BLUNT POINTE™ Sterile Cartridge Unit is suitable for substances to be administered intravenously only. It is intended for use with injection sets specifically manufactured as "needle-less" injection systems. TUBEX® BLUNT POINTE™ is compatible with Abbott's LifeShield® prepierced reseal injection site, Baxter's InterLink® Injection Site, and B. Braun Medical's SafSite® Reflux Valve. Consult manufacturer's recommendations regarding "Directions for Use" of the "needle-less" system. It is also intended for admixture with, and convenient administration of, various medicaments when using Drug Vial Adapters for "needle-less" injection systems.

The TUBEX® Sterile Cartridge-Needle Unit is suitable for substances to be administered intravenously and intramuscularly.

HOW SUPPLIED

TORADOL[IV/IM] for intramuscular or intravenous use is available in a TUBEX® Cartridge-Needle Unit:
15 mg: 15 mg/mL, 1 mL TUBEX® Sterile Cartridge-Needle Unit (22 gauge × 1-1/4 inch needle) box of 10 (NDC 0004-6921-06).
30 mg: 30 mg/mL, 1 mL TUBEX® Sterile Cartridge-Needle Unit (22 gauge × 1-1/4 inch needle) box of 10 (NDC 0004-6923-06).
For IM Single-Dose Use Only—60 mg: 30 mg/mL, 2 mL TUBEX® Sterile Cartridge-Needle Unit (22 gauge × 1-1/4 inch needle) box of 1 (NDC 0004-6924-09).
TORADOL[IV] for intravenous use is available in a TUBEX® BLUNT POINTE™ Sterile Cartridge Unit:
15 mg: 15 mg/mL, 1 mL TUBEX® BLUNT POINTE™ Sterile Cartridge Unit, box of 10 (NDC 0004-6920-06).
30 mg: 30 mg/mL, 1 mL TUBEX® BLUNT POINTE™ Sterile Cartridge Unit, box of 10 (NDC 0004-6922-06).

Manufactured by Wyeth Laboratories, Inc., Philadelphia, PA 19101 for Hoffmann-La Roche Inc., Nutley, NJ 07110.
Store at 15° to 30°C (59° to 86°F) with protection from light.
TORADOL^{ORAL} 10 mg tablets are available in bottles of 100 tablets (NDC 0033-2435-42).
Store bottles at 15° to 30°C (59° to 86°F).
Manufactured by Syntex Puerto Rico, Inc., Humacao, PR 00791

TUBEX® Injector
NOTE: The TUBEX® Injector is reusable: do not discard.
TUBEX® Sterile Cartridge-Needle Unit
DIRECTIONS FOR USE

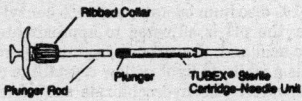

TUBEX® BLUNT POINTE™ Sterile Cartridge Unit
DIRECTIONS FOR USE:

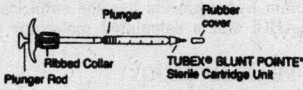

TUBEX® BLUNT POINTE™ Sterile Cartridge Unit is intended for use with injection sets specifically manufactured as "needle-less" injection systems.
TUBEX® BLUNT POINTE™ Sterile Cartridge Unit is compatible with Abbott's LifeShield® prepierced reseal injection site, Baxter's InterLink® Injection Site and B. Braun Medical's SafSite® Reflux Valve. Consult manufacturer's recommendations regarding "Directions for Use" of the "needle-less" injection system.

To load a TUBEX® Sterile Cartridge Unit into the TUBEX® Injector
1. Turn the ribbed collar to the "OPEN" position until it stops.

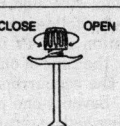

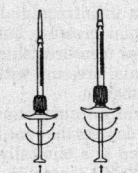

2. Hold the Injector with the open end up and fully insert the TUBEX® Sterile Cartridge Unit.
Firmly tighten the ribbed collar in the direction of the "CLOSE" arrow.
3. Thread the plunger rod into the plunger of the TUBEX® Sterile Cartridge Unit until slight resistance is felt. The Injector is now ready for use in the usual manner.

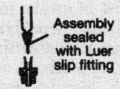

To administer TUBEX® Sterile Cartridge-Needle Units
Method of administration is the same as with conventional syringe. Remove needle cover by grasping it securely; twist and pull. Introduce needle into patient, aspirate by pulling back slightly on the plunger, and inject.

To administer TUBEX® BLUNT POINTE™ Sterile Cartridge Units
"Needle-less" IV set administration is similar to administration with conventional syringes. Remove rubber cover by grasping it securely; twist and pull. For B. Braun Medical's SafSite® Reflux Valves, aseptically swab the luer slip fitting of the BLUNT POINTE™ sterile cartridge tip assembly with a sterile, individually wrapped, saturated 70% Isopropyl Alcohol swab. This action will remove the lubricant coating from the tip to facilitate a tight seal. Introduce TUBEX® BLUNT POINTE™ Sterile Cartridge Unit into the "needle-less" IV set as per manufacturer's "Directions for Use."

To remove the empty TUBEX® Cartridge Unit and dispose into a vertical disposal container
1. Do not recap the needle/point.
Disengage the plunger rod.

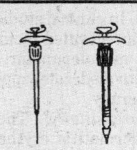

2. Hold the Injector, needle/point down, over a vertical disposal container and loosen the ribbed collar. TUBEX® Cartridge Unit will drop into the container.

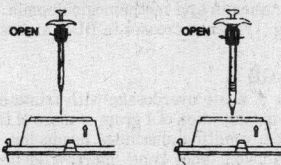

3. Discard the cover.

To remove the empty TUBEX® Cartridge Unit and dispose into a horizontal (mailbox) disposal container
1. Do not recap the needle/point. Disengage the plunger rod.
2. Open the horizontal (mailbox) disposal container. Insert TUBEX® Cartridge Unit, needle/point pointing down, halfway into container. Close the container lid on cartridge. Loosen ribbed collar; TUBEX® Cartridge Unit will drop into the container.
3. Discard the cover.
The TUBEX® Injector is reusable and should not be discarded.
Used TUBEX® Cartridge Units should not be employed for successive injections or as multiple-dose containers. They are intended to be used only once and discarded.
NOTE: Any graduated markings on TUBEX® Sterile Cartridge Units are to be used only as a guide in mixing, withdrawing, or administering measured doses.

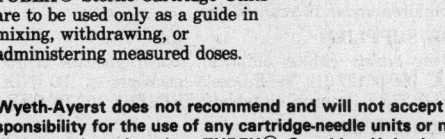

Wyeth-Ayerst does not recommend and will not accept responsibility for the use of any cartridge-needle units or needle-less units other than TUBEX® Cartridge Units in the TUBEX® Injector.

Revised July 1995
Shown in Product Identification Guide, page 332

TRIMPEX®   ℞
[trim 'pex]
brand of trimethoprim
TABLETS

The following text is complete prescribing information based on official labeling in effect June 1996.

DESCRIPTION

Trimpex (trimethoprim) is a synthetic antibacterial available as 100-mg tablets for oral administration. Each tablet also contains lactose, magnesium stearate, sodium starch glycolate and pregelatinized starch.
Trimethoprim is 2,4-diamino-5-(3,4,5-trimethoxybenzyl) pyrimidine. It is a white to light yellow, odorless, bitter compound with a molecular weight of 290.3.

CLINICAL PHARMACOLOGY

Trimethoprim is rapidly absorbed following oral administration. It exists in the blood as unbound, protein-bound and metabolized forms. Ten percent to 20% of trimethoprim is metabolized, primarily in the liver; the remainder is excreted unchanged in the urine. The principal metabolites of trimethoprim are the 1- and 3-oxides and the 3'- and 4'-hydroxy derivatives. The free form is considered to be the therapeutically active form. Approximately 44% of trimethoprim is bound to plasma proteins.
Mean peak plasma concentrations of approximately 1 mcg/mL occur 1 to 4 hours after oral administration of a single 100-mg dose. A single 200-mg dose will result in plasma concentrations approximately twice as high. The half-life of trimethoprim ranges from 8 to 10 hours. However, patients with severely impaired renal function exhibit an increase in half-life of trimethoprim, which requires either dosage regimen adjustment or not using the drug in such patients (see DOSAGE AND ADMINISTRATION section). During a 13-week study of trimethoprim administered at a dosage of 50 mg qid, the mean minimum steady-state concentration of the

---

drug was 1.1 mcg/mL. Steady-state concentrations were achieved within 2 to 3 days of chronic administration and were maintained throughout the experimental period.
Excretion of trimethoprim is primarily by the kidneys through glomerular filtration and tubular secretion. Urine concentrations of trimethoprim are considerably higher than are the concentrations in the blood. After a single oral dose of 100 mg, urine concentrations of trimethoprim ranged from 30 to 160 mcg/mL during the 0- to 4-hour period and declined to approximately 18 to 91 mcg/mL during the 8- to 24-hour period. A 200-mg single oral dose will result in trimethoprim urine concentrations approximately twice as high. After oral administration, 50% to 60% of trimethoprim is excreted in urine within 24 hours, approximately 80% of this being unmetabolized trimethoprim.
Since normal vaginal and fecal flora are the source of most pathogens causing urinary tract infections, it is relevant to consider the distribution of trimethoprim into these sites. Concentrations of trimethoprim in vaginal secretions are consistently greater than those found simultaneously in the serum, being typically 1.6 times the concentrations of simultaneously obtained serum samples. Sufficient trimethoprim is excreted in the feces to markedly reduce or eliminate trimethoprim-susceptible organisms from the fecal flora. The dominant non-*Enterobacteriaceae* fecal organisms, *Bacteroides* spp. and *Lactobacillus* spp., are not susceptible to trimethoprim concentrations obtained with the recommended dosage.
Trimethoprim also passes the placental barrier and is excreted in breast milk.
Microbiology: Trimpex blocks the production of tetrahydrofolic acid from dihydrofolic acid by binding to and reversibly inhibiting the required enzyme, dihydrofolate reductase. This binding is very much stronger for the bacterial enzyme than for the corresponding mammalian enzyme. Thus, Trimpex selectively interferes with bacterial biosynthesis of nucleic acids and proteins.
In vitro serial dilution tests have shown that the spectrum of antibacterial activity of Trimpex includes the common urinary tract pathogens with the exception of *Pseudomonas aeruginosa.*

Representative Minimum Inhibitory Concentrations for Trimethoprim-Susceptible Organisms

Bacteria	Trimethoprim MIC— mcg/mL (Range)
Escherichia coli	0.05—1.5
Proteus mirabilis	0.5—1.5
Klebsiella pneumoniae	0.5—5.0
Enterobacter species	0.5—5.0
Staphylococcus species (coagulase-negative)	0.15—5.0

The recommended quantitative disc susceptibility method[1,2] may be used for estimating the susceptibility of bacteria to Trimpex. With this procedure, reports from the laboratory giving results using the 5-mcg trimethoprim disc should be interpreted according to the following criteria: Organisms producing zones of 16 mm or greater are classified as susceptible, whereas those producing zones of 11 to 15 mm are classified as having intermediate susceptibility. A report from the laboratory of "Susceptible to trimethoprim" or "Intermediate susceptibility to trimethoprim" indicates that the infection is likely to respond when, as in uncomplicated urinary tract infections, effective therapy is dependent upon the urine concentration of trimethoprim. Organisms producing zones of 10 mm or less are reported as resistant, indicating that other therapy should be selected.
Dilution methods for determining susceptibility are also used, and results are reported as the minimum drug concentration inhibiting microbial growth (MIC).[3] If the MIC is 8 mcg per mL or less, the microorganism is considered "susceptible." If the MIC is 16 mcg per mL or greater, the microorganism is considered "resistant."

INDICATIONS AND USAGE

For the treatment of initial episodes of uncomplicated urinary tract infections due to susceptible strains of the following organisms: *Escherichia coli, Proteus mirabilis, Klebsiella pneumoniae, Enterobacter* species and coagulase-negative *Staphylococcus* species, including *S. saprophyticus.*
Cultures and susceptibility tests should be performed to determine the susceptibility of the bacteria to trimethoprim. Therapy may be initiated prior to obtaining the results of these tests.

CONTRAINDICATIONS

Trimpex is contraindicated in individuals hypersensitive to trimethoprim and in those with documented megaloblastic anemia due to folate deficiency.

Continued on next page

Roche Laboratories—Cont.

WARNINGS

Serious hypersensitivity reactions have been reported rarely in patients on trimethoprim therapy. Trimethoprim has been reported rarely to interfere with hematopoiesis, especially when administered in large doses and/or for prolonged periods.

The presence of clinical signs such as sore throat, fever, pallor or purpura may be early indications of serious blood disorders.

PRECAUTIONS

General: Trimethoprim should be given with caution to patients with possible folate deficiency. Folates may be administered concomitantly without interfering with the antibacterial action of trimethoprim. Trimethoprim should also be given with caution to patients with impaired renal or hepatic function. If any clinical signs of a blood disorder are noted in a patient receiving trimethoprim, a complete blood count should be obtained and the drug discontinued if a significant reduction in the count of any formed blood element is found.

Drug Interactions: Trimpex may inhibit the hepatic metabolism of phenytoin. Trimethoprim, given at a common clinical dosage, increased the phenytoin half-life by 51% and decreased the phenytoin metabolic clearance rate by 30%. When administering these drugs concurrently, one should be alert for possible excessive phenytoin effect.

Drug/Laboratory Test Interactions: Trimethoprim can interfere with a serum methotrexate assay as determined by the competitive binding protein technique (CBPA) when a bacterial dihydrofolate reductase is used as the binding protein. No interference occurs, however, if methotrexate is measured by a radioimmunoassay (RIA).

The presence of trimethoprim may also interfere with the Jaffé alkaline picrate reaction assay for creatinine resulting in overestimations of about 10% in the range of normal values.

Carcinogenesis, Mutagenesis, Impairment of Fertility:
Carcinogenesis: Long-term studies in animals to evaluate carcinogenic potential have not been conducted with trimethoprim.

Mutagenesis: Trimethoprim was demonstrated to be non-mutagenic in the Ames assay. No chromosomal damage was observed in human leukocytes cultured *in vitro* with trimethoprim; the concentration used exceeded blood levels following therapy with Trimpex.

Impairment of fertility: No adverse effects on fertility or general reproductive performance were observed in rats given trimethoprim in oral dosages as high as 70 mg/kg/day for males and 14 mg/kg/day for females.

Pregnancy: Teratogenic Effects: Pregnancy Category C. Trimethoprim has been shown to be teratogenic in the rat when given in doses 40 times the human dose. In some rabbit studies, the overall increase in fetal loss (dead and resorbed and malformed conceptuses) was associated with doses 6 times the human therapeutic dose.

While there are no large well-controlled studies on the use of trimethoprim in pregnant women, Brumfitt and Pursell,[4] in a retrospective study, reported the outcome of 186 pregnancies during which the mother received either placebo or trimethoprim in combination wih sulfamethoxazole. The incidence of congenital abnormalities was 4.5% (3 of 66) in those who received placebo and 3.3% (4 of 120) in those receiving trimethoprim plus sulfamethoxazole. There were no abnormalities in the 10 children whose mothers received the drug during the first trimester. In a separate survey, Brumfitt and Pursell also found no congenital abnormalities in 35 children whose mothers had received trimethoprim plus sulfamethoxazole at the time of conception or shortly thereafter.

Because trimethoprim may interfere with folic acid metabolism, Trimpex should be used during pregnancy only if the potential benefit justifies the potential risk to the fetus.

Nonteratogenic Effects: The oral administration of trimethoprim to rats at a dose of 70 mg/kg/day commencing with the last third of gestation and continuing through parturition and lactation caused no deleterious effects on gestation or pup growth and survival.

Nursing Mothers: Trimethoprim is excreted in human milk. Because trimethoprim may interfere with folic acid metabolism, caution should be exercised when Trimpex is administered to a nursing woman.

Pediatric Use: The safety of trimethoprim in infants under two months of age has not been demonstrated. The effectiveness of trimethoprim has not been established in children under 12 years of age.

ADVERSE REACTIONS

The adverse effects encountered most often with trimethoprim were rash and pruritus. Other adverse effects reported involved the gastrointestinal and hematopoietic systems.

Dermatologic: Rash, pruritus and phototoxic skin eruptions. At the recommended dosage regimens of 100 mg bid or 200 mg qd, each for 10 days, the incidence of rash is 2.9% to 6.7%. In clinical studies which employed high doses of Trimpex, an elevated incidence of rash was noted. These rashes were maculopapular, morbilliform, pruritic and generally mild to moderate, appearing 7 to 14 days after the initiation of therapy.

Hypersensitivity: There have been rare reports of exfoliative dermatitis, erythema multiforme, Stevens-Johnson syndrome, Lyell syndrome, anaphylaxis and aseptic meningitis.

Gastrointestinal: Epigastric distress, nausea, vomiting and glossitis. Elevation of serum transaminase and bilirubin.

Hematologic: Thrombocytopenia, leukopenia, neutropenia, megaloblastic anemia and methemoglobinemia.

Miscellaneous: Fever, increases in BUN and serum creatinine levels.

OVERDOSAGE

Acute: Signs of acute overdosage with trimethoprim may appear following ingestion of 1 gram or more of the drug and include nausea, vomiting, dizziness, headaches, mental depression, confusion and bone marrow depression (see CHRONIC OVERDOSAGE).

Treatment consists of gastric lavage and general supportive measures. Acidification of the urine will increase renal elimination of trimethoprim. Peritoneal dialysis is not effective and hemodialysis only moderately effective in eliminating the drug.

Chronic: Use of trimethoprim at high doses and/or for extended periods of time may cause bone marrow depression manifested as thrombocytopenia, leukopenia and/or megaloblastic anemia. If signs of bone marrow depression occur, trimethoprim should be discontinued and the patient should be given leucovorin, 3 to 6 mg intramuscularly daily for 3 days, or as required to restore normal hematopoiesis.

DOSAGE AND ADMINISTRATION

The usual oral adult dosage is 100 mg (one tablet) every 12 hours or 200 mg (2 tablets) every 24 hours, each for 10 days. The use of trimethoprim in patients with a creatinine clearance of less than 15 mL/min is not recommended. For patients with a creatinine clearance of 15 to 30 mL/min, the dose should be 50 mg every 12 hours.

The effectiveness of trimethoprim has not been established in children under 12 years of age.

HOW SUPPLIED

100-mg tablets (white, elliptical, scored)—bottles of 100 (NDC 0004-0127-01); Tel-E-Dose® packages of 100 (NDC 0004-0127-49). Imprint on tablets: TRIMPEX 100 ROCHE.

REFERENCES

1. Bauer AW, Kirby WMM, Sherris JC, Turck M. Antibiotic Susceptibility Testing by Standardized Single Disk Method. *Am J Clin Pathol.* 1996; 45:493–496.
2. Approved Standard ASM-2 Performance Standards for Antimicrobial Disc Susceptibility Test; National Committee for Clinical Laboratory Standards, 771 East Lancaster Avenue, Villanova, Pennsylvania 19085.
3. Ericsson HM, Sherris JC. Antibiotic Sensitivity Testing. Report of an International Collaborative Study. *Acta Pathol Microbiol Scand.* 1971; [B] (Suppl 217): 1–90.
4. Brumfitt W, Pursell R: Trimethoprim/Sulfamethoxazole in the Treatment of Bacteriuria in Women, *J Infect Dis.* 1973; 128 (Suppl):S657–S663.
Revised: August 1993
Shown in Product Identification Guide, page 332

VERSED®
[ver-sed ']
midazolam HCl
INJECTION

The following text is complete prescribing information based on official labeling in effect June 1996.

Intravenous VERSED has been associated with respiratory depression and respiratory arrest, especially when used for conscious sedation. In some cases, where this was not recognized promptly and treated effectively, death or hypoxic encephalopathy has resulted. Intravenous VERSED should be used only in hospital or ambulatory care settings, including physicians' offices, that provide for continuous monitoring of respiratory and cardiac function. Immediate availability of resuscitative drugs and equipment and personnel trained in their use should be assured. (See WARNINGS.)
The initial intravenous dose for conscious sedation may be as little as 1 mg, but should not exceed 2.5 mg in a normal healthy adult. Lower doses are necessary for older (over 60 years) or debilitated patients and in patients receiving concomitant narcotics or other CNS depressants. The initial dose and all subsequent doses should never be given as a bolus; administer over at least 2 minutes and allow an additional 2 or more minutes to fully evaluate the sedative effect. The use of the 1 mg/mL formulation or dilution of the 1 mg/mL or 5 mg/mL formulation is recommended to facilitate slower injection. See DOSAGE AND ADMINISTRATION for complete dosing information.

DESCRIPTION

VERSED (midazolam hydrochloride) is a water-soluble benzodiazepine available as a sterile, nonpyrogenic parenteral dosage form for intravenous or intramuscular injection. Each mL contains midazolam hydrochloride equivalent to 1 mg or 5 mg midazolam compounded with 0.8% sodium chloride and 0.01% disodium edetate, with 1% benzyl alcohol as preservative; the pH is adjusted to approximately 3 with hydrochloric acid and, if necessary, sodium hydroxide.

Midazolam is a white to light yellow crystalline compound, insoluble in water. The hydrochloride salt of midazolam, which is formed *in situ*, is soluble in aqueous solutions. Chemically, midazolam HCl is 8-chloro-6-(2-fluorophenyl)-1-methyl-4H-imidazo[1,5-a][1,4] benzodiazepine hydrochloride. Midazolam hydrochloride has the empirical formula $C_{18}H_{13}ClFN_3 \cdot HCl$ and a calculated molecular weight of 362.25.

CLINICAL PHARMACOLOGY

VERSED is a short-acting benzodiazepine central nervous system depressant.

The effects of VERSED on the CNS are dependent on the dose administered, the route of administration, and the presence or absence of other premedications. Onset time of sedative effects after IM administration was 15 minutes, with peak sedation occurring 30 to 60 minutes following injection. In one study, when tested the following day, 73% of the patients who received VERSED intramuscularly had no recall of memory cards shown 30 minutes following drug administration; 40% had no recall of the memory cards shown 60 minutes following drug administration.

Sedation after IV injection was achieved within 3 to 5 minutes; the time of onset is affected by total dose administered and the concurrent administration of narcotic premedication. Seventy-one percent of the patients in the endoscopy studies had no recall of introduction of the endoscope; 82% of the patients had no recall of withdrawal of the endoscope.

When VERSED is given intravenously as an anesthetic induction agent, induction of anesthesia occurs in approximately 1.5 minutes when narcotic premedication has been administered and in 2 to 2.5 minutes without narcotic premedication or with sedative premedication. Some impairment in a test of memory was noted in 90% of the patients studied.

VERSED, used as directed, does not delay awakening from general anesthesia. Gross tests of recovery after awakening (orientation, ability to stand and walk, suitability for discharge from the recovery room, return to baseline Trieger competency) usually indicate recovery within 2 hours but recovery may take up to 6 hours in some cases. When compared with patients who received thiopental, patients who received midazolam generally recovered at a slightly slower rate.

In patients without intracranial lesions, induction with VERSED is associated with a moderate decrease in cerebrospinal fluid pressure (lumbar puncture measurements), similar to that seen following use of thiopental. Preliminary data in intracranial surgical patients with normal intracranial pressure but decreased compliance (subarachnoid screw measurements) show comparable elevations of intracranial pressure with VERSED and with thiopental during intubation.

Usual intramuscular premedicating doses of VERSED do not depress the ventilatory response to carbon dioxide stimulation to a clinically significant extent. Induction doses of VERSED depress the ventilatory response to carbon dioxide stimulation for 15 minutes or more beyond the duration of ventilatory depression following administration of thiopental. Impairment of ventilatory response to carbon dioxide is more marked in patients with chronic obstructive pulmonary disease (COPD). Sedation with intravenous VERSED does not adversely affect the mechanics of respiration (resistance, static recoil, most lung volume measurements); total lung capacity and peak expiratory flow decrease significantly but static compliance and maximum expiratory flow at 50% of awake total lung capacity (Vmax) increase.

In cardiac hemodynamic studies, induction with VERSED was associated with a slight to moderate decrease in mean arterial pressure, cardiac output, stroke volume and systemic vascular resistance. Slow heart rates (less than 65/minute), particularly in patients taking propranolol for angina, tended to rise slightly; faster heart rates (eg, 85/minute) tended to slow slightly.

The following preliminary pharmacokinetic data for midazolam have been reported. In normal subjects and healthy patients intravenous midazolam exhibited an elimination half-life of 1.2 to 12.3 hours, a large volume of distribution (0.95 to 6.6 L/kg) and a plasma clearance of 0.15 to 0.77 L/hr/kg. Clinical effects of VERSED do not directly correlate with the blood concentrations of midazolam.

Following intravenous administration, less than 0.03% of the dose is excreted in the urine as intact midazolam. Midazolam is rapidly metabolized to 1-hydroxymethyl midazolam, which is conjugated, with subsequent excretion in the urine. Approximately 45% to 57% of the dose is excreted in the urine as the conjugate of 1-hydroxymethyl midazolam, the major metabolite of midazolam. The half-life of elimination of 1-hydroxymethyl midazolam is similar to the parent compound. The concentration of midazolam is 10- to 30-fold greater than that of 1-hydroxymethyl midazolam after single IV administration.

In a small group of patients (n=11) with congestive heart failure, there appeared to be a 2- to 3-fold increase in the elimination half-life and volume of distribution of midazolam; however, the total body clearance of midazolam appeared to remain unchanged at a single 5-mg intravenous dose. There was no apparent change in the pharmacokinetic profile following the intravenous administration of 5 mg of midazolam to a small group of patients (n=12) with hepatic dysfunction. There was a 1.5- to 2-fold increase in elimination half-life, total body clearance and volume of distribution in a small group of patients (n=15) with chronic renal failure.

In a small group (n=12) of surgical patients, aged 49 to 60 years old, given 0.2 mg/kg midazolam intravenously, there appeared to be a small increase in the volume of distribution and elimination half-life with little change in total body clearance compared to an equal number of younger surgical patients (aged 18 to 30).

The mean absolute bioavailability of midazolam following intramuscular administration is greater than 90%. The mean time of maximum midazolam plasma concentrations following intramuscular dosing occurs within 45 minutes postadministration. Peak concentrations of midazolam as well as 1-hydroxymethyl midazolam after intramuscular administration are about one-half of those achieved after equivalent intravenous doses. The pharmacokinetic profile of elimination after intramuscularly administered midazolam is comparable to that observed following intravenous administration of the drug. Dose-linearity relationships have not been adequately defined.

Midazolam is approximately 97% plasma protein-bound in normal subjects and patients with renal failure. In animals, midazolam has been shown to cross the blood-brain barrier. In animals and in humans, midazolam has been shown to cross the placenta and enter into fetal circulation. Midazolam is excreted in human milk. (See PRECAUTIONS: *Nursing Mothers*).

INDICATIONS

Injectable VERSED is indicated—
- intramuscularly for preoperative sedation (induction of sleepiness or drowsiness and relief of apprehension) and to impair memory of perioperative events;
- intravenously as an agent for conscious sedation prior to short diagnostic, therapeutic or endoscopic procedures, such as bronchoscopy, gastroscopy, cystoscopy, coronary angiography and cardiac catheterization, either alone or with a narcotic;
- intravenously for induction of general anesthesia, before administration of other anesthetic agents. With the use of narcotic premedication, induction of anesthesia can be attained within a relatively narrow dose range and in a short period of time. Intravenous VERSED can also be used as a component of intravenous supplementation of nitrous oxide and oxygen (balanced anesthesia) *for short surgical procedures;* longer procedures have not been studied.

When used intravenously, VERSED is associated with a high incidence of partial or complete impairment of recall for the next several hours. (See CLINICAL PHARMACOLOGY.)

CONTRAINDICATIONS

Injectable VERSED is contraindicated in patients with a known hypersensitivity to the drug. Benzodiazepines are contraindicated in patients with acute narrow angle glaucoma. Benzodiazepines may be used in patients with open angle glaucoma only if they are receiving appropriate therapy. Measurements of intraocular pressure in patients without eye disease show a moderate lowering following induction with VERSED; patients with glaucoma have not been studied.

VERSED is not intended for intrathecal or epidural administration due to the presence of the preservative benzyl alcohol in the dosage form.

WARNINGS

VERSED must never be used without individualization of dosage. Prior to the intravenous administration of VERSED in any dose, the immediate availability of oxygen, resuscitative equipment and skilled personnel for the maintenance of a patent airway and support of ventilation should be ensured. Patients should be continuously monitored for early signs of underventilation or apnea, which can lead to hypoxia/cardiac arrest unless effective countermeasures are taken immediately. Vital signs should continue to be monitored during the recovery period. Because intravenous

VERSED depresses respiration (see CLINICAL PHARMACOLOGY) and because opioid agonists and other sedatives can add to this depression, VERSED should be administered as an induction agent only by a person trained in general anesthesia and should be used for conscious sedation only in the presence of personnel skilled in early detection of underventilation, maintaining a patent airway and supporting ventilation. **When used for conscious sedation, VERSED should not be administered by rapid or single bolus intravenous administration.**

Serious cardiorespiratory adverse events have occurred. These have included respiratory depression, apnea, respiratory arrest and/or cardiac arrest, sometimes resulting in death. There have also been rare reports of hypotensive episodes requiring treatment during or after diagnostic or surgical manipulations in patients who have received VERSED. Hypotension occurred more frequently in the conscious sedation studies in patients premedicated with a narcotic.

Reactions such as agitation, involuntary movements (including tonic/clonic movements and muscle tremor), hyperactivity and combativeness have been reported. These reactions may be due to inadequate or excessive dosing or improper administration of VERSED; however, consideration should be given to the possibility of cerebral hypoxia or true paradoxical reactions. Should such reactions occur, the response to each dose of VERSED and all other drugs, including local anesthetics, should be evaluated before proceeding.

Concomitant use of barbiturates, alcohol or other central nervous system depressants may increase the risk of underventilation or apnea and may contribute to profound and/or prolonged drug effect. Narcotic premedication also depresses the ventilatory response to carbon dioxide stimulation.

Higher risk surgical patients, elderly patients and debilitated patients require lower dosages, whether premedicated or not. Patients with chronic obstructive pulmonary disease are unusually sensitive to the respiratory depressant effect of VERSED. Patients with chronic renal failure and patients with congestive heart failure eliminate midazolam more slowly. (See CLINICAL PHARMACOLOGY.) Because elderly patients frequently have inefficient function of one or more organ systems, and because dosage requirements have been shown to decrease with age, reduced initial dosage of VERSED is recommended and the possibility of profound and/or prolonged effect should be considered.

Injectable VERSED should not be administered to patients in shock or coma, or in acute alcohol intoxication with depression of vital signs. Particular care should be exercised in the use of intravenous VERSED in patients with uncompensated acute illnesses, such as severe fluid or electrolyte disturbances.

The hazards of intra-arterial injection of VERSED solutions in humans are unknown; therefore, precautions against unintended intra-arterial injection should be taken. Extravasation should also be avoided.

The safety and efficacy of VERSED following non-intravenous and non-intramuscular routes of administration have not been established. VERSED should only be administered intramuscularly or intravenously.

The decision as to when patients who have received injectable VERSED, particularly on an outpatient basis, may again engage in activities requiring complete mental alertness, operate hazardous machinery or drive a motor vehicle must be individualized. Gross tests of recovery from the effects of VERSED (see CLINICAL PHARMACOLOGY) cannot be relied upon alone to predict reaction time under stress. This drug is never used alone during anesthesia and the contribution of other perioperative drugs and events can vary. It is recommended that no patient operate hazardous machinery or a motor vehicle until the effects of the drug, such as drowsiness, have subsided or until the day after anesthesia and surgery, whichever is longer.

Usage in Pregnancy: An increased risk of congenital malformations associated with the use of benzodiazepine drugs (diazepam and chlordiazepoxide) has been suggested in several studies. If this drug is used during pregnancy, the patient should be apprised of the potential hazard to the fetus.

PRECAUTIONS

General: Intravenous doses of VERSED should be decreased for elderly and for debilitated patients. (See WARNINGS and DOSAGE AND ADMINISTRATION.) These patients will also probably take longer to recover completely after VERSED administration for the induction of anesthesia.

VERSED does not protect against the increase in intracranial pressure or against the heart rate rise and/or blood pressure rise associated with endotracheal intubation under light general anesthesia.

Use in Preoperative Sedation, Conscious Sedation, and Monitored Anesthesia Care (MAC): Both the efficacy and safety of midazolam in clinical use are a function of the dose administered and the clinical status of the individual patient. Anticipated effects range from mild sedation to deep levels of sedation where the patient may require external support of vital functions. Care must be taken to individualize the dose to the patient's conditions, administer to the desired effect

and have the personnel and facilities available for monitoring and intervention (see BOX WARNING, WARNINGS and DOSAGE AND ADMINISTRATION sections.)

Information for Patients: To assure safe and effective use of benzodiazepines, the following information and instructions should be communicated to the patient when appropriate:
1. Inform your physician about any alcohol consumption and medicine you are now taking, including drugs you buy without a prescription. Alcohol has an increased effect when consumed with benzodiazepines; therefore, caution should be exercised regarding simultaneous ingestion of alcohol during benzodiazepine treatment.
2. Inform your physician if you are pregnant or are planning to become pregnant.
3. Inform your physician if you are nursing.

Drug Interactions: The sedative effect of intravenous VERSED is accentuated by premedication, particularly narcotics (eg, morphine, meperidine and fentanyl) and also secobarbital and Innovar (fentanyl and droperidol). Consequently, the dosage of VERSED should be adjusted according to the type and amount of premedication administered. (See DOSAGE AND ADMINISTRATION.)

A moderate reduction in induction dosage requirements of thiopental (about 15%) has been noted following use of intramuscular VERSED for premedication.

The intravenous administration of VERSED decreases the minimum alveolar concentration (MAC) of halothane required for general anesthesia. This decrease correlates with the dose of VERSED administered.

Although the possibility of minor interactive effects has not been fully studied, VERSED and pancuronium have been used together in patients without noting clinically significant changes in dosage, onset or duration. VERSED does not protect against the characteristic circulatory changes noted after administration of succinylcholine or pancuronium and does not protect against the increased intracranial pressure noted following administration of succinylcholine. VERSED does not cause a clinically significant change in dosage, onset or duration of a single intubating dose of succinylcholine.

No significant adverse interactions with commonly used premedications or drugs used during anesthesia and surgery (including atropine, scopolamine, glycopyrrolate, diazepam, hydroxyzine, d-tubocurarine, succinylcholine and nondepolarizing muscle relaxants) or topical local anesthetics (including lidocaine, dyclonine HCl and Cetacaine) have been observed.

Caution is advised when midazolam is administered to patients receiving erythromycin since this may result in a decrease in the plasma clearance of midazolam.

The clearance of midazolam and certain other benzodiazepines may be delayed with the concomitant administration of cimetidine (but not ranitidine). The clinical significance of this interaction is unclear.

Drug/Laboratory Test Interactions: Midazolam has not been shown to interfere with results obtained in clinical laboratory tests.

Carcinogenesis, Mutagenesis, Impairment of Fertility:
Carcinogenesis: Midazolam maleate was administered with diet in mice and rats for 2 years at dosages of 1, 9 and 80 mg/kg/day. In female mice in the highest dose group there was a marked increase in the incidence of hepatic tumors. In high dose male rats there was a small but statistically significant increase in benign thyroid follicular cell tumors. Dosages of 9 mg/kg/day of midazolam maleate (25 times a human dose of 0.35 mg/kg) do not increase the incidence of tumors. The pathogenesis of induction of these tumors is not known. These tumors were found after chronic administration, whereas human use will ordinarily be of single or several doses.

Mutagenesis: Midazolam did not have mutagenic activity in *Salmonella typhimurium* (5 bacterial strains), Chinese hamster lung cells (V79), human lymphocytes, or in the micronucleus test in mice.

Impairment of Fertility: A reproduction study in male and female rats did not show any impairment of fertility at dosages up to 10 times the human IV dose of 0.35 mg/kg.

Pregnancy: Teratogenic Effects: Pregnancy Category D. See WARNINGS section.

Segment II teratology studies, performed with midazolam maleate injectable in rabbits and rats at 5 and 10 times the human dose of 0.35 mg/kg, did not show evidence of teratogenicity.

Nonteratogenic Effects: Studies in rats showed no adverse effects on reproductive parameters during gestation and lactation. Dosages tested were approximately 10 times the human dose of 0.35 mg/kg.

Labor and Delivery: In humans, measurable levels of midazolam were found in maternal venous serum, umbilical venous and arterial serum and amniotic fluid, indicating placental transfer of the drug. Following intramuscular administration of 0.05 mg/kg of midazolam, both the venous and the umbilical arterial serum concentrations were lower than maternal concentrations.

Continued on next page

Roche Laboratories—Cont.

The use of injectable VERSED in obstetrics has not been evaluated in clinical studies. Because midazolam is transferred transplacentally and because other benzodiazepines given in the last weeks of pregnancy have resulted in neonatal CNS depression, VERSED is not recommended for obstetrical use.

Nursing Mothers: Midazolam is excreted in human milk. VERSED is not recommended for use in nursing mothers.

Pediatric Use: Safety and effectiveness of VERSED in children below the age of 18 years have not been established.

ADVERSE REACTIONS

See WARNINGS concerning serious cardiorespiratory events and possible paradoxical reactions. Fluctuations in vital signs were the most frequently seen findings following parenteral administration of VERSED and included decreased tidal volume and/or respiratory rate decrease (23.3% of patients following IV and 10.8% of patients following IM administration) and apnea (15.4% of patients following IV administration), as well as variations in blood pressure and pulse rate.

The following additional adverse reactions were reported after intramuscular administration:

headache (1.3%)

Local effects at IM injection site
pain (3.7%)
induration (0.5%)
redness (0.5%)
muscle stiffness (0.3%)

Administration of IM VERSED to elderly and/or higher risk surgical patients has been associated with rare reports of death under circumstances compatible with cardiorespiratory depression. In most of these cases, the patients also received other central nervous system depressants capable of depressing respiration, especially narcotics (see DOSAGE AND ADMINISTRATION).

The following additional adverse reactions were reported subsequent to intravenous administration:

hiccoughs (3.9%)
nausea (2.8%)
vomiting (2.6%)
coughing (1.3%)
"oversedation" (1.6%)
headache (1.5%)
drowsiness (1.2%)

Local effects at the IV site
tenderness (5.6%)
pain during injection (5.0%)
redness (2.6%)
induration (1.7%)
phlebitis (0.4%)

Other adverse experiences, observed mainly following IV injection and occurring at an incidence of less than 1.0%, are as follows:

Respiratory: Laryngospasm, bronchospasm, dyspnea, hyperventilation, wheezing, shallow respirations, airway obstruction, tachypnea.

Cardiovascular: Bigeminy, premature ventricular contractions, vasovagal episode, bradycardia, tachycardia, nodal rhythm.

Gastrointestinal: Acid taste, excessive salivation, retching.

CNS/Neuromuscular: Retrograde amnesia, euphoria, hallucination, confusion, argumentativeness, nervousness, anxiety, grogginess, restlessness, emergence delirium or agitation, prolonged emergence from anesthesia, dreaming during emergence, sleep disturbance, insomnia, nightmares, athetoid movements, seizure-like activity, ataxia, dizziness, dysphoria, slurred speech, dysphonia, paresthesia.

Special Sense: Blurred vision, diplopia, nystagmus, pinpoint pupils, cyclic movements of eyelids, visual disturbance, difficulty focusing eyes, ears blocked, loss of balance, lightheadedness.

Integumentary: Hive-like elevation at injection site, swelling or feeling of burning, warmth or coldness at injection site.

Hypersensitivity: Allergic reactions including anaphylactoid reactions, hives, rash, pruritus.

Miscellaneous: Yawning, lethargy, chills, weakness, toothache, faint feeling, hematoma.

DRUG ABUSE AND DEPENDENCE

Midazolam is subject to Schedule IV control under the Controlled Substances Act of 1970.

Midazolam was actively self-administered in primate models used to assess the positive reinforcing effects of psychoactive drugs.

Midazolam produced physical dependence of a mild to moderate intensity in cynomolgus monkeys after 5 to 10 weeks of administration. Available data concerning the drug abuse and dependence potential of midazolam suggest that its abuse potential is at least equivalent to that of diazepam.

OVERDOSAGE

While there is insufficient human data on overdosage with VERSED, the manifestations of VERSED overdosage are expected to be similar to those observed with other benzodiazepines and include sedation, somnolence, confusion, impaired coordination, diminished reflexes, coma and untoward effects on vital signs. No evidence of specific organ toxicity from VERSED overdosage would be expected.

Treatment of Overdosage: Treatment of injectable VERSED overdosage is the same as that followed for overdosage with other benzodiazepines. Respiration, pulse rate and blood pressure should be monitored and general supportive measures should be employed. Attention should be given to the maintenance of a patent airway and support of ventilation. An intravenous infusion should be started. Should hypotension develop, treatment may include intravenous fluid therapy, repositioning, judicious use of vasopressors appropriate to the clinical situation, if indicated, and other appropriate countermeasures. There is no information as to whether peritoneal dialysis, forced diuresis or hemodialysis are of any value in the treatment of midazolam overdosage.

Flumazenil, a specific benzodiazepine-receptor antagonist, is indicated for the complete or partial reversal of the sedative effects of benzodiazepines and may be used in situations when an overdose with a benzodiazepine is known or suspected. Prior to the administration of flumazneil, necessary measures should be instituted to secure airway, ventilation, and intravenous access. Flumazenil is intended as an adjunct to, not as a substitute for, proper management of benzodiazepine overdose. Patients treated with flumazenil should be monitored for resedation, respiratory depression and other residual benzodiazepine effects for an appropriate period after treatment. The prescriber should be aware of a risk of seizure in association with flumazenil treatment, particularly in long-term benzodiazepine users and in cyclic antidepressant overdose. The complete flumazenil package insert, including CONTRAINDICATIONS, WARNINGS, and PRECAUTIONS, should be consulted prior to use.

DOSAGE AND ADMINISTRATION

VERSED is a potent sedative agent used for preoperative sedation, conscious sedation and monitored anesthesia care (MAC), which requires slow administration and individualization of dosage. Clinical experience has shown VERSED to be 3 to 4 times as potent per mg as diazepam. BECAUSE SERIOUS AND LIFE-THREATENING CARDIORESPIRATORY ADVERSE EVENTS HAVE BEEN REPORTED, PROVISION FOR MONITORING, DETECTION AND CORRECTION OF THESE REACTIONS MUST BE MADE FOR EVERY PATIENT TO WHOM VERSED INJECTION IS ADMINISTERED, REGARDLESS OF AGE OR HEALTH STATUS. Excess doses or rapid or single bolus intravenous administration may result in respiratory depression and/or arrest. (See WARNINGS.)

Reactions such as agitation, involuntary movements, hyperactivity and combativeness have been reported. Should such reactions occur, caution should be exercised before continuing administration of VERSED. (See WARNINGS.)

VERSED should only be administered IM or IV (See WARNINGS.)

Care should be taken to avoid intra-arterial injection or extravasation. (See WARNINGS.)

VERSED Injection may be mixed in the same syringe with the following frequently used premedications: morphine sulfate, meperidine, atropine sulfate or scopolamine. VERSED, at a concentration of 0.5 mg/mL, is compatible with 5% dextrose in water and 0.9% sodium chloride for up to 24 hours and with lactated Ringer's solution for up to 4 hours. Both the 1 mg/mL and 5 mg/mL formulations of VERSED may be diluted with 0.9% sodium chloride or 5% dextrose in water.

INTRAMUSCULARLY

For preoperative sedation (induction of sleepiness or drowsiness and relief of apprehension) and to impair memory of perioperative events.

For intramuscular use, VERSED should be injected deep in a large muscle mass.

USUAL ADULT DOSE

The recommended premedication dose of VERSED for good risk (ASA Physical Status I & II) adult patients below the age of 60 years is 0.07 to 0.08 mg/kg IM (approximately 5 mg IM) administered approximately 1 hour before surgery.

The dose must be individualized and reduced when IM VERSED is administered to patients with chronic obstructive pulmonary disease, other higher risk surgical patients, patients 60 or more years of age, and patients who have received concomitant narcotics or other CNS depressants (see ADVERSE REACTIONS). In a study of patients 60 years or older, who did not receive concomitant administration of narcotics, 2 to 3 mg (0.02 to 0.05 mg/kg) of VERSED produced adequate sedation during the preoperative period. The dose of 1 mg IM VERSED may suffice for some older patients if the anticipated intensity and duration of sedation is less critical.

INTRAVENOUSLY

Conscious Sedation
(See INDICATIONS): Narcotic premedication results in less variability in patient response and a reduction in dosage of VERSED. For peroral procedures, the use of an appropriate topical anesthetic is recommended. For bronchoscopic procedures, the use of narcotic premedication is recommended. VERSED 1 mg/mL formulation is recommended for conscious sedation, to facilitate slower injection. Both the 1 mg/mL and the 5 mg/mL formulations may be diluted with 0.9% sodium chloride or 5% dextrose in water.

As with any potential respiratory depressant, these patients require observation for signs of cardiorespiratory depression after receiving IM VERSED.

Onset is within 15 minutes, peaking at 30 to 60 minutes. It can be administered concomitantly with atropine sulfate or scopolamine hydrochloride and reduced doses of narcotics.

When used for conscious sedation, dosage must be individualized and titrated. VERSED should not be administered by rapid or single bolus intravenous administration. Individual response will vary with age, physical status and concomitant medications, but may also vary independent of these factors. (See WARNINGS concerning cardiac/respiratory arrest.)

1. *Healthy Adults Below the Age of 60:*
Titrate *slowly* to the desired effect, eg. the initiation of slurred speech. Some patients may respond to as little as 1 mg. No more than 2.5 mg should be given over a period of at least 2 minutes. Wait an additional 2 or more minutes to fully evaluate the sedative effect. If further titration is necessary, continue to titrate, using small increments, to the appropriate level of sedation. Wait an additional 2 or more minutes after each increment to fully evaluate the sedative effect. A total dose greater than 5 mg is not usually necessary to reach the desired endpoint.

If narcotic premedication or other CNS depressants are used, patients will require approximately 30% less VERSED than unpremedicated patients.

2. *Patients Age 60 or Older, and Debilitated or Chronically Ill Patients:*
Because the danger of underventilation or apnea is greater in elderly patients and those with chronic disease states or decreased pulmonary reserve, and because the peak effect may take longer in these patients, increments should be smaller and the rate of injection slower.

Titrate *slowly* to the desired effect, eg, the initiation of slurred speech. Some patients may respond to as little as 1 mg. No more than 1.5 mg should be given over a period of no less than 2 minutes. Wait an additional 2 or more minutes to fully evaluate the sedative effect. If additional titration is necessary, it should be given at a rate of no more than 1 mg over a period of 2 minutes, waiting an additional 2 or more minutes each time to fully evaluate the sedative effect. Total doses greater than 3.5 mg are not usually necessary.

If concomitant CNS depressant premedications are used in these patients, they will require at least 50% less VERSED than healthy young unpremedicated patients.

Induction of Anesthesia:
For induction of general anesthesia, before administration of other anesthetic agents.

3. *Maintenance Dose:*
Additional doses to maintain the desired level of sedation may be given in increments of 25% of the dose used to first reach the sedative endpoint, but again only by slow titration, especially in the elderly and chronically ill or debilitated patient. These additional doses should be given *only* after a thorough clinical evaluation clearly indicates the need for additional sedation.
Individual response to the drug is variable, particularly when a narcotic premedication is not used. The dosage should be titrated to the desired effect according to the patient's age and clinical status.
When VERSED is used before other intravenous agents for induction of anesthesia, the initial dose of each agent may be significantly reduced, at times to as low as 25% of the usual initial dose of the individual agents.
Unpremedicated Patients:
In the absence of premedication, an average adult under the age of 55 years will usually require an initial dose of 0.3 to 0.35 mg/kg for induction, administered over 20 to 30 seconds and allowing 2 minutes for effect. If needed to complete induction, increments of approximately 25% of the patient's initial dose may be used; induction may instead be completed with volatile liquid inhalational anesthetics. In resistant cases, up to 0.6 mg/kg total dose may be used for induction, but such larger doses may prolong recovery.
Unpremedicated patients over the age of 55 years usually require less VERSED for induction; an initial dose of 0.3 mg/kg is recommended.
Unpremedicated patients with severe systemic disease or other debilitation usually require less VERSED for induction. An initial dose of 0.2 to 0.25 mg/kg will usually suffice; in some cases, as little as 0.15 mg/kg may suffice.
Premedicated Patients:
When the patient has received sedative or narcotic premedication, particularly narcotic premedication, the range of recommended doses is 0.15 to 0.35 mg/kg.
In average adults below the age of 55 years, a dose of 0.25 mg/kg, administered over 20 to 30 seconds and allowing 2 minutes for effect, will usually suffice.
The initial dose of 0.2 mg/kg is recommended for good risk (ASA I & II) surgical patients over the age of 55 years.
In some patients with severe systemic disease or debilitation, as little as 0.15 mg/kg may suffice.
Narcotic premedication frequently used during clinical trials included fentanyl (1.5 to 2 μg/kg IV, administered 5 minutes before induction), morphine (dosage individualized, up to 0.15 mg/kg IM), meperidine (dosage individualized, up to 1 mg/kg IM) and Innovar (0.02 mL/kg IM). Sedative premedications were

hydroxyzine pamoate (100 mg orally) and sodium secobarbital (200 mg orally). Except for intravenous fentanyl, administered 5 minutes before induction, all other premedications should be administered approximately 1 hour prior to the time anticipated for VERSED induction.
Incremental injections of approximately 25% of the induction dose should be given in response to signs of lightening of anesthesia and repeated as necessary.

Injectable VERSED can also be used during maintenance of anesthesia, *for short surgical procedures,* as a component of balanced anesthesia. Effective narcotic premedication is especially recommended in such cases. Long surgical procedures have not been studied.
Note: Parenteral drug products should be inspected visually for particulate matter and discoloration prior to administration, whenever solution and container permit.

HOW SUPPLIED
Package configurations containing midazolam hydrochloride equivalent to **5 mg midazolam/mL:**
1-mL vials (5 mg)—boxes of 10 (NDC 0004-1974-01);*
2-mL vials (10 mg)—boxes of 10 (NDC 0004-1973-01);†
5-mL vials (25 mg)—boxes of 10 (NDC 0004-1975-01);†
10-mL vials (50 mg)—boxes of 10 (NDC 0004-1946-01);†
2-mL Tel-E-Ject® disposable syringes (10 mg)—boxes of 10 (NDC 0004-1947-01).*
Package configurations containing midazolam hydrochloride equivalent to **1 mg midazolam/mL:**
2-mL vials (2 mg)—boxes of 10 (NDC 0004-1998-06);†
5-mL vials (5 mg)—boxes of 10 (NDC 0004-1999-01);†
10-mL vials (10 mg)—boxes of 10 (NDC 0004-2000-06).†
Store at 59° to 86°F (15° to 30°C).
* Manufactured and distributed by Hoffmann-LaRoche Inc., Nutley, New Jersey 07110.
† Manufactured by Roche Pharma, Inc., Manati, Puerto Rico 00674 or Hoffmann-LaRoche Inc., Nutley, New Jersey 07110. Distributed by Hoffmann-LaRoche Inc., Nutley, New Jersey 07110.
Revised: June 1994

VESANOID® ℞
[ves 'ă noid]
(tretinoin)
CAPSULES

WARNINGS:

1. *Experienced Physician and Institution:* Patients with acute promyelocytic leukemia (APL) are at high risk in general and can have severe adverse reactions to VESANOID (tretinoin). VESANOID should therefore be administered under the supervision of a physician who is experienced in the management of patients with acute leukemia and in a facility with laboratory and supportive services sufficient to monitor drug tolerance and protect and maintain a patient compromised by drug toxicity, including respiratory compromise. Use of VESANOID requires that the physician concludes that the possible benefit to the patient outweighs the following known adverse effects of the therapy.

2. *Retinoic Acid-APL Syndrome:* About 25% of patients with APL treated with VESANOID have experienced a syndrome called the retinoic-acid-APL (RA-APL) syndrome characterized by fever, dyspnea, weight gain, radiographic pulmonary infiltrates and pleural or pericardial effusions. This syndrome has occasionally been accompanied by impaired myocardial contractility and episodic hypotension. It has been observed with or without concomitant leukocytosis. Endotracheal intubation and mechanical ventilation have been required in some cases due to progressive hypoxemia, and several patients have expired with multiorgan failure. The syndrome generally occurs during the first month of treatment, with some cases reported following the first dose of VESANOID.
The management of the syndrome has not been defined rigorously, but high-dose steroids given at the first suspicion of the RA-APL syndrome appear to reduce morbidity and mortality. At the first signs suggestive of the syndrome (unexplained fever, dyspnea and/or weight gain, abnormal chest auscultatory findings or radiographic abnormalities), high-dose steroids (dexamethasone 10 mg intravenously administered every 12 hours for 3 days or until the

resolution of symptoms) should be immediately initiated, irrespective of the leukocyte count. The majority of patients do not require termination of VESANOID therapy during treatment of the RA-APL syndrome.

3. *Leukocytosis at Presentation and Rapidly Evolving Leukocytosis During VESANOID Treatment:* During VESANOID treatment about 40% of patients will develop rapidly evolving leukocytosis. Patients who present with high WBC at diagnosis ($>5 \times 10^9$/L) have an increased risk of a further rapid increase in WBC counts. Rapidly evolving leukocytosis is associated with a higher risk of life-threatening complications.
If signs and symptoms of the RA-APL syndrome are present together with leukocytosis, treatment with high-dose steroids should be initiated immediately. Some investigators routinely add chemotherapy to VESANOID treatment in the case of patients presenting with a WBC count of $>5 \times 10^9$/L or in the case of a rapid increase in WBC count for patients leukopenic at start of treatment, and have reported a lower incidence of the RA-APL syndrome. Consideration could be given to adding full-dose chemotherapy (including an anthracycline if not contraindicated) to the VESANOID therapy on day 1 or 2 for patients presenting with a WBC count of $>5 \times 10^9$/L, or immediately, for patients presenting with a WBC count of $<5 \times 10^9$/L, if the WBC count reaches $\geq 6 \times 10^9$/L by day 5, or $\geq 10 \times 10^9$/L by day 10, or $\geq 15 \times 10^9$/L by day 28.

4. *Teratogenic Effects. Pregnancy Category D—see WARNINGS.* There is a high risk that a severely deformed infant will result if VESANOID is administered during pregnancy. If, nonetheless, it is determined that VESANOID represents the best available treatment for a pregnant woman or a woman of childbearing potential, it must be assured that the patient has received full information and warnings of the risk to the fetus if she were to be pregnant and of the risk of possible contraception failure and has been instructed in the need to use two reliable forms of contraception simultaneously during therapy and for 1 month following discontinuation of therapy, and has acknowledged her understanding of the need for using dual contraception, unless abstinence is the chosen method.
Within 1 week prior to the institution of VESANOID therapy, the patient should have blood or urine collected for a serum or urine pregnancy test with a sensitivity of at least 50 mIU/L. When possible VESANOID therapy should be delayed until a negative result from this test is obtained. When a delay is not possible the patient should be placed on two reliable forms of contraception. Pregnancy testing and contraception counseling should be repeated monthly throughout the period of VESANOID treatment.

DESCRIPTION
VESANOID (tretinoin) is a retinoid that induces maturation of acute promyelocytic leukemia (APL) cells in culture. It is available in a 10 mg soft gelatin capsule for oral administration. Each capsule also contains beeswax, butylated hydroxyanisole, edetate disodium, hydrogenated soybean oil flakes, hydrogenated vegetable oils and soybean oil. The gelatin capsule shell contains glycerin, yellow iron oxide, red iron oxide, titanium dioxide, methylparaben and propylparaben. Chemically, tretinoin is all-*trans* retinoic acid and is related to retinol (Vitamin A). It is a yellow to light orange crystalline powder with a molecular weight of 300.44.

CLINICAL PHARMACOLOGY
Mechanism of Action: Tretinoin is not a cytolytic agent but instead induces cytodifferentiation and decreased proliferation of APL cells in culture and in vivo. In APL patients, tretinoin treatment produces an initial maturation of the primitive promyelocytes derived from the leukemic clone, followed by a repopulation of the bone marrow and peripheral blood by normal, polyclonal hematopoietic cells in patients achieving complete remission (CR). The exact mechanism of action of tretinoin in APL is unknown.

PHARMACOKINETICS
Tretinoin activity is primarily due to the parent drug. In human pharmacokinetics studies, orally administered drug was well absorbed into the systemic circulation, with approximately two-thirds of the administered radiolabel recovered in the urine. The terminal elimination half-life of tretinoin following initial dosing is 0.5 to 2 hours in patients with APL. There is evidence that tretinoin induces its own metabolism. Plasma tretinoin concentrations decrease on average to one-third of their day 1 values during 1 week of continuous therapy. Mean ± SD peak tretinoin concentrations decreased

Continued on next page

Roche Laboratories—Cont.

from 394 ± 89 to 138 ± 139 ng/mL, while area under the curve (AUC) values decreased from 537 ± 191 ng·h/mL to 249 ± 185 ng·h/mL during 45 mg/m^2 daily dosing in 7 APL patients. Increasing the dose to "correct" for this change has not increased response.

Absorption: A single 45 mg/m^2 (~80 mg) oral dose to APL patients resulted in a mean ± SD peak tretinoin concentration of 347 ± 266 ng/mL. Time to reach peak concentration was between 1 and 2 hours.

Distribution: The apparent volume of distribution of tretinoin has not been determined. Tretinoin is greater than 95% bound in plasma, predominately to albumin. Plasma protein binding remains constant over the concentration range of 10 to 500 ng/mL.

Metabolism: Tretinoin metabolites have been identified in plasma and urine. Cytochrome P450 (CYP) enzymes have been implicated in the oxidative metabolism of tretinoin. Metabolites include 13-*cis* retinoic acid, 4-oxo *trans* retinoic acid, 4-oxo *cis* retinoic acid, and 4-oxo *trans* retinoic acid glucuronide. In APL patients, daily administration of a 45 mg/m^2 dose of tretinoin resulted in an approximately tenfold increase in the urinary excretion of 4-oxo *trans* retinoic acid glucuronide after 2 to 6 weeks of continuous dosing, when compared to baseline values.

Excretion: Studies with radiolabeled drug have demonstrated that after the oral administration of 2.75 and 50 mg doses of tretinoin, greater than 90% of the radioactivity was recovered in the urine and feces. Based upon data from 3 subjects, approximately 63% of radioactivity was recovered in the urine within 72 hours and 31% appeared in the feces within 6 days.

Special Populations: The pharmacokinetics of tretinoin have not been separately evaluated in women, in members of different ethnic groups, or in individuals with renal or hepatic insufficiency.

Drug-Drug Interactions: In 13 patients who had received daily doses of tretinoin for 4 consecutive weeks, administration of ketoconazole (400 to 1200 mg oral dose) 1 hour prior to the administration of the tretinoin dose on day 29 led to a 72% increase (218 ± 224 versus 375 ± 285 ng·h/mL) in tretinoin mean plasma AUC. The precise CYP system involved in these interactions has not been specified; CYP, 3A4, 2C8 and 2E have been implicated in various preliminary reports.

Clinical Studies: VESANOID has been investigated in 114 previously treated APL patients and in 67 previously untreated ("de novo") patients in one open-label, uncontrolled single investigator clinical study (Memorial Sloan-Kettering Cancer Center [MSKCC]) and in two cohorts of compassionate cases treated by multiple investigators under the auspices of the National Cancer Institute (NCI). All patients received 45 mg/m^2/day as a divided oral dose for up to 90 days or 30 days beyond the day that CR was reached. Results are shown in the following table:

[See table below.]

The median time to CR was between 40 and 50 days (range: 2 to 120 days). Most patients in these studies received cytotoxic chemotherapy during the remission phase. These results compare to the 30% to 50% CR rate and ≤6 month median survival reported for cytotoxic chemotherapy of APL in the treatment of relapse.

Ten of 15 pediatric cases achieved CR (8 of 10 males and 2 of 5 females). There were insufficient patients of black, Hispanic or Asian derivation to estimate relative response rates in these groups, but responses were seen in each category.

Responses were seen in 3 of 4 patients for whom cytogenetic analysis failed to detect the t(15;17) translocation typically seen in APL. The t(15;17) translocation results in the PML/RARα gene, which appears necessary for this disease. Molecular genetic studies were not conducted in these cases, but it is likely they represent cases with a masked translocation giving rise to PML/RARα. Responses to tretinoin have not been observed in cases in which PML/RARα fusion has been shown to be absent.

INDICATIONS AND USAGE

VESANOID (tretinoin) capsules are indicated for the induction of remission in patients with acute promyelocytic leukemia (APL), French-American-British (FAB) classification M3 (including the M3 variant), characterized by the presence of the t(15;17) translocation and/or the presence of the PML/RARα gene who are refractory to, or who have relapsed from, anthracycline chemotherapy, or for whom anthracycline-based chemotherapy is contraindicated. VESANOID is for the induction of remission only. The optimal consolidation or maintenance regimens have not been defined, but all patients should receive an accepted form of remission consolidation and/or maintenance therapy for APL after completion of induction therapy with VESANOID.

CONTRAINDICATIONS

VESANOID is contraindicated in patients with a known hypersensitivity to retinoids. VESANOID should not be given to patients who are sensitive to parabens, which are used as preservatives in the gelatin capsule.

WARNINGS

Pregnancy Category D—see boxed WARNINGS: Tretinoin has teratogenic and embryotoxic effects in mice, rats, hamsters, rabbits and pigtail monkeys, and may be expected to cause fetal harm when administered to a pregnant woman. Tretinoin causes fetal resorptions and a decrease in live fetuses in all animals studied. Gross external, soft tissue and skeletal alterations occurred at doses higher than 0.7 mg/kg/day in mice, 2 mg/kg/day in rats, 7 mg/kg/day in hamsters, and at a dose of 10 mg/kg/day, the only dose tested, in pigtail monkeys (about 1/20, 1/4, and 1/2 and 4 times the human dose, respectively, on a mg/m^2 basis).

There are no adequate and well controlled studies in pregnant women. Although experience with humans administered VESANOID is extremely limited, increased spontaneous abortions and major human fetal abnormalities related to the use of other retinoids have been documented in humans.

Reported defects include abnormalities of the CNS, musculoskeletal system, external ear, eye, thymus and great vessels; and facial dysmorphia, cleft palate, and parathyroid hormone deficiency. Some of these abnormalities were fatal. Cases of IQ scores less than 85, with or without obvious CNS abnormalities, have also been reported. All fetuses exposed during pregnancy can be affected and at the present time there is no antepartum means of determining which fetuses are and are not affected.

Effective contraception must be used by all females during VESANOID therapy and for 1 month following discontinuation of therapy. Contraception must be used even when there is a history of infertility or menopause, unless a hysterectomy has been performed. Whenever contraception is required, it is recommended that two reliable forms of contraception be used simultaneously, unless abstinence is the chosen method. If pregnancy does occur during treatment, the physician and patient should discuss the desirability of continuing or terminating the pregnancy.

Patients without the t(15;17) Translocation: Initiation of therapy with VESANOID may be based on the morphological diagnosis of acute promyelocytic leukemia. Confirmation of the diagnosis of APL should be sought by detection of the t(15;17) genetic marker by cytogenetic studies. If these are negative, PML/RARα fusion should be sought using molecular diagnostic techniques. The response rate of other AML subtypes to VESANOID has not been demonstrated; therefore, patients who lack the genetic marker should be considered for alternative treatment.

Retinoic Acid-APL (RA-APL) Syndrome: In up to 25% of patients with APL treated with VESANOID, a syndrome occurs which can be fatal (see boxed WARNINGS and ADVERSE REACTIONS).

Leukocytosis at Presentation and Rapidly Evolving Leukocytosis During VESANOID Treatment: (see boxed WARNINGS).

Pseudotumor Cerebri: Retinoids, including VESANOID, have been associated with pseudotumor cerebri (benign intracranial hypertension), especially in pediatric patients. Early signs and symptoms of pseudotumor cerebri include papilledema, headache, nausea and vomiting and visual disturbances. Patients with these symptoms should be evaluated for pseudotumor cerebri, and, if present, appropriate care should be instituted in concert with neurological assessment.

Lipids: Up to 60% of patients experienced hypercholesterolemia and/or hypertriglyceridemia, which were reversible upon completion of treatment. The clinical consequences of temporary elevation of triglycerides and cholesterol are unknown, but venous thrombosis and myocardial infarction have been reported in patients who ordinarily are at low risk for such complications.

Elevated Liver Function Test Results: Elevated liver function test results occur in 50% to 60% of patients during treatment. Liver function test results should be carefully monitored during treatment and consideration be given to a temporary withdrawal of VESANOID if test results reach greater than five times the upper limit of normal values. However, the majority of these abnormalities resolve without interruption of VESANOID or after completion of treatment.

PRECAUTIONS

General: VESANOID has potentially significant toxic side effects in APL patients. Patients undergoing therapy should be closely observed for signs of respiratory compromise and/or leukocytosis (see boxed WARNINGS). Supportive care appropriate for APL patients; eg, prophylaxis for bleeding, prompt therapy for infection, should be maintained during therapy with VESANOID.

Laboratory Tests: The patient's hematologic profile, coagulation profile, liver function test results, and triglyceride and cholesterol levels should be monitored frequently.

Drug Interactions: Limited clinical data on potential drug interactions are available. As VESANOID is metabolized by the hepatic CYP system, there is a potential for alteration of pharmacokinetics parameters in patients administered concomitant medications that are also inducers or inhibitors of this system. Medications that generally induce hepatic CYP enzymes include rifampicin, glucocorticoids, phenobarbital and pentobarbital. Medications that generally inhibit hepatic CYP enzymes include ketoconazole, cimetidine, erythromycin, verapamil, diltiazem and cyclosporin. To date there are no data to suggest that co-use with these medications increases or decreases either efficacy or toxicity of VESANOID.

Effect of Food: No data on the effect of food on the absorption of VESANOID are available. The absorption of retinoids as a class has been shown to be enhanced when taken together with food.

Carcinogenesis, Mutagenesis and Impairment of Fertility: No long-term carcinogenicity studies with tretinoin have been conducted. In short-term carcinogenicity studies, tretinoin at a dose of 30 mg/kg/day (about 2 times the human dose on a mg/m^2 basis) was shown to increase the rate of diethylnitrosamine (DEN)-induced mouse liver adenomas and carcinomas. Tretinoin was negative when tested in the Ames and Chinese hamster V79 cell HGPRT assays for mutagenicity. A twofold increase in the sister chromatid exchange (SCE) has been demonstrated in human diploid fibroblasts, but other chromosome aberration assays, including an in vitro assay in human peripheral lymphocytes and an in vivo mouse micronucleus assay, did not show a clastogenic or aneuploidogenic effect. Adverse effects on fertility and reproductive performance were not observed in studies conducted in rats at doses up to 5 mg/kg/day (about 2/3 the human dose on a mg/m^2 basis). In a 6-week toxicology study in dogs, minimal to marked testicular degeneration, with increased numbers of immature spermatozoa, were observed at 10 mg/kg/day (about 4 times the equivalent human dose in mg/m^2).

Nursing Mothers: It is not known whether this drug is excreted in human milk. Because many drugs are excreted in human milk, and because of the potential for serious adverse reactions from VESANOID in nursing infants, mothers should discontinue nursing prior to taking this drug.

Pediatric Use: There are limited clinical data on the pediatric use of VESANOID. Of 15 pediatric patients (age range: 1 to 16 years) treated with VESANOID, the incidence of complete remission was 67%. Safety and effectiveness in pediatric patients below the age of 1 year have not been established. Some pediatric patients experience severe headache and pseudotumor cerebri, requiring analgesic treatment and lumbar puncture for relief. Increased caution is recommended in the treatment of pediatric patients. Dose reduction may be considered for pediatric patients experiencing serious and/or intolerable toxicity; however, the efficacy and safety of VESANOID at doses lower than 45 mg/m^2/day have not been evaluated in the pediatric population.

ADVERSE REACTIONS

Virtually all patients experience some drug related toxicity, especially headache, fever, weakness, and fatigue. These adverse effects are seldom permanent or irreversible nor do they usually require interruption of therapy. Some of the adverse events are common in patients with APL, including hemorrhage, infections, gastrointestinal hemorrhage, disseminated intravascular coagulation, pneumonia, septicemia, and cerebral hemorrhage. The following describes the adverse events, regardless of drug relationship, that were observed in patients treated with VESANOID.

	MSKCC		NCI Cohort 1		NCI Cohort 2	
	Relapsed n=20	De Novo n=15	Relapsed* n=48	De Novo n=14	Relapsed n=46	De Novo† n=38
Complete Remission	16 (80%)	11 (73%)	24 (50%)	5 (36%)	24 (52%)	26 (68%)
Median Survival (Mo)	10.8	NR	5.8	0.5	8.8	NR
Median Follow-up (Mo)	9.9	42.9	5.6	1.2	8.0	13.1
RA-APL Syndrome	4 (20%)	5 (33%)	10 (21%)	6 (43%)	NA	NA

NR = Not Reached
NA = Not Available
*Including 9 chemorefractory patients
†Including 8 patients who received chemotherapy but failed to enter remission

Typical Retinoid Toxicity: The most frequently reported adverse events were similar to those described in patients taking high doses of vitamin A and included headache (86% of patients), fever (83%), skin/mucous membrane dryness (77%), bone pain (77%), nausea/vomiting (57%), rash (54%), mucositis (26%), pruritus (20%), increased sweating (20%), visual disturbances (17%), ocular disorders (17%), alopecia (14%), skin changes (14%), changed visual acuity (6%), bone inflammation (3%), visual field defects (3%).
RA-APL Syndrome: APL patients treated with VESANOID have experienced a syndrome characterized by fever, dyspnea, weight gain, radiographic pulmonary infiltrates and pleural or pericardial effusions. This syndrome has occasionally been accompanied by impaired myocardial contractility and episodic hypotension and has been observed with or without concomitant leukocytosis. Some patients have expired due to progressive hypoxemia and multiorgan failure. The syndrome generally occurs during the first month of treatment, with some cases reported following the first dose of VESANOID. The management of the syndrome has not been defined rigorously, but high-dose steroids given at the first signs of the syndrome appear to reduce morbidity and mortality. Treatment with dexamethasone, 10 mg intravenously administered every 12 hours for 3 days or until resolution of symptoms, should be initiated without delay at the first suspicion of symptoms (one or more of the following: fever, dyspnea, weight gain, abnormal chest auscultatory findings or radiographic abnormalities). Sixty percent or more of patients treated with VESANOID may require high-dose steroids because of these symptoms. The majority of patients do not require termination of VESANOID therapy during treatment of the syndrome.
Body as a Whole: General disorders related to VESANOID administration and/or associated with APL included malaise (66%), shivering (63%), hemorrhage (60%), infections (58%), peripheral edema (52%), pain (37%), chest discomfort (32%), edema (29%), disseminated intravascular coagulation (26%), weight increase (23%), injection site reactions (17%), anorexia (17%), weight decrease (17%), myalgia (14%), flank pain (9%), cellulitis (8%), face edema (6%), fluid imbalance (6%), pallor (6%), lymph disorders (6%), acidosis (3%), hypothermia (3%), ascites (3%).
Respiratory System Disorders: Respiratory system disorders were commonly reported in APL patients administered VESANOID. The majority of these events are symptoms of the RA-APL syndrome (see boxed WARNING). Respiratory system adverse events included upper respiratory tract disorders (63%), dyspnea (60%), respiratory insufficiency (26%), pleural effusion (20%), pneumonia (14%), rales (14%), expiratory wheezing (14%), lower respiratory tract disorders (9%), pulmonary infiltration (6%), bronchial asthma (3%), pulmonary edema (3%), larynx edema (3%), unspecified pulmonary disease (3%).
Ear Disorders: Ear disorders were consistently reported, with earache or feeling of fullness in the ears reported by 23% of the patients. Hearing loss and other unspecified auricular disorders were observed in 6% of patients, with infrequent (<1%) reports of irreversible hearing loss.
Gastrointestinal Disorders: GI disorders included GI hemorrhage (34%), abdominal pain (31%), other gastrointestinal disorders (26%), diarrhea (23%), constipation (17%), dyspepsia (14%), abdominal distention (11%), hepatosplenomegaly (9%), hepatitis (3%), ulcer (3%), unspecified liver disorder (3%).
Cardiovascular and Heart Rate and Rhythm Disorders: Arrhythmias (23%), flushing (23%), hypotension (14%), hypertension (11%), phlebitis (11%), cardiac failure (6%) and for 3% of patients: cardiac arrest, myocardial infarction, enlarged heart, heart murmur, ischemia, stroke, myocarditis, pericarditis, pulmonary hypertension, secondary cardiomyopathy.
Central and Peripheral Nervous System Disorders and Psychiatric: Dizziness (20%), paresthesias (17%), anxiety (17%), insomnia (14%), depression (14%), confusion (11%), cerebral hemorrhage (9%), intracranial hypertension (9%), agitation (9%), hallucination (6%) and for 3% of patients: abnormal gait, agnosia, aphasia, asterixis, cerebellar edema, cerebellar disorders, convulsions, coma, CNS depression, dysarthria, encephalopathy, facial paralysis, hemiplegia, hyporeflexia, hypotaxia, no light reflex, neurologic reaction, spinal cord disorder, tremor, leg weakness, unconsciousness, dementia, forgetfulness, somnolence, slow speech.
Urinary System Disorders: Renal insufficiency (11%), dysuria (9%), acute renal failure (3%), micturition frequency (3%), renal tubular necrosis (3%), enlarged prostate (3%).
Miscellaneous Adverse Events: Isolated cases of erythema nodosum, basophilia and hyperhistaminemia, Sweet's syndrome, organomegaly, hypercalcemia, pancreatitis and myositis have been reported.

OVERDOSAGE

There has been no experience with acute overdosage in humans. The maximal tolerated dose in patients with myelodysplastic syndrome or solid tumors was 195 mg/m^2/day. The maximal tolerated dose in pediatric patients was lower at 60 mg/m^2/day. Overdosage with other retinoids has been associated with transient headache, facial flushing, cheilosis, abdominal pain, dizziness and ataxia. These symptoms have quickly resolved without apparent residual effects.

DOSAGE AND ADMINISTRATION

The recommended dose is 45 mg/m^2/day administered as two evenly divided doses until complete remission is documented. Therapy should be discontinued 30 days after achievement of complete remission or after 90 days of treatment, whichever occurs first.
If after initiation of treatment of VESANOID the presence of the t(15;17) translocation is not confirmed by cytogenetics and/or by polymerase chain reaction studies and the patient has not responded to VESANOID, alternative therapy appropriate for acute myelogenous leukemia should be considered.
VESANOID is for the induction of remission only. Optimal consolidation or maintenance regimens have not been determined. All patients should therefore receive a standard consolidation and/or maintenance chemotherapy regimen for APL after induction therapy with VESANOID, unless otherwise contraindicated.

HOW SUPPLIED

VESANOID is supplied as 10 mg capsules, two-tone (lengthwise), orange-yellow and reddish-brown and imprinted VESANOID 10 ROCHE. Supplied in high density polyethylene, opaque Prescription Pak Bottles of 100 capsules with child-resistant closure (NDC 0004-0250-01).
Store at 15°C to 30°C (59°F to 86°F). Protect from light.

Issued: November 1995

Shown in Product Identification Guide, page 332

EDUCATIONAL MATERIAL

Please contact your Roche representative concerning availability of educational programs and material.

Roche Products Inc.
Manati, Puerto Rico 00674

Direct Medical Inquiries to:
Roche Laboratories
(800) 526-6367
Direct Customer Service (Distribution) Inquiries to:
Roche Laboratories
(800) 526-0625

DALMANE® Ⓒ
[dal 'mane]
brand of flurazepam hydrochloride
CAPSULES

The following text is complete prescribing information based on official labeling in effect June 1996.

DESCRIPTION

Dalmane is available as capsules containing 15 mg or 30 mg flurazepam hydrochloride. Each 15-mg capsule also contains corn starch, lactose, magnesium stearate and talc; gelatin capsule shells may contain methyl and propyl parabens and potassium sorbate, with the following dye systems: D&C Red No. 28, FD&C Red No. 40, FD&C Yellow No. 6 and D&C Yellow No. 10. Each 30-mg capsule also contains corn starch, lactose and magnesium stearate; gelatin capsule shells may contain methyl and propyl parabens and potassium sorbate, with the following dye systems: FD&C Blue No. 1, FD&C Yellow No. 6, D&C Yellow No. 10 and either FD&C Red No. 3 or FD&C Red No. 40.
Flurazepam hydrochloride is chemically 7-chloro-1-[2-(diethylamino)ethyl]-5-(*o*-fluorophenyl)-1, 3-dihydro-2*H*-1, 4-benzodiazepin-2-one dihydrochloride. It is a pale yellow, crystalline compound, freely soluble in USP alcohol and very soluble in water. It has a molecular weight of 460.826.

CLINICAL PHARMACOLOGY

Flurazepam hydrochloride is rapidly absorbed from the GI tract. Flurazepam is rapidly metabolized and is excreted primarily in the urine. Following a single oral dose, peak flurazepam plasma concentrations ranging from 0.5 to 4.0 ng/mL occur at 30 to 60 minutes post-dosing. The harmonic mean apparent half-life of flurazepam is 2.3 hours. The blood level profile of flurazepam and its major metabolites was determined in man following the oral administration of 30 mg daily for 2 weeks. The N_1-hydroxyethyl-flurazepam was measurable only during the early hours after a 30-mg dose and was not detectable after 24 hours. The major metabolite in blood was N_1-desalkyl-flurazepam, which reached steady-state (plateau) levels after 7 to 10 days of dosing, at levels approximately 5- to 6-fold greater than the 24-hour levels observed on Day 1. The half-life of elimination of N_1-desalkyl-flurazepam ranged from 47 to 100 hours. The major urinary metabolite is conjugated N_1-hydroxyethyl-flurazepam which accounts for 22% to 55% of the dose. Less than 1% of the dose is excreted in the urine as N_1-desalkyl-flurazepam.
This pharmacokinetic profile may be responsible for the clinical observation that flurazepam is increasingly effective on the second or third night of consecutive use and that for 1 or 2 nights after the drug is discontinued both sleep latency and total wake time may still be decreased.

INDICATIONS

Dalmane is a hypnotic agent useful for the treatment of insomnia characterized by difficulty in falling asleep, frequent nocturnal awakenings, and/or early morning awakening. Dalmane can be used effectively in patients with recurring insomnia or poor sleeping habits, and in acute or chronic medical situations requiring restful sleep. Sleep laboratory studies have objectively determined that Dalmane is effective for at least 28 consecutive nights of drug administration. Since insomnia is often transient and intermittent, short-term use is usually sufficient. Prolonged use of hypnotics is usually not indicated and should only be undertaken concomitantly with appropriate evaluation of the patient.

CONTRAINDICATIONS

Dalmane is contraindicated in patients with known hypersensitivity to the drug.
Usage in Pregnancy: Benzodiazepines may cause fetal damage when administered during pregnancy. An increased risk of congenital malformations associated with the use of diazepam and chlordiazepoxide during the first trimester of pregnancy has been suggested in several studies.
Dalmane is contraindicated in pregnant women. Symptoms of neonatal depression have been reported; a neonate whose mother received 30 mg of Dalmane nightly for insomnia during the 10 days prior to delivery appeared hypotonic and inactive during the first 4 days of life. Serum levels of N_1-desalkyl-flurazepam in the infant indicated transplacental circulation and implicate this long-acting metabolite in this case. If there is a likelihood of the patient becoming pregnant while receiving flurazepam, she should be warned of the potential risks to the fetus. Patients should be instructed to discontinue the drug prior to becoming pregnant. The possibility that a woman of childbearing potential may be pregnant at the time of institution of therapy should be considered.

WARNINGS

Patients receiving Dalmane should be cautioned about possible combined effects with alcohol and other CNS depressants. Also, caution patients that an additive effect may occur if alcoholic beverages are consumed during the day following the use of Dalmane for nighttime sedation. The potential for this interaction continues for several days following discontinuance of flurazepam, until serum levels of psychoactive metabolites have declined.
Patients should also be cautioned about engaging in hazardous occupations requiring complete mental alertness such as operating machinery or driving a motor vehicle after ingesting the drug, including potential impairment of the performance of such activities which may occur the day following ingestion of Dalmane.
Usage in Children: Clinical investigations of Dalmane have not been carried out in children. Therefore, the drug is not currently recommended for use in persons under 15 years of age.
Withdrawal symptoms of the barbiturate type have occurred after the discontinuation of benzodiazepines. (See DRUG ABUSE AND DEPENDENCE section.)

PRECAUTIONS

Since the risk of the development of oversedation, dizziness, confusion and/or ataxia increases substantially with larger doses in elderly and debilitated patients, it is recommended that in such patients the dosage be limited to 15 mg. If Dalmane is to be combined with other drugs having known hypnotic properties or CNS-depressant effects, due consideration should be given to potential additive effects.
The usual precautions are indicated for severely depressed patients or those in whom there is any evidence of latent depression; particularly the recognition that suicidal tendencies may be present and protective measures may be necessary.
The usual precautions should be observed in patients with impaired renal or hepatic function and chronic pulmonary insufficiency.
Information for Patients: To assure the safe and effective use of benzodiazepines, patients should be informed that since benzodiazepines may produce psychological and physical dependence, it is advisable that they consult with their

Continued on next page

Roche Products—Cont.

physician before either increasing the dose or abruptly discontinuing this drug.

ADVERSE REACTIONS

Dizziness, drowsiness, light-headedness, staggering, ataxia and falling have occurred, particularly in elderly or debilitated persons. Severe sedation, lethargy, disorientation and coma, probably indicative of drug intolerance or overdosage, have been reported.
Also reported were headache, heartburn, upset stomach, nausea, vomiting, diarrhea, constipation, gastrointestinal pain, nervousness, talkativeness, apprehension, irritability, weakness, palpitations, chest pains, body and joint pains and genitourinary complaints. There have also been rare occurrences of leukopenia, granulocytopenia, sweating, flushes, difficulty in focusing, blurred vision, burning eyes, faintness, hypotension, shortness of breath, pruritus, skin rash, dry mouth, bitter taste, excessive salivation, anorexia, euphoria, depression, slurred speech, confusion, restlessness, hallucinations, and elevated SGOT, SGPT, total and direct bilirubins, and alkaline phosphatase. Paradoxical reactions, eg, excitement, stimulation and hyperactivity, have also been reported in rare instances.

DRUG ABUSE AND DEPENDENCE

Withdrawal symptoms, similar in character to those noted with barbiturates and alcohol (convulsions, tremor, abdominal and muscle cramps, vomiting and sweating), have occurred following abrupt discontinuance of benzodiazepines. The more severe withdrawal symptoms have usually been limited to those patients who had received excessive doses over an extended period of time. Generally milder withdrawal symptoms (eg, dysphoria and insomnia) have been reported following abrupt discontinuance of benzodiazepines taken continuously at therapeutic levels for several months. Consequently, after extended therapy, abrupt discontinuation should generally be avoided and a gradual dosage tapering schedule followed. Addiction-prone individuals (such as drug addicts or alcoholics) should be under careful surveillance when receiving flurazepam or other psychotropic agents because of the predisposition of such patients to habituation and dependence.

DOSAGE AND ADMINISTRATION

Dosage should be individualized for maximal beneficial effects. The usual adult dosage is 30 mg before retiring. In some patients, 15 mg may suffice. In elderly and/or debilitated patients, 15 mg is usually sufficient for a therapeutic response and it is therefore recommended that therapy be initiated with this dosage.

OVERDOSAGE

Manifestations of Dalmane overdosage include somnolence, confusion and coma. Respiration, pulse and blood pressure should be monitored as in all cases of drug overdosage. General supportive measures should be employed, along with immediate gastric lavage. Intravenous fluids should be administered and an adequate airway maintained. Hypotension and CNS depression may be combated by judicious use of appropriate therapeutic agents. The value of dialysis has not been determined. If excitation occurs in patients following Dalmane overdosage, barbiturates should not be used. As with the management of intentional overdosage with any drug, it should be borne in mind that multiple agents may have been ingested.
Flumazenil, a specific benzodiazepine-receptor antagonist, is indicated for the complete or partial reversal of the sedative effects of benzodiazepines and may be used in situations when an overdose with a benzodiazepine is known or suspected. Prior to the administration of flumazenil, necessary measures should be instituted to secure airway ventilation and intravenous access. Flumazenil is intended as an adjunct to, not as a substitute for, proper management of benzodiazepine overdose. Patients treated with flumazenil should be monitored for resedation, respiratory depression and other residual benzodiazepine effects for an appropriate period after treatment. **The prescriber should be aware of a risk of seizure in association with flumazenil treatment, particularly in long-term benzodiazepine users and in cyclic antidepressant overdose.** The complete flumazenil package insert, including CONTRAINDICATIONS, WARNINGS and PRECAUTIONS, should be consulted prior to use.

HOW SUPPLIED

Dalmane (flurazepam hydrochloride) capsules—15 mg, orange and ivory; 30 mg, red and ivory—bottles of 100 and 500.
Revised: March 1994

Shown in Product Identification Guide, page 332

LIBRAX® ℞

[lib 'rax]
CAPSULES

The following text is complete prescribing information based on official labeling in effect June 1996.

DESCRIPTION

Librax combines in a single capsule formulation the antianxiety action of Librium (chlordiazepoxide hydrochloride) and the anticholinergic/spasmolytic effects of Quarzan (clidinium bromide), both exclusive developments of Roche research.
Each Librax capsule contains 5 mg chlordiazepoxide hydrochloride and 2.5 mg clidinium bromide. Each capsule also contains corn starch, lactose and talc. Gelatin capsule shells may contain methyl and propyl parabens and potassium sorbate, with the following dye systems: D&C Yellow No. 10 and either FD&C Blue No. 1 or FD&C Green No. 3.
Librium (chlordiazepoxide hydrochloride) is a versatile, therapeutic agent of proven value for the relief of anxiety and tension. It is indicated when anxiety, tension or apprehension are significant components of the clinical profile. It is among the safer of the effective psychopharmacologic compounds.
Chlordiazepoxide hydrochloride is 7-chloro-2-methylamino-5-phenyl-3H-1, 4-benzodiazepine 4-oxide hydrochloride. A colorless, crystalline substance, it is soluble in water. It is unstable in solution and the powder must be protected from light. The molecular weight is 336.22.
Quarzan (clidinium bromide) is a synthetic anticholinergic agent which has been shown in experimental and clinical studies to have a pronounced antispasmodic and antisecretory effect on the gastrointestinal tract.

ANIMAL PHARMACOLOGY

Chlordiazepoxide hydrochloride has been studied extensively in many species of animals and these studies are suggestive of action on the limbic system of the brain,[1,2,3] which recent evidence indicates is involved in emotional responses.[4,5]
Hostile monkeys were made tame by oral drug doses which did not cause sedation. Chlordiazepoxide hydrochloride revealed a "taming" action with the elimination of fear and aggression.[6] The taming effect of chlordiazepoxide hydrochloride was further demonstrated in rats made vicious by lesions in the septal area of the brain. The drug dosage which effectively blocked the vicious reaction was well below the dose which caused sedation in these animals.[6]
The oral LD_{50} of single doses of chlordiazepoxide hydrochloride, calculated according to the method of Miller and Tainter,[7] is 720 ± 51 mg/kg as determined in mice observed over a period of five days following dosage.
Clidinium bromide is an effective anticholinergic agent with activity approximating that of atropine sulfate against acetylcholine-induced spasms in isolated intestinal strips. On oral administration in mice it proved an effective antisialagogue in preventing pilocarpine-induced salivation. Spontaneous intestinal motility in both rats and dogs is reduced following oral dosing with 0.1 to 0.25 mg/kg. Potent cholinergic ganglionic blocking effects (vagal) are produced with intravenous usage in anesthetized dogs.
Oral doses of 2.5 mg/kg to dogs produced signs of nasal dryness and slight pupillary dilation. In two other species, monkeys and rabbits, doses of 5 mg/kg, p.o., given three times daily for 5 days did not produce apparent secretory or visual changes.
The oral LD_{50} of single doses of clidinium bromide is 860 ± 57 mg/kg as determined in mice observed over a period of 5 days following dosage; the calculations were made according to the method of Miller and Tainter.[7]
Effects on Reproduction: Reproduction studies in rats fed chlordiazepoxide hydrochloride, 10, 20 and 80 mg/kg daily, and bred through one or two matings showed no congenital anomalies, nor were there adverse effects on lactation of the dams or growth of the newborn. However, in another study at 100 mg/kg daily there was noted a significant decrease in the fertilization rate and a marked decrease in the viability and body weight of offspring which may be attributable to sedative activity, thus resulting in lack of interest in mating and lessened maternal nursing and care of the young.[8,9] One neonate in each of the first and second matings in the rat reproduction study at the 100 mg/kg dose exhibited major skeletal defects. Further studies are in progress to determine the significance of these findings.
Two series of reproduction experiments with clidinium bromide were carried out in rats, employing dosages of 2.5 and 10 mg/kg daily in each experiment. In the first experiment clidinium bromide was administered for a 9-week interval prior to mating; no untoward effect on fertilization or gestation was noted. The offspring were taken by caesarean section and did not show a significant incidence of congenital anomalies when compared to control animals. In the second experiment adult animals were given clidinium bromide for ten days prior to and through two mating cycles. No significant effects were observed on fertility, gestation, viability of offspring or lactation, as compared to control animals, nor was there a significant incidence of congenital anomalies in the offspring derived from these experiments.
A reproduction study of Librax was carried out in rats through two successive matings. Oral daily doses were administered in two concentrations: 2.5 mg/kg chlordiazepoxide hydrochloride with 1.25 mg/kg clidinium bromide, or 25 mg/kg chlordiazepoxide hydrochloride with 12.5 mg/kg clidinium bromide. In the first mating no significant differences were noted between the control or the treated groups, with the exception of a slight decrease in the number of animals surviving during lactation among those receiving the highest dosage. As with all anticholinergic drugs, an inhibiting effect on lactation may occur. In the second mating similar results were obtained except for a slight decrease in the number of pregnant females and in the percentage of offspring surviving until weaning. No congenital anomalies were observed in both matings in either the control or treated groups. Additional animal reproduction studies are in progress.

INDICATIONS

Based on a review of this drug by the National Academy of Sciences—National Research Council and/or other information, FDA has classified the indications as follows:
"Possibly" effective: as adjunctive therapy in the treatment of peptic ulcer and in the treatment of the irritable bowel syndrome (irritable colon, spastic colon, mucous colitis) and acute enterocolitis.
Final classification of the less-than-effective indications requires further investigation.

CONTRAINDICATIONS

Librax is contraindicated in the presence of glaucoma (since the anticholinergic component may produce some degree of mydriasis) and in patients with prostatic hypertrophy and benign bladder neck obstruction. It is contraindicated in patients with known hypersensitivity to chlordiazepoxide hydrochloride and/or clidinium bromide.

WARNINGS

As in the case of other preparations containing CNS-acting drugs, patients receiving Librax should be cautioned about possible combined effects with alcohol and other CNS depressants. For the same reason, they should be cautioned against hazardous occupations requiring complete mental alertness such as operating machinery or driving a motor vehicle.

Usage in Pregnancy: **An increased risk of congenital malformations associated with the use of minor tranquilizers (chlordiazepoxide, diazepam and meprobamate) during the first trimester of pregnancy has been suggested in several studies. Because use of these drugs is rarely a matter of urgency, their use during this period should almost always be avoided. The possibility that a woman of childbearing potential may be pregnant at the time of institution of therapy should be considered. Patients should be advised that if they become pregnant during therapy or intend to become pregnant they should communicate with their physicians about the desirability of discontinuing the drug.**

As with all anticholinergic drugs, an inhibiting effect on lactation may occur. (See Animal Pharmacology.)
Management of Overdosage: Manifestations of Librium (chlordiazepoxide hydrochloride) overdosage include somnolence, confusion, coma and diminished reflexes. Respiration, pulse and blood pressure should be monitored, as in all cases of drug overdosage, although, in general, these effects have been minimal following Librium (chlordiazepoxide hydrochloride) overdosage.
While the signs and symptoms of Librax overdosage may be produced by either of its components, usually such symptoms will be overshadowed by the anticholinergic actions of Quarzan (clidinium bromide). The symptoms of overdosage of Quarzan (clidinium bromide) are excessive dryness of mouth, blurring of vision, urinary hesitancy and constipation.
General supportive measures should be employed, along with immediate gastric lavage. Administer physostigmine (Antilirium) 0.5 to 2 mg at a rate of no more than 1 mg per minute. This may be repeated in 1 to 4 mg doses if arrhythmias, convulsions or deep coma recur. Intravenous fluids should be administered and an adequate airway maintained. Hypotension may be combated by the use of Levophed® (levarterenol) or Aramine (metaraminol). Ritalin (methylphenidate) or caffeine and sodium benzoate may be given to combat CNS-depressive effects. Dialysis is of limited value. Should excitation occur, barbiturates should not be used. As with the management of intentional overdosage with any drug, it should be borne in mind that multiple agents may have been ingested.
Withdrawal symptoms of the barbiturate type have occurred after the discontinuation of benzodiazepines. (See DRUG ABUSE AND DEPENDENCE section.)

PRECAUTIONS

In elderly and debilitated patients, it is recommended that the dosage be limited to the smallest effective amount to preclude the development of ataxia, oversedation, or confusion (not more than two Librax capsules per day initially, to be increased gradually as needed and tolerated). In general, the concomitant administration of Librax and other psychotropic agents is not recommended. If such combination therapy seems indicated, careful consideration should be given to the pharmacology of the agents to be employed—particularly when the known potentiating compounds such as the MAO inhibitors and phenothiazines are to be used. The usual precautions in treating patients with impaired renal or hepatic function should be observed.

Paradoxical reactions to chlordiazepoxide hydrochloride, *e.g.*, excitement, stimulation and acute rage, have been reported in psychiatric patients and should be watched for during Librax therapy. The usual precautions are indicated when chlordiazepoxide hydrochloride is used in the treatment of anxiety states where there is any evidence of impending depression; it should be borne in mind that suicidal tendencies may be present and protective measures may be necessary. Although clinical studies have not established a cause and effect relationship, physicians should be aware that variable effects on blood coagulation have been reported very rarely in patients receiving oral anticoagulants and Librium (chlordiazepoxide hydrochloride).

Information for Patients: To assure the safe and effective use of benzodiazepines, patients should be informed that, since benzodiazepines may produce psychological and physical dependence, it is advisable that they consult with their physician before either increasing the dose or abruptly discontinuing this drug.

ADVERSE REACTIONS[10]

No side effects or manifestations not seen with either compound alone have been reported with the administration of Librax. However, since Librax contains chlordiazepoxide hydrochloride and clidinium bromide, the possibility of untoward effects which may be seen with either of these two compounds cannot be excluded.

When chlordiazepoxide hydrochloride has been used alone the necessity of discontinuing therapy because of undesirable effects has been rare.[11] Drowsiness,[12] ataxia[13] and confusion[9] have been reported in some patients—particularly the elderly and debilitated.[9] While these effects can be avoided in almost all instances by proper dosage adjustment, they have occasionally been observed at the lower dosage ranges. In a few instances syncope has been reported.[14]

Other adverse reactions reported during therapy with Librium (chlordiazepoxide hydrochloride) include isolated instances of skin eruptions,[12] edema,[15] minor menstrual irregularities,[12] nausea and constipation,[16] extrapyramidal symptoms,[9] as well as increased and decreased libido. Such side effects have been infrequent and are generally controlled with reduction of dosage. Changes in EEG patterns (low-voltage fast activity) have been observed in patients during and after Librium (chlordiazepoxide hydrochloride) treatment.[17]

Blood dyscrasias,[10] including agranulocytosis,[18] jaundice and hepatic dysfunction[19] have occasionally been reported during therapy with Librium (chlordiazepoxide hydrochloride). When Librium (chlordiazepoxide hydrochloride) treatment is protracted, periodic blood counts and liver function tests are advisable.

Adverse effects reported with use of *Librax* are those typical of anticholinergic agents, *i.e.*, dryness of the mouth, blurring of vision, urinary hesitancy and constipation. Constipation has occurred most often when Librax therapy has been combined with other spasmolytic agents and/or a low residue diet.

DRUG ABUSE AND DEPENDENCE

Withdrawal symptoms, similar in character to those noted with barbiturates and alcohol (convulsions, tremor, abdominal and muscle cramps, vomiting and sweating), have occurred following abrupt discontinuance of chlordiazepoxide. The more severe withdrawal symptoms have usually been limited to those patients who had received excessive doses over an extended period of time. Generally milder withdrawal symptoms (*e.g.*, dysphoria and insomnia) have been reported following abrupt discontinuance of benzodiazepines taken continuously at therapeutic levels for several months. Consequently, after extended therapy, abrupt discontinuation should generally be avoided and a gradual dosage tapering schedule followed. Addiction-prone individuals (such as drug addicts or alcoholics) should be under careful surveillance when receiving chlordiazepoxide or other psychotropic agents because of the predisposition of such patients to habituation and dependence.

DOSAGE

Because of the varied individual responses to tranquilizers and anticholinergics, the optimum dosage of Librax varies with the diagnosis and response of the individual patient. The dosage, therefore, should be individualized for maximum beneficial effects. The usual maintenance dose is 1 or 2 capsules, 3 or 4 times a day administered before meals and at bedtime.

HOW SUPPLIED

Librax is available in green capsules, each containing 5 mg chlordiazepoxide hydrochloride (Librium®) and 2.5 mg clidinium bromide (Quarzan®)—bottles of 100 (NDC 0140-0007-01) and 500 (NDC 0140-0007-14); Tel-E-Dose® packages of 100 (NDC 0140-0007-49).

REFERENCES

1. Schallek, W., *et al: Arch. Int. Pharmacodyn. 149*:467-483, 1964.
2. Himwich, H. E., *et al: J. Neuropsych. 3* (Suppl. 1):S15-S26, Aug. 1962.
3. Morillo, A., *et al: Psychopharmacologia 3* (No. 5):386-394, 1962.
4. MacLean, P. D.: *Psychosomatic Med. 17:* 355-366, Sept. 1955.
5. Morgan, C. T.: Physiological Psychology, 3rd Ed.; New York, McGraw-Hill, 1965.
6. Randall, L. O. *et al: J. Pharm. Exper. Therap. 129*:163-171, June 1960.
7. Miller, L. C. and Tainter, M. C.: *Proc. Soc. Exp. Biol. & Med. 57*:261, 1944.
8. Zbinden, G., *et al: Toxicology and Applied Pharmacology 3*:619-637, Nov. 1961.
9. Data on file, Hoffmann-La Roche Inc., Nutley, N.J.
10. Bibliography and References available on request from Roche Laboratories.
11. Rickels, K. *et al: Med. Times 93*:238-245, Mar. 1965.
12. Tobin, J. M. *et al: J. Amer. Med. Assoc. 174:* 1242-1249, Nov. 1960.
13. Jenner, F. A., *et al: J. Ment. Sci. 107*:575-582, May 1961.
14. Robinson, R. C. V.: *Dis. Nerv. System 21*:43-45, Mar. 1960.
15. Rose, J. T.: *Amer. J. Psychiat. 120*:899-900, Mar. 1964.
16. Hines, L. R.: *Curr. Therap. Res. 2*:227-236, June 1960.
17. Gibbs, F. A. and Gibbs, E. L.: *J. Neuropsych., 3* (Suppl. 1):S73-S78, Aug. 1962.
18. Kaelbling, R., *et al: J. Amer. Med. Assoc. 174*:1863-1865, Dec. 1960.
19. Cacioppo, J., *et al: Amer. J. Psychiat. 117*:1040-1041, May 1961.

Revised: February 1988

Shown in Product Identification Guide, page 332

LIBRIUM® ℂ

[*lib'ree-um*]

brand of chlordiazepoxide HCl

CAPSULES

The following text is complete prescribing information based on official labeling in effect June 1996.

DESCRIPTION

Librium, the original chlordiazepoxide HCl and prototype for the benzodiazepine compounds, was synthesized and developed at Hoffmann-La Roche Inc. It is a versatile therapeutic agent of proven value for the relief of anxiety. Librium is among the safer of the effective psychopharmacologic compounds available, as demonstrated by extensive clinical evidence.

Librium is available as capsules containing 5 mg, 10 mg or 25 mg chlordiazepoxide HCl. Each capsule also contains corn starch, lactose and talc. Gelatin capsule shells may contain methyl and propyl parabens and potassium sorbate, with the following dye systems: 5-mg capsules—FD&C Yellow No. 6 plus D&C Yellow No. 10 and either FD&C Blue No. 1 or FD&C Green No. 3. 10-mg capsules—FD&C Yellow No. 6 plus D&C Yellow No. 10 and either FD&C Blue No. 1 plus FD&C Red No. 3 or FD&C Green No. 3 plus FD&C Red No. 40. 25-mg capsules—D&C Yellow No. 10 and either FD&C Green No. 3 or FD&C Blue No. 1.

Chlordiazepoxide hydrochloride is 7-chloro-2-(methylamino)-5-phenyl-3H-1,4-benzodiazepine 4-oxide hydrochloride. A white to practically white crystalline substance, it is soluble in water. It is unstable in solution and the powder must be protected from light. The molecular weight is 336.22.

ACTIONS

Librium (chlordiazepoxide HCl) has antianxiety, sedative, appetite-stimulating and weak analgesic actions. The precise mechanism of action is not known. The drug blocks EEG arousal from stimulation of the brain stem reticular formation. It takes several hours for peak blood levels to be reached and the half-life of the drug is between 24 and 48 hours. After the drug is discontinued plasma levels decline slowly over a period of several days. Chlordiazepoxide is excreted in the urine, with 1% to 2% unchanged and 3% to 6% as a conjugate.

Animal Pharmacology: The drug has been studied extensively in many species of animals and these studies are suggestive of action on the limbic system of the brain, which recent evidence indicates is involved in emotional responses. Hostile monkeys were made tame by oral drug doses which did not cause sedation. Chlordiazepoxide HCl revealed a "taming" action with the elimination of fear and aggression. The taming effect of chlordiazepoxide HCl was further demonstrated in rats made vicious by lesions in the septal area of the brain. The drug dosage which effectively blocked the vicious reaction was well below the dose which caused sedation in these animals.

The LD_{50} of parenterally administered chlordiazepoxide HCl was determined in mice (72 hours) and rats (5 days), and calculated according to the method of Miller and Tainter, with the following results: mice, IV, 123 $\pm$12 mg/kg; mice, IM, 366 $\pm$7 mg/kg; rats, IV, 120 $\pm$7 mg/kg; rats, IM, $>$160 mg/kg.

Effects on Reproduction: Reproduction studies in rats fed 10, 20 and 80 mg/kg daily and bred through one or two matings showed no congenital anomalies, nor were there adverse effects on lactation of the dams or growth of the newborn. However, in another study at 100 mg/kg daily there was noted a significant decrease in the fertilization rate and a marked decrease in the viability and body weight of offspring which may be attributable to sedative activity, thus resulting in lack of interest in mating and lessened maternal nursing and care of the young. One neonate in each of the first and second matings in the rat reproduction study at the 100 mg/kg dose exhibited major skeletal defects. Further studies are in progress to determine the significance of these findings.

INDICATIONS

Librium is indicated for the management of anxiety disorders or for the short-term relief of symptoms of anxiety, withdrawal symptoms of acute alcoholism, and preoperative apprehension and anxiety. Anxiety or tension associated with the stress of everyday life usually does not require treatment with an anxiolytic.

The effectiveness of Librium in long-term use, that is, more than 4 months, has not been assessed by systematic clinical studies. The physician should periodically reassess the usefulness of the drug for the individual patient.

CONTRAINDICATIONS

Librium is contraindicated in patients with known hypersensitivity to the drug.

WARNINGS

Chlordiazepoxide HCl may impair the mental and/or physical abilities required for the performance of potentially hazardous tasks such as driving a vehicle or operating machinery. Similarly, it may impair mental alertness in children. The concomitant use of alcohol or other central nervous system depressants may have an additive effect. PATIENTS SHOULD BE WARNED ACCORDINGLY.

Usage in Pregnancy: An increased risk of congenital malformations associated with the use of minor tranquilizers (chlordiazepoxide, diazepam and meprobamate) during the first trimester of pregnancy has been suggested in several studies. Because use of these drugs is rarely a matter of urgency, their use during this period should almost always be avoided. The possibility that a woman of childbearing potential may be pregnant at the time of institution of therapy should be considered. Patients should be advised that if they become pregnant during therapy or intend to become pregnant they should communicate with their physicians about the desirability of discontinuing the drug.

Withdrawal symptoms of the barbiturate type have occurred after the discontinuation of benzodiazepines. (See DRUG ABUSE AND DEPENDENCE section.)

PRECAUTIONS

In elderly and debilitated patients, it is recommended that the dosage be limited to the smallest effective amount to preclude the development of ataxia or oversedation (10 mg or less per day initially, to be increased gradually as needed and tolerated). In general, the concomitant administration of Librium and other psychotropic agents is not recommended. If such combination therapy seems indicated, careful consideration should be given to the pharmacology of the agents to be employed — particularly when the known potentiating compounds such as the MAO inhibitors and phenothiazines are to be used. The usual precautions in treating patients with impaired renal or hepatic function should be observed.

Paradoxical reactions, eg, excitement, stimulation and acute rage, have been reported in psychiatric patients and in hyperactive aggressive children, and should be watched for during Librium therapy. The usual precautions are indicated when Librium is used in the treatment of anxiety states where there is any evidence of impending depression; it should be borne in mind that suicidal tendencies may be present and protective measures may be necessary. Although clinical studies have not established a cause and effect relationship, physicians should be aware that variable

Continued on next page

Roche Products—Cont.

effects on blood coagulation have been reported very rarely in patients receiving oral anticoagulants and Librium. In view of isolated reports associating chlordiazepoxide with exacerbation of porphyria, caution should be exercised in prescribing chlordiazepoxide to patients suffering from this disease.

Information for Patients: To assure the safe and effective use of benzodiazepines, patients should be informed that, since benzodiazepines may produce psychological and physical dependence it is advisable that they consult with their physician before either increasing the dose or abruptly discontinuing this drug.

ADVERSE REACTIONS

The necessity of discontinuing therapy because of undesirable effects has been rare. Drowsiness, ataxia and confusion have been reported in some patients — particularly the elderly and debilitated. While these effects can be avoided in almost all instances by proper dosage adjustment, they have occasionally been observed at the lower dosage ranges. In a few instances syncope has been reported.

Other adverse reactions reported during therapy include isolated instances of skin eruptions, edema, minor menstrual irregularities, nausea and constipation, extrapyramidal symptoms, as well as increased and decreased libido. Such side effects have been infrequent and are generally controlled with reduction of dosage. Changes in EEG patterns (low-voltage fast activity) have been observed in patients during and after Librium treatment.

Blood dyscrasias (including agranulocytosis), jaundice and hepatic dysfunction have occasionally been reported during therapy. When Librium treatment is protracted, periodic blood counts and liver function tests are advisable.

DRUG ABUSE AND DEPENDENCE

Chlordiazepoxide hydrochloride capsules are classified by the Drug Enforcement Administration as a Schedule IV controlled substance.

Withdrawal symptoms, similar in character to those noted with barbiturates and alcohol (convulsions, tremor, abdominal and muscle cramps, vomiting and sweating), have occurred following abrupt discontinuance of chlordiazepoxide. The more severe withdrawal symptoms have usually been limited to those patients who had received excessive doses over an extended period of time. Generally milder withdrawal symptoms (eg, dysphoria and insomnia) have been reported following abrupt discontinuance of benzodiazepines taken continuously at therapeutic levels for several months. Consequently, after extended therapy, abrupt discontinuation should generally be avoided and a gradual dosage tapering schedule followed. Addiction-prone individuals (such as drug addicts or alcoholics) should be under careful surveillance when receiving chlordiazepoxide or other psychotropic agents because of the predisposition of such patients to habituation and dependence.

OVERDOSAGE

Manifestations of Librium overdosage include somnolence, confusion, coma and diminished reflexes. Respiration, pulse and blood pressure should be monitored, as in all cases of drug overdosage, although, in general, these effects have been minimal following Librium overdosage. General supportive measures should be employed, along with immediate gastric lavage. Intravenous fluids should be administered and an adequate airway maintained. Hypotension may be combated by the use of Levophed® (norepinephrine) or Aramine (metaraminol). Dialysis is of limited value. There have been occasional reports of excitation in patients following chlordiazepoxide HCl overdosage; if this occurs barbiturates should not be used. As with the management of intentional overdosage with any drug, it should be borne in mind that multiple agents may have been ingested.

Flumazenil, a specific benzodiazepine-receptor antagonist, is indicated for the complete or partial reversal of the sedative effects of benzodiazepines and may be used in situations when an overdose with a benzodiazepine is known or suspected. Prior to the administration of flumazenil, necessary measures should be instituted to secure airway, ventilation and intravenous access. Flumazenil is intended as an adjunct to, not as a substitute for, proper management of benzodiazepine overdose. Patients treated with flumazenil should be monitored for resedation, respiratory depression and other residual benzodiazepine effects for an appropriate period after treatment. **The prescriber should be aware of a risk of seizure in association with flumazenil treatment, particularly in long-term benzodiazepine users and in cyclic antidepressant overdose.** The complete flumazenil package insert, including CONTRAINDICATIONS, WARNINGS and PRECAUTIONS, should be consulted prior to use.

DOSAGE AND ADMINISTRATION

Because of the wide range of clinical indications for Librium, the optimum dosage varies with the diagnosis and response of the individual patient. The dosage, therefore, should be individualized for maximum beneficial effects.

ADULTS	*USUAL DAILY DOSE*
Relief of Mild and Moderate Anxiety Disorders and Symptoms of Anxiety	5 mg or 10 mg, 3 or 4 times daily
Relief of Severe Anxiety Disorders and Symptoms of Anxiety	20 mg or 25 mg, 3 or 4 times daily
Geriatric Patients, or in the presence of debilitating disease	5 mg, 2 to 4 times daily

Preoperative Apprehension and Anxiety:
On days preceding surgery, 5 to 10 mg orally, 3 or 4 times daily. If used as preoperative medication, 50 to 100 mg IM* 1 hour prior to surgery.

CHILDREN	*USUAL DAILY DOSE*
Because of the varied response of children to CNS-acting drugs, therapy should be initiated with the lowest dose and increased as required. Since clinical experience in children under 6 years of age is limited, the use of the drug in this age group is not recommended.	5 mg, 2 to 4 times daily (may be increased in some children to 10 mg, 2 to 3 times daily)

For the relief of withdrawal symptoms of acute alcoholism, the parenteral form* is usually used initially. If the drug is administered orally, the suggested initial dose is 50 to 100 mg, to be followed by repeated doses as needed until agitation is controlled — up to 300 mg per day. Dosage should then be reduced to maintenance levels.

* See package insert for Injectable Librium (chlordiazepoxide HCl).

HOW SUPPLIED

Librium (chlordiazepoxide HCl) capsules—5 mg, green and yellow; 10 mg, green and black; 25 mg, green and white—bottles of 100 and 500; Tel-E-Dose® packages of 100, available in boxes of 4 reverse-numbered cards of 25, and in boxes containing 10 strips of 10.

Revised: June 1993

Shown in Product Identification Guide, page 332

LIBRIUM® INJECTABLE Ⓒ

[lib 'ree-um]

brand of chlordiazepoxide HCl

The following text is complete prescribing information based on official labeling in effect June 1996.

DESCRIPTION

Librium is a versatile therapeutic agent of proven value for the relief of anxiety and tension.

Librium is the first of a new class, unrelated chemically and pharmacologically to other types of tranquilizers. Librium promptly relieves anxiety and is among the safer of the effective psychopharmacologic compounds available.

Chlordiazepoxide HCl is 7-chloro-2-methylamino-5-phenyl-3H-1,4-benzodiazepine 4-oxide hydrochloride. A colorless, crystalline substance, it is soluble in water. It is unstable in solution and the powder must be protected from light. The molecular weight is 336.22.

ANIMAL PHARMACOLOGY

The drug has been studied extensively in many species of animals and these studies are suggestive of action on the limbic system of the brain, which recent evidence indicates is involved in emotional responses.

Hostile monkeys were made tame by oral drug doses which did not cause sedation. Librium revealed a "taming" action with the elimination of fear and aggression. The taming effect of Librium was further demonstrated in rats made vicious by lesions in the septal area of the brain. The drug dosage which effectively blocked the vicious reaction was well below the dose which caused sedation in these animals.

The LD_{50} of parenterally administered chlordiazepoxide HCl was determined in mice (72 hours) and rats (5 days), and calculated according to the method of Miller and Tainter, with the following results: mice, IV, 123 $\pm$ 12 mg/kg; mice, IM, 366 $\pm$ 7 mg/kg; rats, IV, 120 $\pm$ 7 mg/kg; rats, IM, $>$160 mg/kg.

Effects on Reproduction: Reproduction studies in rats fed 10, 20 and 80 mg/kg daily and bred through one or two matings showed no congenital anomalies, nor were there adverse effects on lactation of the dams or growth of the newborn. However, in another study at 100 mg/kg daily there was noted a significant decrease in the fertilization rate and a marked decrease in the viability and body weight of offspring which may be attributable to sedative activity, thus resulting in lack of interest in mating and lessened maternal nursing and care of the young. One neonate in each of the first and second matings in the rat reproduction study at the 100 mg/kg dose exhibited major skeletal defects. Further studies are in progress to determine the significance of these findings.

INDICATIONS

Injectable Librium is indicated for the management of anxiety disorders or for the short-term relief of symptoms of anxiety, withdrawal symptoms of acute alcoholism, and preoperative apprehension and anxiety. Anxiety or tension associated with the stress of everyday life usually does not require treatment with an anxiolytic.

CONTRAINDICATIONS

Librium is contraindicated in patients with known hypersensitivity to the drug.

WARNINGS

As in the case of other CNS-acting drugs, patients receiving Librium should be cautioned about possible combined effects with alcohol and other CNS depressants.

As is true of all preparations containing CNS-acting drugs, patients receiving Librium should be cautioned against hazardous occupations requiring complete mental alertness such as operating machinery or driving a motor vehicle.

Usage in Pregnancy: **An increased risk of congenital malformations associated with the use of minor tranquilizers (chlordiazepoxide, diazepam and meprobamate) during the first trimester of pregnancy has been suggested in several studies. Because use of these drugs is rarely a matter of urgency, their use during this period should almost always be avoided. The possibility that a woman of childbearing potential may be pregnant at the time of institution of therapy should be considered. Patients should be advised that if they become pregnant during therapy or intend to become pregnant they should communicate with their physicians about the desirability of discontinuing the drug.**

Management of Overdosage: Manifestations of Librium overdosage include somnolence, confusion, coma and diminished reflexes. Respiration, pulse and blood pressure should be monitored, as in all cases of drug overdosage, although, in general, these effects have been minimal following Librium overdosage. General supportive measures should be employed, along with immediate gastric lavage.

Intravenous fluids should be administered and an adequate airway maintained. Hypotension may be combated by the use of Levophed® (levarterenol) or Aramine (metaraminol). Dialysis is of limited value. There have been occasional reports of excitation in patients following Librium overdosage; if this occurs barbiturates should not be used. As with the management of intentional overdosage with any drug, it should be borne in mind that multiple agents may have been ingested.

Flumazenil, a specific benzodiazepine-receptor antagonist, is indicated for the complete or partial reversal of the sedative effects of benzodiazepines and may be used in situations when an overdose with a benzodiazepine is known or suspected. Prior to the administration of flumazenil, necessary measures should be instituted to secure airway, ventilation and intravenous access. Flumazenil is intended as an adjunct to, not as a substitute for, proper management of benzodiazepine overdose. Patients treated with flumazenil should be monitored for resedation, respiratory depression and other residual benzodiazepine effects for an appropriate period after treatment. **The prescriber should be aware of a risk of seizure in association with flumazenil treatment, particularly in long-term benzodiazepine users and in cyclic antidepressant overdose.** The complete flumazenil package insert, including CONTRAINDICATIONS, WARNINGS and PRECAUTIONS, should be consulted prior to use.

Withdrawal symptoms of the barbiturate type have occurred after the discontinuation of benzodiazepines. (See DRUG ABUSE AND DEPENDENCE section.)

PRECAUTIONS

Injectable Librium (intramuscular or intravenous) is indicated primarily in acute states, and patients receiving this form of therapy should be kept under observation, preferably in bed, for a period of up to 3 hours. Ambulatory patients should not be permitted to operate a vehicle following an injection. Injectable Librium should not be given to patients in shock or comatose states. Reduced dosage (usually 25 to 50 mg) should be used for elderly or debilitated patients, and for children age 12 or older. In general, the concomitant administration of Librium and other psychotropic agents is not recommended. If such combination therapy seems indicated, careful consideration should be given to the pharmacology of the agents to be employed—particularly when the known potentiating compounds such as the MAO inhibitors and phenothiazines are to be used. The usual precautions in treating patients with impaired renal or hepatic function should be observed.

Paradoxical reactions, eg, excitement, stimulation and acute rage, have been reported in psychiatric patients and in hyperactive aggressive children, and should be watched for during Librium therapy. The usual precautions are indicated when Librium is used in the treatment of anxiety states where there is any evidence of impending depression; it should be borne in mind that suicidal tendencies may be present and protective measures may be necessary. Although clinical studies have not established a cause and effect relationship, physicians should be aware that variable effects on blood coagulation have been reported very rarely in patients receiving oral anticoagulants and Librium. In view of isolated reports associating chlordiazepoxide with exacerbation of porphyria, caution should be exercised in prescribing chlordiazepoxide to patients suffering from this disease.

ADVERSE REACTIONS

The necessity of discontinuing therapy because of undesirable effects has been rare. Drowsiness, ataxia and confusion are more commonly seen in the elderly and debilitated. Other adverse reactions reported during therapy include isolated instances of syncope, hypotension, tachycardia, skin eruptions, edema, minor menstrual irregularities, nausea and constipation, extrapyramidal symptoms, blurred vision, as well as increased and decreased libido. Such side effects have been infrequent and are generally controlled with reduction of dosage. Similarly, hypotension associated with spinal anesthesia has occurred. Pain following intramuscular injection has been reported. Changes in EEG patterns (low-voltage fast activity) have been observed in patients during and after Librium treatment.

Blood dyscrasias (including agranulocytosis), jaundice and hepatic dysfunction, have occasionally been reported during therapy. When Librium treatment is protracted, periodic blood counts and liver function tests are advisable.

DRUG ABUSE AND DEPENDENCE

Withdrawal symptoms, similar in character to those noted with barbiturates and alcohol (convulsions, tremor, abdominal and muscle cramps, vomiting and sweating), have occurred following abrupt discontinuance of chlordiazepoxide. The more severe withdrawal symptoms have usually been limited to those patients who had received excessive doses over an extended period of time. Generally milder withdrawal symptoms (eg, dysphoria and insomnia) have been reported following abrupt discontinuance of benzodiazepines taken continuously at therapeutic levels for several months. Consequently, after extended therapy, abrupt discontinuation should generally be avoided and a gradual dosage tapering schedule followed. Addiction-prone individuals (such as drug addicts or alcoholics) should be under careful surveillance when receiving chlordiazepoxide or other psychotropic agents because of the predisposition of such patients to habituation and dependence.

PREPARATION AND ADMINISTRATION OF SOLUTIONS

Solutions of Librium for intramuscular or intravenous use should be prepared aseptically. Sterilization by heating should not be attempted.

Intramuscular: Add 2 mL of *Special Intramuscular Diluent* to contents of 5-mL dry-filled amber ampul of Librium Sterile Powder (100 mg). Avoid excessive pressure in injecting this special diluent into the ampul containing the powder since bubbles will form on the surface of the solution. Agitate gently until completely dissolved. Solution should be prepared immediately before administration. Any unused solution should be discarded. Deep intramuscular injection should be given *slowly* into the upper outer quadrant of the gluteus muscle.

Caution: Librium solution made with the Special Intramuscular Diluent should not be given intravenously because of the air bubbles which form when the intramuscular diluent is added to the Librium powder. Do not use diluent solution if it is opalescent or hazy.

Intravenous: In most cases, intramuscular injection is the preferred route of administration of Injectable Librium since beneficial effects are usually seen within 15 to 30 minutes. When, in the judgment of the physician, even more rapid action is mandatory, Injectable Librium may be administered intravenously. A suitable solution for intravenous administration may be prepared as follows: Add 5 mL of *sterile physiological saline* or *sterile water for injection* to contents of 5-mL dry-filled amber ampul of Librium Sterile Powder (100 mg). Agitate gently until thoroughly dissolved. Solution should be prepared immediately before administration. Any unused portion should be discarded. *Intravenous injection should be given slowly over a 1-minute period.*

Caution: Librium solution made with physiological saline or sterile water for injection should not be given intramuscularly because of pain on injection.

DOSAGE

Dosage should be individualized according to the diagnosis and the response of the patient. While 300 mg may be given

during a 6-hour period, this dose should not be exceeded in any 24-hour period.

INDICATION	ADULT DOSAGE*
Withdrawal Symptoms of Acute Alcoholism	50 to 100 mg IM or IV initially; repeat in 2 to 4 hours, if necessary
Acute or Severe Anxiety Disorders or Symptoms of Anxiety	50 to 100 mg IM or IV initially; then 25 to 50 mg 3 or 4 times daily, if necessary
Preoperative Apprehension and Anxiety	50 to 100 mg IM 1 hour prior to surgery

* Lower doses (usually 25 to 50 mg) should be used for elderly or debilitated patients, and for older children. Since clinical experience in children under 12 years of age is limited, the use of the drug in this age group is not recommended.

In most cases, acute symptoms may be rapidly controlled by parenteral administration so that subsequent treatment, if necessary, may be given orally. (See package insert for Oral Librium.)

HOW SUPPLIED

For Parenteral Administration: Ampuls—Duplex package consisting of a 5-mL dry-filled ampul containing 100 mg chlordiazepoxide HCl in dry crystalline form, and a 2-mL ampul of Special Intramuscular Diluent (for intramuscular administration) compounded with 1.5% benzyl alcohol, 4% polysorbate 80, 20% propylene glycol, 1.6% maleic acid and sodium hydroxide to adjust pH to approximately 3. Boxes of 10.

CAUTION

Before preparing solution for intramuscular or intravenous administration, please read instructions for PREPARATION AND ADMINISTRATION OF SOLUTIONS.
Manufactured by Hoffmann-La Roche Inc., Nutley, NJ 07110
Revised: June 1993

LIMBITROL®   ℞

[lim 'bit-roll]
(chlordiazepoxide and amitriptyline HCl)
DS (double strength) TABLETS
TABLETS
Tranquilizer—Antidepressant

DESCRIPTION

Limbitrol combines for oral administration, chlordiazepoxide, an agent for the relief of anxiety and tension, and amitriptyline, an antidepressant. It is available in DS (double strength) white, film-coated tablets, each containing 10 mg chlordiazepoxide and 25 mg amitriptyline (as the hydrochloride salt); and in blue, film-coated tablets, each containing 5 mg chlordiazepoxide and 12.5 mg amitriptyline (as the hydrochloride salt). Each tablet also contains corn starch, hydroxypropyl cellulose, hydroxypropyl methylcellulose, lactose, magnesium stearate, polyethylene glycol, povidone and propylene glycol; Limbitrol tablets contain the following colorant system—FD&C Blue No. 1 aluminum lake and titanium dioxide; Limbitrol DS tablets contain titanium dioxide.

Chlordiazepoxide is a benzodiazepine with the formula 7-chloro-2-(methylamino)-5-phenyl-3H-1,4-benzodiazepine 4-oxide. It is a slightly yellow crystalline material and is insoluble in water. The molecular weight is 299.76.

Amitriptyline is a dibenzocycloheptadiene derivative. The formula is 10,11-dihydro-N,N-dimethyl-5H -dibenzo[a,d] cycloheptene-$\Delta^{5,\gamma}$ -propylamine hydrochloride. It is a white or practically white crystalline compound that is freely soluble in water. The molecular weight is 313.87.

ACTIONS

Both components of Limbitrol exert their action in the central nervous system. Extensive studies with chlordiazepoxide in many animal species suggest action in the limbic system. Recent evidence indicates that the limbic system is involved in emotional response. Taming action was observed in some species. The mechanism of action of amitriptyline in man is not known, but the drug appears to interfere with the reuptake of norepinephrine into adrenergic nerve endings. This action may prolong the sympathetic activity of biogenic amines.

INDICATIONS

Limbitrol is indicated for the treatment of patients with moderate to severe depression associated with moderate to severe anxiety.

The therapeutic response to Limbitrol occurs earlier and with fewer treatment failures than when either amitriptyline or chlordiazepoxide is used alone.

Symptoms likely to respond in the first week of treatment include: insomnia, feelings of guilt or worthlessness, agita-

tion, psychic and somatic anxiety, suicidal ideation and anorexia.

CONTRAINDICATIONS

Limbitrol is contraindicated in patients with hypersensitivity to either benzodiazepines or tricyclic antidepressants. It should not be given concomitantly with a monoamine oxidase inhibitor. Hyperpyretic crises, severe convulsions and deaths have occurred in patients receiving a tricyclic antidepressant and a monoamine oxidase inhibitor simultaneously. When it is desired to replace a monoamine oxidase inhibitor with Limbitrol, a minimum of 14 days should be allowed to elapse after the former is discontinued. Limbitrol should then be initiated cautiously with gradual increase in dosage until optimum response is achieved.

This drug is contraindicated during the acute recovery phase following myocardial infarction.

WARNINGS

Because of the atropine-like action of the amitriptyline component, great care should be used in treating patients with a history of urinary retention or angle-closure glaucoma. In patients with glaucoma, even average doses may precipitate an attack. Severe constipation may occur in patients taking tricyclic antidepressants in combination with anticholinergic-type drugs.

Patients with cardiovascular disorders should be watched closely. Tricyclic antidepressant drugs, particularly when given in high doses, have been reported to produce arrhythmias, sinus tachycardia and prolongation of conduction time. Myocardial infarction and stroke have been reported in patients receiving drugs of this class.

Because of the sedative effects of Limbitrol, patients should be cautioned about combined effects with alcohol or other CNS depressants. The additive effects may produce a harmful level of sedation and CNS depression.

Patients receiving Limbitrol should be cautioned against engaging in hazardous occupations requiring complete mental alertness, such as operating machinery or driving a motor vehicle.

Usage in Pregnancy: Safe use of Limbitrol during pregnancy and lactation has not been established. Because of the chlordiazepoxide component, please note the following:

An increased risk of congenital malformations associated with the use of minor tranquilizers (chlordiazepoxide, diazepam and meprobamate) during the first trimester of pregnancy has been suggested in several studies. Because use of these drugs is rarely a matter of urgency, their use during this period should almost always be avoided. The possibility that a woman of childbearing potential may be pregnant at the time of institution of therapy should be considered. Patients should be advised that if they become pregnant during therapy or intend to become pregnant they should communicate with their physicians about the desirability of discontinuing the drug.

Withdrawal symptoms of the barbiturate type have occurred after the discontinuation of benzodiazepines. (See DRUG ABUSE AND DEPENDENCE section.)

PRECAUTIONS

General: Use with caution in patients with a history of seizures.

Close supervision is required when Limbitrol is given to hyperthyroid patients or those on thyroid medication.

The usual precautions should be observed when treating patients with impaired renal or hepatic function.

Patients with suicidal ideation should not have easy access to large quantities of the drug. The possibility of suicide in depressed patients remains until significant remission occurs.

Essential Laboratory Tests: Patients on prolonged treatment should have periodic liver function tests and blood counts.

Drug and Treatment Interactions: Because of its amitriptyline component, Limbitrol may block the antihypertensive action of guanethidine or compounds with a similar mechanism of action.

Drugs Metabolized by P450 2D6: The biochemical activity of the drug metabolizing isozyme cytochrome P450 2D6 (debrisoquin hydroxylase) is reduced in a subset of the caucasian population (about 7% to 10% of caucasians are so called "poor metabolizers"); reliable estimates of the prevalence of reduced P450 2D6 isozyme activity among Asian, African and other populations are not yet available. Poor metabolizers have higher than expected plasma concentrations of tricyclic antidepressants (TCAs) when given usual doses. Depending on the fraction of drug metabolized by P450 2D6, the increase in plasma concentration may be small or quite large (8-fold increase in plasma AUC of the TCA).

In addition, certain drugs inhibit the activity of this isozyme and make normal metabolizers resemble poor metabolizers. An individual who is stable on a given dose of TCA may become abruptly toxic when given one of these inhibiting drugs as concomitant therapy. The drugs that inhibit cytochrome P450 2D6 include some that are not metabolized by the enzyme (quinidine; cimetidine) and many that are substrates for P450 2D6 (many other antidepressants, phenothiazines,

Continued on next page

Roche Products—Cont.

and the type 1c antiarrhythmics propafenone and flecainide). While all the selective serotonin reuptake inhibitors (SSRIs), eg, fluoxetine, sertraline and paroxetine, inhibit P450 2D6, they may vary in the extent of inhibition. The extent to which SSRI TCA interactions may pose clinical problems will depend on the degree of inhibition and the pharmacokinetics of the SSRI involved. Nevertheless, caution is indicated in the coadministration of TCAs with any of the SSRIs and also in switching from one class to the other. Of particular importance, sufficient time must elapse before initiating TCA treatment in a patient being withdrawn from fluoxetine, given the long half-life of the parent and active metabolite (at least 5 weeks may be necessary).

Concomitant use of tricyclic antidepressants with drugs that can inhibit cytochrome P450 2D6 may require lower doses than usually prescribed for either the tricyclic antidepressant or the other drug. Furthermore, whenever one of these other drugs is withdrawn from cotherapy, an increased dose of tricyclic antidepressant may be required. It is desirable to monitor TCA plasma levels whenever a TCA is going to be coadministered with another drug known to be an inhibitor of P450 2D6.

The effects of concomitant administration of Limbitrol and other psychotropic drugs have not been evaluated. Sedative effects may be additive.

Cimetidine is reported to reduce hepatic metabolism of certain tricyclic antidepressants and benzodiazepines, thereby delaying elimination and increasing steady-state concentrations of these drugs. Clinically significant effects have been reported with the tricyclic antidepressants when used concomitantly with cimetidine (Tagamet).

The drug should be discontinued several days before elective surgery.

Concurrent administration of ECT and Limbitrol should be limited to those patients for whom it is essential.

Pregnancy: See WARNINGS section.

Nursing Mothers: It is not known whether this drug is excreted in human milk. As a general rule, nursing should not be undertaken while a patient is on a drug, since many drugs are excreted in human milk.

Pediatric Use: Safety and effectiveness in children below the age of 12 years have not been established.

Elderly Patients: In elderly and debilitated patients it is recommended that dosage be limited to the smallest effective amount to preclude the development of ataxia, oversedation, confusion or anticholinergic effects.

Information for Patients: To assure the safe and effective use of benzodiazepines, patients should be informed that, since benzodiazepines may produce psychological and physical dependence, it is advisable that they consult with their physician before either increasing the dose or abruptly discontinuing this drug.

ADVERSE REACTIONS

Adverse reactions to Limbitrol are those associated with the use of either component alone. Most frequently reported were drowsiness, dry mouth, constipation, blurred vision, dizziness and bloating. Other side effects occurring less commonly included vivid dreams, impotence, tremor, confusion and nasal congestion. Many symptoms common to the depressive state, such as anorexia, fatigue, weakness, restlessness and lethargy, have been reported as side effects of treatment with both Limbitrol and amitriptyline.

Granulocytopenia, jaundice and hepatic dysfunction of uncertain etiology have also been observed rarely with Limbitrol. When treatment with Limbitrol is prolonged, periodic blood counts and liver function tests are advisable.

Note: Included in the listing which follows are adverse reactions which have not been reported with Limbitrol. However, they are included because they have been reported during therapy with one or both of the components or closely related drugs.

Cardiovascular: Hypotension, hypertension, tachycardia, palpitations, myocardial infarction, arrhythmias, heart block, stroke.

Psychiatric: Euphoria, apprehension, poor concentration, delusions, hallucinations, hypomania and increased or decreased libido.

Neurologic: Incoordination, ataxia, numbness, tingling and paresthesias of the extremities, extrapyramidal symptoms, syncope, changes in EEG patterns.

Anticholinergic: Disturbance of accommodation, paralytic ileus, urinary retention, dilatation of urinary tract.

Allergic: Skin rash, urticaria, photosensitization, edema of face and tongue, pruritus.

Hematologic: Bone marrow depression including agranulocytosis, eosinophilia, purpura, thrombocytopenia.

Gastrointestinal: Nausea, epigastric distress, vomiting, anorexia, stomatitis, peculiar taste, diarrhea, black tongue.

Endocrine: Testicular swelling and gynecomastia in the male, breast enlargement, galactorrhea and minor menstrual irregularities in the female, elevation and lowering of blood sugar levels, and syndrome of inappropriate ADH (antidiuretic hormone) secretion.

Other: Headache, weight gain or loss, increased perspiration, urinary frequency, mydriasis, jaundice, alopecia, parotid swelling.

DRUG ABUSE AND DEPENDENCE

Withdrawal symptoms, similar in character to those noted with barbiturates and alcohol (convulsions, tremor, abdominal and muscle cramps, vomiting and sweating), have occurred following abrupt discontinuance of chlordiazepoxide. The more severe withdrawal symptoms have usually been limited to those patients who had received excessive doses over an extended period of time. Generally milder withdrawal symptoms (eg, dysphoria and insomnia) have been reported following abrupt discontinuance of benzodiazepines taken continuously at therapeutic levels for several months. Withdrawal symptoms (eg, nausea, headache and malaise) have also been reported in association with abrupt amitriptyline discontinuation. Consequently, after extended therapy, abrupt discontinuation should generally be avoided and a gradual dosage tapering schedule followed. Addiction-prone individuals (such as drug addicts or alcoholics) should be under careful surveillance when receiving chlordiazepoxide or other psychotropic agents because of the predisposition of such patients to habituation and dependence.

OVERDOSAGE*

Deaths may occur from overdosage with this class of drugs. Multiple drug ingestion (including alcohol) is common in deliberate tricyclic antidepressant overdose. As the management is complex and changing, it is recommended that the physician contact a poison control center for current information on treatment. Signs and symptoms of toxicity develop rapidly after tricyclic antidepressant overdose; therefore, hospital monitoring is required as soon as possible.

Manifestations: Critical manifestations of overdose include: cardiac dysrhythmias, severe hypotension, convulsions and CNS depression, including coma. Changes in the electrocardiogram, particularly in QRS axis or width, are clinically significant indicators of tricyclic antidepressant toxicity.

Other signs of overdose may include: confusion, disturbed concentration, transient visual hallucinations, dilated pupils, agitation, hyperactive reflexes, stupor, drowsiness, muscle rigidity, vomiting, hypothermia, hyperpyrexia or any of the symptoms listed under ADVERSE REACTIONS.

Management: *General:* Obtain an ECG and immediately initiate cardiac monitoring. Protect the patient's airway, establish an intravenous line and initiate gastric decontamination. A minimum of 6 hours of observation with cardiac monitoring and observation for signs of CNS or respiratory depression, hypotension, cardiac dysrhythmias and/or conduction blocks, and seizures is necessary. If signs of toxicity occur at any time during this period, extended monitoring is required. *There are case reports of patients succumbing to fatal dysrhythmias late after overdose; these patients had clinical evidence of significant poisoning prior to death and most received inadequate gastrointestinal decontamination.* Monitoring of plasma drug levels should not guide management of the patient.

Gastrointestinal Decontamination: All patients suspected of tricyclic antidepressant overdose should receive gastrointestinal decontamination. This should include large volume gastric lavage followed by activated charcoal. If consciousness is impaired, the airway should be secured prior to lavage. Emesis is contraindicated.

Cardiovascular: A maximal limb-lead QRS duration of ≥ 0.10 seconds may be the best indication of the severity of the overdose. Serum alkalinization, to a pH of 7.45 to 7.56, using intravenous sodium bicarbonate and hyperventilation (as needed) should be instituted for patients with dysrhythmias and/or QRS widening. A pH > 7.60 or a pCO_2 < 20 mm Hg is undesirable. Dysrhythmias unresponsive to sodium bicarbonate therapy/hyperventilation may respond to lidocaine, bretylium or phenytoin. Type *1A and 1C* antiarrhythmics are generally contraindicated (eg, quinidine, disopyramide and procainamide).

In rare instances, hemoperfusion may be beneficial in acute refractory cardiovascular instability in patients with acute toxicity. However, hemodialysis, peritoneal dialysis, exchange transfusions and forced diuresis generally have been reported as ineffective in tricyclic antidepressant poisoning.

CNS: In patients with CNS depression, early intubation is advised because of the potential for abrupt deterioration. Seizures should be controlled with benzodiazepines, or if these are ineffective, other anticonvulsants (eg, phenobarbital, phenytoin). *Physostigmine is not recommended except to treat life-threatening symptoms that have been unresponsive to other therapies,* and then only in consultation with a poison control center.

Psychiatric Follow-up: Since overdosage is often deliberate, patients may attempt suicide by other means during the recovery phase. Psychiatric referral may be appropriate.

Pediatric Management: The principles of management of child and adult overdosages are similar. It is strongly recommended that the physician contact the local poison control center for specific pediatric treatment.

*Poisindex® Toxicologic Management. Topic: Antidepressants, Tricyclic. *Micromedex Inc.* Vol. 85.

Chlordiazepoxide Overdosage: Manifestations of benzodiazepine overdosage include somnolence, confusion, coma and diminished reflexes. Dialysis is of limited value. There have been occasional reports of excitation in patients following benzodiazepine overdosage; if this occurs, barbiturates should not be used. Withdrawal symptoms of the barbiturate type have occurred after the discontinuation of benzodiazepines (see DRUG ABUSE AND DEPENDENCE section).

Since Limbitrol contains amitriptyline, it is important to note that use of the benzodiazepine antagonist flumazenil is contraindicated in patients who are showing signs of serious cyclic antidepressant overdose.

DOSAGE AND ADMINISTRATION

Optimum dosage varies with the severity of the symptoms and the response of the individual patient. When a satisfactory response is obtained, dosage should be reduced to the smallest amount needed to maintain the remission. The larger portion of the total daily dose may be taken at bedtime. In some patients, a single dose at bedtime may be sufficient. In general, lower dosages are recommended for elderly patients.

Limbitrol DS (double strength) Tablets are recommended in an initial dosage of 3 or 4 tablets daily in divided doses; this may be increased to 6 tablets daily as required. Some patients respond to smaller doses and can be maintained on 2 tablets daily.

Limbitrol Tablets in an initial dosage of 3 or 4 tablets daily in divided doses may be satisfactory in patients who do not tolerate higher doses.

HOW SUPPLIED

DS (double strength) Tablets, containing 10 mg chlordiazepoxide and 25 mg amitriptyline (as the hydrochloride salt)—bottles of 100 and 500.

Tablets, containing 5 mg chlordiazepoxide and 12.5 mg amitriptyline (as the hydrochloride salt)—bottles of 100 and 500.

Revised: June 1996

Shown in Product Identification Guide, page 332

Tel-E-Ject® ℞

Available in the following product: Valium® (diazepam) disposable syringes, 2 mL.

Shown in Product Identification Guide, page 332

VALIUM® Injectable Ⓒ

[val'ee-um]

brand of diazepam

The following text is complete prescribing information based on official labeling in effect June 1996.

DESCRIPTION

Each mL contains 5 mg diazepam compounded with 40% propylene glycol, 10% ethyl alcohol, 5% sodium benzoate and benzoic acid as buffers, and 1.5% benzyl alcohol as preservative.

Diazepam is a benzodiazepine derivative developed through original Roche research. Chemically, diazepam is 7-chloro-1, 3-dihydro-1-methyl-5-phenyl-2H-1,4-benzodiazepin-2-one. It is a colorless crystalline compound, insoluble in water and has a molecular weight of 284.74.

ACTIONS

In animals, diazepam appears to act on parts of the limbic system, the thalamus and hypothalamus, and induces calming effects. Diazepam, unlike chlorpromazine and reserpine, has no demonstrable peripheral autonomic blocking action, nor does it produce extrapyramidal side effects; however, animals treated with diazepam do have a transient ataxia at higher doses. Diazepam was found to have transient cardiovascular depressor effects in dogs. Long-term experiments in rats revealed no disturbances of endocrine function. Injections into animals have produced localized irritation of tissue surrounding injection sites and some thickening of veins after intravenous use.

INDICATIONS

Valium is indicated for the management of anxiety disorders or for the short-term relief of the symptoms of anxiety. Anxiety or tension associated with the stress of everyday life usually does not require treatment with an anxiolytic.

In acute alcohol withdrawal, Valium may be useful in the symptomatic relief of acute agitation, tremor, impending or acute delirium tremens and hallucinosis.

As an adjunct prior to endoscopic procedures if apprehension, anxiety or acute stress reactions are present, and to diminish the patient's recall of the procedures. (See WARNINGS.)

Valium is a useful adjunct for the relief of skeletal muscle spasm due to reflex spasm to local pathology (such as inflammation of the muscles or joints, or secondary to trauma); spasticity caused by upper motor neuron disorders (such as cerebral palsy and paraplegia); athetosis; stiff-man syndrome; and tetanus.

Injectable Valium is a useful adjunct in status epilepticus and severe recurrent convulsive seizures.

Valium is a useful premedication (the IM route is preferred) for relief of anxiety and tension in patients who are to undergo surgical procedures. Intravenously, prior to cardioversion for the relief of anxiety and tension and to diminish the patient's recall of the procedure.

CONTRAINDICATIONS

Injectable Valium is contraindicated in patients with a known hypersensitivity to this drug; acute narrow angle glaucoma; and open angle glaucoma unless patients are receiving appropriate therapy.

WARNINGS

When used intravenously, the following procedures should be undertaken to reduce the possibility of venous thrombosis, phlebitis, local irritation, swelling, and, rarely, vascular impairment: the solution should be injected slowly, taking at least 1 minute for each 5 mg (1 mL) given; do not use small veins, such as those on the dorsum of the hand or wrist; extreme care should be taken to avoid intra-arterial administration or extravasation.

Do not mix or dilute Valium with other solutions or drugs in syringe or infusion flask. If it is not feasible to administer Valium directly IV, it may be injected slowly through the infusion tubing as close as possible to the vein insertion.

Extreme care must be used in administering Injectable Valium, particularly by the IV route, to the elderly, to very ill patients and to those with limited pulmonary reserve because of the possibility that apnea and/or cardiac arrest may occur. Concomitant use of barbiturates, alcohol or other central nervous system depressants increases depression with increased risk of apnea. Resuscitative equipment including that necessary to support respiration should be readily available.

When Valium is used with a narcotic analgesic, the dosage of the narcotic should be reduced by at least one-third and administered in small increments. In some cases the use of a narcotic may not be necessary.

Injectable Valium should not be administered to patients in shock, coma or in acute alcoholic intoxication with depression of vital signs. As is true of most CNS-acting drugs, patients receiving Valium should be cautioned against engaging in hazardous occupations requiring complete mental alertness, such as operating machinery or driving a motor vehicle.

Tonic status epilepticus has been precipitated in patients treated with IV Valium for petit mal status or petit mal variant status.

Usage in Pregnancy: **An increased risk of congenital malformations associated with the use of minor tranquilizers (diazepam, meprobamate and chlordiazepoxide) during the first trimester of pregnancy has been suggested in several studies. Because use of these drugs is rarely a matter of urgency, their use during this period should almost always be avoided. The possibility that a woman of childbearing potential may be pregnant at the time of institution of therapy should be considered. Patients should be advised that if they become pregnant during therapy or intend to become pregnant they should communicate with their physicians about the desirability of discontinuing the drug.**

In humans, measurable amounts of diazepam were found in maternal and cord blood, indicating placental transfer of the drug. Until additional information is available, Valium Injectable is not recommended for obstetrical use.

Use in Children: Efficacy and safety of parenteral Valium has not been established in the neonate (30 days or less of age).

Prolonged central nervous system depression has been observed in neonates, apparently due to inability to biotransform Valium into inactive metabolites.

In pediatric use, in order to obtain maximal clinical effect with the minimum amount of drug and thus to reduce the risk of hazardous side effects, such as apnea or prolonged periods of somnolence, it is recommended that the drug be given slowly over a 3-minute period in a dosage not to exceed 0.25 mg/kg. After an interval of 15 to 30 minutes the initial dosage can be safely repeated. If, however, relief of symptoms is not obtained after a third administration, adjunctive therapy appropriate to the condition being treated is recommended.

Withdrawal symptoms of the barbiturate type have occurred after the discontinuation of benzodiazepines. (See DRUG ABUSE AND DEPENDENCE section.)

PRECAUTIONS

Although seizures may be brought under control promptly, a significant proportion of patients experience a return to seizure activity, presumably due to the short-lived effect of Valium after IV administration. The physician should be prepared to readminister the drug. However, Valium is not recommended for maintenance, and once seizures are brought under control, consideration should be given to the administration of agents useful in longer term control of seizures.

If Valium is to be combined with other psychotropic agents or anticonvulsant drugs, careful consideration should be given to the pharmacology of the agents to be employed—particularly with known compounds which may potentiate the action of Valium, such as phenothiazines, narcotics, barbiturates, MAO inhibitors and other antidepressants. In highly anxious patients with evidence of accompanying depression, particularly those who may have suicidal tendencies, protective measures may be necessary. The usual precautions in treating patients with impaired hepatic function should be observed. Metabolites of Valium are excreted by the kidney; to avoid their excess accumulation, caution should be exercised in the administration to patients with compromised kidney function.

Since an increase in cough reflex and laryngospasm may occur with peroral endoscopic procedures, the use of a topical anesthetic agent and the availability of necessary countermeasures are recommended.

Until additional information is available, injectable diazepam is not recommended for obstetrical use.

Injectable Valium has produced hypotension or muscular weakness in some patients particularly when used with narcotics, barbiturates or alcohol.

Lower doses (usually 2 mg to 5 mg) should be used for elderly and debilitated patients.

The clearance of Valium and certain other benzodiazepines can be delayed in association with Tagamet (cimetidine) administration. The clinical significance of this is unclear.

ADVERSE REACTIONS

Side effects most commonly reported were drowsiness, fatigue and ataxia; venous thrombosis and phlebitis at the site of injection. Other adverse reactions less frequently reported include: *CNS:* confusion, depression, dysarthria, headache, hypoactivity, slurred speech, syncope, tremor, vertigo. *G.I.:*

	USUAL ADULT DOSAGE	DOSAGE RANGE IN CHILDREN (IV administration should be made slowly)
Moderate Anxiety Disorders and Symptoms of Anxiety.	2 mg to 5 mg, IM or IV. Repeat in 3 to 4 hours, if necessary.	
Severe Anxiety Disorders and Symptoms of Anxiety.	5 mg to 10 mg, IM or IV. Repeat in 3 to 4 hours, if necessary.	
Acute Alcohol Withdrawal: As an aid in symptomatic relief of acute agitation, tremor, impending or acute delirium tremens and hallucinosis.	10 mg, IM or IV initially, then 5 mg to 10 mg in 3 to 4 hours, if necessary.	
Endoscopic Procedures: Adjunctively, if apprehension, anxiety or acute stress reactions are present prior to endoscopic procedures. Dosage of narcotics should be reduced by at least a third and in some cases may be omitted. See *Precautions* for peroral procedures.	Titrate IV dosage to desired sedative response, such as slurring of speech, with slow administration immediately prior to the procedure. Generally 10 mg or less is adequate, but up to 20 mg IV may be given, particularly when concomitant narcotics are omitted. If IV cannot be used, 5 mg to 10 mg IM approximately 30 minutes prior to the procedure.	
Muscle Spasm: Associated with local pathology, cerebral palsy, athetosis, stiff-man syndrome or tetanus.	5 mg to 10 mg, IM or IV initially, then 5 mg to 10 mg in 3 to 4 hours, if necessary. For tetanus, larger doses may be required.	For tetanus in infants over 30 days of age, 1 mg to 2 mg IM or IV, slowly, repeated every 3 to 4 hours as necessary. In children 5 years or older, 5 mg to 10 mg repeated every 3 to 4 hours may be required to control tetanus spasms. Respiratory assistance should be available.
Status Epilepticus and Severe Recurrent Convulsive Seizures: In the convulsing patient, the IV route is by far preferred. This injection should be administered slowly. However, if IV administration is impossible, the IM route may be used.	5 mg to 10 mg initially (IV preferred). This injection may be repeated if necessary at 10 to 15 minute intervals up to a maximum dose of 30 mg. If necessary, therapy with Valium may be repeated in 2 to 4 hours; however, residual active metabolites may persist, and readministration should be made with this consideration. Extreme caution must be exercised with individuals with chronic lung disease or unstable cardiovascular status.	Infants over 30 days of age and children under 5 years, 0.2 mg to 0.5 mg slowly every 2 to 5 minutes up to a maximum of 5 mg (IV preferred). Children 5 years or older, 1 mg every 2 to 5 minutes up to a maximum of 10 mg (slow IV administration preferred). Repeat in 2 to 4 hours if necessary. EEG monitoring of the seizure may be helpful.
Preoperative Medication: To relieve anxiety and tension. (If atropine, scopolamine or other premedications are desired, they must be administered in separate syringes.)	10 mg, IM (preferred route), before surgery.	
Cardioversion: To relieve anxiety and tension and to reduce recall of procedure.	5 mg to 15 mg, IV, within 5 to 10 minutes prior to the procedure.	

Continued on next page

Roche Products—Cont.

constipation, nausea. *G.U.:* incontinence, changes in libido, urinary retention. *Cardiovascular:* bradycardia, cardiovascular collapse, hypotension. *EENT:* blurred vision, diplopia, nystagmus. *Skin:* urticaria, skin rash. *Other:* hiccups, changes in salivation, neutropenia, jaundice. Paradoxical reactions such as acute hyperexcited states, anxiety, hallucinations, increased muscle spasticity, insomnia, rage, sleep disturbances and stimulation have been reported; should these occur, use of the drug should be discontinued. Minor changes in EEG patterns, usually low-voltage fast activity, have been observed in patients during and after Valium therapy and are of no known significance.

In peroral endoscopic procedures, coughing, depressed respiration, dyspnea, hyperventilation, laryngospasm and pain in throat or chest have been reported.

Because of isolated reports of neutropenia and jaundice, periodic blood counts and liver function tests are advisable during long-term therapy.

DRUG ABUSE AND DEPENDENCE

Withdrawal symptoms, similar in character to those noted with barbiturates and alcohol (convulsions, tremor, abdominal and muscle cramps, vomiting and sweating), have occurred following abrupt discontinuance of diazepam. The more severe withdrawal symptoms have usually been limited to those patients who had received excessive doses over an extended period of time. Generally milder withdrawal symptoms (eg, dysphoria and insomnia) have been reported following abrupt discontinuance of benzodiazepines taken continuously at therapeutic levels for several months. Consequently, after extended therapy, abrupt discontinuation should generally be avoided and a gradual dosage tapering schedule followed. Addiction-prone individuals (such as drug addicts or alcoholics) should be under careful surveillance when receiving diazepam or other psychotropic agents because of the predisposition of such patients to habituation and dependence.

DOSAGE AND ADMINISTRATION

Dosage should be individualized for maximum beneficial effect. The usual recommended dose in older children and adults ranges from 2 mg to 20 mg IM or IV, depending on the indication and its severity. In some conditions, eg, tetanus, larger doses may be required. (See dosage for specific indications.) In acute conditions the injection may be repeated within 1 hour although an interval of 3 to 4 hours is usually satisfactory. Lower doses (usually 2 mg to 5 mg) and slow increase in dosage should be used for elderly or debilitated patients and when other sedative drugs are administered. (See WARNINGS and ADVERSE REACTIONS.)

For dosage in infants above the age of 30 days and children, see the specific indications below. When intravenous use is indicated, facilities for respiratory assistance should be readily available.

Intramuscular: Injectable Valium should be injected deeply into the muscle.

Intravenous Use: (See WARNINGS, particularly for use in children.) The solution should be injected slowly, taking at least 1 minute for each 5 mg (1 mL) given. Do not use small veins, such as those on the dorsum of the hand or wrist. Extreme care should be taken to avoid intra-arterial administration or extravasation.

Do not mix or dilute Valium with other solutions or drugs in syringe or infusion flask. If it is not feasible to administer Valium directly IV, it may be injected slowly through the infusion tubing as close as possible to the vein insertion.

[See table on preceding page.]

Once the acute symptomatology has been properly controlled with Injectable Valium, the patient may be placed on oral therapy with Valium if further treatment is required.

Management of Overdosage:

Manifestations of Valium overdosage include somnolence, confusion, coma and diminished reflexes. Respiration, pulse and blood pressure should be monitored, as in all cases of drug overdosage, although, in general, these effects have been minimal. General supportive measures should be employed, along with intravenous fluids, and an adequate airway maintained. Hypotension may be combated by the use of Levophed® (levarterenol) or Aramine (metaraminol). Dialysis is of limited value.

Flumazenil, a specific benzodiazepine-receptor antagonist, is indicated for the complete or partial reversal of the sedative effects of benzodiazepines and may be used in situations when an overdose with a benzodiazepine is known or suspected. Prior to the administration of flumazenil, necessary measures should be instituted to secure airway, ventilation and intravenous access. Flumazenil is intended as an adjunct to, not as a substitute for, proper management of benzodiazepine overdose. Patients treated with flumazenil should be monitored for resedation, respiratory depression and other residual benzodiazepine effects for an appropriate period after treatment. **The prescriber should be aware of a risk of seizure in association with flumazenil treatment, particularly in long-term benzodiazepine users and cyclic antidepressant overdose.** The complete flumazenil package insert, including CONTRAINDICATIONS, WARNINGS and PRECAUTIONS, should be consulted prior to use.

HOW SUPPLIED

Ampuls, 2 mL, boxes of 10; *Vials,* 10 mL, boxes of 1. *Tel-E-Ject* ® (disposable syringes), 2 mL, boxes of 10.

ANIMAL PHARMACOLOGY

Oral LD_{50} of diazepam is 720 mg/kg in mice and 1240 mg/kg in rats. Intraperitoneal administration of 400 mg/kg to a monkey resulted in death on the sixth day.

Reproduction Studies: A series of rat reproduction studies was performed with diazepam in oral doses of 1, 10, 80 and 100 mg/kg given for periods ranging from 60 to 228 days prior to mating. At 100 mg/kg there was a decrease in the number of pregnancies and surviving offspring in these rats. These effects may be attributable to prolonged sedative activity, resulting in lack of interest in mating and lessened maternal nursing and care of the young. Neonatal survival of rats at doses lower than 100 mg/kg was within normal limits. Several neonates, both controls and experimentals, in these rat reproduction studies showed skeletal or other defects. Further studies in rats at doses up to and including 80 mg/kg/day did not reveal significant teratological effects on the offspring. Rabbits were maintained on doses of 1, 2, 5 and 8 mg/kg from day 6 through day 18 of gestation. No adverse effects on reproduction and no teratological changes were noted.

Manufactured by Hoffmann-La Roche Inc., Nutley N.J. 07110

Revised: June 1993

VALIUM® Ⓒ

[*val 'ee-um*]
brand of diazepam
TABLETS

The following text is complete prescribing information based on official labeling in effect June 1996.

DESCRIPTION

Valium (diazepam) is a benzodiazepine derivative developed through original Roche research. Chemically, diazepam is 7-chloro-1,3-dihydro-1-methyl -5- phenyl-2H-1,4-benzodiazepin-2-one. It is a colorless crystalline compound, insoluble in water and has a molecular weight of 284.74.

Valium 5-mg tablets contain FD&C Yellow No. 6 and D&C Yellow No. 10 dyes. Valium 10-mg tablets contain FD&C Blue No. 1 dye. Valium 2-mg tablets contain no dye.

PHARMACOLOGY

In animals, Valium appears to act on parts of the limbic system, the thalamus and hypothalamus, and induces calming effects. Valium, unlike chlorpromazine and reserpine, has no demonstrable peripheral autonomic blocking action, nor does it produce extrapyramidal side effects; however, animals treated with Valium do have a transient ataxia at higher doses. Valium was found to have transient cardiovascular depressor effects in dogs. Long-term experiments in rats revealed no disturbances of endocrine function.

Oral LD_{50} of diazepam is 720 mg/kg in mice and 1240 mg/kg in rats. Intraperitoneal administration of 400 mg/kg to a monkey resulted in death on the sixth day.

Reproduction Studies: A series of rat reproduction studies was performed with diazepam in oral doses of 1, 10, 80 and 100 mg/kg. At 100 mg/kg there was a decrease in the number of pregnancies and surviving offspring in these rats. Neonatal survival of rats at doses lower than 100 mg/kg was within normal limits. Several neonates in these rat reproduction studies showed skeletal or other defects. Further studies in rats at doses up to and including 80 mg/kg/day did not reveal teratological effects on the offspring.

In humans, measurable blood levels of Valium were obtained in maternal and cord blood, indicating placental transfer of the drug.

INDICATIONS

Valium is indicated for the management of anxiety disorders or for the short-term relief of the symptoms of anxiety. Anxiety or tension associated with the stress of everyday life usually does not require treatment with an anxiolytic.

In acute alcohol withdrawal, Valium may be useful in the symptomatic relief of acute agitation, tremor, impending or acute delirium tremens and hallucinosis.

Valium is a useful adjunct for the relief of skeletal muscle spasm due to reflex spasm to local pathology (such as inflammation of the muscles or joints, or secondary to trauma); spasticity caused by upper motor neuron disorders (such as cerebral palsy and paraplegia); athetosis; and stiff-man syndrome.

Oral Valium may be used adjunctively in convulsive disorders, although it has not proved useful as the sole therapy.

The effectiveness of Valium in long-term use, that is, more than 4 months, has not been assessed by systematic clinical studies. The physician should periodically reassess the usefulness of the drug for the individual patient.

CONTRAINDICATIONS

Valium is contraindicated in patients with a known hypersensitivity to this drug and, because of lack of sufficient clinical experience, in children under 6 months of age. It may be used in patients with open angle glaucoma who are receiving appropriate therapy, but is contraindicated in acute narrow angle glaucoma.

WARNINGS

Valium is not of value in the treatment of psychotic patients and should not be employed in lieu of appropriate treatment.

As is true of most preparations containing CNS-acting drugs, patients receiving Valium should be cautioned against engaging in hazardous occupations requiring complete mental alertness such as operating machinery or driving a motor vehicle.

As with other agents which have anticonvulsant activity, when Valium is used as an adjunct in treating convulsive disorders, the possibility of an increase in the frequency and/or severity of grand mal seizures may require an increase in the dosage of standard anticonvulsant medication. Abrupt withdrawal of Valium in such cases may also be associated with a temporary increase in the frequency and/or severity of seizures.

Since Valium has a central nervous system depressant effect, patients should be advised against the simultaneous ingestion of alcohol and other CNS-depressant drugs during Valium therapy.

Usage in Pregnancy: **An increased risk of congenital malformations associated with the use of minor tranquilizers (diazepam, meprobamate and chlordiazepoxide) during the first trimester of pregnancy has been suggested in several studies. Because use of these drugs is rarely a matter of urgency, their use during this period should almost always be avoided. The possibility that a woman of childbearing potential may be pregnant at the time of institution of therapy should be considered. Patients should be advised that if they become pregnant during therapy or intend to become pregnant they should communicate with their physicians about the desirability of discontinuing the drug.**

Management of Overdosage: Manifestations of Valium overdosage include somnolence, confusion, coma and diminished reflexes. Respiration, pulse and blood pressure should be monitored, as in all cases of drug overdosage, although, in general, these effects have been minimal following overdosage. General supportive measures should be employed, along with immediate gastric lavage. Intravenous fluids should be administered and an adequate airway maintained. Hypotension may be combated by the use of Levophed® (levarterenol) or Aramine (metaraminol). Dialysis is of limited value.

As with the management of intentional overdosage with any drug, it should be borne in mind that multiple agents may have been ingested.

Flumazenil, a specific benzodiazepine-receptor antagonist, is indicated for the complete or partial reversal of the sedative effects of benzodiazepines and may be used in situations when an overdose with a benzodiazepine is known or suspected. Prior to the administration of flumazenil, necessary measures should be instituted to secure airway, ventilation, and intravenous access. Flumazenil is intended as an adjunct to, not as a substitute for, proper management of benzodiazepine overdose. Patients treated with flumazenil should be monitored for resedation, respiratory depression and other residual benzodiazepine effects for an appropriate period after treatment. **The prescriber should be aware of a risk of seizure in association with flumazenil treatment, particularly in long-term benzodiazepine users and in cyclic antidepressant overdose.** The complete flumazenil package insert, including CONTRAINDICATIONS, WARNINGS and PRECAUTIONS, should be consulted prior to use.

Withdrawal symptoms of the barbiturate type have occurred after the discontinuation of benzodiazepines. (See DRUG ABUSE AND DEPENDENCE section.)

PRECAUTIONS

If Valium is to be combined with other psychotropic agents or anticonvulsant drugs, careful consideration should be given to the pharmacology of the agents to be employed—particularly with known compounds which may potentiate the action of Valium, such as phenothiazines, narcotics, barbiturates, MAO inhibitors and other antidepressants. The usual precautions are indicated for severely depressed patients or those in whom there is any evidence of latent de-

pression; particularly the recognition that suicidal tendencies may be present and protective measures may be necessary. The usual precautions in treating patients with impaired renal or hepatic function should be observed.

In elderly and debilitated patients, it is recommended that the dosage be limited to the smallest effective amount to preclude the development of ataxia or oversedation (2 mg to 2½ mg once or twice daily, initially, to be increased gradually as needed and tolerated).

The clearance of Valium and certain other benzodiazepines can be delayed in association with Tagamet (cimetidine) administration. The clinical significance of this is unclear.

Information for Patients: To assure the safe and effective use of benzodiazepines, patients should be informed that, since benzodiazepines may produce psychological and physical dependence, it is advisable that they consult with their physician before either increasing the dose or abruptly discontinuing this drug.

ADVERSE REACTIONS

Side effects most commonly reported were drowsiness, fatigue and ataxia. Infrequently encountered were confusion, constipation, depression, diplopia, dysarthria, headache, hypotension, incontinence, jaundice, changes in libido, nausea, changes in salivation, skin rash, slurred speech, tremor, urinary retention, vertigo and blurred vision. Paradoxical reactions such as acute hyperexcited states, anxiety, hallucinations, increased muscle spasticity, insomnia, rage, sleep disturbances and stimulation have been reported; should these occur, use of the drug should be discontinued.

Because of isolated reports of neutropenia and jaundice, periodic blood counts and liver function tests are advisable during long-term therapy. Minor changes in EEG patterns, usually low-voltage fast activity, have been observed in patients during and after Valium therapy and are of no known significance.

DRUG ABUSE AND DEPENDENCE

Withdrawal symptoms, similar in character to those noted with barbiturates and alcohol (convulsions, tremor, abdominal and muscle cramps, vomiting and sweating), have occurred following abrupt discontinuance of diazepam. The more severe withdrawal symptoms have usually been limited to those patients who had received excessive doses over an extended period of time. Generally milder withdrawal symptoms (eg, dysphoria and insomnia) have been reported following abrupt discontinuation of benzodiazepines taken continuously at therapeutic levels for several months. Consequently, after extended therapy, abrupt discontinuation should generally be avoided and a gradual dosage tapering schedule followed. Addiction-prone individuals (such as drug addicts or alcoholics) should be under careful surveillance when receiving diazepam or other psychotropic agents because of the predisposition of such patients to habituation and dependence.

DOSAGE AND ADMINISTRATION

Dosage should be individualized for maximum beneficial effect. While the usual daily dosages given below will meet the needs of most patients, there will be some who may require higher doses. In such cases dosage should be increased cautiously to avoid adverse effects.

	USUAL DAILY DOSE
ADULTS:	
Management of Anxiety Disorders and Relief of Symptoms of Anxiety.	Depending upon severity of symptoms—2 mg to 10 mg, 2 to 4 times daily
Symptomatic Relief in Acute Alcohol Withdrawal.	10 mg, 3 or 4 times during the first 24 hours, reducing to 5 mg, 3 or 4 times daily as needed
Adjunctively for Relief of Skeletal Muscle Spasm.	2 mg to 10 mg, 3 or 4 times daily
Adjunctively in Convulsive Disorders.	2 mg to 10 mg, 2 to 4 times daily
Geriatric Patients, or in the presence of debilitating disease.	2 mg to 2½ mg, 1 or 2 times daily initially; increase gradually as needed and tolerated
CHILDREN: Because of varied responses to CNS-acting drugs, initiate therapy with lowest dose and increase as required. Not for use in children under 6 months.	1 mg to 2½ mg, 3 or 4 times daily initially; increase gradually as needed and tolerated

HOW SUPPLIED

For oral administration, round, scored tablets with a cut out "V" design—2 mg, white; 5 mg, yellow; 10 mg, blue—bottles of 100 and 500. Tel-E-Dose® packages of 100, available in boxes of 4 reverse-numbered cards of 25, and in boxes containing 10 strips of 10.

Imprint on tablets:

2 mg:
2 VALIUM® (front)
ROCHE (scored side)

5 mg:
5 VALIUM® (front)
ROCHE (scored side)

10 mg:
10 VALIUM® (front)
ROCHE (scored side)

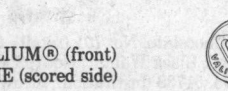

Revised: June 1993
Shown in Product Identification Guide, page 332

Roerig Division
see Pfizer Inc

Ross Products Division
**ABBOTT LABORATORIES
COLUMBUS, OH 43215-1724**

Direct Inquiries to:
1-800-227-5767

ADVERA®   OTC
[ad-ver'ah]
Specialized, Complete Nutrition

USAGE

To provide specialized, complete nutrition uniquely designed for the dietary management of people with HIV/AIDS. Advera is a calorie- and nutrient-dense formula that is low in fat with a fat source abundant in n-3 (omega-3) fatty acids and contains specialized peptides and fiber. It may be used as an oral supplement, a meal replacement or as a sole source of nutrition, either orally or by tube feeding.
Not for parenteral use.

AVAILABILITY
Ready To Use:
8-fl-oz cans; 24 per case; Chocolate, No. 51304 (retail), Chocolate, No. 51800 (institution); Vanilla, No. 52452 (retail); Vanilla, No. 52450 (institution).

COMPOSITION
Ready To Use Vanilla (Chocolate flavor has similar composition. For specific information, see product labels.)

INGREDIENTS
Ⓤ-D Water, Maltodextrin, Soy Protein Hydrolysate, Sugar (sucrose), Canola Oil, Sodium Caseinate, Soy Fiber (a source of dietary fiber), Medium-Chain Triglycerides (Fractionated Coconut Oil), Natural and Artificial Flavors, Refined Deodorized Sardine Oil, Calcium Phosphate Tribasic, Sodium Citrate, Diacetyl Tartaric Acid Esters of Mono-diglycerides (an emulsifier), Ascorbic Acid, Calcium Carbonate, Magnesium Phosphate Dibasic, Carrageenan, Choline Chloride, Taurine, L-Carnitine, Ferrous Sulfate, Zinc Sulfate, Sodium Chloride, Alpha-Tocopheryl Acetate, Niacinamide, Calcium Pantothenate, Beta-Carotene, Cupric Sulfate, Magnanese Sulfate, Thiamine Chloride Hydrochloride, Pyridoxine Hydrochloride, Riboflavin, Vitamin A Palmitate, Folic Acid, Biotin, Potassium Iodide, Sodium Selenate, Cyanocobalamin, Phylloquinone and Vitamin D_3.
Nutrients (grams/8 fl oz): Protein, 14.2; Fat, 5.4; Carbohydrate, 51.1*; L-carnitine, 0.03; Taurine, 0.05; Water, 190. Calories per mL, 1.28; Calories per fl oz, 37.9.
*Includes soy fiber that provides 5.8 Calories and 2.1 g total dietary fiber.
(FAN 7027-01)

ALIMENTUM®   OTC
[al"ah-men'tum]
**Protein Hydrolysate Formula
With Iron**
● **Ready To Feed**

For most current information, refer to product labels.

ALITRAQ®   OTC
[al'ah-trak']
**Specialized Elemental Nutrition
With Glutamine**

USAGE
A complete, elemental feeding designed for metabolically stressed patients with impaired GI function. AlitraQ helps maintain nutritional status and provides supplemental glutamine to nourish the GI tract and restore glutamine depleted during catabolic states. Five servings (1500 Calories) meet or exceed 100% of the RDI for vitamins and minerals.
Not for parenteral use.

AVAILABILITY
Powder:
2.68 oz (76 g) packets; 24 packets per case; Vanilla, No. 50630.

COMPOSITION
INGREDIENTS
Ⓤ-D Maltodextrin, Soy Hydrolysate, Sugar (Sucrose), L-Glutamine, Fructose, Medium-Chain Triglycerides (Fractionated Coconut Oil), Safflower Oil, Whey Protein Concentrate, Lactalbumin Hydrolysate, Magnesium Sulfate, L-Arginine, Tricalcium Phosphate Dibasic, L-Leucine, L-Valine, L-Lysine, Potassium Phosphate Dibasic, Potassium Citrate, L-Phenylalanine, Sodium Citrate, L-Isoleucine, L-Threonine, L-Tyrosine, L-Methionine, Sodium Chloride, Ascorbic Acid, L-Histidine, Choline Chloride, Natural and Artificial Flavors, L-Tryptophan, Taurine, L-Carnitine, Carrageenan, Alpha-Tocopheryl Acetate, Niacinamide, D-Calcium Pantothenate, Zinc Sulfate, Ferrous Sulfate, Vitamin A Palmitate, Thiamine Chloride Hydrochloride, Pyridoxine Hydrochloride, Manganese Sulfate, Riboflavin, Cupric Sulfate, Folic Acid, Biotin, Potassium Iodide, Sodium Molybdate, Phylloquinone, Chromium Chloride, Sodium Selenite, Vitamin D_3 and Cyanocobalamin.

Nutrients (grams)	Per 300 Calories* (1 packet)
Protein	15.8
Fat	4.65
Carbohydrate	49.5

*In standard dilution (76 g of AlitraQ powder mixed in 250 mL of water)
(FAN 7003-01)

CLEAR EYES®   OTC
[klēr īz]
Lubricant Eye Redness Reliever Drops

(See PDR For Nonprescription Drugs or PDR For Ophthalmology.)

CLEAR EYES® ACR   OTC
[klēr īz]
Astringent/Lubricant Eye Redness Reliever Drops

(See PDR For Nonprescription Drugs or PDR For Ophthalmology.)

CLEAR EYES® CLR   OTC
[Klēr īz]
**Soothing drops
Contact Lens Relief**

(See PDR For Nonprescription Drugs or PDR For Ophthalmology.)

EAR DROPS BY MURINE®   OTC
**See Murine Ear Wax Removal
System/Murine Ear Drops**

(See PDR For Nonprescription Drugs.)

ENSURE® High Protein   OTC
[en-shur']
Complete, Balanced Nutrition™

USAGE
For complete, balanced nutrition. Ensure High Protein is a concentrated oral supplement for patients who require additional protein, calories, vitamins and minerals, such as pa-

Continued on next page

Ross Laboratories—Cont.

tients recovering from general surgery or hip fractures, patients at risk of pressure ulcers and patients on modified fat diets. Ensure High Protein can be used as a low-residue feeding. Ensure High Protein can be used on sodium-restricted, low-cholesterol, lactose-restricted or gluten-free diets. Ensure High Protein provides 25% of the RDI for 24 key vitamins and minerals in an 8-fl-oz serving.

Not for parenteral use.

AVAILABILITY

Ready To Use:
8-fl-oz cans; 24 per case; Vanilla Supreme, No. 52070 (retail), Vanilla Supreme, No. 52100 (institution); Chocolate Royal, No. 52068 (retail), Chocolate Royal, No. 52098 (institution); Wild Berry, No. 52072; Banana, No. 52064.

COMPOSITION

Ready To Use Vanilla Supreme (Other flavors have similar composition and nutrient values. For specific information, see product labels.)

INGREDIENTS

Ⓤ-D Water, Sugar (Sucrose), Maltodextrin, Calcium and Sodium Caseinates, High-Oleic Safflower Oil, Soy Protein Isolate, Canola Oil, Soy Oil, Potassium Citrate, Calcium Phosphate Dibasic, Magnesium Chloride, Sodium Citrate, Artificial Flavor, Magnesium Phosphate Dibasic, Sodium Chloride, Soy Lecithin, Choline Chloride, Ascorbic Acid, Carrageenan, Calcium Carbonate, Zinc Sulfate, Ferrous Sulfate, Alpha-Tocopheryl Acetate, Niacinamide, Calcium Pantothenate, Manganese Sulfate, Cupric Sulfate, Vitamin A Palmitate, Thiamine Chloride Hydrochloride, Pyridoxine Hydrochloride, Riboflavin, Folic Acid, Biotin, Sodium Molybdate, Chromium Chloride, Potassium Iodide, Sodium Selenate, Phylloquinone, Cyanocobalamin and Vitamin D_3.
Nutrients per 8 fl oz: Calories, 225; Protein, 12 g; Carbohydrate, 30.8 g; Fat, 6 g; Sodium, 290 mg; Potassium, 500 mg.
(FAN 7047-04)

ENSURE® LIGHT   OTC
[en-shur']
Complete, Balanced Nutrition™

USAGE

For complete, balanced nutrition. Ensure Light can be used for supplemental use between or with meals. Ensure Light can be used for normal-weight or overweight patients who need extra nutrition in a lower calorie, lower fat supplement. Ensure Light contains 25% of the RDI for 24 key vitamins and minerals in an 8-fl-oz serving.

Not for parenteral use.

AVAILABILITY

Ready To Use:
8-fl-oz cans; 24 per case; French Vanilla, No. 52770; Chocolate Supreme, No. 52768; Strawberry Swirl, No. 52686.

COMPOSITION

Ready To Use French Vanilla (Other flavors have similar composition and nutrient values. For specific information, see product labels.)

INGREDIENTS

Ⓤ-D Water, Maltodextrin, Sugar (Sucrose), Calcium Caseinate, High-Oleic Safflower Oil, Canola Oil, Magnesium Chloride, Sodium Citrate, Potassium Citrate, Potassium Phosphate Dibasic, Magnesium Phosphate, Natural and Artificial Flavor, Calcium Phosphate Tribasic, Cellulose Gel, Choline Chloride, Soy Lecithin, Carrageenan, Sodium Chloride, Ascorbic Acid, Cellulose Gum, Ferrous Sulfate, Alpha-Tocopheryl Acetate, Zinc Sulfate, Niacinamide, Manganese Sulfate, Calcium Pantothenate, Cupric Sulfate, Thiamine Chloride Hydrochloride, Vitamin A Palmitate, Pyridoxine Hydrochloride, Riboflavin, Chromium Chloride, Folic Acid, Sodium Molybdate, Biotin, Potassium Iodide, Sodium Selenate, Phylloquinone, Vitamin D_3 and Cyanocobalamin.
Nutrients per 8 fl oz: Calories, 200; Protein, 10 g; Carbohydrate, 33 g; Fat, 3 g; Sodium, 200 mg; Potassium, 370 mg.
(FAN 7063-01)

ENSURE®   OTC
[en-shur']
Complete, Balanced Nutrition™

USAGE

For complete, balanced nutrition. Ensure can be used as a supplement with or between meals or as a meal replacement. Ensure can be used for patients requiring a low-residue diet. Ensure can be used on sodium-restricted, low-cholesterol, lactose-restricted or gluten-free diets. Ensure may be fed orally or by tube. Ensure is useful whenever the patient's

medical, surgical or psychological state causes inadequate dietary intake. An 8-fl-oz serving of Ensure provides at least 25% of the RDI for 24 key vitamins and minerals.

Not for parenteral use.

AVAILABILITY

Ready To Use:
8-fl-oz cans; 24 per case; Chocolate, No. 701 (retail), Chocolate, No. 50462 (institution); Black Walnut, No. 703; Coffee, No. 704 (retail), Coffee, No. 51738 (institution); Strawberry, No. 705 (retail), Strawberry, No. 50648 (institution); Eggnog, No. 710 (retail), Eggnog, No. 51744 (institution); Vanilla, No. 711 (retail), Vanilla, No. 50460 (institution); Butter Pecan, No. 51784 (retail), Butter Pecan, No. 51892 (institution).
32-fl-oz cans; 6 per case; Vanilla, No. 733; Chocolate, No. 799.

Powder:
14-oz (400 g) cans; 6 per case; Vanilla, No. 750.

COMPOSITION

Ready To Use Vanilla (Other flavors have similar composition and nutrient values. For specific information, see product labels.)

Ensure is also available in powder form; however, formulation differs. See product label for more specific information.

INGREDIENTS

Ⓤ-D Water, Corn Syrup, Maltodextrin, Sugar (Sucrose), Sodium and Calcium Caseinates, High-Oleic Safflower Oil, Canola Oil, Soy Protein Isolate, Whey Protein Concentrate, Corn Oil, Calcium Phosphate Tribasic, Potassium Citrate, Magnesium Phosphate Dibasic, Soy Lecithin, Magnesium Chloride, Natural and Artificial Flavor, Sodium Chloride, Carrageenan, Choline Chloride, Potassium Chloride, Ascorbic Acid, Sodium Citrate, Ferrous Sulfate, Alpha-Tocopheryl Acetate, Zinc Sulfate, Niacinamide, Calcium Pantothenate, Manganese Sulfate, Cupric Sulfate, Vitamin A Palmitate, Thiamine Chloride Hydrochloride, Pyridoxine Hydrochloride, Riboflavin, Folic Acid, Biotin, Chromium Chloride, Sodium Molybdate, Sodium Selenate, Potassium Iodide, Phylloquinone, Cyanocobalamin and Vitamin D_3.
Nutrients per 8 fl oz: Calories, 250; Protein, 8.8 g; Carbohydrate, 40 g; Fat, 6.1 g; Sodium, 200 mg; Potassium, 370 mg.
(FAN 7044-01)

ENSURE PLUS®   OTC
[en-shur']
High-Calorie, Complete Nutrition™

USAGE

As a high-calorie liquid food providing complete, balanced nutrition. Caloric density is 1500 Calories per liter. Ensure Plus is intended for use when extra calories and correspondingly higher concentrations of protein and most other nutrients are needed to achieve a required calorie intake in a limited volume. When used to provide total nutrition, Ensure Plus can deliver the high-calorie intakes required by patients who are nutritionally depleted, and who may not be able to tolerate large-volume intakes. As a supplement to a diet, Ensure Plus can supply extra calories and protein for those patients unable to consume adequate nutrition. Can be used on sodium restricted, low-cholesterol, lactose-restricted or gluten-free diets.

Not for parenteral use.

AVAILABILITY

Ready To Use:
8-fl-oz cans; 24 per case; Chocolate, No. 702 (retail), Chocolate, No. 50466 (institution); Vanilla, No. 707 (retail), Vanilla, No. 50464 (institution); Eggnog, No. 716 (retail), Eggnog, No. 51742 (institution); Coffee, No. 717 (retail), Coffee, No. 51740 (institution); Strawberry, No. 718 (retail), Strawberry, No. 50646 (institution); Butter Pecan, No. 51786 (retail), Butter Pecan, No. 51894 (institution).
32-fl-oz cans; 6 per case; Vanilla, No. 688; Chocolate, No. 698; Strawberry, No. 51172.
1-liter Ross Ready-To-Hang® Enteral Feeding Containers; 8 per case; No. 50340.

COMPOSITION

Ready To Use Vanilla (Other flavors and Ready-To-Hang have similar composition. For specific information, see product labels.)

INGREDIENTS

Ⓤ-D Water, corn syrup, maltodextrin, corn oil, sodium and calcium caseinates, sugar (sucrose), soy protein isolate, magnesium chloride, potassium citrate, calcium phosphate tribasic, soy lecithin, natural and artificial flavor, sodium citrate, potassium chloride, choline chloride, ascorbic acid, carrageenan, zinc sulfate, ferrous sulfate, alpha-tocopheryl acetate, niacinamide, calcium pantothenate, manganese sulfate, cupric sulfate, thiamine chloride hydrochloride, pyridoxine hydrochloride, riboflavin, vitamin A palmitate, folic acid, biotin, sodium molybdate, chromium chloride, potassium iodide, sodium selenite, phylloquinone, cyanocobalamin and vitamin D_3.

Nutrients per 8 fl oz: Calories, 355; Protein, 13 g; Carbohydrate, 47.3 g; Fat, 12.6 g; Cholesterol, < 5 mg; Sodium, 250 mg; Potassium, 460 mg.
(FAN 3120-04)

ENSURE® WITH FIBER   OTC
[en-shur']
Complete, Balanced Nutrition™

USAGE

As a fiber-containing, nutritionally complete liquid food, Ensure With Fiber is useful for persons who can benefit from increased dietary fiber and supplemental nutrition. Ensure With Fiber is suitable for persons who do not require a low-residue diet. Although intended primarily as an oral feeding, Ensure With Fiber may be fed by tube. Can be used on low-cholesterol and low-sodium diets.

Not for parenteral use.

AVAILABILITY

Ready To Use:
8-fl-oz cans; 24 per case; Vanilla, No. 759 (retail), Vanilla, No. 50650 (institution); Chocolate, No. 756; Butter Pecan, No. 51782.
32-fl-oz cans; 6 per case; Vanilla, No. 706.

COMPOSITION

Vanilla (Other flavors have similar composition. For specific information, see product label.)

INGREDIENTS

Ⓤ-D Water, Maltodextrin, Sugar (Sucrose), Corn Oil, Sodium and Calcium Caseinates, Soy Fiber (A Source of Dietary Fiber), Soy Protein Isolate, Potassium Citrate, Magnesium Chloride, Calcium Phosphate Tribasic, Soy Lecithin, Sodium Citrate, Natural and Artificial Flavors, Potassium Chloride, Choline Chloride, Ascorbic Acid, Zinc Sulfate, Ferrous Sulfate, Alpha-Tocopheryl Acetate, Niacinamide, Calcium Pantothenate, Manganese Sulfate, Cupric Sulfate, Thiamine Chloride Hydrochloride, Pyridoxine Hydrochloride, Riboflavin, Vitamin A Palmitate, Folic Acid, Biotin, Chromium Chloride, Sodium Molybdate, Potassium Iodide, Sodium Selenite, Phylloquinone, Cyanocobalamin And Vitamin D_3.
Nutrients per 8 fl oz: Calories, 260; Protein, 9.4 g; Carbohydrate, 38.3 g; Fat, 8.8 g; Sodium, 200 mg; Potassium, 400 mg.

(FAN 3113-05)

GLUCERNA®   OTC
[glu-ser'nah]
Specialized Nutrition with Fiber for Patients with Abnormal Glucose Tolerance

USAGE

A reduced-carbohydrate, modified-fat, fiber-containing formula providing complete nutrition for patients with abnormal glucose tolerance. Glucerna has a unique formulation designed to maintain or improve nutritional status, yet enhance blood glucose control. Glucerna can be used as a tube feeding or oral supplement in persons with type I or type II diabetes mellitus or stress-induced hyperglycemia.

Not for parenteral use.

AVAILABILITY

Ready To Use:
8-fl-oz cans; 24 per case; Vanilla, No. 50240. 1-liter Ross Ready-To-Hang® Enteral Feeding Containers; 8 per case; No. 51206 and 1500-mL Ready-To-Hang Containers; 6 per case; No. 52602.

INGREDIENTS

Ⓤ-D Water, Maltodextrin, High-Oleic Safflower Oil, Sodium and Calcium Caseinates, Soy Fiber (A Source of Dietary Fiber), Fructose, Canola Oil, Soy Lecithin, Magnesium Chloride, Calcium Phosphate Tribasic, Sodium Citrate, Natural and Artificial Flavor, M-Inositol, Potassium Citrate, Potassium Phosphate Dibasic, Potassium Chloride, Choline Chloride, Ascorbic Acid, L-Carnitine, Taurine, Zinc Sulfate, Alpha-Tocopheryl Acetate, Ferrous Sulfate, Niacinamide, Calcium Pantothenate, Manganese Sulfate, Cupric Sulfate, Thiamine Chloride Hydrochloride, Pyridoxine Hydrochloride, Riboflavin, Vitamin A Palmitate, Beta-Carotene, Folic Acid, Biotin, Chromium Chloride, Sodium Molybdate, Potassium Iodide, Sodium Selenate, Phylloquinone, Cyanocobalamin and Vitamin D_3.
Nutrients (Grams/8 fl oz): Protein, 9.9; Fat, 12.9; Carbohydrate, 22.7*; L-carnitine, 0.034; Taurine, 0.025; m-Inositol, 0.20; Water, 202. Calories per mL, 1.0; Calories per fl oz, 29.6.

*Includes soy fiber
U.S. Patent 4,921,877
(FAN 7059-03)

ISOMIL®   OTC
[ī′sō-mil]
Soy Formula With Iron
● Powder
● Concentrated Liquid
● Ready To Feed

For most current information, refer to product labels.

ISOMIL® DF   OTC
Soy Formula For Diarrhea

● Ready To Feed
For most current information, refer to product labels.

ISOMIL® SF   OTC
[ī′sō-mil]
Sucrose-Free Soy Formula With Iron
● Concentrated Liquid

For most current information, refer to product labels.

JEVITY®   OTC
[jev′ə-tē″]
Isotonic Liquid Nutrition with Fiber

USAGE
As a fiber-containing, isotonic, high-nitrogen, nutritionally complete liquid food for tube feeding, Jevity helps patients maintain normal bowel function. 1400 Cal provides at least 100% of the RDI for vitamins and minerals. The high-nitrogen and concentrated vitamin/mineral content of Jevity makes it ideal for patients with increased nutrient needs and/or reduced caloric requirements. Because it is fortified with selenium, chromium, molybdenum, carnitine and taurine, Jevity can be used as the sole source of nutrition for extended periods of time.
Not for parenteral use.

AVAILABILITY
Ready To Use:
8-fl-oz cans; 24 per case; No. 143.
32-fl-oz cans; 6 per case; No. 50330.
1-liter Ross Ready-To-Hang® Enteral Feeding Containers; 8 per case; No. 682.
1500 mL Ross Ready–To–Hang® Enteral Feeding Containers; 6 per case; No. 52604.

COMPOSITION
Ready To Use (Ready-To-Hang has similar composition. For specific information, see product label.)

INGREDIENTS
Ⓤ-D Water, Maltodextrin, Sodium and Calcium Caseinates, Corn Syrup, Soy Fiber (A Source of Dietary Fiber), High-Oleic Safflower Oil, Canola Oil, Medium-Chain Triglycerides (Fractionated Coconut Oil), Calcium Phosphate Tribasic, Magnesium Chloride, Potassium Citrate, Soy Lecithin, Sodium Citrate, Ascorbic Acid, Potassium Chloride, Choline Chloride, Magnesium Sulfate, Carrageenan, Taurine, L-Carnitine, Zinc Sulfate, Ferrous Sulfate, Alpha-Tocopheryl Acetate, Niacinamide, Calcium Pantothenate, Manganese Sulfate, Cupric Sulfate, Vitamin A Palmitate, Thiamine Chloride Hydrochloride, Pyridoxine Hydrochloride, Riboflavin, Folic Acid, Biotin, Sodium Molybdate, Chromium Chloride, Potassium Iodide, Sodium Selenate, Phylloquinone, Cyanocobalamin and Vitamin D_3.
Nutrients (grams/8 fl oz): Protein, 10.5; Fat, 8.2; Carbohydrate, 36.4*; L-carnitine, 0.027; Taurine, 0.027; Water, 197. Calories per mL, 1.06; Calories per fl oz, 31.3.

*Includes soy fiber (a source of dietary fiber that provides 10 Calories and 3.4 g total dietary fiber).
(FAN 3135-05)

JEVITY® PLUS   OTC
[jev′ə-tē″]
1.2 Cal/mL, High-Nitrogen Liquid Nutrition
With Patented Fiber Blend

USAGE
As a 1.2 Cal/mL, high-nitrogen, fiber-fortified liquid food for long- or short-term tube feeding. Jevity Plus contains a patented four-fiber blend to provide both insoluble and soluble fiber and fructooligosaccharides. 1200 Calories provides at least 100% of the RDI for vitamins and minerals. Jevity Plus is ideal for patients who would benefit from a moderate increase in protein intake and caloric density. Jevity Plus also contains added beta-carotene.
Not for parenteral use.

AVAILABILITY
Ready To Use:
8-fl-oz cans; 24 per case; No. 53118.
1-liter Ross Ready-To-Hang® Enteral Feeding Containers; 8 per case; No. 53124.
1500 mL Ross Ready-To-Hang® Enteral Feeding Containers; 6 per case; No. 53114.

COMPOSITION
Ready To Use (Ready-To-Hang has similar composition. For specific information, see product label.)

INGREDIENTS
Ⓤ-D Water, Corn Syrup, Maltodextrin, Sodium and Calcium Caseinate, High-Oleic Safflower Oil, Canola Oil, Fructooligo-saccharides, Medium-Chain Triglycerides (Fractionated Coconut Oil), Oat Fiber, Soy Fiber, Calcium Phosphate Tribasic, Gum Arabic, Sodium Citrate, Soy Lecithin, Magnesium Phosphate Dibasic, Potassium Citrate, Potassium Chloride, Sodium Carboxymethylcellulose, Magnesium Chloride, Ascorbic Acid, Choline Chloride, Potassium Phosphate Dibasic, L-Carnitine, Taurine, Zinc Sulfate, Iron Sulfate, Alpha-Tocopheryl Acetate, Niacinamide, Manganese Sulfate, Beta-Carotene, Cupric Sulfate, Thiamine Chloride Hydrochloride, Pyridoxine Hydrochloride, Riboflavin, Calcium Pantothenate, Vitamin A Palmitate, Folic Acid, Biotin, Chromium Chloride, Sodium Molybdate, Potassium Iodide, Sodium Selenate, Cyanocobalamin, Vitamin D_3 and Phylloquinone.
Nutrients (grams/8 fl oz): Protein, 13.2; Fat, 9.3; Carbohydrate, 41.5*; L-carnitine, 0.036; Taurine, 0.036; Water, 193. Calories per mL, 1.2; Calories per fl oz, 35.6.

*Includes 2.37 g of fructooligosaccharides and 3.42 g of a patented fiber blend that provides 2.85 g total dietary fiber.
(FAN 7069-01)

MURINE TEARS™   OTC
[mur′ēn]
Lubricant Eye Drops

(See PDR For Nonprescription Drugs or PDR For Ophthalmology.)

MURINE TEARS™ PLUS   OTC
[mur′ēn]
Lubricant Redness Reliever Eye Drops

(See PDR For Nonprescription Drugs or PDR For Ophthalmology.)

MURINE® EAR WAX REMOVAL   OTC
SYSTEM/MURINE® EAR DROPS
[mur′ēn]
Carbamide Peroxide Ear Wax Removal Aid

(See PDR For Nonprescription Drugs.)

NEPRO®   OTC
[nep′rō]
Specialized Liquid Nutrition
for renal patients requiring electrolyte and fluid restrictions

USAGE
As a moderate-protein, low-electrolyte, low-fluid, high-calorie formula, Nepro is designed to provide balanced nutrition for dialyzed patients with chronic or acute renal failure. Nepro may be fed orally or by tube. It can be used as a primary or supplemental source of nutrition for dialyzed renal patients under medical supervision.
Not for parenteral use.

AVAILABILITY
Ready To Use
8-fl-oz cans; 24 per case; Vanilla, No. 50632.

COMPOSITION
INGREDIENTS
Ⓤ-D Water, Corn Syrup, High-Oleic Safflower Oil, Calcium, Magnesium and Sodium Caseinates, Sugar (Sucrose), Soy Oil, Soy Lecithin, Natural and Artificial Flavors, Calcium Carbonate, Potassium Citrate, Sodium Chloride, Sodium Citrate, Choline Chloride, Magnesium Hydroxide, Calcium Hydroxide, Ascorbic Acid, L-Carnitine, Taurine, Zinc Sulfate, Alpha-Tocopheryl Acetate, Ferrous Sulfate, Niacinamide, Calcium Pantothenate, Manganese Sulfate, Pyridoxine Hydrochloride, Cupric Sulfate, Thiamine Chloride Hydrochloride, Riboflavin, Folic Acid, Vitamin A Palmitate, Biotin, Potassium Iodide, Sodium Selenite, Phylloquinone, Cyanocobalamin and Vitamin D_3.

Nutrients (Grams/8 fl oz): Protein, 16.6; Fat, 22.7; Carbohydrate, 51.1; L-carnitine, 0.062; Taurine, 0.038; Water, 167. Calories per mL, 2.0; Calories per fl oz, 59.4.
(FAN 3079-02)

OSMOLITE®   OTC
[oz′mō-līt]
Isotonic Liquid Nutrition

USAGE
As an isotonic liquid food providing complete, balanced nutrition. Osmolite is useful for patients sensitive to hyperosmotic feedings. Osmolite may be used as a tube feeding (nasogastric, nasoduodenal or jejunal) or as an oral feeding. Two quarts (2000 Calories) of Osmolite meet or surpass 100% of the RDIs for vitamins and minerals for adults and children 4 or more years of age.
Not for parenteral use.

AVAILABILITY
Ready To Use:
8-fl-oz bottles; 24 per case; No. 715.
8-fl-oz cans; 24 per case; No. 709.
32-fl-oz cans; 6 per case; No. 738.
1-liter Ross Ready-To-Hang® Enteral Feeding Containers; 8 per case; No. 50350.

COMPOSITION
Ready To Use (Ready-To-Hang has similar composition. For specific information, see product label.)

INGREDIENTS
Ⓤ-D Water, Maltodextrin, Sodium and Calcium Caseinates, High-Oleic Safflower Oil, Canola Oil, Medium-Chain Triglycerides (Fractionated Coconut Oil), Soy Protein Isolate, Potassium Citrate, Soy Lecithin, Magnesium Chloride, Calcium Phosphate Tribasic, Carrageenan, Choline Chloride, Ascorbic Acid, Magnesium Sulfate, Sodium Citrate, Taurine, L-Carnitine, Zinc Sulfate, Ferrous Sulfate, Alpha-Tocopheryl Acetate, Niacinamide, Calcium Pantothenate, Manganese Sulfate, Thiamine Chloride Hydrochloride, Cupric Sulfate, Pyridoxine Hydrochloride, Vitamin A Palmitate, Riboflavin, Folic Acid, Biotin, Sodium Molybdate, Chromium Chloride, Potassium Iodide, Sodium Selenate, Phylloquinone, Cyanocobalamin and Vitamin D_3.
Nutrients (Grams/8 fl oz): Protein, 8.8; Fat, 8.2; Carbohydrate, 35.6; L-carnitine, 0.019; Taurine, 0.019; Water, 199. Calories per mL, 1.06; Calories per fl oz, 31.3.
(FAN 3135-08)

OSMOLITE® HN   OTC
[oz′mō-līt]
High-Nitrogen Isotonic Liquid Nutrition

USAGE
As a high-nitrogen, isotonic liquid food providing complete, balanced nutrition. Osmolite HN is designed to meet the needs of tube-fed patients with decreased energy requirements or increased protein needs with intolerance to hyperosmolar feedings. Osmolite HN helps tube-fed patients get the vitamins, minerals and protein they need when their volume intake is low. Osmolite HN may be used as a tube feeding (nasogastric, nasoduodenal or jejunal).
Not for parenteral use.

AVAILABILITY
Ready To Use:
8-fl-oz bottles; 24 per case; No. 736.
8-fl-oz cans; 24 per case; No. 735.
32-fl-oz cans; 6 per case; No. 739.
1-liter Ross Ready-To-Hang® Enteral Feeding Containers; 8 per case; No. 668.
1500 mL Ross Ready–To–Hang® Enteral Feeding Containers; 6 per case; No. 52600.

COMPOSITION
Ready To Use (Ready-To-Hang has similar composition. For specific information, see product label.)

INGREDIENTS
Ⓤ-D Water, Maltodextrin, Sodium and Calcium Caseinates, High-Oleic Safflower Oil, Canola Oil, Soy Protein Isolate, Medium-Chain Triglycerides (Fractionated Coconut Oil), Potassium Citrate, Soy Lecithin, Magnesium Chloride, Calcium Phosphate Tribasic, Sodium Citrate, Choline Chloride, Ascorbic Acid, Carrageenan, Potassium Chloride, Potassium Phosphate Dibasic, Taurine, L-Carnitine, Zinc Sulfate, Ferrous Sulfate, Alpha-Tocopheryl Acetate, Niacinamide, Calcium Pantothenate, Manganese Sulfate, Cupric Sulfate, Vitamin A Palmitate, Thiamine Chloride Hydrochloride, Pyridoxine Hydrochloride, Riboflavin, Folic Acid, Biotin, Sodium Molybdate, Chromium Chloride, Potassium

Continued on next page

Ross Laboratories—Cont.

Iodide, Sodium Selenate, Phylloquinone, Cyanocobalamin and Vitamin D₃.
Nutrients (Grams/8 fl oz): Protein, 10.5; Fat, 8.2; Carbohydrate, 33.9; L-carnitine, 0.027; Taurine, 0.027; Water, 199. Calories per mL, 1.06; Calories per fl oz, 31.3.
(FAN 7045-08)

OSMOLITE® HN PLUS
OTC

[oz' mō-lĭt]
1.2 Cal/mL, High-Nitrogen Liquid Nutrition

USAGE
As a calorically-dense, high-nitrogen, low-residue liquid food for tube-fed patients who could benefit from a moderate increase in caloric density and protein intake. 1200 Calories provides at least 100% of the RDI for vitamins and minerals. Osmolite HN Plus also contains added beta-carotene.
Not for parenteral use.

AVAILABILITY
Ready To Use:
8-fl-oz cans: 24 per case; No. 53120.
1-liter Ross Ready-To-Hang® Enteral Feeding Containers; 8 per case; No. 53122.
1500 mL Ross Ready-To-Hang® Enteral Feeding Containers; 6 per case: No. 53116.

COMPOSITION
Ready To Use (Ready-To-Hang has similar composition. For specific information, see product label.)

INGREDIENTS
Ⓤ-D Water, Maltodextrin, Sodium Caseinate, High-Oleic Safflower Oil, Calcium Caseinate, Canola Oil, Medium-Chain Triglycerides (Fractionated Coconut Oil), Calcium Phosphate Tribasic, Sodium Citrate, Soy Lecithin, Magnesium Phosphate, Potassium Citrate, Potassium Chloride, Magnesium Chloride, Cellulose Gel, Ascorbic Acid, Choline Chloride, Potassium Phosphate Dibasic, Taurine, L-Carnitine, Zinc Sulfate, Ferrous Sulfate, Alpha-Tocopheryl Acetate, Niacinamide, Calcium Pantothenate, Manganese Sulfate, Beta-Carotene, Cupric Sulfate, Vitamin A Palmitate, Thiamine Chloride Hydrochloride, Pyridoxine Hydrochloride, Riboflavin, Folic Acid, Biotin, Chromium Chloride, Sodium Molybdate, Potassium Iodide, Sodium Selenate, Phylloquinone, Cyanocobalamin and Vitamin D₃.
Nutrients (grams/8 fl oz): Protein, 13.2; Fat, 9.3; Carbohydrate, 37.5; L-carnitine, 0.036; Taurine, 0.036; Water, 195. Calories per mL, 1.2; Calories per fl oz, 35.6.
(FAN 7069–01)

PEDIALYTE®
OTC

[pē 'dē-ah-līt "]
Oral Electrolyte Maintenance Solution

USAGE
To quickly restore fluid and minerals lost in diarrhea and vomiting; for maintenance of water and electrolytes following corrective parenteral therapy for severe diarrhea. Pedialyte is designed to promote fluid absorption more effectively than common household beverages.
Features:
● Ready To Use—no mixing or dilution necessary.
● Balanced electrolytes to replace stool losses and provide maintenance requirements.
● Provides glucose to promote sodium and water absorption.
● Unflavored form available for young infants; fruit-flavored, bubble gum-flavored and grape-flavored forms available to enhance compliance in older infants and children.
● Plastic liter bottles are resealable and easy to pour.
● Widely available in grocery, drug and discount stores.

AVAILABILITY
Ready To Use:
1 Qt 1.8 fl oz (1 L) plastic bottles; 8 per case; Unflavored, No. 00336; Fruit Flavor, No. 00365; Bubble Gum Flavor, No. 51752; Grape Flavor, No. 00240.
8-fl-oz (237 mL) bottles; 4 six-packs per case; Unflavored, No. 00160. For hospital use, Pedialyte is available in the Ross Hospital Formula System.

DOSAGE
Administration Guide to restore fluid and minerals lost in diarrhea and vomiting (Pedialyte Unflavored, Fruit Flavor, Bubble Gum Flavor or Grape Flavor) and management of mild to moderate dehydration secondary to moderate to severe diarrhea (Rehydralyte® Oral Electrolyte Rehydration Solution).

Pedialyte, Rehydralyte Administration Guide*

For Infants and Young Children

Age	2 Weeks	3 Months	6 Months	9 Months	1	1½	2	2½ Years	3	3½	4	5	6
Approximate Weight†													
(lb)	7	13	17	20	23	25	28	30	32	35	38	41	46
(kg)	3.2	6.0	7.8	9.2	10.2	11.4	12.6	13.6	14.6	16.0	17.0	18.7	20.7
PEDIALYTE UNFLAVORED, FRUIT FLAVOR, BUBBLE GUM FLAVOR OR GRAPE FLAVOR fl oz/day for maintenance**	13 to 16	28 to 32	34 to 40	38 to 44	41 to 46	45 to 50	48 to 53	51 to 56	54 to 58	56 to 60	57 to 62	59 to 66	62 to 69
REHYDRALYTE fl oz/day for Replacement for 5% Dehydration (including maintenance)**	18 to 21	38 to 42	47 to 53	53 to 59	58 to 63	64 to 69	69 to 74	74 to 79	78 to 82	83 to 87	85 to 90	90 to 97	96 to 104
REHYDRALYTE fl oz/day for Replacement for 10% Dehydration (including maintenance)**	23 to 26	48 to 52	60 to 66	68 to 74	75 to 80	83 to 88	90 to 95	97 to 102	102 to 106	110 to 114	113 to 118	121 to 128	131 to 138

*Administration Guide does not apply to infants less than 1 week of age. For children over 6 years, maintenance intakes may exceed 2 liters daily.

**Fluid intake in guide is total fluid requirement from oral electrolyte solution, formula or other fluids, but does not take into account ongoing stool losses. Fluid loss in the stool should be replaced by consumption of an amount of Pedialyte or Rehydralyte equal to stool losses in addition to fluid maintenance requirement in this Administration Guide.

†Weight based on the 50th percentile of weight for age of the National Center for Health Statistics (NCHS) reference growth data. Hamill PVV, Drizd TA, Johnson CL, et al: Physical growth: National Center for Health Statistics percentiles. *Am J Clin Nutr* 1979;32:607-629.

1. Extrapolated from Barness L: Nutrition and nutritional disorders, in Behrman RE, Kliegman RM, Nelson WE, Vaughan VC III: *Nelson Textbook of Pediatrics*, ed 14. Philadelphia: WB Saunders Co, 1992, pp 105-107.

Pedialyte (Unflavored, Fruit Flavor, Bubble Gum Flavor or Grape Flavor) or Rehydralyte should be offered frequently in amounts tolerated. Total daily intake should be adjusted to meet individual needs, based on thirst and response to therapy. The following suggested intakes for maintenance are based on water requirements for ordinary energy expenditure.[1] For dehydrated children, the suggested intakes are for replacement and for maintenance, based on a fluid deficit of 5% or 10% of body weight (including maintenance requirement). The fluid deficit should be replaced as quickly as possible, usually in the first 4 to 6 hours.
[See table above.]

COMPOSITION
Unflavored Pedialyte (Fruit Flavor, Bubble Gum Flavor and Grape Flavor Pedialyte have similar composition and nutrient values. Fruit Flavor and Grape Flavor Pedialyte contain fructose. For specific information including artificial colors in flavored products, see product labels.)

INGREDIENTS
(Pareve, Ⓤ) Water, dextrose, potassium citrate, sodium chloride and sodium citrate.

Provides:	Per 8 Fl Oz	Per Liter
Sodium (mEq)	10.6	45
Potassium (mEq)	4.7	20
Chloride (mEq)	8.3	35
Citrate (mEq)	7.1	30
Dextrose (g)	5.9	25
Calories	24	100

(FAN 3250-01)

PEDIAZOLE® (8030)
℞

erythromycin ethylsuccinate and sulfisoxazole acetyl for oral suspension

DESCRIPTION
Pediazole is a combination of erythromycin ethylsuccinate, USP, and sulfisoxazole acetyl, USP. When reconstituted with water as directed on the label, the granules form a white, strawberry-banana flavor suspension that provides the equivalent of 200 mg erythromycin activity and the equivalent of 600 mg of sulfisoxazole activity per teaspoonful (5 mL).
Erythromycin is produced by a strain of *Saccaropolyspora erythraea* and belongs to the macrolide group of antibiotics. It is basic and readily forms salts and esters. Erythromycin ethylsuccinate is the 2'-ethylsuccinyl ester of erythromycin.

It is essentially a tasteless form of the antibiotic suitable for oral administration, particularly in suspension dosage forms. The chemical name is erythromycin 2'-(ethyl succinate). Erythromycin ethylsuccinate has the following structural formula:

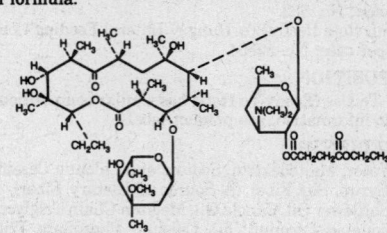

Sulfisoxazole acetyl or N^1-acetyl sulfisoxazole is an ester of sulfisoxazole. Chemically, sulfisoxazole is N-(3,4-Dimethyl-5-isoxazolyl)-N-sulfanilylacetamide. Sulfisoxazole acetyl has the following structural formula:

Inactive Ingredients: Citric acid, magnesium aluminum silicate, poloxamer, sodium carboxymethylcellulose, sodium citrate, sucrose and artificial flavoring.

CLINICAL PHARMACOLOGY
Orally administered erythromycin ethylsuccinate suspensions are readily and reliably absorbed. Erythromycin ethylsuccinate products have demonstrated rapid and consistent absorption in both fasting and nonfasting conditions. However, higher serum concentrations are obtained when these products are given with food. Bioavailability data are available from Ross Products Division. Erythromycin is largely bound to plasma proteins. After absorption, erythromycin diffuses readily into most body fluids. In the absence of meningeal inflammation, low concentrations are normally achieved in the spinal fluid, but the passage of the drug across the blood-brain barrier increases in meningitis. Erythromycin crosses the placental barrier and is excreted in human milk. Erythromycin is not removed by peritoneal dialysis or hemodialysis.
In the presence of normal hepatic function, erythromycin is concentrated in the liver and is excreted in the bile; the effect of hepatic dysfunction on biliary excretion of erythro-

mycin is not known. After oral administration, less than 5% of the administered dose can be recovered in the active form in the urine.

Wide variation in blood levels may result following identical doses of a sulfonamide. Blood levels should be measured in patients receiving these drugs for serious infections. Free sulfonamide blood levels of 50 to 150 mcg/mL may be considered therapeutically effective for most infections, with blood levels of 120 to 150 mcg/mL being optimal for serious infections. The maximum sulfonamide level should be 200 mcg/mL, because adverse reactions occur more frequently above this concentration.

Following oral administration, sulfisoxazole is rapidly and completely absorbed; the small intestine is the major site of absorption, but some of the drug is absorbed from the stomach. Sulfonamides are present in the blood as free, conjugated (acetylated and possibly other forms), and protein-bound forms. The amount present as "free" drug is considered to be the therapeutically active form. Approximately 85% of a dose of sulfisoxazole is bound to plasma proteins, primarily to albumin; 65% to 72% of the unbound portion is in the nonacetylated form.

Maximum plasma concentrations of intact sulfisoxazole following a single 2-g oral dose of sulfisoxazole to healthy adult volunteers ranged from 127 to 211 mcg/mL (mean, 169 mcg/mL), and the time of peak plasma concentration ranged from 1 to 4 hours (mean, 2.5 hours). The elimination half-life of sulfisoxazole ranged from 4.6 to 7.8 hours after oral administration. The elimination of sulfisoxazole has been shown to be slower in elderly subjects (63 to 75 years) with diminished renal function (creatine clearance 37 to 68 mL/min).[1] After multiple-dose oral administration of 500 mg q.i.d. to healthy volunteers, the average steady-state plasma concentrations of intact sulfisoxazole ranged from 49.9 to 88.8 mcg/mL (mean, 63.4 mcg/mL).[2]

Sulfisoxazole and its acetylated metabolites are excreted primarily by the kidneys through glomerular filtration. Concentrations of sulfisoxazole are considerably higher in the urine than in the blood. The mean urinary recovery following oral administration of sulfisoxazole is 97% within 48 hours; 52% of this is intact drug, and the remainder is the N[4]-acetylated metabolite.

Sulfisoxazole is distributed only in extracellular body fluids. It is excreted in human milk. It readily crosses the placental barrier. In healthy subjects, cerebrospinal fluid concentrations of sulfisoxazole vary; in patients with meningitis, however, concentrations of free drug in cerebrospinal fluid as high as 94 mcg/mL have been reported.

Microbiology:
Pediazole has been formulated to contain sulfisoxazole for concomitant use with erythromycin.

Erythromycin acts by inhibition of protein synthesis by binding 50 S ribosomal subunits of susceptible organisms. It does not affect nucleic acid synthesis. Antagonism has been demonstrated in vitro between erythromycin and clindamycin, lincomycin, and chloramphenicol.

The sulfonamides are bacteriostatic agents, and the spectrum of activity is similar for all. Sulfonamides inhibit bacterial synthesis of dihydrofolic acid by preventing the condensation of the pteridine with para-aminobenzoic acid through competitive inhibition of the enzyme dihydropteroate synthetase. Resistant strains have altered dihydropteroate synthetase with reduced affinity for sulfonamides or produce increased quantities of para-aminobenzoic acid.

Susceptibility Testing:
Quantitative methods that require measurement of zone diameter give the most precise estimates of the susceptibility of bacteria to antimicrobial agents. One such standardized single-disc procedure[3] has been recommended for use with discs to test susceptibility to erythromycin and sulfisoxazole. Interpretation involves correlation of the zone diameters obtained in the disc test with minimal inhibitory concentration (MIC) values for erythromycin.

If the standardized procedure of disc susceptibility is used, a 15-mcg erythromycin disc should give a zone diameter of at least 18 mm when tested against an erythromycin-susceptible bacterial strain, and a 250-300 mcg sulfisoxazole disc should give a zone diameter of at least 17 mm when tested against a sulfisoxazole-susceptible bacterial strain.

In vitro sulfonamide susceptibility tests are not always reliable because media containing excessive amounts of thymidine are capable of reversing the inhibitory effect of sulfonamides, which may result in false resistant reports. The tests must be carefully coordinated with bacteriological and clinical responses. When the patient is already taking sulfonamides, follow-up cultures should have aminobenzoic acid added to the isolation media but not to subsequent susceptibility test media.

INDICATIONS AND USAGE
For treatment of ACUTE OTITIS MEDIA in children that is caused by susceptible strains of Haemophilus influenzae.

CONTRAINDICATIONS
Pediazole is contraindicated in the following patient populations:

Patients with a known hypersensitivity to either of its components, children younger than 2 months, pregnant women at term, and mothers nursing infants less than 2 months of age.

Use in pregnant women at term, in children less than 2 months of age, and in mothers nursing infants less than 2 months of age is contraindicated because sulfonamides may promote kernicterus in the newborn by displacing bilirubin from plasma proteins.

Erythromycin is contraindicated in patients taking terfenadine. (See PRECAUTIONS—Drug Interactions.)

WARNINGS
FATALITIES ASSOCIATED WITH THE ADMINISTRATION OF SULFONAMIDES, ALTHOUGH RARE, HAVE OCCURRED DUE TO SEVERE REACTIONS INCLUDING STEVENS-JOHNSON SYNDROME, TOXIC EPIDERMAL NECROLYSIS, FULMINANT HEPATIC NECROSIS, AGRANULOCYTOSIS, APLASTIC ANEMIA, AND OTHER BLOOD DYSCRASIAS.

SULFONAMIDES, INCLUDING SULFONAMIDE-CONTAINING PRODUCTS SUCH AS PEDIAZOLE, SHOULD BE DISCONTINUED AT THE FIRST APPEARANCE OF SKIN RASH OR ANY SIGN OF ADVERSE REACTION. In rare instances, a skin rash may be followed by a more severe reaction, such as Stevens-Johnson syndrome, toxic epidermal necrolysis, hepatic necrosis, and serious blood disorders. (See PRECAUTIONS.)

Clinical signs such as sore throat, fever, pallor, rash, purpura, or jaundice may be early indications of serious reactions.

There have been reports of hepatic dysfunction with or without jaundice, occurring in patients receiving oral erythromycin products.

Cough, shortness of breath, and pulmonary infiltrates are hypersensitivity reactions of the respiratory tract that have been reported in association with sulfonamide treatment.

The sulfonamides should not be used for the treatment of group A beta-hemolytic streptococcal infections. In an established infection, they will not eradicate the streptococcus and, therefore, will not prevent sequelae such as rheumatic fever.

Pseudomembranous colitis has been reported with nearly all antibacterial agents, including Pediazole, and may range in severity from mild to life-threatening. Therefore, it is important to consider this diagnosis in patients who present with diarrhea subsequent to the administration of antibacterial agents.

Treatment with antibacterial agents alters the normal flora of the colon and may permit overgrowth of clostridia. Studies indicate that a toxin produced by Clostridium difficile is one primary cause of "antibiotic-associated colitis."

After diagnosis of pseudomembranous colitis has been established, therapeutic measures should be initiated. Mild cases of pseudomembranous colitis usually respond to drug discontinuation alone. In moderate to severe cases, consideration should be given to management with fluids and electrolytes, protein supplementation, and treatment with an antibacterial drug clinically effective against Clostridium difficile colitis.

There have been reports suggesting that erythromycin does not reach the fetus in adequate concentration to prevent congenital syphilis. Infants born to women treated during pregnancy with erythromycin for early syphilis should be treated with an appropriate penicillin regimen.

Rhabdomyolysis with or without renal impairment has been reported in seriously ill patients receiving erythromycin concomitantly with lovastatin. Therefore, patients receiving concomitant lovastatin and erythromycin should be carefully monitored for creatine kinase (CK) and serum transaminase levels. (See package insert for lovastatin.)

PRECAUTIONS
General: Erythromycin is principally excreted by the liver. Caution should be exercised when erythromycin is administered to patients with impaired hepatic function. (See CLINICAL PHARMACOLOGY and WARNING sections.)

Prolonged or repeated use of erythromycin may result in an overgrowth of nonsusceptible bacteria or fungi. If superinfection occurs, erythromycin should be discontinued and appropriate therapy instituted.

There have been reports that erythromycin may aggravate the weakness of patients with myasthenia gravis.

When indicated, incision and drainage or other surgical procedures should be performed in conjunction with antibiotic therapy.

Sulfonamides should be given with caution to patients with impaired renal or hepatic function and to those with severe allergy or bronchial asthma. In glucose-6-phosphate dehydrogenase-deficient individuals, hemolysis may occur; this reaction is frequently dose-related.

Information for Patients: Patients should maintain an adequate fluid intake to prevent crystalluria and stone formation.

Laboratory Tests: Complete blood counts should be done frequently in patients receiving sulfonamides. If a signifi-

cant reduction in the count of any formed blood element is noted, Pediazole should be discontinued. Urinalysis with careful microscopic examination and renal function tests should be performed during therapy, particularly for those patients with impaired renal function. Blood levels should be measured in patients receiving a sulfonamide for serious infections. (See INDICATIONS AND USAGE.)

Drug/laboratory Test Interactions: Erythromycin interferes with the fluorometric determination of urinary catecholamines.

Drug Interactions: Erythromycin use in patients who are receiving high doses of theophylline may be associated with an increase in serum theophylline levels and potential theophylline toxicity. In case of theophylline toxicity and/or elevated serum theophylline levels, the dose of theophylline should be reduced while the patient is receiving concomitant erythromycin therapy.

Concomitant administration of erythromycin and digoxin has been reported to result in elevated digoxin serum levels. There have been reports of increased anticoagulant effects when erythromycin and oral anticoagulants were used concomitantly. Increased anticoagulation effects due to this drug may be more pronounced in the elderly.

Concurrent use of erythromycin and ergotamine or dihydroergotamine has been associated in some patients with acute ergot toxicity characterized by severe peripheral vasospasm and dysesthesia.

Erythromycin has been reported to decrease the clearance of triazolam and midazolam and thus may increase the pharmacologic effect of these benzodiazepines.

The use of erythromycin in patients concurrently taking drugs metabolized by the cytochrome P450 system may be associated with elevations in serum levels of these other drugs. There have been reports of interactions of erythromycin with carbamazepine, cyclosporine, hexobarbital, phenytoin, alfentanil, diisopyramide, lovastatin, and bromocriptine. Serum concentrations of drugs metabolized by the cytochrome P450 system should be monitored closely in patients concurrently receiving erythromycin.

Erythromycin significantly alters the metabolism of terfenadine when taken concomitantly. Rare cases of serious cardiovascular adverse events, including death, cardiac arrest, torsades de pointes, and other ventricular arrhythmias, have been observed. (See CONTRAINDICATIONS.)

It has been reported that sulfisoxazole may prolong the prothrombin time in patients who are receiving the anticoagulant warfarin. This interaction should be kept in mind when Pediazole is given to patients already on anticoagulant therapy, and the coagulation time should be reassessed.

It has been proposed that sulfisoxazole competes with thiopental for plasma protein binding. In one study involving 48 patients, intravenous sulfisoxazole resulted in a decrease in the amount of thiopental required for anesthesia and in a shortening of the awakening time. It is not known whether chronic oral doses of sulfisoxazole have a similar effect. Until more is known about this interaction, physicians should be aware that patients receiving sulfisoxazole might require less thiopental for anesthesia.

Sulfonamides can displace methotrexate from plasma protein binding sites, thus increasing free methotrexate concentrations. Studies in man have shown sulfisoxazole infusions to decrease plasma protein-bound methotrexate by one fourth.

Sulfisoxazole can also potentiate the blood-sugar-lowering activity of sulfonylureas.

Carcinogenesis, Mutagenesis, Impairment of Fertility:
Carcinogenesis: Pediazole has not undergone adequate trials relating to carcinogenicity; each component, however, has been evaluated separately. Long-term (21 month) oral studies conducted in rats with erythromycin ethylsuccinate did not provide evidence of tumorigenicity. Sulfisoxazole was not carcinogenic in either sex when administered to mice by gavage for 103 weeks at dosages up to approximately 18 times the recommended human dose or to rats at 4 times the human dose. Rats appear to be especially susceptible to the goitrogenic effects of sulfonamides, and long-term administration of sulfonamides has resulted in thyroid malignancies in this species.

Mutagenesis: There are no studies available that adequately evaluate the mutagenic potential of Pediazole or either of its components. However, sulfisoxazole was not observed to be mutagenic in E. coli Sd-4-73 when tested in the absence of a metabolic activating system. There was no apparent effect on male or female fertility in rats fed erythromycin (base) at levels up to 0.25% of diet.

Impairment of Fertility: Pediazole has not undergone adequate trials relating to impairment of fertility. In a reproduction study in rats given 7 times the human dose per day of sulfisoxazole, no effects were observed regarding mating behavior, conception rate or fertility index (percent pregnant).

Pregnancy: Teratogenic Effects. Pregnancy Category C. At dosages 7 times the human daily dose, sulfisoxazole was not

Continued on next page

Ross Laboratories—Cont.

teratogenic in either rats or rabbits. However, in two other teratogenicity studies, cleft palates developed in both rats and mice after administration of 5 to 9 times the human therapeutic dose of sulfisoxazole.

There is no evidence of teratogenicity or any other adverse effect on reproduction in female rats fed erythromycin base (up to 0.25% of diet) prior to and during mating, during gestation, and through weaning of two successive litters. There are, however, no adequate and well-controlled studies in pregnant women. Because animal reproduction studies are not always predictive of human response, this drug should be used during pregnancy only if clearly needed. Erythromycin has been reported to cross the placental barrier in humans, but fetal plasma levels are generally low.

There are no adequate or well-controlled studies of Pediazole in either laboratory animals or in pregnant women. It is not known whether Pediazole can cause fetal harm when administered to a pregnant woman prior to term or can affect reproduction capacity. Pediazole should be used during pregnancy only if the potential benefit justifies the potential risk to the fetus.

Nonteratogenic Effects: Kernicterus may occur in the newborn as a result of treatment of a pregnant woman *at term* with sulfonamides. **(See CONTRAINDICATIONS.)**

Labor and Delivery: The effects of erythromycin and sulfisoxazole on labor and delivery are unknown.

Nursing Mothers: Both erythromycin and sulfisoxazole are excreted in human milk. **Because of the potential for the development of kernicterus in neonates due to the displacement of bilirubin from plasma proteins by sulfisoxazole, a decision should be made whether to discontinue nursing or discontinue the drug, taking into account the importance of the drug to the mother. (See CONTRAINDICATIONS.)**

Pediatric Use: **See INDICATIONS AND USAGE and DOSAGE AND ADMINISTRATION** sections. Not for use in children under 2 months of age. **(See CONTRAINDICATIONS.)**

ADVERSE REACTIONS

Erythromycin ethylsuccinate: The most frequent side effects of oral erythromycin preparations are gastrointestinal and are dose-related. They include nausea, vomiting, abdominal pain, diarrhea and anorexia. Symptoms of hepatic dysfunction and/or abnormal liver-function test results may occur **(see WARNINGS section).** Pseudomembranous colitis has been rarely reported in association with erythromycin therapy.

Allergic reactions ranging from urticaria and mild skin eruptions to anaphylaxis have occurred.

There have been isolated reports of reversible hearing loss occurring chiefly in patients with renal insufficiency and in patients receiving high doses of erythromycin.

Onset of pseudomembranous colitis symptoms may occur during or after antibiotic treatment. **(See WARNINGS.)**

Sulfisoxazole acetyl: Included in the listing that follows are adverse reactions that have been reported with other sulfonamide products: pharmacologic similarities require that each of the reactions be considered with Pediazole administration.

Allergic/Dermatologic: Anaphylaxis, erythema multiforme (Stevens-Johnson syndrome), toxic epidermal necrolysis (Lyell's syndrome), exfoliative dermatitis, angioedema, arteritis, vasculitis, allergic myocarditis, serum sickness, rash, urticaria, pruritus, photosensitivity, and conjunctival and scleral injection. In addition, periarteritis nodosa and systemic lupus erythematosus have been reported. **(See WARNINGS.)**

Cardiovascular: Tachycardia, palpitations, syncope, and cyanosis.

Rarely, erythromycin has been associated with the production of ventricular arrhythmias, including ventricular tachycardia and torsade de pointes, in individuals with prolonged QT intervals.

Endocrine: The sulfonamides bear certain chemical similarities to some goitrogens, diuretics (acetazolamide and the thiazides) and oral hypoglycemic agents. Cross-sensitivity may exist with these agents. Developments of goiter, diuresis, and hypoglycemia have occurred rarely in patients receiving sulfonamides.

Gastrointestinal: Hepatitis, hepatocellular necrosis, jaundice, pseudomembranous colitis, nausea, emesis, anorexia, abdominal pain, diarrhea, gastrointestinal hemorrhage, melena, flatulence, glossitis, stomatitis, salivary gland enlargement, and pancreatitis. Onset of pseudomembranous colitis symptoms may occur during or after treatment with sulfisoxazole, a component of Pediazole. **(See WARNINGS.)**

The sulfisoxazole acetyl component of Pediazole has been reported to cause increased elevation of liver-associated enzymes in patients with hepatitis.

Genitourinary: Crystalluria, hematuria, BUN and creatinine elevations, nephritis, and toxic nephrosis with oliguria and anuria. Acute renal failure and urinary retention have also been reported.

The frequency of renal complications, commonly associated with some sulfonamides, is lower in patients receiving the more soluble sulfonamides such as sulfisoxazole.

Hematologic: Leukopenia, agranulocytosis, aplastic anemia, thrombocytopenia, purpura, hemolytic anemia, eosinophilia, clotting disorders including hypoprothrombinemia and hypofibrinogenemia, sulfhemoglobinemia, and methemoglobinemia.

Neurologic: Headache, dizziness, peripheral neuritis, paresthesia, convulsions, tinnitus, vertigo, ataxia, and intracranial hypertension.

Psychiatric: Psychosis, hallucinations, disorientation, depression, and anxiety.

Respiratory: Cough, shortness of breath, and pulmonary infiltrates. **(See WARNINGS.)**

Vascular: Angioedema, arteritis, and vasculitis.

Miscellaneous: Edema (including periorbital), pyrexia, drowsiness, weakness, fatigue, lassitude, rigors, flushing, hearing loss, insomnia, and pneumonitis.

OVERDOSAGE

No information is available on a specific result of overdose with Pediazole. Overdosage of erythromycin should be handled with the prompt elimination of unabsorbed drug and all other appropriate measures. Erythromycin is not removed by peritoneal dialysis or hemodialysis.

The amount of a single dose of sulfisoxazole that is either associated with symptoms of overdosage or is likely to be life-threatening has not been reported. Signs and symptoms of overdosage reported with sulfonamides include anorexia, colic, nausea, vomiting, dizziness, headache, drowsiness and unconsciousness. Pyrexia, hematuria and crystalluria may be noted. Blood dyscrasias and jaundice are potential late manifestations of overdosage.

General principles of treatment include the immediate discontinuation of the drug, instituting gastric lavage or emesis, forcing oral fluids, and administering intravenous fluids if urine output is low and renal function is normal. The patient should be monitored with blood counts and appropriate blood chemistries, including electrolytes. If the patient becomes cyanotic, the possibility of methemoglobinemia should be considered and, if present, the condition should be treated appropriately with intravenous 1% methylene blue. If a significant blood dyscrasia or jaundice occurs, specific therapy should be instituted for these complications. Peritoneal dialysis is not effective, and hemodialysis is only moderately effective in removing sulfonamides.

The acute toxicity of sulfisoxazole in animals is as follows:

Species	$LD_{50} \pm$ S.E. (mg/kg)
mouse	5700 ± 235
rats	> 10,000
rabbits	> 2000

DOSAGE AND ADMINISTRATION

PEDIAZOLE SHOULD NOT BE ADMINISTERED TO INFANTS UNDER 2 MONTHS OF AGE BECAUSE OF CONTRAINDICATIONS OF SYSTEMIC SULFONAMIDES IN THIS AGE GROUP.

For Acute Otitis Media in Children: The dose of Pediazole can be calculated based on the erythromycin component (50 mg/kg/day) or the sulfisoxazole component (150 mg/kg/day to a maximum of 6 g/day). The total daily dose of Pediazole should be administered in equally divided doses three or four times a day for 10 days. Pediazole may be administered without regard to meals.

The following approximate dosage schedules are recommended for using Pediazole:

Children: Two months of age or older

FOUR-TIMES-A-DAY SCHEDULE

Weight	Dose—every 6 hours
Less than 8 kg (<18 lbs)	Adjust dosage by body weight
8 kg (18 lbs)	1/2 teaspoonful (2.5 mL)
16 kg (35 lbs)	1 teaspoonful (5 mL)
24 kg (53 lbs)	1 1/2 teaspoonfuls (7.5 mL)
Over 32 kg (over 70 lbs)	2 teaspoonfuls (10 mL)

THREE-TIMES-A-DAY SCHEDULE

Weight	Dose—every 8 hours
Less than 6 kg (<13 lbs)	Adjust dosage by body weight
6 kg (13 lbs)	1/2 teaspoonful (2.5 mL)
12 kg (26 lbs)	1 teaspoonful (5 mL)
18 kg (40 lbs)	1 1/2 teaspoonfuls (7.5 mL)
24 kg (53 lbs)	2 teaspoonfuls (10 mL)
Over 30 kg (over 66 lbs)	2 1/2 teaspoonfuls (12.5 mL)

TO PATIENT: Shake before using. Oversize bottle provides shake space. Keep tightly closed. Store in the refrigerator. Use within 14 days. Unused portion should be discarded after 14 days.

HOW SUPPLIED

Pediazole Suspension is available for teaspoon dosage in 100-mL (**NDC** 0074-8030-13), 150-mL (**NDC** 0074-8030-43), 200-mL (**NDC** 0074-8030-53) and 250-mL (**NDC** 0074-8030-73) bottles, in the form of granules to be reconstituted with water. The suspension provides erythromycin ethylsuccinate equivalent to 200 mg erythromycin activity and sulfisoxazole acetyl equivalent to 600 mg sulfisoxazole per teaspoonful (5 mL).

Before mixing, store below 86°F (30°C).

REFERENCES

1. Biovert A, Barbeau G, Belanger PM: Pharmacokinetics of sulfisoxazole in young and elderly subjects. *Gerontology* 1984; 30:125-131.
2. Oie S, Gambertoglio JG, Fleckenstein L: Comparison of the disposition of total and unbound sulfisoxazole after single and multiple dosing. *J Pharmacokinet Biopharm* 1982; 10:157-172.
3. National Committee for Clinical Laboratory Standards: *Performance Standards for Antimicrobial Disk Susceptibility Tests*, ed. 4. Approved Standard NCCLS Document M2-A4, Vol 10, No. 7. Villanova, Pa: NCCLS, 1990.

July 1994

PEDIASURE® OTC

[*pē 'dē-ah-shur "*]

Complete Liquid Nutrition

USAGE

As a nutritionally complete, balanced, isotonic enteral formula especially designed for tube or oral feeding of children 1 to 10 years of age. May be used as the sole source of nutrition or as a supplement. PediaSure meets or exceeds 100% of the NAS-NRC RDAs for protein, vitamins and minerals for children 1 to 6 years of age in 1000 mL (approx. 34 fl oz), and for children 7 to 10 years of age in 1300 mL (approx. 44 fl oz). Calcium/phosphorus ratio of 1.2:1 meets recommendations by the American Academy of Pediatrics Committee on Nutrition (AAP-CON) for growing children. Fortified with biotin, choline, inositol, taurine and carnitine.

Not for parenteral use.

Not intended for infants under 1 year of age unless specified by a physician.

AVAILABILITY

Ready To Use:

8-fl-oz (237 mL) cans: 24 per case; Vanilla, No. 00373 (retail), Vanilla, No. 51804 (institution); Chocolate, No. 51812 (retail), Chocolate, No. 51882 (institution); Strawberry, No. 51810 (retail), Strawberry, No. 51880 (institution); Banana Cream, No. 51808 (retail), Banana Cream, No. 51884 (institution).

COMPOSITION

Ready To Use Vanilla. (Other flavors have similar composition and nutrient values. For specific information, see product labels.)

INGREDIENTS

Ⓤ-D Water, Hydrolyzed Cornstarch, Sugar (Sucrose), Sodium Caseinate, High-Oleic Safflower Oil, Soy Oil, Fractionated Coconut Oil (Medium-Chain Triglycerides), Whey Protein Concentrate, Calcium Phosphate Tribasic, Natural and Artificial Flavor, Potassium Citrate, Magnesium Chloride, Potassium Phosphate Dibasic, Potassium Chloride, Soy Lecithin, Mono- and Diglycerides, Choline Chloride, Carrageenan, Ascorbic Acid, M-Inositol, Taurine, Ferrous Sulfate, Zinc Sulfate, Niacinamide, Alpha-Tocopheryl Acetate, L-Carnitine, Calcium Pantothenate, Manganese Sulfate, Thiamine Chloride Hydrochloride, Pyridoxine Hydrochloride, Riboflavin, Cupric Sulfate, Vitamin A Palmitate, Folic Acid, Biotin, Potassium Iodide, Sodium Selenite, Sodium Molybdate, Phylloquinone, Vitamin D_3 and Cyanocobalamin.

NUTRIENTS (GRAMS/8 FL OZ):

Protein	7.1	g
Fat	11.8	g
Carbohydrate	26	g
L-Carnitine	0.004	g
Taurine	0.017	g
Water	200	g
Calories		
Per mL	1.0	
Per FL OZ	29.6	

VITAMINS/MINERALS PER 8 FL OZ:

Vitamin A	610	IU
Vitamin D	120	IU
Vitamin E	5.4	IU
Vitamin K_1	9.0	mcg
Vitamin C	24	mg

Folic Acid	88	mcg
Thiamin (Vit B$_1$)	0.64	mg
Riboflavin (Vit B$_2$)	0.50	mg
Vitamin B$_6$	0.62	mg
Vitamin B$_{12}$	1.4	mcg
Niacin	4.0	mg
Choline	71	mg
Biotin	76	mcg
Pantothenic Acid	2.4	mg
Inositol	19	mg
Sodium	90	mg
Potassium	310	mg
Chloride	240	mg
Calcium	230	mg
Phosphorus	190	mg
Magnesium	47	mg
Iodine	23	mcg
Manganese	0.59	mg
Copper	0.24	mg
Zinc	2.8	mg
Iron	3.3	mg
Chromium	7.1	mcg
Molybdenum	8.5	mcg
Selenium	5.4	mcg

(FAN 3139-02)

PEDIASURE® WITH FIBER   OTC
[pē′dē-ah-shur″]
Complete Liquid Nutrition

USAGE
As a fiber-containing, nutritionally complete, balanced, isotonic enteral formula especially designed for tube or oral feeding of children 1 to 10 years of age. The fiber level in PediaSure With Fiber helps normalize bowel function. May be used as the sole source of nutrition or as a supplement. PediaSure With Fiber meets or exceeds 100% of the NAS-NRC RDAs for protein, vitamins and minerals for children 1 to 6 years of age in 1000 mL (approx. 34 fl. oz.), and for children 7 to 10 years of age in 1300 mL (approx. 44 fl. oz.). Calcium/phosphorus ratio of 1.2:1 meets recommendations by the American Academy of Pediatrics Committee on Nutrition (AAP-CON) for growing children. Fortified with biotin, choline, inositol, taurine and carnitine.
Not for parenteral use.
Not intended for infants under 1 year of age unless specified by a physician.

AVAILABILITY
Ready To Use:
8-fl-oz (237 mL) cans: 24 per case; Vanilla, No. 50652 (retail), Vanilla, No. 51806 (institution).

INGREDIENTS
Ⓤ-D Water, Hydrolyzed Cornstarch, Sugar (Sucrose), Sodium Caseinate, High-Oleic Safflower Oil, Soy Oil, Fractionated Coconut Oil (Medium-Chain Triglycerides), Whey Protein Concentrate, Soy Fiber, Calcium Phosphate Tribasic, Natural and Artificial Flavor, Potassium Citrate, Magnesium Chloride, Potassium Phosphate Dibasic, Potassium Chloride, Soy Lecithin, Mono- and Diglycerides, Choline Chloride, Carrageenan, Ascorbic Acid, M-Inositol, Taurine, Ferrous Sulfate, Zinc Sulfate, Niacinamide, Alpha-Tocopheryl Acetate, L-Carnitine, Calcium Pantothenate, Manganese Sulfate, Thiamine Chloride Hydrochloride, Pyridoxine Hydrochloride, Riboflavin, Cupric Sulfate, Vitamin A Palmitate, Folic Acid, Biotin, Potassium Iodide, Sodium Selenite, Sodium Molybdate, Phylloquinone, Vitamin D$_3$ and Cyanocobalamin.

NUTRIENTS (GRAMS/8 FL OZ):

Protein	7.1	g
Fat	11.8	g
Carbohydrate	26.9	g*
L-Carnitine	0.004	g
Taurine	0.017	g
Water	200	g
Calories		
Per mL	1.0	
Per FL OZ	29.6	

* Includes soy fiber (a source of dietary fiber that provides 3.4 calories and 1.2 g of total dietary fiber).

VITAMINS/MINERALS PER 8 FL OZ:

Vitamin A	610	IU
Vitamin D	120	IU
Vitamin E	5.4	IU
Vitamin K$_1$	9.0	mcg
Vitamin C	24	mg
Folic Acid	88	mcg
Thiamin (Vit B$_1$)	0.64	mg
Riboflavin (Vit B$_2$)	0.50	mg
Vitamin B$_6$	0.62	mg
Vitamin B$_{12}$	1.4	mcg
Niacin	4.0	mg
Choline	71	mg

Biotin	76	mcg
Pantothenic Acid	2.4	mg
Inositol	19	mg
Sodium	90	mg
Potassium	310	mg
Chloride	240	mg
Calcium	230	mg
Phosphorus	190	mg
Magnesium	47	mg
Iodine	23	mcg
Manganese	0.59	mg
Copper	0.24	mg
Zinc	2.8	mg
Iron	3.3	mg
Chromium	7.1	mcg
Molybdenum	8.5	mcg
Selenium	5.4	mcg

(FAN 3139-01)

PERATIVE®   OTC
[per′ah-tiv]
Specialized Liquid Nutrition
with partially hydrolyzed proteins for metabolically stressed patients

USAGE
As complete, balanced nutrition for use in the nutritional management of metabolically stressed patients with injuries such as multiple fractures, wounds, burns, surgery and the associated conditions of hypermetabolism, catabolism and susceptibility to sepsis.
Not for parenteral use.

AVAILABILITY
Ready To Use:
8-fl-oz cans; 24 cans per case; No. 50628.
1-liter Ross Ready-To-Hang® Enteral Feeding Containers; 8 per case; No. 51948.

COMPOSITION
INGREDIENTS
Ⓤ-D Water, maltodextrin, partially hydrolyzed sodium caseinate, lactalbumin hydrolysate, canola oil, medium-chain triglycerides (fractionated coconut oil), L-arginine, corn oil, magnesium chloride, potassium citrate, calcium phosphate tribasic, citric acid, soy lecithin, ascorbic acid, potassium phosphate dibasic, choline chloride, carrageenan, potassium chloride, taurine, L-carnitine, zinc sulfate, ferrous sulfate, alpha-tocopheryl acetate, niacinamide, calcium pantothenate, manganese sulfate, beta-carotene, cupric sulfate, thiamine chloride hydrochloride, pyridoxine hydrochloride, riboflavin, vitamin A palmitate, folic acid, biotin, sodium molybdate, chromium chloride, potassium iodide, sodium selenite, phylloquinone, cyanocobalamin and vitamin D$_3$.
Nutrients (Grams/8 fl oz): Protein, 15.8; Fat, 8.8; Carbohydrate, 42.0; L-carnitine, 0.031; Taurine, 0.031; Water, 187. Calories per fl oz, 38.5.
(FAN 3124-01)

POLYCOSE®   OTC
[pol′ē-kōs]
Glucose Polymers

USAGE
As a source of calories (derived solely from carbohydrate) for persons with increased caloric needs or those unable to meet their caloric needs with their normal diet. Polycose is particularly useful in supplying carbohydrate calories for protein-, electrolyte- and fat-restricted diets. Polycose is minimally sweet and mixes readily with most foods and beverages.

PRECAUTIONS
NOT FOR PARENTERAL USE.
Polycose is nutritionally incomplete and should not be used as the sole source of nutrition. Polycose is for enteral use only and should be used as directed by a health care professional.
FOR INFANT USE: Not to be fed undiluted. USE ONLY AS SPECIFICALLY DIRECTED BY A PHYSICIAN.

AVAILABILITY
Powder: 12.3 oz (350g) cans: 6 per case; No. 00746.
Liquid: (43% solution): 4.2-fl-oz bottles; 48 per case; No. 00431.

COMPOSITION
Powder: (Pareve, Ⓤ) Glucose Polymers derived from controlled hydrolysis of Cornstarch.
Nutrients (per 100 grams):

Carbohydrate		94 g
Water		6 g
Calcium	Does not exceed	30 mg (1.5 mEq)
Sodium	Does not exceed	110 mg (4.8 mEq)
Potassium	Does not exceed	10 mg (0.3 mEq)

Chloride	Does not exceed	223 mg (6.3 mEq)
Phosphorus	Does not exceed	5 mg
Calories		380

Approximate Caloric Equivalents:
1 level teaspoonful (2 g) = 8 Calories; 1 level tablespoonful (6 g) = 23 Calories; ¼ cup (25 g) = 95 Calories; ⅓ cup (33 g) = 125 Calories; ½ cup (50 g) = 190 Calories; 1 cup (100 g) = 380 Calories.
(FAN 366-01)

COMPOSITION
Liquid: (Pareve, Ⓤ) Water and Glucose Polymers derived from controlled hydrolysis of Cornstarch.
Nutrients (per 100 mL):

Carbohydrate		50 g
Water		70 g
Calcium	Does not exceed	20 mg (1.0 mEq)
Sodium	Does not exceed	70 mg (3.0 mEq)
Potassium	Does not exceed	6 mg (0.15 mEq)
Chloride	Does not exceed	140 mg (3.9 mEq)
Phosphorus	Does not exceed	3 mg
Calories		200

Approximate Caloric Equivalents:
1 mL = 2 Calories; 1 fl oz = 60 Calories; 100 mL = 200 Calories.
(FAN 3079-01)

PROMOTE®   OTC
[pruh-mōt]
High-Protein Liquid Nutrition

USAGE
As a high-protein, nutritionally complete liquid food, Promote is designed for patients who may benefit from an increased protein intake. It has a low nutrient base and permits nonambulatory patients, with energy requirements as low as 1000 Calories, to meet 100% of the RDIs for vitamins and minerals. Promote also contains added beta-carotene. Promote has a mild vanilla flavor, making it useful as a high-protein oral supplement.
Not for parenteral use.

AVAILABILITY
Ready To Use:
8-fl-oz cans; 24 cans per case; No. 50774.
1-liter Ross Ready-To-Hang® Enteral Feeding Containers; 8 per case; No. 51616.

COMPOSITION
INGREDIENTS
Ⓤ-D Water, hydrolyzed cornstarch, sodium and calcium caseinates, high-oleic safflower oil, sucrose, canola oil, medium-chain triglycerides (fractionated coconut oil), soy protein isolate, magnesium phosphate, natural and artificial flavors, sodium citrate, potassium chloride, calcium citrate, potassium citrate, soy lecithin, ascorbic acid, choline chloride, calcium carbonate, potassium phosphate dibasic, calcium phosphate dibasic, carrageenan, taurine, L-carnitine, zinc sulfate, ferrous sulfate, alpha-tocopheryl acetate, niacinamide, calcium pantothenate, manganese sulfate, cupric sulfate, vitamin A palmitate, thiamine chloride hydrochloride, pyridoxine hydrochloride, beta-carotene, riboflavin, folic acid, biotin, chromium chloride, sodium molybdate, potassium iodide, sodium selenate, phylloquinone, cyanocobalamin and vitamin D$_3$.
Nutrients (Grams/8 fl oz): Protein, 14.8; Fat, 6.2; Carbohydrate, 30.8; L-carnitine, 0.036; Taurine, 0.036; Water, 198. Calories per mL, 1.0; Calories per fl oz, 29.6.
(FAN 3079-03)

PROMOTE® WITH FIBER   OTC
[pruh-mōt]
High-Protein Liquid Nutrition

USAGE
As a fiber-containing, high-protein, nutritionally complete liquid food, Promote With Fiber is designed for patients who may benefit from fiber and an increased protein intake. It has a low nutrient base and permits nonambulatory patients with energy requirements as low as 1000 Calories to meet 100% of the RDI for vitamins and minerals. Promote With Fiber also contains added beta-carotene. Promote With Fiber has a mild vanilla flavor, making it useful as a high-protein oral supplement.
Not for parenteral use.

AVAILABILITY
Ready To Use:
8-fl-oz cans; 24 per case; Vanilla, No. 51872.
1-liter Ross Ready-To-Hang® Enteral Feeding Containers; 8 per case; No. 51874.

Continued on next page

Ross Laboratories—Cont.

COMPOSITION

Ready To Use (Ready-To-Hang has similar composition. For specific information, see product label.)

INGREDIENTS

Ⓤ-D Water, Hydrolyzed Cornstarch, Sodium and Calcium Caseinates, Sucrose, Oat Fiber, High-Oleic Safflower Oil, Canola Oil, Medium-Chain Triglycerides (Fractionated Coconut Oil), Natural and Artificial Flavors, Soy Fiber, Magnesium Phosphate, Soy Lecithin, Potassium Chloride, Calcium Phosphate Dibasic, Sodium Citrate, Calcium Citrate, Calcium Carbonate, Ascorbic Acid, Choline Chloride, Potassium Phosphate Dibasic, Potassium Citrate, Taurine, L-Carnitine, Zinc Sulfate, Ferrous Sulfate, Alpha-Tocopheryl Acetate, Niacinamide, Calcium Pantothenate, Manganese Sulfate, Cupric Sulfate, Vitamin A Palmitate, Thiamine Chloride Hydrochloride, Pyridoxine Hydrochloride, Beta-Carotene, Riboflavin, Folic Acid, Biotin, Chromium Chloride, Sodium Molybdate, Potassium Iodide, Sodium Selenate, Phylloquinone, Cyanocobalamin and Vitamin D₃.

Nutrients (grams/8 fl oz): Protein, 14.8; Fat, 6.7; Carbohydrate, 33.0*; L-carnitine, 0.036; Taurine, 0.036; Water, 197. Calories per mL, 1.0; Calories per fl oz, 29.6.

*Includes 3.9 g oat fiber and soy fiber (sources of dietary fiber that provide 2 Calories and 3.4 g total dietary fiber).

(FAN 7018-01)

PULMOCARE®   OTC
[pul'mō-kār]
Specialized Nutrition for Pulmonary Patients

USAGE

For the dietary management of respiratory insufficiency, the high-fat and low-carbohydrate content of Pulmocare is designed to reduce carbon dioxide production, respiratory quotient and ventilatory requirements. It has a unique fat blend with n-3 fatty acids and MCT oil and is fortified with the antioxidants vitamin E and beta-carotene (imparts color) and with carnitine and taurine. Pulmocare can be used for enteral tube feeding or oral supplementation and is appropriate for ambulatory or ventilator-dependent patients.
Not for parenteral use.

AVAILABILITY

8-fl-oz cans; 24 per case; Vanilla, No. 699; Strawberry, No. 50180.
1-liter Ross Ready-To-Hang® Enteral Feeding Containers; 8 per case; No. 51204.

COMPOSITION

Vanilla (Strawberry flavor has similar composition. For specific information, see product label.)

INGREDIENTS

Ⓤ-D Water, Sodium and Calcium Caseinates, Sugar (Sucrose), Canola Oil, Maltodextrin, Medium-Chain Triglycerides (Fractionated Coconut Oil), Corn Oil, High-Oleic Safflower Oil, Magnesium Chloride, Calcium Phosphate Tribasic, Soy Lecithin, Potassium Citrate, Natural and Artificial Flavors, Sodium Citrate, Potassium Phosphate Dibasic, Choline Chloride, Ascorbic Acid, Taurine, L-Carnitine, Sodium Chloride, Zinc Sulfate, d-Alpha-Tocopheryl Acetate, Ferrous Sulfate, Niacinamide, Carrageenan, Calcium Pantothenate, Beta-Carotene, Manganese Sulfate, Cupric Sulfate, Thiamine Chloride Hydrochloride, Vitamin A Palmitate, Pyridoxine Hydrochloride, Riboflavin, Folic Acid, Biotin, Sodium Molybate, Chromium Chloride, Potassium Iodide, Sodium Selenite, Phylloquinone, Cyanocobalamin and Vitamin D₃.

Nutrients (Grams/8 fl oz): Protein, 14.8; Fat, 22.1; Carbohydrate, 25.0; L-carnitine, 0.036; Taurine, 0.036; Water, 186. Calories per mL, 1.5; Calories per fl oz, 44.4.

(FAN 7017-05)

REHYDRALYTE®   OTC
[rē-hī'drə-līt"]
Oral Electrolyte Rehydration Solution

USAGE

To quickly restore fluid and minerals lost during moderate to severe diarrhea.

FEATURES

- Ready To Use—no mixing or dilution necessary.
- Safe, economical alternative to IV therapy.
- 75 mEq of sodium per liter for effective replacement of fluid deficits.
- 2½% Glucose solution to promote sodium and water absorption and provide energy.
- Available in pharmacies.

AVAILABILITY

8-fl-oz (237 mL) bottles; 4 six-packs per case; No. 00162.

DOSAGE

(See Administration Guide under Pedialyte®)

INGREDIENTS

(Pareve, Ⓤ) Water, Dextrose, Sodium Chloride, Potassium Citrate and Sodium Citrate.

Provides:	Per 8 Fl Oz	Per Liter
Sodium (mEq)	17.7	75
Potassium (mEq)	4.7	20
Chloride (mEq)	15.4	65
Citrate (mEq)	7.1	30
Dextrose (g)	5.9	25
Calories	24	100

(FAN 3333-01)

ROSS HOSPITAL FORMULA SYSTEM
Products for hospital nursery use

ALIMENTUM® (20 Cal/fl oz)
Protein Hydrolysate Formula With Iron
  Availability: Ready To Feed
    3.5-fl-oz (103 mL) glass bottles; 48 per case; No. 51516.

ISOMIL® 20 (20 Cal/fl oz)
Soy Formula With Iron
  Availability: Ready To Feed
    2-fl-oz (59 mL) plastic bottles; 48 per case; No. 51018.
    4-fl-oz (118 mL) glass bottles; 48 per case; No. 00406.

PEDIALYTE®
Oral Electrolyte Maintenance Solution
  Availability: Ready To Use
    4-fl-oz (118 mL) glass bottles; 48 per case; No. 51856.

SIMILAC® 20 (20 Cal/fl oz)
Low-Iron Infant Formula
  Availability: Ready To Feed
    2-fl-oz (59 mL) plastic bottles; 48 per case; No. 51008.
    4-fl-oz (118 mL) glass bottles; 48 per case; No. 00415.

SIMILAC® WITH IRON 20 (20 Cal/fl oz)
Infant Formula
  Availability: Ready To Feed
    2-fl-oz (59 mL) plastic bottles; 48 per case; No. 51014.
    4-fl-oz (118 mL) glass bottles; 48 per case; No. 00426.

SIMILAC® 24 (24 Cal/fl oz)
Low-Iron Infant Formula
  Availability: Ready To Feed
    2-fl-oz (59 mL) plastic bottles; 48 per case; No. 51010.
    4-fl-oz (118 mL) glass bottles; 48 per case; No. 00404.

SIMILAC® WITH IRON 24 (24 Cal/fl oz)
Infant Formula
  Availability: Ready To Feed
    2-fl-oz (59 mL) plastic bottles; 48 per case; No. 51016.
    4-fl-oz (118 mL) glass bottles; 48 per case; No. 00403.

SIMILAC® 27 (27 Cal/fl oz)
Low-Iron Infant Formula
  Availability: Ready To Feed
    2-fl-oz (59 mL) plastic bottles; 48 per case; No. 51012.
    4-fl-oz (118 mL) glass bottles; 48 per case; No. 00427.

SIMILAC NATURAL CARE® (24 Cal/fl oz)
Low-Iron Human Milk Fortifier
  Availability: Ready To Use
    4-fl-oz (118 mL) glass bottles; 48 per case; No. 00443.

SIMILAC NEOCARE® (22 Cal/fl oz)
Infant Formula With Iron
  Availability: Ready To Feed
    4-fl-oz (118 mL) glass bottles; 48 per case; No. 51848.

SIMILAC® PM 60/40 (20 Cal/fl oz)
Low-Iron Infant Formula
  Availability: Ready To Feed
    4-fl-oz (118 mL) glass bottles; 48 per case; No. 00424.

SIMILAC® SPECIAL CARE® 20 (20 Cal/fl oz)
Low-Iron Premature Infant Formula
  Availability: Ready To Feed
    2-fl-oz (59 mL) plastic bottles; 48 per case; No. 51020.
    4-fl-oz (118 mL) glass bottles; 48 per case; No. 00439.

SIMILAC® SPECIAL CARE® WITH IRON 20 (20 Cal/fl oz)
Premature Infant Formula
  Availability: Ready To Feed
    2-fl-oz (59 mL) plastic bottles; 48 per case; No. 52418.
    4-fl-oz (118 mL) glass bottles; 48 per case; No. 50588.

SIMILAC® SPECIAL CARE® 24 (24 Cal/fl oz)
Low-Iron Premature Infant Formula
  Availability: Ready To Feed
    2-fl-oz (59 mL) plastic bottles; 48 per case; No. 51022.
    4-fl-oz (118 mL) glass bottles; 48 per case; No. 00433.

SIMILAC® SPECIAL CARE® WITH IRON 24 (24 Cal/fl oz)
Premature Infant Formula
  Availability: Ready To Feed
    2-fl-oz (59 mL) plastic bottles; 48 per case; No. 51024.
    4-fl-oz (118 mL) glass bottles; 48 per case; No. 00478.

STERILIZED WATER
For Oral Use Only
  Availability: Ready To Feed
    2-fl-oz (59 mL) plastic bottles; 48 per case; No. 51000.
    4-fl-oz (118 mL) glass bottles; 48 per case; No. 00432.

SIMILAC® 5% GLUCOSE WATER
For Oral Use Only
  Availability: Ready To Feed
    2-fl-oz (59 mL) plastic bottles; 48 per case; No. 51002.
    4-fl-oz (118 mL) glass bottles; 48 per case; No. 00405.

SIMILAC® 10% GLUCOSE WATER
For Oral Use Only
  Availability: Ready To Feed
    2-fl-oz (59 mL) plastic bottles; 48 per case; No. 51004.
    4-fl-oz (118 mL) glass bottles; 48 per case; No. 00410.

ROSS METABOLIC FORMULA SYSTEM

CALCILO XD®
Low-Calcium/Vitamin D-Free Infant Formula With Iron
USAGE:
For use in the nutrition support of infants with hypercalcemia, as may occur in infants with Williams syndrome, or in management of infants with osteopetrosis and when a low-calcium/vitamin D-free formula is needed.
Powder: 14.1-oz (400-g) cans; measuring scoop enclosed; 6 per case; No. 00378.

CYCLINEX®-1
Amino Acid-Modified Medical Food With Iron
USAGE:
When a nonessential amino acid-free medical food is needed for nutrition support of infants and toddlers with a defect in a urea cycle enzyme or with gyrate atrophy of the choroid and retina.
Powder: 12.3-oz (350-g) cans; 6 per case; No. 51144.

CYCLINEX®-2
Amino Acid-Modified Medical Food
USAGE:
When a nonessential amino acid-free medical food is needed for nutrition support of children and adults with a defect in a urea cycle enzyme or with gyrate atrophy of the choroid and retina.
Powder: 11.4-oz (325-g) cans; 6 per case; No. 51146.

FLAVONEX® Flavored Energy Supplement
USAGE:
With amino acid-modified medical foods for children and adults.
Powder: Red Punch, 21.1-oz (600-g) cans; 6 per case; No. 51530. Grapefruit, 21.1-oz (600-g) cans; 6 per case; No. 51280.

GLUTAREX®-1
Amino Acid-Modified Medical Food With Iron
USAGE:
When a lysine- and tryptophan-free medical food is needed for nutrition support of infants and toddlers with glutaric aciduria type I.
Powder: 12.3-oz (350-g) cans; 6 per case; No. 51140.

GLUTAREX®-2
Amino Acid-Modified Medical Food
USAGE:
When a lysine- and tryptophan-free medical food is needed for nutrition support of children and adults with glutaric aciduria type I.
Powder: 11.4-oz (325-g) cans; 6 per case; No. 51142.

HOMINEX®-1
Amino Acid-Modified Medical Food With Iron
USAGE:
When a methionine-free medical food is needed for nutrition support of infants and toddlers with vitamin B₆-nonresponsive homocystinuria or hypermethioninemia.
Powder: 12.3-oz (350-g) cans; 6 per case; No. 51116.

HOMINEX®-2
Amino Acid-Modified Medical Food
USAGE:
When a methionine-free medical food is needed for nutrition support of children and adults with vitamin B₆-nonresponsive homocystinuria or hypermethioninemia.
Powder: 11.4-oz (325-g) cans; 6 per case; No. 51118.

I-VALEX®-1
Amino Acid-Modified Medical Food With Iron
USAGE:
When a leucine-free medical food is needed for nutrition support of infants and toddlers with isovaleric acidemia or other disorders of leucine catabolism.
Powder: 12.3-oz (350-g) cans; 6 per case; No. 51136.

I-VALEX®-2
Amino Acid-Modified Medical Food
USAGE:
When a leucine-free medical food is needed for nutrition support of children and adults with isovaleric acidemia or other disorders of leucine catabolism.
Powder: 11.4-oz (325-g) cans; 6 per case; No. 51138.

KETONEX®-1
Amino Acid-Modified Medical Food With Iron
USAGE:
When a branched-chain amino acid-free medical food is needed for nutrition support of infants and toddlers with branched-chain ketoaciduria (maple syrup urine disease—MSUD).
Powder: 12.3-oz (350-g) cans; 6 per case; No. 51112.

KETONEX®-2
Amino Acid-Modified Medical Food
USAGE:
When a branched-chain amino acid-free medical food is needed for nutrition support of children and adults with branched-chain ketoaciduria (maple syrup urine disease—MSUD).
Powder: 11.4-oz (325-g) cans; 6 per case; No. 51114.

PHENEX™-1
Amino Acid-Modified Medical Food With Iron
USAGE:
When a phenylalanine-free medical food is needed for nutrition support of infants and toddlers with phenylketonuria (PKU) or hyperphenylalaninemia.
Powder: 12.3-oz (350-g) cans; 6 per case; No. 51120.

PHENEX™-2
Amino Acid-Modified Medical Food
USAGE:
When a phenylalanine-free medical food is needed for nutrition support of children and adults with phenylketonuria (PKU) or hyperphenylalaninemia.
Powder: 11.4-oz (325-g) cans; 6 per case; No. 51122.

PRO-PHREE®
Protein-Free Energy Module With Iron, Vitamins & Minerals
USAGE:
When a protein-free medical food is indicated for nutrition support of infants and toddlers requiring reduced protein intake, specific mixture of L-amino acids or increased energy, minerals and vitamins.
Powder: 12.3-oz (350-g) cans; 6 per case; No. 51148.

PROPIMEX®-1
Amino Acid-Modified Medical Food With Iron
USAGE:
When a methionine- and valine-free, low-isoleucine and low-threonine medical food is needed for nutrition support of infants and toddlers with propionic or methylmalonic acidemia.
Powder: 12.3-oz (350-g) cans; 6 per case; No. 51132.

PROPIMEX®-2
Amino Acid-Modified Medical Food
USAGE:
When a methionine- and valine-free, low-isoleucine and low-threonine medical food is needed for nutrition support of children and adults with propionic or methylmalonic acidemia.
Powder: 11.4-oz (325-g) cans; 6 per case; No. 51134.

PROVIMIN®
Protein-Vitamin-Mineral
Formula Component With Iron
USAGE:
For use as the protein base in the preparation of liquid diets for feeding infants and children with chronic diarrhea and other malabsorptive disorders that require restriction of fat and carbohydrate intake.
Powder: 5.3-oz (150-g) cans; 6 per case; No. 50260.

RCF®
Ross Carbohydrate Free
Soy Formula Base With Iron
USAGE:
For use in the dietary management of persons unable to tolerate the type or amount of carbohydrate in milk or conventional infant formulas; many of these patients have intractable diarrhea and are not able to tolerate other formulas. This product has been formulated to contain no carbohydrate, which must be added before feeding.
Concentrated Liquid: 13-fl-oz (384-mL) cans; 12 per case; No. 00108.

SIMILAC® PM 60/40
[sim 'e-lak]
Low-Iron Infant Formula
USAGE:
For infants in the lower range of homeostatic capacity; those who are predisposed to hypocalcemia; and those whose renal, digestive or cardiovascular functions would benefit from lowered mineral levels.
Powder: 1-lb (454-g) cans, measuring scoop enclosed; 6 per case; No. 00850.
For hospital use, Ready To Feed Similac PM 60/40 in disposable nursing bottles is available in the Ross Hospital Formula System. (Ready To Feed has similar composition and nutrient values as Powder. For specific information see bottle tray.)

TYROMEX®-1
Amino Acid-Modified Medical Food With Iron
USAGE:
When a phenylalanine-, tyrosine- and methionine-free medical food is needed for nutrition support of infants and toddlers with tyrosinemia type I.
Powder: 12.3-oz (350-g) cans; 6 per case; No. 51128.

TYREX®-2
Amino Acid-Modified Medical Food
USAGE:
When a phenylalanine- and tyrosine-free medical food is needed for nutrition support of children and adults with tyrosinemia type II.
Powder: 11.4-oz (325-g) cans; 6 per case; No. 51126.

SELSUN® Rx ℞
[sel 'sun]
(2.5% selenium sulfide lotion, USP)

DESCRIPTION
A liquid antiseborrheic, antifungal preparation for topical application. Contains: Selenium sulfide 2 ½% w/v in aqueous suspension; also contains: bentonite, lauric diethanolamide, ethylene glycol monostearate, titanium dioxide, amphoteric-2, sodium lauryl sulfate, sodium phosphate (monobasic), glyceryl monoricinoleate, citric acid, captan and perfume.

CLINICAL PHARMACOLOGY
Selenium sulfide appears to have a cytostatic effect on cells of the epidermis and follicular epithelium, reducing corneocyte production.

INDICATIONS AND USAGE
Treatment of tinea versicolor, seborrheic dermatitis of scalp and treatment of dandruff.

CONTRAINDICATIONS
Not to be used by patients allergic to ingredients.

PRECAUTIONS
General: Not to be used when inflammation or exudation is present as increased absorption may occur.
Information for Patients: See Warnings and Precautions section under Application Instructions.
Carcinogenesis: Dermal application of 25% and 50% solutions of 2.5% selenium sulfide lotion on mice over an 88 week period, indicated no carcinogenic effects.
Pregnancy: WHEN USED FOR THE TREATMENT OF TINEA VERSICOLOR, SELSUN IS CLASSIFIED AS PREGNANCY CATEGORY C. Animal reproduction studies have not been conducted with SELSUN. It is also not known whether SELSUN can cause fetal harm when applied to body surfaces of a pregnant woman or can affect reproduction capacity. Under ordinary circumstances SELSUN should not be used for the treatment of tinea versicolor in pregnant women.
Pediatric Use: Safety and effectiveness in infants have not been established.

ADVERSE REACTIONS
In decreasing order of severity: skin irritation; occasional reports of increase in normal hair loss; discoloration of hair (can be avoided or minimized by thorough rinsing of hair

after treatment). As with other shampoos, oiliness or dryness of hair and scalp may occur.

OVERDOSAGE
Accidental Oral Ingestion:
No documented reports of serious toxicity in humans resulting from acute ingestion of SELSUN, however, acute toxicity studies in animals suggest that ingestion of large amounts could result in potential human toxicity. Evacuation of the stomach contents should be considered in cases of acute oral ingestion.

DOSAGE AND ADMINISTRATION
See application instructions.
Treatment of tinea versicolor: Apply to affected areas and lather with a small amount of water. Allow product to remain on skin for 10 minutes, then rinse thoroughly. Repeat procedure once a day for 7 days.
Treatment of seborrheic dermatitis and dandruff: Usually two applications each week for two weeks will afford control. After this, may be used at less frequent intervals —weekly, every two weeks, or every 3 or 4 weeks in some cases. Should not be applied more frequently than required to maintain control.
APPLICATION INSTRUCTIONS: Keep tightly capped.
Shake well before using. Product may damage jewelry; remove jewelry before use.
For treatment of tinea versicolor:
1. Apply to affected areas and lather with a small amount of water.
2. Allow to remain on skin for 10 minutes.
3. Rinse body thoroughly.
4. Repeat this procedure once a day for 7 days.
For treatment of dandruff and seborrheic dermatitis of the scalp:
1. Massage about 1 or 2 teaspoonfuls of shampoo into wet scalp.
2. Allow to remain on scalp for 2 to 3 minutes.
3. Rinse scalp thoroughly.
4. Repeat application and rinse thoroughly.
5. After treatment, wash hands well.
6. Repeat treatments as directed by physician.
WARNINGS AND PRECAUTIONS:
For External Use Only. Do not use on broken skin or inflamed areas. If allergic reactions occur, discontinue use. Avoid getting shampoo in eyes or in contact with genital area and skin folds as it may cause irritation and burning. These areas should be thoroughly rinsed after application. Keep this and all medicines out of reach of children.
Store below 86°F (30°C).

HOW SUPPLIED
4-fl-oz bottles (NDC 0074-2660-04).
(.2960)

SELSUN BLUE® OTC
[sel 'sun]
Dandruff Shampoo
(selenium sulfide lotion, 1%)

(See PDR For Nonprescription Drugs)

SIMILAC® OTC
[sim 'e-lak]
Low-Iron Infant Formula
● **Powder**
● **Concentrated Liquid**
● **Ready To Feed**

For most current information, refer to product labels.

SIMILAC NEOCARE® OTC
[sim 'e-lak nēo 'ka(ə)r]
Infant Formula With Iron
● **Powder**

For most current information, refer to product labels.

SIMILAC® SPECIAL CARE® OTC
WITH IRON 24
Premature Infant Formula
● **Ready To Feed**

For most current information, refer to product labels.

Continued on next page

Ross Laboratories—Cont.

SIMILAC® WITH IRON   OTC
[sim 'e-lak]
Infant Formula
- **Powder**
- **Concentrated Liquid**
- **Ready To Feed**

For most current information, refer to product labels.

SUPLENA®   OTC
[suh-plĕn 'ah]
Specialized Liquid Nutrition
for patients requiring protein, electrolyte
and fluid restrictions

USAGE
For patients requiring protein, electrolyte and fluid restrictions. Suplena is a high-calorie, low-protein, low-electrolyte liquid food. In the dietary management of patients prone to uremia, Suplena helps maintain nutritional status while minimizing accumulation of nitrogenous wastes, fluid and electrolytes. Suplena may be fed orally or by tube. It can be used as a supplement to the prescribed diet or as the sole source of nutrition under medical supervision.
Not for parenteral use.

AVAILABILITY
Ready To Use:
8-fl-oz cans; 24 per case; Vanilla, No. 50164.

COMPOSITION
INGREDIENTS
Ⓓ-D Water, Maltodextrin, Hi-Oleic Safflower Oil, Sodium and Calcium Caseinates, Sugar (Sucrose), Soy Oil, Soy Lecithin, Natural and Artificial Flavors, Calcium Carbonate, Potassium Citrate, Magnesium Phosphate Dibasic, Calcium Phosphate Tribasic, Choline Chloride, Sodium Chloride, Ascorbic Acid, Taurine, L-Carnitine, Potassium Chloride, Carrageenan, Zinc Sulfate, Alpha-Tocopheryl Acetate, Ferrous Sulfate, Niacinamide, Calcium Pantothenate, Manganese Sulfate, Pyridoxine Hydrochloride, Cupric Sulfate, Thiamine Chloride Hydrochloride, Riboflavin, Folic Acid, Vitamin A Palmitate, Biotin, Potassium Iodide, Sodium Selenite, Phylloquinone, Cyanocobalamin and Vitamin D₃.
Nutrients (Grams/8 fl oz): Protein, 7.1; Fat, 22.7; Carbohydrate, 60.6; L-carnitine, 0.038; Taurine, 0.038; Water, 169. Calories per mL, 2.0; Calories per fl oz, 59.4.
(FAN 3079-03)

SURVANTA®   ℞
beractant
intratracheal suspension

Sterile Suspension
For Intratracheal Use Only

DESCRIPTION
SURVANTA® (beractant) Intratracheal Suspension is a sterile, non-pyrogenic pulmonary surfactant intended for intratracheal use only. It is a natural bovine lung extract containing phospholipids, neutral lipids, fatty acids, and surfactant-associated proteins to which colfosceril palmitate (dipalmitoylphosphatidylcholine), palmitic acid, and tripalmitin are added to standardize the composition and to mimic surface-tension lowering properties of natural lung surfactant. The resulting composition provides 25 mg/mL phospholipids (including 11.0-15.5 mg/mL disaturated phosphatidylcholine), 0.5-1.75 mg/mL triglycerides, 1.4-3.5 mg/mL free fatty acids, and less than 1.0 mg/mL protein. It is suspended in 0.9% sodium chloride solution, and heat-sterilized. SURVANTA contains no preservatives. Its protein content consists of two hydrophobic, low molecular weight, surfactant-associated proteins commonly known as SP-B and SP-C. It does not contain the hydrophilic, large molecular weight surfactant-associated protein known as SP-A.
Each mL of SURVANTA contains 25 mg of phospholipids. It is an off-white to light brown liquid supplied in single-use glass vials containing 8 mL (200 mg phospholipids).

CLINICAL PHARMACOLOGY
Endogenous pulmonary surfactant lowers surface tension on alveolar surfaces during respiration and stabilizes the alveoli against collapse at resting transpulmonary pressures. Deficiency of pulmonary surfactant causes Respiratory Distress Syndrome (RDS) in premature infants. SURVANTA replenishes surfactant and restores surface activity to the lungs of these infants.
Activity
In vitro, SURVANTA reproducibly lowers minimum surface tension to less than 8 dynes/cm as measured by the pulsating bubble surfactometer and Wilhelmy Surface Balance. *In situ*, SURVANTA restores pulmonary compliance to excised rat lungs artificially made surfactant-deficient. *In vivo*, single SURVANTA doses improve lung pressure-volume measurements, lung compliance, and oxygenation in premature rabbits and sheep.
Animal Metabolism
SURVANTA is administered directly to the target organ, the lungs, where biophysical effects occur at the alveolar surface. In surfactant-deficient premature rabbits and lambs, alveolar clearance of radio-labelled lipid components of SURVANTA is rapid. Most of the dose becomes lung-associated within hours of administration, and the lipids enter endogenous surfactant pathways of reutilization and recycling. In surfactant-sufficient adult animals, SURVANTA clearance is more rapid than in premature and young animals. There is less reutilization and recycling of surfactant in adult animals.
Limited animal experiments have not found effects of SURVANTA on endogenous surfactant metabolism. Precursor incorporation and subsequent secretion of saturated phosphatidylcholine in premature sheep are not changed by SURVANTA treatments.
No information is available about the metabolic fate of the surfactant-associated proteins in SURVANTA. The metabolic disposition in humans has not been studied.
Clinical Studies
Clinical effects of SURVANTA were demonstrated in six single-dose and four multiple-dose randomized, multicenter, controlled clinical trials involving approximately 1700 infants. Three open trials, including a Treatment IND, involved more than 8500 infants. Each dose of SURVANTA in all studies was 100 mg phospholipids/kg birth weight and was based on published experience with Surfactant TA, a lyophilized powder dosage form of SURVANTA having the same composition.
Prevention Studies
Infants of 600-1250 g birth weight and 23 to 29 weeks estimated gestational age were enrolled in two *multiple-dose* studies. A dose of SURVANTA was given within 15 minutes of birth to prevent the development of RDS. Up to three additional doses in the first 48 hours, as often as every 6 hours, were given if RDS subsequently developed and infants required mechanical ventilation with an FiO₂ ≥ 0.30. Results of the studies at 28 days of age are shown in Table 1.

TABLE 1

Study 1

	SURVANTA	Control	P-Value
Number infants studied	119	124	
Incidence of RDS (%)	27.6	63.5	< 0.001
Death due to RDS (%)	2.5	19.5	< 0.001
Death or BPD due to RDS (%)	48.7	52.8	0.536
Death due to any cause (%)	7.6	22.8	0.001
Air Leaks[a] (%)	5.9	21.7	0.001
Pulmonary interstitial emphysema (%)	20.8	40.0	0.001

Study 2[b]

	SURVANTA	Control	P-Value
Number infants studied	91	96	
Incidence of RDS (%)	28.6	48.3	0.007
Death due to RDS (%)	1.1	10.5	0.006
Death or BPD due to RDS (%)	27.5	44.2	0.018
Death due to any cause[c] (%)	16.5	13.7	0.633
Air Leaks[a] (%)	14.5	19.6	0.374
Pulmonary interstitial emphysema (%)	26.5	33.2	0.298

[a] Pneumothorax or pneumopericardium
[b] Study discontinued when Treatment IND initiated
[c] No cause of death in the SURVANTA group was significantly increased; the higher number of deaths in this group was due to the sum of all causes.

Rescue Studies
Infants of 600-1750 g birth weight with RDS requiring mechanical ventilation and an FiO₂ ≥ 0.40 were enrolled in two *multiple-dose* rescue studies. The initial dose of SURVANTA was given after RDS developed and before 8 hours of age. Infants could receive up to three additional doses in the first 48 hours, as often as every 6 hours, if they required mechanical ventilation and an FiO₂ ≥ 0.30. Results of the studies at 28 days of age are shown in Table 2.

TABLE 2

Study 3[a]

	SURVANTA	Control	P-Value
Number infants studied	198	193	
Death due to RDS (%)	11.6	18.1	0.071
Death or BPD due to RDS (%)	59.1	66.8	0.102
Death due to any cause (%)	21.7	26.4	0.285
Air Leaks[b] (%)	11.8	29.5	< 0.001
Pulmonary interstitial emphysema (%)	16.3	34.0	< 0.001

Study 4

	SURVANTA	Control	P-Value
Number infants studied	204	203	
Death due to RDS (%)	6.4	22.3	< 0.001
Death or BPD due to RDS (%)	43.6	63.4	< 0.001
Death due to any cause (%)	15.2	28.2	0.001
Air Leaks[b] (%)	11.2	22.2	0.005
Pulmonary interstitial emphysema (%)	20.8	44.4	< 0.001

[a] Study discontinued when Treatment IND initiated
[b] Pneumothorax or pneumopericardium

Acute Clinical Effects
Marked improvements in oxygenation may occur within minutes of administration of SURVANTA.
All controlled clinical studies with SURVANTA provided information regarding the acute effects of SURVANTA on the arterial-alveolar oxygen ratio (a/APO₂), FiO₂, and mean airway pressure (MAP) during the first 48 to 72 hours of life. Significant improvements in these variables were sustained for 48-72 hours in SURVANTA-treated infants in four single-dose and two multiple-dose rescue studies and in two multiple-dose prevention studies. In the single-dose prevention studies, FiO₂ improved significantly.

INDICATIONS AND USAGE
SURVANTA is indicated for prevention and treatment ("rescue") of Respiratory Distress Syndrome (RDS) (hyaline membrane disease) in premature infants. SURVANTA significantly reduces the incidence of RDS, mortality due to RDS and air leak complications.
Prevention
In premature infants less than 1250 g birth weight or with evidence of surfactant deficiency, give SURVANTA as soon as possible, preferably within 15 minutes of birth.
Rescue
To treat infants with RDS confirmed by x-ray and requiring mechanical ventilation, give SURVANTA as soon as possible, preferably by 8 hours of age.

CONTRAINDICATIONS
None known.

WARNINGS
SURVANTA is intended for intratracheal use only.
SURVANTA CAN RAPIDLY AFFECT OXYGENATION AND LUNG COMPLIANCE. Therefore, its use should be restricted to a highly supervised clinical setting with immediate availability of clinicians experienced with intubation, ventilator management, and general care of premature infants. Infants receiving SURVANTA should be frequently monitored with arterial or transcutaneous measurement of systemic oxygen and carbon dioxide.
DURING THE DOSING PROCEDURE, TRANSIENT EPISODES OF BRADYCARDIA AND DECREASED OXYGEN SATURATION HAVE BEEN REPORTED. If these occur, stop the dosing procedure and initiate appropriate measures to alleviate the condition. After stabilization, resume the dosing procedure.

PRECAUTIONS
General
Rales and moist breath sounds can occur transiently after administration. Endotracheal suctioning or other remedial action is not necessary unless clear-cut signs of airway obstruction are present.
Increased probability of post-treatment nosocomial sepsis in SURVANTA-treated infants was observed in the controlled clinical trials (Table 3). The increased risk for sepsis among SURVANTA-treated infants was not associated with increased mortality among these infants. The causative organisms were similar in treated and control infants. There was no significant difference between groups in the rate of post-treatment infections other than sepsis.
Use of SURVANTA in infants less than 600 g birth weight or greater than 1750 g birth weight has not been evaluated in controlled trials. There is no controlled experience with use of SURVANTA in conjunction with experimental therapies for RDS (eg, high-frequency ventilation or extracorporeal membrane oxygenation).
No information is available on the effects of doses other than 100 mg phospholipids/kg, more than four doses, dosing more frequently than every 6 hours, or administration after 48 hours of age.

Carcinogenesis, Mutagenesis, Impairment of Fertility
Carcinogenicity studies have not been performed with SURVANTA. SURVANTA was negative when tested in the Ames test for mutagenicity. Using the maximum feasible dose volume, SURVANTA up to 500 mg phospholipids/kg/day (approximately one-third the premature infant dose based on mg/m^2/day) was administered subcutaneously to newborn rats for 5 days. The rats reproduced normally and there were no observable adverse effects in their offspring.

ADVERSE REACTIONS

The most commonly reported adverse experiences were associated with the dosing procedure. In the multiple-dose controlled clinical trials, each dose of SURVANTA was divided into four quarter-doses which were instilled through a catheter inserted into the endotracheal tube by briefly disconnecting the endotracheal tube from the ventilator. Transient bradycardia occurred with 11.9% of *doses*. Oxygen desaturation occurred with 9.8% of *doses*.

Other reactions during the dosing procedure occurred with fewer than 1% of doses and included endotracheal tube reflux, pallor, vasoconstriction, hypotension, endotracheal tube blockage, hypertension, hypocarbia, hypercarbia, and apnea. No deaths occurred during the dosing procedure, and all reactions resolved with symptomatic treatment.

The occurrence of concurrent illnesses common in premature infants was evaluated in the controlled trials. The rates in all controlled studies are in Table 3.

TABLE 3

	All Controlled Studies		
Concurrent Event	SURVANTA (%)	Control (%)	*P*-Value[a]
Patent ductus arteriosus	46.9	47.1	0.814
Intracranial hemorrhage	48.1	45.2	0.241
Severe intracranial hemorrhage	24.1	23.3	0.693
Pulmonary air leaks	10.9	24.7	<0.001
Pulmonary interstitial emphysema	20.2	38.4	<0.001
Necrotizing enterocolitis	6.1	5.3	0.427
Apnea	65.4	59.6	0.283
Severe apnea	46.1	42.5	0.114
Post-treatment sepsis	20.7	16.1	0.019
Post-treatment infection	10.2	9.1	0.345
Pulmonary hemorrhage	7.2	5.3	0.166

[a] *P*-value comparing groups in controlled studies

When all controlled studies were pooled, there was no difference in intracranial hemorrhage. However, in one of the single-dose rescue studies and one of the multiple-dose prevention studies, the rate of intracranial hemorrhage was significantly higher in SURVANTA patients than control patients (63.3% *v* 30.8%, *P*=0.001; and 48.8% *v* 34.2%, *P*=0.047, respectively). The rate in a Treatment IND involving approximately 8100 infants was lower than in the controlled trials.

In the controlled clinical trials, there was no effect of SURVANTA on results of common laboratory tests: white blood cell count and serum sodium, potassium, bilirubin, creatinine.

More than 4300 pretreatment and posttreatment serum samples from approximately 1500 patients were tested by Western Blot Immunoassay for antibodies to surfactant-associated proteins SP-B and SP-C. No IgG or or IgM antibodies were detected.

Several other complications are known to occur in premature infants. The following conditions were reported in the controlled clinical studies. The rates of the complications were not different in treated and control infants, and none of the complications were attributed to SURVANTA.

Respiratory: lung consolidation, blood from the endotracheal tube, deterioration after weaning, respiratory decompensation, subglottic stenosis, paralyzed diaphragm, respiratory failure.

Cardiovascular: hypotension, hypertension, tachycardia, ventricular tachycardia, aortic thrombosis, cardiac failure, cardio-respiratory arrest, increased apical pulse, persistent fetal circulation, air embolism, total anomalous pulmonary venous return.

Gastrointestinal: abdominal distention, hemorrhage, intestinal perforations, volvulus, bowel infarct, feeding intolerance, hepatic failure, stress ulcer.

Renal: renal failure, hematuria.

Hematologic: coagulopathy, thrombocytopenia, disseminated intravascular coagulation.

Central Nervous System: seizures.

Endocrine/Metabolic: adrenal hemorrhage, inappropriate ADH secretion, hyperphosphatemia.

Musculoskeletal: inguinal hernia.

Systemic: fever, deterioration.

Follow-Up Evaluations
To date, no long-term complications or sequelae of SURVANTA therapy have been found.

Single-Dose Studies
Six-month adjusted-age follow-up evaluations of 232 infants (115 treated) demonstrated no clinically important differences between treatment groups in pulmonary and neurologic sequelae, incidence or severity of retinopathy of prematurity, rehospitalizations, growth, or allergic manifestations.

Multiple-Dose Studies
Six-month adjusted age follow-up evaluations have been completed in 631 (345 treated) of 916 surviving infants. There were significantly less cerebral palsy and need for supplemental oxygen in SURVANTA infants than controls. Wheezing at the time of examination was significantly more frequent among SURVANTA infants, although there was no difference in bronchodilator therapy.

Final twelve-month follow-up data from the multiple-dose studies are available from 521 (272 treated) of 909 surviving infants. There was significantly less wheezing in SURVANTA infants than controls, in contrast to the six-month results. There was no difference in the incidence of cerebral palsy at twelve months.

Twenty-four month adjusted age evaluations were completed in 429 (226 treated) of 906 surviving infants. There were significantly fewer SURVANTA infants with rhonchi, wheezing, and tachypnea at the time of examination. No other differences were found.

OVERDOSAGE

Overdosage with SURVANTA has not been reported. Based on animal data, overdosage might result in acute airway obstruction. Treatment should be symptomatic and supportive.

Rales and moist breath sounds can transiently occur after SURVANTA is given, and do not indicate overdosage. Endotracheal suctioning or other remedial action is not required unless clear-cut signs of airway obstruction are present.

DOSAGE AND ADMINISTRATION

FOR INTRATRACHEAL ADMINISTRATION ONLY.

SURVANTA should be administered by or under the supervision of clinicians experienced in intubation, ventilator management, and general care of premature infants.

Marked improvements in oxygenation may occur within minutes of administration of SURVANTA. Therefore, frequent and careful clinical observation and monitoring of systemic oxygenation are essential to avoid hyperoxia.

Review of audiovisual instructional materials describing dosage and administration procedures is recommended before using SURVANTA. Materials are available upon request from Ross Products Division.

Dosage
Each dose of SURVANTA is 100 mg of phospholipids/kg birth weight (4 mL/kg). The SURVANTA DOSING CHART shows the total dosage for a range of birth weights.

SURVANTA DOSING CHART

WEIGHT (grams)	TOTAL DOSE (mL)	WEIGHT (grams)	TOTAL DOSE (mL)
600- 650	2.6	1301-1350	5.4
651- 700	2.8	1351-1400	5.6
701- 750	3.0	1401-1450	5.8
751- 800	3.2	1451-1500	6.0
801- 850	3.4	1501-1550	6.2
851- 900	3.6	1551-1600	6.4
901- 950	3.8	1601-1650	6.6
951-1000	4.0	1651-1700	6.8
1001-1050	4.2	1701-1750	7.0
1051-1100	4.4	1751-1800	7.2
1101-1150	4.6	1801-1850	7.4
1151-1200	4.8	1851-1900	7.6
1201-1250	5.0	1901-1950	7.8
1251-1300	5.2	1951-2000	8.0

Four doses of SURVANTA can be administered in the first 48 hours of life. Doses should be given no more frequently than every 6 hours.

Directions for Use
SURVANTA should be inspected visually for discoloration prior to administration. The color of SURVANTA is off-white to light brown. If settling occurs during storage, swirl the vial gently (DO NOT SHAKE) to redisperse. Some foaming at the surface may occur during handling and is inherent in the nature of the product.

SURVANTA is stored refrigerated (2-8°C). Before administration, SURVANTA should be warmed by standing at room temperature for at least 20 minutes or warmed in the hand for at least 8 minutes. ARTIFICIAL WARMING METHODS SHOULD NOT BE USED. If a prevention dose is to be given, preparation of SURVANTA should begin before the infant's birth.

Unopened, unused vials of SURVANTA that have been warmed to room temperature may be returned to the refrigerator within 8 hours of warming, and stored for future use. Drug should not be warmed and returned to the refrigerator more than once. Each single-use vial of SURVANTA should be entered only once. Used vials with residual drug should be discarded.

SURVANTA DOES NOT REQUIRE RECONSTITUTION OR SONICATION BEFORE USE.

Dosing Procedures

General
SURVANTA is administered intratracheally by instillation through a 5 French end-hole catheter. The catheter can be inserted into the infant's endotracheal tube without interrupting ventilation by passing the catheter through a neonatal suction valve attached to the endotracheal tube. Alternatively, SURVANTA can be instilled through the catheter by briefly disconnecting the endotracheal tube from the ventilator.

The neonatal suction valve used for administering SURVANTA should be a type that allows entry of the catheter into the endotracheal tube without interrupting ventilation and also maintains a closed airway circuit system by sealing the valve around the catheter.

If the neonatal suction valve is used, the catheter should be rigid enough to pass easily into the endotracheal tube. A very soft and pliable catheter may twist or curl within the neonatal suction valve. The length of the catheter should be shortened so that the tip of the catheter protrudes just beyond the end of the endotracheal tube above the infant's carina. SURVANTA should not be instilled into a mainstem bronchus.

To ensure homogenous distribution of SURVANTA throughout the lungs, each dose is divided into *four quarter-doses*.

Each quarter-dose is administered with the infant in a different position. The recommended positions are:

- Head and body inclined 5–10° down, head turned to the right
- Head and body inclined 5–10° down, head turned to the left
- Head and body inclined 5–10° up, head turned to the right
- Head and body inclined 5–10° up, head turned to the left

The dosing procedure is facilitated if one person administers the dose while another person positions and monitors the infant.

First Dose
Determine the total dose of SURVANTA from the SURVANTA DOSING CHART based on the infant's birth weight. Slowly withdraw the entire contents of the vial into a plastic syringe through a large-gauge needle (eg, at least 20 gauge). DO NOT FILTER SURVANTA AND AVOID SHAKING.

Attach the premeasured 5 French end-hole catheter to the syringe. Fill the catheter with SURVANTA. Discard excess SURVANTA through the catheter so that only the total dose to be given remains in the syringe.

BEFORE ADMINISTERING SURVANTA, assure proper placement and patency of the endotracheal tube. At the discretion of the clinician, the endotracheal tube may be suctioned before administering SURVANTA. The infant should be allowed to stabilize before proceeding with dosing.

In the prevention strategy, weigh, intubate and stabilize the infant. Administer the dose as soon as possible after birth, preferably within 15 minutes. Position the infant appropriately and gently inject the first quarter-dose through the catheter over 2-3 seconds.

After administration of the first quarter-dose, remove the catheter from the endotracheal tube. Manually ventilate with a hand-bag with sufficient oxygen to prevent cyanosis, at a rate of 60 breaths/minute, and sufficient positive pressure to provide adequate air exchange and chest wall excursion.

In the rescue strategy, the first dose should be given as soon as possible after the infant is placed on a ventilator for management of RDS. In the clinical trials, immediately before instilling the first quarter-dose, the infant's ventilator settings were changed to rate 60/minute, inspiratory time 0.5 second, and FiO_2 1.0.

Position the infant appropriately and gently inject the first quarter-dose through the catheter over 2–3 seconds. After administration of the first quarter-dose, remove the catheter from the endotracheal tube and continue mechanical ventilation.

In both strategies, ventilate the infant for at least 30 seconds or until stable. Reposition the infant for instillation of the next quarter-dose.

Instill the remaining quarter-doses using the same procedures. After instillation of each quarter-dose, remove the catheter and ventilate for at least 30 seconds or until the infant is stabilized. After instillation of the final quarter-dose, remove the catheter without flushing it. Do not suction the infant for 1 hour after dosing unless signs of significant airway obstruction occur.

Continued on next page

Ross Laboratories—Cont.

AFTER COMPLETION OF THE DOSING PROCEDURE, RESUME USUAL VENTILATOR MANAGEMENT AND CLINICAL CARE.

Repeat Doses

The dosage of SURVANTA for repeat doses is also 100 mg phospholipids/kg and is based on the infant's birth weight. The infant should not be reweighed for determination of the SURVANTA dosage. Use the SURVANTA DOSING CHART to determine the total dosage.

The need for additional doses of SURVANTA is determined by evidence of continuing respiratory distress. Using the following criteria for redosing, significant reductions in mortality due to RDS were observed in the multiple-dose clinical trials with SURVANTA.

Dose no sooner than 6 hours after the preceding dose if the infant remains intubated and requires at least 30% inspired oxygen to maintain a PaO_2 less than or equal to 80 torr.

Radiographic confirmation of RDS should be obtained before administering additional doses to those who received a prevention dose.

Prepare SURVANTA and position the infant for administration of each quarter-dose as previously described. After instillation of each quarter-dose, remove the dosing catheter from the endotracheal tube and ventilate the infant for at least 30 seconds or until stable.

In the clinical studies, ventilator settings used to administer repeat doses were different than those used for the first dose. For repeat doses, the FiO_2 was increased by 0.20 or an amount sufficient to prevent cyanosis. The ventilator delivered a rate of 30/minute with an inspiratory time less than 1.0 second. If the infant's pretreatment rate was 30 or greater, it was left unchanged during SURVANTA instillation.

Manual hand-bag ventilation should not be used to administer repeat doses. DURING THE DOSING PROCEDURE, VENTILATOR SETTINGS MAY BE ADJUSTED AT THE DISCRETION OF THE CLINICIAN TO MAINTAIN APPROPRIATE OXYGENATION AND VENTILATION. AFTER COMPLETION OF THE DOSING PROCEDURE, RESUME USUAL VENTILATOR MANAGEMENT AND CLINICAL CARE.

Dosing Precautions

If an infant experiences bradycardia or oxygen desaturation during the dosing procedure, stop the dosing procedure and initiate appropriate measures to alleviate the condition. After the infant has stabilized, resume the dosing procedure. Rales and moist breath sounds can occur transiently after administration of SURVANTA. Endotracheal suctioning or other remedial action is unnecessary unless clear-cut signs of airway obstruction are present.

HOW SUPPLIED

SURVANTA (beractant) Intratracheal Suspension is supplied in single-use glass vials containing 8 mL of SURVANTA (NDC 0074-1040-08). Each milliliter contains 25 mg of phospholipids (200 mg phospholipids/8 mL) suspended in 0.9% sodium chloride solution. The color is off-white to light brown.

Store unopened vials at refrigeration temperature (2-8°C). Protect from light. Store vials in carton until ready for use. Vials are for single use only. Upon opening, discard unused drug.

April, 1995

TODDLER'S BEST™   OTC
[täd 'lərs best]
Nutritional Beverage With Iron

- Milk-Based
- For Toddlers Over 12 Months Old
- Ready To Use 8-fl-oz (237 mL) drink box
- Flavors: Vanilla and Chocolate
- Serve instead of milk or juice

For most current information, refer to product labels.

TODDLER'S BEST™   OTC
[täd ' lars best]
Lactose-Free Nutritional Beverage With Iron

- Soy-Based
- For Toddlers Over 12 Months Old
- Ready To Use 8-fl-oz (237 mL) drink box
- Vanilla Flavor
- Serve instead of milk or juice

For most current information, refer to product labels.

TRONOLANE®   OTC
[tron 'e-lān]
**Anesthetic Cream for Hemorrhoids
Hemorrhoidal Suppositories**

(See PDR For Nonprescription Drugs.)

PEDIAFLOR® Drops   ℞
Sodium Fluoride Oral Solution, USP
1.7 fl oz (50 mL) bottles, calibrated dropper

PRAMILET® FA   ℞
Prenatal Vitamin/Mineral Preparation with Folic Acid
100 Tablet Bottles

VI-DAYLIN® ADC VITAMINS Drops   OTC
Dietary Supplement of Vitamins A,D, and C
50 mL Spil-gard bottles, calibrated dropper

VI-DAYLIN® ADC VITAMINS + IRON Drops   OTC
Dietary Supplement of Vitamins A,D, and C with Iron
50 mL Spil-gard bottles, calibrated dropper

VI-DAYLIN® MULTIVITAMIN DROPS   OTC
Multivitamin Supplement
50 mL Spil-gard Bottles, calibrated dropper

VI-DAYLIN® MULTIVITAMIN + IRON Drops   OTC
Multivitamin/Iron Supplement
50 mL Spil-gard bottles, calibrated dropper

VI-DAYLIN®/F ADC VITAMINS   ℞
Drops With Fluoride
ADC Vitamins/Fluoride
50 mL Spil-gard bottles, calibrated dropper

VI-DAYLIN®/F ADC VITAMINS + IRON   ℞
Drops With Fluoride
ADC Vitamins/Fluoride/Iron Supplement
50 mL Spil-gard bottles, calibrated dropper

VI-DAYLIN®/F MULTIVITAMIN   ℞
Drops With Fluoride
Multivitamins/Fluoride
50 mL Spil-gard bottles, calibrated dropper

VI-DAYLIN®/F MULTIVITAMIN + IRON   ℞
Drops With Fluoride
Multivitamins/Fluoride/Iron Supplement
50 mL Spil-gard bottles, calibrated dropper

VI-DAYLIN® MULTIVITAMIN   OTC
Chewable Tablets
Multivitamin Supplement
100 tablet bottles

VI-DAYLIN® MULTIVITAMIN + IRON   OTC
Chewable Tablets
Multivitamin/Iron Supplement
100 tablet bottles

VI-DAYLIN®/F MULTIVITAMIN   ℞
Chewable Tablets With Fluoride
Multivitamins/Fluoride
100 tablet bottles

VI-DAYLIN®/F MULTIVITAMIN + IRON   ℞
Chewable Tablets With Fluoride
Multivitamins/Fluoride/Iron
100 tablet bottles

VI-DAYLIN® MULTIVITAMIN Liquid   OTC
Multivitamin Supplement
16-fl-oz (473 mL) bottles
8-fl-oz (237 mL) bottles

VI-DAYLIN® MULTIVITAMIN + IRON   OTC
Liquid
Multivitamin/Iron Supplement
16-fl-oz (473 mL) bottles
8-fl-oz (237 mL) bottles

VITAL® HIGH NITROGEN   OTC
[vi'tel]
**Nutritionally Complete
Partially Hydrolyzed Diet**

USAGE

As a source of total or supplemental nutrition for patients with limited digestion/absorption. VITAL HIGH NITROGEN may be used as a tube feeding (nasogastric, nasoduodenal or jejunal) or as an oral feeding. Five servings (1500 Calories) meet or exceed 100% of the RDI for vitamins and minerals.
Not for parenteral use.

AVAILABILITY

Powder: 2.79 oz (79 g) packets; 24 packets per case; Vanilla, No. 766.

COMPOSITION
INGREDIENTS

Hydrolyzed cornstarch, protein components (partially hydrolyzed whey, meat and soy), sucrose, safflower oil, medium-chain triglycerides (fractionated coconut oil), artificial and natural flavor, magnesium sulfate, calcium phosphate tribasic, potassium phosphate dibasic, L-tyrosine, magnesium chloride, L-leucine, L-valine, sodium chloride, L-isoleucine, L-phenylalanine, L-histidine, choline chloride, ascorbic acid, L-methionine, L-threonine, soy lecithin, mono- and diglycerides, L-tryptophan, zinc sulfate, ferrous sulfate, niacinamide, alpha-tocopheryl acetate, calcium pantothenate, manganese sulfate, thiamine chloride hydrochloride, cupric sulfate, pyridoxine hydrochloride, riboflavin, vitamin A palmitate, potassium citrate, folic acid, biotin, sodium molybdate, chromium chloride, potassium iodide, sodium selenite, phylloquinone, cyanocobalamin and vitamin D_3.

Nutrients: (grams)	Per 300 Calories* (1 packet)	Per 1500 Calories* (5 packets)
Protein	12.5	62.5
Fat	3.25	16.25
Carbohydrate	55.4	277
Water (Max)	5.2	26.0

* In standard dilution (79 g of Vital High Nitrogen Powder mixed in 255 mL of water).
(FAN 3075-04)

EDUCATIONAL MATERIAL

A complete program of educational services for health professionals and patients is available.
Contact your local Ross representative.

Roxane Laboratories, Inc.
**P.O. 16532
COLUMBUS, OH 43216-6532**

Direct Inquiries to:
Professional Services Department
P.O. 16532
Columbus, OH 43216-6532
(800) 848-0120
(614) 276-4000

HOSPITAL UNIT DOSE

Hospital Unit Dose—Roxane, was developed to aid in improved drug distribution and administration. With Hospital Unit Dose, each single unit of medication moves from our quality controlled production lines to the patient's bedside in tamper resistant containers, labeled for positive identification, thus protecting dosage integrity to the point of administration.

The following products are currently available in Hospital Unit Dose:

Acetaminophen Oral Solution USP (lime) 325mg/10.15mL, 650mg/20.3mL
Acetaminophen Oral Solution USP (cherry) 160mg/5mL, 325mg/10.15mL, 650mg/20.3mL
Acetaminophen Tablets USP 325mg, 500mg, 650mg
Acetaminophen 120mg and Codeine Phosphate 12mg Oral Solution USP
Acetaminophen 300mg and Codeine Phosphate 30mg Tablets USP
Acetylcysteine Solution USP 10% 4 mL, 20% 4mL
Alprazolam Tablets, USP 0.25mg, 0.5mg, 1mg
Aluminum Hydroxide Gel USP (Flavored) 2700mg/30mL
Aluminum Hydroxide, Concentrate, 2700mg/20mL, 4050mg/30mL
Alumina and Magnesia Oral Suspension USP 30 mL
Alumina, Magnesia, and Simethicone Oral Suspension USP I 15mL, 30mL
Aminophylline Tablets USP 100mg, 200mg
Aminophylline Oral Solution USP 210mg/10mL, 315mg/15mL
Aromatic Cascara Fluidextract USP 5mL
Aromatic Castor Oil USP 30mL, 60mL
Azathioprine Tablets, USP 50mg
Calcium Carbonate Tablets USP 1250mg
Calcium Carbonate Oral Suspension 1250mg/5mL
Calcium Gluconate Tablets USP 500mg
Castor Oil USP 30mL, 60mL
Cimetidine Tablets USP 300mg, 400mg, 800mg

Cocaine Hydrochloride Topical Solution 4%/4mL, 10%/4mL
Cocaine Hydrochloride Topical Solution (STERILE) 4%/mL, 10%/mL
Cocaine Hydrochloride Viscous Topical Solution 4%/4mL, 10%/4mL
Codeine Phosphate Oral Solution 15mg/5mL
Codeine Sulfate Tablets USP 15mg, 30mg, 60mg
Dexamethasone Oral Solution 0.5mg/5mL, 2mg/20mL
Dexamethasone Tablets USP 0.5mg, 0.75mg, 1mg, 1.5mg, 2mg, 4mg, 6mg
Diazepam Oral Solution 5 mg/5 mL, 10 mg/10 mL
Diclofenac Sodium Tablets 25mg, 50mg, 75mg
Diflunisal Tablets, USP 250mg, 500mg
Digoxin Elixir USP 0.125mg/2.5mL, 0.25mg/5mL
DHT (Dihydrotachysterol) Tablets USP 0.125mg, 0.2mg
Diluent (Flavored) for Oral Use 15mL
Diphenhydramine Hydrochloride Elixir USP 25mg/10mL
Diphenoxylate Hydrochloride and Atropine Sulfate Oral Solution USP 5mL, 10mL
Docusate Sodium Syrup USP 50mg/15mL, 100mg/30mL
Ferrous Sulfate Oral Solution USP 300mg/5mL
Ferrous Sulfate Tablets USP 300mg
Furosemide Oral Solution 40mg/5mL, 80mg/10mL
Furosemide Tablets USP 20mg, 40mg, 80mg
Guaifenesin Syrup USP 100mg/5mL, 200mg/10mL, 300mg/15mL
Haloperidol Tablets USP 0.5 mg, 1 mg, 2 mg, 5 mg, 10 mg and 20 mg
Hydromorphone Hydrochloride Tablets USP 2mg, 4mg
Hydroxyurea Capsules USP 500mg
Ipecac Syrup USP 15mL, 30mL
Isoetharine Inhalation Solution USP 0.1%, 2.5mL
Isoetharine Inhalation Solution USP 0.125%, 4mL
Isoetharine Inhalation Solution USP 0.167%, 3mL
Isoetharine Inhalation Solution USP 0.2%, 2.5mL
Isoetharine Inhalation Solution USP 0.25%, 2mL
Kaolin-Pectin Suspension 30mL
Lactulose Solution USP 10gm/15mL
Leucovorin Calcium Tablets 5mg. 10mg, 15mg, 25mg
Levorphanol Tartrate Tablets USP 2 mg
Lidocaine Viscous 2% 20mL
Lithium Carbonate Capsules USP 150mg, 300mg, 600mg
Lithium Carbonate Tablets USP 300mg
Lithium Citrate Syrup USP 8mEq per 5mL, 16mEq per 10mL
Loperamide Hydrochloride Capsules USP 2mg
Loperamide Hydrochloride Oral Solution 1mg/5mL, 2mg/10mL, 4mg/20mL
Methadone Hydrochloride Tablets USP 5mg, 10mg
Methotrexate Tablets USP, 2.5mg
Metoclopramide Oral Solution USP 10mg/10mL
Mexiletine Hydrochloride Capsules, USP 150mg, 200mg, 250mg
Milk of Magnesia USP 30mL
Milk of Magnesia Concentrated Flavored 10mL,
Milk of Magnesia—Cascara Suspension Concentrated 15mL
Milk of Magnesia—Mineral Oil Emulsion 30mL
Milk of Magnesia—Mineral Oil Emulsion (Flavored) 30mL
Mineral Oil, Topical Light, USP 10mL, 30mL
Mineral Oil USP 30mL
Morphine Sulfate Tablets 15mg, 30mg
Morphine Sulfate Oral Solution 10mg/5mL, 20mg/10mL
Naproxen Sodium Tablets USP 275mg, 550mg
Naproxen Tablets USP 250mg, 375mg, 500mg
Neomycin Sulfate Tablets USP 500mg
Nystatin Oral Suspension USP 100,000 USP units per mL 5mL
Oramoprh SR Tablets (Morphine sulfate sustained release tablets) 15mg, 30mg, 60mg, 100mg
Phenobarbital Elixir USP 20mg/5mL, 30mg/7.5mL
Phenobarbital Tablets USP 15mg, 30mg, 60mg, 100mg
Potassium Chloride Oral Solution USP 10% (15mEq/11.25mL), (20mEq/15mL), (30mEq/22.5mL), (40mEq/30mL)
Prednisone Oral Solution 5mg/5mL
Prednisone Tablets USP 1mg, 2.5mg, 5mg, 10mg, 20mg, 50mg
Propantheline Bromide Tablets USP 15mg
Propranolol Hydrochloride Oral Solution 20mg/5mL and 40mg/5 mL
Pseudoephedrine Hydrochloride Tablets USP 30mg, 60mg
Quinidine Sulfate Tablets USP 200mg, 300mg
Roxanol Suppositories 10mg, 20mg, 30mg
Roxicet Oral Solution (Oxycodone Hydrochloride 5mg and Acetaminophen 325mg/5mL)
Roxicet Tablets (Oxycodone and Acetaminophen Tablets USP 5mg/325mg)
Roxicet 5/500 Caplets (Oxycodone and Acetaminophen Tablets USP, 5mg/500mg)
Roxicodone Oral Solution (Oxycodone Hydrochloride Oral Solution USP 5mg/5mL)
Roxicodone Tablets (Oxycodone Tablets USP 5mg)
Roxiprin Tablets (Oxycodone Hydrochloride 4.5mg, Oxycodone Terephthalate 0.38mg, and Aspirin 325mg Tablets USP)
Saliva Substitute
Sodium Chloride Inhalation Solution USP (Normal Saline) Sterile 0.9% 3mL, 5mL
Sodium Polystyrene Sulfonate Suspension 60mL, and 120mL Enema Package, 200 mL Enema Package
Sulfamethoxazole and Trimethoprim Tablets USP (Regular Strength) 400mg Sulfamethoxazole and 80mg Trimethoprim, (Double Strength) 800mg Sulfamethoxazole and 160 mg Trimethoprim
Theophylline Oral Solution 80mg/15mL, 100mg/18.75mL, 160mg/30mL
Torecan Tablets (thiethylperazine maleate tablets USP) 10mg
Triazolam Tablets USP, 0.125mg, 0.25mg

As research continues, new Roxane Laboratories' products will be available in Hospital Unit Dose packages.

AZATHIOPRINE ℞
TABLETS USP 50 MG
COMPLETE PRESCRIBING INFORMATION

> **WARNING:** Chronic immunosuppression with this purine antimetabolite increases *risk of neoplasia* in humans. Physicians using this drug should be very familiar with this risk as well as with the mutagenic potential to both men and women and with possible hematologic toxicities. See **WARNINGS**.

DESCRIPTION
Azathioprine, an immunosuppressive antimetabolite, is available in tablet form for oral administration. Each scored tablet contains 50 mg azathioprine and the inactive ingredients anhydrous lactose, starch (corn), povidone, magnesium stearate and stearic acid.

Azathioprine is chemically 6-[(1-methyl-4-nitroimidazol-5-yl)thio]purine. The structural formula of azathioprine is:

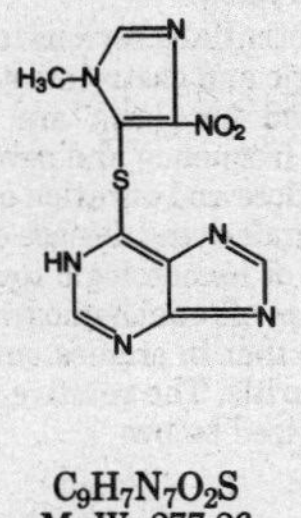

$C_9H_7N_7O_2S$
M. W. 277.26

It is an imidazolyl derivative of 6-mercaptopurine and many of its biological effects are similar to those of the parent compound.

Azathioprine is insoluble in water, but may be dissolved with addition of one molar equivalent of alkali. The sodium salt of azathioprine is sufficiently soluble to make a 10 mg/mL water solution which is stable for 24 hours of 59° to 77°F (15° to 25°C). Azathioprine is stable in solution at neutral or acid pH but hydrolysis to mercaptopurine occurs in excess sodium hydroxide (0.1N), especially on warming. Conversion to mercaptopurine also occurs in the presence of sulfhydryl compounds such as cysteine, glutathione and hydrogen sulfide.

CLINICAL PHARMACOLOGY AND ACTIONS
Metabolism[1]: Azathioprine is well absorbed following oral administration. Maximum serum radioactivity occurs at one to two hours after oral ^{35}S-azathioprine and decays with a half-life of five hours. This is not an estimate of the half-life of azathioprine itself but is the decay rate of all ^{35}S-containing metabolites of the drug. Because of extensive metabolism, only a fraction of the radioactivity is present as azathioprine. Usual doses produce blood levels of azathioprine, and of mercaptopurine derived from it, which are low (<1 μg/mL). Blood levels are of little predictive value for therapy since the magnitude and duration of clinical effects correlate with thiopurine nucleotide levels in tissues rather than with plasma drug levels. Azathioprine and mercaptopurine are moderately bound to serum proteins (30%) and are partially dialyzable.

Azathioprine is cleaved *in vito* to mercaptopurine. Both compounds are rapidly eliminated from blood and are oxidized or methylated in erythrocytes and liver; no azathioprine or mercaptopurine is detectable in urine after eight hours. Conversion to inactive 6-thiouric acid by xanthine oxidase is an important degradative pathway, and the inhibition of this pathway in patients receiving allopurinol is the basis for the azathioprine dosage reduction required in these patients (see **Drug Interactions** under **PRECAUTIONS**). Proportions of metabolites are different in individual patients, and this presumably accounts for variable magnitude and duration of drug effects. Renal clearance is probably not important in predicting biological effectiveness or toxicities, although dose reduction is practiced in patients with poor renal function.

Homograft Survival[1,2]: Summary information from transplant centers and registries indicates relatively universal use of azathioprine with or without other immunosuppressive agents.[3,4,5] Although the use of azathioprine for inhibition of renal homograft rejection is well established, the mechanism(s) for this action are somewhat obscure. The drug suppresses hypersensitivities of the cell-mediated type and causes variable alterations in antibody production. Suppression of T-cells effects, including ablation of T-cell suppression is dependent on the temporal relationship to antigenic stimulus or engraftment. This agent has little effect on established graft rejections or secondary responses.

Alterations in specific immune responses or immunologic functions in transplant recipients are difficult to relate specifically to immunosuppression by azathioprine. These patients have subnormal responses to vaccines, low numbers of T-cells, and abnormal phagocytosis by peripheral blood cells, but their mitogenic responses, serum immunoglobulins and secondary antibody responses are usually normal.

Immunoinflammatory Response: Azathioprine suppresses disease manifestations as well as underlying pathology in animal models of auto-immune disease. For example, the severity of adjuvant arthritis is reduced by azathioprine.

The mechanisms whereby azathioprine affects auto-immune diseases are not known. Azathioprine is immunosuppressive, delayed hypersensitivity and cellular cytotoxicity tests being suppressed to a greater degree than are antibody responses. In the rat model of adjuvant arthritis, azathioprine has been shown to inhibit the lymph node hyperplasia which preceded the onset of the signs of the disease. Both the immunosuppressive and therapeutic effects in animal models are dose-related. Azathioprine is considered a slow-acting drug and effects may persist after the drug has been discontinued.

INDICATIONS AND USAGE
Azathioprine is indicated as an adjunct for the prevention of rejection in renal homotransplantation. It is also indicated for the management of severe, active rheumatoid arthritis unresponsive to rest, aspirin or other nonsteroidal anti-inflammatory drugs, or to agents in the class of which gold is an example.

Renal Homotransplantation: Azathioprine is indicated as an adjunct for the prevention of rejection in renal homotransplantation. Experience with over 16,000 transplants shows a five-year patient survival of 35% to 55%, but this is dependent on donor, match of HLA antigens, antidonor or anti B-cell alloantigen antibody and other variables. The effect of azathioprine on these variables has not been tested in controlled trials.

Rheumatoid Arthritis[6,7]: Azathioprine is indicated only in adult patients meeting criteria for classic or definite rheumatoid arthritis as specified by the American Rheumatism Association.[8] Azathioprine should be restricted to patients with severe, active and erosive disease not responsive to conventional management including rest, aspirin or other nonsteroidal drugs or to agents in the class of which gold is an example. Rest, physiotherapy and salicylates should be continued while azathioprine is given, but it may be possible to reduce the dose of corticosteroids in patients on azathioprine. The combined use of azathioprine with gold, antimalarials or penicillamine has not been studied for either added benefit or unexpected adverse effects. The use azathioprine with these agents cannot be recommended.

CONTRAINDICATIONS
Azathioprine should not be given to patients who have shown hypersensitivity to the drug.

Azathioprine should not be used to treating rheumatoid arthritis in pregnant women.

Patients with rheumatoid arthritis previously treated with alkylating agents (cyclophosphamide, chlorambucil, melphalan or others) may have a prohibitive risk of neoplasia if treated with azathioprine.[9]

WARNINGS
Severe *leukopenia and/or thrombocytopenia* may occur in patients on azathioprine. Macrocytic anemia and severe bone marrow depression may also occur. Hematologic toxicities are dose related and may be more severe in renal transplant patients whose homograft is undergoing rejection. It is suggested that patients on azathioprine have complete blood counts, including platelet counts, weekly during the first month, twice monthly for the second and third months of treatment, then monthly or more frequently if dosage alterations or other therapy changes are necessary. Delayed hematologic suppression may occur. Prompt reduction in dos-

Continued on next page

Roxane Laboratories—Cont.

age or temporary withdrawal of the drug may be necessary if there is a rapid fall in, or persistently low leukocyte count or other evidence of bone marrow depression. Leukopenia does not correlate with therapeutic effect; therefore the dose should not be increased intentionally to lower the white blood cell count.

Serious infections are a constant hazard for patients on chronic immunosuppression, especially for homograft recipients. Fungal, viral, bacterial and protozoal infections may be fatal and should be treated vigorously. Reduction of azathioprine dosage and/or use of other drugs should be considered.

Azathioprine is mutagenic in animals and humans, carcinogenic in animals, and may increase the patient's *risk of neoplasia*. Renal transplant patients are known to have an increased risk of malignancy, predominantly skin cancer and reticulum cell or lymphomatous tumors.[10] The risk of post-transplant lymphomas may be increased in patients who receive aggressive treatment with immunosuppressive drugs.[11] The degree of immunosuppression is determined not only by the immunosuppressive regimen but also by a number of other patient factors. The number of immunosuppressive agents may not necessarily increase the risk of post-transplant lymphomas. However, transplant patients who receive multiple immunosuppressive agents may be at risk for over-immunosuppression; therefore, immunosuppressive drug therapy should be maintained at the lowest effective levels. Information is available on the spontaneous neoplasia risk in rheumatoid arthritis,[12,13] and on neoplasia following immunosuppressive therapy of other autoimmune diseases.[14,15] It has not been possible to define the precise risk of neoplasia due to azathioprine.[16] The data suggest the risk may be elevated in patients with rheumatoid arthritis, though lower than for renal transplant patients.[11,13] However, acute myelogenous leukemia as well as solid tumors have been reported in patients with rheumatoid arthritis who have received azathioprine. Data on neoplasia in patients receiving azathioprine can be found under **ADVERSE REACTIONS**.

Azathioprine has been reported to cause temporary depression in spermatogenesis and reduction in sperm viability and sperm count in mice at doses 10 times the human therapeutic dose[17]; a reduced percentage of fertile matings occurred when animals received 5 mg/kg.[18]

Pregnancy: "Pregnancy Category D": Azathioprine can cause fetal harm when administered to a pregnant woman. Azathioprine should not be given during pregnancy without careful weighing of risk versus benefit. Whenever possible, use of azathioprine in pregnant patients should be avoided. This drug should not be used for treating rheumatoid arthritis in pregnant women.[19]

Azathioprine is teratogenic in rabbits and mice when given in doses equivalent to the human dose (5 mg/kg daily). Abnormalities included skeletal malformations and visceral anomalies.[18]

Limited immunologic and other abnormalities have occurred in a few infants born of renal allograft recipients on azathioprine. In a detailed case report,[20] documented lymphopenia, diminished IgG and IgM levels, CMV infection, and a decreased thymic shadow were noted in an infant born to a mother receiving 150 mg azathioprine and 30 mg prednisone daily throughout pregnancy. At ten weeks most features were normalized. DeWitte et al[21] reported pancytopenia and severe immune deficiency in a pre-term infant whose mother received 125 mg azathioprine and 12.5 mg prednisone daily. There have been two published reports of abnormal physical findings. Williamson and Karp[22] described an infant born with preaxial polydactyly whose mother received azathioprine 200 mg daily and prednisone 20 mg every other day during pregnancy. Tallent et al[23] described an infant with a large myelomeringocele in the upper lumbar region, bilateral dislocated hips, and bilateral talipes equinovarus. The father was on long-term azathioprine therapy.

Benefit versus risk must be weighed carefully before use of azathioprine in patients of reproductive potential. There are no adequate and well-controlled studies in pregnant women. If this drug is used during pregnancy or if the patient becomes pregnant while taking this drug, the patient should be apprised of the potential hazard to the fetus. Women of childbearing age should be advised to avoid becoming pregnant.

PRECAUTIONS

General: A gastrointestinal hypersensitivity reaction characterized by severe nausea and vomiting has been reported.[24,25,26] These symptoms may also be accompanied by diarrhea, rash, fever, malaise, myalgias, elevations in liver enzymes, and occasionally, hypotension. Symptoms of gastrointestinal toxicity most often develop within the first several weeks of azathioprine therapy and are reversible upon discontinuation of the drug. The reaction can recur within hours after rechallenge with a single dose of azathioprine.

Information for Patients:

Patients being started on azathioprine should be informed of the necessity of periodic blood counts while they are receiving the drug and should be encouraged to report any unusual bleeding or bruising to their physician. They should be informed of the danger of infection while receiving azathioprine and encouraged to report signs and symptoms of infection to their physician. Careful dosage instructions should be given to the patient, especially when azathioprine is being administered in the presence of impaired renal function or concomitantly with allopurinol (see **DOSAGE AND ADMINISTRATION** and **Drug Interactions** under **PRECAUTIONS**). Patients should be advised of the potential risks of the use of azathioprine during pregnancy and during the nursing period. The increased risk of neoplasia following azathioprine therapy should be explained to the patient.

Laboratory Tests: See **WARNINGS** and **ADVERSE REACTIONS**.

Drug Interactions:

Use with Allopurinol: The principal pathway for detoxification of azathioprine is inhibited by allopurinol. Patients receiving azathioprine and allopurinol concomitantly should have a dose reduction of azathioprine, to approximately 1/3 to 1/4 the usual dose.

Use with Other Agents Affecting Myelopoesis: Drugs which may effect leukocyte production, including co-trimoxazole, may lead to exaggerated leukopenia, especially in renal transplant recipients.[27]

Use with Angiotensin Converting Enzyme Inhibitors: The use of angiotensin converting enzyme inhibitors to control hypertension in patients on azathioprine has been reported to induce severe leukopenia.[28]

Carcinogenesis, Mutagenesis, Impairment of Fertility: See **WARNINGS** section.

Pregnancy: Teratogenic Effect. Pregnancy Category D. See **WARNINGS** section.

Nursing Mothers: The use of azathioprine in nursing mothers is not recommended. Azathioprine or its metabolites are transferred at low levels, both transplacentally and in breast milk.[29,30,31] Because of the potential for tumorigenicity shown for azathioprine, a decision should be made whether to discontinue nursing or discontinue the drug, taking into account the importance of the drug to the mother.

Pediatric Use: Safety and efficacy of azathioprine in children have not been established.

ADVERSE REACTIONS

The principal and potentially serious toxic effects of azathioprine are hematologic and gastrointestinal. The risks of secondary infection and neoplasia are also significant (see **WARNINGS**). The frequency and severity of adverse reactions depend on the dose and duration of azathioprine as well as on the patient's underlying disease or concomitant therapies. The incidence of hematologic toxicities and neoplasia encountered in groups of renal hemograft recipients is significantly higher than that in studies employing azathioprine for rheumatoid arthritis. The relative incidences in clinical studies are summarized below:

Toxicity	Renal Homograft	Rheumatoid Arthritis
Leukopenia		
Any Degree	> 50%	28%
< 2500/mm³	16%	5.3%
Infections	20%	< 1%
Neoplasia		
Lymphoma	0.5%	
Others	2.8%	

*Data on the rate and risk of neoplasia among persons with rheumatoid arthritis treated with azathioprine are limited. The incidence of lymphoproliferative disease in patients with RA appears to be significantly higher than that in the general population.[12] In one completed study, the rate of lymphoproliferative disease in RA patients receiving higher than recommended doses of azathioprine (5 mg/kg/day) was 1.8 cases per 1000 patient years of follow-up compared with 0.8 cases per 1000 patient years of follow-up, in those not receiving azathioprine.[13] However, the proportion of the increased risk attributable to the azathioprine dosage or to other therapies (i.e., alkylating agents) received by azathioprine-treated patients cannot be determined.

Hematologic: Leukopenia and/or thrombocytopenia are dose dependent and may occur late in the course of azathioprine therapy. Dose reduction or temporary withdrawal allows reversal of these toxicities. Infection may occur as a secondary manifestation of bone marrow suppression or leukopenia, but the incidence of infection in renal homotransplantation is 30 to 60 times that in rheumatoid arthritis. Macrocytic anemia and/or bleeding have been reported in two patients on azathioprine.

Gastrointestinal: Nausea and vomiting may occur within the first few months of azathioprine therapy, and occurred in approximately 12% of 676 rheumatoid arthritis patients. The frequency of gastric disturbance can be reduced by administration of the drug in divided doses and/or after meals. However, in some patients, nausea and vomiting may be severe and may be accompanied by symptoms such as diarrhea, fever, malaise, and myalgias (see **PRECAUTIONS**). Vomiting with abdominal pain may occur rarely with a hypersensitivity pancreatitis. Hepatotoxicity manifest by elevation of serum alkaline phosphatase, bilirubin and/or serum transaminases is known to occur following azathioprine use, primarily in allograft recipients. Hepatotoxicity has been uncommon (less than 1%) in rheumatoid arthritis patients. Hepatotoxicity following transplantation most often occurs within 6 months of transplantation and is generally reversible after interruption of azathioprine. A rare, but life-threatening hepatic veno-occlusive disease associated with chronic administration of azathioprine has been described in transplant patients and in one patient receiving azathioprine for panuveitis.[32,33,34] Periodic measurement of serum transaminases, alkaline phosphatase and bilirubin is indicated for early detection of hepatotoxicity. If hepatic veno-occlusive disease is clinically suspected, azathioprine should be permanently withdrawn.

Others: Additional side effects of low frequency have been recorded. These include skin rashes (approximately 2%), alopecia, fever, arthralgias, diarrhea, steatorrhea and negative nitrogen balance (all less than 1%).

OVERDOSAGE

The oral LD_{50}s for single doses of azathioprine in mice and rats are 2500 mg/kg and 400 mg/kg, respectively. Very large doses of this antimetabolite may lead to marrow hypoplasia, bleeding, infection, and death. About 30% of azathioprine is bound to serum proteins, but approximately 45% is removed during an 8 hour hemodialysis.[35] A single case has been reported of a renal transplant patient who ingested a single dose of 7500 mg azathioprine. The immediate toxic reactions were nausea, vomiting, and diarrhea, followed by mild leukopenia, and mild abnormalities in liver function. The white blood cell count, SGOT, and bilirubin returned to normal six days after the overdose.

DOSAGE AND ADMINISTRATION

Renal Homotransplantation: The dose of azathioprine required to prevent rejection and minimize toxicity will vary with individual patients; this necessitates careful management. Initial dose is usually 3 to 5 mg/kg daily, beginning at the time of transplant. Azathioprine is usually given as a single daily dose on the day of, and in a minority of cases one to three days before, transplantation. Azathioprine is often initiated with the intravenous administration of the sodium salt, with subsequent use of tablets (at the same dose level) after the post-operative period. Intravenous administration of the sodium salt is indicated only in patients unable to tolerate oral medications. Dose reduction to maintenance levels of 1 to 3 mg/kg daily is usually possible. The dose of azathioprine should not be increased to toxic levels because of threatened rejection. Discontinuation may be necessary for severe hematologic or other toxicity, even if rejection of the homograft may be a consequence of drug withdrawal.

Rheumatoid Arthritis: Azathioprine is usually given on a daily basis. The initial dose should be approximately 1.0 mg/kg (50 to 100 mg) given as a single dose or on a twice daily schedule. The dose may be increased, beginning at six to eight weeks and thereafter by steps at four-week intervals, if there are no serious toxicities and if initial response is unsatisfactory. Dose increments should be 0.5 mg/kg daily, up to a maximum dose of 2.5 mg/kg/day. Therapeutic response occurs after several weeks of treatment, usually six to eight; an adequate trial should be a minimum of 12 weeks. Patients not improved after twelve weeks can be considered refractory. Azathioprine may be continued long-term in patients with clinical response, but patients should be monitored carefully, and gradual dosage reduction should be attempted to reduce risk of toxicities.

Maintenance therapy should be at the lowest effective dose, and the dose given can be lowered decrementally with changes of 0.5 mg/kg or approximately 25 mg daily every four weeks while other therapy is kept constant. The optimum duration of maintenance azathioprine has not been determined. Azathioprine can be discontinued abruptly, but delayed effects are possible.

Use in Renal Dysfunction: Relatively oliguric patients, especially those with tubular necrosis in the immediate post-cadaveric transplant period, may have delayed clearance of azathioprine or its metabolites, may be particularly sensitive to this drug and may require lower doses.

Procedures for proper handling and disposal of this immunosuppressive antimetabolite drug should be considered. Several guidelines on this subject have been published.[36-42] There is no general agreement that all of the procedures recommended in the guidelines are necessary or appropriate.

HOW SUPPLIED

Azathioprine Tablets USP, 50 mg

Yellow, round, scored tablets (identified 54 043)

NDC 0054-8084-25: Unit dose, 10 tablets per strip, 10 strips per shelf pack, 10 shelf packs per shipper.

NDC 0054-4084-25: Bottles of 100 tablets.

Caution: Federal law prohibits dispensing without prescription.
Store between 15°C–25°C (59°–77°F)
Protect From Light
Protect From Moisture
Dispense in tight, light resistant container as defined in the USP/NF.

REFERENCES

1. Elion GB, Hitchings GH. Azathioprine In: Sartorelli AC, Johns DG, eds. *Antineoplastic and Immunosuppressive Agents Pt II.* New York, NY:Springer Verlag; 1975:chap 48.
2. McIntosh J, Hansen P, Ziegler J, Penny R. Defective immune and phagocytic functions in uraemia and renal transplantation. *Int Arch Allergy Appl Immunol.* 1976;15:544-549.
3. Renal Transplant Registry Advisory Committee. The 12th report of the Human Renal Transplant Registry. JAMA. 1975;233:787-796.
4. McGeown M. Immunosuppression for kidney transplantation. *Lancet.* 1973;1:310-312.
5. Simmons RL, Thompson EJ, Yunis EJ, et al. 115 Patients with first cadaver kidney transplants followed two to seven and a half years: a multifactorial analysis. *Am J Med.* 1977;62:234-242.
6. Fye K, Talal N. Cytotoxic drugs in the treatment of rheumatoid arthritis. *Ration Drug Ther.* 1975;9(4):1-5.
7. Davis JD, Muss HB, Turner RA. Cytotoxic agents in the treatment of rheumatoid arthritis. *South Med J.* 1978;71:58-64.
8. McEwen C. the diagnosis and differential diagnosis of rheumatoid arthritis. In: Hollander JL, ed. *Arthritis and Allied Conditions: A Textbook of Rheumatology.* 8th ed. Philadelphia, PA: Lea and Febiger; 1972:403-418.
9. Hoover R, Fraumeni, JF. Drug-induced cancer. *Cancer.* 1981;47(5):1071-1080.
10. Hoover R, Fraumeni JF Jr. Risk of cancer in renal transplant recipients. *Lancet.* 1973;2:55-57.
11. Wilkenson AH, Smith JL, Hunsicker LG, et al. Increased frequency of post-transplant lymphomas in patients treated with cyclosporine, azathioprine, and prednisone. *Transplantation.* 1989;47:293-296.
12. Prior P, Symmons DP, Hawkins CF, et al. Cancer morbidity in rheumatoid arthritis. *Ann Rheum Dis* 1984;43:128-131.
13. Silman AJ, Petrie J, Hazelman B, et al. Lymphoproliferative cancer and other malignancy in patients with rheumatoid arthritis treated with azathioprine: a 20 year follow up study. *Ann Rheum Dis.* 1988;47:988-992.
14. Louie S, Schwartz RS. Immunodeficiency and pathogenesis of lymphoma and leukemia. *Semin Hematol.* 1978;15:117-138.
15. Wang KK, Czaja AJ, Beaver SJ, et al. Extra hepatic malignancy following long-term immunosuppressive therapy of severe hepatitis B surface antigen-negative chronic active hepatitis. *Hepatology.* 1989;10:39-43.
16. Sieber SM, Adamson RH. Toxicity of antineoplastic agents in man: chromosomal aberrations, antifertility effects, congenital malformations and carcinogenic potential. In: Klein G, Weinhouse S, eds. *Advances in Cancer Research,* v.22. New York, NY: Academic Press; 1975:57-155.
17. Clark JM. The mutagenicity of azathioprine in mice, *Drosophila Melanogaster* and *Neurospora Crassa. Mut Res.* 1975;28(1):87-99.
18. Data on file at Burroughs Wellcome Co.
19. Tagatz GE, Simmons RL. Pregnancy after renal transplantation. *Ann Intern Med.* 1975;82:113-114, Editorial Notes.
20. Coté CJ, Meuwissen HJ, Pickering RJ. Effects on the neonate of prednisone and azathioprine administered to the mother during pregnancy. *J Pediatr.* 1974;85(3):324-328.
21. DeWitte DB, Buick MK, Stephen EC, et al. Neonatal pancytopenia and severe combined immunodeficiency associated with antenatal administration of azathioprine and prednisone. *J Pediatr.* 1984;105(4):625-628.
22. Williamson RA, Karp LE. Azathioprine teratogenicity: review of the literature and case report. *Obstet Gynecol.* 1981;58:247-250.
23. Tallent MB, Simmons RL, Najarian JS. Birth defects in child of male recipient of kidney transplant. *JAMA.* 1970;211(11):1854-1855.
24. Assini JF, Hamilton R, Strosberg JM. Adverse reactions to azathioprine mimicking gastroenteritis. *J Rheumatol.* 1986;13:1117-1118.
25. Cochrane D, Adamson AR, Halsey JP. Adverse reactions to azathioprine mimicking gastroenteritis. *J Rheumatol.* 1987;14:1075.
26. Cox J, Daneshmend JK, Hawkey CJ, et al. Devastating diarrhea caused by azathioprine: management difficulty in inflammatory bowel disease. *Gut.* 1988;29(5):686-688.
27. Bradley PP, Warden GD, Maxwell JG, et al. Neutropenia and thrombocytopenia in renal allograft recipients treated with trimethoprim-sulfamethoxazole. *Ann Int Med.* 1980;93:560-562.
28. Kirchertz EJ, Grone HJ, Rieger J, et al. Successful low dose captopril rechallenge following drug-induced leucopenia. *Lancet.* 1981;8234:1362-1363.
29. Nelson D, Bugge C. Data on file, Burroughs Wellcome Co.
30. Saarikoski S, Seppälä M. Immunosuppression during pregnancy: transmission of azathioprine and its metabolites from the mother to the fetus. *Am J Obstet Gynecol.* 1973;115:1100-1106.
31. Coulam CB, Moyer TP, Jiang NS, et al. Breast-feeding after renal transplantation. *Transplant Proc.* 1982;14:605-609.
32. Read AE, Wiesner RH, LaBrecque DR, et al. Hepatic veno-occlusive disease associated with renal transplantation and azathioprine therapy. *Ann Intern Med.* 1986;104:651-655.
33. Katzka DA, Saul SH, Jorkasky D, Sigal H, Reynolds JC, Soloway RD. Azathioprine and hepatic venocclusive disease in renal transplant patients. *Gastroenterology.* 1986;90:446-454.
34. Weitz H, Gokel JM, Loeschke K, et al. Veno-occlusive disease of the liver in patients receiving immunosuppressive therapy. *Virchows Arch A.* 1982;395:245-256.
35. Schusziarra V, Ziekursch V, Schlamp R, et al. Pharmacokinetics of azathioprine under haemodialysis. *Int J Clin Pharmacol Biopharm.* 1976;14(4):298-302.
36. Recommendations for the safe handling of parenteral antineoplastic drugs. Washington, DC: Division of Safety, National Institutes of Health; 1983. US Dept of Health and Human Service publication NIH 83-2621.
37. AMA Council on Scientific Affairs. Guidelines for handling parenteral antineoplastics. *JAMA* 1985;253:1590-1591.
38. National Studv Commission on Cytotoxic Exposure. Recommendations for handling cytotoxic agents. 1984. Available from Louis P. Jeffrey, ScD, Director of Pharmacy Services, Rhode Island Hospital, 593 Eddy Street, Providence, Rhode Island 02902.
39. Clinical Oncological Society of Australia. Guidelines and recommendations for safe handling of antineoplastic agents. *Med J Australia.* 1983;1:426-428.
40. Jones RB, Frank R, Mass T. Safe handling of chemotherapeutic agents: a report from the Mount Sinai Medical Center. *CA-A Cancer J for Clin.* 1983;33(Sept/Oct):258-263.
41. American Society of Hospital Pharmacists. ASHP technical assistance bulletin on handling cytotoxic and hazardous drugs. *Am J Hosp Pharm.* 1990;47:1033-1049.
42. Yodaiken RE, Bennett D. OSHA work-practice guidelines for personnel dealing with cytotoxic (antineoplastic) drugs. *Am J Hosp Pharm.* 1986;43:1193-1204.

4042500 Revised October 1995
105

Roxane Laboratories, Inc.
Columbus, Ohio 43216

DHT™ ℞
Dihydrotachysterol
Tablets USP and Intensol

DESCRIPTION

Each tablet contains:
Dihydrotachysterol .... 0.125 mg, 0.2 mg, or 0.4 mg
Each mL of Intensol contains:
Dihydrotachysterol .... 0.2 mg
Dihydrotachysterol is a synthetic reduction product of tachysterol, a close isomer of vitamin D. Chemically Dihydrotachysterol is *9,10- Secoergosta-5,7,22-tri-en-3β- ol.*
Dihydrotachysterol acts as a blood calcium regulator.

CLINICAL PHARMACOLOGY

Dihydrotachysterol is hydroxylated in the liver to 25-hydroxydihydrotachysterol, which is the major circulating active form of the drug. It does not undergo further hydroxylation by the kidney and therefore is the analogue of 1,25-dihydroxyvitamin D. Dihydrotachysterol is effective in the elevation of serum calcium by stimulating intestinal calcium absorption and mobilizing bone calcium in the absence of parathyroid hormone and of functioning renal tissue. Dihydrotachysterol also increases renal phosphate excretion. In contrast to parathyroid extract, Dihydrotachysterol is active when taken orally, exerts a slow but persistent effect, and may be used for long periods without increasing the dosage or causing tolerance. Dihydrotachysterol is faster-acting than pharmacologic doses of vitamin D and is less persistent after cessation of treatment, thus decreasing the risk of accumulation and of hypercalcemia.

INDICATIONS AND USAGE

Dihydrotachysterol is indicated for the treatment of acute, chronic, and latent forms of postoperative tetany, idiopathic tetany, and hypoparathyroidism.

CONTRAINDICATIONS

Contraindicated in patients with hypercalcemia, abnormal sensitivity to the effects of vitamin D, and hypervitaminosis D.

PRECAUTIONS

General: The difference between therapeutic dose and intoxicating dose may be small in any patient and therefore dosage must be individualized and periodically reevaluated.
In patients with renal osteodystrophy accompanied by hyperphosphatemia, maintenance of a normal serum phosphorus level by dietary phosphate restriction and/or administration of aluminum gels as intestinal phosphate binders is essential to prevent metastatic calcification.
Because of its effect on serum calcium, Dihydrotachysterol should be administered to pregnant patients or to patients with renal stones only when, in the judgment of the physician, the potential benefits outweigh the possible hazards.
Laboratory tests: **To prevent hypercalcemia, treatment should always be controlled by regular determinations of blood calcium level, which should be maintained within the normal range.**
Drug interactions: Administration of thiazide diuretics to hypoparathyroid patients who are concurrently being treated with Dihydrotachysterol may cause hypercalcemia.
Pregnancy: Teratogenic effects —Pregnancy Category C: Animal reproduction studies have shown fetal abnormalities in several species associated with hypervitaminosis D. These are similar to the supravalvular aortic stenosis syndrome described in infants by Black in England (1963). This syndrome was characterized by supravalvular aortic stenosis, elfin facies, and mental retardation.
There are no adequate and well-controlled studies in pregnant women. Dihydrotachysterol should be used during pregnancy only if the potential benefit justifies the potential risk to the fetus.
Nursing mothers: It is not known whether this drug is excreted in human milk. Because many drugs are excreted in human milk, caution should be exercised when Dihydrotachysterol is administered to a nursing woman.

OVERDOSAGE

The effects of Dihydrotachysterol can persist for up to one month after cessation of treatment.
Manifestations: Toxicity associated with Dihydrotachysterol is similar to that seen with large doses of vitamin D. Overdosage is manifested by symptoms of hypercalcemia, i.e., weakness, headache, anorexia, nausea, vomiting, abdominal cramps, diarrhea, constipation, vertigo, tinnitus, ataxia, hypotonia, lethargy, depression, amnesia, disorientation, hallucinations, syncope, and coma. Impairment of renal function may result in polyuria, polydipsia, and albuminuria. Widespread calcification of soft tissues, including heart, blood vessels, kidneys, and lungs, can occur. Death can result from cardiovascular or renal failure.
Treatment: Treatment of overdosage consists of withdrawal of Dihydrotachysterol, bed rest, liberal intake of fluids, a low-calcium diet, and administration of a laxative. Hypercalcemic crisis with dehydration, stupor, coma, and azotemia requires more vigorous treatment. The first step should be hydration of the patient. Intravenous saline may quickly and significantly increase urinary calcium excretion. A loop diuretic (furosemide or ethacrynic acid) may be given with the saline infusion to further increase renal calcium excretion. Other reported therapeutic measures include dialysis or the administration of citrates, sulfates, phosphates, corticosteroids, EDTA (ethylenediaminetetraacetic acids), and mithramycin via appropriate regimens.

DOSAGE AND ADMINISTRATION

The dosage depends on the nature and seriousness of the disorder and should be adapted to each individual patient. Serum calcium levels should be maintained between 9 to 10 mg per 100 mL.
The following dosage schedule will serve as a guide:
Initial dose: 0.8 mg to 2.4 mg daily for several days.
Maintenance dose: 0.2 mg to 1.0 mg daily as required for normal serum calcium levels. The average maintenance dose is 0.6 mg daily. This dose may be supplemented with 10 to 15 grams of calcium lactate or gluconate by mouth daily.

HOW SUPPLIED

0.125 mg white tablets.
NDC 0054-8172-25: Unit dose, 10 tablets per strip, 10 strips per shelf pack, 10 shelf packs per shipper.
NDC 0054-4190-19: Bottles of 50 tablets.
0.2 mg pink tablets.
NDC 0054-8182-25: Unit dose, 10 tablets per strip, 10 strips per shelf pack, 10 shelf packs per shipper.
NDC 0054-4189-25: Bottles of 100 tablets.
0.4 mg white tablets.
NDC 0054-4191-19: Bottles of 50 tablets.

Continued on next page

Roxane Laboratories—Cont.

Intensol 0.2 mg/mL
NDC 0054-3170-44: Bottles of 30 mL with calibrated dropper (graduated 0.25 mL to 1.0 mL)
4049201
104   Revised October 1994

DOLOPHINE® HYDROCHLORIDE
Methadone Hydrochloride
Tablets USP 5 mg, 10 mg
Methadone Hydrochloride
Injection USP 10 mg per mL

(Warning: May be habit forming)

DESCRIPTION
Chemically, Methadone Hydrochloride is 3-Heptanone, 6-(dimethylamino)-4,4-diphenyl-, hydrochloride, which can be represented by the following structural formula:

$C_{21}H_{27}NO \cdot HCl$ M.W. 345.91

Each tablet for oral administration contains:
Methadone Hydrochloride .... 5 mg, 10 mg
(Warning: May be habit forming)
Each mL contains methadone hydrochloride 10 mg (0.029 mmol) and sodium chloride 0.9%. Sodium hydroxide and/or hydrochloric acid may have been added during manufacture to adjust the pH. The 20 mL vials also contain chlorobutanol (chloroform derivative), 0.5%, as a preservative.
Inactive Ingredients:
The tablets contain magnesium stearate, cellulose, starch (corn), lactose, sucrose and talc. The 10 mg tablet also contains acacia.

HOW SUPPLIED
DOLOPHINE HYDROCHLORIDE®
(Methadone Hydrochloride Tablets USP)
5 mg tablets (Identified 54 162).
NDC 0054-4216-25: Bottles of 100 tablets.
10 mg tablets (Identified 54 549).
NDC 0054-4217-25: Bottles of 100 tablets.
DOLOPHINE HYDROCHLORIDE®
(Methadone Hydrochloride Injection USP)
10 mg per mL, Multiple-Dose Vials.
NDC 0054-1218-42: Single 20 mL multiple-dose vials.
Store at Controlled Room Temperature 15°–30°C (59°–86°F)
Protect from light.
Dispense in a tight, light-resistant container as defined in the USP/NF.
Caution: Federal law prohibits dispensing without prescription.
March 1995

IPRATROPIUM BROMIDE
INHALATION SOLUTION, 0.02%

Prescribing Information

DESCRIPTION
The active ingredient, ipratropium bromide monohydrate, is an anticholinergic bronchodilator chemically described as 8-azoniabicyclo [3.2.1]-octane, 3-(3-hydroxy-1-oxo-2-phenyl-propoxy)-8-methyl-8-(1-methylethyl)-, bromide, monohydrate (*endo, syn*), (±); a synthetic quarternary ammonium compound, chemically related to atropine.

Ipratropium Bromide $C_{20}H_{30}BrNO_3 \cdot H_2O$
                       Mol. Wt. 430.4

Ipratropium bromide is a white crystalline substance, freely soluble in water and lower alcohols. It is a quarternary ammonium compound and thus exists in an ionized state in aqueous solutions. It is relatively insoluble in non-polar media.
Ipratropium Bromide Inhalation Solution is administered by oral inhalation with the aid of a nebulizer. It contains ipratropium bromide 0.02% (anhydrous basis) in a sterile, preservative-free, isotonic saline solution, pH-adjusted to 3.4 (3 to 4) with hydrochloric acid.

HOW SUPPLIED
Ipratropium Bromide Inhalation Solution Unit-Dose Vial is supplied as a 0.02% clear, colorless solution containing 2.5 mL with 25 vials per foil pouch (NDC 0054-8402-11).
2.5 mL with 30 vials per foil pouch (NDC 0054-8402-13).
Each vial is made from a low-density polyethylene (LDPE) resin.
Store between 59°F (15°C) and 86°F (30°C).
Protect from light.
Store unused vials in the foil pouch.
ATTENTION PHARMACIST: Detach "Patient's Instructions for Use" from Package Insert and dispense with solution.
Caution: Federal law prohibits dispensing without prescription.
Licensed from Boehringer Ingelheim International GmbH
Manufactured by
Roxane Laboratories, Inc., Columbus OH 43228
Distributed by
Roxane Laoratories, Inc.
Columbus, Ohio 43216
4054320   Revised March 1996
036
©RLI, 1996

LITHIUM CARBONATE   ℞
CAPSULES USP 150 mg, 300 mg, and 600 mg
TABLETS USP 300 mg

WARNING
Lithium toxicity is closely related to serum lithium levels, and can occur at doses close to therapeutic levels. Facilities for prompt and accurate serum lithium determinations should be available before initiating therapy.

DESCRIPTION
Each tablet for oral administration contains:
    Lithium Carbonate .... 300 mg
Each capsule for oral administration contains:
    Lithium Carbonate .... 150 mg, 300 mg, or 600 mg
Inactive Ingredients:
The capsules contain talc, gelatin, FD&C Red No. 40, titanium dioxide, and the imprinting ink contains FD&C Blue No. 2, FD&C Yellow No. 6, FD&C Red No. 40, synthetic black iron oxide, and pharmaceutical glaze. The tablets contain calcium stearate, microcrystalline cellulose, povidone, sodium lauryl sulfate, and sodium starch glycolate.
Lithium Carbonate is a white, light alkaline powder with molecular formula Li_2CO_3 and molecular weight 73.89. Lithium is an element of the alkali-metal group with atomic number 3, atomic weight 6.94 and an emission line at 671 nm on the flame photometer. Lithium acts as an antimanic.

CLINICAL PHARMACOLOGY
Preclinical studies have shown that lithium alters sodium transport in nerve and muscle cells and effects a shift toward intraneuronal metabolism of catecholamines, but the specific biochemical mechanism of lithium action in mania is unknown.

INDICATIONS AND USAGE
Lithium carbonate is indicated in the treatment of manic episodes of Bipolar Disorder. Bipolar Disorder, Manic (DSM-III) is equivalent to Manic Depressive illness, Manic, in the older DSM-II terminology.
Lithium is also indicated as a maintenance treatment for individuals with a diagnosis of Bipolar Disorder. Maintenance therapy reduces the frequency of manic episodes and diminishes the intensity of those episodes which may occur.
Typical symptoms of mania include pressure of speech, motor hyperactivity, reduced need for sleep, flight of ideas, grandiosity, or poor judgment, aggressiveness, and possibly hostility. When given to a patient experiencing a manic episode, lithium may produce a normalization of symptomatology within 1 to 3 weeks.

CONTRAINDICATIONS
Lithium should generally not be given to patients with significant renal or cardiovascular disease, severe debilitation or dehydration, or sodium depletion, and to patients receiving diuretics, since the risk of lithium toxicity is very high in such patients. If the psychiatric indication is life-threatening, and if such a patient fails to respond to other measures, lithium treatment may be undertaken with extreme caution, including daily serum lithium determinations and adjustment to the usually low doses ordinarily tolerated by these individuals. In such instances, hospitalization is a necessity.

WARNINGS
Lithium may cause fetal harm when administered to a pregnant woman. There have been reports of lithium having adverse effects on nidation in rats, embryo viability in mice, and metabolism in-vitro of rat testis and human spermatozoa have been attributed to lithium, as have teratogenicity in submammalian species and cleft palates in mice. Studies in rats, rabbits and monkeys have shown no evidence of lithium-induced teratology. Data from lithium birth registries suggest an increase in cardiac and other anomalies, especially Ebstein's anomaly. If the patient becomes pregnant while taking lithium, she should be apprised of the potential risk to the fetus. If possible, lithium should be withdrawn for at least the first trimester unless it is determined that this would seriously endanger the mother.
Chronic lithium therapy may be associated with diminution of renal concentrating ability, occasionally presenting as nephrogenic diabetes insipidus, with polyuria and polydipsia. Such patients should be carefully managed to avoid dehydration with resulting lithium retention and toxicity. This condition is usually reversible when lithium is discontinued. Morphologic changes with glomerular and interstitial fibrosis and nephron-atrophy have been reported in patients on chronic lithium therapy. Morphologic changes have been seen in bipolar patients never exposed to lithium. The relationship between renal functional and morphologic changes and their association with lithium therapy has not been established. To date, lithium in therapeutic doses has not been reported to cause end-stage renal disease.
When kidney function is assessed, for baseline data prior to starting lithium therapy or thereafter, routine urinalysis and other tests may be used to evaluate tubular function (e.g., urine specific gravity or osmolality following a period of water deprivation, or 24-hour urine volume) and glomerular function (e.g., serum creatinine or creatinine clearance). During lithium therapy, progressive or sudden changes in renal function, even within the normal range, indicate the need for reevaluation of treatment.
Lithium toxicity is closely related to serum lithium levels, and can occur at doses close to therapeutic levels (see DOSAGE AND ADMINISTRATION).

PRECAUTIONS
General: The ability to tolerate lithium is greater during the acute manic phase and decreases when manic symptoms subside (See DOSAGE AND ADMINISTRATION).
The distribution space of lithium approximates that of total body water. Lithium is primarily excreted in urine with insignificant excretion in feces. Renal excretion of lithium is proportional to its plasma concentration. The half-life of elimination of lithium is approximately 24 hours. Lithium decreases sodium reabsorption by the renal tubules which could lead to sodium depletion. Therefore, it is essential for the patient to maintain a normal diet, including salt, and an adequate fluid intake (2500-3000 mL) at least during the initial stabilization period. Decreased tolerance to lithium has been reported to ensue from protracted sweating or diarrhea and, if such occur, supplemental fluid and salt should be administered.
In addition to sweating and diarrhea, concomitant infection with elevated temperatures may also necessitate a temporary reduction or cessation of medication.
Previously existing underlying thyroid disorders do not necessarily constitute a contraindication to lithium treatment; where hypothyroidism exists, careful monitoring of thyroid function during lithium stabilization and maintenance allows for correction of changing thyroid parameters, if any. Where hypothyroidism occurs during lithium stabilization and maintenance, supplemental thyroid treatment may be used.
Information for the patients: Outpatients and their families should be warned that the patient must discontinue lithium therapy and contact his physician if such clinical signs of lithium toxicity as diarrhea, vomiting, tremor, mild ataxia, drowsiness, or muscular weakness occur.
Lithium may impair mental and/or physical abilities. Caution patients about activities requiring alertness (e.g., operating vehicles or machinery).
Drug interactions: Combined use of haloperidol and lithium: An encephalopathic syndrome (characterized by weakness, lethargy, fever, tremulousness and confusion, extrapyramidal symptoms, leucocytosis, elevated serum enzymes, BUN and FBS) followed by irreversible brain damage has occurred in a few patients treated with lithium plus haloperidol. A causal relationship between these events and the concomitant administration of lithium and haloperidol has not been established; however, patients receiving such combined therapy should be monitored closely for early evidence of neurological toxicity and treatment discontinued promptly if such signs appear.
The possibility of similar adverse interactions with other antipsychotic medication exists.
Lithium may prolong the effects of neuromuscular blocking agents. Therefore, neuromuscular blocking agents should be given with caution to patients receiving lithium.

Indomethacin and piroxicam have been reported to increase significantly steady state plasma lithium levels. In some cases lithium toxicity has resulted from such interactions. There is also evidence that other non-steroidal, anti-inflammatory agents may have a similar effect. When such combinations are used, increased plasma lithium level monitoring is recommended.

Caution should be used when lithium and diuretics or angiotensin converting enzyme (ACE) inhibitors are used concomitantly because sodium loss may reduce the renal clearance of lithium and increase serum lithium levels with risk of lithium toxicity. When such combinations are used, the lithium dosage may need to be decreased, and more frequent monitoring of lithium plasma levels is recommended.

Pregnancy: Teratogenic effects—Pregnancy Category D, See "Warnings" section.

Nursing mothers: Lithium is excreted in human milk. Nursing should not be undertaken during lithium therapy except in rare and unusual circumstances where, in the view of the physician, the potential benefits to the mother outweigh possible hazards to the child.

Usage in Children: Since information regarding the safety and effectiveness of lithium in children under 12 years of age is not available, its use in such patients is not recommended at this time. There has been a report of a transient syndrome of acute dystonia and hyperreflexia occurring in a 15 kg child who ingested 300 mg lithium carbonate.

ADVERSE REACTIONS

Lithium toxicity: The likelihood of toxicity increases with increasing serum lithium levels. Serum lithium levels greater than 1.5 mEq/l carry a greater risk than lower levels. However, patients sensitive to lithium may exhibit toxic signs at serum levels below 1.5 mEq/l.

Diarrhea, vomiting, drowsiness, muscular weakness and lack of coordination may be early signs of lithium toxicity, and can occur at lithium levels below 2.0 mEq/l. At higher levels, giddiness, ataxia, blurred vision, tinnitus and a large output of dilute urine may be seen. Serum lithium levels above 3.0 mEq/l may produce a complex clinical picture involving multiple organs and organ systems. Serum lithium levels should not be permitted to exceed 2.0 mEq/l during the acute treatment phase.

Fine hand tremor, polyuria and mild thirst may occur during initial therapy for the acute manic phase, and may persist throughout treatment. Transient and mild nausea and general discomfort may also appear during the first few days of lithium administration.

These side effects are an inconvenience rather than a disabling condition, and usually subside with continued treatment or a temporary reduction or cessation of dosage. If persistent, a cessation of dosage is indicated.

The following adverse reactions have been reported and do not appear to be directly related to serum lithium levels.

Neuromuscular: tremor, muscle hyperirritability (fasciculations, twitching, clonic movements of whole limbs), ataxia, choreo-athetotic movements, hyperactive deep tendon reflexes.

Central Nervous System: Blackout spells, epileptiform seizures, slurred speech, dizziness, vertigo, incontinence of urine or feces, somnolence, psychomotor retardation, restlessness, confusion, stupor, coma, acute dystonia, downbeat nystagmus.

Cardiovascular: cardiac arrhythmia, hypotension, peripheral circulatory collapse.

Neurological: Cases of pseudotumor cerebri (increased intracranial pressure and papilledema) have been reported with lithium use. If undetected, this condition may result in enlargement of the blind spot, constriction of visual fields and eventual blindness due to optic atrophy. Lithium should be discontinued, if clinically possible, if this syndrome occurs.

Gastrointestinal: anorexia, nausea, vomiting, diarrhea.

Genitourinary: albuminuria, oliguria, polyuria, glycosuria.

Dermatologic: drying and thinning of hair, anesthesia of skin, chronic folliculitis, xerosis cutis, alopecia and exacerbation of psoriasis.

Autonomic Nervous System: blurred vision, dry mouth.

Thyroid Abnormalities: euthyroid goiter and/or hypothyroidism (including myxedema) accompanied by lower T_3 and T_4. Iodine 131 uptake may be elevated. (See PRECAUTIONS). Paradoxically, rare cases of hyperthyroidism have been reported.

EEG Changes: diffuse slowing, widening of frequency spectrum, potentiation and disorganization of background rhythm.

EKG Changes: reversible flattening, isoelectricity or inversion of T-waves.

Miscellaneous: fatigue, lethargy, transient scotomata, dehydration, weight loss, tendency to sleep.

Miscellaneous reactions unrelated to dosage are: transient electroencephalographic and electrocardiographic changes, leucocytosis, headache, diffuse nontoxic goiter with or without hypothyroidism, transient hyperglycemia, generalized pruritis with or without rash, cutaneous ulcers, albuminuria, worsening of organic brain syndromes, excessive weight gain, edematous swelling of ankles or wrists, and thirst or polyuria, sometimes resembling diabetes insipidus, and metallic taste.

A single report has been received of the development of painful discoloration of fingers and toes and coldness of the extremities within one day of the starting of treatment of lithium. The mechanism through which these symptoms (resembling Raynaud's Syndrome) developed is not known. Recovery followed discontinuance.

OVERDOSAGE

The toxic levels for lithium are close to the therapeutic levels. It is therefore important that patients and their families be cautioned to watch for early symptoms and to discontinue the drug and inform the physician should they occur. Toxic symptoms are listed in detail under ADVERSE REACTIONS.

Treatment: No specific antidote for lithium poisoning is known. Early symptoms of lithium toxicity can usually be treated by reduction or cessation of dosage of the drug and resumption of the treatment at a lower dose after 24 to 48 hours. In severe cases of lithium poisoning, the first and foremost goal of treatment consists of elimination of this ion from the patient.

Treatment is essentially the same as that used in barbiturate poisoning: 1) gastric lavage, 2) correction of fluid and electrolyte imbalance and 3) regulation of kidney functioning. Urea, mannitol, and aminophylline all produce significant increases in lithium excretion. Hemodialysis is an effective and rapid means of removing the ion from the severely toxic patient. Infection prophylaxis, regular chest X-rays, and preservation of adequate respiration are essential.

DOSAGE AND ADMINISTRATION

Acute Mania: Optimal patient response to Lithium Carbonate usually can be established and maintained with 600 mg t.i.d. Such doses will normally produce an effective serum lithium level ranging between 1.0 and 1.5 mEq/l. Dosage must be individualized according to serum levels and clinical response. Regular monitoring of the patient's clinical state and of serum lithium levels is necessary. Serum levels should be determined twice per week during the acute phase, and until the serum level and clinical condition of the patient have been stabilized.

Long-term Control: The desirable serum lithium levels are 0.6 to 1.2 mEq/l. Dosage will vary from one individual to another, but usually 300 mg t.i.d. or q.i.d. will maintain this level. Serum lithium levels in uncomplicated cases receiving maintenance therapy during remission should be monitored at least every two months.

Patients abnormally sensitive to lithium may exhibit toxic signs at serum levels of 1.0 to 1.5 mEq/l. Elderly patients often respond to reduced dosage, and may exhibit signs of toxicity at serum levels ordinarily tolerated by other patients.

N.B.: Blood samples for serum lithium determination should be drawn immediately prior to the next dose when lithium concentrations are relatively stable (i.e., 8–12 hours after the previous dose.) Total reliance must not be placed on serum levels alone. Accurate patient evaluation requires both clinical and laboratory analysis.

HOW SUPPLIED

Lithium Carbonate Tablets USP

300 mg white, scored tablets (Identified 54 452)

NDC 0054-8528-25: Unit dose, 10 tablets per strip, 10 strips per shelf pack, 10 shelf packs per shipper.
(For Institutional Use Only).
NDC 0054-4527-25: Bottles of 100 tablets.
NDC 0054-4527-31: Bottles of 1000 tablets.

Lithium Carbonate Capsules USP

150 mg white opaque colored capsules (size 4) (Identified 54 213).

NDC 0054-8526-25: Unit dose, 10 capsules per strip, 10 strips per shelf pack, 10 shelf packs per shipper.
(For Institutional Use Only).
NDC 0054-2526-25: Bottles of 100 capsules.

300 mg flesh-colored capsules (size 2) (Identified 54 463).

NDC 0054-8527-25: Unit dose, 10 capsules per strip, 10 strips per shelf pack, 10 shelf packs per shipper.
(For Institutional Use Only).
NDC 0054-2527-25: Bottles of 100 capsules.
NDC 0054-2527-31: Bottles of 1000 capsules.

600 mg white opaque/flesh colored capsules (size 0) (Identified 54 702).

NDC 0054-8531-25: Unit dose, 10 capsules per strip, 10 strips per shelf pack, 10 shelf packs per shipper.
(For Institutional Use Only.)
NDC 0054-2531-25: Bottles of 100 capsules.
NDC 0054-2531-31: Bottles of 1000 capsules.

Caution: Federal law prohibits dispensing without prescription.

4055500 Revised March 1994
034

LITHIUM CITRATE SYRUP USP ℞

8 mEq of Lithium per 5 mL, 16mEq of Lithium per 10 mL
SUGAR FREE
FOR ORAL ADMINISTRATION ONLY

DESCRIPTION

Lithium Citrate Syrup is a palatable oral dosage form of lithium ion. Lithium citrate is prepared in solution from lithium hydroxide and citric acid in a ratio approximating di-lithium citrate:

Each 5 mL of Lithium Citrate Syrup contains 8 mEq of lithium ion ($Li+$), equivalent to the amount of lithium in 300 mg of lithium carbonate and alcohol 0.3% v/v.

Inactive ingredients:

The syrup contains alcohol, sorbitol, flavoring, water, and other ingredients.

Lithium is an element of the alkali-metal group with atomic number 3, atomic weight 6.94, and an emission line at 671 nm on the flame photometer.

HOW SUPPLIED

Lithium Citrate Syrup, 8 mEq per 5 mL

NDC 0054-8529-04: Unit dose Patient Cup™ filled to deliver 5 mL, ten 5 mL Patient Cups™ per shelf pack, ten shelf packs per shipper. (For Institutional Use Only).
NDC 0054-3527-63: Bottles of 500 mL.

Lithium Citrate Syrup, 16 mEq per 10 mL

NDC 0054-8530-04: Unit dose Patient Cup™ filled to deliver 10 mL, ten 10 mL Patient Cups™ per shelf pack, ten shelf packs per shipper. (For Institutional Use Only).

Refer to Lithium Carbonate Capsules and Tablets heading for complete text.

MARINOL® Ⓒ ℞

(Dronabinol)
Capsules

(WARNING: May be habit forming)

DESCRIPTION

Dronabinol is a cannabinoid designated chemically as (6a*R*-*trans*)-6a,7,8,10a-tetrahydro-6,6,9-trimethyl-3-pentyl-6*H* -dibenzo[b,*d*]pyran-1-ol. Dronabinol has the following empirical and structural formulas:

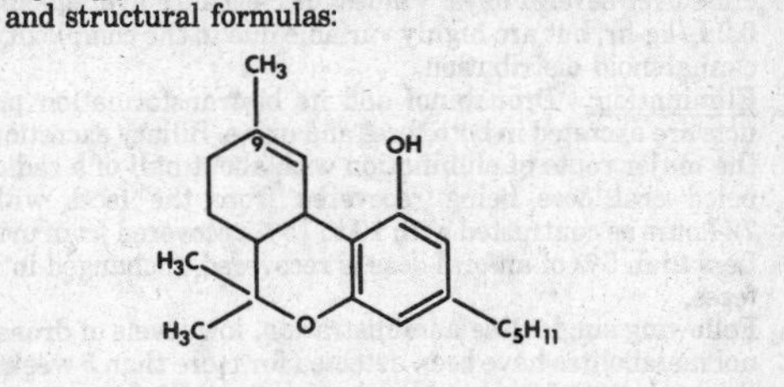

$C_{21}H_{30}O_2$ (molecular weight = 314.47)

Dronabinol, delta-9-tetrahydrocannabinol (delta-9-THC), is naturally-occurring and has been extracted from *Cannabis sativa* L. (marijuana).

Dronabinol is also chemically synthesized and is a light-yellow resinous oil that is sticky at room temperature and hardens upon refrigeration. Dronabinol is insoluble in water and is formulated in sesame oil. It has a pK_a of 10.6 and an octanol-water partition coefficient: 6,000:1 at pH7.

Capsules for oral administration: Marinol is supplied as round, soft gelatin capsules containing either 2.5 mg, 5 mg, or 10 mg dronabinol. Each Marinol capsule is formulated with the following inactive ingredients: sesame oil, gelatin, glycerin, methylparaben, propylparaben, and titanium dioxide.

CLINICAL PHARMACOLOGY

Dronabinol is an orally active cannabinoid which, like other cannabinoids, has complex effects on the central nervous system (CNS), including central sympathomimetic activity. Cannabinoid receptors have been discovered in neural tissues. These receptors may play a role in mediating the effects of dronabinol and other cannabinoids.

Pharmacodynamics: Dronabinol-induced sympathomimetic activity may result in tachycardia and/or conjunctival injection. Its effects on blood pressure are inconsistent, but occasional subjects have experienced orthostatic hyptotension and/or syncope upon abrupt standing.

Dronabinol also demonstrates reversible effects on appetite, mood, cognition, memory, and perception. These phenomena appear to be dose-related, increasing in frequency with higher dosages, and subject to great interpatient variability.

After oral administration, dronabinol has an onset of action of approximately 0.5 to 1 hours and peak effect at 2 to 4 hours. Duration of action for psychoactive effects is 4 to 6 hours, but the appetite stimulant effect of dronabinol may continue for 24 hours or longer after administration.

Continued on next page

Roxane Laboratories—Cont.

Tachyphylaxis and tolerance develop to some of the pharmacologic effects of dronabinol and other cannabinoids with chronic use, suggesting an indirect effect on sympathetic neurons. In a study of the pharmacodynamics of chronic dronabinol exposure, healthy male volunteers (N=12) received 210 mg/day dronabinol, administered orally in divided doses, for 16 days. An initial tachycardia induced by dronabinol was replaced successively by normal sinus rhythm and then bradycardia. A decrease in supine blood pressure, made worse by standing, was also observed initially. These volunteers developed tolerance to the cardiovascular and subjective adverse CNS effects of dronabinol within 12 days of treatment initiation.

Tachyphylaxis and tolerance do not, however, appear to develop to the appetite stimulant effect of Marinol. In studies involving patients with Acquired Immune Deficiency Syndrome (AIDS), the appetite stimuant effect of Marinol has been sustained for up to five months in clinical trials, at dosages ranging from 2.5 mg/day to 20 mg/day.

Pharmacokinetics:

Absorption and Distribution: Marinol (dronabinol) is almost completely absorbed (90 to 95%) after single oral doses. Due to the combined effects of first pass hepatic metabolism and high lipid solubility, only 10 to 20% of the administered dose reaches the systemic circulation. Dronabinol has a large apparent volume of distribution, approximately 10 L/kg, because of its lipid solubility. The plasma protein binding of dronabinol and its metabolites is approximately 97%.

The elimination phase of dronabinol can be described using a two compartment model with an initial (alpha) half-life of about 4 hours and a terminal (beta) half-life of 25 to 36 hours. Because of its large volume of distribution, dronabinol and its metabolites may be excreted at low levels for prolonged periods of time.

Metabolism: Dronabinol undergoes extensive first-pass hepatic metabolism, primarily by microsomal hydroxylation, yielding both active and inactive metabolites. Dronabinol and its principal active metabolite, 11-OH-delta-9-THC, are present in approximately equal concentrations in plasma. Concentrations of both parent drug and metabolite peak at approximately 2 to 4 hours after oral dosing and decline over several days. Values for clearance average about 0.2 L/kg-hr, but are highly variable due to the complexity of cannabinoid distribution.

Elimination: Dronabinol and its biotransformation products are excreted in both feces and urine. Biliary excretion is the major route of elimination with about half of a radiolabeled oral dose being recovered from the feces within 72 hours as contrasted with 10 to 15% recovered from urine. Less than 5% of an oral dose is recovered unchanged in the feces.

Following single dose administration, low levels of dronabinol metabolites have been detected for more than 5 weeks in the urine and feces.

In a study of Marinol involving AIDS patients, urinary cannabinoid/creatinine concentration ratios were studied biweekly over a six week period. The urinary cannabinoid/creatinine ratio was closely correlated with dose. No increase in the cannabinoid/creatinine ratio was observed after the first two weeks of treatment, indicating that steady-state cannabinoid levels had been reached. This conclusion is consistent with predictions based on the observed terminal half-life of dronabinol.

Special Populations: The pharmacokinetic profile of Marinol has not been investigated in either pediatric or geriatric patients.

CLINICAL TRIALS

Appetite Stimulation: The appetite stimulant effect of Marinol (dronabinol) in the treatment of AIDS-related anorexia associated with weight loss was studied in a randomized, double-blind, placebo-controlled study involving 139 patients. The initial dosage of Marinol in all patients was 5 mg/day, administered in doses of 2.5 mg one hour before lunch and one hour before supper. In pilot studies, early morning administration of Marinol appeared to have been associated with an increased frequency of adverse experiences, as compared to dosing later in the day. The effect of Marinol on appetite, weight, mood, and nausea was measured at scheduled intervals during the six-week treatment period. Side effects (feeling high, dizziness, confusion, somnolence) occurred in 13 to 72 patients (18%) at this dosage level and the dosage was reduced to 2.5 mg/day, administered as a single dose at supper or bedtime.

As compared to placebo, Marinol treatment resulted in a statistically significant improvement in appetite as measured by visual analog scale (see figure). Trends toward improved body weight and mood, and decreases in nausea were also seen.

After completing the 6-week study, patients were allowed to continue treatment with Marinol in an open-label study, in which there was a sustained improvement in appetite.

[See Figure at top of next column.]

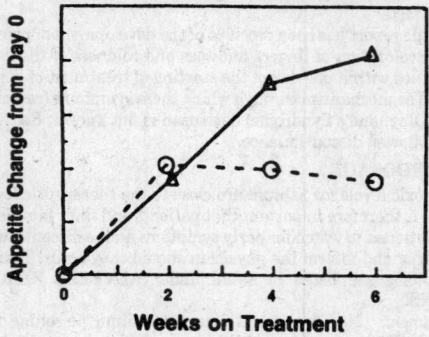

Appetite Change from Baseline

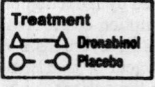

Treatment
△—△ Dronabinol
○--○ Placebo

Antiemetic: Marinol (dronabinol) treatment of chemotherapy-induced emesis was evaluated in 454 patients with cancer, who received a total of 750 courses of treatment of various malignancies. The antiemetic efficacy of Marinol was greatest in patients receiving cytotoxic therapy with MOPP for Hodgkin's and non-Hodgkin's lymphomas. Marinol dosages ranged from 2.5 mg/day to 40 mg/day, administered in equally divided doses every four to six hours (four times daily). As indicated in the following table, escalating the Marinol dose above 7 mg/m² increased the frequency of adverse experiences, with no additional antiemetic benefit.

Marinol Dose: Response Frequency and Adverse Experiences*
(N=750 treatment courses)

Marinol Dose	Response Frequency (%)			Adverse Events Frequency (%)		
	Complete	Partial	Poor	None	Nondysphoric	Dysphoric
<7 mg/m²	36	32	32	23	65	12
>7 mg/m²	33	31	36	13	58	28

* Nondysphoric events consisted of drowsiness, tachycardia, etc.

Combination antiemetic therapy with Marinol and a phenothiazine (prochlorperazine) may result in synergistic or additive antiemetic effects and attenuate the toxicities associated with each of the agents.

INDIVIDUALIZATION OF DOSAGES

The pharmacologic effects of Marinol (dronabinol) are dose-related and subject to considerable interpatient variability. Therefore, dosage individualization is critical in achieving the maximum benefit of Marinol treatment.

Appetite Stimulation: In the clinical trials, the majority of patients were treated with 5 mg/day Marinol, although the dosages ranged from 2.5 to 20 mg/day. For an adult:

1. Begin with 2.5 mg before lunch and 2.5 mg before supper. If CNS symptoms (feeling high, dizziness, confusion, somnolence) do occur, they usually resolve in 1 to 3 days with continued dosage.
2. If CNS symptoms are severe or persistent, reduce the dose to 2.5 mg before supper. If symptoms continue to be a problem, taking the single dose in the evening or at bedtime may reduce their severity.
3. When adverse effects are absent or minimal and further therapeutic effect is desired, increase the dose to 2.5 mg before lunch and 5 mg before supper or 5 and 5 mg. Although most patients respond to 2.5 mg twice daily, 10 mg twice daily has been tolerated in about half of the patients in appetite stimulation studies.

The pharmacologic effects of Marinol are reversible upon treatment cessation.

Antiemetic: Most patients respond to 5 mg three or four times daily. Dosage may be escalated during a chemotherapy cycle or at subsequent cycles, based upon initial results. Therapy should be initiated at the lowest recommended dosage and titrated to clinical response. Administration of Marinol with phenothiazines, such as prochlorperazine, has resulted in improved efficacy as compared to either drug alone, without additional toxicity.

Pediatrics: Marinol is not recommended for AIDS-related anorexia in pediatric patients because it has not been studied in this population. The pediatric dosage for the treatment of chemotherapy-induced emesis is the same as in adults. Caution is recommended in prescribing Marinol for children because of the psychoactive effects.

Geriatrics: Caution is advised in prescribing Marinol in elderly patients because they are generally more sensitive to the psychoactive effects of drugs. In antiemetic studies, no difference in tolerance or efficacy was apparent in patients >55 years old.

INDICATIONS AND USAGE

Marinol (dronabinol) is indicated for the treatment of:
1. anorexia associated with weight loss in patients with AIDS; and
2. nausea and vomiting associated with cancer chemotherapy in patients who have failed to respond adequately to conventional antiemetic treatments.

CONTRAINDICATIONS

Marinol (dronabinol) is contraindicated in any patient who has a history of hypersensitivity to any cannabinoid or sesame oil.

WARNINGS

Marinol (dronabinol) is a medication with a potential for abuse. Physicians and pharmacists should use the same care in prescribing and accounting for Marinol as they would with morphine or other drugs controlled under Schedule II (CII) of the Controlled Substances Act. Because of the risk of diversion, it is recommended that prescriptions be limited to the amount necessary for the period between clinic visits. Patients receiving treatment with Marinol should be specifically warned not to drive, operate machinery, or engage in any hazardous activity until it is established that they are able to tolerate the drug and to perform such tasks safely.

PRECAUTIONS

General: The risk/benefit ratio of Marinol (dronabinol) use should be carefully evaluated in patients with the following medical conditions because of individual variation in response and tolerance to the effects of Marinol.

Marinol should be used with caution in patients with cardiac disorders because of occasional hypotension, possible hypertension, syncope, or tachycardia (see CLINICAL PHARMACOLOGY).

Marinol should be used with caution in patients with a history of substance abuse, including alcohol abuse or dependence, because they may be more prone to abuse Marinol as well. Multiple substance abuse is common and marijuana, which contains the same active compound, is a frequently abused substance.

Marinol should be used with caution and careful psychiatric monitoring in patients with mania, depression, or schizophrenia because Marinol may exacerbate these illnesses.

Marinol should be used with caution in patients receiving concomitant therapy with sedatives, hypnotics or other psychoactive drugs because of the potential for additive or synergistic CNS effects.

Marinol should be used with caution in pregnant patients, nursing mothers, or pediatric patients because it has not been studied in these patient populations.

Marinol should be used with caution for treatment of anorexia and weight loss in elderly patients with AIDS because they may be more sensitive to the psychoactive effects and because its use in these patients has not been studied.

Information for Patients: Patients receiving treatment with Marinol (dronabinol) should be alerted to the potential for additive central nervous system depression if Marinol is used concomitantly with alcohol or other CNS depressants such as benzodiazepines and barbiturates.

Patients receiving treatment with Marinol should be specifically warned not to drive, operate machinery, or engage in any hazardous activity until it is established that they are able to tolerate the drug and to perform such tasks safely. Patients using Marinol should be advised of possible changes in mood and other adverse behavioral effects of the drug so as to avoid panic in the event of such manifestations. Patients should remain under the supervision of a responsible adult during initial use of Marinol and following dosage adjustments.

Drug Interactions: In studies involving patients with AIDS and/or cancer, Marinol (dronabinol) has been co-administered with a variety of medications (e.g., cytotoxic agents, anti-infective agents, sedatives, or opioid analgesics) without resulting in any clinically significant drug/drug interactions. Although no drug/drug interactions were discovered during the clincial trials of Marinol, cannabinoids may interact with other medications through both metabolic and pharmacodynamic mechanisms. Dronabinol is highly protein bound to plasma proteins, and therefore, might displace other protein-bound drugs. Although this displacement has not been confirmed *in vivo*, practitioners should monitor patients for a change in dosage requirements when administering dronabinol to patients receiving other highly protein-bound drugs. Published reports of drug/drug interactions involving cannabinoids are summarized in the following table.

CONCOMITANT DRUG	CLINICAL EFFECT(S)
Amphetamines, cocaine, other sympathomimetic agents	Additive hypertension, tachycardia possibly cardiotoxicity

Atropine, scopolamine, antihistamines, other anticholinergic agents	Additive or super-additive tachycardia, drowsiness
Amitriptyline, amoxapine, desipramine, other tricyclic antidepressants	Additive tachycardia, hypertension, drowsiness
Barbiturates, benzodiazepines, ethanol, lithium, opioids, buspirone, antihistamines, muscle relaxants, other CNS depressants	Additive drowsiness and CNS depression
Disulfiram	A reversible hypomanic reaction was reported in a 28 y/o man who smoked marijuana; confirmed by dechallenge and rechallenge
Fluoxetine	A 21 y/o female with depression and bulimia receiving 20 mg/day fluoxetine × 4 wks became hypomanic after smoking marijuana; symptoms resolved after 4 days
Antipyrine, barbiturates	Decreased clearance of these agents, presumably via competitive inhibition of metabolism
Theophylline	Increased theophylline metabolism reported with smoking of marijuana; effect similar to that following smoking tobacco

Carcinogenesis, Mutagenesis, Impairment of Fertility: Carcinogenicity studies have not been performed with dronabinol. Mutagenicity testing of dronabinol was negative in an Ames test. In a long-term study (77 days) in rats, oral administration of dronabinol at doses of 30 to 150 mg/m^2, equivalent to 0.3 to 1.5 times maximum recommended human dose (MRHD) of 90 mg/m^2/day in cancer patients or 2 to 10 times MRHD of 15 mg/m^2/day in AIDS patients, reduced ventral prostate, seminal vesicle and epididymal weights and caused a decrease in seminal fluid volume. Decreases in spermatogenesis, number of developing germ cells, and number of Leydig cells in the testis were also observed. However, sperm count, mating success and testosterone levels were not affected. The significance of these animal findings in humans is not known.

Pregnancy: Pregnancy Category C. Reproduction studies with dronabinol have been performed in mice at 15 to 450 mg/m^2, equivalent to 0.2 to 5 times maximum recommended human dose (MRHD) of 90 mg/m^2/day in cancer patients or 1 to 30 times MRHD of 15 mg/m^2/day in AIDS patients, and in rats at 74 to 295 mg/m^2 (equivalent to 0.8 to 3 times MRHD of 90 mg/m^2 in cancer patients or 5 to 20 times MRHD of 15 mg/m^2/day in AIDS patients). These studies have revealed no evidence of teratogenicity due to dronabinol. At these dosages in mice and rats, dronabinol decreased maternal weight gain and number of viable pups and increased fetal mortality and early resorptions. Such effects were dose dependent and less apparent at lower doses which produced less maternal toxicity. There are no adequate and well-controlled studies in pregnant women. Dronabinol should be used only if the potential benefit justifies the potential risk to the fetus.

Nursing Mothers: Use of Marinol is not recommended in nursing mothers since, in addition to the secretion of HIV virus in breast milk, dronabinol is concentrated in and secreted in human breast milk and is absorbed by the nursing baby.

ADVERSE REACTIONS

Adverse experiences information summarized in the tables below was derived from well-controlled clinical trials conducted in the US and US territories involving 474 patients exposed to Marinol (dronabinol). Studies of AIDS-related weight loss included 157 patients receiving dronabinol at a dose of 2.5 mg twice daily and 67 receiving placebo. Studies of different durations were combined by considering the first occurrence of events during the first 28 days. Studies of nausea and vomiting related to cancer chemotherapy included 317 patients receiving dronabinol and 68 receiving placebo.

A cannabinoid dose-related "high" (easy laughing, elation and heightened awareness) has been reported by patients receiving Marinol in both the antiemetic (24%) and the lower dose appetite stimulant clinical trials (8%) (see CLINICAL TRIALS).

The most frequently reported adverse experiences in patients with AIDS during placebo-controlled clinical trials involved the CNS and were reported by 33% of patients receiving Marinol. About 25% of patients reported a minor CNS adverse event during the first 2 weeks and about 4% reported such an event each week for the next 6 weeks thereafter.

PROBABLY CAUSALLY RELATED: Incidence greater than 1%.

Rates derived from clinical trials in AIDS-related anorexia (N=157) and chemotherapy-related nausea (N=317). Rates were generally higher in the anti-emetic use (given in parentheses).

Body as a whole: Asthenia.
Cardiovascular. Palpitations, tachycardia, vasodilation/facial flush.
Digestive: Abdominal pain*, nausea*, vomiting*.
Nervous system: (Amnesia), anxiety/nervousness, (ataxia), confusion, depersonalization, dizziness*, euphoria*, (hallucination), paranoid reaction*, somnolence*, thinking abnormal*.

*Incidence of events 3% to 10%

PROBABLY CAUSALLY RELATED: Incidence less than 1%.
Event rates derived from clinical trials in AIDS-related anorexia (N=157) and chemotherapy-related nausea (N=317).

Cardiovascular: Conjunctivitis*, hypotension*.
Digestive: Diarrhea*, fecal incontinence.
Musculoskeletal: Myalgias.
Nervous system: Depression, nightmares, speech difficulties, tinnitus.
Skin and Appendages: Flushing*.
Special senses: Vision difficulties.

*Incidence of events 0.3% to 1%.

CAUSAL RELATIONSHIP UNKNOWN: Incidence less than 1%.
The clinical significance of the association of these events with Marinol treatment is unknown, but they are reported as alerting information for the clinician.

Body as a whole: Chills, headache, malaise.
Digestive: Anorexia, hepatic enzyme elevation.
Respiratory: Cough, rhinitis, sinusitis.
Skin and Appendages: Sweating.

DRUG ABUSE AND DEPENDENCE

Marinol (dronabinol) is one of the psychoactive compounds present in cannabis, and is abusable and controlled Schedule II (CII) under the Controlled Substances Act. Both psychological and physiological dependence have been noted in healthy individuals receiving dronabinol, but addiction is uncommon and has only been seen after prolonged high dose administration.

Chronic abuse of cannabis has been associated with decrements in motivation, cognition, judgement, and perception. The etiology of these impairments is unknown, but may be associated with the complex process of addiction rather than an isolated effect of the drug. No such decrements in psychological, social or neurological status have been associated with the administration of Marinol for therapeutic purposes. In an open-label study in patients with AIDS who received Marinol for up to five months, no abuse, diversion or systematic change in personality or social functioning were observed despite the inclusion of a substantial number of patients with a past history of drug abuse.

An abstinence syndrome has been reported after the abrupt discontinuation of dronabinol in volunteers receiving dosages of 210 mg/day for 12 to 16 consecutive days. Within 12 hours after discontinuation, these volunteers manifested symptoms such as irritability, insomnia, and restlessness. By approximately 24 hours post-dronabinol discontinuation, withdrawal symptoms intensified to include "hot flashes", sweating, rhinorrhea, loose stools, hiccoughs and anorexia. These withdrawal symptoms gradually dissipated over the next 48 hours. Electroencephalographic changes consistent with the effects of drug withdrawal (hyperexcitation) were recorded in patients after abrupt dechallenge. Patients also complained of disturbed sleep for several weeks after discontinuing therapy with high dosages of dronabinol.

OVERDOSAGE

Signs and symptoms following MILD Marinol (dronabinol) intoxication include drowsiness, euphoria, heightened sensory awareness, altered time perception, reddened conjunctiva, dry mouth and tachycardia; following MODERATE intoxication include memory impairment, depersonalization, mood alteration, urinary retention, and reduced bowel motility; and following SEVERE intoxication include decreased motor coordination, lethargy, slurred speech, and postural hypotension. Apprehensive patients may experience panic reactions and seizures may occur in patients with existing seizure disorders.

The estimated lethal human dose of intravenous dronabinol is 30 mg/kg (2100 mg/70kg). Significant CNS symptoms in antiemetic studies followed oral doses of 0.4 mg/kg (28 mg/70 kg) of Marinol.

Management: A potentially serious oral ingestion, if recent, should be managed with gut decontamination. In unconscious patients with a secure airway, instill activated charcoal (30 to 100 g in adults, 1 to 2 g/kg in infants) via a nasogastric tube. A saline cathartic or sorbitol may be added to the first dose of activated charcoal. Patients experiencing depressive, hallucinatory or psychotic reactions should be placed in a quiet area and offered reassurance. Benzodiazepines (5 to 10 mg diazepam *po*) may be used for treatment of extreme agitation. Hypotension usually responds to Trendelenburg position and IV fluids. Pressors are rarely required.

DOSAGE AND ADMINISTRATION

Appetite stimulation: Initially, 2.5 mg Marinol (dronabinol) should be administered orally twice daily (b.i.d.) before lunch and supper. For patients unable to tolerate this 5 mg/day dosage of Marinol, the dosage can be reduced to 2.5 mg/day, administered as a single dose in the evening or at bedtime. If clinically indicated and in the absence of significant adverse effects, the dosage may be gradually increased to a maximum of 20 mg/day Marinol, administered in divided oral doses. Caution should be exercised in escalating the dosage of Marinol because of the increased frequency of dose-related adverse experiences at higher dosages (see PRECAUTIONS).

Antiemetic: Marinol is best administered at an initial dose of 5 mg/m^2, given 1 to 3 hours prior to the administration of chemotherapy, then every 2 to 4 hours after chemotherapy is given, for a total of 4 to 6 doses/day. Should the 5 mg/m^2 dose prove to be ineffective, and in the absence of significant side effects, the dose may be escalated by 2.5 mg/m^2 increments to a maximum of 15 mg/m^2 per dose. Caution should be exercised in dose escalation, however, as the incidence of disturbing psychiatric symptoms increases significantly at maximum dose (see PRECAUTIONS).

SAFETY AND HANDLING

Marinol (dronabinol) should be packaged in a well-closed container and stored in a cool environment between 8° and 15°C (46° and 59°F). Protect from freezing. No particular hazard to health care workers handling the capsules has been identified.

Access to abusable drugs such as Marinol presents an occupational hazard for addiction in the health care industry. Routine procedures for handling controlled substances developed to protect the public may not be adequate to protect health care workers. Implementation of more effective accounting procedures and measures to appropriately restrict access to drugs of this class may minimize the risk of self-administration by health care providers.

HOW SUPPLIED

MARINOL® CAPSULES (dronabinol solution in sesame oil in soft gelatin capsules)
2.5 mg white capsules (Identified RL).
NDC 0054-2601-11: Bottles of 25 capsules.
NDC 0054-2601-21: Bottles of 60 capsules.
NDC 0054-2601-25: Bottles of 100 capsules.
5 mg dark brown capsules (Identified RL).
NDC 0054-2602-11: Bottles of 25 capsules.
NDC 0054-2602-25: Bottles of 100 capsules.
10 mg orange capsules (Identified RL).
NDC 0054-2603-11: Bottles of 25 capsules.

MARINOL® is a registered trademark of Unimed Pharmaceuticals Inc. and is marketed by Roxane Laboratories, Inc. under license from Unimed Pharmaceuticals, Inc.
Manufactured by Banner Gelatin Products Corporation, Chatsworth CA 91311

DEA ORDER FORM REQUIRED
Caution: Federal law prohibits dispensing without prescription.

4056050 Revised December 1994
124

Roxane
Laboratories, Inc.
Columbus, Ohio 43216
Shown in Product Identification Guide, page 332

METHADONE HYDROCHLORIDE Ⓒ℞

[*mĕth′ă-dōn hī-drō- klō-rīd*]
DISKETS® (dispersible tablets)
Tablets, USP
(*See also* **Dolophine® Hydrochloride**)

DESCRIPTION

Each tablet for oral administration contains:
Methadone Hydrochloride .... 40 mg
(Warning: May be habit forming)

Continued on next page

Roxane Laboratories—Cont.

Inactive Ingredients:
The dispersible tablets contain magnesium stearate, microcrystalline cellulose, and starch (corn). The Diskets® contain cellulose, FD&C Yellow No. 6, flavors, magnesium stearate, potassium phosphate, silicon dioxide, cornstarch, and stearic acid.
Methadone hydrochloride is a white crystalline material which is water soluble. However, the methadone hydrochloride dispersible tablets have been specially formulated with insoluble excipients to deter the use of this drug by injection.
Chemically, Methadone Hydrochloride is 6-(Dimethylamino)-4,4-diphenyl-3-heptanone hydrochloride, which can be represented by the following structural formula:

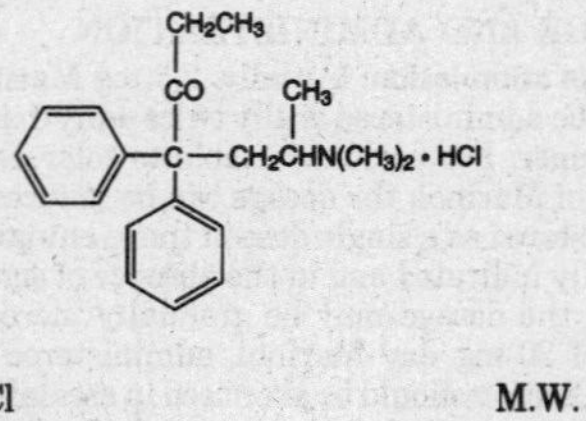

$C_{21}H_{27}NO \cdot HCl$ M.W. 345.91

HOW SUPPLIED

Methadone Hydrochloride
Tablets USP (Dispersible), 40 mg
40 mg white cross-scored tablets (identified 54 843).
NDC 0054-8547-25: Unit dose, 20 tablets per card (reverse numbered), 5 cards per shipper.
NDC 0054-4547-25: Bottles of 100 tablets.
Methadone Hydrochloride
Tablets USP, 40 mg Diskets®
40 mg peach-colored, cross-scored tablets (identified 54 883).
NDC 0054-4538-25: Bottles of 100 tablets.
Store at Controlled Room Temperature
15°–30°C (59°–86°F)
Dispense in a well-closed container as defined in the USP/NF, with a child-resistant closure.
Caution: Federal law prohibits dispensing without prescription.
4056070

Revised
025 February 1995

METHADONE HYDROCHLORIDE ℂ ℞

Oral Concentrate USP
10 mg per mL
For Methadone Treatment Programs Only

(Warning: May be habit forming)

CONDITIONS FOR DISTRIBUTION
AND USE OF METHADONE PRODUCTS:
Code of Federal Regulations,
Title 21, Sec. 291.505

METHADONE PRODUCTS, WHEN USED FOR TREATMENT OF NARCOTIC ADDICTION IN DETOXIFICATION OR MAINTENANCE PROGRAMS, SHALL BE DISPENSED ONLY BY APPROVED HOSPITAL PHARMACIES, APPROVED COMMUNITY PHARMACIES, AND MAINTENANCE PROGRAMS APPROVED BY THE FOOD AND DRUG ADMINISTRATION AND THE DESIGNATED STATE AUTHORITY.
APPROVED MAINTENANCE PROGRAMS SHALL DISPENSE AND USE METHADONE IN ORAL FORM ONLY AND ACCORDING TO THE TREATMENT REQUIREMENTS STIPULATED IN THE FEDERAL METHADONE REGULATIONS (21 CFR 291.505).
FAILURE TO ABIDE BY THE REQUIREMENTS IN THESE REGULATIONS MAY RESULT IN CRIMINAL PROSECUTION, SEIZURE OF THE DRUG SUPPLY, REVOCATION OF THE PROGRAM APPROVAL, AND INJUNCTION PRECLUDING OPERATION OF THE PROGRAM.

DESCRIPTION

Each mL for oral administration contains:
Methadone Hydrochloride .... 10 mg
(Warning: May be habit forming)
Each mL, for oral administration, contains 10 mg of (methadone hydrochloride. *Inactive ingredients:* sodium benzoate, citric acid, and water.

CLINICAL PHARMACOLOGY

Methadone Hydrochloride is a synthetic narcotic analgesic with multiple actions quantitatively similar to those of morphine, the most prominent of which involve the central nervous system and organs composed of smooth muscle. The principal actions of therapeutic value are analgesia and sedation, detoxification or maintenance in narcotic addiction. The methadone abstinence syndrome, although qualitatively similar to that of morphine, differs in that the onset is slower, the course is more prolonged, and the symptoms are less severe.
When administered orally, methadone is approximately one-half as potent as when given parenterally. Oral administration results in a delay of the onset, a lowering of the peak, and an increase in the duration of analgesic effect.

INDICATIONS AND USAGE

1. Detoxification treatment of narcotic addiction (heroin or other morphine-like drugs).
2. Maintenance treatment of narcotic addiction (heroin or other morphine-like drugs), in conjunction with appropriate social and medical services.

NOTE
If methadone is administered for treatment of heroin dependence for more than three weeks, the procedure passes from treatment of the acute withdrawal syndrome (detoxification) to maintenance therapy. Maintenance treatment is permitted to be undertaken only by approved methadone programs. This does not preclude the maintenance treatment of an addict who is hospitalized for medical conditions other than addiction and who requires temporary maintenance during the critical period of his stay or whose enrollment has been verified in a program which has approval for maintenance treatment with methadone.

CONTRAINDICATIONS

Hypersensitivity to methadone.

WARNINGS

Methadone Hydrochloride Oral Concentrate is for oral administration only. This preparation must not be injected. It is recommended that Methadone Hydrochloride Oral Concentrate, if dispensed, be packaged in child-resistant containers and kept out of the reach of children to prevent accidental ingestion.

Methadone Hydrochloride, a narcotic, is a Schedule II controlled substance under the Federal Controlled Substances Act. Appropriate security measures should be taken to safeguard stocks of methadone against diversion.
DRUG DEPENDENCE-METHADONE CAN PRODUCT DRUG DEPENDENCE OF THE MORPHINE TYPE AND, THEREFORE, HAS THE POTENTIAL FOR BEING ABUSED. PSYCHIC DEPENDENCE, PHYSICAL DEPENDENCE, AND TOLERANCE MAY DEVELOP UPON REPEATED ADMINISTRATION OF METHADONE, AND IT SHOULD BE PRESCRIBED AND ADMINISTERED WITH THE SAME DEGREE OF CAUTION APPROPRIATE TO THE USE OF MORPHINE.
Interaction with Other Central-Nervous-System Depressants—Methadone should be used with caution and in reduced dosage in patients who are concurrently receiving other narcotic analgesics, general anesthetics, phenothiazines, other tranquilizers, sedative-hyponotics, tricyclic antidepressants, and other C.N.S. depressants (including alcohol). Respiratory depression, hypotension, and profound sedation or coma may result.
Anxiety—Since methadone, as used by tolerant subjects at a constant maintenance dosage, is not a tranquilizer, patients who are maintained on this drug will react to life problems and stresses with the same symptoms of anxiety as do other individuals. The physician should not confuse such symptoms with those of narcotic abstinence and should not attempt to treat anxiety by increasing the dosage of methadone. The action of methadone in maintenance treatment is limited to the control of narcotic symptoms and is ineffective for relief of general anxiety.
Head Injury and Increased Intracranial Pressure—The respiratory depressant effects of methadone and its capacity to elevate cerebrospinal-fluid pressure may be markedly exaggerated in the presence of increased intracranial pressure. Furthermore, narcotics produce side effects that may obscure the clinical course of patients with headinjuries. In such patients, methadone must be used with caution and only if it is deemed essential.
Asthma and Other Respiratory Conditions—Methadone should be used with caution in patients having an acute asthmatic attack, in those with chronic obstructive pulmonary disease or cor pulmonale, and in individuals with a substantially decreased respiratory reserve, preexisting respiratory depression, hypoxia, or hypercapnia. In such patients, even usual therapeutic doses of narcotics may decrease respiratory drive while simultaneously increasing airway resistance to the point of apnea.
Hypotensive Effect—The administration of methadone may result in severe hypotension in an individual whose ability to maintain his blood pressure has already been compromised by a depleted blood volume or concurrent administration of such drugs as the phenothiazines or certain anesthetics.
Use in Ambulatory Patients—Methadone may impair the mental and/or physical abilities required for the performance of potentially hazardous tasks, such as driving a car or operating machinery. The patient should be cautioned accordingly.
Methadone, like other narcotics, may produce orthostatic hypotension in ambulatory patients.
Use in Pregnancy—Safe use in pregnancy has not been established in relation to possible adverse effects on fetal development. Therefore, methadone should not be used in pregnant women unless, in the judgment of the physician, the potential benefits outweigh the possible hazards.

PRECAUTIONS

Interaction with Pentazocine—Patients who are addicted to heroin or who are on the methadone maintenance program may experience withdrawal symptoms when given pentazocine.
Interaction with Rifampin—The concurrent administration of rifampin may possibly reduce the blood concentration of methadone to a degree sufficient to produce withdrawal symptoms. The mechanism by which rifampin may decrease blood concentrations of methadone is not fully understood although enhanced microsomal drug-metabolized enzymes may influence drug disposition.
Interaction with Monoamine Oxidase (MAO) Inhibitors—Therapeutic doses of meperidine have precipitated severe reactions in patients concurrently receiving monoamine oxidase inhibitors or those who have received such agents within 14 days. Similar reactions thus far have not been reported with methadone; but if the use of methadone is necessary in such patients, a sensitivity test should be performed in which repeated small incremental doses are administered over the course of several hours while the patient's condition and vital signs are under careful observation.
Acute Abdominal Conditions—The administration of methadone or other narcotics may obscure the diagnosis or clinical course of patients with acute abdominal conditions.
Special-Risk Patients—Methadone should be given with caution and the initial dose should be reduced in certain patients, such as the elderly or debilitated and those with severe impairment of hepatic or renal function, hypothyroidism, Addison's disease, prostatic hypertrophy, or urethral stricture.

ADVERSE REACTIONS

Heroin Withdrawal—During the induction phase of methadone maintenance treatment, patients are being withdrawn from heroin and may therefore show typical withdrawal symptoms, which should be differentiated from methadone-induced side effects. They may exhibit some or all of the following symptoms associated with acute withdrawal from heroin or other opiates: lacrimation, rhinorrhea, sneezing, yawning, excessive perspiration, goose-flesh, fever, chilliness alternating with flushing, restlessness, irritability, "sleepy yen", weakness, anxiety, depression, dilated pupils, tremors, tachycardia, abdominal cramps, body aches, involuntary twitching and kicking movements, anorexia, nausea, vomiting, diarrhea, intestinal spasms, and weight loss.
Initial Administration—Initially, the dosage of methadone should be carefully titrated to the individual. Induction too rapid for the patient's sensitivity is more likely to produce the following effects.
THE MAJOR HAZARDS OF METHADONE, AS OF OTHER NARCOTIC ANALGESICS, ARE RESPIRATORY DEPRESSION AND, TO A LESSER DEGREE, CIRCULATORY DEPRESSION. RESPIRATORY ARREST, SHOCK, AND CARDIAC ARREST HAVE OCCURRED.
The most frequently observed adverse reactions include lightheadedness, dizziness, sedation, nausea, vomiting, and sweating. These effects seem to be more prominent in ambulatory patients and in those who are not suffering severe chronic pain. In such individuals, lower doses are advisable. Some adverse reactions may be alleviated in the ambulatory patient if he lies down.
Other adverse reactions include the following:
Central Nervous System—Euphoria, dysphoria, weakness, headache, insomnia, agitation, disorientation, and visual disturbances.
Gastrointestinal—Dry mouth, anorexia, constipation and biliary tract spasm.
Cardiovascular—Flushing of the face, bradycardia, palpitation, faintness, and syncope.
Genito-Urinary—Urinary retention or hesitancy, antidiuretic effect, and reduced libido and/or potency.
Allergic—Pruritus, urticaria, other skin rashes, edema, and, rarely hemorrhagic urticaria.
Maintenance on a Stabilized Dose—During prolonged administration of methadone, as in a methadone maintenance

treatment program, there is a gradual, yet progressive disappearance of side effects over a period of several weeks. However, constipation and sweating often persist.

OVERDOSAGE

Symptoms—Serious overdosage of methadone is characterized by respiratory depression (a decrease in respiratory rate and/or tidal volume, Cheyne-Stokes respiration, cyanosis), extreme somnolence progressing to stupor or coma, maximally constricted pupils, skeletal-muscle flaccidity, cold and clammy skin, and, sometimes, bradycardia and hypotension. In severe overdosage, particularly by the intravenous route, apnea, circulatory collapse, cardiac arrest, and death may occur.

Treatment—Primary attention should be given to the reestablishment of adequate respiratory exchange through provision of a patent airway and institution of assisted or controlled ventilation. If a non-tolerant person, especially a child, takes a large dose of methadone, effective narcotic antagonists are available to counter-act the potentially lethal respiratory depression. THE PHYSICIAN MUST REMEMBER, HOWEVER, THAT METHADONE IS A LONG-ACTING DEPRESSANT (THIRTY-SIX TO FORTY-EIGHT HOURS), WHEREAS THE ANTAGONISTS ACT FOR MUCH SHORTER PERIODS (ONE TO THREE HOURS). The patient must, therefore, be monitored continuously for recurrence of respiratory depression and treated repeatedly with the narcotic antagonist as needed. If the diagnosis is correct and respiratory depression is due only to overdosage of methadone, the use of respiratory stimulants is not indicated.

An antagonist should not be administered in the absence of clinically significant respiratory or cardiovascular depression. Intravenously administered narcotic antagonists, naloxone hydrochloride, nalorphine hydrochloride, or levallorphan tartrate are the drugs of choice to reverse signs of intoxication. These agents should be given repeatedly until the patient's status remains satisfactory. The hazard that the narcotic antagonist will further depress respiration is less likely with the use of naloxone.

Oxygen, intravenous fluids, vasopressors, and other supportive measures should be employed as indicated.

NOTE: IN AN INDIVIDUAL PHYSICALLY DEPENDENT ON NARCOTICS, THE ADMINISTRATION OF THE USUAL DOSE OF A NARCOTIC ANTAGONIST WILL PRECIPITATE AN ACUTE WITHDRAWAL SYNDROME. THE SEVERITY OF THIS SYNDROME WILL DEPEND ON THE DEGREE OF PHYSICAL DEPENDENCE AND THE DOSE OF THE ANTAGONIST ADMINISTERED. THE USE OF A NARCOTIC ANTAGONIST IN SUCH A PERSON SHOULD BE AVOIDED IF POSSIBLE. IF IT MUST BE USED TO TREAT SERIOUS RESPIRATORY DEPRESSION IN THE PHYSICALLY DEPENDENT PATIENT, THE ANTAGONIST SHOULD BE ADMINISTERED WITH EXTREME CARE AND BY TITRATION WITH SMALLER THAN USUAL DOSES OF THE ANTAGONIST.

DOSAGE AND ADMINISTRATION

For Detoxification Treatment—THE DRUG SHALL BE ADMINISTERED DAILY UNDER CLOSE SUPERVISION AS FOLLOWS:

A detoxification treatment course shall not exceed 21 days and may not be repeated earlier than four weeks after completion of the preceding course.

In detoxification, the patient may receive methadone when there are significant symptoms of withdrawal. The dosage schedules indicated below are recommended but could be varied in accordance with clinical judgment. Initially, a single oral dose of 15 to 20 mg of methadone will often be sufficient to suppress withdrawal symptoms. Additional methadone may be provided if withdrawal symptoms are not suppressed or if symptoms reappear. When patients are physically dependent on high doses, it may be necessary to exceed these levels. Forty mg per day in single or divided doses will usually constitute an adequate stabilizing dosage level. Stabilization can be continued for two to three days, and then the amount of methadone normally will be gradually decreased. The rate at which methadone is decreased will be determined separately with each patient. The dose of methadone can be decreased on a daily basis or at two-day intervals, but the amount of intake shall always be sufficient to keep withdrawal symptoms at a tolerable level. In hospitalized patients, a daily reduction of 20 percent of the total daily dose may be tolerated and may cause little discomfort. In ambulatory patients, a somewhat slower schedule may be needed. If methadone is administered for more than three weeks, the procedure is considered to have progressed from detoxification or treatment of the acute withdrawal syndrome to maintenance treatment, even though the goal and intent may be eventual total withdrawal.

For Maintenance Treatment—In maintenance treatrespiratory depression, or other effects of acute intoxication. It is important that the initial dosage be adjusted on an individual basis to the narcotic tolerance of the new patient. If such a patient has been a heavy user of heroin up to the day of admission, he/she may be given 20 mg 4 to 8 hours later or 40 mg in a single oral dose. If the patient enters treatment with little or no narcotic tolerance (e.g., if he/she has recently been released from jail or other confinement), the initial dosage may be one-half these quantities. When there is any doubt, the smaller dose should be used initially. The patient should then be kept under observation, and, if symptoms of abstinence are distressing, additional 10 mg doses may be administered as needed. Subsequently, the dosage should be adjusted individually, as tolerated and required, up to a level of 120 mg daily. The patient will initially ingest the drug under observation daily, or at least 6 days a week, for the first 3 months. After demonstrating satisfactory adherence to the program regulations for at least 3 months, the patient may be permitted to reduce to 3 times weekly the occasions when he/she must ingest the drug under observation. The patient shall receive no more than a 2-day take-home supply. With continuing adherence to the program's requirements for at least 2 years, he/she may then be permitted twice-weekly visits to the program for drug ingestion under observation, with a 3-day take-home supply. A daily dose of 120 mg or more shall be justified in the medical record. Prior approval from state authority and the Food and Drug Administration is required for any dose above 120 mg administered at the clinic and for any dose above 100 mg to be taken at home. A regular review of dosage level should be made by the responsible physician, with careful consideration given to reduction of dosage as indicated on an individual basis. A new dosage level is only a test level until stability is achieved.

Special Considerations for a Pregnant Patient–Caution shall be taken in the maintenance treatment of pregnant patients. Dosage levels should be kept as low as possible if continued methadone treatment is deemed necessary. It is the responsibility of the program sponsor to assure that each female patient be fully informed concerning the possible risks to a pregnant woman or her unborn child from the use of methadone.

Special Limitations-

Treatment of Patients Under Age 18

1. The safety and effectiveness of methadone for use in the treatment of adolescents have not been proved by adequate clinical study. Special procedures are therefore necessary to assure that patients under age 16 will not be admitted to a program and that patients between 16 and 18 years of age will be admitted to maintenance treatment only under limited conditions.
2. Patients between 16 and 18 years of age who were enrolled and under treatment in approved programs on December 15, 1972, may continue in maintenance treatment. No new patients between 16 and 18 years of age may be admitted to a maintenance treatment program after March 15, 1973, unless a parent, legal guardian, or responsible adult designated by the state authority completes and signs Form FD 2635, "Consent for Methadone Treatment".
   Methadone treatment of new patients between the ages of 16 and 18 years will be permitted after December 15, 1972, only with a documented history of 2 or more unsuccessful attempts at detoxification and a documented history of dependence on heroin or other morphine-like drugs beginning 2 years or more prior to application for treatment. No patient under age 16 may be continued or started on methadone treatment after December 15, 1972, but these patients may be detoxified and retained in the program in a drug-free state for follow-up and aftercare.
3. Patients under age 18 who are not placed on maintenance treatment may be detoxified. Detoxification may not exceed 3 weeks. A repeat episode of detoxification may not be initiated until 4 weeks after the completion of the previous detoxification.

HOW SUPPLIED

Methadone Hydrochloride Oral Concentrate USP
10 mg per mL
Clear, flavorless solution.
NDC 0054-3553-67: Bottles of 32 fluid ounces (1 quart).
Store at Controlled Room Temperature
15°-30°C (59°-86°F)
Protect from light.
Dispense in a tight, light-resistant container as defined in the USP/NF.

Caution: Federal law prohibits dispensing without prescription.

4056321 Revised June 1994
064

Roxane Laboratories, Inc.
Columbus, Ohio 43216

METHADONE HYDROCHLORIDE ORAL SOLUTION USP TABLETS USP

Ⓒ℞

(WARNING: May be habit forming)

CONDITIONS FOR DISTRIBUTION AND USE OF METHADONE PRODUCTS:
Code of Federal Regulations,
Title 21, Sec. 291.505

METHADONE PRODUCTS, WHEN USED FOR TREATMENT OF NARCOTIC ADDICTION IN DETOXIFICATION OR MAINTENANCE PROGRAMS, SHALL BE DISPENSED ONLY BY APPROVED HOSPITAL PHARMACIES, APPROVED COMMUNITY PHARMACIES, AND MAINTENANCE PROGRAMS APPROVED BY THE FOOD AND DRUG ADMINISTRATION AND THE DESIGNATED STATE AUTHORITY.

APPROVED MAINTENANCE PROGRAMS SHALL DISPENSE AND USE METHADONE IN ORAL FORM ONLY AND ACCORDING TO THE TREATMENT REQUIREMENTS STIPULATED IN THE FEDERAL METHADONE REGULATIONS (21 CFR 291.505).

FAILURE TO ABIDE BY THE REQUIREMENTS IN THESE REGULATIONS MAY RESULT IN CRIMINAL PROSECUTION, SEIZURE OF THE DRUG SUPPLY, REVOCATION OF THE PROGRAM APPROVAL, AND INJUNCTION PRECLUDING OPERATION OF THE PROGRAM.

A METHADONE PRODUCT, WHEN USED AS AN ANALGESIC, MAY BE DISPENSED IN ANY LICENSED PHARMACY.

DESCRIPTION

Each 5 mL of Methadone Hydrochloride Oral Solution contains:
Methadone Hydrochloride .... 5 mg or 10 mg
(**Warning:** May be habit forming)
Alcohol 8%
Each tablet for oral administration contains:
Methadone Hydrochloride .... 5 mg or 10 mg
(**Warning:** May be habit forming)

Inactive Ingredients:
The oral solution contains alcohol, FD&C Red No. 40, FD&C Yellow No. 6, flavoring, glycol, sorbitol, water, and other ingredients.
The tablets contain magnesium stearate, microcrystalline cellulose, and starch (corn).
Chemically, Methadone Hydrochloride is 3-Heptanone, 6-(dimethylamino)-4,4-diphenyl-, hydrochloride.
Methadone Hydrochloride acts as a narcotic analgesic.

CLINICAL PHARMACOLOGY

Methadone Hydrochloride is a synthetic narcotic analgesic with multiple actions quantitatively similar to those of morphine, the most prominent of which involve the central nervous system and organs composed of smooth muscle. The principal actions of therapeutic value are analgesia and sedation and detoxification or temporary maintenance in narcotic addiction. The methadone abstinence syndrome, although qualitatively similar to that of morphine, differs in that the onset is slower, the course is more prolonged, and the symptoms are less severe.

When administered orally, methadone is approximately one-half as potent as when given parenterally. Oral administration results in a delay of the onset, a lowering of the peak, and an increase in the duration of analgesic effect.

INDICATIONS AND USAGE

Methadone Hydrochloride is indicated for relief of severe pain, for detoxification treatment of narcotic addiction, and for temporary maintenance treatment of narcotic addiction.

Note

If methadone is administered for treatment of heroin dependence for more than three weeks, the procedure passes from treatment of the acute withdrawal syndrome (detoxification) to maintenance therapy. Maintenance treatment is permitted to be undertaken only by approved methadone programs. This does not preclude the maintenance treatment of an addict who is hospitalized for medical conditions other than addiction and who requires temporary maintenance during the critical period of his stay or whose enrollment has been verified in a program which has approval for maintenance treatment with methadone.

CONTRAINDICATIONS

Hypersensitivity to methadone.

Continued on next page

Roxane Laboratories—Cont.

WARNINGS

> Methadone Hydrochloride Tablets are for oral administration only and *must not* be used for injection. It is recommended that Methadone Hydrochloride Tablets, if dispensed, be packaged in child-resistant containers and kept out of the reach of children to prevent accidental ingestion.

Methadone Hydrochloride, a narcotic, is a Schedule II controlled substance under the Federal Controlled Substances Act. Appropriate security measures should be taken to safeguard stocks of methadone against diversion.

DRUG DEPENDENCE — METHADONE CAN PRODUCE DRUG DEPENDENCE OF THE MORPHINE TYPE AND, THEREFORE, HAS THE POTENTIAL FOR BEING ABUSED. PSYCHIC DEPENDENCE, PHYSICAL DEPENDENCE, AND TOLERANCE MAY DEVELOP UPON REPEATED ADMINISTRATION OF METHADONE, AND IT SHOULD BE PRESCRIBED AND ADMINISTERED WITH THE SAME DEGREE OF CAUTION APPROPRIATE TO THE USE OF MORPHINE.

Interaction with Other Central-Nervous-System Depressants —Methadone should be used with caution and in reduced dosage in patients who are concurrently receiving other narcotic analgesics, general anesthetics, phenothiazines, other tranquilizers, sedative-hypnotics, tricyclic antidepressants, and other C.N.S. depressants (including alcohol). Respiratory depression, hypotension, and profound sedation or coma may result.

Anxiety —Since methadone, as used by tolerant subjects at a constant maintenance dosage, is not a tranquilizer, patients who are maintained on this drug will react to life problems and stresses with the same symptoms of anxiety as do other individuals. The physician should not confuse such symptoms with those of narcotic abstinence and should not attempt to treat anxiety by increasing the dosage of methadone. The action of methadone in maintenance treatment is limited to the control of narcotic symptoms and is ineffective for relief of general anxiety.

Head Injury and Increased Intracranial Pressure —The respiratory depressant effects of methadone and its capacity to elevate cerebrospinal-fluid pressure may be markedly exaggerated in the presence of increased intracranial pressure. Furthermore, narcotics produce side effects that may obscure the clinical course of patients with head injuries. In such patients, methadone must be used with caution and only if it is deemed essential.

Asthma and Other Respiratory Conditions— Methadone should be used with caution in patients having an acute asthmatic attack, in those with chronic obstructive pulmonary disease or cor pulmonale, and in individuals with a substantially decreased respiratory reserve, preexisting respiratory depression, hypoxia, or hypercapnia. In such patients, even usual therapeutic doses of narcotics may decrease respiratory drive while simultaneously increasing airway resistance to the point of apnea.

Hypotensive Effect —The administration of methadone may result in severe hypotension in an individual whose ability to maintain his blood pressure has already been compromised by a depleted blood volume or concurrent administration of such drugs as the phenothiazines or certain anesthetics.

Use in Ambulatory Patients —Methadone may impair the mental and/or physical abilities required for the performance of potentially hazardous tasks, such as driving a car or operating machinery. The patient should be cautioned accordingly.

Methadone, like other narcotics, may produce orthostatic hypotension in ambulatory patients.

Use in Pregnancy —Safe use in pregnancy has not been established in relation to possible adverse effects on fetal development. Therefore, methadone should not be used in pregnant women unless, in the judgment of the physician, the potential benefits outweigh the possible hazards.

Methadone is not recommended for obstetric analgesia because its long duration of action increases the probability of respiratory depression in the newborn.

Use in Children —Methadone is not recommended for use as an analgesic in children, since documented clinical experience has been insufficient to establish a suitable dosage regimen for the pediatric age group.

PRECAUTIONS

***Interaction with Pentazocine* —Patients who are addicted to heroin or who are on the methadone maintenance program may experience withdrawal symptoms when given pentazocine.**

Interaction with Rifampin —The concurrent administration of rifampin may possibly reduce the blood concentration of methadone. The mechanism by which rifampin may decrease blood concentrations of methadone is not fully understood, although enhanced microsomal drug-metabolized enzymes may influence drug disposition.

Acute Abdominal Conditions —The administration of methadone or other narcotics may obscure the diagnosis or clinical course in patients with acute abdominal conditions.

Interaction with Monoamine Oxidase (MAO) Inhibitors — Therapeutic doses of meperidine have precipitated severe reactions in patients concurrently receiving monoamine oxidase inhibitors or those who have received such agents within 14 days. Similar reactions thus far have not been reported with methadone; but if the use of methadone is necessary in such patients, a sensitivity test should be performed in which repeated small incremental doses are administered over the course of several hours while the patient's condition and vital signs are under careful observation.

Special-Risk Patients —Methadone should be given with caution and the initial dose should be reduced in certain patients, such as the elderly or debilitated and those with severe impairment of hepatic or renal function, hypothyroidism, Addison's disease, prostatic hypertrophy, or urethral stricture.

ADVERSE REACTIONS

THE MAJOR HAZARDS OF METHADONE, AS OF OTHER NARCOTIC ANALGESICS, ARE RESPIRATORY DEPRESSION AND, TO A LESSER DEGREE, CIRCULATORY DEPRESSION. RESPIRATORY ARREST, SHOCK, AND CARDIAC ARREST HAVE OCCURRED.

The most frequently observed adverse reactions include lightheadedness, dizziness, sedation, nausea, vomiting, and sweating. These effects seem to be more prominent in ambulatory patients and in those who are not suffering severe chronic pain. In such individuals, lower doses are advisable. Some adverse reactions may be alleviated in the ambulatory patient if he lies down.

Other adverse reactions include the following:

Central Nervous System —Euphoria, dysphoria, weakness, headache, insomnia, agitation, disorientation, and visual disturbances.

Gastrointestinal —Dry mouth, anorexia, constipation, and biliary tract spasm.

Cardiovascular —Flushing of the face, bradycardia, palpitation, faintness, and syncope.

Genitourinary —Urinary retention or hesitancy, antidiuretic effect, and reduced libido and/or potency.

Allergic —Pruritus, urticaria, other skin rashes, edema, and, rarely, hemorrhagic urticaria.

ADMINISTRATION AND DOSAGE

For relief of Severe Pain —Dosage should be adjusted according to the severity of the pain and the response of the patient. Occasionally it may be necessary to exceed the usual dosage recommended in cases of exceptionally severe chronic pain or in those patients who have become tolerant to the analgesic effect of narcotics.

For severe acute pain, the usual adult dose is 2.5 mg to 10 mg every three to four hours as necessary.

For Detoxification Treatment —THE DRUG SHALL BE ADMINISTERED DAILY UNDER CLOSE SUPERVISION AS FOLLOWS:

A detoxification treatment course shall not exceed 21 days and may not be repeated earlier than four weeks after completion of the preceding course.

The oral form of administration is preferred. However, if the patient is unable to ingest oral medication, he may be started on the parenteral form initially.

In detoxification, the patient may receive methadone when there are significant symptoms of withdrawal. The dosage schedules indicated below are recommended but could be varied in accordance with clinical judgment. Initially, a single dose of 15 to 20 mg of methadone will often be sufficient to suppress withdrawal symptoms. Additional methadone may be provided if withdrawal symptoms are not suppressed or if symptoms reappear. When patients are physically dependent on high doses, it may be necessary to exceed these levels. Forty mg per day in single or divided doses will usually constitute an adequate stabilizing dosage level. Stabilization can be continued for two to three days, and then the amount of methadone normally will be gradually decreased. The rate at which methadone is decreased will be determined separately for each patient. The dose of methadone can be decreased on a daily basis or at two-day intervals, but the amount of intake shall always be sufficient to keep withdrawal symptoms at a tolerable level. In hospitalized patients, a daily reduction of 20 percent of the total dose may be tolerated and may cause little discomfort. In ambulatory patients, a somewhat slower schedule may be needed. If methadone is administered for more than three weeks, the procedure is considered to have progressed from detoxification or treatment of the acute withdrawal syndrome to maintenance treatment, even though the goal and intent may be eventual total withdrawal.

OVERDOSAGE

Symptoms —Serious overdosage of methadone is characterized by respiratory depression (a decrease in respiratory rate and/or tidal volume, Cheyne-Stokes respiration, cyanosis), extreme somnolence progressing to stupor or coma, maximally constricted pupils, skeletal-muscle flaccidity, cold and clammy skin, and sometimes, bradycardia and hypotension. In severe overdosage, particularly by the intravenous route, apnea, circulatory collapse, cardiac arrest, and death may occur.

Treatment —Primary attention should be given to the reestablishment of adequate respiratory exchange through provision of a patent airway and institution of assisted or controlled ventilation. If a nontolerant person, especially a child, takes a large dose of methadone, effective narcotic antagonists are available to counteract the potentially lethal respiratory depression. **The physician must remember, however, that methadone is a long-acting depressant (36 to 48 hours), whereas the antagonists act for much shorter periods (one to three hours).** The patient must, therefore, be monitored continuously for recurrence of respiratory depression and treated repeatedly with the narcotic antagonist as needed. If the diagnosis is correct and respiratory depression is due only to overdosage of methadone, the use of other respiratory stimulants is not indicated.

An antagonist should not be administered in the absence of clinically significant respiratory or cardiovascular depression. Intravenously administered narcotic antagonists (naloxone and nalorphine) are the drugs of choice to reverse signs of intoxication. These agents should be given repeatedly until the patient's status remains satisfactory. The hazard that the narcotic agent will further depress respiration is less likely with the use of naloxone.

Oxygen, intravenous fluids, vasopressors, and other supportive measures should be employed as indicated.

> **Note**
>
> IN AN INDIVIDUAL PHYSICALLY DEPENDENT ON NARCOTICS, THE ADMINISTRATION OF THE USUAL DOSE OF A NARCOTIC ANTAGONIST WILL PRECIPITATE AN ACUTE WITHDRAWAL SYNDROME. THE SEVERITY OF THIS SYNDROME WILL DEPEND ON THE DEGREE OF PHYSICAL DEPENDENCE AND THE DOSE OF THE ANTAGONIST ADMINISTERED. THE USE OF A NARCOTIC ANTAGONIST IN SUCH A PERSON SHOULD BE AVOIDED IF POSSIBLE. IF IT MUST BE USED TO TREAT SERIOUS RESPIRATORY DEPRESSION IN THE PHYSICALLY DEPENDENT PATIENT, THE ANTAGONIST SHOULD BE ADMINISTERED WITH EXTREME CARE AND BY TITRATION WITH SMALLER THAN USUAL DOSES OF THE ANTAGONIST.

HOW SUPPLIED

Methadone Hydrochloride Oral Solution USP

Clear, orange-colored, citrus-flavored solution

5 mg per 5 mL

NDC 0054-3555-63: Bottles of 500 mL

10 mg per 5 mL

NDC 0054-3556-63: Bottles of 500 mL

Methadone Hydrochloride Tablets USP

5 mg white, scored identified (54 210) tablets.

NDC 0054-4570-25: Bottle of 100 tablets.

NDC 0054-8553-24: Unit dose, 25 tablets per card (reverse numbered), 4 cards per shipper.

10 mg white, scored identified (54 142) tablets.

NDC 0054-4571-25: Bottle of 100 tablets.

NDC 0054-8554-24: Unit dose, 25 tablets per card (reverse numbered), 4 cards per shipper.

Caution: Federal law prohibits dispensing without prescription.

4056301

054 Revised May 1994

MORPHINE SULFATE IMMEDIATE RELEASE ORAL SOLUTION Ⓒ℞

(WARNING: May be habit forming.)

MORPHINE SULFATE IMMEDIATE RELEASE TABLETS Ⓒ℞

(WARNING: May be habit forming.)

DESCRIPTION

Each 5 mL of Morphine Sulfate Oral Solution contains:

Morphine Sulfate .... 10 or 20 mg

(WARNING: May be habit forming.)

Each tablet for oral administration contains:

Morphine Sulfate .... 15 or 30 mg

(WARNING: May be habit forming.)

HOW SUPPLIED

Morphine Sulfate Oral Solution

(Unflavored).

10 mg per 5 mL.

NDC 0054-8585-16: Unit dose Patient Cup™ filled to deliver 5 mL (10 mg Morphine Sulfate), ten 5 mL Patient Cups™ per shelf pack, four shelf packs per shipper.

NDC 0054-8586-16: Unit dose Patient Cup™ filled to deliver 10 mL (20 mg Morphine Sulfate), ten 10 mL Patient Cups™ per shelf pack, four shelf packs per shipper.
NDC 0054-3785-49: 100 mL "Unit of use" calibrated bottle.
NDC 0054-3785-63: Bottles of 500 mL.
20 mg per 5 mL.
NDC 0054-3786-49: 100 mL "Unit of Use" calibrated bottle.
NDC 0054-3786-63: Bottles of 500 mL.
Tablets
15 mg white scored, identified (54/733) tablets.
NDC 0054-8582-24: Unit dose, 25 tablets per card (reverse numbered), 4 cards per shipper.
NDC 0054-4582-25: Bottles of 100 tablets.
30 mg white scored, identified (54/262) tablets.
NDC 0054-8583-24: Unit dose, 25 tablets per card (reverse numbered), 4 cards per shipper.
NDC 0054-4583-25: Bottles of 100 Tablets.
DEA Order Form Required

ORAMORPH SR™   © ℞
(MORPHINE SULFATE)
SUSTAINED RELEASE TABLETS
15 mg, 30 mg, 60 mg, 100 mg
(WARNING: May be habit forming.)

> **NOTE**
> THIS IS A SUSTAINED RELEASE DOSAGE FORM. PATIENT SHOULD BE INSTRUCTED TO SWALLOW THE TABLET AS A WHOLE; THE TABLE SHOULD NOT BE BROKEN IN HALF, NOR SHOULD IT BE CRUSHED OR CHEWED.
> THE SUSTAINED RELEASE OF MORPHINE FROM ORAMORPH SR SHOULD BE TAKEN INTO CONSIDERATION IN EVENT OF ADVERSE REACTIONS OR OVERDOSAGE.

DESCRIPTION

Each tablet for oral administration contains:
Morphine sulfate .... 15 mg, 30 mg, 60 mg, or 100 mg
(WARNING: May be habit forming)
in a tablet that provides for sustained release of the medication.
Morphine sulfate occurs as white, feathery, silky crystals, cubical masses of crystals, or white crystalline powder; it is soluble in water and slightly soluble in alcohol. Morphine has a pKa of 7.9, with an octanol/water partition coefficient of 1.42 at pH 7.4. At this pH, the tertiary amino group is mostly ionized, making the molecule water-soluble. Morphine is significantly more water-soluble than any other opioid in clinical use.
Chemically, morphine sulfate is 7,8-didehydro-4,5α-epoxy-17-methyl-morphinian-3,6α-diol sulfate (2:1)(salt) pentahydrate, and has the following structural formula:

Each ORAMORPH SR Tablet contains 15 mg, 30 mg, 60 mg, or 100 mg Morphine Sulfate USP. Inactive ingredients: Lactose, Hydroxypropyl Methylcellulose, Colloidal Silicon Dioxide, and Stearic Acid.

CLINICAL PHARMACOLOGY

Morphine is the prototype of many narcotic drugs that interact predominantly with the opioid μ-receptor. These μ-binding sites are discretely distributed in the human brain, with high densities in the posterior amygdala, hypothalamus, thalamus, nucleus caudatus, putamen, and certain cortical areas. They are also found on the terminal axons of primary afferents with laminae I and II (substantia gelatinosa) of the spinal cord and in the spinal nucleus of the trigeminal nerve.
In clinical settings, morphine exerts its principal pharmacological effect on the central nervous system and gastrointestinal tract. Its primary actions of therapeutic value are analgesia and sedation. Morphine appears to increase the patient's tolerance for pain and to decrease discomfort, although the presence of the pain itself may still be recognized. In addition to analgesia, alterations in mood, euphoria and dysphoria, and drowsiness commonly occur.
Morphine depresses various respiratory centers, depresses the cough reflex, and constricts the pupils. Analgesically effective blood levels of morphine may cause nausea and vomiting directly by stimulating the chemoreceptor trigger zone, but nausea and vomiting are significantly more common in ambulatory than in recumbent patients, as is postural syncope.
Morphine increases the tone and decreases the propulsive contractions of the smooth muscle of the gastrointestinal tract. The resultant prolongation in gastrointestinal transit time is responsible for the constipating effect of morphine. Because morphine may increase biliary-tract pressure, some patients with biliary colic may experience worsening rather than relief of pain.
While morphine generally increases the tone of urinary-tract smooth muscle, the net effect tends to be variable, in some cases producing urinary urgency, in others, difficulty in urination.
In therapeutic doses, morphine does not usually exert major effects on the cardiovascular system. Some patients, however, exhibit a propensity to develop orthostatic hypotension and fainting. Rapid intravenous injection is more likely to precipitate a fall in blood pressure than oral dosing. Morphine can cause histamine release, which appears to be responsible for dilation of cutaneous blood vessels, with resulting flushing of the face and neck, pruritus, and sweating.

PHARMACOKINETICS

ORAMORPH SR Tablets are a sustained release oral dosage form of morphine sulfate. Only about 40% of the administered dose reaches the central compartment because of first-pass effect (i.e., metabolism in the gut wall and liver). Once absorbed, morphine is distributed to skeletal muscle, kidneys, liver, intestinal tract, lungs, spleen and brain. Morphine also crosses the placental membrane and has been found in breast milk.
For all practical purposes, virtually all morphine is converted to glucuronide metabolites; only a small fraction (less than 5%) of absorbed morphine is demethylated. Among these glucuronide metabolites, morphine-3-glucuronide is present in the highest plasma concentration following oral administration; a smaller fraction is converted to morphine-6-glucuronide, which has the greater analgesic activity of these two metabolites.
The glucuronide system has a high capacity and is not easily saturated, even in disease. Therefore, the rate of delivery of morphine to the gut and liver does not influence the total and/or the relative quantities of the various metabolites formed.
The pharmacokinetic parameters following oral administration of ORAMORPH SR, presented in the table below, show considerable inter-subject variation, but are representative of average values reported in the literature. The volume of distribution (Vd) for morphine is 4 liters per kilogram (L/kg), and the terminal elimination half-life is approximately 2 to 4 hours.
[See table above.]
Following the administration of conventional, immediate-release, oral morphine products, approximately 50% of the morphine that will ever reach the central compartment, reaches it within 30 minutes. Following the administration of an equal amount of ORAMORPH SR to normal volunteers, however, 50% of absorption occurs, on average, after 1.5 hours.
The possible effect of food upon the systemic bioavailability of ORAMORPH SR has not been evaluated.
Although variation in the physico-mechanical properties of a formulation of an oral morphine drug product can affect both its absolute bioavailability and its absorption rate constant (k_a), morphine distribution and clearance are unchanged, as they are fundamental properties of morphine in the organism. However, in chronic use, the possibility of shifts in metabolite-to-parent drug ratios cannot be excluded.
When immediate-release oral morphine or ORAMORPH SR is given on a fixed dosing regimen, steady-state is achieved in about one or two days.
For a given dose and dosing interval, the Area-Under-the-Curve (AUC) and average blood concentration of morphine at steady-state (C_{SS}) will be independent of the type of oral formulation administered, as long as the formulations have the same absolute bioavailability. The absorption rate of a formulation will, however, affect the maximum (C_{max}) and minimum (C_{min}) plasma concentrations and the time between administration and their occurrence. For any fixed dose and dosing interval, ORAMORPH SR will have, at steady-state, a lower C_{max} and a higher C_{min} than conventional immediate-release morphine, which might be a therapeutic advantage in chronic pain control (see also PHARMACODYNAMICS).
The clearance of morphine occurs primarily as renal excretion of morphine-3-glucuronide. A small amount of the glucuronide conjugate is excreted in the bile, and there is some minor enterohepatic recycling; about 10% of the glucuronide conjugate is excreted in the feces. Because morphine is essentially metabolized in the liver, the effects of renal disease on morphine's clearance are not likely to be pronounced. As with any drug, however, caution should be taken to guard against unanticipated accumulation if renal and/or hepatic function is seriously impaired.

PHARMACODYNAMICS

In clinical settings, morphine's primary actions of therapeutic value are analgesia and sedation. Opiate analgesia involves at least three anatomical areas of the central nervous system: the periaqueductal-periventricular gray matter, the ventromedial medulla, and the spinal cord. Morphine appears to increase the patient's tolerance for pain, and to decrease the discomfort, although the presence of pain itself may still be recognized.
While there is considerable variability in the relationship between morphine blood concentration and analgesic response, effective analgesia probably will not occur below some minimum blood level in a given patient. The minimum effective blood level for analgesia will vary among patients, especially among patients who have been previously treated with potent μ-agonist opioids. Similarly, there is a considerable variability in the relationship between morphine plasma concentration and untoward clinical responses, but higher concentrations are more likely to be toxic.
In contrast to immediate-release morphine, after dosing with ORAMORPH SR, the morphine blood levels show reduced fluctuation between peak and trough plasma levels; that means that they are more centered within the theoretical 'therapeutic window'. On the other hand, the reduced fluctuation in morphine plasma concentration might conceivably affect other phenomena, as for example, the rate of tolerance induction.
ORAMORPH SR is an analgesic intended for patients who require chronic morphine analgesia and who will have, in consequence, markedly different degrees of pharmacodynamic tolerance for opioid drugs. Morphine and similar opioids induce tolerance to their effects, so that a shortening of the duration of satisfactory analgesia may be the first sign of an increase in tolerance.
Once patients are started on morphine, the dose required for satisfactory analgesia will rise, with the rate of development of tolerance varying, depending on the patient's prior nar-

TABLE OF APPROXIMATE[1] AVERAGE PHARMACOKINETIC PARAMETERS FOLLOWING ORAL DOSING OF ORAMORPH SR ™

Pharmacokinetic Parameter (scientific notation) (unit)		Dose of 2 × 15 mg	Dose of ORAMORPH SR 30 mg	Dose of ORAMORPH SR 60 mg	Dose of ORAMORPH SR 100 mg
Bioavailability (oral compared to injectable)			approximately 40%		
Time-to-peak plasma concentration $\{T_{max}\}$ (h)	mean (range)	3.7 (1–6)	3.8 (1–7)	3.8 (2–7)	3.6 (1.5–12)
Peak plasma concentration $\{C_{max}\}$ (ng/mL) [single dose]	mean (range)	11.1 (6.5–16.2)	9.9 (5.0–18.6)	16.1 (10.0–25.3)	27.4 (14.1–46.1)
Volume of distribution (calculated from mean clearance and terminal half-life) $\{Vd(\beta)\}$ (L/kg)	mean	.... 4 L/kg			

Dose metabolized = approximately 90%
Morphine metabolites (%) = morphine-3-glucuronide (55–75%),
morphine-6-glucuronide (1–5%)
[1]Derived from pharmacokinetic studies in 24 normal volunteers

Continued on next page

Roxane Laboratories—Cont.

cotic use, level of pain, degree of anxiety, use of other CNS-active drugs, circulatory status, total daily dose, and the dosing interval.

INDICATIONS AND USAGE

ORAMORPH SR is indicated for the relief of pain in patients who require opioid analgesics for more than a few days.

CONTRAINDICATIONS

ORAMORPH SR is contraindicated in patients with respiratory depression in the absence of resuscitative equipment, in patients with acute or severe bronchial asthma and in patients with known hypersensitivity to morphine.

ORAMORPH SR is contraindicated in any patient who has or is suspected of having a paralytic ileus.

WARNINGS

IMPAIRED RESPIRATION:

Respiratory depression is the chief hazard of all morphine preparations. Respiratory depression occurs more frequently in the elderly and debilitated patients, as well as in those suffering from conditions accompanied by hypoxia or hypercapnia when even moderate therapeutic doses may dangerously decrease pulmonary ventiliation.

Morphine should be used with extreme caution in patients who have a decreased respiratory reserve (e.g., emphysema, severe obesity, kyphoscoliosis, or paralysis of the phrenic nerve). ORAMORPH SR should not be given in cases of chronic asthma, upper airway obstruction, or in any other chronic pulmonary disorder without due consideration of the known risk of acute respiratory failure following morphine administration in such patients.

DRUG ABUSE AND DEPENDENCE

CONTROLLED SUBSTANCE:

Morphine sulfate is a Schedule II narcotic under the United States Controlled Substance Act (21 U.S.C. 801–886).

Morphine is the most commonly cited prototype for narcotic substances that possess an addiction-forming or addition-sustaining liability. A patient may be at risk for developing a dependence to morphine if used improperly or for overly long periods of time. As with all potent opioids which are μ-agonists, tolerance as well as psychological and physical dependence to morphine may develop irrespective of the route of administration (oral, intravenous, intramuscular, intrathecal, epidural). Individuals with a prior history of opioid or other substance abuse or dependence, being more apt to respond to eurphorogenic and reinforcing properties of morphine, would be considered to be at greater risk.

Care must be taken to avert withdrawal symptoms when morphine is discontinued abruptly or upon administration of a narcotic antagonist.

PRECAUTIONS

General Precautions:

Selection of patients for treatment with ORAMORPH SR should be governed by the same principles that apply to the use of morphine or other potent opioid analgesics. Narcotic analgesics are drugs that have a narrow therapeutic index in the old, the sick, and the infirm, i.e., the very population in which their use is indicated. Physicians should individualize treatment with ORAMORPH SR in every case, weighing the need for analgesia against the risk of serious or fatal reactions to the drug.

Use in Patients with Increased Intracranial Pressure or with Head Injury:

ORAMORPH SR should be used with extreme caution in patients with increased intracranial pressure or with head injury. The respiratory depressant effects of morphine (increased pCO_2) may result in elevation of cerebrospinal fluid pressure and may thus be markedly exaggerated in the presence of head injury, other intracranial lesions, or a pre-existing increased intracranial pressure. Morphine produces effects which may obscure neurologic signs of further increases in pressure in patients with head injuries. Pupillary changes (miosis), associated with morphine, may conceal the existence, extent, and course of intracranial pathology.

Use in Hepatic or Renal Disease:

The clearance of morphine may be reduced in patients with hepatic dysfunction, while the clearance of its metabolites may be decreased in renal dysfunction. This will be manifested by both, a prolonged elimination half-life and the accumulation of levels of either morphine or its metabolites in excess of those produced in normals, with the potential for an increase of adverse effects (see WARNINGS and ADVERSE REACTIONS). These changes in morphine pharmacodynamics, in patients with hepatic or renal dysfunctions, should be considered when adjusting the dose and dosage intervals, taking also into account the slow-release character of ORAMORPH SR.

Drug Interactions:

Use with Other Central Nervous System Depressants:

The depressant effects of morphine are potentiated by the presence of other CNS depressants such as alcohol, sedatives, antihistaminics, or psychotropic drugs. Use of neuroleptics in conjunction with oral morphine may increase the risk of respiratory depression, hypotension and profound sedation or coma.

Interaction with Mixed Agonist/Antagonist Opioid Analgesics:

Agonist/antagonist analgesics (i.e., pentazocine, nalbuphine, butorphanol, or buprenorphine) should NOT be administered to patients who have received or are receiving a course of therapy with a pure opioid agonist analgesic. In these patients, the mixed agonist/antagonist may alter the analgesic effect or may precipitate withdrawal symptoms.

Carcinogenesis, Mutagenesis, Impairment of Fertility:

Studies of morphine sulfate in animals to evaluate the drug's carcinogenic and mutagenic potential or the effect on fertility have not been conducted.

Pregnancy:

Teratogenic Effects—Category C: There are no well-controlled studies in women, but marketing experience does not include any evidence of adverse effects on the fetus following routine (short-term) clinical use of morphine sulfate products. Although there is no clearly defined risk, such experience cannot exclude the possibility of infrequent or subtle damage to the human fetus.

ORAMORPH SR should be used in pregnant women only when clearly needed. (See also: PRECAUTIONS: Labor and Delivery, and DRUG ABUSE AND DEPENDENCE CONTROLLED SUBSTANCE.)

Nonteratogenic Effects:

Infants born from mothers who have been taking morphine chronically may exhibit withdrawal symptoms.

Labor and Delivery:

ORAMORPH SR is not recommended for use in women during and immediately prior to labor. Occasionally, opioid analgesics may prolong labor through actions which temporarily reduce the strength, duration and frequency of uterine contractions.

Neonates, whose mothers received opioid analgesics during labor, should be observed closely for signs of respiratory depression. A specific narcotic antagonist, naloxone, should be available for reversal of narcotic-induced respiratory depression in the neonate.

Nursing Mothers:

ORAMORPH SR should not be given to nursing mothers because morphine is excreted in maternal milk. Effects on the nursing infant are not known, but withdrawal symptoms can occur in breast-fed infants when maternal administration of morphine sulfate is stopped.

Pediatric Use:

ORAMORPH SR has not been evaluated in children. Its use in the pediatric population is, therefore, not recommended.

Use in the Aged:

The pharmacodynamic effects of morphine in the aged are more variable than in the younger population. Patients will vary widely in the effective initial dose, rate of development of tolerance, and the frequency and magnitude of associated adverse effects as the dose is increased. Individualization of doses must receive careful attention in elderly patients.

Information for Patients:

If clinically advisable, patients receiving ORAMORPH SR brand or morphine sulfate sustained release tablets, should be given the following instructions by the physician:

1. Morphine may produce psychological and/or physical dependence. For this reason, the dose of the drug should not be increased without consulting a physician.
2. Morphine may impair mental and/or physical ability required for the performance of potentially hazardous tasks (e.g., driving, operating machinery).
3. Morphine should not be taken with alcohol or other CNS depressants (sleep aids, tranquilizers) because additive effects, including CNS depression, may occur. A physician should be consulted if other prescription and/or over-the-counter medications are currently being used or are prescribed for future use.
4. For women of childbearing potential, who become or are planning to become pregnant, a physician should be consulted regarding analgesics and other drug use.

ADVERSE REACTIONS

> **NOTE:** THE SUSTAINED RELEASE OF MORPHINE FROM ORAMORPH SR SHOULD BE TAKEN INTO CONSIDERATION IN THE EVENT OF OCCURRING ADVERSE REACTIONS.

Adverse reactions caused by morphine are essentially those observed with other opioid analgesics. They include the following *major hazards:* **respiratory depression**, and less frequently, **circulatory depression, apnea, shock** and **cardiac arrest** secondary to respiratory and/or circulatory depression.

Most Frequently Observed Reactions:

Constipation, nausea, vomiting, lightheadedness, dizziness sedation, dysphoria, euphoria, and sweating. Some of these effects seem to be more prominent in ambulatory patients and in those not experiencing severe pain. Some adverse reactions in ambulatory patients may be alleviated if the patient is in a supine position.

Less Frequently Observed Reactions:

Body as a Whole: Edema, antidiuretic effect, chills, muscle tremor, muscle rigidity.

Cardiovascular: Flushing of the face, tachycardia, bradycardia, palpitation, faintness, syncope, hypotension, hypertension.

Gastrointestinal: Dry mouth, biliary tract spasm, laryngospasm, anorexia, diarrhea, cramps, taste alterations.

Genitourinary: Urine retention or hesitance, reduced libido and/or potency.

Nervous System: Weakness, headache, agitation, tremor, uncoordinated muscle movements, seizure, paresthesia, alterations of mood (nervousness, apprehension, depression, floating feelings), dreams, transient hallucination and disorientation, visual disturbances, insomnia, increased intracranial pressure.

Skin: Pruritus, urticaria and other skin rashes.

Special Senses: Blurred vision, nystagmus, diplopia, miosis.

DRUG ABUSE AND DEPENDENCE

Opioid analgesics may cause psychological and physical dependence (see WARNINGS). Physical dependence results in withdrawal symptoms in patients who abruptly discontinue the drug, or these symptoms may be precipitated through the administration of drugs with antagonistic activity, e.g., naloxone or mixed agonist/antagonist analgesics (pentazocine, etc.; see also OVERDOSAGE). Physical dependence usually does not occur, to a clinically significant degree, until several weeks of continued opioid usage. Tolerance, in which increasingly larger doses are required to produce the same degree of analgesia, is initially manifested by a shortened duration of a analgesic effect and, subsequently, by decreases in the intensity of analgesia. In patients with chronic pain, as well as in opioid-tolerant cancer patients, the administration of ORAMORPH SR (morphine sulfate) should be guided by the degree of tolerance manifested. Physical dependence, *per se*, is not ordinarily a concern when one is dealing with opioid-tolerant patients whose pain and suffering is associated with an irreversible illness.

If ORAMORPH SR is abruptly discontinued, an abstinence syndrome may occur. Withdrawal symptoms, in patients dependent on morphine, begin shortly before the time of the next scheduled dose, reaching a peak at 36 to 72 hours after the last dose, and then slowly subside over a period of 7 to 10 days. Symptoms include yawning, sweating, lacrimation, rhinorrhea, restless sleep, dilated pupils, gooseflesh, irritability, tremor, nausea, vomiting, and diarrhea.

Treatment of the abstinence syndrome is primarily symptomatic and supportive, including maintenance of proper fluid and electrolyte balance. If withdrawal has inadvertently been precipitated in a patient who requires narcotics for pain management, the withdrawal syndrome can be terminated rapidly by the administration of an appropriate dose of a pure agonist opioid, such as morphine. The degree of physical dependence of a patient on ORAMORPH SR can be intentionally reduced by a gradual reduction of dosage and symptomatic treatment of withdrawal symptomatology.

OVERDOSAGE

> **NOTE:** THE SUSTAINED RELEASE OF MORPHINE FROM **ORAMORPH SR** SHOULD BE TAKEN INTO CONSIDERATION IN THE EVENT OF AN OVERDOSAGE.

Overdosage of morphine is characterized by respiratory depression, with or without concomitant CNS depression. Since respiratory arrest may result either through direct depression of the respiratory center, or as the result of hypoxia, primary attention should be given to the establishment of adequate respiratory exchange through provision of a patent airway and institution of assisted, or controlled, ventilation. The narcotic antagonist, naloxone, is a specific antidote. An initial dose of 0.4 to 2 mg of naloxone should be administered intravenously, simultaneously with respiratory resuscitation. If the desired degree of counteraction and improvement in respiratory function is not obtained, naloxone may be repeated at 2 to 3 minute intervals. If no response is observed after 10 mg of naloxone has been administered, the diagnosis of narcotic-induced, or partial narcotic-induced, toxicity should be questioned. Intramuscular or subcutaneous administration may be used if the intravenous route is not available.

As the duration of effect of naloxone is considerably shorter than that of ORAMORPH SR, repeated administration may be necessary. Patients should be closely observed for evidence of renarcotization.

> NOTE: In a individual physically dependent on opioids, administration of the usual dose of the antagonist will precipitate an acute withdrawal syndrome. The severity of the withdrawal syndrome produced will depend on the degree of physical dependence and the dose of the

antagonist administered. Use of a narcotic antagonist in such a person should be avoided. If necessary to treat serious respiratory depression in a physically dependent patient, the antagonist should be administered with extreme care and by titration with smaller than usual dose of the antagonist.

When indicated, gut decontamination should be performed via emesis and/or activated charcoal (60 to 100 g in adults, 1 to 2 g/kg in children) with cathartic. Since ORAMORPH SR is a sustained release product, absorption may be expected to continue for many hours, particularly following an overdose, combined with decreased peristaltic activity of the gastrointestinal tract.

Supportive measures (including oxygen, vasopressors) should be employed in the management of circulatory shock and pulmonary edema accompanying overdose as indicated. Cardiac arrest or arrhythmias may require cardiac massage or defibrillation.

DOSAGE AND ADMINISTRATION

(See also: CLINICAL PHARMACOLOGY, WARNINGS and PRECAUTIONS sections.)

NOTE: ORAMORPH SR TABLET MUST BE SWALLOWED WHOLE. DO NOT BREAK THE TABLET IN HALF. DO NOT CRUSH OR CHEW. TAKING BROKEN, CHEWED OR CRUSHED TABLETS COULD LEAD TO THE RAPID RELEASE AND ABSORPTION OF A POTENTIALLY TOXIC DOSE OF MORPHINE.

ORAMORPH SR is intended for use in patients who require more than several days of continuous treatment with a potent opioid analgesic. The sustained release nature of the formulation allows it to be administered on a more convenient schedule than conventional immediate-release oral morphine products (see CLINICAL PHARMACOLOGY—PHARMACOKINETICS). However, ORAMORPH SR does not release morphine continuously over the course of a dosing interval. The administration of single doses of ORAMORPH SR on a q12h dosing schedule will result in peak and trough plasma levels similar to those following an identical daily dose of morphine administered using conventional oral formulations on a q4h regimen. If pain is not controlled for a full 12 hours, then the dosing interval should be shortened, but to no less than 8 hours.

As with any potent opioid, it is critical to adjust the dosing regimen for each patient individually, taking into account the patient's prior analgesic treatment experience. Although it is not possible to enumerate every condition that is important to the selection of the initial dose and dosing interval of ORAMORPH SR, attention should be given to (1) the daily dose, potency and characteristics of a pure agonist, or mixed agonist-antagonist, the patient has been taking previously, (2) the reliability of the relative potentcy estimate to calculate the dose of morphine needed [N.B.: potency estimates may vary with the route of administration], (3) the fact that roughly only 40% of the morphine sulfate in ORAMORPH SR becomes available after pre-systemic metabolization in the intestinal wall and liver, (4) the degree of opioid tolerance, and (5) the general condition and medical status of the patient.

The following dosing recommendation for ORAMORPH SR therefore, can only be considered suggested approaches to the series of clinical decisions in the management of pain of an individual patient.

Conversion from Conventional Immediate-Release Oral Morphine to ORAMORPH SR:

A patient's daily morphine requirement is established by using the Daily Oral Morphine Requirement of the immediate-release formulation which gives the Daily Oral Morphine Requirement for ORAMORPH SR. Since ORAMORPH SR is given on an 'every 12 hour' schedule, the single dose of ORAMORPH SR is half of the Daily Oral Morphine Requirement. Dose and dosing interval is adjusted as needed (see discussion below). For initial conversion, the 30 mg tablet strength is recommended for patients with a daily morphine requirement of 120 mg or less.

Conversion from Parental Morphine or Other Opioid Analgesics (parental or oral) to ORAMORPH SR:

Because of uncertainty about relative estimates of opioid potency and cross tolerance, as well as intersubject variation, initial dosing regimens should be conservative, i.e., an underestimation of the 24-hour oral morphine requirement is preferred to an overestimate. To this end, initial individual doses of ORAMORPH SR should be estimated conservatively. In patients whose daily morphine requirements are expected to be less than or equal to 120 mg per day, the 30 mg tablet strength is recommended for the initial titration period. Once a stable dose regimen is reached, the patient can be converted to the 60 mg or 100 mg tablet strength, as appropriate.

Estimates of the relative potency of opioids are only approximate, and are influenced by route of administration, individual patient differences, and possibly, by the patient's medical condition. Consequently, it is difficult to recommend any precise rule for converting a patient to ORAMORPH SR directly. However, the following general points should be considered:

1. *Parenteral to oral morphine ratio:* Estimates of the oral-to-parenteral potency of morphine vary. Some authorities suggest that a dose of morphine only 3 times the daily parenteral morphine requirement may be sufficient in chronic use settings. (3 times the Daily Parenteral Morphine Requirement = the Daily Oral Morphine Requirement)
2. *Oral parenteral or oral opioids to oral morphine:* Because of a lack of reliable relative potency assays, specific recommendations are not possible. In general, it is safer to underestimate the Total Daily Dose of ORAMORPH SR required and rely upon *ad hoc* supplementation to deal with inadequate analgesia (see discussion which follows).

Use of ORAMORPH SR as the First Opioid Analgesic:

There has been no systematic evaluation of ORAMORPH SR as an initial opioid analgesic in the management of pain. Because it may be more difficult to titrate a patient using a sustained release morphine, it is ordinarily advisable to begin treatment using an immediate release formulation.

Considerations in the Adjustment of Dosing Regimens.

Whatever the approach, if signs of excessive opioid effects are observed early in a dosing interval, the next dose should be reduced. If this adjustment leads to inadequate analgesia, i.e., 'breakthrough' pain occurs late in the dosing interval, the dosing interval may be shortened. Alternatively, a supplemental dose of a short-acting analgesic may be given.

As experience is gained, adjustments can be made to obtain an appropriate balance between pain relief, opioid side effects and the convenience of the dosing schedule.

In adjusting dose requirements, it is recommended that the dosing interval never be extended beyond 12 hours, because the administration of very large single doses of ORAMORPH SR may lead to acute overdosage.

For patients with low daily morphine requirements, the 15 mg tablet should be used. In this regard, adjustment in dose should NOT be attempted by breaking or crushing the tablets. ORAMORPH SR tablets are intended to be swallowed whole.

Conversion from ORAMORPH SR to Parenteral Opioids:

When converting a patient from ORAMORPH SR to parenteral opioids, it is best to assume that the parenteral to oral potency relationship is high. NOTE THAT THIS IS THE CONVERSE OF THE STRATEGY USED WHEN THE DIRECTION OF CONVERSION IS FROM THE PARENTERAL TO ORAL FORMULATIONS. IN BOTH CASES, HOWEVER, THE AIM IS TO ESTIMATE THE NEW DOSE CONSERVATIVELY. For example, to estimate the required 24-hour dose of morphine for IM use, one could employ a conversion of 1 mg of morphine IM for every 6 mg of morphine as ORAMORPH SR. Of course, the IM 24-hour dose would have to be divided by six and administered on a q4h regimen. This approach is recommended because it is least likely to cause overdosage.

NOTE: ORAMORPH SR TABLET MUST BE SWALLOWED WHOLE. DO NOT BREAK THE TABLET IN HALF. DO NOT CRUSH OR CHEW.

HOW SUPPLIED

ORAMORPH SR™ (Morphine Sulfate)
Sustained Release Tablets
15 mg white tablets (Identified 54 782)
[Embossed with 15]

NDC 0054-8790-24: Unit dose, 25 tablets per card (reverse numbered), 4 cards per shipper.
NDC 0054-4790-25: Bottles of 100 tablets.
NDC 0054-4790-29: Bottles of 500 tablets.

30 mg white tablets (Identified 54 409)
[Embossed with 30]

NDC 0054-8805-24: Unit dose, 25 tablets per card (reverse numbered), 4 cards per shipper.
NDC 0054-4805-19: Bottles of 50 tablets.
NDC 0054-4805-25: Bottles of 100 tablets.
NDC 0054-4805-27: Bottles of 250 tablets.

60 mg white tablets (Identified 54 933)
[Embossed with 60]

NDC 0054-8792-11: Unit dose, 25 tablets per card (reverse numbered), 1 card per shipper.
NDC 0054-4792-25: Bottles of 100 tablets.

100 mg white tablets (Identified 54 862)
[Embossed with 100]

NDC 0054-8793-11: Unit dose, 25 tablets per card (reverse numbered), 1 card per shipper.
NDC 0054-4793-25: Bottles of 100 tablets.

DEA Order Form Required.

Dispense in a tight, light-resistant container.

Storage: ORAMORPH SR Tablets should be stored in unopened containers at or below room temperature.

Caution: Federal law prohibits dispensing without prescription. Federal law prohibits the transfer of this drug to any person other than the patient for whom it was prescribed.

Safety and Handling Instructions:

ORAMORPH SR is supplied as tablets that pose little risk of direct exposure to health care personnel and should be handled and disposed of in accordance with hospital policy. Patients and their families should be instructed to dispose of ORAMORPH SR tablets, that are no longer needed, down the toilet.

4073305 Revised February 1995
025

Roxane
Laboratories, Inc.
Columbus, Ohio 43216

Shown in Product Identification Guide, page 332

ORLAAM® Ⓒ℞

Levomethadyl Acetate Hydrochloride Oral Solution
Warning: May be habit forming.

CONDITIONS FOR DISTRIBUTION AND USE OF ORLAAM (21 CFR 291.505)

ORLAAM, used for the treatment of narcotic addiction, shall be dispensed only by treatment programs approved by FDA, DEA and the designated state authority. Approved treatment programs shall dispense and use ORLAAM in oral form only and according to the treatment requirements stipulated in Federal regulations. Failure to abide by these requirements may result in injunction precluding operation of the program, seizure of the drug supply, revocation of the program approval, and possible criminal prosecution.

ORLAAM has no recommended uses outside of the treatment of opiate addiction.

DESCRIPTION

ORLAAM (brand of levomethadyl acetate hydrochloride) is a synthetic opiate agonist. Chemically, it is levo-alpha-6-dimethylamino-4, 4-diphenyl-3-heptyl acetate hydrochloride, $C_{23}H_{31}NO_2 \bullet HCl$. It is also known as levo-alpha-acetymethadol hydrochloride (LAAM). The structural formula is:

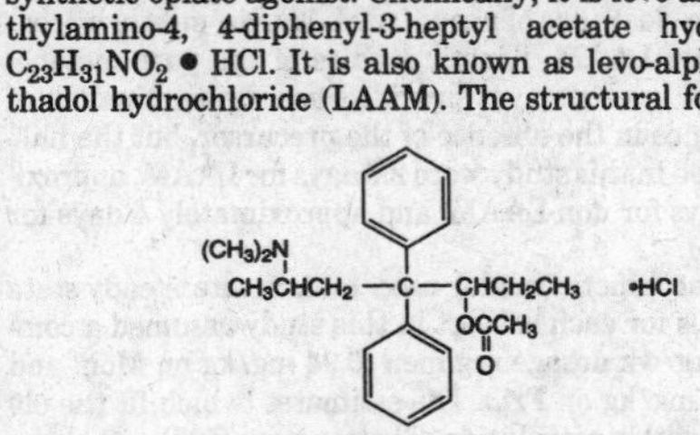

The compound is a white crystalline powder, soluble in water (> 15 mg/mL), ethanol, and methyl ethyl ketone. The octanol:water partition coefficient of LAAM is 405:1 at physiologic pH. Doses of ORLAAM (LAAM) are always expressed as the weight of the hydrochloride salt (molecular weight 389.95).

ORLAAM is an aqueous solution which is diluted for oral administration. Each one mL of ORLAAM contains:
Levomethadyl acetate hydrochloride (LAAM) 10 mg.
Inactive ingredients:

Methylparaben	1.8 mg
Propylparaben	0.2 mg

CLINICAL PHARMACOLOGY

LAAM is a synthetic opioid agonist with actions qualitatively similar to morphine (a prototypic mu agonist) and affecting the central nervous system (CNS) and smooth muscle. Principal actions include analgesia and sedation. Tolerance to these effects develops with repeated use. An abstinence syndrome generally occurs upon cessation of chronic administration similar to that observed with other opiates, but with slower onset, more prolonged course, and less severe symptoms.

LAAM exerts its clinical effects in the treatment of opiate abuse through two mechanisms. First, LAAM cross-substitutes for opiates of the morphine-type, suppressing symptoms of withdrawal in opiate-dependent individuals. Second, chronic oral administration of LAAM can produce sufficient tolerance to block the subjective "high" of usual doses of parenterally administered opiates.

LAAM is metabolized by N-demethylation to nor-LAAM and dinor-LAAM, which are also opioid agonists. These metabolities are more potent than the parent drug. The opiod effect which occurs when LAAM is administered is slower in onset and longer in duration (72 hours) than that of methadone (24 hours). This extended duration of action allows three-times-weekly administration (see CLINCAL TRIALS).

PHARMACODYNAMICS

The duration of action of a single dose of LAAM is due to the sum of the opioid activity of the parent drug and its metabolites. A single dose of orally administered LAAM has an onset of opioid effects averaging 2 to 4 hours of ingestion and a duration of action of 48 to 72 hours (as measured by pupillary constriction and suppression of abstinence signs). LAAM

Continued on next page

Roxane Laboratories—Cont.

cross-substitutes for opiates like morphine in opiate-dependent individuals, suppressing symptom of withdrawal from these compounds. Single oral doses of 30 to 60 mg of LAAM eliminate signs of abstinence for 24 to 48 hours in individuals maintained on high doses of morphine who are abruptly withdrawn. At higher doses (80 mg and above), suppression of withdrawal can increase to 48 to 72 hours in most individuals.

Repeated oral administration of LAAM can produce sufficient tolerance to block the effects of parenterally administered opiates. Chronic oral administration of 70 to 100 mg of LAAM three times weekly produces tolerance which blocks the "high" of a 25 mg dose of intravenously administered heroin for up to 72 hours; maintenance on lower does (50 mg) of LAAM produces only partial blockage for the same period.

PHARMACOKINETICS

Absorption

LAAM is rapidly absorbed from an oral solution. Plasma levels are detectable within 15 to 30 minutes after ingestion and reach their peak within 1.5 to 2 hours at steady-state. LAAM undergoes first-pass metabolism to its demethylated metabolite nor-LAAM, which is sequentially N-demethylated to dinor-LAAM. Both metabolites are active and contribute to the extent and duration of ORLAAM's clinical activity (see PHARMACODYNAMICS).

Pharmacokinetic Model

The steady-state pharmacokinetics of LAAM were modeled from a study in 25 health adult addicts using three-times-a-week dosing over a 15-day observation period. LAAM and its metabolites were found to follow a multu-compartment model with extensive tissue distribution (Vd - 20 L/kg). LAAM had a clearance of about 0.22 L/kg/hr, mostly by conversion to nor-LAAM. Kinetic studies of the pure metabolites in man have not yet provided accurate estimates of their clearance in the absence of the precursor, but the half-lives observed in this study were 2.6 days for LAAM, approximately 2 days for non-LAAM, and approximately 4 days for dinor-LAAM.

The pharmacokinetic model used to estimate steady-state plasma levels for each subject in this study assumed a common 3 mg/kg/wk dosage regimen (0.94 mg/kg on Mon. and Wed., 1.125 mg/kg on Fri.). The estimates (which fit the observed data with a correlation of better than 0.95) revealed a large inter-patient variability. There was at least a 5-fold range in peak plasma concentrations for LAAM and its metabolites across the 25 subjects over the 72-hoiur interval from Friday to Monday on a 3-times-a-week dosage regimen. Table 1 contains these estimates of peak and trough plasma concentrations of LAAM, nor-LAAM, and dinor-LAAM.

Table 1: Peak and Trough Estimated Steady-State Plasma Concentrations During the 72 Hour Interval (Friday to Monday) for 65-kg Patient Given 3 mg/kg/Week on Mon./Wed./Fri.

	LAAM	Nor-LAAM	Dinor-LAAM
(Cmax(ng/mL)*	204 (34%)	173 (34%)	114 (28%)
Cmin(ng/mL)**	36 (62%)	85 (58%)	96 (34%)

* Following Friday Morning Does
** Prior to Monday Morning Dose

Figure 1: Simulated Steady-State Plasma Concentrations of LAAM, Nor-LAAM and Dinor-LAAM following Thrice Weekly Dosing with ORLAAM

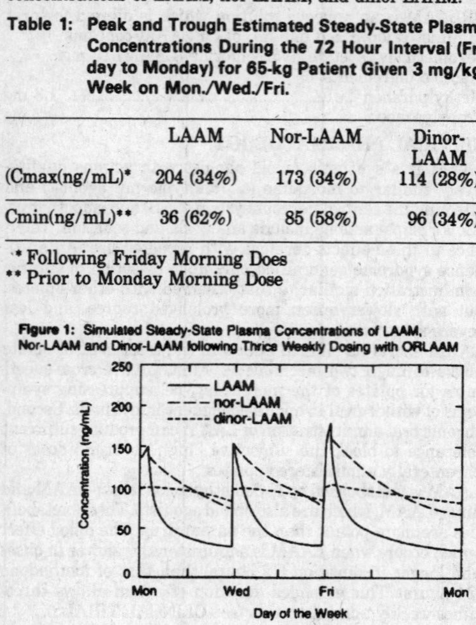

Metabolism and Elimination

As noted above, the information of nor-LAAM and dinor-LAAM is by sequential demethylation, such that dinor-LAAM is formed from nor-LAAM, not directly from LAAM. While N-demethylation is the primary route of metabolism, minor pathways of elimination include direct excretion and deacetylation to methadol, nor-methadol, and dinor-methadol.

Special Populations

Gender

An analysis of the data from the above study showed some differences in the plasma clearance of LAAM in 8 females versus 17 males. Males showed a trend toward a slower conversion of LAAM to nor-LAAM, which may alter the plasma concentration profile of LAAM and its active opioid metabolites. Although this effect was much smaller than the observed inter-individual differences, physicians should be alert to a possible gender difference (see INDIVIDUALIZATION OF DOSAGE).

Hepatic and Renal Disease

At the present time no pharmacokinetics studies have been carried out in subjects with clinically significant hepatic insufficiency or serious renal impairment. Since both the pharmacokinetics and pharmacodynamics of opiate agonists may be altered in these subjects, and any additional risks of ORLAAM therapy are not well understood in such patients, physicians may choose to manage such patients with methadone due to its simpler metabolic profile.

CLINICAL TRIALS

ORLAAM has been studied in 2666 street addicts and 3319 methadone maintenance patients, including 5697 males and 288 females. During the course of 27 studies, 4610 patients received orally administered ORLAAM for up to three years in thrice-weekly doses ranging from 10 to 140 mg. Twenty-one studies provide the primary evidence upon which the dosing recommendations for ORLAAM are based.

The vast majority of patients who received ORLAAM were treated on a thrice-weekly basis, typically on Mondays, Wednesdays and Fridays (Mon./Wed./Fri.), although every-other-day dosing schedules were used in some settings. Most of the sites dosing patients with LAAM on a 3-times-a-week (Mon./Wed./Fri. or Tues./Thurs./Sat.) schedule increased the dose prior to the 72-hour inter-dose interval by 20 to 40% to obtain coverage for the full 72 hours.

In controlled clinical trials, treatment with ORLAAM was found to be comparable to treatment with methadone with respect to reduction in use of illicit opioids. ORLAAM doses in the range of 60 to 100 mg 3-times-a-week reduced the average frequency of urine samples positive for opiates to 15–20%, as did therapy with 50 to 100 mg a day of methadone. There was a trend for more patients to drop out of ORLAAM therapy than methadone therapy in the first 4 weeks of treatment (16% dropouts for ORLAAM v. 12% for methadone), but the dropout rates for both treatments rapidly declined and both were in the range of 1 to 2% per week for the remaining patients by the third month of the studies. Global ratings of patient acceptability and response to treatment were similar for both LAAM and methadone.

In the Phase III studies, ORLAAM tended to be more effective in patients perceived by staff to benefit from a reduced frequency of clinic visits and less effective in patients perceived as needing the added support of daily clinic visits.

Four independent studies were concerned with other research objectives, including induction regimens, methadone-to-ORLAAM (and ORLAAM-to-methadone) crossover ratios, and detoxification. This research involved 800 adults (including 11 females), approximately 440 of whom were methadone maintenance patients. The results of these studies, as well as the results of a nationwide Phase III usage study of 623 patients (including 204 females) in 25 representative clinics across the country, are reflected in the dosing recommendations.

INDIVIDUALIZATION OF DOSAGE

ORLAAM is intended for use as part of a comprehensive treatment plan for narcotic dependence of the opioid type. Supplying narcotic drugs to narcotic addicts for the treatment of addiction without appropriate medical evaluation, treatment planning, and counseling has not been shown to be effective, and is a violation of the law except in special circumstances.

The therapeutic goal early in treatment with ORLAAM is to reduce illicit opioid use. The dose of ORLAAM should be chosen and adjusted as needed to provide a dose that is high enough to suppress drug withdrawal, illicit drug seeking and usage, and related high-risk behavior. If opioid side effects persist once illicit dry use is controlled, the dose of ORLAAM may require further adjustment later in treatment to minimize adverse effects.

Physicians should be alert to patient differences in levels of opioid tolerance and inter-patient variability in the absorption, distribution and metabolism of both ORLAAM and its metabolites. As with methadone, an important contribution to continued abuse of illicit drugs is an inadequate dose of the treatment medication.

Initial dosage adjustment with ORLAAM is complex due to its delayed onset of action. If the starting dose is too high or if the dose is escalated too rapidly for the patient's level of tolerance, symptoms characteristic of excessive opioid effect may occur, i.e., poor concentration, sedation, and orthostatic hypotension. Patients should be watched for such symptoms, and the dose should be lowered if they appear. In rare instances, serious symptoms of narcotic overdosage may occur, leading to profound CNS and respiratory depression.

ORLAAM and its metabolites quickly accumulate to toxic levels if the doses intended for 3-times-a-week dosing are given too frequently. The recommended doses are intended for every-other-day or 3-times-a-week dosing and **should not be given daily.**

The recommended initial dose for patients with low or unknown tolerance to opioids is 20 to 40 mg **three-times-a-week** or **every-other-day**. Successive doses may be increased by 5 to 10 mg. At least two weeks are needed to achieve a clinical plateau after a dosage adjustment. Adjustment to a dosing schedule is dependent upon the rate at which an individual develops tolerance to the increaseing level of ORLAAM (and its metabolites) as well as the time required for ORLAAM and its metabolites to accumulate to steady-state levels.

The goal of dosage titration is to suppress narcotic withdrawal while avoiding excessive opioid effects due to the build-up of long-acting metabolites. It may be safer to provide extra counseling and support rather than to attempt to completely suppress a patient's withdrawal or narcotic hunger during the first week or two of therapy. On the other hand, there is the ever-present danger that patients who receive sub-therapeutic starting doses will supplement with street drugs, resulting in overdose. Patients should be strongly warned against this practice. Later in the titration process, dosage adjustments are better made on a weekly basis whenever possible.

For patients on methadone maintenance whose level of tolerance is known, the recommended initial dose of ORLAAM is 1.2 to 1.3 times the patient's daily dose of methadone, not to exceed 120 mg. Care should be taken not to adjust the dose too frequently thereafter (usually 5 to 10 mg changes every second or third dose) since increasing the dose too rapidly may result in oversedation.

One major advantage of ORLAAM therapy is reduction in need for daily clinic visits and for take-home medication. In some patients, ORLAAM may not provide adequate suppression of withdrawal for a full 72 hours. For such individuals, several therapeutic options are available: (1) extra support and an explanation of reasons for the effect, (2) increasing the dose given prior to the 72-hour interval, (3) switching to an every-other-day dosing schedule, (4) dispensing a supplemental methadone dose.

Most patients do not experience withdrawal during 72-hour inter-dose interval after reaching pharmacological steady-state **with** or **without** adjustment of the Friday dose. If additional opioids are required, small doses of supplemental methadone should be given rather than giving ORLAAM on two consecutive days. Take-home doses of methadone always pose a risk in this setting and physicians should carefully weigh the potential therapeutic benefit against the risk of diversion (see DOSAGE AND ADMINISTRATION).

Patients should receive extra support and counseling and be warned against supplementing street drugs as they make the switch from methadone to ORLAAM. The variability in the clearance of LAAM, nor-LAAM, and dinor-LAAM and clinical experience suggest that there will be a small number of patients who require either lower or higher doses than those recommended.

DURATION OF ORLAAM THERAPY

There is no information from controlled clinical trials as to the appropriate duration of ORLAAM therapy. There are reports from investigators that some patients on ORLAAM may experience less variation in opioid effects and have less drug craving than with methadone, so ORLAAM should be considered for patients who need long-term maintenance during social and vocational rehabilitation.

When a patient has eliminated illicit drug use, achieved social and occupational stability, and made lifestyle changes to reduce the risk of relapse, consideration may be given to discontinuation of ORLAAM therapy. Such a decision should be carefully considered as part of an individualized treatment plan. Stable long-term ORLAAM therapy is preferable to repeated cycles of premature discontinuation of medication followed by relapse to uncontrolled addiction.

A patient is most likely to remain abstinent if discontinuation of medication is attempted after the achievement of behavioral objectives and is accompanied by appropriate non-pharmacological support. The rate of dose reduction should vary according to patient's response. Discontinuation of ORLAAM therapy for administrative reasons or because of adverse reactions to the drug should be managed as described below under DOSAGE AND ADMINISTRATION.

INDICATIONS

ORLAAM is indicated for the management of opiate dependence.

CONTRAINDICATIONS

The only known contraindication in the treatment of opiate dependence is hypersensitivity to LAAM.

ORLAAM is not recommended for any use other than for the treatment of opioid dependence (see WARNINGS).

WARNINGS

> Administration of ORLAAM on a daily basis has led to excessive drug accumulation and risk of fatal overdose. ORLAAM has only been studied on a thrice-weekly or every-other-day dosing regimen. Routine daily dosing after a patient has been inducted onto ORLAAM treatment is not allowed by current treatment regulations. Any decision to administer ORLAAM more frequently than every other day for any reason should be approached with extreme caution. Even then only very small doses (5 to 10 mg) should be considered.

Risk of Overdose: Analysis of some of the deaths from overdose observed in the development of ORLAAM has shown that when ORLAAM is diverted into channels of abuse, the uninformed addict can become impatient with the slow onset of ORLAAM (2 to 4 hours) and take illicit drugs, resulting in a potentially lethal combined overdose when the peak ORLAAM effect develops. Due to these risks of diversion and accidental death, ORLAAM has been approved for use only when **dispensed** by a licensed facility and is not given in take-home doses.

Use of Narcotic Antagonist: In an individual receiving ORLAAM, the administration of the usual dose of a narcotic antagonist may precipitate an acute withdrawal syndrome. The severity of this syndrome depends on the dose of the antagonist administered and the patient's level of physical dependence. Narcotic antagonist should be used in patients receiving ORLAAM only if needed. If a narcotic antagonist is used to treat respiratory depression in the physically dependent patient, it should be administered with care and titration should begin with much smaller-than-usual doses (0.1 to 0.2 mg recommended). If the desired effect is not achieved, escalating doses may be administered every 2 to 3 minutes. If a cumulative dose of 10 mg of naloxone has been given without effect, further administration is unlikely to be of benefit (see OVERDOSAGE).

If the patient does respond to narcotic antagonist, physicians should remember that naloxone has a much shorter duration of action than ORLAAM. Such patients should remain under prolonged observation rather than being allowed to leave emergency treatment, since ORLAAM's action will outlast naloxone-induced reversal, putting the unsupervised patient at risk of relapse, a return of respiratory depression and possible death if continuing medical attention is not available. Use of other parenteral opioid antagonists may be appropriate in some cases, but only if the dosage of such drugs can be readily titrated. Oral naltrexone would not be appropriate for the treatment of ORLAAM overdose, as it has been associated with the precipitation of prolonged opioid withdrawal symptoms when used in overdose settings.

Warnings to Patients:

> Patients must be warned that the peak activity of ORLAAM is not immediate, and that use or abuse of other psychoactive drugs, including alcohol, may result in **fatal** overdose, especially with the first few doses of ORLAAM, either during initation of treatment of after a lapse in treatment.

Use in High Risk Patients: Suicide attempts with opiates, especially in combination with tricyclic antidepressants, alcohol, and other CNS active agents, are part of the clinical pattern of addiction. Although outpatient therapy with ORLAAM and other drugs of this class is usually associated with a reduction in the risk of suicide, such risk is not eliminated. Individualized evaluation and treatment planning, including hospitalization, should be considered for patients who continue to exhibit uncontrolled drug use and persistent high-risk behavior despite adequate pharmacotherapy.

PRECAUTIONS

Initial Administration and Dosage Adjustment: Due to the long half-lives of ORLAAM and its metabolites, patients will not feel the full effects of the medication for at least several days. Consequently, extra care is needed when starting patients on ORLAAM and when making initial dosage adjustments (see INDIVIDUALIZATION OF DOSAGE and DOSAGE AND ADMINISTRATION)

Use In Ambulatory Patients: Initiation of therapy or excessive doses of ORLAAM may impair the mental and/or physical abilities required for performance of potentially hazardous tasks, such as driving a car or operating machinery. Patients should be warned not to engage in such activities if their alertness and behavior are affected. Most patients show no detectable impairment of ordinary tasks on ORLAAM therapy.

Head Injury and Increased Intracranial Pressure: The respiratory depressant effects of narcotics and their capacity to elevate cerebrospinal fluid pressure may be markedly exaggerated in the presence of increased intracranial pressure. Furthermore, narcotics produce side effects that may make it difficult to evaluate the clinical course of patients with head injuries. In view of LAAM's profile as a mu agonist, it should be used with extreme caution and only if deemed essential in such patients.

Asthma and Other Respiratory Conditions: ORLAAM, as with other opioids, should be used with caution in patients with asthma, in those with chronic obstructive pulmonary disease or cor pulmonale, and in individuals with a substantially decreased respiratory reserve, preexisting respiratory depression, hypoxia, or hypercapnea. In such patients, even usual therapeutic doses of narcotics may decrease respiratory drive while simultaneously increasing airway resistance to the point of apnea.

Special Risk Patients: Opioids should be given with caution and at reduced initial dose in certain patients, such as the elderly or debilitated and those with significant hepatic or renal dysfunction, hypothyroidism, Addison's Disease, prostatic hypertrophy, or urethral stricture.

Effects on Cardiac Conduction: ORLAAM has been shown to prolong the ST segment of the electrocardiogram in beagle dogs dosed five days a week. Serial EKGs performed in a pharmacokinetics study showed a prolongation of the QTc interval in some patients which was not associated with dose. Such a prolongation of the QTc interval has been seen with other opioids, and it is not known if this is an effect specific to a LAAM or if it is also seen with methadone. In either case, careful monitoring is recommended when using ORLAAM in patients with a history of known cardiac conduction defects, those taking medications affecting cardiac conduction and in other cases where an unusual risk of dysrhythmia is suggested by history or physical examination. This information is provided to alert the prescribing physician, and is not intended to deter the appropriate use of opioid agonists in patients with a history of cardiac disease. No adverse cardiac events have been associated with ORLAAM therapy in clinical study of the drug, and the risk of morbidity from treatment with either methadone or LAAM is less than the risk of morbidity from untreated addiction.

Acute Abdominal Conditions: As with other mu agonists, treatment with ORLAAM may obscure the diagnosis or clinical course in patients with acute abdominal conditions.

DRUG INTERACTIONS

Polydrug and Alcohol Abusers—Patients who are known to abuse sedatives, tranquilizers, propoxyphene, antidepressants, benzodiazepines, and alcohol should be warned of the risk of serious overdose if these substances are taken while on ORAAM maintenance.

Interaction with Narcotic Antagonists, Mixed Agonists/Antagonists, Partial Agonists, and Pure Agonists—As with other mu agonists, patients maintained on ORLAAM may experience withdrawal symptoms when administered pure narcotic antagonists, mixed agonist/antagonists or partial agonists such as naloxone, naltrexone, pentazocine, nalbuphine, butorphanol, and buprenorphine.

In addition, agonists such as meperidine and propoxyphene, which are N-demethylated to long-acting, excitatory metabolites, should not be used by patients taking ORLAAM because they would be ineffective unless given in such high doses that the risk of toxic effects of the metabolites becomes unacceptable.

Anesthesia and Analgesia—Patients receiving ORLAAM will develop a similar level of tolerance for opioids as patients receiving methadone. Anesthetists and other practitioners should be prepared to adjust their management of these patients accordingly.

Other Drug Interactions—The anti-tuberculosis drug rifampin has been found to produce a marked (50%) reduction in serum methadone levels, leading to the appearance of symptoms of withdrawal in well-stabilized methadone maintenance patients. Similar effects on serum methadone levels have been observed for carbamazepine, phenobarbital, and phenytoin, The presumed mechanism for this effect is the induction of methadone metabolizing enzymes. Since ORLAAM is metabolized into a **more** active metabolite, nor-LAAM, administration of these drugs may **increase** ORLAAM's peak activity and/or **shorten** its duration of action.

Conversely, drugs like erythromycin, cimetidine, and antifungal drugs like ketoconazole that inhibit hepatic metabolism, may **slow** the onset, **lower** the activity, and/or **increase** the duration of action of ORLAAM. Caution and close observation of patients receiving these drugs are advised to allow early detection of any need to adjust the dose or dosing interval.

Information for Patients:

Patients should be provided the patient package insert for ORLAAM if they are new to the drug, and in addition should be advised that:

ORLAAM, unlike methadone, is not to be taken daily, and daily use of the usual doses will lead to serious overdose.

ORLAAM is slow acting and patients should be alerted to the risk of abusing any psychoactive drug, including alcohol, while on ORLAAM therapy. This is particularly important during the first 7 to 10 days of treatment, before ORLAAM has had time to exert its full pharmacologic effect.

In addition to being warned of the delay in onset of ORLAAM, patients who are transferring from ORLAAM to methadone should be informed that they should wait 48 hours after the last dose of ORLAAM before ingesting their first dose of methadone or other narcotic (see DOSAGE AND ADMINISTRATION)

Patients should inform their adult family members that, in the event of overdose, the treating physician or emergency room staff should be told that the patient is being treated with ORLAAM, a long-acting opioid which is likely to outlast naloxone-induced reversal and which requires prolonged observation and careful monitoring. In addition, the treating physician or emergency room staff should be informed that the patient is physically dependent on narcotics and that naloxone should be administered with care so as to minimize any precipitated abstinence syndrome.

As with most mu agonists, ORLAAM may interact with other CNS depressants and should be used with caution, and in reduced dosage, in patients concurrently receiving other narcotic analgesics, antihistamines, benzodiazepines, phenothiazines or other major tranquilizers, anxiolytics, sedative-hypnotics, tricyclic antidepressants, and other CNS depressants, including alcohol. Patients should be warned of the importance of reporting the use of any of these compounds to their physicians, as serious side effects could result, including respiratory depression, hypotension, profound sedation or coma.

Carcinogenesis, Mutagenesis and Impairment of Fertility: Two-year carcinogenicity studies with LAAM in rats at 13 mg/kg (77 mg/m^2) and in mice at 30 mg/kg (90 mg/m^2) given orally in the diet did not show carcinogenic changes. LAAM is not mutagenic in the Ames test, the unscheduled DNA synthesis and repair test mouse lymphoma cells in vitro, or chromosal aberration tests in rats in vivo. LAAM tested positive in the forward mutation assay in N. crassa at 150 μg/mL in vitro and in the heritable translocation assay in mice at 21 mg/kg (63 mg/m^2). The clinical significance of these findings is not known.

Chronic treatment with LAAM at 80 mg three times a week did not produce chromosomal aberrations in peripheral human lymphocytes. Effects of LAAM on fertility in animals has not been fully evaluated.

Use in Pregnancy: Pregnancy Category C

Animal reproduction studies are not complete and there are no clinical data on the safety of ORLAAM in pregnancy. For these reasons, ORLAAM is not recommended for use in pregnancy. Women who may become pregnant should be advised of the risks of ORLAAM therapy and of the desirability of discontinuing ORLAAM prior to a planned pregnancy. Current regulations mandate monthly pregnancy tests in female patients of childbearing potential who are using ORLAAM. If a female patient becomes pregnant on ORLAAM despite these precautions, it is recommended she be transferred to methadone for the remainder of the pregnancy (see TRANSFER FROM ORLAAM TO METHADONE, in DOSAGE AND ADMINISTRATION). If it appears wiser to continue a specific patient on ORLAAM, the physician should be alert to possible respiratory depression of the newborn and other perinatal complications (see Labor and Delivery).

Labor and Delivery: The effects of ORLAAM on labor and delivery are not known. Like other mu agonist opioids, however, ORLAAM is expected to produce respiratory depression and a possible neonatal dependence syndrome with a delayed emergence of withdrawal symptoms. Use of ORLAAM in labor and delivery is not recommended unless, in the opinion of the treating physician, the potential benefits outweigh the possible hazards.

Nursing Mothers: The effects of LAAM on infants of nursing mothers have not been studied. It is not known if LAAM is excreted in human milk in sufficient concentration to affect an infant. Use of ORLAAM in nursing mothers is not recommended unless, in the opinion of the treating physician, the potential benefits outweigh the possible hazards.

Pediatric Use: The use of ORLAAM in addicts under 18 years of age has not been studied. Its use is not recommended and is contrary to current regulations.

ADVERSE REACTIONS

Physicians should be alert to palpitations, syncope, or other symptoms suggestive of episodes of irregular cardiac rhythm in patients taking ORLAAM and promptly evaluate such cases (see Effects on Cardiac Conduction in PRECAUTIONS).

Heroin or Methadone Withdrawal Reactions—Patients presenting for ORLAAM treatment are frequently in withdrawal from heroin or other opiates. They may display typical withdrawal symptoms which should be differentiated from ORLAAM's side effects. Patients may exhibit some or all of the following signs and symptoms associated with withdrawal from opiates: lacrimation, rhinorrhea, sneezing, yawning, perspiration, gooseflesh, fever, chilliness alternating with flushing, restlessness, irritability, insomnia, weakness, anxiety, depression, dilated pupils, tremors, tachycardia, abdominal cramps, body aches, anorexia, nausea, vomit-

Continued on next page

Roxane Laboratories—Cont.

ing, diarrhea, and weight loss. Control of such symptoms is a primary goal of therapy. However, because of the slow onset and long half-lives of ORLAAM, nor-LAAM and dinor-LAAM, overly aggresive increases in dosage to control these withdrawal symptoms with ORLAAM may result in overdose (see INDIVIDUALIZATION OF DOSAGE).

Signs and Symptoms of ORLAAM Excess—The interaction between the development and maintenance of opioid tolerance and ORLAAM dose can be complex. Dose reduction is recommended in cases where patients develop signs and symptoms of excessive ORLAAM effect, characterized by complaints of "feeling wired", poor concentration, drowsiness, and possibly dizziness on standing.

ORLAAM Withdrawal—Patients may experience withdrawal symptoms (nasal congestion, abdominal symptoms, diarrhea, muscle aches, anxiety) over the 72-hour dosing interval if the dose of ORLAAM is too low. This may be managed as described under INDIVIDUALIZATION OF DOSAGE, but physicians should be alert to the possible need for dose or dose schedule adjustments if patients complain of weekend withdrawal symptoms in the last day of the 72-hour dosing interval.

Adverse Reactions on Stable Therapy:
The following adverse events were observed in the 25-site, 623-patient usage study in male and female opiate addicts (see CLINICAL TRIALS). These signs and symptoms were reported during the second and third months of treatment with ORLAAM, and were considered severe enough to require medical evaluation. In this study, both questionnaires and spontaneous reports were used to gather information. Questionnaire-elicited symptom frequencies were about five times as frequent as the spontaneous reporting frequencies given below.

Incidence greater than 1%, Probably Causally Related

Body of a Whole—	Asthenia*, back pain chills, edema, hot flashes (males 2:1), flu syndrome and malaise (11%).
Gastrointestinal—	Abdominal pain*, constipation*, diarrhea, dry mouth, nausea and vomiting.
Musculoskeletal—	Arthralgia*
Nervous System—	Abnormal dreams, anxiety, decreased sex drive, depression, euphoria, headache, hypesthesia, insomnia (9.1%), nervousness*, somnolence.
Respiratory—	Cough, rhinitis, and yawning.
Skin/appendages—	Rash, sweating*.
Special Senses—	Blurred vision.
Urogenital—	Difficult ejaculation*, impotence*.

*Reactions in 3–9% of patients; reactions in 1–3% are unmarked.

Incidence less than 1%, Probably Causally Related

Cardiovascular—	Postural hypotension.
Musculoskeletal—	Myalgia.
Special Senses—	Tearing.

Causal Relationship Unknown
These reactions were reported with low frequency in controlled and uncontrolled studies of LAAM, are not known to be causally related to the administration of the drug, and are provided as alerting information for physicians.

Cardiovascular—	Hypertension, prolongation of the QT interval, non-specific ST-T wave changes.
Hepatic—	Hepatitis and abnormal liver function tests.
Urogenital—	Amenorrhea, pyuria.

DRUG DEPENDENCE

ORLAAM is a Schedule II controlled substance under the Federal Controlled Substances Act. ORLAAM produces dependence of the morphine-type and has potential for abuse. Tolerance and physical dependence will develop upon repeated administration. As with methadone and any other narcotic administered to narcotic addicts. ORLAAM is at risk for diversion and illicit use, and should be handled accordingly (see WARNINGS).

OVERDOSE

Signs and Symptoms: All but a few cases of ORLAAM overdose have involved multiple drugs. Overdose on ORLAAM alone is rare and has always been the result of too frequent (daily) dosing. Overdose is primarily of concern in persons not tolerant to opiates, since in such individuals a dose of 20 to 40 mg of ORLAAM may cause somnolence, and a larger initial dose may cause serious overdose. Tolerant individuals will generally not show symptoms unless higher doses are administered.

In ORLAAM overdose, as with other mu agonist opioids, the following signs and symptoms should be anticipated: respiratory depression (decrease in respiratory rate and/or tidal volume. Cheyne-Stokes respiration, cyanosis), extreme somnolence progressing to stupor or coma, maximally constricted pupils, skeletal muscle flaccidity, cold and clammy skin, bradycardia, and hypotension. In severe overdose, apnea, circulatory collapse, pulmonary edema, cardiac arrest and death may occur.

Treatment: In the case of ORLAAM overdose, protect the patient's airway and support ventilation and circulation. Absorption of ORLAAM from the gastrointestinal tract may be decreased by gastric emptying and/or administration of activated charcoal. (Safeguard the patient's airway when employing gastric emptying or administering charcoal in any patient with diminished consciousness). Forced diuresis, peritoneal dialysis, hemodialysis, or charcoal hemoperfusion are unlikely to be beneficial for ORLAAM overdose due to its high lipid solubility and large volume of distribution.

In managing ORLAAM overdose, the physician should consider the possibility of multiple drugs, the interaction between drugs, and any unusual drug kinetics in the patient. Naloxone may be given to antagonize opiate effects, but the airway must be secured as vomiting may ensue. If possible, naloxone should be titrated to clinical effect rather than given as a large single bolus, since rapid reversal of opioid effects by large naloxone doses can cause severe precipitated withdrawal effects that may include cardiac instability. If a patient has received a total of 10 mg of naloxone without clinical response, the diagnosis of opioid overdose is unlikely. If the patient does respond to naloxone, the physician should remember that the duration of ORLAAM activity is much longer (days) than that of naloxone (minutes) and repeated dosing with or continuous intravenous infusion of naloxone is likely to be required. Use of oral naltrexone in this setting is not recommended because it may precipitate prolonged opioid withdrawal symptoms (see Use of Narcotic Antagonists).

DOSAGE AND ADMINISTRATION

ORLAAM produces opioid effects and a high degree of opioid tolerance that inhibits drug-seeking behavior and blocks the euphoria produced by the usual doses of heroin. The dose of ORLAAM in each patient should be adjusted to achieve the optimal therapeutic benefit with acceptable adverse opioid effects (see INDIVIDUALIZATION OF DOSAGE).

ORLAAM must always be diluted before administration, and should be mixed with diluent prior to dispensing. To avoid confusion between prepared doses of ORLAAM and methadone, the liquid used to dilute ORLAAM should be a different color from that used to dilute methadone in any specific clinic setting.

ORLAAM DOSING

Dosing Schedules:
ORLAAM is usually administered three times a week, either on Monday, Wednesday and Friday, or on Tuesday, Thursday and Saturday. If withdrawal is a problem during the 72-hour inter-dose interval, the preceding dose may be increased. In some cases, an every-other-day schedule may be appropriate (see INDIVIDUALIZATION OF DOSAGE). The usual doses of ORLAAM must not be given on consecutive days because of the risk of fatal overdose. No dose mentioned in this label is **ever** meant to be given as a daily dose (see WARNINGS).

INDUCTION
The initial dose of ORLAAM for street addicts should be 20 to 40 mg. Each subsequent dose, administered at 48- or 72-hour intervals, may be adjusted in increments of 5 to 10 mg until a pharmacokinetic and pharmacodynamic steady-state is reached, usually within 1 or 2 weeks (see INDIVIDUALIZATION OF DOSAGE).

Patients dependent on methadone may require higher initial doses of ORLAAM. The suggested initial 3-times-a-week dose of ORLAAM for such patients is 1.2 to 1.3 times the daily methadone maintenance dose being replaced. This initial dose should not exceed 120 mg and subsequent doses, administered at 48- or 72-hour intervals, should be adjusted according to clinical response.

Most patients can tolerate the 72-hour inter-dose interval during the induction period. Some patients may require additional intervention (see INDIVIDUALIZATION OF DOSAGE). If additional opioids are required, supplemental methadone in small doses should be given rather than giving ORLAAM on two consecutive days. Take-home doses of methadone always pose a risk in this setting and physicians should carefully weigh the potential therapeutic benefit against the risk of diversion.

In some cases, where the degree of tolerance is unknown, patients can be started on methadone to facilitate more rapid titration to an effective dose, then converted to ORLAAM after a few weeks of methadone therapy.

The crossover from methadone to ORLAAM should be accomplished in a single dose; complete transfer to ORLAAM is simpler and preferable to more complex regimens involving escalating doses of ORLAAM and decreasing doses of methadone.

Dosage should be carefully titrated to the individual; induction too rapid for the patient's level of tolerance may result in overdose. Serious hazards, as seen in association with all narcotic analgesics, are respiratory depression and, to a lesser extent, circulatory depression.

MAINTENANCE
Most patients will be stabilized on doses in the range of 60 to 90 mg, 3-times-a-week. Doses as low as 10 mg and as high as 140 mg three times a week have been given in clinical studies.

Supplemental dosing over the 72-hour inter-dose interval (weekend) is rarely needed. For example, if a patient on a Mon./Wed./Fri. schedule complains of withdrawal on Sundays, the recommended dosage adjustment is to increase the Friday dose in 5 to 10 mg increments up to 40% over the Mon./Wed. dose or to a maximum of 140 mg.

If withdrawal symptoms persist after adjustment of dose, consideration may be given to every-other-day dosing if clinic hours permit. If the clinic is not opern seven days a week and every-other day dosing is not practical, the patient's schedule may be adjusted so the 72-hour interval occurrs during the week and the patient can come to the clinic to receive a supplemental dose of methadone (see INDIVIDUALIZATION OF DOSAGE).

The maximum **total** amount of ORLAAM recommended for any patient is 140-140-140 mg or 130-130-180 mg on a thrice-weekly schedule or 140 mg every other day.

PLANNED TEMPORARY INTERRUPTION OF ORLAAM MAINTENANCE

ORLAAM take-home doses are not permitted by regulation. Thus, several circumstances may cause the planned temporary discontinuation of treatment with ORLAAM. Patients eligible for one or more take-home doses of methadone, who are unable to attend the clinic for their next regularly scheduled ORLAAM dose because of illness, personal or family crisis, other hardships, travel and/or state/federal holidays, may be temporarily transferred directly to methadone.

Patients meeting these criteria may receive one or more methadone doses. Methadone doses should be 80% of the patient's Monday/Wednesday ORLAAM dose (e.g., patients receiving 80-80-100 mg of ORLAAM on a Monday/Wednesday/Friday regimen would be transferred to a daily methadone dose of 64 mg). The first dose of methadone should be ingested no sooner than 48 hours after the last ORLAAM dose. The number of takehome methadone doses should be **two less** than the number of days of expected absence and should not exceed, in any case, the number of take-homes allowed in the methadone regulations.

Upon return to clinic, patients should resume ORLAAM maintenance following the same dosage regimen used prior to the temporary interruption (see above). If more than 48 hours has elapsed since their last methadone dose, patients should be reinducted on ORLAAM at a dose determined by clinical and/or toxicological evaluation of the patient by the physician.

REINDUCTION AFTER AN UNPLANNED LAPSE IN DOSING:

Following a lapse of one ORLAAM dose:

1) If a patient comes to the clinic to be dosed **on the day following a missed scheduled dose** (misses Monday, arrives Tuesday), the regular Monday dose should be administered on Tuesday, with the scheduled Wednesday dose administered on Thursday and the Friday dose given on Saturday. The patient's regular schedule may be resumed the following Monday (misses Wednesday, receives the regular dose on Thursday and Saturday, and returns to the regular Monday/Wednesday/Friday dosing schedule the next week).
2) If a patient misses one dose and comes to the clinic **on the day of the next scheduled dose** (misses Monday, arrives Wednesday), the usual dose will be well tolerated in most instances, although a reduced dose may be appropriate in selected cases.

Following a lapse of more than one ORLAAM dose:
Patients should be reinducted at an initial dose of $^1/_2$ or $^3/_4$ their previous ORLAAM dose, followed by increases of 5 to 10 mg every dosing day (48- or 72-hours intervals) until their previous maintenance dose is achieved. Patients who have been off of ORLAAM treatment for more than a week should be reinducted.

TRANSFER FROM ORLAAM TO METHADONE
Patients maintained on ORLAAM may be transferred directly to methadone. Because of the difference between the two compounds' metabolites and their pharmacological half-lives, it is recommended that methadone be started on a daily dose at 80% of the ORLAAM dose being replaced; the initial methadone dose must be given no sooner than 48 hours after the last ORLAAM dose. Subsequent increases or decreases of 5 to 10 mg in the daily methadone dose may be given to control symptoms or withdrawal or, less likely, symptoms of excessive sedation, in accordance with clinical observations.

DETOXIFICATION FROM ORLAAM
There is a limited experience with detoxifying patients from ORLAAM in a systematic manner, and both gradual reduction (5 to 10% a week) and abrupt withdrawal schedules have been used successfully. The decision to discontinue ORLAAM therapy should be made as part of a comprehensive treatment plan (see INDIVIDUALIZATION OF DOSAGE).

SAFETY AND HANDLING

ORLAAM is a solution of a potent narcotic (LAAM). There are no known specific hazards associated with dermal and aerosol exposure to ORLAAM. In case of accidental dermal exposure, promptly remove contaminated clothing and rinse the affected skin with cool water.

For the first six to twelve months, sales of ORLAAM will be restricted to clinics that have received training in its use, until there is general knowledge about how to use the drug safely. Since ORLAAM can be potentially dangerous if diverted, appropriate security measures should be taken to safeguard stock of ORLAAM as required by 21 CFR 1301.74 & 1304.28.

HOW SUPPLIED

ORLAAM Oral Solution (10 mg/mL) is a clear, colorless liquid supplied in plastic bottles as follows:
One pint (474 mL) per bottle, NDC 0054-3639-62
Store at controlled room temperature, 15-30°C (59-86°F). Protect from direct sunlight. Retain in original carton until needed for use.
ORLAAM is compatible with the materials used in most dispensing systems. Information about obtaining appropriate dispensing systems suitable for use with ORLAAM is available from the manufacturer upon request.
Manufactured
Roxane Laboratories, Inc.
Columbus Ohio 43216
Revised March 1995
035
© RLI, 1995

PREDNISONE TABLETS USP ℞
1 mg, 2.5 mg, 5 mg, 10 mg, 20 mg, or
50 mg

HOW SUPPLIED

1 mg white, scored tablets, gluten-free (Identified 54 092).
NDC 0054-8739-25: Unit dose, 10 tablets per strip, 10 strips per shelf pack, 10 shelf packs per shipper.
NDC 0054-4741-25: Bottles of 100 tablets.
2.5 mg white, scored tablets, gluten-free (Identified 54 339).
NDC 0054-8740-25: Unit dose, 10 tablets per strip, 10 strips per shelf pack, 10 shelf packs per shipper.
NDC 0054-4742-25: Bottles of 100 tablets.
5 mg white, scored tablets, gluten-free (Identified 54 612).
NDC 0054-8724-25: Unit dose, 10 tablets per strip, 10 strips per shelf pack, 10 shelf packs per shipper.
NDC 0054-4728-25: Bottles of 100 tablets.
NDC 0054-4728-31: Bottles of 1000 tablets.
10 mg white, scored tablets, gluten-free (Identified 54 899).
NDC 0054-8725-25: Unit dose, 10 tablets per strip, 10 strips per shelf pack, 10 shelf packs per shipper.
NDC 0054-4730-25: Bottles of 100 tablets.
NDC 0054-4730-29: Bottles of 500 tablets.
20 mg white, scored tablets, gluten-free (Identified 54 760).
NDC 0054-8726-25: Unit dose, 10 tablets per strip, 10 strips per shelf pack, 10 shelf packs per shipper.
NDC 0054-4729-25: Bottles of 100 tablets.
NDC 0054-4729-29: Bottles of 500 tablets.
50 mg white, scored tablets, gluten-free (Identified 54 343).
NDC 0054-8729-25: Unit dose, 10 tablets per strip, 10 strips per shelf pack, 10 shelf packs per shipper.
NDC 0054-4733-25: Bottles of 100 tablets.

ROXANOL™ Ⓒ ℞
[rox´-ĕ-nŭl]
Morphine Sulfate Immediate Release, Concentrated Oral Solution
20 mg per mL
(WARNING: May be habit forming.)

ROXANOL 100™
Morphine Sulfate Immediate Release, Concentrated Oral Solution
100 mg per 5 mL
(WARNING: May be habit forming.)

DESCRIPTION
Each mL of Roxanol™ contains:
Morphine Sulfate .... 20 mg
(Warning: May be habit forming.)
Each 5 mL of Roxanol 100™ contains:
Morphine Sulfate .... 100 mg
(Warning: May be habit forming.)
Chemically, Morphine Sulfate is, Morphinan-3,6-diol, 7,8-didehydro-4,5-epoxy-17-methyl-, (5α,6α)-, sulfate (2:1) (salt), pentahydrate.
Morphine Sulfate acts as a narcotic analgesic.

CLINICAL PHARMACOLOGY
The major effects of morphine are on the central nervous system and the bowel. Opioids act as agonists, interacting with stereospecific and saturable binding sites or receptors in the brain and other tissues.
Morphine is about two-thirds absorbed from the gastrointestinal tract with the maximum analgesic effect occurring 60 minutes post administration.

INDICATIONS AND USAGE
Morphine is indicated for the relief of severe acute and severe chronic pain.

CONTRAINDICATIONS
Hypersensitivity to morphine; respiratory insufficiency or depression; severe CNS depression; attack of bronchial asthma; heart failure secondary to chronic lung disease; cardiac arrhythmias; increased intracranial or cerebrospinal pressure; head injuries; brain tumor; acute alcoholism; delirium tremens; convulsive disorders; after biliary tract surgery; suspected surgical abdomen; surgical anastomosis; concomitantly with MAO inhibitors or within 14 days of such treatment.

WARNINGS
Morphine can cause tolerance, psychological and physical dependence. Withdrawal will occur on abrupt discontinuation or administration of a narcotic antagonist.
Interaction with Other Central-Nervous-System Depressants —Morphine should be used with caution and in reduced dosage in patients who are concurrently receiving other narcotic analgesics, general anesthetics, phenothiazines, other tranquilizers, sedative-hypnotics, tricyclic antidepressants, and other CNS depressants (including alcohol). Respiratory depression, hypotension, and profound sedation or coma may result.

PRECAUTIONS
General:
Head Injury and Increased Intracranial Pressure —The respiratory depressant effects of morphine and its capacity to elevate cerebrospinal-fluid pressure may be markedly exaggerated in the presence of increased intracranial pressure. Furthermore, narcotics produce side effects that may obscure the clinical course of patients with head injuries. In such patients, morphine must be used with caution and only if it is deemed essential.
Asthma and Other Respiratory Conditions —Morphine should be used with caution in patients having an acute asthmatic attack, in those with chronic obstructive pulmonary disease or cor pulmonale, and in individuals with a substantially decreased respiratory reserve, preexisting respiratory depression, hypoxia, or hypercapnia. In such patients, even usual therapeutic doses of narcotics may decrease respiratory drive while simultaneously increasing airway resistance to the point of apnea.
Hypotensive Effect —The administration of morphine may result in severe hypotension in an individual whose ability to maintain his blood pressure has already been compromised by a depleted blood volume or concurrent administration of such drugs as the phenothiazines or certain anesthetics.
Special-Risk Patients —Morphine should be given with caution and the initial dose should be reduced in certain patients, such as the elderly or debilitated and those with severe impairment of hepatic or renal function, hypothyroidism, Addison's disease, prostatic hypertrophy, or urethral stricture.
Acute Abdominal Conditions —The administration of morphine or other narcotics may obscure the diagnosis or clinical course in patients with acute abdominal conditions.
Information for patients:
Use in Ambulatory Patients —Morphine may impair the mental and/or physical abilities required for the performance of potentially hazardous tasks, such as driving a car or operating machinery. The patient should be cautioned accordingly.
Morphine, like other narcotics, may produce orthostatic hypotension in ambulatory patients.
Patients should be cautioned about the combined effects of alcohol or other central nervous system depressants with morphine.
Drug interactions:
Generally, effects of morphine may be potentiated by alkalizing agents and antagonized by acidifying agents. Analgesic effect of morphine is potentiated by chlorpromazine and methocarbamol. CNS depressants such as anaesthetics, hypnotics, barbiturates, phenothiazines, chloral hydrate, glutethimide, sedatives, MAO inhibitors (including procarbazine hydrochloride), antihistamines, β-blockers (propranolol), alcohol, furazolidone and other narcotics may enhance the depressant effects of morphine.
Morphine may increase anticoagulant activity of coumarin and other anticoagulants.
Carcinogenicity/Mutagenicity:
Long-term studies to determine the carcinogenic and mutagenic potential of morphine are not available.
Pregnancy:
Teratogenic Effects —Pregnancy Category C: Animal production studies have not been conducted with morphine. It is also not known whether morphine can cause fetal harm when administered to a pregnant woman or can affect reproduction capacity. Morphine should be given to a pregnant woman only if clearly needed.
Labor and Delivery:
Morphine readily crosses the placental barrier and, if administered during labor, may lead to respiratory depression in the neonate.
Nursing Mothers:
Morphine has been detected in human milk. For this reason, caution should be exercised when morphine is administered to a nursing woman.
Pediatric Usage:
Safety and effectiveness in children have not been established.

ADVERSE REACTIONS
THE MAJOR HAZARDS OF MORPHINE AS OF OTHER NARCOTIC ANALGESICS, ARE RESPIRATORY DEPRESSION AND, TO A LESSER DEGREE, CIRCULATORY DEPRESSION, RESPIRATORY ARREST, SHOCK, AND CARDIAC ARREST HAVE OCCURRED.
The most frequently observed adverse reactions include lightheadedness, dizziness, sedation, nausea, vomiting, and sweating. These effects seem to be more prominent in ambulatory patients and in those who are not suffering severe pain. In such individuals, lower doses are advisable. Some adverse reactions may be alleviated in the ambulatory patient if he lies down.
Other adverse reactions include the following:
Central Nervous System —Euphoria, dysphoria, weakness, headache, insomnia, agitation, disorientation, and visual disturbances.
Gastrointestinal —Dry mouth, anorexia, constipation, and biliary tract spasm.
Cardiovascular —Flushing of the face, bradycardia, palpitation, faintness, and syncope.
Genitourinary —Urinary retention or hesitancy, anti-diuretic effect, and reduced libido and/or potency.
Allergic —Pruritus, urticaria, other skin rashes, edema, and, rarely hemorrhagic urticaria.
Treatment of the most frequent adverse reactions:
Constipation —Ample intake of water or other liquids should be encouraged. Concomitant administration of a stool softener and a peristaltic stimulant with the narcotic analgesic can be an effective preventive measure for those patients in need of therapeutics. If elimination does not occur for two days, an enema should be administered to prevent impaction.
In the event diarrhea occurs, seepage around a fecal impaction is a possible cause to consider before antidiarrheal measures are employed.
Nausea and Vomiting —Phenothiazines and antihistamines can be effective treatments for nausea of the medullary and vestibular sources respectively. However, these drugs may potentiate the side effects of the narcotics or the antinauseant.
Drowsiness (sedation) —Once pain control is achieved, undesirable sedation can be minimized by titrating the dosage to a level that just maintains a tolerable pain or pain free state.

DRUG ABUSE AND DEPENDENCE
Morphine Sulfate, narcotic, is a Schedule II controlled substance under the Federal Controlled Substance Act. As with other narcotics, some patients may develop a physical and psychological dependence on morphine. They may increase dosage without consulting a physician and subsequently may develop a physical dependence on the drug. In such cases, abrupt discontinuance may precipitate typical withdrawal symptoms, including convulsions. Therefore the drug should be withdrawn gradually from any patient known to be taking excessive dosages over a long period of time.
In treating the terminally ill patient the benefit of pain relief may outweigh the possibility of drug dependence. *The chance of drug dependence is substantially reduced when the patient is placed on scheduled narcotic programs instead of a "pain to relief-of-pain" cycle typical of a PRN regimen.*

OVERDOSAGE
Signs and Symptoms: Serious overdose with morphine is characterized by respiratory depression (a decrease in respiratory rate and/or tidal volume, Cheyne-Stokes respiration, cyanosis), extreme somnolence progressing to stupor or coma, skeletal muscle flaccidity, cold or clammy skin, and sometimes bradycardia and hypotension. In severe overdosage, apnea, circulatory collapse, cardiac arrest and death may occur.
Treatment: Primary attention should be given to the reestablishment of adequate respiratory exchange through provision of a patent airway and the institution of assisted or controlled ventilation. The narcotic antagonist naloxone is a specific antidote against respiratory depression which may result from overdosage or unusual sensitivity to narcotics, including morphine. Therefore, an appropriate dose of naloxone (usual initial adult dose: 0.4 mg) should be administered, preferably by the intravenous route and simultaneously

Continued on next page

Roxane Laboratories—Cont.

with efforts at respiratory resuscitation. Since the duration of action of morphine may exceed that of the antagonist, the patient should be kept under continued surveillance and repeated doses of the antagonist should be administered as needed to maintain adequate respiration.

An antagonist should not be administered in the absence of clinically significant respiratory or cardiovascular depression.

Oxygen, intravenous fluids, vasopressors and other supportive measures should be employed as indicated.

Gastric emptying may be useful in removing unabsorbed drug.

DOSAGE AND ADMINISTRATION

ROXANOL™ and ROXANOL 100™—Usual Adult Oral Dose: 10 to 30 mg every 4 hours or as directed by physician. Dosage is a patient dependent variable, therefore increased dosage may be required to achieve adequate analgesia.

For control of chronic, agonizing pain in patients with certain terminal disease, this drug should be administered on a regularly scheduled basis, every 4 hours, at the lowest dosage level that will achieve adequate analgesia.

Note: Medication may suppress respiration in the elderly, the very ill, and those patients with respiratory problems, therefore lower doses may be required.

Morphine Dosage Reduction: During the first two to three days of effective pain relief, the patient may sleep for many hours. This can be misinterpreted as the effect of excessive analgesic dosing rather than the first sign of relief in a pain exhausted patient. The dose, therefore, should be maintained for at least three days before reduction, if respiratory activity and other vital signs are adequate.

Following successful relief of severe pain, periodic attempts to reduce the narcotic dose should be made. Smaller doses or complete discontinuation of the narcotic analgesic may become feasible due to a physiologic change or the improved mental state of the patient.

HOW SUPPLIED

Roxanol™
Morphine Sulfate (Immediate Release)
Concentrated Oral Solution
20 mg per mL
NDC 0054-3751-44: Bottles of 30 mL with calibrated dropper.
NDC 0054-3751-50: Bottles of 120 mL with calibrated dropper.
Roxanol 100™
Morphine Sulfate (Immediate Release)
Concentrated Oral Solution
100 mg per 5 mL
NDC 0054-3751-58: Bottles of 240 mL with calibrated patient spoon.
Morphine Sulfate (Immediate Release)
Concentrated Oral Solution
30 mg per 1.5 mL
NDC 0054-8788-11: Unit dose vial of 1.5 mL (30 mg Morphine Sulfate), 25 reverse number vials per carton.
DEA Order Form Required
4073001
054
©RLI, 1994.   Revised May 1994
Shown in Product Identification Guide, page 332

ROXICET™ Tablets   © ℞
[*rox-ē-cĕt*]
Oxycodone and Acetaminophen Tablets USP
(Oxycodone Hydrochloride 5 mg and Acetaminophen 325 mg)
    (WARNING: May be habit forming)

ROXICET™ Oral Solution   © ℞
Oxycodone and Acetaminophen Oral Solution
(Oxycodone Hydrochloride 5 mg and Acetaminophen 325 mg Oral Solution per 5 mL)
    (WARNING: May be habit forming)

ROXICET 5/500™ Caplet   © ℞
Oxycodone and Acetaminophen Tablets USP
(Oxycodone Hydrochloride 5 mg and Acetaminophen 500 mg)
    (WARNING: May be habit forming)

DESCRIPTION

Each tablet contains:
Oxycodone Hydrochloride+ .... 5 mg
            (Warning: May Be Habit Forming)
Acetaminophen .... 325 mg
Each 5 mL contains:
Oxycodone Hydrochloride+ .... 5 mg
            (Warning: May Be Habit Forming)
Acetaminophen .... 325 mg
Alcohol 0.4%

Each caplet contains:
Oxycodone Hydrochloride+ .... 5 mg
            Warning: May be Habit Forming)
Acetaminophen .... 500 mg
(+5 mg Oxycodone HCl is equivalent to 4.4815 mg Oxycodone.)

HOW SUPPLIED

ROXICET™ Tablets, Oxycodone and Acetaminophen Tablets USP (Oxycodone Hydrochloride 5 mg and Acetaminophen 325 mg) white scored tablets (Identified 54 543).
NDC 0054-8650-24: Unit dose, 25 tablets per card (reverse numbered), 4 cards per shipper.
NDC 0054-4650-25: Bottles of 100 tablets.
NDC 0054-4650-29: Bottles of 500 tablets.
ROXICET™ Oral Solution,
Oxycodone and Acetaminophen Oral Solution (Oxycodone Hydrochloride 5 mg and Acetaminophen 325 mg Oral Solution per 5 mL)
NDC 0054-8648-16: Unit dose Patient Cups™ filled to deliver 5 mL (Oxycodone Hydrochloride 5 mg, Acetaminophen 325 mg), ten 5 mL Patient Cups™ per shelf pack, 4 shelf packs per shipper.
NDC 0054-3686-63: Bottles of 500 mL.
ROXICET 5/500™ Caplets,
Oxycodone and Acetaminophen Tablets USP (Oxycodone Hydrochloride 5 mg and Acetaminophen 500 mg), white scored capsule-shaped tablets (Identified 54 730).
NDC 0054-8784-24: Unit dose, 25 caplets per card (reverse numbered), 4 cards per shipper.
NDC 0054-4784-25: Bottles of 100 caplets.
Store at Controlled Room Temperature (15°–30°C (59°–86°F).
DEA Order Form Required.
Caution: Federal law prohibits dispensing without prescription.

ROXICODONE™   © ℞
[*rox-ē-cō-dōne*]
(oxycodone hydrochloride)
Tablets USP, Oral Solution USP, and Intensol™

DESCRIPTION

Each tablet contains:
Oxycodone Hydrochloride .... 5 mg
            (WARNING: May be habit forming)
Each 5 mL Oral Solution contains:
Oxycodone Hydrochloride .... 5 mg
            (WARNING: May be habit forming)
Each mL Intensol™ contains:
Oxycodone Hydrochloride .... 20 mg
            (WARNING: May be habit forming)
Inactive Ingredients:
The tablets contain microcrystalline cellulose and stearic acid.
The oral solution contains alcohol, FD&C Red No. 40, flavoring, glycol, sorbitol, water, and other ingredients.
The Intensol™ contains citric acid, sodium benzoate, and water.
Oxycodone is 14-hydroxydihydrocodeinone, a white odorless crystalline powder which is derived from the opium alkaloid, thebaine.

ACTIONS

The analgesic ingredient, oxycodone, is a semisynthetic narcotic with multiple actions qualitatively similar to those of morphine; the most prominent of these involve the central nervous system and organs composed of smooth muscle. The principal actions of therapeutic value of oxycodone are analgesia and sedation.

Oxycodone is similar to codeine and methadone in that it retains at least one half of its analgesic activity when administered orally.

INDICATIONS

For the relief of moderate to moderately severe pain.

CONTRAINDICATIONS

Hypersensitivity to oxycodone.

WARNINGS

Drug Dependence: Oxycodone can produce drug dependence of the morphine type, and therefore, has the potential for being abused. Psychic dependence, physical dependence and tolerance may develop upon repeated administration of this drug, and it should be prescribed and administered with the same degree of caution appropriate to the use of other oral narcotic-containing medications. Like other narcotic-containing medications, this drug is subject to the Federal Controlled Substances Act.

Usage in Ambulatory Patients: Oxycodone may impair the mental and/or physical abilities required for the performance of potentially hazardous tasks such as driving a car or operating machinery. The patient using this drug should be cautioned accordingly.

Interaction with Other Central Nervous System Depressants: Patients receiving other narcotic analgesics, general

---

anesthetics, phenothiazines, other tranquilizers, sedative-hypnotics or other CNS depressants (including alcohol) concomitantly with oxycodone hydrochloride may exhibit an additive CNS depression. When such combined therapy is contemplated, the dose of one or both agents should be reduced.

Usage In Pregnancy: Safe use in pregnancy has not been established relative to possible adverse effects on fetal development. Therefore, this drug should not be used in pregnant women unless, in the judgment of the physician, the potential benefits outweigh the possible hazards.

Usage In Children: This drug should not be administered to children.

PRECAUTIONS

Head Injury and Increased Intracranial Pressure: The respiratory depressant effects of narcotics and their capacity to elevate cerebrospinal fluid pressure may be markedly exaggerated in the presence of head injury, other intracranial lesions or a pre-existing increase in intracranial pressure. Furthermore, narcotics produce adverse reactions which may obscure the clinical course of patients with head injuries.

Acute Abdominal Conditions: The administration of this drug or other narcotics may obscure the diagnosis or clinical course in patients with acute abdominal conditions.

Special Risk Patients: This drug should be given with caution to certain patients such as the elderly, or debilitated, and those with severe impairment of hepatic or renal function, hypothyroidism, Addison's disease and prostatic hypertrophy or urethral stricture.

ADVERSE REACTIONS

The most frequently observed adverse reactions include light headedness, dizziness, sedation, nausea and vomiting. These effects seem to be more prominent in ambulatory than in nonambulatory patients, and some of these adverse reactions may be alleviated if the patient lies down.

Other adverse reactions include euphoria, dysphoria, constipation, skin rash and pruritus.

DOSAGE AND ADMINISTRATION

The usual adult oral dose is 10 to 30 mg every 4 hours as needed for pain or as directed by physician. The dose must be individually adjusted according to severity of pain, patient response and patient size. More severe pain may require 30 mg or more every 4 hours. If the pain increases in severity, analgesia is not adequate or tolerance occurs, a gradual increase in dosage may be required.

For control of severe, chronic pain in patients with certain terminal diseases, this drug should be administered on a regularly scheduled basis, every 4 hours, at the lowest dosage level that will achieve adequate analgesia.

DRUG INTERACTIONS

The CNS depressant effects of oxycodone hydrochloride may be additive with that of other CNS depressants. See WARNINGS.

MANAGEMENT OF OVERDOSAGE

Signs and Symptoms: Serious overdose of oxycodone hydrochloride is characterized by respiratory depression (a decrease in respiratory rate and/or tidal volume, Cheyne-Stokes respiration, cyanosis), extreme somnolence progressing to stupor or coma, skeletal muscle flaccidity, cold and clammy skin, and sometimes bradycardia and hypotension. In severe overdosage, apnea, circulatory collapse, cardiac arrest and death may occur.

Treatment: Primary attention should be given to the reestablishment of adequate respiratory exchange through provision of a patent airway and the institution of assisted or controlled ventilation. The narcotic antagonist naloxone is a specific antidote against respiratory depression which may result from overdosage or unusual sensitivity to narcotics, including oxycodone. Therefore, an appropriate dose of naloxone (usual initial adult dose: 0.4 mg) should be administered, preferably by the intravenous route, simultaneously with efforts at respiratory resuscitation. Since the duration of action of oxycodone may exceed that of the antagonist, the patient should be kept under continued surveillance and repeated doses of the antagonist should be administered as needed to maintain adequate respiration.

An antagonist should not be administered in the absence of clinically significant respiratory or cardiovascular depression.

Oxygen, intravenous fluids, vasopressors and other supportive measures should be employed as indicated.

Gastric emptying may be useful in removing unabsorbed drug.

HOW SUPPLIED

5 mg white scored tablets. (Identified 54 582).
NDC 0054-8657-24: Unit dose, 25 tablets per card (reverse numbered), 4 cards per shipper.

NDC 0054-4657-25: Bottles of 100 tablets.

5 mg per 5 mL Oral Solution.

NDC 0054-8545-16: Unit dose Patient Cups™ filled to deliver 5 mL (oxycodone hydrochloride 5 mg), ten 5 mL Patient Cups™ per shelf pack, 4 shelf packs per shipper.

NDC 0054-3682-63: Bottles of 500 mL.

20 mg per mL Intensol™

(Concentrated Oral Solution)

NDC 0054-3683-44: Bottles of 30 mL with calibrated dropper [graduations of 0.25 mL (5 mg), 0.5 mL (10 mg), 0.75 mL (15 mg), and 1 mL (20 mg) on the dropper].

DEA Order Form Required

Revised May 1994

4064400 © RLI, 1994.

054

SODIUM POLYSTYRENE SULFONATE SUSPENSION USP ℞

CATION-EXCHANGE RESIN

DESCRIPTION

Sodium Polystyrene Sulfonate Suspension USP can be administered orally or in an enema and contains the following per 60 mL:

Sodium Polystyrene Sulfonate USP	15 g
Sorbitol USP	14.1 g
Alcohol	0.1%

The suspension is carmel-cherry-flavored and also contains Propylene Glycol USP, Microcrystalline Cellulose and Carboxymethylcellulose Sodium, Methylparaben NF, Propylparaben NF, Saccharin Sodium USP, Flavors and Purified Water USP.

Sodium Polystyrene Sulfonate is a benzene, diethenyl-, polymer with ethenylbenzene, sulfonated, sodium salt.

The sodium content of the suspension is 1500 mg (65 mEq) per 60 mL. It is a brown, slightly viscous suspension with an *in-vitro* exchange capacity of approximately 3.1 mEq (*in-vivo* approximately 1 mEq) of potassium per 4 mL (1 gram) of suspension.

CLINICAL PHARMACOLOGY

As the resin passes along the intestine or is retained in the colon after administration by enema, the sodium ions are partially released and are replaced by potassium ions. For the most part, this action occurs in the large intestine, which excretes potassium ions to a greater degree than does the small intestine. The efficiency of this process is limited and unpredictably variable. It commonly approximates the order of 33%, but the range is so large that definite indices of electrolyte balance must be clearly monitored. Metabolic data are unavailable.

INDICATIONS AND USAGE

Sodium Polystyrene Sulfonate suspension is indicated to treatment of hyperkalemia.

CONTRAINDICATIONS

Sodium Polystyrene Sulfonate suspension is contraindicated in patients with hypokalema or those patients who are hypersensitive to it.

WARNINGS

Alternative Therapy in Severe Hyperkalemia:

Since the effective lowering of serum potassium with Sodium Polystyrene Sulfonate may take hours to days, treatment with this drug alone may be insufficient to rapidly correct severe hyperkalemia associated with states of rapid tissue breakdown (e.g., burns and renal failure) or hyperkalemia so marked as to constitute a medical emergency. Therefore, other definite measures, including dialysis, should always be considered and may be imperative.

Hypokalemia:

Serious potassium deficiency can occur from Sodium Polystyrene Sulfonate therapy. The effect must be carefully controlled by frequent serum potassium determination within each 24 hour period. Since intracellular potassium deficiency is not always reflected by serum potassium levels, the level at which treatment with Sodium Polystyrene Sulfonate should be discontinued must be determined individually for each patient. Important aids in making this determination are the patient's clinical condition and electrocardiogram. Early clinical signs of severe hypokalemia include a pattern of irritable confusion and delayed thought processes. Electocardiographically, severe hypokalemia is often associated with a lengthened Q-T interval, widening, flattening, or inversion of the T wave, and prominent U waves. Also, cardiac arrhythmias may occur, such as premature atrial, nodal, and ventricular contractions, and supraventricular and ventricular tachycardias. The toxic effects of digitalis are likely to be exaggerated. Marked hypokalemia can also be manifested by severe muscle weakness, at times extending into frank paralysis.

Electrolyte Disturbances:

Like all cation-exchange resins, Sodium Polystyrene Sulfonate is not totally selective (for potassium) in its actions, and small amounts of other cations such as magnesium and calcium can also be lost during treatment. Accordingly, patients receiving Sodium Polystyrene Sulfonate should be monitored for all applicable electrolyte disturbances.

Systemic Alkalosis:

Systemic alkalosis has been reported after cation-exchange resins were administered orally in combination with nonabsorbable cation-donating antacids and laxatives such as magnesium hydroxide and aluminum carbonate. Magnesium hydroxide should not be administered with Sodium Polystyrene Sulfonate. One case of grand mal seizure has been reported in a patient with chronic hypocalcemia of renal failure who was given Sodium Polystyrene Sulfonate with magnesium hydroxide as a laxative. (See PRECAUTIONS, Drug Interactions).

PRECAUTIONS

Caution is advised when Sodium Polystyrene Sulfonate is administered to patients who cannot tolerate even a small increase in sodium loads (i.e., severe congestive heart failure, severe hypertension, or marked edema). In such instances compensatory restriction of sodium intake from other sources may be indicated.

If constipation occurs, patients should be treated with sorbitol (from 10 to 20 mL of 70% syrup every 2 hours or as needed to produce 1 to 2 watery stools daily) a measure which also reduces any tendency to fecal impaction.

Drug Interactions:

Antacids: The simultaneous oral administration of Sodium Polystyrene Sulfonate suspension with nonabsorbable cation-donating antacids and laxatives may reduce the resin's potassium exchange capability.

Systemic alkalosis has been reported after cation-exchange resins were administered orally in combination with nonabsorbable cation-donating antacids and laxatives such as magnesium hydroxide and aluminum carbonate. Magnesium hydroxide should not be administered with Sodium Polystyrene Sulfonate suspension. One case of grand mal seizure has been reported in a patient with chronic hypocalcemia of renal failure who was given Sodium Polystyrene Sulfonate with magnesium hydroxide as a laxative. Intestinal obstruction due to concretions of aluminum hydroxide when used in combination with Sodium Polystyrene Sulfonate has been reported.

Digitalis: The toxic effects of digitalis on the heart, especially various ventricular arrhythmias and A-V nodal dissociation, are likely to be exaggerated by hypokalemia, even in the face of serum digoxin concentrations in the "normal range". (See WARNINGS.)

Carcinogenesis, Mutagenesis, Impairment of Fertility:

Studies have not been performed.

Pregnancy Category C: Animal reproduction studies have not been conducted with Sodium Polystyrene Sulfonate. It is also not known whether Sodium Polystyrene Sulfonate can cause fetal harm when administered to a pregnant woman or can affect reproduction capacity. Sodium Polystyrene Sulfonate should be given to a pregnant woman only if clearly needed.

Nursing Mothers: It is not known whether this drug is excreted in human milk. Because many drugs are excreted in human milk, caution should be exercised when Sodium Polystyrene Sulfonate is administered to a nursing woman.

ADVERSE REACTIONS

Sodium Polystyrene Sulfonate may cause some degree of gastric irritation. Anorexia, nausea, vomiting, and constipation may occur especially if high doses are given. Also, hypokalemia, hypocalcemia, and significant sodium retention may occur. Occasionally diarrhea develops. Large doses in elderly individuals may cause fecal impaction (see PRECAUTIONS). This effect may be obviated through usage of the resin in enemas as described under DOSAGE AND ADMINISTRATION. Rare instances of colonic necrosis have been reported. Intestinal obstruction due to concretions of aluminum hydroxide, when used in combination with Sodium Polystyrene Sulfonate, has been reported.

DOSAGE AND ADMINISTRATION

Oral Administration

The average daily adult dose is 15 g (60 mL) to 60 g (240 mL) of suspension. This is best provided by administering 15 g (60 mL) of Sodium Polystyrene Sulfonate suspension one to four times daily. Each 60 mL of Sodium Polystyrene Sulfonate suspension contains 1500 mg (65 mEq) of sodium. Since the *in-vivo* efficiency of sodium-potassium exchange resins is approximately 33%, about one-third of the resin's actual sodium content is being delivered to the body.

In smaller children and infants, lower doses should be employed by using as a guide a rate of 1 mEq of potassium per gram of resin as the basis of calculation.

The suspension may be introduced into the stomach through a plastic tube and, if desired, mixed with a diet appropriate for a patient in renal failure.

Rectal Administration:

The suspension may also be given, although with less effective results, as a retention enema for adults of 30 g (120 mL) to 50 g (200 mL) every six hours. The enema should be retained as long as possible and followed by a cleansing enema. After an initial cleansing enema, a soft, large size (French 28) rubber tube is inserted into the rectum for a distance of 20 cm, with the tip well into the sigmoid colon and taped in place. The suspension is introduced at body temperature by gravity. The suspension is flushed with 50 or 100 mL of fluid, following which the tube is clamped and left in place. If back leakage occurs, the hips are elevated on pillows or a knee-chest position is taken temporarily. The suspension is kept in the sigmoid colon for several hours, if possible. Then the colon is irrigated with a nonsodium-containing solution at body temperature in order to remove the resin. Two quarts of flushing solution may be necessary. The returns are drained constantly through a Y tube connection. Particular attention should be paid to this cleansing enema when sorbitol has been used.

The intensity and duration of therapy depend upon the severity and resistance of hyperkalemia.

HOW SUPPLIED

Sodium Polystyrene Sulfonate Suspension USP, 15 g per 60 mL (an amber-colored, cherry/caramel-flavored suspension)

NDC 0054-8816-11: Unit dose bottle filled to deliver 60 mL, 10 bottles per shipper.

NDC 0054-8815-01: Unit dose enema bottle filled to contain 120 mL (for use in delivering the suspension rectally through appropriate tubing).

NDC 0054-8817-55: Unit dose enema bottle filled to contain 200 mL (for use in delivering the suspension rectally through appropriate tubing).

NDC 0054-3805-63: Bottle of 500 mL.

Note: Sodium Polystyrene Sulfonate suspension should not be heated for to do so may alter the exchange properties of the resin.

SHAKE WELL BEFORE USING

Dispense in a tight container as defined in the USP/NF.

Store at Controlled Room Temperature 15°–30°C (59°–86°F).

Caution: Federal law prohibits dispensing without prescription.

4073701 **Revised May 1994**

054

Roxane

Laboratories, Inc. © RLI, 1994.

Columbus, Ohio 43216

TORECAN® ℞

(thiethylperazine maleate tablets USP)

(thiethylperazine malate injection USP)

(for intramuscular use only)

Caution: Federal law prohibits dispensing without prescription.

DESCRIPTION

Torecan® (thiethylperazine) is a phenothiazine. Thiethylperazine is characterized by a substituted thioethyl group at position 2 in the phenothiazine nucleus, and a piperazine moiety in the side chain. The chemical designation is: 2-ethyl-mercapto-10-[3'(1''-methyl-piperazinyl-4'')-propyl-1']phenothiazine. Thiethylperazine has the following structural formula:

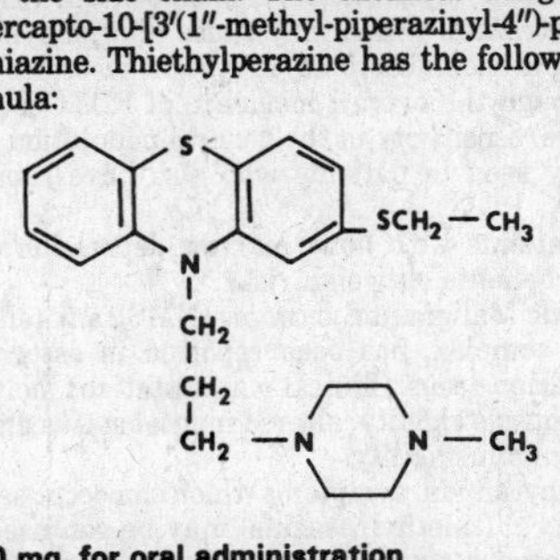

Tablet, 10 mg, for oral administration

ACTIVE INGREDIENT: thiethylperazine maleate USP, 10 mg. *INACTIVE INGREDIENTS:* acacia, carnauba wax, FD&C Yellow No. 5 aluminum lake (tartrazine), FD& C Yellow No. 6 aluminum lake, gelatin, lactose, magnesium stearate, povidone, sodium benzoate, sorbitol, starch, stearic acid, sucrose, talc, titanium dioxide.

Ampul, 2 ml, for intramuscular administration

ACTIVE INGREDIENT: thiethylperazine malate USP, 10 mg per 2 ml. *INACTIVE INGREDIENTS:* sodium metabisulfite NF, 0.5 mg; ascorbic acid USP, 2.0 mg; sorbitol NF, 40 mg; carbon dioxide gas q.s.; water for injection USP, q.s. to 2 ml.

Continued on next page

Roxane Laboratories—Cont.

ACTIONS
The pharmacodynamic action of Torecan® (thiethylperazine) in humans is unknown. However, a direct action of Torecan on both the CTZ and the vomiting center may be concluded from induced vomiting experiments in animals.

INDICATIONS
Torecan® (thiethylperazine) is indicated for the relief of nausea and vomiting.

CONTRAINDICATIONS
Severe central nervous system (CNS) depression and comatose states.
In patients who have demonstrated a hypersensitivity reaction (e.g., blood dyscrasias, jaundice) to phenothiazines.
Because severe hypotension has been reported after the intravenous administration of phenothiazines, this route of administration is contraindicated.
Usage in Pregnancy: Torecan® (thiethylperazine) is contraindicated in pregnancy.

WARNINGS
Torecan® (thiethylperazine) injection contains sodium metabisulfite, a sulfite that may cause allergic-type reactions including anaphylactic symptoms and life-threatening or less severe asthmatic episodes in certain susceptible people. The overall prevalence of sulfite sensitivity in the general population is unknown and probably low. Sulfite sensitivity is seen more frequently in asthmatic than in nonasthmatic people.
Phenothiazines are capable of potentiating CNS depressants (e.g., anesthetics, opiates, alcohol, etc.) as well as atropine and phosphorus insecticides.
Since Torecan® (thiethylperazine) may impair mental and/or physical ability required in the performance of potentially hazardous tasks such as driving a car or operating machinery, it is recommended that patients be warned accordingly.
Postoperative Nausea and Vomiting: With the use of this drug to control postoperative nausea and vomiting occurring in patients undergoing elective surgical procedures, restlessness and postoperative CNS depression during anesthesia recovery may occur. Possible postoperative complications of a severe degree of any of the known reactions of this class of drug must be considered. Postural hypotension may occur after an initial injection, rarely with the tablet or suppository.
The administration of epinephrine should be avoided in the treatment of drug-induced hypotension in view of the fact that phenothiazines may induce a reversed epinephrine effect on occasion.
Should a vasoconstrictive agent be required, the most suitable are norepinephrine bitartrate and phenylephrine.
The use of this drug has not been studied following intracardiac and intracranial surgery.

PRECAUTIONS
Abnormal movements such as extrapyramidal symptoms (E.P.S.) (e.g., dystonia, torticollis, dysphasia, oculogyric crises, akathisia) have occurred. Convulsions have also been reported. The varied symptom complex is more likely to occur in young adults and children. Extrapyramidal effects must be treated by reduction of dosage or cessation of medication.
Torecan® (thiethylperazine) tablets contain FD&C Yellow No. 5 (tartrazine) which may cause allergic-type reactions (including bronchial asthma) in certain susceptible individuals. Although the overall incidence of FD&C Yellow No. 5 (tartrazine) sensitivity in the general population is low, it is frequently seen in patients who also have aspirin hypersensitivity.
Use in patients with bone marrow depression only when potential benefits outweigh risks.
Neuroleptic Malignant Syndrome (NMS), a potentially fatal symptom complex, has been reported in association with phenothiazine drugs. Clinical manifestations include: hyperpyrexia, muscle rigidity, altered mental status and evidence of autonomic instability.
The extrapyramidal symptoms which can occur secondary to TORECAN® (thiethylperazine) may be confused with the central nervous system signs of an undiagnosed primary disease responsible for the vomiting, e.g., Reye's Syndrome or other encephalopathy. The use of TORECAN® (thiethylperazine) and other potential hepatotoxins should be avoided in children and adolescents whose signs and symptoms suggest Reye's Syndrome.
Phenothiazine drugs may cause elevated prolactin levels that persist during chronic administration. Since approximately one-third of human breast cancers are prolactin-dependent *in vitro*, this elevation is of potential importance if phenothiazine drug administration is contemplated in a patient with a previously-detected breast cancer. Neither clinical nor epidemiologic studies to date, however, have shown an association between the chronic administration of phenothiazine drugs and mammary tumorigenesis.
Postoperative Nausea and Vomiting: When used in the treatment of the nausea and/or vomiting associated with anesthesia and surgery, it is recommended that Torecan® (thiethylperazine) should be administered by deep intramuscular injection at or shortly before the termination of anesthesia.
Information for Patients: Patients receiving TORECAN® (thiethylperazine) should be cautioned about possible combined effects with alcohol and other CNS depressants. Patients should be cautioned not to operate machinery or drive a motor vehicle after ingesting the drug.
Drug Interactions: Phenothiazines are capable of potentiating CNS depressants (e.g., barbiturates, anesthetics, opiates, alcohol, etc.) as well as atropine and phosphorus insecticides.
Laboratory Test Interactions: The usual precautions should be observed in patients with impaired renal or hepatic function.
Nursing Mothers: Information is not available concerning the excretion of TORECAN® (thiethylperazine) in the milk of nursing mothers. As a general rule, nursing should not be undertaken while the patient is on a drug, since many drugs are excreted in human milk.
Pediatric Use: The safety and efficacy of TORECAN® (thiethylperazine) in children under 12 years of age has not been established.

ADVERSE REACTIONS
Central Nervous System: Serious: Convulsions have been reported. Extrapyramidal symptoms (E.P.S.) may occur, such as dystonia, torticollis, oculogyric crises, akathisia and gait disturbances. Others: Occasional cases of dizziness, headache, fever and restlessness have been reported.
Drowsiness may occur on occasion, following an initial injection. Generally this effect tends to subside with continued therapy or is usually alleviated by a reduction in dosage.
Autonomic Nervous System: Dryness of the mouth and nose, blurred vision, tinnitus. An occasional case of sialorrhea together with altered gustatory sensation has been observed.
Endocrine System: Peripheral edema of the arms, hands and face.
Hepatotoxicity: An occasional case of cholestatic jaundice has been observed.
Other: An occasional case of cerebral vascular spasm and trigeminal neuralgia has been reported.
Phenothiazine Derivatives: The physician should be aware that the following have occurred with one or more phenothiazines and should be considered whenever one of these drugs is used:
Blood Dyscrasias Serious—Agranulocytosis, leukopenia, thrombocytopenia, aplastic anemia, pancytopenia. Other—Eosinophilia, leukocytosis.
Autonomic Reactions Miosis, obstipation, anorexia, paralytic ileus.
Cutaneous Reactions Serious—Erythema, exfoliative dermatitis, contact dermatitis.
Hepatotoxicity Serious—Jaundice, biliary stasis.
Cardiovascular Effects Serious—Hypotension, rarely leading to cardiac arrest; electrocardiographic (ECG) changes.
Extrapyramidal Symptoms Serious—Akathisia, agitation, motor restlessness, dystonic reactions, trismus, torticollis, opisthotonos, oculogyric crises, tremor, muscular rigidity, akinesia—some of which have persisted for several months or years especially in patients of advanced age with brain damage.
Endocrine Disturbances Menstrual irregularities, altered libido, gynecomastia, weight gain. False positive pregnancy tests have been reported.
Urinary Disturbances Retention, incontinence.
Allergic Reactions Serious—Fever, laryngeal edema, angioneurotic edema, asthma.
Others: Hyperpyrexia, Behavioral effects suggestive of a paradoxical reaction have been reported. These include excitement, bizarre dreams, aggravation of psychoses and toxic confusional states. While there is no evidence at present that ECG changes observed in patients receiving phenothiazines are in any way precursors of any significant disturbance of cardiac rhythm, it should be noted that sudden and unexpected deaths apparently due to cardiac arrest have been reported in a few instances in hospitalized psychotic patients previously showing characteristic ECG changes. A peculiar skin-eye syndrome has also been recognized as a side effect following long-term treatment with certain phenothiazines. This reaction is marked by progressive pigmentation of areas of the skin or conjunctiva and/or accompanied by discoloration of the exposed sclera and cornea. Opacities of the anterior lens and cornea described as irregular or stellate in shape have also been reported.

DOSAGE AND ADMINISTRATION
Adult: Usual daily dose range is 10 mg to 30 mg. *ORAL:* One tablet one to three times daily. *INTRAMUSCULAR:* 2 ml IM, one to three times daily. (See PRECAUTIONS.)
Children: Appropriate dosage of Torecan® (thiethylperazine) has not been determined in children.

HOW SUPPLIED
Tablets Each tablet contains 10 mg thiethylperazine maleate, USP.
NDC 0054-8748-25: Unit dose tablets, 10 tablets per strip, 10 strips per shelf pack.
NDC 0054-4748-25: Bottles of 100 tablets.
Ampuls: Each 2 ml ampul contains in aqueous solution 10 mg thiethylperazine malate, USP. Boxes of 20 and 100.
Storage: Below 86°F; protect from light.
Administer only if clear and colorless.
Manufactured by
Sandoz Pharmaceuticals Corporation
East Hanover, NJ 07936
Distributed by
Roxane Laboratories Inc.
Columbus OH 43216
Revised 11/92

VIRAMUNE® (nevirapine) Tablets ℞

WARNING
VIRAMUNE® (NEVIRAPINE) IS INDICATED FOR USE IN COMBINATION WITH NUCLEOSIDE ANALOGUES FOR THE TREATMENT OF HIV-1 INFECTED ADULTS WHO HAVE EXPERIENCED CLINICAL AND/OR IMMUNOLOGIC DETERIORATION. THIS INDICATION IS BASED ON ANALYSIS OF CHANGES IN SURROGATE ENDPOINTS IN STUDIES OF UP TO 48 WEEKS DURATION. AT PRESENT, THERE ARE NO RESULTS FROM CONTROLLED CLINICAL TRIALS EVALUATING THE EFFECT OF VIRAMUNE® WITH NUCLEOSIDE ANALOGUES ON THE CLINICAL PROGRESSION OF HIV-1 INFECTION, SUCH AS INCIDENCE OF OPPORTUNISTIC INFECTIONS OR SURVIVAL.
THE DURATION OF BENEFIT FROM ANTIRETROVIRAL THERAPY MAY BE LIMITED. ALTERATION OF ANTIRETROVIRAL THERAPIES SHOULD BE CONSIDERED IF DISEASE PROGRESSION OCCURS WHILE PATIENTS ARE RECEIVING VIRAMUNE®.
RESISTANT VIRUS EMERGES RAPIDLY AND UNIFORMLY WHEN VIRAMUNE® IS ADMINISTERED AS MONOTHERAPY. THEREFORE, VIRAMUNE® SHOULD ALWAYS BE ADMINISTERED IN COMBINATION WITH AT LEAST ONE ADDITIONAL ANTIRETROVIRAL AGENT.
VIRAMUNE® HAS BEEN ASSOCIATED WITH SEVERE RASH, WHICH IN SOME CASES HAVE BEEN LIFE-THREATENING. WHEN SEVERE RASH OCCURS, VIRAMUNE® MUST BE DISCONTINUED.

DESCRIPTION
VIRAMUNE® is the brand name for nevirapine (NVP), a non-nucleoside reverse transcriptase inhibitor with activity against Human Immunodeficiency Virus Type 1 (HIV-1). Nevirapine is structurally a member of the dipyridodiazepinone chemical class of compounds.
VIRAMUNE® is available as tablets for oral administration. Each tablet contains 200 mg of nevirapine and the inactive ingredients microcrystalline cellulose, lactose monohydrate, povidone, sodium starch glycolate, colloidal silicon dioxide and magnesium stearate.
The chemical name of nevirapine is 11-cyclopropyl-5,11-dihydro- 4-methyl-6H-dipyrido[3,2-b:2',3'-e][1,4]diazepin-6-one. Nevirapine is a white to off-white crystalline powder with the molecular weight of 266.3 and the molecular formula $C_{15}H_{14}N_4O$. Nevirapine has the following structural formula:

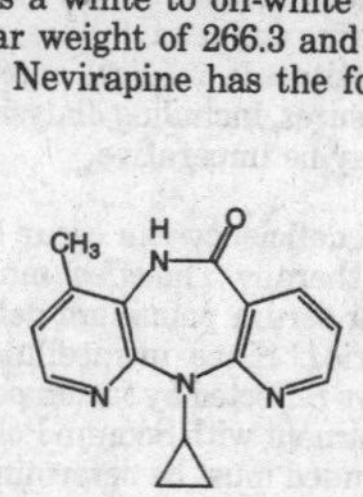

MICROBIOLOGY ***Mechanism of Action:*** Nevirapine is a non-nucleoside reverse transcriptase inhibitor (NNRTI) of HIV-1. Nevirapine binds directly to reverse transcriptase (RT) and blocks the RNA-dependent and DNA-dependent DNA polymerase activities by causing a disruption of the enzyme's catalytic site. The activity of nevirapine does not compete with template or nucleoside triphosphates. HIV-2 RT and eukaryotic DNA polymerases (such as human DNA polymerases α, β, γ, or δ) are not inhibited by nevirapine.
In Vitro HIV Susceptibility: The relationship between *in vitro* susceptibility of HIV-1 to nevirapine and the inhibition

of HIV-1 replication in humans has not been established. The *in vitro* antiviral activity of nevirapine was measured in peripheral blood mononuclear cells, monocyte derived macrophages, and lymphoblastoid cell lines. IC_{50} values (50% inhibitory concentration) ranged from 10-100 nM against laboratory and clinical isolates of HIV-1. In cell culture, nevirapine demonstrated additive to synergistic activity against HIV in drug combination regimens with zidovudine (ZDV), didanosine (ddI), stavudine (d4T), lamivudine (3TC) and saquinavir.

Resistance: HIV isolates with reduced susceptibility (100-250-fold) to nevirapine emerge *in vitro*. Genotypic analysis showed mutations in the HIV RT gene at amino acid positions 181 and/or 106 depending upon the virus strain and cell line employed. Time to emergence of nevirapine resistance *in vitro* was not altered when selection included nevirapine in combination with several other NNRTIs.

Phenotypic and genotypic changes in HIV-1 isolates from patients treated with either nevirapine (n=24) or nevirapine and ZDV (n=14) were monitored in Phase I/II trials over 1 to ≥12 weeks. After 1 week of nevirapine monotherapy, isolates from 3/3 patients had decreased susceptibility to nevirapine *in vitro*; one or more of the RT mutations at amino acid positions 103, 106, 108, 181, 188 and 190 were detected in some patients as early as 2 weeks after therapy initiation. By week eight of nevirapine monotherapy, 100% of the patients tested (n=24) had HIV isolates with a >100-fold decrease in susceptibility to nevirapine *in vitro* compared to baseline, and had one or more of the nevirapine-associated RT resistance mutations; 19 of 24 patients (80%) had isolates with a position 181 mutation regardless of dose. Nevirapine+ZDV combination therapy did not alter the emergence rate of nevirapine-resistant virus or the magnitude of nevirapine resistance *in vitro*; however, a different RT mutation pattern, predominantly distributed amongst amino acid positions 103, 106, 188, and 190, was observed. In patients (6 of 14) whose baseline isolates possessed a wild type RT gene, nevirapine+ZDV combination therapy did not appear to delay emergence of ZDV-resistant RT mutations. The clinical relevance of phenotypic and genotypic changes associated with nevirapine therapy has not been established.

Cross-resistance: Rapid emergence of HIV strains which are cross-resistant to NNRTIs has been observed *in vitro*. Data on cross-resistance between the NNRTI nevirapine and nucleoside analogue RT inhibitors are very limited. In four patients, ZDV-resistant isolates tested *in vitro* retained susceptibility to nevirapine and in six patients, nevirapine-resistant isolates were susceptible to ZDV and ddI. Cross-resistance between nevirapine and HIV protease inhibitors is unlikely because the enzyme targets involved are different.

ANIMAL PHARMACOLOGY Animal studies have shown that nevirapine is widely distributed to nearly all tissues and readily crosses the blood-brain barrier.

CLINICAL PHARMACOLOGY

Absorption and Bioavailability in Adults: Nevirapine is readily absorbed (>90%) after oral administration in healthy volunteers and in adults with HIV-1 infection. Absolute bioavailability in 12 healthy adults following single-dose administration was 93 ± 9% (mean ± SD) for a 50 mg tablet and 91 ± 8% for an oral solution. Peak plasma nevirapine concentrations of 2 ± 0.4 μg/mL (7.5 μM) were attained by 4 hours following a single 200 mg dose. Following multiple doses, nevirapine peak concentrations appear to increase linearly in the dose range of 200 to 400 mg/day. Steady state trough nevirapine concentrations of 4.5 ± 1.9 μg/mL (17 ± 7 μM), (n=242) were attained at 400 mg/day.

When VIRAMUNE® (200 mg) was administered to 24 healthy adults (12 female, 12 male), with either a high fat breakfast (857 kcal, 50 g fat, 53% of calories from fat) or antacid (Maalox® 30 mL), the extent of nevirapine absorption (AUC) was comparable to that observed under fasting conditions. In a separate study in HIV-1-infected patients (n=6), nevirapine steady-state systemic exposure (AUCт) was not significantly altered by ddI, which is formulated with an alkaline buffering agent. VIRAMUNE® may be administered with or without food, antacid or ddI.

Distribution: Nevirapine is highly lipophilic and is essentially nonionized at physiologic pH. Following intravenous administration to healthy adults, the apparent volume of distribution (Vdss) of nevirapine was 1.21 ± 0.09 L/kg, suggesting that nevirapine is widely distributed in humans. Nevirapine readily crosses the placenta and is found in breast milk. (see PRECAUTIONS, *Nursing Mothers*) Nevirapine is about 60% bound to plasma proteins in the plasma concentration range of 1–10 μg/mL. Nevirapine concentrations in human cerebrospinal fluid (n=6) were 45% (±5%) of the concentrations in plasma; this ratio is approximately equal to the fraction not bound to plasma protein.

Metabolism/Elimination: *In vivo* studies in humans and *in vitro* studies with human liver microsomes have shown that nevirapine is extensively biotransformed via cytochrome P450 (oxidative) metabolism to several hydroxylated metabolites. *In vitro* studies with human liver microsomes suggest that oxidative metabolism of nevirapine is mediated primarily by cytochrome P450 isozymes from the CYP3A family, although other isozymes may have a secondary role. In a mass balance/excretion study in eight healthy male volunteers dosed to steady state with nevirapine 200 mg given twice daily followed by a single 50 mg dose of ^{14}C-nevirapine, approximately 91.4 ± 10.5% of the radiolabeled dose was recovered, with urine (81.3 ± 11.1%) representing the primary route of excretion compared to feces (10.1 ± 1.5%). Greater than 80% of the radioactivity in urine was made up of glucuronide conjugates of hydroxylated metabolites. Thus cytochrome P450 metabolism, glucuronide conjugation, and urinary excretion of glucuronidated metabolites represent the primary route of nevirapine biotransformation and elimination in humans. Only a small fraction (<5%) of the radioactivity in urine (representing <3% of the total dose) was made up of parent compound; therefore, renal excretion plays a minor role in elimination of the parent compound.

Nevirapine has been shown to be an inducer of hepatic cytochrome P450 metabolic enzymes. The pharmacokinetics of autoinduction are characterized by an approximately 1.5 to 2 fold increase in the apparent oral clearance of nevirapine as treatment continues from a single dose to two-to-four weeks of dosing with 200–400 mg/day. Autoinduction also results in a corresponding decrease in the terminal phase half-life of nevirapine in plasma from approximately 45 hours (single dose) to approximately 25–30 hours following multiple dosing with 200–400 mg/day.

Special Populations: Renal/Hepatic Dysfunction: The pharmacokinetics of nevirapine have not been evaluated in patients with either renal or hepatic dysfunction.

Gender: In one Phase I study in healthy volunteers (15 females, 15 males), the weight-adjusted apparent volume of distribution (Vdss/F) of nevirapine was higher in the female subjects (1.54 L/kg) compared to the males (1.38 L/kg), suggesting that nevirapine was distributed more extensively in the female subjects. However, this difference was offset by a slightly shorter terminal-phase half-life in the females resulting in no significant gender difference in nevirapine oral clearance or plasma concentrations following either single- or multiple-dose administration(s).

Race: An evaluation of nevirapine plasma concentrations (pooled data from several clinical trials) from HIV-1-infected patients (27 Black, 24 Hispanic, 189 Caucasian) revealed no marked difference in nevirapine steady-state trough concentrations (median Cminss=4.7 μg/mL Black, 3.8 μg/mL Hispanic, 4.3 μg/mL Caucasian) with long-term nevirapine treatment at 400 mg/day. However, the pharmacokinetics of nevirapine have not been evaluated specifically for the effects of ethnicity.

Age: Nevirapine pharmacokinetics in HIV-1-infected adults do not appear to change with age (range 18–68 years); however, nevirapine has not been extensively evaluated in patients beyond the age of 55 years. Nevirapine is metabolized more rapidly in pediatric patients than in adults. (see PRECAUTIONS, *Pediatric Use*)

Drug Interactions: No dosage adjustments are required when VIRAMUNE® is taken in combination with ZDV, ddI, or ddC. When the ZDV data were pooled from two studies (n=33) in which HIV-1-infected patients received VIRAMUNE® 400 mg/day either alone or in combination with 200–300 mg/day ddI or 0.375 to 0.75 mg/day ddC on a background of ZDV therapy, nevirapine produced a non-significant decline of 13% in ZDV AUC and a non-significant increase of 5.8% in ZDV Cmax. In a subset of patients (n=6) who were administered nevirapine 400 mg/day and ddI on a background of ZDV therapy, nevirapine produced a significant decline of 32% in ZDV AUC and a non-significant decline of 27% in ZDV Cmax. Paired data suggest that ZDV had no effect on the pharmacokinetics of nevirapine. In one crossover study, nevirapine had no effect on the steady-state pharmacokinetics of either ddI (n=18) or ddC (n=6).

Available data on the potential interactions between nevirapine and other CYP3A substrates are limited and preliminary; therefore, recommendations for dose adjustments cannot be made. (see PRECAUTIONS, *Drug Interactions*, for recommendations regarding rifampin, rifabutin, protease inhibitors and oral contraceptives)

In vitro: Studies using human liver microsomes indicated that the formation of nevirapine hydroxylated metabolites was not affected by the presence of dapsone, rifabutin, rifampin, and trimethoprim/sulfamethoxazole. Ketoconazole significantly inhibited the formation of nevirapine hydroxylated metabolites.

In vivo: Monitoring of steady-state nevirapine trough plasma concentrations in patients who received long-term VIRAMUNE® treatment in combination with ketoconazole (n=11) revealed no evidence of a significant inhibitory effect on nevirapine metabolism. Steady-state nevirapine trough plasma concentrations were elevated in patients who received cimetidine (+21%, n=11) and macrolides (+12%, n=24), known inhibitors of CYP3A.

Steady-state nevirapine trough concentrations were reduced in patients who received rifabutin (−16%, n=19) and rifampin (−37%, n=3), known inducers of CYP3A. Nevirapine is an inducer of CYP3A, with maximal induction occurring within 2–4 weeks of initiating multiple-dose therapy. Other compounds that are substrates of CYP3A may have decreased plasma concentrations when co-administered with VIRAMUNE®. Therefore, careful monitoring of the therapeutic effectiveness of CYP3A-metabolized drugs is recommended when taken in combination with VIRAMUNE®. (see PRECAUTIONS)

INDICATIONS AND USAGE

VIRAMUNE® (nevirapine) in combination with nucleoside analogues is indicated for the treatment of HIV-1 infected adults who have experienced clinical and/or immunologic deterioration. This indication is based on analysis of changes in surrogate endpoints in studies of up to 48 weeks duration. At present, there are no results from controlled clinical trials evaluating the effect of VIRAMUNE® with nucleoside analogues on the clinical progression of HIV-1 infection, such as the incidence of opportunistic infections or survival. The duration of benefit from antiretroviral therapy may be limited. Alteration of antiretroviral therapy should be considered if disease progression occurs while patients are receiving VIRAMUNE®.

Resistant virus emerges rapidly and uniformly when VIRAMUNE® is administered as monotherapy. Therefore, VIRAMUNE® should always be administered in combination with at least one additional antiretroviral agent.

Description of Clinical Studies:

Patients with a prior history of nucleoside therapy:

ACTG 241 compared treatment with VIRAMUNE® +ZDV+ddI versus ZDV+ddI in 398 HIV-1-infected patients (median age 38 years, 74% Caucasian, 80% male) with CD4+cell counts ≤350 cells/mm³ (mean 153 cells/mm³) and a mean baseline plasma HIV-1 RNA concentration of 4.59 $\log_{10}$ copies/mL (38,905 copies/mL), who had received at least 6 months of nucleoside therapy prior to enrollment (median 115 weeks). Treatment doses were VIRAMUNE®, 200 mg daily for two weeks, followed by 200 mg twice daily, or placebo; ZDV, 200 mg three times daily; ddI, 200 mg twice daily. Mean changes in CD4+ cell counts are shown in Figure 1. For 198 patients in the virology sub-study, mean HIV-1 RNA concentration changes from baseline are shown in Figure 2.

Figure 1: Mean Change from Baseline for CD4+ Cell Count (absolute number of CD4+ cells/mm³), Trial ACTG 241

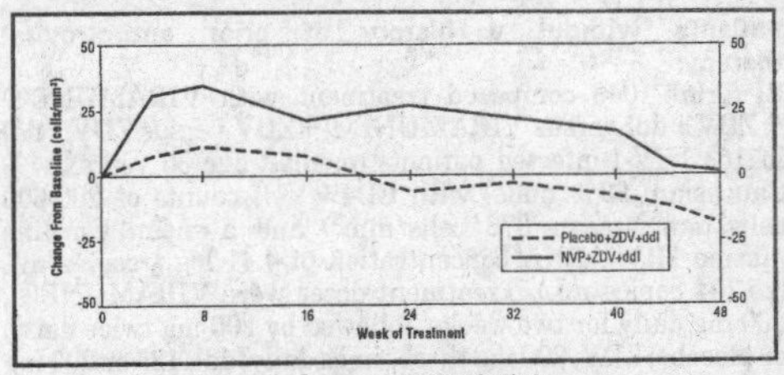

Number of patients with CD4 cell counts at each timepoint

	Baseline	Week 16	Week 32	40-48 Weeks
NVP+ZDV+ddI	196	177	157	161
Placebo+ZDV+ddI	196	176	160	167

Figure 2: Mean Change from Baseline in HIV-1 RNA* Concentrations ($\log_{10}$ copies/mL), Virology Sub-study of Trial ACTG 241

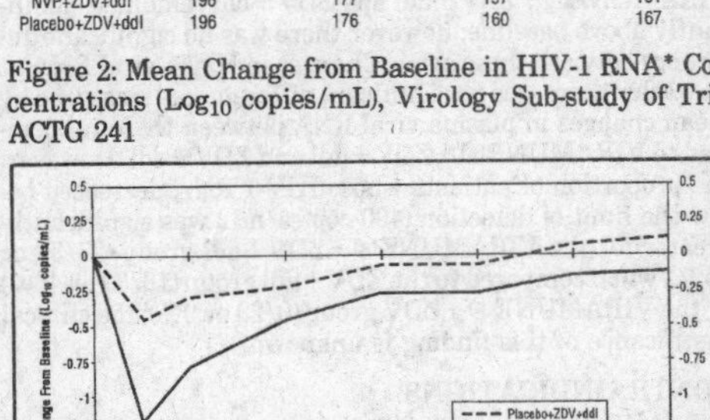

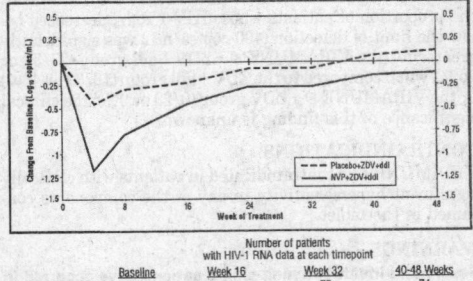

Number of patients with HIV-1 RNA data at each timepoint

	Baseline	Week 16	Week 32	40-48 Weeks
NVP+ZDV+ddI	95	84	75	74
Placebo+ZDV+ddI	93	82	75	75

* the clinical significance of changes in serum viral RNA measurements during treatment with VIRAMUNE® has not been established

Trial BI 1037 compared treatment with VIRAMUNE® +ZDV versus ZDV in 60 HIV-1-infected patients (median age 33 years, 70% Caucasian, 93% male) with CD4+ cell counts between 200 and 500 cells/mm³ (mean 373 cells/mm³) and a mean baseline plasma HIV-1 RNA concentra-

Continued on next page

Roxane Laboratories—Cont.

tion of 4.24 $\log_{10}$ copies/mL (17,378 copies/mL), who had received between 3 and 24 months of prior ZDV therapy (median 35 weeks). Treatment doses were VIRAMUNE® 200 mg daily for 2 weeks, followed by 200 mg twice daily, or placebo; ZDV, 500–600 mg/day. Mean changes in CD4+ cell counts are shown in Figure 3. Mean HIV-1 RNA concentration changes from baseline are shown in Figure 4.

Figure 3: Mean Change from Baseline for CD4+ Cell Count (absolute number of CD4+ cells/mm³), Trial BI 1037

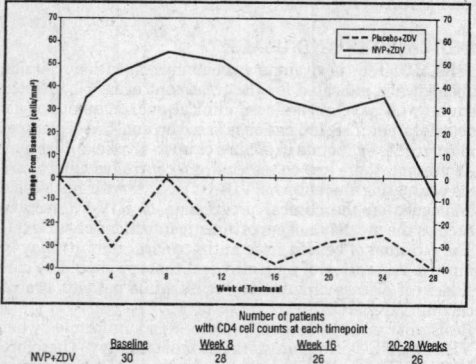

	Baseline	Week 8	Week 16	20-28 Weeks
NVP+ZDV	30	28	26	26
Placebo+ZDV	30	30	28	29

Figure 4: Mean Change from Baseline in HIV-1 RNA Concentrations ($\log_{10}$ copies/mL), Trial BI 1037

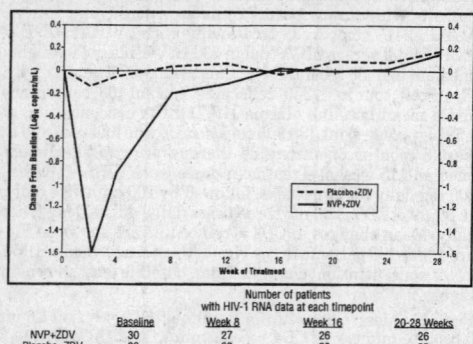

Number of patients with HIV-1 RNA data at each timepoint

	Baseline	Week 8	Week 16	20-28 Weeks
NVP+ZDV	30	27	26	26
Placebo+ZDV	30	29	28	29

Patients without a history of prior antiretroviral therapy:
BI Trial 1046 compared treatment with VIRAMUNE® +ZDV+ddl versus VIRAMUNE® +ZDV versus ZDV+ddl in 151 HIV-1-infected patients (median age 36 years, 94% Caucasian, 93% male) with CD4+ cell counts of 200-600 cells/mm³ (mean 376 cells/mm³) and a mean baseline plasma HIV-1 RNA concentration of 4.41 $\log_{10}$ copies/mL (25,704 copies/mL). Treatment doses were VIRAMUNE®, 200 mg daily for two weeks, followed by 200 mg twice daily, or placebo; ZDV, 200 mg three times daily; ddl, 125 or 200 mg twice daily. Changes in CD4+ cell counts at 24 weeks: mean levels of CD4+ cell counts in those randomized to VIRAMUNE® +ZDV+ddl and ZDV+ddl remained significantly above baseline; however there was no significant difference between these arms. Changes in HIV-1 viral RNA at 24 weeks: there was no significant difference as measured by mean changes in plasma viral RNA between those randomized to VIRAMUNE® +ZDV+ddl and ZDV+ddl. However, the proportion of patients whose HIV-1 RNA decreased below the limit of detection (400 copies/mL) was significantly greater for the VIRAMUNE® +ZDV+ddl group (27/36 or 75%), when compared to the ZDV+ddl group (18/39 or 46%) or the VIRAMUNE® +ZDV group (0/28 or 0%); the clinical significance of this finding is unknown.

CONTRAINDICATIONS

VIRAMUNE® is contraindicated in patients with clinically significant hypersensitivity to any of the components contained in the tablet.

WARNINGS

Severe and life-threatening skin reactions have occurred in patients treated with VIRAMUNE®, including Stevens-Johnson syndrome (SJS). VIRAMUNE® must be discontinued in patients developing a severe rash or a rash accompanied by constitutional symptoms such as fever, blistering, oral lesions, conjunctivitis, swelling, muscle or joint aches, or general malaise. (see PRECAUTIONS, Information for Patients; ADVERSE REACTIONS)

VIRAMUNE® therapy must be initiated with a 14-day lead-in period of 200 mg/day, which has been shown to reduce the frequency of rash. Dose escalation should not occur if rash is

Table 1: Percentage of patients with rashes in controlled trials[a]

	ACTG 241[b]		BI 1037		BI 1011		COMBINED DATA	
	NVP+ZDV +ddl	ZDV+ddl	NVP+ZDV	ZDV	NVP+ZDV	ZDV	NVP	CONTROL
n	197	201	30	30	25	24	252	255
Rash events of all Grades and all causality	39.6%	23.9%	26.7%	6.7%	32.0%	4.2%	37.3%	20.0%
Grade 3 or 4 rash events; all causality	8.1%	1.5%	3.3%	0%	8.0%	0%	7.6%	1.2%

[a] At recommended dose of one 200 mg tablet daily for the first 14 days followed by one 200 mg tablet twice daily
[b] Trial ACTG 241 was designed to report Grade 3/4 (severe or life-threatening) events; except for several pre-specified events including rash for which all grades are reported

observed during this lead-in period until the rash has resolved. (see DOSAGE AND ADMINISTRATION)

PRECAUTIONS

General: When administering VIRAMUNE® as part of an antiretroviral treatment regimen, the complete product information for each therapeutic component should be consulted before initiation of treatment.
While nevirapine is extensively metabolized by the liver and nevirapine metabolites are extensively eliminated by the kidney, the pharmacokinetics of nevirapine have not been evaluated in patients with either hepatic or renal dysfunction. Therefore, VIRAMUNE® should be used with caution in these patient populations.
Abnormal liver function tests have been reported with VIRAMUNE®, some in the first few weeks of therapy, including cases of hepatitis. VIRAMUNE® administration should be interrupted in patients experiencing moderate or severe liver function test abnormalities until liver function tests return to baseline values. VIRAMUNE® treatment should be permanently discontinued if liver function abnormalities recur on readministration.

Drug Interactions: Although clinical studies have not been conducted, induction of CYP3A by nevirapine may result in lower plasma concentrations of other concomitantly administered drugs that are extensively metabolized by CYP3A. (see CLINICAL PHARMACOLOGY) Thus, if a patient has been stabilized on a dosage regimen for a drug metabolized by CYP3A, and begins treatment with VIRAMUNE®, dose adjustments may be necessary.

Rifampin/Rifabutin: There are insufficient data to assess whether dose adjustments are necessary when nevirapine and rifampin or rifabutin are coadministered. Therefore, these drugs should only be used in combination if clearly indicated and with careful monitoring.

Protease Inhibitors: Nevirapine may decrease plasma concentrations of protease inhibitors. Therefore, until clinical data are available that evaluate the need for dose adjustments, these drugs should not be administered concomitantly with VIRAMUNE®.

Oral Contraceptives: There are no clinical data on the effects of nevirapine on the pharmacokinetics of oral contraceptives. Nevirapine may decrease plasma concentrations of oral contraceptives (also other hormonal contraceptives); therefore, these drugs should not be administered concomitantly with VIRAMUNE®.

Information for Patients: Patients should be informed that VIRAMUNE® is not a cure for HIV-1 infection, and that they may continue to experience illnesses associated with advanced HIV-1 infection, including opportunistic infections. Treatment with VIRAMUNE® has not been shown to reduce the incidence or frequency of such illnesses, and patients should be advised to remain under the care of a physician when using VIRAMUNE®.
Patients should be informed that the long-term effects of VIRAMUNE® are unknown at this time. They should also be informed that VIRAMUNE® therapy has not been shown to reduce the risk of transmission of HIV-1 to others through sexual contact or blood contamination.

Patients should be instructed that the major toxicity of VIRAMUNE® is rash and should be advised to promptly notify their physician of any rash. The majority of rashes associated with VIRAMUNE® occur within the first 6 weeks of initiation of therapy. Therefore, patients should be monitored carefully for the appearance of rash during this period. Patients should be instructed that dose escalation is not to occur if any rash occurs during the two-week lead-in dosing period, until the rash resolves. Any patient experiencing severe rash or a rash accompanied by constitutional symptoms such as fever, blistering, oral lesions, conjunctivitis, swelling, muscle or joint aches, or general malaise should discontinue medication and consult a physician.

Patients should be informed to take VIRAMUNE® every day as prescribed. Patients should not alter the dose without consulting their doctor. If a dose is missed, patients should take the next dose as soon as possible. However, if a dose is skipped, the patient should not double the next dose.
VIRAMUNE® may interact with some drugs; therefore, patients should be advised to report to their doctor the use of any other medications.
Patients should be instructed that oral contraceptives and other hormonal methods of birth control should not be used as a method of contraception in women taking VIRAMUNE®

Carcinogenesis, Mutagenesis, Impairment of Fertility: Long-term carcinogenicity studies of nevirapine in animals are currently in progress. In genetic toxicology assays, nevirapine showed no evidence of mutagenic or clastogenic activity in a battery of *in vitro* and *in vivo* assays including microbial assays for gene mutation (Ames: Salmonella strains and *E. coli*), mammalian cell gene mutation assays (CHO/HGPRT), cytogenetic assays using a Chinese hamster ovary cell line and a mouse bone marrow micronucleus assay following oral administration. In reproductive toxicology studies, evidence of impaired fertility was seen in female rats at doses providing systemic exposure, based on AUC, approximately equivalent to that provided with the recommended clinical dose of VIRAMUNE®.

Pregnancy: Pregnancy Category C: No observable teratogenicity was detected in reproductive studies performed in pregnant rats and rabbits. In rats, a significant decrease in fetal body weight occurred at doses providing systemic exposure approximately 50% higher, based on AUC, than that seen at the recommended human clinical dose. The maternal and developmental no-observable-effect level dosages in rats and rabbits produced systemic exposures approximately equivalent to or approximately 50% higher, respectively, than those seen at the recommended daily human dose, based on AUC. There are no adequate and well-controlled studies in pregnant women. VIRAMUNE® should be used during pregnancy only if the potential benefit justifies the potential risk to the fetus.

Nursing Mothers: Preliminary results from an ongoing pharmacokinetic study (ACTG 250) of 10 HIV-1-infected pregnant women who were administered a single oral dose of 100 or 200 mg VIRAMUNE® at a median of 5.8 hours before delivery, indicate that nevirapine readily crosses the placenta and is found in breast milk. Consistent with the recommendation by the U.S. Public Health Service Centers for Disease Control and Prevention that HIV-infected mothers not breast-feed their infants to avoid risking postnatal transmission of HIV, mothers should discontinue nursing if they are receiving VIRAMUNE®.

Pediatric Use: Safety and effectiveness of VIRAMUNE® in pediatric patients have not been established.

VIRAMUNE® has been studied in two open-label, uncontrolled trials (BI 882, BI 892) in 37 HIV-1-infected pediatric patients with a median age of 0.9 years (range: 0.1 to 15 years) who were treated for a median duration of 20.7 months. Seven patients developed rashes while receiving VIRAMUNE®. In an ongoing, controlled trial of VIRAMUNE® combination therapy in HIV-1-infected pediatric patients (ACTG 245), one of approximately 288 patients treated with VIRAMUNE® experienced Stevens-Johnson syndrome.

Because there are no data on multi-dose pharmacokinetics in children, no recommendation on dosing can be made. Based on single-dose pharmacokinetics in 9 HIV-1-infected pediatric patients (age 9 mos. to 14 years) who were administered nevirapine in a suspension formulation, it appears that oral clearance is approximately 2-fold greater in children when compared to adults.

Table 2: Comparative Incidence of Selected Drug-Related Events in Controlled Trials

	ACTG 241		Trial BI 1037 and BI 1011	
	Grade 3/4 events		All severities	
	NVP+ZDV+ddl	ZDV+ddl	NVP+ZDV	ZDV alone
Number of patients	197	201	55	30
Overall incidence of related adverse events	31%	23%	42%	33%
Rash	8	2	20	3
Fever	3	3	11	3
Nausea	5	4	9	3
Headache	3	3	11	0
Diarrhea	2	2	0	0
Abdominal pain	1	2	2	0
Ulcerative stomatitis	0	0	4	0
Peripheral Neuropathy	0	2	0	0
Paraesthesia	1	0	2	0
Myalgia	1	0	2	7
Hepatitis	1	0	4	0

ADVERSE REACTIONS

The most frequently reported adverse events related to VIRAMUNE® therapy were rash, fever, nausea, headache, and abnormal liver function tests.

The major clinical toxicity of VIRAMUNE® is rash, with VIRAMUNE®-attributable rash occurring in 17% of patients in combination regimens in Phase II/III controlled studies. Thirty-seven percent of patients treated with VIRAMUNE® experienced rash compared with 20% of patients treated in control groups of either ZDV+ddl or ZDV alone (Table 1). Severe or life-threatening rash occurred in 7.6% of VIRAMUNE®-treated patients compared with 1.2% of patients treated in the control groups.

Rashes are usually mild to moderate, maculopapular erythematous cutaneous eruptions, with or without pruritus, located on the trunk, face and extremities. The majority of severe rashes occurred within the first 28 days of treatment; 25% of the patients with severe rashes required hospitalization; and one patient required surgical intervention. All patients recovered. Overall, 7% of patients discontinued VIRAMUNE® due to rash.

[See table 1 on preceding page.]

Table 2 lists treatment-related clinical adverse events that occurred in patients receiving VIRAMUNE® in ACTG 241 and in Trials BI 1037 and BI 1011.

[See table 2 above.]

Laboratory Abnormalities: Table 3 summarizes marked laboratory abnormalities occurring in three controlled studies.

Table 3: Percentage of patients with marked laboratory abnormalities

	Data combined for controlled trials ACTG 241, BI 1037 & BI 1011	
	VIRAMUNE® n=252	Control n=255
Hematology		
Decreased Hg (<8.0 g/dL)	1.2%	2.0%
Decreased platelets (<50,000/mm³)	0.8	0.8
Decreased neutrophils (<750/mm³)	11.1	10.2
Blood chemistry		
Increased ALT (>250 U/L)	3.4	3.5
Increased AST (>250 U/L)	2.0	2.4
Increased GGT (>450 U/L)	2.4	1.2
Increased total bilirubin (>2.5 mg/dL)	0.4	1.2

Asymptomatic elevations in GGT levels are more frequent in VIRAMUNE® recipients than in controls. Because hepatitis has occasionally been reported in VIRAMUNE®-treated patients, monitoring of liver function tests should be considered.

OVERDOSAGE

There is no known antidote for VIRAMUNE® overdosage. No acute toxicities or sequelae were reported for one patient who ingested 800 mg of VIRAMUNE® for one day.

DOSAGE AND ADMINISTRATION

The recommended dose for VIRAMUNE® is one 200 mg tablet daily for the first 14 days (**this lead-in period should be used because it has been found to lessen the frequency of rash**), followed by one 200 mg tablet twice daily, in combination with nucleoside analogue antiretroviral agents. For concomitantly administered nucleoside therapy, the manufacturer's recommended dosage and monitoring should be followed.

Monitoring Of Patients: Clinical chemistry tests, which include liver function tests, should be performed prior to initiating VIRAMUNE® therapy and at appropriate intervals during therapy.

Dosage Adjustment: **VIRAMUNE® should be discontinued if patients experience severe rash or a rash accompanied by constitutional findings (see WARNINGS). Patients experiencing rash during the 14-day lead-in period of 200 mg/day should not have their VIRAMUNE® dose increased until the rash has resolved. (see PRECAUTIONS, Information for Patients)**

VIRAMUNE® administration should be interrupted in patients experiencing moderate or severe liver function test abnormalities (excluding GGT), until the liver function test elevations have returned to baseline. VIRAMUNE® may then be restarted at half the previous dose level. VIRAMUNE® should be permanently discontinued if moderate or severe liver function test abnormalities recur. (see PRECAUTIONS)

Patients who interrupt VIRAMUNE® dosing for more than 7 days should restart the recommended dosing, using one 200 mg tablet daily for the first 14 days (lead-in) followed by one 200 mg tablet twice daily.

No data are available to recommend a dosage of VIRAMUNE® in patients with hepatic dysfunction, renal insufficiency, or undergoing dialysis.

HOW SUPPLIED

VIRAMUNE® (nevirapine) Tablets, 200 mg, are white, oval, biconvex tablets, 9.3 mm × 19.1 mm. One side is embossed with "54 193", with a single bisect separating the "54" and "193". The opposite side has a single bisect.

VIRAMUNE® Tablets are supplied in bottles of 100 (NDC 0054-4647-25) and individually blister-sealed unit-dose cartons of 100 tablets as 10 × 10 cards (NDC 0054-8647-25). Store at 15°C–30°C (59°F–86°F). The bottles should be kept tightly closed.

Manufactured by: Boehringer Ingelheim Pharmaceuticals, Inc.
Ridgefield, CT 06877

Distributed by: Roxane Laboratories, Inc.
Columbus, OH 43216

CAUTION FEDERAL LAW PROHIBITS DISPENSING WITHOUT PRESCRIPTION

Roxane
Laboratories, Inc.
A Boehringer Ingelheim Company
Shown in Product Identification Guide, page 332

EDUCATIONAL MATERIAL

Booklets
"Oral Morphine in Advanced Cancer," Robert G. Twycross and Sylvia A. Lack. Practical guidelines on the considerations which must be taken into account when initiating oral morphine therapy, free to physicians and pharmacists.
"Oral Morphine—Information for Patients, Families, and Friends," Robert G. Twycross and Sylvia A. Lack. free to physicians, pharmacists, and patients.

Rystan Company, Inc.
47 CENTER AVENUE
P.O. BOX 214
LITTLE FALLS, NJ 07424-0214

Direct Inquiries to:
Professional Services Department
(201) 256-3737

CHLORESIUM®   OTC
[klor-eez'ium]
Ointment and Solution
Healing and Deodorizing Agent

COMPOSITION
Ointment: 0.5% Chlorophyllin Copper Complex Sodium, USP in a hydrophilic base. Solution: 0.2% Chlorophyllin Copper Complex Sodium, USP in isotonic saline solution.

ACTIONS AND USES
To promote healing and to relieve itching and discomfort of minor wounds, burns, surface ulcers, cuts, abrasions and skin irritations. To reduce malodors in wounds and surface ulcers.

ADMINISTRATION AND DOSAGE
Ointment: Apply generously and cover with an appropriate dressing, or as directed by physician. Dressings preferably changed no more often than every 48 to 72 hours. Solution: Apply full strength as continuous wet dressing, or as directed by physician.

SIDE EFFECTS
CHLORESIUM Ointment and Solution are soothing and nontoxic. Sensitivity reactions are extremely rare, and only a few instances of slight itching or irritation have been reported.

HOW SUPPLIED
Ointment: 1 oz and 4 oz tubes, 1 lb. jars (NDC 0263-5155-01 and -04, -16). Solution: 8 fl oz and 32 fl oz bottles (NDC 0263-5158-08 and -32).

DERIFIL® Tablets   OTC
[der'ah-fil]
Internal Deodorant

COMPOSITION
100 mg Chlorophyllin Copper Complex Sodium, USP per tablet.

INDICATIONS
Oral deodorant for internal use: 1. An aid to reduce fecal odor due to incontinence, 2. An aid to reduce odor from a colostomy or ileostomy.

DIRECTIONS
Adults and children 12 years of age and over: Oral dosage is one to two tablets daily in divided doses as required. If odor is not controlled, take up to an additional tablet daily in divided doses as required. The smallest effective dose should be used. Do not exceed 3 tablets daily. Children under 12 years of age: consult a doctor. In ostomies, tablets may be either taken by mouth or placed in the appliance.

SIDE EFFECTS
When used as directed, no toxic effects have been reported. As with any drug, do not exceed the recommended dosage. A temporary mild laxative effect may be noted, and the fecal discharge is commonly stained dark green.

WARNING
If cramps or diarrhea occurs, reduce the dosage. If symptoms persist, consult your doctor.

HOW SUPPLIED
Dark green, round, film-coated tablet with "R" on one side and score on other. Each tablet contains 100 mg Chlorophyllin Copper Complex Sodium, USP. Bottles of 30 (NDC 0263-5001-03), 100 (NDC 0263-5001-10), 1000 tablets (NDC 0263-5001-11) and blister pack of 40 tablets (NDC 0263-5001-04).

Continued on next page

Rystan—Cont.

PANAFIL® Ointment ℞
[pan 'ah-fil]
Papain-Urea-Chlorophyllin Copper Complex Sodium
Debriding-Healing Ointment

CAUTION
Federal law prohibits dispensing without prescription.

DESCRIPTION
PANAFIL® Ointment is an enzymatic debriding-healing ointment which contains standardized Papain, USP 10%, Urea USP 10% and Chlorophyllin Copper Complex Sodium, USP 0.5% in a hydrophilic base. Inactive ingredients are Purified Water, USP; Propylene Glycol, USP; White Petrolatum, USP; Stearyl Alcohol, NF; Polyoxyl 40 Stearate, NF; Sorbitan Monostearate, NF: Boric Acid, NF; Chlorobutanol (Anhydrous), NF as a preservative; Sodium Borate, NF.

CLINICAL PHARMACOLOGY
Papain, the proteolytic enzyme derived from the fruit of carica papaya, is a potent digestant of nonviable protein matter, but is harmless to viable tissue. It has the unique advantage of being active over a wide pH range, 3 to 12. Despite its recognized value as a digestive agent, papain is relatively ineffective when used alone as a debriding agent, primarily because it requires the presence of activators to exert its digestive function.
In PANAFIL® Ointment, Urea is combined with papain to provide two supplementary chemical actions: 1) to expose by solvent action the activators of papain (sulfhydryl groups) which are always present, but not necessarily accessible, in the nonviable tissue or debris of lesions, and 2) to denature the nonviable protein matter in lesions and thereby render it more susceptible to enzymatic digestion. In pharmacologic studies involving digestion of beef powder, Miller[1] showed that the combination of papain and urea produced twice as much digestion as papain alone.
Chlorophyllin Copper Complex Sodium adds healing action to the cleansing action of the proteolytic papain-urea combination. The basic wound-healing properties of Chlorophyllin Copper Complex Sodium are promotion of healthy granulations, control of local inflammation and reduction of wound odors.[2] Specifically, Chlorophyllin Copper Complex Sodium inhibits the hemagglutinating and inflammatory properties of protein degradation products in the wound, including the products of enzymatic digestion, thus providing an additional protective factor.[1,3] The incorporation of Chlorophyllin Copper Complex Sodium in PANAFIL® Ointment permits its continuous use for as long as desired to help produce and then maintain a clean wound base and to promote healing.

INDICATIONS AND USES
PANAFIL® Ointment is suggested for treatment of acute and chronic lesions such as varicose, diabetic and decubitus ulcers, burns, postoperative wounds, pilonidal cyst wounds, carbuncles and miscellaneous traumatic or infected wounds. PANAFIL® Ointment is applied continuously throughout treatment of these conditions (1) for enzymatic debridement of necrotic tissue and liquefaction of fibrinous, purulent debris, (2) to keep the wound clean, and simultaneously (3) to promote normal healing.

CONTRAINDICATIONS
None known.

PRECAUTIONS
See Dosage and Administration.
Not to be used in eyes.

ADVERSE REACTIONS
PANAFIL® Ointment is generally well tolerated and nonirritating. A small percentage of patients may experience a transient "burning" sensation on application of the ointment. Occasionally, the profuse exudate resulting from enzymatic digestion may cause irritation. In such cases, more frequent changes of dressings until exudate diminishes will alleviate discomfort.

DOSAGE AND ADMINISTRATION
Apply PANAFIL® Ointment directly to lesion and cover with appropriate dressing. When practicable, daily or twice daily changes of dressings are preferred. Longer intervals between redressings (two or three days) have proved satisfactory, and PANAFIL® Ointment may be applied under pressure dressings. At each redressing, the lesion should be irrigated with isotonic saline solution or other mild cleansing solution (except hydrogen peroxide solution, which may inactivate the papain) to remove any accumulation of liquefied necrotic material.

NOTE
Papain may also be inactivated by the salts of heavy metals (lead, silver, mercury, etc.). Contact with medications containing these metals should be avoided.

HOW SUPPLIED
Available on prescription only in 1 oz tube (NDC 0263-5145-01) and 1 lb. jar (NDC 0263-5145-16).

REFERENCES
1–3. Data on file.   9/92

PANAFIL®-WHITE ℞
[pan' ah-fil]
Papain-Urea Debriding Ointment

CAUTION
Federal law prohibits dispensing without prescription.

DESCRIPTION
PANAFIL-WHITE Ointment is an enzymatic debriding ointment containing standardized Papain, USP (10,000 Rystan Units of enzyme activity per gm of ointment) and Urea USP 10% in a hydrophilic base. One Rystan Unit is that quantity which under specified conditions will clot 10 microliters of milk substrate in 1 minute at 40°C. Inactive ingredients are Purified Water, USP; Propylene Glycol, USP; White Petrolatum, USP; Stearyl Alcohol, NF; Sorbitan Monostearate, NF; Polyoxyl 40 Stearate, NF; Boric Acid, NF; Sodium Borate, NF; Chlorobutanol (Anhydrous), NF as a preservative.

CLINICAL PHARMACOLOGY
Papain, the proteolytic enzyme from the fruit of carica papaya, is a potent digestant of nonviable protein matter, but is harmless to viable tissue. It has the unique advantage of being active over a wide pH range, 3 to 12. Despite its recognized value as a digestive agent, papain is relatively ineffective when used alone as a debriding agent, primarily because it requires the presence of activators to exert its digestive function.
In PANAFIL-WHITE, urea is combined with papain to provide two supplementary chemical actions: 1) to expose by solvent action the activators of papain (sulfhydryl groups) which are always present, but not necessarily accessible, in the nonviable tissue or debris of lesions, and 2) to denature the nonviable protein matter in lesions and thereby render it more susceptible to enzymatic digestion. In pharmacologic studies involving digestion of beef powder, Miller[1] showed that the combination of papain and urea produced twice as much digestion as papain alone.

INDICATIONS AND USES
PANAFIL-WHITE is indicated for debridement of necrotic tissue and liquefaction of pus in acute and chronic lesions such as decubitus, varicose and diabetic ulcers, burns, postoperative wounds, pilonidal cyst wounds, carbuncles and miscellaneous traumatic or infected wounds.

CONTRAINDICATIONS
None known

PRECAUTIONS
See Dosage and Administration.
Not to be used in eyes.

ADVERSE REACTIONS
PANAFIL-WHITE is generally well tolerated and nonirritating. A small percentage of patients may experience a transient "burning" sensation on application of the ointment. Occasionally, the profuse exudate resulting from enzymatic digestion may cause irritation. In such cases, more frequent changes of dressings until exudate diminishes will alleviate discomfort.

DOSAGE AND ADMINISTRATION
Apply PANAFIL-WHITE directly to lesion and cover with appropriate dressing. Daily or twice daily changes of dressings are preferred. At each redressing, the lesion should be irrigated with isotonic saline solution, or other mild cleansing solution (except hydrogen peroxide solution, which may inactivate the papain) to remove any accumulation of liquefied necrotic material.

NOTE
Papain may also be inactivated by the salts of heavy metals (lead, silver, mercury, etc.). Contact with medications containing these metals should be avoided.

HOW SUPPLIED
Available on prescription only in 1 oz tubes. (NDC 0263-5148-01)

REFERENCE
1. Data on file.
                                                       9/92

PROPHYLLIN® CCC   OTC
[pro-fil 'in]
Topical, Emollient Ointment

ACTIVE INGREDIENT white petrolatum, USP. **Other ingredients:** purified water, USP; stearyl alcohol, NF; propylene glycol, USP; sodium propionate, NF; polyoxyl 40 stearate, NF; methylparaben, NF: fragrance and chlorophyllin copper complex sodium, USP.

INDICATIONS
Helps prevent and temporarily protects chafed, chapped, cracked, or windburned skin and lips. Soothes irritated skin.

DIRECTIONS
Spread generously over area several times daily and upon retiring.

WARNING
For external use only. Avoid contact with the eyes. If condition worsens, or does not improve within seven days, consult a physician. Not to be applied over deep or puncture wounds, infections or lacerations; consult a physician. Keep this and all drugs out of reach of children. In case of accidental ingestion, contact a poison control center or a physician immediately.

HOW SUPPLIED
1 oz tube, (NDC 0263-5085-01)
11/93   Made in U.S.A.

SCS Pharmaceuticals
BOX 5110
CHICAGO, IL 60680

Direct Inquiries to:
(800) 323-1603

For Medical Information Contact:
Generally:
G.D. Searle & Co.
Healthcare Information Services
5200 Old Orchard Road
Skokie, IL 60077

In Emergencies:
Outside IL:
(800) 323-4204 (business hours)
(708) 982-7000 (at other times)
Within IL:
(708) 982-7000

Sales and Ordering:
(800) 323-1603

Alphabetic Product Listing
<u>Product, ID #, (NDC*), Form, Strength</u>
Flagyl, I.V., 1804, Vial (partial fill, lyoph. pwd.), 500 mg
Flagyl I.V. RTU, 1847, Plastic Container, 500 mg/100 ml
Levora® (levonorgestrel and ethinyl estradiol tablets 0.15 mg/30 mg)
Piroxicam USP, 5752, Tablet, 10 mg
Piroxicam USP, 5762, Tablet, 20 mg

---

* When the product ID # is not the same as the NDC #, the NDC # appears in parentheses.

<u>Product Information Available on Request</u>
Levora® (levonorgestrel and ethinyl estradiol tablets USP)
Piroxicam Tablets USP   ℞

* When the product ID # is not the same as the NDC #, the NDC # appears in parentheses.

FLAGYL® I.V. ℞
[flaj'yl]
(metronidazole hydrochloride)
FLAGYL® I.V. RTU® ℞
(metronidazole injection USP) Ready-to-Use
STERILE
For Intravenous Infusion Only

> **WARNING**
> Metronidazole has been shown to be carcinogenic in mice and rats (see *Precautions*). Its use, therefore, should be reserved for the conditions described in the *Indications and Usage* section below.

DESCRIPTION

Flagyl I.V., sterile (metronidazole hydrochloride), and Flagyl I.V. RTU, sterile (metronidazole), are parenteral dosage forms of the synthetic antibacterial agents 1-(β-hydroxyethyl)-2-methyl-5-nitroimidazole hydrochloride and 1-(β-hydroxyethyl)-2-methyl-5-nitroimidazole, respectively.

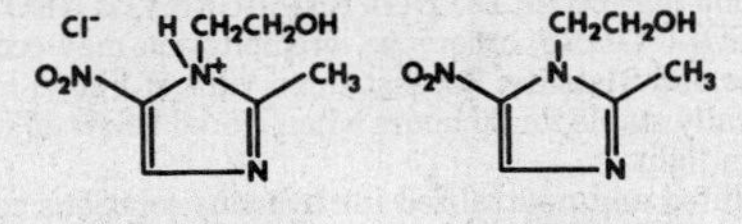

metronidazole hydrochloride   metronidazole

Each single-dose vial of lyophilized Flagyl I.V. contains sterile, nonpyrogenic metronidazole hydrochloride, equivalent to 500 mg metronidazole, and 415 mg mannitol.

Each Flagyl I.V. RTU 100-ml single-dose plastic container contains a sterile, nonpyrogenic, isotonic, buffered solution of 500 mg metronidazole, 47.6 mg sodium phosphate, 22.9 mg citric acid, and 790 mg sodium chloride in Water for Injection USP. Flagyl I.V. RTU has a tonicity of 310 mOsm/L and a pH of 5 to 7. Each container contains 14 mEq of sodium.

The plastic container is fabricated from a specially formulated polyvinyl chloride plastic. Water can permeate from inside the container into the overwrap in amounts insufficient to affect the solution significantly. Solutions in contact with the plastic container can leach out certain of its chemical components in very small amounts within the expiration period, eg, di 2-ethylhexyl phthalate (DEHP), up to 5 parts per million. However, the safety of the plastic has been confirmed in tests in animals according to USP biological tests for plastic containers as well as by tissue culture toxicity studies.

CLINICAL PHARMACOLOGY

Metronidazole is a synthetic antibacterial compound. Disposition of metronidazole in the body is similar for both oral and intravenous dosage forms, with an average elimination half-life in healthy humans of eight hours.

The major route of elimination of metronidazole and its metabolites is via the urine (60–80% of the dose), with fecal excretion accounting for 6–15% of the dose. The metabolites that appear in the urine result primarily from side-chain oxidation [1-(β-hydroxyethyl)-2-hydroxymethyl-5-nitroimidazole and 2-methyl-5-nitroimidazole-1-yl-acetic acid] and glucuronide conjugation, with unchanged metronidazole accounting for approximately 20% of the total. Renal clearance of metronidazole is approximately 10 ml/min/1.73 m^2.

Metronidazole is the major component appearing in the plasma, with lesser quantities of the 2-hydroxymethyl metabolite also being present. Less than 20% of the circulating metronidazole is bound to plasma proteins. Both the parent compound and the metabolite possess *in vitro* bactericidal activity against most strains of anaerobic bacteria.

Metronidazole appears in cerebrospinal fluid, saliva, and breast milk in concentrations similar to those found in plasma. Bactericidal concentrations of metronidazole have also been detected in pus from hepatic abscesses.

Plasma concentrations of metronidazole are proportional to the administered dose. An eight-hour intravenous infusion of 100–4,000 mg of metronidazole in normal subjects showed a linear relationship between dose and peak plasma concentration.

In patients treated with Flagyl I.V., using a dosage regimen of 15 mg/kg loading dose followed six hours later by 7.5 mg/kg every six hours, peak steady-state plasma concentrations of metronidazole averaged 25 mcg/ml with trough (minimum) concentrations averaging 18 mcg/ml.

Decreased renal function does not alter the single-dose pharmacokinetics of metronidazole. However, plasma clearance of metronidazole is decreased in patients with decreased liver function.

In one study newborn infants appeared to demonstrate diminished capacity to eliminate metronidazole. The elimination half-life, measured during the first three days of life, was inversely related to gestational age. In infants whose gestational ages were between 28 and 40 weeks, the corresponding elimination half-lives ranged from 109 to 22.5 hours.

Microbiology: Metronidazole is active *in vitro* against most obligate anaerobes, but does not appear to possess any clinically relevant activity against facultative anaerobes or obligate aerobes. Against susceptible organisms, metronidazole is generally bactericidal at concentrations equal to or slightly higher than the minimal inhibitory concentrations. Metronidazole has been shown to have *in vitro* and clinical activity against the following organisms:

Anaerobic gram-negative bacilli, including:
Bacteroides species, including the *Bacteroides fragilis* group (*B. fragilis, B. distasonis, B. ovatus, B. thetaiotaomicron, B. vulgatus*)
Fusobacterium species.
Anaerobic gram-positive bacilli, including:
Clostridium species and susceptible strains of *Eubacterium*
Anaerobic gram-positive cocci, including:
Peptococcus species
Peptostreptococcus species

Susceptibility Tests: Bacteriologic studies should be performed to determine the causative organisms and their susceptibility to metronidazole; however, the rapid, routine susceptibility testing of individual isolates of anaerobic bacteria is not always practical, and therapy may be started while awaiting these results.

Quantitative methods give the most accurate estimates of susceptibility to antibacterial drugs. A standardized agar dilution method and a broth microdilution method are recommended.[1]

Control strains are recommended for standardized susceptibility testing. Each time the test is performed, one or more of the following strains should be included: *Clostridium perfringens* ATCC 13124, *Bacteroides fragilis* ATCC 25285, and *Bacteroides thetaiotaomicron* ATCC 29741. The mode metronidazole MICs for those three strains are reported to be 0.25, 0.25, and 0.5 mcg/ml, respectively.

A clinical laboratory test is considered under acceptable control if the results of the control strains are within one doubling dilution of the mode MICs reported for metronidazole.

A bacterial isolate may be considered susceptible if the MIC value for metronidazole is not more than 16 mcg/ml. An organism is considered resistant if the MIC is greater than 16 mcg/ml. A report of "resistant" from the laboratory indicates that the infecting organism is not likely to respond to therapy.

INDICATIONS AND USAGE

Treatment of Anaerobic Infections

Flagyl I.V. (metronidazole hydrochloride) and Flagyl I.V. RTU (metronidazole) are indicated in the treatment of serious infections caused by susceptible anaerobic bacteria. Indicated surgical procedures should be performed in conjunction with Flagyl I.V. or Flagyl I.V. RTU therapy. In a mixed aerobic and anaerobic infection, antibiotics appropriate for the treatment of the aerobic infection should be used in addition to Flagyl I.V. or Flagyl I.V. RTU.

Flagyl I.V. and Flagyl I.V. RTU are effective in *Bacteroides fragilis* infections resistant to clindamycin, chloramphenicol, and penicillin.

INTRA-ABDOMINAL INFECTIONS, including peritonitis, intra-abdominal abscess, and liver abscess, caused by *Bacteroides* species including the *B. fragilis* group (*B. fragilis, B. distasonis, B. ovatus, B. thetaiotaomicron, B. vulgatus*), *Clostridium* species, *Eubacterium* species, *Peptococcus* species, and *Peptostreptococcus* species.

SKIN AND SKIN STRUCTURE INFECTIONS caused by *Bacteroides* species including the *B. fragilis* group, *Clostridium* species, *Peptococcus* species, *Peptostreptococcus* species, and *Fusobacterium* species.

GYNECOLOGIC INFECTIONS, including endometritis, endomyometritis, tubo-ovarian abscess, and postsurgical vaginal cuff infection, caused by *Bacteroides* species including the *B. fragilis* group, *Clostridium* species, *Peptococcus* species, and *Peptostreptococcus* species.

BACTERIAL SEPTICEMIA caused by *Bacteroides* species including the *B. fragilis* group, and *Clostridium* species.

BONE AND JOINT INFECTIONS, as adjunctive therapy, caused by *Bacteroides* species including the *B. fragilis* group.

CENTRAL NERVOUS SYSTEM (CNS) INFECTIONS, including meningitis and brain abscess, caused by *Bacteroides* species including the *B. fragilis* group.

LOWER RESPIRATORY TRACT INFECTIONS, including pneumonia, empyema, and lung abscess, caused by *Bacteroides* species including the *B. fragilis* group.

ENDOCARDITIS caused by *Bacteroides* species including the *B. fragilis* group.

Prophylaxis

The prophylactic administration of Flagyl I.V. or Flagyl I.V. RTU preoperatively, intraoperatively, and postoperatively may reduce the incidence of postoperative infection in patients undergoing elective colorectal surgery which is classified as contaminated or potentially contaminated.

Prophylactic use of Flagyl I.V. or Flagyl I.V. RTU should be discontinued within 12 hours after surgery. If there are signs of infection, specimens for cultures should be obtained for the identification of the causative organism(s) so that appropriate therapy may be given (see *Dosage and Administration*).

CONTRAINDICATIONS

Flagyl I.V. and Flagyl I.V. RTU are contraindicated in patients with a prior history of hypersensitivity to metronidazole or other nitroimidazole derivatives.

WARNINGS

Convulsive Seizures and Peripheral Neuropathy: Convulsive seizures and peripheral neuropathy, the latter characterized mainly by numbness or paresthesia of an extremity, have been reported in patients treated with metronidazole. The appearance of abnormal neurologic signs demands the prompt evaluation of the benefit/risk ratio of the continuation of therapy.

PRECAUTIONS

General: Patients with severe hepatic disease metabolize metronidazole slowly, with resultant accumulation of metronidazole and its metabolites in the plasma. Accordingly, for such patients, doses below those usually recommended should be administered cautiously.

Administration of solutions containing sodium ions may result in sodium retention. Care should be taken when administering Flagyl I.V. RTU to patients receiving corticosteroids or to patients predisposed to edema.

Known or previously unrecognized candidiasis may present more prominent symptoms during therapy with Flagyl I.V. or Flagyl I.V. RTU and requires treatment with a candicidal agent.

Laboratory Tests: Metronidazole is a nitroimidazole, and Flagyl I.V. or Flagyl I.V. RTU should be used with care in patients with evidence of or history of blood dyscrasia. A mild leukopenia has been observed during its administration; however, no persistent hematologic abnormalities attributable to metronidazole have been observed in clinical studies. Total and differential leukocyte counts are recommended before and after therapy.

Drug Interactions: Metronidazole has been reported to potentiate the anticoagulant effect of warfarin and other oral coumarin anticoagulants, resulting in a prolongation of prothrombin time. This possible drug interaction should be considered when Flagyl I.V. or Flagyl I.V. RTU is prescribed for patients on this type of anticoagulant therapy.

The simultaneous administration of drugs that induce microsomal liver enzymes, such as phenytoin or phenobarbital, may accelerate the elimination of metronidazole, resulting in reduced plasma levels; impaired clearance of phenytoin has also been reported.

The simultaneous administration of drugs that decrease microsomal liver enzyme activity, such as cimetidine, may prolong the half-life and decrease plasma clearance of metronidazole.

Alcoholic beverages should not be consumed during metronidazole therapy because abdominal cramps, nausea, vomiting, headaches, and flushing may occur.

Psychotic reactions have been reported in alcoholic patients who are using metronidazole and disulfiram concurrently. Metronidazole should not be given to patients who have taken disulfiram within the last two weeks.

Drug/Laboratory Test Interactions: Metronidazole may interfere with certain types of determinations of serum chemistry values, such as aspartate aminotransferase (AST, SGOT), alanine aminotransferase (ALT, SGPT), lactate dehydrogenase (LDH), triglycerides, and hexokinase glucose. Values of zero may be observed. All of the assays in which interference has been reported involve enzymatic coupling of the assay to oxidation-reduction of nicotine adenine dinucleotide ($NAD^+ \rightleftarrows NADH$). Interference is due to the similarity in absorbance peaks of NADH (340 nm) and metronidazole (322 nm) at pH 7.

Carcinogenesis, Mutagenesis, Impairment of Fertility: Tumorigenicity in Rodents—Metronidazole has shown evidence of carcinogenic activity in studies involving chronic, oral administration in mice and rats, but similar studies in the hamster gave negative results. Also, metronidazole has shown mutagenic activity in a number of *in vitro* assay systems, but studies in mammals (*in vivo*) failed to demonstrate a potential for genetic damage.

Pregnancy: Teratogenic Effects—Pregnancy Category B. Metronidazole crosses the placental barrier and enters the fetal circulation rapidly. Reproduction studies have been performed in rats at doses up to five times the human dose and have revealed no evidence of impaired fertility or harm to the fetus due to metronidazole. Metronidazole administered intraperitoneally to pregnant mice at approximately the human dose caused fetotoxicity; administered orally to pregnant mice, no fetotoxicity was observed. There are, however, no adequate and well-controlled studies in pregnant women. Because animal reproduction studies are not always

Continued on next page

SCS—Cont.

predictive of human response, and because metronidazole is a carcinogen in rodents, these drugs should be used during pregnancy only if clearly needed.

Nursing Mothers: Because of the potential for tumorigenicity shown for metronidazole in mouse and rat studies, a decision should be made whether to discontinue nursing or to discontinue the drug, taking into account the importance of the drug to the mother. Metronidazole is secreted in breast milk in concentrations similar to those found in plasma.

Pediatric Use: Safety and effectiveness in children have not been established.

ADVERSE REACTIONS

Two serious adverse reactions reported in patients treated with Flagyl I.V. or Flagyl I.V. RTU have been convulsive seizures and peripheral neuropathy, the latter characterized mainly by numbness or paresthesia of an extremity. Since persistent peripheral neuropathy has been reported in some patients receiving prolonged oral administration of Flagyl® (metronidazole), patients should be observed carefully if neurologic symptoms occur and a prompt evaluation made of the benefit/risk ratio of the continuation of therapy.

The following reactions have also been reported during treatment with Flagyl I.V. (metronidazole hydrochloride) or Flagyl I.V. RTU (metronidazole):

Gastrointestinal: Nausea, vomiting, abdominal discomfort, diarrhea, and an unpleasant metallic taste.
Hematopoietic: Reversible neutropenia (leukopenia).
Dermatologic: Erythematous rash and pruritus.
Central Nervous System: Headache, dizziness, syncope, ataxia, and confusion.
Local Reactions: Thrombophlebitis after intravenous infusion. This reaction can be minimized or avoided by avoiding prolonged use of indwelling intravenous catheters.
Other: Fever. Instances of a darkened urine have also been reported, and this manifestation has been the subject of a special investigation. Although the pigment which is probably responsible for this phenomenon has not been positively identified, it is almost certainly a metabolite of metronidazole and seems to have no clinical significance.

The following adverse reactions have been reported during treatment with oral Flagyl (metronidazole):

Gastrointestinal: Nausea, sometimes accompanied by headache, anorexia, and occasionally vomiting; diarrhea, epigastric distress, abdominal cramping, and constipation.
Mouth: A sharp, unpleasant metallic taste is not unusual. Furry tongue, glossitis, and stomatitis have occurred; these may be associated with a sudden overgrowth of *Candida* which may occur during effective therapy.
Hematopoietic: Reversible neutropenia (leukopenia); rarely, reversible thrombocytopenia.
Cardiovascular: Flattening of the T-wave may be seen in electrocardiographic tracings.
Central Nervous System: Convulsive seizures, peripheral neuropathy, dizziness, vertigo, incoordination, ataxia, confusion, irritability, depression, weakness, and insomnia.
Hypersensitivity: Urticaria, erythematous rash, flushing, nasal congestion, dryness of the mouth (or vagina or vulva), and fever.
Renal: Dysuria, cystitis, polyuria, incontinence, a sense of pelvic pressure, and darkened urine.
Other: Proliferation of *Candida* in the vagina, dyspareunia, decrease of libido, proctitis, and fleeting joint pains sometimes resembling "serum sickness." If patients receiving metronidazole drink alcoholic beverages, they may experience abdominal distress, nausea, vomiting, flushing, or headache. A modification of the taste of alcoholic beverages has also been reported. Rare cases of pancreatitis, which abated on withdrawal of the drug, have been reported.

Crohn's disease patients are known to have an increased incidence of gastrointestinal and certain extraintestinal cancers. There have been some reports in the medical literature of breast and colon cancer in Crohn's disease patients who have been treated with metronidazole at high doses for extended periods of time. A cause and effect relationship has not been established. Crohn's disease is not an approved indication for Flagyl I.V. or Flagyl I.V. RTU.

OVERDOSAGE

Use of dosages of Flagyl I.V. (metronidazole hydrochloride) higher than those recommended has been reported. These include the use of 27 mg/kg three times a day for 20 days, and the use of 75 mg/kg as a single loading dose followed by 7.5 mg/kg maintenance doses. No adverse reactions were reported in either of the two cases.

Single oral doses of metronidazole, up to 15 g, have been reported in suicide attempts and accidental overdoses. Symptoms reported include nausea, vomiting, and ataxia.

Oral metronidazole has been studied as a radiation sensitizer in the treatment of malignant tumors. Neurotoxic effects, including seizures and peripheral neuropathy, have been reported after 5 to 7 days of doses of 6 to 10.4 g every other day.

Treatment: There is no specific antidote for overdose; therefore, management of the patient should consist of symptomatic and supportive therapy.

DOSAGE AND ADMINISTRATION

In elderly patients the pharmacokinetics of metronidazole may be altered and therefore monitoring of serum levels may be necessary to adjust the metronidazole dosage accordingly.

Treatment of Anaerobic Infections
The recommended dosage schedule for *adults* is:
Loading dose:
15 mg/kg infused over one hour (approximately 1 g for a 70-kg adult).
Maintenance Dose:
7.5 mg/kg infused over one hour every six hours (approximately 500 mg for a 70-kg adult). The first maintenance dose should be instituted six hours following the initiation of the loading dose.

Parenteral therapy may be changed to oral Flagyl (metronidazole) when conditions warrant, based upon the severity of the disease and the response of the patient to Flagyl I.V. or Flagyl I.V. RTU (metronidazole) treatment. The usual adult oral dosage is 7.5 mg/kg every six hours.

A maximum of 4 g should not be exceeded during a 24-hour period.

Patients with severe hepatic disease metabolize metronidazole slowly, with resultant accumulation of metronidazole and its metabolites in the plasma. Accordingly, for such patients, doses below those usually recommended should be administered cautiously. Close monitoring of plasma metronidazole levels[2] and toxicity is recommended.

In patients receiving Flagyl I.V. or Flagyl I.V. RTU in whom gastric secretions are continuously removed by nasogastric aspiration, sufficient metronidazole may be removed in the aspirate to cause a reduction in serum levels.

The dose of Flagyl I.V. or Flagyl I.V. RTU should not be specifically reduced in anuric patients since accumulated metabolites may be rapidly removed by dialysis.

The usual duration of therapy is 7 to 10 days; however, infections of the bone and joint, lower respiratory tract, and endocardium may require longer treatment.

Prophylaxis
For surgical prophylactic use, to prevent postoperative infection in contaminated or potentially contaminated colorectal surgery, the recommended dosage schedule for adults is:
a. 15 mg/kg infused over 30 to 60 minutes and completed approximately one hour before surgery; followed by
b. 7.5 mg/kg infused over 30 to 60 minutes at 6 and 12 hours after the initial dose.

It is important that (1) administration of the initial preoperative dose be completed approximately one hour before surgery so that adequate drug levels are present in the serum and tissues at the time of initial incision, and (2) Flagyl I.V. or Flagyl I.V. RTU be administered, if necessary, at 6-hour intervals to maintain effective drug levels. Prophylactic use of Flagyl I.V. or Flagyl I.V. RTU should be limited to the day of surgery only, following the above guidelines.

CAUTION: Flagyl I.V. (metronidazole hydrochloride) or Flagyl I.V. RTU (metronidazole) is to be administered by slow intravenous drip infusion only, either as a continuous or intermittent infusion. I.V. admixtures containing metronidazole and other drugs should be avoided. Additives should not be introduced into the Flagyl I.V. RTU solution. If used with a primary intravenous fluid system, the primary solution should be discontinued during metronidazole infusion. DO NOT USE EQUIPMENT CONTAINING ALUMINUM (EG, NEEDLES, CANNULAE) THAT WOULD COME IN CONTACT WITH THE DRUG SOLUTION.

FLAGYL I.V.
Flagyl I.V. cannot be given by direct intravenous injection (I.V. bolus) because of the low pH (0.5 to 2.0) of the reconstituted product. FLAGYL I.V. MUST BE FURTHER DILUTED AND NEUTRALIZED FOR I.V. INFUSION.
Flagyl I.V. is prepared for use in two steps:
NOTE: ORDER OF MIXING IS IMPORTANT
A. Reconstitution
B. Dilution in intravenous solution followed by pH neutralization with sodium bicarbonate injection into the dilution.

Reconstitution: To prepare the solution, add 4.4 ml of one of the following diluents and mix thoroughly: Sterile Water for Injection, USP; Bacteriostatic Water for Injection, USP; 0.9% Sodium Chloride Injection, USP; or Bacteriostatic 0.9% Sodium Chloride Injection, USP. The resultant approximate withdrawal volume is 5.0 ml with an approximate concentration of 100 mg/ml.

The pH of the reconstituted product will be in the range of 0.5 to 2.0. Reconstituted Flagyl I.V. is clear, and pale yellow to yellow-green in color.

Dilution in Intravenous Solutions: Properly reconstituted Flagyl I.V. (metronidazole hydrochloride) may be added to a glass or plastic I.V. container not to exceed a concentration of 8 mg/ml. Any of the following intravenous solutions may be used: 0.9% Sodium Chloride Injection, USP; 5% Dextrose Injection, USP; or Lactated Ringer's Injection, USP.
NEUTRALIZATION IS REQUIRED PRIOR TO ADMINISTRATION.
The final product should be mixed thoroughly and used within 24 hours.

Neutralization For Intravenous Infusion: Neutralize the intravenous solution containing Flagyl I.V. with approximately 5 mEq of sodium bicarbonate injection for each 500 mg of Flagyl I.V. used. Mix thoroughly. The pH of the neutralized intravenous solution will be approximately 6.0 to 7.0. Carbon dioxide gas will be generated with neutralization. It may be necessary to relieve gas pressure within the container.

Note: When the contents of one vial (500 mg) are diluted and neutralized to 100 ml, the resultant concentration is 5 mg/ml. Do not exceed an 8 mg/ml concentration of Flagyl I.V. in the neutralized intravenous solution, since neutralization will decrease the aqueous solubility and precipitation may occur. DO NOT REFRIGERATE NEUTRALIZED SOLUTIONS; otherwise, precipitation may occur.

Storage and Stability: Reconstituted vials of Flagyl I.V. are chemically stable for 96 hours when stored below 86°F (30°C) in room light.

Use diluted and neutralized intravenous solutions containing Flagyl I.V. within 24 hours of mixing.

FLAGYL I.V. RTU
Flagyl I.V. RTU is a ready-to-use isotonic solution. **NO DILUTION OR BUFFERING IS REQUIRED.** Do not refrigerate. Each container of Flagyl I.V. RTU contains 14 mEq of sodium.

Directions for use of plastic container:
CAUTION: Do not use plastic containers in series connections. Such use could result in air embolism due to residual air (approximately 15 ml) being drawn from the primary container before administration of the fluid from the secondary container is complete.

To open. Tear overwrap down side at slit and remove solution container. Some opacity of the plastic due to moisture absorption during the sterilization process may be observed. This is normal and does not affect the solution quality or safety. The opacity will diminish gradually. Check for minute leaks by squeezing inner bag firmly. If leaks are found discard solution as sterility may be impaired.

Preparation for administration:
1. Suspend container from eyelet support.
2. Remove plastic protector from outlet port at bottom of container.
3. Attach administration set. Refer to complete directions accompanying set.

Parenteral drug products should be inspected visually for particulate matter and discoloration prior to administration, whenever solution and container permit. Do not use if cloudy or precipitated or if the seal is not intact.

Use sterile equipment. It is recommended that the intravenous administration apparatus be replaced at least once every 24 hours.

HOW SUPPLIED

FLAGYL I.V.
Flagyl I.V., sterile (metronidazole hydrochloride), is supplied in single-dose lyophilized vials each containing 500 mg metronidazole equivalent, individually packaged in cartons of 10 vials.

Flagyl I.V., prior to reconstitution, should be stored below 86°F (30°C) and protected from light.

FLAGYL I.V. RTU
Flagyl I.V. RTU, sterile (metronidazole), is supplied in 100-ml single-dose plastic containers, each containing an isotonic, buffered solution of 500 mg metronidazole, individually packaged in boxes of 24.

Flagyl I.V. RTU should be stored at controlled room temperature, 59° to 86° F (15° to 30°C), and protected from light during storage.

1. Proposed standard: PSM-11—Proposed Reference Dilution Procedure for Antimicrobic Susceptibility Testing of Anaerobic Bacteria, National Committee for Clinical Laboratory Standards; and Sutter, et al.: Collaborative Evaluation of a Proposed Reference Dilution Method of Susceptibility Testing of Anaerobic Bacteria, Antimicrob. Agents Chemother. 16: 495–502 (Oct.) 1979; and Tally, et al.: *In Vitro* Activity of Thienamycin, Antimicrob. Agents Chemother. 14: 436–438 (Sept.) 1978.
2. Ralph, E.D., and Kirby, W.M.M.: Bioassay of Metronidazole With Either Anaerobic or Aerobic Incubation, J. Infect. Dis. 132: 587–591 (Nov.) 1975; or Gulaid, et al.: Determination of Metronidazole and Its Major Metabolites in Biological Fluids by High Pressure Liquid Chromatography, Br. J Clin. Pharmacol. 6: 430–432, 1978.

2/18/93●A05034-7

Sandoz Pharmaceuticals/ Consumer Division
59 RT. 10
EAST HANOVER, NJ 07936

Direct Inquiries to:
(201) 503-7500
FAX: (201) 503-8265

For Medical Information Contact:
Medical Department
Sandoz Pharmaceuticals
East Hanover, NJ 07936
(201) 503-7500

BiCozene® Skin Medicine   OTC
External Analgesic

(See PDR For Nonprescription Drugs.)

DORCOL® CHILDREN'S COUGH SYRUP   OTC
[door'call]

(See PDR For Nonprescription Drugs.)

EX-LAX® LAXATIVE Pills   OTC
Regular Strength Ex-Lax,
Extra Gentle Ex-Lax,
Maximum Relief Formula Ex-Lax
Gentle Nature Stimulant-Free Stool Softner Caplets

(See PDR For Nonprescription Drugs.)

EX-LAX® CHOCOLATED LAXATIVE   OTC
Tablets

(See PDR For Nonprescription Drugs.)

GAS-X® REGULAR STRENGTH ANTI-GAS CHEWABLE TABLETS   OTC
**GAS-X EXTRA STRENGTH ®
ANTI-GAS CHEWABLE TABLETS
GAS-X EXTRA STRENGTH ANTI-GAS SOFTGELS**
Simethicone - Anti-Gas

(See PDR For Nonprescription Drugs.)

TAVIST-D® Tablets   OTC
12 Hour Relief
Antihistamine/Nasal Decongestant

(See PDR For Nonprescription Drugs.)

TAVIST-1® Tablets   OTC
12 Hour Relief
Antihistamine

(See PDR For Nonprescription Drugs.)

THERAFLU®   OTC
Flu and Cold Hot Liquid Medicine
Flu, Cold & Cough Hot Liquid Medicine
Maximum Strength NightTime Flu, Cold & Cough Hot Liquid Medicine
Maximum Strength Non-Drowsy Flu, Cold & Cough Hot Liquid Medicine
Maximum Strength Apple Cinnamon Sore Throat Flu & Cold Hot Liquid Medicine
Maximum Strength Non-Drowsy Flu, Cold & Cough Caplets
Maximum Strength Non-Drowsy Sinus Caplets
Maximum Strength NightTime Flu, Cold & Cough Caplets

(See PDR For Nonprescription Drugs.)

TRIAMINIC® AM COUGH AND DECONGESTANT FORMULA   OTC
[tri"ah-min'ic]

(See PDR for Nonprescription Drugs.)

TRIAMINIC® AM DECONGESTANT FORMULA   OTC
[tri"ah-min'ic]

(See PDR For Nonprescription Drugs.)

TRIAMINIC® EXPECTORANT   OTC
[tri"ah-min'ic]
The Congestion Medicine

(See PDR For Nonprescription Drugs.)

TRIAMINIC® EXPECTORANT DH   CIII
[tri"ah-min'ic]

DESCRIPTION
Each teaspoonful (5 mL) of TRIAMINIC Expectorant DH contains:
hydrocodone bitartrate 1.67 mg (Warning: May be habit forming), phenylpropanolamine hydrochloride 12.5 mg, pheniramine maleate 6.25 mg, pyrilamine maleate 6.25 mg, and guaifenesin 100 mg.
Other ingredients:
alcohol (5%), benzoic acid, Blue 1, flavors, ethyl vanillin, menthol, purified water, sorbitol, spearmint oil, sucrose, Yellow 10, Yellow 6.

HOW SUPPLIED
TRIAMINIC Expectorant DH (green) is available in pint bottles. Store at room temperature. TRIAMINIC Expectorant DH is a Schedule III controlled substance.

TRIAMINIC TRIAMINICOL® MULTI-SYMPTOM RELIEF SYRUP   OTC
[tri"ah-min'i-call]
When the Cold Comes With a Cough

(See PDR For Nonprescription Drugs.)

TRIAMINIC® NightTime   OTC
Nighttime Cough and Cold Medicine for Children
[tri"ah-min'ic]

(See PDR For Nonprescription Drugs.)

TRIAMINIC® Rx PEDIATRIC ORAL SOLUTION
[tri"ah-min'ic]
(Formerly Triaminic Oral Infant Drops)

DESCRIPTION
Each ml of TRIAMINIC Rx Pediatric Oral Solution contains:
phenylpropanolamine hydrochloride 20 mg, pheniramine maleate 10 mg, and pyrilamine maleate 10 mg.
Other ingredients:
benzoic acid, flavor, glycerin, purified water, Red 33, sorbitol, sucrose, Yellow 6.

HOW SUPPLIED
TRIAMINIC Rx Pediatric Oral Solution is available in a 15 ml plastic squeeze bottle that delivers approximately 24 drops per ml. Store at room temperature.

TRIAMINIC® SORE THROAT FORMULA   OTC

(See PDR For Nonprescription Drugs.)

TRIAMINIC® SYRUP   OTC
[tri"ah-min'ic]
For Colds and Allergies

(See PDR For Nonprescription Drugs.)

TRIAMINIC®DM SYRUP   OTC
[tri"ah-min'ic]
Cough Relief

(See PDR For Nonprescription Drugs.)

Sandoz Pharmaceuticals Corporation
Dorsey Division
Sandoz Division
ROUTE 10, EAST HANOVER, NJ 07936

For Medical Information Contact:
Medical Services
(201)503-7500

BELLERGAL-S®   Rx
[bel'er-gal]
TABLETS

CAUTION: Federal law prohibits dispensing without prescription.
The following prescribing information is based on official labeling in effect on August 1, 1996.

Autonomic Stabilizer

DESCRIPTION
Each Bellergal-S® tablet contains:
phenobarbital, USP, (Warning: May be habit-forming), 40 mg; ergotamine tartrate, USP, 0.6 mg; Bellafoline® (levorotatory alkaloids of belladonna), 0.2 mg.
Inactive Ingredients: colloidal silicon dioxide, color additives including FD&C Blue #1, FD&C Red #40, FD&C Yellow #5, FD&C Yellow #6 (Sunset Yellow), gelatin, lactose, magnesium stearate, malic acid, polyvinyl acetate resins, stearic acid, sucrose, and tartaric acid.

CLINICAL PHARMACOLOGY
Based on the concept that functional disorders frequently involve hyperactivity of both the sympathetic and parasympathetic nervous systems, the ingredients in Bellergal-S® are combined to provide a balanced preparation designed to correct imbalance of the autonomic nervous system. The integrated action of Bellergal-S® is effected through the combined administration of ergotamine and the levorotatory alkaloids of belladonna, specific inhibitors of the sympathetic and parasympathetic respectively, reinforced by the synergistic action of phenobarbital in dampening the cortical centers. It should be noted that on a weight basis the levorotatory alkaloids of belladonna have approximately twice the pharmacological effects as do the usual racemic mixtures.

INDICATIONS AND USAGE
Bellergal-S® is employed in the management of disorders characterized by nervous tension and exaggerated autonomic response: *Menopausal disorders* with hot flushes, sweats, restlessness and insomnia; *cardiovascular disorders* with palpitation, tachycardia, chest oppression and vasomotor disturbances; *gastrointestinal disorders* with hypermotility, hypersecretion, "nervous stomach," and alternately diarrhea and constipation; interval treatment of *recurrent, throbbing headache.*

CONTRAINDICATIONS
Peripheral vascular disease, coronary heart disease, hypertension, impaired hepatic or renal function, sepsis, pregnancy, nursing mothers and glaucoma. The concomitant administration of ergotamine and dopamine should be avoided, due to the increased potential for ischemic vasoconstriction. Phenobarbital is contraindicated in patients with a history of manifest or latent porphyria. Phenobarbital is contraindicated in those patients in whom the drug produces restlessness and/or excitement. Bellergal-S® is contraindicated in patients with a demonstrated hypersensitivity to any of the components.

WARNINGS
Total weekly dosage of ergotamine tartrate should not exceed 10 mg. (This dosage corresponds to 16 Bellergal-S® tablets.) Due to the presence of a barbiturate, may be habit-forming.

PRECAUTIONS
Even though the ergotamine tartrate content of this product is low and untoward effects have been rare and of minor significance, caution should be exercised if large or prolonged dosage is contemplated, and physicians should be alert to possible peripheral vascular complications in patients sensitive to ergot. Due to the presence of the anticholinergic

Continued on next page

Sandoz—Cont.

agent, special caution should be exercised in the use of this drug in patients with bronchial asthma or obstructive uropathy.

Bellergal-S® contains FD&C Yellow #5 (tartrazine) which may cause allergic-type reactions (including bronchial asthma) in certain susceptible individuals. Although the overall incidence of FD&C Yellow #5 (tartrazine) sensitivity in the general population is low, it is frequently seen in patients who also have aspirin hypersensitivity.

Information for Patients

Patients on large or prolonged dosage should be asked to report numbness or tingling of extremities, claudication or other symptoms of peripheral vasoconstriction.

Drug Interaction

Oral Anticoagulants: Phenobarbital may lower the plasma levels of dicumarol (name previously used: bishydroxycoumarin) and may cause a decrease in anticoagulant activity as measured by the prothrombin time. More frequent monitoring of prothrombin time responses is indicated whenever phenobarbital is initiated or discontinued, and the dosage of anticoagulants should be adjusted accordingly.

CNS Depressants: Combined administration of phenobarbital and CNS depressants such as alcohol, tricyclic antidepressants, phenothiazines and narcotic analgesics may result in a potentiation of the depressant action.

Beta Adrenergic Blocking Agents: Although proof is lacking, several reports in the literature suggest a possible interaction between ergot alkaloids and beta adrenergic blocking agents. This interaction may result in excessive vasoconstriction. Although many patients can apparently take propranolol and ergot alkaloids without ill effects, there is enough evidence of an interaction to dictate closer surveillance of patients so treated.

Hepatic Metabolism: Through the mechanism of enzyme induction caused by phenobarbital, a number of substances have been shown to be metabolized at an increased rate. In these cases, clinical responses should be closely monitored and appropriate dosage adjustments made. Included are such substances as griseofulvin, quinidine, doxycycline and estrogen. Although the meaning of published reports regarding the effects of phenobarbital on estrogen metabolism are unclear at this time, if avoidance of pregnancy is critical, consideration should be given to alternative methods of contraception.

Phenytoin, Sodium Valproate, Valproic Acid: The effect of barbiturates on the metabolism of phenytoin appears to be variable. Some investigators report an accelerating effect, while others report no effect. Because the effect of barbiturates on the metabolism of phenytoin is not predictable, phenytoin and barbiturate blood levels should be monitored more frequently if these drugs are given concurrently. Sodium valproate and valproic acid appear to decrease barbiturate metabolism; therefore, barbiturate blood levels should be monitored and appropriate dosage adjustments made as indicated.

Tricyclic Antidepressants: Due to the presence of levorotatory alkaloids of belladonna, concomitant administration of tricyclic antidepressants may result in additive anticholinergic effects.

Carcinogenesis

No data are available on the long-term potential for carcinogenicity in animals or humans.

Pregnancy

Pregnancy Category X—due to the potential uterotonic effects of the ergot alkaloids, the use of Bellergal-S® during pregnancy is contraindicated. See *CONTRAINDICATIONS.*

Nursing Mothers

A number of ergot alkaloids inhibit the secretion of prolactin. Therefore, Bellergal-S® is contraindicated in nursing mothers. See *CONTRAINDICATIONS.*

Pediatric Use

Safety and effectiveness in pediatric patients have not been established.

ADVERSE REACTIONS

Tingling and other paresthesias of the extremities, blurred vision, palpitations, dry mouth, decreased sweating, decreased gastrointestinal motility, urinary retention, tachycardia, flushing, and drowsiness occur rarely.

DRUG ABUSE AND DEPENDENCE

Barbiturates may be habit-forming. Tolerance, psychological dependence, and physical dependence may occur especially following prolonged use of high doses. Daily administration in excess of 400 mg of pentobarbital or secobarbital for approximately 90 days is likely to produce some degree of physical dependence. By way of comparison, the phenobarbital component of Bellergal-S® at the highest recommended daily dosage amounts to 80 mg.

OVERDOSAGE

Management of Overdosage: While severe symptoms of overdosage with Bellergal-S® have not been reported, theoretically they could occur. It is imperative to note that overdosage symptoms with Bellergal-S® may be attributable to any one or more of the three active ingredients. Which toxic manifestation might predominate in any individual case would be impossible to predict but one should be alert to the various possibilities. When anticholinergic/antispasmodic drugs are taken in sufficient overdose to produce such severe symptoms, prompt treatment should be instituted. Gastric lavage and other measures to limit intestinal absorption should be initiated without delay.

Cholinesterase inhibitors administered parenterally may be necessary for treatment of the serious manifestations of anticholinergic overdosage. Additionally, symptomatic therapy, including oxygen, sedatives and control of hyperthermia may be necessary.

Acute barbiturate overdosage symptoms with Bellergal-S®, while possible, have not been reported. While the usual procedures for handling barbiturate poisoning should be employed, keep in mind the possibility of anticholinergic overdosing effects.

Acute ergot overdosage symptoms with Bellergal-S®, while possible, have not been reported. The usual procedures for handling ergot overdosage include the administration of a peripheral vasodilator to counteract the vasospasm.

DOSAGE AND ADMINISTRATION

One tablet in the morning and one tablet in the evening.

HOW SUPPLIED

Bellergal-S® Tablets

Compressed tablets of tri-colored pattern: dark green, orange and light lemon yellow, cruciform on one side, embossed "78-31" on other side.

Bottles of 100 (NDC 0078-0031-05)

Store and Dispense

Below 77°F (25°C); tight, light-resistant container.

[REV: FEBRUARY 1996 30108902]

Shown in Product Identification Guide, page 332

CAFERGOT® ℞

[kaf'er-got]

(ergotamine tartrate and caffeine) TABLETS, USP
(ergotamine tartrate and caffeine) SUPPOSITORIES, USP

CAUTION: Federal law prohibits dispensing without prescription.

The following prescribing information is based on official labeling in effect on August 1, 1996.

DESCRIPTION

CAFERGOT®

(ergotamine tartrate and caffeine) Tablet

ergotamine tartrate USP	1 mg
caffeine USP	100 mg

Inactive Ingredients: acacia, carnauba wax, lactose, methylparaben, povidone, propylparaben, sodium benzoate, sorbitol, starch, stearic acid, sucrose, synthetic black ferric oxide, synthetic red ferric oxide, synthetic yellow ferric oxide, talc, tartaric acid, and titanium dioxide.

CAFERGOT®

(ergotamine tartrate and caffeine) Suppository

ergotamine tartrate USP	2 mg
caffeine USP	100 mg

Inactive Ingredients: cocoa butter NF and tartaric acid NF.

CAFERGOT® (ergotamine tartrate and caffeine) suppositories are *sealed* in foil to afford protection from cocoa butter leakage. If an unavoidable period of exposure to heat softens the suppository, it should be chilled in ice-cold water to solidify it before removing the foil.

CLINICAL PHARMACOLOGY

Ergotamine is an alpha adrenergic blocking agent with a direct stimulating effect on the smooth muscle of peripheral and cranial blood vessels and produces depression of central vasomotor centers. The compound also has the properties of serotonin antagonism. In comparison to hydrogenated ergotamine, the adrenergic blocking actions are less pronounced and vasoconstrictive actions are greater.

Caffeine, also a cranial vasoconstrictor, is added to further enhance the vasoconstrictive effect without the necessity of increasing ergotamine dosage.

Many migraine patients experience excessive nausea and vomiting during attacks, making it impossible for them to retain any oral medication. In such cases, therefore, the only practical means of medication is through the rectal route where medication may reach the cranial vessels directly, evading the splanchnic vasculature and the liver.

INDICATIONS AND USAGE

CAFERGOT® (ergotamine tartrate and caffeine)

Indicated as therapy to abort or prevent vascular headache, e.g., migraine, migraine variants or so-called "histaminic cephalalgia".

CONTRAINDICATIONS

CAFERGOT® (ergotamine tartrate and caffeine) may cause fetal harm when administered to pregnant women. CAFERGOT® (ergotamine tartrate and caffeine) is contraindicated in women who are or may become pregnant. If this drug is used during pregnancy or if the patient becomes pregnant while taking this product, the patient should be apprised of the potential hazard to the fetus.

Peripheral vascular disease, coronary heart disease, hypertension, impaired hepatic or renal function and sepsis.

Hypersensitivity to any of the components.

PRECAUTIONS

General

Although signs and symptoms of ergotism rarely develop even after long term intermittent use of the orally or rectally administered drugs, care should be exercised to remain within the limits of recommended dosage.

Ergotism is manifested by intense arterial vasoconstriction, producing signs and symptoms of peripheral vascular ischemia. Ergotamine induces vasoconstriction by a direct action on vascular smooth muscle. In chronic intoxication with ergot derivatives, headache, intermittent claudication, muscle pains, numbness, coldness and pallor of the digits may occur. If the condition is allowed to progress untreated, gangrene can result.

While most cases of ergotism associated with ergotamine treatment result from frank overdosage, some cases have involved apparent hypersensitivity. There are few reports of ergotism among patients taking doses within the recommended limits or for brief periods of time. In rare instances, patients, particularly those who have used the medication indiscriminately over long periods of time, may display withdrawal symptoms consisting of rebound headache upon discontinuation of the drug.

Rare cases of a solitary rectal or anal ulcer have occurred from abuse of ergotamine suppositories usually in higher than recommended doses or with continual use at the recommended dose for many years. Spontaneous healing occurs within usually 4-8 weeks after drug withdrawal.

Information for Patients

Patients should be advised that two tablets or one suppository of CAFERGOT® (ergotamine tartrate and caffeine) should be taken at the first sign of a migraine headache. No more than 6 tablets or 2 suppositories should be taken for any single migraine attack. No more than 10 tablets or 5 suppositories should be taken during any 7-day period. CAFERGOT® (ergotamine tartrate and caffeine) should be used only for migraine headaches. It is not effective for other types of headaches and it lacks analgesic properties. Patients should be advised to report to the physician immediately any of the following: numbness or tingling in the fingers and toes, muscle pain in the arms and legs, weakness in the legs, pain in the chest or temporary speeding or slowing of the heart rate, swelling or itching.

Drug Interactions

CAFERGOT® (ergotamine tartrate and caffeine) should not be administered with other vasoconstrictors. Use with sympathomimetics (pressor agents) may cause extreme elevation of blood pressure. The beta-blocker Inderal (propranolol) has been reported to potentiate the vasoconstrictive action of CAFERGOT® (ergotamine tartrate and caffeine) by blocking the vasodilating property of epinephrine. Nicotine may provoke vasoconstriction in some patients, predisposing to a greater ischemic response to ergot therapy.

The blood levels of ergotamine-containing drugs are reported to be elevated by the concomitant administration of macrolide antibiotics and vasospastic reactions have been reported with therapeutic doses of the ergotamine-containing drugs when coadministered with these antibiotics.

Pregnancy

Teratogenic Effects

Pregnancy Category X: There are no studies on the placental transfer or teratogenicity of the combined products of CAFERGOT® (ergotamine tartrate and caffeine). Caffeine is known to cross the placenta and has been shown to be teratogenic in animals. Ergotamine crosses the placenta in small amounts, although it does not appear to be embryotoxic in this quantity. However, prolonged vasoconstriction of the uterine vessels and/or increased myometrial tone leading to reduced myometrial and placental blood flow may have contributed to fetal growth retardation observed in animals. (*See CONTRAINDICATIONS*)

Nonteratogenic Effects

CAFERGOT® (ergotamine tartrate and caffeine) is contraindicated in pregnancy due to the oxytocic effects of ergotamine. (*See CONTRAINDICATIONS*)

Labor and Delivery

CAFERGOT® (ergotamine tartrate and caffeine) is contraindicated in labor and delivery due to its oxytocic effect which is maximal in the third trimester. (*See CONTRAINDICATIONS*)

Nursing Mothers

Ergot drugs are known to inhibit prolactin but there are no reports of decreased lactation with CAFERGOT® (ergotamine tartrate and caffeine). Ergotamine is excreted in breast milk and may cause symptoms of vomiting, diarrhea, weak pulse and unstable blood pressure in nursing infants. Because of the potential for serious adverse reactions in nursing infants from CAFERGOT® (ergotamine tartrate

and caffeine), a decision should be made whether to discontinue nursing or discontinue the drug, taking into account the importance of the drug to the mother.

Pediatric Use

Safety and effectiveness in children have not been established.

ADVERSE REACTIONS

Cardiovascular: Vasoconstrictive complications of a serious nature may occur at times. These include ischemia, cyanosis, absence of pulse, cold extremities, gangrene, precordial distress and pain, EKG changes and muscle pains. Although these effects occur most commonly with long-term therapy at relatively high doses, they have also been reported with short-term or normal doses. Other cardiovascular adverse effects include transient tachycardia or bradycardia and hypertension.

Gastrointestinal: Nausea and vomiting; rectal or anal ulcer (from overuse of suppositories).

Neurological: paresthesias, numbness, weakness, and vertigo.

Allergic: Localized edema and itching.

Fibrotic Complications: There have been a few reports of patients on CAFERGOT® (ergotamine tartrate and caffeine) therapy developing retroperitoneal and/or pleuropulmonary fibroses. There have also been rare reports of fibrotic thickening of the aortic, mitral, tricuspid, and/or pulmonary valves with long-term, continuous use of CAFERGOT® (ergotamine tartrate and caffeine).

DRUG ABUSE AND DEPENDENCE

There have been reports of drug abuse and psychological dependence in patients on CAFERGOT® (ergotamine tartrate and caffeine) therapy. Due to the chronicity of vascular headaches, it is imperative that patients be advised not to exceed recommended dosages with long-term use to avoid ergotism. (*See PRECAUTIONS*)

OVERDOSAGE

The toxic effects of an acute overdosage of CAFERGOT® (ergotamine tartrate and caffeine) are due primarily to the ergotamine component. The amount of caffeine is such that its toxic effects will be overshadowed by those of ergotamine. Symptoms include vomiting, numbness, tingling, pain and cyanosis of the extremities associated with diminished or absent peripheral pulses; hypertension or hypotension; drowsiness, stupor, coma, convulsions and shock. A case has been reported of reversible bilateral papillitis with ring scotomata in a patient who received five times the recommended daily adult dose over a period of 14 days.

Treatment consists of removal of the offending drug by induction of emesis, gastric lavage, and catharsis. Maintenance of adequate pulmonary ventilation, correction of hypotension, and control of convulsions and blood pressure are important considerations. Treatment of peripheral vasospasm should consist of warmth, but not heat, and protection of the ischemic limbs. Vasodilators may be beneficial but caution must be exercised to avoid aggravating an already existent hypotension.

DOSAGE AND ADMINISTRATION

Procedure

For the best results, dosage should start at the first sign of an attack.

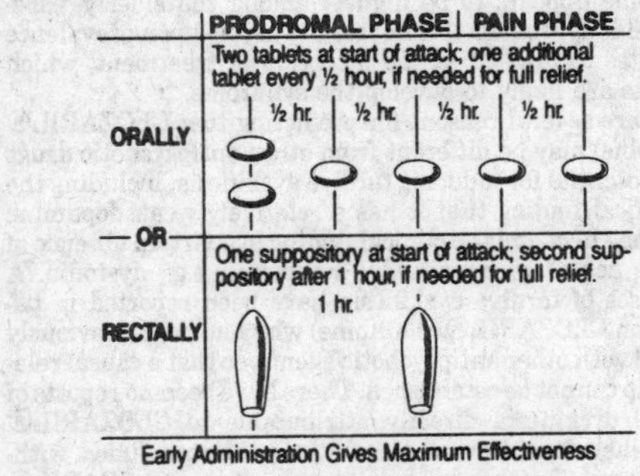
PRODROMAL PHASE | PAIN PHASE
Two tablets at start of attack; one additional tablet every ½ hour, if needed for full relief.
½ hr.
½ hr.
½ hr.
½ hr.
ORALLY
— OR —
One suppository at start of attack; second suppository after 1 hour, if needed for full relief.
1 hr.
RECTALLY
Early Administration Gives Maximum Effectiveness

MAXIMUM ADULT DOSAGE

Orally

Total dose for any one attack should not exceed 6 tablets.

Rectally

Two suppositories is the maximum dose for an individual attack.

Total weekly dosage should not exceed 10 tablets or 5 suppositories.

In carefully selected patients, with due consideration of maximum dosage recommendations, administration of the drug at bedtime may be an appropriate short-term preventive measure.

HOW SUPPLIED

CAFERGOT®

(ergotamine tartrate and caffeine) Tablets

Shell pink colored, sugar coated, imprinted "CAFERGOT" on one side, " △ " on other side.

Bottles of 90 (NDC 0078-0034-34).

Bottles of 250 (NDC 0078-0034-28).

Cartons of three SigPak® (dispensing unit) packages, each containing 30 tablets in individual blisters (NDC 0078-0034-42).

Store and Dispense

Below 77°F (25°C); tight, light-resistant container.

CAFERGOT®

(ergotamine tartrate and caffeine) Suppositories

Sealed in fuchsia-colored aluminum foil, imprinted " △ CAFERGOT® SUPPOSITORY 78-33 SANDOZ".

Boxes of 12 (NDC 0078-0033-02).

Store and Dispense

Below 77°F (25°C); tight container (sealed foil).

[REV: MAY 1993 30113902]

CLOZARIL® ℞

[klō'ză-ril]

(clozapine) Tablets

Caution: Federal law prohibits dispensing without prescription.

The following prescribing information is based on official labeling in effect on August 1, 1996.

DESCRIPTION

CLOZARIL® (clozapine), an atypical antipsychotic drug, is a tricyclic dibenzodiazepine derivative, 8-chloro-11-(4-methyl-1-piperazinyl)-5*H*-dibenzo [*b,e*] [1,4] diazepine.

The structural formula is:

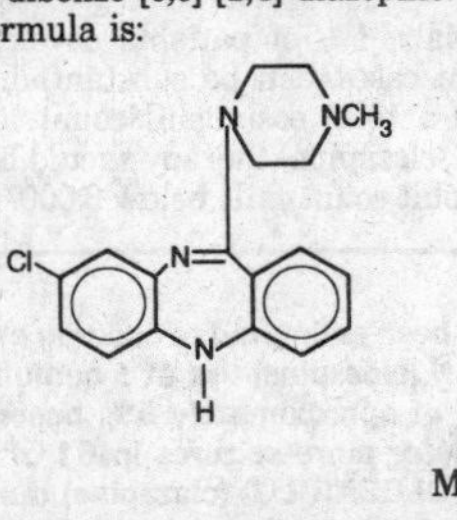
N
NCH3
Cl
N
N
H

$C_{18}H_{19}ClN_4$ Mol. wt. 326.83

CLOZARIL® (clozapine) is available in pale yellow tablets of 25 mg and 100 mg for oral administration.

25 mg and 100 mg Tablets

Active Ingredient: clozapine is a yellow, crystalline powder, very slightly soluble in water.

Inactive Ingredients: colloidal silicon dioxide, NF; lactose, NF; magnesium stearate, NF; povidone, USP; starch, NF; and talc, USP.

CLINICAL PHARMACOLOGY

Pharmacodynamics

CLOZARIL® (clozapine) is classified as an 'atypical' antipsychotic drug because its profile of binding to dopamine receptors and its effects on various dopamine mediated behaviors differ from those exhibited by more typical antipsychotic drug products. In particular, although CLOZARIL® (clozapine) does interfere with the binding of dopamine at both D-1 and D-2 receptors, it does not induce catalepsy nor inhibit apomorphine-induced stereotypy. This evidence, consistent with the view that CLOZARIL® (clozapine) is preferentially more active at limbic than at striatal dopamine receptors, may explain the relative freedom of CLOZARIL® (clozapine) from extrapyramidal side effects.

CLOZARIL® (clozapine) also acts as an antagonist at adrenergic, cholinergic, histaminergic and serotonergic receptors.

Absorption, Distribution, Metabolism and Excretion

In man, CLOZARIL® (clozapine) tablets (25 mg and 100 mg) are equally bioavailable relative to a clozapine solution. Following a dosage of 100 mg b.i.d., the average steady state peak plasma concentration was 319 ng/mL (range: 102–771 ng/mL), occurring at the average of 2.5 hours (range: 1–6 hours) after dosing. The average minimum concentration at steady state was 122 ng/mL (range: 41–343 ng/mL), after 100 mg b.i.d. dosing. Food does not appear to affect the systemic bioavailability of CLOZARIL® (clozapine). Thus, CLOZARIL® (clozapine) may be administered with or without food.

Clozapine is approximately 97% bound to serum proteins. The interaction between CLOZARIL® (clozapine) and other highly protein-bound drugs has not been fully evaluated but may be important. *(See PRECAUTIONS)*

Clozapine is almost completely metabolized prior to excretion and only trace amounts of unchanged drug are detected in the urine and feces. Approximately 50% of the administered dose is excreted in the urine and 30% in the feces. The demethylated, hydroxylated and N-oxide derivatives are components in both urine and feces. Pharmacological testing has shown the desmethyl metabolite to have only limited activity, while the hydroxylated and N-oxide derivatives were inactive.

The mean elimination half-life of clozapine after a single 75 mg dose was 8 hours (range: 4-12 hours), compared to a mean elimination half-life, after achieving steady state with 100 mg b.i.d. dosing, of 12 hours (range: 4-66 hours). A comparison of single-dose and multiple-dose administration of clozapine showed that the elimination half-life increased significantly after multiple dosing relative to that after single-dose administration, suggesting the possibility of concentration dependent pharmacokinetics. However, at steady state, linearly dose-proportional changes with respect to AUC (area under the curve), peak and minimum clozapine plasma concentrations were observed after administration of 37.5 mg, 75 mg, and 150 mg b.i.d.

Human Pharmacology

In contrast to more typical antipsychotic drugs, CLOZARIL® (clozapine) therapy produces little or no prolactin elevation.

As is true of more typical antipsychotic drugs, clinical EEG studies have shown that CLOZARIL® (clozapine) increases delta and theta activity and slows dominant alpha frequencies. Enhanced synchronization occurs, and sharp wave activity and spike and wave complexes may also develop. Patients, on rare occasions, may report an intensification of dream activity during CLOZARIL® (clozapine) therapy. REM sleep was found to be increased to 85% of the total sleep time. In these patients, the onset of REM sleep occurred almost immediately after falling asleep.

INDICATIONS AND USAGE

CLOZARIL® (clozapine) is indicated for the management of severely ill schizophrenic patients who fail to respond adequately to standard antipsychotic drug treatment. Because of the significant risk of agranulocytosis and seizure associated with its use, CLOZARIL® (clozapine) should be used only in patients who have failed to respond adequately to treatment with appropriate courses of standard antipsychotic drugs, either because of insufficient effectiveness or the inability to achieve an effective dose due to intolerable adverse effects from those drugs. *(See WARNINGS)*

The effectiveness of CLOZARIL® (clozapine) in a treatment resistant schizophrenic population was demonstrated in a 6-week study comparing CLOZARIL® (clozapine) and chlorpromazine. Patients meeting DSM-III criteria for schizophrenia and having a mean BPRS total score of 61 were demonstrated to be treatment resistant by history and by open, prospective treatment with haloperidol before entering into the double-blind phase of the study. The superiority of CLOZARIL® (clozapine) to chlorpromazine was documented in statistical analyses employing both categorical and continuous measures of treatment effect.

Because of the significant risk of agranulocytosis and seizure, events which both present a continuing risk over time, the extended treatment of patients failing to show an acceptable level of clinical response should ordinarily be avoided. In addition, the need for continuing treatment in patients exhibiting beneficial clinical responses should be periodically re-evaluated.

CONTRAINDICATIONS

CLOZARIL® (clozapine) is contraindicated in patients with myeloproliferative disorders, uncontrolled epilepsy, or a history of CLOZARIL® (clozapine) induced agranulocytosis or severe granulocytopenia. As with more typical antipsychotic drugs, CLOZARIL® (clozapine) is contraindicated in severe central nervous system depression or comatose states from any cause.

CLOZARIL® (clozapine) should not be used simultaneously with other agents having a well-known potential to cause agranulocytosis or otherwise suppress bone marrow function. The mechanism of CLOZARIL® (clozapine) induced agranulocytosis is unknown; nonetheless, it is possible that causative factors may interact synergistically to increase the risk and/or severity of bone marrow suppression.

WARNINGS

General

BECAUSE OF THE SIGNIFICANT RISK OF AGRANULOCYTOSIS, A POTENTIALLY LIFE-THREATENING ADVERSE EVENT *(SEE FOLLOWING),* CLOZARIL® (clozapine) SHOULD BE RESERVED FOR USE IN THE TREATMENT OF SEVERELY ILL SCHIZOPHRENIC PATIENTS WHO FAIL TO SHOW AN ACCEPTABLE RESPONSE TO ADEQUATE COURSES OF STANDARD ANTIPSYCHOTIC DRUG TREATMENT, EITHER BECAUSE OF INSUFFICIENT EFFECTIVENESS OR THE INABILITY TO ACHIEVE AN EFFECTIVE DOSE DUE TO INTOLERABLE ADVERSE EFFECTS FROM THOSE DRUGS. CONSEQUENTLY, BEFORE INITIATING TREATMENT WITH CLOZARIL® (clozapine), IT IS STRONGLY RECOMMENDED THAT A PATIENT BE GIVEN AT LEAST 2 TRIALS, EACH WITH A DIFFERENT STANDARD ANTIPSYCHOTIC DRUG PRODUCT, AT AN ADEQUATE DOSE, AND FOR AN ADEQUATE DURATION.

Continued on next page

Sandoz—Cont.

PATIENTS WHO ARE BEING TREATED WITH CLOZARIL® (clozapine) MUST HAVE A BASELINE WHITE BLOOD CELL (WBC) AND DIFFERENTIAL COUNT BEFORE INITIATION OF TREATMENT, AND A WBC COUNT EVERY WEEK THROUGHOUT TREATMENT, AND FOR 4 WEEKS AFTER THE DISCONTINUATION OF CLOZARIL® (clozapine). CLOZARIL® (clozapine) IS AVAILABLE ONLY THROUGH A DISTRIBUTION SYSTEM THAT ENSURES WEEKLY WBC TESTING PRIOR TO DELIVERY OF THE NEXT WEEK'S SUPPLY OF MEDICATION.

Agranulocytosis

Agranulocytosis, defined as an absolute neutrophil count (ANC) of less than 500/mm^3, has been estimated to occur in association with CLOZARIL® (clozapine) use at a cumulative incidence at 1 year of approximately 1.3%, based on the occurrence of 15 US cases out of 1743 patients exposed to CLOZARIL® (clozapine) during its clinical testing prior to domestic marketing. All of these cases occurred at a time when the need for close monitoring of WBC counts was already recognized. This reaction could prove fatal if not detected early and therapy interrupted. Of the 149 cases of agranulocytosis reported worldwide in association with CLOZARIL® (clozapine) use as of December 31, 1989, 32% were fatal. However, few of these deaths occurred since 1977, at which time the knowledge of CLOZARIL® (clozapine) induced agranulocytosis became more widespread, and close monitoring of WBC counts more widely practiced. Nevertheless, it is unknown at present what the case fatality rate will be for CLOZARIL® (clozapine) induced agranulocytosis, despite strict adherence to the recommendation for weekly monitoring of WBC counts. In the US, under a weekly WBC monitoring system with CLOZARIL® (clozapine), there have been 317 cases of agranulocytosis as of January 1, 1994; 11 were fatal. During this period, over 68,000 patients received CLOZARIL® (clozapine).

Because of the substantial risk of agranulocytosis in association with CLOZARIL® (clozapine) use, which may persist over an extended period of time, patients must have a blood sample drawn for a WBC count before initiation of treatment with CLOZARIL® (clozapine), and must have subsequent WBC counts done at least weekly for the duration of therapy, as well as for 4 weeks thereafter. The distribution of CLOZARIL® (clozapine) is contingent upon performance of the required blood tests.

Treatment should not be initiated if the WBC count is less than 3500/mm^3, or if the patient has a history of a myeloproliferative disorder, or previous CLOZARIL® (clozapine) induced agranulocytosis or granulocytopenia. Patients should be advised to report immediately the appearance of lethargy, weakness, fever, sore throat or any other signs of infection. If, after the initiation of treatment, the total WBC count has dropped below 3500/mm^3 or it has dropped by a substantial amount from baseline, even if the count is above 3500/mm^3, or if immature forms are present, a repeat WBC count and a differential count should be done. A substantial drop is defined as a single drop of 3,000 or more in the WBC count or a cumulative drop of 3,000 or more within 3 weeks. If subsequent WBC counts and the differential count reveal a total WBC count between 3000 and 3500/mm^3 and an ANC above 1500/mm^3, twice weekly WBC counts and differential counts should be performed.

If the total WBC count falls below 3000/mm^3 or the ANC below 1500/mm^3, CLOZARIL® (clozapine) therapy should be interrupted, WBC count and differential should be performed daily, and patients should be carefully monitored for flu-like symptoms or other symptoms suggestive of infection. CLOZARIL® (clozapine) therapy may be resumed if no symptoms of infection develop, and if the total WBC count returns to levels above 3000/mm^3 and the ANC returns to levels above 1500/mm^3. However, in this event, twice-weekly WBC counts and differential counts should continue until total WBC counts return to levels above 3500/mm^3. If the total WBC count falls below 2000/mm^3 or the ANC falls below 1000/mm^3, bone marrow aspiration should be considered to ascertain granulopoietic status. Protective isolation with close observation may be indicated if granulopoiesis is determined to be deficient. Should evidence of infection develop, the patient should have appropriate cultures performed and an appropriate antibiotic regimen instituted.

Patients whose total WBC counts fall below 2000/mm^3, or ANCs below 1000/mm^3 during CLOZARIL® (clozapine) therapy should have daily WBC count and differential. These patients should not be re-challenged with CLOZARIL® (clozapine). Patients discontinued from CLOZARIL® (clozapine) therapy due to significant WBC suppression have been found to develop agranulocytosis upon re-challenge, often with a shorter latency on re-exposure. To reduce the chances of re-challenge occurring in patients who have experienced significant bone marrow suppression during CLOZARIL® (clozapine) therapy, a single, national master file will be maintained confidentially.

Except for evidence of significant bone marrow suppression during initial CLOZARIL® (clozapine) therapy, there are no established risk factors, based on worldwide experience, for the development of agranulocytosis in association with CLOZARIL® (clozapine) use. However, a disproportionate number of the US cases of agranulocytosis occurred in patients of Jewish background compared to the overall proportion of such patients exposed during domestic development of CLOZARIL® (clozapine). Most of the US cases occurred within 4-10 weeks of exposure, but neither dose nor duration is a reliable predictor of this problem. No patient characteristics have been clearly linked to the development of agranulocytosis in association with CLOZARIL® (clozapine) use, but agranulocytosis associated with other antipsychotic drugs has been reported to occur with a greater frequency in women, the elderly and in patients who are cachectic or have serious underlying medical illness; such patients may also be at particular risk with CLOZARIL® (clozapine).

To reduce the risk of agranulocytosis developing undetected, CLOZARIL® (clozapine) is available only through a distribution system that ensures weekly WBC testing prior to delivery of the next week's supply of medication.

Eosinophilia

In clinical trials, 1% of patients developed eosinophilia, which, in rare cases, can be substantial. If a differential count reveals a total eosinophil count above 4,000/mm^3, CLOZARIL® (clozapine) therapy should be interrupted until the eosinophil count falls below 3,000/mm^3.

Seizures

Seizure has been estimated to occur in association with CLOZARIL® (clozapine) use at a cumulative incidence at one year of approximately 5%, based on the occurrence of one or more seizures in 61 of 1743 patients exposed to CLOZARIL® (clozapine) during its clinical testing prior to domestic marketing (i.e., a crude rate of 3.5%). Dose appears to be an important predictor of seizure, with a greater likelihood of seizure at the higher CLOZARIL® (clozapine) doses used.

Caution should be used in administering CLOZARIL® (clozapine) to patients having a history of seizures or other predisposing factors. Because of the substantial risk of seizure associated with CLOZARIL® (clozapine) use, patients should be advised not to engage in any activity where sudden loss of consciousness could cause serious risk to themselves or others, e.g., the operation of complex machinery, driving an automobile, swimming, climbing, etc.

Adverse Cardiovascular and Respiratory Effects

Orthostatic hypotension with or without syncope can occur with CLOZARIL® (clozapine) treatment and may represent a continuing risk in some patients. Rarely (approximately 1 case per 3,000 patients), collapse can be profound and be accompanied by respiratory and/or cardiac arrest. Orthostatic hypotension is more likely to occur during initial titration in association with rapid dose escalation and may even occur on first dose. In one report, initial doses as low as 12.5 mg were associated with collapse and respiratory arrest. When restarting patients who have had even a brief interval off CLOZARIL® (clozapine), i.e., 2 days or more since the last dose, it is recommended that treatment be reinitiated with one-half of a 25 mg tablet (12.5 mg) once or twice daily (see DOSAGE AND ADMINISTRATION).

Some of the cases of collapse/respiratory arrest/cardiac arrest during initial treatment occurred in patients who were being administered benzodiazepines; similar events have been reported in patients taking other psychotropic drugs or even CLOZARIL® (clozapine) by itself. Although it has not been established that there is an interaction between CLOZARIL® (clozapine) and benzodiazepines or other psychotropics, caution is advised when clozapine is initiated in patients taking a benzodiazepine or any other psychotropic drug.

Tachycardia, which may be sustained, has also been observed in approximately 25% of patients taking CLOZARIL® (clozapine), with patients having an average increase in pulse rate of 10-15 bpm. The sustained tachycardia is not simply a reflex response to hypotension, and is present in all positions monitored. Either tachycardia or hypotension may pose a serious risk for an individual with compromised cardiovascular function.

A minority of CLOZARIL® (clozapine) treated patients experience ECG repolarization changes similar to those seen with other antipsychotic drugs, including S-T segment depression and flattening or inversion of T waves, which all normalize after discontinuation of CLOZARIL® (clozapine). The clinical significance of these changes is unclear. However, in clinical trials with CLOZARIL® (clozapine), several patients experienced significant cardiac events, including ischemic changes, myocardial infarction, arrhythmias and sudden death. In addition there have been postmarketing reports of congestive heart failure, myocarditis, with or without eosinophilia, and pericarditis/pericardial effusions in association with CLOZARIL® (clozapine) use. Causality assessment was difficult in many of these cases because of serious preexisting cardiac disease and plausible alternative causes. Rare instances of sudden death have been reported in psychiatric patients, with or without associated antipsychotic drug treatment, and the relationship of these events to antipsychotic drug use is unknown.

CLOZARIL® (clozapine) should be used with caution in patients with known cardiovascular and/or pulmonary disease, and the recommendation for gradual titration of dose should be carefully observed.

Neuroleptic Malignant Syndrome (NMS)

A potentially fatal symptom complex sometimes referred to as Neuroleptic Malignant Syndrome (NMS) has been reported in association with antipsychotic drugs. Clinical manifestations of NMS are hyperpyrexia, muscle rigidity, altered mental status and evidence of autonomic instability (irregular pulse or blood pressure, tachycardia, diaphoresis, and cardiac dysrhythmias).

The diagnostic evaluation of patients with this syndrome is complicated. In arriving at a diagnosis, it is important to identify cases where the clinical presentation includes both serious medical illness (e.g., pneumonia, systemic infection, etc.) and untreated or inadequately treated extrapyramidal signs and symptoms (EPS). Other important considerations in the differential diagnosis include central anticholinergic toxicity, heat stroke, drug fever and primary central nervous system (CNS) pathology.

The management of NMS should include 1) immediate discontinuation of antipsychotic drugs and other drugs not essential to concurrent therapy, 2) intensive symptomatic treatment and medical monitoring, and 3) treatment of any concomitant serious medical problems for which specific treatments are available. There is no general agreement about specific pharmacological treatment regimens for uncomplicated NMS.

If a patient requires antipsychotic drug treatment after recovery from NMS, the potential reintroduction of drug therapy should be carefully considered. The patient should be carefully monitored, since recurrences of NMS have been reported.

There have been several reported cases of NMS in patients receiving CLOZARIL® (clozapine) alone or in combination with lithium or other CNS-active agents.

Tardive Dyskinesia

A syndrome consisting of potentially irreversible, involuntary, dyskinetic movements may develop in patients treated with antipsychotic drugs. Although the prevalence of the syndrome appears to be highest among the elderly, especially elderly women, it is impossible to rely upon prevalence estimates to predict, at the inception of treatment, which patients are likely to develop the syndrome.

There are several reasons for predicting that CLOZARIL® (clozapine) may be different from other antipsychotic drugs in its potential for inducing tardive dyskinesia, including the preclinical finding that it has a relatively weak dopamine blocking effect and the clinical finding of a virtual absence of certain acute extrapyramidal symptoms, e.g., dystonia. A few cases of tardive dyskinesia have been reported in patients on CLOZARIL® (clozapine) who had been previously treated with other antipsychotic agents, so that a causal relationship cannot be established. There have been no reports of tardive dyskinesia directly attributable to CLOZARIL® (clozapine) alone. Nevertheless, it cannot be concluded, without more extended experience, that CLOZARIL® (clozapine) is incapable of inducing this syndrome.

Both the risk of developing the syndrome and the likelihood that it will become irreversible are believed to increase as the duration of treatment and the total cumulative dose of antipsychotic drugs administered to the patient increase. However, the syndrome can develop, although much less commonly, after relatively brief treatment periods at low doses. There is no known treatment for established cases of tardive dyskinesia, although the syndrome may remit, partially or completely, if antipsychotic drug treatment is withdrawn. Antipsychotic drug treatment, itself, however, may suppress (or partially suppress) the signs and symptoms of the syndrome and thereby may possibly mask the under-

lying process. The effect that symptom suppression has upon the long-term course of the syndrome is unknown.

Given these considerations, CLOZARIL® (clozapine) should be prescribed in a manner that is most likely to minimize the occurrence of tardive dyskinesia. As with any antipsychotic drug, chronic CLOZARIL® (clozapine) use should be reserved for patients who appear to be obtaining substantial benefit from the drug. In such patients, the smallest dose and the shortest duration of treatment should be sought. The need for continued treatment should be reassessed periodically.

If signs and symptoms of tardive dyskinesia appear in a patient on CLOZARIL® (clozapine), drug discontinuation should be considered. However, some patients may require treatment with CLOZARIL® (clozapine) despite the presence of the syndrome.

PRECAUTIONS

General

Because of the significant risk of agranulocytosis and seizure, both of which present a continuing risk over time, the extended treatment of patients failing to show an acceptable level of clinical response should ordinarily be avoided. In addition, the need for continuing treatment in patients exhibiting beneficial clinical responses should be periodically re-evaluated. Although it is not known whether the risk would be increased, it is prudent either to avoid CLOZARIL® (clozapine) or use it cautiously in patients with a previous history of agranulocytosis induced by other drugs.

Fever

During CLOZARIL® (clozapine) therapy, patients may experience transient temperature elevations above 100.4°F (38°C), with the peak incidence within the first 3 weeks of treatment. While this fever is generally benign and self limiting, it may necessitate discontinuing patients from treatment. On occasion, there may be an associated increase or decrease in WBC count. Patients with fever should be carefully evaluated to rule out the possibility of an underlying infectious process or the development of agranulocytosis. In the presence of high fever, the possibility of Neuroleptic Malignant Syndrome (NMS) must be considered. There have been several reports of NMS in patients receiving CLOZARIL® (clozapine), usually in combination with lithium or other CNS-active drugs. [*See Neuroleptic Malignant Syndrome (NMS), under WARNINGS*]

Anticholinergic Toxicity

CLOZARIL® (clozapine) has very potent anticholinergic effects and great care should be exercised in using this drug in the presence of prostatic enlargement or narrow angle glaucoma. In addition, CLOZARIL® (clozapine) use has been associated with varying degrees of impairment of intestinal peristalsis, ranging from constipation to intestinal obstruction, fecal impaction and paralytic ileus *(see ADVERSE REACTIONS)*. On rare occasions, these cases have been fatal. Constipation should be initially treated by ensuring adequate hydration, and use of ancillary therapy such as bulk laxatives. Consultation with a gastroenterologist is advisable in more serious cases.

Interference with Cognitive and Motor Performance

Because of initial sedation, CLOZARIL® (clozapine) may impair mental and/or physical abilities, especially during the first few days of therapy. The recommendations for gradual dose escalation should be carefully adhered to, and patients cautioned about activities requiring alertness.

Use in Patients with Concomitant Illness

Clinical experience with CLOZARIL® (clozapine) in patients with concomitant systemic diseases is limited. Nevertheless, caution is advisable in using CLOZARIL® (clozapine) in patients with hepatic, renal or cardiac disease.

Use in Patients Undergoing General Anesthesia

Caution is advised in patients being administered general anesthesia because of the CNS effects of CLOZARIL® (clozapine). Check with the anesthesiologist regarding continuation of CLOZARIL® (clozapine) therapy in a patient scheduled for surgery.

Information for Patients

Physicians are advised to discuss the following issues with patients for whom they prescribe CLOZARIL® (clozapine):

—Patients who are to receive CLOZARIL® (clozapine) should be warned about the significant risk of developing agranulocytosis. They should be informed that weekly blood tests are required to monitor for the occurrence of agranulocytosis, and that CLOZARIL® (clozapine) tablets will be made available only through a special program designed to ensure the required blood monitoring. Patients should be advised to report immediately the appearance of lethargy, weakness, fever, sore throat, malaise, mucous membrane ulceration or other possible signs of infection. Particular attention should be paid to any flu-like complaints or other symptoms that might suggest infection.

—Patients should be informed of the significant risk of seizure during CLOZARIL® (clozapine) treatment, and they should be advised to avoid driving and any other potentially hazardous activity while taking CLOZARIL® (clozapine).

—Patients should be advised of the risk of orthostatic hypotension, especially during the period of initial dose titration.

—Patients should be informed that if they stop taking CLOZARIL® (clozapine) for more than 2 days, they should not restart their medication at the same dosage, but should contact their physician for dosing instructions.

—Patients should notify their physician if they are taking, or plan to take, any prescription or over-the-counter drugs or alcohol.

—Patients should notify their physician if they become pregnant or intend to become pregnant during therapy.

—Patients should not breast feed an infant if they are taking CLOZARIL® (clozapine).

Drug Interactions

The risks of using CLOZARIL® (clozapine) in combination with other drugs have not been systematically evaluated. The mechanism of CLOZARIL® (clozapine) induced agranulocytosis is unknown; nonetheless, the possibility that causative factors may interact synergistically to increase the risk and/or severity of bone marrow suppression warrants consideration. Therefore, CLOZARIL® (clozapine) should not be used with other agents having a well-known potential to suppress bone marrow function.

Given the primary CNS effects of CLOZARIL® (clozapine), caution is advised in using it concomitantly with other CNS-active drugs or alcohol.

Orthostatic hypotension in patients taking clozapine can, in rare cases (approximately 1 case per 3,000 patients), be accompanied by profound collapse and respiratory and/or cardiac arrest. Some of the cases of collapse/respiratory arrest/cardiac arrest during initial treatment occurred in patients who were being administered benzodiazepines; similar events have been reported in patients taking other psychotropic drugs or even CLOZARIL® (clozapine) by itself. Although it has not been established that there is an interaction between CLOZARIL® (clozapine) and benzodiazepines or other psychotropics, caution is advised when clozapine is initiated in patients taking a benzodiazepine or any other psychotropic drug.

Because CLOZARIL® (clozapine) is highly bound to serum protein, the administration of CLOZARIL® (clozapine) to a patient taking another drug which is highly bound to protein (e.g., warfarin, digitoxin) may cause an increase in plasma concentrations of these drugs, potentially resulting in adverse effects. Conversely, adverse effects may result from displacement of protein-bound CLOZARIL® (clozapine) by other highly bound drugs.

Cimetidine may increase plasma levels of CLOZARIL® (clozapine), potentially resulting in adverse effects. Although concomitant use of CLOZARIL® (clozapine) and carbamazepine is not recommended, it should be noted that discontinuation of concomitant carbamazepine administration may result in an increase in CLOZARIL® (clozapine) plasma levels. Phenytoin may decrease CLOZARIL® (clozapine) plasma levels, resulting in a decrease in effectiveness of a previously effective CLOZARIL® (clozapine) dose.

A subset (3%-10%) of the population has reduced activity of certain drug metabolizing enzymes such as the cytochrome P450 isozyme P450 2D6. Such individuals are referred to as "poor metabolizers" of drugs such as debrisoquin, dextromethorphan, the tricyclic antidepressants, and clozapine. These individuals may develop higher than expected plasma concentrations of clozapine when given usual doses. In addition, certain drugs that are metabolized by this isozyme, including many antidepressants (clozapine, selective serotonin reuptake inhibitors, and others), may inhibit the activity of this isozyme, and thus may make normal metabolizers resemble poor metabolizers with regard to concomitant therapy with other drugs metabolized by this enzyme system, leading to drug interaction.

Concomitant use of clozapine with other drugs metabolized by cytochrome P450 2D6 may require lower doses than usually prescribed for either clozapine or the other drug. Therefore, co-administration of clozapine with other drugs that are metabolized by this isozyme, including antidepressants, phenothiazines, carbamazepine, and Type 1C antiarrhythmics (e.g., propafenone, flecainide and encainide), or that inhibit this enzyme (e.g., quinidine), should be approached with caution.

CLOZARIL® (clozapine) may also potentiate the hypotensive effects of antihypertensive drugs and the anticholinergic effects of atropine-type drugs. The administration of epinephrine should be avoided in the treatment of drug induced hypotension because of a possible reverse epinephrine effect.

Carcinogenesis, Mutagenesis, Impairment of Fertility

No carcinogenic potential was demonstrated in long-term studies in mice and rats at doses approximately 7 times the typical human dose on a mg/kg basis. Fertility in male and female rats was not adversely affected by clozapine. Clozapine did not produce genotoxic or mutagenic effects when assayed in appropriate bacterial and mammalian tests.

Pregnancy Category B

Reproduction studies have been performed in rats and rabbits at doses of approximately 2-4 times the human dose and have revealed no evidence of impaired fertility or harm to the fetus due to clozapine. There are, however, no adequate and well-controlled studies in pregnant women. Because animal reproduction studies are not always predictive of human response, and in view of the desirability of keeping the administration of all drugs to a minimum during pregnancy, this drug should be used only if clearly needed.

Nursing Mothers

Animal studies suggest that clozapine may be excreted in breast milk and have an effect on the nursing infant. Therefore, women receiving CLOZARIL® (clozapine) should not breast feed.

Pediatric Use

Safety and effectiveness in pediatric patients have not been established.

ADVERSE REACTIONS

Associated with Discontinuation of Treatment

Sixteen percent of 1080 patients who received CLOZARIL® (clozapine) in premarketing clinical trials discontinued treatment due to an adverse event, including both those that could be reasonably attributed to CLOZARIL® (clozapine) treatment and those that might more appropriately be considered intercurrent illness. The more common events considered to be causes of discontinuation included: CNS, primarily drowsiness/sedation, seizures, dizziness/syncope; cardiovascular, primarily tachycardia, hypotension and ECG changes; gastrointestinal, primarily nausea/vomiting; hematologic, primarily leukopenia/granulocytopenia/agranulocytosis; and fever. None of the events enumerated accounts for more than 1.7% of all discontinuations attributed to adverse clinical events.

Commonly Observed

Adverse events observed in association with the use of CLOZARIL® (clozapine) in clinical trials at an incidence of greater than 5% were: central nervous system complaints, including drowsiness/sedation, dizziness/vertigo, headache and tremor; autonomic nervous system complaints, including salivation, sweating, dry mouth and visual disturbances; cardiovascular findings, including tachycardia, hypotension and syncope; and gastrointestinal complaints, including constipation and nausea; and fever. Complaints of drowsiness/sedation tend to subside with continued therapy or dose reduction. Salivation may be profuse, especially during sleep, but may be diminished with dose reduction.

Incidence in Clinical Trials

The following table enumerates adverse events that occurred at a frequency of 1% or greater among CLOZARIL® (clozapine) patients who participated in clinical trials. These rates are not adjusted for duration of exposure.

Treatment-Emergent Adverse Experience Incidence Among Patients Taking CLOZARIL® (clozapine) in Clinical Trials (N = 842) (Percentage of Patients Reporting)

Body System Adverse Event[a]	Percent
Central Nervous System	
Drowsiness/Sedation	39
Dizziness/Vertigo	19
Headache	7
Tremor	6
Syncope	6
Disturbed sleep/Nightmares	4
Restlessness	4
Hypokinesia/Akinesia	4
Agitation	4
Seizures (convulsions)	3[b]
Rigidity	3
Akathisia	3
Confusion	3
Fatigue	2
Insomnia	2
Hyperkinesia	1
Weakness	1
Lethargy	1
Ataxia	1
Slurred speech	1
Depression	1
Epileptiform movements/Myoclonic jerks	1
Anxiety	1
Cardiovascular	
Tachycardia	25[b]
Hypotension	9
Hypertension	4
Chest pain/Angina	1
ECG change/Cardiac abnormality	1

Continued on next page

Sandoz—Cont.

Gastrointestinal	
Constipation	14
Nausea	5
Abdominal discomfort/Heartburn	4
Nausea/Vomiting	3
Vomiting	3
Diarrhea	2
Liver test abnormality	1
Anorexia	1
Urogenital	
Urinary abnormalities	2
Incontinence	1
Abnormal ejaculation	1
Urinary urgency/frequency	1
Urinary retention	1
Autonomic Nervous System	
Salivation	31
Sweating	6
Dry mouth	6
Visual disturbances	5
Integumentary (Skin)	
Rash	2
Musculoskeletal	
Muscle weakness	1
Pain (back, neck, legs)	1
Muscle spasm	1
Muscle pain, ache	1
Respiratory	
Throat discomfort	1
Dyspnea, shortness of breath	1
Nasal congestion	1
Hemic/Lymphatic	
Leukopenia/Decreased WBC/Neutropenia	3
Agranulocytosis	1[b]
Eosinophilia	1
Miscellaneous	
Fever	5
Weight gain	4
Tongue numb/sore	1

[a] Events reported by at least 1% of CLOZARIL® (clozapine) patients are included.

[b] Rate based on population of approximately 1700 exposed during premarket clinical evaluation of CLOZARIL® (clozapine).

Other Events Observed During the Premarketing Evaluation of CLOZARIL® (clozapine)

This section reports additional, less frequent adverse events which occurred among the patients taking CLOZARIL® (clozapine) in clinical trials. Various adverse events were reported as part of the total experience in these clinical studies; a causal relationship to CLOZARIL® (clozapine) treatment cannot be determined in the absence of appropriate controls in some of the studies. The table above enumerates adverse events that occurred at a frequency of at least 1% of patients treated with CLOZARIL® (clozapine). The list below includes all additional adverse experiences reported as being temporally associated with the use of the drug which occurred at a frequency less than 1%, enumerated by organ system.

Central Nervous System: loss of speech, amentia, tics, poor coordination, delusions/hallucinations, involuntary movement, stuttering, dysarthria, amnesia/memory loss, histrionic movements, libido increase or decrease, paranoia, shakiness, Parkinsonism, and irritability.

Cardiovascular System: edema, palpitations, phlebitis/thrombophlebitis, cyanosis, premature ventricular contraction, bradycardia, and nose bleed.

Gastrointestinal System: abdominal distention, gastroenteritis, rectal bleeding, nervous stomach, abnormal stools, hematemesis, gastric ulcer, bitter taste, and eructation.

Urogenital System: dysmenorrhea, impotence, breast pain/discomfort, and vaginal itch/infection.

Autonomic Nervous System: numbness, polydypsia, hot flashes, dry throat, and mydriasis.

Integumentary (Skin): pruritus, pallor, eczema, erythema, bruise, dermatitis, petechiae, and urticaria.

Musculoskeletal System: twitching and joint pain.

Respiratory System: coughing, pneumonia/pneumonia-like symptoms, rhinorrhea, hyperventilation, wheezing, bronchitis, laryngitis, and sneezing.

Hemic and Lymphatic System: anemia and leukocytosis.

Miscellaneous: chills/chills with fever, malaise, appetite increase, ear disorder, hypothermia, eyelid disorder, bloodshot eyes, and nystagmus.

Postmarketing Clinical Experience

Postmarketing experience has shown an adverse experience profile similar to that presented above. Voluntary reports of adverse events temporally associated with CLOZARIL® (clozapine) not mentioned above that have been received since market introduction and that may have no causal relationship with the drug include the following:

Central Nervous System: delirium; EEG abnormal; exacerbation of psychosis; myoclonus; overdose; paresthesia; possible mild cataplexy; and status epilepticus.

Cardiovascular System: atrial or ventricular fibrillation and periorbital edema.

Gastrointestinal System: acute pancreatitis; dysphagia; fecal impaction; hepatitis; intestinal obstruction/paralytic ileus; jaundice; and salivary gland swelling.

Hepatic System: cholestasis.

Urogenital System: acute interstitial nephritis and priapism.

Integumentary (Skin): hypersensitivity reactions: photosensitivity, vasculitis, erythema multiforme, and Stevens-Johnson Syndrome.

Musculoskeletal System: myasthenic syndrome and rhabdomyolysis.

Respiratory System: aspiration and pleural effusion.

Hemic and Lymphatic System: deep vein thrombosis; elevated hemoglobin/hematocrit; ESR increased; pulmonary embolism; sepsis; thrombocytosis; and thrombocytopenia.

Miscellaneous: CPK elevation; hyperglycemia; hyperuricemia; hyponatremia; and weight loss.

DRUG ABUSE AND DEPENDENCE

Physical and psychological dependence have not been reported or observed in patients taking CLOZARIL® (clozapine).

OVERDOSAGE

Human Experience

The most commonly reported signs and symptoms associated with CLOZARIL® (clozapine) overdose are: altered states of consciousness, including drowsiness, delirium and coma; tachycardia; hypotension; respiratory depression or failure; hypersalivation. Aspiration pneumonia and cardiac arrhythmias have also been reported. Seizures have occurred in a minority of reported cases. Fatal overdoses have been reported with CLOZARIL® (clozapine), generally at doses above 2500 mg. There have also been reports of patients recovering from overdoses well in excess of 4 g.

Management of Overdose

Establish and maintain an airway; ensure adequate oxygenation and ventilation. Activated charcoal, which may be used with sorbitol, may be as or more effective than emesis or lavage, and should be considered in treating overdosage. Cardiac and vital signs monitoring is recommended along with general symptomatic and supportive measures. Additional surveillance should be continued for several days because of the risk of delayed effects. Avoid epinephrine and derivatives when treating hypotension, and quinidine and procainamide when treating cardiac arrhythmia.

There are no specific antidotes for CLOZARIL® (clozapine). Forced diuresis, dialysis, hemoperfusion and exchange transfusion are unlikely to be of benefit.

In managing overdosage, the physician should consider the possibility of multiple drug involvement.

Up-to-date information about the treatment of overdose can often be obtained from a certified Regional Poison Control Center. Telephone numbers of certified Poison Control Centers are listed in the Physicians' Desk Reference® (PDR).*

DOSAGE AND ADMINISTRATION

In order to minimize the risk of agranulocytosis, CLOZARIL® (clozapine) is available only through a distribution system that ensures weekly WBC testing prior to delivery of the next week's supply of medication. Upon initiation of CLOZARIL® (clozapine) therapy, up to a 1 week supply of additional CLOZARIL® (clozapine) tablets may be provided to the patient to be held for emergencies (e.g., weather, holidays).

Initial Treatment

It is recommended that treatment with CLOZARIL® (clozapine) begin with one-half of a 25 mg tablet (12.5 mg) once or twice daily and then be continued with daily dosage increments of 25-50 mg/day, if well-tolerated, to achieve a target dose of 300-450 mg/day by the end of 2 weeks. Subsequent dosage increments should be made no more than once or twice-weekly, in increments not to exceed 100 mg. Cautious titration and a divided dosage schedule are necessary to minimize the risks of hypotension, seizure, and sedation.

In the multicenter study that provides primary support for the effectiveness of CLOZARIL® (clozapine) in patients resistant to standard antipsychotic drug treatment, patients were titrated during the first 2 weeks up to a maximum dose of 500 mg/day, on a t.i.d. basis, and were then dosed in a total daily dose range of 100-900 mg/day, on a t.i.d. basis thereafter, with clinical response and adverse effects as guides to correct dosing.

Therapeutic Dose Adjustment

Daily dosing should continue on a divided basis as an effective and tolerable dose level is sought. While many patients may respond adequately at doses between 300-600 mg/day, it may be necessary to raise the dose to the 600-900 mg/day range to obtain an acceptable response. [Note: In the multicenter study providing the primary support for the superiority of CLOZARIL® (clozapine) in treatment resistant patients, the mean and median CLOZARIL® (clozapine) doses were both approximately 600 mg/day.]

Because of the possibility of increased adverse reactions at higher doses, particularly seizures, patients should ordinarily be given adequate time to respond to a given dose level before escalation to a higher dose is contemplated.

Dosing should not exceed 900 mg/day.

Because of the significant risk of agranulocytosis and seizure, events which both present a continuing risk over time, the extended treatment of patients failing to show an acceptable level of clinical response should ordinarily be avoided.

Maintenance Treatment

While the maintenance effectiveness of CLOZARIL® (clozapine) in schizophrenia is still under study, the effectiveness of maintenance treatment is well established for many other antipsychotic drugs. It is recommended that responding patients be continued on CLOZARIL® (clozapine), but at the lowest level needed to maintain remission. Because of the significant risk associated with the use of CLOZARIL® (clozapine), patients should be periodically reassessed to determine the need for maintenance treatment.

Discontinuation of Treatment

In the event of planned termination of CLOZARIL® (clozapine) therapy, gradual reduction in dose is recommended over a 1-2 week period. However, should a patient's medical condition require abrupt discontinuation (e.g., leukopenia), the patient should be carefully observed for the recurrence of psychotic symptoms.

Reinitiation of Treatment in Patients Previously Discontinued

When restarting patients who have had even a brief interval off CLOZARIL® (clozapine), i.e., 2 days or more since the last dose, it is recommended that treatment be reinitiated with one-half of a 25 mg tablet (12.5 mg) once or twice daily *(see WARNINGS)*. If that dose is well tolerated, it may be feasible to titrate patients back to a therapeutic dose more quickly than is recommended for initial treatment. However, any patient who has previously experienced respiratory or cardiac arrest with initial dosing, but was then able to be successfully titrated to a therapeutic dose, should be re-titrated with extreme caution after even 24 hours of discontinuation.

Certain additional precautions seem prudent when reinitiating treatment. The mechanisms underlying CLOZARIL® (clozapine) induced adverse reactions are unknown. It is conceivable, however, that re-exposure of a patient might enhance the risk of an untoward event's occurrence and increase its severity. Such phenomena, for example, occur when immune mediated mechanisms are responsible. Consequently, during the reinitiation of treatment, additional caution is advised. Patients discontinued for WBC counts below 2000/mm^3 or an ANC below 1000/mm^3 must *not* be restarted on CLOZARIL® (clozapine). *(See WARNINGS)*

HOW SUPPLIED

CLOZARIL® (clozapine) is available only through a distribution system that ensures weekly WBC testing prior to delivery of the next week's supply of medication.

CLOZARIL® (clozapine) is available as 25 mg and 100 mg round, pale-yellow, uncoated tablets with a facilitated score.

CLOZARIL® (clozapine) Tablets

25 mg

Engraved with "CLOZARIL" once on the periphery of one side. Engraved with a facilitated score and "25" once on the other side.

Bottle of 100 (NDC 0078-0126-05).

SandoPak® unit-dose packages of 100: 2 × 5 strips, 10 blisters per strip (NDC 0078-0126-06).

100 mg

Engraved with "CLOZARIL" once on the periphery of one side. Engraved with a facilitated score and "100" once on the other side.

Bottle of 100 (NDC 0078-0127-05).

SandoPak® unit-dose packages of 100: 2 × 5 strips, 10 blisters per strip (NDC 0078-0127-06).

Store and Dispense

Storage temperature should not exceed 86°F (30°C). Drug dispensing should not ordinarily exceed a weekly supply. Dispensing should be contingent upon the results of a WBC count.

*Trademark of Medical Economics Data Production Company.

[REV: MARCH 1996 30118904]

Shown in Product Identification Guide, page 332

D.H.E. 45®* ℞
(dihydroergotamine mesylate) injection, USP

Caution: Federal law prohibits dispensing without prescription.
The following prescribing information is based on official labeling in effect on August 1, 1996.

DESCRIPTION
D.H.E. 45® is ergotamine hydrogenated in the 9, 10 position as the mesylate salt. D.H.E. 45® is known chemically as ergotaman- 3′,6′,18-trione,9,10-dihydro- 12′-hydroxy-2′-methyl-5′-(phenylmethyl)-,(5′α,10α)-, monomethanesulfonate (salt). Its structure is as follows:

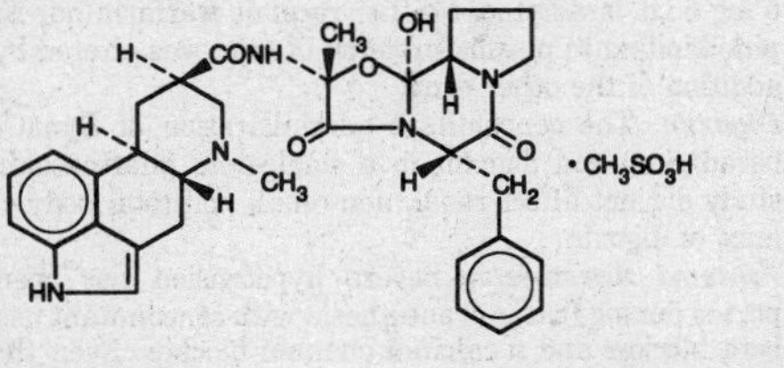

$C_{33}H_{37}N_5O_5 \cdot CH_4O_3S$ Mol. wt. 679.79

D.H.E. 45® (dihydroergotamine mesylate) is a clear, colorless solution supplied in sterile ampuls for I.V. or I.M. administration containing per mL:

dihydroergotamine mesylate, USP	1 mg
methanesulfonic acid/ sodium hydroxide, qs to	pH 3.6 ±0.4
alcohol, USP	6.1% by vol.
glycerin, USP	15% by wt.
water for injection, USP, qs to	1 mL

ACTIONS
Dihydroergotamine is an alpha adrenergic blocking agent with a direct stimulating effect on the smooth muscle of peripheral and cranial blood vessels, and produces depression of central vasomotor centers. The compound also has the properties of serotonin antagonism. In comparison to ergotamine, the adrenergic blocking actions are more pronounced, the vasoconstrictive actions somewhat less pronounced, and there is reduced incidence and degree of nausea and vomiting.
Onset of action occurs in 15-30 minutes following intramuscular administration and persists for 3-4 hours.
Repeated dosage at 1 hour intervals up to 3 hours may be required to obtain maximal effect.

INDICATIONS
D.H.E. 45® (dihydroergotamine mesylate) injection, USP, therapy is indicated to abort or prevent vascular headache, e.g., migraine, migraine variants, or so-called "histaminic cephalalgia" when rapid control is desired or when other routes of administration are not feasible.
For best results, treatment should commence at the first symptom or sign of a migraine headache attack.

CONTRAINDICATIONS
Dihydroergotamine mesylate is contraindicated in patients who have previously shown hypersensitivity to ergot alkaloids.
The drug is also contraindicated in patients having conditions predisposing to vasospastic reactions such as known peripheral arterial disease, coronary artery disease (in particular, unstable or vasospastic angina), sepsis, shock, vascular surgery, uncontrolled hypertension, and severely impaired hepatic or renal function.
Dihydroergotamine possesses oxytocic properties and, therefore, should not be administered during pregnancy.
Dihydroergotamine should not be used in nursing mothers *(see PRECAUTIONS).*
Dihydroergotamine should not be used with vasoconstrictors because the combination may result in extreme elevation of blood pressure.

WARNINGS
Vasospasm
Dihydroergotamine, like other ergot alkaloids, can cause vasospastic reactions, including angina, although it seems to do so less frequently than other ergots. This action appears to be dose related; however, some patients may demonstrate individual sensitivity to the agent.
Vasospastic reactions are manifested by intense arterial vasoconstriction, producing signs and symptoms of peripheral vascular ischemia (e.g., muscle pains, numbness, coldness, and pallor or cyanosis of the digits), angina or unusual syndromes, such as mesenteric ischemia. Because persistent vasospasm can result in gangrene or death, D.H.E. 45® (dihydroergotamine mesylate) injection, USP, should be discontinued immediately if signs or symptoms of vasoconstriction develop.

PRECAUTIONS
Information for Patients
No more than 3 mL intramuscularly or 2 mL intravenously should be injected for any single migraine attack. No more than 6 mL should be injected during any 7-day period.
D.H.E. 45® (dihydroergotamine mesylate) injection, USP, should be used only for vascular headaches of the migraine type. It is not effective for other types of headaches and it lacks analgesic properties. Patients should be advised to report to the physician immediately any of the following: numbness or tingling in the fingers and toes, muscle pain in the arms and legs, weakness in the legs, pain in the chest, or temporary speeding or slowing of the heart rate, swelling, or itching.
Drug Interactions
Vasoconstrictors
D.H.E. 45® (dihydroergotamine mesylate) injection, USP, should not be administered with vasoconstrictors or sympathomimetics (pressor agents) because the combination may cause extreme elevation of blood pressure.
Beta Blockers
There have been reports that propranolol may potentiate the vasoconstrictive action of ergotamine by blocking the vasodilating property of epinephrine.
Nicotine
Nicotine may provoke vasoconstriction in some patients, predisposing to a greater ischemic response to ergot therapy.
Macrolide Antibiotics (e.g., Erythromycin)
Agents of the ergot alkaloid class, of which D.H.E. 45® (dihydroergotamine mesylate) injection, USP, is a member, have been shown to interact with antibiotics of the macrolide class, resulting in increased plasma levels of unchanged alkaloids and peripheral vasoconstriction. Vasospastic reactions have been reported with therapeutic doses of ergotamine-containing drugs when coadministered with these antibiotics.
Pregnancy
Teratogenic Effects
Pregnancy Category X: Animal reproductive (teratogenic) studies in rats, rabbits, and nonhuman primates, employing oral D.H.E. 45® (dihydroergotamine mesylate) at doses of 1, 3, 10, and 30 mg/kg/day (approximately 12, 36, 120, and 360 times the maximum recommended daily dose based on a 50 kg man) did not produce any evidence of adverse reproductive effects. There are no studies on the placental transfer or teratogenicity of D.H.E. 45® (dihydroergotamine mesylate). Ergotamine crosses the placenta in small amounts, although it does not appear to be embryotoxic. However, prolonged vasoconstriction of the uterine vessels and/or increased myometrial tone leading to reduced myometrial and placenta blood flow may contribute to fetal growth retardation in animals. *(See CONTRAINDICATIONS.)*
Nursing Mothers
Ergot drugs are known to inhibit prolactin. It is likely that D.H.E. 45® (dihydroergotamine mesylate) is excreted in human milk. However, there are no data on the concentration of dihydroergotamine in human milk. It is known that ergotamine is excreted in breast milk and may cause vomiting, diarrhea, weak pulse and unstable blood pressure in nursing infants. Because of the potential for these serious adverse reactions in nursing infants from D.H.E. 45® (dihydroergotamine mesylate), nursing should not be undertaken during the use of D.H.E. 45® (dihydroergotamine mesylate).
Pediatric Use
Safety and effectiveness in pediatric patients have not been established.

ADVERSE REACTIONS
Numbness and tingling of fingers and toes, muscle pains in the extremities, weakness in the legs, precordial distress and pain, transient tachycardia or bradycardia, nausea, vomiting, localized edema, itching, and injection site reactions.
In studies with normal volunteers, doses of D.H.E. 45® (dihydroergotamine mesylate) injection, USP, of 2-3 mg resulted in an increased frequency of headache, leg cramps and soreness, nausea, and vomiting.
There have been reports of pleural and retroperitoneal fibrosis in patients following prolonged use of dihydroergotamine.
Postmarketing Clinical Experience
The following events derived from postmarketing experience have been occasionally reported in patients receiving D.H.E. 45® (dihydroergotamine mesylate) injection: vasospasm, paraesthesia, hypertension, dizziness, anxiety, dyspnea, headache, flushing, diarrhea, rash, increased sweating; and pleural and retroperitoneal fibrosis after long-term use of dihydroergotamine. Extremely rare cases of myocardial infarction and cerebral vascular accident have been reported. A causal relationship has not been established.

DRUG ABUSE AND DEPENDENCE
Abuse and Dependence
Currently available data have not demonstrated drug abuse and psychological dependence with dihydroergotamine. However, cases of drug abuse and psychological dependence in patients on other forms of ergot therapy have been reported. Thus, due to the chronicity of vascular headaches, it is imperative that patients be advised not to exceed recommended dosages.

OVERDOSAGE
To date, there have been no reports of acute overdosage with this drug. Due to the risk of vascular spasm, exceeding the recommended dosages of D.H.E. 45® (dihydroergotamine mesylate) injection, USP, is to be avoided. Excessive doses of dihydroergotamine may result in peripheral signs and symptoms of ergotism. Treatment includes discontinuance of the drug, local application of warmth to the affected area, the administration of vasodilators (e.g., sodium nitroprusside or phentolamine), and nursing care to prevent tissue damage.
In general, the symptoms of an acute D.H.E. 45® (dihydroergotamine mesylate) overdose are similar to those of an ergotamine overdose, although there is less pronounced nausea and vomiting with D.H.E. 45® (dihydroergotamine mesylate). The symptoms of an ergotamine overdose include the following: numbness, tingling, pain, and cyanosis of the extremities associated with diminished or absent peripheral pulses; respiratory depression; an increase and/or decrease in blood pressure, usually in that order; confusion, delirium, convulsions, and coma; and/or some degree of nausea; vomiting; and abdominal pain.

DOSAGE AND ADMINISTRATION
D.H.E. 45® (dihydroergotamine mesylate) should be administered in a dose of 1 mL intramuscularly at the first warning sign of headache, and repeated at 1 hour intervals to a total dose of 3 mL. Optimal results are obtained by titrating the dose over the course of several headaches to find the minimal effective dose for each patient; this dose should then be employed at onset of subsequent attacks. Where more rapid effect is desired, the intravenous route may be employed to a maximum of 2 mL. Total weekly dosage should not exceed 6 mL.

HOW SUPPLIED
D.H.E. 45® (dihydroergotamine mesylate) injection, USP
Available as a clear, colorless, sterile solution in single 1 mL sterile ampuls containing 1 mg of dihydroergotamine mesylate per mL, in packages of 10 (NDC 0078-0041-01).
Store and Dispense
To assure constant potency, protect the ampuls from light and heat. Store and dispense below 77°F (25°C), in light-resistant containers. Administer only if clear and colorless.
[REV: MAY 1996 30220905]
* Also known as Dyhydergot®

DYNACIRC® ℞
[*dī-nă serk*]
(isradipine) CAPSULES

CAUTION: Federal law prohibits dispensing without prescription.
The following prescribing information is based on official labeling in effect on August 1, 1996.

DESCRIPTION
DynaCirc® (isradipine) is a calcium antagonist available for oral administration in capsules containing 2.5 mg or 5 mg. The structural formula of isradipine is:

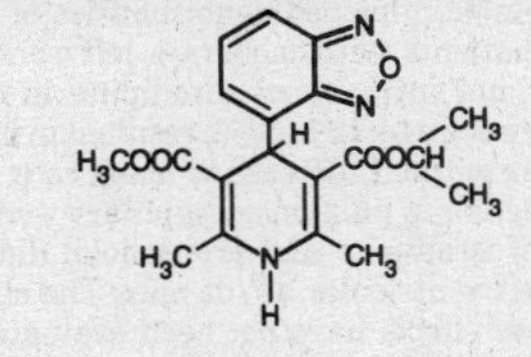

$C_{19}H_{21}N_3O_5$ Mol. wt. 371.39

Chemically, isradipine is 3,5-Pyridinedicarboxylic acid, 4-(4-benzofurazanyl)-1,4-dihydro-2,6-dimethyl-, methyl 1-methylethyl ester. Isradipine is a yellow, fine crystalline powder which is odorless or has a faint characteristic odor. Isradipine is practically insoluble in water (< 10 mg/L at 37°C), but is soluble in ethanol and freely soluble in acetone, chloroform and methylene chloride.
Active Ingredient: isradipine
Inactive Ingredients: colloidal silicon dioxide, D&C Red No. 7 Calcium Lake, FD&C Red No. 40 (5 mg capsule only), FD&C Yellow No. 6 Aluminum Lake, gelatin, lactose, starch, titanium dioxide and other ingredients.
The 2.5 mg and 5 mg capsules may also contain: benzyl alcohol, butylparaben, edetate calcium disodium, methylparaben, propylparaben, sodium propionate.

Continued on next page

Sandoz—Cont.

CLINICAL PHARMACOLOGY

Mechanism of Action

Isradipine is a dihydropyridine calcium channel blocker. It binds to calcium channels with high affinity and specificity and inhibits calcium flux into cardiac and smooth muscle. The effects observed in mechanistic experiments *in vitro* and studied in intact animals and man are compatible with this mechanism of action and are typical of the class.

Except for diuretic activity, the mechanism of which is not clearly understood, the pharmacodynamic effects of isradipine observed in whole animals can also be explained by calcium channel blocking activity, especially dilating effects in arterioles which reduce systemic resistance and lower blood pressure, with a small increase in resting heart rate. Although like other dihydropyridine calcium channel blockers, isradipine has negative inotropic effects *in vitro*, studies conducted in intact anesthetized animals have shown that the vasodilating effect occurs at doses lower than those which affect contractility. In patients with normal ventricular function, isradipine's afterload reducing properties lead to some increase in cardiac output.

Effects in patients with impaired ventricular function have not been fully studied.

Clinical Effects

Dose-related reductions in supine and standing blood pressure are achieved within 2-3 hours following single oral doses of 2.5 mg, 5 mg, 10 mg, and 20 mg DynaCirc® (isradipine), with a duration of action (at least 50% of peak response) of more than 12 hours following administration of the highest dose.

DynaCirc® (isradipine) has been shown in controlled, double-blind clinical trials to be an effective antihypertensive agent when used as monotherapy, or when added to therapy with thiazide-type diuretics. During chronic administration, divided doses (b.i.d.) in the range of 5-20 mg daily have been shown to be effective, with response at trough (prior to next dose) over 50% of the peak blood pressure effect. The response is dose-related between 5-10 mg daily. DynaCirc® (isradipine) is equally effective in reducing supine, sitting, and standing blood pressure.

On chronic administration, increases in resting pulse rate averaged about 3-5 beats/min. These increases were not dose-related.

Hemodynamics

In man, peripheral vasodilation produced by DynaCirc® (isradipine) is reflected by decreased systemic vascular resistance and increased cardiac output. Hemodynamic studies conducted in patients with normal left ventricular function produced, following intravenous isradipine administration, increases in cardiac index, stroke volume index, coronary sinus blood flow, heart rate, and peak positive left ventricular dP/dt. Systemic, coronary, and pulmonary vascular resistance were decreased. These studies were conducted with doses of isradipine which produced clinically significant decreases in blood pressure. The clinical consequences of these hemodynamic effects, if any, have not been evaluated.

Effects on heart rate are variable, dependent upon rate of administration and presence of underlying cardiac condition. While increases in both peak positive dP/dt and LV ejection fraction are seen when intravenous isradipine is given, it is impossible to conclude that these represent a positive inotropic effect due to simultaneous changes in preload and afterload. In patients with coronary artery disease undergoing atrial pacing during cardiac catheterization, intravenous isradipine diminished abnormalities of systolic performance. In patients with moderate left ventricular dysfunction, oral and intravenous isradipine in doses which reduce blood pressure by 12%-30%, resulted in improvement in cardiac index without increase in heart rate, and with no change or reduction in pulmonary capillary wedge pressure. Combination of isradipine and propranolol did not significantly affect left ventricular dP/dt max. The clinical consequences of these effects have not been evaluated.

Electrophysiologic Effects

In general, no detrimental effects on the cardiac conduction system were seen with the use of DynaCirc® (isradipine). Electrophysiologic studies were conducted on patients with normal sinus and atrioventricular node function. Intravenous isradipine in doses which reduce systolic blood pressure did not affect PR, QRS, AH* or HV* intervals.

No changes were seen in Wenckebach cycle length, atrial, and ventricular refractory periods. Slight prolongation of QT_c interval of 3% was seen in one study. Effects on sinus node recovery time (CSNRT) were mild or not seen.

In patients with sick sinus syndrome, at doses which significantly reduced blood pressure, intravenous isradipine resulted in no depressant effect on sinus and atrioventricular node function.

*AH = conduction time from low right atrium to His bundle deflection, or AV nodal conduction time; HV = conduction time through His bundle and the bundle branch-Purkinje system.

Pharmacokinetics and Metabolism

Isradipine is 90%-95% absorbed and is subject to extensive first-pass metabolism, resulting in a bioavailability of about 15%-24%. Isradipine is detectable in plasma within 20 minutes after administration of single oral doses of 2.5-20 mg, and peak concentrations of approximately 1 ng/mL/mg dosed occur about 1.5 hours after drug administration. Administration of DynaCirc® (isradipine) with food significantly increases the time to peak by about an hour, but has no effect on the total bioavailability (area under the curve) of the drug. Isradipine is 95% bound to plasma proteins. Both peak plasma concentration and AUC exhibit a linear relationship to dose over the 0-20 mg dose range. The elimination of isradipine is biphasic with an early half-life of $1^1/_2$-2 hours, and a terminal half-life of about 8 hours. The total body clearance of isradipine is 1.4 L/min and the apparent volume of distribution is 3 L/kg.

Isradipine is completely metabolized prior to excretion, and no unchanged drug is detected in the urine. Six metabolites have been characterized in blood and urine, with the mono acids of the pyridine derivative and a cyclic lactone product accounting for >75% of the material identified. Approximately 60%-65% of an administered dose is excreted in the urine and 25%-30% in the feces. Mild renal impairment (creatinine clearance 30-80 mL/min) increases the bioavailability (AUC) of isradipine by 45%. Progressive deterioration reverses this trend, and patients with severe renal failure (creatinine clearance <10 mL/min) who have been on hemodialysis show a 20%-50% lower AUC than healthy volunteers. No pharmacokinetic information is available on drug therapy during hemodialysis. In elderly patients, C_{max} and AUC are increased by 13% and 40%, respectively; in patients with hepatic impairment, C_{max} and AUC are increased by 32% and 52%, respectively *(see DOSAGE AND ADMINISTRATION)*.

INDICATIONS AND USAGE

Hypertension

DynaCirc® (isradipine) is indicated in the management of hypertension. It may be used alone or concurrently with thiazide-type diuretics.

CONTRAINDICATIONS

DynaCirc® (isradipine) is contraindicated in individuals who have shown hypersensitivity to any of the ingredients in the formulation.

WARNINGS

None

PRECAUTIONS

General

Blood Pressure: Because DynaCirc® (isradipine) decreases peripheral resistance, like other calcium blockers DynaCirc® (isradipine) may occasionally produce symptomatic hypotension. However, symptoms like syncope and severe dizziness have rarely been reported in hypertensive patients administered DynaCirc® (isradipine), particularly at the initial recommended doses *(see DOSAGE AND ADMINISTRATION)*.

Use in Patients with Congestive Heart Failure: Although acute hemodynamic studies in patients with congestive heart failure have shown that DynaCirc® (isradipine) reduced afterload without impairing myocardial contractility, it has a negative inotropic effect at high doses *in vitro*, and possibly in some patients. Caution should be exercised when using the drug in congestive heart failure patients, particularly in combination with a beta-blocker.

Drug Interactions

Nitroglycerin: DynaCirc® (isradipine) has been safely coadministered with nitroglycerin.

Hydrochlorothiazide: A study in normal healthy volunteers has shown that concomitant administration of DynaCirc® (isradipine) and hydrochlorothiazide does not result in altered pharmacokinetics of either drug. In a study in hypertensive patients, addition of isradipine to existing hydrochlorothiazide therapy did not result in any unexpected adverse effects, and isradipine had an additional antihypertensive effect.

Propranolol: In a single dose study in normal volunteers, coadministration of propranolol had a small effect on the rate but no effect on the extent of isradipine bioavailability. Significant increases in AUC (27%) and C_{max} (58%) and decreases in t_{max} (23%) of propranolol were noted in this study. However, concomitant administration of 5 mg b.i.d. isradipine and 40 mg b.i.d. propranolol to healthy volunteers under steady-state conditions had no relevant effect on either drug's bioavailability. AUC and C_{max} differences were <20% between isradipine given singly and in combination with propranolol, and between propranolol given singly and in combination with isradipine.

Cimetidine: In a study in healthy volunteers, a one-week course of cimetidine at 400 mg b.i.d. with a single 5 mg dose of isradipine on the sixth day showed an increase in isradipine mean peak plasma concentrations (36%) and significant increase in area under the curve (50%). If isradipine therapy is initiated in a patient currently receiving cimetidine, care-

ful monitoring for adverse reactions is advised and downward dose adjustment may be required.

Rifampicin: In a study in healthy volunteers, a six-day course of rifampicin at 600 mg/day followed by a single 5 mg dose of isradipine resulted in a reduction in isradipine levels to below detectable limits. If rifampicin therapy is required, isradipine concentrations and therapeutic effects are likely to be markedly reduced or abolished as a consequence of increased metabolism and higher clearance of isradipine.

Warfarin: In a study in healthy volunteers, no clinically relevant pharmacokinetic or pharmacodynamic interaction between isradipine and racemic warfarin was seen when two single oral doses of warfarin (0.7 mg/kg body weight) were administered during 11 days of multiple-dose treatment with 5 mg b.i.d. isradipine. Neither racemic warfarin nor isradipine binding to plasma proteins *in vitro* was altered by the addition of the other drug.

Digoxin: The concomitant administration of DynaCirc® (isradipine) and digoxin in a single-dose pharmacokinetic study did not affect renal, non-renal, and total body clearance of digoxin.

Fentanyl Anesthesia: Severe hypotension has been reported during fentanyl anesthesia with concomitant use of a beta blocker and a calcium channel blocker. Even though such interactions have not been seen in clinical studies with DynaCirc® (isradipine), an increased volume of circulating fluids might be required if such an interaction were to occur.

Carcinogenesis, Mutagenesis, Impairment of Fertility

Treatment of male rats for 2 years with 2.5, 12.5, or 62.5 mg/kg/day isradipine admixed with the diet (approximately 6, 31, and 156 times the maximum recommended daily dose based on a 50 kg man) resulted in dose dependent increases in the incidence of benign Leydig cell tumors and testicular hyperplasia relative to untreated control animals. These findings, which were replicated in a subsequent experiment, may have been indirectly related to an effect of isradipine on circulating gonadotropin levels in the rats; a comparable endocrine effect was not evident in male patients receiving therapeutic doses of the drug on a chronic basis. Treatment of mice for two years with 2.5, 15, or 80 mg/kg/day isradipine in the diet (approximately 6, 38, and 200 times the maximum recommended daily dose based on a 50 kg man) showed no evidence of oncogenicity. There was no evidence of mutagenic potential based on the results of a battery of mutagenic tests. No effect on fertility was observed in male and female rats treated with up to 60 mg/kg/day isradipine.

Pregnancy

Pregnancy Category C: Isradipine was administered orally to rats and rabbits during organogenesis. Treatment of pregnant rats with doses of 6, 20, or 60 mg/kg/day produced a significant reduction in maternal weight gain during treatment with the highest dose (150 times the maximum recommended human daily dose) but with no lasting effects on the mother or the offspring. Treatment of pregnant rabbits with doses of 1, 3, or 10 mg/kg/day (2.5, 7.5, and 25 times the maximum recommended human daily dose) produced decrements in maternal body weight gain and increased fetal resorptions at the two higher doses. There was no evidence of embryotoxicity at doses which were not maternotoxic and no evidence of teratogenicity at any dose tested. In a peri/postnatal administration study in rats, reduced maternal body weight gain during late pregnancy at oral doses of 20 and 60 mg/kg/day isradipine was associated with reduced birth weights and decreased peri and postnatal pup survival. There are no adequate and well controlled studies in pregnant women. The use of DynaCirc® (isradipine) during pregnancy should only be considered if the potential benefit outweighs potential risks.

Nursing Mothers

It is not known whether DynaCirc® (isradipine) is excreted in human milk. Because many drugs are excreted in human milk, and because of the potential for adverse effects of DynaCirc® (isradipine) on nursing infants, a decision should be made as to whether to discontinue nursing or discontinue the drug, taking into account the importance of the drug to the mother.

Pediatric Use

Safety and effectiveness in pediatric patients have not been established.

ADVERSE REACTIONS

In multiple dose U.S. studies in hypertension, 1228 patients received DynaCirc® (isradipine) alone or in combination with other agents, principally a thiazide diuretic, 934 of them in controlled comparisons with placebo or active agents. An additional 652 patients (which includes 374 normal volunteers) received DynaCirc® (isradipine) in U.S. studies of conditions other than hypertension, and 1321 patients received DynaCirc® (isradipine) in non-U.S. studies. About 500 patients received DynaCirc® (isradipine) in long-term hypertension studies, 410 of them for at least 6 months. The adverse reaction rates given below are principally based on controlled hypertension studies, but rarer serious events are derived from all exposures to DynaCirc® (isradipine), including foreign marketing experience.

Most adverse reactions were mild and related to the vasodilatory effects of DynaCirc® (dizziness, edema, palpitations, flushing, tachycardia), and many were transient. About 5% of isradipine patients left studies prematurely because of adverse reactions (vs. 3% of placebo patients and 6% of active control patients), principally due to headache, edema, dizziness, palpitations, and gastrointestinal disturbances.

The following table shows the most common adverse reactions, volunteered or elicited, considered by the investigator to be at least possibly drug related. The results for the DynaCirc® (isradipine) treated patients are presented for all doses pooled together (reported by 1% or greater of patients receiving any dose of isradipine), and also for the two treatment regimens most applicable to the treatment of hypertension with DynaCirc® (isradipine): (1) initial and maintenance dose of 2.5 mg b.i.d., and (2) initial dose of 2.5 mg b.i.d. followed by maintenance dose of 5.0 mg b.i.d. [See table at right.]

Except for headache, which is not clearly drug-related (see previous table), the more frequent adverse reactions listed show little change, or increase slightly, in frequency over time, as shown in the following table:
[See table below.]

Edema, palpitations, fatigue, and flushing appear to be dose-related, especially at the higher doses of 15-20 mg/day.

In open-label, long-term studies of up to two years in duration, the adverse events reported were generally the same as those reported in the short-term controlled trials. The overall frequencies of these adverse events were slightly higher in the long-term than in the controlled studies, but as in the controlled trials most adverse reactions were mild and transient.

The following adverse experiences were reported in 0.5-1.0% of the isradipine-treated patients in hypertension studies, or are rare. More serious events from this and other data sources, including postmarketing exposure, are shown in italics. The relationship of these adverse events to isradipine administration is uncertain.

Skin: pruritus, *urticaria*

Musculoskeletal: cramps of legs/feet

Respiratory: cough

Cardiovascular: shortness of breath, hypotension, *atrial fibrillation, ventricular fibrillation, myocardial infarction, heart failure*

Gastrointestinal: abdominal discomfort, constipation, diarrhea

Urogenital: nocturia

Nervous System: drowsiness, insomnia, lethargy, nervousness, impotence, decreased libido, depression, *syncope, paresthesia* (which includes numbness and tingling), *transient ischemic attack, stroke*

Autonomic: hyperhidrosis, visual disturbance, dry mouth, numbness

Miscellaneous: throat discomfort, *leukopenia, elevated liver function tests*

OVERDOSAGE

Minimal empirical data are available on DynaCirc® (isradipine) overdosage. Three individual suicide attempts with dosages of isradipine reported to be from 20 mg up to 100 mg resulted in lethargy, sinus tachycardia and, in the case of the person ingesting 100 mg, transient hypotension which responded to fluid therapy. A foreign report of the ingestion of 200 mg of isradipine with ethanol resulted only in flushing, tachycardia with ST depression on ECG, and hypotension, all of which were reversible. The ingestion of 5 mg of isradipine by a 22-month old child and the accidental

	DynaCirc® (isradipine)					Active
	All Doses	2.5 mg b.i.d.	5 mg b.i.d.†	10 mg b.i.d.††	Placebo	Controls*
N=	934	199	150	59	297	414
Adverse Experience	%	%	%	%	%	%
Headache	13.7	12.6	10.7	22.0	14.1	9.4
Dizziness	7.3	8.0	5.3	3.4	4.4	8.2
Edema	7.2	3.5	8.7	8.5	3.0	2.9
Palpitations	4.0	1.0	4.7	5.1	1.4	1.5
Fatigue	3.9	2.5	2.0	8.5	0.3	6.3
Flushing	2.6	3.0	2.0	5.1	0.0	1.2
Chest Pain	2.4	2.5	2.7	1.7	2.4	2.9
Nausea	1.8	1.0	2.7	5.1	1.7	3.1
Dyspnea	1.8	0.5	2.7	3.4	1.0	2.2
Abdominal Discomfort	1.7	0.0	3.3	1.7	1.7	3.9
Tachycardia	1.5	1.0	1.3	3.4	0.3	0.5
Rash	1.5	1.5	2.0	1.7	0.3	0.7
Pollakiuria	1.5	2.0	1.3	3.4	0.0	<1.0
Weakness	1.2	0.0	0.7	0.0	0.0	1.2
Vomiting	1.1	1.0	1.3	0.0	0.3	0.2
Diarrhea	1.1	0.0	2.7	3.4	2.0	1.9

† Initial dose of 2.5 mg b.i.d. followed by maintenance dose of 5.0 mg b.i.d.
†† Initial dose of 2.5 mg b.i.d. followed by sequential titration to 5.0 mg b.i.d., 7.5 mg b.i.d., and maintenance dose of 10.0 mg b.i.d.
* Propranolol, prazosin, hydrochlorothiazide, enalapril, captopril.

ingestion of 100 mg of isradipine by a 58-year old female did not result in any sequelae.

Available data suggest that, as with other dihydropyridines, overdosage with DynaCirc® (isradipine) might result in excessive peripheral vasodilatation with subsequent marked and probably prolonged systemic hypotension, and tachycardia. Emesis, gastric lavage, administration of activated charcoal followed in 30 minutes by a saline cathartic would be reasonable therapy. Isradipine is highly protein-bound and *not* removed by hemodialysis. Overdosage characterized by clinically significant hypotension should be treated with active cardiovascular support including monitoring of cardiac and respiratory function, elevation of lower extremities, and attention to circulating fluid volume and urine output. A vasoconstrictor (such as epinephrine, norepinephrine, or levarterenol) may be helpful in restoring a normotensive state, provided that there is no contraindication to its use. Refractory hypotension or AV conduction disturbances may be treated with intravenous calcium salts, or glucagon. Cimetidine should be withheld in such instances due to the risk of further increasing plasma isradipine levels. Significant lethality was observed in mice given oral doses of over 200 mg/kg and rabbits given about 50 mg/kg of isradipine. Rats tolerated doses of over 2000 mg/kg without effects on survival.

DOSAGE AND ADMINISTRATION

The dosage of DynaCirc® (isradipine) should be individualized. The recommended initial dose of DynaCirc® (isradipine) is 2.5 mg b.i.d. alone or in combination with a thiazide diuretic. An antihypertensive response usually occurs within 2-3 hours. Maximal response may require 2-4 weeks. If a satisfactory reduction in blood pressure does not occur after this period, the dose may be adjusted in incre-

ments of 5 mg/day at 2-4 week intervals up to a maximum of 20 mg/day. Most patients, however, show no additional response to doses above 10 mg/day, and adverse effects are increased in frequency above 10 mg/day.

The bioavailability of DynaCirc® (increased AUC) is increased in elderly patients (above 65 years of age), patients with hepatic functional impairment, and patients with mild renal impairment. Ordinarily, the starting dose should still be 2.5 mg b.i.d. in these patients.

HOW SUPPLIED

DynaCirc® (isradipine) Capsules

2.5 mg
White, imprinted twice with the DynaCirc® (isradipine) logo and "DynaCirc" on one end, and "2.5" and "△" on the other.
Bottles of 100 capsules (NDC 0078-0226-05)
Bottles of 60 capsules (NDC 0078-0226-44)

5 mg
Light pink, imprinted twice with the DynaCirc® (isradipine) logo and "DynaCirc" on one end, and "5" and "△" on the other.
Bottles of 100 capsules (NDC 0078-0227-05)
Bottles of 60 capsules (NDC 0078-0227-44)

Store and Dispense
Below 86°F (30°C) in a tight container. Protect from light.
[REV: MARCH 1996   30119906]
Shown in Product Identification Guide, page 332

DYNACIRC CR®
(isradipine)
Controlled Release Tablets   ℞

Caution: Federal law prohibits dispensing without prescription.

The following prescribing information is based on official labeling in effect on August 1, 1996

DESCRIPTION

DynaCirc CR® contains isradipine, a calcium antagonist. It is available for once-daily oral administration as a controlled release 5 mg and 10 mg tablet for DynaCirc CR® (isradipine). DynaCirc CR® is a registered trademark for isradipine GITS (Gastrointestinal Therapeutic System) tablets. The structural formula of isradipine is:

$C_{19}H_{21}N_3O_5$ Mol. wt. 371.39

Incidence Rates for DynaCirc® (isradipine) (All Doses) by Week (%)

Week	1	2	3	4	5	6
N	694	906	649	847	432	494
Adverse Reaction						
Headache	6.5	6.1	5.2	5.2	5.8	4.5
Dizziness	1.6	1.9	1.7	2.2	2.3	2.0
Edema	1.2	2.5	3.2	3.2	5.3	5.5
Palpitations	1.2	1.3	1.4	1.9	2.1	1.4
Fatigue	0.4	1.0	1.4	1.4	1.2	1.6
Flushing	1.2	1.3	2.0	1.4	2.1	1.4

Week	7	8	9	10	11	12
N	153	377	261	362	107	105
Adverse Reaction						
Headache	2.0	2.7	1.9	2.8	2.8	3.8
Dizziness	2.0	1.9	2.3	3.9	4.7	3.8
Edema	5.9	5.0	4.6	4.7	3.8	3.8
Palpitations	1.3	0.8	0.8	1.7	1.9	2.9
Fatigue	2.0	2.7	1.5	1.4	0.9	1.9
Flushing	3.3	1.3	1.1	0.8	0.0	0.0

Continued on next page

Sandoz—Cont.

Chemically, isradipine is 3,5-Pyridinedicarboxylic acid, 4-(4-benzofurazanyl)-1,4-dihydro-2,6-dimethyl-,methyl 1-methylethyl ester. Isradipine is a yellow, fine crystalline powder which is odorless or has a faint characteristic odor. Isradipine is practically insoluble in water (< 10 mg/L at 37°C), but is soluble in ethanol and freely soluble in acetone, chloroform and methylene chloride.

Active Ingredient: isradipine

Inactive Ingredients: butylated hydroxytoluene; cellulose acetate; hydroxypropyl methylcellulose; magnesium stearate; polyethylene glycol; polyethylene oxide; polysorbate 80; propylene glycol; red ferric oxide; silicon dioxide; sodium chloride; titanium dioxide; yellow ferric oxide.

System Components and Performance

Isradipine is delivered from the DynaCirc CR® (isradipine) Controlled Release Tablet as follows: a semipermeable membrane surrounds an osmotically active drug core. The core is composed of two layers: an "active" layer containing the drug, and a pharmacologically inert but osmotically active "push" layer. After ingestion, the tablet overcoating is quickly dissipated in the gastrointestinal tract, allowing water to enter the tablet through the semipermeable membrane. The polyethylene oxide polymer swells in the osmotic ("push") layer and exerts pressure against the "active" drug layer, releasing isradipine as a fine suspension through the laser-drilled tablet orifice which has been positioned on the "active" drug layer side. Drug delivery is essentially constant as long as the osmotic gradient remains constant and, after either 5 mg or 10 mg of isradipine is released, gradually falls to a negligible amount. The controlled rate of drug delivery into the gastrointestinal lumen is independent of pH or gastrointestinal motility. The delivery of isradipine in DynaCirc CR® (isradipine) Controlled Release Tablets depends on the existence of an osmotic gradient between the contents of the bilayer core and the fluid in the GI tract. The biologically inert core of the tablet remains intact and, unless it becomes trapped, is eliminated in the feces.

CLINICAL PHARMACOLOGY

Mechanism of Action

Isradipine is a dihydropyridine calcium channel blocker. It binds to calcium channels with high affinity and specificity and inhibits calcium flux into cardiac and smooth muscle. The effects observed in mechanistic experiments *in vitro* and studied in intact animals and man are compatible with this mechanism of action and are typical of the class.

Except for diuretic activity, the mechanism of which is not clearly understood, the pharmacodynamic effects of isradipine observed in whole animals can also be explained by calcium channel blocking activity, especially dilating effects in arterioles which reduce systemic resistance and lower blood pressure, with a small increase in resting heart rate. Although like other dihydropyridine calcium channel blockers, isradipine has negative inotropic effects *in vitro*, studies conducted in intact anesthetized animals have shown that the vasodilating effect occurs at doses lower than those which affect contractility. In patients with normal ventricular function, isradipine's afterload reducing properties lead to some increase in cardiac output.

Effects in patients with impaired ventricular function have not been fully studied.

Clinical Effects

In randomized, placebo-controlled, double-blind, clinical trials, DynaCirc CR® (isradipine) Controlled Release Tablets have been shown to have antihypertensive effects proportional to doses between 5 and 20 mg, administered once daily. DynaCirc CR® (isradipine) produced statistically significant reductions in supine and standing blood pressure, compared with placebo, 24 hours postdose. The endpoint results of one parallel group dose-ranging trial showed mean responses 24 hours after ingestion of DynaCirc CR® (isradipine) (systolic/diastolic) -5.2/-2.8, -13.4/-9.7, -15.6/-10.2 and -15.5/-11.8 mmHg, for 5, 10, 15 and 20 mg doses, respectively, change from baseline greater than concurrent placebo. The antihypertensive effect of any one dose begins in about 2 hours and reaches a peak at about 8–10 hours postdose. At the recommended starting dose (5 mg) the trough response (24 hours after dosing) was about 76% that of the peak. At doses of 10, 15 and 20 mg, the trough blood pressure response was about equal to that at peak effect. In association with the fall in blood pressure, resting heart rate is slightly increased, on average from 1–3 beats/minute. The antihypertensive response to DynaCirc CR® (isradipine) has not been detected to be influenced by gender or age.

Hemodynamics

In man, peripheral vasodilation produced by immediate-release DynaCirc® (isradipine) is reflected by decreased systemic vascular resistance and increased cardiac output. Hemodynamic studies conducted in patients with normal left ventricular function produced, following intravenous isradipine administration, increases in cardiac index, stroke volume index, coronary sinus blood flow, heart rate and peak

positive left ventricular dP/dt. Systemic, coronary, and pulmonary vascular resistance was decreased. These studies were conducted with doses of isradipine which produced clinically significant decreases in blood pressure. The clinical consequences of these hemodynamic effects, if any, have not been evaluated.

Effects on heart rate are variable, dependent upon rate of administration and presence of underlying cardiac condition. While increases in both peak positive dP/dt and LV ejection fraction are seen when intravenous isradipine is given, it is impossible to conclude that these represent a positive inotropic effect due to simultaneous changes in preload and afterload. In patients with coronary artery disease undergoing atrial pacing during cardiac catheterization, intravenous isradipine diminished abnormalities of systolic performance. In patients with moderate left ventricular dysfunction, oral and intravenous isradipine in doses which reduce blood pressure by 12%–30%, resulted in improvement in cardiac index without increase in heart rate, and with no change or reduction in pulmonary capillary wedge pressure. Combination of isradipine and propranolol did not significantly affect left ventricular dP/dt max. The clinical consequences of these effects have not been evaluated.

Electrophysiologic Effects

In general, no detrimental effects on the cardiac conduction system were seen with the use of immediate-release DynaCirc® (isradipine). Electrophysiologic studies were conducted on patients with normal sinus and atrioventricular node function. Intravenous isradipine in doses which reduce systolic blood pressure did not affect PR, QRS, AH* or HV* intervals.

No changes were seen in Wenckebach cycle length, atrial, and ventricular refractory periods. Slight prolongation of QT_c interval of 3% was seen in one study. Effects on sinus node recovery time (CSNRT) were mild or not seen.

In patients with sick sinus syndrome, at doses which significantly reduced blood pressure, intravenous isradipine resulted in no depressant effect on sinus and atrioventricular node function.

*AH = conduction time from low right atrium to His bundle deflection, or AV nodal conduction time; HV = conduction time through His bundle and the bundle branch-Purkinje system.

Pharmacokinetics and Metabolism

With the immediate-release formulation DynaCirc® (isradipine) Capsules, 90%–95% of the orally administered dose is absorbed. Because of the biotransformation of isradipine during its first-pass through the portal circulation, the bioavailability of DynaCirc CR® (isradipine) ranges from 15%–24%. Isradipine is 95% bound to plasma proteins.

Peak concentrations of approximately 1 ng/mL/mg dosed occur about 1.5 hours after DynaCirc® (isradipine) Capsules administration. The elimination of isradipine is biphasic with an early half-life of $1^1/_2$-2 hours, and a terminal half-life of about 8 hours, resulting in trough concentrations of about 0.1 ng/mL/mg dosed of immediate-release DynaCirc® (isradipine) Capsules.

In single dose studies of DynaCirc CR® (isradipine) Controlled Release Tablets, after a 2–3 hour lag time, concentrations of isradipine plateau between 7 and 18 hours post-dosing (reaching a C_{max} of 3–4 ng/mL with an AUC of 62–73 ng·h/mL for a 10 mg dose) and then a concentration > 50% of the peak exists for 17–20 hours.

There is no evidence of dose dumping either in the presence or absence of food. Food has been shown to decrease the extent of bioavailability of DynaCirc CR® (isradipine) by up to 25%.

The pharmacokinetics of DynaCirc CR® (isradipine) Controlled Release Tablets are linear over the dose range of 5–20 mg, in that the plasma drug concentrations are proportional to the dose administered.

Isradipine is completely metabolized prior to excretion, and no unchanged drug is detected in the urine. The major routes of isradipine metabolism are ring oxidation of the dihydropyridine moiety to give the corresponding pyridine, and ester cleavage, with or without concomitant oxidation of the dihydropyridine moiety, giving the corresponding carboxylic acids. The cytochrome P-450 IIIA4 system is implicated in the formation of these metabolites, which are hemodynamically inactive. Approximately 60%–65% of an administered dose is excreted in the urine and 25%–30% in the feces. With immediate-release DynaCirc® (isradipine), mild renal impairment (creatinine clearance 30–80 mL/min) increases the AUC of isradipine by 45%. Progressive deterioration reverses this trend, and patients with severe renal failure (creatinine clearance < 10 mL/min) who have been on hemodialysis show a 20%–50% lower AUC than healthy volunteers. In elderly patients administered DynaCirc® (isradipine) Capsules, C_{max} and AUC are increased by 13% and 40%, respectively; in patients with hepatic impairment, C_{max} and AUC are increased by 32% and 52%, respectively (*see DOSAGE AND ADMINISTRATION*).

INDICATIONS AND USAGE

Hypertension

DynaCirc CR® (isradipine) is indicated in the management of hypertension. It may be used alone or concurrently with thiazide-type diuretics.

CONTRAINDICATIONS

DynaCirc CR® (isradipine) is contraindicated in individuals who have shown hypersensitivity to any of the ingredients in the formulation.

WARNINGS

None

PRECAUTIONS

General

Blood Pressure: Because DynaCirc CR® (isradipine) decreases peripheral resistance, like other calcium blockers DynaCirc CR® (isradipine) may occasionally produce symptomatic hypotension. However, symptoms like syncope and severe dizziness have rarely been reported in hypertensive patients administered DynaCirc CR® (isradipine), particularly at the initial recommended doses (*see DOSAGE AND ADMINISTRATION*).

Use in Patients with Congestive Heart Failure: Although acute hemodynamic studies in patients with congestive heart failure have shown that immediate-release DynaCirc® (isradipine) reduced afterload without impairing myocardial contractility, it has a negative inotropic effect at high doses *in vitro* and possibly in some patients. Caution should be exercised when using DynaCirc CR® (isradipine) in congestive heart failure patients, particularly in combination with a beta-blocker.

Peripheral Edema: Peripheral edema, when it occurs, is usually mild to moderate in severity. It is a localized phenomenon thought to be associated with vasodilation of arterioles and other small blood vessels, and not due to left ventricular dysfunction or generalized fluid retention. Peripheral edema is dose-related with an incidence ranging from approximately 9% at 5 mg; 13% at 10 mg; 16% at 15 mg; and 36% at the highest dose studied (20 mg once-daily). With patients whose hypertension is complicated by congestive heart failure, care should be taken to differentiate this edema from the effects of decreasing left ventricular function. Although the frequency of edema is correlated with dose, no DynaCirc CR® (isradipine) treated patients discontinued the short-term (6 weeks or less), placebo-controlled hypertension studies as a result of edema. Less than 5% of DynaCirc CR® (isradipine) treated patients in long-term studies discontinued due to edema.

Other: As with any other non-deformable material, caution should be used when administering DynaCirc CR® (isradipine) in patients with pre-existing severe gastrointestinal narrowing (pathologic or iatrogenic). There have been reports of obstructive symptoms in patients with known strictures associated with ingestion of other GITS products.

Information for Patients: DynaCirc CR® (isradipine) Controlled Release Tablets should be swallowed whole. Do not chew, divide or crush tablets. Do not be concerned if you occasionally notice in your stool something resembling a tablet. In DynaCirc CR® (isradipine), the medication is contained within a nonabsorbable shell that has been specially designed to slowly release the drug for your body to absorb. When this process is completed, the empty tablet shell is eliminated in the stool.

Drug Interactions

Nitroglycerin: Immediate-release DynaCirc® (isradipine) has been safely coadministered with nitroglycerin.

Hydrochlorothiazide: A study in normal healthy volunteers has shown that concomitant administration of immediate-release DynaCirc® (isradipine) and hydrochlorothiazide does not result in altered pharmacokinetics of either drug. In a study in hypertensive patients, addition of isradipine to existing hydrochlorothiazide therapy did not result in any unexpected adverse effects, and isradipine had an additional antihypertensive effect.

Propranolol: In a single dose study in normal volunteers using immediate-release DynaCirc® (isradipine), co-administration of propranolol had a small effect on the rate but no effect on the extent of isradipine bioavailability. Significant increases in AUC (27%) and C_{max} (58%) and decreases in t_{max} (23%) of propranolol were noted in this study.

Digoxin: The concomitant administration of immediate-release DynaCirc® (isradipine) and digoxin in a single-dose pharmacokinetic study did not affect renal, non-renal and total body clearance of digoxin.

Fentanyl Anesthesia: Severe hypotension has been reported during fentanyl anesthesia with concomitant use of a beta blocker and a calcium channel blocker. An increased volume of circulating fluids might be required if such an interaction were to occur.

Carcinogenesis, Mutagenesis, Impairment of Fertility

Treatment of male rats for 2 years with 2.5, 12.5, or 62.5 mg/kg/day isradipine admixed with the diet (approximately 6, 31, and 156 times the maximum recommended daily dose based on a 50 kg man) resulted in dose dependent increases

DynaCirc® (isradipine)

Adverse Experience	All Doses	2.5 mg b.i.d.	5 mg b.i.d.†	10 mg b.i.d.††	Placebo (N=297) %	Active Controls* (N=414) %
Headache	13.7	12.6	10.7	22.0	14.1	9.4
Dizziness	7.3	8.0	5.3	3.4	4.4	8.2
Edema	7.2	3.5	8.7	8.5	3.0	2.9
Palpitations	4.0	1.0	4.7	5.1	1.4	1.5
Fatigue	3.9	2.5	2.0	8.5	0.3	6.3
Flushing	2.6	3.0	2.0	5.1	0.0	1.2
Chest Pain	2.4	2.5	2.7	1.7	2.4	2.9
Nausea	1.8	1.0	2.7	5.1	1.7	3.1
Dyspnea	1.8	0.5	2.7	3.4	1.0	2.2
Abdominal Discomfort	1.7	0.0	3.3	1.7	1.7	3.9
Tachycardia	1.5	1.0	1.3	3.4	0.3	0.5
Rash	1.5	1.5	2.0	1.7	0.3	0.7
Pollakiuria	1.5	2.0	1.3	3.4	0.0	<1.0
Weakness	1.2	0.0	0.7	0.0	0.0	1.2
Vomiting	1.1	1.0	1.3	0.0	0.3	0.2
Diarrhea	1.1	0.0	2.7	3.4	2.0	1.9

† Initial dose of 2.5 mg b.i.d. followed by maintenance dose of 5.0 mg b.i.d.
†† Initial dose of 2.5 mg b.i.d. followed by sequential titration to 5.0 mg b.i.d., 7.5 mg b.i.d., and maintenance dose of 10.0 mg b.i.d.
* Propranolol, prazosin, hydrochlorothiazide, enalapril, captopril.

in the incidence of benign Leydig cell tumors and testicular hyperplasia relative to untreated control animals. These findings, which were replicated in a subsequent experiment, may have been indirectly related to an effect of isradipine on circulating gonadotropin levels in the rats; a comparable endocrine effect was not evident in male patients receiving therapeutic doses of the drug on a chronic basis. Treatment of mice for two years with 2.5, 15, or 80 mg/kg/day isradipine in the diet (approximately 6, 38, and 200 times the maximum recommended dose based on a 50 kg man) showed no evidence of oncogenicity. There was no evidence of mutagenic potential based on the results of a battery of mutagenic tests. No effect on fertility was observed in male and female rats treated with up to 60 mg/kg/day isradipine.

Pregnancy
Pregnancy Category C: Isradipine was administered orally to rats and rabbits during organogenesis. Treatment of pregnant rats with doses of 6, 20, or 60 mg/kg/day produced a significant reduction in maternal weight gain during treatment with the highest dose (150 times the maximum recommended human daily dose) but with no lasting effects on the mother or the offspring. Treatment of pregnant rabbits with doses of 1, 3, or 10 mg/kg/day (2.5, 7.5, and 25 times the maximum recommended human daily dose) produced decrements in maternal body weight gain and increased fetal resorption at the two higher doses. There was no evidence of embryotoxicity at doses which were not maternotoxic and no evidence of teratogenicity at any dose tested. In a peri/postnatal administration study in rats, reduced maternal body weight gain during late pregnancy at oral doses of 20 and 60 mg/kg/day isradipine was associated with reduced birth weights and decreased peri and postnatal pup survival.
There are no adequate and well controlled studies in pregnant women. The use of DynaCirc CR® (isradipine) during pregnancy should only be considered if the potential benefit outweighs potential risks.

Nursing Mothers
It is not known whether DynaCirc® (isradipine) is excreted in human milk. Because many drugs are excreted in human milk, and because of the potential for adverse effects of DynaCirc® (isradipine) on nursing infants, a decision should be made as to whether to discontinue nursing or discontinue the drug, taking into account the importance of the drug to the mother.

Pediatric Use
Safety and effectiveness have not been established in children.

ADVERSE REACTIONS
In a controlled clinical trial with DynaCirc CR® (isradipine), dose-related edema occurred at an incidence of approximately 9% at 5 mg; 13% at 10 mg; 16% at 15 mg; and 36% at the highest dose studied (20 mg), was mild to moderate in severity, and was not related to age or gender.
The incidences of elicited or volunteered adverse reactions (excluding non-drug related) in the following tables are based on 6-week multicenter, placebo-controlled, double-blind hypertension studies. Less than 1% of DynaCirc CR® (isradipine) or placebo-treated patients discontinued from these studies due to adverse reactions.
The most common adverse experiences (≥1.0%) reported with DynaCirc CR® (isradipine) in a dose-response study are shown in the following table. There were no discontinuations

of patients treated with DynaCirc CR® (isradipine) in this study due to these common side effects.

Most Frequently Reported Newly-Occurring Adverse Reactions in Dose-Response Study

DynaCirc CR® (isradipine)

Adverse Reactions (Excluding Non-Drug Related)	5 mg (N=79)	10 mg (N=79)	15 mg (N=82)	20 mg (N=78)	Placebo Group (N=83)
Headache	13.9%	12.7%	18.3%	10.3%	15.7%
Edema	8.9%	12.7%	15.9%	35.9%	3.6%
Dizziness	5.1%	6.3%	3.7%	6.4%	2.4%
Constipation	3.8%	1.3%	1.2%	2.6%	0.0%
Fatigue	2.5%	7.6%	3.7%	3.8%	2.4%
Flushing	2.5%	3.8%	1.2%	1.3%	1.2%
Abdominal Discomfort	1.3%	5.1%	3.7%	5.1%	1.2%
Rash	1.3%	1.3%	0.0%	2.6%	0.0%

The table below shows elicited or volunteered adverse experiences for DynaCirc CR® (isradipine) treated patients in two 6-week, placebo-controlled, multicenter studies, at doses from 5-20 mg, and considered by the investigator to be at least possibly drug related. The results for DynaCirc CR® (isradipine) treated patients are presented for all doses pooled together (reported by at least 1.0% of active drug treated patients). The incidence of adverse reactions are listed below:

Adverse Reactions (Excluding Non-Drug Related)	DynaCirc CR® (isradipine) (N=422)	Placebo (N=186)
Edema	15.2%	2.2%
Headache	13.0%	12.4%
Dizziness	4.7%	2.7%
Fatigue	4.3%	2.2%
Abdominal Discomfort	2.8%	0.5%
Flushing	1.9%	0.5%
Constipation	1.7%	0.0%
Palpitations	1.2%	0.0%
Nausea	1.2%	1.6%
Abdominal Distention	1.2%	0.0%

The following adverse experiences were reported in 0.5%-1.0% or less of DynaCirc CR® (isradipine) or immediate-release DynaCirc® (isradipine) treated patients in hypertensive studies, or were noted in postmarketing experience with immediate-release DynaCirc® (isradipine) Capsules. More serious events are shown in italics. The relationship of these adverse experiences to isradipine administration is uncertain.
Skin: pruritus, *urticaria*
Musculoskeletal: backache/pain, joint pain, neck pain/sore/stiff, legs ache/pain, cramps of legs/feet
Respiratory: dyspnea, nasal congestion, cough
Cardiovascular: epistaxis, tachycardia, chest pain, shortness of breath, hypotension, *syncope, atrial or ventricular fibrillation, myocardial infarction, heart failure*

Gastrointestinal: diarrhea, vomiting, appetite increased or decreased
Urogenital: pollakiuria, impotence, dysuria, nocturia
Central Nervous: drowsiness, insomnia, lethargy, nervousness, libido decrease/frigidity, impotence, depression, *paresthesia* (which includes numbness and tingling), *transient ischemic attack, stroke*
Autonomic: dry mouth, hyperhidrosis, visual disturbance
Miscellaneous: weight gain, throat discomfort, *drug fever, leukopenia, elevated liver function tests*
No gastrointestinal bleeding has been reported in clinical trials with DynaCirc CR® (isradipine) Controlled Release Tablets.
In a long-term (one-year) DynaCirc CR® (isradipine) open-label, hypertension trial, the adverse events reported were generally the same as those seen in the short-term placebo-controlled studies. About 6% of DynaCirc CR® (isradipine) treated patients discontinued the long-term trial due to adverse reactions.
With immediate-release DynaCirc® (isradipine) Capsules, most of the adverse experiences were transient, mild, and related to vasodilatory effects. The following table shows the most common adverse events reported in U.S. clinical trials for immediate-release DynaCirc® (isradipine) Capsules, volunteered or elicited, and considered by the investigator to be at least possibly drug related.

[See table above.]
In open-label, long-term studies of up to two years in duration with immediate-release DynaCirc® (isradipine) Capsules, the adverse experiences reported were generally the same as those reported in the short-term controlled trials. The overall frequencies of these adverse events were slightly higher in the long-term than in the controlled studies, but in the controlled studies most adverse reactions were mild and transient.

OVERDOSAGE
Although there is no well documented experience with DynaCirc® (isradipine) overdosage, available data suggest that, as with other dihydropyridines, gross overdosage would result in excessive peripheral vasodilation with subsequent marked and probably prolonged systemic hypotension. Clinically significant hypotension overdosage calls for active cardiovascular support including monitoring of cardiac and respiratory function, elevation of lower extremities and attention to circulating fluid volume and urine output. A vasoconstrictor (such as epinephrine, norepinephrine, or levarterenol) may be helpful in restoring vascular tone and blood pressure, provided that there is no contraindication to its use. Since isradipine is highly protein bound, dialysis is not likely to be of benefit.
Significant lethality was observed in mice given oral doses of over 200 mg/kg and rabbits given about 50 mg/kg of isradipine. Rats tolerated doses of over 2000 mg/kg without effects on survival.

DOSAGE AND ADMINISTRATION
The dosage of DynaCirc CR® (isradipine) Controlled Release Tablets should be individualized. The recommended initial dose of DynaCirc CR® (isradipine) is 5 mg once-daily as monotherapy or in combination with a thiazide diuretic. An antihypertensive response usually occurs within 2 hours, with the peak antihypertensive response occurring 8–10 hours post-dose; blood pressure reduction is maintained for at least 24 hours following drug administration. If necessary, the dose may be adjusted in increments of 5 mg at 2–4 week intervals up to a maximum dose of 20 mg/day. Adverse experiences are increased in frequency above 10 mg/day. DynaCirc CR® (isradipine) Controlled Release Tablets should be swallowed whole and should not be bitten or divided.
The bioavailability (increased AUC) of immediate-release DynaCirc® (isradipine) is increased in elderly patients (above 65 years of age), patients with hepatic functional impairment, and patients with mild renal impairment. Ordinarily, a starting dose of DynaCirc CR® (isradipine) 5 mg once-daily should be used in these patients.

HOW SUPPLIED
DynaCirc CR® (isradipine) Controlled Release Tablets
5 mg
Light pink, standard biconvex, round tablet, imprinted in red with "DynaCirc CR" on one side and "5" on the other.
Bottles of 100 controlled release tablets (NDC 0078-0235-05)
Bottles of 30 controlled release tablets (NDC 0078-0235-15)
10 mg
Beige, standard biconvex, round tablet, imprinted in red with "DynaCirc CR" on one side and "10" on the other.
Bottles of 100 controlled release tablets (NDC 0078-0236-05)
Bottles of 30 controlled release tablets (NDC 0078-0236-15)
Store and Dispense
Below 86°F (30°C) in a tight container, protected from moisture and humidity.
[REV: JUNE 1996   37022903]
Shown in Product Identification Guide, page 332

Continued on next page

Sandoz—Cont.

FIORICET® ℞
[fē-ōr'i-set]
(Butalbital, Acetaminophen, and Caffeine Tablets, USP)

Caution: Federal law prohibits dispensing without prescription.
The following prescribing information is based on official labeling in effect on August 1, 1996.

DESCRIPTION
Fioricet® (Butalbital, Acetaminophen, and Caffeine Tablets, USP) is supplied in tablet form for oral administration. Each tablet contains:

butalbital*, USP .... 50 mg
*Warning: May be habit-forming.
acetaminophen, USP .... 325 mg
caffeine, USP .... 40 mg

Active Ingredients: butalbital, USP, acetaminophen, USP, and caffeine, USP.
Inactive Ingredients: crospovidone, FD&C Blue #1, magnesium stearate, microcrystalline cellulose, povidone, pregelatinized starch, and stearic acid.
Butalbital (5-allyl-5-isobutylbarbituric acid), is a short to intermediate-acting barbiturate. It has the following structural formula:

$C_{11}H_{16}N_2O_3$ Mol. wt. 224.26

Acetaminophen (4'-hydroxyacetanilide), is a non-opiate, non-salicylate analgesic and antipyretic. It has the following structural formula:

$C_8H_9NO_2$ Mol. wt. 151.16

Caffeine (1,3,7-trimethylxanthine), is a central nervous system stimulant. It has the following structural formula:

$C_8H_{10}N_4O_2$ Mol. wt. 194.19

CLINICAL PHARMACOLOGY
This combination drug product is intended as a treatment for tension headache.
It consists of a fixed combination of butalbital, acetaminophen and caffeine. The role each component plays in the relief of the complex of symptoms known as tension headache is incompletely understood.

Pharmacokinetics
The behavior of the individual components is described below.

Butalbital
Butalbital is well absorbed from the gastrointestinal tract and is expected to distribute to most tissues in the body. Barbiturates in general may appear in breast milk and readily cross the placental barrier. They are bound to plasma and tissue proteins to a varying degree and binding increases directly as a function of lipid solubility.
Elimination of butalbital is primarily via the kidney (59% to 88% of the dose) as unchanged drug or metabolites. The plasma half-life is about 35 hours. Urinary excretion products include parent drug (about 3.6% of the dose), 5-isobutyl-5-(2, 3-dihydroxypropyl) barbituric acid (about 24% of the dose), 5-allyl-5(3-hydroxy-2-methyl-1-propyl) barbituric acid (about 4.8% of the dose), products with the barbituric acid ring hydrolyzed with excretion of urea (about 14% of the dose), as well as unidentified materials. Of the material excreted in the urine, 32% is conjugated.
See *OVERDOSAGE* for toxicity information.

Acetaminophen
Acetaminophen is rapidly absorbed from the gastrointestinal tract and is distributed throughout most body tissues. The plasma half-life is 1.25 to 3 hours, but may be increased by liver damage and following overdosage. Elimination of acetaminophen is principally by liver metabolism (conjugation) and subsequent renal excretion of metabolites. Approximately 85% of an oral dose appears in the urine within 24 hours of administration, most as the glucuronide conjugate, with small amounts of other conjugates and unchanged drug.
See *OVERDOSAGE* for toxicity information.

Caffeine
Like most xanthines, caffeine is rapidly absorbed and distributed in all body tissues and fluids, including the CNS, fetal tissues, and breast milk.
Caffeine is cleared through metabolism and excretion in the urine. The plasma half-life is about 3 hours. Hepatic biotransformation prior to excretion results in about equal amounts of 1-methylxanthine and 1-methyluric acid. Of the 70% of the dose that is recovered in the urine, only 3% is unchanged drug.
See *OVERDOSAGE* for toxicity information.

INDICATIONS AND USAGE
Fioricet® (Butalbital, Acetaminophen, and Caffeine Tablets) is indicated for the relief of the symptom complex of tension (or muscle contraction) headache.
Evidence supporting the efficacy and safety of this combination product in the treatment of multiple recurrent headaches is unavailable. Caution in this regard is required because butalbital is habit-forming and potentially abusable.

CONTRAINDICATIONS
This product is contraindicated under the following conditions:
—Hypersensitivity or intolerance to any component of this product
—Patients with porphyria.

WARNINGS
Butalbital is habit-forming and potentially abusable. Consequently, the extended use of this product is not recommended.

PRECAUTIONS
General
Butalbital, acetaminophen and caffeine tablets should be prescribed with caution in certain special-risk patients, such as the elderly or debilitated, and those with severe impairment or renal or hepatic function, or acute abdominal conditions.

Information for Patients
This product may impair mental and/or physical abilities required for the performance of potentially hazardous tasks such as driving a car or operating machinery. Such tasks should be avoided while taking this product.
Alcohol and other CNS depressants may produce an additive CNS depression, when taken with this combination product, and should be avoided.
Butalbital may be habit-forming. Patients should take the drug only for as long as it is prescribed, in the amounts prescribed, and no more frequently than prescribed.

Laboratory Tests
In patients with severe hepatic or renal disease, effects of therapy should be monitored with serial liver and/or renal function tests.

Drug Interactions
The CNS effects of butalbital may be enhanced by monoamine oxidase (MAO) inhibitors.
Butalbital, acetaminophen and caffeine may enhance the effects of: other narcotic analgesics, alcohol, general anesthetics, tranquilizers such as chlordiazepoxide, sedative-hypnotics, or other CNS depressants, causing increased CNS depression.

Drug/Laboratory Test Interactions
Acetaminophen may produce false-positive test results for urinary 5-hydroxyindoleacetic acid.

Carcinogenesis, Mutagenesis, Impairment of Fertility
No adequate studies have been conducted in animals to determine whether acetaminophen or butalbital have a potential for carcinogenesis, mutagenesis or impairment of fertility.

Pregnancy
Teratogenic Effects
Pregnancy Category C: Animal reproduction studies have not been conducted with this combination product. It is also not known whether butalbital, acetaminophen and caffeine can cause fetal harm when administered to a pregnant woman or can affect reproduction capacity. This product should be given to a pregnant woman only when clearly needed.

Nonteratogenic Effects
Withdrawal seizures were reported in a two-day-old male infant whose mother had taken a butalbital-containing drug during the last two months of pregnancy. Butalbital was found in the infant's serum. The infant was given phenobarbital 5 mg/kg, which was tapered without further seizure or other withdrawal symptoms.

Nursing Mothers
Caffeine, barbiturates and acetaminophen are excreted in breast milk in small amounts, but the significance of their effects on nursing infants is not known. Because of potential for serious adverse reactions in nursing infants from butalbital, acetaminophen and caffeine, a decision should be made whether to discontinue nursing or to discontinue the drug, taking into account the importance of the drug to the mother.

Pediatric Use
Safety and effectiveness in pediatric patients have not been established.

ADVERSE REACTIONS
Frequently Observed
The most frequently reported adverse reactions are drowsiness, lightheadedness, dizziness, sedation, shortness of breath, nausea, vomiting, abdominal pain, and intoxicated feeling.

Infrequently Observed
All adverse events tabulated below are classified as infrequent.
Central Nervous: headache, shaky feeling, tingling, agitation, fainting, fatigue, heavy eyelids, high energy, hot spells, numbness, sluggishness, seizure. Mental confusion, excitement or depression can also occur due to intolerance, particularly in elderly or debilitated patients, or due to overdosage of butalbital.
Autonomic Nervous: dry mouth, hyperhidrosis.
Gastrointestinal: difficulty swallowing, heartburn, flatulence, constipation.
Cardiovascular: tachycardia.
Musculoskeletal: leg pain, muscle fatigue.
Genitourinary: diuresis.
Miscellaneous: pruritus, fever, earache, nasal congestion, tinnitus, euphoria, allergic reactions.
Several cases of dermatological reactions, including toxic epidermal necrolysis and erythema multiforme, have been reported.
The following adverse drug events may be borne in mind as potential effects of the components of this product. Potential effects of high dosage are listed in the *OVERDOSAGE* section.
Acetaminophen: allergic reactions, rash, thrombocytopenia, agranulocytosis.
Caffeine: cardiac stimulation, irritability, tremor, dependence, nephrotoxicity, hyperglycemia.

DRUG ABUSE AND DEPENDENCE
Abuse and Dependence
Butalbital
Barbiturates may be habit-forming: Tolerance, psychological dependence, and physical dependence may occur especially following prolonged use of high doses of barbiturates. The average daily dose for the barbiturate addict is usually about 1500 mg. As tolerance to barbiturates develops, the amount needed to maintain the same level of intoxication increases; tolerance to a fatal dosage, however, does not increase more than two-fold. As this occurs, the margin between an intoxication dosage and fatal dosage becomes smaller. The lethal dose of a barbiturate is far less if alcohol is also ingested. Major withdrawal symptoms (convulsions and delirium) may occur within 16 hours and last up to 5 days after abrupt cessation of these drugs. Intensity of withdrawal symptoms gradually declines over a period of approximately 15 days. Treatment of barbiturate dependence consists of cautious and gradual withdrawal of the drug. Barbiturate-dependent patients can be withdrawn by using a number of different withdrawal regimens. One method involves initiating treatment at the patient's regular dosage level and gradually decreasing the daily dosage as tolerated by the patient.

OVERDOSAGE
Following an acute overdosage of butalbital, acetaminophen and caffeine, toxicity may result from the barbiturate or the acetaminophen. Toxicity due to caffeine is less likely, due to the relatively small amounts in this formulation.

Signs and Symptoms
Toxicity from *barbiturate* poisoning include drowsiness, confusion, and coma; respiratory depression; hypotension; and hypovolemic shock.
In *acetaminophen* overdosage: dose-dependent, potentially fatal hepatic necrosis is the most serious adverse effect. Renal tubular necroses, hypoglycemic coma and thrombocytopenia may also occur. Early symptoms following a potentially hepatotoxic overdose may include: nausea, vomiting, diaphoresis and general malaise. Clinical and laboratory evidence of hepatic toxicity may not be apparent until 48 to 72 hours post-ingestion. In adults hepatic toxicity has rarely been reported with acute overdoses of less than 10 grams, or fatalities with less than 15 grams.
Acute *caffeine* poisoning may cause insomnia, restlessness, tremor, and delirium, tachycardia and extrasystoles.

Treatment
A single or multiple overdose with this combination product is a potentially lethal polydrug overdose, and consultation with a regional poison control center is recommended. Immediate treatment includes support of cardiorespiratory function and measures to reduce drug absorption. Vomiting should be induced mechanically, or with syrup of ipecac, if the patient is alert (adequate pharyngeal and laryngeal reflexes). Oral activated charcoal (1 g/kg) should follow gastric emptying. The first dose should be accompanied by an appro-

priate cathartic. If repeated doses are used, the cathartic might be included with alternate doses as required. Hypotension is usually hypovolemic and should respond to fluids. Pressors should be avoided. A cuffed endotracheal tube should be inserted before gastric lavage of the unconscious patient and, when necessary, to provide assisted respiration. If renal function is normal, forced diuresis may aid in the elimination of the barbiturate. Alkalinization of the urine increases renal excretion of some barbiturates, especially phenobarbital.

Meticulous attention should be given to maintaining adequate pulmonary ventilation. In severe cases of intoxication, peritoneal dialysis,. or preferably hemodialysis may be considered. If hypoprothrombinemia occurs due to acetaminophen overdose, vitamin K should be administered intravenously.

If the dose of acetaminophen may have exceeded 140 mg/kg, acetylcysteine should be administered as early as possible. Serum acetaminophen levels should be obtained, since levels four or more hours following ingestion help predict acetaminophen toxicity. Do not await acetaminophen assay results before initiating treatment. Hepatic enzymes should be obtained initially, and repeated at 24-hour intervals. Methemoglobinemia over 30% should be treated with methylene blue by slow intravenous administration.

Toxic Doses (for adults)

Butalbital:	toxic dose	1.0 g	(20 tablets)
Acetaminophen:	toxic dose	10.0 g	(30 tablets)
Caffeine:	toxic dose	1.0 g	(25 tablets)

DOSAGE AND ADMINISTRATION

One or 2 tablets every 4 hours as needed. Total daily dosage should not exceed 6 tablets.

Extended and repeated use of this product is not recommended because of the potential for physical dependence.

HOW SUPPLIED

Fioricet®

(Butalbital, Acetaminophen, and Caffeine Tablets, USP)

Containing 50 mg butalbital, 325 mg acetaminophen, and 40 mg caffeine. Available as light-blue, round compressed tablets, engraved "FIORICET" and "△" on one side, three-head profile "⟨⟨⟨⟩⟩" on other side. Bottles of 100 (NDC 0078-0084-05) and 500 (NDC 0078-0084-08).

SandoPak® (unit-dose) packages of 100, 10 blister strips of 10 tablets (NDC 0078-0084-06).

Store and Dispense

Store below 86°F (30°C); dispense in a tight container.
[REV: MARCH 1996   30131903]
Shown in Product Identification Guide, page 332

FIORICET® with CODEINE   Ⓒ℞

[fē -ōr' ĭ-set]
(butalbital, acetaminophen, caffeine, and codeine phosphate)
Capsules

Caution: Federal law prohibits dispensing without prescription.

The following prescribing information is based on official labeling in effect on August 1, 1996.

DESCRIPTION

Fioricet® with Codeine (butalbital, acetaminophen, caffeine, and codeine phosphate) is supplied in capsule form for oral administration.

Each capsule contains:

codeine phosphate, USP .... 30 mg (½ gr)
　Warning: May be habit-forming.
butalbital, USP .... 50 mg
　Warning: May be habit-forming.
caffeine, USP .... 40 mg
acetaminophen, USP .... 325 mg

Codeine phosphate [morphine-3-methyl ether phosphate (1:1) (salt) hemihydrate, $C_{18}H_{24}NO_7P$, anhydrous mw 397.37], a white crystalline powder, is a narcotic analgesic and antitussive.

Butalbital (5-allyl-5-isobutylbarbituric acid, $C_{11}H_{16}N_2O_3$, mw 224.26), a slightly bitter, white crystalline powder, is a short-to intermediate-acting barbiturate.

Caffeine (1,3,7-trimethylxanthine, $C_8H_{10}N_4O_2$, mw 194.19), a bitter, white crystalline powder, is a central nervous system stimulant.

Acetaminophen (4'-hydroxyacetanilide, $C_8H_9NO_2$, mw 151.16), a slightly bitter white crystalline powder, is a non-opiate, non-salicylate analgesic and antipyretic.

Active Ingredients: codeine phosphate, USP, butalbital, USP, caffeine, USP, and acetaminophen, USP.

Inactive Ingredients: black iron oxide, colloidal silicon dioxide, D&C Red #7 (calcium lake), D&C Red #33, FD&C Blue #1, FD&C Blue #1 (aluminum lake), gelatin, magnesium stearate, pregelatinized starch, red iron oxide, sodium lauryl sulfate, and titanium dioxide.

May also include: benzyl alcohol, butylparaben, carboxymethylcellulose sodium, edetate calcium disodium, methylparaben, propylparaben, silicon dioxide, and sodium propionate.

CLINICAL PHARMACOLOGY

Fioricet® with Codeine is a combination drug product intended as a treatment for tension headache.

Fioricet® consists of a fixed combination of butalbital 50 mg, acetaminophen 325 mg and caffeine 40 mg. The role each component plays in the relief of the complex of symptoms known as tension headache is incompletely understood.

Pharmacokinetics

The behavior of the individual components is described below.

Codeine

Codeine is readily absorbed from the gastrointestinal tract. It is rapidly distributed from the intravascular spaces to the various body tissues, with preferential uptake by parenchymatous organs such as the liver, spleen and kidney. Codeine crosses the blood-brain barrier, and is found in fetal tissue and breast milk. The plasma concentration does not correlate with brain concentration or relief of pain; however, codeine is not bound to plasma proteins and does not accumulate in body tissues.

The plasma half-life is about 2.9 hours. The elimination of codeine is primarily via the kidneys, and about 90% of an oral dose is excreted by the kidneys within 24 hours of dosing. The urinary secretion products consist of free and glucuronide conjugated codeine (about 70%), free and conjugated norcodeine (about 10%), free and conjugated morphine (about 10%), normorphine (4%), and hydrocodone (1%). The remainder of the dose is excreted in the feces.

At therapeutic doses, the analgesic effect reaches a peak within 2 hours and persists between 4 and 6 hours.

See *OVERDOSAGE* for toxicity information.

Butalbital

Butalbital is well absorbed from the gastrointestinal tract and is expected to distribute to most tissues in the body. Barbiturates in general may appear in breast milk and readily cross the placental barrier. They are bound to plasma and tissue proteins to a varying degree and binding increases directly as a function of lipid solubility.

Elimination of butalbital is primarily via the kidney (59%–88% of the dose) as unchanged drug or metabolites. The plasma half-life is about 35 hours. Urinary excretion products include parent drug (about 3.6% of the dose), 5-isobutyl-5-(2,3-dihydroxypropyl) barbituric acid (about 24% of the dose), 5-allyl-5(3-hydroxy-2-methyl-1-propyl) barbituric acid (about 4.8% of the dose), products with the barbituric acid ring hydrolyzed with excretion of urea (about 14% of the dose), as well as unidentified materials. Of the material excreted in the urine, 32% is conjugated.

See *OVERDOSAGE* for toxicity information.

Caffeine

Like most xanthines, caffeine is rapidly absorbed and distributed in all body tissues and fluids, including the CNS, fetal tissues, and breast milk.

Caffeine is cleared through metabolism and excretion in the urine. The plasma half-life is about 3 hours. Hepatic biotransformation prior to excretion results in about equal amounts of 1-methyl-xanthine and 1-methyluric acid. Of the 70% of the dose that is recovered in the urine, only 3% is unchanged drug.

See *OVERDOSAGE* for toxicity information.

Acetaminophen

Acetaminophen is rapidly absorbed from the gastrointestinal tract and is distributed throughout most body tissues. The plasma half-life is 1.25–3 hours, but may be increased by liver damage and following overdosage. Elimination of acetaminophen is principally by liver metabolism (conjugation) and subsequent renal excretion of metabolites. Approximately 85% of an oral dose appears in the urine within 24 hours of administration, most as the glucuronide conjugate, with small amounts of other conjugates and unchanged drug.

See *OVERDOSAGE* for toxicity information.

INDICATIONS

Fioricet® with Codeine is indicated for the relief of the symptom complex of tension (or muscle contraction) headache.

Evidence supporting the efficacy and safety of Fioricet® with Codeine in the treatment of multiple recurrent headaches is unavailable. Caution in this regard is required because codeine and butalbital are habit-forming and potentially abusable.

CONTRAINDICATIONS

Fioricet® with Codeine is contraindicated under the following conditions:

—Hypersensitivity or intolerance to acetaminophen, caffeine, butalbital, or codeine.

—Patients with porphyria.

WARNINGS

In the presence of head injury or other intracranial lesions, the respiratory depressant effects of codeine and other narcotics may be markedly enhanced, as well as their capacity for elevating cerebrospinal fluid pressure. Narcotics also produce other CNS depressant effects, such as drowsiness, that may further obscure the clinical course of the patients with head injuries.

Codeine or other narcotics may obscure signs on which to judge the diagnosis or clinical course of patients with acute abdominal conditions.

Butalbital and codeine are both habit-forming and potentially abusable. Consequently, the extended use of Fioricet® with Codeine is not recommended.

PRECAUTIONS

General

Fioricet® with Codeine should be prescribed with caution in certain special-risk patients such as the elderly or debilitated, and those with severe impairment of renal or hepatic function, head injuries, elevated intracranial pressure, acute abdominal conditions, hypothyroidism, urethral stricture, Addison's disease, or prostatic hypertrophy.

Information for Patients

Fioricet® with Codeine may impair mental and/or physical abilities required for the performance of potentially hazardous tasks such as driving a car or operating machinery. Such tasks should be avoided while taking Fioricet® with Codeine.

Alcohol and other CNS depressants may produce an additive CNS depression, when taken with Fioricet® with Codeine, and should be avoided.

Codeine and butalbital may be habit-forming. Patients should take the drug only for as long as it is prescribed, in the amounts prescribed, and no more frequently than prescribed.

Laboratory Tests

In patients with severe hepatic or renal disease, effects of therapy should be monitored with serial liver and/or renal function tests.

Drug Interactions

The CNS effects of butalbital may be enhanced by monoamine oxidase (MAO) inhibitors.

Fioricet® with Codeine may enhance the effects of:

—Other narcotic analgesics, alcohol, general anesthetics, tranquilizers such as chlordiazepoxide, sedative-hypnotics, or other CNS depressants, causing increased CNS depression.

Drug/Laboratory Test Interactions

Codeine

Codeine may increase serum amylase levels.

Acetaminophen

Acetaminophen may produce false-positive test results for urinary 5-hydroxyindoleacetic acid.

Carcinogenesis, Mutagenesis, Impairment of Fertility

No adequate studies have been conducted in animals to determine whether acetaminophen, codeine and butalbital have a potential for carcinogenesis or mutagenesis. No adequate studies have been conducted in animals to determine whether acetaminophen and butalbital have a potential for impairment of fertility.

Pregnancy

Teratogenic Effects

Pregnancy Category C: Animal reproduction studies have not been conducted with Fioricet® with Codeine. It is also not known whether Fioricet® with Codeine can cause fetal harm when administered to a pregnant woman or can affect reproduction capacity. Fioricet® with Codeine should be given to a pregnant woman only when clearly needed.

Nonteratogenic Effects

Withdrawal seizures were reported in a two-day-old male infant whose mother had taken a butalbital-containing drug during the last 2 months of pregnancy. Butalbital was found in the infant's serum. The infant was given phenobarbital 5 mg/kg, which was tapered without further seizure or other withdrawal symptoms.

Labor and Delivery

Use of codeine during labor may lead to respiratory depression in the neonate.

Nursing Mothers

Caffeine, barbiturates, acetaminophen and codeine are excreted in breast milk in small amounts, but the significance of their effects on nursing infants is not known. Because of potential for serious adverse reactions in nursing infants from Fioricet® with Codeine (butalbital, acetaminophen, caffeine, and codeine phosphate), a decision should be made whether to discontinue nursing or to discontinue the drug, taking into account the importance of the drug to the mother.

Pediatric Use

Safety and effectiveness in children below the age of 12 have not been established.

Continued on next page

Sandoz—Cont.

ADVERSE REACTIONS

Frequently Observed
The most frequently reported adverse reactions are drowsiness, lightheadedness, dizziness, sedation, shortness of breath, nausea, vomiting, abdominal pain, and intoxicated feeling.

Infrequently Observed
All adverse events tabulated below are classified as infrequent.
Central Nervous: headache, shaky feeling, tingling, agitation, fainting, fatigue, heavy eyelids, high energy, hot spells, numbness, sluggishness, seizure. Mental confusion, excitement or depression can also occur due to intolerance, particularly in elderly or debilitated patients, or due to overdosage of butalbital.
Autonomic Nervous: dry mouth, hyperhidrosis.
Gastrointestinal: difficulty swallowing, heartburn, flatulence, constipation.
Cardiovascular: tachycardia.
Musculoskeletal: leg pain, muscle fatigue.
Genitourinary: diuresis.
Miscellaneous: pruritus, fever, earache, nasal congestion, tinnitus, euphoria, allergic reactions.
The following adverse reactions have been voluntarily reported as temporally associated with Fiorinal® with Codeine, a related product containing aspirin, butalbital, caffeine, and codeine.
Central Nervous: abuse, addiction, anxiety, disorientation, hallucination, hyperactivity, insomnia, libido decrease, nervousness, neuropathy, psychosis, sexual activity increase, slurred speech, twitching, unconsciousness, vertigo.
Autonomic Nervous: epistaxis, flushing, miosis, salivation.
Gastrointestinal: anorexia, appetite increased, diarrhea, esophagitis, gastroenteritis, gastrointestinal spasms, hiccup, mouth burning, pyloric ulcer.
Cardiovascular: chest pain, hypotensive reaction, palpitations, syncope.
Skin: erythema, erythema multiforme, exfoliative dermatitis, hives, rash, toxic epidermal necrolysis.
Urinary: kidney impairment, urinary difficulty.
Miscellaneous: allergic reaction, anaphylactic shock, cholangiocarcinoma, drug interaction with erythromycin (stomach upset), edema.
The following adverse drug events may be borne in mind as potential effects of the components of Fioricet® with Codeine. Potential effects of high dosage are listed in the OVERDOSAGE section.
Acetaminophen: allergic reactions, rash, thrombocytopenia, agranulocytosis.
Caffeine: cardiac stimulation, irritability, tremor, dependence, nephrotoxicity, hyperglycemia.
Codeine: nausea, vomiting, drowsiness, lightheadedness, constipation, pruritus.
Several cases of dermatological reactions, including toxic epidermal necrolysis and erythema multiforme, have been reported for Fioricet® (Butalbital, Acetaminophen, and Caffeine Tablets, USP).

DRUG ABUSE AND DEPENDENCE

Controlled Substance
Fioricet® with Codeine is controlled by the Drug Enforcement Administration and is classified under Schedule III.
Abuse and Dependence
Codeine
Codeine can produce drug dependence of the morphine type and, therefore, has the potential for being abused. Psychological dependence, physical dependence, and tolerance may develop upon repeated administration and it should be prescribed and administered with the same degree of caution appropriate to the use of other oral narcotic medications.
Butalbital
Barbiturates may be habit-forming: Tolerance, psychological dependence, and physical dependence may occur especially following prolonged use of high doses of barbiturates. The average daily dose for the barbiturate addict is usually about 1,500 mg. As tolerance to barbiturates develops, the amount needed to maintain the same level of intoxication increases; tolerance to a fatal dosage, however, does not increase more than two-fold. As this occurs, the margin between an intoxication dosage and fatal dosage becomes smaller. The lethal dose of a barbiturate is far less if alcohol is also ingested. Major withdrawal symptoms (convulsions and delirium) may occur within 16 hours and last up to 5 days after abrupt cessation of these drugs. Intensity of withdrawal symptoms gradually declines over a period of approximately 15 days. Treatment of barbiturate dependence consists of cautious and gradual withdrawal of the drug. Barbiturate-dependent patients can be withdrawn by using a number of different withdrawal regimens. One method involves initiating treatment at the patient's regular dosage level and gradually decreasing the daily dosage as tolerated by the patient.

OVERDOSAGE

Following an acute overdosage of Fioricet® with Codeine, toxicity may result from the barbiturate, the codeine, or the acetaminophen. Toxicity due to the caffeine is less likely, due to the relatively small amounts in this formulation.
Signs and Symptoms
Toxicity from *barbiturate* poisoning include drowsiness, confusion, and coma; respiratory depression; hypotension; and hypovolemic shock. Toxicity from *codeine* poisoning includes the opioid triad of: pinpoint pupils, depression of respiration, and loss of consciousness. Convulsions may occur. In *acetaminophen* overdosage: dose-dependent, potentially fatal hepatic necrosis is the most serious adverse effect. Renal tubular necroses, hypoglycemic coma, and thrombocytopenia may also occur. Early symptoms following a potentially hepatotoxic overdose may include: nausea, vomiting, diaphoresis, and general malaise. Clinical and laboratory evidence of hepatic toxicity may not be apparent until 48–72 hours post-ingestion. In adults hepatic toxicity has rarely been reported with acute overdoses of less than 10 grams, or fatalities with less than 15 grams. Acute *caffeine* poisoning may cause insomnia, restlessness, tremor, and delirium, tachycardia, and extrasystoles.
Treatment
A single or multiple overdose with Fioricet® with Codeine is a potentially lethal polydrug overdose, and consultation with a regional poison control center is recommended. Immediate treatment includes support of cardiorespiratory function and measures to reduce drug absorption. Vomiting should be induced mechanically, or with syrup of ipecac, if the patient is alert (adequate pharyngeal and laryngeal reflexes). Oral activated charcoal (1 g/kg) should follow gastric emptying. The first dose should be accompanied by an appropriate cathartic. If repeated doses are used, the cathartic might be included with alternate doses as required. Hypotension is usually hypovolemic and should respond to fluids. Pressors should be avoided. A cuffed endotracheal tube should be inserted before gastric lavage of the unconscious patient and, when necessary, to provide assisted respiration. If renal function is normal, forced diuresis may aid in the elimination of the barbiturate. Alkalinization of the urine increases renal excretion of some barbiturates, especially phenobarbital.
Meticulous attention should be given to maintaining adequate pulmonary ventilation. In severe cases of intoxication, peritoneal dialysis, or preferably hemodialysis may be considered. If hypoprothrombinemia occurs due to acetaminophen overdose, vitamin K should be administered intravenously.
Naloxone, a narcotic antagonist, can reverse respiratory depression and coma associated with opioid overdose. Naloxone 0.4–2 mg is given parenterally. Since the duration of action of codeine may exceed that of the naloxone, the patient should be kept under continuous surveillance and repeated doses of the antagonist should be administered as needed to maintain adequate respiration. A narcotic antagonist should not be administered in the absence of clinically significant respiratory or cardiovascular depression.
If the dose of acetaminophen may have exceeded 140 mg/kg, N-acetyl-cysteine should be administered as early as possible. Serum acetaminophen levels should be obtained, since levels 4 or more hours following ingestion help predict acetaminophen toxicity. Do not await acetaminophen assay results before initiating treatment. Hepatic enzymes should be obtained initially, and repeated at 24-hour intervals. Methemoglobinemia over 30% should be treated with methylene blue by slow intravenous administration.

Toxic doses (for adults)

Butalbital:	toxic dose 1.0 g	
	(20 capsules of Fioricet® with Codeine)	
Acetaminophen:	toxic dose 10 g	
	(30 capsules of Fioricet® with Codeine)	
Caffeine:	toxic dose 1.0 g	
	(25 capsules of Fioricet® with Codeine)	
Codeine:	toxic dose 240 mg	
	(8 capsules of Fioricet® with Codeine)	

DOSAGE AND ADMINISTRATION
One or 2 capsules every 4 hours. Total daily dosage should not exceed 6 capsules.
Extended and repeated use of this product is not recommended because of the potential for physical dependence.

HOW SUPPLIED
Fioricet® with Codeine Capsules
Dark blue, opaque cap with a grey, opaque body. Cap is imprinted twice in light-blue with "FIORICET" and "CODEINE". Body is imprinted twice with four-head profile " 〰️ "in red.
Bottle of 100 (NDC 0078-0243-05)
ControlPak® unit-dose package of 25; continuous reverse-numbered roll of sealed blisters (NDC 0078-0243-13).

Store and Dispense
Below 86°F (30°C); tight container.
[REV: APRIL 1993   30132901]
Shown in Product Identification Guide, page 333

FIORINAL®   Ⓒ Ⅲ ℞
(butalbital, aspirin, and caffeine)
Tablets/Capsules, USP

Caution: Federal law prohibits dispensing without prescription.
The following information is based on official labeling in effect on August 1, 1996.

DESCRIPTION
Each Fiorinal® (butalbital, aspirin, and caffeine) Tablet/Capsule for oral administration contains: butalbital, USP, 50 mg (Warning: May be habit-forming); aspirin, USP, 325 mg; caffeine, USP, 40 mg.
Butalbital, 5-allyl-5-isobutyl-barbituric acid, has an empirical formula of $C_{11}H_{16}N_2O_3$ and a molecular weight of 224.26.
Aspirin, benzoic acid, 2-(acetyloxy)-, has an empirical formula of $C_9H_8O_4$ and a molecular weight of 180.16.
Caffeine, 1, 3, 7-trimethylxanthine, has an empirical formula of $C_8H_{10}N_4O_2$ and a molecular weight of 194.19.
Tablets
Active Ingredients: aspirin, USP, butalbital, USP, and caffeine, USP.
Inactive Ingredients: alginic acid, lactose, microcrystalline cellulose, povidone, stearic acid, and another ingredient.
Capsules
Active Ingredients: aspirin, USP, butalbital, USP, and caffeine, USP.
Inactive Ingredients: D&C Yellow #10, gelatin, microcrystalline cellulose, sodium lauryl sulfate, starch, and talc.
May Also Include: benzyl alcohol, butylparaben, color additives including FD&C Blue #1, FD&C Green #3, FD&C Yellow #6, edetate calcium disodium, methylparaben, propylparaben, silicon dioxide, and sodium propionate.

CLINICAL PHARMACOLOGY
Pharmacologically, Fiorinal® (butalbital, aspirin, and caffeine) combines the analgesic properties of aspirin with the anxiolytic and muscle relaxant properties of butalbital.
The clinical effectiveness of Fiorinal® (butalbital, aspirin, and caffeine) in tension headache has been established in double-blind, placebo-controlled, multi-clinic trials. A factorial design study compared Fiorinal® (butalbital, aspirin, and caffeine) with each of its major components. This study demonstrated that each component contributes to the efficacy of Fiorinal® (butalbital, aspirin, and caffeine) in the treatment of the target symptoms of tension headache (headache pain, psychic tension, and muscle contraction in the head, neck, and shoulder region). For each symptom and the symptom complex as a whole, Fiorinal® (butalbital, aspirin, and caffeine) was shown to have significantly superior clinical effects to either component alone.
Pharmacokinetics
The behavior of the individual components is described below.
Aspirin
The systemic availability of aspirin after an oral dose is highly dependent on the dosage form, the presence of food, the gastric emptying time, gastric pH, antacids, buffering agents, and particle size. These factors affect not necessarily the extent of absorption of total salicylates but more the stability of aspirin prior to absorption.
During the absorption process and after absorption, aspirin is mainly hydrolyzed to salicylic acid and distributed to all body tissues and fluids, including fetal tissues, breast milk, and the central nervous system (CNS). Highest concentrations are found in plasma, liver, renal cortex, heart, and lung. In plasma, about 50%–80% of the salicylic acid and its metabolites are loosely bound to plasma proteins.
The clearance of total salicylates is subject to saturable kinetics; however, first-order elimination kinetics are still a good approximation for doses up to 650 mg. The plasma half-life for aspirin is about 12 minutes and for salicylic acid and/or total salicylates is about 3.0 hours.
The elimination of therapeutic doses is through the kidneys either as salicylic acid or other biotransformation products. The renal clearance is greatly augmented by an alkaline urine as is produced by concurrent administration of sodium bicarbonate or potassium citrate.
The biotransformation of aspirin occurs primarily in the hepatocytes. The major metabolites are salicyluric acid (75%), the phenolic and acyl glucuronides of salicylate (15%), and gentisic and gentisuric acid (1%). The bioavailability of the aspirin component of Fiorinal® (butalbital, aspirin, and caffeine) is equivalent to that of a solution except for a slower rate of absorption. A peak concentration of 8.80 µg/mL was obtained at 40 minutes after a 650 mg dose.
See *OVERDOSAGE* for toxicity information.

Butalbital
Butalbital is well absorbed from the gastrointestinal tract and is expected to distribute to most of the tissues in the body. Barbiturates, in general, may appear in breast milk and readily cross the placental barrier. They are bound to plasma and tissue proteins to a varying degree and binding increases directly as a function of lipid solubility.
Elimination of butalbital is primarily via the kidney (59%–88% of the dose) as unchanged drug or metabolites. The plasma half-life is about 35 hours. Urinary excretion products included parent drug (about 3.6% of the dose), 5-isobutyl-5-(2,3-dihydroxypropyl) barbituric acid (about 24% of the dose), 5-allyl-5(3-hydroxy-2-methyl-1-propyl) barbituric acid (about 4.8% of the dose), products with the barbituric acid ring hydrolyzed with excretion of urea (about 14% of the dose), as well as unidentified materials. Of the material excreted in the urine, 32% was conjugated.
The bioavailability of the butalbital component of Fiorinal® (butalbital, aspirin, and caffeine) is equivalent to that of a solution except for a decrease in the rate of absorption. A peak concentration of 2020 ng/mL is obtained at about 1.5 hours after a 100 mg dose.
The *in vitro* plasma protein binding of butalbital is 45% over the concentration range of 0.5–20 μg/mL. This falls within the range of plasma protein binding (20%–45%) reported with other barbiturates such as phenobarbital, pentobarbital, and secobarbital sodium. The plasma-to-blood concentration ratio was almost unity indicating that there is no preferential distribution of butalbital into either plasma or blood cells.
See *OVERDOSAGE* for toxicity information.

Caffeine
Like most xanthines, caffeine is rapidly absorbed and distributed in all body tissues and fluids, including the CNS, fetal tissues, and breast milk.
Caffeine is cleared rapidly through metabolism and excretion in the urine. The plasma half-life is about 3.0 hours. Hepatic biotransformation prior to excretion results in about equal amounts of 1-methyl-xanthine and 1-methyluric acid. Of the 70% of the dose that has been recovered in the urine, only 3% was unchanged drug.
The bioavailability of the caffeine component for Fiorinal® (butalbital, aspirin, and caffeine) is equivalent to that of a solution except for a slightly longer time to peak. A peak concentration of 1660 ng/mL was obtained in less than an hour for an 80 mg dose.
See *OVERDOSAGE* for toxicity information.

INDICATIONS
Fiorinal® (butalbital, aspirin, and caffeine) is indicated for the relief of the symptom complex of tension (or muscle contraction) headache. Evidence supporting the efficacy and safety of Fiorinal® (butalbital, aspirin, and caffeine) in the treatment of multiple recurrent headaches is unavailable. Caution in this regard is required because butalbital is habit-forming and potentially abusable.

CONTRAINDICATIONS
Fiorinal® (butalbital, aspirin, and caffeine) is contraindicated under the following conditions:
1. Hypersensitivity or intolerance to aspirin, caffeine, or butalbital.
2. Patients with a hemorrhagic diathesis (e.g., hemophilia, hypoprothrombinemia, von Willebrand's disease, the thrombocytopenias, thrombasthenia and other ill-defined hereditary platelet dysfunctions, severe vitamin K deficiency and severe liver damage).
3. Patients with the syndrome of nasal polyps, angioedema and bronchospastic reactivity to aspirin or other nonsteroidal anti-inflammatory drugs. Anaphylactoid reactions have occurred in such patients.
4. Peptic ulcer or other serious gastrointestinal lesions.
5. Patients with porphyria.

WARNINGS
Therapeutic doses of aspirin can cause anaphylactic shock and other severe allergic reactions. It should be ascertained if the patient is allergic to aspirin, although a specific history of allergy may be lacking.
Significant bleeding can result from aspirin therapy in patients with peptic ulcer or other gastrointestinal lesions, and in patients with bleeding disorders. Aspirin administered preoperatively may prolong the bleeding time. Butalbital is habit-forming and potentially abusable. Consequently, the extended use of Fiorinal® (butalbital, aspirin, and caffeine) is not recommended. Results from epidemiologic studies indicate an association between aspirin and Reye's Syndrome. Caution should be used in administering this product to children, including teenagers, with chicken pox or flu.

PRECAUTIONS
General
Fiorinal® (butalbital, aspirin, and caffeine) should be prescribed with caution for certain special-risk patients such as the elderly or debilitated, and those with severe impairment of renal or hepatic function, coagulation disorders, head injuries, elevated intracranial pressure, acute abdominal conditions, hypothyroidism, urethral stricture, Addison's disease, or prostatic hypertrophy.
Aspirin should be used with caution in patients on anticoagulant therapy and in patients with underlying hemostatic defects, and extreme caution in the presence of peptic ulcer.
Precautions should be taken when administering salicylates to persons with known allergies. Hypersensitivity to aspirin is particularly likely in patients with nasal polyps, and relatively common in those with asthma.

Information for Patients
Patients should be informed that Fiorinal® (butalbital, aspirin, and caffeine) contains aspirin and should not be taken by patients with an aspirin allergy.
Fiorinal® (butalbital, aspirin, and caffeine) may impair the mental and/or physical abilities required for performance of potentially hazardous tasks such as driving a car or operating machinery. Such tasks should be avoided while taking Fiorinal® (butalbital, aspirin, and caffeine).
Alcohol and other CNS depressants may produce an additive CNS depression when taken with Fiorinal® (butalbital, aspirin, and caffeine) and should be avoided.
Butalbital may be habit-forming. Patients should take the drug only for as long as it is prescribed, in the amounts prescribed, and no more frequently than prescribed.

Laboratory Tests
In patients with severe hepatic or renal disease, effects of therapy should be monitored with serial liver and/or renal function tests.

Drug Interactions
The CNS effects of butalbital may be enhanced by monoamine oxidase (MAO) inhibitors.
In patients receiving concomitant corticosteroids and chronic use of aspirin, withdrawal of corticosteroids may result in salicylism because corticosteroids enhance renal clearance of salicylates and their withdrawal is followed by return to normal rates of renal clearance.
Fiorinal® (butalbital, aspirin, and caffeine) may enhance the effects of:
1. Oral anticoagulants, causing bleeding by inhibiting prothrombin formation in the liver and displacing anticoagulants from plasma protein binding sites.
2. Oral antidiabetic agents and insulin, causing hypoglycemia by contributing an additive effect, if dosage of Fiorinal® (butalbital, aspirin, and caffeine) exceeds maximum recommended daily dosage.
3. 6-mercaptopurine and methotrexate, causing bone marrow toxicity and blood dyscrasias by displacing these drugs from secondary binding sites, and, in the case of methotrexate, also reducing its excretion.
4. Non-steroidal anti-inflammatory agents, increasing the risk of peptic ulceration and bleeding by contributing additive effects.
5. Other narcotic analgesics, alcohol, general anesthetics, tranquilizers such as chlordiazepoxide, sedative-hypnotics, or other CNS depressants, causing increased CNS depression.

Fiorinal® (butalbital, aspirin, and caffeine) may diminish the effects of:
Uricosuric agents such as probenecid and sulfinpyrazone, reducing their effectiveness in the treatment of gout. Aspirin competes with these agents for protein binding sites.

Drug/Laboratory Test Interactions
Aspirin: Aspirin may interfere with the following laboratory determinations in blood: serum amylase, fasting blood glucose, cholesterol, protein, serum glutamic-oxaloacetic transaminase (SGOT), uric acid, prothrombin time and bleeding time. Aspirin may interfere with the following laboratory determinations in urine: glucose, 5-hydroxyindoleacetic acid, Gerhardt ketone, vanillylmandelic acid (VMA), uric acid, diacetic acid, and spectrophotometric detection of barbiturates.

Carcinogenesis, Mutagenesis, Impairment of Fertility
Adequate long-term studies have been conducted in mice and rats with aspirin, alone or in combination with other drugs, in which no evidence of carcinogenesis was seen. No adequate studies have been conducted in animals to determine whether aspirin has a potential for mutagenesis or impairment of fertility. No adequate studies have been conducted in animals to determine whether butalbital has a potential for carcinogenesis, mutagenesis, or impairment of fertility.

Usage in Pregnancy
Teratogenic Effects:
Pregnancy Category C. Animal reproduction studies have not been conducted with Fiorinal® (butalbital, aspirin, and caffeine). It is also not known whether Fiorinal® (butalbital, aspirin, and caffeine) can cause fetal harm when administered to a pregnant woman or can affect reproduction capacity. Fiorinal® (butalbital, aspirin, and caffeine) should be given to a pregnant woman only when clearly needed.
Nonteratogenic Effects:
Withdrawal seizures were reported in a two-day-old male infant whose mother had taken a butalbital-containing drug during the last 2 months of pregnancy. Butalbital was found in the infant's serum. The infant was given phenobarbital 5mg/kg, which was tapered without further seizure or other withdrawal symptoms.
Studies of aspirin use in pregnant women have not shown that aspirin increases the risk of abnormalities when administered during the first trimester of pregnancy. In controlled studies involving 41,337 pregnant women and their offspring, there was no evidence that aspirin taken during pregnancy caused stillbirth, neonatal death or reduced birth weight. In controlled studies of 50,282 pregnant women and their offspring, aspirin administration in moderate and heavy doses during the first four lunar months of pregnancy showed no teratogenic effect.
Therapeutic doses of aspirin in pregnant women close to term may cause bleeding in mother, fetus, or neonate. During the last 6 months of pregnancy, regular use of aspirin in high doses may prolong pregnancy and delivery.

Labor and Delivery
Ingestion of aspirin prior to delivery may prolong delivery or lead to bleeding in the mother or neonate.

Nursing Mothers
Aspirin, caffeine, and barbiturates are excreted in breast milk in small amounts, but the significance of their effects on nursing infants is not known. Because of potential for serious adverse reactions in nursing infants from Fiorinal® (butalbital, aspirin, and caffeine), a decision should be made whether to discontinue nursing or to discontinue the drug, taking into account the importance of the drug to the mother.

Pediatric Use
Safety and effectiveness in pediatric patients have not been established.

ADVERSE REACTIONS
The most frequent adverse reactions are drowsiness and dizziness. Less frequent adverse reactions are lightheadedness and gastrointestinal disturbances including nausea, vomiting, and flatulence. A single incidence of bone marrow suppression has been reported with the use of Fiorinal® (butalbital, aspirin, and caffeine). Several cases of dermatological reactions including toxic epidermal necrolysis and erythema multiforme have been reported.

DRUG ABUSE AND DEPENDENCE
Controlled Substance
Fiorinal® (butalbital, aspirin, and caffeine) is controlled by the Drug Enforcement Administration and is classified under Schedule III.

Abuse and Dependence
Butalbital
Barbiturates may be habit-forming: Tolerance, psychological dependence, and physical dependence may occur especially following prolonged use of high doses of barbiturates. The average daily dose for the barbiturate addict is usually about 1,500 mg. As tolerance to barbiturates develops, the amount needed to maintain the same level of intoxication increases; tolerance to a fatal dosage, however, does not increase more than twofold. As this occurs, the margin between an intoxication dosage and fatal dosage becomes smaller. The lethal dose of a barbiturate is far less if alcohol is also ingested. Major withdrawal symptoms (convulsions and delirium) may occur within 16 hours and last up to 5 days after abrupt cessation of these drugs. Intensity of withdrawal symptoms gradually declines over a period of approximately 15 days. Treatment of barbiturate dependence consists of cautious and gradual withdrawal of the drug. Barbiturate-dependent patients can be withdrawn by using a number of different withdrawal regimens. One method involves initiating treatment at the patient's regular dosage level and gradually decreasing the daily dosage as tolerated by the patient.

OVERDOSAGE
The toxic effects of acute overdosage of Fiorinal® (butalbital, aspirin, and caffeine) are attributable mainly to its barbiturate component, and, to a lesser extent, aspirin. Because toxic effects of caffeine occur in very high dosages only, the possibility of significant caffeine toxicity from Fiorinal® (butalbital, aspirin, and caffeine) overdosage is unlikely.

Signs and Symptoms
Symptoms attributable to ***acute barbiturate poisoning*** include drowsiness, confusion, and coma; respiratory depression; hypotension; hypovolemic shock. Symptoms attributable to ***acute aspirin poisoning*** include hyperpnea; acid-base disturbances with development of metabolic acidosis; vomiting and abdominal pain; tinnitus; hyperthermia; hypoprothrombinemia; restlessness; delirium; convulsions. ***Acute caffeine poisoning*** may cause insomnia, restlessness, tremor, and delirium; tachycardia and extrasystoles.

Treatment
Treatment consists primarily of management of barbiturate intoxication and the correction of the acid-base imbalance due to salicylism. Vomiting should be induced mechanically or with emetics in the conscious patient. Gastric lavage may be used if the pharyngeal and laryngeal reflexes are present and if less than 4 hours have elapsed since ingestion. A cuffed endotracheal tube should be inserted before gastric

Continued on next page

Sandoz—Cont.

lavage of the unconscious patient and when necessary to provide assisted respiration. Diuresis, alkalinization of the urine, and correction of electrolyte disturbances should be accomplished through administration of intravenous fluids such as 1% sodium bicarbonate in 5% dextrose in water. Meticulous attention should be given to maintaining adequate pulmonary ventilation. The value of vasopressor agents such as Norepinephrine or Phenylephrine Hydrochloride in treating hypotension is questionable since they increase vasoconstriction and decrease blood flow. However, if prolonged support of blood pressure is required, Norepinephrine Bitartrate (Levophed®)* may be given I.V. with the usual precautions and serial blood pressure monitoring. In severe cases of intoxication, peritoneal dialysis, hemodialysis, or exchange transfusion may be lifesaving. Hypoprothrombinemia should be treated with Vitamin K, intravenously.

Up-to-date information about the treatment of overdose can often be obtained from a Certified Regional Poison Control Center. Telephone numbers of Certified Regional Poison Control Centers are listed in the Physicians' Desk Reference®.**

Toxic and Lethal Doses

Butalbital: toxic dose 1.0 g (20 tablets/capsules of Fiorinal®)

Aspirin: toxic blood level greater than 30 mg/100 mL; lethal dose 10-30 g

Caffeine: toxic dose 1.0 g (25 tablets/capsules of Fiorinal®)

DOSAGE AND ADMINISTRATION

One or 2 tablets or capsules every 4 hours. Total daily dose should not exceed 6 tablets or capsules.

Extended and repeated use of this product is not recommended because of the potential for physical dependence.

HOW SUPPLIED

Fiorinal® (butalbital, aspirin, and caffeine) Tablets/Capsules, USP

Tablets

White, round compressed tablet, engraved "FIORINAL" on one side, "SANDOZ" on other side.

Packages of 100 (NDC 0078-0104-05)
Packages of 1000 (NDC 0078-0104-09)
SandoPak® (unit-dose) package of 100 tablets individually blister-sealed (NDC 0078-0104-06)

Capsules

Bright kelly green cap with a lime green body, imprinted "FIORINAL 78-103" on each half of capsule.

Packages of 100 (NDC 0078-0103-05)
Packages of 500 (NDC 0078-0103-08)
ControlPak® package, 25 capsules (continuous reverse-numbered roll of sealed blisters) (NDC 0078-0103-13)

Store and Dispense

Below 77 °F (25 °C), tight container.

*Levophed is a registered Trademark of Sanofi Winthrop Pharmaceuticals.

**Trademark of Medical Economics Data Production Company.

[REV: FEBRUARY 1996 30130903]

Shown in Product Identification Guide, page 333

FIORINAL® with CODEINE ℂ℞

[fē-or'ĭ-nol]

(butalbital, aspirin, caffeine, and codeine phosphate)

Capsules, USP

CAUTION: Federal law prohibits dispensing without prescription.

The following prescribing information is based on official labeling in effect on August 1, 1996.

DESCRIPTION

Fiorinal® with Codeine (butalbital, aspirin, caffeine, and codeine phosphate) is supplied in capsule form for oral administration.

Each capsule contains:

codeine phosphate, USP ....30 mg (1/2 gr)
  Warning: May be habit-forming.
butalbital, USP ....50 mg
  Warning: May be habit-forming.
caffeine, USP ....40 mg
aspirin, USP ....325 mg

Codeine phosphate [morphine-3-methyl ether phosphate (1:1) (salt) hemihydrate. $C_{18}H_{24}NO_7P$, anhydrous mw 397.37], is a narcotic analgesic and antitussive.

Butalbital (5-allyl-5-isobutylbarbituric acid, $C_{11}H_{16}N_2O_3$, mw 224.26), is a short- to intermediate-acting barbiturate.

Caffeine (1,3,7-trimethylxanthine, $C_8H_{10}N_4O_2$, mw 194.19), is a central nervous stimulant.

Aspirin is benzoic acid, 2-*(acetyloxy)*-, $C_9H_8O_4$, mw 180.16, is an analgesic, antipyretic, anti-inflammatory.

Inactive Ingredients: D&C Yellow #10, FD&C Blue #1, FD&C Red #3, FD&C Yellow #6, gelatin, microcrystalline cellulose, sodium lauryl sulfate, starch, talc, titanium dioxide.

May Also Include: benzyl alcohol, butylparaben, edetate calcium disodium, glycerin, methylparaben, propylparaben, silicon dioxide, sodium propionate.

CLINICAL PHARMACOLOGY

Fiorinal® with Codeine (butalbital, aspirin, caffeine, and codeine phosphate) is a combination drug product intended as a treatment for tension headache.

Fiorinal® (butalbital, aspirin, and caffeine) consists of a fixed combination of caffeine 40 mg, butalbital 50 mg, and aspirin 325 mg. The role each component plays in the relief of the complex of symptoms known as tension headache is incompletely understood.

Pharmacokinetics

Bioavailability: The bioavailability of the components of the fixed combination of Fiorinal® with Codeine (butalbital, aspirin, caffeine, and codeine phosphate) is identical to their bioavailability when Fiorinal® (butalbital, aspirin, and caffeine) and Codeine are administered separately in equivalent molar doses.

The behavior of the individual components is described below.

Aspirin

The systemic availability of aspirin after an oral dose is highly dependent on the dosage form, the presence of food, the gastric emptying time, gastric pH, antacids, buffering agents, and particle size. These factors affect not necessarily the extent of absorption of total salicylates but more the stability of aspirin prior to absorption.

During the absorption process and after absorption, aspirin is mainly hydrolyzed to salicylic acid and distributed to all body tissues and fluids, including fetal tissues, breast milk, and the central nervous system (CNS). Highest concentrations are found in plasma, liver, renal cortex, heart, and lung. In plasma, about 50%-80% of the salicylic acid and its metabolites are loosely bound to plasma proteins.

The clearance of total salicylates is subject to saturable kinetics; however, first-order elimination kinetics are still a good approximation for doses up to 650 mg. The plasma half-life for aspirin is about 12 minutes and for salicylic acid and/or total salicylates is about 3.0 hours.

The elimination of therapeutic doses is through the kidneys either as salicylic acid or other biotransformation products. The renal clearance is greatly augmented by an alkaline urine as is produced by concurrent administration of sodium bicarbonate or potassium citrate.

The biotransformation of aspirin occurs primarily in the hepatocytes. The major metabolites are salicyluric acid (75%), the phenolic and acyl glucuronides of salicylate (15%), and gentisic and gentisuric acid (1%). The bioavailability of the aspirin component of Fiorinal® with Codeine (butalbital, aspirin, caffeine, and codeine phosphate) capsules is equivalent to that of a solution except for a slower rate of absorption. A peak concentration of 8.80 μg/mL was obtained at 40 minutes after a 650 mg dose.

See *OVERDOSAGE* for toxicity information.

Codeine

Codeine is readily absorbed from the gastrointestinal tract. It is rapidly distributed from the intravascular spaces to the various body tissues, with preferential uptake by parenchymatous organs such as the liver, spleen, and kidney. Codeine crosses the blood-brain barrier, and is found in fetal tissue and breast milk. The plasma concentration does not correlate with brain concentration or relief of pain, however, codeine is not bound to plasma proteins and does not accumulate in body tissues.

The plasma half-life is about 2.9 hours. The elimination of codeine is primarily via the kidneys, and about 90% of an oral dose is excreted by the kidneys within 24 hours of dosing. The urinary secretion products consist of free and glucuronide-conjugated codeine (about 70%), free and conjugated norcodeine (about 10%), free and conjugated morphine (about 10%), normorphine (4%), and hydrocodone (1%). The remainder of the dose is excreted in the feces.

At therapeutic doses, the analgesic effect reaches a peak within 2 hours and persists between 4 and 6 hours.

The bioavailability of the codeine component of Fiorinal® with Codeine (butalbital, aspirin, caffeine, and codeine phosphate) capsules is equivalent to that of a solution. Peak concentrations of 198 ng/mL were obtained at 1 hour after a 60 mg dose.

See *OVERDOSAGE* for toxicity information.

Butalbital

Butalbital is well absorbed from the gastrointestinal tract and is expected to distribute to most of the tissues in the body. Barbiturates, in general, may appear in breast milk and readily cross the placental barrier. They are bound to plasma and tissue proteins to a varying degree and binding increases directly as a function of lipid solubility.

Elimination of butalbital is primarily via the kidney (59%-88% of the dose) as unchanged drug or metabolites. The plasma half-life is about 35 hours. Urinary excretion products included parent drug (about 3.6% of the dose), 5-isobutyl-5-(2,3-dihydroxypropyl) barbituric acid (about 24% of the dose), 5-allyl-5(3-hydroxy-2-methyl-1-propyl) barbituric acid (about 4.8% of the dose), products with the barbituric acid ring hydrolyzed with excretion of urea (about 14% of the dose), as well as unidentified materials. Of the material excreted in the urine, 32% was conjugated.

The bioavailability of the butalbital component of Fiorinal® with Codeine (butalbital, aspirin, caffeine, and codeine phosphate) capsules is equivalent to that of a solution except for a decrease in the rate of absorption. A peak concentration of 2020 ng/mL is obtained at about 1.5 hours after a 100 mg dose.

The *in vitro* plasma protein binding of butalbital is 45% over the concentration range of 0.5–20 μg/mL. This falls within the range of plasma protein binding (20%–45%) reported with other barbiturates such as phenobarbital, pentobarbital, and secobarbital sodium. The plasma-to-blood concentration ratio was almost unity indicating that there is no preferential distribution of butalbital into either plasma or blood cells.

See *OVERDOSAGE* for toxicity information.

Caffeine

Like most xanthines, caffeine is rapidly absorbed and distributed in all body tissues and fluids, including the CNS, fetal tissues, and breast milk.

Caffeine is cleared rapidly through metabolism and excretion in the urine. The plasma half-life is about 3 hours. Hepatic biotransformation prior to excretion results in about equal amounts of 1-methyl-xanthine and 1-methyluric acid. Of the 70% of the dose that has been recovered in the urine, only 3% was unchanged drug.

The bioavailability of the caffeine component for Fiorinal® with Codeine (butalbital, aspirin, caffeine, and codeine phosphate) capsules is equivalent to that of a solution except for a slightly longer time to peak. A peak concentration of 1660 ng/mL was obtained in less than an hour for an 80 mg dose.

See *OVERDOSAGE* for toxicity information.

INDICATIONS

Fiorinal® with Codeine (butalbital, aspirin, caffeine, and codeine phosphate) is indicated for the relief of the symptom complex of tension (or muscle contraction) headache.

Evidence supporting the efficacy of Fiorinal® with Codeine (butalbital, aspirin, caffeine, and codeine phosphate) is derived from 2 multi-clinic trials that compared patients with tension headache randomly assigned to 4 parallel treatments: Fiorinal® with Codeine (butalbital, aspirin, caffeine, and codeine phosphate), codeine, Fiorinal® (butalbital, aspirin, and caffeine), and placebo. Response was assessed over the course of the first 4 hours of each of 2 distinct headaches, separated by at least 24 hours. Fiorinal® with Codeine (butalbital, aspirin, caffeine, and codeine phosphate) proved statistically significantly superior to each of its components (Fiorinal®, codeine) and to placebo on measures of pain relief.

Evidence supporting the efficacy and safety of Fiorinal® with Codeine (butalbital, aspirin, caffeine, and codeine phosphate) in the treatment of multiple recurrent headaches is unavailable. Caution in this regard is required because codeine and butalbital are habit-forming and potentially abusable.

CONTRAINDICATIONS

Fiorinal® with Codeine (butalbital, aspirin, caffeine, and codeine phosphate) is contraindicated under the following conditions:

1. Hypersensitivity or intolerance to aspirin, caffeine, butalbital or codeine.
2. Patients with a hemorrhagic diathesis (e.g., hemophilia, hypoprothrombinemia, von Willebrand's disease, the thrombocytopenias, thrombasthenia and other ill-defined hereditary platelet dysfunctions, severe vitamin K deficiency and severe liver damage.)
3. Patients with the syndrome of nasal polyps, angioedema and bronchospastic reactivity to aspirin or other non-steroidal anti-inflammatory drugs. Anaphylactoid reactions have occurred in such patients.
4. Peptic ulcer or other serious gastrointestinal lesions.
5. Patients with porphyria.

WARNINGS

Therapeutic doses of aspirin can cause anaphylactic shock and other severe allergic reactions. It should be ascertained if the patient is allergic to aspirin, although a specific history of allergy may be lacking.

Significant bleeding can result from aspirin therapy in patients with peptic ulcer or other gastrointestinal lesions, and in patients with bleeding disorders.

Aspirin administered pre-operatively may prolong the bleeding time.

In the presence of head injury or other intracranial lesions, the respiratory depressant effects of codeine and other narcotics may be markedly enhanced, as well as their capacity for elevating cerebrospinal fluid pressure. Narcotics also produce other CNS depressant effects, such as drowsiness, that may further obscure the clinical course of patients with head injuries.

Codeine or other narcotics may obscure signs on which to judge the diagnosis or clinical course of patients with acute abdominal conditions.

Butalbital and codeine are both habit-forming and potentially abusable. Consequently, the extended use of Fiorinal® with Codeine (butalbital, aspirin, caffeine, and codeine phosphate) is not recommended.

Results from epidemiologic studies indicate an association between aspirin and Reye's Syndrome. Caution should be used in administering this product to children, including teenagers, with chicken pox or flu.

PRECAUTIONS

General

Fiorinal® with Codeine, (butalbital, aspirin, caffeine, and codeine phosphate) should be prescribed with caution for certain special-risk patients such as the elderly or debilitated, and those with severe impairment of renal or hepatic function, coagulation disorders, or head injuries, elevated intracranial pressure, acute abdominal conditions, hypothyroidism, urethral stricture, Addison's disease, prostatic hypertrophy, and peptic ulcer.

Aspirin should be used with caution in patients on anticoagulant therapy and in patients with underlying hemostatic defects.

Precautions should be taken when administering salicylates to persons with known allergies. Hypersensitivity to aspirin is particularly likely in patients with nasal polyps, and relatively common in those with asthma.

Information for Patients

Patients should be informed that Fiorinal® with Codeine (butalbital, aspirin, caffeine, and codeine phosphate) contains aspirin and should not be taken by patients with an aspirin allergy.

Fiorinal® with Codeine (butalbital, aspirin, caffeine, and codeine phosphate) may impair the mental and/or physical abilities required for performance of potentially hazardous tasks such as driving a car or operating machinery. Such tasks should be avoided while taking Fiorinal® with Codeine (butalbital, aspirin, caffeine, and codeine phosphate).

Alcohol and other CNS depressants may produce an additive CNS depression when taken with Fiorinal® with Codeine (butalbital, aspirin, caffeine, and codeine phosphate), and should be avoided.

Codeine and butalbital may be habit-forming. Patients should take the drug only for as long as it is prescribed, in the amounts prescribed, and no more frequently than prescribed.

Laboratory Tests

In patients with severe hepatic or renal disease, effects of therapy should be monitored with serial liver and/or renal function tests.

Drug Interactions

The CNS effects of butalbital may be enhanced by monoamine oxidase (MAO) inhibitors.

In patients receiving concomitant corticosteroids and chronic use of aspirin, withdrawal of corticosteroids may result in salicylism because corticosteroids enhance renal clearance of salicylates and their withdrawal is followed by return to normal rates of renal clearance.

Fiorinal® with Codeine (butalbital, aspirin, caffeine, and codeine phosphate) may enhance the effects of:

1. Oral anticoagulants, causing bleeding by inhibiting prothrombin formation in the liver and displacing anticoagulants from plasma protein binding sites.
2. Oral antidiabetic agents and insulin, causing hypoglycemia by contributing an additive effect, if dosage of Fiorinal® with Codeine (butalbital, aspirin, caffeine, and codeine phosphate) exceeds maximum recommended daily dosage.
3. 6-mercaptopurine and methotrexate, causing bone marrow toxicity and blood dyscrasias by displacing these drugs from secondary binding sites, and, in the case of methotrexate, also reducing its excretion.
4. Non-steroidal anti-inflammatory agents, increasing the risk of peptic ulceration and bleeding by contributing additive effects.
5. Other narcotic analgesics, alcohol, general anesthetics, tranquilizers such as chlordiazepoxide, sedative-hypnotics, or other CNS depressants, causing increased CNS depression.

Fiorinal® with Codeine (butalbital, aspirin, caffeine, and codeine phosphate) may diminish the effects of:

Uricosuric agents such as probenecid and sulfinpyrazone, reducing their effectiveness in the treatment of gout. Aspirin competes with these agents for protein binding sites.

Drug/Laboratory Test Interactions

Aspirin: Aspirin may interfere with the following laboratory determinations in blood: serum amylase, fasting blood glucose, cholesterol, protein, serum glutamic-oxalacetic transaminase (SGOT), uric acid, prothrombin time and bleeding time. Aspirin may interfere with the following laboratory determinations in urine: glucose, 5-hydroxyindoleacetic acid, Gerhardt ketone, vanillylmandelic acid (VMA), uric acid, diacetic acid, and spectrophotometric detection of barbiturates.

Codeine: Codeine may increase serum amylase levels.

Carcinogenesis, Mutagenesis, Impairment of Fertility

Adequate long-term studies have been conducted in mice and rats with aspirin, alone or in combination with other drugs, in which no evidence of carcinogenesis was seen. No adequate studies have been conducted in animals to determine whether aspirin has a potential for mutagenesis or impairment of fertility. No adequate studies have been conducted in animals to determine whether butalbital has a potential for carcinogenesis, mutagenesis, or impairment of fertility.

Usage in Pregnancy

Teratogenic Effects:

Pregnancy Category C. Animal reproduction studies have not been conducted with Fiorinal® with Codeine (butalbital, aspirin, caffeine, and codeine phosphate). It is also not known whether Fiorinal® with Codeine (butalbital, aspirin, caffeine, and codeine phosphate) can cause fetal harm when administered to a pregnant woman or can affect reproduction capacity. Fiorinal® with Codeine (butalbital, aspirin, caffeine, and codeine phosphate) should be given to a pregnant woman only when clearly needed.

Nonteratogenic Effects:

Although Fiorinal® with Codeine (butalbital, aspirin, caffeine, and codeine phosphate) was not implicated in the birth defect, a female infant was born with lissencephaly, pachygyria and heterotopic gray matter. The infant was born 8 weeks prematurely to a woman who had taken an average of 90 Fiorinal® with Codeine (butalbital, aspirin, caffeine, and codeine phosphate) capsules each month from the first few days of pregnancy. The child's development was mildly delayed and from one year of age she had partial simple motor seizures.

Withdrawal seizures were reported in a two-day-old male infant whose mother had taken a butalbital-containing drug during the last 2 months of pregnancy. Butalbital was found in the infant's serum. The infant was given phenobarbital 5mg/kg, which was tapered without further seizure or other withdrawal symptoms.

Studies of aspirin use in pregnant women have not shown that aspirin increases the risk of abnormalities when administered during the first trimester of pregnancy. In controlled studies involving 41,337 pregnant women and their offspring, there was no evidence that aspirin taken during pregnancy caused stillbirth, neonatal death or reduced birth weight. In controlled studies of 50,282 pregnant women and their offspring, aspirin administration in moderate and heavy doses during the first four lunar months of pregnancy showed no teratogenic effect.

Reproduction studies have been performed in rabbits and rats at doses up to 150 times the human dose and have revealed no evidence of impaired fertility or harm to the fetus due to codeine.

Therapeutic doses of aspirin in pregnant women close to term may cause bleeding in mother, fetus, or neonate. During the last 6 months of pregnancy, regular use of aspirin in high doses may prolong pregnancy and delivery.

Labor and Delivery

Ingestion of aspirin prior to delivery may prolong delivery or lead to bleeding in the mother or neonate. Use of codeine during labor may lead to respiratory depression in the neonate.

Nursing Mothers

Aspirin, caffeine, barbiturates and codeine are excreted in breast milk in small amounts, but the significance of their effects on nursing infants is not known. Because of potential for serious adverse reactions in nursing infants from Fiorinal® with Codeine (butalbital, aspirin, caffeine, and codeine phosphate), a decision should be made whether to discontinue nursing or to discontinue the drug, taking into account the importance of the drug to the mother.

Pediatric Use

Safety and effectiveness in pediatric patients have not been established.

ADVERSE REACTIONS

Commonly Observed

The most commonly reported adverse events associated with the use of Fiorinal® with Codeine (butalbital, aspirin, caffeine, and codeine phosphate) and not reported at an equivalent incidence by placebo-treated patients were nausea and/or abdominal pain, drowsiness, and dizziness.

Associated with Treatment Discontinuation

Of the 382 patients treated with Fiorinal® with Codeine (butalbital, aspirin, caffeine, and codeine phosphate) in controlled clinical trials, three (0.8%) discontinued treatment with Fiorinal® with Codeine (butalbital, aspirin, caffeine, and codeine phosphate) because of adverse events. One patient each discontinued treatment for the following reasons: gastrointestinal upset; lightheadedness and heavy eyelids; and drowsiness and generalized tingling.

Incidence in Controlled Clinical Trials

The following table summarizes the incidence rates of the adverse events reported by at least 1% of the Fiorinal® with Codeine (butalbital, aspirin, caffeine, and codeine phosphate) treated patients in controlled clinical trials comparing Fiorinal® with Codeine (butalbital, aspirin, caffeine, and codeine phosphate) to placebo, and provides a comparison to the incidence rates reported by the placebo-treated patients.

The prescriber should be aware that these figures cannot be used to predict the incidence of side effects in the course of usual medical practice where patient characteristics and other factors differ from those that prevailed in the clinical trials. Similarly, the cited frequencies cannot be compared with figures obtained from other clinical investigations involving different treatments, uses, and investigators.

Adverse Events Reported by at Least 1% of Fiorinal® with Codeine (butalbital, aspirin, caffeine, and codeine phosphate) Treated Patients During Placebo Controlled Clinical Trials

Body System/ Adverse Event	Incidence Rate of Adverse Events: Fiorinal®/Codeine (butalbital, aspirin, caffeine, and codeine phosphate) (N=382)	Placebo (N=377)
Central Nervous		
Drowsiness	2.4%	0.5%
Dizziness/ Lightheadedness	2.6%	0.5%
Intoxicated Feeling	1.0%	0%
Gastrointestinal		
Nausea/ Abdominal Pain	3.7%	0.8%

Other Adverse Events Reported During Controlled Clinical Trials

The listing that follows represents the proportion of the 382 patients exposed to Fiorinal® with Codeine (butalbital, aspirin, caffeine, and codeine phosphate) while participating in the controlled clinical trials who reported, on at least one occasion, an adverse event of the type cited. All reported adverse events, except those already presented in the previous table, are included. It is important to emphasize that, although the adverse events reported did occur while the patient was receiving Fiorinal® with Codeine (butalbital, aspirin, caffeine, and codeine phosphate), the adverse events were not necessarily caused by Fiorinal® with Codeine (butalbital, aspirin, caffeine, and codeine phosphate).

Adverse events are classified by body system and frequency. "Frequent" is defined as an adverse event which occurred in at least 1/100 (1%) of the patients; all adverse events listed in the previous table are frequent. "Infrequent" is defined as an adverse event that occurred in less than 1/100 patients but at least 1/1000 patients. All adverse events tabulated below are classified as infrequent.

Central Nervous: headache, shaky feeling, tingling, agitation, fainting, fatigue, heavy eyelids, high energy, hot spells, numbness, and sluggishness.

Autonomic Nervous: dry mouth and hyperhidrosis.

Gastrointestinal: vomiting, difficulty swallowing, and heartburn.

Cardiovascular: tachycardia.

Musculoskeletal: leg pain and muscle fatigue.

Genitourinary: diuresis.

Miscellaneous: pruritus, fever, earache, nasal congestion, and tinnitus.

Voluntary reports of adverse drug events, temporally associated with Fiorinal® with Codeine (butalbital, aspirin, caffeine, and codeine phosphate), that have been received since market introduction and that were not reported in clinical trials by the patients treated with Fiorinal® with Codeine (butalbital, aspirin, caffeine, and codeine phosphate), are listed below. Many or most of these events may have no causal relationship with the drug and are listed according to body system.

Central Nervous: Abuse, addiction, anxiety, depression, disorientation, hallucination, hyperactivity, insomnia, libido decrease, nervousness, neuropathy, psychosis, sedation, sexual activity increase, slurred speech, twitching, unconsciousness, vertigo.

Autonomic Nervous: epistaxis, flushing, miosis, salivation.

Gastrointestinal: anorexia, appetite increased, constipation, diarrhea, esophagitis, gastroenteritis, gastrointestinal spasm, hiccup, mouth burning, pyloric ulcer.

Cardiovascular: chest pain, hypotensive reaction, palpitations, syncope.

Skin: erythema, erythema multiforme, exfoliative dermatitis, hives, rash, toxic epidermal necrolysis.

Continued on next page

Sandoz—Cont.

Urinary: kidney impairment, urinary difficulty.

Miscellaneous: allergic reaction, anaphylactic shock, cholangiocarcinoma, drug interaction with erythromycin (stomach upset), edema.

The following adverse drug events may be borne in mind as potential effects of the components of Fiorinal® with Codeine (butalbital, aspirin, caffeine, and codeine phosphate). Potential effects of high dosage are listed in the *OVERDOSAGE* section of this insert.

Aspirin: occult blood loss, hemolytic anemia, iron deficiency anemia, gastric distress, heartburn, nausea, peptic ulcer, prolonged bleeding time, acute airway obstruction, renal toxicity when taken in high doses for prolonged periods, impaired urate excretion, hepatitis.

Caffeine: cardiac stimulation, irritability, tremor, dependence, nephrotoxicity, hyperglycemia.

Codeine: nausea, vomiting, drowsiness, lightheadedness, constipation, pruritus.

DRUG ABUSE AND DEPENDENCE

Controlled Substance

Fiorinal® with Codeine (butalbital, aspirin, caffeine, and codeine phosphate) is controlled by the Drug Enforcement Administration and is classified under Schedule III.

Abuse and Dependence

Codeine

Codeine can produce drug dependence of the morphine type and, therefore, has the potential for being abused. Psychological dependence, physical dependence, and tolerance may develop upon repeated administration and it should be prescribed and administered with the same degree of caution appropriate to the use of other oral narcotic medications.

Butalbital

Barbiturates may be habit-forming: Tolerance, psychological dependence, and physical dependence may occur especially following prolonged use of high doses of barbiturates. The average daily dose for the barbiturate addict is usually about 1,500 mg. As tolerance to barbiturates develops, the amount needed to maintain the same level of intoxication increases; tolerance to a fatal dosage, however, does not increase more than twofold. As this occurs, the margin between an intoxication dosage and fatal dosage becomes smaller. The lethal dose of a barbiturate is far less if alcohol is also ingested. Major withdrawal symptoms (convulsions and delirium) may occur within 16 hours and last up to 5 days after abrupt cessation of these drugs. Intensity of withdrawal symptoms gradually declines over a period of approximately 15 days. Treatment of barbiturate dependence consists of cautious and gradual withdrawal of the drug. Barbiturate-dependent patients can be withdrawn by using a number of different withdrawal regimens. One method involves initiating treatment at the patient's regular dosage level and gradually decreasing the daily dosage as tolerated by the patient.

OVERDOSAGE

The toxic effects of acute overdosage of Fiorinal® with Codeine (butalbital, aspirin, caffeine, and codeine phosphate) capsules are attributable mainly to the barbiturate and codeine components, and, to a lesser extent, aspirin. Because toxic effects of caffeine occur in very high dosages only, the possibility of significant caffeine toxicity from Fiorinal® with Codeine (butalbital, aspirin, caffeine, and codeine phosphate) overdosage is unlikely.

Signs and Symptoms

Symptoms attributable to ***acute barbiturate poisoning*** include drowsiness, confusion, and coma; respiratory depression; hypotension; hypovolemic shock. Symptoms attributable to ***acute aspirin poisoning*** include hyperpnea; acid-base disturbances with development of metabolic acidosis; vomiting and abdominal pain; tinnitus, hyperthermia; hypoprothrombinemia; restlessness; delirium; convulsions. ***Acute caffeine poisoning*** may cause insomnia, restlessness, tremor, and delirium; tachycardia and extrasystoles. Symptoms of ***acute codeine poisoning*** include the opioid triad of: pinpoint pupils, marked depression of respiration, and loss of consciousness. Convulsions may occur.

Treatment

The following paragraphs describe one approach to the treatment of overdose with Fiorinal® with Codeine (butalbital, aspirin, caffeine, and codeine phosphate). However, because strategies for the management of an overdose continually evolve, consultation with a regional poison control center is strongly encouraged.

Treatment consists primarily of management of barbiturate intoxication, reversal of the effects of codeine, and the correction of the acid-base imbalance due to salicylism. Vomiting should be induced mechanically or with emetics in the conscious patient. Gastric lavage may be used if the pharyngeal and laryngeal reflexes are present and if less than 4 hours have elapsed since ingestion. A cuffed endotracheal tube should be inserted before gastric lavage of the unconscious patient and when necessary to provide assisted respiration. Diuresis, alkalinization of the urine, and correction of electrolyte disturbances should be accomplished through administration of intravenous fluids such as 1% sodium bicarbonate and 5% dextrose in water.

Meticulous attention should be given to maintaining adequate pulmonary ventilation. The value of vasopressor agents such as Norepinephrine or Phenylephrine Hydrochloride in treating hypotension is questionable since they increase vasoconstriction and decrease blood flow. However, if prolonged support of blood pressure is required, Norepinephrine Bitartrate (Levophed®)* may be given I.V. with the usual precautions and serial blood pressure monitoring. In severe cases of intoxication, peritoneal dialysis, hemodialysis, or exchange transfusion may be lifesaving. Hypoprothrombinemia should be treated with vitamin K, intravenously.

Methemoglobinemia over 30% should be treated with methylene blue by slow intravenous administration.

Naloxone, a narcotic antagonist, can reverse respiratory depression and coma associated with opioid overdose. Typically, a dose of 0.4–2.0 mg is given parenterally and may be repeated if an adequate response is not achieved. Since the duration of action of codeine may exceed that of the antagonist, the patient should be kept under continued surveillance and repeated doses of the antagonist should be administered as needed to maintain adequate respiration. A narcotic antagonist should not be administered in the absence of clinically significant respiratory or cardiovascular depression.

Up-to-date information about the treatment of overdose can be obtained from a Certified Regional Poison Control Center. Telephone numbers of Certified Regional Poison Control Centers are listed in the Physicians' Desk Reference®.**

Toxic and Lethal Doses

Butalbital:	toxic dose 1.0 g (adult); lethal dose 2.0–5.0 g (20 capsules of Fiorinal® with Codeine)
Aspirin:	toxic blood level greater than 30 mg/100 mL; lethal dose 10–30 g (adult)
Caffeine:	toxic dose greater than 1.0 g; (25 capsules of Fiorinal® with Codeine); lethal dose unknown
Codeine:	toxic dose 240 mg (8 capsules of Fiorinal® with Codeine); lethal dose 0.5–1.0 g (adult)

DOSAGE AND ADMINISTRATION

One or 2 capsules every 4 hours. Total daily dosage should not exceed 6 capsules.

Extended and repeated use of this product is not recommended because of the potential for physical dependence.

HOW SUPPLIED

Fiorinal® with Codeine
(butalbital, aspirin, caffeine, and codeine phosphate)
Capsules, USP

Imprinted " F-C" on one half, "SANDOZ 78-107" other half, color is blue and yellow.

Bottles of 100 (NDC 0078-0107-05)

ControlPak® package of 25: continuous reverse-numbered roll of sealed blisters (NDC 0078-0107-13)

Store and Dispense

Below 77°F (25°C); tight container.

*Levophed is a registered Trademark of Sanofi Winthrop Pharmaceuticals.

** Trademark of Medical Economics Data Production Company.

[REV: FEBRUARY 1996 30133903]

Shown in Product Identification Guide, page 333

HYDERGINE® ℞

[*hī′der-jēn*]

(ergoloid mesylates) tablets, USP (ORAL)
(ergoloid mesylates) liquid, USP

HYDERGINE® LC ℞

(ergoloid mesylates, USP) liquid capsules

CAUTION: Federal law prohibits dispensing without prescription.

The following prescribing information is based on official labeling in effect on August 1, 1996.

DESCRIPTION

Hydergine® Tablet 1 mg
and Hydergine® LC Liquid Capsule 1 mg

Each contains ergoloid mesylates, USP as follows: dihydroergocornine mesylate 0.333 mg, dihydroergocristine mesylate 0.333 mg, and dihydroergocryptine (dihydro-alpha-ergocryptine and dihydro-beta-ergocryptine in the proportion of 2:1) mesylate 0.333 mg, representing a total of 1 mg.

Inactive Ingredients

Oral Tablets: lactose, povidone, starch, stearic acid, and talc.

Liquid Capsules: ascorbic acid, gelatin, glycerin, methylparaben, polyethylene glycol, propylparaben, propylene glycol, sorbitol, and titanium dioxide.

Hydergine® Liquid 1 mg/mL

Each mL contains ergoloid mesylates, USP as follows: dihydroergocornine mesylate 0.333 mg, dihydroergocristine mesylate 0.333 mg, and dihydroergocryptine (dihydro-alpha-ergocryptine and dihydro-beta-ergocryptine in the proportion of 2:1) mesylate 0.333 mg, representing a total of 1 mg; alcohol, 28.5% by volume.

Inactive Ingredients: alcohol, glycerin, propylene glycol, and purified water

Pharmacokinetic Properties

Pharmacokinetic studies have been performed in normal volunteers with the help of radiolabelled drug as well as employing a specific radioimmunoassay technique. From the urinary excretion quotient of orally and intravenously administered tritium-labelled Hydergine® (ergoloid mesylates) the absorption of ergoloid was calculated to be 25%. Following oral administration, peak levels of 0.5 ng Eq/mL/mg were achieved within 1.5-3 hr. Bioavailability studies with the specific radioimmunoassay confirm that ergoloid is rapidly absorbed from the gastrointestinal tract, with mean peak levels of 0.05-0.13 ng/mL/mg (with extremes of 0.03 and 0.18 ng/mL/mg) achieved within 0.6-1.3 hr (with extremes of 0.4 and 2.8 hr). The finding of lower peak levels of ergoloid compared to the total drug-metabolite composite is consistent with a considerable first pass liver metabolism, with less than 50% of the therapeutic moiety reaching the systemic circulation. The elimination of radioactivity, representing ergoloid plus metabolites bearing the radiolabel, was biphasic with half-lives of 4 and 13 hr. The mean half-life of unchanged ergoloid in plasma is about 2.6-5.1 hr; after 3 half-lives ergoloid plasma levels are less than 10% of radioactivity levels, and by 24 hr no ergoloid is detectable.

Bioequivalence studies were performed comparing Hydergine® (ergoloid mesylates) oral tablets (administered orally) with Hydergine® (ergoloid mesylates) sublingual tablets (administered sublingually), Hydergine® (ergoloid mesylates) oral tablets with Hydergine® (ergoloid mesylates) liquid and Hydergine® (ergoloid mesylates) oral tablets with Hydergine® LC (ergoloid mesylates, USP) liquid capsules. The oral tablet, sublingual tablet, and liquid capsule oral forms were shown to be bioequivalent. Within the bioequivalence limits, the liquid capsule showed a statistically significant (12%) greater bioavailability than the oral tablet. In the study comparing the oral tablet and liquid forms, both forms tested showed an equivalent rate of absorption and an equivalent peak plasma concentration (C_{max}).

ACTIONS

There is no specific evidence which clearly establishes the mechanism by which Hydergine® (ergoloid mesylates) preparations produce mental effects, nor is there conclusive evidence that the drug particularly affects cerebral arteriosclerosis or cerebrovascular insufficiency.

INDICATIONS

A proportion of individuals over sixty who manifest signs and symptoms of an idiopathic decline in mental capacity (i.e., cognitive and interpersonal skills, mood, self-care, apparent motivation) can experience some symptomatic relief upon treatment with Hydergine® (ergoloid mesylates) preparations. The identity of the specific trait(s) or condition(s), if any, which would usefully predict a response to Hydergine® (ergoloid mesylates) therapy is not known. It appears, however, that those individuals who do respond come from groups of patients who would be considered clinically to suffer from some ill-defined process related to aging or to have some underlying dementing condition (i.e., primary progressive dementia, Alzheimer's dementia, senile onset, multi-infarct dementia).

Before prescribing Hydergine® (ergoloid mesylates), the physician should exclude the possibility that the patient's signs and symptoms arise from a potentially reversible and treatable condition. Particular care should be taken to exclude delirium and dementiform illness secondary to systemic disease, primary neurological disease, or primary disturbance of mood. Hydergine® (ergoloid mesylates) preparations are not indicated in the treatment of acute or chronic psychosis, regardless of etiology (*see CONTRAINDICATIONS*).

The decision to use Hydergine® (ergoloid mesylates) in the treatment of an individual with a symptomatic decline in mental capacity of unknown etiology should be continually reviewed since the presenting clinical picture may subsequently evolve sufficiently to allow a specific diagnosis and a specific alternative treatment. In addition, continued clinical evaluation is required to determine whether any initial benefit conferred by Hydergine® (ergoloid mesylates) therapy persists with time.

The efficacy of Hydergine® (ergoloid mesylates) was evaluated using a special rating scale known as the SCAG (Sandoz Clinical Assessment-Geriatric). The specific items on this scale on which modest but statistically significant changes were observed at the end of twelve weeks include: mental alertness, confusion, recent memory, orientation, emotional lability, self-care, depression, anxiety/fears, cooperation,

sociability, appetite, dizziness, fatigue, bothersome(ness), and an overall impression of clinical status.

CONTRAINDICATIONS

Hydergine® (ergoloid mesylates) preparations are contraindicated in individuals who have previously shown hypersensitivity to the drug. Hydergine® (ergoloid mesylates) preparations are also contraindicated in patients who have psychosis, acute or chronic, regardless of etiology.

PRECAUTIONS

Practitioners are advised that because the target symptoms are of unknown etiology, careful diagnosis should be attempted before prescribing Hydergine® (ergoloid mesylates) preparations.

ADVERSE REACTIONS

Hydergine® (ergoloid mesylates) preparations have not been found to produce serious side effects. Transient nausea, and gastric disturbances have been reported. Hydergine® (ergoloid mesylates) preparations do not possess the vasoconstrictor properties of the natural ergot alkaloids.

DOSAGE AND ADMINISTRATION

1 mg three times daily.

Alleviation of symptoms is usually gradual and results may not be observed for 3–4 weeks.

HOW SUPPLIED

Hydergine® (ergoloid mesylates) Tablets, USP (Oral)

1 mg

Round, white, engraved "HYDERGINE 1" on one side, " " other side.

NDC 0078-0070-05: bottles of 100
NDC 0078-0070-06: SandoPak® unit-dose packages of 100
NDC 0078-0070-08: bottles of 500

Store and Dispense

Below 77°F (25°C); tight, light-resistant container.

Hydergine® (ergoloid mesylates) Liquid, USP

1 mg/mL

Supplied with an accompanying dropper graduated to deliver 1 mg.

NDC 0078-0100-36: bottles of 100 mL

Store and Dispense

Below 86°F (30°C); tight, amber glass bottle.

Hydergine® LC (ergoloid mesylates, USP) Liquid Capsules

1 mg

Oblong, off-white, branded "HYDERGINE LC 1 mg" on one side, " " other side.

NDC 0078-0101-05: bottles of 100
NDC 0078-0101-06: SandoPak® unit-dose packages of 100
NDC 0078-0101-08: bottles of 500

Store and Dispense

Between 59° and 77°F (15° and 25°C); tight, light-resistant container. DO NOT FREEZE.

(Encapsulated by
R.P. Scherer, N.A., Clearwater, Florida 33518)

[REV: FEBRUARY 1996 30135905]

Shown in Product Identification Guide, page 333

LAMISIL® CREAM, 1% ℞

[lə″ mə ′səl]

(terbinafine hydrochloride cream)

FOR TOPICAL DERMATOLOGIC USE ONLY — NOT FOR OPHTHALMIC, ORAL, OR INTRAVAGINAL USE.

Caution: Federal (USA) law prohibits dispensing without a prescription.

The following prescribing information is based on official labeling in effect on August 1, 1996.

DESCRIPTION

Lamisil® Cream, 1%, contains the synthetic antifungal compound, terbinafine hydrochloride. It is intended for topical dermatologic use only.

Chemically, terbinafine hydrochloride is (E)-*N*-(6,6-dimethyl-2-hepten-4-ynyl)-*N*-methyl-1-naphthalenemethanamine hydrochloride. The compound has the empirical formula $C_{21}H_{26}ClN$, a molecular weight of 327.90, and the following structural formula:

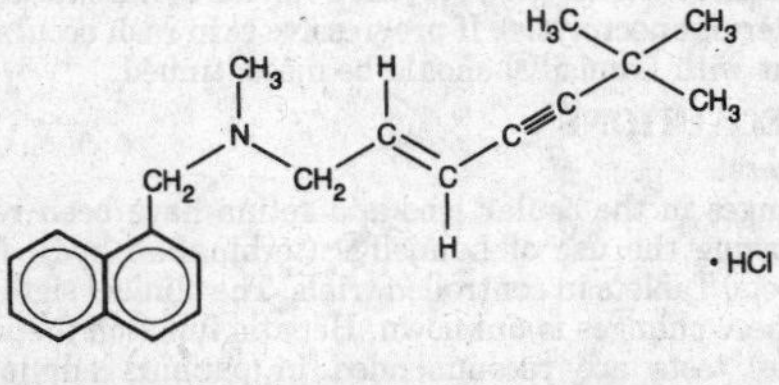

Terbinafine hydrochloride is a white to off-white fine crystalline powder. It is freely soluble in methanol and methylene chloride, soluble in ethanol, and slightly soluble in water. Each gram of Lamisil® Cream, 1%, contains 10 mg of terbinafine hydrochloride in a white cream base of benzyl alcohol NF, cetyl alcohol NF, cetyl palmitate, isopropyl myristate NF, polysorbate 60 NF, purified water USP, sodium hydroxide NF, sorbitan monostearate NF, and stearyl alcohol NF.

CLINICAL PHARMACOLOGY

Pharmacokinetics

Following a single application of 100 μL of Lamisil® Cream, 1% (terbinafine hydrochloride cream) (containing 1 mg of ^{14}C-terbinafine) to a 30 cm^2 area of the ventral forearm of 6 healthy subjects, the recovery of radioactivity in urine and feces averaged 3.5% of the administered dose.

In a study of 16 healthy subjects, 8 of whose skin was artificially compromised by stripping the stratum corneum to the viable layer, single and multiple applications (average 0.1 mg/cm^2 B.I.D. for 5 days) of terbinafine as Lamisil® Cream, 1% (terbinafine hydrochloride cream) were made to various sites. In this study, systemic absorption was highly variable. The maximum measured plasma concentration of terbinafine was 11.4 ng/mL, and the maximum measured plasma concentration of the de-methylated metabolite was 11.0 ng/mL. In many patients there were no detectable plasma levels of either parent compound or metabolite. Urinary excretion accounted for up to 9% of the topically applied dose; the majority excreted less than 4%. No measurement of fecal drug content was performed.

In a study of 10 patients with tinea cruris, once daily application of Lamisil® Cream, 1% (terbinafine hydrochloride cream) for 7 days resulted in plasma concentrations of terbinafine of 0–11 ng/mL on day 7. Plasma concentrations of the metabolites of terbinafine ranged from 11–80 ng/mL in these patients.

Approximately 75% of cutaneously absorbed terbinafine is eliminated in the urine predominantly as metabolites.

Microbiology

Terbinafine hydrochloride is a synthetic allylamine derivative. Terbinafine hydrochloride exerts its antifungal effect by inhibiting squalene epoxidase, a key enzyme in sterol biosynthesis in fungi. This action results in a deficiency in ergosterol and a corresponding accumulation of squalene within the fungal cell and causes fungal cell death.

Terbinafine has been shown to be active against most strains of the following organisms both *in vitro* and in clinical infections at indicated body sites *(See INDICATIONS AND USAGE):*

Epidermophyton floccosum
Trichophyton mentagrophytes
Trichophyton rubrum

The following *in vitro* data are available; ***however, their clinical significance is unknown.*** Terbinafine exhibits satisfactory *in vitro* MIC's against most strains of the following organisms; however, the safety and efficacy of terbinafine in treating clinical infections due to these organisms have not been established in adequate and well-controlled clinical trials.

Microsporum canis
Microsporum gypseum
Microsporum nanum
Trichophyton verrucosum

INDICATIONS AND USAGE

Lamisil® Cream, 1% (terbinafine hydrochloride cream) is indicated for the topical treatment of the following dermatologic infections: interdigital tinea pedis (athlete's foot), tinea cruris (jock itch), or tinea corporis (ringworm) due to *Epidermophyton floccosum, Trichophyton mentagrophytes, or Trichophyton rubrum (See DOSAGE AND ADMINISTRATION).*

Diagnosis of the disease should be confirmed either by direct microscopic examination of scrapings from infected tissue mounted in a solution of potassium hydroxide or by culture.

CONTRAINDICATIONS

Lamisil® Cream, 1% (terbinafine hydrochloride cream) is contraindicated in individuals who have known or suspected hypersensitivity to terbinafine or any other of its components.

WARNINGS

Lamisil® Cream, 1% (terbinafine hydrochloride cream) is not for ophthalmic, oral, or intravaginal use.

PRECAUTIONS

General

If irritation or sensitivity develops with the use of Lamisil® Cream, 1% (terbinafine hydrochloride cream), treatment should be discontinued and appropriate therapy instituted.

Information for Patients

The patient should be told to:

1. Use Lamisil® Cream, 1% (terbinafine hydrochloride cream) as directed by the physician and avoid contact with the eyes, nose, mouth, or other mucous membranes,
2. Use the medication for the treatment time recommended by the physician,
3. Inform the physician if the area of application shows signs of increased irritation or possible sensitization (redness, itching, burning, blistering, swelling, or oozing).
4. Avoid the use of occlusive dressings unless otherwise directed by the physician.

Drug Interactions

Potential interactions between Lamisil® Cream, 1% (terbinafine hydrochloride cream) and other drugs have not been systematically evaluated.

Carcinogenesis, Mutagenesis, Impairment of Fertility

In a 2-year oral carcinogenicity study in mice, a 4% incidence of splenic hemangiosarcomas and a 6% incidence of leiomyosarcoma-like tumors of the seminal vesicles were observed in males at the highest dose level, 156 mg/kg/day (equivalent to at least 390 times the maximum potential exposure at the recommended human topical dose*). In a carcinogenicity study in rats at the highest dose level, 69 mg/kg/day (equivalent to at least 173 times the maximum potential exposure at the recommended human topical dose*), a 6% incidence of both liver tumors and skin lipomas were observed in males. In rats, the formation of liver tumors was associated with peroxisomal proliferation.

A battery of *in vitro* and *in vivo* genotoxicity tests, including Ames assay, mutagenicity evaluation in Chinese hamster ovarian cells, chromosome aberration test, sister chromatid exchanges, and mouse micronucleus test revealed no evidence for a mutagenic or clastogenic potential for the drug.

Reproductive studies in rats administered up to 300 mg/kg/day orally (equivalent to at least 750 times the maximum potential exposure at the recommended human topical dose*) did not reveal any adverse effects on fertility or other reproductive parameters. Intravaginal mucosal application of terbinafine hydrochloride at 150 mg/day in pregnant rabbits did not increase the incidence of abortions or premature deliveries or affect fetal parameters.

Pregnancy

Pregnancy Category B: Oral doses of terbinafine hydrochloride, up to 300 mg/kg/day (equivalent to at least 750 times the maximum potential exposure at the recommended human topical dose*), during organogenesis in rats and rabbits were not teratogenic. Similarly, a subcutaneous study in rats at doses up to 100 mg/kg/day (equivalent to at least 250 times the maximum potential exposure at the recommended human topical dose*) and a percutaneous study in rabbits, including doses up to 150 mg/kg/day (equivalent to at least 350 times the maximum potential exposure at the recommended human topical dose*) did not reveal any teratogenic potential.

There are, however, no adequate and well-controlled studies in pregnant women. Because animal reproduction studies are not always predictive of human response, this drug should be used only if clearly indicated during pregnancy.

*The above comparisons between oral animal doses and maximum potential exposure at the recommended human topical doses are based upon the application to human skin of 0.1 mg of terbinafine/cm^2, the assumption of average human cutaneous exposure of 100 cm^2 [assuming the use of 1 gram of Lamisil® Cream, 1% (terbinafine hydrochloride cream) per dose], and the ***theoretical*** worst case scenario of 100% human cutaneous absorption. At present, comparative animal and human systemic exposure pharmacokinetic data are not available.

Nursing Mothers

After a single ***oral*** dose of 500 mg of terbinafine hydrochloride to 2 volunteers, the total dose of terbinafine hydrochloride secreted in human milk during the 72-hour post-dosing period was 0.65 mg in one person and 0.15 mg in the other. The total excretion of terbinafine in human milk was 0.13% and 0.03% of the administered dose, respectively. The concentrations of the 1 metabolite measured in the human milk of these 2 volunteers were below the detection limit of the assay used (150 ng/mL of milk).

Because of the small amount of data on human neonatal exposure, a decision should be made whether to discontinue nursing or to discontinue the drug, taking into account the importance of the drug to the mother, as well as the findings of tumors in male mice and rats following ***oral*** administration of terbinafine hydrochloride and the lack of data on carcinogenicity in neonatal animals.

Nursing mothers should avoid application of Lamisil® Cream, 1% (terbinafine hydrochloride cream) to the breast.

Pediatric Use

Safety and efficacy in children or infants below the age of 12 years have not been established.

ADVERSE REACTIONS

Clinical Trials

In clinical trials, 6 (0.2%) of 2265 patients treated with Lamisil® Cream, 1% (terbinafine hydrochloride cream) discontinued therapy due to adverse events and 52 (2.3%) reported adverse reactions thought to be possibly, probably, or definitely related to drug therapy. These reactions included irritation (1%), burning (0.8%), itching (0.2%), and dryness (0.2%).

OVERDOSAGE

Overdosage of terbinafine hydrochloride in humans has not been reported to date. Acute overdosage with topical application of terbinafine hydrochloride is unlikely due to the lim-

Continued on next page

Sandoz—Cont.

Successful Outcomes

Therapy	1 Week Therapy			4 Weeks Therapy	
	At 1 wk (end of Rx)	At 4 wks (3 wk f/up)	At 6 wks (5 wk f/up)	At 4 wks (end of Rx)	At 6 wks (2 wk f/up)
Lamisil®	14% (11/79)	51% (40/78)	65% (51/78)	71% (94/133)	73% (97/132)
Vehicle	6% (5/79)	13% (10/75)	12% (8/69)	ND	ND
Active Control	ND	ND	ND	63% (84/133)	59% (79/134)

ited absorption of topically applied drug and would not be expected to lead to a life threatening situation.

Overdosage in rats and mice by the oral and intravenous routes of drug administration has produced sedation, drowsiness, ataxia, dyspnea, exophthalmus, and piloerection. The majority of deaths in animals occurred following oral administration of doses exceeding 3 grams/kilogram or following 200 mg/kg administered intravenously. In rabbits, overdosage produced erythema, edema, and scale formation following topical administration of doses in excess of 1.5 grams/kilogram.

When terbinafine hydrochloride cream, 1% was administered as a single oral dose at 10 and 25 mL/kg (100 and 250 mg/kg, respectively) to rats and mice, no deaths or other drug-related toxicities were observed.

DOSAGE AND ADMINISTRATION

In the treatment of interdigital tinea pedis (athlete's foot), Lamisil® Cream, 1% (terbinafine hydrochloride cream) should be applied to cover the affected and immediately surrounding areas twice daily *until clinical signs and symptoms are significantly improved.* In many patients this occurs by day 7 of drug therapy. The duration of drug therapy should be for a minimum of 1 week and should not exceed 4 weeks. (See CLINICAL STUDIES and following Note.)

In the treatment of tinea cruris (jock itch) or tinea corporis (ringworm), Lamisil® Cream, 1% (terbinafine hydrochloride cream) should be applied to cover the affected and immediately surrounding areas once or twice daily *until clinical signs and symptoms are significantly improved.* In many patients this occurs by day 7 of drug therapy. The duration of drug therapy should be for a minimum of 1 week and should not exceed 4 weeks. (See CLINICAL STUDIES and following Note.)

Note:

Many patients treated with shorter durations of therapy (1–2 weeks) continue to improve during the 2–4 weeks after drug therapy has been completed. As a consequence, patients should not be considered therapeutic failures until they have been observed for a period of 2–4 weeks off therapy. (See CLINICAL STUDIES).

If successful outcome is not achieved during the post-treatment observation period, the diagnosis should be reviewed.

HOW SUPPLIED

Lamisil® Cream, 1% (terbinafine hydrochloride cream)
Tubes of 15 grams (NDC 0078-0170-40)
Tubes of 30 grams (NDC 0078-0170-46)
Store between 5° and 30°C (41°and 86°F).

CLINICAL STUDIES

In the following data presentations, the term "successful outcome" refers to those patients evaluated at a specific time point, who had both negative mycological results (culture and KOH preparation) and a *total* clinical score of less than 2. The clinical score is the sum of the scores of each sign and symptom graded on a scale from 0=absent to 3=severe. Mean clinical scores at entry ranged from 8–11 in the pivotal clinical trials. All studies included, at a minimum, clinical evaluation of erythema, desquamation, and pruritus.

A. Tinea Pedis

In 3 studies of Lamisil® Cream, 1% (terbinafine hydrochloride cream) used B.I.D. in the treatment of tinea pedis, 2 (combined in the table below) were vehicle-controlled (placebo) evaluations of 1 week treatment duration. The third study (see following table) was of 4 weeks therapy compared to another active drug.

[See table on top of page.]

B. Tinea Corporis/Cruris

Two studies (combined below) compared Lamisil® Cream, 1% (terbinafine hydrochloride cream) to vehicle (placebo), applied once daily for 1 week in the treatment of tinea corporis/cruris.

In the following table, sites of infection are separated into 2 groups: (1) tinea corporis and (2) tinea cruris. Patients with mixed tinea corporis/cruris are included in both groups.

[See table in next column.]

Successful Outcomes after 1 Week of Therapy

Disease	Drug	At 1 wk (end of Rx)	At 4 wks (3 wk f/up)
Corporis	Lamisil®	21% (7/33)	83% (25/30)
	Vehicle	0% (0/31)	31% (4/13)
Cruris	Lamisil®	43% (21/49)	92% (45/49)
	Vehicle	9% (5/58)	25% (7/28)

[REV: JUNE 1993 38052901]

LAMISIL®   ℞
(terbinafine hydrochloride tablets)
Tablets

Caution: Federal law prohibits dispensing without prescription.

The following prescribing information is based on official labeling in effect on August 1, 1996.

DESCRIPTION

Lamisil® (terbinafine hydrochloride tablets) Tablets contain the synthetic allylamine antifungal compound terbinafine hydrochloride.

Chemically, terbinafine hydrochloride is (E)-N-(6,6-dimethyl-2-hepten-4-ynyl)-N-methyl-1-naphthalenemethanamine hydrochloride. The empirical formula $C_{21}H_{26}CIN$ with a molecular weight of 327.90, and the following structural formula:

Terbinafine hydrochloride is a white to off-white fine crystalline powder. It is freely soluble in methanol and methylene chloride, soluble in ethanol, and slightly soluble in water.

Each tablet contains:

Active Ingredients: terbinafine hydrochloride (equivalent to 250 mg base)

Inactive Ingredients: colloidal silicon dioxide, NF; hydroxypropyl methylcellulose, USP; magnesium stearate, NF; microcrystalline cellulose, NF; sodium starch glycolate, NF

CLINICAL PHARMACOLOGY
Pharmacokinetics

Following oral administration, terbinafine is well absorbed (>70%) and the bioavailability of Lamisil® (terbinafine hydrochloride tablets) Tablets as a result of first-pass metabolism is approximately 40%. Peak plasma concentrations of 1 μg/mL appear within 2 h after a single 250 mg dose; the AUC (area under the curve) is approximately 4.56 μg·h/mL. An increase in the AUC of terbinafine of less than 20% is observed when Lamisil® is administered with food. No clinically relevant age-dependent changes in steady-state plasma concentrations of terbinafine have been reported. In patients with renal impairment (creatinine clearance ≤50 mL/min) or hepatic cirrhosis, the clearance of terbinafine is decreased by approximately 50% compared to normal volunteers. No effect of gender on the blood levels of terbinafine was detected in clinical trials. In plasma, terbinafine is >99% bound to plasma proteins and there are no specific binding sites. At steady-state, in comparison to a single dose, the peak concentration of terbinafine is 25% higher and plasma AUC increases by a factor of 2.5; the increase in plasma AUC

is consistent with an effective half-life of ~36 hours. Terbinafine is distributed to the sebum and skin. A terminal half-life of 200-400 h may represent the slow elimination of terbinafine from tissues such as skin and adipose. Prior to excretion, terbinafine is extensively metabolized. No metabolites have been identified that have antifungal activity similar to terbinafine. Approximately 70% of the administered dose is eliminated in the urine.

Microbiology

Terbinafine hydrochloride is a synthetic allylamine derivative. Terbinafine hydrochloride exerts its antifungal effect by inhibiting squalene epoxidase, a key enzyme in sterol biosynthesis in fungi. This action results in a deficiency in ergosterol and a corresponding accumulation of sterol within the fungal cell. Depending on the concentration of the drug and the fungal species tested in vitro, terbinafine hydrochloride may be fungicidal; however, the clinical significance of these data is unknown. In vitro, mammalian squalene epoxidase is only inhibited at higher (4,000-fold) concentrations. Terbinafine has been shown to be active against most strains of the following organisms both in vitro and in clinical infections of the nail.

Trichophyton rubrum
Trichophyton mentagrophytes

Blood and tissue levels of terbinafine following oral dosing with Lamisil® 250 mg QD exceed in vitro MIC's against most strains of the following organisms which can infect the nail; however, the efficacy of terbinafine in treating nail infections due to these organisms has not been studied in controlled clinical trials.

Epidermophyton floccosum
Microsporum gypseum
Microsporum nanum
Trichophyton verrucosum
Candida albicans
Scopulariopsis brevicaulis

CLINICAL STUDIES

The efficacy of Lamisil® (terbinafine hydrochloride tablets) Tablets in the treatment of onychomycosis is illustrated by the response of patients with toenail and/or fingernail infections who participated in two US/Canadian placebo-controlled clinical trials.

Results of the toenail study, as assessed at week 48 (12 weeks of treatment with 36 weeks follow-up after completion of therapy), demonstrated mycological cure, defined as simultaneous occurrence of negative KOH plus negative culture, in 70% of patients. Fifty-nine percent (59%) of patients experienced effective treatment (mycological cure plus 0% nail involvement or >5mm of new unaffected nail growth); 38% of patients demonstrated mycological cure plus clinical cure (0% nail involvement).

Results of the fingernail study, as assessed at week 24 (6 weeks of treatment with 18 weeks follow-up after completion of therapy), demonstrated mycological cure in 79% of patients, effective treatment in 75% of the patients, and mycological cure plus clinical cure in 59% of the patients.

The mean time to overall success was approximately 10 months for the toenail study and 4 months for the fingernail study. In the toenail study, for patients evaluated at least six months after achieving clinical cure and at least one year after completing Lamisil® therapy, the clinical relapse rate was approximately 15%.

INDICATIONS AND USAGE

Lamisil® (terbinafine hydrochloride tablets) Tablets are indicated for the treatment of onychomycosis of the toenail or fingernail due to dermatophytes (tinea unguium) (see DOSAGE AND ADMINISTRATION).

CONTRAINDICATIONS

Lamisil® (terbinafine hydrochloride tablets) Tablets are contraindicated in individuals with hypersensitivity to terbinafine.

WARNINGS

Rare cases of symptomatic hepatobiliary dysfunction including cholestatic hepatitis have been reported. Treatment with Lamisil® (terbinafine hydrochloride tablets) Tablets should be discontinued if hepatobiliary dysfunction develops (see PRECAUTIONS). There have been isolated reports of serious skin reactions (e.g., Stevens-Johnson Syndrome and toxic epidermal necrolysis). If progressive skin rash occurs, treatment with Lamisil® should be discontinued.

PRECAUTIONS
General

Changes in the ocular lens and retina have been reported following the use of Lamisil® (terbinafine hydrochloride tablets) Tablets in controlled trials. The clinical significance of these changes is unknown. Hepatic function (hepatic enzyme) tests are recommended in patients administered Lamisil® for more than six weeks (see WARNINGS).

In patients with either pre-existing liver disease or renal impairment (creatinine clearance ≤50 mL/min), the use of Lamisil® has not been adequately studied, and therefore, is not recommended (see CLINICAL PHARMACOLOGY, Pharmacokinetics).

Transient decreases in absolute lymphocyte counts (ALC) have been observed in controlled clinical trials. In placebo-controlled trials, 8/465 Lamisil®-treated patients (1.7%) and 3/137 placebo-treated patients (2.2%) had decreases in ALC to below 1000/mm^3 on two or more occasions. The clinical significance of this observation is unknown. However, in patients with known or suspected immunodeficiency, physicians should consider monitoring complete blood counts in individuals using Lamisil® therapy for greater than six weeks.
Isolated cases of severe neutropenia have been reported. These were reversible upon discontinuation of Lamisil®, with or without supportive therapy. If clinical signs and symptoms suggestive of secondary infection occur, a complete blood count should be obtained. If the neutrophil count is $\leq$1,000 cells/mm^3, Lamisil® should be discontinued and supportive management started.

Drug Interactions

In vitro studies with human liver microsomes showed that terbinafine does not inhibit the metabolism of tolbutamide, ethinylestradiol, ethoxycoumarin, and cyclosporine. *In vivo* drug-drug interaction studies conducted in normal volunteer subjects showed that terbinafine does not affect the clearance of antipyrine, digoxin, and the antihistamine terfenadine.
Terbinafine does not affect the clearance of warfarin or warfarin's effect on prothrombin time. Terbinafine decreases the clearance of intravenously administered caffeine by 19%. Terbinafine increases the clearance of cyclosporine by 15%.
Terbinafine clearance is increased 100% by rifampin, a CyP450 enzyme inducer, and decreased 33% by cimetidine, a CyP450 enzyme inhibitor. Terbinafine clearance is decreased 16% by terfenadine. Terbinafine clearance is unaffected by cyclosporine.
There is no information available from prospectively conducted drug interaction studies with the following classes of drugs: oral contraceptives, hormone replacement therapies, hypoglycemics, theophyllines, phenytoins, thiazide diuretics, beta blockers, and calcium channel blockers.

Carcinogenesis, Mutagenesis, Impairment of Fertility

In a 28-month oral carcinogenicity study in rats, a marginal increase in the incidence of liver tumors was observed in males at the highest dose level, 69 mg/kg/day [13.8× the maximum recommended human dose (MRHD) based on body weight (BW) and 3.6× the MRHD based on body surface area (BSA)]. There was no dose-related trend and the mid-dose male rats (20 mg/kg/day; 4.0× the MRHD based on BW and 1.0× the MRHD based on BSA) did not have any tumors. No increased incidence in liver tumors was noted in female rats at dose levels up to 97 mg/kg/day (19.4× the MRHD based on BW and 4.5× the MRHD based on BSA) or in male or female mice treated orally for 23 months at doses up to 156 mg/kg/day (31.2× the MRHD based on BW and 3.9× the MRHD based on BSA).
A wide range of *in vivo* studies in mice, rats, dogs, and monkeys, and *in vitro* studies using rat, monkey, and human hepatocytes suggest that the development of liver tumors in the high-dose male rats may be associated with peroxisome proliferation, and support the conclusion that this is a rat-specific finding. *In vivo* investigations included evaluations of the effects of Lamisil® on liver weight, morphology, and ultrastructure; hepatic cytochrome P450; and peroxisome proliferation assessed morphologically and biochemically (peroxisomal enzymes) in mice, rats, dogs, and monkeys. The effects of Lamisil® and two known metabolites on hepatic morphology and peroxisomal and P450 enzyme activities were also evaluated *in vivo* in male rats and *in vitro* in primary hepatocyte cultures from male rats and humans and from monkeys. The results of the *in vivo* investigations indicated that oral administration of Lamisil® (500 mg/kg/day) resulted in peroxisome proliferation in rats, and that these effects did not occur in mice, dogs, or monkeys. Further, *in vitro* studies indicated that peroxisome proliferation occurred in rat hepatocytes, but not in monkey or human hepatocytes.
Systemic exposure to Lamisil®, assessed by the steady-state plasma unbound fraction area under the curve (AUC) for terbinafine and metabolites, was 7.7 and 9.7 μg·h/mL for male and female rats, respectively, and 11.2 and 13.1 μg·h/mL for male and female mice, respectively, at doses comparable to the high doses in the carcinogenicity studies. In human subjects at the MRHD (a daily dose of 250 mg of Lamisil®), the unbound AUC was 0.466 μg·h/mL. The resulting safety margins for humans, based on relative systemic exposure (AUC unbound), in rats and mice were 17 to 21 and 24 to 28, respectively.
The results of a variety of *in vitro* and *in vivo* genotoxicity tests gave no evidence of a mutagenic or clastogenic potential, and demonstrated the absence of tumor-initiating or cell-proliferating activity.
Oral reproduction studies in rats at doses up to 300 mg/kg/day (60× the MRHD based on BW and approximately 12× the MRHD based on BSA) did not reveal any specific effects on fertility or other reproductive parameters. Intravaginal application of terbinafine hydrochloride at 150 mg/day in pregnant rabbits did not increase the incidence of abortions or premature deliveries nor affect fetal parameters.

Pregnancy

Pregnancy Category B: Oral reproduction studies have been performed in rabbits and rats at doses up to 300 mg/kg/day (60× the MRHD based on BW and 9× to 12× the MRHD, in rabbits and rats, respectively, based on BSA) and have revealed no evidence of impaired fertility or harm to the fetus due to terbinafine. There are, however, no adequate and well-controlled studies in pregnant women. Because animal reproduction studies are not always predictive of human response, and because treatment of onychomycosis can be postponed until after pregnancy is completed, it is recommended that Lamisil® not be initiated during pregnancy.

Nursing Mothers

After oral administration, terbinafine is present in breast milk of nursing mothers. The ratio of terbinafine in milk to plasma is 7:1. Treatment with Lamisil® is not recommended in nursing mothers.

Pediatric Use

The safety and efficacy of Lamisil® have not been established in pediatric patients.

ADVERSE REACTIONS

The most frequently reported adverse events observed in the 3 US/Canadian placebo-controlled trials are listed in the table below. The adverse events reported encompass gastrointestinal symptoms (including diarrhea, dyspepsia, and abdominal pain), liver test abnormalities, rashes, urticaria, pruritus, and taste disturbances. In general, the adverse events were mild, transient, and did not lead to discontinuation from study participation.

	Adverse Event		Discontinuation	
	Lamisil® (%) n=465	Placebo (%) n=137	Lamisil® (%) n=465	Placebo (%) n=137
Headache	12.9	9.5	0.2	0.0
Gastrointestinal Symptoms:				
Diarrhea	5.6	2.9	0.6	0.0
Dyspepsia	4.3	2.9	0.4	0.0
Abdominal Pain	2.4	1.5	0.4	0.0
Nausea	2.6	2.9	0.2	0.0
Flatulence	2.2	2.2	0.0	0.0
Dermatological Symptoms:				
Rash	5.6	2.2	0.9	0.7
Pruritus	2.8	1.5	0.2	0.0
Urticaria	1.1	0.0	0.0	0.0
Liver Enzyme Abnormalities*	3.3	1.4	0.2	0.0
Taste Disturbance	2.8	0.7	0.2	0.0
Visual Disturbance	1.1	1.5	0.9	0.0

*Liver enzyme abnormalities ≥2× the upper limit of the normal range.

Rare adverse events, based on worldwide experience with Lamisil® (terbinafine hydrochloride tablets) Tablets use, include: symptomatic idiosyncratic hepatobiliary dysfunction (including cholestatic hepatitis) (*see WARNINGS and PRECAUTIONS*), serious skin reactions (see *WARNINGS*), severe neutropenia (*see PRECAUTIONS*), and allergic reactions (including anaphylaxis). Rarely, Lamisil® may cause taste disturbance (including taste loss) which usually recovers within several weeks after discontinuation of the drug.

OVERDOSAGE

There is no information on human overdosage with Lamisil® (terbinafine hydrochloride tablets) Tablets. Single oral doses in rats and mice up to 400 times the therapeutic dose produce sedation, drowsiness, ataxia, dyspnea, exophthalmus, and piloerection; animal mortality was less than 50% at this dose level.

DOSAGE AND ADMINISTRATION

Lamisil® (terbinafine hydrochloride tablets) Tablets, one 250 mg tablet, should be taken once daily for 6 weeks by patients with fingernail onychomycosis. Lamisil®, one 250 mg tablet, should be taken once daily for 12 weeks by patients with toenail onychomycosis. The optimal clinical effect is seen some months after mycological cure and cessation of treatment. This is related to the period required for outgrowth of healthy nail.

HOW SUPPLIED

Lamisil®
(terbinafine hydrochloride tablets)
Tablets

Supplied as white to yellow-tinged white circular, bi-convex, bevelled tablets containing 250 mg of terbinafine imprinted with "LAMISIL" in circular form on one side and code "250" on the other.
Bottles of 100 tablets
NDC 0078-0179-05
Bottles of 30 tablets
NDC 0078-0179-15
Store tablets below 25°C (77°F); in a tight container. Protect from light.

[APRIL 1996 37051901]

Shown in Product Identification Guide, page 333

LESCOL® ℞

(fluvastatin sodium)
Capsules

Caution: Federal law prohibits dispensing without prescription.
The following prescribing information is based on official labeling in effect on August 1, 1996.

DESCRIPTION

Lescol® (fluvastatin sodium) is a water soluble cholesterol lowering agent which acts through the inhibition of 3-hydroxy-3-methylglutaryl-coenzyme A (HMG-CoA) reductase.
Fluvastatin sodium is [R^*,S^*-(E)]-(±)-7-[3-(4-fluorophenyl)-1-(1-methylethyl)-1H-indol-2-yl]-3,5-dihydroxy-6-heptenoic acid, monosodium salt. The structural formula is:

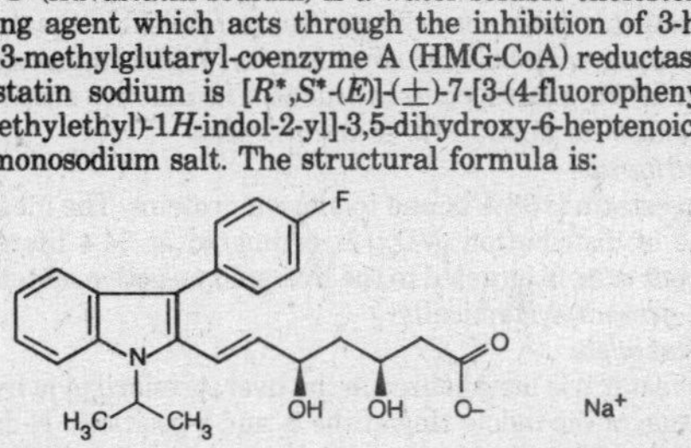

$C_{24}H_{25}FNO_4 \cdot Na$ Mol. wt. 433.46

This molecular entity is the first entirely synthetic HMG-CoA reductase inhibitor, and is in part structurally distinct from the fungal derivatives of this therapeutic class.
Fluvastatin sodium is a white to pale yellow, hygroscopic powder soluble in water, ethanol and methanol. Lescol® (fluvastatin sodium) is supplied as capsules containing fluvastatin sodium, equivalent to 20 mg or 40 mg of fluvastatin, for oral administration.
Active Ingredient: fluvastatin sodium
Inactive Ingredients: gelatin, magnesium stearate, microcrystalline cellulose, pregelatinized starch, red iron oxide, sodium lauryl sulfate, talc, titanium dioxide, yellow iron oxide, and other ingredients.
May Also Include: benzyl alcohol, black iron oxide, butylparaben, carboxymethylcellulose sodium, edetate calcium disodium, methylparaben, propylparaben, silicon dioxide and sodium propionate.

CLINICAL PHARMACOLOGY

A variety of clinical studies have demonstrated that elevated levels of total cholesterol (Total-C), low density lipoprotein cholesterol (LDL-C), and apolipoprotein B (a membrane transport complex for LDL-C) promote human atherosclerosis. Similarly, decreased levels of HDL-cholesterol (HDL-C) and its transport complex, apolipoprotein A, are associated with the development of atherosclerosis. Epidemiologic investigations have established that cardiovascular morbidity and mortality vary directly with the level of Total-C and LDL-C and inversely with the level of HDL-C. The Lipid Research Clinics Coronary Primary Prevention Trial (LRC-CPPT) was a multicenter, randomized, double-blind study involving 3806 asymptomatic middle-aged men in the United States with Type II hyperlipoproteinemia treated with diet and cholestyramine. Results of this trial demonstrated that a statistically significant reduction of 19% in the incidence of definite myocardial infarction and/or coronary heart disease death was associated with an 8% decrease in blood cholesterol and 11% decrease in LDL-C levels. In other multicenter clinical trials, those pharmacologic and/or nonpharmacologic interventions that simultaneously lowered LDL-C and increased HDL-C also have reduced the rate of cardiovascular events (both fatal and nonfatal myocardial infarctions).
In patients with hypercholesterolemia, treatment with Lescol® (fluvastatin sodium) reduced Total-C, LDL-C, and apolipoprotein B. Lescol® (fluvastatin sodium) also moderately reduced triglycerides (TG) while producing an increase in HDL-C of variable magnitude. The agent had no consistent effect on either Lp(a) or fibrinogen. The effect of Lescol® (fluvastatin sodium)-induced changes in lipoprotein

Continued on next page

Sandoz—Cont.

levels, including reduction of serum cholesterol, on cardiovascular morbidity or mortality has not been determined.

Mechanism of Action

Lescol® (fluvastatin sodium) is competitive inhibitor of HMG-CoA reductase, which is responsible for the conversion of 3-hydroxyl-3-methylglutaryl-coenzyme A (HMG-CoA) to mevalonate, a precursor of sterols, including cholesterol. The inhibition of cholesterol biosynthesis reduces the cholesterol in hepatic cells, which stimulates the synthesis of LDL receptors and thereby increases the uptake of LDL particles. The end result of these biochemical processes is a reduction of the plasma cholesterol concentration.

Pharmacokinetics/Metabolism

Oral Absorption

Fluvastatin is absorbed rapidly and completely following oral administration, with peak concentrations reached in less than 1 hour. Following administration of a 10 mg dose, the absolute bioavailability is 24% (range 9%–50%). Administration with food reduces the rate but not the extent of absorption. At steady-state, administration of fluvastatin with the evening meal results in a two-fold decrease in C_{max} and more than two-fold increase in t_{max} as compared to administration 4 hours after the evening meal. No significant difference in extent of absorption or in the lipid-lowering effects were observed between the two administrations. After single or multiple doses above 20 mg, fluvastatin exhibits saturable first-pass metabolism resulting in higher-than-expected plasma fluvastatin concentrations. The inactive enantiomer accounts for about 60% of the increase.

Distribution

Fluvastatin is 98% bound to plasma proteins. The mean volume of distribution (VD_{ss}) is estimated at 34.4 liters. The parent drug is targeted to the liver and no active metabolites are present systemically.

Metabolism

Fluvastatin is metabolized in the liver, primarily via hydroxylation of the indole ring at the 5- and 6-positions. N-dealkylation and beta-oxidation of the side-chain also occurs. The hydroxy metabolites have some pharmacologic activity, but do not circulate in the blood. Both enantiomers of fluvastatin are metabolized in a similar manner.

Elimination

Fluvastatin is primarily (about 90%) eliminated in the feces as metabolites, with less than 2% present as unchanged drug.

Special Populations

Renal Insufficiency: No significant (<6%) renal excretion of fluvastatin occurs in humans.

Hepatic Insufficiency: Fluvastatin is subject to saturable first-pass metabolism/sequestration by the liver and is eliminated primarily via the biliary route. Therefore, the potential exists for drug accumulation in patients with hepatic insufficiency. Caution should therefore be exercised when fluvastatin sodium is administered to patients with a history of liver disease or heavy alcohol ingestion (*see WARNINGS*).

Age: Plasma levels of fluvastatin are not affected by age.

Gender: Women tend to have slightly higher (but statistically insignificant) fluvastatin concentrations than men. This is most likely due to body weight differences, as adjusting for body weight decreases the magnitude of the differences seen.

Pediatric: No data are available. Fluvastatin is not indicated for use in the pediatric population.

Steady-state plasma concentrations show no evidence of accumulation of fluvastatin following administration of up to 80 mg daily, as evidenced by a beta-elimination half-life of less than 3 hours. However, under conditions of maximum rate of absorption (i.e., fasting) systemic exposure to fluvastatin is increased 33% to 53% compared to a single 20 mg or 40 mg dose.

Single-dose and steady-state pharmacokinetic parameters in 33 subjects with hypercholesterolemia are summarized below:

[See table below.]

	C_{max} (ng/mL) mean±SD (range)	AUC (ng·h/mL) mean±SD (range)	t_{max} (hr) mean±SD (range)	CL/F (L/hr) mean±SD (range)	$t_{1/2}$ (hr) mean±SD (range)
20 mg single dose (n=17)	166±106 (48.9–517)	207±65 (111–288)	0.9±0.4 (0.5–2.0)	107±38.1 (69.5–181)	2.5±1.7 (0.5–6.6)
20 mg b.i.d. (n=17)	200±86 (71.8–366)	275±111 (91.6–467)	1.2±0.9 (0.5–4.0)	87.8±45 (42.8–218)	2.8±1.7 (0.9–6.0)
40 mg single dose (n=16)	273±189 (72.8–812)	456±259 (207–1221)	1.2±0.7 (0.75–3.0)	108±44.7 (32.8–193)	2.7±1.3 (0.8–5.9)
40 mg b.i.d. (n=16)	432±236 (119–990)	697±275 (359–1559)	1.2±0.6 (0.5–2.5)	64.2±21.1 (25.7–111)	2.7±1.3 (0.7–5.0)

Clinical Studies

Lescol® (fluvastatin sodium) has been studied in 19 controlled studies worldwide for patients with Type IIa or IIb hyperlipoproteinemia. Lescol® (fluvastatin sodium) alone was administered to 2326 patients in daily dose regimens of 20 mg, 40 mg, and 80 mg (40 mg b.i.d.) in trials from 6–36 weeks in duration. In the largest single randomized study with Lescol® (fluvastatin sodium) (n=292), treatment at a dose of 20 mg QPM resulted in a highly significant decrease in LDL-C of 22% after nine weeks of study. In the largest single study (n=210) of patients randomized to 40 mg daily and limited to FH patients, a mean LDL-C reduction of 24% was observed. This effect was observed after 4 weeks of treatment and was maintained during the additional 8 weeks of fluvastatin administration. In the largest single controlled study (N=266) of patients randomized to 80 mg (40 mg b.i.d.) daily, a mean LDL-C reduction of 35% was observed during the initial evaluation period (average of 4 and 8 weeks exposure) and a mean LDL-C reduction of 32% was observed at endpoint (28 weeks exposure). In a long term open-label free titration study, after 96 weeks LDL-C decreases of 25% (20 mg, N=68), 31% (40 mg, N=298), and 34% (80 mg, N=209) were observed. Reductions in Apo B were also seen as a result of treatment with Lescol® (fluvastatin sodium). Small but statistically significant increases in HDL-C and corresponding decreases in TG were also noted. No consistent effect on Lp(a) was found.

INDICATIONS AND USAGE

Lescol® (fluvastatin sodium) is indicated as an adjunct to diet in the treatment of elevated total cholesterol (Total-C) and LDL-C levels in patients with primary hypercholesterolemia (Type IIa and IIb) whose response to dietary restriction of saturated fat and cholesterol and other nonpharmacological measures has not been adequate.

Therapy with lipid-altering agents should be considered only after secondary causes for hyperlipidemia such as poorly controlled diabetes mellitus, hypothyroidism, nephrotic syndrome, dysproteinemias, obstructive liver disease, other medication, or alcoholism, have been excluded. Prior to initiation of fluvastatin sodium, a lipid profile should be performed to measure Total-C, HDL-C and TG. For patients with TG <400 mg/dL (<4.5 mmol/L), LDL-C can be estimated using the following equation:

$$\text{LDL-C} = \text{Total-C} - \text{HDL-C} - 1/5\ \text{TG}$$

For TG levels >400 mg/dL (>4.5 mmol/L), this equation is less accurate and LDL-C concentrations should be determined by ultracentrifugation. In many hypertriglyceridemic patients LDL-C may be low or normal despite elevated Total-C. In such cases, Lescol® (fluvastatin sodium) is not indicated.

Lipid determinations should be performed at intervals of no less than 4 weeks and dosage adjusted according to the patient's response to therapy.

The National Cholesterol Education Program (NCEP) Treatment Guidelines are summarized below:

LDL-Cholesterol		mg/dL (mmol/L)	
Definite Atherosclerotic Disease*	Two or More Other Risk Factors**	Initiation Level	Goal
NO	NO	≥190 (≥4.9)	<160 (<4.1)
NO	YES	≥160 (≥4.1)	<130 (<3.4)
YES	YES or NO	≥130 (≥3.4)	≤100 (≤2.6)

* Coronary heart disease or peripheral vascular disease (including symptomatic carotid artery disease).

** Other risk factors for coronary heart disease (CHD) include: age (males: ≥45 years; females: ≥55 years or premature menopause without estrogen replacement therapy); family history of premature CHD; current cigarette smoking; hypertension; confirmed HDL-C <35 mg/dL (<0.91 mmol/L); and diabetes mellitus. Subtract one risk factor if HDL-C is ≥60 mg/dL (≥1.6 mmol/L).

Since the goal of treatment is to lower LDL-C, the NCEP recommends that the LDL-C levels be used to initiate and assess treatment response. Only if LDL-C levels are not available, should the Total-C be used to monitor therapy.

Classification of Hyperlipoproteinemias

Type	Lipoproteins Elevated	Lipid Elevations Major	Lipid Elevations Minor
I (rare)	Chylomicrons	TG	↑ → C
IIa	LDL	C	—
IIb	LDL, VLDL	C	TG
III (rare)	IDL	C/TG	—
IV	VLDL	TG	↑ → C
V (rare)	Chylomicrons, VLDL	TG	↑ → C

C = cholesterol, TG = triglycerides, LDL = low density lipoprotein, VLDL = very low density lipoprotein, IDL = intermediate density lipoprotein

Lescol® (fluvastatin sodium) has not been studied in conditions where the major abnormality is elevation of chylomicrons, VLDL, or IDL (i.e., hyperlipoproteinemia Types I, III, IV, or V).

CONTRAINDICATIONS

Hypersensitivity to any component of this medication. Lescol® (fluvastatin sodium) is contraindicated in patients with active liver disease or unexplained, persistent elevations in serum transaminases (*see WARNINGS*).

Pregnancy and Lactation

Atherosclerosis is a chronic process and discontinuation of lipid-lowering drugs during pregnancy should have little impact on the outcome of long-term therapy of primary hypercholesterolemia. Cholesterol and other products of cholesterol biosynthesis are essential components for fetal development (including synthesis of steroids and cell membranes). Since HMG-CoA reductase inhibitors decrease cholesterol synthesis and possibly the synthesis of other biologically active substances derived from cholesterol, they may cause fetal harm when administered to pregnant women. Therefore, HMG-CoA reductase inhibitors are contraindicated during pregnancy and in nursing mothers. **Fluvastatin sodium should be administered to women of childbearing age only when such patients are highly unlikely to conceive and have been informed of the potential hazards.** If the patient becomes pregnant while taking this class of drug, therapy should be discontinued and the patient apprised of the potential hazard to the fetus.

WARNINGS

Liver Enzymes

Biochemical abnormalities of liver function have been associated with HMG-CoA reductase inhibitors and other lipid-lowering agents. A small number of patients treated with Lescol® (fluvastatin sodium) in worldwide controlled trials (N=25, 1.1%) developed dose-related, persistent elevations of transaminase levels to more than 3 times the upper limit of normal. Fourteen of these patients (0.6%) were discontinued from therapy. In all clinical trials, a total of 33/2969 patients (1.1%) had persistent transaminase elevations with an average fluvastatin exposure of approximately 71.2 weeks; 19 of these patients (0.6%) were discontinued. The majority of patients with these abnormal biochemical findings were asymptomatic.

It is recommended that liver function tests be performed before the initiation of treatment, at 6 and 12 weeks after initiation of therapy or elevation in dose, and periodically thereafter (e.g., semiannually). Liver enzyme changes generally occur in the first 3 months of treatment with Lescol® (fluvastatin sodium). Patients who develop increased transaminase levels should be monitored with a second liver function evaluation to confirm the finding and be followed thereafter with frequent liver function tests until the abnormality(ies) return to normal. Should an increase in AST or ALT of three times the upper limit of normal or greater persist, withdrawal of fluvastatin sodium therapy is recommended. Active liver disease or unexplained transaminase elevations are contraindications to the use of Lescol® (fluvastatin sodium) (see CONTRAINDICATIONS). Caution should be exercised when fluvastatin sodium is administered to patients with a history of liver disease or heavy alcohol ingestion (*see CLINICAL PHARMACOLOGY: Pharmacokinetics/Metabolism*). Such patients should be closely monitored.

Skeletal Muscle

Rhabdomyolysis with renal dysfunction secondary to myoglobinuria has been reported with fluvastatin and with other drugs in this class. Myopathy, defined as muscle aching or muscle weakness in conjunction with increases in creatine phosphokinase (CPK) values to greater than 10 times the upper limit of normal, has been reported rarely.

Myopathy should be considered in any patients with diffuse myalgias, muscle tenderness or weakness, and/or marked elevation of CPK. Patients should be advised to report promptly unexplained muscle pain, tenderness or weakness, particularly if accompanied by malaise or fever. Fluvastatin

sodium therapy should be discontinued if markedly elevated CPK levels occur or myopathy is diagnosed or suspected. Fluvastatin sodium therapy should also be temporarily withheld in any patient experiencing an acute or serious condition predisposing to the development of renal failure secondary to rhabdomyolysis, e.g., sepsis; hypotension; major surgery; trauma; severe metabolic, endocrine, or electrolyte disorders; or uncontrolled epilepsy.

The risk of myopathy and or rhabdomyolysis during treatment with HMG-CoA reductase inhibitors has been reported to be increased if therapy with either cyclosporine, gemfibrozil, erythromycin, or niacin is administered concurrently. Myopathy was not observed in a clinical trial in 74 patients involving patients who were treated with fluvastatin sodium together with niacin.

Uncomplicated myalgia has been observed infrequently in patients treated with Lescol® (fluvastatin sodium) at rates indistinguishable from placebo.

The use of fibrates alone may occasionally be associated with myopathy. The combined use of HMG-CoA inhibitors and fibrates should generally be avoided.

PRECAUTIONS

General

Before instituting therapy with Lescol® (fluvastatin sodium), an attempt should be made to control hypercholesterolemia with appropriate diet, exercise, and weight reduction in obese patients, and to treat other underlying medical problems (*see INDICATIONS AND USAGE*).

The HMG-CoA reductase inhibitors may cause elevation of creatine phosphokinase and transaminase levels (*see WARNINGS and ADVERSE REACTIONS*). This should be considered in the differential diagnosis of chest pain in a patient on therapy with fluvastatin sodium.

Homozygous Familial Hypercholesterolemia

HMG-CoA reductase inhibitors are reported to be less effective in patients with rare homozygous familial hypercholesterolemia, possibly because these patients have few functional LDL receptors.

Information for Patients

Patients should be advised to report promptly unexplained muscle pain, tenderness or weakness, particularly if accompanied by malaise or fever.

Women should be informed that if they become pregnant while receiving Lescol® (fluvastatin sodium) the drug should be discontinued immediately to avoid possible harmful effects on a developing fetus from a relative deficit of cholesterol and biological products derived from cholesterol. In addition, Lescol® (fluvastatin sodium) should not be taken during nursing.

(See CONTRAINDICATIONS)

Drug Interactions

Immunosuppressive Drugs, Gemfibrozil, Niacin (Nicotinic Acid), Erythromycin: *See WARNINGS: Skeletal Muscle.*

Antipyrine: Administration of fluvastatin sodium does not influence the metabolism and excretion of antipyrine, either by induction or inhibition. Antipyrine is a model for drugs metabolized by the microsomal hepatic enzyme system; therefore, interactions with other drugs metabolized by this mechanism are not expected.

Niacin/Propranolol: Concomitant administration of fluvastatin sodium with niacin or propranolol has no effect on the bioavailability of fluvastatin sodium.

Cholestyramine: Administration of fluvastatin sodium concomitantly with, or up to 4 hours after cholestyramine, results in fluvastatin decreases of more than 50% for AUC and 50%-80% for C_{max}. However, administration of fluvastatin sodium 4 hours after cholestyramine resulted in a clinically significant additive effect compared with that achieved with either component drug.

Digoxin: In a crossover study involving 18 patients chronically receiving digoxin, a single 40 mg dose of fluvastatin had no effect on digoxin AUC, but had an 11% increase in digoxin C_{max} and small increase in digoxin urinary clearance. Patients taking digoxin should be monitored appropriately when fluvastatin therapy is initiated.

Cimetidine/Ranitidine/Omeprazole: Concomitant administration of fluvastatin sodium with cimetidine, ranitidine and omeprazole results in a significant increase in the fluvastatin C_{max} (43%, 70% and 50%, respectively) and AUC (24%–33%), with an 18%–23% decrease in plasma clearance.

Rifampicin: Administration of fluvastatin sodium to subjects pretreated with rifampicin results in significant reduction in C_{max} (59%) and AUC (51%), with a large increase (95%) in plasma clearance.

Warfarin: *In vitro* protein binding studies demonstrated no interaction at therapeutic concentrations. Concomitant administration of a single dose of warfarin (30 mg) in young healthy males receiving fluvastatin sodium (40 mg/day × 8 days) resulted in no elevation of racemic warfarin concentration. There was also no effect on prothrombin complex activity when compared to concomitant administration of placebo and warfarin. However, bleeding and/or increased prothrombin times have been reported in patients taking coumarin anticoagulants concomitantly with other HMG-CoA reductase inhibitors. Therefore, patients receiving warfarin-type anticoagulants should have their prothrombin times closely monitored when fluvastatin sodium is initiated or the dosage of fluvastatin sodium is changed.

Other Concomitant Therapy: Although specific interaction studies were not performed, in clinical studies, fluvastatin sodium was used concomitantly with angiotensin-converting enzyme (ACE) inhibitors, beta blockers, calcium-channel blockers, diuretics and nonsteroidal anti-inflammatory drugs (NSAIDs) without evidence of clinically significant adverse interactions.

Endocrine Function

HMG-CoA reductase inhibitors interfere with cholesterol synthesis and lower circulating cholesterol levels and, as such, might theoretically blunt adrenal or gonadal steroid hormone production.

Fluvastatin exhibited no effect upon non-stimulated cortisol levels and demonstrated no effect upon thyroid metabolism as assessed by TSH. Small declines in total testosterone have been noted in treated groups, but no commensurate elevation in LH occurred, suggesting that the observation was not due to a direct effect upon testosterone production. No effect upon FSH in males was noted. Due to the limited number of premenopausal females studied to date, no conclusions regarding the effect of fluvastatin upon female sex hormones may be made.

Two clinical studies in patients receiving fluvastatin at doses up to 80 mg daily for periods of 24 to 28 weeks demonstrated no effect of treatment upon the adrenal response to ACTH stimulation. A clinical study evaluated the effect of fluvastatin at doses up to 80 mg daily for 28 weeks upon the gonadal response to HCG stimulation. Although the mean total testosterone response was significantly reduced ($p < 0.05$) relative to baseline in the 80 mg group, it was not significant in comparison to the changes noted in groups receiving either 40 mg of fluvastatin or placebo.

Patients treated with fluvastatin sodium who develop clinical evidence of endocrine dysfunction should be evaluated appropriately. Caution should be exercised if an HMG-CoA reductase inhibitor or other agent used to lower cholesterol levels is administered to patients receiving other drugs (e.g., ketoconazole, spironolactone, or cimetidine) that may decrease the levels of endogenous steroid hormones.

CNS Toxicity

CNS effects, as evidenced by decreased activity, ataxia, loss of righting reflex, and ptosis were seen in the following animal studies: the 18-month mouse carcinogenicity study at 50 mg/kg/day, the 6-month dog study at 36 mg/kg/day, the 6-month hamster study at 40 mg/kg/day, and in acute, high-dose studies in rats and hamsters (50 mg/kg), rabbits (300 mg/kg) and mice (1500 mg/kg). CNS toxicity in the acute high-dose studies was characterized (in mice) by conspicuous vacuolation in the ventral white columns of the spinal cord at a dose of 5000 mg/kg and (in rat) by edema with separation of myelinated fibers of the ventral spinal tracts and sciatic nerve at a dose of 1500 mg/kg. CNS toxicity, characterized by periaxonal vacuolation, was observed in the medulla of dogs that died after treatment for 5 weeks with 48 mg/kg/day; this finding was not observed in the remaining dogs when the dose level was lowered to 36 mg/kg/day. CNS vascular lesions, characterized by perivascular hemorrhages, edema, and mononuclear cell infiltration of perivascular spaces, have been observed in dogs treated with other members of this class. No CNS lesions have been observed after chronic treatment for up to 2 years with fluvastatin in the mouse (at doses up to 350 mg/kg/day), rat (up to 24 mg/kg/day), or dog (up to 16 mg/kg/day).

Prominent bilateral posterior Y suture lines in the ocular lens were seen in dogs after treatment with 1, 8, and 16 mg/kg/day for 2 years.

Carcinogenesis, Mutagenesis, Impairment of Fertility

A 2-year study was performed in rats at dose levels of 6, 9, and 18-24 (escalated after 1 year) mg/kg/day. These treatment levels represented plasma drug levels of approximately 9, 13, and 26-35 times the mean human plasma drug concentration after a 40 mg oral dose. A low incidence of forestomach squamous papillomas and 1 carcinoma of the forestomach at the 24 mg/kg/day dose level was considered to reflect the prolonged hyperplasia induced by direct contact exposure to fluvastatin sodium rather than to a systemic effect of the drug. In addition, an increased incidence of thyroid follicular cell adenomas and carcinomas was recorded for males treated with 18–24 mg/kg/day. The increased incidence of thyroid follicular cell neoplasm in male rats with fluvastatin sodium appears to be consistent with findings from other HMG-CoA reductase inhibitors. In contrast to other HMG-CoA reductase inhibitors, no hepatic adenomas or carcinomas were observed.

The carcinogenicity study conducted in mice at dose levels of 0.3, 15 and 30 mg/kg/day revealed, as in rats, a statistically significant increase in forestomach squamous cell papillomas in males and females at 30 mg/kg/day and in females at 15 mg/kg/day. These treatment levels represented plasma drug levels of approximately 0.05, 2, and 7 times the mean human plasma drug concentration after a 40 mg oral dose.

No evidence of mutagenicity was observed*in vitro*, with or without rat-liver metabolic activation, in the following studies: microbial mutagen tests using mutant strains of *Salmonella typhimurium* or *Escherichia coli*; malignant transformation assay in BALB/3T3 cells; unscheduled DNA synthesis in rat primary hepatocytes; chromosomal aberrations in V79 Chinese Hamster cells; HGPRT V79 Chinese Hamster cells. In addition, there was no evidence of mutagenicity *in vivo* in either a rat or mouse micronucleus test.

In a study in rats at dose levels for females of 0.6, 2 and 6 mg/kg/day and at dose levels for males of 2, 10 and 20 mg/kg/day, fluvastatin sodium had no adverse effects on the fertility or reproductive performance.

Seminal vesicles and testes were small in hamsters treated for 3 months at 20 mg/kg (approximately three times the 40 milligram human daily dose based on surface area, mg/m^2). There was tubular degeneration and aspermatogenesis in testes as well as vesiculitis of seminal vesicles. Vesiculitis of seminal vesicles and edema of the testes were also seen in rats treated for 2 years at 18 mg/kg (approximately 4 times the human C_{max} achieved with a 40 milligram daily dose).

Pregnancy

Pregnancy Category X

See CONTRAINDICATIONS.

Fluvastatin sodium produced delays in skeletal development in rats at doses of 12 mg/kg and in rabbits at doses of 10 mg/kg. Malaligned thoracic vertebrae were seen in rats at 36 mg/kg, a dose that produced maternal toxicity. These doses resulted in 2 times (rat at 12 mg/kg) or 5 times (rabbit at 10 mg/kg) the 40 mg human exposure based on mg/m^2 surface area. A study in which female rats were dosed during the third trimester at 12 and 24 mg/kg/day resulted in maternal mortality at or near term and postpartum. In addition, fetal and neonatal lethality were apparent. No effects on the dam or fetus occurred at 2 mg/kg/day. A second study at levels of 2, 6, 12 and 24 mg/kg/day confirmed the findings in the first study with neonatal mortality beginning at 6 mg/kg. A modified Segment III study was performed at dose levels of 12 or 24 mg/kg/day with or without the presence of concurrent supplementation with mevalonic acid, a product of HMG-CoA reductase which is essential for cholesterol biosynthesis. The concurrent administration of mevalonic acid completely prevented the maternal and neonatal mortality but did not prevent low body weights in pups at 24 mg/kg on days 0 and 7 post-partum. Therefore, the maternal and neonatal lethality observed with fluvastatin sodium reflect its exaggerated pharmacologic effect during pregnancy. There are no data with fluvastatin sodium in pregnant women. However, rare reports of congenital anomalies have been received following intrauterine exposure to other HMG-CoA reductase inhibitors. There has been one report of severe congenital bony deformity, tracheo-esophageal fistula, and anal atresia (VATER association) in a baby born to a woman who took another HMG-CoA reductase inhibitor with dextroamphetamine sulfate during the first trimester of pregnancy. **Lescol® (fluvastatin sodium) should be administered to women of child-bearing potential only when such patients are highly unlikely to conceive and have been informed of the potential hazards.** If a woman becomes pregnant while taking Lescol® (fluvastatin sodium), the drug should be discontinued and the patient advised again as to the potential hazards to the fetus.

Nursing Mothers

Based on preclinical data, drug is present in breast milk in a 2:1 ratio (milk:plasma). Because of the potential for serious adverse reactions in nursing infants, nursing women should not take Lescol® (fluvastatin sodium) (*see CONTRAINDICATIONS*).

Pediatric Use

Safety and effectiveness in individuals less than 18 years old have not been established. Treatment in patients less than 18 years of age is not recommended at this time.

Geriatric Use

The effect of age on the pharmacokinetics of fluvastatin sodium was evaluated. Results indicate that for the general patient population plasma concentrations of fluvastatin sodium do not vary either as a function of age or gender. (*See also CLINICAL PHARMACOLOGY: Pharmacokinetics/Metabolism.*) Elderly patients (≥ 65 years of age) demonstrated a greater treatment response in respect to LDL-C, Total-C and LDL/HDL ratio than patients < 65 years of age.

ADVERSE REACTIONS

In all clinical studies, 1.0% (32/2969) of fluvastatin treated patients were discontinued due to adverse experiences attributed to study drug (mean exposure approximately 16 months ranging in duration from 1 to > 36 months). This results in controlled studies in an exposure adjusted rate of 0.8% (32/4051) per patient year in fluvastatin patients compared to an incidence of 1.1% (4/355) in placebo patients. Adverse reactions have usually been of mild to moderate severity.

Continued on next page

Sandoz—Cont.

Adverse experiences occurring in controlled studies with a frequency > 2% regardless of causality include the following:

Adverse Event	Lescol® (fluvastatin sodium) (%) (N = 2326)	Placebo (%) (N = 960)
Integumentary		
Rash	2.3	2.4
Musculoskeletal		
Back Pain	5.7	6.6
Myalgia	5.0	4.5
Arthralgia	4.0	4.1
Arthritis	2.1	2.0
Respiratory		
Upper Respiratory Tract Infection	16.2	16.5
Pharyngitis	3.8	3.8
Rhinitis	4.7	4.9
Sinusitis	2.6	1.9
Coughing	2.4	2.9
Gastrointestinal		
Dyspepsia	7.9	3.2
Diarrhea	4.9	4.2
Abdominal Pain	4.9	3.8
Nausea	3.2	2.0
Constipation	3.1	3.3
Flatulence	2.6	2.5
Misc. Tooth Disorder	2.1	1.7
Central Nervous System		
Dizziness	2.2	2.5
Psychiatric Disorders		
Insomnia	2.7	1.4
Miscellaneous		
Headache	8.9	7.8
Influenza-Like Symptoms	5.1	5.7
Accidental Trauma	5.1	4.8
Fatigue	2.7	2.3
Allergy	2.3	2.2

The following effects have been reported with drugs in this class. Not all the effects listed below have necessarily been associated with fluvastatin sodium therapy.

Skeletal: muscle cramps, myalgia, myopathy, rhabdomyolysis, arthralgias.

Neurological: dysfunction of certain cranial nerves (including alteration of taste, impairment of extra-ocular movement, facial paresis), tremor, dizziness, vertigo, memory loss, paresthesia, peripheral neuropathy, peripheral nerve palsy, psychic disturbances, anxiety, insomnia, depression.

Hypersensitivity Reactions: An apparent hypersensitivity syndrome has been reported rarely which has included one or more of the following features: anaphylaxis, angioedema, lupus erythematosus-like syndrome, polymyalgia rheumatica, vasculitis, purpura, thrombocytopenia, leukopenia, hemolytic anemia, positive ANA, ESR increase, eosinophilia, arthritis, arthralgia, urticaria, asthenia, photosensitivity, fever, chills, flushing, malaise, dyspnea, toxic epidermal necrolysis, erythema multiforme, including Stevens-Johnson syndrome.

Gastrointestinal: pancreatitis, hepatitis, including chronic active hepatitis, cholestatic jaundice, fatty change in liver, and, rarely, cirrhosis, fulminant hepatic necrosis, and hepatoma; anorexia, vomiting.

Skin: alopecia, pruritus. A variety of skin changes (e.g., nodules, discoloration, dryness of skin/mucous membranes, changes to hair/nails) have been reported.

Reproductive: gynecomastia, loss of libido, erectile dysfunction.

Eye: progression of cataracts (lens opacities), ophthalmoplegia.

Laboratory Abnormalities: elevated transaminases, alkaline phosphatase, γ-glutamyl transpeptidase, and bilirubin; thyroid function abnormalities.

Concomitant Therapy
Fluvastatin sodium has been administered concurrently with cholestyramine and nicotinic acid. No adverse reactions unique to the combination or in addition to those previously reported for this class of drugs alone have been reported. Myopathy and rhabdomyolysis (with or without acute renal failure) have been reported when another HMG-CoA reductase inhibitor was used in combination with immunosuppressive drugs, gemfibrozil, erythromycin, or lipid-lowering doses of nicotinic acid. Concomitant therapy with HMG-CoA reductase inhibitors and these agents is generally not recommended. (*See WARNINGS: Skeletal Muscle.*)

OVERDOSAGE
The approximate oral LD$_{50}$ is greater than 2 g/kg in mice and greater than 0.7 g/kg in rats.

The maximum single oral dose received by healthy volunteers was 60 mg. No clinically significant adverse experiences were seen at this dose. There has been a single report of 2 children, one 2 years old and the other 3 years of age, either of whom may have possibly ingested fluvastatin sodium. The maximum amount of fluvastatin sodium that could have been ingested was 80 mg (4 × 20 mg capsules). Vomiting was induced by ipecac in both children and no capsules were noted in their emesis. Neither child experienced any adverse symptoms and both recovered from the incident without problems.

Should an accidental overdose occur, treat symptomatically and institute supportive measures as required. The dialyzability of fluvastatin sodium and of its metabolites in humans is not known at present.

Information about the treatment of overdose can often be obtained from a certified Regional Poison Control Center. Telephone numbers of certified Regional Poison Control Centers are listed in the Physicians' Desk Reference®.*

DOSAGE AND ADMINISTRATION
The patient should be placed on a standard cholesterol-lowering diet before receiving Lescol® (fluvastatin sodium) and should continue on this diet during treatment with Lescol® (fluvastatin sodium). (See NCEP Treatment Guidelines for details on dietary therapy.)

The recommended starting dose for the majority of patients is 20-40 mg once daily at bedtime. The recommended dosing range is 20-80 mg/day. The daily regimen of 80 mg should be administered in divided doses, i.e., 40 mg b.i.d., and should be reserved for those whose LDL-cholesterol response is inadequate at 40 mg/day. Lescol® (fluvastatin sodium) may be taken without regard to meals, since there are no apparent differences in the lipid-lowering effects of fluvastatin sodium administered with the evening meal or 4 hours after the evening meal. Since the maximal reductions in LDL-C of a given dose are seen within 4 weeks, periodic lipid determinations should be performed and dosage adjustment made according to the patient's response to therapy and established treatment guidelines. The therapeutic effect of Lescol® (fluvastatin sodium) is maintained with prolonged administration.

Concomitant Therapy
Lipid-lowering effects on total cholesterol and LDL cholesterol are additive when Lescol® (fluvastatin sodium) is combined with a bile-acid binding resin or niacin. When administering a bile-acid resin (e.g., cholestyramine) and fluvastatin sodium, Lescol® (fluvastatin sodium) should be administered at bedtime, at least 2 hours following the resin to avoid a significant interaction due to drug binding to resin. (*See also ADVERSE REACTIONS: Concomitant Therapy.*)

Dosage in Patients with Renal Insufficiency
Since fluvastatin sodium is cleared hepatically with less than 6% of the administered dose excreted into the urine, dose adjustments for mild to moderate renal impairment are not necessary. Caution should be exercised with severe impairment.

HOW SUPPLIED
Lescol® (fluvastatin sodium) Capsules
20 mg
Brown and light brown imprinted twice with "△." and "20" on one half and "LESCOL" and the Lescol® (fluvastatin sodium) logo twice on the other half of the capsule.
Bottles of 100 capsules (NDC 0078-0176-05)
Bottles of 30 capsules (NDC 0078-0176-15)
40 mg
Brown and gold imprinted twice with "△" and "40" on one half and "LESCOL" and the Lescol® (fluvastatin sodium) logo twice on the other half of the capsule.
Bottles of 100 capsules (NDC 0078-0234-05)
Bottles of 30 capsules (NDC 0078-0234-15)
Store and Dispense
Below 86°F (30°C) in a tight container. Protect from light.
*Trademark of Medical Economics Data Production Company.

[REV: MARCH 1996   30353904]
Shown in Product Identification Guide, page 333

MELLARIL®*   ℞
[*mel 'ah-ril "*]
(thioridazine HCl) Tablets, USP
(thioridazine HCl) Oral Solution, USP
MELLARIL-S®   ℞
(thioridazine) Oral Suspension, USP

For Oral Administration

CAUTION: Federal law prohibits dispensing without prescription.
The following prescribing information is based on official labeling in effect on August 1, 1996.

DESCRIPTION
Mellaril® (thioridazine) is 2-methylmercapto-10-[2-(N-methyl-2-piperidyl) ethyl] phenothiazine.
The presence of a thiomethyl radical (S-CH$_3$) in position 2, conventionally occupied by a halogen, is unique and could

*Also known as Mellerettes and Mallorol.

account for the greater toleration obtained with recommended doses of thioridazine as well as a greater specificity of psychotherapeutic action.

$C_{21}H_{26}N_2S_2$ Mol. wt. 370.57
10 mg, 15 mg, 25 mg, 50 mg, 100 mg, 150 mg, and 200 mg Tablets
Active Ingredient: thioridazine HCl, USP
10 mg Tablets
Inactive Ingredients: acacia, calcium sulfate dihydrate, carnauba wax, D&C Yellow #10, FD&C Blue #1, FD&C Yellow #6, gelatin, lactose, methylparaben, povidone, propylparaben, sodium benzoate, starch, stearic acid, sucrose, synthetic black iron oxide, talc, titanium dioxide, and other ingredients.
15 mg Tablets
Inactive Ingredients: acacia, calcium sulfate dihydrate, carnauba wax, D&C Red #7, gelatin, lactose, methylparaben, povidone, propylparaben, starch, stearic acid, sucrose, synthetic black iron oxide, talc, titanium dioxide, and other ingredients.
25 mg Tablets
Inactive Ingredients: acacia, calcium sulfate dihydrate, carnauba wax, gelatin, lactose, methylparaben, povidone, propylparaben, sodium benzoate, starch, stearic acid, sucrose, synthetic black iron oxide, synthetic iron oxide, talc, titanium dioxide, and other ingredients.
50 mg Tablets
Inactive Ingredients: acacia, calcium sulfate dihydrate, carnauba wax, gelatin, lactose, sodium benzoate, starch, stearic acid, sucrose, synthetic black iron oxide, talc, titanium dioxide, and other ingredients.
100 mg Tablets
Inactive Ingredients: acacia, calcium sulfate dihydrate, carnauba wax, D&C Yellow #10, FD&C Blue #2, FD&C Yellow #6, lactose, methylparaben, povidone, propylparaben, sodium benzoate, sorbitol, starch, stearic acid, sucrose, synthetic black iron oxide, talc, titanium dioxide, and other ingredients.
150 mg Tablets
Inactive Ingredients: acacia, calcium sulfate dihydrate, carnauba wax, D&C Yellow #10, FD&C Green #3, FD&C Yellow #6, lactose, methylparaben, povidone, propylparaben, sodium benzoate, starch, stearic acid, sucrose, synthetic black iron oxide, talc, titanium dioxide, and other ingredients.
200 mg Tablets
Inactive Ingredients: acacia, ammonium calcium alginate, calcium sulfate dihydrate, carnauba wax, colloidal silicon dioxide, D&C Red #7, lactose, magnesium stearate, methylparaben, povidone, propylparaben, sodium benzoate, starch, stearic acid, sucrose, synthetic black iron oxide, talc, titanium dioxide, and other ingredients.
30 mg and 100 mg Concentrate
Active Ingredient: thioridazine HCl, USP
30 mg Concentrate
Inactive Ingredients: alcohol, 3.0%, flavor, methylparaben, propylparaben, purified water, and sorbitol solution. May contain sodium hydroxide or hydrochloric acid to adjust the pH.
100 mg Concentrate
Inactive Ingredients: alcohol, 4.2%, flavor, glycerin, methylparaben, propylparaben, purified water, sorbitol solution, and sucrose. May contain sodium hydroxide or hydrochloric acid to adjust pH.
25 mg and 100 mg Oral Suspension
Active Ingredient: each 5 mL contains thioridazine, USP, equivalent to 25 mg and 100 mg thioridazine HCl, USP respectively.
25 mg Oral Suspension
Inactive Ingredients: carbomer 934, flavor, polysorbate 80, purified water, sodium hydroxide, and sucrose.
100 mg Oral Suspension
Inactive Ingredients: carbomer 934, D&C Yellow #10, FD&C Yellow #6, flavor, polysorbate 80, purified water, sodium hydroxide, and sucrose.

CLINICAL PHARMACOLOGY
Mellaril® (thioridazine) is effective in reducing excitement, hypermotility, abnormal initiative, affective tension, and agitation through its inhibitory effect on psychomotor functions. Successful modification of such symptoms is the prerequisite for, and often the beginning of, the process of recovery in patients exhibiting mental and emotional disturbances.

Thioridazine's basic pharmacological activity is similar to that of other phenothiazines, but certain specific qualities have come to light which support the observation that the clinical spectrum of this drug shows significant differences from those of the other agents of this class. Minimal antiemetic activity and minimal extrapyramidal stimulation, notably pseudoparkinsonism, are distinctive features of this drug.

INDICATIONS

For the management of manifestations of psychotic disorders.

For the short-term treatment of moderate to marked depression with variable degrees of anxiety in adult patients and for the treatment of multiple symptoms such as agitation, anxiety, depressed mood, tension, sleep disturbances, and fears in geriatric patients.

For the treatment of severe behavioral problems in children marked by combativeness and/or explosive hyperexcitable behavior (out of proportion to immediate provocations), and in the short-term treatment of hyperactive children who show excessive motor activity with accompanying conduct disorders consisting of some or all of the following symptoms: impulsivity, difficulty sustaining attention, aggressivity, mood lability, and poor frustration tolerance.

CONTRAINDICATIONS

In common with other phenothiazines, Mellaril® (thioridazine) is contraindicated in severe central nervous system depression or comatose states from any cause including drug induced central nervous system depression (*see WARNINGS*). It should also be noted that hypertensive or hypotensive heart disease of extreme degree is a contraindication of phenothiazine administration.

WARNINGS

Tardive Dyskinesia

Tardive dyskinesia, a syndrome consisting of potentially irreversible, involuntary, dyskinetic movements may develop in patients treated with neuroleptic (antipsychotic) drugs. Although the prevalence of the syndrome appears to be highest among the elderly, especially elderly women, it is impossible to rely upon prevalence estimates to predict, at the inception of neuroleptic treatment, which patients are likely to develop the syndrome. Whether neuroleptic drug products differ in their potential to cause tardive dyskinesia is unknown.

Both the risk of developing the syndrome and the likelihood that it will become irreversible are believed to increase as the duration of treatment and the total cumulative dose of neuroleptic drugs administered to the patient increase. However, the syndrome can develop, although much less commonly, after relatively brief treatment periods at low doses. There is no known treatment for established cases of tardive dyskinesia, although the syndrome may remit, partially or completely, if neuroleptic treatment is withdrawn. Neuroleptic treatment itself, however, may suppress (or partially suppress) the signs and symptoms of the syndrome and thereby may possibly mask the underlying disease process. The effect that symptomatic suppression has upon the long-term course of the syndrome is unknown.

Given these considerations, neuroleptics should be prescribed in a manner that is most likely to minimize the occurrence of tardive dyskinesia. Chronic neuroleptic treatment should generally be reserved for patients who suffer from a chronic illness that, 1) is known to respond to neuroleptic drugs, and, 2) for whom alternative, equally effective, but potentially less harmful treatments are *not* available or appropriate. In patients who do require chronic treatment, the smallest dose and the shortest duration of treatment producing a satisfactory clinical response should be sought. The need for continued treatment should be reassessed periodically.

If signs and symptoms of tardive dyskinesia appear in a patient on neuroleptics, drug discontinuation should be considered. However, some patients may require treatment despite the presence of the syndrome.

(For further information about the description of tardive dyskinesia and its clinical detection, please refer to the sections on *Information for Patients* and *ADVERSE REACTIONS*.)

It has been suggested in regard to phenothiazines in general, that people who have demonstrated a hypersensitivity reaction (e.g., blood dyscrasias, jaundice) to one may be more prone to demonstrate a reaction to others. Attention should be paid to the fact that phenothiazines are capable of potentiating central nervous system depressants (e.g., anesthetics, opiates, alcohol, etc.) as well as atropine and phosphorus insecticides. Physicians should carefully consider benefit versus risk when treating less severe disorders.

Reproductive studies in animals and clinical experience to date have failed to show a teratogenic effect with Mellaril® (thioridazine). However, in view of the desirability of keeping the administration of all drugs to a minimum during pregnancy, Mellaril® (thioridazine) should be given only when the benefits derived from treatment exceed the possible risks to mother and fetus.

Neuroleptic Malignant Syndrome (NMS)

A potentially fatal symptom complex sometimes referred to as Neuroleptic Malignant Syndrome (NMS) has been reported in association with antipsychotic drugs. Clinical manifestations of NMS are hyperpyrexia, muscle rigidity, altered mental status, and evidence of autonomic instability (irregular pulse or blood pressure, tachycardia, diaphoresis, and cardiac dysrhythmias).

The diagnostic evaluation of patients with this syndrome is complicated. In arriving at a diagnosis, it is important to identify cases where the clinical presentation includes both serious medical illness (e.g., pneumonia, systemic infection, etc.) and untreated or inadequately treated extrapyramidal signs and symptoms (EPS). Other important considerations in the differential diagnosis include central anticholinergic toxicity, heat stroke, drug fever, and primary central nervous system (CNS) pathology.

The management of NMS should include, 1) immediate discontinuation of antipsychotic drugs and other drugs not essential to concurrent therapy, 2) intensive symptomatic treatment and medical monitoring, and 3) treatment of any concomitant serious medical problems for which specific treatments are available. There is no general agreement about specific pharmacological treatment regimens for uncomplicated NMS.

If a patient requires antipsychotic drug treatment after recovery from NMS, the potential reintroduction of drug therapy should be carefully considered. The patient should be carefully monitored, since recurrences of NMS have been reported.

Central Nervous System Depressants

As in the case of other phenothiazines, Mellaril® (thioridazine) is capable of potentiating central nervous system depressants (e.g., alcohol, anesthetics, barbiturates, narcotics, opiates, other psychoactive drugs, etc.) as well as atropine and phosphorus insecticides. Severe respiratory depression and respiratory arrest have been reported when a patient was given a phenothiazine and a concomitant high dose of a barbiturate.

PRECAUTIONS

Leukopenia and/or agranulocytosis and convulsive seizures have been reported but are infrequent. Mellaril® (thioridazine) has been shown to be helpful in the treatment of behavioral disorders in epileptic patients, but anticonvulsant medication should also be maintained. Pigmentary retinopathy, which has been observed primarily in patients taking larger than recommended doses, is characterized by diminution of visual acuity, brownish coloring of vision, and impairment of night vision; examination of the fundus discloses deposits of pigment. The possibility of this complication may be reduced by remaining within the recommended limits of dosage.

Where patients are participating in activities requiring complete mental alertness (e.g., driving) it is advisable to administer the phenothiazines cautiously and to increase the dosage gradually. Female patients appear to have a greater tendency to orthostatic hypotension than male patients. The administration of epinephrine should be avoided in the treatment of drug-induced hypotension in view of the fact that phenothiazines may induce a reversed epinephrine effect on occasion. Should a vasoconstrictor be required, the most suitable are levarterenol and phenylephrine.

Neuroleptic drugs elevate prolactin levels; the elevation persists during chronic administration. Tissue culture experiments indicate that approximately one-third of human breast cancers are prolactin dependent *in vitro*, a factor of potential importance if the prescription of these drugs is contemplated in a patient with a previously detected breast cancer. Although disturbances such as galactorrhea, amenorrhea, gynecomastia, and impotence have been reported, the clinical significance of elevated serum prolactin levels is unknown for most patients. An increase in mammary neoplasms has been found in rodents after chronic administration of neuroleptic drugs. Neither clinical studies nor epidemiologic studies conducted to date, however, have shown an association between chronic administration of these drugs and mammary tumorigenesis; the available evidence is considered too limited to be conclusive at this time.

Concurrent administration of propranolol (100-800 mg daily) has been reported to produce increases in plasma levels of thioridazine (approximately 50%-400%) and its metabolites (approximately 80%-300%).

Pindolol: Concurrent administration of pindolol and thioridazine have resulted in moderate, dose-related increases in the serum levels of thioridazine and two of its metabolites, as well as higher than expected serum pindolol levels.

It is recommended that a daily dose in excess of 300 mg be reserved for use only in severe neuropsychiatric conditions.

Information for Patients: Given the likelihood that some patients exposed chronically to neuroleptics will develop tardive dyskinesia, it is advised that all patients in whom chronic use is contemplated be given, if possible, full information about this risk. The decision to inform patients and/or their guardians must obviously take into account the clini-

cal circumstances and the competency of the patient to understand the information provided.

ADVERSE REACTIONS

In the recommended dosage ranges with Mellaril® (thioridazine) most side effects are mild and transient.

Central Nervous System: Drowsiness may be encountered on occasion, especially where large doses are given early in treatment. Generally, this effect tends to subside with continued therapy or a reduction in dosage. Pseudoparkinsonism and other extrapyramidal symptoms may occur but are infrequent. Nocturnal confusion, hyperactivity, lethargy, psychotic reactions, restlessness, and headache have been reported but are extremely rare.

Autonomic Nervous System: Dryness of mouth, blurred vision, constipation, nausea, vomiting, diarrhea, nasal stuffiness, and pallor have been seen.

Endocrine System: Galactorrhea, breast engorgement, amenorrhea, inhibition of ejaculation, and peripheral edema have been described.

Skin: Dermatitis and skin eruptions of the urticarial type have been observed infrequently. Photosensitivity is extremely rare.

Cardiovascular System: ECG changes have been reported. (*See Phenothiazine Derivatives: Cardiovascular Effects*)

Other: Rare cases described as parotid swelling have been reported following administration of Mellaril® (thioridazine).

Post Introduction Reports

These are voluntary reports of adverse events temporally associated with Mellaril® (thioridazine) that were received since marketing, and there may be no causal relationship between Mellaril® (thioridazine) use and these events: priapism.

Phenothiazine Derivatives

It should be noted that efficacy, indications, and untoward effects have varied with the different phenothiazines. It has been reported that old age lowers the tolerance for phenothiazines. The most common neurological side effects in these patients are parkinsonism and akathisia. There appears to be an increased risk of agranulocytosis and leukopenia in the geriatric population. The physician should be aware that the following have occurred with one or more phenothiazines and should be considered whenever one of these drugs is used:

Autonomic Reactions: Miosis, obstipation, anorexia, paralytic ileus.

Cutaneous Reactions: Erythema, exfoliative dermatitis, contact dermatitis.

Blood Dyscrasias: Agranulocytosis, leukopenia, eosinophilia, thrombocytopenia, anemia, aplastic anemia, pancytopenia.

Allergic Reactions: Fever, laryngeal edema, angioneurotic edema, asthma.

Hepatotoxicity: Jaundice, biliary stasis.

Cardiovascular Effects: Changes in the terminal portion of the electrocardiogram, including prolongation of the Q-T interval, lowering and inversion of the T-wave, and appearance of a wave tentatively identified as a bifid T or a U wave have been observed in some patients receiving the phenothiazine tranquilizers, including Mellaril® (thioridazine). To date, these appear to be due to altered repolarization and not related to myocardial damage. They appear to be reversible. While there is no evidence at present that these changes are in any way precursors of any significant disturbance of cardiac rhythm, it should be noted that several sudden and unexpected deaths apparently due to cardiac arrest have occurred in patients previously showing characteristic electrocardiographic changes while taking the drug. The use of periodic electrocardiograms has been proposed but would appear to be of questionable value as a predictive device. Hypotension, rarely resulting in cardiac arrest.

Extrapyramidal Symptoms: Akathisia, agitation, motor restlessness, dystonic reactions, trismus, torticollis, opisthotonus, oculogyric crises, tremor, muscular rigidity, akinesia.

Tardive Dyskinesia: Chronic use of neuroleptics may be associated with the development of tardive dyskinesia. The salient features of this syndrome are described in the *WARNINGS* section and subsequently.

The syndrome is characterized by involuntary choreoathetoid movements which variously involve the tongue, face, mouth, lips, or jaw (e.g., protrusion of the tongue, puffing of cheeks, puckering of the mouth, chewing movements), trunk, and extremities. The severity of the syndrome and the degree of impairment produced vary widely.

The syndrome may become clinically recognizable either during treatment, upon dosage reduction, or upon withdrawal of treatment. Movements may decrease in intensity and may disappear altogether if further treatment with neuroleptics is withheld. It is generally believed that reversibility is more likely after short rather than long-term neuroleptic exposure. Consequently, early detection of tardive dyskinesia is important. To increase the likelihood of detecting the syndrome at the earliest possible time, the dosage

Continued on next page

Sandoz—Cont.

of neuroleptic drug should be reduced periodically (if clinically possible) and the patient observed for signs of the disorder. This maneuver is critical, for neuroleptic drugs may mask the signs of the syndrome.

Neuroleptic Malignant Syndrome (NMS): Chronic use of neuroleptics may be associated with the development of Neuroleptic Malignant Syndrome. The salient features of this syndrome are described in the *WARNINGS* section and subsequently. Clinical manifestations of NMS are hyperpyrexia, muscle rigidity, altered mental status, and evidence of autonomic instability (irregular pulse or blood pressure, tachycardia, diaphoresis, and cardiac dysrhythmias).

Endocrine Disturbances: Menstrual irregularities, altered libido, gynecomastia, lactation, weight gain, edema. False positive pregnancy tests have been reported.

Urinary Disturbances: Retention, incontinence.

Others: Hyperpyrexia. Behavioral effects suggestive of a paradoxical reaction have been reported. These include excitement, bizarre dreams, aggravation of psychoses, and toxic confusional states. More recently, a peculiar skin-eye syndrome has been recognized as a side effect following long-term treatment with phenothiazines. This reaction is marked by progressive pigmentation of areas of the skin or conjunctiva and/or accompanied by discoloration of the exposed sclera and cornea. Opacities of the anterior lens and cornea described as irregular or stellate in shape have also been reported. Systemic lupus erythematosus-like syndrome.

OVERDOSAGE

Many of the symptoms observed are extensions of the side effects described under *ADVERSE REACTIONS*. Mellaril® (thioridazine) can be toxic in overdose, with cardiac toxicity being of particular concern. Frequent ECG and vital sign monitoring of overdosed patients is recommended. Observation for several days may be required because of the risk of delayed effects.

Signs and Symptoms

Effects and clinical complications of acute overdose involving phenothiazines may include:

Cardiovascular: Cardiac arrhythmias, hypotension, shock, ECG changes, increased QT and PR intervals, non-specific ST and T wave changes, bradycardia, sinus tachycardia, atrioventricular block, ventricular tachycardia, ventricular fibrillation, Torsade de pointes, myocardial depression.

Central Nervous System: Sedation, extrapyramidal effects, confusion, agitation, hypothermia, hyperthermia, restlessness, seizures, areflexia, coma.

Autonomic Nervous System: Mydriasis, miosis, dry skin, dry mouth, nasal congestion, urinary retention, blurred vision.

Respiratory: Respiratory depression, apnea, pulmonary edema.

Gastrointestinal: Hypomotility, constipation, ileus.

Renal: Oliguria, uremia.

Toxic dose and blood concentration ranges for the phenothiazines have not been firmly established. It has been suggested that the toxic blood concentration range for thioridazine begins at 1.0 mg/dL, and 2–8 mg/dL is the lethal concentration range.

Treatment

In managing overdosage, the physician should always consider the possibility of multiple drug involvement. Treatment is essentially symptomatic and supportive. Gastric lavage and repeated doses of activated charcoal should be considered. Induction of emesis is less preferable to gastric lavage because of the risk of dystonia and the potential for aspiration of vomitus. Emesis should not be induced in patients expected to deteriorate rapidly, or those with impaired consciousness.

General management of the overdosed patient should be followed including observation and monitoring of vital signs, central nervous system function, and cardiovascular integrity.

An airway must be established and maintained. Adequate oxygenation and ventilation must be ensured.

Treatment of hypotension may require intravenous fluids, and vasopressors. Phenylephrine, levarterenol, or metaraminol are the appropriate pressor agents for use in the management of refractory hypotension. The potent α adrenergic blocking properties of the phenothiazines makes the use of vasopressors with mixed α and β adrenergic agonist properties inappropriate, including epinephrine and dopamine. Paradoxical vasodilation may result.

Acute extrapyramidal symptoms may be treated with diphenhydramine hydrochloride or benztropine mesylate.

The exact treatment of cardiac arrhythmias depends upon the clinical findings and physician judgement. Treatment may include one or more of the following therapeutic interventions: correction of electrolyte abnormalities and acid-base balance, lidocaine, phenytoin, isopropterenol, ventricular pacing, and defibrillation. Use of procainamide, quinidine, and disopyramide should be avoided, as Mellaril® (thioridazine) itself has a quinidine-like antiarrhythmic effect on the heart. Caution must be exercised when administering lidocaine, as it may increase the risk of developing seizures.

Avoid the use of barbiturates when treating seizures, as they may potentiate phenothiazine-induced respiratory depression.

Forced diuresis, hemoperfusion, hemodialysis and manipulation of urine pH are of unlikely benefit in the treatment of phenothiazine overdose due to their large volume of distribution and extensive plasma protein binding.

Up-to-date information about the treatment of overdose can often be obtained from a certified Regional Poison Control Center. Telephone numbers of certified Regional Poison Control Centers are listed in the Physicians' Desk Reference®.

DOSAGE

Dosage must be individualized according to the degree of mental and emotional disturbance. In all cases, the smallest effective dosage should be determined for each patient.

Adults

Psychotic manifestations: The usual starting dose is 50-100 mg three times a day, with a gradual increment to a maximum of 800 mg daily if necessary. Once effective control of symptoms has been achieved, the dosage may be reduced gradually to determine the minimum maintenance dose. The total daily dosage ranges from 200-800 mg, divided into two to four doses.

For the short-term treatment of moderate to marked depression with variable degrees of anxiety in adult patients and for the treatment of multiple symptoms such as agitation, anxiety, depressed mood, tension, sleep disturbances, and fears in geriatric patients: The usual starting dose is 25 mg three times a day. Dosage ranges from 10 mg two to four times a day in milder cases to 50 mg three or four times a day for more severely disturbed patients. The total daily dosage range is from 20 mg to a maximum of 200 mg.

Children

Mellaril® (thioridazine) is not intended for children under 2 years of age. For children aged 2-12 the dosage of thioridazine hydrochloride ranges from 0.5 mg to a maximum of 3.0 mg/Kg/day. For children with moderate disorders, 10 mg two or three times a day is the usual starting dose. For hospitalized, severely disturbed, or psychotic children, 25 mg two or three times daily is the usual starting dose. Dosage may be increased gradually until optimum therapeutic effect is obtained or the maximum has been reached.

HOW SUPPLIED

Mellaril® (thioridazine HCl) Tablets

10 mg

Bright chartreuse, coated tablets; " " imprinted on one side, "78-2" imprinted on the other side, in black.
Bottle of 100 (NDC 0078-0002-05)
Bottle of 1000 (NDC 0078-0002-09)
SandoPak® package of 100 (NDC 0078-0002-06)

15 mg

Pink, coated tablets; " " imprinted on one side, "78-8" imprinted on the other side, in black.
Bottle of 100 (NDC 0078-0008-05)

25 mg

Light tan, coated tablets; " " imprinted on one side, "MELLARIL 25" imprinted on the other side, in black.
Bottle of 100 (NDC 0078-0003-05)
Bottle of 1000 (NDC 0078-0003-09)
SandoPak® package of 100 (NDC 0078-0003-06)

50 mg

White, coated tablets; " " imprinted on one side, "MELLARIL 50" imprinted on the other side, in black.
Bottle of 100 (NDC 0078-0004-05)
Bottle of 1000 (NDC 0078-0004-09)
SandoPak® package of 100 (NDC 0078-0004-06)

100 mg

Light green, coated tablets; " " imprinted on one side, "MELLARIL 100" imprinted on the other side, in black.
Bottle of 100 (NDC 0078-0005-05)
Bottle of 1000 (NDC 0078-0005-09)
SandoPak® package of 100 (NDC 0078-0005-06)

150 mg

Yellow, coated tablets; " " imprinted on one side, "MELLARIL 150" imprinted on the other side, in black.
Bottle of 100 (NDC 0078-0006-05)

200 mg

Pink, coated tablets; " " imprinted on one side, "MELLARIL 200" imprinted on the other side, in black.
Bottle of 100 (NDC 0078-0007-05)
SandoPak® package of 100 (NDC 0078-0007-06)

Store and Dispense

Below 86°F (30°C); tight container.

Mellaril® (thioridazine HCl) Concentrate

30 mg/mL

A clear, straw-yellow liquid with a cherry-like odor. Each mL contains 30 mg thioridazine hydrochloride, USP, alcohol, 3.0% by volume. Immediate container: amber glass bottles of 4 fl. oz. (118 mL) as follows: 4 fl. oz. bottles, in cartons of 12 bottles, with an accompanying dropper graduated to deliver 10 mg, 25 mg, and 50 mg of thioridazine hydrochloride, USP (NDC 0078-0001-31).

100 mg/mL

A clear, light-yellow liquid with a strawberry-like odor. Each mL contains 100 mg thioridazine hydrochloride, USP, alcohol, 4.2% by volume. Immediate container: amber glass bottles of 4 fl. oz. (118 mL), in cartons of 12 bottles, with an accompanying dropper graduated to deliver 100 mg, 150 mg, and 200 mg of thioridazine hydrochloride, USP (NDC 0078-0009-31).

Store and Dispense

Below 86°F (30°C); tight, amber glass bottle.

The concentrate may be diluted with distilled water, acidified tap water, or suitable juices. Each dose should be so diluted just prior to administration—preparation and storage of bulk dilutions is not recommended.

Mellaril-S® (thioridazine) Oral Suspension

25 mg/5 mL

An off-white suspension with a buttermint taste and a peppermint odor. Each 5 mL contains thioridazine, USP, equivalent to 25 mg thioridazine hydrochloride, USP. Buttermint-flavored in pint bottles (NDC 0078-0068-33).

100 mg/5 mL

A yellow suspension with a buttermint taste and a peppermint odor. Each 5 mL contains thioridazine, USP, equivalent to 100 mg thioridazine hydrochloride, USP. Buttermint-flavored in pint bottles (NDC 0078-0069-33).

Store and Dispense

Below 77°F (25°C); tight, amber glass bottle.

Additional information available to physicians.

REV: FEBRUARY 1995 30160903

Shown in Product Identification Guide, page 333

MESANTOIN®* ℞

[*meh-san 'toyn*]

(mephenytoin) tablets, USP

CAUTION: Federal law prohibits dispensing without prescription.

The following prescribing information is based on official labeling in effect on August 1, 1996.

DESCRIPTION

Mesantoin® (mephenytoin) is 3-methyl 5,5-phenyl-ethyl-hydantoin. It may be considered to be the hydantoin homolog of the barbiturate mephobarbital. Mesantoin® (mephenytoin) has the following structure:

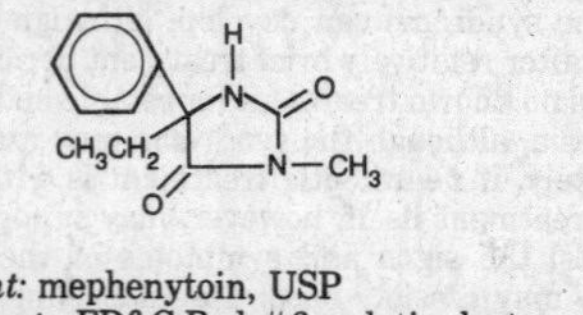

Active Ingredient: mephenytoin, USP

Inactive Ingredients: FD&C Red #3, gelatin, lactose, starch, stearic acid, and sucrose.

ACTIONS

Mephenytoin exhibits pharmacologic effects similar to both diphenylhydantoin and the barbiturates in antagonizing experimental seizures in laboratory animals. Mephenytoin produces behavioral and electroencephalographic effects in man which are similar to those produced by barbiturates.

INDICATIONS

For the control of grand mal, focal, Jacksonian, and psychomotor seizures in those patients who have been refractory to less toxic anticonvulsants.

CONTRAINDICATIONS

Hypersensitivity to hydantoin products.

WARNINGS

Mephenytoin should be used only after safer anticonvulsants have been given an adequate trial and have failed.

As with all anticonvulsants, dose reduction must be gradual so as to minimize the risk of precipitating seizures.

Patients should be cautioned about possible additive effects of alcohol and other CNS depressants. Acute alcohol intoxication may increase the anticonvulsant effect due to decreased metabolic breakdown. Chronic alcohol abuse may result in decreased anticonvulsant effect due to enzyme induction.

Usage in Pregnancy

The effects of mephenytoin in human pregnancy and nursing infants are unknown.

Recent reports suggest an association between the use of anticonvulsant drugs by women with epilepsy and an elevated incidence of birth defects in children born to these women. Data are more extensive with respect to diphenylhydantoin and phenobarbital, but these are also the most commonly prescribed anticonvulsants; less systematic or anec-

*Also known as Sedantoinal

dotal reports suggest a possible similar association with the use of all known anticonvulsant drugs.

The reports suggesting an elevated incidence of birth defects in children of drug-treated epileptic women cannot be regarded as adequate to prove a definite cause and effect relationship. There are intrinsic methodologic problems in obtaining adequate data on drug teratogenicity in humans; the possibility also exists that other factors, e.g., genetic factors or the epileptic condition itself, may be more important than drug therapy in leading to birth defects. The great majority of mothers on anticonvulsant medication deliver normal infants. It is important to note that anticonvulsant drugs should not be discontinued in patients in whom the drug is administered to prevent major seizures because of the strong possibility of precipitating status epilepticus with attendant hypoxia and threat to life. In individual cases where the severity and frequency of the seizure disorder are such that the removal of medication does not pose a serious threat to the patient, discontinuation of the drug may be considered prior to and during pregnancy, although it cannot be said with any confidence that even minor seizures do not pose some hazards to the developing embryo or fetus.

The prescribing physician will wish to weigh these considerations in treating or counseling epileptic women of childbearing potential.

PRECAUTIONS

The patient taking Mesantoin® (mephenytoin) must be kept under close medical supervision at all times since serious adverse reactions may emerge.

Because the primary site of degradation is the liver, it is recommended that screening tests of liver function precede introduction of the drug.

Some patients may show side reactions as the result of individual sensitivity. These reactions can be broken down into three types respectively according to severity: 1) blood dyscrasias; 2) skin and mucous membrane manifestations; and 3) central effects. The blood, skin and mucous membrane manifestations are the more important since they can be more serious in nature. Since mephenytoin has been reported to produce blood dyscrasia in certain instances, the patient must be instructed that in the event any unusual symptoms develop (e.g., sore throat, fever, mucous membrane bleeding, glandular swelling, cutaneous reaction), he/she must discontinue the drug and report for examination immediately. It is recommended that blood examinations be made (total white cell count and differential count) during the initial phase of administration. Such tests are best made: a) before starting medication; b) after 2 weeks on a low dosage; c) again after 2 weeks when full dosage is reached; d) thereafter, monthly for a year; e) from then on, every 3 months. If the neutrophils drop to between 2500 and 1600/cu.mm., counts are made every 2 weeks. Stop medication if the count drops to 1600.

ADVERSE REACTIONS

A number of side effects and toxic reactions have been reported with Mesantoin® (mephenytoin) as well as with other hydantoin compounds. Many of these appear to be dose related while others seem to be a manifestation of a hypersensitivity reaction to these drugs.

Blood Dyscrasias

Leukopenia, neutropenia, agranulocytosis, thrombocytopenia and pancytopenia have occurred. Eosinophilia, monocytosis, and leukocytosis have been described. Simple anemia, hemolytic anemia, megaloblastic anemia and aplastic anemia have occurred but are uncommon.

Skin and Mucous Membrane Manifestations

Maculopapular, morbilliform, scarlatiniform, urticarial, purpuric (associated with thrombocytopenia) and non-specific skin rashes have been reported. Exfoliative dermatitis, erythema multiforme (Stevens-Johnson Syndrome), toxic epidermal necrolysis and fatal dermatitides have been described on rare occasions. Skin pigmentation and rashes associated with a lupus erythematosus syndrome have also been reported.

Central Effects

Drowsiness is dose-related and may be reduced by a reduction in dose. Ataxia, diplopia, nystagmus, dysarthria, fatigue, irritability, choreiform movements, depression, and tremor have been encountered.

Nervousness, nausea, vomiting, sleeplessness and dizziness may occur during the initial stages of therapy. Generally, these symptoms are transient, often disappearing with continued treatment.

Mental confusion and psychotic disturbances and increased seizures have been reported, but a definite causal relationship with the drug is uncertain.

Miscellaneous

Hepatitis, jaundice and nephrosis have been reported but a definite cause and effect relationship between the drug and these effects has not been established.

Alopecia, weight gain, edema, photophobia, conjunctivitis, and gum hyperplasia have been encountered.

Polyarthropathy, pulmonary fibrosis, lupus erythematosus syndrome and lymphadenopathy which simulates Hodgkin's Disease have also been observed.

DOSAGE AND ADMINISTRATION

Dosage of antiepileptic therapy should be adjusted to the needs of the individual patient. Maintenance dosage is that smallest amount of antiepileptic necessary to suppress seizures completely or reduce their frequency. Optimum dosage is attained by starting with $^1/_2$ or 1 tablet of Mesantoin® (mephenytoin) per day during the first week and thereafter increasing the daily dose by $^1/_2$ or 1 tablet at weekly intervals. No dose should be increased until it has been taken for at least 1 week.

The average dose of Mesantoin® (mephenytoin) for adults ranges from 2–6 tablets (0.2–0.6 Gm.) daily. In some instances it may be necessary to administer as much as 8 tablets or more daily in order to obtain full seizure control. Children usually require from 1–4 tablets (0.1–0.4 Gm.) according to nature of seizures and age.

When the physician wishes to replace the anticonvulsant now being employed with Mesantoin® (mephenytoin), he/she should give $^1/_2$–1 tablet of Mesantoin® (mephenytoin) daily during the first week and gradually increase the daily dose at weekly intervals while gradually reducing that of the drug being discontinued. The transition can be made smoothly over a period of 3–6 weeks. If seizures are not completely controlled with the dose so attained, the daily dose should then be increased by a one-tablet increment at weekly intervals to the point of maximum effect. If the patient had also been receiving phenobarbital, it is well to continue it until the transition is completed, at which time gradual withdrawal of the phenobarbital may be tried.

HOW SUPPLIED

Mesantoin® (mephenytoin) Tablets, USP

100 mg, speckled, pale pink, round, uncoated tablets embossed "78/52" and scored on one side, " " on the other side. Tablets are scored to permit half-dosage.

Packages of 100 (NDC 0078-0052-05)

Store and Dispense

Below 86°F (30°C); tight container.

[Rev: February 1996 30163902]

METHERGINE® ℞

(methylergonovine maleate) Tablets, USP
(methylergonovine maleate) Injection, USP

Caution: Federal law prohibits dispensing without prescription.

The following prescribing information is based on official labeling in effect on August 1, 1996.

DESCRIPTION

Methergine® (methylergonovine maleate) is a semi-synthetic ergot alkaloid used for the prevention and control of postpartum hemorrhage.

Methergine® (methylergonovine maleate) is available in sterile ampuls of 1 mL, containing 0.2 mg methylergonovine maleate for intramuscular or intravenous injection and in tablets for oral ingestion containing 0.2 mg methylergonovine maleate.

Tablets

Active Ingredient: methylergonovine maleate USP, 0.2 mg
Inactive Ingredients: acacia, carnauba wax, D&C Red #7, FD&C Blue #1, gelatin special, lactose, maleic acid, mixed parabens, povidone, sodium benzoate, sodium hydroxide, starch, stearic acid, sucrose, talc, and titanium dioxide.

Ampuls, 1 mL, clear, colorless solution

Active Ingredient: methylergonovine maleate USP, 0.2 mg
Inactive Ingredients: sodium chloride USP 3 mg, tartaric acid NF 0.25 mg, water for injection USP qs to 1 mL.

Chemically, methylergonovine maleate is designated as ergoline-8-carboxamide, 9,10-didehydro-*N*-[1-(hydroxymethyl) propyl]-6-methyl-, [8*β*(*S*)]-, (*Z*)-2-butenedioate (1:1) (salt).

Its structural formula is:

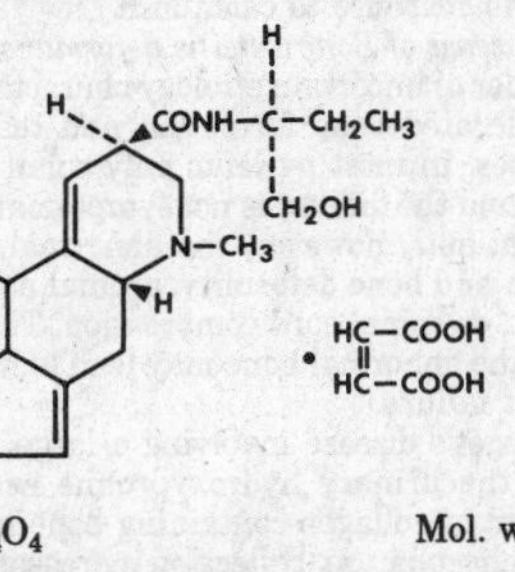

$C_{20}H_{25}N_3O_2 \cdot C_4H_4O_4$ Mol. wt. 455.51

CLINICAL PHARMACOLOGY

Methergine® (methylergonovine maleate) acts directly on the smooth muscle of the uterus and increases the tone, rate, and amplitude of rhythmic contractions. Thus, it induces a rapid and sustained tetanic uterotonic effect which shortens the third stage of labor and reduces blood loss. The onset of action after i.v. administration is immediate; after i.m. administration, 2–5 minutes, and after oral administration, 5–10 minutes.

Pharmacokinetic studies following an i.v. injection have shown that methylergonovine is rapidly distributed from plasma to peripheral tissues within 2–3 minutes or less. The bioavailability after oral administration was reported to be about 60% with no accumulation after repeated doses. During delivery, with intramuscular injection, bioavailability increased to 78%. Ergot alkaloids are mostly eliminated by hepatic metabolism and excretion, and the decrease in bioavailability following oral administration is probably a result of first-pass metabolism in the liver.

Bioavailability studies conducted in fasting healthy female volunteers have shown that oral absorption of a 0.2 mg methylergonovine tablet was fairly rapid with a mean peak plasma concentration of 3243 ± 1308 pg/mL observed at 1.12 ± 0.82 hours. For a 0.2 mg intramuscular injection, a mean peak plasma concentration of 5918 ± 1952 pg/mL was observed at 0.41 ± 0.21 hours. The extent of absorption of the tablet, based upon methylergonovine plasma concentrations, was found to be equivalent to that of the i.m. solution given orally, and the extent of oral absorption of the i.m. solution was proportional to the dose following administration of 0.1, 0.2, and 0.4 mg. When given intramuscularly, the extent of absorption of Methergine® (methylergonovine maleate) solution was about 25% greater than the tablet. The volume of distribution (Vd_{ss}/F) of methylergonovine was calculated to be 56.1 ± 17.0 liters, and the plasma clearance (CLp/F) was calculated to be 14.4 ± 4.5 liters per hour. The plasma level decline was biphasic with a mean elimination half-life of 3.39 hours (range 1.5 to 12.7 hours). A delayed gastrointestinal absorption (T_{max} about 3 hr) or Methergine® (methylergonovine maleate) tablet might be observed in postpartum women during continuous treatment with this oxytocic agent.

INDICATIONS AND USAGE

For routine management after delivery of the placenta; postpartum atony and hemorrhage; subinvolution. Under full obstetric supervision, it may be given in the second stage of labor following delivery of the anterior shoulder.

CONTRAINDICATIONS

Hypertension; toxemia; pregnancy; and hypersensitivity.

WARNINGS

This drug should not be administered i.v. routinely because of the possibility of inducing sudden hypertensive and cerebrovascular accidents. If i.v. administration is considered essential as a lifesaving measure, Methergine® (methylergonovine maleate) should be given slowly over a period of no less than 60 seconds with careful monitoring of blood pressure. Intraarterial or periarterial injection should be strictly avoided.

PRECAUTIONS

General

Caution should be exercised in the presence of sepsis, obliterative vascular disease, hepatic or renal involvement. Also use with caution during the second stage of labor. The necessity for manual removal of a retained placenta should occur only rarely with proper technique and adequate allowance of time for its spontaneous separation.

Drug Interactions

Caution should be exercised when Methergine® (methylergonovine maleate) is used concurrently with other vasoconstrictors or ergot alkaloids.

Carcinogenesis, Mutagenesis, Impairment of Fertility

No long-term studies have been performed in animals to evaluate carcinogenic potential. The effect of the drug on mutagenesis or fertility has not been determined.

Pregnancy

Category C. Animal reproductive studies have not been conducted with Methergine® (methylergonovine maleate). It is also not known whether methylergonovine maleate can cause fetal harm or can affect reproductive capacity. Use of Methergine® (methylergonovine maleate) is contraindicated during pregnancy because of its uterotonic effects. *(See INDICATIONS AND USAGE)*

Labor and Delivery

The uterotonic effect of Methergine® (methylergonovine maleate) is utilized after delivery to assist involution and decrease hemorrhage, shortening the third stage of labor.

Nursing Mothers

Methergine® (methylergonovine maleate) may be administered orally for a maximum of 1 week postpartum to control uterine bleeding. Recommended dosage is 1 tablet (0.2 mg) 3 or 4 times daily. At this dosage level a small quantity of drug appears in mothers' milk. Caution should be exercised when Methergine® (methylergovine maleate) is administered to a nursing woman.

Continued on next page

Sandoz—Cont.

ADVERSE REACTIONS

The most common adverse reaction is hypertension associated in several cases with seizure and/or headache. Hypotension has also been reported. Nausea and vomiting have occurred occasionally. Rarely observed reactions have included, in order of severity: acute myocardial infarction, transient chest pains, dyspnea, hematuria, thrombophlebitis, water intoxication, hallucinations, leg cramps, dizziness, tinnitus, nasal congestion, diarrhea, diaphoresis, palpitation, and foul taste.[3]

There have been rare isolated reports of anaphylaxis, without a proven causal relationship to the drug product.

DRUG ABUSE AND DEPENDENCE

Methergine® (methylergonovine maleate) has not been associated with drug abuse or dependence of either a physical or psychological nature.

OVERDOSE

Symptoms of acute overdose may include: nausea, vomiting, abdominal pain, numbness, tingling of the extremities, rise in blood pressure, in severe cases followed by hypotension, respiratory depression, hypothermia, convulsions, and coma. Because reports of overdosage with Methergine® (methylergonovine maleate) are infrequent, the lethal dose in humans has not been established. The oral LD$_{50}$ (in mg/kg) for the mouse is 187, the rat 93, and the rabbit 4.5.[4] Several cases of accidental Methergine® (methylergonovine maleate) injection in newborn infants have been reported, and in such cases 0.2 mg represents an overdose of great magnitude. However, recovery occurred in all but one case following a period of respiratory depression, hypothermia, hypertonicity with jerking movements, and, in one case, a single convulsion.

Also, several children 1–3 years of age have accidentally ingested up to 10 tablets (2 mg) with no apparent ill effects. A postpartum patient took 4 tablets at one time in error and reported paresthesias and clamminess as her only symptoms.

Treatment of acute overdosage is symptomatic and includes the usual procedures of:

1. removal of offending drug by inducing emesis, gastric lavage, catharsis, and supportive diuresis.
2. maintenance of adequate pulmonary ventilation, especially if convulsions or coma develop.
3. correction of hypotension with pressor drugs as needed.
4. control of convulsions with standard anticonvulsant agents.
5. control of peripheral vasospasm with warmth to the extremities if needed.[5]

DOSAGE AND ADMINISTRATION

Parenteral drug products should be inspected visually for particulate matter and discoloration prior to administration.

Intramuscularly

1 mL, 0.2 mg, after delivery of the anterior shoulder, after delivery of the placenta, or during the puerperium. May be repeated as required, at intervals of 2–4 hours.

Intravenously

Dosage same as intramuscular. *(See WARNINGS)*

Orally

One tablet, 0.2 mg, 3 or 4 times daily in the puerperium for a maximum of 1 week.

HOW SUPPLIED

Tablets

0.2 mg round, coated, orchid, branded "78-54" one side, "SANDOZ" other side.

Bottles of 100 (NDC 0078-0054-05)

Bottles of 1000 (NDC 0078-0054-09)

SandoPak® (unit dose) packages of 100, 10 blister strips of 10 tablets (NDC 0078-0054-06)

Ampuls

1 mL size

Boxes of 20 (NDC 0078-0053-03)

Boxes of 50 (NDC 0078-0053-04)

Store and Dispense

Tablets: Below 77°F (25°C); tight, light-resistant container.

Ampuls: Below 77°F (25°C); protect from light—administer only if solution is clear and colorless.

References

1. Mantyla, R. and Kants, J.: Clinical Pharmacokinetics of Methylergometrine (Methylergonovine). Int. J. Clin. Pharmacol. Ther. Toxicol. 19(9): 386-391, 1981
2. Iwamura, S. and Kambegawa, A.: Determination of Methylergometrine and Dihydroergotoxine in Biological Fluids. J. Pharm. Dyn. 4: 275-281, 1981
3. Information on Adverse Reactions supplied by Medical Services Dept., Sandoz Pharmaceuticals, E. Hanover, N.J., based on computerized clinical reports.
4. Berde, B. and Schild, H.O.: *Ergot Alkaloids and Related Compounds,* Springer-Verlag, New York, 1978, p. 810

5. Treatment of Acute Overdosage. Sandoz Dorsey Rx Products. Sandoz Inc., Medical Services Department.
[REV MARCH 1995   30165903]

MIACALCIN®   ℞

[mī"ă-kal'sin]

(calcitonin-salmon) INJECTION, SYNTHETIC

CAUTION: Federal law prohibits dispensing without prescription.

The following prescribing information is based on official labeling in effect on August 1, 1996.

DESCRIPTION

Calcitonin is a polypeptide hormone secreted by the parafollicular cells of the thyroid gland in mammals and by the ultimobranchial gland of birds and fish.

Miacalcin® (calcitonin-salmon) Injection, Synthetic is a synthetic polypeptide of 32 amino acids in the same linear sequence that is found in calcitonin of salmon origin. This is shown by the following graphic formula:

H—Cys—Ser—Asn—Leu—Ser—Thr—Cys—Val—Leu—
      1   2   3   4   5   6   7   8   9

Gly—Lys—Leu—Ser—Gln—Glu—Leu—His—Lys—Leu—
10   11   12   13   14   15   16   17   18   19

Gln—Thr—Tyr—Pro—Arg—Thr—Asn—Thr—Gly—Ser—
20   21   22   23   24   25   26   27   28   29

Gly—Thr—Pro—NH$_2$
30   31   32

It is provided in sterile solution for subcutaneous or intramuscular injection. Each milliliter contains: calcitonin-salmon 200 I.U.; acetic acid, USP, 2.25 mg; phenol, USP, 5.0 mg; sodium acetate trihydrate, USP, 2.0 mg; sodium chloride, USP, 7.5 mg; water for injection, USP, qs to 1.0 mL. The activity of Miacalcin® (calcitonin-salmon) is stated in International Units based on bioassay in comparison with the International Reference Preparation of calcitonin-salmon for Bioassay, distributed by the National Institute for Biological Standards and Control, Holly Hill, London.

CLINICAL PHARMACOLOGY

Calcitonin acts primarily on bone, but direct renal effects and actions on the gastrointestinal tract are also recognized. Calcitonin-salmon appears to have actions essentially identical to calcitonins of mammalian origin, but its potency per mg is greater and it has a longer duration of action. The actions of calcitonin on bone and its role in normal human bone physiology are still incompletely understood.

Bone—Single injections of calcitonin cause a marked transient inhibition of the ongoing bone resorptive process. With prolonged use, there is a persistent, smaller decrease in the rate of bone resorption. Histologically, this is associated with a decreased number of osteoclasts and an apparent decrease in their resorptive activity. Decreased osteocytic resorption may also be involved. There is some evidence that initially bone formation may be augmented by calcitonin through increased osteoblastic activity. However, calcitonin will probably not induce a long-term increase in bone formation. Animal studies indicate that endogenous calcitonin, primarily through its action on bone, participates with parathyroid hormone in the homeostatic regulation of blood calcium. Thus, high blood calcium levels cause increased secretion of calcitonin which, in turn, inhibits bone resorption. This reduces the transfer of calcium from bone to blood and tends to return blood calcium to the normal level. The importance of this process in humans has not been determined. In normal adults, who have a relatively low rate of bone resorption, the administration of exogenous calcitonin results in only a slight decrease in serum calcium. In normal children and in patients with generalized Paget's disease, bone resorption is more rapid and decreases in serum calcium are more pronounced in response to calcitonin.

Paget's Disease of Bone (osteitis deformans)—Paget's disease is a disorder of uncertain etiology characterized by abnormal and accelerated bone formation and resorption in one or more bones. In most patients only small areas of bone are involved and the disease is not symptomatic. In a small fraction of patients, however, the abnormal bone may lead to bone pain and bone deformity, cranial and spinal nerve entrapment, or spinal cord compression. The increased vascularity of the abnormal bone may lead to high output congestive heart failure.

Active Paget's disease involving a large mass of bone may increase the urinary hydroxyproline excretion (reflecting breakdown of collagen-containing bone matrix) and serum alkaline phosphatase (reflecting increased bone formation). Calcitonin-salmon, presumably by an initial blocking effect on bone resorption, causes a decreased rate of bone turnover with a resultant fall in the serum alkaline phosphatase and urinary hydroxyproline excretion in approximately 2/3 of patients treated. These biochemical changes appear to correspond to changes toward more normal bone, as evidenced by a small number of documented examples of: 1) radiologic regression of Pagetic lesions, 2) improvement of impaired auditory nerve and other neurologic function, 3) decreases (measured) in abnormally elevated cardiac output. These improvements occur extremely rarely, if ever, spontaneously (elevated cardiac output may disappear over a period of years when the disease slowly enters a sclerotic phase; in the cases treated with calcitonin, however, the decreases were seen in less than one year.)

Some patients with Paget's disease who have good biochemical and/or symptomatic responses initially, later relapse. Suggested explanations have included the formation of neutralizing antibodies and the development of secondary hyperparathyroidism, but neither suggestion appears to explain adequately the majority of relapses.

Although the parathyroid hormone levels do appear to rise transiently during each hypocalcemic response to calcitonin, most investigators have been unable to demonstrate persistent hypersecretion of parathyroid hormone in patients treated chronically with calcitonin-salmon.

Circulating antibodies to calcitonin after 2-18 months' treatment have been reported in about half of the patients with Paget's disease in whom antibody studies were done, but calcitonin treatment remained effective in many of these cases. Occasionally, patients with high antibody titers are found. These patients usually will have suffered a biochemical relapse of Paget's disease and are unresponsive to the acute hypocalcemic effects of calcitonin.

Hypercalcemia—In clinical trials, calcitonin-salmon has been shown to lower the elevated serum calcium of patients with carcinoma (with or without demonstrated metastases), multiple myeloma or primary hyperparathyroidism (lesser response). Patients with higher values for serum calcium tend to show greater reduction during calcitonin therapy. The decrease in calcium occurs about 2 hours after the first injection and lasts for about 6-8 hours. Calcitonin-salmon given every 12 hours maintained a calcium lowering effect for about 5-8 days, the time period evaluated for most patients during the clinical studies. The average reduction of 8-hour post-injection serum calcium during this period was about 9 percent.

Kidney—Calcitonin increases the excretion of filtered phosphate, calcium, and sodium by decreasing their tubular reabsorption. In some patients, the inhibition of bone resorption by calcitonin is of such magnitude that the consequent reduction of filtered calcium load more than compensates for the decrease in tubular reabsorption of calcium. The result in these patients is a decrease rather than an increase in urinary calcium.

Transient increases in sodium and water excretion may occur after the initial injection of calcitonin. In most patients, these changes return to pretreatment levels with continued therapy.

Gastrointestinal Tract—Increasing evidence indicates that calcitonin has significant actions on the gastrointestinal tract. Short-term administration results in marked transient decreases in the volume and acidity of gastric juice and in the volume and the trypsin and amylase content of pancreatic juice. Whether these effects continue to be elicited after each injection of calcitonin during chronic therapy has not been investigated.

Metabolism—The metabolism of calcitonin-salmon has not yet been studied clinically. Information from animal studies with calcitonin-salmon and from clinical studies with calcitonins of porcine and human origin suggest that calcitonin-salmon is rapidly metabolized by conversion to smaller inactive fragments, primarily in the kidneys, but also in the blood and peripheral tissues. A small amount of unchanged hormone and its inactive metabolites are excreted in the urine.

It appears that calcitonin-salmon cannot cross the placental barrier and its passage to the cerebrospinal fluid or to breast milk has not been determined.

INDICATIONS AND USAGE

Miacalcin® (calcitonin-salmon) Injection, Synthetic is indicated for the treatment of symptomatic Paget's disease of bone, for the treatment of hypercalcemia, and for the treatment of postmenopausal osteoporosis.

Paget's Disease—At the present time, effectiveness has been demonstrated principally in patients with moderate to severe disease characterized by polyostotic involvement with elevated serum alkaline phosphatase and urinary hydroxyproline excretion.

In these patients, the biochemical abnormalities were substantially improved (more than 30% reduction) in about 2/3 of patients studied, and bone pain was improved in a similar fraction. A small number of documented instances of reversal of neurologic deficits has occurred, including improvement in the basilar compression syndrome, and improvement of spinal cord and spinal nerve lesions. At present, there is too little experience to predict the likelihood of improvement of any given neurologic lesion. Hearing loss, the most common neurologic lesion of Paget's disease, is im-

proved infrequently (4 of 29 patients studied audiometrically).

Patients with increased cardiac output due to extensive Paget's disease have had measured decreases in cardiac output while receiving calcitonin. The number of treated patients in this category is still too small to predict how likely such a result will be.

The large majority of patients with localized, especially monostotic disease do not develop symptoms and most patients with mild symptoms can be managed with analgesics. There is no evidence that the prophylactic use of calcitonin is beneficial in asymptomatic patients, although treatment may be considered in exceptional circumstances in which there is extensive involvement of the skull or spinal cord with the possibility of irreversible neurologic damage. In these instances, treatment would be based on the demonstrated effect of calcitonin on Pagetic bone, rather than on clinical studies in the patient population in question.

Hypercalcemia —Miacalcin® (calcitonin-salmon) Injection, Synthetic is indicated for early treatment of hypercalcemic emergencies, along with other appropriate agents, when a rapid decrease in serum calcium is required, until more specific treatment of the underlying disease can be accomplished. It may also be added to existing therapeutic regimens for hypercalcemia such as intravenous fluids and furosemide, oral phosphate or corticosteroids, or other agents.

Postmenopausal Osteoporosis —Miacalcin® (calcitonin-salmon) Injection, Synthetic is indicated for the treatment of postmenopausal osteoporosis in conjunction with adequate calcium and vitamin D intake to prevent the progressive loss of bone mass. No evidence currently exists to indicate whether or not Miacalcin® (calcitonin-salmon) decreases the risk of vertebral crush fractures or spinal deformity. A recent controlled study, which was discontinued prior to completion because of questions regarding its design and implementation, failed to demonstrate any benefit of salmon calcitonin on fracture rate. No adequate controlled trials have examined the effect of salmon calcitonin injection on vertebral bone mineral density beyond 1 year of treatment. Two placebo-controlled studies with salmon calcitonin have shown an increase in total body calcium at 1 year, followed by a trend to decreasing total body calcium (still above baseline) at 2 years. The minimum effective dose of Miacalcin® (calcitonin-salmon) for prevention of vertebral bone mineral density loss has not been established. It has been suggested that those postmenopausal patients having increased rates of bone turnover may be more likely to respond to antiresorptive agents such as Miacalcin® (calcitonin-salmon).

CONTRAINDICATIONS
Clinical allergy to synthetic calcitonin-salmon.

WARNINGS
Allergic Reactions
Because calcitonin is protein in nature, the possibility of a systemic allergic reaction exists. **Administration of calcitonin-salmon has been reported in a few cases to cause serious allergic-type reactions (e.g. bronchospasm, swelling of the tongue or throat, and anaphylactic shock), and in one case, death attributed to anaphylaxis.** The usual provisions should be made for the emergency treatment of such a reaction should it occur. Allergic reactions should be differentiated from generalized flushing and hypotension.

Skin testing should be considered prior to treatment with calcitonin, particularly for patients with suspected sensitivity to calcitonin. The following procedure is suggested: Prepare a dilution of 10 I.U. per mL by withdrawing 1/20 mL (0.05 mL) in a tuberculin syringe and filling it to 1.0 mL with Sodium Chloride Injection, USP. Mix well, discard 0.9 mL and inject intracutaneously 0.1 mL (approximately 1 I.U.) on the inner aspect of the forearm. Observe the injection site 15 minutes after injection. The appearance of more than mild erythema or wheal constitutes a positive response.

The incidence of osteogenic sarcoma is known to be increased in Paget's disease. Pagetic lesions, with or without therapy, may appear by X-ray to progress markedly, possibly with some loss of definition of periosteal margins. Such lesions should be evaluated carefully to differentiate these from osteogenic sarcoma.

PRECAUTIONS
1. General
The administration of calcitonin possibly could lead to hypocalcemic tetany under special circumstances although no cases have yet been reported. Provisions for parenteral calcium administration should be available during the first several administrations of calcitonin.

2. Laboratory Tests
Periodic examinations of urine sediment of patients on chronic therapy are recommended.

Coarse granular casts and casts containing renal tubular epithelial cells were reported in young adult volunteers at bed rest who were given calcitonin-salmon to study the effect of immobilization on osteoporosis. There was no other evidence of renal abnormality and the urine sediment became normal after calcitonin was stopped. Urine sediment abnormalities have not been reported by other investigators.

3. Instructions for the Patient
Careful instruction in sterile injection technique should be given to the patient, and to other persons who may administer Miacalcin® (calcitonin-salmon) Injection, Synthetic.

4. Carcinogenesis, Mutagenesis, and Impairment of Fertility
An increased incidence of pituitary adenomas has been observed in one-year toxicity studies in Sprague-Dawley rats administered calcitonin-salmon at dosages of 20 and 80 I.U./kg/day and in Fisher 344 rats given 80 I.U./kg/day. The relevance of these findings to humans is unknown. Calcitonin-salmon was not mutagenic in tests using *Salmonella typhimurium, Escherichia coli,* and Chinese Hamster V79 cells.

5. Pregnancy: Teratogenic Effects
Category C
Calcitonin-salmon has been shown to cause a decrease in fetal birth weights in rabbits when given in doses 14-56 times the dose recommended for human use. Since calcitonin does not cross the placental barrier, this finding may be due to metabolic effects on the pregnant animal. There are no adequate and well-controlled studies in pregnant women. Miacalcin® (calcitonin-salmon) Injection, Synthetic should be used during pregnancy only if the potential benefit justifies the potential risk to the fetus.

6. Nursing Mothers
It is not known whether this drug is excreted in human milk. As a general rule, nursing should not be undertaken while a patient is on this drug since many drugs are excreted in human milk. Calcitonin has been shown to inhibit lactation in animals.

7. Pediatric Use
Disorders of bone in children referred to as juvenile Paget's disease have been reported rarely. The relationship of these disorders to adult Paget's disease has not been established and experience with the use of calcitonin in these disorders is very limited. There are no adequate data to support the use of Miacalcin® (calcitonin-salmon) Injection, Synthetic in children.

ADVERSE REACTIONS
Gastrointestinal System
Nausea with or without vomiting has been noted in about 10% of patients treated with calcitonin. It is most evident when treatment is first initiated and tends to decrease or disappear with continued administration.

Dermatologic/Hypersensitivity
Local inflammatory reactions at the site of subcutaneous or intramuscular injection have been reported in about 10% of patients. Flushing of face or hands occurred in about 2-5% of patients. Skin rashes, nocturia, pruritus of the ear lobes, feverish sensation, pain in the eyes, poor appetite, abdominal pain, edema of feet, and salty taste have been reported in patients treated with calcitonin-salmon. Administration of calcitonin-salmon has been reported in a few cases to cause serious allergic-type reactions (e.g. bronchospasm, swelling of the tongue or throat, and anaphylactic shock), and in one case, death attributed to anaphylaxis [see *Warnings*].

OVERDOSAGE
A dose of 1000 I.U. subcutaneously may produce nausea and vomiting as the only adverse effects. Doses of 32 units per kg per day for 1-2 days demonstrate no other adverse effects. Data on chronic high dose administration are insufficient to judge toxicity.

DOSAGE AND ADMINISTRATION
Paget's Disease —The recommended starting dose of calcitonin-salmon in Paget's disease is 100 I.U. (0.5 mL) per day administered subcutaneously (preferred for outpatient self-administration) or intramuscularly. Drug effect should be monitored by periodic measurement of serum alkaline phosphatase and 24-hour urinary hydroxyproline (if available) and evaluations of symptoms. A decrease toward normal of the biochemical abnormalities is usually seen, if it is going to occur, within the first few months. Bone pain may also decrease during that time. Improvement of neurologic lesions, when it occurs, requires a longer period of treatment, often more than one year.

In many patients, doses of 50 I.U. (0.25 mL) per day or every other day are sufficient to maintain biochemical and clinical improvement. At the present time, however, there are insufficient data to determine whether this reduced dose will have the same effect as the higher dose on forming more normal bone structure. It appears preferable, therefore, to maintain the higher dose in any patient with serious deformity or neurological involvement.

In any patient with a good response initially who later relapses, either clinically or biochemically, the possibility of antibody formation should be explored. The patient may be tested for antibodies by an appropriate specialized test or evaluated for the possibility of antibody formation by critical clinical evaluation.

Patient compliance should also be assessed in the event of relapse.

In patients who relapse, whether because of antibodies or for unexplained reasons, a dosage increase beyond 100 I.U. per day does not usually appear to elicit an improved response.

Hypercalcemia —The recommended starting dose of Miacalcin® (calcitonin-salmon) Injection, Synthetic in hypercalcemia is 4 I.U./kg body weight every 12 hours by subcutaneous or intramuscular injection. If the response to this dose is not satisfactory after one or two days, the dose may be increased to 8 I.U./kg every 12 hours. If the response remains unsatisfactory after two more days, the dose may be further increased to a maximum of 8 I.U./kg every 6 hours.

Postmenopausal Osteoporosis —The minimum effective dose of salmon calcitonin for the prevention of vertebral bone mineral density loss has not been established. Data from a single one-year placebo-controlled study with salmon calcitonin injection suggested that 100 I.U. (subcutaneously or intramuscularly) every other day might be effective in preserving vertebral bone mineral density. Baseline and interval monitoring of biochemical markers of bone resorption/turnover (e.g., fasting AM, second-voided urine hydroxyproline to creatinine ratio) and of bone mineral density may be useful in achieving the minimum effective dose. Patients should also receive supplemental calcium such as calcium carbonate 1.5 g daily and an adequate vitamin D intake (400 units daily). An adequate diet is also essential.

If the volume of Miacalcin® (calcitonin-salmon) Injection, Synthetic to be injected exceeds 2 mL, intramuscular injection is preferable and multiple sites of injection should be used.

Parenteral drug products should be inspected visually for particulate matter and discoloration prior to administration whenever solution and container permit.

HOW SUPPLIED
Miacalcin® (calcitonin-salmon) Injection, Synthetic is available as a sterile solution in individual 2 mL vials containing 200 I.U. per mL (NDC 0078-0149-23).
Store in Refrigerator—Between 2°-8°C (36°-46°F).
Manufactured by
Schering-Plough Products, Inc.
Manati, Puerto Rico for
Sandoz Pharmaceuticals Corporation
East Hanover, NJ 07936
[REV: MAY 1993   38567901]

MIACALCIN®   ℞
(calcitonin-salmon)
Nasal Spray

Caution: Federal law prohibits dispensing without prescription.
The following prescribing information is based on official labeling in effect on August 1, 1996.

DESCRIPTION
Calcitonin is a polypeptide hormone secreted by the parafollicular cells of the thyroid gland in mammals and by the ultimobranchial gland of birds and fish.
Miacalcin® (calcitonin-salmon) Nasal Spray is a synthetic polypeptide of 32 amino acids in the same linear sequence that is found in calcitonin of salmon origin. This is shown by the following graphic formula:

```
H—Cys—Ser—Asn—Leu—Ser—Thr—Cys—Val—Leu—
    1    2    3    4    5    6    7    8    9

Gly—Lys—Leu—Ser—Gln—Glu—Leu—His—Lys—Leu—
 10   11   12   13   14   15   16   17   18   19

Gln—Thr—Tyr—Pro—Arg—Thr—Asn—Thr—Gly—Ser—
 20   21   22   23   24   25   26   27   28   29

Gly—Thr—Pro—NH₂
 30   31   32
```

It is provided in 2 mL fill glass bottles as a solution for nasal administration. This is sufficient medication for 14 doses. Each milliliter contains calcitonin-salmon 2200 I.U. (corresponding to 200 I.U. per 0.09 mL actuation), sodium chloride 8.5 mg, benzalkonium chloride 0.10 mg, nitrogen, hydrochloric acid (added as necessary to adjust pH) and purified water. The activity of Miacalcin® (calcitonin-salmon) Nasal Spray is stated in International Units based on bioassay in comparison with the International Reference Preparation of calcitonin-salmon for Bioassay, distributed by the National Institute of Biologic Standards and Control, Holly Hill, London.

CLINICAL PHARMACOLOGY
Calcitonin acts primarily on bone, but direct renal effects and actions on the gastrointestinal tract are also recognized. Calcitonin-salmon appears to have actions essentially identical to calcitonins of mammalian origin, but its potency per mg is greater and it has a longer duration of action.
The information below, describing the clinical pharmacology of calcitonin, has been derived from studies with *injectable* calcitonin. The mean bioavailability of Miacalcin® (calcitonin-salmon) Nasal Spray is approximately 3% of that

Continued on next page

Sandoz—Cont.

of injectable calcitonin in normal subjects and, therefore, the conclusions concerning the *CLINICAL PHARMACOLOGY* of this preparation may be different.

The actions of calcitonin on bone and its role in normal human bone physiology are still not completely elucidated, although calcitonin receptors have been discovered in osteoclasts and osteoblasts.

Single injections of calcitonin cause a marked transient inhibition of the ongoing bone resorptive process. With prolonged use, there is a persistent, smaller decrease in the rate of bone resorption. Histologically, this is associated with a decreased number of osteoclasts and an apparent decrease in their resorptive activity. *In vitro* studies have shown that calcitonin-salmon causes inhibition of osteoclast function with loss of the ruffled osteoclast border responsible for resorption of bone. This activity resumes following removal of calcitonin-salmon from the test system. There is some evidence from the *in vitro* studies that bone formation may be augmented by calcitonin through increased osteoblastic activity.

Animal studies indicate that endogenous calcitonin, primarily through its action on bone, participates with parathyroid hormone in the homeostatic regulation of blood calcium. Thus, high blood calcium levels cause increased secretion of calcitonin which, in turn, inhibits bone resorption. This reduces the transfer of calcium from bone to blood and tends to return blood calcium towards the normal level. The importance of this process in humans has not been determined. In normal adults, who have a relatively low rate of bone resorption, the administration of exogenous calcitonin results in only a slight decrease in serum calcium in the limits of the normal range. In normal children and in patients with Paget's disease in whom bone resorption is more rapid, decreases in serum calcium are more pronounced in response to calcitonin.

Bone biopsy and radial bone mass studies at baseline and after 26 months of daily injectable calcitonin indicate that calcitonin therapy results in formation of normal bone.

Postmenopausal Osteoporosis—Osteoporosis is a disease characterized by low bone mass and architectural deterioration of bone tissue leading to enhanced bone fragility and a consequent increase in fracture risk as patients approach or fall below a bone mineral density associated with increased frequency of fracture. The most common type of osteoporosis occurs in postmenopausal females. Osteoporosis is a result of a disproportionate rate of bone resorption compared to bone formation which disrupts the structural integrity of bone, rendering it more susceptible to fracture. The most common sites of these fractures are the vertebrae, hip, and distal forearm (Colles' fractures). Vertebral fractures occur with the highest frequency and are associated with back pain, spinal deformity and a loss of height.

Calcitonin, given by the intranasal route, has been shown to increase spinal bone mass in postmenopausal women with established osteoporosis but not in early postmenopausal women.

Calcium Homeostasis—In two clinical studies designed to evaluate the pharmacodynamic response to Miacalcin® (calcitonin-salmon) Nasal Spray, administration of 100–1600 I.U. to healthy volunteers resulted in rapid and sustained small decreases (but still within the normal range) in both total serum calcium and serum ionized calcium. Single doses greater than 400 I.U. did not produce any further biological response to the drug. The development of hypocalcemia has not been reported in studies in healthy volunteers or postmenopausal females.

Kidney—Studies with injectable calcitonin show increases in the excretion of filtered phosphate, calcium, and sodium by decreasing their tubular reabsorption. Comparable studies have not been carried out with Miacalcin® (calcitonin-salmon) Nasal Spray.

Gastrointestinal Tract—Some evidence from studies with injectable preparations suggest that calcitonin may have significant actions on the gastrointestinal tract. Short-term administration of injectable calcitonin results in marked transient decreases in the volume and acidity of gastric juice and in the volume and the trypsin and amylase content of pancreatic juice. Whether these effects continue to be elicited after each injection of calcitonin during chronic therapy has not been investigated. These studies have not been conducted with Miacalcin® (calcitonin-salmon) Nasal Spray.

Pharmacokinetics and Metabolism

The data on bioavailability of Miacalcin® (calcitonin-salmon) Nasal Spray obtained by various investigators using different methods show great variability. Miacalcin® (calcitonin-salmon) Nasal Spray is absorbed rapidly by the nasal mucosa. Peak plasma concentrations of drug appear 31–39 minutes after nasal administration compared to 16–25 minutes following parenteral dosing. In normal volunteers approximately 3% (range 0.3%-30.6%) of a nasally administered dose is bioavailable compared to the same dose administered by intramuscular injection. The half-life of elimina-

tion of calcitonin-salmon is calculated to be 43 minutes. There is no accumulation of the drug on repeated nasal administration at 10 hour intervals for up to 15 days. Absorption of nasally administered calcitonin has not been studied in postmenopausal women.

INDICATIONS AND USAGE

Postmenopausal Osteoporosis—Miacalcin® (calcitonin-salmon) Nasal Spray is indicated for the treatment of postmenopausal osteoporosis in females greater than 5 years post-menopause with low bone mass relative to healthy premenopausal females. Miacalcin® (calcitonin-salmon) Nasal Spray should be reserved for patients who refuse or cannot tolerate estrogens or in whom estrogens are contraindicated. Use of Miacalcin® (calcitonin-salmon) Nasal Spray is recommended in conjunction with an adequate calcium (at least 1000 mg elemental calcium per day) and vitamin D (400 I.U. per day) intake to retard the progressive loss of bone mass. The evidence of efficacy is based on increases in spinal bone mineral density observed in clinical trials.

Two randomized, placebo controlled trials were conducted in 325 postmenopausal females [227 Miacalcin® (calcitonin-salmon) Nasal Spray treated and 98 placebo treated] with spinal, forearm or femoral bone mineral density (BMD) at least one standard deviation below normal for healthy premenopausal females. These studies conducted over two years demonstrated that 200 I.U. daily of Miacalcin® (calcitonin-salmon) Nasal Spray increases lumbar vertebral BMD relative to baseline and relative to placebo in osteoporotic females who were greater than 5 years postmenopause. Miacalcin® (calcitonin-salmon) Nasal Spray produced statistically significant increases in lumbar vertebral BMD compared to placebo as early as six months after initiation of therapy with persistence of this level for up to 2 years of observation.

No effects of Miacalcin® (calcitonin-salmon) Nasal Spray on cortical bone of the forearm or hip were demonstrated. However, in one study, BMD of the hip showed a statistically significant increase compared with placebo in a region composed of predominantly trabecular bone after one year of treatment changing to a trend at 2 years that was no longer statistically significant.

CONTRAINDICATIONS

Clinical allergy to calcitonin-salmon.

WARNINGS

Allergic Reactions

Because calcitonin is a polypeptide, the possibility of a systemic allergic reaction exists. In clinical trials with Miacalcin® (calcitonin-salmon) Nasal Spray and foreign marketing experience, no serious allergic-type adverse reactions have been reported. However, with injectable calcitonin-salmon there have been a few reports of serious allergic-type reactions (e.g., bronchospasm, swelling of the tongue or throat, anaphylactic shock, and in one case death attributed to anaphylaxis). The usual provisions should be made for the emergency treatment of such a reaction should it occur. Allergic reactions should be differentiated from generalized flushing and hypotension.

Skin testing should be considered prior to treatment with nasal calcitonin for patients with suspected sensitivity to calcitonin. The following procedure is suggested: Prepare a dilution of 10 I.U. per mL by withdrawing 1/20 mL (0.05 mL) of injectable calcitonin-salmon in a tuberculin syringe and filling it to 1.0 mL with Sodium Chloride Injection, USP. Mix well, discard 0.9 mL and inject intracutaneously 0.1 mL (approximately 1 I.U.) on the inner aspect of the forearm. Observe the injection site 15 minutes after injection. The appearance of more than mild erythema or wheal constitutes a positive response.

PRECAUTIONS

1. Drug Interactions

Formal studies designed to evaluate drug interactions with calcitonin-salmon have not been done. No drug interaction studies have been performed with Miacalcin® (calcitonin-salmon) Nasal Spray ingredients.

Currently, no drug interactions with calcitonin-salmon have been observed. The effects of prior use of diphosphonates in postmenopausal osteoporosis patients have not been assessed; however, in patients with Paget's Disease prior diphosphonate use appears to reduce the anti-resorptive response to Miacalcin® (calcitonin-salmon) Nasal Spray.

2. Periodic Nasal Examinations

Periodic nasal examinations with visualization of the nasal mucosa, turbinates, septum and mucosal blood vessel status are recommended.

The development of mucosal alterations or transient nasal conditions occurred in up to 9% of patients who received Miacalcin® (calcitonin-salmon) Nasal Spray and in up to 12% of patients who received placebo nasal spray in studies in postmenopausal females. The majority of patients (approximately 90%) in whom nasal abnormalities were noted also reported nasally related complaints/symptoms as adverse events. Therefore, a nasal examination should

be performed prior to start of treatment with nasal calcitonin and at any time nasal complaints occur.

In all postmenopausal patients treated with Miacalcin® (calcitonin-salmon) Nasal Spray, the most commonly reported nasal adverse events included rhinitis (12%), epistaxis (3.5%), and sinusitis (2.3%). Smoking was shown not to have any contributory effect on the occurrence of nasal adverse events. One patient (0.3%) treated with Miacalcin® (calcitonin-salmon) Nasal Spray who was receiving 400 I.U. daily developed a small nasal wound. In clinical trials in another disorder (Paget's Disease), 2.8% of patients developed nasal ulcerations.

If severe ulceration of the nasal mucosa occurs, as indicated by ulcers greater than 1.5 mm in diameter or penetrating below the mucosa, or those associated with heavy bleeding, Miacalcin® (calcitonin-salmon) Nasal Spray should be discontinued. Although smaller ulcers often heal without withdrawal of Miacalcin® (calcitonin-salmon) Nasal Spray, medication should be discontinued temporarily until healing occurs.

3. Information for Patients

Careful instructions on pump assembly, priming of the pump and nasal introduction of Miacalcin® (calcitonin-salmon) Nasal Spray should be given to the patient. Although instructions for patients are supplied with individual bottles, procedures for use should be demonstrated to each patient. Patients should notify their physician if they develop significant nasal irritation.

Patients should be advised of the following:
- Store new, unassembled bottles in the refrigerator between 36°-46°F (2°-8°C).
- Protect the product from freezing.
- Before priming the pump and using a new bottle, allow it to reach room temperature.
- After a new bottle is assembled, it should be stored at room temperature in an upright position. Each bottle contains 14 doses.
- Discard all unrefrigerated bottles after 30 days.
- See *DOSAGE AND ADMINISTRATION, Priming (Activation) of Pump* for complete instructions on priming the pump and administering Miacalcin® (calcitonin-salmon) Nasal Spray.

4. Carcinogenicity, Mutagenicity, and Impairment of Fertility

An increased incidence of non-functioning pituitary adenomas has been observed in one-year toxicity studies in Sprague-Dawley and Fischer 344 Rats administered (subcutaneously) calcitonin-salmon at dosages of 80 I.U. per kilogram per day (16–19 times the recommended human parenteral dose and about 130–160 times the human intranasal dose based on body surface area). The findings suggest that calcitonin-salmon reduced the latency period for development of pituitary adenomas that do not produce hormones, probably through the perturbation of physiologic processes involved in the evolution of this commonly occurring endocrine lesion in the rat. Although administration of calcitonin-salmon reduces the latency period of the development of nonfunctional proliferative lesions in rats, it did not induce the hyperplastic/neoplastic process.

Calcitonin-salmon was tested for mutagenicity using *Salmonella typhimurium* (5 strains) and *Escherichia coli* (2 strains), with and without rat liver metabolic activation, and found to be non-mutagenic. The drug was also not mutagenic in a chromosome aberration test in mammalian V79 cells of the Chinese Hamster *in vitro*.

5. Laboratory Tests

Urine sediment abnormalities have not been reported in ambulatory volunteers treated with Miacalcin® (calcitonin-salmon) Nasal Spray. Coarse granular casts containing renal tubular epithelial cells were reported in young adult volunteers at bed rest who were given injectable calcitonin-salmon to study the effect of immobilization on osteoporosis. There was no evidence of renal abnormality and the urine sediment became normal after calcitonin was stopped. Periodic examinations of urine sediment should be considered.

6. Pregnancy

Teratogenic Effects

Category C

Calcitonin-salmon has been shown to cause a decrease in fetal birth weights in rabbits when given by injection in doses 8-33 times the parenteral dose and 70-278 times the intranasal dose recommended for human use based on body surface area.

Since calcitonin does not cross the placental barrier, this finding may be due to metabolic effects on the pregnant animal. There are no adequate and well controlled studies in pregnant women with calcitonin-salmon. Miacalcin® (calcitonin-salmon) Nasal Spray is *not* indicated for use in pregnancy.

7. Nursing Mothers

It is not known whether this drug is excreted in human milk. As a general rule, nursing should not be undertaken while a patient is on this drug since many drugs are ex-

creted in human milk. Calcitonin has been shown to inhibit lactation in animals.

8. Geriatric Use

Clinical trials using Miacalcin® (calcitonin-salmon) Nasal Spray have included postmenopausal patients up to 77 years of age. No unusual adverse events or increased incidence of common adverse events have been noted in patients over 65 years of age.

9. Pediatric Use

There are no data to support the use of Miacalcin® (calcitonin-salmon) Nasal Spray in children. Disorders of bone in children referred to as idiopathic juvenile osteoporosis have been reported rarely. The relationship of these disorders to postmenopausal osteoporosis has not been established and experience with the use of calcitonin in these disorders is very limited.

ADVERSE REACTIONS

The incidence of adverse reactions reported in studies involving postmenopausal osteoporotic patients chronically exposed to Miacalcin® (calcitonin-salmon) Nasal Spray (N=341) and to placebo nasal spray (N=131) and reported in greater than 3% of Miacalcin® (calcitonin-salmon) Nasal Spray treated patients are presented below in the following table. Most adverse reactions were mild to moderate in severity. Nasal adverse events were most common with 70% mild, 25% moderate, and 5% severe in nature (placebo rates were 71% mild, 27% moderate, and 2% severe).

Adverse Reactions Occurring in at Least 3% of Postmenopausal Patients Treated Chronically

Adverse Reaction	Miacalcin® (calcitonin-salmon) Nasal Spray N=341 % of Patients	Placebo N=131 % of Patients
Rhinitis	12.0	6.9
Symptom of Nose†	10.6	16.0
Back Pain	5.0	2.3
Arthralgia	3.8	5.3
Epistaxis	3.5	4.6
Headache	3.2	4.6

†Symptom of nose includes: nasal crusts, dryness, redness or erythema, nasal sores, irritation, itching, thick feeling, soreness, pallor, infection, stenosis, runny/blocked, small wound, bleeding wound, tenderness, uncomfortable feeling and sore across bridge of nose.

In addition, the following adverse events were reported in fewer than 3% of patients during chronic therapy with Miacalcin® (calcitonin-salmon) Nasal Spray. Adverse events reported in 1%–3% of patients are identified with an asterisk(*). The remainder occurred in less than 1% of patients. Other than flushing, nausea, possible allergic reactions, and possible local irritative effects in the respiratory tract, a relationship to Miacalcin® (calcitonin-salmon) Nasal Spray has not been established.

Body as a whole—General Disorders: influenza-like symptoms*, fatigue*, periorbital edema, fever

Integumentary: erythematous rash*, skin ulceration, eczema, alopecia, pruritus, increased sweating

Musculoskeletal/Collagen: arthrosis*, myalgia*, arthritis, polymyalgia rheumatica, stiffness

Respiratory/Special Senses: sinusitis*, upper respiratory tract infection*, bronchospasm*, pharyngitis, bronchitis, pneumonia, coughing, dyspnea, taste perversion, parosmia

Cardiovascular: hypertension*, angina pectoris*, tachycardia, palpitation, bundle branch block, myocardial infarction

Gastrointestinal: dyspepsia*, constipation*, abdominal pain*, nausea*, diarrhea*, vomiting, flatulence, increased appetite, gastritis, dry mouth

Liver/Metabolic: cholelithiasis, hepatitis, thirst, weight increase

Endocrine: goiter, hyperthyroidism

Urinary System: cystitis*, pyelonephritis, hematuria, renal calculus

Central and Peripheral Nervous System: dizziness*, paresthesia*, vertigo, migraine, neuralgia, agitation

Hearing/Vestibular: tinnitus, hearing loss, earache

Vision: abnormal lacrimation*, conjunctivitis*, blurred vision, vitreous floater

Vascular: flushing, cerebrovascular accident, thrombophlebitis

Hematologic/Resistance Mechanisms: lymphadenopathy*, infection*, anemia

Psychiatric: depression*, insomnia, anxiety, anorexia

Common adverse reactions associated with the use of injectable calcitonin-salmon occurred less frequently in patients treated with Miacalcin® (calcitonin-salmon) Nasal Spray than in those patients treated with injectable calcitonin. Nausea, with or without vomiting, which occurred in 1.8% of patients treated with the nasal spray (and 1.5% of those receiving placebo nasal spray) occurs in about 10% of patients who take injectable calcitonin-salmon. Flushing, which occurred in less than 1% of patients treated with the Nasal Spray, occurs in 2%-5% of patients treated with injectable calcitonin-salmon. Although the administered dosages of injectable and nasal spray calcitonin-salmon are comparable (50-100 units daily of injectable versus 200 units daily of nasal spray), the nasal dosage form has a mean bioavailability of about 3% (range 0.3%-30.6%) and therefore provides less drug to the systemic circulation, possibly accounting for the decrease in frequency of adverse reactions.

The collective foreign marketing experience with Miacalcin® (calcitonin-salmon) Nasal Spray does not show evidence of any notable difference in the incidence profile of reported adverse reactions when compared with that seen in the clinical trials.

OVERDOSAGE

No instances of overdose with Miacalcin® (calcitonin-salmon) Nasal Spray have been reported and no serious adverse reactions have been associated with high doses. There is no known potential for drug abuse for calcitonin-salmon. Single doses of Miacalcin® (calcitonin-salmon) Nasal Spray up to 1600 I.U., doses up to 800 I.U. per day for three days and chronic administration of doses up to 600 I.U. per day have been studied without serious adverse effects. A dose of 1000 I.U. of Miacalcin® (calcitonin-salmon) injectable solution given subcutaneously may produce nausea and vomiting. A dose of Miacalcin® (calcitonin-salmon) injectable solution of 32 I.U. per kg per day for one or two days demonstrated no additional adverse effects.

There have been no reports of hypocalcemic tetany. However, the pharmacologic actions of Miacalcin® (calcitonin-salmon) Nasal Spray suggest that this could occur in overdose. Therefore, provisions for parenteral administration of calcium should be available for the treatment of overdose.

DOSAGE AND ADMINISTRATION

The recommended dose of Miacalcin® (calcitonin-salmon) Nasal Spray in postmenopausal osteoporotic females is one spray (200 I.U.) per day administered intranasally, alternating nostrils daily.

Drug effect may be monitored by periodic measurements of lumbar vertebral bone mass to document stabilization of bone loss or increases in bone density. Effects of Miacalcin® (calcitonin-salmon) Nasal Spray on biochemical markers of bone turnover have not been consistently demonstrated in studies in postmenopausal osteoporosis. Therefore, these parameters should not be solely utilized to determine clinical response to Miacalcin® (calcitonin-salmon) Nasal Spray therapy in these patients.

Priming (Activation) of Pump

Before the first dose and administration, Miacalcin® (calcitonin-salmon) Nasal Spray should be at room temperature. To prime the pump, the bottle should be held upright and the two white side arms of the pump depressed toward the bottle until a full spray is produced. The pump is primed once the first full spray is emitted. To administer, the nozzle should be carefully placed into the nostril with the head in the upright position, and the pump firmly depressed toward the bottle. The pump should not be primed before each daily dose.

HOW SUPPLIED

Miacalcin® (calcitonin-salmon) Nasal Spray

Available as a metered dose solution in 2 mL fill glass bottles. It is available in a dosage strength of 200 I.U. per activation (0.09 mL/spray). A screw-on pump is provided. This pump, following priming, will deliver 0.09 mL of solution. Miacalcin® (calcitonin-salmon) Nasal Spray contains 2200 I.U./mL calcitonin-salmon and is provided in individual boxes containing one glass bottle and one screw-on pump (NDC 0078-0149-75).

Store and Dispense

Store unopened in refrigerator between 36°-46°F (2°-8°C). Protect from freezing.

Opened bottles must be maintained at room temperature (for up to 30 days) in an upright position. Each bottle, after priming, contains 14 doses.

[REV: APRIL 1996 30367902]

Shown in Product Identification Guide, page 333

NEORAL® Soft Gelatin Capsules ℞

(cyclosporine capsules for microemulsion)

NEORAL® Oral Solution

(cyclosporine oral solution for microemulsion)

[nē ō′răl]

Caution: Federal law prohibits dispensing without prescription.

The following prescribing information is based on official labeling in effect on Aug. 1, 1996.

WARNING

Only physicians experienced in immunosuppressive therapy and management of organ transplant patients should prescribe Neoral®. Patients receiving the drug should be managed in facilities equipped and staffed with adequate laboratory and supportive medical resources. The physician responsible for maintenance therapy should have complete information requisite for the follow-up of the patient.

Neoral® may be administered with other immunosuppressive agents. Increased susceptibility to infection and the possible development of lymphoma and other neoplasms may result from the degree of immunosuppression.

Neoral® Soft Gelatin Capsules (cyclosporine capsules for microemulsion) and Neoral® Oral Solution (cyclosporine oral solution for microemulsion) have increased bioavailability in comparison to Sandimmune® Soft Gelatin Capsules (cyclosporine capsules, USP) and Sandimmune® Oral Solution (cyclosporine oral solution, USP). Neoral® and Sandimmune® are not bioequivalent and cannot be used interchangeably without physician supervision. It is recommended that cyclosporine blood concentrations be monitored in patients taking Neoral® and that dose adjustments be made in order to avoid toxicity due to high concentrations and possible organ rejection due to low concentrations. For a given trough concentration, cyclosporine exposure will be greater with Neoral® than with Sandimmune®. If a patient who is receiving exceptionally high doses of Sandimmune® is converted to Neoral®, particular caution should be exercised. Comparison of blood concentrations in the published literature with blood concentrations obtained using current assays must be done with detailed knowledge of the assay methods employed. *(See Blood Concentration Monitoring under DOSAGE AND ADMINISTRATION)*

DESCRIPTION

Neoral® is an oral formulation of cyclosporine that immediately forms a microemulsion in an aqueous environment.

Cyclosporine, the active principle in Neoral®, is a cyclic polypeptide immunosuppressant agent consisting of 11 amino acids. It is produced as a metabolite by the fungus species *Beauveria nivea.*

Chemically, cyclosporine is designated as [*R*-[*R**,*R**-(*E*)]]-cyclic- (L-alanyl-D-alanyl- *N*- methyl- L-leucyl -*N*- methyl-L-leucyl-*N*-methyl-L-valyl-3-hydroxy-*N*,4-dimethyl -L-2-amino-6-octenoyl- L-α-amino-butyryl- *N*-methylglycyl-*N*-methyl-L-leucyl-L-valyl- *N*-methyl-L-leucyl).

Neoral® Soft Gelatin Capsules (cyclosporine capsules for microemulsion) are available in 25 mg and 100 mg strengths.

Each 25 mg capsule contains:

cyclosporine	25 mg
alcohol, USP dehydrated	9.5% wt/vol.

Each 100 mg capsule contains:

cyclosporine	100 mg
alcohol, USP dehydrated	9.5% wt/vol.

Inactive Ingredients: Corn oil-mono-di-triglycerides, polyoxyl 40 hydrogenated castor oil NF, DL-α-tocopherol USP, gelatin NF, glycerol, iron oxide black, propylene glycol USP, titanium dioxide USP, carmine, and other ingredients.

Neoral® Oral Solution (cyclosporine oral solution for microemulsion) is available in 50 mL bottles.

Each mL contains:

cyclosporine	100 mg/mL
alcohol, USP dehydrated	9.5% wt/vol.

Inactive Ingredients: Corn oil-mono-di-triglycerides, polyoxyl 40 hydrogenated castor oil NF, DL-α-tocopherol USP, propylene glycol USP.

The chemical structure of cyclosporine (also known as cyclosporin A) is:

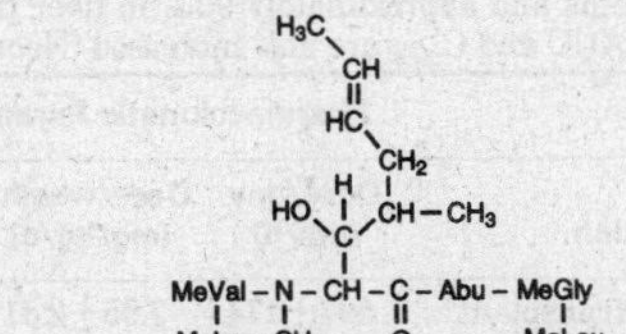

$C_{62}H_{111}N_{11}O_{12}$ Mol. Wt. 1202.63

CLINICAL PHARMACOLOGY

Cyclosporine is a potent immunosuppressive agent that in animals prolongs survival of allogeneic transplants involving skin, kidney, liver, heart, pancreas, bone marrow, small intestine, and lung. Cyclosporine has been demonstrated to suppress some humoral immunity and to a greater extent, cell-mediated immune reactions such as allograft rejection,

Continued on next page

Sandoz—Cont.

delayed hypersensitivity, experimental allergic encephalo-myelitis, Freund's adjuvant arthritis, and graft vs. host disease in many animal species for a variety of organs.

The effectiveness of cyclosporine results from specific and reversible inhibition of immunocompetent lymphocytes in the G_0- and G_1-phase of the cell cycle. T-lymphocytes are preferentially inhibited. The T-helper cell is the main target, although the T-suppressor cell may also be suppressed. Cyclosporine also inhibits lymphokine production and release including interleukin-2.

No effects on phagocytic function (changes in enzyme secretions, chemotactic migration of granulocytes, macrophage migration, carbon clearance *in vivo*) or tumor cells (growth rate, metastasis) have been detected in animals. Cyclosporine does not cause bone marrow suppression in animal models or man.

Pharmacokinetics

The immunosuppressive activity of cyclosporine is primarily due to parent drug. Following oral administration, absorption of cyclosporine is incomplete. The extent of absorption of cyclosporine is dependent on the individual patient, the patient population, and the formulation. Elimination of cyclosporine is primarily biliary with only 6% of the dose (parent drug and metabolites) excreted in urine. The disposition of cyclosporine from blood is generally biphasic, with a terminal half-life of approximately 8.4 hours (range 5 to 18 hours). Following intravenous administration, the blood clearance of cyclosporine (assay: HPLC) is approximately 5 to 7 mL/min/kg in adult recipients of renal or liver allografts. Blood cyclosporine clearance appears to be slightly slower in cardiac transplant patients.

The Neoral® Soft Gelatin Capsules (cyclosporine capsules for microemulsion) and Neoral® Oral Solution (cyclosporine oral solution for microemulsion) are bioequivalent.

The relationship between administered dose and exposure (area under the concentration versus time curve, AUC) is linear within the therapeutic dose range. The intersubject variability (total, %CV) of cyclosporine exposure (AUC) when Neoral® or Sandimmune® is administered ranges from approximately 20% to 50% in renal transplant patients. This intersubject variability contributes to the need for individualization of the dosing regimen for optimal therapy (*see DOSAGE AND ADMINISTRATION*). Intrasubject variability of AUC in renal transplant recipients (%CV) was 9–21% for Neoral® and 19–26% for Sandimmune®. In the same studies, intrasubject variability of trough concentrations (%CV) was 17–30% for Neoral® and 16–38% for Sandimmune®.

Absorption

Neoral® has increased bioavailability compared to Sandimmune®. The absolute bioavailability of cyclosporine administered as Sandimmune® is dependent on the patient population, estimated to be less than 10% in liver transplant patients and as great as 89% in renal patients. The increased bioavailability of Neoral® relative to Sandimmune® varies across patient populations; however, the absolute bioavailability of cyclosporine administered as Neoral® has not been determined in adults. In crossover studies where stable renal transplant patients received both Neoral® and Sandimmune®, the mean relative AUC of Neoral® to Sandimmune® ranged from 1.24 ± 0.34 to 1.51 ± 0.59. The dose normalized AUC in *de novo* renal transplant patients dosed with Neoral® was 23% greater than in those patients dosed with Sandimmune®. The dose normalized AUC in *de novo* liver transplant patients administered Neoral® 28 days after transplantation was 50% greater than in those patients administered Sandimmune®. The increase in AUC is accompanied by an increase in peak blood cyclosporine concentration (C_{max}) in the range of 40% to 106% in renal transplant patients and approximately 90% in liver transplant patients. AUC and C_{max} are also increased (Neoral®

relative to Sandimmune®) in heart transplant patients, but data are very limited. Although the AUC and C_{max} values are higher on Neoral® relative to Sandimmune®, the pre-dose trough concentrations (dose-normalized) are similar for the two formulations.

Following oral administration of Neoral®, the time to peak blood cyclosporine concentrations (T_{max}) ranged from 1.5 to 2.0 hours in renal transplant patients. The administration of food with Neoral® decreases the AUC and C_{max} of cyclosporine. A high fat meal (669 kcal, 45 grams fat) consumed within one-half hour before Neoral® administration decreased the AUC by 13% and C_{max} by 33%. The effects of a low fat meal (667 kcal, 15 grams fat) were similar.

The effect of T-tube diversion of bile on the absorption of cyclosporine from Neoral® was investigated in eleven *de novo* liver transplant patients. When the patients were administered Neoral® with and without T-tube diversion of bile, very little difference in absorption was observed, as measured by the change in maximal cyclosporine blood concentrations from pre-dose values with the T-tube closed relative to when it was open: $6.9\pm41\%$ (range -55% to 68%). [See table below.]

Distribution

Cyclosporine is distributed largely outside the blood volume. The steady state volume of distribution during intravenous dosing has been reported as 3–5 L/kg in solid organ transplant recipients. In blood, the distribution is concentration dependent. Approximately 33–47% is in plasma, 4–9% in lymphocytes, 5–12% in granulocytes, and 41–58% in erythrocytes. At high concentrations, the binding capacity of leukocytes and erythrocytes becomes saturated. In plasma, approximately 90% is bound to proteins, primarily lipoproteins. Cyclosporine is excreted in human milk. (*See PRECAUTIONS*)

Metabolism

Cyclosporine is extensively metabolized by the cytochrome P-450 III-A enzyme system in the liver, and to a lesser degree in the gastrointestinal tract, and the kidney. At least 25 metabolites have been identified from human bile, feces, blood, and urine. The biological activity of the metabolites and their contributions to toxicity are considerably less than those of the parent compound. The major metabolites (M1, M9, and M4N) result from oxidation at the 1-beta, 9-gamma, and 4-N-desmethylated positions, respectively. At steady state following the oral administration of Sandimmune®, the mean AUCs for blood concentrations of M1, M9 and M4N are about 70%, 21%, and 7.5% of the AUC for blood cyclosporine concentrations, respectively. Based on blood concentration data from stable renal transplant patients (13 pa-

tients administered Neoral® and Sandimmune® in a crossover study), and bile concentration data from *de novo* liver transplant patients (4 administered Neoral®, 3 administered Sandimmune®), the percentage of dose present as M1, M9, and M4N metabolites is similar when either Neoral® or Sandimmune® is administered.

Excretion

Only 0.1% of a cyclosporine dose is excreted unchanged in the urine. Elimination is primarily biliary with only 6% of the dose (parent drug and metabolites) excreted in the urine. Neither dialysis nor renal failure alter cyclosporine clearance significantly.

Pediatric Population

Pharmacokinetic data from pediatric patients administered Neoral® or Sandimmune® are very limited. In 15 renal transplant patients aged 3–16 years, cyclosporine whole blood clearance after IV administration of Sandimmune® was 10.6 ± 3.7 mL/min/kg (assay: Cyclo-trac specific RIA). In a study of 7 renal transplant patients aged 2–16, the cyclosporine clearance ranged from 9.8 to 15.5 mL/min/kg. In 9 liver transplant patients aged 0.6 to 5.6 years, clearance was 9.3 ± 5.4 mL/min/kg (assay: HPLC).

In the pediatric population, Neoral® also demonstrates an increased bioavailability as compared to Sandimmune®. In 7 liver *de novo* transplant patients aged 1.4 to 10 years, the absolute bioavailability of Neoral® was 43% (range 30% to 68%) and for Sandimmune® in the same individuals absolute bioavailability was 28% (range 17% to 42%). [See table above.]

INDICATIONS AND USAGE

Neoral® is indicated for the prophylaxis of organ rejection in kidney, liver, and heart allogeneic transplants. Neoral® has been used in combination with azathioprine and corticosteroids.

CONTRAINDICATIONS

Neoral® is contraindicated in patients with a hypersensitivity to cyclosporine or to any of the ingredients of the formulation.

WARNINGS

(See boxed WARNINGS)

Cyclosporine, the active ingredient of Neoral®, can cause nephrotoxicity and hepatotoxicity when used in high doses. It is not unusual for serum creatinine and BUN levels to be elevated during cyclosporine therapy. These elevations in renal transplant patients do not necessarily indicate rejection, and each patient must be fully evaluated before dosage adjustment is initiated.

Based on the historical Sandimmune® experience with oral solution, nephrotoxicity associated with cyclosporine had been noted in 25% of cases of renal transplantation, 38% of cases of cardiac transplantation, and 37% of cases of liver transplantation. Mild nephrotoxicity was generally noted 2–3 months after renal transplant and consisted of an arrest in the fall of the pre-operative elevations of BUN and creatinine at a range of 35–45 mg/dl and 2.0–2.5 mg/dl respectively. These elevations were often responsive to cyclosporine dosage reduction.

More overt nephrotoxicity was seen early after transplantation and was characterized by a rapidly rising BUN and creatinine. Since these events are similar to renal rejection episodes, care must be taken to differentiate between them. This form of nephrotoxicity is usually responsive to cyclosporine dosage reduction.

Although specific diagnostic criteria which reliably differentiate renal graft rejection from drug toxicity have not been found, a number of parameters have been significantly associated with one or the other. It should be noted however, that

Pediatric Pharmacokinetic Parameters (mean±SD)

Patient Population	Dose/day (mg/d)	Dose/weight (mg/kg/d)	AUC[1] (ng·hr/mL)	C_{max} (ng/mL)	CL/F (mL/min)	CL/F (mL/min/kg)
[2] Stable liver transplant Age 2–8, Dosed TID (N=9)	101 ± 25	5.95 ± 1.32	2163 ± 801	629 ± 219	285 ± 94	16.6 ± 4.3
Age 8–15, Dosed BID (N=8)	188 ± 55	4.96 ± 2.09	4272 ± 1462	975 ± 281	378 ± 80	10.2 ± 4.0
[3] Stable liver transplant Age 3, Dosed BID (N=1)	120	8.33	5832	1050	171	11.9
Age 8–15, Dosed BID (N=5)	158 ± 55	5.51 ± 1.91	4452 ± 2475	1013 ± 635	328 ± 121	11.0 ± 1.9
[3] Stable renal transplant Age 7–15, Dosed BID (N=5)	328 ± 83	7.37 ± 4.11	6922 ± 1988	1827 ± 487	418 ± 143	8.7 ± 2.9

[1] AUC was measured over one dosing interval
[2] Assay: Cyclo-trac specific monoclonal radioimmunoassay
[3] Assay: TDx specific monoclonal fluorescence polarization immunoassay

Pharmacokinetic Parameters in Adult Patients (mean±SD)

Patient Population	Dose/day (mg/d)	Dose/weight (mg/kg/d)	AUC[1] (ng·hr/mL)	C_{max} (ng/mL)	Trough[2] (ng/mL)	CL/F (mL/min)	CL/F (mL/min/kg)
[3]*De novo* renal transplant Week 4 (N=37)	597 ± 174	7.95 ± 2.81	8772 ± 2089	1802 ± 428	361 ± 129	593 ± 204	7.8 ± 2.9
[3]Stable renal transplant (N=55)	344 ± 122	4.10 ± 1.58	6035 ± 2194	1333 ± 469	251 ± 116	492 ± 140	5.9 ± 2.1
[4]*De novo* liver transplant Week 4 (N=18)	458 ± 190	6.89 ± 3.68	7187 ± 2816	1555 ± 740	268 ± 101	577 ± 309	8.6 ± 5.7

[1] AUC was measured over one dosing interval
[2] Trough concentrations was measured just prior to the morning Neoral® dose, approximately 12 hours after the previous dose
[3] Assay: TDx specific monoclonal fluorescence polarization immunoassay
[4] Assay: Cyclo-trac specific monoclonal radioimmunoassay

up to 20% of patients may have simultaneous nephrotoxicity and rejection.
[See table at right.]

A form of a cyclosporine-associated nephropathy is characterized by serial deterioration in renal function and morphologic changes in the kidneys. From 5% to 15% of transplant recipients who have received cyclosporine will fail to show a reduction in rising serum creatinine despite a decrease or discontinuation of cyclosporine therapy. Renal biopsies from these patients will demonstrate one or several of the following alterations: tubular vacuolization, tubular microcalcifications, peritubular capillary congestion, arteriolopathy, and a striped form of interstitial fibrosis with tubular atrophy. Though none of these morphologic changes is entirely specific, a diagnosis of cyclosporine-associated structural nephrotoxicity requires evidence of these findings.

When considering the development of cyclosporine-associated nephropathy, it is noteworthy that several authors have reported an association between the appearance of interstitial fibrosis and higher cumulative doses or persistently high circulating trough levels of cyclosporine. This is particularly true during the first 6 posttransplant months when the dosage tends to be highest and when, in kidney recipients, the organ appears to be most vulnerable to the toxic effects of cyclosporine. Among other contributing factors to the development of interstitial fibrosis in these patients are prolonged perfusion time, warm ischemia time, as well as episodes of acute toxicity, and acute and chronic rejection. The reversibility of interstitial fibrosis and its correlation to renal function have not yet been determined. Reversibility of arteriolopathy has been reported after stopping cyclosporine or lowering the dosage.

Impaired renal function at any time requires close monitoring, and frequent dosage adjustment may be indicated.

In the event of severe and unremitting rejection, when rescue therapy with pulse steroids and monoclonal antibodies fail to reverse the rejection episode, it may be preferable to switch to alternative immunosuppressive therapy rather than increase the Neoral® dose to excessive levels.

Occasionally patients have developed a syndrome of thrombocytopenia and microangiopathic hemolytic anemia which may result in graft failure. The vasculopathy can occur in the absence of rejection and is accompanied by avid platelet consumption within the graft as demonstrated by Indium 111 labeled platelet studies. Neither the pathogenesis nor the management of this syndrome is clear. Though resolution has occurred after reduction or discontinuation of cyclosporine and 1) administration of streptokinase and heparin or 2) plasmapheresis, this appears to depend upon early detection with Indium 111 labeled platelet scans. (See ADVERSE REACTIONS)

Significant hyperkalemia (sometimes associated with hyperchloremic metabolic acidosis) and hyperuricemia have been seen occasionally in individual patients.

Hepatotoxicity associated with cyclosporine use had been noted in 4% of cases of renal transplantation, 7% of cases of cardiac transplantation, and 4% of cases of liver transplantation. This was usually noted during the first month of therapy when high doses of cyclosporine were used and consisted of elevations of hepatic enzymes and bilirubin. The chemistry elevations usually decreased with a reduction in dosage.

As in patients receiving other immunosuppressants, those patients receiving cyclosporine are at increased risk for development of lymphomas and other malignancies, particularly those of the skin. The increased risk appears related to the intensity and duration of immunosuppression rather than to the use of specific agents. Because of the danger of oversuppression of the immune system resulting in increased risk of infection or malignancy, a treatment regimen containing multiple immunosuppressants should be used with caution.

There have been reports of convulsions in adult and pediatric patients receiving cyclosporine, particularly in combination with high dose methylprednisolone.

Care should be taken in using cyclosporine with nephrotoxic drugs. (See PRECAUTIONS)

Because Neoral® is not bioequivalent to Sandimmune®, conversion from Neoral® to Sandimmune® using a 1:1 ratio (mg/kg/day) may result in lower cyclosporine blood concentrations. Conversion from Neoral® to Sandimmune® should be made with increased monitoring to avoid the potential of underdosing.

PRECAUTIONS
General
Cyclosporine is the active ingredient of Neoral®. Hypertension is a common side effect of cyclosporine therapy. (See ADVERSE REACTIONS) Mild or moderate hypertension is encountered more frequently than severe hypertension and the incidence decreases over time. Antihypertensive therapy may be required. Control of blood pressure can be accomplished with any of the common antihypertensive agents. However, since cyclosporine may cause hyperkalemia, potassium-sparing diuretics should not be used. Calcium antagonists can be effective agents in treating cyclosporine-associated hypertension. However, care should be taken

Nephrotoxicity vs Rejection

Parameter	Nephrotoxicity	Rejection
History	Donor >50 years old or hypotensive Prolonged kidney preservation Prolonged anastomosis time Concomitant nephrotoxic drugs	Antidonor immune response Retransplant patient
Clinical	Often >6 weeks postop[b] Prolonged initial nonfunction (acute tubular necrosis)	Often <4 weeks postop[b] Fever >37.5°C Weight gain >0.5 kg Graft swelling and tenderness Decrease in daily urine volume >500 mL (or 50%)
Laboratory	CyA serum trough level >200 ng/mL Gradual rise in Cr (<0.15 mg/dl/day)[a] Cr plateau <25% above baseline BUN/Cr ≥ 20	CyA serum trough level <150 ng/mL Rapid rise in Cr (>0.3 mg/dl/day)[a] Cr >25% above baseline BUN/Cr <20
Biopsy	Arteriolopathy (medial hypertrophy[a], hyalinosis, nodular deposits, intimal thickening, endothelial vacuolization, progressive scarring) Tubular atrophy, isometric vacuolization, isolated calcifications Minimal edema Mild focal infiltrates[c] Diffuse interstitial fibrosis, often striped form	Endovasculitis[c] (proliferation[a], intimal arteritis[b], necrosis, sclerosis) Tubulitis with RBC[b] and WBC[b] casts, some irregular vacuolization Interstitial edema[c] and hemorrhage[b] Diffuse moderate to severe mononuclear infiltrates[d] Glomerulitis (mononuclear cells)[c]
Aspiration Cytology	CyA deposits in tubular and endothelial cells Fine isometric vacuolization of tubular cells	Inflammatory infiltrate with mononuclear phagocytes, macrophages, lymphoblastoid cells, and activated T-cells These strongly express HLA-DR antigens
Urine Cytology	Tubular cells with vacuolization and granularization	Degenerative tubular cells, plasma cells, and lymphocyturia >20% of sediment
Manometry	Intracapsular pressure <40 mm Hg[b]	Intracapsular pressure >40 mm Hg[b]
Ultrasonography	Unchanged graft cross sectional area	Increase in graft cross sectional area AP diameter ≥ Transverse diameter
Magnetic Resonance Imagery	Normal appearance	Loss of distinct corticomedullary junction, swelling image intensity of parachyma approaching that of psoas, loss of hilar fat
Radionuclide Scan	Normal or generally decreased perfusion Decrease in tubular function ([131]l-hippuran) > decrease in perfusion (^{99m}Tc DTPA)	Patchy arterial flow Decrease in perfusion > decrease in tubular function Increased uptake of Indium 111 labeled platelets or Tc-99m in colloid
Therapy	Responds to decreased cyclosporine	Responds to increased steroids or antilymphocyte globulin

[a]p <0.05, [b]p <0.01, [c]p <0.001, [d]p <0.0001

---

since interference with cyclosporine metabolism may require a dosage adjustment. (See Drug Interactions)

During treatment with cyclosporine, vaccination may be less effective; and the use of live attenuated vaccines should be avoided.

Information for Patients
Patients should be advised that any change of cyclosporine formulation should be made cautiously and only under physician supervision because it may result in the need for a change in dosage.

Patients should be informed of the necessity of repeated laboratory tests while they are receiving the drug. Patients should be advised of the potential risks during pregnancy and informed of the increased risk of neoplasia.

Patients should be given careful dosage instructions. Neoral® Oral Solution (cyclosporine oral solution for microemulsion) should be diluted, preferably with orange or apple juice that is at room temperature. Grapefruit and grapefruit juice affect metabolism of cyclosporine and should be avoided. The combination of Neoral® Oral Solution (cyclosporine oral solution for microemulsion) with milk can be unpalatable.

Patients should be advised to take Neoral® on a consistent schedule with regard to time of day and relation to meals.

Laboratory Tests
Renal and liver functions should be assessed repeatedly by measurement of BUN, serum creatinine, serum bilirubin, and liver enzymes.

Drug Interactions
All of the individual drugs cited below are well substantiated to interact with cyclosporine.

Drugs That May Potentiate Renal Dysfunction
Antibiotics
gentamicin
tobramycin
vancomycin
trimethoprim with sulfamethoxazole
Antineoplastics
melphalan
Antifungals
amphotericin B
ketoconazole
Anti-inflammatory Drugs
azapropazon
diclofenac

Gastrointestinal Agents
cimetidine
ranitidine
Immunosuppressives
tacrolimus
Careful monitoring of renal function should be practiced when Neoral® is used with nephrotoxic drugs.

Drugs That Alter Cyclosporine Levels
Cyclosporine is extensively metabolized. Cyclosporine concentrations may be influenced by drugs that affect microsomal enzymes, particularly cytochrome P-450 III-A. Substances that inhibit this enzyme could decrease metabolism and increase cyclosporine concentrations. Substances that are inducers of cytochrome P-450 activity could increase metabolism and decrease cyclosporine concentrations. Monitoring of circulating cyclosporine concentrations and appropriate Neoral® dosage adjustment are essential when these drugs are used concomitantly. (See Blood Concentration Monitoring)

Drugs That Increase Cyclosporine Concentrations
Calcium Channel Blockers
diltiazem
nicardipine
verapamil
Antifungals
fluconazole
itraconazole
ketoconazole
Antibiotics
clarithromycin
erythromycin
Glucocorticoids
methylprednisolone
Other Drugs
allopurinol
bromocriptine
danazol
metoclopramide

Drugs That Decrease Cyclosporine Concentrations
Antibiotics
nafcillin
rifampin

Continued on next page

Sandoz—Cont.

Anticonvulsants
carbamazepine
phenobarbital
phenytoin
Other Drugs
octreotide
ticlopidine

Rifabutin is known to increase the metabolism of other drugs metabolized by the cytochrome P-450 system. The interaction between rifabutin and cyclosporine has not been studied. Care should be exercised when these two drugs are administered concomitantly.

Other Drug Interactions

Reduced clearance of prednisolone, digoxin, and lovastatin has been observed when these drugs are administered with cyclosporine. In addition, a decrease in the apparent volume of distribution of digoxin has been reported after cyclosporine administration. Severe digitalis toxicity has been seen within days of starting cyclosporine in several patients taking digoxin. Cyclosporine should not be used with potassium-sparing diuretics because hyperkalemia can occur. During treatment with cyclosporine, vaccination may be less effective. The use of live vaccines should be avoided. Myositis has occurred with concomitant lovastatin, frequent gingival hyperplasia with nifedipine, and convulsions with high dose methylprednisolone. Further information on drugs that have been reported to interact with cyclosporine is available from Sandoz Pharmaceuticals Corporation.

Carcinogenesis, Mutagenesis, and Impairment of Fertility

Cyclosporine gave no evidence of mutagenic or teratogenic effects in appropriate test systems. Only at dose levels toxic to dams, were adverse effects seen in reproduction studies in rats. (See *Pregnancy*)

Carcinogenicity studies were carried out in male and female rats and mice. In the 78-week mouse study, evidence of a statistically significant trend was found for lymphocytic lymphomas in females, and the incidence of hepatocellular carcinomas in mid-dose males significantly exceeded the control value. In the 24-month rat study, pancreatic islet cell adenomas significantly exceeded the control rate in the low dose level. Doses used in the mouse and rat studies were 0.01 to 0.16 times the clinical maintenance dose. The hepatocellular carcinomas and pancreatic islet cell adenomas were not dose related.

No impairment in fertility was demonstrated in studies in male and female rats.

Cyclosporine has not been found to be mutagenic/genotoxic in the Ames Test, the V79-HGPRT Test, the micronucleus test in mice and Chinese hamsters, the chromosome-aberration tests in Chinese hamster bone-marrow, the mouse dominant lethal assay, and the DNA-repair test in sperm from treated mice. A recent study analyzing sister chromatid exchange (SCE) induction by cyclosporine using human lymphocytes *in vitro* gave indication of a positive effect (i.e., induction of SCE), at high concentrations in this system.

An increased incidence of malignancy is a recognized complication of immunosuppression in recipients of organ transplants. The most common forms of neoplasms are non-Hodgkin's lymphoma and carcinomas of the skin. The risk of malignancies in cyclosporine recipients is higher than in the normal, healthy population but similar to that in patients receiving other immunosuppressive therapies. Reduction or discontinuance of immunosuppression may cause the lesions to regress.

Pregnancy

Pregnancy Category C. Cyclosporine has been shown to be embryo- and fetotoxic in rats and rabbits following oral administration at maternally toxic doses. Fetal toxicity was noted in rats at 0.8 and rabbits at 5.4 times the human maintenance dose of 6.0 mg/kg, where dose corrections are based on body surface area. Cyclosporine was embryo- and fetotoxic as indicated by increased pre- and postnatal mortality and reduced fetal weight together with related skeletal retardations.

There are no adequate and well-controlled studies in pregnant women. Neoral® should be used during pregnancy only if the potential benefit justifies the potential risk to the fetus.

The following data represent the reported outcomes of 116 pregnancies in women receiving cyclosporine during pregnancy, 90% of whom were transplant patients, and most of whom received cyclosporine throughout the entire gestational period. The only consistent patterns of abnormality were premature birth (gestational period of 28 to 36 weeks) and low birth weight for gestational age. Sixteen fetal losses occurred. Most of the pregnancies (85 of 100) were complicated by disorders, including pre-eclampsia, eclampsia, premature labor, abruptio placentae, oligohydramnios, Rh incompatibility and fetoplacental dysfunction. Preterm delivery occurred in 47%. Seven malformations were reported in 5 viable infants and in 2 cases of fetal loss. Twenty-eight per-

cent of the infants were small for gestational age. Neonatal complications occurred in 27%. Therefore, the risks and benefits of using Neoral® during pregnancy should be carefully weighed.

Nursing Mothers

Since cyclosporine is excreted in human milk, nursing should be avoided.

Pediatric Use

Although no adequate and well controlled studies have been completed in children, patients as young as one year of age have received Neoral® with no unusual adverse effects.

ADVERSE REACTIONS

The principal adverse reactions of cyclosporine therapy are renal dysfunction, tremor, hirsutism, hypertension, and gum hyperplasia.

Hypertension, which is usually mild to moderate, may occur in approximately 50% of patients following renal transplantation and in most cardiac transplant patients.

Glomerular capillary thrombosis has been found in patients treated with cyclosporine and may progress to graft failure. The pathologic changes resemble those seen in the hemolytic-uremic syndrome and include thrombosis of the renal microvasculature, with platelet-fibrin thrombi occluding glomerular capillaries and afferent arterioles, microangiopathic hemolytic anemia, thrombocytopenia, and decreased renal function. Similar findings have been observed when other immunosuppressives have been employed post-transplantation.

Hypomagnesemia has been reported in some, but not all, patients exhibiting convulsions while on cyclosporine therapy. Although magnesium-depletion studies in normal subjects suggest that hypomagnesemia is associated with neurologic disorders, multiple factors, including hypertension, high dose methylprednisolone, hypocholesterolemia, and nephrotoxicity associated with high plasma concentrations of cyclosporine appear to be related to the neurological manifestations of cyclosporine toxicity.

In controlled studies, the nature, severity and incidence of the adverse events that were observed in 493 transplanted patients treated with Neoral® were comparable with those observed in 208 transplanted patients who received Sandimmune® in these same studies when the dosage of the two drugs was adjusted to achieve the same cyclosporine blood trough concentrations.

Based on the historical experience with Sandimmune®, the following reactions occurred in 3% or greater of 892 patients involved in clinical trials of kidney, heart, and liver transplants.

[See first table above.]

Among 705 kidney transplant patients treated with cyclosporine oral solution (Sandimmune®) in clinical trials, the reason for treatment discontinuation was renal toxicity in 5.4%, infection in 0.9%, lack of efficacy in 1.4%, acute tubular necrosis in 1.0%, lymphoproliferative disorders in 0.3%, hypertension in 0.3%, and other reasons in 0.7%.

The following reactions occurred in 2% or less of Sandimmune®-treated patients: allergic reactions, anemia, anorexia, confusion, conjunctivitis, edema, fever, brittle fingernails, gastritis, hearing loss, hiccups, hyperglycemia, muscle pain, peptic ulcer, thrombocytopenia, tinnitus.

The following reactions occurred rarely: anxiety, chest pain, constipation, depression, hair breaking, hematuria, joint pain, lethargy, mouth sores, myocardial infarction, night sweats, pancreatitis, pruritus, swallowing difficulty, tingling, upper GI bleeding, visual disturbance, weakness, weight loss.

[See second table above.]

OVERDOSAGE

There is a minimal experience with cyclosporine overdosage. Forced emesis can be of value up to 2 hours after administration of Neoral®. Transient hepatotoxicity and nephrotoxicity may occur which should resolve following drug withdrawal. General supportive measures and symptomatic treatment should be followed in all cases of overdosage. Cyclosporine is not dialyzable to any great extent, nor is it cleared well by charcoal hemoperfusion. The oral dosage at which half of experimental animals are estimated to die is 31 times, 39 times and > 54 times the human maintenance dose

Body System/ Adverse Reactions	Randomized Kidney Patients		Cyclosporine Patients (Sandimmune®)		
	Sandimmune® (N=227) %	Azathioprine (N=228) %	Kidney (N=705) %	Heart (N=112) %	Liver (N=75) %
Genitourinary					
Renal Dysfunction	32	6	25	38	37
Cardiovascular					
Hypertension	26	18	13	53	27
Cramps	4	<1	2	<1	0
Skin					
Hirsutism	21	<1	21	28	45
Acne	6	8	2	2	1
Central Nervous System					
Tremor	12	0	21	31	55
Convulsions	3	1	1	4	5
Headache	2	<1	2	15	4
Gastrointestinal					
Gum Hyperplasia	4	0	9	5	16
Diarrhea	3	<1	3	4	8
Nausea/Vomiting	2	<1	4	10	4
Hepatotoxicity	<1	<1	4	7	4
Abdominal Discomfort	<1	0	<1	7	0
Autonomic Nervous System					
Paresthesia	3	0	1	2	1
Flushing	<1	0	4	0	4
Hematopoietic					
Leukopenia	2	19	<1	6	0
Lymphoma	<1	0	1	6	1
Respiratory					
Sinusitis	<1	0	4	3	7
Miscellaneous					
Gynecomastia	<1	0	<1	4	3

Infectious Complications in Historical Randomized Studies in Renal Transplant Patients Using Sandimmune®

Complication	Cyclosporine Treatment (N=227) % of Complications	Azathioprine with Steroids* (N=228) % of Complications
Septicemia	5.3	4.8
Abscesses	4.4	5.3
Systemic Fungal Infection	2.2	3.9
Local Fungal Infection	7.5	9.6
Cytomegalovirus	4.8	12.3
Other Viral Infections	15.9	18.4
Urinary Tract Infections	21.1	20.2
Wound and Skin Infections	7.0	10.1
Pneumonia	6.2	9.2

* Some patients also received ALG.

(6mg/kg: corrections based on body surface area) in mice, rats, and rabbits.

DOSAGE AND ADMINISTRATION

Neoral® Soft Gelatin Capsules
(cyclosporine capsules for microemulsion) and
Neoral® Oral Solution
(cyclosporine oral solution for microemulsion)

Neoral® has increased bioavailability in comparison to Sandimmune®. Neoral® and Sandimmune® are not bioequivalent and cannot be used interchangeably without physician supervision.

The daily dose of Neoral® should always be given in two divided doses (BID). It is recommended that Neoral® be administered on a consistent schedule with regard to time of day and relation to meals.

Newly Transplanted Patients

The initial oral dose of Neoral® can be given 4–12 hours prior to transplantation or be given postoperatively. The initial dose of Neoral® varies depending on the transplanted organ and the other immunosuppressive agents included in the immunosuppressive protocol. In newly transplanted patients, the initial oral dose of Neoral® is the same as the initial oral dose of Sandimmune®. Suggested initial doses are available from the results of a 1994 survey of the use of Sandimmune® in US transplant centers. The mean ±SD initial doses were 9±3 mg/kg/day for renal transplant patients (75 centers), 8±4 mg/kg/day for liver transplant patients (30 centers), and 7±3 mg/kg/day for heart transplant patients (24 centers). Total daily doses were divided into two equal daily doses. The Neoral® dose is subsequently adjusted to achieve a pre-defined cyclosporine blood concentration. *(See Blood Concentration Monitoring below)* If cyclosporine trough blood concentrations are used, the target range is the same for Neoral® as for Sandimmune®. Using the same trough concentration target range for Neoral® as for Sandimmune® results in greater cyclosporine exposure when Neoral® is administered. *(See Pharmacokinetics, Absorption)* Dosing should be titrated based on clinical assessments of rejection and tolerability. Lower Neoral® doses may be sufficient as maintenance therapy.

Adjunct therapy with adrenal corticosteroids is recommended initially. Different tapering dosage schedules of prednisone appear to achieve similar results. A representative dosage schedule based on the patient's weight started with 2.0 mg/kg/day for the first 4 days tapered to 1.0 mg/kg/day by 1 week, 0.6 mg/kg/day by 2 weeks, 0.3 mg/kg/day by 1 month, and 0.15 mg/kg/day by 2 months and thereafter as a maintenance dose. Steroid doses may be further tapered on an individualized basis depending on status of patient and function of graft. Adjustments in dosage of prednisone must be made according to the clinical situation.

Conversion from Sandimmune ® to Neoral ®

In transplanted patients who are considered for conversion to Neoral® from Sandimmune®, Neoral® should be started with the same daily dose as was previously used with Sandimmune® (1:1 dose conversion). The Neoral® dose should subsequently be adjusted to attain the pre-conversion cyclosporine blood trough concentration. Using the same trough concentration target range for Neoral® as for Sandimmune® results in greater cyclosporine exposure when Neoral® is administered. *(See Pharmacokinetics, Absorption)* Patients with suspected poor absorption of Sandimmune® require different dosing strategies. *(See Patients with Poor Absorption of Sandimmune®, below)* In some patients, the increase in blood trough concentration is more pronounced and may be of clinical significance.

Until the blood trough concentration attains the pre-conversion value, it is strongly recommended that the cyclosporine blood trough concentration be monitored every 4 to 7 days after conversion to Neoral®. In addition, clinical safety parameters such as serum creatinine and blood pressure should be monitored every two weeks during the first two months after conversion. If the blood trough concentrations are outside the desired range and/or if the clinical safety parameters worsen, the dosage of Neoral® must be adjusted accordingly.

Patients with Poor Absorption of Sandimmune ®

Patients with lower than expected cyclosporine blood trough concentrations in relation to the oral dose of Sandimmune® may have poor or inconsistent absorption of cyclosporine from Sandimmune®. After conversion to Neoral®, patients tend to have higher cyclosporine concentrations. **Due to the increase in bioavailability of cyclosporine following conversion to Neoral®, the cyclosporine blood trough concentration may exceed the target range. Particular caution should be exercised when converting patients to Neoral® at doses greater than 10 mg/kg/day.** The dose of Neoral® should be titrated individually based on cyclosporine trough concentrations, tolerability, and clinical response. In this population the cyclosporine blood trough concentration should be measured more frequently, at least twice a week (daily, if initial dose exceeds 10 mg/kg/day) until the concentration stabilizes within the desired range.

Neoral® Oral Solution
(cyclosporine oral solution for microemulsion) —
Recommendations for Administration

To make Neoral® Oral Solution (cyclosporine oral solution for microemulsion) more palatable, it should be diluted preferably with orange or apple juice that is at room temperature. Grapefruit juice affects metabolism of cyclosporine and should be avoided. The combination of Neoral® Oral Solution (cyclosporine oral solution for microemulsion) with milk can be unpalatable.

Take the prescribed amount of Neoral® Oral Solution (cyclosporine oral solution for microemulsion) from the container using the dosing syringe supplied, after removal of the protective cover, and transfer the solution to a glass of orange or apple juice. Stir well and drink at once. Do not allow diluted oral solution to stand before drinking. Use a glass container (not plastic). Rinse the glass with more diluent to ensure that the total dose is consumed. After use, dry the outside of the dosing syringe with a clean towel and replace the protective cover. Do not rinse the dosing syringe with water or other cleaning agents. If the syringe requires cleaning, it must be completely dry before resuming use.

Blood Concentration Monitoring

Transplant centers have found blood concentration monitoring of cyclosporine to be an essential component of patient management. Of importance to blood concentration analysis are the type of assay used, the transplanted organ, and other immunosuppressant agents being administered. While no fixed relationship has been established, blood concentration monitoring may assist in the clinical evaluation of rejection and toxicity, dose adjustments, and the assessment of compliance.

Various assays have been used to measure blood concentrations of cyclosporine. Older studies using a non-specific assay often cited concentrations that were roughly twice those of specific assays, thus comparison of the concentrations in published literature to patient concentrations using current assays must be made with detailed knowledge of the assay methods employed. Current assay results are also not interchangeable and their use should be guided by their approved labeling. A discussion of the different assay methods is contained in *Annals of Clinical Biochemistry* 1994;31:420–446. While several assays and assay matrices are available, there is a consensus that parent-compound-specific assays correlate best with clinical events. Of these, HPLC is the standard reference, but the monoclonal antibody RIAs and the monoclonal antibody FPIA offer sensitivity, reproducibility, and convenience. Most clinicians base their monitoring on trough cyclosporine concentrations. *Applied Pharmacokinetics, Principles of Therapeutic Drug Monitoring* (1992) contains a broad discussion of cyclosporine pharmacokinetics and drug monitoring techniques. Blood concentration monitoring is not a replacement for renal function monitoring or tissue biopsies.

HOW SUPPLIED

Neoral® Soft Gelatin Capsules
(cyclosporine capsules for microemulsion)

25 mg

Oval, blue-gray imprinted in red. "NEORAL" over "25 mg." Packages of 30 unit-dose blisters (NDC 0078-0246-15).

100 mg

Oblong, blue-gray imprinted in red, "NEORAL" over "100 mg."
Packages of 30 unit-dose blisters (NDC 0078-0248-15).

Store and Dispense

In the original unit-dose container at controlled room temperature 77°F (25°C).

Neoral® Oral Solution
(cyclosporine oral solution for microemulsion)

A clear, yellow liquid supplied in 50 mL bottles containing 100 mg/mL (NDC 0078-0274-22).

Store and Dispense

In the original container at controlled room temperature 77°F (25°C). Do not store in the refrigerator. Once opened, the contents must be used within two months. At temperatures below 68°F (20°C) the solution may gel; light flocculation or the formation of a light sediment may also occur. There is no impact on product performance or dosing using the syringe provided. Allow to warm to room temperature 77°F (25°C) to reverse these changes.

Neoral® Soft Gelatin Capsules
(cyclosporine capsules for microemulsion)
Manufactured by R.P. Scherer GmbH
EBERBACH/BADEN, GERMANY
Manufactured for Sandoz Pharmaceuticals Corporation
East Hanover, NJ 07936

Neoral® Oral Solution
(cyclosporine oral solution for microemulsion)
Manufactured by SANDOZ PHARMA LTD.
Basle, Switzerland
Manufactured for Sandoz Pharmaceuticals Corporation
East Hanover, NJ 07936

Sandoz Pharmaceuticals Corporation
East Hanover, New Jersey 07936

[SEPTEMBER 1995 38371902]
Shown in Product Identification Guide, page 333

PAMELOR® ℞

[pam 'ah-lar"]
(nortriptyline HCl) CAPSULES, USP
(nortriptyline HCl) ORAL SOLUTION, USP

CAUTION: Federal law prohibits dispensing without prescription.

The following prescribing information is based on official labeling in effect on August 1, 1996.

DESCRIPTION

Pamelor® (nortriptyline HCl) is 1-Propanamine, 3-(10,11-dihydro-5*H*-dibenzo[*a,d*]cyclohepten-5-ylidene)-*N*-methyl-, hydrochloride.

The structural formula is as follows:

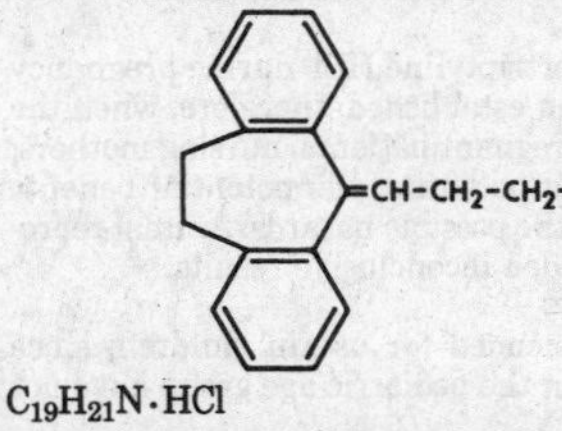

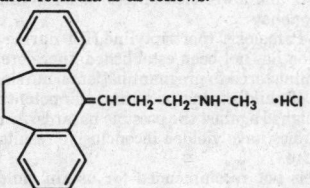

$C_{19}H_{21}N \cdot HCl$ Mol. wt. 299.8

10 mg, 25 mg, 50 mg, and 75 mg Capsules

Active Ingredient: nortriptyline HCl, USP

10 mg, 25 mg, and 75 mg Capsules

Inactive Ingredients: D&C Yellow #10, FD&C Yellow #6, gelatin, silicone fluid, sodium lauryl sulfate, starch, and titanium dioxide.

May Also Include: benzyl alcohol, butylparaben, edetate calcium disodium, methylparaben, propylparaben, silicon dioxide, and sodium propionate.

50 mg Capsules

Inactive Ingredients: gelatin, silicone fluid, sodium lauryl sulfate, starch, and titanium dioxide.

May Also Include: benzyl alcohol, butylparaben, edetate calcium disodium, methylparaben, propylparaben, silicon dioxide, sodium bisulfite (capsule shell only), and sodium propionate.

Solution

Active Ingredient: nortriptyline HCl, USP

Inactive Ingredients: alcohol, benzoic acid, flavoring, purified water, and sorbitol.

ACTIONS

The mechanism of mood elevation by tricyclic antidepressants is at present unknown. Pamelor® (nortriptyline HCl) is not a monoamine oxidase inhibitor. It inhibits the activity of such diverse agents as histamine, 5-hydroxytryptamine, and acetylcholine. It increases the pressor effect of norepinephrine but blocks the pressor response of phenethylamine. Studies suggest that Pamelor® (nortriptyline HCl) interferes with the transport, release, and storage of catecholamines. Operant conditioning techniques in rats and pigeons suggest that Pamelor® (nortriptyline HCl) has a combination of stimulant and depressant properties.

INDICATIONS

Pamelor® (nortriptyline HCl) is indicated for the relief of symptoms of depression. Endogenous depressions are more likely to be alleviated than are other depressive states.

CONTRAINDICATIONS

The use of Pamelor® (nortriptyline HCl) or other tricyclic antidepressants concurrently with a monoamine oxidase (MAO) inhibitor is contraindicated. Hyperpyretic crises, severe convulsions, and fatalities have occurred when similar tricyclic antidepressants were used in such combinations. It is advisable to have discontinued the MAO inhibitor for at least two weeks before treatment with Pamelor® (nortriptyline HCl) is started. Patients hypersensitive to Pamelor® (nortriptyline HCl) should not be given the drug. Cross-sensitivity between Pamelor® (nortriptyline HCl) and other dibenzazepines is a possibility.

Pamelor® (nortriptyline HCl) is contraindicated during the acute recovery period after myocardial infarction.

WARNINGS

Patients with cardiovascular disease should be given Pamelor® (nortriptyline HCl) only under close supervision because of the tendency of the drug to produce sinus tachycardia and to prolong the conduction time. Myocardial infarction, arrhythmia, and strokes have occurred. The antihypertensive action of guanethidine and similar agents may be blocked. Because of its anticholinergic activity, Pamelor® (nortriptyline HCl) should be used with great caution in patients who have glaucoma or a history of urinary retention.

Continued on next page

Sandoz—Cont.

Patients with a history of seizures should be followed closely when Pamelor® (nortriptyline HCl) is administered, inasmuch as this drug is known to lower the convulsive threshold. Great care is required if Pamelor® (nortriptyline HCl) is given to hyperthyroid patients or to those receiving thyroid medication, since cardiac arrhythmias may develop. Pamelor® (nortriptyline HCl) may impair the mental and/or physical abilities required for the performance of hazardous tasks, such as operating machinery or driving a car; therefore, the patient should be warned accordingly. Excessive consumption of alcohol in combination with nortriptyline therapy may have a potentiating effect, which may lead to the danger of increased suicidal attempts or overdosage, especially in patients with histories of emotional disturbances or suicidal ideation.

The concomitant administration of quinidine and nortriptyline may result in a significantly longer plasma half-life, higher AUC, and lower clearance of nortriptyline.

Use in Pregnancy
Safe use of Pamelor® (nortriptyline HCl) during pregnancy and lactation has not been established; therefore, when the drug is administered to pregnant patients, nursing mothers, or women of childbearing potential, the potential benefits must be weighed against the possible hazards. Animal reproduction studies have yielded inconclusive results.

Pediatric Use
This drug is not recommended for use in children, since safety and effectiveness in the pediatric age group have not been established.

PRECAUTIONS
The use of Pamelor® (nortriptyline HCl) in schizophrenic patients may result in an exacerbation of the psychosis or may activate latent schizophrenic symptoms. If the drug is given to overactive or agitated patients, increased anxiety and agitation may occur. In manic-depressive patients, Pamelor® (nortriptyline HCl) may cause symptoms of the manic phase to emerge.

Troublesome patient hostility may be aroused by the use of Pamelor® (nortriptyline HCl). Epileptiform seizures may accompany its administration, as is true of other drugs of its class.

When it is essential, the drug may be administered with electroconvulsive therapy, although the hazards may be increased. Discontinue the drug for several days, if possible, prior to elective surgery.

The possibility of a suicidal attempt by a depressed patient remains after the initiation of treatment; in this regard, it is important that the least possible quantity of drug be dispensed at any given time.

Both elevation and lowering of blood sugar levels have been reported.

Drug Interactions
Administration of reserpine during therapy with a tricyclic antidepressant has been shown to produce a "stimulating" effect in some depressed patients.

Close supervision and careful adjustment of the dosage are required when Pamelor® (nortriptyline HCl) is used with other anticholinergic drugs and sympathomimetic drugs.

Concurrent administration of cimetidine and tricyclic antidepressants can produce clinically significant increases in the plasma concentrations of the tricyclic antidepressant. The patient should be informed that the response to alcohol may be exaggerated.

A case of significant hypoglycemia has been reported in a type II diabetic patient maintained on chlorpropamide (250 mg/day), after the addition of nortriptyline (125 mg/day).

Drugs Metabolized by P450 2D6 – The biochemical activity of the drug metabolizing isozyme cytochrome P450 2D6 (debrisoquin hydroxylase) is reduced in a subset of the caucasian population (about 7%-10% of caucasians are so called "poor metabolizers"); reliable estimates of the prevalence of reduced P450 2D6 isozyme activity among Asian, African and other populations are not yet available. Poor metabolizers have higher than expected plasma concentrations of tricyclic antidepressants (TCAs) when given usual doses. Depending on the fraction of drug metabolized by P450 2D6, the increase in plasma concentration may be small, or quite large (8 fold increase in plasma AUC of the TCA).

In addition, certain drugs inhibit the activity of this isozyme and make normal metabolizers resemble poor metabolizers. An individual who is stable on a given dose of TCA may become abruptly toxic when given one of these inhibiting drugs as concomitant therapy. The drugs that inhibit cytochrome P450 2D6 include some that are not metabolized by the enzyme (quinidine; cimetidine) and many that are substrates for P450 2D6 (many other antidepressants, phenothiazines, and the Type 1C antiarrhythmics propafenone and flecainide). While all the selective serotonin reuptake inhibitors (SSRIs), e.g., fluoxetine, sertraline, and paroxetine, inhibit P450 2D6, they may vary in the extent of inhibition. The extent to which SSRI TCA interactions may pose clinical

problems will depend on the degree of inhibition and the pharmacokinetics of the SSRI involved. Nevertheless, caution is indicated in the co-administration of TCAs with any of the SSRIs and also in switching from one class to the other. Of particular importance, sufficient time must elapse before initiating TCA treatment in a patient being withdrawn from fluoxetine, given the long half-life of the parent and active metabolite (at least 5 weeks may be necessary).

Concomitant use of tricyclic antidepressants with drugs that can inhibit cytochrome P450 2D6 may require lower doses than usually prescribed for either the tricyclic antidepressant or the other drug. Furthermore, whenever one of these other drugs is withdrawn from co-therapy, an increased dose of tricyclic antidepressant may be required. It is desirable to monitor TCA plasma levels whenever a TCA is going to be co-administered with another drug known to be an inhibitor of P450 2D6.

ADVERSE REACTIONS
Note: Included in the following list are a few adverse reactions that have not been reported with this specific drug. However, the pharmacologic similarities among the tricyclic antidepressant drugs require that each of the reactions be considered when nortriptyline is administered.

Cardiovascular – Hypotension, hypertension, tachycardia, palpitation, myocardial infarction, arrhythmias, heart block, stroke.

Psychiatric – Confusional states (especially in the elderly) with hallucinations, disorientation, delusions; anxiety, restlessness, agitation; insomnia, panic, nightmares; hypomania; exacerbation of psychosis.

Neurologic – Numbness, tingling, paresthesias of extremities; incoordination, ataxia, tremors; peripheral neuropathy; extrapyramidal symptoms; seizures, alteration in EEG patterns; tinnitus.

Anticholinergic – Dry mouth and, rarely, associated sublingual adenitis; blurred vision, disturbance of accommodation, mydriasis; constipation, paralytic ileus; urinary retention, delayed micturition, dilation of the urinary tract.

Allergic – Skin rash, petechiae, urticaria, itching, photosensitization (avoid excessive exposure to sunlight); edema (general or of face and tongue), drug fever, cross-sensitivity with other tricyclic drugs.

Hematologic – Bone marrow depression, including agranulocytosis; eosinophilia; purpura; thrombocytopenia.

Gastrointestinal – Nausea and vomiting, anorexia, epigastric distress, diarrhea, peculiar taste, stomatitis, abdominal cramps, blacktongue.

Endocrine – Gynecomastia in the male, breast enlargement and galactorrhea in the female; increased or decreased libido, impotence; testicular swelling; elevation or depression of blood sugar levels; syndrome of inappropriate ADH (antidiuretic hormone) secretion.

Other – Jaundice (simulating obstructive), altered liver function; weight gain or loss; perspiration; flushing; urinary frequency, nocturia; drowsiness, dizziness, weakness, fatigue; headache; parotid swelling; alopecia.

Withdrawal Symptoms – Though these are not indicative of addiction, abrupt cessation of treatment after prolonged therapy may produce nausea, headache, and malaise.

DOSAGE AND ADMINISTRATION
Pamelor® (nortriptyline HCl) is not recommended for children.

Pamelor® (nortriptyline HCl) is administered orally in the form of capsules or liquid. Lower than usual dosages are recommended for elderly patients and adolescents. Lower dosages are also recommended for outpatients than for hospitalized patients who will be under close supervision. The physician should initiate dosage at a low level and increase it gradually, noting carefully the clinical response and any evidence of intolerance. Following remission, maintenance medication may be required for a longer period of time at the lowest dose that will maintain remission.

If a patient develops minor side effects, the dosage should be reduced. The drug should be discontinued promptly if adverse effects of a serious nature or allergic manifestations occur.

Usual Adult Dose —25 mg three or four times daily; dosage should begin at a low level and be increased as required. As an alternate regimen, the total daily dosage may be given once a day. When doses above 100 mg daily are administered, plasma levels of nortriptyline should be monitored and maintained in the optimum range of 50-150 ng/mL. Doses above 150 mg/day are not recommended.

Elderly and Adolescent Patients —30-50 mg/day, in divided doses, or the total daily dosage may be given once a day.

OVERDOSAGE
Deaths may occur from overdosage with this class of drugs. Multiple drug ingestion (including alcohol) is common in deliberate tricyclic antidepressant overdose. As the management is complex and changing, it is recommended that the physician contact a poison control center for current information on treatment. Signs and symptoms of toxicity develop rapidly after tricyclic antidepressant overdose, therefore, hospital monitoring is required as soon as possible.

Manifestations:
Critical manifestations of overdose include: cardiac dysrhythmias, severe hypotension, shock, congestive heart failure, pulmonary edema, convulsions, and CNS depression, including coma. Changes in the electrocardiogram, particularly in QRS axis or width, are clinically significant indicators of tricyclic antidepressant toxicity.

Other signs of overdose may include: confusion, restlessness, disturbed concentration, transient visual hallucinations, dilated pupils, agitation, hyperactive reflexes, stupor, drowsiness, muscle rigidity, vomiting, hypothermia, hyperpyrexia, or any of the acute symptoms listed under ADVERSE REACTIONS. There have been reports of patients recovering from nortriptyline overdoses of up to 525 mg.

Management:
General: Obtain an ECG and immediately initiate cardiac monitoring. Protect the patient's airway, establish an intravenous line and initiate gastric decontamination. A minimum of six hours of observation with cardiac monitoring and observation for signs of CNS or respiratory depression, hypotension, cardiac dysrhythmias and/or conduction blocks, and seizures is necessary. If signs of toxicity occur at any time during this period, extended monitoring is required. There are case reports of patients succumbing to fatal dysrhythmias late after overdose; these patients had clinical evidence of significant poisoning prior to death and most received inadequate gastrointestinal decontamination. Monitoring of plasma drug levels should not guide management of the patient.

Gastrointestinal Decontamination: All patients suspected of tricyclic antidepressant overdose should receive gastrointestinal decontamination. This should include large volume gastric lavage followed by activated charcoal. If consciousness is impaired, the airway should be secured prior to lavage. EMESIS IS CONTRAINDICATED.

Cardiovascular: A maximal limb-lead QRS duration of ≥ 0.10 seconds may be the best indication of the severity of the overdose. Intravenous sodium bicarbonate shoud be used to maintain the serum pH in the range of 7.45 to 7.55. If the pH response is inadequate, hyperventilation may also be used. Concomitant use of hyperventilation and sodium bicarbonate should be done with extreme caution, with frequent pH monitoring. A pH > 7.60 or a pCO_2 < 20 mm Hg is undesirable. Dysrhythmias unresponsive to sodium bicarbonate therapy/hyperventilation may respond to lidocaine, bretylium or phenytoin. Type 1A and 1C antiarrhythmics are generally contraindicated (e.g., quinidine, disopyramide, and procainamide).

In rare instances, hemoperfusion may be beneficial in acute refractory cardiovascular instability in patients with acute toxicity. However, hemodialysis, peritoneal dialysis, exchange transfusions, and forced diuresis generally have been reported as ineffective in tricyclic antidepressant poisoning.

CNS: In patients with CNS depression, early intubation is advised because of the potential for abrupt deterioration. Seizures should be controlled with benzodiazepines, or if these are ineffective, other anticonvulsants (e.g., phenobarbital, phenytoin). Physostigmine is not recommended except to treat life-threatening symptoms that have been unresponsive to other therapies, and then only in consultation with a poison control center.

Psychiatric Follow-up: Since overdosage is often deliberate, patients may attempt suicide by other means during the recovery phase. Psychiatric referral may be appropriate.

Pediatric Management: The principles of management of child and adult overdosages are similar. It is strongly recommended that the physician contact the local poison control center for specific pediatric treatment.

HOW SUPPLIED
Pamelor®(nortriptyline HCl) Capsules, USP
Pamelor® (nortriptyline HCl) Capsules, USP, equivalent to 10 mg, 25 mg, 50 mg, and 75 mg base, are available in bottles of 100 (10 mg: NDC 0078-0086-05; 25 mg: NDC 0078-0087-05; 50 mg: NDC 0078-0078-05; 75 mg: NDC 0078-0079-05). 10 mg, 25 mg, and 50 mg are available in SandoPak® (unit-dose) box of 100 individually labeled blisters, each containing 1 capsule (10 mg: NDC 0078-0086-06; 25 mg: NDC 0078-0087-06; 50 mg: NDC 0078-0078-06). Pamelor® (nortriptyline HCl) Capsules, USP 25 mg is also available in bottles of 500 (NDC 0078-0087-08).

10 mg capsules branded "⚕SANDOZ" on one half, "◗PAMELOR 10 mg" other half; 25 mg capsules branded "⚕SANDOZ" on one half, "◗PAMELOR 25 mg" other half; 50 mg capsules branded "⚕SANDOZ" on one half, "◗PAMELOR 50 mg" other half; and 75 mg capsules branded "⚕SANDOZ" on one half, "◗PAMELOR 75 mg" other half.

Store and Dispense: Below 86°F (30°C); tight container.
Pamelor®(nortriptyline HCl) Solution, USP
Pamelor® (nortriptyline HCl) Solution, USP, equivalent to 10 mg base per 5 mL, is supplied in 16-fluid-ounce bottles (NDC 0078-0016-33). Alcohol content 4%.

Store and Dispense: Below 86°F (30°C); tight, light-resistant container.

[REV: APRIL 1996 30175904]

Shown in Product Identification Guide, page 333

PARLODEL® ℞

[par'lō-del"]

SnapTabs®

(bromocriptine mesylate) tablets, USP

(bromocriptine mesylate) capsules, USP

CAUTION: Federal law prohibits dispensing without prescription.

The following prescribing information is based on official labeling in effect on August 1, 1996.

DESCRIPTION

Parlodel® (bromocriptine mesylate) is an ergot derivative with potent dopamine receptor agonist activity. Each Parlodel® (bromocriptine mesylate) SnapTabs® tablet for oral administration contains $2^1/_2$ mg and each capsule contains 5 mg bromocriptine (as the mesylate). Parlodel® (bromocriptine mesylate) is chemically designated as Ergotaman-3',6',18-trione, 2-bromo-12'-hydroxy-2'-(1-methylethyl)-5'-(2-methylpropyl)-, (5'α)-monomethanesulfonate (salt).

The structural formula is:

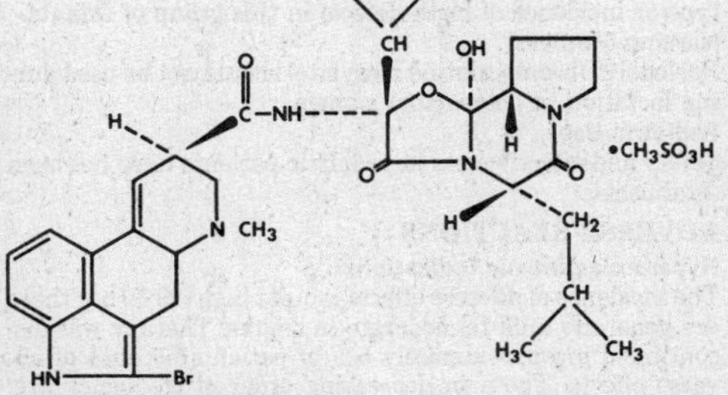

$C_{32}H_{40}BrN_5O_5 \cdot CH_4SO_3$ Mol. wt. 750.70

$2^1/_2$ mg SnapTabs®

Active Ingredient: bromocriptine mesylate, USP

Inactive Ingredients: colloidal silicon dioxide, lactose, magnesium stearate, povidone, starch, and another ingredient

5 mg Capsules

Active Ingredient: bromocriptine mesylate, USP

Inactive Ingredients: colloidal silicon dioxide, gelatin, lactose, magnesium stearate, red iron oxide, silicon dioxide, sodium lauryl sulfate, starch, titanium dioxide, yellow iron oxide, and another ingredient

CLINICAL PHARMACOLOGY

Parlodel® (bromocriptine mesylate) is a dopamine receptor agonist, which activates post-synaptic dopamine receptors. The dopaminergic neurons in the tuberoinfundibular process modulate the secretion of prolactin from the anterior pituitary by secreting a prolactin inhibitory factor (thought to be dopamine); in the corpus striatum the dopaminergic neurons are involved in the control of motor function. Clinically, Parlodel® (bromocriptine mesylate) significantly reduces plasma levels of prolactin in patients with physiologically elevated prolactin as well as in patients with hyperprolactinemia. The inhibition of physiological lactation as well as galactorrhea in pathological hyperprolactinemic states is obtained at dose levels that do not affect secretion of other tropic hormones from the anterior pituitary. Experiments have demonstrated that bromocriptine induces long lasting stereotyped behavior in rodents and turning behavior in rats having unilateral lesions in the substantia nigra. These actions, characteristic of those produced by dopamine, are inhibited by dopamine antagonists and suggest a direct action of bromocriptine on striatal dopamine receptors.

Parlodel® (bromocriptine mesylate) is a nonhormonal, nonestrogenic agent that inhibits the secretion of prolactin in humans, with little or no effect on other pituitary hormones, except in patients with acromegaly, where it lowers elevated blood levels of growth hormone in the majority of patients.

In about 75% of cases of amenorrhea and galactorrhea, Parlodel® (bromocriptine mesylate) therapy suppresses the galactorrhea completely, or almost completely, and reinitiates normal ovulatory menstrual cycles.

Menses are usually reinitiated prior to complete suppression of galactorrhea; the time for this on average is 6 - 8 weeks. However, some patients respond within a few days, and others may take up to 8 months.

Galactorrhea may take longer to control depending on the degree of stimulation of the mammary tissue prior to therapy. At least a 75% reduction in secretion is usually observed after 8 - 12 weeks. Some patients may fail to respond even after 12 months of therapy.

In many acromegalic patients, Parlodel® (bromocriptine mesylate) produces a prompt and sustained reduction in circulating levels of serum growth hormone.

Parlodel® (bromocriptine mesylate) produces its therapeutic effect in the treatment of Parkinson's disease, a clinical condition characterized by a progressive deficiency in dopamine synthesis in the substantia nigra, by directly stimulating the dopamine receptors in the corpus striatum. In contrast, levodopa exerts its therapeutic effect only after conversion to dopamine by the neurons of the substantia nigra, which are known to be numerically diminished in this patient population.

Pharmacokinetics

The pharmacokinetics and metabolism of bromocriptine in human subjects were studied with the help of radioactively labeled drug. Twenty-eight percent of an oral dose was absorbed from the gastrointestinal tract. The blood levels following a $2^1/_2$ mg dose were in the range of 2 - 3 ng equivalents/mL. Plasma levels were in the range of 4 - 6 ng equivalents/mL indicating that the red blood cells did not contain appreciable amounts of drug and/or metabolites. *In vitro* experiments showed that the drug was 90% - 96% bound to serum albumin.

Bromocriptine was completely metabolized prior to excretion. The major route of excretion of absorbed drug was via the bile. Only 2.5% - 5.5% of the dose was excreted in the urine. Almost all (84.6%) of the administered dose was excreted in the feces in 120 hours.

INDICATIONS AND USAGE

Hyperprolactinemia-Associated Dysfunctions

Parlodel® (bromocriptine mesylate) is indicated for the treatment of dysfunctions associated with **hyperprolactinemia** including **amenorrhea** with or without **galactorrhea, infertility or hypogonadism.** Parlodel® (bromocriptine mesylate) treatment is indicated in patients with **prolactin-secreting adenomas,** which may be the basic underlying endocrinopathy contributing to the above clinical presentations. **Reduction in tumor size** has been demonstrated in both male and female patients with macroadenomas. In cases where adenectomy is elected, a course of Parlodel® (bromocriptine mesylate) therapy may be used to reduce the tumor mass prior to surgery.

Acromegaly

Parlodel® (bromocriptine mesylate) therapy is indicated in the treatment of acromegaly. Parlodel® (bromocriptine mesylate) therapy, alone or as adjunctive therapy with pituitary irradiation or surgery, reduces serum growth hormone by 50% or more in approximately $^1/_2$ of patients treated, although not usually to normal levels.

Since the effects of external pituitary radiation may not become maximal for several years, adjunctive therapy with Parlodel® (bromocriptine mesylate) offers potential benefit before the effects of irradiation are manifested.

Parkinson's Disease

Parlodel® (bromocriptine mesylate) SnapTabs® or capsules are indicated in the treatment of the signs and symptoms of idiopathic or postencephalitic Parkinson's disease. As adjunctive treatment to levodopa (alone or with a peripheral decarboxylase inhibitor), Parlodel® (bromocriptine mesylate) therapy may provide additional therapeutic benefits in those patients who are currently maintained on optimal dosages of levodopa, those who are beginning to deteriorate (develop tolerance) to levodopa therapy, and those who are experiencing "end of dose failure" on levodopa therapy. Parlodel® (bromocriptine mesylate) therapy may permit a reduction of the maintenance dose of levodopa and, thus may ameliorate the occurrence and/or severity of adverse reactions associated with long-term levodopa therapy such as abnormal involuntary movements (e.g., dyskinesias) and the marked swings in motor function ("on-off" phenomenon). Continued efficacy of Parlodel® (bromocriptine mesylate) therapy during treatment of more than 2 years has not been established.

Data are insufficient to evaluate potential benefit from treating newly diagnosed Parkinson's disease with Parlodel® (bromocriptine mesylate). Studies have shown, however, significantly more adverse reactions (notably nausea, hallucinations, confusion and hypotension) in Parlodel® (bromocriptine mesylate) treated patients than in levodopa/carbidopa treated patients. Patients unresponsive to levodopa are poor candidates for Parlodel® (bromocriptine mesylate) therapy.

CONTRAINDICATIONS

Uncontrolled hypertension and sensitivity to any ergot alkaloids. In patients being treated for hyperprolactinemia Parlodel® (bromocriptine mesylate) should be withdrawn when pregnancy is diagnosed *(see PRECAUTIONS, Hyperprolactinemic States).* In the event that Parlodel® (bromocriptine mesylate) is reinstituted to control a rapidly expanding macroadenoma *(see PRECAUTIONS, Hyperprolactinemic States)* and a patient experiences a hypertensive disorder of pregnancy, the benefit of continuing Parlodel® (bromocriptine mesylate) must be weighed against the possible risk of its use during a hypertensive disorder of pregnancy. When Parlodel® (bromocriptine mesylate) is being used to treat acromegaly, prolactinoma, or Parkinson's disease in patients who subsequently become pregnant, a decision should be made as to whether the therapy continues to be medically necessary or can be withdrawn. If it is continued, the drug should be withdrawn in those who may experience hypertensive disorders of pregnancy (including eclampsia, preeclampsia, or pregnancy-induced hypertension) unless withdrawal of Parlodel® (bromocriptine mesylate) is considered to be medically contraindicated.

The drug should not be used during the post-partum period in women with a history of coronary artery disease and other severe cardiovascular conditions unless withdrawal is considered medically contraindicated. If the drug is used in the post-partum period the patient should be observed with caution.

WARNINGS

Since hyperprolactinemia with amenorrhea/galactorrhea and infertility has been found in patients with pituitary tumors, a complete evaluation of the pituitary is indicated before treatment with Parlodel® (bromocriptine mesylate).

If pregnancy occurs during Parlodel® (bromocriptine mesylate) administration, careful observation of these patients is mandatory. Prolactin-secreting adenomas may expand and compression of the optic or other cranial nerves may occur, emergency pituitary surgery becoming necessary. In most cases, the compression resolves following delivery. Reinitiation of Parlodel® (bromocriptine mesylate) treatment has been reported to produce improvement in the visual fields of patients in whom nerve compression has occurred during pregnancy. The safety of Parlodel® (bromocriptine mesylate) treatment during pregnancy to the mother and fetus has not been established.

Symptomatic hypotension can occur in patients treated with Parlodel® (bromocriptine mesylate) for any indication. In postpartum studies with Parlodel® (bromocriptine mesylate), decreases in supine systolic and diastolic pressures of greater than 20 mm and 10 mm Hg, respectively, have been observed in almost 30% of patients receiving Parlodel® (bromocriptine mesylate). On occasion, the drop in supine systolic pressure was as much as 50-59 mm of Hg.

While hypotension during the start of therapy with Parlodel® (bromocriptine mesylate) occurs in some patients, in postmarketing experience in the U.S. in postpartum patients 89 cases of hypertension have been reported, sometimes at the initiation of therapy, but often developing in the second week of therapy; seizures have been reported in 72 cases (including 4 cases of status epilepticus), both with and without the prior development of hypertension; 30 cases of stroke have been reported mostly in postpartum patients whose prenatal and obstetric courses had been uncomplicated. Many of these patients experiencing seizures and/or strokes reported developing a constant and often progressively severe headache hours to days prior to the acute event. Some cases of strokes and seizures were also preceded by visual disturbances (blurred vision, and transient cortical blindness). Nine cases of acute myocardial infarction have been reported.

Although a causal relationship between Parlodel® (bromocriptine mesylate) administration and hypertension, seizures, strokes, and myocardial infarction in postpartum women has not been established, use of the drug for prevention of physiological lactation, or in patients with uncontrolled hypertension is not recommended. In patients being treated for hyperprolactinemia Parlodel® (bromocriptine mesylate) should be withdrawn when pregnancy is diagnosed *(see PRECAUTIONS, Hyperprolactinemic States).* In the event that Parlodel® (bromocriptine mesylate) is reinstituted to control a rapidly expanding macroadenoma *(see PRECAUTIONS, Hyperprolactinemia States)* and a patient experiences a hypertensive disorder of pregnancy, the benefit of continuing Parlodel® (bromocriptine mesylate) must be weighed against the possible risk of its use during a hypertensive disorder of pregnancy. When Parlodel® (bromocriptine mesylate) is being used to treat acromegaly or Parkinson's disease in patients who subsequently become pregnant, a decision should be made as to whether the therapy continues to be medically necessary or can be withdrawn. If it is continued, the drug should be withdrawn in those who may experience hypertensive disorders of pregnancy (including eclampsia, preeclampsia, or pregnancy-induced hypertension) unless withdrawal of Parlodel® (bromocriptine mesylate) is considered to be medically contraindicated. Because of the possibility of an interaction between Parlodel® (bromocriptine mesylate) and other ergot alkaloids, the concomitant use of these medications is not recommended. Particular attention should be paid to patients who have recently received other drugs that can alter the blood pressure. Periodic monitoring of the blood pressure, particularly during the first weeks of therapy is prudent. If hypertension, severe, progressive, or unremitting headache (with or without visual disturbance), or evidence of

Continued on next page

Sandoz—Cont.

CNS toxicity develops, drug therapy should be discontinued and the patient should be evaluated promptly.

Long-term treatment (6-36 months) with Parlodel® (bromocriptine mesylate) in doses ranging from 20-100 mg/day has been associated with pulmonary infiltrates, pleural effusion and thickening of the pleura in a few patients. In those instances in which Parlodel® (bromocriptine mesylate) treatment was terminated, the changes slowly reverted towards normal.

PRECAUTIONS

General

Safety and efficacy of Parlodel® (bromocriptine mesylate) have not been established in patients with renal or hepatic disease. Care should be exercised when administering Parlodel® (bromocriptine mesylate) therapy concomitantly with other medications known to lower blood pressure.

The drug should be used with caution in patients with a history of psychosis or cardiovascular disease. If acromegalic patients or patients with prolactinoma or Parkinson's disease are being treated with Parlodel® (bromocriptine mesylate) during pregnancy, they should be cautiously observed, particularly during the post-partum period if they have a history of cardiovascular disease.

Hyperprolactinemic States

The relative efficacy of Parlodel® (bromocriptine mesylate) versus surgery in preserving visual fields is not known. Patients with rapidly progressive visual field loss should be evaluated by a neurosurgeon to help decide on the most appropriate therapy. Since pregnancy is often the therapeutic objective in many hyperprolactinemic patients presenting with amenorrhea/galactorrhea and hypogonadism (infertility), a careful assessment of the pituitary is essential to detect the presence of a prolactin-secreting adenoma. Patients not seeking pregnancy, or those harboring large adenomas, should be advised to use contraceptive measures, other than oral contraceptives, during treatment with Parlodel® (bromocriptine mesylate). Since pregnancy may occur prior to reinitiation of menses, a pregnancy test is recommended at least every 4 weeks during the amenorrheic period, and, once menses are reinitiated, every time a patient misses a menstrual period. Treatment with Parlodel® (bromocriptine mesylate) SnapTabs® or capsules should be discontinued as soon as pregnancy has been established. Patients must be monitored closely throughout pregnancy for signs and symptoms that may signal the enlargement of a previously undetected or existing prolactin-secreting tumor. Discontinuation of Parlodel® (bromocriptine mesylate) treatment in patients with known macroadenomas has been associated with rapid regrowth of tumor and increase in serum prolactin in most cases.

Acromegaly

Cold sensitive digital vasospasm has been observed in some acromegalic patients treated with Parlodel® (bromocriptine mesylate). The response, should it occur, can be reversed by reducing the dose of Parlodel® (bromocriptine mesylate) and may be prevented by keeping the fingers warm. Cases of severe gastrointestinal bleeding from peptic ulcers have been reported, some fatal. Although there is no evidence that Parlodel® (bromocriptine mesylate) increases the incidence of peptic ulcers in acromegalic patients, symptoms suggestive of peptic ulcer should be investigated thoroughly and treated appropriately. Patients with a history of peptic ulcer or gastrointestinal bleeding should be observed carefully during treatment with Parlodel® (bromocriptine mesylate). Possible tumor expansion while receiving Parlodel® (bromocriptine mesylate) therapy has been reported in a few patients. Since the natural history of growth hormone secreting tumors is unknown, all patients should be carefully monitored and, if evidence of tumor expansion develops, discontinuation of treatment and alternative procedures considered.

Parkinson's Disease

Safety during long-term use for more than 2 years at the doses required for parkinsonism has not been established. As with any chronic therapy, periodic evaluation of hepatic, hematopoietic, cardiovascular, and renal function is recommended. Symptomatic hypotension can occur and, therefore, caution should be exercised when treating patients receiving antihypertensive drugs.

High doses of Parlodel® (bromocriptine mesylate) may be associated with confusion and mental disturbances. Since parkinsonian patients may manifest mild degrees of dementia, caution should be used when treating such patients. Parlodel® (bromocriptine mesylate) administered alone or concomitantly with levodopa may cause hallucinations visual or auditory). Hallucinations usually resolve with dosage reduction; occasionally, discontinuation of Parlodel® (bromocriptine mesylate) is required. Rarely, after high doses, hallucinations have persisted for several weeks following discontinuation of Parlodel® (bromocriptine mesylate). As with levodopa, caution should be exercised when administering Parlodel® (bromocriptine mesylate) to patients with

a history of myocardial infarction who have a residual atrial, nodal, or ventricular arrhythmia.

Retroperitoneal fibrosis has been reported in a few patients receiving long-term therapy (2 - 10 years) with Parlodel® (bromocriptine mesylate) in doses ranging from 30 - 140 mg daily.

Information For Patients

When initiating therapy, all patients receiving Parlodel® (bromocriptine mesylate) should be cautioned with regard to engaging in activities requiring rapid and precise responses, such as driving an automobile or operating machinery since dizziness (8% - 16%), drowsiness (8%), faintness, fainting (8%), and syncope (less than 1%) have been reported early in the course of therapy. Patients receiving Parlodel® (bromocriptine mesylate) for hyperprolactinemic states associated with macroadenoma or those who have had previous transsphenoidal surgery, should be told to report any persistent watery nasal discharge to their physician. Patients receiving Parlodel® (bromocriptine mesylate) for treatment of a macroadenoma should be told that discontinuation of drug may be associated with rapid regrowth of the tumor and recurrence of their original symptoms.

Drug Interactions

The risk of using Parlodel® (bromocriptine mesylate) in combination with other drugs has not been systematically evaluated, but alcohol may potentiate the side effects of Parlodel® (bromocriptine mesylate). Parlodel® (bromocriptine mesylate) may interact with dopamine antagonists, butyrophenones, and certain other agents. Compounds in these categories result in a decreased efficacy of Parlodel® (bromocriptine mesylate): phenothiazines, haloperidol, metoclopramide, pimozide. Concomitant use of Parlodel® (bromocriptine mesylate) with other ergot alkaloids is not recommended.

Carcinogenesis, Mutagenesis, Impairment of Fertility

A 74-week study was conducted in mice using dietary levels of bromocriptine mesylate equivalent to oral doses of 10 and 50 mg/kg/day. A 100-week study in rats was conducted using dietary levels equivalent to oral doses of 1.7, 9.8, and 44 mg/kg/day. The highest doses tested in mice and rats were approximately 2.5 and 4.4 times, respectively, the maximum human dose administered in controlled clinical trials (100 mg/day) based on body surface area. Malignant uterine tumors, endometrial and myometrial, were found in rats as follows: 0/50 control females, 2/50 females given 1.7 mg/kg daily, 7/49 females given 9.8 mg/kg daily, and 9/50 females given 44 mg/kg/daily. The occurrence of these neoplasms is probably attributable to the high estrogen/progesterone ratio which occurs in rats as a result of the prolactin-inhibiting action of bromocriptine mesylate. The endocrine mechanisms believed to be involved in the rats are not present in humans. There is no known correlation between uterine malignancies occurring in bromocriptine-treated rats and human risk. In contrast to the findings in rats, the uteri from mice killed after 74 weeks treatment did not exhibit evidence of drug-related changes.

Bromocriptine mesylate was evaluated for mutagenic potential in the battery of tests that included Ames bacterial mutation assay, mutagenic activity in vitro on V79 Chinese hamster fibroblasts, cytogenetic analysis of Chinese hamster bone marrow cells following in vivo treatment, and an in vivo micronucleus test for mutagenic potential in mice.

No mutagenic effects were obtained in any of these tests. Fertility and reproductive performance in female rats were not influenced adversely by treatment with bromocriptine beyond the predicted decrease in the weight of pups due to suppression of lactation. In males treated with 50 mg/kg of this drug, mating and fertility were within the normal range. Increased perinatal loss was produced in the subgroups of dams, sacrificed on day 21 postpartum (p.p.) after mating with males treated with the highest does (50 mg/kg).

Pregnancy

Category B: Administration of 10 - 30 mg/kg of bromocriptine to 2 strains of rats on days 6 - 15 post coitum (p.c.) as well as a single dose of 10 mg/kg on day 5 p.c., interfered with nidation. Three mg/kg given on days 6 - 15 were without effect on nidation, and did not produce any anomalies. In animals treated from day 8 - 15 p.c., i.e., after implantation, 30 mg/kg produced increased prenatal mortality in the form of increased incidence of embryonic resorption. One anomaly, aplasia of spinal vertebrae and ribs, was found in the group of 262 fetuses derived from the dams treated with 30 mg/kg bromocriptine. No fetotoxic effects were found in offspring of dams treated during the peri- or post-natal period.

Two studies were conducted in rabbits (2 strains) to determine the potential to interfere with nidation. Dose levels of 100 or 300 mg/kg/day from day 1 to day 6 p.c. did not adversely affect nidation. The high dose was approximately 63 times the maximum human dose administered in controlled clinical trials (100 mg/day), based on body surface area. In New Zealand white rabbits some embryo mortality occurred at 300 mg/kg which was a reflection of overt maternal toxicity. Three studies were conducted in 2 strains of rabbits to determine the teratological potential of bromocriptine at dose levels of 3, 10, 30, 100, and 300 mg/kg given

from day 6 to day 18 p.c. In 2 studies with the Yellow-silver strain, cleft palate was found in 3 and 2 fetuses at maternally toxic doses of 100 and 300 mg/kg, respectively. One control fetus also exhibited this anomaly. In the third study conducted with New Zealand white rabbits using an identical protocol, no cleft palates were produced.

No teratological or embryo-toxic effects of bromocriptine were produced in any of 6 offspring from 6 monkeys at a dose level of 2 mg/kg.

Information concerning 1276 pregnancies in women taking bromocriptine has been collected. In the majority of cases, bromocriptine was discontinued within 8 weeks into pregnancy (mean 28.7 days), however, 8 patients received the drug continuously throughout pregnancy. The mean daily dose for all patients was 5.8 mg (range 1 - 40 mg).

Of these 1276 pregnancies, there were 1088 full term deliveries (4 stillborn), 145 spontaneous abortions (11.4%), and 28 induced abortions (2.2%). Moreover, 12 extrauterine gravidities and 3 hydatidiform moles (twice in the same patient) caused early termination of pregnancy. These data compare favorably with the abortion rate (11%–25%) cited for pregnancies induced by clomiphene citrate, menopausal gonadotropin, and chorionic gonadotropin.

Although spontaneous abortions often go unreported, especially prior to 20 weeks of gestation, their frequency has been estimated to be 15%.

The incidence of birth defects in the population at large ranges from 2%–4.5%. The incidence in 1109 live births from patients receiving bromocriptine is 3.3%.

There is no suggestion that bromocriptine contributed to the type or incidence of birth defects in this group of infants.

Nursing Mothers

Parlodel® (bromocriptine mesylate) should not be used during lactation in postpartum women.

Pediatric Use

Safety and effectiveness in pediatric patients have not been established.

ADVERSE REACTIONS

Hyperprolactinemic Indications

The incidence of adverse effects is quite high (69%) but these are generally mild to moderate in degree. Therapy was discontinued in approximately 5% of patients because of adverse effects. These in decreasing order of frequency are: nausea (49%), headache (19%), dizziness (17%), fatigue (7%), lightheadedness (5%), vomiting (5%), abdominal cramps (4%), nasal congestion (3%), constipation (3%), diarrhea (3%) and drowsiness (3%).

A slight hypotensive effect may accompany Parlodel® (bromocriptine mesylate) treatment. The occurrence of adverse reactions may be lessened by temporarily reducing dosage to 1/2 SnapTabs® tablet 2 or 3 times daily. A few cases of cerebrospinal fluid rhinorrhea have been reported in patients receiving Parlodel® (bromocriptine mesylate) for treatment of large prolactinomas. This has occurred rarely, usually only in patients who have received previous transsphenoidal surgery, pituitary radiation, or both, and who were receiving Parlodel® (bromocriptine mesylate) for tumor recurrence. It may also occur in previously untreated patients whose tumor extends into the sphenoid sinus.

Acromegaly

The most frequent adverse reactions encountered in acromegalic patients treated with Parlodel® (bromocriptine mesylate) were: nausea (18%), constipation (14%), postural/orthostatic hypotension (6%), anorexia (4%), dry mouth/nasal stuffiness (4%), indigestion/dyspepsia (4%), digital vasospasm (3%), drowsiness/tiredness (3%) and vomiting (2%).

Less frequent adverse reactions (less than 2%) were: gastrointestinal bleeding, dizziness, exacerbation of Raynaud's Syndrome, headache and syncope. Rarely (less than 1%) hair loss, alcohol potentiation, faintness, lightheadedness, arrhythmia, ventricular tachycardia, decreased sleep requirement, visual hallucinations, lassitude, shortness of breath, bradycardia, vertigo, paresthesia, sluggishness, vasovagal attack, delusional psychosis, paranoia, insomnia, heavy headedness, reduced tolerance to cold, tingling of ears, facial pallor and muscle cramps have been reported.

Parkinson's Disease

In clinical trials in which bromocriptine was administered with concomitant reduction in the dose of levodopa/carbidopa, the most common newly appearing adverse reactions were: nausea, abnormal involuntary movements, hallucinations, confusion, "on-off" phenomenon, dizziness, drowsiness, faintness/fainting, vomiting, asthenia, abdominal discomfort, visual disturbance, ataxia, insomnia, depression, hypotension, shortness of breath, constipation, and vertigo. Less common adverse reactions which may be encountered include: anorexia, anxiety, blepharospasm, dry mouth, dysphagia, edema of the feet and ankles, erythromelalgia, epileptiform seizure, fatigue, headache, lethargy, mottling of skin, nasal stuffiness, nervousness, nightmares, paresthesia, skin rash, urinary frequency, urinary incontinence, urinary retention, and rarely, signs and symptoms of ergotism such as tingling of fingers, cold feet, numbness, muscle cramps of feet and legs or exacerbation of Raynaud's Syndrome.

Abnormalities in laboratory tests may include elevations in blood urea nitrogen, SGOT, SGPT, GGPT, CPK, alkaline phosphatase and uric acid, which are usually transient and not of clinical significance.

Adverse Events Observed in Other Conditions

Postpartum Patients

In postpartum studies with Parlodel®(bromocriptine mesylate) 23 percent of postpartum patients treated had at least 1 side effect, but they were generally mild to moderate in degree. Therapy was discontinued in approximately 3% of patients. The most frequently occurring adverse reactions were: headache (10%), dizziness (8%), nausea (7%), vomiting (3%), fatigue (1.0%), syncope (0.7%), diarrhea (0.4%), and cramps (0.4%). Decreases in blood pressure (≥20 mm Hg systolic and ≥10 mm Hg diastolic) occurred in 28% of patients at least once during the first 3 postpartum days; these were usually of a transient nature. Reports of fainting in the puerperium may possibly be related to this effect. In postmarketing experience in the U.S. serious adverse reactions reported include 72 cases of seizures (including 4 cases of status epilepticus), 30 cases of stroke, and 9 cases of myocardial infarction among postpartum patients. Seizure cases were not necessarily accompanied by the development of hypertension. An unremitting and often progressively severe headache, sometimes accompanied by visual disturbance, often preceded by hours to days many cases of seizure and/or stroke. Most patients had shown no evidence of any of the hypertensive disorders of pregnancy including eclampsia, preeclampsia, or pregnancy induced hypertension. One stroke case was associated with sagittal sinus thrombosis, and another was associated with cerebral and cerebellar vasculitis. One case of myocardial infarction was associated with unexplained disseminated intravascular coagulation and a second occurred in conjunction with use of another ergot alkaloid. The relationship of these adverse reactions to Parlodel® (bromocriptine mesylate) administration has not been established.

OVERDOSAGE

The most commonly reported signs and symptoms associated with acute Parlodel® (bromocriptine mesylate) overdose are: nausea, vomiting, constipation, diaphoresis, dizziness, pallor, severe hypotension, malaise, confusion, lethargy, drowsiness, delusions, hallucinations, and repetitive yawning. The lethal dose has not been established and the drug has a very wide margin of safety. However, one death occurred in a patient who committed suicide with an unknown quantity of Parlodel® (bromocriptine mesylate) and chloroquine.

Treatment of overdose consists of removal of the drug by emesis (if conscious), gastric lavage, activated charcoal, or saline catharsis. Careful supervision and recording of fluid intake and output is essential. Hypotension should be treated by placing the patient in the Trendelenburg position and administering I.V. fluids. If satisfactory relief of hypotension cannot be achieved by using the above measures to their fullest extent, vasopressors should be considered.

DOSAGE AND ADMINISTRATION

General

It is recommended that Parlodel® (bromocriptine mesylate) be taken with food. Patients should be evaluated frequently during dose escalation to determine the lowest dosage that produces a therapeutic response.

Hyperprolactinemic Indications

The initial dosage of Parlodel® (bromocriptine mesylate) is $^1/_2$ to one $2^1/_2$ mg SnapTabs® tablet daily. An additional $2^1/_2$ mg SnapTabs® tablet may be added to the treatment regimen as tolerated every 3 - 7 days until an optimal therapeutic response is achieved. The therapeutic dosage usually is 5 - 7.5 mg and ranges from 2.5 - 15 mg/day.

In order to reduce the likelihood of prolonged exposure to Parlodel® (bromocriptine mesylate) should an unsuspected pregnancy occur, a mechanical contraceptive should be used in conjunction with Parlodel® (bromocriptine mesylate) therapy until normal ovulatory menstrual cycles have been restored. Contraception may then be discontinued in patients desiring pregnancy.

Thereafter, if menstruation does not occur within 3 days of the expected date, Parlodel® (bromocriptine mesylate) therapy should be discontinued and a pregnancy test performed.

Acromegaly

Virtually all acromegalic patients receiving therapeutic benefit from Parlodel® (bromocriptine mesylate) also have reductions in circulating levels of growth hormone. Therefore, periodic assessment of circulating levels of growth hormone will, in most cases, serve as a guide in determining the therapeutic potential of Parlodel® (bromocriptine mesylate). If, after a brief trial with Parlodel® (bromocriptine mesylate) therapy, no significant reduction in growth hormone levels has taken place, careful assessment of the clinical features of the disease should be made, and if no change has occurred, dosage adjustment or discontinuation of therapy should be considered.

The initial recommended dosage is $^1/_2$ to one $2^1/_2$ mg Parlodel® (bromocriptine mesylate) SnapTabs® tablet on retiring (with food) for 3 days. An additional $^1/_2$ to 1 SnapTabs® tablet should be added to the treatment regimen as tolerated every 3 - 7 days until the patient obtains optimal therapeutic benefit. Patients should be reevaluated monthly and the dosage adjusted based on reductions of growth hormone or clinical response. The usual optimal therapeutic dosage range of Parlodel® (bromocriptine mesylate) varies from 20 - 30 mg/day in most patients. The maximal dosage should not exceed 100 mg/day.

Patients treated with pituitary irradiation should be withdrawn from Parlodel® (bromocriptine mesylate) therapy on a yearly basis to assess both the clinical effects of radiation on the disease process as well as the effects of Parlodel® (bromocriptine mesylate) therapy. Usually a 4 - 8 week withdrawal period is adequate for this purpose. Recurrence of the signs/symptoms or increases in growth hormone indicate the disease process is still active and further courses of Parlodel® (bromocriptine mesylate) should be considered.

Parkinson's Disease

The basic principle of Parlodel® (bromocriptine mesylate) therapy is to initiate treatment at a low dosage and, on an individual basis, increase the daily dosage slowly until a maximum therapeutic response is achieved. The dosage of levodopa during this introductory period should be maintained, if possible. The initial dose of Parlodel® (bromocriptine mesylate) is $^1/_2$ of a $2^1/_2$ mg SnapTabs® tablet twice daily with meals. Assessments are advised at 2-week intervals during dosage titration to ensure that the lowest dosage producing an optimal therapeutic response is not exceeded. If necessary, the dosage may be increased every 14 - 28 days by $2^1/_2$ mg/day with meals. Should it be advisable to reduce the dosage of levodopa because of adverse reactions, the daily dosage of Parlodel® (bromocriptine mesylate), if increased, should be accomplished gradually in small ($2^1/_2$ mg) increments.

The safety of Parlodel® (bromocriptine mesylate) has not been demonstrated in dosages exceeding 100 mg/day.

HOW SUPPLIED

Parlodel (bromocriptine mesylate) SnapTabs®

$2^1/_2$ mg

Round, white, scored SnapTabs® each containing $2^1/_2$ mg bromocriptine (as the mesylate). Engraved "PARLODEL $2^1/_2$" on one side and scored on reverse side.

Packages of 30 (NDC 0078-0017-15)
Packages of 100 (NDC 0078-0017-05)

Parlodel (bromocriptine mesylate) Capsules

5 mg

Caramel and white capsules, each containing 5 mg bromocriptine (as the mesylate). Imprinted "PARLODEL 5 mg" on one half and " " on other half.

Packages of 30 (NDC 0078-0102-15)
Packages of 100 (NDC 0078-0102-05)

Store and Dispense

Below 77°F (25°C); tight, light-resistant container.

[REV: FEBRUARY 1996 30177906]

Shown in Product Identification Guide, page 333

RESTORIL® Ⓒ ℞

[res'tah-ril"]

(temazepam) capsules, USP

CAUTION: Federal law prohibits dispensing without prescription.

The following prescribing information is based on official labeling in effect on August 1, 1996.

DESCRIPTION

Restoril® (temazepam) is a benzodiazepine hypnotic agent. The chemical name is 7-chloro-1,3-dihydro-3-hydroxy-1-methyl-5-phenyl-2*H*-1,4-benzodiazepin-2-one, and the structural formula is:

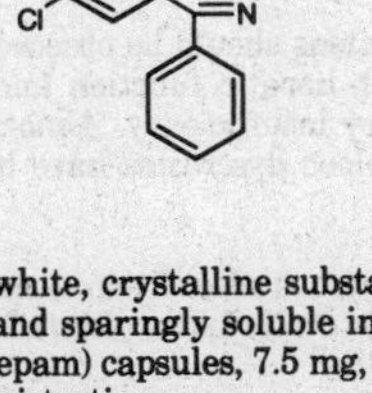

$C_{16}H_{13}ClN_2O_2$ Mol. wt. 300.74

Temazepam is a white, crystalline substance, very slightly soluble in water and sparingly soluble in alcohol, USP.

Restoril® (temazepam) capsules, 7.5 mg, 15 mg, and 30 mg, are for oral administration.

7.5 mg, 15 mg, and 30 mg Capsules

Active Ingredient: temazepam, USP

7.5 mg Capsules

Inactive Ingredients: FD&C Blue #1, FD&C Red #3, gelatin, lactose, magnesium stearate, sodium lauryl sulfate, synthetic red ferric oxide, titanium dioxide, and other ingredients.

May also include: benzyl alcohol, butylparaben, carboxymethylcellulose sodium, edetate calcium disodium, methylparaben, propylparaben, silicon dioxide, and sodium propionate.

15 mg Capsules

Inactive Ingredients: FD&C Blue #1, FD&C Red #3, gelatin, lactose, magnesium stearate, sodium lauryl sulfate, synthetic red ferric oxide, titanium dioxide, and other ingredients.

May also include: benzyl alcohol, butylparaben, carboxymethylcellulose sodium, edetate calcium disodium, methylparaben, propylparaben, silicon dioxide, and sodium propionate.

30 mg Capsules

Inactive Ingredients: FD&C Blue #1, FD&C Red #3, gelatin, lactose, magnesium stearate, sodium lauryl sulfate, titanium dioxide, and other ingredients.

May also include: benzyl alcohol, butylparaben, carboxymethylcellulose sodium, edetate calcium disodium, methylparaben, propylparaben, silicon dioxide, and sodium propionate.

CLINICAL PHARMACOLOGY

Pharmacokinetics

In a single and multiple dose absorption, distribution, metabolism, and excretion (ADME) study, using ^3H labeled drug, Restoril® (temazepam) was well absorbed and found to have minimal (8%) first pass metabolism. There were no active metabolites formed and the only significant metabolite present in blood was the O-conjugate. The unchanged drug was 96% bound to plasma proteins. The blood level decline of the parent drug was biphasic with the short half-life ranging from 0.4–0.6 hours and the terminal half-life from 3.5–18.4 hours (mean 8.8 hours), depending on the study population and method of determination. Metabolites were formed with a half-life of 10 hours and excreted with a half-life of approximately 2 hours. Thus, formation of the major metabolite is the rate limiting step in the biodisposition of temazepam. There is no accumulation of metabolites. A dose-proportional relationship has been established for the area under the plasma concentration/time curve over the 15–30 mg dose range.

Temazepam was completely metabolized through conjugation prior to excretion; 80%–90% of the dose appeared in the urine. The major metabolite was the O-conjugate of temazepam (90%); the O-conjugate of N-desmethyl temazepam was a minor metabolite (7%).

Bioavailability, Induction, and Plasma Levels

Following ingestion of a 30 mg Restoril® (temazepam) capsule, measurable plasma concentrations were achieved 10–20 minutes after dosing with peak plasma levels ranging from 666–982 ng/mL (mean 865 ng/mL) occurring approximately 1.2–1.6 hours (mean 1.5 hours) after dosing.

In a 7 day study, in which subjects were given a 30 mg Restoril® (temazepam) capsule 1 hour before retiring, steady-state (as measured by the attainment of maximal trough concentrations) was achieved by the third dose. Mean plasma levels of temazepam (for days 2–7) were 260±210 ng/mL at 9 hours and 75±80 ng/mL at 24 hours after dosing. A slight trend toward declining 24 hour plasma levels was seen after day 4 in the study, however, the 24 hour plasma levels were quite variable.

At a dose of 30 mg once-a-day for 8 weeks, no evidence of enzyme induction was found in man.

Elimination Rate of Benzodiazepine Hypnotics and Profile of Common Untoward Effects

The type and duration of hypnotic effects and the profile of unwanted effects during administration of benzodiazepine hypnotics may be influenced by the biologic half-life of the administered drug and for some hypnotics, the half-life of any active metabolites formed. Benzodiazepine hypnotics have a spectrum of half-lives from short (<4 hours) to long (>20 hours). When half-lives are long, drug (and for some drugs their active metabolites) may accumulate during periods of nightly administration and be associated with impairments of cognitive and/or motor performance during waking hours; the possibility of interaction with other psychoactive drugs or alcohol will be enhanced. In contrast, if half-lives are shorter, drug (and, where appropriate, its active metabolites) will be cleared before the next dose is ingested, and carry-over effects related to excessive sedation or CNS depression should be minimal or absent. However, during nightly use for an extended period, pharmacodynamic tolerance or adaptation to some effects of benzodiazepine hypnotics may develop. If the drug has a short elimination half-life, it is possible that a relative deficiency of the drug, or, if appropriate, its active metabolites (i.e., in relationship to the receptor site) may occur at some point in the interval between each night's use. This sequence of events may account for 2 clinical findings reported to occur after several weeks of nightly use of rapidly eliminated benzodiazepine hypnotics, namely, increased wakefulness during the last third of the night, and the appearance of increased signs of daytime anxiety.

Continued on next page

Sandoz—Cont.

Controlled Trials Supporting Efficacy

Restoril® (temazepam) improved sleep parameters in clinical studies. Residual medication effects ("hangover") were essentially absent. Early morning awakening, a particular problem in the geriatric patient, was significantly reduced. Patients with chronic insomnia were evaluated in 2 week, placebo controlled sleep laboratory studies with Restoril® (temazepam) at doses of 7.5 mg, 15 mg, and 30 mg, given 30 minutes prior to bedtime. There was a linear dose-response improvement in total sleep time and sleep latency, with significant drug-placebo differences at 2 weeks occurring only for total sleep time at the 2 higher doses, and for sleep latency only at the highest dose.

In these sleep laboratory studies, REM sleep was essentially unchanged and slow wave sleep was decreased. No measurable effects on daytime alertness or performance occurred following Restoril® (temazepam) treatment or during the withdrawal period, even though a transient sleep disturbance in some sleep parameters was observed following withdrawal of the higher doses. There was no evidence of tolerance development in the sleep laboratory parameters when patients were given Restoril® (temazepam) nightly for at least 2 weeks.

In addition, normal subjects with transient insomnia associated with first night adaptation to the sleep laboratory were evaluated in 24 hour, placebo controlled sleep laboratory studies with Restoril® (temazepam) at doses of 7.5 mg, 15 mg, and 30 mg, given 30 minutes prior to bedtime. There was a linear dose-response improvement in total sleep time, sleep latency and number of awakenings, with significant drug-placebo differences occurring for sleep latency at all doses, for total sleep time at the 2 higher doses and for number of awakenings only at the 30 mg dose.

INDICATIONS AND USAGE

Restoril® (temazepam) is indicated for the short-term treatment of insomnia (generally 7–10 days). For patients in whom the drug is used for more than 2-3 weeks, periodic reevaluation is recommended to determine whether there is a continuing need. *(See WARNINGS)*

For patients with short-term insomnia, instructions in the prescription should indicate that Restoril® (temazepam) should be used for short periods of time (7–10 days).

Restoril® (temazepam) should not be prescribed in quantities exceeding a 1-month supply.

Insomnia is characterized by complaints of difficulty in falling asleep, frequent nocturnal awakenings, and/or early morning awakenings. Both sleep laboratory and outpatient studies provide support for the effectiveness of Restoril® (temazepam) administered 30 minutes before bedtime in decreasing sleep latency and improving sleep maintenance in patients with chronic insomnia. In addition, sleep laboratory studies have confirmed similar effects in normal subjects with transient insomnia *(see CLINICAL PHARMACOLOGY)*.

CONTRAINDICATIONS

Benzodiazepines may cause fetal damage when administered during pregnancy. An increased risk of congenital malformations associated with the use of diazepam and chlordiazepoxide during the first trimester of pregnancy has been suggested in several studies. Transplacental distribution has resulted in neonatal CNS depression following the ingestion of therapeutic doses of a benzodiazepine hypnotic during the last weeks of pregnancy.

Reproduction studies in animals with temazepam were performed in rats and rabbits. In a perinatal-postnatal study in rats, oral doses of 60 mg/kg/day resulted in increasing nursling mortality. Teratology studies in rats demonstrated increased fetal resorptions at doses of 30 and 120 mg/kg in one study and increased occurrence of rudimentary ribs, which are considered skeletal variants, in a second study at doses of 240 mg/kg or higher. In rabbits, occasional abnormalities such as exencephaly and fusion or asymmetry of ribs were reported without dose relationship. Although these abnormalities were not found in the concurrent control group, they have been reported to occur randomly in historical controls. At doses of 40 mg/kg or higher, there was an increased incidence of the 13th rib variant when compared to the incidence in concurrent and historical controls.

Restoril® (temazepam) is contraindicated in pregnant women. If there is a likelihood of the patient becoming pregnant while receiving temazepam, she should be warned of the potential risk to the fetus. Patients should be instructed to discontinue the drug prior to becoming pregnant. The possibility that a woman of childbearing potential may be pregnant at the time of institution of therapy should be considered.

WARNINGS

Sleep disturbance may be the presenting manifestation of an underlying physical and/or psychiatric disorder. Consequently, a decision to initiate symptomatic treatment of insomnia should only be made after the patient has been carefully evaluated.

The failure of insomnia to remit after 7–10 days of treatment may indicate the presence of a primary psychiatric and/or medical illness.

Worsening of insomnia may be the consequence of an unrecognized psychiatric or physical disorder as may the emergence of new abnormalities of thinking or behavior. Such abnormalities have also been reported to occur in association with the use of drugs with central nervous system depressant activity, including those of the benzodiazepine class. Some of these changes may be characterized by decreased inhibition, e.g., aggressiveness and extroversion that seem out of character, similar to that seen with alcohol. Other kinds of behavioral changes can also occur, for example, bizarre behavior, agitation, hallucinations, depersonalization, and, in primarily depressed patients, the worsening of depression, including suicidal thinking. In controlled clinical trials involving 1076 patients on Restoril® (temazepam) and 783 patients on placebo, reports of hallucinations, agitation, and overstimulation occurred at rates less than 1 in 100 patients. Hallucinations were reported in 2 Restoril® (temazepam) patients and 1 placebo patient; agitation was reported in 1 Restoril® (temazepam) patient; 2 Restoril® (temazepam) patients reported overstimulation. There were no reports of worsening of depression or suicidal ideation, aggressiveness, extroversion, bizarre behavior or depersonalization in these controlled clinical trials.

It can rarely be determined with certainty whether a particular instance of the abnormal behaviors listed above is drug induced, spontaneous in origin, or a result of an underlying psychiatric or physical disorder. Nonetheless, the emergence of any new behavioral sign or symptom of concern requires careful and immediate evaluation.

Because some of the worrisome adverse effects of benzodiazepines, including Restoril® (temazepam), appear to be dose related *(see PRECAUTIONS and DOSAGE AND ADMINISTRATION)*, it is important to use the lowest possible effective dose. Elderly patients are especially at risk.

Patients receiving Restoril® (temazepam) should be cautioned about possible combined effects with alcohol and other CNS depressants.

Withdrawal symptoms (of the barbiturate type) have occurred after the abrupt discontinuation of benzodiazepines *(see DRUG ABUSE AND DEPENDENCE)*.

PRECAUTIONS

General

Since the risk of the development of oversedation, dizziness, confusion, and/or ataxia increases substantially with larger doses of benzodiazepines in elderly and debilitated patients, 7.5 mg of Restoril® (temazepam) is recommended as the initial dosage for such patients.

Restoril® (temazepam) should be administered with caution in severely depressed patients or those in whom there is any evidence of latent depression; it should be recognized that suicidal tendencies may be present and protective measures may be necessary.

The usual precautions should be observed in patients with impaired renal or hepatic function and in patients with chronic pulmonary insufficiency.

If Restoril® (temazepam) is to be combined with other drugs having known hypnotic properties or CNS-depressant effects, consideration should be given to potential additive effects.

The possibility of a synergistic effect exists with the co-administration of Restoril® (temazepam) and diphenhydramine. One case of stillbirth at term has been reported 8 hours after a pregnant patient received Restoril® (temazepam) and diphenhydramine. A cause and effect relationship has not yet been determined. *(See CONTRAINDICATIONS)*

Information for Patients

The text of a patient package insert is printed at the end of this insert. To assure safe and effective use of Restoril® (temazepam), the information and instructions provided in this patient package insert should be discussed with patients.

Laboratory Tests

The usual precautions should be observed in patients with impaired renal or hepatic function and in patients with chronic pulmonary insufficiency. Abnormal liver function tests as well as blood dyscrasias have been reported with benzodiazepines.

Drug Interactions

The pharmacokinetic profile of temazepam does not appear to be altered by orally administered cimetidine dosed according to labeling.

Carcinogenesis, Mutagenesis, Impairment of Fertility

Carcinogenicity studies were conducted in rats at dietary temazepam doses up to 160 mg/kg/day for 24 months and in mice at dietary dose of 160 mg/kg/day for 18 months. No evidence of carcinogenicity was observed although hyperplastic liver nodules were observed in female mice exposed to the highest dose. The clinical significance of this finding is not known.

Fertility in male and female rats was not adversely affected by Restoril® (temazepam).

No mutagenicity tests have been done with temazepam.

Pregnancy

Pregnancy Category X *(see CONTRAINDICATIONS)*.

Nursing Mothers

It is not known whether this drug is excreted in human milk. Because many drugs are excreted in human milk, caution should be exercised when Restoril® (temazepam) is administered to a nursing woman.

Pediatric Use

Safety and effectiveness in children below the age of 18 years have not been established.

ADVERSE REACTIONS

During controlled clinical studies in which 1076 patients received Restoril® (temazepam) at bedtime, the drug was well tolerated. Side effects were usually mild and transient. Adverse reactions occurring in 1% or more of patients are presented in the following table:

	Restoril® (temazepam) % Incidence (n = 1076)	Placebo % Incidence (n = 783)
Drowsiness	9.1	5.6
Headache	8.5	9.1
Fatigue	4.8	4.7
Nervousness	4.6	8.2
Lethargy	4.5	3.4
Dizziness	4.5	3.3
Nausea	3.1	3.8
Hangover	2.5	1.1
Anxiety	2.0	1.5
Depression	1.7	1.8
Dry Mouth	1.7	2.2
Diarrhea	1.7	1.1
Abdominal Discomfort	1.5	1.9
Euphoria	1.5	0.4
Weakness	1.4	0.9
Confusion	1.3	0.5
Blurred Vision	1.3	1.3
Nightmares	1.2	1.7
Vertigo	1.2	0.8

The following adverse events have been reported less frequently (0.5–0.9%):

Central Nervous System — anorexia, ataxia, equilibrium loss, tremor, increased dreaming
Cardiovascular — dyspnea, palpitations
Gastrointestinal — vomiting
Musculoskeletal — backache
Special Senses — hyperhidrosis, burning eyes

Amnesia, hallucinations, horizontal nystagmus, and paradoxical reactions including restlessness, overstimulation and agitation were rare (less than 0.5%).

DRUG ABUSE AND DEPENDENCE

Controlled Substance

Restoril® (temazepam) is a controlled substance in Schedule IV.

Abuse and Dependence

Withdrawal symptoms, similar in character to those noted with barbiturates and alcohol (convulsions, tremor, abdominal, and muscle cramps, vomiting, and sweating), have occurred following abrupt discontinuance of benzodiazepines. The more severe withdrawal symptoms have usually been limited to those patients who received excessive doses over an extended period of time. Generally milder withdrawal symptoms (e.g., dysphoria and insomnia) have been reported following abrupt discontinuance of benzodiazepines taken continuously at therapeutic levels for several months. Consequently, after extended therapy at doses higher than 15 mg, abrupt discontinuation should generally be avoided and a gradual dosage tapering schedule followed. As with any hypnotic, caution must be exercised in administering Restoril® (temazepam) to individuals known to be addiction-prone or to those whose history suggests they may increase the dosage on their own initiative. It is desirable to limit repeated prescriptions without adequate medical supervision.

OVERDOSAGE

Manifestations of acute overdosage of Restoril® (temazepam) can be expected to reflect the CNS effects of the drug and include somnolence, confusion, and coma, with reduced or absent reflexes, respiratory depression, and hypotension. The oral LD$_{50}$ of Restoril® (temazepam) was 1963 mg/kg in mice, 1833 mg/kg in rats, and >2400 mg/kg in rabbits.

Treatment

If the patient is conscious, vomiting should be induced mechanically or with emetics. Gastric lavage should be employed utilizing concurrently a cuffed endotracheal tube if the patient is unconscious to prevent aspiration and pulmonary complications. Maintenance of adequate pulmonary

ventilation is essential. The use of pressor agents intravenously may be necessary to combat hypotension. Fluids should be administered intravenously to encourage diuresis. The value of dialysis has not been determined. If excitation occurs, barbiturates should not be used. It should be borne in mind that multiple agents may have been ingested.
Flumazenil (Romazicon®)*, a specific benzodiazepine receptor antagonist, is indicated for the complete or partial reversal of the sedative effects of benzodiazepines and may be used in situations when an overdose with a benzodiazepine is known or suspected. Prior to the administration of flumazenil, necessary measures should be instituted to secure airway, ventilation, and intravenous access. Flumazenil is intended as an adjunct to, not as a substitute for, proper management of benzodiazepine overdose. Patients treated with flumazenil should be monitored for re-sedation, respiratory depression, and other residual benzodiazepine effects for an appropriate period after treatment. **The prescriber should be aware of a risk of seizure in association with flumazenil treatment, particularly in long-term benzodiazepine users and in cyclic antidepressant overdose.** The complete flumazenil package insert including CONTRAINDICATIONS, WARNINGS, and PRECAUTIONS should be consulted prior to use.
Up-to-date information about the treatment of overdose can often be obtained from a certified Regional Poison Control Center. Telephone numbers of certified Regional Poison Control Centers are listed in the Physicians' Desk Reference.

DOSAGE AND ADMINISTRATION

While the recommended usual adult dose is 15 mg before retiring, 7.5 mg may be sufficient for some patients, and others may need 30 mg. In transient insomnia, a 7.5 mg dose may be sufficient to improve sleep latency. In elderly or debilitated patients, it is recommended that therapy be initiated with 7.5 mg until individual responses are determined.

HOW SUPPLIED

Restoril® (temazepam) Capsules, USP

7.5 mg
Blue and pink, imprinted "Restoril 7.5 mg" and "FOR SLEEP" twice on each capsule. Bottle of 100, NDC 0078-0140-05; and SandoPak® (unit-dose) package of 100 individually labeled blisters, each containing one capsule, NDC 0078-0140-06.

15 mg
Maroon and pink capsule imprinted "Restoril 15 mg" and "FOR SLEEP" twice on each capsule. Bottle of 100, NDC 0078-0098-05; bottle of 500, NDC 0078-0098-08; and SandoPak® (unit-dose) package of 100 individually labeled blisters, each containing one capsule, NDC 0078-0098-06.

30 mg
Maroon and blue capsule, imprinted "Restoril 30 mg" and "FOR SLEEP" twice on each capsule. Bottle of 100, NDC 0078-0099-05; bottle of 500, NDC 0078-0099-08; and SandoPak® (unit-dose) package of 100 individually labeled blisters, each containing one capsule, NDC 0078-0099-06.

Store and Dispense
Store in a tight, light-resistant container, below 86°F (30°C).

PATIENT INFORMATION

Introduction
Your doctor has prescribed Restoril® (temazepam) to help you sleep. The following information is intended to guide you in the safe use of this medicine. It is not meant to take the place of your doctor's instructions. If you have any questions about Restoril® (temazepam) capsules be sure to ask your doctor or pharmacist.
Restoril® (temazepam) is used to treat different types of sleep problems, such as:
- trouble falling asleep
- waking up too early in the morning
- waking up often during the night

Some people may have more than one of these problems.
Restoril® (temazepam) belongs to a group of medicines known as the "benzodiazepines." There are many different benzodiazepine medicines used to help people sleep better. Sleep problems are usually temporary, requiring treatment for only a short time, usually 7–10 days. However, if your sleep problems continue, consult your doctor. He/she will determine whether other measures are needed to overcome your sleep problems. Some people have chronic sleep problems that may require more prolonged use of sleep medicine. However, you should not use these medicines for long periods without talking with your doctor about the risks and benefits of prolonged use.

SIDE EFFECTS

Common Side Effects
All medicines have side effects. The most common side effects of benzodiazepine sleeping medicines include:
- drowsiness
- dizziness
- lightheadedness
- difficulty with coordination

You may find that these medicines make you sleepy during the day. How drowsy you feel depends upon how your body reacts to the medicine, which benzodiazepine sleeping medicine you are taking, and how large a dose your doctor has prescribed. Day-time drowsiness is best avoided by taking the lowest dose possible that will still help you to sleep at night. Your doctor will work with you to find the dose of Restoril® (temazepam) that is best for you.

To manage these side effects while you are taking this medicine:
- Use extreme care while doing anything that requires complete alertness, such as driving a car, operating machinery, or piloting an aircraft. As with any medicines used to help people sleep better, you should be very careful when you first start taking Restoril® (temazepam) until you know how the medicine will affect you.
- NEVER drink alcohol while you are being treated with Restoril® (temazepam) or any benzodiazepine medicine. Alcohol can increase the side effects of Restoril® (temazepam) or any other benzodiazepine medicine.
- Do not take any other medicines without asking your doctor first. This includes medicines you can buy without a prescription. Some medicines can cause drowsiness and are best avoided while taking Restoril® (temazepam).
- Always take the exact dose of Restoril® (temazepam) prescribed by your doctor. Never change your dose without talking to your doctor first.

SPECIAL CONCERNS
There are some special problems that may occur while taking benzodiazepine sleeping medicines.

Memory Problems
Benzodiazepine sleeping medicines may cause a special type of memory loss or "amnesia". When this occurs, a person may not remember what has happened for several hours after taking the medicine. This is usually not a problem since most people fall asleep after taking the medicine.
Memory loss can be a problem, however, when sleeping medicines are taken while traveling, such as during an airplane flight and the person wakes up before the effect of the medicine is gone. This has been called "traveler's amnesia".
Memory problems were noticed in fewer than 1 in 100 patients taking Restoril® (temazepam) in clinical trials. Memory problems can be avoided if you take Restoril® (temazepam) only when you are able to get a full night's sleep (7–8 hours) before you need to be active again. Be sure to talk to your doctor if you think you are having memory problems.

Tolerance
When benzodiazepine sleeping medicines are used every night for more than a few weeks, they may lose their effectiveness to help you sleep. This is known as "tolerance".
If tolerance to the medicine develops, other effects may occur depending upon which benzodiazepine sleeping medicine you are taking. Tolerance to benzodiazepine sleeping medicines that are shorter-acting may cause you to:
- wake up during the last third of the night
- become anxious or nervous while you are awake

These effects are less common with Restoril® (temazepam) because it is intermediate-acting.

Dependence
All the benzodiazepine sleeping medicines can cause dependence, especially when these medicines are used regularly for longer than a few weeks or at high doses. Some people develop a need to continue taking their medicines. This is known as dependence or "addiction."
When people develop dependence, they may have difficulty stopping the benzodiazepine sleeping medicine. If the medicine is suddenly stopped, the body is not able to function normally and unpleasant symptoms may occur *(see Withdrawal).* They may find they have to keep taking the medicine either at the prescribed dose or at increasing doses just to avoid withdrawal symptoms.
All people taking benzodiazepine sleeping medicines have some risk of becoming dependent on the medicine. However, people who have been dependent on alcohol or other drugs in the past may have a higher chance of becoming addicted to benzodiazepine medicines. This possibility must be considered before using these medicines for more than a few weeks.
If you have been addicted to alcohol or drugs in the past, it is important to tell your doctor before starting Restoril® (temazepam) or any benzodiazepine sleeping medicine.

Withdrawal
Withdrawal symptoms may occur when a benzodiazepine sleeping medicine is stopped suddenly after being used daily for a long time. But these symptoms can occur even if the medicine has been used for only a week or two.
In mild cases, withdrawal symptoms may include unpleasant feelings. In more severe cases, abdominal and muscle cramps, vomiting, sweating, shakiness, and rarely, seizures may occur. These more severe withdrawal symptoms are very uncommon.
Another problem that may occur when benzodiazepine sleeping medicines are stopped is known as "rebound insomnia". This means that a person may have more trouble sleeping the first few nights after the medicine is stopped than before starting the medicine. If you should experience rebound insomnia, do not get discouraged. This problem usually goes away on its own after 1 or 2 nights.
If you have been taking Restoril® (temazepam) or any other benzodiazepine sleeping medicine for more than 1 or 2 weeks, do not stop taking it on your own. Your doctor may give you special directions on how to gradually decrease your dose before stopping the medicine. Always follow your doctor's directions.

Changes in Behavior and Thinking
Some people using benzodiazepine sleeping medicines have experienced unusual changes in their thinking and/or behavior, including: more outgoing or aggressive behavior than normal; loss of personal identity; confusion; strange behavior; agitation; hallucinations; worsening of depression; and suicidal thoughts.
How often these effects occur depends on several factors, such as a person's general health or the use of other medicines. Clinical studies with Restoril® (temazepam) revealed that unusual behavior changes occurred in less than 1 in 100 patients.
It is also important to realize that it is rarely clear whether these behavior changes are caused by the medicine, an illness, or occur on their own. In fact, sleep problems that do not improve may be due to illnesses that were present before the medicine was used. If you or your family notice any changes in your behavior, or if you have any unusual or disturbing thoughts, call your doctor immediately.

Pregnancy
Certain benzodiazepines have been linked to birth defects when taken by a pregnant woman in the early months of pregnancy. These medicines can also cause sedation of the unborn baby when used during the last weeks of pregnancy. Restoril® (temazepam) should not be taken at any time during pregnancy. Be sure to tell your doctor if you are pregnant, if you are planning to become pregnant, or if you become pregnant while taking Restoril® (temazepam).

SAFE USE OF BENZODIAZEPINE SLEEPING MEDICINES
To ensure the safe and effective use of Restoril® (temazepam) or any other benzodiazepine sleeping medicine, you should observe the following cautions:
1. Restoril® (temazepam) is a prescription medicine and should be used ONLY as directed by your doctor. Follow your doctor's instructions about how to take, when to take, and how long to take Restoril® (temazepam).
2. Never use Restoril® (temazepam) or any other benzodiazepine sleeping medicine for longer than 1 or 2 weeks without first asking your doctor.
3. If you notice any unusual or disturbing thoughts or behavior during treatment with Restoril® (temazepam) or any other benzodiazepine sleeping medicine, contact your doctor.
4. Tell your doctor about any medicines you may be taking, including medicines you may buy without a prescription. You should also tell your doctor if you drink alcohol. DO NOT use alcohol while taking Restoril® (temazepam) or any other benzodiazepine sleeping medicine.
5. Do not take Restoril® (temazepam) or any other benzodiazepine sleeping medicine unless you are able to get a full night's sleep before you must be active again. For example, Restoril® (temazepam) or any other benzodiazepine sleeping medicine should not be taken on an overnight airplane flight of less than 7–8 hours since "traveler's amnesia" may occur.
6. Do not increase the prescribed dose of Restoril® (temazepam) or any other benzodiazepine sleeping medicine unless instructed by your doctor.
7. Use extreme care while doing anything that requires complete alertness, such as driving a car, operating machinery, or piloting an aircraft when you first start taking Restoril® (temazepam) or any other benzodiazepine sleeping medicine until you know whether the medicine will still have some carryover effect in you the next day.
8. Be aware that you may have more sleeping problems (rebound insomnia) the first night or two after stopping Restoril® (temazepam) or any other benzodiazepine sleeping medicine.
9. Be sure to tell your doctor if you are pregnant, if you are planning to become pregnant, or if you become pregnant while taking Restoril® (temazepam). Restoril® (temazepam) or any other benzodiazepine sleeping medicine should not be taken at any time during pregnancy.
10. As with all prescription medicines, never share Restoril® (temazepam) or any other benzodiazepine sleeping medicine with anyone else. Always store

*Romazicon is the registered trademark of Roche Laboratories.

Continued on next page

Sandoz—Cont.

Restoril® (temazepam) or any other benzodiazepine sleeping medicine in the original container out of reach of children.

[REV: DECEMBER 1994 30282901]

Shown in Product Identification Guide, page 333

SANDIMMUNE® Soft Gelatin Capsules ℞
(cyclosporine capsules, USP)

SANDIMMUNE® Oral Solution ℞
(cyclosporine oral solution, USP)

SANDIMMUNE® Injection ℞
(cyclosporine concentrate for injection, USP)
FOR INFUSION ONLY

Caution: Federal law prohibits dispensing without prescription.

The following prescribing information is based on official labeling in effect on August 1, 1996.

WARNING

Only physicians experienced in immunosuppressive therapy and management of organ transplant patients should prescribe Sandimmune® (cyclosporine). Patients receiving the drug should be managed in facilities equipped and staffed with adequate laboratory and supportive medical resources. The physician responsible for maintenance therapy should have complete information requisite for the follow-up of the patient.

Sandimmune® (cyclosporine) should be administered with adrenal corticosteroids but not with other immunosuppressive agents. Increased susceptibility to infection and the possible development of lymphoma may result from immunosuppression.

Sandimmune® soft gelatin capsules (cyclosporine capsules, USP) and Sandimmune® oral solution (cyclosporine oral solution, USP) have decreased bioavailability in comparison to Neoral® soft gelatin capsules (cyclosporine capsules for microemulsion) and Neoral® oral solution (cyclosporine oral solution for microemulsion).

Sandimmune® and Neoral® are not bioequivalent and cannot be used interchangeably without physician supervision.

The absorption of cyclosporine during chronic administration of Sandimmune® soft gelatin capsules and oral solution was found to be erratic. It is recommended that patients taking the soft gelatin capsules or oral solution over a period of time be monitored at repeated intervals for cyclosporine blood levels and subsequent dose adjustments be made in order to avoid toxicity due to high levels and possible organ rejection due to low absorption of cyclosporine. This is of special importance in liver transplants. Numerous assays are being developed to measure blood levels of cyclosporine. Comparison of levels in published literature to patient levels using current assays must be done with detailed knowledge of the assay methods employed. *(See Blood Level Monitoring under DOSAGE AND ADMINISTRATION)*

DESCRIPTION

Cyclosporine, the active principle in Sandimmune® (cyclosporine) is a cyclic polypeptide immunosuppressant agent consisting of 11 amino acids. It is produced as a metabolite by the fungus species *Beauveria nivea.*

Chemically, cyclosporine is designated as *[R-[R*,R*-(E)]]*-cyclic(L-alanyl-D-alanyl-*N*-methyl-L-leucyl-*N*-methyl-L-leucyl-*N*-methyl -L- valyl -3- hydroxy - *N*, 4-dimethyl-L-2-amino -6- octenoyl-L -*α*- amino-butyryl- *N*-methylglycyl- *N*-methyl-L-leucyl-L-valyl-*N*-methyl-L-leucyl).

Sandimmune® soft gelatin capsules (cyclosporine capsules, USP) are available in 25 mg, 50 mg, and 100 mg strengths.

Each 25 mg capsule contains:
cyclosporine, USP .... 25 mg
alcohol, USP dehydrated .... max 12.7% by volume

Each 50 mg capsule contains:
cyclosporine, USP .... 50 mg
alcohol, USP dehydrated .... max 12.7% by volume

Each 100 mg capsule contains:
cyclosporine, USP .... 100 mg
alcohol, USP dehydrated .... max 12.7% by volume

Inactive Ingredients: corn oil, gelatin, glycerol, Labrafil M 2125 CS (polyoxyethylated glycolysed glycerides), red iron oxide (25 mg and 100 mg capsules only), sorbitol, titanium dioxide, yellow iron oxide (50 mg capsule only), and other ingredients.

Sandimmune® oral solution (cyclosporine oral solution, USP) is available in 50 mL bottles.

Each mL contains:
cyclosporine, USP .... 100 mg
alcohol, Ph. Helv. .... 12.5% by volume
dissolved in an olive oil, Ph. Helv./Labrafil M 1944 CS (polyoxyethylated oleic glycerides) vehicle which must be further diluted with milk, chocolate milk, or orange juice before oral administration.

Sandimmune® injection (cyclosporine concentrate for injection, USP) is available in a 5 mL sterile ampul for I.V. administration.

Each mL contains:
cyclosporine, USP .... 50 mg
*Cremophor® EL
(polyoxyethylated castor oil) .... 650 mg
alcohol, Ph. Helv. .... 32.9% by volume
nitrogen .... qs
which must be diluted further with 0.9% Sodium Chloride Injection or 5% Dextrose Injection before use.

The chemical structure of cyclosporine (also known as cyclosporin A) is:

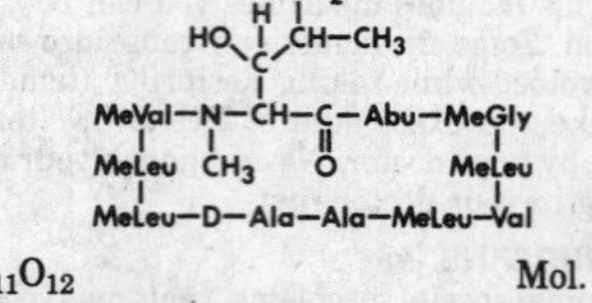

$C_{62}H_{111}N_{11}O_{12}$ Mol. Wt. 1202.63

CLINICAL PHARMACOLOGY

Sandimmune® (cyclosporine) is a potent immunosuppressive agent which in animals prolongs survival of allogeneic transplants involving skin, heart, kidney, pancreas, bone marrow, small intestine, and lung. Sandimmune® (cyclosporine) has been demonstrated to suppress some humoral immunity and to a greater extent, cell-mediated reactions such as allograft rejection, delayed hypersensitivity, experimental allergic encephalomyelitis, Freund's adjuvant arthritis, and graft vs. host disease in many animal species for a variety of organs.

Successful kidney, liver, and heart allogeneic transplants have been performed in man using Sandimmune® (cyclosporine).

The exact mechanism of action of Sandimmune® cyclosporine) is not known. Experimental evidence suggests that the effectiveness of cyclosporine is due to specific and reversible inhibition of immunocompetent lymphocytes in the G_0- or G_1-phase of the cell cycle. T-lymphocytes are preferentially inhibited. The T-helper cell is the main target, although the T-suppressor cell may also be suppressed. Sandimmune® (cyclosporine) also inhibits lymphokine production and release including interleukin-2 or T-cell growth factor (TCGF).

No functional effects on phagocytic (changes in enzyme secretions not altered, chemotactic migration of granulocytes, macrophage migration, carbon clearance *in vivo*) or tumor cells (growth rate, metastasis) can be detected in animals. Sandimmune® (cyclosporine) does not cause bone marrow suppression in animal models or man.

The absorption of cyclosporine from the gastrointestinal tract is incomplete and variable. Peak concentrations (C_{max}) in blood and plasma are achieved at about 3.5 hours. C_{max} and area under the plasma or blood concentration/time curve (AUC) increase with the administered dose; for blood the relationship is curvilinear (parabolic) between 0 and 1400 mg. As determined by a specific assay, C_{max} is approximately 1.0 ng/mL/mg of dose for plasma and 2.7-1.4 ng/mL/mg of dose for blood (for low to high doses). Compared to an intravenous infusion, the absolute bioavailability of the oral solution is approximately 30% based upon the results in 2 patients. The bioavailability of Sandimmune® soft gelatin capsules (cyclosporine capsules, USP) is equivalent to Sandimmune® oral solution, (cyclosporine oral solution, USP).

Cyclosporine is distributed largely outside the blood volume. In blood the distribution is concentration dependent. Approximately 33%-47% is in plasma, 4%-9% in lymphocytes, 5%-12% in granulocytes, and 41%-58% in erythrocytes. At high concentrations, the uptake by leukocytes and erythrocytes becomes saturated. In plasma, approximately 90% is bound to proteins, primarily lipoproteins.

The disposition of cyclosporine from blood is biphasic with a terminal half-life of approximately 19 hours (range: 10-27 hours). Elimination is primarily biliary with only 6% of the dose excreted in the urine.

Cyclosporine is extensively metabolized but there is no major metabolic pathway. Only 0.1% of the dose is excreted in the urine as unchanged drug. Of 15 metabolites characterized in human urine, 9 have been assigned structures. The major pathways consist of hydroxylation of the Cγ-carbon of 2 of the leucine residues, Cη-carbon hydroxylation, and cyclic ether formation (with oxidation of the double bond) in the side chain of the amino acid 3-hydroxyl-*N*,4-dimethyl-L-2-amino-6-octenoic acid and *N*-demethylation of *N*-methyl leucine residues. Hydrolysis of the cyclic peptide chain or conjugation of the aforementioned metabolites do not appear to be important biotransformation pathways.

*Cremophor is the registered trademark of BASF Aktiengesellschaft.

INDICATIONS AND USAGE

Sandimmune® (cyclosporine) is indicated for the prophylaxis of organ rejection in kidney, liver, and heart allogeneic transplants. It is always to be used with adrenal corticosteroids. The drug may also be used in the treatment of chronic rejection in patients previously treated with other immunosuppressive agents.

Because of the risk of anaphylaxis, Sandimmune® injection (cyclosporine concentrate for injection, USP) should be reserved for patients who are unable to take the soft gelatin capsules or oral solution.

CONTRAINDICATIONS

Sandimmune® injection (cyclosporine concentrate for injection, USP) is contraindicated in patients with a hypersensitivity to Sandimmune® (cyclosporine) and/or Cremophor® EL (polyoxyethylated castor oil).

[See table at top of next page.]

WARNINGS

(See boxed WARNINGs)

Sandimmune® (cyclosporine), when used in high doses, can cause hepatotoxicity and nephrotoxicity.

It is not unusual for serum creatinine and BUN levels to be elevated during Sandimmune® (cyclosporine) therapy. These elevations in renal transplant patients do not necessarily indicate rejection, and each patient must be fully evaluated before dosage adjustment is initiated.

Nephrotoxicity has been noted in 25% of cases of renal transplantation, 38% of cases of cardiac transplantation, and 37% of cases of liver transplantation. Mild nephrotoxicity was generally noted 2-3 months after transplant and consisted of an arrest in the fall of the preoperative elevations of BUN and creatinine at a range of 35-45 mg/dl and 2.0-2.5 mg/dl respectively. These elevations were often responsive to dosage reduction.

More overt nephrotoxicity was seen early after transplantation and was characterized by a rapidly rising BUN and creatinine. Since these events are similar to rejection episodes care must be taken to differentiate between them. This form of nephrotoxicity is usually responsive to Sandimmune® (cyclosporine) dosage reduction.

Although specific diagnostic criteria which reliably differentiate renal graft rejection from drug toxicity have not been found, a number of parameters have been significantly associated to one or the other. It should be noted however, that up to 20% of patients may have simultaneous nephrotoxicity and rejection.

A form of chronic progressive cyclosporine-associated nephrotoxicity is characterized by serial deterioration in renal function and morphologic changes in the kidneys. From 5%-15% of transplant recipients will fail to show a reduction in a rising serum creatinine despite a decrease or discontinuation of cyclosporine therapy. Renal biopsies from these patients will demonstrate an interstitial fibrosis with tubular atrophy. In addition, toxic tubulopathy, peritubular capillary congestion, arteriolopathy, and a striped form of interstitial fibrosis with tubular atrophy may be present. Though none of these morphologic changes is entirely specific, a histologic diagnosis of chronic progressive cyclosporine-associated nephrotoxicity requires evidence of these.

When considering the development of chronic nephrotoxicity it is noteworthy that several authors have reported an association between the appearance of interstitial fibrosis and higher cumulative doses or persistently high circulating trough levels of cyclosporine. This is particularly true during the first 6 post-transplant months when the dosage tends to be highest and when, in kidney recipients, the organ appears to be most vulnerable to the toxic effects of cyclosporine. Among other contributing factors to the development of interstitial fibrosis in these patients must be included, prolonged perfusion time, warm ischemia time, as well as episodes of acute toxicity, and acute and chronic rejection. The reversibility of interstitial fibrosis and its correlation to renal function have not yet been determined.

Impaired renal function at any time requires close monitoring, and frequent dosage adjustment may be indicated. In patients with persistent high elevations of BUN and creatinine who are unresponsive to dosage adjustments, consideration should be given to switching to other immunosuppressive therapy. In the event of severe and unremitting rejection, it is preferable to allow the kidney transplant to be rejected and removed rather than increase the Sandimmune® (cyclosporine) dosage to a very high level in an attempt to reverse the rejection.

Occasionally patients have developed a syndrome of thrombocytopenia and microangiopathic hemolytic anemia which

may result in graft failure. The vasculopathy can occur in the absence of rejection and is accompanied by avid platelet consumption within the graft as demonstrated by Indium 111 labeled platelet studies. Neither the pathogenesis nor the management of this syndrome is clear. Though resolution has occurred after reduction or discontinuation of Sandimmune® (cyclosporine) and 1) administration of streptokinase and heparin or 2) plasmapheresis, this appears to depend upon early detection with Indium 111 labeled platelet scans. (See ADVERSE REACTIONS)

Significant hyperkalemia (sometimes associated with hyperchloremic metabolic acidosis) and hyperuricemia have been seen occasionally in individual patients.

Hepatotoxicity has been noted in 4% of cases of renal transplantation, 7% of cases of cardiac transplantation, and 4% of cases of liver transplantation. This was usually noted during the first month of therapy when high doses of Sandimmune® (cyclosporine) were used and consisted of elevations of hepatic enzymes and bilirubin. The chemistry elevations usually decreased with a reduction in dosage.

As in patients receiving other immunosuppressants, those patients receiving Sandimmune® (cyclosporine) are at increased risk for development of lymphomas and other malignancies, particularly those of the skin. The increased risk appears related to the intensity and duration of immunosuppression rather than to the use of specific agents. Because of the danger of oversuppression of the immune system, which can also increase susceptibility to infection, Sandimmune® (cyclosporine) should not be administered with other immunosuppressive agents except adrenal corticosteroids. The efficacy and safety of cyclosporine in combination with other immunosuppressive agents have not been determined.

There have been reports of convulsions in adult and pediatric patients receiving cyclosporine, particularly in combination with high dose methylprednisolone.

Rarely (approximately 1 in 1000), patients receiving Sandimmune® injection (cyclosporine concentrate for injection, USP) have experienced anaphylactic reactions. Although the exact cause of these reactions is unknown, it is believed to be due to the Cremophor® EL (polyoxyethylated castor oil) used as the vehicle for the I.V. formulation. These reactions have consisted of flushing of the face and upper thorax, acute respiratory distress with dyspnea and wheezing, blood pressure changes, and tachycardia. One patient died after respiratory arrest and aspiration pneumonia. In some cases, the reaction subsided after the infusion was stopped.

Patients receiving Sandimmune® injection (cyclosporine concentrate for injection, USP) should be under continuous observation for at least the first 30 minutes following the start of the infusion and at frequent intervals thereafter. If anaphylaxis occurs, the infusion should be stopped. An aqueous solution of epinephrine 1:1000 should be available at the bedside as well as a source of oxygen.

Anaphylactic reactions have not been reported with the soft gelatin capsules or oral solution which lack Cremophor® EL (polyoxyethylated castor oil). In fact, patients experiencing anaphylactic reactions have been treated subsequently with the soft gelatin capsules or oral solution without incident. Care should be taken in using Sandimmune® (cyclosporine) with nephrotoxic drugs. (See PRECAUTIONS)

Because Sandimmune® is not bioequivalent to Neoral®, conversion from Neoral® to Sandimmune® using a 1:1 ratio (mg/kg/day) may result in a lower cyclosporine blood concentration. Conversion from Neoral® to Sandimmune® should be made with increased blood concentration monitoring to avoid the potential of underdosing.

PRECAUTIONS

General

Patients with malabsorption may have difficulty in achieving therapeutic levels with Sandimmune® soft gelatin capsules or oral solution.

Hypertension is a common side effect of Sandimmune® (cyclosporine) therapy. (See ADVERSE REACTIONS) Mild or moderate hypertension is more frequently encountered than severe hypertension and the incidence decreases over time. Antihypertensive therapy may be required. Control of blood pressure can be accomplished with any of the common antihypertensive agents. However, since cyclosporine may cause hyperkalemia, potassium-sparing diuretics should not be used. While calcium antagonists can be effective agents in treating cyclosporine-associated hypertension, care should be taken since interference with cyclosporine metabolism may require a dosage adjustment. (See Drug Interactions) During treatment with Sandimmune® (cyclosporine), vaccination may be less effective; and the use of live attenuated vaccines should be avoided.

Information for Patients

Patients should be advised that any change of cyclosporine formulation should be made cautiously and only under physician supervision because it may result in the need for a change in dosage.

Patients should be informed of the necessity of repeated laboratory tests while they are receiving the drug. They should be given careful dosage instructions, advised of the potential risks during pregnancy, and informed of the increased risk of neoplasia.

Patients using cyclosporine oral solution with its accompanying syringe for dosage measurement should be cautioned not to rinse the syringe either before or after use. Introduction of water into the product by any means will cause variation in dose.

Laboratory Tests

Renal and liver functions should be assessed repeatedly by measurement of BUN, serum creatinine, serum bilirubin, and liver enzymes.

Drug Interactions

All of the individual drugs cited below are well substantiated to interact with Sandimmune® (cyclosporine).

Drugs That Exhibit Nephrotoxic Synergy

gentamicin	cimetidine
tobramycin	ranitidine
vancomycin	diclofenac
amphotericin B	trimethoprim
ketoconazole	with sulfamethoxazole
melphalan	azapropazon

Careful monitoring of renal function should be practiced when Sandimmune® (cyclosporine) is used with nephrotoxic drugs.

Drugs That Alter Cyclosporine Levels

Cyclosporine is extensively metabolized by the liver. Therefore, circulating cyclosporine levels may be influenced by drugs that affect hepatic microsomal enzymes, particularly the cytochrome P-450 system. Substances known to inhibit these enzymes will decrease hepatic metabolism and increase cyclosporine levels. Substances that are inducers of cytochrome P-450 activity will increase hepatic metabolism and decrease cyclosporine levels. Monitoring of circulating cyclosporine levels and appropriate Sandimmune® (cyclosporine) dosage adjustment are essential when these drugs are used concomitantly (see Blood Level Monitoring).

Drugs That Increase Cyclosporine Levels

diltiazem	danazol
nicardipine	bromocriptine
verapamil	metoclopramide
ketoconazole	erythromycin
fluconazole	methylprednisolone
intraconazole	

Drugs That Decrease Cyclosporine Levels

rifampin	phenobarbital
phenytoin	carbamazepine

Other Drug Interactions

Reduced clearance of prednisolone, digoxin, and lovastatin has been observed when these drugs are administered with Sandimmune® (cyclosporine). In addition, a decrease in the apparent volume of distribution of digoxin has been reported after Sandimmune® (cyclosporine) administration. Severe digitalis toxicity has been seen within days of starting cyclosporine in several patients taking digoxin. Sandimmune® (cyclosporine) should not be used with potassium-sparing diuretics because hyperkalemia can occur. During treatment with Sandimmune® (cyclosporine), vaccination may be less effective; and the use of live vaccines should be avoided. Myositis has occurred with concomitant lovastatin, frequent gingival hyperplasia with nifedipine, and convulsions with high dose methylprednisolone. Further information on drugs that have been reported to interact with Sandimmune® (cyclosporine) is available from Sandoz Pharmaceuticals Corporation.

Carcinogenesis, Mutagenesis, and Impairment of Fertility

Cyclosporine gave no evidence of mutagenic or teratogenic effects in appropriate test systems. Only at dose levels toxic to dams, were adverse effects seen in reproduction studies in rats. (See Pregnancy)

Carcinogenicity studies were carried out in male and female rats and mice. In the 78-week mouse study, at doses of 1, 4, and 16 mg/kg/day, evidence of a statistically significant trend was found for lymphocytic lymphomas in females, and the incidence of hepatocellular carcinomas in mid-dose males significantly exceeded the control value. In the 24-month rat study, conducted at 0.5, 2, and 8 mg/kg/day, pancreatic islet cell adenomas significantly exceeded the control rate in the low dose level. The hepatocellular carcinomas and pancreatic islet cell adenomas were not dose related.

Nephrotoxicity vs Rejection

Parameter	Nephrotoxicity	Rejection
History	Donor >50 years old or hypotensive Prolonged kidney preservation Prolonged anastomosis time Concomitant nephrotoxic drugs	Antidonor immune response Retransplant patient
Clinical	Often >6 weeks postop[b] Prolonged initial nonfunction (acute tubular necrosis)	Often <4 weeks postop[b] Fever >37.5°C Weight gain >0.5 kg Graft swelling and tenderness Decrease in daily urine volume >500 mL (or 50%)
Laboratory	CyA serum trough level >200 ng/mL Gradual rise in Cr (<0.15 mg/dl/day)[a] Cr plateau <25% above baseline BUN/Cr ≥ 20	CyA serum trough level <150 ng/mL Rapid rise in Cr (>0.3 mg/dl/day)[a] Cr >25% above baseline BUN/Cr <20
Biopsy	Arteriolopathy (medial hypertrophy[a], hyalinosis, nodular deposits, intimal thickening, endothelial vacuolization, progressive scarring) Tubular atrophy, isometric vacuolization, isolated calcifications Minimal edema Mild focal infiltrates[c] Diffuse interstitial fibrosis, often striped form	Endovasculitis[c] (proliferation[a], intimal arteritis[b], necrosis, sclerosis) Tubulitis with RBC[b] and WBC[b] casts, some irregular vacuolization Interstitial edema[c] and hemorrhage[b] Diffuse moderate to severe mononuclear infiltrates[d] Glomerulitis (mononuclear cells)[c]
Aspiration Cytology	CyA deposits in tubular and endothelial cells Fine isometric vacuolization of tubular cells	Inflammatory infiltrate with mononuclear phagocytes, macrophages, lymphoblastoid cells, and activated T-cells These strongly express HLA-DR antigens
Urine Cytology	Tubular cells with vacuolization and granularization	Degenerative tubular cells, plasma cells, and lymphocyturia >20% of sediment
Manometry	Intracapsular pressure <40 mm Hg[b]	Intracapsular pressure >40 mm Hg[b]
Ultrasonography	Unchanged graft cross sectional area	Increase in graft cross sectional area AP diameter ≥ Transverse diameter
Magnetic Resonance Imagery	Normal appearance	Loss of distinct corticomedullary junction, swelling image intensity of parachyma approaching that of psoas, loss of hilar fat
Radionuclide Scan	Normal or generally decreased perfusion Decrease in tubular function (^{131}I-hippuran) >decrease in perfusion (^{99m}Tc DTPA)	Patchy arterial flow Decrease in perfusion >decrease in tubular function Increased uptake of Indium 111 labeled platelets or Tc-99m in colloid
Therapy	Responds to decreased Sandimmune® (cyclosporine)	Responds to increased steroids or antilymphocyte globulin

[a]$p < 0.05$, [b]$p < 0.01$, [c]$p < 0.001$, [d]$p < 0.0001$

Continued on next page

Sandoz—Cont.

No impairment in fertility was demonstrated in studies in male and female rats.

Cyclosporine has not been found mutagenic/genotoxic in the Ames Test, the V79-HGPRT Test, the micronucleus test in mice and Chinese hamsters, the chromosome-aberration tests in Chinese hamster bone-marrow, the mouse dominant lethal assay, and the DNA-repair test in sperm from treated mice. A recent study analyzing sister chromatid exchange (SCE) induction by cyclosporine using human lymphocytes *in vitro* gave indication of a positive effect (i.e., induction of SCE), at high concentrations in this system.

An increased incidence of malignancy is a recognized complication of immunosuppression in recipients of organ transplants. The most common forms of neoplasms are non-Hodgkin's lymphoma and carcinomas of the skin. The risk of malignancies in cyclosporine recipients is higher than in the normal, healthy population but similar to that in patients receiving other immunosuppressive therapies. It has been reported that reduction or discontinuance of immunosuppression may cause the lesions to regress.

Pregnancy

Pregnancy Category C. Sandimmune® oral solution (cyclosporine oral solution, USP) has been shown to be embryo- and fetotoxic in rats and rabbits when given in doses 2-5 times the human dose. At toxic doses (rats at 30 mg/kg/day and rabbits at 100 mg/kg/day), Sandimmune® oral solution (cyclosporine oral solution, USP) was embryo- and fetotoxic as indicated by increased pre- and postnatal mortality and reduced fetal weight together with related skeletal retardations. In the well-tolerated dose range (rats at up to 17 mg/kg/day and rabbits at up to 30 mg/kg/day), Sandimmune® oral solution (cyclosporine oral solution, USP) proved to be without any embryolethal or teratogenic effects.

There are no adequate and well-controlled studies in pregnant women. Sandimmune® (cyclosporine) should be used during pregnancy only if the potential benefit justifies the potential risk to the fetus.

The following data represent the reported outcomes of 116 pregnancies in women receiving Sandimmune® (cyclosporine) during pregnancy, 90% of whom were transplant patients, and most of whom received Sandimmune® (cyclosporine) throughout the entire gestational period. Since most of the patients were not prospectively identified, the results are likely to be biased toward negative outcomes. The only consistent patterns of abnormality were premature birth (gestational period of 28 to 36 weeks) and low birth weight for gestational age. It is not possible to separate the effects of Sandimmune® (cyclosporine) on these pregnancies from the effects of the other immunosuppressants, the underlying maternal disorders, or other aspects of the transplantation milieu. Sixteen fetal losses occurred. Most of the pregnancies (85 of 100) were complicated by disorders; including, pre-eclampsia, eclampsia, premature labor, abruptio placentae, oligohydramnios, Rh incompatibility and fetoplacental dysfunction. Preterm delivery occurred in 47%. Seven malformations were reported in 5 viable infants and in 2 cases of fetal loss. Twenty-eight percent of the infants were small for gestational age. Neonatal complications occurred in 27%. In a report of 23 children followed up to 4 years, postnatal development was said to be normal. More information on cyclosporine use in pregnancy is available from Sandoz Pharmaceuticals Corporation.

Nursing Mothers

Since Sandimmune® (cyclosporine) is excreted in human milk, nursing should be avoided.

Pediatric Use

Although no adequate and well controlled studies have been conducted in children, patients as young as 6 months of age have received the drug with no unusual adverse effects.

ADVERSE REACTIONS

The principal adverse reactions of Sandimmune® (cyclosporine) therapy are renal dysfunction, tremor, hirsutism, hypertension, and gum hyperplasia.

Hypertension, which is usually mild to moderate, may occur in approximately 50% of patients following renal transplantation and in most cardiac transplant patients.

Glomerular capillary thrombosis has been found in patients treated with cyclosporine and may progress to graft failure. The pathologic changes resemble those seen in the hemolytic-uremic syndrome and include thrombosis of the renal microvasculature, with platelet-fibrin thrombi occluding glomerular capillaries and afferent arterioles, microangiopathic hemolytic anemia, thrombocytopenia, and decreased renal function. Similar findings have been observed when other immunosuppressives have been employed post-transplantation.

Hypomagnesemia has been reported in some, but not all, patients exhibiting convulsions while on cyclosporine therapy. Although magnesium-depletion studies in normal subjects suggest that hypomagnesemia is associated with neurologic disorders, multiple factors, including hypertension, high dose methylprednisolone, hypocholesterolemia, and nephrotoxicity associated with high plasma concentrations of cyclosporine appear to be related to the neurological manifestations of cyclosporine toxicity.

The following reactions occurred in 3% or greater of 892 patients involved in clinical trials of kidney, heart, and liver transplants:
[See table below.]

The following reactions occurred in 2% or less of patients: allergic reactions, anemia, anorexia, confusion, conjunctivitis, edema, fever, brittle fingernails, gastritis, hearing loss, hiccups, hyperglycemia, muscle pain, peptic ulcer, thrombocytopenia, tinnitus.

The following reactions occurred rarely: anxiety, chest pain, constipation, depression, hair breaking, hematuria, joint pain, lethargy, mouth sores, myocardial infarction, night sweats, pancreatitis, pruritus, swallowing difficulty, tingling, upper GI bleeding, visual disturbance, weakness, weight loss.

[See table above.]
[See table at top of next page.]

Cremophor® EL (polyoxyethylated castor oil) is known to cause hyperlipemia and electrophoretic abnormalities of lipoproteins. These effects are reversible upon discontinuation of treatment but are usually not a reason to stop treatment.

OVERDOSAGE

There is a minimal experience with overdosage. Because of the slow absorption of Sandimmune® soft gelatin capsules or oral solution, forced emesis would be of value up to 2 hours after administration. Transient hepatotoxicity and nephrotoxicity may occur which should resolve following drug withdrawal. General supportive measures and symptomatic treatment should be followed in all cases of overdosage. Sandimmune® (cyclosporine) is not dialyzable to any great extent, nor is it cleared well by charcoal hemoperfusion. The oral LD_{50} is 2329 mg/kg in mice, 1480 mg/kg in rats, and >1000 mg/kg in rabbits. The I.V. LD_{50} is 148 mg/kg in mice, 104 mg/kg in rats, and 46 mg/kg in rabbits.

DOSAGE AND ADMINISTRATION

Sandimmune® Soft Gelatin Capsules (cyclosporine capsules, USP) and Sandimmune® Oral Solution (cyclosporine oral solution, USP)

Sandimmune® soft gelatin capsules (cyclosporine capsules, USP) and Sandimmune® oral solution (cyclosporine oral solution, USP) have decreased bioavailability in comparison to Neoral® soft gelatin capsules (cyclosporine capsules for microemulsion) and Neoral® oral solution (cyclosporine oral solution for microemulsion). Sandimmune® and Neoral® are not bioequivalent and cannot be used interchangeably without physician supervision.

The initial oral dose of Sandimmune® (cyclosporine) should be given 4-12 hours prior to transplantation as a single dose of 15 mg/kg. Although a daily single dose of 14-18 mg/kg was used in most clinical trials, few centers continue to use the highest dose, most favoring the lower end of the scale. There is a trend towards use of even lower initial doses for renal transplantation in the ranges of 10-14 mg/kg/day. The initial single daily dose is continued postoperatively for 1-2 weeks and then tapered by 5% per week to a maintenance dose of 5-10 mg/kg/day. Some centers have successfully tapered the maintenance dose to as low as 3 mg/kg/day in selected *renal* transplant patients without an apparent rise in rejection rate.

(See Blood Level Monitoring below)

In pediatric usage, the same dose and dosing regimen may be used as in adults although in several studies children have required and tolerated higher doses than those used in adults.

Adjunct therapy with adrenal corticosteroids is recommended. Different tapering dosage schedules of prednisone appear to achieve similar results. A dosage schedule based on the patient's weight started with 2.0 mg/kg/day for the first 4 days tapered to 1.0 mg/kg/day by 1 week, 0.6 mg/kg/day by 2 weeks, 0.3 mg/kg/day by 1 month, and 0.15 mg/kg/day by 2 months and thereafter as a maintenance dose. Another center started with an initial dose of 200 mg tapered by 40 mg/day until reaching 20 mg/day. After 2 months at this dose, a further reduction to 10 mg/day was made. Adjustments in dosage of prednisone must be made according to the clinical situation.

To make Sandimmune® oral solution (cyclosporine oral solution, USP) more palatable, the oral solution may be diluted with milk, chocolate milk, or orange juice preferably at

Renal Transplant Patients in Whom Therapy Was Discontinued

| | Randomized Patients | | All Sandimmune® Patients |
Reason for Discontinuation	Sandimmune® (N=227) %	Azathioprine (N=228) %	(N=705) %
Renal Toxicity	5.7	0	5.4
Infection	0	0.4	0.9
Lack of Efficacy	2.6	0.9	1.4
Acute Tubular Necrosis	2.6	0	1.0
Lymphoma/Lymphoproliferative Disease	0.4	0	0.3
Hypertension	0	0	0.3
Hematological Abnormalities	0	0.4	0
Other	0	0	0.7

Sandimmune® (cyclosporine) was discontinued on a temporary basis and then restarted in 18 additional patients.

Body System/ Adverse Reactions	Randomized Kidney Patients		All Sandimmune® (cyclosporine) Patients		
	Sandimmune® (N=227) %	Azathioprine (N=228) %	Kidney (N=705) %	Heart (N=112) %	Liver (N=75) %
Genitourinary					
Renal Dysfunction	32	6	25	38	37
Cardiovascular					
Hypertension	26	18	13	53	27
Cramps	4	<1	2	<1	0
Skin					
Hirsutism	21	<1	21	28	45
Acne	6	8	2	2	1
Central Nervous System					
Tremor	12	0	21	31	55
Convulsions	3	1	1	4	5
Headache	2	<1	2	15	4
Gastrointestinal					
Gum Hyperplasia	4	0	9	5	16
Diarrhea	3	<1	3	4	8
Nausea/Vomiting	2	<1	4	4	10
Hepatotoxicity	<1	<1	4	7	4
Abdominal Discomfort	<1	0	<1	7	0
Autonomic Nervous System					
Paresthesia	3	0	1	2	1
Flushing	<1	0	4	0	4
Hematopoietic					
Leukopenia	2	19	<1	6	0
Lymphoma	<1	0	1	6	1
Respiratory					
Sinusitis	<1	0	4	3	7
Miscellaneous					
Gynecomastia	<1	0	<1	4	3

Infectious Complications in the Randomized Renal Transplant Patients

Complication	Sandimmune® Treatment (N=227) % of Complications	Standard Treatment* (N=228) % of Complications
Septicemia	5.3	4.8
Abscesses	4.4	5.3
Systemic Fungal Infection	2.2	3.9
Local Fungal Infection	7.5	9.6
Cytomegalovirus	4.8	12.3
Other Viral Infections	15.9	18.4
Urinary Tract Infections	21.1	20.2
Wound and Skin Infections	7.0	10.1
Pneumonia	6.2	9.2

* Some patients also received ALG.

room temperature. Patients should avoid switching diluents frequently. Sandimmune® soft gelatin capsules and oral solution should be administered on a consistent schedule with regard to time of day and relation to meals.

Take the prescribed amount of Sandimmune® (cyclosporine) from the container using the dosage syringe supplied after removal of the protective cover, and transfer the solution to a glass of milk, chocolate milk, or orange juice. Stir well and drink at once. Do not allow to stand before drinking. It is best to use a glass container and rinse it with more diluent to ensure that the total dose is taken. After use, replace the dosage syringe in the protective cover. Do not rinse the dosage syringe with water or other cleaning agents either before or after use. If the dosage syringe requires cleaning, it must be completely dry before resuming use. Introduction of water into the product by any means will cause variation in dose.

Sandimmune® Injection (cyclosporine concentrate for injection, USP)
FOR INFUSION ONLY
Note: Anaphylactic reactions have occurred with Sandimmune® injection (cyclosporine concentrate for injection, USP). *(See WARNINGS)*
Patients unable to take Sandimmune® soft gelatin capsules or oral solution pre- or postoperatively may be treated with the I.V. concentrate. **Sandimmune® injection (cyclosporine concentrate for injection, USP) is administered at $^1/_3$ the oral dose.** The initial dose of Sandimmune® injection (cyclosporine concentrate for injection, USP) should be given 4-12 hours prior to transplantation as a single I.V. dose of 5-6 mg/kg/day. This daily single dose is continued postoperatively until the patient can tolerate the soft gelatin capsules or oral solution. Patients should be switched to Sandimmune® soft gelatin capsules or oral solution as soon as possible after surgery. In pediatric usage, the same dose and dosing regimen may be used, although higher doses may be required.
Adjunct steroid therapy is to be used. *(See aforementioned)*
Immediately before use, the I.V. concentrate should be diluted 1 mL Sandimmune® injection (cyclosporine concentrate for injection, USP) in 20 mL-100 mL 0.9% Sodium Chloride Injection or 5% Dextrose Injection and given in a slow intravenous infusion over approximately 2-6 hours. Diluted infusion solutions should be discarded after 24 hours.
The Cremophor® EL (polyoxyethylated castor oil) contained in the concentrate for intravenous infusion can cause phthalate stripping from PVC.
Parenteral drug products should be inspected visually for particulate matter and discoloration prior to administration, whenever solution and container permit.

Blood Level Monitoring
Several study centers have found blood level monitoring of cyclosporine useful in patient management. While no fixed relationships have yet been established, in one series of 375 consecutive cadaveric renal transplant recipients, dosage was adjusted to achieve specific whole blood 24-hour trough levels of 100-200 ng/mL as determined by high-pressure liquid chromatography (HPLC).
Of major importance to blood level analysis is the type of assay used. The above levels are specific to the parent cyclosporine molecule and correlate directly to the new monoclonal specific radioimmunoassays (mRIA-sp). Nonspecific assays are also available which detect the parent compound molecule and various of its metabolites. Older studies often cited levels using a nonspecific assay which were roughly twice those of specific assays. Assay results are not interchangeable and their use should be guided by their approved labeling. If plasma specimens are employed, levels will vary with the temperature at the time of separation from whole blood. Plasma levels may range from $^1/_2$-$^1/_5$ of whole blood levels. Refer to individual assay labeling for complete instructions. In addition, *Transplantation Proceedings* (June 1990) contains position papers and a broad consensus generated at the Cyclosporine-Therapeutic Drug Monitoring conference that year. Blood level monitoring is not a replacement for renal function monitoring or tissue biopsies.

HOW SUPPLIED
Sandimmune® Soft Gelatin Capsules (cyclosporine capsules, USP)
25 mg
Oblong, pink, branded "S78/240". SandoPak® unit-dose packages of 30 capsules, 3 blister cards of 10 capsules (NDC 0078-0240-15).
50 mg
Oblong, corn-yellow, branded "S78/242". SandoPak® unit-dose packages of 30 capsules, 3 blister cards of 10 capsules (NDC 0078-0242-15).
100 mg
Oblong, dusty rose, branded "S78/241". SandoPak® unit-dose packages of 30 capsules, 3 blister cards of 10 capsules (NDC 0078-0241-15).
Store and Dispense
In the original unit-dose container at temperatures below 86°F (30°C). An odor may be detected upon opening the unit-dose container, which will dissipate shortly thereafter. This odor does not affect the quality of the product.
Sandimmune® Oral Solution (cyclosporine oral solution, USP)
Supplied in 50 mL bottles containing 100 mg of cyclosporine per mL (NDC 0078-0110-22). A dosage syringe is provided for dispensing.
Store and Dispense
In the original container at temperatures below 86°F (30°C). Do not store in the refrigerator. Protect from freezing. Once opened, the contents must be used within 2 months.
Sandimmune® Injection (cyclosporine concentrate for injection, USP)
FOR INTRAVENOUS INFUSION
Supplied as a 5 mL sterile ampul containing 50 mg of cyclosporine per mL, in boxes of 10 ampuls (NDC 0078-0109-01).
Store and Dispense
At temperatures below 86°F (30°C) and protected from light.
Sandimmune® Soft Gelatin Capsules (cyclosporine capsules, USP)
Manufactured by
R.P. Scherer GmbH, EBERBACH/BADEN, GERMANY
Manufactured for
Sandoz Pharmaceuticals Corporation,
East Hanover, NJ 07936
Sandimmune® Oral Solution (cyclosporine oral solution, USP) and Sandimmune® Injection (cyclosporine concentrate for injection, USP)
FOR INFUSION ONLY
Manufactured by
SANDOZ PHARMA LTD., Basle, Switzerland
Manufactured for
Sandoz Pharmaceuticals Corporation,
East Hanover, NJ 07936
[REV: MAY 1996   37925910]
Shown in Product Identification Guide, page 333

IMMUNE GLOBULIN INTRAVENOUS (HUMAN) SANDOGLOBULIN®
Lyophilized Preparation
℞

CAUTION: US Federal law prohibits dispensing without prescription.
The following prescribing information is based on official labeling in effect on August 1, 1996.

DESCRIPTION
Immune Globulin Intravenous (Human)*, Sandoglobulin®, is a sterile, highly purified polyvalent antibody product containing in concentrated form all the IgG antibodies which regularly occur in the donor population (1). This immunoglobulin preparation is produced by cold alcohol fractionation from the plasma of over 16,000 volunteer US donors. Part of the fractionation may be performed by another US-licensed manufacturer. Sandoglobulin® (IGIV) is made

suitable for intravenous use by treatment at acid pH in the presence of trace amounts of pepsin (2,3). The preparation contains at least 96% of IgG and after reconstitution with a neutral unbuffered diluent has a pH of 6.6 $\pm$ 0.2. Most of the immunoglobulins are monomeric (7 S) IgG; the remainder consists of dimeric IgG and a small amount of polymeric IgG, traces of IgA and IgM and immunoglobulin fragments (4). The distribution of IgG subclasses corresponds to that of normal serum (5,6,7,8). Final container lyophilized units are prepared so as to contain 1, 3, 6, or 12 g protein with 1.67 g sucrose and less than 20 mg NaCl per gram of protein. The lyophilized preparation is devoid of any preservatives and may be reconstituted with sterile water, 5% dextrose or 0.9% saline to a solution with protein concentrations ranging from 3%-12%. The patient's fluid, electrolyte and caloric requirements should be considered in selecting an appropriate diluent and concentration.
*Hereinafter referred to as IGIV.

Table 1
Calculated Sandoglobulin® (IGIV) Osmolality (mOsm/kg)

Diluent	Concentration			
	3%	6%	9%	12%
0.9% NaCl	498	690	882	1074
5% Dextrose	444	636	828	1020
Sterile Water	192	384	576	768

CLINICAL PHARMACOLOGY
This product contains a broad spectrum of antibody specificities against bacterial, viral, parasitic, and mycoplasma antigens, that are capable of both opsonization and neutralization of microbes and toxins. The 3 week half-life of Immune Globulin Intravenous (Human), Sandoglobulin®, corresponds to that of Immune Globulin (Human) for intramuscular use, although individual variations in half-life have been observed (9,10). Appropriate doses of Sandoglobulin® (IGIV) restore abnormally low immunoglobulin G levels to the normal range. One hundred percent of the infused dose is available in the recipient's circulation immediately after infusion. After approximately 6 days, an equilibrium is reached between the intra- and extravascular compartments, with immunoglobulin G being distributed approximately 50% intravascular and 50% extravascular. In comparison, after the intramuscular injection of immune globulin, the IgG requires 2-5 days to reach its maximum concentration in the intravascular compartment. This concentration corresponds to about 40% of the injected dose (10).
While Sandoglobulin® (IGIV) has been shown to be effective in some cases of idiopathic thrombocytopenic purpura (ITP) *(see INDICATIONS AND USAGE)*, the mechanism of action in ITP has not been fully elucidated.
Toxicity from overdose has not been observed on regimens of 0.4 g/kg body weight each day for 5 days (11,12,13). Sucrose is added to Sandoglobulin® (IGIV) for reasons of stability, solubility, and safety.
The intravenous administration of the sucrose used for for stabilizing Immune Globulin Intravenous (Human), Sandoglobulin®, is considered to be innocuous (14). Because sucrose is excreted unchanged in the urine when given intravenously, Immune Globulin Intravenous (Human), Sandoglobulin® may be given to diabetics without compensatory changes in insulin dosage regimen.

INDICATIONS AND USAGE
Immunodeficiency
Sandoglobulin® (IGIV) is indicated for the maintenance treatment of patients with primary immunodeficiencies, e.g., in common variable immunodeficiency, severe combined immunodeficiency, and primary immunoglobulin deficiency syndromes such as X-linked agammaglobulinemia (12,15,16,17). Sandoglobulin® (IGIV) is preferable to intramuscular Immune Globulin (Human) preparations in treating patients who require an immediate and large increase in the intravascular immunoglobulin level (10), in patients with limited muscle mass, and in patients with bleeding tendencies for whom intramuscular injections are contraindicated. The infusions must be repeated at regular intervals.

Idiopathic Thrombocytopenic Purpura (ITP)
Acute
A controlled study was performed in children in which Sandoglobulin® (IGIV) was compared with steroids for the treatment of acute (defined as less than 6 months duration) ITP. In this study sequential platelet levels of 30,000, 100,000, and 150,000/μl were all achieved faster with Sandoglobulin® (IGIV) than with steroids and without any of the side effects associated with steroids (11,18). However,

Continued on next page

Sandoz—Cont.

it should be noted that many cases of acute ITP in childhood resolve spontaneously within weeks to months. Immune Globulin Intravenous (Human), Sandoglobulin®, has been used with good results in the treatment of acute ITP in adult patients (19,20,21). In a study involving 10 adults with ITP of less than 16 weeks duration, Sandoglobulin® (IGIV) therapy raised the platelet count to the normal range after a 5 day course. This effect lasted a mean of over 173 days, ranging from 30-372 days (22).

Chronic

Children and adults with chronic (defined as greater than 6 months duration) ITP have also shown an increase (sometimes temporary) in platelet counts upon administration of Immune Globulin Intravenous (Human), Sandoglobulin® (18,22,23,24,25,26). Therefore, in situations that require a rapid rise in platelet count, for example prior to surgery or to control excessive bleeding, use of Sandoglobulin® (IGIV) should be considered. In children with chronic ITP, Sandoglobulin® (IGIV) therapy resulted in a mean rise in platelet count of 312,000/μl with a duration of increase ranging from 2-6 months (23,26). Sandoglobulin® (IGIV) therapy may be considered as a means to defer or avoid splenectomy (25,26,27). In adults, Sandoglobulin® (IGIV) therapy has been shown to be effective in maintaining the platelet count in an acceptable range with or without periodic booster therapy. The mean rise in platelet count was 93,000/μl and the average duration of the increase was 20-24 days (22,23). However, it should be noted that not all patients will respond. Even in those patients who do respond, this treatment should not be considered to be curative.

CONTRAINDICATIONS

As with all blood products containing IgA, Sandoglobulin® (IGIV) is contraindicated in patients with selective IgA deficiency, who possess antibody to IgA. It may also be contraindicated in patients who have had severe systemic reactions to the intravenous or intramuscular administration of human immune globulin.

WARNINGS

Patients with agamma- or extreme hypogammaglobulinemia who have never before received immunoglobulin substitution treatment or whose time from last treatment is greater than 8 weeks, may be at risk of developing inflammatory reactions on rapid infusion of Immune Globulin Intravenous (Human), Sandoglobulin®, (over 20 drops [1 mL] per minute). These reactions are manifested by a rise in temperature, chills, nausea, and vomiting. The patient's vital signs should be monitored continuously and he should be carefully observed throughout the infusion, since these reactions on rare occasions may lead to shock. Epinephrine should be available for treatment of an acute anaphylactic reaction. Particular care should be exercised when Immune Globulin Intravenous (Human), Sandoglobulin®, is administered to patients with paraproteins (17).

PRECAUTIONS

Please see *DOSAGE AND ADMINISTRATION* below, for important information on Sandoglobulin® (IGIV) compatibility with other medications or fluids.

Pregnancy

Pregnancy Category C: Animal reproduction studies have not been conducted with Sandoglobulin® (IGIV). It is also not known whether Sandoglobulin® (IGIV) can cause fetal harm when administered to a pregnant woman or can affect reproduction capacity. Sandoglobulin® (IGIV) should be given to a pregnant woman only if clearly needed (21). Intact immune globulins such as those contained in Sandoglobulin® (IGIV) cross the placenta from maternal circulation increasingly after 30 weeks gestation (28,29). In cases of maternal ITP where Sandoglobulin® (IGIV) was administered to the mother prior to delivery, the platelet response and clinical effect were similar in the mother and neonate (21,29-38).

Pediatric Use

High dose administration of Immune Globulin Intravenous (Human), Sandoglobulin®, in children with acute or chronic idiopathic thrombocytopenic purpura did not reveal any pediatric-specific hazard (11).

Antibodies in Immune Globulin Intravenous (Human) may interfere with the response to live viral vaccines such as measles, mumps, and rubella. Immunizing physicians should be informed of recent therapy with Immune Globulin Intravenous (Human) so that appropriate precautions may be taken.

Aseptic Meningitis Syndrome

An aseptic meningitis syndrome (AMS) has been reported to occur infrequently in association with Immune Globulin Intravenous (Human) (IGIV) treatment. The syndrome usually begins within several hours to two days following IGIV treatment. It is characterized by symptoms and signs including severe headache, nuchal rigidity, drowsiness, fever, photophobia, painful eye movements, and nausea and vomiting. Cerebrospinal fluid studies are frequently positive with pleo-

cytosis up to several thousand cells per cu.mm., predominantly from the granulocytic series, and elevated protein levels up to several hundred mg/dl. Patients exhibiting such symptoms and signs should receive a thorough neurological examination, including CSF studies, to rule out other causes of meningitis. AMS may occur more frequently in association with high dose (2 g/kg) IGIV treatment. Discontinuation of IGIV treatment has resulted in remission of AMS within several days without sequelae.

ADVERSE REACTIONS

Adverse reactions to Sandoglobulin® (IGIV) are rare and occur in less than 1% of patients who are not immunodeficient. Agammaglobulinemic and hypogammaglobulinemic patients who have never received immunoglobulin substitution therapy before or whose time from last treatment is greater than 8 weeks may show adverse reactions if the initial infusion rate exceeds 20 drops (1 mL) per minute. This occurs in approximately 10% of such cases.

These reactions, which generally become apparent only 30 minutes to 1 hour after the beginning of the infusion, are as follows: flushing of the face, feelings of tightness in the chest, chills, fever, dizziness, nausea, diaphoresis, and hypotension. In such cases the infusion should be temporarily stopped until the symptoms have subsided. Immediate anaphylactoid and hypersensitivity reactions due to previous sensitization of the recipient to certain antigens, most commonly IgA, may be observed in exceptional cases, described under *CONTRAINDICATIONS* (12,13,39).

In patients with ITP, who receive higher doses (0.4 g/kg/day or greater) 2.9% of infusions may result in adverse reactions (18). Headache, generally mild, is the most common symptom noted, occurring during or following 2% of infusions.

DOSAGE AND ADMINISTRATION

It is generally advisable not to dilute plasma derivatives with other infusable drugs. Immune Globulin Intravenous (Human), Sandoglobulin®, should be given by a separate infusion line. No other medications or fluids should be mixed with the Sandoglobulin® (IGIV) preparation.

Adult and Child Substitution Therapy

The usual dose of Sandoglobulin® (IGIV) in immunodeficiency syndromes is 0.2 g/kg of body weight administered once a month by intravenous infusion. If the clinical response is inadequate, the dose may be increased to 0.3 g/kg of body weight or the infusion may be repeated more frequently than once a month (12,15,16,17).

The first infusion of Immune Globulin Intravenous (Human), Sandoglobulin®, in previously untreated agammaglobulinemic or hypogammaglobulinemic patients must be given as a 3% immunoglobulin solution (use the total volume of fluid provided, or see *Table 2*, to reconstitute the lyophilized product). Start with a flow rate of 10-20 drops (0.5-1.0 mL) per minute. After 15-30 minutes the rate of infusion may be further increased to 30-50 drops (1.5-2.5 mL) per minute.

After the first bottle of 3% solution is infused and the patient shows good tolerance, subsequent infusions may be administered at a higher rate or concentration. Such increases should be made gradually allowing 15-30 minutes before each increment.

Infusion of Immune Globulin Intravenous (Human), Sandoglobulin®, at rates up to 30 mg/kg/min has been achieved without any increase in the number or degree of adverse reactions observed (13). The first infusion of Sandoglobulin® (IGIV) in previously untreated agammaglobulinemic and hypogammaglobulinemic patients may lead to systemic side effects. Some of the effects may occur as a result of the reaction between the antibodies administered and free antigens in the blood and tissues of the immunodeficient recipient (39,41). When free antigen is no longer present, further administration of Sandoglobulin® (IGIV) to immunodeficient patients as well as to normal individuals usually does not cause further untoward side effects.

Therapy of Idiopathic Thrombocytopenic Purpura (ITP)

Induction

0.4 g/kg of body weight on 2-5 consecutive days.

Acute ITP-Childhood

In acute ITP of childhood, if an initial platelet count response to the first two doses is adequate (30-50,000/μl), therapy may be discontinued after the second day of the 5 day course (18).

Maintenance-Chronic ITP

In adults and children, if after induction therapy the platelet count falls to less than 30,000/μl and/or the patient manifests clinically significant bleeding, 0.4 g/kg of body weight may be given as a single infusion. If an adequate response does not result, the dose can be increased to 0.8-1.0 g/kg of body weight given as a single infusion (19, 40).

Reconstitution

For a 3% solution from the Sandoglobulin® (IGIV) kit

1. Tear off the protective caps from the bottle containing the solvent and the Immune Globulin Intravenous (Human), Sandoglobulin®. Disinfect both rubber stoppers with alcohol.

2. Remove the protective cover from one end of the transfer set and insert the needle through the rubber stopper into the bottle containing the solvent.

3. Remove the cover from the other needle and plunge the inverted Immune Globulin Intravenous (Human), Sandoglobulin®, bottle onto it, as shown in 3.

4. Invert the two bottles so that the solvent flows into the Sandoglobulin® (IGIV) bottle.

5. Discard the empty solvent bottle and the transfer set.

For a 6% solution from the Sandoglobulin® (IGIV) kit

1. Follow steps 1-3 aforementioned.

2. Invert the two bottles so that the solvent flows into the Immune Globulin Intravenous (Human), Sandoglobulin®, bottle. Use half the solvent by removing the solvent bottle with transfer needle as soon as the fluid reaches the 6% mark printed on the Sandoglobulin® (IGIV) label.

3. Discard any unused solvent and the transfer set.

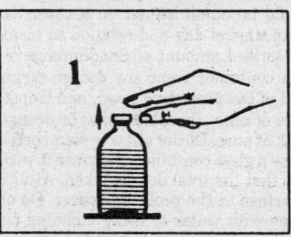

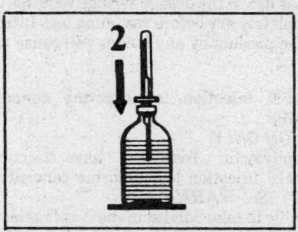

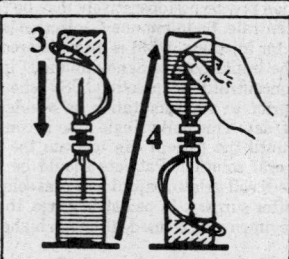

To reconstitute Sandoglobulin® (IGIV) from the multivial bulk pack, or when using other diluents or higher concentrations, *Table 2* indicates the volume of sterile diluent required. Observing aseptic technique, this volume should be drawn into a sterile hypodermic syringe and needle. The diluent is then injected into the corresponding Immune Globulin Intravenous (Human), Sandoglobulin®, vial size.

Table 2
Required Diluent Volume

Concentration	1 g Vial	3 g Vial	6 g Vial	12 g Vial
3%	33.0 cc	100 cc	200 cc	*
6%	16.5 cc	50 cc	100 cc	200 cc
9%	11.0 cc	33 cc	66 cc	132 cc
12%	8.3 cc	25 cc	50 cc	100 cc

*Container not large enough to permit this concentration

If large doses of Sandoglobulin® (IGIV) are to be administered, several reconstituted vials of identical concentration and diluent may be pooled in an empty sterile glass or plastic i.v. infusion container using aseptic technique.

Sandoglobulin® (IGIV) normally dissolves within a few minutes, though in exceptional cases it may take up to 20 minutes.

DO NOT SHAKE! Excessive shaking will cause foaming. Any undissolved particles should respond to careful rotation of the bottle. Avoid foaming. Parenteral drug products should be inspected visually for particulate matter and discoloration prior to administration, whenever solution and container permit.

Filtering of Immune Globulin Intravenous (Human), Sandoglobulin®, is acceptable but not required. Pore sizes of 15 microns or larger will be less likely to slow infusion, especially with higher Sandoglobulin® (IGIV) concentrations. Antibacterial filters (0.2 microns) may be used.

When reconstitution of Sandoglobulin® (IGIV) occurs outside of sterile laminar air flow conditions, administration

must begin promptly with partially used vials discarded. When reconstitution is carried out in a sterile laminar flow hood using aseptic technique, administration may begin within 24 hours provided the solution has been refrigerated during that time. Do not freeze Sandoglobulin® (IGIV) solution.

PROCEED WITH INFUSION ONLY IF SOLUTION IS CLEAR AND AT APPROXIMATELY ROOM TEMPERATURE!

HOW SUPPLIED

Immune Globulin Intravenous (Human), Sandoglobulin®, is available as a white lyophilized powder in 1, 3, 6, and 12 g size vials; it may be supplied with or without diluent. The only diluents which may be used to reconstitute the product are sterile (0.9%) Sodium Chloride Injection USP, 5% Dextrose, or Sterile Water.

Sandoglobulin® (IGIV) is available in bulk packs of ten vials (without diluent), and *either* individual vial packages (without diluent) or Kits [which contain the lyophilized preparation, diluent (sterile Sodium Chloride Injection USP), and one double-ended spike for reconstitution].

1 g

- Individual vial package (NDC 0078-0120-94) *or* Kit: Sandoglobulin® (NDC 0078-0120-58) and 33 mL Sodium Chloride Injection USP (NDC 0078-0125-39)

3 g

- Bulk pack (NDC 0078-0122-19)
- Individual vial package (NDC 0078-0122-95) *or* Kit: Sandoglobulin® (NDC 0078-0122-59) and 100 mL Sodium Chloride Injection USP (NDC 0078-0125-36)

6 g

- Bulk pack (NDC 0078-0124-19)
- Individual vial package (NDC 0078-0124-96) *or* Kit: Sandoglobulin® (NDC 0078-0124-60) and 200 mL Sodium Chloride Injection USP (NDC 0078-0125-37)

12 g

- Bulk pack (NDC 0078-0244-19)
- Individual vial package (NDC 0078-0244-93)

Please see *Table 1* for Calculated Sandoglobulin® (IGIV) Osmolality (mOsm/kg).

Store and Dispense

Immune Globulin Intravenous (Human), Sandoglobulin®, should be stored at room temperature not exceeding 30°C (86°F). The preparation should not be used after the expiration date printed on the label.

References

1. Gardi A: Quality control in the production of an immunoglobulin for intravenous use. *Blut* **48**:337–344, 1984.
2. Römer J, Morgenthaler JJ, Scherz R, et al: Characterization of various immunoglobulin-preparations for intravenous application. I. Protein composition and antibody content. *Vox Sang* **42**:62-73, 1982.
3. Römer J, Späth PJ, Skvaril F, et al: Characterization of various immunoglobulin preparations for intravenous application. II. Complement activation and binding to Staphylococcus protein A. *Vox Sang* **42**:74-80, 1982.
4. Römer J, Späth PJ: Molecular composition of immunoglobulin preparations and its relation to complement activation, in Nydegger UE (ed): *Immunohemotherapy: A Guide to Immunoglobulin Prophylaxis and Therapy.* London, Academic Press, 1981, p 123.
5. Skvaril F, Roth-Wicky B, and Barandun S: IgG subclasses in human-γ-globulin preparations for intravenous use and their reactivity with Staphylococcus protein A. *Vox Sang* **38**:147, 1980.
6. Skvaril F: Qualitative and quantitative aspects of IgG subclasses in i.v. immunoglobulin preparations, in Nydegger UE (ed): *Immunohemotherapy: A Guide to Immunoglobulin Prophylaxis and Therapy.* London, Academic Press, 1981, p 113.
7. Skvaril F, and Barandun S: In vitro characterization of immunoglobulins for intravenous use, in Alving BM, Finlayson JS (eds): *Immunoglobulins: Characteristics and Uses of Intravenous Preparations,* DHHS Publication No. (FDA)-80-9005. US Government Printing Office, 1980, pp 201-206.
8. Burckhardt JJ, Gardi A, Oxelius V, et al: Immunoglobulin G subclass distribution in three human intravenous immunoglobulin preparations. *Vox Sang* **57**:10-14, 1989.
9. Morell A, and Skvaril F: Struktur und biologische Eigenschaften von Immunoglobulinen und γ-Globulin-Präparaten. II. Eigenschaften von γ-Globulin-Präparaten. *Schweiz Med Wochenschr* **110**:80, 1980.
10. Morell A, Schürch B, Ryser D, et al: In vivo behavior of gamma globulin preparations. *Vox Sang* **38**:272, 1980.
11. Imbach P, Barandun S, d'Apuzzo V, et al: High-dose intravenous gamma globulin for idiopathic thrombocytopenic purpura in childhood. *Lancet* **1**:1228, 1981.
12. Barandun S, Morell A, Skvaril F: Clinical experiences with immunoglobulin for intravenous use, in Alving BM, Finlayson JS (eds): *Immunoglobulins: Characteristics and Uses of Intravenous Preparations.* DHHS Publication No. (FDA)-80-9005. US Government Printing Office, 1980, pp 31-35.
13. Schiff R, Sedlak D, Buckley R: Rapid infusion of Sandoglobulin® in patients with primary humoral immunodeficiency. *J Allergy Clin Immunol* **88**:61, 1991.
14. Wade A (ed): *Martindale: The Extra Pharmacopoeia,* ed 27. London, The Pharmaceutical Press, 1979, p 65.
15. Joller PW, Barandun S, Hitzig WH: Neue Möglichkeiten der Immunoglobulin-Ersatztherapie bei Antikörpermangel. Syndrom. *Schweiz Med Wochenschr* **110**:1451, 1980.
16. Barandun S, Imbach P, Morell A, et al: Clinical indications for immunoglobulin infusion, in Nydegger UE (ed): *Immunohemotherapy: A Guide to Immunoglobulin Prophylaxis and Therapy.* London, Academic Press, 1981, p 275.
17. Cunningham-Rundles C, Smithwick EM, Siegal FP, et al: Treatment of primary humoral immunodeficiency disease with intravenous (pH 4.0 treated) gamma globulin, in Nydegger UE (ed): *Immunohemotherapy: A Guide to Immunoglobulin Prophylaxis and Therapy.* London, Academic Press, 1981, p 283.
18. Imbach P, Wagner HP, Berchtold W, et al: Intravenous immunoglobulin versus oral corticosteroids in acute immune thrombocytopenic purpura in childhood. *Lancet* **2**:464, 1985.
19. Fehr J, Hofmann V, Kappeler U: Transient reversal of thrombocytopenia in idiopathic thrombocytopenic purpura by high-dose intravenous gamma globulin. *N Engl J Med* **306**:1254, 1982.
20. Müeller-Eckhardt C, Küenzlen E, Thilo-Körner D, et al: High-dose intravenous immunoglobulin for posttransfusion purpura. *N Engl J Med* **308**:287, 1983.
21. Wenske G, Gaedicke G, Küenzlen E, et al: Treatment of idiopathic thrombocytopenic purpura in pregnancy by high-dose intravenous immunoglobulin. *Blut* **46**:347-353, 1983.
22. Newland AC, Treleaven JG, Minchinton B, et al: High-dose intravenous IgG in adults with autoimmune thrombocytopenia. *Lancet* **1**:84-87, 1983.
23. Bussel JB, Kimberly RP, Inman RD, et al: Intravenous gammaglobulin for chronic idiopathic thrombocytopenic purpura. *Blood* **62**:480-486, 1983.
24. Abe T, Matsuda J, Kawasugi K, et al: Clinical effect of intravenous immunoglobulin in chronic idiopathic thrombocytopenic purpura. *Blut* **47**:69-75, 1983.
25. Bussel JB, Schulman I, Hilgartner MW, et al: Intravenous use of gamma globulin in the treatment of chronic immune thrombocytopenic purpura as a means to defer splenectomy. *J Pediatr* **103**:651-654, 1983.
26. Imholz B, et al: Intravenous immunoglobulin (i.v. IgG) for previously treated acute or for chronic idiopathic thrombocytopenic purpura (ITP) in childhood: A prospective multicenter study. *Blut* **56**:63-68, 1988.
27. Lusher JM, and Warrier I: Use of intravenous gamma globulin in children with idiopathic thrombocytopenic purpura and other immune thrombocytopenias. *Am J Med* **83(suppl 4A)**:10-16, 1987.
28. Hammarstrom L, and Smith CI: Placental transfer of intravenous immunoglobulin. *Lancet* **1**:681, 1986.
29. Sidiropoulos D, et al: Transplacental passage of intravenous immunoglobulin in the last trimester of pregnancy. *J Pediatr* **109**:505-508, 1986.
30. Wenske G, et al: Idiopathic thrombocytopenic purpura in pregnancy and neonatal period. *Blut* **48**:377-382, 1984.
31. Fabris P, et al: Successful treatment of a steroid-resistant form of idiopathic thrombocytopenic purpura in pregnancy with high doses of intravenous immunoglobulins. *Acta Haemat* **77**:107-110, 1987.
32. Coller BS, et al: Management of severe ITP during pregnancy with intravenous immunoglobulin (IVIgG). *Clin Res* **33**:545A, 1985.
33. Tchernia G, et al: Management of immune thrombocytopenia in pregnancy: Response to infusions of immunoglobulins. *Am J Obstet Gynecol* **148**:225-226, 1984.
34. Newland AC, et al: Intravenous IgG for autoimmune thrombocytopenia in pregnancy. *N Engl J Med* **310**:261-262, 1984.
35. Morgenstern GR, et al: Autoimmune thrombocytopenia in pregnancy: New approach to management. *Br Med J* **287**:584, 1983.
36. Ciccimarra F, et al: Treatment of neonatal passive immune thrombocytopenia. *J Pediat* **105**:677-678, 1984.
37. Rose VL, and Gordon LI: Idiopathic thrombocytopenic purpura in pregnancy. Successful management with immunoglobulin infusion. *JAMA* **254**:2626-2628, 1985.
38. Gounder MP, et al: Intravenous gammaglobulin therapy in the management of a patient with idiopathic thrombocytopenic purpura and a warm autoimmune erythrocyte panagglutinin during pregnancy. *Obstet Gynecol* **67**:741-746, 1986.
39. Cunningham-Rundles C, Day NK, Wahn V, et al: Reactions to intravenous gamma globulin infusions and immune complex formation, in Nydegger UE (ed): *Immunohemotherapy: A Guide to Immunoglobulin Prophylaxis and Therapy.* London, Academic Press, 1981, p 447.
40. Bussel JB, Pham LC, Hilgartner MW, et al: Long-term maintenance of adults with ITP using intravenous gamma globulin. Abstract, *American Society of Hematology.* New Orleans, December, 1985.
41. Barandun S, Morell A: Adverse reactions to immunoglobulin preparations, in Nydegger UE (ed): *Immunohemotherapy: A Guide to Immunoglobulin Prophylaxis and Therapy.* London, Academic Press, 1981, p 223.

Manufactured by:
CENTRAL LABORATORY
BLOOD TRANSFUSION SERVICE
SWISS RED CROSS
Wankdorfstrasse 10, 3000 Berne 22
Switzerland
US License No. 647
Distributed by:
SANDOZ PHARMACEUTICALS CORPORATION
East Hanover, NJ 07936
[REV: JUNE 1995 30484902]

SANDOSTATIN® ℞

octreotide acetate/SANDOZ
INJECTION

CAUTION: Federal law prohibits dispensing without a prescription.

The following prescribing information is based on official labeling in effect on August 1, 1996.

DESCRIPTION

Sandostatin® (octreotide acetate) Injection, a cyclic octapeptide prepared as a clear sterile solution of octreotide, acetate salt, in buffered sodium chloride for administration by deep subcutaneous (intrafat) or intravenous injection. Octreotide acetate, known chemically as L-Cysteinamide, D-phenylalanyl-L-cysteinyl -L- phenylalanyl -D- tryptophyl-L-lysyl -L- threonyl -N- [2- hydroxy -1- (hydroxymethyl) propyl]-,cyclic (2→7)-disulfide; [R-(R*, R*)] acetate salt, is a long-acting octapeptide with pharmacologic actions mimicking those of the natural hormone somatostatin.

Sandostatin® (octreotide acetate) Injection is available as: sterile 1 mL ampuls in 3 strengths, containing 50, 100, or 500 mcg octreotide (as acetate), and sterile 5 mL multi-dose vials in 2 strengths, containing 200 and 1000 mcg/mL of octreotide (as acetate).

Each ampul also contains:

acetic acid, glacial, USP	2.0 mg
sodium acetate trihydrate, USP	2.0 mg
sodium chloride, USP	7.0 mg
water for injection, qs to	1.0 mL

Each mL of the multi-dose vials also contains:

acetic acid, glacial, USP	2.0 mg
sodium acetate trihydrate, USP	2.0 mg
sodium chloride, USP	7.0 mg
phenol, USP	5.0 mg
water for injection, qs to	1.0 mL

Acetic acid and sodium acetate trihydrate are added to provide a buffered solution, pH 4.2 ± 0.3.

The molecular weight of octreotide acetate is 1019.3 (free peptide, $C_{49}H_{66}N_{10}O_{10}S_2$) and its amino acid sequence is:

H-D-Phe-Cys-Phe-D-Trp-Lys-Thr-Cys-Thr-ol,
x CH_3COOH where x = 1.4 to 2.5

CLINICAL PHARMACOLOGY

Sandostatin® (octreotide acetate) exerts pharmacologic actions similar to the natural hormone, somatostatin. It is an even more potent inhibitor of growth hormone, glucagon, and insulin than somatostatin. Like somatostatin, it also suppresses LH response to GnRH, decreases splanchnic blood flow, and inhibits release of serotonin, gastrin, vasoactive intestinal peptide, secretin, motilin, and pancreatic polypeptide.

By virtue of these pharmacological actions, Sandostatin® (octreotide acetate) has been used to treat the symptoms associated with metastatic carcinoid tumors (flushing and diarrhea), and Vasoactive Intestinal Peptide (VIP) secreting adenomas (watery diarrhea).

Sandostatin® (octreotide acetate) substantially reduces growth hormone and/or IGF-I (somatomedin C) levels in patients with acromegaly.

Single doses of Sandostatin (octreotide acetate) have been shown to inhibit gallbladder contractility and to decrease bile secretion in normal volunteers. In controlled clinical trials the incidence of gallstone or biliary sludge formation was markedly increased (*See WARNINGS*).

Sandostatin® (octreotide acetate) suppresses secretion of thyroid stimulating hormone (TSH).

Continued on next page

Sandoz—Cont.

Pharmacokinetics

After subcutaneous injection, octreotide is absorbed rapidly and completely from the injection site. Peak concentrations of 5.2 ng/mL (100 mcg dose) were reached 0.4 hours after dosing. Using a specific radioimmunoassay, intravenous and subcutaneous doses were found to be bioequivalent. Peak concentrations and area under the curve values were dose proportional both after subcutaneous or intravenous single doses up to 400 mcg and with multiple doses of 200 mcg t.i.d. (600 mcg/day). Clearance was reduced by about 66% suggesting non-linear kinetics of the drug at daily doses of 600 mcg/day as compared to 150 mcg/day. The relative decrease in clearance with doses above 600 mcg/day is not defined.

In healthy volunteers the distribution of octreotide from plasma was rapid ($t\alpha^{1}/_{2}=0.2$ h), the volume of distribution (Vdss) was estimated to be 13.6 L, and the total body clearance was 10 L/hr.

In blood, the distribution into the erythrocytes was found to be negligible and about 65% was bound in the plasma in a concentration-independent manner. Binding was mainly to lipoprotein and, to a lesser extent, to albumin.

The elimination of octreotide from plasma had an apparent half-life of 1.7 hours compared with 1-3 minutes with the natural hormone. The duration of action of Sandostatin® (octreotide acetate) is variable but extends up to 12 hours depending upon the type of tumor. About 32% of the dose is excreted unchanged into the urine. In an elderly population, dose adjustments may be necessary due to a significant increase in the half-life (46%) and a significant decrease in the clearance (26%) of the drug.

In patients with acromegaly, the pharmacokinetics differ somewhat from those in healthy volunteers. A mean peak concentration of 2.8 ng/mL (100 mcg dose) was reached in 0.7 hours after subcutaneous dosing. The volume of distribution (Vdss) was estimated to be 21.6 ± 8.5 L and the total body clearance was increased to 18 L/h. The mean percent of the drug bound was 41.2%. The disposition and elimination half-lives were similar to normals.

In patients with severe renal failure requiring dialysis, clearance was reduced to about half that found in normal subjects (from approximately 10 L/h to 4.5 L/h). The effect of hepatic diseases on the disposition of octreotide is unknown.

INDICATIONS AND USAGE

Acromegaly

Sandostatin® (octreotide acetate) is indicated to reduce blood levels of growth hormone and IGF-I (somatomedin C) in acromegaly patients who have had inadequate response to or cannot be treated with surgical resection, pituitary irradiation, and bromocriptine mesylate at maximally tolerated doses. The goal is to achieve normalization of growth hormone and IGF-I (somatomedin C) levels (See DOSAGE AND ADMINISTRATION). In patients with acromegaly, Sandostatin® (octreotide acetate) reduces growth hormone to within normal ranges in 50% of patients and reduces IGF-I (somatomedin C) to within normal ranges in 50%-60% of patients. Since the effects of pituitary irradiation may not become maximal for several years, adjunctive therapy with Sandostatin® (octreotide acetate) to reduce blood levels of growth hormone and IGF-I (somatomedin C) offers potential benefit before the effects of irradiation are manifested.

Improvement in clinical signs and symptoms or reduction in tumor size or rate of growth were not shown in clinical trials performed with Sandostatin® (octreotide acetate); these trials were not optimally designed to detect such effects.

Carcinoid Tumors

Sandostatin® (octreotide acetate) is indicated for the symptomatic treatment of patients with metastatic carcinoid tumors where it suppresses or inhibits the severe diarrhea and flushing episodes associated with the disease.

Sandostatin® (octreotide acetate) studies were not designed to show an effect on the size, rate of growth or development of metastases.

Vasoactive Intestinal Peptide Tumors (VIPomas)

Sandostatin® (octreotide acetate) is indicated for the treatment of the profuse watery diarrhea associated with VIP-secreting tumors. Sandostatin® (octreotide acetate) studies were not designed to show an effect on the size, rate of growth or development of metastases.

CONTRAINDICATIONS

Sensitivity to this drug or any of its components.

WARNINGS

Single doses of Sandostatin® (octreotide acetate) have been shown to inhibit gallbladder contractility and decrease bile secretion in normal volunteers. In clinical trials (primarily patients with acromegaly or psoriasis), the incidence of biliary tract abnormalities was 63% (27% gallstones, 24% sludge without stones, 12% biliary duct dilatation). The incidence of stones or sludge in patients who received Sandostatin® (octreotide acetate) for 12 months or longer

was 52%. Less than 2% of patients treated with Sandostatin® (octreotide acetate) for 1 month or less developed gallstones. The incidence of gallstones did not appear related to age, sex or dose. Like patients without gallbladder abnormalities, the majority of patients developing gallbladder abnormalities on ultrasound had gastrointestinal symptoms. The symptoms were not specific for gallbladder disease. A few patients developed acute cholecystitis, ascending cholangitis, biliary obstruction, cholestatic hepatitis, or pancreatitis during Sandostatin® (octreotide acetate) therapy or following its withdrawal. One patient developed ascending cholangitis during Sandostatin® (octreotide acetate) therapy and died.

PRECAUTIONS

General

Sandostatin® (octreotide acetate) alters the balance between the counterregulatory hormones, insulin, glucagon and growth hormone, which may result in hypoglycemia or hyperglycemia. Sandostatin® (octreotide acetate) also suppresses secretion of thyroid stimulating hormone, which may result in hypothyroidism. Cardiac conduction abnormalities have also occurred during treatment with Sandostatin® (octreotide acetate). However, the incidence of these adverse events during long-term therapy was determined vigorously only in acromegaly patients who, due to their underlying disease and/or the subsequent treatment they receive, are at an increased risk for the development of diabetes mellitus, hypothyroidism, and cardiovascular disease. Although the degree to which these abnormalities are related to Sandostatin® (octreotide acetate) therapy is not clear, new abnormalities of glycemic control, thyroid function and ECG developed during Sandostatin® (octreotide acetate) therapy as described below.

The hypoglycemia or hyperglycemia which occurs during Sandostatin® (octreotide acetate) therapy is usually mild, but may result in overt diabetes mellitus or necessitate dose changes in insulin or other hypoglycemic agents. Hypoglycemia and hyperglycemia occurred on Sandostatin® (octreotide acetate) in 3% and 16% of acromegalic patients, respectively. Severe hyperglycemia, subsequent pneumonia, and death following initiation of Sandostatin® (octreotide acetate) therapy was reported in one patient with no history of hyperglycemia.

In acromegalic patients, 12% developed biochemical hypothyroidism only, 8% developed goiter, and 4% required initiation of thyroid replacement therapy while receiving Sandostatin® (octreotide acetate). Baseline and periodic assessment of thyroid function (TSH, total and/or free T_4) is recommended during chronic therapy.

In acromegalics, bradycardia (<50 bpm) developed in 25%; conduction abnormalities occurred in 10% and arrhythmias occurred in 9% of patients during Sandostatin® (octreotide acetate) therapy. Other EKG changes observed included QT prolongation, axis shifts, early repolarization, low voltage, R/S transition, and early R wave progression. These ECG changes are not uncommon in acromegalic patients. Dose adjustments in drugs such as beta-blockers that have bradycardia effects may be necessary. In one acromegalic patient with severe congestive heart failure, initiation of Sandostatin® (octreotide acetate) therapy resulted in worsening of CHF with improvement when drug was discontinued. Confirmation of a drug effect was obtained with a positive rechallenge.

Several cases of pancreatitis have been reported in patients receiving Sandostatin® (octreotide acetate) therapy.

Sandostatin® (octreotide acetate) may alter absorption of dietary fats in some patients.

In patients with severe renal failure requiring dialysis, the half-life of Sandostatin® (octreotide acetate) may be increased, necessitating adjustment of the maintenance dosage.

Depressed vitamin B_{12} levels and abnormal Schilling's tests have been observed in some patients receiving Sandostatin® (octreotide acetate) therapy, and monitoring of vitamin B_{12} levels is recommended during chronic Sandostatin® (octreotide acetate) therapy.

Information for Patients

Careful instruction in sterile subcutaneous injection technique should be given to the patients and to other persons who may administer Sandostatin® (octreotide acetate) Injection.

Laboratory Tests

Laboratory tests that may be helpful as biochemical markers in determining and following patient response depend on the specific tumor. Based on diagnosis, measurement of the following substances may be useful in monitoring the progress of therapy:

Acromegaly: Growth Hormone, IGF-I (somatomedin C)

Responsiveness to Sandostatin® (octreotide acetate) may be evaluated by determining growth hormone levels at 1-4 hour intervals for 8-12 hours post dose. Alternatively, a single measurement of IGF-I (somatomedin C) level

may be made two weeks after drug initiation or dosage change.

Carcinoid: 5-HIAA (urinary 5-hydroxyindole acetic acid), plasma serotonin, plasma Substance P

VIPoma: VIP (plasma vasoactive intestinal peptide)

Baseline and periodic total and/or free T_4 measurements should be performed during chronic therapy (see PRECAUTIONS — General).

Drug Interactions

Sandostatin® (octreotide acetate) has been associated with alterations in nutrient absorption, so it may have an effect on absorption of orally administered drugs. Concomitant administration of Sandostatin® (octreotide acetate) with cyclosporine may decrease blood levels of cyclosporine and result in transplant rejection.

Patients receiving insulin, oral hypoglycemic agents, beta blockers, calcium channel blockers, or agents to control fluid and electrolyte balance, may require dose adjustments of these therapeutic agents.

Drug Laboratory Test Interactions

No known interference exists with clinical laboratory tests, including amine or peptide determinations.

Carcinogenesis/Mutagenesis/Impairment of Fertility

Studies in laboratory animals have demonstrated no mutagenic potential of Sandostatin® (octreotide acetate).

No carcinogenic potential was demonstrated in mice treated subcutaneously for 85-99 weeks at doses up to 2000 mcg/kg/day (8× the human exposure based on body surface area). In a 116-week subcutaneous study in rats, a 27% and 12% incidence of injection site sarcomas or squamous cell carcinomas was observed in males and females, respectively, at the highest dose level of 1250 mcg/kg/day (10× the human exposure based on body surface area) compared to an incidence of 8%-10% in the vehicle control groups. The increased incidence of injection site tumors was most probably caused by irritation and the high sensitivity of the rat to repeated subcutaneous injections at the same site. Rotating injection sites would prevent chronic irritation in humans. There have been no reports of injection site tumors in patients treated with Sandostatin® (octreotide acetate) for up to 5 years. There was also a 15% incidence of uterine adenocarcinomas in the 1250 mcg/kg/day females compared to 7% in the saline control females and 0% in the vehicle control females. The presence of endometritis coupled with the absence of corpora lutea, the reduction in mammary fibroadenomas, and the presence of uterine dilatation suggest that the uterine tumors were associated with estrogen dominance in the aged female rats which does not occur in humans.

Sandostatin® (octreotide acetate) did not impair fertility in rats at doses up to 1000 mcg/kg/day, which represents 7× the human exposure based on body surface area.

Pregnancy Category B

Reproduction studies have been performed in rats and rabbits at doses up to 16 times the highest human dose based on body surface area and have revealed no evidence of impaired fertility or harm to the fetus due to Sandostatin® (octreotide acetate). There are, however, no adequate and well-controlled studies in pregnant women. Because animal reproduction studies are not always predictive of human response, this drug should be used during pregnancy only if clearly needed.

Nursing Mothers

It is not known whether this drug is excreted in human milk. Because many drugs are excreted in milk, caution should be exercised when Sandostatin® (octreotide acetate) is administered to a nursing woman.

Pediatric Use

Experience with Sandostatin® (octreotide acetate) in the pediatric population is limited. The youngest patient to receive the drug was 1 month old. Doses of 1-10 mcg/kg body weight were well tolerated in the young patients. A single case of an infant (nesidioblastosis) was complicated by a seizure thought to be independent of Sandostatin® (octreotide acetate) therapy.

ADVERSE REACTIONS

Gallbladder Abnormalities

Gallbladder abnormalities, especially stones and/or biliary sludge, frequently develop in patients on chronic Sandostatin® (octreotide acetate) therapy (See WARNINGS).

Cardiac

In acromegalics, sinus bradycardia (<50 bpm) developed in 25%; conduction abnormalities occurred in 10% and arrhythmias developed in 9% of patients during Sandostatin® (octreotide acetate) therapy (See PRECAUTIONS— General).

Gastrointestinal

Diarrhea, loose stools, nausea and abdominal discomfort were each seen in 34%-61% of acromegalic patients in US studies although only 2.6% of the patients discontinued ther-

apy due to these symptoms. These symptoms were seen in 5%-10% of patients with other disorders.

The frequency of these symptoms was not dose-related, but diarrhea and abdominal discomfort generally resolved more quickly in patients treated with 300 mcg/day than in those treated with 750 mcg/day. Vomiting, flatulence, abnormal stools, abdominal distention, and constipation were each seen in less than 10% of patients.

Hypo/Hyperglycemia

Hypoglycemia and hyperglycemia occurred in 3% and 16% of acromegalic patients, respectively, but only in about 1.5% of other patients. Symptoms of hypoglycemia were noted in approximately 2% of patients.

Hypothyroidism

In acromegalics, biochemical hypothyroidism alone occurred in 12% while goiter occurred in 6% during Sandostatin® (octreotide acetate) therapy (*See PRECAUTIONS — General*). In patients without acromegaly, hypothyroidism has only been reported in several isolated patients and goiter has not been reported.

Other Adverse Events

Pain on injection was reported in 7.7%, headache in 6% and dizziness in 5%.

Other Adverse Events 1%–4%

Other events (relationship to drug not established), each observed in 1%-4% of patients, included fatigue, weakness, pruritus, joint pain, backache, urinary tract infection, cold symptoms, flu symptoms, injection site hematoma, bruise, edema, flushing, blurred vision, pollakiuria, fat malabsorption, hair loss, visual disturbance and depression.

Other Adverse Events < 1%

Events reported in less than 1% of patients and for which relationship to drug is not established are listed: *Gastrointestinal:* hepatitis, jaundice, increase in liver enzymes, GI bleeding, hemorrhoids, appendicitis, gastric/peptic ulcer, gallbladder polyp; *Integumentary:* rash, cellulitis, petechiae, urticaria, basal cell carcinoma; *Musculoskeletal:* arthritis, joint effusion, muscle pain, Raynaud's phenomenon; *Cardiovascular:* chest pain, shortness of breath, thrombophlebitis, ischemia, congestive heart failure, hypertension, hypertensive reaction, palpitations, orthostatic BP decrease, tachycardia; *CNS:* anxiety, libido decrease, syncope, tremor, seizure, vertigo, Bell's Palsy, paranoia, pituitary apoplexy, increased intraocular pressure, amnesia, hearing loss, neuritis; *Respiratory:* pneumonia, pulmonary nodule, status asthmaticus; *Endocrine:* galactorrhea, hypoadrenalism, diabetes insipidus, gynecomastia, amenorrhea, polymenorrhea, oligomenorrhea, vaginitis; *Urogenital:* nephrolithiasis, hematuria; *Hematologic:* anemia, iron deficiency, epistaxis; *Miscellaneous:* otitis, allergic reaction, increased CK, weight loss.

Evaluation of 20 patients treated for at least 6 months has failed to demonstrate titers of antibodies exceeding background levels. However, antibody titers to Sandostatin® (octreotide acetate) were subsequently reported in three patients and resulted in prolonged duration of drug action in two patients. Anaphylactoid reactions, including anaphylactic shock, have been reported in several patients receiving Sandostatin® (octreotide acetate).

OVERDOSAGE

No frank overdose has occurred in any patient to date. Intravenous bolus doses of 1 mg (1000 mcg) given to healthy volunteers and of 30 mg (30,000 mcg) IV over 20 minutes and of 120 mg (120,000 mcg) IV over 8 hours to research patients have not resulted in serious ill effects.

Up-to-date information about the treatment of overdose can often be obtained from a certified Regional Poison Control Center. Telephone numbers of certified Regional Poison Control Centers are listed in the Physicians' Desk Reference® (PDR).*

Mortality occurred in mice and rats given 72 mg/kg and 18 mg/kg IV, respectively.

*Trademark of Medical Economics Company Inc.

Drug Abuse and Dependence

There is no indication that Sandostatin® (octreotide acetate) has potential for drug abuse or dependence. Sandostatin® (octreotide acetate) levels in the central nervous system are negligible, even after doses up to 30,000 mcg.

DOSAGE AND ADMINISTRATION

Sandostatin® (octreotide acetate) may be administered subcutaneously or intravenously. Subcutaneous injection is the usual route of administration of Sandostatin® (octreotide acetate) for control of symptoms. Pain with subcutaneous administration may be reduced by using the smallest volume that will deliver the desired dose. Multiple subcutaneous injections at the same site within short periods of time should be avoided. Sites should be rotated in a systematic manner.

Parenteral drug products should be inspected visually for particulate matter and discoloration prior to administration. **Do not use if particulates and/or discoloration are observed.** Proper sterile technique should be used in the preparation of parenteral admixtures to minimize the possibility of microbial contamination. **Sandostatin® (octreotide acetate) is not compatible in Total Parenteral Nutrition (TPN) solutions because of the formation of a glycosyl octreotide conjugate which may decrease the efficacy of the product.**

Sandostatin® (octreotide acetate) is stable in sterile isotonic saline solutions or sterile solutions of dextrose 5% in water for 24 hours. It may be diluted in volumes of 50-200 mL and infused intravenously over 15-30 minutes or administered by IV push over 3 minutes. In emergency situations (e.g.: carcinoid crisis) it may be given by rapid bolus.

The initial dosage is usually 50 mcg administered twice or three times daily. Upward dose titration is frequently required. Dosage information for patients with specific tumors follows.

Acromegaly

Dosage may be initiated at 50 mcg t.i.d. Beginning with this low dose may permit adaptation to adverse gastrointestinal effects for patients who will require higher doses. IGF-I (somatomedin C) levels every 2 weeks can be used to guide titration. Alternatively, multiple growth hormone levels at 0-8 hours after Sandostatin® (octreotide acetate) administration permit more rapid titration of dose. The goal is to achieve growth hormone levels less than 5 ng/mL or IGF-I (somatomedin C) levels less than 1.9 U/mL in males and less than 2.2 U/mL in females. The dose most commonly found to be effective is 100 mcg t.i.d., but some patients require up to 500 mcg t.i.d. for maximum effectiveness. Doses greater than 300 mcg/day seldom result in additional biochemical benefit, and if an increase in dose fails to provide additional benefit, the dose should be reduced. IGF-I (somatomedin C) or growth hormone levels should be reevaluated at 6 month intervals.

Sandostatin® (octreotide acetate) should be withdrawn yearly for approximately 4 weeks from patients who have received irradiation to assess disease activity. If growth hormone or IGF-I (somatomedin C) levels increase and signs and symptoms recur, Sandostatin® (octreotide acetate) therapy may be resumed.

Carcinoid Tumors

The suggested daily dosage of Sandostatin® (octreotide acetate) during the first 2 weeks of therapy ranges from 100–600 mcg/day in 2-4 divided doses (mean daily dosage is 300 mcg). In the clinical studies, the **median** daily maintenance dosage was approximately 450 mcg, but clinical and biochemical benefits were obtained in some patients with as little as 50 mcg, while others required doses up to 1500 mcg/day. However, experience with doses above 750 mcg/day is limited.

VIPomas

Daily dosages of 200-300 mcg in 2-4 divided doses are recommended during the initial 2 weeks of therapy (range 150-750 mcg) to control symptoms of the disease. On an individual basis, dosage may be adjusted to achieve a therapeutic response, but usually doses above 450 mcg/day are not required.

HOW SUPPLIED

Sandostatin® (octreotide acetate) Injection is available in 1 mL ampuls and 5 mL multi-dose vials as follows:

Ampuls

50 mcg/mL octreotide (as acetate)
Package of 20 ampuls (NDC 0078-0180-03)
Package of 50 ampuls (NDC 0078-0180-04)

100 mcg/mL octreotide (as acetate)
Package of 20 ampuls (NDC 0078-0181-03)
Package of 50 ampuls (NDC 0078-0181-04)

500 mcg/mL octreotide (as acetate)
Package of 20 ampuls (NDC 0078-0182-03)
Package of 50 ampuls (NDC 0078-0182-04)

Multi-Dose Vials

200 mcg/mL octreotide (as acetate)
Box of one (NDC 0078-0183-25)

1000 mcg/mL octreotide (as acetate)
Box of one (NDC 0078-0184-25)

Storage

For prolonged storage, Sandostatin® (octreotide acetate) ampuls and multi-dose vials should be stored at refrigerated temperatures 2°-8°C (36°-46°F) and protected from light. At room temperature, (20°-30°C or 70°-86°F), Sandostatin® (octreotide acetate) is stable for 14 days if protected from light. The solution can be allowed to come to room temperature prior to administration. Do not warm artificially. After initial use, multiple dose vials should be discarded within 14 days. Ampuls should be opened just prior to administration and the unused portion discarded.

The ampuls are manufactured by
SANDOZ PHARMA LTD., Basle, Switzerland for
SANDOZ PHARMACEUTICALS CORPORATION,
East Hanover, New Jersey 07936
The multi-dose vials are manufactured by
SCHERING-PLOUGH PRODUCTS, INC.,
Manati, Puerto Rico for
SANDOZ PHARMACEUTICALS CORPORATION,
East Hanover, New Jersey 07936

[REV: DECEMBER 1995 30283902]

SANOREX® C ℞

[san 'ō-rex"]

(mazindol) tablets, USP

Caution: Federal law prohibits dispensing without prescription.

The following prescribing information is based on official labeling in effect on August 1, 1996.

DESCRIPTION

Sanorex® (mazindol) is an imidazoisoindole anorectic agent. It is chemically designated as 5-(4-chlorophenyl)-2,5-dihydro-3H-imidazo[2,1-a]isoindol-5-ol, a tautomeric form of 2-[(2′)-(p-chlorobenzoyl) phenyl]-2-imidazoline, and has the following structure:

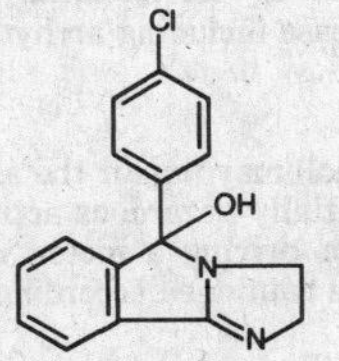

$C_{16}H_{13}ClN_2O$ Mol. wt. 284.74

1 mg and 2 mg Tablets

Active Ingredient: mazindol, USP.

Inactive Ingredients: calcium sulfate dihydrate, NF; lactose, NF; magnesium stearate, NF; povidone, USP; starch, NF; and talc, USP.

ACTIONS

Sanorex® (mazindol), although an isoindole, has pharmacologic activity similar in many ways to the prototype drugs used in obesity, the amphetamines. Actions include central nervous system stimulation in humans and animals, as well as such amphetamine-like effects in animals as the production of stereotyped behavior. Animal experiments also suggest certain differences from phenethylamine anorectic drugs, e.g., amphetamine, with respect to site and mechanism of action; for example, mazindol appears to exert its primary effects on the limbic system. The significance of these differences for humans is uncertain. It does not cause brain norepinephrine depletion in animals; on the other hand, it does appear to inhibit storage site uptake of norepinephrine as is suggested by its marked potentiation of the effect of exogenous norepinephrine on blood pressure in dogs (*see WARNINGS*) and on smooth muscle contraction *in vitro*.

Tolerance has been demonstrated with all drugs of this class in which this phenomenon has been studied.

Drugs used in obesity are commonly known as "anorectics" or "anorexigenics." It has not been established, however, that the action of such drugs in treating obesity is exclusively one of appetite suppression. Other central nervous system actions, or metabolic effects may be involved as well.

Adult obese subjects instructed in dietary management and treated with anorectic drugs, lose more weight on the average than those treated with placebo and diet, as determined in relatively short-term clinical trials.

The average magnitude of increased weight loss of drug-treated patients over placebo-treated patients in studies of anorectics in general is ordinarily only a fraction of a pound a week. The rate of weight loss is greatest in the first weeks of therapy for both drug and placebo subjects and tends to decrease in succeeding weeks.

The amount of weight loss associated with the use of Sanorex® (mazindol), as with other anorectic drugs, varies from trial to trial, and the increased weight loss appears to be related in part to variables other than the drugs prescribed, such as the interaction between physician-investigator and the patient, the population treated, and the diet prescribed. The importance of non-drug factors in such weight loss has not been elucidated.

The natural history of obesity is measured in years, whereas, most studies cited are restricted to a few weeks' duration; thus, the total impact of drug-induced weight loss over that of diet alone must be considered clinically limited.

INDICATIONS AND USAGE

Sanorex® (mazindol) is indicated in the management of exogenous obesity as a short-term (a few weeks) adjunct in a regimen of weight reduction based on caloric restriction. The limited usefulness of agents of this class (*see ACTIONS*) should be measured against possible risk factors inherent in their use, such as those described below.

CONTRAINDICATIONS

Glaucoma; hypersensitivity or idiosyncrasy to Sanorex® (mazindol).

Continued on next page

Sandoz—Cont.

Agitated states.
Patients with a history of drug abuse.
During or within 14 days following the administration of monoamine oxidase inhibitors, (hypertensive crises may result).

WARNINGS

Tolerance to the effect of many anorectic drugs may develop within a few weeks; if this occurs, the recommended dose should not be exceeded in an attempt to increase the effect; rather, the drug should be discontinued.
Sanorex® (mazindol) is not recommended for severely hypertensive patients or for patients with symptomatic cardiovascular disease including arrhythmias.

PRECAUTIONS

General
Sanorex® (mazindol) may impair the ability of the patient to engage in potentially hazardous activities such as operating machinery or driving a motor vehicle; the patient should therefore be cautioned accordingly.

Drug Interactions
Sanorex® (mazindol) may decrease the hypotensive effect of guanethidine or similar substances; patients should be monitored accordingly.
Sanorex® (mazindol) may markedly potentiate the pressor effect of exogenous catecholamines. If it should be necessary to give a pressor amine agent (e.g., levarterenol or isoproterenol) to a patient in shock (e.g., from a myocardial infarction) who has recently been taking Sanorex® (mazindol), extreme care should be taken in monitoring blood pressure at frequent intervals and initiating pressor therapy with a low initial dose and careful titration.
It should be recognized that reduction in carbohydrate intake may require reduced insulin dosage. However, in diabetic patients treated with insulin and given Sanorex® (mazindol) for 12 weeks, no change in insulin requirement was noted.
Sanorex® (mazindol) may potentiate blood pressure increases in those patients taking sympathomimetic medications.

Pregnancy
Sanorex® (mazindol) was studied in reproduction experiments in rats and rabbits and an increase in neonatal mortality and a possible increased incidence of rib anomalies in rats were observed at relatively high doses.
Although these studies have not indicated important adverse effects, use of mazindol by women who are or may become pregnant requires that the potential benefit be weighed against the possible hazard to mother and infant.

Nursing Mothers
The extent to which Sanorex® (mazindol) may be transferred in breast milk is not known. Therefore, mothers who are nursing should not receive this drug.

Pediatric Use
Safety and effectiveness in pediatric patients have not been established.

ADVERSE REACTIONS

The most common adverse effects of Sanorex® (mazindol) are dry mouth, tachycardia, constipation, nervousness and insomnia.
Cardiovascular: Palpitation, tachycardia, edema.
Central Nervous System: Overstimulation, restlessness, dizziness, insomnia, dysphoria, tremor, headache, depression, drowsiness, weakness.
Gastrointestinal: Dryness of the mouth, unpleasant taste, diarrhea, constipation, nausea, vomiting, abdominal discomfort.
Skin: Rash, excessive sweating, clamminess.
Endocrine: Impotence, changes in libido have rarely been observed with Sanorex® (mazindol).
Eye: Treatment of dogs with high doses of Sanorex® (mazindol) for long periods resulted in some corneal opacities, reversible on cessation of medication. No such effect has been observed in humans.
Autonomic: Blurred vision, fainting sensation, hot/cold flashes, hyperdipsia, paresthesia.
Genitourinary: Dysuria, pollakiuria.

DRUG ABUSE AND DEPENDENCE

Controlled Studies
Sanorex® (mazindol) is controlled by the Drug Enforcement Administration and is classified under Schedule IV.

Abuse or Dependence
In preliminary chronic safety studies in humans, dosages of 2 mg Sanorex® (mazindol) t.i.d. were administered for 24 consecutive weeks. Two to three days following abrupt withdrawal of medication the subjects were interviewed and no subject requested or required reinstitution of active medication, and no evidence suggestive of dependence was observed.
In widespread clinical use of Sanorex® (mazindol) in the United States since 1973, Sandoz Pharmaceuticals has received no reports of development of physical or psychological dependence, drug tolerance, habituation, chronic abuse, or symptoms of withdrawal or abstinence.

OVERDOSAGE

The minimum lethal dose for humans is not known. The oral LD_{50}, expressed in mg/kg, is 106 for the mouse, 180-320 for the rat, 98 for the rabbit, and 9-20 for the dog. Fewer than 2 dozen cases of Sanorex® (mazindol) overdosage in humans have been reported, and all but 1 of these recovered completely. A 25-year-old female died after ingesting a massive dose of 200 mg of Sanorex® (mazindol) and an undetermined amount of ethanol.
The maximum overdosage of Sanorex® (mazindol) on record from which the patient recovered is 80 mg. A 20-year-old female ingested 40 Sanorex® (mazindol) tablets (2 mg each) and 75-125 mg phenmetrazine in a suicide attempt. The patient was alert during hospitalization and the only clinical finding was frequent premature ventricular contractions. The patient was treated with Lidocaine and recovered completely.
Approximately half of the overdosage cases involved accidental ingestion in children 1-4 years of age. The reported doses ingested ranged from 4-40 mg. All recovered.
In cases in which overdosages have been reported, the symptoms listed below were cited: irritability, agitation, hyperactivity, tachycardia, arrhythmia (premature ventricular contractions occurred in the patient also taking phenmetrazine), tachypnea.
The following symptomatic treatment may include:
Emesis—If the patient is conscious, vomiting should be induced with ipecac syrup (15-30 cc).
Gastric Lavage—Patients should have pharyngeal and laryngeal reflexes. In unconscious patients gastric lavage should not be attempted unless cuffed endotracheal intubation has been performed to prevent aspiration and pulmonary complications.
Sedation—Chlorpromazine (0.5-1 mg/kg, IM) may be given every 30 minutes as needed to control symptoms of central nervous (CNS) overstimulation. A short-acting barbiturate is generally considered the second best choice. Lidocaine may be administered to counteract cardiac arrhythmias.
Forced Acid Diuresis—Sufficient fluids should be given to maintain a urine output of 5-7 L/m^2/day or 2-4 times normal excretion. A 15% solution of mannitol (2.5 mg/kg) given IV every 4-6 hours or whenever the urine specific gravity falls below 1.025 is usually sufficient to produce an acid urine in young people. If necessary, methenamine mandelate or ammonium chloride can be used to acidify the urine. During prolonged forced diuresis, serum electrolytes must be evaluated frequently to avoid hyponatremia or hypokalemia.
Data about treating acute Sanorex® (mazindol) overdosage with hemodialysis or peritoneal dialysis are not available. However, Sanorex® (mazindol) is soluble only in acid so dialysis with basic or neutral solvents would not remove the drug.

DOSAGE AND ADMINISTRATION

To determine the lowest effective dose, therapy with Sanorex® (mazindol) may be initiated at 1 mg once a day and adjusted to the need and response of the patient. Dosage may be increased to a maximum of 3 mg/day given in divided doses with meals.

HOW SUPPLIED

Sanorex® (mazindol) tablets, USP
Sanorex® (mazindol) is available in 1 mg (NDC 0078-0071-05) elliptical, white tablets, engraved "SANOREX" one side, "78-71" other side; and in 2 mg (NDC 0078-0066-05) round, white scored tablets, engraved "78/66" one side, "SANDOZ" other side, in packages of 100.
Store and Dispense
Below 77°F (25°C); tight container.
[REV: APRIL 1996 30185902]

SANSERT® ℞

[san'surt]
(methysergide maleate) tablets, USP

Caution: Federal law prohibits dispensing without prescription.
The following prescribing information is based on official labeling in effect on August 1, 1996.

> **WARNING**
> **Retroperitoneal Fibrosis, Pleuropulmonary Fibrosis and Fibrotic Thickening of Cardiac Valves May Occur in Patients Receiving Long-term Methysergide Maleate Therapy. Therefore, This Preparation Must Be Reserved for Prophylaxis in Patients Whose Vascular Headaches Are Frequent and/or Severe and Uncontrollable and Who Are Under Close Medical Supervision.**
> ***(See also WARNINGS section)***

DESCRIPTION

Sansert® (methysergide maleate) is a partially synthetic compound structurally related to lysergic acid butanolamide, well-known as methylergonovine in obstetrical practice as an oxytocic agent.
Chemically, methysergide maleate is designated as ergoline-8-carboxamide,9,10-didehydro-*N*-[1-(hydroxymethyl)propyl]-1,6-dimethyl-, (8β)-, (*Z*)-2-butenedioate (1:1) (salt).
Its structural formula is:

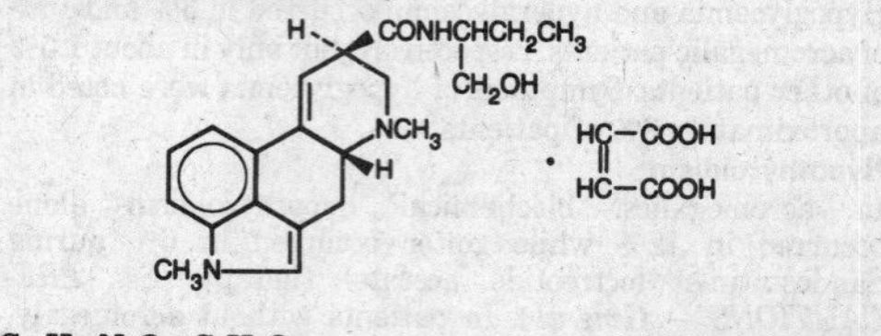

$C_{21}H_{27}N_3O_2 \cdot C_4H_4O_4$ Mol. wt. 469.54

Methylation in the number 1 position of the ring structure enormously enhances the antagonism to serotonin which is present to a much lesser degree in the partially methylated compound (methylergonovine maleate) as well as profoundly altering other pharmacologic properties.
Active Ingredient: methysergide maleate, USP.
Inactive Ingredients: acacia, carnauba wax, colloidal silicon dioxide, FD&C Blue #1, FD&C Yellow #5, gelatin, lactose, malic acid, povidone, sodium benzoate, starch, stearic acid, sucrose, synthetic black iron oxide, talc, and titanium dioxide.

ACTIONS

Sansert® (methysergide maleate) has been shown, *in vitro* and *in vivo*, to inhibit or block the effects of serotonin, a substance which may be involved in the mechanism of vascular headaches. Serotonin has been variously described as a central neurohumoral agent or chemical mediator, as a "headache substance" acting directly or indirectly to lower pain threshold (others in this category include tyramine; polypeptides, such as bradykinin; histamine; and acetylcholine), as an intrinsic "motor hormone" of the gastrointestinal tract, and as a "hormone" involved in connective tissue reparative processes. Suggestions have been made by investigators as to the mechanism whereby methysergide produces its clinical effects, but this has not been finally established.

INDICATIONS

For the prevention or reduction of intensity and frequency of vascular headaches in the following kinds of patients:
1. Patients suffering from one or more severe vascular headaches per week.
2. Patients suffering from vascular headaches that are uncontrollable or so severe that preventive therapy is indicated regardless of the frequency of the attack.

CONTRAINDICATIONS

Hypersensitivity to the drug, pregnancy, peripheral vascular disease, severe arteriosclerosis, severe hypertension, coronary artery disease, phlebitis or cellulitis of the lower limbs, pulmonary disease, collagen diseases or fibrotic processes, impaired liver or renal function, valvular heart disease, debilitated states and serious infections.

WARNINGS

With long-term, uninterrupted administration, retroperitoneal fibrosis or related conditions—pleuropulmonary fibrosis and cardiovascular disorders with murmurs or vascular bruits have been reported. Patients must be warned to report immediately the following symptoms and to discontinue the drug: cold, numb, and painful hands and feet; leg cramps on walking; any type of girdle, flank, or chest pain, shortness of breath, or any associated symptomatology. Should any of these symptoms develop, methysergide should be discontinued. Continuous administration should not exceed 6 months. There must be a drug-free interval of 3-4 weeks after each 6-month course of treatment. The dosage should be reduced gradually during the last 2-3 weeks of each treatment course to avoid "headache rebound."
The drug is not recommended for use in children.

PRECAUTIONS

General
All patients receiving Sansert® (methysergide maleate) should remain under constant supervision of the physician and be examined regularly for the development of fibrotic or vascular complications. *(See ADVERSE REACTIONS)*
The manifestations of retroperitoneal fibrosis, pleuropulmonary fibrosis, and vascular shutdown have shown a high incidence of regression once Sansert® (methysergide maleate) is withdrawn. These facts should be borne in mind to avoid unnecessary surgical intervention. Cardiac murmurs, which may indicate endocardial fibrosis, have shown varying degrees of regression, with complete disappearance in some and persistence in others.
Sansert® (methysergide maleate) has been specifically designed for the prophylaxis of vascular headache and has no place in the management of the acute attack.

Sansert® (methysergide maleate) tablets contain FD&C Yellow No. 5 (tartrazine) which may cause allergic-type reactions (including bronchial asthma) in certain susceptible individuals. Although the overall incidence of FD&C Yellow No. 5 (tartrazine) sensitivity in the general population is low, it is frequently seen in patients who also have aspirin hypersensitivity.

Information for Patients

Sansert® (methysergide maleate) is intended for use as a preventive agent in the treatment of vascular headaches. It should not be used for acute migraine attacks. If, after a 3-week trial period, Sansert® (methysergide maleate) has not been effective in decreasing the frequency or intensity of headaches, it is unlikely that longer administration of Sansert® (methysergide maleate) will be beneficial.

Patients should be advised to report the following symptoms immediately and to discontinue the drug: cold, numb, and painful hands and feet; leg cramps on walking; any type of girdle, flank, or chest pain; shortness of breath; or any associated symptomatology. There must be a drug-free interval of 3–4 weeks after each 6-month course of treatment.

Sansert® (methysergide maleate) should be taken with meals. Weight gain may necessitate modification of diet.

Drug Interactions

Methysergide may reverse the analgesic activity of narcotic analgesics.

Pregnancy Category X

Sansert® (methysergide maleate) is contraindicated in pregnancy due to its oxytocic actions.

Nursing Mothers

There are no specific studies on the use of Sansert® (methysergide maleate) in nursing mothers. Ergot alkaloids, in general, appear in mothers' milk.

Sansert® (methysergide maleate) is a semi-synthetic compound structurally related to ergotamine, and thus it may appear in breast milk. Ergot alkaloids have been reported to cause nausea, vomiting, diarrhea and weakness in the nursing infant and suppression of prolactin secretion and lactation in the mother.

Because of the potential for serious adverse reactions in nursing infants from Sansert® (methysergide maleate), a decision should be made whether to discontinue nursing or to discontinue the drug, taking into account the importance of the drug to the mother.

Pediatric Use

Safety and effectiveness in children have not been established.

ADVERSE REACTIONS

Within the recommended dose levels, the following side effects have been reported:

1) Fibrotic Complications

Fibrotic changes have been observed in the retroperitoneal, pleuropulmonary, cardiac, and other tissues, either singly or, very rarely, in combination.

Retroperitoneal Fibrosis

This nonspecific fibrotic process is usually confined to the retroperitoneal connective tissue above the pelvic brim and may present clinically with one or more symptoms such as general malaise, fatigue, weight loss, backache, low grade fever (elevated sedimentation rate), urinary obstruction (girdle or flank pain, dysuria, polyuria, oliguria, elevated BUN), vascular insufficiency of the lower limbs (leg pain, Leriche syndrome, edema of legs, thrombophlebitis). The single most useful diagnostic procedure in suspected cases of retroperitoneal fibrosis is intravenous pyelography. Typical deviation and obstruction of one or both ureters may be observed.

Pleuropulmonary Complications

A similar nonspecific fibrotic process, limited to the pleural and immediately subjacent pulmonary tissues, usually presents clinically with dyspnea, tightness and pain in the chest, pleural friction rubs, and pleural effusion. These findings may be confirmed by chest X-ray.

Cardiac Complications

Nonrheumatic fibrotic thickenings of the aortic root and of the aortic and mitral valves usually present clinically with cardiac murmurs and dyspnea.

Other Fibrotic Complications

Several cases of fibrotic plaques, simulating Peyronie's Disease have been described.

2) Cardiovascular Complications

Encroachment of retroperitoneal fibrosis on the aorta, inferior vena cava and their common iliac branches may result in vascular insufficiency of the lower limbs, the presenting features of which are mentioned under *Retroperitoneal Fibrosis*.

Intrinsic vasoconstriction of large and small arteries, involving one or more vessels or merely a segment of a vessel, may occur at any stage of therapy. Depending on the vessel involved, this complication may present with chest pain, abdominal pain, or cold, numb, painful extremities with or without paresthesias and diminished or absent pulses. Progression to ischemic tissue damage has rarely been reported. Prompt withdrawal of the drug at the first signs of impaired

circulation is recommended (see *WARNINGS*) to obviate such effects.

Postural hypotension and tachycardia have also been observed.

3) Gastrointestinal Symptoms

Nausea, vomiting, diarrhea, heartburn, abdominal pain. These effects tend to appear early and can frequently be obviated by gradual introduction of the medication and by administration of the drug with meals. Constipation and elevation of gastric HCl have also been reported.

4) CNS Symptoms

Seizure, insomnia, drowsiness, mild euphoria, dizziness, ataxia, lightheadedness, hyperesthesia, unworldly feelings (described variously as "dissociation", "hallucinatory experiences", etc.). Some of these symptoms may be associated with vascular headaches, per se, and may, therefore, be unrelated to the drug.

5) Dermatological Manifestations

Facial flush, telangiectasia, and nonspecific rashes have rarely been reported. Increased hair loss may occur, but in many instances the tendency has abated despite continued therapy.

6) Edema

Peripheral edema, and, more rarely, localized brawny edema may occur.

Dependent edema has responded to lowered doses, salt restriction, or diuretics.

7) Weight Gain

Weight gain may be a reason to caution patients regarding their caloric intake.

8) Hematological Manifestations

Neutropenia, eosinophilia, and thrombocytopenia.

9) Miscellaneous

Weakness, arthralgia, myalgia, fever, and mydriasis.

OVERDOSAGE

Few cases of acute Sansert® (methysergide maleate) intoxication have been reported. The possible symptom complex is therefore not fully known. The following symptoms are based on these few case reports. Euphoria, hyperactivity, tachycardia, dilated pupils, and dizziness have been reported in a child with a dose of 20–24 mg of Sansert® (methysergide maleate). In adults, peripheral vasospasm, with diminished or absent pulses, coldness, mottling and cyanosis, has been observed at a dose of 200 mg. Ischemic tissue damage has not been reported in acute overdosage with Sansert® (methysergide maleate).

Treatment consists of removal of the offending drug by induction of emesis, gastric lavage and catharsis. There is no evidence that forced diuresis accelerates the elimination of Sansert® (methysergide maleate). However, as a general supportive measure, I.V. fluids may be given for supportive therapy.

Treatment of peripheral vasospasm should consist of warmth, but not heat, and protection of the ischemic limbs. In reported cases of Sansert® (methysergide maleate) overdosage, the use of vasodilators has not been necessary. However, if vasospasm is persistent, or there is evidence of impending ischemic tissue damage, these agents may be beneficial.

Up-to-date information about the treatment of overdose can often be obtained from a certified Regional Poison Control Center. Telephone numbers of certified Regional Poison Control Centers are listed in the Physicians' Desk Reference.

DOSAGE AND ADMINISTRATION

Usual adult dose 4-8 mg daily. Tablets to be given with meals.

Note: There must be a medication-free interval of 3-4 weeks after every 6-month course of treatment. (See WARNINGS) No pediatric dosage has been established.

If, after a 3-week trial period, efficacy has not been demonstrated, longer administration of Sansert® (methysergide maleate) is unlikely to be of benefit.

HOW SUPPLIED

Sansert® (methysergide maleate) tablets, USP

Bottles of 100 tablets (NDC 0078-0058-05), each tablet containing 2 mg of methysergide maleate, USP. Imprinted "78-58" on one side, "SANDOZ" other side.

Store and dispense

Below 86°F (30°C); tight container.

[REV: JUNE 1995   30186902]

SYNTOCINON®   ℞

[sin "tō'si-non]

(oxytocin) injection, USP

Caution: Federal law prohibits dispensing without prescription.

The following prescribing information is based on official labeling in effect on August 1, 1996.

DESCRIPTION

Syntocinon® (oxytocin) is a synthetic, (1-6) cyclic nonapeptide. Chemically, oxytocin is designated as Glycinamide,

L- cysteinyl -L- tyrosyl -L- isoleucyl -L- glutaminyl-L-asparaginyl-L-cysteinyl-L-prolyl-L-leucyl-, cyclic (1-6)-disulfide.

The structural formula is:

$$\text{H–Cys–Tyr–Ile–Glu(NH}_2\text{)–Asp(NH}_2\text{)–Cys–Pro–Leu–Gly–NH}_2$$
$$1 \quad 2 \quad 3 \quad 4 \qquad 5 \qquad 6 \quad 7 \quad 8 \quad 9$$

$C_{43}H_{66}N_{12}O_{12}S_2$ Mol. wt. 1007.19

Syntocinon® (oxytocin) injection is provided as a sterile solution for intravenous or intramuscular administration. Each 1 mL of solution contains 10 USP or International Units of oxytocin and the following inactive ingredients:

acetic acid, NF, qs to	pH 4 ± 0.3
alcohol, USP	0.61% by vol.
chlorobutanol, NF	0.5%
sodium acetate, USP	1 mg
sodium chloride, USP	0.017 mg
water for injection, USP, qs to	1 mL

CLINICAL PHARMACOLOGY

The pharmacologic and clinical properties of Syntocinon® (oxytocin) are identical with the naturally occurring oxytocic principle of the posterior lobe of the pituitary. Syntocinon® (oxytocin) injection does not contain the amino acids characteristic of vasopressin, and therefore has fewer and less severe cardiovascular effects. Syntocinon® (oxytocin) exerts a selective action on the smooth musculature of the uterus, particularly toward the end of pregnancy, during labor and immediately following delivery. Oxytocin stimulates rhythmic contractions of the uterus, increases the frequency of existing contractions, and raises the tone of the uterine musculature.

Syntocinon® (oxytocin), when given in appropriate doses during pregnancy, is capable of eliciting graded increases in uterine motility from a moderate increase in the rate and force of spontaneous motor activity to sustained tetanic contraction.

Syntocinon® (oxytocin) is promptly effective after parenteral administration. Following intramuscular injection, the myotonic effect on the uterus appears in 3–7 minutes, and persists for 30–60 minutes. With intravenous injection, the uterine effect appears within 1 minute and is of more brief duration.

INDICATIONS AND USAGE

Important Notice

Syntocinon® (oxytocin) injection is indicated for the medical rather than the elective induction of labor. Available data and information are inadequate to define the benefits to risk considerations in the use of the drug product for elective induction. Elective induction of labor is defined as the initiation of labor for convenience in an individual with a term pregnancy who is free of medical indications.

Antepartum

Syntocinon® (oxytocin) is indicated for the initiation or improvement of uterine contractions, where this is desirable and considered suitable, in order to achieve early vaginal delivery for fetal or maternal reasons. It is indicated for (1) induction of labor in patients with a medical indication for the initiation of labor, such as Rh problems, maternal diabetes, pre-eclampsia at or near term, when delivery is in the best interest of mother and fetus or when membranes are prematurely ruptured and delivery is indicated; (2) stimulation or reinforcement of labor, as in selected cases of uterine inertia; (3) as adjunctive therapy in the management of incomplete or inevitable abortion. In the first trimester, curettage is generally considered primary therapy. In the second trimester abortion, oxytocin infusion will often be successful in emptying the uterus. Other means of therapy, however, may be required in such cases.

Postpartum

Syntocinon® (oxytocin) injection is indicated to produce uterine contractions during the third stage of labor and to control postpartum bleeding or hemorrhage.

CONTRAINDICATIONS

Syntocinon® (oxytocin) injection is contraindicated in any of the following conditions: Significant cephalopelvic disproportion; unfavorable fetal positions or presentations which are undeliverable without conversion prior to delivery (transverse lies); i.e., in obstetrical emergencies where the benefit-to-risk ratio for either the fetus or the mother favors surgical intervention; in cases of fetal distress where delivery is not imminent; prolonged use in uterine inertia or severe toxemia; hypertonic uterine patterns; patients with hypersensitivity to the drug; induction or augmentation of labor in those cases where vaginal delivery is contraindicated, such as cord presentation or prolapse, total placental previa, and vasa previa.

Continued on next page

Sandoz—Cont.

WARNINGS

Syntocinon® (oxytocin), when given for induction or stimulation of labor, must be administered only by the intravenous route and with adequate medical supervision in a hospital.

PRECAUTIONS

General

All patients receiving intravenous oxytocin must be under continuous observation by trained personnel with a thorough knowledge of the drug and qualified to identify complications. A physician qualified to manage any complications should be immediately available.

When properly administered, oxytocin should stimulate uterine contractions similar to those seen in normal labor. Overstimulation of the uterus by improper administration can be hazardous to both mother and fetus. Even with proper administration and adequate supervision, hypertonic contractions can occur in patients whose uteri are hypersensitive to oxytocin.

Except in unusual circumstances, oxytocin should not be administered in the following conditions: prematurity, borderline cephalopelvic disproportion, previous major surgery on the cervix or uterus including cesarean section, overdistention of the uterus, grand multiparity, or invasive cervical carcinoma. Because of the variability of the combinations of factors which may be present in the conditions listed above, the definition of "unusual circumstances" must be left to the judgment of the physician. The decision can only be made by carefully weighing the potential benefits which oxytocin can provide in a given case against rare but definite potential for the drug to produce hypertonicity or tetanic spasm.

Maternal deaths due to hypertensive episodes, subarachnoid hemorrhage, rupture of the uterus, and fetal deaths due to various causes have been reported associated with the use of parenteral oxytocic drugs for induction of labor or for augmentation in the first and second stages of labor.

Oxytocin has been shown to have an intrinsic antidiuretic effect, acting to increase water reabsorption from the glomerular filtrate. Consideration should, therefore, be given to the possibility of water intoxication, particularly when oxytocin is administered continuously by infusion and the patient is receiving fluids by mouth.

Drug Interactions

Severe hypertension has been reported when oxytocin was given 3-4 hours following prophylactic administration of a vasoconstrictor in conjunction with caudal block anesthesia. Cyclopropane anesthesia may modify oxytocin's cardiovascular effects, so as to produce unexpected results such as hypotension. Maternal sinus bradycardia with abnormal atrioventricular rhythms has also been noted when oxytocin was used concomitantly with cyclopropane anesthesia.

Carcinogenesis, Mutagenesis, Impairment of Fertility

There are no animal or human studies on the carcinogenicity and mutagenicity of this drug, nor is there any information on its effect on fertility.

Pregnancy

Teratogenic Effects: Animal reproduction studies have not been conducted with oxytocin. There are no known indications for use in the first trimester of pregnancy other than in relation to spontaneous or induced abortion. Based on the wide experience with this drug and its chemical structure and pharmacological properties, it would not be expected to present a risk of fetal abnormalities when used as indicated.

Nonteratogenic Effects: *See ADVERSE REACTIONS in the fetus or infant.*

Labor and Delivery

See INDICATIONS AND USAGE.

Nursing Mothers

Syntocinon® (oxytocin) may be found in small quantities in mother's milk. If a patient requires the drug postpartum to control severe bleeding, she should not commence nursing until the day after Syntocinon® (oxytocin) has been discontinued.

Pediatric Use

Safety and effectiveness in pediatric patients have not been established.

ADVERSE REACTIONS

The following adverse reactions have been reported in the mother: Anaphylactic reaction, Postpartum hemorrhage, Cardiac arrhythmia, Fatal afibrinogenemia, Nausea, Vomiting, Premature ventricular contractions, and Pelvic hematoma.

Excessive dosage or hypersensitivity to the drug may result in uterine hypertonicity, spasm, tetanic contraction, or rupture of the uterus.

The possibility of increased blood loss and afibrinogenemia should be kept in mind when administering the drug.

Severe water intoxication with convulsions and coma has occurred, associated with a slow oxytocin infusion over a 24-hour period. Maternal death due to oxytocin-induced water intoxication has been reported.

The following adverse reactions have been reported in the fetus or infant:

Due to induced uterine motility: Bradycardia, Premature ventricular contractions and other arrhythmias, Permanent CNS or brain damage, and Fetal death.

Due to use of oxytocin in the mother: Low Apgar scores at 5 minutes, Neonatal jaundice, and Neonatal retinal hemorrhage.

DRUG ABUSE AND DEPENDENCE

There is no evidence that Syntocinon® (oxytocin) has been abused or has provoked drug dependence.

OVERDOSAGE

Overdosage with oxytocin depends essentially on uterine hyperactivity, whether or not due to hypersensitivity to this agent. Hyperstimulation with strong (hypertonic) or prolonged (tetanic) contractions, or a resting tone of 15-20 mm H_2O or more between contractions can lead to tumultuous labor, uterine rupture, cervical and vaginal lacerations, postpartum hemorrhage, uteroplacental hypoperfusion, and variable deceleration of fetal heart, fetal hypoxia, hypercapnia, or death. Water intoxication with convulsions, which is caused by the inherent antidiuretic effect of oxytocin, is a serious complication that may occur if large doses (40-50 mL/minute) are infused for long periods. Treatment of water intoxication consists of discontinuation of oxytocin, restriction of fluid intake, diuresis, IV hypertonic saline solution, correction of electrolyte imbalance, control of convulsions with judicious use of a barbiturate, and special nursing care for the comatose patient.

DOSAGE AND ADMINISTRATION

Dosage of oxytocin is determined by uterine response. The following dosage information is based upon the various regimens and indications in general use. Parenteral drug products should be inspected visually for particulate matter and discoloration prior to administration, wherever solution and container permit.

A. Induction or Stimulation of Labor

Intravenous infusion (drip method) is the only acceptable method of administration for the induction or stimulation of labor.

Accurate control of the rate of infusion flow is essential. An infusion pump or other such device and frequent monitoring of strength of contractions and fetal heart rate are necessary for the safe administration of oxytocin for the induction or stimulation of labor. If uterine contractions become too powerful, the infusion can be abruptly stopped, and oxytocin stimulation of the uterine musculature will soon wane.

1. An intravenous infusion of non-oxytocin containing solution should be started. Physiologic electrolyte solution should be used except under unusual circumstances.
2. To prepare the usual solution for infusion, the contents of one 1-mL ampul are combined aseptically with 1,000 mL of nonhydrating diluent. The combined solution, rotated in the infusion bottle to insure thorough mixing, contains 10 mU/mL. Add the container with dilute oxytocin solution to the system through use of a constant infusion pump or other such device, to control accurately the rate of infusion.
3. The initial dose should be no more than 1–2 mU/minute. The dose may be gradually increased in increments of no more than 1–2 mU/minute, until a contraction pattern has been established, which is similar to normal labor.
4. The fetal heart rate, resting uterine tone, and the frequency, duration, and force of contractions should be monitored.
5. The oxytocin infusion should be discontinued immediately in the event of uterine hyperactivity or fetal distress. Oxygen should be administered to the mother. The mother and the fetus must be evaluated by the responsible physician.

B. Control of Postpartum Uterine Bleeding

1. *Intravenous Infusion (Drip Method):* To control postpartum bleeding, 10–40 units of oxytocin may be added to 1,000 mL of a non-hydrating diluent and run at a rate necessary to control uterine atony.
2. *Intramuscular Administration:* 1 mL (10 units) of oxytocin can be given after delivery of the placenta.

C. Treatment of Incomplete or Inevitable Abortion

Intravenous infusion with physiologic saline solution, 500 mL, or 5% dextrose in physiologic saline solution to which 10 units of Syntocinon® (oxytocin) have been added should be infused at a rate of 20–40 drops/minute.

HOW SUPPLIED

Syntocinon® (oxytocin) injection, USP

Available as a 1 mL sterile ampul containing 10 USP or International Units of oxytocin. SandoPak® unit dose packages of 50 ampuls (NDC 0078-0060-04).

Store and dispense

Below 77°F (25°C); DO NOT FREEZE.

[REV: MAY 1996 30288904]

TAVIST® ℞

(clemastine fumarate) Syrup

Caution: Federal law prohibits dispensing without prescription.

The following prescribing information is based on official labeling in effect on August 1, 1996.

Tavist® (clemastine) Syrup 0.5 mg/5 mL
(present as clemastine fumarate 0.67 mg/5 mL)

DESCRIPTION

Each teaspoonful (5 mL) of Tavist® (clemastine fumarate) Syrup for oral administration contains clemastine 0.5 mg (present as clemastine fumarate 0.67 mg). Other ingredients: alcohol 5.5%, flavors, methylparaben, propylene glycol, propylparaben, purified water, saccharin sodium, sorbitol in a buffered solution. Tavist® (clemastine fumarate) belongs to the benzhydryl ether group of antihistaminic compounds. The chemical name is (+) - (2R)-2-[2-[[(R)-p-Chloro-α-methyl-α-phenylbenzyl]-oxy]ethyl]-1-methylpyrrolidine fumarate* and has the following structural formula:

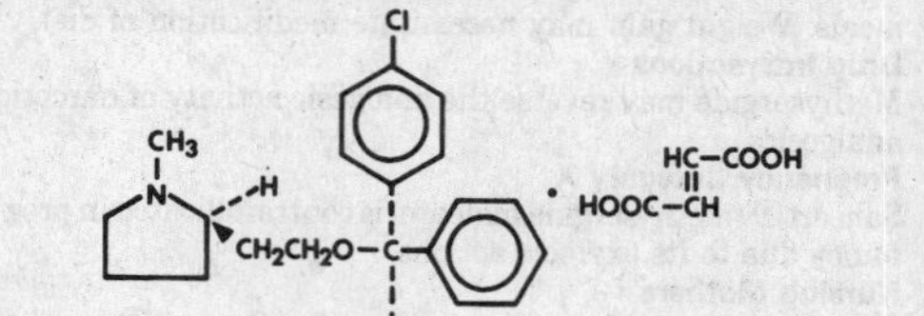

CAS Registration Number 14976-57-9
*U.S. Patent No. 3,097,212

Clemastine fumarate occurs as a colorless to faintly yellow, practically odorless, crystalline powder. Tavist® (clemastine fumarate) Syrup has an approximate pH of 6.2.

CLINICAL PHARMACOLOGY

Tavist® (clemastine fumarate) is an antihistamine with anticholinergic (drying) and sedative side effects. Antihistamines competitively antagonize various physiological effects of histamine including increased capillary permeability and dilatation, the formation of edema, the "flare" and "itch" response, and gastrointestinal and respiratory smooth muscle constriction. Within the vascular tree, H_1-receptor antagonists inhibit both the vasoconstrictor and vasodilator effects of histamine. Depending on the dose, H_1-receptor antagonists can produce CNS stimulation or depression. Most antihistamines exhibit central and/or peripheral anticholinergic activity. Antihistamines act by competitively blocking H_1-receptor sites. Antihistamines do not pharmacologically antagonize or chemically inactivate histamine, nor do they prevent the release of histamine.

PHARMACOKINETICS

Antihistamines are well-absorbed following oral administration. Chlorpheniramine maleate, clemastine fumarate, and diphenhydramine hydrochloride achieve peak blood levels within 2-5 hours following oral administration. The absorption of antihistamines is often partially delayed by the use of controlled release dosage forms. In these instances, plasma concentrations from identical doses of the immediate and controlled release dosage forms will not be similar. Tissue distribution of the antihistamines in humans has not been established.

Antihistamines appear to be metabolized in the liver chiefly via mono- and didemethylation and glucuronide conjugation. Antihistamine metabolites and small amounts of unchanged drug are excreted in the urine. Small amounts of the drugs may also be excreted in breast milk.

In normal human subjects who received histamine injections over a 24-hour period, the antihistaminic activity of Tavist® (clemastine fumarate) reached a peak at 5-7 hours, persisted for 10-12 hours and, in some cases, for as long as 24 hours. Pharmacokinetic studies in man utilizing ^3H and ^{14}C labeled compound demonstrates that: Tavist® (clemastine fumarate) is rapidly absorbed from the gastrointestinal tract, peak plasma concentrations are attained in 2-4 hours, and urinary excretion is the major mode of elimination.

INDICATIONS AND USAGE

Tavist® (clemastine fumarate) Syrup is indicated for the relief of symptoms associated with allergic rhinitis such as sneezing, rhinorrhea, pruritus and lacrimation. Tavist® (clemastine fumarate) Syrup is indicated for use in pediatric populations (age 6 years through 12) and adults (see *DOSAGE AND ADMINISTRATION*).

It should be noted that Tavist® (clemastine fumarate) is indicated for the relief of mild uncomplicated allergic skin manifestations of urticaria and angioedema at the 2 mg dosage level only.

CONTRAINDICATIONS

Antihistamines are contraindicated in patients hypersensitive to the drug or to other antihistamines of similar chemical structure (*see PRECAUTIONS —Drug Interactions*).

Antihistamines ***should not*** be used ***in newborn or premature infants.*** Because of the higher risk of antihistamines for infants generally and for newborns and prematures in particular, antihistamine therapy is contraindicated ***in nursing mothers*** (*see PRECAUTIONS —Nursing Mothers*).

WARNINGS

Antihistamines should be used with considerable caution in patients with: narrow angle glaucoma, stenosing peptic ulcer, pyloroduodenal obstruction, symptomatic prostatic hypertrophy, and bladder neck obstruction.

Use with CNS Depressants: Tavist® (clemastine fumarate) has additive effects with alcohol and other CNS depressants (hypnotics, sedatives, tranquilizers, etc.).

Use in Activities Requiring Mental Alertness: Patients should be warned about engaging in activities requiring mental alertness such as driving a car or operating appliances, machinery, etc.

Use in the Elderly (approximately 60 years or older): Antihistamines are more likely to cause dizziness, sedation, and hypotension in elderly patients.

PRECAUTIONS

General

Tavist® (clemastine fumarate) should be used with caution in patients with: history of bronchial asthma, increased intraocular pressure, hyperthyroidism, cardiovascular disease, and hypertension.

Information for Patients

Patients taking antihistamines should receive the following information and instructions:

1. Antihistamines are prescribed to reduce allergic symptoms.
2. Patients should be questioned regarding a history of glaucoma, peptic ulcer, urinary retention, or pregnancy before starting antihistamine therapy.
3. Patients should be told not to take alcohol, sleeping pills, sedatives, or tranquilizers while taking antihistamines.
4. Antihistamines may cause drowsiness, dizziness, dry mouth, blurred vision, weakness, nausea, headache, or nervousness in some patients.
5. Patients should avoid driving a car or working with hazardous machinery until they assess the effects of this medicine.
6. Patients should be told to store this medicine in a tightly closed container in a dry, cool place away from heat or direct sunlight and out of the reach of children.

Drug Interactions

Additive CNS depression may occur when antihistamines are administered concomitantly with other CNS depressants including barbiturates, tranquilizers, and alcohol. Patients receiving antihistamines should be advised against the concurrent use of other CNS depressant drugs.

Monoamine oxidase (MAO) inhibitors prolong and intensify the anticholinergic effects of antihistamines.

Carcinogenesis, Mutagenesis, Impairment of Fertility

Carcinogenesis and Mutagenesis: In a 2-year oral study in the rat at a dose of 84 mg/kg (about 500 times the adult human dose) and an 85-week oral study in the mouse at 206 mg/kg (about 1300 times the adult human dose), clemastine fumarate showed no evidence of carcinogenesis. No mutagenic studies have been conducted with clemastine fumarate.

Impairment of Fertility: Oral doses of clemastine fumarate in the rat produced a decrease in mating ability of the male at 312 times the adult human dose. This effect was not found at 156 times the adult human dose.

Pregnancy

Pregnancy Category B: Oral reproduction studies performed with clemastine fumarate in rats and rabbits at doses up to 312 and 188 times the adult human doses respectively, have revealed no evidence of teratogenic effects.

There are no adequate and well-controlled studies of Tavist® (clemastine fumarate) Syrup in pregnant women. Because animal reproduction studies are not always predictive of human response, this drug should be used in pregnancy only if clearly needed.

Nursing Mothers

Although quantitative determinations of antihistaminic drugs in breast milk have not been reported, qualitative tests have documented the excretion of diphenhydramine, pyrilamine, and tripelennamine in human milk.

Because of the potential for adverse reactions in nursing infants from antihistamines, a decision should be made whether to discontinue nursing or to discontinue the drug.

Pediatric Use

The safety and efficacy of Tavist® (clemastine fumarate) Syrup has been confirmed in the pediatric population (age 6 years through 12). Safety and dose tolerance studies have confirmed children 6 through 11 years tolerated dosage ranges of 0.75 to 2.25 mg clemastine. In infants and children particularly, antihistamines in overdosage may produce hallucinations, convulsions, and death. Symptoms of antihistamine toxicity in children may include fixed dilated pupils, flushed face, dry mouth, fever, excitation, hallucinations, ataxia, incoordination, athetosis, tonic-clonic convulsions, and postictal depression (see *OVERDOSAGE*).

ADVERSE REACTIONS

The most frequent adverse reactions are underlined:

Nervous System: Sedation, sleepiness, dizziness, disturbed coordination, fatigue, confusion, restlessness, excitation, nervousness, tremor, irritability, insomnia, euphoria, paresthesia, blurred vision, diplopia, vertigo, tinnitus, acute labyrinthitis, hysteria, neuritis, convulsions.

Gastrointestinal System: Epigastric distress, anorexia, nausea, vomiting, diarrhea, constipation.

Respiratory System: Thickening of bronchial secretions, tightness of chest and wheezing, nasal stuffiness.

Cardiovascular System: Hypotension, headache, palpitations, tachycardia, extrasystoles.

Hematologic System: Hemolytic anemia, thrombocytopenia, agranulocytosis.

Genitourinary System: Urinary frequency, difficult urination, urinary retention, early menses.

General: Urticaria, drug rash, anaphylactic shock, photosensitivity, excessive perspiration, chills, dryness of mouth, nose and throat.

OVERDOSAGE

Antihistamine overdosage reactions may vary from central nervous system depression to stimulation. In children, stimulation predominates initially in a syndrome which may include excitement, hallucinations, ataxia, incoordination, muscle twitching, athetosis, hyperthermia, cyanosis convulsions, tremors, and hyperreflexia followed by postictal depression and cardio-respiratory arrest. Convulsions in children may be preceded by mild depression. Dry mouth, fixed dilated pupils, flushing of the face, and fever are common. In adults, CNS depression, ranging from drowsiness to coma, is more common. The convulsant dose of antihistamines lies near the lethal dose. Convulsions indicate a poor prognosis. In both children and adults, coma and cardiovascular collapse may occur. Deaths are reported especially in infants and children.

There is no specific therapy for acute overdosage with antihistamines. The latent period from ingestion to appearance of toxic effects is characteristically short (½-2 hours). General symptomatic and supportive measures should be instituted promptly and maintained for as long as necessary.

Since overdoses of other classes of drugs (i.e., tricyclic antidepressants) may also present anticholinergic symptomatology, appropriate toxicological analysis should be performed as soon as possible to identify the causative agent.

In the conscious patient, vomiting should be induced even though it may have occurred spontaneously. If vomiting cannot be induced, gastric lavage is indicated. Adequate precautions must be taken to protect against aspiration, especially in infants and children. Charcoal slurry or other suitable agents should be instilled into the stomach after vomiting or lavage. Saline cathartics or milk of magnesia may be of additional benefit.

In the unconscious patient, the airway should be secured with a cuffed endotracheal tube before attempting to evacuate the gastric contents. Intensive supportive and nursing care is indicated, as for any comatose patient.

If breathing is significantly impaired, maintenance of an adequate airway and mechanical support of respiration is the most effective means of providing adequate oxygenation.

Hypotension is an early sign of impending cardiovascular collapse and should be treated vigorously. Although general supportive measures are important, specific treatment with intravenous infusion of a vasopressor titrated to maintain adequate blood pressure may be necessary.

Do not use with CNS stimulants.

Convulsions should be controlled by careful administration of diazepam or a short-acting barbiturate, repeated as necessary. Physostigmine may also be considered for use in controlling centrally mediated convulsions.

Ice packs and cooling sponge baths, not alcohol, can aid in reducing the fever commonly seen in children. A more detailed review of antihistamine toxicology and overdose management is available in Gosselin, R.E., et al., "Clinical Toxicology of Commercial Products."

DOSAGE AND ADMINISTRATION

DOSAGE SHOULD BE INDIVIDUALIZED ACCORDING TO THE NEEDS AND RESPONSE OF THE PATIENT.

Pediatric: Children aged 6 to 12 years

For Symptoms of Allergic Rhinitis—The starting dose is 1 teaspoonful (0.5 mg clemastine) twice daily. Since single doses of up to 2.25 mg clemastine were well tolerated by this age group, dosage may be increased as required, but not to exceed 6 teaspoonsful daily (3 mg clemastine).

For Urticaria and Angioedema—The starting dose is 2 teaspoonsful (1 mg clemastine) twice daily, not to exceed 6 teaspoonsful daily (3 mg clemastine).

Adults and Children 12 Years and Over

For Symptoms of Allergic Rhinitis—The starting dose is 2 teaspoonsful (1.0 mg clemastine) twice daily. Dosage may be increased as required, but not to exceed 12 teaspoonsful daily (6 mg clemastine).

For Urticaria and Angioedema—The starting dose is 4 teaspoonsful (2 mg clemastine) twice daily, not to exceed 12 teaspoonsful daily (6 mg clemastine).

HOW SUPPLIED

Tavist® (clemastine fumarate) Syrup

Clemastine 0.5 mg/5 mL (present as clemastine fumarate 0.67mg/5 mL). A clear, colorless liquid with a citrus flavor, in 4 fl. oz. bottle (NDC 0078-0222-31).

Store and Dispense

Below 77°F (25°C) tight, amber glass bottle. Store in an upright position.

[REV: MARCH 1994 38191901]

TAVIST 1® OTC

CLEMASTINE FUMARATE TABLETS, USP, 1.34 MG

TAVIST® ℞

CLEMASTINE FUMARATE TABLETS, USP, 2.68 MG

Caution: Federal law prohibits dispensing without prescription.

The following prescribing information is based on official labeling in effect on August 1, 1996.

DESCRIPTION

TAVIST® (clemastine fumarate, USP) belongs to the benzhydryl ether group of antihistaminic compounds. The chemical name is (+)-2-[-2-[(p-chloro-α-methyl-α-phenylbenzyl) oxy]ethyl]-1-methyl-pyrrolidine* hydrogen fumarate.

Its structural formula is:

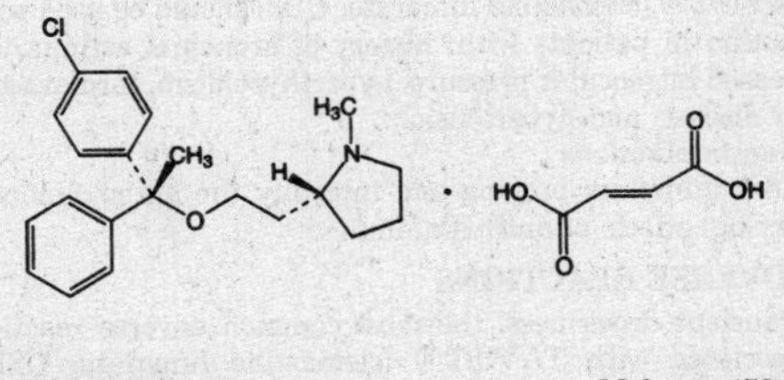

$C_{21}H_{26}ClNO \cdot C_4H_4O_4$ Mol. wt. 459.97

*US Patent No. 3,097,212

1.34 mg and 2.68 mg Tablets

Active Ingredient: clemastine fumarate, USP

Inactive Ingredients: lactose, povidone, starch, stearic acid, and talc

ACTIONS

TAVIST® is an antihistamine with anticholinergic (drying) and sedative side effects. Antihistamines appear to compete with histamine for cell receptor sites on effector cells. The inherently long duration of antihistaminic effects of TAVIST® has been demonstrated in wheal and flare studies. In normal human subjects who received histamine injections over a 24-hour period, the antihistaminic activity of TAVIST® reached a peak at 5-7 hours, persisted for 10-12 hours and, in some cases, for as long as 24 hours. Pharmacokinetic studies in man utilizing ^3H and ^{14}C labeled compound demonstrates that: TAVIST® (clemastine fumarate, USP) is rapidly and nearly completely absorbed from the gastrointestinal tract, peak plasma concentrations are attained in 2-4 hours, and urinary excretion is the major mode of elimination.

INDICATIONS

TAVIST-1® Tablets, 1.34 mg are indicated for the relief of symptoms associated with allergic rhinitis such as sneezing, rhinorrhea, pruritus, and lacrimation.

TAVIST® Tablets 2.68 mg are indicated for the relief of symptoms associated with allergic rhinitis such as sneezing, rhinorrhea, pruritus, and lacrimation. TAVIST® Tablets 2.68 mg are also indicated for the relief of mild, uncomplicated allergic skin manifestations of urticaria and angioedema.

It should be noted that TAVIST® (clemastine fumarate, USP) is indicated for the dermatologic indications at the 2.68 mg dosage level only.

CONTRAINDICATIONS

Use in Nursing Mothers

Because of the higher risk of antihistamines for infants generally and for newborns and prematures in particular, antihistamine therapy is contraindicated in nursing mothers.

Continued on next page

Sandoz—Cont.

Use in Lower Respiratory Disease
Antihistamines *should not* be used to treat lower respiratory tract symptoms including asthma.
Antihistamines are also contraindicated in the following conditions:

Hypersensitivity to TAVIST® (clemastine fumarate, USP) or other antihistamines of similar chemical structure.

Monamine oxidase inhibitor therapy. *(See Drug Interactions Section)*

WARNINGS

Antihistamines should be used with considerable caution in patients with: narrow angle glaucoma, stenosing peptic ulcer, pyloroduodenal obstruction, symptomatic prostatic hypertrophy, and bladder neck obstruction.
Pediatric Use
Safety and efficacy of TAVIST® have not been established in children under the age of 12.
Use in Pregnancy
Experience with this drug in pregnant women is inadequate to determine whether there exists a potential for harm to the developing fetus.
Use with CNS Depressants
TAVIST® has additive effects with alcohol and other CNS depressants (hypnotics, sedatives, tranquilizers, etc.).
Use in Activities Requiring Mental Alertness
Patients should be warned about engaging in activities requiring mental alertness such as driving a car or operating appliances, machinery, etc.
Use in the Elderly (approximately 60 years or older)
Antihistamines are more likely to cause dizziness, sedation, and hypotension in elderly patients.

PRECAUTIONS

TAVIST® (clemastine fumarate, USP) should be used with caution in patients with: history of bronchial asthma, increased intraocular pressure, hyperthyroidism, cardiovascular disease, and hypertension.
Drug Interactions
MAO inhibitors prolong and intensify the anticholinergic (drying) effects of antihistamines.

ADVERSE REACTIONS

Transient drowsiness, the most common adverse reaction associated with TAVIST® (clemastine fumarate, USP), occurs relatively frequently and may require discontinuation of therapy in some instances.
Antihistaminic Compounds
It should be noted that the following reactions have occurred with one or more antihistamines and, therefore, should be kept in mind when prescribing drugs belonging to this class, including TAVIST®. The most frequent adverse reactions are underlined.

1. *General:* Urticaria, drug rash, anaphylactic shock, photosensitivity, excessive perspiration, chills, dryness of mouth, nose, and throat.
2. *Cardiovascular System:* Hypotension, headache, palpitations, tachycardia, extrasystoles.
3. *Hematologic System:* Hemolytic anemia, thrombocytopenia, agranulocytosis.
4. *Nervous System:* <u>Sedation, sleepiness, dizziness, disturbed coordination,</u> fatigue, confusion, restlessness, excitation, nervousness, tremor, irritability, insomnia, euphoria, parasthesias, blurred vision, diplopia, vertigo, tinnitus, acute labyrinthitis, hysteria, neuritis, convulsions.
5. *GI System:* <u>Epigastric distress,</u> anorexia, nausea, vomiting, diarrhea, constipation.
6. *GU System:* Urinary frequency, difficult urination, urinary retention, early menses.
7. *Respiratory System:* Thickening of bronchial secretions, tightness of chest and wheezing, nasal stuffiness.

OVERDOSAGE

Antihistamine overdosage reactions may vary from central nervous system depression to stimulation. Stimulation is particularly likely in children. Atropine-like signs and symptoms: dry mouth; fixed, dilated pupils; flushing; and gastrointestinal symptoms may also occur.
If vomiting has not occurred spontaneously the conscious patient should be induced to vomit. This is best done by having him drink a glass of water or milk after which he should be made to gag. Precautions against aspiration must be taken, especially in infants and children.
If vomiting is unsuccessful gastric lavage is indicated within 3 hours after ingestion and even later if large amounts of milk or cream were given beforehand. Isotonic and $^1/_2$ isotonic saline is the lavage solution of choice.
Saline cathartics, such as milk of magnesia, by osmosis draw water into the bowel and therefore, are valuable for their action in rapid dilution of bowel content.
Stimulants should *not* be used.
Vasopressors may be used to treat hypotension.

DOSAGE AND ADMINISTRATION

DOSAGE SHOULD BE INDIVIDUALIZED ACCORDING TO THE NEEDS AND RESPONSE OF THE PATIENT.
TAVIST-1® Tablets 1.34 mg
The recommended starting dose is one tablet twice daily. Dosage may be increased as required, but not to exceed six tablets daily.
TAVIST® Tablets 2.68 mg
The maximum recommended dosage is one tablet three times daily. Many patients respond favorably to a single dose which may be repeated as required, but not to exceed three tablets daily.

HOW SUPPLIED

TAVIST-1® clemastine fumarate tablets, USP, *1.34 mg*
White, capsule shaped, compressed, scored tablet, engraved "TAVIST 1" on both sides. Packages of 100.
TAVIST® clemastine fumarate tablets, USP, *2.68 mg*
White, round, compressed tablet, engraved "78/72" and scored on one side, "TAVIST" on other. Packages of 100.
Store and Dispense
Controlled room temperature, between 59°-86°F (15°-30°C); tight, light-resistant container.
[REV: MAY 1996 30190901]
Shown in Product Identification Guide, page 333

VISKEN® ℞
[*vis'kin*]
(pindolol) tablets, USP

Caution: Federal law prohibits dispensing without prescription.
The following prescribing information is based on official labeling in effect on August 1, 1996.

DESCRIPTION

Visken® (pindolol), a synthetic beta-adrenergic receptor blocking agent with intrinsic sympathomimetic activity is 1-(Indol-4-yloxy)-3-(isopropylamino)-2-propanol.
Its structural formula is:

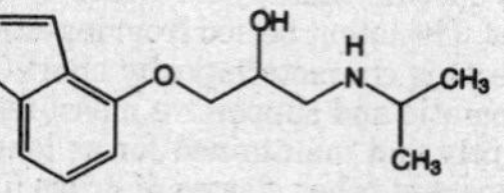

$C_{14}H_{20}N_2O_2$ Mol. wt. 248.33

Pindolol is a white to off-white odorless powder soluble in organic solvents and aqueous acids. Visken® (pindolol) is intended for oral administration.
5 mg and 10 mg Tablets
Active Ingredient: pindolol
Inactive Ingredients: colloidal silicon dioxide, magnesium stearate, microcrystalline cellulose, and pregelatinized starch.

CLINICAL PHARMACOLOGY

Visken® (pindolol) is a non-selective beta-adrenergic antagonist (beta-blocker) which possesses intrinsic sympathomimetic activity (ISA) in therapeutic dosage ranges but does not possess quinidine-like membrane stabilizing activity.

PHARMACODYNAMICS

In standard pharmacologic tests in man and animals, Visken® (pindolol) attenuates increases in heart rate, systolic blood pressure, and cardiac output resulting from exercise and isoproterenol administration, thus confirming its beta-blocking properties. The ISA or partial agonist activity of Visken® (pindolol) is mediated directly at the adrenergic receptor sites and may be blocked by other beta-blockers. In catecholamine-depleted animal experiments, ISA is manifested as an increase in the inotropic and chronotropic activity of the myocardium. In man, ISA is manifested by a smaller reduction in the resting heart rate (4-8 beats/min) than is seen with drugs lacking ISA. There is also a smaller reduction in resting cardiac output. The clinical significance of this observation has not been evaluated and there is no evidence, or reason to believe, that exercise cardiac output is less affected by Visken® (pindolol).
Visken® (pindolol) has been shown in controlled, double-blind clinical studies to be an effective antihypertensive agent when used as monotherapy, or when added to therapy with thiazide-type diuretics. Divided dosages in the range of 10-60 mg daily have been shown to be effective. As monotherapy, Visken® (pindolol) is as effective as propranolol, α-methyldopa, hydrochlorothiazide, and chlorthalidone in reducing systolic and diastolic blood pressure. The effect on blood pressure is not orthostatic, i.e. Visken® (pindolol) was equally effective in reducing the supine and standing blood pressure.
In open, long-term studies up to 4 years, no evidence of diminution of the blood pressure-lowering response was observed.
An average 3-pound increase in body weight has been noted in patients treated with Visken® (pindolol) alone, a larger increase than was observed with propranolol or placebo. The weight gain appeared unrelated to blood pressure response and was not associated with an increased risk of heart failure, although edema was more common than in control patients. Visken® (pindolol) does not have a consistent effect on plasma renin activity.
The mechanism of the antihypertensive effects of beta-blocking agents has not been established, but several mechanisms have been postulated: 1) an effect on the central nervous system resulting in a reduced sympathetic outflow to the periphery, 2) competitive antagonism of catecholamines at peripheral (especially cardiac) adrenergic receptor sites, leading to decreased cardiac output, 3) an inhibition of renin release. These mechanisms appear less likely for pindolol than other beta-blockers in view of the modest effect on resting cardiac output and renin.
Beta-blockade therapy is useful when it is necessary to suppress the effects of beta-adrenergic agonists in order to achieve therapeutic goals. However, in certain clinical situations, (e.g., cardiac failure, heart block, bronchospasm), the preservation of an adequate sympathetic tone may be necessary to maintain vital functions. Although a beta-antagonist with ISA such as Visken® (pindolol) does not eliminate sympathetic tone entirely, there is no controlled evidence that it is safer than other beta-blockers in such conditions as heart failure, heart block, or bronchospasm or is less likely to cause those conditions. In single dose studies of the effects of beta-blockers on FEV_1, Visken® (pindolol) was indistinguishable from other non-cardioselective agents in its reduction of FEV_1, and its reduction in the effectiveness of an exogenous beta agonist.
Exacerbation of angina and, in some cases, myocardial infarction and ventricular dysrhythmias have been reported after abrupt discontinuation of therapy with beta-adrenergic blocking agents in patients with coronary artery disease. Abrupt withdrawal of these agents in patients without coronary artery disease has resulted in transient symptoms, including tremulousness, sweating, palpitation, headache, and malaise. Several mechanisms have been proposed to explain these phenomena, among them increased sensitivity to catecholamines because of increased numbers of beta receptors.

PHARMACOKINETICS AND METABOLISM
Visken® (pindolol) is rapidly and reproducibly absorbed (greater than 95%), achieving peak plasma concentrations within 1 hour of drug administration. Visken® (pindolol) has no significant first-pass effect. The blood concentrations are proportional in a linear manner to the administered dose in the range of 5-20 mg. Upon repeated administration to the same subject, variation is minimal. After a single dose, intersubject variation for peak plasma concentrations was about 4 fold (e.g., 45-167 ng/mL for a 20 mg dose). Upon multiple dosing, intersubject variation decreased to 2-2.5 fold. Visken® (pindolol) is only 40% bound to plasma proteins and is evenly distributed between plasma and red cells. The volume of distribution in healthy subjects is about 2 L/kg.
Visken® (pindolol) undergoes extensive metabolism in animals and man. In man, 35%-40% is excreted unchanged in the urine and 60%-65% is metabolized primarily to hydroxy-metabolites which are excreted as glucuronides and ethereal sulfates. The polar metabolites are excreted with a half-life of approximately 8 hours and thus multiple dosing therapy (q.8H) results in a less than 50% accumulation in plasma. About 6%-9% of an administered intravenous dose is excreted by the bile into the feces.
The disposition of Visken® (pindolol) after oral administration is monophasic with a half-life in healthy subjects or hypertensive patients with normal renal function of approximately 3-4 hours. Following t.i.d. administration (q.8H), no significant accumulation of Visken® (pindolol) is observed.
In elderly hypertensive patients with normal renal function, the half-life of Visken® (pindolol) is more variable, averaging about 7 hours, but with values as high as 15 hours.
In hypertensive patients with renal diseases, the half-life is within the range expected for healthy subjects. However, a significant decrease (50%) in volume of distribution (V_D) is observed in uremic patients and V_D appears to be directly correlated to creatinine clearance. Therefore, renal drug clearance is significantly reduced in uremic patients, resulting in a significant decrease in urinary excretion of unchanged drug. Uremic patients with a creatinine clearance of less than 20 mL/min generally excreted less than 15% of the administered dose unchanged in the urine.
In patients with histologically diagnosed cirrhosis of the liver, the elimination of Visken® (pindolol) was more variable in rate and generally significantly slower than in healthy subjects. The total body clearance of Visken® (pindolol) in cirrhotic patients ranged from about 50-300 mL/min and was directly correlated to antipyrine clearance. The half-life ranges from 2.5 hours to greater than 30 hours. These findings strongly suggest that caution should be exercised in dosage adjustments of Visken® (pindolol) in such patients.

The bioavailability of Visken® (pindolol) is not significantly affected by co-administration of food, hydralazine, hydrochlorothiazide or aspirin. Visken® (pindolol) has no effect on warfarin activity or the clinical effectiveness of digoxin, although small transient decreases in plasma digoxin concentrations were noted.

INDICATIONS AND USAGE

Visken® (pindolol) is indicated in the management of hypertension. It may be used alone or concomitantly with other antihypertensive agents, particularly with a thiazide-type diuretic.

CONTRAINDICATIONS

Visken® (pindolol) is contraindicated in: 1) bronchial asthma; 2) overt cardiac failure; 3) cardiogenic shock; 4) second and third degree heart block; 5) severe bradycardia. *(See WARNINGS)*

WARNINGS

Cardiac Failure

Sympathetic stimulation may be a vital component supporting circulatory function in patients with congestive heart failure, and its inhibition by beta-blockade may precipitate more severe failure. Although beta-blockers should be avoided in overt congestive heart failure, if necessary, Visken® (pindolol) can be used with caution in patients with a history of failure who are well-compensated, usually with digitalis and diuretics. Beta-adrenergic blocking agents do not abolish the inotropic action of digitalis on heart muscle.

In Patients Without History of Cardiac Failure

In patients with latent cardiac insufficiency, continued depression of the myocardium with beta-blocking agents over a period of time can in some cases lead to cardiac failure. At the first sign or symptom of impending cardiac failure, patients should be fully digitalized and/or be given a diuretic, and the response observed closely. If cardiac failure continues, despite adequate digitalization and diuretic, Visken® (pindolol) therapy should be withdrawn (gradually if possible).

Exacerbation of Ischemic Heart Disease Following Abrupt Withdrawal

Hypersensitivity to catecholamines has been observed in patients withdrawn from beta-blocker therapy; exacerbation of angina and, in some cases, myocardial infarction have occurred after *abrupt* discontinuation of such therapy. When discontinuing chronically administered Visken® (pindolol), particularly in patients with ischemic heart disease, the dosage should be gradually reduced over a period of 1-2 weeks and the patient should be carefully monitored. If angina markedly worsens or acute coronary insufficiency develops, Visken® (pindolol) administration should be reinstituted promptly, at least temporarily, and other measures appropriate for the management of unstable angina should be taken. Patients should be warned against interruption or discontinuation of therapy without the physician's advice. Because coronary artery disease is common and may be unrecognized, it may be prudent not to discontinue Visken® (pindolol) therapy abruptly even in patients treated only for hypertension.

Nonallergic Bronchospasm (e.g., chronic bronchitis, emphysema) – Patients with Bronchospastic Diseases Should in General Not Receive Beta-Blockers

Visken® (pindolol) should be administered with caution since it may block bronchodilation produced by endogenous or exogenous catecholamine stimulation of beta$_2$ receptors.

Major Surgery

Because beta blockade impairs the ability of the heart to respond to reflex stimuli and may increase the risks of general anesthesia and surgical procedures, resulting in protracted hypotension or low cardiac output, it has generally been suggested that such therapy should be gradually withdrawn several days prior to surgery. Recognition of the increased sensitivity to catecholamines of patients recently withdrawn from beta-blocker therapy, however, has made this recommendation controversial. If possible, beta-blockers should be withdrawn well before surgery takes place. In the event of emergency surgery, the anesthesiologist should be informed that the patient is on beta-blocker therapy.

The effects of Visken® (pindolol) can be reversed by administration of beta-receptor agonists such as isoproterenol, dopamine, dobutamine, or levarterenol. Difficulty in restarting and maintaining the heart beat has also been reported with beta-adrenergic receptor blocking agents.

Diabetes and Hypoglycemia

Beta-adrenergic blockade may prevent the appearance of premonitory signs and symptoms (e.g., tachycardia and blood pressure changes) of acute hypoglycemia. This is especially important with labile diabetics. Beta-blockade also reduces the release of insulin in response to hyperglycemia; therefore, it may be necessary to adjust the dose of antidiabetic drugs.

Thyrotoxicosis

Beta-adrenergic blockade may mask certain clinical signs (e.g., tachycardia) of hyperthyroidism. Patients suspected of developing thyrotoxicosis should be managed carefully to avoid abrupt withdrawal of beta-blockade which might precipitate a thyroid crisis.

Adverse Reactions Which Were Volunteered or Elicited (and at least possibly drug related)

Body System/Adverse Reactions	Visken® (pindolol) (N = 322) %	Active Controls* (N = 188) %	Placebo (N = 78) %
Central Nervous System			
Bizarre or Many Dreams	5	0	6
Dizziness	9	11	1
Fatigue	8	4	4
Hallucinations	<1	0	0
Insomnia	10	3	10
Nervousness	7	3	5
Weakness	4	2	1
Autonomic Nervous System			
Paresthesia	3	1	6
Cardiovascular			
Dyspnea	5	4	6
Edema	6	3	1
Heart Failure	<1	<1	0
Palpitations	<1	1	0
Musculoskeletal			
Chest Pain	3	1	3
Joint Pain	7	4	4
Muscle Cramps	3	1	0
Muscle Pain	10	9	8
Gastrointestinal			
Abdominal Discomfort	4	4	5
Nausea	5	2	1
Skin			
Pruritus	1	<1	0
Rash	<1	<1	1

* Active Controls: Patients received either propranolol, α-methyldopa or a diuretic (hydrochlorothiazide or chlorthalidone).

PRECAUTIONS

Impaired Renal or Hepatic Function

Beta-blocking agents should be used with caution in patients with impaired hepatic or renal function. Poor renal function has only minor effects on Visken® (pindolol) clearance, but poor hepatic function may cause blood levels of Visken® (pindolol) to increase substantially.

Information for Patients

Patients, especially those with evidence of coronary artery insufficiency, should be warned against interruption or discontinuation of Visken® (pindolol) therapy without the physician's advice. Although cardiac failure rarely occurs in properly selected patients, patients being treated with beta-adrenergic blocking agents should be advised to consult the physician at the first sign or symptom of impending failure.

Drug Interactions

Catecholamine-depleting drugs (e.g., reserpine) may have an additive effect when given with beta-blocking agents. Patients receiving Visken® (pindolol) plus a catecholamine-depleting agent should, therefore, be closely observed for evidence of hypotension and/or marked bradycardia which may produce vertigo, syncope, or postural hypotension.

Visken® (pindolol) has been used with a variety of antihypertensive agents, including hydrochlorothiazide, hydralazine, and guanethidine without unexpected adverse interactions.

Visken® (pindolol) has been shown to increase serum thioridazine levels when both drugs are co-administered. Visken® (pindolol) levels may also be increased with this combination.

Risk of Anaphylactic Reaction: While taking beta blockers, patients with a history of severe anaphylactic reaction to a variety of allergens may be more reactive to repeated challenge, either accidental, diagnostic, or therapeutic. Such patients may be unresponsive to the usual doses of epinephrine used to treat allergic reaction.

Carcinogenesis, Mutagenesis, Impairment of Fertility

In chronic oral toxicologic studies (1-2 years) in mice, rats, and dogs, Visken® (pindolol) did not produce any significant toxic effects. In 2-year oral carcinogenicity studies in rats and mice in doses as high as 59 mg/kg/day and 124 mg/kg/day (50 and 100 times the maximum recommended human dose), respectively, Visken® (pindolol) did not produce any neoplastic, preneoplastic, or nonneoplastic pathologic lesions. In fertility and general reproductive performance studies in rats, Visken® (pindolol) caused no adverse effects at a dose of 10 mg/kg.

In the male fertility and general reproductive performance test in rats, definite toxicity characterized by mortality and decreased weight gain was observed in the group given 100 mg/kg/day. At 30 mg/kg/day, decreased mating was associated with testicular atrophy and/or decreased spermatogenesis. This response is not clearly drug related, however, as there was no dose response relationship within this experiment and no similar effect on testes of rats administered Visken® (pindolol) as a dietary admixture for 104 weeks. There appeared to be an increase in prenatal mortality in males given 100 mg/kg but development of offspring was not impaired.

In females administered Visken® (pindolol) prior to mating through day 21 of lactation, mating behavior was decreased at 100 mg/kg and 30 mg/kg. At these dosages there also was increased mortality of offspring. Prenatal mortality was increased at 10 mg/kg but there was not a clear dose response relationship in this experiment. There was an increased resorption rate at 100 mg/kg observed in females necropsied on the 15th day of gestation.

Pregnancy

Category B: Studies in rats and rabbits exceeding 100 times the maximum recommended human doses, revealed no embryotoxicity or teratogenicity. Since there are no adequate and well-controlled studies in pregnant women, and since animal reproduction studies are not always predictive of human response, Visken® (pindolol), as with any drug, should be employed during pregnancy only if the potential benefit justifies the potential risk to the fetus.

Nursing Mothers

Since Visken® (pindolol) is secreted in human milk, nursing should not be undertaken by mothers receiving the drug.

Pediatric Use

Safety and effectiveness in pediatric patients have not been established.

CLINICAL LABORATORY

Minor persistent elevations in serum transaminases (SGOT, SGPT) have been noted in 7% of patients during Visken® (pindolol) administration, but progressive elevations were not observed. These elevations were not associated with any other abnormalities that would suggest hepatic impairment, such as decreased serum albumin and total proteins. During more than a decade of worldwide marketing, there have been no reports in the medical literature of overt hepatic injury. Alkaline phosphatase, lactic acid dehydrogenase (LDH), and uric acid are also elevated on rare occasions. The significance of these findings is unknown.

ADVERSE REACTIONS

Most adverse reactions have been mild. The incidences listed in the following table are derived from 12-week comparative double-blind, parallel design trials in hypertensive patients given Visken® (pindolol) as monotherapy, given various active control drugs as monotherapy, or given placebo. Data for Visken® (pindolol) and the positive controls were pooled from several trials because no striking differences were seen in the individual studies, with 1 exception. When considering all adverse reactions reported, the frequency of edema was noticeably higher in positive control trials [16% Visken® (pindolol) vs. 9% positive control] than in placebo controlled trials [6% Visken® (pindolol) vs. 3% placebo]. The table includes adverse reactions either volunteered or elicited, and at least possibly drug related, which were reported in greater than 2% of Visken® (pindolol) patients and other selected important reactions.

[See table above.]

The following selected (potentially important) adverse reactions were seen in 2% or fewer patients and their relation-

Continued on next page

Sandoz—Cont.

ship to Visken® (pindolol) is uncertain. CENTRAL NERVOUS SYSTEM: anxiety, lethargy; AUTONOMIC NERVOUS SYSTEM: visual disturbances, hyperhidrosis; CARDIOVASCULAR: bradycardia, claudication, cold extremities, heart block, hypotension, syncope, tachycardia, weight gain; GASTROINTESTINAL: diarrhea, vomiting; RESPIRATORY: wheezing; UROGENITAL: impotence, pollakiuria; MISCELLANEOUS: eye discomfort or burning eyes.

POTENTIAL ADVERSE EFFECTS

In addition, other adverse effects not aforementioned have been reported with other beta-adrenergic blocking agents and should be considered potential adverse effects of Visken® (pindolol).

Central Nervous System: Reversible mental depression progressing to catatonia; an acute reversible syndrome characterized by disorientation for time and place, short-term memory loss, emotional lability, slightly clouded sensorium, and decreased performance on neuropsychometrics.

Cardiovascular: Intensification of AV block. *(See CONTRAINDICATIONS)*

Allergic: Erythematous rash; fever combined with aching and sore throat; laryngospasm; respiratory distress.

Hematologic: Agranulocytosis; thrombocytopenic and nonthrombocytopenic purpura.

Gastrointestinal: Mesenteric arterial thrombosis; ischemic colitis.

Miscellaneous: Reversible alopecia; Peyronie's disease.

The oculomucocutaneous syndrome associated with the betablocker practolol has not been reported with Visken® (pindolol) during investigational use and extensive foreign experience amounting to over 4 million patient-years.

OVERDOSAGE

No specific information on emergency treatment of overdosage is available. Therefore, on the basis of the pharmacologic actions of Visken® (pindolol), the following general measures should be employed as appropriate in addition to gastric lavage:

Excessive Bradycardia: administer atropine; if there is no response to vagal blockade, administer isoproterenol cautiously.

Cardiac Failure: digitalize the patient and/or administer diuretic. It has been reported that glucagon may be useful in this situation.

Hypotension: administer vasopressors, e.g., epinephrine or levarterenol, with serial monitoring of blood pressure. (There is evidence that epinephrine may be the drug of choice.)

Bronchospasm: administer a beta$_2$ stimulating agent such as isoproterenol and/or a theophylline derivative.

A case of an acute overdosage has been reported with an intake of 500 mg of Visken® (pindolol) by a hypertensive patient. Blood pressure increased and heart rate was ≥ 80 beats/min. Recovery was uneventful. In another case, 250 mg of Visken® (pindolol) was taken with 150 mg diazepam and 50 mg nitrazepam, producing coma and hypotension. The patient recovered in 24 hours.

DOSAGE AND ADMINISTRATION

The dosage of Visken® (pindolol) should be individualized. The recommended initial dose of Visken® (pindolol) is 5 mg b.i.d. alone or in combination with other antihypertensive agents. An antihypertensive response usually occurs within the first week of treatment. Maximal response, however, may take as long as or occasionally longer than 2 weeks. If a satisfactory reduction in blood pressure does not occur within 3-4 weeks, the dose may be adjusted in increments of 10 mg/day at these intervals up to a maximum of 60 mg/day.

HOW SUPPLIED

Visken® (pindolol) tablets, USP

White, uncoated, heart-shaped tablets; 5 mg and 10 mg, packages of 100. 5 mg tablets engraved "VISKEN 5" on one side, and embossed "V" on other side (NDC 0078-0111-05). 10 mg tablets engraved "VISKEN 10" on one side, and embossed "V" on other side (NDC 0078-0073-05).

Store and Dispense

Below 86°F (30°C); tight, light-resistant container.

[REV: APRIL 1996   30195902]

Shown in Product Identification Guide, page 333

Check the **PINK** section
to find a particular **BRAND**.

Sanofi Winthrop Pharmaceuticals
90 PARK AVENUE
NEW YORK, NY 10016

Direct Inquiries to:
(212) 551-4000

For Medical Information Contact:
Product Information Services
(800) 446-6267

Sales and Ordering:
East Coast: (800) 223-1062
West Coast: (800) 223-5511

ARALEN® Hydrochloride
brand of chloroquine hydrochloride
injection, USP   ℞

**For Malaria and
Extraintestinal Amebiasis**

> WARNING: PHYSICIANS SHOULD COMPLETELY FAMILIARIZE THEMSELVES WITH THE COMPLETE CONTENTS OF THIS LEAFLET BEFORE PRESCRIBING ARALEN.

DESCRIPTION

Parenteral solution, each mL containing 50 mg of the dihydrochloride salt equivalent to 40 mg of chloroquine base. ARALEN hydrochloride, a 4-aminoquinoline compound, is chemically 7- (Chloro - 4 - [[4 - diethylamino) - 1 - methylbutyl] amino]-quinoline dihydrochloride, a white, crystalline substance, freely soluble in water.

ACTIONS

The compound is a highly active antimalarial and amebicidal agent.

ARALEN hydrochloride has been found to be highly active against the erythrocytic forms of *Plasmodium vivax* and *malariae* and most strains of *Plasmodium falciparum* (but not the gametocytes of *P. falciparum)*. The precise mechanism of action of the drug is not known.

ARALEN hydrochloride does not prevent relapses in patients with vivax or malariae malaria because it is not effective against exoerythrocytic forms of the parasite, nor will it prevent vivax or malariae infection when administered as a prophylactic. It is highly effective as a suppressive agent in patients with vivax or malariae malaria, in terminating acute attacks, and significantly lengthening the interval between treatment and relapse. In patients with falciparum malaria it abolishes the acute attack and effects complete cure of the infection, unless due to a resistant strain of *P. falciparum.*

INDICATIONS

ARALEN hydrochloride is indicated for the treatment of extraintestinal amebiasis and for treatment of acute attacks of malaria due to *P. vivax, P. malariae, P. ovale,* and susceptible strains of *P. falciparum* when oral therapy is not feasible.

CONTRAINDICATIONS

Use of this drug is contraindicated in the presence of retinal or visual field changes either attributable to 4- aminoquinoline compounds or to any other etiology, and in patients with known hypersensitivity to 4-aminoquinoline compounds. However, in the treatment of acute attacks of malaria caused by susceptible strains of plasmodia, the physician may elect to use this drug after carefully weighing the possible benefits and risks to the patient.

WARNINGS

Children and infants are extremely susceptible to adverse effects from an overdose of parenteral ARALEN and sudden deaths have been recorded after such administration. In no instance should the single dose of parenteral ARALEN administered to infants or children exceed 5 mg base per kg.

In recent years it has been found that certain strains of *P. falciparum* have become resistant to 4-aminoquinoline compounds (including chloroquine and hydroxychloroquine) as shown by the fact that normally adequate doses have failed to prevent or cure clinical malaria or parasitemia. Treatment with quinine or other specific forms of therapy is therefore advised for patients infected with a resistant strain of parasites.

Use of ARALEN should be avoided in patients with psoriasis, for it may precipitate a severe attack of psoriasis. Some authors consider the use of 4-aminoquinoline compounds con-

---

traindicated in patients with porphyria since the condition may be exacerbated.

Irreversible retinal damage has been observed in some patients who had received long-term or high-dosage 4-aminoquinoline therapy. Retinopathy has been reported to be dose related.

If there is any indication (past or present) of abnormality in the visual acuity, visual field, or retinal macular areas (such as pigmentary changes, loss of foveal reflex), or any visual symptoms (such as light flashes and streaks) which are not fully explainable by difficulties of accommodation or corneal opacities, the drug should be discontinued immediately and the patient closely observed for possible progression. Retinal changes (and visual disturbances) may progress even after cessation of therapy.

Usage in Pregnancy. Usage of this drug during pregnancy should be avoided except in the suppression or treatment of malaria when in the judgment of the physician the benefit outweighs the possible hazard. It should be noted that radioactively tagged chloroquine administered intravenously to pregnant pigmented CBA mice passed rapidly across the placenta, accumulated selectively in the melanin structures of the fetal eyes and was retained in the ocular tissues for five months after the drug had been eliminated from the rest of the body.[1]

PRECAUTIONS

Since the drug is known to concentrate in the liver, it should be used with caution in patients with hepatic disease or alcoholism or in conjunction with known hepatotoxic drugs.

The drug should be administered with caution to patients having G-6-PD (glucose-6-phosphate dehydrogenase) deficiency.

ADVERSE REACTIONS

Respiratory depression, cardiovascular collapse, shock, convulsions, and death have been reported with overdoses of ARALEN hydrochloride, brand of chloroquine hydrochloride injection, especially in infants and children.

Any of the adverse reactions associated with short-term oral administration of chloroquine phosphate must be considered a possibility with chloroquine hydrochloride. Cardiovascular effects, such as hypotension and electrocardiographic changes (particularly inversion or depression of the T-wave, widening of the QRS complex), have rarely been noted in patients receiving usual antimalarial doses of the drug. Mild and transient headache, pruritus, psychic stimulation, visual disturbances (blurring of vision and difficulty of focusing or accommodation), pleomorphic skin eruptions, and gastrointestinal complaints (anorexia, nausea, vomiting, diarrhea, abdominal cramps) have been observed.

Instances of convulsive seizures associated with oral chloroquine therapy in patients with extraintestinal amebiasis have been reported.

A few cases of a nerve type of deafness have been reported after prolonged therapy, usually in high doses. Tinnitus and reduced hearing have been reported, in a patient with preexistent auditory damage, after administration of only 500 mg once a week for a few months. Since neuromyopathy, blood dyscrasias, lichen planus-like eruptions, and skin and mucosal pigmentary changes have been noted during prolonged oral therapy, their occurrence with this dosage form is possible.

Patients with retinal changes may be asymptomatic, especially in early cases, or may complain of nyctalopia and scotomatous vision with field defects of paracentral, pericentral ring types, and typically temporal scotomas, eg, difficulty in reading with words tending to disappear, seeing only half an object, misty vision, and fog before the eyes. Rarely scotomatous vision may occur without observable retinal changes.

DOSAGE AND ADMINISTRATION

Malaria — Adult Dose. An initial dose of 4 mL or 5 mL (160 mg to 200 mg chloroquine base) may be injected intramuscularly and repeated in 6 hours if necessary. The total parenteral dosage in the first 24 hours should not exceed 800 mg chloroquine base. Treatment by mouth should be started as soon as practicable and continued until a course of approximately 1.5 g of base in 3 days is completed.

Pediatric Dose. Infants and children are extremely susceptible to overdosage of parenteral ARALEN. Severe reactions and deaths have occurred. In the pediatric age range, parenteral ARALEN dosage should be calculated in proportion to the adult dose based upon body weight. The recommended single dose in infants and children is 5 mg base per kg. This dose may be repeated in 6 hours; however, the total dose in any 24 hour period should not exceed 10 mg base per kg of body weight. Parenteral administration should be terminated and oral therapy instituted as soon as possible.

Extraintestinal Amebiasis—In adult patients not able to tolerate oral therapy, from 4 mL to 5 mL (160 mg to 200 mg chloroquine base) may be injected daily for 10 to 12 days. Oral administration should be substituted or resumed as soon as possible.

OVERDOSAGE

Inadvertent toxic doses may produce respiratory depression or shock with hypotension. Respiratory depression is treated by artificial respiration and administration of oxygen. In shock with hypotension, a potent vasopressor, such as NEO-SYNEPHRINE® hydrochloride, brand of phenylephrine hydrochloride, USP, should be given intramuscularly in doses of 2 mg to 5 mg.

HOW SUPPLIED

Ampuls of 5 mL, box of 5 (NDC 0024-0074-01)

REFERENCE

Ullberg S, Lindquist N G, Sjostrand S E: Accumulation of chorio-retinotoxic drugs in the foetal eye. *Nature* 1970; 227:1257.

AW-100-H

ARALEN® Phosphate
brand of chloroquine phosphate tablets, USP

℞

For Malaria and Extraintestinal Amebiasis

> **WARNING**
> PHYSICIANS SHOULD COMPLETELY FAMILIAR-IZE THEMSELVES WITH THE COMPLETE CONTENTS OF THIS LEAFLET BEFORE PRESCRIBING ARALEN.

DESCRIPTION

ARALEN phosphate, brand of chloroquine phosphate, USP, is a 4-aminoquinoline compound for oral administration. It is a white, odorless, bitter tasting, crystalline substance, freely soluble in water.

ARALEN phosphate is an antimalarial and amebicidal drug. Chemically, it is 7-chloro- 4-[[4- (diethylamino) -1-methyl-butyl]amino] quinoline phosphate (1:2).

Inactive Ingredients: Carnauba Wax, Colloidal Silicon Dioxide, D&C Red No 27, Dibasic Calcium Phosphate, Hydroxypropyl Methylcellulose, Magnesium Stearate, Microcrystalline Cellulose, Polyethylene Glycol, Polysorbate 80, Pregelatinized Starch, Sodium Starch Glycolate, Stearic Acid, Titanium Dioxide.

CLINICAL PHARMACOLOGY

ARALEN phosphate has been found to be highly active against the erythrocytic forms of *Plasmodium vivax* and *Plasmodium malariae* and most strains of *Plasmodium falciparum* (but not the gametocytes of *P. falciparum*).

The mechanism of plasmodicidal action of chloroquine is not completely certain. While the drug can inhibit certain enzymes, its effect is believed to result, at least in part, from its interaction with DNA.

Chloroquine is rapidly and almost completely absorbed from the gastrointestinal tract, and only a small proportion of the administered dose is found in the stools. Approximately 55% of the drug in the plasma is bound to nondiffusible plasma constituents. Excretion of chloroquine is quite slow, but is increased by acidification of the urine. Chloroquine is deposited in the tissues in considerable amounts. In animals, from 200 to 700 times the plasma concentration may be found in the liver, spleen, kidney, and lung; leukocytes also concentrate the drug. The brain and spinal cord, in contrast, contain only 10 to 30 times the amount present in plasma.

Chloroquine undergoes appreciable degradation in the body. The main metabolite is desethylchloroquine, which accounts for one fourth of the total material appearing in the urine; bisdesethylchloroquine, a carboxylic acid derivative, and other metabolic products as yet uncharacterized are found in small amounts. Slightly more than half of the urinary drug products can be accounted for as unchanged chloroquine.

Microbiology

ARALEN phosphate has been found to be highly active against the erythrocytic forms of *Plasmodium vivax* and *malariae* and most strains of *Plasmodium falciparum* (but not the gametocytes of *P. falciparum*). The precise mechanism of action of the drug is not known.

In vitro studies with trophozoites of *Entamoeba histolytica* have demonstrated that ARALEN phosphate also possesses amebicidal activity comparable to that of emetine.

INDICATIONS AND USAGE

ARALEN phosphate, brand of chloroquine phosphate, is indicated for the suppressive treatment and for acute attacks of malaria due to *P. vivax, P. malariae, P. ovale,* and susceptible strains of *P. falciparum.* The drug is also indicated for the treatment of extraintestinal amebiasis.

ARALEN phosphate does not prevent relapses in patients with vivax or malariae malaria because it is not effective against exoerythrocytic forms of the parasite, nor will it prevent vivax or malariae infection when administered as a prophylactic. It is highly effective as a suppressive agent in patients with vivax or malariae malaria, in terminating acute attacks, and significantly lengthening the interval between treatment and relapse. In patients with falciparum malaria it abolishes the acute attack and effects complete cure of the infection, unless due to a resistant strain of *P. falciparum.*

CONTRAINDICATIONS

Use of this drug is contraindicated in the presence of retinal or visual field changes either attributable to 4-aminoquinoline compounds or to any other etiology, and in patients with known hypersensitivity to 4-aminoquinoline compounds. However, in the treatment of acute attacks of malaria caused by susceptible strains of plasmodia, the physician may elect to use this drug after carefully weighing the possible benefits and risks to the patient.

WARNINGS

In recent years it has been found that certain strains of *P. falciparum* have become resistant to 4-aminoquinoline compounds (including chloroquine and hydroxychloroquine) as shown by the fact that normally adequate doses have failed to prevent or cure clinical malaria or parasitemia. Treatment with quinine or other specific forms of therapy is therefore advised for patients infected with a resistant strain of parasites.

Irreversible retinal damage has been observed in some patients who had received long-term or high-dosage 4-aminoquinoline therapy. Retinopathy has been reported to be dose related.

When prolonged therapy with any antimalarial compound is contemplated, initial (base line) and periodic ophthalmologic examinations (including visual acuity, expert slit-lamp, funduscopic, and visual field tests) should be performed.

If there is any indication (past or present) of abnormality in the visual acuity, visual field, or retinal macular areas (such as pigmentary changes, loss of foveal reflex), or any visual symptoms (such as light flashes and streaks) which are not fully explainable by difficulties of accommodation or corneal opacities, the drug should be discontinued immediately and the patient closely observed for possible progression. Retinal changes (and visual disturbances) may progress even after cessation of therapy.

All patients on long-term therapy with this preparation should be questioned and examined periodically, including testing knee and ankle reflexes, to detect any evidence of muscular weakness. If weakness occurs, discontinue the drug.

A number of fatalities have been reported following the accidental ingestion of chloroquine, sometimes in relatively small doses (0.75 g or 1 g chloroquine phosphate in one 3-year-old child). Patients should be strongly warned to keep this drug out of the reach of children because they are especially sensitive to the 4-aminoquinoline compounds.

Use of ARALEN phosphate, brand of chloroquine phosphate tablets, in patients with psoriasis may precipitate a severe attack of psoriasis. When used in patients with porphyria the condition may be exacerbated. The drug should not be used in these conditions unless in the judgment of the physician the benefit to the patient outweighs the possible hazard.

PRECAUTIONS

General

If any severe blood disorder appears which is not attributable to the disease under treatment, discontinuance of the drug should be considered.

Since this drug is known to concentrate in the liver, it should be used with caution in patients with hepatic disease or alcoholism or in conjunction with known hepatotoxic drugs.

The drug should be administered with caution to patients having G-6-PD (glucose-6-phosphate dehydrogenase) deficiency.

Laboratory Tests

Complete blood cell counts should be made periodically if patients are given prolonged therapy.

Nursing Mothers

Because of the potential for serious adverse reactions in nursing infants from chloroquine, a decision should be made whether to discontinue nursing or to discontinue the drug, taking into account the importance of the drug to the mother.

Pediatric Use

See WARNINGS and DOSAGE AND ADMINISTRATION.

ADVERSE REACTIONS

Ocular reactions: Irreversible retinal damage in patients receiving long-term or high-dosage 4-aminoquinoline therapy; visual disturbances (blurring of vision and difficulty of focusing or accommodation); nyctalopia; scotomatous vision with field defects of paracentral, pericentral ring types, and typically temporal scotomas, eg, difficulty in reading with words tending to disappear, seeing half an object, misty vision, and fog before the eyes.

Neuromuscular reactions: Convulsive seizures.

Auditory reactions: Nerve type deafness; tinnitus, reduced hearing in patients with preexisting auditory damage.

Gastrointestinal reactions: Anorexia, nausea, vomiting, diarrhea, abdominal cramps.

Dermatologic reactions: Pleomorphic skin eruptions, skin and mucosal pigmentary changes; lichen planus-like eruptions, pruritus, and hair loss.

CNS reactions: Mild and transient headache, psychic stimulation.

Cardiovascular reactions: Rarely, hypotension, electrocardiographic change.

OVERDOSAGE

Symptoms: Chloroquine is very rapidly and completely absorbed after ingestion. Toxic doses of chloroquine can be fatal. As little as 1 g may be fatal in children. Toxic symptoms can occur within minutes. These consist of headache, drowsiness, visual disturbances, nausea and vomiting, cardiovascular collapse, and convulsions followed by sudden and early respiratory and cardiac arrest. The electrocardiogram may reveal atrial standstill, nodal rhythm, prolonged intraventricular conduction time, and progressive bradycardia leading to ventricular fibrillation and/or arrest.

Treatment: Treatment is symptomatic and must be prompt with immediate evacuation of the stomach by emesis (at home, before transportation to the hospital) or gastric lavage until the stomach is completely emptied. If finely powdered, activated charcoal is introduced by stomach tube, after lavage, and within 30 minutes after ingestion of the antimalarial, it may inhibit further intestinal absorption of the drug. To be effective, the dose of activated charcoal should be at least five times the estimated dose of chloroquine ingested. Convulsions, if present, should be controlled before attempting gastric lavage. If due to cerebral stimulation, cautious administration of an ultra short-acting barbiturate may be tried but, if due to anoxia, it should be corrected by oxygen administration and artificial respiration. In shock with hypotension, a potent vasopressor should be administered. Because of the importance of supporting respiration, tracheal intubation or tracheostomy, followed by gastric lavage, may also be necessary. Peritoneal dialysis and exchange transfusions have also been suggested to reduce the level of the drug in the blood.

A patient who survives the acute phase and is asymptomatic should be closely observed for at least six hours. Fluids may be forced, and sufficient ammonium chloride (8 g daily in divided doses for adults) may be administered for a few days to acidify the urine to help promote urinary excretion in cases of both overdosage or sensitivity.

DOSAGE AND ADMINISTRATION

The dosage of chloroquine phosphate is often expressed or calculated as the base. Each 500 mg tablet of ARALEN phosphate, brand of chloroquine phosphate, is equivalent to 300 mg base. In infants and children the dosage is preferably calculated on the body weight.

Malaria: Suppression—**Adult Dose:** 500 mg (= 300 mg base) on exactly the same day of each week.

Pediatric Dose: The weekly suppressive dosage is 5 mg calculated as base, per kg of body weight, but should not exceed the adult dose regardless of weight.

If circumstances permit, suppressive therapy should begin two weeks prior to exposure. However, failing this in adults, an initial double (loading) dose of 1 g (= 600 mg base), or in children 10 mg base/kg may be taken in two divided doses, six hours apart. The suppressive therapy should be continued for eight weeks after leaving the endemic area.

For Treatment of Acute Attack

Adults: An initial dose of 1 g (= 600 mg base) followed by an additional 500 mg (= 300 mg base) after six to eight hours and a single dose of 500 mg (= 300 mg base) on each of two consecutive days. This represents a total dose of 2.5 g chloroquine phosphate or 1.5 g base in three days.

The dosage for adults may also be calculated on the basis of body weight; this method is preferred for infants and children. A total dose representing 25 mg of base per kg of body weight is administered in three days, as follows:

First dose: 10 mg base per kg (but not exceeding a single dose of 600 mg base).

Second dose: 5 mg base per kg (but not exceeding a single dose of 300 mg base) 6 hours after first dose.

Third dose: 5 mg base per kg 18 hours after second dose.

Fourth dose: 5 mg base per kg 24 hours after third dose.

For radical cure of *vivax* and *malariae* malaria concomitant therapy with an 8-aminoquinoline compound is necessary.

Continued on next page

This product information was prepared in September 1996. On these and other products of Sanofi Winthrop Pharmaceuticals, detailed information may be obtained on a current basis by direct inquiry to Product Information Services, 90 Park Avenue, New York, NY 10016 (toll free 1-800-446-6267).

Sanofi Winthrop—Cont.

Extraintestinal Amebiasis: Adults, 1 g (600 mg base) daily for two days, followed by 500 mg (300 mg base) daily for at least two to three weeks. Treatment is usually combined with an effective intestinal amebicide.

HOW SUPPLIED

Tablets of 500 mg (= 300 mg base), bottles of 25 (NDC 0024-0084-01).

Pink, film-coated convex tablets, ½ inch in diameter with an uncoated core, containing 500 mg chloroquine phosphate, equivalent to 300 mg of chloroquine base.

ASW-2

Shown in Product Identification Guide, page 333

BRONKOSOL® ℞

brand of isoetharine inhalation solution, USP, 1%
BRONCHODILATOR SOLUTION FOR ORAL INHALATION

DESCRIPTION

Isoetharine hydrochloride, USP, 1% also contains: Acetone Sodium Bisulfite, Glycerin, Parabens, Purified Water, Sodium Chloride, and Sodium Citrate.

BRONKOMETER® ℞

brand of isoetharine mesylate inhalation aerosol, USP

DESCRIPTION

BRONKOMETER is a complete pocket nebulizer containing isoetharine mesylate 0.61% (w/w) with alcohol 30% (w/w), ascorbic acid 0.1% (w/w), (as preservative), fluorochlorohydrocarbons (as gaseous propellants), menthol and saccharin.

The BRONKOMETER unit is designed to contain 20 metered doses per mL of solution (eg, 200 doses per 10 mL) and to deliver 340 μg isoetharine mesylate at the mouthpiece per actuation.

Isoetharine mesylate is a sympathomimetic amine which provides therapeutic bronchodilation is a metered dose inhaler.

Chemically, isoetharine mesylate is 3.4-Dihydroxy-α-[1-(isopropylamino)propyl]benzyl alcohol methanesulfonate (salt).

CLINICAL PHARMACOLOGY

Isoetharine is a sympathomimetic amine with preferential affinity for $Beta_2$ adrenergic receptor sites of bronchial and certain arteriolar musculature, and a lower order of affinity for $Beta_1$ adrenergic receptors. Its activity in symptomatic relief of bronchospasm is rapid and of relatively long duration. By relieving bronchospasm, BRONKOSOL and BRONKOMETER help give prompt relief and significantly increases the FVC, FEV_1, and $FEF_{25\%-75\%}$.

Recent studies in laboratory animals (minipigs, rodents, and dogs) recorded the occurrence of cardiac arrhythmias and sudden death (with histologic evidence of myocardial necrosis) when beta agonists and methylxanthines were administered concurrently. The significance of these findings when applied to humans is currently unknown.

INDICATIONS AND USAGE

BRONKOSOL and BRONKOMETER are indicated for use as bronchodilators for bronchial asthma and for reversible bronchospasm that may occur in association with bronchitis and emphysema.

CONTRAINDICATION

BRONKOSOL and BRONKOMETER should not be administered to patients who are hypersensitive to any of their ingredients.

WARNINGS

Excessive use of an adrenergic aerosol should be discouraged as it may lose its effectiveness. Occasional patients have been reported to develop severe paradoxical airway resistance with repeated excessive use of an aerosol adrenergic inhalation preparation. The cause of this refractory state is unknown. It is advisable that in such instances the use of the aerosol adrenergic be discontinued immediately and alternative therapy instituted, since in the reported cases the patients did not respond to other forms of therapy until the drug was withdrawn. Cardiac arrest has been noted in several instances.

BRONKOSOL and BRONKOMETER should not be administered along with epinephrine or other sympathomimetic amines, since these drugs are direct cardiac stimulants and may cause excessive tachycardia. They may, however, be alternated if desired.

PRECAUTIONS

Dosage must be carefully adjusted in patients with hyperthyroidism, hypertension, acute coronary disease, cardiac asthma, limited cardiac reserve, and in individuals sensitive to sympathomimetic amines, since overdosage may result in tachycardia, palpitation, nausea, headache, or epinephrine-like side effects.

Information For Patients: Do not inhale more often than directed by your physician. Read enclosed instructions before using (see attachment to insert). Do not exceed the dose prescribed by your physician. If difficulty in breathing persists, contact your physician immediately. Avoid spraying in eyes. Contents under pressure. Do not break or incinerate. Store at controlled room temperature 15°C to 30°C (59°F to 86°F). Keep out of the reach of children.

Drug Interactions: BRONKOSOL and BRONKOMETER should not be administered along with epinephrine or other sympathomimetic amines, since these drugs are direct cardiac stimulants and may cause excessive tachycardia. They may, however, be alternated if desired.

Carcinogenesis, Mutagenesis, Impairment of Fertility: Chronic toxicity studies up to twelve months in dogs with doses up to 20 mg/kg/day (equivalent to approximately 200 times the human dose based on a 70 kg individual) and chronic toxicity studies in rats with doses up to 45 mg/kg/day (equivalent to approximately 450 times the human dose, based on a 70 kg individual) revealed no evidence of carcinogenicity due to isoetharine. No animal studies have been conducted for evaluating the potential for mutagenesis and impairment of fertility of BRONKOSOL and BRONKOMETER.

Pregnancy Category C: Animal reproduction studies have not been conducted with isoetharine mesylate. It is also not known whether isoetharine mesylate can cause fetal harm when administered to a pregnant woman or can affect reproduction capacity, although there is no evidence of such harm or effects. Isoetharine mesylate should be given to a pregnant woman only if clearly needed.

Nursing Mothers: It is not known whether this drug is excreted in human milk. Because many drugs are excreted in human milk, caution should be exercised when isoetharine mesylate is administered to a nursing woman.

Pediatric Use: The safety and efficacy of this product in children under the age of 12 have not been established.

ADVERSE REACTIONS

Although BRONKOSOL and BRONKOMETER are relatively free of toxic side effects, too frequent use may cause the following reactions, as is the case with other sympathomimetic amines:

Cardiovascular: Tachycardia, palpitations, changes in blood pressure.
Gastrointestinal: Nausea.
CNS: Headache, restlessness, insomnia, anxiety, tension, dizziness, excitement.
Other: Tremor, weakness.

OVERDOSAGE

Overdosage of BRONKOSOL and BRONKOMETER may produce signs and symptoms typical of excessive sympathomimetic effects, including tachycardia, palpitations, nausea, headache, blood pressure changes, anxiety, restlessness, insomnia, tremor, weakness, dizziness, and excitation. Excessive use of adrenergic aerosols may result in loss of effectiveness or severe paradoxical airway resistance. Cardiac arrest has been noted in several instances. In all cases of overdose or excessive use of BRONKOSOL and BRONKOMETER, the drug should be discontinued immediately and vital functions supported until the patient is stabilized. It is not known whether isoetharine mesylate is dialyzable.

The single dose amount of drug that may be toxic or life threatening is highly variable according to patient characteristics and drug history. The acute oral LD_{50} in mice is 2000 mg/kg.

DOSAGE AND ADMINISTRATION

BRONKOSOL can be administered by hand nebulizer, oxygen aerosolization, or intermittent positive pressure breathing (IPPB). Usually treatment need not be repeated more often than every four hours, although in severe cases more frequent administration may be necessary.

Method of Administration	Usual Dose	Range	Usual Dilution
Hand nebulizer	4 inhalations	3-7 inhalations	undiluted
Oxygen aerosolization*	½ mL	¼-½ mL	1:3 with saline or other diluent
IPPB†	½ mL	¼-1 mL	1:3 with saline or other diluent

* Administered with oxygen flow adjusted to 4 to 6 liters/minute over a period of 15 to 20 minutes.
† Usually an inspiratory flow rate of 15 liters/minute at a cycling pressure of 15 cm H_2O is recommended. It may be necessary, according to patient and type of IPPB apparatus, to adjust flow rate to 6 to 30 liters per minute, cycling pressure to 10 to 15 cm H_20, and further dilution according to needs of patient.

BRONKOMETER®

DOSAGE AND ADMINISTRATION

The average adult dose is one or two inhalations. Occasionally, more may be required. It is important, however, to wait one full minute after the initial one or two inhalations in order to be certain whether another is necessary. In most cases, inhalations need not be repeated more often than every four hours, although more frequent administration may be necessary in severe cases.

HOW SUPPLIED

BRONKOMETER is supplied in a white coated glass container with a white HDPE actuator which is designed to contain 20 metered doses per mL of solution (eg, 200 doses per 10 mL). Each actuation delivers 340 μg isoetharine mesylate from the mouthpiece.

Vial of 10 mL, with oral nebulizer (NDC 0024-1040-01)
Refill only, 10 mL (NDC 0024-1041-01)
Vial of 15 mL, with oral nebulizer (NDC 0024-1040-03)
Refill only, 15 mL (NDC 0024-1041-03)

The bronchodilator isoetharine is also available in a convenient solution for use with conventional nebulizers, by oxygen aerosolization, and in IPPB machines as BRONKOSOL, brand of isoetharine inhalation solution, 1%. It is supplied as follows:

Bottle of 10 mL (NDC 0024-1071-10)
Bottle of 30 mL (NDC 0024-1071-30)

Store at controlled room temperature 15°C to 30°C (59°F to 86°F). Protect from light.

Caution: Federal law prohibits dispensing without prescription.

Note: The indented statement below is required by the Federal government's Clean Air Act for all products containing or manufactured with chlorofluorocarbons (CFC's).

> **WARNING: Contains dichlorodifluoromethane and dichlorotetrafluoroethane, substances which harm public health and environment by destroying ozone in the upper atmosphere.**

A notice similar to the above WARNING has been placed in the information for the patient of this product pursuant to EPA regulations.

CARBOCAINE® ℞

mepivacaine hydrochloride injection, USP

THESE SOLUTIONS ARE NOT INTENDED FOR SPINAL ANESTHESIA OR DENTAL USE

DESCRIPTION

Mepivacaine hydrochloride is 2-Piperidinecarboxamide, *N*-(2,6-dimethylphenyl)-1-methyl-, monohydrochloride.

It is a white crystalline odorless powder, soluble in water, but very resistant to both acid and alkaline hydrolysis.

CARBOCAINE is a local anesthetic available as sterile isotonic solutions (clear, colorless) in concentrations of 1%, 1.5%, and 2% for injection via local infiltration, peripheral nerve block, and caudal and lumbar epidural blocks.

Mepivacaine hydrochloride is related chemically and pharmacologically to the amide-type local anesthetics. It contains an amide linkage between the aromatic nucleus and the amino group.

[See table at top of next page.]

The pH of the solutions is adjusted between 4.5 and 6.8 with sodium hydroxide or hydrochloric acid.

CLINICAL PHARMACOLOGY

Local anesthetics block the generation and the conduction of nerve impulses, presumably by increasing the threshold for electrical excitation in the nerve, by slowing the propagation of the nerve impulse, and by reducing the rate of rise of the action potential. In general, the progression of anesthesia is related to the diameter, myelination, and conduction velocity of affected nerve fibers. Clinically, the order of loss of nerve function is as follows: pain, temperature, touch, proprioception, and skeletal muscle tone.

Systemic absorption of local anesthetics produces effects on the cardiovascular and central nervous systems. At blood concentrations achieved with normal therapeutic doses, changes in cardiac conduction, excitability, refractoriness, contractility, and peripheral vascular resistance are minimal. However, toxic blood concentrations depress cardiac conduction and excitability, which may lead to atrioventricular block and ultimately to cardiac arrest. In addition, myocardial contractility is depressed and peripheral vasodilation occurs, leading to decreased cardiac output and arterial blood pressure.

Following systemic absorption, local anesthetics can produce central nervous system stimulation, depression, or both. Apparent central stimulation is manifested as restlessness, tremors, and shivering, progressing to convulsions, followed by depression and coma progressing ultimately to respira-

tory arrest. However, the local anesthetics have a primary depressant effect on the medulla and on higher centers. The depressed stage may occur without a prior excited stage.

Pharmacokinetics

The rate of systemic absorption of local anesthetics is dependent upon the total dose and concentration of drug administered, the route of administration, the vascularity of the administration site, and the presence or absence of epinephrine in the anesthetic solution. A dilute concentration of epinephrine (1:200,000 or 5 mcg/mL) usually reduces the rate of absorption and plasma concentration of CARBOCAINE, however, it has been reported that vasoconstrictors do not significantly prolong anesthesia with CARBOCAINE.

Onset of anesthesia with CARBOCAINE is rapid, the time of onset for sensory block ranging from about 3 to 20 minutes depending upon such factors as the anesthetic technique, the type of block, the concentration of the solution, and the individual patient. The degree of motor blockade produced is dependent on the concentration of the solution. A 0.5% solution will be effective in small superficial nerve blocks while the 1% concentration will block sensory and sympathetic conduction without loss of motor function. The 1.5% solution will provide extensive and often complete motor block and the 2% concentration of CARBOCAINE will produce complete sensory and motor block of any nerve group.

The duration of anesthesia also varies depending upon the technique and type of block, the concentration, and the individual. Mepivacaine will normally provide anesthesia which is adequate for 2 to 2½ hours of surgery.

Local anesthetics are bound to plasma proteins in varying degrees. Generally, the lower the plasma concentration of drug, the higher the percentage of drug bound to plasma. Local anesthetics appear to cross the placenta by passive diffusion. The rate and degree of diffusion is governed by the degree of plasma protein binding, the degree of ionization, and the degree of lipid solubility. Fetal/maternal ratios of local anesthetics appear to be inversely related to the degree of plasma protein binding, because only the free, unbound drug is available for placental transfer. CARBOCAINE is approximately 75% bound to plasma proteins. The extent of placental transfer is also determined by the degree of ionization and lipid solubility of the drug. Lipid soluble, nonionized drugs readily enter the fetal blood from the maternal circulation.

Depending upon the route of administration, local anesthetics are distributed to some extent to all body tissues, with high concentrations found in highly perfused organs such as the liver, lungs, heart, and brain.

Various pharmacokinetic parameters of the local anesthetics can be significantly altered by the presence of hepatic or renal disease, addition of epinephrine, factors affecting urinary pH, renal blood flow, the route of drug administration, and the age of the patient. The half-life of CARBOCAINE in adults is 1.9 to 3.2 hours and in neonates 8.7 to 9 hours.

Mepivacaine, because of its amide structure, is not detoxified by the circulating plasma esterases. It is rapidly metabolized, with only a small percentage of the anesthetic (5 percent to 10 percent) being excreted unchanged in the urine. The liver is the principal site of metabolism, with over 50% of the administered dose being excreted into the bile as metabolites. Most of the metabolized mepivacaine is probably resorbed in the intestine and then excreted into the urine since only a small percentage is found in the feces. The principal route of excretion is via the kidney. Most of the anesthetic and its metabolites are eliminated within 30 hours. It has been shown that hydroxylation and N-demethylation, which are detoxification reactions, play important roles in the metabolism of the anesthetic. Three metabolites of mepivacaine have been identified from human adults: two phenols, which are excreted almost exclusively as their glucuronide conjugates, and the N-demethylated compound (2′, 6′-pipecoloxylidide).

Mepivacaine does not ordinarily produce irritation or tissue damage, and does not cause methemoglobinemia when administered in recommended doses and concentrations.

INDICATIONS AND USAGE

CARBOCAINE is indicated for production of local or regional analgesia and anesthesia by local infiltration, peripheral nerve block techniques, and central neural techniques including epidural and caudal blocks.

The routes of administration and indicated concentrations for CARBOCAINE are:

local infiltration	0.5% (via dilution) or 1%
peripheral nerve blocks	1% and 2%
epidural block	1%, 1.5%, 2%
caudal block	1%, 1.5%, 2%

See DOSAGE AND ADMINISTRATION for additional information. Standard textbooks should be consulted to determine the accepted procedures and techniques for the administration of CARBOCAINE.

Composition of Available Solutions*

	1% Single-Dose 30 mL Vial mg/mL	1% Multiple-Dose 50 mL Vial mg/mL	1.5% Single-Dose 30 mL Vial mg/mL	2% Single-Dose 20 mL Vial mg/mL	2% Multiple-Dose 50 mL Vial mg/mL
Mepivacaine hydrochloride	10	10	15	20	20
Sodium chloride	6.6	7	5.6	4.6	5
Potassium chloride	0.3		0.3	0.3	
Calcium chloride	0.33		0.33	0.33	
Methylparaben		1			1

*In Water for Injection

CONTRAINDICATIONS

CARBOCAINE is contraindicated in patients with a known hypersensitivity to it or to any local anesthetic agent of the amide-type or to other components of solutions of CARBOCAINE.

WARNINGS

LOCAL ANESTHETICS SHOULD ONLY BE EMPLOYED BY CLINICIANS WHO ARE WELL VERSED IN DIAGNOSIS AND MANAGEMENT OF DOSE-RELATED TOXICITY AND OTHER ACUTE EMERGENCIES WHICH MIGHT ARISE FROM THE BLOCK TO BE EMPLOYED, AND THEN ONLY AFTER INSURING THE IMMEDIATE AVAILABILITY OF OXYGEN, OTHER RESUSCITATIVE DRUGS, CARDIOPULMONARY RESUSCITATIVE EQUIPMENT, AND THE PERSONNEL RESOURCES NEEDED FOR PROPER MANAGEMENT OF TOXIC REACTIONS AND RELATED EMERGENCIES. (See also ADVERSE REACTIONS and PRECAUTIONS.) DELAY IN PROPER MANAGEMENT OF DOSE-RELATED TOXICITY, UNDERVENTILATION FROM ANY CAUSE, AND/OR ALTERED SENSITIVITY MAY LEAD TO THE DEVELOPMENT OF ACIDOSIS, CARDIAC ARREST AND, POSSIBLY, DEATH.

Local anesthetic solutions containing antimicrobial preservatives (i.e., those supplied in multiple-dose vials) should not be used for epidural or caudal anesthesia because safety has not been established with regard to intrathecal injection, either intentionally or inadvertently, of such preservatives. It is essential that aspiration for blood or cerebrospinal fluid (where applicable) be done prior to injecting any local anesthetic, both the original dose and all subsequent doses, to avoid intravascular or subarachnoid injection. However, a negative aspiration does not ensure against an intravascular or subarachnoid injection.

Reactions resulting in fatality have occurred on rare occasions with the use of local anesthetics.

CARBOCAINE with epinephrine or other vasopressors should not be used concomitantly with ergot-type oxytocic drugs, because a severe persistent hypertension may occur. Likewise, solutions of CARBOCAINE containing a vasoconstrictor, such as epinephrine, should be used with extreme caution in patients receiving monoamine oxidase inhibitors (MAOI) or antidepressants of the triptyline or imipramine types, because severe prolonged hypertension may result. Local anesthetic procedures should be used with caution when there is inflammation and/or sepsis in the region of the proposed injection.

Mixing or the prior or intercurrent use of any local anesthetic with CARBOCAINE cannot be recommended because of insufficient data on the clinical use of such mixtures.

PRECAUTIONS

General

The safety and effectiveness of local anesthetics depend on proper dosage, correct technique, adequate precautions, and readiness for emergencies. Resuscitative equipment, oxygen, and other resuscitative drugs should be available for immediate use. (See WARNINGS and ADVERSE REACTIONS.) During major regional nerve blocks, the patient should have IV fluids running via an indwelling catheter to assure a functioning intravenous pathway. The lowest dosage of local anesthetic that results in effective anesthesia should be used to avoid high plasma levels and serious adverse effects. Injections should be made slowly, with frequent aspirations before and during the injection to avoid intravascular injection. Current opinion favors fractional administration with constant attention to the patient, rather than rapid bolus injection. Syringe aspirations should also be performed before and during each supplemental injection in continuous (intermittent) catheter techniques. An intravascular injection is still possible even if aspirations for blood are negative. During the administration of epidural anesthesia, it is recommended that a test dose be administered initially and the effects monitored before the full dose is given. When using a "continuous" catheter technique, test doses should be given prior to both the original and all reinforcing doses, because plastic tubing in the epidural space can migrate into a blood vessel or through the dura. When clinical conditions permit, an effective test dose should contain epinephrine (10 mcg to 15 mcg have been suggested) to serve as a warning of unintended intravascular injection. If injected into a blood

vessel, this amount of epinephrine is likely to produce an "epinephrine response" within 45 seconds, consisting of an increase of pulse and blood pressure, circumoral pallor, palpitations, and nervousness in the unsedated patient. The sedated patient may exhibit only a pulse rate increase of 20 or more beats per minute for 15 or more seconds. Therefore, following the test dose, the heart rate should be monitored for a heart rate increase. The test dose should also contain 45 mg to 50 mg of CARBOCAINE to detect an unintended intrathecal administration. This will be evidenced within a few minutes by signs of spinal block (e.g., decreased sensation of the buttocks, paresis of the legs, or, in the sedated patient, absent knee jerk).

Injection of repeated doses of local anesthetics may cause significant increases in plasma levels with each repeated dose due to slow accumulation of the drug or its metabolites or to slow metabolic degradation. Tolerance to elevated blood levels varies with the status of the patient. Debilitated, elderly patients, and acutely ill patients should be given reduced doses commensurate with their age and physical status. Local anesthetics should also be used with caution in patients with severe disturbances of cardiac rhythm, shock, heart block, or hypotension.

Careful and constant monitoring of cardiovascular and respiratory (adequacy of ventilation) vital signs, and the patient's state of consciousness should be performed after each local anesthetic injection. It should be kept in mind at such times that restlessness, anxiety, incoherent speech, lightheadedness, numbness and tingling of the mouth and lips, metallic taste, tinnitus, dizziness, blurred vision, tremors, twitching, depression, or drowsiness may be early warning signs of central nervous system toxicity.

Local anesthetic solutions containing a vasoconstrictor should be used cautiously and in carefully restricted quantities in areas of the body supplied by end arteries or having otherwise compromised blood supply such as digits, nose, external ear, penis. Patients with hypertensive vascular disease may exhibit exaggerated vasoconstrictor response. Ischemic injury or necrosis may result.

Mepivacaine should be used with caution in patients with known allergies and sensitivities.

Because amide-type local anesthetics such as CARBOCAINE are metabolized by the liver and excreted by the kidneys, these drugs, especially repeat doses, should be used cautiously in patients with hepatic and renal disease. Patients with severe hepatic disease, because of their inability to metabolize local anesthetics normally, are at a greater risk of developing toxic plasma concentrations. Local anesthetics should also be used with caution in patients with impaired cardiovascular function because they may be less able to compensate for functional changes associated with the prolongation of AV conduction produced by these drugs.

Serious dose-related cardiac arrhythmias may occur if preparations containing a vasoconstrictor such as epinephrine are employed in patients during or following the administration of potent inhalation anesthetics. In deciding whether to use these products concurrently in the same patient, the combined action of both agents upon the myocardium, the concentration and volume of vasoconstrictor used, and the time since injection, when applicable, should be taken into account.

Many drugs used during the conduct of anesthesia are considered potential triggering agents for familial malignant hyperthermia. Because it is not known whether amide-type local anesthetics may trigger this reaction and because the need for supplemental general anesthesia cannot be predicted in advance, it is suggested that a standard protocol for management should be available. Early unexplained signs of tachycardia, tachypnea, labile blood pressure, and metabolic acidosis may precede temperature elevation. Successful out-

Continued on next page

This product information was prepared in September 1996. On these and other products of Sanofi Winthrop Pharmaceuticals, detailed information may be obtained on a current basis by direct inquiry to Product Information Services, 90 Park Avenue, New York, NY 10016 (toll free 1-800-446-6267).

Sanofi Winthrop—Cont.

come is dependent on early diagnosis, prompt discontinuance of the suspect triggering agent(s), and institution of treatment, including oxygen therapy, indicated supportive measures, and dantrolene. (Consult dantrolene sodium intravenous package insert before using.)

Use in Head and Neck Area

Small doses of local anesthetics injected into the head and neck area may produce adverse reactions similar to systemic toxicity seen with unintentional intravascular injections of larger doses. The injection procedures require the utmost care.

Confusion, convulsions, respiratory depression, and/or respiratory arrest, and cardiovascular stimulation or depression have been reported. These reactions may be due to intra-arterial injection of the local anesthetic with retrograde flow to the cerebral circulation. Patients receiving these blocks should have their circulation and respiration monitored and be constantly observed. Resuscitative equipment and personnel for treating adverse reactions should be immediately available. Dosage recommendations should not be exceeded.

Information for Patients

When appropriate, patients should be informed in advance that they may experience temporary loss of sensation and motor activity, usually in the lower half of the body, following proper administration of caudal or epidural anesthesia. Also, when appropriate, the physician should discuss other information including adverse reactions listed in the package insert on CARBOCAINE.

Clinically Significant Drug Interactions

The administration of local anesthetic solutions containing epinephrine or norepinephrine to patients receiving monoamine oxidase inhibitors or tricyclic antidepressants may produce severe, prolonged hypertension. Concurrent use of these agents should generally be avoided. In situations when concurrent therapy is necessary, careful patient monitoring is essential.

Concurrent administration of vasopressor drugs and of ergot-type oxytocic drugs may cause severe, persistent hypertension or cerebrovascular accidents.

Phenothiazines and butyrophenones may reduce or reverse the pressor effect of epinephrine.

Carcinogenesis, Mutagenesis, and Impairment of Fertility

Long-term studies in animals of most local anesthetics including mepivacaine to evaluate the carcinogenic potential have not been conducted. Mutagenic potential or the effect on fertility has not been determined. There is no evidence from human data that CARBOCAINE may be carcinogenic or mutagenic or that it impairs fertility.

Pregnancy Category C

Animal reproduction studies have not been conducted with mepivacaine. There are no adequate and well-controlled studies in pregnant women of the effect of mepivacaine on the developing fetus. Mepivacaine hydrochloride should be used during pregnancy only if the potential benefit justifies the potential risk to the fetus. This does not preclude the use of CARBOCAINE at term for obstetrical anesthesia or analgesia. (See *Labor and Delivery*.)

CARBOCAINE has been used for obstetrical analgesia by the epidural, caudal, and paracervical routes without evidence of adverse effects on the fetus when no more than the maximum safe dosages are used and strict adherence to technique is followed.

Labor and Delivery

Local anesthetics rapidly cross the placenta, and when used for epidural, paracervical, caudal, or pudendal block anesthesia, can cause varying degrees of maternal, fetal, and neonatal toxicity. (See *Pharmacokinetics*—CLINICAL PHARMACOLOGY.) The incidence and degree of toxicity depend upon the procedure performed, the type and amount of drug used, and the technique of drug administration. Adverse reactions in the parturient, fetus, and neonate involve alterations of the central nervous system, peripheral vascular tone, and cardiac function.

Maternal hypotension has resulted from regional anesthesia. Local anesthetics produce vasodilation by blocking sympathetic nerves. Elevating the patient's legs and positioning her on her left side will help prevent decreases in blood pressure. The fetal heart rate also should be monitored continuously and electronic fetal monitoring is highly advisable.

Epidural, paracervical, caudal, or pudendal anesthesia may alter the forces of parturition through changes in uterine contractility or maternal expulsive efforts. In one study, paracervical block anesthesia was associated with a decrease in the mean duration of first stage labor and facilitation of cervical dilation. Epidural anesthesia has been reported to prolong the second stage of labor by removing the parturient's reflex urge to bear down or by interfering with motor function. The use of obstetrical anesthesia may increase the need for forceps assistance.

The use of some local anesthetic drug products during labor and delivery may be followed by diminished muscle strength

and tone for the first day or two of life. The long-term significance of these observations is unknown.

Fetal bradycardia may occur in 20 to 30 percent of patients receiving paracervical block anesthesia with the amide-type local anesthetics and may be associated with fetal acidosis. Fetal heart rate should always be monitored during paracervical anesthesia. Added risk appears to be present in prematurity, postmaturity, toxemia of pregnancy, and fetal distress. The physician should weigh the possible advantages against dangers when considering paracervical block in these conditions. Careful adherence to recommended dosage is of the utmost importance in obstetrical paracervical block. Failure to achieve adequate analgesia with recommended doses should arouse suspicion of intravascular or fetal intracranial injection.

Cases compatible with unintended fetal intracranial injection of local anesthetic solution have been reported following intended paracervical or pudendal block or both. Babies so affected present with unexplained neonatal depression at birth which correlates with high local anesthetic serum levels and usually manifest seizures within six hours. Prompt use of supportive measures combined with forced urinary excretion of the local anesthetic has been used successfully to manage this complication.

Case reports of maternal convulsions and cardiovascular collapse following use of some local anesthetics for paracervical block in early pregnancy (as anesthesia for elective abortion) suggest that systemic absorption under these circumstances may be rapid. The recommended maximum dose of the local anesthetic should not be exceeded. Injection should be made slowly and with frequent aspiration. Allow a five-minute interval between sides.

It is extremely important to avoid aortocaval compression by the gravid uterus during administration of regional block to parturients. To do this, the patient must be maintained in the left lateral decubitus position or a blanket roll or sandbag may be placed beneath the right hip and the gravid uterus displaced to the left.

Nursing Mothers

It is not known whether local anesthetic drugs are excreted in human milk. Because many drugs are excreted in human milk, caution should be exercised when local anesthetics are administered to a nursing woman.

Pediatric Use

Guidelines for the administration of mepivacaine to children are presented in DOSAGE AND ADMINISTRATION.

ADVERSE REACTIONS

Reactions to CARBOCAINE are characteristic of those associated with other amide-type local anesthetics. A major cause of adverse reactions to this group of drugs is excessive plasma levels, which may be due to overdosage, inadvertent intravascular injection, or slow metabolic degradation.

Systemic

The most commonly encountered acute adverse experiences which demand immediate countermeasures are related to the central nervous system and the cardiovascular system. These adverse experiences are generally dose related and due to high plasma levels which may result from overdosage, rapid absorption from the injection site, diminished tolerance, or from unintentional intravascular injection of the local anesthetic solution. In addition to systemic dose-related toxicity, unintentional subarachnoid injection of drug during the intended performance of caudal or lumbar epidural block or nerve blocks near the vertebral column (especially in the head and neck region) may result in underventilation or apnea ("Total or High Spinal"). Also, hypotension due to loss of sympathetic tone and respiratory paralysis or underventilation due to cephalad extension of the motor level of anesthesia may occur. This may lead to secondary cardiac arrest if untreated. Factors influencing plasma protein binding, such as acidosis, systemic diseases which alter protein production, or competition of other drugs for protein binding sites, may diminish individual tolerance.

Central Nervous System Reactions

These are characterized by excitation and/or depression. Restlessness, anxiety, dizziness, tinnitus, blurred vision, or tremors may occur, possibly proceeding to convulsions. However, excitement may be transient or absent, with depression being the first manifestation of an adverse reaction. This may quickly be followed by drowsiness merging into unconsciousness and respiratory arrest. Other central nervous system effects may be nausea, vomiting, chills, and constriction of the pupils.

The incidence of convulsions associated with the use of local anesthetics varies with the procedure used and the total dose administered. In a survey of studies of epidural anesthesia, overt toxicity progressing to convulsions occurred in approximately 0.1% of local anesthetic administrations.

Cardiovascular Reactions

High doses or, inadvertent intravascular injection, may lead to high plasma levels and related depression of the myocardium, decreased cardiac output, heart block, hypotension (or sometimes hypertension), bradycardia, ventricular arrhythmias, and possibly cardiac arrest). (See WARNINGS, PRECAUTIONS, and OVERDOSAGE sections.)

Allergic

Allergic-type reactions are rare and may occur as a result of sensitivity to the local anesthetic or to other formulation ingredients, such as the antimicrobial preservative methylparaben, contained in multiple-dose vials. These reactions are characterized by signs such as urticaria, pruritus, erythema, angioneurotic edema (including laryngeal edema), tachycardia, sneezing, nausea, vomiting, dizziness, syncope, excessive sweating, elevated temperature, and possibly, anaphylactoid-like symptomatology (including severe hypotension). Cross sensitivity among members of the amide-type local anesthetic group has been reported. The usefulness of screening for sensitivity has not been definitely established.

Neurologic

The incidences of adverse neurologic reactions associated with the use of local anesthetics may be related to the total dose of local anesthetic administered and are also dependent upon the particular drug used, the route of administration, and the physical status of the patient. Many of these effects may be related to local anesthetic techniques, with or without a contribution from the drug.

In the practice of caudal or lumbar epidural block, occasional unintentional penetration of the subarachnoid space by the catheter or needle may occur. Subsequent adverse effects may depend partially on the amount of drug administered intrathecally and the physiological and physical effects of a dural puncture. A high spinal is characterized by paralysis of the legs, loss of consciousness, respiratory paralysis, and bradycardia.

Neurologic effects following epidural or caudal anesthesia may include spinal block of varying magnitude (including high or total spinal block); hypotension secondary to spinal block; urinary retention; fecal and urinary incontinence; loss of perineal sensation and sexual function; persistent anesthesia, paresthesia, weakness, paralysis of the lower extremities, and loss of sphincter control all of which may have slow, incomplete, or no recovery; headache; backache; septic meningitis; meningismus; slowing of labor; increased incidence of forceps delivery; cranial nerve palsies due to traction on nerves from loss of cerebrospinal fluid.

Neurologic effects following other procedures or routes of administration may include persistent anesthesia, paresthesia, weakness, paralysis, all of which may have slow, incomplete, or no recovery.

OVERDOSAGE

Acute emergencies from local anesthetics are generally related to high plasma levels encountered during therapeutic use of local anesthetics or to unintended subarachnoid injection of local anesthetic solution. (See ADVERSE REACTIONS, WARNINGS, and PRECAUTIONS.)

Management of Local Anesthetic Emergencies

The first consideration is prevention, best accomplished by careful and constant monitoring of cardiovascular and respiratory vital signs and the patient's state of consciousness after each local anesthetic injection. At the first sign of change, oxygen should be administered.

The first step in the management of systemic toxic reactions, as well as underventilation or apnea due to unintentional subarachnoid injection of drug solution, consists of immediate attention to the establishment and maintenance of a patent airway and effective assisted or controlled ventilation with 100% oxygen with a delivery system capable of permitting immediate positive airway pressure by mask. This may prevent convulsions if they have not already occurred.

If necessary, use drugs to control the convulsions. A 50 mg to 100 mg bolus IV injection of succinylcholine will paralyze the patient without depressing the central nervous or cardiovascular systems and facilitate ventilation. A bolus IV dose of 5 mg to 10 mg of diazepam or 50 mg to 100 mg of thiopental will permit ventilation and counteract central nervous system stimulation, but these drugs also depress central nervous system, respiratory, and cardiac function, add to postictal depression and may result in apnea. Intravenous barbiturates, anticonvulsant agents, or muscle relaxants should only be administered by those familiar with their use. Immediately after the institution of these ventilatory measures, the adequacy of the circulation should be evaluated. Supportive treatment of circulatory depression may require administration of intravenous fluids, and when appropriate, a vasopressor dictated by the clinical situation (such as ephedrine or epinephrine to enhance myocardial contractile force).

Endotracheal intubation, employing drugs and techniques familiar to the clinician may be indicated after initial administration of oxygen by mask, if difficulty is encountered in the maintenance of a patent airway or if prolonged ventilatory support (assisted or controlled) is indicated.

Recent clinical data from patients experiencing local anesthetic induced convulsions demonstrated rapid development of hypoxia, hypercarbia, and acidosis within a minute of the onset of convulsions. These observations suggest that oxygen consumption and carbon dioxide production are greatly increased during local anesthetic convulsions and emphasize

Recommended Concentrations and Doses of CARBOCAINE

Procedure	Concentration	Total Dose mL	Total Dose mg	Comments
Cervical, brachial, intercostal, pudendal nerve block	1%	5–40	50–400	Pudendal block: one half of total dose injected each side.
	2%	5–20	100–400	
Transvaginal block (paracervical plus pudendal)	1%	up to 30 (both sides)	up to 300 (both sides)	One half of total dose injected each side. See PRECAUTIONS.
Paracervical block	1%	up to 20 (both sides)	up to 200 (both sides)	One half of total dose injected each side. This is maximum recommended dose per 90-minute period in obstetrical and non-obstetrical patients. Inject slowly, 5 minutes between sides. See PRECAUTIONS.
Caudal and Epidural block	1%	15–30	150–300	Use only single-dose vials which do not contain a preservative.
	1.5%	10–25	150–375	
	2%	10–20	200–400	
Infiltration	1%	up to 40	up to 400	An equivalent amount of a 0.5% solution (prepared by diluting the 1% solution with Sodium Chloride Injection, USP) may be used for large areas.
Therapeutic block (pain management)	1%	1–5	10–50	
	2%	1–5	20–100	

Unused portions of solutions not containing preservatives should be discarded.

the importance of immediate and effective ventilation with oxygen which may avoid cardiac arrest.

If not treated immediately, convulsions with simultaneous hypoxia, hypercarbia, and acidosis, plus myocardial depression from the direct effects of the local anesthetic may result in cardiac arrhythmias, bradycardia, asystole, ventricular fibrillation, or cardiac arrest. Respiratory abnormalities, including apnea, may occur. Underventilation or apnea due to unintentional subarachnoid injection of local anesthetic solution may produce these same signs and also lead to cardiac arrest if ventilatory support is not instituted. If cardiac arrest should occur, standard cardiopulmonary resuscitative measures should be instituted and maintained for a prolonged period if necessary. Recovery has been reported after prolonged resuscitative efforts.

The supine position is dangerous in pregnant women at term because of aortocaval compression by the gravid uterus. Therefore during treatment of systemic toxicity, maternal hypotension, or fetal bradycardia following regional block, the parturient should be maintained in the left lateral decubitus position if possible, or manual displacement of the uterus off the great vessels be accomplished.

The mean seizure dosage of mepivacaine in rhesus monkeys was found to be 18.8 mg/kg with mean arterial plasma concentration of 24.4 mcg/mL. The intravenous and subcutaneous LD_{50} in mice is 23 mg/kg to 35 mg/kg and 280 mg/kg respectively.

DOSAGE AND ADMINISTRATION

The dose of any local anesthetic administered varies with the anesthetic procedure, the area to be anesthetized, the vascularity of the tissues, the number of neuronal segments to be blocked, the depth of anesthesia and degree of muscle relaxation required, the duration of anesthesia desired, individual tolerance and the physical condition of the patient. The smallest dose and concentration required to produce the desired result should be administered. Dosages of CARBOCAINE should be reduced for elderly and debilitated patients and patients with cardiac and/or liver disease. The rapid injection of a large volume of local anesthetic solution should be avoided and fractional doses should be used when feasible.

For specific techniques and procedures, refer to standard textbooks.

The recommended single **adult** dose (or the total of a series of doses given in one procedure) of CARBOCAINE for unsedated, healthy, normal-sized individuals should not usually exceed 400 mg. The recommended dosage is based on requirements for the average adult and should be reduced for elderly or debilitated patients.

While maximum doses of 7 mg/kg (550 mg) have been administered without adverse effect, these are not recommended, except in exceptional circumstances and under no circumstances should the administration be repeated at intervals of less than 1½ hours. The total dose for any 24-hour period should not exceed 1,000 mg because of a slow accumulation of the anesthetic or its derivatives or slower than normal metabolic degradation or detoxification with repeat administration (see CLINICAL PHARMACOLOGY and PRECAUTIONS).

Children tolerate the local anesthetic as well as adults. However, the pediatric dose should be *carefully measured* as a percentage of the total adult dose *based on weight*, and should not exceed 5 mg/kg to 6 mg/kg (2.5 mg/lb to 3 mg/lb) in children, especially those weighing less than 30 lb. In children *under 3 years of age or weighing less than 30 lb* concentrations less than 2% (eg, 0.5% to 1.5%) should be employed. **Unused portions of solutions not containing preservatives, ie, those supplied in single-dose vials, should be discarded following initial use.**

This product should be inspected visually for particulate matter and discoloration prior to administration whenever solution and container permit. Solutions which are discolored or which contain particulate matter should not be administered.

[See table above.]

HOW SUPPLIED

Single-dose vials and multiple-dose vials of CARBOCAINE may be sterilized by autoclaving at 15 pound pressure, 121°C (250°F) for 15 minutes. Solutions of CARBOCAINE may be reautoclaved when necessary. Do not administer solutions which are discolored or which contain particulate matter. THESE SOLUTIONS ARE NOT INTENDED FOR SPINAL ANESTHESIA OR DENTAL USE.

1% Single-dose vials of 30 mL (NDC 0024-0231-01)
1% Multiple-dose vials of 50 mL (NDC 0024-0232-01)
1.5% Single-dose vials of 30 mL (NDC 0024-0234-01)
2% Single-dose vials of 20 mL (NDC 0024-0236-01)
2% Multiple-dose vials of 50 mL (NDC 0024-0237-01)
Store at controlled room temperature between 15°C to 30°C (59°F to 86°F); brief exposure up to 40°C (104°F) does not adversely affect the product.
Caution: Federal law prohibits dispensing without prescription.

CSW-2A

CARPUJECT® sterile cartridge unit ℞

Sanofi Winthrop Pharmaceuticals offers a broad line of injectable drug products in unit of use pre-filled cartridges. Each cartridge is clearly labelled by medication name and dosage calibrations.

The cartridges are packaged in a unique DETECTO-SEAL® tamper detection package specially designed to discourage narcotic diversion and allow for easy inventory analysis.

This package contains a sturdy aluminum shield to prevent plunger end diversion.

Prior to injection the pre-filled cartridges are placed in a unique sturdy plastic holder. This full-length holder provides secure, stable injections and is lightweight, durable, and reusable in design.

In addition, the holder utilized for CARPUJECT products has an open-ended barrel allowing for release of used needles into most any disposal bin. This holder is designed with nursing personnel in mind to eliminate the need for recapping needles and minimize the potential for needle stick injuries.

Product	Units/Package
CODEINE Phosphate Injection, USP ℃II	
30 mg (22 G × 1¼″) 0024-0272-02	10 (2 mL)
60 mg (22 G × 1¼″) 0024-0274-02	10 (2 mL)
DEMEROL® ℃II	
meperidine HCl injection, USP	
with Luer Lock	
25 mg 0024-0324-23	1 mL fill in 2 mL
50 mg 0024-0325-33	1 mL fill in 2 mL
75 mg 0024-0326-33	1 mL fill in 2 mL
100 mg 0024-0328-33	1 mL fill in 2 mL
DEMEROL® ℃II	
meperidine HCl injection, USP	
25 mg (22 G × 1¼″) 0024-0324-02	10 (1 mL fill in 2 mL)
50 mg (22 G × 1¼″) 0024-0325-02	10 (1 mL fill in 2 mL)
75 mg (22 G × 1¼″) 0024-0326-02	10 (1 mL fill in 2 mL)
100 mg (22 G × 1¼″) 0024-0328-02	10 (1 mL fill in 2 mL)
DEMEROL®	
meperidine HCl injection, USP	
With InterLink® System Cannula[1]	
25 mg 0024-0324-42	10 (1 mL fill in 2 mL)
50 mg 0024-0325-43	10 (1 mL fill in 2 mL)
75 mg 0024-0326-44	10 (1 mL fill in 2 mL)
100 mg 0024-0328-45	10 (1 mL fill in 1 mL)
DIAZEPAM Injection ℃IV	
with Luer Lock	
5 mg/mL 0024-0376-20	2 mL fill in 2 mL
DIAZEPAM Injection, USP ℃IV	
10 mg/2 mL (22 G × 1¼″) 0024-0376-02	10 (2 mL)
FENTANYL Citrate Injection, USP ℃II	
with Luer Lock	
50 mcg/mL 0024-0682-33	2 mL
50 mcg/mL 0024-0682-34	5 mL
FENTANYL Citrate Injection, USP ℃II	
100 mcg/2 mL (22 G × 1¼″) 0024-0682-02	10 (2 mL)
250 mcg/5 mL (22 G × 1¼″) 0024-0682-05	10 (5 mL)
FUROSEMIDE Injection, USP	
10 mg/mL (22 G × 1¼″) 0024-0611-03	10 (2 mL)
10 mg/mL (22 G × 1¼″) 0024-0609-40	10 (4 mL fill in 5 mL)

Continued on next page

This product information was prepared in September 1996. On these and other products of Sanofi Winthrop Pharmaceuticals, detailed information may be obtained on a current basis by direct inquiry to Product Information Services, 90 Park Avenue, New York, NY 10016 (toll free 1-800-446-6267).

Sanofi Winthrop—Cont.

FUROSEMIDE Injection, USP
With InterLink System Cannula
10 mg/mL   10 (2 mL)
0024-0611-13
10 mg/mL   10 (4 mL fill in 5 mL)
0024-0609-23

HEP-PAK® Convenience Package[2]
10 USP heparin U/mL   50 × 3
(25 G × ⅝") 0024-0725-03
100 USP heparin U/mL   50 × 3
(25 G × ⅝") 0024-0736-03

HEP-PAK® CVC Convenience Package[3]
10 USP heparin U/2 mL   30 × 3
(25 G × ⅝") 0024-0725-02
100 USP heparin U/2 mL   30 × 3
(25 G × ⅝") 0024-0736-02

HEPARIN LOCK FLUSH Solution, USP
with Luer Lock
10 USP heparin U/mL   1 mL fill in 2 mL
0024-0721-01
10 USP heparin U/mL   2 mL fill in 2 mL
0024-0721-02
10 USP heparin U/mL   3 mL fill in 5 mL
0024-0721-18
10 USP heparin U/mL   5 mL fill in 5 mL
0024-0721-20
100 USP heparin U/mL   1 mL fill in 2 mL
0024-0722-26
100 USP heparin U/mL   2 mL fill in 2 mL
0024-0722-27
100 USP heparin U/mL   3 mL fill in 5 mL
0024-0722-21
100 USP heparin U/mL   5 mL fill in 5 mL
0024-0722-22

HEPARIN LOCK FLUSH Solution, USP
10 USP heparin U/mL   50 (1 mL fill in 2 mL)
(25 G × ⅝") 0024-0721-12
10 USP heparin U/mL   50 (2 mL)
(25 G × ⅝") 0024-0721-13
10 USP heparin U/mL   25 (3 mL fill in 5 mL)
(25 G × ⅝") 0024-0721-14
10 USP heparin U/mL   25 (5 mL)
(25 G × ⅝") 0024-0721-15
100 USP heparin U/mL   50 (1 mL fill in 2 mL)
(25 G × ⅝") 0024-0722-12
100 USP heparin U/mL   50 (2 mL)
(25 G × ⅝") 0024-0722-13
100 USP heparin U/mL   25 (3 mL fill in 5 mL)
(25 G × ⅝") 0024-0722-14
100 USP heparin U/mL   25 (5 mL)
(25 G × ⅝") 0024-0722-15

HEPARIN LOCK FLUSH Solution, USP
With InterLink System Cannula:
10 USP heparin U/mL   50 (1 mL fill in 2 mL)
0024-0721-16
10 USP heparin U/mL   50 (2 mL)
0024-0721-17
10 USP heparin U/mL   25 (3 mL fill in 5 mL)
0024-0721-32
10 USP heparin U/mL   25 (5 mL)
0024-0721-34
100 USP heparin U/mL   25 (3 mL fill in 5 mL)
0024-0722-33
100 USP heparin U/mL   25 (5 mL)
0024-0722-35
100 USP heparin U/mL   50 (1 mL fill in 2 mL)
0024-0722-16
100 USP heparin U/mL   50 (2 mL)
0024-0722-17

HEPARIN Sodium Injection, USP
Preservative-Free
2500 USP heparin U/0.25 mL   10 (0.25 mL fill in 2 mL)
(25 G × ⅝") 0024-0733-03
5000 USP heparin U/0.5 mL   10 (0.5 mL fill in 2 mL)
(25 G × ⅝") 0024-0733-05
5000 USP heparin, U/0.5 mL   50 (0.5 mL fill in 2 mL)
(25 G × ⅝") 0024-0733-15
7500 USP heparin U/0.75 mL   10 (0.75 mL fill in 2 mL)
(25 G × ⅝") 0024-0733-04
10,000 USP heparin U/mL   10 (1 mL fill in 2 mL)
(25 G × ⅝") 0024-0733-02
10,000 USP heparin U/mL   50 (1 mL fill in 2 mL)
(25 G × ⅝") 0024-0733-12

HEPARIN Sodium Injection, USP
5000 USP heparin U/mL   10 (1 mL fill in 2 mL)
(25 G × ⅝") 0024-0793-02
5000 USP heparin U/mL   50 (1 mL fill in 2 mL)
(25 G × ⅝") 0024-0793-12

HYDROMORPHONE Hydrochloride   C-II
Injection, USP
with Luer Lock
1 mg   1 mL fill in 2 mL
0024-0726-22
2 mg   1 mL fill in 2 mL
0024-0728-22
4 mg   1 mL fill in 2 mL
0024-0727-22

HYDROMORPHONE Hydrochloride   C-II
Injection, USP
1 mg (22 G × 1¼")   10 (1 mL fill in 2 mL)
0024-0726-02
2 mg (22 G × 1¼")   10 (1 mL fill in 2 mL)
0024-0728-02
4 mg (22 G × 1¼")   10 (1 mL fill in 2 mL)
0024-0727-02

HYDROXYZINE Hydrochloride Injection, USP
25 mg (22 G × 1¼")   10 (1 mL fill in 2 mL)
0024-0711-02
50 mg (22 G × 1¼")   10 (1 mL fill in 2 mL)
0024-0712-02
100 mg (22 G × 1¼")   10 (2 mL)
0024-0713-02

LORAZEPAM Injection, USP   C-IV
with Luer Lock
2 mg   1 mL fill in 2 mL
0024-1155-30
4 mg   1 mL fill in 2 mL
0024-1156-30

LORAZEPAM Injection, USP   C-IV
2 mg/mL (22 G × 1¼")   10 (1 mL fill in 2 mL)
0024-1155-10
4 mg/mL (22 G × 1¼")   10 (1 mL fill in 2 mL)
0024-1156-10

MORPHINE Sulfate Injection, USP   C-II
2 mg (25 G × ⅝")   10 (1 mL fill in 2 mL)
0024-1257-02
4 mg (25 G × ⅝")   10 (1 mL fill in 2 mL)
0024-1258-02
8 mg (22 G × 1¼")   10 (1 mL fill in 2 mL)
0024-1259-02
8 mg (25 G × ⅝")   10 (1 mL fill in 2 mL)
0024-1260-02
10 mg (22 G × 1¼")   10 (1 mL fill in 2 mL)
0024-1261-02
10 mg (25 G × ⅝")   10 (1 mL fill in 2 mL)
0024-1263-02
15 mg (22 G × 1¼")   10 (1 mL fill in 2 mL)
0024-1262-02
15 mg (25 G × ⅝")   10 (1 mL fill in 2 mL)
0024-1264-02

MORPHINE Sulfate Injection, USP   C-II
with Luer Lock
2 mg   1 mL fill in 2 mL
0024-1257-21
4 mg   1 mL fill in 2 mL
0024-1258-23
8 mg   1 mL fill in 2 mL
0024-1260-27
10 mg   1 mL fill in 2 mL
0024-1261-28
15 mg   1 mL fill in 2 mL
0024-1263-20

MORPHINE Sulfate Injection, USP   C-II
With InterLink System Cannula
2 mg   10 (1 mL fill in 2 mL)
0024-1257-01
4 mg   10 (1 mL fill in 2 mL)
0024-1258-03
8 mg   10 (1 mL fill in 2 mL)
0024-1260-07
10 mg   10 (1 mL fill in 2 mL)
0024-1263-08
15 mg   10 (1 mL fill in 2 mL)
0024-1264-10

NALOXONE Hydrochloride Injection, USP
0.4 mg/mL (22 G × 1¼")   10 (1 mL fill in 2 mL)
0024-1313-02
0.02 mg/mL (Neonatal)   10 (2 mL fill in 2 mL)
(25 G × ⅝")
0024-0314-02

NALOXONE Hydrochloride Injection, USP
With InterLink System Cannula
0.4 mg/mL   10 (1 mL fill in 2 mL)
0024-1313-26
0.02 mg/mL (Neonatal)   10 (2 mL fill in 2 mL)
0024-0314-27

NEO-SYNEPHRINE® Hydrochloride
brand of phenylephrine HCl injection, USP
10 mg (22 G × 1¼")   50 (1 mL fill in 2 mL)
0024-1340-02

PHENYTOIN Sodium Injection, USP
100 mg/2 mL (22 G × 1¼")   10 (2 mL)
0024-1549-01
250 mg/5 mL (22 G × 1¼")   10 (5 mL)
0024-1549-05
250 mg/5mL (22 G × 1¼")   50 (5 mL)
0024-1549-25

PHENYTOIN Sodium Injection, USP
With InterLink System Cannula
100 mg/2 mL   10 (2 mL)
0024-1549-72
250 mg/5 mL   25 (5 mL)
0024-1549-78

PRIMACOR®
brand of milrinone lactate injection, USP
5 mg/mL (22 G × 1¼")   10 (5 mL)
0023-1200-05

PRIMACOR®
brand of milrinone lactate injection, USP
With InterLink System Cannula
5 mg/mL   10 (5 mL)
0024-1200-06

PROCAINAMIDE Hydrochloride, USP
500 mg/mL   10 (2 mL)
(22 G × 1¼")
0024-1526-02

PROCHLORPERAZINE Edisylate Injection, USP
10 mg/2 mL (22 G × 1¼")   10 (2 mL)
0024-1598-01

PROCHLORPERAZINE Edisylate Injection, USP
With InterLink System Cannula
10 mg/2 mL   10 (2 mL)
0024-1598-04

SODIUM Chloride Injection, USP, 0.9%
(22 G × 1¼")   50 (2 mL)
0024-1811-02
(22 G × 1¼")   25 (5 mL)
0024-1811-05
(25 G × ⅝")   50 (2 mL)
0024-1815-02
(25 G × ⅝")   25 (3 mL fill in 5 mL)
0024-1815-03
(25 G × ⅝")   25 (5 mL)
0024-1815-05

SODIUM Chloride Injection, USP, 0.9%
With InterLink System Cannula
0024-1812-02   50 (2 mL)
0024-1812-03   25 (3 mL fill in 5 mL)
0024-1812-05   25 (5 mL)
0024-1812-07   10 (5 mL)

SODIUM Chloride Injection, USP, 0.9%
With Luer Lock
0024-1816-02   50 (2 mL)
0024-1816-03   25 (3 mL in 5 mL fill)
0024-1816-05   25 (5 mL)

SAL-PAK™ 2 Convenience Package[4]
0024-1811-20
(25 G × 1¼")   50 (2 mL)
0024-1815-20

TALWIN® Injection   C-IV
pentazocine lactate Injection, USP
30 mg (22 G × 1¼")   10 (1 mL fill in 2 mL)
0024-1917-02
60 mg (22 G × 1¼")   10 (2 mL)
0024-1919-02

TRIMETHOBENZAMIDE
Hydrochloride Injection, USP
200 mg (22 G × 1¼")   10 (2 mL)
0024-1955-03

VERAPAMIL Hydrochloride
5 mg (22 G × 1¼″) 10 (2 mL)
0024-2110-03

VERAPAMIL Hydrochloride
With Interlink System Cannula
5 mg 10 (2 mL)
0024-2110-41

EMPTY STERILE CARPUJECT
(22 G × 1¼″) 10 (2 mL)
(25 G × ⅝″) 10 (2 mL)

1 InterLink is a trademark of Baxter Healthcare Corp. U.S.
2 Each HEP-PAK® contains one cartridge of Heparin Lock Flush Solution, USP (10 U/mL or 100 U/mL) with two cartridges of Sodium Chloride Injection, USP, 0.9% (2 mL).
3 Each HEP-PAK® CVC Convenience Package contains one cartridge of Heparin Lock Flush Solution 2 mL fill (20 or 200 U/2 mL) with two cartridges of Sodium Chloride Injection, USP, 0.9% (2 mL).
4 Each SAL-PAK™ contains 2 cartridges of Sodium Chloride Injection, USP, 0.9%, (2 mL fill in 2 mL cartridge).

DANOCRINE® ℞
DANAZOL, USP

DESCRIPTION

DANOCRINE, brand of danazol, is a synthetic steroid derived from ethisterone. It is a white to pale yellow crystalline powder, practically insoluble or insoluble in water, and sparingly soluble in alcohol. Chemically, danazol is 17α-Pregna-2,4-dien-20-yno [2,3-*d*]-isoxazol-17-ol. The molecular formula is $C_{22}H_{27}NO_2$. It has a molecular weight of 337.46 and the following structural formula:

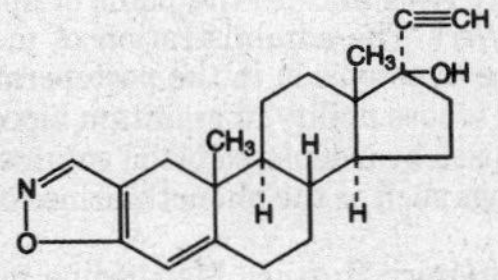

Danocrine capsules for oral administration contain 50 mg, 100 mg or 200 mg danazol.

Inactive Ingredients: Corn Starch, Lactose, Magnesium Stearate, Talc. Capsules 50 mg, 100 mg and 200 mg contain D&C Yellow #10, FD&C Red #40, Gelatin, Silicon Dioxide, Sodium Lauryl Sulfate, Titanium Dioxide. The 50 mg and 200 mg capsules also contain D&C Red #28.

CLINICAL PHARMACOLOGY

DANOCRINE suppresses the pituitary-ovarian axis. This suppression is probably a combination of depressed hypothalamic-pituitary response to lowered estrogen production, the alteration of sex steroid metabolism, and interaction of danazol with sex hormone receptors. The only other demonstrable hormonal effect is weak androgenic activity. DANOCRINE depresses the output of both follicle-stimulating hormone (FSH) and luteinizing hormone (LH).

Recent evidence suggests a direct inhibitory effect at gonadal sites and a binding of DANOCRINE to receptors of gonadal steroids at target organs. In addition, DANOCRINE has been shown to significantly decrease IgG, IgM and IgA levels, as well as phospholipid and IgG isotope autoantibodies in patients with endometriosis and associated elevations of autoantibodies, suggesting this could be another mechanism by which it facilitates regression of the disease.

Bioavailability studies indicate that blood levels do not increase proportionally with increases in the administered dose. When the dose of DANOCRINE is doubled the increase in plasma levels is only about 35% to 40%.

Separate single dosing of 100 mg and 200 mg capsules of DANOCRINE to female volunteers showed that both the extent of availability and the maximum plasma concentration increased by three-to-four fold, respectively, following a meal (> 30 grams of fat), when compared to the fasted state. Further, food also delayed mean time to peak concentration of DANOCRINE by about 30 minutes.

In the treatment of endometriosis, DANOCRINE alters the normal and ectopic endometrial tissue so that it becomes inactive and atrophic. Complete resolution of endometrial lesions occurs in the majority of cases.

Changes in vaginal cytology and cervical mucus reflect the suppressive effect of DANOCRINE on the pituitary-ovarian axis.

In the treatment of fibrocystic breast disease, DANOCRINE usually produces partial to complete disappearance of nodularity and complete relief of pain and tenderness. Changes in the menstrual pattern may occur.

Generally, the pituitary-suppressive action of DANOCRINE is reversible. Ovulation and cyclic bleeding usually return within 60 to 90 days when therapy with DANOCRINE is discontinued.

In the treatment of hereditary angioedema, DANOCRINE at effective doses prevents attacks of the disease characterized by episodic edema of the abdominal viscera, extremities, face, and airway which may be disabling and, if the airway is involved, fatal. In addition, DANOCRINE corrects partially or completely the primary biochemical abnormality of hereditary angioedema by increasing the levels of the deficient C1 esterase inhibitor (C1EI). As a result of this action the serum levels of the C4 component of the complement system are also increased.

INDICATIONS AND USAGE

Endometriosis. DANOCRINE is indicated for the treatment of endometriosis amenable to hormonal management.

Fibrocystic Breast Disease. Most cases of symptomatic fibrocystic breast disease may be treated by simple measures (e.g., padded brassieres and analgesics).

In infrequent patients, symptoms of pain and tenderness may be severe enough to warrant treatment by suppression of ovarian function. DANOCRINE is usually effective in decreasing nodularity, pain, and tenderness. It should be stressed to the patient that this treatment is not innocuous in that it involves considerable alterations of hormone levels and that recurrence of symptoms is very common after cessation of therapy.

Hereditary Angioedema. DANOCRINE is indicated for the prevention of attacks of angioedema of all types (cutaneous, abdominal, laryngeal) in males and females.

CONTRAINDICATIONS

DANOCRINE should not be administered to patients with:

1. Undiagnosed abnormal genital bleeding.
2. Markedly impaired hepatic, renal, or cardiac function.
3. Pregnancy. (See WARNINGS.)
4. Breast feeding.
5. Porphyria—DANOCRINE can induce ALA synthetase activity and hence porphyrin metabolism.

WARNINGS

Use of danazol in pregnancy is contraindicated. A sensitive test (e.g., beta subunit test if available) capable of determining early pregnancy is recommended immediately prior to start of therapy. Additionally a non-hormonal method of contraception should be used during therapy. If a patient becomes pregnant while taking danazol, administration of the drug should be discontinued and the patient should be apprised of the potential risk to the fetus. Exposure to danazol in utero may result in androgenic effects on the female fetus; reports of clitoral hypertrophy, labial fusion, urogenital sinus defect, vaginal atresia, and ambiguous genitalia have been received. (See PRECAUTIONS: Pregnancy, Teratogenic Effects.)

Thromboembolism, thrombotic and thrombophlebitic events including sagittal sinus thrombosis and life-threatening or fatal strokes have been reported.

Experience with long-term therapy with danazol is limited. Peliosis hepatis and benign hepatic adenoma have been observed with long-term use. Peliosis hepatis and hepatic adenoma may be silent until complicated by acute, potentially life-threatening intra-abdominal hemorrhage. The physician therefore should be alert to this possibility. Attempts should be made to determine the lowest dose that will provide adequate protection. If the drug was begun at a time of exacerbation of hereditary angioneurotic edema due to trauma, stress or other cause, periodic attempts to decrease or withdraw therapy should be considered.

Danazol has been associated with several cases of benign intracranial hypertension also known as pseudotumor cerebri. Early signs and symptoms of benign intracranial hypertension include papilledema, headache, nausea and vomiting, and visual disturbances. Patients with these symptoms should be screened for papilledema and, if present, the patients should be advised to discontinue danazol immediately and be referred to a neurologist for further diagnosis and care.

A temporary alteration of lipoproteins in the form of decreased high density lipoproteins and possibly increased low density lipoproteins has been reported during danazol therapy. These alterations may be marked, and prescribers should consider the potential impact on the risk of atherosclerosis and coronary artery disease in accordance with the potential benefit of the therapy to the patient.

Before initiating therapy of fibrocystic breast disease with DANOCRINE, carcinoma of the breast should be excluded. However, nodularity, pain, tenderness due to fibrocystic breast disease may prevent recognition of underlying carcinoma before treatment is begun. Therefore, if any nodule persists or enlarges during treatment, carcinoma should be considered and ruled out.

Patients should be watched closely for signs of androgenic effects some of which may not be reversible even when drug administration is stopped.

PRECAUTIONS

Because DANOCRINE may cause some degree of fluid retention, conditions that might be influenced by this factor, such as epilepsy, migraine, or cardiac or renal dysfunction, require careful observation.

Since hepatic dysfunction manifested by modest increases in serum transaminase levels has been reported in patients treated with DANOCRINE, periodic liver function tests should be performed (see WARNINGS and ADVERSE REACTIONS).

Administration of danazol has been reported to cause exacerbation of the manifestations of acute intermittent porphyria. (See CONTRAINDICATIONS.)

Drug Interactions: Prolongation of prothrombin time occurs in patients stabilized on warfarin. Therapy with danazol may cause an increase in carbamazepine levels in patients taking both drugs.

Laboratory Tests: Danazol treatment may interfere with laboratory determinations of testosterone, androstenedione and dehydroepiandrosterone.

Carcinogenesis, Mutagenesis, Impairment of Fertility: No valid studies have been performed to assess the carcinogenicity of DANOCRINE.

Pregnancy, Teratogenic Effects: (See CONTRAINDICATIONS.) Pregnancy Category X. DANOCRINE administered orally to pregnant rats from the 6th through the 15th day of gestation at doses up to 250 mg/kg/day (7–15 times the human dose) did not result in drug-induced embryotoxicity or teratogenicity, nor difference in litter size, viability or weight of offspring compared to controls. In rabbits, the administration of DANOCRINE on days 6–18 of gestation at doses of 60 mg/kg/day and above (2–4 times the human dose) resulted in inhibition of fetal development.

Nursing Mothers: (See CONTRAINDICATIONS.)

Pediatric Use: Safety and effectiveness in children have not been established.

ADVERSE REACTIONS

The following events have been reported in association with the use of DANOCRINE:

Androgen like effects include weight gain, acne and seborrhea. Mild hirsutism, edema, hair loss, voice change, which may take the form of hoarseness, sore throat or of instability or deepening of pitch, may occur and may persist after cessation of therapy. Hypertrophy of the clitoris is rare.

Other possible endocrine effects include menstrual disturbances in the form of spotting, alteration of the timing of the cycle and amenorrhea. Although cyclical bleeding and ovulation usually return within 60–90 days after discontinuation of therapy with DANOCRINE, persistent amenorrhea has occasionally been reported.

Flushing, sweating, vaginal dryness and irritation and reduction in breast size, may reflect lowering of estrogen. Nervousness and emotional lability have been reported. In the male a modest reduction in spermatogenesis may be evident during treatment. Abnormalities in semen volume, viscosity, sperm count, and motility may occur in patients receiving long-term therapy.

Hepatic dysfunction, as evidenced by reversible elevated serum enzymes and/or jaundice, has been reported in patients receiving a daily dosage of DANOCRINE of 400 mg or more. It is recommended that patients receiving DANOCRINE be monitored for hepatic dysfunction by laboratory tests and clinical observation. Serious hepatic toxicity including cholestatic jaundice, peliosis hepatis, and hepatic adenoma have been reported. (See WARNINGS and PRECAUTIONS.)

Abnormalities in laboratory tests may occur during therapy with DANOCRINE including CPK, glucose tolerance, glucagon, thyroid binding globulin, sex hormone binding globulin, other plasma proteins, lipids and lipoproteins.

The following reactions have been reported, a causal relationship to the administration of DANOCRINE has neither been confirmed nor refuted; *allergic:* urticaria, pruritus and rarely, nasal congestion; *CNS effects:* headache, nervousness and emotional lability, dizziness and fainting, depression, fatigue, sleep disorders, tremor, paresthesias, weakness,

Continued on next page

This product information was prepared in September 1996. On these and other products of Sanofi Winthrop Pharmaceuticals, detailed information may be obtained on a current basis by direct inquiry to Product Information Services, 90 Park Avenue, New York, NY 10016 (toll free 1-800-446-6267).

Sanofi Winthrop—Cont.

visual disturbances, and rarely, benign intracranial hypertension, anxiety, changes in appetite, chills, and rarely convulsions, Guillain-Barre syndrome; *gastrointestinal:* gastroenteritis, nausea, vomiting, constipation, and rarely, pancreatitis; *musculoskeletal:* muscle cramps or spasms, or pains, joint pain, joint lockup, joint swelling, pain in back, neck, or extremities, and rarely, carpal tunnel syndrome which may be secondary to fluid retention; *genitourinary:* hematuria, prolonged posttherapy amenorrhea; *hematologic:* an increase in red cell and platelet count. Reversible erythrocytosis, leukocytosis or polycythemia may be provoked. Eosinophilia, leukopenia and thrombocytopenia have also been noted. *Skin:* rashes (maculopapular, vesicular, papular, purpuric, petechial), and rarely, sun sensitivity, Stevens-Johnson syndrome; *other:* increased insulin requirements in diabetic patients, change in libido, elevation in blood pressure, and rarely, cataracts, bleeding gums, fever, pelvic pain, nipple discharge. Malignant liver tumors have been reported in rare instances, after long-term use.

DOSAGE AND ADMINISTRATION

Endometriosis. In moderate to severe disease, or in patients infertile due to endometriosis, a starting dose of 800 mg given in two divided doses is recommended. Amenorrhea and rapid response to painful symptoms is best achieved at this dosage level. Gradual downward titration to a dose sufficient to maintain amenorrhea may be considered depending upon patient response. For mild cases, an initial daily dose of 200 mg to 400 mg given in two divided doses is recommended and may be adjusted depending on patient response. **Therapy should begin during menstruation. Otherwise, appropriate tests should be performed to ensure that the patient is not pregnant while on therapy with DANOCRINE. (See CONTRAINDICATIONS and WARNINGS.) It is essential that therapy continue uninterrupted for 3 to 6 months but may be extended to 9 months if necessary.** After termination of therapy, if symptoms recur, treatment can be reinstituted.

Fibrocystic Breast Disease. The total daily dosage of DANOCRINE for fibrocystic breast disease ranges from 100 mg to 400 mg given in two divided doses depending upon patient response. **Therapy should begin during menstruation. Otherwise, appropriate tests should be performed to ensure that the patient is not pregnant while on therapy with DANOCRINE.** A nonhormonal method of contraception is recommended when DANOCRINE is administered at this dose, since ovulation may not be suppressed.

In most instances, breast pain and tenderness are significantly relieved by the first month and eliminated in 2 to 3 months. Usually elimination of nodularity requires 4 to 6 months of uninterrupted therapy. Regular menstrual patterns, irregular menstrual patterns, and amenorrhea each occur in approximately one-third of patients treated with 100 mg of DANOCRINE. Irregular menstrual patterns and amenorrhea are observed more frequently with higher doses. Clinical studies have demonstrated that 50% of patients may show evidence of recurrence of symptoms within one year. In this event, treatment may be reinstated.

Hereditary Angioedema. The dosage requirements for continuous treatment of hereditary angioedema with DANOCRINE should be individualized on the basis of the clinical response of the patient. It is recommended that the patient be started on 200 mg, two or three times a day. After a favorable initial response is obtained in terms of prevention of episodes of edematous attacks, the proper continuing dosage should be determined by decreasing the dosage by 50% or less at intervals of one to three months or longer if frequency of attacks prior to treatment dictates. If an attack occurs, the daily dosage may be increased by up to 200 mg. During the dose adjusting phase, close monitoring of the patient's response is indicated, particularly if the patient has a history of airway involvement.

HOW SUPPLIED

Capsules of 200 mg (orange), bottles of 60 (NDC 0024-0305-60).

Capsules of 200 mg (orange), bottles of 100 (NDC 0024-0305-06).

Capsules of 100 mg (yellow), bottles of 100 (NDC 0024-0304-06).

Capsules of 50 mg (orange and white), bottles of 100 (NDC 0024-0303-06).

Store at controlled room temperature, 15° C to 30° C (59° F to 86° F).

Caution: Federal law prohibits dispensing without prescription.

DSW-5 D (O)

Shown in Product Identification Guide, page 333

DEMEROL® Ⓒ℞

MEPERIDINE HYDROCHLORIDE, USP

WARNING: May be habit forming

DESCRIPTION

Meperidine hydrochloride is ethyl 1-methyl-4-phenylisonipecotate hydrochloride, a white crystalline substance with a melting point of 186° C to 189° C. It is readily soluble in water and has a neutral reaction and a slightly bitter taste. The solution is not decomposed by a short period of boiling. The syrup is a pleasant-tasting, nonalcoholic, banana-flavored solution containing 50 mg of DEMEROL, brand of meperidine hydrochloride, per 5 mL teaspoon (25 drops contain 13 mg of DEMEROL). The tablets contain 50 mg or 100 mg of the analgesic.

DEMEROL injectable is supplied in **Carpuject®**, **CARPUJECT** with InterLink® and **CARPUJECT** with Luer Lock of 2.5% (25 mg/1 mL), 5% (50 mg/1 mL), 7.5% (75 mg/1 mL), and 10% (100 mg/1 mL). Uni-Amp® unit dose pak-ampuls of 5% solution (25 mg/0.5 mL), (50 mg/1 mL), (75 mg/1.5 mL), (100 mg/2 mL), and 10% solution (100 mg/1 mL). Uni-Nest™ ampul pak-ampuls of 5% solution (25 mg/0.5 mL), (50 mg/1 mL), (75 mg/1.5 mL), (100 mg/2 mL), and 10% solution (100 mg/1 mL). Multiple-dose vials of 5% and 10% solutions contain metacresol 0.1% as preservative.

The pH of DEMEROL solutions is adjusted between 3.5 and 6 with sodium hydroxide or hydrochloric acid.

DEMEROL, brand of meperidine hydrochloride, 5 percent solution has a specific gravity of 1.0086 at 20° C and 10 percent solution, a specific gravity of 1.0165 at 20° C.

Inactive Ingredients—TABLETS: Calcium Sulfate, Dibasic Calcium Phosphate, Starch, Stearic Acid, Talc. SYRUP: Benzoic Acid, Flavor, Liquid Glucose, Purified Water, Saccharin Sodium.

CLINICAL PHARMACOLOGY

Meperidine hydrochloride is a narcotic analgesic with multiple actions qualitatively similar to those of morphine; the most prominent of these involve the central nervous system and organs composed of smooth muscle. The principal actions of therapeutic value are analgesia and sedation.

There is some evidence which suggests that meperidine may produce less smooth muscle spasm, constipation, and depression of the cough reflex than equianalgesic doses of morphine. Meperidine, in 60 mg to 80 mg parenteral doses, is approximately equivalent in analgesic effect to 10 mg of morphine. The onset of action is slightly more rapid than with morphine, and the duration of action is slightly shorter. Meperidine is significantly less effective by the oral than by the parenteral route, but the exact ratio of oral to parenteral effectiveness is unknown.

INDICATIONS AND USAGE

For the relief of moderate to severe pain (parenteral and oral forms)

For preoperative medication (parenteral form only)

For support of anesthesia (parenteral form only)

For obstetrical analgesia (parenteral form only)

CONTRAINDICATIONS

Hypersensitivity to meperidine.

Meperidine is contraindicated in patients who are receiving monoamine oxidase (MAO) inhibitors or those who have recently received such agents. Therapeutic doses of meperdine have occasionally precipitated unpredictable, severe, and occasionally fatal reactions in patients who have received such agents within 14 days. The mechanism of these reactions is unclear, but may be related to a preexisting hyperphenylalaninemia. Some have been characterized by coma, severe respiratory depression, cyanosis, and hypotension, and have resembled the syndrome of acute narcotic overdose. In other reactions the predominant manifestations have been hyperexcitability, convulsions, tachycardia, hyperpyrexia, and hypertension. Although it is not known that other narcotics are free of the risk of such reactions, virtually all of the reported reactions have occurred with meperidine. If a narcotic is needed in such patients, a sensitivity test should be performed in which repeated, small, incremental doses of morphine are administered over the course of several hours while the patient's condition and vital signs are under careful observation. (Intravenous hydrocortisone or prednisolone have been used to treat severe reactions, with the addition of intravenous chlorpromazine in those cases exhibiting hypertension and hyperpyrexia. The usefulness and safety of narcotic antagonists in the treatment of these reactions is unknown.)

Solutions of DEMEROL and barbituates are chemically incompatible.

WARNINGS

Drug Dependence. Meperidine can produce drug dependence of the morphine type and therefore has the potential for being abused. Psychic dependence, physical dependence, and tolerance may develop upon repeated administration of meperidine, and it should be prescribed and administered with the same degree of caution appropriate to the use of morphine. Like other narcotics, meperidine is subject to the provisions of the Federal narcotic laws.

Interaction with Other Central Nervous System Depressants. MEPERIDINE SHOULD BE USED WITH GREAT CAUTION AND IN REDUCED DOSAGE IN PATIENTS WHO ARE CONCURRENTLY RECEIVING OTHER NARCOTIC ANALGESICS, GENERAL ANESTHETICS, PHENOTHIAZINES, OTHER TRANQUILIZERS (SEE DOSAGE AND ADMINISTRATION), SEDATIVE-HYPNOTICS (INCLUDING BARBITUATES), TRICYCLIC ANTIDEPRESSANTS AND OTHER CNS DEPRESSANTS (INCLUDING ALCOHOL). RESPIRATORY DEPRESSION, HYPOTENSION, AND PROFOUND SEDATION OR COMA MAY RESULT.

Head Injury and Increased Intracranial Pressure. The respiratory depressant effects of meperidine and its capacity to elevate cerebrospinal fluid pressure may be markedly exaggerated in the presence of head injury, other intracranial lesions, or a preexisting increase in intracranial pressure. Furthermore, narcotics produce adverse reactions which may obscure the clinical course of patients with head injuries. In such patients, meperidine must be used with extreme caution and only if its use is deemed essential.

Intravenous Use. If necessary, meperidine may be given intravenously, but the injection should be given very slowly, preferably in the form of a diluted solution. Rapid intravenous injection of narcotic analgesics, including meperidine, increases the incidence of adverse reactions; severe respiratory depression, apnea, hypotension, peripheral circulatory collapse, and cardiac arrest have occurred. Meperidine should not be administered intravenously unless a narcotic antagonist and the facilities for assisted or controlled respiration are immediately available. When meperidine is given parenterally, especially intravenously, the patient should be lying down.

Asthma and Other Respiratory Conditions. Meperidine should be used with extreme caution in patients having an acute asthmatic attack, patients with chronic obstructive pulmonary disease or cor pulmonale, patients having a substantially decreased respiratory reserve, and patients with preexisting respiratory depression, hypoxia, or hypercapnia. In such patients, even usual therapeutic doses of narcotics may decrease respiratory drive while simultaneously increasing airway resistance to the point of apnea.

Hypotensive Effect. The administration of meperidine may result in severe hypotension in the postoperative patient or any individual whose ability to maintain blood pressure has been compromised by a depleted blood volume or the administration of drugs such as the phenothiazines or certain anesthetics.

Usage in Ambulatory Patients. Meperidine may impair the mental and/or physical abilities required for the performance of potentially hazardous tasks such as driving a car or operating machinery. The patient should be cautioned accordingly.

Meperidine, like other narcotics, may produce orthostatic hypotension in ambulatory patients.

Usage in Pregnancy and Lactation. Meperidine should not be used in pregnant women prior to the labor period, unless in the judgment of the physician the potential benefits outweigh the possible hazards, because safe use in pregnancy prior to labor has not been established relative to possible adverse effects on fetal development.

When used as an obstetrical analgesic, meperidine crosses the placental barrier and can produce depression of respiration and psychophysiologic functions in the newborn. Resuscitation may be required (see section on OVERDOSAGE).

Meperidine appears in the milk of nursing mothers receiving the drug.

PRECAUTIONS

As with all intramuscular preparations, DEMEROL intramuscular injection should be injected well within the body of a large muscle.

Supraventricular Tachycardias. Meperidine should be used with caution in patients with atrial flutter and other supraventricular tachycardias because of a possible vagolytic action which may produce a significant increase in the ventricular response rate.

Convulsions. Meperidine may aggravate preexisting convulsions in patients with convulsive disorders. If dosage is escalated substantially above recommended levels because of tolerance development, convulsions may occur in indivduals without a history of convulsive disorders.

Acute Abdominal Conditions. The administration of meperidine or other narcotics may obscure the diagnosis or clinical course in patients with acute abdominal conditions.

Special Risk Patients. Meperidine should be given with caution and the initial dose should be reduced in certain patients such as the elderly or debilitated, and those with severe impairment of hepatic or renal function, hypothyroidism, Addison's disease, and prostatic hypertrophy or urethral stricture.

ADVERSE REACTIONS

The major hazards of meperidine, as with other narcotic analgesics, are respiratory depression and, to a lesser degree,

circulatory depression; respiratory arrest, shock, and cardiac arrest have occurred.
The most frequently observed adverse reactions include lightheadedness, dizziness, sedation, nausea, vomiting, and sweating. These effects seem to be more prominent in ambulatory patients and in those who are not experiencing severe pain. In such individuals, lower doses are advisable. Some adverse reactions in ambulatory patients may be alleviated if the patient lies down.
Other adverse reactions include:
Nervous System. Euphoria, dysphoria, weakness, headache, agitation, tremor, uncoordinated muscle movements, severe convulsions, transient hallucinations and disorientation, visual disturbances. Inadvertent injection about a nerve trunk may result in sensory-motor paralysis which is usually, though not always, transitory.
Gastrointestinal. Dry mouth, constipation, biliary tract spasm.
Cardiovascular. Flushing of the face, tachycardia, bradycardia, palpitation, hypotension (see WARNINGS), syncope, phlebitis following intravenous injection.
Genitourinary. Urinary retention.
Allergic. Pruritus, urticaria, other skin rashes, wheal and flare over the vein with intravenous injection.
Other. Pain at injection site; local tissue irritation and induration following subcutaneous injection, particularly when repeated; antidiuretic effect.

DOSAGE AND ADMINISTRATION

For Relief of Pain
Dosage should be adjusted according to the severity of the pain and the response of the patient. While subcutaneous administration is suitable for occasional use, intramuscular administration is preferred when repeated doses are required. If intravenous administration is required, dosage should be decreased and the injection made very slowly, preferably utilizing a diluted solution. Meperidine is less effective orally than on parenteral administration. The dose of DEMEROL should be proportionately reduced (usually by 25 to 50 percent) when administered concomitantly with phenothiazines and many other tranquilizers since they potentiate the action of DEMEROL.
Adults. The usual dosage is 50 mg to 150 mg intramuscularly, subcutaneously, or orally, every 3 or 4 hours as necessary.
Children. The usual dosage is 0.5 mg/lb to 0.8 mg/lb intramuscularly, subcutaneously, or orally up to the adult dose, every 3 or 4 hours as necessary.
Each dose of the syrup should be taken in one-half glass of water, since if taken undiluted, it may exert a slight topical anesthetic effect on mucous membranes.

For Preoperative Medication
Adults. The usual dosage is 50 mg to 100 mg intramuscularly or subcutaneously, 30 to 90 minutes before the beginning of anesthesia.
Children. The usual dosage is 0.5 mg/lb to 1 mg/lb intramuscularly or subcutaneously up to the adult dose, 30 to 90 minutes before the beginning of anesthesia.

For Support of Anesthesia
Repeated slow intravenous injections of fractional doses (e.g., 10 mg/mL) or continuous intravenous infusion of a more dilute solution (e.g., 1 mg/mL) should be used. The dose should be titrated to the needs of the patient and will depend on the premedication and type of anesthesia being employed, the characteristics of the particular patient, and the nature and duration of the operative procedure.

For Obstetrical Analgesia
The usual dosage is 50 mg to 100 mg intramuscularly or subcutaneously when pain becomes regular, and may be repeated at 1-to 3-hour intervals.

OVERDOSAGE

Symptoms. Serious overdosage with meperidine is characterized by respiratory depression (a decrease in respiratory rate and/or tidal volume, Cheyne-Stokes respiration, cyanosis), extreme somnolence progressing to stupor or coma, skeletal muscle flaccidity, cold and clammy skin, and sometimes bradycardia and hypotension. In severe overdosage, particularly by the intravenous route, apnea, circulatory collapse, cardiac arrest, and death may occur.
Treatment. Primary attention should be given to the reestablishment of adequate respiratory exchange through provision of a patent airway and institution of assisted or controlled ventilation. The narcotic antagonist, naloxone hydrochloride, is a specific antidote against respiratory depression which may result from overdosage or unusual sensitivity to narcotics, including meperidine. Therefore, an appropriate dose of this antagonist should be administered, preferably by the intravenous route, simultaneously with efforts at respiratory resuscitation.
An antagonist should not be administered in the absence of clinically significant respiratory or cardiovascular depression.
Oxygen, intravenous fluids, vasopressors, and other supportive measures should be employed as indicated.
In cases of overdosage with DEMEROL tablets, the stomach should be evacuated by emesis or gastric lavage.
NOTE: In an individual physically dependent on narcotics, the administration of the usual dose of a narcotic antagonist will precipitate an acute withdrawal syndrome. The severity of this syndrome will depend on the degree of physical dependence and the dose of antagonist administered. The use of narcotic antagonists in such individuals should be avoided if possible. If a narcotic antagonist must be used to treat serious respiratory depression in the physically dependent patient, the antagonist should be administered with extreme care and only one-fifth to one-tenth the usual initial dose administered.

HOW SUPPLIED

For Parenteral Use
Solutions of DEMEROL for parenteral use are clear and colorless and are available as follows:
CARPUJECT sterile cartridge unit in Detecto-Seal® tamper detection package:
WITH 22 GAUGE 1¹/₄ INCH NEEDLE:
2.5 percent (25 mg per mL) NDC 0024-0324-02,
5 percent (50 mg per mL) NDC 0024-0325-02,
7.5 percent (75 mg per mL) NDC 0024-0326-02,
10 percent (100 mg per mL) NDC 0024-0328-02,
all in boxes of 10.
WITH INTERLINK® SYSTEM CANNULA
2.5 percent (25 mg per mL) NDC 0024-0324-42,
5 percent (50 mg per mL) NDC 0024-0325-43,
7.5 percent (75 mg per mL) NDC 0024-0326-44,
10 percent (100 mg per mL) NDC 0024-0328-45,
all in boxes of 10.
WITH LUER LOCK
2.5 percent (25 per mL) NDC 0024-0324-23,
5 percent (50 mg per mL) NDC 0024-0325-33,
7.5 percent (75 mg per mL) NDC 0024-0326-33,
10 percent (100 mg per mL) NDC 0024-0328-33,
all in boxes of 10.
Uni-Amp® unit dose pak-
5 percent solution, ampuls:
0.5 mL (25 mg) NDC 0024-0361-04,
1 mL (50 mg) NDC 0024-0362-04,
1.5 mL (75 mg) NDC 0024-0363-04,
2 mL (100 mg) NDC 0024-0364-04,
all in boxes of 25.
10 percent solution, ampuls
1 mL (100 mg) NDC 0024-0365-04,
in boxes of 25.
Uni-Nest™ ampul pak-
5 percent solution, ampuls:
0.5 mL (25 mg) NDC 0024-0371-04,
1 mL (50 mg) NDC 0024-0372-04,
1.5 mL (75 mg) NDC 0024-0373-04,
and 2 mL (100 mg) NDC 0024-0374-04,
all in boxes of 25.
10 percent solution, ampuls
1 mL (100 mg) NDC 0024-0375-04,
in boxes of 25.
Vials
5 percent multiple-dose vials of 30 mL NDC 0024-0329-01,
10 percent multiple-dose vials of 20 mL NDC 0024-0331-01,
all in boxes of 1.
Note: The pH of DEMEROL solutions is adjusted between 3.5 and 6 with sodium hydroxide or hydrochloric acid. Multiple-dose vials contain metacresol 0.1 percent as preservative. No preservatives are added to the ampuls or **CARPUJECT** sterile cartridge units.
For Oral Use
Tablets are white, round and convex: the 50 mg tablet is scored.
Tablets

50 mg:	bottles of 100 (NDC 0024-0335-04),
	bottles of 500 (NDC 0024-0335-06),
	Hospital Blister Pak of 25 (NDC 0024-0335-02).
100 mg:	bottles of 100 (NDC 0024-0337-04),
	bottles of 500 (NDC 0024-0337-06),
	Hospital Blister Pak of 25 (NDC 0024-0337-02).

Syrup
Nonalcoholic, banana-flavored 50 mg per 5 mL teaspoon, bottles of 16 fl oz (NDC 0024-0332-06).
Store at room temperature up to 25° C (77° F). Tablets in Hospital Blister Paks may be stored at controlled room temperature 25° C to 30° C (59° F to 86° F).
CAUTION: Federal law prohibits dispensing without prescription.
InterLink® is a Trademark of Baxter International, Inc.
U.S. Pat. Nos. 5, 158,554; 5, 171,234; 5, 188,620; Pat. Pending
DSW-3 D
Shown in Product Identification Guide, page 333

INOCOR® ℞

AMRINONE LACTATE INJECTION
Sterile Intravenous Solution

DESCRIPTION

INOCOR, brand of amrinone lactate injection, represents a new class of cardiac inotropic agents distinct from digitalis glycosides or catecholamines. Amrinone lactate is designated chemically as 5-Amino[3,4′-bipyridin]-6(1*H*)-one 2-hydroxypropanate and has the following structure:

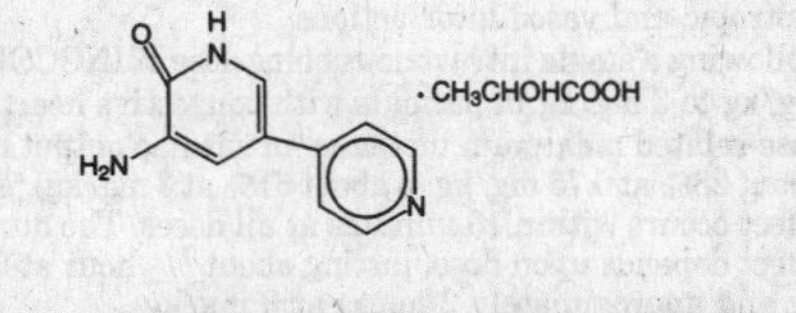

Amrinone is a pale yellow crystalline compound with a molecular weight of 187.2 and an empirical formula of $C_{10}H_9N_3O$. Each mole of lactic acid has a molecular weight of 90.08 and an empirical formula of $C_3H_6O_3$. The solubilities of amrinone at pH's 4.1, 6.0, and 8.0 are 25, 0.9, and 0.7 mg/mL, respectively.
INOCOR is a clear yellow sterile solution available in 20 mL ampuls for intravenous administration. Each mL contains amrinone lactate equivalent to 5 mg of base and 0.25 mg of sodium metabisulfite added as a preservative in Water for Injection. All dosages expressed in the package insert are expressed in terms of the base, amrinone. The pH is adjusted to between 3.2 to 4.0 with lactic acid or sodium hydroxide. The total concentration of lactic acid can vary between 5 mg/mL and 7.5 mg/mL.

CLINICAL PHARMACOLOGY

INOCOR is a positive inotropic agent with vasodilator activity, different in structure and mode of action from either digitalis glycosides or catecholamines.
The mechanism of its inotropic and vasodilator effects has not been fully elucidated.
With respect to its inotropic effect, experimental evidence indicates that it is not a beta-adrenergic agonist. It inhibits myocardial cyclic adenosine monophosphate (c-AMP) phosphodiesterase activity and increases cellular levels of c-AMP. Unlike digitalis, it does not inhibit sodium-potassium adenosine triphosphatase activity.
With respect to its vasodilatory activity, INOCOR reduces afterload and preload by its direct relaxant effect on vascular smooth muscle.

Pharmacokinetics
Following intravenous bolus (1 to 2 minutes) injection of 0.68 mg/kg to 1.2 mg/kg to normal volunteers, INOCOR had a volume of distribution of 1.2 liters/kg, and following a distributive phase half-life of about 4.6 minutes in plasma, had a mean apparent first-order terminal elimination half-life of about 3.6 hours. In patients with congestive heart failure receiving infusions of INOCOR the mean apparent first-order terminal elimination half-life was about 5.8 hours.
Amrinone has been shown in one study to be 10% to 22% bound to human plasma protein by ultrafiltration in vitro, and in another study 35% to 49% bound by either ultrafiltration or equilibrium dialysis.
The primary route of excretion in man is *via* the urine as both amrinone and several metabolites (N-glycolyl, N-acetate, O-glucuronide and N-glucuronide). In normal volunteers, approximately 63% of an oral dose of ^{14}C-labelled amrinone was excreted in the urine over a 96–hour period. In the first 8 hours, 51% of the radioactivity in the urine was amrinone with 5% as the N-acetate, 8% as the N-glycolate, and less than 5% for each glucuronide. Approximately 18% of the administered dose was excreted in the feces in 72 hours.
In a 24-hour nonradioactive intravenous study, 10% to 40% of the dose was excreted in urine as unchanged amrinone with the N-acetyl metabolite representing less than 2% of the dose.
In congestive heart failure patients, after a loading bolus dose, steady-state plasma levels of about 2.4 mcg/mL were able to be maintained by an infusion of 5 mcg/kg/min to 10 mcg/kg/min. In some congestive heart failure patients, with associated compromised renal and hepatic perfusion, it is possible that plasma levels of amrinone may rise during the infusion period; therefore, in these patients, it may be necessary to monitor the hemodynamic response and/or drug

Continued on next page

This product information was prepared in September 1996. On these and other products of Sanofi Winthrop Pharmaceuticals, detailed information may be obtained on a current basis by direct inquiry to Product Information Services, 90 Park Avenue, New York, NY 10016 (toll free 1-800-446-6267).

Sanofi Winthrop—Cont.

level. The principal measures of patient response include cardiac index, pulmonary capillary wedge pressure, central venous pressure, and their relationship to plasma concentrations. Additionally, measurements of blood pressure, urine output, and body weight may prove useful, as may such clinical symptoms as orthopnea, dyspnea, and fatigue.

Pharmacodynamics

In patients with depressed myocardial function, INOCOR produces a prompt increase in cardiac output due to its inotropic and vasodilator actions.

Following a single intravenous bolus dose of INOCOR of 0.75 mg/kg to 3 mg/kg in patients with congestive heart failure, dose-related maximum increases in cardiac output occur (of about 28% at 0.75 mg/kg to about 61% at 3 mg/kg). The peak effect occurs within 10 minutes at all doses. The duration of effect depends upon dose, lasting about $1/2$ hour at 0.75 mg/kg and approximately 2 hours at 3 mg/kg.

Over the same range of doses, pulmonary capillary wedge pressure and total peripheral resistance show dose-related decreases (mean maximum decreases of 29% in pulmonary capillary wedge pressure and 29% in systemic vascular resistance). At doses up to 3 mg/kg dose-related decreases in diastolic pressure (up to 13%) have been observed. Mean arterial pressure decreases (9.7%) at a dose of 3 mg/kg. The heart rate is generally unchanged.

The changes in hemodynamic parameters are maintained during continuous intravenous infusion and for several hours thereafter.

INOCOR is effective in fully digitalized patients without causing signs of cardiac glycoside toxicity. Its inotropic effects are additive to those of digitalis. In cases of atrial flutter/fibrillation, it is possible that INOCOR may increase ventricular response rate because of its slight enhancement of AV conduction. In these cases, prior treatment with digitalis is recommended.

Improvement in left ventricular function and relief of congestive heart failure in patients with ischemic heart disease have been observed. The improvement has occurred without inducing symptoms or electrocardiographic signs of myocardial ischemia.

At constant heart rate and blood pressure, increases in cardiac output occur without measurable increases in myocardial oxygen consumption or changes in arteriovenous oxygen difference.

Inotropic activity is maintained following repeated intravenous doses of INOCOR. INOCOR administration produces hemodynamic and symptomatic benefits to patients not satisfactorily controlled by conventional therapy with diuretics and cardiac glycosides.

INDICATIONS AND USAGE

INOCOR is indicated for the short-term management of congestive heart failure. Because of limited experience and potential for serious adverse effects (see ADVERSE REACTIONS), INOCOR should be used only in patients who can be closely monitored and who have not responded adequately to digitalis, diuretics, and/or vasodilators. Although most patients have been studied hemodynamically for periods only up to 24 hours, some patients were studied for longer periods and demonstrated consistent hemodynamic and clinical effects. The duration of therapy should depend on patient responsiveness.

CONTRAINDICATIONS

INOCOR is contraindicated in patients who are hypersensitive to it.

It is also contraindicated in those patients known to be hypersensitive to bisulfites.

WARNING

Contains sodium metabisulfite, a sulfite that may cause allergic-type reactions including anaphylactic symptoms and life-threatening or less severe asthmatic episodes in certain susceptible people. The overall prevalence of sulfite sensitivity in the general population is unknown and probably low. Sulfite sensitivity is seen more frequently in asthmatic than in nonasthmatic people.

PRECAUTIONS

General

INOCOR should not be used in patients with severe aortic or pulmonic valvular disease in lieu of surgical relief of the obstruction. Like other inotropic agents, it may aggravate outflow tract obstruction in hypertrophic subaortic stenosis. During intravenous therapy with INOCOR, blood pressure and heart rate should be monitored and the rate of infusion slowed or stopped in patients showing excessive decreases in blood pressure.

Patients who have received vigorous diuretic therapy may have insufficient cardiac filling pressure to respond adequately to INOCOR, in which case cautious liberalization of fluid and electrolyte intake may be indicated.

Supraventricular and ventricular arrhythmias have been observed in the very high-risk population treated. While amrinone per se has not been shown to be arrhythmogenic, the potential for arrhythmia, present in congestive heart failure itself, may be increased by any drug or combination of drugs.

Thrombocytopenia and hepatotoxicity have been noted (see ADVERSE REACTIONS).

USE IN ACUTE MYOCARDIAL INFARCTION

No clinical trials have been carried out in patients in the acute phase of postmyocardial infarction. Therefore, INOCOR is not recommended in these cases.

Laboratory Tests

Fluid and Electrolytes: Fluid and electrolyte changes and renal function should be carefully monitored during amrinone lactate therapy. Improvement in cardiac output with resultant diuresis may necessitate a reduction in the dose of diuretic. Potassium loss due to excessive diuresis may predispose digitalized patients to arrhythmias. Therefore, hypokalemia should be corrected by potassium supplementation in advance of or during amrinone use.

Drug Interactions

In a relatively limited experience, no untoward clinical manifestations have been observed in patients in which INOCOR was used concurrently with the following drugs: digitalis glycosides; lidocaine, quinidine; metoprolol, propranolol; hydralazine, prazosin; isosorbide dinitrate, nitrogycerine; chlorthalidone, ethacrynic acid, furosemide, hydrochlorothiazide, spironolactone; captopril; heparin, warfarin; potassium supplements; insulin; diazepam.

One case report of excessive hypotension has been reported when amrinone was used concurrently with disopyramide. Unit additional experience is available, concurrent administration with NORPACE® (disopyramide) should be undertaken with caution.

Chemical Interactions

A chemical interaction occurs slowly over a 24-hour period when the intravenous solution of INOCOR is mixed <u>directly</u> with dextrose (glucose)-containing solutions. **THEREFORE, INOCOR SHOULD NOT BE DILUTED WITH SOLUTIONS THAT CONTAIN DEXTROSE (GLUCOSE) PRIOR TO INJECTION.**

A chemical interaction occurs immediately, which is evidenced by the formation of a precipitate when furosemide is injected into an intravenous line of an infusion of amrinone. Therefore, furosemide should not be administered in intravenous lines containing amrinone.

Carcinogenesis, Mutagenesis, Impairment of Fertility

There was no suggestion of a carcinogenic potential with amrinone when administered orally for up to two years to rats and mice at dose levels up to the maximally tolerated dose of 80 mg/kg/day.

The mouse micronucleus test (at 7.5 to 10 times the maximum human dose) and the Chinese hamster ovary chromosome aberration assay were positive indicating both clastogenic potential and suppression of the number of polychromatic erythrocytes. However, the Ames Salmonella assay, mouse lymphoma study, and cultured human lymphocyte metaphase analysis were all negative. The clastogenic effects are in contrast to negative results obtained in the rat male and female fertility studies, and a three-generation study in rats, both oral dosing.

Slight prolongation of the rat gestation period was seen in these studies at dose levels of 50 mg/kg/day and 100 mg/kg/day. Dystocia occurred in dams receiving 100 mg/kg/day resulting in increased numbers of stillbirths, decreased litter size, and poor pup survival.

Pregnancy Category C

In New Zealand white rabbits, amrinone has been shown to produce fetal skeletal and gross external malformations at oral doses of 16 mg/kg and 50 mg/kg which were toxic for the rabbit. Studies in French Hy/Cr rabbits using oral doses up to 32 mg/kg/day did not confirm this finding. No malformations were seen in rats receiving amrinone intravenously at the maximum dose used, 15 mg/kg/day (approximately the recommended daily intravenous dose for patients with congestive heart failure). There are no adequate and well-controlled studies in pregnant women. Amrinone should be used during pregnancy only if the potential benefit justifies the potential risk to the fetus.

Nursing Mothers

Caution should be exercised when amrinone is administered to nursing women, since it is not known whether it is excreted in human milk.

Pediatric Use

Safety and effectiveness in children have not been established.

ADVERSE REACTIONS

Thrombocytopenia: Intravenous INOCOR resulted in platelet count reductions to below 100,000/mm³ or normal limits in 2.4 percent of the patients.

It is more common in patients receiving prolonged therapy. To date, in closely-monitored clinical trials, in patients whose platelet counts were not allowed to remain depressed, no bleeding phenomena have been observed.

Platelet reduction is dose dependent and appears due to a decrease in platelet survival time. Several patients who developed thrombocytopenia while receiving amrinone had bone marrow examinations which were normal. There is no evidence relating platelet reduction to immune response or to a platelet activating factor.

Gastrointestinal Effects: Gastrointestinal adverse reactions reported with INOCOR during clinical use included nausea (1.7%), vomiting (0.9%), abdominal pain (0.4%), and anorexia (0.4%).

Cardiovascular Effects: Cardiovascular adverse reactions reported with INOCOR include arrhythmia (3%) and hypotension (1.3%).

Hepatic Toxicity: In dogs, at IV doses between 9 mg/kg/day and 32 mg/kg/day, amrinone showed dose-related hepatotoxicity manifested either as enzyme elevation or hepatic cell necrosis or both. Hypatotoxicity has been observed in man following long-term oral dosing and has been observed, in a limited experience (0.2%), following intravenous administration of amrinone. There have also been rare reports of enzyme and bilirubin elevation and jaundice.

Hypersensitivity: There have been reports of several apparent hypersensitivity reactions in patients treated with oral amrinone for about two weeks. Signs and symptoms were variable but included pericarditis, pleuritis and ascites (1 case), myositis with interstitial shadowing on chest x-ray and elevated sedimentation rate (1 case) and vasculitis with nodular pulmonary densities, hypoxemia, and jaundice (1 case). The first patient died, not necessarily of the possible reaction, while the last two resolved with discontinuation of therapy. None of the cases were rechallenged so that attribution to amrinone is not certain, but possible hypersensitivity reactions should be considered in any patient maintained for a prolonged period on amrinone.

General: Additional adverse reactions observed in intravenous amrinone clinical studies include fever (0.9%), chest pain (0.2%), and burning at the site of injection (0.2%).

Management of Adverse Reactions

Platelet Count Reduction: Asymptomatic platelet count reduction (to < 150,000/mm³) may be reversed within one week of a decrease in drug dosage. Further, with no change in drug dosage, the count may stabilize at lower than pre-drug levels without any clinical sequelae. Pre-drug platelet counts and frequent platelet counts during therapy are recommended to assist in decisions regarding dosage modifications.

Should a platelet count less than 150,000/mm³ occur, the following actions may be considered.

- Maintain total daily dose unchanged, since in some cases counts have either stabilized or returned to pretreatment levels.
- Decrease total daily dose.
- Discontinue amrinone, if, in the clinical judgment of the physician, risk exceeds the potential benefit.

Gastrointestinal Side Effects: While gastrointestinal side effects were seen infrequently with intravenous therapy, should severe or debilitating ones occur, the physician may wish to reduce dosage or discontinue the drug based on the usual benefit-to-risk considerations.

Hepatic Toxicity: In clinical experience to date with intravenous administration, hepatotoxicity has been observed rarely. If acute market alterations in liver enzymes occur together with clinical symptoms suggesting an idiosyncratic hypersensitivity reaction, amrinone therapy should be promptly discontinued.

If less than marked enzyme alterations occur without clinical symptoms, these nonspecific changes should be evaluated on an individual basis. The clinician may wish to continue amrinone, reduce dosage, or discontinue the drug based on the usual benefit/risk considerations.

OVERDOSAGE

A death has been reported with a massive accidental overdose (840 mg over three hours by initial bolus and infusion) of amrinone, although causal relation is uncertain. Diligence should be exercised during product preparation and administration.

Doses of INOCOR may produce hypotension because of its vasodilator effect. If this occurs, amrinone administration should be reduced or discontinued. No specific antidote is known, but general measures for circulatory support should be taken.

In rats, the LD₅₀ of amrinone, as the lactate salt, was 102 mg/kg or 130 mg/kg intravenously in two different studies and 132 mg/kg orally (intragastrically); as a suspension in aqueous gum tragacanth the oral LD₅₀ was 239 mg/kg.

DOSAGE AND ADMINISTRATION

Loading doses of INOCOR should be administered as supplied (undiluted). Infusions of INOCOR may be administered in normal or half normal saline solution to a concentration of 1 mg/mL to 3 mg/mL. Diluted solutions should be used within 24 hours.

INOCOR may be injected into running dextrose (glucose) infusions through a Y-Connector or directly into the tubing where preferable.

LOADING DOSE DETERMINATION
0.75 mg/kg (undiluted)

Patient Weight in kg	30	40	50	60	70	80	90	100	110	120
mL of undiluted INOCOR Inj	4.5	6.0	7.5	9.0	10.5	12.0	13.5	15.0	16.5	18.0

INOCOR IV (amrinone) INFUSION RATE (mL/hr) CHART
Using 2.5 mg/mL Infusion Concentration*

Patient Weight in kg	30	40	50	60	70	80	90	100	110	120
Dosage: 5.0 mcg/kg/min		4	5	6	7	8	10	11	12	13	14
7.5 mcg/kg/min		5	7	9	11	13	14	16	18	20	22
10.0 mcg/kg/min		7	10	12	14	17	19	22	24	26	29

Example: A 70 kg patient would require a loading dose of 10.5 mL of undiluted INOCOR. If the physician selects a dose of 7.5 mcg/kg/min for the infusion, the flow rate would be 13 mL/hr at the 2.5 mg/mL concentration of INOCOR.

*Dilution: To prepare the 2.5 mg/mL concentration recommended for infusion mix INOCOR with an equal volume of diluent. For example, mix three 20 mL ampuls of INOCOR (3×20 mL=60 mL) with 60 mL of diluent for a total volume of 120 mL of the final 2.5 mg/mL solution of INOCOR.

Chemical Interactions

A chemical interaction occurs slowly over a 24-hour period when the intravenous solution of INOCOR is mixed directly with dextrose (glucose)-containing solutions. **THEREFORE, INOCOR SHOULD NOT BE DILUTED WITH SOLUTIONS THAT CONTAIN DEXTROSE (GLUCOSE) PRIOR TO INJECTION.**

A chemical interaction occurs immediately, which is evidenced by the formation of a precipitate when furosemide is injected into an intravenous line of an infusion of amrinone. Therefore, furosemide should not be administered in intravenous lines containing amrinone.

The following procedure is recommended for the administration of INOCOR:

1. Initiate therapy with a 0.75 mg/kg loading dose given slowly over 2 to 3 minutes.
[See first table above.]

2. Continue therapy with a maintenance infusion between 5 mcg/kg/min and 10 mcg/kg/min.

3. Based on clinical response, an additional loading dose of 0.75 mg/kg may be given 30 minutes after the initiation of therapy.

4. The rate of infusion usually ranges from 5 mcg/kg/min to 10 mcg/kg/min such that the recommended total daily dose (including loading doses) does not exceed 10 mg/kg. A limited number of patients studied at higher doses support a dosage regimen up to 18 mg/kg/day for shortened durations of therapy.

The following infusion rate chart may be used to assure that the calculations are made correctly.

To utilize the chart, the concentration of amrinone infusion solution used must be 2.5 mg/mL (2500 mcg/mL). This concentration is prepared by mixing the amrinone solution with an equal volume of diluent (normal or half normal saline).

[See second table above.]

5. The rate of administration and the duration of therapy should be adjusted according to the response of the patient. The physician may wish to reduce or titrate the infusion downward based on clinical responsiveness or untoward effects.

The above dosing regimens can be expected to place most patients' plasma concentration of amrinone at approximately 3 mcg/mL. Increases in cardiac index show a linear relationship to plasma concentration of a range of 0.5 mcg/mL to 7 mcg/mL. No observations have been made of greater plasma concentrations.

Patient improvement may be reflected by increases in cardiac output, reduction in pulmonary capillary wedge pressure, and such clinical responses as a lessening of dyspnea and an improvement in other symptoms of heart failure, such as orthopnea and fatigue.

Monitoring central venous pressure (CVP) may be valuable in the assessment of hypotension and fluid balance management. Prior correction or adjustment of fluid/electrolytes is essential to obtain satisfactory response with amrinone. Parenteral drug products should be inspected visually and should not be used if particulate matter or discoloration is observed.

HOW SUPPLIED

Ampuls of 20 mL sterile, clear yellow solution containing INOCOR 5 mg/mL, box of 5 (NDC 0024-0888-20). Each mL contains amrinone lactate equivalent to 5 mg base and 0.25 mg sodium metabisulfite in Water for Injection. The pH of INOCOR is adjusted to a range of 3.2 to 4.0 with lactic acid or sodium hydroxide.

Protect INOCOR ampuls from light. Ampul packaging is light resistant for protection during storage.

Store at controlled room temperature 15°C to 30°C (59°F to 86°F).
Caution: Federal law prohibits dispensing without prescription.
NORPACE, trademark, G. D. Searle & Co.
FOR MEDICAL INFORMATION ON INOCOR CALL TOLL FREE 1-800-446-6267.

ISUPREL®
ISOPROTERENOL HYDROCHLORIDE INJECTION, USP
sterile injection 1:5000

Ŗ

DESCRIPTION

Isoproterenol hydrochloride is 3,4-Dihydroxy-α-[(isopropylamino)methyl] benzyl alcohol hydrochloride, a synthetic sympathomimetic amine that is structurally related to epinephrine but acts almost exclusively on beta receptors. The molecular formula is $C_{11}H_{17}NO_3 \cdot HCl$. It has a molecular weight of 247.72 and the following structural formula:

Isoproterenol hydrochloride is a racemic compound.
Each milliliter of the sterile 1:5000 solution contains:
ISUPREL, brand of isoproterenol hydrochloride injection, USP ... 0.2 mg
Lactic Acid ... 0.12 mg
Sodium Chloride ... 7.0 mg
Sodium Lactate ... 1.8 mg
Sodium Metabisulfite (as preservative) ... 1.0 mg
Water for Injection qs ad ... 1.0 mL
The pH is adjusted between 2.5 and 4.5 with hydrochloric acid. The air in the ampuls has been displaced by nitrogen gas.
The sterile 1:5000 solution is non-pyrogenic and can be administered by the intravenous, intramuscular, subcutaneous, or intracardiac routes.

CLINICAL PHARMACOLOGY

Isoproterenol is a potent nonselective beta-adrenergic agonist with very low affinity for alpha-adrenergic receptors. Intravenous infusion of isoproterenol in man lowers peripheral vascular resistance, primarily in skeletal muscle but also in renal and mesenteric vascular beds. Diastolic pressure falls. Renal blood flow is decreased in normotensive subjects but is increased markedly in shock. Systolic blood pressure may remain unchanged or rise, although mean arterial pressure typically falls. Cardiac output is increased because of the positive inotropic and chronotropic effects of the drug in the face of diminished peripheral vascular resistance. The cardiac effects of isoproterenol may lead to palpitations, sinus tachycardia, and more serious arrhythmias; large doses of isoproterenol may cause myocardial necrosis in animals.

Isoproterenol relaxes almost all varieties of smooth muscle when the tone is high, but this action is most pronounced on bronchial and gastrointestinal smooth muscle. It prevents or relieves bronchoconstriction, but tolerance to this effect develops with overuse of the drug.

In man, isoproterenol causes less hyperglycemia than does epinephrine. Isoproterenol and epinephrine are equally effective in stimulating the release of free fatty acids and energy production.

Absorption, Fate, and Excretion. Isoproterenol is readily absorbed when given parenterally or as an aerosol. It is metabolized primarily in the liver and other tissues by COMT. Isoproterenol is a relatively poor substrate for MAO and is not taken up by sympathetic neurons to the same extent as are epinephrine and norepinephrine. The duration of action of isoproterenol may therefore be longer than that of epinephrine, but is still brief.

INDICATIONS AND USAGE

Isoproterenol hydrochloride injection is indicated:

- For mild or transient episodes of heart block that do not require electric shock or pacemaker therapy.
- For serious episodes of heart block and Adams-Stokes attacks (except when caused by ventricular tachycardia or fibrillation). (See CONTRAINDICATIONS.)
- For use in cardiac arrest until electric shock or pacemaker therapy, the treatments of choice, is available. (See CONTRAINDICATIONS.)
- For bronchospasm occurring during anesthesia.
- As an adjunct to fluid and electrolyte replacement therapy and the use of other drugs and procedures in the treatment of hypovolemic and septic shock, low cardiac output (hypoperfusion) states, congestive heart failure, and cardiogenic shock. (See WARNINGS.)

CONTRAINDICATIONS

Use of isoproterenol hydrochloride injection is contraindicated in patients with tachyarrhythmias; tachycardia or heart block caused by digitalis intoxication; ventricular arrhythmias which require inotropic therapy; and angina pectoris.

WARNINGS

Isoproterenol hydrochloride injection, by increasing myocardial oxygen requirements while decreasing effective coronary perfusion, may have a deleterious effect on the injured or failing heart. Most experts discourage its use as the initial agent in treating cardiogenic shock following myocardial infarction. However, when a low arterial pressure has been elevated by other means, isoproterenol hydrochloride injection may produce beneficial hemodynamic and metabolic effects.

In a few patients, presumably with organic disease of the AV node and its branches, isoproterenol hydrochloride injection has paradoxically been reported to worsen heart block or to precipitate Adams-Stokes attacks during normal sinus rhythm or transient heart block.

Contains sodium metabisulfite, a sulfite that may cause allergic-type reactions including anaphylactic symptoms and life-threatening or less severe asthmatic episodes in certain susceptible people. The overall prevalence of sulfite sensitivity in the general population is unknown and probably low. Sulfite sensitivity is seen more frequently in asthmatic than in nonasthmatic people.

PRECAUTIONS

General

Isoproterenol hydrochloride injection should generally be started at the lowest recommended dose. This may be gradually increased if necessary while carefully monitoring the patient. Doses sufficient to increase the heart rate to more than 130 beats per minute may increase the likelihood of inducing ventricular arrhythmias. Such increases in heart rate will also tend to increase cardiac work and oxygen requirements which may adversely affect the failing heart or the heart with a significant degree of arteriosclerosis.

Particular caution is necessary in administering isoproterenol hydrochloride injection to patients with coronary artery disease, coronary insufficiency, diabetes, hyperthyroidism, and sensitivity to sympathomimetic amines.

Adequate filling of the intravascular compartment by suitable volume expanders is of primary importance in most cases of shock and should precede the administration of vasoactive drugs. In patients with normal cardiac function, determination of central venous pressure is a reliable guide during volume replacement. If evidence of hypoperfusion persists after adequate volume replacement, isoproterenol hydrochloride injection may be given.

In addition to the routine monitoring of systemic blood pressure, heart rate, urine flow, and the electrocardiograph, the response to therapy should also be monitored by frequent determination of the central venous pressure and blood gases. Patients in shock should be closely observed during isoproterenol hydrochloride injection administration. If the

Continued on next page

This product information was prepared in September 1996. On these and other products of Sanofi Winthrop Pharmaceuticals, detailed information may be obtained on a current basis by direct inquiry to Product Information Services, 90 Park Avenue, New York, NY 10016 (toll free 1-800-446-6267).

Sanofi Winthrop—Cont.

Recommended dosage for adults with heart block, Adams-Stokes attacks, and cardiac arrest:

Route of Administration	Preparation of Dilution	Initial Dose	Subsequent Dose Range*
Bolus Intravenous injection	Dilute 1 mL (0.2 mg) to 10 mL with Sodium Chloride Injection, USP, or 5% Dextrose Injection, USP	0.02 mg to 0.06 mg (1 mL to 3 mL of diluted solution)	0.01 mg to 0.2 mg (0.5 mL to 10 mL of diluted solution)
Intravenous infusion	Dilute 10 mL (2 mg) in 500 mL of 5% Dextrose Injection, USP	5 mcg/min. (1.25 mL of diluted solution per minute)	
Intramuscular	Use Solution 1:5000 undiluted	0.2 mg (1 mL)	0.02 mg to 1 mg (0.1 mL to 5 mL)
Subcutaneous	Use Solution 1:5000 undiluted	0.2 mg (1 mL)	0.15 mg to 0.2 mg (0.75 mL to 1 mL)
Intracardiac	Use Solution 1:5000 undiluted	0.02 mg (0.1 mL)	

*Subsequent dosage and method of administration depend on the ventricular rate and the rapidity with which the cardiac pacemaker can take over when the drug is gradually withdrawn.

Recommended dosage for adults with shock and hypoperfusion states:

Route of Administration	Preparation of Dilution†	Infusion Rate††
Intravenous infusion	Dilute 5 mL (1 mg) in 500 mL of 5% Dextrose Injection, USP	0.5 mcg to 5 mcg per minute (0.25 mL to 2.5 mL of diluted solution)

† Concentrations up to 10 times greater have been used when limitation of volume is essential.

†† Rates over 30 mcg per minute have been used in advanced stages of shock. The rate of infusion should be adjusted on the basis of heart rate, central venous pressure, systemic blood pressure, and urine flow. If the heart rate exceeds 110 beats per minute, it may be advisable to decrease or temporarily discontinue the infusion.

Recommended dosage for adults with bronchospasm occurring during anesthesia:

Route of Administration	Preparation of Dilution	Initial Dose	Subsequent Dose
Bolus intravenous injection	Dilute 1 mL (0.2 mg) to 10 mL with Sodium Chloride Injection, USP, or 5% Dextrose Injection, USP	0.01 mg to 0.02 mg (0.5 mL to 1 mL of diluted solution)	The initial dose may be repeated when necessary

heart rate exceeds 110 beats per minute, it may be advisable to decrease the infusion rate or temporarily discontinue the infusion. Determinations of cardiac output and circulation time may also be helpful. Appropriate measures should be taken to ensure adequate ventilation. Careful attention should be paid to acid-base balance and to the correction of electrolyte disturbances. In cases of shock associated with bacteremia, suitable antimicrobial therapy is, of course, imperative.

Drug Interactions
Isoproterenol hydrochloride injection and epinephrine should not be administered simultaneously because both drugs are direct cardiac stimulants and their combined effects may induce serious arrhythmias. The drugs may, however, be administered alternately provided a proper interval has elapsed between doses.
ISUPREL should be used with caution, if at all, when potent inhalational anesthetics such as halothane are employed because of potential to sensitize the myocardium to effects of sympathomimetic amines.

Carcinogenesis, Mutagenesis, Impairment of Fertility
Long-term studies in animals to evaluate the carcinogenic potential of isoproterenol hydrochloride have not been done. Mutagenic potential and effect on fertility have not been determined. There is no evidence from human experience that isoproterenol hydrochloride injection may be carcinogenic or mutagenic or that it impairs fertility.

Pregnancy Category C
Animal reproduction studies have not been conducted with isoproterenol hydrochloride. It is also not known whether isoproterenol hydrochloride can cause fetal harm when administered to a pregnant woman or can affect reproduction capacity. Isoproterenol hydrochloride should be given to a pregnant woman only if clearly needed.

Nursing Mothers
It is not known whether this drug is excreted in human milk. Because many drugs are excreted in human milk, caution should be exercised when isoproterenol hydrochloride injection is administered to a nursing woman.

ADVERSE REACTIONS
The following reactions to isoproterenol hydrochloride injection have been reported:
CNS: Nervousness, headache, dizziness.

Cardiovascular: Tachycardia, palpitations, angina, Adams-Stokes attacks, pulmonary edema, hypertension, hypotension, ventricular arrhythmias, tachyarrhythmias.
In a few patients, presumably with organic disease of the AV node and its branches, isoproterenol hydrochloride injection has been reported to precipitate Adams-Stokes seizures during normal sinus rhythm or transient heart block.
Other: Flushing of the skin, sweating, mild tremors, weakness.

OVERDOSAGE
The acute toxicity of isoproterenol hydrochloride in animals is much less than that of epinephrine. Excessive doses in animals or man can cause a striking drop in blood pressure, and repeated large doses in animals may result in cardiac enlargement and focal myocarditis.
In case of accidental overdosage as evidenced mainly by tachycardia or other arrhythmias, palpitations, angina, hypotension, or hypertension, reduce rate of administration or discontinue isoproterenol hydrochloride injection until patient's condition stabilizes. Blood pressure, pulse, respiration, and EKG should be monitored.
It is not known whether isoproterenol hydrochloride is dialyzable.
The oral LD_{50} of isoproterenol hydrochloride in mice is 3,850 mg/kg $\pm$ 1,190 mg/kg of pure drug in solution.

DOSAGE AND ADMINISTRATION
ISUPREL injection 1:5000 should generally be started at the lowest recommended dose and the rate of administration gradually increased if necessary while carefully monitoring the patient. The usual route of administration is by intravenous infusion or bolus intravenous injection. In dire emergencies, the drug may be administered by intracardiac injection. If time is not of the utmost importance, initial therapy by intramuscular or subcutaneous injection is preferred.
[See first table above.]
There are no well-controlled studies in children to establish appropriate dosing; however, the American Heart Association recommends an initial infusion rate of 0.1 mcg/kg/min, with the usual range being 0.1 mcg/kg/min to 1.0 mcg/kg/min.
[See second table above.]
Parenteral drug products should be inspected visually for particulate matter and discoloration prior to administration,

whenever solution and container permit. Such solution should not be used.

HOW SUPPLIED
Ampuls of 1 mL (0.2 mg) UNI-NEST PAK™ of 25 (NDC 0024-0866-25)
Ampuls of 5 mL (1 mg) box of 10 (NDC 0024-0866-02)
Protect from light. Keep in opaque container until used.
Store in a cool place between 8° C to 15° C (46° F to 59° F).
Do not use if the injection is pinkish to darker than slightly yellow or contains a precipitate.
Caution: Federal law prohibits dispensing without prescription.
ISW-5 B

ISUPREL®   ℞
brand of isoproterenol hydrochloride inhalation aerosol, USP
MISTOMETER®

Potent Bronchodilator

DESCRIPTION
ISUPREL MISTOMETER is a beta agonist sympathomimetic bronchodilator. It is a complete nebulizing unit consisting of a plastic-coated vial of aerosol solution, detachable plastic mouthpiece with built-in nebulizer, and protective cap. The vial contains isoproterenol hydrochloride 0.25% (w/w) with inert ingredients of alcohol 33% (w/w) and ascorbic acid 0.1% (w/w) and, as propellants, dichlorodifluoromethane and dichlorotetrafluoroethane.
Chemically, isoproterenol hydrochloride is 3,4-Dihydroxy-α-[(isopropylamino)methyl]benzyl alcohol hydrochloride.
The contents permit the delivery of not less than 200 actuations from the 11.2 g (10 mL) vial and not less than 300 actuations from the 16.8 g (15 mL) vial. The MISTOMETER delivers a measured dose of 131 μg of the bronchodilator in a fine, even mist for inhalation.

CLINICAL PHARMACOLOGY
ISUPREL relaxes bronchial spasm and facilitates expectoration of pulmonary secretions by acting almost exclusively on beta receptors. It is frequently effective when epinephrine and other drugs fail, and it has a wide margin of safety. ISUPREL is readily absorbed when given as an aerosol. It is metabolized primarily in the liver and other tissues by catechol-O-methyltransferase (COMT).
Recent studies in laboratory animals (minipigs, rodents, and dogs) recorded the occurrence of cardiac arrhythmias and sudden death (with histologic evidence of myocardial necrosis) when beta agonists and methylxanthines were concomitantly administered. The significance of these findings when applied to human usage is currently unknown.

INDICATIONS AND USAGE
ISUPREL is indicated for the relief of bronchospasm associated with acute and chronic asthma and reversible bronchospasm which may be associated with chronic bronchitis or emphysema.

CONTRAINDICATIONS
Use of isoproterenol in patients with preexisting cardiac arrhythmias associated with tachycardia is generally considered contraindicated because the cardiac stimulant effect of the drug may aggravate such disorders. The use of this medication is contraindicated in those patients who have a known hypersensitivity to isoproterenol or to any of the other components of this drug.

WARNINGS
Excessive use of an adrenergic aerosol should be discouraged as it may lose its effectiveness.
In patients with status asthmaticus and abnormal blood gas tensions, improvement in vital capacity and in blood gas tensions may not accompany apparent relief of bronchospasm. Facilities for administering oxygen mixtures and ventilatory assistance are necessary for such patients.
Occasional patients have been reported to develop severe paradoxical airway resistance with repeated, excessive use of isoproterenol inhalation preparations. The cause of this refractory state is unknown. It is advisable that in such instances the use of this preparation be discontinued immediately and alternative therapy instituted, since in the reported cases the patients did not respond to other forms of therapy until the drug was withdrawn.
Deaths have been reported following excessive use of isoproterenol inhalation preparations and the exact cause is unknown. Cardiac arrest was noted in several instances.

PRECAUTIONS
General
Isoproterenol should be used with caution in patients with cardiovascular disorders including coronary insufficiency, diabetes, or hyperthyroidism, and in persons sensitive to sympathomimetic amines.
A single treatment with the ISUPREL MISTOMETER is usually sufficient for controlling isolated attacks of asthma. Any patient who requires more than three aerosol treat-

ments within a 24-hour period should be under the close supervision of a physician. Further therapy with the bronchodilator aerosol alone is inadvisable when three to five treatments within six to twelve hours produce minimal or no relief.

Information for Patients
Do not inhale more often than directed by your physician. Read enclosed instructions before using (see attachment to insert). Do not exceed the dose prescribed by your physician. If difficulty in breathing persists, contact your physician immediately. Avoid spraying in eyes. Contents under pressure. Do not break or incinerate. Do not store at temperatures above 120°F. Keep out of reach of children.

Drug Interactions
Epinephrine should not be administered concomitantly with ISUPREL, as both drugs are direct cardiac stimulants and their combined effects may induce serious arrhythmia. If desired they may, however, be alternated, provided an interval of at least four hours has elapsed.

Carcinogenesis, Mutagenesis, Impairment of Fertility
Long-term chronic toxicity studies in animals have not been done to evaluate isoproterenol in these areas.

Pregnancy Category C
Animal reproduction studies have not been conducted with isoproterenol hydrochloride. It is also not known whether isoproterenol hydrochloride can cause fetal harm when administered to a pregnant woman or can affect reproduction capacity. Isoproterenol hydrochloride should be given to a pregnant woman only if clearly needed.

Nursing Mothers
It is not known whether this drug is excreted in human milk. Because many drugs are excreted in human milk, caution should be exercised when isoproterenol hydrochloride is administered to a nursing woman.

Pediatric Use
In general, the technique of ISUPREL MISTOMETER in administration to children is similar to that of adults, since children's smaller ventilatory exchange capacity automatically provides proportionally smaller aerosol intake.

ADVERSE REACTIONS
The mist from the ISUPREL MISTOMETER contains alcohol but is generally very well tolerated. An occasional patient may experience some transient throat irritation which has been attributed to the alcohol content.
Serious reactions to ISUPREL, brand of isoproterenol hydrochloride inhalation aerosol, are infrequent. The following reactions, however, have been reported:
CNS: Nervousness, headache, dizziness, weakness.
Gastrointestinal: Nausea, vomiting.
Cardiovascular: Tachycardia, palpitations, precordial distress, anginal-type pain.
Other: Flushing of the skin, tremor, and sweating.
The inhalation route is usually accompanied by a minimum of side effects. These untoward reactions disappear quickly and do not, as a rule, inconvenience the patient to the extent that the drug must be discontinued. No cumulative effects have been reported.

OVERDOSAGE
Overdosage of ISUPREL may produce signs and symptoms typical of excessive sympathomimetic effects, including tachycardia, palpitations, nervousness, nausea, and vomiting. Excessive use of adrenergic aerosols may result in loss of effectiveness or severe paradoxical airway resistance. Cardiac arrest has been noted in several instances. In all cases of overdose or excessive use of ISUPREL, the drug should be discontinued immediately and vital functions supported until the patient is stabilized. It is not known whether isoproterenol hydrochloride is dialyzable.
The acute oral LD$_{50}$ in mice is 3,850 mg/kg $\pm$ 1,190 mg/kg of pure drug in solution (isoproterenol hydrochloride). In dogs, the toxic dose is 1,000 times the therapeutic dose. Converted to the amount used clinically in man, this would be about 2,500 times the therapeutic dose.

DOSAGE AND ADMINISTRATION
Acute Bronchial Asthma: Hold the MISTOMETER in an inverted position. Close lips and teeth around open end of mouthpiece. Breathe out, expelling as much air from the lungs as possible; then inhale deeply while pressing down on the bottle to activate spray mechanism. Try to hold breath for a few seconds before exhaling. Wait one full minute in order to determine the effect before considering a second inhalation. A treatment may be repeated up to 5 times daily if necessary. (See PRECAUTIONS.) If carefully instructed, children quickly learn to keep the stream of mist clear of the teeth and tongue, thereby assuring inhalation into the lungs. Occlusion of the nares of very young children may be advisable to make inhalation certain.
Warm water should be run through the mouthpiece once daily to wash it and prevent clogging.
The mouthpiece may also be sanitized by immersion in alcohol.
Bronchospasm in Chronic Obstructive Lung Disease: The MISTOMETER provides a convenient aerosol method for delivering ISUPREL, brand of isoproterenol hydrochloride inhalation aerosol. The treatment described above for Acute Bronchial Asthma may be repeated at not less than 3 to 4 hour intervals as part of a programmed regimen of treatment of obstructive lung disease complicated by a reversible bronchospastic component. One application from the MISTOMETER may be regarded as equivalent in effectiveness to 5 to 7 operations of a hand-bulb nebulizer using a 1:100 solution.

Children's Dosage
In general, the technique of ISUPREL MISTOMETER in administration to children is similar to that of adults, since children's smaller ventilatory exchange capacity automatically provides proportionally smaller aerosol intake.

HOW SUPPLIED
ISUPREL MISTOMETER is supplied as a metered dose aerosol providing 131 µg of isoproterenol hydrochloride per actuation.
  Vial of 11.2 g (10 mL) with oral nebulizer
  (NDC 0024-0878-05)
  Vial of 16.8 g (15 mL) with oral nebulizer
  (NDC 0024-0878-01)
  Refill only, 16.8 g (15 mL)
  (NDC 0024-0879-01)
Store at controlled room temperature 15°C to 30°C (59°F to 86°F).
Caution: Federal law prohibits dispensing without prescription.
Note: The indented statement below is required by the Federal government's Clean Air Act for all products containing or manufactured with chlorofluorocarbons (CFC's).
  WARNING: Contains dichlorodifluoromethane and dichlorotetrafluoroethane, substances which harm public health and environment by destroying ozone in the upper atmosphere.
A notice similar to the above WARNING has been placed in the information for the patient of this product pursuant to EPA regulations.

ISW-4A

ISUPREL® Hydrochloride ℞
brand of isoproterenol
inhalation solution, USP
SOLUTION 1:200
SOLUTION 1:100

Potent Bronchodilator

DESCRIPTION
ISUPREL hydrochloride, brand of isoproterenol inhalation solution, is a beta agonist sympathomimetic bronchodilator.
Solution 1:200 contains isoproterenol hydrochloride 5 mg/mL.
Inactive Ingredients: Chlorobutanol 0.5 percent and Sodium Metabisulfite 0.3 percent as preservatives, Citric Acid, Glycerin, Purified Water, and Sodium Chloride.
Solution 1:100 contains isoproterenol hydrochloride 10 mg/mL.
Inactive Ingredients: Chlorobutanol 0.5 percent and Sodium Metabisulfite 0.3 percent as preservatives, Citric Acid, Purified Water, Saccharin Sodium, Sodium Chloride, and Sodium Citrate.
Isoproterenol hydrochloride is soluble in water (1 g isoproterenol hydrochloride dissolves in 3 mL H$_2$O). The solutions have a pH range of 3 to 4.5.
Isoproterenol hydrochloride is a racemic compound with a molecular weight of 247.72 and the molecular formula C$_{11}$H$_{17}$NO$_3$·HCl.
Chemically, isoproterenol hydrochloride is 3,4-Dihydroxy-α-[(isopropylamino)methyl]benzyl alcohol hydrochloride.
The air in the bottles has been displaced by nitrogen gas.

CLINICAL PHARMACOLOGY
ISUPREL relaxes bronchial spasm and facilitates expectoration of pulmonary secretions by acting almost exclusively on beta receptors.
ISUPREL is readily absorbed when given as an aerosol. It is metabolized primarily in the liver and other tissues by catechol-0-methyltransferase (COMT).
Recent studies in laboratory animals (minipigs, rodents, and dogs) recorded the occurrence of cardiac arrhythmias and sudden death (with histologic evidence of myocardial necrosis) when beta agonists and methylxanthines were concomitantly administered. The significance of these findings when applied to human usage is currently unknown.

INDICATIONS AND USAGE
ISUPREL is indicated for the relief of bronchospasm associated with acute and chronic asthma and reversible bronchospasm which may be associated with chronic bronchitis or emphysema.

CONTRAINDICATION
Use of isoproterenol in patients with preexisting cardiac arrhythmias associated with tachycardia is generally considered contraindicated because the cardiac stimulant effect of the drug may aggravate such disorders.

WARNINGS
Excessive use of an adrenergic aerosol should be discouraged as it may lose its effectiveness.
Isoproterenol administration as a solution for nebulization has been associated with a decrease in arterial pO$_2$ in asthmatic patients as a result of ventilation-perfusion abnormalities despite improvement in airway obstruction. The clinical significance of this relative hypoxemia is unclear.
As with other inhaled beta adrenergic agonists, ISUPREL can produce paradoxical bronchospasm, that can be life threatening. If this occurs, the product should be discontinued immediately and alternative therapy instituted.
Deaths have been reported following excessive use of isoproterenol inhalation preparations and the exact cause is unknown. Cardiac arrest was noted in several instances. It is therefore essential that the physician instruct the patient in the need for further evaluation if his/her asthma worsens.
Contains sodium metabisulfite, a sulfite that may cause allergic-type reactions including anaphylactic symptoms and life-threatening or less severe asthmatic episodes in certain susceptible people. The overall prevalence of sulfite sensitivity in the general population is unknown and probably low. Sulfite sensitivity is seen more frequently in asthmatic than in nonasthmatic people.

PRECAUTIONS
ISUPREL, as with all sympathomimetic amines, should be used with caution in patients with cardiovascular disorders, especially coronary insufficiency, cardiac arrhythmias, and hypertension; in patients with convulsive disorders, hyperthyroidism, or diabetes mellitus; and in patients who are unusually responsive to sympathomimetic amines. Clinically significant changes in systolic and diastolic blood pressure have been seen in some patients after use of any beta adrenergic bronchodilator.
Any patient who requires more than three aerosol treatments within a 24-hour period should be under the close supervision of his physician. Further therapy with the bronchodilator aerosol alone is inadvisable when three to five treatments within six to twelve hours produce minimal or no relief.
When compressed oxygen is employed as the aerosol propellant, the percentage of oxygen used should be determined by the patient's individual requirements to avoid depression of respiratory drive.
Drug Interactions: Other sympathomimetic aerosol bronchodilators or epinephrine should not be used concomitantly with ISUPREL. If additional adrenergic drugs are to be administered by any route to the patient using ISUPREL, they should be used with caution to avoid deleterious cardiovascular effects.
Beta adrenergic agonists should be administered with caution to patients being treated with MAO inhibitors or tricyclic antidepressants since the action of the beta adrenergic agonists on the vascular system may be potentiated.
Beta receptor blocking agents and ISUPREL inhibit the effects of each other.
Carcinogenesis, Mutagenesis, Impairment of Fertility: Long-term chronic toxicity studies in animals have not been done to evaluate isoproterenol in these areas.
Pregnancy Category C: Animal reproduction studies have not been conducted with isoproterenol hydrochloride. It is also not known whether isoproterenol hydrochloride can cause fetal harm when administered to a pregnant woman or can affect reproduction capacity. Isoproterenol hydrochloride should be given to a pregnant woman only if clearly needed.
Nursing Mothers: It is not known whether this drug is excreted in human milk. Because many drugs are excreted in human milk, caution should be exercised when isoproterenol hydrochloride is administered to a nursing woman.
Pediatric Use: In general, the technique of isoproterenol hydrochloride solution in administration to children is similar to that of adults, since children's smaller ventilatory exchange capacity automatically provides proportionally smaller aerosol intake. However, it is generally recommended that the 1:200 solution (rather than the 1:100) be used for an acute attack of bronchospasm, and no more than 0.25 mL of the 1:200 solution should be used for each 10 to 15 minute programmed treatment in chronic bronchospastic disease.

Continued on next page

This product information was prepared in September 1996. On these and other products of Sanofi Winthrop Pharmaceuticals, detailed information may be obtained on a current basis by direct inquiry to Product Information Services, 90 Park Avenue, New York, NY 10016 (toll free 1-800-446-6267).

Sanofi Winthrop—Cont.

ADVERSE REACTIONS

Serious reactions to ISUPREL are infrequent. The following reactions, however, have been reported:

CNS: Nervousness, headache, dizziness, weakness.

Gastrointestinal: Nausea, vomiting.

Cardiovascular: Tachycardia, palpitations, precordial distress, anginal-type pain.

Other: Flushing of the skin, tremor, and sweating.

The inhalation route is usually accompanied by a minimum of side effects. These untoward reactions disappear quickly and do not as a rule, inconvenience the patient to the extent that the drug must be discontinued. No cumulative effects have been reported.

OVERDOSAGE

Overdosage of ISUPREL may produce signs and symptoms typical of excessive sympathomimetic effects, including tachycardia, palpitations, nervousness, nausea, and vomiting. Excessive use of adrenergic aerosols may result in loss of effectiveness or severe paradoxical airway resistance. Cardiac arrest has been noted in several instances. In all cases of overdose or excessive use of ISUPREL, the drug should be discontinued immediately and vital functions supported until the patient is stabilized. It is not known whether isoproterenol hydrochloride is dialyzable.

The acute oral LD_{50} in mice is 3,850 mg/kg ± 1,190 mg/kg of pure drug in solution (isoproterenol hydrochloride). In dogs, the toxic dose is 1,000 times the therapeutic dose. Converted to the amount used clinically in man, this would be about 2,500 times the therapeutic dose.

DOSAGE AND ADMINISTRATION

ISUPREL hydrochloride solutions can be administered as an aerosol mist by hand-bulb nebulizer, compressed air or oxygen operated nebulizer, or by intermittent positive pressure breathing (IPPB) devices. The method of delivery, and the treatment regimen employed in the management of the reversible bronchospastic element accompanying bronchial asthma, chronic bronchitis, and chronic obstructive lung diseases, will depend on such factors as the severity of the bronchospasm, patient age, tolerance to the medication, complicating cardiopulmonary conditions, and whether therapy is for an intermittent acute attack of bronchospasm or is part of a programmed treatment regimen for constant bronchospasm.

Acute Bronchial Asthma. *Hand-Bulb Nebulizer*—Depending on the frequency of treatment and the type of nebulizer used, a volume of solution of ISUPREL, sufficient for not more than one day's treatment, should be placed in the nebulizer using the dropper provided. In time, the patient can learn to adjust the volume required. For adults and children, the 1:200 solution is administered by hand-bulb nebulization in a dosage of 5 to 15 deep inhalations (using an all glass or plastic nebulizer). In adults, the 1:100 solution may be used if a stronger solution seems to be indicated. The dose is 3 to 7 deep inhalations. If after about 5 to 10 minutes inadequate relief is observed, these doses may be repeated one more time. If the acute attack recurs, treatments may be repeated up to 5 times daily if necessary. (See PRECAUTIONS.)

Bronchospasm in Chronic Obstructive Lung Disease. *Hand-Bulb Nebulizer*—A solution of 1:200 or 1:100 of ISUPREL may be administered daily at not less than 3 to 4 hour intervals for subacute bronchospastic attacks or as part of a programmed treatment regimen in patients with chronic obstructive lung disease with a reversible bronchospastic component. An adequate dose is usually 5 to 15 deep inhalations, using the 1:200 solution. Some patients with severe attacks of bronchospasm may require 3 to 7 deep inhalations using the 1:100 solution of ISUPREL.

Nebulization by Compressed Air or Oxygen—A method often used in patients with severe chronic obstructive lung disease is to deliver the isoproterenol mist *in more dilute form over a longer period of time.* The purpose is, not so much to increase the dose supplied, as to achieve progressively deeper bronchodilatation and thus insure that the mist achieves maximum penetration of the finer bronchioles. In this method, 0.5 mL of a 1:200 solution of ISUPREL is diluted to 2 mL to 2.5 mL with water or isotonic saline to achieve a use concentration of 1:800 to 1:1000. If desired, 0.25 mL of the 1:100 solution may be similarly diluted to achieve the same use concentration. The diluted solution is placed in a nebulizer (eg, DeVilbiss #640 unit) connected to either a source of compressed air or oxygen. The flow rate is regulated to suit the particular nebulizer so that the diluted solution of ISUPREL will be delivered over approximately 10 to 20 minutes. A treatment may be repeated up to 5 times daily if necessary. Although the total delivered dose of ISUPREL is somewhat higher than with the treatment regimen employing the hand-bulb nebulizer, patients usually tolerate it well because of the greater dilution and longer application-time factors.

Intermittent Positive Pressure Breathing (IPPB)—Diluted solutions of 1:200 or 1:100 of ISUPREL are used in a programmed regimen for the treatment of reversible bronchospasm in patients with chronic obstructive lung disease who require intermittent positive pressure breathing therapy. These devices generally have a small nebulizer, usually of 3 mL to 5 mL capacity, on a patient-operated side arm. The effectiveness of IPPB therapy is greatly enhanced by the simultaneous use of aerosolized bronchodilators. As with compressed air or oxygen operated nebulizers, the usual regimen is to place 0.5 mL of 1:200 solution of ISUPREL diluted to 2 mL to 2.5 mL with water or isotonic saline in the nebulizer cup and follow the IPPB manufacturer's operating instructions. IPPB-bronchodilator treatments are usually administered over 15 to 20 minutes, up to 5 times daily if necessary.

Children's Dosage: In general, the technique of isoproterenol hydrochloride solution in administration to children is similar to that of adults, since children's smaller ventilatory exchange capacity automatically provides proportionally smaller aerosol intake. However, it is generally recommended that the 1:200 solution (rather than the 1:100) be used for an acute attack of bronchospasm, and no more than 0.25 mL of the 1:200 solution should be used for each 10 to 15 minute programmed treatment in chronic bronchospastic disease.

HOW SUPPLIED

Solution 1:100 contains isoproterenol hydrochloride 1% (10 mg/mL).

Solution 1:200 contains isoproterenol hydrochloride 0.5% (5 mg/mL).

Solution 1:100
  bottle of 10 mL NDC 0024-0873-01
Solution 1:200
  bottle of 10 mL NDC 0024-0871-01
  bottle of 60 mL NDC 0024-0871-03

Protect from light. Do not use the inhalation solutions if their color is pinkish to brownish or if they contain a precipitate. Although solutions of ISUPREL left in nebulizers will remain clear and potent for many days, for sanitary reasons it is recommended that they be changed daily.

Store at controlled room temperature 15°C to 30°C (59°F to 86°F).

ISW-3

KAYEXALATE® ℞
brand of sodium polystyrene sulfonate, USP

> Cation-Exchange Resin

DESCRIPTION

KAYEXALATE, brand of sodium polystyrene sulfonate, is a benzene, diethenyl-, polymer with ethenylbenzene, sulfonated, sodium salt.

The drug is a light brown to brown, finely ground, powdered form of sodium polystyrene sulfonate, a cation-exchange resin prepared in the sodium phase with an in vitro exchange capacity of approximately 3.1 mEq (in vivo approximately 1 mEq) of potassium per gram. The sodium content is approximately 100 mg (4.1 mEq) per gram of the drug. It can be administered orally or in an enema.

CLINICAL PHARMACOLOGY

As the resin passes along the intestine or is retained in the colon after administration by enema, the sodium ions are partially released and are replaced by potassium ions. For the most part, this action occurs in the large intestine, which excretes potassium ions to a greater degree than does the small intestine. The efficiency of this process is limited and unpredictably variable. It commonly approximates the order of 33 percent but the range is so large that definitive indices of electrolyte balance must be clearly monitored.

Metabolic data are unavailable.

INDICATION AND USAGE

KAYEXALATE is indicated for the treatment of hyperkalemia.

CONTRAINDICATIONS

KAYEXALATE is contraindicated in patients with hypokalemia or those patients who are hypersensitive to it.

WARNINGS

Alternative Therapy in Severe Hyperkalemia:
Since effective lowering of serum potassium with KAYEXALATE may take hours to days, treatment with this drug alone may be insufficient to rapidly correct severe hyperkalemia associated with states of rapid tissue breakdown (eg, burns and renal failure) or hyperkalemia so marked as to constitute a medical emergency. Therefore, other definitive measures, including dialysis, should always be considered and may be imperative.

Hypokalemia: Serious potassium deficiency can occur from therapy with KAYEXALATE. The effect must be carefully controlled by frequent serum potassium determinations within each 24-hour period. Since intracellular potassium deficiency is not always reflected by serum potassium levels, the level at which treatment with KAYEXALATE should be discontinued must be determined individually for each patient. Important aids in making this determination are the patient's clinical condition and electrocardiogram. Early clinical signs of severe hypokalemia include a pattern of irritable confusion and delayed thought processes. Electrocardiographically, severe hypokalemia is often associated with a lengthened Q-T interval, widening, flattening, or inversion of the T wave, and prominent U waves. Also, cardiac arrhythmias may occur, such as premature atrial, nodal, and ventricular contractions, and supraventricular and ventricular tachycardias. The toxic effects of digitalis are likely to be exaggerated. Marked hypokalemia can also be manifested by severe muscle weakness, at times extending into frank paralysis.

Electrolyte Disturbances: Like all cation-exchange resins, KAYEXALATE is not totally selective (for potassium) in its actions, and small amounts of other cations such as magnesium and calcium can also be lost during treatment. Accordingly, patients receiving KAYEXALATE should be monitored for all applicable electrolyte disturbances.

Systemic Alkalosis: Systemic alkalosis has been reported after cation-exchange resins were administered orally in combination with nonabsorbable cation-donating antacids and laxatives such as magnesium hydroxide and aluminum carbonate. Magnesium hydroxide should not be administered with KAYEXALATE. One case of grand mal seizure has been reported in a patient with chronic hypocalcemia of renal failure who was given KAYEXALATE with magnesium hydroxide as laxative. (See PRECAUTIONS, Drug Interactions.)

PRECAUTIONS

Caution is advised when KAYEXALATE is administered to patients who cannot tolerate even a small increase in sodium loads (ie, severe congestive heart failure, severe hypertension, or marked edema). In such instances compensatory restriction of sodium intake from other sources may be indicated.

If constipation occurs, patients should be treated with sorbitol (from 10 mL to 20 mL of 70 percent syrup every two hours or as needed to produce one or two watery stools daily), a measure which also reduces any tendency to fecal impaction.

Drug Interactions

Antacids: The simultaneous oral administration of KAYEXALATE with nonabsorbable cation-donating antacids and laxatives may reduce the resin's potassium exchange capability.

Systemic alkalosis has been reported after cation-exchange resins were administered orally in combination with nonabsorbable cation-donating antacids and laxatives such as magnesium hydroxide and aluminum carbonate. Magnesium hydroxide should not be administered with KAYEXALATE. One case of grand mal seizure has been reported in a patient with chronic hypocalcemia of renal failure who was given KAYEXALATE with magnesium hydroxide as a laxative. Intestinal obstruction due to concretions of aluminum hydroxide when used in combination with KAYEXALATE has been reported.

Digitalis: The toxic effects of digitalis on the heart, especially various ventricular arrhythmias and A-V nodal dissociation, are likely to be exaggerated by hypokalemia, even in the face of serum digoxin concentrations in the "normal range". (See WARNINGS.)

Carcinogenesis, Mutagenesis, Impairment of Fertility
Studies have not been performed.

Pregnancy Category C
Animal reproduction studies have not been conducted with KAYEXALATE. It is also not known whether KAYEXALATE can cause fetal harm when administered to a pregnant woman or can affect reproduction capacity. KAYEXALATE should be given to a pregnant woman only if clearly needed.

Nursing Mothers
It is not known whether this drug is excreted in human milk. Because many drugs are excreted in human milk, caution should be exercised when KAYEXALATE is administered to a nursing woman.

ADVERSE REACTIONS

KAYEXALATE may cause some degree of gastric irritation. Anorexia, nausea, vomiting, and constipation may occur especially if high doses are given. Also, hypokalemia, hypocalcemia, and significant sodium retention may occur. Occasionally diarrhea develops. Large doses in elderly individuals may cause fecal impaction (see PRECAUTIONS). This effect may be obviated through usage of the resin in enemas as described under DOSAGE AND ADMINISTRATION. Rare instances of colonic necrosis have been reported. Intestinal obstruction due to concretions of aluminum hydroxide, when used in combination with KAYEXALATE, has been reported.

DOSAGE AND ADMINISTRATION

Suspension of this drug should be freshly prepared and not stored beyond 24 hours.

The average daily adult dose of the resin is 15 g to 60 g. This is best provided by administering 15 g (approximately 4 *level* teaspoons) of KAYEXALATE one to four times daily. One gram of KAYEXALATE contains 4.1 mEq of sodium; one level teaspoon contains approximately 3.5 g of KAYEXALATE and 15 mEq of sodium. (A heaping teaspoon may contain as much as 10 g to 12 g of KAYEXALATE, brand of sodium polystyrene sulfonate.) Since the in vivo efficiency of sodium-potassium exchange resins is approximately 33 percent, about one third of the resin's actual sodium content is being delivered to the body.

In smaller children and infants, lower doses should be employed by using as a guide a rate of 1 mEq of potassium per gram of resin as the basis for calculation.

Each dose should be given as a suspension in a small quantity of water or, for greater palatability, in syrup. The amount of fluid usually ranges from 20 mL to 100 mL, depending on the dose, or may be simply determined by allowing 3 mL to 4 mL per gram of resin. Sorbitol may be administered in order to combat constipation.

The resin may be introduced into the stomach through a plastic tube and, if desired, mixed with a diet appropriate for a patient in renal failure.

The resin may also be given, although with less effective results, in an enema consisting (for adults) of 30 g to 50 g every six hours. Each dose is administered as a warm emulsion (at body temperature) in 100 mL of aqueous vehicle, such as sorbitol. The emulsion should be agitated gently during administration. The enema should be retained as long as possible and followed by a cleansing enema.

After an initial cleansing enema, a soft, large size (French 28) rubber tube is inserted into the rectum for a distance of about 20 cm, with the tip well into the sigmoid colon, and taped in place. The resin is then suspended in the appropriate amount of aqueous vehicle at body temperature and introduced by gravity, while the particles are kept in suspension by stirring. The suspension is flushed with 50 mL or 100 mL of fluid, following which the tube is clamped and left in place. If back leakage occurs, the hips are elevated on pillows or a knee-chest position is taken temporarily. A somewhat thicker suspension may be used, but care should be taken that no paste is formed, because the latter has a greatly reduced exchange surface and will be particularly ineffective if deposited in the rectal ampulla. The suspension is kept in the sigmoid colon for several hours, if possible. Then, the colon is irrigated with nonsodium containing solution at body temperature in order to remove the resin. Two quarts of flushing solution may be necessary. The returns are drained constantly through a Y tube connection. Particular attention should be paid to this cleansing enema when sorbitol has been used.

The intensity and duration of therapy depend upon the severity and resistance of hyperkalemia.

HOW SUPPLIED

Store at room temperature.

KAYEXALATE should not be heated for to do so may alter the exchange properties of the resin.

Caution: Federal law prohibits dispensing without prescription.

KAYEXALATE is available as a powder in jars of 1 pound (453.6 g), **NDC** 0024-1075-01.

KSW-1

LEVOPHED® Bitartrate ℞

brand of norepinephrine bitartrate injection, USP

DESCRIPTION

Norepinephrine (sometimes referred to as *l-arterenol/Levarterenol* or *l-norepinephrine*) is a sympathomimetic amine which differs from epinephrine by the absence of a methyl group on the nitrogen atom.

Norepinephrine Bitartrate is (-)-α-(aminomethyl)-3,4-dihydroxybenzyl alcohol tartrate (1:1) (salt) monohydrate.

LEVOPHED is supplied in sterile aqueous solution in the form of the bitartrate salt to be administered by intravenous infusion following dilution. Norepinephrine is sparingly soluble in water, very slightly soluble in alcohol and ether, and readily soluble in acids. Each mL of LEVOPHED bitartrate injection contains the equivalent of 1 mg base of LEVOPHED, sodium chloride for isotonicity, and not more than 2 mg of sodium metabisulfite as an antioxidant. It has a pH of 3 to 4.5. The air in the ampuls has been displaced by nitrogen gas.

CLINICAL PHARMACOLOGY

LEVOPHED functions as a peripheral vasoconstrictor (alpha-adrenergic action) and as an inotropic stimulator of the heart and dilator of coronary arteries (beta-adrenergic action).

INDICATIONS AND USAGE

For blood pressure control in certain acute hypotensive states (eg, pheochromocytomectomy, sympathectomy, poliomyelitis, spinal anesthesia, myocardial infarction, septicemia, blood transfusion, and drug reactions).

As an adjunct in the treatment of cardiac arrest and profound hypotension.

CONTRAINDICATIONS

LEVOPHED should not be given to patients who are hypotensive from blood volume deficits except as an emergency measure to maintain coronary and cerebral artery perfusion until blood volume replacement therapy can be completed. If LEVOPHED is continuously administered to maintain blood pressure in the absence of blood volume replacement, the following may occur: severe peripheral and visceral vasoconstriction, decreased renal perfusion and urine output, poor systemic blood flow despite "normal" blood pressure, tissue hypoxia, and lactate acidosis.

LEVOPHED should also not be given to patients with mesenteric or peripheral vascular thrombosis (because of the risk of increasing ischemia and extending the area of infarction) unless, in the opinion of the attending physician, the administration of LEVOPHED is necessary as a life-saving procedure.

Cyclopropane and halothane anesthetics increase cardiac autonomic irritability and therefore seem to sensitize the myocardium to the action of intravenously administered epinephrine or norepinephrine. Hence, the use of LEVOPHED during cyclopropane and halothane anesthesia is generally considered contraindicated because of the risk of producing ventricular tachycardia or fibrillation.

The same type of cardiac arrhythmias may result from the use of LEVOPHED in patients with profound hypoxia or hypercarbia.

WARNINGS

LEVOPHED should be used with extreme caution in patients receiving monoamine oxidase inhibitors (MAOI) or antidepressants of the triptyline or imipramine types, because severe, prolonged hypertension may result.

LEVOPHED Bitartrate Injection contains sodium metabisulfite, a sulfite that may cause allergic-type reactions including anaphylactic symptoms and life-threatening or less severe asthmatic episodes in certain susceptible people. The overall prevalence of sulfite sensitivity in the general population is unknown. Sulfite sensitivity is seen more frequently in asthmatic than in nonasthmatic people.

PRECAUTIONS

General

Avoid Hypertension: Because of the potency of LEVOPHED and because of varying response to pressor substances, the possibility always exists that dangerously high blood pressure may be produced with overdoses of this pressor agent. It is desirable, therefore, to record the blood pressure every two minutes from the time administration is started until the desired blood pressure is obtained, then every five minutes if administration is to be continued.

The rate of flow must be watched constantly, and the patient should never be left unattended while receiving LEVOPHED. Headache may be a symptom of hypertension due to overdosage.

Site of Infusion: Whenever possible, infusions of LEVOPHED should be given into a large vein, particularly an antecubital vein because, when administered into this vein, the risk of necrosis of the overlying skin from prolonged vasoconstriction is apparently very slight. Some authors have indicated that the femoral vein is also an acceptable route of administration. A catheter tie-in technique should be avoided, if possible, since the obstruction to blood flow around the tubing may cause stasis and increased local concentration of the drug. Occlusive vascular diseases (for example, atherosclerosis, arteriosclerosis, diabetic endarteritis, Buerger's disease) are more likely to occur in the lower than in the upper extremity. Therefore, one should avoid the veins of the leg in elderly patients or in those suffering from such disorders. Gangrene has been reported in a lower extremity when infusions of LEVOPHED were given in an ankle vein.

Extravasation: The infusion site should be checked frequently for free flow. Care should be taken to avoid extravasation of LEVOPHED (norepinephrine) into the tissues, as local necrosis might ensue due to the vasoconstrictive action of the drug. Blanching along the course of the infused vein, sometimes without obvious extravasation, has been attributed to vasa vasorum constriction with increased permeability of the vein wall, permitting some leakage.

This also may progress on rare occasions to superficial slough, particularly during infusion into leg veins in elderly patients or in those suffering from obliterative vascular disease. Hence, if blanching occurs, consideration should be given to the advisability of changing the infusion site at intervals to allow the effects of local vasoconstriction to subside.

IMPORTANT—Antidote for Extravasation Ischemia: To prevent sloughing and necrosis in areas in which extravasation has taken place, the area should be infiltrated as soon as possible with 10 mL to 15 mL of saline solution containing from 5 mg to 10 mg of **Regitine® (brand of phentolamine)**, an adrenergic blocking agent. A syringe with a fine hypodermic needle should be used, with the solution being infiltrated liberally throughout the area, which is easily identified by its cold, hard, and pallid appearance. Sympathetic blockade with phentolamine causes immediate and conspicuous local hyperemic changes if the area is infiltrated within 12 hours. Therefore, phentolamine should be given as soon as possible after the extravasation is noted.

Drug Interactions: Cyclopropane and halothane anesthetics increase cardiac automatic irritability and therefore seem to sensitize the myocardium to the action of intravenously administered epinephrine or norepinephrine. Hence, the use of LEVOPHED, brand of norepinephrine bitartrate injection, during cyclopropane and halothane anesthesia is generally considered contraindicated because of the risk of producing ventricular tachycardia or fibrillation. The same type of cardiac arrhythmias may result from the use of LEVOPHED in patients with profound hypoxia or hypercarbia.

LEVOPHED should be used with extreme caution in patients receiving monoamine oxidase inhibitors (MAOI) or antidepressants of the triptyline or imipramine types, because severe, prolonged hypertension may result.

Carcinogenesis, Mutagenesis, Impairment of Fertility: Studies have not been performed.

Pregnancy Category C: Animal reproduction studies have not been conducted with LEVOPHED. It is also not known whether LEVOPHED can cause fetal harm when administered to a pregnant woman or can affect reproduction capacity. LEVOPHED should be given to a pregnant woman only if clearly needed.

Nursing Mothers: It is not known whether this drug is excreted in human milk. Because many drugs are excreted in human milk, caution should be exercised when LEVOPHED is administered to a nursing woman.

Pediatric Use: Safety and effectiveness in children have not been established.

ADVERSE REACTIONS

The following reactions can occur:

Body As A Whole: Ischemic injury due to potent vasoconstrictor action and tissue hypoxia.

Cardiovascular System: Bradycardia, probably as a reflex result of a rise in blood pressure, arrhythmias.

Nervous System: Anxiety, transient headache.

Respiratory System: Respiratory difficulty.

Skin and Appendages: Extravasation necrosis at injection site.

Prolonged administration of any potent vasopressor may result in plasma volume depletion which should be continuously corrected by appropriate fluid and electrolyte replacement therapy. If plasma volumes are not corrected, hypotension may recur when LEVOPHED is discontinued, or blood pressure may be maintained at the risk of severe peripheral and visceral vasoconstriction (eg, decreased renal perfusion) with diminution in blood flow and tissue perfusion with subsequent tissue hypoxia and lactic acidosis and possible ischemic injury. Gangrene of extremities has been rarely reported.

Overdoses or conventional doses in hypersensitive persons (eg, hyperthyroid patients) cause severe hypertension with violent headache, photophobia, stabbing retrosternal pain, pallor, intense sweating, and vomiting.

OVERDOSAGE

Overdosage with LEVOPHED may result in headache, severe hypertension, reflex bradycardia, marked increase in peripheral resistance, and decreased cardiac output. In case of accidental overdosage, as evidenced by excessive blood pressure elevation, discontinue LEVOPHED until the condition of the patient stabilizes.

DOSAGE AND ADMINISTRATION

Norepinephrine Bitartrate Injection is a concentrated, potent drug which must be diluted in dextrose containing solutions prior to infusion. An infusion of LEVOPHED should be given into a large vein (see PRECAUTIONS).

Continued on next page

This product information was prepared in September 1996. On these and other products of Sanofi Winthrop Pharmaceuticals, detailed information may be obtained on a current basis by direct inquiry to Product Information Services, 90 Park Avenue, New York, NY 10016 (toll free 1-800-446-6267).

Sanofi Winthrop—Cont.

Restoration of Blood Pressure
In Acute Hypotensive States
Blood volume depletion should always be corrected as fully as possible before any vasopressor is administered. When, as an emergency measure, intra-aortic pressures must be maintained to prevent cerebral or coronary artery ischemia, LEVOPHED bitartrate, brand of norepinephrine bitartrate injection, can be administered before and concurrently with blood volume replacement.
Diluent: LEVOPHED should be diluted in 5 percent dextrose injection or 5 percent dextrose and sodium chloride injections. These dextrose containing fluids are protection against significant loss of potency due to oxidation. **Administration in saline solution alone is not recommended.** Whole blood or plasma, if indicated to increase blood volume, should be administered separately (for example, by use of a Y-tube and individual containers if given simultaneously).
Average Dosage: Add a 4 mL ampul (4 mg) of LEVOPHED to 1000 mL of a 5 percent dextrose containing solution. Each 1 mL of this dilution contains 4 µg of the base of LEVOPHED. Give this solution by intravenous infusion. Insert a plastic intravenous catheter through a suitable bore needle well advanced centrally into the vein and securely fixed with adhesive tape, avoiding, if possible, a catheter tie-in technique as this promotes stasis. An IV drip chamber or other suitable metering device is essential to permit an accurate estimation of the rate of flow in drops per minute. After observing the response to an initial dose of 2 mL to 3 mL (from 8 µg to 12 µg of base) per minute, adjust the rate of flow to establish and maintain a low normal blood pressure (usually 80 mm Hg to 100 mm Hg systolic) sufficient to maintain the circulation to vital organs. In previously hypertensive patients, it is recommended that the blood pressure should be raised no higher than 40 mm Hg below the preexisting systolic pressure. The average maintenance dose ranges from 0.5 mL to 1 mL per minute (from 2 µg to 4 µg of base).
High Dosage: Great individual variation occurs in the dose required to attain and maintain an adequate blood pressure. In all cases, dosage of LEVOPHED should be titrated according to the response of the patient. Occasionally much larger or even enormous daily doses (as high as 68 mg base or 17 ampuls) may be necessary if the patient remains hypotensive, but occult blood volume depletion should always be suspected and corrected when present. Central venous pressure monitoring is usually helpful in detecting and treating this situation.
Fluid Intake: The degree of dilution depends on clinical fluid volume requirements. If large volumes of fluid (dextrose) are needed at a flow rate that would involve an excessive dose of the pressor agent per unit of time, a solution more dilute than 4 µg per mL should be used. On the other hand, when large volumes of fluid are clinically undesirable, a concentration greater than 4 µg per mL may be necessary.
Duration of Therapy: The infusion should be continued until adequate blood pressure and tissue perfusion are maintained without therapy. Infusions of LEVOPHED should be reduced gradually, avoiding abrupt withdrawal. In some of the reported cases of vascular collapse due to acute myocardial infarction, treatment was required for up to six days.
Adjunctive Treatment in Cardiac Arrest
Infusions of LEVOPHED are usually administered intravenously during cardiac resuscitation to restore and maintain an adequate blood pressure after an effective heartbeat and ventilation have been established by other means. [LEVOPHED'S powerful beta-adrenergic stimulating action is also thought to increase the strength and effectiveness of systolic contractions once they occur.]
Average Dosage: To maintain systemic blood pressure during the management of cardiac arrest, LEVOPHED bitartrate, brand of norepinephrine bitartrate injection, is used in the same manner as described under Restoration of Blood Pressure in Acute Hypotensive States.
Parenteral drug products should be inspected visually for particulate matter and discoloration prior to use, whenever solution and container permit.

HOW SUPPLIED
LEVOPHED Bitartrate (norepinephrine injection, USP), contains the equivalent of 4 mg base of LEVOPHED per each 4 mL ampul.
Do not use the solution if its color is pinkish or darker than slightly yellow or if it contains a precipitate.
Avoid contact with iron salts, alkalis, or oxidizing agents.
Supplied as:
Ampuls of 4 mL in boxes of 10, NDC 0024-1123-02.
Store at room temperature. Protect from light.
Caution: Federal law prohibits dispensing without prescription.

Regitine, trademark, CIBA Pharmaceutical Company
LSW-5

MARCAINE® ℞
bupivacaine hydrochloride injection, USP

MARCAINE® ℞
WITH EPINEPHRINE 1:200,000 (AS BITARTRATE)
bupivacaine hydrochloride and epinephrine injection, USP

DESCRIPTION
Bupivacaine hydrochloride is 2-Piperidinecarboxamide, 1-butyl-*N*-(2,6-dimethylphenyl)-, monohydrochloride, monohydrate, a white crystalline powder that is freely soluble in 95 percent ethanol, soluble in water, and slightly soluble in chloroform or acetone.
Epinephrine is (-)-3, 4-Dihydroxy-α-[(methylamino)methyl] benzyl alcohol.
MARCAINE is available in sterile isotonic solutions with and without epinephrine (as bitartrate) 1:200,000 for injection via local infiltration, peripheral nerve block, and caudal and lumbar epidural blocks. Solutions of MARCAINE may be autoclaved if they do not contain epinephrine. Solutions are clear and colorless.
Bupivacaine is related chemically and pharmacologically to the aminoacyl local anesthetics. It is a homologue of mepivacaine and is chemically related to lidocaine. All three of these anesthetics contain an amide linkage between the aromatic nucleus and the amino, or piperidine group. They differ in this respect from the procaine-type local anesthetics, which have an ester linkage.
MARCAINE—Sterile isotonic solutions containing sodium chloride. In multiple-dose vials, each mL also contains 1 mg methylparaben as antiseptic preservative. The pH of these solutions is adjusted to between 4 and 6.5 with sodium hydroxide or hydrochloric acid.
MARCAINE with epinephrine 1:200,000 (as bitartrate)—Sterile isotonic solutions containing sodium chloride. Each mL contains bupivacaine hydrochloride and 0.0091 mg epinephrine bitartrate, with 0.5 mg sodium metabisulfite, 0.001 mL monothioglycerol, and 2 mg ascorbic acid as antioxidants, 0.0017 mL 60% sodium lactate buffer, and 0.1 mg edetate calcium disodium as stabilizer. In multiple-dose vials, each mL also contains 1 mg methylparaben as antiseptic preservative. The pH of these solutions is adjusted to between 3.4 and 4.5 with sodium hydroxide or hydrochloric acid. The specific gravity of MARCAINE 0.5% with epinephrine 1:200,000 (as bitartrate) at 25° C is 1.008 and at 37° C is 1.008.

CLINICAL PHARMACOLOGY
Local anesthetics block the generation and the conduction of nerve impulses, presumably by increasing the threshold for electrical excitation in the nerve, by slowing the propagation of the nerve impulse, and by reducing the rate of rise of the action potential. In general, the progression of anesthesia is related to the diameter, myelination, and conduction velocity of affected nerve fibers. Clinically, the order of loss of nerve function is as follows: (1) pain, (2) temperature, (3) touch, (4) proprioception, and (5) skeletal muscle tone.
Systemic absorption of local anesthetics produces effects on the cardiovascular and central nervous systems (CNS). At blood concentrations achieved with normal therapeutic doses, changes in cardiac conduction, excitability, refractoriness, contractility, and peripheral vascular resistance are minimal. However, toxic blood concentrations depress cardiac conduction and excitability, which may lead to atrioventricular block, ventricular arrhythmias, and cardiac arrest, sometimes resulting in fatalities. In addition, myocardial contractility is depressed and peripheral vasodilation occurs, leading to decreased cardiac output and arterial blood pressure. Recent clinical reports and animal research suggest that these cardiovascular changes are more likely to occur after unintended intravascular injection of bupivacaine. Therefore, incremental dosing is necessary.
Following systemic absorption, local anesthetics can produce central nervous system stimulation, depression, or both. Apparent central stimulation is manifested as restlessness, tremors and shivering progressing to convulsions, followed by depression and coma progressing ultimately to respiratory arrest. However, the local anesthetics have a primary depressant effect on the medulla and on higher centers. The depressed stage may occur without a prior excited state.
Pharmacokinetics: The rate of systemic absorption of local anesthetics is dependent upon the total dose and concentration of drug administered, the route of administration, the vascularity of the administration site, and the presence or absence of epinephrine in the anesthetic solution. A dilute concentration of epinephrine (1:200,000 or 5 mcg/mL) usually reduces the rate of absorption and peak plasma concentration of MARCAINE, permitting the use of moderately larger total doses and sometimes prolonging the duration of action.
The onset of action with MARCAINE is rapid and anesthesia is long lasting. The duration of anesthesia is significantly longer with MARCAINE than with any other commonly used local anesthetic. It has also been noted that there is a period of analgesia that persists after the return of sensa-

tion, during which time the need for strong analgesics is reduced.
The onset of action following dental injections is usually 2 to 10 minutes and anesthesia may last two or three times longer than lidocaine and mepivacaine for dental use, in many patients up to 7 hours. The duration of anesthetic effect is prolonged by the addition of epinephrine 1:200,000. Local anesthetics are bound to plasma proteins in varying degrees. Generally, the lower the plasma concentration of drug the higher the percentage of drug bound to plasma proteins.
Local anesthetics appear to cross the placenta by passive diffusion. The rate and degree of diffusion is governed by (1) the degree of plasma protein binding, (2) the degree of ionization, and (3) the degree of lipid solubility. Fetal/maternal ratios of local anesthetics appear to be inversely related to the degree of plasma protein binding, because only the free, unbound drug is available for placental transfer. MARCAINE with a high protein binding capacity (95%) has a low fetal/maternal ratio (0.2 to 0.4). The extent of placental transfer is also determined by the degree of ionization and lipid solubility of the drug. Lipid soluble, nonionized drugs readily enter the fetal blood from the maternal circulation. Depending upon the route of administration, local anesthetics are distributed to some extent to all body tissues, with high concentrations found in highly perfused organs such as the liver, lungs, heart, and brain.
Pharmacokinetic studies on the plasma profile of MARCAINE after direct intravenous injection suggest a three-compartment open model. The first compartment is represented by the rapid intravascular distribution of the drug. The second compartment represents the equilibration of the drug throughout the highly perfused organs such as the brain, myocardium, lungs, kidneys, and liver. The third compartment represents an equilibration of the drug with poorly perfused tissues, such as muscle and fat. The elimination of drug from tissue distribution depends largely upon the ability of binding sites in the circulation to carry it to the liver where it is metabolized.
After injection of MARCAINE for caudal, epidural, or peripheral nerve block in man, peak levels of bupivacaine in the blood are reached in 30 to 45 minutes, followed by a decline to insignificant levels during the next three to six hours.
Various pharmacokinetic parameters of the local anesthetics can be significantly altered by the presence of hepatic or renal disease, addition of epinephrine, factors affecting urinary pH, renal blood flow, the route of drug administration, and the age of the patient. The half-life of MARCAINE in adults is 2.7 hours and in neonates 8.1 hours.
Amide-type local anesthetics such as MARCAINE are metabolized primarily in the liver via conjugation with glucuronic acid. Patients with hepatic disease, especially those with severe hepatic disease, may be more susceptible to the potential toxicities of the amide-type local anesthetics. Pipecoloxylidine is the major metabolite of MARCAINE. The kidney is the main excretory organ for most local anesthetics and their metabolites. Urinary excretion is affected by urinary perfusion and factors affecting urinary pH. Only 6% of bupivacaine is excreted unchanged in the urine.
When administered in recommended doses and concentrations, MARCAINE does not ordinarily produce irritation or tissue damage and does not cause methemoglobinemia.

INDICATIONS AND USAGE
MARCAINE is indicated for the production of local or regional anesthesia or analgesia for surgery, dental and oral surgery procedures, diagnostic and therapeutic procedures, and for obstetrical procedures. Only the 0.25% and 0.5% concentrations are indicated for obstetrical anesthesia. (See WARNINGS.)
Experience with nonobstetrical surgical procedures in pregnant patients is not sufficient to recommend use of 0.75% concentration of MARCAINE in these patients.
MARCAINE is not recommended for intravenous regional anesthesia (Bier Block). See WARNINGS.
The routes of administration and indicated MARCAINE concentrations are:

● local infiltration	0.25%
● peripheral nerve block	0.25% and 0.5%
● retrobulbar block	0.75%
● sympathetic block	0.25%
● lumbar epidural	0.25%, 0.5%, and 0.75% (0.75% not for obstetrical anesthesia)
● caudal	0.25% and 0.5%
● epidural test dose	0.5% with epinephrine 1:200,000
● dental blocks	0.5% with epinephrine 1:200,000

(See DOSAGE AND ADMINISTRATION for additional information.)
Standard textbooks should be consulted to determine the accepted procedures and techniques for the administration of MARCAINE.

CONTRAINDICATIONS

MARCAINE is contraindicated in obstetrical paracervical block anesthesia. Its use in this technique has resulted in fetal bradycardia and death.

MARCAINE is contraindicated in patients with a known hypersensitivity to it or to any local anesthetic agent of the amide-type or to other components of MARCAINE solutions.

WARNINGS

THE 0.75% CONCENTRATION OF MARCAINE IS NOT RECOMMENDED FOR OBSTETRICAL ANESTHESIA. THERE HAVE BEEN REPORTS OF CARDIAC ARREST WITH DIFFICULT RESUSCITATION OR DEATH DURING USE OF MARCAINE FOR EPIDURAL ANESTHESIA IN OBSTETRICAL PATIENTS. IN MOST CASES, THIS HAS FOLLOWED USE OF THE 0.75% CONCENTRATION. RESUSCITATION HAS BEEN DIFFICULT OR IMPOSSIBLE DESPITE APPARENTLY ADEQUATE PREPARATION AND APPROPRIATE MANAGEMENT. CARDIAC ARREST HAS OCCURRED AFTER CONVULSIONS RESULTING FROM SYSTEMIC TOXICITY, PRESUMABLY FOLLOWING UNINTENTIONAL INTRAVASCULAR INJECTION. THE 0.75% CONCENTRATION SHOULD BE RESERVED FOR SURGICAL PROCEDURES WHERE A HIGH DEGREE OF MUSCLE RELAXATION AND PROLONGED EFFECT ARE NECESSARY.

LOCAL ANESTHETICS SHOULD ONLY BE EMPLOYED BY CLINICIANS WHO ARE WELL VERSED IN DIAGNOSIS AND MANAGEMENT OF DOSE-RELATED TOXICITY AND OTHER ACUTE EMERGENCIES WHICH MIGHT ARISE FROM THE BLOCK TO BE EMPLOYED, AND THEN ONLY AFTER INSURING THE *IMMEDIATE* AVAILABILITY OF OXYGEN, OTHER RESUSCITATIVE DRUGS, CARDIOPULMONARY RESUSCITATIVE EQUIPMENT, AND THE PERSONNEL RESOURCES NEEDED FOR PROPER MANAGEMENT OF TOXIC REACTIONS AND RELATED EMERGENCIES. (See also ADVERSE REACTIONS, PRECAUTIONS, and OVERDOSAGE.) DELAY IN PROPER MANAGEMENT OF DOSE-RELATED TOXICITY, UNDERVENTILATION FROM ANY CAUSE, AND/OR ALTERED SENSITIVITY MAY LEAD TO THE DEVELOPMENT OF ACIDOSIS, CARDIAC ARREST AND, POSSIBLY, DEATH.

Local anesthetic solutions containing antimicrobial preservatives, i.e., those supplied in multiple-dose vials, should not be used for epidural or caudal anesthesia because safety has not been established with regard to intrathecal injection, either intentionally or unintentionally, of such preservatives.

It is essential that aspiration for blood or cerebrospinal fluid (where applicable) be done prior to injecting any local anesthetic, both the original dose and all subsequent doses, to avoid intravascular or subarachnoid injection. However, a negative aspiration does *not* ensure against an intravascular or subarachnoid injection.

MARCAINE with epinephrine 1:200,000 or other vasopressors should not be used concomitantly with ergot-type oxytocic drugs, because a severe persistent hypertension may occur. Likewise, solutions of MARCAINE containing a vasoconstrictor, such as epinephrine, should be used with extreme caution in patients receiving monoamine oxidase inhibitors (MAOI) or antidepressants of the triptyline or imipramine types, because severe prolonged hypertension may result.

Until further experience is gained in children younger than 12 years, administration of MARCAINE in this age group is not recommended.

Mixing or the prior or intercurrent use of any other local anesthetic with MARCAINE cannot be recommended because of insufficient data on the clinical use of such mixtures.

There have been reports of cardiac arrest and death during the use of MARCAINE for intravenous regional anesthesia (Bier Block). Information on safe dosages and techniques of administration of MARCAINE in this procedure is lacking. Therefore, MARCAINE is not recommended for use in this technique.

MARCAINE with epinephrine 1:200,000 contains sodium metabisulfite, a sulfite that may cause allergic-type reactions including anaphylactic symptoms and life-threatening or less severe asthmatic episodes in certain susceptible people. The overall prevalence of sulfite sensitivity in the general population is unknown and probably low. Sulfite sensitivity is seen more frequently in asthmatic than in nonasthmatic people. Single-dose ampuls and single-dose vials of ***MARCAINE*** without epinephrine do not contain sodium metabisulfite.

PRECAUTIONS

General: The safety and effectiveness of local anesthetics depend on proper dosage, correct technique, adequate precautions, and readiness for emergencies. Resuscitative equipment, oxygen, and other resuscitative drugs should be available for immediate use. (See WARNINGS, ADVERSE REACTIONS, and OVERDOSAGE.) During major regional nerve blocks, the patient should have IV fluids running via an indwelling catheter to assure a functioning intravenous pathway. The lowest dosage of local anesthetic that results in effective anesthesia should be used to avoid high plasma levels and serious adverse effects. The rapid injection of a large volume of local anesthetic solution should be avoided and fractional (incremental) doses should be used when feasible.

Epidural Anesthesia: During epidural administration of MARCAINE, 0.5% and 0.75% solutions should be administered in incremental doses of 3 mL to 5 mL with sufficient time between doses to detect toxic manifestations of unintentional intravascular or intrathecal injection. Injections should be made slowly, with frequent aspirations before and during the injection to avoid intravascular injection. Syringe aspirations should also be performed before and during each supplemental injection in continuous (intermittent) catheter techniques. An intravascular injection is still possible even if aspirations for blood are negative.

During the administration of epidural anesthesia, it is recommended that a test dose be administered initially and the effects monitored before the full dose is given. When using a "continuous" catheter technique, test doses should be given prior to both the original and all reinforcing doses, because plastic tubing in the epidural space can migrate into a blood vessel or through the dura. When clinical conditions permit, the test dose should contain epinephrine (10 mcg to 15 mcg has been suggested) to serve as a warning of unintended intravascular injection. If injected into a blood vessel, this amount of epinephrine is likely to produce a transient "epinephrine response" within 45 seconds, consisting of an increase in heart rate and/or systolic blood pressure, circumoral pallor, palpitations, and nervousness in the unsedated patient. The sedated patient may exhibit only a pulse rate increase of 20 or more beats per minute for 15 or more seconds. Therefore, following the test dose, the heart rate should be monitored for a heart rate increase. Patients on beta-blockers may not manifest changes in heart rate, but blood pressure monitoring can detect a transient rise in systolic blood pressure. The test dose should also contain 10 mg to 15 mg of MARCAINE or an equivalent amount of another local anesthetic to detect an unintended intrathecal administration. This will be evidenced within a few minutes by signs of spinal block (e.g., decreased sensation of the buttocks, paresis of the legs, or, in the sedated patient, absent knee jerk). The Test Dose formulation of MARCAINE contains 15 mg of bupivacaine and 15 mcg of epinephrine in a volume of 3 mL. An intravascular or subarachnoid injection is still possible even if results of the test dose are negative. The test dose itself may produce a systemic toxic reaction, high spinal or epinephrine-induced cardiovascular effects.

Injection of repeated doses of local anesthetics may cause significant increases in plasma levels with each repeated dose due to slow accumulation of the drug or its metabolites, or to slow metabolic degradation. Tolerance to elevated blood levels varies with the status of the patient. Debilitated, elderly patients and acutely ill patients should be given reduced doses commensurate with their age and physical status. Local anesthetics should also be used with caution in patients with hypotension or heartblock.

Careful and constant monitoring of cardiovascular and respiratory (adequacy of ventilation) vital signs and the patient's state of consciousness should be performed after each local anesthetic injection. It should be kept in mind at such times that restlessness, anxiety, incoherent speech, lightheadedness, numbness and tingling of the mouth and lips, metallic taste, tinnitus, dizziness, blurred vision, tremors, twitching, depression, or drowsiness may be early warning signs of central nervous system toxicity.

Local anesthetic solutions containing a vasoconstrictor should be used cautiously and in carefully restricted quantities in areas of the body supplied by end arteries or having otherwise compromised blood supply such as digits, nose, external ear, or penis. Patients with hypertensive vascular disease may exhibit exaggerated vasoconstrictor response. Ischemic injury or necrosis may result.

Because amide-type local anesthetics such as MARCAINE are metabolized by the liver, these drugs, especially repeat doses, should be used cautiously in patients with hepatic disease. Patients with severe hepatic disease, because of their inability to metabolize local anesthetics normally, are at a greater risk of developing toxic plasma concentrations. Local anesthetics should also be used with caution in patients with impaired cardiovascular function because they may be less able to compensate for functional changes associated with the prolongation of AV conduction produced by these drugs.

Serious dose-related cardiac arrhythmias may occur if preparations containing a vasoconstrictor such as epinephrine are employed in patients during or following the administration of potent inhalation anesthetics. In deciding whether to use these products concurrently in the same patient, the combined action of both agents upon the myocardium, the concentration and volume of vasoconstrictor used, and the time since injection, when applicable, should be taken into account.

Many drugs used during the conduct of anesthesia are considered potential triggering agents for familial malignant hyperthermia. Because it is not known whether amide-type local anesthetics may trigger this reaction and because the need for supplemental general anesthesia cannot be predicted in advance, it is suggested that a standard protocol for management should be available. Early unexplained signs of tachycardia, tachypnea, labile blood pressure, and metabolic acidosis may precede temperature elevation. Successful outcome is dependent on early diagnosis, prompt discontinuance of the suspect triggering agent(s) and prompt institution of treatment, including oxygen therapy, indicated supportive measures and dantrolene. (Consult dantrolene sodium intravenous package insert before using.)

Use in Head and Neck Area: Small doses of local anesthetics injected into the head and neck area, including retrobulbar, dental, and stellate ganglion blocks, may produce adverse reactions similar to systemic toxicity seen with unintentional intravascular injections of larger doses. The injection procedures require the utmost care. Confusion, convulsions, respiratory depression, and/or respiratory arrest, and cardiovascular stimulation or depression have been reported. These reactions may be due to intra-arterial injection of the local anesthetic with retrograde flow to the cerebral circulation. They may also be due to puncture of the dural sheath of the optic nerve during retrobulbar block with diffusion of any local anesthetic along the subdural space to the midbrain. Patients receiving these blocks should have their circulation and respiration monitored and be constantly observed. Resuscitative equipment and personnel for treating adverse reactions should be immediately available. Dosage recommendations should not be exceeded. (See DOSAGE AND ADMINISTRATION.)

Use in Ophthalmic Surgery: Clinicians who perform retrobulbar blocks should be aware that there have been reports of respiratory arrest following local anesthetic injection. Prior to retrobulbar block, as with all other regional procedures, the immediate availability of equipment, drugs, and personnel to manage respiratory arrest or depression, convulsions, and cardiac stimulation or depression should be assured (see also WARNINGS and *Use in Head and Neck Area,* above). As with other anesthetic procedures, patients should be constantly monitored following ophthalmic blocks for signs of these adverse reactions, which may occur following relatively low total doses. A concentration of 0.75% bupivacaine is indicated for retrobulbar block; however, this concentration is not indicated for any other peripheral nerve block, including the facial nerve, and not indicated for local infiltration, including the conjunctiva (see INDICATIONS and PRECAUTIONS, *General*). Mixing MARCAINE with other local anesthetics is not recommended because of insufficient data on the clinical use of such mixtures.

When MARCAINE 0.75% is used for retrobulbar block, complete corneal anesthesia usually precedes onset of clinically acceptable external ocular muscle akinesia. Therefore, presence of akinesia rather than anesthesia alone should determine readiness of the patient for surgery.

Use in Dentistry: Because of the long duration of anesthesia, when MARCAINE 0.5% with epinephrine is used for dental injections, patients should be cautioned about the possibility of inadvertent trauma to tongue, lips, and buccal mucosa and advised not to chew solid foods or test the anesthetized area by biting or probing.

Information for Patients: When appropriate, patients should be informed in advance that they may experience temporary loss of sensation and motor activity, usually in the lower half of the body, following proper administration of caudal or epidural anesthesia. Also, when appropriate, the physician should discuss other information including adverse reactions in the package insert of MARCAINE.

Patients receiving dental injections of MARCAINE should be cautioned not to chew solid foods or test the anesthetized area by biting or probing until anesthesia has worn off (up to 7 hours).

Clinically Significant Drug Interactions: The administration of local anesthetic solutions containing epinephrine or norepinephrine to patients receiving monoamine oxidase inhibitors or tricyclic antidepressants may produce severe, prolonged hypertension. Concurrent use of these agents should generally be avoided. In situations when concurrent therapy is necessary, careful patient monitoring is essential.

Continued on next page

This product information was prepared in September 1996. On these and other products of Sanofi Winthrop Pharmaceuticals, detailed information may be obtained on a current basis by direct inquiry to Product Information Services, 90 Park Avenue, New York, NY 10016 (toll free 1-800-446-6267).

Sanofi Winthrop—Cont.

Concurrent administration of vasopressor drugs and of ergot-type oxytocic drugs may cause severe, persistent hypertension or cerebrovascular accidents.

Phenothiazines and butyrophenones may reduce or reverse the pressor effect of epinephrine.

Carcinogenesis, Mutagenesis, Impairment of Fertility: Long-term studies in animals of most local anesthetics including bupivacaine to evaluate the carcinogenic potential have not been conducted. Mutagenic potential or the effect on fertility has not been determined. There is no evidence from human data that MARCAINE may be carcinogenic or mutagenic or that it impairs fertility.

Pregnancy Category C: Decreased pup survival in rats and an embryocidal effect in rabbits have been observed when bupivacaine hydrochloride was administered to these species in doses comparable to nine and five times respectively the maximum recommended daily human dose (400 mg). There are no adequate and well-controlled studies in pregnant women of the effect of bupivacaine on the developing fetus. Bupivacaine hydrochloride should be used during pregnancy only if the potential benefit justifies the potential risk to the fetus. This does not exclude the use of MARCAINE at term for obstetrical anesthesia or analgesia. (See *Labor and Delivery*.)

Labor and Delivery: SEE BOXED WARNING REGARDING OBSTETRICAL USE OF 0.75% MARCAINE. MARCAINE is contraindicated for obstetrical paracervical block anesthesia.

Local anesthetics rapidly cross the placenta, and when used for epidural, caudal, or pudendal block anesthesia, can cause varying degrees of maternal, fetal, and neonatal toxicity. (See *Pharmacokinetics* in CLINICAL PHARMACOLOGY.) The incidence and degree of toxicity depend upon the procedure performed, the type, and amount of drug used, and the technique of drug administration. Adverse reactions in the parturient, fetus, and neonate involve alterations of the central nervous system, peripheral vascular tone, and cardiac function.

Maternal hypotension has resulted from regional anesthesia. Local anesthetics produce vasodilation by blocking sympathetic nerves. Elevating the patient's legs and positioning her on her left side will help prevent decreases in blood pressure. The fetal heart rate also should be monitored continuously and electronic fetal monitoring is highly advisable.

Epidural, caudal, or pudendal anesthesia may alter the forces of parturition through changes in uterine contractility or maternal expulsive efforts. Epidural anesthesia has been reported to prolong the second stage of labor by removing the parturient's reflex urge to bear down or by interfering with motor function. The use of obstetrical anesthesia may increase the need for forceps assistance.

The use of some local anesthetic drug products during labor and delivery may be followed by diminished muscle strength and tone for the first day or two of life. This has not been reported with bupivacaine.

It is extremely important to avoid aortocaval compression by the gravid uterus during administration of regional block to parturients. To do this, the patient must be maintained in the left lateral decubitus position or a blanket roll or sandbag may be placed beneath the right hip and gravid uterus displaced to the left.

Nursing Mothers: It is not known whether local anesthetic drugs are excreted in human milk. Because many drugs are excreted in human milk, caution should be exercised when local anesthetics are administered to a nursing woman.

Pediatric Use: Until further experience is gained in children younger than 12 years, administration of MARCAINE in this age group is not recommended. Continuous infusions of bupivacaine in children have been reported to result in high systemic levels of bupivacaine and seizures; high plasma levels may also be associated with cardiovascular abnormalities. (See WARNINGS, PRECAUTIONS, and OVERDOSAGE.)

ADVERSE REACTIONS

Reactions to MARCAINE are characteristic of those associated with other amide-type local anesthetics. A major cause of adverse reactions to this group of drugs is excessive plasma levels, which may be due to overdosage, unintentional intravascular injection, or slow metabolic degradation.

The most commonly encountered acute adverse experiences which demand immediate countermeasures are related to the central nervous system and the cardiovascular system. These adverse experiences are generally dose related and due to high plasma levels which may result from overdosage, rapid absorption from the injection site, diminished tolerance, or from unintentional intravascular injection of the local anesthetic solution. In addition to systemic dose-related toxicity, unintentional subarachnoid injection of drug during the intended performance of caudal or lumbar epidural block or nerve blocks near the vertebral column (especially in the head and neck region) may result in underventilation

or apnea ("Total or High Spinal"). Also, hypotension due to loss of sympathetic tone and respiratory paralysis or underventilation due to cephalad extension of the motor level of anesthesia may occur. This may lead to secondary cardiac arrest if untreated. Factors influencing plasma protein binding, such as acidosis, systemic diseases which alter protein production, or competition of other drugs for protein binding sites, may diminish individual tolerance.

Central Nervous System Reactions: These are characterized by excitation and/or depression. Restlessness, anxiety, dizziness, tinnitus, blurred vision, or tremors may occur, possibly proceeding to convulsions. However, excitement may be transient or absent, with depression being the first manifestation of an adverse reaction. This may quickly be followed by drowsiness merging into unconsciousness and respiratory arrest. Other central nervous system effects may be nausea, vomiting, chills, and constriction of the pupils. The incidence of convulsions associated with the use of local anesthetics varies with the procedure used and the total dose administered. In a survey of studies of epidural anesthesia, overt toxicity progressing to convulsions occurred in approximately 0.1% of local anesthetic administrations.

Cardiovascular System Reactions: High doses or unintentional intravascular injection may lead to high plasma levels and related depression of the myocardium, decreased cardiac output, heartblock, hypotension, bradycardia, ventricular arrhythmias, including ventricular tachycardia and ventricular fibrillation, and cardiac arrest. (See WARNINGS, PRECAUTIONS, and OVERDOSAGE sections.)

Allergic: Allergic-type reactions are rare and may occur as a result of sensitivity to the local anesthetic or to other formulation ingredients, such as the antimicrobial preservative methylparaben contained in multiple-dose vials or sulfites in epinephrine-containing solutions. These reactions are characterized by signs such as urticaria, pruritus, erythema, angioneurotic edema (including laryngeal edema), tachycardia, sneezing, nausea, vomiting, dizziness, syncope, excessive sweating, elevated temperature, and possibly, anaphylactoid-like symptomatology (including severe hypotension). Cross sensitivity among members of the amide-type local anesthetic group has been reported. The usefulness of screening for sensitivity has not been definitely established.

Neurologic: The incidences of adverse neurologic reactions associated with the use of local anesthetics may be related to the total dose of local anesthetic administered and are also dependent upon the particular drug used, the route of administration, and the physical status of the patient. Many of these effects may be related to local anesthetic techniques, with or without a contribution from the drug.

In the practice of caudal or lumbar epidural block, occasional unintentional penetration of the subarachnoid space by the catheter or needle may occur. Subsequent adverse effects may depend partially on the amount of drug administered intrathecally and the physiological and physical effects of a dural puncture. A high spinal is characterized by paralysis of the legs, loss of consciousness, respiratory paralysis, and bradycardia.

Neurologic effects following epidural or caudal anesthesia may include spinal block of varying magnitude (including high or total spinal block); hypotension secondary to spinal block; urinary retention; fecal and urinary incontinence; loss of perineal sensation and sexual function; persistent anesthesia, paresthesia, weakness, paralysis of the lower extremities and loss of sphincter control all of which may have slow, incomplete, or no recovery; headache; backache; septic meningitis; meningismus; slowing of labor; increased incidence of forceps delivery; and cranial nerve palsies due to traction on nerves from loss of cerebrospinal fluid.

Neurologic effects following other procedures or routes of administration may include persistent anesthesia, paresthesia, weakness, paralysis, all of which may have slow, incomplete, or no recovery.

OVERDOSAGE

Acute emergencies from local anesthetics are generally related to high plasma levels encountered during therapeutic use of local anesthetics or to unintended subarachnoid injection of local anesthetic solution. (See ADVERSE REACTIONS, WARNINGS, and PRECAUTIONS.)

Management of Local Anesthetic Emergencies: The first consideration is prevention, best accomplished by careful and constant monitoring of cardiovascular and respiratory vital signs and the patient's state of consciousness after each local anesthetic injection. At the first sign of change, oxygen should be administered.

The first step in the management of systemic toxic reactions, as well as underventilation or apnea due to unintentional subarachnoid injection of drug solution, consists of immediate attention to the establishment and maintenance of a patent airway and effective assisted or controlled ventilation with 100% oxygen with a delivery system capable of permitting immediate positive airway pressure by mask. This may prevent convulsions if they have not already occurred.

If necessary, use drugs to control the convulsions. A 50 mg to 100 mg bolus IV injection of succinylcholine will paralyze the patient without depressing the central nervous or cardio-

vascular systems and facilitate ventilation. A bolus IV dose of 5 mg to 10 mg of diazepam or 50 mg to 100 mg of thiopental will permit ventilation and counteract central nervous system stimulation, but these drugs also depress central nervous system, respiratory, and cardiac function, add to postictal depression and may result in apnea. Intravenous barbiturates, anticonvulsant agents, or muscle relaxants should only be administered by those familiar with their use. Immediately after the institution of these ventilatory measures, the adequacy of the circulation should be evaluated. Supportive treatment of circulatory depression may require administration of intravenous fluids, and when appropriate, a vasopressor dictated by the clinical situation (such as ephedrine or epinephrine to enhance myocardial contractile force).

Endotracheal intubation, employing drugs and techniques familiar to the clinician, may be indicated after initial administration of oxygen by mask if difficulty is encountered in the maintenance of a patent airway, or if prolonged ventilatory support (assisted or controlled) is indicated.

Recent clinical data from patients experiencing local anesthetic-induced convulsions demonstrated rapid development of hypoxia, hypercarbia, and acidosis with bupivacaine within a minute of the onset of convulsions. These observations suggest that oxygen consumption and carbon dioxide production are greatly increased during local anesthetic convulsions and emphasize the importance of immediate and effective ventilation with oxygen which may avoid cardiac arrest.

If not treated immediately, convulsions with simultaneous hypoxia, hypercarbia, and acidosis plus myocardial depression from the direct effects of the local anesthetic may result in cardiac arrhythmias, bradycardia, asystole, ventricular fibrillation, or cardiac arrest. Respiratory abnormalities, including apnea, may occur. Underventilation or apnea due to unintentional subarachnoid injection of local anesthetic solution may produce these same signs and also lead to cardiac arrest if ventilatory support is not instituted. *If cardiac arrest should occur, successful outcome may require prolonged resuscitative efforts.*

The supine position is dangerous in pregnant women at term because of aortocaval compression by the gravid uterus. Therefore during treatment of systemic toxicity, maternal hypotension or fetal bradycardia following regional block, the parturient should be maintained in the left lateral decubitus position if possible, or manual displacement of the uterus off the great vessels be accomplished.

The mean seizure dosage of bupivacaine in rhesus monkeys was found to be 4.4 mg/kg with mean arterial plasma concentration of 4.5 mcg/mL. The intravenous and subcutaneous LD_{50} in mice is 6 mg/kg to 8 mg/kg and 38 mg/kg to 54 mg/kg respectively.

DOSAGE AND ADMINISTRATION

The dose of any local anesthetic administered varies with the anesthetic procedure, the area to be anesthetized, the vascularity of the tissues, the number of neuronal segments to be blocked, the depth of anesthesia and degree of muscle relaxation required, the duration of anesthesia desired, individual tolerance, and the physical condition of the patient. The smallest dose and concentration required to produce the desired result should be administered. Dosages of MARCAINE should be reduced for elderly and debilitated patients and patients with cardiac and/or liver disease. The rapid injection of a large volume of local anesthetic solution should be avoided and fractional (incremental) doses should be used when feasible.

For specific techniques and procedures, refer to standard textbooks.

In recommended doses, MARCAINE produces complete sensory block, but the effect on motor function differs among the three concentrations.

0.25%—when used for caudal, epidural, or peripheral nerve block, produces incomplete motor block. Should be used for operations in which muscle relaxation is not important, or when another means of providing muscle relaxation is used concurrently. Onset of action may be slower than with the 0.5% or 0.75% solutions.

0.5%—provides motor blockade for caudal, epidural, or nerve block, but muscle relaxation may be inadequate for operations in which complete muscle relaxation is essential.

0.75%—produces complete motor block. Most useful for epidural block in abdominal operations requiring complete muscle relaxation, and for retrobulbar anesthesia. Not for obstetrical anesthesia.

The duration of anesthesia with MARCAINE is such that for most indications, a single dose is sufficient.

Maximum dosage limit must be individualized in each case after evaluating the size and physical status of the patient, as well as the usual rate of systemic absorption from a particular injection site. Most experience to date is with single doses of MARCAINE up to 225 mg with epinephrine 1:200,000 and 175 mg without epinephrine; more or less drug may be used depending on individualization of each case.

Table 1. Recommended Concentrations and Doses of MARCAINE

Type of Block	Conc.	Each Dose (mL)	(mg)	Motor Block[1]
Local infiltration	0.25%[4]	up to max.	up to max.	—
Epidural	0.75%[2,4]	10–20	75–150	complete
	0.5%[4]	10–20	50–100	moderate to complete
	0.25%[4]	10–20	25–50	partial to moderate
Caudal	0.5%[4]	15–30	75–150	moderate to complete
	0.25%[4]	15–30	37.5–75	moderate
Peripheral nerves	0.5%[4]	5 to max.	25 to max.	moderate to complete
	0.25%[4]	5 to max.	12.5 to max.	moderate to complete
Retrobulbar[3]	0.75%[4]	2–4	15–30	complete
Sympathetic	0.25%	20–50	50–125	—
Dental[3]	0.5% w/epi	1.8–3.6 per site	9–18 per site	—
Epidural[3] Test Dose	0.5% w/epi	2–3	10–15 (10–15 micrograms epinephrine)	—

[1]With continuous (intermittent) techniques, repeat doses increase the degree of motor block. The first repeat dose of 0.5% may produce complete motor block. Intercostal nerve block with 0.25% may also produce complete motor block for intra-abdominal surgery.

[2]For single-dose use, not for intermittent epidural technique. Not for obstetrical anesthesia.

[3]See PRECAUTIONS.

[4]Solutions with or without epinephrine.

These doses may be repeated up to once every three hours. In clinical studies to date, total daily doses have been up to 400 mg. Until further experience is gained, this dose should not be exceeded in 24 hours. The duration of anesthetic effect may be prolonged by the addition of epinephrine.

The dosages in Table 1 have generally proved satisfactory and are recommended as a guide for use in the average adult. These dosages should be reduced for elderly or debilitated patients. Until further experience is gained, MARCAINE is not recommended for children younger than 12 years. MARCAINE is contraindicated for obstetrical paracervical blocks, and is not recommended for intravenous regional anesthesia (Bier Block).

Use in Epidural Anesthesia: During epidural administration of MARCAINE, 0.5% and 0.75% solutions should be administered in incremental doses of 3 mL to 5 mL with sufficient time between doses to detect toxic manifestatons of unintentional intravascular or intrathecal injection. In obstetrics, only the 0.5% and 0.25% concentrations should be used; incremental doses of 3 mL to 5 mL of the 0.5% solution not exceeding 50 mg to 100 mg at any dosing interval are recommended. Repeat doses should be preceded by a test dose containing epinephrine if not contraindicated. Use only the single-dose ampuls and single-dose vials for caudal or epidural anesthesia; the multiple-dose vials contain a preservative and therefore should not be used for these procedures.

Test Dose for Caudal and Lumbar Epidural Blocks: The Test Dose of MARCAINE (0.5% bupivacaine with 1:200,000 epinephrine in a 3 mL ampul) is recommended for use as a test dose when clinical conditions permit prior to caudal and lumbar epidural blocks. This may serve as a warning of unintended intravascular or subarachnoid injection. (See PRECAUTIONS.) The pulse rate and other signs should be monitored carefully immediately following each test dose administration to detect possible intravascular injection, and adequate time for onset of spinal block should be allotted to detect possible intrathecal injection. An intravascular or subarachnoid injection is still possible even if results of the test dose are negative. The test dose itself may produce a systemic toxic reaction, high spinal or cardiovascular effects from the epinephrine. (See WARNINGS and OVERDOSAGE.)

Use in Dentistry: The 0.5% concentration with epinephrine is recommended for infiltration and block injection in the maxillary and mandibular area when a longer duration of local anesthetic action is desired, such as for oral surgical procedures generally associated with significant postoperative pain. The average dose of 1.8 mL (9 mg) per injection site will usually suffice; an occasional second dose of 1.8 mL (9 mg) may be used if necessary to produce adequate anesthesia after making allowance for 2 to 10 minutes onset time. (See CLINICAL PHARMACOLOGY.) The lowest effective dose should be employed and time should be allowed between injections; it is recommended that the total dose for all injection sites, *spread out* over a single dental sitting, should not ordinarily exceed 90 mg for a healthy adult patient (ten 1.8 mL injections of 0.5% MARCAINE with epinephrine). Injections should be made slowly and with frequent aspirations. Until further experience is gained, MARCAINE in dentistry is not recommended for children younger than 12 years.

Unused portions of solution not containing preservatives, i.e., those supplied in single-dose ampuls and single-dose vials, should be discarded following initial use.

This product should be inspected visually for particulate matter and discoloration prior to administration whenever solution and container permit. Solutions which are discolored or which contain particulate matter should not be administered.

[See Table 1 above.]

HOW SUPPLIED

These solutions are not for spinal anesthesia.

Store at controlled room temperature, between 15° C and 30° C (59° F and 86° F).

MARCAINE — Solutions of MARCAINE that do not contain epinephrine may be autoclaved. Autoclave at 15-pound pressure, 121° C (250° F) for 15 minutes.

0.25%—Contains 2.5 mg bupivacaine hydrochloride per mL.
Single-dose ampuls of 50 mL, box of 5
NDC 0024-1212-02
Single-dose vials of 10 mL, box of 10
NDC 0024-1212-10
Single-dose vials of 30 mL, box of 10
NDC 0024-1212-30
Multiple-dose vials of 50 mL, box of 1
NDC 0024-1217-01

0.5%—Contains 5 mg bupivacaine hydrochloride per mL.
Single-dose ampuls of 30 mL, box of 5
NDC 0024-1213-02
Single-dose vials of 10 mL, box of 10
NDC 0024-1213-10
Single-dose vials of 30 mL, box of 10
NDC 0024-1213-30
Multiple-dose vials of 50 mL, box of 1
NDC 0024-1218-01

0.75%—Contains 7.5 mg bupivacaine hydrochloride per mL.
Single-dose ampuls of 30 mL, box of 5
NDC 0024-1214-02
Single-dose vials of 10 mL, box of 10
NDC 0024-1214-10
Single-dose vials of 30 mL, box of 10
NDC 0024-1214-30

MARCAINE with epinephrine 1:200,000 (as bitartrate)— Solutions of MARCAINE that contain epinephrine should not be autoclaved and should be protected from light. Do not use the solution if its color is pinkish or darker than slightly yellow or if it contains a precipitate.

0.25%—with epinephrine 1:200,000
Contains 2.5 mg bupivacaine hydrochloride per mL.
Single-dose ampuls of 50 mL, box of 5
NDC 0024-1222-02
Single-dose vials of 10 mL, box of 10
NDC 0024-1222-10
Single-dose vials of 30 mL, box of 10
NDC 0024-1222-30
Multiple-dose vials of 50 mL, box of 1
NDC 0024-1227-01

0.5%—with epinephrine 1:200,000
Contains 5 mg bupivacaine hydrochloride per mL.
Single-dose ampuls of 3 mL, box of 10
NDC 0024-1223-03
Single-dose ampuls of 30 mL, box of 5
NDC 0024-1223-02
Single-dose vials of 10 mL, box of 10
NDC 0024-1223-10
Single-dose vials of 30 mL, box of 10
NDC 0024-1223-30
Multiple-dose vials of 50 mL, box of 1
NDC 0024-1228-01

0.75%—with epinephrine 1:200,000
Contains 7.5 mg bupivacaine hydrochloride per mL.
Single-dose ampuls of 30 mL, box of 5
NDC 0024-1224-02

CAUTION: Federal law prohibits dispensing without prescription.

MSW-6 B

MARCAINE® Spinal ℞
brand of bupivacaine hydrochloride in dextrose injection, USP

STERILE HYPERBARIC SOLUTION FOR SPINAL ANESTHESIA

DESCRIPTION

Bupivacaine hydrochloride is 2-Piperidinecarboxamide, 1-butyl-*N*-(2,6-dimethylphenyl)-, monohydrochloride, monohydrate, a white crystalline powder that is freely soluble in 95 percent ethanol, soluble in water, and slightly soluble in chloroform or acetone.

Dextrose is D-glucopyranose monohydrate.

MARCAINE Spinal is available in sterile hyperbaric solution for subarachnoid injection (spinal block).

Bupivacaine hydrochloride is related chemically and pharmacologically to the aminoacyl local anesthetics. It is a homologue of mepivacaine and is chemically related to lidocaine. All three of these anesthetics contain an amide linkage between the aromatic nucleus and the amino or piperidine group. They differ in this respect from the procaine-type local anesthetics, which have an ester linkage.

Each 1 mL of MARCAINE Spinal contains 7.5 mg bupivacaine hydrochloride and 82.5 mg dextrose. The pH of this solution is adjusted to between 4.0 and 6.5 with sodium hydroxide or hydrochloric acid.

The specific gravity of MARCAINE Spinal is between 1.030 and 1.035 at 25° C and 1.03 at 37° C.

MARCAINE Spinal does not contain any preservatives.

CLINICAL PHARMACOLOGY

Local anesthetics block the generation and the conduction of nerve impulses, presumably by increasing the threshold for electrical excitation in the nerve, by slowing the propagation of the nerve impulse, and by reducing the rate of rise of the action potential. In general, the progression of anesthesia is related to the diameter, myelination, and conduction velocity of affected nerve fibers. Clinically, the order of loss of nerve function is as follows: (1) pain, (2) temperature, (3) touch, (4) proprioception, and (5) skeletal muscle tone.

Systemic absorption of local anesthetics produces effects on the cardiovascular and central nervous systems (CNS). At blood concentrations achieved with normal therapeutic doses, changes in cardiac conduction, excitability, refractoriness, contractility, and peripheral vascular resistance are minimal. However, toxic blood concentrations depress cardiac conduction and excitability, which may lead to atrioventricular block, ventricular arrhythmias, and cardiac arrest, sometimes resulting in fatalities. In addition, myocardial contractility is depressed and peripheral vasodilation occurs, leading to decreased cardiac output and arterial blood pressure. Recent clinical reports and animal research suggest that these cardiovascular changes are more likely to occur after unintended direct intravascular injection of bupivacaine. Therefore, when epidural anesthesia with bupivacaine hydrochloride is considered, incremental dosing is necessary.

Following systemic absorption, local anesthetics can produce central nervous system stimulation, depression, or both. Apparent central stimulation is manifested as restlessness, tremors and shivering, progressing to convulsions, followed by depression and coma progressing ultimately to respiratory arrest. However, the local anesthetics have a primary depressant effect on the medulla and on higher centers. The depressed stage may occur without a prior excited stage.

Pharmacokinetics: The rate of systemic absorption of local anesthetics is dependent upon the total dose and concentration of drug administered, the route of administration, the

Continued on next page

This product information was prepared in September 1996. On these and other products of Sanofi Winthrop Pharmaceuticals, detailed information may be obtained on a current basis by direct inquiry to Product Information Services, 90 Park Avenue, New York, NY 10016 (toll free 1-800-446-6267).

Consult 1997 supplements and future editions for revisions

Sanofi Winthrop—Cont.

vascularity of the administraton site, and the presence or absence of epinephrine in the anesthetic solution. A dilute concentration of epinephrine (1:200,000 or 5 μg/mL) usually reduces the rate of absorption and peak plasma concentration of MARCAINE, permitting the use of moderately larger total doses and sometimes prolonging the duration of action.

The onset of action with MARCAINE is rapid and anesthesia is long lasting. The duration of anesthesia is significantly longer with MARCAINE than with any other commonly used local anesthetic. It has also been noted that there is a period of analgesia that persists after the return of sensation, during which time the need for strong analgesics is reduced.

The onset of sensory blockade following spinal block with MARCAINE Spinal is very rapid (within one minute); maximum motor blockade and maximum dermatome level are achieved within 15 minutes in most cases. Duration of sensory blockade (time to return of complete sensation in the operative site or regression of two dermatomes) following a 12 mg dose averages 2 hours with or without 0.2 mg epinephrine. The time to return of complete motor ability with 12 mg MARCAINE Spinal averages 3½ hours without the addition of epinephrine and 4½ hours if 0.2 mg epinephrine is added. When compared to equal milligram doses of hyperbaric tetracaine, the duration of sensory blockade was the same but the time to complete motor recovery was significantly longer for tetracaine. Addition of 0.2 mg epinephrine significantly prolongs the motor blockade and time to first postoperative narcotic with MARCAINE Spinal.

Local anesthetics appear to cross the placenta by passive diffusion. The rate and degree of diffusion is governed by (1) the degree of plasma protein binding, (2) the degree of ionization, and (3) the degree of lipid solubility. Fetal/maternal ratios of local anesthetics appear to be inversely related to the degree of plasma protein binding, because only the free, unbound drug is available for placental transfer. MARCAINE with a high protein binding capacity (95%) has a low fetal/maternal ratio (0.2 to 0.4). The extent of placental transfer is also determined by the degree of ionization and lipid solubility of the drug. Lipid soluble, nonionized drugs readily enter the fetal blood from the maternal circulation.

Depending upon the route of administration, local anesthetics are distributed to some extent to all body tissues, with high concentrations found in highly perfused organs such as the liver, lungs, heart, and brain.

Pharmacokinetic studies on the plasma profiles of MARCAINE after direct intravenous injection suggest a three-compartment open model. The first compartment is represented by the rapid intravascular distribution of the drug. The second compartment represents the equilibration of the drug throughout the highly perfused organs such as the brain, myocardium, lungs, kidneys, and liver. The third compartment represents an equilibration of the drug with poorly perfused tissues, such as muscle and fat. The elimination of drug from tissue distribution depends largely upon the ability of binding sites in the circulation to carry it to the liver where it is metabolized.

Various pharmacokinetic parameters of the local anesthetics can be significantly altered by the presence of hepatic or renal disease, addition of epinephrine, factors affecting urinary pH, renal blood flow, the route of drug administration, and the age of the patient. The half-life of MARCAINE in adults is 2.7 hours and in neonates 8.1 hours.

Amide-type local anesthetics such as MARCAINE are metabolized primarily in the liver via conjugation with glucuronic acid. Patients with hepatic disease, especially those with severe hepatic disease, may be more susceptible to the potential toxicities of the amide-type local anesthetics. Pipecolylxylidine is the major metabolite of MARCAINE.

The kidney is the main excretory organ for most local anesthetics and their metabolites. Urinary excretion is affected by urinary perfusion and factors affecting urinary pH. Only 6% of bupivacaine is excreted unchanged in the urine.

When administered in recommended doses and concentrations, MARCAINE does not ordinarily produce irritation or tissue damage and does not cause methemoglobinemia.

INDICATIONS AND USAGE

MARCAINE Spinal, brand of bupivacaine hydrochloride in dextrose injection, is indicated for the production of subarachnoid block (spinal anesthesia).

Standard textbooks should be consulted to determine the accepted procedures and techniques for the administration of spinal anesthesia.

CONTRAINDICATIONS

MARCAINE Spinal is contraindicated in patients with a known hypersensitivity to it or to any local anesthetic agent of the amide-type.

The following conditions preclude the use of spinal anesthesia:

1. Severe hemorrhage, severe hypotension or shock and arrhythmias, such as complete heart block, which severely restrict cardiac output.
2. Local infection at the site of proposed lumbar puncture.
3. Septicemia.

WARNINGS

LOCAL ANESTHETICS SHOULD ONLY BE EMPLOYED BY CLINICIANS WHO ARE WELL VERSED IN DIAGNOSIS AND MANAGEMENT OF DOSE-RELATED TOXICITY AND OTHER ACUTE EMERGENCIES WHICH MIGHT ARISE FROM THE BLOCK TO BE EMPLOYED, AND THEN ONLY AFTER INSURING THE **IMMEDIATE** AVAILABILITY OF OXYGEN, OTHER RESUSCITATIVE DRUGS, CARDIOPULMONARY RESUSCITATIVE EQUIPMENT, AND THE PERSONNEL RESOURCES NEEDED FOR PROPER MANAGEMENT OF TOXIC REACTIONS AND RELATED EMERGENCIES. (See also ADVERSE REACTIONS and PRECAUTIONS.) DELAY IN PROPER MANAGEMENT OF DOSE-RELATED TOXICITY, UNDERVENTILATION FROM ANY CAUSE AND/OR ALTERED SENSITIVITY MAY LEAD TO THE DEVELOPMENT OF ACIDOSIS, CARDIAC ARREST, AND, POSSIBLY, DEATH.

Spinal anesthetics should not be injected during uterine contractions, because spinal fluid current may carry the drug further cephalad than desired.

A free flow of cerebrospinal fluid during the performance of spinal anesthesia is indicative of entry into the subarachnoid space. However, aspiration should be performed before the anesthetic solution is injected to confirm entry into the subarachnoid space and to avoid intravascular injection.

MARCAINE solutions containing epinephrine or other vasopressors should not be used concomitantly with ergot-type oxytocic drugs, because a severe persistent hypertension may occur. Likewise, solutions of MARCAINE containing a vasoconstrictor, such as epinephrine, should be used with extreme caution in patients receiving monoamine oxidase inhibitors (MAOI) or antidepressants of the triptyline or imipramine types, because severe prolonged hypertension may result.

Until further experience is gained in patients younger than 18 years, administration of MARCAINE in this age group is not recommended.

Mixing or the prior or intercurrent use of any other local anesthetic with MARCAINE cannot be recommended because of insufficient data on the clinical use of such mixtures.

PRECAUTIONS

General: The safety and effectiveness of spinal anesthetics depend on proper dosage, correct technique, adequate precautions, and readiness for emergencies. Resuscitative equipment, oxygen, and other resuscitative drugs should be available for immediate use. (See WARNINGS and ADVERSE REACTIONS.) The patient should have IV fluids running via an indwelling catheter to assure a functioning intravenous pathway. The lowest dosage of local anesthetic that results in effective anesthesia should be used. Aspiration for blood should be performed before injection and injection should be made slowly. Tolerance varies with the status of the patient. Elderly patients and acutely ill patients may require reduced doses. Reduced doses may also be indicated in patients with increased intra-abdominal pressure (including obstetrical patients), if otherwise suitable for spinal anesthesia.

There should be careful and constant monitoring of cardiovascular and respiratory (adequacy of ventilation) vital signs and the patient's state of consciousness after local anesthetic injection. Restlessness, anxiety, incoherent speech, lightheadedness, numbness and tingling of the mouth and lips, metallic taste, tinnitus, dizziness, blurred vision, tremors, depression, or drowsiness may be early warning signs of central nervous system toxicity.

Spinal anesthetics should be used with caution in patients with severe disturbances of cardiac rhythm, shock, or heart block.

Sympathetic blockade occurring during spinal anesthesia may result in peripheral vasodilation and hypotension, the extent depending on the number of dermatomes blocked. Blood pressure should, therefore, be carefully monitored especially in the early phases of anesthesia. Hypotension may be controlled by vasoconstrictors in dosages depending on the severity of hypotension and response of treatment. The level of anesthesia should be carefully monitored because it is not always controllable in spinal techniques.

Because amide-type local anesthetics such as MARCAINE are metabolized by the liver, these drugs, especially repeat doses, should be used cautiously in patients with hepatic disease. Patients with severe hepatic disease, because of their inability to metabolize local anesthetics normally, are at a greater risk of developing toxic plasma concentrations. Local anesthetics should also be used with caution in patients with impaired cardiovascular function because they may be less able to compensate for functional changes associated with the prolongation of AV conduction produced by these drugs. However, dosage recommendations for spinal anesthesia are much lower than dosage recommendations for other major blocks and most experience regarding hepatic and cardiovascular disease dose-related toxicity is derived from these other major blocks.

Serious dose-related cardiac arrhythmias may occur if preparations containing a vasoconstrictor such as epinephrine are employed in patients during or following the administration of potent inhalation agents. In deciding whether to use these products concurrently in the same patient, the combined action of both agents upon the myocardium, the concentration and volume of vasoconstrictor used, and the time since injection, when applicable, should be taken into account.

Many drugs used during the conduct of anesthesia are considered potential triggering agents for familial malignant hyperthermia. Because it is not known whether amide-type local anesthetics may trigger this reaction and because the need for supplemental general anesthesia cannot be predicted in advance, it is suggested that a standard protocol for management should be available. Early unexplained signs of tachycardia, tachypnea, labile blood pressure, and metabolic acidosis may precede temperature elevation. Successful outcome is dependent on early diagnosis, prompt discontinuance of the suspect triggering agent(s) and institution of treatment, including oxygen therapy, indicated supportive measures, and dantrolene. (Consult dantrolene sodium intravenous package insert before using.)

The following conditions may preclude the use of spinal anesthesia, depending upon the physician's evaluation of the situation and ability to deal with the complications or complaints which may occur:

- Preexisting diseases of the central nervous system, such as those attributable to pernicious anemia, poliomyelitis, syphilis, or tumor.
- Hematological disorders predisposing to coagulopathies or patients on anticoagulant therapy. Trauma to a blood vessel during the conduct of spinal anesthesia may, in some instances, result in uncontrollable central nervous system hemorrhage or soft tissue hemorrhage.
- Chronic backache and preoperative headache.
- Hypotension and hypertension.
- Technical problems (persistent paresthesias, persistent bloody tap).
- Arthritis or spinal deformity.
- Extremes of age.
- Psychosis or other causes of poor cooperation by the patient.

Information for Patients: When appropriate, patients should be informed in advance that they may experience temporary loss of sensation and motor activity, usually in the lower half of the body, following proper administration of spinal anesthesia. Also, when appropriate, the physician should discuss other information including adverse reactions in the MARCAINE Spinal package insert.

Clinically Significant Drug Interactions: The administration of local anesthetic solutions containing epinephrine or norepinephrine to patients receiving monoamine oxidase inhibitors or tricyclic antidepressants may produce severe, prolonged hypertension. Concurrent use of these agents should generally be avoided. In situations when concurrent therapy is necessary, careful patient monitoring is essential. Concurrent administration of vasopressor drugs and of ergot-type oxytocic drugs may cause severe persistent hypertension or cerebrovascular accidents.

Phenothiazines and butyrophenones may reduce or reverse the pressor effect of epinephrine.

Carcinogenesis, Mutagenesis, and Impairment of Fertility: Long-term studies in animals of most local anesthetics including bupivacaine hydrochloride to evaluate the carcinogenic potential have not been conducted. Mutagenic potential or the effect on fertility have not been determined. There is no evidence from human data that MARCAINE Spinal, brand of bupivacaine hydrochloride in dextrose injection, may be carcinogenic or mutagenic or that it impairs fertility.

Pregnancy Category C: Decreased pup survival in rats and an embryocidal effect in rabbits have been observed when bupivacaine hydrochloride was administered to these species in doses comparable to 230 and 130 times respectively the maximum recommended human spinal dose. There are no adequate and well-controlled studies in pregnant women of the effect of bupivacaine hydrochloride on the developing fetus. Bupivacaine hydrochloride should be used during pregnancy only if the potential benefit justifies the potential risk to the fetus. This does not exclude the use of MARCAINE Spinal at term for obstetrical anesthesia. (See ***Labor and Delivery.***)

Labor and Delivery: Spinal anesthesia has a recognized use during labor and delivery. Bupivacaine hydrochloride, when administered properly, via the epidural route in doses 10 to 12 times the amount used in spinal anesthesia has been used for obstetrical analgesia and anesthesia without evidence of adverse effects on the fetus.

Maternal hypotension has resulted from regional anesthesia. Local anesthetics produce vasodilation by blocking sympathetic nerves. Elevating the patient's legs and positioning her on her left side will help prevent decreases in blood pres-

sure. The fetal heart rate also should be monitored continuously and electronic fetal monitoring is highly advisable.
It is extremely important to avoid aortocaval compression by the gravid uterus during administrations of regional block to parturients. To do this, the patient must be maintained in the left lateral decubitus position or a blanket roll or sandbag may be placed beneath the right hip and the gravid uterus displaced to the left.
Spinal anesthesia may alter the forces of parturition through changes in uterine contractility or maternal expulsive efforts. Spinal anesthesia has also been reported to prolong the second stage of labor by removing the parturient's reflex urge to bear down or by interfering with motor function. The use of obstetrical anesthesia may increase the need for forceps assistance.
The use of some local anesthetic drug products during labor and delivery may be followed by diminished muscle strength and tone for the first day or two of life. This has not been reported with bupivacaine.
There have been reports of cardiac arrest during use of MARCAINE 0.75% solution for epidural anesthesia in obstetrical patients. The package insert for MARCAINE hydrochloride for epidural, nerve block, etc, has a more complete discussion of preparation for, and management of, this problem. These cases are compatible with systemic toxicity following unintended intravascular injection of the much larger doses recommended for epidural anesthesia and have not occurred within the dose range of bupivacaine hydrochloride 0.75% recommended for spinal anesthesia in obstetrics. The 0.75% concentration of MARCAINE is therefore not recommended for obstetrical epidural anesthesia. MARCAINE Spinal, brand of bupivacaine hydrochloride in dextrose injection, is recommended for spinal anesthesia in obstetrics.
Nursing Mothers: It is not known whether local anesthetic drugs are excreted in human milk. Because many drugs are excreted in human milk, caution should be exercised when local anesthetics are administered to a nursing woman.
Pediatric Use: Until further experience is gained in patients younger than 18 years, administration of MARCAINE Spinal in this age group is not recommended.

ADVERSE REACTIONS

Reactions to bupivacaine hydrochloride are characteristic of those associated with other amide-type local anesthetics.
The most commonly encountered acute adverse experiences which demand immediate countermeasures following the administration of spinal anesthesia are hypotension due to loss of sympathetic tone and respiratory paralysis or underventilation due to cephalad extension of the motor level of anesthesia. These may lead to cardiac arrest if untreated. In addition, dose-related convulsions and cardiovascular collapse may result from diminished tolerance, rapid absorption from the injection site, or from unintentional intravascular injection of a local anesthetic solution. Factors influencing plasma protein binding, such as acidosis, systemic diseases which alter protein production, or competition of other drugs for protein binding sites, may diminish individual tolerance.
Respiratory System: Respiratory paralysis or underventilation may be noted as a result of upward extension of the level of spinal anesthesia and may lead to secondary hypoxic cardiac arrest if untreated. Preanesthetic medication, intraoperative analgesics and sedatives, as well as surgical manipulation, may contribute to underventilation. This will usually be noted within minutes of the injection of spinal anesthetic solution, but because of differing maximal onset times, differing intercurrent drug usage and differing surgical manipulation, it may occur at any time during surgery or the immediate recovery period.
Cardiovascular System: Hypotension due to loss of sympathetic tone is a commonly encountered extension of the clinical pharmacology of spinal anesthesia. This is more commonly observed in patients with shrunken blood volume, shrunken interstitial fluid volume, cephalad spread of the local anesthetic, and/or mechanical obstruction of venous return. Nausea and vomiting are frequently associated with hypotensive episodes following the administration of spinal anesthesia. High doses, or inadvertent intravascular injection, may lead to high plasma levels and related depression of the myocardium, decreased cardiac output, bradycardia, heart block, ventricular arrhythmias, and, possibly, cardiac arrest. (See **WARNINGS, PRECAUTIONS,** and **OVERDOSAGE** sections.)
Central Nervous System: Respiratory paralysis or underventilation secondary to cephalad spread of the level of spinal anesthesia (see *Respiratory System*) and hypotension for the same reason (see *Cardiovascular System*) are the two most commonly encountered central nervous system-related adverse observations which demand immediate countermeasures.
High doses or inadvertent intravascular injection may lead to high plasma levels and related central nervous system toxicity characterized by excitement and/or depression. Restlessness, anxiety, dizziness, tinnitus, blurred vision, or tremors may occur, possibly proceeding to convulsions. However, excitement may be transient or absent, with depression being the first manifestation of an adverse reaction. This may quickly be followed by drowsiness merging into unconsciousness and respiratory arrest.
Neurologic: The incidences of adverse neurologic reactions associated with the use of local anesthetics may be related to the total dose of local anesthetic administered and are also dependent upon the particular drug used, the route of administration, and the physical status of the patient. Many of these effects may be related to local anesthetic techniques, with or without a contribution from the drug.
Neurologic effects following spinal anesthesia may include loss of perineal sensation and sexual function; persistent anesthesia, paresthesia, weakness and paralysis of the lower extremities, and loss of sphincter control all of which may have slow, incomplete, or no recovery; hypotension; high or total spinal block; urinary retention; headache; backache; septic meningitis; meningismus; arachnoiditis; slowing of labor; increased incidence of forceps delivery; shivering; cranial nerve palsies due to traction on nerves from loss of cerebrospinal fluid; and fecal and urinary incontinence.
Allergic: Allergic-type reactions are rare and may occur as a result of sensitivity to the local anesthetic. These reactions are characterized by signs such as urticaria, pruritus, erythema, angioneurotic edema (including laryngeal edema), tachycardia, sneezing, nausea, vomiting, dizziness, syncope, excessive sweating, elevated temperature, and, possibly, anaphylactoid-like symptomatology (including severe hypotension). Cross sensitivity among members of the amide-type local anesthetic group has been reported. The usefulness of screening for sensitivity has not been definitely established.
Other: Nausea and vomiting may occur during spinal anesthesia.

OVERDOSAGE

Acute emergencies from local anesthetics are generally related to high plasma levels encountered during therapeutic use or to underventilation (and perhaps apnea) secondary to upward extension of spinal anesthesia. Hypotension is commonly encountered during the conduct of spinal anesthesia due to relaxation of sympathetic tone, and sometimes, contributory mechanical obstruction of venous return.
Management of Local Anesthetic Emergencies: The first consideration is prevention, best accomplished by careful and constant monitoring of cardiovascular and respiratory vital signs and the patient's state of consciousness after each local anesthetic injection. At the first sign of change, oxygen should be administered.
The first step in the management of systemic toxic reactions, as well as underventilation or apnea due to a high or total spinal, consists of ***immediate*** *attention to the establishment and maintenance of a patent airway and effective assisted or controlled ventilation with 100% oxygen with a delivery system capable of permitting immediate positive airway pressure by mask.* This may prevent convulsions if they have not already occurred.
If necessary, use drugs to control the convulsions. A 50 mg to 100 mg bolus IV injection of succinylcholine will paralyze the patient without depressing the central nervous or cardiovascular systems and facilitate ventilation. A bolus IV dose of 5 mg to 10 mg of diazepam or 50 mg to 100 mg of thiopental will permit ventilation and counteract central nervous system stimulation, but these drugs also depress central nervous system, respiratory and cardiac function, add to postictal depression and may result in apnea. Intravenous barbiturates, anticonvulsant agents, or muscle relaxants should only be administered by those familiar with their use. Immediately after the institution of these ventilatory measures, the adequacy of the circulation should be evaluated. Supportive treatment of circulatory depression may require administration of intravenous fluids, and, when appropriate, a vasopressor dictated by the clinical situation (such as ephedrine or epinephrine to enhance myocardial contractile force).
Hypotension due to sympathetic relaxation may be managed by giving intravenous fluids (such as isotonic saline or lactated Ringer's solution), in an attempt to relieve mechanical obstruction of venous return, or by using vasopressors (such as ephedrine which increases the force of myocardial contractions) and, if indicated, by giving plasma expanders or whole blood.
Endotracheal intubation, employing drugs and techniques familiar to the clinician, may be indicated after initial administration of oxygen by mask if difficulty is encountered in the maintenance of a patent airway, or if prolonged ventilatory support (assisted or controlled) is indicated.
Recent clinical data from patients experiencing local anesthetic-induced convulsions demonstrated rapid development of hypoxia, hypercarbia, and acidosis with bupivacaine hydrochloride within a minute of the onset of convulsions. These observations suggest that oxygen consumption and carbon dioxide production are greatly increased during local anesthetic convulsions and emphasize the importance of immediate and effective ventilation with oxygen which may avoid cardiac arrest.
If not treated immediately, convulsions with simultaneous hypoxia, hypercarbia, and acidosis plus myocardial depression from the direct effects of the local anesthetic may result in cardiac arrhythmias, bradycardia, asystole, ventricular fibrillation, or cardiac arrest. Respiratory abnormalities, including apnea, may occur. Underventilation or apnea due to a high or total spinal may produce these same signs and also lead to cardiac arrest if ventilatory support is not instituted. If cardiac arrest should occur, standard cardiopulmonary resuscitative measures should be instituted and maintained for a prolonged period if necessary. Recovery has been reported after prolonged resuscitative efforts.
The supine position is dangerous in pregnant women at term because of aortocaval compression by the gravid uterus. Therefore during treatment of systemic toxicity, maternal hypotension, or fetal bradycardia following regional block, the parturient should be maintained in the left lateral decubitus position if possible, or manual displacement of the uterus off the great vessels be accomplished.
The mean seizure dosage of bupivacaine in rhesus monkeys was found to be 4.4 mg/kg with mean arterial plasma concentration of 4.5 µg/mL. The intravenous and subcutaneous LD_{50} in mice is 6 mg/kg to 8 mg/kg and 38 mg/kg to 54 mg/kg respectively.

DOSAGE AND ADMINISTRATION

The dose of any local anesthetic administered varies with the anesthetic procedure, the area to be anesthetized, the vascularity of the tissues, the number of neuronal segments to be blocked, the depth of anesthesia and degree of muscle relaxation required, the duration of anesthesia desired, individual tolerance, and the physical condition of the patient. The smallest dose and concentration required to produce the desired result should be administered. Dosages of MARCAINE Spinal, brand of bupivacaine hydrochloride in dextrose injection, should be reduced for elderly and debilitated patients and patients with cardiac and/or liver disease.
For specific techniques and procedures, refer to standard textbooks.
The extent and degree of spinal anesthesia depend upon several factors including dosage, specific gravity of the anesthetic solution, volume of solution used, force of injection, level of puncture, and position of the patient during and immediately after injection.
Seven and one-half mg (7.5 mg or 1.0 mL) MARCAINE Spinal has generally proven satisfactory for spinal anesthesia for lower extremity and perineal procedures including TURP and vaginal hysterectomy. Twelve mg (12.0 mg or 1.6 mL) has been used for lower abdominal procedures such as abdominal hysterectomy, tubal ligation, and appendectomy. These doses are recommended as a guide for use in the average adult and may be reduced for the elderly or debilitated patients. Because experience with MARCAINE Spinal is limited in patients below the age of 18 years, dosage recommendations in this age group cannot be made.
Obstetrical Use: Doses as low as 6 mg bupivacaine hydrochloride have been used for vaginal delivery under spinal anesthesia. The dose range of 7.5 mg to 10.5 mg (1 mL to 1.4 mL) bupivacaine hydrochloride has been used for Cesarean section under spinal anesthesia.
In recommended doses, MARCAINE Spinal produces complete motor and sensory block.
Unused portions of solutions should be discarded following initial use.
MARCAINE Spinal should be inspected visually for discoloration and particulate matter prior to administration; solutions which are discolored or which contain particulate matter should not be administered.

HOW SUPPLIED

Single-dose ampuls of 2 mL (15 mg bupivacaine hydrochloride with 165 mg dextrose), in Uni-Nest™ Unit Dose Pak of 10 (NDC 0024-1229-10)
Store at controlled room temperature, between 15° C and 30° C (59° F and 86° F).
MARCAINE Spinal solution may be autoclaved once at 15 pound pressure, 121° C (250° F) for 15 minutes. Do not administer any solution which is discolored or contains particulate matter.

MSW-7

Continued on next page

This product information was prepared in September 1996. On these and other products of Sanofi Winthrop Pharmaceuticals, detailed information may be obtained on a current basis by direct inquiry to Product Information Services, 90 Park Avenue, New York, NY 10016 (toll free 1-800-446-6267).

Sanofi Winthrop—Cont.

MEBARAL® ℂ ℞
brand of mephobarbital tablets, USP

DESCRIPTION

Mephobarbital, 5-Ethyl-1-methyl-5-phenylbarbituric acid, is a barbiturate with sedative, hypnotic, and anticonvulsant properties. It occurs as a white, nearly odorless, tasteless powder and is slightly soluble in water and in alcohol.
MEBARAL is available as tablets for oral administration.
Inactive Ingredients: Lactose, Starch, Stearic Acid, Talc.

CLINICAL PHARMACOLOGY

Barbiturates are capable of producing all levels of CNS mood alteration from excitation to mild sedation, to hypnosis, and deep coma. Overdosage can produce death. In high enough therapeutic doses, barbiturates induce anesthesia.
Barbiturates depress the sensory cortex, decrease motor activity, alter cerebellar function, and produce drowsiness, sedation, and hypnosis.
Barbiturates are respiratory depressants. The degree of respiratory depression is dependent upon dose. With hypnotic doses, respiratory depression produced by barbiturates is similar to that which occurs during physiologic sleep with slight decrease in blood pressure and heart rate.
Studies in laboratory animals have shown that barbiturates cause reduction in the tone and contractility of the uterus, ureters, and urinary bladder. However, concentrations of the drugs required to produce this effect in humans are not reached with sedative-hypnotic doses.
Barbiturates do not impair normal hepatic function, but have been shown to induce liver microsomal enzymes, thus increasing and/or altering the metabolism of barbiturates and other drugs. (See PRECAUTIONS—Drug Interactions.)
MEBARAL exerts a strong sedative and anticonvulsant action but has a relatively mild hypnotic effect. It reduces the incidence of epileptic seizures in grand mal and petit mal. MEBARAL usually causes little or no drowsiness or lassitude. Hence, when it is used as a sedative or anticonvulsant, patients usually become more calm, more cheerful, and better adjusted to their surroundings without clouding of mental faculties. MEBARAL is reported to produce less sedation than does phenobarbital.
Barbiturates are weak acids that are absorbed and rapidly distributed to all tissues and fluids with high concentrations in the brain, liver, and kidneys. Lipid solubility of the barbiturates is the dominant factor in their distribution within the body. Barbiturates are bound to plasma and tissue proteins to a varying degree with the degree of binding increasing directly as a function of lipid solubility.
Approximately 50% of an oral dose of mephobarbital is absorbed from the gastrointestinal tract. Therapeutic plasma concentrations for mephobarbital have not been established nor has the half-life been determined. Following oral administration, the onset of action of the drug is 30 to 60 minutes and the duration of action is 10 to 16 hours. The primary route of mephobarbital metabolism is N-demethylation by the microsomal enzymes of the liver to form phenobarbital. Phenobarbital may be excreted in the urine unchanged or further metabolized to *p*-hydroxyphenobarbital and excreted in the urine as glucuronide or sulfate conjugates. About 75% of a single oral dose of mephobarbital is converted to phenobarbital in 24 hours.
Therefore, chronic administration of mephobarbital may lead to an accumulation of phenobarbital (not mephobarbital) in plasma. It has not been determined whether mephobarbital or phenobarbital is the active agent during long-time mephobarbital therapy.

INDICATIONS AND USAGE

MEBARAL is indicated for use as a sedative for the relief of anxiety, tension, and apprehension, and as an anticonvulsant for the treatment of grand mal and petit mal epilepsy.

CONTRAINDICATIONS

Hypersensitivity to any barbiturate. Manifest or latent porphyria.

WARNINGS

Habit Forming
Barbiturates may be habit forming. Tolerance, psychological, and physical dependence may occur with continued use. (See DRUG ABUSE AND DEPENDENCE and CLINICAL PHARMACOLOGY.) Patients who have psychological dependence on barbiturates may increase the dosage or decrease the dosage interval without consulting a physician and may subsequently develop a physical dependence on barbiturates. To minimize the possibility of overdosage or the development of dependence, the prescribing and dispensing of sedative-hypnotic barbiturates should be limited to the amount required for the interval until the next appointment. Abrupt cessation after prolonged use in the dependent person may result in withdrawal symptoms, including delirium, convulsions, and possibly death. Barbiturates should be withdrawn gradually from any patient known to be taking excessive dosage over long periods of time. (See DRUG ABUSE AND DEPENDENCE.)

Acute or Chronic Pain
Caution should be exercised when barbiturates are administered to patients with acute or chronic pain, because paradoxical excitement could be induced or important symptoms could be masked. However, the use of barbiturates as sedatives in the postoperative surgical period and as adjuncts to cancer chemotherapy is well established.

Use in Pregnancy
Barbiturates can cause fetal damage when administered to a pregnant woman. Retrospective, case-controlled studies have suggested a connection between the maternal consumption of barbiturates and a higher than expected incidence of fetal abnormalities. Following oral or parenteral administration, barbiturates readily cross the placental barrier and are distributed throughout fetal tissues with highest concentrations found in the placenta, fetal liver, and brain. Fetal blood levels approach maternal blood levels following parenteral administration.
Withdrawal symptoms occur in infants born to mothers who receive barbiturates throughout the last trimester of pregnancy. (See DRUG ABUSE AND DEPENDENCE.) If this drug is used during pregnancy, or if the patient becomes pregnant while taking this drug, the patient should be apprised of the potential hazard to the fetus.

Synergistic Effects
The concomitant use of alcohol or other CNS depressants may produce additive CNS depressant effects.

PRECAUTIONS

General
Barbiturates may be habit forming. Tolerance and psychological and physical dependence may occur with continuing use. (See DRUG ABUSE AND DEPENDENCE.) Barbiturates should be administered with caution, if at all, to patients who are mentally depressed, have suicidal tendencies, or a history of drug abuse.
Elderly or debilitated patients may react to barbiturates with marked excitement, depression, and confusion. In some persons, barbiturates repeatedly produce excitement rather than depression.
In patients with hepatic damage, barbiturates should be administered with caution and initially in reduced doses. Barbiturates should not be administered to patients showing the premonitory signs of hepatic coma.
Status epilepticus may result from the abrupt discontinuation of MEBARAL, even when administered in small daily doses in the treatment of epilepsy.
Caution and careful adjustment of dosage are required when MEBARAL, brand of mephobarbital tablets, is used in patients with impaired renal, cardiac, or respiratory function and in patients with myasthenia gravis and myxedema. The least quantity feasible should be prescribed or dispensed at any one time in order to minimize the possibility of acute or chronic overdosage.
Vitamin D Deficiency: MEBARAL may increase vitamin D requirements, possibly by increasing vitamin D metabolism via enzyme induction. Rarely, rickets and osteomalacia have been reported following prolonged use of barbiturates.
Vitamin K: Bleeding in the early neonatal period due to coagulation defects may follow exposure to anticonvulsant drugs *in utero;* therefore, vitamin K should be given to the mother before delivery or to the child at birth.

Information for the Patient
Practitioners should give the following information and instructions to patients receiving barbiturates.
1. The use of barbiturates carries with it an associated risk of psychological and/or physical dependence. The patient should be warned against increasing the dose of the drug without consulting a physician.
2. Barbiturates may impair mental and/or physical abilities required for the performance of potentially hazardous tasks (eg, driving, operating machinery, etc).
3. Alcohol should not be consumed while taking barbiturates. Concurrent use of the barbiturates with other CNS depressants (eg, alcohol, narcotics, tranquilizers, and antihistamines) may result in additional CNS depressant effects.

Laboratory Tests
Prolonged therapy with barbiturates should be accompanied by periodic laboratory evaluation of organ systems, including hematopoietic, renal, and hepatic systems. (See PRECAUTIONS [General] and ADVERSE REACTIONS.)

Drug Interactions
Most reports of clinically significant drug interactions occurring with the barbiturates have involved phenobarbital. However, the application of these data to other barbiturates appears valid and warrants serial blood level determinations of the relevant drugs when there are multiple therapies.
1. *Anticoagulants.* Phenobarbital lowers the plasma levels of dicumarol (name previously used: bishydroxycoumarin) and causes a decrease in anticoagulant activity as measured by the prothrombin time. Barbiturates can induce hepatic microsomal enzymes resulting in increased metabolism and decreased anticoagulant response of oral anticoagulants (eg, warfarin, acenocoumarol, dicumarol, and phenprocoumon). Patients stabilized on anticoagulant therapy may require dosage adjustments if barbiturates are added to or withdrawn from their dosage regimen.
2. *Corticosteroids.* Barbiturates appear to enhance the metabolism of exogenous corticosteroids probably through the induction of hepatic microsomal enzymes. Patients stabilized on corticosteroid therapy may require dosage adjustments if barbiturates are added to or withdrawn from their dosage regimen.
3. *Griseofulvin.* Phenobarbital appears to interfere with the absorption of orally administered griseofulvin, thus decreasing its blood level. The effect of the resultant decreased blood levels of griseofulvin on therapeutic response has not been established. However, it would be preferable to avoid concomitant administration of these drugs.
4. *Doxycycline.* Phenobarbital has been shown to shorten the half-life of doxycycline for as long as 2 weeks after barbiturate therapy is discontinued.
This mechanism is probably through the induction of hepatic microsomal enzymes that metabolize the antibiotic. If phenobarbital and doxycycline are administered concurrently, the clinical response to doxycycline should be monitored closely.
5. *Phenytoin, Sodium Valproate, Valproic Acid.* The effect of barbiturates on the metabolism of phenytoin appears to be variable. Some investigators report an accelerating effect, while others report no effect. Because the effect of barbiturates on the metabolism of phenytoin is not predictable, phenytoin and barbiturate blood levels should be monitored more frequently if these drugs are given concurrently. Sodium valproate and valproic acid appear to decrease barbiturate metabolism; therefore, barbiturate blood levels should be monitored and appropriate dosage adjustments made as indicated.
6. *Central Nervous System Depressants.* The concomitant use of other central nervous system depressants, including other sedatives or hypnotics, antihistamines, tranquilizers, or alcohol, may produce additive depressant effects.
7. *Monoamine Oxidase Inhibitors (MAOI).* MAOI prolong the effects of barbiturates probably because metabolism of the barbiturate is inhibited.
8. *Estradiol, Estone, Progesterone, and other Steroidal Hormones.* Pretreatment with or concurrent administration of phenobarbital may decrease the effect of estradiol by increasing its metabolism. There have been reports of patients treated with antiepileptic drugs (eg, phenobarbital) who become pregnant while taking oral contraceptives. An alternant contraceptive method might be suggested to women taking phenobarbital.

Carcinogenesis
Animal Data. Phenobarbital sodium is carcinogenic in mice and rats after lifetime administration. In mice, it produced benign and malignant liver cell tumors. In rats, benign liver cell tumors were observed very late in life. Phenobarbital is the major metabolite of MEBARAL.
Human Data. In a 29-year epidemiological study of 9,136 patients who were treated on an anticonvulsant protocol which included phenobarbital, results indicated a higher than normal incidence of hepatic carcinoma. Previously, some of these patients were treated with thorotrast, a drug which is known to produce hepatic carcinomas. Thus, this study did not provide sufficient evidence that phenobarbital sodium is carcinogenic in humans. Phenobarbital is the major metabolite of MEBARAL, brand of mephobarbital tablets.
A retrospective study of 84 children with brain tumors matched to 73 normal controls and 78 cancer controls (malignant disease other than brain tumors) suggested an association between exposure to barbiturates prenatally and an increased incidence of brain tumors.

Pregnancy
Teratogenic Effects. Pregnancy Category D—See WARNINGS—Use in Pregnancy.
Nonteratogenic Effects. Reports of infants suffering from long-term barbiturate exposure *in utero* included the acute withdrawal syndrome of seizures and hyperirritability from birth to a delayed onset of up to 14 days. (See DRUG ABUSE AND DEPENDENCE.)

Labor and Delivery.
Hypnotic doses of these barbiturates do not appear to significantly impair uterine activity during labor. Full anesthetic doses of barbiturates decrease the force and frequency of uterine contractions. Administration of sedative-hypnotic barbiturates to the mother during labor may result in respiratory depression in the newborn. Premature infants are particularly susceptible to the depressant effects of barbiturates. If barbiturates are used during labor and delivery, resuscitation equipment should be available.
Data are currently not available to evaluate the effect of these barbiturates when forceps delivery or other intervention is necessary. Also, data are not available to determine the effect of these barbiturates on the later growth, development, and functional maturation of the child.

Nursing Mothers.
Caution should be exercised when a barbiturate is administered to a nursing woman since small amounts of barbiturates are excreted in the milk.

ADVERSE REACTIONS

The following adverse reactions and their incidence were compiled from surveillance of thousands of hospitalized patients. Because such patients may be less aware of certain of the milder adverse effects of barbiturates, the incidence of these reactions may be somewhat higher in fully ambulatory patients.
More than 1 in 100 Patients. The most common adverse reaction estimated to occur at a rate of 1 to 3 patients per 100 is:
Nervous System: Somnolence.
Less than 1 in 100 Patients. Adverse reactions estimated to occur at a rate of less than 1 in 100 patients listed below, grouped by organ system, and by decreasing order of occurrence are:
Nervous System: Agitation, confusion, hyperkinesia, ataxia, CNS depression, nightmares, nervousness, psychiatric disturbance, hallucinations, insomnia, anxiety, dizziness, thinking abnormality.
Respiratory System: Hypoventilation, apnea.
Cardiovascular System: Bradycardia, hypotension, syncope.
Digestive System: Nausea, vomiting, constipation.
Other Reported Reactions: Headache, hypersensitivity reactions (angioedema, skin rashes, exfoliative dermatitis), fever, liver damage, megaloblastic anemia following chronic phenobarbital use.

DRUG ABUSE AND DEPENDENCE

Mephobarbital is a controlled substance in Narcotic Schedule IV. Barbiturates may be habit forming. Tolerance, psychological dependence, and physical dependence may occur especially following prolonged use of high doses of barbiturates. As tolerance to barbiturates develops, the amount needed to maintain the same level of intoxication increases; tolerance to a fatal dosage, however, does not increase more than two-fold. As this occurs, the margin between an intoxicating dosage and fatal dosage becomes smaller.
Symptoms of acute intoxication with barbiturates include unsteady gait, slurred speech, and sustained nystagmus. Mental signs of chronic intoxication include confusion, poor judgment, irritability, insomnia, and somatic complaints.
Symptoms of barbiturate dependence are similar to those of chronic alcoholism. If an individual appears to be intoxicated with alcohol to a degree that is radically disproportionate to the amount of alcohol in his or her blood the use of barbiturates should be suspected. The lethal dose of a barbiturate is far less if alcohol is also ingested.
The symptoms of barbiturate withdrawal can be severe and may cause death. Minor withdrawal symptoms may appear 8 to 12 hours after the last dose of a barbiturate. These symptoms usually appear in the following order: anxiety, muscle twitching, tremor of hands and fingers, progressive weakness, dizziness, distortion in visual perception, nausea, vomiting, insomnia, and orthostatic hypotension. Major withdrawal symptoms (convulsions and delirium) may occur within 16 hours and last up to 5 days after abrupt cessation of these drugs. Intensity of withdrawal symptoms gradually declines over a period of approximately 15 days. Individuals susceptible to a barbiturate abuse and dependence include alcoholics and opiate abusers, as well as other sedative-hypnotic and amphetamine abusers.
Drug dependence to barbiturates arises from repeated administration of a barbiturate or agent with barbiturate-like effect on a continuous basis, generally in amounts exceeding therapeutic dose levels. The characteristics of drug dependence to barbiturates include: (a) a strong desire or need to continue taking the drug; (b) a tendency to increase the dose; (c) a psychic dependence on the effects of the drug related to subjective and individual appreciation of those effects; and (d) a physical dependence on the effects of the drug requiring its presence for maintenance of homeostasis and resulting in a definite, characteristic, and self-limited abstinence syndrome when the drug is withdrawn.
Treatment of barbiturate dependence consists of cautious and gradual withdrawal of the drug. Barbiturate-dependent patients can be withdrawn by using a number of different withdrawal regimens. In all cases withdrawal takes an extended period of time. One method involves substituting a 30 mg dose of phenobarbital for each 100 mg to 200 mg dose of barbiturate that the patient has been taking. The total daily amount of phenobarbital is then administered in 3 to 4 divided doses, not to exceed 600 mg daily. Should signs of withdrawal occur on the first day of treatment, a loading dose of 100 mg to 200 mg of phenobarbital may be administered IM in addition to the oral dose. After stabilization on phenobarbital, the total daily dose is decreased by 30 mg a day as long as withdrawal is proceeding smoothly. A modification of this regimen involves initiating treatment at the patient's regular dosage level and decreasing the daily dosage by 10% if tolerated by the patient.
Infants physically dependent on barbiturates may be given phenobarbital 3 mg/kg/day to 10 mg/kg/day. After withdrawal symptoms (hyperactivity, disturbed sleep, tremors, hyperreflexia) are relieved, the dosage of phenobarbital should be gradually decreased and completely withdrawn over a 2-week period.

OVERDOSAGE

The toxic dose of barbiturates varies considerably. In general, an oral dose of 1 g of most barbiturates produces serious poisoning in an adult. Death commonly occurs after 2 g to 10 g of ingested barbiturate. Barbiturate intoxication may be confused with alcoholism, bromide intoxication, and with various neurological disorders.
Acute overdosage with barbiturates is manifested by CNS and respiratory depression which may progress to Cheyne-Stokes respiration, areflexia, constriction of the pupils to a slight degree (though in severe poisoning they may show paralytic dilation), oliguria, tachycardia, hypotension, lowered body temperature, and coma. Typical shock syndrome (apnea, circulatory collapse, respiratory arrest, and death) may occur.
In extreme overdose, all electrical activity in the brain may cease, in which case a "flat" EEG normally equated with clinical death cannot be accepted. This effect is fully reversible unless hypoxic damage occurs. Consideration should be given to the possibility of barbiturate intoxication even in situations that appear to involve trauma.
Complications such as pneumonia, pulmonary edema, cardiac arrhythmias, congestive heart failure, and renal failure may occur. Uremia may increase CNS sensitivity to barbiturates if renal function is impaired. Differential diagnosis should include hypoglycemia, head trauma, cerebrovascular accidents, convulsive states, and diabetic coma.
Treatment of overdosage is mainly supportive and consists of the following:

1. Maintenance of an adequate airway, with assisted respiration and oxygen administration as necessary.
2. Monitoring of vital signs and fluid balance.
3. If the patient is conscious and has not lost the gag reflex, emesis may be induced with ipecac. Care should be taken to prevent pulmonary aspiration of vomitus. After completion of vomiting, 30 g activated charcoal in a glass of water may be administered.
4. If emesis is contraindicated, gastric lavage may be performed with a cuffed endotracheal tube in place with the patient in the face down position. Activated charcoal may be left in the emptied stomach and a saline cathartic administered.
5. Fluid therapy and other standard treatment for shock, if needed.
6. If renal function is normal, forced diuresis may aid in the elimination of the barbiturate. Alkalinization of the urine increases renal excretion of some barbiturates, including mephobarbital (which is metabolized to phenobarbital).
7. Although not recommended as a routine procedure, hemodialysis may be used in severe barbiturate intoxications or if the patient is anuric or in shock.
8. Patient should be rolled from side to side every 30 minutes.
9. Antibiotics should be given if pneumonia is suspected.
10. Appropriate nursing care to prevent hypostatic pneumonia, decubiti aspiration, and other complications of patients with altered states of consciousness.

DOSAGE AND ADMINISTRATION

Epilepsy: Average dose for adults: 400 mg to 600 mg (6 grains to 9 grains) daily; children under 5 years: 16 mg to 32 mg ($^1/_4$ grain to $^1/_2$ grain) three or four times daily; children over 5 years: 32 mg to 64 mg ($^1/_2$ grain to 1 grain) three or four times daily. MEBARAL is best taken at bedtime if seizures generally occur at night, and during the day if attacks are diurnal. Treatment should be started with a small dose which is gradually increased over four or five days until the optimum dosage is determined. If the patient has been taking some other antiepileptic drug, it should be tapered off as the doses of MEBARAL are increased, to guard against the temporary marked attacks that may occur when any treatment for epilepsy is changed abruptly. Similarly, when the dose is to be lowered to a maintenance level or to be discontinued, the amount should be reduced gradually over four or five days.
Special Patient Population. Dosage should be reduced in the elderly or debilitated because these patients may be more sensitive to barbiturates. Dosage should be reduced for patients with impaired renal function or hepatic disease.
Combination with Other Drugs: MEBARAL may be used in combination with phenobarbital, either in the form of alternating courses or concurrently. When the two drugs are used at the same time, the dose should be about one-half the amount of each used alone. The average daily dose for an adult is from 50 mg to 100 mg ($^3/_4$ grain to $1^1/_2$ grains) of phenobarbital and from 200 mg to 300 mg (3 grains to $4^1/_2$ grains) of MEBARAL, brand of mephobarbital tablets.
MEBARAL may also be used with phenytoin sodium; in some cases, combined therapy appears to give better results than either agent used alone, since phenytoin sodium is particularly effective for the psychomotor types of seizure but relatively ineffective for petit mal. When the drugs are employed concurrently, a reduced dose of phenytoin sodium is advisable, but the full dose of MEBARAL may be given. Satisfactory results have been obtained with an average daily dose of 230 mg ($3^1/_2$ grains) of phenytoin sodium plus about 600 mg (9 grains) of MEBARAL.
Sedation: Adults: 32 mg to 100 mg ($^1/_2$ grain to $1^1/_2$ grains) —optimum dose, 50 mg ($^3/_4$ grain)—three to four times daily. Children: 16 mg to 32 mg ($^1/_4$ grain to $^1/_2$ grain) three to four times daily.

HOW SUPPLIED

Tablets
32 mg ($^1/_2$ grain), bottles of 250
(NDC 0024-1231-05)
50 mg ($^3/_4$ grain), bottles of 250
(NDC 0024-1232-05)
100 mg ($1^1/_2$ grains), bottles of 250
(NDC 0024-1233-05)

MSW-9

NegGram® ℞
NALIDIXIC ACID, USP

DESCRIPTION

NegGram®, brand of nalidixic acid, is a quinolone antibacterial agent for oral administration. Nalidixic acid is 1-ethyl-1, 4-dihydro-7-methyl-4-oxo-1, 8-naphthyridine-3-carboxylic acid. It a pale yellow, crystalline substance and a very weak organic acid.
Nalidixic acid has the following structural formula:

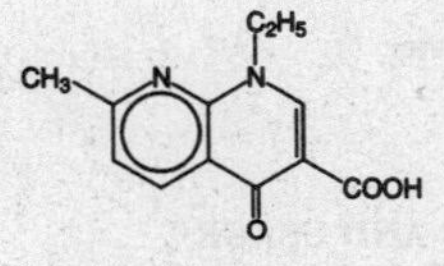

Inactive Ingredients—SUSPENSION: Carbomer 934P, FD&C Red #40, Flavor, Parabens, Purified Water, Saccharin Sodium, Sodium Chloride, Sorbitol Solution. CAPLETS: Hydrogenated Vegetable Oil, Methylcellulose, Microcrystalline Cellulose, Sodium Lauryl Sulfate, Yellow Ferric Oxide.

CLINICAL PHARMACOLOGY

Following oral administration, NegGram is rapidly absorbed from the gastrointestinal tract, partially metabolized in the liver, and rapidly excreted through the kidneys. Unchanged nalidixic acid appears in the urine along with an active metabolite, hydroxynalidixic acid, which has antibacterial activity similar to that of nalidixic acid. Other metabolites include glucuronic acid conjugates of nalidixic acid and hydroxy nalidixic acid, and the dicarboxylic acid derivative. The hydroxy metabolite represents 30 percent of the biologically active drug in the blood and 85 percent in the urine. Peak serum levels of active drug average approximately 20 mcg to 40 mcg per mL (90 percent protein bound), one to two hours after administration of a 1 g dose to a fasting normal individual, with a half-life of about 90 minutes. Peak urine levels of active drug average approximately 150 mcg to 200 mcg per mL, three to four hours after administration, with a half-life of about six hours. Approximately four percent of NegGram is excreted in the feces. Traces of nalidixic acid were found in blood and urine of an infant whose mother had received the drug during the last trimester of pregnancy. (See PRECAUTIONS—Drug Interactions.)
Microbiology
NegGram has marked antibacterial activity against gram-negative bacteria including *Enterobacter* species, *Escherichia coli, Morganella Morganii; Proteus Mirabilis, Proteus vulgaris,* and *Providencia rettgeri. Pseudomonas* species are generally resistant to the drug. NegGram is bactericidal and is effective over the entire urinary pH range. Conventional chromosomal resistance to NegGram taken in full dosage has been reported to emerge in approximately 2 to 14 percent of patients during treatment; however, bacterial resistance to NegGram has not been shown to be transferable via R factor.

Continued on next page

This product information was prepared in September 1996. On these and other products of Sanofi Winthrop Pharmaceuticals, detailed information may be obtained on a current basis by direct inquiry to Product Information Services, 90 Park Avenue, New York, NY 10016 (toll free 1-800-446-6267).

Sanofi Winthrop—Cont.

Susceptibility Test

Diffusion Techniques: Quantitative methods that require measurement of zone diameters give the most precise estimates of antibacterial susceptibility. One such procedure recommended for use with a disc containing 30 mcg of nalidixic acid is the National Committee for Clinical Laboratory Standards (NCCLS) approved procedure. Only organisms from urinary tract infections should be tested. Results of laboratory tests using 30 mcg nalidixic acid discs should be interpreted using the following criteria:

Zone Diameter (mm)	Interpretation
≥19	(S) Susceptible
14–18	(I) Intermediate
≤13	(R) Resistant

Dilution Techniques: Broth and agar dilution methods, such as those recommended by the NCCLS, may be used to determine the minimum inhibitory concentration (MIC) of nalidixic acid. MIC test results should be interpreted according to the following criteria:

MIC (mcg/mL)	Interpretation
≤16	(S) Susceptible
≥32	(R) Resistant

For any susceptibility test, a report of "susceptible" indicates that the pathogen is likely to respond to nalidixic acid therapy. A report of "resistant" indicates that the pathogen is not likely to respond. A report of "intermediate" generally indicates that the test result is equivocal.
The Quality Control strains should have the following assigned daily ranges for nalidixic acid:

QC Strains
E. Coli
(ATCC 25922)

Disc Zone Diameter
22–28

MIC (mcg/mL)
1.0–4.0

INDICATIONS AND USAGE

NegGram is indicated for the treatment of urinary tract infections caused by susceptible gram-negative microorganisms, including the majority of *E. Coli, Enterobacter* species, *Klebsiella* species, and *Proteus* species. Disc susceptibility testing with the 30 mcg disc should be performed prior to administration of the drug, and during treatment if clinical response warrants.

CONTRAINDICATIONS

NegGram is contraindicated in patients with known hypersensitivity to nalidixic acid and in patients with a history of convulsive disorders.

WARNINGS

Central Nervous System (CNS) effects including convulsions, increased intracranial pressure, and toxic psychosis have been reported with nalidixic acid therapy. Convulsive seizures have been reported with other drugs in this class. Quinolones may also cause CNS stimulation which may lead to tremor, restlessness, lightheadedness, confusion, and hallucinations. Therefore, nalidixic acid should be used with caution in patients with known or suspected CNS disorders, such as, cerebral arteriosclerosis or epilepsy, or other factors which predispose seizures. (See ADVERSE REACTIONS.) If these reactions occur in patients receiving nalidixic acid, the drug should be discontinued and appropriate measures instituted.
Serious and occasionally fatal hypersensitivity (anaphylactoid) reactions, some following the first dose, have been reported in patients receiving quinolone therapy. Some reactions were accompanied by cardiovascular collapse, loss of consciousness, tingling, pharyngeal or facial edema, dyspnea, urticaria, and itching. Only a few patients had a history of hypersensitivity reactions. Serious anaphylactoid reactions required immediate emergency treatment with epinephrine. Oxygen, intravenous steroids, and airway management, including intubation, should be administered as indicated.
Nalidixic acid and other members of the quinolone drug class have been shown to cause arthropathy in juvenile animals. (See PRECAUTIONS and ANIMAL PHARMACOLOGY.)
Pseudomembranous colitis has been reported with nearly all antibacterial agents, including quinolones, and may range in severity from mild to life-threatening. Therefore, it is important to consider this diagnosis in patients who present with diarrhea subsequent to the administration of antibacterial agents.
Treatment with antibacterial agents alters the normal flora of the colon and may permit overgrowth of clostridia. Studies indicate that a toxin produced by *Clostridium difficile* is one primary cause of "antibiotic-associated colitis".
After the diagnosis of pseudomembranous colitis has been established, therapeutic measures should be initiated. Mild cases of pseudomembranous colitis usually respond to drug discontinuation alone. In moderate to severe cases, consideration should be given to management with fluids and electrolytes, protein supplementation, and treatment with an antibacterial drug clinically effective against *C. difficile* colitis.

PRECAUTIONS

General
Blood counts and renal and liver function tests should be performed periodically if treatment is continued for more than two weeks. NegGram should be used with caution in patients with liver disease, epilepsy, or severe cerebral arteriosclerosis. (See WARNINGS.) While caution should be used in patients with severe renal failure, therapeutic concentrations of NegGram in the urine, without increased toxicity due to drug accumulation in the blood, have been observed in patients on full dosage with creatinine clearances as low as 2 mL/minute to 8 mL/minute.
Moderate to severe phototoxicity reactions have been observed in patients who are exposed to direct sunlight while receiving NegGram or other members of this drug class. Excessive sunlight should be avoided. Therapy should be discontinued if phototoxicity occurs.
If bacterial resistance to NegGram emerges during treatment, it usually does so within 48 hours, permitting rapid change to another antimicrobial. Therefore, if the clinical response is unsatisfactory or if relapse occurs, cultures and sensitivity tests should be repeated. Underdosage with NegGram during initial treatment (with less than 4 g per day for adults) may predispose to emergence of bacterial resistance. (See DOSAGE AND ADMINISTRATION.)

Information for Patients
Patients should be advised NegGram may be taken with or without meals. Patients should be advised to drink fluids liberally and not take antacids.
Patients should be advised that quinolones may be associated with hypersensitivity reactions, even following a single dose, and to discontinue the drug at the first sign of a skin rash or other allergic reactions.
Quinolones may cause dizziness and lightheadedness, therefore, patients should know how they react to NegGram before they operate an automobile or machinery or engage in activities requiring mental alertness or coordination.
Patients should be advised that quinolones may increase the effects of theophylline and caffeine. There is a possibility of caffeine accumulation when products containing caffeine are consumed while taking quinolones. Patients should be advised to avoid excessive sunlight or artificial ultraviolet light while receiving nalidixic acid and to discontinue therapy if phototoxicity occurs.

Drug Interactions
Elevated plasma levels of theophylline have been reported with concomitant quinolone use. There have been reports of theophylline-related side effects in patients on concomitant therapy with quinolones and theophylline. Therefore, monitoring of theophylline plasma levels should be considered and dosage of theophylline adjusted, as required.
Quinolones have been shown to interfere with the metabolism of caffeine. This may lead to reduced clearance of caffeine and the prolongation of its plasma half-life.
Quinolones, including nalidixic acid, may enhance the effects of the oral anticoagulant warfarin or its derivatives. When these products are administered concomitantly, prothrombin time or other suitable coagulation test should be closely monitored.
Nitrofurantoin interferes with the therapeutic action of nalidixic acid.
Antacids containing magnesium, aluminum, or calcium; sucralfate or divalent or trivalent cations such as iron; and multivitamins containing zinc may substantially interfere with the absorption of quinolones, resulting in urine levels considerably lower than desired. They should not be given concomitantly or within two hours of the administration of quinolones.
Elevated serum levels of cyclosporine have been reported with the concomitant use of some quinolones and cyclosporine. Therefore, cyclosporine serum levels should be monitored and appropriate cyclosporine dosage adjustments made when these drugs are used concomitantly.

Drug Laboratory Test Interactions
When Benedict's or Fehling's solution or Clinitest® Reagent Tablets are used to test the urine of patients taking NegGram, a false-positive reaction for glucose may be obtained, due to the liberation of glucuronic acid from the metabolites excreted. However, a colorimetric test for glucose based on an enzyme reaction (e.g., with Clinistix® Reagent Strips or Tes-Tape®) does not give a false-positive reaction to the liberated glucuronic acid.
Incorrect values may be obtained for urinary 17-keto and ketogenic steroids in patients receiving NegGram, because of an interaction between the drug and the *m*-dinitrobenzene used in the usual assay method. In such cases, the Porter-Silber test for 17-hydroxycorticoids may be used.

Carcinogenesis, Mutagenesis, Impairment of Fertility
In lifetime studies in the rat given nalidixic acid in the diet, there was an increased incidence of preputial gland neoplasms in the treated males and clitoral gland neoplasms in the treated females. Studies in mice in which nalidixic acid was administered in the feed for two years, or was given in the feed for 76 weeks followed by no treatment for 9 weeks, gave equivocal evidence of carcinogenic activity.
Nalidixic acid was tested in the Ames bacterial mutagenicity test (maximum dose 33 mcg/plate) and the mouse lymphoma assay (L5178Y/TK; maximum dose 100 mcg/mL) with and without metabolic activation, and results were negative.

Pregnancy: Teratogenic Effects.
Pregnancy Category C.
NegGram has been shown to be teratogenic and embryocidal in rats when given in oral doses six times the human dose. NegGram also prolonged the duration of pregnancy especially at four times the clinical dose. There are no adequate and well-controlled studies in pregnant women. Since nalidixic acid, like other drugs in this class, causes arthropathy in immature animals, NegGram should be used during pregnancy only if the potential benefit justifies the potential risk to the fetus. (See WARNINGS and ANIMAL PHARMACOLOGY.)

Nursing Mothers
It is not known whether NegGram is excreted in human milk. Because other drugs are excreted in human milk and because of the potential for serious adverse reactions in nursing infants from NegGram, a decision should be made whether to discontinue nursing or to discontinue the drug taking into account the importance of the drug to the mother.

Pediatric Use
Safety and effectiveness in infants below the age of three months have not been established.

Usage in Patients Under 18 Years of Age
Toxicological studies have shown that nalidixic acid and related drugs can produce erosions of the cartilage in weight-bearing joints and other signs of arthropathy in immature animals of most species tested. No such joint lesions have been reported in humans to date. Nevertheless, until the significance of this finding is clarified, this drug should only be used in patients under 18 years of age when the potential benefit justifies the potential risk. (See WARNINGS and ANIMAL PHARMACOLOGY.)

ADVERSE REACTIONS

Reactions reported after oral administration of NegGram include the following.
CNS effects: drowsiness, weakness, headache, and dizziness and vertigo. Reversible subjective visual disturbances without objective findings have occurred infrequently (generally with each dose during the first few days of treatment). These reactions include overbrightness of lights, change in color perception, difficulty in focusing, decrease in visual acuity, and double vision. They usually disappeared promptly when dosage was reduced or therapy was discontinued. Toxic psychosis or brief convulsions have been reported rarely, usually following excessive doses. In general, the convulsions have occurred in patients with predisposing factors such as epilepsy or cerebral arteriosclerosis. In infants and children receiving therapeutic doses of NegGram, increased intracranial pressure with bulging anterior fontanel, papilledema, and headache has occasionally been observed. A few cases of 6th cranial nerve palsy have been reported. Although the mechanisms of these reactions are unknown, the signs and symptoms usually disappeared rapidly with no sequelae when treatment was discontinued.
Gastrointestinal: abdominal pain, nausea, vomiting, and diarrhea.
Allergic: rash, pruritus, urticaria, angioedema, eosinophilia, arthralgia with joint stiffness and swelling, and anaphylactoid reaction. Erythema Multiforme and Stevens-Johnson syndrome have been reported with nalidixic acid and other drugs in this class. Rash was the most frequently reported adverse reaction. Photosensitivity reactions consisting of erythema and bullae on exposed skin surfaces usually resolve completely in 2 weeks to 2 months after NegGram is discontinued; however, bullae may continue to appear with successive exposures to sunlight or with mild skin trauma for up to 3 months after discontinuation of drug. (See PRECAUTIONS.)
Other: rarely, cholestasis, paresthesia, metabolic acidosis, thrombocytopenia, leukopenia, or hemolytic anemia, sometimes associated with glucose 6-phosphate dehydrogenase deficiency.

OVERDOSAGE

Manifestations: Toxic psychosis, convulsions, increased intracranial pressure, or metabolic acidosis may occur in patients taking more than the recommended dosage. Vomiting, nausea, and lethargy may also occur following overdosage.
Treatment: Reactions are short-lived (two or three hours) because the drug is rapidly excreted. If overdosage is noted early, gastric lavage is indicated. If absorption has occurred, increased fluid administration is advisable and supportive measures such as oxygen and means of artificial respiration should be available. Although anticonvulsant therapy has

not been used in the few instances of overdosage reported, it may be indicated in a severe case.

DOSAGE AND ADMINISTRATION

Adults. The recommended dosage for initial therapy in adults is 1 g administered four times daily for one or two weeks (total daily dose, 4 g). For prolonged therapy, the total daily dose may be reduced to 2 g after the initial treatment period. Underdosage during initial treatment may predispose to emergence of bacterial resistance.

Children. Until further experience is gained, NegGram should not be administered to infants younger than three months. Dosage in children 12 years of age and under should be calculated on the basis of body weight. The recommended total daily dosage for initial therapy is 25 mg/lb/day (55 mg/kg/day), administered in four equally divided doses. For prolonged therapy, the total daily dose may be reduced to 15 mg/lb/day (33 mg/kg/day). NegGram Suspension or NegGram Caplets of 250 mg may be used. One 250 mg tablet is equivalent to one teaspoon (5 mL) of the Suspension.

HOW SUPPLIED

Suspension (250 mg/5 mL tsp), raspberry flavored, bottles of 1 pint (NDC 0024-1318-06)

Caplets of 1 g, light buff-colored capsule-shaped tablets, bottles of 100 (NDC 0024-1323-04)

Caplets of 500 mg, light buff-colored capsule-shaped tablets, bottles of 56 (NDC 0024-1322-03) 500 (NDC 0024-1322-06)

Caplets of 250 mg, light buff-colored capsule-shaped tablets, bottles of 56 (NDC 0024-1321-03)

Store suspension at room temperature up to 25° C (77° F).

Store caplets at room temperature, up to 30° C (86° F).

Caution: Federal law prohibits dispensing without prescription.

ANIMAL PHARMACOLOGY

NegGram (nalidixic acid) and related drugs have been shown to cause arthropathy in juvenile animals of most species tested. (See WARNINGS.)

Long-term administration of nalidixic acid to rats resulted in retinal degeneration and cataracts.

Hydroxynalidixic acid, the principal metabolite of NegGram, did not produce any oculotoxic effects at any dosage level in seven species of animals including three primate species. However, oral administration of this metabolite in high doses has been shown to have oculotoxic potential, namely in dogs and cats where it produced retinal degeneration upon prolonged administration leading, in some cases, to blindness.

In experiments with NegGram itself, little if any such activity could be elicited in either dogs or cats. Sensitivity to CNS side effects in these species limited the doses of NegGram that could be used; this factor, together with a low conversion rate to the hydroxy metabolite in these species, may explain the absence of these effects.

NSW-6 C (0)

Shown in Product Identification Guide, page 333

NEO-SYNEPHRINE® Hydrochloride ℞

brand of phenylephrine hydrochloride injection, USP
1% INJECTION

Well-Tolerated Vasoconstrictor and Pressor

WARNING: PHYSICIANS SHOULD COMPLETELY FAMILIARIZE THEMSELVES WITH THE COMPLETE CONTENTS OF THIS LEAFLET BEFORE PRESCRIBING NEO-SYNEPHRINE.

DESCRIPTION

NEO-SYNEPHRINE hydrochloride, brand of phenylephrine hydrochloride injection, is a vasoconstrictor and pressor drug chemically related to epinephrine and ephedrine.

NEO-SYNEPHRINE hydrochloride is a synthetic sympathomimetic agent in sterile form for parenteral injection. Chemically, phenylephrine hydrochloride is (−)-*m*-Hydroxy-α-[(methylamino) methyl] benzyl alcohol hydrochloride.

CLINICAL PHARMACOLOGY

NEO-SYNEPHRINE hydrochloride produces vasoconstriction that lasts longer than that of epinephrine and ephedrine. Responses are more sustained than those to epinephrine, lasting 20 minutes after intravenous and as long as 50 minutes after subcutaneous injection. Its action on the heart contrasts sharply with that of epinephrine and ephedrine, in that it slows the heart rate and increases the stroke output, producing no disturbance in the rhythm of the pulse.

Phenylephrine is a powerful postsynaptic alpha-receptor stimulant with little effect on the beta receptors of the heart. In therapeutic doses, it produces little if any stimulation of either the spinal cord or cerebrum. A singular advantage of this drug is the fact that repeated injections produce comparable effects.

The predominant actions of phenylephrine are on the cardiovascular system. Parenteral administration causes a rise in systolic and diastolic pressures in man and other species. Accompanying the pressor response to phenylephrine is a marked reflex bradycardia that can be blocked by atropine; after atropine, large doses of the drug increase the heart rate only slightly. In man, cardiac output is slightly decreased and peripheral resistance is considerably increased. Circulation time is slightly prolonged, and venous pressure is slightly increased; venous constriction is not marked. Most vascular beds are constricted; renal splanchnic, cutaneous, and limb blood flows are reduced but coronary blood flow is increased. Pulmonary vessels are constricted, and pulmonary arterial pressure is raised.

The drug is a powerful vasoconstrictor, with properties very similar to those of norepinephrine but almost completely lacking the chronotropic and inotropic actions on the heart. Cardiac irregularities are seen only very rarely even with large doses.

INDICATIONS AND USAGE

NEO-SYNEPHRINE is intended for the maintenance of an adequate level of blood pressure during spinal and inhalation anesthesia and for the treatment of vascular failure in shock, shocklike states, and drug-induced hypotension, or hypersensitivity. It is also employed to overcome paroxysmal supraventricular tachycardia, to prolong spinal anesthesia, and as a vasoconstrictor in regional analgesia.

CONTRAINDICATIONS

NEO-SYNEPHRINE hydrochloride should not be used in patients with severe hypertension, ventricular tachycardia, or in patients who are hypersensitive to it.

WARNINGS

If used in conjunction with oxytocic drugs, the pressor effect of sympathomimetic pressor amines is potentiated (see Drug Interaction). The obstetrician should be warned that some oxytocic drugs may cause severe persistent hypertension and that even a rupture of a cerebral blood vessel may occur during the postpartum period.

Contains sodium metabisulfite, a sulfite that may cause allergic-type reactions including anaphylactic symptoms and life-threatening or less severe asthmatic episodes in certain susceptible people. The overall prevalence of sulfite sensitivity in the general population is unknown and probably low. Sulfite sensitivity is seen more frequently in asthmatic than in nonasthmatic people.

PRECAUTIONS

NEO-SYNEPHRINE hydrochloride should be employed only with extreme caution in elderly patients or in patients with hyperthyroidism, bradycardia, partial heart block, myocardial disease, or severe arteriosclerosis.

Drug Interactions—Vasopressors, particularly metaraminol, may cause serious cardiac arrhythmias during halothane anesthesia and therefore should be used only with great caution or not at all.

MAO Inhibitors—The pressor effect of sympathomimetic pressor amines is markedly potentiated in patients receiving monoamine oxidase inhibitors (MAOI). Therefore, when initiating pressor therapy in these patients, the initial dose should be small and used with due caution. The pressor response of adrenergic agents may also be potentiated by tricyclic antidepressants.

Carcinogenesis, Mutagenesis, Impairment of Fertility—No long-term animal studies have been done to evaluate the potential of NEO-SYNEPHRINE in these areas.

Pregnancy Category C—Animal reproduction studies have not been conducted with NEO-SYNEPHRINE. It is also not known whether NEO-SYNEPHRINE can cause fetal harm when administered to a pregnant woman or can affect reproduction capacity. NEO-SYNEPHRINE should be given to a pregnant woman only if clearly needed.

Labor and Delivery—If vasopressor drugs are either used to correct hypotension or added to the local anesthetic solution, the obstetrician should be cautioned that some oxytocic drugs may cause severe persistent hypertension and that even a rupture of a cerebral blood vessel may occur during the postpartum period (see WARNINGS).

Nursing Mother—It is not known whether this drug is excreted in human milk. Because many are excreted in human milk, caution should be exercised when NEO-SYNEPHRINE hydrochloride, brand of phenylephrine hydrochloride injection, is administered to a nursing woman.

Pediatric Use—To combat hypotension during spinal anesthesia in children, a dose of 0.5 mg to 1 mg per 25 pounds body weight, administered subcutaneously or intramuscularly, is recommended.

ADVERSE REACTIONS

Headache, reflex bradycardia, excitability, restlessness, and rarely arrhythmias.

OVERDOSAGE

Overdosage may induce ventricular extrasystoles and short paroxysms of ventricular tachycardia, a sensation of fullness in the head and tingling of the extremities.

Should an excessive elevation of blood pressure occur, it may be immediately relieved by an α-adrenergic blocking agent, eg, phentolamine.

The oral LD_{50} in the rat is 350 mg/kg, in the mouse 120 mg/kg.

DOSAGE AND ADMINISTRATION

NEO-SYNEPHRINE is generally injected subcutaneously, intramuscularly, slowly intravenously, or in dilute solution as a continuous intravenous infusion. In patients with paroxysmal supraventricular tachycardia and, if indicated, in case of emergency, NEO-SYNEPHRINE is administered directly intravenously. The dose should be adjusted according to the pressor response.

Dosage Calculations

Dose Required	Use NEO-SYNEPHRINE 1%
10 mg	1 mL
5 mg	0.5 mL
1 mg	0.1 mL

For convenience in intermittent intravenous administration, dilute 1 mL NEO-SYNEPHRINE 1% with 9 mL Sterile Water for Injection, USP, to yield 0.1% NEO-SYNEPHRINE.

Dose Required	Use Diluted NEO-SYNEPHRINE (0.1%)
0.1 mg	0.1 mL
0.2 mg	0.2 mL
0.5 mg	0.5 mL

Mild or Moderate Hypotension

Subcutaneously or Intramuscularly: Usual dose, from 2 mg to 5 mg. Range, from 1 mg to 10 mg. Initial dose should not exceed 5 mg.

Intravenously: Usual dose, 0.2 mg. Range, from 0.1 mg to 0.5 mg. Initial dose should not exceed 0.5 mg.

Injections should not be repeated more often than every 10 to 15 minutes. A 5 mg intramuscular dose should raise blood pressure for one to two hours. A 0.5 mg intravenous dose should elevate the pressure for about 15 minutes.

Severe Hypotension and Shock—Including Drug-Related Hypotension

Blood volume depletion should always be corrected as fully as possible before any vasopressor is administered. When, as an emergency measure, intraaortic pressures must be maintained to prevent cerebral or coronary artery ischemia, NEO-SYNEPHRINE hydrochloride, brand of phenylephrine hydrochloride injection, can be administered before and concurrently with blood volume replacement.

Hypotension and occasionally severe shock may result from overdosage or idiosyncrasy following the administration of certain drugs, especially adrenergic and ganglionic blocking agents, rauwolfia and veratrum alkaloids, and phenothiazine tranquilizers. Patients who receive a phenothiazine derivative as preoperative medication are especially susceptible to these reactions. As an adjunct in the management of such episodes, NEO-SYNEPHRINE hydrochloride is a suitable agent for restoring blood pressure.

Higher initial and maintenance doses of NEO-SYNEPHRINE are required in patients with persistent or untreated severe hypotension or shock. Hypotension produced by powerful peripheral adrenergic blocking agents, chlorpromazine, or pheochromocytomectomy may also require more intensive therapy.

Continuous Infusion—Add 10 mg of the drug (1 mL of 1 percent solution) to 500 mL of Dextrose Injection, USP, or Sodium Chloride Injection, USP (providing a 1:50,000 solution). To raise the blood pressure rapidly, start the infusion at about 100 μg to 180 μg per minute (based on 20 drops per mL this would be 100 to 180 drops per minute). When the blood pressure is stabilized (at a low normal level for the individual), a maintenance rate of 40 μg to 60 μg per minute usually suffices (based on 20 drops per mL this would be 40 to 60 drops per minute). If the drop size of the infusion system varies from the 20 drops per mL, the dose must be adjusted accordingly.

If a prompt initial pressor response is not obtained, additional increments of NEO-SYNEPHRINE (10 mg or more) are added to the infusion bottle. The rate of flow is then adjusted until the desired blood pressure level is obtained. (In some cases, a more potent vasopressor, such as norepinephrine bitartrate, may be required.) Hypertension should be avoided. The blood pressure should be checked frequently. Headache and/or bradycardia may indicate hypertension. Arrhythmias are rare.

Continued on next page

This product information was prepared in September 1996. On these and other products of Sanofi Winthrop Pharmaceuticals, detailed information may be obtained on a current basis by direct inquiry to Product Information Services, 90 Park Avenue, New York, NY 10016 (toll free 1-800-446-6267).

Sanofi Winthrop—Cont.

Spinal Anesthesia—Hypotension

Routine parenteral use of NEO-SYNEPHRINE has been recommended for the prophylaxis and treatment of hypotension during spinal anesthesia. It is best administered subcutaneously or intramuscularly three or four minutes before injection of the spinal anesthetic. The total requirement for high anesthetic levels is usually 3 mg, and for lower levels, 2 mg. For hypotensive emergencies during spinal anesthesia, NEO-SYNEPHRINE may be injected intravenously, using an initial dose of 0.2 mg. Any subsequent dose should not exceed the previous dose by more than 0.1 mg to 0.2 mg and no more than 0.5 mg should be administered in a single dose. To combat hypotension during spinal anesthesia in children, a dose of 0.5 mg to 1 mg per 25 pounds body weight, administered subcutaneously or intramuscularly, is recommended.

Prolongation of Spinal Anesthesia

The addition of 2 mg to 5 mg of NEO-SYNEPHRINE hydrochloride to the anesthetic solution increases the duration of motor block by as much as approximately 50 percent without any increase in the incidence of complications such as nausea, vomiting, or blood pressure disturbances.

Vasoconstrictor for Regional Analgesia

Concentrations about ten times those employed when epinephrine is used as a vasoconstrictor are recommended. The optimum strength is 1:20,000 (made by adding 1 mg of NEO-SYNEPHRINE hydrochloride to every 20 mL of local anesthetic solution). Some pressor responses can be expected when 2 mg or more are injected.

Paroxysmal Supraventricular Tachycardia

Rapid intravenous injection (within 20 to 30 seconds) is recommended; the initial dose should not exceed 0.5 mg, and subsequent doses, which are determined by the initial blood pressure response, should not exceed the preceding dose by more than 0.1 mg to 0.2 mg, and should never exceed 1 mg.

HOW SUPPLIED

Solution 1 percent

Each 1 mL contains 10 mg of NEO-SYNEPHRINE hydrochloride, 3.5 mg of sodium chloride, 4 mg of sodium citrate, 1 mg of citric acid monohydrate, and not more than 2 mg of sodium metabisulfite.

Uni-Nest™ ampuls of 1 mL, box of 25
(NDC 0024-1342-04).

CARPUJECT® Sterile Cartridge-Needle Unit, 10 mg/mL (1 mL fill in 2 mL cartridge), 22-gauge, 1¼ inch needle, dispensing bins of 50
(NDC 0024-1340-02).

The air in all ampuls and Cartridge-Needle Units has been displaced by nitrogen gas.

Protect from light if removed from carton or dispensing bin.

NSW-2

NEO-SYNEPHRINE® Hydrochloride ℞

brand of phenylephrine hydrochloride ophthalmic solution, USP
Vasoconstrictor and Mydriatic
SOLUTIONS 2.5% AND 10%
VISCOUS SOLUTION 10%

For Use in Ophthalmology

> WARNING: PHYSICIANS SHOULD COMPLETELY FAMILIARIZE THEMSELVES WITH THE COMPLETE CONTENTS OF THIS LEAFLET BEFORE PRESCRIBING NEO-SYNEPHRINE.

DESCRIPTION

NEO-SYNEPHRINE hydrochloride, brand of phenylephrine hydrochloride ophthalmic solution, is a sterile solution used as a vasoconstrictor and mydriatic for use in ophthalmology.

NEO-SYNEPHRINE hydrochloride is a synthetic sympathomimetic compound structurally similar to epinephrine and ephedrine.

Phenylephrine hydrochloride is (–)-*m* -Hydroxy-α-[(methylamino)methyl] benzyl alcohol hydrochloride.

CLINICAL PHARMACOLOGY

NEO-SYNEPHRINE possesses predominantly α-adrenergic effects. In the eye, phenylephrine acts locally as a potent vasoconstrictor and mydriatic, by constricting ophthalmic blood vessels and the radial muscle of the iris.

The ophthalmologic usefulness of NEO-SYNEPHRINE hydrochloride is due to its rapid effect and moderately prolonged action, as well as to the fact that it produces no compensatory vasodilatation.

The action of different concentrations of ophthalmic solutions of NEO-SYNEPHRINE hydrochloride is shown in the following table:

Strength of solution (%)	Mydriasis: Maximal (minutes)	Mydriasis: Recovery time (hours)	Paralysis of accommodation
2.5	15-60	3	trace
10	10-60	6	slight

Although rare, systemic absorption of sufficient quantities of phenylephrine may lead to systemic α-adrenergic effects, such as rise in blood pressure which may be accompanied by a reflex atropine-sensitive bradycardia.

INDICATIONS AND USAGE

NEO-SYNEPHRINE hydrochloride is recommended for use as a decongestant and vasoconstrictor and for pupil dilatation in uveitis (posterior synechiae), wide angle glaucoma, prior to surgery, refraction, ophthalmoscopic examination, and diagnostic procedures.

CONTRAINDICATIONS

Ophthalmic solutions of NEO-SYNEPHRINE hydrochloride are contraindicated in persons with narrow angle glaucoma (and in those individuals who are hypersensitive to NEO-SYNEPHRINE). NEO-SYNEPHRINE hydrochloride 10 percent ophthalmic solutions are contraindicated in infants and in patients with aneurysms.

WARNINGS

There have been rare reports associating the use of NEO-SYNEPHRINE 10 percent ophthalmic solutions with the development of serious cardiovascular reactions, including ventricular arrhythmias and myocardial infarctions. These episodes, some ending fatally, have usually occurred in elderly patients with preexisting cardiovascular diseases.

PRECAUTIONS

Exceeding recommended dosages or applying NEO-SYNEPHRINE hydrochloride ophthalmic solutions to the instrumented, traumatized, diseased or postsurgical eye or adnexa, or to patients with suppressed lacrimation, as during anesthesia, may result in the absorption of sufficient quantities of phenylephrine to produce a systemic vasopressor response.

A significant elevation in blood pressure is rare but has been reported following conjunctival instillation of recommended doses of NEO-SYNEPHRINE 10 percent ophthalmic solutions. Caution, therefore, should be exercised in administering the 10 percent solutions to children of low body weight, the elderly, and patients with insulin-dependent diabetes, hypertension, hyperthyroidism, generalized arteriosclerosis, or cardiovascular disease. The posttreatment blood pressure of these patients, and any patients who develop symptoms, should be carefully monitored.

Ordinarily, any mydriatic, including NEO-SYNEPHRINE hydrochloride, brand of phenylephrine hydrochloride ophthalmic solution, is contraindicated in patients with glaucoma, since it may occasionally raise intraocular pressure. However, when temporary dilatation of the pupil may free adhesions or when vasoconstriction of intrinsic vessels may lower intraocular tension, these advantages may temporarily outweigh the danger from coincident dilatation of the pupil.

Rebound miosis has been reported in older persons one day after receiving NEO-SYNEPHRINE hydrochloride ophthalmic solutions, and reinstillation of the drug produced a reduction in mydriasis. This may be of clinical importance in dilating the pupils of older subjects prior to retinal detachment or cataract surgery.

Due to a strong action of the drug on the dilator muscle, older individuals may also develop transient pigment floaters in the aqueous humor 30 to 45 minutes following the administration of NEO-SYNEPHRINE hydrochloride ophthalmic solutions. The appearance may be similar to anterior uveitis or to a microscopic hyphema.

To prevent pain, a drop of suitable topical anesthetic may be applied before using the 10 percent ophthalmic solution.

Drug Interaction: As with all other adrenergic drugs, when NEO-SYNEPHRINE 10 percent ophthalmic solutions or 2.5 percent ophthalmic solution is administered simultaneously with, or up to 21 days after, administration of monoamine oxidase (MAO) inhibitors, careful supervision and adjustment of dosages are required since exaggerated adrenergic effects may occur. The pressor response of adrenergic agents may also be potentiated by tricyclic antidepressants, propranolol, reserpine, guanethidine, methyldopa, and atropine-like drugs.

It has been reported that the concomitant use of NEO-SYNEPHRINE 10 percent ophthalmic solutions and systemic beta blockers has caused acute hypertension and, in one case, the rupture of a congenital cerebral aneurysm. NEO-SYNEPHRINE may potentiate the cardiovascular depressant effects of potent inhalation anesthetic agents.

Carcinogenesis, Mutagenesis, Impairment of Fertility: No long-term animal studies have been done to evaluate the potential of NEO-SYNEPHRINE in these areas.

Pregnancy Category C: Animal reproduction studies have not been conducted with NEO-SYNEPHRINE. It is also not known whether NEO-SYNEPHRINE can cause fetal harm when administered to a pregnant woman or can affect reproduction capacity. NEO-SYNEPHRINE should be given to a pregnant woman only if clearly needed.

Nursing Mothers: It is not known whether this drug is excreted in milk; many are. Caution should be exercised when NEO-SYNEPHRINE hydrochloride ophthalmic solution is administered to a nursing woman.

Pediatric Use: NEO-SYNEPHRINE hydrochloride 10 percent ophthalmic solutions are contraindicated in infants. (See CONTRAINDICATIONS.) For use in older children see DOSAGE AND ADMINISTRATION.

Exceeding recommended dosages or applying NEO-SYNEPHRINE hydrochloride ophthalmic solutions to the instrumented, traumatized, diseased or postsurgical eye or adnexa, or to patients with suppressed lacrimation, as during anesthesia, may result in the absorption of sufficient quantities of phenylephrine to produce a systemic vasopressor response.

The hypertensive effects of phenylephrine may be treated with an alpha-adrenergic blocking agent such as phentolamine mesylate, 5 mg to 10 mg intravenously, repeated as necessary.

The oral LD_{50} of phenylephrine in the rat: 350 mg/kg, in the mouse: 120 mg/kg.

DOSAGE AND ADMINISTRATION

Prolonged exposure to air or strong light may cause oxidation and discoloration. Do not use if solution is brown or contains a precipitate.

Vasoconstriction and Pupil Dilatation

NEO-SYNEPHRINE hydrochloride 10 percent ophthalmic solutions are especially useful when rapid and powerful dilatation of the pupil and reduction of congestion in the capillary bed are desired. A drop of a suitable topical anesthetic may be applied, followed in a few minutes by 1 drop of the NEO-SYNEPHRINE hydrochloride 10 percent ophthalmic solutions on the upper limbus. The anesthetic prevents stinging and consequent dilution of the solution by lacrimation. It may occasionally be necessary to repeat the instillation after one hour, again preceded by the use of the topical anesthetic.

Uveitis: Posterior Synechiae

NEO-SYNEPHRINE hydrochloride 10 percent ophthalmic solutions may be used in patients with uveitis when synechiae are present or may develop. The formation of synechiae may be prevented by the use of the 10 percent ophthalmic solutions and atropine to produce wide dilatation of the pupil. It should be emphasized, however, that the vasoconstrictor effect of NEO-SYNEPHRINE hydrochloride may be antagonistic to the increase of local blood flow in uveal infection.

To free recently formed posterior synechiae, 1 drop of the 10 percent ophthalmic solutions may be applied to the upper surface of the cornea. On the following day, treatment may be continued if necessary. In the interim, hot compresses should be applied for five or ten minutes three times a day, with 1 drop of a 1 or 2 percent solution of atropine sulfate before and after each series of compresses.

Glaucoma

In certain patients with glaucoma, temporary reduction of intraocular tension may be attained by producing vasoconstriction of the intraocular vessels; this may be accomplished by placing 1 drop of the 10 percent ophthalmic solutions on the upper surface of the cornea. This treatment may be repeated as often as necessary.

NEO-SYNEPHRINE hydrochloride, brand of phenylephrine hydrochloride ophthalmic solution, may be used with miotics in patients with wide angle glaucoma. It reduces the difficulties experienced by the patient because of the small field produced by miosis, and still it permits and often supports the effect of the miotic in lowering the intraocular pressure. Hence, there may be marked improvement in visual acuity after using NEO-SYNEPHRINE hydrochloride in conjunction with miotic drugs.

Surgery

When a short-acting mydriatic is needed for wide dilatation of the pupil before intraocular surgery, the 10 percent ophthalmic solutions or 2.5 percent ophthalmic solution may be applied topically from 30 to 60 minutes before the operation.

Refraction

Prior to determination of refractive errors, NEO-SYNEPHRINE hydrochloride 2.5 percent ophthalmic solution may be used effectively with homatropine hydrobromide, atropine sulfate, or a combination of homatropine and cocaine hydrochloride.

For *adults,* a drop of the preferred cycloplegic is placed in each eye, followed in five minutes by 1 drop of NEO-SYNEPHRINE hydrochloride 2.5 percent ophthalmic solution and in ten minutes by another drop of the cycloplegic. In 50 to 60 minutes, the eyes are ready for refraction.

For *children*, a drop of atropine sulfate 1 percent is placed in each eye, followed in 10 to 15 minutes by 1 drop of NEO-SYNEPHRINE hydrochloride 2.5 percent ophthalmic solution and in five to ten minutes by a second drop of atropine sulfate 1 percent. In one to two hours, the eyes are ready for refraction.

For a "one application method," NEO-SYNEPHRINE hydrochloride 2.5 percent ophthalmic solution may be combined with a cycloplegic to elicit synergistic action. The additive effect varies depending on the patient. Therefore, when using a "one application method," it may be desirable to increase the concentration of the cycloplegic.

Ophthalmoscopic Examination

One drop of NEO-SYNEPHRINE hydrochloride 2.5 percent ophthalmic solution is placed in each eye. Sufficient mydriasis to permit examination is produced in 15 to 30 minutes. Dilatation lasts from one to three hours.

Diagnostic Procedures

Provocative Test for Angle Block in Patients with Glaucoma: The 2.5 percent ophthalmic solution may be used as a provocative test when latent increased intraocular pressure is suspected. Tension is measured before application of NEO-SYNEPHRINE hydrochloride and again after dilatation. A 3 to 5 mm of mercury rise in pressure suggests the presence of angle block in patients with glaucoma; however, failure to obtain such a rise does not preclude the presence of glaucoma from other causes.

Shadow Test (Retinoscopy): When dilatation of the pupil without cycloplegic action is desired for the shadow test, the 2.5 percent ophthalmic solution may be used alone.

Blanching Test: One or 2 drops of the 2.5 percent ophthalmic solution should be applied to the injected eye. After five minutes, examine for perilimbal blanching. If blanching occurs, the congestion is superficial and probably does not indicate iritis.

HOW SUPPLIED

In Mono-Drop ® (plastic dropper) bottle:
Low surface tension solutions
2.5 percent ophthalmic solution — NEO-SYNEPHRINE hydrochloride, brand of phenylephrine hydrochloride ophthalmic solution, 2.5 percent in a sterile, isotonic, buffered, low surface tension vehicle with sodium phosphate, sodium biphosphate, boric acid, and, as antiseptic preservative, benzalkonium chloride, NF, 1:7500. The pH is adjusted with phosphoric acid or sodium hydroxide.
Bottles of 15 mL (NDC 0024-1358-01)
10 percent ophthalmic solution — NEO-SYNEPHRINE hydrochloride 10 percent in a sterile, buffered, low surface tension vehicle with sodium phosphate, sodium biphosphate, and, as antiseptic preservative, benzalkonium chloride 1:10,000. The pH is adjusted with phosphoric acid or sodium hydroxide.
Bottles of 5 mL (NDC 0024-1359-01)
Viscous solution
10 percent ophthalmic solution — NEO-SYNEPHRINE hydrochloride 10 percent in a sterile, buffered, viscous vehicle with sodium phosphate, sodium biphosphate, methylcellulose, and, as antiseptic preservative, benzalkonium chloride 1:10,000. The pH is adjusted with phosphoric acid or sodium hydroxide.
Bottles of 5 mL (NDC 0024-1362-01)

NSW-5-A

NOVOCAIN® ℞
brand of procaine hydrochloride
injection, USP

DESCRIPTION

Procaine hydrochloride is benzoic acid, 4-amino-, 2-(diethylamino)ethyl ester, monohydrochloride, the ester of diethylaminoethanol and aminobenzoic acid.
It is a white crystalline, odorless powder that is freely soluble in water, but less soluble in alcohol.

HOW SUPPLIED

NOVOCAIN Solution 1 percent
Uni-Nest™ ampul pak, single-dose ampuls of 2 mL, box of 25
NDC 0024-1381-25
Single-dose ampuls of 6 mL, box of 50 **NDC 0024-1381-05**
Multiple-dose vials of 30 mL, box of 1 **NDC 0024-1385-01**
NOVOCAIN Solution 2 percent
Multiple-dose vials of 30 mL, box of 1 **NDC 0024-1386-01**
Store at room temperature up to 30° C (86° F).
Caution: Federal law prohibits dispensing without prescription.
For complete prescribing information, see package insert or contact Product Information Services.

NSW-8 A

NOVOCAIN® ℞
brand of procaine hydrochloride
injection, USP
10% Solution for Spinal Anesthesia

DESCRIPTION

NOVOCAIN, brand of procaine hydrochloride, is benzoic acid, 4-amino-, 2-(diethylamino) ethyl ester, monohydrochloride, the ester of diethylaminoethanol and aminobenzoic acid.
It is a white crystalline, odorless powder that is freely soluble in water, but less soluble in alcohol. Each mL contains 100 mg procaine hydrochloride and 4 mg acetone sodium bisulfite as antioxidant. DO NOT USE SOLUTIONS IF CRYSTALS, CLOUDINESS, OR DISCOLORATION IS OBSERVED. EXAMINE SOLUTIONS CAREFULLY BEFORE USE. REAUTOCLAVING INCREASES LIKELIHOOD OF CRYSTAL FORMATION.

CLINICAL PHARMACOLOGY

NOVOCAIN stabilizes the neuronal membrane and prevents the initiation and transmission of nerve impulses, thereby effecting local anesthesia. NOVOCAIN lacks surface anesthetic activity. The onset of action is rapid (2 to 5 minutes) and the duration of action is relatively short (average 1 to $1^1/_2$ hours), depending upon the anesthetic technique, the type of block, the concentration, and the individual patient.
NOVOCAIN is readily absorbed following parenteral administration and is rapidly hydrolyzed by plasma cholinesterase to aminobenzoic acid and diethylaminoethanol.
A vasoconstrictor may be added to the solution of NOVOCAIN to promote local hemostasis, delay systemic absorption, and increase duration of anesthesia.

INDICATIONS AND USAGE

NOVOCAIN is indicated for spinal anesthesia.

CONTRAINDICATIONS

Spinal anesthesia with NOVOCAIN is contraindicated in patients with generalized septicemia: sepsis at the proposed injection site; certain diseases of the cerebrospinal system, eg, meningitis, syphilis; and a known hypersensitivity to the drug, drugs of a similar chemical configuration, or aminobenzoic acid or its derivatives.
The decision as to whether or not spinal anesthesia should be used in an individual case should be made by the physician after weighing the advantages with the risks and possible complications.

WARNINGS

RESUSCITATIVE EQUIPMENT AND DRUGS SHOULD BE IMMEDIATELY AVAILABLE WHENEVER ANY LOCAL ANESTHETIC DRUG IS USED. Spinal anesthesia should only be administered by those qualified to do so.
Large doses of local anesthetics should not be used in patients with heart block.
Reactions resulting in fatality have occurred on rare occasions with the use of local anesthetics, even in the absence of a history of hypersensitivity.
Usage in Pregnancy. Safe use of NOVOCAIN has not been established with respect to adverse effects on fetal development. Careful consideration should be given to this fact before administering this drug to women of childbearing potential particularly during early pregnancy. This does not exclude the use of the drug at term for obstetrical analgesia.
Vasopressor agents (administered for the treatment of hypotension or added to the anesthetic solution for vasoconstriction) should be used with extreme caution in the presence of oxytocic drugs as they may produce severe, persistent hypertension with possible rupture of a cerebral blood vessel.
Solutions which contain a vasoconstrictor should be used with extreme caution in patients receiving drugs known to produce alterations in blood pressure (ie, monoamine oxidase inhibitors (MAOI), tricyclic antidepressants, phenothiazines, etc), as either severe sustained hypertension or hypotension may occur.
Local anesthetic procedures should be used with caution when there is inflammation and/or sepsis in the region of the proposed injection.
Contains acetone sodium bisulfite, a sulfite that may cause allergic-type reactions including anaphylactic symptoms and life-threatening or less severe asthmatic episodes in certain susceptible people The overall prevalence of sulfite sensitivity in the general population is unknown and probably low. Sulfite sensitivity is seen more frequently in asthmatic than in nonasthmatic people.

PRECAUTIONS

Standard textbooks should be consulted for specific techniques and precautions for various spinal anesthetic procedures.
The safety and effectiveness of a spinal anesthetic depend upon proper dosage, correct technique, adequate precautions, and readiness for emergencies. The lowest dosage that results in effective anesthesia should be used to avoid high plasma levels and possible adverse effects. Tolerance varies

---

with the status of the patient. Debilitated, elderly patients, or acutely ill patients should be given reduced doses commensurate with their weight and physical status. Reduced dosages are also indicated for obstetric delivery and patients with increased intra-abdominal pressure.
The decision whether or not to use spinal anesthesia in the following disease states depends on the physician's appraisal of the advantages as opposed to the risk: cardiovascular disease (ie, shock, hypertension, anemia, etc), pulmonary disease, renal impairment, metabolic or endocrine disorders, gastrointestinal disorders (ie, intestinal obstruction, peritonitis, etc), or complicated obstetrical deliveries.
NOVOCAIN SHOULD BE USED WITH CAUTION IN PATIENTS WITH KNOWN DRUG ALLERGIES AND SENSITIVITIES. A thorough history of the patient's prior experience with NOVOCAIN or other local anesthetics as well as concomitant or recent drug use should be taken (see CONTRAINDICATIONS). NOVOCAIN should not be used in any condition in which a sulfonamide drug is being employed since aminobenzoic acid inhibits the action of sulfonamides. Solutions containing a vasopressor should be used with caution in the presence of diseases which may adversely affect the cardiovascular system.
NOVOCAIN should be used with caution in patients with severe disturbances of cardiac rhythm, shock or heart block.

ADVERSE REACTIONS

Systemic adverse reactions involving the central nervous system and the cardiovascular system usually result from high plasma levels due to excessive dosage, rapid absorption, or inadvertent intravascular injection. In addition, use of inappropriate doses or techniques may result in extensive spinal blockade leading to hypotension and respiratory arrest.
A small number of reactions may result from hypersensitivity, idiosyncrasy, or diminished tolerance to normal dosage.
Excitatory CNS effects (nervousness, dizziness, blurred vision, tremors) commonly represent the initial signs of local anesthetic systemic toxicity. However, these reactions may be very brief or absent in some patients in which case the first manifestation of toxicity may be drowsiness or convulsions merging into unconsciousness and respiratory arrest.
Cardiovascular system reactions include depression of the myocardium, hypotension (or sometimes hypertension), bradycardia, and even cardiac arrest.
Allergic reactions are characterized by cutaneous lesions of delayed onset, or urticaria, edema, and other manifestations of allergy. The detection of sensitivity by skin testing is of limited value. As with other local anesthetics, hypersensitivity, idiosyncrasy and anaphylactoid reactions have occurred rarely. The reaction may be abrupt and severe and is not usually dose related.
The following adverse reactions may occur with spinal anesthesia: *Central Nervous System:* postspinal headache, meningismus, arachnoiditis, palsies, or spinal nerve paralysis. *Cardiovascular:* hypotension due to vasomotor paralysis and pooling of the blood in the venous bed. *Respiratory:* respiratory impairment or paralysis due to the level of anesthesia extending to the upper thoracic and cervical segments. *Gastrointestinal:* nausea and vomiting.
Treatment of Reactions. Toxic effects of local anesthetics require symptomatic treatment: there is no specific cure. The physician should be prepared to maintain an airway and to support ventilation with oxygen and assisted or controlled respiration as required. Supportive treatment of the cardiovascular system includes intravenous fluids and, when appropriate, vasopressors (preferably those that stimulate the myocardium, such as ephedrine). Convulsions may be controlled with oxygen and by the intravenous administration of diazepam or ultrashort-acting barbiturates or a short-acting muscle relaxant (succinylcholine). Intravenous anticonvulsant agents and muscle relaxants should only be administered by those familiar with their use and only when ventilation and oxygenation are assured. In spinal and epidural anesthesia, sympathetic blockade also occurs as a pharmacological reaction, resulting in peripheral vasodilation and often *hypotension*. The extent of the hypotension will usually depend on the number of dermatomes blocked. The blood pressure should therefore be monitored in the early phases of anesthesia. If hypotension occurs, it is readily controlled by vasoconstrictors administered either by the intramuscular or the intravenous route, the dosage of which would depend on the severity of the hypotension and the response to treatment.

Continued on next page

This product information was prepared in September 1996. On these and other products of Sanofi Winthrop Pharmaceuticals, detailed information may be obtained on a current basis by direct inquiry to Product Information Services, 90 Park Avenue, New York, NY 10016 (toll free 1-800-446-6267).

Sanofi Winthrop—Cont.

RECOMMENDED DOSAGE FOR SPINAL ANESTHESIA

	NOVOCAIN 10% Solution			
Extent of Anesthesia	Volume of 10% Solution (mL)	Volume of Diluent (mL)	Total Dose (mg)	Site of Injection (lumbar interspace)
Perineum	0.5	0.5	50	4th
Perineum and lower extremities	1	1	100	3rd or 4th
Up to costal margin	2	1	200	2nd, 3rd or 4th

DOSAGE AND ADMINISTRATION

As with all local anesthetics, the dose of NOVOCAIN varies and depends upon the area to be anesthetized, the vascularity of the tissues, the number of neuronal segments to be blocked, individual tolerance, and the technique of anesthesia. The lowest dose needed to provide effective anesthesia should be administered. For specific techniques and procedures, refer to standard textbooks.

[See table above.]

The diluent may be sterile normal saline, sterile distilled water, spinal fluid; and for hyperbaric technique, sterile dextrose solution.

The usual rate of injection is 1 mL per 5 seconds. Full anesthesia and fixation usually occur in 5 minutes.

STERILIZATION

The drug in intact ampuls is sterile. The preferred method of destroying bacteria on the exterior of ampuls before opening is heat sterilization (autoclaving). Immersion in antiseptic solution is not recommended.

Autoclave at 15-pound pressure, at 121° C (250° F), for 15 minutes. The diluent dextrose may show some brown discoloration due to caramelization.

HOW SUPPLIED

Uni-Nest™—ampuls of 2 mL (200 mg), box of 25 (NDC 0024-1384-25).
The air in the ampuls has been displaced by nitrogen gas. Protect solutions from light.
Store at room temperature up to 30° C (86° F).
Caution: Federal law prohibits dispensing without prescription.

NSW-7 A

PEDIACOF®   C R

DESCRIPTION

Each teaspoon (5 mL) contains:
Codeine phosphate, USP .... 5.0 mg
  (Warning: May be habit forming.)
Phenylephrine hydrochloride, USP .... 2.5 mg
Chlorpheniramine maleate, USP .... 0.75 mg
Potassium iodide, USP .... 75.0 mg
with sodium benzoate 0.2% as preservative and alcohol 5%.
Inactive Ingredients: Alcohol, Citric Acid, FD&C Red #40, Flavor, Glycerin, Liquid Glucose, Purified Water, Saccharin Sodium, Sodium Benzoate.

HOW SUPPLIED

Bottle of 16 fl oz   (NDC 0024-1509-06)
Available on prescription only.
For complete prescribing information see package insert or contact Product Information Services.

PSW-10

---

pHisoHex®   R
brand of hexachlorophene detergent cleanser

sudsing antibacterial soapless skin cleanser

DESCRIPTION

pHisoHex, brand of hexachlorophene detergent cleanser, is an antibacterial sudsing emulsion for topical administration. pHisoHex contains a colloidal dispersion of hexachlorophene 3% (w/w) in a stable emulsion consisting of entsufon sodium, petrolatum, lanolin cholesterols, methylcellulose, polyethylene glycol, polyethylene glycol monostearate, lauryl myristyl diethanolamide, sodium benzoate, and water. pH is adjusted with hydrochloric acid. Entsufon sodium is a synthetic detergent.
Chemically, hexachlorophene is Phenol, 2,2'-methylenebis[3,4,6-trichloro-].

CLINICAL PHARMACOLOGY

pHisoHex is a bacteriostatic cleansing agent. It cleanses the skin thoroughly and has bacteriostatic action against staphylococci and other gram-positive bacteria. Cumulative antibacterial action develops with repeated use. Cleansing with alcohol or soaps containing alcohol removes the antibacterial residue.
Detectable blood levels of hexachlorophene following absorption through intact skin have been found in subjects who regularly scrubbed with hexachlorophene emulsion 3%. (See WARNINGS for additional information.)
pHisoHex has the same slight acidity as normal skin (pH value 5.0 to 6.0).

INDICATIONS AND USAGE

pHisoHex is indicated for use as a surgical scrub and a bacteriostatic skin cleanser. It may also be used to control an outbreak of gram-positive infection where other infection control procedures have been unsuccessful. Use only as long as necessary for infection control.

CONTRAINDICATIONS

pHisoHex should not be used on burned or denuded skin. It should not be used as an occlusive dressing, wet pack, or lotion.
It should not be used routinely for prophylactic total body bathing.
It should not be used as a vaginal pack or tampon, or on any mucous membranes.
pHisoHex should not be used on persons with sensitivity to any of its components. It should not be used on persons who have demonstrated primary light sensitivity to halogenated phenol derivatives because of the possibility of cross-sensitivity to hexachlorophene.

WARNINGS

RINSE THOROUGHLY AFTER EACH USE. Patients should be closely monitored and use should be immediately discontinued at the first sign of any of the symptoms described below.
Rapid absorption of hexachlorophene may occur with resultant toxic blood levels when preparations containing hexachlorophene are applied to skin lesions such as ichthyosis congenita, the dermatitis of Letterer-Siwe's syndrome, or other generalized dermatological conditions. Application to burns has also produced neurotoxicity and death.
pHisoHex SHOULD BE DISCONTINUED PROMPTLY IF SIGNS OR SYMPTOMS OF CEREBRAL IRRITABILITY OCCUR.
Infants, especially premature infants or those with dermatoses, are particularly susceptible to hexachlorophene absorption. Systemic toxicity may be manifested by signs of stimulation (irritation) of the central nervous system, sometimes with convulsions.
Infants have developed dermatitis, irritability, generalized clonic muscular contractions and decerebrate rigidity following application of a 6 percent hexachlorophene powder. Examination of brainstems of those infants revealed vacuolization like that which can be produced in newborn experimental animals following repeated topical application of 3 percent hexachlorophene. Moreover, a study of histologic sections of premature infants who died of unrelated causes has shown a positive correlation between hexachlorophene baths and lesions in white matter of brains.

PRECAUTIONS

General
Avoid accidental contact of pHisoHex with the eyes.
If contact occurs, promptly rinse thoroughly with water. To assist in the detection of ocular irritation, applications to the head and periorbital skin areas should be performed only in responsive patients with unanesthetized eyes.
RINSE THOROUGHLY AFTER USE, especially from sensitive areas such as the scrotum and perineum.
pHisoHex is intended for external use only. If swallowed, pHisoHex is harmful, especially to infants and children.
pHisoHex should not be poured into measuring cups, medicine bottles, or similar containers since it may be mistaken for baby formula or other medications.

Carcinogenesis, Mutagenesis, Impairment of Fertility

Carcinogenicity studies in animals: Hexachlorophene was tested in one experiment in rats by oral administration; it had no carcinogenic effect.
Hexachlorophene was not mutagenic in *Salmonella typhimurium* and was negative in a dominant lethal assay in male mice. Cytogenetic tests with cultured human lymphocytes were also negative.
Human data: No case reports or epidemiological studies were available.
Impairment of fertility: Topical exposure of neonatal rats to 3% hexachlorophene solution caused reduced fertility in 7-month-old males, due to inability to ejaculate.

Embryotoxicity and Teratogenicity

Placental transfer of hexachlorophene has been demonstrated in rats.
Hexachlorophene is embryotoxic and produces some teratogenic effects.

Pregnancy Category C

There are no adequate and well-controlled studies in pregnant women. Hexachlorophene should be used during pregnancy only if the potential benefit justifies potential risk to the fetus.
Hexachlorophene has been shown to be teratogenic and embryotoxic in rats when given by mouth or instilled into the vagina in large doses.
Administration of 500 mg/kg diet or 20 to 30 mg/kg bw/day by gavage to rats caused some malformations (angulated ribs, cleft palate, micro- and anophthalmia) and reduction in litter size.
Placental transfer and excretion in milk of hexachlorophene has been demonstrated in rats.
In another study, doses of up to 50 mg/kg diet failed to produce any effects in 3 generations of rats. Hexachlorophene did not interfere with reproduction in hamsters.

Nursing Mothers

It is not known whether this drug is excreted in human milk. Because many drugs are excreted in human milk and because of the potential for serious adverse reactions in nursing infants from hexachlorophene, a decision should be made whether to discontinue nursing or to discontinue the drug taking into account the importance of the drug to the mother.

Pediatric Use

pHisoHex, brand of hexachlorophene detergent cleanser, should not be used routinely for bathing infants. See WARNINGS. For premature infants: see WARNINGS.

ADVERSE REACTIONS

Adverse reactions to pHisoHex may include dermatitis and photosensitivity. Sensitivity to hexachlorophene is rare; however, persons who have developed photoallergy to similar compounds also may become sensitive to hexachlorophene.
In persons with highly sensitive skin the use of pHisoHex may at times produce a reaction characterized by redness and/or mild scaling or dryness, especially when it is combined with such mechanical factors as excessive rubbing or exposure to heat or cold.

OVERDOSAGE

The accidental ingestion of pHisoHex in amounts from 1 oz to 4 oz has caused anorexia, vomiting, abdominal cramps, diarrhea, dehydration, convulsions, hypotension, and shock, and in several reported instances, fatalities.
If patients are seen early, the stomach should be evacuated by emesis or gastric lavage. Olive oil or vegetable oil (60 mL or 2 fl oz) may then be given to delay absorption of hexachlorophene, followed by a saline cathartic to hasten removal. Treatment is symptomatic and supportive; intravenous fluids (5 percent dextrose in physiologic saline solution) may be given for dehydration. Any other electrolyte derangement should be corrected. If marked hypotension occurs, vasopressor therapy is indicated. Use of opiates may be considered if gastrointestinal symptoms (cramping, diarrhea) are severe. Scheduled medical or surgical procedures should be postponed until the patient's condition has been evaluated and stabilized.

DOSAGE AND ADMINISTRATION

Surgical Hand Scrub
1. Wet hands and forearms with water. Apply approximately 5 mL of pHisoHex over the hands and rub into a copious lather by adding small amounts of water. Spread suds over hands and forearms and scrub well with a wet brush for 3 minutes. Pay particular attention to the nails and interdigital spaces. A separate nail cleaner may be used. *Rinse thoroughly* under running water.
2. Apply 5 mL of pHisoHex to hands again and scrub as above for another 3 minutes. *Rinse thoroughly* with running water and dry.
3. For repeat surgical scrubs during the day, scrub thoroughly with the same amount of pHisoHex for 3 minutes only. *Rinse thoroughly* with water and dry.

Bacteriostatic Cleansing

Wet hands with water. Dispense approximately 5 mL of pHisoHex into the palm, work up a lather with water and apply to area to be cleansed.

Rinse thoroughly after each washing.

INFANT CARE: pHisoHex should not be used routinely for bathing infants. See **WARNINGS.**

PREMATURE INFANTS: See **WARNINGS.**

Use of baby skin products containing alcohol may decrease the antibacterial action of pHisoHex, brand of hexachlorophene detergent cleanser.

HOW SUPPLIED

pHisoHex is available in plastic squeeze bottle of 5 ounces (NDC 0024-1535-02) and 1 pint (NDC 0024-1535-06); in plastic bottle of 1 gallon (NDC 0024-1535-08) and 1/4 oz (8 mL) unit packets, box of 50 (NDC 0024-1535-05).

The following, specially constructed, refillable dispensers made with metals and plastics compatible with pHisoHex can also be supplied: 16 oz hand operated wall dispensers; 30 oz pedal operated wall dispensers; 30 oz pedal operated wall dispenser with stand; portable stand with two 30 oz pedal operated dispensers.

Prolonged direct exposure of pHisoHex to strong light may cause brownish surface discoloration but does not affect its antibacterial or detergent properties. Shaking will disperse the color. If pHisoHex is spilled or splashed on porous surfaces, rinse off to avoid discoloration.

pHisoHex should not be dispensed from, or stored in, containers with ordinary metal parts. A special type of stainless steel must be used or undesirable discoloration of the product or oxidation of metal may occur. Specially designed dispensers for hospital or office use may be obtained through your local dealer.

Directions for Cleaning Dispensers: Before initial installation and use, run an antiseptic, such as an aqueous solution of benzalkonium chloride, NF, 1:500 to 1:750, or alcohol, through the working parts; rinse with sterile water. At weekly intervals thereafter, remove dispenser and pour off remainder of pHisoHex emulsion. Rinse empty dispenser with water. Run water through the working parts by operating the dispenser. Sanitize as described above. Rinse thoroughly with sterile water.

ANIMAL TOXICITY

The oral LD_{50} of hexachlorophene in male rats is 66 mg/kg bw, in females 56 mg/kg bw, and in weanling rats 120 mg/kg bw.

In suckling rats (10-days old), it is 9 mg/kg bw.

PSW-9B

PLAQUENIL® Sulfate ℞

brand of hydroxychloroquine sulfate tablets, USP

WARNING
PHYSICIANS SHOULD COMPLETELY FAMILIARIZE THEMSELVES WITH THE COMPLETE CONTENTS OF THIS LEAFLET BEFORE PRESCRIBING HYDROXYCHLOROQUINE.

DESCRIPTION

The compound is a colorless crystalline solid, soluble in water to at least 20 percent; chemically the drug is 2-[[4-[(7-Chloro-4- quinolyl) amino] pentyl] ethylamino] ethanol sulfate (1:1).

Inactive Ingredients: Dibasic Calcium Phosphate, Magnesium Stearate, Starch.

ACTIONS

The drug possesses antimalarial actions and also exerts a beneficial effect in lupus erythematosus (chronic discoid or systemic) and acute or chronic rheumatoid arthritis. The precise mechanism of action is not known.

INDICATIONS

PLAQUENIL is indicated for the suppressive treatment and treatment of acute attacks of malaria due to *Plasmodium vivax, P. malariae, P. ovale,* and susceptible strains of *P. falciparum.* It is also indicated for the treatment of discoid and systemic lupus erythematosus, and rheumatoid arthritis.

CONTRAINDICATIONS

Use of this drug is contraindicated (1) in the presence of retinal or visual field changes attributable to any 4-aminoquinoline compound, (2) in patients with known hypersensitivity to 4-aminoquinoline compounds, and (3) for long-term therapy in children.

WARNINGS, General

PLAQUENIL is not effective against chloroquine-resistant strains of *P. falciparum.*

Children are especially sensitive to the 4-aminoquinoline compounds. A number of fatalities have been reported following the accidental ingestion of chloroquine, sometimes in relatively small doses (0.75 g or 1 g in one 3- year-old child). Patients should be strongly warned to keep these drugs out of the reach of children.

Use of PLAQUENIL in patients with psoriasis may precipitate a severe attack of psoriasis. When used in patients with porphyria the condition may be exacerbated. The preparation should not be used in these conditions unless in the judgment of the physician the benefit to the patient outweighs the possible hazard.

Usage in Pregnancy—Usage of this drug during pregnancy should be avoided except in the suppression or treatment of malaria when in the judgment of the physician the benefit outweighs the possible hazard. It should be noted that radioactively-tagged chloroquine administered intravenously to pregnant, pigmented CBA mice passed rapidly across the placenta. It accumulated selectively in the melanin structures of the fetal eyes and was retained in the ocular tissues for five months after the drug had been eliminated from the rest of the body.

PRECAUTIONS, General

Antimalarial compounds should be used with caution in patients with hepatic disease or alcoholism or in conjunction with known hepatotoxic drugs.

Periodic blood cell counts should be made if patients are given prolonged therapy. If any severe blood disorder appears which is not attributable to the disease under treatment, discontinuation of the drug should be considered. The drug should be administered with caution in patients having G-6-PD (glucose-6-phosphate dehydrogenase) deficiency.

OVERDOSAGE

The 4-aminoquinoline compounds are very rapidly and completely absorbed after ingestion, and in accidental overdosage, or rarely with lower doses in hypersensitive patients, toxic symptoms may occur within 30 minutes. These consist of headache, drowsiness, visual disturbances, cardiovascular collapse, and convulsions, followed by sudden and early respiratory and cardiac arrest. The electrocardiogram may reveal atrial standstill, nodal rhythm, prolonged intraventricular conduction time, and progressive bradycardia leading to ventricular fibrillation and/or arrest. Treatment is symptomatic and must be prompt with immediate evacuation of the stomach by emesis (at home, before transportation to the hospital) or gastric lavage until the stomach is completely emptied. If finely powdered, activated charcoal is introduced by the stomach tube, after lavage, and within 30 minutes after ingestion of the tablets, it may inhibit further intestinal absorption of the drug. To be effective, the dose of activated charcoal should be at least five times the estimated dose of hydroxychloroquine ingested. Convulsions, if present, should be controlled before attempting gastric lavage. If due to cerebral stimulation, cautious administration of an ultrashort-acting barbiturate may be tried but, if due to anoxia, it should be corrected by oxygen administration, artificial respiration or, in shock with hypotension, by vasopressor therapy. Because of the importance of supporting respiration, tracheal intubation or tracheostomy, followed by gastric lavage, may also be necessary. Exchange transfusions have been used to reduce the level of 4-aminoquinoline drug in the blood.

A patient who survives the acute phase and is asymptomatic should be closely observed for at least six hours. Fluids may be forced, and sufficient ammonium chloride (8 g daily in divided doses for adults) may be administered for a few days to acidify the urine to help promote urinary excretion in cases of both overdosage and sensitivity.

MALARIA

ACTIONS

Like chloroquine phosphate, USP, PLAQUENIL sulfate is highly active against the erythrocytic forms of *P. vivax* and *malariae* and most strains of *P. falciparum* (but not the gametocytes of *P. falciparum).*

PLAQUENIL sulfate does not prevent relapses in patients with *vivax* or *malariae* malaria because it is not effective against exo-erythrocytic forms of the parasite, nor will it prevent *vivax* or *malariae* infection when administered as a prophylactic. It is highly effective as a suppressive agent in patients with *vivax* or *malariae* malaria, in terminating acute attacks, and significantly lengthening the interval between treatment and relapse. In patients with *falciparum* malaria, it abolishes the acute attack and effects complete cure of the infection, unless due to a resistant strain of *P. falciparum.*

INDICATIONS

PLAQUENIL sulfate, brand of hydroxychloroquine sulfate tablets, is indicated for the treatment of acute attacks and suppression of malaria.

WARNING

In recent years, it has been found that certain strains of *P. falciparum* have become resistant to 4-aminoquinoline compounds (including hydroxychloroquine) as shown by the fact that normally adequate doses have failed to prevent or cure clinical malaria or parasitemia. Treatment with quinine or other specific forms of therapy is therefore advised for patients infected with a resistant strain of parasites.

ADVERSE REACTIONS

Following the administration in doses adequate for the treatment of an acute malarial attack, mild and transient headache, dizziness, and gastrointestinal complaints (diarrhea, anorexia, nausea, abdominal cramps and, on rare occasions, vomiting) may occur.

DOSAGE AND ADMINISTRATION

One tablet of 200 mg of hydroxychloroquine sulfate is equivalent to 155 mg base.

Malaria: Suppression—*In adults,* 400 mg (=310 mg base) on exactly the same day of each week. *In infants and children,* the weekly suppressive dosage is 5 mg, calculated as base, per kg of body weight, but should not exceed the adult dose regardless of weight.

If circumstances permit, suppressive therapy should begin two weeks prior to exposure. However, failing this, in adults an initial double (loading) dose of 800 mg (= 620 mg base), or in children 10 mg base/kg may be taken in two divided doses, six hours apart. The suppressive therapy should be continued for eight weeks after leaving the endemic area.

Treatment of the acute attack—*In adults,* an initial dose of 800 mg (= 620 mg base) followed by 400 mg (= 310 mg base) in six to eight hours and 400 mg (310 mg base) on each of two consecutive days (total 2 g hydroxychloroquine sulfate or 1.55 g base). An alternative method, employing a single dose of 800 mg (= 620 mg base), has also proved effective.

The dosage for adults may also be calculated on the basis of body weight; this method is preferred for infants and children. A total dose representing 25 mg of base per kg of body weight is administered in three days, as follows:

First dose: 10 mg base per kg (but not exceeding a single dose of 620 mg base).

Second dose: 5 mg base per kg (but not exceeding a single dose of 310 mg base) 6 hours after first dose.

Third dose: 5 mg base per kg 18 hours after second dose.

Fourth dose: 5 mg base per kg 24 hours after third dose.

For radical cure of *vivax* and *malariae* malaria concomitant therapy with an 8-aminoquinoline compound is necessary.

LUPUS ERYTHEMATOSUS AND RHEUMATOID ARTHRITIS

INDICATIONS

PLAQUENIL is useful in patients with the following disorders who have not responded satisfactorily to drugs with less potential for serious side effects: lupus erythematosus (chronic discoid and systemic) and acute or chronic rheumatoid arthritis.

WARNINGS

PHYSICIANS SHOULD COMPLETELY FAMILIARIZE THEMSELVES WITH THE COMPLETE CONTENTS OF THIS LEAFLET BEFORE PRESCRIBING PLAQUENIL.

Irreversible retinal damage has been observed in some patients who had received long-term or high-dosage 4-aminoquinoline therapy for discoid and systemic lupus erythematosus, or rheumatoid arthritis. Retinopathy has been reported to be dose related.

When prolonged therapy with any antimalarial compound is contemplated, initial (base line) and periodic (every three months) ophthalmologic examinations (including visual acuity, expert slit-lamp, funduscopic, and visual field tests) should be performed.

If there is any indication of abnormality in the visual acuity, visual field, or retinal macular areas (such as pigmentary changes, loss of foveal reflex), or any visual symptoms (such as light flashes and streaks) which are not fully explainable by difficulties of accommodation or corneal opacities, the drug should be discontinued immediately and the patient closely observed for possible progression. Retinal changes (and visual disturbances) may progress even after cessation of therapy.

All patients on long-term therapy with this preparation should be questioned and examined periodically, including the testing of knee and ankle reflexes, to detect any evidence

Continued on next page

This product information was prepared in September 1996. On these and other products of Sanofi Winthrop Pharmaceuticals, detailed information may be obtained on a current basis by direct inquiry to Product Information Services, 90 Park Avenue, New York, NY 10016 (toll free 1-800-446-6267).

Sanofi Winthrop—Cont.

of muscular weakness. If weakness occurs, discontinue the drug.

In the treatment of rheumatoid arthritis, if objective improvement (such as reduced joint swelling, increased mobility) does not occur within six months, the drug should be discontinued. Safe use of the drug in the treatment of juvenile arthritis has not been established.

PRECAUTIONS

Dermatologic reactions to PLAQUENIL sulfate, brand of hydroxychloroquine sulfate tablets, may occur and, therefore, proper care should be exercised when it is administered to any patient receiving a drug with a significant tendency to produce dermatitis.

The methods recommended for early diagnosis of "chloroquine retinopathy" consist of (1) funduscopic examination of the macula for fine pigmentary disturbances or loss of the foveal reflex and (2) examination of the central visual field with a small red test object for pericentral or paracentral scotoma or determination of retinal thresholds to red. Any unexplained visual symptoms, such as light flashes or streaks should also be regarded with suspicion as possible manifestations of retinopathy.

If serious toxic symptoms occur from overdosage or sensitivity, it has been suggested that ammonium chloride (8 g daily in divided doses for adults) be administered orally three or four days a week for several months after therapy has been stopped, as acidification of the urine increases renal excretion of the 4-aminoquinoline compounds by 20 to 90 percent. However, caution must be exercised in patients with impaired renal function and/or metabolic acidosis.

ADVERSE REACTIONS

Not all of the following reactions have been observed with every 4-aminoquinoline compound during long-term therapy, but they have been reported with one or more and should be borne in mind when drugs of this class are administered. Adverse effects with different compounds vary in type and frequency.

CNS Reactions: Irritability, nervousness, emotional changes, nightmares, psychosis, headache, dizziness, vertigo, tinnitus, nystagmus, nerve deafness, convulsions, ataxia.

Neuromuscular Reactions: Extraocular muscle palsies, skeletal muscle weakness, absent or hypoactive deep tendon reflexes.

Ocular Reactions:

A. *Ciliary body:* Disturbance of accommodation with symptoms of blurred vision. This reaction is dose related and reversible with cessation of therapy.

B. *Cornea:* Transient edema, punctate to lineal opacities, decreased corneal sensitivity. The corneal changes, with or without accompanying symptoms (blurred vision, halos around lights, photophobia), are fairly common, but reversible. Corneal deposits may appear as early as three weeks following initiation of therapy.

The incidence of corneal changes and visual side effects appears to be considerably lower with hydroxychloroquine than with chloroquine.

C. *Retina:*

Macula: Edema, atrophy, abnormal pigmentation (mild pigment stippling to a "bull's-eye" appearance), loss of foveal reflex, increased macular recovery time following exposure to a bright light (photo-stress test), elevated retinal threshold to red light in macular, paramacular and peripheral retinal areas.

Other fundus changes include optic disc pallor and atrophy, attenuation of retinal arterioles, fine granular pigmentary disturbances in the peripheral retina and prominent choroidal patterns in advanced stage.

D. *Visual field defects:* pericentral or paracentral scotoma, central scotoma with decreased visual acuity, rarely field constriction.

The most common visual symptoms attributed to the retinopathy are: reading and seeing difficulties (words, letters, or parts of objects missing), photophobia, blurred distance vision, missing or blacked out areas in the central or peripheral visual field, light flashes and streaks.

Retinopathy appears to be dose related and has occurred within several months (rarely) to several years of daily therapy; a small number of cases have been reported several years after antimalarial drug therapy was discontinued. It has not been noted during prolonged use of weekly doses of the 4-aminoquinoline compounds for suppression of malaria. Patients with retinal changes may have visual symptoms or may be asymptomatic (with or without visual field changes). Rarely scotomatous vision or field defects may occur without obvious retinal change.

Retinopathy may progress even after the drug is discontinued. In a number of patients, early retinopathy (macular pigmentation sometimes with central field defects) diminished or regressed completely after therapy was discontinued. Paracentral scotoma to red targets (sometimes called "premaculopathy") is indicative of early retinal dysfunction which is usually reversible with cessation of therapy.

A small number of cases of retinal changes have been reported as occurring in patients who received only hydroxychloroquine. These usually consisted of alteration in retinal pigmentation which was detected on periodic ophthalmologic examination; visual field defects were also present in some instances. A case of delayed retinopathy has been reported with loss of vision starting one year after administration of hydroxychloroquine had been discontinued.

Dermatologic Reactions: Bleaching of hair, alopecia, pruritus, skin and mucosal pigmentation, skin eruptions (urticarial, morbilliform, lichenoid, maculopapular, purpuric, erythema annulare centrifugum and exfoliative dermatitis).

Hematologic Reactions: Various blood dyscrasias such as aplastic anemia, agranulocytosis, leukopenia, thrombocytopenia (hemolysis in individuals with glucose-6-phosphate dehydrogenase (G-6-PD) deficiency).

Gastrointestinal Reactions: Anorexia, nausea, vomiting, diarrhea, and abdominal cramps.

Miscellaneous Reactions: Weight loss, lassitude, exacerbation or precipitation of porphyria and nonlight-sensitive psoriasis.

Cardiomyopathy has been rarely reported and the relationship to hydroxychloroquine is unclear.

DOSAGE AND ADMINISTRATION

One tablet of hydroxychloroquine sulfate, 200 mg, is equivalent to 155 mg base.

Lupus erythematosus—Initially, the average *adult* dose is 400 mg (=310 mg base) once or twice daily. This may be continued for several weeks or months, depending on the response of the patient. For prolonged maintenance therapy, a smaller dose, from 200 mg to 400 mg (= 155 mg to 310 mg base) daily will frequently suffice.

The incidence of retinopathy has been reported to be higher when this maintenance dose is exceeded.

Rheumatoid arthritis—The compound is cumulative in action and will require several weeks to exert its beneficial therapeutic effects, whereas minor side effects may occur relatively early. Several months of therapy may be required before maximum effects can be obtained. If objective improvement (such as reduced joint swelling, increased mobility) does not occur within six months, the drug should be discontinued. Safe use of the drug in the treatment of juvenile rheumatoid arthritis has not been established.

Initial dosage—In *adults*, from 400 mg to 600 mg (=310 mg to 465 mg base) daily, each dose to be taken with a meal or a glass of milk. In a small percentage of patients, troublesome side effects may require temporary reduction of the initial dosage. Later (usually from five to ten days), the dose may gradually be increased to the optimum response level, often without return of side effects.

Maintenance dosage—When a good response is obtained (usually in four to twelve weeks), the dosage is reduced by 50 percent and continued at a usual maintenance level of 200 mg to 400 mg (=155 mg to 310 mg base) daily, each dose to be taken with a meal or a glass of milk. The incidence of retinopathy has been reported to be higher when this maintenance dose is exceeded.

Should a relapse occur after medication is withdrawn, therapy may be resumed or continued on an intermittent schedule if there are no ocular contraindications.

Corticosteroids and salicylates may be used in conjunction with this compound, and they can generally be decreased gradually in dosage or eliminated after the drug has been used for several weeks. When gradual reduction of steroid dosage is indicated, it may be done by reducing every four to five days the dose of cortisone by no more than from 5 mg to 15 mg; of hydrocortisone from 5 mg to 10 mg; of prednisolone and prednisone from 1 mg to 2.5 mg; of methylprednisolone and triamcinolone from 1 mg to 2 mg; and of dexamethasone from 0.25 mg to 0.5 mg.

HOW SUPPLIED

Tablets of 200 mg (equivalent to 155 mg of base), bottle of 100 (**NDC** 0024-1562-10)

PSW-5

Shown in Product Identification Guide, page 333

PONTOCAINE® Hydrochloride
brand of tetracaine hydrochloride, USP

℞

Prolonged Spinal Anesthesia

DESCRIPTION

Tetracaine hydrochloride is 2-(Dimethylamino)ethyl *p*-(butylamino) benzoate monohydrochloride. It is a white crystalline, odorless powder that is readily soluble in water, physiologic saline solution, and dextrose solution.

Tetracaine hydrochloride is a local anesthetic of the ester-linkage type, related to procaine.

PONTOCAINE hydrochloride is supplied in two forms for prolonged spinal anesthesia: Niphanoid® and 1% Solution.

NIPHANOID: A sterile, instantly soluble form consisting of a network of extremely fine, highly purified particles, resembling snow.

1% Solution: A sterile, isotonic, isobaric solution, each 1 mL containing 10 mg tetracaine hydrochloride, 6.7 mg sodium chloride, and not more than 2 mg acetone sodium bisulfite. The air in the ampuls has been displaced by nitrogen gas. The pH is 3.2 to 6.

These formulations do not contain preservatives.

CLINICAL PHARMACOLOGY

Parenteral administration of PONTOCAINE stabilizes the neuronal membrane and prevents initiation and transmission of nerve impulses thereby effecting local anesthesia. The onset of action is rapid, and the duration prolonged (up to two or three hours or longer of surgical anesthesia). PONTOCAINE is detoxified by plasma esterases to aminobenzoic acid and diethylaminoethanol.

INDICATIONS AND USAGE

PONTOCAINE is indicated for the production of spinal anesthesia for procedures requiring two to three hours.

CONTRAINDICATIONS

Spinal anesthesia with PONTOCAINE is contraindicated in patients with known hypersensitivity to tetracaine hydrochloride or to drugs of a similar chemical configuration (ester-type local anesthetics), or aminobenzoic acid or its derivatives; and in patients for whom spinal anesthesia as a technique is contraindicated.

The decision as to whether or not spinal anesthesia should be used for an individual patient should be made by the physician after weighing the advantages with the risks and possible complications. Contraindications to spinal anesthesia as a technique can be found in standard reference texts, and usually include generalized septicemia, infection at the site of injection, certain diseases of the cerebrospinal system, uncontrolled hypotension, etc.

WARNINGS

RESUSCITATIVE EQUIPMENT AND DRUGS SHOULD BE IMMEDIATELY AVAILABLE WHENEVER ANY LOCAL ANESTHETIC DRUG IS USED.

Large doses of local anesthetics should not be used in patients with heartblock.

Reactions resulting in fatality have occurred on rare occasions with the use of local anesthetics, even in the absence of a history of hypersensitivity.

Contains acetone sodium bisulfite, a sulfite that may cause allergic-type reactions including anaphylactic symptoms and life-threatening or less severe asthmatic episodes in certain susceptible people. The overall prevalence of sulfite sensitivity in the general population is unknown and probably low. Sulfite sensitivity is seen more frequently in asthmatic than in nonasthmatic people.

PRECAUTIONS

The safety and effectiveness of any spinal anesthetic depend upon proper dosage, correct technique, adequate precautions, and readiness for emergencies. The lowest dosage that results in effective anesthesia should be used to avoid high plasma levels and serious systemic side effects. Tolerance varies with the status of the patient; debilitated, elderly patients or acutely ill patients should be given reduced doses commensurate with their weight, age, and physical status. Reduced doses are also indicated for obstetric patients and those with increased intra-abdominal pressure.

Caution should be used in administering PONTOCAINE to patients with abnormal or reduced levels of plasma esterases.

Blood pressure should be frequently monitored during spinal anesthesia and hypotension immediately corrected.

Spinal anesthetics should be used with caution in patients with severe disturbances of cardiac rhythm, shock, or heartblock.

Drug Interactions: PONTOCAINE should not be used if the patient is being treated with a sulfonamide because aminobenzoic acid inhibits the action of sulfonamides.

Carcinogenesis, Mutagenesis, Impairment of Fertility: Long-term animal studies to evaluate carcinogenic potential and reproduction studies in animals have not been performed. There is no evidence from human data that PONTOCAINE may be carcinogenic or that it impairs fertility.

Pregnancy Category C: Animal reproduction studies have not been conducted with PONTOCAINE. It is not known whether PONTOCAINE can cause fetal harm when administered to a pregnant woman or can affect reproduction capacity. PONTOCAINE should be given to a pregnant woman only if clearly needed and the potential benefits outweigh the risk.

Labor and Delivery: Vasopressor agents administered for the treatment of hypotension resulting from spinal anesthesia may result in severe persistent hypertension and/or rupture of cerebral blood vessels if oxytocic drugs have also been administered; therefore, vasopressors should be used with extreme caution in the presence of oxytocic drugs.

SUGGESTED DOSAGE FOR SPINAL ANESTHESIA

| Extent of anesthesia | Using NIPHANOID | | | Using 1% Solution | | Site of injection (lumbar interspace) |
	Dose of NIPHANOID (mg)	Volume of spinal fluid (mL)	Dose of solution (mL)	Volume of spinal fluid (mL)		
Perineum	5*	1	0.5 (=5 mg)*	0.5		4th
Perineum and lower extremities	10	2	1 (=10 mg)	1		3d or 4th
Up to costal margin	15 to 20†	3	1.5 to 2 (=15 mg to 20 mg)†	1.5 to 2		2d, 3d, or 4th

* For vaginal delivery (saddle block), from 2 mg to 5 mg in dextrose.
† Doses exceeding 15 mg are rarely required and should be used only in exceptional cases. Inject solution at rate of about 1 mL per 5 seconds.

PONTOCAINE has a recognized use during labor and delivery; the effect of the drug on duration of labor, incidence of forceps delivery, status of the newborn, and later growth and development of the child have not been studied.

Nursing Mothers: It is not known whether PONTOCAINE is excreted in human milk; however, it is rapidly metabolized following absorption into the plasma. Because many drugs are excreted in human milk, caution should be exercised when PONTOCAINE, brand of tetracaine hydrochloride, is administered to a nursing woman.

Pediatric Use: Safety and effectiveness of PONTOCAINE in children have not been established.

ADVERSE REACTIONS

Systemic adverse reactions to PONTOCAINE are characteristic of those associated with other local anesthetics and can involve the central nervous system and the cardiovascular system. Systemic reactions usually result from high plasma levels due to excessive dosage, rapid absorption, or inadvertent intravascular injection.

A small number of reactions to PONTOCAINE may result from hypersensitivity, idiosyncrasy, or diminished tolerance to normal dosage.

Central nervous system effects are characterized by excitation or depression. The first manifestation may be nervousness, dizziness, blurred vision, or tremors, followed by drowsiness, convulsions, unconsciousness and possibly respiratory and cardiac arrest. Since excitement may be transient or absent, the first manifestation may be drowsiness, sometimes merging into unconsciousness and respiratory and cardiac arrest. Other central nervous system effects may be nausea, vomiting, chills, constriction of the pupils, or tinnitus.

Cardiovascular system reactions include depression of the myocardium, blood pressure changes (usually hypotension), and cardiac arrest.

Allergic reactions, which may be due to hypersensitivity, idiosyncrasy, or diminished tolerance, are characterized by cutaneous lesions (eg, urticaria), edema, and other manifestations of allergy. Detection of sensitivity by skin testing is of limited value. Severe allergic reactions including anaphylaxis have occurred rarely and are not usually dose-related.

Reactions Associated with Spinal Anesthesia Techniques: *Central Nervous System:* post-spinal headache, meningismus, arachnoiditis, palsies, or spinal nerve paralysis. *Cardiovascular:* hypotension due to vasomotor paralysis and pooling of the blood in the venous bed. *Respiratory:* respiratory impairment or paralysis due to the level of anesthesia extending to the upper thoracic and cervical segments. *Gastrointestinal:* nausea and vomiting.

Treatment of Reactions: Toxic effects of local anesthetics require symptomatic treatment; there is no specific cure. The most important measure is oxygenation of the patient by maintaining an airway and supporting ventilation. Supportive treatment of the cardiovascular system includes intravenous fluids and, when appropriate, vasopressors (preferably those that stimulate the myocardium). Convulsions are usually controlled with adequate oxygenation alone but intravenous administration in small increments of a barbiturate (preferably an ultrashort-acting barbiturate such as thiopental and thiamylal) or diazepam can be utilized. Intravenous barbiturates or anticonvulsant agents should only be administered by those familiar with their use and only if ventilation and oxygenation have first been assured. In spinal anesthesia, sympathetic blockade also occurs as a pharmacological action, resulting in peripheral vasodilation and often hypotension. The extent of the hypotension will usually depend on the number of dermatomes blocked. The blood pressure should therefore be monitored in the early phases of anesthesia. If hypotension occurs, it is readily controlled by vasoconstrictors administered either by the intramuscular or the intravenous route, the dosage of which would depend on the severity of the hypotension and the response to treatment.

DOSAGE AND ADMINISTRATION

As with all anesthetics, the dosage varies and depends upon the area to be anesthetized, the number of neuronal segments to be blocked, individual tolerance, and the technique of anesthesia. The lowest dosage needed to provide effective anesthesia should be administered. For specific techniques and procedures, refer to standard textbooks.
[See table above.]

The extent and degree of spinal anesthesia depend upon dosage, specific gravity of the anesthetic solution, volume of solution used, force of the injection, level of puncture, position of the patient during and immediately after injection, etc.

When spinal fluid is added to either the NIPHANOID or solution, some turbidity results, the degree depending on the pH of the spinal fluid, the temperature of the solution during mixing, as well as the amount of drug and diluent employed. This cloudiness is due to the release of the *base* from the hydrochloride. Liberation of base (which is completed within the spinal canal) is held to be essential for satisfactory results with any spinal anesthetic.

The specific gravity of spinal fluid at 25°C/25°C varies under normal conditions from 1.0063 to 1.0075. A solution of the instantly soluble form (NIPHANOID) in spinal fluid has only a slightly greater specific gravity. The 1% concentration in saline solution has a specific gravity of 1.0060 to 1.0074 at 25°C/25°C.

A hyperbaric solution may be prepared by mixing equal volumes of the 1% Solution and Dextrose Solution 10% (which is available in ampuls of 3 mL).

If the NIPHANOID form is preferred, it is first dissolved in Dextrose Solution 10% in a ratio of 1 mL dextrose to 10 mg of the anesthetic. Further dilution is made with an equal volume of spinal fluid. The resulting solution now contains 5% dextrose with 5 mg of anesthetic agent per milliliter.

A hypobaric solution may be prepared by dissolving the NIPHANOID in Sterile Water for Injection, USP (1 mg per milliliter). The specific gravity of this solution is essentially the same as that of water, 1.000 at 25°C/25°C.

Examine ampuls carefully before use. Do not use solution if crystals, cloudiness, or discoloration is observed.

These formulations of tetracaine hydrochloride do not contain preservatives; therefore, unused portions should be discarded and the reconstituted NIPHANOID should be used immediately.

STERILIZATION OF AMPULS

The drug in intact ampuls is sterile. The preferred method of destroying bacteria on the exterior of ampuls before opening is heat sterilization (autoclaving). Immersion in antiseptic solution is not recommended.

Autoclave at 15-pound pressure, at 121°C (250°F), for 15 minutes. The NIPHANOID form may also be autoclaved in the same way but may lose its snowlike appearance and tend to adhere to the sides of the ampul. This may slightly decrease the rate at which the drug dissolves but does not interfere with its anesthetic potency.

Autoclaving increases likelihood of crystal formation. Unused autoclaved ampuls should be discarded. Under no circumstance should unused ampuls which have been autoclaved be returned to stock.

HOW SUPPLIED

Protect ampuls from light and store solution under refrigeration.

NIPHANOID (instantly soluble): Ampuls of 20 mg, box of 100.
NDC 0024-1577-06
Uni-Nest ™—1% isotonic isobaric solution: Ampuls of 2 mL, box of 25.
NDC 0024-1574-25

PSW-6

PRIMACOR® ℞
MILRINONE LACTATE INJECTION

DESCRIPTION

PRIMACOR, brand of milrinone lactate injection, is a member of a new class of bipyridine inotropic/vasodilator agents with phosphodiesterase inhibitor activity, distinct from digitalis glycosides or catecholamines. PRIMACOR (milrinone lactate) is designated chemically as 1,6-dihydro-2-methyl-6-oxo-[3,4'-bipyridine]-5-carbonitrile lactate and has the following structure:

Milrinone is an off-white to tan crystalline compound with a molecular weight of 211.2 and an empirical formula of $C_{12}H_9N_3O$. It is slightly soluble in methanol, and very slightly soluble in chloroform and in water. As the lactate salt, it is stable and colorless to pale yellow in solution. PRIMACOR is available as sterile aqueous solutions of the lactate salt of milrinone for injection or infusion intravenously.

Sterile, single-dose vials: Single-dose vials of 10 and 20 mL contain in each mL milrinone lactate equivalent to 1 mg milrinone and 47 mg Dextrose, Anhydrous, USP, in Water for Injection, USP. The pH is adjusted to between 3.2 and 4.0 with lactic acid or sodium hydroxide. The total concentration of lactic acid can vary between 0.95 mg/mL and 1.29 mg/mL. These vials require preparation of dilutions prior to administration to patients intravenously.

Pre-Mix Flexible Container: The Flexible Container provides a ready-to-use dilution of milrinone in a volume of 100 mL of 5% Dextrose Injection. Each mL contains milrinone lactate equivalent to 200 mcg milrinone. The nominal concentration of lactic acid is 0.282 mg/mL. Each mL also contains 49.4 mg Dextrose, Anhydrous, USP. The pH is adjusted to between 3.2 and 4.0 with lactic acid or sodium hydroxide. The flexible plastic container is comprised of polyvinyl chloride with a foil overwrap. Water can permeate the plastic into the overwrap, but the amount is insufficient to significantly affect the pre-mix solution.

CLINICAL PHARMACOLOGY

PRIMACOR is a positive inotrope and vasodilator, with little chronotropic activity different in structure and mode of action from either the digitalis glycosides or catecholamines. PRIMACOR, at relevant inotropic and vasorelaxant concentrations, is a selective inhibitor of peak III cAMP phosphodiesterase isozyme in cardiac and vascular muscle. This inhibitory action is consistent with cAMP mediated increases in intracellular ionized calcium and contractile force in cardiac muscle, as well as with cAMP dependent contractile protein phosphorylation and relaxation in vascular muscle. Additional experimental evidence also indicates that PRIMACOR is not a beta-adrenergic agonist nor does it in-

Continued on next page

This product information was prepared in September 1996. On these and other products of Sanofi Winthrop Pharmaceuticals, detailed information may be obtained on a current basis by direct inquiry to Product Information Services, 90 Park Avenue, New York, NY 10016 (toll free 1-800-446-6267).

Sanofi Winthrop—Cont.

hibit sodium-potassium adenosine triphosphatase activity as do the digitalis glycosides.

Clinical studies in patients with congestive heart failure have shown that PRIMACOR produces dose-related and plasma drug concentration-related increases in the maximum rate of increase of left ventricular pressure. Studies in normal subjects have shown that PRIMACOR produces increases in the slope of the left ventricular pressure-dimension relationship, indicating a direct inotropic effect of the drug. PRIMACOR also produces dose-related and plasma concentration-related increases in forearm blood flow in patients with congestive heart failure, indicating a direct arterial vasodilator activity of the drug.

Both the inotropic and vasodilatory effects have been observed over the therapeutic range of plasma milrinone concentrations of 100 ng/mL to 300 ng/mL.

In addition to increasing myocardial contractility, PRIMACOR improves diastolic function as evidenced by improvements in left ventricular diastolic relaxation.

A further clinical perspective was obtained in a single, multicenter, double-blind trial of the chronic administration of oral milrinone. Patients with New York Heart Association Class III and IV heart failure and left ventricular ejection fraction of less than 35% were randomized to placebo (N=527) or oral milrinone (40 mg daily, N=561) and followed for a median of six months. The oral milrinone treatment group had statistically significantly increased all-cause mortality and cardiovascular mortality. This finding in patients on oral milrinone was not apparent during the initial period of chronic treatment (15 days) in either the overall patient population or in the NYHA Class IV subgroup.

The acute administration of intravenous milrinone has also been evaluated in clinical trials in excess of 1600 patients, with chronic heart failure, associated with cardiac surgery, and heart failure associated with myocardial infarction. The total number of deaths, either on therapy or shortly thereafter (24 hours) was 15, less than 0.9%, few of which were thought to be drug-related.

Pharmacokinetics

Following intravenous injections of 12.5 mcg/kg to 125 mcg/kg to congestive heart failure patients, PRIMACOR had a volume of distribution of 0.38 liters/kg, a mean terminal elimination half-life of 2.3 hours, and a clearance of 0.13 liters/kg/hr. Following intravenous infusions of 0.20 mcg/kg/min to 0.70 mcg/kg/min to congestive heart failure patients, the drug had a volume of distribution of about 0.45 liters/kg, a mean terminal elimination half-life of 2.4 hours, and a clearance of 0.14 liters/kg/hr. These pharmacokinetic parameters were not dose-dependent, and the area under the plasma concentration versus time curve following injections was significantly dose-dependent.

PRIMACOR has been shown (by equilibrium dialysis) to be approximately 70% bound to human plasma protein.

The primary route of excretion of PRIMACOR in man is via the urine. The major urinary excretions of orally administered PRIMACOR in man are milrinone (83%) and its 0-glucuronide metabolite (12%). Elimination in normal subjects via the urine is rapid, with approximately 60% recovered within the first two hours following dosing and approximately 90% recovered within the first eight hours following dosing. The mean renal clearance of PRIMACOR is approximately 0.3 liters/min, indicative of active secretion.

Pharmacodynamics

In patients with depressed myocardial function, PRIMACOR produced a prompt increase in cardiac output and decreases in pulmonary capillary wedge pressure and vascular resistance, without a significant increase in heart rate or myocardial oxygen consumption. These hemodynamic improvements were dose and plasma milrinone concentration related. Hemodynamic improvement during intravenous therapy with PRIMACOR was accompanied by clinical symptomatic improvement, as measured by changes in New York Heart Association classification. The great majority of patients experience improvements in hemodynamic function within 5 to 15 minutes of the initiation of therapy.

In studies in congestive heart failure patients, PRIMACOR when administered as a loading injection followed by a maintenance infusion produced significant mean initial increases in cardiac index of 25 percent, 38 percent, and 42 percent at dose regimens of 37.5 mcg/kg/0.375 mcg/kg/min, 50 mcg/kg/0.50 mcg/kg/min, and 75 mcg/kg/0.75 mcg/kg/min, respectively. Over the same range of loading injections and maintenance infusions, pulmonary capillary wedge pressure significantly decreased by 20 percent, 23 percent, and 36 percent, respectively, while systemic vascular resistance significantly decreased by 17 percent, 21 percent, and 37 percent. The heart rate was generally unchanged (increases of 3, 3 and 10 percent, respectively). Mean arterial pressure fell by up to 5 percent at the two lower dose regimens, but by 17 percent at the highest dose. Patients evaluated for 48 hours maintained improvements in hemodynamic function, with no evidence of diminished response (tachyphylaxis). A

smaller number of patients have received infusions of PRIMACOR for periods up to 72 hours without evidence of tachyphylaxis.

The duration of therapy should depend upon patient responsiveness. Patients have been maintained on infusions of PRIMACOR for up to 5 days.

PRIMACOR has a favorable inotropic effect in fully digitalized patients without causing signs of glycoside toxicity. Theoretically, in cases of atrial flutter/fibrillation, it is possible that PRIMACOR may increase ventricular response rate because of its slight enhancement of AV node conduction. In these cases, digitalis should be considered prior to the institution of therapy with PRIMACOR.

Improvement in left ventricular function in patients with ischemic heart disease has been observed. The improvement has occurred without inducing symptoms or electrocardiographic signs of myocardial ischemia.

The steady-state plasma milrinone concentrations after approximately 6 to 12 hours of unchanging maintenance infusion of 0.50 mcg/kg/min are approximately 200 ng/mL. Near maximum favorable effects of PRIMACOR on cardiac output and pulmonary capillary wedge pressure are seen at plasma milrinone concentrations in the 150 ng/mL to 250 ng/mL range.

INDICATIONS AND USAGE

PRIMACOR is indicated for the short-term intravenous therapy of congestive heart failure. The majority of experience with intravenous PRIMACOR has been in patients receiving digoxin and diuretics.

In some patients injections of PRIMACOR and oral PRIMACOR have been shown to increase ventricular ectopy, including nonsustained ventricular tachycardia. Patients receiving PRIMACOR should be closely monitored during infusion.

CONTRAINDICATIONS

PRIMACOR is contraindicated in patients who are hypersensitive to it.

PRECAUTIONS

General

PRIMACOR should not be used in patients with severe obstructive aortic or pulmonic valvular disease in lieu of surgical relief of the obstruction. Like other inotropic agents, it may aggravate outflow tract obstruction in hypertrophic subaortic stenosis.

Supraventricular and ventricular arrhythmias have been observed in the high-risk population treated. In some patients, injections of PRIMACOR and oral PRIMACOR have been shown to increase ventricular ectopy, including nonsustained ventricular tachycardia. The potential for arrhythmia, present in congestive heart failure itself, may be increased by many drugs or combinations of drugs. Patients receiving PRIMACOR should be closely monitored during infusion.

PRIMACOR produces a slight shortening of AV node conduction time, indicating a potential for an increased ventricular response rate in patients with atrial flutter/fibrillation which is not controlled with digitalis therapy.

During therapy with PRIMACOR, blood pressure and heart rate should be monitored and the rate of infusion slowed or stopped in patients showing excessive decreases in blood pressure.

If prior vigorous diuretic therapy is suspected to have caused significant decreases in cardiac filling pressure, PRIMACOR should be cautiously administered with monitoring of blood pressure, heart rate, and clinical symptomatology.

USE IN ACUTE MYOCARDIAL INFARCTION

No clinical studies have been conducted in patients in the acute phase of post myocardial infarction. Until further clinical experience with this class of drugs is gained, PRIMACOR is not recommended in these patients.

Laboratory Tests

Fluid and Electrolytes: Fluid and electrolyte changes and renal function should be carefully monitored during therapy with PRIMACOR. Improvement in cardiac output with resultant diuresis may necessitate a reduction in the dose of diuretic. Potassium loss due to excessive diuresis may predispose digitalized patients to arrhythmias. Therefore, hypokalemia should be corrected by potassium supplementation in advance of or during use of PRIMACOR.

Drug Interactions

No untoward clinical manifestations have been observed in limited experience with patients in whom PRIMACOR was used concurrently with the following drugs: digitalis glycosides; lidocaine, quinidine; hydralazine, prazosin; isosorbide dinitrate, nitroglycerin; chlorthalidone, furosemide, hydrochlorothiazide, spironolactone; captopril; heparin, warfarin, diazepam, insulin; and potassium supplements.

Chemical Interactions

There is an immediate chemical interaction which is evidenced by the formation of a precipitate when furosemide is injected into an intravenous line of an infusion of PRIMACOR. Therefore, furosemide should not be administered in intravenous lines containing PRIMACOR.

Carcinogenesis, Mutagenesis, Impairment of Fertility

Twenty-four months of oral administration of PRIMACOR to mice at doses up to 40 mg/kg/day (about 50 times the human oral therapeutic dose in a 50 kg patient) was unassociated with evidence of carcinogenic potential. Neither was there evidence of carcinogenic potential when PRIMACOR was orally administered to rats at doses up to 5 mg/kg/day (about 6 times the human oral therapeutic dose) for twenty-four months or at 25 mg/kg/day (about 30 times the human oral therapeutic dose) for up to 18 months in males and 20 months in females. Whereas the Chinese Hamster Ovary Chromosome Aberration Assay was positive in the presence of a metabolic activation system, results from the Ames Test, the Mouse Lymphoma Assay, the Micronucleus Test, and the in vivo Rat Bone Marrow Metaphase Analysis indicated an absence of mutagenic potential. In reproductive performance studies in rats, PRIMACOR had no effect on male or female fertility at oral doses up to 32 mg/kg/day.

Animal Toxicity

Oral and intravenous administration of toxic dosages of PRIMACOR to rats and dogs resulted in myocardial degeneration/fibrosis and endocardial hemorrhage, principally affecting the left ventricular papillary muscles. Coronary vascular lesions characterized by periarterial edema and inflammation have been observed in dogs only. The myocardial/endocardial changes are similar to those produced by beta-adrenergic receptor agonists such as isoproterenol, while the vascular changes are similar to those produced by minoxidil and hydralazine. Doses within the recommended clinical dose range (up to 1.13 mg/kg/day) for congestive heart failure patients have not produced significant adverse effects in animals.

Pregnancy Category C

Oral administration of PRIMACOR to pregnant rats and rabbits during organogenesis produced no evidence of teratogenicity at dose levels up to 40 mg/kg/day and 12 mg/kg/day, respectively. PRIMACOR did not appear to be teratogenic when administered intravenously to pregnant rats at doses up to 3 mg/kg/day (about 2.5 times the maximum recommended clinical intravenous dose) or pregnant rabbits at doses up to 12 mg/kg/day, although an increased resorption rate was apparent at both 8 mg/kg/day, 12 mg/kg/day (intravenous) in the latter species. There are no adequate and well-controlled studies in pregnant women. PRIMACOR should be used during pregnancy only if the potential benefit justifies the potential risk to the fetus.

Nursing Mothers

Caution should be exercised when PRIMACOR is administered to nursing women, since it is not known whether it is excreted in human milk.

Pediatric Use

Safety and effectiveness in children have not been established.

Use in Elderly Patients

There are no special dosage recommendations for the elderly patient. Ninety percent of all patients administered PRIMACOR in clinical studies were within the age range of 45 to 70 years, with a mean age of 61 years. Patients in all age groups demonstrated clinically and statistically significant responses. No age-related effects on the incidence of adverse reactions have been observed. Controlled pharmacokinetic studies have not disclosed any age-related effects on the distribution and elimination of PRIMACOR.

ADVERSE REACTIONS

Cardiovascular Effects: In patients receiving PRIMACOR in Phase II and III clinical trials, ventricular arrhythmias were reported in 12.1%: Ventricular ectopic activity, 8.5%; nonsustained ventricular tachycardia, 2.8%; sustained ventricular tachycardia, 1% and ventricular fibrillation, 0.2% (2 patients experienced more than one type of arrhythmia). Holter recordings demonstrated that in some patients injection of PRIMACOR increased ventricular ectopy, including nonsustained ventricular tachycardia. Life-threatening arrhythmias were infrequent and when present have been associated with certain underlying factors such as preexisting arrhythmias, metabolic abnormalities (e.g. hypokalemia), abnormal digoxin levels and catheter insertion. PRIMACOR was not shown to be arrhythmogenic in an electrophysiology study. Supraventricular arrhythmias were reported in 3.8% of the patients receiving PRIMACOR. The incidence of both supraventricular and ventricular arrhythmias has not been related to the dose or plasma milrinone concentration.

Other cardiovascular adverse reactions include hypotension, 2.9% and angina/chest pain, 1.2%.

CNS Effects

Headaches, usually mild to moderate in severity, have been reported in 2.9% of patients receiving PRIMACOR.

Other Effects

Other adverse reactions reported, but not definitely related to the administration of PRIMACOR include hypokalemia, 0.6%; tremor, 0.4%; and thrombocytopenia, 0.4%. Isolated spontaneous reports of bronchospasm have been received.

OVERDOSAGE

Doses of PRIMACOR may produce hypotension because of its vasodilator effect. If this occurs, administration of PRIMACOR should be reduced or temporarily discontinued until the patient's condition stabilizes. No specific antidote is known, but general measures for circulatory support should be taken.

DOSAGE AND ADMINISTRATION

PRIMACOR should be administered with a loading dose followed by a continuous infusion (maintenance dose) according to the following guidelines:

LOADING DOSE

50 mcg/kg: Administer slowly over 10 minutes
The table below shows the loading dose in milliliters (mL) of PRIMACOR (1 mg/mL) by patient body weight (kg).

Loading Dose (mL) Using 1 mg/mL Concentration

Patient Body Weight (kg)

kg	30	40	50	60	70	80	90	100	110	120
mL	1.5	2.0	2.5	3.0	3.5	4.0	4.5	5.0	5.5	6.0

The loading dose may be given undiluted, but diluting to a rounded total volume of 10 or 20 mL (see Maintenance Dose for diluents) may simplify the visualization of the injection rate.

[See table on top of page.]

PRIMACOR drawn from vials should be diluted prior to maintenance dose administration. The diluents that may be used are 0.45% Sodium Chloride Injection USP, 0.9% Sodium Chloride Injection USP, or 5% Dextrose Injection USP. The table below shows the volume of diluent in milliliters (mL) that must be used to achieve concentrations recommended for infusion, 100 mcg/mL, 150 mcg/mL, or 200 mcg/mL, and the resultant total volumes.

Desired Infusion Concentration mcg/mL	PRIMACOR 1 mg/mL (mL)	Diluent (mL)	Total Volume (mL)
100	10	90	100
100	20	180	200
150	10	56.7	66.7
150	20	113	133
200	10	40	50
200	20	80	100

The infusion rate should be adjusted according to hemodynamic and clinical response. Patients should be closely monitored. In controlled clinical studies, most patients showed an improvement in hemodynamic status as evidenced by increases in cardiac output and reductions in pulmonary capillary wedge pressure.

Note: See "**Dosage Adjustment in Renally Impaired Patients.**" Dosage may be titrated to the maximum hemodynamic effect and should not exceed 1.13 mg/kg/day. Duration of therapy should depend upon patient responsiveness. The maintenance dose in mL/hr by patient body weight (kg) may be determined by reference to one of the following three tables.

[See tables on bottom of page.]

When administering PRIMACOR (milrinone lactate) by continuous infusion, it is advisable to use a calibrated electronic infusion device.

The Flexible Container has a concentration of milrinone equivalent to 200 mcg/mL in 5% Dextrose Injection and is more convenient to use than dilutions prepared from the vials. To use the Flexible Container, tear the overwrap at the notch and remove the Pre-Mix solution container. Squeeze the container firmly to check for leaks. Discard the container if leaks are found since the sterility of the product could be affected. Do not add supplementary medication. To prepare the container for administration of PRIMACOR intravenously, use aseptic techniques.

1) The flow control clamp of the administration set is closed.
2) The cover of the outlet port at the bottom of the container is removed.
3) Noting the full directions on the administration set carton, the piercing pin of the set is inserted into the port with a twisting motion until it is firmly seated.
4) The container is suspended on the hanger.
5) The drip chamber is squeezed and released to establish the fill level.
6) The flow control clamp is opened to expel air from the set, and then closed.
7) The set is attached to the venipuncture device, primed, and if not indwelling, the venipuncture is performed.
8) The rate of administration is controlled with the flow control clamp. WARNING- DO NOT USE IN SERIES CONNECTIONS. Caution: Do not use plastic containers in series connections. Such use could result in air embolism due to residual air being drawn from the primary container before administration of the fluid from the secondary container is complete.

Intravenous drug products should be inspected visually and should not be used if particulate matter or discoloration is present.

Dosage Adjustment in Renally Impaired Patients

Data obtained from patients with severe renal impairment (creatinine clearance = 0 to 30 mL/min) but without congestive heart failure have demonstrated that the presence of renal impairment significantly increases the terminal elimination half-life of PRIMACOR. Reductions in infusion rate may be necessary in patients with renal impairment. For patients with clinical evidence of renal impairment, the recommended infusion rate can be obtained from the following table:

Creatinine Clearance (mL/min/1.73 m²)	Infusion Rate (mcg/kg/min)
5	0.20
10	0.23
20	0.28
30	0.33
40	0.38
50	0.43

MAINTENANCE DOSE

	Infusion Rate	Total Daily Dose (24 Hours)	
Minimum	0.375 mcg/kg/min	0.59 mg/kg	Administer as a
Standard	0.50 mcg/kg/min	0.77 mg/kg	continuous
Maximum	0.75 mcg/kg/min	1.13 mg/kg	intravenous infusion.

HOW SUPPLIED

PRIMACOR is supplied as 10 mL (1 mg/mL) NDC 0024-1200-10, box of 10 and 20 mL (1 mg/mL) NDC 0024-1200-20, box of 10 single-dose vials containing a sterile, clear, colorless to pale yellow solution. Each mL contains milrinone lactate equivalent to 1 mg milrinone.

PRIMACOR is also supplied as Carpuject® Sterile Cartridge Unit with InterLink® System Cannula, 5 mL (1 mg/mL) NDC 0024-1200-06 in 5 mL cartridges, box of 10. Each mL contains milrinone lactate equivalent to 1 mg milrinone.

PRIMACOR is also supplied as **CARPUJECT** Sterile Cartridge Unit (22-gauge, 1 ¼ Inch Needle) 5 mL (1 mg/mL) NDC 0024-1200-05 in 5 mL cartridges, box of 10. Each mL contains milrinone lactate equivalent to 1 mg milrinone. Store at controlled room temperature 15° C to 30° C (59° F to 86° F). Avoid freezing.

The following **PRIMACOR Flexible Container** containing 100 mL is also supplied:

200 mcg/mL NDC 0024-1203-01 in 5% Dextrose Injection. Exposure of pharmaceutical products to heat should be minimized. Avoid excessive heat. Protect from freezing. It is recommended that the Flexible Containers be stored at room temperature, 25° C (77° F), however, brief exposure up to 40° C (104° F) does not adversely affect the product.

Caution: Federal law prohibitis dispensing without prescription.

InterLink® is a Trademark of Baxter International, Inc.
U.S. Pat. Nos. 5,158,554; 5,171,234; 5,188,620; Pat. Pending
PRIMACOR FLEXIBLE CONTAINER is manufactured for Sanofi Winthrop by Abbott Laboratories, North Chicago, IL 60064

PSW-1K

PRIMACOR Infusion Rate (mL/hr) Using 100 mcg/mL Concentration

Maintenance Dose	Patient Body Weight (kg)									
mcg/kg/min	30	40	50	60	70	80	90	100	110	120
0.375	6.8	9.0	11.3	13.5	15.8	18.0	20.3	22.5	24.8	27.0
0.400	7.2	9.6	12.0	14.4	16.8	19.2	21.6	24.0	26.4	28.8
0.500	9.0	12.0	15.0	18.0	21.0	24.0	27.0	30.0	33.0	36.0
0.600	10.8	14.4	18.0	21.6	25.2	28.8	32.4	36.0	39.6	43.2
0.700	12.6	16.8	21.0	25.2	29.4	33.6	37.8	42.0	46.2	50.4
0.750	13.5	18.0	22.5	27.0	31.5	36.0	40.5	45.0	49.5	54.0

PRIMACOR Infusion Rate (mL/hr) Using 150 mcg/mL Concentration

Maintenance Dose	Patient Body Weight (kg)									
(mcg/kg/min)	30	40	50	60	70	80	90	100	110	120
0.375	4.5	6.0	7.5	9.0	10.5	12.0	13.5	15.0	16.5	18.0
0.400	4.8	6.4	8.0	9.6	11.2	12.8	14.4	16.0	17.6	19.2
0.500	6.0	8.0	10.0	12.0	14.0	16.0	18.0	20.0	22.0	24.0
0.600	7.2	9.6	12.0	14.4	16.8	19.2	21.6	24.0	26.4	28.8
0.700	8.4	11.2	14.0	16.8	19.6	22.4	25.2	28.0	30.8	33.6
0.750	9.0	12.0	15.0	18.0	21.0	24.0	27.0	30.0	33.0	36.0

Note: PRIMACOR supplied in 100 mL Flexible Containers (200 mcg/mL in 5% Dextrose Injection) need not be diluted prior to use.

PRIMACOR Infusion Rate (mL/hr) Using 200 mcg/mL Concentration

Maintenance Dose	Patient Body Weight (kg)									
(mcg/kg/min)	30	40	50	60	70	80	90	100	110	120
0.375	3.4	4.5	5.6	6.8	7.9	9.0	10.1	11.3	12.4	13.5
0.400	3.6	4.8	6.0	7.2	8.4	9.6	10.8	12.0	13.2	14.4
0.500	4.5	6.0	7.5	9.0	10.5	12.0	13.5	15.0	16.5	18.0
0.600	5.4	7.2	9.0	10.8	12.6	14.4	16.2	18.0	19.8	21.6
0.700	6.3	8.4	10.5	12.6	14.7	16.8	18.9	21.0	23.1	25.2
0.750	6.8	9.0	11.3	13.5	15.8	18.0	20.3	22.5	24.8	27.0

Continued on next page

This product information was prepared in September 1996. On these and other products of Sanofi Winthrop Pharmaceuticals, detailed information may be obtained on a current basis by direct inquiry to Product Information Services, 90 Park Avenue, New York, NY 10016 (toll free 1-800-446-6267).

Sanofi Winthrop—Cont.

TALACEN® Ⓒ℞
Pentazocine hydrochloride, USP, equivalent to 25 mg base and acetaminophen, USP, 650 mg

DESCRIPTION
TALACEN is a combination of pentazocine hydrochloride, USP, equivalent to 25 mg base and acetaminophen, USP, 650 mg.
Pentazocine is a member of the benzazocine series (also known as the benzomorphan series). Chemically, pentazocine is 1,2,3,4,5,6-hexahydro-6,11-dimethyl-3-(3-methyl-2-butenyl)-2,6-methano-3-benzazocin-8-ol, a white, crystalline substance soluble in acidic aqueous solutions.
Chemically, acetaminophen is Acetamide, *N*- (4-hydroxyphenyl)-.
Pentazocine is an analgesic and acetaminophen is an analgesic and antipyretic.
TALACEN is a pale blue, scored caplet for oral administration.
Inactive Ingredients: Colloidal Silicon Dioxide, FD&C Blue #1, Gelatin, Microcrystalline Cellulose, Potassium Sorbate, Pregelatinized Starch, Sodium Lauryl Sulfate, Sodium Metabisulfite, Sodium Starch Glycolate, Stearic Acid.

CLINICAL PHARMACOLOGY
TALACEN is an analgesic possessing antipyretic actions.
Pentazocine is an analgesic with agonist/antagonist action which when administered orally is approximately equivalent on a mg for mg basis in analgesic effect to codeine.
Acetaminophen is an analgesic and antipyretic.
Onset of significant analgesia with pentazocine usually occurs between 15 and 30 minutes after oral administration, and duration of action is usually three hours or longer. Onset and duration of action and the degree of pain relief are related both to dose and the severity of pretreatment pain. Pentazocine weakly antagonizes the analgesic effects of morphine, meperidine, and phenazocine; in addition, it produces incomplete reversal of cardiovascular, respiratory, and behavioral depression induced by morphine and meperidine. Pentazocine has about 1/50 the antagonistic activity of nalorphine. It also has sedative activity.
Pentazocine is well absorbed from the gastrointestinal tract. Plasma levels closely correspond to the onset, duration, and intensity of analgesia. The time to mean peak concentration in 24 normal volunteers was 1.7 hours (range 0.5 to 4 hours) after oral administration and the mean plasma elimination half-life was 3.6 hours (range 1.5 to 10 hours).
The action of pentazocine is terminated for the most part by biotransformation in the liver with some free pentazocine excreted in the urine. The products of the oxidation of the terminal methyl groups and glucuronide conjugates are excreted by the kidney. Elimination of approximately 60% of the total dose occurs within 24 hours. Pentazocine passes the placental barrier.
Onset of significant analgesic and antipyretic activity of acetaminophen when administered orally occurs within 30 minutes and is maximal at approximately $2^1/_2$ hours. The pharmacological mode of action of acetaminophen is unknown at this time.
Acetaminophen is rapidly and almost completely absorbed from the gastrointestinal tract. In 24 normal volunteers the time to mean peak plasma concentration was 1 hour (range 0.25 to 3 hours) after oral administration and the mean plasma elimination half-life was 2.8 hours (range 2 to 4 hours).
The effect of pentazocine on acetaminophen plasma protein binding or vice versa has not been established. For acetaminophen there is little or no plasma protein binding at normal therapeutic doses. When toxic doses of acetaminophen are ingested and drug plasma levels exceed 90 mcg/mL, plasma binding may vary from 8% to 43%.
Acetaminophen is conjugated in the liver with glucuronic acid and to a lesser extent with sulfuric acid. Approximately 80% of acetaminophen is excreted in the urine after conjugation and about 3% is excreted unchanged. The drug is also conjugated to a lesser extent with cysteine and additionally metabolized by hydroxylation.
If TALACEN is taken every 4 hours over an extended period of time, accumulation of pentazocine and to a lesser extent, acetaminophen, may occur.

INDICATIONS AND USAGE
TALACEN is indicated for the relief of mild to moderate pain.

CONTRAINDICATIONS
TALACEN should not be administered to patients who are hypersensitive to either pentazocine or acetaminophen.

WARNINGS
Contains sodium metabisulfite, a sulfite that may cause allergic-type reactions including anaphylactic symptoms and life-threatening or less severe asthmatic episodes in certain susceptible people. The overall prevalence of sulfite sensitivity in the general population is unknown and probably low. Sulfite sensitivity is seen more frequently in asthmatic than in nonasthmatic people.
Head Injury and Increased Intracranial Pressure. As in the case of other potent analgesics, the potential of pentazocine for elevating cerebrospinal fluid pressure may be attributed to CO_2 retention due to the respiratory depressant effects of the drug. These effects may be markedly exaggerated in the presence of head injury, other intracranial lesions, or a preexisting increase in intracranial pressure. Furthermore, pentazocine can produce effects which may obscure the clinical course of patients with head injuries. In such patients, TALACEN must be used with extreme caution and only if its use is deemed essential.
Acute CNS Manifestations. Patients receiving therapeutic doses of pentazocine have experienced hallucinations (usually visual), disorientation, and confusion which have cleared spontaneously within a period of hours. The mechanism of this reaction is not known. Such patients should be closely observed and vital signs checked. If the drug is reinstituted, it should be done with caution since these acute CNS manifestations may recur.
There have been instances of psychological and physical dependence on parenteral pentazocine in patients with a history of drug abuse, and rarely, in patients without such a history. (See DRUG ABUSE AND DEPENDENCE.)
Due to the potential for increased CNS depressant effects, alcohol should be used with caution in patients who are currently receiving pentazocine.
Pentazocine may precipitate opioid abstinence symptoms in patients receiving courses of opiates for pain relief.

PRECAUTIONS
In prescribing TALACEN for chronic use, the physician should take precautions to avoid increases in dose by the patient.
Myocardial Infarction. As with all drugs, TALACEN should be used with caution in patients with myocardial infarction who have nausea or vomiting.
Certain Respiratory Conditions. Although respiratory depression has rarely been reported after oral administration of pentazocine, the drug should be administered with caution to patients with respiratory depression from any cause, severely limited respiratory reserve, severe bronchial asthma and other obstructive respiratory conditions, or cyanosis.
Impaired Renal or Hepatic Function. Decreased metabolism of the drug by the liver in extensive liver disease may predispose to accentuation of side effects. Although laboratory tests have not indicated that pentazocine causes or increases renal or hepatic impairment, the drug should be administered with caution to patients with such impairment. Since acetaminophen is metabolized by the liver, the question of the safety of its use in the presence of liver disease should be considered.
Biliary Surgery. Narcotic drug products are generally considered to elevate biliary tract pressure for varying periods following their administration. Some evidence suggests that pentazocine may differ from other marketed narcotics in this respect (i.e., it causes little or no elevation in biliary tract pressures). The clinical significance of these findings, however, is not yet known.
CNS Effect. Caution should be used when TALACEN is administered to patients prone to seizures; seizures have occurred in a few such patients in association with the use of pentazocine although no cause and effect relationship has been established.
Information for Patients. Since sedation, dizziness, and occasional euphoria have been noted, ambulatory patients should be warned not to operate machinery, drive cars, or unnecessarily expose themselves to hazards. Pentazocine may cause physical and psychological dependence when taken alone and may have additive CNS depressant properties when taken in combination with alcohol or other CNS depressants.
Drug Interactions. Pentazocine is a mild narcotic antagonist. Some patients previously given narcotics, including methadone for the daily treatment of narcotic dependence, have experienced withdrawal symptoms after receiving pentazocine.
Carcinogenesis, Mutagenesis, Impairment of Fertility. Carcinogenesis, mutagenesis, and impairment of fertility studies have not been done with this combination product.
Pentazocine, when administered orally or parenterally, had no adverse effect on either the reproductive capabilities or the course of pregnancy in rabbits and rats. Embryotoxic effects on the fetuses were not shown.
The daily administration of 4 mg/kg to 20 mg/kg pentazocine subcutaneously to female rats during a 14 day pre-mating period and until the 13th day of pregnancy did not have any adverse effects on the fertility rate.
There is no evidence in long-term animal studies to demonstrate that pentazocine is carcinogenic.
Pregnancy Category C. Animal reproduction studies have not been conducted with TALACEN. It is also not known whether TALACEN can cause fetal harm when administered to pregnant women or can affect reproduction capacity. TALACEN should be given to pregnant women only if clearly needed. However, animal reproduction studies with pentazocine have not demonstrated teratogenic or embryotoxic effects.
Nonteratogenic Effects. There has been no experience in this regard with the combination pentazocine and acetaminophen. However, there have been rare reports of possible abstinence syndromes in newborns after prolonged use of pentazocine during pregnancy.
Labor and Delivery. Patients receiving pentazocine during labor have experienced no adverse effects other than those that occur with commonly used analgesics. TALACEN should be used with caution in women delivering premature infants. The effect of TALACEN on the mother and fetus, the duration of labor or delivery, the possibility that forceps delivery or other intervention or resuscitation of the newborn may be necessary, or the effect of TALACEN, on the later growth, development, and functional maturation of the child are unknown at the present time.
Nursing Mothers. It is not known whether this drug is excreted in human milk. Because many drugs are excreted in human milk, caution should be exercised when TALACEN is administered to a nursing woman.
Pediatric Use. Safety and effectiveness in children below the age of 12 have not been established.

ADVERSE REACTIONS
Clinical experience with TALACEN has been insufficient to define all possible adverse reactions with this combination. However, reactions reported after oral administration of pentazocine hydrochloride in 50 mg dosage include *gastrointestinal:* nausea, vomiting, infrequently constipation; and rarely abdominal distress, anorexia, diarrhea. *CNS effects:* dizziness, lightheadedness, hallucinations, sedation, euphoria, headache, confusion, disorientation; infrequently weakness, disturbed dreams, insomnia, syncope, visual blurring and focusing difficulty, depression; and rarely tremor, irritability, excitement, tinnitus. *Autonomic:* sweating; infrequently flushing; and rarely chills. *Allergic:* infrequently rash; and rarely urticaria, edema of the face. *Cardiovascular:* infrequently decrease in blood pressure, tachycardia. *Hematologic:* rarely depression of white blood cells (especially granulocytes), which is usually reversible, moderate transient eosinophilia. *Other:* rarely respiratory depression, urinary retention, paresthesia, toxic epidermal necrolysis, and in one instance, an apparent anaphylactic reaction has been reported.
Numerous clinical studies have shown that acetaminophen, when taken in recommended doses, is relatively free of adverse effects in most age groups, even in the presence of a variety of disease states.
A few cases of hypersensitivity to acetaminophen have been reported, as manifested by skin rashes, thrombocytopenic purpura, rarely hemolytic anemia and agranulocytosis. Occasional individuals respond to ordinary doses with nausea and vomiting and diarrhea.

DRUG ABUSE AND DEPENDENCE
Controlled Substance. TALACEN is a Schedule IV controlled substance.
Abuse and Dependence. There have been some reports of dependence and of withdrawal symptoms with orally administered pentazocine. There have been recorded instances of psychological and physical dependence in patients using parenteral pentazocine. Abrupt discontinuance following the extended use of parenteral pentazocine has resulted in withdrawal symptoms. Patients with a history of drug dependence should be under close supervision while receiving TALACEN. There have been rare reports of possible abstinence syndromes in newborns after prolonged use of pentazocine during pregnancy.
Some tolerance to the analgesic and subjective effects of pentazocine develops with frequent and repeated use.
Drug addicts who are given closely spaced doses of pentazocine (e.g., 60 mg to 90 mg every 4 hours) develop physical dependence which is demonstrated by abrupt withdrawal or by administration of naloxone. The withdrawal symptoms exhibited after chronic doses of more than 500 mg of pentazocine per day have similar characteristics, but to a lesser degree, of opioid withdrawal and may be associated with drug seeking behavior.

OVERDOSAGE
Manifestations. Clinical experience with TALACEN has been insufficient to define the signs of overdosage with this product. It may be assumed that signs and symptoms of TALACEN overdose would be a combination of those observed with pentazocine overdose and acetaminophen overdose.
For pentazocine alone in single doses above 60 mg there have been reports of the occurrence of nalorphine-like psychotomimetic effects such as anxiety, nightmares, strange thoughts, and hallucinations. Marked respiratory depression associated with increased blood pressure and tachycardia have also resulted from excessive doses as have dizziness, nausea, vomiting, lethargy, and paresthesias. The respira-

tory depression is antagonized by naloxone (see *Treatment*). In acute acetaminophen overdosage, dose-dependent, potentially fatal hepatic necrosis is the most serious adverse effect. Renal tubular necrosis, hypoglycemic coma, and thrombocytopenia may also occur.

In adults, a single dose of 10 g to 15 g (200 mg/kg to 250 mg/kg) of acetaminophen may cause hepatotoxicity. A dose of 25 g or more is potentially fatal. The potential seriousness of the intoxication may not be evident during the first two days of acute acetaminophen poisoning. During the first 24 hours, nausea, vomiting, anorexia, and abdominal pain occur. These may persist for a week or more. Liver injury may become evident the second day, initial signs being elevation of serum transaminase and lactic dehydrogenase activity, increased serum bilirubin concentration, and prolongation of prothrombin time. Serum albumin concentration and alkaline phosphatase activity may remain normal. The hepatotoxicity may lead to encephalopathy, coma, and death. Transient azotemia is evident in a majority of patients and acute renal failure occurs in some.

There have been reports of glycosuria and impaired glucose tolerance, but hypoglycemia may also occur. Metabolic acidosis and metabolic alkalosis have been reported. Cerebral edema and nonspecific myocardial depression have also been noted. Biopsy reveals centrolobular necrosis with sparing of the periportal area. The hepatic lesions are reversible over a period of weeks or months in nonfatal cases.

The severity of the liver injury can be determined by measurement of the plasma half-time of acetaminophen during the first day of acute poisoning. If the half-time exceeds 4 hours, hepatic necrosis is likely and if the half-time is greater than 12 hours, hepatic coma will probably occur. Only minimal liver damage has developed when the serum concentration was below 120 mcg/mL at 12 hours after ingestion of the drug. If serum bilirubin concentration is greater than 4 mg/100 mL during the first 5 days, encephalopathy may occur.

The seven day oral LD_{50} value for TALACEN in mice is 3570 mg/kg.

Treatment. Oxygen, intravenous fluids, vasopressors, and other supportive measures should be employed as indicated. Assisted or controlled ventilation should also be considered. For respiratory depression due to overdosage or unusual sensitivity to TALACEN, parenteral naloxone is a specific and effective antagonist.

The toxic effects of acetaminophen may be prevented or minimized by antidotal therapy with N-acetylcysteine. In order to obtain the best possible results, N-acetylcysteine should be administered within approximately 16 hours of ingestion of the overdose.

For complete prescribing information for the approved use of acetylcysteine in the treatment of acetaminophen overdose, see package insert for MUCOMYST® (acetylcysteine) Bristol-Myers Squibb.

Vigorous supportive therapy is required in severe intoxication. Procedures to limit the continuing absorption of the drug must be readily performed since the hepatic injury is dose dependent and occurs early in the course of intoxication. Induction of vomiting or gastric lavage, followed by oral administration of activated charcoal should be done in all cases.

If hemodialysis can be initiated within the first 12 hours, it is advocated for patients with a plasma acetaminophen concentration exceeding 120 mcg/mL at 4 hours after ingestion of the drug.

DOSAGE AND ADMINISTRATION

Adult. The usual adult dose is 1 caplet every 4 hours as needed for pain relief, up to a maximum of 6 caplets per day. The usual duration of therapy is dependent upon the condition being treated but in any case should be reviewed regularly by the physician. The effect of meals on the rate and extent of bioavailability of both pentazocine and acetaminophen has not been documented.

HOW SUPPLIED

Caplets, pale blue, scored, each containing pentazocine hydrochloride equivalent to 25 mg base and acetaminophen 650 mg.

Bottles of 100 (NDC 0024-1937-04).

Unit Dose Dispenser Package of 250 (NDC 0024-1937-14), 10 sleeves of 25 CAPLETS each.

Store at controlled room temperature 15° C to 30° C (59° F to 86° F).

Caution: Federal law prohibits dispensing without prescription.

TSW-6 A

Shown in Product Identification Guide, page 333

TALWIN® Injection   ℂ ℞
brand of pentazocine lactate injection, USP

Analgesic for Parenteral Use

DESCRIPTION

TALWIN injection, brand of pentazocine lactate injection, is a member of the benzazocine series (also known as the benzo-morphan series). Chemically, pentazocine lactate is 1, 2, 3, 4, 5, 6-hexahydro-6, 11-dimethyl-3-(3-methyl-2-butenyl)-2,6-methano-3- benzazocin-8-ol lactate, a white, crystalline substance soluble in acidic aqueous solutions.

CLINICAL PHARMACOLOGY

TALWIN is a potent analgesic and 30 mg is usually as effective an analgesic as morphine 10 mg or meperidine 75 mg to 100 mg; however, a few studies suggest the TALWIN to morphine ratio may range from 20 mg to 40 mg TALWIN to 10 mg morphine. The duration of analgesia may sometimes be less than that of morphine. Analgesia usually occurs within 15 to 20 minutes after intramuscular or subcutaneous injection and within 2 to 3 minutes after intravenous injection. TALWIN weakly antagonizes the analgesic effects of morphine, meperidine, and phenazocine; in addition, it produces incomplete reversal of cardiovascular, respiratory, and behavioral depression induced by morphine and meperidine. TALWIN has about 1/50 the antagonistic activity of nalorphine. It also has sedative activity.

INDICATIONS AND USAGE

For the relief of moderate to severe pain. TALWIN may also be used for preoperative or preanesthetic medication and as a supplement to surgical anesthesia.

CONTRAINDICATION

TALWIN should not be administered to patients who are hypersensitive to it.

WARNINGS

Drug Dependence. *Special care should be exercised in prescribing pentazocine for emotionally unstable patients and for those with a history of drug misuse. Such patients should be closely supervised when greater than 4 or 5 days of therapy is contemplated. There have been instances of psychological and physical dependence on TALWIN in patients with such a history and, rarely, in patients without such a history. Extended use of parenteral TALWIN may lead to physical or psychological dependence in some patients. When TALWIN is abruptly discontinued, withdrawal symptoms such as abdominal cramps, elevated temperature, rhinorrhea, restlessness, anxiety, and lacrimation may occur. However, even when these have occurred, discontinuance has been accomplished with minimal difficulty. In the rare patient in whom more than minor difficulty has been encountered, reinstitution of parenteral TALWIN with gradual withdrawal has ameliorated the patient's symptoms. Substituting methadone or other narcotics for TALWIN in the treatment of the pentazocine abstinence syndrome should be avoided. There have been rare reports of possible abstinence syndromes in newborns after prolonged use of TALWIN during pregnancy.*

In prescribing parenteral TALWIN for chronic use, particularly if the drug is to be self-administered, the physician should take precautions to avoid increases in dose and frequency of injection by the patient.

Just as with all medication, the oral form of TALWIN is preferable for chronic administration.

Tissue Damage at Injection Sites. Severe sclerosis of the skin, subcutaneous tissues, and underlying muscle have occurred at the injection sites of patients who have received multiple doses of pentazocine lactate. Constant rotation of injection sites is, therefore, essential. In addition, animal studies have demonstrated that TALWIN is tolerated less well subcutaneously than intramuscularly. (See DOSAGE AND ADMINISTRATION.)

Head Injury and Increased Intracranial Pressure. As in the case of other potent analgesics, the potential of TALWIN injection for elevating cerebrospinal fluid pressure may be attributed to CO_2 retention due to the respiratory depressant effects of the drug. These effects may be markedly exaggerated in the presence of head injury, other intracranial lesions, or a preexisting increase in intracranial pressure. Furthermore, TALWIN can produce effects which may obscure the clinical course of patients with head injuries. In such patients, TALWIN must be used with extreme caution and only if its use is deemed essential.

Usage in Pregnancy. Safe use of TALWIN during pregnancy (other than labor) has not been established. Animal reproduction studies have not demonstrated teratogenic or embryotoxic effects. However, TALWIN should be administered to pregnant patients (other than labor) only when, in the judgment of the physician, the potential benefits outweigh the possible hazards. Patients receiving TALWIN during labor have experienced no adverse effects other than those that occur with commonly used analgesics. TALWIN should be used with caution in women delivering premature infants.

Acute CNS Manifestations. Patients receiving therapeutic doses of pentazocine have experienced hallucinations (usually visual), disorientation, and confusion which have cleared spontaneously within a period of hours. The mechanism of this reaction is not known. Such patients should be closely observed and vital signs checked. If the drug is rein-stituted, it should be done with caution since these acute CNS manifestations may recur.

Due to the potential for increased CNS depressant effects, alcohol should be used with caution in patients who are currently receiving pentazocine.

Usage in Children. Because clinical experience in children under twelve years of age is limited, the use of TALWIN in this age group is not recommended.

Ambulatory Patients. Since sedation, dizziness, and occasional euphoria have been noted, ambulatory patients should be warned not to operate machinery, drive cars, or unnecessarily expose themselves to hazards.

Myocardial Infarction. Caution should be exercised in the intravenous use of pentazocine for patients with acute myocardial infarction accompanied by hypertension or left ventricular failure. Data suggest that intravenous administration of pentazocine increases systemic and pulmonary arterial pressure and systemic vascular resistance in patients with acute myocardial infarction.

NOTE: Acetone sodium bisulfite, a sulfite that may cause allergic-type reactions including anaphylactic symptoms and life-threatening or less severe asthmatic episodes in certain susceptible people, is contained in both Carpuject® Sterile Cartridge-Needle Unit and multiple-dose vials. The overall prevalence of sulfite sensitivity in the general population is unknown and probably low. Sulfite sensitivity is seen more frequently in asthmatic than in nonasthmatic people.

The ampuls in the Uni-Amp® Pak and the Uni-Nest™ Pak do not contain acetone sodium bisulfite.

PRECAUTIONS

Certain Respiratory Conditions. The possibility that TALWIN may cause respiratory depression should be considered in treatment of patients with bronchial asthma. TALWIN injection, brand of pentazocine lactate injection, should be administered only with caution and in low dosage to patients with respiratory depression (eg, from other medication, uremia, or severe infection), severely limited respiratory reserve, obstructive respiratory conditions, or cyanosis.

Impaired Renal or Hepatic Function. Although laboratory tests have not indicated that TALWIN causes or increases renal or hepatic impairment, the drug should be administered with caution to patients with such impairment. Extensive liver disease appears to predispose to greater side effects (eg, marked apprehension, anxiety, dizziness, sleepiness) from the usual clinical dose, and may be the result of decreased metabolism of the drug by the liver.

Biliary Surgery. Narcotic drug products are generally considered to elevate biliary tract pressure for varying periods following their administration. Some evidence suggests that pentazocine may differ from other marketed narcotics in this respect (ie, it causes little or no elevation in biliary tract pressures). The clinical significance of these findings, however, is not yet known.

Patients Receiving Narcotics. TALWIN is a mild narcotic antagonist. Some patients previously given narcotics, including methadone for the daily treatment of narcotic dependence, have experienced withdrawal symptoms after receiving TALWIN.

CNS Effect. Caution should be used when TALWIN is administered to patients prone to seizures; seizures have occurred in a few such patients in association with the use of TALWIN although no cause and effect relationship has been established.

Use in Anesthesia. Concomitant use of CNS depressants with parenteral TALWIN may produce additive CNS depression. Adequate equipment and facilities should be available to identify and treat systemic emergencies should they occur.

ADVERSE REACTIONS

The most commonly occurring reactions are: nausea, dizziness or lightheadedness, vomiting, euphoria.

Dermatologic Reactions: Soft tissue induration, nodules, and cutaneous depression can occur at injection sites. Ulceration (sloughing) and severe sclerosis of the skin and subcutaneous tissues (and, rarely, underlying muscle) have been reported after multiple doses. Other reported dermatologic reactions include diaphoresis, sting on injection, flushed skin including plethora, dermatitis including pruritus.

Infrequently occurring reactions are—*respiratory:* respiratory depression, dyspnea, transient apnea in a small number of newborn infants whose mothers received TALWIN during labor; *cardiovascular:* circulatory depression, shock, hypertension; *CNS effects:* dizziness, lightheadedness, hallucinations, sedation, euphoria, headache, confusion, disorienta-

Continued on next page

This product information was prepared in September 1996. On these and other products of Sanofi Winthrop Pharmaceuticals, detailed information may be obtained on a current basis by direct inquiry to Product Information Services, 90 Park Avenue, New York, NY 10016 (toll free 1-800-446-6267).

Sanofi Winthrop—Cont.

tion; infrequently weakness, disturbed dreams, insomnia, syncope, visual blurring and focusing difficulty, depression; and rarely tremor, irritability, excitement, tinnitus. *Gastrointestinal:* constipation, dry mouth; *other:* urinary retention, headache, paresthesia, alterations in rate or strength of uterine contractions during labor.
Rarely reported reactions include—*neuromuscular and psychiatric:* muscle tremor, insomnia, disorientation, hallucinations; *gastrointestinal:* taste alteration, diarrhea and cramps; *ophthalmic:* blurred vision, nystagmus, diplopia, miosis; *hematologic:* depression of white blood cells (especially granulocytes), which is usually reversible, moderate transient eosinophilia; *other:* tachycardia, weakness or faintness, chills, allergic reactions including edema of the face, toxic epidermal necrolysis.
See **Acute CNS Manifestations** and **Drug Dependence** under **WARNINGS.**

DOSAGE AND ADMINISTRATION

Adults, Excluding Patients in Labor. The recommended single parenteral dose is 30 mg by intramuscular, subcutaneous, or intravenous route. This may be repeated every 3 to 4 hours. Doses in excess of 30 mg intravenously or 60 mg intramuscularly or subcutaneously are not recommended. Total daily dosage should not exceed 360 mg.
The subcutaneous route of administration should be used only when necessary because of possible severe tissue damage at injection sites (see WARNINGS). When frequent injections are needed, the drug should be administered intramuscularly. In addition, constant rotation of injection sites (eg, the upper outer quadrants of the buttocks, mid-lateral aspects of the thighs, and the deltoid areas) is essential.
Patients in Labor. A single, intramuscular 30 mg dose has been most commonly administered. An intravenous 20 mg dose has given adequate pain relief to some patients in labor when contractions become regular, and this dose may be given two or three times at two-to three-hour intervals, as needed.
Children Under 12 Years of Age. Since clinical experience in children under twelve years of age is limited, the use of TALWIN in this age group is not recommended.
CAUTION. TALWIN should not be mixed in the same syringe with soluble barbiturates because precipitation will occur.

OVERDOSAGE

Manifestations: Clinical experience with TALWIN overdosage has been insufficient to define the signs of this condition.
Treatment: Oxygen, intravenous fluids, vasopressors, and other supportive measures should be employed as indicated. Assisted or controlled ventilation should also be considered. For respiratory depression due to overdosage or unusual sensitivity to TALWIN, brand of pentazocine lactate injection, parenteral naloxone is a specific and effective antagonist.

HOW SUPPLIED

UNI-AMP—Individual unit dose ampuls of 1 mL (30 mg) **NDC 0024-1924-04**, *1.5 mL (45 mg)* **NDC 0024-1925-04**, *and 2 mL (60 mg)* **NDC 0024-1926-04** in box of 25.
UNI-NEST ampuls of 1 mL (30 mg) **NDC 0024-1924-14** *and 2 mL (60 mg)* **NDC 0024-1926-14** in box of 25.
Each 1 mL contains pentazocine lactate equivalent to 30 mg base and 2.8 mg sodium chloride, in Water for Injection.
Detecto-Seal ®—**Carpuject Sterile Cartridge-Needle Unit**, *1 mL (30 mg)* **NDC 0024-1917-02**, *1.5 mL (45 mg)* **NDC 0024-1918-02**, *and 2 mL (60 mg)* **NDC 0024-1919-02, all in 2 mL cartridges,** box of 10. Each 1 mL contains pentazocine lactate equivalent to 30 mg base, 1 mg acetone sodium bisulfite, and 2.2 mg sodium chloride, in Water for Injection.
CARPUJECT Sterile Cartridge-Needle Unit, **SmartPak™** Injection Delivery System *1 mL (30 mg)* **NDC 0024-1917-01** and *2 mL (60 mg)* **NDC 0024-1919-06, each in a 2 mL cartridge,** box of 10. Each 1 mL contains pentazocine lactate equivalent to 30 mg base, 1 mg acetone sodium bisulfite, and 2.2 mg sodium chloride in Water for Injection.
Multiple-dose vials of 10 mL **NDC 0024-1916-01**, box of 1. Each 1 mL contains pentazocine lactate equivalent to 30 mg base, 2 mg acetone sodium bisulfite, 1.5 mg sodium chloride, and 1 mg methylparaben as preservative, in Water for Injection.
The pH of TALWIN solutions is adjusted between 4 and 5 with lactic acid or sodium hydroxide. The air in the ampuls, vials, and Cartridge-Needle Units has been displaced by nitrogen gas.

TSW-3A

TALWIN® Compound ©️ ℞
pentazocine hydrochloride and aspirin, USP

DESCRIPTION

TALWIN Compound is a combination of pentazocine hydrochloride, USP, equivalent to 12.5 mg base and aspirin, USP, 325 mg.
Pentazocine is a member of the benzazocine series (also known as the benzomorphan series). Chemically, pentazocine is 1, 2, 3, 4, 5, 6 -hexahydro - 6, 11-dimethyl-3-(3-methyl-2-butenyl)-2, 6-methano-3-benzazocin-8-ol, a white, crystalline substance soluble in acidic aqueous solutions.
Chemically, aspirin is Benzoic acid, 2-(acetyloxy)-,.
Inactive Ingredients: Magnesium Stearate, Microcrystalline Cellulose, Sodium Lauryl Sulfate, Starch.

CLINICAL PHARMACOLOGY

Pentazocine is a potent analgesic which when administered orally is approximately equivalent, on a mg for mg basis, in analgesic effect to codeine. Two caplets of TALWIN Compound when administered orally have the additive analgesic effect equivalent to 25 mg of TALWIN plus 650 mg of aspirin. TALWIN Compound provides the analgesic effects of pentazocine and the analgesic, anti-inflammatory, and antipyretic actions of aspirin.
Onset of significant analgesia usually occurs between 15 and 30 minutes after oral administration, and duration of action is usually three hours or longer. Onset and duration of action and the degree of pain relief are related both to dose and the severity of pretreatment pain. Pentazocine weakly antagonizes the analgesic effects of morphine, meperidine, and phenazocine; in addition, it produces incomplete reversal of cardiovascular, respiratory, and behavioral depression induced by morphine and meperidine. Pentazocine has about $^1/_{50}$ the antagonistic activity of nalorphine. It also has sedative activity.

INDICATION AND USAGE

For the relief of moderate pain

CONTRAINDICATIONS

TALWIN Compound should not be administered to patients who are hypersensitive to either pentazocine or salicylates, or in any situation where aspirin is contraindicated.

WARNINGS

Drug Dependence. There have been instances of psychological and physical dependence on parenteral pentazocine in patients with a history of drug abuse, and rarely, in patients without such a history. Abrupt discontinuance following the extended use of parenteral pentazocine has resulted in withdrawal symptoms. There have been a few reports of dependence and of withdrawal symptoms with orally administered pentazocine. Patients with a history of drug dependence should be under close supervision while receiving TALWIN Compound orally. There have been rare reports of possible abstinence syndromes in newborns after prolonged use of pentazocine during pregnancy.
In prescribing TALWIN Compound for chronic use, the physician should take precautions to avoid increases in dose by the patient and to prevent the use of the drug in anticipation of pain rather than for the relief of pain.
Head Injury and Increased Intracranial Pressure. The respiratory depressant effects of pentazocine and its potential for elevating cerebrospinal fluid pressure may be markedly exaggerated in the presence of head injury, other intracranial lesions, or a preexisting increase in intracranial pressure. Furthermore, pentazocine can produce effects which may obscure the clinical course of patients with head injuries. In such patients, TALWIN Compound must be used with extreme caution and only if its use is deemed essential.
Usage in Pregnancy. Safe use of pentazocine during pregnancy (other than labor) has not been established. Animal reproduction studies have not demonstrated teratogenic or embryotoxic effects. However, TALWIN Compound should be administered to pregnant patients (other than labor) only when, in the judgment of the physician, the potential benefits outweigh the possible hazards. Patients receiving pentazocine during labor have experienced no adverse effects other than those that occur with commonly used analgesics. TALWIN Compound, should be used with caution in women delivering premature infants.
Acute CNS Manifestations. Patients receiving therapeutic doses of pentazocine have experienced hallucinations (usually visual), disorientation, and confusion which have cleared spontaneously within a period of hours. The mechanism of this reaction is not known. Such patients should be closely observed and vital signs checked. If the drug is reinstituted it should be done with caution since these acute CNS manifestations may recur.
Due to the potential for increased CNS depressant effects, alcohol should be used with caution in patients who are currently receiving pentazocine.
Usage in Children. Because clinical experience in children under 12 years of age is limited, administration of TALWIN Compound in this age group is not recommended.
Ambulatory Patients. Since sedation, dizziness, and occasional euphoria have been noted, ambulatory patients should be warned not to operate machinery, drive cars, or unnecessarily expose themselves to hazards.
Other. Because of its aspirin content, TALWIN Compound should be used with caution in the presence of peptic ulcer, in conjunction with anticoagulant therapy, or in any situation where the effects of aspirin may be deleterious.

PRECAUTIONS

Certain Respiratory Conditions. Although respiratory depression has rarely been reported after oral administration of pentazocine, TALWIN Compound, should be administered with caution to patients with respiratory depression from any cause, severely limited respiratory reserve, severe bronchial asthma and other obstructive respiratory conditions, or cyanosis.
Impaired Renal or Hepatic Function. Decreased metabolism of the drug by the liver in extensive liver disease may predispose to accentuation of side effects. Although laboratory tests have not indicated that pentazocine causes or increases renal or hepatic impairment, TALWIN Compound should be administered with caution to patients with such impairment.
Myocardial Infarction. As with all drugs, TALWIN Compound should be used with caution in patients with myocardial infarction who have nausea or vomiting.
Biliary Surgery. Narcotic drug products are generally considered to elevate biliary tract pressure for varying periods following administration. Some evidence suggests that pentazocine may differ in this respect (i.e., it causes little or no elevation in biliary tract pressures). The clinical significance of these findings, however, is not yet known.
Patients Receiving Narcotics. Pentazocine is a mild narcotic antagonist. Some patients previously given narcotics, including methadone for the daily treatment of narcotic dependence, have experienced withdrawal symptoms after receiving pentazocine.
CNS Effect. Caution should be used when pentazocine is administered to patients prone to seizures. Seizures have occurred in a few such patients in association with the use of pentazocine although no cause and effect relationship has been established.

ADVERSE REACTIONS

Reactions reported after oral administration of pentazocine or TALWIN Compound include *Gastrointestinal:* nausea, vomiting; infrequently constipation; and rarely abdominal distress, anorexia, diarrhea. *CNS Effects:* dizziness, lightheadedness, hallucinations, sedation, euphoria, headache, confusion, disorientation; infrequently weakness, disturbed dreams, insomnia, syncope, visual blurring and focusing difficulty, depression; and rarely tremor, irritability, excitement, tinnitus. *Autonomic:* sweating; infrequently flushing; and rarely chills. *Allergic:* infrequently rash; and rarely urticaria, edema of the face, and angioneurotic edema. *Cardiovascular:* infrequently decrease in blood pressure, tachycardia. *Hematologic:* rarely depression of white blood cells (especially granulocytes), which is usually reversible, moderate transient eosinophilia. *Other:* rarely respiratory depression, urinary retention, paresthesia, toxic epidermal necrolysis, and angioneurotic edema.

DOSAGE AND ADMINISTRATION

Adults. The usual adult dose is 2 caplets three or four times a day.
Children Under 12 Years of Age. Since clinical experience in children under 12 years of age is limited, administration of TALWIN Compound in this age group is not recommended.
Duration of Therapy. Patients with chronic pain who receive pentazocine orally for prolonged periods have only rarely been reported to experience withdrawal symptoms when administration was abruptly discontinued (see WARNINGS). Tolerance to the analgesic effect of pentazocine has also been reported only rarely. Significant abnormalities of liver and kidney function tests have not been reported, even after prolonged administration of pentazocine.

OVERDOSAGE

Manifestations: Clinical experience with pentazocine overdosage has been insufficient to define the signs of this condition. Signs of salicylate overdosage include headache, dizziness, confusion, tinnitus, diaphoresis, thirst, nausea, vomiting, diarrhea, tachycardia, tachypnea, Kussmaul breathing, convulsions, and coma. Death is usually from respiratory failure.
Treatment: Treatment for overdosage of TALWIN Compound, should include treatment for salicylate poisoning as outlined in standard references.
Oxygen, intravenous fluids, vasopressors, and other supportive measures should be employed as indicated. Assisted or controlled ventilation should also be considered. For respiratory depression due to overdosage or unusual sensitivity to pentazocine, parenteral naloxone is a specific and effective antagonist.

HOW SUPPLIED

Caplets, white, each containing pentazocine hydrochloride equivalent to 12.5 mg base and aspirin 325 mg. Bottles of 100 (NDC 0024-1927-04).
Store at room temperature up to 30° C (86° F).
Caution: Federal law prohibits dispensing without prescription.

TSW-5 A

TALWIN® Nx Ⓒ℞
pentazocine and naloxone hydrochlorides USP

Analgesic for Oral Use Only

> TALWIN® Nx is intended for oral use only. Severe, potentially lethal, reactions may result from misuse of TALWIN® Nx by injection either alone or in combination with other substances. (See DRUG ABUSE AND DEPENDENCE section.)

DESCRIPTION

TALWIN Nx contains pentazocine hydrochloride, USP, equivalent to 50 mg base and is a member of the benzazocine series (also known as the benzomorphan series), and naloxone hydrochloride, USP, equivalent to 0.5 mg base.
TALWIN Nx is an analgesic for oral administration.
Chemically, pentazocine hydrochloride is 1,2,3,4,5,6-Hexahydro -6,11 -dimethyl -3-(3-methyl-2-butenyl)-2, 6-methano-3-benzazocin-8-ol hydrochloride, a white, crystalline substance soluble in acidic aqueous solutions.
Chemically, naloxone hydrochloride is Morphinan-6-one, 4, 5-epoxy-3, 14-dihydroxy-17-(2-propenyl)-, hydrochloride, (5α)-. It is a slightly off-white powder, and is soluble in water and dilute acids.
Inactive Ingredients: Colloidal Silicon Dioxide, Dibasic Calcium Phosphate, D&C Yellow #10, FD&C Yellow #6, Magnesium Stearate, Microcrystalline Cellulose, Sodium Lauryl Sulfate, Starch.

CLINICAL PHARMACOLOGY

Pentazocine is a potent analgesic which when administered orally in a 50 mg dose appears equivalent in analgesic effect to 60 mg (1 grain) of codeine. Onset of significant analgesia usually occurs between 15 and 30 minutes after oral administration, and duration of action is usually three hours or longer. Onset and duration of action and the degree of pain relief are related both to dose and the severity of pretreatment pain. Pentazocine weakly antagonizes the analgesic effects of morphine and meperidine; in addition, it produces incomplete reversal of cardiovascular, respiratory, and behavioral depression induced by morphine and meperidine. Pentazocine has about 1/50 the antagonistic activity of nalorphine. It also has sedative activity.
Pentazocine is well absorbed from the gastrointestinal tract. Concentrations in plasma coincide closely with the onset, duration, and intensity of analgesia; peak values occur 1 to 3 hours after oral administration. The half-life in plasma is 2 to 3 hours.
Pentazocine is metabolized in the liver and excreted primarily in the urine. Pentazocine passes into the fetal circulation.
Naloxone when administered orally at 0.5 mg has no pharmacologic activity. Naloxone hydrochloride administered parenterally at the same dose is an effective antagonist to pentazocine and a pure antagonist to narcotic analgesics.
TALWIN Nx is a potent analgesic when administered orally. However, the presence of naloxone in TALWIN Nx will prevent the effect of pentazocine if the product is misused by injection.
Studies in animals indicate that the presence of naloxone does not affect pentazocine analgesia when the combination is given orally. If the combination is given by injection the action of pentazocine is neutralized.

INDICATIONS AND USAGE

> TALWIN® Nx is intended for oral use only. Severe, potentially lethal, reactions may result from misuse of TALWIN® Nx by injection either alone or in combination with other substances. (See DRUG ABUSE AND DEPENDENCE section.)

TALWIN Nx is indicated for the relief of moderate to severe pain.
TALWIN Nx is indicated for oral use only.

CONTRAINDICATIONS

TALWIN Nx should not be administered to patients who are hypersensitive to either pentazocine or naloxone.

WARNINGS

> TALWIN® Nx is intended for oral use only. Severe, potentially lethal, reactions may result from misuse of TALWIN® Nx by injection either alone or in combination with other substances. (See DRUG ABUSE AND DEPENDENCE section.)

Drug Dependence. Pentazocine can cause a physical and psychological dependence. (See DRUG ABUSE AND DEPENDENCE.)
Head Injury and Increased Intracranial Pressure. As in the case of other potent analgesics, the potential of pentazocine for elevating cerebrospinal fluid pressure may be attributed to CO_2 retention due to the respiratory depressant effects of the drug. These effects may be markedly exaggerated in the presence of head injury, other intracranial lesions, or a preexisting increase in intracranial pressure. Furthermore, pentazocine can produce effects which may obscure the clinical course of patients with head injuries. In such patients, pentazocine must be used wth extreme caution and only if its use is deemed essential.
Usage with Alcohol. Due to the potential for increased CNS depressant effects, alcohol should be used with caution in patients who are currently receiving pentazocine.
Patients Receiving Narcotics. Pentazocine is a mild narcotic antagonist. Some patients previously given narcotics, including methadone for the daily treatment of narcotic dependence, have experienced withdrawal symptoms after receiving pentazocine.
Certain Respiratory Conditions. Although respiratory depression has rarely been reported after oral administration of pentazocine, the drug should be administered with caution to patients with respiratory depression from any cause, severely limited respiratory reserve, severe bronchial asthma, and other obstructive respiratory conditions, or cyanosis.
Acute CNS Manifestations. Patients receiving therapeutic doses of pentazocine have experienced hallucinations (usually visual), disorientation, and confusion which have cleared spontaneously within a period of hours. The mechanism of this reaction is not known. Such patients should be very closely observed and vital signs checked. If the drug is reinstituted, it should be done with caution since these acute CNS manifestations may recur.

PRECAUTIONS

CNS Effect. Caution should be used when pentazocine is administered to patients prone to seizures; seizures have occurred in a few such patients in association with the use of pentazocine though no cause and effect relationship has been established.
Impaired Renal or Hepatic Function. Decreased metabolism of pentazocine by the liver in extensive liver disease may predispose to accentuation of side effects. Although laboratory tests have not indicated that pentazocine causes or increases renal or hepatic impairment, the drug should be administered with caution to patients with such impairment.
In prescribing pentazocine for long-term use, the physician should take precautions to avoid increases in dose by the patient.
Biliary Surgery. Narcotic drug products are generally considered to elevate biliary tract pressure for varying periods following their administration. Some evidence suggests that pentazocine may differ from other marketed narcotics in this respect (i.e., it causes little or no elevation in biliary tract pressures). The clinical significance of these findings, however, is not yet known.
Information for Patients. Since sedation, dizziness, and occasional euphoria have been noted, ambulatory patients should be warned not to operate machinery, drive cars, or unnecessarily expose themselves to hazards. Pentazocine may cause physical and psychological dependence when taken alone and may have additive CNS depressant properties when taken in combination with alcohol or other CNS depressants.
Myocardial Infarction. As with all drugs, pentazocine should be used with caution in patients with myocardial infarction who have nausea or vomiting.
Drug Interactions. Usage with Alcohol: See WARNINGS.
Carcinogenesis, Mutagenesis, Impairment of Fertility. No long-term studies in animals to test for carcinogenesis have been performed with the components of TALWIN Nx.
Pregnancy Category C. Animal reproduction studies have not been conducted with TALWIN Nx. It is also not known whether TALWIN Nx can cause fetal harm when administered to pregnant women or can affect reproduction capacity. TALWIN Nx should be given to pregnant women only if clearly needed. However, animal reproduction studies with pentazocine have not demonstrated teratogenic or embryotoxic effects.
Labor and Delivery. Patients receiving pentazocine during labor have experienced no adverse effects other than those that occur with commonly used analgesics. TALWIN Nx should be used with caution in women delivering premature infants. The effect of TALWIN Nx on the mother and fetus, the duration of labor or delivery, the possibility that forceps delivery or other intervention or resuscitation of the newborn may be necessary, or the effect of TALWIN Nx on the later growth, development, and functional maturation of the child are unknown at the present time.
Nursing Mothers. It is not known whether this drug is excreted in human milk. Because many drugs are excreted in human milk, caution should be exercised when TALWIN Nx is administered to a nursing woman.
Pediatric Use. Safety and effectiveness in children below the age of 12 years have not been established.

ADVERSE REACTIONS

Cardiovascular. Hypotension, tachycardia, syncope.
Respiratory. Rarely, respiratory depression.
Acute CNS Manifestations. Patients receiving therapeutic doses of pentazocine have experienced hallucinations (usually visual), disorientation, and confusion which have cleared spontaneously within a period of hours. The mechanism of this reaction is not known. Such patients should be closely observed and vital signs checked. If the drug is reinstituted it should be done with caution since these acute CNS manifestations may recur.
Other CNS Effects. Dizziness, lightheadedness, hallucinations, sedation, euphoria, headache, confusion, disorientation; infrequently weakness, disturbed dreams, insomnia, syncope, visual blurring and focusing difficulty, depression; and rarely tremor, irritability, excitement, tinnitus.
Autonomic. Sweating; infrequently flushing; and rarely chills.
Gastrointestinal. Nausea, vomiting, constipation, diarrhea, anorexia, rarely abdominal distress.
Allergic. Edema of the face; dermatitis, including pruritus; flushed skin, including plethora; infrequently rash, and rarely urticaria.
Ophthalmic. Visual blurring and focusing difficulty.
Hematologic. Depression of white blood cells (especially granulocytes), which is usually reversible, moderate transient eosinophilia.
Other. Headache, chills, insomnia, weakness, urinary retention, paresthesia.

DRUG ABUSE AND DEPENDENCE

Controlled Substance. TALWIN Nx is a Schedule IV controlled substance.
There have been some reports of dependence and of withdrawal symptoms with orally administered pentazocine. Patients with a history of drug dependence should be under close supervision while receiving pentazocine orally. There have been rare reports of possible abstinence syndromes in newborns after prolonged use of pentazocine during pregnancy.
There have been instances of psychological and physical dependence on parenteral pentazocine in patients with a history of drug abuse and rarely, in patients without such a history. Abrupt discontinuance following the extended use of parenteral pentazocine has resulted in withdrawal symptoms.
In prescribing pentazocine for chronic use, the physician should take precautions to avoid increases in dose by the patient.
The amount of naloxone present in TALWIN Nx (0.5 mg per tablet) has no action when taken orally and will not interfere with the pharmacologic action of pentazocine. However, this amount of naloxone given by injection has profound antagonistic action to narcotic analgesics.
Severe, even lethal, consequences may result from misuse of tablets by injection either alone or in combination with other substances, such as pulmonary emboli, vascular occlusion, ulceration and abscesses, and withdrawal symptoms in narcotic dependent individuals.
TALWIN Nx contains an opioid antagonist, naloxone (0.5 mg). Naloxone is inactive when administered orally at this dose, and its inclusion in TALWIN Nx is intended to curb a form of misuse of oral pentazocine. Parenterally, naloxone is an active narcotic antagonist. Thus, TALWIN Nx has a lower potential for parenteral misuse than the previous oral pentazocine formulation TALWIN® 50, (pentazocine hydrochloride tablets, USP). However, it is still subject to patient misuse and abuse by the oral route.

OVERDOSAGE

Manifestations. Clinical experience of overdosage with this oral medication has been insufficient to define the signs of this condition.

Continued on next page

This product information was prepared in September 1996. On these and other products of Sanofi Winthrop Pharmaceuticals, detailed information may be obtained on a current basis by direct inquiry to Product Information Services, 90 Park Avenue, New York, NY 10016 (toll free 1-800-446-6267).

Sanofi Winthrop—Cont.

Treatment. Oxygen, intravenous fluids, vasopressors, and other supportive measures should be employed as indicated. Assisted or controlled ventilation should also be considered. For respiratory depression due to overdosage or unusual sensitivity to pentazocine, parenteral naloxone is a specific and effective antagonist.

DOSAGE AND ADMINISTRATION

> TALWIN® Nx is intended for oral use only. Severe, potentially lethal, reactions may result from misuse of TALWIN® Nx by injection either alone or in combination with other substances. (See DRUG ABUSE AND DEPENDENCE section.)

Adults. The usual initial adult dose is 1 tablet every three or four hours. This may be increased to 2 tablets when needed. Total daily dosage should not exceed 12 tablets.
When anti-inflammatory or antipyretic effects are desired in addition to analgesia, aspirin can be administered concomitantly with this product.
Children Under 12 Years of Age. Since clinical experience in children under 12 years of age is limited, administration of this product in this age group is not recommended.
Duration of Therapy. Patients with chronic pain who receive TALWIN Nx orally for prolonged periods have only rarely been reported to experience withdrawal symptoms when administration was abruptly discontinued (see WARNINGS). Tolerance to the analgesic effect of pentazocine has also been reported only rarely. However, there is no long-term experience with the oral administration of TALWIN Nx.

HOW SUPPLIED

Tablets (oblong), yellow, scored, each containing pentazocine hydrochloride equivalent to 50 mg base and naloxone hydrochloride equivalent to 0.5 mg base.
Bottles of 100 (NDC 0024-1951-04).
Unit Dose Dispenser Package of 250 (NDC 0024-1951-24), 10 sleeves of 25 tablets each.
Store at controlled room temperature 15° C to 30° C (59° F to 80° F).
Caution: Federal law prohibits dispensing without prescription.

TSW-4 A

Shown in Product Identification Guide, page 333

TRANCOPAL® ℞

brand of chlormezanone
Nonhypnotic Antianxiety Agent

DESCRIPTION

TRANCOPAL, brand of chlormezanone, is [2-(*p*-Chlorophenyl)tetrahydro-3-methyl-4*H*-1, 3-thiazin-4-one 1, 1-dioxide], a white, virtually tasteless, crystalline powder with a solubility of less than 0.25 percent w/v in water.
Inactive Ingredients—Caplets® **100 mg:** Dibasic Calcium Phosphate, FD&C Yellow #6, Magnesium Stearate, Saccharin Sodium, Starch; CAPLETS **200 mg:** Dibasic Calcium Phosphate, D&C Yellow #10, FD&C Blue #1, Magnesium Stearate, Saccharin Sodium, Starch.

CLINICAL PHARMACOLOGY

TRANCOPAL improves the emotional state by allaying mild anxiety, usually without impairing clarity of consciousness.
The relief of symptoms is often apparent in fifteen to thirty minutes after administration and may last up to six hours or longer.

INDICATIONS AND USAGE

TRANCOPAL is indicated for the treatment of mild anxiety and tension states.
The effectiveness of chlormezanone in long-term use, that is, more than 4 months, has not been assessed by systematic clinical studies. The physician should periodically reassess the usefulness of the drug for the individual patient.

CONTRAINDICATION

Contraindicated in patients with a history of a previous hypersensitivity reaction to chlormezanone.

WARNINGS

Should drowsiness occur, the dose should be reduced. As with other CNS-acting drugs, patients receiving chlormezanone should be warned against performing potentially hazardous tasks which require complete mental alertness, such as operating a motor vehicle or dangerous machinery. Patients should also be warned of the possible additive effects which may occur when the drug is taken with alcohol or other CNS-acting drugs.
Usage in Pregnancy. Safe use of this preparation in pregnancy or lactation has not been established, as no animal reproduction studies have been performed; therefore, use of the drug in pregnancy, lactation, or in women of childbearing age requires that the potential benefit of the drug be weighed against its possible hazards to the mother and fetus.

ADVERSE REACTIONS

Adverse effects reported to occur with TRANCOPAL include drowsiness, drug rash, dizziness, flushing, nausea, depression, edema, inability to void, weakness, excitement, tremor, confusion, and headache. Rare instances of erythema multiforme, Stevens-Johnson syndrome, and toxic epidermal necrolysis have been reported. Medication should be discontinued or modified as the case demands.
Jaundice, apparently of the cholestatic type, has been reported as occurring rarely during the use of chlormezanone, but was reversible on discontinuance of therapy.

OVERDOSAGE

Overdose with amounts as low as 7 grams has resulted in coma, hypotension, absence of reflexes, and flaccidity. Ingestion of higher doses may also result in alternation between coma and excitement.

DOSAGE AND ADMINISTRATION

The usual **adult** dosage is 200 mg orally three or four times daily but in some patients 100 mg may suffice. The dosage for **children from 5 to 12 years** is 50 mg to 100 mg three or four times daily. Since the effect of CNS-acting drugs varies, treatment, particularly in children, should begin with the lowest dosage which may be increased as needed.

HOW SUPPLIED

100 mg (peach colored, scored CAPLETS)
bottle of 100 (NDC 0024-1973-04)
200 mg (green colored, scored CAPLETS)
bottle of 100 (NDC 0024-1974-04)

TSW-7

WINSTROL® Ⓒ ℞

brand of stanozolol tablets, USP
For Oral Administration

DESCRIPTION

WINSTROL, brand of stanozolol tablets, is an anabolic steroid, a synthetic derivative of testosterone. Each tablet contains 2 mg of stanozolol. It is designated chemically as 17-methyl-2′*H*-5α-androst-2-eno[3,2-*c*]pyrazol-17β-ol.
Inactive Ingredients: Dibasic Calcium Phosphate, D&C Red #28, FD&C Red #40, Lactose, Magnesium Stearate, Starch.

CLINICAL PHARMACOLOGY

Anabolic steroids are synthetic derivatives of testosterone. Certain clinical effects and adverse reactions demonstrate the androgenic properties of this class of drugs. Complete dissociation of anabolic and androgenic effects has not been achieved. The actions of anabolic steroids are therefore similar to those of male sex hormones with the possibility of causing serious disturbances of growth and sexual development if given to young children. They suppress the gonadotropic functions of the pituitary and may exert a direct effect upon the testes.
WINSTROL has been found to increase low-density lipoproteins and decrease high-density lipoproteins. These changes are not associated with any increase in total cholesterol or triglyceride levels and revert to normal on discontinuation of treatment.
Hereditary angioedema (HAE) is an autosomal dominant disorder caused by a deficient or nonfunctional C1 esterase inhibitor (C1 INH) and clinically characterized by episodes of swelling of the face, extremities, genitalia, bowel wall, and upper respiratory tract.
In small scale clinical studies, stanozolol was effective in controlling the frequency and severity of attacks of angioedema and in increasing serum levels of C1 INH and C4. WINSTROL is not effective in stopping HAE attacks while they are under way. The effect of WINSTROL on increasing serum levels of C1 INH and C4 may be related to an increase in protein anabolism.

INDICATIONS AND USAGE

Hereditary Angioedema. WINSTROL is indicated prophylactically to decrease the frequency and severity of attacks of angioedema.

CONTRAINDICATIONS

The use of WINSTROL is contraindicated in the following:

1. Male patients with carcinoma of the breast, or with known or suspected carcinoma of the prostate.
2. Carcinoma of the breast in females with hypercalcemia; androgenic anabolic steroids may stimulate osteolytic resorption of bone.
3. Nephrosis or the nephrotic phase of nephritis.
4. WINSTROL can cause fetal harm when administered to a pregnant woman.

WINSTROL is contraindicated in women who are or may become pregnant. If this drug is used during pregnancy, or if the patient becomes pregnant while taking this drug, the patient should be apprised of the potential hazard to the fetus.

WARNINGS

> PELIOSIS HEPATIS, A CONDITION IN WHICH LIVER AND SOMETIMES SPLENIC TISSUE IS REPLACED WITH BLOOD-FILLED CYSTS, HAS BEEN REPORTED IN PATIENTS RECEIVING ANDROGENIC ANABOLIC STEROID THERAPY. THESE CYSTS ARE SOMETIMES PRESENT WITH MINIMAL HEPATIC DYSFUNCTION, BUT AT OTHER TIMES THEY HAVE BEEN ASSOCIATED WITH LIVER FAILURE. THEY ARE OFTEN NOT RECOGNIZED UNTIL LIFE-THREATENING LIVER FAILURE OR INTRA-ABDOMINAL HEMORRHAGE DEVELOPS. WITHDRAWAL OF DRUG USUALLY RESULTS IN COMPLETE DISAPPEARANCE OF LESIONS.
> LIVER CELL TUMORS ARE ALSO REPORTED. MOST OFTEN THESE TUMORS ARE BENIGN AND ANDROGEN-DEPENDENT, BUT FATAL MALIGNANT TUMORS HAVE BEEN REPORTED. WITHDRAWAL OF DRUG OFTEN RESULTS IN REGRESSION OR CESSATION OF PROGRESSION OF THE TUMOR. HOWEVER, HEPATIC TUMORS ASSOCIATED WITH ANDROGENS OR ANABOLIC STEROIDS ARE MUCH MORE VASCULAR THAN OTHER HEPATIC TUMORS AND MAY BE SILENT UNTIL LIFE-THREATENING INTRA-ABDOMINAL HEMORRHAGE DEVELOPS.
> BLOOD LIPID CHANGES THAT ARE KNOWN TO BE ASSOCIATED WITH INCREASED RISK OF ATHEROSCLEROSIS ARE SEEN IN PATIENTS TREATED WITH ANDROGENS AND ANABOLIC STEROIDS. THESE CHANGES INCLUDE DECREASED HIGH-DENSITY LIPOPROTEIN AND SOMETIMES INCREASED LOW-DENSITY LIPOPROTEIN. THE CHANGES MAY BE VERY MARKED AND COULD HAVE A SERIOUS IMPACT ON THE RISK OF ATHEROSCLEROSIS AND CORONARY ARTERY DISEASE.

Cholestatic hepatitis and jaundice occur with 17-alpha-alkylated androgens at relatively low doses. If cholestatic hepatitis with jaundice appears, the anabolic steroid should be discontinued. If liver function tests become abnormal, the patient should be monitored closely and the etiology determined. Generally, the anabolic steroid should be discontinued although in cases of mild abnormalities, the physician may elect to follow the patient carefully at a reduced drug dosage.
In patients with breast cancer, anabolic steroid therapy may cause hypercalcemia by stimulating osteolysis. In this case, the drug should be discontinued.
Edema with or without congestive heart failure may be a serious complication in patients with preexisting cardiac, renal, or hepatic disease. Concomitant administration of adrenal cortical steroids or ACTH may add to the edema.
Geriatric male patients treated with androgenic anabolic steroids may be at an increased risk for the development of prostatic hypertrophy and prostatic carcinoma.
In children, anabolic steroid treatment may accelerate bone maturation without producing compensatory gain in linear growth. This adverse effect may result in compromised adult stature. The younger the child, the greater the risk of compromising final mature height. The effect on bone maturation should be monitored by assessing bone age of the wrist and hand every six months.
Anabolic steroids have not been shown to enhance athletic ability.

PRECAUTIONS

General

Anabolic steroids may cause suppression of clotting factors II, V, VII, and X, and an increase in prothrombin time.
Women should be observed for signs of virilization (deepening of the voice, hirsutism, acne, and clitoromegaly). To prevent irreversible change, drug therapy must be discontinued, or the dosage significantly reduced when mild virilism is first detected. Such virilization is usual following androgenic anabolic steroid use at high doses. Some virilizing changes in women are irreversible even after prompt discontinuance of therapy and are not prevented by concomitant use of estrogens. Menstrual irregularities may also occur.
The insulin or oral hypoglycemic dosage may need adjustment in diabetic patients who receive anabolic steroids.
Information for the Patient. The physician should instruct patients to report any of the following side effects of androgens:
Adult or Adolescent Males. Too frequent or persistent erections of the penis, appearance or aggravation of acne.
Women. Hoarseness, acne, changes in menstrual periods, or more hair on the face.

All Patients. Any nausea, vomiting, changes in skin color, or ankle swelling.

Laboratory Tests. Women with disseminated breast carcinoma should have frequent determination of urine and serum calcium levels during the course of androgenic anabolic steroid therapy (see WARNINGS).

Because of the hepatotoxicity associated with the use of 17-alpha-alkylated androgens, liver function tests should be obtained periodically.

Periodic (every 6 months) x-ray examinations of bone age should be made during treatment of prepubertal patients to determine the rate of bone maturation and the effects of androgenic anabolic steroid therapy on the epiphyseal centers.

In common with other anabolic steroids, WINSTROL, brand of stanozolol tablets, has been reported to lower the level of high-density lipoproteins and raise the level of low-density lipoproteins. These changes usually revert to normal on discontinuation of treatment. Increased low-density lipoproteins and decreased high-density lipoproteins are considered cardiovascular risk factors. Serum lipids and high-density lipoprotein cholesterol should be determined periodically.

Hemoglobin and hematocrit should be checked periodically for polycythemia in patients who are receiving high doses of anabolic steroids.

Drug Interaction. Anabolic steroids may increase sensitivity to anticoagulants; therefore, dosage of an anticoagulant may have to be decreased in order to maintain the prothrombin time at the desired therapeutic level.

Drug/Laboratory Test Interferences. Therapy with androgenic anabolic steroids may decrease levels of thyroxine-binding globulin resulting in decreased total T_4 serum levels and increase resin uptake of T_3 and T_4. Free thyroid hormone levels remain unchanged and there is no clinical evidence of thyroid dysfunction.

Carcinogenesis, Mutagenesis, Impairment of Fertility.
Animal data: Testosterone has been tested by subcutaneous injection and implantation in mice and rats. The implant induced cervical-uterine tumors in mice, which metastasized in some cases. There is suggestive evidence that injection of testosterone into some strains of female mice increases their susceptibility to hepatoma. Testosterone is also known to increase the number of tumors and decrease the degree of differentiation of chemically-induced carcinomas of the liver in rats.

Human data: There are rare reports of hepatocellular carcinoma in patients receiving long-term therapy with androgens in high doses. Withdrawal of the drugs did not lead to regression of the tumors in all cases.

Geriatric patients treated with androgens may be at an increased risk of developing prostatic hypertrophy and prostatic carcinoma although conclusive evidence to support this concept is lacking.

This compound has not been tested for mutagenic potential. However, as noted above, cacinogenic effects have been attributed to treatment with androgenic hormones. The potential carcinogenic effects likely occur through a hormonal mechanism rather than by a direct chemical interaction mechanism.

Impairment of fertility was not tested directly in animal species. However, as noted below under ADVERSE REACTIONS, oligospermia in males and amenorrhea in females are potential adverse effects of treatment with WINSTROL Tablets. Therefore, impairment of fertility is a possible outcome of treatment with WINSTROL.

Pregnancy Category X. See CONTRAINDICATIONS section.

Nursing Mothers. It is not known whether anabolic steroids are excreted in human milk. Many drugs are excreted in human milk and because of the potential for adverse reactions in nursing infants from WINSTROL, a decision should be made whether to discontinue nursing or discontinue the drug, taking into account the importance of the drug to the mother.

Pediatric Use. Anabolic agents may accelerate epiphyseal maturation more rapidly than linear growth in children, and the effect may continue for 6 months after the drug has been stopped. Therefore, therapy should be monitored by x-ray studies at 6 month intervals in order to avoid the risk of compromising the adult height. The safety and efficacy of WINSTROL in children with hereditary angioedema have not been established.

ADVERSE REACTIONS

Hepatic: Cholestatic jaundice with, rarely, hepatic necrosis and death. Hepatocellular neoplasms and peliosis hepatis have been reported in association with long-term androgenic-anabolic steroid therapy (see WARNINGS). Reversible changes in liver function tests also occur including increased bromsulphalein (BSP) retention and increases in serum bilirubin, glutamic oxaloacetic transaminase (SGOT), and alkaline phosphatase.

Genitourinary System: *In men. Prepubertal:* Phallic enlargement and increased frequency of erections.
Postpubertal: Inhibition of testicular function, testicular atrophy and oligospermia, impotence, chronic priapism, epididymitis and bladder irritability.
In women: Clitoral enlargement, menstrual irregularities.
In both sexes: Increased or decreased libido.

CNS: Habituation, excitation, insomnia, depression.
Gastrointestinal: Nausea, vomiting, diarrhea.
Hematologic: Bleeding in patients on concomitant anticoagulant therapy.
Breast: Gynecomastia.
Larynx: Deepening of the voice in women.
Hair: Hirsutism and male pattern baldness in women.
Skin: Acne (especially in women and prepubertal boys).
Skeletal: Premature closure of epiphyses in children (see PRECAUTIONS, **Pediatric Use**).
Fluid and Electrolytes: Edema, retention of serum electrolytes (sodium, chloride, potassium, phosphate, calcium).
Metabolic/Endocrine: Decreased glucose tolerance (see PRECAUTIONS), increased serum levels of low-density lipoproteins and decreased levels of high-density lipoproteins (see PRECAUTIONS, **Laboratory Tests**), increased creatine and creatinine excretion, increased serum levels of creatinine phosphokinase (CPK).

Some virilizing changes in women are irreversible even after prompt discontinuance of therapy and are not prevented by concomitant use of estrogens (see PRECAUTIONS).

DRUG ABUSE AND DEPENDENCE

Controlled Substance Class: WINSTROL is classified as a controlled substance under the Anabolic Steroids Control Act of 1990 and has been assigned to Schedule III.

DOSAGE AND ADMINISTRATION

The use of anabolic steroids may be associated with serious adverse reactions, many of which are dose related; therefore, patients should be placed on the lowest possible effective dose.

Hereditary Angioedema. The dosage requirements for continuous treatment of hereditary angioedema with WINSTROL should be individualized on the basis of the clinical response of the patient. It is recommended that the patient be started on 2 mg, three times a day. After a favorable initial response is obtained in terms of prevention of episodes of edematous attacks, the proper continuing dosage should be determined by decreasing the dosage at intervals of one to three months to a maintenance dosage of 2 mg a day. Some patients may be successfully managed on a 2 mg alternate day schedule. During the dose adjusting phase, close monitoring of the patient's response is indicated, particularly if the patient has a history of airway involvement.

The prophylactic dose of WINSTROL, brand of stanozolol tablets, to be used prior to dental extraction, or other traumatic or stressful situations has not been established and may be substantially larger.

Attacks of hereditary angioedema are generally infrequent in childhood and the risks from stanozolol administration are substantially increased. Therefore, long-term prophylactic therapy with this drug is generally not recommended in children, and should only be undertaken with due consideration of the benefits and risks involved (see PRECAUTIONS, **Pediatric Use**).

HOW SUPPLIED

Tablets of 2 mg, scored, bottle of 100 (NDC 0024-2253-04)

WSW-1-A(O)

Shown in Product Identification Guide, page 333

Savage Laboratories®

a division of Altana Inc.
60 BAYLIS ROAD
MELVILLE, NY 11747

Direct Inquiries to:
Customer Service
(800) 231-0206
FAX: (516) 454-0732

For Medical Information Contact:
Dr. Arnold Yeadon
(516) 454-9071
FAX: (516) 454-6389

AXOCET® ℞

(Butalbital and Acetaminophen Capsules)

DESCRIPTION

AXOCET® (butalbital and acetaminophen capsules) is supplied in capsule form for oral administration.

Butalbital (5-allyl-5-isobutylbarbituric acid), a slightly bitter, white, odorless, crystalline powder, is a short to intermediate-acting barbiturate. It has the following structural formula:

[See chemical structure at top of next column.]

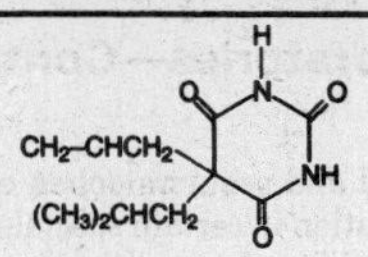

$C_{11}H_{16}N_2O_3$ Molecular Weight: 224.26

Acetaminophen (4'-hydroxyacetanilide), a slightly bitter, white, odorless, crystalline powder, is a non-opiate, non-salicylate analgesic and antipyretic. It has the following structural formula:

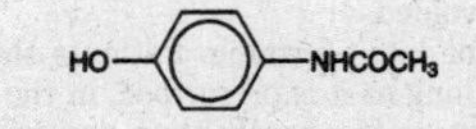

$C_8H_9NO_2$ Molecular Weight: 151.16

Each capsule contains:
Butalbital, USP .... 50 mg
(WARNING-May be habit forming)
Acetaminophen, USP .... 650 mg

In addition each capsule contains the following inactive ingredients: Gelatin, synthetic iron oxide black, titanium dioxide, sodium lauryl sulfate, benzyl alcohol, sodium propionate, edetate calcium disodium, carboxymethylcellulose sodium, butylparaben, propylparaben and methylparaben.

CLINICAL PHARMACOLOGY

This combination drug product is intended as a treatment for tension headache.

It consists of a fixed combination of butalbital and acetaminophen. The role each component plays in the relief of the complex of symptoms known as tension headache is incompletely understood.

PHARMACOKINETICS

The behavior of the individual components is described below.

Butalbital:
Butalbital is well absorbed from the gastrointestinal tract and is expected to distribute to most tissues in the body. Barbiturates in general may appear in breast milk and readily cross the placental barrier. They are bound to plasma and tissue proteins to a varying degree and binding increases directly as a function of lipid solubility.

Elimination of butalbital is primarily via the kidney (59% to 88% of the dose) as unchanged drug or metabolites. The plasma half-life is about 35 hours. Urinary excretion products include parent drug (about 3.6% of the dose), 5-isobutyl-5-(2,3-dihydroxypropyl)-barbituric acid (about 24% of the dose), 5-allyl-5-(3-hydroxy-2-methyl-1-propyl)-barbituric acid (about 4.8% of the dose), products with the barbituric acid ring hydrolyzed with excretion of urea (about 14% of the dose), as well as unidentified materials. Of the material excreted in the urine, 32% is conjugated.

See **OVERDOSAGE** for toxicity information.

Acetaminophen:
Acetaminophen is rapidly absorbed from the gastrointestinal tract and is distributed throughout most body tissues. The plasma half-life is 1.25 to 3 hours, but may be increased by liver damage and following overdosage. Elimination of acetaminophen is principally by liver metabolism (conjugation) and subsequent renal excretion of metabolites. Approximately 85% of an oral dose appears in the urine within 24 hours of administration, most as the glucuronide conjugate, with small amounts of other conjugates and unchanged drug.

See **OVERDOSAGE** for toxicity information.

INDICATIONS AND USAGE

Butalbital and acetaminophen capsules are indicated for the relief of the symptom complex of tension (or muscle contraction) headache.

Evidence supporting the efficacy and safety of this combination product in the treatment of multiple recurrent headaches is unavailable. Caution in this regard is required because butalbital is habit-forming and potentially abusable.

CONTRAINDICATIONS

This product is contraindicated under the following conditions:

- Hypersensitivity or intolerance to any component of this product.
- Patients with porphyria.

WARNINGS

Butalbital is habit-forming and potentially abusable. Consequently, the extended use of this product is not recommended.

Continued on next page

Savage Laboratories—Cont.

PRECAUTIONS

General: Butalbital and acetaminophen capsules should be prescribed with caution in certain special-risk patients, such as the elderly or debilitated, and those with severe impairment of renal or hepatic function, or acute abdominal conditions.

Information for Patients: This product may impair mental and/or physical abilities required for the performance of potentially hazardous tasks such as driving a car or operating machinery. Such tasks should be avoided while taking this product.

Alcohol and other CNS depressants may produce an additive CNS depression, when taken with this combination product, and should be avoided.

Butalbital may be habit-forming. Patients should take the drug only for as long as it is prescribed, in the amounts prescribed, and no more frequently than prescribed.

Laboratory Tests: In patients with severe hepatic or renal disease, effects of therapy should be monitored with serial liver and/or renal function tests.

Drug Interactions: The CNS effects of butalbital may be enhanced by monoamine oxidase (MAO) inhibitors.

Butalbital and acetaminophen may enhance the effects of: other narcotic analgesics, alcohol, general anesthetics, tranquilizers such as chlordiazepoxide, sedative-hypnotics, or other CNS depressants, causing increased CNS depression.

Drug/Laboratory Test Interactions: Acetaminophen may produce false-positive test results for urinary 5-hydroxyindoleacetic acid.

Carcinogenesis, Mutagenesis, Impairment of Fertility: No adequate studies have been conducted in animals to determine whether acetaminophen or butalbital have a potential for carcinogenesis, mutagenesis or impairment of fertility.

Pregnancy: *Teratogenic Effects:* Pregnancy Category C: Animal reproduction studies have not been conducted with this combination product. It is also not known whether butalbital and acetaminophen can cause fetal harm when administered to a pregnant woman or can affect reproduction capacity. This product should be given to a pregnant woman only when clearly needed.

Nonteratogenic Effects: Withdrawal seizures were reported in a two-day-old male infant whose mother had taken a butalbital-containing drug during the last two months of pregnancy. Butalbital was found in the infant's serum. The infant was given phenobarbital 5 mg/kg, which was tapered without further seizure or other withdrawal symptoms.

Nursing Mothers: Barbiturates and acetaminophen are excreted in breast milk in small amounts, but the significance of their effects on nursing infants is not known. Because of potential for serious adverse reactions in nursing infants from butalbital and acetaminophen, a decision should be made whether to discontinue nursing or to discontinue the drug, taking into account the importance of the drug to the mother.

Pediatric Use: Safety and effectiveness in children below the age of 12 have not been established.

ADVERSE REACTIONS

Frequently Observed: The most frequently reported adverse reactions are drowsiness, lightheadedness, dizziness, sedation, shortness of breath, nausea, vomiting, abdominal pain, and intoxicated feeling.

Infrequently Observed: All adverse events tabulated below are classified as infrequent.

Central Nervous: Headache, shaky feeling, tingling, agitation, fainting, fatigue, heavy eyelids, high energy, hot spells, numbness, sluggishness, seizure. Mental confusion, excitement or depression can also occur due to intolerance, particularly in elderly or debilitated patients, or due to overdosage of butalbital.

Autonomic Nervous: dry mouth, hyperhidrosis.

Gastrointestinal: difficulty swallowing, heartburn, flatulence, constipation.

Cardiovascular: tachycardia.

Musculoskeletal: leg pain, muscle fatigue.

Genitourinary: diuresis.

Miscellaneous: pruritus, fever, earache, nasal congestion, tinnitus, euphoria, allergic reactions.

Several cases of dermatological reactions, including toxic epidermal necrolysis and erythema multiforme, have been reported.

The following adverse drug events may be borne in mind as potential effects of the components of the product. Potential effects of high dosage are listed in the OVERDOSAGE section.

Acetaminophen: Allergic reactions, rash, thrombocytopenia, agranulocytosis.

DRUG ABUSE AND DEPENDENCE

Abuse and Dependence: Butalbital: *Barbiturates may be habit forming:* Tolerance, psychological dependence, and physical dependence may occur especially following prolonged use of high doses of barbiturates. The average daily dose for the barbiturate addict is usually about 1500 mg. As

tolerance to barbiturates develops, the amount needed to maintain the same level of intoxication increases; tolerance to a fatal dosage, however, does not increase more than twofold. As this occurs, the margin between an intoxication dosage and fatal dosage becomes smaller. The lethal dose of a barbiturate is far less if alcohol is also ingested. Major withdrawal symptoms (convulsions and delirium) may occur within 16 hours and last up to 5 days after abrupt cessation of these drugs. Intensity of withdrawal symptoms gradually declines over a period of approximately 15 days. Treatment of barbiturate dependence consists of cautious and gradual withdrawal of the drug. Barbiturate-dependent patients can be withdrawn by using a number of different withdrawal regimens. One method involves initiating treatment at the patient's regular dosage level and gradually decreasing the daily dosage as tolerated by the patient.

OVERDOSAGE

Following an acute overdosage of butalbital and acetaminophen, toxicity may result from the barbiturate or the acetaminophen.

Signs and Symptoms: Toxicity from <u>barbiturate</u> poisoning include drowsiness, confusion, and coma; respiratory depression; hypotension; and hypovolemic shock.

In <u>acetaminophen</u> overdosage: dose-dependent, potentially fatal hepatic necrosis is the most serious adverse effect. Renal tubular necrosis, hypoglycemic coma and thrombocytopenia may also occur. Early symptoms following a potentially hepatotoxic overdose may include: nausea, vomiting, diaphoresis and general malaise. Clinical and laboratory evidence of hepatic toxicity may not be apparent until 48 to 72 hours post-ingestion. In adults hepatic toxicity has rarely been reported with acute overdoses of less than 10 grams, or fatalities with less than 15 grams.

Treatment: A single or multiple overdose with this combination product is a potentially lethal polydrug overdose, and consultation with a regional poison control center is recommended.

Immediate treatment includes support of cardiorespiratory function and measures to reduce drug absorption. Vomiting should be induced mechanically, or with syrup of ipecac, if the patient is alert (adequate pharyngeal and laryngeal reflexes). Oral activated charcoal (1 g/kg) should follow gastric emptying. The first dose should be accompanied by an appropriate cathartic. If repeated doses are used, the cathartic might be included with alternate doses as required. Hypotension is usually hypovolemic and should respond to fluids. Pressors should be avoided. A cuffed endotracheal tube should be inserted before gastric lavage of the unconscious patient and, when necessary, to provide assisted respiration. If renal function is normal, forced diuresis may aid in the elimination of the barbiturate. Alkalinization of the urine increases renal excretion of some barbiturates, especially phenobarbital.

Meticulous attention should be given to maintaining adequate pulmonary ventilation. In severe cases of intoxication, peritoneal dialysis, or preferably hemodialysis may be considered. If hypoprothrombinemia occurs due to acetaminophen overdose, vitamin K should be administered intravenously.

If the dose of acetaminophen may have exceeded 140 mg/kg, acetylcysteine should be administered as early as possible. Serum acetaminophen levels should be obtained, since levels four or more hours following ingestion help predict acetaminophen toxicity. Do not await acetaminophen assay results before initiating treatment. Hepatic enzymes should be obtained initially, and repeated at 24-hour intervals. Methemoglobinemia over 30% should be treated with methylene blue by slow intravenous administration.

Toxic Doses (for adults):

Butalbital:	toxic dose 1 g	(20 capsules)
Acetaminophen:	toxic dose 10 g	(15 capsules)

DOSAGE AND ADMINISTRATION

One capsule every four hours. Total daily dosage should not exceed 6 capsules.

Extended and repeated use of this product is not recommended because of the potential for physical dependence.

HOW SUPPLIED

Each AXOCET® capsule contains: butalbital 50 mg (WARNING-May be habit forming) and acetaminophen 650 mg. AXOCET® is supplied in bottles of 100 opaque grey capsules imprinted with Savage logo and 0198, NDC 0281-0198-17.

Dispense in a tight, light-resistant container.

Store at controlled room temperature 15°-30°C (59°-86°F).

CAUTION: Federal law prohibits dispensing without prescription.

Manufactured by: D.M. Graham Laboratories, Inc., Hobart, NY 13788

Distributed by:

SAVAGE LABORATORIES®
a division of Altana Inc.
MELVILLE, NEW YORK 11747   R4/94

Shown in Product Identification Guide, page 333

BREXIN® L.A. Capsules   ℞
(chlorpheniramine maleate, pseudoephedrine hydrochloride)

DESCRIPTION

A red and clear colored capsule containing red and blue colored beads. Each capsule for oral administration contains: chlorpheniramine maleate 8 mg, pseudoephedrine hydrochloride 120 mg in a specially prepared base to provide prolonged action.

HOW SUPPLIED

NDC 0281-1934-53, bottle of 100 capsules.

CHROMAGEN®   ℞
[kro "mah-jen]
Soft Gelatin Capsules

DESCRIPTION

CONTENTS: Each maroon soft gelatin capsule contains: ferrous fumarate USP 200 mg, ascorbic acid USP 250 mg, cyanocobalamin USP 10 mcg, desiccated stomach substance 100 mg.

DISCUSSION: The amount of elemental iron and the absorption of the iron components of commercial iron preparations vary widely. It is further established that certain "accessory components" may be included to enhance absorption and utilization of iron. Chromagen® Capsules are formulated to provide the essential factors for a complete, versatile hematinic.

ACTIONS

HIGH ELEMENTAL IRON CONTENT: Ferrous fumarate, used in Chromagen® Capsules, is an organic iron complex which has a higher elemental iron content than any other hematinic salt—33%. This compares with 20% for ferrous sulfate and 12% for ferrous gluconate.[1,2]

MORE COMPLETE ABSORPTION: It has been repeatedly shown that ascorbic acid, when given in sufficient amounts, can increase the absorption of ferrous iron from the gastrointestinal tract.[3,4,5,6,7,8,9] The absorption-promoting effect is mainly due to the reducing action of ascorbic acid within the gastrointestinal lumen, which helps to prevent or delay the formation of insoluble or less dissociated ferric compounds.[3] Iron absorption has been shown to increase sharply with increasing amounts of ascorbic acid, showing a gain in absorption of approximately 40% at 250 mg. Above 250 mg, the gain becomes insignificant, with an additional gain of only approximately 8% at 500 mg.[3] Each Chromagen® Capsule contains 250 mg of ascorbic acid, believed to be the optimal amount.

PROMOTES MOVEMENT OF PLASMA IRON: Ascorbic acid also plays an important role in the movement of plasma iron to storage depots in the tissues.[10] The action, which leads to the transport of plasma iron to ferritin, presumably involves its reducing effect, converting transferrin iron from the ferric to the ferrous state.[5] There is also evidence that ascorbic acid improves iron utilization, presumably as a further result of its reducing action,[6,9] and some evidence that it may have a direct effect upon erythropoiesis. Ascorbic acid is further alleged to enhance the conversion of folic acid to a more physiologically active form, folinic acid, which would make it even more important in the treatment of anemia since it would aid in the utilization of dietary folic acid.[11]

EXCELLENT ORAL TOLERATION: Ferrous fumarate is used in Chromagen® Capsules because it is less likely to cause the gastric disturbances so often associated with oral iron therapy. Ferrous fumarate has a low ionization constant and high solubility in the entire pH range of the gastrointestinal tract. It does not precipitate proteins or have the astringency of more ionizable forms of iron, and does not interfere with proteolytic or diastatic activities of the digestive system. Because of excellent oral toleration, Chromagen® Capsules can usually be administered between meals when iron absorption is maximal.

FACILITATES ABSORPTION OF VITAMIN B$_{12}$: It is now known that "Intrinsic Factor" is essential for the adequate alimentary absorption of vitamin B$_{12}$.[12,13,14,15] The chemical structure of intrinsic factor is still undetermined and it has not yet been isolated in pure form;[16] however, the inclusion of desiccated stomach substance with oral vitamin B$_{12}$ will furnish sufficient intrinsic factor to assure absorption of the vitamin.

TOXICITY: Ferrous fumarate was found to be the least toxic of three popular oral iron salts, with an oral LD$_{50}$ of 630 mg/kg. In the same report, the LD$_{50}$ of ferrous gluconate was reported to be 320 mg/kg and ferrous sulfate 230 mg/kg.[1,17]

INDICATIONS

For the treatment of all anemias responsive to oral iron therapy, such as hypochromic anemia associated with pregnancy, chronic or acute blood loss, dietary restriction, metabolic disease and post-surgical convalescence.

CONTRAINDICATIONS
Hemochromatosis and hemosiderosis are contraindications to iron therapy.

SIDE EFFECTS
Average capsule doses in sensitive individuals or excessive dosage may cause nausea, skin rash, vomiting, diarrhea, precordial pain, or flushing of the face and extremities.

DOSAGE AND ADMINISTRATION
Usual adult dose is 1 soft gelatin capsule daily or as recommended by physician.

HOW SUPPLIED
Chromagen® Capsules:
NDC **0281-4285-53**, bottle of 100
NDC **0281-4285-56**, bottle of 500
Store at controlled room temperature 15°–30°C (59°–86°F).
CAUTION: Federal law prohibits dispensing without prescription.

BIBLIOGRAPHY
[1]Berk, M.S. and Novich, M.A.: "Treatment of Iron Deficiency Anemia With Ferrous Fumarate," Am. J. Obst. & Gynec., 203–206, 1962. [2]Shapleigh, J.B., and Montgomery, A.; Am. Pract & Dig. Treat 10–461, 1959. [3]Brise, H. and Hallberg. L.: "Effect of Ascorbic Acid on Iron Absorption," Acta. Med. Scand. 171:376, 51–58, 1962. [4]New Drugs, p.309, AMA, Chicago, 1966. [5]Mazur, A., Green, S. and Carleton, A.: "Mechanism of Plasma Iron Incorporation into Hepatic Ferritin," J. of Bio. Chem. 3:595–603, 1960. [6]Greenberg, S.M., Tucker, A.E., Mathues, H. and J.D.: "Iron Absorption and Metabolism, I. Interrelationship of Ascorbic Acid and Vitamin E", J. Nutrition 63:19–31, 1957. [7]Moore, C.V., and Dubach, R.: "Observations on the Absorption of Iron From Foods Tagged with Radioiron," Trans. Assoc. Amer. Physic. 64:245, 1951. [8]Steinkamp, R., Dubach, R. and Moore, C.V.: "Studies in Iron Transportation and Metabolism," Arch. Int. Med. 95:181, 1955. [9]Gorten, M.K. and Bradley, J.E.: "The Treatment of Nutritional Anemia in Infancy and Childhood with Oral Iron and Ascorbic Acid," J. Pediatrics, 45:1, 1954. [10]Mazur, A.: "Role of Ascorbic Acid in the Incorportion of Plasma Iron into Ferritin," An. N.Y. Acad. Sci. 92:223–229, 1961. [11]Cox, E.V. et al.: "The Anemia of Scurvy," Amer. J. Med. 42:220–227, 1967. [12]Berk, L. et al.: "Observations on the Etiologic Relationship of Achylia Gastrica to Pernicious Anemia, X," N. Eng. J. Med. 239:911–913, 1948. [13]Hall, B.E.: "Studies on the Nature of the Intrinsic Factor of Castle," Brit. Med. J. 2:585–589, 1950. [14]Wallerstein, R.O. et al.: "Observations on the Etiologic Relationship of Achylia Gastrica to Pernicious Anemia, XV," J. Lab & Clin. Med. 41:363–375, 1953. [15]Castle, W.B.: "Observations on the Etiologic Relationship of Achylia Gastrica to Pernicious Anemia, 1," Am. J. Med. Sc. 178:748–764, 1929. [16]Goodman, L.S. and Gilman, A.: The Pharmacological Basis of Therapeutics, 2 ed., P. 1482, N.Y., 1958. [17]Berenbaum, M.C. et al.: Blood, 15:540, 1960.

Manufactured by R.P. Scherer Corporation, St. Petersburg, Florida 33702
Distributed by
SAVAGE LABORATORIES®
a division of Altana Inc.
MELVILLE, NEW YORK 11747 R/11/90
Shown in Product Identification Guide, page 333

CHROMAGEN® FA ℞
Soft Gelatin Capsules

DESCRIPTION
CONTENTS: Each maroon and brown soft gelatin capsule contains: ferrous fumarate USP, 200 mg (elemental iron 66 mg), ascorbic acid USP, 250 mg, folic acid USP, 1 mg, cyanocobalamin USP, 10 mcg.
DISCUSSION: The amount of elemental iron and the absorption of the iron components of commercial iron preparations vary widely. It is further established that certain "accessory components" may be included to enhance absorption and utilization of iron. Chromagen® FA Capsules are formulated to provide the essential factors for a complete, versatile hematinic.

ACTIONS
HIGH ELEMENTAL IRON CONTENT: Ferrous fumarate, used in Chromagen® FA Capsules is an organic iron complex which has the highest elemental iron content of any hematinic salt-33%. This compares with 20% for ferrous sulfate (heptahydrate) and 13% for ferrous gluconate.[1,2]
MORE COMPLETE ABSORPTION: It has been repeatedly shown that ascorbic acid, when given in sufficient amounts, can increase the absorption of ferrous iron from the gastrointestinal tract.[3,4,5,6,7,8,9] The absorption-promoting effect is mainly due to the reducing action of ascorbic acid within the gastrointestinal lumen, which helps to prevent or delay the formation of insoluble or less dissociated ferric compounds.[3] Iron absorption has been shown to increase sharply with increasing amounts of ascorbic acid, showing a gain in absorption of approximately 40% at 250 mg. Above 250 mg, the gain becomes insignificant, with an additional gain of only approximately 8% at 500 mg.[3] Each Chromagen® FA Capsule contains 250 mg of ascorbic acid, believed to be the optimal amount.
PROMOTES MOVEMENT OF PLASMA IRON: Ascorbic acid also plays an important role in the movement of plasma iron to storage depots in the tissues.[10] The action, which leads to the transport of plasma iron to ferritin presumably involves its reducing effect, converting transferrin iron from the ferric to the ferrous state.[5] There is also evidence that ascorbic acid improves iron utilization, presumably as a further result of its reducing action,[6,9] and some evidence that it may have a direct effect upon erythropoiesis. Ascorbic acid is further alleged to enhance the conversion of folic acid to a more physiologically active form, folinic acid, which would make it even more important in the treatment of anemia since it would aid in the utilization of dietary folic acid.[11]
EXCELLENT ORAL TOLERATION: Ferrous fumarate is used in Chromagen® FA Capsules because it is less likely to cause the gastric disturbances so often associated with oral iron therapy. Ferrous fumarate has a low ionization constant and high solubility in the entire pH range of the gastrointestinal tract. It does not precipitate proteins or have the astringency of more ionizable forms of iron, and does not interfere with proteolytic or diastatic activities of the digestive system. Because of excellent oral toleration, Chromagen® FA Capsules can usually be administered between meals when iron absorption is maximal.
FOLIC ACID SUPPLEMENTATION: The use of supplemental folic acid may be indicated in patients with increased requirements for this vitamin, such as iron deficiency anemia. Folic acid administration can reduce the risk of neural tube defects in the developing fetus.[12] Folic acid has also been shown to reduce circulating homocysteine levels in the blood.[15,16] Folate as 5-methyltetrahydrofolate and B_{12} as methylcobalamin are involved in the remethylation reaction of homocysteine to methionine.[17,18] Elevated homocysteine plasma levels are associated with increase risk of preeclampsia, neural tube defects, myocardial infarction and artherosclerosis.[19–23]
TOXICITY: Ferrous fumarate was found to be the least toxic of three popular oral salts, with an oral LD_{50} of 630 mg/kg. In the same report, the LD_{50} of ferrous gluconate was reported to be 320 mg/kg and ferrous sulfate 230 mg/kg.[1,13]

INDICATIONS
For the treatment of all anemias responsive to oral iron therapy, such as hylpochromic anemia with pregnancy, chronic or acute blood loss, dietary restriction, metabolic disease and post-surgical convalescence.

CONTRAINDICATIONS
Hemochromatosis and hemosiderosis are contraindications to iron therapy. Folic acid is contraindicated in patients with pernicious anemia (see **PRECAUTIONS**).

SIDE EFFECTS
Average capsule doses in sensitive individuals or excessive dosage may cause nausea, skin rash, vomiting, diarrhea, precordial pain, or flushing of the face and extremities.

PRECAUTIONS
Folic acid should not be prescribed until the diagnosis of pernicious anemia has been eliminated, since it can alleviate the hematologic manifestations, while allowing neurological damage to continue undetected.[14]

DOSAGE AND ADMINISTRATION
Usual adult dose is 1 soft gelatin capsule daily.

HOW SUPPLIED
Capsules: NDC 0281-0259-53, Bottle of 100
NDC 0281-0259-56, Bottle of 500
CAUTION: Federal law prohibits dispensing without prescription.

BIBLIOGRAPHY
[1]Berk, M.S. and Novich, M.A.: "Treatment of Iron Deficiency Anemia With Ferrous Fumarate," Am. J. Obst. & Gynec., 203–206, 1962. [2]Shapleigh, J.B., and Montgomery, A.: Am. Pract. & Dig. Treat. 10–461, 1959. [3]Brise, H. And Hallberg, L.: "Effect of Ascorbic Acid on Iron Absorption," Acta. Med. Scand.171:376, 51-58, 1962. [4]New Drugs, p. 309, AMA, Chicago, 1966. [5]Mazur, A., Green, S. and Carleton, A,: "Mechanism of Plasma Iron Incorporation into Hepatic Ferritin," J. Bio. Chem. 3:595-603, 1960. [6]Greenberg, S.M., Tucker, A. E., Mathues, H and J.D.: "Iron Absorption and Metabolism, I. Interrelationship of Ascorbic Acid and Vitamin E," J. Nutrition 63:19–31, 1957. [7]Moore, C.V. and Dubach, R. "Observations on the Absorption of Iron from Foods Tagged with Radioiron" Trans. Assoc. Amer. Physic. 64:245, 1951. [8]Steinkamp, R. Dubach, R. And Moore, C.V.: "Studies in Iron Transportation and Metabolism,"Arch. Int. Med. 95:181, 1955. [9]Gorten, M. K. And Bradley, J. E.: "The Treatment of Nutritional Anemia in Infancy and Childhood with Oral Iron and Ascorbic Acid," J. Pediatrics, 45:1, 1954. [10]Mazur, A.: "Role of Ascorbic Acid in the Incorporation of Plasma Iron into Ferritin," Ann. N.Y. Acad. Sci, 92:223–229, 1961. [11]Cox, E.V. et al.: "The Anemia of Scurvy," Amer. J. Med. 42:220-227, 1967. [12]McEvoy, G.K., Ed.: AHFS Drug Information p. 2667–2669, Am. Soc. Hosp. Pharm., Bethesda, 1996. [13]Berenbaum, M.C. et al.: Blood, 15:540, 1960. [14]Drug Information for the Health Care Professional, p. 1365–1368, U. S. Pharmacopeial Conven., Rockville, 1995. [15]Franken DG, Boers GH, Blom HJ, Trijbels JM. Effect of various regimens of vitamin B_6 and folic acid on mild hyperhomocysteinaemia in vascular patients. J Inherit Metab Dis 1994; 17:159–62. [16]Brattstrom L, Israelsson B, Norving B, et al. Impaired homocysteine metabolism in early-onset cerebral and peripheral occlusive disease—effects of pyridoxine and folic acid treatment. Atherosclerosis 1990; 81:2004–6. [17]Kang S. Wong PWK, Norusis M. Homocysteinemia due to folate deficiency. Metabolism 1987; 36: 458–62. [18]Allen RH, Stabler SP, Savage DG, Lindernbaum J. Diagnosis of cobalamin deficiency. IL usefulness of serum methylmalonic acid and total homocysteine concentrations. AM J Hematol 1990; 34: 90–98. [19]Dekker GA, de Vries Jl, Doelitzsch PM, Huijgens PC, von Blomberg BM, Jakobs, C, van Geijn HP. 1985. Underlying disorder associated with severe early-onset preeclampsia. Am. J. Obstet Gynecol. 173: 1042–1048. [20]Mills JL, McPartlin JM, Kirke PN, Lee YJ, Conley MR, Weir DG, Scott JM. 1995. Homocysteine metabolism in pregnancies complicated by neural-tube defects. Lancet, 345: 149–151. [21]Steegers-Theunissen RP, Boers GH, Blom HJ, Nijhuis JG, Thomas CM, Borm GF, Eskes TK. 1995. Neural tube defects and elevated homocysteine levels in amniotic fluid. Am. J. Obstet Gynecol. 172: 1436–1441. [22]Landgren F, Israelsson B, Lindgren A, Hultberg B, Andersson A, Brattstrom L. 1995. Plasma homocysteine in acute myocardial infarction: Homocysteine-lowering effect of folic acid. J Intern Med. 237: 381–388. [23]Mayer EL, Jacobsen DW, Robinson K. 1996. Homocysteine and Coronary Atherosclerosis. J. Am. Coll. Cardiol. 27: 517–27.

Manufactured for:
SAVAGE LABORATORIES®
a division of Altana Inc.
MELVILLE, NEW YORK 11747
by: R.P. Scherer Corporation, St. Petersburg, Florida 33702
IF70259
R7/96
Shown in Product Identification Guide, page 333

CHROMAGEN® FORTE ℞
SOFT GELATIN CAPSULES

DESCRIPTION
Contents: Each brown soft gelatin capsule contains: ferrous fumarate USP, 460 mg (151 mg elemental iron), ascorbic acid USP, 60 mg, folic acid USP, 1 mg, cyanocobalamin USP, 10 mcg.
Discussion: The amount of elemental iron and the absorption of the iron components of commercial iron preparations vary widely. It is further established that certain "accessory components" may be included to enhance absorption and utilization of iron. Chromagen® Forte Capsules are formulated to provide the essential factors for a complete, versatile hematinic.
High Elemental Iron Content: Ferrous fumarate, used in Chromagen® Forte Capsules is an organic iron complex which has the highest elemental iron content of any hematinic salt – 33%. This compares with 20% for ferrous sulfate (heptahydrate) and 13% for ferrous gluconate.[1,2] Chromagen® Forte contains 151 mg of elemental iron.
More Complete Absorption: It has been repeatedly shown that ascorbic acid when given in sufficient amounts, can increase the absorption of ferrous iron from the gastrointestinal tract.[3,4,5,6,7,8,9] The absorption-promoting effect is mainly due to the reducing action of ascorbic acid within the gastrointestinal lumen, which helps to prevent or delay the formation of insoluble or less dissociated ferric compounds.[3]
Promotes Movement Of Plasma Iron: Ascorbic acid also plays an important role in the movement of plasma iron to storage depots in the tissues.[10] The action, which leads to the transport of plasma iron to ferritin, presumably involves its reducing effect, converting transferrin iron from the ferric to the ferrous state.[5] There is also evidence that ascorbic acid improves iron utilization, presumably as a further result of its reducing action,[6,9] and some evidence that it may have a direct effect upon erythropoiesis. Ascorbic acid is further alleged to enhance the conversion of folic acid to a more physiologically active form, folinic acid, which would make it even more important in the treatment of anemia since it would aid in the utilization of dietary folic acid.[11]
Excellent Oral Toleration: Ferrous fumarate is used in Chromagen® Forte Capsules because it is less likely to cause the gastric disturbances so often associated with oral iron therapy. Ferrous fumarate has a low ionization constant and high solubility in the entire pH range of the gastrointestinal tract. It does not precipitate proteins or have the astringency

Continued on next page

Savage Laboratories—Cont.

of more ionizable forms of iron, and does not interfere with proteolytic or diastatic activities of the digestive system. Because of excellent oral toleration, Chromagen® Forte Capsules can usually be administered between meals when iron absorption is maximal.

Folic Acid Supplementation: The use of supplemental folic acid may be indicated in patients with increased requirements for this vitamin, such as iron deficiency anemia. Folic acid administration can reduce the risk of neural tube defects in the developing fetus.[12] Folic acid has also been shown to reduce circulating homocysteine levels in the blood.[15,16] Folate as 5-methyltetrahydrofolate and B_{12} as methylcobalamin are involved in the remethylation reaction of homocysteine to methionine.[17,18] Elevated homocysteine plasma levels are associated with increase risk of preeclampsia, neural tube defects, myocardial infarction and artherosclerosis.[19–23]

Toxicity: Ferrous fumarate was found to be the least toxic of three popular oral iron salts, with an oral LD_{50} of 630 mg/kg. In the same report, the LD_{50} of ferrous gluconate was reported to be 320 mg/kg and ferrous sulfate 230 mg/kg.[1,13]

INDICATIONS
For the treatment of all anemias responsive to oral iron therapy, such as hypochromic anemia associated with pregnancy, chronic or acute blood loss, dietary restriction, metabolic disease and post-surgical convalescence.

CONTRAINDICATIONS
Hemochromatosis and hemosiderosis are contraindications to iron therapy. Folic acid is contraindicated in patients with pernicious anemia (see **PRECAUTIONS**).

SIDE EFFECTS
Average capsule doses in sensitive individuals or excessive dosage may cause nausea, skin rash, vomiting, diarrhea, precordial pain, or flushing of the face and extremities.

PRECAUTIONS
Folic acid should not be prescribed until the diagnosis of pernicious anemia has been eliminated, since it can alleviate the hematologic manifestations, while allowing neurological damage to continue undetected.[14]

DOSAGE AND ADMINISTRATION
Usual adult dose is 1 soft gelatin capsule daily.

HOW SUPPLIED
Capsules: NDC 0281-0262-53, Bottle of 100
NDC 0281-0262-56, Bottle of 500
CAUTION: Federal law prohibits dispensing without prescription.

BIBLIOGRAPHY

[1]Berk, M.S. and Novich, M.A.: "Treatment of Iron Deficiency Anemia With Ferrous Fumarate," Am. J. Obst. & Gynec., 203-206, 1962. [2]Shapleigh, J.B., and Montgomery, A.:Am. Pract. & Dig. Treat. 10-461 1959. [3]Brise, H. And Hallberg, L.: "Effect of Ascorbic Acid on Iron Absorption," Acta. Med. Scand. 171:376, 51-58, 1962. [4]New Drugs, p. 309, AMA, Chicago, 1966. [5]Mazur, A., Green, S. and Carleton, A,: "Mechanism of Plasma Iron Incorporation into Hepatic Ferritin," J. Bio. Chem. 3:595-603, 1960. [6]Greenberg, S.M., Tucker, A.E., Mathues, H and J.D.: "Iron Absorption and Metabolism, I. Interrelationship of Ascorbic Acid and Vitamin E," J. Nutrition 63:19-31, 1957. [7]Moore, C.V. and Dubach, R. "Observations on the Absorption of Iron from Foods Tagged with Radioiron" Trans. Assoc. Amer. Physic. 64:245, 1951. [8]Steinkamp, R. Dubach, R. And Moore, C.V.: "Studies in Iron Transportation and Metabolism," Arch. Int. Med. 95:181, 1955. [9]Gorten, M.K. And Bradley, J.E.: "The Treatment of Nutritional Anemia in Infancy and Childhood with Oral Iron and Ascorbic Acid," J. Pediatrics, 45:1, 1954. [10]Mazur, A.: "Role of Ascorbic Acid in the Incorporation of Plasma Iron into Ferritin," Ann. N.Y. Acad. Sci, 92:223-229, 1961. [11]Cox, E.V. et al.: "The Anemia of Scurvy," Amer. J. Med. 42:220-227, 1967. [12]McEvoy, G.K., Ed.: AHFS Drug Information, p. 2667-2669, Am. Soc. Hosp. Pharm., Bethesda, 1996. [13]Berenbaum, M.C. et al.: Blood, 15:540, 1960. [14]Drug Information for the Health Care Professional, p. 1365-1368, U.S. Pharmacopeial Conven., Rockville, 1995. [15]Franken DG, Boers GH, Blom HJ, Trijbels JM. Effect of various regimens of vitamin B[6] and folic acid on mild hyperhomocysteinaemia in vascular patients. J Inherit Metab Dis 1994; 17:159-62. [16]Brattstrom L, Israelsson B, Norrving B, et al. Impaired homocysteine metabolism in early-onset cerebral and peripheral occlusive disease—effects of pyridoxine and folic acid treatment. Atherosclerosis 1990; 81: 2004-6. [17]Kang S. Wong PWK, Norusis M. Homocysteinemia due to folate deficiency. Metabolism 1987; 36: 458-62. [18]Allen RH, Stabler SP, Savage DG, Lindernbaum J. Diagnosis of cobalamin deficiency. IL usefulness of serum methylmalonic acid and total homocysteine concentrations. AM J Hematol 1990; 34: 90-98. [19]Dekker GA, de Vries JI, Doelitzsch PM, Huijgens PC, von Blomberg BM, Jakobs, C, van Geijn HP. 1985. Underlying disorder associated with severe early-onset preeclampsia. Am. J. Obstet Gynecol. 173: 1042-1048. [20]Mills JL, McPartin JM, Kirke PN, Lee YJ, Conley MR, Weir DG, Scott JM. 1995. Homocysteine metabolism in pregnancies complicated by neural-tube defects. Lancet. 345: 149-151. [21]Steegers-Theunissen RP, Boers GH, Blom HJ, Nijhuis JG, Thomas CM, Borm GF, Eskes TK, 1995. Neural tube defects and elevated homocysteine levels in amniotic fluid. Am. J. Obstet Gynecol. 172: 1436-1441. [22]Landgren F, Israelsson B, Lindgren A, Hultberg B, Andersson A, Brattstrom L. 1995. Plasma homocysteine in acute myocardial infarction: Homocysteine-lowering effect of folic acid. J Intern Med. 237: 381-388. [23]Mayer EL, Jacobsen DW, Robinson K. 1996. Homocysteine and Coronary Atherosclerosis. J. Am. Coll. Cardiol. 27: 517-27.

Manufactured for:
SAVAGE LABORATORIES®
a division of Altana Inc.
MELVILLE, NEW YORK 11747
by: R.P. Scherer Corporation,
St. Petersburg, Florida 33702 IF70262
R6/96

Shown in Product Identification Guide, page 333

DILOR® Tablets ℞
(dyphylline tablets USP)

DESCRIPTION
Dyphylline [(±-7-(2,3-dihydroxypropyl)theophylline] [$C_{10}H_{14}N_4O_4$] is a white, extremely bitter, amorphous solid, freely soluble in water and soluble to the extent of 2g/100 mL alcohol.

HOW SUPPLIED
Dilor® Tablets

200 mg–	NDC 0281-1115-53, Bottle of 100.
	NDC 0281-1115-57, Bottle of 1000.
	NDC 0281-1115-63, Unit dose, Box of 100
400 mg–	NDC 0281-1116-53, Bottle of 100.
	NDC 0281-1116-57, Bottle of 1000.
	NDC 0281-1116-63, Unit dose, Box of 100

ALSO AVAILABLE
Dilor® Elixir, dyphylline USP 160 mg/15 mL; and Dilor® Injection, dyphylline USP 250 mg/mL.

DILOR-G® ℞
(dyphylline and guaifenesin tablets USP)

DESCRIPTION
Each tablet contains dyphylline USP 200 mg and guaifenesin USP 200 mg. Also contains the following inactive ingredients:
Colloidal silicon dioxide, corn starch, food starch, povidone, stearic acid, and artificial coloring.
Dyphylline is a molecular modification, rather than a salt or complex of theophylline, therefore, the usual side effects of theophylline are diminished without affecting activity. The result is less gastric upset than with other theophyllines.

HOW SUPPLIED
Dilor-G® Tablets
NDC 0281-1124-53, Tablets, Bottle of 100.
NDC 0281-1124-57, Tablets, Bottle of 1000.
NDC 0281-1124-63, Unit dose, Box of 100.
Dilor-G® Liquid
NDC 0281-1127-74, pint.
NDC 0281-1127-76, gallon.

ETHIODOL® ℞
BRAND OF ETHIODIZED OIL INJECTION
A Low Viscosity Radio-Opaque Diagnostic Agent

NOT FOR INTRAVASCULAR, INTRATHECAL OR INTRABRONCHIAL USE

DESCRIPTION
Ethiodol, brand of ethiodized oil, is a sterile injectable radio-opaque diagnostic agent for use in hysterosalpingography and lymphography. It contains 37% iodine (475 mg/ml) organically combined with ethyl esters of the fatty acids (primarily as ethyl monoiodostearate and ethyl diiodostearate) of poppyseed oil. Stabilized with poppyseed oil, 1%. The precise structure of Ethiodol is unknown at this time. Ethiodol is a straw to amber colored, oily fluid, which because of simplified molecular structure, possesses a greatly reduced viscosity (1.280 specific gravity at 15 degrees C yields viscosity of 0.5–1.0 poise). This high fluidity provides a new flexibility for radiographic exploration.

CLINICAL PHARMACOLOGY
There has been little detailed investigation of the metabolic fate of Ethiodol in either man or animals. However, the fate of Ethiodol following lymphangiography in dogs has been reported. [1]Koehler et al. employed I^{131}–tagged Ethiodol for lymphangiography in dogs and analyses of individual organs at various time intervals were done. The investigators reported an average of only 25% of the injected medium was retained in the lymphatics at the end of three days. An average of 50% was recovered from the lungs. They found the remainder of injected activity was fairly uniformly distributed throughout the body. Urinary excretion in the form of inorganic iodine was revealed as the chief mode of iodine loss from the system.

INDICATIONS
Ethiodol is indicated for use as a radio-opaque medium for hysterosalpingography and lymphography.

IN HYSTEROSALPINGOGRAPHY

CONTRAINDICATIONS
Ethiodol is contraindicated in patients hypersensitive to it. Ethiodol should not be injected intrathecally or intravascularly, or used in bronchography. A history of sensitivity to iodine contraindicates the use of Ethiodol; iodine is split off from fatty compounds and becomes free iodine in the body. Hysterosalpingography is contraindicated in intrauterine pregnancy, acute pelvic inflammatory disease, marked cervical erosion, endocervicitis in the presence of intrauterine bleeding, in the immediate pre- or postmenstrual phase, or within 30 days of curettage or conization.

WARNINGS
Ethiodol is not intended for use in bronchography and, therefore, is not to be introduced into the bronchial tree. A history of sensitivity to iodine or to other contrast materials is not an absolute contraindication to Ethiodol, but calls for extreme caution. All procedures utilizing contrast media carry a definite risk of adverse reactions. While most reactions are minor, life threatening and fatal reactions may occur without warning. The risk/benefit factor should always be carefully evaluated. At all times a fully equipped emergency cart and resuscitation equipment should be readily available, and personnel competent in recognizing and treating reactions of all severity should be on hand.

PRECAUTIONS
General: Since iodine-containing contrast materials may alter the results of certain thyroid function tests, such tests, if indicated, should be performed prior to the administration of this drug. Pulmonary embolization of the contrast material may occur if hysterosalpingography is performed under conditions which may lead to intravasation of the contrast materials. These conditions include uterine bleeding, recent curettage or conization and injection of the contrast material under excessive pressure.

Carcinogenesis, Mutagenesis, and Impairment of Fertility: Long-term studies in animals have not been performed to evaluate carcinogenic potential, mutagenesis, or whether Ethiodol can affect fertility in males or females.

Pregnancy Category C: Animal reproduction studies have not been conducted with Ethiodol. It is also not known whether Ethiodol can cause fetal harm when administered to a pregnant woman or can affect reproduction capacity. Ethiodol should be administered to a pregnant woman only if clearly needed.

Nursing Mothers: It is not known whether this drug is excreted in human milk. Because many drugs are excreted in human milk and because of the potential for serious adverse reactions in nursing infants from Ethiodol, a decision should be made whether to discontinue nursing or to discontinue the drug, taking into account the importance of the drug to the mother.

ADVERSE REACTIONS
Hypersensitivity reactions, foreign body reactions and exacerbation of pelvic inflammatory disease, although infrequent, have been reported. In an occasional patient, abdominal pains may occur. Such pains may be the result of tubal torsion, or possibly due to too rapid a rate of instillation or excessive pressure, or both. The condition is usually only transitory, lasting one or two hours at most, and may be relieved by the administration of any of the commonly used analgesics.

DOSAGE AND ADMINISTRATION
The hysterosalpingogram is preferably taken during the patient's preovulatory phase (as determined from her basal body temperature record) and not less than two days after cessation of her menstrual flow. It has been frequently observed that some bleeding will occur during or after the onset of pregnancy which cannot be distinguished by the patient from a normal menstrual period. In such cases a basal body temperature record will reveal a sustained high temperature phase, and thus enable an operator to avoid hysterosalpingography when a pregnancy may exist. Salpingography should not be performed if the blood is exuding

from the cervical os (which occasionally occurs without the patient being aware of it) or if any gross evidence of endocervicitis exists.

Careful aseptic technique should be employed as for any operative procedure in which the uterus is entered. A self-retaining cannula should be used thereby permitting removal of the vaginal speculum so that the outline of the cervical canal may be seen in the film. The use of a radio-opaque aluminum speculum may be employed in patients where a lacerated or patulous cervix does not permit the use of a retaining cannula.

The radio-opaque agent is introduced under pressure and preferably with fluoroscopic control. A preliminary film is exposed and a skiagram is made after the injection of 5 ml of the agent. The pressure is raised to 80–90 mm Hg. In cases of normal bilateral tubal patency, the pressure falls immediately to below 60 mm Hg. The wet film may be viewed immediately and if both tubes are seen to "fill", the apparatus is removed and the procedure is finished, except for the 24 hour follow-up to establish whether or not "spill" into the peritoneal cavity has occurred.

Increments of 2 ml of the agent are injected and successive films exposed until tubal patency is established or until the patient's limit of tolerance to discomfort is reached. Few patients will complain of discomfort at pressures under 200 mm Hg.

IN LYMPHOGRAPHY

CONTRAINDICATIONS

Ethiodol is contraindicated in patient's hypersensitive to it. Ethiodol should not be injected intrathecally or intravascularly or introduced into the bronchial tree. Patients with known sensitivity to iodine should not have lymphography performed. Iodine is split off from fatty compounds and becomes free iodine in the body. Lymphography is contraindicated in patients with a right to left cardiac shunt, in patients with advanced pulmonary disease, especially those with alveolar-capillary block, and in patients who have had radiotherapy to the lungs.

WARNINGS

The use of intralymphatic Ethiodol presents a significant hazard in patients with pre-existing pulmonary disease characterized by a decrease in pulmonary diffusing capacity and/or pulmonary blood flow. A few fatalities have been noted in such patients. With reference to this potential complication, recent studies indicate a significant decrease in both pulmonary diffusing capacity and pulmonary capillary blood flow following Ethiodol lymphography without appreciable concomitant clinical manifestations. Also, care should be exercised in patients with other types of pulmonary disease in view of the more frequent incidence of overt pulmonary complications such as pulmonary infarction, in these groups. However, it is to be noted that pulmonary infarction, although rare, has occurred in patients without evidence of pre-existing pulmonary disease.

The safety of intralymphatic Ethiodol has not been established in pregnant women, and accordingly, its use should be restricted to such situations where it is deemed necessary.

PRECAUTIONS

General: Although subclinical pulmonary embolization occurs in a majority of patients following Ethiodol lymphography, clinical evidence of such embolization is infrequent and is usually of a transient nature. Such clinical manifestations are usually immediate, but may be delayed from a few hours to days. It would appear that it is advantageous to use the smallest volume of Ethiodol necessary for radiographic visualization. For this reason, and to prevent inadvertent venous administration, radiographic monitoring of patients is recommended during the injection of Ethiodol.

The timing and choice of anesthesia following Ethiodol injection may be influenced by consideration of the above noted decrease in pulmonary and capillary blood flow and diffusing capacity. It should be noted that although an average of 2 to 3 days was required for complete reversibility for such tests, an occasional patient required up to 12 days to return to baseline values.

PBI determination of thyroid uptake studies should be carried out prior to the lymphographic procedure because interference with these tests may be anticipated for as long as one year. In the presence of known iodine sensitivity, Ethiodol lymphography should be carried out with greatest precaution.

Carcinogenesis, Mutagenesis, and Impairment of Fertility: Long-term studies in animals have not been performed to evaluate carcinogenic potential, mutagenesis, or whether Ethiodol can affect fertility in males or females.

Pregnancy Category C: Animal reproduction studies have not been conducted with Ethiodol. It is also not known whether Ethiodol can cause fetal harm when administered to a pregnant woman or can affect reproduction capacity. Ethiodol should be administered in a pregnant woman only if clearly needed.

Nursing Mothers: It is not known whether this drug is excreted in human milk. Because many drugs are excreted in human milk and because of the potential for serious adverse reactions in nursing infants from Ethiodol, a decision should be made whether to discontinue nursing or discontinue the drug, taking into account the importance of the drug to the mother.

ADVERSE REACTIONS

The occasional observation of pulmonary Ethiodol embolization (infarction) several hours after injection has been reported. This was noticed more frequently when excessive amounts of Ethiodol have been injected, in the presence of marked lymphatic obstruction or through accidental intravenous injection. Radiologic manifestations are fine, granular stippling throughout both lung fields. The clinical symptoms usually noted have been mild, consisting of moderate temperature elevation, dyspnea, and cough. However, severe acute symptoms developed in two patients both of whom were severely ill and required extensive care.[2] Fuchs[3] experienced 1 severe and 3 minor complications in a series of 20 bilateral procedures. Two are described by the author as cardiovascular collapse occurring at two hours respectively following the completion of the procedure. It was postulated that minute emboli may have been causative. Recovery was rapid and complete in both instances.

The occurrence of pulmonary invasion may be minimized if radiographic confirmation of intralymphatic (rather than venous) injection is secured, and the procedure discontinued when the medium becomes visible in the thoracic duct or the presence of lymphatic obstruction is noticed.

While rare, other side effects reported include transient fever, lymphangitis, iodism (headache, soreness of mouth and pharynx, coryza and skin rash), allergic dermatitis, and lipogranuloma formation. Delayed wound healing at the site of incision and secondary infection are occasionally seen, and can be prevented or minimized by adhering to a strict sterile technique.

Transient edema or temporary exacerbation of preexisting lymphedema, as well as thrombophlebitis have also been reported. In the extremely rare presence of concomitant lymphatic and inferior vena cava obstruction the contrast medium may be shunted partially to the liver, resulting in hepatic embolization. Also, when accidental intravenous administration of Ethiodol results in a considerable amount of this medium entering the circulation, embolization other than pulmonary may occur as reported in 2 cases.[4] Both cases developed a transient, psychotic-like manifestation, which in all probability stemmed from the entrance of fine oil droplets into the cerebral circulation. Recovery was uneventful and complete without evidence of neurological sequelae.

DOSAGE AND ADMINISTRATION

This method applies for both the upper and lower extremities. A lymphatic vessel is selected for cannulization.

The patient should be comfortably arranged in a supine position on a portable stretcher or an x-ray table. When available, a radiolucent pad will add to the patient's comfort during the one to two hours required for completion of the examination. It is important that the patient be in a cooperative state. Premedication might be advisable in the unusually apprehensive patient.

In the unusually restless patient, the extremities should be immobilized during the entire procedure to prevent displacement of the needle. Thomas splints have been satisfactorily employed for the legs and simple arm boards for the upper extremities. The cut-down and injection instruments and materials include the following:

Sterile pediatric cut-down set
Sterile towels for draping, sponges, etc.
Local anesthetic, such a procaine hydrochloride, and a syringe
Bactericidal painting solution
20 ml syringe containing 15 ml of Ethiodol with an 18 inch catheter to which is affixed a 27 or 30 gauge needle. (If bilateral lymphography is scheduled, two syringes should be prepared.)
A manually driven or motorized unit (a pressure regulated pump) to provide for slow injection.

Under local infiltration anesthesia, a transverse, curvilinear or longitudinal small skin incision should be made near the ankle or wrist (just lateral and distal to the first metatarsal head on the dorsum of the foot, or just over the "snuff-box" in the dorsum of the hand).

Upon superficial dissection (but not penetrating the subcutaneous layer of tissue) lymph vessels will be noted in the immediate subcutaneous tissue, while larger lymph vessel trunks are found in the extrafascial plane. The deeper lymph trunks will be easier to cannulate.

One lymph vessel is then exposed, avoiding circumferential dissection. The less manipulation performed, the better the results that will be obtained. The lymphatic, thus isolated, is then cannulated with a 27 or 30 gauge ⅝ inch needle, depending upon the size of the lymphatic selected for injection. It is rarely possible to cannulate with a needle greater than 27 gauge. Insertion of the needle through the skin flap before cannulating the lymphatic serves to reduce the movement of the needle with the vessel. Additional security of the needle

in the lymphatic is obtained by strapping, with sterile tape, the polyethylene tubing to the patient's foot.

The injection should be started at a slow rate, i.e., 0.1 ml to 0.2 ml per minute. Radiographic monitoring either by fluoroscopy or serial radiographs after 1 ml to 2 ml has been injected, will confirm the proper intralymphatic placement of the needle, rule out accidental intravenous injection or extravasation of the medium by perforation or rupture of the lymphatic. Monitoring will also permit prompt termination of the procedure in the event that lymphatic blockage is present. In such situations, continuation of the injection will result in unnecessary introduction of contrast material in the venous system via the lymphovenous communication channels. If the injection is satisfactory, approximately 6 to 8 ml. are then injected. However, as soon as it becomes radiographically evident that Ethiodol has entered the thoracic duct, the procedure should be terminated to minimize entry of the contrast material into the subclavian vein. Two to four ml of Ethiodol injected into the upper extremity will suffice to demonstrate the axillary and supraclavicular nodes. In penile lymphography approximately 2 to 3 ml of Ethiodol is required. In infants and children, a minimum of 1 ml to a maximum of 6 ml should be employed.

The rate of speed at which the contrast material may be introduced varies and is dependent upon receptivity of the lymphatics in the individual patient. If the injection is proceeding at too rapid a rate, extravasation will be noted and the patient may refer to pain in the foot, leg or arm.

At the completion of the injection, anteroposterior roentgenograms are obtained of the legs or arms, thighs, pelvis, abdomen and chest (dorsal spine technique). Lateral or oblique views as well as laminograms are obtained when indicated. Follow-up films at 24 or 48 hours provide better demonstration of lymph nodes and permit more concise evaluation of nodal architecture.

As a general rule, the smallest possible amount of Ethiodol should be employed according to the anatomical area to be visualized. Therefore, and to prevent inadvertent venous administration, fluoroscopic monitoring or serial radiographic guidance of patients is recommended during the injection of Ethiodol.

Average dose in the adult patient for unilateral lymphography of the upper extremities is 2 to 4 ml; of lower extremities, 6 to 8 ml; of penile lymphography, 2 to 3 ml; of cervical lymphography, 1 to 2 ml.

In the pedatric patient, a minimum of 1 ml to a maximum of 6 ml may be employed according to the anatomical area to be visualized.

SUMMARY OF STEPS TO AVOID COMPLICATIONS IN LYMPHOGRAPHY[5]

1. Contraindicate patients:
A. With a known hypersensitivity to Ethiodol
B. With a right to left cardiac shunt
C. With advanced pulmonary disease, especially those with alveolar-capillary block. Pulmonary gas diffusion studies should be done if in doubt.
D. Who have had radiation therapy to the lungs
2. Proceed with caution:
A. Patients having markedly advanced neoplastic disease with expected lymphatic obstruction.
B. Patients having undergone previous surgery interrupting the lymphatic system.
C. Patients having had deep radiation therapy to the examined area.
   If in those cases in which extreme caution should be exercised, lymphography is still necessary, a smaller dose of oily contrast medium with protracted injection time with less pressure and careful monitoring is required.
3. Skin testing should be done on all patients before submitting them to lymphography. Be aware of possible hypersensitivity to local anesthetics and skin disinfectants. Careful history taking is important.
4. Technique of cannulation: extravasation is to be avoided and/or detected early. The injection site should be included on the "scout film" or observed under image amplification fluoroscopy. The needle tip must remain visible in the incision wound.
5. Oily contrast materials: once opened, ampules should be discarded. Ampules of Ethiodol should not be used if the color has darkened or if particulate matter is present. The average dose for each foot in an adult is 5 to 6 ml; one-half as much for the upper extremity. The amount for children should be determined by careful monitoring. It should stay below 0.25 ml/kg.
6. Injection pressure should be regulated to deliver the average dose of no less than 1¼ hours. Continuous monitoring helps to determine the speed most appropriate for each individual. Sensation of pain is a warning of too high pressure.
7. Scout roentgenograms: if scout roentgenograms are used for monitoring, they should be developed and viewed immediately in order to apply corrective measures when needed; e.g., discontinuation of the study when one sees

Continued on next page

Savage Laboratories—Cont.

intravenous injection or lymphatico-venous anastomosis. Reduction of injection speed is needed if evidence of collateral circulation occurs or if the higher abdomino-aortic nodes do not opacify in spite of the usual injection pressure. This is highly suggestive of lymphatic obstruction. Scout roentgenograms should be taken more frequently in such cases.

8. Surgical technique: strict aseptic surgical technique is followed including the wearing of a face mask. Before suturing the incision wound, the remnants of the lymphatic vessels and loose tissue are removed and the wound well washed with saline to remove any possible oil. In case of reflux type lymphedema, the cannulated large lymphatic vessel may have to be closed by catgut to avoid development of a lymphocyst.

The patient is instructed to elevate the legs as often as possible to promote healing. The sutures are removed from the feet on the 10th day, and on the 5th or 6th from the hands.

HOW SUPPLIED
Ethiodol (ethiodized oil for injection) is supplied in a box of two 10 ml ampules. NDC 0281-7062-37.
Store at controlled room temperature 15°–30°C (59°–86°F). Protect from light. Remove from carton only upon use.
Parenteral drug products should be inspected visually for particulate matter and discoloration prior to administration, whenever solution and container permit. Ethiodol brand of ethiodized oil for injection is straw to amber color under normal conditions. (See Description).
Caution: Federal law prohibits dispensing without prescription.
A development of Guerbet Laboratories.

BIBLIOGRAPHY
1. P. Ruben Koehler, M.D. et al.: "Body Distribution of Ethiodol Following Lymphangiography", Radiology, 1964, 82, 5 866–871.
2. Bronk, et al.: "Oil Embolism in Lymphography", Radiation, 80:194, February 1963.
3. Fuchs, S.A., "Complications in Lymphography With Oily Contrast Media", Acta Radiol., 57:247, November 1962.
4. Viamonte, M. Jr., University of Miami, Jackson Memorial Hospital, Miami, Florida, Private Communication.
5. Kuisk, H., "Techniques of Lymphography and Principles of Interpretation", 1971, Warren H. Green, Inc., St. Louis, Missouri, 63105.

SAVAGE LABORATORIES
a division of Altana Inc.
MELVILLE, NEW YORK 11747

R 7/93

EVAC-Q-KWIK®   OTC

DESCRIPTION
A bowel evacuant system comprised of three separate products that are intended to be administered sequentially at intervals intended to minimize the overlap of pharmacological activity.
Evac-Q-Mag®—(saline cathartic)
Electrolyte content of 250 mEq of magnesium, 21 mEq of potassium, and .95 mEq of sodium.
Evac-Q-Tabs®—(oral stimulant laxative)
Each tablet containing 130 mg of phenolphthalein.
Evac-Q-Kwik® suppository—Each containing 10 mg of bisacodyl.
To promote the flushing of the G.I. tract. Together the products and the liquid comprise the bowel evacuant system.

HOW SUPPLIED
One 10 fl oz Evac-Q-Mag
Two tablets Evac-Q-Tabs
One Evac-Q-Kwik suppository (NDC 0281-2189-76)

ILOPAN—CHOLINE® TABLETS   ℞
Dexpanthenol 50 mg and Choline Bitartrate 25 mg

DESCRIPTION
Each tablet of Ilopan-choline contains dexpanthenol 50 mg and choline bitartrate 25 mg. ILOPAN-CHOLINE is an antiflatulent.
Dexpanthenol is a derivative of pantothenic acid, a member of the B-Complex vitamins.

HOW SUPPLIED
Bottle of 100 (NDC 0281-2311-17)

ILOPAN® INJECTION   ℞
Dexpanthenol Preparation USP

DESCRIPTION
ILOPAN® (dexpanthenol preparation USP) is a derivative of pantothenic acid, a member of the B complex vitamins. ILOPAN INJECTION is a sterile aqueous solution for use as a gastrointestinal stimulant.

HOW SUPPLIED
Each milliliter of ILOPAN INJECTION contains dexpanthenol preparation USP 250 mg in water for injection.
ILOPAN INJECTION is available as follows:
ILOPAN INJECTION NDC 0281-2356-95 2 mL Ampuls, Box of 25
ILOPAN STAT-PAK® (unit dose) NDC 0281-2366-95 Disposable Syringe 2 mL, Box of 25
Protect from freezing or excessive heat (40°C).

KAOCHLOR® 10% LIQUID   ℞
(Contains sugar)
(Potassium Chloride Liquid)

DESCRIPTION
Potassium chloride oral solution, USP 10% liquid. Each 15 mL (one tablespoonful) supplies 20 mEq of potassium and chloride (as potassium chloride, 1.5 g) with sugar, saccharin and flavoring. Alcohol 5%.

HOW SUPPLIED
480 mL (pint) bottle (NDC 0281-3103-51).

KAOCHLOR® S-F 10% LIQUID (SUGAR FREE) ℞
(Potassium Chloride Liquid)

DESCRIPTION
Potassium chloride oral solution, USP 10% liquid. Each 15 mL (one tablespoonful) supplies 20 mEq of potassium and chloride (as potassium chloride 1.5 g) with saccharin and flavoring. Alcohol 5%.

HOW SUPPLIED
480 mL (pint) bottle (NDC 0281-3093-51)

KAON-CL® 8   ℞

DESCRIPTION
KAON-CL® Extended-release Tablets, USP are a solid oral dosage form of potassium chloride. Each contains 600 mg of potassium chloride equivalent to 8 mEq of potassium in a wax matrix tablet. This formulation is intended to slow the release of potassium so that the likelihood of a high localized concentration of potassium chloride within the gastrointestinal tract is reduced.
KAON-CL® Extended-release Tablets are an electrolyte replenisher. The chemical name is potassium chloride, and the structural formula is KCl. Potassium chloride USP occurs as a white, granular or as colorless crystals. It is odorless and has asaline taste. It's solutions are neutral to litmus. It is freely soluble in water and insoluble in alcohol.
Inactive Ingredients: Castor oil, hydroxypropyl methylcellulose 2910, magnesium stearate, polyethylene glycol 3350, propylene glycol, synthetic iron oxide, titanium dioxide, and other ingredients. Dark blue tablets also contain FD&C Blue No. 1 aluminum lake.

HOW SUPPLIED
Film coated, imprinted with Savage logo and 212 round dark blue tablets containing:
   600 mg potassium chloride (equivalent to 8mEq)
   NDC 0281-0212-17, bottles of 100
   NDC 0281-0212-21, bottles of 500
   NDC 0281-0212-23, bottles of 1000
   NDC 0281-0212-18, unit dose packages of 100
Protect from light and moisture. Store at controlled room temperature, 59°-86°F (15°-30°C). Dispense in container with child-resistant closure.

KAON-CL® 10   ℞
(Potassium Chloride Extended-Release Tablets, USP) 10 mEq

DESCRIPTION
KAON-CL® 10 Extended-release Tablets, USP are a solid oral dosage form of potassium chloride. Each contains 750 mg of potassium chloride equivalent to 10 mEq of potassium in a wax matrix tablet. This formulation is intended to slow the release of potassium so that the likelihood of a high local-

---

ized concentration of potassium chloride within the gastrointestinal tract is reduced.
Inactive Ingredients: Castor oil, hydroxypropylmethylcellulose 2910, magnesium stearate, polyethylene glycol 3350, propylene glycol, synthetic iron oxide, titanium dioxide, and other ingredients.

HOW SUPPLIED
Film coated imprinted round white tablets containing:
750 mg potassium chloride (equivalent to 10mEq)
NDC 0281-3131-17, bottles of 100
NDC 0281-3131-21, bottles of 500
NDC 0281-3131-23, bottles of 1000
NDC 0281-3131-18, unit dose packages of 100

KAON-CL® 20% LIQUID   ℞
(Potassium Chloride Liquid)

Potassium chloride oral solution, USP, sugar free. Each 15 mL (one tablespoonful) supplies 40 mEq of potassium chloride, 3.0 g with saccharin and flavoring. Alcohol 5%.

HOW SUPPLIED
480 mL (pint) bottle (NDC 0281-3113-51).

KAON® GRAPE ELIXIR   ℞
(Sugar free)
(Potassium Gluconate Liquid)

DESCRIPTION
Potassium gluconate. Each 15 mL (one tablespoonful) supplies 20 mEq of potassium (as potassium gluconate 4.68 g) with saccharin and aromatics. Alcohol 5%.

HOW SUPPLIED
480 mL (pint) bottle (NDC 0281-3203-51).

MAGAN® 545 MG TABLET   ℞
Magnesium Salicylate

DESCRIPTION
Contains 545 mg of magnesium salicylate, USP (equivalent to 500 mg of salicylate). Magnesium Salicylate is a non-steroidal, anti-inflammatory agent with antipyretic and analgesic properties.

HOW SUPPLIED
Bottle of 100 (NDC 0281-4121-17).

MODANE® BULK POWDER   OTC

DESCRIPTION
A powdered mixture of equivalent parts of psyllium, a bulking agent and dextrose, as a dispersing agent. Each rounded teaspoonful contains approximately 3.5 g psyllium, 3.5 g dextrose, 2 mg sodium and 37 mg potassium. Provides 14 calories.
For treatment of constipation resulting from a diet low in residue. It is also used as an adjunctive therapy in patients with diverticular disease, spastic or irritable colon, hemorrhoids, in pregnancy and in convalescent and senile patients.

HOW SUPPLIED
(13oz) 369 g (NDC 0281-5035-13).

MODANE® SOFT 100MG CAPSULE   OTC
100mg of docusate sodium

DESCRIPTION
Stool Softener

HOW SUPPLIED
Bottle of 30 (NDC 0281-5111-13).

MODANE® TABLET   OTC

DESCRIPTION
Contains 130 mg of phenolphthalein, a stimulant laxative.

HOW SUPPLIED
Bottles of 10 (NDC 0281-5131-07), 30 (NDC 0281-5131-13), and 100 (NDC 0281-5131-17).

MODANE® PLUS TABLET OTC

DESCRIPTION
Contains 65 mg of phenolphthalein and 100 mg of docusate sodium. Acts as a stimulant laxative with a stool softener.

HOW SUPPLIED
Bottle of 30 (NDC 0281-5151-13).

MYTREX® ℞
(nystatin and triamcinolone acetonide)
Cream USP and Ointment USP

DESCRIPTION
MYTREX® (nystatin and triamcinolone acetonide) Cream USP and Ointment USP contain the antifungal agent nystatin and the synthetic corticosteroid triamcinolone acetonide.
Each gram of MYTREX® (nystatin and triamcinolone acetonide) Cream USP contains 100,000 USP Nystatin Units and 1 mg of triamcinolone acetonide in a cream base containing polyoxyethylene fatty alcohol ether, white petrolatum, glyceryl monostearate, polyethylene glycol 400 monostearate, sorbitol solution, simethicone emulsion, propylene glycol, aluminum hydroxide gel, polysorbate 60, titanium dioxide, and purified water with benzyl alcohol as a preservative. Hydrochloric acid or sodium hydroxide to adjust pH.
Each gram of MYTREX® (nystatin and triamcinolone acetonide) Ointment USP contains 100,000 USP Nystatin Units and 1 mg of triamcinolone acetonide in a base of polyethylene and mineral oil.

HOW SUPPLIED
MYTREX® Cream
(Nystatin and triamcinolone acetonide cream, USP)
12 × 1.5 Gram Foilpac—NDC 0281-0081-08
15 Gram Tube—NDC 0281-0081-15
30 Gram Tube—NDC 0281-0081-30
60 Gram Tube—NDC 0281-0081-60
MYTREX® Ointment
(Nystatin and triamcinolone acetonide ointment, USP)
15 gram tube—NDC 0281-0089-15
30 gram tube—NDC 0281-0089-30

NITROL® OINTMENT ℞
APPLI-KIT®
(2% nitroglycerin ointment, USP) with
Appli-Tape® adhesive dosage covers

DESCRIPTION
Nitroglycerin is 1,2,3 propanetriol trinitrate, an organic nitrate, whose structural formula is

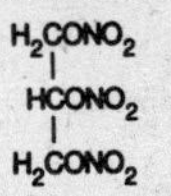

and whose molecular weight is 227.09. The organic nitrates are vasodilators, active on both arteries and veins.
NITROL® Ointment contains lactose and 2% nitroglycerin in a base of lanolin and white petrolatum. Each inch (2.5 cm), as squeezed from the tube, contains approximately 15 mg of nitroglycerin.

HOW SUPPLIED:
(NDC 0281-5804-56) 60 gram 6 Pack
(NDC 0281-5804-59) Titratable Unit Dose—50 × 3g tubes
NITROL® Ointment Appli-Kit®
(Packages include a supply of Appli-Tape® for convenient application)
(NDC 0281-5804-46) 30 gram tube Appli-Kit
(NDC 0281-5804-47) 60 gram tube Appli-Kit
(NDC 0281-5804-48) Titratable Unit Dose—50 × 3g tubes Appli-Kit
Keep tube tightly closed and store at controlled room temperature 15°-30°C (59°-86°F).
Caution: Federal law prohibits dispensing without prescription.

PANDEL® ℞
(hydrocortisone buteprate)
Cream, 0.1%
For Dermatologic Use Only
Not for Ophthalmic Use

DESCRIPTION
PANDEL Cream contains hydrocortisone buteprate, a non-halogenated synthetic adrenocorticosteroid, for dermatologic use. The topical corticosteroids constitute a class of primarily synthetic steroids used as anti-inflammatory and anti-pruritic agents.
Hydrocortisone buteprate is a tasteless and odorless white crystalline powder practically insoluble in hexane or water, slightly soluble in ether, and very soluble in dichloromethane, methanol and acetone. Chemically, it is 11β,17,21-trihydroxypregn-4-ene-3,20-dione 17-butyrate 21-propionate. The structural formula is:

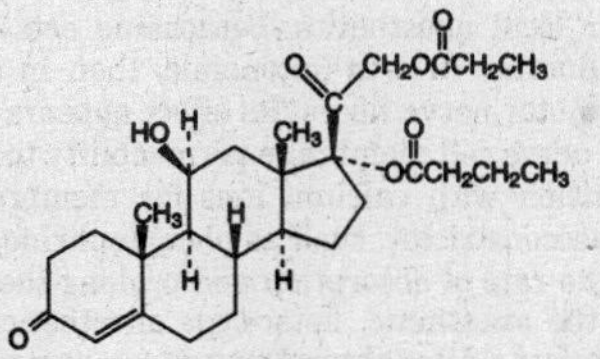

Molecular Formula: $C_{28}H_{40}O_7$ Molecular Weight: 488.62

Each gram of PANDEL (hydrocortisone buteprate) Cream, 0.1% contains: 1 mg of hydrocortisone buteprate in a cream base of propylene glycol, white petrolatum, light mineral oil, stearyl alcohol, polysorbate 60, sorbitan monostearate, glyceryl monostearate, PEG-20 stearate, glyceryl stearate SE, methylparaben, butylparaben, citric acid anhydrous, sodium citrate anhydrous, and purified water.

CLINICAL PHARMACOLOGY
Topical corticosteroids share anti-inflammatory, anti-pruritic and vasoconstrictive actions. The mechanism of anti-inflammatory activity of the topical corticosteroids is unclear. However, corticosteroids are thought to act by the induction of phospholipase A_2 inhibitory proteins, collectively called lipocortins. It is postulated that these proteins control the biosynthesis of potent mediators of inflammation such as prostaglandins and leukotrienes by inhibiting the release of their common precursor arachidonic acid. Arachidonic acid is released from membrane phospholipids by phospholipase A_2.
Pharmacokinetics: The extent of percutaneous absorption of topical corticosteroids is determined by many factors, including the vehicle and the integrity of the epidermal barrier. Use of occlusive dressings with hydrocortisone for up to 24 hours have not been shown to increase penetration; however, occlusion of hydrocortisone for 96 hours does markedly enhance penetration. Topical corticosteroids can be absorbed from normal intact skin. Inflammation and/or other disease processes in the skin increase percutaneous absorption.
Studies performed with PANDEL Cream indicate that it is in the medium range of potency compared with other topical corticosteroids.

INDICATIONS AND USAGE
PANDEL Cream is a medium potency corticosteroid indicated for the relief of the inflammatory and pruritic manifestations of corticosteroid-responsive dermatoses in patients 18 years of age and older.

CONTRAINDICATIONS
PANDEL Cream is contraindicated in those patients who are hypersensitive to hydrocortisone buteprate or to any of the components of the preparation.

PRECAUTIONS
General: Systemic absorption of topical corticosteroids has produced reversible hypothalamic-pituitary-adrenal (HPA) axis suppression with the potential for glucocorticosteroid insufficiency after withdrawal of treatment. Manifestations of Cushing's syndrome, hyperglycemia, and glucosuria can also be produced in some patients by systemic absorption of topical corticosteroids while on treatment.
Patients applying a topical steroid to a large surface area or to areas under occlusion should be evaluated periodically for evidence of HPA axis suppression. This may be done by using the ACTH stimulation, A.M. plasma cortisol or urinary free cortisol tests.
If HPA axis suppression is noted, an attempt should be made to withdraw the drug, to reduce the frequency of application, or to substitute a less potent steroid. Recovery of HPA axis function is generally prompt and complete upon discontinuation of the drug. Infrequently, signs and symptoms of steroid withdrawal may occur, requiring supplemental systemic corticosteroids. For information on systemic supplementation, see prescribing information for those products.
Pediatric patients may be more susceptible to systemic toxicity from equivalent doses due to their larger skin surface to body mass ratios. (See **PRECAUTIONS Pediatric Use**).
If irritation develops, PANDEL Cream should be discontinued and appropriate therapy instituted. Allergic contact dermatitis with corticosteroids is usually diagnosed by observing a failure to heal rather than noting a clinical exacerbation, as observed with most topical products not containing corticosteroids. If concomitant skin infections are present or develop, an appropriate antifungal or antibacterial agent should be used. If a favorable response does not occur promptly, use of PANDEL Cream should be discontinued until the infection has been adequately controlled.
Information for Patients: Patients using PANDEL Cream should receive the following information and instructions:
1. This medication is to be used as directed by the physician. It is for external use only. Avoid contact with the eyes.
2. This medication should not be used for any disorder other than that for which it was prescribed.
3. The treated skin area should not be bandaged or otherwise covered or wrapped so as to be occlusive, unless directed by the physician.
4. Patients should report to their physician any signs of local adverse reactions.
5. Parents of pediatric patients should be advised not to use PANDEL Cream in the treatment of diaper dermatitis. PANDEL Cream should not be applied in the diaper area as diapers or plastic pants may constitute occlusive dressings (See **DOSAGE AND ADMINISTRATION**).
6. This medication should not be used on the face, underarms, or groin areas unless directed by the physician.
7. As with other corticosteroids, therapy should be discontinued when control is achieved. If no improvement is seen within two weeks, contact the physician.

Laboratory Tests: The following tests may be helpful in evaluating if HPA axis suppression does occur:
ACTH stimulation test
A.M. plasma cortisol test
Urinary free cortisol test
Carcinogenesis, Mutagenesis and Impairment of Fertility: Long-term animal studies have not been performed to evaluated the carcinogenic potential or the effect on fertility of topical corticosteroids.
Studies to determine mutagenicity with prednisolone and hydrocortisone have revealed negative results.
Pregnancy: Teratogenic Effects—*Pregnancy Category C.* Corticosteroids are generally teratogenic in laboratory animals when administered systemically at relatively low dosage levels. Some corticosteroids have been shown to be teratogenic after dermal application in laboratory animals.
Hydrocortisone buteprate has not been tested for teratogenicity when applied topically; however, it is absorbed percutaneously, and studies in Wistar rats using the subcutaneous route resulted in teratogenicity at dose levels greater than 1 mg/kg. Abnormalities seen included delayed ossification of the caudal vertebrae and other skeletal variations, cleft palate, umbilical hernia, edema and exencephalia. In rabbits, hydrocortisone buteprate given by the subcutaneous route was teratogenic at doses greater than 0.1 mg/kg. Abnormalities seen included delayed ossification of the caudal vertebrae and other skeletal abnormalities, cleft palate and increased fetal mortality.
There are no adequate and well-controlled studies in pregnant women on teratogenic effects from topically applied corticosteroids. Therefore, PANDEL Cream should be used during pregnancy only if the potential benefit justifies the potential risk to the fetus.
Nursing Mothers: Systemically administered corticosteroids appear in human milk and could suppress growth, interfere with endogenous corticosteroid production, or cause other untoward effects. It is not known whether topical administration of corticosteroids could result in sufficient systemic absorption to produce detectable quantities in human milk. Because many drugs are excreted in human milk, caution should be exercised when PANDEL Cream is administered to a nursing woman.
Pediatric Use: Safety and effectiveness in pediatric patients have not been established. Because of a higher ratio of skin surface area to body mass, pediatric patients are at a greater risk than adults of HPA axis suppression and Cushing's syndrome when they are treated with topical corticosteroids. They are therefore also at a greater risk of adrenal insufficiency during and/or after withdrawal of treatment. Adverse effects including striae have been reported with inappropriate use of topical corticosteroids in infants and children.
Hypothalamic-pituitary-adrenal (HPA) axis suppression, Cushing's syndrome, linear growth retardation, delayed weight gain, and intracranial hypertension have been reported in children receiving topical corticosteroids. Manifestations of adrenal suppression in children include low plasma cortisol levels and an absence of response to ACTH stimulation. Manifestations of intracranial hypertension include bulging fontanelles, headaches, and bilateral papilledema.

ADVERSE REACTIONS
The most frequent adverse reactions reported for PANDEL Cream have included burning in 4, stinging in 2, and moderate paresthesia in 1 out of 226 patients.
The following local adverse reactions are reported with topical corticosteroids, and they may occur more frequently with the use of occlusive dressings. These reactions are listed in an approximate decreasing order of occurrence: burning,

Continued on next page

Savage Laboratories—Cont.

itching, irritation, dryness, folliculitis, hypertrichosis, acneiform eruptions, hypopigmentation, perioral dermatitis, allergic contact dermatitis, secondary infections, skin atrophy, striae, miliaria.

OVERDOSAGE

Topically applied corticosteroids can be absorbed in sufficient amounts to produce systemic effects. (See PRECAUTIONS.)

DOSAGE AND ADMINISTRATION

Apply a thin film of PANDEL Cream to the affected area once or twice a day depending on the severity of the condition. Massage gently until the medication disappears.

Occlusive dressings may be used for the management of refractory lesions of psoriasis and other deep-seated dermatoses, such as localized neurodermatitis (lichen simplex chronicus).

As with other corticosteroids, therapy should be discontinued when control is achieved. If no improvement is seen within 2 weeks, reassessment of the diagnosis may be necessary.

PANDEL Cream should not be used with occlusive dressings unless directed by the physician. PANDEL Cream should not be applied in the diaper area if the child still requires diapers or plastic pants as these garments may constitute occlusive dressing.

HOW SUPPLIED

PANDEL (hydrocortisone buteprate) Cream, 0.1%, a white to off-white opaque cream is supplied as follows:
15 g tubes (NDC 0281-0153-15)
45 g tubes (NDC 0281-0153-46)
Store at controlled room temperature 15°–30°C (59°–86°F).
CAUTION: Federal law prohibits dispensing without prescription.

SAVAGE LABORATORIES®
a division of Altana Inc.
MELVILLE, NEW YORK 11747   REV 8/96
Shown in Product Identification Guide, page 333

TYMPAGESIC® OTIC SOLUTION   ℞
(Analgesic-Decongestant Ear Drops)

DESCRIPTION

TYMPAGESIC® Otic Solution, analgesic-decongestant ear drops, contains phenylephrine hydrochloride USP 0.25%, antipyrine USP 5% and benzocaine USP 5% w/v in propylene glycol USP.

Phenylephrine hydrochloride is a sympathomimetic amine with local vasoconstriction or decongestant action. It is chemically (R)-3-hydroxy-α[(methylamino)methyl] benzenemethanol hydrochloride and has the following structure:

$C_9H_{13}NO_2HCl$ M.W. 203.67

It occurs as white crystals, has bitter taste and is freely soluble in water and alcohol.

Antipyrine is an analgesic with local anesthetic action. It is chemically 2:3-dimethyl-1-phenyl-3-pyrazolin-5-one and has the following structure:

$C_{11}H_{12}N_2O$ M.W. 188.23

Antipyrine occurs as colorless crystals or white powder, has a slightly bitter taste and is soluble in water and alcohol.
Benzocaine is a local anesthetic. It is chemically ethyl p-aminobenzoate and has the following structure:

$C_9H_{11}NO_2$ M.W. 165.19

It occurs as white crystals or white crystalline powder and is slightly soluble in water and soluble in organic solvents.

CLINICAL PHARMACOLOGY

Topical application of phenylephrine produces vasoconstriction mainly by a direct effect on α-adrenergic receptors. The effects of phenylephrine are similar to those of epinephrine. However, phenylephrine is considered less CNS and cardiostimulatory than epinephrine. Phenylephrine, after its absorption, is metabolized in the liver and the intestine by the enzyme monoamine oxidase (MAO). The type, route and rate of excretion of metabolites have not been defined.

Like other local anesthetics, benzocaine acts by blocking nerve conduction first in autonomic, then in sensory and finally in motor nerve fibers. Its effect appears to be due to decreased nerve cell membrane permeability to sodium ions or competition with calcium ions for membrane binding sites. A vasoconstrictor, such as phenylephrine, is added to decrease the rate of absorption and prolong the duration of action of the anesthetic. Ester-type anesthetics, which include benzocaine, after absorption are comparatively rapidly degraded by esterases mainly in the liver and excreted in the urine as metabolites and in small amounts as the unchanged drug.

Antipyrine is believed to have analgesic and local anesthetic effects on the nerve endings. After absorption, it is slowly metabolized in the liver by oxidation and conjugation with glucuronic acid and is excreted in the urine mainly in the conjugated form.

INDICATIONS AND USAGE

TYMPAGESIC® Otic Solution may be used as a topical anesthetic in the external auditory canal to relieve ear pain. It may be used concomitantly with systemic antibiotics as in the treatment of acute otitis media.

CONTRAINDICATIONS

TYMPAGESIC® or any medication for use in the external ear canal is contraindicated in the presence of a perforated tympanic membrane or ear discharge and in individuals with a history of hypersensitivity to any of its ingredients.

WARNINGS

As with all drugs containing a sympathomimetic or an anesthetic, systemic reactions may occur after local application. Phenylephrine may cause blanching and feeling of coolness in the skin. Allergic and idiosyncratic reactions to local anesthetics have been observed infrequently. Such reactions are unlikely because absorption from the skin of the ear drum or the external ear canal is minimal.

Discontinue promptly if sensitization or irritation occurs. Cross-sensitivity reactions between members of the *caine* group of local anesthetics have been reported.

Contains *sodium metabisulfite*, a sulfite that may cause allergic-type reactions including anaphylactic symptoms and life-threatening or less severe asthmatic episodes in certain susceptible people. The overall prevalence of sulfite sensitivity in the general population is unknown and probably low. Sulfite sensitivity is seen more frequently in asthmatic than nonasthmatic people.

PRECAUTIONS

General—Drugs containing a sympathomimetic should be used with caution in the elderly and in patients with hypertension, increased intraocular pressure, diabetes mellitus, ischemic heart disease, hyperthyroidism and prostatic hypertrophy. High plasma levels of benzocaine and antipyrine may cause CNS stimulation with nausea and vomiting. Such levels, however, are unlikely to be attained following local application in the external ear.

Drug Interactions—MAO inhibitors and β-adrenergic blockers enhance the effects of sympathomimetics. Benzocaine is hydrolyzed in the body to p-aminobenzoic acid which competes with the antibacterial action of sulfonamides. However, these are unlikely to occur because of limited absorption from the external ear canal.

Carcinogenesis, Mutagenesis, Impairment of Fertility—There have been no studies in animals or humans to evaluate the carcinogenesis, mutagenesis or impairment of fertility for TYMPAGESIC.®

Pregnancy—Category C. Animal reproduction studies have not been conducted with TYMPAGESIC. It is also not known whether TYMPAGESIC can cause fetal harm when administered to a pregnant woman or can effect reproduction capacity. TYMPAGESIC should be given to a pregnant woman only if clearly needed.

Nursing Mothers—It is not known whether this drug is excreted in human milk. Because many drugs are excreted in human milk, caution should be exercised when TYMPAGESIC is administered to a nursing woman.

Pediatric Use—Safety and effectiveness in children below the age of 12 has not been established.

ADVERSE REACTIONS

Following its absorption, phenylephrine may produce a pressor response or cause restlessness, anxiety, nervousness, weakness, pallor, headache and dizziness. Absorption of benzocaine and antipyrine in the plasma may cause chills, nausea, vomiting, tinnitus and agranulocytosis. Such reactions

are unlikely following application of TYMPAGESIC on the external ear canal.

Benzocaine can cause a hypersensitivity reaction consisting of rash, urticaria and edema. Individuals frequently exposed to ester-type local anesthetics can develop contact dermatitis characterized by erythema and pruritus which may progress to vesiculation and oozing.

OVERDOSAGE

It is more likely to be associated with accidental or deliberate ingestion rather than cutaneous absorption. Phenylephrine present in a bottle (13 mL) of TYMPAGESIC, if absorbed, may cause hyperextension, headache, vomiting and palpitations. Effects of benzocaine overdosage may include yawning, restlessness, excitement, nausea and vomiting. Antipyrine overdosage may cause giddiness, tremor, sweating, and skin eruptions.

Treatment is symptomatic. If ingestion of the contents of a bottle or more of TYMPAGESIC is recent or food is present in the stomach, induction of emesis with ipecac syrup, gastric emptying and lavage and introduction of activated charcoal may be recommended.

DOSAGE AND ADMINISTRATION

Using the dropper, instill TYMPAGESIC Otic Solution in the external ear canal allowing the solution to run into the canal until filled. Insert a cotton pledget into the meatus after moistening with otic solution. Repeat every 2 to 4 hours if necessary, until pain is relieved.
Replace dropper in bottle without rinsing.

HOW SUPPLIED

TYMPAGESIC Otic Solution is supplied in 13 mL amber glass dropper bottles (NDC 0281-7363-39).
Store at 15°–30°C (59°–86°F).
Shown in Product Identification Guide, page 333

Scandipharm, Inc.
22 INVERNESS CENTER PARKWAY
BIRMINGHAM, AL 35242

Direct Inquiries to:
Dale Brakhage, Director of Marketing
(205) 991-8085
FAX: (205) 991-9547
For Medical Emergencies Contact:
John R. Booth, R.Ph.
(205) 991-8085
FAX: (205) 991-9547

ULTRASE®   ℞
[*ul'trāce*]
(pancrelipase) Capsules
Enteric-Coated Microspheres

Prescribing Information

DESCRIPTION

ULTRASE® (pancrelipase) Capsules are orally administered capsules containing enteric-coated microspheres of porcine pancreatic enzyme concentrate, predominantly pancreatic lipase, amylase, and protease.
Each ULTRASE ® capsule contains:

Lipase	4,500 U.S.P. Units
Amylase	20,000 U.S.P. Units
Protease	25,000 U.S.P. Units

Inactive ingredients: povidone, talc, sugar, methacrylic acid copolymer (Type C), triethyl citrate, simethicone emulsion.

CLINICAL PHARMACOLOGY

ULTRASE® (pancrelipase) Capsules are designed to prevent inactivation by gastric acid thereby resulting in the delivery of high levels of biologically active enzymes into the duodenum. The enzymes catalyze the hydrolysis of fats into glycerol and fatty acids, starch into dextrins and sugars, and protein into proteoses and derived substances.

INDICATIONS AND USAGE

ULTRASE® (pancrelipase) Capsules are indicated for patients with partial or complete exocrine pancreatic insufficiency caused by:
● Cystic fibrosis
● Chronic pancreatitis due to alcohol use or other causes
● Surgery (pancreatico-duodenectomy or Whipple's procedure, with or without Wirsung duct injection, total pancreatectomy)
● Obstruction (pancreatic and biliary duct lithiasis, pancreatic and duodenal neoplasms, ductal stenosis)
● Other pancreatic disease (hereditary, post traumatic and allograft pancreatitis, hemochromatosis, Schwachman's Syndrome, lipomatosis, hyperparathyroidism)

- Poor mixing (Billroth II gastrectomy, other types of gastric bypass surgery, gastrinoma)

Pancrelipase capsules are effective in controlling steatorrhea.[1-9]

CONTRAINDICATIONS

Pancrelipase capsules are contraindicated in patients known to be hypersensitive to pork protein. Pancrelipase capsules are contraindicated in patients with acute pancreatitis or with acute exacerbations of chronic pancreatic diseases.

WARNINGS

Should hypersensitivity occur, discontinue medication and treat symptomatically.

PRECAUTIONS

General

TO PROTECT ENTERIC COATING, MICROSPHERES MUST NOT BE CRUSHED OR CHEWED. Where swallowing of capsules is difficult, they may be opened and the microspheres added to a small quantity of a soft food (e.g. applesauce, gelatin, etc.) that does not require chewing, and swallowed immediately. Contact of the microsphere with foods having a pH greater than 5.5 can dissolve the protective enteric shell.

Carcinogenesis, Mutagenesis, Impairment of Fertility

Long-term studies in animals have not been performed to evaluate carcinogenic potential. Methacrylic acid, a minor component of the methacrylic acid copolymer enteric-coating contained in ULTRASE® (pancrelipase) Capsules, has been reported to act as a teratogen in rat embryo cultures. However, the copolymer enteric-coating of ULTRASE® (pancrelipase) Capsules was not mutagenic by the Ames test, and it did not produce chromosome damage in a test for unscheduled DNA synthesis in rat hepatocytes.

Pregnancy: Category C.

Animal reproduction studies have not been conducted with ULTRASE® (pancrelipase) Capsules. It is not known whether ULTRASE® (pancrelipase) Capsules can cause fetal harm when administered to a pregnant woman or can affect reproduction capacity. ULTRASE® (pancrelipase) Capsules should be given to a pregnant woman only if the potential benefit outweighs the potential risk to the fetus.

Nursing Mothers

It is not known whether ULTRASE® (pancrelipase) is excreted in human milk. Because many drugs are excreted in human milk, caution should be exercised when ULTRASE® (pancrelipase) Capsules are administered to a nursing mother.

ADVERSE REACTIONS

The most frequently reported adverse reactions to products containing pancrelipase are gastrointestinal in nature. Less frequently, allergic-type reactions have also been observed. Extremely high doses of exogenous pancreatic enzymes have been associated with hyperuricosuria and hyperuricemia when the preparations given were pancrelipase in powdered or capsule form, or pancreatin in tablet form.

Colonic strictures have been reported in cystic fibrosis patients treated with both high- and lower-strength enzyme supplements.[10] A causal relationship has not been established. The possibility of bowel stricture should be considered if symptoms suggestive of gastrointestinal obstruction occur. Since impaired fluid secretion may be a factor in the development of intestinal obstruction, care should be taken to maintain adequate hydration, particularly in warm weather.[11]

"Fibrosing colonopathy" is a term used to describe a condition seen in patients with CF who have taken high amounts of pancreatic enzyme supplements (>6,000 lipase U/kg/meal). At its most advanced, this condition leads to colonic strictures.

1. In whom should one consider the diagnosis of fibrosing colonopathy?
a. Patients with cystic fibrosis who have evidence of partial or complete obstruction, bloody diarrhea or chylous ascites.
b. Patients who have two of the following three symptoms:
  abdominal pain
  ongoing diarrhea
  poor weight gain
  ESPECIALLY if they have:
  taken >6,000 lipase U/kg/meal
  age less than twelve years
  history of meconium ileus
  prior intestinal surgery
  history of recurrent DIOS
  "inflammatory bowel disease"[12]

DOSAGE AND ADMINISTRATION

The enzymatic activity of ULTRASE® (pancrelipase) Capsules is expressed in U.S.P. units. The smallest effective dose should be used. Dosage should be adjusted according to the severity of the exocrine pancreatic insufficiency. Begin therapy with one or two capsules with meals or snacks and adjust dosage according to symptoms.

The number of capsules or capsule strength given with meals and/or snacks should be estimated by assessing which dose

---

minimizes steatorrhea and maintains good nutritional status. Dosages should be adjusted according to the response of the patient. Where swallowing of capsules is difficult, they may be opened and the microspheres added to a small quantity of a soft food (e.g. applesauce, gelatin, etc.) that does not require chewing, and swallowed immediately.

It is recommended that the total dose of pancrelipase being ingested for a meal or snack be dispersed equally (with fluids) before, during, and after the meal or snack.

SUGGESTION FOR THE USE OF PANCREATIC ENZYMES IN CYSTIC FIBROSIS [12]

1. Patients should be receiving optimal diet for age and clinical status, recognizing that those with failure to thrive or malnutrition require additional calories and other nutrients for catch-up growth.
2. Nutrition assessment should be a part of routine clinical evaluations.
3. Initial dosing of pancreatic enzyme supplements should begin with 500 lipase U/kg/meal using enteric-coated microcapsule products.
4. Patients should be reassessed 2–4 weeks after initiation of therapy. The following items should be assessed:
  Clinical status, e.g. abdominal symptoms and exam
  Nutritional intake and growth (height, weight, head circumference)
  Character of stools—greasy, oily (for information, not for decision making)
  Quantitative 72-hr fecal fat when indicated (perform on a normal diet for age)
  Fat soluble vitamin measures.
5. Corollaries to dosing suggestions:
  a. Dose may be increased in a stepwise fashion.
  b. Dose approaching 2,000 lipase U/kg/meal would indicate the need for further investigation (see below). Patients presently on higher doses should be reevaluated; either immediately decrease the dose or titrate down to a lower dose range at, or below, 2,000 lipase U/kg/meal. Doses >6,000 lipase U/kg/meal have been associated with colonic strictures.
  c. Pancreatic supplements mixed with applesauce or other acidic food substances should be administered immediately, not stored.
  d. Enteric-coated microcapsules should not be crushed.
  e. Enzyme doses (as lipase U/kg/meal) tend to decrease with advancing age.
  f. Patients should accept only product brands prescribed by CF Center staff.
  g. Adjustment of dosage is the responsibility of the CF Center staff. Patients should be advised not to adjust doses without consulting the CF Center staff. Changes in product may require an adjustment period.
  h. Complaints transmitted by phone should be investigated before dose is adjusted.
  i. Pancreatic supplements should be stored in a cool dry place and checked regularly for expiration date.

HOW SUPPLIED

ULTRASE ® (pancrelipase) Capsules

Gelatin capsules (opaque white and opaque white), imprinted ULTRASE MS4. Bottles of 50 (NDC 58914-045-05), bottles of 100 (NDC 58914-045-10), bottles of 250 (NDC 58914-045-25), and bottles of 500 (NDC 58914-045-50).

Store at controlled room temperature, between 15°C and 30°C (59°F and 86°F), in a dry place. Do not refrigerate.

REFERENCES

1. Delchier JC, Vidon N. *et al.* Fate of orally ingested enzymes in pancreatic insufficiency: comparison of two pancreatic enzyme preparations. *Aliment Pharmacol Therap.* 1991;5:365-378.
2. Duhamel JP, Vidailhet M, *et al.* Étude multicentrique comparative d'une nouvelle présentation de pancréatine en microgranules gastrorésistants dans l'insuffisance pancréatique exocrine de la mucoviscidose chez l'enfant. *Ann Pediatr.* 1988;35:69-74.
3. Dutta SK, Tilley DK. The pH-sensitive enteric-coated pancreatic enzyme preparations: an evaluation of therapeutic efficacy in adult patients with pancreatic insufficiency. *J Clin Gastroenterol.* 1983;5:51-54.
4. Dutta SK, Rubin J. Harvey J. Comparative evaluation of the therapeutic efficacy of a pH-sensitive enteric-coated pancreatic enzyme preparation with conventional pancreatic enzyme therapy in the treatment of exocrine pancreatic insufficiency. *Gastroenterol.* 1983;84:476-482.
5. Gouerou H, Dain MP, *et al.* Alipase versus nonenteric-coated enzymes in pancreatic insufficiency. *Int J Pancreatol.* 1989;5:45-50.
6. Mischler EH, Parrell S, *et al.* Comparison of effectiveness of pancreatic enzyme preparations in cystic fibrosis. *Am J Dis Child.* 1982;136:1060-1063.
7. Salen G, Prakash A. Evaluation of enteric-coated microspheres for enzyme replacement therapy in adults with pancreatic insufficiency. *Cur Ther Res.* 1979;25:650-656.
8. Schneider MU, Knoll-Ruzicka ML, *et al.* Pancreatic enzyme replacement therapy: comparative effects of conventional and enteric-coated microspheric pancreatin

---

and acid-stable fungal enzyme preparations on steatorrhea in chronic pancreatitis. *Hepato-gastroenterol.* 1985;32:97-102.
9. Halgreen H, Thorsgaard Pedersen N, Worning H. Symptomatic effect of pancreatic enzyme therapy in patients with chronic pancreatitis. *Scand J Gastroenterol.* 1986;21:104-108.
10. Smyth RL, van Velzen D, *et al.* Strictures of ascending colon in cystic fibrosis and high-strength pancreatic enzymes. *The Lancet.* 1994;343:85-86.
11. Lands L, Zinman R, *et al.* Pancreatic function testing in meconium disease in CF: two case reports. *J Ped Gastroenterol and Nut.* 1988;7:276-279.
12. Cystic Fibrosis Foundation Conference on Pancreatic Enzyme Supplementation in the Context of Fibrosing Colonopathy; Washington, D.C., March 23-24, 1995.

Manufactured by:
Eurand International
Milan, Italy
Marketed by:
Scandipharm, Inc.
22 Inverness Center Parkway
Birmingham, AL 35242
U.S.A.

CAUTION
Federal Law prohibits dispensing without a prescription.
Rev.4/95.
ULTRASE® is a registered trademark of Scandipharm, Inc.

Shown in Product Identification Guide, page 333

ULTRASE® MT ℞
[ul'trāce]
(pancrelipase) Capsules
Enteric-Coated Minitablets

Prescribing Information

DESCRIPTION

ULTRASE® MT (pancrelipase) Capsules are orally administered capsules containing enteric-coated minitablets of porcine pancreatic enzyme concentrate, predominantly pancreatic lipase, amylase, and protease.

Each ULTRASE ® MT12 Capsule contains:

Lipase	12,000 U.S.P. Units
Amylase	39,000 U.S.P. Units
Protease	39,000 U.S.P. Units

Each ULTRASE ® MT18 Capsule contains:

Lipase	18,000 U.S.P. Units
Amylase	58,500 U.S.P. Units
Protease	58,500 U.S.P. Units

Each ULTRASE ® MT20 Capsule contains:

Lipase	20,000 U.S.P. Units
Amylase	65,000 U.S.P. Units
Protease	65,000 U.S.P. Units

ULTRASE® MT (pancrelipase) Capsules contain an amount of pancrelipase equivalent to but not more than 125% of the labeled lipase activity expressed in U.S.P. Units.

Inactive ingredients: hydrogenated castor oil, silicon dioxide, sodium carboxymethylcellulose, magnesium stearate, microcrystalline cellulose, methacrylic acid copolymer (Type C), talc, simethicone, triethylcitrate, iron oxides and titanium oxide.

CLINICAL PHARMACOLOGY

ULTRASE® MT (pancrelipase) Capsules are designed to prevent inactivation by gastric acid thereby resulting in the delivery of high levels of biologically active enzymes into the duodenum. The enzymes catalyze the hydrolysis of fats into glycerol and fatty acids, starch into dextrins and sugars, and protein into proteoses and derived substances.

INDICATIONS AND USAGE

ULTRASE® MT (pancrelipase) Capsules are indicated for patients with partial or complete exocrine pancreatic insufficiency caused by:

- Cystic fibrosis
- Chronic pancreatitis due to alcohol use or other causes
- Surgery (pancreatico-duodenectomy or Whipple's procedure, with or without Wirsung duct injection, total pancreatectomy)
- Obstruction (pancreatic and biliary duct lithiasis, pancreatic and duodenal neoplasms, ductal stenosis)
- Other pancreatic disease (hereditary, post traumatic and allograft pancreatitis, hemochromatosis, Schwachman's Syndrome, lipomatosis, hyperparathyroidism)
- Poor mixing (Billroth II gastrectomy, other types of gastric bypass surgery, gastrinoma)

Pancrelipase capsules are effective in controlling steatorrhea.[1-9]

CONTRAINDICATIONS

Pancrelipase capsules are contraindicated in patients known to be hypersensitive to pork protein. Pancrelipase capsules

Continued on next page

Scandipharm—Cont.

are contraindicated in patients with acute pancreatitis or with acute exacerbations of chronic pancreatic diseases.

WARNINGS

Should hypersensitivity occur, discontinue medication and treat symptomatically.

PRECAUTIONS

General
TO PROTECT ENTERIC COATING, MINITABLETS MUST NOT BE CRUSHED OR CHEWED. Where swallowing of capsules is difficult, they may be opened and the minitablets added to a small quantity of a soft food (e.g. applesauce, gelatin, etc.) that does not require chewing, and swallowed immediately. Contact of the minitablet with foods having a pH greater than 5.5 can dissolve the protective enteric shell.
Carcinogenesis, Mutagenesis, Impairment of Fertility
Long-term studies in animals have not been performed to evaluate carcinogenic potential. Methacrylic acid, a minor component of the methacrylic acid copolymer enteric-coating contained in ULTRASE® MT (pancrelipase) Capsules, has been reported to act as a teratogen in rat embryo cultures. However, ULTRASE® MT (pancrelipase) Capsules have been shown to contain <0.001% of methacrylic acid, and the mammalian teratology studies in the rat and rabbit were negative.
The copolymer enteric-coating of ULTRASE® MT (pancrelipase) Capsules was not mutagenic by the Ames test, and it did not produce chromosome damage in a test for unscheduled DNA synthesis in rat hepatocytes.
Pregnancy: Category C.
Animal reproduction studies have not been conducted with ULTRASE® MT (pancrelipase) Capsules. It is not known whether ULTRASE® MT (pancrelipase) Capsules can cause fetal harm when administered to a pregnant woman or can affect reproduction capacity. ULTRASE® MT (pancrelipase) Capsules should be given to a pregnant woman only if the potential benefit outweighs the potential risk to the fetus.
Nursing Mothers
It is not known whether ULTRASE® MT (pancrelipase) is excreted in human milk. Because many drugs are excreted in human milk, caution should be exercised when ULTRASE® MT (pancrelipase) Capsules are administered to a nursing mother.

ADVERSE REACTIONS

The most frequently reported adverse reactions to pancrelipase-containing products are gastrointestinal in nature. Less frequently, allergic-type reactions have also been observed. Extremely high doses of exogenous pancreatic enzymes have been associated with hyperuricosuria and hyperuricemia when the preparations given were pancrelipase in powdered or capsule form, or pancreatin in tablet form.
In two clinical studies with ULTRASE® MT in 193 patients with cystic fibrosis, the adverse events described were all gastrointestinal in nature and may actually represent symptoms of the underlying disease, such as abdominal pain/cramps (5.7%), diarrhea (3.6%), and greasy stools and flatulence (1.5% each). In a postmarketing trial with another enteric-coated formulation, 160 adverse events occurred in the 15,711 patients (0.97%) evaluated.[10] The most frequent events reported were diarrhea, skin reaction, and abdominal discomfort (0.2% each).
Colonic strictures have been reported in cystic fibrosis patients treated with both high- and lower-strength enzyme supplements.[11] A causal relationship has not been established. The possibility of bowel stricture should be considered if symptoms suggestive of gastrointestinal obstruction occur. Since impaired fluid secretion may be a factor in the development of intestinal obstruction, care should be taken to maintain adequate hydration, particularly in warm weather.[12]
"Fibrosing colonopathy" is a term used to describe a condition seen in patients with CF who have taken high amounts of pancreatic enzyme supplements (>6,000 lipase U/kg/meal). At its most advanced, this condition leads to colonic strictures.
1. In whom should one consider the diagnosis of fibrosing colonopathy?
a. Patients with cystic fibrosis who have evidence of partial or complete obstruction, bloody diarrhea or chylous ascites.
b. Patients who have two of the following three symptoms:
  abdominal pain
  ongoing diarrhea
  poor weight gain
  ESPECIALLY if they have:
  taken >6,000 lipase U/kg/meal
  age less than twelve years
  history of meconium ileus
  prior intestinal surgery
  history of recurrent DIOS
  "inflammatory bowel disease"[13]

DOSAGE AND ADMINISTRATION

The enzymatic activity of ULTRASE® MT (pancrelipase) Capsules is expressed in U.S.P. units. Each capsule contains the labeled amount of lipase activity and an overage of not more than 25%.
The smallest effective dose should be used. Dosage should be adjusted according to the severity of the exocrine pancreatic insufficiency. Begin therapy with one or two capsules with meals or snacks and adjust dosage according to symptoms. The number of capsules or capsule strength given with meals and/or snacks should be estimated by assessing which dose minimizes steatorrhea and maintains good nutritional status. Dosages should be adjusted according to the response of the patient. Where swallowing of capsules is difficult, they may be opened and the minitablets added to a small quantity of a soft food (e.g. applesauce, gelatin, etc.) that does not require chewing, and swallowed immediately.
It is recommended that the total dose of pancrelipase being ingested for a meal or snack be dispersed equally (with fluids) before, during, and after the meal or snack.
SUGGESTIONS FOR THE USE OF PANCREATIC ENZYMES IN CYSTIC FIBROSIS[13]
1. Patients should be receiving optimal diet for age and clinical status, recognizing that those with failure to thrive or malnutrition require additional calories and other nutrients for catch-up growth.
2. Nutrition assessment should be a part of routine clinical evaluations.
3. Initial dosing of pancreatic enzyme supplements should begin with 500 lipase U/kg/meal using enteric-coated microcapsule products.
4. Patients should be reassessed 2–4 weeks after initiation of therapy.
  The following items should be assessed:
  Clinical status, e.g. abdominal symptoms and exam
  Nutritional intake and growth (height, weight, head circumference)
  Character of stools—greasy, oily (for information, not for decision making)
  Quantitative 72-hr fecal fat when indicated (perform on a normal diet for age)
  Fat soluble vitamin measures.
5. Corollaries to dosing suggestions:
  a. Dose may be increased in a stepwise fashion.
  b. Dose approaching 2,000 lipase U/kg/meal would indicate the need for further investigation (see below). Patients presently on higher doses should be reevaluated; either immediately decrease the dose or titrate down to a lower dose range at, or below, 2,000 lipase U/kg/meal. Doses >6,000 lipase U/kg/meal have been associated with colonic strictures.
  c. Pancreatic supplements mixed with applesauce or other acidic food substances should be administered immediately, not stored.
  d. Enteric-coated microcapsules should not be crushed.
  e. Enzyme doses (as lipase U/kg/meal) tend to decrease with advancing age.
  f. Patient should accept only product brands prescribed by CF Center staff.
  g. Adjustment of dosage is the responsibility of the CF Center staff. Patients should be advised not to adjust doses without consulting the CF Center staff. Changes in product may require an adjustment period.
  h. Complaints transmitted by phone should be investigated before dose is adjusted.
  i. Pancreatic supplements should be stored in a cool dry place and checked regularly for expiration date.

HOW SUPPLIED

ULTRASE® MT12 (pancrelipase) Capsules
Gelatin capsules (white and yellow), imprinted ULTRASE MT12. Bottles of 50 (NDC 58914-002-05), bottles of 100 (NDC 58914-002-10), and bottles of 500 (NDC 58914-002-50).

ULTRASE® MT18 (pancrelipase) Capsules
Gelatin capsules (gray and white), imprinted ULTRASE MT18. Bottles of 50 (NDC 58914-018-05), bottles of 100 (NDC 58914-018-10), and bottles of 500 (NDC 58914-018-50).
ULTRASE® MT20 (pancrelipase) Capsules
Gelatin capsules (light gray and yellow), imprinted ULTRASE MT20. Bottles of 50 (NDC 58914-004-05), bottles of 100 (NDC 58914-004-10), and bottles of 500 (NDC 58914-004-50).
Store at controlled room temperature, between 15°C and 30°C (59°F and 86°F), in a dry place. Do not refrigerate.

REFERENCES

1. Delchier JC, Vidon N, *et al.* Fate of orally ingested enzymes in pancreatic insufficiency: comparison of two pancreatic enzyme preparations. *Aliment Pharmacol Therap.* 1991;5:365–378.
2. Duhamel JP, Vidailhet M, *et al.* Étude multicentrique comparative d'une nouvelle présentation de pancréatine en microgranules gastrorésistants dans l'insuffisance pancréatique exocrine de la mucoviscidose chez l'enfant. *Ann Pediatr.* 1988;35:69–74.
3. Dutta SK, Tilley DK. The pH-sensitive enteric-coated pancreatic enzyme preparations: an evaluation of therapeutic efficacy in adult patients with pancreatic insufficiency. *J Clin Gastroenterol.* 1983;5:51–54.
4. Dutta SK, Rubin J, Harvey J. Comparative evaluation of the therapeutic efficacy of a pH-sensitive enteric-coated pancreatic enzyme preparation with conventional pancreatic enzyme therapy in the treatment of exocrine pancreatic insufficiency. *Gastroenterol.* 1983;84:476–482.
5. Gouerou H, Dain MP, *et al.* Alipase versus nonenteric-coated enzymes in pancreatic insufficiency. *Int J Pancreatol.* 1989;5:45–50.
6. Mischler EH, Parrell S, *et al.* Comparison of effectiveness of pancreatic enzyme preparations in cystic fibrosis. *Am J Dis Child.* 1982;136:1060–1063.
7. Salen G, Prakash A. Evaluation of enteric-coated microspheres for enzyme replacement therapy in adults with pancreatic insufficiency. *Cur Ther Res.* 1979;25:650–656.
8. Schneider MU, Knoll-Ruzicka ML, *et al.* Pancreatic enzyme replacement therapy: comparative effects of conventional and enteric-coated microspheric pancreatin and acid-stable fungal enzyme preparations on steatorrhea in chronic pancreatitis. *Hepato-gastroenterol.* 1985;32:97–102.
9. Halgreen H, Thorsgaard Pedersen N, Worning H. Symptomatic effect of pancreatic enzyme therapy in patients with chronic pancreatitis. *Scand J Gastroenterol.* 1986;21:104–108.
10. Gretzmacher I, Rüther HG. Maldigestion. *Therapiewoche.* 1983;33:6776–6782.
11. Smyth RL, van Velzen D, *et al.* Strictures of ascending colon in cystic fibrosis and high-strength pancreatic enzymes. *The Lancet.* 1994;343:85–86.
12. Lands L, Zinman R, *et al.* Pancreatic function testing in meconium disease in CF: two case reports. *J Ped Gastroenterol and Nut.* 1988;7:276–279.
13. Cystic Fibrosis Foundation Conference on Pancreatic Enzyme Supplementation in the Context of Fibrosing Colonopathy; Washington, D.C., March 23–24, 1995.

Manufactured by:
Eurand International
Milan, Italy
Marketed by:
Scandipharm, Inc.
22 Inverness Center Parkway
Birmingham, AL 35242
U.S.A.

CAUTION

Federal Law prohibits dispensing without a prescription.
Rev. 5/96.
ULTRASE® is a registered trademark of Scandipharm, Inc.
Shown in Product Identification Guide, page 334

Schein Pharmaceutical, Inc.
100 CAMPUS DRIVE
FLORHAM PARK, NJ 07932

Direct Inquiries to:
Customer Service
(800) 356-5790
FAX: 201-593-5945

For Medical Information Contact:
(800) 548-6236 (24 Hours)

INFeD®   ℞
(IRON DEXTRAN INJECTION, USP)

> **WARNING**
> THE PARENTERAL USE OF COMPLEXES OF IRON AND CARBOHYDRATES HAS RESULTED IN ANAPHYLACTIC-TYPE REACTIONS. DEATHS ASSOCIATED WITH SUCH ADMINISTRATION HAVE BEEN REPORTED. THEREFORE, INFeD SHOULD BE USED ONLY IN THOSE PATIENTS IN WHOM THE INDICATIONS HAVE BEEN CLEARLY ESTABLISHED AND LABORATORY INVESTIGATIONS CONFIRM AN IRON DEFICIENT STATE NOT AMENABLE TO ORAL IRON THERAPY.

DESCRIPTION

INFeD (iron dextran injection, USP) is a dark brown, slightly viscous sterile liquid complex of ferric hydroxide and dextran for intravenous or intramuscular use.
Each mL contains the equivalent of 50 mg of elemental iron (as an iron dextran complex), approximately 0.9% sodium chloride, in water for injection. Sodium hydroxide and/or

hydrochloric acid may have been used to adjust pH. The pH of the solution is between 5.2 and 6.5.
The iron dextran complex has an average apparent molecular weight of 165,000.
Therapeutic Class: Hematinic

CLINICAL PHARMACOLOGY

General: After intramuscular injection, iron dextran is absorbed from the injection site into the capillaries and the lymphatic system. Circulating iron dextran is removed from the plasma by cells of the reticuloendothelial system, which split the complex into its components of iron and dextran. The iron is immediately bound to the available protein moieties to form hemosiderin or ferritin, the physiological forms of iron, or to a lesser extent to transferrin. This iron which is subject to physiological control replenishes hemoglobin and depleted iron stores.
Dextran, a polyglucose, is either metabolized or excreted. Negligible amounts of iron are lost via the urinary or alimentary pathways after administration of iron dextran.
The major portion of intramuscular injections of iron dextran is absorbed within 72 hours; most of the remaining iron is absorbed over the ensuing 3 to 4 weeks.
Various studies involving intravenously administered ^{59}Fe iron dextran to iron deficient subjects, some of whom had coexisting diseases, have yielded half-life values ranging from 5 hours to more than 20 hours. The 5-hour value was determined for ^{59}Fe iron dextran from a study that used laboratory methods to separate the circulating ^{59}Fe iron dextran from the transferrin-bound ^{59}Fe. The 20-hour value reflects a half-life determined by measuring total ^{59}Fe, both circulating and bound. It should be understood that these half-life values do not represent clearance of iron from the body. Iron is not easily eliminated from the body and accumulation of iron can be toxic.

INDICATIONS AND USAGE

Intravenous or intramuscular injections of iron dextran are indicated for treatment of patients with documented iron deficiency in whom oral administration is unsatisfactory or impossible.

CONTRAINDICATIONS

Hypersensitivity to the product. All anemias not associated with iron deficiency.

WARNINGS

See BOXED WARNING.
A risk of carcinogenesis may attend the intramuscular injection of iron-carbohydrate complexes. Such complexes have been found under experimental conditions to produce sarcoma when large doses or small doses injected repeatedly at the same site were given to rats, mice, and rabbits, and possibly in hamsters.
The long latent period between the injection of a potential carcinogen and the appearance of a tumor makes it impossible to measure accurately the risk in man. There have, however, been several reports in the literature describing tumors at the injection site in humans who had previously received intramuscular injections of iron-carbohydrate complexes.
Large intravenous doses, such as used with total dose infusions (TDI), have been associated with an increased incidence of adverse effects. The adverse effects frequently are delayed (1–2 days) reactions typified by one or more of the following symptoms; arthralgia, backache, chills, dizziness, moderate to high fever, headache, malaise, myalgia, nausea, and vomiting. The onset is usually 24–48 hours after administration and symptoms generally subside within 3–4 days. These symptoms have also been reported following intramuscular injection and generally subside within 3–7 days. The etiology of these reactions is not known. The potential for a delayed reaction must be considered when estimating the risk/benefit of treatment.
The maximum daily dose should not exceed 2 mL undiluted iron dextran.
This preparation should be used with extreme care in patients with serious impairment of liver function.
It should not be used during the acute phase of infectious kidney disease.
Adverse reactions experienced following administration of INFeD may exacerbate cardiovascular complications in patients with pre-existing cardiovascular disease.

PRECAUTIONS

General: Unwarranted therapy with parenteral iron will cause excess storage of iron with the consequent possibility of exogenous hemosiderosis. Such iron overload is particularly apt to occur in patients with hemoglobinopathies and other refractory anemias that might be erroneously diagnosed as iron deficiency anemias.
INFeD should be used with caution in individuals with histories of significant allergies and/or asthma.
Anaphylaxis and other hypersensitivity reactions have been reported after uneventful test doses as well as therapeutic doses of iron dextran injection. Therefore, administration of subsequent test doses during therapy should be considered. (See DOSAGE AND ADMINISTRATION: Administration.)

$$\frac{\text{mg blood iron}}{\text{lb body weight}} = \frac{\text{mL blood}}{\text{lb body weight}} \times \frac{\text{g hemoglobin}}{\text{mL blood}} \times \frac{\text{mg iron}}{\text{g hemoglobin}}$$

a) Blood volume	65 mL/kg body weight
b) Normal hemoglobin (males and females)	
over 15 kg (33 lbs)	14.8 g/dl
15 kg (33 lbs) or less	12.0 g/dl
c) Iron content of hemoglobin	0.34%
d) Hemoglobin deficit	
e) Weight	

Based on the above factors, individuals with normal hemoglobin levels will have approximately 33 mg of blood iron per kilogram of body weight (15 mg/lb).
Note: The table and accompanying formula are applicable for dosage determinations only in patients with iron deficiency anemia; they are not to be used for dosage determinations in patients requiring iron replacement for blood loss.

Epinephrine should be immediately available in the event of acute hypersensitivity reactions. (Usual adult dose: 0.5 mL of a 1:1000 solution, by subcutaneous or intramuscular injection.)
Note: Patients using beta-blocking agents may not respond adequately to epinephrine. Isoproterenol or similar beta-agonist agents may be required in these patients.
Patients with rheumatoid arthritis may have an acute exacerbation of joint pain and swelling following the administration of INFeD.
Reports in the literature from countries outside the United States (in particular, New Zealand) have suggested that the use of intramuscular iron dextran in neonates has been associated with an increased incidence of gram-negative sepsis, primarily due to *E. Coli.*
Information For Patients: Patients should be advised of the potential adverse reactions associated with the use of INFeD.
Drug/Laboratory Test Interactions: Large doses of iron dextran (5 mL or more) have been reported to give a brown color to serum from a blood sample drawn 4 hours after administration.
The drug may cause falsely elevated values of serum bilirubin and falsely decreased values of serum calcium.
Serum iron determinations (especially by colorimetric assays) may not be meaningful for 3 weeks following the administration of iron dextran.
Serum ferritin peaks approximately 7 to 9 days after an intravenous dose of INFeD and slowly returns to baseline after about 3 weeks.
Examination of the bone marrow for iron stores may not be meaningful for prolonged periods following iron dextran therapy because residual iron dextran may remain in the reticuloendothelial cells.
Bone scans involving 99m Tc-diphosphonate have been reported to show a dense, crescentic area of activity in the buttocks, following the contour of the iliac crest, 1 to 6 days after intramuscular injections of iron dextran.
Bone scans with 99m Tc-labeled bone seeking agents, in the presence of high serum ferritin levels or following iron dextran infusions, have been reported to show reduction of bony uptake, marked renal activity, and excessive blood pool and soft tissue accumulation.
Carcinogenesis, Mutagenesis, Impairment Of Fertility: See WARNINGS.
Pregnancy: *Pregnancy Category C:* Iron dextran has been shown to be teratogenic and embryocidal in mice, rats, rabbits, dogs, and monkeys when given in doses of about 3 times the maximum human dose.
No consistent adverse fetal effects were observed in mice, rats, rabbits, dogs and monkeys at doses of 50 mg iron/kg or less. Fetal and maternal toxicity has been reported in monkeys at a total intravenous dose of 90 mg iron/kg over a 14 day period. Similar effects were observed in mice and rats on administration of a single dose of 125 mg iron/kg. Fetal abnormalities in rats and dogs were observed at doses of 250 mg iron/kg and higher. The animals used in these tests were not iron deficient. There are no adequate and well-controlled studies in pregnant women. INFeD should be used during pregnancy only if the potential benefit justifies the potential risk to the fetus.
Placental Transfer: Various animal studies and studies in pregnant humans have demonstrated inconclusive results with respect to the placental transfer of iron dextran as iron dextran. It appears that some iron does reach the fetus, but the form in which it crosses the placenta is not clear.
Nursing Mothers: Caution should be exercised when INFeD is administered to a nursing woman. Traces of unmetabolized iron dextran are excreted in human milk.
Pediatric Use: Not recommended for use in infants under 4 months of age (See DOSAGE AND ADMINISTRATION.)

ADVERSE REACTIONS

Severe/Fatal: Anaphylactic reactions have been reported with the use of iron dextran injection; on occasions these reactions have been fatal. Such reactions, which occur most often within the first several minutes of administration, have been generally characterized by sudden onset of respiratory difficulty and/or cardiovascular collapse. (See boxed WARNING and PRECAUTIONS: General, pertaining to immediate availability of epinephrine.)
Cardiovascular: Chest pain, chest tightness, shock, hypotension, hypertension, tachycardia, flushing, arrhythmias. (Flushing and hypotension may occur from too rapid injections by the intravenous route.)
Dermatologic: Urticaria, pruritus, purpura, rash.
Gastrointestinal: Abdominal pain, nausea, vomiting, diarrhea.
Hematologic/lymphatic: Leucocytosis, lymphadenopathy.
Musculoskeletal/soft tissue: Arthralgia, arthritis (may represent reactivation in patients with quiescent rheumatoid arthritis—See PRECAUTIONS: General), myalgia; backache; sterile abscess, atrophy/fibrosis (intramuscular injection site); brown skin and/or underlying tissue discoloration (staining), soreness or pain at or near intramuscular injection sites; cellulitis; swelling; inflammation; local phlebitis at or near intravenous injection site.
Neurologic: Convulsions, seizures, syncope, headache, weakness, unresponsiveness, paresthesia, febrile episodes, chills, dizziness, disorientation, numbness.
Respiratory: Respiratory arrest, dyspnea, bronchospasm.
Urologic: Hematuria.
Delayed reactions: Arthralgia, backache, chills, dizziness, fever, headache, malaise, myalgia, nausea, vomiting (See WARNINGS.).
Miscellaneous: Febrile episodes, sweating, shivering, chills, malaise, altered taste.

OVERDOSAGE

Overdosage with iron dextran is unlikely to be associated with any acute manifestations. Dosages of iron dextran in excess of the requirements for restoration of hemoglobin and replenishment of iron stores may lead to hemosiderosis. Periodic monitoring of serum ferritin levels may be helpful in recognizing a deleterious progressive accumulation of iron resulting from impaired uptake of iron from the reticuloendothelial system in concurrent medical conditions such as chronic renal failure, Hodgkin's disease, and rheumatoid arthritis. The LD_{50} of iron dextran is not less than 500 mg/kg in the mouse.

DOSAGE AND ADMINISTRATION

Oral iron should be discontinued prior to administration of INFeD.
Dosage:
I. ***Iron Deficiency Anemia:*** Periodic hematologic determination (hemoglobin and hematocrit) is a simple and accurate technique for monitoring hematological response, and should be used as a guide in therapy. It should be recognized that iron storage may lag behind the appearance of normal blood morphology. Serum iron, total iron binding capacity (TIBC) and percent saturation of transferrin are other important tests for detecting and monitoring the iron deficient state.
After administration of iron dextran complex, evidence of a therapeutic response can be seen in a few days as an increase in the reticulocyte count.
Although serum ferritin is usually a good guide to body iron stores, the correlation of body iron stores and serum ferritin may not be valid in patients on chronic renal dialysis who are also receiving iron dextran complex.
Although there are significant variations in body build and weight distribution among males and females, the accompanying table and formula represent a convenient means for estimating the total iron required. This total iron requirement reflects the amount of iron needed to restore hemoglobin concentration to normal or near normal levels plus an additional allowance to provide adequate replenishment of iron stores in most individuals with moderately or severely reduced levels of hemoglobin. It should be remembered that iron deficiency anemia will not appear until essentially all iron stores have been depleted. Therapy, thus, should aim at not only replenishment of hemoglobin iron but iron stores as well.
Factors contributing to the formula are shown below.
[See table above.]
[See table at bottom of next page.]
The total amount of INFeD in mL required to treat the anemia and replenish iron stores may be approximated as follows:

Continued on next page

Schein Pharmaceutical—Cont.

Adults and Children over 15 kg (33 lbs): See Dosage Table. Alternatively the total dose may be calculated:

Dose (mL) = 0.0442 (Desired Hb − Observed Hb) × LBW + (0.26 × LBW)

Based on: Desired Hb = the target Hb in g/dl.

Observed Hb = the patient's current hemoglobin in g/dl.

LBW = Lean body weight in kg. A patient's lean body weight (or actual body weight if less than lean body weight) should be utilized when determining dosage.

For males: LBW = 50 kg + 2.3 kg for each inch of patient's height over 5 feet

For females: LBW = 45.5 kg + 2.3 kg for each inch of patient's height over 5 feet

To calculate a patient's weight in kg when lbs are known:

$$\frac{\text{patient's weight in pounds}}{2.2} = \text{weight in kilograms}$$

Children 5–15 kg (11–33 lbs): See Dosage Table.

INFeD should not normally be given in the first four months of life. (See PRECAUTIONS: Pediatric Use.)

Alternatively the total dose may be calculated:

Dose (mL) = 0.0442 (Desired Hb − Observed Hb) × W + (0.26 × W)

Based on: Desired Hb = the target Hb in g/dl. (Normal Hb for Children 15 kg or less is 12 g/dl.)

W = Weight in kg.

To calculate a patient's weight in kg when lbs are known:

$$\frac{\text{patient's weight in pounds}}{2.2} = \text{weight in kilograms}$$

II. Iron Replacement for Blood Loss: Some individuals sustain blood losses on an intermittent or repetitive basis. Such blood losses may occur periodically in patients with hemorrhagic diatheses (familial telangiectasia; hemophilia; gastrointestinal bleeding) and on a repetitive basis from procedures such as renal hemodialysis.

Iron therapy in these patients should be directed toward replacement of the equivalent amount of iron represented in the blood loss. The table and formula described under **I.** *Iron Deficiency Anemia* are *not* applicable for simple iron replacement values.

Quantitative estimates of the individual's periodic blood loss and hematocrit during the bleeding episode provide a convenient method for the calculation of the required iron dose. The formula shown below is based on the approximation that 1 mL of normocytic, normochromic red cells contains 1 mg of elemental iron:

Replacement iron (in mg) = Blood loss (in mL) × hematocrit

Example: Blood loss of 500 mL with 20% hematocrit

Replacement Iron = 500 × 0.20 = 100 mg

$$\text{INFeD dose} = \frac{100 \text{ mg}}{50} = 2 \text{ mL}$$

Administration: The total amount of INFeD required for the treatment of iron deficiency anemia or iron replacement for blood loss is determined from the table or appropriate formula. (See Dosage.)

1. *Intravenous Injection*—PRIOR TO RECEIVING THEIR FIRST INFeD THERAPEUTIC DOSE, ALL PATIENTS SHOULD BE GIVEN AN INTRAVENOUS TEST DOSE OF 0.5 mL. (See PRECAUTIONS: General.) THE TEST DOSE SHOULD BE ADMINISTERED AT A GRADUAL RATE OVER AT LEAST 30 SECONDS. Although anaphylactic reactions known to occur following INFeD administration are usually evident within a few minutes, or sooner, it is recommended that a period of an hour or longer elapse before the remainder of the initial therapeutic dose is given. Individual doses of 2 mL or less may be given on a daily basis until the calculated total amount required has been reached. INFeD is given undiluted at a **slow gradual rate** not to exceed 50 mg (1 mL) per minute.

2. *Intramuscular Injection*—PRIOR TO RECEIVING THEIR FIRST INFeD THERAPEUTIC DOSE, ALL PATIENTS SHOULD BE GIVEN AN INTRAMUSCULAR TEST DOSE OF 0.5 mL. (See PRECAUTIONS: General.) The test dose should be administered in the same recommended test site and by the same technique as described in the last paragraph of this section. Although anaphylactic reactions known to occur following INFeD administration are usually evident within a few minutes or sooner, it is recommended that at least an hour or longer elapse before the remainder of the initial therapeutic dose is given.

If no adverse reactions are observed, INFeD can be given according to the following schedule until the calculated total amount required has been reached. Each day's dose should ordinarily not exceed 0.5 mL (25 mg of iron) for infants under 5 kg (11 lbs); 1.0 mL (50 mg of iron) for children under 10 kg (22 lbs); and 2.0 mL (100 mg of iron) for other patients.

INFeD should be injected only into the muscle mass of the upper outer quadrant of the buttock—never into the arm or other exposed areas—and should be injected deeply, with a 2-inch or 3-inch 19 or 20 gauge needle. If the patient is standing, he/she should be bearing his/her weight on the leg opposite the injection site, or if in bed, he/she should be in the lateral position with injection site uppermost. To avoid injection or leakage into the subcutaneous tissue, a Z-track technique (displacement of the skin laterally prior to injection) is recommended.

NOTE: Do not mix INFeD with other medications or add to parenteral nutrition solutions for intravenous infusion. Parenteral drug products should be inspected visually for particulate matter and discoloration prior to administration, whenever the solution and container permit.

HOW SUPPLIED

INFeD® (Iron Dextran Injection, USP) containing 50 mg of elemental iron per mL, is available in 2 mL single dose amber vials (for intramuscular or intravenous use) in cartons of 10 (NDC 0364-3012-47).

Store at controlled room temperature 15°–30°C (59°–86°F).

CAUTION: Federal law prohibits dispensing without prescription.

Literature revised: July 1995

Product No.: 1001-02

SCHEIN PHARMACEUTICAL, INC.
Florham Park, NJ 07932 USA

Shown in Product Identification Guide, page 334

Schering Corporation
a wholly-owned subsidiary of Schering-Plough Corporation
GALLOPING HILL ROAD
KENILWORTH, NJ 07033

Direct Inquiries to:
(908) 298-4000
CUSTOMER SERVICE:
(800) 222-7579
FAX: (908) 820-6400

For Medical Information Contact:
Schering Laboratories
Drug Information Services
2000 Galloping Hill Road
Kenilworth, NJ 07033
(800) 526-4099
FAX: (908) 298-2188

Product Identification Codes

To provide quick and positive identification of Schering Products, we have imprinted the product identification number of the National Drug Code on most tablets and capsules. In some cases, identification letters also appear.

Additionally, the following telephone numbers are provided for inquiries:

Professional Services Department
9:00 AM to 5:00 PM EST
1-800-526-4099

After regular hours and on weekends: (908) 298-4000

CEDAX® ℞
(ceftibuten capsules)
and
(ceftibuten for oral suspension)
FOR ORAL USE ONLY

DESCRIPTION

CEDAX (ceftibuten capsules) and (ceftibuten for oral suspension) contain the active ingredient ceftibuten as ceftibuten dihydrate. Ceftibuten dihydrate is a semisynthetic cephalosporin antibiotic for oral administration. Chemically, it is (+)-(6R,7R)-7-[(Z)-2-(2-Amino-4-thiazolyl)-4-carboxycrotonamido]-8-oxo-5-thia-1-azabicyclo[4.2.0]oct-2-ene-2-carboxylic acid, dihydrate. Its molecular formula is $C_{15}H_{14}N_4O_6S_2 \bullet 2H_2O$. Its molecular weight is 446.43 as the dihydrate.

Ceftibuten dihydrate has the following structural formula:

CEDAX Capsules contain ceftibuten dihydrate equivalent to 400 mg of ceftibuten. Inactive ingredients contained in the capsule formulation include: magnesium stearate, microcrystalline cellulose, and sodium starch glycolate. The capsule shell and/or band contains gelatin, sodium lauryl sulfate, titanium dioxide, and polysorbate 80. The capsule shell may also contain benzyl alcohol, sodium propionate, edetate calcium disodium, butylparaben, propylparaben, and methylparaben.

CEDAX Oral Suspension after reconstitution contains ceftibuten dihydrate equivalent to either 90 mg of ceftibuten per 5 mL or 180 mg of ceftibuten per 5 mL. CEDAX Oral Sus-

TOTAL INFeD® REQUIREMENT FOR HEMOGLOBIN RESTORATION AND IRON STORES REPLACEMENT*

PATIENT LEAN BODY WEIGHT		Milliliter Requirement of INFeD Based On Observed Hemoglobin of							
kg	lb	3 (g/dl)	4 (g/dl)	5 (g/dl)	6 (g/dl)	7 (g/dl)	8 (g/dl)	9 (g/dl)	10 (g/dl)
5	11	3	3	3	3	2	2	2	2
10	22	7	6	6	5	5	4	4	3
15	33	10	9	9	8	7	7	6	5
20	44	16	15	14	13	12	11	10	9
25	55	20	18	17	16	15	14	13	12
30	66	23	22	21	19	18	17	15	14
35	77	27	26	24	23	21	20	18	17
40	88	31	29	28	26	24	22	21	19
45	99	35	33	31	29	27	25	23	21
50	110	39	37	35	32	30	28	26	24
55	121	43	41	38	36	33	31	28	26
60	132	47	44	42	39	36	34	31	28
65	143	51	48	45	42	39	36	34	31
70	154	55	52	49	45	42	39	36	33
75	165	59	55	52	49	45	42	39	35
80	176	63	59	55	52	48	45	41	38
85	187	66	63	59	55	51	48	44	40
90	198	70	66	62	58	54	50	46	42
95	209	74	70	66	62	57	53	49	45
100	220	78	74	69	65	60	56	52	47
105	231	82	77	73	68	63	59	54	50
110	242	86	81	76	71	67	62	57	52
115	253	90	85	80	75	70	64	59	54
120	264	94	88	83	78	73	67	62	57

* Table values were calculated based on a normal adult hemoglobin of 14.8 g/dl for weights greater than 15 kg (33 lbs) and a hemoglobin of 12.0 g/dl for weights less than or equal to 15 kg (33 lbs).

pension is cherry flavored and contains the inactive ingredients: cherry flavoring, polysorbate 80, silicon dioxide, simethicone, sodium benzoate, sucrose (approximately 1 g/5 mL), titanium dioxide, and xanthan gum.

CLINICAL PHARMACOLOGY

PHARMACOKINETICS

Absorption:

CEDAX CAPSULES

Ceftibuten is rapidly absorbed after oral administration of CEDAX Capsules. The plasma concentrations and pharmacokinetic parameters of ceftibuten after a single 400-mg dose of CEDAX Capsules to 12 healthy adult male volunteers (20 to 39 years of age) are displayed in the table below. When CEDAX Capsules were administered once daily for 7 days, the average C_{max} was 17.9 μg/mL on day 7. Therefore, ceftibuten accumulation in plasma is about 20% at steady state.

CEDAX ORAL SUSPENSION

Ceftibuten is rapidly absorbed after oral administration of CEDAX Oral Suspension. The plasma concentrations and pharmacokinetic parameters of ceftibuten after a single 9-mg/kg dose of CEDAX Oral Suspension to 32 fasting pediatric patients (6 months to 12 years of age) are displayed in the following table:

[See table above.]

Parameter	Average Plasma Concentration (in μg/mL of ceftibuten after a single 400-mg dose) and Derived Pharmacokinetic Parameters (± 1 SD) (n=12 healthy adult males)	Average Plasma Concentration (in μg/mL of ceftibuten after a single 9-mg/kg dose) and Derived Pharmacokinetic Parameters (± 1 SD) (n=32 pediatric patients)
1.0 h	6.1 (5.1)	9.3 (6.3)
1.5 h	9.9 (5.9)	8.6 (4.4)
2.0 h	11.3 (5.2)	11.2 (4.6)
3.0 h	13.3 (3.0)	9.0 (3.4)
4.0 h	11.2 (2.9)	6.6 (3.1)
6.0 h	5.8 (1.6)	3.8 (2.5)
8.0 h	3.2 (1.0)	1.6 (1.3)
12.0 h	1.1 (0.4)	0.5 (0.4)
C_{max}, μg/mL	15.0 (3.3)	13.4 (4.9)
T_{max}, h	2.6 (0.9)	2.0 (1.0)
AUC, μg • h/mL	73.7 (16.0)	56.0 (16.9)
$T^1/_2$, h	2.4 (0.2)	2.0 (0.6)
Total body clearance (CI/F) mL/min/kg	1.3 (0.3)	2.9 (0.7)

The absolute bioavailability of CEDAX Oral Suspension has not been determined. The plasma concentrations of ceftibuten in pediatric patients are dose proportional following single doses of CEDAX Capsules of 200 mg and 400 mg and of CEDAX Oral Suspension between 4.5 mg/kg and 9 mg/kg.

Distribution:

CEDAX CAPSULES

The average apparent volume of distribution (V/F) of ceftibuten in 6 adult subjects is 0.21 L/kg (± 1 SD=0.03 L/kg).

CEDAX ORAL SUSPENSION

The average apparent volume of distribution (V/F) of ceftibuten in 32 fasting pediatric patients is 0.5 L/kg (± 1 SD=0.2 L/kg).

Protein Binding:

Ceftibuten is 65% bound to plasma proteins. The protein binding is independent of plasma ceftibuten concentration.

Tissue Penetration:

Bronchial secretions: In a study of 15 adults administered a single 400-mg dose of ceftibuten and scheduled to undergo bronchoscopy, the mean concentrations in epithelial lining fluid and bronchial mucosa were 15% and 37%, respectively, of the plasma concentrations.

Sputum: Ceftibuten sputum levels average approximately 7% of the concomitant plasma ceftibuten level. In a study of 24 adults administered ceftibuten 200 mg bid or 400 mg qd, the average C_{max} in sputum (1.5 μg/mL) occurred at 2 hours postdose and the average C_{max} in plasma (17 μg/mL) occurred at 2 hours postdose.

Middle-ear fluid (MEF): Ceftibuten middle-ear fluid levels average approximately 50% of the concomitant plasma ceftibuten level. In a study of 30 children administered 9 mg/kg of ceftibuten, the average C_{max} in MEF (2.9 ± 0.9 μg/mL) occurred at 4 hours postdose and the average C_{max} in plasma (6.7 ± 1.9 μg/mL) occurred at 2 hours postdose.

Tonsillar tissue: Data on ceftibuten penetration into tonsillar tissue are not available.

Cerebrospinal fluid: Data on ceftibuten penetration into cerebrospinal fluid are not available.

Metabolism and Excretion:

A study with radiolabeled ceftibuten administered to 6 healthy adult male volunteers demonstrated that *cis*-ceftibuten is the predominant component in both plasma and urine. About 10% of ceftibuten is converted to the *trans*-isomer. The *trans*-isomer is approximately $^1/_8$ as antimicrobially potent as the *cis*-isomer.

Ceftibuten is excreted in the urine; 95% of the administered radioactivity was recovered either in urine or feces. In 6 healthy adult male volunteers, approximately 56% of the administered dose of ceftibuten was recovered from urine and 39% from the feces within 24 hours. Because renal excretion is a significant pathway of elimination, patients with renal dysfunction and patients undergoing hemodialysis require dosage adjustment (see **DOSAGE AND ADMINISTRATION**).

Food Effect on Absorption:

Food affects the bioavailability of ceftibuten from CEDAX Capsules and CEDAX Oral Suspension.

The effect of food on the bioavailability of CEDAX Capsules was evaluated in 26 healthy adult male volunteers who ingested 400 mg of CEDAX Capsules after an overnight fast or immediately after a standardized breakfast. Results showed that food delays the time of C_{max} by 1.75 hours, decreases the C_{max} by 18%, and decreases the extent of absorption (AUC) by 8%.

The effect of food on the bioavailability of CEDAX Oral Suspension was evaluated in 18 healthy adult male volunteers who ingested 400 mg of CEDAX Oral Suspension after an overnight fast or immediately after a standardized breakfast. Results obtained demonstrated a decrease in C_{max} of 26% and an AUC of 17% when CEDAX Oral Suspension was administered with a high-fat breakfast, and a decrease in C_{max} of 17% and in AUC of 12% when CEDAX Oral Suspension was administered with a low-calorie nonfat breakfast (see **PRECAUTIONS**).

Bioequivalence of Dosage Formulations:

A study in 18 healthy adult male volunteers demonstrated that a 400-mg dose of CEDAX Capsules produced equivalent concentrations to a 400-mg dose of CEDAX Oral Suspension. Average C_{max} values were 15.6 (3.1) μg/mL for the capsule and 17.0 (3.2) μg/mL for the suspension. Average AUC values were 80.1 (14.4) μg • hr/mL for the capsule and 87.0 (12.2) μg • hr/mL for the suspension.

Special Populations:

Geriatric patients: Ceftibuten pharmacokinetics have been investigated in elderly (65 years of age and older) men (n=8) and women (n=4). Each volunteer received ceftibuten 200-mg capsules twice daily for $3^1/_2$ days. The average C_{max} was 17.5 (3.7) μg/mL after $3^1/_2$ days of dosing compared to 12.9 (2.1) μg/mL after the first dose; ceftibuten accumulation in plasma was 40% at steady state. Information regarding the renal function of these volunteers was not available; therefore, the significance of this finding for clincial use of CEDAX Capsules in elderly patients is not clear. Ceftibuten dosage adjustment in elderly patients may be necessary (see **DOSAGE AND ADMINISTRATION**).

Patients with renal insufficiency: Ceftibuten pharmacokinetics have been investigated in adult patients with renal dysfunction. The ceftibuten plasma half-life increased and apparent total clearance (Cl/F) decreased proportionately with increasing degree of renal dysfunction. In 6 patients with moderate renal dysfunction (creatinine clearance 30 to 49 mL/min), the plasma half-life of ceftibuten increased to 7.1 hours and Cl/F decreased to 30 mL/min. In 6 patients with severe renal dysfunction (creatinine clearance 5 to 29 mL/min), the half-life increased to 13.4 hours and Cl/F decreased to 16 mL/min. In 6 functionally anephric patients (creatinine clearance <5 mL/min), the half-life increased to 22.3 hours and Cl/F decreased to 11 mL/min (a 7- to 8-fold change compared to healthy volunteers). Hemodialysis removed 65% of the drug from the blood in 2 to 4 hours. These changes serve as the basis for dosage adjustment recommendations in adult patients with mild to severe renal dysfunction (see **DOSAGE AND ADMINISTRATION**).

Microbiology:

Ceftibuten exerts its bactericidal action by binding to essential target proteins of the bacterial cell wall. This binding leads to inhibition of cell-wall synthesis.

Ceftibuten is stable in the presence of most plasmid-mediated beta-lactamases, but it is not stable in the presence of chromosomally-mediated cephalosporinases produced in organisms such as *Bacteroids, Citrobacter, Enterobacter, Morganella,* and *Serratia.* Like other beta-lactam agents, ceftibuten should not be used against strains resistant to betalactams due to general mechanisms such as permeability or penicillin-binding protein changes like penicillin-resistant *S. pneumoniae.*

Ceftibuten has been shown to be active against most strains of the following organisms both *in vitro* and in clinical infections (see **INDICATIONS AND USAGE**):

Gram-positive aerobes:

Streptococcus pneumoniae (penicillin-susceptible strains only)

Streptococcus pyogenes

Gram-negative aerobes:

Haemophilus influenzae (including β-lactamase-producing strains)

Moraxella catarrhalis (including β-lactamase-producing strains)

There are no known organisms which are potential pathogens in the indications approved for ceftibuten for which ceftibuten exhibits *in vitro* activity but for which the safety and efficacy of ceftibuten in treating clinical infections due to these organisms, have not been established in adequate and well-controlled trials.

NOTE: Ceftibuten is INACTIVE *in vitro* against *Acinetobacter, Bordetella, Campylobacter, Enterobacter, Enterococcus, Flavobacterium, Hafnia, Listeria, Pseudomonas, Staphylococcus,* and *Streptococcus* (except *pneumoniae* and *pyogenes*) species. In addition, it shows little *in vitro* activity against most anaerobes, including most species of *Bacteroides.*

Susceptibility Testing:

Dilution Techniques: Quantitative methods are used to determine antimicrobial minimal inhibitory concentrations (MICs). These MICs provide estimates of the susceptibility of bacteria to antimicrobial compounds. The MICs should be determined using a standardized procedure. Standardized procedures are based on a dilution method (broth, agar, or microdilution) or equivalent with standardized inoculum concentrations and standardized concentrations of ceftibuten powder. The MIC values should be interpreted according to the following criteria when testing *Haemophilus* species using Haemophilus Test Media (HTM):

MIC (μg/mL)	Interpretation
≤2	(S) Susceptible

The current absence of resistant strains precludes defining any categories other than "Susceptible". Strains yielding results suggestive of a "Nonsusceptible" category should be submitted to a reference laboratory for further testing.

A report of "Susceptible" implies that an infection due to the strain may be appropriately treated with the dosage of antimicrobial agent recommended for that type of infection and infecting species, unless otherwise contraindicated.

Ceftibuten is indicated for penicillin-susceptible only strains of *Streptococcus pneumoniae.* A pneumococcal isolate that is susceptible to penicillin (MIC ≤0.06 μg/mL) can be considered susceptible to ceftibuten for approved indications. Testing of ceftibuten against penicillin-intermediate or penicillin-resistant isolates is not recommended. Reliable interpretive criteria for ceftibuten are not currently available. Physicians should be informed that clinical response rates with ceftibuten may be lower in strains that are not penicillin-susceptible.

Standardized susceptibility test procedures require the use of laboratory control microorganisms to control the technical aspect of laboratory procedures. Standard ceftibuten powder should provide the following MIC values:

Organism	MIC range (μg/mL)
Haemophilus influenzae ATCC 49274	0.25–1.0

Diffusion Techniques: Quantitative methods that require measurement of zone diameters also provide estimates of the susceptibility of bacteria to antimicrobial compounds. One such standardized procedure requires the use of standardized inoculum concentrations. This procedure uses paper disks impregnated with 30 μg of ceftibuten to test the susceptibility of microorganisms to ceftibuten.

Reports from the laboratory providing results of the standard single-disk susceptibility test with a 30-μg ceftibuten disk should be interpreted according to the following criteria when testing *Haemophilus* species using Haemophilus Test Media (HTM):

Zone diameter (mm)	Interpretation
≥28	(S) Susceptible

The current absence of resistant strains precludes defining any categories other than "Susceptible". Strains yielding

Continued on next page

Information on Schering products appearing on these pages is effective as of August 15, 1996.

Consult 1997 supplements and future editions for revisions

Schering—Cont.

results suggestive of a "Nonsusceptible" category should be submitted to a reference laboratory for further testing.
Interpretation should be as stated above for results using dilution techniques.
Ceftibuten is indicated for penicillin-susceptible only strains of *Streptococcus pneumoniae.*
Pneumococcal isolates with oxacillin zone sizes of ≥20 mm are susceptible to penicillin and can be considered susceptible for approved indications. Reliable disk diffusion tests for ceftibuten do not yet exist.
As with standardized dilution techniques, diffusion methods require the use of laboratory control microorganisms that are used to control the technical aspects of the laboratory procedures. For the diffusion technique, the 30-μg ceftibuten disk should provide the following zone diameters in these laboratory test quality control strains:

Organism	Zone diameter (mm)
Haemophilus influenzae ATCC 49247	29–35

Cephalosporin-class disks should not be used to test for susceptibility to ceftibuten.

INDICATIONS AND USAGE

CEDAX (ceftibuten) is indicated for the treatment of individuals with mild-to-moderate infections caused by susceptible strains of the designated microorganisms in the specific conditions listed below (see **DOSAGE AND ADMINISTRATION** and **CLINICAL STUDIES** sections).
Acute Bacterial Exacerbations of Chronic Bronchitis due to *Haemophilus influenzae* (including β-lactamase-producing strains). *Moraxella catarrhalis* (including β-lactamase-producing strains), or *Streptococcus pneumoniae* (penicillin-susceptible strains only).
NOTE: In acute bacterial exacerbations of chronic bronchitis clinical trials where *Moraxella catarrhalis* was isolated from infected sputum at baseline, ceftibuten clinical efficacy was 22% less than control.
Acute Bacterial Otitis Media due to *Haemophilus influenzae* (including β-lactamase-producing strains), *Moraxella catarrhalis* (including β-lactamase-producing strains), or *Streptococcus pyogenes.*
NOTE: Although ceftibuten used empirically was equivalent to comparators in the treatment of clinically and/or microbiologically documented acute otitis media, the efficacy against *Streptococcus pneumoniae* was 23% less than control. Therefore, ceftibuten should be given empirically only when adequate antimicrobial coverage against *Streptococcus pneumoniae* has been previously administered.
Pharyngitis and Tonsillitis due to *Streptococcus pyogenes.*
NOTE: Only penicillin by the intramuscular route of administration has been shown to be effective in the prophylaxis of rheumatic fever. Ceftibuten is generally effective in the eradication of *Streptococcus pyogenes* from the oropharynx; however, data establishing the efficacy of CEDAX for the prophylaxis of subsequent rheumatic fever are not available.

CONTRAINDICATIONS

CEDAX (ceftibuten) is contraindicated in patients with known allergy to the cephalosporin group of antibiotics.

WARNINGS

BEFORE THERAPY WITH CEDAX IS INSTITUTED, CAREFUL INQUIRY SHOULD BE MADE TO DETERMINE WHETHER THE PATIENT HAS HAD PREVIOUS HYPERSENSITIVITY REACTIONS TO CEDAX, OTHER CEPHALOSPORINS, PENICILLINS, OR OTHER DRUGS. IF THIS PRODUCT IS TO BE GIVEN TO PENICILLIN-SENSITIVE PATIENTS, CAUTION SHOULD BE EXERCISED BECAUSE CROSS HYPERSENSITIVITY AMONG BETA-LACTAM ANTIBIOTICS HAS BEEN CLEARLY DOCUMENTED AND MAY OCCUR IN UP TO 10% OF PATIENTS WITH A HISTORY OF PENICILLIN ALLERGY. IF AN ALLERGIC REACTION TO CEDAX OCCURS, DISCONTINUE THE DRUG. SERIOUS ACUTE HYPERSENSITIVITY REACTIONS MAY REQUIRE TREATMENT WITH EPINEPHRINE AND OTHER EMERGENCY MEASURES, INCLUDING OXYGEN, INTRAVENOUS FLUIDS, INTRAVENOUS ANTIHISTAMINES, CORTICOSTEROIDS, PRESSOR AMINES, AND AIRWAY MANAGEMENT, AS CLINICALLY INDICATED.
Pseudomembranous colitis has been reported with nearly all antibacterial agents, including ceftibuten, and may range in severity from mild to life threatening. Therefore, it is important to consider this diagnosis in patients who present with diarrhea subsequent to the adminsitration of antibacterial agents.
Treatment with antibacterial agents alters normal flora of the colon and may permit overgrowth of clostridia. Studies indicate that a toxin produced by *Clostridium difficile* is one primary cause of "antibiotic-associated colitis".
After the diagnosis of pseudomembranous colitis has been established, appropriate therapeutic measures should be initiated. Mild cases of pseudomembranous colitis usually respond to drug discontinuation alone. In moderate to severe cases, consideration should be given to management with fluids and electrolytes, protein supplementation, and treatment with an antibacterial drug clinically effective against *Clostridium difficile.*

PRECAUTIONS

General:
As with other broad-spectrum antibiotics, prolonged treatment may result in the possible emergence and overgrowth of resistant organisms. Careful observation of the patient is essential. If superinfection occurs during therapy, appropriate measures should be taken.
The dose of ceftibuten may require adjustment in patients with varying degrees of renal insufficiency, particularly in patients with creatinine clearance less than 50 mL/min or undergoing hemodialysis (see **DOSAGE AND ADMINISTRATION**). Ceftibuten is readily dialyzable. Dialysis patients should be monitored carefully, and administration of ceftibuten should occur immediately following dialysis.
Ceftibuten should be prescribed with caution to individuals with a history of gastrointestinal disease, particularly colitis.
Information to Patients:
Patients should be informed that:
- If the patient is diabetic, he/she should be informed that CEDAX Oral Suspension contains 1 gram sucrose per teaspoon of suspension.
- CEDAX Oral Suspension should be taken at least 2 hours before a meal or at least 1 hour after a meal (see **CLINICAL PHARMACOLOGY, Food Effect on Absorption**).

Drug Interactions:
Theophylline: Twelve healthy male volunteers were administered one 200-mg ceftibuten capsule twice daily for 6 days. With the morning dose of ceftibuten on day 6, each volunteer received a single intravenous infusion of theophylline (4 mg/kg). The pharmacokinetics of theophylline were not altered. The effect of ceftibuten on the pharmacokinetics of theophylline administered orally has not been investigated.
Antacids or H_2-receptor antagonists: The effect of increased gastric pH on the bioavailability of ceftibuten was evaluated in 18 healthy adult volunteers. Each volunteer was administered one 400-mg ceftibuten capsule. A single dose of liquid antacid did not affect the C_{max} or AUC of ceftibuten; however, 150 mg of ranitidine q12h for 3 days increased the ceftibuten C_{max} by 23% and ceftibuten AUC by 16%. The clinical relevance of these increases is not known.
Drug/Laboratory Test Interactions:
There have been no chemical or laboratory test interactions with ceftibuten noted to date. False-positive direct Coombs' tests have been reported during treatment with other cephalosporins. Therefore, it should be recognized that a positive Coombs' test could be due to the drug. The results of assays using red cells from healthy subjects to determine whether ceftibuten would cause direct Coombs' reactions *in vitro* showed no positive reaction at ceftibuten concentrations as high as 40 μg/mL.
Carcinogenesis, Mutagenesis, Impairment of Fertility:
Long-term animal studies have not been performed to evaluate the carcinogenic potential of ceftibuten. No mutagenic effects were seen in the following studies: *in vitro* chromosome assay in human lymphocytes, *in vivo* chromosome assay in mouse bone marrow cells, Chinese Hamster Ovary (CHO) cell point mutation assay at the hypoxanthine-guanine phosphoribosyl transferase (HGPRT) locus, and in a bacterial reversion point mutation test (Ames). No impairment of fertility occurred when rats were administered ceftibuten orally up to 2000 mg/kg/day (approximately 43 times the human dose based on $mg/m^2/day$).
Pregnancy: Teratogenic effects: Pregnancy Category B:
Ceftibuten was not teratogenic in the pregnant rat at oral doses up to 400 mg/kg/day (approximately 8.6 times the human dose based on $mg/m^2/day$). Ceftibuten was not teratogenic in the pregnant rabbit at oral doses up to 40 mg/kg/day (approximately 1.5 times the human dose based on $mg/m^2/day$) and has revealed no evidence of harm to the fetus. There are no adequate and well-controlled studies in pregnant women. Because animal reproduction studies are not always predictive of human response, this drug should be used during pregnancy only if clearly needed.
Labor and Delivery:
Ceftibuten has not been studied for use during labor and delivery. Its use during such clinical situations should be weighed in terms of potential risk and benefit to both mother and fetus.
Nursing Mothers:
It is not known whether ceftibuten (at recommended dosages) is excreted in human milk. Because many drugs are excreted in human milk, caution should be exercised when ceftibuten is administered to a nursing woman.
Pediatric Use:
The safety and efficacy of ceftibuten in infants less than 6 months of age has not been established.
Geriatric Patients:
The usual adult dosage recommendation may be followed for patients in this age group. However, these patients should be monitored closely, particularly their renal function, as dosage adjustment may be required.

ADVERSE EVENTS

Clinical Trials:

CEDAX CAPSULES (adult patients)

In clinical trials, 1728 adult patients (1092 US and 636 international) were treated with the recommended dose of ceftibuten capsules (400 mg per day). There were no deaths or permanent disabilities thought due to drug toxicity in any of the patients in these studies. Thirty-six of 1728 (2%) patients discontinued medication due to adverse events thought by the investigators to be possibly, probably, or almost certainly related to drug toxicity. The discontinuations were primarily for gastrointestinal disturbances, usually diarrhea, vomiting, or nausea. Six of 1728 (0.3%) patients were discontinued due to rash or pruritus thought related to ceftibuten administration.
In the US trials, the following adverse events were thought by the investigators to be possibly, probably, or almost certainly related to ceftibuten capsules in multiple-dose clinical trials (n=1092 ceftibuten-treated patients).

ADVERSE REACTIONS
CEFTIBUTEN CAPSULES
US CLINICAL TRIALS IN ADULT PATIENTS (n=1092)

Incidence equal to or greater than 1%	Nausea	4%
	Headache	3%
	Diarrhea	3%
	Dyspepsia	2%
	Dizziness	1%
	Abdominal pain	1%
	Vomiting	1%
Incidence less than 1% but greater than 0.1%	Anorexia	
	Constipation	
	Dry mouth	
	Dyspnea	
	Dysuria	
	Eructation	
	Fatigue	
	Flatulence	
	Loose stools	
	Moniliasis	
	Nasal congestion	
	Paresthesia	
	Pruritus	
	Rash	
	Somnolence	
	Taste perversion	
	Urticaria	
	Vaginitis	

LABORATORY VALUE CHANGES*
CEFTIBUTEN CAPSULES
US CLINICAL TRIALS IN ADULT PATIENTS

Incidence equal to or greater than 1%	↑BUN	4%
	↑Eosinophils	3%
	↓Hemoglobin	2%
	↑ALT (SGPT)	1%
	↑Bilirubin	1%
Incidence less than 1% but greater than 0.1%	↑Alk phosphatase	
	↑Creatinine	
	↑Platelets	
	↓Platelets	
	↓Leukocytes	
	↑AST (SGOT)	

*Changes in laboratory values with possible clinical significance regardless of whether or not the investigator thought that the change was due to drug toxicity.

CEDAX ORAL SUSPENSION (pediatric patients)

In clinical trials, 1152 pediatric patients (772 US and 380 international), 97% of whom were younger than 12 years of age, were treated with the recommended dose of ceftibuten (9 mg/kg once daily up to a maximum dose of 400 mg per day) for 10 days. There were no deaths, life-threatening adverse events, or permanent disabilities in any of the patients in these studies. Eight of 1152 (<1%) patients discontinued medication due to adverse events thought by the investigators to be possibly, probably, or almost certainly related to drug toxicity. The discontinuations were primarily (7 out of 8) for gastrointestinal disturbances, usually diarrhea or vomiting. One patient was discontinued due to a cutaneous rash thought possibly related to ceftibuten administration.
In the US trials, the following adverse events were thought by the investigators to be possibly, probably, or almost certainly related to ceftibuten oral suspension in multiple-dose clinical trials (n=772 ceftibuten-treated patients).

ADVERSE REACTIONS
CEFTIBUTEN ORAL SUSPENSION
US CLINCIAL TRIALS IN PEDIATRIC PATIENTS (n=772)

Incidence equal to or greater than 1%	Diarrhea*	4%
	Vomiting	2%
	Abdominal pain	2%
	Loose stools	2%
Incidence less than 1% but greater than 0.1%	Agitation	
	Anorexia	
	Dehydration	
	Diaper dermatitis	
	Dizziness	
	Dyspepsia	
	Fever	
	Headache	
	Hematuria	
	Hyperkinesia	
	Insomnia	
	Irritability	
	Nausea	
	Pruritus	
	Rash	
	Rigors	
	Urticaria	

*NOTE: The incidence of diarrhea in children ≤2 years old was 8% (23/301) compared with 2% (9/471) in children >2 years old.

LABORATORY VALUE CHANGES*
CEFTIBUTEN ORAL SUSPENSION
US CLINICAL TRIALS IN PEDIATRIC PATIENTS

Incidence equal to or greater than 1%	↑Eosinophils	3%
	↑BUN	2%
	↓Hemoglobin	1%
	↑Platelets	1%
Incidence less than 1% but greater than 0.1%	↑ALT (SGPT)	
	↑AST (SGOT)	
	↑Alk phosphatase	
	↑Bilirubin	
	↑Creatinine	

*Changes in laboratory values with possible clinical significance regardless of whether or not the investigator thought that the change was due to drug toxicity.

In Post-marketing Experience:
In addition to the events reported during clinical trials with ceftibuten, the following adverse experiences have been reported during worldwide post-marketing surveillance:
CEDAX CAPSULES: Aphasia, jaundice, psychosis, stridor, toxic epidermal necrolysis.
CEDAX ORAL SUSPENSION: Melena.

Cephalosporin-class Adverse Reactions:
In addition to the adverse reactions listed above that have been observed in patients treated with ceftibuten capsules, the following adverse events and altered laboratory tests have been reported for cephalosporin-class antibiotics:
allergic reactions, anaphylaxis, drug fever, Stevens-Johnson syndrome, renal dysfunction, toxic nephropathy, hepatic cholestasis, aplastic anemia, hemolytic anemia, hemorrhage, false-positive test for urinary glucose, neutropenia, pancytopenia, and agranulocytosis. Pseudomembranous colitis; onset of symptoms may occur during or after antibiotic treatment (see **WARNINGS**).
Several cephalosporins have been implicated in triggering seizures, particularly in patients with renal impairment when the dosage was not reduced (see **DOSAGE AND ADMINISTRATION** and **OVERDOSAGE**). If seizures associated with drug therapy occur, the drug should be discontinued. Anticonvulsant therapy can be given if clinically indicated.

OVERDOSAGE
Overdosage of cephalosporins can cause cerebral irritation leading to convulsions. Ceftibuten is readily dialyzable and significant quantities (65% of plasma concentrations) can be removed from the circulation by a single hemodialysis session. Information does not exist with regard to removal of ceftibuten by peritoneal dialysis.

DOSAGE AND ADMINISTRATION
The recommended doses of CEDAX Oral Suspension are presented in the table below. **CEDAX Suspension must be administered at least 2 hours before or 1 hour after a meal.**
[See first table at top right of page.]

Type of infection (as qualified in the INDICATIONS AND USAGE section of this labeling)	Daily Maximum Dose	Dose and Frequency	Duration
ADULTS (12 years of age and older): Acute Bacterial Exacerbations of Chronic Bronchitis due to *H. influenzae* (including β-lactamase-producing strains), *M. catarrhalis* (including β-lactamase-producing strains), or *Streptococcus pneumoniae* (penicillin-susceptible strains only). (See INDICATIONS AND USAGE—NOTE) Pharyngitis and tonsillitis due to *S. pyogenes*. Acute Bacterial Otitis Media due to *H. influenzae* (including β-lactamase-producing strains), *M. catarrhalis* (including β-lactamase-producing strains), or *S. pyogenes*. (See INDICATIONS AND USAGE—NOTE)	400 mg	400 mg QD	10 days
CHILDREN: Pharyngitis and tonsillitis due to *S. pyogenes*. Acute Bacterial Otitis Media due to *H. influenzae* (including β-lactamase-producing strains), and *M. catarrhalis* (including β-lactamase-producing strains), or *S. pyogenes*. (See INDICATIONS AND USAGE—NOTE)	400 mg	9 mg/kg QD	10 days

DIRECTIONS FOR MIXING CEDAX ORAL SUSPENSION

Final Concentration	Bottle Size	Amount of Water	Directions
90 mg per 5 mL	30 mL	Suspend in 28 mL of water	First tap the bottle to loosen powder. Then add water in two portions, shaking well after each aliquot.
	60 mL	Suspend in 53 mL of water	
	120 mL	Suspend in 103 mL of water	
180 mg per 5 mL	30 mL	Suspend in 28 mL of water	
	60 mL	Suspend in 53 mL of water	
	120 mL	Suspend in 103 mL of water	

CLINICAL AND BACTERIOLOGICAL OUTCOME
ACUTE BACTERIAL EXACERBATIONS OF CHRONIC BRONCHITIS

	Ceftibuten 400 mg QD	Control
Clinical Cure Rates	171/271 (63%)	147/216 (68%)

The 95% confidence interval around the difference in the means is (−14%, +4%).

Bacteriological Eradication Rates		
Haemophilus influenzae	45/62 (73%)	26/36 (72%)
H. parainfluenzae	10/10	4/6
Moraxella catarrhalis	33/46 (72%)	32/34 (94%)
Streptococcus pneumoniae	23/35 (66%)	14/20 (70%)

CLINICAL AND BACTERIOLOGICAL OUTCOME
ACUTE BACTERIAL OTITIS MEDIA

	Ceftibuten 9 mg/kg QD	Control
Clinical Cure Rates	266/365 (73%)	174/226 (77%)

The 95% confidence interval around the difference in the means is (−12%, +4%).

Bacteriological Eradication Rates		
Haemophilus influenzae	56/67 (81%)	29/38 (76%)
Moraxella catarrhalis	20/26 (77%)	13/17 (77%)
Streptococcus pneumoniae	68/105 (65%)	35/40 (88%)
Streptococcus pyogenes	13/15 (87%)	5/5

CEFTIBUTEN ORAL SUSPENSION PEDIATRIC DOSAGE CHART

CHILD'S WEIGHT		90 mg/5 mL	180 mg/5 mL
10 kg	22 lbs	1 tsp QD	1/2 tsp QD
20 kg	44 lbs	2 tsp QD	1 tsp QD
40 kg	88 lbs	4 tsp QD	2 tsp QD

Children weighing more than 45 kg should receive the maximum daily dose of 400 mg.

Renal Impairment:
CEDAX Capsules and CEDAX Oral Suspension may be administered at normal doses in the presence of impaired renal function with creatinine clearance of 50 mL/min or greater. The recommendations for dosing in patients with varying degrees of renal insufficiency are presented in the following table.

Creatinine Clearance (mL/min)	Recommended Dosing Schedules
>50	9 mg/kg or 400 mg Q24h (normal dosing schedule)
30–49	4.5 mg/kg or 200 mg Q24h
5–29	2.25 mg/kg or 100 mg Q24h

Hemodialysis Patients:
In patients undergoing hemodialysis two or three times weekly, a single 400-mg dose of ceftibuten capsules or a single dose of 9 mg/kg (maximum of 400 mg of ceftibuten) oral suspension may be administered at the end of each hemodialysis session.

Directions for Mixing CEDAX Oral Suspension:
[See second table above.]
After mixing, the suspension may be kept for 14 days and must be stored in the refrigerator. Keep tightly closed. Shake well before each use. Discard any unused portion after 14 days.

HOW SUPPLIED
CEDAX Capsules, containing 400 mg of ceftibuten (as ceftibuten dihydrate) are white, opaque capsules imprinted with the product name and strength, are available as follows:
20 Capsules/Bottle (NDC 0085-0691-01)
100 Capsules/Bottle (NDC 0085-0691-02)
Unit-dose dispensing (10 strips of 4 capsules each) (NDC 0085-0691-03)
Store the capsules between 2° and 25°C (36° and 77°F). Replace cap securely after each opening.
CEDAX Oral Suspension is an off-white to cream-colored powder that, when reconstituted as directed, contains either ceftibuten equivalent to 90 mg/5 mL or 180 mg/5 mL, supplied as follows: *Continued on next page*

Information on Schering products appearing on these pages is effective as of August 15, 1996.

Schering—Cont.

90 mg/5 mL
18 mg/mL 30-mL Bottle (NDC 0085-0777-03)
18 mg/mL 60-mL Bottle (NDC 0085-0777-01)
18 mg/mL 120-mL Bottle (NDC 0085-0777-02)
180 mg/5 mL
36 mg/mL 30-mL Bottle (NDC 0085-0834-03)
36 mg/mL 60-mL Bottle (NDC 0085-0834-01)
36 mg/mL 120-mL Bottle (NDC 0085-0834-02)
Prior to reconstitution, the powder must be stored between 2° and 25°C (36° and 77°F). Once it is reconstituted, the oral suspension is stable for 14 days when stored in the refrigerator between 2° and 8°C (36° and 46°F).

CLINICAL STUDIES

Acute Bacterial Exacerbations of Chronic Bronchitis:
Three clinical trials (two domestic, the third abroad) have been conducted testing ceftibuten in the treatment of acute exacerbations of chronic bronchitis (AECB). Overall, the clinical outcome among patients who had signs and symptoms of AECB, who had a gram stain showing a predominance of PMNs and few epithelial cells, and who were evaluated at approximately 1 to 2 weeks after completing therapy is presented in the table below. The bacterial eradication rates of specific pathogens from these three trials are also presented:
[See third table at top right of preceding page.]
Acute Bacterial Otitis Media:
Four clinical trials (three domestic, the fourth abroad) have been conducted testing ceftibuten in the treatment of acute bacterial otitis media. Overall, the clinical outcome among patients who had signs and symptoms of acute bacterial otitis media and who were evaluated approximately 1 to 2 weeks after completing therapy is presented in the table below. Tympanocentesis was performed on patients in three of the above-mentioned studies; the bacterial eradication rates of specific pathogens from these three trials are also presented:
[See fourth table at top right of preceding page.]

REFERENCES

1. National Committee for Clinical Laboratory Standards. Methods for Dilution Antimicrobial Susceptibility Tests for Bacteria that Grow Aerobically—Third Edition. Approved Standard NCCLS Document M7-A3, Vol. 13, No. 25, NCCLS, Villanova, PA. December, 1993.
2. National Committee for Clinical Laboratory Standards. Performance Standards for Antimicrobial Disk Susceptibility Tests—Fifth Edition. Approved Standard NCCLS Document M2-A5, Vol. 13, No. 24, NCCLS, Villanova, PA. December, 1993.

Schering Corporation
Kenilworth, NJ 07033 USA
Copyright © 1995, Schering Corporation.
All rights reserved.
11/95

18890909T
Shown in Product Identification Guide, page 334

CELESTONE® SOLUSPAN®*   ℞

brand of
sterile betamethasone sodium
phosphate and betamethasone
acetate Suspension, USP
6 mg per mL
*brand of rapid and repository injectable.

DESCRIPTION

Each mL of CELESTONE SOLUSPAN* Suspension contains: 3.0 mg betamethasone as betamethasone sodium phosphate; 3.0 mg betamethasone acetate; 7.1 mg dibasic sodium phosphate; 3.4 mg monobasic sodium phosphate; 0.1 mg edetate disodium; and 0.2 mg benzalkonium chloride. It is a sterile, aqueous suspension with a pH between 6.8 and 7.2. The formula for betamethasone sodium phosphate is $C_{22}H_{28}FNa_2O_8P$ with a molecular weight of 516.41. Chemically it is 9-Fluoro-11β,17,21-trihydroxy-16β-methylpregna-1,4-diene-3,20-dione 21-(disodium phosphate).
The formula for betamethasone acetate is $C_{24}H_{31}FO_6$ with a molecular weight of 434.50. Chemically it is 9-Fluoro-11β,17,21-trihydroxy-16β-methylpregna-1,4-diene-3,20-dione 21-acetate.
The chemical structures for betamethasone sodium phosphate and betamethasone acetate are as follows:

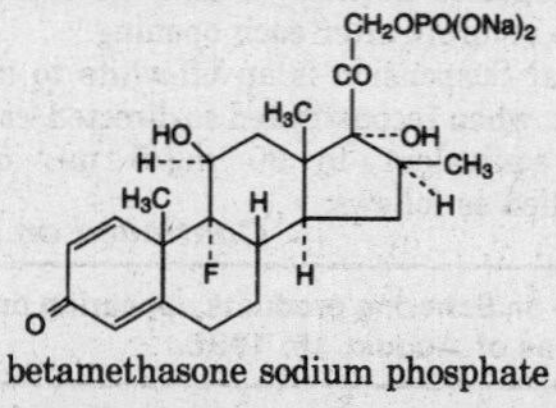

betamethasone sodium phosphate

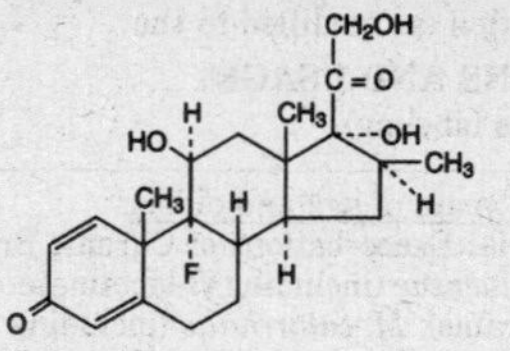

betamethasone acetate

Betamethasone sodium phosphate is a white to practically white, odorless powder, and is hygroscopic. It is freely soluble in water and in methanol, but is practically insoluble in acetone and in chloroform.
Betamethasone acetate is a white to creamy white, odorless powder that sinters and resolidifies at about 165°C, and remelts at about 200°C–220°C with decomposition. It is practically insoluble in water, but freely soluble in acetone, and is soluble in alcohol and in chloroform.

ACTIONS

Naturally occurring glucocorticoids (hydrocortisone), which also have salt-retaining properties, are used as replacement therapy in adrenocortical deficiency states. Their synthetic analogs are primarily used for their potent anti-inflammatory effects in disorders of many organ systems.
Betamethasone sodium phosphate, a soluble ester, provides prompt activity, while betamethasone acetate is only slightly soluble and affords sustained activity.
Glucocorticoids cause profound and varied metabolic effects. In addition, they modify the body's immune responses to diverse stimuli.

INDICATIONS

When oral therapy is not feasible and the strength, dosage form, and route of administration of the drug reasonably lend the preparation to the treatment of the condition, CELESTONE SOLUSPAN Suspension for intramuscular use is indicated as follows:

Endocrine disorders: Primary or secondary adrenocortical insufficiency (hydrocortisone or cortisone is the drug of choice; synthetic analogs may be used in conjunction with mineralocorticoids where applicable; in infancy mineralocorticoid supplementation is of particular importance). Acute adrenocortical insufficiency (hydrocortisone or cortisone is the drug of choice; mineralocorticoid supplementation may be necessary, particularly when synthetic analogs are used); preoperatively and in the event of serious trauma or illness, in patients with known adrenal insufficiency or when adrenocortical reserve is doubtful; shock unresponsive to conventional therapy if adrenocortical insufficiency exists or is suspected; congenital adrenal hyperplasia; nonsuppurative thyroiditis; hypercalcemia associated with cancer.

Rheumatic disorders: As adjunctive therapy for short-term administration (to tide the patient over an acute episode or exacerbation) in: post-traumatic osteoarthritis; synovitis of osteoarthritis; rheumatoid arthritis, including juvenile rheumatoid arthritis (selected cases may require low-dose maintenance therapy); acute and subacute bursitis; epicondylitis; acute non-specific tenosynovitis; acute gouty arthritis; psoriatic arthritis; ankylosing spondylitis.

Collagen diseases: During an exacerbation or as maintenance therapy in selected cases of systemic lupus erythematosus, acute rheumatic carditis.

Dermatologic diseases: Pemphigus, severe erythema multiforme (Stevens-Johnson syndrome), exfoliative dermatitis, bullous dermatitis herpetiformis, severe seborrheic dermatitis, severe psoriasis, mycosis fungoides.

Allergic states: Control of severe or incapacitating allergic conditions intractable to adequate trials of conventional treatment in: bronchial asthma, contact dermatitis, atopic dermatitis, serum sickness, seasonal or perennial allergic rhinitis, drug hypersensitivity reactions, urticarial transfusion reactions, acute noninfectious laryngeal edema (epinephrine is the drug of first choice).

Ophthalmic diseases: Severe acute and chronic allergic and inflammatory processes involving the eye, such as: herpes zoster ophthalmicus, iritis and iridocyclitis, chorioretinitis, diffuse posterior uveitis and choroiditis, optic neuritis, sympathetic ophthalmia, anterior segment inflammation, allergic conjunctivitis, allergic corneal marginal ulcers, keratitis.

Gastrointestinal diseases: To tide the patient over a critical period of disease in: ulcerative colitis—(systemic therapy), regional enteritis—(systemic therapy).

Respiratory diseases: Symptomatic sarcoidosis, berylliosis, fulminating or disseminated pulmonary tuberculosis when used concurrently with appropriate antituberculous chemotherapy, Loeffler's syndrome not manageable by other means, aspiration pneumonitis.

Hematologic disorders: Acquired (autoimmune) hemolytic anemia, secondary thrombocytopenia in adults, erythroblastopenia (RBC anemia), congenital (erythroid) hypoplastic anemia.

Neoplastic diseases: For palliative management of: leukemias and lymphomas in adults, acute leukemia of childhood.

Edematous states: To induce diuresis or remission of proteinuria in the nephrotic syndrome, without uremia, of the idiopathic type or that due to lupus erythematosus.

Miscellaneous: Tuberculous meningitis with subarachnoid block or impending block when used concurrently with appropriate antituberculous chemotherapy, trichinosis with neurologic or myocardial involvement.
When the strength and dosage form of the drug lend the preparation to the treatment of the condition, the **intra-articular or soft tissue administration** of CELESTONE SOLUSPAN Suspension is indicated as adjunctive therapy for short-term administration (to tide the patient over an acute episode or exacerbation) in: synovitis of osteoarthritis, rheumatoid arthritis, acute and subacute bursitis, acute gouty arthritis, epicondylitis, acute nonspecific tenosynovitis, post-traumatic osteoarthritis.
When the strength and dosage form of the drug lend the preparation to the treatment of the condition, the **intralesional administration** of CELESTONE SOLUSPAN Suspension is indicated for: keloids; localized hypertrophic, infiltrated, inflammatory lesions of: lichen planus, psoriatic plaques, granuloma annulare, and lichen simplex chronicus (neurodermatitis); discoid lupus erythematosus; necrobiosis lipoidica diabeticorum; alopecia areata.
CELESTONE SOLUSPAN Suspension may also be useful in cystic tumors of an aponeurosis or tendon (ganglia).

CONTRAINDICATIONS

CELESTONE SOLUSPAN Suspension is contraindicated in systemic fungal infections.

WARNINGS

CELESTONE SOLUSPAN Suspension should <u>not</u> be administered intravenously.
In patients on corticosteroid therapy subjected to any unusual stress, increased dosage of rapidly acting corticosteroids before, during, and after the stressful situation is indicated.
Corticosteroids may mask some signs of infection, and new infections may appear during their use. There may be decreased resistance and inability to localize infection when corticosteroids are used.
Prolonged use of corticosteroids may produce posterior subcapsular cataracts, glaucoma with possible damage to the optic nerves, and may enhance the establishment of secondary ocular infections due to fungi or viruses.
CELESTONE SOLUSPAN Suspension contains two betamethasone esters one of which, betamethasone sodium phosphate, disappears rapidly from the injection site. The potential for systemic effect produced by the soluble portion of CELESTONE SOLUSPAN Suspension should therefore be taken into account by the physician when using the drug.
Average and large doses of cortisone or hydrocortisone can cause elevation of blood pressure, salt and water retention, and increased excretion of potassium. These effects are less likely to occur with the synthetic derivatives except when used in large doses. Dietary salt restriction and potassium supplementation may be necessary. All corticosteroids increase calcium excretion.
While on corticosteroid therapy patients should not be vaccinated against smallpox. Other immunization procedures should not be undertaken in patients who are on corticosteroids, especially in high doses, because of possible hazards of neurological complications and lack of antibody response.
Persons who are on drugs which suppress the immune system are more susceptible to infections than healthy individuals. Chickenpox and measles, for example, can have a more serious or even fatal course in non-immune children or adults on corticosteroids. In such children, or adults who have not had these diseases, particular care should be taken to avoid exposure. How the dose, route, and duration of corticosteroid administration affects the risk of developing a disseminated infection is not known. The contribution of the underlying disease and/or prior corticosteroid treatment to the risk is also not known. If exposed to chickenpox, prophylaxis with varicella-zoster immune globulin (VZIG) may be indicated. If exposed to measles, prophylaxis with pooled intramuscular immunoglobulin (IG) may be indicated. (See the respective package inserts for complete VZIG and IG prescribing information.) If chickenpox develops, treatment with antiviral agents may be considered.
Similarly, corticosteroids should be used with great care in patients with known or suspected *Strongyloides* (threadworm) infestation. In such patients, corticosteroid-induced

immunosuppression may lead to *Strongyloides* hyperinfection and dissemination with widespread larval migration, often accompanied by severe enterocolitis and potentially fatal gram-negative septicemia.
The use of CELESTONE SOLUSPAN Suspension in active tuberculosis should be restricted to those cases of fulminating or disseminated tuberculosis in which the corticosteroid is used for the management of the disease in conjunction with appropriate antituberculous regimen.
If corticosteroids are indicated in patients with latent tuberculosis or tuberculin reactivity, close observation is necessary as reactivation of the disease may occur. During prolonged corticosteroid therapy, these patients should receive chemoprophylaxis.
Because rare instances of anaphylactoid reactions have occurred in patients receiving parenteral corticosteroid therapy, appropriate precautionary measures should be taken prior to administration, especially when the patient has a history of allergy to any drug.
Usage in pregnancy: Since adequate human reproduction studies have not been done with corticosteroids, the use of these drugs in pregnancy, nursing mothers, or women of childbearing potential requires that the possible benefits of the drug be weighed against the potential hazards to the mother and embryo or fetus. Infants born of mothers who have received substantial doses of corticosteroids during pregnancy should be carefully observed for signs of hypoadrenalism.

PRECAUTIONS

Information for Patients: Persons who are on immunosuppressant doses of corticosteroids should be warned to avoid exposure to chickenpox or measles. Patients should also be advised that if they are exposed, medical advice should be sought without delay.
General: Drug-induced secondary adrenocortical insufficiency may be minimized by gradual reduction of dosage. This type of relative insufficiency may persist for months after discontinuation of therapy; therefore, in any situation of stress occurring during that period, hormone therapy should be reinstituted. Since mineralocorticoid secretion may be impaired, salt and/or a mineralocorticoid should be administered concurrently.
There is an enhanced effect of corticosteroids in patients with hypothyroidism and in those with cirrhosis.
Corticosteroids should be used cautiously in patients with ocular herpes simplex for fear of corneal perforation.
The lowest possible dose of corticosteroid should be used to control the condition under treatment, and when reduction in dosage is possible, the reduction must be gradual.
Psychic derangements may appear when corticosteroids are used, ranging from euphoria, insomnia, mood swings, personality changes, and severe depression to frank psychotic manifestations. Also, existing emotional instability or psychotic tendencies may be aggravated by corticosteroids.
Aspirin should be used cautiously in conjunction with corticosteroids in hypoprothrombinemia.
Steroids should be used with caution in nonspecific ulcerative colitis, if there is a probability of impending perforation, abscess or other pyogenic infection, also in diverticulitis, fresh intestinal anastomoses, active or latent peptic ulcer, renal insufficiency, hypertension, osteoporosis, and myasthenia gravis.
Growth and development of infants and children on prolonged corticosteroid therapy should be carefully followed.
The following additional precautions also apply for parenteral corticosteroids. **Intra-articular injection of a corticosteroid may produce systemic as well as local effects.**
Appropriate examination of any joint fluid present is necessary to exclude a septic process.
A marked increase in pain accompanied by local swelling, further restriction of joint motion, fever, and malaise are suggestive of septic arthritis. If this complication occurs and the diagnosis of sepsis is confirmed, appropriate antimicrobial therapy should be instituted.
Local injection of a steroid into a previously infected joint is to be avoided.
Corticosteroids should not be injected into unstable joints.
The slower rate of absorption by intramuscular administration should be recognized.

ADVERSE REACTIONS

Fluid and electrolyte disturbances: sodium retention, fluid retention, congestive heart failure in susceptible patients, potassium loss, hypokalemic alkalosis, hypertension.
Musculoskeletal: muscle weakness, steroid myopathy, loss of muscle mass, osteoporosis, vertebral compression fractures, aseptic necrosis of femoral and humeral heads, pathologic fracture of long bones.
Gastrointestinal: peptic ulcer with possible subsequent perforation and hemorrhage, pancreatitis, abdominal distention, ulcerative esophagitis.
Dermatologic: impaired wound healing, thin fragile skin, petechiae and ecchymoses, facial erythema, increased sweating, may suppress reactions to skin tests.
Neurological: convulsions, increased intracranial pressure with papilledema (pseudotumor cerebri) usually after treatment, vertigo, headache.
Endocrine: menstrual irregularities; development of cushingoid state; suppression of growth in children; secondary adrenocortical and pituitary unresponsiveness, particularly in times of stress, as in trauma, surgery, or illness: decreased carbohydrate tolerance; manifestations of latent diabetes mellitus; increased requirements for insulin or oral hypoglycemic agents in diabetics.
Ophthalmic: posterior subcabsular cataracts, increased intraocular pressure, glaucoma, exophthalmos.
Metabolic: negative nitrogen balance due to protein catabolism.
The following *additional* adverse reactions are related to parenteral corticosteroid therapy: rare instances of blindness associated with intralesional therapy around the face and head, hyperpigmentation or hypopigmentation, subcutaneous and cutaneous atrophy, sterile abscess, post-injection flare (following intra-articular use), charcot-like arthropathy.

DOSAGE AND ADMINISTRATION

The initial dosage of CELESTONE SOLUSPAN Suspension may vary from 0.5 to 9.0 mg per day depending on the specific disease entity being treated. In situations of less severity, lower doses will generally suffice while in selected patients higher initial doses may be required. Usually the parenteral dosage ranges are one-third to one-half the oral dose given every 12 hours. However, in certain overwhelming, acute, life-threatening situations, administration in dosages exceeding the usual dosages may be justified and may be in multiples of the oral dosages.
The initial dosage should be maintained or adjusted until a satisfactory response is noted. If after a reasonable period of time there is a lack of satisfactory clinical response, CELESTONE SOLUSPAN Suspension should be discontinued and the patient transferred to other appropriate therapy. *It Should Be Emphasized That Dosage Requirements Are Variable and Must Be Individualized on the Basis of the Disease Under Treatment and the Response of the Patient.* After a favorable response is noted, the proper maintenance dosage should be determined by decreasing the initial drug dosage in small decrements at appropriate time intervals until the lowest dosage which will maintain an adequate clinical response is reached. It should be kept in mind that constant monitoring is needed in regard to drug dosage. Included in the situations which may make dosage adjustments necessary are changes in clinical status secondary to remissions or exacerbations in the disease process, the patient's individual drug responsiveness, and the effect of patient exposure to stressful situations not directly related to the disease entity under treatment; in this latter situation it may be necessary to increase the dosage of CELESTONE SOLUSPAN Suspension for a period of time consistent with the patient's condition. If after long-term therapy the drug is to be stopped, it is recommended that it be withdrawn gradually rather than abruptly.
If coadministration of a local anesthetic is desired, CELESTONE SOLUSPAN Suspension may be mixed with 1% or 2% lidocaine hydrochloride, using the formuations which do not contain parabens. Similar local anesthetics may also be used. Diluents containing methylparaben, propylparaben, phenol, etc., should be avoided since these compounds may cause flocculation of the steroid. The required dose of CELESTONE SOLUSPAN Suspension is first withdrawn from the vial into the syringe. The local anesthetic is then drawn in, and the syringe shaken briefly. **Do not inject local anesthetics into the vial of CELESTONE SOLUSPAN Suspension.**
Bursitis, tenosynovitis, peritendinitis. In acute subdeltoid, subacromial, olecranon, and prepatellar bursitis, one intrabursal injection of 1.0 mL CELESTONE SOLUSPAN Suspension can relieve pain and restore full range of movement. Several intrabursal injections of corticosteroids are usually required in recurrent acute bursitis and in acute exacerbations of chronic bursitis. Partial relief of pain and some increase in mobility can be expected in both conditions after one or two injections. Chronic bursitis may be treated with reduced dosage once the acute condition is controlled. In tenosynovitis and tendinitis, three or four local injections at intervals of 1 to 2 weeks between injections are given in most cases. Injections should be made into the affected tendon sheaths rather than into the tendons themselves. In ganglions of joint capsules and tendon sheaths, injection of 0.5 mL directly into the ganglion cysts has produced marked reduction in the size of the lesions.
Rheumatoid arthritis and osteoarthritis. Following intra-articular administration of 0.5 to 2.0 mL of CELESTONE SOLUSPAN Suspension, relief of pain, soreness, and stiffness may be experienced. Duration of relief varies widely in both diseases. Intra-articular Injection—CELESTONE SOLUSPAN Suspension is well tolerated in joints and periarticular tissues. There is virtually no pain on injection, and the "secondary flare" that sometimes occurs a few hours after intra-articular injection of corticosteroids has not been reported with CELESTONE SOLUSPAN Suspension. Using sterile technique, a 20- to 24-gauge needle on an empty syringe is inserted into the synovial cavity, and a few drops of synovial fluid are withdrawn to confirm that the needle is in the joint. The aspirating syringe is replaced by a syringe containing CELESTONE SOLUSPAN Suspension and injection is then made into the joint.

Recommended Doses for Intra-articular Injection

Size of joint	Location	Dose (mL)
Very Large	Hip	1.0–2.0
Large	Knee, Ankle, Shoulder	1.0
Medium	Elbow, Wrist	0.5–1.0
Small (Metacarpophalangeal, interphalangeal) (Sternoclavicular)	Hand Chest	0.25–0.5

A portion of the administered dose of CELESTONE SOLUSPAN Suspension is absorbed systemically following intra-articular injection. In patients being treated concomitantly with oral or parenteral corticosteroids, especially those receiving large doses, the systemic absorption of the drug should be considered in determining intra-articular dosage.
Dermatologic conditions. In intralesional treatment, 0.2 mL/sq cm of CELESTONE SOLUSPAN Suspension is injected intradermally (not subcutaneously) using a tuberculin syringe with a 25-gauge, 1/2-inch needle. Care should be taken to deposit a uniform depot of medication intradermally. A total of no more than 1.0 mL at weekly intervals is recommended.
Disorders of the foot. A tuberculin syringe with a 25-gauge, 3/4-inch needle is suitable for most injections into the foot. The following doses are recommended at intervals of 3 days to a week.

Diagnosis	CELESTONE SOLUSPAN Suspension Dose (mL)
Bursitis	
under heloma durum or heloma molle	0.25–0.5
under calcaneal spur	0.5
over hallux rigidus or digiti quinti varus	0.5
Tenosynovitis, periostitis of cuboid	0.5
Acute gouty arthritis	0.5–1.0

HOW SUPPLIED

CELESTONE SOLUSPAN Suspension, 5 mL multiple-dose vial; box of one (NDC 0085-0566-05).
Shake well before using.
Store between 2° and 25°C (36° and 77°F).
Protect from light.
Schering Corporation
Kenilworth, NJ 07033
Copyright © 1969, 1993, 1994, 1995, Schering Corporation. All rights reserved.
Rev. 10/95 10229782

CLARITIN® ℞
brand of loratadine
TABLETS
Long-Acting Antihistamine

DESCRIPTION

CLARITIN Tablets contain 10 mg micronized loratadine, an antihistamine, to be administered orally. They also contain the following inactive ingredients: corn starch, lactose, and magnesium stearate.
Loratadine is a white to off-white powder not soluble in water, but very soluble in acetone, alcohol, and chloroform. It has a molecular weight of 382.89, and empirical formula of $C_{22}H_{23}ClN_2O_2$; its chemical name is ethyl 4-(8-chloro-5,6-dihydro-11*H*-benzo[5,6]cyclohepta[1,2-*b*]pyridin-11-ylidene)-1-piperidinecarboxylate and has the following structural formula:

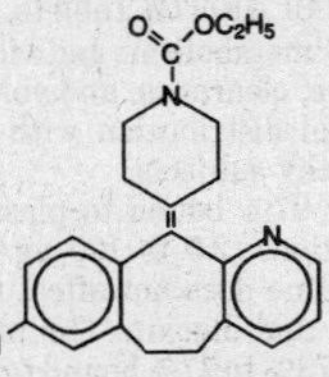

Continued on next page

Information on Schering products appearing on these pages is effective as of August 15, 1996.

Schering—Cont.

CLINICAL PHARMACOLOGY

Loratadine is a long-acting tricyclic antihistamine with selective peripheral histamine H_1-receptor antagonistic activity.

Human histamine skin wheal studies following single and repeated 10 mg oral doses of CLARITIN Tablets have shown that the drug exhibits an antihistaminic effect beginning within 1 to 3 hours, reaching a maximum at 8 to 12 hours and lasting in excess of 24 hours. There was no evidence of tolerance to this effect after 28 days of dosing with CLARITIN Tablets.

Pharmacokinetic studies following single and multiple oral doses of loratadine in 115 volunteers showed that loratadine is rapidly absorbed and extensively metabolized to an active metabolite (descarboethoxyloratadine). Approximately 80% of the total dose administered can be found equally distributed between urine and feces in the form of metabolic products after 10 days. The mean elimination half-lives found in studies in normal adult subjects (n=54) were 8.4 hours (range=3 to 20 hours) for loratadine and 28 hours (range=8.8 to 92 hours) for the major active metabolite (descarboethoxyloratadine). In nearly all patients, exposure (AUC) to the metabolite is greater than exposure to parent loratadine. Loratadine and descarboethoxyloratadine reached steady-state in most patients by approximately the fifth dosing day. The pharmacokinetics of loratadine and descarboethoxyloratadine are dose independent over the dose range of 10 to 40 mg and are not significantly altered by the duration of treatment.

In vitro studies with human liver microsomes indicate that loratadine is metabolized to descarboethoxyloratadine predominantly by P450 CYP3A4 and, to a lesser extent, by P450 CYP2D6. In the presence of a CYP3A4 inhibitor ketoconazole, loratadine is metabolized to descarboethoxyloratadine predominantly by CYP2D6. Concurrent administration of loratadine with either ketoconazole, erythromycin (both CYP3A4 inhibitors), or cimetidine (CYP2D6 and CYP3A4 inhibitor) to healthy volunteers was associated with significantly increased plasma concentrations of loratadine (see **Drug Interactions** section).

In a study involving twelve healthy geriatric subjects (66 to 78 years old), the AUC and peak plasma levels (Cmax) of both loratadine and descarboethoxyloratadine were significantly higher (approximately 50% increased) than in studies of younger subjects. The mean elimination half-lives for the elderly subjects were 18.2 hours (range=6.7 to 37 hours) for loratadine and 17.5 hours (range=11 to 38 hours) for the active metabolite.

In the clinical efficacy studies, CLARITIN Tablets were administered before meals. In a single-dose study, food increased the AUC of loratadine by approximately 40% and of descarboethoxyloratadine by approximately 15%. The time to peak plasma concentration (Tmax) of loratadine and descarboethoxyloratadine was delayed by 1 hour with a meal.

In patients with chronic renal impairment (creatinine clearance ≤30 mL/min) both the AUC and peak plasma levels (Cmax) increased on average by approximately 73% for loratadine; and approximately by 120% for descarboethoxyloratadine, compared to individuals with normal renal function. The mean elimination half-lives of loratadine (7.6 hours) and descarboethoxyloratadine (23.9 hours) were not significantly different from that observed in normal subjects. Hemodialysis does not have an effect on the pharmacokinetics of loratadine or its active metabolite (descarboethoxyloratadine) in subjects with chronic renal impairment.

In patients with chronic alcoholic liver disease the AUC and peak plasma levels (Cmax) of loratadine were double while the pharmacokinetic profile of the active metabolite (descarboethoxyloratadine) was not significantly changed from that in normals. The elimination half-lives for loratadine and descarboethoxyloratadine were 24 hours and 37 hours, respectively, and increased with increasing severity of liver disease.

There was considerable variability in the pharmacokinetic data in all studies of CLARITIN Tablets, probably due to the extensive first-pass metabolism. Individual histograms of area under the curve, clearance, and volume of distribution showed a log normal distribution with a 25-fold range in distribution in healthy subjects.

Loratadine is about 97% bound to plasma proteins at the expected concentrations (2.5 to 100 ng/mL) after a therapeutic dose. Loratadine does not affect the plasma protein binding of warfarin and digoxin. The metabolite descarboethoxyloratadine is 73% to 77% bound to plasma proteins (at 0.5 to 100 ng/mL).

Whole body autoradiographic studies in rats and monkeys, radiolabeled tissue distribution studies in mice and rats, and *in vivo* radioligand studies in mice have shown that neither loratadine nor its metabolites readily cross the blood-brain barrier. Radioligand binding studies with guinea pig pulmonary and brain H_1-receptors indicate that there was preferential binding to peripheral versus central nervous system H_1-receptors.

Clinical trials of CLARITIN Tablets involved over 10,700 patients who received either CLARITIN Tablets or another anithistamine and/or placebo in double-blind randomized controlled studies. In placebo-controlled trials, 10 mg once daily of CLARITIN Tablets was superior to placebo and similar to clemastine (1 mg BID) or terfenadine (60 mg BID) in effects on nasal and non-nasal symptoms of allergic rhinitis. In these studies, somnolence occurred less frequently with CLARITIN Tablets than with clemastine and at about the same frequency as terfenadine or placebo. In studies with CLARITIN Tablets at doses 2 to 4 times higher than the recommended dose of 10 mg, a dose-related increase in the incidence of somnolence was observed. Therefore, some patients, particularly those with hepatic or renal impairment and the elderly, may experience somnolence.

Among those patients involved in double-blind, randomized controlled studies of CLARITIN Tablets, approximately 1000 patients were enrolled in studies of idiopathic chronic urticaria. In placebo-controlled clinical trials, CLARITIN Tablets 10 mg once daily were superior to placebo in the management of idiopathic chronic urticaria, as demonstrated by reduction of associated itching, erythema, and hives. In these studies, the incidence of somnolence seen with CLARITIN Tablets was similar to that seen with placebo.

In a study in which CLARITIN Tablets were administered at 4 times the clinical dose for 90 days, no clinically significant increase in the QT_c was seen on ECGs.

INDICATIONS AND USAGE

CLARITIN Tablets are indicated for the relief of nasal and non-nasal symptoms of seasonal allergic rhinitis and for the management of idiopathic chronic urticaria.

CONTRAINDICATIONS

CLARITIN Tablets are contraindicated in patients who are hypersensitive to this medication or to any of its ingredients.

PRECAUTIONS

General: Patients with liver impairment or renal insufficiency (GFR <30 mL/min) should be given a lower initial dose (10 mg every other day) because they have reduced clearance of CLARITIN Tablets.

Drug Interactions: Loratadine (10 mg once daily) has been safely coadministered with therapeutic doses of erythromycin, cimetidine, and ketoconazole in controlled clinical pharmacology studies. Although increased plasma concentrations (AUC 0–24 hrs) of loratadine and/or descarboethoxyloratadine were observed following coadministration of loratadine with each of these drugs in normal volunteers (n=24 in each study), there were no clinically relevant changes in the safety profile of loratadine, as assessed by electrocardiographic parameters, clinical laboratory tests, vital signs, and adverse events. There were no significant effects on QT_c intervals, and no reports of sedation or syncope. No effects on plasma concentrations of cimetidine or ketoconazole were observed. Plasma concentrations (AUC 0–24 hrs) of erythromycin decreased 15% with coadministration of loratadine relative to that observed with erythromycin alone. The clinical relevance of this difference is unknown. These above findings are summarized in the following table:

Effects on Plasma Concentrations (AUC 0–24 hrs) of Loratadine and Descarboethoxyloratadine After 10 Days of Coadministration (Loratadine 10 mg) in Normal Volunteers

	Loratadine	Descarboethoxyloratadine
Erythromycin (500 mg Q8h)	+ 40%	+46%
Cimetidine (300 mg QID)	+103%	+ 6%
Ketoconazole (200 mg Q12h)	+307%	+73%

There does not appear to be an increase in adverse events in subjects who received oral contraceptives and loratadine.

Carcinogenesis, Mutagenesis, and Impairment of Fertility: In an 18-month oncogenicity study in mice and a 2-year study in rats, loratadine was administered in the diet at doses up to 40 mg/kg (mice) and 25 mg/kg (rats). In the carcinogenicity studies, pharmacokinetic assessments were carried out to determine animal exposure to the drug. AUC data demonstrated that the exposure of mice given 40 mg/kg of loratadine was 3.6 (loratadine) and 18 (active metabolite) times higher than a human given 10 mg/day. Exposure of rats given 25 mg/kg of loratadine was 28 (loratadine) and 67 (active metabolite) times higher than a human given 10 mg/day. Male mice given 40 mg/kg had a significantly higher incidence of hepatocellular tumors (combined adenomas and carcinomas) than concurrent controls. In rats, a significantly higher incidence of hepatocellular tumors (combined adenomas and carcinomas) was observed in males given 10 mg/kg and males and females given 25 mg/kg. The clinical significance of these findings during long-term use of CLARITIN Tablets is not known.

In mutagenicity studies, there was no evidence of mutagenic potential in reverse (Ames) or forward point mutation (CHO-HGPRT) assays, or in the assay for DNA damage (Rat Primary Hepatocyte Unscheduled DNA Assay) or in two assays for chromosomal aberrations (Human Peripheral Blood Lymphocyte Clastogenesis Assay and the Mouse Bone Marrow Erythrocyte Micronucleus Assay). In the Mouse Lymphoma Assay, a positive finding occurred in the nonactivated but not the activated phase of the study.

Loratadine administration produced hepatic microsomal enzyme induction in the mouse at 40 mg/kg and rat at 25 mg/kg, but not at lower doses.

Decreased fertility in male rats, shown by lower female conception rates, occurred at approximately 64 mg/kg and was reversible with cessation of dosing. Loratadine had no effect on male or female fertility or reproduction in the rat at doses of approximately 24 mg/kg.

Pregnancy Category B: There was no evidence of animal teratogenicity in studies performed in rats and rabbits at oral doses up to 96 mg/kg (75 times and 150 times, respectively, the recommended daily human dose on a mg/m^2 basis). There are, however, no adequate and well-controlled studies in pregnant women. Because animal reproduction studies are not always predictive of human response, CLARITIN Tablets should be used during pregnancy only if clearly needed.

Nursing Mothers: Loratadine and its metabolite, descarboethoxyloratadine, pass easily into breast milk and achieve concentrations that are equivalent to plasma levels with an AUC_{milk}/AUC_{plasma} ratio of 1.17 and 0.85 for the parent and active metabolite, respectively. Following a single oral dose of 40 mg, a small amount of loratadine and metabolite was excreted into the breast milk (approximately 0.03% of 40 mg over 48 hours). A decision should be made whether to discontinue nursing or to discontinue the drug, taking into account the importance of the drug to the mother. Caution should be exercised when CLARITIN Tablets are administered to a nursing woman.

Pediatric Use: Safety and effectiveness in children below the age of 12 years have not been established.

ADVERSE REACTIONS

Approximately 90,000 patients received CLARITIN Tablets 10 mg once daily in controlled and uncontrolled studies. Placebo-controlled clincial trials at the recommended dose of 10 mg once a day varied from 2 weeks' to 6 months' duration. The rate of premature withdrawal from these trials was approximately 2% in both the treated and placebo groups. [See table below.]

Adverse events reported in placebo-controlled idiopathic chronic urticaria trials were similar to those reported in allergic rhinitis studies.

Adverse event rates did not appear to differ significantly based on age, sex, or race, although the number of non-white subjects was relatively small.

In addition to those adverse events reported above, the following adverse events have been reported in 2% or fewer patients.

Autonomic Nervous System: Altered lacrimation, altered salivation, flushing, hypoesthesia, impotence, increased sweating, thirst.

Body As A Whole: Angioneurotic edema, asthenia, back pain, blurred vision, chest pain, conjunctivitis, earache, eye pain, fever, leg cramps, malaise, rigors, tinnitus, upper respiratory infection, weight gain.

REPORTED ADVERSE EVENTS WITH AN INCIDENCE OF MORE THAN 2% IN PLACEBO-CONTROLLED ALLERGIC RHINITIS CLINICAL TRIALS
PERCENT OF PATIENTS REPORTING

	LORATADINE 10 mg QD n=1926	PLACEBO n=2545	CLEMASTINE 1 mg BID n=536	TERFENADINE 60 mg BID n=684
Headache	12	11	8	8
Somnolence	8	6	22	9
Fatigue	4	3	10	2
Dry Mouth	3	2	4	3

Cardiovascular System: Hypertension, hypotension, palpitations, syncope, tachycardia.
Central and Peripheral Nervous System: Blepharospasm, dizziness, dysphonia, hyperkinesia, migraine, paresthesia, tremor, vertigo.
Gastrointestinal System: Abdominal distress, altered taste, anorexia, constipation, diarrhea, dyspepsia, flatulence, gastritis, increased appetite, nausea, stomatitis, toothache, vomiting.
Musculoskeletal System: Arthralgia, myalgia.
Psychiatric: Agitation, amnesia, anxiety, confusion, decreased libido, depression, impaired concentration, insomnia, nervousness, paroniria.
Reproductive System: Breast pain, dysmenorrhea, menorrhagia, vaginitis.
Respiratory System: Bronchitis, bronchospasm, coughing, dyspnea, epistaxis, hemoptysis, laryngitis, nasal congestion, nasal dryness, pharyngitis, sinusitis, sneezing.
Skin and Appendages: Dermatitis, dry hair, dry skin, photosensitivity reaction, pruritus, purpura, rash, urticaria.
Urinary System: Altered micturition, urinary discoloration.
In addition, the following spontaneous adverse events have been reported rarely during the marketing of loratadine: abnormal hepatic function, including jaundice, hepatitis, and hepatic necrosis; alopecia; anaphylaxis; breast enlargement; erythema multiforme; peripheral edema; seizures; and supraventricular tachyarrhythmias.

DRUG ABUSE AND DEPENDENCE

There is no information to indicate that abuse or dependency occurs with CLARITIN Tablets.

OVERDOSAGE

Somnolence, tachycardia, and headache have been reported with overdoses greater than 10 mg (40 to 180 mg). In the event of overdosage, general symptomatic and supportive measures should be instituted promptly and maintained for as long as necessary.
Treatment of overdosage would reasonably consist of emesis (ipecac syrup), except in patients with impaired consciousness, followed by the administration of activated charcoal to absorb any remaining drug. If vomiting is unsuccessful, or contraindicated, gastric lavage should be performed with normal saline. Saline cathartics may also be of value for rapid dilution of bowel contents. Loratadine is not eliminated by hemodialysis. It is not known if loratadine is eliminated by peritoneal dialysis.
Oral LD_{50} values for loratadine were greater than 5000 mg/kg in rats and mice. Doses as high as 10 times the recommended clinical doses showed no effects in rats, mice, and monkeys.

DOSAGE AND ADMINISTRATION

Adults and children 12 years of age and over: One 10 mg tablet daily.
In patients with liver failure or renal insufficiency (GFR < 30 mL/min), 10 mg every other day should be the starting dose.

HOW SUPPLIED

CLARITIN Tablets, 10 mg, white to off-white compressed tablets; impressed with the product identification number "458" on one side; and "CLARITIN 10" on the other; high density polyethylene plastic bottles of 100 (NDC 0085-0458-03) and 500 (NDC 0085-0458-06). Also available, CLARITIN Unit-of-Use packages of 14 tablets (7 tablets per blister card) (NDC 0085-0458-01) and 30 tablets (10 tablets per blister card) (NDC 0085-0458-05); and 10 × 10 tablet Unit Dose-Hospital Pack (NDC 0085-0458-04).
Protect Unit-of-Use packaging and Unit Dose-Hospital Pack from excessive moisture. Store between 2° and 30°C (36° and 86°F).
Schering Corporation
Kenilworth, NJ 07033 USA
Rev. 9/95 **18779501T**
Copyright© 1992, 1995, Schering Corporation. All rights reserved.
Shown in Product Identification Guide, page 334

CLARITIN®-D ℞

brand of loratadine and pseudoephedrine sulfate, USP
Long-Acting Antihistamine/
Extended Release Decongestant Tablets

CAUTION: Federal Law Prohibits Dispensing Without Prescription

DESCRIPTION

CLARITIN-D Long-Acting Antihistamine/Extended Release Decongestant Tablets contain 5 mg loratadine in the tablet coating for immediate release and 120 mg pseudoephedrine sulfate, USP equally distributed between the tablet coating for immediate release and the barrier-coated extended release core.
Loratadine is a white to off-white powder, not soluble in water, but very soluble in acetone, alcohol, and chloroform. Loratadine has a molecular weight of 382.89 and empirical formula of $C_{22}H_{23}ClN_2O_2$; the chemical name, ethyl 4-(8-chloro-5,6-dihydro-11*H*-benzo[5,6]cyclohepta[1,2-*b*]pyridin-11-ylidene)-1-piperidinecarboxylate; and has the following chemical structure:

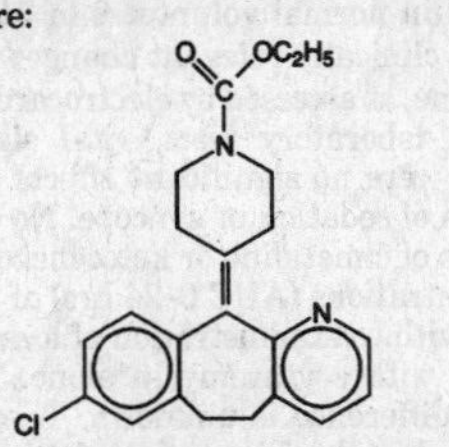

Pseudoephedrine sulfate is the synthetic salt of one of the naturally occurring dextrorotatory diastereomers of ephedrine and is classified as an indirect sympathomimetic amine. The empirical formula for pseudoephedrine sulfate is $(C_{10}H_{15}NO)_2 \cdot H_2SO_4$; the chemical name is [S-(R*,R*)]-α-[1(methylamino)ethyl] benzenemethanol sulfate (2:1) (salt), and the following chemical structure:

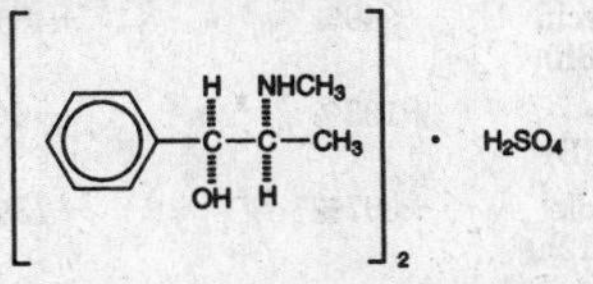

The molecular weight of pseudoephedrine sulfate is 428.54. It is a white powder, freely soluble in water and methanol and sparingly soluble in chloroform.
The inactive ingredients for CLARITIN-D Tablets are acacia, butylparaben, calcium sulfate, carnauba wax, corn starch, lactose, magnesium stearate, microcrystalline cellulose, neutral soap, oleic acid, povidone, rosin, sugar, talc, titanium dioxide, white wax, and zein.

CLINICAL PHARMACOLOGY

The following information is based upon studies of loratadine alone or pseudoephedrine alone, except as indicated.
Loratadine is a long-acting tricyclic antihistamine with selective peripheral histamine H_1-receptor antagonistic activity.
Human histamine skin wheal studies following single and repeated oral doses of loratadine have shown that the drug exhibits an antihistaminic effect beginning within 1 to 3 hours, reaching a maximum at 8 to 12 hours and lasting in excess of 24 hours. There was no evidence of tolerance to this effect developing after 28 days of dosing with loratadine.
Pharmacokinetic studies following single and multiple oral doses of loratadine in 115 volunteers showed that loratadine is rapidly absorbed and extensively metabolized to an active metabolite (descarboethoxyloratadine). Approximately 80% of the total dose administered can be found equally distributed between urine and feces in the form of metabolic products after 10 days. The mean elimination half-lives found in studies in normal adult subjects (n=54) were 8.4 hours (range=3 to 20 hours) for loratadine and 28 hours (range=8.8 to 92 hours) for the major active metabolite (descarboethoxyloratadine). In nearly all patients, exposure (AUC) to the metabolite is greater than exposure to parent loratadine. Loratadine and descarboethoxyloratadine reached steady-state in most patients by approximately the fifth dosing day. The pharmacokinetics of loratadine and descarboethoxyloratadine are dose independent over the dose range of 10 to 40 mg and are not significantly altered by the duration of treatment.
In vitro studies with human liver microsomes indicate that loratadine is metabolized to descarboethoxyloratadine predominantly by P450 CYP3A4 and, to a lesser extent, by P450 CYP2D6. In the presence of a CYP3A4 inhibitor ketoconazole, loratadine is metabolized to descarboethoxyloratadine predominantly by CYP2D6. Concurrent administration of loratadine with either ketoconazole, erythromycin (both CYP3A4 inhibitors), or cimetidine (CYP2D6 and CYP3A4 inhibitor) to healthy volunteers was associated with significantly increased plasma concentrations of loratadine (see **Drug Interactions** section).
In a study involving twelve healthy geriatric subjects (66 to 78 years old), the AUC and peak plasma levels (C_{max}) of both loratadine and descarboethoxyloratadine were significantly higher (approximately 50% increased) than in studies of younger subjects. The mean elimination half-lives for the elderly subjects were 18.2 hours (range=6.7 to 37 hours) for loratadine and 17.5 hours (range=11 to 38 hours) for the active metabolite.
In the clinical efficacy studies, loratadine was administered before meals. In a single-dose study, food increased the AUC of loratadine by approximately 40% and of descarboethoxyloratadine by approximately 15%. The time of peak plasma concentration (T_{max}) of loratadine and descarboethoxyloratadine was delayed by 1 hour with a meal. Although these differences would not be expected to be clinically important, loratadine should be administered on an empty stomach.
In patients with chronic renal impairment (creatinine clearance ≤ 30 mL/min) both the AUC and peak plasma levels (C_{max}) increased on average by approximately 73% for loratadine; and approximately by 120% for descarboethoxyloratadine, compared to individuals with normal renal function. The mean elimination half-lives of loratadine (7.6 hours) and descarboethoxyloratadine (23.9 hours) were not significantly different from that observed in normal subjects. Hemodialysis does not have an effect on the pharmacokinetics of loratadine or its active metabolite (descarboethoxyloratadine) in subjects with chronic renal impairment.
In patients with chronic alcoholic liver disease the AUC and peak plasma levels (C_{max}) of loratadine were double while the pharmacokinetic profile of the active metabolite (descarboethoxyloratadine) was not significantly changed from that in normals. The elimination half-lives for loratadine and descarboethoxyloratadine were 24 hours and 37 hours, respectively, and increased with increasing severity of liver disease.
There was considerable variability in the pharmacokinetic data in all studies of loratadine, probably due to the extensive first-pass metabolism. Individual histograms of area under the curve, clearance, and volume of distribution showed a log normal distribution with a 25-fold range in distribution in healthy subjects.
Loratadine is about 97% bound to plasma proteins at the expected concentrations (2.5 to 100 ng/mL) after a therapeutic dose. Loratadine does not affect the plasma protein binding of warfarin and digoxin. The metabolite descarboethoxyloratadine is 73% to 77% bound to plasma proteins (at 0.5 to 100 ng/mL).
Whole body autoradiographic studies in rats and monkeys, radiolabeled tissue distribution studies in mice and rats, and *in vivo* radioligand studies in mice have shown that neither loratadine nor its metabolites readily cross the blood-brain barrier. Radioligand binding studies with guinea pig pulmonary and brain H_1-receptors indicate that there was preferential binding to peripheral versus central nervous system H_1-receptors.
In a study in which loratadine alone was administered at four times the clinical dose for 90 days, no clinically significant increase in the QT_c was seen on ECGs.
Pseudoephedrine sulfate (d-isoephedrine sulfate) is an orally active sympathomimetic amine which exerts a decongestant action on the nasal mucosa. It is recognized as an effective agent for the relief of nasal congestion due to allergic rhinitis. Pseudoephedrine produces peripheral effects similar to those of ephedrine and central effects similar to, but less intense than, amphetamines. It has the potential for excitatory side effects.
The pseudoephedrine component of CLARITIN-D Tablets was absorbed at a similar rate and was equally available from the combination tablet as from a pseudoephedrine sulfate repetabs 120 mg tablet. Mean (%CV) steady-state peak plasma concentration of 464 ng/mL (22) was attained at 3.9 hours (50). The terminal half-life of pseudoephedrine from the combination tablet administered twice daily was 6.3 hours (23). The ingestion of food was found not to affect the absorption of pseudoephedrine from CLARITIN-D Tablets. Loratadine and pseudoephedrine sulfate do not influence the pharmacokinetics of each other when administered concomitantly.
Clinical Studies: Clinical trials of CLARITIN-D Tablets in seasonal allergic rhinitis involved approximately 3700 patients who received either the combination product, a comparative treatment, or placebo, in double-blind, randomized controlled studies. Four of the largest studies involved approximately 1600 patients in comparisons of the combination product, loratadine (5 mg bid), pseudoephedrine sulfate (120 mg bid), and placebo. Improvement in symptoms of seasonal allergic rhinitis for patients receiving CLARITIN-D Tablets was significantly greater than the improvement in those patients who received the individual components or placebo. The combination reduced the intensity of sneezing, rhinorrhea, nasal pruritus, and eye tearing more than pseudoephedrine and reduced the intensity of nasal congestion more than loratadine, demonstrating a contribution of each of the components. The onset of antihistamine and nasal decongestant actions occurred after the first dose of CLARITIN-D Tablets. CLARITIN-D Tablets were well tolerated, with a frequency of sedation similar to that seen with placebo, and an adverse event profile clinically similar to that of pseudoephedrine.

Continued on next page

Information on Schering products appearing on these pages is effective as of August 15, 1996.

Schering—Cont.

INDICATIONS AND USAGE

CLARITIN-D Tablets are indicated for the relief of symptoms of seasonal allergic rhinitis. CLARITIN-D Tablets should be administered when both the antihistaminic properties of CLARITIN (loratadine) and the nasal decongestant activity of pseudoephedrine are desired (see **CLINICAL PHARMACOLOGY**).

CONTRAINDICATIONS

CLARITIN-D Tablets are contraindicated in patients who are hypersensitive to this medication or to any of its ingredients.

This product, due to its pseudoephedrine component, is contraindicated in patients with narrow-angle glaucoma or urinary retention, and in patients receiving monoamine oxidase (MAO) inhibitor therapy or within fourteen (14) days of stopping such treatment (see **Drug Interactions** section). It is also contraindicated in patients with severe hypertension, severe coronary artery disease, and in those who have shown hypersensitivity or idiosyncrasy to its components, to adrenergic agents, or to other drugs of similar chemical structures. Manifestations of patient idiosyncrasy to adrenergic agents include: insomnia, dizziness, weakness, tremor, or arrhythmias.

WARNINGS

CLARITIN-D Tablets should be used with caution in patients with hypertension, diabetes mellitus, ischemic heart disease, increased intraocular pressure, hyperthyroidism, renal impairment, or prostatic hypertrophy. Central nervous system stimulation with convulsions or cardiovascular collapse with accompanying hypotension may be produced by sympathomimetic amines.

Use in Patients Approximately 60 years and Older: The safety and efficacy of CLARITIN-D Tablets in patients greater than 60 years old have not been investigated in placebo-controlled clinical trials. The elderly are more likely to have adverse reactions to sympathomimetic amines.

PRECAUTIONS

General: Because the doses of this fixed combination product cannot be individually titrated and hepatic insufficiency results in a reduced clearance of loratadine to a much greater extent than pseudoephedrine, CLARITIN-D Tablets should generally be avoided in patients with hepatic insufficiency. Patients with renal insufficiency (GFR < 30 mL/min) should be given a lower initial dose (one tablet per day) because they have reduced clearance of loratadine and pseudoephedrine.

Information for Patients: Patients taking CLARITIN-D Tablets should receive the following information: CLARITIN-D Tablets are prescribed for the relief of symptoms of seasonal allergic rhinitis. Patients should be instructed to take CLARITIN-D Tablets only as prescribed and not to exceed the prescribed dose. Patients should also be advised against the concurrent use of CLARITIN-D Tablets with over-the-counter antihistamines and decongestants.

This product should not be used by patients who are hypersensitive to it or to any of its ingredients. Due to its pseudoephedrine component, this product should not be used by patients with narrow-angle glaucoma, urinary retention, or by patients receiving a monoamine oxidase (MAO) inhibitor or within 14 days of stopping use of an MAO inhibitor. It also should not be used by patients with severe hypertension or severe coronary artery disease.

Patients who are or may become pregnant should be told that this product should be used in pregnancy or during lactation only if the potential benefit justifies the potential risk to the fetus or nursing infant.

Patients should be instructed not to break or chew the tablet.

Drug Interactions: No specific interaction studies have been conducted with CLARITIN-D Tablets. How-

ever, loratadine (10 mg once daily) has been safely coadministered with therapeutic doses of erythromycin, cimetidine, and ketoconazole in controlled clinical pharmacology studies. Although increased plasma concentrations (AUC 0–24 hrs) of loratadine and/or descarboethoxyloratadine were observed following coadministration of loratadine with each of these drugs in normal volunteers (n = 24 in each study), there were no clinically relevant changes in the safety profile of loratadine, as assessed by electrocardiographic parameters, clinical laboratory tests, vital signs, and adverse events. There were no significant effects on QT_c intervals, and no reports of sedation or syncope. No effects on plasma concentrations of cimetidine or ketoconazole were observed. Plasma concentrations (AUC 0–24 hrs) of erythromycin decreased 15% with coadministration of loratadine relative to that observed with erythromycin alone. The clinical relevance of this difference is unknown. These above findings are summarized in the following table:

Effects on Plasma Concentrations (AUC 0—24 hrs) of Loratadine and Descarboethoxyloratadine After 10 Days of Coadministration (Loratadine 10 mg) in Normal Volunteers

	Loratadine	Descarboethoxyloratadine
Erythromycin (500 mg Q8h)	+40%	+46%
Cimetidine (300 mg QID)	+103%	+ 6%
Ketoconazole (200 mg Q12h)	+307%	+73%

There does not appear to be an increase in adverse events in subjects who received oral contraceptives and loratadine. CLARITIN-D Tablets (pseudoephedrine component) are contraindicated in patients taking monoamine oxidase inhibitors and for 2 weeks after stopping use of an MAO inhibitor. The antihypertensive effects of beta-adrenergic blocking agents, methyldopa, mecamylamine, reserpine, and veratrum alkaloids may be reduced by sympathomimetics. Increased ectopic pacemaker activity can occur when pseudoephedrine is used concomitantly with digitalis.

Drug/Laboratory Test Interactions: The *in vitro* addition of pseudoephedrine to sera containing the cardiac isoenzyme MB of serum creatinine phosphokinase progressively inhibits the activity of the enzyme. The inhibition becomes complete over 6 hours.

Carcinogenesis, Mutagenesis, Impairment of Fertility: There are no animal or laboratory studies on the combination product loratadine and pseudoephedrine sulfate to evaluate carcinogenesis, mutagenesis, or impairment of fertility.

In an 18-month oncogenicity study in mice and a 2-year study in rats loratadine was administered in the diet at doses up to 40 mg/kg (mice) and 25 mg/kg (rats). In the carcinogenicity studies pharmacokinetic assessments were carried out to determine animal exposure to the drug. AUC data demonstrated that the exposure of mice given 40 mg/kg of loratadine was 3.6 (loratadine) and 18 (active metabolite) times higher than a human given 10 mg/day. Exposure of rats given 25 mg/kg of loratadine was 28 (loratadine) and 67 (active metabolite) times higher than a human given 10 mg/day. Male mice given 40 mg/kg had a significantly higher incidence of hepatocellular tumors (combined adenomas and carcinomas) than concurrent controls. In rats, a significantly higher incidence of hepatocellular tumors (combined adenomas and carcinomas) was observed in males given 10 mg/kg and males and females given 25 mg/kg. The clinical significance of these findings during long-term use of loratadine is not known.

In mutagenicity studies with loratadine alone, there was no evidence of mutagenic potential in reverse (Ames) or forward point mutation (CHO-HGPRT) assays, or in the assay for DNA damage (Rat Primary Hepatocyte Unscheduled DNA Assay) or in two assays for chromosomal aberrations (Hu-

man Peripheral Blood Lymphocyte Clastogenesis Assay and the Mouse Bone Marrow Erythrocyte Micronucleus Assay). In the Mouse Lymphoma Assay, a positive finding occurred in the nonactivated but not the activated phase of the study. Loratadine administration produced hepatic microsomal enzyme induction in the mouse at 40 mg/kg and rat at 25 mg/kg, but not at lower doses.

Decreased fertility in male rats, shown by lower female conception rates, occurred at approximately 64 mg/kg of loratadine and was reversible with cessation of dosing. Loratadine had no effect on male or female fertility or reproduction in the rat at doses approximately 24 mg/kg.

Pregnancy Category B: There was no evidence of animal teratogenicity in reproduction studies performed on rats and rabbits with this combination at oral doses up to 150 mg/kg ($885 mg/m^2$ or 5 times the recommended daily human dosage of 250 mg or $185 mg/m^2$), and 120 mg/kg ($1416 mg/m^2$ or 8 times the recommended daily human dosage), respectively. There are, however, no adequate and well-controlled studies in pregnant women. Because animal reproduction studies are not always predictive of human response, CLARITIN-D Tablets should be used during pregnancy only if clearly needed.

Nursing Mothers: It is not known if this combination product is excreted in human milk. However, loratadine when administered alone and its metabolite descarboethoxyloratadine pass easily into breast milk and achieve concentrations that are equivalent to plasma levels, with an AUC_{milk}/AUC_{plasma} ratio of 1.17 and 0.85 for the parent and active metabolite, respectively. Following a single oral dose of 40 mg, a small amount of loratadine and metabolite was excreted into the breast milk (approximately 0.03% of 40 mg after 48 hours). Pseudoephedrine administered alone also distributes into breast milk of the lactating human female. Pseudoephedrine concentrations in milk are consistently higher than those in plasma. The total amount of drug in milk as judged by the area under the curve (AUC) is 2 to 3 times greater than in plasma. The fraction of a pseudoephedrine dose excreted in milk is estimated to be 0.4% to 0.7%. A decision should be made whether to discontinue nursing or to discontinue the drug, taking into account the importance of the drug to the mother. Caution should be exercised when CLARITIN-D Tablets are administered to a nursing woman.

Pediatric Use: Safety and effectiveness in children below the age of 12 years have not been established.

ADVERSE REACTIONS

Experience from controlled and uncontrolled clinical studies involving approximately 10,000 patients who received the combination of loratadine and pseudoephedrine sulfate for a period of up to 1 month provides information on adverse reactions. The usual dose was one tablet every 12 hours for up to 28 days.

In controlled clinical trials using the recommended dose of one tablet every 12 hours, the incidence of reported adverse events was similar to those reported with placebo, with the exception of insomnia (16%) and dry mouth (14%).

[See table below.]

Adverse event rates did not appear to differ significantly based on age, sex, or race, although the number of nonwhite subjects was relatively small.

In addition to those adverse events reported above (≥2%), the following less frequent adverse events have been reported in at least one CLARITIN-D treated patient:

Autonomic Nervous System: Abnormal lacrimation, dehydration, flushing, hypoesthesia, increased sweating, mydriasis.

Body As A Whole: Asthenia, back pain, blurred vision, chest pain, conjunctivitis, earache, ear infection, eye pain, fever, flu-like symptoms, leg cramps, lymphadenopathy, malaise, photophobia, rigors, tinnitus, viral infection, weight gain.

Cardiovascular System: Hypertension, hypotension, palpitations, peripheral edema, syncope, tachycardia, ventricular extrasystoles.

Central and Peripheral Nervous System: Dysphonia, hyperkinesia, hypertonia, migraine, paresthesia, tremors, vertigo.

Gastrointestinal System: Abdominal distension, abdominal distress, abdominal pain, altered taste, constipation, diarrhea, eructation, flatulence, gastritis, gingival bleeding, hemorrhoids, increased appetite, stomatitis, taste loss, tongue discoloration, toothache, vomiting.

Liver and Biliary System: Hepatic function abnormal.

Musculoskeletal System: Arthralgia, myalgia, torticollis.

Psychiatric: Aggressive reaction, agitation, anxiety, apathy, confusion, decreased libido, depression, emotional lability, euphoria, impaired concentration, irritability, paroniria.

Reproductive System: Dysmenorrhea, impotence, intermenstrual bleeding, vaginitis.

Respiratory System: Bronchitis, bronchospasm, chest congestion, coughing, dry throat, dyspnea, epistaxis, halitosis, nasal congestion, nasal irritation, sinusitis, sneezing, sputum increased, upper respiratory infection, wheezing.

Skin and Appendages: Acne, bacterial skin infection, dry skin, eczema, edema, epidermal necrolysis, erythema, hematoma, pruritus, rash, urticaria.

REPORTED ADVERSE EVENTS WITH AN INCIDENCE OF ≥2% ON CLARITIN-D IN PLACEBO-CONTROLLED CLINICAL TRIALS
PERCENT OF PATIENTS REPORTING

	CLARITIN-D n=1023	Loratadine n=543	Pseudoephedrine n=548	Placebo n=922
Headache	19	18	17	19
Insomnia	16	4	19	3
Dry Mouth	14	4	9	3
Somnolence	7	8	5	4
Nervousness	5	3	7	2
Dizziness	4	1	5	2
Fatigue	4	6	3	3
Dyspepsia	3	2	3	1
Nausea	3	2	3	2
Pharyngitis	3	3	2	3
Anorexia	2	1	2	1
Thirst	2	1	2	1

Urinary System: Dysuria, micturition frequency, nocturia, polyuria, urinary retention.

The following additional adverse events have been reported with the use of CLARITIN Tablets: alopecia, altered salivation, amnesia, anaphylaxis, angioneurotic edema, blepharospasm, breast enlargement, breast pain, dermatitis, dry hair, erythema multiforme, hemoptysis, hepatic necrosis, hepatitis, jaundice, laryngitis, menorrhagia, nasal dryness, photosensitivity reaction, purpura, seizures, supraventricular tachyarrhythmias, and urinary discoloration.

Pseudoephedrine may cause mild CNS stimulation in hypersensitive patients. Nervousness, excitability, restlessness, dizziness, weakness, or insomnia may occur. Headache, drowsiness, tachycardia, palpitation, pressor activity, and cardiac arrhythmias have been reported. Sympathomimetic drugs have also been associated with other untoward effects, such as fear, anxiety, tenseness, tremor, hallucinations, seizures, pallor, respiratory difficulty, dysuria, and cardiovascular collapse.

DRUG ABUSE AND DEPENDENCE

There is no information to indicate that abuse or dependency occurs with loratadine or the combination of loratadine and pseudoephedrine. Pseudoephedrine, like other central nervous system stimulants, has been abused. At high doses, subjects commonly experience an elevation of mood, a sense of increased energy and alertness, and decreased appetite. Some individuals become anxious, irritable, and loquacious. In addition to the marked euphoria, the user experiences a sense of markedly enhanced physical strength and mental capacity. With continued use, tolerance develops, the user increases the dose, and toxic signs and symptoms appear. Depression may follow rapid withdrawal.

OVERDOSAGE

In the event of overdosage, general symptomatic and supportive measures should be instituted promptly and maintained for as long as necessary. Treatment of overdosage would reasonably consist of emesis (ipecac syrup), except in patients with impaired consciousness, followed by the administration of activated charcoal to absorb any remaining drug. If vomiting is unsuccessful, or contraindicated, gastric lavage should be performed with normal saline. Saline cathartics may also be of value for rapid dilution of bowel contents. Loratadine is not eliminated by hemodialysis. It is not known if loratadine is eliminated by peritoneal dialysis.

Somnolence, tachycardia, and headache have been reported with doses of 40 to 180 mg of CLARITIN Tablets. In large doses, sympathomimetics may give rise to giddiness, headache, nausea, vomiting, sweating, thirst, tachycardia, precordial pain, palpitations, difficulty in micturition, muscular weakness and tenseness, anxiety, restlessness, and insomnia. Many patients can present a toxic psychosis with delusions and hallucinations. Some may develop cardiac arrhythmias, circulatory collapse, convulsions, coma, and respiratory failure.

The oral LD_{50} values for the mixture of the two drugs were greater than 525 and 1839 mg/kg in mice and rats, respectively. Oral LD_{50} values for loratadine were greater than 5000 mg/kg in rats and mice. Doses of loratadine as high as 10 times the recommended daily clinical dose showed no effect in rats, mice, and monkeys.

DOSAGE AND ADMINISTRATION

Adults and children 12 years of age and over: one tablet twice a day (every 12 hours) on an empty stomach. Because the doses of this fixed combination product cannot be individually titrated and hepatic insufficiency results in a reduced clearance of loratadine to a much greater extent than pseudoephedrine, CLARITIN-D Tablets should generally be avoided in patients with hepatic insufficiency. Patients with renal insufficiency (GFR < 30 mL/min) should be given a lower initial dose (one tablet per day) because they have reduced clearance of loratadine and pseudoephedrine.

HOW SUPPLIED

CLARITIN-D Tablets contain 5 mg loratadine and 120 mg pseudoephedrine sulfate. CLARITIN-D Tablets are white tablets branded in green with "CLARITIN-D", which are supplied in high density polyethylene bottles of 100 (NDC 0085-0635-01). Also available are CLARITIN-D Unit-of-Use packages of 30 tablets (3 packs of 10 tablets each) (NDC 0085-0635-05); and 10 × 10 tablets Unit Dose-Hospital Pack (NDC 0085-0635-04).

Keep Unit-of-Use packaging and Unit Dose-Hospital Pack in a dry place.

Store between 2° and 25°C (36° and 77°F).

Rev. 1/95 17798626

Copyright © 1994, 1995, Schering Corporation.
All rights reserved.

Shown in Product Identification Guide, page 334

DIPROLENE® AF ℞

brand of augmented
betamethasone dipropionate*
CREAM 0.05%
(potency expressed as betamethasone)
***Vehicle augments the penetration of the steroid.**
For Dermatologic Use Only–Not for Ophthalmic Use

DESCRIPTION

DIPROLENE® AF Cream contains betamethasone dipropionate, USP, a synthetic adrenocorticosteroid, for dermatologic use in an emollient base. Betamethasone, an analog of prednisolone, has a high degree of corticosteroid activity and a slight degree of mineralocorticoid activity. Betamethasone dipropionate is the 17,21-dipropionate ester of betamethasone.

Chemically, betamethasone dipropionate is 9-fluoro-11β, 17,21-trihydroxy-16β-methylpregna-1,4-diene-3,20-dione 17, 21-dipropionate, with the empirical formula $C_{28}H_{37}FO_7$, a molecular weight of 504.6, and the following structural formula:

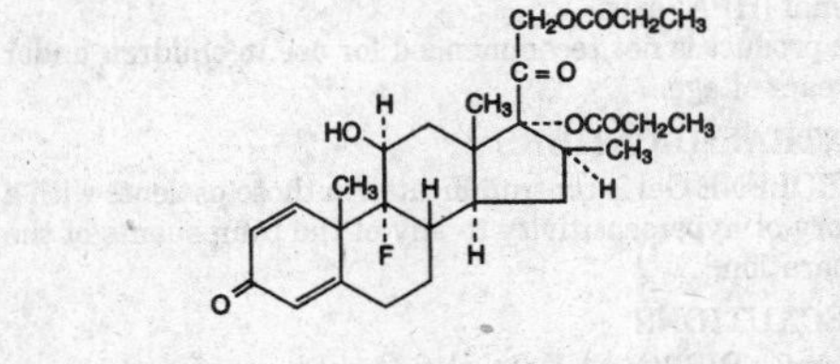

Betamethasone dipropionate is a white to creamy white, odorless crystalline powder, insoluble in water.

Each gram of DIPROLENE AF Cream 0.05% contains: 0.64 mg betamethasone dipropionate, USP (equivalent to 0.5 mg betamethasone) in an emollient cream base of purified water, chlorocresol, propylene glycol, white petrolatum, white wax, cyclomethicone, sorbitol solution, glyceryl monooleate, ceteareth-30, carbomer 940 and sodium hydroxide.

CLINICAL PHARMACOLOGY

The corticosteroids are a class of compounds comprising steroid hormones secreted by the adrenal cortex and their synthetic analogs. In pharmacologic doses, corticosteroids are used primarily for their anti-inflammatory and/or immunosuppressive effects.

Topical corticosteroids, such as betamethasone dipropionate, are effective in the treatment of corticosteroid-responsive dermatoses primarily because of their anti-inflammatory, anti-pruritic, and vasoconstrictive actions. However, while the physiologic, pharmacologic, and clinical effects of the corticosteroids are well-known, the exact mechanisms of their actions in each disease are uncertain. Betamethasone dipropionate, a corticosteroid, has been shown to have topical (dermatologic) and systemic pharmacologic and metabolic effects characteristic of this class of drugs.

Pharmacokinetics: The extent of percutaneous absorption of topical corticosteroids is determined by many factors including the vehicle, the integrity of the epidermal barrier, and the use of occlusive dressings. (See **DOSAGE AND ADMINISTRATION** section.)

Topical corticosteroids can be absorbed through normal intact skin. Inflammation and/or other disease processes in the skin may increase percutaneous absorption. Occlusive dressings substantially increase the percutaneous absorption of topical corticosteroids. (See **DOSAGE AND ADMINISTRATION** section.)

Once absorbed through the skin, topical corticosteroids enter pharmacokinetic pathways similar to systemically administered corticosteroids. Corticosteroids are bound to plasma proteins in varying degrees, are metabolized primarily in the liver and excreted by the kidneys. Some of the topical corticosteroids and their metabolites are also excreted into the bile.

DIPROLENE AF Cream was applied once daily at 7 grams per day for one week to diseased skin, in patients with psoriasis or atopic dermatitis, to study its effects on the hypothalamic-pituitary-adrenal (HPA) axis. The results suggested that the drug caused a slight lowering of adrenal corticosteroid secretion, although in no case did plasma cortisol levels go below the lower limit of the normal range.

INDICATIONS AND USAGE

DIPROLENE AF Cream is indicated for relief of the inflammatory and pruritic manifestations of corticosteroid-responsive dermatoses.

CONTRAINDICATIONS

DIPROLENE AF Cream is contraindicated in patients who are hypersensitive to betamethasone dipropionate, to other corticosteroids, or to any ingredient in this preparation.

PRECAUTIONS

General: Systemic absorption of topical corticosteroids has produced reversible HPA axis suppression, manifestations of Cushing's syndrome, hyperglycemia, and glucosuria in some patients.

Conditions which augment systemic absorption include the application of the more potent corticosteroids, use over large surface areas, prolonged use, and the addition of occlusive dressings. (See **DOSAGE AND ADMINISTRATION** section.)

Therefore, patients receiving a large dose of a potent topical steroid applied to a large surface area should be evaluated periodically for evidence of HPA axis suppression by using the urinary free cortisol and ACTH stimulation tests. If HPA axis suppression is noted, an attempt should be made to withdraw the drug, to reduce the frequency of application, or to substitute a less potent steroid.

Recovery of HPA axis function is generally prompt and complete upon discontinuation of the drug. Infrequently, signs and symptoms of steroid withdrawal may occur, requiring supplemental systemic corticosteroids.

Children may absorb proportionally larger amounts of topical corticosteroids and thus be more susceptible to systemic toxicity. (See **PRECAUTIONS—Pediatric Use.**)

If irritation develops, topical corticosteroids should be discontinued and appropriate therapy instituted.

In the presence of dermatological infections, the use of an appropriate antifungal or antibacterial agent should be instituted. If a favorable response does not occur promptly, the corticosteroid should be discontinued until the infection has been adequately controlled.

Information for Patients: Patients using topical corticosteroids should receive the following information and instructions. This information is intended to aid in the safe and effective use of this medication. It is not a disclosure of all possible adverse or intended effects.

1. This medication is to be used as directed by the physician and should not be used longer than the prescribed time period. It is for external use only. Avoid contact with the eyes.
2. Patients should be advised not to use this medication for any disorder other than that for which it was prescribed.
3. The treated skin areas should not be bandaged or otherwise covered or wrapped as to be occlusive. (See **DOSAGE AND ADMINISTRATION** section.)
4. Patients should report any signs of local adverse reactions.

Laboratory Tests: The following tests may be helpful in evaluating HPA axis suppression:

Urinary free cortisol test
ACTH stimulation test

Carcinogenesis, Mutagenesis, and Impairment of Fertility: Long-term animal studies have not been performed to evaluate the carcinogenic potential or the effect on fertility of topically applied corticosteroids.

Studies to determine mutagenicity with prednisolone and hydrocortisone have revealed negative results.

Pregnancy Category C: Corticosteroids are generally teratogenic in laboratory animals when administered systemically at relatively low dosage levels. The more potent corticosteroids have been shown to be teratogenic after dermal application in laboratory animals. There are no adequate and well-controlled studies of the teratogenic effects of topically applied corticosteroids in pregnant women. Therefore, topical corticosteroids should be used during pregnancy only if the potential benefit justifies the potential risk to the fetus. Drugs of this class should not be used extensively on pregnant patients, in large amounts, or for prolonged periods of time.

Nursing Mothers: It is not known whether topical administration of corticosteroids can result in sufficient systemic absorption to produce detectable quantities in breast milk. Systemically administered corticosteroids are secreted into breast milk in quantities not likely to have a deleterious effect on the infant. Nevertheless, a decision should be made whether to discontinue nursing or to discontinue the drug, taking into account the importance of the drug to the mother.

Pediatric Use: Use of DIPROLENE AF Cream in children under 12 years is not recommended.

Pediatric patients may demonstrate greater susceptibility to topical corticosteroid-induced HPA axis suppression and Cushing's syndrome than mature patients because of a larger skin surface area to body weight ratio.

Hypothalamic-pituitary-adrenal (HPA) axis suppression, Cushing's syndrome, and intracranial hypertension have been reported in children receiving topical corticosteroids. Manifestations of adrenal suppression in children include linear growth retardation, delayed weight gain, low plasma cortisol levels, and absence of response to ACTH stimulation. Manifestations of intracranial hypertension include bulging fontanelles, headaches, and bilateral papilledema. Chronic

Continued on next page

Information on Schering products appearing on these pages is effective as of August 15, 1996.

Schering—Cont.

corticosteroid therapy may interfere with the growth and development of children.

ADVERSE REACTIONS

The only local adverse reaction reported to be possibly or probably related to treatment with DIPROLENE AF Cream during controlled clinical studies was stinging. It occurred in 0.4% of the 242 patients or subjects involved in the studies.

The following local adverse reactions are reported infrequently when topical corticosteroids are used as recommended. These reactions are listed in approximate decreasing order of occurrence: burning, itching, irritation, dryness, folliculitis, hypertrichosis, acneiform eruptions, hypopigmentation, perioral dermatitis, allergic contact dermatitis, maceration of the skin, secondary infection, skin atrophy, striae, miliaria.

OVERDOSAGE

Topically applied corticosteroids can be absorbed in sufficient amounts to produce systemic effects. (See **PRECAUTIONS**.)

DOSAGE AND ADMINISTRATION

Apply a thin film of DIPROLENE AF Cream to the affected skin areas once or twice daily. Treatment with DIPROLENE AF Cream should be limited to 45 g per week.

DIPROLENE AF Cream is not to be used with occlusive dressings.

HOW SUPPLIED

DIPROLENE AF Cream 0.05% is supplied in 15 g (NDC 0085-0517-01), and 50 g (NDC 0085-0517-04) tubes; boxes of one.

Store between 2° and 30°C (36° and 86°F).

Schering Corporation
Kenilworth, NJ 07033 USA
Rev. 7/95

18670305T

Copyright © 1987, 1991, 1994, 1995, Schering Corporation. All rights reserved.

DIPROLENE® ℞
brand of augmented betamethasone dipropionate*
Gel 0.05%
(potency expressed as betamethasone)
***Vehicle augments the penetration of the steroid.**
For Dermatologic Use Only—
Not for Ophthalmic Use

DESCRIPTION

DIPROLENE® Gel contains betamethasone dipropionate, USP, a synthetic fluorinated corticosteroid for topical dermatologic use. Betamethasone dipropionate is included in a class of compounds consisting primarily of synthetic corticosteroids for use topically as anti-inflammatory and anti-pruritic agents.

Chemically, betamethasone dipropionate is 9-fluoro-11β, 17,21-trihydroxy-16β-methylpregna-1,4-diene-3,20-dione 17, 21-dipropionate, with the empirical formula $C_{28}H_{37}FO_7$ and a molecular weight of 504.6,

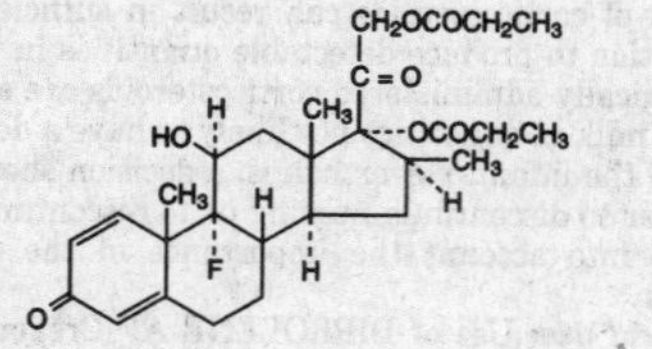

Betamethasone dipropionate is a white to creamy white, odorless crystalline powder, insoluble in water.

Each gram of DIPROLENE Gel contains: 0.64 mg betamethasone dipropionate, USP (equivalent to 0.5 mg betamethasone), in an augmented gel base of purified water, propylene glycol, carbomer 940, and sodium hydroxide.

CLINICAL PHARMACOLOGY

Like other topical corticosteroids, betamethasone dipropionate has anti-inflammatory, anti-pruritic, and vasoconstrictive properties. The mechanism of the anti-inflammatory activity of the topical steroids, in general, is unclear. However, corticosteroids are thought to act by the induction of phospholipase A_2 inhibitory proteins, collectively called lipocortins. It is postulated that these proteins control the biosynthesis of potent mediators of inflammation, such as prostaglandins and leukotrienes, by inhibiting the release of their common precursor, arachidonic acid. Arachidonic acid is released from membrane phospholipids by phospholipase A_2.

Pharmacokinetics: The extent of percutaneous absorption of topical corticosteroids is determined by many factors including the vehicle and the integrity of the epidermal barrier. Occlusive dressings with hydrocortisone for up to 24 hours have not been demonstrated to increase penetration; however, occlusion of hydrocortisone for 96 hours markedly enhances penetration. Topical corticosteroids can be absorbed from normal intact skin. In addition, inflammation and/or other disease processes in the skin may increase percutaneous absorption. Studies performed with DIPROLENE (augmented betamethasone dipropionate) Gel indicate that it is in the super-high range of potency as compared with other topical corticosteroids.

INDICATIONS AND USAGE

DIPROLENE Gel is a super-high potency corticosteroid indicated for the relief of the inflammatory and pruritic manifestations of corticosteroid-responsive dermatoses. Treatment beyond two consecutive weeks is not recommended, and the total dose should not exceed 50 g per week because of potential for the drug to suppress the hypothalamic-pituitary-adrenal (HPA) axis.

This product is not recommended for use in children under 12 years of age.

CONTRAINDICATIONS

DIPROLENE Gel is contraindicated in those patients with a history of hypersensitivity to any of the components of the preparation.

PRECAUTIONS

General: DIPROLENE Gel should not be used in the treatment of rosacea or perioral dermatitis, and it should not be used on the face, groin, or in the axillae.

Systemic absorption of topical corticosteroids can produce reversible hypothalamic-pituitary-adrenal (HPA) axis suppression with the potential for glucocorticosteroid insufficiency after withdrawal of treatment. Manifestations of Cushing's syndrome, hyperglycemia, and glucosuria can also be produced in some patients by systemic absorption of topical corticosteroids while on treatment.

At 7 g per day (applied once daily or as 3.5 g twice daily), DIPROLENE Gel was shown to cause inhibition of the HPA axis following application for one, two or three weeks to diseased skin in some patients with psoriasis or atopic dermatitis. These effects were reversible upon discontinuation of treatment.

Patients receiving DIPROLENE Gel applied to large areas should be evaluated periodically for evidence of HPA axis suppression. This may be done by using the ACTH-stimulation, morning plasma cortisol and urinary free-cortisol tests. Patients should not be treated with DIPROLENE Gel for more than 2 weeks at a time, and amounts greater than 50 g per week should not be used because of the potential for the drug to suppress the HPA axis.

If HPA axis suppression is noted, an attempt should be made to withdraw the drug, to reduce the frequency of application, or to substitute a less potent corticosteroid. Recovery of HPA axis function is generally prompt and complete upon discontinuation of topical corticosteroids. Infrequently, signs and symptoms of glucocorticosteroid insufficiency may occur, requiring supplemental systemic corticosteroids. For information on systemic supplementation, see prescribing information for systemic corticosteroids.

Children may be more susceptible to systemic toxicity from equivalent doses due to their larger skin surface to body mass ratios (see **PRECAUTIONS**—Pediatric Use).

If irritation develops, DIPROLENE Gel should be discontinued and appropriate therapy instituted. Allergic contact dermatitis with corticosteroids is usually diagnosed by observing failure to heal rather than noting clinical exacerbation as with most topical products not containing corticosteroids. Such an observation should be corroborated with appropriate diagnostic patch testing.

If concomitant fungal and/or bacterial skin infections are present or develop, an appropriate antifungal or antibacterial agent should be used. If a favorable response does not occur promptly, use of DIPROLENE Gel should be discontinued until the infection has been adequately controlled.

Information for Patients: Patients using topical corticosteroids should receive the following information and instructions:

1. The medication is to be used as directed by the physician. It is for external use only. Avoid contact with the eyes.
2. The medication should not be used for any disorder other than that for which it was prescribed.
3. The treated skin area should not be bandaged or otherwise covered or wrapped so as to be occlusive.
4. Patients should report to their physician any signs of local adverse reactions.

Laboratory Tests: The following tests may be helpful in evaluating patients for HPA axis suppression:

ACTH-stimulation test
Morning plasma-cortisol test
Urinary free-cortisol test

Carcinogenesis, Mutagenesis, and Impairment of Fertility: Long-term animal studies have not been performed to evaluate the carcinogenic potential of betamethasone dipropionate.

Studies in rabbits, mice and rats using intramuscular doses up to 1.0, 33 and 2.0 mg/kg, respectively, resulted in dose related increases in fetal resorptions in the rabbits and mice.

Pregnancy: Teratogenic Effects: Pregnancy Category C: Corticosteroids have been shown to be teratogenic in laboratory animals when administered systemically at relatively low dosage levels. Some corticosteroids have been shown to be teratogenic after dermal application to laboratory animals.

Betamethasone dipropionate has been shown to be teratogenic in rabbits when given by the intramuscular route at doses of 0.05 mg/kg. This dose is approximately 26 times the human topical dose of DIPROLENE Gel assuming human percutaneous absorption of approximately 3% and the use in a 70 kg person of 7 g per day. The abnormalities observed included umbilical hernias, cephalocele and cleft palate.

There are no adequate and well-controlled studies of the teratogenic potential of betamethasone dipropionate in pregnant women. Therefore, DIPROLENE Gel should be used during pregnancy only if the potential benefit justifies the potential risk to the fetus.

Nursing Mothers: Systemically administered corticosteroids appear in human milk and could suppress growth, interfere with endogenous corticosteroid production, or cause other untoward effects. It is not known whether topical administration of corticosteroids could result in sufficient systemic absorption to produce detectable quantities in human milk. Because many drugs are excreted in human milk, caution should be exercised when DIPROLENE Gel is administered to a nursing woman.

Pediatric Use: Safety and effectiveness of DIPROLENE Gel in children have not been established, therefore its use in children under 12 is not recommended. *Because of a higher ratio of skin surface area to body mass, children are at a greater risk than adults of HPA axis suppression when they are treated with topical corticosteroids. They are, therefore, also at greater risk of glucocorticosteroid insufficiency after withdrawal of treatment and of Cushing's syndrome while on treatment.* Adverse effects, including striae, have been reported with inappropriate use of topical corticosteroids in infants and children.

HPA axis suppression, Cushing's syndrome, and intracranial hypertension have been reported in children receiving topical corticosteroids. Manifestations of adrenal suppression in children include linear growth retardation, delayed weight gain, low plasma cortisol levels, and absence of response to ACTH stimulation. Manifestations of intracranial hypertension include bulging fontanelles, headaches, and bilateral papilledema.

ADVERSE REACTIONS

In controlled clinical trials, the total incidence of adverse events associated with the use of DIPROLENE (augmented betamethasone dipropionate) Gel was 10%. These included stinging or burning in 6% of patients, dry skin in 4% of patients, and pruritus in 2% of patients. Less frequently reported adverse reactions were irritation, skin atrophy, telangiectasia, erythema, cracking/tightening of the skin, follicular rash, and allergic contact dermatitis.

The following additional local adverse reactions are reported infrequently with topical corticosteroids, but may occur more frequently with super-high potency corticosteroids, such as DIPROLENE Gel. These reactions are listed in approximate decreasing order of occurrence: acneiform eruptions, hypopigmentation, perioral dermatitis, secondary infection, striae and miliaria.

OVERDOSAGE

Topically applied DIPROLENE Gel can be absorbed in sufficient amounts to produce systemic effects (see **PRECAUTIONS**).

DOSAGE AND ADMINISTRATION

Apply a thin layer of DIPROLENE Gel to the affected skin once or twice daily and rub in gently and completely.

DIPROLENE Gel is a super-high potency topical corticosteroid; therefore, treatment should be limited to two weeks, and amounts greater than 50 g per week should not be used.

DIPROLENE Gel should not be used with occlusive dressings.

HOW SUPPLIED

DIPROLENE Gel 0.05% is supplied in 15 g (NDC 0085-0634-01), and 50 g (NDC 0085-0634-03) tubes; boxes of one.

Store between 2° and 25°C (36° and 77°F).

Schering Corporation
Kenilworth, NJ 07033 USA
Rev. 6/95 **18671409T**

Copyright© 1991, 1996, Schering Corporation. All rights reserved.

DIPROLENE® ℞
brand of augmented
betamethasone dipropionate*
Lotion 0.05%
(potency expressed as betamethasone)

*Vehicle augments the penetration of the steroid.
For Dermatologic Use Only—Not for Ophthalmic Use

DESCRIPTION

DIPROLENE® Lotion contains betamethasone dipropionate, USP, a synthetic adrenocorticosteroid, for dermatologic use. Betamethasone, an analog of prednisolone, has a high degree of corticosteroid activity and a slight degree of mineralocorticoid activity. Betamethasone dipropionate is the 17, 21-dipropionate ester of betamethasone.

Chemically, betamethasone dipropionate is 9-fluoro-11 β, 17,21-trihydroxy -16β- methylpregna-1,4-diene-3,20-dione 17,21-dipropionate, with the empirical formula $C_{28}H_{37}FO_7$, a molecular weight of 504.6, and the following structural formula:

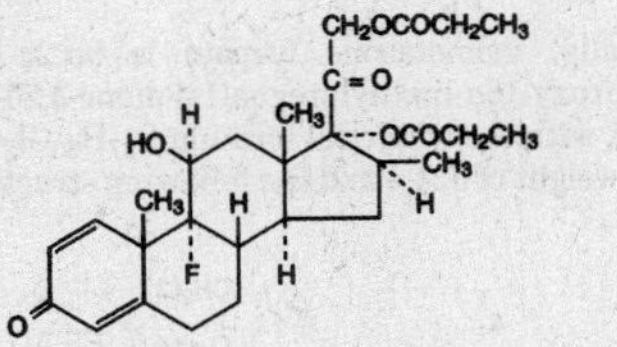

Betamethasone dipropionate is a white to creamy white, odorless crystalline powder, insoluble in water.

Each gram of DIPROLENE Lotion 0.05% contains: 0.64 mg betamethasone dipropionate, USP (equivalent to 0.5 mg betamethasone), in a lotion base of purified water, isopropyl alcohol (30%), hydroxypropylcellulose, propylene glycol, sodium phosphate; phosphoric acid and sodium hydroxide used to adjust the pH to 4.5.

CLINICAL PHARMACOLOGY

The corticosteroids are a class of compounds comprising steroid hormones secreted by the adrenal cortex and their synthetic analogs. In pharmacologic doses, corticosteroids are used primarily for their anti-inflammatory and/or immunosuppressive effects.

Topical corticosteroids, such as betamethasone dipropionate, are effective in the treatment of corticosteroid-responsive dermatoses primarily because of their anti-inflammatory, anti-pruritic, and vasoconstrictive actions. However, while the physiologic, pharmacologic, and clinical effects of the corticosteroids are well-known, the exact mechanisms of their actions in each disease are uncertain. Betamethasone dipropionate, a corticosteroid, has been shown to have topical (dermatologic) and systemic pharmacologic and metabolic effects characteristic of this class of drugs.

Pharmacokinetics The extent of percutaneous absorption of topical corticosteroids is determined by many factors including the vehicle, the integrity of the epidermal barrier, and the use of occlusive dressings. (See **DOSAGE AND ADMINISTRATION** section.)

Topical corticosteroids can be absorbed through normal intact skin. Inflammation and/or other disease processes in the skin may increase percutaneous absorption. Occlusive dressings substantially increase the percutaneous absorption of topical corticosteroids. (See **DOSAGE AND ADMINISTRATION** section.)

Once absorbed through the skin, topical corticosteroids enter pharmacokinetic pathways similar to systemically administered corticosteroids. Corticosteroids are bound to plasma proteins in varying degrees, are metabolized primarily in the liver and excreted by the kidneys. Some of the topical corticosteroids and their metabolites are also excreted into the bile.

DIPROLENE Lotion was applied once daily at 7 mL per day for 21 days to diseased skin (in patients with scalp psoriasis), to study its effects on the hypothalamic-pituitary-adrenal (HPA) axis. In 2 out of 11 patients, the drug lowered plasma cortisol levels below normal limits. Adrenal depression in these patients was transient, and returned to normal within a week. In one of these patients, plasma cortisol levels returned to normal while treatment continued.

INDICATIONS AND USAGE

DIPROLENE Lotion is indicated for treatment of the inflammatory and pruritic manifestations of moderate to severe corticosteroid-responsive dermatoses.

Treatment beyond two weeks is not recommended, and the total dosage should not exceed 50 mL per week because of potential for the drug to suppress the hypothalamic-pituitary-adrenal axis.

CONTRAINDICATIONS

DIPROLENE Lotion is contraindicated in patients who are hypersensitive to betamethasone dipropionate, to other corticosteroids, or to any ingredient in this preparation.

PRECAUTIONS

General DIPROLENE Lotion is a highly potent topical corticosteroid that has been shown to suppress the HPA axis at 7 mL per day.

Systemic absorption of topical corticosteroids has produced reversible HPA axis suppression, manifestations of Cushing's syndrome, hyperglycemia, and glucosuria in some patients.

Conditions which augment systemic absorption include the application of the more potent corticosteroids such as DIPROLENE, use over large surface areas, prolonged use, and the addition of occlusive dressings. (See **DOSAGE AND ADMINISTRATION** section.)

Therefore, patients receiving large doses of a potent topical steroid applied to a large surface area should be evaluated periodically for evidence of HPA axis suppression by using the urinary free cortisol and ACTH stimulation tests. If HPA axis suppression is noted, an attempt should be made to withdraw the drug, to reduce the frequency of application, or to substitute a less potent steroid.

Recovery of HPA axis function is generally prompt and complete upon discontinuation of the drug. Infrequently, signs and symptoms of steroid withdrawal may occur, requiring supplemental systemic corticosteroids.

Children may absorb proportionally larger amounts of topical corticosteroids and thus be more susceptible to systemic toxicity. (See **PRECAUTIONS—Pediatric Use.**)

If irritation develops, topical corticosteroids should be discontinued and appropriate therapy instituted.

In the presence of dermatological infections, the use of an appropriate antifungal or antibacterial agent should be instituted. If a favorable response does not occur promptly, the corticosteroid should be discontinued until the infection has been adequately controlled.

Information for Patients Patients using topical corticosteroids should receive the following information and instructions. This information is intended to aid in the safe and effective use of this medication. It is not a disclosure of all possible adverse or intended effects.

1. This medication is to be used as directed by the physician and should not be used longer than the prescribed time period. It is for external use only. Avoid contact with the eyes.
2. Patients should be advised not to use this medication for any disorder other than that for which it was prescribed.
3. The treated skin areas should not be bandaged or otherwise covered or wrapped so as to be occlusive. (See **DOSAGE AND ADMINISTRATION** section.)
4. Patients should report any sign of local adverse reactions.

Laboratory Tests The following tests may be helpful in evaluating HPA axis suppression:
Urinary free cortisol test
ACTH stimulation test

Carcinogenesis, Mutagenesis, and Impairment of Fertility Long-term animal studies have not been performed to evaluate the carcinogenic potential or the effect on fertility of topically applied corticosteroids.

Studies to determine mutagenicity with prednisolone and hydrocortisone have revealed negative results.

Pregnancy Category C Corticosteroids are generally teratogenic in laboratory animals when administered systemically at relatively low dosage levels. The more potent corticosteroids have been shown to be teratogenic after dermal application in laboratory animals.

Betamethasone dipropionate has not been tested for teratogenicity by this route; however, it appears to be fairly well-absorbed percutaneously. There are no adequate and well-controlled studies of the teratogenic effects of topically applied corticosteroids in pregnant women. Therefore, topical corticosteroids should be used during pregnancy only if the potential benefit justifies the potential risk to the fetus. Drugs of this class should not be used extensively on pregnant patients, in large amounts, or for prolonged periods of time.

Nursing Mothers It is not known whether topical administration of corticosteroids can result in sufficient systemic absorption to produce detectable quantities in breast milk. Systemically administered corticosteroids are secreted into breast milk in quantities not likely to have a deleterious effect on the infant. Nevertheless, a decision should be made whether to discontinue nursing or to discontinue the drug, taking into account the importance of the drug to the mother.

Pediatric Use The safety and efficacy of DIPROLENE Lotion when used in children under 12 years of age have not been established.

Pediatric patients may demonstrate greater susceptibility to topical corticosteroid-induced HPA axis suppression and Cushing's syndrome than mature patients because of a larger skin surface area to body weight ratio.

Hypothalamic-pituitary-adrenal (HPA) axis suppression. Cushing's syndrome, and intracranial hypertension have been reported in children receiving topical corticosteroids. Manifestations of adrenal suppression in children include linear growth retardation, delayed weight gain, low plasma cortisol levels, and absence of response to ACTH stimulation. Manifestations of intracranial hypertension include bulging fontanelles, headaches, and bilateral papilledema. Chronic corticosteroid therapy may interfere with the growth and development of children.

ADVERSE REACTIONS

The overall incidence of drug-related adverse reactions in the DIPROLENE Lotion clinical studies was 5%. The adverse reactions that were reported to be possibly or probably related to treatment with DIPROLENE Lotion during controlled clinical studies involving 327 patients or normal volunteers, were as follows: folliculitis occurred in 2%, burning and acneiform papules each occurred in 1%, and hyperesthesia and irritation each occurred in less than 1% of patients.

The following adverse reactions are also reported infrequently when topical corticosteroids are used as recommended. These reactions are listed in approximate decreasing order of occurrence: itching, dryness, hypertrichosis, hypopigmentation, perioral dermatitis, allergic contact dermatitis, maceration of the skin, secondary infection, skin atrophy, striae, miliaria.

OVERDOSAGE

Topically applied corticosteroids can be absorbed in sufficient amounts to produce systemic effects. (See **PRECAUTIONS**.)

DOSAGE AND ADMINISTRATION

Apply a few drops of DIPROLENE Lotion to the affected area once or twice daily and massage lightly until the lotion disappears.

Treatment must be limited to 14 days, and amounts greater than 50 mL per week should not be used.

DIPROLENE Lotion is not to be used with occlusive dressings.

HOW SUPPLIED

DIPROLENE Lotion 0.05% is supplied in 30 mL (29 g) (NDC 0085-0962-01), and 60 mL (58 g) (NDC 0085-0962-02), plastic squeeze bottles; boxes of one.

Store between 2° and 25°C (36° and 77°F).

Shering Corporation
Kenilworth, NJ 07033 USA
Rev. 11/91 16566012

DIPROLENE® ℞
brand of augmented
betamethasone dipropionate*
Ointment 0.05%
(potency expressed as betamethasone)
***Vehicle augments the penetration of the steroid.**
For Dermatologic Use Only–
Not for Ophthalmic Use

DESCRIPTION

DIPROLENE Ointment contains betamethasone dipropionate. USP, a synthetic adrenocorticosteroid, for dermatologic use. Betamethasone, an analog of prednisolone, has a high degree of corticosteroid activity and a slight degree of mineralocorticoid activity. Betamethasone dipropionate is the 17,21 - dipropionate ester of betamethasone.

Chemically, betamethasone dipropionate is 9-fluoro-11β, 17,21-trihydroxy -16β - methyl-pregna-1,4-diene -3,20- dione 17,21-dipropionate, with the empirical formula $C_{28}H_{37}FO_7$, a molecular weight of 504.6, and the following structural formula:

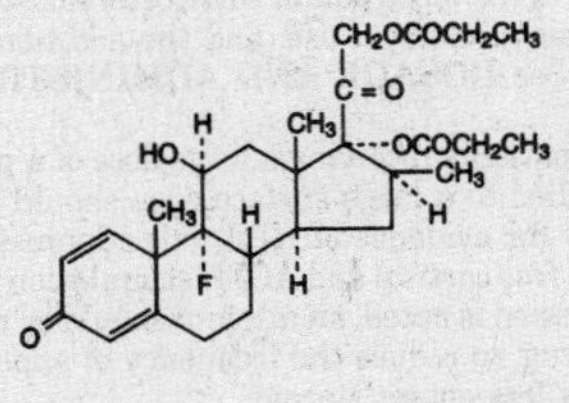

Betamethasone dipropionate is a white to creamy white, odorless crystalline powder, insoluble in water.

Each gram of DIPROLENE Ointment 0.05% contains: 0.64 mg betamethasone dipropionate, USP (equivalent to 0.5 mg betamethasone), in ACTIBASE®, an optimized vehicle of propylene glycol, propylene glycol stearate, white wax, and white petrolatum.

Continued on next page

Information on Schering products appearing on these pages is effective as of August 15, 1996.

Schering—Cont.

CLINICAL PHARMACOLOGY

The corticosteroids are a class of compounds comprising steroid hormones secreted by the adrenal cortex and their synthetic analogs. In pharmacologic doses, corticosteroids are used primarily for their anti-inflammatory and/or immunosuppressive effects.

Topical corticosteroids, such as betamethasone dipropionate, are effective in the treatment of corticosteroid-responsive dermatoses primarily because of their anti-inflammatory, anti-pruritic, and vasoconstrictive actions. However, while the physiologic, pharmacologic, and clinical effects of the corticosteroids are well known, the exact mechanisms of their actions in each disease are uncertain. Betamethasone dipropionate, a corticosteroid, has been shown to have topical (dermatologic) and systemic pharmacologic and metabolic effects characteristic of this class of drugs.

Pharmacokinetics The extent of percutaneous absorption of topical corticosteroids is determined by many factors including the vehicle, the integrity of the epidermal barrier, and the use of occlusive dressing. (See **DOSAGE AND ADMINISTRATION** section.)

Topical corticosteroids can be absorbed from normal intact skin. Inflammation and/or other disease processes in the skin may increase percutaneous absorption. Occlusive dressings substantially increase the percutaneous absorption of topical corticosteroids. (See **DOSAGE AND ADMINISTRATION** section.)

Once absorbed through the skin, topical corticosteroids enter pharmacokinetic pathways similar to systemically administered corticosteroids. Corticosteroids are bound to plasma proteins in varying degrees. Corticosteroids are metabolized primarily in the liver and are then excreted by the kidneys. Some of the topical corticosteroids and their metabolites are also excreted into the bile.

At 14 g per day, DIPROLENE Ointment was shown to depress the plasma levels of adrenal cortical hormones following repeated application to diseased skin in patients with psoriasis. Adrenal depression in these patients was transient, and rapidly returned to normal upon cessation of treatment. At 7 g per day (3.5 g bid), DIPROLENE Ointment was shown to cause minimal inhibition of the hypothalamic-pituitary-adrenal (HPA) axis when applied two times daily for 2 to 3 weeks, in normal patients and in patients with psoriasis and eczematous disorders.

With 6 to 7 g of DIPROLENE Ointment applied once daily for 3 weeks, no significant inhibition of the HPA axis was observed in patients with psoriasis and atopic dermatitis, as measured by plasma cortisol and 24-hour urinary 17-hydroxycorticosteroid levels.

INDICATIONS AND USAGE

DIPROLENE Ointment is indicated for relief of the inflammatory and pruritic manifestations of corticosteroid-responsive dermatoses.

CONTRAINDICATIONS

DIPROLENE Ointment is contraindicated in patients who are hypersensitive to betamethasone dipropionate, to other corticosteroids, or to any ingredient in this preparation.

PRECAUTIONS

General Systemic absorption of topical corticosteroids has produced reversible HPA axis suppression, manifestations of Cushing's syndrome, hyperglycemia, and glucosuria in some patients.

Conditions which augment systemic absorption include the application of the more potent corticosteroids, use over large surface areas, prolonged use, and the addition of occlusive dressings. (See **DOSAGE AND ADMINISTRATION** section.)

Therefore, patients receiving a large dose of a potent topical steroid applied to a large surface area should be evaluated periodically for evidence of HPA axis suppression by using the urinary free cortisol and ACTH stimulation tests. If HPA axis suppression is noted, an attempt should be made to withdraw the drug, to reduce the frequency of application, or to substitute a less potent steroid.

Recovery of HPA axis function is generally prompt and complete upon discontinuation of the drug. Infrequently, signs and symptoms of steroid withdrawal may occur, requiring supplemental systemic corticosteroids.

Children may absorb proportionally larger amounts of topical corticosteroids and thus be more susceptible to systemic toxicity. (See **PRECAUTIONS–Pediatric Use.**)

If irritation develops, topical corticosteroids should be discontinued and appropriate therapy instituted.

In the presence of dermatological infections, the use of an appropriate antifungal or antibacterial agent should be instituted. If a favorable response does not occur promptly, the corticosteroid should be discontinued until the infection has been adequately controlled.

Information for Patients Patients using topical corticosteroids should receive the following information and instructions:

1. This medication is to be used as directed by the physician and should not be used longer than the prescribed time period. It is for external use only. Avoid contact with the eyes.
2. Patients should be advised not to use this medication for any disorder other than that for which it was prescribed.
3. The treated skin area should not be bandaged or otherwise covered or wrapped as to be occlusive. (See **DOSAGE AND ADMINISTRATION** section.)
4. Patients should report any signs of local adverse reactions.

Laboratory Tests The following tests may be helpful in evaluating HPA axis suppression:

Urinary free cortisol test
ACTH stimulation test

Carcinogenesis, Mutagenesis, and Impairment of Fertility Long-term animal studies have not been performed to evaluate the carcinogenic potential or the effect on fertility of topically applied corticosteroids.

Studies to determine mutagenicity with prednisolone have revealed negative results.

Pregnancy Category C Corticosteroids are generally teratogenic in laboratory animals when administered systemically at relatively low dosage levels. The more potent corticosteroids have been shown to be teratogenic after dermal application in laboratory animals. There are no adequate and well-controlled studies of the teratogenic effects of topically applied corticosteroids in pregnant women. Therefore, topical corticosteroids should be used during pregnancy only if the potential benefit justifies the potential risk to the fetus. Drugs of this class should not be used extensively on pregnant patients, in large amounts, or for prolonged periods of time.

Nursing Mothers It is not known whether topical administration of corticosteroids could result in sufficient systemic absorption to produce detectable quantities in breast milk. Systemically administered corticosteroids are secreted into breast milk in quantities not likely to have a deleterious effect on the infant. Nevertheless, caution should be exercised when topical corticosteroids are prescribed for a nursing woman.

Pediatric Use Use of DIPROLENE Ointment in children under 12 years is not recommended.

Pediatric patients may demonstrate greater susceptibility to topical corticosteroid-induced HPA axis suppression and Cushing's syndrome than mature patients because of a larger skin surface area to body weight ratio.

Hypothalamic-pituitary-adrenal (HPA) axis suppression, Cushing's syndrome, and intracranial hypertension have been reported in children receiving topical corticosteroids. Manifestations of adrenal suppression in children include linear growth retardation, delayed weight gain, low plasma cortisol levels, and absence of response to ACTH stimulation. Manifestations of intracranial hypertension include bulging fontanelles, headaches, and bilateral papilledema.

Administration of topical corticosteroids to children should be limited to the least amount compatible with an effective therapeutic regimen. Chronic corticosteroid therapy may interfere with the growth and development of children.

ADVERSE REACTIONS

The local adverse reactions were reported with DIPROLENE Ointment applied either once or twice a day during clinical studies are as follows: erythema, 3 per 767 patients; folliculitis, 2 per 767 patients; pruritus, 2 per 767 patients; vesiculation, 1 per 767 patients.

The following local adverse reactions are reported infrequently when topical corticosteroids are used as recommended. These reactions are listed in an approximate decreasing order of occurrence: burning, itching, irritation, dryness, folliculitis, hypertrichosis, acneiform eruptions, hypopigmentation, perioral dermatitis, allergic contact dermatitis, maceration of the skin, secondary infection, skin atrophy, striae, miliaria.

Systemic absorption of topical corticosteroids has produced reversible HPA axis suppression, manifestations of Cushing's syndrome, hyperglycemia, and glucosuria in some patients.

OVERDOSAGE

Topically applied corticosteroids can be absorbed in sufficient amounts to produce systemic effects. (See **PRECAUTIONS.**)

DOSAGE AND ADMINISTRATION

Apply a thin film of DIPROLENE Ointment to the affected skin areas once or twice daily. Treatment with DIPROLENE Ointment should be limited to 45 g per week.

DIPROLENE Ointment is not to be used with occlusive dressings.

HOW SUPPLIED

DIPROLENE Ointment 0.05% is supplied in 15 g (NDC 0085-0575-02), and 50 g (NDC 0085-0575-05) tubes; boxes of one.

Store between 2° and 25°C (36° and 77°F).

Schering Corporation
Kenilworth, NJ 07033 USA
Rev. 7/95

18670500T

ELOCON® ℞

brand of mometasone furoate cream
Cream 0.1%
For Dermatologic Use Only
Not for Ophthalmic Use

DESCRIPTION

ELOCON® (mometasone furoate cream) Cream contains mometasone furoate for dermatologic use. Mometasone furoate is a synthetic corticosteroid with anti-inflammatory activity.

Chemically, mometasone furoate is 9α,21-Dichloro-11β, 17-dihydroxy-16α-methylpregna-1,4-diene-3,20-dione 17-(2-furoate), with the empirical formula $C_{27}H_{30}Cl_2O_6$, and a molecular weight of 521.4 and the following structural formula:

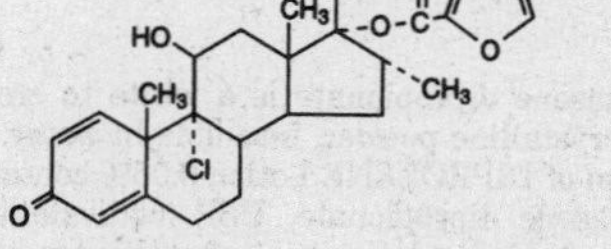

Mometasone furoate is a white to off-white powder practically insoluble in water, slightly soluble in octanol, and moderately soluble in ethyl alcohol

Each gram of ELOCON Cream 0.1% contains: 1 mg mometasone furoate in a cream base of hexylene glycol, phosphoric acid, propylene glycol stearate, stearyl alcohol and ceteareth-20, titanium dioxide, aluminum starch octenyl-succinate, white wax, white petrolatum, and purified water.

CLINICAL PHARMACOLOGY

Like other topical corticosteroids, mometasone furoate has anti-inflammatory, antipruritic, and vasoconstrictive properties. The mechanism of the anti-inflammatory activity of the topical steroids, in general, is unclear. However, corticosteroids are thought to act by the induction of phospholipase A_2 inhibitory proteins, collectively called lipocortins. It is postulated that these proteins control the biosynthesis of potent mediators of inflammation such as prostaglandins and leukotrienes by inhibiting the release of their common precursor arachidonic acid. Arachidonic acid is released from membrane phospholipids by phospholipase A_2.

Pharmacokinetics The extent of percutaneous absorption of topical corticosteroids is determined by many factors including the vehicle and the integrity of the epidermal barrier. Occlusive dressings with hydrocortisone for up to 24 hours have not been demonstrated to increase penetration; however, occlusion of hydrocortisone for 96 hours markedly enhances penetration. Studies in humans indicate that approximately 0.4% of the applied dose of ELOCON Cream 0.1% enters the circulation after 8 hours of contact on normal skin without occlusion. Inflammation and/or other disease processes in the skin may increase percutaneous absorption.

Studies performed with ELOCON Cream indicate that it is in the medium range of potency as compared with other topical corticosteroids.

In a pediatric trial, 24 atopic dermatitis patients, of which 19 patients were age 2 to 12 years, were treated with ELOCON Cream 0.1% once daily. The majority of patients cleared within 3 weeks.

INDICATIONS AND USAGE

ELOCON Cream 0.1% is a medium potency corticosteroid indicated for the relief of the inflammatory and pruritic manifestations of corticosteroid-responsive dermatoses.

ELOCON (mometasone furoate cream) Cream may be used in pediatric patients 2 years of age or older, although the safety and efficacy of drug use for longer than 3 weeks have not been established (see **PRECAUTIONS–Pediatric Use**). Since safety and efficacy of ELOCON Cream have not been established in pediatric patients below 2 years of age, its use in this age group is not recommended.

CONTRAINDICATIONS

ELOCON Cream is contraindicated in those patients with a history of hypersensitivity to any of the components in the preparation.

PRECAUTIONS

General Systemic absorption of topical corticosteroids can produce reversible hypothalamic-pituitary-adrenal (HPA) axis suppression with the potential for glucocorticosteroid insufficiency after withdrawal of treatment. Manifestations of Cushing's syndrome, hyperglycemia, and glucosuria can also be produced in some patients by systemic absorption of topical corticosteroids while on treatment.

Patients applying a topical steroid to a large surface area or to areas under occlusion should be evaluated periodically for evidence of HPA axis suppression. This may be done by using the ACTH stimulation, A.M. plasma cortisol, and urinary free cortisol tests.

In a study evaluating the effects of mometasone furoate cream on the hypothalamic-pituitary-adrenal (HPA) axis, 15 grams were applied twice daily for 7 days to six adult patients with psoriasis or atopic dermatitis. The cream was applied without occlusion to at least 30% of the body surface. The results show that the drug caused a slight lowering of adrenal corticosteroid secretion.

If HPA axis suppression is noted, an attempt should be made to withdraw the drug, to reduce the frequency of application, or to substitute a less potent corticosteroid. Recovery of HPA axis function is generally prompt upon discontinuation of topical corticosteroids. Infrequently, signs and symptoms of glucocorticosteroid insufficiency may occur requiring supplemental systemic corticosteroids. For information on systemic supplementation, see Prescribing Information for those products.

Pediatric patients may be more susceptible to systemic toxicity from equivalent doses due to their larger skin surface to body mass ratios (see **PRECAUTIONS–Pediatric Use**).

If irritation develops, ELOCON Cream should be discontinued and appropriate therapy instituted. Allergic contact dermatitis with corticosteroids is usually diagnosed by observing a failure to heal rather than noting a clinical exacerbation as with most topical products not containing corticosteroids. Such an observation should be corroborated with appropriate diagnostic patch testing.

If concomitant skin infections are present or develop, an appropriate antifungal or antibacterial agent should be used. If a favorable response does not occur promptly, use of ELOCON Cream should be discontinued until the infection has been adequately controlled.

Information for Patients Patients using topical corticosteroids should receive the following information and instructions:

1. This medication is to be used as directed by the physician. It is for external use only. Avoid contact with the eyes.
2. This medication should not be used for any disorder other than that for which it was prescribed.
3. The treated skin area should not be bandaged or otherwise covered or wrapped so as to be occlusive unless directed by the physician.
4. Patients should report to their physician any signs of local adverse reactions.
5. Parents of pediatric patients should be advised not to use ELOCON Cream in the treatment of diaper dermatitis. ELOCON Cream should not be applied in the diaper area as diapers or plastic pants may constitute occlusive dressing (see **DOSAGE AND ADMINISTRATION**).
6. This medication should not be used on the face, underarms, or groin areas unless directed by the physician.
7. As with other corticosteroids, therapy should be discontinued when control is achieved. If no improvement is seen within 2 weeks, contact the physician.

Laboratory Tests The following tests may be helpful in evaluating patients for HPA axis suppression:

ACTH stimulation test
A.M. plasma cortisol test
Urinary free cortisol test

Carcinogenesis, Mutagenesis, and Impairment of Fertility In studies of the effect of mometasone furoate on fertility, pregnancy, and postnatal development in rats and rabbits, 25 rats were treated with doses up to 1.2 mg/kg of drug topically, and 15 rabbits with doses up to 0.3 mg/kg of drug topically. The drugs were left on the skin for 6 hours daily during gestation. At the highest dosage, the rat dams lost weight. One of the rabbit dams at the highest dosage had wrinkled skin, muscle wasting and aborted 5 fetuses.

Genetic toxicity studies with mometasone furoate, which included the Ames test, mouse lymphoma assay, and a micronucleus test did not reveal any mutagenic potential.

Long term animal studies have not been performed to evaluate the carcinogenic potential of ELOCON (mometasone furoate cream) Cream.

Pregnancy Teratogenic effects: Pregnancy Category C Corticosteroids have been shown to be teratogenic in laboratory animals when administered systemically at relatively low dosage levels. Some corticosteroids have been shown to be teratogenic after dermal application in laboratory animals.

Rat offspring of dams treated with 1.2 mg/kg of mometasone furoate topically (4 times the maximum dose in a 50 kg individual) displayed umbilical hernias, unossified sternebrae and vertebrae, and wavy ribs, as well as markedly depressed fetal growth. Rabbit offspring of dams treated with up to 0.3 mg/kg of mometasone furoate topically (the same dose as the maximum dose in a 50 kg individual) displayed flexed paws, umbilical hernias, and cleft palate. A 50 kg female using 1 gram of ELOCON Cream would apply approximately 0.023 mg/kg.

There are no adequate and well-controlled studies of the teratogenic potential of mometasone furoate in pregnant women. ELOCON Cream should be used during pregnancy only if the potential benefit justifies the potential risk to the fetus.

Nursing Mothers Systemtically administered corticosteroids appear in human milk and could suppress growth, interfere with endogenous corticosteroid production, or cause other untoward effects. It is not known whether topical administration of corticosteroids could result in sufficient systemic absorption to produce detectable quantities in human milk. Because many drugs are excreted in human milk, caution should be exercised when ELOCON Cream is administered to a nursing woman.

Pediatric Use ELOCON Cream may be used with caution in pediatric patients 2 years of age or older, although the safety and efficacy of drug use for longer than 3 weeks have not been established. Use of ELOCON Cream is supported by results from adequate and well-controlled studies in pediatric patients with corticosteroid-responsive dermatoses. Since safety and efficacy of ELOCON Cream have not been established in pediatric patients below 2 years of age, its use in this age group is not recommended. Because of a higher ratio of skin surface area to body mass, pediatric patients are at a greater risk than adults of HPA axis suppression and Cushing's syndrome when they are treated with topical corticosteroids. They are, therefore, also at greater risk of adrenal insufficiency during and/or after withdrawal of treatment. Pediatric patients may be more susceptible than adults to skin atrophy, including striae, when they are treated with topical corticosteroids. Pediatric patients applying topical corticosteroids to greater than 20% of body surface are at higher risk of HPA axis suppression.

HPA axis suppression, Cushing's syndrome, linear growth retardation, delayed weight gain, and intracranial hypertension have been reported in pediatric patients receiving topical corticosteroids. Manifestations of adrenal suppression in children include low plasma cortisol levels, and an absence of response to ACTH stimulation. Manifestations of intracranial hypertension include bulging fontanelles, headaches, and bilateral papilledema.

ELOCON (mometasone furoate cream) Cream should not be used in the treatment of diaper dermatitis.

ADVERSE REACTIONS

In controlled clinical studies involving 319 patients, the incidence of adverse reactions associated with the use of ELOCON Cream was 1.6%. Reported reactions included burning, pruritus, and skin atrophy. Reports of rosacea associated with the use of ELOCON Cream have also been received. In controlled clinical studies (n=74) involving pediatric patients 2 to 12 years of age, the incidence of adverse experiences associated with the use of ELOCON Cream was approximately 7%. Reported reactions included stinging, pruritus, and furunculosis.

The following additional local adverse reactions have been reported infrequently with topical corticosteroids, but may occur more frequently with the use of occlusive dressings. These reactions are listed in an approximate decreasing order of occurrence: irritation, dryness, folliculitis, hypertrichosis, acneiform eruptions, hypopigmentation, perioral dermatitis, allergic contact dermatitis, secondary infection, striae, and miliaria.

OVERDOSAGE

Topically applied ELOCON Cream can be absorbed in sufficient amounts to produce systemic effects (see **PRECAUTIONS**).

DOSAGE AND ADMINISTRATION

Apply a thin film of ELOCON Cream to the affected skin areas once daily.

ELOCON Cream may be used in pediatric patients 2 years of age or older. Safety and efficacy of ELOCON Cream in pediatric patients for more than 3 weeks of use have not been established. Use in pediatric patients under 2 years of age is not recommended.

As with other corticosteroids, therapy should be discontinued when control is achieved. If no improvement is seen within 2 weeks, reassessment of diagnosis may be necessary. ELOCON Cream should not be used with occlusive dressings unless directed by a physician. ELOCON Cream should not be applied in the diaper area if the child still requires diapers or plastic pants as these garments may constitute occlusive dressing.

HOW SUPPLIED

ELOCON Cream 0.1% is supplied in 15 g (NDC 0085-0567-01) and 45 g (NDC 0085-0567-02) tubes; boxes of one.

Store ELOCON Cream between 2° and 25°C (36° and 77°F).

Schering Corporation
Kenilworth, NJ 07033 USA
Revised 8/95

18724308T

ELOCON® ℞

brand of mometasone furoate
Lotion 0.1%
For Dermatologic Use Only
Not for Ophthalmic Use

DESCRIPTION

ELOCON Lotion 0.1% contains mometasone furoate for dermatologic use. Mometasone furoate is a synthetic corticosteroid with anti-inflammatory activity.

Chemically, mometasone furoate is 9α, 21-Dichloro-11β, 17-dihydroxy-16α-methylpregna-1, 4-diene-3, 20 dione 17-(2-furoate), with the empirical formula $C_{27}H_{30}Cl_2O_6$, a molecular weight of 521.4 and the following structural formula:

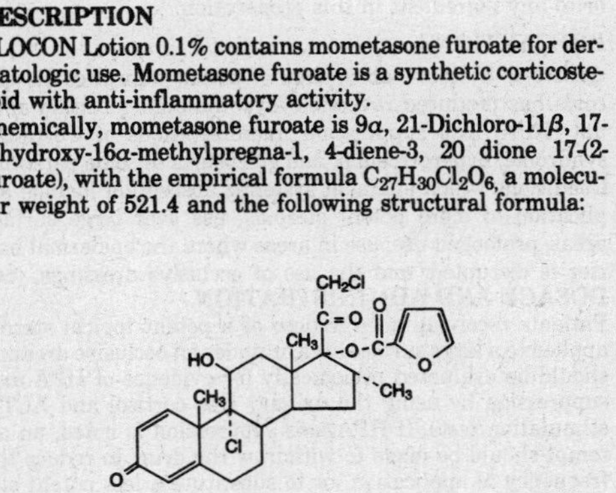

Mometasone furoate is a white to off-white powder practically insoluble in water, slightly soluble in octanol, and moderately soluble in ethyl alcohol.

Each gram of ELOCON Lotion 0.1% contains: 1 mg of mometasone furoate in a lotion base of isopropyl alcohol (40%), propylene glycol, hydroxypropylcellulose, sodium phosphate and water. May also contain phosphoric acid and sodium hydroxide used to adjust the pH to approximately 4.5.

CLINICAL PHARMACOLOGY

The corticosteroids are a class of compounds comprising steroid hormones secreted by the adrenal cortex and their synthetic analogs. In pharmacologic doses corticosteroids are used primarily for their anti-inflammatory and/or immunosuppressive effects.

Topical corticosteroids, such as mometasone furoate, are effective in the treatment of corticosteroid-responsive dermatoses primarily because of their anti-inflammatory, antipruritic, and vasoconstrictive actions. However, while the physiologic, pharmacologic, and clinical effects of the corticosteroids are well known, the exact mechanisms of their actions in each disease are uncertain. Mometasone furoate has been shown to have topical (dermatologic) and systemic pharmacologic and metabolic effects characteristic of this class of drugs.

Pharmacokinetics The extent of percutaneous absorption of topical corticosteroids is determined by many factors including the vehicle, the integrity of the epidermal barrier, and the use of occlusive dressings. (See **DOSAGE AND ADMINISTRATION.**) Topical corticosteroids can be absorbed from normal intact skin.

A study using a radio-labelled ^3H mometasone furoate ointment (0.1%) formulation was performed in man to measure systemic absorption and excretion. Results showed that approximately 0.7% of the steroid was absorbed during 8 hours of contact, without occlusion, with intact skin of normal volunteers. A similar minimal degree of absorption of the corticosteroid from the lotion formulation would be anticipated. Inflammation and/or disease processes in the skin increase percutaneous absorption. Occlusive dressings substantially increase the percutaneous absorption of topical corticosteroids. (See **DOSAGE AND ADMINISTRATION.**)

Mometasone furoate lotion was applied at 15 mL twice daily (30 mL per day) to diseased skin (patients with scalp and body psoriasis) of four patients for seven days, to study its effects on the hypothalamic-pituitary-adrenal (HPA) axis. Plasma cortisol levels for each of the four patients remained well within the normal range and changed little from baseline.

Once absorbed through the skin, topical corticosteroids are handled through pharmacokinetic pathways similar to systemically administered corticosteroids. Corticosteroids are

Continued on next page

Information on Schering products appearing on these pages is effective as of August 15, 1996.

Schering—Cont.

bound to plasma proteins in varying degrees. Corticosteroids are metabolized primarily in the liver and are then excreted by the kidneys. Some of the topical corticosteroids and their metabolites are also excreted into the bile.

INDICATIONS AND USAGE

ELOCON Lotion is indicated for the relief of the inflammatory and pruritic manifestations of corticosteroid-responsive dermatoses.

CONTRAINDICATIONS

ELOCON Lotion is contraindicated in patients who are hypersensitive to mometasone furoate, to other corticosteroids, or to any ingredient in this preparation.

PRECAUTIONS

General Systemic absorption of potent topical corticosteroids has produced reversible hypothalamic-pituitary-adrenal (HPA) axis suppression, manifestations of Cushing's syndrome, hyperglycemia, and glucosuria in some patients. Conditions which augment systemic absorption include application of more potent steroids, use over large surface areas, prolonged use, use in areas where the epidermal barrier is disrupted, and the use of occlusive dressings. (See **DOSAGE AND ADMINISTRATION**.)

Patients receiving a large dose of a potent topical steroid applied to a large surface area or under an occlusive dressing should be evaluated periodically for evidence of HPA axis suppression by using the urinary free cortisol and ACTH stimulation tests. If HPA axis suppression is noted, an attempt should be made to withdraw the drug, to reduce the frequency of application, or to substitute a less potent steroid.

Recovery of HPA axis function is generally prompt and complete upon discontinuation of the drug. Infrequently, signs and symptoms of steroid withdrawal may occur, requiring supplemental systemic corticosteroids.

Children may absorb proportionally larger amounts of topical corticosteroids and thus be more susceptible to systemic toxicity. (See **PRECAUTIONS—Pediatric Use.**)

If irritation develops, topical corticosteroids should be discontinued and appropriate therapy instituted.

In the presence of dermatological infections, use of an appropriate antifungal or antibacterial agent should be instituted. If a favorable response does not occur promptly, the corticosteroid should be discontinued until the infection has been adequately controlled.

Information for Patients Patients using topical corticosteroids should receive the following information and instructions. This information is intended to aid in the safe and effective use of this medication. It is not a disclosure of all possible adverse or intended effects.

1. This medication is to be used as directed by the physician. It is for external use only. Avoid contact with the eyes.
2. Patients should be advised not to use this medication for any disorder other than that for which it was prescribed.
3. The treated skin area should not be bandaged or otherwise covered or wrapped as to be occlusive unless directed by the physician. (See **DOSAGE AND ADMINISTRATION**.)
4. Patients should report any signs of local adverse reactions.
5. Parents of pediatric patients should be advised not to use tight-fitting diapers or plastic pants on a child being treated in the diaper area, as these garments may constitute occlusive dressing. (See **DOSAGE AND ADMINISTRATION**.)

Laboratory Tests The following tests may be helpful in evaluating HPA axis suppression:

Urinary free cortisol test

ACTH stimulation test

Carcinogenesis, Mutagenesis, and Impairment of Fertility Long-term animal studies have not been performed to evaluate the carcinogenic potential or the effect on fertility of topical corticosteroids.

Genetic toxicity studies with mometasone furoate, which included the Ames test, mouse lymphoma assay, and a micronucleus test, did not reveal any mutagenic potential.

Pregnancy Category C Corticosteroids are generally teratogenic in laboratory animals when administered systemically at relatively low dosage levels. Corticosteroids have been shown to be teratogenic after dermal application in laboratory animals. There are no adequate and well-controlled studies of teratogenic effects from topically applied corticosteroids in pregnant women. Therefore, topical corticosteroids should be used during pregnancy only if the potential benefit justifies the potential risk to the fetus. Drugs of this class should not be used extensively on pregnant patients, in large amounts, or for prolonged periods.

Nursing Mothers It is not known whether topical administration of corticosteroids could result in sufficient systemic absorption to produce detectable quantities in breast milk. Systemically administered corticosteroids are secreted into breast milk in quantities not likely to have a deleterious effect on the infant. Nevertheless, a decision should be made whether to discontinue nursing or to discontinue the drug, taking into account the importance of the drug to the mother.

Pediatric Use Pediatric patients may demonstrate greater susceptibility to topical corticosteroid-induced HPA axis suppression and Cushing's syndrome than mature patients because of a larger skin surface area to body weight ratio.

Hypothalamic-pituitary-adrenal (HPA) axis suppression, Cushing's syndrome, and intracranial hypertension have been reported in children receiving topical corticosteroids. Manifestations of adrenal suppression in children include linear growth retardation, delayed weight gain, low plasma cortisol levels, and absence of response to ACTH stimulation. Manifestations of intracranial hypertenson include bulging fontanelles, headaches, and bilateral papilledema. Administration of topical corticosteroids to children should be limited to the least amount compatible with an effective therapeutic regimen. Chronic corticosteroid therapy may interfere with the growth and development of children.

ADVERSE REACTIONS

The following local adverse reactions were reported with ELOCON Lotion during clinical studies with 209 patients: acneiform reaction, 2; burning, 4; and itching, 1. In an irritation/sensitization study with 156 normal subjects, folliculitis was reported in 4.

The following local adverse reactions have been reported infrequently when other topical dermatologic corticosteroids have been used as recommended. These reactions are listed in an approximate decreasing order of occurrence: burning, itching, irritation, dryness, folliculitis, hypertrichosis, acneiform eruptions, hypopigmentation, perioral dermatitis, allergic contact dermatitis, maceration of the skin, secondary infection, skin atrophy, striae, miliaria.

OVERDOSAGE

Topically applied corticosteroids can be absorbed in sufficient amounts to produce systemic effects. (See **PRECAUTIONS**.)

DOSAGE AND ADMINISTRATION

Apply a few drops of ELOCON Lotion to the affected areas once daily and massage lightly until it disappears. For the most effective and economical use, hold the nozzle of the bottle very close to the affected areas and gently squeeze.

HOW SUPPLIED

ELOCON Lotion 0.1% is supplied in 30 mL (27.5 g) (NDC-0085-0854-01) and 60 mL (55 g) (NDC-0085-0854-02) bottles; boxes of one.

Store ELOCON Lotion between 2° and 30°C (36° and 86°F).

Schering Corporation
Kenilworth, NJ 07033 USA
Rev. 11/93
17980904

Copyright © 1989, 1991, 1994, Schering Corporation.
All rights reserved.

ELOCON® ℞

brand of mometasone furoate ointment
Ointment 0.1%
For Dermatologic Use Only
Not for Ophthalmic Use

DESCRIPTION

ELOCON® (mometasone furoate ointment) Ointment contains mometasone furoate for dermatologic use. Mometasone furoate is a synthetic corticosteroid with anti-inflammatory activity.

Chemically, mometasone furoate is 9α,21-Dichloro-11β, 17-dihydroxy-16α-methylpregna- 1,4-diene-3,20-dione 17-(2-furoate), with the empirical formula $C_{27}H_{30}Cl_2O_6$, a molecular weight of 521.4 and the following structural formula:

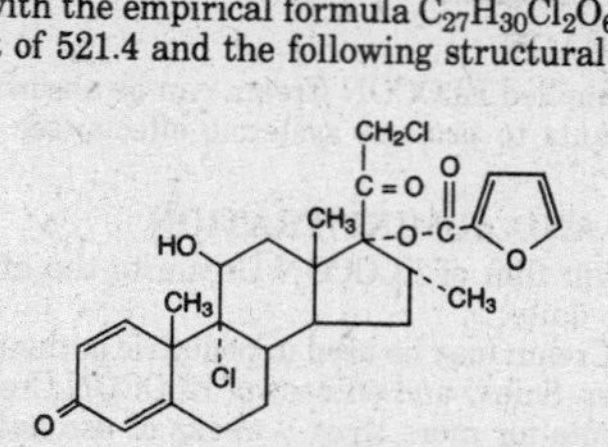

Mometasone furoate is a white to off-white powder practically insoluble in water, slightly soluble in octanol, and moderately soluble in ethyl alcohol.

Each gram of ELOCON Ointment 0.1% contains: 1 mg mometasone furoate in an ointment base of hexylene glycol, phosphoric acid, propylene glycol stearate, white wax, white petrolatum, and purified water.

CLINICAL PHARMACOLOGY

Like other topical corticosteroids, mometasone furoate has anti-inflammatory, antipruritic, and vasoconstrictive properties. The mechanism of the anti-inflammatory activity of the topical steroids, in general, is unclear. However, corticosteroids are thought to act by the induction of phospholipase A_2 inhibitory proteins, collectively called lipocortins. It is postulated that these proteins control the biosynthesis of potent mediators of inflammation such as prostaglandins and leukotrienes by inhibiting the release of their common precursor arachidonic acid. Arachidonic acid is released from membrane phospholipids by phospholipase A_2.

Pharmacokinetics The extent of percutaneous absorption of topical corticosteroids is determined by many factors including the vehicle and the integrity of the epidermal barrier. Occlusive dressings with hydrocortisone for up to 24 hours have not been demonstrated to increase penetration; however, occlusion of hydrocortisone for 96 hours markedly enhances penetration. Studies in humans indicate that approximately 0.7% of the applied dose of ELOCON Ointment 0.1% enters the circulation after 8 hours of contact on normal skin without occlusion. Inflammation and/or other disease processes in the skin may increase percutaneous absorption.

Studies performed with ELOCON Ointment indicate that it is in the medium range of potency as compared with other topical corticosteroids.

In a pediatric trial, 24 atopic dermatitis patients, of which 19 patients were age 2 to 12 years, were treated with ELOCON Cream 0.1% once daily. The majority of patients cleared within 3 weeks.

INDICATIONS AND USAGE

ELOCON Ointment 0.1% is a medium potency corticosteroid indicated for the relief of the inflammatory and pruritic manifestations of corticosteroid-responsive dermatoses.

ELOCON (mometasone furoate ointment) Ointment may be used in pediatric patients 2 years of age or older, although the safety and efficacy of drug use for longer than 3 weeks have not been established (see **PRECAUTIONS—Pediatric Use**). Since safety and efficacy of ELOCON Ointment have not been established in pediatric patients below 2 years of age, its use in this age group is not recommended.

CONTRAINDICATIONS

ELOCON Ointment is contraindicated in those patients with a history of hypersensitivity to any of the components in the preparation.

PRECAUTIONS

General Systemic absorption of topical corticosteroids can produce reversible hypothalamic-pituitary-adrenal (HPA) axis suppression with the potential for glucocorticosteriod insufficiency after withdrawal of treatment. Manifestations of Cushing's syndrome, hyperglycemia, and glucosuria can also be produced in some patients by systemic absorption of topical corticosteroids while on treatment.

Patients applying a topical steroid to a large surface area or areas under occlusion should be evaluated periodically for evidence of HPA axis suppression. This may be done by using the ACTH stimulation, A.M. plasma cortisol, and urinary free cortisol tests.

In a study evaluating the effects of mometasone furoate ointment on the hypothalamic-pituitary-adrenal (HPA) axis, 15 grams were applied twice daily for 7 days to six adult patients with psoriasis or atopic dermatitis. The ointment was applied without occlusion to at least 30% of the body surface. The results show that the drug caused a slight lowering of adrenal corticosteroid secretion.

If HPA axis suppression is noted, an attempt should be made to withdraw the drug, to reduce the frequency of application, or to substitute a less potent corticosteroid. Recovery of HPA axis function is generally prompt upon discontinuation of topical corticosteroids. Infrequently, signs and symptoms of glucocorticosteroid insufficiency may occur requiring supplemental systemic corticosteroids. For information on systemic supplementation, see Prescribing Information for those products.

Pediatric patients may be more susceptible to systemic toxicity from equivalent doses due to their larger skin surface to body mass ratios (see **PRECAUTIONS -Pediatric Use**).

If irritation develops, ELOCON Ointment should be discontinued and appropriate therapy instituted. Allergic contact dermatitis with corticosteroids is usually diagnosed by observing failure to heal rather than noting a clinical exacerbation as with most topical products not containing corticosteroids. Such an observation should be corroborated with appropriate diagnostic patch testing.

If concomitant skin infections are present or develop, an appropriate antifugal or antibacterial agent should be used. If a favorable response does not occur promptly, use of ELOCON Ointment should be discontinued until the infection has been adequately controlled.

Information for Patients Patients using topical corticosteroids should receive the following information and instructions:

1. This medication is to be used as directed by the physician. It is for external use only. Avoid contact with the eyes.
2. This medication should not be used for any disorder other than that for which it was prescribed.
3. The treated skin area should not be bandaged or otherwise covered or wrapped so as to be occlusive unless directed by the physician.

4. Patients should report to their physician any signs of local adverse reactions.
5. Parents of pediatric patients should be advised not to use ELOCON Ointment in the treatment of diaper dermatitis. ELOCON Ointment should not be applied in the diaper area as diapers or plastic pants may constitute occlusive dressing (see **DOSAGE AND ADMINISTRATION**).
6. This medication should not be used on the face, underarms, or groin areas unless directed by the physician.
7. As with other corticosteroids, therapy should be discontinued when control is achieved. If no improvement is seen within 2 weeks, contact the physician.

Laboratory Tests The following tests may be helpful in evaluating patients for HPA axis suppression:
ACTH stimulation test
A.M. plasma cortisol test
Urinary free cortisol test

Carcinogenesis, Mutagenesis, and Impairment of Fertility In studies of the effect of mometasone furoate on fertility, pregnancy, and postnatal development in rats and rabbits, 25 rats were treated with doses up to 1.2 mg/kg of drug topically, and 15 rabbits with doses up to 0.3 mg/kg of drug topically. The drugs were left on the skin for 6 hours daily during gestation. At the highest dosage, the rat dams lost weight. One of the rabbit dams at the highest dosage had wrinkled skin, muscle wasting and aborted 5 fetuses.
Genetic toxicity studies with mometasone furoate, which included the Ames test, mouse lymphoma assay, and a micronucleus test did not reveal any mutagenic potential.
Long term animal studies have not been performed to evaluate the carcinogenic potential of ELOCON (mometasone furoate ointment) Ointment.

Pregnancy Teratogenic effects: Pregnancy C Corticosteroids have been shown to be teratogenic in laboratory animals when administered systemically at relatively low dosage levels. Some corticosteroids have been shown to be teratogenic after dermal application in laboratory animals.
Rat offspring of dams treated with 1.2 mg/kg of mometasone furoate topically (4 times the maximum dose in a 50 kg individual) displayed umbilical hernias, unossified sternebrae and vertebrae, and wavy ribs, as well as markedly depressed fetal growth. Rabbit offspring of dams treated with up to 0.3 mg/kg of mometasone furoate topically (the same dose as the maximum dose in a 50 kg individual) displayed flexed paws, umbilical hernias, and cleft palate. A 50 kg female using 1 gram of ELOCON Ointment would apply approximately 0.023 mg/kg.
There are no adequate and well-controlled studies of the teratogenic potential of mometasone furoate in pregnant women. Therefore, ELOCON Ointment should be used during pregnancy only if the potential benefit justifies the potential risk to the fetus.

Nursing Mothers Systemically administered corticosteroids appear in human milk and could suppress growth, interfere with endogenous corticosteroid production, or cause other untoward effects. It is not known whether topical administration of corticosteroids could result in sufficient systemic absorption to produce detectable quantities in human milk. Because many drugs are excreted in human milk, caution should be exercised when ELOCON Ointment is administered to a nursing woman.

Pediatric Use ELOCON Ointment may be used with caution in pediatric patients 2 years of age or older, although the safety and efficacy of drug use for longer than 3 weeks have not been established. Use of ELOCON Ointment is supported by results from adequate and well-controlled studies in pediatric patients with corticosteroid-responsive dermatoses. Since safety and efficacy of ELOCON Ointment have not been established in pediatric patients below 2 years of age, its use in this age group is not recommended. Because of a higher ratio of skin surface area to body mass, pediatric patients are at a greater risk than adults of HPA axis supression and Cushing's syndrome when they are treated with topical corticosteroids. They are, therefore, also at greater risk of glucocorticosteroid insufficiency during and/or after withdrawal of treatment. Pediatric patients may be more susceptible than adults to skin atrophy, including striae, when they are treated with topical corticosteroids. Pediatric patients applying topical corticosteroids to greater than 20% of body surface are at a higher risk of HPA axis supression. HPA axis supression, Cushing's syndrome, linear growth retardation, delayed weight gain, and intracranial hypertension have been reported in children receiving topical corticosteroids. Manifestations of adrenal suppression in children include low plasma cortisol levels, and absence of response to ACTH stimulation. Manifestations of intracranial hypertension include bulging fontanelles, headaches, and bilateral papilledema.
ELOCON (mometasone furoate ointment) Ointment should not be used in the treatment of diaper dermatitis.

ADVERSE REACTIONS

In controlled clinical studies involving 812 patients, the incidence of adverse reactions associated with the use of ELOCON Ointment was 4.8%. Reported reactions included burning, pruritus, skin atrophy, tingling/stinging, and furunculosis. Reports of rosacea associated with the use of ELOCON Ointment have been received. In controlled clinical studies (n=74) involving pediatric patients 2 to 12 years of age, the incidence of adverse experiences associated with the use of ELOCON Cream is approximately 7%. Reported reactions included stinging, pruritus, and furunculosis.
The following additional local adverse reactions have been reported infrequently with topical corticosteroids, but may occur more frequently with the use of occlusive dressings. These reactions are listed in an approximate decreasing order of occurence: irritation, dryness, folliculitis, hypertrichosis, acneiform eruptions, hypopigmentation, perioral dermatitis, allergic contact dermatitis, secondary infection, striae, and miliaria.

OVERDOSAGE

Topically applied ELOCON Ointment can be absorbed in sufficient amounts to produce systemic effects (see **PRECAUTIONS**).

DOSAGE AND ADMINISTRATION

Apply a thin film of ELOCON Ointment to the affected skin areas once daily. ELOCON Ointment may be used in pediatric patients 2 years of age or older. Safety and efficacy of ELOCON Ointment in pediatric patients for more than 3 weeks have not been established. Use in pediatric patients under 2 years of age is not recommended.
As with other corticosteroids, therapy should be discontinued when control is achieved. If no improvement is seen within 2 weeks, reassessment of diagnosis may be necessary. ELOCON Ointment should not be used with occlusive dressings unless directed by a physician. ELOCON Ointment should not be applied in the diaper area if the child still requires diapers or plastic pants as these garments may constitute occlusive dressing.

HOW SUPPLIED

ELOCON Ointment 0.1% is supplied in 15 g (NDC 0085–0370–01) and 45 g (NDC 0085–0370–02) tubes; boxes of one.
Store ELOCON Ointment between 2° and 30°C (36° and 86°F).
Schering Corporation
Kenilworth, NJ 07033 USA
Revised 8/95

18724200T

ETRAFON® ℞

brand of perphenazine and amitriptyline hydrochloride
ETRAFON 2-10 TABLETS (2-10), USP
ETRAFON TABLETS (2-25), USP
ETRAFON-FORTE TABLETS (4-25), USP

DESCRIPTION

ETRAFON Tablets contain perphenazine, USP and amitriptyline hydrochloride, USP. Perphenazine is a piperazinyl phenothiazine having the chemical formula, $C_{21}H_{26}ClN_3OS$. Amitriptyline hydrochloride is a dibenzocycloheptadiene derivative having the chemical formula, $C_{20}H_{23}N.HCl$.
ETRAFON Tablets are available in multiple strengths to afford dosage flexibility for optimum management. They are available as ETRAFON 2-10 Tablets, 2 mg perphenazine and 10 mg amitriptyline hydrochloride; ETRAFON Tablets, 2 mg perphenazine and 25 mg amitriptyline hydrochloride; ETRAFON-Forte Tablets, 4 mg perphenazine and 25 mg amitriptyline hydrochloride.
The inactive ingredients for ETRAFON 2-10 Tablets (2-10) include: acacia, butylparaben, calcium phosphate, calcium sulfate, carnauba wax, corn starch, D&C Yellow No. 10 Al Lake, FD&C Yellow No. 6 Al Lake, gelatin, lactose, magnesium stearate, potato starch, sugar, and white wax. May also contain talc.
The inactive ingredients for ETRAFON Tablets (2-25) include: acacia, butylparaben, calcium phosphate, calcium sulfate, carnauba wax, corn starch, D&C Red No. 30 Al Lake, FD&C Yellow No. 6 Al Lake, gelatin, lactose, magnesium stearate, potato starch, sugar, and white wax. May also contain talc.
The inactive ingredients for ETRAFON-Forte Tablets (4-25) include: acacia, butylparaben, calcium phosphate, calcium sulfate, carnauba wax, corn starch, FD&C Red No. 40 Al Lake, FD&C Yellow No. 6 Al Lake, gelatin, lactose, magnesium stearate, potato starch, sugar, and white wax. May also contain talc.

ACTIONS

ETRAFON Tablets combine the tranquilizing action of perphenazine with the antidepressant properties of amitriptyline hydrochloride. Perphenazine acts on the central nervous system, and has a greater behavioral potency than other phenothiazine derivatives whose side chains do not contain a piperazine moiety. Amitriptyline hydrochloride is a tricyclic antidepressant. While its mechanism of action in man is not known, it does not act primarily by stimulation of the central nervous system, and is not a monoamine oxidase inhibitor.

INDICATIONS

ETRAFON Tablets are indicated for the treatment of patients with moderate to severe anxiety and/or agitation and depressed mood; patients with depression in whom anxiety and/or agitation are moderate or severe; patients with anxiety and depression associated with chronic physical disease; patients in whom depression and anxiety cannot be clearly differentiated.
Schizophrenic patients who have associated symptoms of depression should be considered for therapy with ETRAFON.

CONTRAINDICATIONS

ETRAFON Tablets are contraindicated in comatose or greatly obtunded patients and in patients receiving large doses of central nervous system depressants (barbiturates, alcohol, narcotics, analgesics, or antihistamines); in the presence of existing blood dyscrasias, bone marrow depression, or liver damage; and in patients who have shown hypersensitivity to ETRAFON Tablets, its components, or related compounds.
ETRAFON Tablets are also contraindicated in patients with suspected or established subcortical brain damage, with or without hypothalamic damage, since a hyperthermic reaction with temperatures in excess of 104°F may occur in such patients, sometimes not until 14 to 16 hours after drug administration. Total body ice-packing is recommended for such a reaction; antipyretics may also be useful.
ETRAFON Tablets should not be given concomitantly with a monoamine oxidase inhibiting compound. Hyperpyretic crises, severe convulsions, and deaths have occurred in patients receiving tricyclic antidepressant and monoamine oxidase inhibiting drugs simultaneously. In patients who have been receiving a monoamine oxidase inhibitor, it is recommended that 2 weeks or longer elapse before the start of treatment with ETRAFON Tablets to permit recovery from the effects of the MAO inhibitor and to avoid possible potentiation. Treatment with ETRAFON Tablets should be initiated cautiously in such patients, with gradual increase in dosage until a satisfactory response is obtained.
Amitriptyline hydrochloride is not recommended for use during the acute recovery phase following myocardial infarction.

WARNINGS

Tardive dyskinesia, a syndrome consisting of potentially irreversible, involuntary, dyskinetic movements, may develop in patients treated with neuroleptic (antipsychotic) drugs. Although the prevalence of the syndrome appears to be highest among the elderly, especially elderly women, it is impossible to rely upon prevalence estimates to predict, at the inception of neuroleptic treatment, which patients are likely to develop the syndrome. Whether neuroleptic drug products differ in their potential to cause tardive dyskinesia is unknown.
Both the risk of developing the syndrome and the likelihood that it will become irreversible are believed to increase as the duration of treatment and the total cumulative dose of neuroleptic drugs administered to the patient increase. However, the syndrome can develop, although much less commonly, after relatively brief treatment periods at low doses.
There is no known treatment for established cases of tardive dyskinesia, although the syndrome may remit, partially or completely, if neuroleptic treatment is withdrawn. Neuroleptic treatment itself, however, may suppress (or partially suppress) the signs and symptoms of the syndrome, and thereby may possibly mask the underlying disease process. The effect that symptomatic suppression has upon the long-term course of the syndrome is unknown.
Given these considerations, neuroleptics should be prescribed in a manner that is most likely to minimize the occurrence of tardive dyskinesia. Chronic neuroleptic treatment should generally be reserved for patients who suffer from a chronic illness that, 1) is known to respond to neuroleptic drugs, and, 2) for whom alternative, equally effective, but potentially less harmful treatments are not available or appropriate. In patients who do require chronic treatment, the smallest dose and the shortest duration of treatment producing a satisfactory clinical response should be sought. The need for continued treatment should be reassessed periodically.
If signs and symptoms of tardive dyskinesia appear in a patient on neuroleptics, drug discontinuation should be consid-

Continued on next page

Information on Schering products appearing on these pages is effective as of August 15, 1996.

Schering—Cont.

ered. However, some patients may require treatment despite the presence of the syndrome.

(For further information about the description of tardive dyskinesia and its clinical detection, please refer to **Information for Patients** and **ADVERSE REACTIONS.**)

NEUROLEPTIC MALIGNANT SYNDROME (NMS)

A potentially fatal symptom complex, sometimes referred to as Neuroleptic Malignant Syndrome (NMS), has been reported in association with antipsychotic drugs. Clinical manifestations of NMS are hyperpyrexia, muscle rigidity, altered mental status, and evidence of autonomic instability (irregular pulse or blood pressure, tachycardia, diaphoresis, and cardiac dysrhythmias).

The diagnostic evaluation of patients with this syndrome is complicated. In arriving at a diagnosis, it is important to identify cases where the clinical presentation includes both serious medical illness (eg, pneumonia, systemic infection, etc.) and untreated or inadequately treated extrapyramidal signs and symptoms (EPS). Other important considerations in the differential diagnosis include central anticholinergic toxicity, heat stroke, drug fever, and primary central nervous system (CNS) pathology.

The management of NMS should include 1) immediate discontinuation of antipsychotic drugs and other drugs not essential to concurrent therapy, 2) intensive symptomatic treatment and medical monitoring, and 3) treatment of any concomitant serious medical problems for which specific treatments are available. There is no general agreement about specific pharmacological treatment regimens for uncomplicated NMS.

If a patient requires antipyschotic drug treatment after recovery from NMS, the reintroduction of drug therapy should be carefully considered. The patient should be carefully monitored since recurrences of NMS have been reported.

Patients with cardiovascular disorders should be watched closely. Tricyclic antidepressant drugs, including amitriptyline hydrochloride, particularly when given in high doses, have been reported to produce arrhythmias, sinus tachycardia, and prolongation of the conduction time. Myocardial infarction and stroke have been reported with drugs of this class.

ETRAFON Tablets should not be given concomitantly with guanethidine or similarly acting compounds, since amitriptyline, like other tricyclic antidepressants, may block the antihypertensive effect of these compounds. If hypotension develops, epinephrine should not be administered since its action is blocked and partially reversed by perphenazine. If a vasopressor is needed, norepinephrine may be used. Severe, acute hypotension has occurred with the use of phenothiazines and is particularly likely to occur in patients with mitral insufficiency or pheochromocytoma. Rebound hypertension may occur in pheochromocytoma patients.

Perphenazine can lower the convulsive threshold in susceptible individuals; it should be used with caution in alcohol withdrawal and in patients with convulsive disorders. If the patient is being treated with an anticonvulsant agent, increased dosage of that agent may be required when ETRAFON Tablets are used concomitantly.

Because of the anticholinergic activity of amitriptyline hydrochloride, ETRAFON Tablets should be used with caution in patients with glaucoma, increased intraocular pressure, and those in whom urinary retention is present or anticipated. In patients with angle-closure glaucoma, even average doses may precipitate an attack.

Close supervision is required when amitriptyline hydrochloride is given to hyperthyroid patients or those receiving thyroid medication.

ETRAFON Tablets may impair the mental and/or physical abilities required for the performance of potentially hazardous tasks, such as driving a car or operating machinery; the patient should be warned accordingly.

Usage in Children: Since a dosage for children has not been established, ETRAFON Tablets are not recommended for use in children.

Use in Pregnancy: Safe use of ETRAFON Tablets during pregnancy and lactation has not been established; therefore, in administering the drug to pregnant patients, nursing mothers, or women who may become pregnant, the possible benefits must be weighed against the possible hazards to mother and child.

PRECAUTIONS

The possibility of suicide in depressed patients remains during treatment and until significant remission occurs. This type of patient should not have access to large quantities of this drug.

Perphenazine

As with all phenothiazine compounds, perphenazine should not be used indiscriminately. Caution should be observed in giving it to patients who have previously exhibited severe adverse reactions to other phenothiazines. Some of the untoward actions of perphenazine tend to appear more frequently when high doses are used. However, as with other phenothiazine compounds, patients receiving perphenazine in any dosage should be kept under close supervision.

Neuroleptic drugs elevate prolactin levels; the elevation persists during chronic administration. Tissue culture experiments indicate that approximately one third of human breast cancers are prolactin dependent *in vitro*, a factor of potential importance if the prescription of these drugs is contemplated in a patient with a previously detected breast cancer. Although disturbances such as galactorrhea, amenorrhea, gynecomastia, and impotence have been reported, the clinical significance of elevated serum prolactin levels is unknown for most patients. An increase in mammary neoplasms has been found in rodents after chronic administration of neuroleptic drugs. Neither clinical studies nor epidemiologic studies conducted to date, however, have shown an association between chronic administration of these drugs and mammary tumorigenesis; the available evidence is considered too limited to be conclusive at this time.

The antiemetic effect of perphenazine may obscure signs of toxicity due to overdosage of other drugs, or render more difficult the diagnosis of disorders such as brain tumors or intestinal obstruction.

A significant, not otherwise explained, rise in body temperature may suggest individual intolerance to perphenazine, in which case ETRAFON Tablets should be discontinued.

Blood counts and hepatic and renal functions should be checked periodically. The appearance of signs of blood dyscrasias requires the discontinuance of the drug and institution of appropriate therapy. If abnormalities in hepatic tests occur, phenothiazine treatment should be discontinued. Renal function in patients on long-term therapy should be monitored; if blood urea nitrogen (BUN) becomes abnormal, treatment with the drug should be discontinued.

The use of phenothiazine derivatives in patients with diminished renal function should be undertaken with caution.

Use with caution in patients suffering from respiratory impairment due to acute pulmonary infections, or in chronic respiratory disorders such as severe asthma or emphysema.

In general, phenothiazines do not produce psychic dependence. Gastritis, nausea and vomiting, dizziness, and tremulousness have been reported following abrupt cessation of high-dose therapy. Reports suggest that these symptoms can be reduced by continuing concomitant antiparkinson agents for several weeks after the phenothiazine is withdrawn.

The possibility of liver damage, corneal and lenticular deposits, and irreversible dyskinesias should be kept in mind when patients are on long-term therapy.

Because photosensitivity has been reported, undue exposure to the sun should be avoided during phenothiazine treatment.

Information for Patients: This information is intended to aid in the safe and effective use of this medication. It is not a disclosure of all possible adverse or intended effects.

Given the likelihood that a substantial proportion of patients exposed chronically to neuroleptics will develop tardive dyskinesia, it is advised that all patients in whom chronic use is contemplated be given, if possible, full information about this risk. The decision to inform patients and/or their guardians must obviously take into account the clinical circumstances and the competency of the patient to understand the information provided.

Amitriptyline Hydrochloride

In manic-depressive psychosis, depressed patients may experience a shift toward the manic phase if they are treated with an antidepressant drug. Patients with paranoid symptomatology may have an exaggeration of such symptoms. The tranquilizing effect of ETRAFON Tablets has seemed to reduce the likelihood of this effect.

Both elevation and lowering of blood sugar levels have been reported.

The usefulness of amitriptyline in the treatment of depression has been amply demonstrated; however, it should be realized that abuse of amitriptyline among a narcotic-dependent population is not uncommon.

Drug Interactions: Drugs Metabolized by P450 2D6—The biochemical activity of the drug metabolizing isozyme cytochrome P450 2D6 (debrisoquin hydroxylase) is reduced in a subset of the Caucasian population (about 7%–10% of Caucasians are so called "poor metabolizers"); reliable estimates of the prevalence of reduced P450 2D6 isozyme activity among Asian, African, and other populations are not yet available. Poor metabolizers have higher than expected plasma concentrations of tricyclic antidepressants (TCAs) when given usual doses. Depending on the fraction of drug metabolized by P450 2D6, the increase in plasma concentration may be small, or quite large (8-fold increase in plasma AUC of the TCA).

In addition, certain drugs inhibit the activity of this isozyme and make normal metabolizers resemble poor metabolizers. An individual who is stable on a given dose of TCA may become abruptly toxic when given one of these inhibiting drugs as concomitant therapy. The drugs that inhibit cytochrome P450 2D6 include some that are not metabolized by the enzyme (quinidine; cimetidine) and many that are substrates for P450 2D6 (many other antidepressants, phenothiazines, and the Type 1C antiarrhythmics propafenone and flecainide). While all the selective serotonin reuptake inhibitors (SSRIs), eg, fluoxetine, sertraline, and paroxetine, inhibit P450 2D6, they may vary in the extent of inhibition. The extent to which SSRI TCA interactions may pose clinical problems will depend on the degree of inhibition and the pharmacokinetics of the SSRI involved. Nevertheless, caution is indicated in the coadministration of TCAs with any of the SSRIs and also in switching from one class to the other. Of particular importance, sufficient time must elapse before initiating TCA treatment in a patient being withdrawn from fluoxetine, given the long half-life of the parent and active metabolite (at least 5 weeks may be necessary).

Concomitant use of tricyclic antidepressants with drugs that can inhibit cytochrome P450 2D6 may require lower doses than usually prescribed for either the tricyclic antidepressant or the other drug. Furthermore, whenever one of these other drugs is withdrawn from cotherapy, an increased dose of tricyclic antidepressant may be required. It is desirable to monitor TCA plasma levels whenever a TCA is going to be coadministered with another drug known to be an inhibitor of P450 2D6.

Perphenazine

Patients on large doses of a phenothiazine drug who are undergoing surgery should be watched carefully for possible hypotensive phenomena. Moreover, reduced amounts of anesthetics or central nervous system depressants may be necessary.

Since phenothiazines and central nervous system depressants (opiates, analgesics, antihistamines, barbiturates) can potentiate each other, less than the usual dosage of the added drug is recommended and caution is advised when they are administered concomitantly.

Use with caution in patients who are receiving atropine or related drugs because of additive anticholinergic effects and also in patients who will be exposed to extreme heat or organic phosphate insecticides.

The use of alcohol should be avoided, since additive effects and hypotension may occur. Patients should be cautioned that their response to alcohol may be increased while they are being treated with ETRAFON Tablets. The risk of suicide and the danger of overdose may be increased in patients who use alcohol excessively due to its potentiation of the drug's effect.

Amitriptyline Hydrochloride

When amitriptyline hydrochloride is given with anticholinergic agents or sympathomimetic drugs, including epinephrine combined with local anesthetics, close supervision and careful adjustment of dosages are required.

Paralytic ileus may occur in patients taking tricyclic antidepressants in combination with anticholinergic-type drugs.

Concurrent use of large doses of ethchlorvynol should be used with caution, since transient delirium has been reported in patients receiving this drug in combination with amitriptyline hydrochloride.

This drug may enhance the response to alcohol and the effects of barbiturates and other CNS depressants.

Concurrent administration of amitriptyline hydrochloride and electroshock therapy may increase the hazards of therapy. Such treatment should be limited to patients for whom it is essential.

Discontinue the drug several days before elective surgery, if possible.

Concurrent administration of cimetidine and tricyclic antidepressants can produce clinically significant increases in the plasma concentrations of the tricyclic antidepressant. Serious anticholinergic symptoms (severe dry mouth, urinary retention, blurred vision) have been associated with elevations in the serum levels of the tricyclic antidepressant when cimetidine is added to the drug regimen. Additionally, higher than expected steady-state serum concentrations of the tricyclic antidepressant have been observed when therapy is initiated in patients taking cimetidine.

Alternatively, decreases in the steady-state serum concentration of the tricyclic antidepressant have been reported in well-controlled patients on concurrent therapy upon discontinuance of cimetidine. The therapeutic efficacy of the tricyclic antidepressant may be compromised in these patients as the cimetidine is discontinued.

ADVERSE REACTIONS

Adverse reactions to ETRAFON Tablets are the same as those to its components, perphenazine and amitriptyline hydrochloride. There have been no reports of effects peculiar to the combination of these components in ETRAFON Tablets.

Perphenazine

Not all of the following adverse reactions have been reported with perphenazine; however, pharmacological similarities among various phenothiazine derivatives require that each be considered. With the piperazine group (of which perphenazine is an example), the extrapyramidal symptoms are more common, and others (eg, sedative effects, jaundice, and blood dyscrasias) are less frequently seen.

CNS Effects: *Extrapyramidal reactions:* opisthotonus, trismus, torticollis, retrocollis, aching and numbness of the limbs, motor restlessness, oculogyric crisis, hyperreflexia,

dystonia, including protrusion, discoloration, aching and rounding of the tongue, tonic spasm of the masticatory muscles, tight feeling in the throat, slurred speech, dysphagia, akathisia, dyskinesia, parkinsonism, and ataxia. Their incidence and severity usually increase with an increase in dosage, but there is considerable individual variation in the tendency to develop such symptoms. Extrapyramidal symptoms can usually be controlled by the concomitant use of effective antiparkinsonian drugs, such as benztropine mesylate, and/or by reduction in dosage. In some instances, however, these extrapyramidal reactions may persist after discontinuation of treatment with perphenazine.

Persistent tardive dyskinesia: As with all antipsychotic agents, tardive dyskinesia may appear in some patients on long-term therapy or may appear after drug therapy has been discontinued. Although the risk appears to be greater in elderly patients on high-dose therapy, especially females, it may occur in either sex and in children. The symptoms are persistent and in some patients appear to be irreversible. The syndrome is characterized by rhythmical, involuntary movements of the tongue, face, mouth, or jaw (eg, protrusion of tongue, puffing of cheeks, puckering of mouth, chewing movements). Sometimes these may be accompanied by involuntary movements of the extremities. There is no known effective treatment for tardive dyskinesia; antiparkinsonism agents usually do not alleviate the symptoms of this syndrome. It is suggested that all antipsychotic agents be discontinued if these symptoms appear. Should it be necessary to reinstitute treatment, increase the dosage of the agent, or switch to a different antipsychotic agent, the syndrome may be masked. It has been reported that fine, vermicular movements of the tongue may be an early sign of the syndrome, and if the medication is stopped at that time the syndrome may not develop.

Other CNS effects include cerebral edema; abnormality of cerebrospinal fluid proteins; convulsive seizures, particularly in patients with EEG abnormalities or a history of such disorders; and headaches.

Neuroleptic malignant syndrome has been reported in patients treated with neuroleptic drugs (see **WARNINGS** section for further information).

Drowsiness may occur, particularly during the first or second week, after which it generally disappears. If troublesome, lower the dosage. Hypnotic effects appear to be minimal, especially in patients who are permitted to remain active.

Adverse behavioral effects include paradoxical exacerbation of psychotic symptoms, catatonic-like states, paranoid reactions, lethargy, paradoxical excitement, restlessness, hyperactivity, nocturnal confusion, bizarre dreams, and insomnia.

Hyperreflexia has been reported in the newborn when a phenothiazine was used during pregnancy.

Autonomic Effects: dry mouth or salivation, nausea, vomiting, diarrhea, anorexia, constipation, obstipation, fecal impaction, urinary retention, frequency or incontinence, polyuria, bladder paralysis, nasal congestion, pallor, myosis, mydriasis, blurred vision, glaucoma, perspiration, hypertension, hypotension, and a change in pulse rate occasionally may occur. Significant autonomic effects have been infrequent in patients receiving less than 24 mg perphenazine daily.

Adynamic ileus occasionally occurs with phenothiazine therapy and if severe, can result in complications and death. It is of particular concern in psychiatric patients, who may fail to seek treatment of the condition.

Allergic Effects: urticaria, erythema, eczema, exfoliative dermatitis, pruritus, photosensitivity, asthma, fever, anaphylactoid reactions, laryngeal edema, and angioneurotic edema; contact dermatitis in nursing personnel administering the drug; and in extremely rare instances, individual idiosyncrasy or hypersensitivity to phenothiazines has resulted in cerebral edema, circulatory collapse, and death.

Endocrine Effects: lactation, galactorrhea, moderate breast enlargement in females and gynecomastia in males on large doses, disturbances in the menstrual cycle, amenorrhea, changes in libido, inhibition of ejaculation, false-positive pregnancy tests, hyperglycemia, hypoglycemia, glycosuria, syndrome of inappropriate ADH (antidiuretic hormone) secretion.

Cardiovascular Effects: Postural hypotension, tachycardia (especially with sudden marked increase in dosage), bradycardia, cardiac arrest, faintness, and dizziness. Occasionally the hypotensive effect may produce a shock-like condition. ECG changes, nonspecific (quinidine-like effect), usually reversible, have been observed in some patients receiving phenothiazine tranquilizers.

Sudden death has occasionally been reported in patients who have received phenothiazines. In some cases, the death was apparently due to cardiac arrest; in others, the cause appeared to be asphyxia due to failure of the cough reflex. In some patients, the cause could not be determined nor could it be established that the death was due to the phenothiazine.

Hematological Effects: agranulocytosis, eosinophilia, leukopenia, hemolytic anemia, thrombocytopenic purpura, and pancytopenia. Most cases of agranulocytosis have occurred between the fourth and tenth weeks of therapy. Patients should be watched closely, especially during that period, for the sudden appearance of sore throat or signs of infection. If white blood cell and differential cell counts show significant cellular depression, discontinue the drug and start appropriate therapy. However, a slightly lowered white count is not in itself an indication to discontinue the drug.

Other Effects: Special considerations in long-term therapy include pigmentation of the skin, occurring chiefly in the exposed areas; ocular changes consisting of deposition of fine particulate matter in the cornea and lens, progressing in more severe cases to star-shaped lenticular opacities; epithelial keratopathies; and pigmentary retinopathy. Also noted: peripheral edema, reversed epinephrine effect, increase in PBI not attributable to an increase in thyroxine, parotid swelling (rare), hyperpyrexia, systemic lupus erythematosus-like syndrome, increases in appetite and weight, polyphagia, photophobia, and muscle weakness.

Liver damage (biliary stasis) may occur. Jaundice may occur, usually between the second and fourth weeks of treatment, and is regarded as a hypersensitivity reaction. Incidence is low. The clinical picture resembles infectious hepatitis but with laboratory features of obstructive jaundice. It is usually reversible; however, chronic jaundice has been reported.

Amitriptyline Hydrochloride

Although activation of latent schizophrenia has been reported with antidepressant drugs, including amitriptyline hydrochloride, it may be prevented with ETRAFON Tablets in some cases because of the antipsychotic effect of perphenazine. A few instances of epileptiform seizures have been reported in chronic schizophrenic patients during treatment with amitriptyline hydrochloride.

Note: Included in the listing which follows are a few adverse reactions which have not been reported with this specific drug. However, pharmacological similarities among the tricyclic antidepressant drugs require that each of the reactions be considered when amitriptyline hydrochloride is administered.

Allergic Effects: Rash, pruritus, urticaria, photosensitization, edema of face and tongue.

Anticholinergic Effects: Dry mouth, blurred vision, disturbance of accommodation, constipation, paralytic ileus, urinary retention, dilatation of urinary tract.

Cardiovascular Effects: Hypotension, hypertension, tachycardia, palpitations, myocardial infarction, arrhythmias, heart block, stroke.

CNS and Neuromuscular Effects: Confusional states, disturbed concentration, disorientation, delusions, hallucinations, excitement, jitteriness, anxiety, restlessness, insomnia, nightmares, numbness, tingling, and paresthesias of the extremities, peripheral neuropathy, incoordination, ataxia, tremors, seizures, alteration in EEG patterns, extrapyramidal symptoms, tinnitus.

Endocrine Effects: Testicular swelling and gynecomastia in the male, breast enlargement and galactorrhea in the female, increased or decreased libido, elevation and lowering of blood sugar levels, syndrome of inappropriate ADH (antidiuretic hormone) secretion.

Gastrointestinal Effects: Nausea, epigastric distress, heartburn, vomiting, anorexia, stomatitis, peculiar taste, diarrhea, jaundice, parotid swelling, black tongue. Rarely hepatitis has occurred (including altered liver function and jaundice).

Hematological Effects: Bone marrow depression, including agranulocytosis, leukopenia, eosinophilia, purpura, thrombocytopenia.

Other Effects: Dizziness, weakness, fatigue, headache, weight gain or loss, increased perspiration, urinary frequency, mydriasis, drowsiness, alopecia.

Withdrawal Symptoms: Abrupt cessation of treatment after prolonged administration may produce nausea, headache, and malaise. These are not indicative of addiction.

DOSAGE AND ADMINISTRATION

Initial Dosage

In psychoneurotic patients whose anxiety and depression warrant combined therapy, one ETRAFON Tablet (2–25) or one ETRAFON-Forte Tablet (4–25) three or four times a day is recommended.

In elderly patients and adolescents, a lower initial dosage may be needed. The dosage may then be adjusted cautiously to produce an adequate response.

In more severely ill patients with schizophrenia, two ETRAFON-Forte Tablets (4–25) three times a day are recommended as the initial dosage. If necessary, a fourth dose may be given at bedtime. The total daily dosage should not exceed eight tablets of any strength.

Maintenance Dosage

Depending on the condition being treated, the onset of therapeutic response may vary from a few days to a few weeks or even longer. After a satisfactory response is noted, dosage should be reduced to the smallest dose which is effective for relief of the symptoms for which ETRAFON Tablets are being administered. A useful maintenance dosage is one ETRAFON Tablet (2–25) or one ETRAFON-Forte Tablet (4–25) two to four times a day. In some patients, maintenance dosage is required for many months.

ETRAFON 2-10 Tablets (2–10) can be used to increase flexibility in adjusting maintenance dosage to the lowest amount consistent with relief of symptoms.

OVERDOSAGE*

Deaths may occur from overdosage with this class of drugs. Multiple drug ingestion (including alcohol) is common in deliberate overdose. As the management is complex and changing, it is recommended that the physician contact a poison control center for current information on treatment. Signs and symptoms of toxicity develop rapidly after overdose, therefore, hospital monitoring is required as soon as possible.

Manifestations: Overdosage of ETRAFON Tablets may cause any of the adverse reactions listed for perphenazine or amitriptyline hydrochloride.

Overdosage of perphenazine usually produces extrapyramidal symptoms such as dyskinesia and dystonia as described under **ADVERSE REACTIONS**, but this may be masked by the anticholinergic effects of amitriptyline. Other symptoms may include stupor or coma; children may have convulsive seizures.

Critical manifestations of tricyclic antidepressant overdose includes: cardiac dysrhythmias, severe hypotension, convulsions, and CNS depression, including coma. Changes in the electrocardiogram, particularly in QRS axis or width, are clinically significant indicators of tricyclic antidepressant toxicity. Other signs of overdose may include: confusion, disturbed concentration, transient visual hallucinations, dilated pupils, agitation, hyperactive reflexes, stupor, drowsiness, muscle rigidity, vomiting, hypothermia, hyperpyrexia, or any of the symptoms listed under **ADVERSE REACTIONS.**

Management: *General:* Obtain an ECG and immediately initiate cardiac monitoring. Protect the patient's airway, establish an intravenous line, and initiate gastric decontamination. A minimum of 6 hours of observation with cardiac monitoring and observation for signs of CNS or respiratory depression, hypotension, cardiac dysrhythmias and/or conduction blocks, and seizures is necessary. If signs of toxicity occur at any time during this period, extended monitoring is required. There are case reports of patients succumbing to fatal dysrhythmias late after overdose; these patients had clinical evidence of significant poisoning prior to death and most received inadequate gastrointestinal decontamination. Monitoring of plasma drug levels should not guide management of the patient.

Gastrointestinal Decontamination: All patients suspected of tricyclic antidepressant overdose should receive gastrointestinal decontamination. This should include large volume gastric lavage followed by activated charcoal. If consciousness is impaired, the airway should be secured prior to lavage. Emesis is contraindicated.

Cardiovascular: A maximal limb-lead QRS duration of ≥ 0.10 seconds may be the best indication of the severity of the overdose. Serum alkalinization, to a pH of 7.45 to 7.55, using intravenous sodium bicarbonate and hyperventilation (as needed) should be instituted for patients with dysrhythmias and/or QRS widening. A pH > 7.60 or a $pCO_2 < 20$ mm Hg is undesirable. Dysrhythmias unresponsive to sodium bicarbonate therapy/hyperventilation may respond to lidocaine, bretylium, or phenytoin. Type 1A and 1C antiarrhythmics are generally contraindicated (eg, quinidine, disopyramide, and procainamide).

In rare instances, hemoperfusion may be beneficial in acute refractory cardiovascular instability in patients with acute toxicity. However, hemodialysis, peritoneal dialysis, exchange transfusions, and forced diuresis generally have been reported as ineffective in tricyclic antidepressant poisoning.

CNS: In patients with CNS depression, early intubation is advised because of the potential for abrupt deterioration. Seizures should be controlled with benzodiazepines, or if these are ineffective, other anticonvulsants (eg, phenobarbital, phenytoin). Physostigmine is not recommended except to treat life-threatening symptoms that have been unresponsive to other therapies, and then only in consultation with a poison control center.

Psychiatric Follow-up: Since overdosage is often deliberate, patients may attempt suicide by other means during the recovery phase. Psychiatric referral may be appropriate.

Pediatric Management: The principles of management of child and adult overdosages are similar. It is strongly recommended that the physician contact the local poison control center for specific pediatric treatment.

HOW SUPPLIED

ETRAFON 2-10 Tablets (perphenazine 2 mg and amitriptyline hydrochloride 10 mg): deep yellow, sugar-coated tablets branded in blue-black with the Schering trademark and either product identification letters, ANA, or number, 287;

Continued on next page

Information on Schering products appearing on these pages is effective as of August 15, 1996.

Schering—Cont.

bottles of 100 (NDC 0085-0287-04), and box of 100 for unit-dose dispensing (10 strips of 10 tablets each) (NDC 0085-0287-08).

ETRAFON Tablets (perphenazine 2 mg and amitriptyline hydrochloride 25 mg): pink, sugar-coated tablets branded in red with the Schering trademark and either product identification letters, ANC, or number, 598; bottles of 100 (NDC 0085-0598-04), and box of 100 for unit-dose dispensing (10 strips of 10 tablets each) (NDC 0085-0598-08).

ETRAFON-Forte Tablets (perphenazine 4 mg and amitriptyline hydrochloride 25 mg): red, sugar-coated tablets branded in blue with the Schering trademark and either product identification letters, ANE, or number, 720; bottles of 100 (NDC 0085-0720-04), and box of 100 for unit-dose dispensing (10 strips of 10 tablets each) (NDC 0085-0720-08).

Store ETRAFON 2-10, 2-25, 4-25 Tablets between 2° and 25°C (36° and 77°F). In addition, protect unit-dose packages from excessive moisture.

* *Poisindex® Toxicologic Management.*
Topic: Antidepressants, Tricyclic.
Micromedex Inc. Vol 85.

ETRAFON®
brand of perphenazine and
amitriptyline hydrochloride
ETRAFON 2-10 TABLETS (2-10), USP
ETRAFON TABLETS (2-25), USP
ETRAFON-FORTE TABLETS (4-25), USP
Schering Corporation
Kenilworth, NJ 07033 USA
Rev. 3/96   16184578
Copyright © 1969, 1994, 1996, Schering Corporation.
All rights reserved.
Shown in Product Identification Guide, page 334

EULEXIN®   ℞
brand of flutamide
Capsules

DESCRIPTION
EULEXIN Capsules contain flutamide, an acetanilid, non-steroidal, orally active antiandrogen having the chemical name, 2-methyl-N-[4-nitro-3-(trifluoromethyl)phenyl] propanamide.

Each capsule contains 125 mg flutamide. The compound is a buff to yellow powder with a molecular weight of 276.2 and the following structural formula:

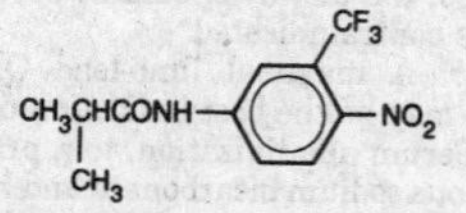

The inactive ingredients for EULEXIN Capsules include: corn starch, lactose, magnesium stearate, povidone, and sodium lauryl sulfate. Gelatin capsule shells may contain methylparaben, propylparaben, butylparaben, and the following dye systems: FD&C Blue 1, FD&C Yellow 6, and either FD&C Red 3 or FD&C Red 40 plus D&C Yellow 10, with titanium dioxide and other inactive ingredients.

CLINICAL PHARMACOLOGY
General: In animal studies, flutamide demonstrates potent antiandrogenic effects. It exerts its antiandrogenic action by inhibiting androgen uptake and/or by inhibiting nuclear binding of androgen in target tissues or both. Prostatic carcinoma is known to be androgen-sensitive and responds to treatment that counteracts the effect of androgen and/or removes the source of androgen, eg, castration. Elevations of plasma testosterone and estradiol levels have been noted following flutamide administration.

Pharmacokinetics:
Absorption: Analysis of plasma, urine, and feces following a single oral 200 mg dose of tritium-labeled flutamide to human volunteers showed that the drug is rapidly and completely absorbed. Following a single 250 mg oral dose to normal adult volunteers, the biologically active alpha-hydroxylated metabolite reaches maximum plasma concentrations in about 2 hours, indicating that it is rapidly formed from flutamide.

Distribution: In male rats neither flutamide nor any of its metabolites is preferentially accumulated in any tissue ex-

cept the prostate after an oral 5 mg/kg dose of ^{14}C-flutamide. Total drug levels were highest 6 hours after drug administration in all tissues. Levels declined at roughly similar rates to low levels at 18 hours. The major metabolite was present at higher concentrations than flutamide in all tissues studied. Following a single 250 mg oral dose to normal adult volunteers, low plasma levels of flutamide were detected. The plasma half-life for the alpha-hydroxylated metabolite of flutamide is about 6 hours. Flutamide, *in vivo*, at steady-state plasma concentrations of 24 to 78 ng/mL, is 94% to 96% bound to plasma proteins. The active metabolite of flutamide, *in vivo*, at steady-state plasma concentrations of 1556 to 2284 ng/mL, is 92% to 94% bound to plasma proteins.

Metabolism: The composition of plasma radioactivity, following a single 200 mg oral dose of tritium-labeled flutamide to normal adult volunteers, showed that flutamide is rapidly and extensively metabolized, with flutamide comprising only 2.5% of plasma radioactivity 1 hour after administration. At least 6 metabolites have been identified in plasma. The major plasma metabolite is a biologically active alpha-hydroxylated derivative which accounts for 23% of the plasma tritium 1 hour after drug administration. The major urinary metabolite is 2-amino-5-nitro-4-(trifluoromethyl) phenol.

Excretion: Flutamide and its metabolites are excreted mainly in the urine with only 4.2% of the dose excreted in the feces over 72 hours.
[See table below.]

Special Populations:
Geriatric: Following multiple oral dosing of 250 mg t.i.d. in normal geriatric volunteers, flutamide and its active metabolite approached steady-state plasma levels (based on pharmacokinetic simulations) after the fourth flutamide dose. The half-life of the active metabolite in geriatric volunteers after a single flutamide dose is about 8.1 hours and at steady state in 9.6 hours.

Race: There are no known alterations in flutamide absorption, distribution, metabolism, or excretion due to race.

Renal Impairment: Following a single 250 mg dose of flutamide administered to subjects with chronic renal insufficiency, there appeared to be no correlation between creatinine clearance and either C_{max} or AUC of flutamide. Renal impairment did not have an effect on the C_{max} or AUC of the biologically active alpha-hydroxylated metabolite of flutamide. In subjects with creatinine clearance of < 29 mL/min, the half-life of the active metabolite was slightly prolonged. Flutamide and its active metabolite were not well dialyzed. Dose adjustment in patients with chronic renal insufficiency is not warranted.

Hepatic Impairment: No information on the pharmacokinetics of flutamide in hepatic impairment is available (see WARNINGS, Hepatic Injury).

Drug-Drug Interactions: Interactions between EULEXIN Capsules and LHRH-agonists have not occurred. Increases in prothrombin have been noted in patients receiving warfarin therapy (see PRECAUTIONS).

Clinical Studies: Flutamide has been demonstrated to interfere with testosterone at the cellular level. This can complement medical castration achieved with LHRH agonists which suppresses testicular androgen production by inhibiting luteinizing hormone secretion.

The effects of combination therapy have been evaluated in two studies. One study evaluated the effects of flutamide and an LHRH agonist as neoadjuvant therapy to radiation in stage B_2-C prostatic carcinoma and the other study evaluated flutamide and an LHRH agonist as the sole therapy in stage D_2 metastatic carcinoma.

Stage B_2-C Prostatic Carcinoma: The effects of hormonal treatment combined with radiation were studied in 466 patients (231 EULEXIN Capsules + LHRH-A + radiation, 235 radiation alone) with bulky primary tumors confined to the prostate (stage B_2) or extending beyond the capsule (stage C), with or without pelvic node involvement.

In this multicentered, controlled trial, administration of EULEXIN Capsules (250 mg t.i.d.) and goserelin acetate (3.6 mg depot) prior to and during radiation was associated with a significantly lower rate of local failure compared to radiation alone (16% vs 33% at 4 years, $P < 0.001$). The combination therapy also resulted in a trend toward reduction in the incidence of distant metastases (27% vs 36% at 4 years, $P = 0.058$). Median disease-free survival was significantly increased in patients who received complete hormonal therapy combined with radiation as compared to those patients who received radiation alone (4.4 vs 2.6 years, $P < 0.001$). Inclusion of normal PSA level as a criterion for disease-free survival also resulted in significantly increased median dis-

ease-free survival in patients receiving the combination therapy (2.7 vs 1.5 years, $P < 0.001$).

Stage D_2 Metastatic Carcinoma: To study the effects of combination therapy in metastatic disease, 617 patients (311 leuprolide + flutamide, 306 leuprolide + placebo) with previously untreated advanced prostatic carcinoma were enrolled in a large multicentered, controlled clinical trial. Three and one-half years after the study was initiated, median survival had been reached. The median actuarial survival time was 34.9 months for patients treated with leuprolide and flutamide versus 27.9 months for patients treated with leuprolide alone. This 7-month increment represents a 25% improvement in overall survival time with the flutamide therapy. Analysis of progression-free survival showed a 2.6 month improvement in patients who received leuprolide plus flutamide, a 19% increment over leuprolide and placebo.

INDICATIONS AND USAGE
EULEXIN Capsules are indicated for use in combination with LHRH agonists for the management of locally confined Stage B_2-C and Stage D_2 metastatic carcinoma of the prostate.

Stage B_2-C Prostatic Carcinoma: Treatment with EULEXIN Capsules and the LHRH agonist should start 8 weeks prior to initiating radiation therapy and continue during radiation therapy.

Stage D_2 Metastatic Carcinoma: To achieve benefit from treatment, EULEXIN Capsules should be initiated with the LHRH agonist and continued until progression.

CONTRAINDICATIONS
EULEXIN Capsules are contraindicated in patients who are hypersensitive to flutamide or any component of this preparation.

WARNINGS
Gynecomastia occurred in 9% of patients receiving flutamide together with medical castration.

Flutamide may cause fetal harm when administered to a pregnant woman. There was decreased 24-hour survival in the offspring of rats treated with flutamide at doses of 30, 100, or 200 mg/kg/day (approximately 3, 9, and 19 times the human dose) during pregnancy. A slight increase in minor variations in the development of the sternebrae and vertebrae was seen in fetuses of rats at the two higher doses. Feminization of the males also occurred at the two higher dose levels. There was a decreased survival rate in the offspring of rabbits receiving the highest dose (15 mg/kg/day; equal to 1.4 times the human dose).

Preclinical data from rats, cats, dogs, and monkeys as well as clinical data in men, demonstrate that one metabolite of flutamide is 4-nitro-3-fluoro-methylaniline. Several toxicities consistent with aniline exposure including methemoglobinemia, hemolytic anemia, and cholestatic jaundice have been observed in animals and humans after flutamide administration. Methemoglobin levels should be monitored in patients susceptible to aniline toxicity (eg, persons with glucose-6-phosphate dehydrogenase deficiency or hemoglobin M disease as well as patients who smoke).

Serious cardiac lesions were observed in 2/10 beagle dogs receiving 25 mg/kg/day for 78 weeks and 3/16 receiving 40 mg/kg/day for 2–4 years. The lesions, indicative of chronic injury and repair processes, including chronic myxomatous degeneration, intra-atrial fibrosis, myocardial acidophilic degeneration, vasculitis, and perivasculitis. The doses at which these lesions occurred were associated with 2-hydroxyflutamide levels that were 1- to 12-fold greater than those observed in humans at therapeutic levels.

Hepatic Injury: Since transaminase abnormalities, cholestatic jaundice, hepatic necrosis, and hepatic encephalopathy have been reported with the use of flutamide, periodic liver function tests should be considered. (See ADVERSE REACTIONS section.) Appropriate laboratory testing should be done at the first symptom/sign of liver dysfunction (eg, pruritus, dark urine, persistent anorexia, jaundice, right upper quadrant tenderness, or unexplained "flu-like" symptoms). If the patient has clinically evident jaundice, in the absence of biopsy-confirmed liver metastases, EULEXIN therapy should be discontinued. In clinically asymptomatic patients, if transaminases increase over 2–3 times the upper limit of normal, treatment should be discontinued. The hepatic injury is usually reversible after discontinuation of therapy, and in some patients, after dosage reduction. However, there have been reports of death following severe hepatic injury associated with use of flutamide.

PRECAUTIONS
Information for Patients: Patients should be informed that EULEXIN Capsules and the drug used for medical castration should be administered concomitantly, and that they should not interrupt their dosing or stop taking these medications without consulting their physician.

Laboratory Tests: Regular assessment of serum Prostate Specific Antigen (PSA) may be helpful in monitoring the patient's response. If PSA levels rise significantly and consistently during EULEXIN therapy the patient should be eval-

---

Plasma Pharmacokinetics of Flutamide and Hydroxyflutamide in Geriatric Volunteers (mean ± S)

	Single Dose		Steady State	
	Flutamide	Hydroxyflutamide	Flutamide	Hydroxyflutamide
C_{max} (ng/mL)	25.2 ± 34.2	894 ± 406	113 ± 213	1629 ± 586
Elimination half-life (hr)	—	8.1 ± 1.3	7.8	9.6 ± 2.5
T_{max} (hr)	1.9 ± 0.7	2.7 ± 1.0	1.3 ± 0.7	1.9 ± 0.6
C_{min} (ng/mL)	—	—	—	673 ± 316

uated for clinical progression. For patients who have objective progression of disease together with an elevated PSA, a treatment-free period of antiandrogen while continuing the LHRH analogue may be considered.

Since transaminase abnormalities, and rarely jaundice, have been reported with the use of EULEXIN Capsules, periodic liver function tests should be considered, eg, when the patient has jaundice or laboratory evidence of liver injury in the absence of liver metastases, EULEXIN therapy should be discontinued. Abnormalities are usually reversible upon discontinuation. See **WARNINGS, Hepatic Injury** above.

Drug Interactions: Increases in prothrombin time have been noted in patients receiving long-term warfarin therapy after flutamide was initiated. Therefore close monitoring of prothrombin time is recommended and adjustment of the anticoagulant dose may be necessary when EULEXIN Capsules are administered concomitantly with warfarin.

Carcinogenesis, Mutagenesis, Impairment of Fertility: In a 1-year dietary study in male rats, interstitial cell adenomas of the testes were present in 49% to 75% of all treated rats (daily oral doses of 10, 30, and 50 mg/kg/day were administered). These produce plasma C_{max} values that are 1, 2-3, and 4-fold, respectively, those associated with therapeutic doses in humans. In male rats similarly dosed for 1 year, tumors were still present after 1 year of a drug-free period, but the incidences were 43% to 47%. In a 2-year carcinogenicity study in male rats, daily administration of flutamide at these same doses produced testicular interstitial cell adenomas in 91% to 95% of all treated rats as opposed to 11% of untreated control rats. Mammary adenomas, adenocarcinomas, and fibroadenomas were increased in treated male rats at exposure levels that were 1- to 4-fold those observed during therapeutic dosing in humans. There are likewise reports of malignant breast neoplasms in men treated with EULEXIN Capsules (see **ADVERSE REACTIONS** section). Flutamide did not demonstrate DNA modifying activity in the Ames *Salmonella*/microsome Mutagenesis Assay. Dominant lethal tests in rats were negative.

Reduced sperm counts were observed during a 6-week study of flutamide monotherapy in normal human volunteers.

Flutamide did not affect estrous cycles or interfere with the mating behavior of male and female rats when the drug was administered at 25 and 75 mg/kg/day prior to mating. Males treated with 150 mg/kg/day (30 times the minimum effective antiandrogenic dose) failed to mate; mating behavior returned to normal after dosing was stopped. Conception rates were decreased in all dosing groups. Suppression of spermatogenesis was observed in rats dosed for 52 weeks at approximately 3, 8, or 17 times the human dose and in dogs dosed for 78 weeks at 1.4, 2.3, and 3.7 times the human dose.

Pregnancy: *Pregnancy Category D.* See **WARNINGS** section.

ADVERSE REACTIONS

Stage B₂-C Prostatic Carcinoma: Treatment with EULEXIN Capsules and the LHRH agonist did not add substantially to the toxicity of radiation treatment alone. The following adverse experiences were reported during a multicenter clinical trial comparing EULEXIN Capsules + LHRH-A + radiation versus radiation alone. The most frequently reported (greater than 5%) adverse experiences are listed below.

[See table above.]

Additional adverse event data was collected for the combination therapy with radiation group over both the hormonal treatment and hormonal treatment plus radiation phases of the study. Adverse experiences occurring in more than 5% of patients in this group, over both parts of the study, were hot flashes (46%), diarrhea (40%), nausea (9%), and skin rash (8%).

Stage D₂ Metastatic Carcinoma: The following adverse experiences were reported during a multicenter clinical trial comparing EULEXIN Capsules + LHRH agonist versus placebo + LHRH agonist.

The most frequently reported (greater than 5%) adverse experiences during treatment with EULEXIN Capsules in combination with an LHRH agonist are listed in the table below. For comparison, adverse experiences seen with an LHRH agonist and placebo are also listed in the following table.

[See table below.]

Adverse Events During Acute Radiation Therapy (within first 90 days of radiation therapy)		
	(n=231) *LHRH-A + EULEXIN Capsules + Radiation* % All	(n=235) *Radiation Only* % All
Rectum/Large Bowel	80	76
Bladder	58	60
Skin	37	37

Adverse Events During Late Radiation Phase (after 90 days of radiation therapy)		
	(n=231) *LHRH-A + EULEXIN Capsules + Radiation* % All	(n=235) *Radiation Only* % All
Diarrhea	36	40
Cystitis	16	16
Rectal Bleeding	14	20
Proctitis	8	8
Hematuria	7	12

As shown in the table, for both treatment groups, the most frequently occurring adverse experiences (hot flashes, impotence, loss of libido) were those known to be associated with low serum androgen levels and known to occur with LHRH agonists alone.

The only notable difference was the higher incidence of diarrhea in the flutamide + LHRH agonist group (12%), which was severe in 5% as opposed to the placebo + LHRH agonist (4%), which was severe in less than 1%.

In addition, the following adverse reactions were reported during treatment with flutamide + LHRH agonist. No causal relatedness of these reactions to drug treatment has been made, and some of the adverse experiences reported are those that commonly occur in elderly patients.

Cardiovascular System: hypertension in 1% of patients.

Central Nervous System: CNS (drowsiness/confusion/depression/anxiety/nervousness) reactions occurred in 1% of patients.

Gastrointestinal System: anorexia 4%, and other GI disorders occurred in 6% of patients.

Hematopoietic System: anemia occurred in 6%, leukopenia in 3%, and thrombocytopenia in 1% of patients.

Liver and Biliary System: hepatitis and jaundice in less than 1% of patients.

Skin: irritation at the injection site and rash occurred in 3% of patients.

Other: edema occurred in 4%, genitourinary and neuromuscular symptoms in 2%, and pulmonary symptoms in less than 1% of patients.

In addition, the following spontaneous adverse experiences have been reported during the marketing of flutamide: hemolytic anemia, macrocytic anemia, methemoglobinemia, photosensitivity reactions (including erythema, ulceration, bullous eruptions, and epidermal necrolysis), and urine discoloration. The urine was noted to change to an amber or yellow-green appearance which can be attributed to the flutamide and/or its metabolites. Also reported were cholestatic jaundice, hepatic encephalopathy, and hepatic necrosis. The hepatic conditions were usually reversible after discontinuing therapy; however, there have been reports of death following severe hepatic injury associated with use of flutamide.

Two reports of malignant breast neoplasms occurring in male patients being dosed with EULEXIN Capsules have been reported. One involved a pre-existing nodule which was first detected 3–4 months before initiation of EULEXIN monotherapy. After excision, this nodule was diagnosed as a poorly differentiated ductal carcinoma. The other report involved gynecomastia and a breast nodule noted 2 and 6 months, respectively, after initiation of EULEXIN monotherapy. The nodule was excised and diagnosed as a moderately differentiated invasive ductal tumor.

Abnormal Laboratory Test Values: Laboratory abnormalities including elevated SGOT, SGPT, bilirubin values, SGGT, BUN, and serum creatinine have been reported.

OVERDOSAGE

In animal studies with flutamide alone, signs of overdose included hypoactivity, piloerection, slow respiration, ataxia, and/or lacrimation, anorexia, tranquilization, emesis, and methemoglobinemia.

Clinical trials have been conducted with flutamide in doses up to 1500 mg per day for periods up to 36 weeks with no serious adverse effects reported. Those adverse reactions reported included gynecomastia, breast tenderness, and some increases in SGOT. The single dose of flutamide ordinarily associated with symptoms of overdose or considered to be life-threatening has not been established.

Since flutamide is highly protein bound, dialysis may not be of any use as treatment for overdose. As in the management of overdose with any drug, it should be borne in mind that multiple agents may have been taken. If vomiting does not occur spontaneously, it should be induced if the patient is alert. General supportive care, including frequent monitoring of the vital signs and close observation of the patient, is indicated.

DOSAGE AND ADMINISTRATION

The recommended dosage is 2 capsules 3 times a day at 8-hour intervals for a total daily dose of 750 mg.

HOW SUPPLIED

EULEXIN Capsules, 125 mg, are available as opaque, two-toned brown capsules, imprinted with "Schering 525". They are supplied as follows:

NDC 0085-0525-05 - Bottles of 500
NDC 0085-0525-03 - Unit Dose packages of 100 (10 × 10's)
NDC 0085-0525-06 - Bottles of 180

Store between 2° and 30°C (36° and 86°F).
Protect the Unit Dose packages from excessive moisture.
Schering Corporation
Kenilworth, NJ 07033 USA
Rev. 6/96

18822415T

Copyright © 1989, 1996, Schering Corporation,
All rights reserved.
Shown in Product Identification Guide, page 334

FULVICIN® P/G ℞
brand of ultramicrosize griseofulvin
Tablets, USP

DESCRIPTION

FULVICIN P/G Tablets contain ultramicrosize crystals of griseofulvin, an antibiotic derived from a species of *Penicillium*. Griseofulvin crystals are partly dissolved in polyethylene glycol 8000 and partly dispersed throughout the tablet matrix.

Each FULVICIN P/G Tablet contains 125 mg or 250 mg griseofulvin ultramicrosize.

The inactive ingredients for FULVICIN P/G Tablets, 125 or 250 mg, include: corn starch, lactose, magnesium stearate, PEG, and sodium lauryl sulfate.

ACTIONS

Microbiology Griseofulvin is fungistatic with *in vitro* activity against various species of *Microsporum, Epidermophyton,* and *Trichophyton*. It has no effect on bacteria or on other genera of fungi.

Human Pharmacology: Following oral administration, griseofulvin is deposited in the keratin precursor cells and has a greater affinity for diseased tissue. The drug is tightly bound to the new keratin which becomes highly resistant to fungal invasions.

Continued on next page

	(n=294) *Flutamide + LHRH agonist* % All	(n=285) *Placebo + LHRH agonist* % All
Hot Flashes	61	57
Loss of Libido	36	31
Impotence	33	29
Diarrhea	12	4
Nausea/Vomiting	11	10
Gynecomastia	9	11
Other	7	9
Other GI	6	4

Schering—Cont.

The efficiency of gastrointestinal absorption of ultramicrocrystalline griseofulvin is approximately one and one-half times that of the conventional microsized griseofulvin. This factor permits the oral intake of two-thirds as much ultramicrocrystalline griseofulvin as the microsize form. However, there is currently no evidence that this lower dose confers any significant clinical differences with regard to safety and/or efficacy.

INDICATIONS

FULVICIN P/G Tablets are indicated for the treatment of ringworm infections of the skin, hair, and nails, namely: tinea corporis, tinea pedis, tinea cruris, tinea barbae, tinea capitis, tinea unguium (onychomycosis) when caused by one or more of the following genera of fungi: *Trichophyton rubrum, Trichophyton tonsurans, Trichophyton mentagrophytes, Trichophyton interdigitale, Trichophyton verrucosum, Trichophyton megninii, Trichophyton gallinae, Trichophyton crateriforme, Trichophyton sulphureum, Trichophyton schoenleinii, Microsporum audouini, Microsporum canis, Microsporum gypseum,* and *Epidermophyton floccosum.*
Note: Prior to therapy, the type of fungi responsible for the infection should be identified.
The use of this drug is not justified in minor or trivial infections which will respond to topical agents alone.
Griseofulvin is not effective in the following: bacterial infections, candidiasis (moniliasis), histoplasmosis, actinomycosis, sporotrichosis, chromoblastomycosis, coccidioidomycosis, North American blastomycosis, cryptococcosis (torulosis), tinea versicolor, and nocardiosis.

CONTRAINDICATIONS

This drug is contraindicated in patients with porphyria, hepatocellular failure, and in individuals with a history of hypersensitivity to griseofulvin.
Rare cases of conjoined twins have been reported in patients taking griseofulvin during the first trimester of pregnancy. Griseofulvin should not be prescribed to pregnant patients or to women contemplating pregnancy.

WARNINGS

Prophylactic Usage: Safety and efficacy of griseofulvin for prophylaxis of fungal infections have not been established. Since griseofulvin has demonstrated harmful effects *in vitro* on the genotype in bacteria, plants, and fungi, males should wait at least six months after completing griseofulvin therapy before fathering a child. Females should avoid risk of pregnancy while receiving griseofulvin therapy.
Animal Toxicology: Chronic feeding of griseofulvin, at levels ranging from 0.5–2.5% of the diet, resulted in the development of liver tumors in several strains of mice, particularly in males. Smaller particle sizes result in an enhanced effect. Lower oral dosage levels have not been tested. Subcutaneous administration of relatively small doses of griseofulvin once a week during the first three weeks of life has also been reported to induce hepatomata in mice. Thyroid tumors, mostly adenomas but some carcinomas, have been reported in male rats receiving griseofulvin at levels of 2.0%, 1.0%, and 0.2% of the diet, and in female rats receiving the two higher dose levels. Although studies in other animal species have not yielded evidence of tumorigenicity, these studies were not of adequate design to form a basis for conclusions in this regard.
In subacute toxicity studies, orally administered griseofulvin produced hepatocellular necrosis in mice, but this has not been seen in other species. Disturbances in porphyrin metabolism have been reported in griseofulvin-treated laboratory animals. Griseofulvin has been reported to have a colchicine-like effect on mitosis and cocarcinogenicity with methylcholanthrene in cutaneous tumor induction in laboratory animals.
Griseofulvin interferes with chromosomal distribution during cell division, causing aneuploidy in plant and mammalian cells. These effects have been demonstrated *in vitro* at concentrations that may be achieved in the serum with the recommended therapeutic dosage.
Usage in Pregnancy: Griseofulvin should not be prescribed to pregnant patients or to women contemplating pregnancy (see **CONTRAINDICATIONS**).
Animal Reproduction Studies: It has been reported in the literature that griseofulvin was found to be embryotoxic and teratogenic on oral administration to pregnant rats. Pups with abnormalities have been reported in the litters of a few bitches treated with griseofulvin.
Suppression of spermatogenesis has been reported to occur in rats, but investigation in man failed to confirm this.

PRECAUTIONS

Patients on prolonged therapy with any potent medication should be under close observation. Periodic monitoring of organ system function, including renal, hepatic, and hematopoietic, should be done.
Since griseofulvin is derived from species of *Penicillium,* the possibility of cross-sensitivity with penicillin exists; however, known penicillin-sensitive patients have been treated without difficulty.
Since a photosensitivity reaction is occasionally associated with griseofulvin therapy, patients should be warned to avoid exposure to intense natural or artificial sunlight.
Lupus erythematosus or lupus-like syndromes, or exacerbation of existing lupus, have been reported in patients receiving griseofulvin.
Drug Interactions
Griseofulvin decreases the activity of warfarin-type anticoagulants so that patients receiving these drugs concomitantly may require dosage adjustment of the anticoagulant during and after griseofulvin therapy.
Barbiturates usually depress griseofulvin activity, and concomitant administration may require a dosage adjustment of the antifungal agent.
The effects of alcohol may be potentiated by griseofulvin, producing such effects as tachycardia and flush.
Griseofulvin may potentiate an increase in hepatic enzymes that metabolize estrogens at an increased rate, including the estrogen component of oral contraceptives, thereby causing possible decreased contraceptive effects and menstrual irregularities.

ADVERSE REACTIONS

When adverse reactions occur, they are most commonly of the hypersensitivity type, such as skin rashes and urticaria; and rarely, angioneurotic edema and epidermal necrolysis (Lyell's syndrome), and may necessitate withdrawal of therapy and appropriate countermeasures. Paresthesias of the hands and feet have been reported rarely after extended therapy. Other side effects reported occasionally are oral thrush, nausea, vomiting, epigastric distress, diarrhea, headache, fatigue, dizziness, insomnia, mental confusion, and impairment of performance of routine activities.
Proteinuria, nephrosis, leukopenia, hepatic toxicity, GI bleeding and menstrual irregularities have been reported rarely. Administration of the drug should be discontinued if granulocytopenia occurs.
When rare, serious reactions occur with griseofulvin, they are usually associated with high dosages, long periods of therapy, or both.

DOSAGE AND ADMINISTRATION

Accurate diagnosis of the infecting organism is essential. Identification should be made either by direct microscopic examination of a mounting of infected tissue in a solution of potassium hydroxide or by culture on an appropriate medium.
Medication must be continued until the infecting organism is completely eradicated as indicated by appropriate clinical or laboratory examination. Representative treatment periods are tinea capitis, 4 to 6 weeks; tinea corporis, 2 to 4 weeks; tinea pedis, 4 to 8 weeks; tinea unguium—depending on rate of growth—fingernails, at least 4 months; toenails, at least 6 months.
General measures in regard to hygiene should be observed to control sources of infection or reinfection. Concomitant use of appropriate topical agents is usually required, particularly in treatment of tinea pedis. In some forms of athlete's foot, yeasts and bacteria may be involved as well as fungi. Griseofulvin will not eradicate the bacterial or monilial infection.
Adults: Daily administration of 375 mg (as a single dose or in divided amounts) will give a satisfactory response in most patients with tinea corporis, tinea cruris, and tinea capitis. For those fungus infections more difficult to eradicate, such as tinea pedis and tinea unguium, a divided dose of 750 mg is recommended.
Children: Approximately 3.3 mg per pound of body weight per day of ultramicrosize griseofulvin is an effective dose for most children. On this basis, the following dosage schedule is suggested: Children weighing 35 to 60 pounds—125 mg to 187.5 mg daily. Children weighing over 60 pounds—187.5 mg to 375 mg daily.
Children 2 years of age and younger—dosage has not been established.
Clinical experience with griseofulvin in children with tinea capitis indicates that a single daily dose is effective. Clinical relapse will occur if the medication is not continued until the infecting organism is eradicated.

HOW SUPPLIED

FULVICIN P/G Tablets, 125 mg, white, compressed, scored tablets impressed with the Schering trademark and product identification numbers, 228; bottle of 100 (NDC 0085-0228-03).
FULVICIN P/G Tablets, 250 mg, white, compressed, scored tablets impressed with the Schering trademark and product identification numbers, 507; bottle of 100 (NDC 0085-0507-03).
Store between 15° and 30°C (59° and 86°F).
Revised 1/93   16184748

Shown in Product Identification Guide, page 334

FULVICIN® P/G 165 and 330
brand of ultramicrosize griseofulvin
   Tablets, USP

℞

DESCRIPTION

FULVICIN P/G Tablets contain ultramicrosize crystals of griseofulvin, an antibiotic derived from a species of *Penicillium.* Griseofulvin crystals are partly dissolved in polyethylene glycol 8000 and partly dispersed throughout the tablet matrix.
Each FULVICIN P/G Tablet contains 165 mg or 330 mg ultramicrosize griseofulvin, USP.
The inactive ingredients for FULVICIN P/G 165 and 330 Tablets include: corn starch, lactose, magnesium stearate, PEG, and sodium lauryl sulfate.

ACTIONS

Microbiology: Griseofulvin is fungistatic with *in vitro* activity against various species of *Microsporum, Epidermophyton,* and *Trichophyton.* It has no effect on bacteria or on other genera of fungi.
Human Pharmacology: Following oral administration, griseofulvin is deposited in the keratin precursor cells and has a greater affinity for diseased tissue. The drug is tightly bound to the new keratin which becomes highly resistant to fungal invasions.
The efficiency of gastrointestinal absorption of ultramicrocrystalline griseofulvin is approximately one and one-half times that of the conventional microsize griseofulvin. This factor permits the oral intake of two-thirds as much ultramicrocrystalline griseofulvin as the microsize form. However, there is currently no evidence that this lower dose confers any significant clinical differences with regard to safety and/or efficacy.

INDICATIONS

FULVICIN P/G Tablets are indicated for the treatment of ringworm infections of the skin, hair, and nails, namely: tinea corporis, tinea pedis, tinea cruris, tinea barbae, tinea capitis, tinea unguium (onychomycosis) when caused by one or more of the following genera of fungi: *Trichophyton rubrum, Trichophyton tonsurans, Trichophyton mentagrophytes, Trichophyton interdigitale, Trichophyton verrucosum, Trichophyton megninii, Trichophyton gallinae, Trichophyton crateriforme, Trichophyton sulphureum, Trichophyton schoenleinii, Microsporum audouini, Microsporum canis, Microsporum gypseum,* and *Epidermophyton floccosum.*
Note: Prior to therapy, the type of fungi responsible for the infection should be identified.
The use of this drug is not justified in minor or trivial infections which will respond to topical agents alone.
Griseofulvin is not effective in the following: bacterial infections, candidiasis (moniliasis), histoplasmosis, actinomycosis, sporotrichosis, chromoblastomycosis, coccidioidomycosis, North American blastomycosis, cryptococcosis (torulosis), tinea versicolor, and nocardiosis.

CONTRAINDICATIONS

This drug is contraindicated in patients with porphyria, hepatocellular failure, and in individuals with a history of hypersensitivity to griseofulvin.
Rare cases of conjoined twins have been reported in patients taking griseofulvin during the first trimester of pregnancy. Griseofulvin should not be prescribed to pregnant patients or to women contemplating pregnancy.

WARNINGS

Prophylactic Usage: Safety and efficacy of griseofulvin for prophylaxis of fungal infections have not been established. Since griseofulvin has demonstrated harmful effects *in vitro* on the genotype in bacteria, plants, and fungi, males should wait at least six months after completing griseofulvin therapy before fathering a child. Females should avoid risk of pregnancy while receiving griseofulvin therapy.
Animal Toxicology: Chronic feeding of griseofulvin, at levels ranging from 0.5–2.5% of the diet, resulted in the development of liver tumors in several strains of mice, particularly in males. Smaller particle sizes result in an enhanced effect. Lower oral dosage levels have not been tested. Subcutaneous administration of relatively small doses of griseofulvin once a week during the first three weeks of life has also been reported to induce hepatomata in mice. Thyroid tumors, mostly adenomas but some carcinomas, have been reported in male rats receiving griseofulvin at levels of 2.0%, 1.0%, and 0.2% of the diet, and in female rats receiving the two higher dose levels. Although studies in other animal species have not yielded evidence of tumorigenicity, these studies were not of adequate design to form a basis for conclusions in this regard.
In subacute toxicity studies, orally administered griseofulvin produced hepatocellular necrosis in mice, but this has not been seen in other species. Disturbances in porphyrin metabolism have been reported in griseofulvin-treated laboratory animals. Griseofulvin has been reported to have a colchicine-like effect on mitosis and cocarcinogenicity with methylcholanthrene in cutaneous tumor induction in laboratory animals.

Griseofulvin interferes with chromosomal distribution during cell division, causing aneuploidy in plant and mammalian cells. These effects have been demonstrated *in vitro* at concentrations that may be achieved in the serum with the recommended therapeutic dosage.

Usage in Pregnancy: Griseofulvin should not be prescribed to pregnant patients or to women contemplating pregnancy (see **CONTRAINDICATIONS**).

Animal Reproduction Studies: It has been reported in the literature that griseofulvin was found to be embryotoxic and teratogenic on oral administration to pregnant rats. Pups with abnormalities have been reported in the litters of a few bitches treated with griseofulvin.

Suppression of spermatogenesis has been reported to occur in rats, but investigation in man failed to confirm this.

PRECAUTIONS

Patients on prolonged therapy with any potent medication should be under close observation. Periodic monitoring of organ system function, including renal, hepatic, and hematopoietic, should be done.

Since griseofulvin is derived from species of *Penicillium*, the possibility of cross-sensitivity with penicillin exists; however, known penicillin-sensitive patients have been treated without difficulty.

Since a photosensitivity reaction is occasionally associated with griseofulvin therapy, patients should be warned to avoid exposure to intense natural or artificial sunlight.

Lupus erythematosus or lupus-like syndromes, or exacerbation of existing lupus, have been reported in patients receiving griseofulvin.

Drug Interactions: Griseofulvin decreases the activity of warfarin-type anticoagulants so that patients receiving these drugs concomitantly may require dosage adjustment of the anticoagulant during and after griseofulvin therapy.

Barbiturates usually depress griseofulvin activity, and concomitant administration may require a dosage adjustment of the antifungal agent.

The effects of alcohol may be potentiated by griseofulvin, producing such effects as tachycardia and flush.

Griseofulvin may potentiate an increase in hepatic enzymes that metabolize estrogens at an increased rate, including the estrogen component of oral contraceptives, thereby causing possible decreased contraceptive effects and menstrual irregularities.

ADVERSE REACTIONS

When adverse reactions occur, they are most commonly of the hypersensitivity type, such as skin rashes and urticaria; and rarely, angioneurotic edema and epidermal necrolysis (Lyell's syndrome), and may necessitate withdrawal of therapy and appropriate countermeasures. Paresthesias of the hands and feet have been reported rarely after extended therapy. Other side effects reported occasionally are oral thrush, nausea, vomiting, epigastric distress, diarrhea, headache, fatigue, dizziness, insomnia, mental confusion, and impairment of performance of routine activities.

Proteinuria, nephrosis, leukopenia, hepatic toxicity, GI bleeding and menstrual irregularities have been reported rarely. Administration of the drug should be discontinued if granulocytopenia occurs.

When rare, serious reactions occur with griseofulvin, they are usually associated with high dosages, long periods of therapy, or both.

DOSAGE AND ADMINISTRATION

Accurate diagnosis of the infecting organism is essential. Identification should be made either by direct microscopic examination of a mounting of infected tissue in a solution of potassium hydroxide or by culture on an appropriate medium.

Medication must be continued until the infecting organism is completely eradicated as indicated by appropriate clinical or laboratory examination. Representative treatment periods are tinea capitis, 4 to 6 weeks; tinea corporis, 2 to 4 weeks; tinea pedis, 4 to 8 weeks; tinea unguium—depending on rate of growth—fingernails, at least 4 months; toenails, at least 6 months.

General measures in regard to hygiene should be observed to control sources of infection or reinfection. Concomitant use of appropriate topical agents is usually required, particularly in treatment of tinea pedis. In some forms of athlete's foot, yeasts and bacteria may be involved as well as fungi. Griseofulvin will not eradicate the bacterial or monilial infection.

Adults: Daily administration of 330 mg (as a single dose or in divided amounts) will give a satisfactory response in most patients with tinea corporis, tinea cruris, and tinea capitis. For those fungus infections more difficult to eradicate, such as tinea pedis and tinea unguium, a divided daily dosage of 660 mg is recommended.

Children: Approximately 3.3 mg per pound of body weight per day is an effective dose for most children. On this basis, the following dosage schedule is suggested: Children weighing 30 to 50 pounds—82.5 mg to 165 mg daily. Children weighing over 50 pounds—165 mg to 330 mg daily.

Children 2 years of age and younger—dosage has not been established.

Clinical experience with griseofulvin in children with tinea capitis indicates that a single daily dose is effective. Clinical relapse will occur if the medication is not continued until the infecting organism is eradicated.

HOW SUPPLIED

FULVICIN P/G 165 Tablets, 165 mg, off-white, oval, compressed, scored tablets impressed with the product name (FULVICIN P/G) and product identification numbers, 654; bottle of 100 (NDC 0085-0654-03).

FULVICIN P/G 330 Tablets, 330 mg, off-white, oval, compressed, scored tablets impressed with the product name (FULVICIN P/G) and product identification numbers, 352; bottle of 100 (NDC 0085-0352-03).

Store between 2° and 30°C (36° and 86°F).

Revised 6/92 16100129

Copyright © 1976, 1989, 1992, Schering Corporation. All rights reserved.

Shown in Product Identification Guide, page 334

GARAMYCIN® ℞

brand of gentamicin sulfate
Cream, USP 0.1% and
Ointment, USP 0.1%
For Dermatologic Use Only–Not For Ophthalmic Use

DESCRIPTION

Each gram of GARAMYCIN **Cream** 0.1% contains 1.7 mg gentamicin sulfate, USP, equivalent to 1.0 mg gentamicin base, with 1.0 mg methylparaben and 4.0 mg butylparaben as preservatives, in a bland, emulsion-type vehicle composed of stearic acid, propylene glycol stearate, isopropyl myristate, propylene glycol, polysorbate 40, sorbitol solution and purified water.

Each gram of GARAMYCIN **Ointment** 0.1% contains 1.7 mg gentamicin sulfate, USP, equivalent to 1.0 mg gentamicin base, with 0.5 mg methylparaben and 0.1 mg propylparaben as preservatives in a bland, unctuous petrolatum base.

ACTIONS

GARAMYCIN, a wide-spectrum antibiotic, provides highly effective topical treatment in primary and secondary bacterial infections of the skin. GARAMYCIN may clear infections that have not responded to other topical antibiotic agents. In impetigo contagiosa and other primary skin infections, treatment three or four times daily with GARAMYCIN usually clears the lesions promptly. In secondary skin infections, GARAMYCIN facilitates the treatment of the underlying dermatosis by controlling the infection. Bacteria susceptible to the action of GARAMYCIN include sensitive strains of streptococci (group A beta-hemolytic, alpha-hemolytic), *Staphylococcus aureus* (coagulase-positive, coagulase-negative, and some penicillinase-producing strains), and the gram-negative bacteria, *Pseudomonas aeruginosa, Aerobacter aerogenes, Escherichia coli, Proteus vulgaris,* and *Klebsiella pneumoniae.*

INDICATIONS

Primary skin infections: Impetigo contagiosa, superficial folliculitis, ecthyma, furunculosis, sycosis barbae, and pyoderma gangrenosum. *Secondary skin infections:* Infectious eczematoid dermatitis, pustular acne, pustular psoriasis, infected seborrheic dermatitis, infected contact dermatitis (including poison ivy), infected excoriations, and bacterial superinfections of fungal or viral infections. Note: GARAMYCIN is a bactericidal agent that is not effective against viruses or fungi in skin infections. GARAMYCIN is useful in the treatment of infected skin cysts and certain other skin abscesses when preceded by incision and drainage to permit adequate contact between the antibiotic and the infecting bacteria. Good results have been obtained in the treatment of infected stasis and other skin ulcers, infected superficial burns, paronychia, infected insect bites and stings, infected lacerations and abrasions, and wounds from minor surgery. Patients sensitive to neomycin can be treated with gentamicin, although regular observation of patients sensitive to topical antibiotics is advisable when such patients are treated with any topical antibiotic. GARAMYCIN **Ointment** helps retain moisture and has been useful in infection on dry eczematous or psoriatic skin. GARAMYCIN **Cream** is recommended for wet, oozing primary infections and greasy, secondary infections, such as pustular acne or infected seborrheic dermatitis. If a water-washable preparation is desired, GARAMYCIN **Cream** is preferable. GARAMYCIN **Ointment** and **Cream** have been used successfully in infants over one year of age, as well as in adults and children.

CONTRAINDICATIONS

This drug is contraindicated in individuals with a history of sensitivity reactions to any of its components.

PRECAUTIONS

Use of topical antibiotics occasionally allows overgrowth of nonsusceptible organisms, including fungi. If this occurs, or if irritation, sensitization, or superinfection develops, treatment with gentamicin should be discontinued and appropriate therapy instituted.

ADVERSE REACTIONS

In patients with dermatoses treated with gentamicin, irritation (erythema and pruritus) that did not usually require discontinuance of treatment has been reported in a small percentage of cases. There was no evidence of irritation or sensitization, however, in any of these patients patch-tested subsequently with gentamicin on normal skin. Possible photosensitization has been reported in several patients but could not be elicited in these patients by reapplication of gentamicin followed by exposure to ultraviolet radiation.

DOSAGE AND ADMINISTRATION

A small amount of GARAMYCIN **Cream** or **Ointment** should be applied gently to the lesions three or four times daily. The area treated may be covered with a gauze dressing if desired. In impetigo contagiosa, the crusts should be removed before application of GARAMYCIN to permit maximum contact between the antibiotic and the infection. Care should be exercised to avoid further contamination of the infected skin. Infected stasis ulcers have responded well to GARAMYCIN under gelatin packing.

HOW SUPPLIED

GARAMYCIN **Cream** 0.1% (NDC-0085-0008-05) and GARAMYCIN **Ointment** 0.1% (NDC-0085-0343-05), 15 g tubes.

Store between 2° and 30°C (36° and 86°F).

Schering Corporation
Kenilworth, NJ 07033 USA
Revised 7/91 11808654

Copyright © 1966, 1991, Schering Corporation. All rights reserved.

GARAMYCIN® ℞

brand of gentamicin sulfate
Ophthalmic Solution, USP—Sterile
Ophthalmic Ointment, USP—Sterile
Each mL or gram contains gentamicin sulfate, USP equivalent to 3.0 mg gentamicin

DESCRIPTION

Gentamicin sulfate is a water-soluble antibiotic of the aminoglycoside group.

Gentamicin Sulfate Ophthalmic Solution is a sterile, aqueous solution buffered to approximately pH 7 for ophthalmic use. Each mL contains gentamicin sulfate, USP (equivalent to 3.0 mg gentamicin), disodium phosphate, monosodium phosphate, sodium chloride, and benzalkonium chloride (0.1 mg) as a preservative.

Gentamicin Sulfate Ophthalmic Ointment is a sterile ointment, each gram containing gentamicin sulfate, USP (equivalent to 3.0 mg gentamicin) in a base of white petrolatum, with methylparaben (0.5 mg) and propylparaben (0.1 mg) as preservatives.

Gentamicin is obtained from cultures of *Micromonospora purpurea.* It is a mixture of the sulfate salts of gentamicin C_1, C_2 and C_{1A}. All three components appear to have similar antimicrobial activities. Gentamicin sulfate occurs as a white powder and is soluble in water and insoluble in alcohol. The structure is as follows:

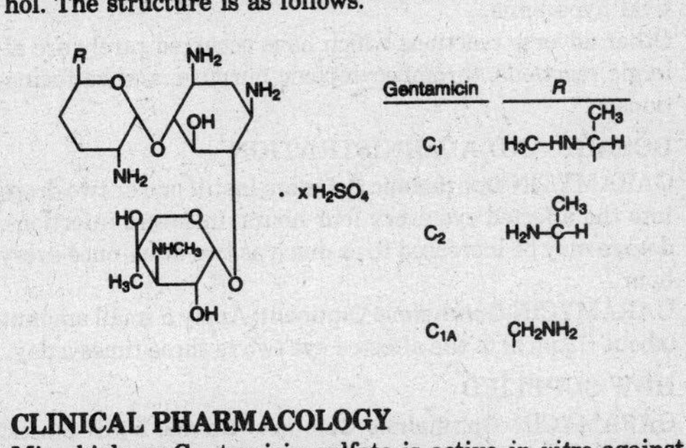

CLINICAL PHARMACOLOGY

Microbiology: Gentamicin sulfate is active *in vitro* against many strains of the following microorganisms: *Staphylococcus aureus, Staphylococcus epidermidis, Streptococcus pyogenes, Streptococcus pneumoniae, Enterobacter aerogenes, Escherichia coli, Haemophilus influenzae, Klebsiella*

Continued on next page

Information on Schering products appearing on these pages is effective as of August 15, 1996.

Schering—Cont.

pneumoniae, Neisseria gonorrhoeae, Pseudomonas aeruginosa, and *Serratia marcescens.*

INDICATIONS AND USAGE

GARAMYCIN Sterile Ophthalmic Solution and Ointment are indicated in the topical treatment of ocular bacterial infections, including conjunctivitis, keratitis, keratoconjunctivitis, corneal ulcers, blepharitis, blepharoconjunctivitis, acute meibomianitis, and dacryocystitis caused by susceptible strains of the following microorganisms:
Staphylococcus aureus, Staphylococcus epidermidis, Streptococcus pyogenes, Streptococcus pneumoniae, Enterobacter aerogenes, Escherichia coli, Haemophilus influenzae, Klebsiella pneumoniae, Neisseria gonorrhoeae, Pseudomonas aeruginosa, and *Serratia marcescens.*

CONTRAINDICATIONS

GARAMYCIN Ophthalmic Solution and Ointment are contraindicated in patients with known hypersensitivity to any of the components.

WARNINGS

NOT FOR INJECTION INTO THE EYE.
Gentamicin Sulfate Ophthalmic Solution and Ointment are not for injection. They should never be injected subconjunctivally, nor should they be directly introduced into the anterior chamber of the eye.

PRECAUTIONS

General: Prolonged use of topical antibiotics may give rise to overgrowth of nonsusceptible organisms including fungi. Bacterial resistance to gentamicin may also develop. If purulent discharge, inflammation or pain becomes aggravated, the patient should discontinue use of the medication and consult a physician.
If irritation or hypersensitivity to any component of the drug develops, the patient should discontinue use of this preparation, and appropriate therapy should be instituted.
Ophthalmic ointments may retard corneal healing.
Information for Patients: To avoid contamination, do not touch tip of container to the eye, eyelid, or any surface.
Carcinogenesis, Mutagenesis, Impairment of Fertility: There are no published carcinogenicity or impairment of fertility studies on gentamicin. Aminoglycoside antibiotics have been found to be non-mutagenic.
Pregnancy: Pregnancy Category C. Gentamicin has been shown to depress body weights, kidney weights, and median glomerular counts in newborn rats when administered systemically to pregnant rats in daily doses approximately 500 times the maximum recommended ophthalmic human dose. There are no adequate and well-controlled studies in pregnant women. Gentamicin should be used during pregnancy only if the potential benefit justifies the potential risk to the fetus.

ADVERSE REACTIONS

Bacterial and fungal corneal ulcers have developed during treatment with gentamicin ophthalmic preparations.
The most frequently reported adverse reactions are ocular burning and irritation upon drug instillation, non-specific conjunctivitis, conjunctival epithelial defects, and conjunctival hyperemia.
Other adverse reactions which have occurred rarely are allergic reactions, thrombocytopenic purpura, and hallucinations.

DOSAGE AND ADMINISTRATION

GARAMYCIN **Ophthalmic Solution:** Instill one or two drops into the affected eye every four hours. In severe infections, dosage may be increased to as much as two drops once every hour.
GARAMYCIN **Ophthalmic Ointment:** Apply a small amount (about $1/2$ inch) to the affected eye two to three times a day.

HOW SUPPLIED

GARAMYCIN **Ophthalmic Solution**—Sterile, 5-mL plastic dropper bottle, box of one (NDC- 0085-0899-05).
GARAMYCIN **Ophthalmic Ointment**—Sterile, 3.5 g tube, box of one (NDC-0085-0151-05).
Store GARAMYCIN **Ophthalmic Ointment and Solution between 2° and 30°C (36° and 86°F).**
Schering Corporation
Kenilworth, NJ 07033 USA
Revised 4/92   13227225
Copyright © 1969, 1992, Schering Corporation. All rights reserved.

GARAMYCIN® Injectable   ℞
brand of gentamicin sulfate injection, USP
40 mg per mL
Each mL contains gentamicin sulfate, USP equivalent to 40 mg gentamicin.
For Parenteral Administration

WARNINGS

Patients treated with aminoglycosides should be under close clinical observation because of the potential toxicity associated with their use.
As with other aminoglycosides, GARAMYCIN Injectable is potentially nephrotoxic. The risk of nephrotoxicity is greater in patients with impaired renal function and in those who receive high dosage or prolonged therapy.
Neurotoxicity manifested by ototoxicity, both vestibular and auditory, can occur in patients treated with GARAMYCIN Injectable, primarily in those with pre-existing renal damage and in patients with normal renal function treated with higher doses and/or for longer periods than recommended. Aminoglycoside-induced ototoxicity is usually irreversible. Other manifestations of neurotoxicity may include numbness, skin tingling, muscle twitching, and convulsions.
Renal and eighth cranial nerve function should be closely monitored, especially in patients with known or suspected reduced renal function at onset of therapy, and also in those whose renal function is initially normal but who develop signs of renal dysfunction during therapy. Urine should be examined for decreased specific gravity, increased excretion of protein, and the presence of cells or casts. Blood urea nitrogen, serum creatinine, or creatinine clearance should be determined periodically. When feasible, it is recommended that serial audiograms be obtained in patients old enough to be tested, particularly high-risk patients. Evidence of ototoxicity (dizziness, vertigo, ataxia, tinnitus, roaring in the ears, or hearing loss) or nephrotoxicity requires dosage adjustment or discontinuance of the drug. As with the other aminoglycosides, on rare occasions changes in renal and eighth cranial nerve function may not become manifest until soon after completion of therapy.
Serum concentrations of aminoglycosides should be monitored when feasible to assure adequate levels and to avoid potentially toxic levels. When monitoring gentamicin peak concentrations, dosage should be adjusted so that prolonged levels above 12 mcg/mL are avoided. When monitoring gentamicin trough concentrations, dosage should be adjusted so that levels above 2 mcg/mL are avoided. Excessive peak and/or trough serum concentrations of aminoglycosides may increase the risk of renal and eighth cranial nerve toxicity. In the event of overdose or toxic reactions, hemodialysis may aid in the removal of gentamicin from the blood, especially if renal function is, or becomes, compromised. The rate of removal of gentamicin is considerably less by peritoneal dialysis than by hemodialysis.
Concurrent and/or sequential systemic or topical use of other potentially neurotoxic and/or nephrotoxic drugs, such as cisplatin, cephaloridine, kanamycin, amikacin, neomycin, polymyxin B, colistin, paromomycin, streptomycin, tobramycin, vancomycin, and viomycin, should be avoided. Other factors which may increase patient risk of toxicity are advanced age and dehydration.
The concurrent use of gentamicin with potent diuretics, such as ethacrynic acid or furosemide, should be avoided, since certain diuretics by themselves may cause ototoxicity. In addition, when administered intravenously, diuretics may enhance aminoglycoside toxicity by altering the antibiotic concentration in serum and tissue.

DESCRIPTION

Gentamicin sulfate, USP, a water-soluble antibiotic of the aminoglycoside group, is derived from *Micromonospora purpurea,* an actinomycete. GARAMYCIN Injectable is a sterile, aqueous solution for parenteral administration. Each mL contains gentamicin sulfate, USP equivalent to 40 mg gentamicin base; 1.8 mg methylparaben and 0.2 mg propylparaben as preservatives; 3.2 mg sodium bisulfite; and 0.1 mg edetate disodium.

CLINICAL PHARMACOLOGY

After intramuscular administration of GARAMYCIN Injectable, peak serum concentrations usually occur between 30 and 60 minutes and serum levels are measurable for 6 to 8 hours. When gentamicin is administered by intravenous infusion over a 2-hour period, the serum concentrations are similar to those obtained by intramuscular administration. In patients with normal renal function, peak serum concentrations of gentamicin (mcg/mL) are usually up to four times

the single intramuscular dose (mg/kg); for example, a 1.0 mg/kg injection in adults may be expected to result in a peak serum concentration up to 4 mcg/mL; a 1.5 mg/kg dose may produce levels up to 6 mcg/mL. While some variation is to be expected due to a number of variables such as age, body temperature, surface area, and physiologic differences, the individual patient given the same dose tends to have similar levels in repeated determinations. Gentamicin administered at 1.0 mg/kg every 8 hours for the usual 7- to 10-day treatment period to patients with normal renal function does not accumulate in the serum.
Gentamicin, like all aminoglycosides, may accumulate in the serum and tissues of patients treated with higher doses and/or for prolonged periods, particularly in the presence of impaired renal function. In adult patients, treatment with gentamicin dosages of 4 mg/kg/day or higher for 7 to 10 days may result in a slight, progressive rise in both peak and trough concentrations. In patients with impaired renal function, gentamicin is cleared from the body more slowly than in patients with normal renal function. The more severe the impairment, the slower the clearance. (Dosage must be adjusted.)
Since gentamicin is distributed in extracellular fluid, peak serum concentrations may be lower than usual in adult patients who have a large volume of this fluid. Serum concentrations of gentamicin in febrile patients may be lower than those in afebrile patients given the same dose. When body temperature returns to normal, serum concentrations of the drug may rise. Febrile and anemic states may be associated with a shorter than usual serum half-life. (Dosage adjustment is usually not necessary.) In severely burned patients, the half-life may be significantly decreased and resulting serum concentrations may be lower than anticipated from the mg/kg dose.
Protein-binding studies have indicated that the degree of gentamicin binding is low; depending upon the methods used for testing, this may be between 0 and 30%.
After initial administration to patients with normal renal function, generally 70% or more of the gentamicin dose is recoverable in the urine in 24 hours; concentrations in urine above 100 mcg/mL may be achieved. Little, if any, metabolic transformation occurs; the drug is excreted principally by glomerular filtration. After several days of treatment, the amount of gentamicin excreted in the urine approaches the daily dose administered. As with other aminoglycosides, a small amount of the gentamicin dose may be retained in the tissues, especially in the kidneys. Minute quantities of aminoglycosides have been detected in the urine weeks after drug administration was discontinued. Renal clearance of gentamicin is similar to that of endogenous creatinine.
In patients with marked impairment of renal function, there is a decrease in the concentration of aminoglycosides in urine and in their penetration into defective renal parenchyma. This decreased drug excretion, together with the potential nephrotoxicity of aminoglycosides, should be considered when treating such patients who have urinary tract infections.
Probenecid does not affect renal tubular transport of gentamicin.
The endogenous creatinine clearance rate and the serum creatinine level have a high correlation with the half-life of gentamicin in serum. Results of these tests may serve as guides for adjusting dosage in patients with renal impairment (see **DOSAGE AND ADMINISTRATION**).
Following parenteral administration, gentamicin can be detected in serum, lymph, tissues, sputum, and in pleural, synovial, and peritoneal fluids. Concentrations in renal cortex sometimes may be eight times higher than the usual serum levels. Concentrations in bile, in general, have been low and have suggested minimal biliary excretion. Gentamicin crosses the peritoneal as well as the placental membranes. Since aminoglycosides diffuse poorly into the subarachnoid space after parenteral administration, concentrations of gentamicin in cerebrospinal fluid are often low and dependent upon dose, rate of penetration, and degree of meningeal inflammation. There is minimal penetration of gentamicin into ocular tissues following intramuscular or intravenous administration.
Microbiology: *In vitro* tests have demonstrated that gentamicin is a bactericidal antibiotic which acts by inhibiting normal protein synthesis in susceptible microorganisms. It is active against a wide variety of pathogenic bacteria including *Escherichia coli, Proteus* species (indole-positive and indole-negative), *Pseudomonas aeruginosa,* species of the *Klebsiella-Enterobacter-Serratia* group. *Citrobacter* species and *Staphylococcus* species (including penicillin- and methicillin-resistant strains). Gentamicin is also active *in vitro* against species of *Salmonella* and *Shigella.* The following bacteria are usually resistant to aminoglycosides: *Streptococcus pneumoniae,* most species of streptococci, particularly group D and anaerobic organisms, such as *Bacteroides* species or *Clostridium* species.
In vitro studies have shown that an aminoglycoside combined with an antibiotic that interferes with cell wall synthesis may act synergistically against some group D streptococcal strains. The combination of gentamicin and penicillin G

has a synergistic bactericidal effect against virtually all strains of *Streptococcus faecalis* and its varieties *(S. faecalis* var. *liquifaciens, S. faecalis* var. *zymogenes), S. faecium* and *S. durans*. An enhanced killing effect against many of these strains has also been shown *in vitro* with combinations of gentamicin and ampicillin, carbenicillin, nafcillin, or oxacillin.

The combined effect of gentamicin and carbenicillin is synergistic for many strains of *Pseudomonas aeruginosa. In vitro* synergism against other gram-negative organisms has been shown with combinations of gentamicin and cephalosporins. Gentamicin may be active against clinical isolates of bacteria resistant to other aminoglycosides. Bacteria resistant to one aminoglycoside may be resistant to one or more other aminoglycosides. Bacterial resistance to gentamicin is generally developed slowly.

Susceptibility Testing: If the disc method of susceptibility testing used is that described by Bauer *et al. (Am J Clin Path* 45:493, 1966; *Federal Register* 37:20525-20529, 1972), a disc containing 10 mcg of gentamicin should give a zone of inhibition of 15mm or more to indicate susceptibility of the infecting organism. A zone of 12mm or less indicates that the infecting organism is likely to be resistant. Zones greater than 12mm and less than 15mm indicate intermediate susceptibility. In certain conditions it may be desirable to do additional susceptibility testing by the tube or agar dilution method; gentamicin substance is available for this purpose.

INDICATIONS AND USAGE

GARAMYCIN Injectable is indicated in the treatment of serious infections caused by susceptible strains of the following microorganisms: *Pseudomonas aeruginosa, Proteus* species (indole-positive and indole-negative), *Escherichia coli, Klebsiella-Enterobacter-Serratia* species, *Citrobacter* species, and *Staphylococcus* species (coagulase-positive and coagulase-negative).

Clinical studies have shown GARAMYCIN Injectable to be effective in bacterial neonatal sepsis; bacterial septicemia; and serious bacterial infections of the central nervous system (meningitis), urinary tract, respiratory tract, gastrointestinal tract (including peritonitis), skin, bone and soft tissue (including burns). Aminoglycosides, including gentamicin, are not indicated in uncomplicated initial episodes of urinary tract infections unless the causative organisms are susceptible to these antibiotics and are not susceptible to antibiotics having less potential for toxicity.

Specimens for bacterial culture should be obtained to isolate and identify causative organisms and to determine their susceptibility to gentamicin.

GARAMYCIN may be considered as initial therapy in suspected or confirmed gram-negative infections, and therapy may be instituted before obtaining results of susceptibility testing. The decision to continue therapy with this drug should be based on the results of susceptibility tests, the severity of the infection, and the important additional concepts contained in the "**WARNINGS** Box". If the causative organisms are resistant to gentamicin, other appropriate therapy should be instituted.

In serious infections when the causative organisms are unknown, GARAMYCIN may be administered as initial therapy in conjunction with a penicillin-type or cephalosporin-type drug before obtaining results of susceptibility testing. If anaerobic organisms are suspected as etiologic agents, consideration should be given to using other suitable antimicrobial therapy in conjunction with gentamicin. Following identification of the organism and its susceptibility, appropriate antibiotic therapy should then be continued.

GARAMYCIN has been used effectively in combination with carbenicillin for the treatment of life-threatening infections caused by *Pseudomonas aeruginosa*. It has also been found effective when used in conjunction with a penicillin-type drug for the treatment of endocarditis caused by group D streptococci.

GARAMYCIN Injectable has also been shown to be effective in the treatment of serious staphylococcal infections. While not the antibiotic of first choice, GARAMYCIN Injectable may be considered when penicillins or other less potentially toxic drugs are contraindicated and bacterial susceptibility tests and clinical judgment indicate its use. It may also be considered in mixed infections caused by susceptible strains of staphylococci and gram-negative organisms.

In the neonate with suspected bacterial sepsis or staphylococcal pneumonia, a penicillin-type drug is also usually indicated as concomitant therapy with gentamicin.

CONTRAINDICATIONS

Hypersensitivity to gentamicin is a contraindication to its use. A history of hypersensitivity or serious toxic reactions to other aminoglycosides may contraindicate use of gentamicin because of the known cross-sensitivity of patients to drugs in this class.

WARNINGS

(See boxed **WARNINGS**.) Aminoglycosides can cause fetal harm when administered to a pregnant woman. Aminoglyco-

side antibiotics cross the placenta, and there have been several reports of total irreversible bilateral congenital deafness in children whose mothers received streptomycin during pregnancy. Serious side effects to mother, fetus, or newborn have not been reported in the treatment of pregnant women with other aminoglycosides. Animal reproduction studies conducted on rats and rabbits did not reveal evidence of impaired fertility or harm to the fetus due to gentamicin sulfate.

It is not known whether gentamicin sulfate can cause fetal harm when administered to a pregnant woman or can affect reproduction capacity. If gentamicin is used during pregnancy or if the patient becomes pregnant while taking gentamicin, she should be apprised of the potential hazard to the fetus.

GARAMYCIN Injectable contains sodium bisulfite, a sulfite that may cause allergic-type reactions including anaphylactic symptoms and life-threatening or less severe asthmatic episodes in certain susceptible people. The overall prevalence of sulfite sensitivity in the general population is unknown and probably low. Sulfite sensitivity is seen more frequently in asthmatic than in nonasthmatic people.

PRECAUTIONS

Neurotoxic and nephrotoxic antibiotics may be absorbed in significant quantities from body surfaces after local irrigation or application. The potential toxic effect of antibiotics administered in this fashion should be considered.

Increased nephrotoxicity has been reported following concomitant administration of aminoglycoside antibiotics and cephalosporins.

Neuromuscular blockade and respiratory paralysis have been reported in the cat receiving high doses (40 mg/kg) of gentamicin. The possibility of these phenomena occurring in man should be considered if aminoglycosides are administered by any route to patients receiving anesthetics, or to patients receiving neuromuscular blocking agents, such as succinylcholine, tubocurarine, or decamethonium, or in patients receiving massive transfusions of citrate-anticoagulated blood. If neuromuscular blockade occurs, calcium salts may reverse it.

Aminoglycosides should be used with caution in patients with neuromuscular disorders, such as myasthenia gravis, since these drugs may aggravate muscle weakness because of their potential curare-like effects on the neuromuscular junction. During or following gentamicin therapy, paresthesias, tetany, positive Chvostek and Trousseau signs, and mental confusion have been described in patients with hypomagnesemia, hypocalcemia, and hypokalemia. When this has occurred in infants, tetany and muscle weakness has been described. Both adults and infants required appropriate corrective electrolyte therapy.

Elderly patients may have reduced renal function which may not be evident in the results of routine screening tests, such as BUN or serum creatinine. A creatinine clearance determination may be more useful. Monitoring of renal function during treatment with gentamicin, as with other aminoglycosides, is particularly important in such patients. A Fanconi-like syndrome, with aminoaciduria and metabolic acidosis, has been reported in some adults and infants being given gentamicin injections.

Cross-allergenicity among aminoglycosides has been demonstrated.

Patients should be well hydrated during treatment.

Although the *in vitro* mixing of gentamicin and carbenicillin results in a rapid and significant inactivation of gentamicin, this interaction has not been demonstrated in patients with normal renal function who received both drugs by different routes of administration. A reduction in gentamicin serum half-life has been reported in patients with severe renal impairment receiving carbenicillin concomitantly with gentamicin.

Treatment with gentamicin may result in overgrowth of nonsusceptible organisms. If this occurs, appropriate therapy is indicated.

See "**WARNINGS** Box" regarding concurrent use of potent diuretics and regarding concurrent and/or sequential use of other neurotoxic and/or nephrotoxic antibiotics and for other essential information.

Usage in Pregnancy—Safety for use in pregnancy has not been established.

ADVERSE REACTIONS

Nephrotoxicity Adverse renal effects, as demonstrated by the presence of casts, cells, or protein in the urine or by rising BUN, NPN, serum creatinine or oliguria, have been reported. They occur more frequently in patients with a history of renal impairment and in patients treated for longer periods or with larger dosage than recommended.

Neurotoxicity Serious adverse effects on both vestibular and auditory branches of the eighth cranial nerve have been reported, primarily in patients with renal impairment (especially if dialysis is required) and in patients on high doses and/or prolonged therapy. Symptoms include dizziness, ver-

tigo, ataxia, tinnitus, roaring in the ears and hearing loss, which, as with the other aminoglycosides, may be irreversible. Hearing loss is usually manifested initially by diminution of high-tone acuity. Other factors which may increase the risk of toxicity include excessive dosage, dehydration, and previous exposure to other ototoxic drugs.

Peripheral neuropathy or encephalopathy, including numbness, skin tingling, muscle twitching, convulsions, and a myasthenia gravis-like syndrome, have been reported.

Note: The risk of toxic reactions is low in patients with normal renal function who do not receive GARAMYCIN Injectable at higher doses or for longer periods of time than recommended.

Other reported adverse reactions possibly related to gentamicin include: respiratory depression, lethargy, confusion, depression, visual disturbances, decreased appetite, weight loss, and hypotension and hypertension; rash, itching, urticaria, generalized burning, laryngeal edema, anaphylactoid reactions, fever, and headache; nausea, vomiting, increased salivation, and stomatitis; purpura, pseudotumor cerebri, acute organic brain syndrome, pulmonary fibrosis, alopecia, joint pain, transient hepatomegaly, and splenomegaly.

Laboratory abnormalities possibly related to gentamicin include: increased levels of serum transaminase (SGOT, SGPT), serum LDH, and bilirubin; decreased serum calcium, magnesium, sodium, and potassium; anemia, leukopenia, granulocytopenia, transient agranulocytosis, eosinophilia, increased and decreased reticulocyte counts, and thrombocytopenia. While clinical laboratory test abnormalities may be isolated findings, they may also be associated with clinically related signs and symptoms. For example, tetany and muscle weakness may be associated with hypomagnesemia, hypocalcemia, and hypokalemia.

While local tolerance of GARAMYCIN Injectable is generally excellent, there has been an occasional report of pain at the injection site. Subcutaneous atrophy or fat necrosis suggesting local irritation has been reported rarely.

OVERDOSAGE

In the event of overdose or toxic reactions, hemodialysis may aid in the removal of gentamicin from the blood, and is especially important if renal function is, or becomes, compromised. The rate of removal of gentamicin is considerably less by peritoneal dialysis than it is by hemodialysis.

DOSAGE AND ADMINISTRATION

GARAMYCIN Injectable may be given intramuscularly or intravenously. The patient's pretreatment body weight should be obtained for calculation of correct dosage. The dosage of aminoglycosides in obese patients should be based on an estimate of the lean body mass. It is desirable to limit the duration of treatment with aminoglycosides to short term.

DOSAGE FOR PATIENTS WITH NORMAL RENAL FUNCTION

Adults: The recommended dosage of GARAMYCIN Injectable for patients with serious infections and normal renal function is 3 mg/kg/day, administered in three equal doses every 8 hours (Table I).

For patients with life-threatening infections, dosages up to 5 mg/kg/day may be administered in three or four equal doses. This dosage should be reduced to 3 mg/kg/day as soon as clinically indicated (Table I).

It is desirable to measure periodically both peak and trough serum concentrations of gentamicin when feasible during therapy to assure adequate but not excessive drug levels. For example, the peak concentration (at 30 to 60 minutes after intramuscular injection) is expected to be in the range of 4 to 6 mcg/mL. When monitoring peak concentrations after intramuscular or intravenous administration, dosage should be adjusted so that prolonged levels above 12 mcg/mL are avoided. When monitoring trough concentrations (just prior to the next dose), dosage should be adjusted so that levels above 2 mcg/mL are avoided. Determination of the adequacy of a serum level for a particular patient must take into consideration the susceptibility of the causative organism, the severity of the infection, and the status of the patient's host-defense mechanisms.

In patients with extensive burns, altered pharmacokinetics may result in reduced serum concentrations of aminoglycosides. In such patients treated with gentamicin, measurement of serum concentrations is recommended as a basis for dosage adjustment.

Continued on next page

Information on Schering products appearing on these pages is effective as of August 15, 1996.

Schering—Cont.

TABLE I
DOSAGE SCHEDULE GUIDE FOR ADULTS WITH NORMAL RENAL FUNCTION
(Dosage at 8-Hour Intervals)
40 mg per mL

Patient's Weight* kg	(lb)	Usual Dose for Serious Infections 1 mg/kg q8h (3 mg/kg/day) mg/dose q8h	mL/dose	Dose For Life-Threatening Infections (Reduce As Soon As Clinically Indicated) 1.7 mg/kg q8h** (5 mg/kg/day) mg/dose q8h	mL/dose
40	(88)	40	1.0	66	1.6
45	(99)	45	1.1	75	1.9
50	(110)	50	1.25	83	2.1
55	(121)	55	1.4	91	2.25
60	(132)	60	1.5	100	2.5
65	(143)	65	1.6	108	2.7
70	(154)	70	1.75	116	2.9
75	(165)	75	1.9	125	3.1
80	(176)	80	2.0	133	3.3
85	(187)	85	2.1	141	3.5
90	(198)	90	2.25	150	3.75
95	(209)	95	2.4	158	4.0
100	(220)	100	2.5	166	4.2

* The dosage of aminoglycosides in obese patients should be based on an estimate of the lean body mass.
** For q6h schedules, dosage should be recalculated.

Children: 6 to 7.5 mg/kg/day. (2.0 to 2.5 mg/kg administered every 8 hours.)

Infants and Neonates: 7.5 mg/kg/day. (2.5 mg/kg administered every 8 hours.)

Premature or Full-Term Neonates One Week of Age or Less: 5 mg/kg/day. (2.5 mg/kg administered every 12 hours.)

For further information concerning the use of gentamicin in infants and children, see GARAMYCIN Pediatric Injectable Product Information.

The usual duration of treatment for all patients is 7 to 10 days. In difficult and complicated infections, a longer course of therapy may be necessary. In such cases, monitoring of renal, auditory, and vestibular functions is recommended, since toxicity is more apt to occur with treatment extended for more than 10 days. Dosage should be reduced if clinically indicated.

For Intravenous Administration

The intravenous administration of gentamicin may be particularly useful for treating patients with bacterial septicemia or those in shock. It may also be the preferred route of administration for some patients with congestive heart failure, hematologic disorders, severe burns, or those with reduced muscle mass. For intermittent intravenous administration in adults, a single dose of GARAMYCIN Injectable may be diluted in 50 to 200 mL of sterile isotonic saline solution or in a sterile solution of dextrose 5% in water; in infants and children, the volume of diluent should be less. The solution may be infused over a period of $^1/_2$ to 2 hours.

The recommended dosage for intravenous and intramuscular administration is identical.

GARAMYCIN Injectable should not be physically premixed with other drugs, but should be administered separately in accordance with the recommended route of administration and dosage schedule.

DOSAGE FOR PATIENTS WITH IMPAIRED RENAL FUNCTION

Dosage must be adjusted in patients with impaired renal function to assure therapeutically adequate, but not excessive, blood levels. Whenever possible, serum concentrations of gentamicin should be monitored. One method of dosage adjustment is to increase the interval between administration of the usual doses. Since the serum creatinine concentration has a high correlation with the serum half-life of gentamicin, this laboratory test may provide guidance for adjustment of the interval between doses. The interval between doses (in hours) may be approximated by multiplying the serum creatinine level (mg/100 mL) by 8. For example, a patient weighing 60 kg with a serum creatinine level of 2.0 mg/100 mL could be given 60 mg (1 mg/kg) every 16 hours (2×8).

In patients with serious systemic infections and renal impairment, it may be desirable to administer the antibiotic more frequently but in reduced dosage. In such patients, serum concentrations of gentamicin should be measured so that adequate but not excessive levels result. A peak and trough concentration measured intermittently during therapy will provide optimal guidance for adjusting dosage. After the usual initial dose, a rough guide for determining reduced dosage at 8-hour intervals is to divide the normally recommended dose by the serum creatinine level (Table II). For example, after an initial dose of 60 mg (1.0 mg/kg), a patient weighing 60 kg with a serum creatinine level of 2.0 mg/100 mL could be given 30 mg every 8 hours (60 ÷ 2). It should be noted that the status of renal function may be changing over the course of the infectious process.

It is important to recognize that deteriorating renal function may require a greater reduction in dosage than that specified in the above guidelines for patients with stable renal impairment.

TABLE II
DOSAGE ADJUSTMENT GUIDE FOR PATIENTS WITH RENAL IMPAIRMENT
(Dosage at 8-Hour Intervals After the Usual Initial Dose)

Serum Creatinine (mg %)	Approximate Creatinine Clearance Rate (mL/min/1.73M²)	Percent of Usual Doses Shown in Table I
≤ 1.0	> 100	100
1.1–1.3	70–100	80
1.4–1.6	55–70	65
1.7–1.9	45–55	55
2.0–2.2	40–45	50
2.3–2.5	35–40	40
2.6–3.0	30–35	35
3.1–3.5	25–30	30
3.6–4.0	20–25	25
4.1–5.1	15–20	20
5.2–6.6	10–15	15
6.7–8.0	< 10	10

In adults with renal failure undergoing hemodialysis, the amount of gentamicin removed from the blood may vary depending upon several factors including the dialysis method used. An 8-hour hemodialysis may reduce serum concentrations of gentamicin by approximately 50%. The recommended dosage at the end of each dialysis period is 1 to 1.7 mg/kg depending upon the severity of infection. In children, a dose of 2 mg/kg may be administered.

The above dosage schedules are not intended as rigid recommendations but are provided as guides to dosage when the measurement of gentamicin serum levels is not feasible.

A variety of methods is available to measure gentamicin concentrations in body fluids; these include microbiologic, enzymatic, and radioimmunoassay techniques.

HOW SUPPLIED

GARAMYCIN Injectable, 40 mg per mL, for parenteral administration, is supplied in 2 mL (80 mg) vials, boxes of 25 (NDC 0085-0069-04).

Also available, GARAMYCIN Pediatric Injectable, 10 mg per mL, for parenteral administration, supplied in 2 mL (20 mg) vials, boxes of 10 (NDC 0085-0013-06).

GARAMYCIN Injectable is a clear, stable solution that requires no refrigeration.

Store between 2° and 30°C (36° and 86°F).

Schering Corporation
Kenilworth, NJ 07033 USA

Copyright © 1968, 1992, 1994, Schering Corporation.
All rights reserved.

Revised 10/93 17150820

HYPERSTAT® I.V. ℞

brand of diazoxide, USP
Injection
For Intravenous Use In Hospitalized Patients Only

DESCRIPTION

HYPERSTAT I.V. Injection is a nondiuretic benzothiadiazine antihypertensive agent. Each ampule (20 ml) contains 300 mg diazoxide, USP, in a clear, sterile, colorless aqueous solution; the pH is adjusted to approximately 11.6 with sodium hydroxide.

Diazoxide has the following structural formula:

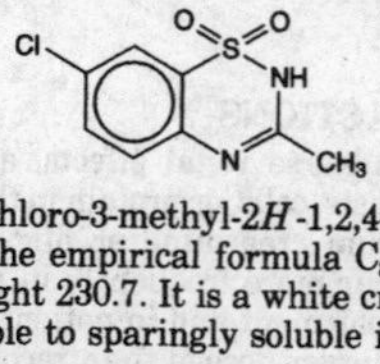

Diazoxide is 7-chloro-3-methyl-2*H*-1,2,4-benzothiadiazine 1,1-dioxide, with the empirical formula $C_8H_7ClN_2O_2S$, and the molecular weight 230.7. It is a white crystalline powder practically insoluble to sparingly soluble in water.

CLINICAL PHARMACOLOGY

HYPERSTAT I.V. Injection produces a prompt reduction of blood pressure in man by relaxing smooth muscle in the peripheral arterioles. Cardiac output is increased as blood pressure is reduced. Studies in animals demonstrate that coronary blood flow is maintained, while renal blood flow is increased after an initial decrease.

Transient hyperglycemia occurs in the majority of patients treated with HYPERSTAT, but usually requires treatment only in patients with diabetes mellitus. It will respond to the usual management measures, including insulin.

Blood glucose levels should be monitored, especially in patients with diabetes and in those requiring multiple injections of diazoxide. Cataracts have been observed in a few animals receiving repeated daily doses of intravenous diazoxide.

Since diazoxide causes sodium retention, repeated injections may precipitate edema and congestive heart failure. Increased volume of extracellular fluid may be a cause of treatment failure in nonresponsive patients. The increase in fluid volume characteristically responds to diuretic agents if adequate renal function exists. Concurrently administered thiazide diuretics may be expected to potentiate the antihypertensive and hyperuricemic actions of diazoxide. (See **Drug Interactions.**)

Diazoxide is extensively bound to serum protein (> 90%). The plasma half-life is 28 ± 8.3 hours; however, the duration of its antihypertensive effect is variable, generally lasting less than 12 hours.

INDICATIONS AND USAGE

HYPERSTAT I.V. Injection is indicated for short-term use in the emergency reduction of blood pressure in severe, nonmalignant and malignant hypertension in hospitalized adults; and in acute severe hypertension in hospitalized children, when prompt and urgent decrease of diastolic pressure is required. Treatment with orally effective antihypertensive agents should not be instituted until blood pressure has stabilized. The use of HYPERSTAT I.V. Injection for longer than 10 days is not recommended.

HYPERSTAT I.V. Injection is ineffective against hypertension due to pheochromocytoma.

CONTRAINDICATIONS

HYPERSTAT I.V. Injection should not be used in the treatment of compensatory hypertension, such as that associated with aortic coarctation or arteriovenous shunt, and should not be used in patients hypersensitive to diazoxide, other thiazides, or other sulfonamide-derived drugs.

WARNINGS

Rapid Decrease of Blood Pressure Caution must be observed when reducing severely elevated blood pressure. Diazoxide should only be administered utilizing the new 150-mg minibolus dosage. The use of a 300-mg intravenous dose of diazoxide has been associated with angina and with myocardial and cerebral infarction. One instance of optic nerve infarction was reported when a 100-mmHg reduction in diastolic pressure occurred over ten minutes following a single 300-mg bolus. In one prospective trial conducted in patients with severe hypertension and coexistent coronary artery disease, a 50% incidence of ischemic changes in the electrocardiogram was observed following single 300-mg bolus injections of diazoxide. The desired blood pressure lowering should therefore be achieved over as long a period of time as is compatible with the patient's status. At least several hours and preferably one or two days is tentatively recommended. Improved safety with equal efficacy can be achieved by administering HYPERSTAT I.V. Injection as a minibolus dose (1 to 3 mg/kg every 5 to 15 minutes up to a maximum of 150 mg in a single injection) until a diastolic blood pressure below 100 mmHg is achieved. HYPERSTAT I.V. Injection should not be administered in a bolus dose of 300 mg since this mode of administration is less predictable and less controllable than the minibolus dosage. If hypotension severe enough to require therapy results from the reduction in blood pressure, it will usually respond to the Trendelenberg maneuver. If necessary, sympathomimetic agents such as dopamine or norepinephrine may be administered.

Special attention is required for patients with diabetes mellitus and those in whom retention of salt and water may present serious problems.

Myocardial Lesions in Animals Intravenous administration of diazoxide in dogs has induced subendocardial necrosis and necrosis of papillary muscles. These lesions, which are also produced by other vasodilator drugs (i.e., hydralazine, minoxidil) and by catecholamines, are presumed to be related to anoxia resulting from a combination of reflex tachycardia and decreased perfusion.

PRECAUTIONS

General: HYPERSTAT (diazoxide) I.V. Injection is an effective antihypertensive agent requiring close monitoring of the patient's blood pressure at frequent intervals. Its administration may occasionally cause hypotension requiring treatment with sympathomimetic drugs. Therefore, HYPERSTAT I.V. Injection should be used primarily in the hospital or where adequate facilities exist to treat such untoward responses.

HYPERSTAT I.V. Injection should be administered only into a peripheral vein. Because the alkalinity of the solution is irritating to tissue, avoid extravascular injection or leak-

age. Subcutaneous administration has produced inflammation and pain without subsequent necrosis. If leakage into subcutaneous tissue occurs, the area should be treated with warm compresses and rest.

HYPERSTAT I.V. Injection should be used with care in patients who have impaired cerebral or cardiac circulation, that is, patients in whom abrupt reduction in blood pressure might be detrimental or those in whom mild tachycardia or decreased blood perfusion may be deleterious (see **WARNINGS**). Prolonged hypotension should be avoided so as not to aggravate preexisting renal failure.

Information for Patients: During and immediately following intravenous injection of HYPERSTAT I.V. Injection, the patient should remain supine.

Laboratory Tests: Diagnostic laboratory tests necessary to establish the patient's condition and status should be carried out prior to treatment with HYPERSTAT I.V. Injection. During and following treatment with HYPERSTAT I.V. Injection, laboratory tests to monitor the effects of treatment with this drug and the patient's condition should be done. Among the tests (not necessarily inclusive) are: hematologic (hematocrit, hemoglobin, white blood cell and platelet counts); metabolic (glucose, uric acid, total protein, albumin); electrolyte (sodium, potassium) and osmolality; renal function (creatinine, urine-protein); electrocardiogram.

Drug Interactions: Diazoxide is highly bound to serum protein. It can be expected to displace other substances which are also bound to protein, such as bilirubin or coumarin and its derivatives, resulting in higher blood levels of these substances.

An undesirable hypotension may result when diazoxide is administered to patients who have received other antihypertensive medication within six hours.

One patient in a clinical study exhibited excessive hypotension after concomitant administration of HYPERSTAT with hydralazine and methyldopa. An episode of maternal hypotension and fetal bradycardia occurred in a patient in labor who received both reserpine and hydralazine prior to administration of diazoxide. Neonatal hyperglycemia following intrapartum administration of HYPERSTAT I.V. Injection has also been reported.

HYPERSTAT I.V. Injection should not be administered within six hours of the administration of: hydralazine, reserpine, alphaprodine, methyldopa, beta-blockers, prazosin, minoxidil, the nitrites and other papaverine-like compounds.

Concomitant administration with thiazides or other commonly used diuretics may be expected to potentiate the hyperuricemic and antihypertensive effects of diazoxide.

Drug/Laboratory Test Interactions: The hyperglycemic and hyperuricemic effects of diazoxide preclude proper assessment of these metabolic states. Increased renin secretion, IgG concentrations and decreased cortisol secretion have also been noted. Diazoxide inhibits glucagon-stimulated insulin release and will cause a false-negative insulin response to glucagon. In the rat, dog, and monkey, diazoxide increased serum free fatty acids and decreased plasma insulin levels.

Carcinogenesis, Mutagenesis, Impairment of Fertility: No long-term animal dosing study has been done to evaluate the carcinogenic potential of diazoxide. No laboratory studies of mutagenic potential or animal studies of effects on fertility have been done.

Pregnancy Category C: Diazoxide has been shown to reduce fetal and/or pup survival; and to reduce fetal growth in rats, rabbits, and dogs at daily doses of 30, 21, or 10 mg/kg, respectively. In rats treated at term, diazoxide, at doses of 10 mg/kg and above, prolonged parturition.

The safety of HYPERSTAT I.V. Injection in pregnancy has not been established.

Nonteratogenic Effects: Diazoxide crosses the placental barrier and appears in cord blood. When given to the mother prior to delivery, the drug may produce fetal or neonatal hyperbilirubinemia, thrombocytopenia, altered carbohydrate metabolism, and possibly other side effects that have occurred in adults.

Labor and Delivery: HYPERSTAT I.V. Injection is not indicated for use in pregnancy. Intravenous administration of the drug during labor may cause cessation of uterine contractions, requiring administration of an oxytocic agent.

Nursing Mothers: Information is not available concerning the passage of HYPERSTAT in breast milk. Because many drugs are excreted in human milk and because of the potential for adverse reactions in nursing infants from diazoxide, a decision should be made whether to discontinue nursing or to discontinue the drug, taking into account the importance of the drug to the mother.

Pediatric Use: See **INDICATIONS AND USAGE.**

ADVERSE REACTIONS

It is reasonable to speculate that the currently recommended minibolus dosing regimen, which has replaced the 300-mg bolus dose in clinical practice, will result in adverse effects which are of similar character but of lesser frequency and severity.

In clinical experience with the rapid bolus administration of 300 mg, the most common adverse reactions reported were: hypotension (7%); nausea and vomiting (4%); dizziness and weakness (2%). Additional adverse reactions reported with bolus administration of 300 mg were as follows:

Cardiovascular: sodium and water retention after repeated injections, especially important in patients with impaired cardiac reserve; hypotension to shock levels; myocardial ischemia, usually transient and manifested by angina, atrial and ventricular arrhythmias, and marked electrocardiographic changes, but occasionally leading to myocardial infarction; optic nerve infarction following too rapid decrease in severely elevated blood pressure; supraventricular tachycardia and palpitation; bradycardia; chest discomfort or nonanginal "tightness in the chest."

Central Nervous System: cerebral ischemia, usually transient but occasionally leading to infarction and manifested by unconsciousness, convulsions, paralysis, confusion, or focal neurological deficit such as numbness of the hands; vasodilative phenomena, such as orthostatic hypotension, sweating, flushing, and generalized or localized sensations of warmth; various transient neurological findings secondary to alteration in regional blood flow to brain, such as headache (sometimes throbbing), dizziness, lightheadedness, sleepiness (also reported as lethargy, somnolence or drowsiness), euphoria or "funny feeling," ringing in the ears and momentary hearing loss, and weakness of short duration; apprehension or anxiety.

Gastrointestinal: rarely, acute pancreatitis; nausea, vomiting and/or abdominal discomfort; anorexia; alteration in taste; parotid swelling; salivation; dry mouth; lacrimation; ileus; constipation and diarrhea.

Other: hyperglycemia in diabetic patients, especially after repeated injections; hyperosmolar coma in an infant; transient hyperglycemia in nondiabetic patients; transient retention of nitrogenous wastes; various respiratory findings secondary to the relaxation of smooth muscle, such as dyspnea, cough and choking sensation; warmth or pain along the injected vein; cellulitis without sloughing and/or phlebitis at the injection site of extravasation; back pain and increased nocturia; hypersensitivity reactions, such as rash, leukopenia and fever; papilledema induced by plasma volume expansion secondary to the administration of diazoxide reported in a patient who had received eleven injections (300 mg/dose) over a 22-day period; malaise and blurred vision; transient cataract in an infant; hirsutism, and decreased libido.

OVERDOSAGE

Overdosage of HYPERSTAT I.V. Injection may cause an undesirable hypotension. Usually, this can be controlled with the Trendelenberg maneuver. If necessary, sympathomimetic agents, such as dopamine or norepinephrine, may be administered. Failure of blood pressure to rise in response to such agents suggests that the hypotension may have been caused by something other than diazoxide. Excessive hyperglycemia resulting from overdosage will respond to conventional therapy of hyperglycemia.

DOSAGE AND ADMINISTRATION

HYPERSTAT I.V. Injection was originally recommended for use by bolus administration of 300 mg. Recent studies have shown that minibolus administration of HYPERSTAT I.V. Injection, i.e., doses of 1 to 3 mg/kg repeated at intervals of 5 to 15 minutes is as effective in reducing blood pressure. Minibolus administration usually provides a more gradual reduction in blood pressure and thus may be expected to reduce the circulatory and neurological risks associated with acute hypotension.

HYPERSTAT I.V. Injection is administered undiluted and rapidly by intravenous injections of 1 to 3 mg/kg up to a maximum of 150 mg in a single injection. This dose may be repeated at intervals of 5 to 15 minutes until a satisfactory reduction in blood pressure (diastolic pressure below 100 mmHg) has been achieved.

With the patient recumbent, the calculated dose of HYPERSTAT I.V. Injection is administered intravenously in 30 seconds or less.

HYPERSTAT I.V. Injection should only be given into a peripheral vein. Do not administer it intramuscularly, subcutaneously, or into body cavities. Avoid extravasation of the drug into subcutaneous tissues.

Following the use of HYPERSTAT I.V. Injection, the blood pressure should be monitored closely until it has stabilized. Thereafter, measurements taken hourly during the balance of the effect should indicate any unusual response. A further decrease in blood pressure 30 minutes or more after injection should be investigated for causes other than the action of HYPERSTAT I.V. Injection. It is preferable that the patient remain supine for at least one hour after injection. In ambulatory patients, the blood pressure should also be measured with the patient standing before surveillance is ended.

Repeated administration of HYPERSTAT I.V. Injection at intervals of 4 to 24 hours usually will maintain the blood pressure below pretreatment levels until a regimen of oral antihypertensive medication can be instituted. The interval between injections may be adjusted by the duration of the response to each injection. It is usually unnecessary to continue treatment with HYPERSTAT I.V. Injection for more than four to five days.

Since repeated administration of HYPERSTAT I.V. Injection can lead to sodium and water retention, administration of a diuretic may be necessary both for maximal blood pressure reduction and to avoid congestive heart failure. (See **CLINICAL PHARMACOLOGY.**)

Parenteral drug products should be inspected visually for particulate matter and discoloration prior to administration, whenever solution and container permit.

HOW SUPPLIED

HYPERSTAT I.V. Injection is supplied in a 20-ml ampule, containing 300 mg diazoxide, in a clear, sterile, colorless, aqueous solution; box of one ampule (NDC 0085-0201-05).

Protect from light and freezing. Store between 2° and 30°C (36° and 86°F).

Revised 2/85 B-11037496

Copyright ©1972, 1984, 1985. Schering Corporation. USA. All rights reserved.

INSPIREASE® * ℞

Drug Delivery System for use with metered dose inhalers
*** U.S. Patent 4,484,577**

Instructions for use and care
Includes Instructions for Universal Mouthpiece and Actuation Aid

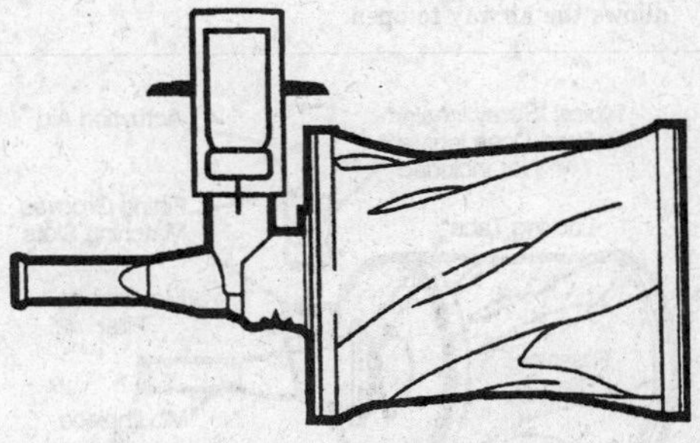

InspirEase® is a portable drug delivery system that helps "spray inhalers" (also known as metered-dose inhalers) deliver medication to the lungs. It is designed to improve the delivery of these medications by making it easier for you to use them.

If you are using a "spray inhaler" alone, you may not be getting all your medication. These "spray inhalers" provide a convenient and effective method for delivering drugs, but it is not easy to use them correctly. You must carefully time each breath while squeezing the "spray inhaler" downward. If your timing is incorrect, the full dose of medication may not be deliverd deep within your lungs.

InspirEase makes it simpler to use your "spray inhaler" correctly. After you press down on your "spray inhaler," medication is released and stored in the compact bag, giving you the chance to breathe in the medication in two breaths. This does away with the need to carefully coordinate taking a breath and releasing the spray.

And InspirEase has a special feature to help teach you better breathing technique. When you are using it correctly (taking a slow, deep breath that helps get the medication deep within your lungs), the bag will collapse and you will *not* hear a whistling sound. However, if you breathe in too fast (a common mistake that can reduce the effectiveness of your treatment), you will hear a whistling sound.

This signals you to breathe slower.

Slow breathing and holding your breath after taking each dose of medication are necessary to obtain more complete relief. See diagram below:

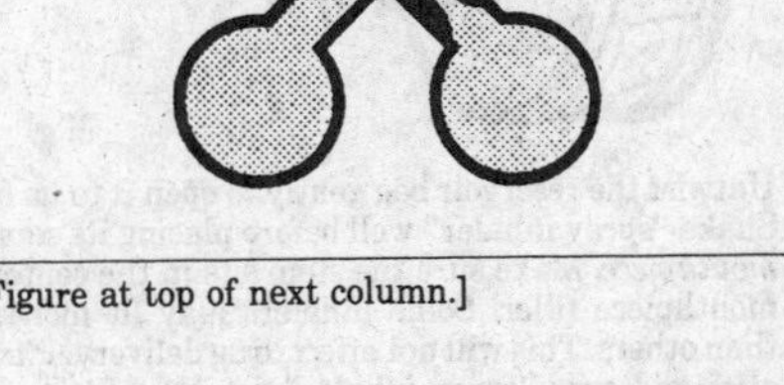
1) Open Airway
Blocked Airway

[See Figure at top of next column.]

Continued on next page

Information on Schering products appearing on these pages is effective as of August 15, 1996.

Schering—Cont.

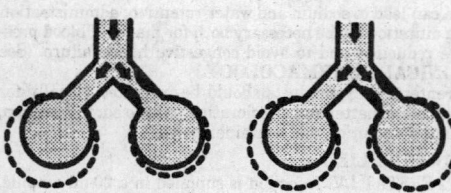

2) Fast breathing causes less lung expansion when you have a blocked airway.

Slow (optimal) breathing causes lung expansion to be more equal even if an airway is blocked.

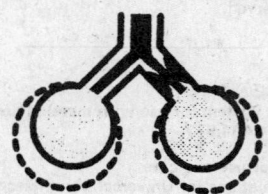

3) Aerosol drug delivered—Settling of drug on blocked airway with slow breathing, followed by breath holding, allows the airway to open.

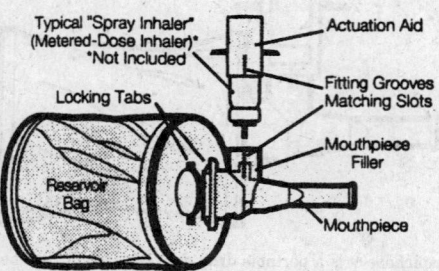

Typical "Spray Inhaler" (Metered-Dose Inhaler)* *Not Included — Actuation Aid — Fitting Grooves Matching Slots — Mouthpiece Filler — Mouthpiece — Locking Tabs — Reservoir Bag

Contents

Your InspirEase® kit includes 3 replaceable reservoir bags, one actuation aid, and a *single universal mouthpiece* which can be used with both metal and white plastic stem inhalers.

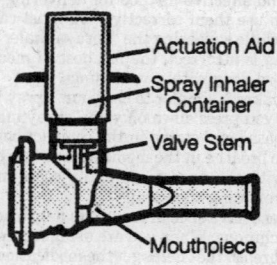

Actuation Aid — Spray Inhaler Container — Valve Stem — Mouthpiece

INSTRUCTIONS FOR USE

1. Connect the mouthpiece to the reservoir bag by lining up the *locking tabs* with the opening in the reservoir bag. Push in and twist to lock.

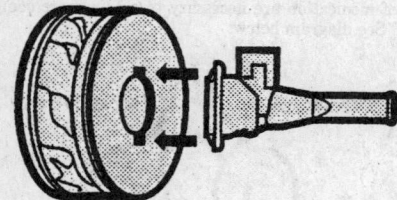

2. Untwist the reservoir bag gently to open it to its full size. Shake "spray inhaler" well before placing its stem in the *mouthpiece*. Make sure the stem sits in the center of the mouthpiece filler. Some inhalers may fit more loosely than others. This will not affect drug delivery. Place actuation aid over "spray inhaler" canister, fitting grooves into matching slots in the mouthpiece. Fingerholds may align either parallel with or across the mouthpiece. Patients with smaller hands may prefer them across.

[See Figure at top of next column.]

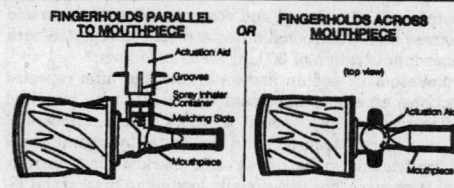

FINGERHOLDS PARALLEL TO MOUTHPIECE — OR — FINGERHOLDS ACROSS MOUTHPIECE

Actuation Aid — Grooves — Spray Inhaler Container — Matching Slots — Mouthpiece — (top view) — Actuation Aid — Mouthpiece

3. Place mouthpiece in mouth and close lips tightly around it.
4. Place fingers on fingerholds with thumb under mouthpiece on thumbhold as shown, and pull down with fingers to release one dose of medication into the bag. Alternatively, two hands may be used to actuate the "spray inhaler" with the actuation aid in the across position.

IMPORTANT NOTE: Follow your physician's instructions regarding the number of doses you should take and when to take them.

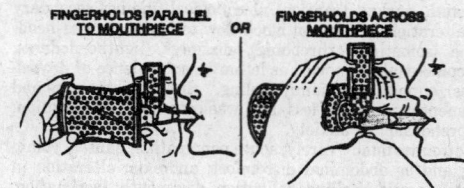

FINGERHOLDS PARALLEL TO MOUTHPIECE — OR — FINGERHOLDS ACROSS MOUTHPIECE

5. Breathe in *slowly* through the mouthpiece. If you hear a whistling sound, breathe slower until no sound can be heard.

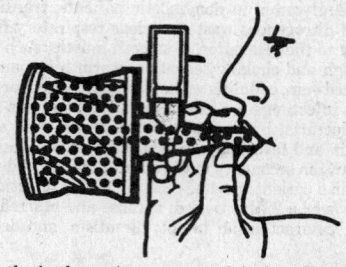

6. Breathe in the entire contents of the bag. You will know to stop when the bag collapses and you cannot breathe in anymore.
7. *Hold your breath while slowly counting to five.*
8. Breathe out slowly into the bag.

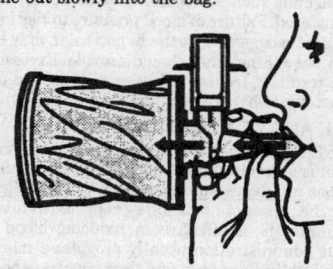

9. Repeat the breathing in and out steps (numbers 5, 6, 7, and 8) a second time, keeping lips tightly closed around the mouthpiece.
10. Remove the mouthpiece from your mouth. Unlock mouthpiece from the bag by untwisting and pulling out and store all components in carrying case.

How to tell if your "spray inhaler" is full or empty

Drop your "spray inhaler" into a pan of water. Its position in the water will tell you how much medication is left. See diagram below.

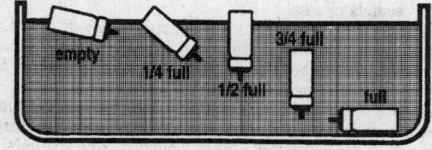

empty — 1/4 full — 1/2 full — 3/4 full — full

Important Instructions

Clean mouthpiece thoroughly with warm (not hot) running water *at least* once a day. *The InspirEase® system is not dishwasher safe. Always clean by hand.*

The clear plastic reed section of the mouthpiece should not be touched due to potential breakage. We recommend a visual inspection of the reed section for signs of breakage prior to each use. If reed breakage occurs, replace mouthpiece immediately; otherwise replace mouthpiece as needed every six months.

After cleaning, wait until mouthpiece is *completely dry* before storing in carrying case. Do not place near artificial heat such as dishwasher or oven.

We recommend that the reservoir bag be replaced every two to three weeks or as needed. *However, if there is a hole or tear in it, replace immediately.*

NOTE: You will need a physician's prescription for replacement bags or a new starter kit.

InspirEase is designed for use with most "spray inhaler" (metered-dose inhaler) containers currently available; for single-patient use and single-drug use.

The usual caution should be exercised in dosing medications and evaluating patient response. The prescribing information for the marketed MDIs varies with respect to dosing, administration, etc. We recommend that these be followed when using InspirEase.

CAUTION: Federal law restricts this device to sale by, or on the order of, a physician.

Distributed by: Key Pharmaceuticals, Inc.
Kenilworth, NJ 07033 USA

INTRON® A   ℞
Interferon alfa-2b, recombinant For Injection

DESCRIPTION

INTRON A Interferon alfa-2b, recombinant for intramuscular, subcutaneous, intralesional, or intravenous Injection is a purified sterile recombinant interferon product.

Powder for Injection The 3 million, 5 million, 18 million, 25 million, and 50 million IU packages are for use by intramuscular or subcutaneous injection. The 10 million IU package is for intramuscular, subcutaneous, intralesional, or intravenous injection. (See **WARNINGS** and **PRECAUTIONS**.)

Solution for Injection The 10 million, 18 million multidose, and 25 million IU packages are for use by intramuscular or subcutaneous injection, and not for intralesional or intravenous use. (See **WARNINGS** and **PRECAUTIONS**.)

Interferon alfa-2b, recombinant for Injection has been classified as an alpha interferon and is a water soluble protein with a molecular weight of 19,271 daltons produced by recombinant DNA techniques. It is obtained from the bacterial fermentation of a strain of *Escherichia coli* bearing a genetically engineered plasmid containing an interferon alfa-2b gene from human leukocytes. The fermentation is carried out in a defined nutrient medium containing the antibiotic tetracycline hydrochloride at a concentration of 5 to 10 mg/L; the presence of this antibiotic is not detectable in the final product. The specific activity of Interferon alfa-2b, recombinant is approximately 2×10^8 IU/mg protein.

Powder for Injection After reconstitution, the 3 million, 5 million, 10 million (1 mL), 18 million, 25 million, and 50 million IU vials contain, respectively, per mL either 3 million, 5 million, 10 million, 18 million, 5 million, or 50 million IU of interferon alfa-2b, recombinant. Each mL also contains 20 mg glycine, 2.3 mg sodium phosphate dibasic, 0.55 mg sodium phosphate monobasic, and 1.0 mg human albumin. Based on the specific activity of approximately 2×10^8 IU/mg protein, the corresponding quantities of interferon alfa-2b, recombinant in the vials described above are approximately 0.015 mg, 0.025 mg, 0.05 mg, 0.90 mg, 0.125 mg, and 0.25 mg protein, respectively. Prior to administration, the INTRON A Powder for Injection is to be reconstituted with the provided Diluent for INTRON A Interferon alfa-2b, recombinant for Injection (bacteriostatic water for injection) containing 0.9% benzyl alcohol as a preservative. (See **DOSAGE AND ADMINISTRATION**.) INTRON A Powder for Injection is a white to cream colored powder.

Solution for Injection Each INTRON A vial contains either 10 million IU of interferon alfa-2b, recombinant per 2 mL (5 million IU/mL), 22.8 million IU of interferon alfa-2b, recombinant per 3.8 mL (6 million IU/mL), or 25 million IU of interferon alfa-2b, recombinant per 5 mL (5 million IU/mL). Each mL also contains 20 mg glycine, 2.3 mg sodium phosphate dibasic, 0.55 mg sodium phosphate monobasic, 1.0 mg human albumin, and 1.2 mg methylparaben and 0.12 mg propylparaben as preservatives. The 18 million IU multidose vial contains a total of 22.8 million IU of interferon alfa-2b, recombinant per 3.8 mL in order to provide the delivery of six 0.5 mL doses, each containing 3 million IU of INTRON A Interferon alfa-2b, recombinant for Injection (for a label strength of 18 million IU). Based on the specific activity of approximately 2×10^8 IU/mg protein, the corresponding quantities of interferon alfa-2b, recombinant in the vials described above are approximately 0.05 mg, 0.114 mg, and 0.125 mg protein, respectively. These packages do not require reconstitution prior to administration. (See **DOSAGE AND ADMINISTRATION**.) INTRON A Solution for Injection is a colorless to light yellow solution.

CLINICAL PHARMACOLOGY

General The interferons are a family of naturally occurring small proteins and glycoproteins with molecular weights of

approximately 15,000 to 27,600 daltons produced and secreted by cells in response to viral infections and to synthetic or biological inducers.

Preclinical Pharmacology Interferons exert their cellular activities by binding to specific membrane receptors on the cell surface. Once bound to the cell membrane, interferons initiate a complex sequence of intracellular events. *In vitro* studies demonstrated that these include the induction of certain enzymes, suppression of cell proliferation, immunomodulating activities such as enhancement of the phagocytic activity of macrophages and augmentation of the specific cytotoxicity of lymphocytes for target cells, and inhibition of virus replication in virus-infected cells.

In a study using human hepatoblastoma cell line, HB 611, the *in vitro* antiviral activity of alpha interferon was demonstrated by its inhibition of hepatitis B virus (HBV) replication.

The correlation between these *in vitro* data and the clinical results is unknown. Any of these activities might contribute to interferon's therapeutic effects.

Pharmacokinetics The pharmacokinetics of INTRON A Interferon alfa-2b, recombinant for Injection were studied in 12 healthy male volunteers following single doses of 5 million IU/m^2 administered intramuscularly, subcutaneously, and as a 30-minute intravenous infusion in a crossover design. INTRON A concentrations were determined using a radioimmunoassay (RIA) with a detection limit equal to 10 IU/mL.

The mean serum INTRON A concentrations following intramuscular and subcutaneous injections were comparable. The maximum serum concentrations obtained via these routes were approximately 18 to 116 IU/mL and occurred 3 to 12 hours after administration. The elimination half-life of INTRON A Interferon alfa-2b, recombinant for Injection following both intramuscular and subcutaneous injections was approximately 2 to 3 hours. Serum concentrations were below the detection limit by 16 hours after the injections.

After intravenous administration, serum INTRON A concentrations peaked (135 to 273 IU/mL) by the end of the 30-minute infusion, then declined at a slightly more rapid rate than after intramuscular or subcutaneous drug administration, becoming undetectable 4 hours after the infusion. The elimination half-life was approximately 2 hours.

Urine INTRON A concentrations following a single dose (5 million IU/m^2) were not detectable after any of the parenteral routes of administration. This result was expected since preliminary studies with isolated and perfused rabbit kidneys have shown that the kidney may be the main site of interferon catabolism.

There are no pharmacokinetic data available for the intralesional route of administration.

Serum Neutralizing Antibodies In INTRON A treated patients tested for antibody activity in clinical trials, serum anti-interferon neutralizing antibodies were detected in 0% (0/90) of patients with hairy cell leukemia, 0.8% (2/260) of patients treated intralesionally for condylomata acuminata, and 4% (1/24) of patients with AIDS-Related Kaposi's Sarcoma. Serum neutralizing antibodies have been detected in <3% of patients treated with higher INTRON A doses in malignancies other than hairy cell leukemia or AIDS-Related Kaposi's Sarcoma. The clinical significance of the appearance of serum anti-interferon neutralizing activity in these indications is not known.

Serum anti-interferon neutralizing antibodies were detected in 15% (7/46) of patients with chronic hepatitis NANB/C and in 13% (6/48) of patients who received INTRON A therapy for chronic hepatitis B at 5 million IU QD for 4 months, and in 3% (1/33) of patients treated at 10 million IU TIW. In patients with chronic hepatitis the titers detected were low (≤1:40) and the appearance of serum anti-interferon neutralizing activity did not appear to affect safety or efficacy.

Hairy Cell Leukemia In clinical trials in patients with hairy cell leukemia, there was depression of hematopoiesis during the first 1 to 2 months of INTRON A treatment, resulting in reduced numbers of circulating red and white blood cells, and platelets. Subsequently, both splenectomized and nonsplenectomized patients achieved substantial and sustained improvements in granulocytes, platelets, and hemoglobin levels in 75% of treated patients and at least some improvement (minor responses) occurred in 90%. INTRON A treatment resulted in a decrease in bone marrow hypercellularity and hairy cell infiltrates. The hairy cell index (HCI), which represents the percent of bone marrow cellularity times the percent of hairy cell infiltrate, was greater than or equal to 50% at the beginning of the study in 87% of patients. The percentage of patients with such an HCI decreased to 25% after 6 months and to 14% after 1 year. These results indicate that even though hematologic improvement had occurred earlier, prolonged INTRON A treatment may be required to obtain maximal reduction in tumor cell infiltrates in the bone marrow.

The percentage of patients with hairy cell leukemia who required red blood cell or platelet transfusions decreased significantly during treatment and the percentage of patients with confirmed and serious infections declined as granulocyte counts improved. Reversal of splenomegaly and of clinically significant hypersplenism was demonstrated in some patients.

A study was conducted to assess the effects of extended INTRON A treatment on duration of response for patients who responded to initial therapy. In this study, 126 responding patients were randomized to receive additional INTRON A treatment for 6 months or observation for a comparable period, after 12 months of initial INTRON A therapy. During this 6-month period, 3% (2/66) of INTRON A treated patients relapsed compared with 18% (11/60) who were not treated. This represents a significant difference in time to relapse in favor of continued INTRON A treatment (p = 0.006/0.01, Log Rank/Wilcoxon). Since a small proportion of the total population had relapsed, median time to relapse could not be estimated in either group. A similar pattern in relapses was seen when all randomized treatment, including that beyond 6 months, and available follow-up data were assessed. The 15% (10/66) relapses among INTRON A patients occurred over a significantly longer period of time than the 40% (24/60) with observation (p = 0.0002/0.0001, Log Rank/Wilcoxon). Median time to relapse was estimated, using the Kaplan-Meier method, to be 6.8 months in the observation group but could not be estimated in the INTRON A group.

Subsequent follow-up with a median time of approximately 40 months demonstrated an overall survival of 87.8%. In a comparable historical control group followed for 24 months, overall median survival was approximately 40%.

Malignant Melanoma The safety and efficacy of INTRON A Interferon alfa-2b, recombinant for Injection was evaluated as adjuvant to surgical treatment in patients with melanoma who were free of disease (post-surgery) but at high risk for systemic recurrence. These included patients with lesions of Breslow thickness >4 mm, or patients with lesions of any Breslow thickness with primary or recurrent nodal involvement. In a randomized controlled trial in 280 patients, 143 patients received INTRON A therapy at 20 million IU/m^2 intravenously five times per week for 4 weeks (induction phase) followed by 10 million IU/m^2 subcutaneously three times per week for 48 weeks (maintenance phase). INTRON A therapy was begun ≤56 days after surgical resection. The remaining 137 patients were observed.

INTRON A therapy produced a significant increase in relapse-free and overall survival. Median time to relapse for the INTRON A treated patients *versus*observation patients was 1.72 years *versus* 0.98 years (p<0.01, stratified Log Rank). The estimated 5-year relapse- free survival rate, using the Kaplan-Meier method, was 37% for INTRON A treated patients *versus* 26% for observation patients. Median overall survival time for INTRON A treated patients *versus* observation patients was 3.82 years *versus* 2.78 years (p=0.047, stratified Log Rank). The estimated 5-year overall survival rate, using the Kaplan-Meier method, was 46% for INTRON A treated patients *versus* 37% for observation patients.

Condylomata Acuminata Condylomata acuminata (venereal or genital warts) are associated with infections of the human papilloma virus (HPV). The safety and efficacy of INTRON A Interferon alfa-2b, recombinant for Injection in the treatment of condylomata acuminata were evaluated in three controlled double-blind clinical trials. In these studies INTRON A doses of 1 million IU per lesion were administered intralesionally three times a week (TIW), in ≤5 lesions per patient for 3 weeks. The patients were observed for up to 16 weeks after completion of the full treatment course.

INTRON A treatment of condylomata was significantly more effective than placebo, as measured by disappearance of lesions, decreases in lesion size, and by an overall change in disease status. Of 192 INTRON A treated patients and 206 placebo treated patients who were evaluable for efficacy at the time of best response during the course of the study, 42% of INTRON A patients *versus* 17% of placebo patients experienced clearing of all treated lesions. Likewise 24% of INTRON A patients *versus* 8% of placebo patients experienced marked (≥75% to <100%) reduction in lesion size, 18% *versus* 9% experienced moderate (≥50% to ≤75%) reduction in lesion size, 10% *versus* 42% had a slight (<50%) reduction in lesion size, 5% *versus* 24% had no change in lesion size, and 0% *versus* 1% experienced exacerbation (p<0.001).

In one of these studies, 43% (54/125) of patients in whom multiple (≤3) lesions were treated, experienced complete clearing of all treated lesions during the course of the study. Of these patients, 81% remained cleared 16 weeks after treatment was initiated.

Patients who did not achieve total clearing of all their treated lesions had these same lesions treated with a second course of therapy. During this second course of treatment, 38% to 67% of patients had clearing of all treated lesions. The overall percentage of patients who had cleared all their treated lesions after 2 courses of treatment ranged from 57% to 85%.

INTRON A treated lesions showed improvement within 2 to 4 weeks after the start of treatment in the above study; maximal response to INTRON A therapy was noted 4 to 8 weeks after initiation of treatment.

The response to INTRON A therapy was better in patients who had condylomata for shorter durations than in patients with lesions for a longer duration.

Another study involved 97 patients in whom three lesions were treated with either an intralesional injection of 1.5 million IU of INTRON A Interferon alfa-2b, recombinant for Injection per lesion followed by a topical application of 25% podophyllin, or a topical application of 25% podophyllin alone. Treatment was given once a week for 3 weeks. The combined treatment of INTRON A Interferon alfa-2b, recombinant for Injection and podophyllin was shown to be significantly more effective than podophyllin alone, as determined by the number of patients whose lesions cleared. This significant difference in response was evident after the second treatment (week 3) and continued through 8 weeks post-treatment. At the time of the patient's best response, 67% (33/49) of the INTRON A Interferon alfa-2b, recombinant for Injection and podophyllin treated patients had all three treated lesions clear while 42% (20/48) of the podophyllin treated patients had all three clear (p = 0.003).

AIDS-Related Kaposi's Sarcoma The safety and efficacy of INTRON A Interferon alfa-2b, recombinant for Injection in the treatment of Kaposi's Sarcoma (KS), a common manifestation of the Acquired Immune Deficiency Syndrome (AIDS), were evaluated in clinical trials in 144 patients.

In one study, INTRON A doses of 30 million IU/m^2 were administered subcutaneously three times per week (TIW), to patients with AIDS-Related KS. Doses were adjusted for patient tolerance. The average weekly dose delivered in the first 4 weeks was 150 million IU; at the end of 12 weeks this averaged 110 million IU/week; and by 24 weeks averaged 75 million IU/week.

Forty-four percent of asymptomatic patients responded *versus* 7% of symptomatic patients. The median time to response was approximately 2 months and 1 month, respectively, for asymptomatic and symptomatic patients. The median duration of response was approximately 3 months and 1 month, respectively, for the asymptomatic and symptomatic patients. Baseline T4/T8 ratios were 0.46 for responders *versus* 0.33 for nonresponders.

In another study, INTRON A doses of 35 million IU were administered subcutaneously, daily (QD), for 12 weeks. Maintenance treatment, with every other day dosing (QOD), was continued for up to 1 year in patients achieving antitumor and antiviral responses. The median time to response was 2 months and the median duration of response was 5 months in the asymptomatic patients.

In all studies, the likelihood of response was greatest in patients with relatively intact immune systems as assessed by baseline CD4 counts (interchangeable with T4 counts). Results at doses of 30 million IU/m^2 TIW and 35 million IU/QD, subcutaneously were similar and are provided together in TABLE 1. This table demonstrates the relationship of response to baseline CD4 count in both asymptomatic and symptomatic patients in the 30 million IU/m^2 TIW and the 35 million IU/QD treatment groups.

In the 30 million IU study group, 7% (5/72) of patients were complete responders and 22% (16/72) of the patients were partial responders. The 35 million IU study had 13% (3/23 patients) complete responders and 17% (4/23) partial responders.

For patients who received 30 million IU TIW, the median survival time was longer in patients with CD4 greater than 200 (30.7 months) than in patients with CD4 less than or equal to 200 (8.9 months). Among responders, the median survival time was 22.6 months *versus* 9.7 months in nonresponders.

TABLE 1

RESPONSE BY BASELINE CD4 COUNT*

IN AIDS-RELATED KS PATIENTS

	30 million IU/m^2 TIW, SC and 35 million IU QD, SC	
	Asymptomatic	*Symptomatic*
CD4<200	4/14 (29%)	0/19 (0%)
200≤CD4≤400	6/12 (50%)	0/5 (0%)
	58%	
CD4>400	5/7 (71%)	0/0 (0%)

* Data for CD4, and asymptomatic and symptomatic classification were not available for all patients.

Chronic Hepatitis Non-A, Non-B/C (NANB/C) The safety and efficacy of INTRON A Interferon alfa-2b, recombinant for Injection in the treatment of chronic hepatitis NANB/C were evaluated in 4 randomized controlled clinical studies in which INTRON A doses of 1, 2, or 3 million IU three times a week (TIW), were administered subcutaneously for 6 months (23 or 24 weeks). The patients were 18 years of age or older and had compensated liver disease. Of the 332 patients evaluable for efficacy, 81% had a history of blood or blood product exposure, 8% had a history of intravenous drug

Continued on next page

Information on Schering products appearing on these pages is effective as of August 15, 1996.

Schering—Cont.

abuse, 2% had a history of surgery without blood products, and the remainder had other exposure. Retrospectively, 86% (172/199) of the patients with blood or blood product exposure who were tested were found to be positive for antibody to hepatitis C virus (HCV).

In each of 3 clinical studies, INTRON A therapy at 3 million IU TIW, resulted in a reduction in serum alanine aminotransferase (ALT) in a statistically significantly greater proportion of patients versus control patients (see TABLE 2). Of the 54% of patients responding to INTRON A therapy at a dose of 3 million IU, 70% achieved reductions in ALT levels to normal, 18% achieved reductions to near normal levels, and 12% achieved partial responses.

Histological improvement was evaluated by comparison of pre- and posttreatment liver biopsies using the semi-quantitative Knodell Histology Activity Index (HAI).[4]

In one of the three studies there was histological improvement in a statistically significantly greater proportion of INTRON A treated patients compared to controls (see TABLE 3). A similar, but not statistically significant trend for improvement was observed in the other two studies.

Subsequent combined analysis of results for the 3 studies showed histological improvement in a statistically significantly greater proportion of patients treated with INTRON A doses of 3 million IU than in control patients (p=0.04). The improvement was due primarily to decreases in severity of necrosis and degeneration in the lobular and periportal regions (Knodell HAI Categories I + II), which were observed in 65% (52/80) of patients treated at 3 million IU compared to 46% (32/70) of controls. Diminution of disease activity in these regions of the liver was accompanied by a reduction or normalization of serum ALT in many patients. Disease activity increased in these regions in only 3% of all INTRON A treated patients, whereas an increase was observed in 16% of the controls. No patient achieving an ALT response with 3 million IU INTRON A therapy showed increased periportal or lobular necrosis and degeneration. Patients were followed for 6 months after the end of INTRON A therapy. During this period the ALT response was maintained in 51% (26/51) of patients who responded at the 3 million IU TIW dose. Of patients who relapsed during the follow-up period and were retreated at this dose, 83% (15/18) responded to retreatment.

TABLE 2
ALT RESPONSES†
IN CHRONIC HEPATITIS NANB/C PATIENTS

Study Number	INTRON A 3 million IU		Controls‡		P§ Value
1[1]	29/55	(53%)	5/55	(9%)	<0.001
2[2]	10/23	(43%)	3/25	(12%)	0.02
3[3]	12/17	(71%)	3/17	(18%)	0.005
All Studies	**51/95**	**(54%)**	**11/97**	**(11%)**	**<0.001**

† Includes reduction in serum ALT to:
  normal,
  near normal (≤ 1.5 times the upper limit of normal), or
  partial response (>50% decrease in serum ALT).
‡ Untreated or Placebo
§ INTRON A 3 million IU TIW, 6 months versus control.

TABLE 3
HISTOLOGICAL IMPROVEMENT¶
IN CHRONIC HEPATITIS NANB/C PATIENTS

Study Number	INTRON A 3 million IU		Controls**		P†† Value
1	29/45	(64%)	18/36	(50%)	0.26
2	12/19	(63%)	10/18	(56%)	0.75
3	14/16	(88%)	8/15	(53%)	0.054
All Studies	**55/80**	**(69%)**	**36/69**	**(52%)**	**0.04**

¶Assessed by the Knodell Histology Activity Index which includes:
  Category I —Periportal necrosis
  Category II —Intralobular degeneration and necrosis
  Category III—Portal inflammation
  Category IV—Fibrosis
**Untreated or Placebo
††INTRON A 3 million IU TIW, 6 months compared to control for improvement versus no improvement.

Chronic Hepatitis B The safety and efficacy of INTRON A Interferon alfa-2b, recombinant for Injection in the treatment of chronic hepatitis B were evaluated in three clinical trials in which INTRON A doses of 30 to 35 million IU per week were administered subcutaneously (SC), as either 5 million IU daily (QD), or 10 million IU three times a week (TIW) for 16 weeks versus no treatment. All patients were 18 years of age or older with compensated liver disease, and had chronic hepatitis B virus (HBV) infection (serum HBsAg positive for at least 6 months) and HBV replication (serum HBeAg positive). Patients were also serum HBV-DNA positive, an additional indicator of HBV replication, as measured by a research assay.[5,6] All patients had elevated serum alanine aminotransferase (ALT) and liver biopsy findings compatible with the diagnosis of chronic hepatitis. Patients with the presence of antibody to human immunodeficiency virus (anti-HIV) or antibody to hepatitis delta virus (anti-HDV) in the serum were excluded from the studies.

Virologic response to treatment was defined in these studies as a loss of serum markers of HBV replication (HBeAg and HBV DNA). Secondary parameters of response included loss of serum HBsAg, decreases in serum ALT, and improvement in liver histology.

In each of two randomized controlled studies, a significantly greater proportion of INTRON A treated patients exhibited a virologic response compared with untreated control patients (see TABLE 4). In a third study without a concurrent control group, a similar response rate to INTRON A therapy was observed. Pretreatment with prednisone, evaluated in two of the studies, did not improve the response rate and provided no additional benefit.

The response to INTRON A therapy was durable. No patient responding to INTRON A therapy at a dose of 5 million IU QD or 10 million IU TIW, relapsed during the follow-up period which ranged from 2 to 6 months after treatment ended. The loss of serum HBeAg and HBV- DNA was maintained in 100% of 19 responding patients followed for 3.5 to 36 months after the end of therapy.

In a proportion of responding patients, loss of HBeAg was followed by the loss of HBsAg. HBsAg was lost in 27% (4/15) of patients who responded to INTRON A therapy at a dose of 5 million IU QD, and 35% (8/23) of patients who responded to 10 million IU TIW. No untreated control patient lost HBsAg in these studies.

In a pilot study, 12 patients responding to INTRON A therapy were followed for 3.8 to 6.6 years after treatment; 100% (12/12) remained serum HBeAg negative and 58% (7/12) lost serum HBsAg.

INTRON A therapy resulted in normalization of serum ALT in a significantly greater proportion of treated patients compared to untreated patients in each of two controlled studies (see TABLE 5). In a third study without a concurrent control group, normalization of serum ALT was observed in 50% (12/24) of patients receiving INTRON A therapy.

Virologic response was associated with a reduction in serum ALT to normal or near normal (≤ 1.5 times the upper limit of normal) in 87% (13/15) of patients responding to INTRON A therapy at 5 million IU QD, and 100% (23/23) of patients responding to 10 million IU TIW.

Improvement in liver histology was evaluated in Studies 1 and 3 by comparison of pre- and 6- month posttreatment

TABLE 4
VIROLOGIC RESPONSE*
IN CHRONIC HEPATITIS B PATIENTS

Study Number	INTRON A 5 million IU QD		INTRON A 10 million IU TIW		Untreated Controls		P** Value
1[5]	15/38	(39%)	—		3/42	(7%)	0.0009
2	—		10/24	(42%)	1/22	(5%)	0.005
3[6]	—		13/24‡	(54%)	2/27	(7%)‡	NA‡
All Studies	**15/38**	**(39%)**	**23/48**	**(48%)**	**6/91**	**(7%)**	**—**

*Loss of HBeAg and HBV DNA by 6 months posttherapy.
¶Patients pretreated with prednisone not shown.
**INTRON A treatment group versus untreated control.
‡Untreated control patients evaluated after 24 week observation period. A subgroup subsequently received INTRON A therapy. A direct comparison is not applicable (NA).

TABLE 5
ALT RESPONSES*
IN CHRONIC HEPATITIS B PATIENTS

Study Number	INTRON A 5 million IU QD		INTRON A 10 million IU TIW		Untreated Controls		P** Value
1	16/38	(42%)	—		8/42	(19%)	0.03
2	—		10/24	(42%)	1/22	(5%)	0.0034
3	—		12/24†	(50%)	2/27	(7%)†	NA†
All Studies	**16/38**	**(42%)**	**22/48**	**(46%)**	**11/91**	**(12%)**	**—**

*Reduction in serum ALT to normal by 6 months posttherapy.
**INTRON A treatment group versus untreated control.
†Untreated control patients evaluated after 24 week observation period. A subgroup subsequently received INTRON A therapy. A direct comparison is not applicable (NA).

liver biopsies using the semi-quantitative Knodell Histology Activity Index.[4] No statistically significant difference in liver histology was observed in treated patients compared to control patients in Study 1. Although statistically significant histological improvement from baseline was observed in treated patients in Study 3 (p≤0.01), there was no control group for comparison. Of those patients exhibiting a virologic response following treatment with 5 million IU QD or 10 million IU TIW, histological improvement was observed in 85% (17/20) compared to 36% (9/25) of patients who were not virologic responders. The histological improvement was due primarily to decreases in severity of necrosis, degeneration, and inflammation in the periportal, lobular, and portal regions of the liver (Knodell Categories I + II + III). Continued histological improvement was observed in four responding patients who lost serum HBsAg and were followed 2 to 4 years after the end of INTRON A therapy.[7]

[See Tables 4 and 5 above.]

INDICATIONS AND USAGE

General INTRON A Interferon alfa-2b, recombinant for Injection is indicated in patients 18 years of age or older for the treatment of hairy cell leukemia, selected cases of condylomata acuminata involving external surfaces of the genital and perianal areas, selected patients with AIDS-Related Kaposi's Sarcoma, chronic hepatitis Non-A, Non-B/C (NANB/C) in patients with compensated liver disease who have a history of blood or blood-product exposure and/or are HCV antibody positive, and chronic hepatitis B in patients with compensated liver disease and HBV replication (serum HBeAg positive), and as adjuvant treatment to surgery in patients with malignant melanoma who are free of disease but at high risk for systemic recurrence.

Hairy Cell Leukemia INTRON A Interferon alfa-2b, recombinant for Injection is indicated for the treatment of patients 18 years of age or older with hairy cell leukemia.

Malignant Melanoma INTRON A Interferon alfa-2b, recombinant for Injection is indicated as adjuvant to surgical treatment in patients 18 years of age or older with malignant melanoma who are free of disease but at high risk for systemic recurrence, within 56 days of surgery.

Condylomata Acuminata INTRON A Interferon alfa-2b, recombinant for Injection is indicated for intralesional treatment of selected patients 18 years of age or older with condylomata acuminata involving external surfaces of the genital and perianal areas (see DOSAGE AND ADMINISTRATION).

In selecting patients for INTRON A treatment, the physician should consider the nature of the patient's lesion and the patient's past treatment history, in addition to the patient's ability to comply with the treatment regimen. INTRON A therapy offers an additional approach to treatment in condylomata and is particularly useful for those patients who do not respond satisfactorily to other treatment modalities (eg, podophyllin resin, surgery, cryotherapy, chemotherapy, and laser therapy), or whose lesions are more

readily treatable by INTRON A Interferon alfa-2b, recombinant for Injection than by other treatments.

The use of this product in adolescents has not been studied. Interferon alpha has been shown to affect the menstrual cycle in nonhuman primates and to decrease serum estradiol and progesterone levels in women. Consideration should be given as to whether the adolescent patient should be treated.

AIDS-Related Kaposi's Sarcoma INTRON A Interferon alfa-2b, recombinant for Injection is indicated for the treatment of selected patients 18 years of age or older with AIDS-Related Kaposi's Sarcoma. Studies have demonstrated a greater likelihood of response to INTRON A therapy in patients who are without systemic symptoms, who have limited lymphadenopathy and who have a relatively intact immune system as indicated by total CD4 count.

Chronic Hepatitis Non-A, Non-B/C (NANB/C) INTRON A Interferon alfa-2b, recombinant for Injection is indicated for the treatment of chronic hepatitis Non-A, Non-B/C (NANB/C) in patients 18 years of age or older with compensated liver disease who have a history of blood or blood product exposure and/or are HCV antibody positive. Studies in these patients demonstrated that INTRON A therapy can produce clinically meaningful effects on this disease, manifested by normalization of serum alanine aminotransferase (ALT) and reduction in liver necrosis and degeneration.

A liver biopsy should be performed to establish the diagnosis of chronic hepatitis. Patients should be tested for the presence of antibody to HCV. Patients with other causes of chronic hepatitis, including autoimmune hepatitis, should be excluded. Prior to initiation of INTRON A therapy, the physician should establish that the patient has compensated liver disease. The following patient entrance criteria for compensated liver disease were used in the clinical studies and should be considered before INTRON A treatment of patients with chronic hepatitis NANB/C:

- No history of hepatic encephalopathy, variceal bleeding, ascites, or other clinical signs of decompensation
- Bilirubin   ≤2 mg/dL
- Albumin   Stable and within normal limits
- Prothrombin Time   <3 seconds prolonged
- WBC   ≥3000/mm³
- Platelets   ≥70,000/mm³

Serum creatinine should be normal or near normal.

Prior to initiation of INTRON A therapy, CBC and platelet counts should be evaluated in order to establish baselines for monitoring potential toxicity. These tests should be repeated at weeks 1 and 2 following initiation of INTRON A therapy, and monthly thereafter. Serum ALT should be evaluated after 2, 16, and 24 weeks of therapy to assess response to treatment (see **DOSAGE AND ADMINISTRATION**).

Patients with preexisting thyroid abnormalities may be treated if thyroid stimulating hormone (TSH) levels can be maintained in the normal range by medication. TSH levels must be within normal limits upon initiation of INTRON A treatment and TSH testing should be repeated at 3 and 6 months (see **PRECAUTIONS—Laboratory Tests**).

Chronic Hepatitis B INTRON A Interferon alfa-2b, recombinant for Injection is indicated for the treatment of chronic hepatitis B in patients 18 years of age or older with compensated liver disease and HBV replication. Patients must be serum HBsAg positive for at least 6 months and have HBV replication (serum HBeAg positive) with elevated serum ALT. Studies in these patients demonstrated that INTRON A therapy can produce virologic remission of this disease (loss of serum HBeAg), and normalization of serum aminotransferases. INTRON A therapy resulted in the loss of serum HBsAg in some responding patients.

Prior to initiation of INTRON A therapy, it is recommended that a liver biopsy be performed to establish the presence of chronic hepatitis and the extent of liver damage. The physician should establish that the patient has compensated liver disease. The following patient entrance criteria for compensated liver disease were used in the clinical studies and should be considered before INTRON A treatment of patients with chronic hepatitis B:

- No history of hepatic encephalopathy, variceal bleeding, ascites, or other signs of clinical decompensation
- Bilirubin   Normal
- Albumin   Stable and within normal limits
- Prothrombin Time   <3 seconds prolonged
- WBC   ≥4000/mm³
- Platelets   ≥100,000/mm³

Patients with causes of chronic hepatitis other than chronic hepatitis B or chronic hepatitis NANB/C should not be treated with INTRON A Interferon alfa-2b, recombinant for Injection. CBC and platelet counts should be evaluated prior to initiation of INTRON A therapy in order to establish baselines for monitoring potential toxicity. These tests should be repeated at treatment weeks 1, 2, 4, 8, 12, and 16. Liver function tests, including serum ALT, albumin, and bilirubin, should be evaluated at treatment weeks 1, 2, 4, 8, 12, and 16. HBeAg, HBsAg, and ALT should be evaluated at the end of therapy, as well as 3 and 6 months posttherapy, since patients may become virologic responders during the 6-month period following the end of treatment. In clinical studies,

39% (15/38) of responding patients lost HBeAg 1 to 6 months following the end of INTRON A therapy. Of responding patients who lost HBsAg, 58% (7/12) did so 1 to 6 months posttreatment.

A transient increase in ALT ≥ 2 times baseline value (flare) can occur during INTRON A therapy for chronic hepatitis B. In clinical trials, this flare generally occurred 8 to 12 weeks after initiation of therapy and was more frequent in responders (63%, 24/38) than in nonresponders (27%, 13/48). However, elevations in bilirubin ≥3 mg/dL occurred infrequently (2%, 2/86) during therapy. When ALT flare occurs, in general, INTRON A therapy should be continued unless signs and symptoms of liver failure are observed. During ALT flare, clinical symptomatology and liver function tests including ALT, prothrombin time, alkaline phosphatase, albumin, and bilirubin, should be monitored at approximately 2-week intervals (see **WARNINGS**).

DOSAGE AND ADMINISTRATION

IMPORTANT: INTRON A Interferon alfa-2b, recombinant for Injection dosing regimens are different for each of the following indications described in this section of the product information sheet.

Hairy Cell Leukemia The recommended dosage of INTRON A Interferon alfa-2b, recombinant for Injection for the treatment of hairy cell leukemia is 2 million IU/m² administered intramuscularly (see **WARNINGS**) or subcutaneously 3 times a week. The 50 million IU strength of the INTRON A Powder for Injection is not to be used for the treatment of hairy cell leukemia. Higher doses are not recommended. The normalization of one or more hematologic variables usually begins within 2 months of initiation of therapy. Improvement in all three hematologic variables may require 6 months or more of therapy. Responding patients may benefit from continued treatment after that time point with fewer relapses and a longer relapse-free interval. If treatment with INTRON A therapy has been interrupted, it should be noted that retreatment with INTRON A therapy has led to response in greater than 90% of patients.

This dosage regimen should be maintained unless the disease progresses rapidly, or severe intolerance is manifested. If severe adverse reactions develop, the dosage should be modified (50% reduction) or therapy should be temporarily discontinued until the adverse reactions abate. If persistent or recurrent intolerance develops following adequate dosage adjustment, or disease progresses, INTRON A treatment should be discontinued. The minimum effective INTRON A dose has not been established.

Malignant Melanoma The recommended INTRON A treatment regimen includes induction treatment 5 consecutive days per week for 4 weeks as an intravenous (IV) infusion at a dose of 20 million IU/m², followed by maintenance treatment 3 times per week for 48 weeks as a subcutaneous (SC) injection, at a dose of 10 million IU/m².

In the clinical trial, the median daily INTRON A doses administered to patients were 19.1 million IU/m² during the induction phase and 9.1 million IU/m² during the maintenance phase.

Regular laboratory testing should be performed to monitor laboratory abnormalities for the purposes of dose modification (see **PRECAUTIONS-Laboratory Tests**). If adverse reactions develop during INTRON A treatment, particularly if granulocytes decrease to <500/mm³ or SGPT/SGOT rises to >5 x upper limit of normal, treatment should be temporarily discontinued until the adverse reactions abate. INTRON A treatment should be restarted at 50% of the previous dose. If intolerance persists after dose adjustments or if granulocytes decrease to <250/mm³ or SGPT/SGOT rises to >10 x upper limit of normal, INTRON A therapy should be discontinued. In the clinical trial, patients were able to achieve clinical benefit in conjunction with appropriate dose modifications. Therapy should be maintained for 1 year unless there is progression of disease.

Condylomata Acuminata The 10 million IU vial of INTRON A Powder for Injection must be reconstituted with 1 mL of Diluent for INTRON A Interferon alfa-2b, recombinant for Injection (bacteriostatic water for injection). Do not reconstitute the 10 million IU vial of INTRON A Powder for Injection with more than 1 mL of diluent since the injection would be subpotent. Do not use the 3 million, 5 million, 18 million, 25 million, or 50 million IU vials of INTRON A Powder for Injection for the treatment of condylomata acuminata since the resulting reconstituted solution would be either hypertonic or an inappropriate concentration. Do not use the 10 million, 18 million multidose, or 25 million IU vials of INTRON A Solution for Injection for the intralesional treatment of condylomata acuminata since the concentrations are inappropriate for such use.

Inject 1.0 million IU of INTRON A Interferon alfa-2b, recombinant for Injection (0.1 mL of reconstituted INTRON A solution) into each lesion three times per week on alternate days, for 3 weeks. The injection should be administered intralesionally using a Tuberculin or similar syringe and a 25–30 gauge needle. The needle should be directed at the center of the base of the wart and at an angle almost parallel to the plane of the skin (approximating that in the commonly

used PPD test). This will deliver the interferon to the dermal core of the lesion, infiltrating the lesion and causing a small wheal. Care should be taken not to go beneath the lesion too deeply; subcutaneous injection should be avoided, since this area is below the base of the lesion. Do not inject too superficially since this will result in possible leakage, infiltrating only the keratinized layer, and not the dermal core. As many as 5 lesions can be treated at one time. To reduce side effects, INTRON A injections may be administered in the evening, when possible. Additionally, acetaminophen may be administered at the time of injection to alleviate some of the potential side effects.

The maximum response usually occurs 4 to 8 weeks after initiation of the first treatment course. If results at 12 to 16 weeks after the initial treatment course has concluded are not satisfactory, a second course of treatment using the above dosage schedule may be instituted providing that clinical symptoms and signs, or changes in laboratory parameters (liver function tests, WBC, and platelets) do not preclude such a course of action.

Patients with six to ten condylomata may receive a second (sequential) course of treatment at the above dosage schedule, to treat up to five additional condylomata per course of treatment. Patients with greater than ten condylomata may receive additional sequences depending on how large a number of condylomata are present.

AIDS-Related Kaposi's Sarcoma The recommended INTRON A dosage is 30 million IU/m² three times a week administered subcutaneously or intramuscularly. The 10 million, 18 million multidose, and 25 million IU vials of the INTRON A Solution for Injection are not to be used for the treatment of condylomata acuminata or AIDS-Related Kaposi's Sarcoma.

The selected dosage regimen should be maintained unless the disease progresses rapidly or severe intolerance is manifested. If severe adverse reactions develop, the dosage should be modified (50% reduction) or therapy should be temporarily discontinued until the adverse reactions abate. When patients initiate therapy at 30 million IU/m² TIW, the average dose tolerated at the end of 12 weeks of therapy is 110 million IU/week and 75 million IU/week at the end of 24 weeks of therapy.

When disease stabilization or a response to treatment occurs, treatment should continue until there is no further evidence of tumor or until discontinuation is required by evidence of a severe opportunistic infection or adverse effect.

Chronic Hepatitis Non-A, Non-B/C (NANB/C) The recommended dosage of INTRON A Interferon alfa-2b, recombinant for Injection for the treatment of chronic hepatitis NANB/C is 3 million IU three times a week (TIW) administered subcutaneously or intramuscularly.

Normalization of serum alanine aminotransferase (ALT) may occur in some patients as early as 2 weeks after initiation of treatment; however, current experience suggests that patients responding to INTRON A therapy with a reduction in serum ALT should complete 6 months (24 weeks) of treatment. The optimal dose and duration of therapy are currently under investigation.

In clinical trials, 54% (51/95) of the patients at a dose of 3 million IU TIW responded with a reduction in serum ALT after 6 months of INTRON A therapy. Since most of these patients (49/51) responded within the first 16 weeks of treatment, consideration could be given to discontinuing INTRON A therapy in patients who fail to respond after 16 weeks. The effect of dose escalation in these patients is under investigation.

If severe adverse reactions develop during INTRON A treatment, the dose should be modified (50% reduction) or therapy should be temporarily discontinued until the adverse reactions abate. If intolerance persists after dose adjustment, INTRON A therapy should be discontinued.

Patients who relapse following INTRON A therapy may be retreated with the same dosage regimen to which they had previously responded.

Chronic Hepatitis B The recommended dosage of INTRON A Interferon alfa-2b, recombinant for Injection for the treatment of chronic hepatitis B is 30 to 35 million IU per week, administered subcutaneously or intramuscularly, either as 5 million IU daily (QD) or as 10 million IU three times a week (TIW) for 16 weeks.

If severe adverse reactions or laboratory abnormalities develop during INTRON A therapy the dose should be modified (50% reduction), or discontinued if appropriate, until the adverse reactions abate. If intolerance persists after dose adjustment, INTRON A therapy should be discontinued.

For patients with decreases in granulocyte or platelet counts, the following guidelines for dose modification were used in the clinical trials:

Continued on next page

Information on Schering products appearing on these pages is effective as of August 15, 1996.

Schering—Cont.

INTRON A Dose	*Granulocyte Count*	*Platelet Count*
Reduce 50%	<750/mm³	<50,000/mm³
Interrupt	<500/mm³	<30,000/mm³

INTRON A therapy was resumed at up to 100% of the initial dose when granulocyte and/or platelet counts returned to normal or baseline values.

At the discretion of the physician, the patient may self-administer the medication. (See illustrated **PATIENT INFORMATION SHEET** for instructions.)

Preparation and Administration of INTRON A Interferon alfa-2b, recombinant Powder for Injection for Intramuscular, Subcutaneous, or Intralesional Administration

Reconstitution of INTRON A Powder for Injection Inject the amount of Diluent for INTRON A Interferon alfa-2b, recombinant for Injection (bacteriostatic water for injection) stated in the appropriate chart below (diluent is supplied in either a vial or syringe, see **HOW SUPPLIED** below), into the INTRON A vial. Swirl gently to hasten complete dissolution of the powder. The appropriate INTRON A dose should then be withdrawn and injected intramuscularly, subcutaneously, or intralesionally. (See **PATIENT INFORMATION SHEET** for detailed instructions.) After preparation and administration of the INTRON A injection, it is essential to follow the procedure for proper disposal of syringes and needles. (See **PATIENT INFORMATION SHEET** for detailed instructions.)

Preparation and Administration of INTRON A Interferon alfa-2b, recombinant Powder for Injection for Intravenous Infusion

The infusion solution should be prepared immediately prior to use. Based on the desired dose, the appropriate vial strength(s) of INTRON A Interferon alfa-2b, recombinant Powder for Injection should be reconstituted with the diluent provided. The appropriate INTRON A dose should then be withdrawn and injected into a 100 mL bag of 0.9% Sodium Chloride Injection, USP. The final concentration of INTRON A Interferon alfa-2b, recombinant for Injection should be not less than 10 million IU/100 mL. The prepared solution should be infused over a 20-minute period.

Hairy Cell Leukemia

Vial Strength	mL Diluent	Final Concentration
3 million IU	1	3 million IU/mL
5 million IU	1	5 million IU/mL
10 million IU	2	5 million IU/mL
25 million IU	5	5 million IU/mL

Condylomata Acuminata

Vial Strength	mL Diluent	Final Concentration
*10 million IU	1	10 million IU/mL

*IMPORTANT: For patients with condylomata acuminata reconstitute the 10 million IU vial with only 1 mL of the diluent provided to reach a final concentration of 10 million IU/mL to be administered intralesionally (see **DOSAGE AND ADMINISTRATION, Condylomata Acuminata**).

AIDS-Related Kaposi's Sarcoma

Vial Strength	mL Diluent	Final Concentration
*50 million IU	1	50 million IU/mL

*IMPORTANT: This vial size is to be used only for treatment of patients with AIDS-Related Kaposi's Sarcoma (see **DOSAGE AND ADMINISTRATION, Aids-Related Kaposi's Sarcoma, Malignant Melanoma**).

[See table on bottom of page.]

Chronic Hepatitis Non-A, Non-B/C

Vial Strength	mL Diluent	Final Concentration
3 million IU	1	3 million IU/mL

Chronic Hepatitis B

Vial Strength	mL Diluent	Final Concentration
5 million IU	1	5 million IU/mL
10 million IU	1	10 million IU/mL

Stability INTRON A Interferon alfa-2b, recombinant Powder for Injection provided in vials ranging from 3 to 50 million IU per vial, is stable at 45°C (113°F) for up to 7 days. After reconstitution with Diluent for INTRON A Interferon alfa-2b, recombinant for Injection (bacteriostatic water for injection) the solution is stable for 1 month at 2° to 8°C (36° to 46°F). The reconstituted solution is clear and colorless to light yellow.

Preparation and Administration of INTRON A Interferon alfa-2b, recombinant Solution for Injection

The 10 million IU vials of INTRON A Solution for Injection are supplied in 2 mL vials. The 18 million multidose and 25 million IU vials of INTRON A Solution for Injection are supplied in 5 mL vials. The solution is colorless to light yellow. These packages do not require reconstitution prior to administration. The appropriate INTRON A dose should be withdrawn from the vial and injected intramuscularly or subcutaneously. (See **PATIENT INFORMATION SHEET** for detailed instructions.) After administration of INTRON A Solution for Injection, it is essential to follow the procedure for proper disposal of syringes and needles. (See **PATIENT INFORMATION SHEET** for detailed instructions.)

Hairy Cell Leukemia

Vial Strength	mL Solution	Final Concentration
10 million IU	2 mL	5 million IU/mL
‡18 million IU multidose	3.8 mL	6 million IU/mL
25 million IU	5 mL	5 million IU/mL

‡ This is a multidose vial which contains a total of 22.8 million IU of interferon alfa-2b, recombinant per 3.8 mL in order to provide the delivery of six 0.5 mL doses, each containing 3 million IU of INTRON A Interferon alfa-2b, recombinant for Injection (for a label strength of 18 million IU).

Chronic Hepatitis Non-A, Non-B/C

Vial Strength	mL Solution	Final Concentration
10 million IU	2 mL	5 million IU/mL
†18 million IU multidose	3.8 mL	6 million IU/mL
25 million IU	5 mL	5 million IU/mL

† This is a multidose vial which contains a total of 22.8 million IU of interferon alfa-2b, recombinant per 3.8 mL in order to provide the delivery of six 0.5 mL doses, each containing 3 million IU of INTRON A Interferon alfa-2b, recombinant for Injection (for a label strength of 18 million IU).

Chronic Hepatitis B

Vial Strength	mL Solution	Final Concentration
10 million IU	2 mL	5 million IU/mL
25 million IU	5 mL	5 million IU/mL

IMPORTANT: The 10 million, 18 million multidose, and 25 million IU strengths of INTRON A Solution for Injection are not to be used for condylomata acuminata or for AIDS-Related Kaposi's Sarcoma. (See **DOSAGE AND ADMINISTRATION, Condylomata Acuminata; DOSAGE AND ADMINISTRATION, AIDS-Related Kaposi's Sarcoma.**)

Parenteral drug products should be inspected visually for particulate matter and discoloration prior to administration, whenever solution and container permit. INTRON A Interferon alfa-2b, recombinant for Injection may be administered using either sterilized glass or plastic disposable syringes.

INTRON A SOLUTION FOR INJECTION IS NOT RECOMMENDED FOR INTRAVENOUS ADMINISTRATION.

CONTRAINDICATIONS

INTRON A Interferon alfa-2b, recombinant for Injection is contraindicated in patients with a history of hypersensitivity to interferon alfa or any component of the injection.

WARNINGS

General Moderate to severe adverse experiences may require modification of the patient's dosage regimen, or in some cases termination of INTRON A therapy. Because of the fever and other "flu-like" symptoms associated with INTRON A administration, it should be used cautiously in patients with debilitating medical conditions, such as those with a history of pulmonary disease (eg, chronic obstructive pulmonary disease), or diabetes mellitus prone to ketoacidosis. Caution should also be observed in patients with coagulation disorders (eg, thrombophlebitis, pulmonary embolism) or severe myelosuppression.

Patients with platelet counts of less than 50,000/mm³ should not be administered INTRON A Interferon alfa-2b, recombinant for Injection intramuscularly, but instead by subcutaneous administration.

INTRON A therapy should be used cautiously in patients with a history of cardiovascular disease such as unstable angina or uncontrolled congestive heart failure. Those patients with a recent history of myocardial infarction and/or previous or current arrhythmic disorder who require INTRON A therapy should be closely monitored (see **Laboratory Tests**). Cardiovascular adverse experiences, which include hypotension, arrhythmia, or tachycardia of 150 beats per minute or greater, and transient reversible cardiomyopathy have been observed in some INTRON A treated patients. Transient reversible cardiomyopathy was reported in approximately 2% of the AIDS-Related Kaposi's Sarcoma patients treated with INTRON A Interferon alfa-2b, recombinant for Injection. The incidence of these complications in patients with preexisting heart disease is unknown. Hypotension may occur during INTRON A administration, or up to 2 days posttherapy, and may require supportive therapy including fluid replacement to maintain intravascular volume. Supraventricular arrhythmias occurred rarely and appeared to be correlated with preexisting conditions and prior therapy with cardiotoxic agents. These adverse experiences were controlled by modifying the dose or discontinuing treatment, but may require specific additional therapy.

DEPRESSION AND SUICIDAL BEHAVIOR INCLUDING SUICIDAL IDEATION, SUICIDAL ATTEMPTS, AND COMPLETED SUICIDES HAVE BEEN REPORTED IN ASSOCIATION WITH TREATMENT WITH ALFA INTERFERONS, INCLUDING INTRON A THERAPY. Patients with a preexisting psychiatric condition, especially depression, or a history of severe psychiatric disorder should not be treated with INTRON A Interferon alfa-2b, recombinant for Injection.[8] INTRON A therapy should be discontinued for any patient developing severe depression or other psychiatric disorder during treatment. Obtundation and coma have also been observed in some patients, usually elderly, treated at higher doses. While these effects are usually rapidly reversible upon discontinuation of therapy, full resolution of symptoms has taken up to 3 weeks in a few severe episodes. Narcotics, hypnotics, or sedatives may be used concurrently with caution and patients should be closely monitored until the adverse effects have resolved.

Patients with preexisting thyroid abnormalities whose thyroid function cannot be maintained in the normal range by medication should not be treated with INTRON A Interferon alfa-2b, recombinant for Injection. Therapy should be discontinued for patients developing thyroid abnormalities during treatment whose thyroid function cannot be normalized by medication.

Hepatotoxicity, including fatality, has been observed rarely in INTRON A treated patients. Any patient developing liver function abnormalities during treatment should be monitored closely and if appropriate, treatment should be discontinued.

Pulmonary infiltrates, pneumonitis and pneumonia, including fatality, have been observed rarely in interferon alfa treated patients, including those treated with INTRON A Interferon alfa-2b, recombinant for Injection. The etiologic explanation for these pulmonary findings has yet to be established. Any patient developing fever, cough, dyspnea, or other respiratory symptoms should have a chest X-ray taken. If the chest X-ray shows pulmonary infiltrates or there is evidence of pulmonary function impairment, the patient should be closely monitored, and, if appropriate, interferon alfa treatment should be discontinued. While this has been reported more often in patients with chronic hepatitis NANB/C treated with interferon alfa, it has also been reported in patients with oncologic diseases treated with interferon alfa.

Retinal hemorrhages, cotton-wool spots, and retinal artery or vein obstruction have been observed rarely in patients treated with interferon alfa, including those treated with INTRON A Interferon alfa-2b, recombinant for Injection. The etiologic explanation for these findings has not yet been established. These events appear to occur after use of the drug for several months, but also have been reported after shorter treatment periods. Diabetes mellitus or hypertension have been present in some patients. Any patient complaining of changes in visual acuity or visual fields, or reporting other ophthalmologic symptoms during treatment with INTRON A Interferon alfa-2b, recombinant for Injection, should have an eye examination. Because the retinal events may have to be differentiated from those seen with diabetic or hypertensive retinopathy, a baseline ocular examination is recommended prior to treatment

Malignant Melanoma

	Vial Strength	mL Diluent	Final Concentration
¶ Induction phase	3 million IU	1	3 million IU/mL
	5 million IU	1	5 million IU/mL
	10 million IU	1	10 million IU/mL
	18 million IU	1	18 million IU/mL
	25 million IU	5	5 million IU/mL
	*50 million IU	1	50 million IU/mL
Maintenance phase	3 million IU	1	3 million IU/mL
	5 million IU	1	5 million IU/mL
	10 million IU	1	10 million IU/mL
	18 million IU	1	18 million IU/mL
	*50 million IU	1	50 million IU/mL

¶Based on the desired dose, the appropriate vial strengths should be reconstituted and administered intravenously.
*IMPORTANT: This vial size is to be used only for treatment of patients with AIDS-Related Kaposi's Sarcoma or for patients with malignant melanoma (See **DOSAGE AND ADMINISTRATION, AIDS-Related Kaposi's Sarcoma, Malignant Melanoma**).

TREATMENT-RELATED ADVERSE EXPERIENCES BY INDICATION
Dosing Regimens
Percentage (%) of Patients*

ADVERSE EXPERIENCE	MALIGNANT MELANOMA 20 MIU/m² Induction (IV) 10 MIU/m² Maintenance (SC) N=143	HAIRY CELL LEUKEMIA 2 million IU/m² TIW/SC N=145	CONDYLOMATA ACUMINATA 1 million IU/lesion N=352	AIDS-RELATED KAPOSI'S SARCOMA 30 million IU/m² TIW/SC N=74	35 million IU/QD/SC N=29	CHRONIC HEPATITIS NANB/C 3 million IU TIW N=159	CHRONIC HEPATITIS B 5 million IU QD N=101	10 million IU TIW N=78
Application-Site Disorders								
injection site inflammation	—	20	—	—	—	7	3	—
other (<5%)	burning, injection site bleeding, injection site pain, injection site reaction, itching							
Blood Disorders (<5%)	anemia, granulocytopenia, hemolytic anemia, leukopenia, thrombocytopenia							
Body as a Whole								
facial edema	—	—	<1	—	10	1	3	1
weight decrease	3	<1	<1	5	3	<1	2	5
other (≤5%)	cachexia, dehydration, earache, hypercalcemia, lymphadenitis, lymphadenopathy, mastitis, periorbital edema, peripheral edema, scrotal/penile edema, thirst, weakness							
Cardiovascular System Disorders (<5%)	angina, arrythmia, atrial fibrillation, bradycardia, cardiac failure, cardiomyopathy, extrasystoles, hypertension, hypotension, palpitations, postural hypotension, tachycardia							
Endocrine System Disorders (<5%)	aggravation of diabetes mellitus, gynecomastia, hypertriglyceridemia, thyroid disorder, virilism							
Flu-like Symptoms								
fever	81	68	56	47	55	43	66	86
headache	62	39	47	36	21	43	61	44
chills	54	46	45	—	—	—	—	—
myalgia	75	39	44	34	28	42	59	40
fatigue	96	61	18	84	48	19	75	69
increased sweating	6	8	2	4	21	3	1	1
asthenia	—	7	—	11	—	24	5	15
rigors	2	—	—	30	14	27	38	42
arthralgia	6	8	9	—	3	19	19	8
dizziness	23	12	9	7	24	9	13	10
influenza-like symptoms	10	37	—	45	79	9	5	—
back pain	—	19	6	1	3	3	—	—
dry mouth	1	19	—	22	28	4	6	5
chest pain	2	<1	<1	1	28	1	4	—
malaise	6	—	14	5	—	3	9	6
pain (unspecified)	15	18	—	3	3	—	—	—
other (<5%)	chest pain substernal, rhinitis, rhinorrhea							
Gastrointestinal System Disorders								
diarrhea	35	18	2	18	45	13	19	8
anorexia	69	19	1	38	41	13	43	53
nausea	66	21	17	28	21	23	50	33
taste alteration	24	13	<1	5	7	1	10	—
abdominal pain	2	<5	1	5	21	6	5	4
loose stools	—	—	<1	—	10	3	2	—
vomiting	†	6	2	11	14	3	7	10
constipation	1	<1	—	1	10	<1	5	—
gingivitis	2‡	—	2	4	14	—	1	—
dyspepsia	—	—	2	4	—	3	3	8
other (<5%)	abdominal ascites, abdominal distention, dysphagia, eructation, esophagitis, flatulence, gallstones, gastric ulcer, gastroenteritis, gastrointestinal hemorrhage, gastrointestinal mucosal discoloration, gingival bleeding, gum hyperplasia, halitosis, increased appetite, increased saliva, melena, oral leukoplakia, rectal bleeding after stool, rectal hemorrhage, stomatitis, stomatitis ulcerative, taste loss							

with interferon in patients with diabetes mellitus or hypertension.

The 50 million IU strength of the INTRON A Powder for Injection is not to be used for the treatment of hairy cell leukemia, condylomata acuminata, chronic hepatitis NANB/C, or chronic hepatitis B. The 3 million, 5 million, 18 million, and 25 million IU strengths of the INTRON A Powder for Injection are not to be used for the intralesional treatment of condylomata acuminata since the dilution required for the intralesional use would result in a hypertonic solution.

The 10 million, 18 million multidose, and 25 million IU strengths of the INTRON A Solution for Injection are not to be used for the treatment of condylomata acuminata, AIDS-Related Kaposi's Sarcoma, or intravenous treatment of malignant melanoma.

AIDS-Related Kaposi's Sarcoma INTRON A therapy should not be used for patients with rapidly progressive visceral disease (see **CLINICAL PHARMACOLOGY**). Also of note, there may be synergistic adverse effects between INTRON A Interferon alfa-2b, recombinant for Injection and zidovudine. Patients receiving concomitant zidovudine have had a higher incidence of neutropenia than that expected with zidovudine alone. Careful monitoring of the WBC count is indicated in all patients who are myelosuppressed and in all patients receiving other myelosuppressive medications. The effects of INTRON A Interferon alfa-2b, recombinant for Injection when combined with other drugs used in the treatment of AIDS-Related disease are unknown.

Chronic Hepatitis Non-A, Non-B/C (NANB/C) and Chronic Hepatitis B Patients with decompensated liver disease, autoimmune hepatitis or a history of autoimmune disease, and patients who are immunosuppressed transplant recipients should not be treated with INTRON A Interferon alfa-2b, recombinant for Injection. There are reports of worsening liver disease, including jaundice, hepatic encephalopathy, hepatic failure, and death following INTRON A therapy in such patients. Therapy should be discontinued for any patient developing signs and symptoms of liver failure.

Chronic hepatitis B patients with evidence of decreasing hepatic synthetic functions, such as decreasing albumin levels or prolongation of prothrombin time, who nevertheless meet the entry criteria to start therapy, may be at increased risk of clinical decompensation if a flare of aminotransferases occurs during INTRON A treatment. In such patients, if increases in ALT occur during INTRON A therapy for chronic hepatitis B, they should be followed carefully including close monitoring of clinical symptomatology and liver function tests, including ALT, prothrombin time, alkaline phosphatase, albumin, and bilirubin. In considering these patients for INTRON A therapy, the potential risks must be evaluated against the potential benefits of treatment.

PRECAUTIONS

General Acute serious hypersensitivity reactions (eg, urticaria, angioedema, bronchoconstriction, anaphylaxis) have been observed rarely in INTRON A treated patients; if such an acute reaction develops, the drug should be discontinued immediately and appropriate medical therapy instituted. Transient rashes have occurred in some patients following injection, but have not necessitated treatment interruption. While fever may be related to the flu-like syndrome reported commonly in patients treated with interferon, other causes of persistent fever should be ruled out.

There have been reports of interferon exacerbating preexisting psoriasis; therefore, INTRON A therapy should be used in these patients only if the potential benefit justifies the potential risk.

Variations in dosage, routes of administration, and adverse reactions exist among different brands of interferon. Therefore, do not use different brands of interferon in any single treatment regimen.

Drug Interactions Interactions between INTRON A Interferon alfa-2b, recombinant for Injection and other drugs have not been fully evaluated. Caution should be exercised when administering INTRON A therapy in combination with other potentially myelosuppressive agents such as zidovudine. Concomitant use of alfa interferon and theophylline decreases theophylline clearance resulting in a 100% increase in serum theophylline levels.

Information for Patients Patients receiving INTRON A treatment should be directed in its appropriate use, informed of benefits and risks associated with treatment, and referred to the **PATIENT INFORMATION SHEET**. This information is intended to aid in the safe and effective use of this medication. It is not a disclosure of all possible adverse or intended effects.

If home use is prescribed, a puncture-resistant container for the disposal of used syringes and needles should be supplied to the patient. Patients should be thoroughly instructed in the importance of proper disposal and cautioned against any reuse of needles and syringes. The full container should be

Continued on next page

Information on Schering products appearing on these pages is effective as of August 15, 1996.

Consult 1997 supplements and future editions for revisions

Schering—Cont.

TREATMENT-RELATED ADVERSE EXPERIENCES BY INDICATION
Dosing Regimens
Percentage (%) of Patients*

ADVERSE EXPERIENCE	MALIGNANT MELANOMA 20 MIU/m² Induction (IV) 10 MIU/m² Maintenance (SC) (N=143)	HAIRY CELL LEUKEMIA 2 million IU/m² TIW/SC N=145	CONDYLOMATA ACUMINATA 1 million IU/ lesion N=352	AIDS-RELATED KAPOSI'S SARCOMA 30 million IU/m² TIW/SC N=74	AIDS-RELATED KAPOSI'S SARCOMA 35 million IU/QD/SC N=29	CHRONIC HEPATITIS NANB/C 3 million IU TIW N=159	CHRONIC HEPATITIS B 5 million IU QD N=101	CHRONIC HEPATITIS B 10 million IU TIW N=78
Liver and Biliary System Disorders (<5%)	*abnormal hepatic function tests, bilirubinemia, increased transaminases (elevated SGOT 63% in malignant melanoma), jaundice, right upper quadrant pain and very rarely, hepatic encephalopathy, hepatic failure, and death							
Musculoskeletal System Disorders								
musculoskeletal pain	—	—	—	—	—	—	9	1
other (<5%)	arthritis, arthrosis, bone pain, carpel tunnel syndrome, leg cramps, muscle weakness							
Nervous System and Psychiatric Disorders								
depression	40	6	3	9	28	8	17	6
paresthesia	13	6	1	3	21	1	6	3
impaired concentration	—	—	<1	3	14	4	8	5
amnesia	**	<5	—	—	14	—	—	—
confusion	8	<5	4	12	10	1	—	—
hypoesthesia	—	<5	1	—	10	—	—	—
irritability	1	—	—	—	—	4	16	12
somnolence	1	<5	3	3	—	1	14	9
anxiety	1	5	<1	—	3	1	2	—
insomnia	5	—	<1	3	3	4	11	6
nervousness	1	—	1	—	3	—	3	—
decreased libido	1	<5	—	—	—	1	5	1
other (<5%)	abnormal coordination, abnormal dreaming, abnormal gait, abnormal thinking, aggravated depression, aggressive reaction, agitation, apathy, aphasia, ataxia, CNS dysfunction, coma, convulsions, dysphonia, emotional lability, extrapyramidal disorder, feeling of ebriety, flushing, hearing disorder, hot flashes, hyperesthesia, hyperkinesia, hypertonia, hypokinesia, impaired consciousness, migraine, neuropathy, neurosis, paresis, paroniria, parosmia, personality disorder, polyneuropathy, speech disorder, stroke, suicide attempt, syncope, tinnitus, tremor, vertigo							
Reproduction System Disorders (<5%)	amenorrhea, impotence, leukorrhea, menorrhagia, menstrual irregularity, pelvic pain, uterine bleeding							
Resistance Mechanism Disorders								
moniliasis	—	—	<1	—	17	—	—	—
herpes simplex	1	—	1	—	3	—	5	—
other (<5%)	abscess, conjunctivitis, fungal infection, hemophilus, herpes zoster, sepsis, stye, trichomonas, viral infection							
Respiratory System Disorders								
dyspnea	15	<1	—	1	34	<1	5	—
coughing	6	<1	—	—	31	<1	4	—
pharyngitis	2	<5	1	1	31	1	7	1
sinusitis	1	—	—	—	21	—	—	—
nonproductive coughing	2	—	—	—	14	—	1	—
nasal congestion	1	—	1	—	10	—	4	—
other (≤5%)	bronchitis, bronchospasm, cyanosis, epistaxis, hemoptysis, lung fibrosis, pleural pain, pneumonia, pneumothorax, sneezing, wheezing							
Skin and Appendages Disorders								
dermatitis	1	8	—	—	—	—	1	—
alopecia	29	8	—	12	31	17	26	38
pruritus	—	11	1	7	—	6	6	4
rash	19	25	—	9	10	6	8	1
dry skin	1	9	—	9	10	<1	3	—
other (<5%)	abnormal hair texture, acne, cellulitis, cyanosis of the hand, cold and clammy skin, dermatitis lichenoides, epidermal necrolysis, erythema, folliculitis, furunculosis, increased hair growth, lacrimal gland disorder, lipoma, melanosis, nail disorders, nonherpetic cold sores, peripheral ischemia, photosensitivity, psoriasis, purpura, skin depigmentation, skin discoloration, urticaria, vitiligo							
Urinary System Disorders (<5%)	albumin/protein in urine, increased BUN, hematuria, incontinence, micturition disorder, micturition frequency, nocturia, polyuria, urinary tract infection							
Vision Disorders (<5%)	abnormal vision, blurred vision, diplopia, dry eyes, eye pain, photophobia							

* Dash (—) indicates not reported
† Vomiting was reported with nausea as a single term
‡ Includes stomatitis/mucositis
** Amnesia was reported with confusion as a single term

disposed of according to the directions provided by the physician (see **PATIENT INFORMATION SHEET**).

Patients should be cautioned not to change brands of interferon without medical consultation as a change in dosage may result.

Patients receiving high INTRON A doses should be cautioned against performing tasks that would require complete mental alertness, such as operating machinery or driving a motor vehicle.

The most common adverse experiences occurring with INTRON A therapy are "flu-like" symptoms, such as fever, headache, fatigue, anorexia, nausea, or vomiting (see **ADVERSE REACTIONS** section) and appear to decrease in severity as treatment continues. Some of these "flu-like" symptoms may be minimized by bedtime administration. Acetaminophen may be used to prevent or partially alleviate the fever and headache. Another common adverse experience is thinning of the hair.

It is advised that patients be well hydrated, especially during the initial stages of treatment.

Laboratory Tests In addition to those tests normally required for monitoring patients, the following laboratory tests are recommended for all patients on INTRON A therapy, prior to beginning treatment and then periodically thereafter.

● Standard hematologic tests—including hemoglobin, complete and differential white blood cell counts, and platelet count.

● Blood chemistries—electrolytes, liver function tests, and TSH.

Those patients who have preexisting cardiac abnormalities and/or are in advanced stages of cancer should have electrocardiograms taken prior to and during the course of treatment.

Mild to moderate leukopenia and elevated serum liver enzyme (SGOT) levels have been reported with intralesional administration of INTRON A Interferon alfa-2b, recombinant for Injection (see **ADVERSE REACTIONS** section); therefore, the monitoring of these laboratory parameters should be considered.

Baseline chest X-rays are suggested and should be repeated if clinically indicated.

For malignant melanoma patients, differential WBC count and liver function tests should be monitored weekly during the induction phase of therapy and monthly during the maintenance phase of therapy.

For specific recommendations in chronic hepatitis NANB/C and chronic hepatitis B, see **INDICATIONS AND USAGE** section.

Carcinogenesis, Mutagenesis, Impairment of Fertility Studies with INTRON A Interferon alfa-2b, recombinant for Injection have not been performed to determine carcinogenicity.

Interferon may impair fertility. In studies of interferon administration in nonhuman primates, menstrual cycle abnormalities have been observed. Decreases in serum estradiol and progesterone concentrations have been reported in women treated with human leukocyte interferon.[9] Therefore, fertile women should not receive INTRON A therapy unless they are using effective contraception during the therapy period. INTRON A therapy should be used with caution in fertile men.

ABNORMAL LABORATORY TEST VALUES BY INDICATION
Dosing Regimens
Percentage (%) of Patients

Laboratory Tests	MALIGNANT MELANOMA 20 MIU/m² Induction (IV) 10 MIU/² Maintenance (SC) N=143	HAIRY CELL LEUKEMIA 2 million IU/m² TIW/SC N=145	CONDYLOMATA ACUMINATA 1 million IU/ lesion N=352	AIDS-RELATED KAPOSI'S SARCOMA 30 million IU/m² TIW/SC N=69–73	35 million IU/QD/SC N=26–28	CHRONIC HEPATITIS NANB/C 3 million IU TIW N=87–158	CHRONIC HEPATITIS B 5 million IU QD N=96–101	10 million IU TIW N=75–103
Hemoglobin	22%	NA	—	1%	15%	15%	32%*	23%*
White Blood Cell Count	**	NA	17%	10%	22%	18%	68%†	34%†
Platelet Count	15%	NA	—	0%	8%	9%	12%‡	5%‡
Serum Creatinine	3%	0%	—	—	—	2%	3%	0%
Alkaline Phosphatase	13%	4%	—	—	—	3%	8%	4%
Lactate Dehydrogenase	1%	0%	—	—	—	—	—	—
Serum Urea Nitrogen	12%	0%	—	—	—	1%	2%	0%
SGOT	63%	4%	12%	11%	41%	—	—	—
SGPT	2%	13%	—	10%	15%	—	—	—
Granulocyte Count								
• Total	92%	NA	—	31%	39%	37%§	75%§	61%§
• 1000 – <1500/mm³	66%	—	—	—	—	—	30%	32%
• 750 – <1000/mm³	—	—	—	—	—	—	24%	18%
• 500 – <750/mm³	25%	—	—	—	—	—	17%	9%
• <500/mm³	1%	—	—	—	—	—	4%	2%

NA—Not Applicable—Patients' initial hematologic laboratory test values were abnormal due to their condition.
* Decrease of ≥ 2 g/dL
† Decrease to <3000/mm³
‡ Decrease to <70,000/mm³
§ Neutrophils plus bands
** White Blood Cell Count was reported as neutropenia

Mutagenicity studies have demonstrated that INTRON A Interferon alfa-2b, recombinant for Injection is not mutagenic.

Studies in mice (0.1, 1.0 million IU/day), rats (4, 20, 100 million IU/kg/day), and cynomolgus monkeys (1.1 million IU/kg/day; 0.25, 0.75, 2.5 million IU/kg/day) injected with INTRON A Interferon alfa-2b, recombinant for Injection for up to 9 days, 3 months, and 1 month, respectively, have revealed no evidence of toxicity. However, in cynomolgus monkeys (4, 20, 100 million IU/kg/day) injected daily for 3 months with INTRON A Interferon alfa-2b, recombinant for Injection toxicity was observed at the mid- and high-doses and mortality was observed at the high dose.

However, due to the known species-specificity of interferon, the effects in animals are unlikely to be predictive of those in man.

Pregnancy Category C INTRON A Interferon alfa-2b, recombinant for Injection has been shown to have abortifacient effects in *Macaca mulatta* (rhesus monkeys) at 7.5, 15, and 30 million IU/kg (90, 180, and 360 times the intramuscular or subcutaneous dose of 2 million IU/m²). Although abortion was observed in all dose groups, it was only statistically significant at the mid- and high-dose groups. There are no adequate and well-controlled studies in pregnant women. INTRON A therapy should be used during pregnancy only if the potential benefit justifies the potential risk to the fetus.

Nursing Mothers It is not known whether this drug is excreted in human milk. However, studies in mice have shown that mouse interferons are excreted into the milk. Because of the potential for serious adverse reactions from the drug in nursing infants, a decision should be made whether to discontinue nursing or to discontinue INTRON A therapy, taking into account the importance of the drug to the mother.

Pediatric Use Safety and effectiveness have not been established in patients below the age of 18 years.

ADVERSE REACTIONS

General The adverse experiences listed below were reported to be possibly or probably related to INTRON A therapy during clinical trials. Most of these adverse reactions were mild to moderate in severity and were manageable. Some were transient and most diminished with continued therapy.

The most frequently reported adverse reactions were flu-like symptoms, particularly fever, headache, chills, myalgia, and fatigue. More severe toxicities are observed generally at higher doses and may be difficult for patients to tolerate.

[See table at top of page 2511.]

[See table at top of page 2512.]

Hairy Cell Leukemia The adverse reactions most frequently reported during clinical trials in 145 patients with hairy cell leukemia were the flu-like symptoms of fever (68%), fatigue (61%), and chills (46%).

Malignant Melanoma The INTRON A dose was modified because of adverse events in 65% (n=93) of the patients. INTRON A therapy was discontinued because of adverse events in 8% of the patients during induction and 18% of the patients during maintenance. The most frequently reported adverse reaction was fatigue which was observed in 96% of patients. Other adverse reactions that were recorded in >20% of INTRON A treated patients included neutropenia

(92%), fever (81%), myalgia (75%), anorexia (69%), vomiting/nausea (66%), increased SGOT (63%), headache (62%), chills (54%), depression (40%), diarrhea (35%), alopecia (29%), altered taste sensation (24%), dizziness/vertigo (23%), and anemia (22%).

Adverse reactions classified as severe or life-threatening (ECOG Toxicity Criteria grade 3 or 4) were recorded in 66% and 14% of INTRON A treated patients, respectively. Severe adverse reactions recorded in >10% of INTRON A treated patients included neutropenia/leukopenia (26%), fatigue (23%), fever (18%), myalgia (17%) headache (17%), chills (16%), and increased SGOT (14%). Grade 4 fatigue was recorded in 4% and grade 4 depression was recorded in 2% of INTRON A treated patients. No other grade 4 AE was reported in more than 2 INTRON A treated patients. Lethal hepatotoxicity occurred in 2 INTRON A treated patients early in the clinical trial. No subsequent lethal hepatotoxicities were observed with adequate monitoring of liver function tests (see **PRECAUTIONS - Laboratory Tests**).

Condylomata Acuminata Eighty-eight percent (311/352) of patients treated with INTRON A Interferon alfa-2b, recombinant for Injection for condylomata acuminata who were evaluable for safety, reported an adverse reaction during treatment. The incidence of the adverse reactions reported increased when the number of treated lesions increased from 1 to 5. All 40 patients who had 5 warts treated, reported some type of adverse reaction during treatment.

Adverse reactions and abnormal laboratory test values reported by patients who were retreated were qualitatively and quantitatively similar to those reported during the initial INTRON A treatment period.

AIDS-Related Kaposi's Sarcoma In patients with AIDS-Related Kaposi's Sarcoma, some type of adverse reaction occurred in 100% of the 74 patients treated with 30 million IU/m² three times a week and in 97% of the 29 patients treated with 35 million IU per day.

Of these adverse reactions, those classified as severe (World Health Organization grade 3 or 4) were reported in 27% to 55% of patients. Severe adverse reactions in the 30 million IU/m² TIW study included: fatigue (20%), influenza-like symptoms (15%), anorexia (12%), dry mouth (4%), headache (4%), confusion (3%), fever (3%), myalgia (3%), and nausea and vomiting (1% each). Severe adverse reactions for patients who received the 35 million IU QD included: fever (24%), fatigue (17%), influenza-like symptoms (14%), dyspnea (14%), headache (10%), pharyngitis (7%), and ataxia, confusion, dysphagia, GI hemorrhage, abnormal hepatic function, increased SGOT, myalgia, cardiomyopathy, face edema, depression, emotional lability, suicide attempt, chest pain, and coughing (1 patient each). Overall, the incidence of severe toxicity was higher among patients who received the 35 million IU per day dose.

Chronic Hepatitis Non-A, Non-B/C (NANB/C) In patients with chronic hepatitis NANB/C, alopecia, injection site reactions, rash, depression, and irritability apparently increased in incidence with continued treatment; residual mild alopecia persisted posttreatment.

Infrequently, patients receiving INTRON A therapy for chronic hepatitis NANB/C developed thyroid abnormalities, either hypothyroid or hyperthyroid. In clinical trials <1% (4/426) developed thyroid abnormalities. The abnormalities were controlled by conventional therapy for thyroid dysfunction. The mechanism by which INTRON A Interferon alfa-

2b, recombinant for Injection may alter thyroid status is unknown. Prior to initiation of INTRON A therapy for the treatment of chronic hepatitis NANB/C, serum TSH should be evaluated. Patients developing symptoms consistent with possible thyroid dysfunction during the course of INTRON A therapy should have their thyroid function evaluated and appropriate treatment instituted. INTRON A treatment may be continued if TSH levels can be maintained in the normal range by medication. Discontinuation of INTRON A therapy has not always reversed thyroid dysfunction occurring during treatment.

Chronic Hepatitis B In patients with chronic hepatitis B, some type of adverse reaction occurred in 98% of the 101 patients treated at 5 million IU QD and 90% of the 78 patients treated at 10 million IU TIW. Most of these adverse reactions were mild to moderate in severity, were manageable, and were reversible following the end of therapy.

Adverse reactions classified as severe (causing a significant interference with normal daily activities or clinical state) were reported in 21% to 44% of patients. The severe adverse reactions reported most frequently were the flu-like symptoms of fever (28%), fatigue (15%), headache (5%), myalgia (4%), and rigors (4%), and other severe flu-like symptoms which occurred in 1% to 3% of patients. Other severe adverse reactions occurring in more than one patient were alopecia (8%), anorexia (6%), depression (3%), nausea (3%), and vomiting (2%).

To manage side effects, the dose was reduced, or INTRON A therapy was interrupted in 25% to 38% of patients. Five percent of patients discontinued treatment due to adverse experiences.

[See table above.]

HOW SUPPLIED

INTRON A Interferon alfa-2b, recombinant Powder for Injection INTRON A Interferon alfa-2b, recombinant Powder for Injection, 3 million IU per vial and Diluent for INTRON A Interferon alfa-2b, recombinant for Injection (bacteriostatic water for injection) 1 mL per vial or syringe; boxes containing 1 INTRON A vial and 1 vial of INTRON A Diluent (NDC 0085-0647-03); boxes containing 1 INTRON A vial and 1 syringe of INTRON A Diluent (NDC 0085-0647-04). INTRON A Interferon alfa-2b, recombinant Powder for Injection INTRON® A, Pak-3, containing 6 INTRON A vials, 3 million IU per vial, and 6 syringes of Diluent for INTRON A Interferon alfa-2b, recombinant for Injection (bacteriostatic water for injection) 1 mL per syringe for Chronic Hepatitis Non-A, Non-B/C (NDC 0085-0647-05). INTRON A Interferon alfa-2b, recombinant Powder for Injection, 5 million IU per vial and Diluent for INTRON A

Continued on next page

Information on Schering products appearing on these pages is effective as of August 15, 1996.

Consult 1997 supplements and future editions for revisions

Schering—Cont.

Interferon alfa-2b, recombinant for Injection (bacteriostatic water for injection) 1 mL per vial; boxes containing 1 INTRON A vial and 1 vial of INTRON A Diluent (NDC 0085-0120-02).

INTRON A Interferon alfa-2b, recombinant Powder for Injection INTRON® A, Pak-5, containing 6 INTRON A vials, 5 million IU per vial, and 6 syringes of Diluent for INTRON A Interferon alfa-2b, recombinant for Injection (bacteriostatic water for injection) 1 mL per syringe for Chronic Hepatitis B (NDC 0085-0120-04).

INTRON A Interferon alfa-2b, recombinant Powder for Injection, 10 million IU per vial and Diluent for INTRON A Interferon alfa-2b, recombinant for Injection (bacteriostatic water for injection) 2 mL per vial; boxes containing 1 INTRON A vial and 1 vial of INTRON A Diluent (NDC 0085-0571-02).

INTRON A Interferon alfa-2b, recombinant Powder for Injection INTRON® A, Pak-10, containing 6 INTRON A vials, 10 million IU per vial, and 6 syringes of Diluent for INTRON A Interferon alfa-2b, recombinant for Injection (bacteriostatic water for injection) 1 mL per syringe for Chronic Hepatitis B (NDC 0085-0571-06).

INTRON A Interferon alfa-2b, recombinant Powder for Injection, 18 million IU per vial and Diluent for INTRON A Interferon alfa-2b, recombinant for Injection (bacteriostatic water for injection) 1 mL per vial; boxes containing 1 vial of INTRON A and 1 vial of INTRON A Diluent (NDC 0085-1110-01).

INTRON A Interferon alfa-2b, recombinant Powder for Injection, 25 million IU per vial and Diluent for INTRON A Interferon alfa-2b, recombinant for Injection (bacteriostatic water for injection) 5 mL per vial; boxes containing 1 INTRON A vial and 1 vial of INTRON A Diluent (NDC 0085-0285-02).

INTRON A Interferon alfa-2b, recombinant Powder for Injection, 50 million IU per vial and Diluent for INTRON A Interferon alfa-2b, recombinant for Injection (bacteriostatic water for injection) 1 mL per vial; boxes containing 1 INTRON A vial and 1 vial of INTRON A Diluent (NDC 0085-0539-01).

Store INTRON A Interferon alfa-2b, recombinant Powder for Injection both before and after reconstitution between 2° and 8°C (36° and 46°F).

INTRON A Interferon alfa-2b, recombinant Solution for Injection INTRON A Interferon alfa-2b, recombinant Solution for Injection, 10 million IU per 2 mL per vial; boxes containing 1 vial of INTRON A Solution for Injection (NDC 0085-0923-01).

INTRON A Interferon alfa-2b, recombinant Solution for Injection, 18 million IU multidose vial (22.8 million IU per 3.8 mL per vial); boxes containing 1 vial of INTRON A Solution for Injection (NDC 0085-0953-01).

INTRON A Interferon alfa-2b, recombinant Solution for Injection, 25 million IU per 5 mL per vial; boxes containing 1 vial of INTRON A Solution for Injection (NDC 0085-0769-01).

Store INTRON A Interferon alfa-2b, recombinant Solution for Injection between 2° and 8°C (36° and 46°F).

REFERENCES

1. Davis G, et al. *N Engl J Med.* 1989;321:1501–1506.
2. Causse X, et al. *Gastroenterology.* 1991;101:497–502.
3. Marcellin P, et al. *Hepatology.* 1991;13:393–397.
4. Knodell R, et al. *Hepatology.* 1981;1:431–435.
5. Perrillo R, et al. *N Engl J Med.* 1990;323:295–301.
6. Perez V, et al. *J Hepatol.* 1990;11:S113–S117.
7. Perrillo R, et al. *Ann Intern Med.* 1991;115:113–115.
8. Renault P, et al. *Arch Intern Med.* 1987;147:1577–1580.
9. Kauppila A, et al. *Int J Cancer.* 1982;29:291–294.

Schering Corporation
Kenilworth, NJ 07033 USA

Rev. 1/96   18766116

U.S. Patents 4,530,901 & 4,496,537

LOTRIMIN®   ℞

brand of clotrimazole
  Cream, USP 1%*
  Lotion, USP 1%*
  Topical Solution, USP 1%*
For Dermatologic Use Only—
Not For Ophthalmic Use
***These preparations are also available without a prescription as LOTRIMIN AF.**

DESCRIPTION

LOTRIMIN products contain clotrimazole, USP, a synthetic antifungal agent having the chemical name 1-(o-Chloro-α,α-diphenylbenzyl)imidazole; the empirical formula, $C_{22}H_{17}ClN_2$; a molecular weight of 344.84; and the chemical structure:

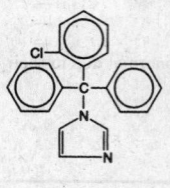

Clotrimazole is an odorless, white crystalline substance. It is practically insoluble in water, sparingly soluble in ether and very soluble in polyethylene glycol 400, ethanol, and chloroform.

Each gram of LOTRIMIN **Cream** contains 10 mg clotrimazole, USP in a vanishing cream base of benzyl alcohol, cetearyl alcohol, cetyl esters wax, octyldodecanol, polysorbate, sorbitan monostearate, and water.

Each gram of LOTRIMIN **Lotion** contains 10 mg clotrimazole, USP dispersed in an emulsion vehicle composed of benzyl alcohol, cetearyl alcohol, cetyl esters wax, octyldodecanol, polysorbate, sodium phosphate, sorbitan monostearate, and water.

Each mL of LOTRIMIN **Topical Solution** contains 10 mg clotrimazole, USP in a nonaqueous vehicle of PEG.

CLINICAL PHARMACOLOGY

Clotrimazole is a broad-spectrum antifungal agent that is used for the treatment of dermal infections caused by various species of pathogenic dermatophytes, yeasts, and *Malassezia furfur*. The primary action of clotrimazole is against dividing and growing organisms.

In vitro, clotrimazole exhibits fungistatic and fungicidal activity against isolates of *Trichophyton rubrum, Trichophyton mentagrophytes, Epidermophyton floccosum, Microsporum canis,* and *Candida* species, including *Candida albicans.* In general, the *in vitro* activity of clotrimazole corresponds to that of tolnaftate and griseofulvin against the mycelia of dermatophytes (*Trichophyton, Microsporum,* and *Epidermophyton*), and to that of the polyenes (amphotericin B and nystatin) against budding fungi (*Candida*). Using an *in vivo* (mouse) and an *in vitro* (mouse kidney homogenate) testing system, clotrimazole and miconazole were equally effective in preventing the growth of the pseudomycelia and mycelia of *Candida albicans.*

Strains of fungi having a natural resistance to clotrimazole are rare. Only a single isolate of *Candida guilliermondi* has been reported to have primary resistance to clotrimazole. No single-step or multiple-step resistance to clotrimazole has developed during successive passages of *Candida albicans* and *Trichophyton mentagrophytes.* No appreciable change in sensitivity was detected after successive passages of isolates of *C. albicans, C. krusei,* or *C. pseudotropicalis* in liquid or solid media containing clotrimazole. Also, resistance could not be developed in chemically induced mutant strains of polyene-resistant isolates of *C. albicans.* Slight, reversible resistance was noted in three isolates of *C. albicans* tested by one investigator. There is a single report that records the clinical emergence of a *C. albicans* strain with considerable resistance to flucytosine and miconazole, and with cross-resistance to clotrimazole; the strain remained sensitive to nystatin and amphotericin B.

In studies of the mechanism of action, the minimum fungicidal concentration of clotrimazole caused leakage of intracellular phosphorus compounds into the ambient medium with concomitant breakdown of cellular nucleic acids and accelerated potassium efflux. Both these events began rapidly and extensively after addition of the drug.

Clotrimazole appears to be well absorbed in humans following oral administration and is eliminated mainly as inactive metabolites. Following topical and vaginal administration, however, clotrimazole appears to be minimally absorbed. Six hours after the application of radioactive clotrimazole 1% cream and 1% solution onto intact and acutely inflamed skin, the concentration of clotrimazole varied from 100 mcg/cm³ in the stratum corneum to 0.5 to 1 mcg/cm³ in the stratum reticulare, and 0.1 mcg/cm³ in the subcutis. No measurable amount of radioactivity (≤0.001 mcg/mL) was found in the serum within 48 hours after application under occlusive dressing of 0.5 mL of the solution or 0.8 g of the cream. Only 0.5% or less of the applied radioactivity was excreted in the urine.

Following intravaginal administration of 100 mg ¹⁴C-clotrimazole vaginal tablets to nine adult females, an average peak serum level, corresponding to only 0.03 μg equivalents/mL of clotrimazole, was reached 1 to 2 days after application. After intravaginal administration of 5 g of 1% ¹⁴C-clotrimazole vaginal cream containing 50 mg active drug, to five subjects (one with candidal colpitis), serum levels corresponding to approximately 0.01 μg equivalents/mL were reached between 8 and 24 hours after application.

INDICATIONS AND USAGE

Prescription LOTRIMIN (clotrimazole cream, lotion, and solution 1%) products are indicated for the topical treatment of candidiasis due to *Candida albicans* and tinea versicolor due to *Malassezia furfur.*

These formulations are also available as the LOTRIMIN AF (clotrimazole cream, lotion, and solution 1%) line of nonprescription products which are indicated for the topical treatment of the following dermal infections: tinea pedis, tinea cruris, and tinea corporis due to *Trichophyton rubrum, Trichophyton mentagrophytes, Epidermophyton floccosum,* and *Microsporum canis.*

CONTRAINDICATIONS

LOTRIMIN products are contraindicated in individuals who have shown hypersensitivity to any of their components.

WARNINGS

LOTRIMIN products are not for ophthalmic use.

PRECAUTIONS

General: If irritation or sensitivity develops with the use of clotrimazole, treatment should be discontinued and appropriate therapy instituted.

Information For Patients: This information is intended to aid in the safe and effective use of this medication. It is not a disclosure of all possible adverse or intended effects.
The patient should be advised to:
1. Use the medication for the full treatment time even though the symptoms may have improved. Notify the physician if there is no improvement after 4 weeks of treatment.
2. Inform the physician if the area of application shows signs of increased irritation (redness, itching, burning, blistering, swelling, oozing) indicative of possible sensitization.
3. Avoid sources of infection or reinfection.

Laboratory Tests: If there is lack of response to clotrimazole, appropriate microbiological studies should be repeated to confirm the diagnosis and rule out other pathogens before instituting another course of antimycotic therapy.

Drug Interactions: Synergism or antagonism between clotrimazole and nystatin, or amphotericin B, or flucytosine against strains of *C. albicans* has not been reported.

Carcinogenesis, Mutagenesis, Impairment of Fertility: An 18-month oral dosing study with clotrimazole in rats has not revealed any carcinogenic effect.
In tests for mutagenesis, chromosomes of the spermatophores of Chinese hamsters which had been exposed to clotrimazole were examined for structural changes during the metaphase. Prior to testing, the hamsters had received five oral clotrimazole doses of 100 mg/kg body weight. The results of this study showed that clotrimazole had no mutagenic effect.

Usage in Pregnancy: Pregnancy Category B: The disposition of ¹⁴C-clotrimazole has been studied in humans and animals. Clotrimazole is very poorly absorbed following dermal application or intravaginal administration to humans. (See **CLINICAL PHARMACOLOGY**.)
In clinical trials, use of vaginally applied clotrimazole in pregnant women in their second and third trimesters has not been associated with ill effects. There are, however, no adequate and well-controlled studies in pregnant women during the first trimester of pregnancy.
Studies in pregnant rats with intravaginal doses up to 100 mg/kg have revealed no evidence of harm to the fetus due to clotrimazole.
High oral doses of clotrimazole in rats and mice ranging from 50 to 120 mg/kg resulted in embryotoxicity (possibly secondary to maternal toxicity), impairment of mating, decreased litter size and number of viable young and decreased pup survival to weaning. However, clotrimazole was not teratogenic in mice, rabbits, and rats at oral doses up to 200, 180,

and 100 mg/kg, respectively. Oral absorption in the rat amounts to approximately 90% of the administered dose.
Because animal reproduction studies are not always predictive of human response, this drug should be used only if clearly indicated during the first trimester of pregnancy.

Nursing Mothers: It is not known whether this drug is excreted in human milk. Because many drugs are excreted in human milk, caution should be exercised when clotrimazole is used by a nursing woman.

Pediatric Use: Safety and effectiveness in children have been established for clotrimazole when used as indicated and in the recommended dosage.

ADVERSE REACTIONS

The following adverse reactions have been reported in connection with the use of clotrimazole: erythema, stinging, blistering, peeling, edema, pruritus, urticaria, burning, and general irritation of the skin.

OVERDOSAGE

Acute overdosage with topical application of clotrimazole is unlikely and would not be expected to lead to a life-threatening situation.

DOSAGE AND ADMINISTRATION

Gently massage sufficient LOTRIMIN into the affected and surrounding skin areas twice a day, in the morning and evening.
Clinical improvement, with relief of pruritus, usually occurs within the first week of treatment with LOTRIMIN. If the patient shows no clinical improvement after 4 weeks of treatment with LOTRIMIN, the diagnosis should be reviewed.

HOW SUPPLIED

LOTRIMIN Cream 1% is supplied in 15, 30, 45, and 90-g tubes (NDC 0085-0613-02, 05, 04, 03, respectively); boxes of one.
Store between 2° and 30°C (36° and 86°F).
LOTRIMIN Lotion 1% is supplied in 30-mL bottles (NDC 0085-0707-02); boxes of one.
Store between 2° and 25°C (36° and 77°F).
Shake well before using.
LOTRIMIN Topical Solution 1% is supplied in 10-mL and 30-mL plastic bottles (NDC 0085-0182-02, 04, respectively); boxes of one.
Store between 2° and 30°C (36° and 86°F).
Rev. 11/93
Copyright © 1984, 1991, 1993, 1994,
Schering Corporation.
All rights reserved.
17981005

LOTRISONE®

℞

brand of clotrimazole and betamethasone dipropionate Cream, USP

**For Dermatologic Use Only—
Not for Ophthalmic Use**

DESCRIPTION

LOTRISONE Cream contains a combination of clotrimazole, USP, a synthetic antifungal agent, and betamethasone dipropionate, USP, a synthetic corticosteroid, for dermatologic use.
Chemically, clotrimazole is 1-(*o*-Chloro-*α*,*α*-diphenyl-benzyl) imidazole, with the empirical formula $C_{22}H_{17}ClN_2$, a molecular weight of 344.8, and the following structural formula:

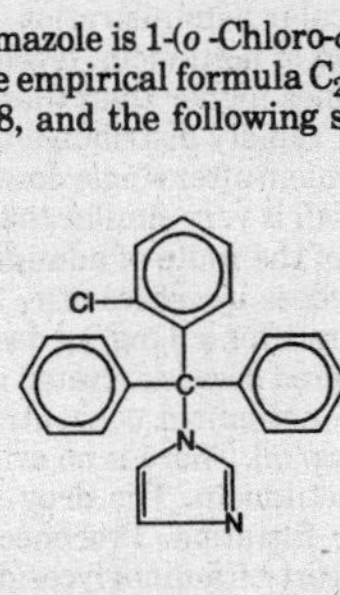

Clotrimazole is an odorless, white crystalline powder, insoluble in water and soluble in ethanol.
Betamethasone dipropionate has the chemical name 9-Fluoro-11*β*, 17,21-trihydroxy-16*β*-methylpregna-1,4-diene-3, 20-dione 17,21-dipropionate, with the empirical formula $C_{28}H_{37}FO_7$, a molecular weight of 504.6, and the following structural formula:
[See chemical structure at top of next column.]
Betamethasone dipropionate is a white to creamy white, odorless crystalline powder, insoluble in water.
Each gram of LOTRISONE Cream contains 10.0 mg clotrimazole, USP, and 0.64 mg betamethasone dipropionate, USP (equivalent to 0.5 mg betamethasone), in a hydrophilic emollient cream consisting of purified water, mineral oil, white petrolatum, cetearyl alcohol, ceteareth-30, propylene

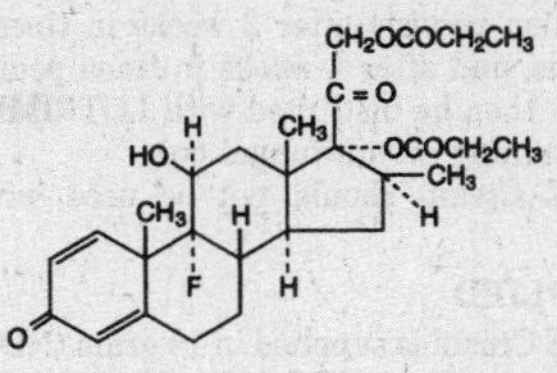

glycol, sodium phosphate monobasic, and phosphoric acid; benzyl alcohol as preservative.
LOTRISONE is a smooth, uniform, white to off-white cream.

CLINICAL PHARMACOLOGY

Clotrimazole

Clotrimazole is a broad-spectrum, antifungal agent that is used for the treatment of dermal infections caused by various species of pathogenic dermatophytes, yeasts, and *Malassezia furfur*. The primary action of clotrimazole is against dividing and growing organisms.
In vitro, clotrimazole exhibits fungistatic and fungicidal activity against isolates of *Trichophyton rubrum*, *Trichophyton mentagrophytes*, *Epidermophyton floccosum*, and *Microsporum canis*. In general, the *in vitro* activity of clotrimazole corresponds to that of tolnaftate and griseofulvin against the mycelia of dermatophytes (*Trichophyton*, *Microsporum*, and *Epidermophyton*).
In vivo studies in guinea pigs infected with *Trichophyton mentagrophytes* have shown no measurable loss of clotrimazole activity due to combination with betamethasone dipropionate.
Strains of fungi having a natural resistance to clotrimazole have not been reported.
No single-step or multiple-step resistance to clotrimazole has developed during successive passages of *Trichophyton mentagrophytes*.
In studies of the mechanism of action in fungal cultures, the minimum fungicidal concentration of clotrimazole caused leakage of intracellular phosphorous compounds into the ambient medium with concomitant breakdown of cellular nucleic acids, and accelerated potassium efflux. Both of these events began rapidly and extensively after addition of the drug to the cultures.
Clotrimazole appears to be minimally absorbed following topical application to the skin. Six hours after the application of radioactive clotrimazole 1% cream and 1% solution onto intact and acutely inflamed skin, the concentration of clotrimazole varied from 100 mcg/cm^3 in the stratum corneum, to 0.5 to 1 mcg/cm^3 in the stratum reticulare, and 0.1 mcg/cm^3 in the subcutis. No measureable amount of radioactivity (< 0.001 mcg/mL) was found in the serum within 48 hours after application under occlusive dressing of 0.5 mL of the solution or 0.8 g of the cream.

Betamethasone dipropionate

Betamethasone dipropionate, a corticosteroid, is effective in the treatment of corticosteroid-responsive dermatoses primarily because of its anti-inflammatory, anti-pruritic, and vasoconstrictive actions. However, while the physiologic, pharmacologic, and clinical effects of corticosteroids are well known, the exact mechanisms of their actions in each disease are uncertain. Betamethasone dipropionate, a corticosteroid, has been shown to have topical (dermatologic) and systemic pharmacologic and metabolic effects characteristic of this class of drugs.

Pharmacokinetics: The extent of percutaneous absorption of topical corticosteroids is determined by many factors including the vehicle, the integrity of the epidermal barrier, and the use of occlusive dressings. (See **DOSAGE AND ADMINISTRATION** section.)
Topical corticosteroids can be absorbed from normal intact skin. Inflammation and/or other disease processes in the skin increase percutaneous absorption. Occlusive dressings substantially increase the percutaneous absorption of topical corticosteroids. (See **DOSAGE AND ADMINISTRATION** section.)
Once absorbed through the skin, topical corticosteroids are handled through pharmacokinetic pathways similar to systemically administered corticosteroids. Corticosteroids are bound to plasma proteins in varying degrees. Corticosteroids are metabolized primarily in the liver and are then excreted by the kidneys. Some of the topical corticosteroids and their metabolites are also excreted into the bile.

Clotrimazole and betamethasone dipropionate

In clinical studies of tinea corporis, tinea cruris, and tinea pedis, patients treated with LOTRISONE Cream showed a better clinical response at the first return visit than patients treated with clotrimazole cream. In tinea corporis and tinea cruris, the patient returned three days after starting treatment, and in tinea pedis, after one week. Mycological cure rates observed in patients treated with LOTRISONE Cream were as good as or better than in those patients treated with clotrimazole cream.
In these same clinical studies, patients treated with LOTRISONE Cream showed statistically significantly better clinical responses and mycological cure rates when compared with patients treated with betamethasone dipropionate cream.

INDICATIONS AND USAGE

LOTRISONE Cream is indicated for the topical treatment of the following dermal infections: tinea pedis, tinea cruris, and tinea corporis due to *Trichophyton rubrum*, *Trichophyton mentagrophytes*, *Epidermophyton floccosum*, and *Microsporum canis*.

CONTRAINDICATIONS

LOTRISONE Cream is contraindicated in patients who are sensitive to clotrimazole, betamethasone dipropionate, other corticosteroids or imidazoles, or to any ingredient in this preparation.

PRECAUTIONS

General: Systemic absorption of topical corticosteroids has produced reversible hypothalamic-pituitary-adrenal (HPA) axis suppression, manifestations of Cushing's syndrome, hyperglycemia, and glucosuria in some patients.
Conditions which augment systemic absorption include the application of the more potent steroids, use over large surface areas, prolonged use, and the addition of occlusive dressings. (See **DOSAGE AND ADMINISTRATION** section.)
Therefore, patients receiving a large dose of a potent topical steroid applied to a large surface area should be evaluated periodically for evidence of HPA axis suppression by using the urinary free cortisol and ACTH stimulation tests. If HPA axis suppression is noted, an attempt should be made to withdraw the drug, to reduce the frequency of application, or to substitute a less potent steroid.
Recovery of HPA axis function is generally prompt and complete upon discontinuation of the drug. Infrequently, signs and symptoms of steroid withdrawal may occur, requiring supplemental systemic corticosteroids.
Children may absorb proportionally larger amounts of topical corticosteroids and thus be more susceptible to systemic toxicity. (See **PRECAUTIONS-Pediatric Use.**)
If irritation or hypersensitivity develops with the use of LOTRISONE Cream, treatment should be discontinued and appropriate therapy instituted.

Information for Patients: Patients using LOTRISONE Cream should receive the following information and instructions:

1. This medication is to be used as directed by the physician. It is for external use only. Avoid contact with the eyes.
2. The medication is to be used for the full prescribed treatment time, even though the symptoms may have improved. Notify the physician if there is no improvement after 1 week of treatment for tinea cruris or tinea corporis, or after 2 weeks for tinea pedis.
3. Patients should be advised not to use this medication for any disorder other than for which it was prescribed.
4. The treated skin areas should not be bandaged or otherwise covered or wrapped as to be occluded. (See **DOSAGE AND ADMINISTRATION** section.)
5. When using this medication in the groin area, patients should be advised to use the medication for 2 weeks only, and to apply the cream sparingly. The physician should be notified if the condition persists after 2 weeks. Patients should also be advised to wear loose fitting clothing. (See **DOSAGE AND ADMINISTRATION** section.)
6. Patients should report any signs of local adverse reactions.
7. Patients should avoid sources of infection or reinfection.

Laboratory Tests: If there is a lack of response to LOTRISONE Cream, appropriate microbiological studies should be repeated to confirm the diagnosis and rule out other pathogens before instituting another course of antimycotic therapy.
The following tests may be helpful in evaluating HPA axis suppression due to the corticosteroid component:
Urinary free cortisol test
ACTH stimulation test

Carcinogenesis, Mutagenesis, Impairment of Fertility: There are no animal or laboratory studies with the combination clotrimazole and betamethasone dipropionate to evaluate carcinogenesis, mutagenesis, or impairment of fertility.
An 18-month oral dosing study with clotrimazole in rats has not revealed any carcinogenic effect.
In tests for mutagenesis, chromosomes of the spermatophores of Chinese hamsters which had been exposed to clotrimazole were examined for structural changes during the metaphase. Prior to testing, the hamsters had received five <u>oral</u> clotrimazole doses of 100 mg/kg body weight. The results of this study showed that clotrimazole had no mutagenic effect.

Continued on next page

Information on Schering products appearing on these pages is effective as of August 15, 1996.

Schering—Cont.

Pregnancy Category C: There have been no teratogenic studies performed with the combination clotrimazole and betamethasone dipropionate.

Studies in pregnant rats with <u>intravaginal</u> doses up to 100 mg/kg have revealed no evidence of harm to the fetus due to clotrimazole.

High <u>oral</u> doses of clotrimazole in rats and mice ranging from 50 to 120 mg/kg resulted in embryotoxicity (possibly secondary to maternal toxicity), impairment of mating, decreased litter size and number of viable young and decreased pup survival to weaning. However, clotrimazole was <u>not</u> teratogenic in mice, rabbits, and rats at oral doses up to 200, 180, and 100 mg/kg, respectively. Oral absorption in the rat amounts to approximately 90% of the administered dose. Corticosteroids are generally teratogenic in laboratory animals when administered systemically at relatively low dosage levels. The more potent corticosteroids have been shown to be teratogenic after dermal application in laboratory animals.

There are no adequate and well-controlled studies in pregnant women on teratogenic effects from a topically applied combination of clotrimazole and betamethasone dipropionate. Therefore, LOTRISONE Cream should be used during pregnancy only if the potential benefit justifies the potential risk to the fetus.

Drugs containing corticosteroids should not be used extensively on pregnant patients, in large amounts, or for prolonged periods of time.

Nursing Mothers: It is not known whether this drug is excreted in human milk. Because many drugs are excreted in human milk, caution should be exercised when LOTRISONE Cream is used by a nursing woman.

Pediatric Use: Safety and effectiveness in children below the age of 12 have not been established with LOTRISONE Cream.

<u>Pediatric patients may demonstrate greater susceptibility to topical corticosteroid-induced HPA axis suppression and Cushing's syndrome than mature patients because of a larger skin surface area to body weight ratio.</u>

Hypothalamic-pituitary-adrenal (HPA) axis suppression, Cushing's syndrome, and intracranial hypertension have been reported in children receiving topical corticosteroids. Manifestations of adrenal suppression in children include linear growth retardation, delayed weight gain, low plasma cortisol levels, and absence of response to ACTH stimulation. Manifestations of intracranial hypertension include bulging fontanelles, headaches, and bilateral papilledema.

Administration of topical dermatologics containing a corticosteroid to children should be limited to the least amount compatible with an effective therapeutic regimen. Chronic corticosteroid therapy may interfere with the growth and development of children.

The use of LOTRISONE Cream in diaper dermatitis is not recommended.

ADVERSE REACTIONS

The following adverse reactions have been reported in connection with the use of LOTRISONE Cream: paresthesia in 5 of 270 patients, maculopapular rash, edema, and secondary infection, each in 1 of 270 patients.

Adverse reactions reported with the use of clotrimazole are as follows: erythema, stinging, blistering, peeling, edema, pruritus, urticaria, and general irritation of the skin.

The following local adverse reactions are reported infrequently when topical corticosteroids are used as recommended. These reactions are listed in an approximate decreasing order of occurrence: burning, itching, irritation, dryness, folliculitis, hypertrichosis, acneiform eruptions, hypopigmentation, perioral dermatitis, allergic contact dermatitis, maceration of the skin, secondary infection, skin atrophy, striae, and miliaria.

OVERDOSAGE

Acute overdosage with topical application of LOTRISONE Cream is unlikely and would not be expected to lead to a life-threatening situation.

Topically applied corticosteroids can be absorbed in sufficient amounts to produce systemic effects. (See **PRECAUTIONS.**)

DOSAGE AND ADMINISTRATION

Gently massage sufficient LOTRISONE Cream into the affected and surrounding skin areas twice a day, in the morning and evening, for 2 weeks in tinea cruris and tinea corporis and for 4 weeks in tinea pedis. The use of LOTRISONE Cream for longer than 4 weeks is not recommended.

Clinical improvement, with relief of erythema and pruritus, usually occurs within 3 to 5 days of treatment. If a patient with tinea cruris or tinea corporis shows no clinical improvement after 1 week of treatment with LOTRISONE Cream, the diagnosis should be reviewed. In tinea pedis, the treatment should be applied for 2 weeks prior to making that decision.

Treatment with LOTRISONE Cream should be discontinued if the condition persists after 2 weeks in tinea cruris and tinea corporis, and after 4 weeks in tinea pedis. Alternate therapy may then be instituted with LOTRIMIN Cream, a product containing an antifungal only.

LOTRISONE Cream should <u>not</u> be used with occlusive dressings.

HOW SUPPLIED

LOTRISONE Cream is supplied in 15-gram (NDC 0085-0924-01), and 45-gram tubes (NDC 0085-0924-02); boxes of one.

Store between 2° and 30°C (36° and 86°F).

Rev. 1/94   17969609

NETROMYCIN®   ℞
brand of netilmicin sulfate
Injection, USP 100 mg/ml

WARNINGS

Patients treated with aminoglycosides should be under close clinical observation because of the potential toxicity associated with the use of these drugs.

Netilmicin has potent neuromuscular blocking potential. Neuromuscular blockade and respiratory paralysis have been reported in animals receiving netilmicin. The possibility of these phenomena occurring in man should be considered if aminoglycosides are administered by any route to patients receiving neuromuscular blocking agents, such as succinylcholine, tubocurarine, or decamethonium, or to patients receiving massive transfusions of citrate-anticoagulated blood. If neuromuscular blockade occurs, calcium salts may lessen it, but mechanical respiratory assistance may also be necessary.

As with other aminoglycosides, netilmicin sulfate injection is potentially nephrotoxic. The risk is greater in patients with impaired renal function, in those who receive high dosage or prolonged therapy, and in the elderly.

Neurotoxicity manifested by ototoxicity, both vestibular and auditory, can occur in patients treated with netilmicin, primarily in those with preexisting renal damage and in patients treated with higher doses and/or for longer periods than recommended. Aminoglycoside-induced ototoxicity is usually irreversible. Other manifestations of aminoglycoside-induced neurotoxicity include numbness, skin tingling, muscle twitching, and convulsions.

Renal and eighth cranial nerve functions should be closely monitored, especially in patients with known or suspected impairment of renal function either at onset of therapy or during therapy. Urine should be examined for increased excretion of protein, the presence of cells or casts, and decreased specific gravity. Serum creatinine concentration or blood urea nitrogen should be determined periodically. A more precise measure of glomerular filtration rate is a carefully conducted determination of creatinine clearance rate or, often more practically, an estimate of creatinine clearance based on published nomograms or equations. (See **DOSAGE AND ADMINISTRATION**.) When feasible it is recommended that serial audiograms be obtained in patients old enough to be tested, particularly in high-risk patients. The dosage of netilmicin should be reduced or administration discontinued if evidence of drug-induced auditory or vestibular toxicity (dizziness, vertigo, tinnitus, nystagmus, or hearing loss) develops during therapy. If evidence of nephrotoxicity occurs, dosage should be adjusted. (See **DOSAGE AND ADMINISTRATION, DOSAGE FOR IMPAIRED RENAL FUNCTION.**) As with the other aminoglycosides, on rare occasions changes in renal and eighth cranial nerve functions may not become manifest until soon after completion of therapy.

Serum concentrations of aminoglycosides should be monitored when feasible to assure adequate levels and to avoid potentially toxic levels. After administration of an appropriate dose of netilmicin, peak serum concentrations occur approximately 30 to 60 minutes after an intramuscular injection or at the end of a one hour intravenous infusion. Dosage should be adjusted so that prolonged peak serum concentrations above 16 mcg/ml are avoided.

When monitoring trough concentrations, dosage should be adjusted so that levels above 4 mcg/ml are avoided. Excessive peak and/or trough serum concentrations of aminoglycosides may increase the risk of renal and eighth cranial nerve toxicity. In the event of overdose or toxic reactions, hemodialysis may aid in removal of netilmicin from the blood, especially if renal function is, or becomes, compromised. Removal of netilmicin by

peritoneal dialysis is at a rate considerably less than by hemodialysis.

Concurrent and/or sequential systemic or topical use of other potentially neurotoxic and/or nephrotoxic drugs, such as: cephaloridine, amphotericin B, streptomycin, kanamycin, acyclovir, gentamicin, tobramycin, amikacin, neomycin, vancomycin, bacitracin, polymixin B, colistin, paromomycin, viomycin, or cisplatin should be avoided. The concurrent use of aminoglycosides with potent diuretics, such as ethacrynic acid or furosemide, should be avoided since certain diuretics by themselves may cause ototoxicity. In addition, when administered intravenously, diuretics may enhance aminoglycoside toxicity by altering the antibiotic concentration in the serum and tissues. Other factors which may increase patient risk of toxicity are advanced age and dehydration.

DESCRIPTION

NETROMYCIN Injection contains netilmicin sulfate, USP in clear, sterile aqueous solution with a pH range of 3.5 to 6.0 for intramuscular or intravenous administration. Netilmicin is a semisynthetic, water-soluble antibiotic of the aminoglycoside group, derived from sisomicin. Its chemical name is: O-3-Deoxy-4-C-methyl-3-(methylamino)-β-L-arabinopyranosyl(1→4)-O-[2,6-diamino-2,3,4,6-tetradeoxy-α-D-$glycero$-hex-4-enopyranosyl-(1→6)]-2-deoxy-N^3-ethyl-L-streptamine sulfate (2:5) (salt), having the following structural formula:

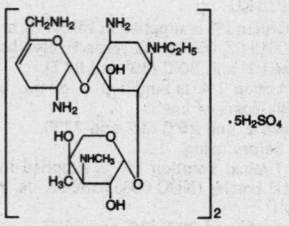

Each ml of NETROMYCIN Injection contains netilmicin sulfate, USP equivalent to 100 mg netilmicin; 10 mg benzyl alcohol as a preservative; 0.1 mg edetate disodium; 2.4 mg sodium metabisulfite; 0.8 mg sodium sulfite; and water for injection, q.s.

CLINICAL PHARMACOLOGY

Netilmicin is rapidly and completely absorbed after intramuscular injection. Peak serum levels, after intramuscular injection, usually occur within 30 to 60 minutes and levels are measurable for 12 hours. In adult volunteers with normal renal function, peak serum concentrations of netilmicin in mcg/ml are usually about 3 to 3.5 times the single intramuscular dose in mg/kg. For example, a dose of 2.0 mg/kg may be expected to result in a peak serum concentration of approximately 7 mcg/ml. At eight or more hours after administration of a dose in the recommended range, serum levels are usually less than 3 mcg/ml. When a single dose of netilmicin is administered by 60-minute intravenous infusion, the peak serum concentrations are similar to those obtained by intramuscular administration. Following a rapid intravenous injection of netilmicin, levels in serum may be transiently 2 to 3 times higher than those of the 60-minute infusion. Netilmicin rapidly distributes to tissues.

The half-life of netilmicin after single doses is usually 2 to 2.5 hours, a half-life which is very similar to that of gentamicin, and is independent of the route of administration. The half-life increases as the dose increases (e.g., 2.2 hours after a 1 mg/kg dose to 3 hours after a 3 mg/kg dose). Approximately 80% of the administered dose is excreted in the urine within 24 hours; the urine netilmicin concentration after a dose often exceeds 100 mcg/ml. There is no evidence of metabolic transformation of netilmicin. The drug is excreted principally by glomerular filtration. Probenecid does not affect renal tubular transport of aminoglycosides. The volume of distribution of netilmicin is approximately 20% of body weight; total body clearance is about 80 ml/min and renal clearance is about 60 ml/min. In multiple-dose studies in volunteers when the drug was administered every 12 hours at doses ranging from 1.0 to 4.0 mg/kg, steady-state levels were obtained by the second day.

The serum levels at steady-state were less than 20% higher than those of the first dose. As with other aminoglycosides, the half-life of netilmicin increases, and its renal clearance decreases with decreasing renal function.

The endogenous creatinine clearance rate and the serum creatinine level have a high correlation with the half-life of netilmicin. Results of these tests can serve as a guide for adjusting dosage in patients with renal impairment.

In patients with marked impairment of renal function, there is a decrease in the concentration of aminoglycosides in

urine and in their penetration into defective renal parenchyma. This should be considered when treating patients with urinary tract infections. In one study of adults with renal failure undergoing hemodialysis, netilmicin serum levels were reduced by approximately 63% over an 8-hour dialysis session. Shorter dialysis sessions will remove less drug. No hemodialysis information is available for children. Aminoglycosides are also removed by peritoneal dialysis but at a rate considerably less than by hemodialysis.

Since netilmicin is distributed in extracellular fluid, peak serum concentrations may be lower than usual in patients whose extracellular fluid volume is expanded (e.g., patients with edema or ascites). Serum concentrations of aminoglycosides in febrile patients may be lower than those in afebrile patients given the same dose. When body temperature returns to normal, serum concentrations of the drug may rise. Both febrile and anemic states may be associated with a shorter than usual half-life. (Dosage adjustment is usually not necessary.)

In severely burned patients, the half-life of aminoglycosides may be significantly decreased, and serum concentrations resulting from a particular dose may be lower than anticipated.

The elimination half-life of netilmicin in neonates during the first week of life is inversely correlated with body weight, ranging from approximately 8 hours for neonates weighing 1.5 to 2.0 kg to approximately 4.5 hours for 3.0 to 4.0 kg neonates. The elimination half-life of infants and children 6 weeks of age and older is 1.5 to 2.0 hours.

Following parenteral administration, aminoglycosides can be detected in serum, tissues, and sputum and in pericardial, pleural, synovial, and peritoneal fluids. A variety of methods are available to measure netilmicin concentrations in body fluids; these include microbiologic, enzymatic, and radioimmunoassay techniques. Concentrations in renal cortex may be markedly higher than the usual serum levels.

Minute quantities of aminoglycosides have been detected in the urine for up to 30 days after discontinuing administration. Hepatic secretion is minimal. As with all aminoglycosides, netilmicin diffuses poorly into the subarachnoid space after parenteral administration. Concentrations of netilmicin in cerebrospinal fluid are often low and dependent upon dose and the degree of meningeal inflammation. Netilmicin crosses the placenta and has been detected in cord blood and in the fetus. Studies in nursing mothers indicate that small amounts of the drug are excreted in breast milk. Netilmicin is poorly absorbed from the intact gastrointestinal tract after oral administration. As with other aminoglycosides, the binding of netilmicin to serum proteins is low (0–30%).

Microbiology: Netilmicin is a rapidly acting, broad-spectrum bactericidal antibiotic which appears to act by inhibiting normal protein synthesis in susceptible microorganisms. Netilmicin is active *in vitro* against a wide variety of pathogenic bacteria, primarily gram-negative bacilli and also a few gram-positive organisms including *Citrobacter, Enterobacter, Escherichia coli, Klebsiella* species, *Proteus mirabilis, Pseudomonas aeruginosa, Salmonella* species, *Shigella* species, and *Staphylococcus* species (penicillin- and methicillin-resistant strains).

Netilmicin is also active *in vitro* against some isolates of *Acinetobacter* and *Neisseria* species, indole-positive *Proteus* species, *Pseudomonas* and *Serratia* species. In addition, netilmicin is active *in vitro* against many strains which have acquired resistance to other aminoglycosides. Such resistance is usually caused by aminoglycoside modifying (inactivating) enzymes. In general, netilmicin is active against organisms which inactivate aminoglycosides by either phosphorylation or adenylylation; it has variable activity against acetylating strains, depending on the specific type. For example, the susceptibility of *Serratia* species producing a combination of adenylylating and acetylating enzymes varies according to the level of acetylating enzyme present. Netilmicin is active *in vitro* against certain strains of gram-negative bacteria resistant to gentamicin and tobramycin: *Citrobacter, Enterobacter* species, *Escherichia coli, Klebsiella, Proteus* (indole-positive), *Pseudomonas, Salmonella,* and *Shigella* species. Netilmicin is active *in vitro* against certain staphylococci resistant to amikacin and tobramycin. Like other aminoglycosides, netilmicin is not active against bacteria with reduced permeability to this class of antibiotics.

Most species of streptococci and anaerobic organisms, such as *Bacteroides* and *Clostridium* species, are resistant to aminoglycosides.

The *in vitro* activity of netilmicin and of other aminoglycosides is affected by media pH, protein content, divalent cation concentration, and inoculum size.

Netilmicin acts synergistically *in vitro* with members of the penicillin class of antibiotics against *Streptococcus faecalis.* It also acts synergistically with those penicillins which are active alone against many strains of *Pseudomonas.* In addition, many, but not all isolates of *Serratia* which are resistant to multiple antibiotics, are inhibited by synergistic combinations of netilmicin with carbenicillin, azlocillin, mezlocillin, cefamandole, cefotaxime, or moxalactam. Tests for antibiotic synergy are necessary.

Susceptibility Testing: Quantitative methods that require measurements of zone diameters give the most precise estimates of antibiotic susceptibility. One such procedure has been recommended for use with discs to test susceptibility to netilmicin. Interpretation involves correlation of the diameters obtained in the disc test with minimal inhibitory concentration (MIC) values for netilmicin.

Reports from the laboratory giving results of the standardized single disc susceptibility test (Bauer, et al. Am J Clin Path 1966; 45:493 and Federal Register 37:20525–20529, 1972), using a 30 mcg netilmicin disc should be interpreted according to the following criteria:

Organisms producing zones of 15 mm or greater, or MIC's of 8.0 mcg or less are considered susceptible, indicating that the tested organism is likely to respond to therapy.

Resistant organisms produce zones of 12 mm or less or MIC's of 16 mcg or greater. A report of "resistant" from the laboratory indicates that the infecting organism is not likely to respond to therapy.

Zones greater than 12 mm and less than 15 mm, or MIC's of greater than 8.0 mcg and less than 16 mcg, indicate intermediate susceptibility. A report of "intermediate" susceptibility suggests that the organism would be susceptible if the infection is confined to tissues and fluids (e.g., urine), in which high antibiotic levels are attained.

Control organisms are recommended for susceptibility testing. Each time the test is performed one or more of the following organisms should be included: *Escherichia coli* ATCC 25922, *Staphylococcus aureus* ATCC 25923, and *Pseudomonas aeruginosa* ATCC 27853. The control organisms should produce zones of inhibition within the following ranges:

Escherichia coli (ATCC 25922) 22–30 mm
Staphylococcus aureus (ATCC 25923) 22–31 mm
Pseudomonas aeruginosa (ATCC 27853) 17–23 mm

In certain circumstances, particularly with strains of *Pseudomonas aeruginosa,* it may be desirable to do additional susceptibility testing by the tube or agar dilution method. Netilmicin sulfate powder, a diagnostic reagent, is available for this purpose.

The MIC values of netilmicin for the control strains are the following:

Escherichia coli (ATCC 25922) 0.25–0.5 mcg/ml
Staphylococcus aureus (ATCC 25923) 0.125–0.25 mcg/ml
Pseudomonas aeruginosa (ATCC 27853) 4–8 mcg/ml in media supplemented with calcium and magnesium.

INDICATIONS AND USAGE

Netilmicin sulfate injection is indicated for the short-term treatment of patients of all ages, including neonates, infants, and children with serious or life-threatening bacterial infections caused by susceptible strains of the designated microorganisms in the diseases listed below:

COMPLICATED URINARY TRACT infections caused by *Escherichia coli, Klebsiella pneumoniae, Pseudomonas aeruginosa, Enterobacter* species, *Proteus mirabilis, Proteus* species (indole-positive), *Serratia** and *Citrobacter* species, and *Staphylococcus aureus.***

SEPTICEMIA caused by *Escherichia coli, Klebsiella pneumoniae, Pseudomonas aeruginosa, Enterobacter* and *Serratia** species, and *Proteus mirabilis.*

SKIN AND SKIN STRUCTURE infections caused by *Escherichia coli, Klebsiella pneumoniae, Pseudomonas aeruginosa, Enterobacter* and *Serratia** species. *Proteus mirabilis, Proteus* species (indole-positive), and *Staphylococcus aureus*** (pencillinase- and non-penicillinase-producing strains).

INTRA-ABDOMINAL infections including peritonitis and intra-abdominal abscess caused by *Escherichia coli, Klebsiella pneumoniae, Pseudomonas aeruginosa, Enterobacter* species, *Proteus mirabilis, Proteus* species (indole-positive), and *Staphylococcus aureus*** (penicillinase- and non-penicillinase-producing strains).

LOWER RESPIRATORY TRACT infections caused by *Escherichia coli, Klebsiella pneumoniae, Pseudomonas aeruginosa, Enterobacter* and *Serratia** species, *Proteus mirabilis, Proteus* species (indole-positive), and *Staphylococcus aureus*** (penicillinase- and non-penicillinase-producing strains).

*(See **Microbiology** Section.)

**While not the antibiotic class of first choice, aminoglycosides, including netilmicin, may be considered for the treatment of serious staphylococcal infections when penicillins or other less potentially toxic drugs are contraindicated and bacterial susceptibility tests and clinical judgment indicate their use. They may also be considered in mixed infections caused by susceptible strains of staphylococci and gram-negative organisms.

Aminoglycosides are indicated for those infections for which less potentially toxic antimicrobial agents are ineffective or contraindicated. They are not indicated in the treatment of uncomplicated initial episodes of urinary tract infection unless the causative organisms are resistant to antimicrobial agents having less potential toxicity.

Netilmicin sulfate injection may be considered as initial therapy in suspected or confirmed gram-negative infections, and therapy may be instituted before obtaining results of

susceptibility testing. The decision to continue therapy with netilmicin should be based on the results of susceptibility tests, the severity of the infection, and the important additional concepts contained in the "WARNINGS Box" above. If the causative organisms are resistant to netilmicin, other appropriate therapy should be instituted.

In serious infections when the causative organisms are unknown, netilmicin may be administered as initial therapy in conjunction with a penicillin-type or cephalosporin-type drug before obtaining results of susceptibility testing. In neonates with suspected sepsis, a penicillin-type drug is also usually indicated as concomitant therapy with netilmicin. If anaerobic organisms are suspected as etiologic agents, other suitable antimicrobial therapy should also be given. Following identification of the organism and its susceptibility, appropriate antibiotic therapy should then be continued. Netilmicin sulfate injection has been used effectively in combination with carbenicillin or ticarcillin for the treatment of life-threatening infections caused by *Pseudomonas aeruginosa.*

Clinical studies have shown that netilmicin has been effective in the treatment of serious infections caused by some organisms resistant to other aminoglycosides, *i.e.,* gentamicin, tobramycin, and/or amikacin.

Specimens for bacterial culture should be obtained to isolate and identify causative organisms and to determine their susceptibility to netilmicin.

CONTRAINDICATION

Hypersensitivity to netilmicin or to any of the ingredients of the preparation is a contraindication to its use. See **WARNINGS** if patient is hypersensitive to another aminoglycoside.

WARNINGS

(See "WARNINGS Box" above.) If the patient has a history of hypersensitivity or serious toxic reaction to another aminoglycoside, netilmicin should be used very cautiously, if at all, because cross-sensitivity to drugs in this class has been reported.

Aminoglycosides can cause fetal harm when administered to a pregnant woman. Aminoglycoside antibiotics cross the placenta and there have been several reports of total irreversible bilateral congenital deafness in children whose mothers received streptomycin during pregnancy. Although serious side effects to fetus or newborn have not been reported in the treatment of pregnant women with other aminoglycosides, the potential for harm exists. Reproduction studies of netilmicin have been performed in rats and rabbits using intramuscular and subcutaneous doses approximately 13–15 times the highest adult human dose and have revealed no evidence of impairment of fertility or harm to the fetus. Moreover, there was no evidence of ototoxicity in the offspring of rats treated subcutaneously with netilmicin throughout pregnancy and during the subsequent lactation period. It is not known whether netilmicin sulfate can cause fetal harm when administered to a pregnant woman or can affect reproduction capacity. However, if this drug is used during pregnancy, or if the patient becomes pregnant while taking this drug, the patient should be apprised of the potential hazard to the fetus.

NETROMYCIN Injection contains sodium metabisulfite and sodium sulfite, which may cause allergic-type reactions including anaphylactic symptoms and life-threatening or less severe asthmatic episodes in certain susceptible people. The overall prevalence of sulfite sensitivity in the general population is unknown and probably low. Sulfite sensitivity is seen more frequently in asthmatic than in nonasthmatic people.

PRECAUTIONS

General: Neurotoxic and nephrotoxic antibiotics may be almost completely absorbed from body surfaces (except the urinary bladder) after local irrigation and after topical application during surgical procedures. The potential toxic effects of antibiotics administered in this fashion (neuromuscular blockade, respiratory paralysis, oto- and nephrotoxicity) should be considered. (See "WARNINGS Box.")

Increased nephrotoxicity has been reported following concomitant administration of aminoglycoside antibiotics with some cephalosporins.

Aminoglycosides should be used with caution in patients with neuromuscular disorders, such as myasthenia gravis, or infant botulism, since these drugs may aggravate muscle weakness because of their potential curare-like effect on the neuromuscular junction.

During or following netilmicin therapy, parasthesias, tetany, positive Chvostek and Trousseau signs, and mental confusion have been described in patients with hypomagnesemia, hypocalcemia, and hypokalemia. When this has occurred in infants, tetany and muscle weakness has been de-

Continued on next page

Information on Schering products appearing on these pages is effective as of August 15, 1996.

Schering—Cont.

scribed. Both adults and infants required appropriate corrective electrolyte therapy.
Elderly patients may have reduced renal function which may not be evident in the results of routine screening tests, such as BUN or serum creatinine levels. Determination of creatinine clearance or an estimate based on published nomograms or equations may be more useful. Monitoring of renal function during treatment with netilmicin, as with other aminoglycosides, is particularly important in such patients. A Fanconi-like syndrome, with aminoaciduria and metabolic acidosis, has been reported in some adults and infants being given netilmicin injections.
Patients should be well hydrated during treatment.
Treatment with netilmicin may result in overgrowth of nonsusceptible organisms. If this occurs, appropriate therapy is indicated.
Laboratory Tests: *Tests of renal function:* Urine should be examined periodically for increased excretion of protein and the presence of cells and casts, keeping in mind the effects of the primary illness on these tests. One or more of the following laboratory measurements should be obtained at the onset of therapy, periodically during therapy, and at, or shortly after, the end of therapy:

- creatinine clearance rate (either carefully measured or estimated from published nomograms or equations based on the patient's age, sex, body weight, and serum creatinine concentration) (preferred over BUN);
- serum creatinine concentration (preferred over BUN);
- blood urea nitrogen (BUN).

More frequent testing is desirable if renal function is changing.
See also "**PRECAUTIONS, General**" above regarding elderly patients.
Test of eighth cranial nerve functions: Serial audiometric tests are suggested, particularly when renal function is impaired and/or prolonged aminoglycoside therapy is required; such tests should also be repeated periodically after treatment if there is evidence of a hearing deficit or vestibular abnormality before or during therapy, or when consecutive or concomitant use of other potentially ototoxic drugs is unavoidable.
Drug Interactions: *In vitro* mixing of an aminoglycoside with beta-lactam-type antibiotics (penicillins or cephalosporins) may result in a significant mutual inactivation. Even when an aminoglycoside and a penicillin-type drug are administered separately by different routes, a reduction in aminoglycoside serum half-life or serum levels has been reported in patients with impaired renal function and in some patients with normal renal function. Usually, such inactivation of the aminoglycoside is clinically significant only in patients with severely impaired renal function. (See also "**Drug/Laboratory Test Interactions.**") See "**WARNINGS** Box" regarding concurrent use of potent diuretics, concurrent and/or sequential use of other neurotoxic and/or nephrotoxic antibiotics, and for other essential information.
See also "**PRECAUTIONS, General.**"
Drug/Laboratory Test Interactions: Concomitant cephalosporin therapy may spuriously elevate creatinine determinations.
The inactivation between aminoglycosides and beta-lactam antibiotics described in "**Drug Interactions**" may continue in specimens of body fluids collected for assay, resulting in inaccurate, false low aminoglycoside readings. Such specimens should be properly handled, *i.e.,* assayed promptly, frozen, or treated with beta-lactamase.
Carcinogenesis, Mutagenesis, Impairment of Fertility: Lifetime carcinogenicity tests have been undertaken in the mouse and rat and no drug-related tumors were observed. Similarly, mutagenesis tests with netilmicin have proven negative, and no impairment in fertility has been observed in the rat.
Pregnancy Category D: (See **WARNINGS** Section.)
Nursing Mothers: Clinical studies in nursing mothers indicate that small amounts of netilmicin are excreted in breast milk. Because of the potential for serious adverse reactions from aminoglycosides in nursing infants, a decision should be made whether to discontinue nursing or to discontinue the drug, taking into account the importance of the drug to the mother.
Pediatric Use: Aminoglycosides should be used with caution in prematures and neonates because of the renal immaturity of these patients and the resulting prolongation of serum half-life of these drugs (also see **DOSAGE AND ADMINISTRATION** for use in Neonates and Children).

ADVERSE REACTIONS

Nephrotoxicity—Adverse renal effects due to netilmicin were reported in 7 per 100 patients.
They were demonstrated by a rise in serum creatinine and may have been accompanied by oliguria; the presence of casts, cells or protein in the urine; by rising levels of BUN; or by decreasing creatinine clearance rates. These effects occurred more frequently in the elderly, in patients with a history of renal impairment, and in patients treated for longer periods or with larger doses than recommended. While permanent impairment of renal function may occur following aminoglycoside therapy, observed renal impairment associated with netilmicin was usually mild and reversible after treatment ended while the drug was being excreted.
Neurotoxicity—Adverse effects on both the auditory and vestibular branches of the eighth cranial nerves have been reported.
Audiometric changes associated with netilmicin occurred in approximately 4 per 100 patients. Subjective netilmicin-related hearing loss occurred in about 1 per 250 patients. Vestibular abnormalities related to netilmicin were seen in 1 per 150 patients. Factors which may increase the risk of aminoglycoside-induced ototoxicity include renal impairment (especially if dialysis is required), excessive dosage, dehydration, concomitant administration of ethacrynic acid or furosemide, or previous exposure to other ototoxic drugs. Peripheral neuropathy or encephalopathy including numbness, skin tingling, muscle twitching, convulsions, and myasthenia gravis-like syndrome have been reported.
Symptoms include dizziness, vertigo, tinnitus, nystagmus, and hearing loss. Aminoglycoside-induced ototoxicity is usually irreversible. Cochlear damage is usually manifested initially by small changes in audiometric test results at the higher frequencies and may not be associated with subjective hearing loss. Vestibular dysfunction is usually manifested by nystagmus, vertigo, nausea, vomiting, or acute Meniere's syndrome.
The risk of toxic reactions is low in patients with normal renal function who do not receive netilmicin injection at higher doses or for longer periods of time than recommended. Some patients who have had previous neurotoxic reactions to other aminoglycosides have been treated with netilmicin without further neurotoxicity.
Neuromuscular blockade manifested as acute muscular paralysis and apnea can occur following treatment with aminoglycosides. (See "**WARNINGS** Box.")
The approximate incidence of other reported adverse reactions to netilmicin injection follows: increased levels of serum transaminase (SGOT or SGPT), alkaline phosphatase, or bilirubin in 15 patients per 1000; rash or itching in 4 or 5 patients per 1000; eosinophilia in 4 patients per 1000; thrombocytosis in 2 patients per 1000; prolonged prothrombin time in 1 patient per 1000; fever in 1 patient per 1000.
Fewer than one patient per 1000 was reported to have netilmicin-related anemia, leukopenia, thrombocytopenia, leukemoid reaction, immature circulating white blood cells, hyperkalemia, vomiting, diarrhea, palpitations, hypotension, headache, disorientation, blurred vision, or paresthesias.
Local tolerance to intramuscular injection and intravenous infusion of netilmicin is generally excellent, but approximately four patients per 1000 have had severe pain, and similar numbers had induration or hematomas.

OVERDOSAGE

In the event of overdosage or toxic reaction, netilmicin can be removed from the blood by hemodialysis, and is especially important if renal function is, or becomes, compromised. Although there is no specific information concerning removal of netilmicin by peritoneal dialysis, other aminoglycosides are known to be removed by this method but at a rate considerably less than by hemodialysis.

DOSAGE AND ADMINISTRATION

Netilmicin injection may be given intramuscularly or intravenously. (See **CLINICAL PHARMACOLOGY.**) The recommended dosage for both methods of administration is identical.
The patient's pretreatment body weight should be obtained for calculation of correct dosage. The dosage of aminoglycosides in obese patients should be based on an estimate of the lean body mass.
The status of renal function should be estimated by measurement of the serum creatinine concentration or calculation of the endogenous creatinine clearance rate. The blood urea nitrogen (BUN) level is much less reliable for this purpose. Reassessment of renal function should be made periodically during therapy.
In patients with extensive body surface burns, altered pharmacokinetics may result in reduced serum concentrations of aminoglycosides. Measurement of netilmicin serum concentrations is particularly important as a basis for dosage adjustment in such patients.
Duration of Treatment: It is desirable to limit the duration of treatment with aminoglycosides to short-term whenever feasible. The usual duration of treatment for all patients is seven to fourteen days. In complicated infections, a longer course of therapy may be necessary. Although prolonged courses of netilmicin injection have been well tolerated, it is particularly important that patients treated for longer than the usual period be carefully monitored for changes in renal, auditory, and vestibular functions. Dosage should be adjusted if clinically indicated.
Measurement of Serum Concentrations: It is desirable to measure both peak and trough serum concentrations of netilmicin to determine the adequacy and safety of the administered dosage.
When such measurements are feasible, they should be carried out periodically during therapy. Peak serum concentrations are expected to range from 4 to 12 mcg/ml. Dosage should be adjusted to attain the desired peak and trough concentrations and to avoid prolonged peak serum concentrations above 16 mcg/ml. When monitoring trough concentrations (just prior to the next dose), dosage should be adjusted so that levels above 4 mcg/ml are avoided. Inter-patient variation of aminoglycoside serum concentrations occurs in patients with normal or abnormal renal function. Generally, desirable peak and trough concentrations will be in the range of 6–10 and 0.5–2 mcg/ml, respectively.
Determination of the adequacy of a serum level for a particular patient must take into consideration the susceptibility of the causative organism, the severity of the infection, and the status of the patient's host-defense mechanisms.
The dosage recommendations which follow are not intended as rigid schedules, but are provided as guides for initial therapy, or for when the measurement of netilmicin serum levels during therapy is not feasible.

DOSAGE FOR PATIENTS WITH NORMAL RENAL FUNCTION

Table I shows the recommended dosage of netilmicin injection for patients of various ages with normal renal function. [See Table I at left.]
Although a causal relationship has not been established, administration of injections preserved with benzyl alcohol has been associated with toxicity in neonates. Caution should be used when NETROMYCIN Injection (100 mg/ml) is administered to neonates and children.

TABLE I
DOSAGE GUIDE FOR ADULTS WITH NORMAL RENAL FUNCTION

Patient's Weight* kg	(lb)	For Complicated Urinary Tract Infections, Give 3.0–4.0 mg/kg/day as 1.5–2.0 mg/kg — EVERY 12 HOURS mg/dose	For Serious Systemic Infections Give 4.0–6.5 mg/kg/day as 1.3–2.2 mg/kg or 2.0–3.25 mg/kg — EVERY 8 HOURS mg/dose	EVERY 12 HOURS mg/dose
40	(88)	60–80	52–88	80–130
45	(99)	68–90	59–99	90–146
50	(110)	75–100	65–110	100–163
55	(121)	83–110	72–121	110–179
60	(132)	90–120	78–132	120–195
65	(143)	98–130	85–143	130–211
70	(154)	105–140	91–154	140–228
75	(165)	113–150	98–165	150–244
80	(176)	120–160	104–176	160–260
85	(187)	128–170	111–187	170–276
90	(198)	135–180	117–198	180–293
95	(209)	143–190	124–209	190–309
100	(220)	150–200	130–220	200–325

*The dosage of aminoglycosides in obese patients should be based on an estimate of the lean body mass.

Neonates (less than 6 weeks): 4.0 to 6.5 mg/kg/day given as 2.0 to 3.25 mg/kg every 12 hours.

Infants and Children (6 weeks through 12 years): 5.5 to 8.0 mg/kg/day given either as 1.8 to 2.7 mg/kg every 8 hours, or as 2.7 to 4.0 mg/kg every 12 hours.

DOSAGE FOR PATIENTS WITH IMPAIRED RENAL FUNCTION

Dosage must be individualized in patients with impaired renal function to ensure therapeutic levels are attained. There are several methods of doing this; however, dosage adjustment based upon the measurement of serum drug concentrations during treatment is the most accurate. If netilmicin serum concentrations are not available and renal function is stable, serum creatinine and creatinine clearance values are the most reliable, readily available indicators of the degree of renal impairment for use as a guide for dosage adjustment.

It is also important to recognize that deteriorating renal function may require a greater reduction in dosage than that specified in the guidelines given below for patients with stable renal impairment.

The initial or loading dose is the same as that for a patient with normal renal function. A number of methods are available to adjust the total daily dosage for the degree of renal impairment. Three suggested methods are:

1) Divide the suggested dosage value for patients with normal renal function from Table I above by the serum creatinine level to obtain the adjusted size of each dose.

2) If the creatinine clearance rate is known or can be estimated from the serum creatinine levels using the formula given below, the adjusted daily dose of netilmicin may be determined by multiplying the dose given in Table I by:

$$\frac{\text{Patient's Creatinine Clearance Rate}}{\text{Normal Creatinine Clearance Rate}}$$

3) Alternatively, the following graph may be used to obtain the percentage of the dose selected from Table I, which should be administered at 8-hour intervals:

REDUCED DOSAGE GRAPH

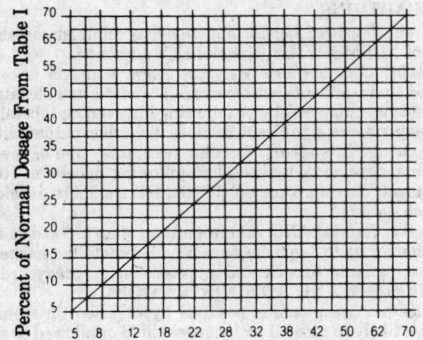

Creatinine Clearance Rate
ml/min/1.73 m²

Creatinine clearance can be estimated from serum creatinine levels by the following formula for adult males; multiply by 0.85 for adult females (Nephron, 1976; 16:31–41):

$$C_{cr} = \frac{(140 - \text{Age})(\text{Wt. Kg})}{72 \times S_{cr}(\text{mg}/100 \text{ ml})}$$

The adjusted total daily dose may be administered as one dose at 24-hour intervals, or as 2 or 3 equally divided doses at 12-hour or 8-hour intervals, respectively. Generally, each individual dose should not exceed 3.25 mg/kg. In adults with renal failure who are undergoing hemodialysis, the amount of netilmicin removed from the blood may vary depending upon the dialysis equipment and methods used. (See CLINICAL PHARMACOLOGY.) In adults, a dose of 2.0 mg/kg at the end of each dialysis period is recommended until the results of tests measuring netilmicin serum levels become available. Dosage should then be appropriately adjusted based on these tests.

ALTERNATE DOSING METHOD FOR PATIENTS WITH NORMAL OR IMPAIRED RENAL FUNCTION

An alternate method of determining a dosage regimen (dose and dosing interval) applicable to all ages and all states of renal function (both normal and abnormal) is to employ pharmacokinetic parameters derived from measurements of serum concentrations.

TABLE II
LARGE VOLUME PARENTERAL SOLUTIONS IN WHICH NETILMICIN SULFATE IS STABLE

Products/Compositions Tested	Other Trade Names and Manufacturers (Solutions of Same Composition)
Sterile Water for Injection	
0.9% Sodium Chloride Injection alone or with	
5% Dextrose	
5% or 10% Dextrose Injection in Water, or 5% Dextrose in Polysal Injection, or 5% Dextrose with Electrolyte #48 or #75	
Ringer's and Lactated Ringer's, and Lactated Ringer's with 5% Dextrose Injection	
10% Travert with Electrolyte #2 or #3 Injection (Travenol)	Electrolyte #3 (Cooke & Crowley's Solution) with 10% Inverted Sugar Injection (Cutter)
Isolyte E, M, or P with 5% Dextrose Injection	
10% Dextran 40 or 6% Dextran 75 in 5% Dextrose Injection	
Plasma-Lyte 56 or 148 Injection with 5% Dextrose (Travenol)	Normosol-M or R in D5-W (Abbott), Isolyte H or S with 5% Dextrose (McGaw), Polyonic R-148 or M-56 with 5% Dextrose (Cutter)
Plasma-Lyte M Injection 5% Dextrose (Travenol)	Polysal M with 5% Dextrose (Cutter)
Ionosol B in D5-W	
5% Amigen Injection alone or with 5% Dextrose	
Normosol-R	Polyonic R-148 (Cutter), Isolyte S (McGaw), Plasma-Lyte 148 Injection in Water (Travenol)
Polysal (Plain)	
Aminosol 5% Injection	
Fre-Amine II 8.5% Injection	
Plasma-Lyte 148 Injection (approx. pH 7.4) (Travenol)	Normosol-R pH 7.4 (Abbott)
10% Fructose Injection	

Following the administration of an initial dose of netilmicin and the determination of drug serum concentrations in post-infusion blood samples, the drug's half-life and the patient's elimination rate constant and volume of distribution can be calculated. Desired peak and trough serum levels for a particular patient are then selected by taking into consideration the susceptibility of the causative organism, the severity of infection, and the status of the patient's host-defense mechanisms. The dosage regimen (dose and dosing interval) is then determined using standardized formulae and the appropriate computer program, and the dosage regimen can be adjusted to the nearest practical interval and amount.

ADDITION OF NETILMICIN SULFATE TO VARIOUS INTRAVENOUS PREPARATIONS

In adults, a single dose of netilmicin injection may be diluted in 50 to 200 ml of one of the parenteral solutions listed below. In infants and children, the volume of diluent should be less according to the fluid requirements of the patient. The solution may be infused over a period of one-half to two hours. Tested at concentrations of 2.1 to 3.0 mg/ml, netilmicin sulfate has been shown to be stable in the following large volume parenteral solutions for up to 72 hours when stored in glass containers, both when refrigerated and at room temperature. Use after this time period is not recommended. [See table above.]

Parenteral drug products should be inspected visually for particulate matter and discoloration prior to administration, whenever solution and container permit.

HOW SUPPLIED
NETROMYCIN Injection 100 mg/ml is supplied in 1.5 ml vials, box of 10 (NDC 0085-0264-02). **Store between 2° and 30°C (36°F and 86°F).**

ANIMAL PHARMACOLOGY AND/OR ANIMAL TOXICOLOGY
Netilmicin sulfate, administered by the intravenous and intramuscular routes, has been compared to kanamycin, sisomicin, gentamicin, amikacin, and tobramycin in studies ranging in duration from two weeks to three months. Among the aminoglycosides, netilmicin is one of the more potent neuromuscular-blocking agents; however, in six different species, netilmicin sulfate has proven to be the least nephrotoxic and ototoxic of these aminoglycosides, using morphological as well as functional end points. In the clinical trials nephrotoxicity and ototoxicity occurred at about the same frequency in netilmicin-treated patients as in those treated with other aminoglycosides.

Schering Biochem Corporation,
Manati, Puerto Rico 00701
An Affiliate of Schering Corporation,
Kenilworth, NJ 07033

Revised 1/87   12759568

NORMODYNE®   ℞
brand of labetalol hydrochloride, USP
Injection

DESCRIPTION
NORMODYNE (labetalol HCl) is an adrenergic receptor blocking agent that has both selective alpha₁- and nonselective beta-adrenergic receptor blocking actions in a single substance.

Labetalol HCl is a racemate, chemically designated as 5-[1-hydroxy-2-[(1-methyl-3-phenylpropyl) amino] ethyl]salicylamide monohydrochloride, and has the following structure:

Labetalol HCl has the empirical formula $C_{19}H_{24}N_2O_3 \cdot$ HCl and a molecular weight of 364.9. It has two asymmetric centers and therefore exists as a molecular complex of two diastereoisomeric pairs. Dilevalol, the R,R' stereoisomer, makes up 25% of racemic labetalol.

Labetalol HCl is a white or off-white crystalline powder, soluble in water.

NORMODYNE (labetalol HCl) Injection is a clear, colorless to light yellow aqueous sterile isotonic solution for intravenous injection. It has a pH range of 3.0 to 4.0. Each mL con-

Continued on next page

Information on Schering products appearing on these pages is effective as of August 15, 1996.

Schering—Cont.

tains 5 mg labetalol HCl, USP, 45 mg anhydrous dextrose, 0.10 mg edetate disodium; 0.80 mg methylparaben and 0.10 mg propylparaben as preservatives; citric acid monohydrate and sodium hydroxide, as necessary, to bring the solution into the pH range.

CLINICAL PHARMACOLOGY

NORMODYNE (labetalol HCl) combines both selective, competitive alpha$_1$-adrenergic blocking and nonselective, competitive beta-adrenergic blocking activity in a single substance. In man, the ratios of alpha- to beta-blockade have been estimated to be approximately 1:3 and 1:7 following oral and intravenous administration, respectively. Beta$_2$-agonist activity has been demonstrated in animals with minimal beta$_1$-agonist (ISA) activity detected. In animals, at doses greater than those required for alpha- or beta-adrenergic blockade, a membrane-stabilizing effect has been demonstrated.

Pharmacodynamics The capacity of labetalol HCl to block alpha receptors in man has been demonstrated by attenuation of the pressor effect of phenylephrine and by a significant reduction of the pressor response caused by immersing the hand in ice-cold water ("cold-pressor test"). Labetalol HCl's beta$_1$-receptor blockade in man was demonstrated by a small decrease in the resting heart rate, attenuation of tachycardia produced by isoproterenol or exercise, and by attenuation of the reflex tachycardia to the hypotension produced by amyl nitrite. Beta$_2$-receptor blockade was demonstrated by inhibition of the isoproterenol-induced fall in diastolic blood pressure. Both the alpha- and beta-blocking actions of orally administered labetalol HCl contribute to a decrease in blood pressure in hypertensive patients. Labetalol HCl consistently, in dose-related fashion, blunted increases in exercise-induced blood pressure and heart rate, and in their double product. The pulmonary circulation during exercise was not affected by labetalol HCl dosing.

Single oral doses of labetalol HCl administered in patients with coronary artery disease had no significant effect on sinus rate, intraventricular conduction, or QRS duration. The AV conduction time was modestly prolonged in 2 of 7 patients. In another study, intravenous labetalol HCl slightly prolonged AV nodal conduction time and atrial effective refractory period with only small changes in heart rate. The effects on AV nodal refractoriness were inconsistent.

Labetalol HCl produces dose-related falls in blood pressure without reflex tachycardia and without significant reduction in heart rate, presumably through a mixture of its alpha-blocking and beta-blocking effects. Hemodynamic effects are variable with small nonsignificant changes in cardiac output seen in some studies but not others, and small decreases in total peripheral resistance. Elevated plasma renins are reduced.

Doses of labetalol HCl that controlled hypertension did not affect renal function in mild to severe hypertensive patients with normal renal function.

Due to the alpha$_1$-receptor blocking activity of labetalol HCl, blood pressure is lowered more in the standing than in the supine position, and symptoms of postural hypotension can occur. During dosing with intravenous labetalol HCl, the contribution of the postural component should be considered when positioning patients for treatment, and patients should not be allowed to move to an erect position unmonitored until their ability to do so is established.

In a clinical pharmacologic study in severe hypertensives, an initial 0.25 mg/kg injection of labetalol HCl, administered to patients in the supine position, decreased blood pressure by an average of 11/7 mmHg. Additional injections of 0.5 mg/kg at 15-minute intervals up to a total cumulative dose of 1.75 mg/kg of labetalol HCl caused further dose-related decreases in blood pressure. Some patients required cumulative doses of up to 3.25 mg/kg. The maximal effect of each dose level occurred within 5 minutes. Following discontinuation of intravenous treatment with labetalol HCl, the blood pressure rose gradually and progressively, approaching pretreatment baseline values within an average of 16–18 hours in the majority of patients.

Similar results were obtained in the treatment of patients with severe hypertension requiring urgent blood pressure reduction with an initial dose of 20 mg (which corresponds to 0.25 mg/kg for an 80 kg patient) followed by additional doses of either 40 or 80 mg at 10-minute intervals to achieve the desired effect or up to a cumulative dose of 300 mg.

Labetalol HCl administered as a continuous intravenous infusion, with a mean dose of 136 mg (27 to 300 mg) over a period of 2 to 3 hours (mean of 2 hours and 39 minutes) lowered the blood pressure by an average of 60/35 mmHg.

Exacerbation of angina and, in some cases, myocardial infarction and ventricular dysrhythmias have been reported after abrupt discontinuation of therapy with beta-adrenergic blocking agents in patients with coronary artery disease. Abrupt withdrawal of these agents in patients without coronary artery disease has resulted in transient symptoms, including tremulousness, sweating, palpitation, headache, and malaise. Several mechanisms have been proposed to explain these phenomena, among them increased sensitivity to catecholamines because of increased numbers of beta receptors.

Although beta-adrenergic receptor blockade is useful in the treatment of angina and hypertension, there are also situations in which sympathetic stimulation is vital. For example, in patients with severely damaged hearts, adequate ventricular function may depend on sympathetic drive. Beta-adrenergic blockade may worsen AV block by preventing the necessary facilitating effects of sympathetic activity on conduction. Beta$_2$- adrenergic blockade results in passive bronchial constriction by interfering with endogenous adrenergic bronchodilator activity in patients subject to bronchospasm and may also interfere with exogenous bronchodilators in such patients.

Pharmacokinetics and Metabolism Following intravenous infusion, the elimination half-life is about 5.5 hours and the total body clearance is approximately 33 mL/min/kg. The plasma half-life of labetalol following oral administration is about 6 to 8 hours. In patients with decreased hepatic or renal function, the elimination half-life of labetalol is not altered; however, the relative bioavailability in hepatically impaired patients is increased due to decreased "first-pass" metabolism.

The metabolism of labetalol is mainly through conjugation to glucuronide metabolites. These metabolites are present in plasma and are excreted in the urine and, via the bile, into the feces. Approximately 55% to 60% of a dose appears in the urine as conjugates or unchanged labetalol within the first 24 hours of dosing.

Labetalol has been shown to cross the placental barrier in humans. Only negligible amounts of the drug crossed the blood-brain barrier in animal studies. Labetalol is approximately 50% protein bound. Neither hemodialysis nor peritoneal dialysis removes a significant amount of labetalol HCl from the general circulation (<1%).

INDICATIONS AND USAGE

NORMODYNE (labetalol HCl) Injection is indicated for control of blood pressure in severe hypertension.

CONTRAINDICATIONS

NORMODYNE (labetalol HCl) Injection is contraindicated in bronchial asthma, overt cardiac failure, greater than first degree heart block, cardiogenic shock, severe bradycardia, other conditions associated with severe and prolonged hypotension, and in patients with a history of hypersensitivity to any component of the product (see **WARNINGS**).

WARNINGS

Hepatic Injury Severe hepatocellular injury, confirmed by rechallenge in at least one case, occurs rarely with labetalol therapy. The hepatic injury is usually reversible, but hepatic necrosis and death have been reported. Injury has occurred after both short- and long-term treatment and may be slowly progressive despite minimal symptomatology. Similar hepatic events have been reported with a related compound, dilevalol HCl, including two deaths. Dilevalol HCl is one of the four isomers of labetalol HCl. Thus, for patients taking labetalol, periodic determination of suitable hepatic laboratory tests would be appropriate. Laboratory testing should also be done at the very first symptom or sign of liver dysfunction (eg, pruritus, dark urine, persistent anorexia, jaundice, right upper quadrant tenderness, or unexplained "flu-like" symptoms). If the patient has jaundice or laboratory evidence of liver injury, labetalol HCl should be stopped and not restarted.

Cardiac Failure Sympathetic stimulation is a vital component supporting circulatory function in congestive heart failure. Beta blockade carries a potential hazard of further depressing myocardial contractility and precipitating more severe failure. Although beta-blockers should be avoided in overt congestive heart failure, if necessary, labetalol HCl can be used with caution in patients with a history of heart failure who are well-compensated. Congestive heart failure has been observed in patients receiving labetalol HCl. Labetalol HCl does not abolish the inotropic action of digitalis on heart muscle.

In Patients Without a History of Cardiac Failure In patients with latent cardiac insufficiency, continued depression of the myocardium with beta-blocking agents over a period of time can lead, in some cases, to cardiac failure. At the first sign or symptom of impending cardiac failure, patients should be fully digitalized and/or be given a diuretic, and the response observed closely. If cardiac failure continues, despite adequate digitalization and diuretic, NORMODYNE (labetalol HCl) therapy should be withdrawn (gradually if possible).

Ischemic Heart Disease Angina pectoris has not been reported upon labetalol HCl discontinuation. However, following abrupt cessation of therapy with some beta-blocking agents in patients with coronary artery disease, exacerbations of angina pectoris and, in some cases, myocardial infarction have been reported. Therefore, such patients should be cautioned against interruption of therapy without the physician's advice. Even in the absence of overt angina pectoris, when discontinuation of NORMODYNE (labetalol HCl) is planned, the patient should be carefully observed and should be advised to limit physical activity. If angina markedly worsens or acute coronary insufficiency develops, NORMODYNE (labetalol HCl) administration should be reinstituted promptly, at least temporarily, and other measures appropriate for the management of unstable angina should be taken.

Nonallergic Bronchospasm (eg, chronic bronchitis and emphysema) Since NORMODYNE (labetalol HCl) Injection at the usual intravenous therapeutic doses has not been studied in patients with nonallergic bronchospastic disease, it should not be used in such patients.

Pheochromocytoma Intravenous labetalol HCl has been shown to be effective in lowering the blood pressure and relieving symptoms in patients with pheochromocytoma; higher than usual doses may be required. However, paradoxical hypertensive responses have been reported in a few patients with this tumor; therefore, use caution when administering labetalol HCl to patients with pheochromocytoma.

Diabetes Mellitus and Hypoglycemia Beta-adrenergic blockade may prevent the appearance of premonitory signs and symptoms (eg, tachycardia) of acute hypoglycemia. This is especially important with labile diabetics. Beta-blockade also reduces the release of insulin in response to hyperglycemia; it may therefore be necessary to adjust the dose of antidiabetic drugs.

Major Surgery The necessity or desirability of withdrawing beta-blocking therapy prior to major surgery is controversial. Protracted severe hypotension and difficulty in restarting or maintaining a heartbeat have been reported with beta-blockers. The effect of labetalol HCl's alpha-adrenergic activity has not been evaluated in this setting.

A synergism between labetalol HCl and halothane anesthesia has been shown (see **PRECAUTIONS—Drug Interactions**).

Rapid Decreases of Blood Pressure Caution must be observed when reducing severely elevated blood pressure. Although such findings have not been reported with intravenous labetalol HCl, a number of adverse reactions, including cerebral infarction, optic nerve infarction, angina and ischemic changes in the electrocardiogram, have been reported with other agents when severely elevated blood pressure was reduced over time courses of several hours to as long as 1 or 2 days. The desired blood pressure lowering should therefore be achieved over as long a period of time as is compatible with the patient's status.

PRECAUTIONS

General: *Impaired Hepatic Function* may diminish metabolism of NORMODYNE (labetalol HCl) Injection.

Following Coronary Artery Bypass Surgery In one uncontrolled study, patients with low cardiac indices and elevated systemic vascular resistance following intravenous labetalol HCl experienced significant declines in cardiac output with little change in systemic vascular resistance. One of these patients developed hypotension following labetalol HCl treatment. Therefore, use of labetalol HCl should be avoided in such patients.

High-Dose Labetalol HCl Administration of up to 3 g/d as an infusion for up to 2 to 3 days has been anecdotally reported; several patients experienced hypotension or bradycardia (see **DOSAGE AND ADMINISTRATION**).

Hypotension Symptomatic postural hypotension (incidence 58%) is likely to occur if patients are tilted or allowed to assume the upright position within 3 hours of receiving NORMODYNE (labetalol HCl) Injection. Therefore, the patient's ability to tolerate an upright position should be established before permitting any ambulation.

Jaundice or Hepatic Dysfunction (see **WARNINGS**).

Information for Patients: The following information is intended to aid in the safe and effective use of this medication. It is not a disclosure of all possible adverse or intended effects. During and immediately following (for up to 3 hours) NORMODYNE (labetalol HCl) Injection, the patient should remain supine. Subsequently, the patient should be advised on how to proceed gradually to become ambulatory, and should be observed at the time of first ambulation.

When the patient is started on NORMODYNE (labetalol HCl) Tablets, following adequate control of blood pressure with NORMODYNE (labetalol HCl) Injection, appropriate directions for titration of dosage should be provided (see **DOSAGE AND ADMINISTRATION**).

As with all drugs with beta-blocking activity, certain advice to patients being treated with labetalol HCl is warranted: While no incident of the abrupt withdrawal phenomenon (exacerbation of angina pectoris) has been reported with labetalol HCl, dosing with NORMODYNE (labetalol HCl) Tablets should not be interrupted or discontinued without a physician's advice. Patients being treated with NORMODYNE (labetalol HCl) Tablets should consult a physician at any signs or symptoms of impending cardiac failure or hepatic dysfunction (see **WARNINGS**). Also, transient scalp tingling may occur, usually when treatment with NORMODYNE (labetalol HCl) Tablets is initiated (see **ADVERSE REACTIONS**).

Labetalol HCl Daily Dose (mg)	200	300	400	600	800	900	1200	1600	2400
Number of Patients	522	181	606	608	503	117	411	242	175
Dizziness (%)	2	3	3	3	5	1	9	13	16
Fatigue	2	1	4	4	5	3	7	6	10
Nausea	<1	0	1	2	4	0	7	11	19
Vomiting	0	0	<1	<1	<1	0	1	2	3
Dyspepsia	1	0	2	1	1	0	2	2	4
Paresthesias	2	0	2	2	1	1	2	5	5
Nasal Stuffiness	1	1	2	2	2	2	4	5	6
Ejaculation Failure	0	2	1	2	3	0	4	3	5
Impotence	1	1	1	1	2	4	3	4	3
Edema	1	0	1	1	1	0	1	2	2

Laboratory Tests: Routine laboratory tests are ordinarily not required before or after intravenous labetalol HCl. In patients with concomitant illnesses, such as impaired renal function, appropriate tests should be done to monitor these conditions.

Drug Interactions: Since NORMODYNE (labetalol HCl) Injection may be administered to patients already being treated with other medications, including other antihypertensive agents, careful monitoring of these patients is necessary to detect and treat promptly any undesired effect from concomitant administration.

In one survey, 2.3% of patients taking labetalol HCl orally in combination with tricyclic antidepressants experienced tremor as compared to 0.7% reported to occur with labetalol HCl alone. The contribution of each of the treatments to this adverse reaction is unknown but the possibility of a drug interaction cannot be excluded.

Drugs possessing beta-blocking properties can blunt the bronchodilator effect of beta-receptor agonist drugs in patients with bronchospasm; therefore, doses greater than the normal anti-asthmatic dose of beta-agonist bronchodilator drugs may be required.

Cimetidine has been shown to increase the bioavailability of labetalol HCl administered orally. Since this could be explained either by enhanced absorption or by an alteration of hepatic metabolism of labetalol HCl, special care should be used in establishing the dose required for blood pressure control in such patients.

Synergism has been shown between halothane anesthesia and intravenously administered labetalol HCl. During controlled hypotensive anesthesia using labetalol HCl in association with halothane, high concentrations (3% or above) of halothane should not be used because the degree of hypotension will be increased and because of the possibility of a large reduction in cardiac output and an increase in central venous pressure. The anesthesiologist should be informed when a patient is receiving labetalol HCl.

Labetalol HCl blunts the reflex tachycardia produced by nitroglycerin without preventing its hypotensive effect. If labetalol HCl is used with nitroglycerin in patients with angina pectoris, additional antihypertensive effects may occur. Care should be taken if labetalol HCl is used concomitantly with calcium antagonists of the verapamil type.

When drug products that are alkaline, such as furosemide, have been administered in combination with labetalol, a white precipitate has been noted. Therefore, these drugs should not be administered in the same infusion line.

Risk of Anaphylactic Reaction While taking beta-blockers, patients with a history of severe anaphylactic reactions to a variety of allergens may be more reactive to repeated challenge, either accidental, diagnostic, or therapeutic. Such patients may be unresponsive to the usual doses of epinephrine used to treat allergic reaction.

Drug/Laboratory Test Interactions: The presence of labetalol metabolites in the urine may result in falsely elevated levels of urinary catecholamines, metanephrine, normetanephrine, and vanillylmandelic acid (VMA) when measured by fluorimetric or photometric methods. In screening patients suspected of having a pheochromocytoma and being treated with labetalol HCl, a specific method, such as high performance liquid chromatographic assay with solid phase extraction (eg, *J Chromatogr* 385:241, 1987) should be employed in determining levels of catecholamines.

Labetalol HCl has also been reported to produce a false-positive test for amphetamine when screening urine for the presence of drugs using the commercially available assay methods Toxi-Lab A® (thin-layer chromatographic assay) and Emit-d.a.u.® (radioenzymatic assay). When patients being treated with labetalol HCl have a positive urine test for amphetamine using these techniques, confirmation should be made by using more specific methods, such as a gas chromatographic-mass spectrometer technique.

Carcinogenesis, Mutagenesis, Impairment of Fertility: Long-term oral dosing studies with labetalol HCl for 18 months in mice and for 2 years in rats showed no evidence of carcinogenesis. Studies with labetalol HCl, using dominant lethal assays in rats and mice, and exposing microorganisms according to modified Ames tests, showed no evidence of mutagenesis.

Pregnancy Category C: Teratogenic studies have been performed with labetalol HCl in rats and rabbits at oral doses up to approximately 6 and 4 times the maximum recommended human dose (MRHD), respectively. No reproducible evidence of fetal malformations was observed. Increased fetal resorptions were seen in both species at doses approximating the MRHD. A teratology study performed with labetalol HCl in rabbits at intravenous doses up to 1.7 times the MRHD revealed no evidence of drug-related harm to the fetus. There are no adequate and well-controlled studies in pregnant women. Labetalol HCl should be used during pregnancy only if the potential benefit justifies the potential risk to the fetus.

Nonteratogenic Effects: Hypotension, bradycardia, hypoglycemia, and respiratory depression have been reported in infants of mothers who were treated with labetalol HCl for hypertension during pregnancy. Oral administration of labetalol to rats during late gestation through weaning at doses of 2 to 4 times the MRHD caused a decrease in neonatal survival.

Labor and Delivery: Labetalol HCl given to pregnant women with hypertension did not appear to affect the usual course of labor and delivery.

Nursing Mothers: Small amounts of labetalol (approximately 0.004% of the maternal dose) are excreted in human milk. Caution should be exercised when NORMODYNE (labetalol HCl) Injection is administered to a nursing woman.

Pediatric Use: Safety and effectiveness in children have not been established.

ADVERSE REACTIONS

NORMODYNE (labetalol HCl) Injection is usually well tolerated. Most adverse effects have been mild and transient and in controlled trials involving 92 patients did not require labetalol HCl withdrawal. Symptomatic postural hypotension (incidence 58%) is likely to occur if patients are tilted or allowed to assume the upright position within 3 hours of receiving NORMODYNE (labetalol HCl) Injection. Moderate hypotension occurred in 1 of 100 patients while supine. Increased sweating was noted in 4 of 100 patients, and flushing occurred in 1 of 100 patients.

The following also were reported with NORMODYNE (labetalol HCl) Injection with the incidence per 100 patients as noted:

Cardiovascular System Ventricular arrhythmia in 1.

Central and Peripheral Nervous Systems Dizziness in 9; tingling of the scalp/skin 7; hypoesthesia (numbness) and vertigo, 1 each.

Gastrointestinal System Nausea in 13; vomiting 4; dyspepsia and taste distortion, 1 each.

Metabolic Disorders Transient increases in blood urea nitrogen and serum creatinine levels occurred in 8 of 100 patients; these were associated with drops in blood pressure, generally in patients with prior renal insufficiency.

Psychiatric Disorders Somnolence/yawning in 3.

Respiratory System Wheezing in 1.

Skin Pruritus in 1.

The incidence of adverse reactions depends upon the dose of labetalol HCl. The largest experience is with oral labetalol HCl (see NORMODYNE (labetalol HCl) Tablet Product Information for details). Certain of the side effects increased with increasing oral dose as shown in the table below which depicts the entire U.S. therapeutic trials data base for adverse reactions that are clearly or possibly dose related.

[See table above.]

In addition, a number of other less common adverse events have been reported:

Cardiovascular Hypotension, and rarely, syncope, bradycardia, heart block.

Liver and Biliary System Hepatic necrosis, hepatitis, cholestatic jaundice, elevated liver function tests.

Hypersensitivity Rare reports of hypersensitivity (eg, rash, urticaria, pruritus, angioedema, dyspnea) and anaphylactoid reactions.

The oculomucocutaneous syndrome associated with the beta-blocker practolol has not been reported with labetalol HCl during investigational use and extensive foreign marketing experience.

Clinical Laboratory Tests: Among patients dosed with NORMODYNE (labetalol HCl) Tablets, there have been reversible increases of serum transaminases in 4% of patients tested, and more rarely, reversible increases in blood urea.

OVERDOSAGE

Overdosage with NORMODYNE (labetalol HCl) Injection causes excessive hypotension that is posture sensitive, and sometimes, excessive bradycardia. Patients should be placed supine and their legs raised if necessary to improve the blood supply to the brain. If overdosage with labetalol HCl follows oral ingestion, gastric lavage or pharmacologically induced emesis (using syrup of ipecac) may be useful for removal of the drug shortly after ingestion. The following additional measures should be employed if necessary: *Excessive bradycardia* —administer atropine or epinephrine. *Cardiac failure* —administer a digitalis glycoside and a diuretic. Dopamine or dobutamine may also be useful. *Hypotension* —administer vasopressors, eg, norepinephrine. There is pharmacological evidence that norepinephrine may be the drug of choice. *Bronchospasm*—administer epinephrine and/or an aerosolized $beta_2$-agonist. *Seizures* —administer diazepam.

In severe beta-blocker overdose resulting in hypotension and/or bradycardia, glucagon has been shown to be effective when administered in large doses (5 to 10 mg rapidly over 30 seconds, followed by continuous infusion of 5 mg/hr that can be reduced as the patient improves).

Neither hemodialysis nor peritoneal dialysis removes a significant amount of labetalol HCl from the general circulation (<1%).

The oral LD_{50} value of labetalol HCl in the mouse is approximately 600 mg/kg and in the rat is greater than 2 g/kg. The intravenous LD_{50} in these species is 50 to 60 mg/kg.

DOSAGE AND ADMINISTRATION

NORMODYNE (labetalol HCl) Injection is intended for intravenous use in hospitalized patients. DOSAGE MUST BE INDIVIDUALIZED depending upon the severity of hypertension and the response of the patient during dosing.

Patients should always be kept in a supine position during the period of intravenous drug administration. A substantial fall in blood pressure on standing should be expected in these patients. The patient's ability to tolerate an upright position should be established before permitting any ambulation, such as using toilet facilities.

Either of two methods of administration of NORMODYNE (labetalol HCl) Injection may be used: a) repeated intravenous injections, b) slow continuous infusion.

Repeated Intravenous Injection: Initially, NORMODYNE (labetalol HCl) Injection should be given in a dose of 20 mg labetalol HCl (which corresponds to 0.25 mg/kg for an 80 kg patient) by slow intravenous injection over a 2-minute period.

Immediately before the injection and at 5 and 10 minutes after injection, supine blood pressure should be measured to evaluate response. Additional injections of 40 mg or 80 mg can be given at 10-minute intervals until a desired supine blood pressure is achieved or a total of 300 mg labetalol HCl has been injected. The maximum effect usually occurs within 5 minutes of each injection.

Slow Continuous Infusion: NORMODYNE (labetalol HCl) Injection is prepared for intravenous continuous infusion by diluting the contents with commonly used intravenous fluids (see below). Examples of methods of preparing the infusion solution are:

The contents of either two 20 mL vials (40 mL), or one 40 mL vial, are added to 160 mL of a commonly used intravenous fluid such that the resultant 200 mL of solution contains 200 mg of labetalol HCl, 1 mg/mL. The diluted solution should be administered at a rate of 2 mL/min to deliver 2 mg/min.

Alternatively, the contents of either two 20 mL vials (40 mL), or one 40 mL vial, of NORMODYNE (labetalol HCl) Injection are added to 250 mL of a commonly used intravenous fluid. The resultant solution will contain 200 mg of labetalol HCl, approximately 2 mg/3 mL. The diluted solution should be administered at a rate of 3 mL/min to deliver approximately 2 mg/min.

The rate of infusion of the diluted solution may be adjusted according to the blood pressure response, at the discretion of the physician. To facilitate a desired rate of infusion, the diluted solution can be infused using a controlled administration mechanism, eg, graduated burette or mechanically driven infusion pump.

Since the half-life of labetalol is 5 to 8 hours, steady-state blood levels (in the face of a constant rate of infusion) would not be reached during the usual infusion time period. The infusion should be continued until a satisfactory response is obtained and should then be stopped and oral labetalol HCl started (see below). The effective intravenous dose is usually in the range of 50 to 200 mg. A total dose of up to 300 mg may be required in some patients.

Blood Pressure Monitoring: The blood pressure should be monitored during and after completion of the infusion or intravenous injections. Rapid or excessive falls in either systolic or diastolic blood pressure during intravenous treatment should be avoided. In patients with excessive systolic

Continued on next page

Information on Schering products appearing on these pages is effective as of August 15, 1996.

Schering—Cont.

hypertension, the decrease in systolic pressure should be used as indicator of effectiveness in addition to the response of the diastolic pressure.

Initiation of Dosing with NORMODYNE (labetalol HCl) Tablets: Subsequent oral dosing with NORMODYNE (labetalol HCl) Tablets should begin when it has been established that the supine diastolic blood pressure has begun to rise. The recommended initial dose is 200 mg, followed in 6–12 hours by an additional dose of 200 or 400 mg, depending on the blood pressure response. Thereafter, *inpatient titration with NORMODYNE (labetalol HCl) Tablets* may proceed as follows:

Inpatient Titration Instructions

Regimen	Daily Dose*
200 mg b.i.d.	400 mg
400 mg b.i.d.	800 mg
800 mg b.i.d.	1600 mg
1200 mg b.i.d.	2400 mg

* If needed, the total daily dose may be given in three divided doses.

While in the hospital, the dosage of NORMODYNE (labetalol HCl) Tablets may be increased at 1-day intervals to achieve the desired blood pressure reduction.

For subsequent outpatient titration or maintenance dosing see NORMODYNE (labetalol HCl) Tablets Product Information **DOSAGE AND ADMINISTRATION** for additional recommendations.

Compatibility with commonly used intravenous fluids: Parenteral drug products should be inspected visually for particulate matter and discoloration prior to administration, whenever solution and container permit.

NORMODYNE (labetalol HCl) Injection was tested for compatibility with commonly used intravenous fluids at final concentrations of 1.25 mg to 3.75 mg labetalol HCl per mL of the mixture. NORMODYNE (labetalol HCl) Injection was found to be compatible with and stable (for 24 hours refrigerated or at room temperature) in mixtures with the following solutions:

Ringers Injection, USP
Lactated Ringers Injection, USP
5% Dextrose and Ringers Injection
5% Lactated Ringers and 5% Dextrose Injection
5% Dextrose Injection, USP
0.9% Sodium Chloride Injection, USP
5% Dextrose and 0.2% Sodium Chloride Injection, USP
2.5% Dextrose and 0.45% Sodium Chloride Injection, USP
5% Dextrose and 0.9% Sodium Chloride Injection, USP
5% Dextrose and 0.33% Sodium Chloride Injection, USP

NORMODYNE (labetalol HCl) Injection was NOT compatible with 5% Sodium Bicarbonate Injection, USP.

HOW SUPPLIED

NORMODYNE (labetalol HCl) Injection, 5 mg/mL, is supplied in:

20 mL (100 mg) (NDC-0085-0362-07) multi-dose vial, box of 1 and
40 mL (200 mg) (NDC-0085-0362-06) multi-dose vial, box of 1
4 mL (20 mg) (NDC-0085-0362-08) single-dose, pre-filled, disposable syringe, box of 1 and
8 mL (40 mg) (NDC-0085-0362-09) single-dose, pre-filled, disposable syringe, box of 1

Store between 2° and 30°C (36° and 86°F). Protect from freezing. Protect syringe from light.

Note: To insure patient safety, the needle and the pre-filled syringes should be handled with care and should be destroyed and discarded if damaged in any manner. If the cannula is bent, no attempt should be made to straighten it. To prevent needle-stick injuries, needles should not be recapped, purposely bent, or broken by hand.

Only the pre-filled syringes are manufactured for Schering Corporation by:

Survival Technology, Inc.,
Rockville, MD 20850

Key Pharmaceuticals, Inc.
Kenilworth, NJ 07033 USA
Revised 10/94 14525670

Copyright © 1984, 1994, 1995, Schering Corporation. All rights reserved.

Shown in Product Identification Guide, page 334

NORMODYNE® ℞

brand of
labetalol hydrochloride
Tablets, USP

DESCRIPTION

NORMODYNE (labetalol HCl) is an adrenergic receptor blocking agent that has both selective alpha$_1$-and nonselective beta-adrenergic receptor blocking actions in a single substance.

Labetalol HCl is a racemate, chemically designated as 5-[1-hydroxy-2-[(1-methyl-3-phenylpropyl) amino] ethyl]salicylamide monohydrochloride, and has the following structure:

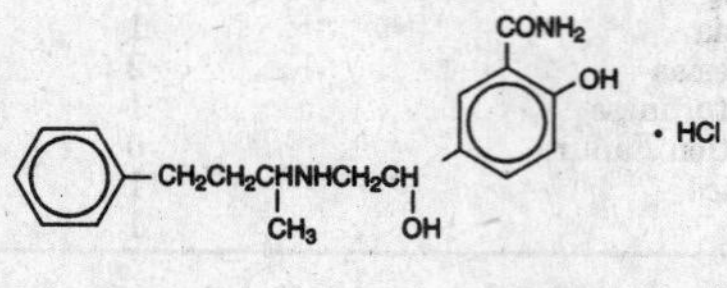

Labetalol HCl has the empirical formula $C_{19}H_{24}N_2O_3 \cdot HCl$ and a molecular weight of 364.9. It has two asymmetric centers and therefore exists as a molecular complex of two diastereoisomeric pairs. Dilevalol, the R,R' stereoisomer, makes up 25% of racemic labetalol.

Labetalol HCl is a white or off-white crystalline powder, soluble in water.

NORMODYNE Tablets contain 100 mg, 200 mg, or 300 mg labetalol HCl, USP and are taken orally.

The inactive ingredients for NORMODYNE Tablets, 100 mg, include: corn starch, FD&C Blue No. 2 Al Lake, FD&C Yellow No. 6 Al Lake, hydroxypropyl methylcellulose, lactose, magnesium stearate, methylparaben, PEG, and propylparaben. May also contain: potato starch and wheat starch.

The inactive ingredients for NORMODYNE Tablets, 200 mg, include: corn starch, hydroxypropyl methylcellulose, lactose, magnesium stearate, methylparaben, PEG, propylparaben, and titanium dioxide. May also contain: potato starch and wheat starch.

The inactive ingredients for NORMODYNE Tablets, 300 mg, include: corn starch, FD&C Blue No. 2 Al Lake, hydroxypropyl methylcellulose, lactose, magnesium stearate, methylparaben, PEG, and propylparaben. May also contain: potato starch and wheat starch.

CLINICAL PHARMACOLOGY

NORMODYNE (labetalol HCl) combines both selective, competitive alpha$_1$-adrenergic blocking and nonselective, competitive beta-adrenergic blocking activity in a single substance. In man, the ratios of alpha- to beta-blockade have been estimated to be approximately 1:3 and 1:7 following oral and intravenous administration, respectively. Beta$_2$-agonist activity has been demonstrated in animals with minimal beta$_1$-agonist (ISA) activity detected. In animals, at doses greater than those required for alpha- or beta-adrenergic blockade, a membrane-stabilizing effect has been demonstrated.

Pharmacodynamics The capacity of labetalol HCl to block alpha receptors in man has been demonstrated by attenuation of the pressor effect of phenylephrine and by a significant reduction of the pressor response caused by immersing the hand in ice-cold water ("cold-pressor test"). Labetalol HCl's beta$_1$-receptor blockade in man was demonstrated by a small decrease in the resting heart rate, attenuation of tachycardia produced by isoproterenol or exercise, and by attenuation of the reflex tachycardia to the hypotension produced by amyl nitrite. Beta$_2$-receptor blockade was demonstrated by inhibition of the isoproterenol-induced fall in diastolic blood pressure. Both the alpha- and beta-blocking actions of orally administered labetalol HCl contribute to a decrease in blood pressure in hypertensive patients. Labetalol HCl consistently, in dose-related fashion, blunted increases in exercise-induced blood pressure and heart rate, and in their double product. The pulmonary circulation during exercise was not affected by labetalol HCl dosing.

Single oral doses of labetalol HCl administered in patients with coronary artery disease had no significant effect on sinus rate, intraventricular conduction, or QRS duration. The AV conduction time was modestly prolonged in 2 of 7 patients. In another study, intravenous labetalol HCl slightly prolonged AV nodal conduction time and atrial effective refractory period with only small changes in heart rate. The effects on AV nodal refractoriness were inconsistent.

Labetalol HCl produces dose-related falls in blood pressure without reflex tachycardia and without significant reduction in heart rate, presumably through a mixture of its alpha-blocking and beta-blocking effects. Hemodynamic effects are variable with small nonsignificant changes in cardiac output seen in some studies but not others, and small decreases in total peripheral resistance. Elevated plasma renins are reduced.

Doses of labetalol HCl that controlled hypertension did not affect renal function in mild to severe hypertensive patients with normal renal function.

Due to the alpha$_1$-receptor blocking activity of labetalol HCl, blood pressure is lowered more in the standing than in the supine position, and symptoms of postural hypotension (2%), including rare instances of syncope, can occur. Following oral administration, when postural hypotension has occurred, it has been transient and is uncommon when the recommended starting dose and titration increments are closely followed (see **DOSAGE AND ADMINISTRATION**). Symptomatic postural hypotension is most likely to occur 2 to 4 hours after a dose, especially following the use of large initial doses or upon large changes in dose.

The peak effects of single oral doses of labetalol HCl occur within 2 to 4 hours. The duration of effect depends upon dose, lasting at least 8 hours following single oral doses of 100 mg and more than 12 hours following single oral doses of 300 mg. The maximum, steady-state blood pressure response upon oral, twice-a-day dosing occurs within 24 to 72 hours.

The antihypertensive effect of labetalol has a linear correlation with the logarithm of labetalol plasma concentration, and there is also a linear correlation between the reduction in exercise-induced tachycardia occurring at 2 hours after oral administration of labetalol HCl and the logarithm of the plasma concentration.

About 70% of the maximum beta-blocking effect is present for 5 hours after the administration of a single oral dose of 400 mg, with suggestion that about 40% remains at 8 hours.

The anti-anginal efficacy of labetalol HCl has not been studied. In 37 patients with hypertension and coronary artery disease, labetalol HCl did not increase the incidence or severity of angina attacks.

Exacerbation of angina and, in some cases, myocardial infarction and ventricular dysrhythmias have been reported after abrupt discontinuation of therapy with beta-adrenergic blocking agents in patients with coronary artery disease. Abrupt withdrawal of these agents in patients without coronary artery disease has resulted in transient symptoms, including tremulousness, sweating, palpitation, headache, and malaise. Several mechanisms have been proposed to explain these phenomena, among them increased sensitivity to catecholamines because of increased numbers of beta receptors.

Although beta-adrenergic receptor blockade is useful in the treatment of angina and hypertension, there are also situations in which sympathetic stimulation is vital. For example, in patients with severely damaged hearts, adequate ventricular function may depend on sympathetic drive. Beta-adrenergic blockade may worsen AV block by preventing the necessary facilitating effects of sympathetic activity on conduction. Beta$_2$-adrenergic blockade results in passive bronchial constriction by interfering with endogenous adrenergic bronchodilator activity in patients subject to bronchospasm and may also interfere with exogenous bronchodilators in such patients.

Pharmacokinetics and Metabolism Labetalol HCl is completely absorbed from the gastrointestinal tract with peak plasma levels occurring 1 to 2 hours after oral administration. The relative bioavailability of labetalol HCl tablets compared to an oral solution is 100%. The absolute bioavailability (fraction of drug reaching systemic circulation) of labetalol when compared to an intravenous infusion is 25%; this is due to extensive "first-pass" metabolism. Despite "first-pass" metabolism there is a linear relationship between oral doses of 100 to 3000 mg and peak plasma levels. The absolute bioavailability of labetalol is increased when administered with food.

The plasma half-life of labetalol following oral administration is about 6 to 8 hours. Steady-state plasma levels of labetalol during repetitive dosing are reached by about the third day of dosing. In patients with decreased hepatic or renal function, the elimination half-life of labetalol is not altered; however, the relative bioavailability in hepatically impaired patients is increased due to decreased "first-pass" metabolism.

The metabolism of labetalol is mainly through conjugation to glucuronide metabolites. These metabolites are present in plasma and are excreted in the urine and, via the bile, into the feces. Approximately 55% to 60% of a dose appears in the urine as conjugates or unchanged labetalol within the first 24 hours of dosing.

Labetalol has been shown to cross the placental barrier in humans. Only negligible amounts of the drug crossed the blood-brain barrier in animal studies. Labetalol is approximately 50% protein bound. Neither hemodialysis nor peritoneal dialysis removes a significant amount of labetalol HCl from the general circulation (<1%).

INDICATIONS AND USAGE

NORMODYNE (labetalol HCl) Tablets are indicated in the management of hypertension. NORMODYNE Tablets may be used alone or in combination with other antihypertensive agents, especially thiazide and loop diuretics.

CONTRAINDICATIONS

NORMODYNE (labetalol HCl) Tablets are contraindicated in bronchial asthma, overt cardiac failure, greater than first degree heart block, cardiogenic shock, severe bradycardia, other conditions associated with severe and prolonged hypotension, and in patients with a history of hypersensitivity to any component of the product (see **WARNINGS**).

WARNINGS

Hepatic Injury Severe hepatocellular injury, confirmed by rechallenge in at least one case, occurs rarely with labetalol therapy. The hepatic injury is usually reversible, but hepatic

necrosis and death have been reported. Injury has occurred after both short- and long-term treatment and may be slowly progressive despite minimal symptomatology. Similar hepatic events have been reported with a related compound, dilevalol HCl, including two deaths. Dilevalol HCl is one of the four isomers of labetalol HCl. Thus, for patients taking labetalol, periodic determination of suitable hepatic laboratory tests would be appropriate. Laboratory testing should also be done at the very first symptom or sign of liver dysfunction (eg, pruritis, dark urine, persistent anorexia, jaundice, right upper quadrant tenderness, or unexplained "flu-like" symptoms). If the patient has jaundice or laboratory evidence of liver injury, labetalol HCl should be stopped and not restarted.

Cardiac Failure Sympathetic stimulation is a vital component supporting circulatory function in congestive heart failure. Beta blockade carries a potential hazard of further depressing myocardial contractility and precipitating more severe failure. Although beta-blockers should be avoided in overt congestive heart failure, if necessary, labetalol HCl can be used with caution in patients with a history of heart failure who are well-compensated. Congestive heart failure has been observed in patients receiving labetalol HCl. Labetalol HCl does not abolish the inotropic action of digitalis on heart muscle.

In Patients Without a History of Cardiac Failure In patients with latent cardiac insufficiency, continued depression of the myocardium with beta-blocking agents over a period of time can, in some cases, lead to cardiac failure. At the first sign or symptom of impending cardiac failure, patients should be fully digitalized and/or be given a diuretic, and the response observed closely. If cardiac failure continues, despite adequate digitalization and diuretic, NORMODYNE (labetalol HCl) therapy should be withdrawn (gradually if possible).

Exacerbation of Ischemic Heart Disease Following Abrupt Withdrawal Angina pectoris has not been reported upon labetalol HCl discontinuation. However, hypersensitivity to catecholamines has been observed in patients withdrawn from beta-blocker therapy; exacerbation of angina and, in some cases, myocardial infarction have occurred after *abrupt* discontinuation of such therapy. When discontinuing chronically administered NORMODYNE (labetalol HCl), particularly in patients with ischemic heart disease, the dosage should be gradually reduced over a period of 1 to 2 weeks and the patient should be carefully monitored. If angina markedly worsens or acute coronary insufficiency develops, NORMODYNE (labetalol HCl) administration should be reinstituted promptly, at least temporarily, and other measures appropriate for the management of unstable angina should be taken. Patients should be warned against interruption or discontinuation of therapy without the physician's advice. Because coronary artery disease is common and may be unrecognized, it may be prudent not to discontinue NORMODYNE (labetalol HCl) therapy abruptly even in patients treated only for hypertension.

Nonallergic bronchospasm (eg, chronic bronchitis and emphysema) patients with bronchospastic disease should, in general, not receive beta-blockers. NORMODYNE (labetalol HCl) may be used with caution, however, in patients who do not respond to, or cannot tolerate, other antihypertensive agents. It is prudent, if NORMODYNE (labetalol HCl) is used, to use the smallest effective dose, so that inhibition of endogenous or exogenous beta-agonists is minimized.

Pheochromocytoma Labetalol HCl has been shown to be effective in lowering the blood pressure and relieving symptoms in patients with pheochromocytoma. However, paradoxical hypertensive responses have been reported in a few patients with this tumor; therefore, use caution when administering labetalol HCl to patients with pheochromocytoma.

Diabetes Mellitus and Hypoglycemia Beta-adrenergic blockade may prevent the appearance of premonitory signs and symptoms (eg, tachycardia) of acute hypoglycemia. This is especially important with labile diabetics. Beta-blockade also reduces the release of insulin in response to hyperglycemia; it may therefore be necessary to adjust the dose of antidiabetic drugs.

Major Surgery The necessity or desirability of withdrawing beta-blocking therapy prior to major surgery is controversial. Protracted severe hypotension and difficulty in restarting or maintaining a heartbeat have been reported with beta-blockers. The effect of labetalol HCl's alpha-adrenergic activity has not been evaluated in this setting.

A synergism between labetalol HCl and halothane anesthesia has been shown (see **PRECAUTIONS–Drug Interactions**).

PRECAUTIONS

General *Impaired Hepatic Function* NORMODYNE (labetalol HCl) Tablets should be used with caution in patients with impaired hepatic function since metabolism of the drug may be diminished.

Jaundice or Hepatic Dysfunction (see **WARNINGS**).

Information for Patients
As with all drugs with beta-blocking activity, certain advice to patients being treated with labetalol HCl is warranted. This information is intended to aid in the safe and effective use of this medication. It is not a disclosure of all possible adverse or intended effects. While no incident of the abrupt withdrawal phenomenon (exacerbation of angina pectoris) has been reported with labetalol HCl, dosing with NORMODYNE (labetalol HCl) Tablets should not be interrupted or discontinued without a physician's advice. Patients being treated with NORMODYNE (labetalol HCl) Tablets should consult a physician at any signs or symptoms of impending cardiac failure or hepatic dysfunction (see **WARNINGS**). Also, transient scalp tingling may occur, usually when treatment with NORMODYNE (labetalol HCl) Tablets is initiated (see **ADVERSE REACTIONS**).

Laboratory Tests
As with any new drug given over prolonged periods, laboratory parameters should be observed over regular intervals. In patients with concomitant illnesses, such as impaired renal function, appropriate tests should be done to monitor these conditions.

Drug Interactions
In one survey, 2.3% of patients taking labetalol HCl in combination with tricyclic antidepressants experienced tremor as compared to 0.7% reported to occur with labetalol HCl alone. The contribution of each of the treatments to this adverse reaction is unknown but the possibility of a drug interaction cannot be excluded.

Drugs possessing beta-blocking properties can blunt the bronchodilator effect of beta-receptor agonist drugs in patients with bronchospasm; therefore, doses greater than the normal anti-asthmatic dose of beta-agonist bronchodilator drugs may be required.

Cimetidine has been shown to increase the bioavailability of labetalol HCl. Since this could be explained either by enhanced absorption or by an alteration of hepatic metabolism of labetalol HCl, special care should be used in establishing the dose required for blood pressure control in such patients. Synergism has been shown between halothane anesthesia and intravenously administered labetalol HCl. During controlled hypotensive anesthesia using labetalol HCl in association with halothane, high concentrations (3% or above) of halothane should not be used because the degree of hypotension will be increased and because of the possibility of a large reduction in cardiac output and an increase in central venous pressure. The anesthesiologist should be informed when a patient is receiving labetalol HCl.

Labetalol HCl blunts the reflex tachycardia produced by nitroglycerin without preventing its hypotensive effect. If labetalol HCl is used with nitroglycerin in patients with angina pectoris, additional antihypertensive effects may occur. Care should be taken if labetalol HCl is used concomitantly with calcium antagonists of the verapamil type.

Risk of Anaphylactic Reaction While taking beta-blockers, patients with a history of severe anaphylactic reaction to a variety of allergens may be more reactive to repeated challenge, either accidental, diagnostic, or therapeutic. Such patients may be unresponsive to the usual doses of epinephrine used to treat allergic reaction.

Drug/Laboratory Test Interactions
The presence of labetalol metabolites in the urine may result in falsely elevated levels of urinary catecholamines, metanephrine, normetanephrine, and vanillylmandelic acid (VMA) when measured by fluorimetric or photometric methods. In screening patients suspected of having a pheochromocytoma and being treated with labetalol HCl, a specific method, such as a high performance liquid chromatographic assay with solid phase extraction (eg, *J Chromatogr* 385:241,1987) should be employed in determining levels of catecholamines.

Labetalol HCl has also been reported to produce a false-positive test for amphetamine when screening urine for the presence of drugs using the commercially available assay methods Toxi-Lab A® (thin-layer chromatographic assay) and Emit-d.a.u.® (radioenzymatic assay). When patients being treated with labetalol HCl have a positive urine test for amphetamine using these techniques, confirmation should be made by using more specific methods, such as a gas chromatographic-mass spectrometer technique.

Carcinogenesis, Mutagenesis, Impairment of Fertility
Long-term oral dosing studies with labetalol HCl for 18 months in mice and for 2 years in rats showed no evidence of carcinogenesis. Studies with labetalol HCl, using dominant lethal assays in rats and mice, and exposing microorganisms according to modified Ames tests, showed no evidence of mutagenesis.

Pregnancy Category C
Teratogenic studies have been performed with labetalol HCl in rats and rabbits at oral doses up to approximately 6 and 4 times the maximum recommended human dose (MRHD), respectively. No reproducible evidence of fetal malformations was observed. Increased fetal resorptions were seen in both species at doses approximating the MRHD. A teratology study performed with labetalol HCl in rabbits at intravenous doses up to 1.7 times the MRHD revealed no evidence of drug-related harm to the fetus. There are no adequate and well-controlled studies in pregnant women. Labetalol HCl should be used during pregnancy only if the potential benefit justifies the potential risk to the fetus.

Nonteratogenic Effects
Hypotension, bradycardia, hypoglycemia, and respiratory depression have been reported in infants of mothers who were treated with labetalol HCl for hypertension during pregnancy. Oral administration of labetalol to rats during late gestation through weaning at doses of 2 to 4 times the MRHD caused a decrease in neonatal survival.

Labor and Delivery
Labetalol HCl given to pregnant women with hypertension did not appear to affect the usual course of labor and delivery.

Nursing Mothers
Small amounts of labetalol (approximately 0.004% of the maternal dose) are excreted in human milk. Caution should be exercised when NORMODYNE (labetalol HCl) Tablets are administered to a nursing woman.

Pediatric Use
Safety and effectiveness in children have not been established.

ADVERSE REACTIONS

Most adverse effects are mild, transient and occur early in the course of treatment. In controlled clinical trials of 3 to 4 months duration, discontinuation of NORMODYNE (labetalol HCl) Tablets due to one or more adverse effects was required in 7% of all patients. In these same trials, beta-blocker control agents led to discontinuation in 8% to 10% of patients, and a centrally acting alpha-agonist in 30% of patients.

The incidence rates of adverse reactions listed in the following table were derived from multicenter controlled clinical trials, comparing labetalol HCl, placebo, metoprolol, and propranolol, over treatment periods of 3 and 4 months. Where the frequency of adverse effects for labetalol HCl and placebo is similar, causal relationship is uncertain. The rates are based on adverse reactions considered probably drug related by the investigator. If all reports are considered, the rates are somewhat higher (eg, dizziness 20%, nausea 14%, fatigue 11%), but the overall conclusions are unchanged.
[See table at top of next page.]

The adverse effects were reported spontaneously and are representative of the incidence of adverse effects that may be observed in a properly selected hypertensive patient population, ie, a group excluding patients with bronchospastic disease, overt congestive heart failure, or other contraindications to beta-blocker therapy.

Clinical trials also included studies utilizing daily doses up to 2400 mg in more severely hypertensive patients. Certain of the side effects increased with increasing dose as shown in the table below which depicts the entire U.S. therapeutic trials data base for adverse reactions that are clearly or possibly drug related.
[See second table at top of next page.]

In addition, a number of other less common adverse events have been reported:

Body as a Whole Fever.
Cardiovascular Hypotension, and rarely, syncope, bradycardia, heart block.
Central and Peripheral Nervous Systems Paresthesias, most frequently described as scalp tingling. In most cases, it was mild, transient and usually occurred at the beginning of treatment.
Collagen Disorders Systemic lupus erythematosus; positive antinuclear factor (ANF).
Eyes Dry eyes.
Immunological System Antimitochondrial antibodies.
Liver and Biliary System Hepatic necrosis; hepatitis; cholestatic jaundice; elevated liver function tests.
Musculoskeletal System Muscle cramps; toxic myopathy.
Respiratory System Bronchospasm.
Skin and Appendages Rashes of various types, such as generalized maculopapular; lichenoid; urticarial; bullous lichen planus; psoriaform; facial erythema; Peyronie's disease; reversible alopecia.
Urinary System Difficulty in micturition, including acute urinary bladder retention.
Hypersensitivity Rare reports of hypersensitivity (eg, rash, urticaria, pruritus, angioedema, dyspnea) and anaphylactoid reactions.

Following approval for marketing in the United Kingdom, a monitored release survey involving approximately 6,800 patients was conducted for further safety and efficacy evaluation of this product. Results of this survey indicate that the type, severity, and incidence of adverse effects were comparable to those cited above.

Potential Adverse Effects
In addition, other adverse effects not listed above have been reported with other beta-adrenergic blocking agents.
Central Nervous System Reversible mental depression progressing to catatonia; an acute reversible syndrome charac-

Continued on next page

Information on Schering products appearing on these pages is effective as of August 15, 1996.

Schering—Cont.

Body as a whole	Labetalol HCl (N=227) %	Placebo (N=98) %	Propranolol (N=84) %	Metoprolol (N=49) %
fatigue	5	0	12	12
asthenia	1	1	1	0
headache	2	1	1	2
Gastrointestinal				
nausea	6	1	1	2
vomiting	<1	0	0	0
dyspepsia	3	1	1	0
abdominal pain	0	0	1	2
diarrhea	<1	0	2	0
taste distortion	1	0	0	0
Central and Peripheral Nervous Systems				
dizziness	11	3	4	4
paresthesias	<1	0	0	0
drowsiness	<1	2	2	2
Autonomic Nervous System				
nasal stuffiness	3	0	0	0
ejaculation failure	2	0	0	0
impotence	1	0	1	3
increased sweating	<1	0	0	0
Cardiovascular				
edema	1	0	0	0
postural hypotension	1	0	0	0
bradycardia	0	0	5	12
Respiratory				
dyspnea	2	0	1	2
Skin				
rash	1	0	0	0
Special Senses				
vision abnormality	1	0	0	0
vertigo	2	1	0	0

Labetalol HCl

Daily Dose (mg)	200	300	400	600	800	900	1200	1600	2400
Number of Patients	522	181	606	608	503	117	411	242	175
Dizziness (%)	2	3	3	3	5	1	9	13	16
Fatigue	2	1	4	4	5	3	7	6	10
Nausea	<1	0	1	2	4	0	7	11	19
Vomiting	0	0	<1	<1	<1	0	1	2	3
Dyspepsia	1	0	2	1	1	0	2	2	4
Paresthesias	2	0	2	2	1	1	2	5	5
Nasal Stuffiness	1	1	2	2	2	2	4	5	6
Ejaculation Failure	0	2	1	2	3	0	4	3	5
Impotence	1	1	1	1	2	4	3	4	3
Edema	1	0	1	1	1	0	1	2	2

terized by disorientation for time and place, short-term memory loss, emotional lability, slightly clouded sensorium, and decreased performance on neuropsychometrics.
Cardiovascular Intensification of AV block (see **CONTRAINDICATIONS**).
Allergic Fever combined with aching and sore throat; laryngospasm; respiratory distress.
Hematologic Agranulocytosis; thrombocytopenic or non-thrombocytopenic purpura.
Gastrointestinal Mesenteric artery thrombosis; ischemic colitis.
The oculomucocutaneous syndrome associated with the beta-blocker practolol has not been reported with labetalol HCl.

Clinical Laboratory Tests
There have been reversible increases of serum transaminases in 4% of patients treated with labetalol HCl and tested, and more rarely, reversible increases in blood urea.

OVERDOSAGE
Overdosage with NORMODYNE (labetalol HCl) Tablets causes excessive hypotension that is posture sensitive, and sometimes, excessive bradycardia. Patients should be placed supine and their legs raised if necessary to improve the blood supply to the brain. If overdosage with labetalol HCl follows oral ingestion, gastric lavage or pharmacologically induced emesis (using syrup of ipecac) may be useful for removal of the drug shortly after ingestion. The following additional measures should be employed if necessary: *Excessive bradycardia*—administer atropine or epinephrine. *Cardic failure*—administer a digitalis glycoside and a diuretic. Dopamine or dobutamine may also be useful. *Hypotension*—administer vasopressors, eg, norepinephrine. There is pharmacological evidence that norepinephrine may be the drug of choice. *Bronchospasm*—administer epinephrine and/or an aerosolized beta₂-agonist. *Seizures*—administer diazepam.
In severe beta-blocker overdose resulting in hypotension and/or bradycardia, glucagon has been shown to be effective when administered in large doses (5 to 10 mg rapidly over 30 seconds, followed by continuous infusion of 5 mg/hr that can be reduced as the patient improves).
Neither hemodialysis nor peritoneal dialysis removes a significant amount of labetalol HCl from the general circulation (<1%).

The oral LD₅₀ value of labetalol HCl in the mouse is approximately 600 mg/kg and in the rat is greater than 2 g/kg. The intravenous LD₅₀ in these species is 50 to 60 mg/kg.

DOSAGE AND ADMINISTRATION
DOSAGE MUST BE INDIVIDUALIZED. The recommended initial dose is 100 mg twice daily whether used alone or added to a diuretic regimen. After 2 or 3 days, using standing blood pressure as an indicator, dosage may be titrated in increments of 100 mg b.i.d. every 2 or 3 days. The usual maintenance dosage of labetalol HCl is between 200 and 400 mg twice daily.
Since the full antihypertensive effect of labetalol HCl is usually seen within the first 1 to 3 hours of the initial dose or dose increment, the assurance of a lack of an exaggerated hypotensive response can be clinically established in the office setting. The antihypertensive effects of continued dosing can be measured at subsequent visits, approximately 12 hours after a dose, to determine whether further titration is necessary.
Patients with severe hypertension may require from 1200 mg to 2400 mg per day, with or without thiazide diuretics. Should side effects (principally nausea or dizziness) occur with these doses administered b.i.d., the same total daily dose administered t.i.d. may improve tolerability and facilitate further titration. Titration increments should not exceed 200 mg b.i.d..
When a diuretic is added, an additive antihypertensive effect can be expected. In some cases this may necessitate a labetalol HCl dosage adjustment. As with most antihypertensive drugs, optimal dosages of NORMODYNE (labetalol HCl) Tablets are usually lower in patients also receiving a diuretic.
When transferring patients from other antihypertensive drugs, NORMODYNE (labetalol HCl) Tablets should be introduced as recommended and the dosage of the existing therapy progressively decreased.

HOW SUPPLIED
NORMODYNE (labetalol HCl) Tablets, 100 mg, light-brown, round, scored, film-coated tablets engraved on one side with Schering and product identification numbers 244, and on the other side the number 100 for the strength and "NORMODYNE"; bottles of 100 (NDC-0085-0244-04), bottles of 500 (NDC-0085-0244-05), bottles of 1000 (NDC-0085-0244-

07), and box of 100 for unit-dose dispensing (NDC-0085-0244-08).
NORMODYNE (labetalol HCl) Tablets, 200 mg, white, round, scored, film-coated tablets engraved on one side with Schering and product identification numbers 752, and on the other side the number 200 for the strength and "NORMODYNE"; bottles of 100 (NDC-0085-0752-04), bottles of 500 (NDC-0085-0752-05), bottles of 1000 (NDC-0085-0752-07), box of 100 for unit-dose dispensing (NDC-0085-0752-08).
NORMODYNE (labetalol HCl) Tablets, 300 mg, blue, round, film-coated tablets engraved on one side with Schering and product identification numbers 438, and on the other side the number 300 for the strength and "NORMODYNE"; bottles of 100 (NDC-0085-0438-03), bottles of 500 (NDC-0085-0438-05), box of 100 for unit-dose dispensing (NDC-0085-0438-06).
NORMODYNE (labetalol HCl) Tablets should be stored between 2° and 30°C (36° and 86°F).
NORMODYNE (labetalol HCl) Tablets in the unit-dose boxes should be protected from excessive moisture.
Key Pharmaceuticals, Inc.
Kenilworth, NJ 07033 USA
Rev. 5/94   16833525
Copyright © 1984, 1992, 1994, Schering Corporation. All rights reserved.
Shown in Product Identification Guide, page 334

PROVENTIL®   ℞
brand of albuterol, USP
Inhalation Aerosol
Bronchodilator Aerosol
FOR ORAL INHALATION ONLY

DESCRIPTION
The active component of PROVENTIL Inhalation Aerosol is albuterol, USP racemic (α¹-[(*tert*-butylamino) methyl]-4-hydroxy-*m*-xylene-α,α'-diol), a relatively selective beta₂-adrenergic bronchodilator, having the chemical structure:

Albuterol is the official generic name in the United States. The World Health Organization recommended name for the drug is salbutamol. The molecular weight of albuterol is 239.3, and the empirical formula is $C_{13}H_{21}NO_3$. Albuterol is a white to off-white crystalline solid. It is soluble in ethanol, sparingly soluble in water, and very soluble in chloroform.
PROVENTIL Inhalation Aerosol is a metered-dose aerosol unit for oral inhalation. It contains a microcrystalline suspension of albuterol in propellants (trichloromonofluoromethane and dichlorodifluoromethane) with oleic acid. Each actuation delivers from the mouthpiece 90 mcg of albuterol, USP. Each canister provides at least 200 inhalations.

CLINICAL PHARMACOLOGY
In vitro studies and *in vivo* pharmacologic studies have demonstrated that albuterol has a preferential effect on beta₂-adrenergic receptors compared with isoproterenol. While it is recognized that beta₂-adrenergic receptors are the predominant receptors in bronchial smooth muscle, recent data indicate that there is a population of beta₂-receptors in the human heart existing in a concentration between 10% and 50%. The precise function of these, however, is not yet established.
The pharmacologic effects of beta-adrenergic agonist drugs, including albuterol, are at least in part attributable to stimulation through beta-adrenergic receptors of intracellular adenyl cyclase, the enzyme which catalyzes the conversion of adenosine triphosphate (ATP) to cyclic-3', 5'-adenosine monophosphate (c-AMP). Increased c-AMP levels are associated with relaxation of bronchial smooth muscle and inhibition of release of mediators of immediate hypersensitivity from cells, especially from mast cells.
Albuterol has been shown in most controlled clinical trials to have more effect on the respiratory tract, in the form of bronchial smooth muscle relaxation, than isoproterenol at comparable doses while producing fewer cardiovascular effects. Controlled clinical studies and other clinical experience have shown that inhaled albuterol, like other beta-adrenergic agonist drugs, can produce a significant cardiovascular effect in some patients, as measured by pulse rate, blood pressure, symptoms, and/or ECG changes.
Albuterol is longer acting than isoproterenol by any route of administration in most patients because it is not a substrate for the cellular uptake processes for catecholamines nor for catechol-O-methyl transferase.
Because of its gradual absorption from the bronchi, systemic levels of albuterol are low after inhalation of recommended

doses. Studies undertaken with four subjects administered tritiated albuterol resulted in maximum plasma concentrations occurring within 2 to 4 hours. Due to the sensitivity of the assay method, the metabolic rate and half-life of elimination of albuterol in plasma could not be determined. However, urinary excretion provided data indicating that albuterol has an elimination half-life of 3.8 hours. Approximately 72% of the inhaled dose is excreted within 24 hours in the urine, and consists of 28% of unchanged drug and 44% as metabolite.
Results of animal studies show that albuterol does not pass the blood-brain barrier.
Recent studies in laboratory animals (minipigs, rodents, and dogs) recorded the occurrence of cardiac arrhythmias and sudden death (with histologic evidence of myocardial necrosis) when beta-agonists and methylxanthines were administered concurrently. The significance of these findings when applied to humans is currently unknown.
The effects of rising doses of albuterol and isoproterenol aerosols were studied in volunteers and asthmatic patients. Results in normal volunteers indicated that albuterol is $^1/_2$ to $^1/_4$ as active as isoproterenol in producing increases in heart rate. In asthmatic patients similar cardiovascular differentiation between the two drugs was also seen.

INDICATIONS AND USAGE

PROVENTIL Inhalation Aerosol is indicated for the prevention and relief of bronchospasm in patients with reversible obstructive airway disease, and for the prevention of exercise-induced bronchospasm.
In controlled clinical trials the onset of improvement in pulmonary function was within 15 minutes, as determined by both maximal midexpiratory flow rate (MMEF) and FEV_1. MMEF measurements also showed that near maximum improvement in pulmonary function generally occurs within 60 to 90 minutes, following 2 inhalations of albuterol and that clinically significant improvement generally continues for 3 to 4 hours in most patients. In clinical trials, some patients with asthma showed a therapeutic response (defined by maintaining FEV_1 values 15% or more above baseline) which was still apparent at 6 hours. Continued effectiveness of albuterol was demonstrated over a 13-week period in these same trials.
In clinical studies, 2 inhalations of albuterol taken approximately 15 minutes prior to exercise prevented exercise-induced bronchospasm, as demonstrated by the maintenance of FEV_1 within 80% of baseline values in the majority of patients. One of these studies also evaluated the duration of the prophylactic effect to repeated exercise challenges, which was evident at 4 hours in the majority of patients, and at 6 hours in approximately one-third of the patients.

CONTRAINDICATIONS

PROVENTIL Inhalation Aerosol is contraindicated in patients with a history of hypersensitivity to any of its components.

WARNINGS

As with other inhaled beta-adrenergic agonists, PROVENTIL Inhalation Aerosol can produce paradoxical bronchospasm that can be life-threatening. If it occurs, the preparation should be discontinued immediately and alternative therapy instituted.
Fatalities have been reported in association with excessive use of inhaled sympathomimetic drugs. The exact cause of death is unknown, but cardiac arrest following the unexpected development of a severe acute asthmatic crisis and subsequent hypoxia is suspected.
Immediate hypersensitivity reactions may occur after administration of albuterol inhalation aerosol, as demonstrated by rare cases of urticaria, angioedema, rash, bronchospasm, anaphylaxis, and oropharyngeal edema.
The contents of PROVENTIL Inhalation Aerosol are under pressure. Do not puncture. Do not use or store near heat or open flame. Exposure to temperatures above 120°F may cause bursting. Never throw container into fire or incinerator. Keep out of reach of children.

PRECAUTIONS

General: Albuterol, as with all sympathomimetic amines, should be used with caution in patients with cardiovascular disorders, especially coronary insufficiency, cardiac arrhythmias, and hypertension; in patients with convulsive disorders, hyperthyroidism, or diabetes mellitus; and in patients who are unusually responsive to sympathomimetic amines.
Large doses of intravenous albuterol have been reported to aggravate preexisting diabetes and ketoacidosis. Additionally, beta-agonists, including albuterol, when given intraveneously may cause a decrease in serum potassium, possibly through intracellular shunting. The relevance of this observation to the use of PROVENTIL Inhalation Aerosol is unknown, since the aerosol dose is much lower than the doses given intravenously.
Although there have been no reports concerning the use of PROVENTIL Inhalation Aerosol during labor and delivery, it has been reported that high doses of albuterol administered intravenously inhibit uterine contractions. Although this effect is extremely unlikely as a consequence of aerosol use, it should be kept in mind.
Information For Patients: The action of PROVENTIL Inhalation Aerosol may last up to 6 hours and therefore it should not be used more frequently than recommended. Increasing the number or frequency of doses without consulting your physician can be dangerous. If recommended dosage does not provide relief of symptoms or symptoms become worse, seek immediate medical attention. While taking PROVENTIL Inhalation Aerosol, other inhaled medicines should not be used unless prescribed.
See Illustrated Patient's Instructions For Use.
Drug Interactions: Other sympathomimetic aerosol bronchodilators should not be used concomitantly with albuterol. If additional adrenergic drugs are to be administered by any route, they should be used with caution to avoid deleterious cardiovascular effects.
Albuterol should be administered with caution to patients being treated with monoamine oxidase inhibitors or tricyclic antidepressants, since the action of albuterol on the vascular system may be potentiated.
Beta-receptor blocking agents and albuterol inhibit the effect of each other.
Since albuterol may lower serum potassium, care should be taken in patients also using other drugs which lower serum potassium as the effects may be additive.
Carcinogenesis, Mutagenesis, and Impairment of Fertility: In a 2-year study in the rat, albuterol sulfate caused a significant dose-related increase in the incidence of benign leiomyomas of the mesovarium at doses corresponding to 111, 555, and 2,800 times the maximum human inhalational dose. In another study this effect was blocked by the coadministration of propranolol. The relevance of these findings to humans is not known. An 18-month study in mice revealed no evidence of tumorigenicity. Studies with albuterol revealed no evidence of mutagenesis. Reproduction studies in rats revealed no evidence of impaired fertility.
Teratogenic Effects — Pregnancy Category C: Albuterol has been shown to be teratogenic in mice when given in doses corresponding to 14 times the human dose. There are no adequate and well-controlled studies in pregnant women. Albuterol should be used during pregnancy only if the potential benefit justifies the potential risk to the fetus. A reproduction study in CD-1 mice with albuterol (0.025, 0.25, and 2.5 mg/kg, corresponding to 1.4, 14, and 140 times the maximum human inhalational dose) showed cleft palate formation in 5 of 111 (4.5%) fetuses at 0.25 mg/kg and in 10 of 108 (9.3 %) fetuses at 2.5 mg/kg. None were observed at 0.025 mg/kg. Cleft palate also occurred in 22 of 72 (30.5%) fetuses treated with 2.5 mg/kg isoproterenol (positive control). A reproduction study in Stride Dutch rabbits revealed cranioschisis in 7 of 19 (37%) fetuses at 50 mg/kg, corresponding to 2,800 times the maximum human inhalational dose of albuterol. During marketing, various congenital anomalies, including cleft palate and limb defects, have been reported in the offspring of patients being treated with albuterol. Some of the mothers were taking multiple medications during their pregnancies. Because no consistent pattern of defects can be discerned, a relationship between albuterol use and congenital anomalies cannot be established.
Nursing Mothers: It is not known whether this drug is excreted in human milk. Because of the potential for tumorigenicity shown for albuterol in animal studies, a decision should be made whether to discontinue nursing or to discontinue the drug, taking into account the importance of the drug to the mother.
Pediatric Use: Safety and effectiveness in children below the age of 12 years have not been established.

ADVERSE REACTIONS

The adverse reactions of albuterol are similar in nature to those of other sympathomimetic agents, although the incidence of certain cardiovascular effects is less with albuterol. A 13-week double-blind study compared albuterol and isoproterenol aerosols in 147 asthmatic patients. The results of this study showed that the incidence of cardiovascular effects was: palpitations, less than 10 per 100 with albuterol and less than 15 per 100 with isoproterenol; tachycardia, 10 per 100 with both albuterol and isoproterenol; and increased blood pressure, less than 5 per 100 with both albuterol and isoproterenol. In the same study, both drugs caused tremor or nausea in less than 15 patients per 100; dizziness or heartburn in less than 5 per 100 patients. Nervousness occurred in less than 10 per 100 patients receiving albuterol and in less than 15 per 100 patients receiving isoproterenol.
Rare cases of urticaria, angioedema, rash, bronchospasm, and oropharyngeal edema have been reported after the use of inhaled albuterol.
In addition, albuterol, like other sympathomimetic agents, can cause adverse reactions such as hypertension, angina, vomiting, vertigo, central nervous system stimulation, insomnia, headache, unusual taste, and drying or irritation of the oropharynx.

OVERDOSAGE

Manifestations of overdosage may include anginal pain, hypertension, hypokalemia, and exaggeration of the pharmacological effects listed in **ADVERSE REACTIONS.**
As with all sympathomimetic aerosol medications, cardiac arrest and even death may be associated with abuse.
The oral LD_{50} in male and female rats and mice was greater than 2,000 mg/kg. The aerosol LD_{50} could not be determined.
Dialysis is not appropriate treatment for overdosage of PROVENTIL Inhalation Aerosol. The judicious use of a cardioselective beta-receptor blocker, such as metoprolol tartrate, is suggested, bearing in mind the danger of inducing an asthmatic attack.

DOSAGE AND ADMINISTRATION

For treatment of acute episodes of bronchospasm or prevention of asthmatic symptoms, the usual dosage for adults and children 12 years and older is 2 inhalations repeated every 4 to 6 hours; in some patients, 1 inhalation every 4 hours may be sufficient. More frequent administration or a larger number of inhalations is not recommended. For maintenance therapy or prevention of exacerbation of bronchospasm, 2 inhalations, 4 times a day should be sufficient.
The use of PROVENTIL Inhalation Aerosol can be continued as medically indicated to control recurring bouts of bronchospasm. During this time most patients gain optimal benefit from regular use of the inhaler. Safe usage for periods extending over several years has been documented.
If a previously effective dosage regimen fails to provide the usual relief, medical advice should be sought immediately, as this is often a sign of seriously worsening asthma which would require reassessment of therapy.
Exercise-Induced Bronchospasm Prevention: The usual dosage for adults and children 12 years and older is 2 inhalations, 15 minutes prior to exercise.
For treatment, see above.

HOW SUPPLIED

PROVENTIL Inhalation Aerosol, 17.0 g canister box of one (NDC-0085-0614-02); and 6.8 g canister for institutional use only, box of one (NDC-0085-0615-10). Each actuation delivers 90 mcg of albuterol from the mouthpiece. Each canister is supplied with an oral adapter and Patient's Instructions. PROVENTIL Inhalation Aerosol REFILL canister, 17.0 g, with Patient's Instructions; box of one (NDC-0085-0614-03).
Store between 15° and 30°C (59° and 86°F). Failure to use the product within this temperature range may result in improper dosing. Shake well before using.
NOTE: The indented statement below is required by the Federal government's Clean Air Act for all products containing or manufactured with chlorofluorocarbons (CFCs).

> **WARNING:** Contains dichlorodifluoromethane (CFC-11) and trichloromonofluoromethane (CFC-12), substances which harm public health and the environment by destroying ozone in the upper atmosphere.

A notice similar to the above WARNING has been placed in the "Patient's Instructions for Use" portion of this package insert pursuant to EPA regulations.

Rev. 10/94 18206811
Shown in Product Identification Guide, page 334

PROVENTIL® ℞

brand of albuterol sulfate, USP
Solution for Inhalation 0.5%*
(*Potency expressed as albuterol)

DESCRIPTION

PROVENTIL Solution for Inhalation contains albuterol sulfate, USP, the racemic form of albuterol and a relatively selective beta$_2$-adrenergic bronchodilator (see **CLINICAL PHARMACOLOGY** section below). Albuterol sulfate has the chemical name α^1-[(*tert*-Butylamino) methyl]-4-hydroxy-*m*-xylene-α,α'-diol sulfate (2:1) (salt), and the following chemical structure:

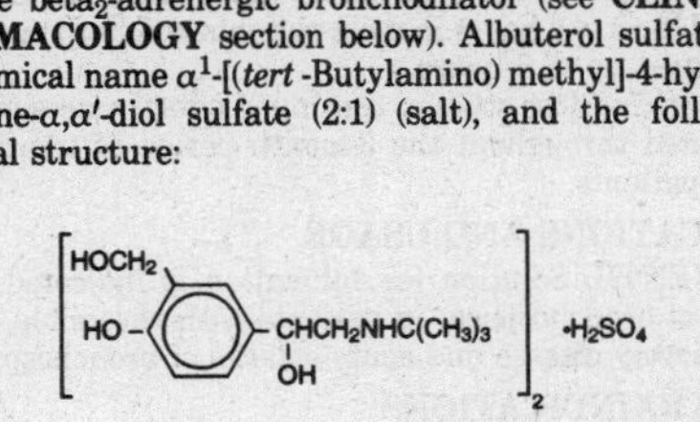
HOCH2
HO
CHCH2NHC(CH3)3
OH
•H2SO4
2

Albuterol sulfate has a molecular weight of 576.7 and the empirical formula $(C_{13}H_{21}NO_3)_2 \cdot H_2SO_4$. Albuterol sulfate is

Continued on next page

Information on Schering products appearing on these pages is effective as of August 15, 1996.

Schering—Cont.

a white crystalline powder, soluble in water and slightly soluble in ethanol.

The World Health Organization's recommended name for albuterol base is salbutamol.

PROVENTIL Solution for Inhalation 0.5% is in concentrated form. Dilute 0.5 mL of the solution to 3 mL with sterile normal saline solution prior to administration.

Each mL of PROVENTIL Solution for Inhalation 0.5% contains 5 mg of albuterol (as 6.0 mg of albuterol sulfate) in an aqueous solution containing benzalkonium chloride; sulfuric acid is used to adjust the pH between 3 and 5. PROVENTIL Solution for Inhalation 0.5% contains no sulfiting agents. It is supplied in 20 mL bottles.

PROVENTIL Solution for Inhalation is a clear, colorless to light yellow solution.

CLINICAL PHARMACOLOGY

The prime action of beta-adrenergic drugs is to stimulate adenyl cyclase, the enzyme which catalyzes the formation of cyclic-3',5'-adenosine monophosphate (cyclic AMP) from adenosine triphosphate (ATP). The cyclic AMP thus formed mediates the cellular responses. *In vitro* studies and *in vivo* pharmacologic studies have demonstrated that albuterol has a preferential effect on $beta_2$-adrenergic receptors compared with isoproterenol. While it is recognized that $beta_2$-adrenergic receptors are the predominant receptors in bronchial smooth muscle, recent data indicate that 10% to 50% of the beta receptors in the human heart may be $beta_2$ receptors. The precise function of these receptors, however, is not yet established. Albuterol has been shown in most controlled clinical trials to have more effect on the respiratory tract, in the form of bronchial smooth muscle relaxation, than isoproterenol at comparable doses while producing fewer cardiovascular effects. Controlled clinical studies and other clinical experience have shown that inhaled albuterol, like other beta-adrenergic agonist drugs, can produce a significant cardiovascular effect in some patients, as measured by pulse rate, blood pressure, symptoms, and/or ECG changes.

Albuterol is longer acting than isoproterenol in most patients by any route of administration because it is not a substrate for the cellular uptake processes for catecholamines nor for catechol-*O*-methyl transferase.

Studies in asthmatic patients have shown that less than 20% of a single albuterol dose was absorbed following either IPPB or nebulizer administration; the remaining amount was recovered from the nebulizer and apparatus and expired air. Most of the absorbed dose was recovered in the urine 24 hours after drug administration. Following a 3.0 mg dose of nebulized albuterol, the maximum albuterol plasma level at 0.5 hour was 2.1 ng/mL (range 1.4 to 3.2 ng/mL). There was a significant dose-related response in FEV_1 and peak flow rate (PFR). It has been demonstrated that following oral administration of 4 mg albuterol, the elimination half-life was 5 to 6 hours.

Animal studies show that albuterol does not pass the blood-brain barrier. Recent studies in laboratory animals (minipigs, rodents, and dogs) recorded the occurrence of cardiac arrhythmias and sudden death (with histologic evidence of myocardial necrosis) when beta-agonists and methylxanthines were administered concurrently. The significance of these findings when applied to humans is currently unknown.

In controlled clinical trials, most patients exhibited an onset of improvement in pulmonary function within 5 minutes as determined by FEV_1. FEV_1 measurements also showed that the maximum average improvement in pulmonary function usually occurred at approximately 1 hour following inhalation of 2.5 mg of albuterol by compressor-nebulizer, and remained close to peak for 2 hours. Clinically significant improvement in pulmonary function (defined as maintenance of a 15% or more increase in FEV_1 over baseline values) continued for 3 to 4 hours in most patients and in some patients continued up to 6 hours.

In repetitive dose studies, continued effectiveness was demonstrated throughout the 3-month period of treatment in some patients.

INDICATIONS AND USAGE

PROVENTIL Solution for Inhalation is indicated for the relief of bronchospasm in patients with reversible obstructive airway disease and acute attacks of bronchospasm.

CONTRAINDICATIONS

PROVENTIL Solution for Inhalation is contraindicated in patients with a history of hypersensitivity to any of its components.

WARNINGS

As with other inhaled beta-adrenergic agonists, PROVENTIL Solution for Inhalation can produce paradoxical bronchospasm, which can be life threatening. If it occurs, the preparation should be discontinued immediately and alternative therapy instituted.

Fatalities have been reported in association with excessive use of inhaled sympathomimetic drugs and with the home use of sympathomimetic nebulizers. It is, therefore, essential that the physician instruct the patient in the need for further evaluation if his/her asthma becomes worse. In individual patients, any $beta_2$-adrenergic agonist, including albuterol inhalation solution and solution for inhalation, may have a clinically significant cardiac effect.

Immediate hypersensitivity reactions may occur after administration of albuterol as demonstrated by rare cases of urticaria, angioedema, rash, bronchospasm, and oropharyngeal edema.

PRECAUTIONS

General: Albuterol, as with all sympathomimetic amines, should be used with caution in patients with cardiovascular disorders, especially coronary insufficiency, cardiac arrhythmias and hypertension, in patients with convulsive disorders, hyperthyroidism or diabetes mellitus, and in patients who are unusually responsive to sympathomimetic amines.

Large doses of intravenous albuterol have been reported to aggravate preexisting diabetes mellitus and ketoacidosis. Additionally, beta-agonists, including albuterol, when given intravenously may cause a decrease in serum potassium, possibly through intracellular shunting. The decrease is usually transient, not requiring supplementation. The relevance of these observations to the use of PROVENTIL Solution for Inhalation is unknown.

To avoid contaminating the multi-dose bottle of PROVENTIL Solution for Inhalation, proper aseptic technique should be used when withdrawing and delivering the dose into the nebulizer.

Information For Patients: The action of PROVENTIL Solution for Inhalation may last up to 6 hours and therefore it should not be used more frequently than recommended. Do not increase the dose or frequency of medication without medical consultation. If symptoms get worse, medical consultation should be sought promptly. While taking PROVENTIL Solution for Inhalation, other anti-asthma medicines should not be used unless prescribed.

Drug stability and safety of PROVENTIL Solution for Inhalation when mixed with other drugs in a nebulizer have not been established.

See illustrated **"Patient's Instructions for Use."**

Drug Interactions: Other sympathomimetic aerosol bronchodilators or epinephrine should not be used concomitantly with albuterol.

Albuterol should be administered with extreme caution to patients being treated with monoamine oxidase inhibitors or tricyclic antidepressants, since the action of albuterol on the vascular system may be potentiated.

Beta-receptor blocking agents and albuterol inhibit the effect of each other.

Since albuterol may lower serum potassium, care should be taken in patients also using other drugs which lower serum potassium as the effects may be additive.

Carcinogenesis, Mutagenesis, and Impairment of Fertility: Albuterol sulfate, like other agents in its class, caused a significant dose-related increase in the incidence of benign leiomyomas of the mesovarium in a 2-year study in the rat, at oral doses corresponding to 10, 50, and 250 times the maximum human nebulizer dose. In another study, this effect was blocked by the coadministration of propranolol. The relevance of these findings to humans is not known. An 18-month study in mice and a lifetime study in hamsters revealed no evidence of tumorigenicity. Studies with albuterol revealed no evidence of mutagenesis. Reproduction studies in rats revealed no evidence of impaired fertility.

Teratogenic Effects—Pregnancy Category C: Albuterol has been shown to be teratogenic in mice when given subcutaneously in doses corresponding to the human nebulization dose. There are no adequate and well-controlled studies in pregnant women. Albuterol should be used during pregnancy only if the potential benefit justifies the potential risk to the fetus. A reproduction study in CD-1 mice with albuterol (0.025, 0.25, and 2.5 mg/kg subcutaneously, corresponding to 0.1, 1, and 12.5 times the maximum human nebulization dose, respectively) showed cleft palate formation in 5 of 111 (4.5%) fetuses at 0.25 mg/kg and in 10 of 108 (9.3%) fetuses at 2.5 mg/kg. None were observed at 0.025 mg/kg. Cleft palate also occurred in 22 of 72 (30.5%) fetuses treated with 2.5 mg/kg isoproterenol (positive control). A reproduction study in Stride Dutch rabbits revealed cranioschisis in 7 of 19 (37%) fetuses at 50 mg/kg, corresponding to 250 times the maximum human nebulization dose. During marketing, various congenital anomalies, including cleft palate and limb defects, have been reported in the offspring of patients being treated with albuterol. Some of the mothers were taking multiple medications during their pregnancies. Because no consistent pattern of defects can be discerned, a relationship between albuterol use and congenital anomalies cannot be established.

Labor and Delivery: Oral albuterol has been shown to delay preterm labor in some reports. There are presently no well-controlled studies which demonstrate that it will stop preterm labor or prevent labor at term. Therefore, cautious use of PROVENTIL Solution for Inhalation is required in pregnant patients when given for relief of bronchospasm so as to avoid interference with uterine contractibility.

Nursing Mothers: It is not known whether this drug is excreted in human milk. Because of the potential for tumorigenicity shown for albuterol in some animal studies, a decision should be made whether to discontinue nursing or to discontinue the drug, taking into account the importance of the drug to the mother.

Pediatric Use: Safety and effectiveness of albuterol inhalation solution and solution for inhalation in children below the age of 12 years have not been established.

ADVERSE REACTIONS

The results of clinical trials with PROVENTIL Solution for Inhalation in 135 patients showed the following side effects which were considered probably or possibly drug related:

Central Nervous System: tremors (20%), dizziness (7%), nervousness (4%), headache (3%), insomnia (1%).

Gastrointestinal: nausea (4%), dyspepsia (1%).

Ear, Nose, Throat: pharyngitis (<1%), nasal congestion (1%).

Cardiovascular: tachycardia (1%), hypertension (1%).

Respiratory: bronchospasm (8%), cough (4%), bronchitis (4%), wheezing (1%).

No clinically relevant laboratory abnormalities related to PROVENTIL Solution for Inhalation administration were determined in these studies.

In comparing the adverse reactions reported for patients treated with PROVENTIL Solution for Inhalation with those of patients treated with isoproterenol during clinical trials of 3 months, the following moderate to severe reactions, as judged by the investigators, were reported. This table does not include mild reactions.

Percent Incidence of Moderate To Severe Adverse Reactions

Reaction	Albuterol N=65	Isoproterenol N=65
Central Nervous System		
Tremors	10.7%	13.8%
Headache	3.1%	1.5%
Insomnia	3.1%	1.5%
Cardiovascular		
Hypertension	3.1%	3.1%
Arrhythmias	0%	3.0%
*Palpitation	0%	22.0%
Respiratory		
†Bronchospasm	15.4%	18.0%
Cough	3.1%	5.0%
Bronchitis	1.5%	5.0%
Wheeze	1.5%	1.5%
Sputum Increase	1.5%	1.5%
Dyspnea	1.5%	1.5%
Gastrointestinal		
Nausea	3.1%	0%
Dyspepsia	1.5%	0%
Systemic		
Malaise	1.5%	0%

*The finding of no arrhythmias and no palpitations after albuterol administration in this clinical study should not be interpreted as indicating that these adverse effects cannot occur after the administration of inhaled albuterol.

†In most cases of bronchospasm, this item was generally used to describe exacerbations in the underlying pulmonary disease.

Rare cases of urticaria, angioedema, rash, bronchospasm, and oropharyngeal edema have been reported after the use of inhaled albuterol.

OVERDOSAGE

Manifestations of overdosage may include anginal pain, hypertension, hypokalemia, and exaggeration of the pharmacological effects listed in **ADVERSE REACTIONS.**

The oral LD_{50} in rats and mice was greater than 2,000 mg/kg. The inhalational LD_{50} could not be determined.

There is insufficient evidence to determine if dialysis is beneficial for overdosage of PROVENTIL Solution for Inhalation.

DOSAGE AND ADMINISTRATION

The usual dosage for adults and children 12 years and older is 2.5 mg of albuterol administered 3 to 4 times daily by nebulization. More frequent administration or higher doses are not recommended. To administer 2.5 mg of albuterol, dilute 0.5 mL of the 0.5% solution for inhalation to a total volume of 3 mL with sterile normal saline solution and administer by nebulization. The flow rate is regulated to suit the particular nebulizer so that the PROVENTIL Solution for Inhalation will be delivered over approximately 5 to 15 minutes.

Drug stability and safety of PROVENTIL Solution for Inhalation when mixed with other drugs in a nebulizer have not been established.

The use of PROVENTIL Solution for Inhalation can be continued as medically indicated to control recurring bouts of

bronchospasm. During treatment, most patients gain optimum benefit from regular use of the nebulizer solution.

If a previously effective dosage regimen fails to provide the usual relief, medical advice should be sought immediately, as this is often a sign of seriously worsening asthma which would require reassessment of therapy.

HOW SUPPLIED

PROVENTIL Solution for Inhalation 0.5%, is a clear, colorless to light yellow solution, and is supplied in amber glass bottles of 20 mL fill (NDC-0085-0208-02) with accompanying calibrated dropper; boxes of one. **Store between 2° and 25°C (36 ° and 77°F).**

Rev 10/94 17979914

Copyright © 1986, 1993, 1995, Schering Corporation.
All rights reserved.

PROVENTIL® ℞

brand of albuterol sulfate, USP
Inhalation Solution 0.083%*
(*Potency expressed as albuterol)

DESCRIPTION

PROVENTIL Inhalation Solution contains albuterol sulfate, USP, the racemic form of albuterol, a relatively selective $beta_2$-adrenergic bronchodilator (see **CLINICAL PHARMACOLOGY** section below). Albuterol sulfate has the chemical name (α^1-[(*tert*-Butylamino) methyl]-4-hydroxy-*m*-xylene-α,α'-diol sulfate (2:1) (salt), and the following chemical structure:

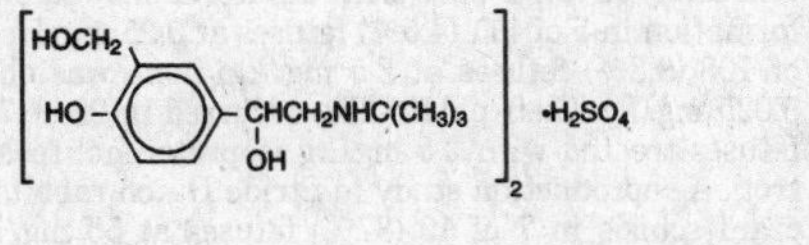

Albuterol sulfate has a molecular weight of 576.7 and the empirical formula $(C_{13}H_{21}NO_3)_2 \cdot H_2SO_4$. Albuterol sulfate is a white crystalline powder, soluble in water and slightly soluble in ethanol.

The World Health Organization recommended name for albuterol base is salbutamol.

Each mL of PROVENTIL Inhalation Solution 0.083% contains 0.83 mg of albuterol (as 1.0 mg of albuterol sulfate) in an isotonic aqueous solution containing sodium chloride and benzalkonium chloride; sulfuric acid is used to adjust the pH between 3 and 5. The 0.083% solution requires no dilution prior to administration. PROVENTIL Inhalation Solution 0.083% contains no sulfiting agents. It is supplied in 3 mL bottles for unit-dose dispensing.

PROVENTIL Inhalation Solution is a clear, colorless to light yellow solution.

CLINICAL PHAMACOLOGY

The prime action of beta-adrenergic drugs is to stimulate adenyl cyclase, the enzyme which catalyzes the formation of cyclic-3',5'-adenosine monophosphate (cyclic AMP) from adenosine triphosphate (ATP). The cyclic AMP thus formed mediates the cellular responses. *In vitro* studies and *in vivo* pharmacologic studies have demonstrated that albuterol has a preferential effect on $beta_2$-adrenergic receptors compared with isoproterenol. While it is recognized that $beta_2$-adrenergic receptors are the predominant receptors in bronchial smooth muscle, recent data indicate that 10% to 50% of the beta receptors in the human heart may be $beta_2$ receptors. The precise function of these receptors, however, is not yet established. Albuterol has been shown in most controlled clinical trials to have more effect on the respiratory tract, in the form of bronchial smooth muscle relaxation, than isoproterenol at comparable doses while producing fewer cardiovascular effects. Controlled clinical studies and other clinical experience have shown that inhaled albuterol, like other beta-adrenergic agonist drugs, can produce a significant cardiovascular effect in some patients, as measured by pulse rate, blood pressure, symptoms, and/or ECG changes.

Albuterol is longer acting than isoproterenol in most patients by any route of administration because it is not a substrate for the cellular uptake processes for catecholamines nor for catechol-*O*-methyl transferase.

Studies in asthmatic patients have shown that less than 20% of a single albuterol dose was absorbed following either IPPB or nebulizer administration; the remaining amount was recovered from the nebulizer and apparatus and expired air. Most of the absorbed dose was recovered in the urine 24 hours after drug administration. Following a 3.0 mg dose of nebulized albuterol, the maximum albuterol plasma level at 0.5 hour was 2.1 ng/mL (range 1.4 to 3.2 ng/mL). There was a significant dose-related response in FEV_1 and peak flow rate (PFR). It has been demonstrated that following oral administration of 4 mg albuterol, the elimination half-life was 5 to 6 hours.

Animal studies show that albuterol does not pass the blood-brain barrier. Recent studies in laboratory animals (minipigs, rodents, and dogs) recorded the occurrence of cardiac arrhythmias and sudden death (with histologic evidence of myocardial necrosis) when beta-agonists and methylxanthines were administered concurrently. The significance of these findings when applied to humans is currently unknown.

In controlled clinical trials, most patients exhibited an onset of improvement in pulmonary function within 5 minutes as determined by FEV_1. FEV_1 measurements also showed that the maximum average improvement in pulmonary function usually occurred at approximately 1 hour following inhalation of 2.5 mg of albuterol by compressor-nebulizer, and remained close to peak for 2 hours. Clinically significant improvement in pulmonary function (defined as maintenance of a 15% or more increase in FEV_1 over baseline values) continued for 3 to 4 hours in most patients and in some patients continued up to 6 hours.

In repetitive dose studies, continued effectiveness was demonstrated throughout the 3-month period of treatment in some patients.

INDICATIONS AND USAGE

PROVENTIL Inhalation Solution is indicated for the relief of bronchospasm in patients with reversible obstructive airway disease and acute attacks of bronchospasm.

CONTRAINDICATIONS

PROVENTIL Inhalation Solution is contraindicated in patients with a history of hypersensitivity to any of its components.

WARNINGS

As with other inhaled beta-adrenergic agonists, PROVENTIL Inhalation Solution can produce paradoxical bronchospasm, which can be life threatening. If it occurs, the preparation should be discontinued immediately and alternative therapy instituted.

Fatalities have been reported in association with excessive use of inhaled sympathomimetic drugs and with the home use of sympathomimetic nebulizers. It is, therefore, essential that the physician instruct the patient in the need for further evaluation if his/her asthma becomes worse. In individual patients, any $beta_2$-adrenergic agonist, including albuterol inhalation solution and solution for inhalation, may have a clinically significant cardiac effect.

Immediate hypersensitivity reactions may occur after administration of albuterol as demonstrated by rare cases of urticaria, angioedema, rash, bronchospasm, and oropharyngeal edema.

PRECAUTIONS

General: Albuterol, as with all sympathomimetic amines, should be used with caution in patients with cardiovascular disorders, especially coronary insufficiency, cardiac arrhythmias and hypertension, in patients with convulsive disorders, hyperthyroidism or diabetes mellitus, and in patients who are unusually responsive to sympathomimetic amines.

Large doses of intravenous albuterol have been reported to aggravate preexisting diabetes mellitus and ketoacidosis. Additionally, beta-agonists, including albuterol, when given intravenously may cause a decrease in serum potassium, possibly through intracellular shunting. The decrease is usually transient, not requiring supplementation. The relevance of these observations to the use of PROVENTIL Inhalation Solution is unknown.

Information For Patients: The action of PROVENTIL Inhalation Solution may last up to 6 hours and therefore it should not be used more frequently than recommended. Do not increase the dose or frequency of medication without medical consultation. If symptoms get worse, medical consultation should be sought promptly. While taking PROVENTIL Inhalation Solution, other anti-asthma medicines should not be used unless prescribed.

Drug stability and safety of PROVENTIL Inhalation Solution when mixed with other drugs in a nebulizer have not been established.

See illustrated **"Patient's Instructions for Use."**

Drug Interactions: Other sympathomimetic aerosol bronchodilators or epinephrine should not be used concomitantly with albuterol.

Albuterol should be administered with extreme caution to patients being treated with monoamine oxidase inhibitors or tricyclic antidepressants, since the action of albuterol on the vascular system may be potentiated.

Beta-receptor blocking agents and albuterol inhibit the effect of each other.

Since albuterol may lower serum potassium, care should be taken in patients also using other drugs which lower serum potassium as the effects may be additive.

Carcinogenesis, Mutagenesis, and Impairment of Fertility: Albuterol sulfate, like other agents in its class, caused a significant dose-related increase in the incidence of benign leiomyomas of the mesovarium in a 2-year study in the rat, at oral doses corresponding to 10, 50, and 250 times the maximum human nebulizer dose. In another study, this effect was blocked by the coadministration of propranolol. The relevance of these findings to humans is not known. An 18-month study in mice and a lifetime study in hamsters revealed no evidence of tumorigenicity. Studies with albuterol revealed no evidence of mutagenesis. Reproduction studies in rats revealed no evidence of impaired fertility.

Teratogenic Effects—Pregnancy Category C: Albuterol has been shown to be teratogenic in mice when given subcutaneously in doses corresponding to the human nebulization dose. There are no adequate and well-controlled studies in pregnant women. Albuterol should be used during pregnancy only if the potential benefit justifies the potential risk to the fetus. A reproduction study in CD-1 mice with albuterol (0.025, 0.25, and 2.5 mg/kg subcutaneously, corresponding to 0.1, 1, and 12.5 times the maximum human nebulization dose, respectively) showed cleft palate formation in 5 of 111 (4.5%) fetuses at 0.25 mg/kg and in 10 of 108 (9.3%) fetuses at 2.5 mg/kg. None were observed at 0.025 mg/kg. Cleft palate also occurred in 22 of 72 (30.5%) fetuses treated with 2.5 mg/kg isoproterenol (positive control). A reproduction study in Stride Dutch rabbits revealed cranioschisis in 7 of 19 (37%) fetuses at 50 mg/kg, corresponding to 250 times the maximum human nebulization dose. During marketing, various congenital anomalies, including cleft palate and limb defects, have been reported in the offspring of patients being treated with albuterol. Some of the mothers were taking multiple medications during their pregnancies. Because no consistent pattern of defects can be discerned, a relationship between albuterol use and congenital anomalies cannot be established.

Labor and Delivery: Oral albuterol has been shown to delay preterm labor in some reports. There are presently no well-controlled studies which demonstrate that it will stop preterm labor or prevent labor at term. Therefore, cautious use of PROVENTIL Inhalation Solution is required in pregnant patients when given for relief of bronchospasm so as to avoid interference with uterine contractibility.

Nursing Mothers: It is not known whether this drug is excreted in human milk. Because of the potential for tumorigenicity shown for albuterol in some animal studies, a decision should be made whether to discontinue nursing or to discontinue the drug, taking into account the importance of the drug to the mother.

Pediatric Use: Safety and effectiveness of albuterol inhalation solution and solution for inhalation in children below the age of 12 years have not been established.

ADVERSE REACTIONS

The results of clinical trials with PROVENTIL Inhalation Solution in 135 patients showed the following side effects which were considered probably or possibly drug related:

Central Nervous System: tremors (20%), dizziness (7%), nervousness (4%), headache (3%), insomnia (1%).
Gastrointestinal: nausea (4%), dyspepsia (1%).
Ear, Nose and Throat: pharyngitis (<1%), nasal congestion (1%).
Cardiovascular: tachycardia (1%), hypertension (1%).
Respiratory: bronchospasm (8%), cough (4%), bronchitis (4%), wheezing (1%).

No clinically relevant laboratory abnormalities related to PROVENTIL Inhalation Solution administration were determined in these studies.

In comparing the adverse reactions reported for patients treated with PROVENTIL Inhalation Solution with those of patients treated with isoproterenol during clinical trials of 3 months, the following moderate to severe reactions, as judged by the investigators, were reported. This table does not include mild reactions.

Incidence of Moderate To Severe Reactions

Reaction	Albuterol N=65	Isoproterenol N=65
Central Nervous System		
Tremors	10.7%	13.8%
Headache	3.1%	1.5%
Insomnia	3.1%	1.5%
Cardiovascular		
Hypertension	3.1%	3.1%
Arrhythmias	0%	3.0%
*Palpitation	0%	22.0%
Respiratory		
**Bronchospasm	15.4%	18.0%
Cough	3.1%	5.0%
Bronchitis	1.5%	5.0%
Wheeze	1.5%	1.5%
Sputum Increase	1.5%	1.5%
Dyspnea	1.5%	1.5%
Gastrointestinal		
Nausea	3.1%	0%
Dyspepsia	1.5%	0%

Continued on next page

Information on Schering products appearing on these pages is effective as of August 15, 1996.

Schering—Cont.

Systemic

Malaise	1.5%	0%

*The finding of no arrhythmias and no palpitations after albuterol administration in this clinical study should not be interpreted as indicating that these adverse effects cannot occur after the administration of inhaled albuterol.

**In most cases of bronchospasm, this term was generally used to describe exacerbations in the underlying pulmonary disease.

Rare cases of urticaria, angioedema, rash, bronchospasm, and oropharyngeal edema have been reported after the use of inhaled albuterol.

OVERDOSAGE

Manifestations of overdosage may include anginal pain, hypertension, hypokalemia, and exaggeration of the pharmacological effects listed in **ADVERSE REACTIONS.**

The oral LD_{50} in rats and mice was greater than 2,000 mg/kg. The inhalational LD_{50} could not be determined.

There is insufficient evidence to determine if dialysis is beneficial for overdosage of PROVENTIL Inhalation Solution.

DOSAGE AND ADMINISTRATION

The usual dosage for adults and children 12 years and older is 2.5 mg of albuterol administered 3 to 4 times daily by nebulization. More frequent administration or higher doses are not recommended. To administer 2.5 mg of albuterol, administer the contents of one unit-dose bottle (3 mL of 0.083% nebulizer solution) by nebulization. The flow rate is regulated to suit the particular nebulizer so that the PROVENTIL Inhalation Solution will be delivered over approximately 5 to 15 minutes.

Drug stability and safety of PROVENTIL Inhalation Solution when mixed with other drugs in a nebulizer have not been established.

The use of PROVENTIL Inhalation Solution can be continued as medically indicated to control recurring bouts of bronchospasm. During treatment, most patients gain optimum benefit from regular use of the nebulizer solution.

If a previously effective dosage regimen fails to provide the usual relief, medical advice should be sought immediately, as this is often a sign of seriously worsening asthma which would require reassessment of therapy.

HOW SUPPLIED

PROVENTIL Inhalation Solution 0.083% is a clear, colorless to light yellow solution, and is supplied in unit-dose HDPE (high density polyethylene) bottles of 3 mL fill each, boxes of 25 (NDC-0085-0209-01). **Store between 2° and 25°C (36° and 77°F).**

Rev. 10/94 17253832

Copyright © 1986, 1993, 1995, Schering Corporation.
All rights reserved.

PROVENTIL® ℞

brand of albuterol sulfate, USP
Syrup

DESCRIPTION

PROVENTIL Syrup contains albuterol sulfate, USP, the racemic form of albuterol and a relatively selective beta$_2$-adrenergic bronchodilator. Albuterol sulfate has the chemical name α^1-[(*tert*-Butylamino)methyl]-4-hydroxy-*m*-xylene-α,α'-diol sulfate (2:1) (salt), and the following chemical structure:

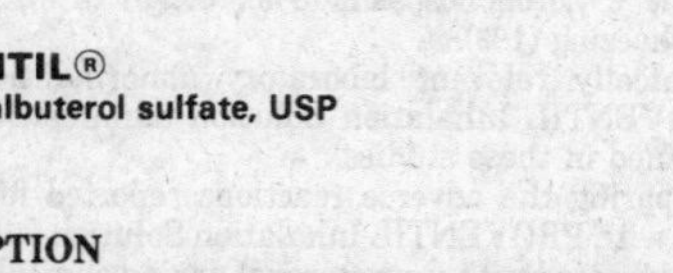

Albuterol sulfate has a molecular weight of 576.7 and the empirical formula $(C_{13}H_{21}NO_3)_2 \cdot H_2SO_4$. Albuterol sulfate is a white crystalline powder, soluble in water and slightly soluble in ethanol.

The World Heatlh Organization recommended name for albuterol base is salbutamol.

PROVENTIL Syrup contains 2 mg of albuterol as 2.4 mg of albuterol sulfate in each teaspoonful (5 mL).

The inactive ingredients for PROVENTIL Syrup include: citric acid, FD&C Yellow No. 6, flavor, hydroxypropyl methylcellulose, saccharin, sodium benzoate, sodium citrate, and water.

CLINICAL PHARMACOLOGY

The prime action of beta-adrenergic drugs is to stimulate adenyl cyclase, the enzyme which catalyzes the formation of cyclic-3',5'-adenosine monophosphate (cyclic AMP) from adenosine triphosphate (ATP). The cyclic AMP thus formed mediates the cellular responses. Based on pharmacologic studies in animals, albuterol appears to exert direct and preferential action on beta$_2$-adrenoceptors including those of the bronchial tree and uterus, and may have less cardiac stimulant effect than isoproterenol, when given in the usual recommended dose.

Albuterol is longer acting than isoproterenol in most patients by any route of administration because it is not a substrate for the cellular uptake processes for catecholamines nor for catechol-*O*-methyl transferase.

After oral administration of 10 mL PROVENTIL Syrup (4 mg albuterol) in normal volunteers, albuterol is rapidly absorbed. Maximum plasma albuterol concentrations of about 18 ng/mL are achieved within 2 hours and the drug is eliminated with a half-life of about 5 hours. In other studies, the analysis of urine samples of patients given 8 mg tritiated albuterol orally showed that 76% of the dose was excreted over 3 days, with the majority of the dose being excreted within the first 24 hours. Sixty percent of this radioactivity was shown to be the metabolite. Feces collected over this period contained 4% of the administered dose.

Animal studies show that albuterol does not pass the blood-brain barrier.

INDICATIONS AND USAGE

PROVENTIL Syrup is indicated for the relief of bronchospasm in adults and in children 2 years of age and older with reversible obstructive airway disease.

In controlled clinical trials in patients with asthma, the onset of improvement in pulmonary function, as measured by maximal midexpiratory flow rate (MMEF) and forced expiratory volume in one second (FEV_1), was within 30 minutes after a dose of PROVENTIL Syrup. Peak improvement of pulmonary function occurred between 2 and 3 hours. In a controlled clinical trial involving 55 children, clinically significant improvement (defined as maintenance of mean values over baseline of 15% or 20% or more in the FEV_1 and MMEF respectively) continued to be recorded up to 6 hours. No decrease in the effectiveness was reported in one uncontrolled study of 32 children who took PROVENTIL Syrup for a 3-month period.

CONTRAINDICATIONS

PROVENTIL Syrup is contraindicated in patients with a history of hypersensitivity to any of its components.

WARNINGS

Immediate hypersensitivity reactions may occur after administration of albuterol, as demonstrated by rare cases of anaphylaxis, angioedema, oropharyngeal edema, bronchospasm, urticaria, and rash.

Rarely, erythema multiforme and Stevens-Johnson syndrome have been associated with the administration of albuterol sulfate syrup in children.

PRECAUTIONS

General: Although albuterol usually has minimal effects on the beta$_1$-adrenoceptors of the cardiovascular system at the recommended dosage, occasionally the usual cardiovascular and CNS stimulatory effects common to all sympathomimetic agents have been seen with patients treated with albuterol necessitating discontinuation. Therefore, albuterol, as with all sympathomimetic amines, should be used with caution in patients with cardiovascular disorders, including coronary insufficiency, cardiac arrhythmias, and hypertension; in patients with convulsive disorders, hyperthyroidism, or diabetes mellitus, and in patients who are unusually responsive to sympathomimetic amines.

Large doses of intravenous albuterol have been reported to aggravate preexisting diabetes mellitus and ketoacidosis. Additionally, albuterol and other beta-agonists, when given intravenously, may cause a decrease in serum potassium, possibly through intracellular shunting. The decrease is usually transient, not requiring supplementation. The relevance of these observations to the use of PROVENTIL Syrup is unknown.

Information for Patients: The action of PROVENTIL Syrup may last up to 6 hours and therefore it should not be taken more frequently than recommended. Do not increase the dose or frequency of medication without medical consultation. If symptoms get worse, medical consultation should be sought promptly. If pregnant or nursing, consult with your physician.

Drug Interactions: The concomitant use of PROVENTIL Syrup and other oral sympathomimetic agents is not recommended since such combined use may lead to deleterious cardiovascular effects. This recommendation does not preclude the judicious use of an aerosol bronchodilator of the adrenergic stimulant type in patients receiving PROVENTIL Syrup. Such concomitant use, however, should be individualized and not given on a routine basis. If regular coadministration is required, then alternative therapy should be considered.

Albuterol should be administered with extreme caution to patients being treated with monoamine oxidase inhibitors or tricyclic antidepressants, since the action of albuterol on the vascular system may be potentiated.

Beta-receptor blocking agents and albuterol inhibit the effect of each other.

Since albuterol may lower serum potassium, care should be taken in patients also using other drugs which lower serum potassium as the effects may be additive.

After single-dose administration of albuterol to normal volunteers who had received digoxin for 10 days, a 16%–22% decrease in serum digoxin levels was demonstrated. The clinical significance of these findings for patients with obstructive airway disease who are receiving albuterol and digoxin on a chronic basis is unclear.

Nevertheless, it would be prudent to carefully evaluate the serum digoxin levels in patients who are concurrently receiving digoxin and albuterol.

Carcinogenesis, Mutagenesis, and Impairment of Fertility: Albuterol sulfate, like other agents in its class, caused a significant dose-related increase in the incidence of benign leiomyomas of the mesovarium in a 2-year study in the rat, at doses corresponding to 2, 9, and 46 times the maximum human (child weighing 21 kg) oral dose. In another study this effect was blocked by the coadministration of propranolol. The relevance of these findings to humans is not known. An 18-month study in mice and a lifetime study in hamsters revealed no evidence of tumorigenicity. Studies with albuterol revealed no evidence of mutagenesis. Reproduction studies in rats revealed no evidence of impaired fertility.

Teratogenic Effects—Pregnancy Category C: Albuterol has been shown to be teratogenic in mice when given subcutaneously in doses corresponding to 0.2 times the maximum human (child weighing 21 kg) oral dose. There are no adequate and well-controlled studies in pregnant women. Albuterol should be used during pregnancy only if the potential benefit justifies the potential risk to the fetus. A reproduction study in CD-1 mice with albuterol showed cleft palate formation in 5 of 111 (4.5%) fetuses at 0.25 mg/kg and in 10 of 108 (9.3%) fetuses at 2.5 mg/kg; none was observed at 0.025 mg/kg. Cleft palate also occurred in 22 of 72 (30.5%) fetuses treated with 2.5 mg/kg isoproterenol (positive control). A reproduction study in Stride Dutch rabbits revealed cranioschisis in 7 of 19 (37%) fetuses at 50 mg/kg, corresponding to 46 times the maximum human (child weighing 21 kg) oral dose of albuterol sulfate. During marketing, various congenital anomalies, including cleft palate and limb defects, have been reported in the offspring of patients being treated with albuterol. Some of the mothers were taking multiple medications during their pregnancies. Because no consistent pattern of defects can be discerned, a relationship between albuterol use and congenital anomalies cannot be established.

Labor and Delivery: Oral albuterol has been shown to delay preterm labor in some reports. There are presently no well-controlled studies which demonstrate that it will stop preterm labor or prevent labor at term. Therefore, cautious use of PROVENTIL Syrup is required in pregnant patients when given for relief of bronchospasm so as to avoid interference with uterine contractibility. Use in such patients should be restricted to those patients in whom the benefits clearly outweigh the risks.

Nursing Mothers: It is not known whether this drug is excreted in human milk. Because of the potential for tumorigenicity shown for albuterol in animal studies, a decision should be made whether to discontinue nursing or to discontinue the drug, taking into account the importance of the drug to the mother.

Pediatric Use: Safety and effectiveness in children below the age of 2 years have not yet been adequately demonstrated.

ADVERSE REACTIONS

The adverse reactions to albuterol are similar in nature to those of other sympathomimetic agents. The most frequent adverse reactions to PROVENTIL Syrup in adults and older children were tremor, 10 of 100 patients; nervousness and shakiness, each 9 of 100 patients. Other reported adverse reactions were headache, 4 of 100 patients; dizziness and increased appetite, each 3 of 100 patients; hyperactivity and excitement, each 2 of 100 patients; tachycardia, epistaxis, irritable behavior, and sleeplessness, each 1 of 100 patients. The following adverse effects occurred in less than 1 of 100 patients each: muscle spasm; disturbed sleep; epigastric pain; cough; palpitations; stomach ache; irritable behavior; dilated pupils; sweating; chest pain; weakness.

In young children 2 to 6 years of age, some adverse reactions were noted more frequently than in adults and older children. Excitement was noted in approximately 20% of patients and nervousness in 15%. Hyperkinesia occurred in 4% of patients; insomnia, tachycardia, and gastrointestinal symptoms in 2% each. Anorexia, emotional lability, pallor, fatigue, and conjunctivitis were seen in 1%.

In addition, albuterol, like other sympathomimetic agents, can cause adverse reactions such as hypertension, angina, vomiting, vertigo, central nervous system stimulation, unusual taste, and drying or irritation of the oropharynx.

The reactions are generally transient in nature, and it is usually not necessary to discontinue treatment with PROVENTIL Syrup. In selected cases, however, dosage may

be reduced temporarily; after the reaction has subsided, dosage should be increased in small increments to the optimal dosage.

OVERDOSAGE

Manifestations of overdosage include anginal pain, hypertension, hypokalemia, and exaggeration of the effects listed in **ADVERSE REACTIONS.**

The oral LD_{50} in rats and mice was greater than 2,000 mg/kg. Dialysis is not appropriate treatment for overdosage of PROVENTIL Syrup. The judicious use of a cardioselective beta-receptor blocker, such as metoprolol tartrate, is suggested, bearing in mind the danger of inducing an asthmatic attack.

DOSAGE AND ADMINISTRATION

The following dosages of PROVENTIL Syrup are expressed in terms of albuterol base.

Usual Dose The usual starting dosage for adults and children over 14 years of age is 2 mg (1 teaspoonful) or 4 mg (2 teaspoonsful) three or four times a day.

The usual starting dosage for children 6 to 14 years of age is 2 mg (1 teaspoonful) three or four times a day.

For children 2 to 6 years of age, dosing should be initiated at 0.1 mg/kg of body weight three times a day. This starting dosage should not exceed 2 mg (1 teaspoonful) three times a day.

Dosage Adjustment For adults and children above age 14, a dosage above 4 mg four times a day should be used *only* when the patient fails to respond. If a favorable response does not occur, the dosage may be cautiously increased stepwise, but the dosage should not exceed 8 mg four times a day.

For children from 6 to 14 years of age who fail to respond to the initial starting dosage of 2 mg four times a day, the dosage may be cautiously increased stepwise, but not to exceed 24 mg per day (given in divided doses).

For children 2 to 6 years of age who do not respond satisfactorily to the initial dosage, the dose may be increased stepwise to 0.2 mg/kg of body weight three times a day, but not to exceed a maximum of 4 mg (2 teaspoonsful) given three times a day.

For elderly patients and those sensitive to beta-adrenergic stimulation, the initial dosage should be restricted to 2 mg three or four times a day and individually adjusted thereafter.

HOW SUPPLIED

PROVENTIL Syrup, a clear orange-yellow liquid with a strawberry flavor, contains 2 mg albuterol as the sulfate per 5 mL; bottles of 16 fluid ounces (NDC 0085-0315-02).

Store between 2° and 30°C (36° and 86°F).

Rev. 10/94 17979329

Copyright © 1982, 1992, 1993, 1995, Schering Corporation. All rights reserved.

PROVENTIL® ℞
brand of albuterol sulfate, USP
REPETABS® brand of
extended-release Tablets
PROVENTIL®
brand of albuterol sulfate, USP
Tablets

DESCRIPTION

PROVENTIL REPETABS Tablets and PROVENTIL Tablets contain albuterol sulfate, USP, the racemic form of albuterol and a relatively selective beta$_2$-adrenergic bronchodilator. Albuterol sulfate has the chemical name α^1-[(*tert*-Butylamino)methyl]-4-hydroxy-*m*-xylene-α, α'-diol sulfate (2:1) (salt), and the following chemical structure:

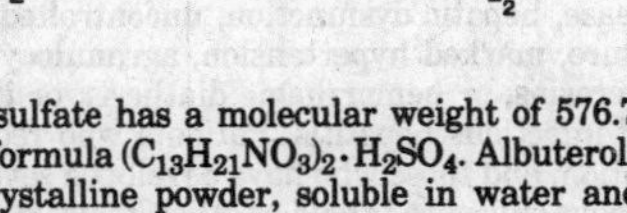

Albuterol sulfate has a molecular weight of 576.7 and the empirical formula $(C_{13}H_{21}NO_3)_2 \cdot H_2SO_4$. Albuterol sulfate is a white crystalline powder, soluble in water and slightly soluble in ethanol.

The World Health Organization recommended name for albuterol base is salbutamol.

Each PROVENTIL REPETABS Tablet contains a total of 4 mg (2 mg in the coating for immediate release and 2 mg in the core for release after several hours) of albuterol as 4.8 mg of albuterol sulfate.

Each PROVENTIL Tablet contains 2 or 4 mg of albuterol as 2.4 and 4.8 mg of albuterol sulfate, respectively.

The inactive ingredients for PROVENTIL REPETABS Tablets include: acacia, butylparaben, calcium phosphate, calcium sulfate, carnauba wax, corn starch, lactose, magnesium stearate, neutral soap, oleic acid, rosin, sugar, talc, titanium dioxide, white wax, and zein.

The inactive ingredients for PROVENTIL Tablets, 2 and 4 mg include: corn starch, lactose, and magnesium stearate.

CLINICAL PHARMACOLOGY

In vitro studies and *in vivo* pharmacologic studies have demonstrated that PROVENTIL has a preferential effect on beta$_2$-adrenergic receptors compared with isoproterenol. While it is recognized that beta$_2$-adrenergic receptors are the predominant receptors in bronchial smooth muscle, recent data indicate that there is a population of beta$_2$-receptors in the human heart, existing in a concentration between 10% and 50%. The precise function of these receptors, however, is not yet established.

Albuterol is longer acting than isoproterenol in most patients by any route of administration because it is not a substrate for the cellular uptake processes for catecholamines nor for catechol-*O*-methyl transferase.

Albuterol is rapidly and well absorbed following oral administration. In studies involving normal volunteers, the mean steady-state peak and trough plasma levels of albuterol were 6.7 and 3.8 ng/mL, respectively, following dosing with a 2 mg PROVENTIL Tablet every 6 hours and 14.8 and 8.6 ng/mL, respectively, following dosing with a 4 mg PROVENTIL Tablet every 6 hours. Maximum albuterol plasma levels are usually obtained between 2 and 3 hours after dosing and the elimination half-life is 5 to 6 hours. These data indicate that albuterol, administered orally, is dose proportional and exhibits dose independent pharmacokinetics.

In other studies, the analysis of urine samples of subjects given tritiated albuterol (4–10 mg) orally showed that 65% to 90% of the dose was excreted over 3 days, with the majority of the dose being excreted within the first 24 hours. Sixty percent of this radioactivity was shown to be the metabolite of albuterol. Feces collected over this period contained 4% of the administered dose.

PROVENTIL REPETABS Tablets have been formulated to provide a duration of action of up to 12 hours. In studies conducted in normal volunteers, the mean steady-state peak and trough plasma levels of albuterol were 6.5 and 3.0 ng/mL, respectively, following dosing with a 4 mg PROVENTIL REPETABS Tablet every 12 hours. In addition, it has been shown that administration of a 4 mg PROVENTIL REPETABS Tablet every 12 hours is bioequivalent to administration of a 2 mg PROVENTIL Tablet every 6 hours.

Animal studies show that albuterol does not pass the blood-brain barrier. Recent studies in laboratory animals (minipigs, rodents, and dogs) recorded the occurrence of cardiac arrhythmias and sudden death (with histologic evidence of myocardial necrosis) when beta-agonists and methylxanthines were administered concurrently. The significance of these findings when applied to humans is currently unknown.

In controlled clinical trials in patients with asthma, the onset of improvement in pulmonary function, as measured by maximal midexpiratory flow rate, MMEF, was noted within 30 minutes after a dose of PROVENTIL Tablets with peak improvement occurring between 2 and 3 hours. In controlled clinical trials, in which measurements were conducted for 6 hours, significant clinical improvement in pulmonary function (defined as maintaining a 15% or more increase in FEV_1 and a 20% or more increase in MMEF over baseline values) was observed in 60% of patients at 4 hours and in 40% at 6 hours. In other single-dose controlled clinical trials, clinically significant improvement was observed in at least 40% of the patients at 8 hours with the 4 mg PROVENTIL Tablet. No decrease in the effectiveness of PROVENTIL Tablets has been reported in patients who received long-term treatment with the drug in uncontrolled studies for periods up to 6 months.

In another controlled clinical study in asthmatic patients, it has been demonstrated that the initiation of therapy with either the 4 mg PROVENTIL REPETABS Tablet dosed every 12 hours, or the 2 mg PROVENTIL Tablet dosed every 6 hours, achieve therapeutically equivalent effects.

INDICATIONS AND USAGE

PROVENTIL REPETABS Tablets and PROVENTIL Tablets are indicated for the relief of bronchospasm in patients with reversible obstructive airway disease.

CONTRAINDICATIONS

PROVENTIL REPETABS Tablets and PROVENTIL Tablets are contraindicated in patients with a history of hypersensitivity to any of their components.

PRECAUTIONS

General: Since albuterol is a sympathomimetic amine, it should be used with caution in patients with cardiovascular disorders, including ischemic heart disease, hypertension, or cardiac arrhythmias, in patients with hyperthyroidism or diabetes mellitus, and in patients who are unusually responsive to sympathomimetic amines or who have convulsive disorders. Significant changes in systolic and diastolic blood pressure could be expected to occur in some patients after use of any beta adrenergic bronchodilator.

Large doses of intravenous albuterol have been reported to aggravate preexisting diabetes mellitus and ketoacidosis. Additionally, albuterol and other beta agonists, when given intravenously, may cause a decrease in serum potassium, possibly through intracellular shunting. The decrease is usually transient, not requiring supplementation. The relevance of these observations to the use of PROVENTIL REPETABS Tablets and PROVENTIL Tablets is unknown.

Information for Patients: Patients being treated with PROVENTIL REPETABS Tablets or PROVENTIL Tablets should receive the following information and instructions. This information is intended to aid in the safe and effective use of this medication. It is not a disclosure of all possible adverse or intended effects.

PROVENTIL REPETABS Tablets and PROVENTIL Tablets should not be taken more frequently than recommended. Do not increase the dose or frequency of medication, or add other medications to your therapy without medical consultation. If symptoms get worse, medical consultation should be sought promptly. If pregnant or nursing, consult with your physician.

Drug Interactions: The concomitant use of PROVENTIL REPETABS Tablets or PROVENTIL Tablets and other oral sympathomimetic agents is not recommended since such combined use may lead to deleterious cardiovascular effects. This recommendation does not preclude the judicious use of an aerosol bronchodilator of the adrenergic stimulant type in patients receiving PROVENTIL REPETABS Tablets or PROVENTIL Tablets. Such concomitant use, however, should be individualized and not given on a routine basis. If regular coadministration is required, then alternative therapy should be considered.

Albuterol should be administered with extreme caution to patients being treated with monoamine oxidase inhibitors or tricyclic antidepressants, since the action of albuterol on the vascular system may be potentiated.

Beta-receptor blocking agents and albuterol inhibit the effect of each other.

Since albuterol may lower serum potassium, care should be taken in patients also using other drugs which lower serum potassium as the effects may be additive.

After single-dose administration of albuterol to normal volunteers who had received digoxin for 10 days, a 16%–22% decrease in serum digoxin levels was demonstrated. The clinical significance of these findings for patients with obstructive airway disease who are receiving albuterol and digoxin on a chronic basis is unclear. Nevertheless, it would be prudent to carefully evaluate the serum digoxin levels in patients who are concurrently receiving digoxin and albuterol.

Carcinogenesis, Mutagenesis, and Impairment of Fertility: Albuterol sulfate, like other agents in its class, caused a significant dose-related increase in the incidence of benign leiomyomas of the mesovarium in a 2-year study in the rat, at doses corresponding to 3, 16, and 78 times the maximum human oral dose. In another study this effect was blocked by the coadministration of propranolol. The relevance of these findings to humans is not known. An 18-month study in mice and a lifetime study in hamsters revealed no evidence of tumorigenicity.

Studies with albuterol revealed no evidence of mutagenesis. Reproduction studies in rats revealed no evidence of impaired fertility.

Teratogenic Effects—Pregnancy Category C: Albuterol has been shown to be teratogenic in mice when given subcutaneously in doses corresponding to 0.4 times the maximum human oral dose. There are no adequate and well-controlled studies in pregnant women. Albuterol should be used during pregnancy only if the potential benefit justifies the potential risk to the fetus. A reproduction study in CD-1 mice with albuterol showed cleft palate formation in 5 of 111 (4.5%) fetuses at 0.25 mg/kg and in 10 of 108 (9.3%) fetuses at 2.5 mg/kg; none were observed at 0.025 mg/kg. Cleft palate also occurred in 22 of 72 (30.5%) fetuses treated with 2.5 mg/kg isoproterenol (positive control). A reproduction study in Stride Dutch rabbits revealed cranioschisis in 7 of 19 (37%) fetuses at 50 mg/kg, corresponding to 78 times the maximum human oral dose of albuterol. During marketing, various congenital anomalies, including cleft palate and limb defects, have been reported in the offspring of patients being treated with albuterol. Some of the mothers were taking multiple medications during their pregnancies. Because no consistent pattern of defects can be discerned, a relationship between albuterol use and congenital anomalies cannot be established.

Labor and Delivery: Oral albuterol has been shown to delay preterm labor in some reports. There are presently no well-controlled studies which demonstrate that it will stop preterm labor or prevent labor at term. Therefore, cautious use of PROVENTIL REPETABS Tablets or PROVENTIL Tablets is required in pregnant patients when given for relief of

Continued on next page

Information on Schering products appearing on these pages is effective as of August 15, 1996.

Schering—Cont.

bronchospasm so as to avoid interference with uterine contractibility.

Nursing Mothers: It is not known whether this drug is excreted in human milk. Because of the potential for tumorigenicity shown for albuterol in some animal studies, a decision should be made whether to discontinue nursing or to discontinue the drug, taking into account the importance of the drug to the mother.

Pediatric Use: Safety and effectiveness in children below the age of 6 years for PROVENTIL Tablets, and below the age of 12 years for PROVENTIL REPETABS Tablets have not been established.

ADVERSE REACTIONS

The adverse reactions to albuterol are similar in nature to those of other sympathomimetic agents. The most frequent adverse reactions to PROVENTIL Tablets were nervousness and tremor, with each occurring in approximately 20 of 100 patients (20%). Other reported reactions were headache, 7 of 100 patients (7%); tachycardia and palpitations, 5 of 100 patients (5%); muscle cramps, 3 of 100 patients (3%); insomnia, nausea, weakness, and dizziness, each occurred in 2 of 100 patients (2%). Drowsiness, flushing, restlessness, irritability, chest discomfort, and difficulty in micturition each occurred in less than 1 of 100 patients (less than 1%).

In a clinical study of 1 week duration comparing a 4 mg PROVENTIL REPETABS Tablet administered every 12 hours to a 2 mg PROVENTIL Tablet administered every 6 hours, the following adverse reactions considered to be possibly or probably treatment related were reported: nervousness in 1 of 50 (2%) and 3 of 50 patients (6%) for PROVENTIL REPETABS and PROVENTIL Tablets, respectively; nausea in 2 of 50 (4%) for both; vomiting in 1 of 50 (2%) and 2 of 50 (4%) for PROVENTIL REPETABS and PROVENTIL Tablets, respectively; somnolence in 1 of 50 (2%) for both. The following adverse reactions were reported for PROVENTIL Tablets only; tremor in 3 of 50 patients (6%), tinnitus, dyspepsia, and rash each occurred in 1 of 50 patients (2%).

Although not reported for PROVENTIL REPETABS Tablets in the above study, there have been reports of tremor in other trials. When all clinical experience is considered, the incidence of tremor is approximately the same as that seen with PROVENTIL Tablets.

In addition to those adverse reactions reported above, albuterol, like other sympathomimetic agents, can cause adverse reactions such as hypertension, angina, vomiting, vertigo, central nervous system stimulation, unusual taste, and drying or irritation of the oropharynx.

The reactions are generally transient in nature, and it is usually not necessary to discontinue treatment with PROVENTIL REPETABS Tablets or PROVENTIL Tablets. In selected cases, however, dosage may be reduced temporarily; after the reaction has subsided, dosage should be increased in small increments to the optimal dosage.

OVERDOSAGE

Manifestations of overdosage include anginal pain, hypertension, hypokalemia, and exaggeration of the pharmacological effects listed in **ADVERSE REACTIONS**.

The oral LD_{50} in rats and mice was greater than 2,000 mg/kg.

There is insufficient evidence to determine if dialysis is beneficial for overdosage of PROVENTIL REPETABS Tablets or PROVENTIL Tablets.

DOSAGE AND ADMINISTRATION

The following dosages of PROVENTIL REPETABS Tablets and PROVENTIL Tablets are expressed in terms of albuterol base.

PROVENTIL REPETABS Tablets

Usual Dose The usual starting dosage of PROVENTIL REPETABS Tablets for adults and children 12 years and over is 4 or 8 mg (one or two tablets) every 12 hours.

Dosage Adjustment Doses of PROVENTIL REPETABS Tablets above 8 mg twice a day should be used only when the patient fails to respond to lower doses. The dose should be increased cautiously stepwise up to a maximum of 16 mg twice a day if a favorable response does not occur with the 4 mg initial dose.

The total daily dose should not exceed 32 mg in adults and children 12 years and over.

Switching to PROVENTIL REPETABS Tablets Patients currently maintained on PROVENTIL Tablets can be switched to PROVENTIL REPETABS Tablets. For example, the administration of a 4 mg PROVENTIL REPETABS Tablet every 12 hours is equivalent to one 2 mg PROVENTIL Tablet every 6 hours. Multiples of this regimen up to the maximum recommended daily dose also apply.

PROVENTIL Tablets

Usual Dose The usual starting dosage for children 6 to 12 years of age is 2 mg three or four times a day.

The usual starting dosage for adults and children 12 years and over is 2 mg or 4 mg three or four times a day.

Dosage Adjustment For children from 6 to 12 years of age who fail to respond to the initial starting dosage of 2 mg four times a day, the dosage may be cautiously increased stepwise, but not to exceed 24 mg per day (given in divided doses). For adults and children 12 years and over, a dosage above 4 mg four times a day should be used only when the patient fails to respond to lower doses. The dose should be increased cautiously stepwise up to a maximum of 8 mg four times a day as tolerated if a favorable response does not occur with the 4 mg initial dose.

Elderly Patients and Those Sensitive to Beta-Adrenergic Stimulators An initial dosage of 2 mg three or four times a day is recommended for elderly patients and for those with a history of unusual sensitivity to beta-adrenergic stimulators. If adequate bronchodilation is not obtained, dosage may be increased gradually to as much as 8 mg three or four times a day.

The total daily dose should not exceed 32 mg in adults and children 12 years and over.

HOW SUPPLIED

PROVENTIL REPETABS Tablets, 4 mg albuterol as the sulfate (2 mg in the coating for immediate release and 2 mg in the core for release after several hours), white, round, coated tablets, branded in red on one side with the Schering trademark and product identification numbers, 431, bottles of 100 (NDC 0085-0431-02) and 500 (NDC 0085-0431-03) and boxes of 100 for unit dose dispensing (NDC 0085-0431-04).

PROVENTIL Tablets, 2 mg albuterol as the sulfate, white, round, compressed tablets, impressed with the product name (PROVENTIL) and the number 2 on one side, and product identification numbers, 252, and scored on the other, bottles of 100 (NDC 0085-0252-02) and 500 (NDC 0085-0252-03).

PROVENTIL Tablets, 4 mg albuterol as the sulfate, white, round, compressed tablets, impressed with the product name (PROVENTIL) and the number 4 on one side, and product identification numbers, 573, and scored on the other, bottles of 100 (NDC 0085-0573-02) and 500 (NDC 0085-0573-03).

Store PROVENTIL REPETABS Tablets between 2° and 25°C (36° and 77°F), and PROVENTIL Tablets between 2° and 30°C (36° and 86°F). Protect PROVENTIL REPETABS Tablets in the unit dose box from excessive moisture.

Rev. 10/94 17543326

Copyright © 1982, 1993, 1995, Schering Corporation. All rights reserved.

Shown in Product Identification Guide, page 334

SOLGANAL® ℞

brand of sterile aurothioglucose
Suspension, USP
FOR INTRAMUSCULAR
INJECTION ONLY—
NOT FOR INTRAVENOUS USE

WARNINGS

Physicians planning to use SOLGANAL Suspension should thoroughly familiarize themselves with its toxicity and its benefits. The possibility of toxic reactions should always be explained to the patient before starting therapy. Patients should be warned to report promptly any symptom suggesting toxicity. Before each injection of SOLGANAL Suspension, the physician should review the results of laboratory work and see the patient to determine the presence or absence of adverse reactions, since some of these can be severe or even fatal.

DESCRIPTION

SOLGANAL is a sterile suspension, for **intramuscular injection only.** SOLGANAL Suspension is an antiarthritic agent which is absorbed gradually following intramuscular injection, producing a therapeutically desired prolonged effect. Each ml contains 50 mg of aurothioglucose, USP in sterile sesame oil with 2% aluminum monostearate; 1 mg propylparaben is added as preservative. Aurothioglucose contains approximately 50% gold by weight.

The empirical formula for aurothioglucose is $C_6H_{11}AuO_5S$; the molecular weight is 392.18. Chemically it is (1-Thio-D-glucopyranosato) gold, with the following structural formula:

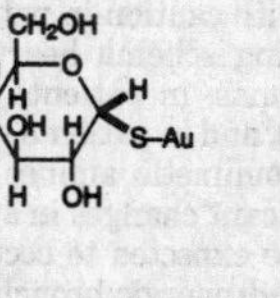

Aurothioglucose is a nearly odorless, yellow powder which is stable in air. An aqueous solution is unstable on long standing. Aurothioglucose is freely soluble in water but practically insoluble in acetone, in alcohol, in chloroform, and in ether.

CLINICAL PHARMACOLOGY

Although the mechanism of action is not well understood, gold compounds have been reported to decrease synovial inflammation and retard cartilage and bone destruction.

Gold is absorbed from injection sites, reaching peak concentration in blood in four to six hours. Following a single intramuscular injection of 50 mg SOLGANAL Suspension in each of two patients, peak serum levels were about 235 mcg/dl in one patient and 450 mcg/dl in the other. In plasma, 95% is bound to the albumin fraction. Approximately 70% of the gold is eliminated in the urine and approximately 30% in the feces. When a standard weekly treatment schedule is followed, approximately 40% of the administered dose is excreted each week, and the remainder is excreted over a longer period. The biological half-life of gold salts following a single 50 mg dose has been reported to range from 3 to 27 days. Following successive weekly doses, the half-life increases and may be 14 to 40 days after the third dose and up to 168 days after the eleventh weekly dose.

After the initial injection, the serum level of gold rises sharply and declines over the next week. Peak levels with aqueous preparations are higher and decline faster than those with oily preparations. Weekly administration produces a continuous rise in the basal value for several months, after which the serum level becomes relatively stable. After a standard weekly dose, considerable individual variation in the levels of gold has been found. A steady decline in gold levels occurs when the interval between injections is lengthened, and small amounts may be found in the serum for months after discontinuance of therapy. The incidence of toxic reactions is apparently unrelated to the plasma level of gold, but it may be related to the cumulative body content of gold.

Storage of gold in human tissues is dependent upon organ mass as well as upon the concentration of gold. Therefore, tissues having the highest gold levels (weight/weight) do not necessarily contain the greatest total amounts of gold. The major depots, in decreasing order of total gold content, are the bone marrow, liver, skin, and bone, accounting for approximately 85% of body gold. The highest concentrations of gold are found in the lymph nodes, adrenal glands, liver, kidneys, bone marrow, and spleen. Relatively small concentrations are found in articular structures.

Gold passes the blood-brain barrier in hamsters.

Transfer of gold across the human placenta at the twentieth week of pregnancy has been documented. The placenta showed numerous gold deposits and smaller amounts were detected in the fetal liver and kidneys; other tissues provided no evidence of gold deposition.

Gold is excreted into human milk in significant amounts and trace amounts can be demonstrated in the blood of nursing infants. (See **PRECAUTIONS**, "*Nursing Mothers.*")

INDICATIONS AND USAGE

SOLGANAL Suspension is indicated for the adjunctive treatment of early active rheumatoid arthritis (both of the adult and juvenile types) not adequately controlled by other anti-inflammatory agents and conservative measures. In chronic, advanced cases of rheumatoid arthritis, gold therapy is less valuable.

Antirheumatic measures such as salicylates and other anti-inflammatory drugs (both steroidal and non-steroidal) may be continued after initiation of gold therapy. After improvement commences, these measures may be discontinued slowly as symptoms permit.

See **PRECAUTIONS**, "*Laboratory Tests*" and **DOSAGE AND ADMINISTRATION**

CONTRAINDICATIONS

A history of known hypersensitivity to any component of SOLGANAL Suspension contraindicates its use. Gold therapy is contraindicated in patients with uncontrolled diabetes mellitus, severe debilitation, systemic lupus erythematosus, renal disease, hepatic dysfunction, uncontrolled congestive heart failure, marked hypertension, agranulocytosis, other blood dyscrasias, or hemorrhagic diathesis; or if there is a history of infectious hepatitis. Patients who recently have had radiation, and those who have developed severe toxicity from previous exposure to gold or other heavy metals should not receive SOLGANAL Suspension.

Urticaria, eczema, and colitis are also contraindications.

Gold therapy is usually contraindicated in pregnancy. (See **PRECAUTIONS**, "*Usage in Pregnancy*".)

Gold salts should not be used with penicillamine, (see **MANAGEMENT OF ADVERSE REACTIONS**) or antimalarials. The safety of coadministration with immunosuppressive agents other than corticosteroids has not been established.

WARNINGS

The following signs should be considered danger signals of gold toxicity, and no additional injection should be given unless further studies reveal some other cause for their presence: rapid reduction of hemoglobin, leukopenia (WBC below

4000/cu mm), eosinophilia above 5%, platelet count below 100,000/cu mm, albuminuria, hematuria, pruritus, dermatitis, stomatitis, jaundice, and petechiae.

Effects that may occur immediately following an injection, or at any time during gold therapy, include: anaphylactic shock, syncope, bradycardia, thickening of the tongue, difficulty in swallowing and breathing, and angioneurotic edema. If such effects are observed, treatment with SOLGANAL Suspension should be discontinued.

Tolerance to gold usually decreases with advancing age. Diabetes mellitus or congestive heart failure should be under control before gold therapy is instituted.

SOLGANAL Suspension should be used with extreme caution in patients with: skin rash, hypersensitivity to other medications, or a history of renal or liver disease.

PRECAUTIONS

General: Before **each** injection, the physician should personally check the patient for adverse reactions and inquiry should be made regarding pruritus, rash, sore mouth, indigestion, and metallic taste. The patient should be observed for at least 15 minutes following each injection. (See also *"Laboratory Tests".*)

Patients with HLA-D locus histocompatibility antigens DRw2 and DRw3 may have a genetic predisposition to develop certain toxic reactions, such as proteinuria, during treatment with gold or D-penicillamine.

SOLGANAL Suspension should be used with caution in patients with compromised cardiovascular or cerebral circulation.

Information for Patients:
1. Promptly report to the physician any unusual symptoms such as pruritus (itching), rash, sore mouth, indigestion, or metallic taste.
2. Increased joint pain may occur for one or two days after an injection and usually subsides after the first few injections.
3. Exposure to sunlight or artificial ultraviolet light should be minimized.
4. Careful oral hygiene is recommended in conjunction with therapy.
5. Patients should be aware of potential hazards if they become pregnant while receiving gold therapy. (See *"Usage in Pregnancy".*)

Laboratory Tests: Before treatment is started, a complete blood count, platelet count, and urinalysis should be done to serve as reference points. Since gold therapy is usually contraindicated in pregnant patients, pregnancy should be ruled out before treatment is started. Throughout the treatment period, urinalysis should be repeated prior to each injection, and complete blood cell and platelet counts should be performed every two weeks. A platelet count is indicated any time that purpura or ecchymosis occurs.

Drug Interactions: Drug interactions have not been reported. (See **CONTRAINDICATIONS.**)

Carcinogenesis, Mutagenesis, and Impairment of Fertility: Renal adenomas developed in rats receiving an injectable gold product similar to SOLGANAL Suspension at doses of 2 mg/kg weekly for 46 weeks, followed by 6 mg/kg daily for 47 weeks. These doses were higher and administered more frequently than the recommended human doses. The adenomas were similar histologically to those produced by chronic administration of other gold compounds and heavy metals, such as lead or nickel.

Renal tubular cell neoplasia consisting of renal adenoma and adenocarcinoma were noted in a dose-response relationship in another study in rats using daily intramuscular doses of 3 mg/kg and 6 mg/kg for up to 2 years. These doses were higher and were administered more frequently than the recommended human doses. In this same study, sarcomas at the injection site occurred in some rats but their numbers were not sufficient to demonstrate a dose-response relationship.

No report of renal adenoma or sarcoma at the injection site in man in association with the use of SOLGANAL Suspension has been received.

Gold compounds have not been studied for evaluation of mutagenesis.

Gold sodium thiomalate given subcutaneously did not adversely affect fertility or reproductive performance.

Usage in Pregnancy: Gold therapy is usually contraindicated in pregnant patients. The patient should be warned about the hazards of becoming pregnant while on gold therapy. Rheumatoid arthritis frequently improves when the patient becomes pregnant, thereby eliminating the need for gold therapy. The potential nephrotoxicity of gold should not be superimposed on the increased renal burden which normally occurs in pregnancy and hence, gold therapy should be discontinued upon recognition of pregnancy unless continued use is required in an individual case. The slow excretion of gold and its persistence in body tissues after discontinuation of treatment should be kept in mind when a woman of child-bearing potential being treated with gold plans to become pregnant.

Pregnancy Category C: Gold sodium thiomalate administered subcutaneously, a route not used clinically, has been shown to be teratogenic during the organogenic period in rats and rabbits when given in doses 140 and 175 times, respectively, the usual human dose. Hydrocephalus and microphthalmia were the malformations observed in rats when gold sodium thiomalate was administered at a dose of 25 mg/kg/day from day 6 through day 15 of gestation. In rabbits, limb defects and gastroschisis were the malformations observed when gold sodium thiomalate was administered at doses of 20 to 45 mg/kg/day from day 6 through day 18 of gestation.

Gold compounds administered orally to rabbits from days 6 through 18 of pregnancy resulted in the occurrence of abdominal defects, such as gastroschisis and umbilical hernia; anomalies of the brain, heart, lung, and skeleton; and microphthalmia.

The administration of excessive doses of gold-containing compounds during pregnancy in the above studies was toxic to the mothers and their embryos; the embryotoxic effects probably were secondary to maternal toxicity. Therefore, the significance of these findings in relation to human use is unknown.

There are no adequate and well-controlled studies with SOLGANAL Suspension in pregnant women. Extensive clinical experience with SOLGANAL Suspension has not demonstrated human teratogenicity.

Nursing Mothers: Gold has been demonstrated in the milk of lactating mothers. In one patient, a total dose of 135 mg of gold thioglucose was given during the postpartum period. Samples of the maternal milk and urine, and samples of red blood cells and serum of the mother and child were evaluated by atomic absorption spectrophotometry. Trace amounts of gold appeared in the serum and red blood cells of the nursing offspring. It has been postulated that this may be the cause of unexplained rashes, nephritis, hepatitis, and hematologic aberrations in the nursing infants of mothers treated with gold. Because of the potential for serious adverse reactions in nursing infants, a decision should be made whether to discontinue nursing or to discontinue the gold therapy, taking into account the importance of the drug to the mother. The slow excretion of gold and its persistence in the mother after discontinuation of treatment should be kept in mind.

Pediatric Use: Safety and effectiveness in children below the age of six years have not been established.

ADVERSE REACTIONS

Adverse reactions to gold therapy may occur at any time during treatment or many months after therapy has been discontinued. The incidence of toxic reactions is apparently unrelated to the plasma level of gold, but it may be related to the cumulative body content of gold. Higher than conventional dosage schedules may increase the occurrence and severity of toxicity. Severe effects are most common after 300 to 500 mg have been administered.

Cutaneous Reactions: Dermatitis is the most common reaction. Pruritus should be considered a warning signal of an impending cutaneous reaction. Erythema and occasionally the more severe reactions such as papular, vesicular, and exfoliative dermatitis leading to alopecia and shedding of the nails may occur. Chrysiasis (gray-to-blue pigmentation) has been reported, especially on photoexposed areas. Gold dermatitis may be aggravated by exposure to sunlight, or an actinic rash may develop.

Mucous Membrane Reactions: Stomatitis is the second most common adverse reaction. Shallow ulcers on the buccal membranes, on the borders of the tongue and on the palate, diffuse glossitis, or gingivitis may be preceded by the sensation of metallic taste. Careful oral hygiene is recommended. Inflammation of the upper respiratory tract, pharyngitis, gastritis, colitis, tracheitis, and vaginitis have also been reported. Conjunctivitis is rare.

Renal Reactions: Nephrotic syndrome or glomerulitis with hematuria, which is usually relatively mild, subsides completely if recognized early and treatment is discontinued. These reactions become severe and chronic if gold therapy is continued after their onset. Therefore, it is important to perform a urinalysis before each injection and to discontinue treatment promptly if proteinuria or hematuria develops.

Hematologic Reactions: Although rare, blood dyscrasias, including granulocytopenia, agranulocytosis, thrombocytopenia with or without purpura, leukopenia, eosinophilia, panmyelopathy, hemorrhagic diathesis, and hypoplastic and aplastic anemia, have been reported. These reactions may occur separately or in combination.

Nitritoid and Allergic Reactions: These reactions, which may rarely occur with SOLGANAL Suspension and which resemble anaphylactoid effects, include flushing, fainting, dizziness, sweating, malaise, weakness, nausea, and vomiting.

Miscellaneous Reactions: On rare occasions, gastrointestinal symptoms, i.e., nausea, vomiting, colic, anorexia, abdominal cramps, diarrhea, ulcerative enterocolitis, and headache have been reported.

There have been rare reports of iritis and corneal ulcers. Transient, asymptomatic gold deposits in the cornea or conjunctiva may occur.

Other reported reactions include encephalitis, immunological destruction of the synovia, EEG abnormalities, intrahepatic cholestasis, hepatitis with jaundice, toxic hepatitis, acute yellow atrophy, peripheral neuritis, gold bronchitis, pulmonary injury manifested by interstitial pneumonitis or fibrosis, fever, and partial or complete hair loss.

Less common but more severe effects that may occur shortly after an injection or at any time during gold therapy include: anaphylactic shock, syncope, bradycardia, thickening of the tongue, difficulty in swallowing and breathing, and angioneurotic edema. If they are observed, treatment with SOLGANAL Suspension should be discontinued.

Arthralgia may occur for one or two days after an injection and usually subsides after the first few injections. The mechanism of the transient increase in rheumatic symptoms after injection of gold (the so-called nonvasomotor postinjection reaction) is unknown. These reactions are usually mild but occasionally may be so severe that treatment is stopped prematurely.

MANAGEMENT OF ADVERSE REACTIONS

In the event of toxic reactions, gold therapy should be discontinued immediately.

In the presence of mild reactions, it may be sufficient to discontinue the administration of SOLGANAL Suspension for a short period and then to resume treatment with smaller doses.

Dermatitis and pruritus may respond to soothing lotions, other appropriate antipruritic treatment, or topical glucocorticoids.

If dermatitis or stomatitis becomes severe or spreads, systemic glucocorticoid treatment may be indicated. For renal, hematologic, and most other adverse reactions, glucocorticoids may be required in larger doses and for a longer time than for dermatologic reactions. Often this treatment may be required for many months because of the slow elimination of gold from the body.

If severe adverse reactions do not improve with steroid treatment in patients who receive large doses of gold, a chelating agent, such as dimercaprol (BAL), may be used. In one case, it was reported that penicillamine was beneficial in the treatment of gold-induced thrombocytopenia. Adjunctive use of an anabolic steroid with other drugs (i.e., BAL, penicillamine, and corticosteroids) may contribute to recovery of bone marrow deficiency.

In the presence of severe or idiosyncratic reactions, treatment with SOLGANAL Suspension should not be reinstituted.

OVERDOSAGE

Overdosage resulting from too rapid increases in dosing with SOLGANAL Suspension will be manifested by rapid appearance of toxic reactions, particularly those relating to renal damage, such as hematuria, proteinuria, and to hematologic effects, such as thrombocytopenia and granulocytopenia. Other toxic effects, including fever, nausea, vomiting, diarrhea, and various skin disorders such as papulovesicular lesions, urticaria, and exfoliative dermatitis, all attended with severe pruritus, may develop. Treatment consists of prompt discontinuation of the medication, and early administration of dimercaprol. Specific supportive therapy should be given for the renal and hematologic complications. (See also **MANAGEMENT OF ADVERSE REACTIONS** above.)

DOSAGE AND ADMINISTRATION

Adults—The usual dosage schedule for the intramuscular administration of SOLGANAL is as follows: first dose, 10 mg; second and third doses, 25 mg; fourth and subsequent doses, 50 mg. The interval between doses is one week. The 50 mg dose is continued at weekly intervals until 0.8 to 1.0 g SOLGANAL has been given. If the patient has improved and has exhibited no sign of toxicity, the 50 mg dose may be continued many months longer, at three- to four-week intervals. A weekly dose above 50 mg is usually unnecessary and contraindicated; the tendency in gold therapy is toward lower dosage. With this in mind, it may eventually be established that a 25 mg dose is the one of choice. If no improvement has been demonstrated after a total administration of 1.0 g of SOLGANAL Suspension, the necessity for gold therapy should be reevaluated.

Children 6 to 12 years—one-fourth of the adult dose, governed chiefly by body weight, not to exceed 25 mg per dose. SOLGANAL Suspension should be injected **intramuscularly**, (preferably intragluteally), **never intravenously.** The patient should be lying down and should remain recumbent for approximately 10 minutes after the injection. The vial should be thoroughly shaken in order to suspend all of the active material. Heating the vial to body temperature (by immersion in warm water) will facilitate drawing the suspension into the syringe. An 18-gauge, $1^1/_2$-inch needle is recommended for depositing the preparation deep into the muscu-

Continued on next page

Information on Schering products appearing on these pages is effective as of August 15, 1996.

Consult 1997 supplements and future editions for revisions

Schering—Cont.

lar tissue. For obese patients, an 18-gauge, 2-inch needle may be used. The site usually selected for injection is the upper outer quadrant of the gluteal region.

NOTE: Shake the vial in horizontal position before the dose is withdrawn. Needle and syringe must be dry. The patient should be observed for at least 15 minutes following each injection.

HOW SUPPLIED
SOLGANAL Suspension is available in 10 ml multiple-dose vials containing 5% (50 mg/ml) aurothioglucose; box of one (NDC-0085-0460-03).

Shake well before using. Store between 0° and 30°C (32° and 86°F). Protect from light. Store in carton until contents are used.

Revised 8/84   13288500

Copyright © 1963, 1984, Schering Corporation. All rights reserved.

TRILAFON®   ℞
brand of perphenazine, USP
   Tablets
   Concentrate
   Injection

DESCRIPTION
TRILAFON products contain perphenazine, USP (4-[3-(2-chlorophenothiazin-10-yl)propyl]-1-piperazineethanol), a piperazinyl phenothiazine having the chemical formula, $C_{21}H_{26}ClN_3OS$. They are available as **Tablets**, 2, 4, 8, and 16 mg; **Concentrate**, 16 mg perphenazine per 5 mL and alcohol less than 0.1%; and **Injection**, perphenazine 5 mg per 1 mL. The inactive ingredients for TRILAFON **Tablets**, 2, 4, 8, and 16 mg. include: acacia, black iron oxide, butylparaben, calcium phosphate, calcium sulfate, carnauba wax, corn starch, gelatin, lactose, magnesium stearate, potato starch, sugar, titanium dioxide, white wax and other ingredients. May also contain talc.

The inactive ingredients for TRILAFON **Concentrate** include: alcohol, citric acid, flavors, menthol, sodium phosphate, sorbitol, sugar, and water.

The inactive ingredients for TRILAFON **Injection** include: citric acid, sodium bisulfite, sodium hydroxide, and water.

ACTIONS
Perphenazine has actions at all levels of the central nervous system, particularly the hypothalamus. However, the site and mechanism of action of therapeutic effect are not known.

INDICATIONS
Perphenazine is indicated for use in the management of the manifestations of psychotic disorders; and for the control of severe nausea and vomiting in adults.

TRILAFON has not been shown effective for the management of behavioral complications in patients with mental retardation.

CONTRAINDICATIONS
TRILAFON products are contraindicated in comatose or greatly obtunded patients and in patients receiving large doses of central nervous system depressants (barbiturates, alcohol, narcotics, analgesics, or antihistamines); in the presence of existing blood dyscrasias, bone marrow depression, or liver damage; and in patients who have shown hypersensitivity to TRILAFON products, their components, or related compounds.

TRILAFON products are also contraindicated in patients with suspected or established subcortical brain damage, with or without hypothalamic damage, since a hyperthermic reaction with temperatures in excess of 104°F may occur in such patients, sometimes not until 14 to 16 hours after drug administration. Total body ice-packing is recommended for such a reaction; antipyretics may also be useful.

WARNINGS
Tardive dyskinesia, a syndrome consisting of potentially irreversible, involuntary, dyskinetic movements, may develop in patients treated with neuroleptic (antipsychotic) drugs. Although the prevalence of the syndrome appears to be highest among the elderly, especially elderly women, it is impossible to rely upon prevalence estimates to predict, at the inception of neuroleptic treatment, which patients are likely to develop the syndrome. Whether neuroleptic drug products differ in their potential to cause tardive dyskinesia is unknown.

Both the risk of developing the syndrome and the likelihood that it will become irreversible are believed to increase as the duration of treatment and the total cumulative dose of neuroleptic drugs administered to the patient increase. However, the syndrome can develop, although much less commonly, after relatively brief treatment periods at low doses.

There is no known treatment for established cases of tardive dyskinesia, although the syndrome may remit, partially or completely, if neuroleptic treatment is withdrawn. Neuroleptic treatment itself, however, may suppress (or partially suppress) the signs and symptoms of the syndrome, and thereby may possibly mask the underlying disease process. The effect that symptomatic suppression has upon the long-term course of the syndrome is unknown.

Given these considerations, neuroleptics should be prescribed in a manner that is most likely to minimize the occurrence of tardive dyskinesia. Chronic neuroleptic treatment should generally be reserved for patients who suffer from a chronic illness that, 1) is known to respond to neuroleptic drugs, and 2) for whom alternative, equally effective, but potentially less harmful treatments are <u>not</u> available or appropriate. In patients who do require chronic treatment, the smallest dose and the shortest duration of treatment producing a satisfactory clinical response should be sought. The need for continued treatment should be reassessed periodically.

If signs and symptoms of tardive dyskinesia appear in a patient on neuroleptics, drug discontinuation should be considered. However, some patients may require treatment despite the presence of the syndrome.

(For further information about the description of tardive dyskinesia and its clinical detection, please refer to **Information for Patients** and **ADVERSE REACTIONS**.)

TRILAFON **Injection** contains sodium bisulfite, a sulfite that may cause allergic-type reactions including anaphylactic symptoms and life-threatening or less severe asthmatic episodes in certain susceptible people. The overall prevalence of sulfite sensitivity is seen more frequently in asthmatic than in nonasthmatic people.

NEUROLEPTIC MALIGNANT SYNDROME (NMS)
A potentially fatal symptom complex sometimes referred to as Neuroleptic Malignant Syndrome (NMS), has been reported in association with antipsychotic drugs. Clinical manifestations of NMS are hyperpyrexia, muscle rigidity, altered mental status and evidence of autonomic instability (irregular pulse or blood pressure, tachycardia, diaphoresis, and cardiac dysrhythmias).

The diagnostic evaluation of patients with this syndrome is complicated. In arriving at a diagnosis, it is important to identify cases where the clinical presentation includes both serious medical illness (e.g., pneumonia, systemic infection, etc.) and untreated or inadequately treated extrapyramidal signs and symptoms (EPS). Other important considerations in the differential diagnosis include central anticholinergic toxicity, heat stroke, drug fever and primary central nervous system (CNS) pathology.

The management of NMS should include 1) immediate discontinuation of antipsychotic drugs and other drugs not essential to concurrent therapy, 2) intensive symptomatic treatment and medical monitoring, and 3) treatment of any concomitant serious medical problems for which specific treatments are available. There is no general agreement about specific pharmacological treatment regimens for uncomplicated NMS.

If a patient requires antipsychotic drug treatment after recovery from NMS, the reintroduction of drug therapy should be carefully considered. The patient should be carefully monitored, since recurrences of NMS have been reported.

If hypotension develops, epinephrine should not be administered since its action is blocked and partially reversed by perphenazine. If a vasopressor is needed, norepinephrine may be used. Severe, acute hypotension has occurred with the use of phenothiazines and is particularly likely to occur in patients with mitral insufficiency or pheochromocytoma. Rebound hypertension may occur in pheochromocytoma patients.

TRILAFON products can lower the convulsive threshold in susceptible individuals; they should be used with caution in alcohol withdrawal and in patients with convulsive disorders. If the patient is being treated with an anticonvulsant agent, increased dosage of that agent may be required when TRILAFON products are used concomitantly.

TRILAFON products should be used with caution in patients with psychic depression.

Perphenazine may impair the mental and/or physical abilities required for the performance of hazardous tasks such as driving a car or operating machinery; therefore, the patient should be warned accordingly.

TRILAFON products are not recommended for children under 12 years of age.

Usage in Pregnancy: Safe use of TRILAFON during pregnancy and lactation has not been established; therefore, in administering the drug to pregnant patients, nursing mothers, or women who may become pregnant, the possible benefits must be weighed against the possible hazards to mother and child.

PRECAUTIONS
The possibility of suicide in depressed patients remains during treatment and until significant remission occurs. This type of patient should not have access to large quantities of this drug.

As with all phenothiazine compounds, perphenazine should not be used indiscriminately. Caution should be observed in giving it to patients who have previously exhibited severe adverse reactions to other phenothiazines. Some of the untoward actions of perphenazine tend to appear more frequently when high doses are used. However, as with other phenothiazine compounds, patients receiving TRILAFON products in any dosage should be kept under close supervision.

Neuroleptic drugs elevate prolactin levels; the elevation persists during chronic administration. Tissue culture experiments indicate that approximately one-third of human breast cancers are prolactin dependent *in vitro*, a factor of potential importance if the prescription of these drugs is contemplated in a patient with a previously detected breast cancer. Although disturbances such as galactorrhea, amenorrhea, gynecomastia, and impotence have been reported, the clinical significance of elevated serum prolactin levels is unknown for most patients. An increase in mammary neoplasms has been found in rodents after chronic administration of neuroleptic drugs. Neither clinical studies nor epidemiologic studies conducted to date, however, have shown an association between chronic administration of these drugs and mammary tumorigenesis; the available evidence is considered too limited to be conclusive at this time.

The antiemetic effect of perphenazine may obscure signs of toxicity due to overdosage of other drugs, or render more difficult the diagnosis of disorders such as brain tumors or intestinal obstruction.

A significant, not otherwise explained, rise in body temperature may suggest individual intolerance to perphenazine, in which case it should be discontinued.

Patients on large doses of a phenothiazine drug who are undergoing surgery should be watched carefully for possible hypotensive phenomena. Moreover, reduced amounts of anesthetics or central nervous system depressants may be necessary.

Since phenothiazines and central nervous system depressants (opiates, analgesics, antihistamines, barbiturates) can potentiate each other, less than the usual dosage of the added drug is recommended and caution is advised when they are administered concomitantly.

Use with caution in patients who are receiving atropine or related drugs because of additive anticholinergic effects and also in patients who will be exposed to extreme heat or phosphorus insecticides.

The use of alcohol should be avoided, since additive effects and hypotension may occur. Patients should be cautioned that their response to alcohol may be increased while they are being treated with TRILAFON products. The risk of suicide and the danger of overdose may be increased in patients who use alcohol excessively due to its potentiation of the drug's effect.

Blood counts and hepatic and renal functions should be checked periodically. The appearance of signs of blood dyscrasias requires the discontinuance of the drug and institution of appropriate therapy. If abnormalities in hepatic tests occur, phenothiazine treatment should be discontinued. Renal function in patients on long-term therapy should be monitored; if blood urea nitrogen (BUN) becomes abnormal, treatment with the drug should be discontinued.

The use of phenothiazine derivatives in patients with diminished renal function should be undertaken with caution.

Use with caution in patients suffering from respiratory impairment due to acute pulmonary infections, or in chronic respiratory disorders such as severe asthma or emphysema.

In general, phenothiazines, including perphenazine, do not produce psychic dependence. Gastritis, nausea and vomiting, dizziness, and tremulousness have been reported following abrupt cessation of high-dose therapy. Reports suggest that these symptoms can be reduced by continuing concomitant antiparkinson agents for several weeks after the phenothiazine is withdrawn.

The possibility of liver damage, corneal and lenticular deposits, and irreversible dyskinesias should be kept in mind when patients are on long-term therapy.

Because photosensitivity has been reported, undue exposure to the sun should be avoided during phenothiazine treatment.

Information for Patients: This information is intended to aid in the safe and effective use of this medication. It is not a disclosure of all possible adverse or intended effects.

Given the likelihood that a substantial proportion of patients exposed chronically to neuroleptics will develop tardive dyskinesia, it is advised that all patients in whom chronic use is contemplated be given, if possible, full information about this risk. The decision to inform patients and/or their guardians must obviously take into account the clinical circumstances and the competency of the patient to understand the information provided.

ADVERSE REACTIONS
Not all of the following adverse reactions have been reported with this specific drug; however, pharmacological similarities among various phenothiazine derivatives require that each be considered. With the piperazine group (of which per-

phenazine is an example), the extrapyramidal symptoms are more common, and others (e.g., sedative effects, jaundice, and blood dyscrasias) are less frequently seen.

CNS Effects: *Extrapyramidal reactions:* opisthotonus, trismus, torticollis, retrocollis, aching and numbness of the limbs, motor restlessness, oculogyric crisis, hyperreflexia, dystonia, including protrusion, discoloration, aching and rounding of the tongue, tonic spasm of the masticatory muscles, tight feeling in the throat, slurred speech, dysphagia, akathisia, dyskinesia, parkinsonism, and ataxia. Their incidence and severity usually increase with an increase in dosage, but there is considerable individual variation in the tendency to develop such symptoms. Extrapyramidal symptoms can usually be controlled by the concomitant use of effective antiparkinsonian drugs, such as benztropine mesylate, and/or by reduction in dosage. In some instances, however, these extrapyramidal reactions may persist after discontinuation of treatment with perphenazine.

Persistent tardive dyskinesia: As with all antipsychotic agents, tardive dyskinesia may appear in some patients on long-term therapy or may appear after drug therapy has been discontinued. Although the risk appears to be greater in elderly patients on high-dose therapy, especially females, it may occur in either sex and in children. The symptoms are persistent and in some patients appear to be irreversible. The syndrome is characterized by rhythmical, involuntary movements of the tongue, face, mouth or jaw (e.g., protrusion of tongue, puffing of cheeks, puckering of mouth, chewing movements). Sometimes these may be accompanied by involuntary movements of the extremities. There is no known effective treatment for tardive dyskinesia; antiparkinsonism agents usually do not alleviate the symptoms of this syndrome. It is suggested that all antipsychotic agents be discontinued if these symptoms appear. Should it be necessary to reinstitute treatment, or increase the dosage of the agent, or switch to a different antipsychotic agent, the syndrome may be masked. It has been reported that fine, vermicular movements of the tongue may be an early sign of the syndrome, and if the medication is stopped at that time the syndrome may not develop.

Other CNS effects include cerebral edema; abnormality of cerebrospinal fluid proteins; convulsive seizures, particularly in patients with EEG abnormalities or a history of such disorders, and headaches.

Neuroleptic malignant syndrome has been reported in patients treated with neuroleptic drugs (see **WARNINGS** for further information).

Drowsiness may occur, particularly during the first or second week, after which it generally disappears. If troublesome, lower the dosage. Hypnotic effects appear to be minimal, especially in patients who are permitted to remain active.

Adverse behavioral effects include paradoxical exacerbation of psychotic symptoms, catatonic-like states, paranoid reactions, lethargy, paradoxical excitement, restlessness, hyperactivity, nocturnal confusion, bizarre dreams, and insomnia.

Hyperreflexia has been reported in the newborn when a phenothiazine was used during pregnancy.

Autonomic Effects: dry mouth or salivation, nausea, vomiting, diarrhea, anorexia, constipation, obstipation, fecal impaction, urinary retention, frequency or incontinence, bladder paralysis, polyuria, nasal congestion, pallor, myosis, mydriasis, blurred vision, glaucoma, perspiration, hypertension, hypotension, and change in pulse rate occasionally may occur. Significant autonomic effects have been infrequent in patients receiving less than 24 mg perphenazine daily.

Adynamic ileus occasionally occurs with phenothiazine therapy and if severe can result in complications and death. It is of particular concern in psychiatric patients, who may fail to seek treatment of the condition.

Allergic Effects: urticaria, erythema, eczema, exfoliative dermatitis, pruritus, photosensitivity, asthma, fever, anaphylactoid reactions, laryngeal edema; and angioneurotic edema; contact dermatitis in nursing personnel administering the drug; and in extremely rare instances, individual idiosyncrasy or hypersensitivity to phenothiazines has resulted in cerebral edema, circulatory collapse, and death.

Endocrine Effects: lactation, galactorrhea, moderate breast enlargement in females and gynecomastia in males on large doses, disturbances in the menstrual cycle, amenorrhea, changes in libido, inhibition of ejaculation, syndrome of inappropriate ADH (antidiuretic hormone) secretion, false positive pregnancy tests, hyperglycemia, hypoglycemia, glycosuria.

Cardiovascular Effects: postural hypotension, tachycardia (especially with sudden marked increase in dosage), bradycardia, cardiac arrest, faintness, and dizziness. Occasionally the hypotensive effect may produce a shock-like condition. ECG changes, nonspecific (quinidine-like effect) usually reversible, have been observed in some patients receiving phenothiazine tranquilizers.

Sudden death has occasionally been reported in patients who have received phenothiazines. In some cases the death was apparently due to cardiac arrest; in others, the cause appeared to be asphyxia due to failure of the cough reflex. In some patients, the cause could not be determined nor could it be established that the death was due to the phenothiazine.

Hematological Effects: agranulocytosis, eosinophilia, leukopenia, hemolytic anemia, thrombocytopenic purpura, and pancytopenia. Most cases of agranulocytosis have occurred between the fourth and tenth weeks of therapy. Patients should be watched closely, especially during that period, for the sudden appearance of sore throat or signs of infection. If white blood cell and differential cell counts show significant cellular depression, discontinue the drug and start appropriate therapy. However, a slightly lowered white count is not in itself an indication to discontinue the drug.

Other Effects: Special considerations in long-term therapy include pigmentation of the skin, occurring chiefly in the exposed areas; ocular changes consisting of deposition of fine particulate matter in the cornea and lens, progressing in more severe cases to star-shaped lenticular opacities; epithelial keratopathies; and pigmentary retinopathy. Also noted: peripheral edema, reversed epinephrine effect, increase in PBI not attributable to an increase in thyroxine, parotid swelling (rare), hyperpyrexia, systemic lupus erythematosus-like syndrome, increases in appetite and weight, polyphagia, photophobia, and muscle weakness.

Liver damage (biliary stasis) may occur. Jaundice may occur, usually between the second and fourth weeks of treatment, and is regarded as a hypersensitivity reaction. Incidence is low. The clinical picture resembles infectious hepatitis but with laboratory features of obstructive jaundice. It is usually reversible; however, chronic jaundice has been reported.

Side effects with intramuscular TRILAFON **Injection** have been infrequent and transient. Dizziness or significant hypotension after treatment with TRILAFON **Injection** is a rare occurrence.

DOSAGE AND ADMINISTRATION

Dosage must be individualized and adjusted according to the severity of the condition and the response obtained. As with all potent drugs, the best dose is the lowest dose that will produce the desired clinical effect. Since extrapyramidal symptoms increase in frequency and severity with increased dosage, it is important to employ the lowest effective dose. These symptoms have disappeared upon reduction of dosage, withdrawal of the drug, or administration of an antiparkinsonian agent.

Prolonged administration of doses exceeding 24 mg daily should be reserved for hospitalized patients or patients under continued observation for early detection and management of adverse reactions. An antiparkinsonian agent, such as trihexyphenidyl hydrochloride or benztropine mesylate, is valuable in controlling drug-induced extrapyramidal symptoms.

TRILAFON **Tablets**

Suggested dosages for **Tablets** for various conditions follow:

Moderately disturbed non-hospitalized psychotic patients: **Tablets** 4 to 8 mg t.i.d. initially; reduce as soon as possible to minimum effective dosage.

Hospitalized psychotic patients: **Tablets** 8 to 16 mg b.i.d. to q.i.d.; avoid dosages in excess of 64 mg daily.

Severe nausea and vomiting in adults: **Tablets** 8 to 16 mg daily in divided doses; 24 mg occasionally may be necessary; early dosage reduction is desirable.

TRILAFON **Injection**—Intramuscular Administration

The injection is used when rapid effect and prompt control of acute or intractable conditions is required or when oral administration is not feasible. TRILAFON **Injection**, administered by deep intramuscular injection, is well tolerated. The injection should be given with the patient seated or recumbent, and the patient should be observed for a short period after administration.

Therapeutic effect is usually evidenced in 10 minutes and is maximal in 1 to 2 hours. The average duration of effective action is 6 hours, occasionally 12 to 24 hours.

Pediatric dosage has not yet been established. Children over 12 years may receive the lowest limit of adult dosage.

The usual initial dose is 5 mg (1 mL). This may be repeated every 6 hours. Ordinarily, the total daily dosage should not exceed 15 mg in ambulatory patients or 30 mg in hospitalized patients. When required for satisfactory control of symptoms in severe conditions, an initial 10-mg intramuscular dose may be given. Patients should be placed on oral therapy as soon as practicable. Generally, this may be achieved within 24 hours. In some instances, however, patients have been maintained on injectable therapy for several months. It has been established that TRILAFON **Injection** is more potent than TRILAFON **Tablets**. Therefore, equal or higher dosage should be used when the patient is transferred to oral therapy after receiving the injection.

Psychotic conditions: While 5 mg of the **Injection** has a definite tranquilizing effect, it may be necessary to use 10-mg doses to initiate therapy in severely agitated states. Most patients will be controlled and amendable to oral therapy within a maximum of 24 to 48 hours. Acute conditions (hysteria, panic reaction) often respond well to a single dose, whereas in chronic conditions, several injections may be required. When transferring patients to oral therapy, it is suggested that increased dosage be employed to maintain adequate clinical control. This should be followed by gradual reduction to the minimal maintenance dose which is effective.

Severe nausea and vomiting in adults: To obtain rapid control of vomiting, administer 5 mg (1 mL); in rare instances it may be necessary to increase the dose to 10 mg; in general, higher doses should be given only to hospitalized patients.

Intravenous Administration

The intravenous administration of TRILAFON **Injection** is seldom required. This route of administration should be used with particular caution and care, and only when absolutely necessary to control severe vomiting, intractable hiccoughs, or acute conditions, such as violent retching during surgery. Its use should be limited to recumbent hospitalized adults in doses not exceeding 5 mg. When employed in this manner, intravenous injection ordinarily should be given as a diluted solution by either fractional injection or a slow drip infusion. In the surgical patient, slow infusion of not more than 5 mg is preferred. When administered in divided doses, TRILAFON **Injection** should be diluted to 0.5 mg/mL (1 mL mixed with 9 mL of physiologic saline solution), and not more than 1 mg per injection given at not less than one- to two-minute intervals. Intravenous injection should be discontinued as soon as symptoms are controlled and should not exceed 5 mg. The possibility of hypotensive and extrapyramidal side effects should be considered and appropriate means for management kept available. Blood pressure and pulse should be monitored continuously during intravenous administration. Pharmacologic and clinical studies indicate that intravenous administration of norepinephrine should be useful in alleviating the hypotensive effect.

TRILAFON **Concentrate**

In hospitalized psychotic patients, the usual dosage range is 8 to 16 mg b.i.d. to q.i.d., depending on the severity of symptoms and individual response. Although a number of investigators have employed higher dosage, a total daily dose of more than 64 mg ordinarily is not required. The **Concentrate** should be diluted only with water, saline, Seven-Up, homogenized milk, carbonated orange drink, and pineapple, apricot, prune, orange. V-8, tomato, and grapefruit juices. Trilafon **Concentrate** should not be mixed with beverages containing caffeine (coffee, cola), tannics (tea), or pectinates (apple juice), since physical incompatibility may result. Suggested dilution is approximately two fluid ounces of diluent for each 5 mL (16 mg) teaspoonful of TRILAFON **Concentrate**. For convenience in measuring smaller doses, a graduated dropper marked to measure 8 mg or 4 mg is supplied with each bottle.

OVERDOSAGE

In the event of overdosage, emergency treatment should be started immediately. All patients suspected of having taken an overdose should be hospitalized as soon as possible.

Manifestations Overdosage of perphenazine primarily involves the extrapyramidal mechanism and produces the same side effects described under **ADVERSE REACTIONS**, but to a more marked degree. It is usually evidenced by stupor or coma; children may have convulsive seizures.

Treatment Treatment is symptomatic and supportive. There is no specific antidote. The patient should be induced to vomit even if emesis has occurred spontaneously. Pharmacologic vomiting by the administration of ipecac syrup is a preferred method. It should be noted that ipecac has a central mode of action in addition to its local gastric irritant properties, and the central mode of action may be blocked by the antiemetic effect of TRILAFON products. Vomiting should not be induced in patients with impaired consciousness. The action of ipecac is facilitated by physical activity and by the administration of 8 to 12 fluid ounces of water. If emesis does not occur within 15 minutes, the dose of ipecac should be repeated. Precautions against aspiration must be taken, especially in infants and children. Following emesis, any drug remaining in the stomach may be adsorbed by activated charcoal administered as a slurry with water. If vomiting is unsuccessful or contraindicated, gastric lavage should be performed. Isotonic and one-half isotonic saline are the lavage solutions of choice. Saline cathartics, such as milk of magnesia, draw water into the bowel by osmosis and therefore, may be valuable for their action in rapid dilution of bowel content.

Standard measures (oxygen, intravenous fluids, corticosteroids) should be used to manage circulatory shock or metabolic acidosis. An open airway and adequate fluid intake should be maintained. Body temperature should be regulated. Hypothermia is expected, but severe hyperthermia may occur and must be treated vigorously. (See **CONTRAINDICATIONS.**)

An electrocardiogram should be taken and close monitoring of cardiac function instituted if there is any sign of abnormality. Cardiac arrhythmias may be treated with neostig-

Continued on next page

Information on Schering products appearing on these pages is effective as of August 15, 1996.

Schering—Cont.

mine, pyridostigmine, or propranolol. Digitalis should be considered for cardiac failure. Close monitoring of cardiac function is advisable for not less than five days. Vasopressors such as norepinephrine may be used to treat hypotension, but epinephrine should NOT be used.

Anticonvulsants (an inhalation anesthetic, diazepam, or paraldehyde) are recommended for control of convulsions, since perphenazine increases the central nervous system depressant action, but not the anticonvulsant action of barbiturates.

If acute parkinson-like symptoms result from perphenazine intoxication, benztropine mesylate or diphenydramine may be administered.

Central nervous system depression may be treated with non-convulsant doses of CNS stimulants. Avoid stimulants that may cause convulsions (e.g., picrotoxin and pentylenetetrazol).

Signs of arousal may not occur for 48 hours.

Dialysis is of no value because of low plasma concentrations of the drug.

Since overdosage is often deliberate, patients may attempt suicide by other means during the recovery phase. Deaths by deliberate or accidental overdosage have occurred with this class of drugs.

HOW SUPPLIED

TRILAFON **Tablets** (2 mg): gray, sugar-coated tablets branded in black with the Schering trademark and either product identification letters, ADH, or numbers, 705, bottles of 100 (NDC 0085-0705-04). **Store between 2° and 25°C (36° and 77°F).**

TRILAFON **Tablets** (4 mg): gray, sugar-coated tablets branded in green with the Schering trademark and either product identification letters, ADK, or numbers, 940; bottles of 100 (NDC 0085-0940-05). **Store between 2° and 25°C (36° and 77°F).**

TRILAFON **Tablets** (8 mg): gray, sugar-coated tablets branded in blue with the Schering trademark and either product identification letters, ADJ, or numbers, 313; bottles of 100 (NDC 0085-0313-05). **Store between 2° and 25°C (36° and 77°F).**

TRILAFON **Tablets** (16 mg): gray, sugar-coated tablets branded in red with the Schering trademark and either product identification letters, ADM, or numbers, 077; bottles of 100 (NDC 0085-0077-05). **Store between 2° and 25°C (36° and 77°F).**

TRILAFON **Concentrate,** 16 mg per 5 mL, 4 fluid ounce (118 mL) bottle with graduated dropper (NDC 0085-0363-02). The **Concentrate** is light-sensitive and should be dispensed in amber bottles. **Protect from light. Store between 2° and 30°C (36° and 86°F). Shake well before using. Store in carton until completely used.**

TRILAFON **Injection,** 5 mg per mL, 1-mL ampul for intramuscular or intravenous use, box of 100 (NDC 0085-0012-04). Keep package closed to protect from light. Exposure may cause discoloration. Slight yellowish discoloration will not alter potency or therapeutic efficacy; if markedly discolored, ampul should be discarded. **Protect from light. Store in carton until completely used.**

TRILAFON®
brand of perphenazine, USP
Tablets, Concentrate,
Injection

Schering Corporation
Kenilworth, NJ 07033 USA
Revised 11/93 17978900

Copyright © 1969, 1991, 1994, Schering Corporation.
All rights reserved.

Shown in Product Identification Guide, page 334

VANCENASE® ℞

brand of beclomethasone dipropionate, USP
POCKETHALER® Nasal Inhaler
For Nasal Inhalation Only

DESCRIPTION

Beclomethasone dipropionate, USP, the active component of VANCENASE POCKETHALER Nasal Inhaler, is an anti-inflammatory steroid having the chemical name, 9-Chloro-11β,17,21-trihydroxy -16β- methylpregna -1,4- diene-3,20-dione 17,21-dipropionate, and the following formula:

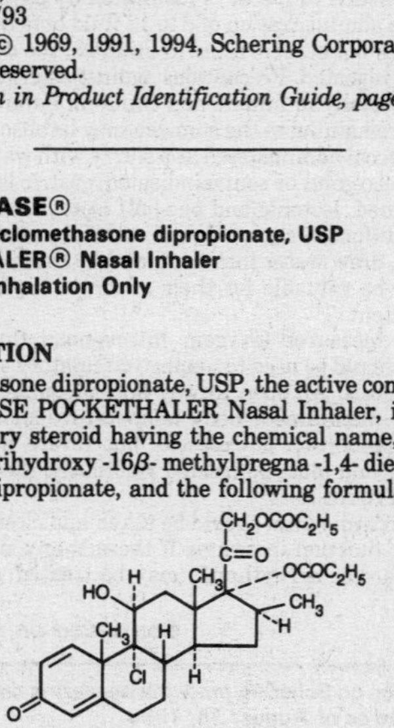

Beclomethasone dipropionate is a white to creamy-white, odorless powder with a molecular weight of 521.25. It is very slightly soluble in water, very soluble in chloroform, and freely soluble in acetone and in alcohol.

VANCENASE POCKETHALER Nasal Inhaler is a metered-dose aerosol unit containing a microcrystalline suspension of beclomethasone dipropionate-trichloromonofluoromethane clathrate in a mixture of propellants (trichloromonofluoromethane and dichlorodifluoromethane) with oleic acid. Each canister contains beclomethasone dipropionate-trichloromonofluoromethane clathrate having a molecular proportion of beclomethasone dipropionate to trichloromonofluoromethane between 3:1 and 3:2. Each actuation delivers from the nasal adapter a quantity of clathrate equivalent to 42 mcg of beclomethasone dipropionate, USP. The contents of one canister provide at least 200 metered doses.

CLINICAL PHARMACOLOGY

Beclomethasone 17,21-dipropionate is a diester of beclomethasone, a synthetic halogenated corticosteroid. Animal studies showed that beclomethasone dipropionate has potent glucocorticoid and weak mineralocorticoid activity. The mechanisms for the anti-inflammatory action of beclomethasone dipropionate are unknown. The precise mechanism of the aerosolized drug's action in the nose is also unknown. Biopsies of nasal mucosa obtained during clinical studies showed no histopathologic changes when beclomethasone dipropionate was administered intranasally.

The effects of beclomethasone dipropionate on hypothalamic-pituitary-adrenal (HPA) function have been evaluated in adult volunteers by other routes of administration. Studies are currently being undertaken with beclomethasone dipropionate by the intranasal route, which may demonstrate that there is more or that there is less absorption by this route of administration. There was no suppression of early morning plasma cortisol concentrations when beclomethasone dipropionate was administered in a dose of 1000 mcg/day for 1 month as an oral aerosol or for 3 days by intramuscular injection. However, partial suppression of plasma cortisol concentration was observed when beclomethasone dipropionate was administered in doses of 2000 mcg/day either by oral aerosol or intramuscularly. Immediate suppression of plasma cortisol concentrations was observed after single doses of 4000 mcg of beclomethasone dipropionate. Suppression of HPA function (reduction of early morning plasma cortisol levels) has been reported in adult patients who received 1600 mcg daily doses of oral beclomethasone dipropionate for one month. In clinical studies using beclomethasone dipropionate intranasally, there was no evidence of adrenal insufficiency.

Beclomethasone dipropionate is sparingly soluble. When given by nasal inhalation in the form of an aqueous or aerosolized suspension, the drug is deposited primarily in the nasal passages. A portion of the drug is swallowed. Absorption occurs rapidly from all respiratory and gastrointestinal tissues. There is no evidence of tissue storage of beclomethasone dipropionate or its metabolites. *In vitro* studies have shown that tissue other than the liver (lung slices) can rapidly metabolize beclomethasone dipropionate to beclomethasone 17-monopropionate and more slowly to free beclomethasone (which has very weak anti-inflammatory activity). However, irrespective of the route of entry, the principal route of excretion of the drug and its metabolites is the feces. In humans, 12% to 15% of an orally administered dose of beclomethasone dipropionate is excreted in the urine as both conjugated and free metabolites of the drug.

Studies have shown that the degree of binding to plasma proteins is 87%.

INDICATIONS AND USAGE

VANCENASE POCKETHALER Nasal Inhaler is indicated for the relief of the symptoms of seasonal or perennial rhinitis in those cases poorly responsive to conventional treatment.

VANCENASE POCKETHALER Nasal Inhaler is also indicated for the prevention of recurrence of nasal polyps following surgical removal.

Clinical studies in seasonal and perennial rhinitis have shown that improvement is usually apparent within a few days. However, symptomatic relief may not occur in some patients for as long as 2 weeks. Although systemic effects are minimal at recommended doses, VANCENASE treatment should not be continued beyond 3 weeks in the absence of significant symptomatic improvement. VANCENASE treatment should not be used in the presence of untreated, localized infection involving the nasal mucosa.

Clinical studies have shown that treatment of the symptoms associated with nasal polyps may have to be continued for several weeks or more before a therapeutic result can be fully assessed. Recurrence of symptoms due to polyps can occur after stopping treatment, depending on the severity of the disease.

CONTRAINDICATIONS

Hypersensitivity to any of the ingredients of this preparation contraindicates its use.

WARNINGS

The replacement of a systemic corticosteroid with VANCENASE POCKETHALER Nasal Inhaler can be accompanied by signs of adrenal insufficiency.

Careful attention must be given when patients, previously treated for prolonged periods with systemic corticosteroids, are transferred to VANCENASE POCKETHALER Nasal Inhaler. This is particularly important in those patients who have associated asthma or other clinical conditions, where too rapid a decrease in systemic corticosteroids may cause a severe exacerbation of their symptoms.

Studies have shown that the combined administration of alternate day prednisone systemic treatment and orally inhaled beclomethasone increased the likelihood of HPA suppression compared to a therapeutic dose of either one alone. Therefore, VANCENASE treatment should be used with caution in patients already on alternate day prednisone regimens for any disease.

If recommended doses of intranasal beclomethasone are exceeded or if individuals are particularly sensitive or predisposed by virtue of recent systemic steroid therapy, symptoms of hypercorticism may occur, including very rare cases of menstrual irregularities, acneiform lesions, and cushingoid features. If such changes occur, VANCENASE POCKETHALER Nasal Inhaler should be discontinued slowly, consistent with accepted procedures for discontinuing oral steroid therapy.

Persons who are on drugs which suppress the immune system are more susceptible to infections than healthy individuals. Chickenpox and measles, for example, can have a more serious or even fatal course in non-immune children or adults on corticosteroids. In such children or adults who have not had these diseases, particular care should be taken to avoid exposure. How the dose, route and duration of corticosteroid administration affects the risk of developing a disseminated infection is not known. The contribution of the underlying disease and/or prior corticosteroid treatment to the risk is also not known. If exposed to chickenpox, prophylaxis with varicella-zoster immune globulin (VZIG) may be indicated. If exposed to measles, prophylaxis with pooled intramuscular immunoglobulin (IG) may be indicated. (See the respective package inserts for complete VZIG and IG prescribing information.) If chickenpox develops, treatment with antiviral agents may be considered.

PRECAUTIONS

General: During withdrawal from oral steroids, some patients may experience symptoms of withdrawal, eg, joint and/or muscular pain, lassitude, and depression.

Extremely rare instances of nasal septum perforation and increased intraocular pressure have been reported following the intranasal application of aerosolized corticosteroids.

In clinical studies with beclomethasone dipropionate administered intranasally, the development of localized infections of the nose and pharynx with *Candida albicans* has occurred only rarely. When such an infection develops, it may require treatment with appropriate local therapy or discontinuance of treatment with VANCENASE POCKETHALER Nasal Inhaler.

Beclomethasone dipropionate is absorbed into the circulation. Use of excessive doses of VANCENASE POCKETHALER Nasal Inhaler may suppress HPA function.

VANCENASE treatment should be used with caution, if at all, in patients with active or quiescent tuberculous infections of the respiratory tract, or in untreated fungal, bacterial, systemic viral infections, or ocular herpes simplex.

For VANCENASE POCKETHALER Nasal Inhaler to be effective in the treatment of nasal polyps, the aerosol must be able to enter the nose. Therefore, treatment of nasal polyps with VANCENASE Nasal Inhaler should be considered adjunctive therapy to surgical removal and/or the use of other medications which will permit effective penetration of the VANCENASE product into the nose. Nasal polyps may recur after any form of treatment.

As with any long-term treatment, patients using VANCENASE treatment over several months or longer should be examined periodically for possible changes in the nasal mucosa.

Because of the inhibitory effect of corticosteroids on wound healing, patients who have experienced recent nasal septum ulcers, nasal surgery, or trauma should not use a nasal corticosteroid until healing has occurred.

Although systemic effects have been minimal with recommended doses, this potential increases with excessive doses. Therefore, larger than recommended doses should be avoided.

Information for Patients: Patients should use VANCENASE POCKETHALER Nasal Inhaler at regular intervals since its effectiveness depends on its regular use. The patient should take the medication as directed. It is not acutely effective and the prescribed dosage should not be increased. Instead, nasal vasoconstrictors or oral antihistamines may be needed until the effects of VANCENASE POCKETHALER Nasal Inhaler are fully manifested. One to

two weeks may pass before full relief is obtained. The patient should contact the doctor if symptoms do not improve, or if the condition worsens, or if sneezing or nasal irritation occurs. For the proper use of this unit and to attain maximum improvement, the patient should read and follow the accompanying PATIENT'S INSTRUCTIONS carefully.

Persons who are on immunosuppressant doses of corticosteroids should be warned to avoid exposure to chickenpox or measles. Patients should also be advised that if they are exposed, medical advice should be sought without delay.

Carcinogenesis, Mutagenesis, Impairment of Fertility: Treatment of rats for a total of 95 weeks, 13 weeks by inhalation and 82 weeks by the oral route, resulted in no evidence of carcinogenic activity. Mutagenic studies have not been performed.

Impairment of fertility, as evidenced by inhibition of the estrus cycle in dogs, was observed following treatment by the oral route. No inhibition of the estrus cycle in dogs was seen following treatment with beclomethasone diproprionate by the inhalation route.

Pregnancy Category C: Like other corticoids, parenteral (subcutaneous) beclomethasone dipropionate has been shown to be teratogenic and embryocidal in the mouse and rabbit when given in doses approximately ten times the human dose. In these studies, beclomethasone was found to produce fetal resorption, cleft palate, agnathia, microstomia, absence of tongue, delayed ossification, and agenesis of the thymus. No teratogenic or embryocidal effects have been seen in the rat when beclomethasone dipropionate was administered by inhalation at ten times the human dose or orally at 1000 times the human dose. There are no adequate and well-controlled studies in pregnant women. Beclomethasone dipropionate should be used during pregnancy only if the potential benefit justifies the potential risk to the fetus.

Nonteratogenic Effects: Hypoadrenalism may occur in infants born of mothers receiving corticosteroids during pregnancy. Such infants should be carefully observed.

Nursing Mothers: It is not known whether beclomethasone dipropionate is excreted in human milk. Because other corticosteroids are excreted in human milk, caution should be exercised when VANCENASE POCKETHALER Nasal Inhaler is administered to nursing women.

Pediatric Use: Safety and effectiveness in children below the age of 6 years have not been established.

ADVERSE REACTIONS

In general, side effects in clinical studies have been primarily associated with the nasal mucous membranes. Adverse reactions reported in controlled clinical trials and in long-term open studies in patients treated with VANCENASE Nasal Inhaler are described below.

Sensations of irritation and burning in the nose (11 per 100 patients) following the use of VANCENASE Nasal Inhaler have been reported. Also, occasional sneezing attacks (10 per 100 patients) have occurred immediately following the use of the intranasal inhaler. This symptom may be more common in children.

Rhinorrhea may occur occasionally (1 per 100 patients).

Localized infections of the nose and pharynx with *Candida albicans* have occurred rarely. (See **PRECAUTIONS.**)

Transient episodes of epistaxis or bloody discharge from the nose have been reported in 2 per 100 patients.

Ulceration of the nasal mucosa has been reported rarely.

Extremely rare instances of nasal septum perforation have been reported following the intranasal application of aerosolized corticosteroids. Rare cases of immediate and delayed hypersensitivity reactions, including urticaria, angioedema, rash, and bronchospasm have been reported following the oral and intranasal inhalation of beclomethasone.

Increased intraocular pressure has been reported rarely. (See **PRECAUTIONS.**)

Systemic corticosteroid side effects were not reported during controlled clinical trials. If recommended doses are exceeded, however, or if individuals are particularly sensitive, symptoms of hypercorticism, ie, Cushing's syndrome could occur.

DOSAGE AND ADMINISTRATION

Adults and Children 12 Years of Age and Over: The usual dosage is one inhalation (42 mcg) in each nostril two to four times a day (total dose 168–336 mcg/day). Patients can often be maintained on a maximum dose of one inhalation in each nostril three times a day (252 mcg/day).

Children 6 to 12 Years of Age: The usual dosage is one inhalation in each nostril three times a day (252 mcg/day). VANCENASE POCKETHALER Nasal Inhaler is not recommended for children below 6 years of age since safety and efficacy studies have not been conducted in this age group.

In patients who respond to VANCENASE POCKETHALER Nasal Inhaler, an improvement of the symptoms of seasonal or perennial rhinitis usually becomes apparent within a few days after the start of VANCENASE POCKETHALER Nasal Inhaler therapy. However, symptomatic relief may not occur in some patients for as long as 2 weeks. VANCENASE POCKETHALER Nasal Inhaler should not be continued beyond 3 weeks in the absence of significant symptomatic improvement.

The therapeutic effects of corticosteroids, unlike those of decongestants, on seasonal or perennial rhinitis or on nasal polyps are not immediate. This should be explained to the patient in advance in order to ensure cooperation and continuation of treatment with the prescribed dosage regimen.

VANCENASE POCKETHALER Nasal Inhaler is not recommended for children below 6 years of age.

In the presence of excessive nasal mucus secretion or edema of the nasal mucosa, the drug may fail to reach the site of intended action. In such cases it is advisable to use a nasal vasoconstrictor during the first 2 to 3 days of VANCENASE POCKETHALER Nasal Inhaler therapy.

Directions for Use: Illustrated PATIENT'S INSTRUCTIONS for proper use accompany each package of VANCENASE POCKETHALER Nasal Inhaler.

CONTENTS UNDER PRESSURE. Do not puncture. Do not use or store near heat or open flame. Exposure to temperatures above 120°F may cause bursting. Never throw container into fire or incinerator. Keep out of reach of children.

OVERDOSAGE

When used at excessive doses, systemic corticosteroid effects such as hypercorticism and adrenal suppression may appear. If such changes occur, VANCENASE POCKETHALER Nasal Inhaler should be discontinued slowly consistent with accepted procedures for discontinuing oral steroid therapy.

The oral LD_{50} of beclomethasone dipropionate is greater than 1 g/kg in rodents. One canister of VANCENASE POCKETHALER Nasal Inhaler contains 8.4 mg of beclomethasone dipropionate; therefore acute overdosage is unlikely.

HOW SUPPLIED

VANCENASE POCKETHALER Nasal Inhaler, 7 g canister: box of one. Supplied with nasal adapter and PATIENT'S INSTRUCTIONS (NDC 0085-0649-02).

Store between 15° and 30°C (59° and 86°F).

Failure to use the product within this temperature range may result in improper dosing. Shake well before using.

Note: The indented statement below is required by the Federal government's Clean Air Act for all products containing or manufactured with chlorofluorocarbons (CFCs).

> **WARNING:** Contains dichlorodifluoromethane (CFC-11) and trichloromonofluoromethane (CFC-12), substances which harm public health and the environment by destroying ozone in the upper atmosphere.

A notice similar to the above WARNING has been placed in the "Patient's Instruction for Use" portion of this package insert pursuant to EPA regulations.

Rev. 7/93

17798103

Shown in Product Identification Guide, page 334

VANCENASE® AQ ℞

brand of beclomethasone dipropionate, monohydrate
Nasal Spray 0.042%*
FOR INTRANASAL USE ONLY
***calculated on the dried basis**

DESCRIPTION

Beclomethasone dipropionate, monohydrate, the active component of VANCENASE AQ Nasal Spray, is an anti-inflammatory steroid having the chemical name, 9-Chloro-11β, 17, 21-trihydroxy-16 β-methylpregna-1, 4-diene-3, 20-dione 17, 21-dipropionate, monohydrate and the following chemical structure:

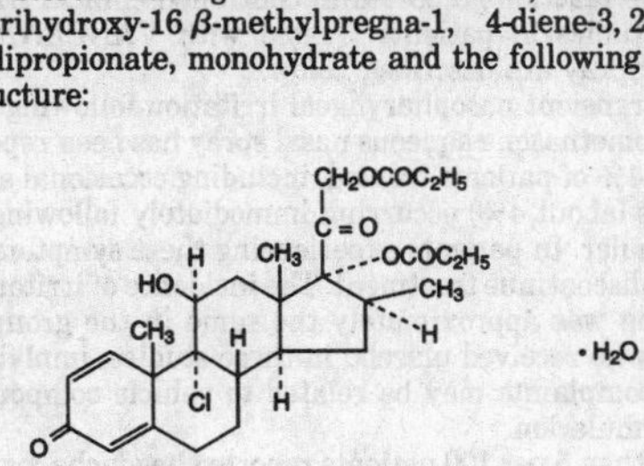

Beclomethasone dipropionate, monohydrate is a white to creamy-white, odorless powder with a molecular weight of 539.06. It is very slightly soluble in water; very soluble in chloroform; and freely soluble in acetone and in alcohol.

VANCENASE AQ Nasal Spray is a metered-dose, manual pump spray unit containing a microcrystalline suspension of beclomethasone dipropionate, monohydrate equivalent to 0.042% w/w beclomethasone dipropionate calculated on the dried basis in an aqueous medium containing microcrystalline cellulose and carboxymethylcellulose sodium, dextrose, benzalkonium chloride, polysorbate 80, and 0.25% v/w phenylethyl alcohol; hydrochloric acid may be added to adjust pH. The pH is between 4.5 and 7.0.

After initial priming (3 to 4 actuations), each actuation of the pump delivers from the nasal adapter 100 mg of suspension containing beclomethasone dipropionate, monohydrate equivalent to 42 mcg beclomethasone dipropionate. Each bottle of VANCENASE AQ Nasal Spray will provide at least 200 metered doses.

CLINICAL PHARMACOLOGY

Beclomethasone 17, 21-dipropionate is a diester of beclomethasone, a synthetic halogenated corticosteroid. Animal studies show that beclomethasone dipropionate has potent glucocorticosteroid and weak mineralocorticosteroid activity. The mechanisms for the anti-inflammatory action of beclomethasone dipropionate are unknown. The precise mechanism of the aerosolized drug's action in the nose is also unknown. Biopsies of nasal mucosa obtained during clinical studies showed no histopathologic changes when beclomethasone dipropionate was administered intranasally.

The effects of beclomethasone dipropionate on hypothalamic-pituitary-adrenal (HPA) function have been evaluated in adult volunteers by other routes of administration. Studies with beclomethasone dipropionate by the intranasal route may demonstrate that there is more or that there is less absorption by this route of administration. There was no suppression of early morning plasma cortisol concentrations when beclomethasone dipropionate was administered in a dose of 1000 mcg/day for 1 month as an oral aerosol or for 3 days by intramuscular injection. However, partial suppression of plasma cortisol concentration was observed when beclomethasone dipropionate was administered in doses of 2000 mcg/day either by oral aerosol or intramuscular injection. Immediate suppression of plasma cortisol concentrations was observed after single doses of 4000 mcg of beclomethasone dipropionate. Suppression of HPA function (reduction of early morning plasma cortisol levels) has been reported in adult patients who received 1600 mcg daily doses of oral beclomethasone dipropionate for 1 month. In clinical studies using beclomethasone dipropionate aerosol intranasally, there was no evidence of adrenal insufficiency. The effect of VANCENASE AQ Nasal Spray on HPA function was not evaluated but would not be expected to differ from intranasal beclomethasone dipropionate aerosol.

In one study in asthmatic children, the administration of inhaled beclomethasone at recommended daily doses for at least 1 year was associated with a reduction in nocturnal cortisol secretion. The clinical significance of this finding is not clear. It reinforces other evidence, however, that topical beclomethasone may be absorbed in amounts that can have systemic effects and that physicians should be alert for evidence of systemic effects, especially in chronically treated patients (see **PRECAUTIONS**).

Beclomethasone dipropionate is sparingly soluble. When given by nasal inhalation in the form of an aqueous or aerosolized suspension, the drug is deposited primarily in the nasal passages. A portion of the drug is swallowed. Absorption occurs rapidly from all respiratory and gastrointestinal tissues. There is no evidence of tissue storage of beclomethasone dipropionate or its metabolites. *In vitro* studies have shown that tissue other than the liver (lung slices) can rapidly metabolize beclomethasone dipropionate to beclomethasone 17-monopropionate and more slowly to free beclomethasone (which has very weak anti-inflammatory activity). However, irrespective of the route of entry the principal route of excretion of the drug and its metabolites is the feces. In humans, 12% to 15% of an orally administered dose of beclomethasone dipropionate is excreted in the urine as both conjugated and free metabolites of the drug.

Studies have shown that the degree of binding to plasma proteins is 87%.

INDICATIONS AND USAGE

VANCENASE AQ Nasal Spray is indicated for the relief of the symptoms of seasonal or perennial allergic and non-allergic (vasomotor) rhinitis. Results from two clinical trials have shown that significant symptomatic relief was obtained within 3 days. However, symptomatic relief may not occur in some patients for as long as 2 weeks. VANCENASE AQ Nasal Spray should not be continued beyond 3 weeks in the absence of significant symptomatic improvement.

VANCENASE AQ Nasal Spray should not be used in the presence of untreated localized infection involving the nasal mucosa.

VANCENASE AQ Nasal Spray is also indicated for the prevention of recurrence of nasal polyps following surgical removal.

Clinical studies have shown that treatment of the symptoms associated with nasal polyps may have to be continued for several weeks or more before a therapeutic result can be

Continued on next page

Information on Schering products appearing on these pages is effective as of August 15, 1996.

Schering—Cont.

fully assessed. Recurrence of symptoms due to polyps can occur after stopping treatment, depending on the severity of the disease.

CONTRAINDICATIONS

Hypersensitivity to any of the ingredients of this preparation contraindicates its use.

WARNINGS

The replacement of a systemic corticosteroid with VANCENASE AQ Nasal Spray can be accompanied by signs of adrenal insufficiency.

When transferred to VANCENASE AQ Nasal Spray, careful attention must be given to patients previously treated for prolonged periods with systemic corticosteroids. This is particularly important in those patients who have associated asthma or other clinical conditions, where too rapid a decrease in systemic corticosteroids may cause a severe exacerbation of their symptoms.

Studies have shown that the combined administration of alternate day prednisone systemic treatment and orally inhaled beclomethasone increased the likelihood of HPA suppression compared to a therapeutic dose of either one alone. Therefore, VANCENASE AQ Nasal Spray treatment should be used with caution in patients already on alternate day prednisone regimens for any disease.

If recommended doses of intranasal beclomethasone are exceeded or if individuals are particularly sensitive or predisposed by virtue of recent systemic steroid therapy, symptoms of hypercorticism may occur, including very rare cases of menstrual irregularities, acneiform lesions, and cushingoid features. If such changes occur, VANCENASE AQ Nasal Spray should be discontinued slowly, consistent with accepted procedures for discontinuing oral steroid therapy.

Persons who are on drugs which suppress the immune system are more susceptible to infections than healthy individuals. Chickenpox and measles, for example, can have a more serious or even fatal course in non-immune children or adults on corticosteroids. In such children or adults who have not had these diseases, particular care should be taken to avoid exposure. How the dose, route and duration of corticosteroid administration affects the risk of developing a disseminated infection is not known. The contribution of the underlying disease and/or prior corticosteroid treatment to the risk is also not known. If exposed to chickenpox, prophylaxis with varicella-zoster immune globulin (VZIG) may be indicated. If exposed to measles, prophylaxis with pooled intramuscular immunoglobulin (IG) may be indicated. (See the respective package inserts for complete VZIG and IG prescribing information.) If chickenpox develops, treatment with antiviral agents may be considered.

PRECAUTIONS

General: During withdrawal from oral steroids, some patients may experience symptoms of withdrawal, eg, joint and/or muscular pain, lassitude, and depression. Rarely, immediate hypersensitivity reactions may occur after the intranasal administration of beclomethasone.

Extremely rare instances of wheezing, nasal septum perforation, and increased intraocular pressure have been reported following the intranasal application of aerosolized corticosteroids. Although these have not been observed in clinical trials with VANCENASE AQ Nasal Spray, vigilance should be maintained.

In clinical studies with beclomethasone dipropionate administered intranasally, the development of localized infections of the nose and pharynx with *Candida albicans* has occurred only rarely. When such an infection develops, it may require treatment with appropriate local therapy or discontinuance of treatment with VANCENASE AQ Nasal Spray.

If persistent nasopharyngeal irritation occurs, it may be an indication for stopping VANCENASE AQ Nasal Spray.

Beclomethasone dipropionate is absorbed into the circulation. Use of excessive doses of VANCENASE AQ Nasal Spray may suppress HPA function.

VANCENASE AQ Nasal Spray should be used with caution, if at all, in patients with active or quiescent tuberculous infections of the respiratory tract, or in untreated fungal, bacterial, systemic viral infections, or ocular herpes simplex.

For VANCENASE AQ Nasal Spray to be effective in the treatment of nasal polyps, the spray must be able to enter the nose. Therefore, treatment of nasal polyps with VANCENASE AQ Nasal Spray should be considered adjunctive therapy to surgical removal and/or the use of other medications which will permit effective penetration of VANCENASE AQ Nasal Spray into the nose. Nasal polyps may recur after any form of treatment.

As with any long-term treatment, patients using VANCENASE AQ Nasal Spray over several months or longer should be examined periodically for possible changes in the nasal mucosa.

Because of the inhibitory effect of corticosteroids on wound healing, patients who have experienced recent nasal septal ulcers, nasal surgery, or trauma should not use a nasal corticosteroid until healing has occurred.

Although systemic effects have been minimal with recommended doses, this potential increases with excessive doses. Therefore, larger than recommended doses should be avoided.

Information for Patients: Patients being treated with VANCENASE AQ Nasal Spray should receive the following information and instructions. This information is intended to aid in the safe and effective use of medication. It is not a disclosure of all possible adverse or intended effects. Patients should use VANCENASE AQ Nasal Spray at regular intervals since its effectiveness depends on its regular use. The patient should take the medication as directed. It is not acutely effective and the prescribed dosage should not be increased. Instead, nasal vasoconstrictors or oral antihistamines may be needed until the effects of VANCENASE AQ Nasal Spray are fully manifested. One to 2 weeks may pass before full relief is obtained. The patient should contact the physician if symptoms do not improve, or if the condition worsens, or if sneezing or nasal irritation occurs. For the proper use of this unit and to attain maximum improvement, the patient should read and follow the accompanying Patient's Instructions carefully.

Patients who are on immunosuppressant doses of corticosteroids should be warned to avoid exposure to chickenpox or measles. Patients should also be advised that if they are exposed, medical advice should be sought without delay.

Carcinogenesis, Mutagenesis, Impairment of Fertility: Treatment of rats for a total of 95 weeks, 13 weeks by inhalation and 82 weeks by the oral route, resulted in no evidence of carcinogenic activity. Mutagenic studies have not been performed.

Impairment of fertility, as evidenced by inhibition of the estrous cycle in dogs, was observed following treatment by the oral route. No inhibition of the estrous cycle in dogs was seen following treatment with beclomethasone dipropionate by the inhalation route.

Pregnancy Category C: Like other corticosteroids, parenteral (subcutaneous) beclomethasone dipropionate has been shown to be teratogenic and embryocidal in the mouse and rabbit when given in doses approximately ten times the human dose. In these studies beclomethasone was found to produce fetal resorption, cleft palate, agnathia, microstomia, absence of tongue, delayed ossification, and agenesis of the thymus. No teratogenic or embryocidal effects have been seen in the rat when beclomethasone dipropionate was administered by inhalation at ten times the human dose or orally at 1000 times the human dose. There are no adequate and well-controlled studies in pregnant women. Beclomethasone dipropionate should be used during pregnancy only if the potential benefit justifies the potential risk to the fetus.

Nonteratogenic Effects: Hypoadrenalism may occur in infants born of mothers receiving corticosteroids during pregnancy. Such infants should be carefully observed.

Nursing Mothers: It is not known whether beclomethasone dipropionate is excreted in human milk. Because other corticosteroids are excreted in human milk, caution should be exercised when VANCENASE AQ Nasal Spray is administered to nursing women.

Pediatric Use: Safety and effectiveness in children below the age of 6 years have not been established.

ADVERSE REACTIONS

In general, side effects in clinical studies have been primarily associated with irritation of the nasal mucous membranes. Rarely, immediate hypersensitivity reactions may occur after the intranasal administration of beclomethasone dipropionate.

Adverse reactions reported in controlled clinical trials and open studies in patients treated with VANCENASE AQ Nasal Spray are described below.

Mild, transient nasopharyngeal irritation following the use of beclomethasone aqueous nasal spray has been reported in up to 24% of patients treated, including occasional sneezing attacks (about 4%) occurring immediately following use of the inhaler. In patients experiencing these symptoms, none had to discontinue treatment. The incidence of irritation and sneezing was approximately the same in the group of patients who received placebo in these studies, implying that these complaints may be related to vehicle components of the formulation.

Fewer than 5 per 100 patients reported headache, nausea, or lightheadedness following the use of VANCENASE AQ (beclomethasone dipropionate, monohydrate) Nasal Spray. Fewer than 3 per 100 patients reported nasal stuffiness, nosebleeds, rhinorrhea, or tearing eyes.

Extremely rare instances of wheezing, nasal septum perforation, and increased intraocular pressure have been reported following the intranasal administration of aerosolized corticosteroids (see **PRECAUTIONS**).

OVERDOSAGE

When used at excessive doses, systemic corticosteroid effects such as hypercorticism and adrenal suppression may appear. If such changes occur, VANCENASE AQ Nasal Spray should be discontinued slowly consistent with accepted procedures for discontinuing oral steroid therapy. The oral LD_{50} of beclomethasone dipropionate is greater than 1 g/kg in rodents. One bottle of VANCENASE AQ Nasal Spray contains beclomethasone dipropionate, monohydrate equivalent to 10.5 mg of beclomethasone dipropionate; therefore, acute overdosage is unlikely.

DOSAGE AND ADMINISTRATION

Adults and Children 6 Years of Age and Over: The usual dosage is 1 or 2 inhalations (42-84 mcg) in each nostril 2 times a day (total dose 168-336 mcg/day).

In patients who respond to VANCENASE AQ Nasal Spray, an improvement of the symptoms of seasonal or perennial rhinitis usually becomes apparent within a few days after the start of VANCENASE AQ Nasal Spray therapy. However, symptomatic relief may not occur in some patients for as long as 2 weeks. VANCENASE AQ Nasal Spray should not be continued beyond 3 weeks in the absence of significant symptomatic improvement.

The therapeutic effects of corticosteroids, unlike those of decongestants on seasonal or perennial rhinitis, or on nasal polyps, are not immediate. This should be explained to the patient in advance in order to ensure cooperation and continuation of treatment with the prescribed dosage regimen.

VANCENASE AQ Nasal Spray is not recommended for children below 6 years of age.

In the presence of excessive nasal mucus secretion or edema of the nasal mucosa, the drug may fail to reach the site of intended action. In such cases it is advisable to use a nasal vasoconstrictor during the first 2 to 3 days of VANCENASE AQ Nasal Spray therapy.

Directions for Use: Illustrated Patient's Instructions for proper use accompany each package of VANCENASE AQ Nasal Spray.

HOW SUPPLIED

VANCENASE AQ (beclomethasone dipropionate, monohydrate) Nasal Spray 0.042%*, 25 g bottle; box of one. Supplied with nasal pump unit and dust cap; and Patient's Instructions (NDC 0085-0259-02).

*calculated on the dried basis

Store between 2° and 25°C (36° and 77°F).

SHAKE WELL BEFORE USING

Rev. 6/94 17905414

Copyright © 1993, 1994, Schering Corporation. All rights reserved.

Shown in Product Identification Guide, page 334

VANCENASE® AQ ℞

84 mcg Double Strength
(beclomethasone dipropionate, monohydrate)
Nasal Spray
FOR INTRANASAL USE ONLY

VANCENASE AQ 84 mcg Double Strength Nasal Spray is a double-strength formulation of VANCENASE AQ 42 mcg Nasal Spray.

DESCRIPTION

Beclomethasone dipropionate, monohydrate, the active component of VANCENASE AQ 84 mcg Double Strength Nasal Spray, is an anti-inflammatory steroid having the chemical name, 9-Chloro-11β, 17,21-trihydroxy-16β-methylpregna-1, 4-diene-3, 20-dione 17,21-dipropionate, monohydrate and the following chemical structure:

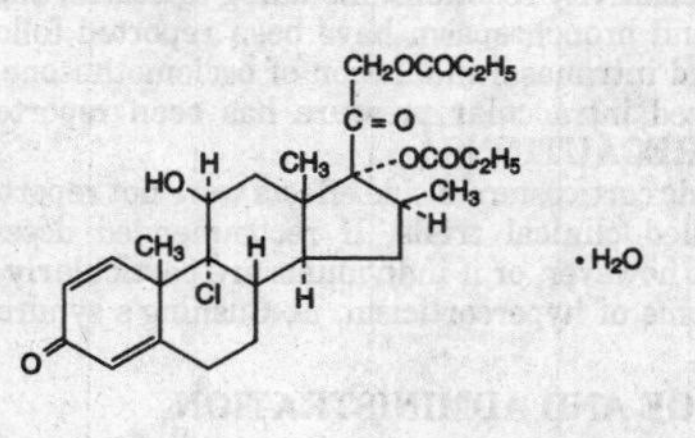

Beclomethasone dipropionate, monohydrate, is a white to creamy-white, odorless powder with a molecular formula of $C_{28}H_{37}ClO_7 \cdot H_2O$ and a molecular weight of 539.06. It is very slightly soluble in water; very soluble in chloroform; and freely soluble in acetone and in alcohol.

VANCENASE AQ 84 mcg Double Strength Nasal Spray is a double-strength formulation of VANCENASE AQ 42 mcg Nasal Spray. After initial priming (at least 6 actuations), each actuation of the pump delivers 100 mg of suspension containing beclomethasone dipropionate, monohydrate equivalent to 84 mcg beclomethasone dipropionate. Each bottle of VANCENASE AQ 84 mcg Double Strength Nasal Spray will provide at least 120 actuations.

VANCENASE AQ 84 mcg Double Strength Nasal Spray is a metered-dose, manual pump spray unit containing a suspension of beclomethasone dipropionate, monohydrate equiva-

lent to 0.084% w/w beclomethasone dipropionate in an aqueous medium containing microcrystalline cellulose, carboxymethylcellulose sodium, dextrose, benzalkonium chloride, polysorbate 80, and phenylethyl alcohol. The suspension is formulated at a target pH of 6.4, with a range of 5.5 to 6.8 over its shelf life.

CLINICAL PHARMACOLOGY

Beclomethasone 17,21-dipropionate is a diester of beclomethasone, a synthetic halogenated corticosteroid. Animal studies show that beclomethasone dipropionate has potent glucocorticosteroid and weak mineralocorticosteroid activity. The mechanisms for the anti-inflammatory action of beclomethasone dipropionate are unknown. The precise mechanism of the aerosolized drug's action in the nose is also unknown. Biopsies of nasal mucosa obtained during clinical studies (duration of treatment from 1 to 6 years at doses up to 336 mcg/day) showed no histopathologic changes when beclomethasone dipropionate was administered intranasally.

In a study evaluating the hypothalamic-pituitary-adrenal (HPA) effects of 336 mcg/day beclomethasone dipropionate administered intranasally for 36 consecutive days via aqueous suspension, there was no statistically significant difference in cortisol suppression between beclomethasone dipropionate 336 mcg once daily, beclomethasone dipropionate 168 mcg twice daily, and placebo. Plasma cortisol response to 6-hour cosyntropin stimulation was attenuated in control patients who received oral prednisone 10 mg daily.

The effects of beclomethasone dipropionate on HPA function have also been evaluated in adult volunteers by other routes of administration. There was no suppression of early morning plasma cortisol concentrations when beclomethasone dipropionate was administered in a dose of 1000 mcg/day for 1 month as an oral aerosol or for 3 days by intramuscular injection. However, partial suppression of plasma cortisol concentration was observed when beclomethasone dipropionate was administered in doses of 2000 mcg/day either by oral aerosol or intramuscular injection. Immediate suppression of plasma cortisol concentrations was observed after single doses of 4000 mcg of beclomethasone dipropionate. Suppression of HPA function (reduction of early morning plasma cortisol levels) has been reported in adult patients who received 1600 mcg daily doses of oral beclomethasone dipropionate for 1 month.

In one study of children with asthma, the administration of inhaled beclomethasone dipropionate at recommended daily doses for at least 1 year was associated with a reduction in nocturnal cortisol secretion. The clinical significance of this finding is not clear. It reinforces other evidence, however, that topical beclomethasone dipropionate may be absorbed in amounts that can have systemic effects and that physicians should be alert for evidence of systemic effects, especially in chronically treated patients (see **PRECAUTIONS**).

Beclomethasone dipropionate is sparingly soluble. When given by nasal inhalation in the form of an aqueous or aerosolized suspension, the drug is deposited primarily in the nasal passages. A portion of the drug is swallowed. Absorption occurs rapidly from all respiratory and gastrointestinal tissues. There is no evidence of tissue storage of beclomethasone dipropionate or its metabolites. *In vitro* studies have shown that tissue other than the liver (lung slices) can rapidly metabolize beclomethasone dipropionate to beclomethasone 17-monopropionate and more slowly to free beclomethasone (which has very weak anti-inflammatory activity). However, irrespective of the route of entry, the principal route of excretion is the feces. In humans, 12% to 15% of an orally administered dose of beclomethasone dipropionate is excreted in the urine. The drug is excreted in both urine and feces as free and conjugated polar metabolites.

Studies have shown that the degree of binding to plasma proteins is 87%.

In clinical trials with VANCENASE AQ 84 mcg Double Strength Nasal Spray in patients with seasonal allergic rhinitis, 336 mcg of beclomethasone dipropionate once daily was superior to placebo with respect to effects on nasal symptoms. In a study comparing VANCENASE AQ 84 mcg Double Strength Nasal Spray once daily with VANCENASE AQ 42 mcg Nasal Spray twice daily, each delivery a total daily dose of 336 mcg beclomethasone dipropionate, both regimens were comparable with respect to effects on physician-rated nasal symptoms. In this study, a significant advantage over placebo was observed for both regimens within 3 days of the start of treatment.

INDICATIONS AND USAGE

VANCENASE AQ 84 mcg Double Strength Nasal Spray is indicated for the relief of symptoms of allergic and nonallergic (vasomotor) rhinitis. Results from clinical trials of intranasal beclomethasone dipropionate in patients with seasonal allergic rhinitis have shown that significant symptom relief was obtained in most patients within 3 days. However, symptom relief may not occur in some patients for as long as 2 weeks. VANCENASE AQ 84 mcg Double Strength Nasal Spray should not be continued beyond 3 weeks in the absence of significant symptom improvement. VANCENASE AQ 84 mcg Double Strength Nasal Spray should not be used in the presence of untreated localized infection involving the nasal mucosa.

VANCENASE AQ 84 mcg Double Strength Nasal Spray is also indicated for the prevention of recurrence of nasal polyps following surgical removal.

Clinical studies with VANCENASE AQ 42 mcg Nasal Spray have shown that treatment of the symptoms associated with nasal polyps may have to be continued for several weeks or more before a therapeutic result can be fully assessed. Recurrence of symptoms due to polyps can occur after stopping treatment. depending on the severity of the disease.

CONTRAINDICATIONS

Hypersensitivity to any of the ingredients of this preparation contraindicates its use.

WARNINGS

The replacement of a systemic corticosteroid with VANCENASE AQ 84 mcg Double Strength Nasal Spray can be accompanied by signs of adrenal insufficiency.

When transferred to VANCENASE AQ 84 mcg Double Strength Nasal Spray, careful attention must be given to patients previously treated for prolonged periods with systemic corticosteroids. This is particularly important in those patients who have associated asthma or other clinical conditions, where too rapid a decrease in systemic corticosteroids may cause a severe exacerbation of their symptoms.

If recommended doses of intranasal beclomethasone dipropionate are exceeded or if individuals are particularly sensitive or predisposed by virtue of recent systemic steroid therapy, symptoms of hypercorticism may occur, including very rare cases of menstrual irregularities, acneiform lesions, and cushingoid features. If such changes occur, VANCENASE AQ 84 mcg Double Strength Nasal Spray should be discontinued slowly, consistent with accepted procedures for discontinuing oral steroid therapy.

Persons who are on drugs which suppress the immune system are more susceptible to infections than healthy individuals. Chickenpox and measles, for example, can have a more serious or even fatal course in nonimmune children or adults on corticosteroids. In such children or adults who have not had these diseases, particular care should be taken to avoid exposure. How the dose, route, and duration of corticosteroid administration affects the risk of developing a disseminated infection is not known. The contribution of the underlying disease and/or prior corticosteroid treatment to the risk is also not known. If exposed to chickenpox, prophylaxis with varicella-zoster immune globulin (VZIG) may be indicated. If exposed to measles, prophylaxis with pooled intramuscular immunoglobulin (IG) may be indicated. (See the respective package inserts for complete VZIG and IG prescribing information.) If chickenpox develops, treatment with antiviral agents may be considered.

PRECAUTIONS

General: During withdrawal from oral steroids, some patients may experience symptoms of withdrawal, e.g., joint and/or muscular pain, lassitude, and depression.

Rarely, immediate hypersensitivity reactions may occur after the intranasal administration of beclomethasone. Rare instances of nasal septum perforation have been reported.

Rare instances of wheezing and increased intraocular pressure have been reported following intranasal application of aerosolized corticosteroids. Although these have not been observed in clinical trials with VANCENASE AQ 84 mcg Double Strength Nasal Spray, vigilance should be maintained.

In clinical studies with beclomethasone dipropionate administered intranasally, the development of localized infections of the nose and pharynx with *Candida albicans* has occurred only rarely. When such an infection develops, use of VANCENASE AQ 84 mcg Double Strength Nasal Spray should be discontinued and appropriate local or systemic therapy instituted, if needed.

If persistent nasopharyngeal irritation occurs, VANCENASE AQ 84 mcg Double Strength Nasal Spray should be discontinued.

Beclomethasone dipropionate is absorbed into the circulation. Use of excessive doses of VANCENASE AQ 84 mcg Double Strength Nasal Spray may suppress HPA function.

VANCENASE AQ 84 mcg Double Strength Nasal Spray should be used with caution, if at all, in patients with active or quiescent tuberculous infections of the respiratory tract, or in untreated fungal, bacterial, systemic viral infections, or ocular herpes simplex.

For VANCENASE AQ 84 mcg Double Strength Nasal Spray to be effective in the treatment of nasal polyps, the spray must be able to enter the nose. Therefore, treatment of nasal polyps with VANCENASE AQ 84 mcg Double Strength Nasal Spray should be considered adjunctive therapy to surgical removal and/or the use of other medications which will permit effective penetration of VANCENASE AQ 84 mcg Double Strength Nasal Spray into the nose. Nasal polyps may recur after any form of treatment.

As with any long-term treatment, patients using VANCENASE AQ 84 mcg Double Strength Nasal Spray over several months or longer should be examined periodically for possible changes in the nasal mucosa.

Because of the inhibitory effect of corticosteroids on wound healing, patients who have experienced recent nasal septum ulcers, nasal surgery, or trauma should not use a corticosteroid intranasally until healing has occurred.

Although systemic effects have been minimal with recommended doses, this potential increases with excessive doses. Therefore, larger than recommended doses should be avoided.

Information for Patients: Patients being treated with VANCENASE AQ 84 mcg Double Strength Nasal Spray should receive the following information and instructions. This information is intended to aid in the safe and effective use of this medication. It is not a disclosure of all possible adverse or intended effects. VANCENASE AQ 84 mcg Double Strength Nasal Spray is a double-strength formulation of VANCENASE AQ 42 mcg Nasal Spray. Patients should use VANCENASE AQ 84 mcg Double Strength Nasal Spray ONLY once daily at a regular interval. Improvement usually becomes apparent within 3 days after the start of therapy. However, 1 to 2 weeks may pass before full relief is obtained. Since VANCENASE AQ 84 mcg Double Strength Nasal Spray is not immediately effective, the prescribed dosage of VANCENASE AQ 84 mcg Double Strength Nasal Spray should not be increased by using it more often than once a day in an attempt to increase its efficacy. Instead, nasal vasoconstrictors or oral anithistamines may be needed until the effects of VANCENASE AQ 84 mcg Double Strength Nasal Spray are fully manifested. The patient should contact the physician if symptoms do not improve, or if the condition worsens, or if sneezing or nasal irritation occurs. For the proper use of this unit and to attain maximum benefit, the patient should read and follow the accompanying Patient's Instructions carefully.

Patients should be warned not to spray VANCENASE AQ 84 mcg Double Strength Nasal Spray into the eyes.

Persons who are on immunosuppressant doses of corticosteroids should be warned to avoid exposure to chickenpox or measles, and patients should also be advised that if they are exposed, medical advice should be sought without delay.

Carcinogenesis, Mutagenesis, Impairment of Fertility: The carcinogenicity of beclomethasone dipropionate was evaluated in rats which were treated for a total of 95 weeks, 13 weeks of inhalation doses up to 0.4 mg/kg/day and the remaining 82 weeks at combined oral and inhalation doses up to 2.4 mg/kg/day (approximately 40 times the maximum recommended human daily intranasal dose on a mg/m^2 basis). There was no evidence of carcinogenicity in this study. Studies to assess the mutagenic potential of beclomethasone dipropionate have not been conducted. Impairment of fertility, as evidenced by inhibition of the estrous cycle in dogs, was observed following treatment by the oral route at a dose of 0.5 mg/kg/day (approximately 40 times the maximum recommended human daily intranasal dose on a mg/m^2 basis). No inhibition of the estrous cycle in dogs was seen following 12 months of exposure to beclomethasone dipropionate by the inhalation route at an estimated weekly dose of 2.3 mg/kg (approximately 26 times the maximum recommended human weekly intranasal dose on a mg/m^2 basis).

Pregnancy Category C: Like other corticosteroids, parenteral (subcutaneous) beclomethasone dipropionate has been shown to be teratogenic and embryocidal in the mouse and rabbit when given at a dose of 0.1 mg/kg/day in mice and at a dose of 0.025 mg/kg/day in rabbits (approximately 1.2 times the maximum recommended human daily intranasal dose on a mg/m^2 basis). No teratogenic or embryocidal effects have been seen in rats treated with beclomethasone by combined inhalation and oral administration at doses of 0.1 mg/kg/day and 10 mg/kg/day, respectively (approximately 250 times the maximum recommended human daily intranasal dose on a mg/m^2 basis). There are no adequate and well-controlled studies in pregnant women. Beclomethasone dipropionate should be used during pregnancy only if the potential benefit justifies the potential risk to the fetus.

Nonteratogenic Effects: Hypoadrenalism may occur in infants born of mothers receiving corticosteroids during pregnancy. Such infants should be carefully observed.

Nursing Mothers: It is not known whether beclomethasone dipropionate is excreted in human milk. Because other corticosteroids are excreted in human milk, caution should be exercised when VANCENASE AQ 84 mcg Double Strength Nasal Spray is administered to nursing women.

Pediatric Use: Safety and effectiveness of VANCENASE AQ 84 mcg Double Strength Nasal Spray in children below the age of 6 years have not been established.

ADVERSE REACTIONS

In clinical studies with intranasally administered beclomethasone dipropionate, adverse effects have primarily been

Continued on next page

Information on Schering products appearing on these pages is effective as of August 15, 1996.

Schering—Cont.

related to irritation of the nasal mucous membranes. Rarely, immediate hypersensitivity reactions may occur after intranasal administration of beclomethasone dipropionate.

Clinical trials of VANCENASE AQ 84 mcg Double Strength Nasal Spray included 187 patients who received VANCENASE AQ 84 mcg Double Strength Nasal Spray, 127 patients who received VANCENASE AQ 42 mcg Nasal Spray, and 192 patients who received vehicle placebo. The incidence and nature of adverse events with VANCENASE AQ 84 mcg Double Strength Nasal Spray (336 mcg beclomethasone dipropionate once daily) was comparable to that seen with VANCENASE AQ 42 mcg Nasal Spray (168 mcg beclomethasone dipropionate twice daily) and with vehicle placebo. Adverse events reported by 2% or more of patients (regardless of relationship to treatment) who received VANCENASE AQ 84 mcg Double Strength Nasal Spray in clinical trials and that were more common with VANCENASE AQ 84 mcg Double Strength Nasal Spray than with placebo are displayed in the table below.

ADVERSE EVENTS FROM CONTROLLED CLINICAL TRIALS IN SEASONAL ALLERGIC RHINITIS

	VANCENASE AQ 84 mcg Double Strength Once daily (N=187)	VANCENASE AQ 42 mcg Twice daily (N=127)	VEHICLE PLACEBO (N=192)
Headache	34%	33%	32%
Pharyngitis	12%	11%	6%
Coughing	6%	6%	5%
Epistaxis	5%	2%	4%
Nasal burning	5%	4%	3%
Pain	4%	2%	1%
Conjunctivitis	2%	2%	1%
Myalgia	2%	1%	1%
Tinnitus	2%	3%	0%

Rare cases of ulceration of the nasal mucosa and instances of nasal septum perforation have been reported following the intranasal administration of beclomethasone dipropionate (see **PRECAUTIONS**).

Rare instances of wheezing and increased intraocular pressure have been reported following the intranasal administration of aerosolized corticosteroids (see **PRECAUTIONS**).

Single cases each of aseptic necrosis of the femoral head and of nasal fungal infection with erosion through the cribriform plate have been reported after long-term administration of beclomethasone dipropionate nasal spray.

OVERDOSAGE

When used at excessive doses, systemic corticosteroid effects such as hypercorticism and adrenal suppression may appear. If such changes occur, VANCENASE AQ 84 mcg Double Strength Nasal Spray should be discontinued slowly consistent with accepted procedures for discontinuing oral steroid therapy. The oral median lethal dose of beclomethasone dipropionate is greater than 1 g/kg in mice and rats (approximately 7000 times and 14,000 times, respectively, the maximum recommended human daily intranasal dose on a mg/m^2 basis). One bottle of VANCENASE AQ 84 mcg Double Strength Nasal Spray contains beclomethasone dipropionate, monohydrate equivalent to 16.0 mg of beclomethasone dipropionate; therefore, acute overdosage is unlikely.

DOSAGE AND ADMINISTRATION

Adults and Children 6 Years of Age and Over: VANCENASE AQ 84 mcg Double Strength Nasal Spray is a double-strength formulation of VANCENASE AQ 42 mcg Nasal Spray. The usual dosage of VANCENASE AQ 84 mcg Double Strength Nasal Spray is 1 or 2 inhalations in each nostril once daily (total dose 168–336 mcg/day).

In patients who respond to VANCENASE AQ 84 mcg Double Strength Nasal Spray, an improvement of the symptoms of allergic rhinitis usually becomes apparent within a few days after the start of therapy. Patients should use VANCENASE AQ 84 mcg Double Strength Nasal Spray ONLY once daily at a regular interval. VANCENASE AQ 84 mcg Double Strength Nasal Spray is not acutely effective, therefore, the prescribed dosage of VANCENASE AQ 84 mcg Double Strength Nasal Spray should not be increased by using it more often than once daily. Symptom relief may not occur in some patients for as long as 2 weeks. VANCENASE AQ 84 mcg Double Strength Nasal Spray should not be continued beyond 3 weeks in the absence of significant symptom improvement.

Since the therapeutic effects of corticosteroids, unlike those of a decongestant on allergic rhinitis or on nasal polyps, are not immediate, this should be explained to the patient in advance in order to ensure cooperation and continuation of treatment with the prescribed dosage regimen.

VANCENASE AQ 84 mcg Double Strength Nasal Spray is not recommended for children below 6 years of age.

In the presence of excessive nasal mucus secretion or edema of the nasal mucosa, the drug may fail to reach the sites of intended action. In such cases it is advisable to use a topical or oral nasal vasoconstrictor/decongestant during the first 2 to 3 days of VANCENASE AQ 84 mcg Double Strength Nasal Spray therapy.

Prior to initial use of VANCENASE AQ 84 mcg Double Strength Nasal Spray, the pump must be primed by actuating six times or until a fine spray appears. If the pump is unused for more than 3 days, it may be necessary to reprime with two sprays or until a fine spray appears. If unused for more than 7 days, reprime fully as described for initial use.

Directions for Use: Illustrated Patient's Instructions for proper use accompany each package of VANCENASE AQ 84 mcg Double Strength Nasal Spray.

HOW SUPPLIED

VANCENASE AQ 84 mcg Double Strength (beclomethasone dipropionate, monohydrate) Nasal Spray, 19 g net weight, 120 actuations, white high-density polyethylene bottle fitted with a white metered-dose nasal spray pump, maroon safety clip, and white dust cap; box of one. Supplied with Patient's Instructions for Use (NDC 0085-1049-01).

Store between 2° and 25°C (36° and 77°F).

SHAKE WELL BEFORE EACH USE.

Schering Corporation
Kenilworth, NJ 07033 USA

Copyright © 1996, Schering Corporation. All rights reserved. Rev. 6/96

18780917T

Shown in Product Identification Guide, page 334

VANCERIL® Inhaler ℞

brand of beclomethasone dipropionate, USP
For Oral Inhalation Only

DESCRIPTION

Beclomethasone dipropionate, USP, the active component of VANCERIL Inhaler, is an anti-inflammatory steroid having the chemical name 9-Chloro-11β,17,21-trihydroxy-16β-methylpregna-1,4-diene-3, 20-dione 17,21-dipropionate.

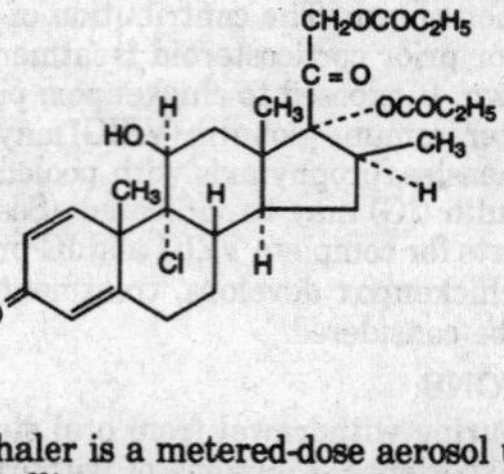

VANCERIL Inhaler is a metered-dose aerosol unit containing a microcrystalline suspension of beclomethasone dipropionate-trichloromonofluoromethane clathrate in a mixture of propellants (trichloromonofluoromethane and dichlorodifluoromethane) with oleic acid. Each canister contains beclomethasone dipropionate-trichloromonofluoromethane clathrate having a molecular proportion of beclomethasone dipropionate, USP, to trichloromonofluoromethane between 3:1 and 3:2. Each actuation delivers from the mouthpiece a quantity of clathrate equivalent to 42 mcg of beclomethasone dipropionate, USP. The contents of one canister provide at least 200 oral inhalations.

CLINICAL PHARMACOLOGY

Beclomethasone 17,21-dipropionate is a diester of beclomethasone, a synthetic corticosteroid which is chemically related to dexamethasone. Beclomethasone differs from dexamethasone only in having a chlorine at the 9-alpha in place of a fluorine and in having a 16β-methyl group instead of a 16 alpha-methyl group. Animal studies showed that beclomethasone dipropionate has potent anti-inflammatory activity. When administered systemically to mice, the anti-inflammatory activity was accompanied by other typical features of glucocorticoid action including thymic involution, liver glycogen deposition, and pituitary-adrenal suppression. However, after systemic administration to rats, the anti-inflammatory action was associated with little or no effect on other tests of glucocorticoid activity.

Beclomethasone dipropionate is sparingly soluble and is poorly mobilized from subcutaneous or intramuscular injection sites. However, systemic absorption occurs after all routes of administration. When given to animals in the form of an aerosolized suspension of the trichloromonofluoromethane clathrate, the drug is deposited in the mouth and nasal passages, the trachea and principal bronchi, and in the lung; a considerable portion of the drug is also swallowed. Absorption occurs rapidly from all respiratory and gastrointestinal tissues, as indicated by the rapid clearance of radioactively labeled drug from local tissues and appearance of tracer in the circulation. There is no evidence of tissue storage of beclomethasone dipropionate or its metabolites. Lung slices can metabolize beclomethasone dipropionate rapidly to beclomethasone 17-monopropionate and more slowly to free beclomethasone (which has very weak anti-inflammatory activity). However, irrespective of the route of administration (injection, oral, or aerosol), the principal route of excretion of the drug and its metabolites is the feces. Less than 10% of the drug and its metabolites is excreted in the urine. In humans, 12% to 15% of an orally administered dose of beclomethasone dipropionate was excreted in the urine as both conjugated and free metabolites of the drug.

The mechanisms responsible for the anti-inflammatory action of beclomethasone dipropionate are unknown. The precise mechanism of the aerosolized drug's action in the lung is also unknown.

INDICATIONS

VANCERIL Inhaler is indicated only for patients who require chronic treatment with corticosteroids for control of the symptoms of bronchial asthma. Such patients would include those already receiving systemic corticosteroids, and selected patients who are inadequately controlled on a nonsteroid regimen and in whom steroid therapy has been withheld because of concern over potential adverse effects.

VANCERIL Inhaler is NOT indicated:

1. For relief of asthma which can be controlled by bronchodilators and other nonsteroid medications.
2. In patients who require systemic corticosteroid treatment infrequently.
3. In the treatment of non-asthmatic bronchitis.

CONTRAINDICATIONS

VANCERIL Inhaler is contraindicated in the primary treatment of status asthmaticus or other acute episodes of asthma where intensive measures are required.

Hypersensitivity to any of the ingredients of this preparation contraindicates its use.

WARNINGS

Particular care is needed in patients who are transferred from systemically active corticosteroids to VANCERIL Inhaler because deaths due to adrenal insufficiency have occurred in asthmatic patients during and after transfer from systemic corticosteroids to aerosol beclomethasone dipropionate. After withdrawal from systemic corticosteroids, a number of months are required for recovery of hypothalamic-pituitary-adrenal (HPA) function. During this period of HPA suppression, patients may exhibit signs and symptoms of adrenal insufficiency when exposed to trauma, surgery or infections, particularly gastroenteritis. Although VANCERIL Inhaler may provide control of asthmatic symptoms during these episodes, it does NOT provide the systemic steroid which is necessary for coping with these emergencies.

During periods of stress or a severe asthmatic attack, patients who have been withdrawn from systemic corticosteroids should be instructed to resume systemic steroids (in large doses) immediately and to contact their physician for further instruction. These patients should also be instructed to carry a warning card indicating that they may need supplementary systemic steroids during periods of stress or a severe asthma attack. To assess the risk of adrenal insufficiency in emergency situations, routine tests of adrenal cortical function, including measurement of early morning resting cortisol levels, should be performed periodically in all patients. An early morning resting cortisol level may be accepted as normal only if it falls at or near the normal mean level.

Localized infections with *Candida albicans* or *Aspergillus niger* have occurred frequently in the mouth and pharynx and occasionally in the larynx. Positive cultures for oral *Candida* may be present in up to 75% of patients. Although the frequency of clinically apparent infection is considerably lower, these infections may require treatment with appropriate antifungal therapy or discontinuance of treatment with VANCERIL Inhaler.

VANCERIL Inhaler is not to be regarded as a bronchodilator and is not indicated for rapid relief of bronchospasm.

Patients should be instructed to contact their physician immediately when episodes of asthma which are not responsive to bronchodilators occur during the course of treatment with VANCERIL. During such episodes, patients may require therapy with systemic corticosteroids.

There is no evidence that control of asthma can be achieved by the administration of VANCERIL in amounts greater than the recommended doses.

Transfer of patients from systemic steroid therapy to VANCERIL Inhaler may unmask allergic conditions previously suppressed by the systemic steroid therapy, eg, rhinitis, conjunctivitis, and eczema.

Persons who are on drugs which suppress the immune system are more susceptible to infections than healthy individuals. Chickenpox and measles, for example, can have a more

serious or even fatal course in nonimmune children or adults on corticosteroids. In such children or adults who have not had these diseases, particular care should be taken to avoid exposure. How the dose, route and duration of corticosteroid administration affects the risk of developing a disseminated infection is not known. The contribution of the underlying disease and/or prior corticosteroid treatment to the risk is also not known. If exposed to chickenpox, prophylaxis with varicella-zoster immune globulin (VZIG) may be indicated. If exposed to measles, prophylaxis with pooled intramuscular immunoglobulin (IG) may be indicated. (See the respective package inserts for complete VZIG and IG prescribing information.) If chickenpox develops, treatment with antiviral agents may be considered.

PRECAUTIONS

During withdrawal from oral steroids, some patients may experience symptoms of systemically active steroid withdrawal, eg, joint and/or muscular pain, lassitude and depression, despite maintenance or even improvement of respiratory function. (See **DOSAGE AND ADMINISTRATION** for details.)

In responsive patients, beclomethasone dipropionate may permit control of asthmatic symptoms without suppression of HPA function, as discussed below. (See **CLINICAL STUDIES**.) Since beclomethasone dipropionate is absorbed into the circulation and can be systemically active, the beneficial effects of VANCERIL Inhaler in minimizing or preventing HPA dysfunction may be expected only when recommended dosages are not exceeded.

The long-term effects of beclomethasone dipropionate in human subjects are still unknown. In particular, the local effects of the agent on developmental or immunologic processes in the mouth, pharynx, trachea, and lung are unknown. There is also no information about the possible long-term systemic effects of the agent.

The potential effects of VANCERIL on acute, recurrent, or chronic pulmonary infections, including active or quiescent tuberculosis, are not known. Similarly, the potential effects of long-term administration of the drug on lung or other tissues are unknown.

Pulmonary infiltrates with eosinophilia may occur in patients on VANCERIL Inhaler therapy. Although it is possible that in some patients this state may become manifest because of systemic steroid withdrawal when inhalational steroids are administered, a causative role for beclomethasone dipropionate and/or its vehicle cannot be ruled out.

Use in Pregnancy: Glucocorticoids are known teratogens in rodent species and beclomethasone dipropionate is no exception.

Teratology studies were done in rats, mice, and rabbits treated with subcutaneous beclomethasone dipropionate. Beclomethasone dipropionate was found to produce fetal resorptions, cleft palate, agnathia, microstomia, absence of tongue, delayed ossification and partial agenesis of the thymus. Well-controlled trials relating to fetal risk in humans are not available. Glucocorticoids are secreted in human milk. It is not known whether beclomethasone dipropionate would be secreted in human milk but it is safe to assume that it is likely. The use of beclomethasone dipropionate in pregnancy, nursing mothers, or women of childbearing potential requires that the possible benefits of the drug be weighed against the potential hazards to the mother, embryo, or fetus. Infants born of mothers who have received substantial doses of corticosteroids during pregnancy should be carefully observed for hypoadrenalism.

Information for Patients: Persons who are on immunosuppressant doses of corticosteroids should be warned to avoid exposure to chickenpox or measles. Patients should also be advised that if they are exposed, medical advice should be sought without delay.

ADVERSE REACTIONS

Deaths due to adrenal insufficiency have occurred in asthmatic patients during and after transfer from systemic corticosteroids to aerosol beclomethasone dipropionate. (See **WARNINGS**.)

Suppression of HPA function (reduction of early morning plasma cortisol levels) has been reported in adult patients who received 1600 mcg daily doses of VANCERIL for 1 month. A few patients on VANCERIL have complained of hoarseness or dry mouth.

Rare cases of immediate and delayed hypersensitivity reactions, including urticaria, angioedema, rash, and bronchospasm have been reported following the oral and intranasal inhalation of beclomethasone.

DOSAGE AND ADMINISTRATION

Adults: The usual recommended dosage is two inhalations (84 mcg) given three or four times a day. Alternatively, four inhalations (168 mcg) given twice daily has been shown to be effective in some patients. In patients with severe asthma, it is advisable to start with 12 to 16 inhalations a day and adjust the dosage downward according to the response of the patient. The maximal daily intake should not exceed 20 inhalations, 840 mcg (0.84 mg), in adults.

Children 6 to 12 Years of Age: The usual recommended dosage is one or two inhalations (42 to 84 mcg) given three or four times a day according to the response of the patient. Alternatively, four inhalations (168 mcg) given twice daily has been shown to be effective in some patients. The maximal daily intake should not exceed ten inhalations, 420 mcg (0.42 mg), in children 6 to 12 years of age. Insufficient clinical data exist with respect to the administration of VANCERIL Inhaler in children below the age of 6.

Rinsing the mouth after inhalation is advised.

Patients receiving bronchodilators by inhalation should be advised to use the bronchodilator before VANCERIL Inhaler in order to enhance penetration of beclomethasone dipropionate into the bronchial tree. After use of an aerosol bronchodilator, several minutes should elapse before use of the VANCERIL Inhaler to reduce the potential toxicity from the inhaled fluorocarbon propellants in the two aerosols.

Different considerations must be given to the following groups of patients in order to obtain the full therapeutic benefit of VANCERIL Inhaler.

Patients Not Receiving Systemic Steroids: The use of VANCERIL Inhaler is straight forward in patients who are inadequately controlled with nonsteroid medications but in whom systemic steroid therapy has been withheld because of concern over potential adverse reactions. In patients who respond to VANCERIL, an improvement in pulmonary function is usually apparent within 1 to 4 weeks after the start of VANCERIL Inhaler.

Patients Receiving Systemic Steroids: In those patients dependent on systemic steroids, transfer to VANCERIL and subsequent management may be more difficult because recovery from impaired adrenal function is usually slow. Such suppression has been known to last for up to 12 months. Clinical studies, however, have demonstrated that VANCERIL may be effective in the management of these asthmatic patients and may permit replacement or significant reduction in the dosage of systemic corticosteroids.

The patient's asthma should be reasonably stable before treatment with VANCERIL Inhaler is started. Initially, the aerosol should be used concurrently with the patient's usual maintenance dose of systemic steroid. After approximately 1 week, gradual withdrawal of the systemic steroid is started by reducing the daily or alternate daily dose. The next reduction is made after an interval of 1 or 2 weeks, depending on the response of the patient. Generally, these decrements should not exceed 2.5 mg of prednisone or its equivalent. A slow rate of withdrawal cannot be overemphasized. During withdrawal, some patients may experience symptoms of systemically active steroid withdrawal, eg, joint and/or muscular pain, lassitude and depression, despite maintenance or even improvement of respiratory function. Such patients should be encouraged to continue with the inhaler but should be watched carefully for objective signs of adrenal insufficiency, such as hypotension and weight loss. If evidence of adrenal insufficiency occurs, the systemic steroid dose should be boosted temporarily and thereafter further withdrawal should continue more slowly.

During periods of stress or a severe asthma attack, transfer patients will require supplementary treatment with systemic steroids. Exacerbations of asthma which occur during the course of treatment with VANCERIL Inhaler should be treated with a short course of systemic steroid which is gradually tapered as these symptoms subside. There is no evidence that control of asthma can be achieved by administration of VANCERIL in amounts greater than the recommended doses.

Directions for Use: Illustrated patient's instructions for proper use accompany each package of VANCERIL Inhaler. CONTENTS UNDER PRESSURE. Do not puncture. Do not use or store near heat or open flame. Exposure to temperatures above 120°F may cause bursting. Never throw container into fire or incinerator. Keep out of reach of children.

HOW SUPPLIED

VANCERIL Inhaler 16.8 g canister supplied with an oral adapter and patient's instructions; box of one (NDC 0085-0736-04).

Institutional Pack for Inpatient Use Only: VANCERIL Inhaler 6.7 g canister supplied with an oral adapter and Patient's Instructions; box of one (NDC 0085-0738-01).

Store between 15° and 30°C (59° and 86°F). Failure to use the product within this temperature range may result in improper dosing. Shake well before using.

Note: The indented statement below is required by the Federal government's Clean Air Act for all products containing or manufactured with chlorofluorocarbons (CFCs).

> **WARNING: Contains dichlorodifluoromethane (CDC-11) and trichloromonofluoromethANE (CFC-12), substances which harm public health and the environment by destroying ozone in the upper atmosphere.**

A notice similar to the above WARNING has been placed in the "Patient's Instructions" portion of this package insert pursuant to EPA regulations.

ANIMAL PHARMACOLOGY AND TOXICOLOGY

Studies in a number of animal species including rats, rabbits, and dogs have shown no unusual toxicity during acute experiments. However, the effects of beclomethasone dipropionate in producing signs of glucocorticoid excess during chronic administration by various routes were dose related.

CLINICAL STUDIES

The effects of beclomethasone dipropionate on hypothalamic-pituitary-adrenal (HPA) function have been evaluated in adult volunteers. There was no suppression of early morning plasma cortisol concentrations when beclomethasone dipropionate was administered in a dose of 1000 mcg/day for 1 month as an aerosol or for 3 days by intramuscular injection. However, partial suppression of plasma cortisol concentration was observed when beclomethasone dipropionate was administered at doses of 2000 mcg/day either intramuscularly or by aerosol. Immediate suppression of plasma cortisol concentrations was observed after single doses of 4000 mcg of beclomethasone dipropionate.

In one study, the effects of beclomethasone dipropionate on HPA function were examined in patients with asthma. There was no change in basal early morning plasma cortisol concentrations or in the cortisol responses to tetracosactrin (ACTH 1:24) stimulation after daily administration of 400, 800, or 1200 mcg of beclomethasone dipropionate for 28 days. After daily administration of 1600 mcg each day for 28 days, there was a slight reduction in basal cortisol concentrations and a statistically significant (p < .01) reduction in plasma cortisol responses to tetracosactrin stimulation. The effects of a more prolonged period of beclomethasone dipropionate administration on HPA function have not been evaluated. However, a number of investigators have noted that when systemic corticosteroid therapy in asthmatic subjects can be replaced with recommended doses of beclomethasone dipropionate, there is gradual recovery of endogenous cortisol concentrations to the normal range. There is still no documented evidence of recovery from other adverse systemic corticosteroid-induced reactions during prolonged therapy of patients with beclomethasone dipropionate.

Clinical experience has shown that some patients with bronchial asthma who require corticosteroid therapy for control of symptoms can be partially or completely withdrawn from systemic corticosteroid if therapy with beclomethasone dipropionate aerosol is substituted. Beclomethasone dipropionate aerosol is not effective for all patients with bronchial asthma or at all stages of the disease in a given patient.

The early clinical experience has revealed several new problems which may be associated with the use of beclomethasone dipropionate by inhalation for treatment of patients with bronchial asthma:

1. There is a risk of adrenal insufficiency when patients are transferred from systemic corticosteroids to aerosol beclomethasone dipropionate. Although the aerosol may provide adequate control of asthma during the transfer period, it does not provide the systemic steroid which is needed during acute stress situations. Deaths due to adrenal insufficiency have occurred in asthmatic patients during and after transfer from systemic corticosteroids to aerosol beclomethasone dipropionate. (See **WARNINGS**.)

2. Transfer of patients from systemic steroid therapy to beclomethasone dipropionate aerosol may unmask allergic conditions which were previously controlled by the systemic steroid therapy, eg, rhinitis, conjunctivitis, and eczema.

3. Localized infections with *Candida albicans* or *Aspergillus niger* have occurred frequently in the mouth and pharynx and occasionally in the larynx. It has been reported that up to 75% of the patients who receive prolonged treatment with beclomethasone dipropionate have positive oral cultures for *Candida albicans*. The incidence of clinically apparent infection is considerably lower but may require therapy with appropriate antifungal agents or discontinuation of treatment with beclomethasone dipropionate aerosol.

The long-term effects of beclomethasone dipropionate in human subjects are still unknown. In particular, the local effects of the agent on developmental or immunologic processes in the mouth, pharynx, trachea, and lung are unknown. There is also no information about the possible long-term systemic effects of the agent. The possible relevance of the data in animal studies to results in human subjects cannot be evaluated.

Rev. 4/95   18443422

Shown in Product Identification Guide, page 334

Information on Schering products appearing on these pages is effective as of August 15, 1996.

Schwarz Pharma, Inc.
5600 W. COUNTY LINE ROAD
P.O. BOX 2038
MILWAUKEE, WI 53201

Direct Inquiries to:
Drug Safety and Information
(414) 238-9994
(800) 558-5114

For Medical Information Contact:
In Emergency:
Drug Safety and Information
(414) 238-9994
(800) 558-5114

CALCIFEROL™ Products
[kal-si 'fur-ol]
CALCIFEROL™ Drops   OTC
(ergocalciferol oral solution USP)
8,000 USP Units/mL
CALCIFEROL™ Tablets   ℞
(ergocalciferol tablets USP)
50,000 USP Units
CALCIFEROL™ in Oil Injection   ℞
(ergocalciferol)
500,000 Units/mL

COLYTE® and COLYTE®-FLAVORED   ℞
(PEG-3350 & Electrolytes) For Oral Solution
For Gastrointestinal Lavage

DESCRIPTION
COLYTE® and COLYTE®-FLAVORED are colon lavage preparations provided as water-soluble components for solution. In solution each COLYTE® and COLYTE®-FLAVORED preparation delivers the following, in grams per liter.

Polyethylene glycol 3350	60.00
Sodium chloride	1.46
Potassium chloride	0.745
Sodium bicarbonate	1.68
Sodium sulfate	5.68
Flavor ingredients (COLYTE®-FLAVORED)	0.463

When dissolved in sufficient water to make 4 liters, the final solution contains 125 mEq/L sodium, 10 mEq/L potassium, 20 mEq/L bicarbonate, 80 mEq/L sulfate, 35 mEq/L chloride and 18 mEq/L polyethylene glycol 3350. The reconstituted solution is isosmotic and has a mildly salty taste. COLYTE® and COLYTE®-FLAVORED are administered orally or via nasogastric tube.

CLINICAL PHARMACOLOGY
COLYTE® and COLYTE®-FLAVORED cleanse the bowel by induction of diarrhea. The osmotic activity of Polyethylene Glycol 3350, in combination with the electrolyte concentration, results in virtually no net absorption or excretion of ions or water. Accordingly, large volumes may be administered without significant changes in fluid and electrolyte balance.

INDICATIONS AND USAGE
COLYTE® and COLYTE®-FLAVORED are indicated for bowel cleansing prior to colonoscopy or barium enema X-ray examination.

CONTRAINDICATIONS
COLYTE® and COLYTE®-FLAVORED are contraindicated in patients with ileus, gastric retention, gastrointestinal obstruction, bowel perforation, toxic colitis and toxic megacolon.

WARNINGS
No additional ingredients (e.g., flavorings) should be added to the solution. COLYTE® and COLYTE®-FLAVORED should be used with caution in patients with severe ulcerative colitis.

PRECAUTIONS
General: Patients with impaired gag reflex, unconscious or semiconscious patients and patients prone to regurgitation or aspiration should be observed during the administration of COLYTE® or COLYTE®-FLAVORED, especially if it is administered via nasogastric tube.
If gastrointestinal obstruction or perforation is suspected appropriate studies should be performed to rule out these conditions before administration of COLYTE® or COLYTE®-FLAVORED.

INFORMATION FOR PATIENTS
COLYTE® and COLYTE®-FLAVORED (PEG-3350 & Electrolytes for Oral Solution) produce a watery stool which cleanses the bowel prior to examination.
For best results, no solid food should be ingested during the 3 to 4 hour period prior to the initiation of COLYTE® or COLYTE®-FLAVORED administration. In no case should solid foods be eaten within 2 hours of drinking COLYTE® or COLYTE®-FLAVORED.
The rate of administration is 240 ml (8 fl. oz.) every 10 minutes. Rapid drinking of each portion is preferred rather than drinking small amounts continuously. The first bowel movement should occur approximately one hour after the start of COLYTE® or COLYTE®-FLAVORED administration. Administration of COLYTE® or COLYTE®-FLAVORED should be continued until the watery stool is clear and free of solid matter. This normally requires the consumption of approximately 3–4 liters (3–4 quarts), although more or less may be required in some patients. The unused portion should be discarded.

DRUG INTERACTIONS
Oral medication administered within one hour of the start of administration of COLYTE® or COLYTE®-FLAVORED may be flushed from the gastrointestinal tract and not absorbed.

CARCINOGENESIS, MUTAGENESIS, IMPAIRMENT OF FERTILITY
Studies to evaluate carcinogenic or mutagenic potential or potential to adversely affect male or female fertility have not been performed.

PREGNANCY
Category C. Animal reproduction studies have not been conducted with COLYTE® or COLYTE®-FLAVORED, and it is not known whether COLYTE® or COLYTE®-FLAVORED can affect reproductive capacity or harm the fetus when administered to a pregnant patient. COLYTE® or COLYTE®-FLAVORED should be given to a pregnant patient only if clearly needed.

PEDIATRIC USE
Safety and effectiveness in pediatric patients have not been established.

ADVERSE REACTIONS
Nausea, abdominal fullness and bloating are the most frequent adverse reactions, occurring in up to 50% of patients. Abdominal cramps, vomiting and anal irritation occur less frequently. These adverse reactions are transient. Isolated cases of urticaria, rhinorrhea and dermatitis have been reported which may represent allergic reactions.

DOSAGE AND ADMINISTRATION
COLYTE® or COLYTE®-FLAVORED can be administered orally or by nasogastric tube. Patients should fast at least 3 hours prior to administration. A one hour waiting period after the appearance of clear liquid stool should be allowed prior to examination to complete bowel evacuation. No foods except clear liquids should be permitted prior to examination after COLYTE® or COLYTE®-FLAVORED administration.

ORAL
The recommended adult oral dose is 240 ml (8 fl. oz.) every 10 minutes (see **INFORMATION FOR PATIENTS**). Lavage is complete when fecal discharge is clear. Lavage is usually complete after the ingestion of 3–4 liters.

NASOGASTRIC TUBE
COLYTE® or COLYTE®-FLAVORED (PEG-3350 & Electrolytes For Oral Solution) is administered at a rate of 20–30 ml per minute (1.2–1.8 L/hour).

PREPARATION OF COLYTE® OR COLYTE®-FLAVORED SOLUTION:
4 Liter: Add tap water to FILL line. Replace cap tightly and mix or shake well until all ingredients have dissolved. (No additional ingredients, e.g., flavorings, should be added to the solution.)
One Gallon: The preparation is made by dissolving the contents of the bottle in a food-grade container, in a sufficient quantity of water to produce the final volume according to package directions. (No additional ingredients, e.g., flavorings, should be added to the solution.) Mix well.

HOW SUPPLIED
COLYTE® and COLYTE®-FLAVORED are supplied in 4 liter (NDC 0091-4401-23 and NDC 0091-4403-05, respectively) and 18 oz. (NDC 0091-4401-49 and NDC 0091-4403-13, respectively) bottles in powdered form, for oral administration as a solution. Each contains the following:
4 liter, (NDC 0091-4401-23 and NDC 0091-4403-05): polyethylene glycol 3350 240 g, sodium chloride 5.84 g, potassium chloride 2.98 g, sodium bicarbonate 6.72 g, sodium sulfate (anhydrous) 22.72 g, flavor ingredients (COLYTE®-FLAVORED only) 1.85 g, in a bottle.
18 oz., (NDC 0091-4401-49 and NDC 0091-4403-13): polyethylene glycol 3350 227.10 g, sodium chloride 5.53 g, potassium chloride 2.82 g, sodium bicarbonate 6.36 g, sodium sulfate (anhydrous) 21.50 g, flavor ingredients (COLYTE®-FLAVORED only) 1.75 g, in a bottle.
Store powder at controlled room temperature 15°–30°C (59°–86°F).

CAUTION
Federal law prohibits dispensing without prescription.
KEEP RECONSTITUTED SOLUTION REFRIGERATED. USE WITHIN 48 HOURS. DISCARD UNUSED PORTION.

Shown in Product Identification Guide, page 334

CORTIFOAM®   ℞
(hydrocortisone acetate) 10%
Rectal Foam

DESCRIPTION
CORTIFOAM® (hydrocortisone acetate) 10% Rectal Foam contains hydrocortisone acetate 10% as the sole active ingredient in 20 g of a foam containing propylene glycol, emulsifying wax, polyoxyethylene-10-stearyl ether, cetyl alcohol, methylparaben and propylparaben, trolamine, purified water and inert propellants, dichlorodifluoromethane and dichlorotetrafluoroethane.
Each application delivers approximately 900 mg of foam containing 80 mg of hydrocortisone (90 mg of hydrocortisone acetate).
Molecular weight: Hydrocortisone acetate 404.50
Solubility of hydrocortisone acetate in water: 1 mg/100 ml
Chemical name: Pregn-4-ene-3,20-dione, 21-(acetyloxy)-11,17-dihydroxy-, (11β)-.

CLINICAL PHARMACOLOGY
CORTIFOAM provides effective topical administration of an anti-inflammatory corticosteroid as adjunctive therapy of ulcerative proctitis.

INDICATIONS
CORTIFOAM is indicated as adjunctive therapy in the topical treatment of ulcerative proctitis of the distal portion of the rectum in patients who cannot retain hydrocortisone or other corticosteroid enemas. Direct observations of methylene blue-containing foam have shown staining about 10 centimeters into the rectum.

CONTRAINDICATIONS
Local contraindications to the use of intrarectal steroids include obstruction, abscess, perforation, peritonitis, fresh intestinal anastomoses, extensive fistulas and sinus tracts. Tuberculosis (active, latent or questionably healed), ocular herpes simplex and acute psychosis are usually considered absolute contraindications to the use of corticosteroids. Relative contraindications include active peptic ulcer, acute glomerulonephritis, myasthenia gravis, osteoporosis, diverticulitis, thrombophlebitis, psychic disturbances, pregnancy, diabetes, hyperthyroidism, acute coronary disease, hypertension, limited cardiac reserve, and local or systemic infections, including fungal or exanthematous diseases. Where these conditions exist, the expected benefits from steroid therapy must be weighed against the risks involved in its use. Pregnancy is a relative contraindication to corticosteroids, particularly during third trimester. If corticosteroids must be administered in pregnancy, watch newborn infant closely for signs of hypoadrenalism, and administer appropriate therapy if needed.

WARNINGS
Do not insert any part of the aerosol container into the anus. Contents of the container are under pressure, but not flammable. Do not burn or puncture the aerosol container. Store at room temperature and not over 120° F. Because CORTIFOAM is not expelled, systemic hydrocortisone absorption may be greater from CORTIFOAM than from corticosteroid enema formulations. If there is not evidence of clinical or proctologic improvement within two or three weeks after starting CORTIFOAM therapy, or if the patient's condition worsens, discontinue the drug.
Persons who are on drugs which suppress the immune system are more susceptible to infections than healthy individuals. Chickenpox and measles, for example, can have a more serious or even fatal course in non-immune pediatric patients or adults on corticosteroids. In such pediatric patients or adults who have not had these diseases, particular care should be taken to avoid exposure. How the dose, route and

duration of corticosteroid administration affects the risk of developing a disseminated infection is not known. The contribution of the underlying disease and/or prior corticosteroid treatment to the risk is also not known. If exposed to chickenpox, prophylaxis with varicella zoster immune globulin (VZIG) may be indicated. If exposed to measles, prophylaxis with pooled intramuscular immunoglobulin (IG) may be indicated. (See the respective package inserts for complete VZIG and IG prescribing information). If chickenpox develops, treatment with antiviral agents may be considered.

PRECAUTIONS

Steroid therapy should be administered with caution in patients with severe ulcerative disease because these patients are predisposed to perforation of the bowel wall. Where surgery is imminent, it is hazardous to wait more than a few days for a satisfactory response to medical treatment. General precautions common to all corticosteroid therapy should be observed during treatment with CORTIFOAM. These include gradual withdrawal of therapy to allow for possible adrenal insufficiency and awareness to possible growth suppression in children. Patients should be kept under close observation, for, as with all drugs, rare individuals may react unfavorably under certain conditions. If severe reactions or idiosyncrasies occur, steroids should be discontinued immediately and appropriate measures instituted. Do not employ in immediate or early postoperative period following ileorectostomy.

Information for patients: Persons who are on immunosuppressant doses of corticosteroids should be warned to avoid exposure to chickenpox or measles. Patients should also be advised that if they are exposed, medical advice should be sought without delay.

ADVERSE REACTIONS

Corticosteroid therapy may produce side effects which include moon face, fluid retention, excessive appetite and weight gain, abnormal fat deposits, mental symptoms, hypertrichosis, acne, ecchymosis, increased sweating, pigmentation, dry scaly skin, thinning scalp hair, thrombophlebitis, decreased resistance to infection, negative nitrogen balance with delayed bone and wound healing, menstrual disorders, neuropathy, peptic ulcer, decreased glucose tolerance, hypopotassemia, adrenal insufficiency, necrotizing angiitis, hypertension, pancreatitis and increased intraocular pressure. In children, suppression of growth may occur. Increased intracranial pressure may occur and possibly account for headache, insomnia and fatigue. Subcapsular cataracts may result from prolonged usage. Long-term use of all corticosteroids results in catabolic effects characterized by negative protein and calcium balance. Osteoporosis, spontaneous fractures and aseptic necrosis of the hip and humerus may occur as part of this catabolic phenomenon. Where hypopotassemia and other symptoms associated with fluid and electrolyte imbalance call for potassium supplementation and salt poor or salt-free diets, these may be instituted and are compatible with diet requirements for ulcerative proctitis.

ADMINISTRATION AND DOSAGE

Usual dose is one applicatorful once or twice daily for two or three weeks, and every second day thereafter, administered rectally. The patient direction package with the applicator describes how to use the aerosol container and applicator. Satisfactory response usually occurs within five to seven days marked by a decrease in symptoms. Symptomatic improvement in ulcerative proctitis should not be used as the sole criterion for evaluating efficacy. Sigmoidoscopy is also recommended to judge dosage adjustment, duration of therapy and rate of improvement.

DIRECTIONS FOR USE

1) Shake foam container vigorously before use. Hold container upright and insert into the opening of the tip of the applicator. **Be sure applicator plunger is drawn all the way out.** Container must be held upright to obtain proper flow of medication. 2) To fill, press down slowly on container cap. When foam reaches fill line in the applicator, it is ready for use. **Caution:** The aerosol container should never be inserted directly into the anus. 3) Remove applicator from container. Allow some foam to remain on the applicator tip. Hold applicator by barrel and gently insert tip into the anus. With applicator in place, push plunger in order to expel foam, then withdraw applicator. (Applicator parts should be pulled apart for thorough cleaning with warm water.)

HOW SUPPLIED

CORTIFOAM (NDC 0021-0695-20) is supplied in an aerosol container with a special rectal applicator. Each applicator delivers approximately 900 mg of foam containing approximately 80 mg of hydrocortisone as 90 mg of hydrocortisone acetate. The aerosol container will deliver a minimum of 14 applications.

Store upright at controlled room temperature 15°–30°C (59°–86°F).

CAUTION

Federal law prohibits dispensing without prescription.

Shown in Product Identification Guide, page 334

DEPONIT® ℞

[*dĕp 'ō-nĭt*]

(nitroglycerin transdermal delivery system)

DESCRIPTION

Nitroglycerin is 1,2,3-propanetriol trinitrate, an organic nitrate whose structural formula is:

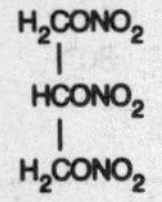
H2CONO2
HCONO2
H2CONO2

and whose molecular weight is 227.09. The organic nitrates are vasodilators, active on both arteries and veins.

The Deponit® transdermal system is a flat unit designed to provide continuous controlled release of nitroglycerin through intact skin. The rate of release of nitroglycerin is linearly dependent upon the area of the applied system; each cm^2 of applied system delivers approximately 0.013 mg of nitroglycerin per hour. Thus, the 16 cm^2 and 32 cm^2 systems deliver approximately 0.2 and 0.4 mg of nitroglycerin per hour, respectively. The remainder of the nitroglycerin in each system serves as a reservoir and is not delivered in normal use. After 12 hours, for example, each system has delivered 15% of its original content of nitroglycerin. Deponit contains nitroglycerin in a matrix composed of lactose, plasticizer, medical adhesive, polyisobutylene and aluminized plastic for controlled release of the active agent through the skin into the systemic circulation. The 16 cm^2 and 32 cm^2 systems contain 16 mg and 32 mg of nitroglycerin, respectively.

The Deponit system is approximately 0.3 mm thick, insoluble in water, and, as illustrated below, consists of two main elements:

1. A flexible, flesh-colored waterproof covering foil.
2. A multilayered adhesive film that constitutes simultaneously the drug reservoir and the release-control system.

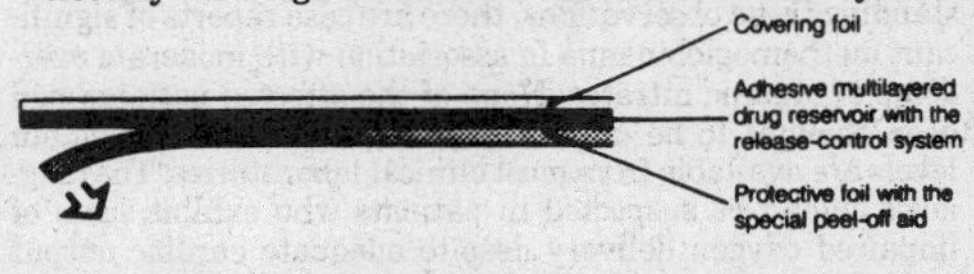
Covering foil
Adhesive multilayered drug reservoir with the release-control system
Protective foil with the special peel-off aid

The system is protected by an aluminum foil which has a patented S-shaped opening to facilitate its removal prior to use of the system. Prior to use, the protective foil is removed from the adhesive surface.

CLINICAL PHARMACOLOGY

The principal pharmacological action of nitroglycerin is relaxation of vascular smooth muscle and consequent dilatation of peripheral arteries and veins, especially the latter. Dilatation of the veins promotes peripheral pooling of blood and decreases venous return to the heart, thereby reducing left ventricular end-diastolic pressure and pulmonary capillary wedge pressure (preload). Arteriolar relaxation reduces systemic vascular resistance, systolic arterial pressure, and mean arterial pressure (afterload). Dilatation of the coronary arteries also occurs. The relative importance of preload reduction, afterload reduction and coronary dilatation remains undefined. Dosing regimens for most chronically used drugs are designed to provide plasma concentrations that are continuously greater than a minimally effective concentration. This strategy is inappropriate for organic nitrates. Several well-controlled clinical trials have used exercise testing to assess the anti-anginal efficacy of continuously-delivered nitrates. In the large majority of these trials, active agents were indistinguishable from placebo after 24 hours (or less) of continuous therapy. Attempts to overcome nitrate tolerance by dose escalation, even to doses far in excess of those used acutely, have consistently failed. Only after nitrates have been absent from the body for several hours has their antianginal efficacy been restored.

Pharmacokinetics: The volume of distribution of nitroglycerin is about 3 L/kg, and nitroglycerin is cleared from this volume at extremely rapid rates, with a resulting serum half-life of about 3 minutes. The observed clearance rates (close to 1 L/kg/min) greatly exceed hepatic blood flow; known sites of extrahepatic metabolism include red blood cells and vascular walls. The first products in the metabolism of nitroglycerin are inorganic nitrate and the 1,2- and 1,3-dinitroglycerols. The dinitrates are less effective vasodilators than nitroglycerin, but they are longer-lived in the serum, and their net contribution to the overall effect of chronic nitroglycerin regimens is not known. The dinitrates are further metabolized to (non-vasoactive) mononitrates and, ultimately, to glycerol and carbon dioxide. To avoid development of tolerance to nitroglycerin, drug-free intervals of 10–12 hours are known to be sufficient; shorter intervals have not been well studied. In one well-controlled clinical trial, subjects receiving nitroglycerin appeared to exhibit a rebound or withdrawal effect, so that their exercise tolerance at the end of the daily drug-free interval was *less* than that exhibited by the parallel group receiving placebo. In healthy volunteers, steady-state plasma concentrations of nitroglycerin are reached by about two hours after application of a patch and are maintained for the duration of wearing the system (observations have been limited to 24 hours). Upon removal of the patch, the plasma concentration declines with a half-life of about an hour.

Clinical trials: Regimens in which nitroglycerin patches were worn for 12 hours daily have been studied in well-controlled trials up to 4 weeks in duration. Starting about 2 hours after application and continuing until 10–12 hours after application, patches that deliver at least 0.4 mg of nitroglycerin per hour have consistently demonstrated greater anti-anginal activity than placebo. Lower-dose patches have not been as well studied, but in one large, well-controlled trial in which higher-dose patches were also studied, patches delivering 0.2 mg/hr had significantly *less* anti-anginal activity than placebo. It is reasonable to believe that the rate of nitroglycerin absorption from patches may vary with the site of application, but this relationship has not been adequately studied. The onset of action of transdermal nitroglycerin is not sufficiently rapid for this product to be useful in aborting an acute anginal episode.

INDICATIONS AND USAGE

Transdermal nitroglycerin is indicated for the prevention of angina pectoris due to coronary artery disease. The onset of action of transdermal nitroglycerin is not sufficiently rapid for this product to be useful in aborting an acute attack.

CONTRAINDICATIONS

Allergic reactions to organic nitrates are extremely rare, but they do occur. Nitroglycerin is contraindicated in patients who are allergic to it. Allergy to the adhesives used in nitroglycerin patches has also been reported, and it similarly constitutes a contraindication to the use of this product.

WARNINGS

The benefits of transdermal nitroglycerin in patients with acute myocardial infarction or congestive heart failure have not been established. If one elects to use nitroglycerin in these conditions, careful clinical or hemodynamic monitoring must be used to avoid the hazards of hypotension and tachycardia. A cardioverter/defibrillator should not be discharged through a paddle electrode that overlies a Deponit patch. The arcing that may be seen in this situation is harmless in itself, but it may be associated with local current concentration that can cause damage to the paddles and burns to the patient.

PRECAUTIONS

General:

Severe hypotension, particularly with upright posture, may occur with even small doses of nitroglycerin. This drug should therefore be used with caution in patients who may be volume depleted or who, for whatever reason, are already hypotensive. Hypotension induced by nitroglycerin may be accompanied by paradoxical bradycardia and increased angina pectoris. Nitrate therapy may aggravate the angina caused by hypertrophic cardiomyopathy. As tolerance to other forms of nitroglycerin develops, the effect of sublingual nitroglycerin on exercise tolerance, although still observable, is somewhat blunted. In industrial workers who have had long-term exposure to unknown (presumably high) doses of organic nitrates, tolerance clearly occurs. Chest pain, acute myocardial infarction, and even sudden death have occurred during temporary withdrawal of nitrates from these workers, demonstrating the existence of true physical dependence. Several clinical trials in patients with angina pectoris have evaluated nitroglycerin regimens which incorporated a 10–12 hour nitrate-free interval. In some of these trials, an increase in the frequency of anginal attacks during the nitrate-free interval was observed in a small number of patients. In one trial, patients demonstrated decreased exercise tolerance at the end of the nitrate-free interval. Hemodynamic rebound has been observed only rarely; on the other hand, few studies were so designed that rebound, if it had occurred, would have been detected. The importance of these observations to the routine, clinical use of transdermal nitroglycerin is unknown.

Information for Patients:

Daily headaches sometimes accompany treatment with nitroglycerin. In patients who get these headaches, the headaches may be a marker of the activity of the drug. Patients should resist the temptation to avoid headaches by altering the schedule of their treatment with nitroglycerin, since loss of headache may be associated with simultaneous loss of antianginal efficacy. Treatment with nitroglycerin may be associated with lightheadedness on standing, especially just after rising from a recumbent or seated position. This effect may be more frequent in patients who have also consumed alcohol. After normal use, there is enough residual nitroglycerin in discarded patches that they are a potential hazard to children and pets. A patient leaflet is supplied with the systems.

Continued on next page

Schwarz Pharma, Inc.—Cont.

Nitroglycerin Transdermal Rated Release in vivo	Total Nitroglycerin in System	System Size	Carton Size	NDC
0.2 mg/hr	16 mg	16 cm²	30	0091-4195-01
			30*	0091-4195-31
			100*	0091-4195-11
0.4 mg/hr	32 mg	32 cm²	30	0091-4196-01
			30*	0091-4196-31
			100*	0091-4196-11

*Institutional Package

Drug Interactions:
The vasodilating effects of nitroglycerin may be additive with those of other vasodilators. Alcohol, in particular, has been found to exhibit additive effects of this variety.
Carcinogenesis, Mutagenesis, Impairment of Fertility:
Studies to evaluate the carcinogenic or mutagenic potential of nitroglycerin have not been performed. Nitroglycerin's effect upon reproductive capacity is similarly unknown.
Pregnancy —Pregnancy Category C:
Animal reproduction studies have not been conducted with nitroglycerin. It is also not known whether nitroglycerin can cause fetal harm when administered to a pregnant woman or whether it can affect reproduction capacity. Nitroglycerin should be given to a pregnant woman only if clearly needed.
Nursing Mothers:
It is not known whether nitroglycerin is excreted in human milk. Because many drugs are excreted in human milk, caution should be exercised when nitroglycerin is administered to a nursing woman.
Pediatric use:
Safety and effectiveness in pediatric patients have not been established.

ADVERSE REACTIONS

Adverse reactions to nitroglycerin are generally dose-related, and almost all of these reactions are the result of nitroglycerin's activity as a vasodilator. Headache, which may be severe, is the most commonly reported side effect. Headache may be recurrent with each daily dose, especially at higher doses. Transient episodes of lightheadedness, occasionally related to blood pressure changes, may also occur. Hypotension occurs infrequently, but in some patients it may be severe enough to warrant discontinuation of therapy. Syncope, crescendo angina, and rebound hypertension have been reported but are uncommon.
Allergic reactions to nitroglycerin are also uncommon, and the great majority of those reported have been cases of contact dermatitis or fixed drug eruptions in patients receiving nitroglycerin in ointments or patches. There have been a few reports of genuine anaphylactoid reactions, and these reactions can probably occur in patients receiving nitroglycerin by any route.
Extremely rarely, ordinary doses of organic nitrates have caused methemoglobinemia in normal-seeming patients; for further discussion of its diagnosis and treatment see OVERDOSAGE.
Application-site irritation may occur but is rarely severe.
In two placebo-controlled trials of intermittent therapy with nitroglycerin patches at 0.2 to 0.8 mg/hr, the most frequent adverse reactions among 307 subjects were as follows:

	placebo	patch
headache	18%	63%
lightheadedness	4%	6%
hypotension and/or syncope	0%	4%
increased angina	2%	2%

OVERDOSAGE:

Hemodynamic Effects:
The ill effects of nitroglycerin overdose are generally the results of nitroglycerin's capacity to induce vasodilatation, venous pooling, reduced cardiac output, and hypotension. These hemodynamic changes may have protean manifestations, including increased intracranial pressure, with any or all of persistent throbbing headache, confusion, and moderate fever, vertigo; palpitations; visual disturbances; nausea and vomiting (possibly with colic and even bloody diarrhea); syncope (especially in the upright posture); air hunger and dyspnea, later followed by reduced ventilatory effort; diaphoresis, with the skin either flushed or cold and clammy; heart block and bradycardia; paralysis; coma; seizures; and death.
Laboratory determinations of serum levels of nitroglycerin and its metabolites are not widely available, and such determinations have, in any event, no established role in the management of nitroglycerin overdose. No data are available to suggest physiological maneuvers (e.g. maneuvers to change the pH of the urine) that might accelerate elimination of nitroglycerin and its active metabolites. Similarly, it is not known which—if any—of these substances can usefully be removed from the body by hemodialysis. No specific antagonist to the vasodilator effects of nitroglycerin is known, and no intervention has been subject to controlled study as a therapy of nitroglycerin overdose. Because the hypotension associated with nitroglycerin overdose is the result of venodilatation and arterial hypovolemia, prudent therapy in this situation should be directed toward increase in central fluid volume. Passive elevation of the patient's legs may be sufficient, but intravenous infusion of normal saline or similar fluid may also be necessary. The use of epinephrine or other arterial vasoconstrictors in this setting is likely to do more harm than good. In patients with renal disease or congestive heart failure, therapy resulting in central volume expansion is not without hazard. Treatment of nitroglycerin overdose in these patients may be subtle and difficult, and invasive monitoring may be required.
Methemoglobinemia:
Nitrate ions liberated during metabolism of nitroglycerin can oxidize hemoglobin into methemoglobin. Even in patients totally without cytochrome b_5 reductase activity, however, and even assuming that the nitrate moieties of nitroglycerin are quantitatively applied to oxidation of hemoglobin, about 1 mg/kg of nitroglycerin should be required before any of these patients manifests clinically significant (≥ 10%) methemoglobinemia. In patients with normal reductase function, significant production of methemoglobin should require even larger doses of nitroglycerin. In one study in which 36 patients received 2–4 weeks of continuous nitroglycerin therapy at 3.1 to 4.4 mg/hr, the average methemoglobin level measured was 0.2%; this was comparable to that observed in parallel patients who received placebo. Notwithstanding these observations, there are case reports of significant methemoglobinemia in association with moderate overdoses of organic nitrates. None of the affected patients had been thought to be unusually susceptible. Methemoglobin levels are available from most clinical laboratories. The diagnosis should be suspected in patients who exhibit signs of impaired oxygen delivery despite adequate cardiac output and adequate arterial pO_2. Classically, methemoglobinemic blood is described as chocolate brown, without color change on exposure to air. When methemoglobinemia is diagnosed, the treatment of choice is methylene blue, 1–2 mg/kg intravenously.

DOSAGE AND ADMINISTRATION

The suggested starting dose is between 0.2 mg/hr and 0.4 mg/hr. Doses between 0.4 mg/hr and 0.8 mg/hr have shown continued effectiveness for 10–12 hours daily for at least one month (the longest period studied) of intermittent administration. Although the minimum nitrate-free interval has not been defined, data show that a nitrate-free interval of 10–12 hrs is sufficient (see CLINICAL PHARMACOLOGY). Thus, an appropriate dosing schedule for nitroglycerin patches would include a daily patch-on period of 12–14 hours and a daily patch-off period of 10–12 hours. Although some well controlled clinical trials using exercise tolerance testing have shown maintenance of effectiveness when patches are worn continuously, the large majority of such controlled trials have shown the development of tolerance (i.e., complete loss of effect) within the first 24 hours after therapy was initiated. Dose adjustment, even to levels much higher than generally used, did not restore efficacy.

HOW SUPPLIED

Deponit® (nitroglycerin transdermal delivery system) is packaged in cartons containing unit doses of flesh-colored systems on aluminum backings. See table below.
[See table above.]
Store at room temperature not above 25° C (77° F). Do not refrigerate.
CAUTION: Federal law prohibits dispensing without prescription.

Shown in Product Identification Guide, page 334

DILATRATE®-SR ℞

[dī'lă-trāt]
(isosorbide dinitrate)
Sustained Release Capsules
40 mg

DESCRIPTION

Isosorbide dinitrate (ISDN) is 1,4:3,6-dianhydro-D-glucitol 2,5 dinitrate, an organic nitrate whose structural formula is
[See chemical structure at top of next column.]
and whose molecular weight is 236.14. The organic nitrates are vasodilators, active on both arteries and veins. Each Dilatrate-SR sustained release capsule contains 40 mg of isosor-

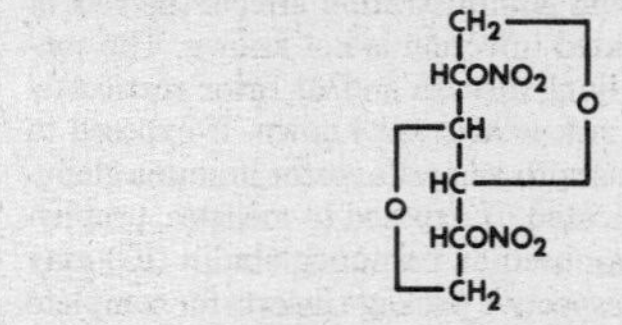

bide dinitrate, in a microdialysis delivery system that causes the active drug to be released over an extended period. Each capsule also contains ethylcellulose, lactose, pharmaceutical glaze, starch, sucrose and talc. The capsule shells contain D&C Red 33, D&C Yellow 10, gelatin and titanium dioxide.

CLINICAL PHARMACOLOGY

The principal pharmacological action of isosorbide dinitrate is relaxation of vascular smooth muscle and consequent dilatation of peripheral arteries and veins, especially the latter. Dilatation of the veins promotes peripheral pooling of blood and decreases venous return to the heart, thereby reducing left ventricular end-diastolic pressure and pulmonary capillary wedge pressure (preload). Arteriolar relaxation reduces systemic vascular resistance, systolic arterial pressure, and mean arterial pressure (afterload). Dilatation of the coronary arteries also occurs. The relative importance of preload reduction, afterload reduction, and coronary dilatation remains undefined.
Dosing regimens for most chronically used drugs are designed to provide plasma concentrations that are continuously greater than a minimally effective concentration. This strategy is inappropriate for organic nitrates. Several well-controlled clinical trials have used exercise testing to assess the antianginal efficacy of continuously-delivered nitrates. In the large majority of these trials, active agents were no more effective than placebo after 24 hours (or less) of continuous therapy. Attempts to overcome nitrate tolerance by dose escalation, even to doses far in excess of those used acutely, have consistently failed. Only after nitrates have been absent from the body for several hours has their antianginal efficacy been restored.
Pharmacokinetics: The kinetics of absorption of isosorbide dinitrate from Dilatrate-SR sustained release capsules have not been well studied. Studies of immediate-release formulations of ISDN have found highly variable bioavailability (10 to 90%), with extensive first-pass metabolism in the liver. Most such studies have observed progressive increases in bioavailability during chronic therapy; it is not known whether similar increases in bioavailability appear during the course of chronic therapy with Dilatrate-SR sustained release capsules.
Once absorbed, the distribution volume of isosorbide dinitrate is 2–4 L/kg and this volume is cleared at the rate of 2–4 L/min, so ISDN's half-life in serum is about an hour. Since the clearance exceeds hepatic blood flow, considerable extrahepatic metabolism must also occur. Clearance is affected primarily by denitration to the 2-mononitrate (15 to 25%) and the 5- mononitrate (75 to 85%).
Both metabolites have biological activity, especially the 5-mononitrate. With an overall half-life of about 5 hours, the 5-mononitrate is cleared from the serum by denitration to isosorbide; glucuronidation to the 5-mononitrate glucuronide; and denitration/hydration to sorbitol. The 2-mononitrate has been less well studied, but it appears to participate in the same metabolic pathways, with a half-life of about 2 hours.
The interdosing interval sufficient to avoid tolerance to ISDN has not been well defined. Studies of nitroglycerin (an organic nitrate with a very short half-life) have shown that dosing intervals of 10–12 hours are usually sufficient to prevent or attenuate tolerance. Dosing intervals that have succeeded in avoiding tolerance during trials of moderate doses (e.g. 30 mg) of immediate release ISDN have generally been somewhat longer (at least 14 hours), but this is consistent with the longer half-lives of ISDN and its active metabolites.
An interdosing interval sufficient to avoid tolerance with Dilatrate-SR has not been demonstrated. In an eccentric dosing study, 40 mg capsules of Dilatrate-SR were administered daily at 0800 and 1400 hours. After two weeks of this regimen, Dilatrate-SR was statistically indistinguishable from placebo. Thus, the necessary interdosing interval sufficient to avoid tolerance remains unknown, but it must be greater than 18 hours.
Few well-controlled clinical trials of organic nitrates have been designed to detect rebound or withdrawal effects. In one such trial, however, subjects receiving nitroglycerin had less exercise tolerance at the end of the daily interdosing interval than the parallel group receiving placebo. The incidence, magnitude, and clinical significance of similar phenomena in patients receiving ISDN have not been studied.
Clinical trials: In clinical trials, extended-release oral isosorbide dinitrate has been administered in a variety of regimens, with total daily doses ranging from 40 to 160 mg. A controlled trial using a single 40 mg sustained-release oral dose of isosorbide dinitrate (Dilatrate-SR) has demonstrated effective reductions in exercise-related angina for up to 8

hours. Antianginal activity is present about 1 hour after dosing.
Adequate multiple-dose trials of Dilatrate-SR sustained release capsules have not been reported.
Most controlled trials of multiple-dose immediate-release oral ISDN taken every 12 hours (or more frequently) for several weeks have shown statistically significant antianginal efficacy for only 2 hours after dosing. Once-daily regimens, and regimens with one daily interdosing interval of at least 14 hours (e.g., a regimen providing doses at 0800, 1400 and 1800 hours), have shown efficacy after the first dose of each day that was similar to that shown in the single dose studies cited above. The efficacy of subsequent doses has not been demonstrated. From large, well-controlled studies of other nitrates, it is reasonable to believe that the maximal achievable daily duration of antianginal effect from isosorbide dinitrate is about 12 hours. No dosing regimen for Dilatrate-SR sustained released capsules has actually been shown to achieve this duration of effect.

INDICATIONS AND USAGE

Dilatrate-SR sustained release capsules are indicated for the prevention of angina pectoris due to coronary artery disease. The onset of action of controlled-release oral isosorbide dinitrate is not sufficiently rapid for this product to be useful in aborting an acute anginal episode.

CONTRAINDICATIONS

Allergic reactions to organic nitrates are extremely rare, but they do occur. Isosorbide dinitrate is contraindicated in patients who are allergic to it.

WARNINGS

The benefits of extended-release oral isosorbide dinitrate in patients with acute myocardial infarction or congestive heart failure have not been established. If one elects to use isosorbide dinitrate in these conditions, careful clinical or hemodynamic monitoring must be used to avoid the hazards of hypotension and tachycardia. Because the effects of extended-release oral isosorbide dinitrate are so difficult to terminate rapidly, this formulation is not recommended in these settings.

PRECAUTIONS

General: Severe hypotension, particularly with upright posture, may occur with even small doses of isosorbide dinitrate. This drug should therefore be used with caution in patients who may be volume depleted or who, for whatever reason, are already hypotensive. Hypotension induced by isosorbide dinitrate may be accompanied by paradoxical bradycardia and increased angina pectoris.
Nitrate therapy may aggravate the angina caused by hypertrophic cardiomyopathy.
As tolerance to isosorbide dinitrate develops, the effect of sublingual nitroglycerin on exercise tolerance, although still observable, is somewhat blunted.
Some clinical trials in angina patients have provided nitroglycerin for about 12 continuous hours of every 24-hour day. During the interdosing intervals in some of these trials, anginal attacks have been more easily provoked than before treatment and patients have demonstrated hemodynamic rebound and decreased exercise tolerance. The importance of these observations to the routine, clinical use of controlled-release oral isosorbide dinitrate is not known.
In industrial workers who have had long-term exposure to unknown (presumably high) doses of organic nitrates, tolerance clearly occurs. Chest pain, acute myocardial infarction, and even sudden death have occurred during temporary withdrawal of nitrates from these workers demonstrating the existence of true physical dependence.
Information for Patients: Patients should be told that the antianginal efficacy of isosorbide dinitrate is strongly related to its dosing regimen, so the prescribed schedule of dosing should be followed carefully. In particular, daily headaches sometimes accompany treatment with isosorbide dinitrate. In patients who get these headaches, the headaches are a marker of the activity of the drug. Patients should resist the temptation to avoid headaches by altering the schedule of their treatment with isosorbide dinitrate, since loss of headache may be associated with simultaneous loss of antianginal efficacy. Aspirin and/or acetaminophen, on the other hand, often successfully relieve isosorbide dinitrate-induced headaches with no deleterious effect on isosorbide dinitrate's antianginal efficacy.
Treatment with isosorbide dinitrate may be associated with lightheadedness on standing, especially just after rising from a recumbent or seated position. This effect may be more frequent in patients who have also consumed alcohol.
Drug Interactions: The vasodilating effects of isosorbide dinitrate may be additive with those of other vasodilators. Alcohol, in particular, has been found to exhibit additive effects of this variety.
Carcinogenesis, Mutagenesis and Impairment of Fertility: No long-term studies in animals have been performed to evaluate the carcinogenic potential of isosorbide dinitrate. In a modified two-litter reproduction study, there was no remarkable gross pathology and no altered fertility or gestation among rats fed isosorbide dinitrate at 25 or 100 mg/kg/day.
Pregnancy Category C: At oral doses 35 and 150 times the daily Maximum Recommended Human Dose (MRHD), isosorbide dinitrate has been shown to cause a dose related increase in embryotoxicity (increase in mummified pups) in rabbits. There are no adequate, well-controlled studies in pregnant women. Isosorbide dinitrate should be used during pregnancy only if the potential benefit justifies the potential risk to the fetus.
Nursing Mothers: It is not known whether isosorbide dinitrate is excreted in human milk. Because many drugs are excreted in human milk, caution should be exercised when isosorbide dinitrate is administered to a nursing woman.
Pediatric Use: Safety and effectiveness in pediatric patients have not been established.

ADVERSE REACTIONS

Adverse reactions to isosorbide dinitrate are generally dose related, and almost all of these reactions are the result of isosorbide dinitrate's activity as a vasodilator. Headache, which may be severe, is the most commonly reported side effect. Headache may be recurrent with each daily dose, especially at higher doses. Transient episodes of lightheadedness, occasionally related to blood pressure changes, may also occur. Hypotension occurs infrequently, but in some patients it may be severe enough to warrant discontinuation of therapy. Syncope, crescendo angina, and rebound hypertension have been reported but are uncommon.
Extremely rarely, ordinary doses of organic nitrates have caused methemoglobinemia in normal-seeming patients. Methemoglobinemia is so infrequent at these doses that further discussion of its diagnosis and treatment is deferred (see OVERDOSAGE).
Data are not available to allow estimation of the frequency of adverse reactions during treatment with Dilatrate-SR sustained release capsules.

OVERDOSAGE

Hemodynamic Effects: The ill effects of isosorbide dinitrate overdose are generally the results of isosorbide dinitrate's capacity to induce vasodilatation, venous pooling, reduced cardiac output, and hypotension. These hemodynamic changes may have protean manifestations, including increased intracranial pressure, with any or all of persistent throbbing headache, confusion, and moderate fever; vertigo; palpitations; visual disturbances; nausea and vomiting (possibly with colic and even bloody diarrhea); syncope (especially in the upright posture); air hunger and dyspnea, later followed by reduced ventilatory effort; diaphoresis, with the skin either flushed or cold and clammy; heart block and bradycardia; paralysis; coma; seizures and death.
Laboratory determinations of serum levels of isosorbide dinitrate and its metabolites are not widely available, and such determinations have, in any event, no established role in the management of isosorbide dinitrate overdose.
There are no data suggesting what dose of isosorbide dinitrate is likely to be life-threatening in humans. In rats, the median acute lethal dose (LD50) was found to be 1100 mg/kg. No data are available to suggest physiological maneuvers (e.g., maneuvers to change the pH of the urine) might accelerate elimination of isosorbide dinitrate and its active metabolites. Similarly, it is not known which, if any, of these substances can usefully be removed from the body by hemodialysis.
No specific antagonist to the vasodilator effects of isosorbide dinitrate is known, and no intervention has been subject to controlled study as a therapy of isosorbide dinitrate overdose. Because the hypotension associated with isosorbide dinitrate overdose is the result of venodilatation and arterial hypovolemia, prudent therapy in this situation should be directed toward increase in central fluid volume. Passive elevation of the patient's legs may be sufficient, but intravenous infusion of normal saline or similar fluid may also be necessary. The use of epinephrine or other arterial vasoconstrictors in this setting is likely to do more harm than good.
In patients with renal disease or congestive heart failure, therapy resulting in central volume expansion is not without hazard. Treatment of isosorbide dinitrate overdose in these patients may be subtle and difficult, and invasive monitoring may be required.
Methemoglobinemia: Nitrate ions liberated during metabolism of isosorbide dinitrate can oxidize hemoglobin into methemoglobin. Even in patients totally without cytochrome b5 reductase activity, however, and even assuming that the nitrate moieties of isosorbide dinitrate are quantitatively applied to oxidation of hemoglobin, about 1 mg/kg of isosorbide dinitrate should be required before any of these patients manifests clinically significant (> 10%) methemoglobinemia. In patients with normal reductase function, significant production of methemoglobin should require even larger doses of isosorbide dinitrate. In one study in which 36 patients received 2–4 weeks of continuous nitroglycerin therapy at 3.1 to 4.4 mg/hr (equivalent, in total administered dose of nitrate ions, to 4.8–6.9 mg of bioavailable isosorbide dinitrate per hour), the average methemoglobin level measured was 0.2%; this was comparable to that observed in parallel patients who received placebo.
Notwithstanding these observations, there are case reports of significant methemoglobinemia in association with moderate overdoses of organic nitrates. None of the affected patients had been thought to be unusually susceptible.
Methemoglobin levels are available from most clinical laboratories. The diagnosis should be suspected in patients who exhibit signs of impaired oxygen delivery despite adequate cardiac output and adequate arterial p02. Classically, methemoglobinemic blood is described as chocolate brown, without color change on exposure to air.
When methemoglobinemia is diagnosed, the treatment of choice is methylene blue, 1–2 mg/kg intravenously.

DOSAGE AND ADMINISTRATION

As noted above (CLINICAL PHARMACOLOGY), multiple studies with ISDN and other nitrates have shown that maintenance of continuous 24-hour plasma levels results in refractory tolerance. Every dosing regimen for organic nitrates including Dilatrate-SR must provide a daily nitrate-free interval to avoid the development of tolerance. To achieve the necessary nitrate-free interval with immediate-release oral ISDN, it appears that at least one of the daily interdose intervals must be at least 14 hours long. The necessary interdose interval for Dilatrate-SR has not been clearly identified, but it must be greater than 18 hours.
As noted under Clinical Pharmacology, only one trial has ever studied the use of extended-release isosorbide dinitrate for more than one dose. In that trial, 40 mg of Dilatrate-SR was administered twice daily in doses given 6 hours apart. After 4 weeks, Dilatrate-SR could not be distinguished from placebo.
Large controlled studies with other nitrates suggest that no dosing regimen with Dilatrate-SR should be expected to provide more than about 12 hours of continuous antianginal efficacy per day.
In clinical trials, immediate-release oral isosorbide dinitrate has been administered in a variety of regimens, with total daily doses ranging from 40 to 160 mg.
Do not exceed 160 mg (4 capsules) per day.

HOW SUPPLIED

Dilatrate®-SR (isosorbide dinitrate) 40 mg Sustained Release Capsules are opaque pink and colorless capsules with white beadlets and are imprinted "Schwarz" and "0920".
They are supplied as follows:

Bottles of 60	NDC 0091-0920-02
Bottles of 100	NDC 0091-0920-01

Store at controlled room temperature 15°–30°C (59°–86°F) in a dry place.
CAUTION: Federal law prohibits dispensing without prescription.

Shown in Product Identification Guide, page 334

EPIFOAM®

℞

topical aerosol
(hydrocortisone acetate 1% and pramoxine hydrochloride 1%)

DESCRIPTION

A topical corticosteroid in an aerosol foam containing hydrocortisone acetate 1% and pramoxine hydrochloride 1% in a base containing: propylene glycol, cetyl alcohol, glyceryl stearate, PEG-100 stearate, laureth-23, polyoxyl-40 stearate, methylparaben, propylparaben, trolamine, hydrochloric acid to adjust pH, purified water and propellants (inert): butane and propane.
EPIFOAM contains a synthetic steroid used as an anti-inflammatory and antipruritic agent, and a local anesthetic.
Hydrocortisone acetate
Molecular weight: 404.50. Solubility of hydrocortisone acetate in water: 1 mg/100 ml. Chemical name: Pregn-4-ene, 3,20-dione, 21-(acetyloxy)-11, 17-dihydroxy- (11β).

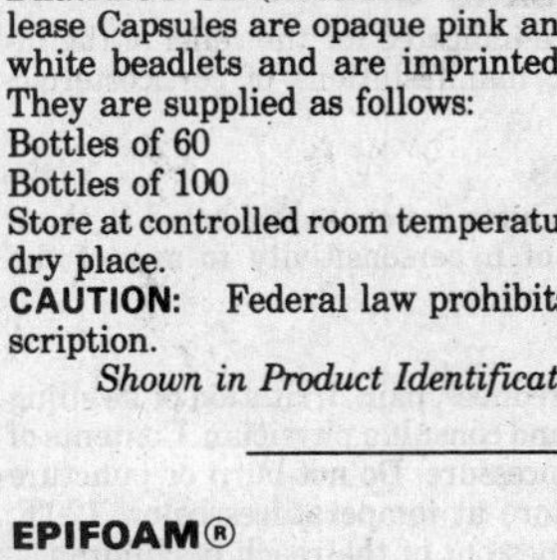

Pramoxine hydrochloride
Molecular weight: 329.87. Pramoxine hydrochloride is freely soluble in water. Chemical names: Morpholine, 4-[3-(4-butoxyphenoxy)propyl]-, hydrochloride, 4-[3-(*p*-butoxyphenoxy) propyl]morpholine hydrochloride.

[See structure at top of next column.]

Continued on next page

Schwarz Pharma, Inc.—Cont.

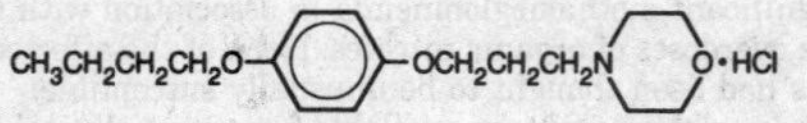

CLINICAL PHARMACOLOGY

Topical corticosteroids share anti-inflammatory, antipruritic and vasoconstrictive actions.
The mechanism of anti-inflammatory activity of the topical corticosteroids is unclear. Various laboratory methods, including vasoconstrictor assays, are used to compare and predict potencies and/or clinical efficacies of the topical corticosteroids. There is some evidence to suggest that a recognizable correlation exists between vasoconstrictor potency and therapeutic efficacy in man.

Pramoxine hydrochloride: A surface or local anesthetic which is not chemically related to the "caine" types of local anesthetics. Its unique chemical structure is likely to minimize the danger of cross-sensitivity reactions in patients allergic to other local anesthetics.

Pharmacokinetics: The extent of percutaneous absorption of topical corticosteroids is determined by many factors including the vehicle, the integrity of the epidermal barrier, and the use of occlusive dressings.
Topical corticosteroids can be absorbed from normal intact skin. Inflammation and/or disease processes in the skin increase the percutaneous absorption of topical corticosteroids. Occlusive dressings substantially increase the percutaneous absorption of topical corticosteroids. Thus, occlusive dressings may be a valuable therapeutic adjunct for treatment of resistant dermatoses. (See DOSAGE AND ADMINISTRATION.)
Once absorbed through the skin, topical corticosteroids are handled through pharmacokinetic pathways similar to systemically administered corticosteroids. Corticosteroids are bound to plasma proteins in varying degrees. Corticosteroids are metabolized primarily in the liver and are then excreted by the kidneys. Some of the topical corticosteroids and their metabolites are also excreted into the bile.

INDICATIONS AND USAGE

Topical corticosteroids are indicated for the relief of the inflammatory and pruritic manifestations of corticosteroid-responsive dermatoses.

CONTRAINDICATIONS

Topical corticosteroid products are contraindicated in those patients with a history of hypersensitivity to any of the components of the preparation.

WARNINGS

Not for prolonged use. If redness, pain, irritation or swelling persists, discontinue use and consult a physician. Contents of the container are under pressure. Do not burn or puncture the aerosol container. Store at temperatures below 120°F. Keep this and all medicines out of the reach of children.

PRECAUTIONS

General: Systemic absorption of topical corticosteroids has produced reversible hypothalamic-pituitary-adrenal (HPA) axis suppression, manifestations of Cushing's syndrome, hyperglycemia and glucosuria in some patients.
Conditions which augment systemic absorption include the application of the more potent steroids, use over large surface areas, prolonged use and the addition of occlusive dressings.
Therefore, patients receiving a large dose of a potent topical steroid applied to a large surface area or under an occlusive dressing should be evaluated periodically for evidence of HPA axis suppression by using the urinary free cortisol and ACTH stimulation tests. If HPA axis suppression is noted, an attempt should be made to withdraw the drug, to reduce the frequency of application, or to substitute a less potent steroid.
Recovery of HPA axis function is generally prompt and complete upon discontinuation of the drug. Infrequently, signs and symptoms of steroid withdrawal may occur, requiring supplemental systemic corticosteroids.
In children, absorption may result in higher blood levels and thus more susceptibility to systemic toxicity. (See PRECAUTIONS—Pediatric Use.)
If irritation develops, topical corticosteroids should be discontinued and appropriate therapy instituted.
In the presence of dermatological infections, the use of an appropriate antifungal or antibacterial agent should be instituted. If a favorable response does not occur promptly, the corticosteroid should be discontinued until the infection has been adequately controlled.

Information for the Patient: Patients using topical corticosteroids should receive the following information and instructions:

1. This medication is to be used as directed by the physician. It is for external use only. Avoid contact with the eyes.
2. Do not use this medication for any disorder other than for which it has been prescribed.
3. The treated skin area should not be bandaged or otherwise covered or wrapped as to be occlusive unless directed by the physician.
4. Report any signs of local adverse reactions especially under occlusive dressings.
5. Do not use any tight fitting diapers or plastic pants on a child being treated in the diaper area, as these garments may constitute occlusive dressings.

Laboratory Tests: The following test may be helpful in evaluating the HPA axis suppression:
Urinary free cortisol test
ACTH stimulation test

Carcinogenesis, Mutagenesis, and Impairment of Fertility: Long-term animal studies have not been performed to evaluate carcinogenic potential or the effect on fertility of topical corticosteroids.
Studies to determine mutagenicity with prednisolone and hydrocortisone have revealed negative results.

Pregnancy Category C: Corticosteroids are generally teratogenic in laboratory animals when administered systemically at relatively low dosage levels. The more potent corticosteroids have been shown to be teratogenic after dermal application in laboratory animals. There are no adequate and well-controlled studies in pregnant women of teratogenic effects from topically applied corticosteroids. Therefore, topical corticosteroids should be used during pregnancy only if the potential benefit justifies the potential risk to the fetus. Drugs of this class should not be used extensively on pregnant patients, in large amounts, or for prolonged periods of time.

Nursing Mothers: It is not known whether topical administration of corticosteroids could result in sufficient systemic absorption to produce detectable quantities in breast milk. Systemically administered corticosteroids are secreted into breast milk in quantities not likely to have a deleterious effect on the infant. Caution should be exercised when any topical corticosteroids are administered to a nursing woman.

Pediatric Use: *Pediatric patients may demonstrate greater susceptibility to topical corticosteroid-induced HPA axis suppression and Cushing's syndrome than mature patients because of a larger skin surface area to body weight ratio.*
Hypothalamic-pituitary-adrenal (HPA) axis suppression, Cushing's syndrome and intracranial hypertension have been reported in children receiving topical corticosteroids. Manifestations of adrenal suppression in children include linear growth retardation, delayed weight gain, low plasma cortisone levels and absence of response to ACTH stimulation. Manifestations of intracranial hypertension include bulging fontanelles, headaches and bilateral papilledema.
Administration of topical corticosteroids to children should be limited to the least amount compatible with an effective therapeutic regimen. Chronic corticosteroid therapy may interfere with the growth and development of children.

ADVERSE REACTIONS

The following local adverse reactions are reported infrequently with topical corticosteroids, but may occur more frequently with the use of occlusive dressings. These reactions are listed in an approximately decreasing order of occurrence: Burning, Itching, Irritation, Dryness, Folliculitis, Hypertrichosis, Acneiform eruptions, Hypopigmentation, Perioral dermatitis, Allergic contact dermatitis, Maceration of the skin, Secondary infection, Skin atrophy, Striae, Miliaria,

OVERDOSAGE

Topically applied corticosteroids can be absorbed in sufficient amounts to produce systemic effects. (See PRECAUTIONS.)

DOSAGE AND ADMINISTRATION

Apply to affected area 3 or 4 times daily.
(NOTE: Refer to the enclosed Directions for Use.):

DIRECTIONS FOR USE

1. Shake foam container vigorously before use.
2. Hold container upright and apply only a small amount directly to affected areas. Alternatively, dispense a small amount onto a pad and apply to affected areas.
3. The container and cap should be disassembled and rinsed with warm water after use.

NOTE: The aerosol container should never be inserted into the vagina or anus.

HOW SUPPLIED

EPIFOAM® (NDC0021-0740-10) is available in 10 g pressurized cans.
Store upright at controlled room temperature 15°–30°C (59°–86°F).

CAUTION

FEDERAL LAW PROHIBITS DISPENSING WITHOUT PRESCRIPTION.

Shown in Product Identification Guide, page 334

ETHAMOLIN® ℞

[eth "am 'o lin]
(ethanolamine oleate)
Injection, 5%
For Local Intravenous Use Only

DESCRIPTION

ETHAMOLIN® (ethanolamine oleate) Injection is a mild sclerosing agent. Chemically it is $C_{17}H_{33}COOH.NH_2CH_2CH_2OH$. It has the following structure:

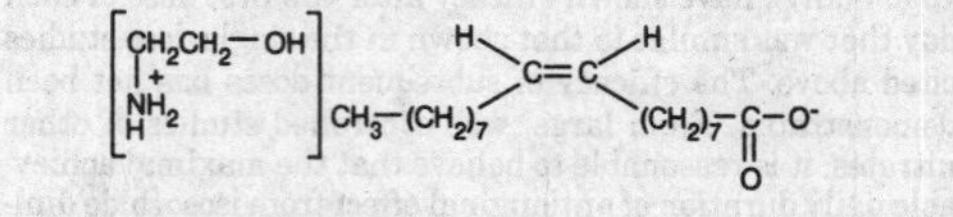

The empirical formula is $C_{20}H_{41}NO_3$, representing a molecular weight of 343.55.
ETHAMOLIN Injection consists of ethanolamine, a basic substance, which when combined with oleic acid forms a clear, straw to pale yellow colored, deliquescent oleate. The pH ranges from 8.0 to 9.0.
ETHAMOLIN Injection is a sterile, apyrogenic, aqueous solution containing in each mL approximately 50 mg of ethanolamine oleate with benzyl alcohol 2% by volume as preservative.

CLINICAL PHARMACOLOGY

When injected intravenously, ETHAMOLIN Injection acts primarily by irritation of the intimal endothelium of the vein and produces a sterile dose-related inflammatory response. This results in fibrosis and possible occlusion of the vein. ETHAMOLIN Injection also rapidly diffuses through the venous wall and produces a dose-related extravascular inflammatory reaction.
The oleic acid component of the ETHAMOLIN Injection is responsible for the inflammatory response, and may also activate coagulation *in vivo* by release of tissue factor and activation of Hageman factor. The ethanolamine component, however, may inhibit fibrin clot formation by chelating calcium, so that a procoagulant action of ETHAMOLIN has not been demonstrated.
After injection, ETHAMOLIN disappears from the injection site within five minutes via the portal vein. When volumes larger than 20 mL are injected, some ETHAMOLIN also flows into the azygos vein through the periesophageal vein. In human autopsy studies it was found that within four days after injection there is neutrophil infiltration of the esophageal wall and hemorrhage within six days. Granulation tissue is first seen at ten days, red thrombi obliterating the varices by twenty days, and sclerosis of the varices by two and a half months. The time course of these findings suggests that sclerosis of esophageal varices will be a delayed rather than an immediate effect of the drug.
The minimum lethal dose of ETHAMOLIN Injection administered intravenously to rabbits is 130 mg/kg.
In dogs, ETHAMOLIN injected into the right atrium at a dose of 1 mL/kg over one minute has been shown to increase extravascular lung water. The maximum recommended human dose is 20 mL, or 0.4 mL/kg for a 50-kg person. The concentration of ETHAMOLIN (ethanolamine oleate) reaching the lung in human treatment will be less than in the dog studies, but pleural effusions, pulmonary edema, pulmonary infiltration and pneumonitis have been reported in clinical trials, and minimizing the total per session dose, especially in patients with concomitant cardiopulmonary disease, is recommended (see PRECAUTIONS).

INDICATIONS AND USAGE

ETHAMOLIN® Injection is indicated for the treatment of patients with esophageal varices that have recently bled, to prevent rebleeding.
ETHAMOLIN is not indicated for the treatment of patients with esophageal varices that have not bled. There is no evidence that treatment of this population decreases the likelihood of bleeding.
Sclerotherapy with ETHAMOLIN has no beneficial effect upon portal hypertension, the cause of esophageal varices, so that recanalization and collateralization may occur, necessitating reinjection.

CONTRAINDICATIONS

ETHAMOLIN® Injection should not be administered to subjects with a known hypersensitivity to ethanolamine, oleic acid, or ethanolamine oleate.

WARNINGS

ETHAMOLIN® Injection should be used in pregnant women only when clearly needed (see PRECAUTIONS).
The practice of injecting varicosities of the leg with ETHAMOLIN Injection is not supported by adequately controlled clinical trials. Therefore, such use is not recommended.

PRECAUTIONS

Fatal anaphylactic shock was reported following injection of a larger than normal volume of ETHAMOLIN® Injection

into a male who had a known allergic disposition. Although there are only three known reports of anaphylaxis, the possibility of an anaphylactic reaction should be kept in mind, and the physician should be prepared to treat it appropriately. In extreme emergencies, 0.25 mL of a 1:1,000 intravenous solution of epinephrine (0.25 mg) should be used and allergic reactions should be controlled with antihistamines.
Acute renal failure with spontaneous recovery followed injection of 15 to 20 mL of ETHAMOLIN Injection into two women.
The physician should bear in mind that severe injection necrosis may result from direct injection of sclerosing agents, especially if excessive volumes are used. At least one fatal case of extensive esophageal necrosis and death has been reported. The drug should be administered by physicians who are familiar with an acceptable injection technique.
Patients in Child Class C are more likely to develop esophageal ulceration than those in Classes A and B. Complications of ulceration, necrosis, and delayed esophageal perforation appear to occur more frequently when ETHAMOLIN® (ethanolamine oleate) Injection is injected submucosally. This route is not recommended.
In patients with concomitant cardiorespiratory disease, careful monitoring and minimization of the total dose per session is recommended.
Fatal aspiration pneumonia has occurred in elderly patients undergoing esophageal variceal sclerotherapy with ETHAMOLIN Injection. This adverse event appears to be procedure-related rather than drug-related, but as aspiration of blood and/or stomach contents is not uncommon in patients with bleeding esophageal varices, special precautions should be taken to prevent its occurrence, especially in the elderly and critically ill subjects.
Pregnancy: ***(Teratogenic Effects: Pregnancy Category C)***: Animal reproduction studies have not been conducted with ETHAMOLIN® Injection. It is also not known whether ETHAMOLIN Injection can cause fetal harm when administered to a pregnant woman or can affect reproduction capacity. ETHAMOLIN Injection should be given to a pregnant woman only if clearly needed.
Nursing Mothers: It is not known whether this drug is excreted in human milk. Because many drugs are excreted in human milk, caution should be exercised when ETHAMOLIN Injection is administered to a nursing woman.
Pediatric Use: Safety and effectiveness in children have not been established.

ADVERSE REACTIONS

The reported frequency of complications/adverse events per injection session was 13%. The most common complications were pleural effusion/infiltration (2.1%), esophageal ulcer (2.1%), pyrexia (1.8%), retrosternal pain (1.6%), esophageal stricture (1.3%), and pneumonia (1.2%).
Other adverse local esophageal reactions have also been reported at rates of 0.1 to 0.4%, including esophagitis, tearing of the esophagus, sloughing of the mucosa overlying the injected varix, ulceration, stricture, necrosis, periesophageal abscess and perforation (see PRECAUTIONS). These complications appear to be dependent upon the dose and the patient's clinical state.
Bacteremia has been observed in patients following injection of esophageal varices with ETHAMOLIN®. Pyrexia and retrosternal pain are not infrequently observed during the post-injection period. Fatal aspiration pneumonia has occurred in patients with esophageal varices who underwent ETHAMOLIN Injection Sclerotherapy (see PRECAUTIONS). Anaphylactic shock and acute renal failure with spontaneous recovery have occurred (see PRECAUTIONS).
A case of disseminated intravascular coagulation has been reported.
Spinal cord paralysis due to occlusion of the anterior spinal artery has been reported in one child eight hours after ETHAMOLIN sclerotherapy.

OVERDOSAGE

Overdosage of ETHAMOLIN® Injection can result in severe intramural necrosis of the esophagus. Complications resulting from such overdosage have resulted in death.

DOSAGE AND ADMINISTRATION

Local ETHAMOLIN® Injection sclerotherapy of esophageal varices should be performed by physicians who are familiar with an acceptable technique. The usual intravenous dose is 1.5 to 5 mL per varix. The maximum dose per treatment session should not exceed 20 mL. Patients with significant liver dysfunction (Child Class C) or concomitant cardiopulmonary disease should usually receive less than the recommended maximum dose. Submucosal injections are not recommended as they are reported more likely to result in ulceration at the site of injection.
To obliterate the varix, injections may be made at the time of the acute bleeding episode and then after one week, six weeks, three months, and six months as indicated.
Note: Parenteral drug products should be inspected visually for particulate matter and discoloration before administration whenever solution and container permit.

HOW SUPPLIED

ETHAMOLIN® (ethanolamine oleate) Injection, 5% is available in 2 mL ampules in boxes of 10 (NDC 0021-4790-06).
Store at Controlled Room Temperature, 15°–30°C (59°–86°F). Protect from light.

CAUTION

Federal law prohibits dispensing without prescription.

FEDAHIST® GYROCAPS® ℞

[fed 'a-hist"]

DESCRIPTION

FEDAHIST® GYROCAPS® contain 65 mg pseudoephedrine hydrochloride USP and 10 mg chlorpheniramine maleate USP in an extended-release formulation designed for oral b.i.d. dosage.
Pseudoephedrine hydrochloride is a nasal decongestant. The empirical formula is $C_{10}H_{15}NO \cdot HCl$ and the molecular weight is 201.70. Chemically, it is benzenemethanol,α-[1-(methylamino)ethyl]- [S-(R*,R*)]-, hydrochloride.
Chlorpheniramine maleate is an antihistamine. The empirical formula is $C_{16}H_{19}ClN_2 \cdot C_4H_4O_4$ and the molecular weight is 390.87. Chemically, it is 2-[p-chloro-α-[2-(dimethylamino) ethyl]benzyl] pyridine maleate (1:1).
Each capsule also contains as inactive ingredients: D&C Yellow #10, FD&C Blue #1, FD&C Blue #2, FD&C Yellow #6, gelatin, pharmaceutical glaze, silicon dioxide, sodium lauryl sulfate, starch, sucrose, titanium dioxide, and other ingredients.

CLINICAL PHARMACOLOGY

Pseudoephedrine is an orally active sympathomimetic amine and exerts a decongestant action on the nasal mucosa. Pseudoephedrine produces peripheral effects similar to those of ephedrine and central effects similar to, but less intense than amphetamines. It has the potential for excitatory side effects. At the recommended oral dosages it has little or no pressor effect in normotensive adults. The serum half-life of pseudoephedrine is approximately 4 to 6 hours. The serum half-life is decreased with increased excretion of drug at urine pH lower than 6 and may be increased with decreased excretion at urine pH higher than 8.
Chlorpheniramine is an antihistamine that possesses anticholinergic and sedative effects. It is considered one of the most effective and least toxic of the histamine antagonists. Chlorpheniramine is a H_1 receptor antagonist. It antagonizes many of the pharmacologic actions of histamine. It prevents released histamine from dilating capillaries and causing edema of the respiratory mucosa. Chlorpheniramine is well absorbed and has a duration of action of 4 to 6 hours (the GYROCAPS formulation provides a continuous therapeutic effect for up to 12 hours). Its half-life in serum is 12-16 hours. Degradation products of chlorpheniramine's metabolic transformation by the liver are almost completely excreted in 24 hours.
FEDAHIST GYROCAPS release 65 mg pseudoephedrine and 10 mg chlorpheniramine at a controlled and predictable rate for 12 hours. Peak blood levels occur in 4 hours for pseudoephedrine and 6 hours for chlorpheniramine. The apparent plasma half-life is approximately 6 hours for pseudoephedrine and 16 hours for chlorpheniramine. The relative bioavailability of a related extended-release formulation is approximately 85% and 100% of the immediate-release dosage forms for pseudoephedrine and chlorpheniramine, respectively.

INDICATIONS AND USAGE

FEDAHIST GYROCAPS are indicated for the relief of nasal congestion and eustachian tube congestion associated with the common cold, sinusitis, and acute upper respiratory infections. FEDAHIST GYROCAPS are also indicated for symptomatic relief of perennial and seasonal allergic rhinitis and vasomotor rhinitis. Decongestants in combination with antihistamines have been used to relieve eustachian tube congestion associated with acute eustachian salpingitis, aerotitis, and serous otitis media.

CONTRAINDICATIONS

Sympathomimetic amines are contraindicated in patients with severe hypertension, severe coronary artery disease and in patients on MAO inhibitor therapy. Antihistamines are contraindicated in patients with narrow-angle glaucoma, urinary retention, peptic ulcer, during an asthmatic attack and in patients receiving MAO inhibitors.
Hypersensitivity: Contraindicated in patients with hypersensitivity or idiosyncrasy to sympathomimetic amines. FEDAHIST GYROCAPS are also contraindicated in patients hypersensitive to chlorpheniramine and other antihistamines of similar chemical structure.
Nursing Mothers: Contraindicated in nursing mothers because of the higher than usual risk for pediatric patients, from birth to two years of age, from sympathomimetic amines.
Newborn or Premature Infants: FEDAHIST GYROCAPS should not be administered to premature or full-term pediatric patients from birth to two years of age.

WARNINGS

Sympathomimetic amines should be used judiciously and sparingly in patients with hypertension, diabetes mellitus, ischemic heart disease, increased intraocular pressure, hyperthyroidism or prostatic hypertrophy (see **CONTRAINDICATIONS**). Sympathomimetics may produce CNS stimulation and convulsions or cardiovascular collapse with accompanying hypotension.
Chlorpheniramine maleate has an atropine-like action and should be used with caution in patients with increased intraocular pressure, cardiovascular disease, hypertension or in patients with a history of bronchial asthma (see **CONTRAINDICATIONS**). Antihistamines may cause excitability, especially in pediatric patients. Do not exceed recommended dosage because at higher doses nervousness, dizziness, or sleeplessness may occur.
Use in the Elderly: The elderly (60 years and older) are more likely to have adverse reactions to sympathomimetics. Overdosage of sympathomimetics in this age group may cause hallucinations, convulsions, central nervous system (CNS) depression and death.

PRECAUTIONS

General:
Should be used with caution in patients with diabetes, hypertension, cardiovascular disease and hyperreactivity to ephedrine. The antihistamine may cause drowsiness, therefore ambulatory patients who operate machinery or motor vehicles should be cautioned accordingly.
Information for Patients:
Antihistamines may impair mental and physical abilities required for the performance of potentially hazardous tasks, such as driving a vehicle or operating machinery, and may impair mental alertness in children.
Drug Interactions:
MAO inhibitors and beta adrenergic blockers increase the effect of sympathomimetics. Sympathomimetics may reduce the antihypertensive effects of methyldopa, mecamylamine, reserpine and veratrum alkaloids. Concomitant use of antihistamines with alcohol, tricyclic antidepressants, barbiturates and other CNS depressants may have an additive effect.
Laboratory Test Interactions:
Antihistamines may suppress the wheal and flare reactions to antigen skin testing. Considerable interindividual variation in the extent and duration of suppression have been reported, depending on the antigen and test technique, antihistamine and dosage regimen, time since the last dose and individual response to testing. In one study, usual oral dosages of chlorpheniramine suppressed the wheal response for about 2 days after the last dose. Whenever possible, antihistamines should be discontinued about 4 days prior to skin testing procedures since they may prevent otherwise positive reactions to dermal reactivity indicators.
Carcinogenesis, Mutagenesis, Impairment of Fertility:
No long-term or reproduction studies in animals have been performed with FEDAHIST GYROCAPS to evaluate its carcinogenic, mutagenic, and impairment of fertility potential.
Pregnancy—Pregnancy Category C:
Animal reproduction studies have not been conducted with FEDAHIST GYROCAPS. It is not known whether the GYROCAPS can cause fetal harm when administered to a pregnant woman or can affect reproduction capacity. FEDAHIST GYROCAPS may be given to a pregnant woman only if clearly needed.
Nursing Mothers:
Pseudoephedrine is contraindicated in nursing mothers because of the higher than usual risk for pediatric patients, from birth to two years of age, from sympathomimetic amines.

ADVERSE REACTIONS

Hyperreactive individuals may display ephedrine-like reactions such as tachycardia, palpitations, headache, dizziness or nausea. Patients sensitive to antihistamines may experience mild sedation.
Sympathomimetic drugs have been associated with certain untoward reactions including fear, anxiety, tenseness, restlessness, tremor, weakness, pallor, respiratory difficulty, dysuria, insomnia, hallucinations, convulsions, CNS depression, arrhythmias, and cardiovascular collapse with hypotension.
Possible side effects of antihistamines are drowsiness, restlessness, dizziness, weakness, dry mouth, anorexia, nausea, headache, nervousness, blurring of vision, heartburn, dysuria, and very rarely, dermatitis. Patient idiosyncrasy to adrenergic agents may be manifested by insomnia, dizziness, weakness, tremor or arrhythmias.

Continued on next page

Schwarz Pharma, Inc.—Cont.

OVERDOSAGE

Symptoms: Manifestations of antihistamine overdosage may vary from CNS depression (sedation, apnea, cardiovascular collapse) to stimulation (insomnia, hallucinations, tremors or convulsions). Other signs and symptoms may be dizziness, tinnitus, ataxia, blurred vision and hypotension. Stimulation is particularly likely in pediatric patients, as are atropine-like signs and symptoms (dry mouth, dilated pupils, flushing, hyperthermia, and gastrointestinal symptoms).

Treatment Recommendations: The patient should be induced to vomit even if emesis has occurred spontaneously; however, vomiting should not be induced in patients with impaired consciousness. Precautions against aspiration should be taken, especially in pediatric patients.

Ipecac Syrup is the preferred method for inducing vomiting. The action of ipecac is facilitated by physical activity and the administration of eight to twelve fluid ounces of water. If emesis does not occur in fifteen minutes, the dose of ipecac should be repeated. Following emesis, any drug remaining in the stomach may be absorbed by activated charcoal administered as a slurry with water.

If vomiting is unsuccessful or contraindicated, gastric lavage should be performed. Isotonic and one-half isotonic saline are the lavage solutions of choice. Saline cathartics, such as milk of magnesia, draw water into the bowel by osmosis and, therefore, may be valuable for their action of rapid dilution of bowel content.

Treatment of the signs and symptoms of overdosage is symptomatic and supportive. Vasopressors may be used to treat hypotension. Short-acting barbiturates, diazepam or paraldehyde may be administered to control seizures. Hyperpyrexia, especially in pediatric patients, may require treatment with tepid water sponge baths or a hypothermic blanket. Apnea is treated with ventilatory support. Stimulants (analeptic agents) should **not** be used.

The LD_{50} for pseudoephedrine is 202 mg/kg delivered intraperitoneally to rats. When given orally to mice, the LD_{50} for chlorpheniramine is 162 mg/kg.

DOSAGE AND ADMINISTRATION

Adults and pediatric patients 12 years of age and older: One CAPSULE every 12 hours not to exceed 2 CAPSULES in 24 hours. Not recommended for pediatric patients under 12 years of age.

HOW SUPPLIED

FEDAHIST GYROCAPS are white and yellow capsules containing white and green beadlets and imprinted with "KREMERS URBAN" AND "053".

    Bottles of 100 capsules   NDC 0091-1053-01

Store at controlled room temperature 15°–30°C (59°–86°F).

CAUTION

Federal law prohibits dispensing without prescription.

   Shown in Product Identification Guide, page 334

KUTRASE® Capsules
[qū 'trās]   ℞

DESCRIPTION

KUTRASE® Capsules contain four standardized digestive enzymes: lipase, amylase, protease, cellulase, and hyoscyamine sulfate USP and phenyltoloxamine citrate. Lipase, amylase, protease and cellulase are derived from fungal, plant and animal sources and are oral digestive enzyme supplements. Hyoscyamine sulfate USP is one of the principal anticholinergic/antispasmodic components of belladonna alkaloids. Phenyltoloxamine citrate is a non-barbiturate sedative. Each capsule contains:

lipase	1,200 USP Units
amylase	30 mg
protease	6 mg
cellulase	2 mg
hyoscyamine sulfate USP	0.0625 mg
phenyltoloxamine citrate	15 mg

Each capsule also contains as inactive ingredients: D&C Yellow #10, ethylcellulose, FD&C Green #3, FD&C Yellow #6, gelatin, lactose, magnesium stearate, titanium dioxide, vanillin and other ingredients.

CLINICAL PHARMACOLOGY

Diminution of secretions from exocrine glands is often a result of the normal aging process. KUTRASE provides a balanced combination of natural proteolytic, amylolytic, cellulolytic and lipolytic enzymes to enhance digestion of proteins, starch and fat in the gastrointestinal tract. These enzymes do not exert any systemic pharmacologic effects. KUTRASE should be considered an enzyme supplement and not an enzyme replacement therapy. Enzymes in KUTRASE are basically derived from fungal and plant sources and possess a broad spectrum of pH activity. Enzymes are promptly released from the capsule and are bioavailable for digestion of

food in the stomach and intestines. Hyoscyamine sulfate provides a potent spasmolytic effect in reducing gastrointestinal hypermotility and intestinal spasm. A mild sedative effect is provided by phenyltoloxamine citrate.

INDICATIONS AND USAGE

KUTRASE is indicated for the relief of the symptoms of functional indigestion devoid of organic pathology commonly referred to as nervous indigestion and colloquially as "butterflies". The symptoms are bloating, gas, and fullness.

CONTRAINDICATIONS

Glaucoma, obstructive uropathy, obstructive disease of the gastrointestinal tract (as in achalasia, pyloroduodenal stenosis); paralytic ileus, intestinal atony of the elderly or debilitated patients; unstable cardiovascular status in acute hemorrhage; severe ulcerative colitis; toxic megacolon complicating ulcerative colitis; myasthenia gravis, or a hypersensitivity to any of the ingredients.

WARNINGS

Do not administer to patients who are allergic to pork products. In the presence of high environmental temperature, heat prostration can occur with drug use (fever and heat stroke due to decreased sweating). Diarrhea may be an early symptom of incomplete intestinal obstruction, especially in patients with ileostomy or colostomy. In this instance, treatment with this drug would be inappropriate. KUTRASE may produce drowsiness or blurred vision. In this event, the patient should be warned not to engage in activities requiring mental alertness such as operating a motor vehicle or other machinery or to perform hazardous work while taking this drug.

PRECAUTIONS

General:

Use with caution in patients with autonomic neuropathy, hyperthyroidism, coronary heart disease, congestive heart failure, cardiac arrhythmias, and hypertension. Investigate any tachycardia before giving any anticholinergic drug since they may increase the heart rate. Use with caution in patients with hiatal hernia associated with reflux esophagitis.

Information for Patients:

If capsules are opened, avoid inhalation of the powder. Sensitive individuals may experience allergic reactions.

Carcinogenesis, Mutagenesis, Impairment of Fertility:

Long-term studies in animals have not been performed to evaluate the carcinogenic, mutagenic or impairment of fertility potential of KUTRASE.

Pregnancy-Pregnancy Category C:

Animal reproduction studies have not been conducted with KUTRASE. It is also not known whether KUTRASE can cause fetal harm when administered to a pregnant woman or can affect reproduction capacity. KUTRASE should be given to a pregnant woman only if clearly needed.

Nursing Mothers:

Hyoscyamine sulfate is excreted in human milk. It is not known whether the enzymes or phenyltoloxamine citrate are excreted in human milk. Caution should be exercised when KUTRASE is administered to a nursing woman.

ADVERSE REACTIONS

Occasionally a slight looseness of the stools may be noticed. If so, dosage should be reduced. Finely powdered pancreatic enzyme may be irritating to the mucous membranes and respiratory tract. Inhalation of the airborne powder may precipitate an asthma attack in sensitive individuals. Other adverse reactions may include dryness of the mouth; urinary hesitancy and retention; blurred vision; tachycardia; palpitations; mydriasis; cycloplegia; increased ocular tension; headache; nervousness; drowsiness; weakness; suppression of lactation; allergic reactions or drug idiosyncrasies; urticaria and other dermal manifestations and decreased sweating.

OVERDOSAGE

The signs and symptoms of overdose are headache, nausea, vomiting, blurred vision, dilated pupils, hot dry skin, dizziness, dryness of the mouth, difficulty in swallowing. Measures to be taken are immediate lavage of the stomach and injection of physostigmine 0.5 to 2 mg intravenously and repeated as necessary up to a total of 5 mg. Fever may be treated symptomatically. Excitement to a degree which demands attention may be managed with sodium thiopental 2% solution given slowly intravenously. In the event of paralysis of the respiratory muscles, artificial respiration should be instituted.

DOSAGE AND ADMINISTRATION

1 or 2 capsules taken with each meal or snack. Dosage may be adjusted according to the conditions and severity of symptoms to assure symptomatic control with a minimum of adverse effects.

HOW SUPPLIED

KUTRASE Capsules are green and white capsules and are imprinted "SCHWARZ" and "475."

    Bottles of 100 capsules   NDC 0091-3475-01

Store at controlled room temperature 15°–30°C (59°–86°F). Protect from high humidity.

CAUTION

Federal law prohibits dispensing without prescription.

   Shown in Product Identification Guide, page 334

KU-ZYME® Capsules
[qū ' zīm]   ℞

DESCRIPTION

KU-ZYME® Capsules contain four standardized enzymes: lipase, amylase, protease and cellulase. They are derived from fungal, plant and animal sources and are designed for oral digestive enzyme supplement therapy.

Each capsule contains:

lipase	1,200 USP Units
amylase	30 mg
protease	6 mg
cellulase	2 mg

Each capsule also contains as inactive ingredients: D&C Yellow #10, FD&C Yellow #6, gelatin, lactose, magnesium stearate, synthetic red iron oxide, titanium dioxide, and vanillin.

CLINICAL PHARMACOLOGY

Diminution of secretions from exocrine glands is often a result of the normal aging process. KU-ZYME provides a balanced combination of natural proteolytic, amylolytic, cellulolytic and lipolytic enzymes to enhance digestion of proteins, starch and fat in the gastrointestinal tract. These enzymes do not exert any systemic pharmacologic effects. KU-ZYME should be considered an enzyme supplement and not an enzyme replacement therapy. Enzymes in KU-ZYME are basically derived from fungal and plant sources and possess a broad spectrum of pH activity. Enzymes are promptly released from the capsule and are bioavailable for digestion of food in the stomach and intestines.

INDICATIONS AND USAGE

For the relief of functional indigestion when due to enzyme deficiency or imbalance. KU-ZYME relieves symptoms due to faulty digestion including the sensation of fullness after meals, dyspepsia, flatulence, abdominal distention and intolerance to certain foods.

CONTRAINDICATIONS

There are no known contraindications to the administration of digestive enzymes. These enzymes do not attack living tissues and do not present any danger to the patient with ulceration or inflammation in the digestive tract.

WARNINGS

Do not administer to patients who are allergic to pork products.

PRECAUTIONS

Information for Patients:

If capsules are opened, avoid inhalation of the powder. Sensitive individuals may experience allergic reactions.

Carcinogenesis, Mutagenesis, Impairment of Fertility:

Long-term studies in animals have not been performed to evaluate carcinogenic, mutagenic or impairment of fertility potential of KU-ZYME.

Pregnancy-Pregnancy Category C:

Animal reproduction studies have not been conducted with KU-ZYME. It is also not known whether KU-ZYME can cause fetal harm when administered to a pregnant woman or can affect reproduction capacity. KU-ZYME should be given to a pregnant woman only if clearly needed.

Nursing Mothers:

It is not known whether KU-ZYME is excreted in human milk. Because many drugs are excreted in human milk, caution should be exercised when KU-ZYME is administered to a nursing woman.

ADVERSE REACTIONS

Virtually unknown. Occasionally, a slight looseness of stools may be noticed. If so, dosage should be reduced. Finely powdered pancreatic enzyme may be irritating to the mucous membranes and respiratory tract. Inhalation of the airborne powder may precipitate an asthma attack in sensitive individuals.

OVERDOSAGE

No systemic toxicity occurs. Excessive dosage may, however, produce a laxative effect.

DOSAGE AND ADMINISTRATION

1 or 2 capsules taken with each meal or snack. Dosage may be adjusted depending on individual requirements for relief of symptoms due to digestive enzyme deficiency. In patients who experience difficulty in swallowing the capsule, it may be opened and the contents sprinkled on the food. When opening the capsules, avoid inhalation of the powder (see PRECAUTIONS and ADVERSE REACTIONS).

HOW SUPPLIED

KU-ZYME Capsules are yellow and white capsules and are imprinted "SCHWARZ" and "522".

Bottles of 100 capsules NDC 0091-3522-01

Store at controlled room temperature 15°–30°C (59°–86°F). Protect from high humidity.

CAUTION

Federal law prohibits dispensing without prescription.

Shown in Product Identification Guide, page 334

KU-ZYME® HP Capsules ℞

[*qū' zīm*]

(pancrelipase capsules USP)

DESCRIPTION

KU-ZYME® HP Capsules (pancrelipase capsules USP) contain standardized lipase, amylase and protease obtained from hog pancreas and are designed for oral digestive enzyme replacement therapy. Each capsule contains:

lipase	8,000 USP Units
protease	30,000 USP Units
amylase	30,000 USP Units

Each capsule also contains as inactive ingredients: gelatin, lactose, magnesium stearate, titanium dioxide and other ingredients.

CLINICAL PHARMACOLOGY

Pancrelipase USP is a pancreatic enzyme concentrate, which hydrolyzes fats to glycerol and fatty acids, changes protein into proteoses and derived substances, and converts starch into dextrins and sugars. The administration of pancrelipase reduces the fat and nitrogen content in the stool. Pancreatic enzymes are normally secreted in great excess. Generally, steatorrhea and malabsorption occur only after a 90 percent or greater reduction in secretion of lipase and proteolytic enzymes. It has been estimated that approximately 8,000 units of lipase per hour should be delivered into the duodenum postprandially. Even if all the enzymes taken orally reached the proximal intestine in active form, ingestion of 24,000 units of lipase (8,000 units per hour) for 3 postprandial hours would be required. If one could deliver sufficient pancreatic enzymes to the small intestine, malabsorption could be corrected. It is rarely possible to achieve complete relief of steatorrhea although major improvement in fat absorption can be achieved in most patients.

INDICATIONS

KU-ZYME HP is effective in patients with deficient exocrine pancreatic secretions. Thus, KU-ZYME HP may be used as enzyme replacement therapy in cystic fibrosis, chronic pancreatitis, post pancreatectomy, in ductal obstructions caused by cancer of the pancreas, pancreatic insufficiency and for steatorrhea of malabsorption syndrome and post gastrectomy (Billroth II and Total). May also be used as a presumptive test for pancreatic function, especially in pancreatic insufficiency due to chronic pancreatitis.

CONTRAINDICATIONS

There are no known contraindications for the use of pancrelipase although sensitivity to pork protein may preclude its use.

WARNINGS

Pancreatic exocrine replacement therapy should not delay or supplant treatment of the primary disorder. Use with caution in patients known to be hypersensitive to pork or enzymes.

PRECAUTIONS

Information for Patients:

If capsules are opened, avoid inhalation of the powder. Sensitive individuals may experience allergic reactions.

Drug Interactions:

The serum iron response to oral iron may be decreased by concomitant administration of pancreatic extracts.

Carcinogenesis, Mutagenesis, and Impairment of Fertility:

Long-term studies in animals have not been performed to evaluate the carcinogenic, mutagenic or impairment of fertility potential of KU-ZYME HP.

Pregnancy-Pregnancy Category C:

Animal reproduction studies have not been conducted with KU-ZYME HP. It is also not known whether KU-ZYME HP can cause fetal harm when administered to a pregnant woman or can affect reproduction capacity. KU-ZYME HP should be given to a pregnant woman only if clearly needed.

Nursing Mothers:

It is not known whether KU-ZYME HP is excreted in human milk. Because many drugs are excreted in human milk, caution should be exercised when KU-ZYME HP is administered to a nursing woman.

ADVERSE REACTIONS

High doses may cause nausea, abdominal cramps and/or diarrhea in certain patients. Finely powdered pancreatic enzyme concentrate may be irritating to the mucous membranes and respiratory tract. Inhalation of the airborne powder may precipitate an asthma attack in sensitive individuals. Extremely high doses of exogenous pancreatic enzymes have been associated with hyperuricemia and hyperuricosuria.

DOSAGE AND ADMINISTRATION

1 to 3 capsules taken with each meal or snack. Dosage may be adjusted depending on individual requirements for control of steatorrhea. In severe deficiencies the dose may be increased to 8 capsules with meals or the frequency of administration may increase to hourly intervals if nausea, cramps and/or diarrhea do not occur.

HOW SUPPLIED

KU-ZYME® HP Capsules (pancrelipase capsules USP) are white opaque capsules and are imprinted "SCHWARZ" and "525."

Bottles of 100 capsules NDC 0091-3525-01

Store at a temperature not exceeding 25°C (77°F).

Protect from high humidity.

CAUTION

Federal law prohibits dispensing without prescription.

Shown in Product Identification Guide, page 334

LEVATOL® ℞

[*lev 'a-tol*]

(penbutolol sulfate) 20 mg

TABLETS

DESCRIPTION

Levatol® (penbutolol sulfate) is a synthetic β-receptor antagonist for oral administration. The chemical name of penbutolol sulfate is (S)-1-tert-butylamino-3-(o-cyclopentylphenoxy)-2-propanol sulfate. It is provided as the levorotatory isomer. The empirical formula for penbutolol sulfate is $C_{36}H_{60}N_2O_8S$. Its molecular weight is 680.94. A dose of 20 mg is equivalent to 29.4 μmol. The structural formula is as follows:

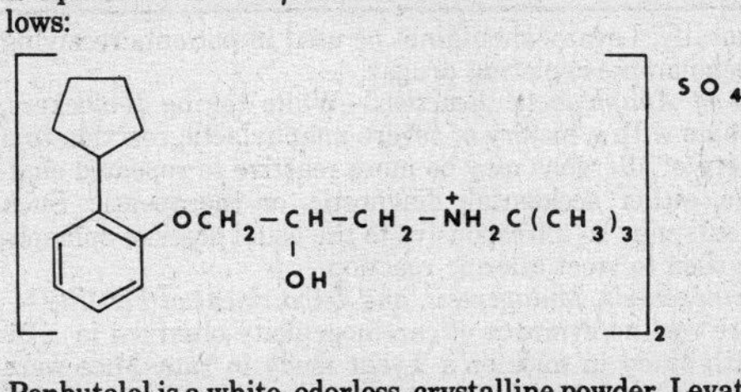
SO4--
OCH2-CH-CH2-NH2C(CH3)3
OH
2

Penbutolol is a white, odorless, crystalline powder. Levatol is available as tablets for oral administration. Each tablet contains 20 mg of penbutolol sulfate. It also contains corn starch, D&C Yellow No. 10, lactose, magnesium stearate, povidone, silicon dioxide, talc, titanium dioxide, and other inactive ingredients.

CLINICAL PHARMACOLOGY

Penbutolol is a β-1, β-2 (nonselective) adrenergic receptor antagonist. Experimental studies showed a dose-dependent increase in heart rate in reserpinized (norepinephrine-depleted) rats given penbutolol intravenously at doses of 0.25 to 1.0 mg/kg, suggesting that penbutolol has some intrinsic sympathomimetic activity. In human studies, however, heart rate decreases have been similar to those seen with propranolol.

Penbutolol antagonizes the heart rate effects of exercise and infused isoproterenol. The β-blocking potency of penbutolol is approximately 4 times that of propranolol. An oral dose of less than 10 mg will reduce exercise-induced tachycardia to one-half its usual level; maximum antagonism follows doses of 10 to 20 mg. The peak effect is between 1.5 and 3 hours after oral administration. The duration of effect exceeds 20 hours during a once-daily dosing regimen. During chronic administration of penbutolol, the duration of antihypertensive effects permits a once-daily dosage schedule.

Acute hemodynamic effects of penbutolol have been studied following single intravenous doses between 0.1 and 4 mg. The cardiovascular responses included significant reductions in heart rate, left ventricular maximum dP/dt, cardiac output, stroke volume index, stroke work, and stroke work index. Systolic pressure and mean arterial pressure were reduced, and total peripheral resistance was increased.

Chronic administration of penbutolol to hypertensive patients results in the hemodynamic pattern typical of β-adrenergic blocking drugs: a reduction in cardiac index, heart rate, systolic and diastolic blood pressures, and the product of heart rate and mean arterial pressure both at rest and with all levels of exercise, without significant change in total peripheral resistance. Penbutolol causes a reduction in left ventricular contractility. Penbutolol decreases glomerular filtration rate, but not significantly.

Clinical trial doses of 10 to 80 mg per day in single daily doses have reduced supine and standing systolic and diastolic blood pressures. In most studies, effects were small, generally a change in blood pressure 5 to 8/3 to 5 mm Hg greater than seen with a placebo measured 24 hours after dosing. It is not clear whether this relatively small effect reflects a characteristic of penbutolol or the particular population studied (the population had relatively mild hypertension but did not appear unusual in others respects). In a direct comparison of penbutolol with adequate doses of twice daily propranolol, no difference in blood pressure effect was seen. In a comparison of placebo and 10-, 20- and 40-mg single daily doses of penbutolol, no significant dose-related difference was seen in response to active drug at 6 weeks, but compared to the 10-mg dose, the two larger doses showed greater effects at 2 and 4 weeks and reached their maximum effect at 2 weeks. In several studies, dose increases from 40 to 80 mg were without additional effect on blood pressure. Response rates to penbutolol are unaffected by sex or age but are greater in caucasians than blacks.

Penbutolol decreases plasma renin activity in normal subjects and in patients with essential and renovascular hypertension. The mechanisms of the antihypertensive actions of β-receptor antagonists have not been established. However, factors that may be involved are: (1) competitive antagonism of catecholamines at peripheral adrenergic receptor sites (especially cardiac) that leads to decreased cardiac output; (2) a central-nervous-system (CNS) action that results in a decrease in tonic sympathetic neural outflow to the periphery; and (3) a reduction of renin secretion through blockade of β-receptors involved in release of renin from the kidneys.

Penbutolol dose dependently increases the RR and QT intervals. There is no influence on the PR, QRS or QT c (corrected) intervals.

Pharmacokinetics—Following oral administration, penbutolol is rapidly and completely absorbed. Peak plasma concentrations of penbutolol occur between 2 and 3 hours after oral administration and are proportional to single and multiple doses between 10 and 40 mg once a day. The average plasma elimination half-life of penbutolol is approximately 5 hours in normal subjects. There is no significant difference in the plasma half-life of penbutolol in healthy elderly persons or patients on renal dialysis. Twelve to 24 hours after oral administration of doses up to 120 mg, plasma concentrations of parent drug are 0% to 10% of the peak level. No accumulation of penbutolol is observed in hypertensive patients after 8 days of therapy at doses of 40 mg daily or 20 mg twice a day. Penbutolol is approximately 80% to 98% bound to plasma proteins.

The metabolism of penbutolol in humans involves conjugation and oxidation. The metabolites are excreted principally in the urine. When radiolabeled penbutolol was administered to humans, approximately 90% of the radioactivity was excreted in the urine. Approximately 1/6 of the dose of penbutolol was recovered as penbutolol conjugate, while the remaining fraction was not identified. Conjugated penbutolol has a plasma elimination half-life of approximately 20 hours in healthy persons, 25 hours in healthy elderly persons and 100 hours in patients on renal dialysis. Thus, accumulation of penbutolol conjugate may be expected upon multiple-dosing in renal insufficiency. An oxidative metabolite of penbutolol, 4-hydroxy penbutolol, has been identified in small quantities in plasma and urine. It is 1/8 to 1/15 times as active as the parent compound in blocking isoproterenol-induced β-adrenergic receptor responses in isolated guinea-pig trachea and is 1/8 to 1 times as potent in anesthetized dogs.

INDICATIONS AND USAGE

Levatol is indicated in the treatment of mild to moderate arterial hypertension. It may be used alone or in combination with other antihypertensive agents, especially thiazide-type diuretics.

CONTRAINDICATIONS

Levatol is contraindicated in patients with cardiogenic shock, sinus bradycardia, second and third degree atrioventricular conduction block, bronchial asthma, and those with known hypersensitivity to this product (*see* WARNINGS).

WARNINGS

Cardiac Failure—Sympathetic stimulation may be essential for supporting circulatory function in patients with heart failure, and its inhibition by β-adrenergic receptor blockade may precipitate more severe failure. Although β-blockers should be avoided in overt congestive heart failure, Levatol can, if necessary, be used with caution in patients with a history of cardiac failure who are well compensated, on treatment with vasodilators, digitalis and/or diuretics. Both digitalis and penbutolol slow AV conduction. Beta-adrenergic receptor antagonists do not inhibit the inotropic action of digitalis on heart muscle. If cardiac failure persists, treatment with Levatol should be discontinued.

Patients Without History of Cardiac Failure—Continued depression of the myocardium with β-blocking agents over a period of time can, in some cases, lead to cardiac failure. At the first evidence of heart failure, patients receiving Levatol

Continued on next page

Schwarz Pharma, Inc.—Cont.

should be given appropriate treatment, and the response should be closely observed. If cardiac failure continues despite adequate intervention with appropriate drugs, Levatol should be withdrawn (gradually, if possible).

Exacerbation of Ischemic Heart Disease Following Abrupt Withdrawal —Hypersensitivity to catecholamines has been observed in patients who were withdrawn from therapy with β-blocking agents; exacerbation of angina, and, in some cases, myocardial infarction have occurred after abrupt discontinuation of such therapy. When discontinuing Levatol, particularly in patients with ischemic heart disease, the dosage should be reduced gradually over a period of 1 to 2 weeks and the patient should be monitored carefully. If angina becomes more pronounced or acute coronary insufficiency develops, administration of Levatol should be reinstated promptly, at least on a temporary basis, and appropriate measures should be taken for the management of unstable angina. Patients should be warned against interruption or discontinuation of therapy without the physician's advice. Because coronary artery disease is common and may not be recognized, it may not be prudent to discontinue Levatol abruptly, even in patients who are being treated only for hypertension.

Nonallergic Bronchospasm (e.g., chronic bronchitis, emphysema) —Levatol is contraindicated in bronchial asthma. In general, patients with bronchospastic diseases should not receive β-blockers. Levatol should be administered with caution because it may block bronchodilation produced by endogenous catecholamine stimulation of β-2 receptors.

Anesthesia and Major Surgery —The necessity, or desirability, of withdrawal of a β-blocking therapy prior to major surgery is controversial. Beta-adrenergic receptor blockade impairs the ability of the heart to respond to β-adrenergically mediated reflex stimuli. Although this might be of benefit in preventing arrhythmic response, the risk of excessive myocardial depression during general anesthesia may be enhanced and difficulty in restarting and maintaining the heart beat has been reported with β-blockers. If treatment is continued, particular care should be taken when using anesthetic agents that depress the myocardium, such as ether, cyclopropane, and trichloroethylene, and it is prudent to use the lowest possible dose of Levatol. Levatol like other β-blockers, is a competitive inhibitor of β-receptor agonists, and its effect on the heart can be reversed by cautious administration of such agents (e.g., dobutamine or isoproterenol—see Overdose). Manifestations of excessive vagal tone (e.g., profound bradycardia, hypotension) may be corrected with atropine 1 to 3 mg IV in divided doses.

Diabetes Mellitus and Hypoglycemia —Beta-adrenergic receptor blockade may prevent the appearance of signs and symptoms of acute hypoglycemia, such as tachycardia and blood pressure changes. This is especially important in patients with labile diabetes. Beta-blockade also reduces the release of insulin in response to hyperglycemia; therefore, it may be necessary to adjust the dose of hypoglycemic drugs. Beta-adrenergic blockade may also impair the homeostatic response to hypoglycemia; in that event, the spontaneous recovery from hypoglycemia may be delayed during treatment with β-adrenergic receptor antagonists.

Thyrotoxicosis —Beta-adrenergic blockade may mask certain clinical signs (e.g., tachycardia) of hyperthyrodism. Patients suspected of developing thyrotoxicosis should be managed carefully to avoid abrupt withdrawal of β-adrenergic receptor blockers that might precipitate a thyroid storm.

PRECAUTIONS

Information for Patients —Patients, especially those with evidence of coronary artery insufficiency, should be warned against interruption or discontinuation of Levatol without the physician's advice. Although cardiac failure rarely occurs in properly selected patients, those being treated with β-adrenergic receptor antagonists should be advised of the symptoms of heart failure and to report such symptoms immediately, should they develop.

Drug Interactions —Levatol has been used in combination with hydrochlorothiazide in at least 100 patients without unexpected adverse reactions.

In one study, the combination of penbutolol and alcohol increased the number of errors in the eye-hand psychomotor function test.

Penbutolol increases the volume of distribution of lidocaine in normal subjects. This could result in a requirement for higher loading doses of lidocaine.

Cimetidine has no effect on the clearance of penbutolol. The major metabolite of penbutolol is a glucuronide, and it has been shown that cimetidine does not inhibit glucoronidation.

Synergistic hypotensive effects, bradycardia, and arrhythmias have been reported in some patients receiving β-adrenergic blocking agents when an oral calcium antagonist was added to the treatment regimen.

Generally, Levatol should not be used in patients receiving catecholamine-depleting drugs.

Risk of Anaphylactic Reaction —While taking β-blockers, patients with a history of severe anaphylactic reaction to a variety of allergens may be more reactive to repeated challenge, either accidental, diagnostic, or therapeutic. Such patients may be unresponsive to the usual doses of epinephrine used to treat allergic reaction.

Carcinogenesis, Mutagenesis, and Impairment of Fertility — There was no evidence of carcinogenicity observed in a 21-month study in mice or a 2-year study in rats. Mice were given penbutolol in the diet for 18 months at doses up to 395 mg/kg/day (about 500 times the Maximum Recommended Human Dose (MRHD) of 40 mg in a 50 kg person). Rats were given 141 mg/kg/ day for the same length of time. Mice were observed for 3 months and rats for 5.5 to 7 months after termination of treatment before necropsy was performed.

No evidence of mutagenic activity of penbutolol was seen in the *Salmonella* mutagenicity test (Ames test), the point mutation induction test (*Saccharomyces*) and the micronucleus test.

Penbutolol had no adverse effects on fertility or general reproductive performance in mice and rats at oral doses up to 172 mg/kg/day.

Pregnancy —Teratogenic Effects: Pregnancy Category C —Teratology studies in rats and rabbits revealed no teratogenic effects related to treatment with penbutolol at oral doses up to 200 mg/kg/day (250 times the MRHD). In rabbits, a slight increase in the intrauterine fetal mortality and a reduced 24-hour offspring survival rate were observed in the groups treated with 125 mg/kg/day (156 times the MRHD) but not in the groups treated with 0.2 and 5 mg (0.25 to 6 times the MRHD).

There are no adequate and well-controlled studies in pregnant women. Levatol should be used during pregnancy only if the potential benefit justifies the potential risk to the fetus.

Nonteratogenic Effects —In a perinatal and postnatal study in rats, the pup body weight and pup survival rate were reduced at the highest dose level of 160 mg/kg/day (200 times the MRHD).

Nursing Mothers —It is not known whether Levatol is excreted in human milk. Because many drugs are excreted in human milk, caution should be exercised when Levatol is administered to a nursing woman.

Pediatric Use —Safety and effectiveness of Levatol in pediatric patients have not been established.

ADVERSE REACTIONS

Levatol is usually well tolerated in properly selected patients. Most adverse effects observed during clinical trials have been mild and reversible.

Table 1.
ADVERSE REACTIONS DURING CONTROLLED U.S. STUDIES

Body System Experience	Penbutolol (N = 628) %	Placebo (N = 212) %	Propranolol (N = 266) %
Body as a Whole			
Asthenia	1.6	0.9	4.9
Pain, chest	2.4	2.8	2.3
Pain, limb	2.4	1.4	1.5
Digestive System			
Diarrhea	3.3	1.9	2.6
Nausea	4.3	0.9	2.3
Dyspepsia	2.7	1.4	5.3
Nervous System			
Dizziness	4.9	2.4	4.2
Fatigue	4.4	1.9	2.6
Headache	7.8	6.1	7.5
Insomnia	1.9	0.9	2.6
Respiratory System			
Cough	2.1	0.5	1.1
Dyspnea	2.1	1.4	3.4
Upper respiratory infection	2.5	3.3	4.9
Skin and Appendages			
Sweating, excessive	1.6	0.5	2.3
Urogenital System			
Impotence, sexual	0.5	0.0	0.8

Table 2.
DISCONTINUATIONS DURING CONTROLLED U.S. STUDIES

Body System Experience	Penbutolol (N = 628) %	Placebo (N = 212) %	Propranolol (N = 266) %
Body as a Whole			
Asthenia	0.6	0.0	0.4
Pain, chest	0.6	1.4	0.4
Digestive System			
Nausea	0.8	0.0	0.8
Nervous System			
Depression	0.6	0.5	0.8
Dizziness	0.6	0.0	0.4
Fatigue	0.5	0.5	0.0
Headache	0.6	0.5	0.4

Table 1 lists the adverse reactions reported from 4 controlled studies conducted in the United States involving once-a-day administration of Levatol (at doses ranging from 10 to 120 mg) as monotherapy or in combination with hydrochlorothiazide. Levatol doses above 40 mg/day are not, however, recommended. The table includes only those events where the prevalence rate in the Levatol group was at least 1.5%, or where the reaction is of particular interest.

Over a dose range from 10 to 40 mg, once a day, fatigue, nausea, and sexual impotence occurred at a greater frequency as the dose was increased.

[See Table 1 above.]

In a double-blind clinical trial comparing Levatol (40 mg and greater once a day) and propranolol (40 mg or more twice a day), heart rates of less than 60 beats/min were recorded at least once in 25% of the patients in the group receiving Levatol and in 37% of the patients in the propranolol group. Corresponding figures for heart rates of less than 50 beats/min were 1.2% and 6%, respectively. No symptoms associated with bradycardia were reported.

Discontinuations of Levatol because of adverse reactions have ranged between 2.4% and 6.9% of patients in double-blind, parallel, controlled clinical trials, as compared to 1.8% to 4.1% in the corresponding control groups that were given placebo. The frequency and severity of adverse reactions have not increased during long-term administration of Levatol. The prevalence of adverse reactions reported from 4 controlled clinical trials (referred to in Table 1) as reasons for discontinuation of therapy by ≥ 0.5% of the Levatol group is listed in Table 2.

[See Table 2 above.]

Potential Adverse Effects —In addition, certain adverse effects not listed above have been reported with other β-blocking agents and should also be considered as potential adverse effects of Levatol.

Central Nervous System —Reversible mental depression progressing to catatonia (an acute syndrome characterized by disorientation for time and place), short-term memory loss, emotional lability, slightly clouded sensorium, and decreased performance (neuropsychometrics).

Cardiovascular —Intensification of AV block (see CONTRAINDICATIONS).

Allergic —Erythematous rash, fever combined with aching and sore throat, laryngospasm, and respiratory distress.

Hematologic —Agranulocytosis, nonthrombocytopenic, and thrombocytopenic purpura.

Gastrointestinal —Mesenteric arterial thrombosis and ischemic colitis.

Miscellaneous —Reversible alopecia and Peyronie's disease. The oculomucocutaneous syndrome associated with the β-blocker practolol has not been reported with Levatol during investigational use and extensive foreign clinical experience.

OVERDOSAGE

There is no actual experience with Levatol overdose. The signs and symptoms that would be expected with overdosage of β-adrenergic receptor antagonists are symptomatic bradycardia, hypotension, bronchospasm, and acute cardiac failure. In addition to discontinuation of Levatol, gastric emptying, and close observation of the patient, the following measures might be considered as appropriate:

Excessive Bradycardia —Administer atropine sulfate to induce vagal blockade. If bradycardia persists, intravenous isoproterenol hydrochloride may be administered cautiously; larger than usual doses may be needed. In refractory cases, the use of a transvenous cardiac pacemaker may be necessary.

Hypotension —Sympathomimetic drug therapy, such as dopamine, dobutamine, or levarterenol, may be considered if hypotension persists despite correction of bradycardia. In refractory cases, administration of glucagon hydrochloride has been reported to be useful.

Bronchospasm —A β-2-agonist or isoproterenol hydrochloride may be administered. Additional therapy with aminophylline may be considered.

Acute Cardiac Failure —Institute conventional therapy immediately. Intravenous administration of dobutamine and glucagon hydrochloride has been reported to be useful.

Heart Block (Second or Third Degree) —Isoproterenol hydrochloride or a transvenous cardiac pacemaker may be used.

DOSAGE AND ADMINISTRATION

The usual starting and maintenance dose of Levatol used alone or in combination with other antihypertensive agents, such as thiazide-type diuretics, is 20 mg given once daily. Doses of 40 mg and 80 mg have been well-tolerated but have not been shown to give a greater antihypertensive effect. The full effect of a 20- or 40-mg dose is seen by the end of 2 weeks. A dose of 10 mg also lowers blood pressure, but the full effect is not seen for 4 to 6 weeks.

HOW SUPPLIED

Levatol® (penbutolol sulfate) 20 mg tablets are yellow, scored, capsule-shaped and engraved "RC22".
Bottles of 100   NDC 0091-4500-15
Store at controlled room temperature 15°–30°C (59°–86°F). Keep tightly closed and protect from light.

CAUTION

Federal law prohibits dispensing without prescription.

ANIMAL TOXICOLOGY

Studies in rats indicated that the combination of penbutolol, triamterene, and hydrochlorothiazide (up to 40, 50 and 25 mg/kg, respectively) increased the incidence and severity of renal tubular dilation and regeneration when compared to that in rats treated only with triamterene and hydrochlorothiazide. Dogs administered the same doses of triamterene and hydrochlorothiazide alone and in combination with penbutolol had an increase in serum alkaline phosphatase and serum alanine transferase, but there were no gross or microscopic abnormalities observed. No significant toxicologic findings were observed in rats and dogs treated with a combination of penbutolol and hydrochlorothiazide.

Shown in Product Identification Guide, page 334

LEVSIN® PRODUCTS   ℞
[lev'sin]
(hyoscyamine sulfate USP)
LEVBID™ Extended-Release Tablets
LEVSIN®/SL Tablets
LEVSIN® Tablets
LEVSIN® Elixir
LEVSIN® Drops (Oral Solution)
LEVSIN® Injection
LEVSINEX™ TIMECAPS™

DESCRIPTION

LEVSIN® (hyoscyamine sulfate USP) is one of the principal anticholinergic/antispasmodic components of belladonna alkaloids. The empirical formula is $(C_{17}H_{23}NO_3)_2 \cdot H_2SO_4 \cdot 2H_2O$ and the molecular weight is 712.85. Chemically, it is benzeneacetic acid, α-(hydroxymethyl)-,8-methyl-8-azabicyclo [3.2.1.] oct-3-yl ester, [3(S)-endo]-, sulfate (2:1), dihydrate.

LEVBID Extended-Release Tablets contain 0.375 mg of hyoscyamine sulfate in a formulation designed for oral b.i.d. dosage. Each LEVBID Extended-Release Tablet also contains as inactive ingredients: lactose, magnesium stearate, FD&C yellow #6 and other ingredients.

LEVSIN/SL Tablets contain 0.125 mg hyoscyamine sulfate formulated for sublingual administration. However, the tablets may also be chewed or taken orally. Each tablet also contains as inactive ingredients: colloidal silicon dioxide, dextrates, FD&C Green #3, flavor, mannitol, and stearic acid.

LEVSIN Tablets contain 0.125 mg hyoscyamine sulfate formulated for oral administration. Each tablet also contains as inactive ingredients: acacia, confectioner's sugar, corn starch, lactose, powdered cellulose and stearic acid.

LEVSIN Elixir contains 0.125 mg hyoscyamine sulfate per 5 mL (teaspoonful) with 20% alcohol for oral administration. LEVSIN Elixir also contains as inactive ingredients: FD&C Red #40, FD&C Yellow #6, flavor, glycerin, purified water, sorbitol solution and sucrose.

LEVSIN Drops, contain 0.125 mg hyoscyamine sulfate per mL with 5% alcohol for oral administration. LEVSIN Drops also contain as inactive ingredients: FD&C Red #40, FD&C Yellow #6, flavor, glycerin, purified water, sodium citrate, sorbitol solution, and sucrose.

LEVSIN Injection is a sterile solution containing 0.5 mg hyoscyamine sulfate per mL. The 1 mL ampuls contain as inactive ingredients: water for injection, pH is adjusted with hydrochloric acid when necessary.

LEVSINEX TIMECAPS contain 0.375 mg hyoscyamine sulfate in an extended-release formulation designed for oral b.i.d. dosage. Each capsule also contains as inactive ingredients: corn starch, D&C Red #28, FD&C Blue #1, FD&C Blue #2, FD&C Red #40, FD&C Yellow #6, gelatin, sucrose, titanium dioxide and other ingredients.

CLINICAL PHARMACOLOGY

LEVSIN inhibits specifically the actions of acetylcholine on structures innervated by postganglionic cholinergic nerves and on smooth muscles that respond to acetylcholine but lack cholinergic innervation. These peripheral cholinergic receptors are present in the autonomic effector cells of the smooth muscle, the cardiac muscle, the sinoatrial node, the atrioventricular node, and the exocrine glands. At therapeutic doses, it is completely devoid of any action on autonomic ganglia. LEVSIN inhibits gastrointestinal propulsive motility and decreases gastric acid secretion. LEVSIN also controls excessive pharyngeal, tracheal and bronchial secretions.

LEVSIN is absorbed totally and completely by sublingual administration as well as oral administration. Once absorbed, LEVSIN disappears rapidly from the blood and is distributed throughout the entire body. The half-life of LEVSIN is 2 to $3^1/_2$ hours. LEVSIN is partly hydrolyzed to tropic acid and tropine but the majority of the drug is excreted in the urine unchanged within the first 12 hours. Only traces of this drug are found in breast milk. LEVSIN passes the blood brain barrier and the placental barrier.

LEVBID releases 0.375 mg hyoscyamine sulfate at a controlled and predictable rate for 12 hours. Peak blood levels occur in approximately 4 hours and the apparent plasma elimination half-life is approximately 9 hours. The relative bioavailability of the extended-release tablet is approximately 92% that of the immediate-release tablet.

LEVSINEX TIMECAPS release 0.375 mg hyoscyamine sulfate at a controlled and predictable rate for 12 hours. Peak blood levels occur in 3 to 4 hours and the apparent plasma elimination half-life is 5 to 6 hours.

INDICATIONS AND USAGE

LEVSIN is effective as adjunctive therapy in the treatment of peptic ulcer. It can also be used to control gastric secretion, visceral spasm, and hypermotility in spastic colitis, spastic bladder, cystitis, pylorospasm, and associated abdominal cramps. May be used in functional intestinal disorders to reduce symptoms such as those seen in mild dysenteries, diverticulitis, and acute enterocolitis. For use as adjunctive therapy in the treatment of irritable bowel syndrome (irritable colon, spastic colon, mucous colitis) and functional gastrointestinal disorders. Also used as adjunctive therapy in the treatment of neurogenic bladder and neurogenic bowel disturbances including the splenic flexure syndrome and neurogenic colon. Also used in the treatment of infant colic (elixir and drops). LEVSIN is indicated along with morphine or other narcotics in symptomatic relief of biliary and renal colic; as a "drying agent" in the relief of symptoms of acute rhinitis; in the therapy of parkinsonism to reduce rigidity and tremors and to control associated sialorrhea and hyperhidrosis. May be used in the therapy of poisoning by anticholinesterase agents.

Parenterally administered LEVSIN is also effective in reducing gastrointestinal motility to facilitate diagnostic procedures such as endoscopy or hypotonic duodenography. LEVSIN may be used to reduce pain and hypersecretion in pancreatitis. LEVSIN may also be used in certain cases of partial heart block associated with vagal activity.

IN ANESTHESIA:

LEVSIN Injection is indicated as a pre-operative antimuscarinic to reduce salivary, tracheobronchial, and pharyngeal secretions; to reduce the volume and acidity of gastric secretions, and to block cardiac vagal inhibitory reflexes during induction of anesthesia and intubation. LEVSIN protects against the peripheral muscarinic effects such as bradycardia and excessive secretions produced by halogenated hydrocarbons and cholinergic agents such as physostigmine, neostigmine, and pyridostigmine given to reverse the actions of curariform agents.

IN UROLOGY:

LEVSIN Injection may also be used intravenously to improve radiologic visibility of the kidneys. It is also indicated along with morphine or other narcotics in symptomatic relief of biliary and renal colic.

CONTRAINDICATIONS

Glaucoma; obstructive uropathy (for example, bladder neck obstruction due to prostatic hypertrophy); obstructive disease of the gastrointestinal tract (as in achalasia, pyloroduodenal stenosis); paralytic ileus, intestinal atony of elderly or debilitated patients; unstable cardiovascular status in acute hemorrhage; severe ulcerative colitis; toxic megacolon complicating ulcerative colitis; myasthenia gravis.

WARNINGS

In the presence of high environmental temperature, heat prostration can occur with drug use (fever and heat stroke due to decreased sweating). Diarrhea may be an early symptom of incomplete intestinal obstruction, especially in patients with ileostomy or colostomy. In this instance, treatment with this drug would be inappropriate and possibly harmful. Like other anticholinergic agents, LEVSIN may produce drowsiness, dizziness or blurred vision. In this event, the patient should be warned not to engage in activities requiring mental alertness such as operating a motor vehicle or other machinery or to perform hazardous work while taking this drug.

Psychosis has been reported in sensitive individuals given anticholinergic drugs. CNS signs and symptoms inlude confusion, disorientation, short term memory loss, hallucinations, dysarthria, ataxia, coma, euphoria, decreased anxiety, fatigue, insomnia, agitation and mannerisms, and inappropriate affect. These CNS signs and symptoms usually resolve within 12 to 48 hours after discontinuation of the drug.

PRECAUTIONS

General:
Use with caution in patients with: autonomic neuropathy, hyperthyroidism, coronary heart disease, congestive heart failure, cardiac arrhythmias, hypertension and renal disease. Investigate any tachycardia before giving any anticholinergic drug since they may increase the heart rate. Use with caution in patients with hiatal hernia associated with reflux esophagitis.

Information for Patients:
Like other anticholinergic agents, LEVSIN may produce drowsiness, dizziness or blurred vision. In this event, the patient should be warned not to engage in activities requiring mental alertness such as operating a motor vehicle or other machinery or to perform hazardous work while taking this drug.

Use of LEVSIN may decrease sweating resulting in heat prostration, fever or heat stroke; febrile patients or those who may be exposed to elevated environmental temperatures should use caution.

Drug Interactions:
Additive adverse effects resulting from cholinergic blockade may occur when LEVSIN is administered concomitantly with other antimuscarinics, amantadine, haloperidol, phenothiazines, monoamine oxidase (MAO) inhibitors, tricyclic antidepressants or some antihistamines.

Antacids may interfere with the absorption of LEVSIN. Administer LEVSIN before meals; antacids after meals.

Carcinogenesis, Mutagenesis, Impairment of Fertility:
No long term studies in animals have been performed to determine the carcinogenic, mutagenic or impairment of fertility potential of LEVSIN; however, 40 years of marketing experience with hyoscyamine sulfate shows no demonstrable evidence of a problem.

Pregnancy—Pregnancy Category C:
Animal reproduction studies have not been conducted with LEVSIN. It is also not known whether LEVSIN can cause fetal harm when administered to a pregnant woman or can affect reproduction capacity. LEVSIN should be given to a pregnant woman only if clearly needed.

Nursing Mothers:
LEVSIN is excreted in human milk. Caution should be exercised when LEVSIN is administered to a nursing woman.

ADVERSE REACTIONS

Not all of the following adverse reactions have been reported with hyoscyamine sulfate. The following adverse reactions have been reported for pharmacologically similar drugs with anticholinergic/antispasmodic action. Adverse reactions may include dryness of the mouth; urinary hesitancy and retention; blurred vision; tachycardia; palpitations; mydriasis; cycloplegia; increased ocular tension; loss of taste; headache; nervousness; drowsiness; weakness; dizziness; insomnia; nausea; vomiting; impotence; suppression of lactation; constipation; bloated feeling; allergic reactions or drug idiosyncrasies; urticaria and other dermal manifestations; ataxia; speech disturbance; some degree of mental confusion and/or excitement (especially in elderly persons); and decreased sweating.

Continued on next page

Schwarz Pharma, Inc.—Cont.

OVERDOSAGE

The signs and symptoms of overdose are headache, nausea, vomiting, blurred vision, dilated pupils, hot dry skin, dizziness, dryness of the mouth, difficulty in swallowing and CNS stimulation.

Measures to be taken are immediate lavage of the stomach and injection of physostigmine 0.5 to 2 mg intravenously and repeated as necessary up to a total of 5 mg. Fever may be treated symptomatically (tepid water sponge baths, hypothermic blanket). Excitement to a degree which demands attention may be managed with sodium thiopental 2% solution given slowly intravenously or chloral hydrate (100–200 mL of a 2% solution) by rectal infusion. In the event of progression of the curare-like effect to paralysis of the respiratory muscles, artificial respiration should be instituted and maintained until effective respiratory action returns.

In rats, the LD_{50} for LEVSIN is 375 mg/kg. LEVSIN is dialyzable.

DOSAGE AND ADMINISTRATION

Dosage may be adjusted according to the conditions and severity of symptoms.

LEVBID Extended-Release Tablets: *Adults and pediatric patients 12 years of age and older:* 1 to 2 tablets every 12 hours. Tablets are scored and may be broken to allow for dose titration if needed. Do not exceed 4 tablets in 24 hours.

LEVSIN/SL Tablets: The tablets may be taken sublingually, orally or chewed. *Adults and pediatric patients 12 years of age and older:* 1 to 2 tablets every four hours or as needed. Do not exceed 12 tablets in 24 hours. *Pediatric patients 2 to under 12 years of age:* 1/2 to 1 tablet every four hours or as needed. Do not exceed 6 tablets in 24 hours.

LEVSIN Tablets: *Adults and pediatric patients 12 years of age and older:* 1 to 2 tablets every four hours or as needed. Do not exceed 12 tablets in 24 hours.

Pediatric patients 2 to under 12 years of age: 1/2 to 1 tablet every four hours or as needed. Do not exceed 6 tablets in 24 hours.

LEVSIN Elixir: *Adults and pediatric patients 12 years of age and older:* 1 to 2 teaspoonfuls every four hours or as needed. Do not exceed 12 teaspoonfuls in 24 hours.

Pediatric patients 2 to under 12 years of age:

Please see the following dosage guide based on body weight. The doses may be repeated every four hours or as needed. Do not exceed 6 teaspoonfuls in 24 hours.

Body Weight	Usual Dose
10 kg (22 lb)	1/4 tsp (1.25 mL)
20 kg (44 lb)	1/2 tsp (2.5 mL)
40 kg (88 lb)	3/4 tsp (3.75 mL)
50 kg (110 lb)	1 tsp (5 mL)

LEVSIN Drops: *Adults and pediatric patients 12 years of age and older:* 1 to 2 mL every four hours or as needed. Do not exceed 12 mL in 24 hours.

Pediatric patients 2 to under 12 years of age: 1/4 to 1 mL every four hours or as needed. Do not exceed 6 mL in 24 hours.

Pediatric patients under 2 years of age: The following dosage guide is based upon body weight. The doses may be repeated every four hours or as needed.

Body Weight	Usual Dose	Do Not Exceed in 24 Hours
3.4 kg (7.5 lb)	4 drops	24 drops
5 kg (11 lb)	5 drops	30 drops
7 kg (15 lb)	6 drops	36 drops
10 kg (22 lb)	8 drops	48 drops

LEVSIN Injection: The dose may be administered subcutaneously, intramuscularly, or intravenously without dilution. As with all parenteral drug products, LEVSIN Injection should be inspected visually for particulate matter and discoloration prior to administration whenever solution and container permit.

Gastrointestinal Disorders: The usual adult recommended dose is 0.5 to 1 mL (0.25 to 0.5 mg). Some patients may need only a single dose; others may require administration two, three, or four times a day at four hour intervals.

Diagnostic Procedures: The usual adult recommended dose is 0.5 to 1 mL (0.25 to 0.5 mg) administered intravenously 5 to 10 minutes prior to the diagnostic procedure.

Anesthesia: Adults and pediatric patients over 2 years of age: As a pre-anesthetic medication, the recommended dose is 5 μg (0.005 mg) per kg of body weight. This dose is usually given 30 to 60 minutes prior to the anticipated time of induction of anesthesia or at the time the pre-anesthetic narcotic or sedative is administered.

LEVSIN Injection may be used during surgery to reduce drug-induced bradycardia. It should be administered intravenously in increments of 0.25 mL and repeated as needed.

To achieve reversal of neuromuscular blockade, the recommended dose is 0.2 mg (0.4 mL) LEVSIN Injection for every 1 mg neostigmine or the equivalent dose of physostigmine or pyridostigmine.

LEVSINEX TIMECAPS: *Adults and pediatric patients 12 years of age and older:* 1 to 2 capsules every 12 hours. Dosage may be adjusted to 1 capsule every 8 hours if needed. Do not exceed 4 capsules in 24 hours.

HOW SUPPLIED

LEVBID Extended-Release Tablets (hyoscyamine sulfate, 0.375 mg) are light orange, capsule-shaped, scored tablets. They are coded SP538.

Bottles of 100 tablets	NDC 0091-3538-01
Bottles of 500 tablets	NDC 0091-3538-05

LEVSIN/SL Tablets (hyoscyamine sulfate tablets USP, 0.125 mg) are pale blue-green, peppermint-flavored, octagonal shaped, scored, and embossed with "SCHWARZ" on one side and "532" on the other.

Bottles of 100 tablets	NDC 0091-3532-01
Bottles of 500 tablets	NDC 0091-3532-05

LEVSIN Tablets (hyoscyamine sulfate tablets USP, 0.125 mg) are white, scored and imprinted with "SCHWARZ" on one side and "531" on the other.

Bottles of 100 tablets	NDC 0091-3531-01
Bottles of 500 tablets	NDC 0091-3531-05

LEVSIN Elixir (hyoscyamine sulfate elixir USP, 0.125 mg/5mL) is orange colored and flavored and contains 20% alcohol.

Pint (473 mL) bottles	NDC 0091-4532-16

LEVSIN Drops (hyoscyamine sulfate oral solution USP, 0.125 mg/mL) are orange colored, orange flavored and contain 5% alcohol.

15 mL Dropper bottles	NDC 0091-4538-15

LEVSIN Injection (hyoscyamine sulfate injection USP, 0.5 mg/mL) is a clear, colorless and sterile solution.

1 mL ampuls-Box of 5	NDC 0091-1536-05

LEVSINEX TIMECAPS (hyoscyamine sulfate USP, 0.375 mg, extended-release) are brown and clear capsules containing brown and white beadlets and imprinted with "SCHWARZ" and "537."

Bottles of 100 capsules	NDC 0091-3537-01
Bottles of 500 capsules	NDC 0091-3537-05

Store at controlled room temperature 15°–30°C (59°–86°F).

CAUTION

Federal law prohibits dispensing without prescription.

Shown in Product Identification Guide, page 334

MONOKET® TABLETS ℞

[mān'-o-ket]

(isosorbide mononitrate)

DESCRIPTION

MONOKET, an organic nitrate, is a vasodilator with effects on both arteries and veins. The empirical formula is $C_6H_9NO_6$ and the molecular weight is 191.14. The chemical name for MONOKET is 1,4:3,6-Dianhydro-D-glucitol 5-nitrate and the compound has the following structural formula:

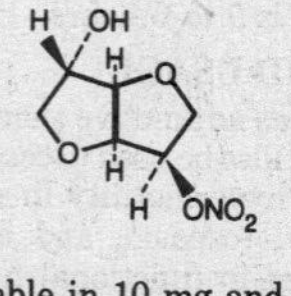

MONOKET is available in 10 mg and 20 mg tablets. Each tablet also contains as inactive ingredients: lactose, talc, colloidal silicon dioxide, starch, microcrystalline cellulose and aluminum stearate.

CLINICAL PHARMACOLOGY

Isosorbide mononitrate is the major active metabolite of isosorbide dinitrate (ISDN), and most of the clinical activity of the dinitrate is attributable to the mononitrate.

The principal pharmacological action of isosorbide mononitrate is relaxation of vascular smooth muscle and consequent dilatation of peripheral arteries and veins, especially the latter. Dilatation of the veins promotes peripheral pooling of blood and decreases venous return to the heart, thereby reducing left ventricular end-diastolic pressure and pulmonary capillary wedge pressure (preload). Arteriolar relaxation reduces systemic vascular resistance, systolic arterial pressure, and mean arterial pressure (afterload). Dilatation of the coronary arteries also occurs. The relative importance of preload reduction, afterload reduction and coronary dilatation remains undefined.

Pharmacodynamics

Dosing regimens for most chronically used drugs are designed to provide plasma concentrations that are continuously greater than a minimally effective concentration. This strategy is inappropriate for organic nitrates. Several well-controlled clinical trials have used exercise testing to assess the antianginal efficacy of continuously-delivered nitrates. In the large majority of these trials, active agents were indistinguishable from placebo after 24 hours (or less) of continuous therapy. Attempts to overcome tolerance by dose escalation, even to doses far in excess of those used acutely, have consistently failed. Only after nitrates have been absent from the body for several hours has their antianginal efficacy been restored.

The drug-free interval sufficient to avoid tolerance to isosorbide mononitrate has not been completely defined. In the only regimen of twice-daily isosorbide mononitrate that has been shown to avoid development of tolerance, the two doses of MONOKET Tablets are given 7 hours apart, so there is a gap of 17 hours between the second dose of each day and the first dose of the next day. Taking account of the relatively long half-life of isosorbide mononitrate this result is consistent with those obtained for other organic nitrates.

The asymmetric twice daily regimen of MONOKET Tablets successfully avoided significant rebound/withdrawal effects. The incidence and magnitude of such phenomena have appeared, in studies of other nitrates, to be highly dependent upon the schedule of nitrate administration.

Pharmacokinetics

MONOKET is rapidly and completely absorbed from the gastrointestinal tract. In humans, MONOKET is not subject to first pass metabolism in the liver. The absolute bioavailability of isosorbide mononitrate from MONOKET Tablets is nearly 100%. Peak plasma concentrations usually occur in about 30–60 minutes. MONOKET exhibits dose proportionality over the recommended dose range. Food does not significantly affect the absorption or bioavailability of MONOKET. Metoprolol coadministration did not change the pharmacokinetics of MONOKET. The volume of distribution is approximately 0.6 L/Kg. Plasma protein binding of MONOKET was found to be less than 5%.

When radiolabelled isosorbide mononitrate was administered to humans in order to elucidate the metabolic fate, about half of the dose was found denitrated and renally excreted as isosorbide and sorbitol. One quarter of the dose was accounted for as conjugates of the parent drug in the urine. None of these metabolites is vasoactive. Only 2% of the dose was excreted as unchanged drug.

The overall elimination half-life of MONOKET is about 5 hours. The rate of clearance is the same in healthy young adults, in patients with various degrees of renal, hepatic or cardiac dysfunction and in the elderly. When radiolabelled isosorbide mononitrate was administered to humans, 93% of the dose was excreted within 48 hours into the urine. Renal excretion was virtually complete after 5 days; fecal excretion amounted to only 1% of the dose.

MONOKET has no known effect on renal and hepatic function. In patients with varying degrees of renal failure, dosage adjustment does not appear necessary. In patients with liver cirrhosis, the pharmacokinetic parameters after a single dose of MONOKET were similar to the values found in healthy volunteers.

Isosorbide mononitrate is significantly removed from the blood during hemodialysis; however, an additional dose to compensate for drug lost is not necessary. In patients undergoing continuous ambulatory peritoneal dialysis, blood levels are similar to patients not on dialysis.

Clinical Trials

The acute and chronic antianginal efficacy of MONOKET has been confirmed in clinical trials. The clinical efficacy of MONOKET was studied in 21 stable angina pectoris patients. After single dose administration of MONOKET, 20 mg, the exercise capacity was increased by 42.7% after one hour, 29.6% after 6 hours and by 25% aftr eight hours when compared to placebo. Controlled trials of single doses of MONOKET Tablets have demonstrated that antianginal activity is present about 1 hour after dosing, with peak effect seen from 1–4 hours after dosing.

In one multicenter placebo controlled trial, MONOKET was found to be safe and effective during acute and chronic (3 weeks) treatment of angina pectoris. Two hundred fourteen (214) patients were enrolled in the trial; 54 patients were randomized to receive placebo and 106 patients were randomized to receive 10 or 20 mg of MONOKET twice daily seven hours apart. The largest effect of MONOKET, compared to placebo, was on day one-dose one. Although 14 hours after the first dose of day 14, the increase in exercise tolerance due to MONOKET was statistically significant, the increase was about half of that seen 2 hours after the first dose of day one. On day 21, two hours after the first dose the effect of MONOKET was 60 to 70% of that seen on day one.

INDICATIONS AND USAGE

MONOKET is indicated for the prevention and treatment of angina pectoris due to coronary artery disease. The onset of action of oral isosorbide mononitrate is not sufficiently rapid for this product to be useful in aborting an acute anginal episode.

CONTRAINDICATIONS

Allergic reactions to organic nitrates are extremely rare, but they do occur. Isosorbide mononitrate is contraindicated in patients who are allergic to it.

WARNINGS

The benefits of isosorbide mononitrate in patients with acute myocardial infarction or congestive heart failure have not been established. Because the effects of isosorbide mononi-

Frequency of Adverse Reactions (Discontinuations)*

6 Placebo Controlled Studies

Dose	Placebo	5 mg	10 mg	20 mg
Patients	160	54	52	159
Headache	6% (0%)	17% (0%)	13% (0%)	35% (5%)
Fatigue	2% (0%)	0% (0%)	4% (0%)	1% (0%)
Upper Respiratory				
Infection	<1% (0%)	0% (0%)	4% (0%)	1% (0%)
Pain	<1% (0%)	4% (0%)	0% (0%)	<1% (0%)
Dizziness	1% (0%)	0% (0%)	0% (0%)	4% (0%)
Nausea	<1% (0%)	0% (0%)	0% (0%)	3% (2%)
Inceased Cough	<1% (0%)	0% (0%)	2% (0%)	<1% (0%)
Rash	0% (0%)	2% (2%)	0% (0%)	<1% (0%)
Abdominal Pain	<1% (0%)	0% (0%)	2% (0%)	0% (0%)
Allergic Reaction	0% (0%)	0% (0%)	2% (0%)	0% (0%)
Cardiovascular				
Disorder	0% (0%)	2% (0%)	0% (0%)	0% (0%)
Chest Pain	<1% (0%)	0% (0%)	2% (0%)	<1% (0%)
Diarrhea	0% (0%)	0% (0%)	2% (0%)	0% (0%)
Flushing	0% (0%)	0% (0%)	2% (0%)	0% (0%)
Emotional Lability	0% (0%)	2% (0%)	0% (0%)	0% (0%)
Pruritus	1% (0%)	2% (2%)	0% (0%)	0% (0%)

*Some individuals discontinued for multiple reasons.

trate are difficult to terminate rapidly, this drug is not recommended in these settings.

If isosorbide mononitrate is used in these conditions, careful clinical or hemodynamic monitoring must be used to avoid the hazards of hypotension and tachycardia.

PRECAUTIONS

General

Severe hypotension, particularly with upright posture, may occur with even small doses of isosorbide mononitrate. This drug should therefore be used with caution in patients who may be volume depleted or who, for whatever reason, are already hypotensive. Hypotension induced by isosorbide mononitrate may be accompanied by paradoxical bradycardia and increased angina pectoris.

Nitrate therapy may aggravate the angina caused by hypertrophic cardiomyopathy.

In industrial workers who have had long-term exposure to unknown (presumably high) doses of organic nitrates, tolerance clearly occurs. Chest pain, acute myocardial infarction, and even sudden death have occurred during temporary withdrawal of nitrates from these workers, demonstrating the existence of true physical dependence. The importance of these observations to the routine, clinical use of oral isosorbide mononitrate is not known.

Information for Patients

Patients should be told that the antianginal efficacy of MONOKET Tablets can be maintained by carefully following the prescribed schedule of dosing (two doses taken seven hours apart). For most patients, this can be accomplished by taking the first dose on awakening and the second dose 7 hours later.

As with other nitrates, daily headaches sometimes accompany treatment with isosorbide mononitrate. In patients who get these headaches, the headaches are a marker of the activity of the drug. Patients should resist the temptation to avoid headaches by altering the schedule of their treatment with isosorbide mononitrate, since loss of headache may be associated with simultaneous loss of antianginal efficacy. Aspirin and/or acetaminophen, on the other hand, often successfully relieve isosorbide mononitrate-induced headaches with no deleterious effect on isosorbide mononitrate's anti-anginal efficacy.

Treatment with isosorbide mononitrate may be associated with light-headedness on standing, especially just after rising from a recumbent or seated position. This effect may be more frequent in patients who have also consumed alcohol.

Drug Interactions

The vasodilating effects of isosorbide mononitrate may be additive with those of other vasodilators. Alcohol, in particular, has been found to exhibit additive effects of this variety. Marked symptomatic orthostatic hypotension has been reported when calcium channel blockers and organic nitrates were used in combination. Dose adjustments of either class of agents may be necessary.

Carcinogenesis, Mutagenesis, Impairment of Fertility

No evidence of carcinogenicity was observed in rats exposed to isosorbide mononitrate in their diets at doses of up to 900 mg/kg/day for the first six months and 500 mg/kg/day for the remaining duration of a study in which males were dosed for up to 121 weeks and females were dosed for up to 137 weeks. No evidence of mutagenicity was seen in vitro in the Salmonella test (Ames test), in human peripheral lymphocytes, in Chinese hamster cells (V79) or, in vivo in the rat micronucleus test. In a study on the fertility and breeding capacity of two generations of rats, MONOKET had no ad-

verse effects on fertility or general reproductive performance with oral doses up to 120 mg/kg/day. A dose of 360 mg/kg/day was associated with increased mortality in treated males and females and a reduced fertility index. (See table at end of Pregnancy section for animal-to-human dosage comparisons.)

Pregnancy

Teratogenic Effects: Pregnancy Category B. Reproduction studies performed in rats and rabbits at doses of up to 540 and 810 mg/kg/day, respectively, have revealed no evidence of harm to the fetus due to isosorbide mononitrate. There are, however, no adequate and well-controlled studies in pregnant women. Because animal reproduction studies are not always predictive of human response, MONOKET should be used during pregnancy only if clearly needed.

Nonteratogenic Effects: Birth weights, neonatal survival and development, and incidence of stillbirths were adversely affected when pregnant rats were administered oral doses of 540 (but not 270) mg isosorbide mononitrate/kg/day during late gestation and lactation. This dose was associated with decreased maternal body weight gain and decreased maternal motor activity.

Species	Daily Dose (mg/kg)	Multiple of MRHD* Based on:	
		Body Weight	Body Surface
Rabbit	810	1013	375
Rat	900	1125	195
	540	675	117
	500	625	108
	360	450	78
	270	338	59

Calculations assume a human weight of 50 kg and human body surface area of 1.46 m², a rabbit weight of 2 kg and rabbit body surface area of 0.163 m², and a rat weight of 150 g and rat body surface area of 0.025 m². *Maximum recommended human dose (MRHD) is 20 mg bid.

Nursing Mothers

It is not known whether isosorbide mononitrate is excreted in human milk. Because many drugs are excreted in human milk, caution should be exercised when isosorbide mononitrate is administered to a nursing woman.

Pediatric Use

Safety and effectiveness of isosorbide mononitrate in pediatric patients have not been established.

ADVERSE REACTIONS

Headache is the most frequent side effect and was the cause of 2% of all dropouts from controlled-clinical trials. Headache decreased in incidence after the first few days of therapy.

The following table shows the frequency of adverse reactions observed in 1% or more of subjects in 6 placebo-controlled trials, conducted in the United States and abroad. The same table shows the frequency of withdrawal for these adverse reactions. In many cases the adverse reactions were of uncertain relation to drug treatment.

[See table on top of page.]

Other adverse reactions, each reported by fewer than 1% of exposed patients, and in many cases of uncertain relation to drug treatment, were:

Cardiovascular: acute myocardial infarction, apoplexy, arrhythmias, bradycardia, edema, hypertension, hypotension, pallor, palpitations, tachycardia.

Dermatologic: sweating.

Gastrointestinal: anorexia, dry mouth, dyspepsia, thirst, vomiting, decreased weight.

Genitourinary: prostatic disorder.

Miscellaneous: amblyopia, back pain, bitter taste, muscle cramps, neck pain, paresthesia, susurrus aurium.

Neurologic: anxiety, impaired concentration, depression, insomnia, nervousness, nightmares, restlessness, tremor, vertigo.

Respiratory: asthma, dyspnea, sinusitis.

Extremely rarely, ordinary doses of organic nitrates have caused methemoglobinemia in normal-seeming patients; for further discussion of its diagnosis and treatment see under Overdosage.

OVERDOSAGE

Hemodynamic Effects

The ill effects of isosorbide mononitrate overdose are generally the results of isosorbide mononitrate's capacity to induce vasodilatation, venous pooling, reduced cardiac output, and hypotension. These hemodynamic changes may have protean manifestations, including increased intracranial pressure, with any or all of persistent throbbing headache, confusion, and moderate fever; vertigo; palpitations; visual disturbances; nausea and vomiting (possibly with colic and even bloody diarrhea); syncope (especially in the upright posture); air hunger and dyspnea, later followed by reduced ventilatory effort; diaphoresis, with the skin either flushed or cold and clammy; heart block and bradycardia; paralysis; coma; seizures and death.

Laboratory determinations of serum levels of isosorbide mononitrate and its metabolites are not widely available, and such determinations have, in any event, no established role in the management of isosorbide mononitrate overdose. There are no data suggesting what dose of isosorbide mononitrate is likely to be life-threatening in humans. In rats and mice, there is significant lethality at oral doses of 1965 mg/kg and 2581 mg/kg, respectively.

No data are available to suggest physiological maneuvers (e.g., maneuvers to change the pH of the urine) that might accelerate elimination of isosorbide mononitrate. Isosorbide mononitrate is significantly removed from the blood during hemodialysis.

No specific antagonist to the vasodilator effects of isosorbide mononitrate is known, and no intervention has been subject to controlled study as a therapy of isosorbide mononitrate overdose. Because the hypotension associated with isosorbide mononitrate overdose is the result of venodilatation and arterial hypovolemia, prudent therapy in this situation should be directed toward an increase in central fluid volume. Passive elevation of the patient's legs may be sufficient, but intravenous infusion of normal saline or similar fluid may also be necessary.

The use of epinephrine or other arterial vasoconstrictors in this setting is likely to do more harm than good.

In patients with renal disease or congestive heart failure, therapy resulting in central volume expansion is not without hazard. Treatment of isosorbide mononitrate overdose in these patients may be subtle and difficult, and invasive monitoring may be required.

Methemoglobinemia

Methemoglobinemia has been reported in patients receiving other organic nitrates, and it probably could also occur as a side effect of isosorbide mononitrate. Certainly nitrate ions liberated during metabolism of isosorbide mononitrate can oxidize hemoglobin into methemoglobin. Even in patients totally without cytochrome b_5 reductase activity, however, and even assuming that the nitrate moiety of isosorbide mononitrate is quantitatively applied to oxidation of hemoglobin, about 2 mg/kg of isosorbide mononitrate should be required before any of these patients manifests clinically significant ($\geq 10\%$) methemoglobinemia. In patients with normal reductase function, significant production of methemoglobin should require even larger doses of isosorbide mononitrate. In one study in which 36 patients received 2–4 weeks of continuous nitroglycerin therapy at 3.1 to 4.4 mg/hr (equivalent, in total administered dose of nitrate ions, to 7.8–11.1 mg of isosorbide mononitrate per hour), the average methemoglobin level measured was 0.2%; this was comparable to that observed in parallel patients who received placebo.

Notwithstanding these observations, there are case reports of significant methemoglobinemia in association with moderate overdoses of organic nitrates. None of the affected patients had been thought to be unusually susceptible.

Methemoglobin levels are available from most clinical laboratories. The diagnosis should be suspected in patients who exhibit signs of impaired oxygen delivery despite adequate cardiac output and adequate arterial pO₂. Classically, methemoglobinemic blood is described as chocolate brown, without color change on exposure to air.

Continued on next page

Schwarz Pharma, Inc.—Cont.

When methemoglobinemia is diagnosed, the treatment of choice is methylene blue, 1–2 mg/kg intravenously.

DOSAGE AND ADMINISTRATION

The recommended regimen of MONOKET Tablets is 20 mg twice daily, with the doses seven hours apart. A starting dose of 5 mg (½ tablet of the 10 mg dosing strength) might be appropriate for persons of particularly small stature but should be increased to at least 10 mg by the second or third day of therapy. Dosage adjustments are not necessary for elderly patients or patients with altered hepatic or renal function.

As noted above (**Clinical Pharmacology**), multiple studies of organic nitrates have shown that maintenance of continuous 24-hour plasma levels results in refractory tolerance. The asymmetric (2 doses, 7 hours apart) dosing regimen for MONOKET Tablets provides a daily nitrate-free interval to minimize the development of tolerance.

As also noted under **Clinical Pharmacology,** well-controlled studies have shown that tolerance to MONOKET Tablets occurs to some extent when using the twice daily regimen in which the two doses are given seven hours apart. This regimen has been shown to have antianginal efficacy beginning one hour after the first dose and lasting at least seven hours after the second dose. The duration (if any) of antianginal activity beyond fourteen hours has not been studied.

In clinical trials, MONOKET has been administered in a variety of regimens and doses. Doses above 20 mg twice a day (with the doses seven hours apart) have not been adequately studied. Doses of 5 mg twice a day are clearly effective (effectiveness based on exercise tolerance) for only the first day of a twice-a-day (with doses 7 hours apart) regimen.

HOW SUPPLIED

MONOKET® (isosorbide mononitrate) 10mg Tablets are white, round, scored and engraved "10" on one side and engraved "SCHWARZ 610" on the other. They are supplied as follows:

Bottles of 100	NDC 0091-3610-01

MONOKET® (isosorbide mononitrate) 20 mg Tablets are white, round, scored and engraved "20" on one side and engraved "SCHWARZ 620" on the other. They are supplied as follows:

Bottles of 60	NDC 0091-3620-60
Bottles of 100	NDC 0091-3620-01
Bottles of 180	NDC 0091-3620-18
Unit Dose Packages of 100	NDC 0091-3620-11

Store at controlled room temperature 15°-30°C (59°-86°F). Keep tightly closed.

CAUTION

Federal law prohibits dispensing without prescription.

Shown in Product Identification Guide, page 334

PROCTOCREAM®•HC 2.5% ℞
(hydrocortisone cream, USP 2.5%)
[topical]

DESCRIPTION

PROCTOCREAM®•HC 2.5% contains Hydrocortisone [Pregn-4-ene-3, 20-dione, 11, 17,21-trihydroxy-, (11β)-], with the molecular formula $C_{21}H_{30}O_5$ and a molecular weight of 362.47. CAS 50-23-7. Each gram for topical administration contains: 25 mg of hydrocortisone in a base of glyceryl monostearate, polyoxyl 40 stearate, glycerin, paraffin, stearyl alcohol, isopropyl palmitate, sorbitan monostearate, benzyl alcohol, potassium sorbate, lactic acid, and purified water.

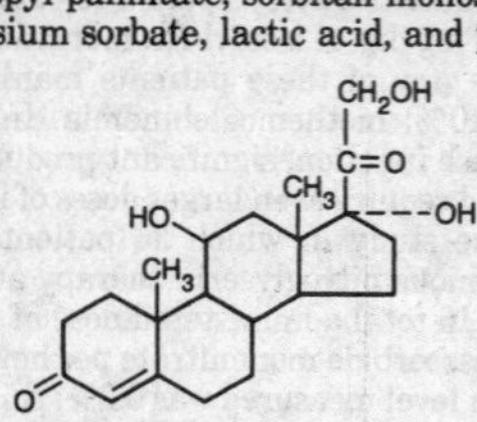

CLINICAL PHARMACOLOGY

Topical corticosteroids share anti-inflammatory, anti-pruritic and vasoconstrictive actions. The mechanism of anti-inflammatory activity of the topical corticosteroids is unclear. Various laboratory methods, including vasoconstrictor assays, are used to compare and predict potencies and/or clinical efficacies of the topical corticosteroids. There is some evidence to suggest that a recognizable correlation exists between vasoconstrictor potency and therapeutic efficacy in man.

Pharmacokinetics: The extent of percutaneous absorption of topical corticosteroids is determined by many factors including the vehicle, the integrity of the epidermal barrier, and the use of occlusive dressings. Topical corticosteroids can be absorbed from normal intact skin. Inflammation and/or other disease processes in the skin increase percutaneous absorption. Occlusive dressings substantially increase the percutaneous absorption of topical corticosteroids. Thus, occlusive dressings may be a valuable therapeutic adjunct for treatment of resistant dermatoses. (See DOSAGE AND ADMINISTRATION). Once absorbed through the skin, topical corticosteroids are handled through pharmacokinetic pathways similar to systemically administered corticosteroids. Corticosteroids are bound to plasma proteins in varying degrees. Corticosteroids are metobolized primarily in the liver and are then excreted by the kidneys. Some of the topical corticosteroids and their metabolites are also excreted into the bile.

INDICATIONS AND USAGE

Topical corticosteroids are indicated for the relief of the inflammatory and pruritic manifestations of corticosteroid-responsive dermatoses.

CONTRAINDICATIONS

Topical corticosteroids are contraindicated in those patients with a history of hypersensitivity to any of the components of the preparation.

PRECAUTIONS

General:

Systemic absorption of topical corticosteroids has produced reversible hypothalamic-pituitary-adrenal (HPA) axis suppression, manifestations Cushing's syndrome, hyperglycemia, and glucosuria in some patients. Conditions which augment systemic absorption include the application of the more potent steroids, use over large surface areas, prolonged use, and the addition of occlusive dressings. Therefore, patients receiving a large dose of a potent topical steroid applied to a large surface area or under an occlusive dressing should be evaluated periodically for evidence of HPA axis suppression by using the urinary free cortisol and ACTH stimulation tests. If HPA axis suppression is noted, an attempt should be made to withdraw the drug, to reduce the frequency of application, or to substitute a less potent steroid. Recovery of HPA axis function is generally prompt and complete upon discontinuation of the drug. Infrequently, signs and symptoms of steroid withdrawal may occur, requiring supplemental systemic corticosteroids. Children may absorb proportionally larger amounts of topical corticosteroids and thus be more susceptible to systemic toxicity (See PRECAUTIONS—Pediatric Use). If irritation develops, topical corticosteroids should be discontinued and appropriate therapy instituted. In the presence of dermatological infections, the use of an appropriate antifungal or antibacterial agent should be instituted. If a favorable response does not occur promptly, the corticosteroid should be discontinued until the infection has been adequately controlled.

Information for the Patient: Patients using topical corticosteroids should receive the following information and instructions:

1. This medication is to be used as directed by the physician. It is for external use only. Avoid contact with the eyes.
2. Patients should be advised not to use this medication for any disorder other than for which it was prescribed.
3. The treated skin area should not be bandaged or otherwise covered or wrapped as to be occlusive unless directed by the physician.
4. Patients should report any signs of local adverses reactions especially under occlusive dressing.
5. Parents of pediatric patients should be advised not to use tight-fitting diapers or plastic pants on a child being treated in the diaper area, as these garments may constitute occlusive dressings.

Laboratory Tests: The following tests may be helpful in evaluating the HPA axis suppression:Urinary free cortisol test; ACTH stimulation test.

Carcinogenesis, Mutagenesis, and Impairment of Fertility: Long-term animal studies have not been performed to evaluate the carcinogenic potential or the effect on fertility of topical corticosteroids. Studies to determine mutagenicity with prednisolone and hydrocortisone have revealed negative results.

Pregnancy: *Teratogenic Effects* — Pregnancy Category C Corticosteroids are generally teratogenic in laboratory animals when administered systemically at relatively low dosage levels. The more potent corticosteroids have been shown to be teratogenic after dermal application in laboratory animals. There are no adequate and well-controlled studies in pregnant women on teratogenic effects from topically applied corticosteroids. Therefore, topical corticosteroids should be used during pregnancy only if the potential benefit justifies the potential risk to the fetus. Drugs of this class should not be used extensively on pregnant patients, in large amounts, or for prolonged periods of time.

Nursing Mothers: It is not known whether topical administration of corticosteroids could result in sufficient systemic absorption to produce detectable quantities in breast milk. Systemically administered corticosteroids are secreted into breast milk in quantities not likely to have a deleterious effect on the infant. Nevertheless, caution should be exercised when topical corticosteroids are administered to a nursing woman.

Pediatric Use: Pediatric patients may demonstrate greater susceptibility to topical corticosteroid-induced hypothalamic-pituitary-adrenal (HPA) axis suppression and Cushing's syndrome than mature patients because of a larger skin surface area to body weight ratio. Hypothalamic-pituitary-adrenal (HPA) axis suppression, Cushing's syndrome, and intracranial hypertension have been reported in pediatric patients receiving topical corticosteroids. Manisfestations of adrenal suppression in pediatric patients include linear growth retardation, delayed weight gain, low plasma cortisol levels, and absence of response to ACTH stimulation. Manifestations of intracranial hypertension include bulging fontanelles, headaches, and bilateral papilledema. Administration of topical corticosteroids to pediatric patients should be limited to the least amount compatible with an effective therapeutic regimen. Chronic corticosteroid therapy may interfere with the growth and development of pediatric patients.

ADVERSE REACTIONS

The following local adverse reactions are reported infrequently with topical corticosteroids, but may occur more frequently with the use of occlusive dressings. These reactions are listed in an approximate decreasing order of occurrence: burning, itching, irritation, dryness, folliculitis, hypertrichosis, acneiform eruptions, hypopigmentation, perioral dermatitis, allergic contact dermatitis, maceration of the skin, secondary infection, skin atrophy, striae and miliaria.

OVERDOSAGE

Topically applied corticosteroids can be absorbed in sufficient amounts to produce systemic effects (See PRECAUTIONS).

DOSAGE AND ADMINISTRATION

Apply to the affected area as a thin film from 2 to 4 times daily depending on the severity of the condition. Occlusive dressings may be used for the management of psoriasis or recalcitrant conditions. If an infection develops, the use of occlusive dressings should be discontinued and appropriate antimicrobial therapy instituted.

HOW SUPPLIED

PROCTOCREAM®•HC 2.5% (hydrocortisone cream USP, 2.5%) is supplied in 30 gram tubes.

30 gram tubes	NDC 0091-4640-24

Store at controlled room temperature 15°-30°C (59°-86°F).

CAUTION: Federal law prohibits dispensing without prescription.

Shown in Product Identification Guide, page 334

PROCTOFOAM®–HC ℞
(hydrocortisone acetate 1%
and pramoxine hydrochloride 1%)
TOPICAL AEROSOL

DESCRIPTION

A topical corticosteroid aerosol foam for anal use containing hydrocortisone acetate 1% and pramoxine hydrochloride 1% in a hydrophilic base of: propylene glycol, ethoxylated cetyl and stearyl alcohols, steareth-10, cetyl alcohol, methylparaben, propylparaben, trolamine, purified water and propellants (inert): dichlorodifluoromethane and dichlorotetrafluoroethane.

PROCTOFOAM®-HC contains a synthetic steroid used as an anti-inflammatory and antipruritic agent, and a local anesthetic.

Hydrocortisone acetate

Molecular weight: 404.50. Solubility of hydrocortisone acetate in water: 1mg/100mL.

Chemical name: Pregn-4-ene-3,20-dione, 21-(acetyloxy)-11, 17-dihydroxy-,(11β).

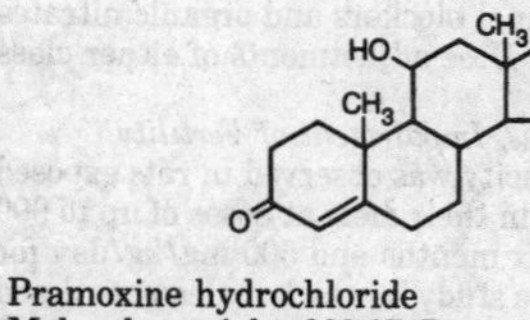

Pramoxine hydrochloride

Molecular weight: 329.87. Pramoxine hydrochloride is freely soluble in water.

Chemical name: Morpholine, 4-[3-(4-butoxyphenoxy) propyl]-, hydrochloride, 4-[3(p-butoxyphenoxy) propyl] morpholine hydrochloride.

[See chemical structure at top of next column.]

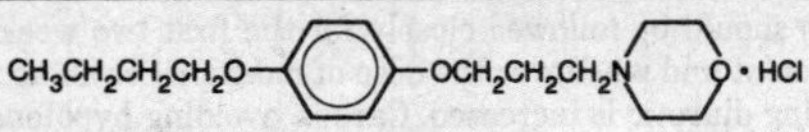

CLINICAL PHARMACOLOGY

Topical corticosteroids share anti-inflammatory, antipruritic and vasoconstrictive actions.

The mechanism of anti-inflammatory activity of the topical corticosteroids is unclear. Various laboratory methods, including vasoconstrictor assays, are used to compare and predict potencies and/or clinical efficacies of the topical corticosteroids. There is some evidence to suggest that a recognizable correlation exists between vasoconstrictor potency and therapeutic efficacy in man.

Pramoxine hydrochloride: A surface or local anesthetic which is not chemically related to the "caine" types of local anesthetics. Its unique chemical structure is likely to minimize the danger of cross-sensitivity reactions in patients allergic to other local anesthetics.

Pharmacokinetics: The extent of percutaneous absorption of topical corticosteroids is determined by many factors including the vehicle, the integrity of the epidermal barrier, and the use of occlusive dressings.

Topical corticosteroids can be absorbed through normal intact skin. Inflammation and/or other disease processes in the skin increase the percutaneous absorption of topical corticosteroids. Occlusive dressings substantially increase the percutaneous absorption of topical corticosteroids. Thus, occlusive dressings may be a valuable therapeutic adjunct for treatment of resistant dermatoses. (See DOSAGE AND ADMINISTRATION.)

Once absorbed through the skin, topical corticosteroids are handled through pharmacokinetic pathways similar to systemically administered corticosteroids. Corticosteroids are bound to plasma proteins in varying degrees. Corticosteroids are metabolized primarily in the liver and are then excreted by the kidneys. Some of the topical corticosteroids and their metabolites are also excreted in the bile.

INDICATIONS AND USAGE

Topical corticosteroids are indicated for the relief of the inflammatory and pruritic manifestations of corticosteroid-responsive dermatoses of the anal region.

CONTRAINDICATIONS

Topical corticosteroid products are contraindicated in those patients with a history of hypersensitivity to any of the components of the preparation.

WARNINGS

Do not insert any part of the aerosol container into the anus. Contents of the container are under pressure. Do not burn or puncture the aerosol container. Store at temperatures below 120°F. If there is no evidence of clinical or proctologic improvement within two or three weeks after therapy, or if the patient's condition worsens, discontinue the drug. Keep this and all medicines out of the reach of children.

PRECAUTIONS

General: Systemic absorption of topical corticosteroids has produced reversible hypothalamic-pituitary-adrenal (HPA) axis suppression, manifestations of Cushing's syndrome, hyperglycemia and glucosuria in some patients.

Conditions which augment systemic absorption include the application of the more potent steroids, use over large surface areas, prolonged use and the addition of occlusive dressings.

Therefore, patients receiving a large dose of a potent topical steroid applied to a large surface area or under an occlusive dressing should be evaluated periodically for evidence of HPA axis suppression by using the urinary free cortisol and ACTH stimulation tests. If HPA axis suppression is noted, an attempt should be made to withdraw the drug, to reduce the frequency of application, or to substitute a less potent steroid.

Recovery of HPA axis function is generally prompt and complete upon discontinuation of the drug. Infrequently, signs and symptoms of steroid withdrawal may occur, requiring supplemental systemic corticosteroids.

In children, absorption may result in higher blood levels and thus more susceptibility to systemic toxicity. (See PRECAUTIONS—Pediatric Use.)

If irritation develops, topical corticosteroids should be discontinued and appropriate therapy instituted.

In the presence of dermatological infections, the use of an appropriate antifungal or antibacterial agent should be instituted. If a favorable response does not occur promptly, the corticosteroid should be discontinued until the infection has been adequately controlled.

Information for the Patient: Patients using topical corticosteroids should receive the following information and instructions:

1. This medication is to be used as directed by the physician. It is for anal or perianal use only. Avoid contact with the eyes.
2. Be advised not to use this medication for any disorder other than for which it has been prescribed.
3. Report any signs of adverse reactions.

Laboratory Tests: The following tests may be helpful in evaluating the HPA axis suppression:
Urinary free cortisol test
ACTH stimulation test

Carcinogenesis, Mutagenesis, and Impairment of Fertility: Long-term animal studies have not been performed to evaluate carcinogenic potential or the effect on fertility of topical corticosteroids.

Studies to determine mutagenicity with prednisolone and hydrocortisone have revealed negative results.

Pregnancy Category C: Corticosteroids are generally teratogenic in laboratory animals when administered systemically at relatively low dosage levels. The more potent corticosteroids have been shown to be teratogenic after dermal application in laboratory animals. There are no adequate and well-controlled studies in pregnant women of teratogenic effects from topically applied corticosteroids. Therefore, topical corticosteroids should be used during pregnancy only if the potential benefit justifies the potential risk to the fetus. Drugs of this class should not be used extensively on pregnant patients, in large amounts, or for prolonged periods of time.

Nursing Mothers: It is not known whether topical administration of corticosteroids could result in sufficient systemic absorption to produce detectable quantities in breast milk. Systemically administered corticosteroids are secreted into breast milk in quantities not likely to have a deleterious effect on the infant. Caution should be exercised when any topical corticosteroids are administered to a nursing woman.

Pediatric Use: *Pediatric patients may demonstrate greater susceptibility to topical corticosteroid-induced HPA axis suppression and Cushing's syndrome than mature patients because of a larger skin surface area to body weight ratio.*

Hypothalamic-pituitary-adrenal (HPA) axis suppression, Cushing's syndrome and intracranial hypertension have been reported in children receiving topical corticosteroids. Manifestations of adrenal suppression in children include linear growth retardation, delayed weight gain, low plasma cortisol levels and absense of response to ACTH stimulation. Manifestations of intracranial hypertension include bulging fontanelles, headaches and bilateral papilledema.

Administration of topical corticosteroids to children should be limited to the least amount compatible with an effective therapeutic regimen. Chronic corticosteroid therapy may interfere with the growth and development of children.

ADVERSE REACTIONS

The following local adverse reactions are reported infrequently with topical corticosteroids, but may occur more frequently with the use of occlusive dressings. These reactions are listed in an approximate decreasing order of occurrence: burning, itching, irritation, dryness, folliculitis, hypertrichosis, acneiform eruptions, hypopigmentation, perioral dermatitis, allergic contact dermatitis, maceration of the skin, secondary infection, skin atrophy, striae and miliaria.

OVERDOSAGE

Topically applied corticosteroids can be absorbed in sufficient amounts to produce systemic effects. (See PRECAUTIONS.)

DOSAGE AND ADMINISTRATION

(NOTE: SEE PACKAGE FOR FULL DIRECTIONS FOR USE.)

Apply to affected areas 3 or 4 times daily. Use the applicator supplied for anal administration. For perianal use, transfer a small quantity to a tissue and rub in gently.

1. Shake foam container vigorously before use. Hold container upright and insert into opening of the tip of the applicator. Be sure applicator plunger is drawn all the way out. **CONTAINER MUST BE HELD UPRIGHT TO OBTAIN PROPER FLOW OF MEDICATION.**
2. To fill, press down slowly on container cap. Repeat until foam reaches fill line in the applicator. CAUTION: Do not insert any part of the aerosol container directly into the anus. Apply to anus only with enclosed applicator. Do not insert any part of applicator past anus into rectum.
3. Remove applicator from container. With applicator in place, push plunger in order to expel foam, then withdraw applicator. (Applicator parts should be pulled apart for thorough cleaning with warm water.)

HOW SUPPLIED

PROCTOFOAM®-HC (hydrocortisone acetate 1% and pramoxine hydrochloride 1%) topical aerosol (NDC 0021-0690-10) is supplied in 10 gram aerosol container with a special anal applicator. **Store upright at controlled room temperature 15°–30°C (59°–86°F).**

When used correctly, the aerosol container will deliver a minimum of 14 applications.

CAUTION

Federal law prohibits dispensing without prescription.

Shown in Product Identification Guide, page 335

UNIVASC® Tablets ℞

[*yü-nə-vask*]

(moexipril hydrochloride)

> **USE IN PREGNANCY**
> **When used in pregnancy during the second and third trimesters, ACE inhibitors can cause injury and even death to the developing fetus.** When pregnancy is detected, UNIVASC should be discontinued as soon as possible. **See WARNINGS, Fetal/Neonatal Morbidity and Mortality.**

DESCRIPTION

UNIVASC (moexipril hydrochloride), the hydrochloride salt of moexipril, has the empirical formula $C_{27}H_{34}N_2O_7 \cdot HCl$ and a molecular weight of 535.04. It is chemically described as [3S-[2[R*(R*)], 3R*]]-2-[2-[[1-(ethoxycarbonyl)-3-phenylpropyl]amino] -1- oxopropyl]-1,2,3,4-tetrahydro -6,7- dimethoxy-3-isoquinolinecarboxylic acid, monohydrochloride. It is a non-sulfhydryl containing precursor of the active angiotensin-converting enzyme (ACE) inhibitor moexiprilat and its structural formula is:

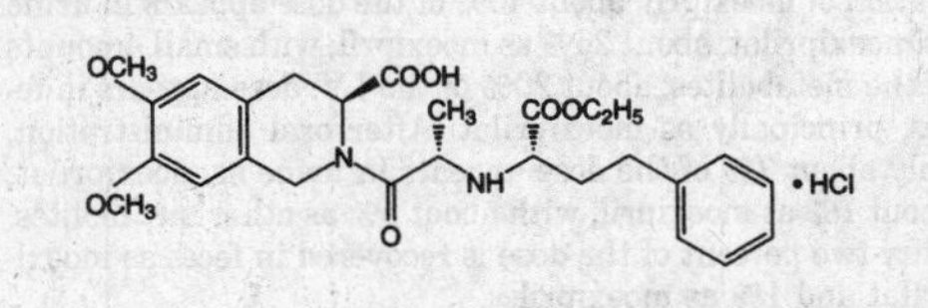

Moexipril hydrochloride is a fine white to off-white powder. It is soluble (about 10% weight-to-volume) in distilled water at room temperature.

UNIVASC is supplied as scored, coated tablets containing 7.5 mg and 15 mg of moexipril hydrochloride for oral administration. In addition to the active ingredient, moexipril hydrochloride, the tablet core contains the following inactive ingredients: lactose, magnesium oxide, crospovidone, magnesium stearate and gelatin. The film coating contains hydroxypropyl methylcellulose, hydroxypropyl cellulose, polyethylene glycol 6000, magnesium stearate, titanium dioxide, and ferric oxide.

CLINICAL PHARMACOLOGY

Mechanism of Action

Moexipril hydrochloride is a prodrug for moexiprilat, which inhibits ACE in humans and animals. The mechanism through which moexiprilat lowers blood pressure is believed to be primarily inhibition of ACE activity. ACE is a peptidyl dipeptidase that catalyzes the conversion of the inactive decapeptide angiotensin I to the vasoconstrictor substance angiotensin II. Angiotensin II is a potent peripheral vasoconstrictor that also stimulates aldosterone secretion by the adrenal cortex and provides negative feedback on renin secretion. ACE is identical to kininase II, an enzyme that degrades bradykinin, an endothelium-dependent vasodilator. Moexiprilat is about 1000 times as potent as moexipril in inhibiting ACE and kininase II. Inhibition of ACE results in decreased angiotensin II formation, leading to decreased vasoconstriction, increased plasma renin activity, and decreased aldosterone secretion. The latter results in diuresis and natriuresis and a small increase in serum potassium concentration (mean increases of about 0.25 mEq/L were seen when moexipril was used alone, see PRECAUTIONS).

Whether increased levels of bradykinin, a potent vasodepressor peptide, play a role in the therapeutic effects of moexipril remains to be elucidated. Although the principal mechanism of moexipril in blood pressure reduction is believed to be through the renin-angiotensin-aldosterone system, ACE inhibitors have some effect on blood pressure even in apparent low-renin hypertension. As is the case with other ACE inhibitors, however, the antihypertensive effect of moexipril is considerably smaller in black patients, a predominantly low-renin population, than in non-black hypertensive patients.

Pharmacokinetics and Metabolism

Pharmacokinetics: Moexipril's antihypertensive activity is almost entirely due to its deesterified metabolite, moexiprilat. Bioavailability of oral moexipril is about 13% compared to intravenous (I.V.) moexipril (both measuring the metabolite moexiprilat), and is markedly affected by food, which reduces the peak plasma level (C_{max}) and AUC (see Absorption). Moexipril should therefore be taken in a fasting state. The time of peak plasma concentration (T_{max}) of moexiprilat is about $1^1/_2$ hours and elimination half-life ($t^1/_2$) is estimated at 2 to 9 hours in various studies, the variability reflecting a complex elimination pattern that is not simply exponential. Like all ACE inhibitors, moexipril has a prolonged terminal elimination phase, presumably reflecting slow release of drug bound to the ACE. Accumulation of mo-

Continued on next page

Schwarz Pharma, Inc.—Cont.

exiprilat with repeated dosing is minimal, about 30%, compatible with a functional elimination $t^1/_2$ of about 12 hours. Over the dose range of 7.5 to 30 mg, pharmacokinetics are approximately dose proportional.

Absorption: Moexipril is incompletely absorbed, with bioavailability as moexiprilat of about 13%. Bioavailability varies with formulation and food intake which reduces C_{max} and AUC by about 70% and 40% respectively after the ingestion of a low-fat breakfast or by 80% and 50% respectively after the ingestion of a high-fat breakfast.

Distribution: The clearance (CL) for moexipril is 441 mL/min and for moexiprilat 232 mL/min with a $t^1/_2$ of 1.3 and 9.8 hours, respectively. Moexiprilat is about 50% protein bound. The volume of distribution of moexiprilat is about 183 liters.

Metabolism and Excretion: Moexipril is relatively rapidly converted to its active metabolite moexiprilat, but persists longer than some other ACE inhibitor prodrugs, such that its $t^1/_2$is over one hour and it has a significant AUC. Both moexipril and moexiprilat are converted to diketopiperazine derivatives and unidentified metabolites. After I.V. administration of moexipril, about 40% of the dose appears in urine as moexiprilat, about 26% as moexipril, with small amounts of the metabolites; about 20% of the I.V. dose appears in feces, principally as moexiprilat. After oral administration, only about 7% of the dose appears in urine as moexiprilat, about 1% as moexipril, with about 5% as other metabolites. Fifty-two percent of the dose is recovered in feces as moexiprilat and 1% as moexipril.

Special Populations:

Decreased Renal Function: The effective elimination $t^1/_2$ and AUC of both moexipril and moexiprilat are increased with decreasing renal function. There is insufficient information available to characterize this relationship fully, but at creatinine clearances in the range of 10 to 40 mL/min, the $t^1/_2$ of moexiprilat is increased by a factor of 3 to 4.

Decreased Hepatic Function: In patients with mild to moderate cirrhosis given single 15 mg doses of moexipril, the C_{max} of moexipril was increased by about 50% and the AUC increased by about 120%, while the C_{max} for moexiprilat was decreased by about 50% and the AUC increased by almost 300%.

Elderly Patients: In elderly male subjects (65–80 years old) with clinically normal renal and hepatic function, the AUC and C_{max} of moexiprilat is about 30% greater than those of younger subjects (19–42 years old).

Pharmacokinetic Interactions With Other Drugs:

No clinically important pharmacokinetic interactions occurred when UNIVASC was administered concomitantly with hydrochlorothiazide, digoxin, or cimetidine.

Pharmacodynamics and Clinical Effect

Single and multiple doses of 15 mg or more of UNIVASC gives sustained inhibition of plasma ACE activity of 80–90%, beginning within 2 hours and lasting 24 hours (80%).

In controlled trials, the peak effects of orally administered moexipril increased with the dose administered over a dose range of 7.5 to 60 mg, given once a day. Antihypertensive effects were first detectable about 1 hour after dosing, with a peak effect between 3 and 6 hours after dosing. Just before dosing (i.e., at trough), the antihypertensive effects were less prominently related to dose and the antihypertensive effect tended to diminish during the 24-hour dosing interval when the drug was administered once a day.

In multiple dose studies in the dose range of 7.5 to 30 mg once daily, UNIVASC lowered sitting diastolic and systolic blood pressure effects at trough by 3 to 6 mmHg and 4 to 11 mmHg, more than placebo, respectively. There was a tendency toward increased response with higher doses over this range. These effects are typical of ACE inhibitors but, to date, there are no trials of adequate size comparing moexipril with other antihypertensive agents.

The trough diastolic blood pressure effects of moexipril were approximately 3 to 6 mmHg in various studies. Generally, higher doses of moexipril leave a greater fraction of the peak blood pressure effect still present at trough. During dose titration, any decision as to the adequacy of a dosing regimen should be based on trough blood pressure measurements. If diastolic blood pressure control is not adequate at the end of the dosing interval, the dose can be increased or given as a divided (BID) regimen.

During chronic therapy, the antihypertensive effect of any dose of UNIVASC is generally evident within 2 weeks of treatment, with maximal reduction after 4 weeks. The antihypertensive effects of UNIVASC have been proven to continue during therapy for up to 24 months.

UNIVASC, like other ACE inhibitors, is less effective in decreasing trough blood pressures in blacks than in non-blacks. Placebo-corrected trough group mean diastolic blood pressure effects in blacks in the proposed dose range varied between +1 to −3 mmHg compared with responses in non-blacks of −4 to −6 mmHg.

The effectiveness of UNIVASC was not significantly influenced by patient age, gender, or weight. UNIVASC has been shown to have antihypertensive activity in both pre and postmenopausal women who have participated in placebo-controlled clinical trials.

Formal interaction studies with moexipril have not been carried out with antihypertensive agents other than thiazide diuretics. In these studies, the added effect of moexipril was similar to its effect as monotherapy. In general, ACE inhibitors have less than additive effects with beta-adrenergic blockers, presumably because both work by inhibiting the renin-angiotensin system.

INDICATIONS AND USAGE

UNIVASC is indicated for treatment of patients with hypertension. It may be used alone or in combination with thiazide diuretics.

In using UNIVASC, consideration should be given to the fact that another ACE inhibitor, captopril, has caused agranulocytosis, particularly in patients with renal impairment or collagen-vascular disease. Available data are insufficient to show that UNIVASC does not have a similar risk (see WARNINGS).

In considering use of UNIVASC, it should be noted that in controlled trials ACE inhibitors have an effect on blood pressure that is less in black patients than in non-blacks. In addition, ACE inhibitors (for which adequate data are available) cause a higher rate of angioedema in black than in non-black patients (see WARNINGS, Angioedema).

CONTRAINDICATIONS

UNIVASC is contraindicated in patients who are hypersensitive to this product and in patients with a history of angioedema related to previous treatment with an ACE inhibitor.

WARNINGS

Anaphylactoid and Possibly Related Reactions

Presumably because angiotensin-converting enzyme inhibitors affect the metabolism of eicosanoids and polypeptides, including endogenous bradykinin, patients recieving ACE inhibitors, including UNIVASC, may be subject to a variety of adverse reactions, some of them serious.

Angioedema: Angioedema involving the face, extremities, lips, tongue, glottis, and/or larynx has been reported in patients treated with ACE inhibitors, including UNIVASC. Symptoms suggestive of angioedema or facial edema occurred in <0.5% of moexipril-treated patients in placebo-controlled trials. None of the cases were considered life-threatening and all resolved either without treatment or with medication (antihistamines or glucocorticoids). One patient treated with hydrochlorothiazide alone experienced laryngeal edema. No instances of angioedema were reported in placebo-treated patients.

In cases of angioedema, treatment should be promptly discontinued and the patient carefully observed until the swelling disappears. In instances where swelling has been confined to the face and lips, the condition has generally resolved without treatment, although antihistamines have been useful in relieving symptoms.

Angioedema associated with involvement of the tongue, glottis, or larynx, may be fatal due to airway obstruction. Appropriate therapy, e.g., subcutaneous epinephrine solution 1:1000 (0.3 to 0.5 mL) and/or measures to ensure a patent airway, should be promptly provided (see ADVERSE REACTIONS).

Anaphylactoid Reactions During Desensitization: Two patients undergoing desensitizing treatment with hymenoptera venom while receiving ACE inhibitors sustained life-threatening anaphylactoid reactions. In the same patients, these reactions did not occur when ACE inhibitors were temporarily withheld, but they reappeared when the ACE inhibitors inadvertently readministered.

Anaphylactoid Reactions During Membrane Exposure: Anaphylactoid reactions have been reported in patients dialyzed with high-flux membranes and treated concomitantly with an ACE inhibitor. Anaphylactoid reactions have also been reported in patients undergoing low-density lipoprotein apheresis with dextran sulfate absorption.

Hypotension

UNIVASC can cause symptomatic hypotension, although, as with other ACE inhibitors, this is unusual in uncomplicated hypertensive patients treated with UNIVASC alone. Symptomatic hypotension was seen in 0.5% of patients given moexipril and led to discontinuation of therapy in about 0.25%. Symptomatic hypotension is most likely to occur in patients who have been salt- and volume-depleted as a result of prolonged diuretic therapy, dietary salt restriction, dialysis, diarrhea, or vomiting. Volume- and salt-depletion should be corrected and, in general, diuretics stopped, before initiating therapy with UNIVASC (see PRECAUTIONS, Drug Interactions, and ADVERSE REACTIONS).

In patients with congestive heart failure, with or without associated renal insufficiency, ACE inhibitor therapy may cause excessive hypotension, which may be associated with oliguria or progressive azotemia, and rarely, with acute renal failure and death. In these patients, UNIVASC therapy should be started under close medical supervision, and patients should be followed closely for the first two weeks of treatment and whenever the dose of moexipril or an accompanying diuretic is increased. Care in avoiding hypotension should also be taken in patients with ischemic heart disease, aortic stenosis, or cerebrovascular disease,in whom an excessive decrease in blood pressure could result in a myocardial infarction or a cerebrovascular accident.

If hypotension occurs, the patient should be placed in a supine position and, if necessary, treated with an intravenous infusion of normal saline. UNIVASC treatment usually can be continued following restoration of blood pressure and volume.

Neutropenia/Agranulocytosis

Another ACE inhibitor, captopril, has been shown to cause agranulocytosis and bone marrow depression, rarely in patients with uncomplicated hypertension, but more frequently in hypertensive patients with renal impairment, especially if they also have a collagen-vascular disease such as systemic lupus erythematosus or scleroderma. Although there were no instances of severe neutropenia (absolute neutrophil count $<500/mm^3$) among patients given UNIVASC, as with other ACE inhibitors, monitoring of white blood cell counts should be considered for patients who have collagen-vascular disease, especially if the disease is associated with impaired renal function. Available data from clinical trials of UNIVASC are insufficient to show that UNIVASC does not cause agranulocytosis at rates similar to captopril.

Fetal/Neonatal Morbidity and Mortality

ACE inhibitors can cause fetal and neonatal morbidity and death when administered to pregnant women. Several dozen cases have been reported in the world literature. When pregnancy is detected, ACE inhibitors should be discontinued as soon as possible.

The use of ACE inhibitors during the second and third trimesters of pregnancy has been associated with fetal and neonatal injury, including hypotension, neonatal skull hypoplasia, anuria, reversible or irreversible renal failure, and death. Oligohydramnios has also been reported, presumably resulting from decreased fetal renal function; oligohydramnios in this setting has been associated with fetal limb contractures, craniofacial deformation, and hypoplastic lung development. Prematurity, intrauterine growth retardation, and patent ductus arteriosus have also been reported, although it is not clear whether these were caused by the ACE inhibitor exposure.

Fetal and neonatal morbidity do not appear to have resulted from intrauterine ACE inhibitor exposure limited to the first trimester. Mothers who have used ACE inhibitors only during the first trimester should be informed of this. Nonetheless, when patients become pregnant, physicians should make every effort to discontinue the use of moexipril as soon as possible. Rarely (probably less often than once in every thousand pregnancies), no alternative to ACE inhibitors will be found. In these rare cases, the mothers should be apprised of the potential hazards to their fetuses, and serial ultrasound examinations should be performed to assess the intraamniotic environment.

If oligohydramnios is observed, moexipril should be discontinued unless it is considered life-saving for the mother. Contraction stress testing (CST), a non-stress test (NST), or biophysical profiling (BPP) may be appropriate, depending upon the week of pregnancy. Patients and physicians should be aware, however, that oligohydramnios may not be detected until after the fetus has sustained irreversible injury.

Infants with histories of *in utero* exposure to ACE inhibitors should be closely observed for hypotension, oliguria, and hyperakalemia. If oliguria occurs, attention should be directed toward support of blood pressure and renal perfusion. Exchange transfusion or peritoneal dialysis may be required as means of reversing hypotension and/or substituting for disordered renal function.

Theoretically, the ACE inhibitor could be removed from the neonatal circulation by exchange transfusion, but no experience with this procedure has been reported.

No embryotoxic, fetotoxic, or teratogenic effects were seen in rats or in rabbits treated with up to 90.9 and 0.7 times, respectively, the Maximum Recommended Human Dose (MRHD) on a mg/m^2 basis.

Hepatic Failure

Rarely, ACE inhibitors have been associated with a syndrome that starts with cholestatic jaundice and progresses to fulminant hepatic necrosis and sometimes death. The mechanism of this syndrome is not understood. Patients receiving ACE inhibitors who develop jaundice or marked elevations of hepatic enzymes should discontinue the ACE inhibitor and receive appropriate medical follow-up.

PRECAUTIONS

General

Impaired Renal Function: As a consequence of inhibition of the reninangiotensin-aldosterone system, changes in renal function may be anticipated in susceptible individuals. There is no clinical experience of UNIVASC in the treatment of hypertension in patients with renal failure.

Some hypertensive patients with no apparent preexisting renal vascular disease have developed increases in blood

urea nitrogen and serum creatinine, usually minor and transient, especially when UNIVASC has been given concomitantly with a thiazide diuretic. This is more likely to occur in patients with preexisting renal impairment. There may be a need for dose adjustment of UNIVASC and/or the discontinuation of the thiazide diuretic.

Evaluation of hypertensive patients should always include assessment of renal function (see DOSAGE AND ADMINISTRATION).

Hypertensive Patients With Congestive Heart Failure: In hypertensive patients with severe congestive heart failure,-whose renal function may depend on the activity of the renin-angiotensin-aldosterone system, treatment with ACE inhibitors, including UNIVASC, may be associated with oliguria and/or progressive azotemia and, rarely, acute renal failure and/or death.

Hypertensive Patients With Renal Artery Stenosis: In hypertensive patients with unilateral or bilateral renal artery stenosis, increases in blood urea nitrogen and serum creatinine have been observed in some patients following ACE inhibitor therapy. These increases were almost always reversible upon discontinuation of the ACE inhibitor and/or diuretic therapy. In such patients, renal function should be monitored during the first few weeks of therapy.

Hyperkalemia: In clinical trials, persistent hyperkalemia (serum potassium above 5.4 mEq/L) occurred in approximately 1.3% of hypertensive patients receiving UNIVASC. Risk factors for the development of hyperkalemia with ACE inhibitors include renal insufficiency, diabetes mellitus, and the concomitant use of potassium-sparing diuretics, potassium supplements, and/or potassium-containing salt substitutes, which should be used cautiously, if at all, with UNIVASC (see PRECAUTIONS, Drug Interactions).

Surgery/Anesthesia: In patients undergoing major surgery or during anesthesia with agents that produce hypotension, moexipril may block the effects of compensatory renin release. If hypotension occurs in this setting and is considered to be due to this mechanism, it can be corrected by volume expansion.

Cough: Presumably due to the inhibition of the degradation of endogenous bradykinin, persistent nonproductive cough has been reported with all ACE inhibitors, always resolving after discontinuation of therapy. ACE inhibitor-induced cough should be considered in the differential diagnosis of cough. In controlled trials with moexipril, cough was present in 6.1% of moexipril patients and 2.2% of patients given placebo.

Information for Patients

Food: Patients should be advised to take moexipril one hour before meals. (see CLINICAL PHARMACOLOGY and DOSAGE AND ADMINISTRATION).

Angioedema: Angioedema, including laryngeal edema, may occur with treatment with ACE inhibitors, usually occuring early in therapy (within the first month). Patients should be so advised and told to report immediately any signs or symptoms suggesting angioedema (swelling of the face, extremities, eyes, lips, tongue, difficulty in breathing) and to take no more UNIVASC until they have consulted with the prescribing physician.

Symptomatic Hypotension: Patients should be cautioned that lightheadedness can occur with UNIVASC, especially during the first few days of therapy. If fainting occurs, the patient should stop taking UNIVASC and consult the prescribing physician.

All patients should be cautioned that excessive perspiration and dehydration may lead to an excessive fall in blood pressure because of reduction in fluid volume. Other causes of volume depletion such as vomiting or diarrhea may also lead to a fall in blood pressure; patients should be advised to consult their physician if they develop these conditions.

Hyperkalemia: Patients should be told not to use potassium supplements or salt substitutes containing potassium without consulting their physician.

Neutropenia: Patients should be told to report promptly any indication of infection (e.g., sore throat, fever) that could be a sign of neutropenia.

Pregnancy: Female patients of childbearing age should be told about the consequences of second- and third- trimester exposure to ACE inhibitors and should also be told that these consequences do not appear to have resulted from intrauterine ACE inhibitor exposure that has been limited to the first trimester. Patients should be asked to report pregnancies to their physicians as soon as possible.

Drug Interactions

Diuretics: Excessive reductions in blood pressure may occur in patients on diuretic therapy when ACE inhibitors are started. The possibility of hypotensive effects with UNIVASC can be minimized by discontinuing diuretic therapy for several days or cautiously increasing salt intake before initiation of treatment with UNIVASC. If this is not possible, the starting dose of moexpril should be reduced. (see WARNINGS and DOSAGE AND ADMINISTRATION).

Potassium Supplements and Potassium-Sparing Diuretics: UNIVASC can increase serum potassium because it decreases aldosterone secretion. Use of potassium-sparing diuretics (spironolactone, triamterene, amiloride) or potassium supplements concomitantly with ACE inhibitors can increase the risk of hyperkalemia. Therefore, if concomitant use of such agents is indicated, they should be given with caution and the patient's serum potassium should be monitored.

Oral Anticoagulants: Interaction studies with warfarin failed to identify any clinically important effect on the serum concentrations of the anticogulant or on its anticoagulant effect.

Lithium: Increased serum lithium levels and symptoms of lithium toxicity have been reported in patients receiving ACE inhibitors during therapy with lithium. These drugs should be coadministered with caution, and frequent monitoring of serum lithium levels is recommended. If a diuretic is also used, the risk of lithium toxicity may be increased.

Other Agents: No clinically important pharmacokinetic interactions occured when UNIVASC was administered concomitantly with hydrochlorothiazide, digoxin, or cimetidine.

UNIVASC has been used in clinical trails concomitantly with calcium-channel-blocking agents, diuretics, H_2 blockers, digoxin, oral hypoglycemic agents, and cholesterol-lowering agents. There was no evidence of clinically important adverse interactions.

Carcinogenesis, Mutagenesis, Impairment of Fertility

No evidence of carcinogenicity was detected in long-term studies in mice and rats at doses up to 14 or 27.3 times the Maximum Recommended Human Dose (MRHD) on a mg/m^2 basis.

No mutagenicity was detected in the Ames test and microbial reverse mutation assay, with and without metabolic activation, or in an *in vivo* nucleus anomaly test. However, increased chromosomal aberration frequency in Chinese hamster ovary cells was detected under metabolic activation conditions at a 20-hour harvest time.

Reproduction studies have been performed in rabbits at oral doses up to 0.7 times the MRHD on a mg/m^2 basis, and in rats up to 90.9 times the MRHD on a mg/m^2 basis. No indication of impaired fertility, reproductive toxicity, or teratogenicity was observed.

Pregnancy

Pregnancy Categories C (first trimester) and D (second and third trimesters). See WARNINGS, Fetal/Neonatal Morbidity and Mortality.

Nursing Mothers

It is not known whether UNIVASC is excreted in human milk. Because many drugs are excreted in human milk, caution should be exercised when UNIVASC is given to a nursing mother.

Geriatric Use

Of the patients who received UNIVASC in controlled clinical studies, 33% were 65 years of age or older. No overall differences in effectiveness or safety were observed between these patients and younger patients. In elderly patients receiving UNIVASC, plasma levels of drug are slightly higher and renal clearance is reduced when compared to younger patients, but this did not have detectable consequences.

Pediatric Use

Safety and effectiveness of UNIVASC in pediatric patients have not been established.

ADVERSE REACTIONS

UNIVASC has been evaluated for safety in more than 2500 patients with hypertension, more than 250 of these patients were treated for approximately one year. The overall incidence of reported adverse events was only slightly greater in patients treated with UNIVASC than patients treated with placebo.

Reported adverse experiences were usually mild and transient, and there were no differences in adverse reaction rates related to gender, race, age, duration of therapy, or total daily dosage within the range of 3.75 mg to 60 mg. Discontinuation of therapy because of adverse experiences was required in 3.4% of patients treated with UNIVASC and in 1.8% of patients treated with placebo. The most common reasons for, discontinutation in patients treated with UNIVASC were cough (0.7%) and dizziness (0.4%).

All adverse experiences considered at least possibly related to treatment that occurred at any dose in placebo-controlled trials of once-daily dosing in more than 1% of patients treated with UNIVASC alone and that were at least as frequent in the UNIVASC group as in the placebo group are shown in the following table:

ADVERSE EVENTS IN PLACEBO-CONTROLLED STUDIES

ADVERSE EVENT	UNIVASC (N=674) N(%)	PLACEBO (N=226) N(%)
Cough Increased	41(6.1)	5(2.2)
Dizziness	29(4.3)	5(2.2)
Diarrhea	21(3.1)	5(2.2)
Flu Syndrome	21(3.1)	0(0)
Fatigue	16(2.4)	4(1.8)
Pharyngitis	12(1.8)	2(0.9)
Flushing	11(1.6)	0(0)
Rash	11(1.6)	2(0.9)
Myalgia	9(1.3)	0(0)

Other adverse events occurring in more than 1% of patients on moexipril that were at least as frequent on placebo include: headache, upper respiratory infection, pain, rhinitis, dyspepsia, nausea, peripheral edema, sinusitis, chest pain, and urinary frequency. See WARNINGS and PRECAUTIONS for discussion of anaphylactoid reactions, angioedema, hypotension, neutropenia/agranulocytosis, second and third trimester fetal/neonatal morbidity and mortality, hyperkalemia, and cough.

Other potentially important adverse experiences reported in controlled or uncontrolled clinical trials in less than 1% of moexipril patients or that have been attributed to other ACE inhibitors include the following:

Cardiovascular: Symptomatic hypotension, postural hypotension, or syncope were seen in 9/1750 (0.51%) patients; these reactions led to discontinuation of therapy in controlled trials in 3/1254 (0.24%) patients who had received UNIVASC monotherapy and in 1/344 (0.3%) patients who had received UNIVASC with hydrochlorothiazide (see PRECAUTIONS and WARNINGS). Other adverse events included angina/myocardial infarction, palpitations, rhythm disturbances, and cerebrovascular accident.

Renal: Of hypertensive patients with no apparent preexisting renal disease, 1% of patients receiving UNIVASC alone and 2% of patients receiving UNIVASC with hydrochlorothiazide experienced increases in serum creatinine to at least 140% of their baseline values (see PRECAUTIONS and DOSAGE AND ADMINISTRATION).

Gastrointestinal: Abdominal pain, constipation, vomiting, appetite/weight change, dry mouth, pancreatitis, hepatitis.

Respiratory: Bronchospasm, dyspnea.

Urogenital: Renal insufficiency, oliguria.

Dermatologic Apparent hypersensitivity reactions manifested by urticaria, rash, pemphigus, pruritus, photosensitivity.

Neurological and Psychiatric: Drowsiness, sleep disturbances, nervousness, mood changes, anxiety.

Other: Angioedema (see WARNINGS), taste disturbances, tinnitus, sweating, malaise, arthralgia, hemolytic anemia.

Clinical Laboratory Test Findings

Creatinine and Blood Urea Nitrogen: As with other ACE inhibitors, minor increases in blood urea nitrogen or serum creatinine, reversible upon disontinuation of therapy, were observed in approximately 1% of patients with essential hypertension who were treated with UNIVASC. Increases are more likely to occur in patients receiving concomitant diuretics and in patients with compromised renal function (see PRECAUTIONS, General).

Other (causal relationship unknown): Clinically important changes in standard laboratory tests were rarely associated with UNIVASC administration.

Elevations of liver enzymes and uric acid have been reported. In trials, less than 1% of moexipril-treated patients discontinued UNIVASC treatment because of laboratory abnormalities. The incidence of abnormal laboratory values with moexipril was similar to that in the placebo-treated group.

OVERDOSAGE

Human overdoses of moexipril have not been reported. In case reports of overdoses with other ACE inhibitors, hypotension has been the principal adverse effect noted. Single oral doses of 2 g/kg moexipril were associated with significant lethality in mice. Rats, however, tolerated single oral doses of up to 3 g/kg.

No data are available to suggest that physiological maneuvers (e.g., maneuvers to change the pH of the urine) would accelerate elimination of moexipril and its metabolites. The dialyzability of moexipril is not known.

Angiotensin II could presumably serve as a specific antagonist-antidote in the setting of moexipril overdose, but angiotensin II is essentially unavailable outside of research facili-

Continued on next page

Schwarz Pharma, Inc.—Cont.

ties. Because the hypotensive effect of moexipril is achieved through vasodilation and effective hypovolemia, it is reasonable to treat moexipril overdose by infusion of normal saline solution. In addition, renal function and serum potassium should be monitored.

DOSAGE AND ADMINISTRATION

Hypertension

The recommended initial dose of UNIVASC in patients not receiving diuretics is 7.5 mg, one hour prior to meals, once daily. Dosage should be adjusted according to blood pressure response. The antihypertensive effect of UNIVASC may diminish towards the end of the dosing interval. Blood pressure should, therefore, be measured just prior to dosing to determine whether satisfactory blood pressure control is obtained. If control is not adequate, increased dose or divided dosing can be tried. The recommended dose range is 7.5 to 30 mg daily, administered in one or two divided doses one hour before meals. Total daily doses above 60 mg a day have not been studied in hypertensive patients.

In patients who are currently being treated with a diuretic, symptomatic hypotension may occasionally occur following the initial dose of UNIVASC. The diuretic should, if possible, be discontinued for 2 to 3 days before therapy with UNIVASC is begun, to reduce the likelihood of hypotension (see WARNINGS). If the patient's blood pressure is not controlled with UNIVASC alone, diuretic therapy may then be reinstituted. If diuretic therapy cannot be discontinued, an initial dose of 3.75 mg of UNIVASC should be used with medical supervision until blood pressure has stabilized (see WARNINGS and PRECAUTIONS, Drug Interactions).

Dosage Adjustment in Renal Impairment

For patients with a creatinine clearance ≤40 mL/min/1.73 m^2, an initial dose of 3.75 mg once daily should be given cautiously. Doses may be titrated upward to a maximum daily dose of 15 mg.

HOW SUPPLIED

UNIVASC (moexipril hydrochloride) 7.5 mg tablets are pink colored, biconvex, film-coated and scored with engraved code **707** on the unscored side and **SP** above and **7.5** below the score. They are supplied as follows:

Bottles of 90 (Unit-of-Use)   NDC 0091-3707-09
Bottles of 100   NDC 0091-3707-01

UNIVASC (moexipril hydrochloride) 15 mg tablets are salmon colored, biconvex, film-coated, and scored with engraved code **715** on the unscored side and **SP** above and **15** below the score. They are supplied as follows:

Bottles of 90 (Unit-of-Use)   NDC 0091-3715-09
Bottles of 100   NDC 0091-3715-01

Store, tightly closed, at controlled room temperature.
Protect from excessive moisture.
If product package is subdivided, dispense in tight containers as described in USP-NF.

Caution: Federal law prohibits dispensing without prescription.

Shown in Product Identification Guide, page 335

G.D. Searle & Co.
BOX 5110
CHICAGO, IL 60680-5110

Direct Inquiries to:
(800) 323-1603

For Medical Information Contact:
Generally:
G.D. Searle & Co.
Healthcare Information Services
5200 Old Orchard Road
Skokie, IL 60077
In Emergencies:
Outside IL:
(800) 323-4204 (business hours)
(847) 982-7000 (at other times)
Within IL:
(847) 982-7000

Sales and Ordering:
(800) 323-1603

Alphabetic Product Listing
Product, ID# (NDC*), Form, Strength
Aldactazide, 1011, Tablet, 25 mg/25 mg
Aldactazide, 1021, Tablet, 50 mg/50 mg
Aldactone, 1001, Tablet, 25 mg
Aldactone, 1041, Tablet, 50 mg
Aldactone, 1031, Tablet, 100 mg
Ambien Ⓒ, 5401, Tablet, 5 mg
Ambien Ⓒ, 5421, Tablet, 10 mg
Brevicon 21-day, (0108), Wallette, Tablet, 0.5 mg/0.035 mg

Brevicon 28-day, (0110), Wallette, Tablet, 0.5 mg/0.035 mg
Calan, 40 (1771), Tablet, 40 mg
Calan, 80 (1851), Tablet, 80 mg
Calan, 120 (1861), Tablet, 120 mg
Calan SR, 120 (1901), Caplet, 120 mg
Calan SR, 180 (1911), Caplet, 180 mg
Calan SR, 240 (1891), Caplet, 240 mg
Covera-HS 180, (2011), Tablets, 180 mg
Covera-HS 240, (2021), Tablets, 240 mg
Cytotec, 1451, Tablet, 100 mcg
Cytotec, 1461, Tablet, 200 mcg
Daypro, 1381, Caplet, 600 mg
Demulen 1/35-21, Compack, 151, Tablet, 1 mg/35 mcg
Demulen 1/35-28, Compack, 151 (0161), Tablet, 1 mg/35 mcg
Demulen 1/50-21, Compack, 71, Tablet, 1 mg/50 mcg
Demulen 1/50-28, Compack, 71 (0081), Tablet, 1 mg/50 mcg
Flagyl, 1831, Tablet, 250 mg
Flagyl 500 (1821), Tablet, 500 mg
Flagyl 375, (1942), Capsule, 375 mg
Kerlone, 10 (5101), Tablet, 10 mg
Kerlone, 20 (5201), Tablet, 20 mg
Lomotil Ⓒ, 61, Tablet, 2.5 mg/0.025 mg
Lomotil Ⓒ, Liquid, 66, 2.5 mg/0.025 mg per 5 ml
Maxaquin, 400, (1651) Tablet, 400 mg
NOR-QD, 0107, Dispensers, Tablets, 0.35 mg
Norinyl 1+35 21-day, (0109), Wallette, Tablets, 1 mg/0.035 mg
Norinyl 1+35 28-day, (0111), Wallette, Tablets, 1 mg/0.035 mg
Norinyl 1+50 21-day, (0100), Wallette, Tablets, 1 mg/0.05 mg
Norinyl 1+50 28-day, (0101), Wallette, Tablets, 1 mg/0.05 mg
Norpace, 2752, Capsule, 100 mg
Norpace, 2762, Capsule, 150 mg
Norpace CR, 2732, Capsule, 100 mg
Norpace CR, 2742, Capsule, 150 mg
Synarel, Liquid, (2260), Bottle, 2 mg/ml
Tri-Norinyl 21-day, (0114), Wallette, Tablets, 0.5 mg/0.035 mg
Tri-Norinyl 28-day, (0115), Wallette, Tablets, 0.5 mg/0.035 mg

* When the product ID # is not the same as the NDC #, the NDC # appears in parentheses.

Product Information Available on Request
Flagyl Tablets

Various educational materials are available for physicians, pharmacists, nurses, physicians' assistants, and patients (through the physician). Please ask your Searle representative for information about these materials.

ALDACTAZIDE®
[al-dac 'tuh "zīde]
(spironolactone with hydrochlorothiazide)

℞

WARNING

Spironolactone, an ingredient of Aldactazide, has been shown to be a tumorigen in chronic toxicity studies in rats (see *Warnings*). Aldactazide should be used only in those conditions described under *Indications and Usage*. Unnecessary use of this drug should be avoided.

Fixed-dose combination drugs are not indicated for initial therapy of edema or hypertension. Edema or hypertension requires therapy titrated to the individual patient. If the fixed combination represents the dosage so determined, its use may be more convenient in patient management. The treatment of hypertension and edema is not static but must be reevaluated as conditions in each patient warrant.

DESCRIPTION

Aldactazide oral tablets contain:

spironolactone .... 25 mg
hydrochlorothiazide .... 25 mg
or
spironolactone .... 50 mg
hydrochlorothiazide .... 50 mg

Spironolactone (Aldactone®), an aldosterone antagonist, is 17- hydroxy-7α-mercapto-3-oxo-17α-pregn-4-ene- 21- carboxylic acid γ-lactone acetate and has the following structural formula:
[See first chemical structure at top of next column.]
Spironolactone is practically insoluble in water, soluble in alcohol, and freely soluble in benzene and in chloroform.

Hydrochlorothiazide, a diuretic and antihypertensive, is 6-chloro-3, 4-dihydro-2H-1,2,4-benzothiadiazine-7-sulfonamide 1,1-dioxide and has the following structural formula:

Hydrochlorothiazide is slightly soluble in water and freely soluble in sodium hydroxide solution.

Inactive ingredients include calcium sulfate, corn starch, flavor, hydroxypropyl cellulose, hydroxypropyl methylcellulose, iron oxide, magnesium stearate, polyethylene glycol, povidone, and titanium dioxide.

CLINICAL PHARMACOLOGY

Mechanism of action: Aldactazide is a combination of two diuretic agents with different but complementary mechanisms and sites of action, thereby providing additive diuretic and antihypertensive effects. Additionally, the spironolactone component helps to minimize the potassium loss characteristically induced by the thiazide component.

The diuretic effect of spironolactone is mediated through its action as a specific pharmacologic antagonist of aldosterone, primarily by competitive binding of receptors at the aldosterone-dependent sodium-potassium exchange site in the distal convoluted renal tubule. Hydrochlorothiazide promotes the excretion of sodium and water primarily by inhibiting their reabsorption in the cortical diluting segment of the distal renal tubule.

Aldactazide is effective in significantly lowering the systolic and diastolic blood pressure in many patients with essential hypertension, even when aldosterone secretion is within normal limits.

Both spironolactone and hydrochlorothiazide reduce exchangeable sodium, plasma volume, body weight, and blood pressure. The diuretic and antihypertensive effects of the individual components are potentiated when spironolactone and hydrochlorothiazide are given concurrently.

Pharmacokinetics: Spironolactone is rapidly and extensively metabolized. Sulfur-containing products are the predominant metabolites and are thought to be primarily responsible, together with spironolactone, for the therapeutic effects of the drug. The following pharmacokinetic data were obtained from 12 healthy volunteers following the administration of 100 mg of spironolactone (Aldactone film-coated tablets) daily for 15 days. On the 15th day, spironolactone was given immediately after a low-fat breakfast and blood was drawn thereafter.

	Accumulation Factor: AUC (0–24 hr, day 15)/AUC (0–24 hr, day 1)	Mean Peak Serum Concentration	Mean (SD) Post-Steady State Half-life
7-α-(thiomethyl) spirolactone (TMS)	1.25	391 ng/mL at 3.2 hr	13.8 hr (6.4) (terminal)
6-β-hydroxy-7-α- (thiomethyl) spirolactone (HTMS)	1.50	125 ng/mL at 5.1 hr	15.0 hr (4.0) (terminal)
Canrenone (C)	1.41	181 ng/mL at 4.3 hr	16.5 hr (6.3) (terminal)
Spironolactone	1.30	80 ng/mL at 2.6 hr	Approximately 1.4 hr (0.5) (β half-life)

The pharmacological activity of spironolactone metabolites in man is not known. However, in the adrenalectomized rat the antimineralocorticoid activities of the metabolites C, TMS, and HTMS, relative to spironolactone, were 1.10, 1.28, and 0.32, respectively. Relative to spironolactone, their binding affinities to the aldosterone receptors in rat kidney slices were 0.19, 0.86, and 0.06, respectively.

In humans the potencies of TMS and 7-α-thiospirolactone in reversing the effects of the synthetic mineralocorticoid, fludrocortisone, on urinary electrolyte composition were 0.33 and 0.26, respectively, relative to spironolactone. However, since the serum concentrations of these steroids were not determined, their incomplete absorption and/or first-pass metabolism could not be ruled out as a reason for their reduced *in vivo* activities.

Both spironolactone and canrenone are more than 90% bound to plasma proteins. The metabolites are excreted primarily in the urine and secondarily in bile.

The effect of food on spironolactone absorption (two 100-mg Aldactone tablets) was assessed in a single dose study of 9 healthy, drug-free volunteers. Food increased the bioavailability of unmetabolized spironolactone by almost 100%. The clinical importance of this finding is not known.

Hydrochlorothiazide is rapidly absorbed following oral administration. Onset of action of hydrochlorothiazide is observed within one hour and persists for 6 to 12 hours. Hydrochlorothiazide plasma concentrations attain peak levels at one to two hours and decline with a half-life of four to five hours. Hydrochlorothiazide undergoes only slight metabolic alteration and is excreted in urine. It is distributed throughout the extracellular space, with essentially no tissue accumulation except in the kidney.

INDICATIONS AND USAGE

Spironolactone, an ingredient of Aldactazide, has been shown to be a tumorigen in chronic toxicity studies in rats (see *Warnings* section). Aldactazide should be used only in those conditions described below. Unnecessary use of this drug should be avoided.

Aldactazide is indicated for:

Edematous conditions for patients with:

Congestive heart failure: For the management of edema and sodium retention when the patient is only partially responsive to, or is intolerant of, other therapeutic measures. The treatment of diuretic-induced hypokalemia in patients with congestive heart failure when other measures are considered inappropriate. The treatment of patients with congestive heart failure taking digitalis when other therapies are considered inadequate or inappropriate.

Cirrhosis of the liver accompanied by edema and/or ascites: Aldosterone levels may be exceptionally high in this condition. Aldactazide is indicated for maintenance therapy together with bed rest and the restriction of fluid and sodium.

The nephrotic syndrome: For nephrotic patients when treatment of the underlying disease, restriction of fluid and sodium intake, and the use of other diuretics do not provide an adequate response.

Essential hypertension

For patients with essential hypertension in whom other measures are considered inadequate or inappropriate. In hypertensive patients for the treatment of a diuretic-induced hypokalemia when other measures are considered inappropriate.

Usage in Pregnancy. The routine use of diuretics in an otherwise healthy woman is inappropriate and exposes mother and fetus to unnecessary hazard. Diuretics do not prevent development of toxemia of pregnancy, and there is no satisfactory evidence that they are useful in the treatment of developing toxemia.

Edema during pregnancy may arise from pathologic causes or from the physiologic and mechanical consequences of pregnancy. Aldactazide is indicated in pregnancy when edema is due to pathologic causes just as it is in the absence of pregnancy (however, see *Warnings* section). Dependent edema in pregnancy, resulting from restriction of venous return by the expanded uterus, is properly treated through elevation of the lower extremities and use of support hose; use of diuretics to lower intravascular volume in this case is unsupported and unnecessary. There is hypervolemia during normal pregnancy which is not harmful to either the fetus or the mother (in the absence of cardiovascular disease), but which is associated with edema, including generalized edema, in the majority of pregnant women. If this edema produces discomfort, increased recumbency will often provide relief. In rare instances, this edema may cause extreme discomfort which is not relieved by rest. In these cases, a short course of diuretics may provide relief and may be appropriate.

CONTRAINDICATIONS

Aldactazide is contraindicated in patients with anuria, acute renal insufficiency, significant impairment of renal excretory function, or hyperkalemia, and in patients who are allergic to thiazide diuretics or to other sulfonamide-derived drugs. Aldactazide may also be contraindicated in acute or severe hepatic failure.

WARNINGS

Potassium supplementation, either in the form of medication or as a diet rich in potassium, should not ordinarily be given in association with Aldactazide therapy. Excessive potassium intake may cause hyperkalemia in patients receiving Aldactazide (see *Precautions* section). Aldactazide should not be administered concurrently with other potassium-sparing diuretics. Spironolactone, when used with ACE inhibitors, even in the presence of a diuretic, has been associated with severe hyperkalemia. Extreme caution should be exercised when Aldactazide is given concomitantly with ACE inhibitors (see *Precautions*).

Sulfonamide derivatives, including thiazides, have been reported to exacerbate or activate systemic lupus erythematosus.

Spironolactone has been shown to be a tumorigen in chronic toxicity studies performed in rats, with its proliferative effects manifested on endocrine organs and the liver. In one study using 25, 75, and 250 times the usual daily human dose (2 mg/kg) there was a statistically significant dose-related increase in benign adenomas of the thyroid and testes. In female rats there was a statistically significant increase in malignant mammary tumors at the mid-dose only. In male rats there was a dose-related increase in proliferative changes in the liver. At the highest dosage level (500 mg/kg), the range of effects included hepatocytomegaly, hyperplastic nodules, and hepatocellular carcinoma; the last was not statistically significant at a value of p = 0.05. A dose-related (above 20 mg/kg/day) incidence of myelocytic leukemia was observed in rats fed daily doses of potassium canrenoate for a period of one year. In long-term (two-year) oral carcinogenicity studies of potassium canrenoate in the rat, myelocytic leukemia and hepatic, thyroid, testicular, and mammary tumors were observed. Potassium canrenoate did not produce a mutagenic effect in tests using bacteria or yeast. It did produce a positive mutagenic effect in several *in vitro* tests in mammalian cells following metabolic activation. In an *in vivo* mammalian system potassium canrenoate was not mutagenic. Canrenone and canrenoic acid are the major metabolites of potassium canrenoate. Spironolactone is also metabolized to canrenone. An increased incidence of leukemia was not observed in chronic rat toxicity studies conducted with spironolactone at doses up to 500 mg/kg/day.

PRECAUTIONS

Patients receiving Aldactazide therapy should be carefully evaluated for possible disturbances of fluid and electrolyte balance. Hyperkalemia may occur in patients with impaired renal function or excessive potassium intake and can cause cardiac irregularities, which may be fatal. Consequently, no potassium supplement should ordinarily be given with Aldactazide. Hyperkalemia can be treated promptly by the rapid intravenous administration of glucose (20% to 50%) and regular insulin, using 0.25 to 0.5 units of insulin per gram of glucose. This is a temporary measure to be repeated as required. Aldactazide use should be discontinued and potassium intake (including dietary potassium) restricted.

Hypokalemia may develop as a result of profound diuresis, particularly when Aldactazide is used concomitantly with loop diuretics, glucocorticoids, or ACTH. Hypokalemia may exaggerate the effects of digitalis therapy. Potassium depletion may induce signs of digitalis intoxication at previously tolerated dosage levels.

Concomitant administration of potassium-sparing diuretics and ACE inhibitors or indomethacin has been associated with severe hyperkalemia.

Warning signs of possible fluid and electrolyte imbalance include dryness of the mouth, thirst, weakness, lethargy, drowsiness, restlessness, muscle pains or cramps, muscular fatigue, hypotension, oliguria, tachycardia, and gastrointestinal symptoms.

Aldactazide therapy may cause a transient elevation of BUN. This appears to represent a concentration phenomenon rather than renal toxicity, since the BUN level returns to normal after use of Aldactazide is discontinued. Progressive elevation of BUN is suggestive of the presence of preexisting renal impairment.

Reversible hyperchloremic metabolic acidosis, usually in association with hyperkalemia, has been reported to occur in some patients with decompensated hepatic cirrhosis, even in the presence of normal renal function.

Dilutional hyponatremia, manifested by dryness of the mouth, thirst, lethargy, and drowsiness, and confirmed by a low serum sodium level, may be induced, especially when Aldactazide is administered in combination with other diuretics. A true low-salt syndrome may rarely develop with Aldactazide therapy and may be manifested by increasing mental confusion similar to that observed with hepatic coma. This syndrome is differentiated from dilutional hyponatremia in that it does not occur with obvious fluid retention. Its treatment requires that diuretic therapy be discontinued and sodium administered.

Gynecomastia may develop in association with the use of spironolactone; physicians should be alert to its possible onset. The development of gynecomastia appears to be related to both dosage level and duration of therapy and is normally reversible when Aldactazide is discontinued. In rare instances some breast enlargement may persist when Aldactazide is discontinued.

Thiazides have been demonstrated to alter the metabolism of uric acid and carbohydrates, with possible development of hyperuricemia, gout, and decreased glucose tolerance. Thiazides may temporarily exaggerate abnormalities of glucose metabolism in diabetic patients or cause abnormalities to appear in patients with latent diabetes.

The antihypertensive effects of hydrochlorothiazide may be enhanced in patients who have undergone sympathectomy.

Pathologic changes in the parathyroid gland with hypercalcemia and hypophosphatemia have been observed in patients on prolonged thiazide therapy. Thiazides may also decrease serum PBI levels without evidence of alteration of thyroid function.

A determination of serum electrolytes to detect possible electrolyte imbalance should be performed at periodic intervals.

Both spironolactone and hydrochlorothiazide reduce the vascular responsiveness to norepinephrine. Therefore, caution should be exercised in the management of patients subjected to regional or general anesthesia while they are being treated with Aldactazide. Thiazides may also increase the responsiveness to tubocurarine.

Spironolactone has been shown to increase the half-life of digoxin. This may result in increased serum digoxin levels and subsequent digitalis toxicity. It may be necessary to reduce the maintenance and digitalization doses when spironolactone is administered, and the patient should be carefully monitored to avoid over- or underdigitalization.

Hydrochlorothiazide may raise the concentration of blood uric acid. Dosage adjustment of antigout medications may be necessary. Hydrochlorothiazide may also raise blood glucose concentrations. Dosage adjustments of insulin or hypoglycemic medications may be necessary. Concurrent use of diuretics with lithium is not recommended as it may produce lithium toxicity.

Several reports of possible interference with digoxin radioimmunoassays by spironolactone, or its metabolites, have appeared in the literature. Neither the extent nor the potential clinical significance of its interference (which may be assay-specific) has been fully established.

Usage in Pregnancy. Spironolactone or its metabolites may, and hydrochlorothiazide does, cross the placental barrier. Therefore, the use of Aldactazide in pregnant women requires that the anticipated benefit be weighed against possible hazards to the fetus. These hazards include fetal or neonatal jaundice, thrombocytopenia, and possible other adverse reactions which have been reported in the adult.

Nursing Mothers. Canrenone, a metabolite of spironolactone, and hydrochlorothiazide appear in breast milk. If use of these drugs is deemed essential, an alternative method of infant feeding should be instituted.

ADVERSE REACTIONS

Gynecomastia is observed not infrequently. A few cases of agranulocytosis have been reported in patients taking spironolactone. Other adverse reactions that have been reported in association with the use of spironolactone are: gastrointestinal symptoms including cramping and diarrhea, drowsiness, lethargy, headache, maculopapular or erythematous cutaneous eruptions, urticaria, mental confusion, drug fever, ataxia, inability to achieve or maintain erection, irregular menses or amenorrhea, postmenopausal bleeding, hirsutism, deepening of the voice, gastric bleeding, ulceration, gastritis, and vomiting. Carcinoma of the breast has been reported in patients taking spironolactone, but a cause and effect relationship has not been established.

Adverse reactions reported in association with the use of thiazides include: gastrointestinal symptoms (anorexia, nausea, vomiting, diarrhea, abdominal cramps), purpura, thrombocytopenia, leukopenia, agranulocytosis, dermatologic symptoms (cutaneous eruptions, pruritus, erythema multiforme), paresthesia, acute pancreatitis, jaundice, dizziness, vertigo, headache, xanthopsia, photosensitivity, necrotizing angiitis, aplastic anemia, orthostatic hypotension, muscle spasm, weakness, restlessness, and hypokalemia.

Adverse reactions are usually reversible upon discontinuation of Aldactazide.

DOSAGE AND ADMINISTRATION

Optimal dosage should be established by individual titration of the components (see Box Warning).

Edema in adults (*congestive heart failure, hepatic cirrhosis, or nephrotic syndrome*). The usual maintenance dose of Aldactazide is 100 mg each of spironolactone and hydrochlorothiazide daily, administered in a single dose or in divided doses, but may range from 25 mg to 200 mg of each component daily depending on the response to the initial titration. In some instances it may be desirable to administer separate tablets of either Aldactone (spironolactone) or hydrochlorothiazide in addition to Aldactazide in order to provide optimal individual therapy.

The onset of diuresis with Aldactazide occurs promptly and, due to prolonged effect of the spironolactone component, persists for two to three days after Aldactazide is discontinued.

Edema in children. The usual daily maintenance dose of Aldactazide should be that which provides 0.75 to 1.5 mg of spironolactone per pound of body weight (1.65 to 3.3 mg/kg).

Essential hypertension. Although the dosage will vary depending on the results of titration of the individual ingredients, many patients will be found to have an optimal response to 50 mg to 100 mg each of spironolactone and hydrochlorothiazide daily, given in a single dose or in divided doses.

Continued on next page

Searle—Cont.

Concurrent potassium supplementation is not recommended when Aldactazide is used in the long-term management of hypertension or in the treatment of most edematous conditions, since the spironolactone content of Aldactazide is usually sufficient to minimize loss induced by the hydrochlorothiazide component.

HOW SUPPLIED

Aldactazide tablets containing 25 mg of spironolactone (Aldactone) and 25 mg of hydrochlorothiazide are round, tan, film coated, with SEARLE and 1011 debossed on one side and ALDACTAZIDE and 25 on the other side, supplied as:

NDC Number	Size
0025-1011-31	bottle of 100
0025-1011-51	bottle of 500
0025-1011-52	bottle of 1000
0025-1011-55	bottle of 2500
0025-1011-34	carton of 100 unit dose

Aldactazide tablets containing 50 mg of spironolactone (Aldactone) and 50 mg of hydrochlorothiazide are oblong, tan, scored, film coated, with SEARLE and 1021 debossed on the scored side and ALDACTAZIDE and 50 on the other side, supplied as:

NDC Number	Size
0025-1021-31	bottle of 100
0025-1021-34	carton of 100 unit dose

Store below 86°F (30°C).

Caution: Federal law prohibits dispensing without prescription.

10/1/92 • A05388-5

Shown in Product Identification Guide, page 335

ALDACTONE® ℞

[al-dac'tone]
(spironolactone)

> **WARNING**
> Spironolactone has been shown to be a tumorigen in chronic toxicity studies in rats (see *Warnings*). Aldactone should be used only in those conditions described under *Indications and Usage.* Unnecessary use of this drug should be avoided.

DESCRIPTION

Aldactone oral tablets contain 25 mg, 50 mg, or 100 mg of the aldosterone antagonist spironolactone, 17-hydroxy-7α-mercapto-3-oxo-17α-pregn-4-ene-21-carboxylic acid γ-lactone acetate, which has the following structural formula:

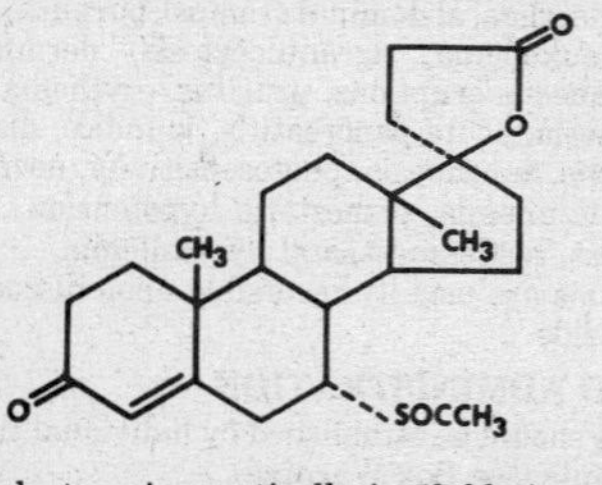

Spironolactone is practically insoluble in water, soluble in alcohol, and freely soluble in benzene and in chloroform.

Inactive ingredients include calcium sulfate, corn starch, flavor, hydroxypropyl methylcellulose, iron oxide, magnesium stearate, polyethylene glycol, povidone, and titanium dioxide.

CLINICAL PHARMACOLOGY

Mechanism of action: Aldactone (spironolactone) is a specific pharmacologic antagonist of aldosterone, acting primarily through competitive binding of receptors at the aldosterone-dependent sodium-potassium exchange site in the distal convoluted renal tubule. Aldactone causes increased amounts of sodium and water to be excreted, while potassium is retained. Aldactone acts both as a diuretic and as an antihypertensive drug by this mechanism. It may be given alone or with other diuretic agents which act more proximally in the renal tubule.

Aldosterone antagonist activity: Increased levels of the mineralocorticoid, aldosterone, are present in primary and secondary hyperaldosteronism. Edematous states in which secondary aldosteronism is usually involved include congestive heart failure, hepatic cirrhosis, and the nephrotic syndrome. By competing with aldosterone for receptor sites, Aldactone provides effective therapy for the edema and ascites in those conditions. Aldactone counteracts secondary aldosteronism induced by the volume depletion and associated sodium loss caused by active diuretic therapy.

Aldactone is effective in lowering the systolic and diastolic blood pressure in patients with primary hyperaldosteronism. It is also effective in most cases of essential hypertension, despite the fact that aldosterone secretion may be within normal limits in benign essential hypertension.

Through its action in antagonizing the effect of aldosterone, Aldactone inhibits the exchange of sodium for potassium in the distal renal tubule and helps to prevent potassium loss.

Aldactone has not been demonstrated to elevate serum uric acid, to precipitate gout, or to alter carbohydrate metabolism.

Pharmacokinetics: Spironolactone is rapidly and extensively metabolized. Sulfur-containing products are the predominant metabolites and are thought to be primarily responsible, together with spironolactone, for the therapeutic effects of the drug. The following pharmacokinetic data were obtained from 12 healthy volunteers following the administration of 100 mg of spironolactone (Aldactone film-coated tablets) daily for 15 days. On the 15th day, spironolactone was given immediately after a low-fat breakfast and blood was drawn thereafter.

	Accumulation Factor: AUC (0–24 hr, day 15)/AUC (0–24 hr, day 1)	Mean Peak Serum Concentration	Mean (SD) Post-Steady State Half-life
7-α-(thiomethyl) spirolactone (TMS)	1.25	391 ng/mL at 3.2 hr	13.8 hr (6.4) (terminal)
6-β-hydroxy-7-α-(thiomethyl) spirolactone (HTMS)	1.50	125 ng/mL at 5.1 hr	15.0 hr (4.0) (terminal)
Canrenone (C)	1.41	181 ng/mL at 4.3 hr	16.5 hr (6.3) (terminal)
Spironolactone	1.30	80 ng/mL at 2.6 hr	Approximately 1.4 hr (0.5) (β half-life)

The pharmacological activity of spironolactone metabolites in man is not known. However, in the adrenalectomized rat the antimineralocorticoid activities of the metabolites C, TMS, and HTMS, relative to spironolactone, were 1.10, 1.28, and 0.32, respectively. Relative to spironolactone, their binding affinities to the aldosterone receptors in rat kidney slices were 0.19, 0.86, and 0.06, respectively.

In humans the potencies of TMS and 7-α-thiospirolactone in reversing the effects of the synthetic mineralocorticoid, fludrocortisone, on urinary electrolyte composition were 0.33 and 0.26, respectively, relative to spironolactone. However, since the serum concentrations of these steroids were not determined, their incomplete absorption and/or first-pass metabolism could not be ruled out as a reason for their reduced *in vivo* activities.

Both spironolactone and canrenone are more than 90% bound to plasma proteins. The metabolites are excreted primarily in the urine and secondarily in bile.

The effect of food on spironolactone absorption (two 100-mg Aldactone tablets) was assessed in a single dose study of 9 healthy, drug-free volunteers. Food increased the bioavailability of unmetabolized spironolactone by almost 100%. The clinical importance of this finding is not known.

INDICATIONS AND USAGE

Aldactone (spironolactone) is indicated in the management of:

Primary hyperaldosteronism for:

Establishing the diagnosis of primary hyperaldosteronism by therapeutic trial.

Short-term preoperative treatment of patients with primary hyperaldosteronism.

Long-term maintenance therapy for patients with discrete aldosterone-producing adrenal adenomas who are judged to be poor operative risks or who decline surgery.

Long-term maintenance therapy for patients with bilateral micro- or macronodular adrenal hyperplasia (idiopathic hyperaldosteronism).

Edematous conditions for patients with:

Congestive heart failure: For the management of edema and sodium retention when the patient is only partially responsive to, or is intolerant of, other therapeutic measures. Aldactone is also indicated for patients with congestive heart failure taking digitalis when other therapies are considered inappropriate.

Cirrhosis of the liver accompanied by edema and/or ascites: Aldosterone levels may be exceptionally high in this condition. Aldactone is indicated for maintenance therapy together with bed rest and the restriction of fluid and sodium.

The nephrotic syndrome: For nephrotic patients when treatment of the underlying disease, restriction of fluid and sodium intake, and the use of other diuretics do not provide an adequate response.

Essential hypertension

Usually in combination with other drugs, Aldactone is indicated for patients who cannot be treated adequately with other agents or for whom other agents are considered inappropriate.

Hypokalemia

For the treatment of patients with hypokalemia when other measures are considered inappropriate or inadequate. Aldactone is also indicated for the prophylaxis of hypokalemia in patients taking digitalis when other measures are considered inadequate or inappropriate.

Usage in Pregnancy. The routine use of diuretics in an otherwise healthy woman is inappropriate and exposes mother and fetus to unnecessary hazard. Diuretics do not prevent development of toxemia of pregnancy, and there is no satisfactory evidence that they are useful in the treatment of developing toxemia.

Edema during pregnancy may arise from pathologic causes or from the physiologic and mechanical consequences of pregnancy.

Aldactone is indicated in pregnancy when edema is due to pathologic causes just as it is in the absence of pregnancy (however, see *Warnings* section). Dependent edema in pregnancy, resulting from restriction of venous return by the expanded uterus, is properly treated through elevation of the lower extremities and use of support hose; use of diuretics to lower intravascular volume in this case is unsupported and unnecessary. There is hypervolemia during normal pregnancy which is not harmful to either the fetus or the mother (in the absence of cardiovascular disease), but which is associated with edema, including generalized edema, in the majority of pregnant women. If this edema produces discomfort, increased recumbency will often provide relief. In rare instances, this edema may cause extreme discomfort which is not relieved by rest. In these cases, a short course of diuretics may provide relief and may be appropriate.

CONTRAINDICATIONS

Aldactone is contraindicated for patients with anuria, acute renal insufficiency, significant impairment of renal excretory function, or hyperkalemia.

WARNINGS

Potassium supplementation, either in the form of medication or as a diet rich in potassium, should not ordinarily be given in association with Aldactone therapy. Excessive potassium intake may cause hyperkalemia in patients receiving Aldactone (see *Precautions* section). Aldactone should not be administered concurrently with other potassium-sparing diuretics. Aldactone, when used with ACE inhibitors, even in the presence of a diuretic, has been associated with severe hyperkalemia. Extreme caution should be exercised when Aldactone is given concomitantly with ACE inhibitors (see *Precautions: Drug interactions*).

Spironolactone has been shown to be a tumorigen in chronic toxicity studies performed in rats, with its proliferative effects manifested on endocrine organs and the liver. In one study using 25, 75, and 250 times the usual daily human dose (2 mg/kg) there was a statistically significant dose-related increase in benign adenomas of the thyroid and testes. In female rats there was a statistically significant increase in malignant mammary tumors at the mid-dose only. In male rats there was a dose-related increase in proliferative changes in the liver. At the highest dosage level (500 mg/kg) the range of effects included hepatocytomegaly, hyperplastic nodules, and hepatocellular carcinoma; the last was not statistically significant at a value of $p = 0.05$. A dose-related (above 20 mg/kg/day) incidence of myelocytic leukemia was observed in rats fed daily doses of potassium canrenoate for a period of one year. In long-term (two-year) oral carcinogenicity studies of potassium canrenoate in the rat, myelocytic leukemia and hepatic, thyroid, testicular, and mammary tumors were observed. Potassium canrenoate did not produce a mutagenic effect in tests using bacteria or yeast. It did produce a positive mutagenic effect in several *in vitro* tests in mammalian cells following metabolic activation. In an *in vivo* mammalian system potassium canrenoate was not mutagenic. Canrenone and canrenoic acid are the major metabolites of potassium canrenoate. Spironolactone is also metabolized to canrenone. An increased incidence of leukemia was not observed in chronic rat toxicity studies conducted with spironolactone at doses up to 500 mg/kg/day.

PRECAUTIONS

General: Because of the diuretic action of Aldactone (spironolactone), patients should be carefully evaluated for possible disturbances of fluid and electrolyte balance. Hyperkalemia may occur in patients with impaired renal function or excessive potassium intake and can cause cardiac irregularities, which may be fatal. Consequently, no potassium supplement should ordinarily be given with Aldactone. Hyperkalemia can be treated promptly by the rapid intravenous administration of glucose (20% to 50%) and regular insulin, using 0.25 to 0.5 units of insulin per gram of glucose. This is a temporary measure to be repeated as required. Aldactone use should be discontinued and potassium intake (including dietary potassium) restricted.

Reversible hyperchloremic metabolic acidosis, usually in association with hyperkalemia, has been reported to occur in some patients with decompensated hepatic cirrhosis, even in the presence of normal renal function.

Hyponatremia, manifested by dryness of the mouth, thirst, lethargy, and drowsiness, and confirmed by a low serum sodium level, may be caused or aggravated, especially when Aldactone is administered in combination with other diuretics.

Gynecomastia may develop in association with the use of spironolactone; physicians should be alert to its possible onset. The development of gynecomastia appears to be related to both dosage level and duration of therapy and is normally reversible when Aldactone is discontinued. In rare instances some breast enlargement may persist when Aldactone is discontinued.

Aldactone therapy may cause a transient elevation of BUN, especially in patients with preexisting renal impairment. Aldactone may cause mild acidosis.

A determination of serum electrolytes to detect possible electrolyte imbalance should be performed at periodic intervals.

Drug interactions: When used in combination with other diuretics or antihypertensive agents, Aldactone potentiates their effects. Therefore, the dosage of such drugs, particularly the ganglionic blocking agents, should be reduced by at least 50% when Aldactone is added to the regimen.

Concomitant administration of potassium-sparing diuretics with ACE inhibitors or indomethacin has been associated with severe hyperkalemia.

Spironolactone reduces the vascular responsiveness to norepinephrine. Therefore, caution should be exercised in the management of patients subjected to regional or general anesthesia while they are being treated with Aldactone.

Spironolactone has been shown to increase the half-life of digoxin. This may result in increased serum digoxin levels and subsequent digitalis toxicity. It may be necessary to reduce the maintenance and digitalization doses when spironolactone is administered, and the patient should be carefully monitored to avoid over- or underdigitalization.

Drug/Laboratory test interactions: Several reports of possible interference with digoxin radioimmunoassays by spironolactone, or its metabolites, have appeared in the literature. Neither the extent nor the potential clinical significance of its interference (which may be assay-specific) has been fully established.

Usage in pregnancy: Spironolactone or its metabolites may cross the placental barrier. Therefore, the use of Aldactone in pregnant women requires that the anticipated benefit be weighed against possible hazard to the fetus.

Nursing mothers: Canrenone, a metabolite of spironolactone, appears in breast milk. If use of the drug is deemed essential, an alternative method of infant feeding should be instituted.

ADVERSE REACTIONS

Gynecomastia is observed not infrequently. A few cases of agranulocytosis have been reported in patients taking spironolactone. Other adverse reactions that have been reported in association with Aldactone are: gastrointestinal symptoms including cramping and diarrhea, drowsiness, lethargy, headache, maculopapular or erythematous cutaneous eruptions, urticaria, mental confusion, drug fever, ataxia, inability to achieve or maintain erection, irregular menses or amenorrhea, postmenopausal bleeding, hirsutism, deepening of the voice, gastric bleeding, ulceration, gastritis, and vomiting. Carcinoma of the breast has been reported in patients taking spironolactone, but a cause and effect relationship has not been established.

Adverse reactions are usually reversible upon discontinuation of the drug.

DOSAGE AND ADMINISTRATION

Primary hyperaldosteronism. Aldactone may be employed as an initial diagnostic measure to provide presumptive evidence of primary hyperaldosteronism while patients are on normal diets.

Long test: Aldactone is administered at a daily dosage of 400 mg for three to four weeks. Correction of hypokalemia and of hypertension provides presumptive evidence for the diagnosis of primary hyperaldosteronism.

Short test: Aldactone is administered at a daily dosage of 400 mg for four days. If serum potassium increases during Aldactone administration but drops when Aldactone is discontinued, a presumptive diagnosis of primary hyperaldosteronism should be considered.

After the diagnosis of hyperaldosteronism has been established by more definitive testing procedures, Aldactone may be administered in doses of 100 to 400 mg daily in preparation for surgery. For patients who are considered unsuitable for surgery, Aldactone may be employed for long-term maintenance therapy at the lowest effective dosage determined for the individual patient.

Edema in adults (*congestive heart failure, hepatic cirrhosis, or nephrotic syndrome*). An initial daily dosage of 100 mg of Aldactone administered in either single or divided doses is recommended, but may range from 25 to 200 mg daily. When given as the sole agent for diuresis, Aldactone should be continued for at least five days at the initial dosage level, after which it may be adjusted to the optimal therapeutic or maintenance level administered in either single or divided daily doses. If, after five days, an adequate diuretic response to Aldactone has not occurred, a second diuretic which acts more proximally in the renal tubule may be added to the regimen. Because of the additive effect of Aldactone when administered concurrently with such diuretics, an enhanced diuresis usually begins on the first day of combined treatment; combined therapy is indicated when more rapid diuresis is desired. The dosage of Aldactone should remain unchanged when other diuretic therapy is added.

Edema in children. The initial daily dosage should provide approximately 1.5 mg of Aldactone per pound of body weight (3.3 mg/kg) administered in either single or divided doses.

Essential hypertension. For adults, an initial daily dosage of 50 to 100 mg of Aldactone administered in either single or divided doses is recommended. Aldactone may also be given with diuretics which act more proximally in the renal tubule or with other antihypertensive agents. Treatment with Aldactone should be continued for at least two weeks, since the maximum response may not occur before this time. Subsequently, dosage should be adjusted according to the response of the patient.

Hypokalemia. Aldactone in a dosage ranging from 25 mg to 100 mg daily is useful in treating a diuretic-induced hypokalemia, when oral potassium supplements or other potassium-sparing regimens are considered inappropriate.

HOW SUPPLIED

Aldactone 25-mg tablets are round, light yellow, film coated, with SEARLE and 1001 debossed on one side and ALDACTONE and 25 on the other side, supplied as:

NDC Number	Size
0025-1001-31	bottle of 100
0025-1001-51	bottle of 500
0025-1001-52	bottle of 1000
0025-1001-55	bottle of 2500
0025-1001-34	carton of 100 unit dose

Aldactone 50-mg tablets are oval, light orange, scored, film coated, with SEARLE and 1041 debossed on the scored side and ALDACTONE and 50 on the other side, supplied as:

NDC Number	Size
0025-1041-31	bottle of 100
0025-1041-34	carton of 100 unit dose

Aldactone 100-mg tablets are round, peach colored, scored, film coated, with SEARLE and 1031 debossed on the scored side and ALDACTONE and 100 on the other side, supplied as:

NDC Number	Size
0025-1031-31	bottle of 100
0025-1031-34	carton of 100 unit dose

Store below 86°F (30°C).

Caution: Federal law prohibits dispensing without prescription.

10/1/92 • A05449-5

Shown in Product Identification Guide, page 335

AMBIEN® Ⓒ ℞

[am 'bē-ən]

(zolpidem tartrate)

DESCRIPTION

Ambien (zolpidem tartrate), is a non-benzodiazepine hypnotic of the imidazopyridine class and is available in 5-mg and 10-mg strength tablets for oral administration.

Chemically, zolpidem is N,N,6-trimethyl-2-p-tolyl-imidazo[1,2-a]pyridine-3-acetamide L-(+)-tartrate (2:1). It has the following structure:

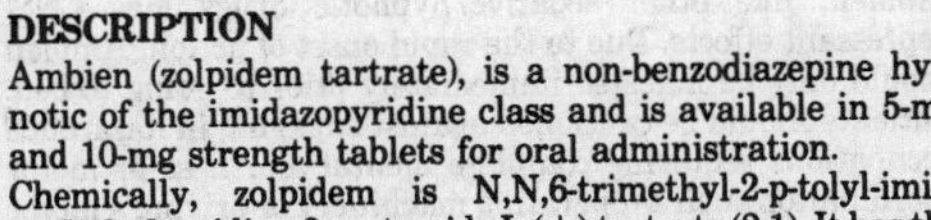

Zolpidem tartrate is a white to off-white crystalline powder that is sparingly soluble in water, alcohol, and propylene glycol. It has a molecular weight of 764.88.

Each Ambien tablet includes the following inactive ingredients: hydroxypropyl methylcellulose, lactose, magnesium stearate, microcrystalline cellulose, polyethylene glycol, sodium starch glycolate, titanium dioxide; the 5-mg tablet also contains FD&C Red No. 40, iron oxide colorant, and polysorbate 80.

CLINICAL PHARMACOLOGY

Pharmacodynamics: Subunit modulation of the $GABA_A$ receptor chloride channel macromolecular complex is hypothesized to be responsible for sedative, anticonvulsant, anxiolytic, and myorelaxant drug properties. The major modulatory site of the $GABA_A$ receptor complex is located on its alpha (α) subunit and is referred to as the benzodiazepine (BZ) or omega (ω) receptor. At least three subtypes of the (ω) receptor have been identified.

While zolpidem is a hypnotic agent with a chemical structure unrelated to benzodiazepines, barbiturates, or other drugs with known hypnotic properties, it interacts with a GABA-BZ receptor complex and shares some of the pharmacological properties of the benzodiazepines. In contrast to the benzodiazepines, which nonselectively bind to and activate all three omega receptor subtypes, zolpidem in vitro binds the (ω_1) receptor preferentially. The (ω_1) receptor is found primarily on the Lamina IV of the sensorimotor cortical regions, substantia nigra (pars reticulata), cerebellum molecular layer, olfactory bulb, ventral thalamic complex, pons, inferior colliculus, and globus pallidus. This selective binding of zolpidem on the (ω_1) receptor is not absolute, but it may explain the relative absence of myorelaxant and anticonvulsant effects in animal studies as well as the preservation of deep sleep (stages 3 and 4) in human studies of zolpidem at hypnotic doses.

Pharmacokinetics: The pharmacokinetic profile of Ambien is characterized by rapid absorption from the GI tract and a short elimination half-life ($T_{1/2}$) in healthy subjects. In a single-dose crossover study in 45 healthy subjects administered 5- and 10-mg zolpidem tartrate tablets, the mean peak concentrations (C_{max}) were 59 (range: 29 to 113) and 121 (range: 58 to 272) ng/mL, respectively, occurring at a mean time (T_{max}) of 1.6 hours for both. The mean Ambien elimination half-life was 2.6 (range: 1.4 to 4.5) and 2.5 (range: 1.4 to 3.8) hours, for the 5- and 10-mg tablets, respectively. Ambien is converted to inactive metabolites that are eliminated primarily by renal excretion. Ambien demonstrated linear kinetics in the dose range of 5 to 20 mg. Total protein binding was found to be 92.5±0.1% and remained constant, independent of concentration between 40 and 790 ng/mL. Zolpidem did not accumulate in young adults following nightly dosing with 20-mg zolpidem tartrate tablets for 2 weeks.

A food-effect study in 30 healthy male volunteers compared the pharmacokinetics of Ambien 10 mg when administered while fasting or 20 minutes after a meal. Results demonstrated that with food, mean AUC and C_{max} were decreased by 15% and 25%, respectively, while mean T_{max} was prolonged by 60% (from 1.4 to 2.2 hr). The half-life remained unchanged. These results suggest that, for faster sleep onset, Ambien should not be administered with or immediately after a meal.

In the elderly, the dose for Ambien should be 5 mg (see *Precautions* and *Dosage and Administration*). This recommendation is based on several studies in which the mean C_{max}, $T_{1/2}$, and AUC were significantly increased when compared to results in young adults. In one study of eight elderly subjects (> 70 years), the means for C_{max}, $T_{1/2}$, and AUC significantly increased by 50% (255 vs 384 ng/mL), 32% (2.2 vs 2.9 hr), and 64% (955 vs 1,562 ng·hr/mL), respectively, as compared to younger adults (20 to 40 years) following a single 20-mg oral zolpidem dose. Ambien did not accumulate in elderly subjects following nightly oral dosing of 10 mg for 1 week.

The pharmacokinetics of Ambien in eight patients with chronic hepatic insufficiency were compared to results in healthy subjects. Following a single 20-mg oral zolpidem dose, mean C_{max} and AUC were found to be two times (250 vs 499 ng/mL) and five times (788 vs 4,203 ng·hr/mL) higher, respectively, in hepatically compromised patients. T_{max} did not change. The mean half-life in cirrhotic patients of 9.9 hr (range: 4.1 to 25.8 hr) was greater than that observed in normals of 2.2 hr (range: 1.6 to 2.4 hr). Dosing should be modified accordingly in patients with hepatic insufficiency (see *Precautions* and *Dosage and Administration*).

The pharmacokinetics of zolpidem tartrate were studied in 11 patients with end-stage renal failure (mean $Cl_{Cr}=6.5\pm1.5$ mL/min) undergoing hemodialysis three times a week, who were dosed with zolpidem 10 mg orally each day for 14 or 21 days. No statistically significant differences were observed for C_{max}, T_{max}, half-life, and AUC between the first and last day of drug administration when baseline concentration adjustments were made. On day 1, C_{max} was 172±29 ng/mL (range: 46 to 344 ng/mL). After repeated dosing for 14 or 21 days, C_{max} was 203±32 ng/mL (range: 28 to 316 ng/mL). On day 1, T_{max} was 1.7±0.3 hr (range: 0.5 to 3.0 hr); after repeated dosing T_{max} was 0.8±0.2 hr (range: 0.5 to 2.0 hr). This variation is accounted for by noting that last-day serum sampling began 10 hours after the previous dose, rather than after 24 hours. This resulted in residual drug concentration and a shorter period to reach maximal serum concentration. On day 1, $T_{1/2}$ was 2.4±0.4 hr (range 0.4 to 5.1 hr). After repeated dosing, $T_{1/2}$ was 2.5±0.4 hr (range: 0.7 to 4.2 hr). AUC was 796±159 ng·hr/mL after the first dose and 818±170 ng·hr/mL after repeated dosing. Zolpidem was not hemodialyzable. No accumulation of unchanged drug appeared after 14 or 21 days. Ambien pharmacokinetics were not significantly different in renally impaired patients. No dosage adjustment is neces-

Continued on next page

Searle—Cont.

sary in patients with compromised renal function. As a general precaution, these patients should be closely monitored.

Postulated relationship between elimination rate of hypnotics and their profile of common untoward effects: The type and duration of hypnotic effects and the profile of unwanted effects during administration of hypnotic drugs may be influenced by the biologic half-life of administered drug and any active metabolites formed. When half-lives are long, drug or metabolites may accumulate during periods of nightly administration and be associated with impairment of cognitive and/or motor performance during waking hours; the possibility of interaction with other psychoactive drugs or alcohol will be enhanced. In contrast, if half-lives, including half-lives of active metabolites, are short, drug and metabolites will be cleared before the next dose is ingested, and carryover effects related to excessive sedation or CNS depression should be minimal or absent. Ambien has a short half-life and no active metabolites. During nightly use for an extended period, pharmacodynamic tolerance or adaptation to some effects of hypnotics may develop. If the drug has a short elimination half-life, it is possible that a relative deficiency of the drug or its active metabolites (ie, in relationship to the receptor site) may occur at some point in the interval between each night's use. This sequence of events may account for two clinical findings reported to occur after several weeks of nightly use of other rapidly eliminated hypnotics, namely, increased wakefulness during the last third of the night, and the appearance of increased signs of daytime anxiety. Increased wakefulness during the last third of the night as measured by polysomnography has not been observed in clinical trials with Ambien.

Controlled trials supporting safety and efficacy
Transient insomnia: Normal adults experiencing transient insomnia (n=462) during the first night in a sleep laboratory were evaluated in a double-blind, parallel group, single-night trial comparing two doses of zolpidem (7.5 and 10 mg) and placebo. Both zolpidem doses were superior to placebo on objective (polysomnographic) measures of sleep latency, sleep duration, and number of awakenings.

Normal elderly adults (mean age 68) experiencing transient insomnia (n = 35) during the first two nights in a sleep laboratory were evaluated in a double-blind, crossover, 2-night trial comparing four doses of zolpidem (5, 10, 15 and 20 mg) and placebo. All zolpidem doses were superior to placebo on the two primary PSG parameters (sleep latency and efficiency) and all four subjective outcome measures (sleep duration, sleep latency, number of awakenings, and sleep quality).

Chronic insomnia: Adult outpatients with chronic insomnia (n=75) were evaluated in a double-blind, parallel group, 5-week trial comparing two doses of zolpidem tartrate (10 and 15 mg) and placebo. On objective (polysomnographic) measures of sleep latency and sleep efficiency, zolpidem 15 mg was superior to placebo for all 5 weeks; zolpidem 10 mg was superior to placebo on sleep latency for the first 4 weeks and on sleep efficiency for weeks 2 and 4. Zolpidem was comparable to placebo on number of awakenings at both doses studied.

Adult outpatients (n=141) with chronic insomnia were evaluated in a double-blind, parallel group, 4-week trial comparing two doses of zolpidem (10 and 15 mg) and placebo. Zolpidem 10 mg was superior to placebo on a subjective measure of sleep latency for all 4 weeks, and on subjective measures of total sleep time, number of awakenings, and sleep quality for the first treatment week. Zolpidem 15 mg was superior to placebo on a subjective measure of sleep latency for the first 3 weeks, on a subjective measure of total sleep time for the first week, and on number of awakenings and sleep quality for the first 2 weeks.

Next-day residual effects: There was no evidence of residual next-day effects seen with Ambien in several studies utilizing the Multiple Sleep Latency Test (MSLT), the Digit Symbol Substitution Test (DSST), and patient ratings of alertness. In one study involving elderly patients, there was a small but statistically significant decrease in one measure of performance, the DSST, but no impairment was seen in the MSLT in this study. In another study involving elderly patients with chronic insomnia, there was no evidence of residual next-day effects utilizing DSST.

Rebound effects: There was no objective (polysomnographic) evidence of rebound insomnia at recommended doses seen in studies evaluating sleep on the nights following discontinuation of Ambien. There was subjective evidence of impaired sleep in the elderly on the first posttreatment night at doses above the recommended elderly dose of 5 mg.

Memory impairment: Controlled studies in adults utilizing objective measures of memory yielded no consistent evidence of next-day memory impairment following the administration of Ambien. However, in one study involving zolpidem doses of 10 and 20 mg, there was a significant decrease in next-morning recall of information presented to subjects during peak drug effect (90 minutes post-dose), ie, these sub-

jects experienced anterograde amnesia. There was also subjective evidence from adverse event data for anterograde amnesia occurring in association with the administration of Ambien, predominantly at doses above 10 mg.

Effects on sleep stages: In studies that measured the percentage of sleep time spent in each sleep stage. Ambien has generally been shown to preserve sleep stages. Sleep time spent in stages 3 and 4 (deep sleep) was found comparable to placebo with only inconsistent, minor changes in REM (paradoxical) sleep at the recommended dose.

INDICATIONS AND USAGE

Ambien (zolpidem tartrate) is indicated for the short-term treatment of insomnia. Hypnotics should generally be limited to 7 to 10 days of use, and reevaluation of the patient is recommended if they are to be taken for more than 2 to 3 weeks.

Ambien should not be prescribed in quantities exceeding a 1-month supply (see *Warnings*).

Ambien has been shown to decrease sleep latency and increase the duration of sleep for up to 5 weeks in controlled clinical studies (see *Clinical Pharmacology*).

CONTRAINDICATIONS

None known.

WARNINGS

Since sleep disturbances may be the presenting manifestation of a physical and/or psychiatric disorder, symptomatic treatment of insomnia should be initiated only after a careful evaluation of the patient. The failure of insomnia to remit after 7 to 10 days of treatment may indicate the presence of a primary psychiatric and/or medical illness which should be evaluated. Worsening of insomnia or the emergence of new thinking or behavior abnormalities may be the consequence of an unrecognized psychiatric or physical disorder. Such findings have emerged during the course of treatment with sedative/hypnotic drugs, including Ambien. Because some of the important adverse effects of Ambien appear to be dose related (see *Precautions* and *Dosage and Administration*), it is important to use the smallest possible effective dose, especially in the elderly.

A variety of abnormal thinking and behavior changes have been reported to occur in association with the use of sedative/hypnotics. Some of these changes may be characterized by decreased inhibition (eg, aggressiveness and extroversion that seemed out of character), similar to effects produced by alcohol and other CNS depressants. Other reported behavioral changes have included bizarre behavior, agitation, hallucinations, and depersonalization. Amnesia and other neuropsychiatric symptoms may occur unpredictably. In primarily depressed patients, worsening of depression, including suicidal thinking, has been reported in association with the use of sedative/hypnotics.

It can rarely be determined with certainty whether a particular instance of the abnormal behaviors listed above are drug induced, spontaneous in origin, or a result of an underlying psychiatric or physical disorder. Nonetheless, the emergence of any new behavioral sign or symptom of concern requires careful and immediate evaluation.

Following the rapid dose decrease or abrupt discontinuation of sedative/hypnotics, there have been reports of signs and symptoms similar to those associated with withdrawal from other CNS-depressant drugs (see *Drug Abuse and Dependence*).

Ambien, like other sedative/hypnotic drugs, has CNS-depressant effects. Due to the rapid onset of action, Ambien should only be ingested immediately prior to going to bed. Patients should be cautioned against engaging in hazardous occupations requiring complete mental alertness or motor coordination such as operating machinery or driving a motor vehicle after ingesting the drug, including potential impairment of the performance of such activities that may occur the day following ingestion of Ambien. Ambien showed additive effects when combined with alcohol and should not be taken with alcohol. Patients should also be cautioned about possible combined effects with other CNS-depressant drugs. Dosage adjustments may be necessary when Ambien is administered with such agents because of the potentially additive effects.

PRECAUTIONS

General
Use in the elderly and/or debilitated patients: Impaired motor and/or cognitive performance after repeated exposure or unusual sensitivity to sedative/hypnotic drugs is a concern in the treatment of elderly and/or debilitated patients. Therefore, the recommended Ambien dosage is 5 mg in such patients (see *Dosage and Administration*) to decrease the possibility of side effects. These patients should be closely monitored.

Use in patients with concomitant illness: Clinical experience with Ambien (zolpidem tartrate) in patients with concomitant systemic illness is limited. Caution is advisable in using Ambien in patients with diseases or conditions that could affect metabolism or hemodynamic responses. Although studies did not reveal respiratory depressant effects

at hypnotic doses of Ambien in normals or in patients with mild to moderate chronic obstructive pulmonary disease (COPD), precautions should be observed if Ambien is prescribed to patients with compromised respiratory function, since sedative/hypnotics have the capacity to depress respiratory drive. Post-marketing reports of respiratory insufficiency, most of which involved patients with pre-existing respiratory impairment, have been received. Data in end-stage renal failure patients repeatedly treated with Ambien did not demonstrate drug accumulation or alterations in pharmacokinetic parameters. No dosage adjustment in renally impaired patients is required; however, these patients should be closely monitored (see *Pharmacokinetics*). A study in subjects with hepatic impairment did reveal prolonged elimination in this group; therefore, treatment should be initiated with 5 mg in patients with hepatic compromise, and they should be closely monitored.

Use in depression: As with other sedative/hypnotic drugs, Ambien should be administered with caution to patients exhibiting signs or symptoms of depression. Suicidal tendencies may be present in such patients and protective measures may be required. Intentional overdosage is more common in this group of patients; therefore, the least amount of drug that is feasible should be prescribed for the patient at any one time.

Information for patients: Patient information is printed at the end of this insert. To assure safe and effective use of Ambien, this information and instructions provided in the patient information section should be discussed with patients.

Laboratory tests: There are no specific laboratory tests recommended.

Drug interactions
CNS-active drugs: Ambien was evaluated in healthy volunteers in single-dose interaction studies for several CNS drugs. A study involving haloperidol and zolpidem revealed no effect of haloperidol on the pharmacokinetics or pharmacodynamics of zolpidem. Imipramine in combination with zolpidem produced no pharmacokinetic interaction other than a 20% decrease in peak levels of imipramine, but there was an additive effect of decreased alertness. Similarly, chlorpromazine in combination with zolpidem produced no pharmacokinetic interaction, but there was an additive effect of decreased alertness and psychomotor performance. The lack of a drug interaction following single-dose administration does not predict a lack following chronic administration.

An additive effect on psychomotor performance between alcohol and zolpidem was demonstrated.

Since the systematic evaluations of Ambien (zolpidem tartrate) in combination with other CNS-active drugs have been limited, careful consideration should be given to the pharmacology of any CNS-active drug to be used with zolpidem. Any drug with CNS-depressant effects could potentially enhance the CNS-depressant effects of zolpidem.

Other drugs: A study involving cimetidine/zolpidem and ranitidine/zolpidem combinations revealed no effect of either drug on the pharmacokinetics or pharmacodynamics of zolpidem. Zolpidem had no effect on digoxin kinetics and did not affect prothrombin time when given with warfarin in normal subjects. Zolpidem's sedative/hypnotic effect was reversed by flumazenil; however, no significant alterations in zolpidem pharmacokinetics were found.

Drug/Laboratory test interactions: Zolpidem is not known to interfere with commonly employed clinical laboratory tests.

Carcinogenesis, mutagenesis, impairment of fertility
Carcinogenesis: Zolpidem was administered to rats and mice for 2 years at dietary dosages of 4, 18, and 80 mg/kg/day. In mice, these doses are 26 to 520 times or 2 to 35 times the maximum 10-mg human dose on a mg/kg or mg/m^2 basis, respectively. In rats these doses are 43 to 876 times or 6 to 115 times the maximum 10-mg human dose on a mg/kg or mg/m^2 basis, respectively. No evidence of carcinogenic potential was observed in mice. Renal liposarcomas were seen in 4/100 rats (3 males, 1 female) receiving 80 mg/kg/day and a renal lipoma was observed in one male rat at the 18 mg/kg/day dose. Incidence rates of lipoma and liposarcoma for zolpidem were comparable to those seen in historical controls and the tumor findings are thought to be a spontaneous occurrence.

Mutagenesis: Zolpidem did not have mutagenic activity in several tests including the Ames test, genotoxicity in mouse lymphoma cells in vitro, chromosomal aberrations in cultured human lymphocytes, unscheduled DNA synthesis in rat hepatocytes in vitro, and the micronucleus test in mice.

Impairment of fertility: In a rat reproduction study, the high dose (100 mg base/kg) of zolpidem resulted in irregular estrus cycles and prolonged precoital intervals, but there was no effect on male or female fertility after daily oral doses of 4 to 100 mg base/kg or 5 to 130 times the recommended human dose in mg/m^2. No effects on any other fertility parameters were noted.

Pregnancy

Teratogenic effects: Pregnancy Category B. Studies to assess the effects of zolpidem on human reproduction and development have not been conducted.

Teratology studies were conducted in rats and rabbits. In rats, adverse maternal and fetal effects occurred at 20 and 100 mg base/kg and included dose-related maternal lethargy and ataxia and a dose-related trend to incomplete ossification of fetal skull bones. Underossification of various fetal bones indicates a delay in maturation and is often seen in rats treated with sedative/hypnotic drugs. There were no teratogenic effects after zolpidem administration. The no-effect dose for maternal or fetal toxicity was 4 mg base/kg or 5 times the maximum human dose on a mg/m^2 basis.

In rabbits, dose-related maternal sedation and decreased weight gain occurred at all doses tested. At the high dose, 16 mg base/kg, there was an increase in postimplantation fetal loss and underossification of sternebrae in viable fetuses. These fetal findings in rabbits are often secondary to reductions in maternal weight gain. There were no frank teratogenic effects. The no-effect dose for fetal toxicity was 4 mg base/kg or 7 times the maximum human dose on a mg/m^2 basis.

Because animal reproduction studies are not always predictive of human response, this drug should be used during pregnancy only if clearly needed.

Nonteratogenic effects: Studies to assess the effects on children whose mothers took zolpidem during pregnancy have not been conducted. However, children born of mothers taking sedative/hypnotic drugs may be at some risk for withdrawal symptoms from the drug during the postnatal period. In addition, neonatal flaccidity has been reported in infants born of mothers who received sedative/hypnotic drugs during pregnancy.

Labor and delivery: Ambien has no established use in labor and delivery.

Nursing mothers: Studies in lactating mothers indicate that the half-life of zolpidem is similar to that in young normal volunteers (2.6±0.3 hr). Between 0.004 and 0.019% of the total administered dose is excreted into milk, but the effect of zolpidem on the infant is unknown.

In addition, in a rat study, zolpidem inhibited the secretion of milk. The no-effect dose was 4 mg base/kg or 6 times the recommended human dose in mg/m^2.

The use of Ambien in nursing mothers is not recommended.

Pediatric use: Safety and effectiveness in children below the age of 18 have not been established.

Geriatric use: A total of 154 patients in U.S. controlled clinical trials and 897 patients in non-U.S. clinical trials who received zolpidem were ≥60 years of age. For a pool of U.S. patients receiving zolpidem at doses of ≤10 mg or placebo, there were three adverse events occurring at an incidence of at least 3% for zolpidem and for which the zolpidem incidence was at least twice the placebo incidence (ie, they could be considered drug related).

Adverse Event	Zolpidem	Placebo
Dizziness	3%	0%
Drowsiness	5%	2%
Diarrhea	3%	1%

A total of 30/1,959 (1.5%) non-U.S. patients receiving zolpidem reported falls, including 28/30 (93%) who were ≥70 years of age. Of these 28 patients, 23 (82%) were receiving zolpidem doses >10 mg. A total of 24/1,959 (1.2%) non-U.S. patients receiving zolpidem reported confusion, including 18/24 (75%) who were ≥70 years of age. Of these 18 patients, 14 (78%) were receiving zolpidem doses >10 mg.

ADVERSE REACTIONS

Associated with discontinuation of treatment: Approximately 4% of 1,701 patients who received zolpidem at all doses (1.25 to 90 mg) in U.S. premarketing clinical trials discontinued treatment because of an adverse clinical event. Events most commonly associated with discontinuation from U.S. trials were daytime drowsiness (0.5%), dizziness (0.4%), headache (0.5%), nausea (0.6%), and vomiting (0.5%).

Approximately 4% of 1,959 patients who received zolpidem at all doses (1 to 50 mg) in similar foreign trials discontinued treatment because of an adverse event. Events most commonly associated with discontinuation from these trials were daytime drowsiness (1.1%), dizziness/vertigo (0.8%), amnesia (0.5%), nausea (0.5%), headache (0.4%), and falls (0.4%).

Incidence in controlled clinical trials

Most commonly observed adverse events in controlled trials: During short-term treatment (up to 10 nights) with Ambien at doses up to 10 mg, the most commonly observed adverse events associated with the use of zolpidem and seen at statistically significant differences from placebo-treated patients were drowsiness (reported by 2% of zolpidem patients), dizziness (1%), and diarrhea (1%). During longer-term treatment (28 to 35 nights) with zolpidem at doses up to 10 mg, the most commonly observed adverse events associated with the use of zolpidem and seen at statistically significant differences

from placebo-treated patients were dizziness (5%) and drugged feelings (3%).

Adverse events observed at an incidence of ≥ 1% in controlled trials: The following tables enumerate treatment-emergent adverse event frequencies that were observed at an incidence equal to 1% or greater among patients with insomnia who received Ambien in U.S. placebo-controlled trials. Events reported by investigators were classified utilizing a modified World Health Organization (WHO) dictionary of preferred terms for the purpose of establishing event frequencies. The prescriber should be aware that these figures cannot be used to predict the incidence of side effects in the course of usual medical practice, in which patient characteristics and other factors differ from those that prevailed in these clinical trials. Similarly, the cited frequencies cannot be compared with figures obtained from other clinical investigators involving related drug products and uses, since each group of drug trials is conducted under a different set of conditions. However, the cited figures provide the physician with a basis for estimating the relative contribution of drug and nondrug factors to the incidence of side effects in the population studied.

The following table was derived from a pool of 11 placebo-controlled short-term U.S. efficacy trials involving zolpidem in doses ranging from 1.25 to 20 mg. The table is limited to data from doses up to and including 10 mg, the highest dose recommended for use.

Incidence of Treatment-Emergent Adverse Experiences in Short-term Placebo-Controlled Clinical Trials
(Percentage of patients reporting)

Body System/ Adverse Event*	Zolpidem (≤10 mg) (N=685)	Placebo (N=473)
Central and Peripheral Nervous System		
Headache	7	6
Drowsiness	2	—
Dizziness	1	—
Gastrointestinal System		
Nausea	2	3
Diarrhea	1	—
Musculoskeletal System		
Myalgia	1	2

*Events reported by at least 1% of Ambien patients are included.

The following table was derived from a pool of three placebo-controlled long-term efficacy trials involving Ambien (zolpidem tartrate). These trials involved patients with chronic insomnia who were treated for 28 to 35 nights with zolpidem at doses of 5, 10, or 15 mg. The table is limited to data from doses up to and including 10 mg, the highest dose recommended for use. The table includes only adverse events occurring at an incidence of at least 1% for zolpidem patients.

Incidence of Treatment-Emergent Adverse Experiences in Long-term Placebo-Controlled Clinical Trials
(Percentage of patients reporting)

Body System/ Adverse Event*	Zolpidem (≤10 mg) (N=152)	Placebo (N=161)
Autonomic Nervous System		
Dry mouth	3	1
Body as a Whole		
Allergy	4	1
Back pain	3	2
Influenza-like symptoms	2	—
Chest pain	1	—
Fatigue	1	2
Cardiovascular System		
Palpitation	2	—
Central and Peripheral Nervous System		
Headache	19	22
Drowsiness	8	5
Dizziness	5	1
Lethargy	3	1
Drugged feeling	3	—
Lightheadedness	2	1
Depression	2	1
Abnormal dreams	1	—
Amnesia	1	—
Anxiety	1	1
Nervousness	1	3
Sleep disorder	1	—
Gastrointestinal System		
Nausea	6	6
Dyspepsia	5	6
Diarrhea	3	2
Abdominal pain	2	2
Constipation	2	1
Anorexia	1	1
Vomiting	1	1
Immunologic System		
Infection	1	1
Musculoskeletal System		
Myalgia	7	7
Arthralgia	4	4
Respiratory System		
Upper respiratory infection	5	6
Sinusitis	4	2
Pharyngitis	3	1
Rhinitis	1	3
Skin and Appendages		
Rash	2	1
Urogenital System		
Urinary tract infection	2	2

*Events reported by at least 1% of patients treated with Ambien.

Dose relationship for adverse events: There is evidence from dose comparison trials suggesting a dose relationship for many of the adverse events associated with zolpidem use, particularly for certain CNS and gastrointestinal adverse events.

Adverse event incidence across the entire preapproval database: Ambien (zolpidem tartrate) was administered to 3,660 subjects in clinical trials throughout the U.S., Canada, and Europe. Treatment-emergent adverse events associated with clinical trial participation were recorded by clinical investigators using terminology of their own choosing. To provide a meaningful estimate of the proportion of individuals experiencing treatment-emergent adverse events, similar types of untoward events were grouped into a smaller number of standardized event categories and classified utilizing a modified World Health Organization (WHO) dictionary of preferred terms. The frequencies presented, therefore, represent the proportions of the 3,660 individuals exposed to zolpidem, at all doses, who experienced an event of the type cited on at least one occasion while receiving zolpidem. All reported treatment-emergent adverse events are included, except those already listed in the table above of adverse events in placebo-controlled studies, those coding terms that are so general as to be uninformative, and those events where a drug cause was remote. It is important to emphasize that, although the events reported did occur during treatment with Ambien, they were not necessarily caused by it.

Adverse events are further classified within body system categories and enumerated in order of decreasing frequency using the following definitions: frequent adverse events are defined as those occurring in greater than 1/100 subjects; infrequent adverse events are those occurring in 1/100 to 1/1,000 patients; rare events are those occurring in less than 1/1,000 patients.

Autonomic nervous system: Infrequent: increased sweating, pallor, postural hypotension, syncope. Rare: abnormal accommodation, altered saliva, flushing, glaucoma, hypotension, impotence, increased saliva, tenesmus.

Body as a whole: Frequent: asthenia. Infrequent: edema, falling, fever, malaise, trauma. Rare: allergic reaction, allergy aggravated, abdominal body sensation, anaphylactic shock, face edema, hot flashes, increased ESR, pain, restless legs, rigors, tolerance increased, weight decrease.

Cardiovascular system: Infrequent: cerebrovascular disorder, hypertension, tachycardia. Rare: angina pectoris, arrhythmia, arteritis, circulatory failure, extrasystoles, hypertension aggravated, myocardial infarction, phlebitis, pulmonary embolism, pulmonary edema, varicose veins, ventricular tachycardia.

Central and peripheral nervous system: Frequent: ataxia, confusion, euphoria, insomnia, vertigo. Infrequent: agitation, decreased cognition, detached, difficulty concentrating, dysarthria, emotional lability, hallucination, hypoesthesia, illusion, leg cramps, migraine, paresthesia, sleeping (after day-time dosing), speech disorder, stupor, tremor. Rare: abnormal gait, abnormal thinking, aggressive reaction, apathy, appetite increased, decreased libido, delusion, dementia, depersonalization, dysphasia, feeling strange, hypokinesia, hypotonia, hysteria, intoxicated feeling, manic reaction, neuralgia, neuritis, neuropathy, neurosis, panic attacks, paresis, personality disorder, somnambulism, suicide attempts, tetany, yawning.

Gastrointestinal system: Frequent: hiccup. Infrequent: constipation, dysphagia, flatulence, gastroenteritis. Rare: enteritis, eructation, esophagospasm, gastritis, hemorrhoids, intestinal obstruction, rectal hemorrhage, tooth caries.

Hematologic and lymphatic system: Rare: anemia, hyperhemoglobinemia, leukopenia, lymphadenopathy, macrocytic anemia, purpura, thrombosis.

Immunologic system: Rare: abscess, herpes simplex, herpes zoster, otitis externa, otitis media.

Liver and biliary system: Infrequent: abnormal hepatic function, increased SGPT. Rare: bilirubinemia, increased SGOT.

Continued on next page

Searle—Cont.

Metabolic and nutritional: Infrequent: hyperglycemia, thirst. Rare: gout, hypercholesteremia, hyperlipidemia, increased alkaline phosphatase, increased BUN, periorbital edema.

Musculoskeletal system: Infrequent: arthritis. Rare: arthrosis, muscle weakness, sciatica, tendinitis.

Reproductive system: Infrequent: menstrual disorder, vaginitis. Rare: breast fibroadenosis, breast neoplasm, breast pain.

Respiratory system: Infrequent: bronchitis, coughing, dyspnea. Rare: bronchospasm, epistaxis, hypoxia, laryngitis, pneumonia.

Skin and appendages: Infrequent: pruritus. Rare: acne, bullous eruption, dermatitis, furunculosis, injection-site inflammation, photosensitivity reaction, urticaria.

Special senses: Frequent: diplopia, vision abnormal. Infrequent: eye irritation, eye pain, scleritis, taste perversion, tinnitus. Rare: conjunctivitis, corneal ulceration, lacrimation abnormal, parosmia, photopsia.

Urogenital system: Infrequent: cystitis, urinary incontinence. Rare: acute renal failure, dysuria, micturition frequency, nocturia, polyuria, pyelonephritis, renal pain, urinary retention.

DRUG ABUSE AND DEPENDENCE

Controlled substance: Zolpidem tartrate is classified as a Schedule IV controlled substance by federal regulation.

Abuse and dependence: Studies of abuse potential in former drug abusers found that the effects of single doses of Ambien (zolpidem tartrate) 40 mg were similar, but not identical, to diazepam 20 mg, while zolpidem tartrate 10 mg was difficult to distinguish from placebo.

Sedative/hypnotics have produced withdrawal signs and symptoms following abrupt discontinuation. These reported symptoms range from mild dysphoria and insomnia to a withdrawal syndrome that may include abdominal and muscle cramps, vomiting, sweating, tremors, and convulsions. The U.S. clinical trial experience from zolpidem does not reveal any clear evidence for withdrawal syndrome. Nevertheless, the following adverse events included in DSM-III-R criteria for uncomplicated sedative/hypnotic withdrawal were reported during U.S. clinical trials following placebo substitution occurring within 48 hours following last zolpidem treatment: fatigue, nausea, flushing, lightheadedness, uncontrolled crying, emesis, stomach cramps, panic attack, nervousness, and abdominal discomfort. These reported adverse events occurred at an incidence of 1% or less. However, available data cannot provide a reliable estimate of the incidence, if any, of dependence during treatment at recommended doses.

Because individuals with a history of addiction to, or abuse of, drugs or alcohol are at risk of habituation and dependence, they should be under careful surveillance when receiving zolpidem or any other hypnotic.

OVERDOSAGE

Signs and symptoms: In European postmarketing reports of overdose with zolpidem alone, impairment of consciousness has ranged from somnolence to light coma. There was one case each of cardiovascular and respiratory compromise. Individuals have fully recovered from zolpidem tartrate overdoses up to 400 mg (40 times the maximum recommended dose). Overdose cases involving multiple CNS-depressant agents, including zolpidem, have resulted in more severe symptomatology, including fatal outcomes.

Recommended treatment: General symptomatic and supportive measures should be used along with immediate gastric lavage where appropriate. Intravenous fluids should be administered as needed. Flumazenil may be useful. As in all cases of drug overdose, respiration, pulse, blood pressure, and other appropriate signs should be monitored and general supportive measures employed. Hypotension and CNS depression should be monitored and treated by appropriate medical intervention. Sedating drugs should be withheld following zolpidem overdosage, even if excitation occurs. The value of dialysis in the treatment of overdosage has not been determined, although hemodialysis studies in patients with renal failure receiving therapeutic doses have demonstrated that zolpidem is not dialyzable.

Poison control center: As with the management of all overdosage, the possibility of multiple drug ingestion should be considered. The physician may wish to consider contacting a poison control center for up-to-date information on the management of hypnotic drug product overdosage.

DOSAGE AND ADMINISTRATION

The dose of Ambien should be individualized.
The recommended dose for adults is 10 mg immediately before bedtime.
Downward dosage adjustment may be necessary when Ambien is administered with agents having known CNS-depressant effects because of the potentially additive effects.

Elderly or debilitated patients may be especially sensitive to the effects of Ambien (zolpidem tartrate). Patients with hepatic insufficiency do not clear the drug as rapidly as normals. An initial 5-mg dose is recommended in these patients (see *Precautions*).
The total Ambien dose should not exceed 10 mg.

HOW SUPPLIED

Ambien 5-mg tablets are capsule-shaped, pink, film coated, identified with markings of AMB 5 on one side and 5401 on the other and supplied as:

NDC Number	Size
0025-5401-31	bottle of 100
0025-5401-34	carton of 100 unit dose

Ambien 10-mg tablets are capsule-shaped, white, film coated, identified with markings of AMB 10 on one side and 5421 on the other and supplied as:

NDC Number	Size
0025-5421-31	bottle of 100
0025-5421-34	carton of 100 unit dose

Store below 86°F (30°C).
Caution: Federal law prohibits dispensing without prescription.

INFORMATION FOR PATIENTS
TAKING AMBIEN

Your doctor has prescribed Ambien to help you sleep. The following information is intended to guide you in the safe use of this medicine. It is not meant to take the place of your doctor's instructions. If you have any questions about Ambien tablets be sure to ask your doctor or pharmacist.
Ambien is used to treat different types of sleep problems, such as:

- trouble falling asleep
- waking up too early in the morning
- waking up often during the night

Some people may have more than one of these problems. Ambien belongs to a group of medicines known as the "sedative/hypnotics," or simply, sleep medicines. There are many different sleep medicines available to help people sleep better. Sleep problems are usually temporary, requiring treatment for only a short time, usually 1 or 2 days up to 1 or 2 weeks. Some people have chronic sleep problems that may require more prolonged use of sleep medicine. However, you should not use these medicines for long periods without talking with your doctor about the risks and benefits of prolonged use.

SIDE EFFECTS

Most common side effects: All medicines have side effects. Most common side effects of sleep medicines include:

- drowsiness
- dizziness
- lightheadedness
- difficulty with coordination

You may find that these medicines make you sleepy during the day. How drowsy you feel depends upon how your body reacts to the medicine, which sleep medicine you are taking, and how large a dose your doctor has prescribed. Daytime drowsiness is best avoided by taking the lowest dose possible that will still help you sleep at night. Your doctor will work with you to find the dose of Ambien that is best for you.
To manage these side effects while you are taking this medicine:

- When you first start taking Ambien or any other sleep medicine until you know whether the medicine will still have some carryover effect in you the next day, use extreme care while doing anything that requires complete alertness, such as driving a car, operating machinery, or piloting an aircraft.
- NEVER drink alcohol while you are being treated with Ambien or any sleep medicine. Alcohol can increase the side effects of Ambien or any other sleep medicine.
- Do not take any other medicines without asking your doctor first. This includes medicines you can buy without a prescription. Some medicines can cause drowsiness and are best avoided while taking Ambien.
- Always take the exact dose of Ambien prescribed by your doctor. Never change your dose without talking to your doctor first.

SPECIAL CONCERNS

There are some special problems that may occur while taking sleep medicines.
Memory problems: Sleep medicines may cause a special type of memory loss or "amnesia." When this occurs, a person may not remember what has happened for several hours after taking the medicine. This is usually not a problem since most people fall asleep after taking the medicine.
Memory loss can be a problem, however, when sleep medicines are taken while traveling, such as during an airplane flight and the person wakes up before the effect of the medicine is gone. This has been called "traveler's amnesia."
Memory problems are not common while taking Ambien. In most instances memory problems can be avoided if you take

Ambien only when you are able to get a full night's sleep (7 to 8 hours) before you need to be active again. Be sure to talk to your doctor if you think you are having memory problems.
Tolerance: When sleep medicines are used every night for more than a few weeks, they may lose their effectiveness to help you sleep. This is known as "tolerance." Sleep medicines should, in most cases, be used only for short periods of time, such as 1 or 2 days and generally no longer than 1 or 2 weeks. If your sleep problems continue, consult your doctor, who will determine whether other measures are needed to overcome your sleep problems.
Dependence: Sleep medicines can cause dependence, especially when these medicines are used regularly for longer than a few weeks or at high doses. Some people develop a need to continue taking their medicines. This is known as dependence or "addiction."
When people develop dependence, they may have difficulty stopping the sleep medicine. If the medicine is suddenly stopped, the body is not able to function normally and unpleasant symptoms (see *Withdrawal*) may occur. They may find they have to keep taking the medicine either at the prescribed dose or at increasing doses just to avoid withdrawal symptoms.
All people taking sleep medicines have some risk of becoming dependent on the medicine. However, people who have been dependent on alcohol or other drugs in the past may have a higher chance of becoming addicted to sleep medicines. This possibility must be considered before using these medicines for more than a few weeks.
If you have been addicted to alcohol or drugs in the past, it is important to tell your doctor before starting Ambien or any sleep medicine.
Withdrawal: Withdrawal symptoms may occur when sleep medicines are stopped suddenly after being used daily for a long time. In some cases, these symptoms can occur even if the medicine has been used for only a week or two.
In mild cases, withdrawal symptoms may include unpleasant feelings. In more severe cases, abdominal and muscle cramps, vomiting, sweating, shakiness, and rarely, seizures may occur. These more severe withdrawal symptoms are very uncommon.
Another problem that may occur when sleep medicines are stopped is known as "rebound insomnia." This means that a person may have more trouble sleeping the first few nights after the medicine is stopped than before starting the medicine. If you should experience rebound insomnia, do not get discouraged. This problem usually goes away on its own after 1 or 2 nights.
If you have been taking Ambien or any other sleep medicine for more than 1 or 2 weeks, do not stop taking it on your own. Always follow your doctor's directions.
Changes in behavior and thinking: Some people using sleep medicines have experienced unusual changes in their thinking and/or behavior. These effects are not common. However, they have included:

- more outgoing or aggressive behavior than normal
- loss of personal identity
- confusion
- strange behavior
- agitation
- hallucinations
- worsening of depression
- suicidal thoughts

How often these effects occur depends on several factors, such as a person's general health, the use of other medicines, and which sleep medicine is being used. Clinical experience with Ambien suggests that it is uncommonly associated with these behavior changes.
It is also important to realize that it is rarely clear whether these behavior changes are caused by the medicine, an illness, or occur on their own. In fact, sleep problems that do not improve may be due to illnesses that were present before the medicine was used. If you or your family notice any changes in your behavior, or if you have any unusual or disturbing thoughts, call your doctor immediately.
Pregnancy: Sleep medicines may cause sedation of the unborn baby when used during the last weeks of pregnancy. Be sure to tell your doctor if you are pregnant, if you are planning to become pregnant, or if you become pregnant while taking Ambien.

SAFE USE OF SLEEPING MEDICINES

To ensure the safe and effective use of Ambien or any other sleep medicine, you should observe the following cautions:

1. Ambien is a prescription medicine and should be used ONLY as directed by your doctor. Follow your doctor's instructions about how to take, when to take, and how long to take Ambien.
2. Never use Ambien or any other sleep medicine for longer than directed by your doctor.
3. If you notice any unusual and/or disturbing thoughts or behavior during treatment with Ambien or any other sleep medicine, contact your doctor.
4. Tell your doctor about any medicines you may be taking, including medicines you may buy without a prescription. You should also tell your doctor if you drink alcohol. DO

NOT use alcohol while taking Ambien or any other sleep medicine.

5. Do not take Ambien or any other sleep medicine unless you are able to get a full night's sleep before you must be active again. For example, Ambien or any other sleep medicine should not be taken on an overnight airplane flight of less than 7 to 8 hours since "traveler's amnesia" may occur.

6. Do not increase the prescribed dose of Ambien or any other sleep medicine unless instructed by your doctor.

7. When you first start taking Ambien or any other sleep medicine until you know whether the medicine will still have some carryover effect in you the next day, use extreme care while doing anything that requires complete alertness, such as driving a car, operating machinery, or piloting an aircraft.

8. Be aware that you may have more sleeping problems the first night or two after stopping Ambien or any other sleep medicine.

9. Be sure to tell your doctor if you are pregnant, if you are planning to become pregnant, or if you become pregnant while taking Ambien.

10. As with all prescription medicines, never share Ambien or any other sleep medicine with anyone else. Always store Ambien or any other sleep medicine in the original container out of reach of children.

11. Ambien works very quickly. You should only take Ambien right before going to bed and are ready to go to sleep.

7/27/95 ● A05211

Manufactured and distributed by
G.D. Searle & Co.
Chicago, IL 60680
by agreement with
Lorex Pharmaceuticals
Skokie, IL

Address medical inquiries to:
G.D. Searle & Co.
Healthcare Information Services
5200 Old Orchard Road
Skokie, IL 60077

Ambien is a registered trademark of Synthelabo.
Shown in Product Identification Guide, page 335

BREVICON®21-DAY Tablets   ℞
(norethindrone and
ethinyl estradiol)

BREVICON® 28-DAY Tablets   ℞
(norethindrone and
ethinyl estradiol)

NORINYL® 1 + 35 21-DAY Tablets   ℞
(norethindrone and
ethinyl estradiol)

NORINYL® 1 + 35 28-DAY Tablets   ℞
(norethindrone and
ethinyl estradiol))

NORINYL® 1 + 50 21-DAY Tablets   ℞
(norethindrone and mestranol)

NORINYL® 1 + 50 28-DAY Tablets   ℞
(norethindrone and mestranol)

PHYSICIAN LABELING

Patients should be counseled that this product does not protect against HIV infection (AIDS) and other sexually transmitted diseases.

ORAL CONTRACEPTIVE AGENTS
DESCRIPTION
BREVICON 21-DAY Tablets provide an oral contraceptive regimen consisting of 21 blue tablets containing norethindrone 0.5 mg and ethinyl estradiol 0.035 mg.
BREVICON 28-DAY Tablets provide a continuous oral contraceptive regimen consisting of 21 blue tablets containing norethindrone 0.5 mg and ethinyl estradiol 0.035 mg and 7 orange tablets containing inert ingredients.
NORINYL 1 + 35 21-DAY Tablets provide an oral contraceptive regimen consisting of 21 yellow-green tablets containing norethindrone 1 mg and ethinyl estradiol 0.035 mg.
NORINYL 1 + 35 28-DAY Tablets provide a continuous oral contraceptive regimen consisting of 21 yellow-green tablets containing norethindrone 1 mg and ethinyl estradiol 0.035 mg followed by 7 orange tablets containing inert ingredients.
NORINYL 1 + 50 21-DAY Tablets provide an oral contraceptive regimen consisting of 21 white tablets containing norethindrone 1 mg and mestranol 0.05 mg.
NORINYL 1 + 50 28-DAY Tablets provide a continuous oral contraceptive regimen consisting of 21 white tablets

---

containing norethindrone 1 mg and mestranol 0.05 mg and 7 orange tablets containing inert ingredients.
Norethindrone is a potent progestational agent with the chemical name 17-Hydroxy-19-Nor-17α-pregn-4-en-20-yn-3-one. Ethinyl estradiol is an estrogen with the chemical name 19-nor-17α-pregna-1, 3, 5(10) -trien-20-yne-3, 17-diol. Mestranol is an estrogen with the chemical name 3-Methoxy-19-nor-17α-pregna-1, 3, 5(10) -trien-20-yn-17-ol. Their structural formulae follow:

NORETHINDRONE

ETHINYL ESTRADIOL

MESTRANOL

The blue BREVICON tablets contain the following inactive ingredients: FD&C Blue No. 1, lactose, magnesium stearate, povidone, and starch.
The yellow-green NORINYL 1 + 35 tablets contain the following inactive ingredients: D&C Green No. 5, D&C Yellow No. 10, lactose, magnesium stearate, povidone, and starch.
The white NORINYL 1 + 50 tablets contain the following inactive ingredients: lactose, magnesium stearate, povidone, and starch.
The inactive orange tablets in the 28-day regimens of BREVICON, NORINYL 1 + 35 and NORINYL 1 + 50 contain the following ingredients: FD&C Yellow No. 6, lactose, magnesium stearate, povidone and starch.

CLINICAL PHARMACOLOGY
Combination oral contraceptives act by suppression of gonadotrophins. Although the primary mechanism of this action is inhibition of ovulation, other alterations include changes in the cervical mucus (which increase the difficulty of sperm entry into the uterus) and the endometrium (which may reduce the likelihood of implantation).

INDICATIONS AND USAGE
Oral contraceptives are indicated for the prevention of pregnancy in women who elect to use these products as a method of contraception.
Oral contraceptives are highly effective. Table I lists the typical accidental pregnancy rates for users of combination oral contraceptives and other methods of contraception.[1] The efficacy of these contraceptive methods, except sterilization, depends upon the reliability with which they are used. Correct and consistent use of methods can result in lower failure rates.

TABLE I: LOWEST EXPECTED AND TYPICAL FAILURE RATES DURING THE FIRST YEAR OF CONTINUOUS USE OF A METHOD
% of Women Experiencing an Accidental Pregnancy in the First Year of Continuous Use

Method	Lowest Expected[a]	Typical[b]
(No contraception)	(85)	(85)
Oral contraceptives		
combined	0.1	N/A[c]
progestogen only	0.5	N/A[c]
Diaphragm with spermicidal cream or jelly	6	18
Spermicides alone (foam, creams, jellies and vaginal suppositories)	3	21
Vaginal sponge		
Nulliparous	6	18
Multiparous	>9	>28
IUD (medicated)	2	3[d]
Condom without spermicides	2	12
Periodic abstinence (all methods)	1–9	20
Injectable progestogen[e]	0.4	0.4
Implants	0.04	0.04
Female sterilization	0.2	0.4
Male sterilization	0.1	0.15

Adapted from J. Trussell, Table 1 [1]
[a] The authors' best guess of the percentage of women expected to experience an accidental pregnancy among couples who initiate a method (not necessarily for the first time) and who use it consistently and correctly during the first year if they do not stop for any other reason.
[b] This term represents "typical" couples who initiate use of a method (not necessarily for the first time), who experience an accidental pregnancy during the first year if they do not stop use for any other reason. The authors derive these data largely from the National Surveys of Family Growth (NSFG), 1976 and 1982.
[c] N/A—Data not available from the NSFG, 1976 and 1982.
[d] Combined typical rate for both medicated and non-medicated IUD. The rate for medicated IUD alone is not available.
[e] All forms.

CONTRAINDICATIONS
Oral contraceptives should not be used in women who have the following conditions:
● Thrombophlebitis or thromboembolic disorders
● A past history of deep vein thrombophlebitis or thromboembolic disorders
● Cerebral vascular or coronary artery disease
● Known or suspected carcinoma of the breast
● Carcinoma of the endometrium, and known or suspected estrogen-dependent neoplasia
● Undiagnosed abnormal genital bleeding
● Cholestatic jaundice of pregnancy or jaundice with prior pill use
● Hepatic adenomas, carcinomas or benign liver tumors
● Known or suspected pregnancy

WARNINGS

Cigarette smoking increases the risk of serious cardiovascular side effects from oral contraceptive use. This risk increases with age and with heavy smoking (15 or more cigarettes per day) and is quite marked in women over 35 years of age. Women who use oral contraceptives are strongly advised not to smoke.

The use of oral contraceptives is associated with increased risks of several serious conditions including myocardial infarction, thromboembolism, stroke, hepatic neoplasia and gallbladder disease, although the risk of serious morbidity and mortality increases significantly in the presence of other underlying risk factors such as hypertension, hyperlipidemias, hypercholesterolemia, obesity and diabetes.[2–5]

Practitioners prescribing oral contraceptives should be familiar with the following information relating to these risks.

The information contained in this package insert is principally based on studies carried out in patients who used oral contraceptives with formulations containing 0.05 mg or higher of estrogen.[6–11] The effects of long-term use with lower dose formulations of both estrogens and progestogens remain to be determined.

Throughout this labeling, epidemiological studies reported are of two types: retrospective or case control studies and prospective or cohort studies. Case control studies provide a measure of the relative risk of a disease. Relative risk, the *ratio* of the incidence of a disease among oral contraceptive users to that among non-users, cannot be assessed directly from case control studies, but the odds ratio obtained is a measure of relative risk. The relative risk does not provide information on the actual clinical occurrence of a disease. Cohort studies provide not only a measure of the relative risk but a measure of attributable risk, which is the *difference* in the incidence of disease between oral contraceptive users and non-users. The attributable risk does provide information about the actual occurrence of a disease in the population.[12–13]

Continued on next page

Searle—Cont.

1. THROMBOEMBOLIC DISORDERS AND OTHER VASCULAR PROBLEMS

a. Myocardial Infarction

An increased risk of myocardial infarction has been attributed to oral contraceptive use. This risk is primarily in smokers or women with other underlying risk factors for coronary artery disease such as hypertension, hypercholesterolemia, morbid obesity and diabetes.[2–5,13] The relative risk of heart attack for current oral contraceptive users has been estimated to be 2 to 6.[2,14–19] The risk is very low under the age of 30. However, there is the possibility of a risk of cardiovascular disease even in very young women who take oral contraceptives.

Smoking in combination with oral contraceptive use has been shown to contribute substantially to the incidence of myocardial infarctions in women 35 or older, with smoking accounting for the majority of excess cases.[20]

Mortality rates associated with circulatory disease have been shown to increase substantially in smokers over the age of 35 and non-smokers over the age of 40 among women who use oral contraceptives (see Table II).[16]

TABLE II: CIRCULATORY DISEASE MORTALITY RATES PER 100,000 WOMAN YEARS BY AGE, SMOKING STATUS AND ORAL CONTRACEPTIVE USE

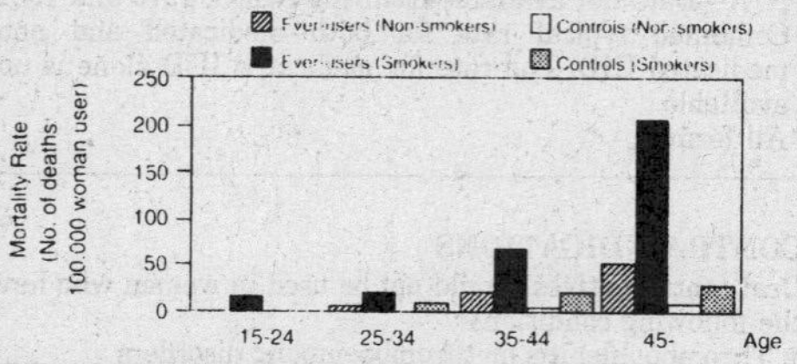

Adapted from P.M. Layde and V. Beral, Table V[16]

Oral contraceptives may compound the effects of well-known risk factors for coronary artery disease, such as hypertension, diabetes, hyperlipidemias, hypercholesterolemia, age and obesity.[3,13,21] In particular, some progestogens are known to decrease HDL cholesterol and impair oral glucose tolerance, while estrogens may create a state of hyperinsulinism.[21–25] Oral contraceptives have been shown to increase blood pressure among users (see **WARNINGS**, section 9). Similar effects on risk factors have been associated with an increased risk of heart disease. Oral contraceptives must be used with caution in women with cardiovascular disease risk factors.

b. Thromboembolism

An increased risk of thromboembolic and thrombotic disease associated with the use of oral contraceptives is well established. Case control studies have found the relative risk of users compared to non-users to be 3 for the first episode of superficial venous thrombosis, 4 to 11 for deep vein thrombosis or pulmonary embolism, and 1.5 to 6 for women with predisposing conditions for venous thromboembolic disease.[12,13,26–31] One cohort study has shown the relative risk to be somewhat lower, about 3 for new cases (subjects with no past history of venous thrombosis or varicose veins) and about 4.5 for new cases requiring hospitalization.[32] The risk of thromboembolic disease due to oral contraceptives is not related to length of use and disappears after pill use is stopped.[12]

A 2- to 6-fold increase in relative risk of post-operative thromboembolic complications has been reported with the use of oral contraceptives.[18] If feasible, oral contraceptives should be discontinued at least 4 weeks prior to and for 2 weeks after elective surgery and during and following prolonged immobilization. Since the immediate postpartum period also is associated with an increased risk of thromboembolism, oral contraceptives should be started no earlier than 4 to 6 weeks after delivery in women who elect not to breast feed.[33]

c. Cerebrovascular diseases

An increase in both the relative and attributable risks of cerebrovascular events (thrombotic and hemorrhagic strokes) has been shown in users of oral contraceptives. In general, the risk is greatest among older (> 35 years), hypertensive women who also smoke. Hypertension was found to be a risk factor for both users and non-users for both types of strokes while smoking interacted to increase the risk for hemorrhagic strokes.[34]

In a large study, the relative risk of thrombotic strokes has been shown to range from 3 for normotensive users to 14 for users with severe hypertension.[35] The relative risk of hemorrhagic stroke is reported to be 1.2 for non-smokers who used oral contraceptives, 2.6 for smokers who did not use oral contraceptives, 7.6 for smokers who used oral contraceptives, 1.8 for normotensive users and 25.7 for users with severe hypertension.[35] The attributable risk also is greater in women 35 or older and among smokers.[13]

d. Dose-related risk of vascular disease from oral contraceptives

A positive association has been observed between the amount of estrogen and progestogen in oral contraceptives and the risk of vascular disease.[36–38] A decline in serum high density lipoproteins (HDL) has been reported with some progestational agents.[22–24] A decline in serum high density lipoproteins has been associated with an increased incidence of ischemic heart disease.[39] Because estrogens increase HDL cholesterol, the net effect of an oral contraceptive depends on a balance achieved between doses of estrogen and progestogen and the nature and absolute amount of progestogens used in the contraceptives. The amount of both hormones should be considered in the choice of an oral contraceptive.[37]

Minimizing exposure to estrogen and progestogen is in keeping with good principles of therapeutics. For any particular estrogen/progestogen combination, the dosage regimen prescribed should be one which contains the least amount of estrogen and progestogen that is compatible with a low failure rate and the needs of the individual patient. New acceptors of oral contraceptive agents should be started on preparations containing the lowest estrogen content that produces satisfactory results for the individual.

e. Persistence of risk of vascular disease

There are three studies which have shown persistence of risk of vascular disease for ever-users of oral contraceptives.[17,34,40] In a study in the United States, the risk of developing myocardial infarction after discontinuing oral contraceptives persists for at least 9 years for women 40–49 years who had used oral contraceptives for 5 or more years, but this increased risk was not demonstrated in other age groups.[17] In another study in Great Britain, the risk of developing cerebrovascular disease persisted for at least 6 years after discontinuation of oral contraceptives, although excess risk was very small.[40] Subarachnoid hemorrhage also has a significantly increased relative risk after termination of use of oral contraceptives.[34] However, these studies were performed with oral contraceptive formulations containing 0.05 mg or higher of estrogen.

2. ESTIMATES OF MORTALITY FROM CONTRACEPTIVE USE

One study gathered data from a variety of sources which have estimated the mortality rates associated with different methods of contraception at different ages (see Table III).[41] These estimates include the combined risk of death associated with contraceptive methods plus the risk attributable to pregnancy in the event of method failure. Each method of contraception has its specific benefits and risks. The study concluded that with the exception of oral contraceptive users 35 and older who smoke and 40 and older who do not smoke, mortality associated with all methods of birth control is low and below that associated with childbirth. The observation of a possible increase in risk of mortality with age for oral contraceptive users is based on data gathered in the 1970's—but not reported in the U.S. until 1983.[16,41] However, current clinical practice involves the use of lower estrogen dose formulations combined with careful restriction of oral contraceptive use to women who do not have the various risk factors listed in this labeling.

Because of these changes in practice and, also, because of some limited new data which suggest that the risk of cardiovascular disease with the use of oral contraceptives may now be less than previously observed,[78,79] the Fertility and Maternal Health Drugs Advisory Committee was asked to review the topic in 1989. The Committee concluded that although cardiovascular disease risks may be increased with oral contraceptive use after age 40 in healthy non-smoking women (even with the newer low-dose formulations), there are greater potential health risks associated with pregnancy in older women and with the alternative surgical and medical procedures which may be necessary if such women do not have access to effective and acceptable means of contraception.

Therefore, the Committee recommended that the benefits of oral contraceptive use by healthy non-smoking women over 40 may outweigh the possible risks. Of course, older women, as all women who take oral contraceptives, should take the lowest possible dose formulation that is effective.[80]

[See Table III below.]

3. CARCINOMA OF THE BREAST AND REPRODUCTIVE ORGANS

Numerous epidemiological studies have been performed on the incidence of breast, endometrial, ovarian and cervical cancer in women using oral contraceptives. The evidence in the literature suggests that use of oral contraceptives is not associated with an increase in the risk of developing breast cancer, regardless of the age and parity of first use or with most of the marketed brands and doses.[42,43] The Cancer and Steroid Hormone study also showed no latent effect on the risk of breast cancer for at least a decade following long-term use.[43] A few studies have shown a slightly increased relative risk of developing breast cancer,[44–47] although the methodology of these studies, which included differences in examination of users and non-users and differences in age at start of use, has been questioned.[47–49] Some studies have reported an increased relative risk of developing breast cancer, particularly at a younger age. This increased relative risk appears to be related to duration of use.[81,82]

Some studies suggest that oral contraceptive use has been associated with an increase in the risk of cervical intraepithelial neoplasia in some populations of women.[50–53] However, there continues to be controversy about the extent to which such findings may be due to differences in sexual behavior and other factors.

In spite of many studies of the relationship between oral contraceptive use and breast or cervical cancers, a cause and effect relationship has not been established.

4. HEPATIC NEOPLASIA

Benign hepatic adenomas are associated with oral contraceptive use although the incidence of benign tumors is rare in the United States. Indirect calculations have estimated the attributable risk to be in the range of 3.3 cases per 100,000 for users, a risk that increases after 4 or more years of use.[54] Rupture of rare, benign, hepatic adenomas may cause death through intra-abdominal hemorrhage.[55–56]

Studies in the United States and Britain have shown an increased risk of developing hepatocellular carcinoma in long-term (> 8 years) oral contraceptive users.[57–59] However, these cancers are extremely rare in the United States and the attributable risk (the excess incidence) of liver cancers in oral contraceptive users is less than 1 per 1,000,000 users.

5. OCULAR LESIONS

There have been clinical case reports of retinal thrombosis associated with the use of oral contraceptives. Oral contraceptives should be discontinued if there is unexplained partial or complete loss of vision; onset of proptosis or diplopia; papilledema; or retinal vascular lesions. Appropriate diagnostic and therapeutic measures should be undertaken immediately.

6. ORAL CONTRACEPTIVE USE BEFORE OR DURING EARLY PREGNANCY

Extensive epidemiological studies have revealed no increased risk of birth defects in women who have used oral contraceptives prior to pregnancy.[60–62] More recent studies do not suggest a teratogenic effect, particularly insofar as cardiac anomalies and limb reduction defects are concerned, when taken inadvertently during early pregnancy.[60,61,63,64]

The administration of oral contraceptives to induce withdrawal bleeding should not be used as a test for pregnancy. Oral contraceptives should not be used during pregnancy to treat threatened or habitual abortion.

It is recommended that for any patient who has missed 2 consecutive periods, pregnancy should be ruled out before continuing oral contraceptive use. If the patient has not adhered to the prescribed schedule, the possibility of pregnancy should be considered at the time of the first missed period. Oral contraceptive use should be discontinued if pregnancy is confirmed.

TABLE III: ESTIMATED ANNUAL NUMBER OF BIRTH-RELATED OR METHOD-RELATED DEATHS ASSOCIATED WITH CONTROL OF FERTILITY PER 100,000 NONSTERILE WOMEN, BY FERTILITY CONTROL METHOD ACCORDING TO AGE

Method of control and outcome	15–19	20–24	25–29	30–34	35–39	40–44
No fertility control methods*	7.0	7.4	9.1	14.8	25.7	28.2
Oral contraceptives non-smoker**	0.3	0.5	0.9	1.9	13.8	31.6
Oral contraceptives smoker**	2.2	3.4	6.6	13.5	51.1	117.2
IUD**	0.8	0.8	1.0	1.0	1.4	1.4
Condom*	1.1	1.6	0.7	0.2	0.3	0.4
Diaphragm/Spermicide*	1.9	1.2	1.2	1.3	2.2	2.8
Periodic abstinence*	2.5	1.6	1.6	1.7	2.9	3.6

* Deaths are birth-related
** Deaths are method-related

Estimates adapted from H.W. Ory, Table 3[41]

7. GALLBLADDER DISEASE

Earlier studies have reported an increased lifetime relative risk of gallbladder surgery in users of oral contraceptives and estrogens.[65-66] More recent studies, however, have shown that the relative risk of developing gallbladder disease among oral contraceptive users may be minimal.[67] The recent findings of minimal risk may be related to the use of oral contraceptive formulations containing lower hormonal doses of estrogens and progestogens.[68]

8. CARBOHYDRATE AND LIPID METABOLIC EFFECTS

Oral contraceptives have been shown to impair oral glucose tolerance.[69] Oral contraceptives containing greater than 0.075 mg of estrogen cause glucose intolerance with impaired insulin secretion, while lower doses of estrogen may produce less glucose intolerance.[70] Progestogens increase insulin secretion and create insulin resistance, this effect varying with different progestational agents.[25,71] However, in the non-diabetic woman, oral contraceptives appear to have no effect on fasting blood glucose.[69] Because of these demonstrated effects, prediabetic and diabetic women should be carefully observed while taking oral contraceptives.

Some women may develop persistent hypertriglyceridemia while on the pill.[72] As discussed earlier (see **WARNINGS**, sections 1a. and 1d.), changes in serum triglycerides and lipoprotein levels have been reported in oral contraceptive users.[23]

9. ELEVATED BLOOD PRESSURE

An increase in blood pressure has been reported in women taking oral contraceptives. The incidence of risk also was reported to increase with continued use and among older women.[66] Data from the Royal College of General Practitioners and subsequent randomized trials have shown that the incidence of hypertension increases with increasing concentrations of progestogens.

Women with a history of hypertension or hypertension-related diseases or renal disease should be encouraged to use another method of contraception. If women elect to use oral contraceptives, they should be monitored closely and if significant elevation of blood pressure occurs oral contraceptives should be discontinued. For most women, elevated blood pressure will return to normal after stopping oral contraceptives and there is no difference in the occurrence of hypertension among ever- and never-users.[73-75]

10. HEADACHE

The onset or exacerbation of migraine or development of headache with a new pattern which is recurrent, persistent or severe requires discontinuation of oral contraceptives and evaluation of the cause.

11. BLEEDING IRREGULARITIES

Breakthrough bleeding and spotting are sometimes encountered in patients on oral contraceptives, especially during the first 3 months of use. Non-hormonal causes should be considered and adequate diagnostic measures taken to rule out malignancy or pregnancy in the event of breakthrough bleeding, as in the case of any abnormal vaginal bleeding. If pathology has been excluded, time or a change to another formulation may solve the problem. In the event of amenorrhea, pregnancy should be ruled out.

Some women may encounter post-pill amenorrhea or oligomenorrhea, especially when such a condition was pre-existent.

PRECAUTIONS

GENERAL

PATIENTS SHOULD BE COUNSELED THAT THIS PRODUCT DOES NOT PROTECT AGAINST HIV (AIDS) AND OTHER SEXUALLY TRANSMITTED DISEASES.

1. PHYSICAL EXAMINATION AND FOLLOW-UP

It is good medical practice for all women to have annual history and physical examinations, including women using oral contraceptives. The physical examination, however, may be deferred until after initiation of oral contraceptives if requested by the woman and judged appropriate by the clinician. The physical examination should include special reference to blood pressure, breasts, abdomen and pelvic organs, including cervical cytology, and relevant laboratory tests. In case of undiagnosed, persistent or recurrent abnormal vaginal bleeding, appropriate measures should be conducted to rule out malignancy. Women with a strong family history of breast cancer or who have breast nodules should be monitored with particular care.

2. LIPID DISORDERS

Women who are being treated for hyperlipidemias should be followed closely if they elect to use oral contraceptives. Some progestogens may elevate LDL levels and may render the control of hyperlipidemias more difficult.

3. LIVER FUNCTION

If jaundice develops in any woman receiving oral contraceptives the medication should be discontinued. Steroid hormones may be poorly metabolized in patients with impaired liver function.

4. FLUID RETENTION

Oral contraceptives may cause some degree of fluid retention. They should be prescribed with caution, and only with careful monitoring, in patients with conditions which might be aggravated by fluid retention.

5. EMOTIONAL DISORDERS

Women with a history of depression should be carefully observed and the drug discontinued if depression recurs to a serious degree.

6. CONTACT LENSES

Contact lens wearers who develop visual changes or changes in lens tolerance should be assessed by an ophthalmologist.

7. DRUG INTERACTIONS

Reduced efficacy and increased incidence of breakthrough bleeding and menstrual irregularities have been associated with concomitant use of rifampin. A similar association though less marked, has been suggested with barbiturates, phenylbutazone, phenytoin sodium, and possibly with griseofulvin, ampicillin and tetracyclines.[76]

8. INTERACTIONS WITH LABORATORY TESTS

Certain endocrine and liver function tests and blood components may be affected by oral contraceptives:

a. Increased prothrombin and factors VII, VIII, IX, and X; decreased antithrombin 3; increased norepinephrine-induced platelet aggregability.

b. Increased thyroid binding globulin (TBG) leading to increased circulating total thyroid hormone, as measured by protein-bound iodine (PBI), T4 by column or by radioimmunoassay. Free T3 resin uptake is decreased, reflecting the elevated TBG. Free T4 concentration is unaltered.

c. Other binding proteins may be elevated in serum.

d. Sex steroid binding globulins are increased and result in elevated levels of total circulating sex steroids and corticoids; however, free or biologically active levels remain unchanged.

e. Triglycerides may be increased.

f. Glucose tolerance may be decreased.

g. Serum folate levels may be depressed by oral contraceptive therapy. This may be of clinical significance if a woman becomes pregnant shortly after discontinuing oral contraceptives.

9. CARCINOGENESIS

See **WARNINGS** section.

10. PREGNANCY

Pregnancy Category X. See **CONTRAINDICATIONS** and **WARNINGS** sections.

11. NURSING MOTHERS

Small amounts of oral contraceptive steroids have been identified in the milk of nursing mothers and a few adverse effects on the child have been reported, including jaundice and breast enlargement. In addition, oral contraceptives given in the postpartum period may interfere with lactation by decreasing the quantity and quality of breast milk. If possible, the nursing mother should be advised not to use oral contraceptives but to use other forms of contraception until she has completely weaned her child.

INFORMATION FOR THE PATIENT

See **PATIENT LABELING** printed below.

ADVERSE REACTIONS

An increased risk of the following serious adverse reactions has been associated with the use of oral contraceptives (see **WARNINGS** section):
- Thrombophlebitis
- Arterial thromboembolism
- Pulmonary embolism
- Myocardial infarction
- Cerebral hemorrhage
- Cerebral thrombosis
- Hypertension
- Gallbladder disease
- Hepatic adenomas, carcinomas or benign liver tumors

There is evidence of an association between the following conditions and the use of oral contraceptives, although additional confirmatory studies are needed:
- Mesenteric thrombosis
- Retinal thrombosis

The following adverse reactions have been reported in patients receiving oral contraceptives and are believed to be drug-related:
- Nausea
- Vomiting
- Gastrointestinal symptoms (such as abdominal cramps and bloating)
- Breakthrough bleeding
- Spotting
- Change in menstrual flow
- Amenorrhea
- Temporary infertility after discontinuation of treatment
- Edema
- Melasma which may persist
- Breast changes: tenderness, enlargement, secretion
- Change in weight (increase or decrease)
- Change in cervical erosion and secretion
- Diminution in lactation when given immediately postpartum
- Cholestatic jaundice
- Migraine
- Rash (allergic)
- Mental depression
- Reduced tolerance to carbohydrates
- Vaginal candidiasis
- Change in corneal curvature (steepening)
- Intolerance to contact lenses

The following adverse reactions have been reported in users of oral contraceptives and the association has been neither confirmed nor refuted:
- Pre-menstrual syndrome
- Cataracts
- Changes in appetite
- Cystitis-like syndrome
- Headache
- Nervousness
- Dizziness
- Hirsutism
- Loss of scalp hair
- Erythema multiforme
- Erythema nodosum
- Hemorrhagic eruption
- Vaginitis
- Porphyria
- Impaired renal function
- Hemolytic uremic syndrome
- Budd-Chiari syndrome
- Acne
- Changes in libido
- Colitis

OVERDOSAGE

Serious ill effects have not been reported following acute ingestion of large doses of oral contraceptives by young children. Overdosage may cause nausea, and withdrawal bleeding may occur in females.

NON-CONTRACEPTIVE HEALTH BENEFITS

The following non-contraceptive health benefits related to the use of oral contraceptives are supported by epidemiological studies which largely utilized oral contraceptive formulations containing estrogen doses exceeding 0.035 mg of ethinyl estradiol or 0.05 mg of mestranol.[6-11]

Effects on menses:
- Increased menstrual cycle regularity
- Decreased blood loss and decreased incidence of iron deficiency anemia
- Decreased incidence of dysmenorrhea

Effects related to inhibition of ovulation:
- Decreased incidence of functional ovarian cysts
- Decreased incidence of ectopic pregnancies

Effects from long-term use:
- Decreased incidence of fibroadenomas and fibrocystic disease of the breast
- Decreased incidence of acute pelvic inflammatory disease
- Decreased incidence of endometrial cancer
- Decreased incidence of ovarian cancer

DOSAGE AND ADMINISTRATION

To achieve maximum contraceptive effectiveness, oral contraceptives must be taken exactly as described and at intervals not exceeding 24 hours.

21-Day Schedule: For a SUNDAY START when menstrual flow begins on or before Sunday, the first tablet (white or yellow-green or blue) is taken on that day. For a Day 5 start, count the first day of menstrual flow as Day 1 and the first tablet (white or yellow-green or blue) is then taken on Day 5. With either a SUNDAY START or DAY 5 START, 1 tablet is taken each day at the same time for 21 days. No tablets are taken for 7 days, then, whether bleeding has stopped or not, a new course is started of 1 tablet a day for 21 days. This institutes a 3 weeks on, 1 week off dosage regimen.

28-Day Schedule: For a SUNDAY START when menstrual flow begins on or before Sunday, the first tablet (white or yellow-green or blue) is taken on that day. For a Day 5 start, count the first day of menstrual flow as Day 1 and the first tablet (white or yellow-green or blue) is then taken on Day 5. With either a SUNDAY START or DAY 5 START, 1 tablet (white or yellow-green or blue) is taken each day at the same time for 21 days. Then the orange tablets are taken for 7 days, whether bleeding has stopped or not. After all 28 tablets have been taken, whether bleeding has stopped or not, the same dosage schedule is repeated beginning on the following day.

INSTRUCTIONS TO PATIENTS

- To achieve maximum contraceptive effectiveness, the oral contraceptive pill must be taken exactly as directed and at intervals not exceeding 24 hours.
- Important: Women should be instructed to use an additional method of protection until after the first 7 days of administration *in the initial cycle.*
- Due to the normally increased risk of thromboembolism occurring postpartum, women should be instructed not to initiate treatment with oral contraceptives earlier than 4 weeks after a full-term delivery. If pregnancy is termi-

Continued on next page

Searle—Cont.

nated in the first 12 weeks, the patient should be instructed to start oral contraceptives immediately or within 7 days. If pregnancy is terminated after 12 weeks, the patient should be instructed to start oral contraceptives after 2 weeks.[33,77]

- If spotting or breakthrough bleeding should occur, the patient should continue the medication according to the schedule. Should spotting or breakthrough bleeding persist, the patient should notify her physician.
- If the patient misses 1 pill, she should be instructed to take it as soon as she remembers and then take the next pill at the regular time. The patient should be advised that missing a pill can cause spotting or light bleeding and that she may be a little sick to her stomach on the days she takes the missed pill with her regularly scheduled pill. If the patient has missed more than one pill, she should not take the missed pills and they should be discarded. She should be advised to take the next pill at the next regular time and continue to take them as scheduled. Furthermore, she should use an additional method of contraception in addition to taking her pills for the remainder of the cycle.
- Use of oral contraceptives in the event of a missed menstrual period:
  1. If the patient has not adhered to the prescribed dosage regimen, the possibility of pregnancy should be considered after the first missed period and oral contraceptives should be withheld until pregnancy has been ruled out.
  2. If the patient has adhered to the prescribed regimen and misses 2 consecutive periods, pregnancy should be ruled out before continuing the contraceptive regimen.

HOW SUPPLIED

BREVICON® 21-DAY Tablets and BREVICON® 28-DAY Tablets (norethindrone and ethinyl estradiol), NORINYL® 1 + 35 21-DAY Tablets and NORINYL® 1 + 35 28-DAY Tablets (norethindrone and ethinyl estradiol), and NORINYL® 1 + 50 21-DAY Tablets and NORINYL® 1 + 50 28-DAY Tablets (norethindrone and mestranol) are available in 21-tablet or 28-tablet blister cards with a WALLETTE® tablet dispenser. Each 28-tablet card contains 7 orange inert tablets.
CAUTION: Federal law prohibits dispensing without prescription.

REFERENCES

1. Trussell, J., et al.: *Stud Fam Plann* 21(1):51–54, 1990 2. Mann, J., et al.: *Br Med J* 2(5956):241–245, 1975. 3. Knopp, R.H.: *J Reprod Med* 31(9):913–921, 1986. 4. Mann, J.I., et al.: *Br Med J* 2:445–447, 1976. 5. Ory, H.: *JAMA* 237:2619–2622, 1977. 6. The Cancer and Steroid Hormone Study of the Centers for Disease Control: *JAMA* 249(2):1596–1599, 1983. 7. The Cancer and Steroid Hormone Study of the Centers for Disease Control: *JAMA* 257(6):796–800, 1987. 8. Ory, H.W.: *JAMA* 228(1):68–69, 1974. 9. Ory, H.W., et al.: *N Engl J Med* 294:419–422, 1976. 10. Ory, H.W.: *Fam Plann Perspect* 14:182–184, 1982. 11. Ory, H.W., et al.: *Making Choices*, New York, The Alan Guttmacher Institute, 1983. 12. Stadel, B.: *N Engl J Med* 305(11):612–618, 1981. 13. Stadel, B.: *N Engl J Med* 305(12):672–677, 1981. 14. Adam, S., et al.: *Br J Obstet Gynaecol* 88:838–845, 1981. 15. Mann, J., et al.: *Br Med J* 2(5965):245–248, 1975. 16. Royal College of General Practitioners' Oral Contraceptive Study: *Lancet* 1:541–546, 1981. 17. Slone, D., et al.: *N Engl J Med* 305(8):420–424, 1981. 18. Vessey, M.P.: *Br J Fam Plann* 6 (Supplement):1–12, 1980. 19. Russell-Briefel, R., et al.: *Prev Med* 15:352–362, 1986. 20. Goldbaum, G., et al.: *JAMA* 258(10):1339–1342, 1987. 21. LaRosa, J.C.: *J Reprod Med* 31(9):906–912, 1986. 22. Krauss, R.M., et al.: *Am J Obstet Gynecol* 145:446–452, 1983. 23. Wahl, P., et al.: *N Engl J Med* 308(15):862–867, 1983. 24. Wynn, V., et al.: *Am J Obstet Gynecol* 142(6):766–771, 1982. 25. Wynn V., et al.: *J Reprod Med* 31(9):892–897, 1986. 26. Inman, W.H., et al.: *Br Med J* 2(5599):193–199, 1968. 27. Maguire, M.G., et al.: *Am J Epidemiol* 110(2):188–195, 1979. 28. Petitti, D., et al.: *JAMA* 242(11):1150–1154, 1979. 29. Vessey, M.P., et al.: *Br Med J* 2(5599):199–205, 1968. 30. Vessey, M.P., et al.: *Br Med J* 2(5658):651–657, 1969. 31. Porter, J.B., et al.: *Obstet Gynecol* 59(3):299–302, 1982. 32. Vessey, M.P., et al.: *J Biosoc Sci* 8:373–427, 1976. 33. Mishell, D.R., et al.: *Reproductive Endocrinology*, Philadelphia, F.A. Davis Co., 1979. 34. Petitti, D.B., et al.: *Lancet* 2:234–236, 1978. 35. Collaborative Group for the Study of Stroke in Young Women: *JAMA* 231(7):718–722, 1975. 36. Inman, W.H., et al.: *Br Med J* 2:203–209, 1970. 37. Meade, T.W., et al.: *Br Med J* 280 (6224):1157–1161, 1980. 38. Kay, C.R.: *Am J Obstet Gynecol* 142(6):762–765, 1982. 39. Gordon, T., et al.: *Am J Med* 62:707–714, 1977. 40. Royal College of General Practitioners' Oral Contraception Study: *J Coll Gen Pract* 33:75–82, 1983. 41. Ory, H.W.: *Fam Plann Perspect* 15(2):57–63, 1983. 42. Paul, C., et al.: *Br Med J* 293:723–725, 1986. 43. The Cancer and Steroid Hormone Study of the Centers for Disease Control: *N Engl J Med* 315(7):405–411, 1986. 44. Pike, M.C., et al.: *Lancet* 2:926–929, 1983. 45. Miller, D.R., et al.: *Obstet Gynecol* 68:863–868, 1986. 46. Olsson, H., et al.: *Lancet* 2:748–749, 1985. 47. McPherson, K., et al.: *Br J Cancer* 56:653–660, 1987. 48. Huggins, G.R., et al.: *Fertil Steril* 47(5):733–761, 1987. 49. McPherson, K., et al.: *Br Med J* 293:709–710, 1986. 50. Ory, H., et al.: *Am J Obstet Gynecol* 124(6):573–577, 1976. 51. Vessey, M.P., et al.: *Lancet*, 2:930, 1983. 52. Brinton, L.A., et al.: *Int J Cancer* 38:339–344, 1986. 53. WHO Collaborative Study of Neoplasia and Steroid Contraceptives: *Br Med J* 290:961–965, 1985. 54. Rooks, J.B., et al.: *JAMA* 242(7):644–648, 1979. 55. Bein, N.N., et al.: *Br J Surg* 64:433–435, 1977. 56. Klatskin, G.: *Gastroenterology* 73:386–394, 1977. 57. Henderson, B.E., et al.: *Br J Cancer* 48:437–440, 1983. 58. Neuberger, J., et al.: *Br Med J* 292:1355–1357, 1986. 59. Forman, D., et al.: *Br Med J* 292:1357–1361, 1986. 60. Harlap, S., et al.: *Obstet Gynecol* 55(4):447–452, 1980. 61. Savolainen, E., et al.: *Am J Obstet Gynecol* 140(5):521–524, 1981. 62. Janerich, D.T., et al.: *Am J Epidemiol* 112(1):73–79, 1980. 63. Ferencz, C., et al.: *Teratology* 21:225–239, 1980. 64. Rothman, K.J., et al.: *Am J Epidemiol* 109(4):433–439, 1979. 65. Boston Collaborative Drug Surveillance Program: *Lancet* 1:1399–1404, 1973. 66. Royal College of General Practitioners: *Oral contraceptives and health*. New York, Pittman, 1974. 67. Rome Group for the Epidemiology and Prevention of Cholelithiasis: *Am J Epidemiol* 119(5):796–805, 1984. 68. Strom, B.L., et al.: *Clin Pharmacol Ther* 39(3):335–341, 1986. 69. Perlman, J.A., et al.: *J Chronic Dis* 38(10):857–864, 1985. 70. Wynn, V., et al.: *Lancet* 1:1045–1049, 1979. 71. Wynn, V.: *Progesterone and Progestin*, New York, Raven Press, 1983. 72. Wynn, V., et al.: *Lancet* 2:720–723, 1966. 73. Fisch, I.R., et al.: *JAMA* 237(23):2499–2503, 1977. 74. Laragh, J.H.: *Am J Obstet Gynecol* 126(1):141–147, 1976. 75. Ramcharan, S., et al.: *Pharmacology of Steroid Contraceptive Drugs*, New York, Raven Press, 1977. 76. Stockley, I.: *Pharm J* 216:140–143, 1976. 77. Dickey, R.P.: *Managing Contraceptive Pill Patients*, Oklahoma, Creative Informatics Inc., 1984. 78. Porter J.B., Hunter J., Jick H., et al: *Obstet Gynecol* 1985;66:1–4. 79. Porter J.B., Hershel J., Walker A.M.: *Obstet Gynecol* 1987;70:29–32. 80. Fertility and Maternal Health Drugs Advisory Committee, F.D.A., October, 1989. 81. Schlesselman J., Stadel B.V., Murray P., Lai S.: *Breast cancer in relation to early use of oral contraceptives*. JAMA 1988;259:1828–1833. 82. Hennekens C.H., Speizer F.E., Lipnick R.J., Rosner B., Bain C., Belanger C., Stampfer M.J., Willett W., Peto R.: *A case-control study of oral contraceptive use and breast cancer*. JNCI 1984:72:39–42.

DETAILED PATIENT LABELING

This product (like all oral contraceptives) is intended to prevent pregnancy. It does not protect against HIV infection (AIDS) and other sexually transmitted diseases.

INTRODUCTION

Any woman who considers using oral contraceptives ("birth control pills" or "the pill") should understand the benefits and risks of using this form of birth control. This leaflet will give you much of the information you will need to make this decision and also will help you determine if you are at risk of developing any of the serious side effects of the pill. It will tell you how to use the pill properly so that it will be as effective as possible. However, this leaflet is not a replacement for a careful discussion between you and your health care provider. You should discuss the information provided in this leaflet with him or her, both when you first start taking the pill and during your regular visits. You also should follow the advice of your health care provider with regard to regular checkups while you are on the pill.

EFFECTIVENESS OF ORAL CONTRACEPTIVES

Oral contraceptives are used to prevent pregnancy and are more effective than other non-surgical methods of birth control. When they are taken correctly, without missing any pills, the chance of becoming pregnant is less than 1% (1 pregnancy per 100 women per year of use). Typical failure rates are actually 3% per year. The chance of becoming pregnant increases with each missed pill during a menstrual cycle.
In comparison, typical failure rates for other nonsurgical methods of birth control during the first year are as follows:
IUD: 3%
Diaphragm with spermicides: 18%
Spermicides alone: 21%
Vaginal sponge: 18 to 28%
Condom alone: 12%
Periodic abstinence: 20%
Injectable progestogen: 0.4%
Implants: 0.04%
No methods: 85%

WHO SHOULD NOT TAKE ORAL CONTRACEPTIVES

> **Cigarette smoking increases the risk of serious cardiovascular side effects from oral contraceptive use. This risk increases with age and with heavy smoking (15 or more cigarettes per day) and is quite marked in women over 35 years of age. Women who use oral contraceptives are strongly advised not to smoke.**

Some women should not use the pill. For example, you should not take the pill if you are pregnant or think you may be pregnant. You also should not use the pill if you have any of the following conditions:

- A history of heart attack or stroke
- Blood clots in the legs (thrombophlebitis), brain (stroke), lungs (pulmonary embolism) or eyes
- A history of blood clots in the deep veins of your legs
- Chest pain (angina pectoris)
- Known or suspected breast cancer or cancer of the lining of the uterus, cervix or vagina
- Unexplained vaginal bleeding (until a diagnosis is reached by your doctor)
- Yellowing of the whites of the eyes or of the skin (jaundice) during pregnancy or during previous use of the pill
- Liver tumor (benign or cancerous)
- Known or suspected pregnancy

Tell your health care provider if you have ever had any of these conditions. Your health care provider can recommend a safer method of birth control.

OTHER CONSIDERATIONS BEFORE TAKING ORAL CONTRACEPTIVES

Tell your health care provider if you have or have had:
- Breast nodules, fibrocystic disease of the breast, an abnormal breast x-ray or mammogram
- Diabetes
- Elevated cholesterol or triglycerides
- High blood pressure
- Migraine or other headaches or epilepsy
- Mental depression
- Gallbladder, heart or kidney disease
- History of scanty or irregular menstrual periods

Women with any of these conditions should be checked often by their health care provider if they choose to use oral contraceptives.
Also, be sure to inform your doctor or health care provider if you smoke or are on any medications.

RISKS OF TAKING ORAL CONTRACEPTIVES

1. Risk of developing blood clots
Blood clots and blockage of blood vessels are the most serious side effects of taking oral contraceptives. In particular, a clot in the legs can cause thrombophlebitis and a clot that travels to the lungs can cause a sudden blocking of the vessel carrying blood to the lungs. Rarely, clots occur in the blood vessels of the eye and may cause blindness, double vision, or impaired vision.
If you take oral contraceptives and need elective surgery, need to stay in bed for a prolonged illness or have recently delivered a baby, you may be at risk of developing blood clots. You should consult your doctor about stopping oral contraceptives three to four weeks before surgery and not taking oral contraceptives for two weeks after surgery or during bed rest. You should also not take oral contraceptives soon after delivery of a baby. It is advisable to wait for at least four weeks after delivery if you are not breast feeding. If you are breast feeding, you should wait until you have weaned your child before using the pill (see **GENERAL PRECAUTIONS, While Breast Feeding**).
2. Heart attacks and strokes
Oral contraceptives may increase the tendency to develop strokes (stoppage or rupture of blood vessels in the brain) and angina pectoris and heart attacks (blockage of blood vessels in the heart). Any of these conditions can cause death or temporary or permanent disability.
Smoking greatly increases the possibility of suffering heart attacks and strokes. Furthermore, smoking and the use of oral contraceptives greatly increase the chances of developing and dying of heart disease.
3. Gallbladder disease
Oral contraceptive users may have a greater risk than nonusers of having gallbladder disease, although this risk may be related to pills containing high doses of estrogen.
4. Liver tumors
In rare cases, oral contraceptives can cause benign but dangerous liver tumors. These benign liver tumors can rupture and cause fatal internal bleeding. In addition, a possible but not definite association has been found with the pill and liver cancers in 2 studies in which a few women who developed these very rare cancers were found to have used oral contraceptives for long periods. However, liver cancers are extremely rare.
5. Cancer of the breast and reproductive organs
There is, at present, no confirmed evidence that oral contraceptives increase the risk of cancer of the reproductive organs in human studies. Several studies have found no overall increase in the risk of developing breast cancer. However, women who use oral contraceptives and have a strong family history of breast cancer or who have breast nodules or abnormal mammograms should be followed closely by their doctors. Some studies have reported an increase in the risk of developing breast cancer, particularly at a younger age. This increased risk appears to be related to duration of use. Some studies have found an increase in the incidence of cancer of the cervix in women who use oral contraceptives. How-

ever, this finding may be related to factors other than the use of oral contraceptives.

ESTIMATED RISK OF DEATH FROM A BIRTH CONTROL METHOD OR PREGNANCY

All methods of birth control and pregnancy are associated with a risk of developing certain diseases which may lead to disability or death. An estimate of the number of deaths associated with different methods of birth control and pregnancy has been calculated and is shown in the following table. [See table at right.]

In the above table, the risk of death from any birth control method is less than the risk of childbirth except for oral contraceptive users over the age of 35 who smoke and pill users over the age of 40 even if they do not smoke. It can be seen from the table that for women aged 15 to 39 the risk of death is highest with pregnancy (7-26 deaths per 100,000 women, depending on age). Among pill users who do not smoke the risk of death is always lower than that associated with pregnancy for any age group, although over the age of 40 the risk increases to 32 deaths per 100,000 women compared to 28 associated with pregnancy at that age. However, for pill users who smoke and are over the age of 35 the estimated number of deaths exceeds those for other methods of birth control. If a woman is over the age of 40 and smokes, her estimated risk of death is 4 times higher (117/100,000 women) than the estimated risk associated with pregnancy (28/100,000 women) in that age group.

The suggestion that women over 40 who don't smoke should not take oral contraceptives is based on information from older high-dose pills and on less selective use of pills than is practiced today. An Advisory Committee of the FDA discussed this issue in 1989 and recommended that the benefits of oral contraceptive use by healthy, non-smoking women over 40 years of age may outweigh the possible risks. However, all women, especially older women, are cautioned to use the lowest dose pill that is effective.

WARNING SIGNALS

If any of these adverse effects occur while you are taking oral contraceptives, call your doctor immediately:

- Sharp chest pain, coughing of blood or sudden shortness of breath (indicating a possible clot in the lung)
- Pain in the calf (indicating a possible clot in the leg)
- Crushing chest pain or heaviness in the chest (indicating a possible heart attack)
- Sudden severe headache or vomiting, dizziness or fainting, disturbances of vision or speech, weakness or numbness in an arm or leg (indicating a possible stroke)
- Sudden partial or complete loss of vision (indicating a possible clot in the eye)
- Breast lumps (indicating possible breast cancer or fibrocystic disease of the breast: ask your doctor or health care provider to show you how to examine your breasts)
- Severe pain or tenderness in the stomach area (indicating a possible ruptured liver tumor)
- Difficulty in sleeping, weakness, lack of energy, fatigue or change in mood (possibly indicating severe depression)
- Jaundice or a yellowing of the skin or eyeballs, accompanied frequently by fever, fatigue, loss of appetite, dark colored urine or light colored bowel movements (indicating possible liver problems)

SIDE EFFECTS OF ORAL CONTRACEPTIVES

1. Vaginal bleeding
Irregular vaginal bleeding or spotting may occur while you are taking the pill. Irregular bleeding may vary from slight staining between menstrual periods to breakthrough bleeding which is a flow much like a regular period. Irregular bleeding occurs most often during the first few months of oral contraceptive use but may also occur after you have been taking the pill for some time. Such bleeding may be temporary and usually does not indicate any serious problem. It is important to continue taking your pills on schedule. If the bleeding occurs in more than 1 cycle or lasts for more than a few days, talk to your doctor or health care provider.

2. Contact lenses
If you wear contact lenses and notice a change in vision or an inability to wear your lenses, contact your doctor or health care provider.

3. Fluid retention
Oral contraceptives may cause edema (fluid retention) with swelling of the fingers or ankles and may raise your blood pressure. If you experience fluid retention, contact your doctor or health care provider.

4. Melasma (Mask of Pregnancy)
A spotty darkening of the skin is possible, particularly of the face.

5. Other side effects
Other side effects may include change in appetite, headache, nervousness, depression, dizziness, loss of scalp hair, rash and vaginal infections.

If any of these side effects occur, contact your doctor or health care provider.

ESTIMATED ANNUAL NUMBER OF BIRTH-RELATED OR METHOD-RELATED DEATHS ASSOCIATED WITH CONTROL OF FERTILITY PER 100,000 NON-STERILE WOMEN, BY FERTILITY CONTROL METHOD ACCORDING TO AGE

Method of control and outcome	15–19	20–24	25–29	30–34	35–39	40–44
No fertility control methods*	7.0	7.4	9.1	14.8	25.7	28.2
Oral contraceptives non-smoker**	0.3	0.5	0.9	1.9	13.8	31.6
Oral contraceptives smoker**	2.2	3.4	6.6	13.5	51.1	117.2
IUD**	0.8	0.8	1.0	1.0	1.4	1.4
Condom*	1.1	1.6	0.7	0.2	0.3	0.4
Diaphragm/Spermicide*	1.9	1.2	1.2	1.3	2.2	2.8
Periodic abstinence*	2.5	1.6	1.6	1.7	2.9	3.6

* Deaths are birth-related
**Deaths are method-related

GENERAL PRECAUTIONS

1. Missed periods and use of oral contraceptives before or during early pregnancy
At times you may not menstruate regularly after you have completed taking a cycle of pills. If you have taken your pills regularly and miss 1 menstrual period, continue taking your pills for the next cycle but be sure to inform your health care provider before doing so. If you have not taken the pills daily as instructed and miss 1 menstrual period, or if you miss 2 consecutive menstrual periods, you may be pregnant. You should stop taking oral contraceptives until you are sure you are not pregnant and continue to use another method of contraception.

There is no conclusive evidence that oral contraceptive use is associated with an increase in birth defects when taken inadvertently during early pregnancy. Previously, a few studies had reported that oral contraceptives might be associated with birth defects but these studies have not been confirmed. Nevertheless, oral contraceptives or any other drugs should not be used during pregnancy unless clearly necessary and prescribed by your doctor. You should check with your doctor about risks to your unborn child from any medication taken during pregnancy.

2. While breast feeding
If you are breast feeding, consult your doctor before starting oral contraceptives. Some of the drug will be passed on to the child in the milk. A few adverse effects on the child have been reported, including yellowing of the skin (jaundice) and breast enlargement. In addition, oral contraceptives may decrease the amount and quality of your milk. If possible, use another method of contraception while breast feeding. You should consider starting oral contraceptives only after you have weaned your child completely.

3. Laboratory tests
If you are scheduled for any laboratory tests, tell your doctor you are taking birth control pills. Certain blood tests may be affected by birth control pills.

4. Drug interactions
Certain drugs may interact with birth control pills to make them less effective in preventing pregnancy or cause an increase in breakthrough bleeding. Such drugs include rifampin; drugs used for epilepsy such as barbiturates (for example phenobarbital) and phenytoin (Dilantin is one brand of this drug); phenylbutazone (Butazolidin is one brand of this drug) and possibly certain antibiotics. You may need to use additional contraception when you take drugs which can make oral contraceptives less effective.

HOW TO TAKE ORAL CONTRACEPTIVES

1. Important points to remember
This product (like all oral contraceptives) is intended to prevent pregnancy. It does not protect against transmission of HIV (AIDS) and other sexually transmitted diseases such as chlamydia, genital herpes, genital warts, gonorrhea, hepatitis B, and syphilis.

Before you start taking your pills:
- Be sure to read these directions:
  Before you start taking your pills.
  Anytime you are not sure what to do.
- The right way to take the Pill is to take one pill every day at the same time. If you miss pills you could get pregnant. The more pills you miss, the more likely you are to get pregnant.
- Many women have spotting or light bleeding while they are taking the Pill, or may feel sick to their stomachs during the first 1-3 packs of pills. If you feel sick to your stomach, do not stop taking the Pill. These problems will usually go away after the first three months. If they do not go away, talk to your doctor or clinic.
- Missing pills can also cause spotting or light bleeding (see the section on MISSED PILLS). You could also feel a little sick to your stomach on the days you take a missed pill with your regularly scheduled pill.
- If you have vomiting or diarrhea, for any reason, or if you take some medicines, including some antibiotics, your pills may not work as well. Use a back-up method of birth control until you check with your doctor or clinic. Talk to your

doctor or clinic about which back-up birth control method is right for you.
- If you have trouble remembering to take the Pill (for example, if you forget to take more than one pill two months in a row), talk to your doctor or clinic about how to make pill-taking easier or about using another method of birth control.
- If you have any questions or are unsure about the information in this leaflet, call your doctor or clinic.

2. Before you start taking your pills
- Decide what time of day you want to take your pill. It is important to take it at about the same time every day.
- Look at your pill pack to see if it has 21 or 28 pills:
  The 21-pill pack has 21 "active" white or yellow-green or blue pills (with hormones) to take for 3 weeks, followed by 1 week without pills.
  The 28-pill pack has 21 "active" white or yellow-green or blue pills (with hormones) to take for 3 weeks, followed by 1 week of "reminder" orange pills (without hormones).
- Also find:
  1) where on the pack to start taking pills.
  2) in what order to take the pills (follow the arrows) and
  3) the days of the week as shown on the pill card.

Brevicon, Norinyl 1 + 35, Norinyl 1 + 50
Active Pill Colors: White or Yellow-Green or Blue

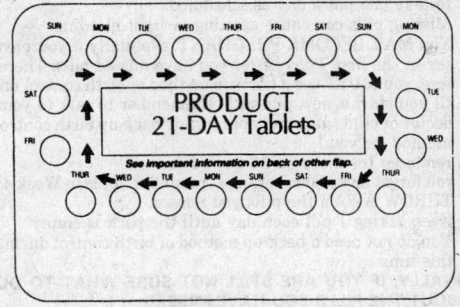

Brevicon, Norinyl 1 + 35, Norinyl 1 + 50
Active Pill Colors: White or Yellow-Green or Blue
Reminder Pill Color: Orange

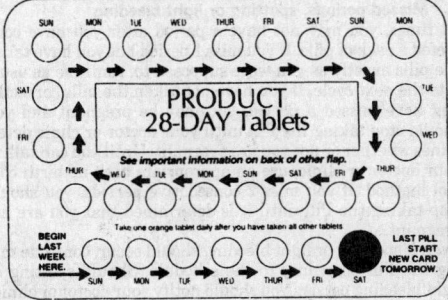

- Be sure you have ready at all times:
  Another kind of birth control to use as a back-up in case you miss pills. (Remember to talk to your doctor or clinic about an appropriate back-up method of birth control for you.) An extra, full pill pack.

3. When to start the first pack of pills
You have a choice of which day to start taking your first pack of pills (Sunday or Day 5 of your period). Decide with your doctor or clinic which is the best day for you to start. Pick a time of day which will be easy to remember.

Sunday Start:
- Take the first pill of the first pack on the Sunday after your period starts, even if you are still bleeding. If your

Continued on next page

Searle—Cont.

period begins on Sunday, take your first pill of the first pack that same day.
* Use another method of birth control as a back-up method if you have sex any time from the Sunday you start your first pack until the next Sunday (7 days). Talk to your doctor about an appropriate back-up method of birth control for you.

Day 5 Start:
* Count the first day of your period as Day 1. Take the first pill of the first pack on the fifth day of your period, even if you are still bleeding.
* Use another method of birth control as a back-up method if you have sex any time during the 7 days after you take your first pill. Talk to your doctor or clinic about an appropriate back-up method of birth control for you.

4. What to do during the month
* Take one pill at the same time every day until the pack is empty.
  Do not skip pills even if you are spotting or have light bleeding between monthly periods or feel sick to your stomach (nausea).
  Do not skip pills even if you do not have sex very often.
* When you finish a pack of pills:
  21 pills: Wait 7 days to start the next pack. You will probably have your period during that week. Be sure that no more than 7 days pass between 21-day packs.
  28 pills: Start the next pack on the day after your last "reminder" pill. Do not wait any days between packs.

5. What to do if you miss pills
If you **MISS 1** "active" white or yellow-green or blue pill:
* Take it as soon as you remember. Take the next pill at your regular time. This means you take 2 pills in 1 day.
* Missing a pill can cause spotting or light bleeding. You could also feel a little sick to your stomach on the days you take a missed pill with your regularly scheduled pill.
* You do not need to use a back-up birth control method if you have sex.
If you **MISS MORE THAN 1** "active" white or yellow-green or blue pill in a row:
* Do not take the missed pills. The missed pills may be discarded. Take the next pill at your regular time. Continue to take one pill a day as scheduled.
* Missing pills can cause spotting or light bleeding.
* You **MAY BECOME PREGNANT**, especially if you have sex in the first 7 days after you have missed pills. Therefore, you **MUST** use a back-up method of birth control until you start a new pill pack. (Remember to talk to your doctor or clinic about an appropriate back-up birth control method for you.)

A reminder for those on 28-day packs:
If you forget any of the 7 orange "reminder" pills in Week 4:
THROW AWAY the pills you missed.
Keep taking 1 pill each day until the pack is empty.
You do not need a back-up method of birth control during this time.

FINALLY, IF YOU ARE STILL NOT SURE WHAT TO DO ABOUT THE PILLS YOU HAVE MISSED:
Use a BACK-UP METHOD OF BIRTH CONTROL anytime you have sex.
KEEP TAKING ONE PILL EACH DAY until you can talk to your doctor or clinic.

6. Missed periods, spotting or light bleeding
At times, you may not have a period after you have completed a pack of pills. If you miss 1 period but you have taken the pills exactly as you were supposed to, continue as usual into the next cycle. If you have not taken the pills correctly, and have missed a period, you may be pregnant and you should stop taking the Pill until your doctor or clinic determines whether or not you are pregnant. Until you can talk to your doctor or clinic, use an appropriate back-up birth control method. If you miss 2 consecutive periods, you should stop taking the Pill until it is determined that you are not pregnant.
Even if spotting or light bleeding should occur, continue taking the Pill according to the schedule. Should spotting or light bleeding persist, you should notify your doctor or clinic.

7. Stopping the pill before surgery or prolonged bed rest
If you are scheduled for surgery or you need to stay in bed for a long period of time you should tell your doctor that you are on the Pill. You should stop taking the Pill four weeks before your operation to avoid an increased risk of blood clots. Talk to your doctor about when you may start taking the Pill again.

8. Starting the pill after pregnancy
After you have a baby it is advisable to wait 4 weeks before starting to take the Pill. Talk to your doctor about when you may start taking the Pill after pregnancy.

9. Pregnancy due to pill failure
When the Pill is taken correctly, the expected pregnancy rate is approximately 1% (i.e., 1 pregnancy per 100 women per year). If pregnancy occurs while taking the Pill, there is little risk to the fetus. The typical failure rate of large num-

bers of pill users is less than 3% when women who have missed pills are included. If you become pregnant, you should discuss your pregnancy with your doctor.

10. Pregnancy after stopping the pill
There may be some delay in becoming pregnant after you stop taking the Pill, especially if you had irregular periods before you started using the Pill. Your doctor may recommend that you delay becoming pregnant until you have had one or more regular periods.
There does not appear to be any increase in birth defects in newborn babies when pregnancy occurs soon after stopping the Pill.

11. Overdosage
There are no reports of serious illness or side effects in young children who have swallowed a large number of pills. In adults, overdosage may cause nausea and/or bleeding in females. In case of overdosage, contact your doctor, clinic or pharmacist.

12. Other information
Your doctor or clinic will take a medical and family history and will examine you before prescribing the Pill. The physical examination may be delayed to another time if you request it and the health care provider believes that it is a good medical practice to postpone it. You should be reexamined at least once a year. Be sure to inform your doctor or clinic if there is a family history of any of the conditions listed previously in this leaflet. Be sure to keep all appointments with your doctor or clinic because this is a time to determine if there are early signs of side effects from using the Pill.
Do not use the Pill for any condition other than the one for which it was prescribed. The Pill has been prescribed specifically for you, do not give it to others who may want birth control pills.
If you want more information about birth control pills, ask your doctor or clinic. They have a more technical leaflet called **PHYSICIAN LABELING** which you might want to read.

NON-CONTRACEPTIVE HEALTH BENEFITS
In addition to preventing pregnancy, use of oral contraceptives may provide certain non-contraceptive health benefits:
* Menstrual cycles may become more regular
* Blood flow during menstruation may be lighter and less iron may be lost. Therefore, anemia due to iron deficiency is less likely to occur
* Pain or other symptoms during menstruation may be encountered less frequently
* Ectopic (tubal) pregnancy may occur less frequently
* Non-cancerous cysts or lumps in the breast may occur less frequently
* Acute pelvic inflammatory disease may occur less frequently
* Oral contraceptive use may provide some protection against developing two forms of cancer: cancer of the ovaries and cancer of the lining of the uterus
Store at controlled room temperature 15–30°C (59–86°F).

BRIEF SUMMARY
PATIENT PACKAGE INSERT
This product (like all oral contraceptives) is intended to prevent pregnancy. It does not protect against HIV infection (AIDS) and other sexually transmitted diseases.
Oral contraceptives, also known as "birth control pills" or "the pill," are taken to prevent pregnancy and, when taken correctly, have a failure rate of about 1% per year when used without missing any pills. The typical failure rate of large numbers of pill users is less than 3% per year when women who miss pills are included. For most women, oral contraceptives are also free of serious or unpleasant side effects. However, forgetting to take oral contraceptives considerably increases the chances of pregnancy.
For the majority of women, oral contraceptives can be taken safely, but there are some women who are at high risk of developing certain serious diseases that can be life-threatening or may cause temporary or permanent disability. The risks associated with taking oral contraceptives increase significantly if you:
* Smoke
* Have high blood pressure, diabetes or high cholesterol
* Have or have had clotting disorders, heart attack, stroke, angina pectoris, cancer of the breast or sex organs, jaundice or malignant or benign liver tumors
You should not take the pill if you suspect you are pregnant or have unexplained vaginal bleeding.

> **Cigarette smoking increases the risk of serious cardiovascular side effects from oral contraceptive use. This risk increases with age and with heavy smoking (15 or more cigarettes per day) and is quite marked in women over 35 years of age. Women who use oral contraceptives are strongly advised not to smoke.**

Most side effects of the pill are not serious. The most common such effects are nausea, vomiting, bleeding between menstrual periods, weight gain, breast tenderness and difficulty

wearing contact lenses. These side effects, especially nausea and vomiting, may subside within the first 3 months of use.

The serious side effects of the pill occur very infrequently, especially if you are in good health and are young. However, you should know that the following medical conditions have been associated with or made worse by the pill:
1. Blood clots in the legs (thrombophlebitis) or lungs (pulmonary embolism), stoppage or rupture of a blood vessel in the brain (stroke), blockage of blood vessels in the heart (heart attack or angina pectoris), eye or other organs of the body. As mentioned above, smoking increases the risk of heart attacks and strokes and subsequent serious medical consequences.
2. Liver tumors, which may rupture and cause severe bleeding. A possible but not definite association has been found with the pill and liver cancer. However, liver cancers are extremely rare.
3. High blood pressure, although blood pressure usually returns to normal when the pill is stopped.
The symptoms associated with these serious side effects are discussed in the detailed leaflet given to you with your supply of pills. Notify your doctor or health care provider if you notice any unusual physical disturbances while taking the pill. In addition, drugs such as rifampin, as well as some anticonvulsants and some antibiotics, may decrease oral contraceptive effectiveness.
Studies to date of women taking the pill have not shown an increase in the incidence of cancer of the breast or cervix. There is, however, insufficient evidence to rule out the possibility that the pill may cause such cancers. Some studies have reported an increase in the risk of developing breast cancer, particularly at a younger age. This increased risk appears to be related to duration of use.
Taking the pill may provide some important non-contraceptive health benefits. These include less painful menstruation, less menstrual blood loss and anemia, fewer acute pelvic infections and fewer cancers of the ovary and the lining of the uterus.
Be sure to discuss any medical condition you may have with your health care provider. Your health care provider will take a medical and family history before prescribing oral contraceptives and will examine you. The physical examination may be delayed to another time if you request it and the health care provider believes that it is a good medical practice to postpone it. You should be reexamined at least once a year while taking oral contraceptives. The detailed patient information leaflet gives you further information which you should read and discuss with your health care provider.
HOW TO TAKE ORAL CONTRACEPTIVES
See full text of How To Take Oral Contraceptives which is printed in full in the Detailed Patient Labeling.
REVISED JUNE 1993
Shown in Product Identification Guide, page 335

CALAN® Tablets ℞
[cal'an]
(verapamil hydrochloride)

PRODUCT OVERVIEW
KEY FACTS
Calan, a calcium ion antagonist, exerts its pharmacologic effects by modulating the influx of ionic calcium across the cell membrane of the arterial smooth muscle as well as in conductile and contractile myocardial cells. Calan increases myocardial oxygen supply, reduces myocardial oxygen consumption, and is a potent inhibitor of coronary artery spasm, making it an effective antianginal agent. By decreasing the influx of calcium, Calan prolongs the effective refractory period within the AV node and slows AV conduction in a rate-related manner, thereby slowing the ventricular rate in patients with chronic atrial flutter or fibrillation. Calan exerts antihypertensive effects by decreasing systemic vascular resistance, usually without orthostatic decreases in blood pressure or reflex tachycardia.

MAJOR USES
Calan Tablets are indicated for: angina at rest, including vasospastic and unstable angina; chronic stable angina; control (in association with digitalis) of ventricular rate at rest and during stress in patients with chronic atrial flutter and/or atrial fibrillation; prophylaxis of repetitive paroxysmal supraventricular tachycardia; management of essential hypertension.

SAFETY INFORMATION
See complete safety information set forth below.

PRESCRIBING INFORMATION
CALAN® Tablets ℞
[cal'an]
(verapamil hydrochloride)

DESCRIPTION

Calan (verapamil HCl) is a calcium ion influx inhibitor (slow-channel blocker or calcium ion antagonist) available for oral administration in film-coated tablets containing 40 mg, 80 mg, or 120 mg of verapamil hydrochloride.
The structural formula of verapamil HCl is

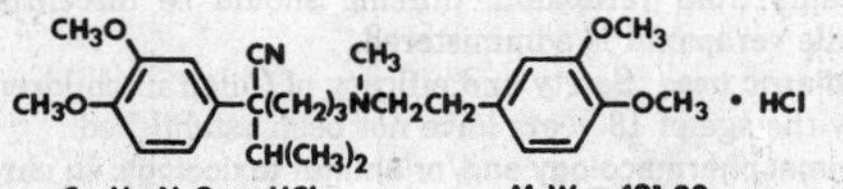

$C_{27}H_{38}N_2O_4 \cdot HCl$ M.W. = 491.08

Benzeneacetonitrile, α-[3-[[2-(3,4-dimethoxyphenyl) ethyl] methylamino]propyl]-3,4-dimethoxy-α-(1-methylethyl) hydrochloride

Verapamil HCl is an almost white, crystalline powder, practically free of odor, with a bitter taste. It is soluble in water, chloroform, and methanol. Verapamil HCl is not chemically related to other cardioactive drugs.
Inactive ingredients include microcrystalline cellulose, corn starch, gelatin, hydroxypropyl cellulose, hydroxypropyl methylcellulose, iron oxide colorant, lactose, magnesium stearate, polyethylene glycol, talc, and titanium dioxide.

CLINICAL PHARMACOLOGY

Calan is a calcium ion influx inhibitor (slow-channel blocker or calcium ion antagonist) that exerts its pharmacologic effects by modulating the influx of ionic calcium across the cell membrane of the arterial smooth muscle as well as in conductile and contractile myocardial cells.

Mechanism of action

Angina: The precise mechanism of action of Calan as an antianginal agent remains to be fully determined, but includes the following two mechanisms:

1. *Relaxation and prevention of coronary artery spasm:* Calan dilates the main coronary arteries and coronary arterioles, both in normal and ischemic regions, and is a potent inhibitor of coronary artery spasm, whether spontaneous or ergonovine-induced. This property increases myocardial oxygen delivery in patients with coronary artery spasm and is responsible for the effectiveness of Calan in vasospastic (Prinzmetal's or variant) as well as unstable angina at rest. Whether this effect plays any role in classical effort angina is not clear, but studies of exercise tolerance have not shown an increase in the maximum exercise rate–pressure product, a widely accepted measure of oxygen utilization. This suggests that, in general, relief of spasm or dilation of coronary arteries is not an important factor in classical angina.
2. *Reduction of oxygen utilization:* Calan regularly reduces the total peripheral resistance (afterload) against which the heart works both at rest and at a given level of exercise by dilating peripheral arterioles. This unloading of the heart reduces myocardial energy consumption and oxygen requirements and probably accounts for the effectiveness of Calan in chronic stable effort angina.

Arrhythmia: Electrical activity through the AV node depends, to a significant degree, upon calcium influx through the slow channel. By decreasing the influx of calcium, Calan prolongs the effective refractory period within the AV node and slows AV conduction in a rate-related manner. This property accounts for the ability of Calan to slow the ventricular rate in patients with chronic atrial flutter or atrial fibrillation.
Normal sinus rhythm is usually not affected, but in patients with sick sinus syndrome, Calan may interfere with sinus-node impulse generation and may induce sinus arrest or sinoatrial block. Atrioventricular block can occur in patients without preexisting conduction defects (see *Warnings*). Calan decreases the frequency of episodes of paroxysmal supraventricular tachycardia.
Calan does not alter the normal atrial action potential or intraventricular conduction time, but in depressed atrial fibers it decreases amplitude, velocity of depolarization, and conduction velocity. Calan may shorten the antegrade effective refractory period of the accessory bypass tract. Acceleration of ventricular rate and/or ventricular fibrillation has been reported in patients with atrial flutter or atrial fibrillation and a coexisting accessory AV pathway following administration of verapamil (see *Warnings*).
Calan has a local anesthetic action that is 1.6 times that of procaine on an equimolar basis. It is not known whether this action is important at the doses used in man.

Essential hypertension: Calan exerts antihypertensive effects by decreasing systemic vascular resistance, usually without orthostatic decreases in blood pressure or reflex tachycardia; bradycardia (rate less than 50 beats/min) is uncommon (1.4%). During isometric or dynamic exercise Calan does not alter systolic cardiac function in patients with normal ventricular function.
Calan does not alter total serum calcium levels. However, one report suggested that calcium levels above the normal range may alter the therapeutic effect of Calan.

Pharmacokinetics and metabolism: More than 90% of the orally administered dose of Calan is absorbed. Because of rapid biotransformation of verapamil during its first pass through the portal circulation, bioavailability ranges from 20% to 35%. Peak plasma concentrations are reached between 1 and 2 hours after oral administration. Chronic oral administration of 120 mg of verapamil HCl every 6 hours resulted in plasma levels of verapamil ranging from 125 to 400 ng/ml, with higher values reported occasionally. A nonlinear correlation between the verapamil dose administered and verapamil plasma levels does exist. No relationship has been established between the plasma concentration of verapamil and a reduction in blood pressure. In early dose titration with verapamil a relationship exists between verapamil plasma concentration and prolongation of the PR interval. However, during chronic administration this relationship may disappear. The mean elimination half-life in single-dose studies ranged from 2.8 to 7.4 hours. In these same studies, after repetitive dosing, the half-life increased to a range from 4.5 to 12.0 hours (after less than 10 consecutive doses given 6 hours apart). Half-life of verapamil may increase during titration. Aging may affect the pharmacokinetics of verapamil. Elimination half-life may be prolonged in the elderly. In healthy men, orally administered Calan undergoes extensive metabolism in the liver. Twelve metabolites have been identified in plasma; all except norverapamil are present in trace amounts only. Norverapamil can reach steady-state plasma concentrations approximately equal to those of verapamil itself. The cardiovascular activity of norverapamil appears to be approximately 20% that of verapamil. Approximately 70% of an administered dose is excreted as metabolites in the urine and 16% or more in the feces within 5 days. About 3% to 4% is excreted in the urine as unchanged drug. Approximately 90% is bound to plasma proteins. In patients with hepatic insufficiency, metabolism is delayed and elimination half-life prolonged up to 14 to 16 hours (see *Precautions*); the volume of distribution is increased and plasma clearance reduced to about 30% of normal. Verapamil clearance values suggest that patients with liver dysfunction may attain therapeutic verapamil plasma concentrations with one third of the oral daily dose required for patients with normal liver function.
After four weeks of oral dosing (120 mg q.i.d.), verapamil and norverapamil levels were noted in the cerebrospinal fluid with estimated partition coefficient of 0.06 for verapamil and 0.04 for norverapamil.

Hemodynamics and myocardial metabolism: Calan reduces afterload and myocardial contractility. Improved left ventricular diastolic function in patients with IHSS and those with coronary heart disease has also been observed with Calan therapy. In most patients, including those with organic cardiac disease, the negative inotropic action of Calan is countered by reduction of afterload, and cardiac index is usually not reduced. However, in patients with severe left ventricular dysfunction (eg, pulmonary wedge pressure above 20 mm Hg or ejection fraction less than 30%), or in patients taking beta-adrenergic blocking agents or other cardiodepressant drugs, deterioration of ventricular function may occur (see *Drug interactions*).

Pulmonary function: Calan does not induce bronchoconstriction and, hence, does not impair ventilatory function.

INDICATIONS AND USAGE

Calan tablets are indicated for the treatment of the following:

Angina

1. Angina at rest, including:
   —Vasospastic (Prinzmetal's variant) angina
   —Unstable (crescendo, pre-infarction) angina
2. Chronic stable angina (classic effort-associated angina)

Arrhythmias

1. In association with digitalis for the control of ventricular rate at rest and during stress in patients with chronic atrial flutter and/or atrial fibrillation (see *Warnings: Accessory bypass tract*)
2. Prophylaxis of repetitive paroxysmal supraventricular tachycardia

Essential hypertension

CONTRAINDICATIONS

Verapamil HCl tablets are contraindicated in:

1. Severe left ventricular dysfunction (see *Warnings*)
2. Hypotension (systolic pressure less than 90 mm Hg) or cardiogenic shock
3. Sick sinus syndrome (except in patients with a functioning artificial ventricular pacemaker)
4. Second- or third-degree AV block (except in patients with a functioning artificial ventricular pacemaker)
5. Patients with atrial flutter or atrial fibrillation and an accessory bypass tract (eg, Wolff-Parkinson-White, Lown-Ganong-Levine syndromes). (See *Warnings*.)
6. Patients with known hypersensitivity to verapamil hydrochloride.

WARNINGS

Heart failure: Verapamil has a negative inotropic effect, which in most patients is compensated by its afterload reduction (decreased systemic vascular resistance) properties without a net impairment of ventricular performance. In clinical experience with 4,954 patients, 87 (1.8%) developed congestive heart failure or pulmonary edema. Verapamil should be avoided in patients with severe left ventricular dysfunction (eg, ejection fraction less than 30%) or moderate to severe symptoms of cardiac failure and in patients with any degree of ventricular dysfunction if they are receiving a beta-adrenergic blocker (see *Drug interactions*). Patients with milder ventricular dysfunction should, if possible, be controlled with optimum doses of digitalis and/or diuretics before verapamil treatment. **(Note interactions with digoxin under *Precautions*.)**

Hypotension: Occasionally, the pharmacologic action of verapamil may produce a decrease in blood pressure below normal levels, which may result in dizziness or symptomatic hypotension. The incidence of hypotension observed in 4,954 patients enrolled in clinical trials was 2.5%. In hypertensive patients, decreases in blood pressure below normal are unusual. Tilt-table testing (60 degrees) was not able to induce orthostatic hypotension.

Elevated liver enzymes: Elevations of transaminases with and without concomitant elevations in alkaline phosphatase and bilirubin have been reported. Such elevations have sometimes been transient and may disappear even with continued verapamil treatment. Several cases of hepatocellular injury related to verapamil have been proven by rechallenge; half of these had clinical symptoms (malaise, fever, and/or right upper quadrant pain), in addition to elevation of SGOT, SGPT, and alkaline phosphatase. Periodic monitoring of liver function in patients receiving verapamil is therefore prudent.

Accessory bypass tract (Wolff-Parkinson-White or Lown-Ganong-Levine): Some patients with paroxysmal and/or chronic atrial fibrillation or atrial flutter and a coexisting accessory AV pathway have developed increased antegrade conduction across the accessory pathway bypassing the AV node, producing a very rapid ventricular response or ventricular fibrillation after receiving intravenous verapamil (or digitalis). Although a risk of this occurring with oral verapamil has not been established, such patients receiving oral verapamil may be at risk and its use in these patients is contraindicated (see *Contraindications*). Treatment is usually DC-cardioversion. Cardioversion has been used safely and effectively after oral Calan.

Atrioventricular block: The effect of verapamil on AV conduction and the SA node may cause asymptomatic first-degree AV block and transient bradycardia, sometimes accompanied by nodal escape rhythms. PR-interval prolongation is correlated with verapamil plasma concentrations especially during the early titration phase of therapy. Higher degrees of AV block, however, were infrequently (0.8%) observed. Marked first-degree block or progressive development to second- or third-degree AV block requires a reduction in dosage or, in rare instances, discontinuation of verapamil HCl and institution of appropriate therapy, depending on the clinical situation.

Patients with hypertrophic cardiomyopathy (IHSS): In 120 patients with hypertrophic cardiomyopathy (most of them refractory or intolerant to propranolol) who received therapy with verapamil at doses up to 720 mg/day, a variety of serious adverse effects were seen. Three patients died in pulmonary edema; all had severe left ventricular outflow obstruction and a past history of left ventricular dysfunction. Eight other patients had pulmonary edema and/or severe hypotension; abnormally high (greater than 20 mm Hg) pulmonary wedge pressure and a marked left ventricular outflow obstruction were present in most of these patients. Concomitant administration of quinidine (see *Drug interactions*) preceded the severe hypotension in 3 of the 8 patients (2 of whom developed pulmonary edema). Sinus bradycardia occurred in 11% of the patients, second-degree AV block in 4%, and sinus arrest in 2%. It must be appreciated that this group of patients had a serious disease with a high mortality rate. Most adverse effects responded well to dose reduction, and only rarely did verapamil use have to be discontinued.

PRECAUTIONS

General

Use in patients with impaired hepatic function: Since verapamil is highly metabolized by the liver, it should be administered cautiously to patients with impaired hepatic function. Severe liver dysfunction prolongs the elimination half-life of verapamil to about 14 to 16 hours; hence, approximately 30% of the dose given to patients with normal liver function should be administered to these patients. Careful monitoring for abnormal prolongation of the PR interval or other signs of excessive pharmacologic effects (see *Overdosage*) should be carried out.

Continued on next page

Searle—Cont.

Use in patients with attenuated (decreased) neuromuscular transmission: It has been reported that verapamil decreases neuromuscular transmission in patients with Duchenne's muscular dystrophy, and that verapamil prolongs recovery from the neuromuscular blocking agent vecuronium. It may be necessary to decrease the dosage of verapamil when it is administered to patients with attenuated neuromuscular transmission.

Use in patients with impaired renal function: About 70% of an administered dose of verapamil is excreted as metabolites in the urine. Verapamil is not removed by hemodialysis. Until further data are available, verapamil should be administered cautiously to patients with impaired renal function. These patients should be carefully monitored for abnormal prolongation of the PR interval or other signs of overdosage (see *Overdosage*).

Drug interactions

Beta-blockers: Controlled studies in small numbers of patients suggest that the concomitant use of Calan and oral beta-adrenergic blocking agents may be beneficial in certain patients with chronic stable angina or hypertension, but available information is not sufficient to predict with confidence the effects of concurrent treatment in patients with left ventricular dysfunction or cardiac conduction abnormalities. Concomitant therapy with beta-adrenergic blockers and verapamil may result in additive negative effects on heart rate, atrioventricular conduction and/or cardiac contractility.

In one study involving 15 patients treated with high doses of propranolol (median dose, 480 mg/day; range, 160 to 1,280 mg/day) for severe angina, with preserved left ventricular function (ejection fraction greater than 35%), the hemodynamic effects of additional therapy with verapamil HCl were assessed using invasive methods. The addition of verapamil to high-dose beta-blockers induced modest negative inotropic and chronotropic effects that were not severe enough to limit short-term (48 hours) combination therapy in this study. These modest cardiodepressant effects persisted for greater than 6 but less than 30 hours after abrupt withdrawal of beta-blockers and were closely related to plasma levels of propranolol. The primary verapamil/beta-blocker interaction in this study appeared to be hemodynamic rather than electrophysiologic.

In other studies verapamil did not generally induce significant negative inotropic, chronotropic, or dromotropic effects in patients with preserved left ventricular function receiving low or moderate doses of propranolol (less than or equal to 320 mg/day); in some patients, however, combined therapy did produce such effects. Therefore, if combined therapy is used, close surveillance of clinical status should be carried out. Combined therapy should usually be avoided in patients with atrioventricular conduction abnormalities and those with depressed left ventricular function.

Asymptomatic bradycardia (36 beats/min) with a wandering atrial pacemaker has been observed in a patient receiving concomitant timolol (a beta-adrenergic blocker) eyedrops and oral verapamil.

A decrease in metoprolol and propranolol clearance has been observed when either drug is administered concomitantly with verapamil. A variable effect has been seen when verapamil and atenolol were given together.

Digitalis: Clinical use of verapamil in digitalized patients has shown the combination to be well tolerated if digoxin doses are properly adjusted. However, chronic verapamil treatment can increase serum digoxin levels by 50% to 75% during the first week of therapy, and this can result in digitalis toxicity. In patients with hepatic cirrhosis the influence of verapamil on digoxin kinetics is magnified. Verapamil may reduce total body clearance and extrarenal clearance of digitoxin by 27% and 29%, respectively. Maintenance and digitalization doses should be reduced when verapamil is administered, and the patient should be reassessed to avoid over- or underdigitalization. Whenever overdigitalization is suspected, the daily dose of digitalis should be reduced or temporarily discontinued. On discontinuation of Calan use, the patient should be reassessed to avoid underdigitalization.

Antihypertensive agents: Verapamil administered concomitantly with oral antihypertensive agents (eg, vasodilators, angiotensin-converting enzyme inhibitors, diuretics, beta-blockers) will usually have an additive effect on lowering blood pressure. Patients receiving these combinations should be appropriately monitored. Concomitant use of agents that attenuate alpha-adrenergic function with verapamil may result in a reduction in blood pressure that is excessive in some patients. Such an effect was observed in one study following the concomitant administration of verapamil and prazosin.

Antiarrhythmic agents:

Disopyramide: Until data on possible interactions between verapamil and disopyramide are obtained, disopyramide should not be administered within 48 hours before or 24 hours after verapamil administration.

Flecainide: A study in healthy volunteers showed that the concomitant administration of flecainide and verapamil may have additive effects on myocardial contractility, AV conduction, and repolarization. Concomitant therapy with flecainide and verapamil may result in additive negative inotropic effect and prolongation of atrioventricular conduction.

Quinidine: In a small number of patients with hypertrophic cardiomyopathy (IHSS), concomitant use of verapamil and quinidine resulted in significant hypotension. Until further data are obtained, combined therapy of verapamil and quinidine in patients with hypertrophic cardiomyopathy should probably be avoided.

The electrophysiologic effects of quinidine and verapamil on AV conduction were studied in 8 patients. Verapamil significantly counteracted the effects of quinidine on AV conduction. There has been a report of increased quinidine levels during verapamil therapy.

Other:

Nitrates: Verapamil has been given concomitantly with short- and long-acting nitrates without any undesirable drug interactions. The pharmacologic profile of both drugs and the clinical experience suggest beneficial interactions.

Cimetidine: The interaction between cimetidine and chronically administered verapamil has not been studied. Variable results on clearance have been obtained in acute studies of healthy volunteers; clearance of verapamil was either reduced or unchanged.

Lithium: Increased sensitivity to the effects of lithium (neurotoxicity) has been reported during concomitant verapamil-lithium therapy with either no change or an increase in serum lithium levels. However, the addition of verapamil has also resulted in the lowering of serum lithium levels in patients receiving chronic stable oral lithium. Patients receiving both drugs must be monitored carefully.

Carbamazepine: Verapamil therapy may increase carbamazepine concentrations during combined therapy. This may produce carbamazepine side effects such as diplopia, headache, ataxia, or dizziness.

Rifampin: Therapy with rifampin may markedly reduce oral verapamil bioavailability.

Phenobarbital: Phenobarbital therapy may increase verapamil clearance.

Cyclosporin: Verapamil therapy may increase serum levels of cyclosporin.

Theophylline: Verapamil may inhibit the clearance and increase the plasma levels of theophylline.

Inhalation anesthetics: Animal experiments have shown that inhalation anesthetics depress cardiovascular activity by decreasing the inward movement of calcium ions. When used concomitantly, inhalation anesthetics and calcium antagonists, such as verapamil, should each be titrated carefully to avoid excessive cardiovascular depression.

Neuromuscular blocking agents: Clinical data and animal studies suggest that verapamil may potentiate the activity of neuromuscular blocking agents (curare-like and depolarizing). It may be necessary to decrease the dose of verapamil and/or the dose of the neuromuscular blocking agent when the drugs are used concomitantly.

Carcinogenesis, mutagenesis, impairment of fertility: An 18-month toxicity study in rats, at a low multiple (6-fold) of the maximum recommended human dose, and not the maximum tolerated dose, did not suggest a tumorigenic potential. There was no evidence of a carcinogenic potential of verapamil administered in the diet of rats for two years at doses of 10, 35, and 120 mg/kg/day or approximately 1, 3.5, and 12 times, respectively, the maximum recommended human daily dose (480 mg/day or 9.6 mg/kg/day).

Verapamil was not mutagenic in the Ames test in 5 test strains at 3 mg per plate with or without metabolic activation.

Studies in female rats at daily dietary doses up to 5.5 times (55 mg/kg/day) the maximum recommended human dose did not show impaired fertility. Effects on male fertility have not been determined.

Pregnancy: Pregnancy Category C. Reproduction studies have been performed in rabbits and rats at oral doses up to 1.5 (15 mg/kg/day) and 6 (60 mg/kg/day) times the human oral daily dose, respectively, and have revealed no evidence of teratogenicity. In the rat, however, this multiple of the human dose was embryocidal and retarded fetal growth and development, probably because of adverse maternal effects reflected in reduced weight gains of the dams. This oral dose has also been shown to cause hypotension in rats. There are no adequate and well-controlled studies in pregnant women. Because animal reproduction studies are not always predictive of human response, this drug should be used during pregnancy only if clearly needed. Verapamil crosses the placental barrier and can be detected in umbilical vein blood at delivery.

Labor and delivery: It is not known whether the use of verapamil during labor or delivery has immediate or delayed adverse effects on the fetus, or whether it prolongs the duration of labor or increases the need for forceps delivery or other obstetric intervention. Such adverse experiences have not been reported in the literature, despite a long history of use of verapamil in Europe in the treatment of cardiac side effects of beta-adrenergic agonist agents used to treat premature labor.

Nursing mothers: Verapamil is excreted in human milk. Because of the potential for adverse reactions in nursing infants from verapamil, nursing should be discontinued while verapamil is administered.

Pediatric use: Safety and efficacy of Calan in children below the age of 18 years have not been established.

Animal pharmacology and/or animal toxicology: In chronic animal toxicology studies verapamil caused lenticular and/or suture line changes at 30 mg/kg/day or greater, and frank cataracts at 62.5 mg/kg/day or greater in the beagle dog but not in the rat. Development of cataracts due to verapamil has not been reported in man.

ADVERSE REACTIONS

Serious adverse reactions are uncommon when Calan therapy is initiated with upward dose titration within the recommended single and total daily dose. See *Warnings* for discussion of heart failure, hypotension, elevated liver enzymes, AV block, and rapid ventricular response. Reversible (upon discontinuation of verapamil) non-obstructive, paralytic ileus has been infrequently reported in association with the use of verapamil. The following reactions to orally administered verapamil occurred at rates greater than 1.0% or occurred at lower rates but appeared clearly drug-related in clinical trials in 4,954 patients:

Constipation	7.3%	Dyspnea	1.4%
Dizziness	3.3%	Bradycardia	
Nausea	2.7%	(HR < 50/min)	1.4%
Hypotension	2.5%	AV block	
Headache	2.2%	total (1°, 2°, 3°)	1.2%
Edema	1.9%	2° and 3°	0.8%
CHF/Pulmonary		Rash	1.2%
edema	1.8%	Flushing	0.6%
Fatigue	1.7%		

Elevated liver enzymes (see *Warnings*)

In clinical trials related to the control of ventricular response in digitalized patients who had atrial fibrillation or flutter, ventricular rates below 50 at rest occurred in 15% of patients and asymptomatic hypotension occurred in 5% of patients.

The following reactions, reported in 1.0% or less of patients, occurred under conditions (open trials, marketing experience) where a causal relationship is uncertain; they are listed to alert the physician to a possible relationship:

Cardiovascular: angina pectoris, atrioventricular dissociation, chest pain, claudication, myocardial infarction, palpitations, purpura (vasculitis), syncope.

Digestive system: diarrhea, dry mouth, gastrointestinal distress, gingival hyperplasia.

Hemic and lymphatic: ecchymosis or bruising.

Nervous system: cerebrovascular accident, confusion, equilibrium disorders, insomnia, muscle cramps, paresthesia, psychotic symptoms, shakiness, somnolence.

Skin: arthralgia and rash, exanthema, hair loss, hyperkeratosis, macules, sweating, urticaria, Stevens-Johnson syndrome, erythema multiforme.

Special senses: blurred vision.

Urogenital: gynecomastia, galactorrhea/hyperprolactinemia, increased urination, spotty menstruation, impotence.

Treatment of acute cardiovascular adverse reactions: The frequency of cardiovascular adverse reactions that require therapy is rare; hence, experience with their treatment is limited. Whenever severe hypotension or complete AV block occurs following oral administration of verapamil, the appropriate emergency measures should be applied immediately; eg, intravenously administered norepinephrine bitartrate, atropine sulfate, isoproterenol HCl (all in the usual doses), or calcium gluconate (10% solution). In patients with hypertrophic cardiomyopathy (IHSS), alpha-adrenergic agents (phenylephrine HCl, metaraminol bitartrate, or methoxamine HCl) should be used to maintain blood pressure, and isoproterenol and norepinephrine should be avoided. If further support is necessary, dopamine HCl or dobutamine HCl may be administered. Actual treatment and dosage should depend on the severity of the clinical situation and the judgment and experience of the treating physician.

OVERDOSAGE

Treat all verapamil overdoses as serious and maintain observation for at least 48 hours (especially Calan SR), preferably under continuous hospital care. Delayed pharmacodynamic consequences may occur with the sustained-release formulation. Verapamil is known to decrease gastrointestinal transit time.

Treatment of overdosage should be supportive. Beta adrenergic stimulation or parenteral administration of calcium solutions may increase calcium ion flux across the slow channel, and have been used effectively in treatment of deliberate overdosage with verapamil. Verapamil cannot be removed

by hemodialysis. Clinically significant hypotensive reactions or high degree AV block should be treated with vasopressor agents or cardiac pacing, respectively. Asystole should be handled by the usual measures including cardiopulmonary resuscitation.

DOSAGE AND ADMINISTRATION

The dose of verapamil must be individualized by titration. The usefulness and safety of dosages exceeding 480 mg/day have not been established; therefore, this daily dosage should not be exceeded. Since the half-life of verapamil increases during chronic dosing, maximum response may be delayed.

Angina: Clinical trials show that the usual dose is 80 mg to 120 mg three times a day. However, 40 mg three times a day may be warranted in patients who may have an increased response to verapamil (eg, decreased hepatic function, elderly, etc). Upward titration should be based on therapeutic efficacy and safety evaluated approximately eight hours after dosing. Dosage may be increased at daily (eg, patients with unstable angina) or weekly intervals until optimum clinical response is obtained.

Arrhythmias: The dosage in digitalized patients with chronic atrial fibrillation (see *Precautions*) ranges from 240 to 320 mg/day in divided (t.i.d. or q.i.d.) doses. The dosage for prophylaxis of PSVT (non-digitalized patients) ranges from 240 to 480 mg/day in divided (t.i.d or q.i.d.) doses. In general, maximum effects for any given dosage will be apparent during the first 48 hours of therapy.

Essential hypertension: Dose should be individualized by titration. The usual initial monotherapy dose in clinical trials was 80 mg three times a day (240 mg/day). Daily dosages of 360 and 480 mg have been used but there is no evidence that dosages beyond 360 mg provided added effect. Consideration should be given to beginning titration at 40 mg three times per day in patients who might respond to lower doses, such as the elderly or people of small stature. The antihypertensive effects of Calan are evident within the first week of therapy. Upward titration should be based on therapeutic efficacy, assessed at the end of the dosing interval.

HOW SUPPLIED

Calan 40-mg tablets are round, pink, film coated, with CALAN debossed on one side and 40 on the other, supplied as:

NDC Number	Size
0025-1771-31	bottle of 100

Calan 80-mg tablets are oval, peach colored, scored, film coated, with CALAN debossed on one side and 80 on the other, supplied as:

NDC Number	Size
0025-1851-31	bottle of 100
0025-1851-51	bottle of 500
0025-1851-52	bottle of 1,000

Calan 120-mg tablets are oval, brown, scored, film coated, with CALAN 120 debossed on one side, supplied as:

NDC Number	Size
0025-1861-31	bottle of 100
0025-1861-52	bottle of 1,000

Store at 59° to 86°F (15° to 30°C) and protect from light. Dispense in tight, light-resistant containers.
Caution: Federal law prohibits dispensing without prescription.

1/24/95 • A05315

Shown in Product Identification Guide, page 335

CALAN® SR ℞
[cal'an ess ar]
(verapamil hydrochloride)
Sustained-Release Oral Caplets

PRODUCT OVERVIEW

KEY FACTS

Calan SR, a calcium ion antagonist designed for sustained release in the gastrointestinal tract, exerts an antihypertensive effect by decreasing systemic vascular resistance, usually without orthostatic decreases in blood pressure or reflex tachycardia.

MAJOR USE

Calan SR is indicated for the management of essential hypertension.

SAFETY INFORMATION

See complete safety information set forth below.

PRESCRIBING INFORMATION

CALAN® SR ℞
[cal'an ess ar]
(verapamil hydrochloride)
Sustained-Release Oral Caplets

DESCRIPTION

Calan SR (verapamil hydrochloride) is a calcium ion influx inhibitor (slow-channel blocker or calcium ion antagonist). Calan SR is available for oral administration as light green, capsule-shaped, scored, film-coated tablets (caplets) containing 240 mg of verapamil hydrochloride; as light pink, oval, scored, film-coated tablets (caplets) containing 180 mg of verapamil hydrochloride; and as light violet, oval, film-coated tablets (caplets) containing 120 mg of verapamil hydrochloride. The caplets are designed for sustained release of the drug in the gastrointestinal tract; sustained-release characteristics are not altered when the caplet is divided in half.

The structural formula of verapamil HCl is

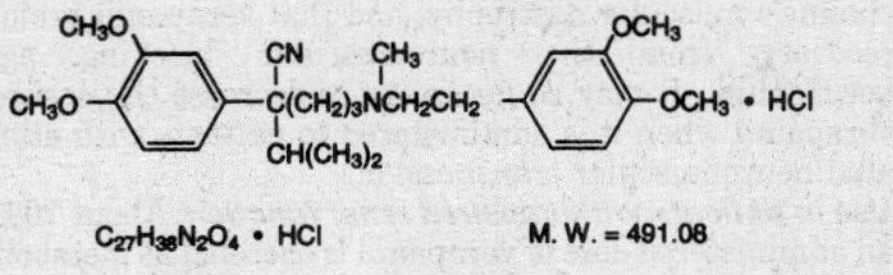

$C_{27}H_{38}N_2O_4 \cdot HCl$ M. W. = 491.08

Benzeneacetonitrile, α-[3-[[2-(3, 4-dimethoxyphenyl) ethyl] methylamino]propyl]-3,4-dimethoxy-α-(1-methylethyl) hydrochloride

Verapamil HCl is an almost white, crystalline powder, practically free of odor, with a bitter taste. It is soluble in water, chloroform, and methanol. Verapamil HCl is not chemically related to other cardioactive drugs.

Inactive ingredients include alginate, carnauba wax, hydroxypropyl methylcellulose, magnesium stearate, microcrystalline cellulose, polyethylene glycol, polyvinyl pyrrolidone, talc, titanium dioxide, and coloring agents: 240-mg—D&C Yellow No. 10 Lake and FD&C Blue No. 2 Lake; 120- and 180-mg—iron oxide.

CLINICAL PHARMACOLOGY

Calan (verapamil HCl) is a calcium ion influx inhibitor (slow-channel blocker or calcium ion antagonist) that exerts its pharmacologic effects by modulating the influx of ionic calcium across the cell membrane of the arterial smooth muscle as well as in conductile and contractile myocardial cells.

Mechanism of action

Essential hypertension: Verapamil exerts antihypertensive effects by decreasing systemic vascular resistance, usually without orthostatic decreases in blood pressure or reflex tachycardia; bradycardia (rate less than 50 beats/min) is uncommon (1.4%). During isometric or dynamic exercise Calan does not alter systolic cardiac function in patients with normal ventricular function.

Calan does not alter total serum calcium levels. However, one report suggested that calcium levels above the normal range may alter the therapeutic effect of Calan.

Other pharmacologic actions of Calan include the following:

Calan dilates the main coronary arteries and coronary arterioles, both in normal and ischemic regions, and is a potent inhibitor of coronary artery spasm, whether spontaneous or ergonovine-induced. This property increases myocardial oxygen delivery in patients with coronary artery spasm and is responsible for the effectiveness of Calan in vasospastic (Prinzmetal's or variant) as well as unstable angina at rest. Whether this effect plays any role in classical effort angina is not clear, but studies of exercise tolerance have not shown an increase in the maximum exercise rate–pressure product, a widely accepted measure of oxygen utilization. This suggests that, in general, relief of spasm or dilation of coronary arteries is not an important factor in classical angina.

Calan regularly reduces the total systemic resistance (afterload) against which the heart works both at rest and at a given level of exercise by dilating peripheral arterioles.

Electrical activity through the AV node depends, to a significant degree, upon calcium influx through the slow channel. By decreasing the influx of calcium, Calan prolongs the effective refractory period within the AV node and slows AV conduction in a rate-related manner.

Normal sinus rhythm is usually not affected, but in patients with sick sinus syndrome, Calan may interfere with sinus-node impulse generation and may induce sinus arrest or sinoatrial block. Atrioventricular block can occur in patients without preexisting conduction defects (see *Warnings*).

Calan does not alter the normal atrial action potential or intraventricular conduction time, but depresses amplitude, velocity of depolarization, and conduction in depressed atrial fibers. Calan may shorten the antegrade effective refractory period of the accessory bypass tract. Acceleration of ventricular rate and/or ventricular fibrillation has been reported in patients with atrial flutter or atrial fibrillation and a coexisting accessory AV pathway following administration of verapamil (see *Warnings*).

Calan has a local anesthetic action that is 1.6 times that of procaine on an equimolar basis. It is not known whether this action is important at the doses used in man.

Pharmacokinetics and metabolism: With the immediate-release formulation, more than 90% of the orally administered dose of Calan is absorbed. Because of rapid biotransformation of verapamil during its first pass through the portal circulation, bioavailability ranges from 20% to 35%. Peak plasma concentrations are reached between 1 and 2 hours after oral administration. Chronic oral administration of 120 mg of verapamil HCl every 6 hours resulted in plasma levels of verapamil ranging from 125 to 400 ng/ml, with higher values reported occasionally. A nonlinear correlation between the verapamil dose administered and verapamil plasma level does exist. In early dose titration with verapamil a relationship exists between verapamil plasma concentration and prolongation of the PR interval. However, during chronic administration this relationship may disappear. The mean elimination half-life in single-dose studies ranged from 2.8 to 7.4 hours. In these same studies, after repetitive dosing, the half-life increased to a range from 4.5 to 12.0 hours (after less than 10 consecutive doses given 6 hours apart). Half-life of verapamil may increase during titration. No relationship has been established between the plasma concentraton of verapamil and a reduction in blood pressure.

Aging may affect the pharmacokinetics of verapamil. Elimination half-life may be prolonged in the elderly. In multiple-dose studies under fasting conditions, the bioavailability, measured by AUC, of Calan SR was similar to Calan (immediate release); rates of absorption were of course different.

In a randomized, single-dose, crossover study using healthy volunteers, administration of 240 mg Calan SR with food produced peak plasma verapamil concentrations of 79 ng/ml; time to peak plasma verapamil concentration of 7.71 hours; and AUC (0–24 hr) of 841 ng·hr/ml). When Calan SR was administered to fasting subjects, peak plasma verapamil concentration was 164 ng/ml; time to peak plasma verapamil concentration was 5.21 hours; and AUC (0–24 hr) was 1,478 ng·hr/ml. Similar results were demonstrated for plasma norverapamil. Food thus produces decreased bioavailability (AUC) but a narrower peak-to-trough ratio. Good correlation of dose and response is not available, but controlled studies of Calan SR have shown effectiveness of doses similar to the effective doses of Calan (immediate release).

In healthy men, orally administered Calan undergoes extensive metabolism in the liver. Twelve metabolites have been identified in plasma; all except norverapamil are present in trace amounts only. Norverapamil can reach steady-state plasma concentrations approximately equal to those of verapamil itself. The cardiovascular activity of norverapamil appears to be approximately 20% that of verapamil. Approximately 70% of an administered dose is excreted as metabolites in the urine and 16% or more in the feces within 5 days. About 3% to 4% is excreted in the urine as unchanged drug. Approximately 90% is bound to plasma proteins. In patients with hepatic insufficiency, metabolism of immediate-release verapamil is delayed and elimination half-life prolonged up to 14 to 16 hours (see *Precautions*); the volume of distribution is increased and plasma clearance reduced to about 30% of normal. Verapamil clearance values suggest that patients with liver dysfunction may attain therapeutic verapamil plasma concentrations with one third of the oral daily dose required for patients with normal liver function.

After four weeks of oral dosing (120 mg q.i.d.), verapamil and norverapamil levels were noted in the cerebrospinal fluid with estimated partition coefficient of 0.06 for verapamil and 0.04 for norverapamil.

Hemodynamics and myocardial metabolism: Calan reduces afterload and myocardial contractility. Improved left ventricular diastolic function in patients with IHSS and those with coronary heart disease has also been observed with Calan. In most patients, including those with organic cardiac disease, the negative inotropic action of Calan is countered by reduction of afterload, and cardiac index is usually not reduced. However, in patients with severe left ventricular dysfunction (eg, pulmonary wedge pressure above 20 mm Hg or ejection fraction less than 30%), or in patients taking beta-adrenergic blocking agents or other cardiodepressant drugs, deterioration of ventricular function may occur (see *Drug interactions*).

Pulmonary function: Calan does not induce bronchoconstriction and, hence, does not impair ventilatory function.

INDICATIONS AND USAGE

Calan SR is indicated for the management of essential hypertension.

CONTRAINDICATIONS

Verapamil HCl caplets are contraindicated in:

1. Severe left ventricular dysfunction (see *Warnings*)

Continued on next page

Searle—Cont.

2. Hypotension (systolic pressure less than 90 mm Hg) or cardiogenic shock

3. Sick sinus syndrome (except in patients with a functioning artificial ventricular pacemaker)

4. Second- or third-degree AV block (except in patients with a functioning artificial ventricular pacemaker)

5. Patients with atrial flutter or atrial fibrillation and an accessory bypass tract (eg, Wolff-Parkinson-White, Lown-Ganong-Levine syndromes). (See *Warnings*.)

6. Patients with known hypersensitivity to verapamil hydrochloride.

WARNINGS

Heart failure: Verapamil has a negative inotropic effect, which in most patients is compensated by its afterload reduction (decreased systemic vascular resistance) properties without a net impairment of ventricular performance. In clinical experience with 4,954 patients, 87 (1.8%) developed congestive heart failure or pulmonary edema. Verapamil should be avoided in patients with severe left ventricular dysfunction (eg, ejection fraction less than 30%) or moderate to severe symptoms of cardiac failure and in patients with any degree of ventricular dysfunction if they are receiving a beta-adrenergic blocker (see *Drug interactions*). Patients with milder ventricular dysfunction should, if possible, be controlled with optimum doses of digitalis and/or diuretics before verapamil treatment. **(Note interactions with digoxin under *Precautions*.)**

Hypotension: Occasionally, the pharmacologic action of verapamil may produce a decrease in blood pressure below normal levels, which may result in dizziness or symptomatic hypotension. The incidence of hypotension observed in 4,954 patients enrolled in clinical trials was 2.5%. In hypertensive patients, decreases in blood pressure below normal are unusual. Tilt-table testing (60 degrees) was not able to induce orthostatic hypotension.

Elevated liver enzymes: Elevations of transaminases with and without concomitant elevations in alkaline phosphatase and bilirubin have been reported. Such elevations have sometimes been transient and may disappear even in the face of continued verapamil treatment. Several cases of hepatocellular injury related to verapamil have been proven by rechallenge; half of these had clinical symptoms (malaise, fever, and/or right upper quadrant pain) in addition to elevation of SGOT, SGPT, and alkaline phosphatase. Periodic monitoring of liver function in patients receiving verapamil is therefore prudent.

Accessory bypass tract (Wolff-Parkinson-White or Lown-Ganong-Levine): Some patients with paroxysmal and/or chronic atrial fibrillation or atrial flutter and a coexisting accessory AV pathway have developed increased antegrade conduction across the accessory pathway bypassing the AV node, producing a very rapid ventricular response or ventricular fibrillation after receiving intravenous verapamil (or digitalis). Although a risk of this occurring with oral verapamil has not been established, such patients receiving oral verapamil may be at risk and its use in these patients is contraindicated (see *Contraindications*). Treatment is usually DC-cardioversion. Cardioversion has been used safely and effectively after oral Calan.

Atrioventricular block: The effect of verapamil on AV conduction and the SA node may cause asymptomatic first-degree AV block and transient bradycardia, sometimes accompanied by nodal escape rhythms. PR-interval prolongation is correlated with verapamil plasma concentrations, especially during the early titration phase of therapy. Higher degrees of AV block, however, were infrequently (0.8%) observed. Marked first-degree block or progressive development to second- or third-degree AV block requires a reduction in dosage or, in rare instances, discontinuation of verapamil HCl and institution of appropriate therapy, depending upon the clinical situation.

Patients with hypertrophic cardiomyopathy (IHSS): In 120 patients with hypertrophic cardiomyopathy (most of them refractory or intolerant to propranolol) who received therapy with verapamil at doses up to 720 mg/day, a variety of serious adverse effects were seen. Three patients died in pulmonary edema; all had severe left ventricular outflow obstruction and a past history of left ventricular dysfunction. Eight other patients had pulmonary edema and/or severe hypotension; abnormally high (greater than 20 mm Hg) pulmonary wedge pressure and a marked left ventricular outflow obstruction were present in most of these patients. Concomitant administration of quinidine (see *Drug interactions*) preceded the severe hypotension in 3 of the 8 patients (2 of whom developed pulmonary edema). Sinus bradycardia occurred in 11% of the patients, second-degree AV block in 4%, and sinus arrest in 2%. It must be appreciated that this group of patients had a serious disease with a high mortality rate. Most adverse effects responded well to dose reduction, and only rarely did verapamil use have to be discontinued.

PRECAUTIONS
General
Use in patients with impaired hepatic function: Since verapamil is highly metabolized by the liver, it should be administered cautiously to patients with impaired hepatic function. Severe liver dysfunction prolongs the elimination half-life of immediate-release verapamil to about 14 to 16 hours; hence, approximately 30% of the dose given to patients with normal liver function should be administered to these patients. Careful monitoring for abnormal prolongation of the PR interval or other signs of excessive pharmacologic effects (see *Overdosage*) should be carried out.

Use in patients with attenuated (decreased) neuromuscular transmission: It has been reported that verapamil decreases neuromuscular transmission in patients with Duchenne's muscular dystrophy, and that verapamil prolongs recovery from the neuromuscular blocking agent vecuronium. It may be necessary to decrease the dosage of verapamil when it is administered to patients with attenuated neuromuscular transmission.

Use in patients with impaired renal function: About 70% of an administered dose of verapamil is excreted as metabolites in the urine. Verapamil is not removed by hemodialysis. Until further data are available, verapamil should be administered cautiously to patients with impaired renal function. These patients should be carefully monitored for abnormal prolongation of the PR interval or other signs of overdosage (see *Overdosage*).

Drug interactions
Beta-blockers: Concomitant therapy with beta-adrenergic blockers and verapamil may result in additive negative effects on heart rate, atrioventricular conduction and/or cardiac contractility. The combination of sustained-release verapamil and beta-adrenergic blocking agents has not been studied. However, there have been reports of excessive bradycardia and AV block, including complete heart block, when the combination has been used for the treatment of hypertension. For hypertensive patients, the risks of combined therapy may outweigh the potential benefits. The combination should be used only with caution and close monitoring.

Asymptomatic bradycardia (36 beats/min) with a wandering atrial pacemaker has been observed in a patient receiving concomitant timolol (a beta-adrenergic blocker) eyedrops and oral verapamil.

A decrease in metroprolol and propranolol clearance has been observed when either drug is administered concomitantly with verapamil. A variable effect has been seen when verapamil and atenolol were given together.

Digitalis: Clinical use of verapamil in digitalized patients has shown the combination to be well tolerated if digoxin doses are properly adjusted. However, chronic verapamil treatment can increase serum digoxin levels by 50% to 75% during the first week of therapy, and this can result in digitalis toxicity. In patients with hepatic cirrhosis the influence of verapamil on digoxin kinetics is magnified. Verapamil may reduce total body clearance and extrarenal clearance of digitoxin by 27% and 29%, respectively. Maintenance digitalis doses should be reduced when verapamil is administered, and the patient should be carefully monitored to avoid over- or underdigitalization. Whenever overdigitalization is suspected, the daily dose of digitalis should be reduced or temporarily discontinued. On discontinuation of Calan use, the patient should be reassessed to avoid underdigitalization.

Antihypertensive agents: Verapamil administered concomitantly with oral antihypertensive agents (eg, vasodilators, angiotensin-converting enzyme inhibitors, diuretics, beta-blockers) will usually have an additive effect on lowering blood pressure. Patients receiving these combinations should be appropriately monitored. Concomitant use of agents that attenuate alpha-adrenergic function with verapamil may result in a reduction in blood pressure that is excessive in some patients. Such an effect was observed in one study following the concomitant administration of verapamil and prazosin.

Antiarrhythmic agents:
Disopyramide: Until data on possible interactions between verapamil and disopyramide phosphate are obtained, disopyramide should not be administered within 48 hours before or 24 hours after verapamil administration.

Flecainide: A study in healthy volunteers showed that the concomitant administration of flecainide and verapamil may have additive effects on myocardial contractility, AV conduction, and repolarization. Concomitant therapy with flecainide and verapamil may result in additive negative inotropic effect and prolongation of atrioventricular conduction.

Quinidine: In a small number of patients with hypertrophic cardiomyopathy (IHSS), concomitant use of verapamil and quinidine resulted in significant hypotension. Until further data are obtained, combined therapy of verapamil and quinidine in patients with hypertrophic cardiomyopathy should probably be avoided.

The electrophysiologic effects of quinidine and verapamil on AV conduction were studied in 8 patients. Verapamil significantly counteracted the effects of quinidine on AV conduction. There has been a report of increased quinidine levels during verapamil therapy.

Other:
Nitrates: Verapamil has been given concomitantly with short- and long-acting nitrates without any undesirable drug interactions. The pharmacologic profile of both drugs and the clinical experience suggest beneficial interactions.

Cimetidine: The interaction between cimetidine and chronically administered verapamil has not been studied. Variable results on clearance have been obtained in acute studies of healthy volunteers; clearance of verapamil was either reduced or unchanged.

Lithium: Increased sensitivity to the effects of lithium (neurotoxicity) has been reported during concomitant verapamil-lithium therapy with either no change or an increase in serum lithium levels. However, the addition of verapamil has also resulted in the lowering of serum lithium levels in patients receiving chronic stable oral lithium. Patients receiving both drugs must be monitored carefully.

Carbamazepine: Verapamil therapy may increase carbamazepine concentrations during combined therapy. This may produce carbamazepine side effects such as diplopia, headache, ataxia, or dizziness.

Rifampin: Therapy with rifampin may markedly reduce oral verapamil bioavailability.

Phenobarbital: Phenobarbital therapy may increase verapamil clearance.

Cyclosporin: Verapamil therapy may increase serum levels of cyclosporin.

Theophylline: Verapamil may inhibit the clearance and increase the plasma levels of theophylline.

Inhalation anesthetics: Animal experiments have shown that inhalation anesthetics depress cardiovascular activity by decreasing the inward movement of calcium ions. When used concomitantly, inhalation anesthetics and calcium antagonists, such as verapamil, should each be titrated carefully to avoid excessive cardiovascular depression.

Neuromuscular blocking agents: Clinical data and animal studies suggest that verapamil may potentiate the activity of neuromuscular blocking agents (curare-like and depolarizing). It may be necessary to decrease the dose of verapamil and/or the dose of the neuromuscular blocking agent when the drugs are used concomitantly.

Carcinogenesis, mutagenesis, impairment of fertility: An 18-month toxicity study in rats, at a low multiple (6-fold) of the maximum recommended human dose, and not the maximum tolerated dose, did not suggest a tumorigenic potential. There was no evidence of a carcinogenic potential of verapamil administered in the diet of rats for two years at doses of 10, 35, and 120 mg/kg/day or approximately 1, 3.5, and 12 times, respectively, the maximum recommended human daily dose (480 mg/day or 9.6 mg/kg/day).

Verapamil was not mutagenic in the Ames test in 5 test strains at 3 mg per plate with or without metabolic activation.

Studies in female rats at daily dietary doses up to 5.5 times (55 mg/kg/day) the maximum recommended human dose did not show impaired fertility. Effects on male fertility have not been determined.

Pregnancy: Pregnancy Category C. Reproduction studies have been performed in rabbits and rats at oral doses up to 1.5 (15 mg/kg/day) and 6 (60 mg/kg/day) times the human oral daily dose, respectively, and have revealed no evidence of teratogenicity. In the rat, however, this multiple of the human dose was embryocidal and retarded fetal growth and development, probably because of adverse maternal effects reflected in reduced weight gains of the dams. This oral dose has also been shown to cause hypotension in rats. There are no adequate and well-controlled studies in pregnant women. Because animal reproduction studies are not always predictive of human response, this drug should be used during pregnancy only if clearly needed. Verapamil crosses the placental barrier and can be detected in umbilical vein blood at delivery.

Labor and delivery: It is not known whether the use of verapamil during labor or delivery has immediate or delayed adverse effects on the fetus, or whether it prolongs the duration of labor or increases the need for forceps delivery or other obstetric intervention. Such adverse experiences have not been reported in the literature, despite a long history of use of verapamil in Europe in the treatment of cardiac side effects of beta-adrenergic agonist agents used to treat premature labor.

Nursing mothers: Verapamil is excreted in human milk. Because of the potential for adverse reactions in nursing infants from verapamil, nursing should be discontinued while verapamil is administered.

Pediatric use: Safety and efficacy of Calan SR in children below the age of 18 years have not been established.

Animal pharmacology and/or animal toxicology: In chronic animal toxicology studies verapamil caused lenticular and/or suture line changes at 30 mg/kg/day or greater, and frank cataracts at 62.5 mg/kg/day or greater in the beagle dog but not in the rat. Development of cataracts due to verapamil has not been reported in man.

ADVERSE REACTIONS

Serious adverse reactions are uncommon when verapamil therapy is initiated with upward dose titration within the recommended single and total daily dose. See *Warnings* for discussion of heart failure, hypotension, elevated liver enzymes, AV block, and rapid ventricular response. Reversible (upon discontinuation of verapamil) non-obstructive, paralytic ileus has been infrequently reported in association with the use of verapamil. The following reactions to orally administered verapamil occurred at rates greater than 1.0% or occurred at lower rates but appeared clearly drug-related in clinical trials in 4,954 patients:

Constipation	7.3%	Dyspnea	1.4%
Dizziness	3.3%	Bradycardia	
Nausea	2.7%	(HR < 50/min)	1.4%
Hypotension	2.5%	AV block	
Headache	2.2%	total (1°, 2°, 3°)	1.2%
Edema	1.9%	2° and 3°	0.8%
CHF, Pulmonary		Rash	1.2%
edema	1.8%	Flushing	0.6%
Fatigue	1.7%		

Elevated liver enzymes (see *Warnings*)

In clinical trials related to the control of ventricular response in digitalized patients who had atrial fibrillation or flutter, ventricular rates below 50/min at rest occurred in 15% of patients and asymptomatic hypotension occurred in 5% of patients.

The following reactions, reported in 1% or less of patients, occurred under conditions (open trials, marketing experience) where a causal relationship is uncertain; they are listed to alert the physician to a possible relationship:

Cardiovascular: angina pectoris, atrioventricular dissociation, chest pain, claudication, myocardial infarction, palpitations, purpura (vasculitis), syncope.

Digestive system: diarrhea, dry mouth, gastrointestinal distress, gingival hyperplasia.

Hemic and lymphatic: ecchymosis or bruising.

Nervous system: cerebrovascular accident, confusion, equilibrium disorders, insomnia, muscle cramps, paresthesia, psychotic symptoms, shakiness, somnolence.

Skin: arthralgia and rash, exanthema, hair loss, hyperkeratosis, macules, sweating, urticaria, Stevens-Johnson syndrome, erythema multiforme.

Special senses: blurred vision.

Urogenital: gynecomastia, galactorrhea/hyperprolactinemia, increased urination, spotty menstruation, impotence.

Treatment of acute cardiovascular adverse reactions: The frequency of cardiovascular adverse reactions that require therapy is rare; hence, experience with their treatment is limited. Whenever severe hypotension or complete AV block occurs following oral administration of verapamil, the appropriate emergency measures should be applied immediately; eg, intravenously administered norepinephrine bitartrate, atropine sulfate, isoproterenol HCl (all in the usual doses), or calcium gluconate (10% solution). In patients with hypertrophic cardiomyopathy (IHSS), alpha-adrenergic agents (phenylephrine HCl, metaraminol bitartrate, or methoxamine HCl) should be used to maintain blood pressure, and isoproterenol and norepinephrine should be avoided. If further support is necessary, dopamine HCl or dobutamine HCl may be administered. Actual treatment and dosage should depend on the severity of the clinical situation and the judgment and experience of the treating physician.

OVERDOSAGE

Treat all verapamil overdoses as serious and maintain observation for at least 48 hours (especially Calan SR), preferably under continuous hospital care. Delayed pharmacodynamic consequences may occur with the sustained-release formulation. Verapamil is known to decrease gastrointestinal transit time.

Treatment of overdosage should be supportive. Beta adrenergic stimulation or parenteral administration of calcium solutions may increase calcium ion flux across the slow channel, and have been used effectively in treatment of deliberate overdosage with verapamil. Verapamil cannot be removed by hemodialysis. Clinically significant hypotensive reactions or high degree AV block should be treated with vasopressor agents or cardiac pacing, respectively. Asystole should be handled by the usual measures including cardiopulmonary resuscitation.

DOSAGE AND ADMINISTRATION

Essential hypertension: The dose of Calan SR should be individualized by titration and the drug should be administered with food. Initiate therapy with 180 mg of sustained-release verapamil HCl, Calan SR, given in the morning. Lower initial doses of 120 mg a day may be warranted in patients who may have an increased response to verapamil (eg, the elderly or small people). Upward titration should be based on therapeutic efficacy and safety evaluated weekly and approximately 24 hours after the previous dose. The antihypertensive effects of Calan SR are evident within the first week of therapy.

If adequate response is not obtained with 180 mg of Calan SR, the dose may be titrated upward in the following manner:

a) 240 mg each morning,
b) 180 mg each morning plus
   180 mg each evening; or
   240 mg each morning plus
   120 mg each evening,
c) 240 mg every 12 hours.

When switching from immediate-release Calan to Calan SR the total daily dose in milligrams may remain the same.

HOW SUPPLIED

Calan SR 240-mg caplets are light green, capsule shaped, scored, film coated, with CALAN debossed on one side and SR 240 on the other, supplied as:

NDC Number	Size
0025-1891-31	bottle of 100
0025-1891-51	bottle of 500
0025-1891-34	carton of 100 unit dose

Calan SR 180-mg caplets are light pink, oval, scored, film coated, with CALAN debossed on one side and SR 180 on the other, supplied as:

NDC Number	Size
0025-1911-31	bottle of 100
0025-1911-34	carton of 100 unit dose

Calan SR 120-mg caplets are light violet, oval, film-coated, with CALAN debossed on one side and SR 120 on the other, supplied as:

NDC Number	Size
0025-1901-31	bottle of 100
0025-1901-34	carton of 100 unit dose

Store at 59° to 77°F (15° to 25°C) and protect from light and moisture. Dispense in tight, light-resistant containers.

Caution: Federal law prohibits dispensing without prescription.

4/25/95 ● A05298-3

Shown in Product Identification Guide, page 335

COVERA-HS™ ℞

[*Cō-ver'-ə*]

(verapamil hydrochloride)
Extended-Release Tablets
Controlled-Onset

DESCRIPTION

Covera-HS (verapamil hydrochloride) is a calcium ion influx inhibitor (slow-channel blocker or calcium ion antagonist). Covera-HS is available for oral administration as pale yellow, round, film-coated tablets containing 240 mg of verapamil hydrochloride and as lavender, round, film-coated tablets containing 180 mg of verapamil hydrochloride. Verapamil is administered as a racemic mixture of the R and S enantiomers. The structural formulae of the verapamil HCl enantiomers are:

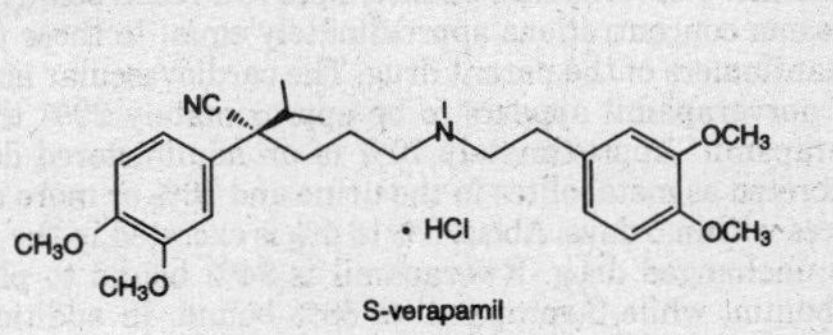

S-verapamil

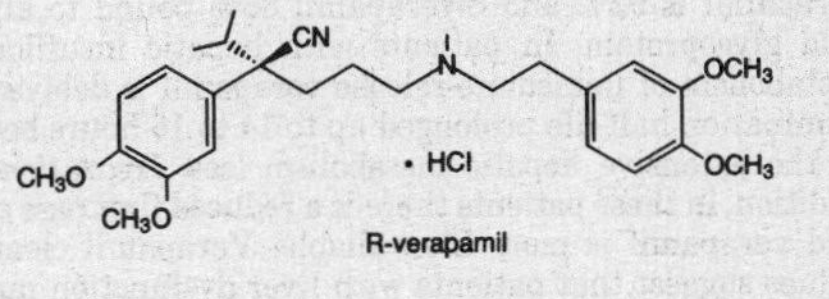

R-verapamil

$C_{27}H_{38}N_2O_4 \cdot HCl$ M.W. = 491.07

Benzeneacetonitrile, (±)-α[3[[2-(3,4-dimethoxyphenyl) ethyl]methylamino]propyl]-3,4-dimethoxy-α-(1-methylethyl) hydrochloride

Verapamil HCl is an almost white, crystalline powder, practically free of odor, with a bitter taste. It is soluble in water, chloroform, and methanol. Verapamil HCl is not chemically related to other cardioactive drugs.

Inactive ingredients are black ferric oxide, BHT, cellulose acetate, hydroxyethyl cellulose, hydroxypropyl cellulose, hydroxypropyl methylcellulose, magnesium stearate, polyethylene glycol, polyethylene oxide, polysorbate 80, povidone, sodium chloride, titanium dioxide, and coloring agents: 240-mg—FD&C Blue No. 2 Lake and D&C Yellow No. 10 Lake; 180-mg—FD&C Blue No. 2 Lake and D&C Red No. 30 Lake.

System components and performance: The Covera-HS formulation has been designed to initiate the release of verapamil 4–5 hours after ingestion. This delay is introduced by a layer between the active drug core and outer semipermeable membrane. As water from the gastrointestinal tract enters the tablet, this delay coating is solubilized and released. As tablet hydration continues, the osmotic layer expands and pushes against the drug layer, releasing drug through precision laser-drilled orifices in the outer membrane at a constant rate. This controlled rate of drug delivery in the gastrointestinal lumen is independent of posture, pH, gastrointestinal motility, and fed or fasting conditions.

The biologically inert components of the delivery system remain intact during GI transit and are eliminated in the feces as an insoluble shell.

CLINICAL PHARMACOLOGY

Covera-HS has a unique delivery system, designed for bedtime dosing, incorporating a 4 to 5-hour delay in drug delivery. The unique controlled-onset, extended-release (COER) delivery system, which is designed for bedtime dosing, results in a maximum plasma concentration (C_{max}) of verapamil in the morning hours.

Verapamil is a calcium ion influx inhibitor (L-type calcium channel blocker or calcium channel antagonist). Verapamil exerts its pharmacologic effects by selectively inhibiting the transmembrane influx of ionic calcium into arterial smooth muscle as well as in conductile and contractile myocardial cells without altering serum calcium concentrations.

Mechanism of Action

In vitro: Verapamil binding is voltage-dependent with affinity increasing as the vascular smooth muscle membrane potential is reduced. In addition, verapamil binding is frequency dependent and apparent affinity increases with increased frequency of depolarizing stimulus.

The L-type calcium channel is an oligomeric structure consisting of five putative subunits designated alpha-1, alpha-2, beta, tau, and epsilon. Biochemical evidence points to separate binding sites for 1,4-dihydropyridines, phenylalkylamines, and the benzothiazepines (all located on the alpha-1 subunit). Although they share a similar mechanism of action, calcium channel blockers represent three heterogeneous categories of drugs with differing vascular-cardiac selectivity ratios.

Essential hypertension: Verapamil produces its antihypertensive effect by a combination of vascular and cardiac effects. It acts as a vasodilator with selectivity for the arterial portion of the peripheral vasculature. As a result the systemic vascular resistence is reduced and usually without orthostatic hypotension or reflex tachycardia. Bradycardia (rate less than 50 beats/min) is uncommon (< 1% with Covera-HS as assessed by ECG). During isometric or dynamic exercise Covera-HS does not alter systolic cardiac function in patients with normal ventricular function.

Covera-HS does not alter total serum calcium levels. However, one report has suggested that calcium levels above the normal range may alter the therapeutic effect of verapamil.

Covera-HS regularly reduces the total systemic resistance (afterload) against which the heart works both at rest and at a given level of exercise by dilating peripheral arterioles.

Effects in hypertension: Covera-HS was evaluated in two placebo-controlled, parallel design, double-blind studies of 382 patients with mild to moderate hypertension.

In clinical trials 287 patients were randomized to placebo, 120 mg, 180 mg, 360 mg, or 540 mg and treated for 8 weeks (the two higher doses were titrated from low doses and maintained for 6 and 4 weeks, respectively). Covera-HS or placebo was given once daily at 10 pm and blood pressure changes were measured with 36-hour ambulatory blood pressure monitoring (ABPM). The results of these studies demonstrate that Covera-HS, at 180–540 mg, is a consistently and significantly more effective antihypertensive agent than placebo in reducing ambulatory blood pressures. Over this dose range, the placebo-subtracted net decreases in diastolic BP at trough (averaged over 6–10 pm) were dose-related, ranged from 4.5 to 11.2 mm Hg after 4–8 weeks of therapy, and correlated well with sitting cuff blood pressures.

These studies demonstrate that clinically and statistically significant blood pressure reductions are achieved with Covera-HS throughout the 24-hour dosing period.

There were no significant treatment differences between patient subgroups of different age (older or younger than 65 years), sex, race (Caucasian and non-Caucasian) and severity of hypertension at baseline (cuff BP below and above 105 mm Hg).

Angina: Verapamil dilates the main coronary arteries and coronary arterioles, both in normal and ischemic regions, and is a potent inhibitor of coronary artery spasm, whether spontaneous or ergonovine-induced. This property increases myocardial oxygen delivery in patients with coronary artery spasm and is responsible for the effectiveness of verapamil in vasospastic (Prinzmetal's or variant) as well as unstable angina at rest. Whether this effect plays any role in classical effort angina is not clear, but studies of exercise tolerance have not shown an increase in the maximum exercise rate-pressure product, a widely associated measure of oxygen

Continued on next page

Searle—Cont.

utilization. This suggests that, in general, relief of spasm or dilation of coronary arteries is not an important factor in classical angina.

Verapamil regularly reduces the total systemic resistance (afterload) against which the heart works both at rest and at a given level of exercise by dilating peripheral arterioles.

Effect in chronic stable angina: Covera-HS was evaluated in two placebo-controlled, parallel design, double-blind studies of 453 patients with chronic stable angina.

In the first clinical trial 277 patients were randomized to placebo, 180 mg, 360 mg, or 540 mg and treated for 4 weeks (the two higher doses were titrated from low doses and maintained for 3 and 2 weeks, respectively). A single dose of 240 mg was compared to placebo in a separate study of 176 patients. In these studies Covera-HS was significantly more effective than placebo in improvement of exercise tolerance. Placebo-adjusted net increases in median exercise times at the end of the dosing interval were 0.1 to 1.0 minute for symptom limited duration, 0.3 to 1.4 minutes for time to angina, and 0.1 to 1.1 minutes for time to ST change. Increases in exercise tolerance were in general greater at higher doses, but dose-response relationship was not well defined due to shorter treatment duration for high doses.

In addition, in the first study, 24 to 34% of patients treated with Covera-HS did not experience exercise-limiting angina on exercise treadmill testing (ETT) versus 12% of patients on placebo.

Electrophysiologic effects: Electrical activity through the AV node depends, to a significant degree, upon the trans-membrane influx of extracellular calcium through the L-type (slow) channel. By decreasing the influx of calcium, verapamil prolongs the effective refractory period within the AV node and slows AV conduction in a rate-related manner.

Normal sinus rhythm is usually not affected, but in patients with sick sinus syndrome, verapamil may interfere with sinus-node impulse generation and may induce sinus arrest or sinoatrial block. Atrioventricular block can occur in patients without preexisting conduction defects (see *Warnings*).

Covera-HS does not alter the normal atrial action potential or intra-ventricular conduction time, but depresses amplitude, velocity of depolarization, and conduction in depressed atrial fibers. Verapamil may shorten the antegrade effective refractory period of the accessory bypass tract. Acceleration of ventricular rate and/or ventricular fibrillation has been reported in patients with atrial flutter or atrial fibrillation and a coexisting accessory AV pathway following administration of verapamil (see *Warnings*).

Verapamil has a local anesthetic action that is 1.6 times that of procaine on an equimolar basis. It is not known whether this action is important at the doses used in man.

Pharmacokinetics and metabolism: Verapamil is administered as a racemic mixture of the R and S enantiomers. The systemic concentrations of R and S enantiomers, as well as overall bioavailability, are dependent upon the route of administration and the rate and extent of release from the dosage forms. Upon oral administration, there is rapid stereoselective biotransformation during the first pass of verapamil through the portal circulation. In a study in 5 subjects with oral immediate-release verapamil, the systemic bioavailability was from 33% to 65% for the R enantiomer and from 13% to 34% for the S enantiomer. The R and S enantiomers have differing levels of pharmacologic activity. In studies in animals and humans, the S enantiomer has 8 to 20 times the activity of the R enantiomer in slowing AV conduction. In animal studies, the S enantiomer has 15 and 50 times the activity of the R enantiomer in reducing myocardial contractility in isolated blood-perfused dog papillary muscle and isolated rabbit papillary muscle, respectively, and twice the effect in reducing peripheral resistance. In isolated septal strip preparations from 5 patients, the S enantiomer was 8 times more potent than the R in reducing myocardial contractility. Dose escalation study data indicate that verapamil concentrations increase disproportionally to dose as measured by relative peak plasma concentrations (C_{max}) or areas under the plasma concentration vs time curves (AUC).

Pharmacokinetic Characteristics of Verapamil Enantiomers After Administration of Escalating Doses

		Total Dose of Racemic Verapamil (mg)			
	Isomer	120	180	360	540
Dose Ratio	—	1	1.5	3	4.5
Relative C_{max}	R	1	1.55	4.47	7.06
	S	1	1.62	5.17	9.21
Relative AUC	R	1	1.59	6.14	11.1
	S	1	1.89	8.17	15.9

Pharmacokinetic Characteristics of Verapamil Enantiomers After Administration of a Single 180 mg Dose and at Steady State

	Isomer	First Dose (Verapamil-naive subject)	Steady State (Current verapamil exposure)
C_{max} (ng/ml)	R	59.4	90.5
	S	11.7	21.2
AUC (0–24h) (ng·hr/ml)	R	644	1,223
	S	111	266

Racemic verapamil is released from Covera-HS at a constant rate following solubilization and release of the delay coat through the tablet orifices. This delay coat produces a lag period in drug release for approximately 4–5 hours. The drug release phase is prolonged with the peak plasma concentration (C_{max}) occurring approximately 11 hours after administration. Trough concentrations occur approximately 4 hours after bedtime dosing while the patient is sleeping. Steady-state pharmacokinetics were determined in healthy volunteers. Steady-state concentration is reached by the third or fourth day of dosing.

Steady-State Pharmacokinetics of Verapamil Enantiomers in Healthy Humans

		Verapamil Dose (mg)	
	Isomer	180	240
Mean C_{max} (ng/ml)	R	90.5	120
	S	21.2	28.7
AUC (0–24h) (ng·hr/ml)	R	1,223	1,470
	S	266	322

In general, bioavailability of Covera-HS is higher and half life longer in older (> 65 yrs) subjects. Lean body weight also affects its pharmacokinetics inversely, but no gender difference was observed in the clinical trials of Covera-HS. However, there are conflicting data in literature suggesting that verapamil clearance decreased with age in women to a greater degree than in men.

Consumption of a high fat meal just prior to dosing at night had no effect on the pharmacokinetics of Covera-HS. The pharmacokinetics were also not affected by whether the volunteers were supine or ambulatory for the 8 hours following dosing. Administering Covera-HS in the morning led to a slower rate of absorption and/or elimination, but did not affect the extent of absorption or extent of metabolism to norverapamil.

Orally administered verapamil undergoes extensive metabolism in the liver. Thirteen metabolites have been identified in urine. Norverapamil enantiomers can reach steady-state plasma concentrations approximately equal to those of the enantiomers of the parent drug. The cardiovascular activity of norverapamil appears to be approximately 20% that of verapamil. Approximately 70% of an administered dose is excreted as metabolites in the urine and 16% or more in the feces within 5 days. About 3% to 4% is excreted in the urine as unchanged drug. R-verapamil is 94% bound to plasma albumin, while S-verapamil is 88% bound. In addition, R-verapamil is 92% and S-verapamil 86% bound to alpha-1 acid glycoprotein. In patients with hepatic insufficiency, metabolism of immediate-release verapamil is delayed and elimination half-life prolonged up to 14 to 16 hours because of the extensive hepatic metabolism (see *Precautions*). In addition, in these patients there is a reduced first pass effect, and verapamil is more bioavailable. Verapamil clearance values suggest that patients with liver dysfunction may attain therapeutic verapamil plasma concentrations with one third of the oral daily dose required for patients with normal liver function.

After four weeks of oral dosing of immediate release verapamil (120 mg q.i.d.), verapamil and norverapamil levels were noted in the cerebrospinal fluid with estimated partition coefficient of 0.06 for verapamil and 0.04 for norverapamil.

Hemodynamics: Verapamil reduces afterload and myocardial contractility. In most patients, including those with organic cardiac disease, the negative inotropic action of verapamil is countered by reduction of afterload and cardiac index remains unchanged. During isometric or dynamic exercise, verapamil does not alter systolic cardiac function in patients with normal ventricular function. Improved left ventricular diastolic function in patients with IHSS and those with coronary heart disease has also been observed with verapamil. In patients with severe left ventricular dysfunction (eg, pulmonary wedge pressure above 20 mm Hg or ejection fraction less than 30%), or in patients taking beta-adrenergic blocking agents or other cardio-depressant drugs,

deterioration of ventricular function may occur (see *Drug interactions*).

Pulmonary function: Verapamil does not induce bronchoconstriction and, hence, does not impair ventilatory function.

Verapamil has been shown to have either a neutral or relaxant effect on bronchial smooth muscle.

INDICATIONS AND USAGE

Covera-HS is indicated for the management of hypertension and angina.

CONTRAINDICATIONS

Covera-HS is contraindicated in:
1. Severe left ventricular dysfunction (see *Warnings*)
2. Hypotension (systolic pressure less than 90 mm Hg) or cardiogenic shock
3. Sick sinus syndrome (except in patients with a functioning artificial ventricular pacemaker)
4. Second- or third-degree AV block (except in patients with a functioning artificial ventricular pacemaker)
5. Patients with atrial flutter or atrial fibrillation and an accessory bypass tract (eg, Wolff-Parkinson-White, Lown-Ganong-Levine syndromes). (See *Warnings*.)
6. Patients with known hypersensitivity to verapamil hydrochloride.

WARNINGS

Heart failure: Verapamil has a negative inotropic effect, which in most patients is compensated by its afterload reduction (decreased systemic vascular resistance) properties without a net impairment of ventricular performance. In previous clinical experience with 4,954 patients primarily with immediate-release verapamil, 1.8% developed congestive heart failure or pulmonary edema. Verapamil should be avoided in patients with severe left ventricular dysfunction (eg, ejection fraction less than 30%) or moderate to severe symptoms of cardiac failure and in patients with any degree of ventricular dysfunction if they are receiving a beta-adrenergic blocker (see *Drug Interactions*). Patients with milder ventricular dysfunction should, if possible, be controlled with optimum doses of digitalis and/or diuretics before verapamil treatment is started. **(Note interactions with digoxin under *Precautions*.)**

Hypotension: Occasionally, the pharmacologic action of verapamil may produce a decrease in blood pressure below normal levels, which may result in dizziness or symptomatic hypotension. In previous verapamil clinical trials the incidence observed in 4,954 patients was 2.5%. In clinical studies of Covera-HS, 0.4% of hypertensive patients and 1.0% of angina patients developed significant hypotension. In hypertensive patients, decreases in blood pressure below normal are unusual. Tilt-table testing (60 degrees) was not able to induce orthostatic hypotension.

Elevated liver enzymes: Elevations of transaminases with and without concomitant elevations in alkaline phosphatase and bilirubin have been reported. Such elevations have sometimes been transient and may disappear even in the face of continued verapamil treatment. Several cases of hepatocellular injury related to verapamil have been proven by rechallenge; half of these had clinical symptoms (malaise, fever, and/or right upper quadrant pain) in addition to elevation of SGOT, SGPT, and alkaline phosphatase. Periodic monitoring of liver function in patients receiving verapamil is therefore prudent.

Accessory bypass tract (Wolff-Parkinson-White or Lown-Ganong-Levine): Some patients with paroxysmal and/or chronic atrial fibrillation or atrial flutter and a coexisting accessory AV pathway have developed increased antegrade conduction across the accessory pathway bypassing the AV node, producing a very rapid ventricular response or ventricular fibrillation after receiving intravenous verapamil (or digitalis). Although a risk of this occurring with oral verapamil has not been established, such patients receiving oral verapamil may be at risk and its use in these patients is contraindicated (see *Contraindications*). Treatment is usually DC-cardioversion. Cardioversion has been used safely and effectively after oral verapamil.

Atrioventricular block: The effect of verapamil on AV conduction and the SA node may cause asymptomatic first-degree AV block and transient bradycardia, sometimes accompanied by nodal escape rhythms. PR-interval prolongation is correlated with verapamil plasma concentrations, especially during the early titration phase of therapy. Higher degrees of AV block, however, were infrequently (0.8%) observed in previous verapamil clinical trials. Marked first-degree block or progressive development to second- or third-degree AV block requires a reduction in dosage or, in rare instances, discontinuation of verapamil HCl and institution of appropriate therapy, depending upon the clinical situation.

Patients with hypertrophic cardiomyopathy (IHSS): In 120 patients with hypertrophic cardiomyopathy (most of them refractory or intolerant to propranolol) who received therapy with verapamil at doses up to 720 mg/day, a variety of serious adverse effects were seen. Three patients died in pulmonary edema; all had severe left ventricular outflow obstruction and a past history of left ventricular dysfunction.

Eight other patients had pulmonary edema and/or severe hypotension; abnormally high (greater than 20 mm Hg) pulmonary wedge pressure and a marked left ventricular outflow obstruction were present in most of these patients. Concomitant administration of quinidine (see *Drug interactions*) preceded the severe hypotension in 3 of the 8 patients (2 of whom developed pulmonary edema). Sinus bradycardia occurred in 11% of the patients, second-degree AV block in 4%, and sinus arrest in 2%. It must be appreciated that this group of patients had a serious disease with a high mortality rate. Most adverse efffects responded well to dose reduction, and only rarely did verapamil use have to be discontinued.

PRECAUTIONS

General

Formulation specific: As with any other non-deformable dosage form caution should be used when administering Covera-HS in patients with preexisting severe gastrointestinal narrowing (pathologic or iatrogenic). In patients with extremely short GI transit time (<7 hrs), pharmacokinetic data are not available and dosage adjustment may be required.

Use in patients with impaired hepatic function: Since verapamil is highly metabolized by the liver, it should be administered cautiously to patients with impaired hepatic function. Severe liver dysfunction prolongs the elimination half-life of immediate-release verapamil to about 14 to 16 hours; hence, approximately 30% of the dose given to patients with normal liver function should be administered to these patients. Careful monitoring for abnormal prolongation of the PR interval or other signs of excessive pharmacologic effects (see *Overdosage*) should be carried out.

Use in patients with attenuated (decreased) neuromuscular transmission: It has been reported that verapamil decreases neuromuscular transmission in patients with Duchenne's muscular dystrophy, and that verapamil prolongs recovery from the neuromuscular blocking agent vecuronium. It may be necessary to decrease the dosage of verapamil when it is administered to patients with attenuated neuromuscular transmission.

Use in patients with impaired renal function: About 70% of an administered dose of verapamil is excreted as metabolites in the urine. Verapamil is not removed by hemodialysis. Until further data are available, verapamil should be administered cautiously to patients with impaired renal function. These patients should be carefully monitored for abnormal prolongation of the PR interval or other signs of overdosage (see *Overdosage*).

Information for patients: Covera-HS tablets should be swallowed whole; do not break, crush, or chew. The medication in the Covera-HS tablet is released slowly through an outer shell that does not dissolve. The patient should not be concerned if they occasionally observe this outer shell in their stool as it passes from the body.

Drug interactions

Alcohol: Verapamil may increase blood alcohol concentrations and prolong its effects.

Beta-blockers: Concomitant therapy with beta-adrenergic blockers and verapamil may result in additive negative effects on heart rate, atrioventricular conduction and/or cardiac contractility. The combination of sustained-release verapamil and beta-adrenergic blocking agents has not been studied. However, there have been reports of excessive bradycardia and AV block, including complete heart block, when the combination has been used for the treatment of hypertension. For hypertensive patients, the risks of combined therapy may outweigh the potential benefits. The combination should be used only with caution and close monitoring.

Asymptomatic bradycardia (36 beats/min) with a wandering atrial pacemaker has been observed in a patient receiving concomitant timolol (a beta-adrenergic blocker) eyedrops and oral verapamil.

A decrease in metoprolol and propranolol clearance has been observed when either drug is administered concomitantly with verapamil. A variable effect has been seen when verapamil and atenolol were given together.

Digitalis: Clinical use of verapamil in digitalized patients has shown the combination to be well tolerated if digoxin doses are properly adjusted. However, chronic verapamil treatment can increase serum digoxin levels by 50% to 75% during the first week of therapy, and this can result in digitalis toxicity. In patients with hepatic cirrhosis the influence of verapamil on digoxin kinetics is magnified. Verapamil may reduce total body clearance and extrarenal clearance of digitoxin by 27% and 29%, respectively. Maintenance and digitalization doses should be reduced when verapamil is administered, and the patient should be reassessed to avoid over- to underdigitalization. Whenever overdigitalization is suspected, the daily dose of digitalis should be reduced or temporarily discontinued. On discontinuation of verapamil use, the patient should be reassessed to avoid underdigitalization. In previous clinical trials with other verapamil formulations related to the control of ventricular response in digitalized patients who had atrial fibrillation or atrial flutter, ventricular rates below 50/min at rest occurred in 15% of patients, and asymptomatic hypotension occurred in 5% of patients.

Antihypertensive agents: Verapamil administered concomitantly with oral antihypertensive agents (eg, vasodilators, angiotensin-converting enzyme inhibitors, diuretics, beta-blockers) will usually have an additive effect on lowering blood pressure. Patients receiving these combinations should be appropriately monitored. Concomitant use of agents that attenuate alpha-adrenergic function with verapamil may result in a reduction in blood pressure that is excessive in some patients. Such an effect was observed in one study following the concomitant administration of verapamil and prazosin.

Antiarrhythmic agents:

Disopyramide: Until data on possible interactions between verapamil and disopyramide are obtained, disopyramide should not be administered within 48 hours before or 24 hours after verapamil administration.

Flecainide: A study in healthy volunteers showed that the concomitant administration of flecainide and verapamil may have additive effects on myocardial contractility, AV conduction, and repolarization. Concomitant therapy with flecainide and verapamil may result in additive negative inotropic effect and prolongation of atrioventricular conduction.

Quinidine: In a small number of patients with hypertrophic cardiomyopathy (IHSS), concomitant use of verapamil and quinidine resulted in significant hypotension. Until further data are obtained, combined therapy of verapamil and quinidine in patients with hypertrophic cardiomyopathy should probably be avoided.

The electrophysiologic effects of quinidine and verapamil on AV conduction were studied in 8 patients. Verapamil significantly counteracted the effects of quinidine on AV conduction. There has been a report of increased quinidine levels during verapamil therapy.

Other:

Nitrates: Verapamil has been given concomitantly with short- and long-acting nitrates without any undesirable drug interactions. The pharmacologic profile of both drugs and clinical experience suggest beneficial interactions.

Cimetidine: The interaction between cimetidine and chronically administered verapamil has not been studied. Variable results on clearance have been obtained in acute studies of healthy volunteers; clearance of verapamil was either reduced or unchanged.

Lithium: Increased sensitivity to the effects of lithium (neurotoxicity) has been reported during concomitant verapamil-lithium therapy with either no change or an increase in serum lithium levels. However, the addition of verapamil has also resulted in the lowering of serum lithium levels in patients receiving chronic stable oral lithium. Patients receiving both drugs must be monitored carefully.

Carbamazepine: Verapamil therapy may increase carbamazepine concentrations during combined therapy. This may produce carbamazepine side effects such as diplopia, headache, ataxia, or dizziness.

Rifampin: Therapy with rifampin may markedly reduce oral verapamil bioavailability.

Phenobarbital: Phenobarbital therapy may increase verapamil clearance.

Cyclosporin: Verapamil therapy may increase serum levels of cyclosporin.

Theophylline: Verapamil may inhibit the clearance and increase the plasma levels of theophylline.

Inhalation anesthetics: Animal experiments have shown that inhalation anesthetics depress cardiovascular activity by decreasing the inward movement of calcium ions. When used concomitantly, inhalation anesthetics and calcium channel blocking agents, such as verapamil, should each be titrated carefully to avoid excessive cardiovascular depression.

Neuromuscular blocking agents: Clinical data and animal studies suggest that verapamil may potentiate the activity of neuromuscular blocking agents (curare-like and depolarizing). It may be necessary to decrease the dose of verapamil and/or the dose of the neuromuscular blocking agent when the drugs are used concomitantly.

Carcinogenesis, mutagenesis, impairment of fertility: An 18-month toxicity study in rats, at a low multiple (6-fold) of the maximum recommended human dose, not the maximum tolerated dose, did not suggest a tumorigenic potential. There was no evidence of a carcinogenic potential of verapamil administered in the diet of rats for two years at doses of 10, 35, and 120 mg/kg/day or approximately 1, 3.5 and 12 times, respectively, the maximum recommended human daily dose (480 mg/day or 9.6 mg/kg/day).

Verapamil was not mutagenic in the Ames test in 5 test strains at 3 mg per plate with or without metabolic activation.

Studies in female rats at daily dietary doses up to 5.5 times (55 mg/kg/day) the maximum recommended human dose did not show impaired fertility. Effects on male fertility have not been determined.

Pregnancy: Pregnancy Category C. Reproduction studies have been performed in rabbits and rats at oral doses up to 1.5 (15 mg/kg/day) and 6 (60 mg/kg/day) times the human oral daily dose, respectively, and have revealed no evidence of teratogenicity. In the rat, however, this multiple of the human dose was embryocidal and retarded fetal growth and development, probably because of adverse maternal effects reflected in reduced weight gains of the dams. This oral dose has also been shown to cause hypotension in rats. There are no adequate and well-controlled studies in pregnant women. Because animal reproduction studies are not always predictive of human response, this drug should be used during pregnancy only if clearly needed. Verapamil crosses the placental barrier and can be detected in umbilical vein blood at delivery.

Labor and delivery: It is not known whether the use of verapamil during labor or delivery has immediate or delayed adverse effects on the fetus, or whether it prolongs the duration of labor or increases the need for forceps delivery or other obstetric intervention. Such adverse experiences have not been reported in the literature, despite a long history of use of verapamil in Europe in the treatment of cardiac side effects of beta-adrenergic agonist agents used to treat premature labor.

Nursing mothers: Verapamil is excreted in human milk. Because of the potential for adverse reactions in nursing infants from verapamil, nursing should be discontinued while verapamil is administered.

Pediatric use: Safety and efficacy of Covera-HS in children below the age of 18 years have not been established.

Elderly use: Dosage adjustment may be required in elderly patients with impaired renal function. Verapamil should be administered cautiously in patients with impaired renal function.

Animal pharmacology and/or animal toxicology: In chronic animal toxicology studies verapamil caused lenticular and/or suture line changes at 30 mg/kg/day or greater, and frank cataracts at 62.5 mg/kg/day or greater in the beagle dog but not in the rat. Development of cataracts due to verapamil has not been reported in man.

ADVERSE REACTIONS

Serious adverse reactions are uncommon when verapamil therapy is initiated with upward dose titration within the recommended single and total daily dose. See *Warnings* for discussion of heart failure, hypotension, elevated liver enzymes, AV block, and rapid ventricular response. Reversible (upon discontinuation of verapamil) non-obstructive, paralytic ileus has been infrequently reported in association with the use of verapamil. The following reactions to orally administered Covera-HS occurred at rates greater than 2.0% or occurred at lower rates but appeared drug-related in clinical trials in hypertension and angina:

	Placebo n=261 %	All doses studied n=572 %
Constipation	2.7	11.7*
Headache	7.3	6.6
Upper respiratory infection	4.6	5.4
Dizziness	2.7	4.7
Fatigue	3.8	4.5
Edema	3.1	3.0
Nausea	1.9	2.1
Av block (1°)	0.0	1.7
Elevated liver enzymes (see *Warnings*)	0.8	1.4
Bradycardia	0.4	1.4
Paresthesia	0.0	1.0
Flushing	0.3	0.8
Hypotension	0.0	0.7
Postural hypotension	0.3	0.4

*Constipation was typically mild, easily manageable, and the incidence usually diminished within about one week. At a typical once-daily dose of 240 mg, the observed incidence was 7.2%.

In previous experience with other formulations of verapamil, the following reactions occurred at rates greater than 1.0% or occurred at lower rates but appeared clearly drug related in clinical trials in 4,954 patients.

Constipation	7.3%
Dizziness	3.3%
Nausea	2.7%
Hypotension	2.5%
Headache	2.2%
Edema	1.9%
CHF/Pulmonary Edema	1.8%
Fatigue	1.7%
Dyspnea	1.4%
Bradycardia (HR<50/min)	1.4%
AV Block (total 1°,2°,3°)	1.2%
AV Block (2° and 3°)	0.8%
Rash	1.2%
Flushing	0.6%

Elevated liver enzymes (see *Warnings*)

Continued on next page

Searle—Cont.

The following reactions, reported with orally administered verapamil in 2% or less of patients, occurred under conditions (open trials, marketing experience) where a causal relationship is uncertain; they are listed to alert the physician to a possible relationship:

Cardiovascular: angina pectoris, AV block (2° & 3°), atrioventricular dissociation, CHF, pulmonary edema, chest pain, claudication, myocardial infarction, palpitations, purpura (vasculitis), syncope.

Digestive system: diarrhea, dry mouth, gastrointestinal distress, gingival hyperplasia.

Hemic and lymphatic: ecchymosis or bruising.

Nervous system: cerebrovascular accident, confusion, equilibrium disorders, insomnia, muscle cramps, psychotic symptoms, shakiness, somnolence.

Skin: arthralgia and rash, exanthema, hair loss, hyperkeratosis, macules, sweating, urticaria, Stevens-Johnson syndrome, erythema multiforme.

Special senses: blurred vision.

Urogenital: gynecomastia, galactorrhea/hyperprolactinemia, increased urination, spotty menstruation, impotence.

Other: allergy aggravated, dyspnea.

Treatment of acute cardiovascular adverse reactions: The frequency of cardiovascular adverse reactions that require therapy is rare; hence, experience with their treatment is limited. Whenever severe hypotension or complete AV block occurs following oral administration of verapamil, the appropriate emergency measures should be applied immediately; eg, intravenously administered norepinephrine bitartrate, atropine sulfate, isoproterenol HCl (all in usual doses), or calcium gluconate (10% solution). In patients with hypertrophic cardiomyopathy (IHSS), alpha-adrenergic agents (phenylephrine HCl, metaraminol bitartrate, or methoxamine HCl) should be used to maintain blood pressure, and isoproterenol and norepinephrine should be avoided. If further support is necessary, dopamine HCl or dobutamine HCl may be administered. Actual treatment and dosage should depend on the severity of the clinical situation and the judgement and experience of the treating physician.

OVERDOSAGE

Treat all verapamil overdoses as serious and maintain observation for at least 48 hours (especially sustained-release verapamil products), preferably under continuous hospital care. Delayed pharmacodynamic consequences may occur with the sustained-release formulations. Verapamil is known to decrease gastrointestinal transit time.

Treatment of overdosage should be supportive. Beta-adrenergic stimulation or parenteral administration of calcium solutions may increase calcium ion flux across the slow channel and have been used effectively in treatment of deliberate overdosage with verapamil. Verapamil cannot be removed by hemodialysis. Clinically significant hypotensive reactions or high degree AV block should be treated with vasopressor agents or cardiac pacing, respectively. Asystole should be handled by the usual measures including cardiopulmonary resuscitation.

DOSAGE AND ADMINISTRATION

Covera-HS should be administered once daily at bedtime. Clinical trials explored dose ranges between 180 mg and 540 mg given at bedtime and found effects to persist throughout the dosing interval.

Covera-HS tablets should be swallowed whole and not chewed, broken, or crushed.

For both hypertension and angina the dose of Covera-HS should be individualized by titration. Initiate therapy with 180 mg of Covera-HS.

If an adequate response is not obtained with 180 mg of Covera-HS, the dose may be titrated upward in the following manner:

a) 240 mg each evening
b) 360 mg each evening (2 × 180 mg)
c) 480 mg each evening (2 × 240 mg)

When Covera-HS is administered at bedtime, office evaluation of blood pressure during morning and early afternoon hours is essentially a measure of peak effect. The usual evaluation of trough effect, which sometimes might be needed to evaluate the appropriateness of any given dose of Covera-HS, would be just prior to bedtime.

HOW SUPPLIED

Covera-HS 240-mg tablets are pale yellow, round, film coated with COVERA-HS 2021 printed on one side, supplied as:

NDC Number	Size
0025-2021-30	bottle of 30
0025-2021-31	bottle of 100
0025-2021-34	carton of 100 unit dose

Covera-HS 180-mg tablets are lavender, round, film coated, with COVERA-HS 2011 printed on one side, supplied as:

NDC Number	Size
0025-2011-30	bottle of 30
0025-2011-31	bottle of 100
0025-2011-34	carton of 100 unit dose

Store at controlled room temperature 20°–25°C (68°–77°F) [see USP]. Dispense in tight, light-resistant containers.

Caution: Federal law prohibits dispensing without prescription.

A05306 ● 2/15/96

Manufactured for
G.D. Searle & Co.
Chicago IL 60680 USA
By Alza Corporation
Palo Alto CA USA
Address medical inquiries to:
G.D. Searle & Co.
Healthcare Information Services
5200 Old Orchard Road
Skokie IL 60077
©1996, G.D. Searle & Co.
Shown in Product Identification Guide, page 335

CYTOTEC® ℞
[sī-tō-tĕc]
(misoprostol)

CONTRAINDICATIONS AND WARNINGS

Cytotec (misoprostol) is contraindicated, because of its abortifacient property, in women who are pregnant. (See *Precautions*.) Patients must be advised of the abortifacient property and warned not to give the drug to others. Anecdotal reports, primarily from Brazil, of congenital anomalies and reports of fetal death subsequent to misuse of misoprostol as an abortifacient have been received. Cytotec should not be used in women of childbearing potential unless the patient requires nonsteroidal anti-inflammatory drug (NSAID) therapy and is at high risk of complications from gastric ulcers associated with use of the NSAID, or is at high risk of developing gastric ulceration. In such patients, Cytotec may be prescribed if the patient

- has had a negative serum pregnancy test within 2 weeks prior to beginning therapy.
- is capable of complying with effective contraceptive measures.
- has received both oral and written warnings of the hazards of misoprostol, the risk of possible contraception failure, and the danger to other women of childbearing potential should the drug be taken by mistake.
- will begin Cytotec only on the second or third day of the next normal menstrual period.

DESCRIPTION

Cytotec oral tablets contain either 100 mcg or 200 mcg of misoprostol, a synthetic prostaglandin E_1 analog.

Misoprostol contains approximately equal amounts of the two diastereomers presented below with their enantiomers indicated by (±):

$C_{22}H_{38}O_5$ M.W. = 382.5

(±) methyl 11α, 16-dihydroxy-16-methyl-9-oxoprost-13E-en-1-oate

Misoprostol is a water-soluble, viscous liquid.

Inactive ingredients of tablets are hydrogenated castor oil, hydroxypropyl methylcellulose, microcrystalline cellulose, and sodium starch glycolate.

CLINICAL PHARMACOLOGY

Pharmacokinetics: Misoprostol is extensively absorbed, and undergoes rapid de-esterification to its free acid, which is responsible for its clinical activity and, unlike the parent compound, is detectable in plasma. The alpha side chain undergoes beta oxidation and the beta side chain undergoes omega oxidation followed by reduction of the ketone to give prostaglandin F analogs.

In normal volunteers, Cytotec (misoprostol) is rapidly absorbed after oral administration with a T_{max} of misoprostol acid of 12 ± 3 minutes and a terminal half-life of 20–40 minutes.

There is high variability of plasma levels of misoprostol acid between and within studies but mean values after single doses show a linear relationship with dose over the range of 200–400 mcg. No accumulation of misoprostol acid was noted in multiple dose studies; plasma steady state was achieved within two days.

Maximum plasma concentrations of misoprostol acid are diminished when the dose is taken with food and total availability of misoprostol acid is reduced by use of concomitant antacid. Clinical trials were conducted with concomitant antacid, however, so this effect does not appear to be clinically important.

Mean ± SD	C_{max}(pg/ml)	AUC (0-4) (pg·hr/ml)	T_{max}(min)
Fasting	811 ± 317	417 ± 135	14 ± 8
With Antacid	689 ± 315	349 ± 108*	20 ± 14
With High Fat Breakfast	303 ± 176*	373 ± 111	64 ± 79*

*Comparisons with fasting results statistically significant, p < 0.05.

After oral administration of radiolabeled misoprostol, about 80% of detected radioactivity appears in urine. Pharmacokinetic studies in patients with varying degrees of renal impairment showed an approximate doubling of $T_{1/2}$, C_{max}, and AUC compared to normals, but no clear correlation between the degree of impairment and AUC. In subjects over 64 years of age, the AUC for misoprostol acid is increased. No routine dosage adjustment is recommended in older patients or patients with renal impairment, but dosage may need to be reduced if the usual dose is not tolerated.

Cytotec does not affect the hepatic mixed function oxidase (cytochrome P-450) enzyme systems in animals.

Drug interaction studies between misoprostol and several nonsteroidal anti-inflammatory drugs showed no effect on the kinetics of ibuprofen or diclofenac, and a 20% decrease in aspirin AUC, not thought to be clinically significant.

Pharmacokinetic studies also showed a lack of drug interaction with antipyrine and propranolol when these drugs were given with misoprostol. Misoprostol given for one week had no effect on the steady state pharmacokinetics of diazepam when the two drugs were administered two hours apart.

The serum protein binding of misoprostol acid is less than 90% and is concentration-independent in the therapeutic range.

Pharmacodynamics: Misoprostol has both antisecretory (inhibiting gastric acid secretion) and (in animals) mucosal protective properties. NSAIDs inhibit prostaglandin synthesis, and a deficiency of prostaglandins within the gastric mucosa may lead to diminishing bicarbonate and mucus secretion and may contribute to the mucosal damage caused by these agents. Misoprostol can increase bicarbonate and mucus production, but in man this has been shown at doses 200 mcg and above that are also antisecretory. It is therefore not possible to tell whether the ability of misoprostol to prevent gastric ulcer is the result of its antisecretory effect, its mucosal protective effect, or both.

In vitro studies on canine parietal cells using tritiated misoprostol acid as the ligand have led to the identification and characterization of specific prostaglandin receptors. Receptor binding is saturable, reversible, and stereospecific. The sites have a high affinity for misoprostol, for its acid metabolite, and for other E type prostaglandins, but not for F or I prostaglandins and other unrelated compounds, such as histamine or cimetidine. Receptor-site affinity for misoprostol correlates well with an indirect index of antisecretory activity. It is likely that these specific receptors allow misoprostol taken with food to be effective topically, despite the lower serum concentrations attained.

Misoprostol produces a moderate decrease in pepsin concentration during basal conditions, but not during histamine stimulation. It has no significant effect on fasting or postprandial gastrin nor on intrinsic factor output.

Effects on gastric acid secretion: Misoprostol, over the range of 50–200 mcg, inhibits basal and nocturnal gastric acid secretion, and acid secretion in response to a variety of stimuli, including meals, histamine, pentagastrin, and coffee. Activity is apparent 30 minutes after oral administration and persists for at least 3 hours. In general, the effects of 50 mcg were modest and shorter lived, and only the 200-mcg dose had substantial effects on nocturnal secretion or on histamine and meal-stimulated secretion.

Uterine effects: Cytotec has been shown to produce uterine contractions that may endanger pregnancy. (See *Contraindications* and *Warnings.*) In studies in women undergoing elective termination of pregnancy during the first trimester, Cytotec caused partial or complete expulsion of the uterine contents in 11% of the subjects and increased uterine bleeding in 41%.

Other pharmacologic effects: Cytotec does not produce clinically significant effects on serum levels of prolactin, gonadotropins, thyroid-stimulating hormone, growth hormone, thyroxine, cortisol, gastrointestinal hormones (somatostatin, gastrin, vasoactive intestinal polypeptide, and motilin), creatinine, or uric acid. Gastric emptying, immunologic competence, platelet aggregation, pulmonary function, or the cardiovascular system are not modified by recommended doses of Cytotec.

Clinical studies: In a series of small short-term (about one week) placebo-controlled studies in healthy human volunteers, doses of misoprostol were evaluated for their ability to prevent NSAID-induced mucosal injury. Studies of 200 mcg q.i.d. of misoprostol with tolmetin and naproxen, and of 100 and 200 mcg q.i.d. with ibuprofen, all showed reduction of the rate of significant endoscopic injury from about 70–75% on placebo to 10–30% on misoprostol. Doses of 25–200 mcg q.i.d. reduced aspirin-induced mucosal injury and bleeding.

Preventing gastric ulcers caused by nonsteroidal anti-inflammatory drugs (NSAIDs): Two 12-week, randomized, double-blind trials in osteoarthritic patients who had gastrointestinal symptoms but no ulcer on endoscopy while taking an NSAID compared the ability of 200 mcg of Cytotec, 100 mcg of Cytotec, and placebo to prevent gastric ulcer (GU) formation. Patients were approximately equally divided between ibuprofen, piroxicam, and naproxen, and continued this treatment throughout the 12 weeks. The 200-mcg dose caused a marked, statistically significant reduction in gastric ulcers in both studies. The lower dose was somewhat less effective, with a significant result in only one of the studies. [See table above.]

In these trials there were no significant differences between Cytotec and placebo in relief of day or night abdominal pain. No effect of Cytotec in preventing duodenal ulcers was demonstrated, but relatively few duodenal lesions were seen.

In another clinical trial, 239 patients receiving aspirin 650–1300 mg q.i.d. for rheumatoid arthritis who had endoscopic evidence of duodenal and/or gastric inflammation were randomized to misoprostol 200 mcg q.i.d. or placebo for eight weeks while continuing to receive aspirin. The study evaluated the possible interference of Cytotec on the efficacy of aspirin in these patients with rheumatoid arthritis by analyzing joint tenderness, joint swelling, physician's clinical assessment, patient's assessment, change in ARA classification, change in handgrip strength, change in duration of morning stiffness, patient's assessment of pain at rest, movement, interference with daily activity, and ESR. Cytotec did not interfere with the efficacy of aspirin in these patients with rheumatoid arthritis.

Prevention of Gastric Ulcers Induced by Ibuprofen, Piroxicam, or Naproxen
[No. of patients with ulcer(s) (%)]

	Therapy Duration			
Therapy	4 weeks	8 weeks	12 weeks	
Study No. 1				
Cytotec 200 mcg q.i.d. (n=74)	1 (1.4)	0	0	1 (1.4)*
Cytotec 100 mcg q.i.d. (n=77)	3 (3.9)	1 (1.3)	1 (1.3)	5 (6.5)*
Placebo (n=76)	11 (14.5)	4 (5.3)	4 (5.3)	19 (25.0)
Study No. 2				
Cytotec 200 mcg q.i.d. (n=65)	1 (1.5)	1 (1.5)	0	2 (3.1)*
Cytotec 100 mcg q.i.d. (n=66)	2 (3.0)	2 (3.0)	1 (1.5)	5 (7.6)
Placebo (n=62)	6 (9.7)	2 (3.2)	3 (4.8)	11 (17.7)
*Studies No. 1 & No. 2***				
Cytotec 200 mcg q.i.d. (n=139)	2 (1.4)	1 (0.7)	0	3 (2.2)*
Cytotec 100 mcg q.i.d. (n=143)	5 (3.5)	3 (2.1)	2 (1.4)	10 (7.0)*
Placebo (n=138)	17 (12.3)	6 (4.3)	7 (5.1)	30 (21.7)

*Statistically significantly different from placebo at the 5% level.
**Combined data from Study No. 1 and Study No. 2.

INDICATIONS AND USAGE

Cytotec (misoprostol) is indicated for the prevention of NSAID (nonsteroidal anti-inflammatory drugs, including aspirin)-induced gastric ulcers in patients at high risk of complications from gastric ulcer, eg, the elderly and patients with concomitant debilitating disease, as well as patients at high risk of developing gastric ulceration, such as patients with a history of ulcer. Cytotec has not been shown to prevent duodenal ulcers in patients taking NSAIDs. Cytotec should be taken for the duration of NSAID therapy. Cytotec has been shown to prevent gastric ulcers in controlled studies of three months' duration. It had no effect, compared to placebo, on gastrointestinal pain or discomfort associated with NSAID use.

CONTRAINDICATIONS

See boxed *CONTRAINDICATIONS AND WARNINGS.*

Cytotec should not be taken by anyone with a history of allergy to prostaglandins.

WARNINGS

See boxed *CONTRAINDICATIONS AND WARNINGS.*

PRECAUTIONS

Information for patients: Cytotec is contraindicated in women who are pregnant, and should not be used in women of childbearing potential unless the patient requires nonsteroidal anti-inflammatory drug (NSAID) therapy and is at high risk of complications from gastric ulcers associated with the use of the NSAID, or is at high risk of developing gastric ulceration. Women of childbearing potential should be told that they must not be pregnant when Cytotec therapy is initiated, and that they must use an effective contraception method while taking Cytotec.

See boxed *CONTRAINDICATIONS AND WARNINGS.*

Patients should be advised of the following:

Cytotec is intended for administration along with nonsteroidal anti-inflammatory drugs (NSAIDs), including aspirin, to decrease the chance of developing an NSAID-induced gastric ulcer.

Cytotec should be taken only according to the directions given by a physician.

If the patient has questions about or problems with Cytotec, the physician should be contacted promptly.

THE PATIENT SHOULD NOT GIVE CYTOTEC TO ANYONE ELSE. Cytotec has been prescribed for the patient's specific condition, may not be the correct treatment for another person, and may be dangerous to the other person if she were to become pregnant.

The Cytotec package the patient receives from the pharmacist will include a leaflet containing patient information. The patient should read the leaflet before taking Cytotec and each time the prescription is renewed because the leaflet may have been revised.

Keep Cytotec out of the reach of children.

SPECIAL NOTE FOR WOMEN: Cytotec must not be used by pregnant women. Cytotec may cause miscarriage. Miscarriages caused by Cytotec may be incomplete, which could lead to potentially dangerous bleeding, hospitalization, surgery, infertility, or maternal or fetal death.

Cytotec is available only as a unit-of-use package that includes a leaflet containing patient information. See *Patient Information* at the end of this labeling.

Drug interactions: See *Clinical Pharmacology.* Cytotec has not been shown to interfere with the beneficial effects of aspirin on signs and symptoms of rheumatoid arthritis. Cytotec does not exert clinically significant effects on the absorption, blood levels, and antiplatelet effects of therapeutic doses of aspirin. Cytotec has no clinically significant effect on the kinetics of diclofenac or ibuprofen.

Animal toxicology: A reversible increase in the number of normal surface gastric epithelial cells occurred in the dog, rat, and mouse. No such increase has been observed in humans administered Cytotec for up to one year.

An apparent response of the female mouse to Cytotec in long-term studies at 100 to 1000 times the human dose was hyperostosis, mainly of the medulla of sternebrae. Hyperostosis did not occur in long-term studies in the dog and rat and has not been seen in humans treated with Cytotec.

Carcinogenesis, mutagenesis, impairment of fertility: There was no evidence of an effect of Cytotec on tumor occurrence or incidence in rats receiving daily doses up to 150 times the human dose for 24 months. Similarly, there was no effect of Cytotec on tumor occurrence or incidence in mice receiving daily doses up to 1000 times the human dose for 21 months. The mutagenic potential of Cytotec was tested in several *in vitro* assays, all of which were negative.

Misoprostol, when administered to breeding male and female rats at doses 6.25 times to 625 times the maximum recommended human therapeutic dose, produced dose-related pre- and post-implantation losses and a significant decrease in the number of live pups born at the highest dose. These findings suggest the possibility of a general adverse effect on fertility in males and females.

Pregnancy: Pregnancy Category X. See boxed *CONTRAINDICATIONS AND WARNINGS.*

Nonteratogenic effects: Cytotec may endanger pregnancy (may cause miscarriage) and thereby cause harm to the fetus when administered to a pregnant woman. Cytotec produces uterine contractions, uterine bleeding, and expulsion of the products of conception. Miscarriages caused by Cytotec may be incomplete. In studies in women undergoing elective termination of pregnancy during the first trimester, Cytotec caused partial or complete expulsion of the products of conception in 11% of the subjects and increased uterine bleeding in 41%. Anecdotal reports, primarily from Brazil, of congenital anomalies and reports of fetal death subsequent to misuse of misoprostol as an abortifacient have been received (see *Contraindications and Warnings*). If a woman is or becomes pregnant while taking this drug, the drug should be discontinued and the patient apprised of the potential hazard to the fetus.

Teratogenic effects: Cytotec is not fetotoxic or teratogenic in rats and rabbits at doses 625 and 63 times the human dose, respectively.

Nursing mothers: See *Contraindications.* It is unlikely that Cytotec is excreted in human milk since it is rapidly metabolized throughout the body. However, it is not known if the active metabolite (misoprostol acid) is excreted in human milk. Therefore, Cytotec should not be administered to nursing mothers because the potential excretion of misoprostol acid could cause significant diarrhea in nursing infants.

Pediatric use: Safety and effectiveness in children below the age of 18 years have not been established.

ADVERSE REACTIONS

The following have been reported as adverse events in subjects receiving Cytotec:

Gastrointestinal: In subjects receiving Cytotec 400 or 800 mcg daily in clinical trials, the most frequent gastrointestinal adverse events were diarrhea and abdominal pain. The incidence of diarrhea at 800 mcg in controlled trials in patients on NSAIDs ranged from 14–40% and in all studies (over 5,000 patients) averaged 13%. Abdominal pain occurred in 13–20% of patients in NSAID trials and about 7% in all studies, but there was no consistent difference from placebo.

Diarrhea was dose related and usually developed early in the course of therapy (after 13 days), usually was self-limiting (often resolving after 8 days), but sometimes required discontinuation of Cytotec (2% of the patients). Rare instances of profound diarrhea leading to severe dehydration have been reported. Patients with an underlying condition such as inflammatory bowel disease, or those in whom dehydration, were it to occur, would be dangerous, should be monitored carefully if Cytotec is prescribed. The incidence of diarrhea can be minimized by administering after meals and at bedtime, and by avoiding coadministration of Cytotec with magnesium-containing antacids.

Gynecological: Women who received Cytotec during clinical trials reported the following gynecological disorders: spotting (0.7%), cramps (0.6%), hypermenorrhea (0.5%), menstrual disorder (0.3%) and dysmenorrhea (0.1%). Postmenopausal vaginal bleeding may be related to Cytotec administration. If it occurs, diagnostic workup should be undertaken to rule out gynecological pathology.

Elderly: There were no significant differences in the safety profile of Cytotec in approximately 500 ulcer patients who were 65 years of age or older compared with younger patients.

Additional adverse events which were reported are categorized as follows:

Incidence greater than 1%: In clinical trials, the following adverse reactions were reported by more than 1% of the subjects receiving Cytotec and may be causally related to the drug: nausea (3.2%), flatulence (2.9%), headache (2.4%), dyspepsia (2.0%), vomiting (1.3%), and constipation (1.1%). However, there were no significant differences between the incidences of these events for Cytotec and placebo.

Causal relationship unknown: The following adverse events were infrequently reported. Causal relationships between Cytotec and these events have not been established but cannot be excluded:

Body as a whole: aches/pains, asthenia, fatigue, fever, rigors, weight changes.

Continued on next page

Searle—Cont.

Skin: rash, dermatitis, alopecia, pallor, breast pain.
Special senses: abnormal taste, abnormal vision, conjunctivitis, deafness, tinnitus, earache.
Respiratory: upper respiratory tract infection, bronchitis, bronchospasm, dyspnea, pneumonia, epistaxis.
Cardiovascular: chest pain, edema, diaphoresis, hypotension, hypertension, arrhythmia, phlebitis, increased cardiac enzymes, syncope.
Gastrointestinal: GI bleeding, GI inflammation/infection, rectal disorder, abnormal hepatobiliary function, gingivitis, reflux, dysphagia, amylase increase.
Hypersensitivity: Anaphylaxis.
Metabolic: glycosuria, gout, increased nitrogen, increased alkaline phosphatase.
Genitourinary: polyuria, dysuria, hematuria, urinary tract infection.
Nervous system/Psychiatric: anxiety, change in appetite, depression, drowsiness, dizziness, thirst, impotence, loss of libido, sweating increase, neuropathy, neurosis, confusion.
Musculoskeletal: arthralgia, myalgia, muscle cramps, stiffness, back pain.
Blood/Coagulation: anemia, abnormal differential, thrombocytopenia, purpura, ESR increased.

OVERDOSAGE

The toxic dose of Cytotec in humans has not been determined. Cumulative total daily doses of 1600 mcg have been tolerated, with only symptoms of gastrointestinal discomfort being reported. In animals, the acute toxic effects are diarrhea, gastrointestinal lesions, focal cardiac necrosis, hepatic necrosis, renal tubular necrosis, testicular atrophy, respiratory difficulties, and depression of the central nervous system. Clinical signs that may indicate an overdose are sedation, tremor, convulsions, dyspnea, abdominal pain, diarrhea, fever, palpitations, hypotension, or bradycardia. Symptoms should be treated with supportive therapy.

It is not known if misoprostol acid is dialyzable. However, because misoprostol is metabolized like a fatty acid, it is unlikely that dialysis would be appropriate treatment for overdosage.

DOSAGE AND ADMINISTRATION

The recommended adult oral dose of Cytotec for the prevention of NSAID-induced gastric ulcers is 200 mcg four times daily with food. If this dose cannot be tolerated, a dose of 100 mcg can be used. (See *Clinical Pharmacology: Clinical studies.*) Cytotec should be taken for the duration of NSAID therapy as prescribed by the physician. Cytotec should be taken with a meal, and the last dose of the day should be at bedtime.

Renal impairment: Adjustment of the dosing schedule in renally impaired patients is not routinely needed, but dosage can be reduced if the 200-mcg dose is not tolerated. (See *Clinical Pharmacology.*)

HOW SUPPLIED

Cytotec 100-mcg tablets are white, round, with SEARLE debossed on one side and 1451 on the other side; supplied as:

NDC Number	Size
0025-1451-60	unit-of-use bottle of 60
0025-1451-20	unit-of-use bottle of 120
0025-1451-34	carton of 100 unit dose

Cytotec 200-mcg tablets are white, hexagonal, with SEARLE debossed above and 1461 debossed below the line on one side and a double stomach debossed on the other side; supplied as:

NDC Number	Size
0025-1461-60	unit-of-use bottle of 60
0025-1461-31	unit-of-use bottle of 100
0025-1461-34	carton of 100 unit dose

Store at or below 25°C (77°F) in a dry area.
Caution: Federal law prohibits dispensing without prescription.

PATIENT INFORMATION

Read this leaflet before taking Cytotec® (misoprostol) and each time your prescription is renewed, because the leaflet may be changed.

Cytotec (misoprostol) is being prescribed by your doctor to decrease the chance of getting stomach ulcers related to the arthritis/pain medication that you take.

Cytotec can cause miscarriage, often associated with potentially dangerous bleeding. This may result in hospitalization, surgery, infertility, or death. **Do not take it if you are pregnant and do not become pregnant while taking this medicine.**

If you become pregnant during Cytotec therapy, stop taking Cytotec and contact your physician immediately. Remember that even if you are on a means of birth control it is still possible to become pregnant. Should this occur, stop taking Cytotec and contact your physician immediately.

Cytotec may cause diarrhea, abdominal cramping, and/or nausea in some people. In most cases these problems develop during the first few weeks of therapy and stop after about a week. You can minimize possible diarrhea by making sure you take Cytotec with food.

Because these side effects are usually mild to moderate and usually go away in a matter of days, most patients can continue to take Cytotec. If you have prolonged difficulty (more than 8 days), or if you have severe diarrhea, cramping and/or nausea, call your doctor.

Take Cytotec only according to the directions given by your physician.

Do not give Cytotec to anyone else. It has been prescribed for your specific condition, may not be the correct treatment for another person, and would be dangerous if the other person were pregnant.

This information sheet does not cover all possible side effects of Cytotec. This patient information leaflet does not address the side effects of your arthritis/pain medication. See your doctor if you have questions.

Keep out of reach of children.

8/8/95 • A05450-1

Shown in Product Identification Guide, page 335

DAYPRO® ℞
[dā-prō]
(oxaprozin)

DESCRIPTION

Daypro (oxaprozin) is a nonsteroidal anti-inflammatory drug (NSAID), chemically designated as 4,5-diphenyl-2-oxazole-propionic acid, and has the following chemical structure:

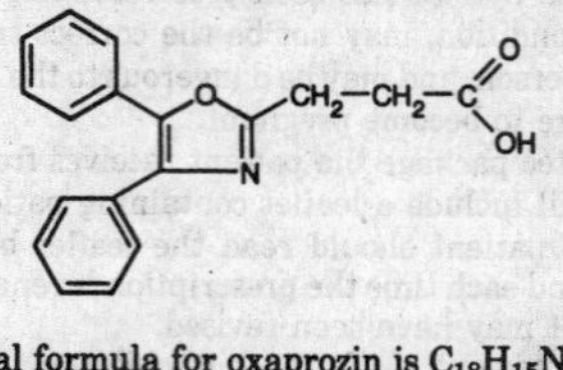

The empirical formula for oxaprozin is $C_{18}H_{15}NO_3$, and the molecular weight is 293. Oxaprozin is a white to off-white powder with a slight odor and a melting point of 162°C to 163°C. It is slightly soluble in alcohol and insoluble in water, with an octanol/water partition coefficient of 4.8 at physiologic pH (7.4). The pK_a in water is 4.3.

Daypro oral caplets contain 600 mg of oxaprozin.

Inactive ingredients in Daypro oral caplets are microcrystalline cellulose, hydroxypropyl methylcellulose, methylcellulose, magnesium stearate, polacrilin potassium, starch, polyethylene glycol, and titanium dioxide.

CLINICAL PHARMACOLOGY

Oxaprozin is a nonsteroidal anti-inflammatory drug (NSAID) that has been shown to have anti-inflammatory, analgesic, and antipyretic properties in animal models. As with other nonsteroidal anti-inflammatory agents, all of the modes of action of oxaprozin are not fully established. Oxaprozin is an inhibitor of several steps along the arachidonic acid pathway of prostaglandin synthesis, and one of its modes of action is presumed to be due to the inhibition of prostaglandin synthesis at the site of inflammation.

Pharmacodynamics: Acute analgesic effects are demonstrable in humans after a single 1200-mg dose of oxaprozin, but anti-inflammatory effects are not reliably achieved after a single dose. Because of the long half-life of oxaprozin, it takes several days of dosing to reach steady state (see *Pharmacokinetics*).

Pharmacokinetics: The pharmacokinetics of oxaprozin have been evaluated in approximately 400 individuals, which have included patients with rheumatoid arthritis, osteoarthritis, healthy elderly volunteers, and patients with cardiac, renal, and hepatic disease.

Oxaprozin demonstrates high oral bioavailability (95%), with peak plasma concentrations occurring between 3 and 5 hours after dosing. Food may reduce the rate of absorption of oxaprozin, but the extent of absorption is unchanged. Antacids have no effect on the rate or extent of oxaprozin absorption.

As is true for most NSAIDs, approximately 99.9% of the oxaprozin present in plasma is bound to albumin. The fraction of the drug present in the tissues across the therapeutic dosage range ranges between 40% and 60% of the total drug in the body and is proportional to dose, since the tissue sites are not saturated with the usual clinical doses.

Figure 1 shows the amount of oxaprozin in the plasma and in the tissue as a function of dose and the concentration of the free drug.

[See Figure at top of next column.]

Unbound oxaprozin is the pharmacologically active component; it is able to distribute into tissues and to be cleared from the body. The average unbound concentration is a function of the tissue-bound and plasma-bound drug, and it increases proportionally with dose.

As the amount of oxaprozin in the tissues increases at higher dose, the plasma concentration of oxaprozin is limited by saturation of plasma protein binding. In addition, the increase in free (unbound) oxaprozin results in an increase in clearance. Both of these contribute to the total plasma concentration of oxaprozin increasing less than proportionately with dose.

Figure 1.
Amount of oxaprozin in plasma and tissue as a function of dose and free (unbound) oxaprozin concentration.

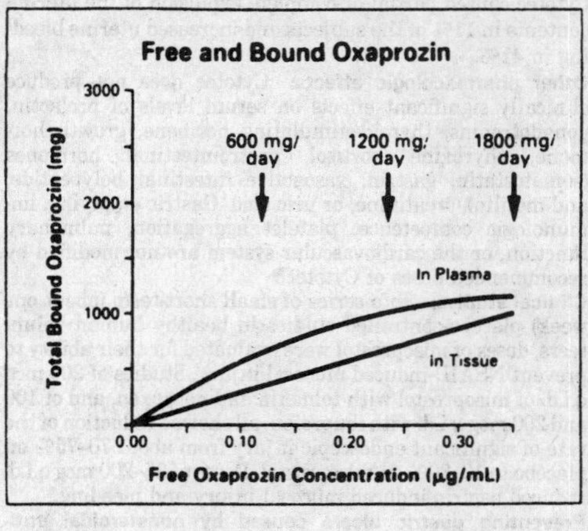

Oxaprozin kinetics were modeled using a two-compartment model with first-order absorption and protein binding that becomes saturable in the clinical dosage range. As the dose is increased from 600 to 1200 mg daily, the steady state clearance of total oxaprozin increases from 0.25 to 0.34 L/hr, the steady state apparent volume of distribution increases from 10 to 12.5 L, and the accumulation half-life decreases from 25 to 21 hours. The terminal elimination half-life is approximately twice as long as the accumulation half-life because of the increased binding and decreased clearance at lower concentrations. Steady state concentrations in clinical usage are achieved in 4 to 7 days.

Plasma levels of total oxaprozin (free and bound drug) in studies of patients taking 600 to 1200 mg/day for several months ranged from 98 to 230 μg/mL, corresponding to estimated levels of free drug ranging from about 0.10 to 0.40 μg/mL.

Oxaprozin is primarily metabolized in the liver, by both microsomal oxidation (65%) and glucuronic acid conjugation (35%). A small amount (<5%) of active phenolic metabolites is produced, but the contribution to overall activity is minimal. All conjugated metabolites are inactive.

Biliary excretion of unchanged oxaprozin is a minor elimination pathway, and enterohepatic recycling of oxaprozin is insignificant. The glucuronide metabolites can be recovered from the urine (65%) and feces (35%), while unchanged oxaprozin is poorly excreted.

Renal dysfunction appears to alter oxaprozin binding and to reduce unbound clearance and unbound volume of distribution; dosage reductions should be made (see *Precautions: General*).

Age, gender, and well-compensated cardiac failure do not affect the plasma protein binding or the pharmacokinetics of oxaprozin.

Like other NSAIDs exhibiting a high degree of protein binding and a primarily metabolic route of elimination, oxaprozin has the potential for drug-drug interactions (see *Precautions: Drug interactions*).

CLINICAL STUDIES

Rheumatoid arthritis: Daypro was evaluated for managing the signs and symptoms of rheumatoid arthritis in placebo and active controlled clinical trials in a total of 646 patients. Daypro was given in single or divided daily doses of 600 to 1800 mg/day and was found to be comparable to 2600 to 3900 mg/day of aspirin. At these doses there was a trend (over all trials) for oxaprozin to be more effective and cause fewer gastrointestinal side effects than aspirin.

Daypro was given as a once-a-day dose of 1200 mg in most of the clinical trials, but larger doses (up to 26 mg/kg or 1800 mg/day) were used in selected patients. In some patients, Daypro may be better tolerated in divided doses. Due to its long half-life, several days of Daypro therapy were needed for the drug to reach its full effect (see *Individualization of Dosage*).

Osteoarthritis: Daypro was evaluated for the management of the signs and symptoms of osteoarthritis in a total of 616 patients in active controlled clinical trials against aspirin (N=464), piroxicam (N=102), and other NSAIDs. Daypro was given both in variable (600 to 1200 mg/day) and in fixed (1200 mg/day) dosing schedules in either single or divided doses. In these trials, oxaprozin was found to be comparable to 2600 to 3200 mg/day doses of aspirin or 20 mg/day doses of piroxicam. Oxaprozin was effective both in once-

daily and in divided dosing schedules. In controlled clinical trials several days of oxaprozin therapy were needed for the drug to reach its full effects (see *Individualization of Dosage*).

INDIVIDUALIZATION OF DOSAGE

Daypro, like other NSAIDs, shows considerable interindividual differences in both pharmacokinetics and clinical response (pharmacodynamics). Therefore, the dosage for each patient should be individualized according to the patient's response to therapy.

The usual starting dose for most normal weight patients with rheumatoid arthritis is 1200 mg, once a day.

The usual starting dose for normal weight patients with mild to moderate osteoarthritis is 600 mg, once a day.

In cases where a quick onset of action is important, the pharmacokinetics of oxaprozin allow therapy to be started with a one-time loading dose of 1200 to 1800 mg (not to exceed 26 mg/kg).

Doses larger than 1200 mg/day should be reserved for patients who weigh more than 50 kg, have normal renal and hepatic function, are at low risk of peptic ulcer, and whose severity of disease justifies maximal therapy. Physicians should ensure that patients are tolerating doses in the 600 to 1200 mg/day range without gastroenterologic, renal, hepatic, or dermatologic adverse effects before advancing to the larger doses.

The maximum recommended total daily dosage is 1800 mg in divided doses.

Most patients will tolerate once-a-day dosing with Daypro, although divided doses may be tried in patients unable to tolerate single doses. As with all drugs of this class, the frequency and severity of adverse events will depend on the dose of the drug, the age and physical condition of the patient, any concurrent medical diagnoses, individual vulnerability, and the duration of therapy. In clinical trials of oxaprozin, no clear dose-response relationship was seen for serious adverse effects, but physicians are cautioned that the reported safety data were developed in patients who had successfully taken lower doses of Daypro before being advanced above 1200 mg/day.

Experience with other NSAIDs has shown that starting therapy with maximal doses in patients at increased risk due to renal or hepatic disease, low body weight, advanced age, a known ulcer diathesis, or known sensitivity to NSAID effects is likely to increase the frequency of adverse events and is not recommended (see *Precautions*).

INDICATIONS AND USAGE

Daypro is indicated for acute and long-term use in the management of the signs and symptoms of osteoarthritis and rheumatoid arthritis.

CONTRAINDICATIONS

Daypro should not be used in patients with previously demonstrated hypersensitivity to oxaprozin or any of its components or in individuals with the complete or partial syndrome of nasal polyps, angioedema, and bronchospastic reactivity to aspirin or other nonsteroidal anti-inflammatory drugs (NSAIDs).

Severe and occasionally fatal asthmatic and anaphylactic reactions have been reported in patients receiving NSAIDs, and there have been rare reports of anaphylaxis in patients taking oxaprozin.

WARNINGS

RISK OF GASTROINTESTINAL (GI) ULCERATION, BLEEDING, AND PERFORATION WITH NONSTEROIDAL ANTIINFLAMMATORY DRUG THERAPY: Serious gastrointestinal toxicity, such as bleeding, ulceration, and perforation, can occur at any time, with or without warning symptoms, in patients treated with NSAIDs. Although minor upper gastrointestinal problems, such as dyspepsia, are common, and usually develop early in therapy, physicians should remain alert for ulceration and bleeding in patients treated chronically with NSAIDs, even in the absence of previous GI tract symptoms. In patients observed in clinical trials for several months to 2 years, symptomatic upper GI ulcers, gross bleeding, or perforation appear to occur in approximately 1% of patients treated for 3 to 6 months, and in about 2% to 4% of patients treated for 1 year. Physicians should inform patients about the signs and/or symptoms of serious GI toxicity and what steps to take if they occur.

Patients at risk for developing peptic ulceration and bleeding are those with a prior history of serious GI events, alcoholism, smoking, or other factors known to be associated with peptic ulcer disease. Elderly or debilitated patients seem to tolerate ulceration or bleeding less well than other individuals, and most spontaneous reports of fatal GI events are in these populations. Studies to date are inconclusive concerning the relative risk of various nonsteroidal anti-inflammatory drugs (NSAIDs) in causing such reactions. High doses of any NSAID probably carry a greater risk of these reactions, and substantial benefit should be anticipated to patients prior to prescribing maximal doses of Daypro.

PRECAUTIONS

General

Hepatic effects: As with other nonsteroidal anti-inflammatory drugs, borderline elevations of one or more liver tests may occur in up to 15% of patients. These abnormalities may progress, remain essentially unchanged, or resolve with continued therapy. The SGPT (ALT) test is probably the most sensitive indicator of liver dysfunction. Meaningful (3 times the upper limit of normal) elevations of SGOT (AST) occurred in controlled clinical trials of Daypro in just under 1% of patients. A patient with symptoms and/or signs suggesting liver dysfunction or in whom an abnormal liver test has occurred should be evaluated for evidence of the development of more severe hepatic reaction while on therapy with this drug. Severe hepatic reactions including jaundice have been reported with Daypro, and there may be a risk of fatal hepatitis with oxaprozin, such as has been seen with other NSAIDs. Although such reactions are rare, if abnormal liver tests persist or worsen, clinical signs and symptoms consistent with liver disease develop, or systemic manifestations occur (eosinophilia, rash, fever), Daypro should be discontinued.

Well-compensated hepatic cirrhosis does not appear to alter the disposition of unbound oxaprozin, so dosage adjustment is not necessary. However, the primary route of elimination of oxaprozin is hepatic metabolism, so caution should be observed in patients with severe hepatic dysfunction.

Renal effects: Acute interstitial nephritis, hematuria, and proteinuria have been reported with Daypro as with other NSAIDs. Long-term administration of some nonsteroidal anti-inflammatory drugs to animals has resulted in renal papillary necrosis and other abnormal renal pathology. This was not observed with oxaprozin, but the clinical significance of this difference is unknown.

A second form of renal toxicity has been seen in patients with preexisting conditions leading to a reduction in renal blood flow, where the renal prostaglandins have a supportive role in the maintenance of renal perfusion. In these patients administration of a nonsteroidal anti-inflammatory drug may cause a dose-dependent reduction in prostaglandin formation and may precipitate overt renal decompensation. Patients at greatest risk of this reaction are those with previously impaired renal function, heart failure, or liver dysfunction, those taking diuretics, and the elderly. Discontinuation of nonsteroidal anti-inflammatory drug therapy is often followed by recovery to the pretreatment state. Those patients at high risk who chronically take oxaprozin should have renal function monitored if they have signs or symptoms that may be consistent with mild azotemia, such as malaise, fatigue, or loss of appetite. As with all NSAID therapy, patients may occasionally develop some elevation of serum creatinine and BUN levels without any signs or symptoms.

The pharmacokinetics of oxaprozin may be significantly altered in patients with renal insufficiency or in patients who are undergoing hemodialysis. Such patients should be started on doses of 600 mg/day, with cautious dosage increases if the desired effect is not obtained. Oxaprozin is not dialyzed because of its high degree of protein binding.

Like other NSAIDs, Daypro may worsen fluid retention by the kidneys in patients with uncompensated cardiac failure due to its effect on prostaglandins. It should be used with caution in patients with a history of hypertension, cardiac decompensation, in patients on chronic diuretic therapy, or in those with other conditions predisposing to fluid retention.

Photosensitivity: Oxaprozin has been associated with rash and/or mild photosensitivity in dermatologic testing. An increased incidence of rash on sun-exposed skin was seen in some patients in the clinical trials.

Recommended laboratory testing: Because serious GI tract ulceration and bleeding can occur without warning symptoms, physicians should follow chronically treated patients for the signs and symptoms of ulceration and bleeding and should inform them of the importance of this follow-up (see *Warnings*).

Anemia may occur in patients receiving oxaprozin or other NSAIDs. This may be due to fluid retention, gastrointestinal blood loss, or an incompletely described effect upon erythrogenesis. Patients on long-term treatment with Daypro should have their hemoglobin or hematocrit values determined at appropriate intervals as determined by the clinical situation.

Oxaprozin, like other NSAIDs, can affect platelet aggregation and prolong bleeding time. Daypro should be used with caution in patients with underlying hemostatic defects or in those who are undergoing surgical procedures where a high degree of hemostasis is needed.

Information for patients: Daypro, like other drugs of its class, nonsteroidal anti-inflammatory drugs (NSAIDs), is not free of side effects. The side effects of these drugs can cause discomfort and, rarely, serious side effects, such as gastrointestinal bleeding, which may result in hospitalization and even fatal outcomes.

NSAIDs are often essential agents in the management of arthritis, but they may also be commonly employed for conditions that are less serious.

Physicians may wish to discuss with their patients the potential risks (see *Warnings, Precautions, and Adverse Reactions*) and likely benefits of Daypro treatment, particularly in less-serious conditions where treatment without Daypro may represent an acceptable alternative to both the patient and the physician.

Patients receiving Daypro may benefit from physician instruction in the symptoms of the more common or serious gastrointestinal, renal, hepatic, hematologic, and dermatologic adverse effects.

Laboratory test interactions: False-positive urine immunoassay screening tests for benzodiazepines have been reported in patients taking Daypro. This is due to lack of specificity of the screening tests. False-positive test results may be expected for several days following discontinuation of Daypro therapy. Confirmatory tests, such as gas chromatography/ mass spectrometry, will distinguish Daypro from benzodiazepines.

Drug interactions

Aspirin: Concomitant administration of Daypro and aspirin is not recommended because oxprozin displaces salicylates from plasma protein binding sites. Coadministration would be expected to increase the risk of salicylate toxicity.

Oral anticoagulants: The anticoagulant effects of warfarin were not affected by the coadministration of 1200 mg/day of Daypro. Nevertheless, caution should be exercised when adding any drug that affects platelet function to the regimen of patients receiving oral anticoagulants.

H_2-*receptor antagonists:* The total body clearance of oxaprozin was reduced by 20% in subjects who concurrently received therapeutic doses of cimetidine or ranitidine; no other pharmacokinetic parameter was affected. A change of clearance of this magnitude lies within the range of normal variation and is unlikely to produce a clinically detectable difference in the outcome of therapy.

Beta-blockers: Subjects receiving 1200 mg Daypro qd with 100 mg metoprolol bid exhibited statistically significant but transient increases in sitting and standing blood pressures after 14 days. Therefore, as with all NSAIDs, routine blood pressure monitoring should be considered in these patients when starting Daypro therapy.

Other drugs: The coadministration of oxaprozin and antacids, acetaminophen, or conjugated estrogens resulted in no statistically significant changes in pharmacokinetic parameters in single- and/or multiple-dose studies. The interaction of oxaprozin with lithium and cardiac glycosides has not been studied.

Carcinogenesis, mutagenesis, impairment of fertility: In oncogenicity studies, oxaprozin administration for 2 years was associated with the exacerbation of liver neoplasms (hepatic adenomas and carcinomas) in male CD mice, but not in female CD mice or rats. The significance of this species-specific finding to man is unknown.

Oxaprozin did not display mutagenic potential. Results from the Ames test, forward mutation in yeast and Chinese hamster ovary (CHO) cells, DNA repair testing in CHO cells, micronucleus testing in mouse bone marrow, chromosomal aberration testing in human lymphocytes, and cell transformation testing in mouse fibroblast all showed no evidence of genetic toxicity or cell-transforming ability.

Oxaprozin administration was not associated with impairment of fertility in male and female rats at oral doses up to 200 mg/kg/day (1180 mg/m²); the usual human dose is 17 mg/kg/day (629 mg/m²). However, testicular degeneration was observed in beagle dogs treated with 37.5 to 150 mg/kg/day (750 to 3000 mg/m²) of oxaprozin for 6 months, or 37.5 mg/kg/day for 42 days, a finding not confirmed in other species. The clinical relevance of this finding is not known.

Pregnancy: Teratogenic Effects—Pregnancy Category C. There are no adequate or well-controlled studies in pregnant women. Teratology studies with oxaprozin were performed in mice, rats, and rabbits. In mice and rats, no drug-related developmental abnormalities were observed at 50 to 200 mg/kg/day of oxaprozin (225 to 900 mg/m²). However, in rabbits, infrequent malformed fetuses were observed in dams treated with 7.5 to 30 mg/kg/day of oxaprozin (the usual human dosage range). Oxaprozin should be used during pregnancy only if the potential benefits justify the potential risks to the fetus.

Labor and delivery: The effect of oxaprozin in pregnant women is unknown. NSAIDs are known to delay parturition, to accelerate closure of the fetal ductus arteriosus, and to be associated with dystocia. Oxaprozin is known to have caused decreases in pup survival in rat studies. Accordingly, the use of oxaprozin during late pregnancy should be avoided.

Nursing mothers: Studies of oxaprozin excretion in human milk have not been conducted; however, oxaprozin was found in the milk of lactating rats. Since the effects of oxaprozin

Continued on next page

Searle—Cont.

on infants are not known, caution should be exercised if oxaprozin is administered to nursing women.

Pediatric use: Safety and effectiveness of Daypro in children have not been established.

Geriatric use: No adjustment of the dose of Daypro is necessary in the elderly for *pharmacokinetic* reasons, although many elderly may need to receive a reduced dose because of low body weight or disorders associated with aging. No significant differences in the pharmacokinetic profile for oxaprozin were seen in studies in the healthy elderly.

Although selected elderly patients in controlled clinical trials tolerated Daypro as well as younger patients, caution should be exercised in treating the elderly, and extra care should be taken when choosing a dose. As with any NSAID, the elderly are likely to tolerate adverse reactions less well than younger patients.

ADVERSE REACTIONS

Adverse reaction data were derived from patients who received Daypro in multidose, controlled, and open-label clinical trials, and from worldwide marketing experience. Rates for events occurring in more than 1% of patients, and for most of the less common events, are based on 2253 patients who took 1200 to 1800 mg Daypro per day in clinical trials. Of these, 1721 were treated for at least 1 month, 971 for at least 3 months, and 366 for more than 1 year. Rates for the rarer events and for events reported from worldwide marketing experience are difficult to estimate accurately and are only listed as less than 1%.

The adverse event rates below refer to the incidence in the first month of use. Most of the events were seen by this time for common adverse reactions. However, the cumulative incidence can be expected to rise with continued therapy, and some events, such as gastrointestinal bleeding (see *Warnings*), seem to occur at a constant or possibly increasing rate over time.

The most frequently reported adverse reactions were related to the gastrointestinal tract. They were nausea (8%) and dyspepsia (8%).

INCIDENCE GREATER THAN 1%: In clinical trials the following adverse reactions occurred at an incidence greater than 1% and are probably related to treatment. Reactions occurring in 3% to 9% of patients treated with Daypro are indicated by an asterisk(*); those reactions occurring in less than 3% of patients are unmarked.

Digestive system: abdominal pain/distress, anorexia, constipation*, diarrhea*, dyspepsia*, flatulence, nausea*, vomiting.

Nervous system: CNS inhibition (depression, sedation, somnolence, or confusion), disturbance of sleep.

Skin and appendages: rash*.

Special senses: tinnitus.

Urogenital system: dysuria or frequency.

INCIDENCE LESS THAN 1%:

Probable causal relationship: The following adverse reactions were reported in clinical trials or from worldwide marketing experience at an incidence of less than 1%. Those reactions reported only from worldwide marketing experience are in *italics*. The probability of a causal relationship exists between the drug and these adverse reactions.

Body as a whole: drug hypersensitivity reactions including anaphylaxis *and serum sickness*.

Cardiovascular system: edema, blood pressure changes.

Digestive system: peptic ulceration and/or GI bleeding (see *Warnings*), liver function abnormalities including *hepatitis* (see *Precautions*), stomatitis, hemorrhoidal or rectal bleeding, *pancreatitis*.

Hematologic system: anemia, thrombocytopenia, leukopenia, ecchymoses.

Metabolic system: weight gain, weight loss.

Nervous system: weakness, malaise.

Respiratory system: symptoms of upper respiratory tract infection.

Skin: pruritus, urticaria, photosensitivity, *pseudoporphyria, exfoliative dermatitis, erythema multiforme, Stevens-Johnson syndrome, toxic epidermal necrolysis (Lyell's syndrome).*

Special senses: blurred vision, conjunctivitis.

Urogenital: *acute interstitial nephritis,* hematuria, renal insufficiency, *acute renal failure,* decreased menstrual flow.

Causal relationship unknown: The following adverse reactions occurred at an incidence of less than 1% in clinical trials, or were suggested from marketing experience, under circumstances where a causal relationship could not be definitely established. They are listed as alerting information for the physician.

Cardiovascular system: palpitations.

Digestive system: alteration in taste.

Respiratory system: sinusitis, pulmonary infections.

Skin and appendages: alopecia.

Special senses: hearing decrease.

Urogenital system: increase in menstrual flow.

DRUG ABUSE AND DEPENDENCE

Daypro is a non-narcotic drug. Usually reliable animal studies have indicated that Daypro has no known addiction potential in humans.

OVERDOSAGE

No patient experienced either an accidental or intentional overdosage of Daypro in the clinical trials of the drug. Symptoms following acute overdose with other NSAIDs are usually limited to lethargy, drowsiness, nausea, vomiting, and epigastric pain and are generally reversible with supportive care. Gastrointestinal bleeding and coma have occurred following NSAID overdose. Hypertension, acute renal failure, and respiratory depression are rare.

Patients should be managed by symptomatic and supportive care following an NSAID overdose. There are no specific antidotes. Gut decontamination may be indicated in patients seen within 4 hours of ingestion with symptoms or following a large overdose (5 to 10 times the usual dose). This should be accomplished via emesis and/or activated charcoal (60 to 100 g in adults, 1 to 2 g/kg in children) with an osmotic cathartic. Forced diuresis, alkalization of the urine, or hemoperfusion would probably not be useful due to the high degree of protein binding of oxaprozin.

DOSAGE AND ADMINISTRATION

Rheumatoid arthritis: The usual daily dose of Daypro in the management of the signs and symptoms of rheumatoid arthritis is 1200 mg (two 600-mg caplets) once a day. Both smaller and larger doses may be required in individual patients (see *Individualization of Dosage*).

Osteoarthritis: The usual daily dose of Daypro for the management of the signs and symptoms of moderate to severe osteoarthritis is 1200 mg (two 600-mg caplets) once a day. For patients of low body weight or with milder disease, an initial dosage of one 600-mg caplet once a day may be appropriate (see *Individualization of Dosage*).

Regardless of the indication, the dosage should be individualized to the lowest effective dose of Daypro to minimize adverse effects, and the maximum recommended total daily dose is 1800 mg (or 26 mg/kg, whichever is <u>lower</u>) in divided doses.

SAFETY AND HANDLING

Daypro is supplied as a solid dosage form in closed containers, is not known to produce contact dermatitis, and poses no known risk to healthcare workers. It may be disposed of in accordance with applicable local regulations governing the disposal of pharmaceuticals.

HOW SUPPLIED

Daypro 600-mg caplets are white, capsule-shaped, scored, film-coated, with DAYPRO debossed on one side and 1381 on the other side.

NDC Number	Size
0025-1381-31	bottle of 100
0025-1381-34	carton of 100 unit dose

Keep bottles tightly closed and store below 86°F (30°C). Dispense in a tight, light-resistant container with a child-resistant closure. Protect the unit dose from light.

Caution: Federal law prohibits dispensing without prescription.

3/13/96 ● A05222-3

Shown in Product Identification Guide, page 335

DEMULEN® 1/35–21
DEMULEN® 1/35–28
DEMULEN® 1/50–21
DEMULEN® 1/50–28 ℞℞℞℞

[*dem 'ū-len*]
(ethynodiol diacetate with ethinyl estradiol)

PRODUCT OVERVIEW

KEY FACTS

The Searle line of oral contraceptives contains two fixed-dose combination oral contraceptives (DEMULEN 1/35-21 and DEMULEN 1/35-28) containing ethynodiol diacetate (1 mg) with ethinyl estradiol (35 mcg) and two fixed-dose combination oral contraceptives (DEMULEN 1/50-21 and DEMULEN 1/50-28) containing ethynodiol diacetate (1 mg) with ethinyl estradiol (50 mcg). DEMULEN 1/35-21 and DEMULEN 1/50-21 are 21-day dosage regimens. DEMULEN 1/35-28 and DEMULEN 1/50-28 are 28-day dosage regimens (including 7 days of inert tablets). These forms are packaged in Compack® tablet dispensers.

MAJOR USE

DEMULEN 1/35 and DEMULEN 1/50 are highly effective in preventing pregnancy.

SAFETY INFORMATION

See complete safety information set forth below.

PRESCRIBING INFORMATION

DEMULEN® 1/35–21
DEMULEN® 1/35–28
DEMULEN® 1/50–21
DEMULEN® 1/50–28 ℞℞℞℞

[*dem 'ū-len*]
(ethynodiol diacetate with ethinyl estradiol)

Patients should be counseled that this product does not protect against HIV infection (AIDS) and other sexually transmitted diseases.

DESCRIPTION

Demulen 1/35-21 and Demulen 1/35-28. Each white tablet contains 1 mg of ethynodiol diacetate and 35 mcg of ethinyl estradiol, and the inactive ingredients include calcium acetate, calcium phosphate, corn starch, hydrogenated castor oil, and povidone. Each blue tablet in the Demulen 1/35-28 package is a placebo containing no active ingredients, and the inactive ingredients include calcium sulfate, corn starch, FD&C Blue No. 1 Lake, magnesium stearate, and sucrose.

Demulen 1/50-21 and Demulen 1/50-28. Each white tablet contains 1 mg of ethynodiol diacetate and 50 mcg of ethinyl estradiol, and the inactive ingredients include calcium acetate, calcium phosphate, corn starch, hydrogenated castor oil, and povidone. Each pink tablet in the Demulen 1/50-28 package is a placebo containing no active ingredients, and the inactive ingredients include calcium sulfate, corn starch, FD&C Red No. 3, FD&C Yellow No. 6, magnesium stearate, and sucrose.

The chemical name for ethynodiol diacetate is 19-nor-17α-pregn-4-en-20-yne-3β, 17-diol diacetate, and for ethinyl estradiol it is 19-nor-17α-pregna-1,3,5(10)-trien-20-yne-3, 17-diol. The structural formulas are as follows:

ethynodiol diacetate

ethinyl estradiol

Therapeutic class: Oral contraceptive.

CLINICAL PHARMACOLOGY

Combination oral contraceptives act primarily by suppression of gonadotropins. Although the primary mechanism of this action is inhibition of ovulation, other alterations in the genital tract, including changes in the cervical mucus (which increase the difficulty of sperm entry into the uterus) and the endometrium (which may reduce the likelihood of implantation) may also contribute to contraceptive effectiveness.

INDICATIONS AND USAGE

Demulen 1/35 and Demulen 1/50 are indicated for the prevention of pregnancy in women who elect to use oral contraceptives as a method of contraception.

Oral contraceptives are highly effective. Table 1 lists the typical accidental pregnancy rates for users of combination oral contraceptives and other methods of contraception. The efficacy of these contraceptive methods, except sterilization and progestogen implants and injections, depends upon the reliability with which they are used. Correct and consistent use of methods can result in lower failure rates.

Table 1. Lowest expected and typical failure rates during the first year of continuous use of a method. Percent of women experiencing an accidental pregnancy in the first year of continuous use.[1,1a]

Method	Lowest Expected*	Typical**
No contraception	85	85
Oral contraceptives		
Combined	0.1	N/A***
Progestogen only	0.5	N/A***
Diaphragm with spermicidal		
cream or jelly	6	18
Spermicides alone (foam,		
creams, jellies and vaginal		
suppositories)	3	21
Vaginal sponge		
Nulliparous	6	18
Parous	9	28

IUD (medicated)		
Progesterone	2	N/A***
Copper T 380A	0.8	N/A***
Condom without spermicides	2	12
Periodic abstinence (all methods)	1–9	20
Progestogen injections	0.3	0.3
Progestogen implants	0.2	0.2
Female sterilization	0.2	0.4
Male sterilization	0.1	0.15

Adapted from Trussell et al.[1]

* The authors' best guess of the percentage of women expected to experience an accidental pregnancy among couples who initiate a method (not necessarily for the first time) and who use it consistently and correctly during the first year if they do not stop for any other reason.

** This term represents "typical" couples who initiate use of a method (not necessarily for the first time), who experience an accidental pregnancy during the first year if they do not stop for any other reason.

*** N/A—Data not available.

CONTRAINDICATIONS

Oral contraceptives should not be used in women who have the following conditions:

- Thrombophlebitis or thromboembolic disorders
- A past history of deep vein thrombophlebitis or thromboembolic disorders
- Cerebral vascular disease, myocardial infarction, or coronary artery disease, or a past history of these conditions
- Known or suspected carcinoma of the breast, or a history of this condition
- Known or suspected carcinoma of the female reproductive organs or suspected estrogen-dependent neoplasia, or a history of these conditions
- Undiagnosed abnormal genital bleeding
- History of cholestatic jaundice of pregnancy or jaundice with prior oral contraceptive use
- Past or present, benign or malignant liver tumors
- Known or suspected pregnancy

WARNINGS

Cigarette smoking increases the risk of serious cardiovascular side effects from oral contraceptive use. This risk increases with age and with heavy smoking (15 or more cigarettes per day) and is quite marked in women over 35 years of age. Women who use oral contraceptives should be strongly advised not to smoke.

The use of oral contraceptives is associated with increased risk of several serious conditions including venous and arterial thromboembolism, thrombotic and hemorrhagic stroke, myocardial infarction, liver tumors or other liver lesions, and gallbladder disease. The risk of morbidity and mortality increases significantly in the presence of other risk factors such as hypertension, hyperlipidemia, obesity, and diabetes mellitus.

Practitioners prescribing oral contraceptives should be familiar with the following information relating to these and other risks.

The information contained herein is principally based on studies carried out in patients who used oral contraceptives with formulations containing higher amounts of estrogens and progestogens than those in common use today. The effect of long-term use of the oral contraceptives with lesser amounts of both estrogens and progestogens remains to be determined.

Throughout this labeling, epidemiological studies reported are of two types: retrospective case-control studies and prospective cohort studies. Case-control studies provide an estimate of the relative risk of a disease, which is defined as the *ratio* of the incidence of a disease among oral contraceptive users to that among nonusers. The relative risk (or odds ratio) does not provide information about the actual clinical occurrence of a disease. Cohort studies provide a measure of both the relative risk and the attributable risk. The latter is the *difference* in the incidence of disease between oral contraceptive users and nonusers. The attributable risk does provide information about the actual occurrence or incidence of a disease in the subject population. For further information, the reader is referred to a text on epidemiological methods.

1. Thromboembolic disorders and other vascular problems.

a. Myocardial infarction. An increased risk of myocardial infarction has been associated with oral contraceptive use.[2–21] This increased risk is primarily in smokers or in women with other underlying risk factors for coronary artery disease such as hypertension, obesity, diabetes, and hypercholesterolemia. The relative risk for myocardial infarction in current oral contraceptive users has been estimated to be 2 to 6. The risk is very low under the age of 30. However, there is the possibility of a risk of cardiovascular disease even in very young women who take oral contraceptives. Smoking in combination with oral contraceptive use has been reported to contribute substantially to the risk of myocardial infarction in women in their mid-thirties or older, with smoking accounting for the majority of excess cases.[22] Mortality rates associated with circulatory disease have been shown to increase substantially in smokers, especially in those 35 years of age and older among women who use oral contraceptives (see Figure 1, Table 2).

Figure 1. Circulatory disease mortality rates per 100,000 woman-years by age, smoking status, and oral contraceptive use.[14]

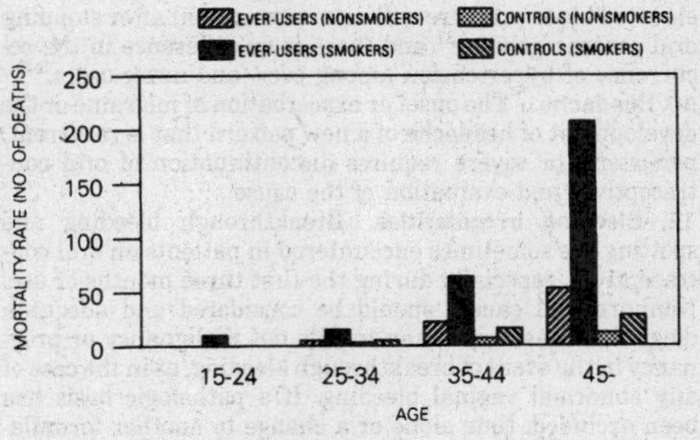

Adapted from Layde and Beral.[14]

Oral contraceptives may compound the effects of well-known cardiovascular risk factors such as hypertension, diabetes, hyperlipidemias, hypercholesterolemia, age, cigarette smoking, and obesity. In particular, some progestogens decrease HDL cholesterol[23–31] and cause glucose intolerance, while estrogens may create a state of hyperinsulinism.[32] Oral contraceptives have been shown to increase blood pressure among some users (see *Warning* No. 9). Similar effects on risk factors have been associated with an increased risk of heart disease.

b. Thromboembolism. An increased risk of thromboembolic and thrombotic disease associated with the use of oral contraceptives is well established.[17,33–51] Case-control studies have estimated the relative risk to be 3 for the first episode of superficial venous thrombosis, 4 to 11 for deep vein thrombosis or pulmonary embolism, and 1.5 to 6 for women with predisposing conditions for venous thromboembolic disease.[34–37,45,46] Cohort studies have shown the relative risk to be somewhat lower, about 3 for new cases (subjects with no past history of venous thrombosis or varicose veins) and about 4.5 for new cases requiring hospitalization.[42,47,48] The risk of venous thromboembolic disease associated with oral contraceptives is not related to duration of use.

A two- to seven-fold increase in relative risk of postoperative thromboembolic complications has been reported with the use of oral contraceptives.[38,39] The relative risk of venous thrombosis in women who have predisposing conditions is about twice that of women without such medical conditions.[43] If feasible, oral contraceptives should be discontinued at least 4 weeks prior to and for 2 weeks after elective surgery of a type associated with an increased risk of thromboembolism, and also during and following prolonged immobilization. Since the immediate postpartum period is also associated with an increased risk of thromboembolism, oral contraceptives should be started no earlier than 4 to 6 weeks after delivery in women who elect not to breast feed.

c. Cerebrovascular diseases. Both the relative and attributable risks of cerebrovascular events (thrombotic and hemorrhagic strokes) have been reported to be increased with oral contraceptive use,[14,17,18,34,42,46,52–59] although, in general, the risk was greatest among older (over 35 years), hypertensive women who also smoked. Hypertension was reported to be a risk factor for both users and nonusers, for both types of strokes, while smoking increased the risk for hemorrhagic strokes.

In one large study,[52] the relative risk for thrombotic stroke was reported as 9.5 times greater in users than in nonusers. It ranged from 3 for normotensive users to 14 for users with severe hypertension.[54] The relative risk for hemorrhagic stroke was reported to be 1.2 for nonsmokers who used oral contraceptives, 1.9 to 2.6 for smokers who did not use oral contraceptives, 6.1 to 7.6 for smokers who used oral contraceptives, 1.8 for normotensive users, and 25.7 for users with severe hypertension. The risk is also greater in older women and among smokers.

d. Dose-related risk of vascular disease with oral contraceptives. A positive association has been reported between the amount of estrogen and progestogen in oral contraceptives and the risk of vascular disease.[41,43,53,59–64] A decline in serum high density lipoproteins (HDL) has been reported with many progestogens.[23–31] A decline in serum high density lipoproteins has been associated with an increased incidence of ischemic heart disease.[65] Because estrogens increase HDL-cholesterol, the net effect of an oral contraceptive depends on the balance achieved between doses of estrogen and progestogen and the nature and absolute amount of progestogens used in the contraceptives. The amount of both steroids should be considered in the choice of an oral contraceptive.

Minimizing exposure to estrogen and progestogen is in keeping with good principles of therapeutics. For any particular estrogen-progestogen combination, the dosage regimen prescribed should be one that contains the least amount of estrogen and progestogen that is compatible with a low failure rate and the needs of the individual patient. New acceptors of oral contraceptives should be started on preparations containing the lowest estrogen content that produces satisfactory results in the individual.

e. Persistence of risk of vascular disease. There are three studies that have shown persistence of risk of vascular disease for users of oral contraceptives. In a study in the United States, the risk of developing myocardial infarction after discontinuing oral contraceptives persisted for at least 9 years for women 40–49 years old who had used oral contraceptives for 5 or more years, but this increased risk was not demonstrated in other age groups.[16] Another American study reported former use of oral contraceptives was significantly associated with increased risk of subarachnoid hemorrhage.[57] In another study, in Great Britain, the risk of developing nonrheumatic heart disease plus hypertension, subarachnoid hemorrhage, cerebral thrombosis, and transient ischemic attacks persisted for at least 6 years after discontinuation of oral contraceptives, although the excess risk was small.[14,18,66] It should be noted that these studies were performed with oral contraceptive formulations containing 50 mcg or more of estrogens.

2. Estimates of mortality from contraceptive use. One study[67] gathered data from a variety of sources that have estimated the mortality rates associated with different methods of contraception at different ages (Table 2). These estimates include the combined risk of death associated with contraceptive methods plus the risk attributable to pregnancy in the event of method failure. Each method of contraception has its specific benefits and risks. The study concluded that, with the exception of oral contraceptive users 35 and older who smoke and 40 or older who do not smoke, mortality associated with all methods of birth control is low and below that associated with childbirth. The observation of a possible increase in risk of mortality with age for oral contraceptive users is based on data gathered in the 1970's, but not reported until 1983.[67] However, current clinical practice involves the use of lower estrogen dose formulations combined with careful restriction of oral contraceptive use to women who do not have the various risk factors listed in this labeling.

Because of these changes in practice and, also, because of some limited new data that suggest that the risk of cardiovascular disease with the use of oral contraceptives may now be less than previously observed,[48,152] the Fertility and Maternal Health Drugs Advisory Committee was asked to review the topic in 1989. The Committee concluded that, although cardiovascular disease risks may be increased with oral contraceptive use after age 40 in healthy nonsmoking women (even with the newer low-dose formulations), there are greater potential health risks associated with pregnancy in older women and with the alternative surgical and medical procedures that may be necessary if such women do not have access to effective and acceptable means of contraception.

Therefore, the Committee recommended that the benefits of oral contraceptive use by healthy nonsmoking women over 40 may outweigh the possible risks. Of course, older women, as all women who take oral contraceptives, should take the lowest dose formulation that is effective.

[See Table 2 at bottom of next page.]

3. Carcinoma of the breast and reproductive organs. Numerous epidemiological studies have been performed on the incidence of breast, endometrial, ovarian, and cervical cancer in women using oral contraceptives. While there are conflicting reports, most studies suggest that the use of oral contraceptives is not associated with an overall increase in the risk of developing breast cancer.[17,40,68–78] Some studies have reported an increased relative risk of developing breast cancer, particularly at a young age.[79–102,151] This increased relative risk appears to be related to duration of use.

Some studies suggested that oral contraceptive use was associated with an increase in the risk of cervical intraepithelial neoplasia, dysplasia, erosion, carcinoma, or microglandular dysplasia in some populations of women.[17,50,103–115] However, there continues to be controversy about the extent to which such findings may be due to differences in sexual behavior and other factors.

In spite of many studies of the relationship between oral contraceptive use and breast and cervical cancers, a cause and effect relationship has not been established.

4. Hepatic neoplasia. Benign hepatic adenomas and other hepatic lesions have been associated with oral contraceptive use,[116–121] although the incidence of such benign tumors is rare in the United States. Indirect calculations have esti-

Continued on next page

Searle—Cont.

mated the attributable risk to be in the range of 3.3 cases per 100,000 for users, a risk that increases after 4 or more years of use.[120] Rupture of benign, hepatic adenomas or other lesions may cause death through intra-abdominal hemorrhage. Therefore, such lesions should be considered in women presenting with abdominal pain and tenderness, abdominal mass, or shock. About one quarter of the cases presented because of abdominal masses; up to one half had signs and symptoms of acute intraperitoneal hemorrhage.[121] Diagnosis may prove difficult.

Studies from the U.S.,[122,150] Great Britain,[123,124] and Italy[125] have shown an increased risk of hepatocellular carcinoma in long-term (> 8 years; relative risk of 7–20) oral contraceptive users. However, these cancers are rare in the United States, and the attributable risk (the excess incidence) of liver cancers in oral contraceptive users approaches less than 1 per 1,000,000 users.

5. Ocular lesions. There have been reports of retinal thrombosis and other ocular lesions associated with the use of oral contraceptives. Oral contraceptives should be discontinued if there is unexplained, gradual or sudden, partial or complete loss of vision; onset of proptosis or diplopia; papilledema; or any evidence of retinal vascular lesions. Appropriate diagnostic and therapeutic measures should be undertaken immediately.

6. Oral contraceptive use before or during pregnancy. Extensive epidemiological studies have revealed no increased risk of birth defects in women who have used oral contraceptives prior to pregnancy.[126,129] The majority of recent studies also do not suggest a teratogenic effect, particularly insofar as cardiac anomalies and limb reduction defects are concerned,[126–129] when the pill is taken inadvertently during early pregnancy.

The administration of oral contraceptives to induce withdrawal bleeding should not be used as a test for pregnancy. Oral contraceptives should not be used during pregnancy to treat threatened or habitual abortion. It is recommended that for any patient who has missed two consecutive periods, pregnancy should be ruled out before continuing oral contraceptive use. If the patient has not adhered to the prescribed schedule, the possibility of pregnancy should be considered at the time of the first missed period and further use of oral contraceptives should be withheld until pregnancy has been ruled out. Oral contraceptive use should be discontinued if pregnancy is confirmed.

7. Gallbladder disease. Earlier studies reported an increased lifetime relative risk of gallbladder surgery in users of oral contraceptives and estrogens.[40,42,53,70] More recent studies, however, have shown that the relative risk of developing gallbladder disease among oral contraceptive users may be minimal.[130–132] The recent findings of minimal risk may be related to the use of oral contraceptive formulations containing lower doses of estrogens and progestogens.

8. Carbohydrate and lipid metabolic effects. Oral contraceptives have been shown to cause a decrease in glucose tolerance in a significant percentage of users.[32] This effect has been shown to be directly related to estrogen dose.[133] Progestogens increase insulin secretion and create insulin resistance, the effect varying with different progestational agents.[32,134] However, in the nondiabetic woman, oral contraceptives appear to have no effect on fasting blood glucose. Because of these demonstrated effects, prediabetic and diabetic women should be carefully observed while taking oral contraceptives.

Some women may have persistent hypertriglyceridemia while on the pill. As discussed earlier (see *Warnings* 1a and 1d), changes in serum triglycerides and lipoprotein levels have been reported in oral contraceptive users.[23–31,135,136]

9. Elevated blood pressure. An increase in blood pressure has been reported in women taking oral contraceptives[50,53,137–139] and this increase is more likely in older oral contraceptive users[137] and with extended duration of use.[53] Data from the Royal College of General Practitioners[138] and subsequent randomized trials have shown that the incidence of hypertension increases with increasing concentrations of progestogens.

Women with a history of hypertension or hypertension-related diseases, or renal disease[139] should be encouraged to use another method of contraception. If such women elect to use oral contraceptives, they should be monitored closely and if significant elevation of blood pressure occurs, oral contraceptives should be discontinued. For most women, elevated blood pressure will return to normal after stopping oral contraceptives,[137] and there is no difference in the occurrence of hypertension among ever- and never-users.[140]

10. Headache. The onset or exacerbation of migraine or the development of headache of a new pattern that is recurrent, persistent, or severe requires discontinuation of oral contraceptives and evaluation of the cause.

11. Bleeding irregularities. Breakthrough bleeding and spotting are sometimes encountered in patients on oral contraceptives, especially during the first three months of use. Nonhormonal causes should be considered and adequate diagnostic measures taken to rule out malignancy or pregnancy in the event of breakthrough bleeding, as in the case of any abnormal vaginal bleeding. If a pathologic basis has been excluded, time alone or a change to another formulation may solve the problem. In the event of amenorrhea, pregnancy should be ruled out.

PRECAUTIONS

1. Physical examination and follow-up. It is good medical practice for all women to have annual history and physical examinations, including women using oral contraceptives. The physical examination, however, may be deferred until after initiation of oral contraceptives if requested by the woman and judged appropriate by the clinician. The physical examination should include special reference to blood pressure, breasts, abdomen, and pelvic organs, including cervical cytology, and relevant laboratory tests. In case of undiagnosed, persistent, or recurrent abnormal vaginal bleeding, appropriate measures should be conducted to rule out malignancy. Women with a strong family history of breast cancer or who have breast nodules should be monitored with particular care.

2. Lipid disorders. Women who are being treated for hyperlipidemias should be followed closely if they elect to use oral contraceptives. Some progestogens may elevate LDL levels and may render the control of hyperlipidemias more difficult.

3. Liver function. If jaundice develops in any woman receiving oral contraceptives, they should be discontinued. Steroids may be poorly metabolized in patients with impaired liver function and should be administered with caution in such patients. Cholestatic jaundice has been reported after combined treatment with oral contraceptives and troleandomycin. Hepatotoxicity following a combination of oral contraceptives and cyclosporine has also been reported.

4. Fluid retention. Oral contraceptives may cause some degree of fluid retention. They should be prescribed with caution, and only with careful monitoring, in patients with conditions that might be aggravated by fluid retention, such as convulsive disorders, migraine syndrome, asthma, or cardiac, hepatic, or renal dysfunction.

5. Emotional disorders. Women with a history of depression should be carefully observed and the drug discontinued if depression recurs to a serious degree.

6. Contact lenses. Contact lens wearers who develop visual changes or changes in lens tolerance should be assessed by an ophthalmologist.

7. Drug interactions. Reduced efficacy and increased incidence of breakthrough bleeding and menstrual irregularities have been associated with concomitant use of rifampin. A similar association, though less marked, has been suggested for barbiturates, phenylbutazone, phenytoin sodium, and possibly with griseofulvin, ampicillin, and tetracyclines.

8. Laboratory test interactions. Certain endocrine and liver function tests and blood components may be affected by oral contraceptives:

a. Increased prothrombin and factors VII, VIII, IX, and X; decreased antithrombin III; increased platelet aggregability.
b. Increased thyroid binding globulin (TBG), leading to increased circulating total thyroid hormone as measured by protein-bound iodine (PBI), T_4 by column or by radioimmunoassay. Free T_3 resin uptake is decreased, reflecting the elevated TBG; free T_4 concentration is unaltered.
c. Other binding proteins may be elevated in the serum.
d. Sex-steroid binding globulins are increased and result in elevated levels of total circulating sex steroids and corticoids; however, free or biologically active levels remain unchanged.
e. Triglycerides and phospholipids may be increased.
f. Glucose tolerance may be decreased.
g. Serum folate levels may be depressed. This may be of clinical significance if a woman becomes pregnant shortly after discontinuing oral contraceptives.
h. Increased sulfobromophthalein and other abnormalities in liver function tests may occur.
i. Plasma levels of trace minerals may be altered.
j. Response to the metyrapone test may be reduced.

9. Carcinogenesis. See *Warnings.*

10. Pregnancy. Pregnancy Category X. See *Contraindications* and *Warnings.*

11. Nursing mothers. Small amounts of oral contraceptive steroids have been identified in the milk of nursing mothers[141–143] and a few adverse effects on the child have been reported, including jaundice and breast enlargement. In addition, oral contraceptives given in the postpartum period may interfere with lactation by decreasing the quantity and quality of breast milk. If possible, the nursing mother should be advised not to use oral contraceptives, but to use other forms of contraception until she has completely weaned her child.

12. Venereal diseases. Oral contraceptives are of no value in the prevention or treatment of venereal disease. The prevalence of cervical *Chlamydia trachomatis* and *Neisseria gonorrhoeae* in oral contraceptive users is increased severalfold.[144,145] It should not be assumed that oral contraceptives afford protection against pelvic inflammatory disease from chlamydia.[144] Patients should be counseled that this product does not protect against HIV infection (AIDS) and other sexually transmitted diseases.

13. General.

a. The pathologist should be advised of oral contraceptive therapy when relevant specimens are submitted.
b. Treatment with oral contraceptives may mask the onset of the climacteric. (See *Warnings* regarding risks in this age group.)

INFORMATION FOR THE PATIENT

See patient labeling printed below.

ADVERSE REACTIONS

An increased risk of the following serious adverse reactions has been associated with the use of oral contraceptives (see *Warnings*):

- Thrombophlebitis and thrombosis
- Arterial thromboembolism
- Pulmonary embolism
- Myocardial infarction and coronary thrombosis
- Cerebral hemorrhage
- Cerebral thrombosis
- Hypertension
- Gallbladder disease
- Benign and malignant liver tumors, and other hepatic lesions

There is evidence of an association between the following conditions and the use of oral contraceptives, although additional confirmatory studies are needed:

- Mesenteric thrombosis
- Neuro-ocular lesions (eg, retinal thrombosis and optic neuritis)

The following adverse reactions have been reported in patients receiving oral contraceptives and are believed to be drug-related:

- Nausea
- Vomiting
- Gastrointestinal symptoms (such as abdominal cramps and bloating)
- Breakthrough bleeding
- Spotting
- Change in menstrual flow
- Amenorrhea during or after use
- Temporary infertility after discontinuation of use
- Edema
- Chloasma or melasma, which may persist
- Breast changes: tenderness, enlargement, secretion
- Change in weight (increase or decrease)

Table 2. Annual number of birth-related or method-related deaths associated with control of fertility per 100,000 nonsterile women, by fertility control method according to age.[67]

	Age					
Method of control	15–19	20–24	25–29	30–34	35–39	40–44
No fertility control methods*	7.0	7.4	9.1	14.8	25.7	28.2
Oral contraceptives						
nonsmoker**	0.3	0.5	0.9	1.9	13.8	31.6
smoker**	2.2	3.4	6.6	13.5	51.1	117.2
IUD**	0.8	0.8	1.0	1.0	1.4	1.4
Condom*	1.1	1.6	0.7	0.2	0.3	0.4
Diaphragm/ spermicide*	1.9	1.2	1.2	1.3	2.2	2.8
Periodic abstinence*	2.5	1.6	1.6	1.7	2.9	3.6

*Deaths are birth-related
**Deaths are method-related
Adapted from Ory.[67]

- Change in cervical erosion or secretion
- Diminution in lactation when given immediately postpartum
- Cholestatic jaundice
- Migraine
- Rash (allergic)
- Mental depression
- Reduced tolerance to carbohydrates
- Vaginal candidiasis
- Change in corneal curvature (steepening)
- Intolerance to contact lenses

The following adverse reactions or conditions have been reported in users of oral contraceptives and the association has been neither confirmed nor refuted:

- Premenstrual syndrome
- Cataracts
- Changes in appetite
- Cystitis-like syndrome
- Headache
- Nervousness
- Dizziness
- Hirsutism
- Loss of scalp hair
- Erythema multiforme
- Erythema nodosum
- Hemorrhagic eruption
- Vaginitis
- Porphyria
- Impaired renal function
- Hemolytic uremic syndrome
- Acne
- Changes in libido
- Colitis
- Budd-Chiari syndrome
- Endocervical hyperplasia or ectropion

OVERDOSAGE

Serious ill effects have not been reported following acute ingestion of large doses of oral contraceptives by young children.[180,181] Overdosage may cause nausea, and withdrawal bleeding may occur in females.

NON-CONTRACEPTIVE HEALTH BENEFITS

The following non-contraceptive health benefits related to the use of oral contraceptives are supported by epidemiological studies that largely utilized oral contraceptive formulations containing estrogen doses exceeding 35 mcg of ethinyl estradiol or 50 mcg of mestranol.[148,149]

Effects on menses:

- Increased menstrual cycle regularity
- Decreased blood loss and decreased risk of iron-deficiency anemia
- Decreased frequency of dysmenorrhea

Effects related to inhibition of ovulation:

- Decreased risk of functional ovarian cysts
- Decreased risk of ectopic pregnancies

Effects from long-term use:

- Decreased risk of fibroadenomas and fibrocystic disease of the breast
- Decreased risk of acute pelvic inflammatory disease
- Decreased risk of endometrial cancer
- Decreased risk of ovarian cancer
- Decreased risk of uterine fibroids

DOSAGE AND ADMINISTRATION

To achieve maximum contraceptive effectiveness, oral contraceptives must be taken exactly as directed and at intervals of 24 hours.

IMPORTANT: If the Sunday start schedule is selected, the patient should be instructed to use an additional method of protection until after the first week of administration *in the initial cycle.* The possibility of ovulation and conception prior to initiation of use should be considered.

Demulen 1/35-21, Demulen 1/35-28, Demulen 1/50-21, and Demulen 1/50-28 Dosage Schedules

The Demulen 1/35-21 and Demulen 1/50-21 Compack® tablet dispensers contain 21 tablets arranged in three numbered rows of 7 tablets each.

The Demulen 1/35-28 and Demulen 1/50-28 tablet dispensers contain 21 white active tablets arranged in three numbered rows of 7 tablets each, followed by a fourth row of 7 pink (blue for Demulen 1/35-28) placebo tablets.

Days of the week are printed above the tablets, starting with Sunday on the left.

Two dosage schedules are described, one of which may be more convenient or suitable than the other for an individual patient.

Schedule #1: Sunday start. The patient begins taking Demulen 1/35-21, Demulen 1/35-28, Demulen 1/50-21, or Demulen 1/50-28 from the first row of her package, one tablet daily, starting on the first Sunday after the onset of menstruation. If the patient's period begins on a Sunday she takes her first tablet that very same day. The 21st tablet or the 28th tablet, depending on whether the patient is taking the 21- or 28-tablet course, will then be taken on a Saturday.

Subsequent cycles:

21-tablet course—The patient begins a new 21-tablet course on the eighth day, Sunday, after taking her last tablet. All subsequent cycles will also begin on Sunday, one tablet being taken each day for 3 weeks followed by a week of no pill-taking.

28-tablet course—The patient begins a new 28-tablet course on the next day, Sunday, and all subsequent cycles will also begin on Sunday, one tablet being taken each and every day.

With a Sunday-start schedule, a woman whose period begins on the day of or 1 to 4 days before taking the first tablet should expect a diminution of flow and fewer menstrual days. The initial cycle will likely be shortened by from 1 to 5 days. Thereafter, cycles should be about 28 days in length.

Schedule #2: Day 1 start. The patient begins taking Demulen 1/35-21 or Demulen 1/50-21 from the first row of her package, one tablet daily, starting with the pill day which corresponds to day 1 of her menstrual cycle; the first day of menstruation is counted as day 1. After the last (Saturday) tablet in row #3 has been taken, if any remain in the first row, the patient completes her 21-tablet schedule starting with Sunday in row #1.

Subsequent cycles: The patient begins a new 21-tablet course on the eighth day after taking her last tablet, again starting the same day of the week on which she began her first course. All subsequent cycles will also begin on that same day, one tablet being taken each day for 3 weeks followed by a week of no pill-taking.

Special notes

Spotting, breakthrough bleeding, or nausea: If spotting (bleeding insufficient to require a pad), breakthrough bleeding (heavier bleeding similar to a menstrual flow), or nausea occurs the patient should continue taking her tablets as directed. The incidence of spotting, breakthrough bleeding, or nausea is minimal, most frequently occurring in the first cycle. Ordinarily spotting or breakthrough bleeding will stop within a week. Usually the patient will begin to cycle regularly within two or three courses of tablet-taking. In the event of spotting or breakthrough bleeding organic causes should be borne in mind. (See *Warning* No. 11.)

Missed menstrual periods. Withdrawal flow will normally occur 2 or 3 days after the last active tablet is taken. Failure of withdrawal bleeding ordinarily does not mean that the patient is pregnant, providing the dosage schedule has been correctly followed. (See *Warning* No. 6.)

If the patient has *not* adhered to the prescribed dosage regimen, the possibility of pregnancy should be considered after the first missed period, and oral contraceptives should be withheld until pregnancy has been ruled out.

If the patient has adhered to the prescribed regimen and misses two consecutive periods, pregnancy should be ruled out before continuing the contraceptive regimen.

The first intermenstrual interval after discontinuing the tablets is usually prolonged; consequently, a patient for whom a 28-day cycle is usual might not begin to menstruate for 35 days or longer. Ovulation in such prolonged cycles will occur correspondingly later in the cycle. Posttreatment cycles after the first one, however, are usually typical for the individual woman prior to taking tablets. (See *Warning* No. 11.)

Missed tablets: If a woman misses taking one active tablet the missed tablet should be taken as soon as it is remembered. In addition, the next tablet should be taken at the usual time. If two consecutive active tablets are missed in week 1 or week 2 of the pack, the dosage should be doubled for the next 2 days. The regular schedule should then be resumed, but an additional method of protection must be used as a backup for the next 7 days if she has sex during that time or she may become pregnant.

If two consecutive active tablets are missed in week 3 of the pack or three consecutive active tablets are missed during any of the first 3 weeks of the pack, direct the patient to do one of the following: Day 1 Starters should discard the rest of the pack and begin a new pack that same day; Sunday Starters should continue to take 1 tablet daily until Sunday, discard the rest of the pack, and begin a new pack that same day. The patient may not have a period this month; however, if she has missed two consecutive periods, pregnancy should be ruled out. An additional method of protection must be used as a backup for the next 7 days after the tablets are missed if she has sex during that time or she may become pregnant.

While there is little likelihood of ovulation if only one active tablet is missed, the possibility of spotting or breakthrough bleeding is increased and should be expected if two or more successive active tablets are missed. However, the possibility of ovulation increases with each successive day that scheduled active tablets are missed.

If one or more placebo tablets of Demulen 1/35-28 or Demulen 1/50-28 are missed, the Demulen 1/35-28 or Demulen 1/50-28 schedule should be resumed on the following Sunday (the eighth day after the last white tablet was taken). Omission of placebo tablets in the 28-tablet courses does not increase the possibility of conception provided that this schedule is followed.

HOW SUPPLIED

Demulen 1/35:

Each white Demulen 1/35 tablet is round in shape, with a debossed SEARLE on one side and 151 and design on the other side, and contains 1 mg of ethynodiol diacetate and 35 mcg of ethinyl estradiol.

Demulen 1/35-21 is packaged in cartons of 6 and 24 Compack tablet dispensers of 21 tablets each.

Demulen 1/35-28 is packaged in cartons of 6 and 24 Compack tablet dispensers. Each Compack contains 21 white Demulen 1/35 tablets and 7 blue placebo tablets. (Placebo tablets have a debossed SEARLE on one side and a "P" on the other side.)

Demulen 1/50:

Each white Demulen 1/50 tablet is round in shape, with a debossed SEARLE on one side and 71 on the other side, and contains 1 mg of ethynodiol diacetate and 50 mcg of ethinyl estradiol.

Demulen 1/50-21 is packaged in cartons of 6 and 24 Compack tablet dispensers of 21 tablets each.

Demulen 1/50-28 is packaged in cartons of 6 and 24 Compack tablet dispensers. Each Compack contains 21 white Demulen 1/50 tablets and 7 pink placebo tablets. (Placebo tablets have a debossed SEARLE on one side and a "P" on the other side.)

Caution: Federal law prohibits dispensing without prescription.

REFERENCES

1. Trussell J, et al. *Stud Fam Plann.* 1987;18(Sept-Oct):237; and 1990;21(Jan-Feb):51. **1a.** *Physicians' Desk Reference.* 47th ed. Oradell, NJ: Medical Economics Co Inc; 1993:2598-2601. **2.** Mann JI, et al. *Br Med J.* 1975;2(May 3):241. **3.** Mann JI, et al. *Br Med J.* 1975;3(Sept 13):631. **4.** Mann JI, et al. *Br Med J.* 1975;2(May 3):245. **5.** Mann JI, et al. *Br Med J.* 1976;2(Aug 21):445. **6.** Arthes FG, et al. *Chest.* 1976;70(Nov):574. **7.** Jain AK. *Am J Obstet Gynecol.* 1976;301(Oct 1):126; and *Stud Fam Plann.* 1977;8(March):50. **8.** Ory HW. *JAMA.* 1977;237(June 13):2619. **9.** Jick H, et al. *JAMA.* 1978;239(April 3):1403, 1407. **10.** Jick H, et al. *JAMA.* 1978;240(Dec 1):2548. **11.** Shapiro S, et al. *Lancet.* 1979;1(April 7):743. **12.** Rosenberg L, et al. *Am J Epidemiol.* 1980;111(Jan):59. **13.** Krueger DE, et al. *Am J Epidemiol.* 1980;111(June):655. **14.** Layde P, et al. *Lancet.* 1981;1(March 7):541. **15.** Adam SA, et al. *Br J Obstet Gynaecol.* 1981;88(Aug):838. **16.** Slone D, et al. *N Engl J Med.* 1981;305(Aug 20):420. **17.** Ramcharan S, et al. *The Walnut Creek Contraceptive Drug Study.* Vol 3. US Govt Ptg Off; 1981; and *J Reprod Med.* 1980;25(Dec):346. **18.** Layde PM, et al. *J R Coll Gen Pract.* 1983;33(Feb):75. **19.** Rosenberg L, et al. *JAMA.* 1985;253(May 24/31):2965. **20.** Mant D, et al. *J Epidemiol Community Health.* 1987;41(Sept):215. **21.** Croft P, et al. *Br Med J.* 1989;298(Jan 21):165. **22.** Goldbaum GM, et al. *JAMA.* 1987;258(Sept 11):1339. **23.** Bradley DD, et al. *N Engl J Med.* 1978;299(July 6):17. **24.** Tikkanen MJ. *J Reprod Med.* 1986;31(Sept suppl):898. **25.** Lipson A, et al. *Contraception.* 1986;34(Aug):121. **26.** Burkman RT, et al. *Obstet Gynecol.* 1988;71(Jan):33. **27.** Knopp RH, *J Reprod Med.* 1986;31(Sept suppl):913. **28.** Krauss RM, et al. *Am J Obstet Gynecol.* 1983; 145(Feb 15):446. **29.** Wahl P, et al. *N Engl J Med.* 1983;308(April 14):862. **30.** Wynn V, et al. *Am J Obstet Gynecol.* 1982;142(March 15):766. **31.** LaRosa JC. *J Reprod Med.* 1986;31(Sept suppl):906. **32.** Wynn V, et al. *J Reprod Med.* 1986;31(Sept suppl):892. **33.** Royal College of General Practitioners. *J R Coll Gen Pract.* 1967;13(May):267. **34.** Inman WHW, et al. *Br Med J.* 1968;2(April 27):193. **35.** Vessey MP, et al. *Br Med J.* 1968;2(April 27):199. **36.** Vessey MP, et al. *Br Med J.* 1969;2(June 14):651. **37.** Sartwell PE, et al. *Am J Epidemiol.* 1969;90(Nov):365. **38.** Vessey MP, et al. *Br Med J.* 1970;3(July 18):123. **39.** Greene GR, et al. *Am J Public Health.* 1972;62(May):680. **40.** Boston Collaborative Drug Surveillance Programme. *Lancet.* 1973;1(June 23):1399. **41.** Stolley PD, et al. *Am J Epidemiol.* 1975;102(Sept):197. **42.** Vessey MP, et al. *J Biosoc Sci.* 1976;8(Oct):373. **43.** Kay CR, *J R Coll Gen Pract.* 1978;28(July):393. **44.** Petitti DB, et al. *Am J Epidemiol.* 1978;108(Dec):480. **45.** Maguire MG, et al. *Am J Epidemiol.* 1979;110(Aug):188. **46.** Petitti DB, et al. *JAMA.* 1979;242(Sept 14):1150. **47.** Porter JB, et al. *Obstet Gynecol.* 1982;59(March):299. **48.** Porter JB, et al. *Obstet Gynecol.* 1985;66(July):1. **49.** Vessey MP, et al. *Br Med J.* 1986;292(Feb 22):526. **50.** Hoover R, et al. *Am J Public Health.* 1978;68(April):335. **51.** Vessey MP. *Br J Fam Plann.* 1980;6(Oct suppl):1. **52.** Collaborative Group for the Study of Stroke in Young Women. *N Engl J Med.* 1973;288(April 26):871. **53.** Royal College of General Practitioners. *Oral Contraceptives and Health.* New York, NY: Pitman Publ Corp; May 1974. **54.** Collaborative Group for the Study of Stroke in Young Women. *JAMA.* 1975;231(Feb 17):718. **55.** Beral V. *Lancet.* 1976;2(Nov 13):1047. **56.** Vessey MP, et al. *Lancet.* 1977;2(Oct 8):731; and 1981;1(March 7):549. **57.** Petitti DB, et al. *Lancet.* 1978;2(July 29):234. **58.** Inman WHW. *Br Med J.* 1979;2(Dec 8):1468. **59.** Vessey MP, et al. *Br Med J.* 1984;289(Sept 1):530. **60.** Inman WHW, et al. *Br Med*

Continued on next page

Searle—Cont.

J. 1970;2(April 25):203. **61.** Meade TW, et al. *Br Med J.* 1980;280(May 10):1157. **62.** Böttiger LE, et al. *Lancet.* 1980;1(May 24):1097. **63.** Kay CR, *Am J Obstet Gynecol.* 1982;142(March 15):762. **64.** Vessey MP, et al. *Br Med J.* 1986;292(Feb 22):526. **65.** Gordon T, et al. *Am J Med.* 1977;62(May): 707. **66.** Beral V, et al. *Lancet.* 1977;2(Oct 8): 727. **67.** Ory H. *Fam Plann Perspect.* 1983;15(March April):57. **68.** Arthes FG, et al. *Cancer.* 1971;28(Dec):1391. **69.** Vessey MP, et al. *Br Med J.* 1972;3(Sept 23):719. **70.** Boston Collaborative Drug Surveillance Program. *N Engl J Med.* 1974;290(Jan 3):15. **71.** Vessey MP, et al. *Lancet.* 1975; 1(April 26):941. **72.** Casagrande J, et al. *J Natl Cancer Inst.* 1976;56(April):839. **73.** Kelsey JL, et al. *Am J Epidemiol.* 1978;107(March):236. **74.** Kay CR, *Br Med J.* 1981;282(June 27):2089. **75.** Vessey MP, et al. *Br Med J.* 1981;282(June 27):2093. **76.** The Cancer and Steroid Hormone Study of the Centers for Disease Control and the National Institute of Child Health and Human Development. Oral contraceptive use and the risk of breast cancer. *N Engl J Med.* 1986;315(Aug 14):405. **77.** Paul C, et al. *Br Med J.* 1986;293(Sept 20):723. **78.** Miller DR, et al. *Obstet Gynecol.* 1986;68(Dec):863. **79.** Pike MC, et al. *Lancet.* 1983;2(Oct 22):926. **80.** McPherson K, et al. *Br J Cancer.* 1987;56(Nov):653. **81.** Hoover R, et al. *N Engl J Med.* 1976;295(Aug 19):401. **82.** Lees AW, et al. *Int J Cancer.* 1978;22(Dec):700. **83.** Brinton LA, et al. *J Natl Cancer Inst.* 1979;62(Jan):37. **84.** Black MM. *Pathol Res Pract.* 1980;166:491; and *Cancer.* 1980;46(Dec):2747; and *Cancer.* 1983;51(June):2147. **85.** Clavel F, et al. *Bull Cancer (Paris).* 1981;68(Dec):449. **86.** Brinton LA, et al. *Int J Epidemiol.* 1982;11(Dec):316. **87.** Harris NV, et al. *Am J Epidemiol.* 1982;116(Oct):643. **88** Jick H, et al. *Am J Epidemiol.* 1980;112(Nov):577. **89.** McPherson K, et al. *Lancet.* 1983;2(Dec 17):1414. **90.** Hoover R, et al. *J Natl Cancer Inst.* 1981;67(Oct):815. **91.** Jick H, et al. *Am J epidemiol.* 1980;112(Nov):586. **92.** Meirik O, et al. *Lancet.* 1986;2(Sept 20):650. **93.** Fasal E, et al. *J Natl Cancer Inst.* 1975;55(Oct):767. **94.** Paffenbarger RS, et al. *Cancer.* 1977; 39(April suppl):1887. **95.** Stadel BV, et al. *Contraception.* 1988;38(Sept):287. **96.** Miller DR, et al. *Am J Epidemiol.* 1989;129(Feb):269. **97.** Kay CR, et al. *Br J Cancer.* 1988;58(Nov):675. **98.** Miller DR, et al. *Obstet Gynecol.* 1986;68(Dec):863. **99.** Olsson H, et al. *Lancet.* 1985;1(March 30):748. **100.** Chilvers C, et al. *Lancet.* 1989;1(May 6):973. **101.** Huggins GR, et al. *Fertil Steril.* 1987;47(May):733. **102.** Pike MC, et al. *Br J Cancer.* 1981;43(Jan):72. **103.** Ory H, et al. *Am J Obstet Gynecol.* 1976;124(March 15):573. **104.** Stern E, et al. *Science.* 1977;196(June 24):1460. **105.** Peritz E, et al. *Am J Epidemiol.* 1977;106(Dec):462. **106.** Ory HW, et al. In: Garattini S, Berendes H, eds. *Pharmacology of Steroid Contraceptive Drugs.* New York, NY: Raven Press; 1977:211–224. **107.** Meisels A, et al. *Cancer.* 1977;40(Dec):3076. **108.** Goldacre MJ, et al. *Br Med J.* 1978;1(March 25):748. **109.** Swan SH, et al. *Am J Obstet Gynecol.* 1981;139(Jan 1):52. **110.** Vessey MP, et al. *Lancet.* 1983;2(Oct 22):930. **111.** Dallenbach-Hellweg G. *Pathol Res Pract.* 1984;179:38. **112.** Thomas DB, et al. *Br Med J.* 1985;290(March 30):961. **113.** Brinton LA, et al. *Int J Cancer.* 1986;38(Sept):339. **114.** Ebeling K, et al. *Int J Cancer.* 1987;39(April):427. **115.** Beral V. et al. *Lancet.* 1988;2(Dec 10):1331. **116.** Baum JK, et al. *Lancet.* 1973;2(Oct 27):926. **117.** Edmondson HA, et al. *N Engl J Med.* 1976;294(Feb 26):470. **118.** Bein NN, et al. *Br J Surg.* 1977;64(June):433. **119.** Klatskin G. *Gastroenterology.* 1977;73(Aug):386. **120.** Rooks JB, et al. *JAMA.* 1979;242(Aug 17):644. **121.** Sturtevant FM. In: Moghissi K, ed. *Controversies in Contraception*, Baltimore, MD; Williams & Wilkins; 1979:93–150. **122.** Henderson BE, et al. *Br J Cancer.* 1983;48(July):437. **123.** Neuberger J, et al. *Br Med J.* 1986;292(May 24):1355. **124.** Forman D, et al. *Br Med J.* 1986;292(May 24):1357. **125.** La Vecchia C, et al. *Br J Cancer.* 1989;59(March):460. **126.** Savolainen E, et al. *Am J Obstet Gynecol.* 1981;140(July 1):521. **127.** Ferencz C, et al. *Teratology.* 1980;21(April):225. **128.** Rothman KJ, et al. *Am J Epidemiol.* 1979;109(April):433. **129.** Harlap S, et al. *Obstet Gynecol.* 1980;55(April):447. **130.** Layde PM, et al. *J Epidemiol Community Health.* 1982;36(Dec):274. **131.** Rome Group for the Epidemiology and Prevention of Cholelithiasis (GREPCO). *Am J Epidemiol.* 1984;119(May):796. **132.** Strom BL, et al. *Clin Pharmacol Ther.* 1986;39(March):335. **133.** Wynn V. In: Bardin CE, et al. eds. *Progesterone and Progestins.* New York, NY: Raven Press; 1983:395–410. **134.** Perlman JA, et al. *J Chron Dis.* 1985;38(Oct):857. **135.** Powell MG, et al. *Obstet Gynecol.* 1984;63(June):764. **136.** Wynn V, et al. *Lancet.* 1966;2(Oct 1):720. **137.** Fisch IR, et al. *JAMA.* 1977;237(June 6):2499. **138.** Kay CR, *Lancet.* 1977;1(March 19):624. **139.** Laragh JH. *Am J Obstet Gynecol.* 1976;126(Sept 1):141. **140.** Ramcharan S. In: Garattini S. Berendes HW, eds. *Pharmacology of Steroid Contraceptive Drugs.* New York, NY: Raven Press; 1977:277–288. **141.** Laumas KR, et al. *Am J Obstet Gynecol.* 1967;98(June 1):411. **142.** Saxena BN, et al. *Contraception.* 1977;16(Dec):605. **143.** Nilsson S, et al. *Contraception.* 1978;17(Feb):131. **144.** Washington AE, et al. *JAMA.* 1985;253(April 19):2246. **145.** Louv WC, et al. *Am J Obstet Gynecol.* 1989;160(Feb):396. **146.** Francis WG, et al. *Can Med Assoc J.* 1965;92(Jan 23):191. **147.** Verhulst HL, et al. *J Clin Pharmacol.* 1967;7(Jan-Feb):9. **148.** Ory HW. *Fam Plann Perspect.* 1982;14(July-Aug):182. **149.** Ory HW, et al. *Making Choices: Evaluating the Health Risks and Benefits of Birth Control Methods.* New York, NY: The Alan Guttmacher Institute; 1983. **150.** Palmer JR, et al. *Am J Epidemiol.* 1989;130(Nov):878. **151.** Romieu I, et al. *J Natl Cancer Inst.* 1989;81(Sept):1313. **152.** Porter JB, et al. *Obstet Gynecol.* 1987;70(July):29.

BRIEF SUMMARY OF PATIENT WARNINGS

This product (like all oral contraceptives) is intended to prevent pregnancy. It does not protect against HIV infection (AIDS) and other sexually transmitted diseases.

> **Cigarette smoking increases the risk of serious adverse effects on the heart and blood vessels from oral contraceptive use. This risk increases with age and with heavy smoking (15 or more cigarettes per day) and is quite marked in women over 35 years of age. Women who use oral contraceptives are strongly advised not to smoke.**

In the detailed leaflet, "What You Should Know About Oral Contraceptives," which you have received, the risks and benefits of oral contraceptives are discussed in much more detail. That leaflet also provides information on other forms of contraception. Please take time to read it carefully for it may have been recently revised.

If you have any questions or problems regarding this information, contact your doctor.

Oral contraceptives, also known as "birth control pills" or "the pill," are taken to prevent pregnancy and, when taken correctly, have a failure rate of about 1% per year when used without missing any pills. The typical failure rate of large numbers of pill users is less than 3% per year when women who miss pills are included. However, forgetting to take pills considerably increases the chances of pregnancy.

For most women, oral contraceptives are free of serious or unpleasant side effects. However, oral contraceptive use is associated with certain serious diseases or conditions that can cause severe disability or death, though rarely. There are some women who are at high risk of developing certain serious diseases that can be life-threatening or may cause temporary or permanent disability. The risks associated with taking oral contraceptives increase significantly if you:

- smoke, or
- have high blood pressure, diabetes, high cholesterol, or are overweight, or
- have or have had clotting disorders, heart attack, stroke, angina pectoris (chest pains on exertion), cancer of the breast or sex organs, jaundice (yellowing of the skin or whites of the eyes), or malignant (cancerous) or benign (noncancerous) liver tumors.

Women should not use oral contraceptives if they suspect they are pregnant or if they have unexplained vaginal bleeding.

Most side effects of the pill are not serious. The most common effects are nausea, vomiting, bleeding between menstrual periods, weight gain, breast tenderness, and difficulty wearing contact lenses. These side effects, especially nausea and vomiting, may subside within the first three months of use.

Proper use of oral contraceptives requires that they be taken under your doctor's continuing supervision, because they can be associated with serious side effects. The serious side effects of the pill occur very infrequently, especially if you are in good health and are young. However, you should know that the following medical conditions have been associated with or made worse by the pill, and that certain of the risks may persist after use of the pill has been discontinued:

1. Blood clots in the legs, arms, lungs, heart (heart attack), eyes, abdomen, or elsewhere in the body. As mentioned above, smoking increases the risk of heart attacks and strokes and subsequent serious medical consequences.
2. Stroke, due to a blood clot, or to bleeding in the brain (hemorrhage) as a result of bursting of a blood vessel. Stroke can lead to paralysis in all or part of the body, or to death.
3. Liver tumors, which may rupture and cause severe bleeding and death. A possible, but not definite, association has also been found with the pill and liver cancer. However, with or without use of the pill, liver cancers are extremely rare in the United States.
4. High blood pressure, although blood pressure ordinarily, but not always, returns to original levels when the pill is stopped.
5. Gallbladder disease, which might require surgery.

The symptoms associated with these serious side effects are discussed in the detailed leaflet given to you with your supply of pills. Notify your doctor or health care provider if you notice any unusual physical disturbances while taking the pill. In addition, you should be aware that drugs such as anti-epileptics, antibiotics (especially rifampin), as well as certain other drugs, may decrease oral contraceptive effectiveness.

There is a conflict among studies regarding breast cancer and oral contraceptive use. Some studies have reported an increase in the risk of developing breast cancer, particularly at a younger age. This increased risk appears to be related to duration of use. The majority of studies have found no overall increase in the risk of developing breast cancer. Some studies have found an increase in the incidence of cancer of the cervix in women who use oral contraceptives. However, this finding may be related to factors other than the use of oral contraceptives. There is insufficient evidence to rule out the possibility that pills may cause such cancers.

Taking the pill may provide some important non-contraceptive benefits. These include less painful menstruation, less menstrual blood loss and anemia, less risk of fibroids, pelvic infections, and noncancerous breast diseases, and less risk of cancer of the ovary and of the lining of the uterus (womb).

Be sure to discuss any medical condition you may have with your health care provider. He or she will take a medical and family history before prescribing oral contraceptives and will also examine you. The physical examination may be delayed to another time if you request it and the health care provider believes that it is a good medical practice to postpone it. You should be reexamined at least once a year while taking oral contraceptives. The detailed patient information leaflet gives you further information that you should read and discuss with your health care provider.

DETAILED PATIENT LABELING: WHAT YOU SHOULD KNOW ABOUT ORAL CONTRACEPTIVES

This product (like all oral contraceptives) is intended to prevent pregnancy. It does not protect against HIV infection (AIDS) and other sexually transmitted diseases.

INTRODUCTION

It is important that any woman who considers using an oral contraceptive understand the risks involved. Although the oral contraceptives have important advantages over other methods of contraception, they have certain risks that no other method has. Only you and your physician can decide whether the advantages are worth these risks. This leaflet will tell you about the most important risks. It will explain how you can help your doctor prescribe the pill as safely as possible by telling him/her about yourself and being alert for the earliest signs of trouble. And it will tell you how to use the pill properly so that it will be as effective as possible. THERE IS MORE DETAILED INFORMATION AVAILABLE IN THE LEAFLET PREPARED FOR DOCTORS. Your pharmacist can show you a copy or you can request one from the manufacturer by phoning toll-free 1-800-323-4204; you may need your doctor's help in understanding parts of it.

This leaflet is not a replacement for a careful discussion between you and your health care provider. You should discuss the information provided in this leaflet with him or her, both when you first start taking the pill and during your revisits. You should also follow your doctor's advice with regard to regular check-ups while you are on the pill.

If you do not have any of the conditions listed below and are thinking about using oral contraceptives, to help you decide, you need information about the advantages and risks of oral contraceptives and of other contraceptive methods as well. This leaflet describes the advantages and risks of oral contraceptives. Except for sterilization, the intrauterine device (IUD), and abortion, which have their own specific risks, the only risks of other methods are those due to pregnancy should the method fail. Your doctor can answer questions you may have with respect to other methods of contraception, and further questions you may have on oral contraceptives after reading this leaflet.

WHAT ARE ORAL CONTRACEPTIVES?

The most common type of oral contraceptive, often simply called "the pill," is a combination of estrogen and progestogen, the two kinds of female hormones. The amount of estrogen and progestogen can vary, but the amount of estrogen is more important because both the effectiveness and some of the dangers of the pill have been related to the amount of estrogen. The pill works principally by preventing release of an egg from the ovary during the cycle in which the pills are taken.

EFFECTIVENESS OF ORAL CONTRACEPTIVES

The pill is one of the most effective methods of birth control. When they are taken correctly, without missing any pills, the chance of becoming pregnant is less than 1% (1 pregnancy per 100 women per year of use) when used perfectly, without missing any pills. Typical failure rates are actually 3% per year. The chance of becoming pregnant increases with each missed pill during a menstrual cycle.

In comparison, typical failure rates for other methods of birth control during the first year of use are as follows:

Progestogen implants: less than 1%
Progestogen injections: less than 1%
Sterilization: less than 1%
IUD: 3%
Diaphragm with spermicides: 18%

Spermicides alone: 21%
Vaginal sponge: 18% to 28%
Condom alone: 12%
Periodic abstinence (rhythm): 20%
No methods: 85%

WHO SHOULD NOT TAKE ORAL CONTRACEPTIVES

Cigarette smoking increases the risk of serious adverse effects on the heart and blood vessels from oral contraceptive use. This risk increases with age and with heavy smoking (15 or more cigarettes per day) and is quite marked in women over 35 years of age. Women who use oral contraceptives are strongly advised not to smoke.

Some women should not use the pill. For example, you should not take the pill if you are pregnant or think you may be pregnant. You should also not use the pill if you have any of the following conditions:

- Heart attack or stroke (blood clot or hemorrhage in the brain), currently or in the past.
- Blood clots in the legs (thrombophlebitis), lungs (pulmonary embolism), eyes, or elsewhere in the body, currently or in the past.
- Chest pain (angina pectoris), currently or in the past.
- Known or suspected breast cancer or cancer of the lining of the uterus (womb), cervix, or vagina, currently or in the past.
- Unexplained vaginal bleeding (until a diagnosis is reached by your doctor).
- Yellowing of the whites of the eyes or of the skin (jaundice) during pregnancy or during previous use of the pill.
- Liver tumor (whether cancerous or not), currently or in the past.
- Known or suspected pregnancy (one or more menstrual periods missed).

Tell your health care provider if you have ever had any of these conditions. He or she can recommend a safer method of birth control.

OTHER CONSIDERATIONS BEFORE TAKING ORAL CONTRACEPTIVES

Tell your health care provider if you have or have had any of the following conditions, as he or she will want to watch them closely or they might cause him or her to suggest using another method of contraception:

- Breast nodules (lumps), fibrocystic disease (breast cysts), abnormal mammograms (x-ray pictures of the breast), or abnormal Pap smears
- Diabetes
- High blood pressure
- High blood cholesterol or triglycerides
- Migraine or other headaches or epilepsy
- Mental depression
- Gallbladder, heart, or kidney disease
- History of scanty or irregular menstrual periods
- Problems during a prior pregnancy
- Fibroid tumors of the womb
- History of jaundice (yellowing of the whites of the eyes or of the skin)
- Varicose veins
- Tuberculosis
- Plans for elective surgery

Women with any of these conditions should be checked often by their health care provider if they choose to use oral contraceptives.

Also, be sure to inform your doctor if you smoke or are on any medications.

RISKS OF TAKING ORAL CONTRACEPTIVES

1. Risk of developing blood clots. Blood clots and blockage of blood vessels are the most serious side effects of taking oral contraceptives. In particular, a clot in the legs can cause thrombophlebitis and a clot that travels to the lungs can cause a sudden blocking of the vessel carrying blood to the lungs. Rarely, clots occur in the blood vessels of the eye and may cause blindness, double vision, or impaired vision.

If you take oral contraceptives and need elective surgery, need to stay in bed for a prolonged illness, or have recently delivered a baby, you may be at risk of developing blood clots. You should consult your doctor about stopping oral contraceptives 3 to 4 weeks before surgery and not taking oral contraceptives for 2 weeks after surgery or during bed rest. You should also not take oral contraceptives soon after delivery of a baby. It is advisable to wait for at least 4 weeks after delivery if you are not breast feeding. If you are breast feeding, you should wait until you have weaned your child before using the pill. (See also the section on Breast feeding in General Precautions.)

The risk of circulatory disease in oral contraceptive users may be higher in users of high-dose pills and may be greater with longer duration of oral contraceptive use. In addition, some of these increased risks may continue for a number of years after stopping oral contraceptives. The risk of abnormal blood clotting increases with age in both users and nonusers of oral contraceptives, but the increased risk from the oral contraceptive appears to be present at all ages. For women aged 20 to 44 it is estimated that about 1 in 2,000 using oral contraceptives will be hospitalized each year because of abnormal clotting. Among nonusers in the same age group, about 1 in 20,000 would be hospitalized each year. For oral contraceptive users in general, it has been estimated that in women between the ages of 15 and 34, the risk of death due to a circulatory disorder is about 1 in 12,000 per year, whereas for nonusers the rate is about 1 in 50,000 per year. In the age group 35 to 44, the risk is estimated to be about 1 in 2,500 per year for oral contraceptive users and about 1 in 10,000 per year for nonusers.

2. Heart attacks and strokes. Oral contraceptives may increase the tendency to develop strokes (stoppage by blood clots or rupture of blood vessels of the brain) and angina pectoris and heart attacks (blockage of blood vessels of the heart). Any of these conditions can cause death or permanent disability.

Smoking greatly increases the possibility of suffering heart attacks and strokes. Furthermore, smoking and the use of oral contraceptives greatly increases the chances of developing and dying of heart disease.

3. Gallbladder disease. Oral contraceptive users probably have a greater risk than nonusers of having gallbladder disease, although this risk may be related to pills containing high doses of estrogens.

4. Liver tumors. In rare cases, oral contraceptives can cause benign but dangerous liver tumors. These benign tumors can rupture and cause fatal internal bleeding. In addition, a possible but not definite association has been found with the pill and liver cancers in several studies, in which a few women who developed these very rare cancers were found to have used oral contraceptives for long periods. However, liver cancers are rare.

5. Cancer of the reproductive organs and breasts. There is conflict among studies regarding breast cancer and oral contraceptive use. Some studies have reported an increase in the risk of developing breast cancer, particularly at a younger age. This increased risk appears to be related to duration of use. The majority of studies have found no overall increase in the risk of developing breast cancer.

Some studies have found an increase in the incidence of cancer of the cervix in women who use oral contraceptives. However, this finding may be related to factors other than the use of oral contraceptives. There is insufficient evidence to rule out the possibility that pills may cause such cancers.

ESTIMATED RISK OF DEATH FROM A BIRTH CONTROL METHOD OR PREGNANCY

All methods of birth control and pregnancy are associated with a risk of developing certain diseases that may lead to disability or death. An estimate of the number of deaths associated with different methods of birth control and pregnancy has been calculated and is shown in the following table.

[See table above.]

Annual number of birth-related or method-related deaths associated with control of fertility per 100,000 nonsterile women, by fertility control method according to age.

	Age					
Method of control	15–19	20–24	25–29	30–34	35–39	40–44
No fertility control methods*	7.0	7.4	9.1	14.8	25.7	28.2
Oral contraceptives non-smoker**	0.3	0.5	0.9	1.9	13.8	31.6
smoker**	2.2	3.4	6.6	13.5	51.1	117.2
IUD**	0.8	0.8	1.0	1.0	1.4	1.4
Condom*	1.1	1.6	0.7	0.2	0.3	0.4
Diaphragm/ spermicide*	1.9	1.2	1.2	1.3	2.2	2.8
Periodic abstinence*	2.5	1.6	1.6	1.7	2.9	3.6

*Deaths are birth-related
**Deaths are method-related

In the above table, the risk of death from any birth control method is less than the risk of childbirth, except for oral contraceptive users over the age of 35 who smoke and pill users over the age of 40 even if they do not smoke. It can be seen in the table that for women aged 15 to 39, the risk of death was highest with pregnancy (7–26 deaths per 100,000 women, depending on age). Among pill users who do not smoke, the risk of death was always lower than that associated with pregnancy for any age group, although over the age of 40, the risk increases to 32 deaths per 100,000 women, compared to 28 associated with pregnancy at that age. However, for pill users who smoke and are over the age of 35, the estimated number of deaths exceeds those for other methods of birth control. If a woman is over the age of 40 and smokes, her estimated risk of death is four times higher (117/100,000 women) than the estimated risk associated with pregnancy (28/100,000) in that age group.

The suggestion that women over 40 who don't smoke should not take oral contraceptives is based on information from older high-dose pills and on less selective use of pills than is practiced today. An Advisory Committee of the FDA discussed this issue in 1989 and recommended that the benefits of oral contraceptive use by healthy, nonsmoking women over 40 years of age may outweigh the possible risks. However, all women, especially older women, are cautioned to use the lowest dose pill that is effective.

WARNING SIGNALS

If any of these adverse effects occur while you are taking oral contraceptives, call your doctor immediately:

- Sharp chest pain, coughing up of blood, or sudden shortness of breath (indicating a possible blood clot in the lung)
- Pain in the calf (indicating a possible blood clot in the leg)
- Crushing chest pain or heaviness in the chest (indicating a possible heart attack)
- Sudden severe headache or vomiting, dizziness or fainting, disturbances of vision or speech, or numbness in an arm or leg (indicating a possible stroke)
- Sudden partial or complete loss of vision (indicating a possible blood clot in the blood vessels of the eye)
- Breast lumps (indicating possible breast cancer or fibrocystic disease of the breast). Ask your doctor or health care provider to show you how to examine your own breasts
- Severe pain or tenderness or a mass in the stomach area (indicating a possibly ruptured liver tumor)
- Difficulty in sleeping, weakness, lack of energy, fatigue, or change in mood (possibly indicating severe depression)
- Jaundice or a yellowing of the skin or eyeballs, accompanied frequently by fever, fatigue, loss of appetite, dark-colored urine, or light-colored bowel movements (indicating possible liver problems)
- Unusual swelling
- Other unusual conditions

SIDE EFFECTS OF ORAL CONTRACEPTIVES

1. Vaginal bleeding

Spotting. This is a slight staining between your menstrual periods that may not even require a pad. Some women spot even though they take their pills exactly as directed. Many women spot although they have never taken the pills. Spotting does not mean that your ovaries are releasing an egg. Spotting may be the result of irregular pill-taking. Getting back on schedule will usually stop it.

If you should spot while taking the pills, you should not be alarmed, because spotting usually stops by itself within a few days. It seldom occurs after the first pill cycle. Consult your doctor if spotting persists for more than a few days or if it occurs after the second cycle.

Unexpected (breakthrough) bleeding. Unexpected (breakthrough) bleeding does not mean that your ovaries have released an egg. It seldom occurs, but when it does happen it is most common in the first pill cycle. It is a flow much like a regular period, requiring the use of a pad or tampon.

If you experience breakthrough bleeding use a pad or tampon and continue with your schedule. Usually your periods will become regular within a few cycles. Breakthrough bleeding will seldom bother you again.

Consult your doctor if breakthrough bleeding is heavy, does not stop within a week, or if it occurs after the second cycle.

2. Contact lenses. If you wear contact lenses and notice a change in vision or an inability to wear your lenses, contact your doctor or health care provider.

3. Fluid retention or raised blood pressure. Oral contraceptives may cause edema (fluid retention), with swelling of the fingers or ankles. If you experience fluid retention, contact your doctor or health care provider. Some women develop high blood pressure while on the pill, which ordinarily, but

Continued on next page

Searle—Cont.

not always, returns to the original levels when the pill is stopped. High blood pressure predisposes one to strokes, heart attacks, kidney disease, and other diseases of the blood vessels.

4. Melasma. A spotty darkening of the skin is possible, particularly of the face. This may persist after the pill is discontinued.

5. Other side effects. Other side effects may include nausea and vomiting, change in appetite, headache, nervousness, depression, dizziness, loss of scalp hair, rash, and vaginal infections.

If any of these, or other, side effects occur, call your doctor or health care provider.

GENERAL PRECAUTIONS

1. Missed periods and use of oral contraceptives before or during early pregnancy. Occasionally women who are taking the pill miss periods. It has been reported to occur as frequently as several times each year in some women, depending on various factors such as age and prior history. (Your doctor is the best source of information about this.) The pill should not be used when you are pregnant or suspect you may be pregnant. Very rarely, women who are using the pill as directed become pregnant. The likelihood of becoming pregnant is higher if you occasionally miss one or two pills. Therefore, if you miss a period you should consult your physician before continuing to take the pill. If you miss a period, especially if you have not taken the pill regularly, you should use an alternative method of contraception until pregnancy has been ruled out; if you have missed more than one pill at any time, you should immediately start using an additional method of contraception and complete your pill cycle.

There is no conclusive evidence that oral contraceptive use is associated with an increase in birth defects when taken inadvertently during early pregnancy. Previously, a few studies had reported that oral contraceptives might be associated with birth defects, but these findings have not been seen in more recent studies. Nevertheless, oral contraceptives or any other drugs should not be used during pregnancy unless clearly necessary and prescribed by your doctor. You should check with your doctor about risks to your unborn child of any medication taken during pregnancy.

2. Breast feeding. If you are breast feeding, consult your doctor before starting oral contraceptives. Some of the drug will be passed on to the child in the milk. A few adverse effects on the child have been reported, including yellowing of the skin (jaundice) and breast enlargement. In addition, oral contraceptives may decrease the amount and quality of your milk. If possible, do not use oral contraceptives while breast feeding. You should use another method of contraception since breast feeding provides only partial protection from becoming pregnant and this partial protection decreases significantly as you breast feed for longer periods of time. You should consider starting oral contraceptives only after you have weaned your child completely.

3. Laboratory tests. If you are scheduled for any laboratory tests, tell your doctor you are taking birth control pills. Certain blood tests may be affected by birth control pills.

4. Drug interactions. Certain drugs may interact with birth control pills to make them less effective in preventing pregnancy or cause an increase in breakthrough bleeding. Such drugs include rifampin, drugs used for epilepsy such as barbiturates (for example, phenobarbital) and phenytoin (Dilantin is one brand of this drug), phenylbutazone (Butazolidin is one brand), and possibly certain antibiotics. You may need to use additional contraception when you take drugs that can make oral contraceptives less effective.

Oral contraceptives may have an influence upon the way other drugs act. Check with your doctor if you are taking *any* other drugs while you are on the pill.

HOW TO TAKE ORAL CONTRACEPTIVES

1. General instructions. You must take your pill every day according to the instructions. Oral contraceptives are most effective if taken 24 hours apart. Take your pill at the same time every day so that you are less likely to forget to take it. You will then maintain an effective dose of the oral contraceptive in your body.

When you first begin to use the pill, you should use an additional method of protection until you have taken your first 7 pills if you are using the Sunday start schedule.

To remove a pill, press down on it. The pill will drop through a hole in the bottom of the Compack.

The two "three weeks on—one week off" schedules. Your Demulen 1/35-21 or Demulen 1/50-21 Compack contains 21 tablets arranged in three numbered rows with the days of the week printed above them.

Day-1 schedule. If you are to begin on day 1, count the day you start to menstruate as day 1 and begin taking your pills that same day. Start in row #1 with the pill under the day that corresponds to the day that your flow began. Continue to take one pill each day on consecutive days of the week.

After the last (Saturday) pill in row #3 has been taken, if any remain in the first row, complete your 21-pill schedule by taking one pill daily starting with Sunday in row #1. Then stop for 1 week before starting to take the pills again. Begin your next pill cycle on the same day of the week that you began the first cycle.

Sunday schedule. Start taking the pills on the first Sunday after your period begins unless your period begins on Sunday. If your period begins on Sunday start taking the pill that very same day.

Begin in row #1 and take your pills, one each day on consecutive days, for 3 weeks (21 days), then stop taking them for 1 week (7 days) before starting to take the pills again on Sunday.

Whether you begin on "day 1" or on Sunday, continue taking your pills as directed, month after month, regardless of whether your flow has or has not ceased, whether you may have experienced spotting or unexpected (breakthrough) bleeding, or whether you feel sick to your stomach during your pill cycle. You will probably have your period about every 28 days.

The "pill-a-day" schedule. Your Demulen 1/35-28 or Demulen 1/50-28 Compack contains 28 pills arranged in four numbered rows of 7 pills each with the days of the week printed above them.

You must take your pills in order, one pill each day. Begin with the Sunday pill in row #1.

1—Start taking the pills on the first Sunday after your period begins unless your period begins on Sunday. *If your period begins on Sunday start taking the pills that very same day.*

2—Continue to take one pill each day on consecutive days of the week.

3—After the Saturday pill in row #1 has been taken begin taking pills in row #2, and so on, until the Saturday pill in row #4 has been taken.

4—Begin a new pill cycle the next day, starting with the Sunday pill in row #1.

You will probably have your period about every 28 days, while you are taking the blue (pink for Demulen 1/50-28) pills.

Continue your pill-a-day schedule, month after month, regardless of whether your flow ceases while you are taking the colored pills, or whether you experience spotting or unexpected (breakthrough) bleeding, or whether you feel sick to your stomach during a cycle.

Take your pill faithfully every "pill day"!
It is important that you take a pill without fail every pill day, at intervals of 24 hours, for two reasons: First, your ovaries may release an egg and therefore you may become pregnant if you do not take your pills regularly. Second, you may spot or start to flow between your periods. This may be inconvenient.

Take your pill at the same time every day!
You are probably wondering why the same time of day is important. By taking your pill at the same time every day it becomes a good habit, and you are much less likely to forget. You may wish to keep your pills in the medicine cabinet near your toothbrush as a reminder to take them when you brush your teeth at night. The best time to take your daily pill may be at bedtime. You may find it helpful to associate your pill-taking with something else you do every day at a particular time.

Another very important reason for you to take your pills as "regular as clockwork" is that you are protected best when you take one every 24 hours; they are made to work that way. Just remember that once every day is not the same as once every 24 hours. Here is why: Suppose you were to take your Monday pill in the morning when you get up, and then not take your Tuesday pill till the evening before you go to bed. True, you will have taken a pill each day, on Monday and on Tuesday—but the time between pill-taking will probably have been more than 36 hours, or more than $1\frac{1}{2}$ days! You might spot. Chances are you would still be protected and would not get pregnant, but why risk it when it is so easy to guarantee yourself maximal protection by taking your pill faithfully every pill day and at the same time every pill day?

If you are scheduled for surgery, or you need prolonged bed rest, you should tell your doctor that you are on the pill and stop taking the pill 4 weeks before surgery to avoid an increased risk of blood clots. It is also advisable not to start oral contraceptives sooner than 4 weeks after delivery of a baby.

2. If you forget to take your pill. If you miss only one white (active) pill in a cycle, the chance of becoming pregnant is small. Take the missed pill as soon as you realize that you have forgotten it and continue to take your tablets for the rest of that cycle as directed. Since the risk of pregnancy increases with each additional pill you skip, it is very important that you take one pill a day.

If you forget your pills (except for the inactive colored pills in Demulen 1/35-28 or Demulen 1/50-28) on 2 consecutive days in week 1 or 2 or the pack, do not be surprised if you spot or start to flow. You should take two pills each day for the next 2 days. You may become pregnant if you have sex in the 7

days after you miss pills. You must use another birth control method (such as condoms, foam, or sponge) as a backup for those 7 days.

If you forget two consecutive active pills in week 3 of the pack or if you forget three consecutive active pills in any of the first 3 weeks of the pack, do one of the following: Day 1 Starters should discard the rest of the pack and begin a new pack that same day; Sunday Starters should continue to take 1 pill daily until Sunday, discard the rest of the pack, and begin a new pack that same day. You may not have a period this month but this is expected. However, if you miss your period 2 months in a row, call your doctor or clinic because you might be pregnant. You may become pregnant if you have sex in the 7 days after you miss pills. You must use another method of birth control as a backup for those 7 days.

If you are using Demulen 1/35-28 or Demulen 1/50-28 and forget to take one or more colored pills, begin a new cycle on the next Sunday; use a new package and start taking the white pills. Missing the colored pills does not increase your chances of getting pregnant providing the white pill schedule has been followed.

3. Pregnancy due to pill failure. The incidence of pill failure resulting in pregnancy is approximately 1% (ie, one pregnancy per 100 women per year) if taken every day as directed, but, because some women fail to follow the daily schedule, more typical failure rates are about 3%. If you become pregnant, you should discuss your pregnancy with your doctor.

4. Pregnancy after stopping the pill. There may be some delay in becoming pregnant after you stop using oral contraceptives, especially if you had irregular menstrual cycles before you used oral contraceptives. It may be advisable to postpone conception until you begin menstruating regularly once you have stopped taking the pill and desire pregnancy.

There does not appear to be any increase in birth defects in newborn babies when pregnancy occurs after stopping the pill.

5. Overdosage. Serious ill effects have not been reported following ingestion of large doses of oral contraceptives by young children. Overdosage may cause nausea and withdrawal bleeding in females. In case of overdosage, contact your health care provider, pharmacist, or Poison Control Center.

6. Other information. Your doctor will take a medical and family history before prescribing oral contraceptives and will also examine you. The physical examination may be delayed to another time if you request it and the health care provider believes that it is a good medical practice to postpone it. You should be reexamined at least once a year. Certain health problems or conditions in your medical or family history may require that your doctor see you more frequently while you are taking the pill. Be sure to keep all appointments with your health care provider because this is a time to determine if there are early signs of side effects of oral contraceptive use.

Do not use the drug for any condition other than the one for which it was prescribed. This drug has been prescribed specifically for you; do not give it to others who may want birth control pills.

This product (like all oral contraceptives) is intended to prevent pregnancy. It does not protect against transmission of HIV (AIDS) and other sexually transmitted diseases such as chlamydia, genital herpes, genital warts, gonorrhea, hepatitis B, and syphilis.

HEALTH BENEFITS FROM ORAL CONTRACEPTIVES

In addition to preventing pregnancy, use of oral contraceptives may provide certain benefits. They are:

- Menstrual cycles may become more regular
- Blood flow during menstruation may be lighter and less iron may be lost. Therefore, anemia due to iron deficiency is less likely to occur.
- Pain or other symptoms during menstruation may be encountered less frequently
- Ectopic (tubal) pregnancy may occur less frequently
- Noncancerous cysts or lumps in the breast may occur less frequently
- Acute pelvic inflammatory disease may occur less frequently
- Fibroids of the uterus (womb) may occur less frequently
- Oral contraceptive use may provide some protection against developing two forms of cancer: cancer of the ovaries and cancer of the lining of the uterus (womb)

If you want more information about birth control pills, ask your doctor or pharmacist. They have a more technical leaflet called the Professional Labeling, which you may wish to read. The Professional Labeling is also published in a book entitled *Physicians' Desk Reference,* available in many book stores and public libraries.

Be certain to read new revisions of this leaflet. You may check the date of the most recent revision by phoning the manufacturer toll-free at 1-800-323-4204, or by writing to the address below.

G.D. Searle & Co.
Healthcare Information Services
5200 Old Orchard Road
Skokie, IL 60077

7/12/94 • A05484-3
Shown in Product Identification Guide, page 335

Flagyl® 375 ℞
[flaj'yl]
(metronidazole capsules)

> **WARNING**
> Metronidazole has been shown to be carcinogenic in mice and rats. (See **PRECAUTIONS.**) Unnecessary use of the drug should be avoided. Its use should be reserved for the conditions described in the **INDICATIONS AND USAGE** section below.

DESCRIPTION

Metronidazole is an oral synthetic antiprotozoal and antibacterial agent, 2-Methyl-5-nitroimidazole-1-ethanol, which has the following structural formula:

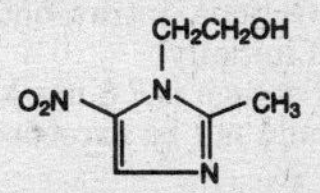

Flagyl® 375 capsules contain 375 mg of metronidazole USP. Inactive ingredients include corn starch, magnesium stearate, gelatin, black iron oxide, titanium dioxide, FD&C Green No. 3, and D&C Yellow No. 10.

CLINICAL PHARMACOLOGY

Disposition of metronidazole in the body is similar for both oral and intravenous dosage forms, with an average elimination half-life in healthy humans of 8 hours.

The major route of elimination of metronidazole and its metabolites is via the urine (60% to 80% of the dose), with fecal excretion accounting for 6% to 15% of the dose. The metabolites that appear in the urine result primarily from side-chain oxidation (1-(β-hydroxyethyl)-2-hydroxymethyl-5-nitroimidazole and 2-methyl-5-nitroimidazole-1-yl-acetic acid] and glucuronide conjugation, with unchanged metronidazole accounting for approximately 20% of the total. Renal clearance of metronidazole is approximately 10 mL/min/1.73m^2.

Metronidazole is the major component appearing in the plasma, with lesser quantities of the 2-hydroxymethyl metabolite also being present. Less than 20% of the circulating metronidazole is bound to plasma proteins. Both the parent compound and the metabolite possess *in vitro* bactericidal activity against most strains of anaerobic bacteria and *in vitro* trichomonacidal activity.

Metronidazole appears in cerebrospinal fluid, saliva, and human milk in concentrations similar to those found in plasma. Bactericidal concentrations of metronidazole have also been detected in pus from hepatic abscesses.

Flagyl® 375 capsules have been shown to have a rate and extent of absorption similar to metronidazole tablets (Flagyl®) and were bioequivalent at an equal single dose of 750 mg. In a study conducted with 23 adult, healthy, female volunteers, oral administration of two 375-mg Flagyl® capsules under fasted conditions produced a mean (± 1 SD) peak plasma concentration (C_{max}) of 21.4 (±2.8) mcg/mL with a mean T_{max} of 1.6 (± 0.7) hours and a mean area under the plasma concentration-time curve (AUC) of 223 (± 44) mcg·hr/mL. In the same study, three 250-mg Flagyl® tablets produced a mean C_{max} of 20.4 (± 3.8) mcg/mL with a mean T_{max} of 1.4 (± 0.4) hours and a mean AUC of 218 (± 50) mcg·hr/mL.

Administration of Flagyl® 375 capsules with food does not affect the extent of absorption of metronidazole; however, the presence of food results in a lower C_{max} and a delayed T_{max} compared to fasted conditions. In a study of 14 healthy, adult, female volunteers, administration of Flagyl® 375 capsules under fasting conditions produced a mean C_{max} of 10.9 (± 1.5) mcg/mL, a mean T_{max} of 1.5 (± 1.4) hours, and a mean AUC of 110 (± 34) mcg·hr/mL compared to a mean C_{max} of 8.6 (± 1.6) mcg/mL, a mean T_{max} of 4.2 (± 1.7) hours, and a mean AUC of 99 (±14) mcg·hr/mL under fed conditions.

Decreased renal function does not alter the single-dose pharmacokinetics of metronidazole. However, plasma clearance of metronidazole is decreased in patients with decreased liver function.

Microbiology:

Metronidazole exerts antimicrobial effects in an anaerobic environment by the following possible mechanism: Once metronidazole enters the organism, the drug is reduced by intracellular electron transport proteins. Because of this alteration to the metronidazole molecule, a concentration gradient is maintained which promotes the drug's intracellular transport. Presumably, free radicals are formed which, in turn, react with cellular components resulting in death of the microorganism.

Metronidazole has been shown to be active against most strains of the following microorganisms both *in vitro* and in clinical infections as described in the **INDICATIONS AND USAGE** section.

Gram-positive anaerobes:
Clostridium species
Eubacterium species
Peptococcus niger
Peptostreptococcus species

Gram-negative anaerobes:
Bacteroides fragilis group (*B. fragilis, B. distasonis, B. ovatus, B. thetaiotaomicron, B. vulgatus*)
Fusobacterium species

Protozoal parasites:
Entamoeba histolytica
Trichomonas vaginalis

The following *in vitro* data are available, **but their clinical significance is unknown:**

Metronidazole exhibits *in vitro* minimal inhibitory concentrations (MIC's) of 8 μg/mL or less against most (≥90%) strains of the following microorganisms; however, the safety and effectiveness of metronidazole in treating clinical infections due to these microorganisms have not been established in adequate and well-controlled clinical trials.

Gram-negative anaerobes:
Bacteroides fragilis group (*B. caccae, B. uniformis*)
Prevotella species (*P. bivia, P. buccae, P. disiens*)

Metronidazole is active against most obligate anaerobes, but does not possess any clinically relevant activity against facultative anaerobes or obligate aerobes.

Susceptibility Tests:

Dilution techniques:

Quantitative methods that are used to determine minimum inhibitory concentrations provide reproducible estimates of the susceptibility of bacteria to antimicrobial compounds. For anaerobic bacteria, the susceptibility to metronidazole can be determined by the reference agar dilution method or by alternate standardized test methods[1]. The MIC values obtained should be interpreted according to the following criteria:

MIC (μg/mL)	Interpretation
≤8	Susceptible (S)
16	Intermediate (I)
≥32	Resistant (R)

For protozoal parasites: Standardized tests do not exist for use in clinical microbiology laboratories.

A report of "Susceptible" indicates that the pathogen is likely to be inhibited by usually achievable concentrations of the antimicrobial compound in the blood. A report of "Intermediate" indicates that the result should be considered equivocal, and, if the microorganism is not fully susceptible to alternative, clinically feasible drugs, the test should be repeated. This category implies possible clinical applicability in body sites where the drug is physiologically concentrated or in situations where high dosage of drug can be used. This category also provides a buffer zone which prevents small uncontrolled technical factors from causing major discrepancies in interpretation. A report of "Resistant" indicates that usually achievable concentrations of the antimicrobial compound in the blood are unlikely to be inhibitory and other therapy should be selected.

Standardized susceptibility test procedures require the use of laboratory control microorganisms that are used to control the technical aspects of the laboratory procedures. Standard metronidazole powder should provide the following MIC values:

Microorganism	MIC (μg/mL)
Bacteroides fragilis ATCC 25285	0.25-1.0
Bacteroides thetaiotaomicron ATCC 29741	0.5-2.0

INDICATIONS AND USAGE

Symptomatic Trichomoniasis. Flagyl® 375 capsules are indicated for the treatment of symptomatic trichomoniasis in females and males when the presence of the trichomonad has been confirmed by appropriate laboratory procedures (wet smears and/or cultures).

Asymptomatic Trichomoniasis. Flagyl® 375 capsules are indicated in the treatment of asymptomatic females when the organism is associated with endocervicitis, cervicitis, or cervical erosion. Since there is evidence that presence of the trichomonad can interfere with accurate assessment of abnormal cytological smears, additional smears should be performed after eradication of the parasite.

Treatment of Asymptomatic Consorts. T. vaginalis infection is a venereal disease. Therefore, asymptomatic sexual partners of treated patients should be treated simultaneously if the organism has been found to be present, in order to prevent reinfection of the partner. The decision as to whether to treat an asymptomatic male partner who has a negative culture or one for whom no culture has been attempted is an individual one. In making this decision, it should be noted that there is evidence that a woman may become reinfected if her consort is not treated. Also, since there can be considerable difficulty in isolating the organism from the asymptomatic male carrier, negative smears and cultures cannot be relied upon in this regard. In any event, the consort should be treated with metronidazole in cases of reinfection.

Amebiasis. Flagyl® 375 capsules are indicated in the treatment of acute intestinal amebiasis (amebic dysentery) and amebic liver abscess.

In amebic liver abscess, metronidazole therapy does not obviate the need for aspiration or drainage of pus.

Anaerobic Bacterial Infections. Flagyl® 375 capsules are indicated in the treatment of serious infections caused by susceptible anaerobic bacteria. Indicated surgical procedures should be performed in conjunction with metronidazole therapy. In a mixed aerobic and anaerobic infection, antimicrobials appropriate for the treatment of the aerobic infection should be used in addition to Flagyl® 375 capsules.

In the treatment of most serious anaerobic infections, intravenous metronidazole is usually administered initially. This may be followed by oral therapy with Flagyl® 375 capsules at the discretion of the physician.

INTRA-ABDOMINAL INFECTIONS, including peritonitis, intra-abdominal abscess, and liver abscess, caused by *Bacteroides* species including the *B, fragilis* group (*B. fragilis, B. distasonis, B. ovatus, B. thetaiotaomicron, B. vulgatus*), *Clostridium* species, *Eubacterium* species, *Peptococcus niger*, or *Peptostreptococcus* species.

SKIN AND SKIN STRUCTURE INFECTIONS caused by *Bacteroides* species including the *B. fragilis* group, *Clostridium* species, *Peptococcus niger, Peptostreptococcus* species, or *Fusobacterium* species.

GYNECOLOGIC INFECTIONS, including endometritis, endomyometritis, tubo-ovarian abscess, and postsurgical vaginal cuff infection, caused by *Bacteroides* species including the *B. fragilis* group, *Clostridium* species, *Peptococcus niger*, or *Peptostreptococcus* species.

BACTERIAL SEPTICEMIA caused by *Bacteroides* species including the *B. fragilis* group or *Clostridium* species.

BONE AND JOINT INFECTIONS (as adjunctive therapy) caused by *Bacteroides* species including the *B. fragilis* group.

CENTRAL NERVOUS SYSTEM (CNS) INFECTIONS, including meningitis and brain abscess, caused by *Bacteroides* species including the *B. fragilis* group.

LOWER RESPIRATORY TRACT INFECTIONS, including pneumonia, empyema, and lung abscess, caused by *Bacteroides* species including the *B. fragilis* group.

ENDOCARDITIS caused by *Bacteroides* species including the *B. fragilis* group.

CONTRAINDICATIONS

Flagyl® 375 capsules are contraindicated in patients with a prior history of hypersensitivity to metronidazole or other nitroimidazole derivatives.

In patients with trichomoniasis, Flagyl® 375 capsules are contraindicated during the first trimester of pregnancy. (See **PRECAUTIONS.**)

WARNINGS

Convulsive seizures and peripheral neuropathy: Convulsive seizures and peripheral neuropathy, the latter characterized mainly by numbness or paresthesia of an extremity, have been reported in patients treated with metronidazole. The appearance of abnormal neurologic signs demands the prompt discontinuation of metronidazole therapy. Metronidazole should be administered with caution to patients with central nervous system diseases.

PRECAUTIONS

General: Patients with severe hepatic disease metabolize metronidazole slowly, with resultant accumulation of metronidazole and its metabolites in the plasma. Accordingly, for such patients, doses below those usually recommended should be administered cautiously. Known or previously unrecognized candidiasis may present more prominent symptoms during therapy with metronidazole and requires treatment with a candidacidal agent.

Information for patients: Alcoholic beverages should be avoided while taking Flagyl® 375 capsules and for at least three days afterward. (See **Drug interactions.**)

Laboratory tests: Metronidazole is a nitroimidazole and should be used with caution in patients with evidence of or history of blood dyscrasia. A mild leukopenia has been observed during its administration; however, no persistent hematologic abnormalities attributable to metronidazole have been observed in clinical studies. Total and differential leukocyte counts are recommended before and after therapy for trichomoniasis and amebiasis, especially if a second

Continued on next page

Searle—Cont.

course of therapy is necessary, and before and after therapy for anaerobic infections.

Drug interactions: Metronidazole has been reported to potentiate the anticoagulant effect of warfarin and other oral coumarin anticoagulants, resulting in a prolongation of prothrombin time. This possible drug interaction should be considered when metronidazole is prescibed for patients on this type of anticoagulant therapy.

The simultaneous administration of drugs that induce microsomal liver enzymes, such as phenytoin or phenobarbital, may accelerate the elimination of metronidazole, resulting in reduced plasma levels; impaired clearance of phenytoin has also been reported.

The simultaneous administration of drugs that decrease microsomal liver enzyme activity, such as cimetidine, may prolong the half-life and decrease plasma clearance of metronidazole. In patients stabilized on relatively high doses of lithium, short-term metronidazole therapy has been associated with elevation of serum lithium and, in a few cases, signs of lithium toxicity. Serum lithium and serum creatinine levels should be obtained several days after beginning metronidazole to detect any increase that may precede clinical symptoms of lithium intoxication.

Alcoholic beverages should not be consumed during metronidazole therapy and for at least three days afterward because abdominal cramps, nausea, vomiting, headaches, and flushing may occur.

Psychotic reactions have been reported in alcoholic patients who are using metronidazole and disulfiram concurrently. Metronidazole should not be given to patients who have taken disulfiram within the last 2 weeks.

Drug/Laboratory test interactions: Metronidazole may interfere with certain types of determinations of serum chemistry values, such as aspartate aminotransferase (AST, SGOT), alanine aminotransferase (ALT, SGPT), lactate dehydrogenase (LDH), triglycerides, and hexokinase glucose. Values of zero may be observed. All of the assays in which interference has been reported involve enzymatic coupling of the assay to oxidation-reduction of nicotinamide adenine dinucleotide ($NAD^+ \rightleftarrows NADH$). Interference is due to the similarity in absorbance peaks of NADH (340 nm) and metronidazole (322 nm) at pH 7.

Carcinogenesis, mutagenesis, impairment of fertility: Metronidazole has shown evidence of carcinogenic activity in a number of studies involving chronic, oral administration in mice and rats, but similar studies in the hamster gave negative results.

Prominent among the effects in the mouse was the promotion of pulmonary tumorigenesis. This has been observed in all six reported studies in that species, including one study in which the animals were dosed on an intermittent schedule (administration during every fourth week only). At very high dose levels (approximately 1500 mg/m^2 which is approximately 3 times the most frequently recommended human dose for a 50 kg adult based on mg/m^2) there was a statistically significant increase in the incidence of malignant liver tumors in males. Also, the published results of one of the mouse studies indicate an increase in the incidence of malignant lymphomas as well as pulmonary neoplasms associated with lifetime feeding of the drug. All these effect are statistically significant.

Several long-term, oral-dosing studies in the rat have been completed. There were statistically significant increases in the incidence of various neoplasms, particularly in mammary and hepatic tumors, among female rats administered metronidazole over those noted in the concurrent female control groups.

Two lifetime tumorigenicity studies in hamsters have been performed and reported to be negative.

Metronidazole has shown mutagenic activity in a number of *in vitro* assay systems. *In vivo* studies have failed to demonstrate a potential for genetic damage.

Fertility studies have been performed in mice at doses up to six times the maximum recommended human dose based on mg/m^2 and have revealed no evidence of impaired fertility.

Pregnancy:

Teratogenic effects: Pregnancy Category B. Metronidazole crosses the placental barrier and enters the fetal circulation rapidly. Reproduction studies have been performed in rats at doses up to five times the human dose and have revealed no evidence of impaired fertility or harm to the fetus due to metronidazole. No fetotoxicity was observed when metronidazole was administered orally to pregnant mice at 60 mg/m^2/day, which is approximately 10% of the human dose when expressed as mg/m^2. However, in a single small study where the drug was administered intraperitoneally, some intrauterine deaths were observed. The relationship of these findings to the drug is unknown. There are, however, no adequate and well-controlled studies in pregnant women. Because animal reproduction studies are not always predictive of human response, and because metronidazole is a carcinogen in rodents, this drug should be used during pregnancy only if clearly needed. (See **CONTRAINDICATIONS.**)

Metronidazole use in the second and third trimesters of pregnancy should be restricted to those patients in whom alternative treatment has been inadequate. Use of metronidazole in the first trimester should be carefully evaluated because metronidazole crosses the placental barrier and its effects on human fetal organogenesis are not known. (See above.)

Nursing mothers: Because of the potential for tumorigenicity shown for metronidazole in mouse and rat studies, a decision should be made whether to discontinue nursing or to discontinue the drug, taking into account the importance of the drug to the mother. Metronidazole is secreted in human milk in concentrations similar to those found in plasma.

Geriatric use: Decreased renal function does not alter the single-dose pharmacokinetics of metronidazole. However, plasma clearance of metronidazole is decreased in patients with decreased liver function. Therefore, in elderly patients, monitoring of serum levels may be necessary to adjust the metronidazole dosage accordingly.

Pediatric use: Safety and effectiveness in children have not been established, except in the treatment of amebiasis.

ADVERSE REACTIONS

The following reactions have also been reported during treatment with metronidazole:

Central Nervous System: Two serious adverse reactions reported in patients treated with metronidazole have been convulsive seizures and peripheral neuropathy, the latter characterized mainly by numbness or paresthesia of an extremity. Since persistent peripheral neuropathy has been reported in some patients receiving prolonged administration of metronidazole, patients should be specifically warned about these reactions and should be told to stop the drug and report immediately to their physicians if any neurologic symptoms occur. In addition, patients have reported dizziness, vertigo, incoordination, ataxia, confusion, irritability, depression, weakness, and insomnia. (See **WARNINGS.**)

Gastrointestinal: The most common adverse reactions reported have been referable to the gastrointestinal tract, particularly nausea reported by about 12% of patients, sometimes accompanied by headache, anorexia, and occasionally vomiting; diarrhea; epigastric distress; and abdominal cramping. Constipation has also been reported.

A sharp, unpleasant metallic taste is not unusual. Furry tongue, glossitis, and stomatitis have occurred; these may be associated with a sudden overgrowth of *Candida* which may occur during therapy. Rare cases of pancreatitis, which generally abated on withdrawal of the drug, have been reported.

Hematopoietic: Reversible neutropenia (leukopenia); rarely, reversible thrombocytopenia.

Cardiovascular: Flattening of the T-wave may be seen in electrocardiographic tracings.

Hypersensitivity: Urticaria, erythematous rash, flushing, nasal congestion, dryness of the mouth (or vagina or vulva), and fever.

Renal: Dysuria, cystitis, polyuria, incontinence, and a sense of pelvic pressure. Instances of darkened urine have been reported by approximately one patient in 100,000. Although the pigment which is probably responsible for this phenomenon has not been positively identified, it is almost certainly a metabolite of metronidazole and seems to have no clinical significance.

Other: Proliferation of *Candida* in the vagina, dyspareunia, decrease of libido, proctitis, and fleeting joint pains sometimes resembling "serum sickness." If patients receiving metronidazole drink alcoholic beverages, they may experience abdominal distress, nausea, vomiting, flushing, or headache. A modification of the taste of alcoholic beverages has also been reported.

Patients with Crohn's disease are known to have an increased incidence of gastrointestinal and certain extraintestinal cancers. There have been some reports in the medical literature of breast and colon cancer in Crohn's disease patients who have been treated with metronidazole at high doses for extended periods of time. A cause and effect relationship has not been established. Crohn's disease is not an approved indication for Flagyl® 375 capsules.

OVERDOSAGE

Single oral doses of metronidazole, up to 15 g, have been reported in suicide attempts and accidental overdoses. Symptoms reported include nausea, vomiting, and ataxia.

Oral metronidazole has been studied as a radiation sensitizer in the treatment of malignant tumors. Neurotoxic effects, including seizures and peripheral neuropathy, have been reported after 5 to 7 days of doses of 6 to 10.4 g every other day.

Treatment: There is no specific antidote for metronidazole overdose; therefore, management of the patient should consist of symptomatic and supportive therapy.

DOSAGE AND ADMINISTRATION

In elderly patients, the pharmacokinetics of metronidazole may be altered, and, therefore, monitoring of serum levels may be necessary to adjust the metronidazole dosage accordingly.

Trichomoniasis:

In the Female:

Seven-day course of treatment—375 mg two times daily for seven consecutive days.

A seven-day course of treatment may minimize reinfection by protecting the patient long enough for the sexual contacts to obtain treatment. Pregnant patients should not be treated during the first trimester. (See **CONTRAINDICATIONS** and **PRECAUTIONS.**)

When repeat courses of the drug are required, it is recommended that an interval of four to six weeks elapse between courses and that the presence of the trichomonad be reconfirmed by appropriate laboratory measures. Total and differential leukocyte counts should be made before and after re-treatments.

In the Male: Treatment should be individualized as for the female.

Amebiasis:

Adults:

For acute intestinal amebiasis (acute amebic dysentery): 750 mg orally three times daily for 5 to 10 days.

For amebic liver abscess: 750 mg orally three times daily for 5 to 10 days.

Children: 35 to 50 mg/kg/24 hours, divided into three doses, orally for 10 days.

Anaerobic Bacterial Infections: In the treatment of most serious anaerobic infections, intravenous metronidazole is usually administered initially.

The usual adult oral dosage is 7.5 mg/kg every 6 hours. A maximum of 4 g should not be exceeded during a 24-hour period.

The usual duration of therapy is 7 to 10 days; however, infections of the bone and joint, lower respiratory tract, and endocardium may require longer treatment.

Patients with severe hepatic disease metabolize metronidazole slowly, with resultant accumulation of metronidazole and its metabolites in the plasma. Accordingly, for such patients, doses below those usually recommended should be administered cautiously. Close monitoring of plasma metronidazole levels[2] and toxicity is recommended.

The dose of metronidazole should not be specifically reduced in anuric patients because accumulated metabolites may be rapidly removed by dialysis.

HOW SUPPLIED

Flagyl® 375 capsules have an iron gray opaque body imprinted with 375 mg and a light green opaque cap imprinted with FLAGYL, supplied as:

NDC Number	Size
0025-1942-50	Bottle of 50
0025-1942-34	Carton of 100 unit dose

Storage and Stability: Store at controlled room temperature 15-30°C (59-86°F). Dispense in a well-closed container with a child-resistant closure.

Caution: Federal law prohibits dispensing without prescription.

REFERENCES

1. National Committee for Clinical Laboratory Standards, Methods for Antimicrobial Susceptibility Testing of Anaerobic Bacteria—Third Edition. Approved Standard NCCLS Document M11-A3, Vol. 13, No. 26, NCCLS, Villanova, PA, December, 1993.

2. Ralph ED, Kirby WMM. Bioassay of metronidazole with either anaerobic or aerobic incubation, *J. Infect. Dis.* 1975; 132(Nov): 587-591 or Gulaid et al. Determination of metronidazole and its major metabolites in biological fluids by high pressure liquid chromatography, *Br. J. Clin. Pharmacol.* 1978; 6:430-432.

Manufactured by
G.D. Searle & Co.
Box 5110
Chicago IL 60680
Address medical inquiries to:
G.D. Searle & Co.
Healthcare Information Services
5200 Old Orchard Road
Skokie IL 60077

10/16/95 •A05712-1

Shown in Product Identification Guide, page 335

KERLONE® ℞

[*kur'lōn*]

(betaxolol hydrochloride)

DESCRIPTION

Kerlone (betaxolol hydrochloride) is a β_1-selective (cardioselective) adrenergic receptor blocking agent available as 10-mg and 20-mg tablets for oral administration. Kerlone is chemically described as 2-propanol, 1-[4-[2-(cyclopropylmethoxy)ethyl]phenoxy]-3-[(1-methylethyl)amino]-, hydrochloride, (±). It has the following chemical structure:

[See chemical structure at top of next column.]

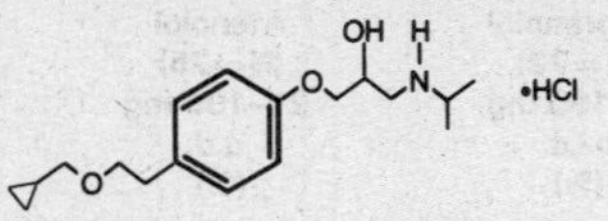

Betaxolol hydrochloride is a water- soluble white crystalline powder with a molecular formula of $C_{18}H_{29}NO_3 \cdot HCl$ and a molecular weight of 343.9. It is freely soluble in water, ethanol, chloroform, and methanol, and has a pKa of 9.4.

The inactive ingredients are hydroxypropyl methylcellulose, lactose, magnesium stearate, polyethylene glycol 400, microcrystalline cellulose, colloidal silicon dioxide, sodium starch glycolate, and titanium dioxide.

CLINICAL PHARMACOLOGY

Kerlone is a β_1-selective (cardioselective) adrenergic receptor blocking agent that has weak membrane-stabilizing activity and no intrinsic sympathomimetic (partial agonist) activity. The preferential effect on β_1 receptors is not absolute, however, and some inhibitory effects on β_2 receptors (found chiefly in the bronchial and vascular musculature) can be expected at higher doses.

Pharmacokinetics and metabolism: In man, absorption of an oral dose is complete. There is a small and consistent first-pass effect resulting in an absolute bioavailability of 89% ± 5% that is unaffected by the concomitant ingestion of food or alcohol. Mean peak blood concentrations of 21.6 ng/ml (range 16.3 to 27.9 ng/ml) are reached between 1.5 and 6 (mean about 3) hours after a single oral dose, in healthy volunteers, of 10 mg of Kerlone. Peak concentrations for 20-mg and 40-mg doses are 2 and 4 times that of a 10-mg dose and have been shown to be linear over the dose range of 5 to 40 mg. The peak to trough ratio of plasma concentrations over 24 hours is 2.7. The mean elimination half-life in various studies in normal volunteers ranged from about 14 to 22 hours after single oral doses and is similar in chronic dosing. Steady state plasma concentrations are attained after 5 to 7 days with once-daily dosing in persons with normal renal function.

Kerlone is approximately 50% bound to plasma proteins. It is eliminated primarily by liver metabolism and secondarily by renal excretion. Following oral administration, greater than 80% of a dose is recovered in the urine as betaxolol and its metabolites. Approximately 15% of the dose administered is excreted as unchanged drug, the remainder being metabolites whose contribution to the clinical effect is negligible.

Steady state studies in normal volunteers and hypertensive patients found no important differences in kinetics. In patients with hepatic disease, elimination half-life was prolonged by about 33%, but clearance was unchanged, leading to little change in AUC. Dosage reductions have not routinely been necessary in these patients. In patients with chronic renal failure undergoing dialysis, mean elimination half-life was approximately doubled, as was AUC, indicating the need for a lower initial dosage (5 mg) in these patients. The clearance of betaxolol by hemodialysis was 0.015 L/h/kg and by peritoneal dialysis, 0.010 L/h/kg. In one study (n=8), patients with stable renal failure, not on dialysis, with mean creatinine clearance of 27 ml/min showed slight increases in elimination half-life and AUC, but no change in C_{max}. In a second study of 30 hypertensive patients with mild to severe renal impairment, there was a reduction in clearance of betaxolol with increasing degrees of renal insufficiency. Inulin clearance (mL/min/1.73 m^2) ranged from 70 to 107 in 7 patients with mild impairment, 41 to 69 in 14 patients with moderate impairment, and 8 to 37 in 9 patients with severe impairment. Clearance following oral dosing was reduced significantly in patients with moderate and severe renal impairment (26% and 35%, respectively) when compared with those with mildly impaired renal function. In the severely impaired group, the mean C_{max} and the mean elimination half-life tended to increase (28% and 24%, respectively) when compared with the mildly impaired group. A starting dose of 5 mg is recommended in patients with severe renal impairment. (See *Dosage and Administration.*)

Studies in elderly patients (n=10) gave inconsistent results but suggest some impairment of elimination, with one small study (n=4) finding a mean half-life of 30 hours. A starting dose of 5 mg is suggested in older patients.

Pharmacodynamics: Clinical pharmacology studies have demonstrated the beta-adrenergic receptor blocking activity of Kerlone by (1) reduction in resting and exercise heart rate, cardiac output, and cardiac work load, (2) reduction of systolic and diastolic blood pressure at rest and during exercise, (3) inhibition of isoproterenol-induced tachycardia, and (4) reduction of reflex orthostatic tachycardia.

The β_1 selectivity of Kerlone in man was shown in three ways: (1) In normal subjects, 10- and 40-mg oral doses of Kerlone, which reduced resting heart rate at least as much as 40 mg of propranolol, produced less inhibition of isoproterenol-induced increases in forearm blood flow and finger tremor than propranolol. In this study, 10 mg of Kerlone was at least comparable to 50 mg of atenolol. Both doses of Kerlone, and the one dose of atenolol, however, had more effect on the isoproterenol-induced changes than placebo (indicating some β_2 effect at clinical doses) and the higher dose of Kerlone was more inhibitory than the lower. (2) In normal subjects, single intravenous doses of betaxolol and propranolol, which produced equal effects on exercise-induced tachycardia, had differing effects on insulin-induced hypoglycemia, with propranolol, but not betaxolol, prolonging the hypoglycemia compared with placebo. Neither drug affected the maximum extent of the hypoglycemic response. (3) In a single-blind crossover study in asthmatics (n=10), intravenous infusion over 30 minutes of low doses of betaxolol (1.5 mg) and propranolol (2 mg) had similar effects on resting heart rate but had differing effects on FEV_1 and forced vital capacity, with propranolol causing statistically significant (10% to 20%) reductions from baseline in mean values for both parameters while betaxolol had no effect on mean values. While blood levels were not measured, the dose of betaxolol used in this study would be expected to produce blood concentrations, at the time of the pulmonary function studies, considerably lower than those achieved during antihypertensive therapy with recommended doses of Kerlone. In a randomized double-blind, placebo-controlled crossover (4×4 Latin Square) study in 10 asthmatics, betaxolol (about 5 or 10 mg IV) had little effect on isoproterenol-induced increases in FEV_1; in contrast, propranolol (about 7 mg IV) inhibited the response.

Consistent with its negative chronotropic effect, due to beta-blockade of the SA node, and lack of intrinsic sympathomimetic activity, Kerlone increases sinus cycle length and sinus node recovery time. Conduction in the AV node is also prolonged.

Significant reductions in blood pressure and heart rate were observed 24 hours after dosing in double-blind, placebo-controlled trials with doses of 5 to 40 mg administered once daily. The antihypertensive response to betaxolol was similar at peak blood levels (3 to 4 hours) and at trough (24 hours). In a large randomized, parallel dose-response study of 5, 10, and 20 mg, the antihypertensive effects of the 5-mg dose were roughly half of the effects of the 20-mg dose (after adjustment for placebo effects) and the 10-mg dose gave more than 80% of the antihypertensive response to the 20-mg dose. The effect of increasing the dose from 10 mg to 20 mg was thus small. In this study, while the antihypertensive response to betaxolol showed a dose-response relationship, the heart rate response (reduction in HR) was not dose related. In other trials, there was little evidence of a greater antihypertensive response to 40 mg than to 20 mg. The maximum effect of each dose was achieved within 1 or 2 weeks. In comparative trials against propranolol, atenolol, and chlorthalidone, betaxolol appeared to be at least as effective as the comparative agent.

Kerlone has been studied in combination with thiazide-type diuretics and the blood pressure effects of the combination appear additive. Kerlone has also been used concurrently with methyldopa, hydralazine, and prazosin.

The mechanism of the antihypertensive effects of beta-adrenergic receptor blocking agents has not been established. Several possible mechanisms have been proposed, however, including: (1) competitive antagonism of catecholamines at peripheral (especially cardiac) adrenergic-neuronal sites, leading to decreased cardiac output, (2) a central effect leading to reduced sympathetic outflow to the periphery, and (3) suppression of renin activity.

The results from long-term studies have not shown any diminution of the antihypertensive effect of Kerlone with prolonged use.

INDICATIONS AND USAGE

Kerlone is indicated in the management of hypertension. It may be used alone or concomitantly with other antihypertensive agents, particularly thiazide-type diuretics.

CONTRAINDICATIONS

Kerlone is contraindicated in patients with known hypersensitivity to the drug.

Kerlone is contraindicated in patients with sinus bradycardia, heart block greater than first degree, cardiogenic shock, and overt cardiac failure (see *Warnings*).

WARNINGS

Cardiac failure: Sympathetic stimulation may be a vital component supporting circulatory function in congestive heart failure, and beta-adrenergic receptor blockade carries the potential hazard of further depressing myocardial contractility and precipitating more severe heart failure. In hypertensive patients who have congestive heart failure controlled by digitalis and diuretics, beta-blockers should be administered cautiously. Both digitalis and beta-adrenergic receptor blocking agents slow AV conduction.

In patients without a history of cardiac failure: Continued depression of the myocardium with beta-blocking agents over a period of time can, in some cases, lead to cardiac failure. Therefore, at the first sign or symptom of cardiac failure, discontinuation of Kerlone should be considered. In some cases beta-blocker therapy can be continued while cardiac failure is treated with cardiac glycosides, diuretics, and other agents, as appropriate.

Exacerbation of angina pectoris upon withdrawal: Abrupt cessation of therapy with certain beta-blocking agents in patients with coronary artery disease has been followed by exacerbations of angina pectoris and, in some cases, myocardial infarction has been reported. Therefore, such patients should be warned against interruption of therapy without the physician's advice. Even in the absence of overt angina pectoris, when discontinuation of Kerlone is planned, the patient should be carefully observed and therapy should be reinstituted, at least temporarily, if withdrawal symptoms occur.

Bronchospastic diseases: PATIENTS WITH BRONCHOSPASTIC DISEASE SHOULD NOT IN GENERAL RECEIVE BETA-BLOCKERS. Because of its relative β_1 selectivity (cardioselectivity), low doses of Kerlone may be used with caution in patients with bronchospastic disease who do not respond to or cannot tolerate alternative treatment. Since β_1 selectivity is not absolute and is inversely related to dose, the lowest possible dose of Kerlone should be used (5 to 10 mg once daily) and a bronchodilator should be made available. If dosage must be increased, divided dosage should be considered to avoid the higher peak blood levels associated with once-daily dosing.

Anesthesia and major surgery: The necessity, or desirability, of withdrawal of a beta-blocking therapy prior to major surgery is controversial. Beta-adrenergic receptor blockade impairs the ability of the heart to respond to beta-adrenergically mediated reflex stimuli. While this might be of benefit in preventing arrhythmic response, the risk of excessive myocardial depression during general anesthesia may be increased and difficulty in restarting and maintaining the heart beat has been reported with beta-blockers. If treatment is continued, particular care should be taken when using anesthetic agents which depress the myocardium, such as ether, cyclopropane, and trichloroethylene, and it is prudent to use the lowest possible dose of Kerlone. Kerlone, like other beta-blockers, is a competitive inhibitor of beta-receptor agonists and its effect on the heart can be reversed by cautious administration of such agents (eg, dobutamine or isoproterenol—see *Overdosage*). Manifestations of excessive vagal tone (eg, profound bradycardia, hypotension) may be corrected with atropine 1 to 3 mg IV in divided doses.

Diabetes and hypoglycemia: Beta-blockers should be used with caution in diabetic patients. Beta-blockers may mask tachycardia occurring with hypoglycemia (patients should be warned of this), although other manifestations such as dizziness and sweating may not be significantly affected. Unlike nonselective beta-blockers, Kerlone does not prolong insulin-induced hypoglycemia.

Thyrotoxicosis: Beta-adrenergic blockade may mask certain clinical signs of hyperthyroidism (eg, tachycardia). Abrupt withdrawal of beta-blockade might precipitate a thyroid storm; therefore, patients known or suspected of being thyrotoxic from whom Kerlone is to be withdrawn should be monitored closely (see *Dosage and Administration: Cessation of therapy*).

PRECAUTIONS

General: Beta-adrenoceptor blockade can cause reduction of intraocular pressure. Since betaxolol hydrochloride is marketed as an ophthalmic solution for treatment of glaucoma, patients should be told that Kerlone may interfere with the glaucoma-screening test. Withdrawal may lead to a return of increased intraocular pressure. Patients receiving beta-adrenergic blocking agents orally and beta-blocking ophthalmic solutions should be observed for potential additive effects either on the intraocular pressure or on the known systemic effects of beta-blockade.

Impaired hepatic or renal function: Kerlone is primarily metabolized in the liver to metabolites that are inactive and then excreted by the kidneys; clearance is somewhat reduced in patients with renal failure but little changed in patients with hepatic disease. Dosage reductions have not routinely been necessary when hepatic insufficiency is present (see *Dosage and Administration*) but patients should be observed. Patients with severe renal impairment and those on dialysis require a reduced dose. (See *Dosage and Administration.*)

Information for patients: Patients, especially those with evidence of coronary artery insufficiency, should be warned against interruption or discontinuation of Kerlone therapy without the physician's advice.

Although cardiac failure rarely occurs in appropriately selected patients, patients being treated with beta-adrenergic blocking agents should be advised to consult a physician at the first sign or symptom of failure.

Patients should know how they react to this medicine before they operate automobiles and machinery or engage in other tasks requiring alertness. Patients should contact their physician if any difficulty in breathing occurs, and before surgery of any type. Patients should inform their physicians or dentists that they are taking Kerlone. Patients with diabetes

Continued on next page

Searle—Cont.

should be warned that beta-blockers may mask tachycardia occurring with hypoglycemia.

Drug interactions: The following drugs have been coadministered with Kerlone and have not altered its pharmacokinetics: cimetidine, nifedipine, chlorthalidone, and hydrochlorothiazide. Concomitant administration of Kerlone with the oral anticoagulant warfarin has been shown not to potentiate the anticoagulant effect of warfarin.

Catecholamine-depleting drugs (eg, reserpine) may have an additive effect when given with beta-blocking agents. Patients treated with a beta-adrenergic receptor blocking agent plus a catecholamine depletor should therefore be closely observed for evidence of hypotension or marked bradycardia, which may produce vertigo, syncope, or postural hypotension.

Should it be decided to discontinue therapy in patients receiving beta-blockers and clonidine concurrently, the beta-blocker should be discontinued slowly over several days before the gradual withdrawal of clonidine.

Literature reports suggest that oral calcium antagonists may be used in combination with beta-adrenergic blocking agents when heart function is normal, but should be avoided in patients with impaired cardiac function. Hypotension, AV conduction disturbances, and left ventricular failure have been reported in some patients receiving beta-adrenergic blocking agents when an oral calcium antagonist was added to the treatment regimen. Hypotension was more likely to occur if the calcium antagonist were a dihydropyridine derivative, eg, nifedipine, while left ventricular failure and AV conduction disturbances, including complete heart block, were more likely to occur with either verapamil or diltiazem.

Risk of anaphylactic reaction: Although it is known that patients on beta-blockers may be refractory to epinephrine in the treatment of anaphylactic shock, beta-blockers can, in addition, interfere with the modulation of allergic reaction and lead to an increased severity and/or frequency of attacks. Severe allergic reactions including anaphylaxis have been reported in patients exposed to a variety of allergens either by repeated challenge, or accidental contact, and with diagnostic or therapeutic agents while receiving beta-blockers. Such patients may be unresponsive to the usual doses of epinephrine used to treat allergic reaction.

Carcinogenesis, mutagenesis, impairment of fertility: Lifetime studies with betaxolol HCl in mice at oral dosages of 6, 20, and 60 mg/kg/day (up to 90 × the maximum recommended human dose [MRHD] based on 60-kg body weight) and in rats at 3, 12, or 48 mg/kg/day (up to 72 × MRHD) showed no evidence of a carcinogenic effect. In a variety of *in vitro* and *in vivo* bacterial and mammalian cell assays, betaxolol HCl was nonmutagenic. Betaxolol did not adversely affect fertility or mating performance of male or female rats at doses up to 256 mg/kg/day (380 × MRHD).

Pregnancy: Pregnancy Category C. In a study in which pregnant rats received betaxolol at doses of 4, 40, or 400 mg/kg/day, the highest dose (600 × MRHD) was associated with increased postimplantation loss, reduced litter size and weight, and an increased incidence of skeletal and visceral abnormalities, which may have been a consequence of drug-related maternal toxicity. Other than a possible increased incidence of incomplete descent of testes and sternebral reductions, betaxolol at 4 mg/kg/day and 40 mg/kg/day (6 × MRHD and 60 × MRHD) caused no fetal abnormalities. In a second study with a different strain of rat, 200 mg betaxolol/kg/day (300 × MRHD) was associated with maternal toxicity and an increase in resorptions, but no teratogenicity. In a study in which pregnant rabbits received doses of 1, 4, 12, or 36 mg betaxolol/kg/day (54 × MRHD), a marked increase in postimplantation loss occurred at the highest dose, but no drug-related teratogenicity was observed. The rabbit is more sensitive to betaxolol than other species because of higher bioavailability resulting from saturation of the first-pass effect. In a peri- and postnatal study in rats at doses of 4, 32, and 256 mg betaxolol/kg/day (380 ×MRHD), the highest dose was associated with a marked increase in total litter loss within 4 days postpartum. In surviving offspring, growth and development were also affected.

There are no adequate and well-controlled studies in pregnant women. Kerlone should be used during pregnancy only if the potential benefit justifies the potential risk to the fetus.

Nursing mothers: Since Kerlone is excreted in human milk in sufficient amounts to have pharmacological effects in the infant, caution should be exercised when Kerlone is administered to a nursing mother.

Pediatric use: Safety and efficacy in children have not been established.

Elderly patients: Kerlone may produce bradycardia more frequently in elderly patients. In general, patients 65 years of age and older had a higher incidence rate of bradycardia

Table 1	Betaxolol (N=509) 5–40 mg q.d.*	Propranolol (N=73) 40–160 mg b.i.d.	Atenolol (N=75) 25–100 mg q.d.	Placebo (N=109)
Dose Range				
Body System/Adverse Reaction	(%)	(%)	(%)	(%)
Cardiovascular				
Bradycardia				
(heart rate <50 BPM)	8.1	4.1	12.0	0
Symptomatic bradycardia	0.8	1.4	0	0
Edema	1.8	0	0	1.8
Central Nervous System				
Headache	6.5	4.1	5.3	15.6
Dizziness	4.5	11.0	2.7	5.5
Fatigue	2.9	9.6	4.0	0
Lethargy	2.8	4.1	2.7	0.9
Psychiatric				
Insomnia	1.2	8.2	2.7	0
Nervousness	0.8	1.4	2.7	0
Bizarre dreams	1.0	2.7	1.3	0
Depression	0.8	2.7	4.0	0
Autonomic				
Impotence	1.2†	0	0	0
Respiratory				
Dyspnea	2.4	2.7	1.3	0.9
Pharyngitis	2.0	0	4.0	0.9
Rhinitis	1.4	0	4.0	0.9
Upper respiratory infection	2.6	0	0	5.5
Gastrointestinal				
Dyspepsia	4.7	6.8	2.7	0.9
Nausea	1.6	1.4	4.0	0
Diarrhea	2.0	6.8	8.0	0.9
Musculoskeletal				
Chest pain	2.4	1.4	2.7	0.9
Arthralgia	3.1	0	4.0	1.8
Skin				
Rash	1.2	0	0	0

* Five patients received 80 mg q.d.
† N = 336 males; impotence is a known possible adverse effect of this pharmacological class.

Table 2	Betaxolol (N=155) 20–40 mg q.d.	Atenolol (N=81) 100 mg q.d.	Placebo (N=60)
Dose Range			
Body System/Adverse Reaction	(%)	(%)	(%)
Cardiovascular			
Bradycardia			
(heart rate <50 BPM)	5.8	5.0	0
Symptomatic bradycardia	1.9	2.5	0
Palpitation	1.9	3.7	1.7
Edema	1.3	1.2	0
Cold extremities	1.9	0	0
Central Nervous System			
Headache	14.8	9.9	23.3
Dizziness	14.8	17.3	15.0
Fatigue	9.7	18.5	0
Asthenia	7.1	0	16.7
Insomnia	5.0	3.7	3.3
Paresthesia	1.9	2.5	0
Gastrointestinal			
Nausea	5.8	1.2	0
Dyspepsia	3.9	7.4	3.3
Diarrhea	1.9	3.7	0
Musculoskeletal			
Chest pain	7.1	6.2	5.0
Joint pain	5.2	4.9	1.7
Myalgia	3.2	3.7	3.3

(heart rate <50 BPM) than younger patients in U.S. clinical trials. In a double-blind study in Europe, 19 elderly patients (mean age = 82) received betaxolol 20 mg daily. Dosage reduction to 10 mg or discontinuation was required for 6 patients due to bradycardia (See *Dosage and Administration*).

ADVERSE REACTIONS

Most adverse reactions have been mild and transient and are typical of beta-adrenergic blocking agents, eg, bradycardia, fatigue, dyspnea, and lethargy. Withdrawal of therapy in U.S. and European controlled clinical trials has been necessary in about 3.5% of patients, principally because of bradycardia, fatigue, dizziness, headache, and impotence. Frequency estimates of adverse events were derived from controlled studies in which adverse reactions were volunteered and elicited in U.S. studies and volunteered and/or elicited in European studies.

In the U.S., the placebo-controlled hypertension studies lasted for 4 weeks, while the active-controlled hypertension studies had a 22- to 24-week double-blind phase. The following doses were studied: betaxolol—5, 10, 20, and 40 mg once daily; atenolol—25, 50, and 100 mg once daily; and propranolol—40, 80, and 160 mg b.i.d.

Kerlone, like other beta-blockers, has been associated with the development of antinuclear antibodies (ANA). In controlled clinical studies, conversion of ANA from negative to positive occurred in 5.3% of the patients treated with betaxolol, 6.3% of the patients treated with atenolol, 4.9% of the patients treated with propranolol, and 3.2% of the patients treated with placebo.

Betaxolol adverse events reported with a 2% or greater frequency, and selected events with lower frequency, in U.S. controlled studies are:

[See Table 1 above.]

Of the above adverse reactions [listed in Table 1] associated with the use of betaxolol, only bradycardia was clearly dose related, but there was a suggestion of dose relatedness for fatigue, lethargy, and dyspepsia.

In Europe, the placebo-controlled study lasted for 4 weeks, while the comparative studies had a 4- to 52-week double-blind phase. The following doses were studied: betaxolol 20 and 40 mg once daily and atenolol 100 mg once daily.

From European controlled hypertension clinical trials, the following adverse events reported by 2% or more patients and selected events with lower frequency are presented:

[See Table 2 above.]

The only adverse event whose frequency clearly rose with increasing dose was bradycardia. Elderly patients were especially susceptible to bradycardia, which in some cases responded to dose-reduction (see *Precautions*).

The following selected (potentially important) adverse events have been reported at an incidence of less than 2% in U.S. controlled and open, long-term clinical studies, European controlled clinical trials, or in marketing experience. It is not known whether a causal relationship exists between betaxolol and these events; they are listed to alert the physician to a possible relationship:

Autonomic: flushing, salivation, sweating.
Body as a whole: allergy, fever, malaise, pain, rigors.
Cardiovascular: angina pectoris, arrhythmia, atrioventricular block, heart failure, hypertension, hypotension, myocardial infarction, thrombosis, syncope.
Central and peripheral nervous system: ataxia, neuralgia, neuropathy, numbness, speech disorder, stupor, tremor, twitching.
Gastrointestinal: anorexia, constipation, dry mouth, increased appetite, mouth ulceration, rectal disorders, vomiting, dysphagia.
Hearing and vestibular: earache, labyrinth disorders, tinnitus, deafness.
Hematologic: anemia, leucocytosis, lymphadenopathy, purpura, thrombocytopenia.
Liver and biliary: increased AST, increased ALT.
Metabolic and nutritional: acidosis, diabetes, hypercholesterolemia, hyperglycemia, hyperkalemia, hyperlipemia, hyperuricemia, hypokalemia, weight gain, weight loss, thirst, increased LDH.
Musculoskeletal: arthropathy, neck pain, muscle cramps, tendonitis.
Psychiatric: abnormal thinking, amnesia, impaired concentration, confusion, emotional lability, hallucinations, decreased libido.
Reproductive disorders: Female: breast pain, breast fibroadenosis, menstrual disorder; Male: Peyronie's disease, prostatitis.
Respiratory: bronchitis, bronchospasm, cough, epistaxis, flu, pneumonia, sinusitis.
Skin: alopecia, eczema, erythematous rash, hypertrichosis, pruritus, skin disorders.
Special senses: abnormal taste, taste loss.
Urinary system: cystitis, dysuria, micturition disorder, oliguria, proteinuria, abnormal renal function, renal pain.
Vascular: cerebrovascular disorder, intermittent claudication, leg cramps, peripheral ischemia, thrombophlebitis.
Vision: abnormal lacrimation, abnormal vision, blepharitis, ocular hemorrhage, conjunctivitis, dry eyes, iritis, cataract, scotoma.

Potential adverse effects: Although not reported in clinical studies with betaxolol, a variety of adverse effects have been reported with other beta-adrenergic blocking agents and may be considered potential adverse effects of betaxolol:
Central nervous system: Reversible mental depression progressing to catatonia, an acute reversible syndrome characterized by disorientation for time and place, short-term memory loss, emotional lability with slightly clouded sensorium, and decreased performance on neuropsychometric tests.
Allergic: Fever combined with aching and sore throat, laryngospasm, respiratory distress.
Hematologic: Agranulocytosis, thrombocytopenic purpura, and nonthrombocytopenic purpura.
Gastrointestinal: Mesenteric arterial thrombosis, ischemic colitis.
Miscellaneous: Raynaud's phenomena. There have been reports of skin rashes and/or dry eyes associated with the use of beta-adrenergic blocking drugs. The reported incidence is small, and in most cases, the symptoms have cleared when treatment was withdrawn. Discontinuation of the drug should be considered if any such reaction is not otherwise explicable. Patients should be closely monitored following cessation of therapy.
The oculomucocutaneous syndrome associated with the beta-blocker practolol has not been reported with Kerlone during investigational use and extensive foreign experience. However, dry eyes have been reported.

OVERDOSAGE

No specific information on emergency treatment of overdosage with Kerlone is available. The most common effects expected are bradycardia, congestive heart failure, hypotension, bronchospasm, and hypoglycemia. In one acute overdosage of betaxolol, a 16-year-old female recovered fully after ingesting 460 mg.
Oral LD_{50}s are 350 to 400 mg betaxolol/kg in mice and 860 to 980 mg/kg in rats.
In the case of overdosage, treatment with Kerlone should be stopped and the patient carefully observed. Hemodialysis or peritoneal dialysis does not remove substantial amounts of the drug. In addition to gastric lavage, the following therapeutic measures are suggested if warranted:
Hypotension: Use sympathomimetic pressor drug therapy, such as dopamine, dobutamine, or norepinephrine. In refractory cases of overdosage of other beta-blockers, the use of glucagon hydrochloride has been reported to be useful.
Bradycardia: Atropine should be administered. If there is no response to vagal blockade, isoproterenol should be administered cautiously. In refractory cases the use of a transvenous cardiac pacemaker may be considered.
Acute cardiac failure: Conventional therapy including digitalis, diuretics, and oxygen should be instituted immediately.
Bronchospasm: Use a β_2-agonist. Additional therapy with aminophylline may be considered.
Heart block (2nd- or 3rd-degree): Use isoproterenol or a transvenous cardiac pacemaker.

DOSAGE AND ADMINISTRATION

The initial dose of Kerlone in hypertension is ordinarily 10 mg once daily either alone or added to diuretic therapy. The full antihypertensive effect is usually seen within 7 to 14 days. If the desired response is not achieved the dose can be doubled after 7 to 14 days. Increasing the dose beyond 20 mg has not been shown to produce a statistically significant additional antihypertensive effect; but the 40-mg dose has been studied and is well tolerated. An increased effect (reduction) on heart rate should be anticipated with increasing dosage. If monotherapy with Kerlone does not produce the desired response, the addition of a diuretic agent or other antihypertensive should be considered (see *Drug interactions*).

Dosage adjustments for specific patients

Patients with renal failure: In patients with renal impairment, clearance of betaxolol declines with decreasing renal function.
In patients with severe renal impairment and those undergoing dialysis the initial dose of Kerlone is 5 mg once daily. If the desired response is not achieved, dosage may be increased by 5 mg/day increments every 2 weeks to a maximum dose of 20 mg/day.
Patients with hepatic disease: Patients with hepatic disease do not have significantly altered clearance. Dosage adjustments are not routinely needed.
Elderly patients: Consideration should be given to reduction in the starting dose to 5 mg in elderly patients. These patients are especially prone to beta-blocker–induced bradycardia, which appears to be dose related and sometimes responds to reductions in dose.
Cessation of therapy: If withdrawal of Kerlone therapy is planned, it should be achieved gradually over a period of about 2 weeks. Patients should be carefully observed and advised to limit physical activity to a minimum.

HOW SUPPLIED

Kerlone 10-mg tablets are round, white, film coated, with KERLONE 10 debossed on one side and scored on the other, supplied as:

NDC Number	Size
0025-5101-31	bottle of 100
0025-5101-34	carton of 100 unit dose

Kerlone 20-mg tablets are round, white, film coated, with KERLONE 20 debossed on one side and β on the other, supplied as:

NDC Number	Size
0025-5201-31	bottle of 100
0025-5201-34	carton of 100 unit dose

Store at controlled room temperature 15°-30°C (59°-86°F).
Caution: Federal law prohibits dispensing without prescription.

Manufactured and distributed by
G.D. Searle & Co.
Chicago, IL 60680
by agreement with
Lorex Pharmaceuticals
Skokie, IL

Kerlone is a registered trademark of Synthelabo.

1/24/95 • A05426

Shown in Product Identification Guide, page 335

LOMOTIL® Liquid Ⓒ
LOMOTIL® Tablets Ⓒ
[lō-mō'til]
(diphenoxylate hydrochloride with atropine sulfate)

DESCRIPTION

Each Lomotil tablet and each 5 ml of Lomotil liquid for oral use contains:
diphenoxylate hydrochloride .... 2.5 mg
(Warning—May be habit forming.)
atropine sulfate .... 0.025 mg

Diphenoxylate hydrochloride, an antidiarrheal, is ethyl 1-(3-cyano-3,3-diphenylpropyl)-4-phenylisonipecotate monohydrochloride and has the following structural formula:

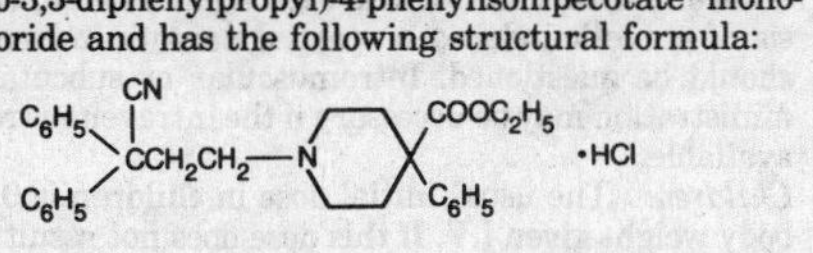

Atropine sulfate, an anticholinergic, is endo-(±)-α-(hydroxymethyl) benzeneacetic acid 8-methyl-8-azabicyclo[3.2.1] oct-3-yl ester sulfate (2:1) (salt) monohydrate and has the following structural formula:

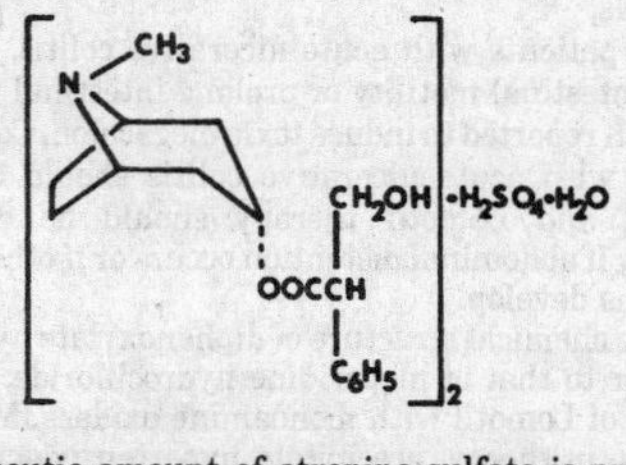

A subtherapeutic amount of atropine sulfate is present to discourage deliberate overdosage.
Inactive ingredients of Lomotil tablets include acacia, corn starch, magnesium stearate, sorbitol, sucrose, and talc. Inactive ingredients of Lomotil liquid include cherry flavor, citric acid, ethyl alcohol 15%, FD&C Yellow No. 6, glycerin, sodium phosphate, sorbitol, and water.

CLINICAL PHARMACOLOGY

Diphenoxylate is rapidly and extensively metabolized in man by ester hydrolysis to diphenoxylic acid (difenoxine), which is biologically active and the major metabolite in the blood. After a 5-mg oral dose of carbon-14 labeled diphenoxylate hydrochloride in ethanolic solution was given to three healthy volunteers, an average of 14% of the drug plus its metabolites was excreted in the urine and 49% in the feces over a four-day period. Urinary excretion of the unmetabolized drug constituted less than 1% of the dose, and diphenoxylic acid plus its glucuronide conjugate constituted about 6% of the dose. In a 16-subject crossover bioavailability study, a linear relationship in the dose range of 2.5 to 10 mg was found between the dose of diphenoxylate hydrochloride (given as Lomotil liquid) and the peak plasma concentration, the area under the plasma concentration-time curve, and the amount of diphenoxylic acid excreted in the urine. In the same study the bioavailability of the tablet compared with an equal dose of the liquid was approximately 90%. The average peak plasma concentration of diphenoxylic acid following ingestion of four 2.5-mg tablets was 163 ng/ml at about 2 hours, and the elimination half-life of diphenoxylic acid was approximately 12 to 14 hours.
In dogs, diphenoxylate hydrochloride has a direct effect on circular smooth muscle of the bowel that conceivably results in segmentation and prolongation of gastrointestinal transit time. The clinical antidiarrheal action of diphenoxylate hydrochloride may thus be a consequence of enhanced segmentation that allows increased contact of the intraluminal contents with the intestinal mucosa.

INDICATIONS AND USAGE

Lomotil is effective as adjunctive therapy in the management of diarrhea.

CONTRAINDICATIONS

Lomotil is contraindicated in patients with
1. Known hypersensitivity to diphenoxylate or atropine.
2. Obstructive jaundice.
3. Diarrhea associated with pseudomembranous enterocolitis or enterotoxin-producing bacteria.

WARNINGS

LOMOTIL IS *NOT* AN INNOCUOUS DRUG AND DOSAGE RECOMMENDATIONS SHOULD BE STRICTLY ADHERED TO, ESPECIALLY IN CHILDREN. LOMOTIL IS NOT RECOMMENDED FOR CHILDREN UNDER 2 YEARS OF AGE. OVERDOSAGE MAY RESULT IN SEVERE RESPIRATORY DEPRESSION AND COMA, POSSIBLY LEADING TO PERMANENT BRAIN DAMAGE OR DEATH (SEE *OVERDOSAGE*). THEREFORE, KEEP THIS MEDICATION OUT OF THE REACH OF CHILDREN.
THE USE OF LOMOTIL SHOULD BE ACCOMPANIED BY APPROPRIATE FLUID AND ELECTROLYTE THERAPY, WHEN INDICATED. IF SEVERE DEHYDRATION OR ELECTROLYTE IMBALANCE IS PRESENT, LOMOTIL SHOULD BE WITHHELD UNTIL APPROPRIATE CORRECTIVE THERAPY HAS BEEN INITIATED. DRUG-INDUCED INHIBITION OF PERISTALSIS MAY RESULT IN FLUID RETENTION IN THE INTESTINE, WHICH MAY FURTHER AGGRAVATE DEHYDRATION AND ELECTROLYTE IMBALANCE.
LOMOTIL SHOULD BE USED WITH SPECIAL CAUTION IN YOUNG CHILDREN BECAUSE THIS AGE GROUP MAY BE PREDISPOSED TO DELAYED DIPHENOXYLATE TOXICITY AND BECAUSE OF THE GREATER VARIABILITY OF RESPONSE IN THIS AGE GROUP.
Antiperistaltic agents may prolong and/or worsen diarrhea associated with organisms that penetrate the intestinal mucosa (toxigenic *E. coli*, *Salmonella*, *Shigella*), and pseudomembranous enterocolitis associated with broad-spectrum

Continued on next page

Searle—Cont.

antibiotics. Antiperistaltic agents should not be used in these conditions.

In some patients with acute ulcerative colitis, agents that inhibit intestinal motility or prolong intestinal transit time have been reported to induce toxic megacolon. Consequently, patients with acute ulcerative colitis should be carefully observed and Lomotil therapy should be discontinued promptly if abdominal distention occurs or if other untoward symptoms develop.

Since the chemical structure of diphenoxylate hydrochloride is similar to that of meperidine hydrochloride, the concurrent use of Lomotil with monoamine oxidase (MAO) inhibitors may, in theory, precipitate hypertensive crisis.

Lomotil should be used with extreme caution in patients with advanced hepatorenal disease and in all patients with abnormal liver function since hepatic coma may be precipitated.

Diphenoxylate hydrochloride may potentiate the action of barbiturates, tranquilizers, and alcohol. Therefore, the patient should be closely observed when any of these are used concomitantly.

PRECAUTIONS

General: Since a subtherapeutic dose of atropine has been added to the diphenoxylate hydrochloride, consideration should be given to the precautions relating to the use of atropine. In children, Lomotil should be used with caution since signs of atropinism may occur even with recommended doses, particularly in patients with Down's syndrome.

Information for patients: INFORM THE PATIENT (PARENT OR GUARDIAN) NOT TO EXCEED THE RECOMMENDED DOSAGE AND TO KEEP LOMOTIL OUT OF THE REACH OF CHILDREN AND IN A CHILD-RESISTANT CONTAINER. INFORM THE PATIENT OF THE CONSEQUENCES OF OVERDOSAGE, INCLUDING SEVERE RESPIRATORY DEPRESSION AND COMA, POSSIBLY LEADING TO PERMANENT BRAIN DAMAGE OR DEATH. Lomotil may produce drowsiness or dizziness. The patient should be cautioned regarding activities requiring mental alertness, such as driving or operating dangerous machinery. Potentiation of the action of alcohol, barbiturates, and tranquilizers with concomitant use of Lomotil should be explained to the patient. The physician should also provide the patient with other information in this labeling, as appropriate.

Drug interactions: Known drug interactions include barbiturates, tranquilizers, and alcohol. Lomotil may interact with MAO inhibitors (see *Warnings*).

In studies with male rats, diphenoxylate hydrochloride was found to inhibit the hepatic microsomal enzyme system at a dose of 2 mg/kg/day. Therefore, diphenoxylate has the potential to prolong the biological half-lives of drugs for which the rate of elimination is dependent on the microsomal drug metabolizing enzyme system.

Carcinogenesis, mutagenesis, impairment of fertility: No long-term study in animals has been performed to evaluate carcinogenic potential. Diphenoxylate hydrochloride was administered to male and female rats in their diets to provide dose levels of 4 and 20 mg/kg/day throughout a three-litter reproduction study. At 50 times the human dose (20 mg/kg/day), female weight gain was reduced and there was a marked effect on fertility as only 4 of 27 females became pregnant in three test breedings. The relevance of this finding to usage of Lomotil in humans is unknown.

Pregnancy: Pregnancy Category C. Diphenoxylate hydrochloride has been shown to have an effect on fertility in rats when given in doses 50 times the human dose (see above discussion). Other findings in this study include a decrease in maternal weight gain of 30% at 20 mg/kg/day and of 10% at 4 mg/kg/day. At 10 times the human dose (4 mg/kg/day), average litter size was slightly reduced.

Teratology studies were conducted in rats, rabbits, and mice with diphenoxylate hydrochloride at oral doses of 0.4 to 20 mg/kg/day. Due to experimental design and small numbers of litters, embryotoxic, fetotoxic, or teratogenic effects cannot be adequately assessed. However, examination of the available fetuses did not reveal any indication of teratogenicity.

There are no adequate and well-controlled studies in pregnant women. Lomotil should be used during pregnancy only if the anticipated benefit justifies the potential risk to the fetus.

Nursing mothers: Caution should be exercised when Lomotil is administered to a nursing woman, since the physicochemical characteristics of the major metabolite, diphenoxylic acid, are such that it may be excreted in breast milk and since it is known that atropine is excreted in breast milk.

Pediatric use: Lomotil may be used as an adjunct to the treatment of diarrhea but should be accompanied by appropriate fluid and electrolyte therapy, if needed. LOMOTIL IS NOT RECOMMENDED FOR CHILDREN UNDER 2 YEARS OF AGE. Lomotil should be used with special caution in young children because of the greater variability of

response in this age group. See *Warnings* and *Dosage and Administration.* In case of accidental ingestion by children, see *Overdosage* for recommended treatment.

ADVERSE REACTIONS

At *therapeutic* doses, the following have been reported; they are listed in decreasing order of severity, but not of frequency:

Nervous system: numbness of extremities, euphoria, depression, malaise/lethargy, confusion, sedation/drowsiness, dizziness, restlessness, headache.

Allergic: anaphylaxis, angioneurotic edema, urticaria, swelling of the gums, pruritus.

Gastrointestinal system: toxic megacolon, paralytic ileus, pancreatitis, vomiting, nausea, anorexia, abdominal discomfort.

The following atropine sulfate effects are listed in decreasing order of severity, but not of frequency: hyperthermia, tachycardia, urinary retention, flushing, dryness of the skin and mucous membranes. These effects may occur, especially in children.

THIS MEDICATION SHOULD BE KEPT IN A CHILD-RESISTANT CONTAINER AND OUT OF THE REACH OF CHILDREN SINCE AN OVERDOSAGE MAY RESULT IN SEVERE RESPIRATORY DEPRESSION AND COMA, POSSIBLY LEADING TO PERMANENT BRAIN DAMAGE OR DEATH.

DRUG ABUSE AND DEPENDENCE

Controlled substance: Lomotil is classified as a Schedule V controlled substance by federal regulation. Diphenoxylate hydrochloride is chemically related to the narcotic analgesic meperidine.

Drug abuse and dependence: In doses used for the treatment of diarrhea, whether acute or chronic, diphenoxylate has not produced addiction.

Diphenoxylate hydrochloride is devoid of morphine-like subjective effects at therapeutic doses. At high doses it exhibits codeine-like subjective effects. The dose which produces antidiarrheal action is widely separated from the dose which causes central nervous system effects. The insolubility of diphenoxylate hydrochloride in commonly available aqueous media precludes intravenous self-administration. A dose of 100 to 300 mg/day, which is equivalent to 40 to 120 tablets, administered to humans for 40 to 70 days, produced opiate withdrawal symptoms. Since addiction to diphenoxylate hydrochloride is possible at high doses, the recommended dosage should not be exceeded.

OVERDOSAGE

RECOMMENDED DOSAGE SCHEDULES SHOULD BE STRICTLY FOLLOWED. THIS MEDICATION SHOULD BE KEPT IN A CHILD-RESISTANT CONTAINER AND OUT OF THE REACH OF CHILDREN, SINCE AN OVERDOSAGE MAY RESULT IN SEVERE, EVEN FATAL, RESPIRATORY DEPRESSION.

Diagnosis: Initial signs of overdosage may include dryness of the skin and mucous membranes, mydriasis, restlessness, flushing, hyperthermia, and tachycardia followed by lethargy or coma, hypotonic reflexes, nystagmus, pinpoint pupils, and respiratory depression. Respiratory depression may be evidenced as late as 30 hours after ingestion and may recur despite an initial response to narcotic antagonists. TREAT ALL POSSIBLE LOMOTIL OVERDOSAGES AS SERIOUS AND MAINTAIN MEDICAL OBSERVATION FOR AT LEAST 48 HOURS, PREFERABLY UNDER CONTINUOUS HOSPITAL CARE.

Treatment: In the event of overdose, induction of vomiting, gastric lavage, establishment of a patent airway, and possibly mechanically assisted respiration are advised. *In vitro* and animal studies indicate that activated charcoal may significantly decrease the bioavailability of diphenoxylate. In noncomatose patients, a slurry of 100 g of activated charcoal can be administered immediately after the induction of vomiting or gastric lavage.

A pure narcotic antagonist (eg, naloxone) should be used in the treatment of respiratory depression caused by Lomotil. When a narcotic antagonist is administered intravenously, the onset of action is generally apparent within two minutes. It may also be administered subcutaneously or intramuscularly, providing a slightly less rapid onset of action but a more prolonged effect.

To counteract respiratory depression caused by Lomotil overdosage, the following dosage schedule for the narcotic antagonist naloxone hydrochloride should be followed:

Adult dosage: An initial dose of 0.4 mg to 2 mg of naloxone hydrochloride may be administered intravenously. If the desired degree of counteraction and improvement in respiratory function is not obtained, it may be repeated at 2- to 3-minute intervals. If no response is observed after 10 mg of naloxone hydrochloride has been administered, the diagnosis of narcotic-induced or partial narcotic-induced toxicity should be questioned. Intramuscular or subcutaneous administration may be necessary if the intravenous route is not available.

Children: The usual initial dose in children is 0.01 mg/kg body weight given I.V. If this dose does not result in the de-

sired degree of clinical improvement, a subsequent dose of 0.1 mg/kg body weight may be administered. If an I.V. route of administration is not available, naloxone hydrochloride may be administered I.M. or S.C. in divided doses. If necessary, naloxone hydrochloride can be diluted with sterile water for injection.

Following initial improvement of respiratory function, repeated doses of naloxone hydrochloride may be required to counteract recurrent respiratory depression. Supplemental intramuscular doses of naloxone hydrochloride may be utilized to produce a longer-lasting effect.

Since the duration of action of diphenoxylate hydrochloride is longer than that of naloxone hydrochloride, improvement of respiration following administration may be followed by recurrent respiratory depression. Consequently, continuous observation is necessary until the effect of diphenoxylate hydrochloride on respiration has passed. This effect may persist for many hours. The period of observation should extend over at least 48 hours, preferably under continuous hospital care. Although signs of overdosage and respiratory depression may not be evident soon after ingestion of diphenoxylate hydrochloride, respiratory depression may occur from 12 to 30 hours later.

DOSAGE AND ADMINISTRATION

DO NOT EXCEED RECOMMENDED DOSAGE.

Adults: The recommended initial dosage is two Lomotil tablets four times daily or 10 ml (two regular teaspoonfuls) of Lomotil liquid four times daily (20 mg per day). Most patients will require this dosage until initial control has been achieved, after which the dosage may be reduced to meet individual requirements. Control may often be maintained with as little as 5 mg (two tablets or 10 ml of liquid) daily.

Clinical improvement of acute diarrhea is usually observed within 48 hours. If clinical improvement of chronic diarrhea after treatment with a maximum daily dose of 20 mg of diphenoxylate hydrochloride is not observed within 10 days, symptoms are unlikely to be controlled by further administration.

Children: Lomotil is not recommended in children under 2 years of age and should be used with special caution in young children (see *Warnings* and *Precautions*). The nutritional status and degree of dehydration must be considered. In children under 13 years of age, use Lomotil liquid. Do not use Lomotil tablets for this age group.

Only the plastic dropper should be used when measuring Lomotil liquid for administration to children.

Dosage schedule for children: The recommended initial total daily dosage of Lomotil liquid for children is 0.3 to 0.4 mg/kg, administered in four divided doses. The following table provides an *approximate* initial daily dosage recommendation for children.

Age (years)	Approximate weight (kg)	(lb)	Dosage in ml (four times daily)
2	11–14	24–31	1.5–3.0
3	12–16	26–35	2.0–3.0
4	14–20	31–44	2.0–4.0
5	16–23	35–51	2.5–4.5
6–8	17–32	38–71	2.5–5.0
9–12	23–55	51–121	3.5–5.0

These pediatric schedules are the best approximation of an average dose recommendation which may be adjusted downward according to the overall nutritional status and degree of dehydration encountered in the sick child. Reduction of dosage may be made as soon as initial control of symptoms has been achieved. Maintenance dosage may be as low as one-fourth of the initial daily dosage. If no response occurs within 48 hours, Lomotil is unlikely to be effective. KEEP THIS AND ALL MEDICATIONS OUT OF THE REACH OF CHILDREN.

HOW SUPPLIED

Tablets—round, white, with SEARLE debossed on one side and 61 on the other side and containing 2.5 mg of diphenoxylate hydrochloride and 0.025 mg of atropine sulfate, supplied as:

NDC Number	Size
0025-0061-31	bottle of 100
0025-0061-51	bottle of 500
0025-0061-52	bottle of 1,000
0025-0061-55	bottle of 2,500
0025-0061-34	carton of 100 unit dose

Liquid—containing 2.5 mg of diphenoxylate hydrochloride and 0.025 mg of atropine sulfate per 5 ml; bottles of 2 fl oz (NDC Number 0025-0066-02). Dispense only in original container.

A plastic dropper calibrated in increments of ½ ml (¼ mg) with a capacity of 2 ml (1 mg) accompanies each 2-oz bottle of Lomotil liquid. Only this plastic dropper should be used when measuring Lomotil liquid for administration to children.

12/9/93 ● A05758-4
Shown in Product Identification Guide, page 335

MAXAQUIN® ℞
[*măx 'ah-kwĭn*]
(lomefloxacin hydrochloride)
Film-coated Tablets

DESCRIPTION

Maxaquin (lomefloxacin HCl) is a synthetic broad-spectrum antimicrobial agent for oral administration. Lomefloxacin HCl, a difluoroquinolone, is the monohydrochloride salt of (±)-1-ethyl-6,8-difluoro-1,4-dihydro-7-(3-methyl-1-piperazinyl)-4-oxo-3-quinolinecarboxylic acid. Its empirical formula is $C_{17}H_{19}F_2N_3O_3 \cdot HCl$, and its structural formula is:

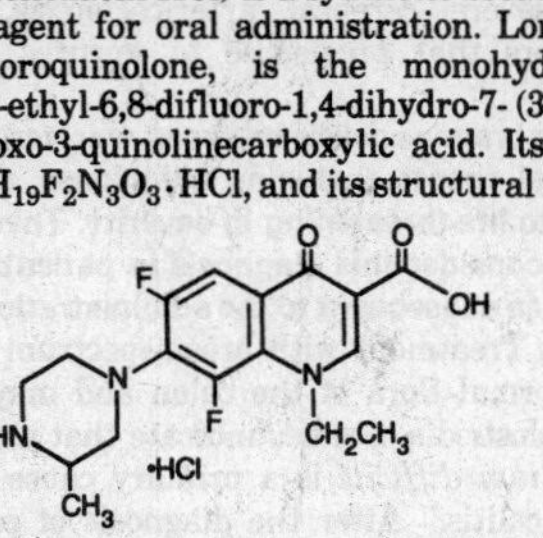

Lomefloxacin HCl is a white to pale yellow powder with a molecular weight of 387.8. It is slightly soluble in water and practically insoluble in alcohol. Lomefloxacin HCl is stable to heat and moisture but is sensitive to light in dilute aqueous solution.
Maxaquin is available as a film-coated tablet formulation containing 400 mg of lomefloxacin base, present as the hydrochloride salt. The base content of the hydrochloride salt is 90.6%. The inactive ingredients are carboxymethylcellulose calcium, hydroxypropyl cellulose, hydroxypropyl methylcellulose, lactose, magnesium stearate, polyethylene glycol, polyoxyl 40 stearate, and titanium dioxide.

CLINICAL PHARMACOLOGY

Pharmacokinetics in healthy volunteers: In 6 fasting healthy male volunteers, approximately 95% to 98% of a single oral dose of lomefloxacin was absorbed. Absorption was rapid following single doses of 200 and 400 mg (T_{max} 0.8 to 1.4 hours). Mean plasma concentration increased proportionally between 100 and 400 mg as shown below.

Dose (mg)	Mean Plasma Concentration (μg/mL)	Area Under Curve (AUC) (μg·h/mL)
100	0.8	5.6
200	1.4	10.9
400	3.2	26.1

In 6 healthy male volunteers administered 400 mg of lomefloxacin on an empty stomach qd for 7 days, the following mean pharmacokinetic parameter values were obtained:

C_{max}	2.8 μg/mL
C_{min}	0.27 μg/mL
$AUC_{0-24\ h}$	25.9 μg·h/mL
T_{max}	1.5 h
$t_{1/2}$	7.75 h

The elimination half-life in 8 subjects with normal renal function was approximately 8 hours. At 24 hours postdose, subjects with normal renal function receiving single doses of 200 or 400 mg had mean plasma lomefloxacin concentrations of 0.10 and 0.24 μg/mL, respectively. Steady-state concentrations were achieved within 48 hours of initiating therapy with one-a-day dosing. There was no drug accumulation with single-daily dosing in patients with normal renal function.
Approximately 65% of an orally administered dose was excreted in the urine as unchanged drug in patients with normal renal function. Following a 400-mg dose of lomefloxacin administered qd for 7 days, the mean urine concentration 4 hours postdose was in excess of 300 μg/mL. The mean urine concentration exceeded 35 μg/mL for at least 24 hours after dosing.
Following a single 400-mg dose, the solubility of lomefloxacin in urine usually exceeded its peak urinary concentration 2- to 6-fold. In this study, urine pH affected the solubility of lomefloxacin with solubilities ranging from 7.8 mg/mL at pH 5.2, to 2.4 mg/mL at pH 6.5, and 3.03 mg/mL at pH 8.12.
The urinary excretion of lomefloxacin was virtually complete within 72 hours after cessation of dosing, with approximately 65% of the dose being recovered as parent drug and 9% as its glucuronide metabolite. The mean renal clearance was 145 mL/min in subjects with normal renal function (GFR = 120 mL/min). This may indicate tubular secretion.
Food effect: When lomefloxacin and food were administered concomitantly, the rate of drug absorption was delayed (T_{max} increased to 2 hours [delayed by 41%], C_{max} decreased by 18%), and the extent of absorption (AUC) was decreased by 12%.
Pharmacokinetics in the geriatric population: In 16 healthy elderly volunteers (61 to 76 years of age) with normal renal function for their age, the half-life of lomefloxacin (mean of 8 hours) and its peak plasma concentration (mean of 4.2 μg/mL) following a single 400-mg dose were similar to those in 8 younger subjects dosed with a single 400-mg dose. Thus, drug absorption appears unaffected in the elderly. Plasma clearance was, however, reduced in this elderly population by approximately 25%, and the AUC was increased by approximately 33%. This slower elimination most likely reflects the decreased renal function normally observed in the geriatric population.
Pharmacokinetics in renally impaired patients: In 8 patients with creatinine clearance (Cl_{Cr}) between 10 and 40 mL/min/1.73 m^2, the mean AUC after a single 400-mg dose of lomefloxacin increased 335% over the AUC demonstrated in patients with a $Cl_{Cr} > 80$ mL/min/1.73 m^2. Also, in these patients, the mean $t_{1/2}$ increased to 21 hours. In 8 patients with $Cl_{Cr} < 10$ mL/min/1.73 m^2, the mean AUC after a single 400-mg dose of lomefloxacin increased 700% over the AUC demonstrated in patients with a $Cl_{Cr} > 80$ mL/min/1.73 m^2. In these patients with $Cl_{Cr} < 10$ mL/min/1.73 m^2, the mean $t_{1/2}$ increased to 45 hours. The plasma clearance of lomefloxacin was closely correlated with creatinine clearance, ranging from 31 mL/min/1.73 m^2 when creatinine clearance was zero to 271 mL/min/1.73 m^2 at a normal creatinine clearance of 110 mL/min/1.73 m^2. Peak lomefloxacin concentrations were not affected by the degree of renal function when single doses of lomefloxacin were administered. Adjustment of dosage schedules for patients with such decreases in renal function is warranted. (See **Dosage and Administration.)**
Pharmacokinetics in patients with cirrhosis: In 12 patients with histologically confirmed cirrhosis, no significant changes in rate or extent of lomefloxacin exposure (C_{max}, T_{max}, $t_{1/2}$, or AUC) were observed when they were administered 400 mg of lomefloxacin as a single dose. No data are available in cirrhotic patients treated with multiple doses of lomefloxacin. Cirrhosis does not appear to reduce the nonrenal clearance of lomefloxacin. There does not appear to be a need for a dosage reduction in cirrhotic patients, provided adequate renal function is present.
Metabolism and pharmacodynamics of lomefloxacin: Lomefloxacin is minimally metabolized although 5 metabolites have been identified in human urine. The glucuronide metabolite is found in the highest concentration and accounts for approximately 9% of the administered dose. The other 4 metabolites together account for <0.5% of the dose.
Approximately 10% of an oral dose was recovered as unchanged drug in the feces.
Serum protein binding of lomefloxacin is approximately 10%.
The following are mean tissue- or fluid-to-plasma ratios of lomefloxacin following oral administration. Studies have not been conducted to assess the penetration of lomefloxacin into human cerebrospinal fluid.

Tissue or Body Fluid	Mean Tissue- or Fluid-to-Plasma Ratio
Bronchial mucosa	2.1
Bronchial secretions	0.6
Prostatic tissue	2.0
Sputum	1.3
Urine	140.0

In two studies including 74 healthy volunteers, the minimal dose of UVA light needed to cause erythema (MED-UVA) was inversely proportional to plasma lomefloxacin concentration. The MED-UVA values (16 hours and 12 hours postdose) were significantly higher than the MED-UVA values 2 hours postdose at steady state. Increasing the interval between lomefloxacin dosing and exposure to UVA light increased the amount of light energy needed for photoreaction.

Microbiology: Lomefloxacin is a bactericidal agent with in vitro activity against a wide range of gram-negative and gram-positive organisms. The bactericidal action of lomefloxacin results from interference with the activity of the bacterial enzyme DNA gyrase, which is needed for the transcription and replication of bacterial DNA. The minimum bactericidal concentration (MBC) generally does not exceed the minimum inhibitory concentration (MIC) by more than a factor of 2, except for staphylococci, which usually have MBCs 2 to 4 times the MIC.
Lomefloxacin has been shown to be active against most strains of the following organisms both in vitro and in clinical infections: (See **Indications and Usage.)**
Gram-positive aerobes
Staphylococcus saprophyticus
Gram-negative aerobes
Citrobacter diversus
Enterobacter cloacae
Escherichia coli
Haemophilus influenzae
Klebsiella pneumoniae
Moraxella (Branhamella) catarrhalis
Proteus mirabilis
Pseudomonas aeruginosa (urinary tract only—See **Indications and Usage** and **Warnings)**
The following in vitro data are available; however, their clinical significance is unknown.
Lomefloxacin exhibits in vitro MICs of 2 μg/mL or less against most strains of the following organisms; however, the safety and effectiveness of lomefloxacin in treating clinical infections due to these organisms have not been established in adequate and well-controlled trials:
Gram-positive aerobes
Staphylococcus aureus (including methicillin-resistant strains)
Staphylococcus epidermidis (including methicillin-resistant strains)
Gram-negative aerobes
Aeromonas hydrophila
Citrobacter freundii
Enterobacter aerogenes
Enterobacter agglomerans
Haemophilus parainfluenzae
Hafnia alvei
Klebsiella oxytoca
Klebsiella ozaenae
Morganella morganii
Proteus vulgaris
Providencia alcalifaciens
Providencia rettgeri
Serratia liquefaciens
Serratia marcescens
Other organisms:
Legionella pneumophila

Beta-lactamase production should have no effect on the in vitro activity of lomefloxacin.
Most group A, B, D, and G streptococci, *Streptococcus pneumoniae, Pseudomonas cepacia, Ureaplasma urealyticum, Mycoplasma hominis,* and anaerobic bacteria are resistant to lomefloxacin.
Lomefloxacin appears slightly less active in vitro when tested at acidic pH. An increase in inoculum size has little effect on the in vitro activity of lomefloxacin. In vitro resistance to lomefloxacin develops slowly (multiple-step mutation). Rapid one-step development of resistance occurs only rarely ($<10^{-9}$) in vitro.
Cross-resistance between lomefloxacin and other quinolone-class antimicrobial agents has been reported; however, cross-resistance between lomefloxacin and members of other classes of antimicrobial agents, such as aminoglycosides, penicillins, tetracyclines, cephalosporins, or sulfonamides has not yet been reported. Lomefloxacin is active in vitro against some strains of cephalosporin- and aminoglycoside-resistant gram-negative bacteria.
Susceptibility tests
Diffusion techniques: Quantitative methods that require measurement of zone diameters give the most precise estimate of the susceptibility of bacteria to antimicrobial agents. One such standardized procedure[1] that has been recommended for use with disks to test the susceptibility of organisms to lomefloxacin uses the 10-μg lomefloxacin disk. Interpretation involves correlation of the diameter obtained in the disk test with the MIC for lomefloxacin.
Reports from the laboratory giving results of the standard single-disk susceptibility test with a 10-μg lomefloxacin disk should be interpreted according to the following criteria:

Zone Diameter (mm)	Interpretation
≥22	Susceptible (S)
19–21	Intermediate (I)
≤18	Resistant (R)

A report of "susceptible" indicates that the pathogen is likely to be inhibited by generally achievable drug concentrations. A report of "intermediate" indicates that the result should be considered equivocal, and, if the organism is not fully susceptible to alternative clinically feasible drugs, the test should be repeated. This category provides a buffer zone that prevents small uncontrolled technical factors from causing major discrepancies in interpretation. A report of "resistant" indicates that achievable drug concentrations are unlikely to be inhibitory, and other therapy should be selected.
Standardized susceptibility test procedures require the use of laboratory control organisms. The 10-μg lomefloxacin disk should give the following zone diameters:

Organism	Zone Diameter (mm)
S aureus (ATCC 25923)	23–29
E coli (ATCC 25922)	27–33
P aeruginosa (ATCC 27853)	22–28

Continued on next page

Searle—Cont.

Dilution techniques: Use a standardized dilution method[2] (broth, agar, or microdilution) or equivalent with lomefloxacin powder. The MIC values obtained should be interpreted according to the following criteria:

MIC (µg/mL)	Interpretation
≤2	Susceptible (S)
4	Intermediate (I)
≥8	Resistant (R)

As with standard diffusion techniques, dilution methods require the use of laboratory control organisms. Standard lomefloxacin powder should provide the following MIC values:

Organism	MIC (µg/mL)
S aureus (ATCC 29213)	0.25–2.0
E coli (ATCC 25922)	0.03–0.12
P aeruginosa (ATCC 27853)	1.0–4.0

INDICATIONS AND USAGE

Treatment:
Maxaquin (lomefloxacin HCl) film-coated tablets are indicated for the treatment of adults with mild to moderate infections caused by susceptible strains of the designated microorganisms in the conditions listed below: (See **Dosage and Administration** for specific dosing recommendations.)

LOWER RESPIRATORY TRACT

Acute Bacterial Exacerbation of Chronic Bronchitis caused by *Haemophilus influenzae* or *Moraxella (Branhamella) catarrhalis.*

NOTE:MAXAQUIN IS NOT INDICATED FOR THE EMPIRIC TREATMENT OF ACUTE BACTERIAL EXACERBATION OF CHRONIC BRONCHITIS WHEN IT IS PROBABLE THAT *S PNEUMONIAE* IS A CAUSATIVE PATHOGEN. *S PNEUMONIAE* EXHIBITS IN VITRO RESISTANCE TO LOMEFLOXACIN, AND THE SAFETY AND EFFICACY OF LOMEFLOXACIN IN THE TREATMENT OF PATIENTS WITH ACUTE BACTERIAL EXACERBATION OF CHRONIC BRONCHITIS CAUSED BY *S PNEUMONIAE* HAVE NOT BEEN DEMONSTRATED. IF LOMEFLOXACIN IS TO BE PRESCRIBED FOR GRAM-STAIN-GUIDED EMPIRIC THERAPY OF ACUTE BACTERIAL EXACERBATION OF CHRONIC BRONCHITIS, IT SHOULD BE USED ONLY IF SPUTUM GRAM STAIN DEMONSTRATES AN ADEQUATE QUALITY OF SPECIMEN (> 25 PMNs/LPF) AND THERE IS BOTH A PREDOMINANCE OF GRAM-NEGATIVE ORGANISMS AND NOT A PREDOMINANCE OF GRAM-POSITIVE ORGANISMS.

URINARY TRACT

Uncomplicated Urinary Tract Infections (cystitis) caused by *Escherichia coli*, *Klebsiella pneumoniae*, *Proteus mirabilis*, or *Staphylococcus saprophyticus*.

Complicated Urinary Tract Infections caused by *Escherichia coli*, *Klebsiella pneumoniae*, *Proteus mirabilis*, *Pseudomonas aeruginosa*, *Citrobacter diversus,** or *Enterobacter cloacae.**

NOTE: In clinical trials with patients experiencing complicated urinary tract infections (UTIs) due to *P aeruginosa*, 12 of 16 patients had the organism eradicated from the urine after therapy with lomefloxacin. No patients had concomitant bacteremia. Serum levels of lomefloxacin do not reliably exceed the MIC of *Pseudomonas* isolates. THE SAFETY AND EFFICACY OF LOMEFLOXACIN IN TREATING PATIENTS WITH *PSEUDOMONAS* BACTEREMIA HAVE NOT BEEN ESTABLISHED.

* Although treatment of infections due to this organism in this organ system demonstrated a clinically acceptable overall outcome, efficacy was studied in fewer than 10 infections.

Appropriate culture and susceptibility tests should be performed before antimicrobial treatment in order to isolate and identify organisms causing infection and to determine their susceptibility to lomefloxacin. In patients with UTIs, therapy with Maxaquin film-coated tablets may be initiated before results of these tests are known; once these results become available, appropriate therapy should be continued. In patients with an acute bacterial exacerbation of chronic bronchitis, therapy should not be started empirically with lomefloxacin when there is a probability the causative pathogen is *S pneumoniae*.

Beta-lactamase production should have no effect on lomefloxacin activity.

Prophylaxis:
Maxaquin (lomefloxacin HCl) film-coated tablets are indicated preoperatively to reduce the incidence of UTIs in the early postoperative period (3 to 5 days postsurgery) in pa-

tients undergoing transurethral surgical procedures. Efficacy in decreasing the incidence of infections other than UTIs in the early postoperative period has not been established. Maxaquin, like all drugs for prophylaxis of transurethral surgical procedures, usually should not be used in minor urologic procedures for which prophylaxis is not indicated (eg, simple cystoscopy or retrograde pyelography).

CONTRAINDICATIONS

Lomefloxacin is contraindicated in patients with a history of hypersensitivity to lomefloxacin or to any of the quinolone group of antimicrobial agents.

WARNINGS

MODERATE TO SEVERE PHOTOTOXIC REACTIONS HAVE OCCURRED IN PATIENTS EXPOSED TO DIRECT OR INDIRECT SUNLIGHT OR TO ARTIFICIAL ULTRAVIOLET LIGHT (eg, sunlamps) DURING OR FOLLOWING TREATMENT WITH LOMEFLOXACIN. THESE REACTIONS HAVE ALSO OCCURRED IN PATIENTS EXPOSED TO SHADED OR DIFFUSE LIGHT, INCLUDING EXPOSURE THROUGH GLASS. PATIENTS SHOULD BE ADVISED TO DISCONTINUE LOMEFLOXACIN THERAPY AT THE FIRST SIGNS OR SYMPTOMS OF A PHOTOTOXICITY REACTION SUCH AS A SENSATION OF SKIN BURNING, REDNESS, SWELLING, BLISTERS, RASH, ITCHING, OR DERMATITIS.

These phototoxic reactions have occurred with and without the use of sunscreens or sunblocks. Single doses of lomefloxacin have been associated with these types of reactions. In a few cases, recovery was prolonged for several weeks. As with some other types of phototoxicity, there is the potential for exacerbation of the reaction on re-exposure to sunlight or artificial ultraviolet light prior to complete recovery from the reaction. In rare cases, reactions have recurred up to several weeks after stopping lomefloxacin therapy.

EXPOSURE TO DIRECT OR INDIRECT SUNLIGHT (EVEN WHEN USING SUNSCREENS OR SUNBLOCKS) SHOULD BE AVOIDED WHILE TAKING LOMEFLOXACIN AND FOR SEVERAL DAYS FOLLOWING THERAPY. LOMEFLOXACIN THERAPY SHOULD BE DISCONTINUED IMMEDIATELY AT THE FIRST SIGNS OR SYMPTOMS OF PHOTOTOXICITY.

THE SAFETY AND EFFICACY OF LOMEFLOXACIN IN CHILDREN, ADOLESCENTS (UNDER THE AGE OF 18 YEARS), PREGNANT WOMEN, AND LACTATING WOMEN HAVE NOT BEEN ESTABLISHED. (See PRECAUTIONS—*Pregnancy; Nursing Mothers;* and *Pediatric Use.*) The oral administration of multiple doses of lomefloxacin to juvenile dogs at 0.3 times and to rats at 5.4 times the recommended adult human dose based on mg/m^2 (0.6 and 34 times the recommended adult human dose based on mg/kg, respectively) caused arthropathy and lameness. Histopathologic examination of the weight-bearing joints of these animals revealed permanent lesions of the cartilage. Other quinolones also produce erosions of cartilage of weight-bearing joints and other signs of arthropathy in juvenile animals of various species. (See **Animal Pharmacology**.)

The safety and efficacy of lomefloxacin in the treatment of acute bacterial exacerbation of chronic bronchitis due to *S pneumoniae* have not been demonstrated. This product should not be used empirically in the treatment of acute bacterial exacerbation of chronic bronchitis when it is probable that *S pneumoniae* is a causative pathogen.

In clinical trials of complicated UTIs due to *P aeruginosa*, 12 of 16 patients had the organism eradicated from the urine after therapy with lomefloxacin. No patients had concomitant bacteremia. Serum levels of lomefloxacin do not reliably exceed the MIC of *Pseudomonas* isolates. THE SAFETY AND EFFICACY OF LOMEFLOXACIN IN TREATING PATIENTS WITH *PSEUDOMONAS* BACTEREMIA HAVE NOT BEEN ESTABLISHED.

Serious and occasionally fatal hypersensitivity (anaphylactoid or anaphylactic) reactions, some following the first dose, have been reported in patients receiving quinolone therapy. Some reactions were accompanied by cardiovascular collapse, loss of consciousness, tingling, pharyngeal or facial edema, dyspnea, urticaria, or itching. Only a few of these patients had a history of previous hypersensitivity reactions. Serious hypersensitivity reactions have also been reported following treatment with lomefloxacin. If an allergic reaction to lomefloxacin occurs, discontinue the drug. Serious acute hypersensitivity reactions may require immediate emergency treatment with epinephrine. Oxygen, intravenous fluids, antihistamines, corticosteroids, pressor amines, and airway management, including intubation, should be administered as indicated.

Convulsions have been reported in patients receiving lomefloxacin. Whether the convulsions were directly related to lomefloxacin administration has not yet been established. However, convulsions, increased intracranial pressure, and toxic psychoses have been reported in patients receiving other quinolones. Quinolones may also cause central nervous system (CNS) stimulation, which may lead to tremors, restlessness, lightheadedness, confusion, and hallucinations. If any of these reactions occurs in patients receiving lomefloxacin, the drug should be discontinued and appropriate measures instituted. No evidence of an effect of lomefloxacin on the electrical activity of the brain has been demonstrated. Lomefloxacin does not alter cerebral blood flow or cerebral glucose uptake in the CNS based on positron emission tomography. However, until more information becomes available, lomefloxacin, like all other quinolones, should be used with caution in patients with known or suspected CNS disorders, such as severe cerebral arteriosclerosis, epilepsy, or other factors that predispose to seizures. (See **Adverse Reactions.**)

Pseudomembranous colitis has been reported with nearly all antibacterial agents, including quinolones, and may range from mild to life-threatening in severity. Therefore, it is important to consider this diagnosis in patients who present with diarrhea subsequent to the administration of antibacterial agents. Treatment with broad-spectrum antibiotics alters the normal flora of the colon and may permit overgrowth of clostridia. Studies indicate that a toxin produced by *Clostridium difficile* is a primary cause of "antibiotic-associated colitis." After the diagnosis of pseudomembranous colitis has been established, therapeutic measures should be initiated. Mild cases of pseudomembranous colitis usually respond to discontinuation of drug alone. In moderate to severe cases, consideration should be given to management with fluids and electrolytes, protein supplementation, and treatment with an antibacterial drug clinically effective against *C difficile* colitis.

PRECAUTIONS

General:
Alteration of the dosage regimen is recommended for patients with impairment of renal function ($\text{Cl}_{Cr} < 40$ mL/min/1.73 m^2). (See **Dosage and Administration**.)

Information for patients:
Patients should be advised

* to avoid to the maximum extent possible direct or indirect sunlight (including exposure through glass and exposure through sunscreens and sunblocks) and artificial ultraviolet light (eg, sunlamps) during treatment with lomefloxacin and for several days after therapy;
* that they may reduce the risk of developing phototoxicity from sunlight by taking the daily dose of lomefloxacin in the evening;
* to discontinue lomefloxacin therapy at the first signs or symptoms of phototoxicity reaction such as a sensation of skin burning, redness, swelling, blisters, rash, itching, or dermatitis;
* that a patient who has experienced a phototoxic reaction should also be advised to avoid re-exposure to sunlight and artificial ultraviolet light until he has completely recovered from the reaction. In rare cases, reactions have recurred up to several weeks after stopping lomefloxacin therapy.
* to drink fluids liberally;
* that lomefloxacin can be taken without regard to meals;
* that mineral supplements or vitamins with iron or minerals should not be taken within the 2-hour period before or after taking lomefloxacin (see **Drug Interactions**);
* that sucralfate or antacids containing magnesium or aluminum should not be taken within 4 hours before or 2 hours after taking lomefloxacin (see **Drug Interactions**);
* that lomefloxacin can cause dizziness and lightheadedness and, therefore, patients should know how they react to lomefloxacin before they operate an automobile or machinery or engage in activities requiring mental alertness and coordination;
* that lomefloxacin may be associated with hypersensitivity reactions, even following the first dose, and to discontinue the drug at the first sign of a skin rash or other allergic reaction.

Drug interactions:
Theophylline: In three pharmacokinetic studies including 46 normal, healthy subjects, theophylline clearance and concentration were not significantly altered by the addition of lomefloxacin. In clinical studies where patients were on chronic theophylline therapy, lomefloxacin had no measurable effect on the mean distribution of theophylline concentrations or the mean estimates of theophylline clearance. Though individual theophylline levels fluctuated, there were no clinically significant symptoms of drug interaction.

Antacids and sucralfate: Sucralfate and antacids containing magnesium or aluminum form chelation complexes with lomefloxacin and interfere with its bioavailability. Sucralfate administered 2 hours before lomefloxacin resulted in a slower rate of absorption (mean C_{max} decreased by 30% and mean T_{max} increased by 1 hour) and a lesser extent of absorption (mean AUC decreased by approximately 25%). Magnesium- and aluminum-containing antacids, administered concomitantly with lomefloxacin, significantly decreased the bioavailability (48%) of lomefloxacin. Separating the doses of antacid and lomefloxacin minimizes this decrease in bioavailability; therefore, administration of these agents should precede lomefloxacin dosing by 4 hours or follow lomefloxacin dosing by at least 2 hours.

Body System	Infection	Unit Dose	Frequency	Duration	Daily Dose
Lower respiratory tract	Acute bacterial exacerbation of chronic bronchitis	400 mg	qd	10 days	400 mg
Urinary tract	Cystitis	400 mg	qd	10 days	400 mg
	Complicated UTIs	400 mg	qd	14 days	400 mg

Caffeine: One hundred mg of caffeine (equivalent to 1 to 3 cups of American coffee) was administered to 16 normal, healthy volunteers who had achieved steady-state blood concentrations of lomefloxacin after being dosed at 400 mg qd. This did not result in any statistically or clinically relevant changes in the pharmacokinetic parameters of either caffeine or lomefloxacin. No data are available on potential interactions in individuals who consume greater than 100 mg of caffeine per day or in those, such as the geriatric population, who are generally believed to be more susceptible to the development of drug-induced CNS-related adverse effects. Other quinolones have demonstrated moderate to marked interference with the metabolism of caffeine, resulting in a reduced clearance, a prolongation of plasma half-life, and an increase in symptoms that accompany high levels of caffeine.

Cimetidine: Cimetidine has been demonstrated to interfere with the elimination of other quinolones. This interference has resulted in significant increases in half-life and AUC. The interaction between lomefloxacin and cimetidine has not been studied.

Cyclosporine: Elevated serum levels of cyclosporine have been reported with concomitant use of cyclosporine with other members of the quinolone class. Interaction between lomefloxacin and cyclosporine has not been studied.

Nonsteroidal anti-inflammatory drugs (NSAIDs): Concomitant administration of the NSAID fenbufen with some quinolones has been reported to increase the risk of CNS stimulation and convulsive seizures.

There was an increase in the incidence of seizures in mice treated with fenbufen, when fenbufen was administered to mice that had been concomitantly treated with a dose of lomefloxacin equivalent to the recommended human dose on a mg/m^2 basis (10 times the recommended human dose on a mg/kg basis). Fenbufen is not presently an approved drug in the United States. (See **Animal Pharmacology**).

Probenecid: Probenecid slows the renal elimination of lomefloxacin. An increase of 63% in the mean AUC and increases of 50% and 4%, respectively, in the mean T_{max} and mean C_{max} were noted in 1 study of 6 individuals.

Warfarin: Quinolones may enhance the effects of the oral anticoagulant, warfarin, or its derivatives. When these products are administered concomitantly, prothrombin or other suitable coagulation tests should be monitored closely.

Carcinogenesis, mutagenesis, impairment of fertility:

Carcinogenesis: Hairless (Skh-1) mice were exposed to UVA light for 3.5 hours five times every 2 weeks for up to 52 weeks while concurrently being administered lomefloxacin. The lomefloxacin doses used in this study caused a phototoxic response. In mice treated with both UVA and lomefloxacin concomitantly, the time to development of skin tumors was 16 weeks. In mice treated concomitantly in this model with both UVA and other quinolones, the times to development of skin tumors ranged from 28 to 52 weeks.

Ninety-two percent (92%) of the mice treated concomitantly with both UVA and lomefloxacin developed well-differentiated squamous cell carcinomas of the skin. These squamous cell carcinomas were nonmetastatic and were endophytic in character. Two-thirds of these squamous cell carcinomas contained large central keratinous inclusion masses and were thought to arise from the vestigial hair follicles in these hairless animals.

In this model, mice treated with lomefloxacin alone did not develop skin or systemic tumors.

There are no data from similar models using pigmented mice and/or fully haired mice.

The clinical significance of these findings to humans is unknown.

Mutagenesis: One in vitro mutagenicity test (CHO/HGPRT assay) was weakly positive at lomefloxacin concentrations ≥ 226 µg/mL and negative at concentrations < 226 µg/mL. Two other in vitro mutagenicity tests (chromosomal aberrations in Chinese hamster ovary cells, chromosomal aberrations in human lymphocytes) and two in vivo mouse micronucleus mutagenicity tests were all negative.

Impairment of fertility: Lomefloxacin did not affect the fertility of male and female rats at oral doses up to 8 times the recommended human dose based on mg/m^2 (34 times the recommended human dose based on mg/kg).

Pregnancy: Teratogenic effects. Pregnancy Category C.

Reproductive function studies have been performed in rats at doses up to 8 times the recommended human dose based on mg/m^2 (34 times the recommended human dose based on mg/kg), and no impaired fertility or harm to the fetus was reported due to lomefloxacin. Increased incidence of fetal loss in monkeys has been observed at approximately 3 to 6 times the recommended human dose based on mg/m^2 (6 to 12 times the recommended human dose based on mg/kg). No teratogenicity has been observed in rats and monkeys at up to 16 times the recommended human dose exposure. In the rabbit, maternal toxicity and associated fetotoxicity, decreased placental weight, and variations of the coccygeal vertebrae occurred at doses 2 times the recommended human exposure based on mg/m^2. There are, however, no adequate and well-controlled studies in pregnant women. Lomefloxacin should be used during pregnancy only if the potential benefit justifies the potential risk to the fetus.

Nursing mothers:

It is not known whether lomefloxacin is excreted in human milk. However, it is known that other drugs of this class are excreted in human milk and that lomefloxacin is excreted in the milk of lactating rats. Because of the potential for serious adverse reactions from lomefloxacin in nursing infants, a decision should be made whether to discontinue nursing or to discontinue the drug, taking into account the importance of the drug to the mother.

Pediatric use:

The safety and effectiveness of lomefloxacin in children and adolescents less than 18 years of age have not been established. Lomefloxacin causes arthropathy in juvenile animals of several species. (See **Warnings and Animal Pharmacology.**)

Geriatric use:

Of the total number of patients in clinical trials of lomefloxacin, 26% were ≥ 65 years of age. No overall differences in effectiveness or safety were observed between these patients and younger patients. (See **Clinical Pharmacology**—*Pharmacokinetics in the Geriatric Population.*)

ADVERSE REACTIONS

In clinical trials, most of the adverse events reported were mild to moderate in severity and transient in nature. During these clinical investigations, 2,869 patients received Maxaquin. In 2.6% of the patients, lomefloxacin was discontinued because of adverse events, primarily involving the gastrointestinal system (0.7%), skin (1.0%), or CNS (0.5%).

Adverse clinical events:

The events with the highest incidence ($\geq$ 1%) in patients, regardless of relationship to drug, were nausea (3.7%), headache (3.2%), photosensitivity (2.4%) [see **Warnings**], dizziness (2.3%), and diarrhea (1.4%).

Additional clinical events reported in less than 1% of patients treated with Maxaquin, regardless of relationship to drug, are listed below:

Autonomic: dry mouth, flushing, increased sweating.

Body as a whole: fatigue, back pain, malaise, asthenia, chest pain, chills, allergic reaction, face edema, influenza-like symptoms, decreased heat tolerance.

Cardiovascular: hypotension, hypertension, edema, syncope, tachycardia, bradycardia, arrhythmia, extrasystoles, cyanosis, cardiac failure, angina pectoris, myocardial infarction, pulmonary embolism, cerebrovascular disorder, cardiomyopathy, phlebitis.

Central nervous system: convulsions, coma, hyperkinesia, tremor, vertigo, paresthesias.

Gastrointestinal: abdominal pain, dyspepsia, vomiting, flatulence, constipation, gastrointestinal inflammation, dysphagia, gastrointestinal bleeding, tongue discoloration.

Hearing: earache, tinnitus.

Hematologic: thrombocytopenia, thrombocythemia, purpura, lymphadenopathy, increased fibrinolysis.

Metabolic: thirst, gout, hypoglycemia.

Musculoskeletal: leg cramps, arthralgia, myalgia.

Ophthalmologic: abnormal vision, conjunctivitis, eye pain.

Psychiatric: somnolence, insomnia, nervousness, anorexia, confusion, anxiety, depression, agitation, increased appetite, depersonalization, paroniria.

Reproductive system: Female: vaginitis, leukorrhea, intermenstrual bleeding, perineal pain, vaginal moniliasis. Male: orchitis, epididymitis.

Respiratory: dyspnea, respiratory infection, epistaxis, respiratory disorder, bronchospasm, cough, increased sputum, stridor.

Skin/Allergic: pruritus, rash, urticaria, eczema, skin exfoliation, skin disorder.

Special senses: taste perversion.

Urinary: dysuria, hematuria, strangury, micturition disorder, anuria.

Adverse laboratory events:

Changes in laboratory parameters, listed as adverse events, without regard to drug relationship include:

Hepatic: elevations of ALT (SGPT) (0.4%), AST (SGOT) (0.3%), bilirubin (0.1%), alkaline phosphatase (0.1%).

Hematologic: monocytosis (0.3%), elevated ESR (0.1%).

Renal: elevated BUN (0.1%), decreased potassium (0.1%).

Additional laboratory changes occurring in $\leq 0.1\%$ in the clinical studies included: elevation of serum gamma glutamyl transferase, decrease in total protein or albumin, prolongation of prothrombin time, anemia, decrease in hemoglobin, leukopenia, eosinophilia, thrombocytopenia, abnormalities of urine specific gravity or serum electrolytes, decrease in blood glucose.

Quinolone-class adverse events:

Adverse events reported from worldwide marketing experience with quinolones, including Maxaquin, are: **anaphylaxis**, cardiopulmonary arrest, laryngeal or pulmonary edema, ataxia, cerebral thrombosis, hallucination, painful oral mucosa, pseudomembranous colitis, hemolytic anemia, hepatitis, tendinitis, diplopia, photophobia, phobia, exfoliative dermatitis, hyperpigmentation, Steven-Johnson syndrome, toxic epidermal necrolysis, dysgeusia, interstitial nephritis, polyuria, renal failure, urinary retention, and vasculitis.

Additional quinolone class adverse events include: erythema nodosum, hepatic necrosis, possible exacerbation of myasthenia gravis, dysphasia, nystagmus, intestinal perforation, manic reaction, renal calculi, acidosis and hiccough.

Laboratory adverse events include: agranulocytosis, elevation of serum triglycerides, elevation of serum cholesterol, elevation of blood glucose, elevation of serum potassium, albuminuria, candiduria, and crystalluria.

OVERDOSAGE

Information on overdosage in humans is limited. In the event of acute overdosage, the stomach should be emptied by inducing vomiting or by gastric lavage, and the patient should be carefully observed and given supportive treatment. Adequate hydration must be maintained. Hemodialysis or peritoneal dialysis is unlikely to aid in the removal of lomefloxacin as $< 3\%$ is removed by these modalities.

Clinical signs of acute toxicity in rodents progressed from salivation to tremors, decreased activity, dyspnea, and clonic convulsions prior to death. These signs were noted in rats and mice as lomefloxacin doses were increased.

DOSAGE AND ADMINISTRATION

Maxaquin (lomefloxacin HCl) may be taken without regard to meals. Risk of reaction to solar UVA light may be reduced by taking Maxaquin in the evening. (See **Clinical Pharmacology.**)

See **Indications and Usage** for information on appropriate pathogens and patient populations.

Treatment:

Patients with normal renal function: The recommended daily dose of Maxaquin is described in the following chart:

[See table above.]

Elderly patients: No dosage adjustment is needed for elderly patients with normal renal function ($Cl_{cr} \geq 40$ mL/min/1.73 m^2).

Patients with impaired renal function: Lomefloxacin is primarily eliminated by renal excretion. (See **Clinical Pharmacology.**) Modification of dosage is recommended in patients with renal dysfunction. In patients with a creatinine clearance > 10 mL/min/1.73m^2 but < 40 mL/min/1.73 m^2, the recommended dosage is an initial loading dose of 400 mg followed by daily maintenance doses of 200 mg ($^1/_2$ tablet) once daily for the duration of treatment. It is suggested that serial determinations of lomefloxacin levels be performed to determine any necessary alteration in the appropriate next dosing interval.

If only the serum creatinine is known, the following formula may be used to estimate creatinine clearance.

$$\text{Men: } \frac{(\text{weight in kg}) \times (140 - \text{age})}{(72) \times \text{serum creatinine (mg/dL)}}$$

$$\text{Women: } (0.85) \times (\text{calculated value for men})$$

Dialysis patients: Hemodialysis removes only a negligible amount of lomefloxacin (3% in 4 hours). Hemodialysis patients should receive an initial loading dose of 400 mg followed by daily maintenance doses of 200 mg ($^1/_2$ tablet) once daily for the duration of treatment.

Patients with cirrhosis: Cirrhosis does not reduce the nonrenal clearance of lomefloxacin. The need for a dosage reduction in this population should be based on the degree of renal

Continued on next page

Searle—Cont.

function of the patient and on the plasma concentrations. (See **Clinical Pharmacology** and **Dosage and Administration**—*Patients with impaired Renal Function.*)

Prophylaxis:

A single dose of 400 mg of Maxaquin should be administered orally 2 to 6 hours prior to surgery when oral preoperative prophylaxis for transurethral surgical procedures is considered appropriate.

HOW SUPPLIED

Maxaquin (lomefloxacin HCl) is supplied as a scored, film-coated tablet containing the equivalent of 400 mg of lomefloxacin base present as the hydrochloride. The tablet is oval, white, and film-coated with "MAXAQUIN 400" debossed on one side and scored on the other side and is supplied in:

NDC Number	Size
0025-1651-20	bottle of 20
0025-1651-34	carton of 100 unit dose

Store at 59° to 86°F (15° to 30°C).

Caution: Federal law prohibits dispensing without prescription.

ANIMAL PHARMACOLOGY

Lomefloxacin and other quinolones have been shown to cause arthropathy in juvenile animals. Arthropathy, involving multiple diarthrodial joints, was observed in juvenile dogs administered lomefloxacin at doses as low as 4.5 mg/kg for 7 to 8 days (0.3 times the recommended human dose based on mg/m^2 or 0.6 times the recommended human dose based on mg/kg). In juvenile rats, no changes were observed in the joints with doses up to 91 mg/kg for 7 days (2 times the recommended human dose based on mg/m^2 or 11 times the recommended human dose based on mg/kg). (See **Warnings.**)

In a 13-week oral rat study, gamma globulin decreased when lomefloxacin was administered at less than the recommended human exposure. Beta globulin decreased when lomefloxacin was administered at 0.6 to 2 times the recommended human dose based on mg/m^2. The A/G ratio increased when lomefloxacin was administered at 6 to 20 times the human dose. Following a 4-week recovery period, beta globulins in the females and A/G ratios in the females returned to control values. Gamma globulin values in the females and beta and gamma globulins and A/G ratios in the males were still statistically significantly different from control values. No effects on globulins were seen in oral studies in dogs or monkeys in the limited number of specimens collected.

Twenty-seven NSAIDs, administered concomitantly with lomefloxacin, were tested for seizure induction in mice at approximately 2 times the recommended human dose based on mg/m^2. At a dose of lomefloxacin equivalent to the recommended human exposure based on mg/m^2 (10 times the human dose based on mg/kg), only fenbufen, when coadministered, produced an increase in seizures.

Crystalluria and ocular toxicity, seen with some related quinolones, were not observed in any lomefloxacin-treated animals, either in studies designed to look for these effects specifically or in subchronic and chronic toxicity studies in rats, dogs, and monkeys.

Long-term, high-dose systemic use of other quinolones in experimental animals has caused lenticular opacities; however, this finding was not observed with lomefloxacin.

REFERENCES

1. National Committee for Clinical Laboratory Standards, *Performance Standards for Antimicrobial Disk Susceptibility Tests*—4th ed. Approved Standard NCCLS Document M2-A4, vol 10, No. 7, NCCLS, Villanova, Pa, 1990. **2.** National Committee for Clinical Laboratory Standards, *Methods for Dilution Antimicrobial Susceptibility Tests for Bacteria that Grow Aerobically*—2nd ed. Approved Standard NCCLS Document M7-A2, vol 10, No. 8, NCCLS, Villanova, Pa, 1990.

2/8/95 ● A05224-1

Shown in Product Identification Guide, page 335

NORPACE® Capsules ℞

[nor′pāce]

(disopyramide phosphate)

NORPACE® CR Capsules ℞

(disopyramide phosphate extended-release)

DESCRIPTION

Norpace (disopyramide phosphate) is an antiarrhythmic drug available for oral administration in immediate-release and controlled-release capsules containing 100 mg or 150 mg of disopyramide base, present as the phosphate. The base content of the phosphate salt is 77.6%. The structural formula of Norpace is:

[See chemical structure at top of next column.]

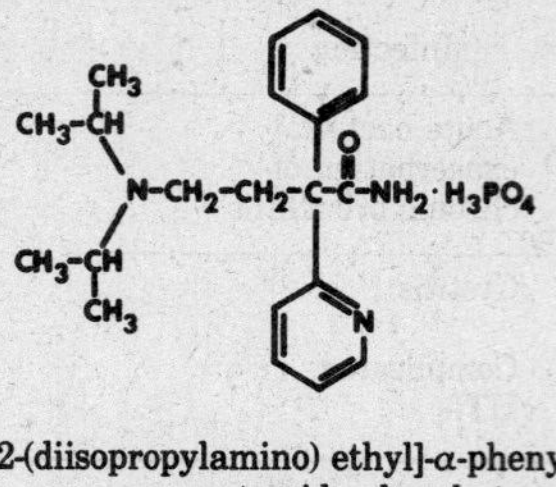

α-[2-(diisopropylamino) ethyl]-α-phenyl-2-pyridine-acetamide phosphate

Norpace is freely soluble in water, and the free base (pKa 10.4) has an aqueous solubility of 1 mg/ml. The chloroform: water partition coefficient of the base is 3.1 at pH 7.2.

Norpace is a racemic mixture of *d*- and *l*-isomers. This drug is not chemically related to other antiarrhythmic drugs.

Norpace CR (controlled-release) capsules are designed to afford a gradual and consistent release of disopyramide. Thus, for maintenance therapy, Norpace CR provides the benefit of less-frequent dosing (every 12 hours) as compared with the every-6-hour dosage schedule of immediate-release Norpace capsules.

Inactive ingredients of Norpace include corn starch, edible ink, FD&C Red No. 3, FD&C Yellow No. 6, gelatin, lactose, talc, and titanium dioxide; the 150-mg capsule also contains FD&C Blue No. 1.

Inactive ingredients of Norpace CR include corn starch, D&C Yellow No. 10, edible ink, ethylcellulose, FD&C Blue No. 1, gelatin, shellac, sucrose, talc, and titanium dioxide; the 150-mg capsule also contains FD&C Red No. 3 and FD&C Yellow No. 6.

CLINICAL PHARMACOLOGY

Mechanisms of Action

Norpace (disopyramide phosphate) is a Type 1 antiarrhythmic drug (ie, similar to procainamide and quinidine). *In animal studies* Norpace decreases the rate of diastolic depolarization (phase 4) in cells with augmented automaticity, decreases the upstroke velocity (phase 0) and increases the action potential duration of normal cardiac cells, decreases the disparity in refractoriness between infarcted and adjacent normally perfused myocardium, and has no effect on alpha- or beta-adrenergic receptors.

Electrophysiology

In man, Norpace at therapeutic plasma levels shortens the sinus node recovery time, lengthens the effective refractory period of the atrium, and has a minimal effect on the effective refractory period of the AV node. Little effect has been shown on AV-nodal and His-Purkinje conduction times or QRS duration. However, prolongation of conduction in accessory pathways occurs.

Hemodynamics

At recommended oral doses, Norpace rarely produces significant alterations of blood pressure in patients without congestive heart failure (see *Warnings*). With intravenous Norpace, either increases in systolic/diastolic or decreases in systolic blood pressure have been reported, depending on the infusion rate and the patient population. Intravenous Norpace may cause cardiac depression with an approximate mean 10% reduction of cardiac output, which is more pronounced in patients with cardiac dysfunction.

Anticholinergic Activity

The *in vitro* anticholinergic activity of Norpace is approximately 0.06% that of atropine; however, the usual dose for Norpace is 150 mg every 6 hours and for Norpace CR 300 mg every 12 hours, compared to 0.4 to 0.6 mg for atropine (see *Warnings* and *Adverse Reactions* for anticholinergic side effects).

Pharmacokinetics

Following oral administration of immediate-release Norpace, disopyramide phosphate is rapidly and almost completely absorbed, and peak plasma levels are usually attained within 2 hours. The usual therapeutic plasma levels of disopyramide base are 2 to 4 mcg/ml, and at these concentrations protein binding varies from 50% to 65%. Because of concentration-dependent protein binding, it is difficult to predict the concentration of the free drug when total drug is measured.

The mean plasma half-life of disopyramide in healthy humans is 6.7 hours (range of 4 to 10 hours). In six patients with impaired renal function (creatinine clearance less than 40 ml/min), disopyramide half-life values were 8 to 18 hours.

After the oral administration of 200 mg of disopyramide to 10 cardiac patients with borderline to moderate heart failure, the time to peak serum concentration of 2.3 ± 1.5 hours (mean $\pm$ SD) was increased, and the mean peak serum concentration of 4.8 ± 1.6 mcg/ml was higher than in healthy volunteers. After intravenous administration in these same patients, the mean elimination half-life was 9.7 ± 4.2 hours (range in healthy volunteers of 4.4 to 7.8 hours). In a second study of the oral administration of disopyramide to 7 patients with heart disease, including left ventricular dysfunction, the mean plasma half-life was slightly prolonged to 7.8 ± 1.9 hours (range of 5 to 9.5 hours).

In healthy men, about 50% of a given dose of disopyramide is excreted in the urine as the unchanged drug, about 20% as the mono-N-dealkylated metabolite, and 10% as the other metabolites. The plasma concentration of the major metabolite is approximately one tenth that of disopyramide. Altering the urinary pH in man does not affect the plasma half-life of disopyramide.

In a crossover study in healthy subjects, the bioavailability of disopyramide from Norpace CR capsules was similar to that from the immediate-release capsules. With a single 300-mg oral dose, peak disopyramide plasma concentrations of 3.23 ± 0.75 mcg/ml (mean $\pm$ SD) at 2.5 ± 2.3 hours were obtained with two 150-mg immediate-release capsules and 2.22 ± 0.47 mcg/ml at 4.9 ± 1.4 hours with two 150-mg Norpace CR capsules. The elimination half-life of disopyramide was 8.31 ± 1.83 hours with the immediate-release capsules and 11.65 ± 4.72 hours with Norpace CR capsules. The amount of disopyramide and mono-N-dealkylated metabolite excreted in the urine in 48 hours was 128 and 48 mg, respectively, with the immediate-release capsules, and 112 and 33 mg, respectively, with Norpace CR capsules. The differences in the urinary excretion of either constituent were not statistically significant.

Following multiple doses, steady-state plasma levels of between 2 and 4 mcg/ml were attained following either 150 mg every-6-hour dosing with immediate-release capsules or 300 mg every-12-hour dosing with Norpace CR capsules.

INDICATIONS AND USAGE

Norpace and Norpace CR are indicated for the treatment of documented ventricular arrhythmias, such as sustained ventricular tachycardia, that, in the judgment of the physician, are life-threatening. Because of the proarrhythmic effects of Norpace and Norpace CR, their use with lesser arrhythmias is generally not recommended. Treatment of patients with asymptomatic ventricular premature contractions should be avoided.

Initiation of Norpace or Norpace CR treatment, as with other antiarrhythmic agents used to treat life-threatening arrhythmias, should be carried out in the hospital. Norpace CR should not be used initially if rapid establishment of disopyramide plasma levels is desired.

Antiarrhythmic drugs have not been shown to enhance survival in patients with ventricular arrhythmias.

CONTRAINDICATIONS

Norpace and Norpace CR are contraindicated in the presence of cardiogenic shock, preexisting second- or third-degree AV block (if no pacemaker is present), congenital Q-T prolongation, or known hypersensitivity to the drug.

WARNINGS

Mortality

In the National Heart, Lung and Blood Institute's Cardiac Arrhythmia Suppression Trial (CAST), a long-term, multi-center, randomized, double-blind study in patients with asymptomatic non-life-threatening ventricular arrhythmias who had had a myocardial infarction more than 6 days but less than 2 years previously, an excessive mortality or non-fatal cardiac arrest rate (7.7%) was seen in patients treated with encainide or flecainide compared with that seen in patients assigned to carefully matched placebo-treated groups (3.0%). The average duration of treatment with encainide or flecainide in this study was 10 months.

The applicability of the CAST results to other populations (eg, those without recent myocardial infarction) is uncertain. Considering the known proarrhythmic properties of Norpace or Norpace CR and the lack of evidence of improved survival for any antiarrhythmic drug in patients without life-threatening arrhythmias, the use of Norpace or Norpace CR as well as other antiarrhythmic agents should be reserved for patients with life-threatening ventricular arrhythmias.

Negative Inotropic Properties:

Heart Failure/Hypotension

Norpace or Norpace CR may cause or worsen congestive heart failure or produce severe hypotension as a consequence of its negative inotropic properties. Hypotension has been observed primarily in patients with primary cardiomyopathy or inadequately compensated congestive heart failure. Norpace or Norpace CR should not be used in patients with uncompensated or marginally compensated congestive heart failure or hypotension unless the congestive heart failure or hypotension is secondary to cardiac arrhythmia. Patients with a history of heart failure may be treated with Norpace or Norpace CR, but careful attention must be given to the maintenance of cardiac function, including optimal digitalization. If hypotension occurs or congestive heart failure worsens, Norpace or Norpace CR should be discontinued and, if necessary, restarted at a

lower dosage only after adequate cardiac compensation has been established.

QRS Widening
Although it is unusual, significant widening (greater than 25%) of the QRS complex may occur during Norpace or Norpace CR administration; in such cases Norpace or Norpace CR should be discontinued.

Q-T Prolongation
As with other Type 1 antiarrhythmic drugs, prolongation of the Q-T interval (corrected) and worsening of the arrhythmia, including ventricular tachycardia and ventricular fibrillation, may occur. Patients who have evidenced prolongation of the Q-T interval in response to quinidine may be at particular risk. As with other Type 1A antiarrhythmics, disopyramide phosphate has been associated with torsade de pointes.

If a Q-T prolongation of greater than 25% is observed and if ectopy continues, the patient should be monitored closely, and consideration be given to discontinuing Norpace or Norpace CR.

Hypoglycemia
In rare instances significant lowering of blood glucose values has been reported during Norpace administration. The physician should be alert to this possibility, especially in patients with congestive heart failure, chronic malnutrition, hepatic, renal, or other diseases, or drugs (eg, beta adrenoceptor blockers, alcohol) which could compromise preservation of the normal glucoregulatory mechanisms in the absence of food. In these patients the blood glucose levels should be carefully followed.

Concomitant Antiarrhythmic Therapy
The concomitant use of Norpace or Norpace CR with other Type 1A antiarrhythmic agents (such as quinidine or procainamide), Type 1C antiarrhythmics (such as encainide, flecainide or propafenone), and/or propranolol should be reserved for patients with life-threatening arrhythmias who are demonstrably unresponsive to single-agent antiarrhythmic therapy. Such use may produce serious negative inotropic effects, or may excessively prolong conduction. This should be considered particularly in patients with any degree of cardiac decompensation or those with a prior history thereof. Patients receiving more than one antiarrhythmic drug must be carefully monitored.

Heart Block
If first-degree heart block develops in a patient receiving Norpace or Norpace CR, the dosage should be reduced. If the block persists despite reduction of dosage, continuation of the drug must depend upon weighing the benefit being obtained against the risk of higher degrees of heart block. Development of second- or third-degree AV block or unifascicular, bifascicular, or trifascicular block requires discontinuation of Norpace or Norpace CR therapy, unless the ventricular rate is adequately controlled by a temporary or implanted ventricular pacemaker.

Anticholinergic Activity
Because of its anticholinergic activity, disopyramide phosphate should not be used in patients with glaucoma, myasthenia gravis, or urinary retention unless adequate overriding measures are taken; these consist of the topical application of potent miotics (eg, pilocarpine) for patients with glaucoma, and catheter drainage or operative relief for patients with urinary retention. Urinary retention may occur in patients of either sex as a consequence of Norpace or Norpace CR administration, but males with benign prostatic hypertrophy are at particular risk. In patients with a family history of glaucoma, intraocular pressure should be measured before initiating Norpace or Norpace CR therapy. Disopyramide phosphate should be used with special care in patients with myasthenia gravis since its anticholinergic properties could precipitate a myasthenic crisis in such patients.

PRECAUTIONS
General
Atrial Tachyarrhythmias
Patients with atrial flutter or fibrillation should be digitalized prior to Norpace or Norpace CR administration to ensure that drug-induced enhancement of AV conduction does not result in an increase of ventricular rate beyond physiologically acceptable limits.

Conduction Abnormalities
Care should be taken when prescribing Norpace or Norpace CR for patients with sick sinus syndrome (bradycardia-tachycardia syndrome), Wolff-Parkinson-White syndrome (WPW), or bundle branch block. The effect of disopyramide phosphate in these conditions is uncertain at present.

Cardiomyopathy
Patients with myocarditis or other cardiomyopathy may develop significant hypotension in response to the usual dosage of disopyramide phosphate, probably due to cardiodepressant mechanisms. Therefore, a loading dose of Norpace should not be given to such patients, and initial dosage and subsequent dosage adjustments should be made under close supervision (see *Dosage and Administration*).

Renal Impairment
More than 50% of disopyramide is excreted in the urine unchanged. Therefore Norpace dosage should be reduced in patients with impaired renal function (see *Dosage and Administration*). The electrocardiogram should be carefully monitored for prolongation of PR interval, evidence of QRS widening, or other signs of overdosage (see *Overdosage*). Norpace CR is not recommended for patients with severe renal insufficiency (creatinine clearance 40 ml/min or less).

Hepatic Impairment
Hepatic impairment also causes an increase in the plasma half-life of disopyramide. Dosage should be reduced for patients with such impairment. The electrocardiogram should be carefully monitored for signs of overdosage (see *Overdosage*).

Patients with cardiac dysfunction have a higher potential for hepatic impairment; this should be considered when administering Norpace or Norpace CR.

Potassium Imbalance
Antiarrhythmic drugs may be ineffective in patients with hypokalemia, and their toxic effects may be enhanced in patients with hyperkalemia. Therefore, potassium abnormalities should be corrected before starting Norpace or Norpace CR therapy.

Drug Interactions
If phenytoin or other hepatic enzyme inducers are taken concurrently with Norpace or Norpace CR, lower plasma levels of disopyramide may occur. Monitoring of disopyramide plasma levels is recommended in such concurrent use to avoid ineffective therapy. Other antiarrhythmic drugs (eg, quinidine, procainamide, lidocaine, propranolol) have occasionally been used concurrently with Norpace. Excessive widening of the QRS complex and/or prolongation of the Q-T interval may occur in these situations (see *Warnings*). In healthy subjects, no significant drug-drug interaction was observed when Norpace was coadministered with either propranolol or diazepam. Concomitant administration of Norpace and quinidine resulted in slight increases in plasma disopyramide levels and slight decreases in plasma quinidine levels. Norpace does not increase serum digoxin levels.

Until data on possible interactions between verapamil and disopyramide phosphate are obtained, disopyramide should not be administered within 48 hours before or 24 hours after verapamil administration.

Carcinogenesis, Mutagenesis, Impairment of Fertility
Eighteen months of Norpace administration to rats, at oral doses up to 400 mg/kg/day (about 30 times the usual daily human dose of 600 mg/day, assuming a patient weight of at least 50 kg), revealed no evidence of carcinogenic potential. An evaluation of mutagenic potential by Ames test was negative. Norpace, at doses up to 250 mg/kg/day, did not adversely affect fertility of rats.

Pregnancy
Teratogenic Effects: Pregnancy Category C. Norpace was associated with decreased numbers of implantation sites and decreased growth and survival of pups when administered to pregnant rats at 250 mg/kg/day (20 or more times the usual daily human dose of 12 mg/kg, assuming a patient weight of at least 50 kg), a level at which weight gain and food consumption of dams were also reduced. Increased resorption rates were reported in rabbits at 60 mg/kg/day (5 or more times the usual daily human dose). Effects on implantation, pup growth, and survival were not evaluated in rabbits. There are no adequate and well-controlled studies in pregnant women. Norpace or Norpace CR should be used during pregnancy only if the potential benefit justifies the potential risk to the fetus.

Nonteratogenic Effects: Norpace has been reported to stimulate contractions of the pregnant uterus. Disopyramide has been found in human fetal blood.

Labor and Delivery
It is not known whether the use of Norpace or Norpace CR during labor or delivery has immediate or delayed adverse effects on the fetus, or whether it prolongs the duration of labor or increases the need for forceps delivery or other obstetric intervention.

Nursing Mothers
Studies in rats have shown that the concentration of disopyramide and its metabolites is between one and three times greater in milk than it is in plasma. Following oral administration, disopyramide has been detected in human milk at a concentration not exceeding that in plasma. Because of the potential for serious adverse reactions in nursing infants from Norpace or Norpace CR, a decision should be made whether to discontinue nursing or to discontinue the drug, taking into account the importance of the drug to the mother.

ADVERSE REACTIONS
The adverse reactions which were reported in Norpace clinical trials encompass observations in 1,500 patients, including 90 patients studied for at least 4 years. The most serious adverse reactions are hypotension and congestive heart failure. The most common adverse reactions, which are dose dependent, are associated with the anticholinergic properties of the drug. These may be transitory, but may be persis-

tent or can be severe. Urinary retention is the most serious anticholinergic effect.

The following reactions were reported in 10% to 40% of patients:
Anticholinergic: dry mouth (32%), urinary hesitancy (14%), constipation (11%)

The following reactions were reported in 3% to 9% of patients:
Anticholinergic: blurred vision, dry nose/eyes/throat
Genitourinary: urinary retention, urinary frequency and urgency
Gastrointestinal: nausea, pain/bloating/gas
General: dizziness, general fatigue/muscle weakness, headache, malaise, aches/pains

The following reactions were reported in 1% to 3% of patients:
Genitourinary: impotence
Cardiovascular: hypotension with or without congestive heart failure, increased congestive heart failure (see *Warnings*), cardiac conduction disturbances (see *Warnings*), edema/weight gain, shortness of breath, syncope, chest pain
Gastrointestinal: anorexia, diarrhea, vomiting
Dermatologic: generalized rash/dermatoses, itching
Central nervous system: nervousness
Other: hypokalemia, elevated cholesterol/triglycerides

The following reactions were reported in less than 1%:
Depression, insomnia, dysuria, numbness/tingling, elevated liver enzymes, AV block, elevated BUN, elevated creatinine, decreased hemoglobin/hematocrit

Hypoglycemia has been reported in association with Norpace administration (see *Warnings*).

Infrequent occurrences of reversible cholestatic jaundice, fever, and respiratory difficulty have been reported in association with disopyramide therapy, as have rare instances of thrombocytopenia, reversible agranulocytosis, and gynecomastia. Some cases of LE (lupus erythematosus) symptoms have been reported; most cases occurred in patients who had been switched to disopyramide from procainamide following the development of LE symptoms. Rarely, acute psychosis has been reported following Norpace therapy, with prompt return to normal mental status when therapy was stopped. The physician should be aware of these possible reactions and should discontinue Norpace or Norpace CR therapy promptly if they occur.

OVERDOSAGE
Symptoms
Deliberate or accidental overdosage of oral disopyramide may be followed by apnea, loss of consciousness, cardiac arrhythmias, and loss of spontaneous respiration. Death has occurred following overdosage.

Toxic plasma levels of disopyramide produce excessive widening of the QRS complex and Q-T interval, worsening of congestive heart failure, hypotension, varying kinds and degrees of conduction disturbance, bradycardia, and finally asystole. Obvious anticholinergic effects are also observed.

The approximate oral LD_{50} of disopyramide phosphate is 580 and 700 mg/kg for rats and mice, respectively.

Treatment
Experience indicates that prompt and vigorous treatment of overdosage is necessary, even in the absence of symptoms. Such treatment may be lifesaving. No specific antidote for disopyramide phosphate has been identified. Treatment should be symptomatic and may include induction of emesis or gastric lavage, administration of a cathartic followed by activated charcoal by mouth or stomach tube, intravenous administration of isoproterenol and dopamine, insertion of an intra-aortic balloon for counterpulsation, and mechanically assisted ventilation. Hemodialysis or, preferably, hemoperfusion with charcoal may be employed to lower serum concentration of the drug.

The electrocardiogram should be monitored, and supportive therapy with cardiac glycosides and diuretics should be given as required.

If progressive AV block should develop, endocardial pacing should be implemented. In case of any impaired renal function, measures to increase the glomerular filtration rate may reduce the toxicity (disopyramide is excreted primarily by the kidney).

The anticholinergic effects can be reversed with neostigmine at the discretion of the physician.

Altering the urinary pH in humans does not affect the plasma half-life or the amount of disopyramide excreted in the urine.

DOSAGE AND ADMINISTRATION
The dosage of Norpace or Norpace CR must be individualized for each patient on the basis of response and tolerance. The usual adult dosage of Norpace or Norpace CR is 400 to 800 mg per day given in divided doses. The recommended dosage for most adults is 600 mg/day given in divided doses (either 150 mg every 6 hours for immediate-release Norpace or 300

Continued on next page

Searle—Cont.

mg every 12 hours for Norpace CR). For patients whose body weight is less than 110 pounds (50 kg), the recommended dosage is 400 mg/day given in divided doses (either 100 mg every 6 hours for immediate-release Norpace or 200 mg every 12 hours for Norpace CR).

For patients with cardiomyopathy or possible cardiac decompensation, a loading dose, as discussed below, should not be given, and initial dosage should be limited to 100 mg of immediate-release Norpace every 6 to 8 hours. Subsequent dosage adjustments should be made gradually, with close monitoring for the possible development of hypotension and/or congestive heart failure (see *Warnings*).

For patients with moderate renal insufficiency (creatinine clearance greater than 40 ml/min) or hepatic insufficiency, the recommended dosage is 400 mg/day given in divided doses (either 100 mg every 6 hours for immediate-release Norpace or 200 mg every 12 hours for Norpace CR).

For patients with severe renal insufficiency (C_{cr} 40 ml/min or less), the recommended dosage regimen of immediate-release Norpace is 100 mg at intervals shown in the table below, with or without an initial loading dose of 150 mg.

IMMEDIATE-RELEASE NORPACE DOSAGE INTERVAL FOR PATIENTS WITH RENAL INSUFFICIENCY

Creatinine clearance (ml/min)	40–30	30–15	less than 15
Approximate maintenance-dosing interval	q 8 hr	q 12 hr	q 24 hr

The above dosing schedules are for Norpace immediate-release capsules; Norpace CR is not recommended for patients with severe renal insufficiency.

For patients in whom rapid control of ventricular arrhythmia is essential, an initial loading dose of 300 mg of immediate-release Norpace (200 mg for patients whose body weight is less than 110 pounds) is recommended, followed by the appropriate maintenance dosage. Therapeutic effects are usually attained 30 minutes to 3 hours after administration of a 300-mg loading dose. If there is no response or evidence of toxicity within 6 hours of the loading dose, 200 mg of immediate-release Norpace every 6 hours may be prescribed instead of the usual 150 mg. If there is no response to this dosage within 48 hours, either Norpace should then be discontinued or the physician should consider hospitalizing the patient for careful monitoring while subsequent immediate-release Norpace doses of 250 mg or 300 mg every 6 hours are given. A limited number of patients with severe refractory ventricular tachycardia have tolerated daily doses of Norpace up to 1600 mg per day (400 mg every 6 hours), resulting in disopyramide plasma levels up to 9 mcg/ml. If such treatment is warranted, it is essential that patients be hospitalized for close evaluation and continuous monitoring.

Norpace CR should not be used initially if rapid establishment of disopyramide plasma levels is desired.

Transferring to Norpace or Norpace CR

The following dosage schedule based on theoretical considerations rather than experimental data is suggested for transferring patients with normal renal function from either quinidine sulfate or procainamide therapy (Type 1 antiarrhythmic agents) to Norpace or Norpace CR therapy:

Norpace or Norpace CR should be started using the regular maintenance schedule **without a loading dose** 6 to 12 hours after the last dose of quinidine sulfate or 3 to 6 hours after the last dose of procainamide.

In patients in whom withdrawal of quinidine sulfate or procainamide is likely to produce life-threatening arrhythmias, the physician should consider hospitalization of the patient. When transferring a patient from immediate-release Norpace to Norpace CR, the maintenance schedule of Norpace CR may be started 6 hours after the last dose of immediate-release Norpace.

Pediatric Dosage

Controlled clinical studies have not been conducted in pediatric patients; however, the following suggested dosage table is based on published clinical experience.

Total daily dosage should be divided and equal doses administered orally every 6 hours or at intervals according to individual patient needs. Disopyramide plasma levels and therapeutic response must be monitored closely. Patients should be hospitalized during the initial treatment period, and dose titration should start at the lower end of the ranges provided below.

SUGGESTED TOTAL DAILY DOSAGE*

Age (years)	Disopyramide (mg/kg body weight/day)
Under 1	10 to 30
1 to 4	10 to 20
4 to 12	10 to 15
12 to 18	6 to 15

* Dosage is expressed in milligrams of disopyramide base. Since Norpace (disopyramide phosphate) 100-mg capsules contain 100 mg of disopyramide base, the pharmacist can readily prepare a 1-mg/ml to 10-mg/ml liquid suspension by adding the entire contents of Norpace capsules to cherry syrup, NF. The resulting suspension, when refrigerated, is stable for one month and should be thoroughly shaken before the measurement of each dose. The suspension should be dispensed in an amber glass bottle with a child-resistant closure.

Norpace CR capsules should not be used to prepare the above suspension.

HOW SUPPLIED

Norpace (disopyramide phosphate) is supplied in hard gelatin capsules containing either 100 mg or 150 mg of disopyramide base, present as the phosphate.

Norpace 100-mg capsules are white and orange, with markings SEARLE, 2752, NORPACE, and 100 MG.

NDC Number	Size
0025-2752-31	bottle of 100
0025-2752-52	bottle of 1,000

Norpace 150-mg capsules are brown and orange, with markings SEARLE, 2762, NORPACE, and 150 MG.

NDC Number	Size
0025-2762-31	bottle of 100
0025-2762-52	bottle of 1,000

Norpace CR (disopyramide phosphate) Controlled-Release is supplied as specially prepared controlled-release beads in hard gelatin capsules containing either 100 mg or 150 mg of disopyramide base, present as the phosphate.

Norpace CR 100-mg capsules are white and light green, with markings SEARLE, 2732, NORPACE CR, and 100 mg.

NDC Number	Size
0025-2732-31	bottle of 100
0025-2732-51	bottle of 500
0025-2732-34	carton of 100 unit dose

Norpace CR 150-mg capsules are brown and light green, with markings SEARLE, 2742, NORPACE CR, and 150 mg.

NDC Number	Size
0025-2742-31	bottle of 100
0025-2742-51	bottle of 500
0025-2742-34	carton of 100 unit dose

Store at controlled room temperature 20°–25°C (68°–77°F) [see USP].

Caution: Federal law prohibits dispensing without prescription.

2/5/96 ● A05855-2

Shown in Product Identification Guide, page 335

NOR-QD® Tablets   ℞
(norethindrone 0.35 mg)

PHYSICIAN LABELING

Patients should be counseled that this product does not protect against HIV infection (AIDS) and other sexually transmitted diseases.

ORAL CONTRACEPTIVE AGENTS

DESCRIPTION

NOR-QD Tablets provide a continuous oral contraceptive regimen of one yellow norethindrone 0.35 mg tablet daily. Norethindrone is a potent progestational agent with the chemical name 17-Hydroxy-19-Nor-17α-pregn-4-en-20-yn-3-one. The structural formula follows:

NORETHINDRONE

The yellow NOR-QD tablets contain the following inactive ingredients: D&C Yellow No. 10, FD&C Yellow No. 6, lactose, magnesium stearate, povidone, and starch.

CLINICAL PHARMACOLOGY

Combination oral contraceptives act by suppression of gonadotrophins. Although the primary mechanism of this action is inhibition of ovulation, other alterations include changes in the cervical mucus (which increase the difficulty of sperm entry into the uterus) and the endometrium (which may reduce the likelihood of implantation).

INDICATIONS AND USAGE

Oral contraceptives are indicated for the prevention of pregnancy in women who elect to use these products as a method of contraception.

Oral contraceptives are highly effective. Table I lists the typical accidental pregnancy rates for users of combination oral contraceptives and other methods of contraception.[1] The efficacy of these contraceptive methods, except sterilization, depends upon the reliability with which they are used. Correct and consistent use of methods can result in lower failure rates.

TABLE I: LOWEST EXPECTED AND TYPICAL FAILURE RATES DURING THE FIRST YEAR OF CONTINUOUS USE OF A METHOD
% of Women Experiencing an Accidental Pregnancy in the First Year of Continuous Use

Method	Lowest Expected[a]	Typical[b]
(No Contraception)	(85)	(85)
Oral contraceptives		3
combined	0.1	N/A[c]
progestogen only	0.5	N/A[c]
Diaphragm with spermicidal cream or jelly	6	18
Spermicides alone (foam, creams, jellies and vaginal suppositories)	3	21
Vaginal Sponge		
Nulliparous	6	18
Multiparous	>9	>28
IUD (medicated)	2	3[d]
Condom without spermicides	2	12
Periodic abstinence (all methods)	1–9	20
Injectable progestogen[e]	0.4	0.4
Implants	0.04	0.04
Female sterilization	0.2	0.4
Male sterilization	0.1	0.15

Adapted from J. Trussell, Table 1 [1]

[a] The authors' best guess of the percentage of women expected to experience an accidental pregnancy among couples who initiate a method (not necessarily for the first time) and who use it consistently and correctly during the first year if they do not stop for any other reason.

[b] This term represents "typical" couples who initiate use of a method (not necessarily for the first time), who experience an accidental pregnancy during the first year if they do not stop use for any other reason. The authors derive these data largely from the National Surveys of Family Growth (NSFG), 1976 and 1982.

[c] N/A—Data not available from the NSFG, 1976 and 1982.

[d] Combined typical rate for both medicated and non-medicated IUD. The rate for medicated IUD alone is not available.

[e] All forms.

CONTRAINDICATIONS

Oral contraceptives should not be used in women who have the following conditions:

- Thrombophlebitis or thromboembolic disorders
- A past history of deep vein thrombophlebitis or thromboembolic disorders
- Cerebral vascular or coronary artery disease
- Known or suspected carcinoma of the breast
- Carcinoma of the endometrium, and known or suspected estrogen-dependent neoplasia
- Undiagnosed abnormal genital bleeding
- Cholestatic jaundice of pregnancy or jaundice with prior pill use
- Hepatic adenomas, carcinomas or benign liver tumors
- Known or suspected pregnancy

WARNINGS

Cigarette smoking increases the risk of serious cardiovascular side effects from oral contraceptive use. This risk increases with age and with heavy smoking (15 or more cigarettes per day) and is quite marked in women over 35 years of age. Women who use oral contraceptives are strongly advised not to smoke.

The use of oral contraceptives is associated with increased risks of several serious conditions including myocardial in-

farction, thromboembolism, stroke, hepatic neoplasia and gallbladder disease, although the risk of serious morbidity and mortality increases significantly in the presence of other underlying risk factors such as hypertension, hyperlipidemias, hypercholesterolemia, obesity and diabetes.[2–5]

Practitioners prescribing oral contraceptives should be familiar with the following information relating to these risks.

The information contained in this package insert is principally based on studies carried out in patients who used oral contraceptives with formulations containing 0.05 mg or higher of estrogen.[6–11] The effects of long-term use with lower dose formulations of both estrogens and progestogens remain to be determined.

Throughout this labeling, epidemiological studies reported are of two types: retrospective or case control studies and prospective or cohort studies. Case control studies provide a measure of the relative risk of a disease. Relative risk, the *ratio* of the incidence of a disease among oral contraceptive users to that among non-users, cannot be assessed directly from case control studies, but the odds ratio obtained is a measure of relative risk. The relative risk does not provide information on the actual clinical occurrence of a disease. Cohort studies provide not only a measure of the relative risk but a measure of attributable risk, which is the *difference* in the incidence of disease between oral contraceptive users and non-users. The attributable risk does provide information about the actual occurrence of a disease in the population.[12–13]

1. THROMBOEMBOLIC DISORDERS AND OTHER VASCULAR PROBLEMS

a. Myocardial Infarction

An increased risk of myocardial infarction has been attributed to oral contraceptive use. This risk is primarily in smokers or women with other underlying risk factors for coronary artery disease such as hypertension, hypercholesterolemia, morbid obesity and diabetes.[2–5,13] The relative risk of heart attack for current oral contraceptive users has been estimated to be 2 to 6.[2,14–19] The risk is very low under the age of 30. However, there is the possibility of a risk of cardiovascular disease even in very young women who take oral contraceptives.

Smoking in combination with oral contraceptive use has been shown to contribute substantially to the incidence of myocardial infarctions in women 35 or older, with smoking accounting for the majority of excess cases.[20]

Mortality rates associated with circulatory disease have been shown to increase substantially in smokers over the age of 35 and non-smokers over the age of 40 among women who use oral contraceptives (see Table II).[16]

TABLE II: CIRCULATORY DISEASE MORTALITY RATES PER 100,000 WOMAN YEARS BY AGE, SMOKING STATUS AND ORAL CONTRACEPTIVE USE

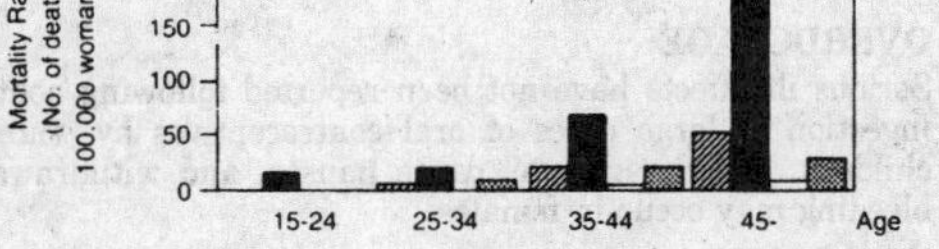

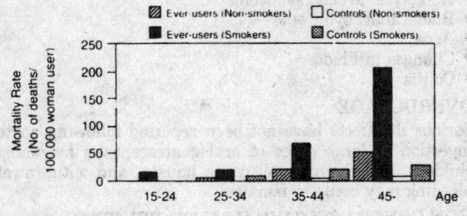

Adapted from P.M. Layde and V. Beral, Table V[16]

Oral contraceptives may compound the effects of well-known risk factors for coronary artery disease, such as hypertension, diabetes, hyperlipidemias, hypercholesterolemia, age and obesity.[3,13,21] In particular, some progestogens are known to decrease HDL cholesterol and impair oral glucose tolerance, while estrogens may create a state of hyperinsulinism.[21–25] Oral contraceptives have been shown to increase blood pressure among users (see **WARNINGS**, section 9). Similar effects on risk factors have been associated with an increased risk of heart disease. Oral contraceptives must be used with caution in women with cardiovascular disease risk factors.

b. Thromboembolism

An increased risk of thromboembolic and thrombotic disease associated with the use of oral contraceptives is well established. Case control studies have found the relative risk of users compared to non-users to be 3 for the first episode of superficial venous thrombosis, 4 to 11 for deep vein thrombosis or pulmonary embolism, and 1.5 to 6 for women with predisposing conditions for venous thromboembolic disease.[12,13,26–31] One cohort study has shown the relative risk to be somewhat lower, about 3 for new cases (subjects with no past history of venous thrombosis or varicose veins) and about 4.5 for new cases requiring hospitalization.[32] The risk of thromboembolic disease due to oral contraceptives is not related to length of use and disappears after pill use is stopped.[12]

A 2- to 6-fold increase in relative risk of post-operative thromboembolic complications has been reported with the use of oral contraceptives.[18] If feasible, oral contraceptives should be discontinued at least 4 weeks prior to and for 2 weeks after elective surgery and during and following prolonged immobilization. Since the immediate postpartum period also is associated with an increased risk of thromboembolism, oral contraceptives should be started no earlier than 4 to 6 weeks after delivery in women who elect not to breast feed.[33]

c. Cerebrovascular diseases

An increase in both the relative and attributable risks of cerebrovascular events (thrombotic and hemorrhagic strokes) has been shown in users of oral contraceptives. In general, the risk is greatest among older (> 35 years), hypertensive women who also smoke. Hypertension was found to be a risk factor for both users and non-users for both types of strokes while smoking interacted to increase the risk for hemorrhagic strokes.[34]

In a large study, the relative risk of thrombotic strokes has been shown to range from 3 for normotensive users to 14 for users with severe hypertension.[35] The relative risk of hemorrhagic stroke is reported to be 1.2 for non-smokers who used oral contraceptives, 2.6 for smokers who did not use oral contraceptives, 7.6 for smokers who used oral contraceptives, 1.8 for normotensive users and 25.7 for users with severe hypertension.[35] The attributable risk also is greater in women 35 or older and among smokers.[13]

d. Dose-related risk of vascular disease from oral contraceptives

A positive association has been observed between the amount of estrogen and progestogen in oral contraceptives and the risk of vascular disease.[36–38] A decline in serum high density lipoproteins (HDL) has been reported with some progestational agents.[22–24] A decline in serum high density lipoproteins has been associated with an increased incidence of ischemic heart disease.[39] Because estrogens increase HDL cholesterol, the net effect of an oral contraceptive depends on a balance achieved between doses of estrogen and progestogen and the nature and absolute amount of progestogens used in the contraceptives. The amount of both hormones should be considered in the choice of an oral contraceptive.[37]

Minimizing exposure to estrogen and progestogen is in keeping with good principles of therapeutics. For any particular estrogen/progestogen combination, the dosage regimen prescribed should be one which contains the least amount of estrogen and progestogen that is compatible with a low failure rate and the needs of the individual patient. New acceptors of oral contraceptive agents should be started on preparations containing the lowest estrogen content that produces satisfactory results for the individual.

e. Persistence of risk of vascular disease

There are three studies which have shown persistence of risk of vascular disease for ever-users of oral contraceptives.[17,34,40] In a study in the United States, the risk of developing myocardial infarction after discontinuing oral contraceptives persists for at least 9 years for women 40–49 years who had used oral contraceptives for 5 or more years, but this increased risk was not demonstrated in other age groups.[17] In another study in Great Britain, the risk of developing cerebrovascular disease persisted for at least 6 years after discontinuation of oral contraceptives, although excess risk was very small.[40] Subarachnoid hemorrhage also has a significantly increased relative risk after termination of use of oral contraceptives.[34] However, these studies were performed with oral contraceptive formulations containing 0.05 mg or higher of estrogen.

2. ESTIMATES OF MORTALITY FROM CONTRACEPTIVE USE

One study gathered data from a variety of sources which have estimated the mortality rates associated with different methods of contraception at different ages (see Table III).[41] These estimates include the combined risk of death associated with contraceptive methods plus the risk attributable to pregnancy in the event of method failure. Each method of contraception has its specific benefits and risks. The study concluded that with the exception of oral contraceptive users 35 and older who smoke and 40 and older who do not smoke, mortality associated with all methods of birth control is low and below that associated with childbirth. The observation of a possible increase in risk of mortality with age for oral contraceptive users is based on data gathered in the 1970s—but not reported in the U.S. until 1983.[16,41] However, current clinical practice involves the use of lower estrogen dose formulations combined with careful restriction of oral contraceptive use to women who do not have the various risk factors listed in this labeling.

Because of these changes in practice and, also, because of some limited new data which suggest that the risk of cardiovascular disease with the use of oral contraceptives may now be less than previously observed,[78,79] the Fertility and Maternal Health Drugs Advisory Committee was asked to review the topic in 1989. The Committee concluded that although cardiovascular disease risks may be increased with oral contraceptive use after age 40 in healthy non-smoking women (even with the newer low-dose formulations), there are greater potential health risks associated with pregnancy in older women and with the alternative surgical and medical procedures which may be necessary if such women do not have access to effective and acceptable means of contraception.

Therefore, the Committee recommended that the benefits of oral contraceptive use by healthy non-smoking women over 40 may outweigh the possible risks. Of course, older women, as all women who take oral contraceptives, should take the lowest possible dose formulation that is effective.[80]

[See table above.]

TABLE III: ESTIMATED ANNUAL NUMBER OF BIRTH-RELATED OR METHOD-RELATED DEATHS ASSOCIATED WITH CONTROL OF FERTILITY PER 100,000 NONSTERILE WOMEN, BY FERTILITY CONTROL METHOD ACCORDING TO AGE

Method of control and outcome	15–19	20–24	25–29	30–34	35–39	40–44
No fertility control methods*	7.0	7.4	9.1	14.8	25.7	28.2
Oral contraceptives non-smoker**	0.3	0.5	0.9	1.9	13.8	31.6
Oral contraceptives smoker**	2.2	3.4	6.6	13.5	51.1	117.2
IUD**	0.8	0.8	1.0	1.0	1.4	1.4
Condom*	1.1	1.6	0.7	0.2	0.3	0.4
Diaphragm/Spermicide*	1.9	1.2	1.2	1.3	2.2	2.8
Periodic abstinence*	2.5	1.6	1.6	1.7	2.9	3.6

* Deaths are birth-related
** Deaths are method-related

Estimates adapted from H.W. Ory, Table 3[41]

3. CARCINOMA OF THE BREAST AND REPRODUCTIVE ORGANS

Numerous epidemiological studies have been performed on the incidence of breast, endometrial, ovarian and cervical cancer in women using oral contraceptives. The evidence in the literature suggests that use of oral contraceptives is not associated with an increase in the risk of developing breast cancer, regardless of the age and parity of first use or with most of the marketed brands and doses.[42,43] The Cancer and Steroid Hormone study also showed no latent effect on the risk of breast cancer for at least a decade following long-term use.[43] A few studies have shown a slightly increased relative risk of developing breast cancer,[44–47] although the methodology of these studies, which included differences in examination of users and non-users and differences in age at start of use, has been questioned.[47–49] Some studies have reported an increased relative risk of developing breast cancer, particularly at a younger age. This increased relative risk appears to be related to duration of use.[81,82]

Some studies suggest that oral contraceptive use has been associated with an increase in the risk of cervical intraepithelial neoplasia in some populations of women.[50–53] However, there continues to be controversy about the extent to which such findings may be due to differences in sexual behavior and other factors.

In spite of many studies of the relationship between oral contraceptive use and breast or cervical cancers, a cause and effect relationship has not been established.

4. HEPATIC NEOPLASIA

Benign hepatic adenomas are associated with oral contraceptive use although the incidence of benign tumors is rare in the United States. Indirect calculations have estimated the attributable risk to be in the range of 3.3 cases per 100,000 for users, a risk that increases after 4 or more years of use.[54] Rupture of rare, benign, hepatic adenomas may cause death through intra-abdominal hemorrhage.[55–56]

Studies in the United States and Britain have shown an increased risk of developing hepatocellular carcinoma in long-term (> 8 years) oral contraceptive users.[57–59] However,

Continued on next page

Searle—Cont.

these cancers are extremely rare in the United States and the attributable risk (the excess incidence) of liver cancers in oral contraceptive users is less than 1 per 1,000,000 users.

5. OCULAR LESIONS

There have been clinical case reports of retinal thrombosis associated with the use of oral contraceptives. Oral contraceptives should be discontinued if there is unexplained partial or complete loss of vision; onset of proptosis or diplopia; papilledema; or retinal vascular lesions. Appropriate diagnostic and therapeutic measures should be undertaken immediately.

6. ORAL CONTRACEPTIVE USE BEFORE OR DURING EARLY PREGNANCY

Extensive epidemiological studies have revealed no increased risk of birth defects in women who have used oral contraceptives prior to pregnancy.[60-62] More recent studies do not suggest a teratogenic effect, particularly insofar as cardiac anomalies and limb reduction defects are concerned, when taken inadvertently during early pregnancy.[60,61,63,64]

The administration of oral contraceptives to induce withdrawal bleeding should not be used as a test for pregnancy. Oral contraceptives should not be used during pregnancy to treat threatened or habitual abortion.

It is recommended that for any patient who has missed 2 consecutive periods, pregnancy should be ruled out before continuing oral contraceptive use. If the patient has not adhered to the prescribed schedule, the possibility of pregnancy should be considered at the time of the first missed period. Oral contraceptive use should be discontinued if pregnancy is confirmed.

7. GALLBLADDER DISEASE

Earlier studies have reported an increased lifetime relative risk of gallbladder surgery in users of oral contraceptives and estrogens.[65-66] More recent studies, however, have shown that the relative risk of developing gallbladder disease among oral contraceptive users may be minimal.[67] The recent findings of minimal risk may be related to the use of oral contraceptive formulations containing lower hormonal doses of estrogens and progestogens.[68]

8. CARBOHYDRATE AND LIPID METABOLIC EFFECTS

Oral contraceptives have been shown to impair oral glucose tolerance.[69] Oral contraceptives containing greater than 0.075 mg of estrogen cause glucose intolerance with impaired insulin secretion, while lower doses of estrogen may produce less glucose intolerance.[70] Progestogens increase insulin secretion and create insulin resistance, this effect varying with different progestational agents.[25,71] However, in the non-diabetic woman, oral contraceptives appear to have no effect on fasting blood glucose.[69] Because of these demonstrated effects, prediabetic and diabetic women should be carefully observed while taking oral contraceptives.

Some women may develop persistent hypertriglyceridemia while on the pill.[72] As discussed earlier (see **WARNINGS**, sections 1a. and 1d.), changes in serum triglycerides and lipoprotein levels have been reported in oral contraceptive users.[23]

9. ELEVATED BLOOD PRESSURE

An increase in blood pressure has been reported in women taking oral contraceptives. The incidence of risk also was reported to increase with continued use and among older women.[66] Data from the Royal College of General Practitioners and subsequent randomized trials have shown that the incidence of hypertension increases with increasing concentrations of progestogens.

Women with a history of hypertension or hypertension-related diseases or renal disease should be encouraged to use another method of contraception. If women elect to use oral contraceptives, they should be monitored closely and if significant elevation of blood pressure occurs oral contraceptives should be discontinued. For most women, elevated blood pressure will return to normal after stopping oral contraceptives and there is no difference in the occurrence of hypertension among ever- and never-users.[73-75]

10. HEADACHE

The onset or exacerbation of migraine or development of headache with a new pattern which is recurrent, persistent or severe requires discontinuation of oral contraceptives and evaluation of the cause.

11. BLEEDING IRREGULARITIES

Breakthrough bleeding and spotting are sometimes encountered in patients on oral contraceptives, especially during the first 3 months of use. Non-hormonal causes should be considered and adequate diagnostic measures taken to rule out malignancy or pregnancy in the event of breakthrough bleeding, as in the case of any abnormal vaginal bleeding. If pathology has been excluded, time or a change to another formulation may solve the problem. In the event of amenorrhea, pregnancy should be ruled out.

Some women may encounter post-pill amenorrhea or oligomenorrhea, especially when such a condition was pre-existent.

PRECAUTIONS

GENERAL

PATIENTS SHOULD BE COUNSELED THAT THIS PRODUCT DOES NOT PROTECT AGAINST HIV (AIDS) AND OTHER SEXUALLY TRANSMITTED DISEASES.

1. PHYSICAL EXAMINATION AND FOLLOW-UP

It is good medical practice for all women to have annual history and physical examinations, including women using oral contraceptives. The physical examination, however, may be deferred until after initiation of oral contraceptives if requested by the woman and judged appropriate by the clinician. The physical examination should include special reference to blood pressure, breasts, abdomen and pelvic organs, including cervical cytology, and relevant laboratory tests. In case of undiagnosed, persistent or recurrent abnormal vaginal bleeding, appropriate measures should be conducted to rule out malignancy. Women with a strong family history of breast cancer or who have breast nodules should be monitored with particular care.

2. LIPID DISORDERS

Women who are being treated for hyperlipidemias should be followed closely if they elect to use oral contraceptives. Some progestogens may elevate LDL levels and may render the control of hyperlipidemias more difficult.

3. LIVER FUNCTION

If jaundice develops in any woman receiving oral contraceptives the medication should be discontinued. Steroid hormones may be poorly metabolized in patients with impaired liver function.

4. FLUID RETENTION

Oral contraceptives may cause some degree of fluid retention. They should be prescribed with caution, and only with careful monitoring, in patients with conditions which might be aggravated by fluid retention.

5. EMOTIONAL DISORDERS

Women with a history of depression should be carefully observed and the drug discontinued if depression recurs to a serious degree.

6. CONTACT LENSES

Contact lens wearers who develop visual changes or changes in lens tolerance should be assessed by an ophthalmologist.

7. DRUG INTERACTIONS

Reduced efficacy and increased incidence of breakthrough bleeding and menstrual irregularities have been associated with concomitant use of rifampin. A similar association though less marked, has been suggested with barbiturates, phenylbutazone, phenytoin sodium, and possibly with griseofulvin, ampicillin and tetracyclines.[76]

8. INTERACTIONS WITH LABORATORY TESTS

Certain endocrine and liver function tests and blood components may be affected by oral contraceptives:

a. Increased prothrombin and factors VII, VIII, IX, and X; decreased antithrombin 3; increased norepinephrine-induced platelet aggregability.

b. Increased thyroid binding globulin (TBG) leading to increased circulating total thyroid hormone, as measured by protein-bound iodine (PBI), T4 by column or by radioimmunoassay. Free T3 resin uptake is decreased, reflecting the elevated TBG. Free T4 concentration is unaltered.

c. Other binding proteins may be elevated in serum.

d. Sex steroid binding globulins are increased and result in elevated levels of total circulating sex steroids and corticoids; however, free or biologically active levels remain unchanged.

e. Triglycerides may be increased.

f. Glucose tolerance may be decreased.

g. Serum folate levels may be depressed by oral contraceptive therapy. This may be of clinical significance if a woman becomes pregnant shortly after discontinuing oral contraceptives.

9. CARCINOGENESIS

See **WARNINGS** section.

10. PREGNANCY

Pregnancy Category X. See **CONTRAINDICATIONS** and **WARNINGS** sections.

11. NURSING MOTHERS

Small amounts of oral contraceptive steroids have been identified in the milk of nursing mothers and a few adverse effects on the child have been reported, including jaundice and breast enlargement. In addition, oral contraceptives given in the postpartum period may interfere with lactation by decreasing the quantity and quality of breast milk. If possible, the nursing mother should be advised not to use oral contraceptives but to use other forms of contraception until she has completely weaned her child.

INFORMATION FOR THE PATIENT

See **PATIENT LABELING** printed below

ADVERSE REACTIONS

An increased risk of the following serious adverse reactions has been associated with the use of oral contraceptives (see **WARNINGS** section):

- Thrombophlebitis
- Arterial thromboembolism
- Pulmonary embolism
- Myocardial infarction
- Cerebral hemorrhage
- Cerebral thrombosis
- Hypertension
- Gallbladder disease
- Hepatic adenomas, carcinomas or benign liver tumors

There is evidence of an association between the following conditions and the use of oral contraceptives, although additional confirmatory studies are needed:

- Mesenteric thrombosis
- Retinal thrombosis

The following adverse reactions have been reported in patients receiving oral contraceptives and are believed to be drug-related:

- Nausea
- Vomiting
- Gastrointestinal symptoms (such as abdominal cramps and bloating)
- Breakthrough bleeding
- Spotting
- Change in menstrual flow
- Amenorrhea
- Temporary infertility after discontinuation of treatment
- Edema
- Melasma which may persist
- Breast changes: tenderness, enlargement, secretion
- Change in weight (increase or decrease)
- Change in cervical erosion and secretion
- Diminution in lactation when given immediately postpartum
- Cholestatic jaundice
- Migraine
- Rash (allergic)
- Mental depression
- Reduced tolerance to carbohydrates
- Vaginal candidiasis
- Change in corneal curvature (steepening)
- Intolerance to contact lenses

The following adverse reactions have been reported in users of oral contraceptives and the association has been neither confirmed nor refuted:

- Pre-menstrual syndrome
- Cataracts
- Changes in appetite
- Cystitis-like syndrome
- Headache
- Nervousness
- Dizziness
- Hirsutism
- Loss of scalp hair
- Erythema multiforme
- Erythema nodosum
- Hemorrhagic eruption
- Vaginitis
- Porphyria
- Impaired renal function
- Hemolytic uremic syndrome
- Budd-Chiari syndrome
- Acne
- Changes in libido
- Colitis

OVERDOSAGE

Serious ill effects have not been reported following acute ingestion of large doses of oral contraceptives by young children. Overdosage may cause nausea, and withdrawal bleeding may occur in females.

NON-CONTRACEPTIVE HEALTH BENEFITS

The following non-contraceptive health benefits related to the use of oral contraceptives are supported by epidemiological studies which largely utilized oral contraceptive formulations containing estrogen doses exceeding 0.035 mg of ethinyl estradiol or 0.05 mg of mestranol.[6-11]

Effects on menses:

- Increased menstrual cycle regularity
- Decreased blood loss and decreased incidence of iron deficiency anemia
- Decreased incidence of dysmenorrhea

Effects related to inhibition of ovulation:

- Decreased incidence of functional ovarian cysts
- Decreased incidence of ectopic pregnancies

Effects from long-term use:

- Decreased incidence of fibroadenomas and fibrocystic disease of the breast
- Decreased incidence of acute pelvic inflammatory disease
- Decreased incidence of endometrial cancer
- Decreased incidence of ovarian cancer

DOSAGE AND ADMINISTRATION

To achieve maximum contraceptive effectiveness, oral contraceptives must be taken exactly as described and at intervals not exceeding 24 hours.

NOR-QD (norethindrone) is administered as a continuous daily dosage regimen starting on the first day of menstruation, i.e., 1 tablet each day, every day. Tablets should be taken at the same time each day and continued daily, with-

out interruption, whether bleeding occurs or not. This is especially important for patients new to progestogen-only oral contraception. The patient should be advised that if prolonged bleeding occurs, she should consult her physician.

INSTRUCTIONS TO PATIENTS

- To achieve maximum contraceptive effectiveness, the oral contraceptive pill must be taken exactly as directed and at intervals not exceeding 24 hours.
- Important: Women should be instructed to use an additional method of protection until after the first 7 days of administration *in the initial cycle*.
- Due to the normally increased risk of thromboembolism occurring postpartum, women should be instructed not to initiate treatment with oral contraceptives earlier than 4 weeks after a full-term delivery. If pregnancy is terminated in the first 12 weeks, the patient should be instructed to start oral contraceptives immediately or within 7 days. If pregnancy is terminated after 12 weeks, the patient should be instructed to start oral contraceptives after 2 weeks.[33,77]
- If spotting or breakthrough bleeding should occur, the patient should continue the medication according to the schedule. Should spotting or breakthrough bleeding persist, the patient should notify her physician.
- If the patient misses 1 pill, she should be instructed to take it as soon as she remembers and then take the next pill at the regular time. The patient should be advised that missing a pill can cause spotting or light bleeding and that she may be a little sick to her stomach on the days she takes the missed pill with her regularly scheduled pill. If the patient has missed more than one pill, she should not take the missed pills and they should be discarded. She should be advised to take the next pill at the next regular time and continue to take them as scheduled. Furthermore, she should use an additional method of contraception in addition to taking her pills for the remainder of the cycle.
- Use of oral contraceptives in the event of a missed menstrual period:
  1. If the patient has not adhered to the prescribed dosage regimen, the possibility of pregnancy should be considered after the first missed period and oral contraceptives should be withheld until pregnancy has been ruled out.
  2. If the patient has adhered to the prescribed regimen and misses 2 consecutive periods, pregnancy should be ruled out before continuing the contraceptive regimen.

HOW SUPPLIED

NOR-QD® (norethindrone) tablets are available in 42-tablet dispensers.

CAUTION: Federal law prohibits dispensing without prescription.

Store at controlled room temperature 15°–30°C (59°–86°F).

REFERENCES

1. Trussell, J., et al.: *Stud Fam Plann* 21(1):51–54, 1990. 2. Mann, J., et al.: *Br Med J* 2(5956):241–245, 1975. 3. Knopp, R.H.: *J Reprod Med* 31(9):913–921, 1986. 4. Mann, J.I., et al.: *Br Med J* 2:445–447, 1976. 5. Ory, H.: *JAMA* 237:2619–2622, 1977. 6. The Cancer and Steroid Hormone Study of the Centers for Disease Control: *JAMA* 249(2):1596–1599, 1983. 7. The Cancer and Steroid Hormone Study of the Centers for Disease Control: *JAMA* 257(6):796–800, 1987. 8. Ory, H.W.: *JAMA* 228(1):68–69, 1974. 9. Ory, H.W., et al.: *N Engl J Med* 294:419–422, 1976. 10. Ory, H.W.: *Fam Plann Perspect* 14:182–184, 1982. 11. Ory, H.W., et al.: *Making Choices*, New York, The Alan Guttmacher Institute, 1983. 12. Stadel, B.: *N Engl J Med* 305(11):612–618, 1981. 13. Stadel, B.: *N Engl J Med* 305(12):672–677, 1981. 14. Adam, S., et al.: *Br J Obstet Gynaecol* 88:838–845, 1981. 15. Mann, J., et al.: *Br Med J* 2(5965):245–248, 1975. 16. Royal College of General Practitioners' Oral Contraceptive Study: *Lancet* 1:541–546, 1981. 17. Slone, D., et al.: *N Engl J Med* 305(8):420–424, 1981. 18. Vessey, M.P.: *Br J Fam Plann* 6 (Supplement):1–12, 1980. 19. Russell-Briefel, R., et al.: *Prev Med* 15:352–362, 1986. 20. Goldbaum, G., et al.: *JAMA* 258(10):1339–1342, 1987. 21. LaRosa, J.C.: *J Reprod Med* 31(9):906–912, 1986. 22. Krauss, R.M., et al.: *Am J Obstet Gynecol* 145:446–452, 1983. 23. Wahl, P., et al.: *N Engl J Med* 308(15):862–867, 1983. 24. Wynn, V., et al.: *Am J Obstet Gynecol* 142(6):766–771, 1982. 25. Wynn V., et al.: *J Reprod Med* 31(9):892–897, 1986. 26. Inman, W.H., et al.: *Br Med J* 2(5599):193–199, 1968. 27. Maguire, M.G., et al.: *Am J Epidemiol* 110(2):188–195, 1979. 28. Petitti, D., et al.: *JAMA* 242(11):1150–1154, 1979. 29. Vessey, M.P., et al.: *Br Med J* 2(5599):199–205, 1968. 30. Vessey, M.P., et al.: *Br Med J* 2(5658):651–657, 1969. 31. Porter, J.B., et al.: *Obstet Gynecol* 59(3):299–302, 1982. 32. Vessey, M.P., et al.: *J Biosoc Sci* 8:373–427, 1976. 33. Mishell, D.R., et al.: *Reproductive Endocrinology*, Philadelphia, F.A. Davis Co., 1979. 34. Petitti, D.B., et al.: *Lancet* 2:234–236, 1978. 35. Collaborative Group for the Study of Stroke in Young Women: *JAMA* 231(7):718–722, 1975. 36. Inman, W.H., et al.: *Br Med J* 2:203–209, 1970. 37. Meade, T.W., et al.: *Br Med J* 280 (6224):1157–1161, 1980. 38. Kay, C.R.: *Am J Obstet Gynecol* 142(6):762–765, 1982. 39. Gordon, T., et al.: *Am J Med* 62:707–714, 1977. 40. Royal College of General Practitioners' Oral Contraception Study: *J Coll Gen Pract* 33:75–82, 1983.

41. Ory, H.W.: *Fam Plann Perspect* 15(2):57–63, 1983. 42. Paul, C., et al.: *Br Med J* 293:723–725, 1986. 43. The Cancer and Steroid Hormone Study of the Centers for Disease Control: *N Engl J Med* 315(7):405–411, 1986. 44. Pike, M.C., et al.: *Lancet* 2:926–929, 1983. 45. Miller, D.R., et al.: *Obstet Gynecol* 68:863–868, 1986. 46. Olsson, H., et al.: *Lancet* 2:748–749, 1985. 47. McPherson, K., et al.: *Br J Cancer* 56:653–660, 1987. 48. Huggins, G.R., et al.: *Fertil Steril* 47(5):733–761, 1987. 49. McPherson, K., et al.: *Br Med J* 293:709–710, 1986. 50. Ory, H., et al.: *Am J Obstet Gynecol* 124(6):573–577, 1976. 51. Vessey, M.P., et al.: *Lancet* 2:930, 1983. 52. Brinton, L.A., et al.: *Int J Cancer* 38:339–344, 1986. 53. WHO Collaborative Study of Neoplasia and Steroid Contraceptives: *Br Med J* 290:961–965, 1985. 54. Rooks, J.B., et al.: *JAMA* 242(7):644–648, 1979. 55. Bein, N.N., et al.: *Br J Surg* 64:433–435, 1977. 56. Klatskin, G.: *Gastroenterology* 73:386–394, 1977. 57. Henderson, B.E., et al.: *Br J Cancer* 48:437–440, 1983. 58. Neuberger, J., et al.: *Br Med J* 292:1355–1357, 1986. 59. Forman, D., et al.: *Br Med J* 292:1357–1361, 1986. 60. Harlap, S., et al.: *Obstet Gynecol* 55(4):447–452, 1980. 61. Savolainen, E., et al.: *Am J Obstet Gynecol* 140(5):521–524, 1981. 62. Janerich, D.T., et al.: *Am J Epidemiol* 112(1):73–79, 1980. 63. Ferencz, C., et al.: *Teratology* 21:225–239, 1980. 64. Rothman, K.J., et al.: *Am J Epidemiol* 109(4):433–439, 1979. 65. Boston Collaborative Drug Surveillance Program: *Lancet* 1:1399–1404, 1973. 66. Royal College of General Practitioners: *Oral contraceptives and health*. New York, Pittman, 1974. 67. Rome Group for the Epidemiology and Prevention of Cholelithiasis: *Am J Epidemiol* 119(5):796–805, 1984. 68. Strom, B.L., et al.: *Clin Pharmacol Ther* 39(3):335–341, 1986. 69. Perlman, J.A., et al.: *J Chronic Dis* 38(10):857–864, 1985. 70. Wynn, V., et al.: *Lancet* 1:1045–1049, 1979. 71. Wynn, V.: *Progesterone and Progestin*, New York, Raven Press, 1983. 72. Wynn, V., et al.: *Lancet* 2:720–723, 1966. 73. Fisch, I.R., et al.: *JAMA* 237(23):2499–2503, 1977. 74. Laragh, J.H.: *Am J Obstet Gynecol* 126(1):141–147, 1976. 75. Ramcharan, S., et al.: *Pharmacology of Steroid Contraceptive Drugs*, New York, Raven Press, 1977. 76. Stockley, I.: *Pharm J* 216:140–143, 1976. 77. Dickey, R.P.: *Managing Contraceptive Pill Patients*, Oklahoma, Creative Informatics Inc., 1984. 78. Porter J.B., Hunter J., Jick H., et al: *Obstet Gynecol* 1985;66:1–4. 79. Porter J.B., Hershel J., Walker A.M.: *Obstet Gynecol* 1987;70:29–32. 80. Fertility and Maternal Health Drugs Advisory Committee, F.D.A., October, 1989. 81. Schlesselman J., Stadel B.V., Murray P., Lai S.: *Breast cancer in relation to early use of oral contraceptives*. JAMA 1988;259:1828–1833. 82. Hennekens C.H., Speizer F.E., Lipnick R.J., Rosner B., Bain C., Belanger C., Stampfer M.J., Willett W., Peto R.: *A case-control study of oral contraceptive use and breast cancer*. JNCI 1984:72:39–42.

DETAILED PATIENT LABELING

This product (like all oral contraceptives) is intended to prevent pregnancy. It does not protect against HIV infection (AIDS) and other sexually transmitted diseases.

INTRODUCTION

Any woman who considers using oral contraceptives ("birth control pills" or "the pill") should understand the benefits and risks of using this form of birth control. This leaflet will give you much of the information you will need to make this decision and also will help you determine if you are at risk of developing any of the serious side effects of the pill. It will tell you how to use the pill properly so that it will be as effective as possible. However, this leaflet is not a replacement for a careful discussion between you and your health care provider. You should discuss the information provided in this leaflet with him or her, both when you first start taking the pill and during your regular visits. You also should follow the advice of your health care provider with regard to regular check-ups while you are on the pill.

EFFECTIVENESS OF ORAL CONTRACEPTIVES

Oral contraceptives are used to prevent pregnancy and are more effective than other non-surgical methods of birth control. When they are taken correctly, without missing any pills, the chance of becoming pregnant is less than 1% (1 pregnancy per 100 women per year of use). Typical failure rates are actually 3% per year. The chance of becoming pregnant increases with each missed pill during a menstrual cycle.

In comparison, typical failure rates for other nonsurgical methods of birth control during the first year are as follows:

IUD: 3%
Diaphragm with spermicides: 18%
Spermicides alone: 21%
Vaginal sponge: 18 to 28%
Condom alone: 12%
Periodic abstinence: 20%
Injectable progestogen: 0.4%
Implants: 0.04%
No methods: 85%

WHO SHOULD NOT TAKE ORAL CONTRACEPTIVES

Cigarette smoking increases the risk of serious cardiovascular side effects from oral contraceptive use. This

risk increases with age and with heavy smoking (15 or more cigarettes per day) and is quite marked in women over 35 years of age. Women who use oral contraceptives are strongly advised not to smoke.

Some women should not use the pill. For example, you should not take the pill if you are pregnant or think you may be pregnant. You also should not use the pill if you have any of the following conditions:

- A history of heart attack or stroke
- Blood clots in the legs (thrombophlebitis), brain (stroke), lungs (pulmonary embolism) or eyes
- A history of blood clots in the deep veins of your legs
- Chest pain (angina pectoris)
- Known or suspected breast cancer or cancer of the lining of the uterus, cervix or vagina
- Unexplained vaginal bleeding (until a diagnosis is reached by your doctor)
- Yellowing of the whites of the eyes or of the skin (jaundice) during pregnancy or during previous use of the pill
- Liver tumor (benign or cancerous)
- Known or suspected pregnancy

Tell your health care provider if you have ever had any of these conditions. Your health care provider can recommend a safer method of birth control.

OTHER CONSIDERATIONS BEFORE TAKING ORAL CONTRACEPTIVES

Tell your health care provider if you have or have had:

- Breast nodules, fibrocystic disease of the breast, an abnormal breast x-ray or mammogram
- Diabetes
- Elevated cholesterol or triglycerides
- High blood pressure
- Migraine or other headaches or epilepsy
- Mental depression
- Gallbladder, heart or kidney disease
- History of scanty or irregular menstrual periods

Women with any of these conditions should be checked often by their health care provider if they choose to use oral contraceptives.

Also, be sure to inform your doctor or health care provider if you smoke or are on any medications.

RISKS OF TAKING ORAL CONTRACEPTIVES

1. Risk of developing blood clots

Blood clots and blockage of blood vessels are the most serious side effects of taking oral contraceptives. In particular, a clot in the legs can cause thrombophlebitis and a clot that travels to the lungs can cause a sudden blocking of the vessel carrying blood to the lungs. Rarely, clots occur in the blood vessels of the eye and may cause blindness, double vision, or impaired vision.

If you take oral contraceptives and need elective surgery, need to stay in bed for a prolonged illness or have recently delivered a baby, you may be at risk of developing blood clots. You should consult your doctor about stopping oral contraceptives three to four weeks before surgery and not taking oral contraceptives for two weeks after surgery or during bed rest. You should also not take oral contraceptives soon after delivery of a baby. It is advisable to wait for at least four weeks after delivery if you are not breast feeding. If you are breast feeding, you should wait until you have weaned your child before using the pill (see **GENERAL PRECAUTIONS, While Breast Feeding**).

2. Heart attacks and strokes

Oral contraceptives may increase the tendency to develop strokes (stoppage or rupture of blood vessels in the brain) and angina pectoris and heart attacks (blockage of blood vessels in the heart). Any of these conditions can cause death or temporary or permanent disability.

Smoking greatly increases the possibility of suffering heart attacks and strokes. Furthermore, smoking and the use of oral contraceptives greatly increase the chances of developing and dying of heart disease.

3. Gallbladder disease

Oral contraceptive users may have a greater risk than non-users of having gallbladder disease, although this risk may be related to pills containing high doses of estrogen.

4. Liver tumors

In rare cases, oral contraceptives can cause benign but dangerous liver tumors. These benign liver tumors can rupture and cause fatal internal bleeding. In addition, a possible but not definite association has been found with the pill and liver cancers in 2 studies in which a few women who developed these very rare cancers were found to have used oral contraceptives for long periods. However, liver cancers are extremely rare.

5. Cancer of the breast and reproductive organs

There is, at present, no confirmed evidence that oral contraceptives increase the risk of cancer of the reproductive organs in human studies. Several studies have found no overall increase in the risk of developing breast cancer. However, women who use oral contraceptives and have a strong family

Continued on next page

Searle—Cont.

history of breast cancer or who have breast nodules or abnormal mammograms should be followed closely by their doctors. Some studies have reported an increase in the risk of developing breast cancer, particularly at a younger age. This increased risk appears to be related to duration of use.

Some studies have found an increase in the incidence of cancer of the cervix in women who use oral contraceptives. However, this finding may be related to factors other than the use of oral contraceptives.

ESTIMATED RISK OF DEATH FROM A BIRTH CONTROL METHOD OR PREGNANCY

All methods of birth control and pregnancy are associated with a risk of developing certain diseases which may lead to disability or death. An estimate of the number of deaths associated with different methods of birth control and pregnancy has been calculated and is shown in the following table.

[See table below.]

In the above table, the risk of death from any birth control method is less than the risk of childbirth except for oral contraceptive users over the age of 35 who smoke and pill users over the age of 40 even if they do not smoke. It can be seen from the table that for women aged 15 to 39 the risk of death is highest with pregnancy (7–26 deaths per 100,000 women, depending on age). Among pill users who do not smoke the risk of death is always lower than that associated with pregnancy for any age group, although over the age of 40 the risk increases to 32 deaths per 100,000 women compared to 28 associated with pregnancy at that age. However, for pill users who smoke and are over the age of 35 the estimated number of deaths exceeds those for other methods of birth control. If a woman is over the age of 40 and smokes, her estimated risk of death is 4 times higher (117/100,000 women) than the estimated risk associated with pregnancy (28/100,000 women) in that age group.

The suggestion that women over 40 who don't smoke should not take oral contraceptives is based on information from older high-dose pills and on less selective use of pills than is practiced today. An Advisory Committee of the FDA discussed this issue in 1989 and recommended that the benefits of oral contraceptive use by healthy, non-smoking women over 40 years of age may outweigh the possible risks. However, all women, especially older women, are cautioned to use the lowest dose pill that is effective.

WARNING SIGNALS

If any of these adverse effects occur while you are taking oral contraceptives, call your doctor immediately:

- Sharp chest pain, coughing of blood or sudden shortness of breath (indicating a possible clot in the lung)
- Pain in the calf (indicating a possible clot in the leg)
- Crushing chest pain or heaviness in the chest (indicating a possible heart attack)
- Sudden severe headache or vomiting, dizziness or fainting, disturbances of vision or speech, weakness or numbness in an arm or leg (indicating a possible stroke)
- Sudden partial or complete loss of vision (indicating a possible clot in the eye)
- Breast lumps (indicating possible breast cancer or fibrocystic disease of the breast: ask your doctor or health care provider to show you how to examine your breasts)
- Severe pain or tenderness in the stomach area (indicating a possible ruptured liver tumor)
- Difficulty in sleeping, weakness, lack of energy, fatigue or change in mood (possibly indicating severe depression)
- Jaundice or a yellowing of the skin or eyeballs, accompanied frequently by fever, fatigue, loss of appetite, dark colored urine or light colored bowel movements (indicating possible liver problems)

SIDE EFFECTS OF ORAL CONTRACEPTIVES

1. Vaginal bleeding

Irregular vaginal bleeding or spotting may occur while you are taking the pill. Irregular bleeding may vary from slight staining between menstrual periods to breakthrough bleeding which is a flow much like a regular period. Irregular bleeding occurs most often during the first few months of oral contraceptive use but may also occur after you have been taking the pill for some time. Such bleeding may be temporary and usually does not indicate any serious problem. It is important to continue taking your pills on schedule. If the bleeding occurs in more than 1 cycle or lasts for more than a few days, talk to your doctor or health care provider.

2. Contact lenses

If you wear contact lenses and notice a change in vision or an inability to wear your lenses, contact your doctor or health care provider.

3. Fluid retention

Oral contraceptives may cause edema (fluid retention) with swelling of the fingers or ankles and may raise your blood pressure. If you experience fluid retention, contact your doctor or health care provider.

4. Melasma (Mask of Pregnancy)

A spotty darkening of the skin is possible, particularly of the face.

5. Other side effects

Other side effects may include change in appetite, headache, nervousness, depression, dizziness, loss of scalp hair, rash and vaginal infections.

If any of these side effects occur, contact your doctor or health care provider.

GENERAL PRECAUTIONS

1. Missed periods and use of oral contraceptives before or during early pregnancy

At times you may not menstruate regularly after you have completed taking a cycle of pills. If you have taken your pills regularly and miss 1 menstrual period, continue taking your pills for the next cycle but be sure to inform your health care provider before doing so. If you have not taken the pills daily as instructed and miss 1 menstrual period, or if you miss 2 consecutive menstrual periods, you may be pregnant. You should stop taking oral contraceptives until you are sure you are not pregnant and continue to use another method of contraception.

There is no conclusive evidence that oral contraceptive use is associated with an increase in birth defects when taken inadvertently during early pregnancy. Previously, a few studies had reported that oral contraceptives might be associated with birth defects but these studies have not been confirmed. Nevertheless, oral contraceptives or any other drugs should not be used during pregnancy unless clearly necessary and prescribed by your doctor. You should check with your doctor about risks to your unborn child from any medication taken during pregnancy.

2. While breast feeding

If you are breast feeding, consult your doctor before starting oral contraceptives. Some of the drug will be passed on to the child in the milk. A few adverse effects on the child have been reported, including yellowing of the skin (jaundice) and breast enlargement. In addition, oral contraceptives may decrease the amount and quality of your milk. If possible, use another method of contraception while breast feeding. You should consider starting oral contraceptives only after you have weaned your child completely.

3. Laboratory tests

If you are scheduled for any laboratory tests, tell your doctor you are taking birth control pills. Certain blood tests may be affected by birth control pills.

4. Drug interactions

Certain drugs may interact with birth control pills to make them less effective in preventing pregnancy or cause an increase in breakthrough bleeding. Such drugs include rifampin; drugs used for epilepsy such as barbiturates (for example phenobarbital) and phenytoin (Dilantin is one brand of this drug); phenylbutazone (Butazolidin is one brand of this drug) and possibly certain antibiotics. You may need to use additional contraception when you take drugs which can make oral contraceptives less effective.

ESTIMATED ANNUAL NUMBER OF BIRTH-RELATED OR METHOD-RELATED DEATHS ASSOCIATED WITH CONTROL OF FERTILITY PER 100,000 NON-STERILE WOMEN, BY FERTILITY CONTROL METHOD ACCORDING TO AGE

Method of control and outcome	15–19	20–24	25–29	30–34	35–39	40–44
No fertility control methods*	7.0	7.4	9.1	14.8	25.7	28.2
Oral contraceptives non-smoker**	0.3	0.5	0.9	1.9	13.8	31.6
Oral contraceptives smoker**	2.2	3.4	6.6	13.5	51.1	117.2
IUD**	0.8	0.8	1.0	1.0	1.4	1.4
Condom*	1.1	1.6	0.7	0.2	0.3	0.4
Diaphragm/Spermicide*	1.9	1.2	1.2	1.3	2.2	2.8
Periodic abstinence*	2.5	1.6	1.6	1.7	2.9	3.6

* Deaths are birth-related

**Deaths are method-related

HOW TO TAKE ORAL CONTRACEPTIVES

1. Important points to remember

This product (like all oral contraceptives) is intended to prevent pregnancy. It does not protect against transmission of HIV (AIDS) and other sexually transmitted diseases such as chlamydia, genital herpes, genital warts, gonorrhea, hepatitis B, and syphilis.

Before you start taking your pills:

- Be sure to read these directions:
  Before you start taking your pills.
  Anytime you are not sure what to do.
- The right way to take the Pill is to take one pill every day at the same time. If you miss pills you could get pregnant. The more pills you miss, the more likely you are to get pregnant.
- Many women have spotting or light bleeding while they are taking the Pill, or may feel sick to their stomachs during the first 1–3 packs of pills. If you feel sick to your stomach, do not stop taking the Pill. These problems will usually go away after the first three months. If they do not go away, talk to your doctor or clinic.
- Missing pills can also cause spotting or light bleeding (see the section on MISSED PILLS). You could also feel a little sick to your stomach on the days you take a missed pill with your regularly scheduled pill.
- If you have vomiting or diarrhea, for any reason, or if you take some medicines, including some antibiotics, your pills may not work as well. Use a back-up method of birth control until you check with your doctor or clinic. Talk to your doctor or clinic about which back-up birth control method is right for you.
- If you have trouble remembering to take the Pill (for example, if you forget to take more than one pill two months in a row), talk to your doctor or clinic about how to make pill-taking easier or about using another method of birth control.
- If you have any questions or are unsure about the information in this leaflet, call your doctor or clinic.

2. Before you start taking your pills

- Decide what time of day you want to take your pill. It is important to take it at about the same time every day.
- The 42-pill pack has 42 yellow pills to take daily, 1 tablet each day, everyday, without interruption.
- Also find:
  1) where on the pack to start taking pills.
  2) in what order to take the pills and
  3) the days of the week as shown on the pill card.

Nor-QD
Pill Color: Yellow

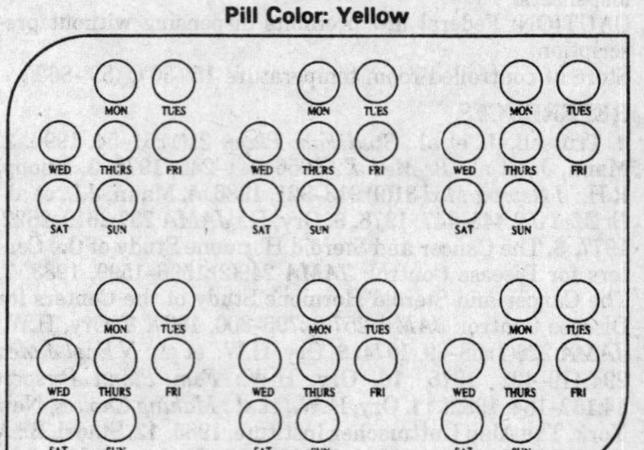

- Be sure you have ready at all times:
  Another kind of birth control to use as a back-up in case you miss pills. (Remember to talk to your doctor or clinic about an appropriate back-up method of birth control for you.)
  An extra, full pill pack.

3. When to start the first pack of pills

- Take the first pill on the first day of the menstrual flow, and take another pill each day, every day until the time for your visit with your physician or health care provider. The pill should be taken at the same time of day, preferably at bedtime, and continued daily without interruption whether bleeding occurs or not. If prolonged bleeding occurs, you should consult your physician.

4. What to do during the month

- **Take one pill at the same time every day until the pack is empty**
  Do not skip pills even if you are spotting or have light bleeding between monthly periods or feel sick to your stomach (nausea).
  Do not skip pills even if you do not have sex very often.
- **When you finish a pack of pills:**
  Start the next pack on the day after your last pill. Do not wait any days between packs.

5. What to do if you miss pills

If you **MISS 1** yellow pill:

- Take it as soon as you remember. Take the next pill at your regular time. This means you take 2 pills in 1 day.

- Missing a pill can cause spotting or light bleeding. You could also feel a little sick to your stomach on the days you take a missed pill with your regularly scheduled pill.
- You do not need to use a back-up birth control method if you have sex.

If you **MISS MORE THAN 1** yellow pill in a row:

- Do not take the missed pills. The missed pills may be discarded. Take the next pill at your regular time. Continue to take one pill a day as scheduled.
- Missing pills can cause spotting or light bleeding.
- You MAY BECOME PREGNANT, especially if you have sex in the first 7 days after you have missed pills. Therefore, you MUST use a back-up method of birth control until you start a new pill pack. (Remember to talk to your doctor or clinic about an appropriate back-up birth control method for you.)

FINALLY, IF YOU ARE STILL NOT SURE WHAT TO DO ABOUT THE PILLS YOU HAVE MISSED:

Use a BACK-UP METHOD OF BIRTH CONTROL anytime you have sex.

KEEP TAKING ONE PILL EACH DAY until you can talk to your doctor or clinic.

6. Missed periods, spotting or light bleeding

At times, you may not have a period after you have completed a pack of pills. If you miss 1 period but you have taken the pills exactly as you were supposed to, continue as usual into the next cycle. If you have not taken the pills correctly, and have missed a period, you may be pregnant and you should stop taking the Pill until your doctor or clinic determines whether or not you are pregnant. Until you can talk to your doctor or clinic, use an appropriate back-up birth control method. If you miss 2 consecutive periods, you should stop taking the Pill until it is determined that you are not pregnant.

Even if spotting or light bleeding should occur, continue taking the Pill according to the schedule. Should spotting or light bleeding persist, you should notify your doctor or clinic.

7. Stopping the pill before surgery or prolonged bed rest

If you are scheduled for surgery or you need to stay in bed for a long period of time you should tell your doctor that you are on the Pill. You should stop taking the Pill four weeks before your operation to avoid an increased risk of blood clots. Talk to your doctor about when you may start taking the Pill again.

8. Starting the pill after pregnancy

After you have a baby it is advisable to wait 4 weeks before starting to take the Pill. Talk to your doctor about when you may start taking the Pill after pregnancy.

9. Pregnancy due to pill failure

When the Pill is taken correctly, the expected pregnancy rate is approximately 1% (i.e., 1 pregnancy per 100 women per year). If pregnancy occurs while taking the Pill, there is little risk to the fetus. The typical failure rate of large numbers of pill users is less than 3% when women who have missed pills are included. If you become pregnant, you should discuss your pregnancy with your doctor.

10. Pregnancy after stopping the pill

There may be some delay in becoming pregnant after you stop taking the Pill, especially if you had irregular periods before you started using the Pill. Your doctor may recommend that you delay becoming pregnant until you have had one or more regular periods.

There does not appear to be any increase in birth defects in newborn babies when pregnancy occurs soon after stopping the Pill.

11. Overdosage

There are no reports of serious illness or side effects in young children who have swallowed a large number of pills. In adults, overdosage may cause nausea and/or bleeding in females. In case of overdosage, contact your doctor, clinic or pharmacist.

12. Other information

Your doctor or clinic will take a medical and family history and will examine you before prescribing the Pill. The physical examination may be delayed to another time if you request it and the health care provider believes that it is a good medical practice to postpone it. You should be reexamined at least once a year. Be sure to inform your doctor or clinic if there is a family history of any of the conditions listed previously in this leaflet. Be sure to keep all appointments with your doctor or clinic because this is a time to determine if there are early signs of side effects from using the Pill.

Do not use the Pill for any condition other than the one for which it was prescribed. The Pill has been prescribed specifically for you, do not give it to others who may want birth control pills.

If you want more information about birth control pills, ask your doctor or clinic. They have a more technical leaflet called **PHYSICIAN LABELING** which you might want to read.

NON-CONTRACEPTIVE HEALTH BENEFITS

In addition to preventing pregnancy, use of oral contraceptives may provide certain non-contraceptive health benefits:

- Menstrual cycles may become more regular
- Blood flow during menstruation may be lighter and less iron may be lost. Therefore, anemia due to iron deficiency is less likely to occur.
- Pain or other symptoms during menstruation may be encountered less frequently
- Ectopic (tubal) pregnancy may occur less frequently
- Non-cancerous cysts or lumps in the breast may occur less frequently
- Acute pelvic inflammatory disease may occur less frequently
- Oral contraceptive use may provide some protection against developing two forms of cancer: cancer of the ovaries and cancer of the lining of the uterus.

Store at controlled room temperature 15°–30°C (59°–86°F).

BRIEF SUMMARY

PATIENT PACKAGE INSERT

This product (like all oral contraceptives) is intended to prevent pregnancy. It does not protect against HIV infection (AIDS) and other sexually transmitted diseases.

Oral contraceptives, also known as "birth control pills" or "the pill," are taken to prevent pregnancy and, when taken correctly, have a failure rate of about 1% per year when used without missing any pills. The typical failure rate of large numbers of pill users is less than 3% per year when women who miss pills are included. For most women, oral contraceptives are also free of serious or unpleasant side effects. However, forgetting to take oral contraceptives considerably increases the chances of pregnancy.

For the majority of women, oral contraceptives can be taken safely, but there are some women who are at high risk of developing certain serious diseases that can be life-threatening or may cause temporary or permanent disability. The risks associated with taking oral contraceptives increase significantly if you:

- Smoke
- Have high blood pressure, diabetes or high cholesterol
- Have or have had clotting disorders, heart attack, stroke, angina pectoris, cancer of the breast or sex organs, jaundice or malignant or benign liver tumors

You should not take the pill if you suspect you are pregnant or have unexplained vaginal bleeding.

Cigarette smoking increases the risk of serious cardiovascular side effects from oral contraceptive use. This risk increases with age and with heavy smoking (15 or more cigarettes per day) and is quite marked in women over 35 years of age. Women who use oral contraceptives are strongly advised not to smoke.

Most side effects of the pill are not serious. The most common such effects are nausea, vomiting, bleeding between menstrual periods, weight gain, breast tenderness and difficulty wearing contact lenses. These side effects, especially nausea and vomiting, may subside within the first 3 months of use.

The serious side effects of the pill occur very infrequently, especially if you are in good health and are young. However, you should know that the following medical conditions have been associated with or made worse by the pill:

1. Blood clots in the legs (thrombophlebitis) or lungs (pulmonary embolism), stoppage or rupture of a blood vessel in the brain (stroke), blockage of blood vessels in the heart (heart attack or angina pectoris), eye or other organs of the body. As mentioned above, smoking increases the risk of heart attacks and strokes and subsequent serious medical consequences.
2. Liver tumors, which may rupture and cause severe bleeding. A possible but not definite association has been found with the pill and liver cancer. However, liver cancers are extremely rare.
3. High blood pressure, although blood pressure usually returns to normal when the pill is stopped.

The symptoms associated with these serious side effects are discussed in the detailed leaflet given to you with your supply of pills. Notify your doctor or health care provider if you notice any unusual physical disturbances while taking the pill. In addition, drugs such as rifampin, as well as some anticonvulsants and some antibiotics, may decrease oral contraceptive effectiveness.

Studies to date of women taking the pill have not shown an increase in the incidence of cancer of the breast or cervix. There is, however, insufficient evidence to rule out the possibility that the pill may cause such cancers. Some studies have reported an increase in the risk of developing breast cancer, particularly at a younger age. This increased risk appears to be related to duration of use.

Taking the pill may provide some important non-contraceptive health benefits. These include less painful menstruation, less menstrual blood loss and anemia, fewer acute pelvic infections and fewer cancers of the ovary and the lining of the uterus.

Be sure to discuss any medical condition you may have with your health care provider. Your health care provider will take a medical and family history before prescribing oral contraceptives and will examine you. The physical examination may be delayed to another time if you request it and the health care provider believes that it is a good medical practice to postpone it. You should be reexamined at least once a year while taking oral contraceptives. The detailed patient information leaflet gives you further information which you should read and discuss with your health care provider.

HOW TO TAKE ORAL CONTRACEPTIVES

See full text of How To Take Oral Contraceptives which is printed in full in the Detailed Patient Labeling.

Revised June 1993

Shown in Product Identification Guide, page 335

SYNAREL® ℞

[sin 'er-el]

(nafarelin acetate)

Nasal Solution 2 mg/mL

(as nafarelin base)

CENTRAL PRECOCIOUS PUBERTY
(FOR ENDOMETRIOSIS, SEE ENDOMETRIOSIS SECTION)

DESCRIPTION

SYNAREL (nafarelin acetate) Nasal Solution is intended for administration as a spray to the nasal mucosa. Nafarelin acetate, the active component of SYNAREL Nasal Solution, is a decapeptide with the chemical name: 5-oxo-L-prolyl-L-histidyl-L-tryptophyl-L-seryl-L-tyrosyl -3- (2-naphthyl)-D-alanyl-L-leucyl-L-arginyl-L-prolyl-glycinamide acetate. Nafarelin acetate is a synthetic analog of the naturally occurring gonadotropin-releasing hormone (GnRH).

Nafarelin acetate has the following chemical structure:

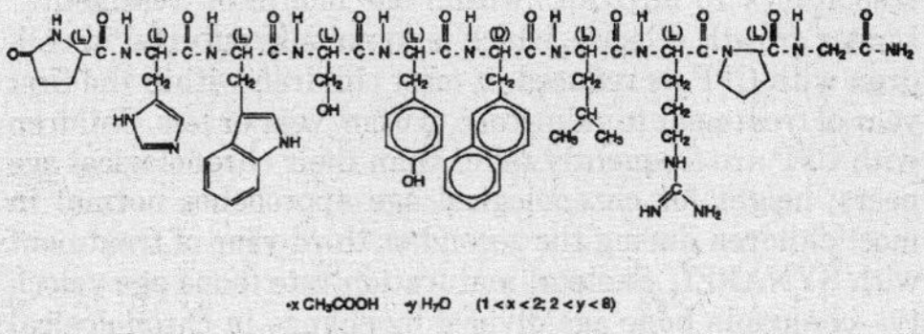

$\cdot x\ CH_3COOH \quad \cdot y\ H_2O \quad (1 < x < 2;\ 2 < y < 8)$

SYNAREL Nasal Solution contains nafarelin acetate (2 mg/mL, content expressed as nafarelin base) in a solution of benzalkonium chloride, glacial acetic acid, sodium hydroxide or hydrochloric acid (to adjust pH), sorbitol, and purified water.

After priming the pump unit for SYNAREL, each actuation of the unit delivers approximately 100 µL of the spray containing approximately 200 µg nafarelin base. The contents of one spray bottle are intended to deliver at least 60 sprays.

CLINICAL PHARMACOLOGY

Nafarelin acetate is a potent agonistic analog of gonadotropin-releasing hormone (GnRH). At the onset of administration, nafarelin stimulates the release of the pituitary gonadotropins, luteinizing hormone (LH) and follicle stimulating hormone (FSH), resulting in a temporary increase of gonadal steroidogenesis. Repeated dosing abolishes the stimulatory effect on the pituitary gland. Twice daily administration leads to decreased secretion of gonadal steroids by about 4 weeks; consequently, tissues and functions that depend on gonadal steroids for their maintenance become quiescent.

In **children**, nafarelin acetate was rapidly absorbed into the systemic circulation after intranasal administration. Maximum serum concentrations (measured by RIA) were achieved between 10 and 45 minutes. Following a single dose of 400 µg base, the observed peak concentration was 2.2 ng/mL, whereas following a single dose of 600 µg base, the observed peak concentration was 6.6 ng/mL. The average serum half-life of nafarelin following intranasal administration of a 400 µg dose was approximately 2.5 hours. It is not known and cannot be predicted what the pharmacokinetics of nafarelin will be in children given a dose above 600 µg.

In **adult women**, nafarelin acetate was rapidly absorbed into the systemic circulation after intranasal administration. Maximum serum concentrations (measured by RIA) were achieved between 10 and 40 minutes. Following a single dose of 200 µg base, the observed average peak concentration was 0.6 ng/mL (range 0.2 to 1.4 ng/mL), whereas following a single dose of 400 µg base, the observed average peak concentration was 1.8 ng/mL (range 0.5 to 5.3 ng/mL). Bioavailability from a 400 µg dose averaged 2.8% (range 1.2 to 5.6%). The average serum half-life of nafarelin following intranasal administration was approximately 3 hours. About 80% of

Continued on next page

Searle—Cont.

nafarelin acetate was bound to plasma proteins at 4°C. Twice daily intranasal administration of 200 or 400 µg of SYNAREL in 18 healthy women for 22 days did not lead to significant accumulation of the drug. Based on the mean C_{min} levels on Days 15 and 22, there appeared to be dose proportionality across the two dose levels.

After subcutaneous administration of ^{14}C-nafarelin acetate to men, 44-55% of the dose was recovered in urine and 18.5-44.2% was recovered in feces. Approximately 3% of the administered dose appeared as unchanged nafarelin in urine. The ^{14}C serum half-life of the metabolites was about 85.5 hours. Six metabolites of nafarelin have been identified of which the major metabolite is Tyr-D(2)-Nal-Leu-Arg-Pro-Gly-NH₂(5-10). The activity of the metabolites, the metabolism of nafarelin by nasal mucosa, and the pharmacokinetics of the drug in hepatically- and renally-impaired patients have not been determined.

There appeared to be no significant effect of rhinitis, i.e., nasal congestion, on the systemic bioavailability of SYNAREL; however, if the use of a nasal decongestant for rhinitis is necessary during treatment with SYNAREL, the decongestant should not be used until at least 2 hours following dosing with SYNAREL.

When used regularly in girls and boys with **central precocious puberty (CPP)** at the recommended dose, SYNAREL suppresses LH and sex steroid hormone levels to prepubertal levels, affects a corresponding arrest of secondary sexual development, and slows linear growth and skeletal maturation. In some cases, initial estrogen withdrawal bleeding may occur, generally within 6 weeks after initiation of therapy. Thereafter, menstruation should cease.

In clinical studies the peak response of LH to GnRH stimulation was reduced from a pubertal response to a prepubertal response (<15 mIU/mL) within one month of treatment. Linear growth velocity, which is commonly pubertal in children with CPP, is reduced in most children within the first year of treatment to values of 5 to 6 cm/year or less. Children with CPP are frequently taller than their chronological age peers; height for chronological age approaches normal in most children during the second or third year of treatment with SYNAREL. Skeletal maturation rate (bone age velocity—change in bone age divided by change in chronological age) is usually abnormal (greater than 1) in children with CPP; in most children, bone age velocity approaches normal (1) during the first year of treatment. This results in a narrowing of the gap between bone age and chronological age, usually by the second or third year of treatment. The mean predicted adult height increases.

In clinical trials, breast development was arrested or regressed in 82% of girls, and genital development was arrested or regressed in 100% of boys. Because pubic hair growth is largely controlled by adrenal androgens, which are unaffected by nafarelin, pubic hair development was arrested or regressed only in 54% of girls and boys.

Reversal of the suppressive effects of SYNAREL has been demonstrated to occur in all children with CPP for whom one-year post- treatment follow-up is available (n=69). This demonstration consisted of the appearance or return of menses, the return of pubertal gonadotropin and gonadal sex steroid levels, and/or the advancement of secondary sexual development. Semen analysis was normal in the two ejaculated specimens obtained thus far from boys who have been taken off therapy to resume puberty. Fertility has not been documented by pregnancies and the effect of long-term use of the drug on fertility is not known.

INDICATIONS AND USAGE FOR CENTRAL PRECOCIOUS PUBERTY
(For Endometriosis, See Endometriosis section)

SYNAREL is indicated for treatment of **central precocious puberty (CPP)** (gonadotropin-dependent precocious puberty) in children of both sexes.

The diagnosis of **central precocious puberty (CPP)** is suspected when premature development of secondary sexual characteristics occurs at or before the age of 8 years in girls and 9 years in boys, and is accompanied by significant advancement of bone age and/or a poor adult height prediction. The diagnosis should be confirmed by pubertal gonadal sex steroid levels and a pubertal LH response to stimulation by native GnRH. Pelvic ultrasound assessment in girls usually reveals enlarged uterus and ovaries, the latter often with multiple cystic formations. Magnetic resonance imaging (MRI) or computed tomography (CT) scanning of the brain is recommended to detect hypothalamic or pituitary tumors, or anatomical changes associated with increased intracranial pressure. Other causes of sexual precocity, such as congenital adrenal hyperplasia, testotoxicosis, testicular tumors and/or other autonomous feminizing or masculinizing disorders, must be excluded by proper clinical hormonal and diagnostic imaging examinations.

CONTRAINDICATIONS
1. Hypersensitivity to GnRH, GnRH agonist analogs or any of the excipients in SYNAREL;
2. Undiagnosed abnormal vaginal bleeding;
3. Use in pregnancy or in women who may become pregnant while receiving the drug. SYNAREL may cause fetal harm when administered to a pregnant woman. Major fetal abnormalities were observed in rats, but not in mice or rabbits, after administration of SYNAREL during the period of organogenesis. There was a dose-related increase in fetal mortality and a decrease in fetal weight in rats (see Pregnancy Section). The effects on rat fetal mortality are expected consequences of the alterations in hormonal levels brought about by the drug. If this drug is used during pregnancy or if the patient becomes pregnant while taking this drug, she should be apprised of the potential hazard to the fetus;
4. Use in women who are breast-feeding (see Nursing Mothers Section).

WARNINGS

The diagnosis of central precocious puberty (CPP) must be established before treatment is initiated. Regular monitoring of CPP patients is needed to assess both patient response as well as compliance. This is particularly important during the first 6 to 8 weeks of treatment to assure that suppression of pituitary-gonadal function is rapid. Testing may include LH response to GnRH stimulation and circulating gonadal sex steroid levels. Assessment of growth velocity and bone age velocity should begin within 3 to 6 months of treatment initiation.

Some patients may not show suppression of the pituitary-gonadal axis by clinical and/or biochemical parameters. This may be due to lack of compliance with the recommended treatment regimen and may be rectified by recommending that the dosing be done by caregivers. If compliance problems are excluded, the possibility of gonadotropin independent sexual precocity should be reconsidered and appropriate examinations should be conducted. If compliance problems are excluded and if gonadotropin independent sexual precocity is not present, the dose of SYNAREL may be increased to 1800 µg/day administered as 600 µg TID.

PRECAUTIONS
General
As with other drugs that stimulate the release of gonadotropins or that induce ovulation, in adult women with endometriosis ovarian cysts have been reported to occur in the first two months of therapy with SYNAREL. Many, but not all, of these events occurred in women with polycystic ovarian disease. These cystic enlargements may resolve spontaneously, generally by about four to six weeks of therapy, but in some cases may require discontinuation of drug and/or surgical intervention. The relevance, if any, of such events in children is unknown.

Information for Patients, Patients' Parents or Guardians
An information pamphlet for patients is included with the product. Patients and their caregivers should be aware of the following information:
1. Reversibility of the suppressive effects of nafarelin has been demonstrated by the appearance or return of menses, by the return of pubertal gonadotropin and gonadal sex steroid levels, and/or by advancement of secondary sexual development. Semen analysis was normal in the two ejaculated specimens obtained thus far from boys who have been taken off therapy to resume puberty. Fertility has not been documented by pregnancies and the effect of long-term use of the drug on fertility is not known.
2. Patients and their caregivers should be adequately counseled to assure full compliance; irregular or incomplete daily doses may result in stimulation of the pituitary-gonadal axis.
3. During the first month of treatment with SYNAREL, some signs of puberty, e.g., vaginal bleeding or breast enlargement, may occur. This is the expected initial effect of the drug. Such changes should resolve soon after the first month. If such resolution does not occur within the first two months of treatment, this may be due to lack of compliance or the presence of gonadotropin independent sexual precocity. If both possibilities are definitively excluded, the dose of SYNAREL may be increased to 1800 µg/day administered as 600 µg TID.
4. Patients with intercurrent rhinitis should consult their physician for the use of a topical nasal decongestant. If the use of a topical nasal decongestant is required during treatment with SYNAREL, the decongestant should not be used until at least 2 hours following dosing with SYNAREL.
5. Sneezing during or immediately after dosing with SYNAREL should be avoided, if possible, since this may impair drug absorption.

Drug Interactions
No pharmacokinetic-based drug-drug interaction studies have been conducted with SYNAREL. However, because nafarelin acetate is a peptide that is primarily degraded by peptidase and not by cytochrome P-450 enzymes, and the drug is only about 80% bound to plasma proteins at 4°C, drug interactions would not be expected to occur.

Carcinogenesis, Mutagenesis, Impairment of Fertility
Carcinogenicity studies of nafarelin were conducted in rats (24 months) at doses up to 100 µg/kg/day and mice (18 months) at doses up to 500 µg/kg/day using intramuscular doses (up to 110 times and 560 times the maximum recommended human intranasal dose, respectively). These multiples of the human dose are based on the relative bioavailability of the drug by the two routes of administration. As seen with other GnRH agonists, nafarelin acetate given to laboratory rodents at high doses for prolonged periods induced proliferative responses (hyperplasia and/or neoplasia) of endocrine organs. At 24 months, there was an increase in the incidence of pituitary tumors (adenoma/carcinoma) in high-dose female rats and a dose-related increase in male rats. There was an increase in pancreatic islet cell adenomas in both sexes, and in benign testicular and ovarian tumors in the treated groups. There was a dose-related increase in benign adrenal medullary tumors in treated female rats. In mice, there was a dose-related increase in Harderian gland tumors in males and an increase in pituitary adenomas in high-dose females. No metastases of these tumors were observed. It is known that tumorigenicity in rodents is particularly sensitive to hormonal stimulation.

Mutagenicity studies were performed with nafarelin acetate using bacterial, yeast, and mammalian systems. These studies provided no evidence of mutagenic potential.

Reproduction studies in male and female rats have shown full reversibility of fertility suppression when drug treatment was discontinued after continuous administration for up to 6 months. The effect of treatment of prepubertal rats on the subsequent reproductive performance of mature animals has not been investigated.

Pregnancy, Teratogenic Effects
Pregnancy Category X. See Contraindications Section. Intramuscular SYNAREL was administered to rats during the period of organogenesis at 0.4, 1.6, and 6.4 µg/kg/day (about 0.5, 2, and 7 times the maximum recommended human intranasal dose based on the relative bioavailability by the two routes of administration). An increase in major fetal abnormalities was observed in 4/80 fetuses at the highest dose. A similar, repeat study at the same doses in rats and studies in mice and rabbits at doses up to 600 µg/kg/day and 0.18 µg/kg/day, respectively, failed to demonstrate an increase in fetal abnormalities after administration during the period of organogenesis. In rats and rabbits, there was a dose-related increase in fetal mortality and a decrease in fetal weight with the highest dose.

Nursing Mothers
It is not known whether SYNAREL is excreted in human milk. Because many drugs are excreted in human milk, and because the effects of SYNAREL on lactation and/or the breastfed child have not been determined, SYNAREL should not be used by nursing mothers.

ADVERSE REACTIONS
In clinical trials of 155 pediatric patients, 2.6% reported symptoms suggestive of drug sensitivity, such as shortness of breath, chest pain, urticaria, rash, and pruritus.

In these 155 patients treated for an average of 41 months and as long as 80 months (6.7 years), adverse events most frequently reported (>3% of patients) consisted largely of episodes occurring during the first 6 weeks of treatment as a result of the transient stimulatory action of nafarelin upon the pituitary-gonadal axis:

    acne (10%)
    transient breast enlargement (8%)
    vaginal bleeding (8%)
    emotional lability (6%)
    transient increase in pubic hair (5%)
    body odor (4%)
    seborrhea (3%)

Hot flashes, common in adult women treated for endometriosis, occurred in only 3% of treated children and were transient. Other adverse events thought to be drug-related, and occurring in >3% of patients were rhinitis (5%) and white or brownish vaginal discharge (3%). Approximately 3% of patients withdrew from clinical trials due to adverse events.

In one male patient with concomitant congenital adrenal hyperplasia, and who had discontinued treatment 8 months previously to resume puberty, adrenal rest tumors were found in the left testis. Relationship to SYNAREL is unlikely.

Regular examinations of the pituitary gland by MRI or CT scanning of children during long-term nafarelin therapy as well as during the post-treatment period have occasionally revealed changes in the shape and size of the pituitary gland. These changes include asymmetry and enlargement of the pituitary gland, and a pituitary micro-adenoma has been suspected in a few children. The relationship of these findings to SYNAREL is not known.

OVERDOSAGE
In experimental animals, a single subcutaneous administration of up to 60 times the recommended human dose (on a

μg/kg basis, not adjusted for bioavailability) had no adverse effects. At present, there is no clinical evidence of adverse effects following overdosage of GnRH analogs.
Based on studies in monkeys, SYNAREL is not absorbed after oral administration.

DOSAGE AND ADMINISTRATION

For the treatment of **central precocious puberty (CPP)**, the recommended daily dose of SYNAREL is 1600 μg. The dose can be increased to 1800 μg daily if adequate suppression cannot be achieved at 1600 μg/day.
The 1600 μg dose is achieved by two sprays (400 μg) into each nostril in the morning (4 sprays) and two sprays into each nostril in the evening (4 sprays), a total of 8 sprays per day. The 1800 μg dose is achieved by 3 sprays (600 μg) into alternating nostrils three times a day, a total of 9 sprays per day. The patient's head should be tilted back slightly, and 30 seconds should elapse between sprays.
If the prescribed therapy has been well tolerated by the patient, treatment of CPP with SYNAREL should continue until resumption of puberty is desired.
There appeared to be no significant effect of rhinitis, i.e., nasal congestion, on the systemic bioavailability of SYNAREL; however, if the use of a nasal decongestant for rhinitis is necessary during treatment with SYNAREL, the decongestant should not be used until at least 2 hours following dosing with SYNAREL.
Sneezing during or immediately after dosing with SYNAREL should be avoided, if possible, since this may impair drug absorption.
At 1600 μg/day, a bottle of SYNAREL provides about a 7-day supply (about 56 sprays). If the daily dose is increased, increase the supply to the patient to ensure uninterrupted treatment for the duration of therapy.

HOW SUPPLIED

Each 0.5 ounce bottle (NDC 0025-0166-10) contains 10 mL SYNAREL (nafarelin acetate) Nasal Solution 2 mg/mL (as nafarelin base) and is supplied with a metered spray pump that delivers 200 μg of nafarelin per spray. A dust cover and a leaflet of patient instructions are also included.
Store upright at room temperature. Avoid heat above 30°C (86°F). Protect from light. Protect from freezing.
CAUTION: Federal law prohibits dispensing without prescription.
U.S. Patent No. 4,234,571.

SEARLE

Manufactured for
G.D. Searle & Co.
Chicago IL 60680 USA — November 1995
By Syntex (U.S.A.) Inc. — ©1995, Searle
Palo Alto CA 94304 — 02-2260-00-00

SYNAREL® ℞
[sin 'er-el]
(nafarelin acetate)
Nasal Solution 2 mg/mL
(as nafarelin base)

ENDOMETRIOSIS
(FOR CENTRAL PRECOCIOUS PUBERTY, SEE CENTRAL PRECOCIOUS PUBERTY SECTION)

DESCRIPTION

SYNAREL (nafarelin acetate) Nasal Solution is intended for administration as a spray to the nasal mucosa. Nafarelin acetate, the active component of SYNAREL Nasal Solution, is a decapeptide with the chemical name: 5-oxo-L-prolyl-L-histidyl-L-tryptophyl-L-seryl-L-tyrosyl- 3- (2-naphthyl) -D-alanyl-L-leucyl-L-arginyl-L-prolyl-glycinamide acetate. Nafarelin acetate is a synthetic analog of the naturally occurring gonadotropin-releasing hormone (GnRH).
Nafarelin acetate has the following chemical structure:

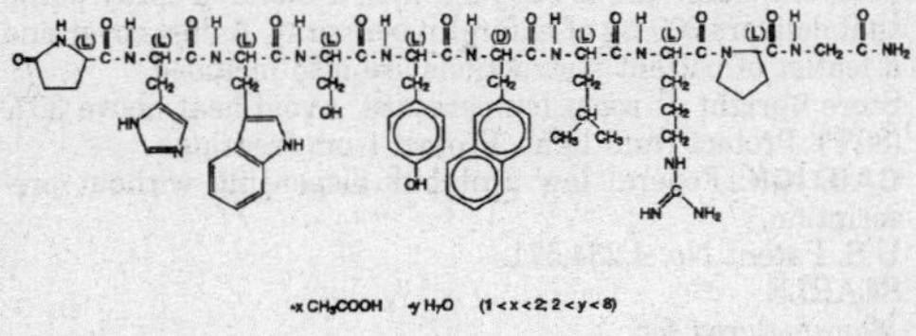

SYNAREL Nasal Solution contains nafarelin acetate (2 mg/mL, content expressed as nafarelin base) in a solution of benzalkonium chloride, glacial acetic acid, sodium hydroxide or hydrochloric acid (to adjust pH), sorbitol, and purified water.
After priming the pump unit for SYNAREL, each actuation of the unit delivers approximately 100 μL of the spray containing approximately 200 μg nafarelin base. The contents of one spray bottle are intended to deliver at least 60 sprays.

CLINICAL PHARMACOLOGY

Nafarelin acetate is a potent agonistic analog of gonadotropin-releasing hormone (GnRH). At the onset of administration, nafarelin stimulates the release of the pituitary gonadotropins, luteinizing hormone (LH) and follicle stimulating hormone (FSH), resulting in a temporary increase of ovarian steroidogenesis. Repeated dosing abolishes the stimulatory effect on the pituitary gland. Twice daily administration leads to decreased secretion of gonadal steroids by about 4 weeks; consequently, tissues and functions that depend on gonadal steroids for their maintenance become quiescent.
In **adult women**, nafarelin acetate is rapidly absorbed into the systemic circulation after intranasal administration. Maximum serum concentrations (measured by RIA) were achieved between 10 and 40 minutes. Following a single dose of 200 μg base, the observed average peak concentration was 0.6 ng/mL (range 0.2 to 1.4 ng/mL), whereas following a single dose of 400 μg base, the observed average peak concentration was 1.8 ng/mL (range 0.5 to 5.3 ng/mL). Bioavailability from a 400 μg dose averaged 2.8% (range 1.2 to 5.6%). The average serum half-life of nafarelin following intranasal administration is approximately 3 hours. About 80% of nafarelin acetate is bound to plasma proteins at 4°C. Twice daily intranasal administration of 200 or 400 μg of SYNAREL in 18 healthy women for 22 days did not lead to significant accumulation of the drug. Based on the mean C_{min} levels on Days 15 and 22, there appeared to be dose proportionality across the two dose levels.
After subcutaneous administration of ^{14}C-nafarelin acetate to men, 44-55% of the dose was recovered in urine and 18.5-44.2% was recovered in feces. Approximately 3% of the administered dose appeared as unchanged nafarelin in urine. The ^{14}C serum half-life of the metabolites was about 85.5 hours. Six metabolites of nafarelin have been identified of which the major metabolite is Tyr-D(2)-Nal-Leu-Arg-Pro-Gly-NH_2(5-10). The activity of the metabolites, the metabolism of nafarelin by nasal mucosa, and the pharmacokinetics of the drug in hepatically- and renally-impaired patients have not been determined.
There appeared to be no significant effect of rhinitis, i.e., nasal congestion, on the systemic bioavailability of SYNAREL; however, if the use of a nasal decongestant for rhinitis is necessary during treatment with SYNAREL, the decongestant should not be used until at least 2 hours following dosing of SYNAREL.
In controlled clinical studies, SYNAREL at doses of 400 and 800 μg/day for 6 months was shown to be comparable to danazol, 800 mg/day, in relieving the clinical symptoms of endometriosis (pelvic pain, dysmenorrhea, and dyspareunia) and in reducing the size of endometrial implants as determined by laparoscopy. The clinical significance of a decrease in endometriotic lesions is not known at this time and, in addition, laparoscopic staging of endometriosis does not necessarily correlate with severity of symptoms.
SYNAREL 400 μg daily induced amenorrhea in approximately 65%, 80%, and 90% of the patients after 60, 90, and 120 days, respectively. In the first, second, and third post-treatment months, normal menstrual cycles resumed in 4%, 82%, and 100%, respectively, of those patients who did not become pregnant.
At the end of treatment, 60% of patients who received SYNAREL, 400 μg/day, were symptom free, 32% had mild symptoms, 7% had moderate symptoms, and 1% had severe symptoms. Of the 60% of patients who had complete relief of symptoms at the end of treatment, 17% had moderate symptoms 6 months after treatment was discontinued, 33% had mild symptoms, 50% remained symptom free, and no patient had severe symptoms.
During the first two months use of SYNAREL, some women experience vaginal bleeding of variable duration and intensity. In all likelihood, this bleeding represents estrogen withdrawal bleeding and is expected to stop spontaneously. If vaginal bleeding continues, the possibility of lack of compliance with the dosing regimen should be considered. If the patient is complying carefully with the regimen, an increase in dose to 400 μg twice a day should be considered.
There is no evidence that pregnancy rates are enhanced or adversely affected by the use of SYNAREL.

INDICATIONS AND USAGE FOR ENDOMETRIOSIS

(For Central Precocious Puberty, See Central Precocious Puberty section)
SYNAREL is indicated for management of endometriosis, including pain relief and reduction of endometriotic lesions. Experience with SYNAREL for the management of endometriosis has been limited to women 18 years of age and older treated for 6 months.

CONTRAINDICATIONS

1. Hypersensitivity to GnRH, GnRH agonist analogs or any of the excipients in SYNAREL;
2. Undiagnosed abnormal vaginal bleeding;
3. Use in pregnancy or in women who may become pregnant while receiving the drug. SYNAREL may cause fetal harm when administered to a pregnant woman. Major fetal abnormalities were observed in rats, but not in mice or rabbits, after administration of SYNAREL during the period of organogenesis. There was a dose-related increase in fetal mortality and a decrease in fetal weight in rats (see Pregnancy Section). The effects on rat fetal mortality are expected consequences of the alterations in hormonal levels brought about by the drug. If this drug is used during pregnancy or if the patient becomes pregnant while taking this drug, she should be apprised of the potential hazard to the fetus;
4. Use in women who are breast-feeding (see Nursing Mothers Section).

WARNINGS

Safe use of nafarelin acetate in pregnancy has not been established clinically. Before starting treatment with SYNAREL, pregnancy must be excluded.
When used regularly at the recommended dose, SYNAREL usually inhibits ovulation and stops menstruation. Contraception is not insured, however, by taking SYNAREL, particularly if patients miss successive doses. Therefore, patients should use nonhormonal methods of contraception. Patients should be advised to see their physician if they believe they may be pregnant. If a patient becomes pregnant during treatment, the drug must be discontinued and the patient must be apprised of the potential risk to the fetus.

PRECAUTIONS

General
As with other drugs that stimulate the release of gonadotropins or that induce ovulation, ovarian cysts have been reported to occur in the first 2 months of therapy with SYNAREL. Many, but not all, of these events occurred in patients with polycystic ovarian disease. These cystic enlargements may resolve spontaneously, generally by about 4 to 6 weeks of therapy, but in some cases may require discontinuation of drug and/or surgical intervention.
Information for Patients
An information pamphlet for patients is included with the product. Patients should be aware of the following information:

1. Since menstruation should stop with effective doses of SYNAREL, the patient should notify her physician if regular menstruation persists. The cause of vaginal spotting, bleeding or menstruation could be noncompliance with the treatment regimen, or it could be that a higher dose of the drug is required to achieve amenorrhea. The patient should be questioned regarding her compliance. If she is careful and compliant, and menstruation persists to the second month, consideration should be given to doubling the dose of SYNAREL. If the patient has missed several doses, she should be counseled on the importance of taking SYNAREL regularly as prescribed.
2. Patients should not use SYNAREL if they are pregnant, breast-feeding, have undiagnosed abnormal vaginal bleeding, or are allergic to any of the ingredients in SYNAREL.
3. Safe use of the drug in pregnancy has not been established clinically. Therefore, a nonhormonal method of contraception should be used during treatment. Patients should be advised that if they miss successive doses of SYNAREL, breakthrough bleeding or ovulation may occur with the potential for conception. If a patient becomes pregnant during treatment, she should discontinue treatment and consult her physician.
4. Those adverse events occurring most frequently in clinical studies with SYNAREL are associated with hypoestrogenism; the most frequently reported are hot flashes, headaches, emotional lability, decreased libido, vaginal dryness, acne, myalgia, and reduction in breast size. Estrogen levels returned to normal after treatment was discontinued. Nasal irritation occurred in about 10% of all patients who used intranasal nafarelin.
5. The induced hypoestrogenic state results in a small loss in bone density over the course of treatment, some of which may not be reversible. During one six-month treatment period, this bone loss should not be important. In patients with major risk factors for decreased bone mineral content such as chronic alcohol and/or tobacco use, strong family history of osteoporosis, or chronic use of drugs that can reduce bone mass such as anticonvulsants or corticosteroids, therapy with SYNAREL may pose an additional risk. In these patients the risks and benefits must be weighed carefully before therapy with SYNAREL is instituted. Repeated courses of treatment with gonadotropin-releasing hormone analogs are not advisable in patients with major risk factors for loss of bone mineral content.

Continued on next page

Searle—Cont.

6. Patients with intercurrent rhinitis should consult their physician for the use of a topical nasal decongestant. If the use of a topical nasal decongestant is required during treatment with SYNAREL, the decongestant should not be used until at least 2 hours following dosing with SYNAREL.

7. Sneezing during or immediately after dosing with SYNAREL should be avoided, if possible, since this may impair drug absorption.

8. Retreatment cannot be recommended since safety data beyond 6 months are not available.

Drug Interactions
No pharmacokinetic-based drug-drug interaction studies have been conducted with SYNAREL. However, because nafarelin acetate is a peptide that is primarily degraded by peptidase and not by cytochrome P-450 enzymes, and the drug is only about 80% bound to plasma proteins at 4°C, drug interactions would not be expected to occur.

Drug/Laboratory Test Interactions
Administration of SYNAREL in therapeutic doses results in suppression of the pituitary-gonadal system. Normal function is usually restored within 4 to 8 weeks after treatment is discontinued. Therefore, diagnostic tests of pituitary gonadotropic and gonadal functions conducted during treatment and up to 4 to 8 weeks after discontinuation of therapy with SYNAREL may be misleading.

Carcinogenesis, Mutagenesis, Impairment of Fertility
Carcinogenicity studies of nafarelin were conducted in rats (24 months) at doses up to 100 µg/kg/day and mice (18 months) at doses up to 500 µg/kg/day using intramuscular doses (up to 110 times and 560 times the maximum recommended human intranasal dose, respectively). These multiples of the human dose are based on the relative bioavailability of the drug by the two routes of administration. As seen with other GnRH agonists, nafarelin acetate given to laboratory rodents at high doses for prolonged periods induced proliferative responses (hyperplasia and/or neoplasia) of endocrine organs. At 24 months, there was an increase in the incidence of pituitary tumors (adenoma/carcinoma) in high-dose female rats and a dose-related increase in male rats. There was an increase in pancreatic islet cell adenomas in both sexes, and in benign testicular and ovarian tumors in the treated groups. There was a dose-related increase in benign adrenal medullary tumors in treated female rats. In mice, there was a dose-related increase in Harderian gland tumors in males and an increase in pituitary adenomas in high-dose females. No metastases of these tumors were observed. It is known that tumorigenicity in rodents is particularly sensitive to hormonal stimulation.
Mutagenicity studies were performed with nafarelin acetate using bacterial, yeast, and mammalian systems. These studies provided no evidence of mutagenic potential.
Reproduction studies in male and female rats have shown full reversibility of fertility suppression when drug treatment was discontinued after continuous administration for up to 6 months. The effect of treatment of prepubertal rats on the subsequent reproductive performance of mature animals has not been investigated.

Pregnancy, Teratogenic Effects
Pregnancy Category X. See Contraindications Section. Intramuscular SYNAREL was administered to rats during the period of organogenesis at 0.4, 1.6, and 6.4 µg/kg/day (about 0.5, 2, and 7 times the maximum recommended human intranasal dose based on the relative bioavailability by the two routes of administration). An increase in major fetal abnormalities was observed in 4/80 fetuses at the highest dose. A similar, repeat study at the same doses in rats and studies in mice and rabbits at doses up to 600 µg/kg/day and 0.18 µg/kg/day, respectively, failed to demonstrate an increase in fetal abnormalities after administration during the period of organogenesis. In rats and rabbits, there was a dose-related increase in fetal mortality and a decrease in fetal weight with the highest dose.

Nursing Mothers
It is not known whether SYNAREL is excreted in human milk. Because many drugs are excreted in human milk, and because the effects of SYNAREL on lactation and/or the breast-fed child have not been determined, SYNAREL should not be used by nursing mothers.

Pediatric Use
Safety and effectiveness of SYNAREL for endometriosis in patients younger than 18 years have not been established.

ADVERSE REACTIONS
As would be expected with a drug which lowers serum estradiol levels, the most frequently reported adverse reactions were those related to hypoestrogenism.
In controlled studies comparing SYNAREL (400 µg/day) and danazol (600 or 800 mg/day), adverse reactions most frequently reported and thought to be drug-related are shown in the figure below:
[See table below.]
In addition, less than 1% of patients experienced paresthesia, palpitations, chloasma, maculopapular rash, eye pain, urticaria, asthenia, lactation, breast engorgement, and arthralgia. In formal clinical trials, immediate hypersensitivity thought to be possibly or probably related to nafarelin occurred in 3 (0.2%) of 1509 healthy subjects or patients.
During postmarketing surveillance of nafarelin, alopecia has been reported by some patients.

Changes in Bone Density
After six months of treatment with SYNAREL, vertebral trabecular bone density and total vertebral bone mass, measured by quantitative computed tomography (QCT), decreased by an average of 8.7% and 4.3%, respectively, compared to pretreatment levels. There was partial recovery of bone density in the post-treatment period; the average trabecular bone density and total bone mass were 4.9% and 3.3% less than the pretreatment levels, respectively. Total vertebral bone mass, measured by dual photon absorptiometry (DPA), decreased by a mean of 5.9% at the end of treatment. Mean total vertebral mass, re-examined by DPA six months after completion of treatment, was 1.4% below pretreatment levels. There was little, if any, decrease in the mineral content in compact bone of the distal radius and second metacarpal. Use of SYNAREL for longer than the recommended six months or in the presence of other known risk factors for decreased bone mineral content may cause additional bone loss.

Changes in Laboratory Values During Treatment
Plasma enzymes. During clinical trials with SYNAREL, regular laboratory monitoring revealed that SGOT and SGPT levels were more than twice the upper limit of normal in only one patient each. There was no other clinical or laboratory evidence of abnormal liver function and levels returned to normal in both patients after treatment was stopped.

Lipids. At enrollment, 9% of the patients in the group taking SYNAREL 400 µg/day and 2% of the patients in the danazol group had total cholesterol values above 250 mg/dL. These patients also had cholesterol values above 250 mg/dL at the end of treatment.
Of those patients whose pretreatment cholesterol values were below 250 mg/dL, 6% in the group treated with SYNAREL and 18% in the danazol group, had post-treatment values above 250 mg/dL.
The mean ($\pm$ SEM) pretreatment values for total cholesterol from all patients were 191.8 (4.3) mg/dL in the group treated with SYNAREL and 193.1 (4.6) mg/dL in the danazol group. At the end of treatment, the mean values for total cholesterol from all patients were 204.5 (4.8) mg/dL in the group treated with SYNAREL and 207.7 (5.1) mg/dL in the danazol group. These increases from the pretreatment values were statistically significant (p < 0.05) in both groups.
Triglycerides were increased above the upper limit of 150 mg/dL in 12% of the patients who received SYNAREL and in 7% of the patients who received danazol.
At the end of treatment, no patients receiving SYNAREL had abnormally low HDL cholesterol fractions (less than 30 mg/dL) compared with 43% of patients receiving danazol. None of the patients receiving SYNAREL had abnormally high LDL cholesterol fractions (greater than 190 mg/dL) compared with 15% of those receiving danazol. There was no increase in the LDL/HDL ratio in patients receiving SYNAREL, but there was approximately a 2-fold increase in the LDL/HDL ratio in patients receiving danazol.
Other changes. In comparative studies, the following changes were seen in approximately 10% to 15% of patients. Treatment with SYNAREL was associated with elevations of plasma phosphorus and eosinophil counts, and decreases in serum calcium and WBC counts. Danazol therapy was associated with an increase of hematocrit and WBC.

OVERDOSAGE
In experimental animals, a single subcutaneous administration of up to 60 times the recommended human dose (on a µg/kg basis, not adjusted for bioavailability) had no adverse effects. At present, there is no clinical evidence of adverse effects following overdosage of GnRH analogs.
Based on studies in monkeys, SYNAREL is not absorbed after oral administration.

DOSAGE AND ADMINISTRATION
For the management of endometriosis, the recommended daily dose of SYNAREL is 400 µg. This is achieved by one spray (200 µg) into one nostril in the morning and one spray into the other nostril in the evening. Treatment should be started between days 2 and 4 of the menstrual cycle.
In an occasional patient, the 400 µg daily dose may not produce amenorrhea. For these patients with persistent regular menstruation after 2 months of treatment, the dose of SYNAREL may be increased to 800 µg daily. The 800 µg dose is administered as one spray into each nostril in the morning (a total of two sprays) and again in the evening.
The recommended duration of administration is six months. Retreatment cannot be recommended since safety data for retreatment are not available. If the symptoms of endometriosis recur after a course of therapy, and further treatment with SYNAREL is contemplated, it is recommended that bone density be assessed before retreatment begins to ensure that values are within normal limits.
There appeared to be no significant effect of rhinitis, i.e., nasal congestion, on the systemic bioavailability of SYNAREL; however, if the use of a nasal decongestant for rhinitis is necessary during treatment with SYNAREL, the decongestant should not be used until at least 2 hours following dosing with SYNAREL.
Sneezing during or immediately after dosing with SYNAREL should be avoided, if possible, since this may impair drug absorption.
At 400 µg/day, a bottle of SYNAREL provides a 30-day (about 60 sprays) supply. If the daily dose is increased, increase the supply to the patient to ensure uninterrupted treatment for the recommended duration of therapy.

HOW SUPPLIED
Each 0.5 ounce bottle (NDC 0025-0166-10) contains 10 mL SYNAREL (nafarelin acetate) Nasal Solution 2 mg/mL (as nafarelin base) and is supplied with a metered spray pump that delivers 200 µg of nafarelin per spray. A dust cover and a leaflet of patient instructions are also included.
Store upright at room temperature. Avoid heat above 30°C (86°F). Protect from light. Protect from freezing.
CAUTION: Federal law prohibits dispensing without prescription.
U.S. Patent No. 4,234,571.
SEARLE
Manufactured for
G.D. Searle & Co.
Chicago IL 60680 USA
by Syntex (U.S.A.) Inc.
Palo Alto CA 94304

November 1995
©1995, Searle
02-2260-00-00

**ADVERSE EVENTS DURING 6 MONTHS TREATMENT
WITH SYNAREL® 400 µg/day vs
DANAZOL 600 OR 800 mg/day**

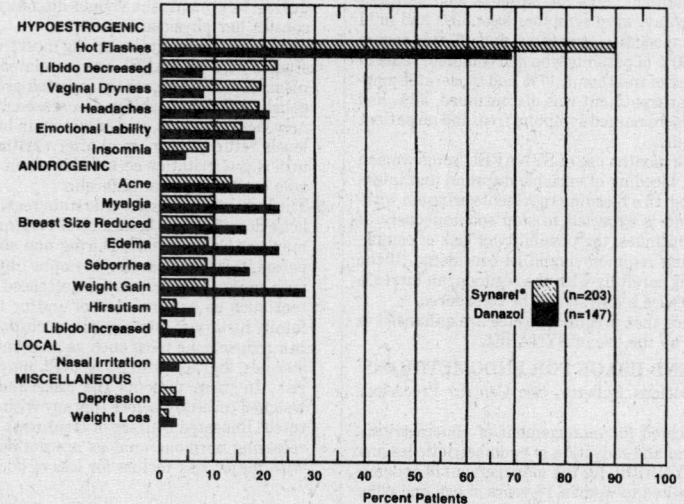

TRI-NORINYL® 21-DAY Tablets ℞
(norethindrone and ethinyl estradiol)

TRI-NORINYL® 28-DAY Tablets ℞
(norethindrone and ethinyl estradiol)

PHYSICIAN LABELING

Patients should be counseled that this product does not protect against HIV infection (AIDS) and other sexually transmitted diseases.

ORAL CONTRACEPTIVE AGENTS

DESCRIPTION

TRI-NORINYL 21-DAY Tablets provide an oral contraceptive regimen of 7 blue tablets followed by 9 yellow-green tablets and 5 more blue tablets. Each blue tablet contains norethindrone 0.5 mg and ethinyl estradiol 0.035 mg and each yellow-green tablet contains norethindrone 1 mg and ethinyl estradiol 0.035 mg.

TRI-NORINYL 28-DAY Tablets provide a continuous oral contraceptive regimen of 7 blue tablets, 9 yellow-green tablets, 5 more blue tablets, and then 7 orange tablets. Each blue tablet contains norethindrone 0.5 mg and ethinyl estradiol 0.035 mg, each yellow-green tablet contains norethindrone 1 mg and ethinyl estradiol 0.035 mg, and each orange tablet contains inert ingredients.

Norethindrone is a potent progestational agent with the chemical name 17-Hydroxy-19-nor-17α-pregn-4-en-20-yn-3-one. Ethinyl estradiol is an estrogen with the chemical name 19-Nor-17α-pregna-1, 3, 5(10) -trien-20-yne-3, 17-diol. Their structural formulae follow:

NORETHINDRONE

ETHINYL ESTRADIOL

The yellow-green TRI-NORINYL tablets contain the following inactive ingredients: D&C Green No. 5, D&C Yellow No. 10, lactose, magnesium stearate, povidone, and starch.

The blue TRI-NORINYL tablets contain the following inactive ingredients: FD&C Blue No. 1, lactose, magnesium stearate, povidone, and starch.

The inactive orange tablets in the 28-day regimen contain the following inactive ingredients: FD&C Yellow No. 6, lactose, magnesium stearate, povidone, and starch.

CLINICAL PHARMACOLOGY

Combination oral contraceptives act by suppression of gonadotrophins. Although the primary mechanism of this action is inhibition of ovulation, other alterations include changes in the cervical mucus (which increase the difficulty of sperm entry into the uterus) and the endometrium (which may reduce the likelihood of implantation).

INDICATIONS AND USAGE

Oral contraceptives are indicated for the prevention of pregnancy in women who elect to use these products as a method of contraception.

Oral contraceptives are highly effective. Table I lists the typical accidental pregnancy rates for users of combination oral contraceptives and other methods of contraception.[1] The efficacy of these contraceptive methods, except sterilization, depends upon the reliability with which they are used. Correct and consistent use of methods can result in lower failure rates.

TABLE I: LOWEST EXPECTED AND TYPICAL FAILURE RATES DURING THE FIRST YEAR OF CONTINUOUS USE OF A METHOD
% of Women Experiencing an Accidental Pregnancy in the First Year of Continuous Use

Method	Lowest Expected[a]	Typical[b]
(No Contraception)	(85)	(85)
Oral contraceptives		3
combined	0.1	N/A[c]
progestogen only	0.5	N/A[c]
Diaphragm with spermicidal cream or jelly	6	18
Spermicides alone (foam, creams, jellies and vaginal suppositories)	3	21
Vaginal Sponge		
Nulliparous	6	18
Multiparous	>9	>28
IUD (medicated)	2	3[d]
Condom without spermicides	2	12
Periodic abstinence (all methods)	1–9	20
Injectable progestogen[e]	0.4	0.4
Implants	0.04	0.04
Female sterilization	0.2	0.4
Male sterilization	0.1	0.15

Adapted from J. Trussell, Table I.[1]

[a] The authors' best guess of the percentage of women expected to experience an accidental pregnancy among couples who initiate a method (not necessarily for the first time) and who use it consistently and correctly during the first year if they do not stop for any other reason.

[b] This term represents "typical" couples who initiate use of a method (not necessarily for the first time), who experience an accidental pregnancy during the first year if they do not stop use for any other reason. The authors derive these data largely from the National Surveys of Family Growth (NSFG), 1976 and 1982.

[c] N/A—Data not available from the NSFG, 1976 and 1982.

[d] Combined typical rate for both medicated and non-medicated IUD. The rate for medicated IUD alone is not available.

[e] All forms.

CONTRAINDICATIONS

Oral contraceptives should not be used in women who have the following conditions:

- Thrombophlebitis or thromboembolic disorders
- A past history of deep vein thrombophlebitis or thromboembolic disorders
- Cerebral vascular or coronary artery disease
- Known or suspected carcinoma of the breast
- Carcinoma of the endometrium, and known or suspected estrogen-dependent neoplasia
- Undiagnosed abnormal genital bleeding
- Cholestatic jaundice of pregnancy or jaundice with prior pill use
- Hepatic adenomas, carcinomas or benign liver tumors
- Known or suspected pregnancy

WARNINGS

> Cigarette smoking increases the risk of serious cardiovascular side effects from oral contraceptive use. This risk increases with age and with heavy smoking (15 or more cigarettes per day) and is quite marked in women over 35 years of age. Women who use oral contraceptives should be strongly advised not to smoke.

The use of oral contraceptives is associated with increased risks of several serious conditions including myocardial infarction, thromboembolism, stroke, hepatic neoplasia and gallbladder disease, although the risk of serious morbidity and mortality increases significantly in the presence of other underlying risk factors such as hypertension, hyperlipidemias, hypercholesterolemia, obesity and diabetes.[2–5]

Practitioners prescribing oral contraceptives should be familiar with the following information relating to these risks.

The information contained in this package insert is principally based on studies carried out in patients who used oral contraceptives with formulations containing 0.05 mg or higher of estrogen.[6–11] The effects of long-term use with lower dose formulations of both estrogens and progestogens remain to be determined.

Throughout this labeling, epidemiological studies reported are of two types: retrospective or case control studies and prospective or cohort studies. Case control studies provide a measure of the relative risk of a disease. Relative risk, the *ratio* of the incidence of a disease among oral contraceptive users to that among non-users, cannot be assessed directly from case control studies, but the odds ratio obtained is a measure of relative risk. The relative risk does not provide information on the actual clinical occurrence of a disease. Cohort studies provide not only a measure of the relative risk but a measure of attributable risk, which is the *difference* in the incidence of disease between oral contraceptive users and non-users. The attributable risk does provide information about the actual occurrence of a disease in the population.[12–13]

1. THROMBOEMBOLIC DISORDERS AND OTHER VASCULAR PROBLEMS

a. Myocardial Infarction

An increased risk of myocardial infarction has been attributed to oral contraceptive use. This risk is primarily in smokers or women with other underlying risk factors for coronary artery disease such as hypertension, hypercholesterolemia, morbid obesity and diabetes.[2–5,13] The relative risk of heart attack for current oral contraceptive users has been estimated to be 2 to 6.[2,14–19] The risk is very low under the age of 30. However, there is the possibility of a risk of cardiovascular disease even in very young women who take oral contraceptives.

Smoking in combination with oral contraceptive use has been shown to contribute substantially to the incidence of myocardial infarctions in women 35 or older, with smoking accounting for the majority of excess cases.[20]

Mortality rates associated with circulatory disease have been shown to increase substantially in smokers over the age of 35 and non-smokers over the age of 40 among women who use oral contraceptives (see Table II).[16]

TABLE II: CIRCULATORY DISEASE MORTALITY RATES PER 100,000 WOMAN YEARS BY AGE, SMOKING STATUS AND ORAL CONTRACEPTIVE USE

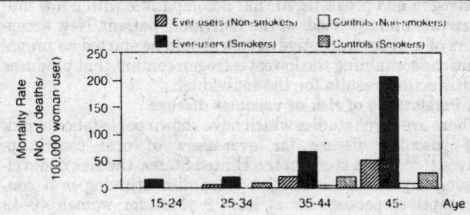

Adapted from P.M. Layde and V. Beral, Table V[16]

Oral contraceptives may compound the effects of well-known risk factors for coronary artery disease, such as hypertension, diabetes, hyperlipidemias, hypercholesterolemia, age and obesity.[3,13,21] In particular, some progestogens are known to decrease HDL cholesterol and impair oral glucose tolerance, while estrogens may create a state of hyperinsulinism.[21–25] Oral contraceptives have been shown to increase blood pressure among users (see **WARNINGS**, section 9). Similar effects on risk factors have been associated with an increased risk of heart disease. Oral contraceptives must be used with caution in women with cardiovascular disease risk factors.

b. Thromboembolism

An increased risk of thromboembolic and thrombotic disease associated with the use of oral contraceptives is well established. Case control studies have found the relative risk of users compared to non-users to be 3 for the first episode of superficial venous thrombosis, 4 to 11 for deep vein thrombosis or pulmonary embolism, and 1.5 to 6 for women with predisposing conditions for venous thromboembolic disease.[12,13,26–31] One cohort study has shown the relative risk to be rather lower, about 3 for new cases (subjects with no past history of venous thrombosis or varicose veins) and about 4.5 for new cases requiring hospitalization.[32] The risk of thromboembolic disease due to oral contraceptives is not related to length of use and disappears after pill use is stopped.[12]

A 2-to 6-fold increase in relative risk of post-operative thromboembolic complications has been reported with the use of oral contraceptives.[18] If feasible, oral contraceptives should be discontinued at least 4 weeks prior to and for 2 weeks after elective surgery and during and following prolonged immobilization. Since the immediate postpartum period also is associated with an increased risk of thromboembolism, oral contraceptives should be started no earlier than 4 to 6 weeks after delivery in women who elect not to breast feed.[33]

c. Cerebrovascular diseases

An increase in both the relative and attributable risks of cerebrovascular events (thrombotic and hemorrhagic strokes) has been shown in users of oral contraceptives. In general, the risk is greatest among older (> 35 years), hypertensive women who also smoke. Hypertension was found to be a risk factor for both users and non-users for both types of strokes while smoking interacted to increase the risk for hemorrhagic strokes.[34]

In a large study, the relative risk of thrombotic strokes has been shown to range from 3 for normotensive users to 14 for users with severe hypertension.[35] The relative risk of hemorrhagic stroke is reported to be 1.2 for non-smokers who used oral contraceptives, 2.6 for smokers who did not use oral contraceptives, 7.6 for smokers who used oral contraceptives, 1.8 for normotensive users and 25.7 for users with severe hypertension.[35] The attributable risk also is greater in women 35 or older and among smokers.[13]

Continued on next page

Searle—Cont.

d. Dose-related risk of vascular disease from oral contraceptives

A positive association has been observed between the amount of estrogen and progestogen in oral contraceptives and the risk of vascular disease.[36-38] A decline in serum high density lipoproteins (HDL) has been reported with some progestational agents.[22-24] A decline in serum high density lipoproteins has been associated with an increased incidence of ischemic heart disease.[39] Because estrogens increase HDL cholesterol, the net effect of an oral contraceptive depends on a balance achieved between doses of estrogen and progestogen and the nature and absolute amount of progestogens used in the contraceptives. The amount of both hormones should be considered in the choice of an oral contraceptive.[37]

Minimizing exposure to estrogen and progestogen is in keeping with good principles of therapeutics. For any particular estrogen/progestogen combination, the dosage regimen prescribed should be one which contains the least amount of estrogen and progestogen that is compatible with a low failure rate and the needs of the individual patient. New acceptors of oral contraceptive agents should be started on preparations containing the lowest estrogen content that produces satisfactory results for the individual.

e. Persistence of risk of vascular disease

There are three studies which have shown persistence of risk of vascular disease for ever-users of oral contraceptives.[17,34,40] In a study in the United States, the risk of developing myocardial infarction after discontinuing oral contraceptives persists for at least 9 years for women 40–49 years who had used oral contraceptives for 5 or more years, but this increased risk was not demonstrated in other age groups.[17] In another study in Great Britain, the risk of developing cerebrovascular disease persisted for at least 6 years after discontinuation of oral contraceptives, although excess risk was very small.[40] Subarachnoid hemorrhage also has a significantly increased relative risk after termination of use of oral contraceptives.[34] However, these studies were performed with oral contraceptive formulations containing 0.05 mg or higher of estrogen.

2. ESTIMATES OF MORTALITY FROM CONTRACEPTIVE USE

One study gathered data from a variety of sources which have estimated the mortality rates associated with different methods of contraception at different ages (see Table III).[41] These estimates include the combined risk of death associated with contraceptive methods plus the risk attributable to pregnancy in the event of method failure. Each method of contraception has its specific benefits and risks. The study concluded that with the exception of oral contraceptive users 35 and older who smoke and 40 and older who do not smoke, mortality associated with all methods of birth control is low and below that associated with childbirth. The observation of a possible increase in risk of mortality with age for oral contraceptive users is based on data gathered in the 1970's—but not reported in the U.S. until 1983.[16,41] However, current clinical practice involves the use of lower estrogen dose formulations combined with careful restriction of oral contraceptive use to women who do not have the various risk factors listed in this labeling.

Because of these changes in practice and, also, because of some limited new data which suggest that the risk of cardiovascular disease with the use of oral contraceptives may now be less than previously observed,[78,79] the Fertility and Maternal Health Drugs Advisory Committee was asked to review the topic in 1989. The Committee concluded that although cardiovascular disease risks may be increased with oral contraceptive use after age 40 in healthy non-smoking women (even with the newer low-dose formulations), there are greater potential health risks associated with pregnancy in older women and with the alternative surgical and medical procedures which may be necessary if such women do not have access to effective and acceptable means of contraception.

Therefore, the Committee recommended that the benefits of oral contraceptive use by healthy non-smoking women over 40 may outweigh the possible risks. Of course, older women, as all women who take oral contraceptives, should take the lowest possible dose formulation that is effective.[80] [See Table III below.]

3. CARCINOMA OF THE BREAST AND REPRODUCTIVE ORGANS

Numerous epidemiological studies have been performed on the incidence of breast, endometrial, ovarian and cervical cancer in women using oral contraceptives. The evidence in the literature suggests that use of oral contraceptives is not associated with an increase in the risk of developing breast cancer, regardless of the age and parity of first use or with most of the marketed brands and doses.[42,43] The Cancer and Steroid Hormone study also showed no latent effect on the risk of breast cancer for at least a decade following long-term use.[43] A few studies have shown a slightly increased relative risk of developing breast cancer,[44-47] although the methodology of these studies, which included differences in examination of users and non-users and differences in age at start of use, has been questioned.[47-49] Some studies have reported an increased relative risk of developing breast cancer, particularly at a younger age. This increased relative risk appears to be related to duration of use.[81,82]

Some studies suggest that oral contraceptive use has been associated with an increase in the risk of cervical intraepithelial neoplasia in some populations of women.[50-53] However, there continues to be controversy about the extent to which such findings may be due to differences in sexual behavior and other factors.

In spite of many studies of the relationship between oral contraceptive use and breast or cervical cancers, a cause and effect relationship has not been established.

4. HEPATIC NEOPLASIA

Benign hepatic adenomas are associated with oral contraceptive use although the incidence of benign tumors is rare in the United States. Indirect calculations have estimated the attributable risk to be in the range of 3.3 cases per 100,000 for users, a risk that increases after 4 or more years of use.[54] Rupture of rare, benign, hepatic adenomas may cause death through intra-abdominal hemorrhage.[55-56]

Studies in the United States and Britain have shown an increased risk of developing hepatocellular carcinoma in long-term (>8 years) oral contraceptive users.[57-59] However, these cancers are extremely rare in the United States and the attributable risk (the excess incidence) of liver cancers in oral contraceptive users is less than 1 per 1,000,000 users.

5. OCULAR LESIONS

There have been clinical case reports of retinal thrombosis associated with the use of oral contraceptives. Oral contraceptives should be discontinued if there is unexplained partial or complete loss of vision; onset of proptosis or diplopia; papilledema; or retinal vascular lesions. Appropriate diagnostic and therapeutic measures should be undertaken immediately.

6. ORAL CONTRACEPTIVE USE BEFORE OR DURING EARLY PREGNANCY

Extensive epidemiological studies have revealed no increased risk of birth defects in women who have used oral contraceptives prior to pregnancy.[60-62] More recent studies do not suggest a teratogenic effect, particularly insofar as cardiac anomalies and limb reduction defects are concerned, when taken inadvertently during early pregnancy.[60,61,63,64]

The administration of oral contraceptives to induce withdrawal bleeding should not be used as a test for pregnancy. Oral contraceptives should not be used during pregnancy to treat threatened or habitual abortion.

It is recommended that for any patient who has missed 2 consecutive periods, pregnancy should be ruled out before continuing oral contraceptive use. If the patient has not adhered to the prescribed schedule, the possibility of pregnancy should be considered at the time of the first missed period.

Oral contraceptive use should be discontinued if pregnancy is confirmed.

7. GALLBLADDER DISEASE

Earlier studies have reported an increased lifetime relative risk of gallbladder surgery in users of oral contraceptives and estrogens.[65-66] More recent studies, however, have shown that the relative risk of developing gallbladder disease among oral contraceptive users may be minimal.[67] The recent findings of minimal risk may be related to the use of oral contraceptive formulations containing lower hormonal doses of estrogens and progestogens.[68]

8. CARBOHYDRATE AND LIPID METABOLIC EFFECTS

Oral contraceptives have been shown to impair oral glucose tolerance.[69] Oral contraceptives containing greater than 0.075 mg of estrogen cause glucose intolerance with impaired insulin secretion, while lower doses of estrogen may produce less glucose intolerance.[70] Progestogens increase insulin secretion and create insulin resistance, this effect varying with different progestational agents.[25,71] However, in the non-diabetic woman, oral contraceptives appear to have no effect on fasting blood glucose.[69] Because of these demonstrated effects, prediabetic and diabetic women should be carefully observed while taking oral contraceptives.

Some women may develop persistent hypertriglyceridemia while on the pill.[72] As discussed earlier (see **WARNINGS**, sections 1a. and 1d.), changes in serum triglycerides and lipoprotein levels have been reported in oral contraceptive users.[23]

9. ELEVATED BLOOD PRESSURE

An increase in blood pressure has been reported in women taking oral contraceptives. The incidence of risk also was reported to increase with continued use and among older women.[66] Data from the Royal College of General Practitioners and subsequent randomized trials have shown that the incidence of hypertension increases with increasing concentrations of progestogens.

Women with a history of hypertension or hypertension-related diseases or renal disease should be encouraged to use another method of contraception. If women elect to use oral contraceptives, they should be monitored closely and if significant elevation of blood pressure occurs oral contraceptives should be discontinued. For most women, elevated blood pressure will return to normal after stopping oral contraceptives and there is no difference in the occurrence of hypertension among ever- and never-users.[73-75]

10. HEADACHE

The onset or exacerbation of migraine or development of headache with a new pattern which is recurrent, persistent or severe requires discontinuation of oral contraceptives and evaluation of the cause.

11. BLEEDING IRREGULARITIES

Breakthrough bleeding and spotting are sometimes encountered in patients on oral contraceptives, especially during the first 3 months of use. Non-hormonal causes should be considered and adequate diagnostic measures taken to rule out malignancy or pregnancy in the event of breakthrough bleeding, as in the case of any abnormal vaginal bleeding. If pathology has been excluded, time or a change to another formulation may solve the problem. In the event of amenorrhea, pregnancy should be ruled out.

Some women may encounter post-pill amenorrhea or oligomenorrhea, especially when such a condition was pre-existent.

PRECAUTIONS
GENERAL
PATIENTS SHOULD BE COUNSELED THAT THIS PRODUCT DOES NOT PROTECT AGAINST HIV (AIDS) AND OTHER SEXUALLY TRANSMITTED DISEASES.

1. PHYSICAL EXAMINATION AND FOLLOW-UP

It is good medical practice for all women to have annual history and physical examinations, including women using oral contraceptives. The physical examination, however, may be deferred until after initiation of oral contraceptives if requested by the woman and judged appropriate by the clinician. The physical examination should include special reference to blood pressure, breasts, abdomen and pelvic organs, including cervical cytology, and relevant laboratory tests. In case of undiagnosed, persistent or recurrent abnormal vaginal bleeding, appropriate measures should be conducted to rule out malignancy. Women with a strong family history of breast cancer or who have breast nodules should be monitored with particular care.

2. LIPID DISORDERS

Women who are being treated for hyperlipidemias should be followed closely if they elect to use oral contraceptives. Some progestogens may elevate LDL levels and may render the control of hyperlipidemias more difficult.

3. LIVER FUNCTION

If jaundice develops in any woman receiving oral contraceptives the medication should be discontinued. Steroid hormones may be poorly metabolized in patients with impaired liver function.

TABLE III: ESTIMATED ANNUAL NUMBER OF BIRTH-RELATED OR METHOD-RELATED DEATHS ASSOCIATED WITH CONTROL OF FERTILITY PER 100,000 NONSTERILE WOMEN, BY FERTILITY CONTROL METHOD ACCORDING TO AGE

Method of control and outcome	15–19	20–24	25–29	30–34	35–39	40–44
No fertility control methods*	7.0	7.4	9.1	14.8	25.7	28.2
Oral contraceptives non-smoker**	0.3	0.5	0.9	1.9	13.8	31.6
Oral contraceptives smoker**	2.2	3.4	6.6	13.5	51.1	117.2
IUD**	0.8	0.8	1.0	1.0	1.4	1.4
Condom*	1.1	1.6	0.7	0.2	0.3	0.4
Diaphragm/Spermicide*	1.9	1.2	1.2	1.3	2.2	2.8
Periodic abstinence*	2.5	1.6	1.6	1.7	2.9	3.6

* Deaths are birth-related
** Deaths are method-related

Estimates adapted from H.W. Ory, Table 3[41]

4. FLUID RETENTION
Oral contraceptives may cause some degree of fluid retention. They should be prescribed with caution, and only with careful monitoring, in patients with conditions which might be aggravated by fluid retention.

5. EMOTIONAL DISORDERS
Women with a history of depression should be carefully observed and the drug discontinued if depression recurs to a serious degree.

6. CONTACT LENSES
Contact lens wearers who develop visual changes or changes in lens tolerance should be assessed by an ophthalmologist.

7. DRUG INTERACTIONS
Reduced efficacy and increased incidence of breakthrough bleeding and menstrual irregularities have been associated with concomitant use of rifampin. A similar association, though less marked, has been suggested with barbiturates, phenylbutazone, phenytoin sodium, and possibly with griseofulvin, ampicillin and tetracyclines.[76]

8. INTERACTIONS WITH LABORATORY TESTS
Certain endocrine and liver function tests and blood components may be affected by oral contraceptives:

a. Increased prothrombin and factors VII, VIII, IX, and X; decreased antithrombin 3; increased norepinephrine-induced platelet aggregability.
b. Increased thyroid binding globulin (TBG) leading to increased circulating total thyroid hormone, as measured by protein-bound iodine (PBI), T4 by column or by radioimmunoassay. Free T3 resin uptake is decreased, reflecting the elevated TBG. Free T4 concentration is unaltered.
c. Other binding proteins may be elevated in serum.
d. Sex steroid binding globulins are increased and result in elevated levels of total circulating sex steroids and corticoids; however, free or biologically active levels remain unchanged.
e. Triglycerides may be increased.
f. Glucose tolerance may be decreased.
g. Serum folate levels may be depressed by oral contraceptive therapy. This may be of clinical significance if a woman becomes pregnant shortly after discontinuing oral contraceptives.

9. CARCINOGENESIS
See **WARNINGS** section.

10. PREGNANCY
Pregnancy Category X. See **CONTRAINDICATIONS** and **WARNINGS** sections.

11. NURSING MOTHERS
Small amounts of oral contraceptive steroids have been identified in the milk of nursing mothers and a few adverse effects on the child have been reported, including jaundice and breast enlargement. In addition, oral contraceptives given in the postpartum period may interfere with lactation by decreasing the quantity and quality of breast milk. If possible, the nursing mother should be advised not to use oral contraceptives but to use other forms of contraception until she has completely weaned her child.

INFORMATION FOR THE PATIENT

See **PATIENT LABELING** printed below.

ADVERSE REACTIONS

An increased risk of the following serious adverse reactions has been associated with the use of oral contraceptives (see **WARNINGS** section):

- Thrombophlebitis
- Arterial thromboembolism
- Pulmonary embolism
- Myocardial infarction
- Cerebral hemorrhage
- Cerebral thrombosis
- Hypertension
- Gallbladder disease
- Hepatic adenomas, carcinomas or benign liver tumors

There is evidence of an association between the following conditions and the use of oral contraceptives, although additional confirmatory studies are needed:

- Mesenteric thrombosis
- Retinal thrombosis

The following adverse reactions have been reported in patients receiving oral contraceptives and are believed to be drug-related:

- Nausea
- Vomiting
- Gastrointestinal symptoms (such as abdominal cramps and bloating)
- Breakthrough bleeding
- Spotting
- Change in menstrual flow
- Amenorrhea
- Temporary infertility after discontinuation of treatment
- Edema
- Melasma which may persist
- Breast changes: tenderness, enlargement, secretion
- Change in weight (increase or decrease)
- Change in cervical erosion and secretion
- Diminution in lactation when given immediately postpartum
- Cholestatic jaundice
- Migraine
- Rash (allergic)
- Mental depression
- Reduced tolerance to carbohydrates
- Vaginal candidiasis
- Change in corneal curvature (steepening)
- Intolerance to contact lenses

The following adverse reactions have been reported in users of oral contraceptives and the association has been neither confirmed nor refuted:

- Pre-menstrual syndrome
- Cataracts
- Changes in appetite
- Cystitis-like syndrome
- Headache
- Nervousness
- Dizziness
- Hirsutism
- Loss of scalp hair
- Erythema multiforme
- Erythema nodosum
- Hemorrhagic eruption
- Vaginitis
- Porphyria
- Impaired renal function
- Hemolytic uremic syndrome
- Budd-Chiari syndrome
- Acne
- Changes in libido
- Colitis

OVERDOSAGE

Serious ill effects have not been reported following acute ingestion of large doses of oral contraceptives by young children. Overdosage may cause nausea, and withdrawal bleeding may occur in females.

NON-CONTRACEPTIVE HEALTH BENEFITS

The following non-contraceptive health benefits related to the use of oral contraceptives are supported by epidemiological studies which largely utilized oral contraceptive formulations containing estrogen doses exceeding 0.035 mg of ethinyl estradiol or 0.05 mg of mestranol.[6–11]

Effects on menses:

- Increased menstrual cycle regularity
- Decreased blood loss and decreased incidence of iron deficiency anemia
- Decreased incidence of dysmenorrhea

Effects related to inhibition of ovulation:

- Decreased incidence of functional ovarian cysts
- Decreased incidence of ectopic pregnancies

Effects from long-term use:

- Decreased incidence of fibroadenomas and fibrocystic disease of the breast
- Decreased incidence of acute pelvic inflammatory disease
- Decreased incidence of endometrial cancer
- Decreased incidence of ovarian cancer

DOSAGE AND ADMINISTRATION

To achieve maximum contraceptive effectiveness, oral contraceptives must be taken exactly as described and at intervals not exceeding 24 hours.

21-Day Regimen Dosage Schedule: The first blue tablet is taken on the first Sunday after menstrual flow begins. If menstrual flow begins on Sunday, the first blue tablet is taken on that day. One blue tablet is taken each evening at bedtime for 7 days, then one yellow-green tablet each evening for 9 days, then one blue tablet each evening for 5 days. No tablets are taken for 7 days; then, whether bleeding has stopped or not, a new sequence of tablets is started for 21 days. This institutes a three weeks on, one week off dosage regimen. For a Day 5 start, the first tablet should be taken on Day 5 of the menstrual cycle, counting the first day of menstrual flow as Day 1, continue to take the pills as described above.

28-Day Regimen Dosage Schedule: The first blue tablet is taken on the first Sunday after menstrual flow begins. If menstrual flow begins on Sunday, the first blue tablet is taken on that day. One blue tablet is taken each evening at bedtime for 7 days, then one yellow-green tablet each evening for 9 days, then one blue tablet each evening for 5 days, then one orange (inert) tablet each evening for 7 days. For a Day 5 start, the first tablet should be taken on Day 5 of the menstrual cycle, counting the first day of menstrual flow as Day 1, continue to take the pills as described above. After all 28 tablets have been taken, whether bleeding has stopped or not, the same dosage schedule is repeated beginning on the following day.

INSTRUCTIONS TO PATIENTS

- To achieve maximum contraceptive effectiveness, the oral contraceptive pill must be taken exactly as directed and at intervals not exceeding 24 hours.
- Important: Women should be instructed to use an additional method of protection until after the first 7 days of administration *in the initial cycle.*
- Due to the normally increased risk of thromboembolism occurring postpartum, women should be instructed not to initiate treatment with oral contraceptives earlier than 4 weeks after a full-term delivery. If pregnancy is terminated in the first 12 weeks, the patient should be instructed to start oral contraceptives immediately or within 7 days. If pregnancy is terminated after 12 weeks, the patient should be instructed to start oral contraceptives after 2 weeks.[33,77]
- If spotting or breakthrough bleeding should occur, the patient should continue the medication according to the schedule. Should spotting or breakthrough bleeding persist, the patient should notify her physician.
- If the patient misses 1 pill, she should be instructed to take it as soon as she remembers and then take the next pill at the regular time. The patient should be advised that missing a pill can cause spotting or light bleeding and that she may be a little sick to her stomach on the days she takes the missed pill with her regularly scheduled pill. If the patient has missed more than one pill, she should not take the missed pills and they should be discarded. She should be advised to take the next pill at the next regular time and continue to take them as scheduled. Furthermore, she should use an additional method of contraception in addition to taking her pills for the remainder of the cycle.
- Use of oral contraceptives in the event of a missed menstrual period:
  1. If the patient has not adhered to the prescribed dosage regimen, the possibility of pregnancy should be considered after the first missed period and oral contraceptives should be withheld until pregnancy has been ruled out.
  2. If the patient has adhered to the prescribed regimen and misses 2 consecutive periods, pregnancy should be ruled out before continuing the contraceptive regimen.

HOW SUPPLIED

TRI-NORINYL® 21-DAY Tablets and TRI-NORINYL® 28-DAY Tablets (norethindrone and ethinyl estradiol) are available in 21-tablet or 28-tablet blister cards with a WALLETTE® tablet dispenser. Each 28-tablet card contains 7 orange inert tablets.

CAUTION: Federal law prohibits dispensing without prescription.

REFERENCES

1. Trussell, J., et al.: *Stud Fam Plann* 21(1):51–54, 1990. **2.** Mann, J., et al.: *Br Med J* 2(5956):241–245, 1975. **3.** Knopp, R.H.: *J Reprod Med* 31(9):913–921, 1986. **4.** Mann, J.I., et al.: *Br Med J* 2:445–447, 1976. **5.** Ory, H.: *JAMA* 237:2619–2622, 1977. **6.** The Cancer and Steroid Hormone Study of the Centers for Disease Control: *JAMA* 249(2):1596–1599, 1983. **7.** The Cancer and Steroid Hormone Study of the Centers for Disease Control: *JAMA* 257(6):796–800, 1987. **8.** Ory, H.W.: *JAMA* 228(1):68–69, 1974. **9.** Ory, H.W., et al.: *N Engl J Med* 294:419–422, 1976. **10.** Ory, H.W.: *Fam Plann Perspect* 14:182–184, 1982. **11.** Ory, H.W., et al.: *Making Choices,* New York, The Alan Guttmacher Institute, 1983. **12.** Stadel, B.: *N Engl J Med* 305(11):612–618, 1981. **13.** Stadel, B: *N Engl J Med* 305(12):672–677, 1981. **14.** Adam, S., et al.: *Br J Obstet Gynaecol* 88:838–845, 1981. **15.** Mann, J., et al.: *Br Med J* 2(5965):245–248, 1975. **16.** Royal College of General Practitioners' Oral Contraceptive Study: *Lancet* 1:541–546, 1981. **17.** Slone, D., et al.: *N Engl J Med* 305(8):420–424, 1981. **18.** Vessey, M.P.: *Br J Fam Plann* 6 (supplement):1–12, 1980. **19.** Russell-Briefel, R., et al.: *Prev Med* 15:352–362, 1986. **20.** Goldbaum, G., et al.: *JAMA* 258(10):1339–1342, 1987. **21.** LaRosa, J.C.: *J Reprod Med* 31(9):906–912, 1986. **22.** Krauss, R.M., et al.: *Am J Obstet Gynecol* 145:446–452, 1983. **23.** Wahl, P., et al.: *N Engl J Med* 308(15):862–867, 1983. **24.** Wynn, V., et al.: *Am J Obstet Gynecol* 142(6):766–771, 1982. **25.** Wynn, V., et al.: *J Reprod Med* 31(9):892–897, 1986. **26.** Inman, W.H., et al.: *Br Med J* 2(5599):193–199, 1968. **27.** Maguire, M.G., et al.: *Am J Epidemiol* 110(2):188–195, 1979. **28.** Petitti, D., et al.: *JAMA* 242(11):1150–1154, 1979. **29.** Vessey, M.P., et al.: *Br Med J* 2(5599):199–205, 1968. **30.** Vessey, M.P., et al.: *Br Med J* 2(5658):651–657, 1969. **31.** Porter, J.B., et al.: *Obstet Gynecol* 59(3):299–302, 1982. **32.** Vessey, M.P., et al.: *J Biosoc Sci* 8:373–427, 1976. **33.** Mishell, D.R., et al.: *Reproductive Endocrinology,* Philadelphia, F.A. Davis Co., 1979. **34.** Petitti, D.B., et al.: *Lancet* 2:234–236, 1978. **35.** Collaborative Group for the Study of Stroke in Young Women: *JAMA* 231(7):718–722, 1975. **36.** Inman, W.H., et al.: *Br Med J* 2:203–209, 1970. **37.** Meade, T.W., et al.: *Br Med J* 280 (6224): 1157–1161, 1980. **38.** Kay, C.R.: *Am J Obstet Gynecol* 142(6):762–765, 1982. **39.** Gordon, T., et al.: *Am J Med* 62:707–714, 1977. **40.** Royal College of General Practitioners' Oral Contraception Study: *J Coll Gen Pract* 33:75–82, 1983. **41.** Ory, H.W.: *Fam Plann Perspect* 15(2):57–63, 1983. **42.** Paul, C., et al.: *Br Med J* 293:723–725, 1986. **43.** The Cancer and Steroid Hormone Study of the Centers for Disease Control: *N Engl J Med* 315(7):405–411, 1986. **44.** Pike, M.C., et al.: *Lancet* 2:926–929, 1983. **45.** Miller, D.R., et al.: *Obstet Gynecol*

Continued on next page

Searle—Cont.

68:863–868, 1986. **46.** Olsson, H., et al.: *Lancet* 2:748–749, 1985. **47.** McPherson, K., et al.: *Br J Cancer* 56:653–660, 1987. **48.** Huggins, G.R., et al.: *Fertil Steril* 47(5):733–761, 1987. **49.** McPherson, K., et al.: *Br Med J* 293:709–710, 1986. **50.** Ory, H., et al.: *Am J Obstet Gynecol* 124(6):573–577, 1976. **51.** Vessey, M.P., et al.: *Lancet,* 2:930, 1983. **52.** Brinton, L.A., et al.: *Int J Cancer* 38:339–344, 1986. **53.** WHO Collaborative Study of Neoplasia and Steroid Contraceptives: *Br Med J* 290:961–965, 1985. **54.** Rooks, J.B., et al.: *JAMA* 242(7):644–648, 1979. **55.** Bein, N.N., et al.: *Br J Surg* 64:433–435, 1977. **56.** Klatskin, G.: *Gastroenterology* 73:386–394, 1977. **57.** Henderson, B.E., et al.: *Br J Cancer* 48:437–440, 1983. **58.** Neuberger, J., et al.: *Br Med J* 292:1355–1357, 1986. **59.** Forman, D., et al.: *Br Med J* 292:1357–1361, 1986. **60.** Harlap, S., et al.: *Obstet Gynecol* 55(4):447–452, 1980. **61.** Savolainen, E., et al.: *Am J Obstet Gynecol* 140(5):521–524, 1981. **62.** Janerich, D.T., et al.: *Am J Epidemiol* 112(1):73–79, 1980. **63.** Ferencz, C., et al.: *Teratology* 21:225–239, 1980. **64.** Rothman, K.J., et al.: *Am J Epidemiol* 109(4):433–439, 1979. **65.** Boston Collaborative Drug Surveillance Program: *Lancet* 1:1399–1404, 1973. **66.** Royal College of General Practitioners: *Oral contraceptives and health.* New York, Pittman, 1974. **67.** Rome Group for the Epidemiology and Prevention of Cholelithiasis: *Am J Epidemiol* 119(5):796–805, 1984. **68.** Strom, B.L., et al.: *Clin Pharmacol Ther* 39(3):335–341, 1986. **69.** Perlman, J.A., et al.: *J Chronic Dis* 38(10):857–864, 1985. **70.** Wynn, V., et al.: *Lancet* 1:1045–1049, 1979. **71.** Wynn, V.: *Progesterone and Progestin,* New York, Raven Press, 1983. **72.** Wynn, V., et al.: *Lancet* 2:720–723, 1966. **73.** Fisch, I.R., et al.: *JAMA* 237(23):2499–2503, 1977. **74.** Laragh, J.H.: *Am J Obstet Gynecol* 126(1):141–147, 1976. **75.** Ramcharan, S., et al.: *Pharmacology of Steroid Contraceptive Drugs,* New York, Raven Press, 1977. **76.** Stockley, I.: *Pharm J* 216:140–143, 1976. **77.** Dickey, R.P.: *Managing Contraceptive Pill Patients,* Oklahoma, Creative Informatics Inc., 1984. **78.** Porter J.B., Hunter J., Jick H., et al: *Obstet Gynecol* 1985;66:1–4. **79.** Porter J.B., Hershel J., Walker A.M.: *Obstet Gynecol* 1987;70:29–32. **80.** Fertility and Maternal Health Drugs Advisory Committee, F.D.A., October, 1989. **81.** Schlesselman J., Stadel B.V., Murray P., Lai S.: *Breast cancer in relation to early use of oral contraceptives.* JAMA 1988;259:1828–1833. **82.** Hennekens C.H., Speizer F.E., Lipnick R.J., Rosner B., Bain C., Belanger C., Stampfer M.J., Willett W., Peto R.: *A case-control study of oral contraceptive use and breast cancer.* JNCl 1984;72:39–42.

DETAILED PATIENT LABELING

This product (like all oral contraceptives) is intended to prevent pregnancy. It does not protect against HIV infection (AIDS) and other sexually transmitted diseases.

INTRODUCTION

Any woman who considers using oral contraceptives ("birth control pills" or "the pill") should understand the benefits and risks of using this form of birth control. This leaflet will give you much of the information you will need to make this decision and also will help you determine if you are at risk of developing any of the serious side effects of the pill. It will tell you how to use the pill properly so that it will be as effective as possible. However, this leaflet is not a replacement for a careful discussion between you and your health care provider. You should discuss the information provided in this leaflet with him or her, both when you first start taking the pill and during your regular visits. You also should follow the advice of your health care provider with regard to regular checkups while you are on the pill.

EFFECTIVENESS OF ORAL CONTRACEPTIVES

Oral contraceptives are used to prevent pregnancy and are more effective than other non-surgical methods of birth control. When they are taken correctly, without missing any pills, the chance of becoming pregnant is less than 1% (1 pregnancy per 100 women per year of use). Typical failure rates are actually 3% per year. The chance of becoming pregnant increases with each missed pill during a menstrual cycle.

In comparison, typical failure rates for other nonsurgical methods of birth control during the first year are as follows:

IUD: 3%
Diaphragm with spermicides: 18%
Spermicides alone: 21%
Vaginal sponge: 18% to 28%
Condom alone: 12%
Periodic abstinence: 20%
Injectable progestogen: 0.4%
Implants: 0.04%
No methods: 85%

WHO SHOULD NOT TAKE ORAL CONTRACEPTIVES

Cigarette smoking increases the risk of serious cardiovascular side effects from oral contraceptive use. This risk increases with age and with heavy smoking (15 or more cigarettes per day) and is quite marked in women over 35 years of age. Women who use oral contraceptives are strongly advised not to smoke.

Some women should not use the pill. For example, you should not take the pill if you are pregnant or think you may be pregnant. You also should not use the pill if you have any of the following conditions:

- A history of heart attack or stroke
- Blood clots in the legs (thrombophlebitis), brain (stroke), lungs (pulmonary embolism) or eyes
- A history of blood clots in the deep veins of your legs
- Chest pain (angina pectoris)
- Known or suspected breast cancer or cancer of the lining of the uterus, cervix or vagina
- Unexplained vaginal bleeding (until a diagnosis is reached by your doctor)
- Yellowing of the whites of the eyes or of the skin (jaundice) during pregnancy or during previous use of the pill
- Liver tumor (benign or cancerous)
- Known or suspected pregnancy

Tell your health care provider if you have ever had any of these conditions. Your health care provider can recommend a safer method of birth control.

OTHER CONSIDERATIONS BEFORE TAKING ORAL CONTRACEPTIVES

Tell your health care provider if you have or have had:

- Breast nodules, fibrocystic disease of the breast, an abnormal breast x-ray or mammogram
- Diabetes
- Elevated cholesterol or triglycerides
- High blood pressure
- Migraine or other headaches or epilepsy
- Mental depression
- Gallbladder, heart or kidney disease
- History of scanty or irregular menstrual periods

Women with any of these conditions should be checked often by their health care provider if they choose to use oral contraceptives.

Also, be sure to inform your doctor or health care provider if you smoke or are on any medications.

RISKS OF TAKING ORAL CONTRACEPTIVES

1. Risk of developing blood clots

Blood clots and blockage of blood vessels are the most serious side effects of taking oral contraceptives. In particular, a clot in the legs can cause thrombophlebitis and a clot that travels to the lungs can cause a sudden blocking of the vessel carrying blood to the lungs. Rarely, clots occur in the blood vessels of the eye and may cause blindness, double vision, or impaired vision.

If you take oral contraceptives and need elective surgery, need to stay in bed for a prolonged illness or have recently delivered a baby, you may be at risk of developing blood clots. You should consult your doctor about stopping oral contraceptives three to four weeks before surgery and not taking oral contraceptives for two weeks after surgery or during bed rest. You should also not take oral contraceptives soon after delivery of a baby. It is advisable to wait for at least four weeks after delivery if you are not breast feeding. If you are breast feeding, you should wait until you have weaned your child before using the pill (see **GENERAL PRECAUTIONS, While Breast Feeding).**

2. Heart attacks and strokes

Oral contraceptives may increase the tendency to develop strokes (stoppage or rupture of blood vessels in the brain) and angina pectoris and heart attacks (blockage of blood vessels in the heart). Any of these conditions can cause death or temporary or permanent disability.

Smoking greatly increases the possibility of suffering heart attacks and strokes. Furthermore, smoking and the use of oral contraceptives greatly increase the chances of developing and dying of heart disease.

3. Gallbladder disease

Oral contraceptive users may have a greater risk than nonusers of having gallbladder disease, although this risk may be related to pills containing high doses of estrogen.

4. Liver tumors

In rare cases, oral contraceptives can cause benign but dangerous liver tumors. These benign liver tumors can rupture and cause fatal internal bleeding. In addition, a possible but not definite association has been found with the pill and liver cancers in 2 studies in which a few women who developed these very rare cancers were found to have used oral contraceptives for long periods. However, liver cancers are extremely rare.

5. Cancer of the breast and reproductive organs

There is, at present, no confirmed evidence that oral contraceptives increase the risk of cancer of the reproductive organs in human studies. Several studies have found no overall increase in the risk of developing breast cancer. However, women who use oral contraceptives and have a strong family history of breast cancer or who have breast nodules or abnormal mammograms should be followed closely by their doctors. Some studies have reported an increase in the risk of developing breast cancer, particularly at a younger age. This increased risk appears to be related to duration of use.

Some studies have found an increase in the incidence of cancer of the cervix in women who use oral contraceptives. However, this finding may be related to factors other than the use of oral contraceptives.

ESTIMATED RISK OF DEATH FROM A BIRTH CONTROL METHOD OR PREGNANCY

All methods of birth control and pregnancy are associated with a risk of developing certain diseases which may lead to disability or death. An estimate of the number of deaths associated with different methods of birth control and pregnancy has been calculated and is shown in the following table.

[See table below.]

In the above table, the risk of death from any birth control method is less than the risk of childbirth except for oral contraceptive users over the age of 35 who smoke and pill users over the age of 40 even if they do not smoke. It can be seen from the table that for women aged 15 to 39 the risk of death is highest with pregnancy (7–26 deaths per 100,000 women, depending on age). Among pill users who do not smoke the risk of death is always lower than that associated with pregnancy for any age group, although over the age of 40 the risk increases to 32 deaths per 100,000 women compared to 28 associated with pregnancy at that age. However, for pill users who smoke and are over the age of 35 the estimated number of deaths exceeds those for other methods of birth control. If a woman is over the age of 40 and smokes, her estimated risk of death is 4 times higher (117/100,000 women) than the estimated risk associated with pregnancy (28/100,000 women) in that age group.

The suggestion that women over 40 who don't smoke should not take oral contraceptives is based on information from older high-dose pills and on less selective use of pills than is practiced today. An Advisory Committee of the FDA discussed this issue in 1989 and recommended that the benefits of oral contraceptive use by healthy, non-smoking women over 40 years of age may outweigh the possible risks. However, all women, especially older women, are cautioned to use the lowest dose pill that is effective.

WARNING SIGNALS

If any of these adverse effects occur while you are taking oral contraceptives, call your doctor immediately:

- Sharp chest pain, coughing of blood or sudden shortness of breath (indicating a possible clot in the lung)
- Pain in the calf (indicating a possible clot in the leg)
- Crushing chest pain or heaviness in the chest (indicating a possible heart attack)
- Sudden severe headache or vomiting, dizziness or fainting, disturbances of vision or speech, weakness or numbness in an arm or leg (indicating a possible stroke)
- Sudden partial or complete loss of vision (indicating a possible clot in the eye)
- Breast lumps (indicating possible breast cancer or fibrocystic disease of the breast: ask your doctor or health care provider to show you how to examine your breasts)

ESTIMATED ANNUAL NUMBER OF BIRTH-RELATED OR METHOD-RELATED DEATHS ASSOCIATED WITH CONTROL OF FERTILITY PER 100,000 NON-STERILE WOMEN, BY FERTILITY CONTROL METHOD ACCORDING TO AGE

Method of control and outcome	15–19	20–24	25–29	30–34	35–39	40–44
No fertility control methods*	7.0	7.4	9.1	14.8	25.7	28.2
Oral contraceptives non-smoker**	0.3	0.5	0.9	1.9	13.8	31.6
Oral contraceptives smoker**	2.2	3.4	6.6	13.5	51.1	117.2
IUD**	0.8	0.8	1.0	1.0	1.4	1.4
Condom*	1.1	1.6	0.7	0.2	0.3	0.4
Diaphragm/Spermicide*	1.9	1.2	1.2	1.3	2.2	2.8
Periodic abstinence*	2.5	1.6	1.6	1.7	2.9	3.6

*Deaths are birth-related
**Deaths are method-related

- Severe pain or tenderness in the stomach area (indicating a possible ruptured liver tumor)
- Difficulty in sleeping, weakness, lack of energy, fatigue or change in mood (possibly indicating severe depression)
- Jaundice or a yellowing of the skin or eyeballs, accompanied frequently by fever, fatigue, loss of appetite, dark colored urine or light colored bowel movements (indicating possible liver problems)

SIDE EFFECTS OF ORAL CONTRACEPTIVES

1. Vaginal bleeding
Irregular vaginal bleeding or spotting may occur while you are taking the pill. Irregular bleeding may vary from slight staining between menstrual periods to breakthrough bleeding which is a flow much like a regular period. Irregular bleeding occurs most often during the first few months of oral contraceptive use but may also occur after you have been taking the pill for some time. Such bleeding may be temporary and usually does not indicate any serious problem. It is important to continue taking your pills on schedule. If the bleeding occurs in more than 1 cycle or lasts for more than a few days, talk to your doctor or health care provider.

2. Contact lenses
If you wear contact lenses and notice a change in vision or an inability to wear your lenses, contact your doctor or health care provider.

3. Fluid retention
Oral contraceptives may cause edema (fluid retention) with swelling of the fingers or ankles and may raise your blood pressure. If you experience fluid retention, contact your doctor or health care provider.

4. Melasma (Mask of Pregnancy)
A spotty darkening of the skin is possible, particularly of the face.

5. Other side effects
Other side effects may include change in appetite, headache, nervousness, depression, dizziness, loss of scalp hair, rash and vaginal infections.
If any of these side effects occurs, contact your doctor or health care provider.

GENERAL PRECAUTIONS

1. Missed periods and use of oral contraceptives before or during early pregnancy
At times you may not menstruate regularly after you have completed taking a cycle of pills. If you have taken your pills regularly and miss 1 menstrual period, continue taking your pills for the next cycle but be sure to inform your health care provider before doing so. If you have not taken the pills daily as instructed and miss 1 menstrual period, or if you miss 2 consecutive menstrual periods, you may be pregnant. You should stop taking oral contraceptives until you are sure you are not pregnant and continue to use another method of contraception.

There is no conclusive evidence that oral contraceptive use is associated with an increase in birth defects when taken inadvertently during early pregnancy. Previously, a few studies had reported that oral contraceptives might be associated with birth defects but these studies have not been confirmed. Nevertheless, oral contraceptives or any other drugs should not be used during pregnancy unless clearly necessary and prescribed by your doctor. You should check with your doctor about risks to your unborn child from any medication taken during pregnancy.

2. While breast feeding
If you are breast feeding, consult your doctor before starting oral contraceptives. Some of the drug will be passed on to the child in the milk. A few adverse effects on the child have been reported, including yellowing of the skin (jaundice) and breast enlargement. In addition, oral contraceptives may decrease the amount and quality of your milk. If possible, use another method of contraception while breast feeding. You should consider starting oral contraceptives only after you have weaned your child completely.

3. Laboratory tests
If you are scheduled for any laboratory tests, tell your doctor you are taking birth control pills. Certain blood tests may be affected by birth control pills.

4. Drug interactions
Certain drugs may interact with birth control pills to make them less effective in preventing pregnancy or cause an increase in breakthrough bleeding. Such drugs include rifampin; drugs used for epilepsy such as barbiturates (for example, phenobarbital) and phenytoin (Dilantin is one brand of this drug); phenylbutazone (Butazolidin is one brand of this drug) and possibly certain antibiotics. You may need to use additional contraception when you take drugs which can make oral contraceptives less effective.

HOW TO TAKE ORAL CONTRACEPTIVES

1. Important points to remember
This product (like all oral contraceptives) is intended to prevent pregnancy. It does not protect against transmission of HIV (AIDS) and other sexually transmitted diseases such as chlamydia, genital herpes, genital warts, gonorrhea, hepatitis B, and syphilis.

Before you start taking your pills:
- Be sure to read these directions:
  Before you start taking your pills.
  Anytime you are not sure what to do.
- The right way to take the Pill is to take one pill every day at the same time. If you miss pills you could get pregnant. The more pills you miss, the more likely you are to get pregnant.
- Many women have spotting or light bleeding while they are taking the Pill, or may feel sick to their stomachs during the first 1–3 packs of pills. If you feel sick to your stomach, do not stop taking the Pill. These problems will usually go away after the first three months. If they do not go away, talk to your doctor or clinic.
- Missing pills can also cause spotting or light bleeding (see the section on MISSED PILLS). You could also feel a little sick to your stomach on the days you take a missed pill with your regularly scheduled pill.
- If you have vomiting or diarrhea, for any reason, or if you take some medicines, including some antibiotics, your pills may not work as well. Use a back-up method of birth control until you check with your doctor or clinic. Talk to your doctor or clinic about which back-up birth control method is right for you.
- If you have trouble remembering to take the Pill (for example, if you forget to take more than one pill two months in a row), talk to your doctor or clinic about how to make pill-taking easier or about using another method of birth control.
- If you have any questions or are unsure about the information in this leaflet, call your doctor or clinic.

2. Before you start taking your pills
- Decide what time of day you want to take your pill. It is important to take it at about the same time every day.
- Look at your pill pack to see if it has 21 or 28 pills:
  The 21-pill pack has 21 "active" blue and yellow-green pills (with hormones) to take for 3 weeks, followed by 1 week without pills.
  The 28-pill pack has 21 "active" blue and yellow-green pills (with hormones) to take for 3 weeks, followed by 1 week of "reminder" orange pills (without hormones).
- Also find:
  1) where on the pack to start taking pills
  2) in what order to take the pills (follow the arrows) and
  3) the days of the week as shown on the pill card.

Active Pill Colors: Blue and Yellow-Green

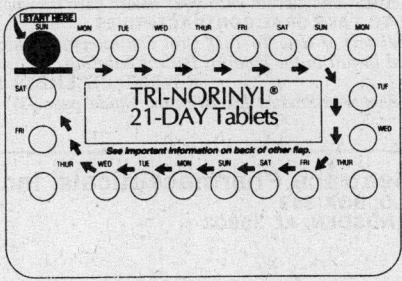

Active Pill Colors: Blue and Yellow-Green
Reminder Pill Color: Orange

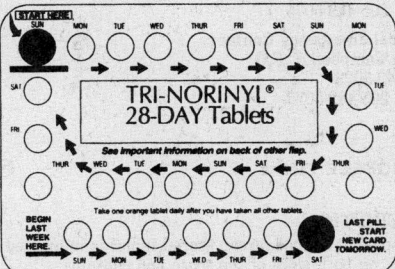

- Be sure you have ready at all times:
  Another kind of birth control to use as a back-up in case you miss pills. (Remember to talk to your doctor or clinic about an appropriate back-up method of birth control for you.)
  An extra, full pill pack.

3. When to start the first pack of pills
You have a choice of which day to start taking your first pack of pills (Sunday or Day 5 of your period). Decide with your doctor or clinic which is the best day for you to start. Pick a time of day which will be easy to remember.

Sunday Start:
- Take the first pill of the first pack on the Sunday after your period starts, even if you are still bleeding. If your period begins on Sunday, take your first pill of the first pack that same day.

- Use another method of birth control as a back-up method if you have sex any time from the Sunday you start your first pack until the next Sunday (7 days). Talk to your doctor about an appropriate back-up method of birth control for you.

Day 5 Start:
- Count the first day of your period as Day 1. Take the first pill of the first pack on the fifth day of your period, even if you are still bleeding.
- Use another method of birth control as a back-up method if you have sex any time during the 7 days after you take your first pill. Talk to your doctor or clinic about an appropriate back-up method of birth control for you.

4. What to do during the month
- **Take one pill at the same time every day until the pack is empty.**
  Do not skip pills even if you are spotting or have light bleeding between monthly periods or feel sick to your stomach (nausea).
  Do not skip pills even if you do not have sex very often.
- **When you finish a pack of pills:**
  21 pills: Wait 7 days to start the next pack. You will probably have your period during that week. Be sure that no more than 7 days pass between 21-day packs.
  28 pills: Start the next pack on the day after your last "reminder" pill. Do not wait any days between packs.

5. What to do if you miss pills
If you **MISS 1** "active" blue or yellow-green pill:
- Take it as soon as you remember. Take the next pill at your regular time. This means you take 2 pills in 1 day.
- Missing a pill can cause spotting or light bleeding. You could also feel a little sick to your stomach on the days you take a missed pill with your regularly scheduled pill.
- You do not need to use a back-up birth control method if you have sex.

If you **MISS MORE THAN 1** "active" blue or yellow-green pill in a row:
- Do not take the missed pills. The missed pills may be discarded. Take the next pill at your regular time. Continue to take one pill a day as scheduled.
- Missing pills can cause spotting or light bleeding.
- You MAY BECOME PREGNANT, especially if you have sex in the first 7 days after you have missed pills. Therefore, you MUST use a back-up method of birth control until you start a new pill pack. (Remember to talk to your doctor or clinic about an appropriate back-up birth control method for you.)

A reminder for those on 28-day packs:
If you forget any of the 7 orange "reminder" pills in Week 4: THROW AWAY the pills you missed.
Keep taking 1 pill each day until the pack is empty.
You do not need a back-up method of birth control during this time.

FINALLY, IF YOU ARE STILL NOT SURE WHAT TO DO ABOUT THE PILLS YOU HAVE MISSED:
Use a BACK-UP METHOD OF BIRTH CONTROL anytime you have sex.
KEEP TAKING ONE PILL EACH DAY until you can talk to your doctor or clinic.

6. Missed periods, spotting or light bleeding
At times, you may not have a period after you have completed a pack of pills. If you miss 1 period but you have taken the pills exactly as you were supposed to, continue as usual into the next cycle. If you have not taken the pills correctly, and have missed a period, you may be pregnant and you should stop taking the Pill until your doctor or clinic determines whether or not you are pregnant. Until you can talk to your doctor or clinic, use an appropriate back-up birth control method. If you miss 2 consecutive periods, you should stop taking the Pill until it is determined that you are not pregnant.
Even if spotting or light bleeding should occur, continue taking the Pill according to the schedule. Should spotting or light bleeding persist, you should notify your doctor or clinic.

7. Stopping the pill before surgery or prolonged bed rest
If you are scheduled for surgery or you need to stay in bed for a long period of time you should tell your doctor that you are on the Pill. You should stop taking the Pill four weeks before your operation to avoid an increased risk of blood clots. Talk to your doctor about when you may start taking the Pill again.

8. Starting the pill after pregnancy
After you have a baby it is advisable to wait 4 weeks before starting to take the Pill. Talk to your doctor about when you may start taking the Pill after pregnancy.

9. Pregnancy due to pill failure
When the Pill is taken correctly, the expected pregnancy rate is approximately 1% (i.e., 1 pregnancy per 100 women per year). If pregnancy occurs while taking the Pill, there is little risk to the fetus. The typical failure rate of large numbers of pill users is less than 3% when women who have missed pills are included. If you become pregnant, you should discuss your pregnancy with your doctor.

Continued on next page

Searle—Cont.

10. Pregnancy after stopping the pill

There may be some delay in becoming pregnant after you stop taking the Pill, especially if you had irregular periods before you started using the Pill. Your doctor may recommend that you delay becoming pregnant until you have had one or more regular periods.

There does not appear to be any increase in birth defects in newborn babies when pregnancy occurs soon after stopping the pill.

11. Overdosage

There are no reports of serious illness or side effects in young children who have swallowed a large number of pills. In adults, overdosage may cause nausea and/or bleeding in females. In case of overdosage, contact your doctor, clinic or pharmacist.

12. Other information

Your doctor or clinic will take a medical and family history and will examine you before prescribing the Pill. The physical examination may be delayed to another time if you request it and the health care provider believes that it is a good medical practice to postpone it. You should be reexamined at least once a year. Be sure to inform your doctor or clinic if there is a family history of any of the conditions listed previously in this leaflet. Be sure to keep all appointments with your doctor or clinic because this is a time to determine if there are early signs of side effects from using the Pill.

Do not use the Pill for any condition other than the one for which it was prescribed. The Pill has been prescribed specifically for you, do not give it to others who may want birth control pills.

If you want more information about birth control pills, ask your doctor or clinic. They have a more technical leaflet called **PHYSICIAN LABELING** which you might want to read.

NON-CONTRACEPTIVE HEALTH BENEFITS

In addition to preventing pregnancy, use of oral contraceptives may provide certain non-contraceptive health benefits:

- Menstrual cycles may become more regular
- Blood flow during menstruation may be lighter and less iron may be lost. Therefore, anemia due to iron deficiency is less likely to occur
- Pain or other symptoms during menstruation may be encountered less frequently
- Ectopic (tubal) pregnancy may occur less frequently
- Non-cancerous cysts or lumps in the breast may occur less frequently
- Acute pelvic inflammatory disease may occur less frequently
- Oral contraceptive use may provide some protection against developing two forms of cancer: cancer of the ovaries and cancer of the lining of the uterus.

Store at controlled room temperature 15–30°C (59–86°F).

BRIEF SUMMARY
PATIENT PACKAGE INSERT

This product (like all oral contraceptives) is intended to prevent pregnancy. It does not protect against HIV infection (AIDS) and other sexually transmitted diseases.

Oral contraceptives, also known as "birth control pills" or "the pill," are taken to prevent pregnancy and, when taken correctly, have a failure rate of about 1% per year when used without missing any pills. The typical failure rate of large numbers of pill users is less than 3% per year when women who miss pills are included. For most women, oral contraceptives are also free of serious or unpleasant side effects. However, forgetting to take oral contraceptives considerably increases the chances of pregnancy.

For the majority of women, oral contraceptives can be taken safely, but there are some women who are at high risk of developing certain serious diseases that can be life-threatening or may cause temporary or permanent disability. The risks associated with taking oral contraceptives increase significantly if you:

- Smoke
- Have high blood pressure diabetes or high cholesterol
- Have or have had clotting disorders, heart attack, stroke, angina pectoris, cancer of the breast or sex organs, jaundice or malignant or benign liver tumors

You should not take the pill if you suspect you are pregnant or have unexplained vaginal bleeding.

Cigarette smoking increases the risk of serious cardiovascular side effects from oral contraceptive use. This risk increases with age and with heavy smoking (15 or more cigarettes per day) and is quite marked in women over 35 years of age. Women who use oral contraceptives are strongly advised not to smoke.

Most side effects of the pill are not serious. The most common such effects are nausea, vomiting, bleeding between menstrual periods, weight gain, breast tenderness and difficulty wearing contact lenses. These side effects, especially nausea and vomiting, may subside within the first 3 months of use.

The serious side effects of the pill occur very infrequently, especially if you are in good health and are young. However, you should know that the following medical conditions have been associated with or made worse by the pill:

1. Blood clots in the legs (thrombophlebitis) or lungs (pulmonary embolism), stoppage or rupture of a blood vessel in the brain (stroke), blockage of blood vessels in the heart (heart attack or angina pectoris), eye or other organs of the body. As mentioned above, smoking increases the risk of heart attacks and strokes and subsequent serious medical consequences.
2. Liver tumors, which may rupture and cause severe bleeding. A possible but not definite association has been found with the pill and liver cancer. However, liver cancers are extremely rare.
3. High blood pressure, although blood pressure usually returns to normal when the pill is stopped.

The symptoms associated with these serious side effects are discussed in the detailed leaflet given to you with your supply of pills. Notify your doctor or health care provider if you notice any unusual physical disturbances while taking the pill. In addition, drugs such as rifampin, as well as some anticonvulsants and some antibiotics, may decrease oral contraceptive effectiveness.

Studies to date of women taking the pill have not shown an increase in the incidence of cancer of the breast or cervix. There is, however, insufficient evidence to rule out the possibility that the pill may cause such cancers. Some studies have reported an increase in the risk of developing breast cancer, particularly at a younger age. This increased risk appears to be related to duration of use.

Taking the pill may provide some important non-contraceptive health benefits. These include less painful menstruation, less menstrual blood loss and anemia, fewer acute pelvic infections and fewer cancers of the ovary and the lining of the uterus.

Be sure to discuss any medical condition you may have with your health care provider. Your health care provider will take a medical and family history before prescribing oral contraceptives and will examine you. The physical examination may be delayed to another time if you request it and the health care provider believes that it is a good medical practice to postpone it. You should be reexamined at least once a year while taking oral contraceptives. The detailed patient information leaflet gives you further information which you should read and discuss with your health care provider.

HOW TO TAKE ORAL CONTRACEPTIVES

See full text of How To Take Oral Contraceptives which is printed in full in the Detailed Patient Labeling.

REVISED DECEMBER 1993
Shown in Product Identification Guide, page 335

Seatrace Pharmaceuticals, Inc.
P.O. BOX 363
GADSDEN, AL 35902

Direct Inquiries to:
Hugh Campbell, C.E.O.
205-442-5023
FAX: 205-442-5075

Medical Emergency Contact:
Hugh Campbell, C.E.O.
205-442-5023
FAX: 205-442-5075

BANOBESE Tablets   ℂⅣ ℞

DESCRIPTION

Each peanut shaped, green scored tablet is imprinted with an "S" on both sides of the score and contains:
Phentermine Hydrochloride   37.5 mg

HOW SUPPLIED

Bottles of 100's (NDC 00551-0194-01).

CETA PLUS Capsule   ℂⅢ ℞

DESCRIPTION

Each opaque white capsule is imprinted in blue with the name "SEATRACE" on both body and cap and contains:
Hydrocodone Bitartrate*   5mg
*(Warning: May be habit forming)
Acetaminophen   500mg

HOW SUPPLIED

Bottles of 100's (NDC 00551-0180-01).

DYLINE GG Liquid   ℞

DESCRIPTION

Slightly red, viscous and clear liquid, peppermint flavored. Each teaspoonful (5ml) contains:
Dyphylline   100mg
Guaifenesin   100mg

HOW SUPPLIED

Bottles of one pint (473ml) (NDC 00551-0124-01).

DYLINE GG Tablets   ℞

DESCRIPTION

Each pink scored tablet imprinted with "0551" on one side of score and "0123" on the other side contains:
Dyphylline   200mg
Guaifenesin   200mg

HOW SUPPLIED

Bottles of 100's (NDC 00551-0123-01).

g-TUSS Liquid   ℞

DESCRIPTION

Colorless, viscous, and clear liquid, peppermint cherry flavored. Each teaspoonful (5ml) contains:
Hydrocodone Bitartrate*   5mg
*(Warning: May be habit forming).
Guaifenesin   100mg

HOW SUPPLIED

Bottles of one pint (473ml) (NDC 00551-0188-01).

GUA-SR Tablets   ℞

DESCRIPTION

Each white sustained release capsule shaped scored tablet imprinted with the name "GSR" on both sides of score and contains:
Guaifenesin   600mg

HOW SUPPLIED

Bottles of 100's (NDC 00551-0189-01).

LOBAC Capsules   ℞

DESCRIPTION

Each opaque, eggshell-colored capsule is imprinted in black with "Seatrace" on cap and body and contains:
Acetaminophen   300mg
Salicylamide   200mg
Phenyltoloxamine Citrate   20mg

HOW SUPPLIED

Bottles of 100's (NDC 00551-0176-01).

LOBAC Tablets   ℞

DESCRIPTION

Each film-coated opaque white, capsule-shaped tablet is imprinted with "SEATRACE" on one side and "LOBAC" on the other and contains:
Acetaminophen   300mg
Salicylamide   200mg
Phenyltoloxamine Dihydrogen Citrate   20mg

HOW SUPPLIED

Bottles of 100's (NDC 00551-0187-01).

MENI-D Capsules   ℞

DESCRIPTION

Each light blue and white capsule is imprinted in black the name "Seatrace" on cap and body and contains:
Meclizine Hydrochloride   25mg

HOW SUPPLIED

Bottles of 100's (NDC 00551-0168-01).

ND CLEAR Capsules ℞

DESCRIPTION

Each clear sustained release capsule containing natural color beads is imprinted in black with the name "ND CLEAR" and "1–AM/PM" and contains:

Chlorpheniramine Maleate	8mg
Pseudoephedrine Hydrochloride	120mg

HOW SUPPLIED

Bottles of 100's (NDC 00551-0147-01).

TENAKE Capsules ℞

DESCRIPTION

Each white capsule is imprinted in green with the name "TENAKE" and "SEATRACE" and contains:

Butalbital*	50mg
*(Warning: May be habit forming)	
Acetaminophen	325mg
Caffeine	40mg

HOW SUPPLIED

Bottles of 100's (NDC 00551-0181-01).

TUSS-DM Liquid ℞

DESCRIPTION

Colorless, viscous, and clear liquid, peach flavored.
Each teaspoonful (5ml) contains:

Dextromethorphan Hydrobromide	10mg
Phenylephrine HCL	5mg
Chlorpheniramine Maleate	2mg

HOW SUPPLIED

Bottles of one pint (473ml) (NDC 00551-0209-01).

TUSS-DS Liquid ℞

DESCRIPTION

Colorless, viscous, and clear liquid, orange vanilla flavored.
Each teaspoonful (5ml) Contains:

Hydrocodone Bitartrate*	5mg	Sugar Free/Dye Free
*(Warning: May be habit forming).		Alcohol Free
Phenylephrine Hydrochloride	5mg	
Chlorpheniramine Maleate	2mg	

HOW SUPPLIED

Bottles of one pint (473ml) (NDC 00551-0182-01).

TUSS-HC Liquid Ⓒ ℞

DESCRIPTION

Colorless, viscous, and clear liquid, cherry vanilla flavored.
Each teaspoonful (5ml) contains:

Hydrocodone Bitartrate*	2.5mg	Sugar Free/Dye Free
*(Warning: May be habit forming).		Alcohol Free
Phenylephrine Hydrochloride	5mg	
Chlorpheniramine Maleate	2mg	

HOW SUPPLIED

Bottles of one pint (473ml) (NDC 0551-0184-01).

TUSS-PD Liquid Ⓒ ℞

DESCRIPTION

Colorless, viscous, and clear liquid, citrus flavored.
Each teaspoonful (5ml) contains:

Hydrocodone Bitartrate*	1.67mg	Sugar Free/Dye Free
*(Warning: May be habit forming).		Alcohol Free
Phenylephrine Hydrochloride	5mg	
Chlorpheniramine Maleate	2mg	

HOW SUPPLIED

Bottles of one pint (473ml) (NDC 00551-0183-01).

V-DEC-M Tablets ℞

DESCRIPTION

Each white round sustained release double scored tablet is imprinted with the name "AM/PM" on the tablet halves and contains:

Pseudoephedrine Hydrochloride	120mg
Guaifenesin	500mg

HOW SUPPLIED

Bottles of 100's (NDC 00551-0170-01).

VERSACAPS Capsules ℞

DESCRIPTION

Each clear sustained release capsule containing natural color beads imprinted in black with the name "VERSACAPS" and "2-AM/PM" and contains:

Psuedoephedrine Hydrochloride	60mg
Guaifenesin	300mg

HOW SUPPLIED

Bottles of 100's (NDC 00551-0173-01).

SEQUUS™ Pharmaceuticals, Inc.
960 Hamilton Court
Menlo Park, CA 94025

Direct Inquiries to:
Dept. of Professional Services
800-323-9049
Medical Emergency Contact:
Ed Schnipper, MD or
Ron Lewis, MD
800-323-9051

DOXIL® ℞
[däk 'sil]
(doxorubicin HCl liposome injection)
FOR INTRAVENOUS INFUSION ONLY
A product of SEQUUS Pharmaceuticals, Inc.

WARNINGS

1. Experience with DOXIL® (doxorubicin HCl liposome injection) at high cumulative doses is too limited to have established its effect on the myocardium. It should therefore be assumed that DOXIL® will have myocardial toxicity similar to conventional formulations of doxorubicin HCl. With these formulations of doxorubicin HCl, serious irreversible myocardial toxicity leading to congestive heart failure often unresponsive to cardiac supportive therapy may be encountered as the total dosage of doxorubicin HCl approaches 550 mg/m^2. Prior use of other anthracyclines or anthracenediones will reduce the total dose of doxorubicin HCl that can be given without cardiac toxicity. Cardiac toxicity also may occur at lower cumulative doses in patients with prior mediastinal irradiation or who are receiving concurrent cyclophosphamide therapy.
   DOXIL® should be administered to patients with a history of cardiovascular disease only when the benefit outweighs the risk to the patient.
2. Acute infusion-associated reactions (flushing, shortness of breath, facial swelling, headache, chills, back pain, tightness in the chest or throat, and/or hypotension) have occurred in about 7% of patients treated with DOXIL®. In most patients, these reactions resolve over the course of several hours to a day once the infusion is terminated. In some patients, the reaction resolves by slowing the infusion rate. (See **WARNINGS—Infusion Reactions.**)
3. Severe myelosuppression may occur.
4. Dosage should be reduced in patients with impaired hepatic function. (See **DOSAGE AND ADMINISTRATION.**)
5. DOXIL® should be administered only under the supervision of a physician who is experienced in the use of cancer chemotherapeutic agents.

DESCRIPTION

DOXIL® (doxorubicin HCl liposome injection) is doxorubicin hydrochloride (HCl) encapsulated in STEALTH® liposomes for intravenous administration.
Note: Liposomal encapsulation can substantially affect a drug's functional properties relative to those of the unencapsulated drug.
In addition, different liposomal drug products may vary from one another in the chemical composition and physical form of the liposomes. Such differences can substantially affect the functional properties of liposomal drug products.
Doxorubicin is a cytotoxic anthracycline antibiotic isolated from *Streptomyces peucetius* var. *caesius*.

Doxorubicin HCl, which is the established name for (8S,10S)-10- [(3-amino-2,3,6 -trideoxy-L-*lyxo*-hexopyranosyl)oxy] -8-glycolyl-7,8,9,10-tetrahydro- 6,8,11-trihydroxy-1-methoxy-5, 12-naphthacenedione hydrochloride, has the following structure:

The molecular formula of the drug is $C_{27} H_{29} NO_{11} \cdot HCl$; its molecular weight is 579.99.
DOXIL® is provided as a sterile, translucent, red liposomal dispersion in 10-mL glass, single use vials. Each vial contains 20 mg doxorubicin HCl at a concentration of 2 mg/mL and a pH of 6.5. The STEALTH® liposome carriers are composed of N-(carbamoyl- methoxypolyethylene glycol 2000)-1,2-distearoyl-sn-glycero-3-phosphoethanolamine sodium salt (MPEG-DSPE), 3.19 mg/mL; fully hydrogenated soy phosphatidylcholine (HSPC), 9.58 mg/mL; and cholesterol, 3.19 mg/mL. Each mL also contains ammonium sulfate, approximately 2 mg; histidine as a buffer; hydrochloric acid and/or sodium hydroxide for pH control; and sucrose to maintain isotonicity. Greater than 90% of the drug is encapsulated in the STEALTH® liposomes.
MPEG-DSPE has the following structural formula:

n=ca. 45

HSPC has the following structural formula:

m, n = 14 or 16

CLINICAL PHARMACOLOGY

Mechanism of Action
The active ingredient of DOXIL® is doxorubicin HCl. The mechanism of action of doxorubicin HCl is thought to be related to its ability to bind DNA and inhibit nucleic acid synthesis. Cell structure studies have demonstrated rapid cell penetration and perinuclear chromatin binding, rapid inhibition of mitotic activity and nucleic acid synthesis, and induction of mutagenesis and chromosomal aberrations.
DOXIL® is doxorubicin HCl encapsulated in long-circulating STEALTH® liposomes. Liposomes are microscopic vesicles composed of a phospholipid bilayer that are capable of encapsulating active drugs. The STEALTH® liposomes of DOXIL® are formulated with surface-bound methoxypolyethylene glycol (MPEG), a process often referred to as pegylation, to protect liposomes from detection by the mononuclear phagocyte system (MPS) and to increase blood circulation time.
Representation of a STEALTH® liposome:
[See Figure at top of next column.]
STEALTH® liposomes have a half-life of approximately 55 hours in humans. They are stable in blood, and direct measurement of liposomal doxorubicin shows that at least 90%

Continued on next page

Sequus—Cont.

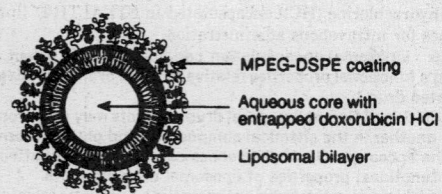

— MPEG-DSPE coating

— Aqueous core with entrapped doxorubicin HCl

— Liposomal bilayer

of the drug (the assay used cannot quantify less than 5–10% free doxorubicin) remains liposome-encapsulated during circulation.

It is hypothesized that because of their small size (ca. 100 nm) and persistence in the circulation the pegylated DOXIL® liposomes are able to penetrate the altered and often compromised vasculature of tumors. This hypothesis is supported by studies using colloidal gold-containing STEALTH® liposomes, which can be visualized microscopically. Evidence of penetration of STEALTH® liposomes from blood vessels and their entry and accumulation in tumors has been seen in mice with C-26 colon carcinoma tumors and in transgenic mice with Kaposi's sarcoma-like lesions. Once the STEALTH® liposomes distribute to the tissue compartment, the encapsulated doxorubicin HCl becomes available. The exact mechanism of release is not understood.

Pharmacokinetics

The plasma pharmacokinetics of DOXIL® were evaluated in 42 patients with AIDS-related Kaposi's sarcoma (KS) who received single doses of 10 or 20 mg/m² administered by a 30-minute infusion. Twenty-three of these patients received single doses of both 10 and 20 mg/m² with a 3-week wash-out period between doses. The pharmacokinetic parameter values of DOXIL®, given for total doxorubicin (most liposomally bound), are presented in the following table.

Pharmacokinetic Parameters of DOXIL® in AIDS Patients with Kaposi's Sarcoma

Parameter (units)	Dose	
	10 mg/m²	20 mg/m²
Peak Plasma Concentration (μg/mL)	4.12 ± 0.215	8.34 ± 0.49
Plasma Clearance (L/h/m²)	0.056 ± 0.01	0.041 ± 0.004
Steady-State Volume of Distribution (L/m²)	2.83 ± 0.145	2.72 ± 0.120
AUC (μg/mL·h)	277 ± 32.9	590 ± 58.7
First Phase (λ_1) Half-Life (h)	4.7 ± 1.1	5.2 ± 1.4
Second Phase (λ_2) Half-Life (h)	52.3 ± 5.6	55.0 ± 4.8

n = 23
Mean ± Standard Error

DOXIL® displayed linear pharmacokinetics. Disposition occurred in two phases after DOXIL® administration, with a relatively short first phase (~5 hours) and a prolonged second phase (~55 hours) that accounted for the majority of the area under the curve (AUC).

Distribution: In contrast to the pharmacokinetics of doxorubicin, which display a large volume of distribution ranging from 700 to 1100 L/m², the steady state volume of distribution of DOXIL® indicated that DOXIL® was confined mostly to the vascular fluid volume. Plasma protein binding of DOXIL® has not been determined; however, the plasma protein binding of doxorubicin is approximately 70%.

Metabolism: Doxorubicinol, the major metabolite of doxorubicin, was detected at very low levels (range: 0.8 to 26.2 ng/mL) in the plasma of patients who received 10 to 20 mg/m² DOXIL®.

Excretion: The plasma clearance of DOXIL® was slow, with a mean clearance value of 0.041 L/h/m² at a dose of 20 mg/m². This is in contrast to doxorubicin, which displays a plasma clearance value ranging from 24 to 35 L/h/m². Because of its slower clearance, the AUC of DOXIL®, primarily representing the circulation of liposome-encapsulated doxorubicin, is approximately two to three orders of magnitude larger than the AUC for a similar dose of conventional doxorubicin HCl as reported in the literature.

Special Populations: The pharmacokinetics of DOXIL® have not been separately evaluated in women, in members of different ethnic groups, or in individuals with renal or hepatic insufficiency.

Drug–Drug Interactions: Although the patient population for the current indication is on various antiviral medications, the drug–drug interactions between DOXIL® and the antiviral drugs have not been evaluated.

Tissue Distribution

Kaposi's sarcoma lesions and normal skin biopsies were obtained at 48 and 96 hours postinfusion of 20 mg/m² DOXIL® in 11 patients. The concentration of DOXIL® in KS lesions was a median of 19 (range, 3–53) times higher than in normal skin at 48 hours posttreatment; however, this was not corrected for likely differences in blood content between KS lesions and normal skin. The corrected ratio may lie between 1 and 22 times. Thus, higher concentrations of DOXIL® are delivered to KS lesions than to normal skin.

Clinical Studies

AIDS-Related Kaposi's Sarcoma

DOXIL® was studied in an open-label, single-arm, multicenter study utilizing DOXIL® at 20 mg/m² by intravenous infusion every three weeks generally until progression or intolerance occurred. In an interim analysis, the treatment history of 383 patients were reviewed, and a cohort of 77 patients was retrospectively identified as having disease progression on prior systemic combination chemotherapy (at least 2 cycles of a regimen containing at least two of three treatments: bleomycin, vincristine or vinblastine, or doxorubicin) or as being intolerant to such therapy. Forty-nine of the 77 (64%) patients had received prior doxorubicin HCl. These 77 patients were predominantly white, homosexual males with a median CD4 count of 10 cells/mm³. Their age ranged from 24 to 54 years, with a mean age of 38 years. Using the ACTG staging criteria,[1] 78% of the patients were at poor risk for tumor burden, 96% at poor risk for immune system, and 58% at poor risk for systemic illness at baseline. Their mean Karnofsky status score was 74%. All 77 patients had cutaneous or subcutaneous lesions, 40% also had oral lesions, 26% pulmonary lesions, and 14% of patients lesions of the stomach/intestine. The majority of these patients had disease progression on prior systemic combination chemotherapy.

The median time on study for these 77 patients was 155 days and ranged from 1 to 456 days. The median cumulative dose was 154 mg/m² and ranged from 20 to 620 mg/m².

Two analyses of tumor response were used to evaluate the effectiveness of DOXIL®: one analysis based on investigator assessment of changes in lesions over the entire body, and one analysis based on changes in indicator lesions.

Investigator Assessment

Investigator response was based on modified ACTG criteria.[1] Partial response was defined as no new lesions, sites of disease, or worsening edema; flattening of ≥ 50% of previously raised lesions or area of indicator lesions decreasing by ≥ 50%; and response lasting at least 21 days with no prior progression.

Indicator Lesion Assessment

A retrospectively defined analysis was conducted based on assessment of the response of up to five prospectively identified representative indicator lesions. A partial response was defined as flattening of ≥ 50% of previously raised indicator lesions, or > 50% decrease in the area of indicator lesions and lasting at least 21 days with no prior progression.

Only patients with adequate documentation of baseline status and follow-up assessments were considered evaluable for response. Patients who received concomitant KS treatment during study, who completed local radiotherapy to sites encompassing one or more of the indicator lesions within two months of study entry, who had less than four indicator lesions, or who had less than three raised indicator lesions at baseline (the latter applies solely to indicator lesion assessment) were considered nonevaluable for response. Of the 77 patients who had disease progression on prior systemic combination chemotherapy or who were intolerant to such therapy, 34 were evaluable for investigator assessment and 42 were evaluable for indicator lesion assessment.

Response is summarized in the table below.

Response in Refractory[a] AIDS-KS

Investigator Assessment	All Evaluable Patients (n = 34)	Evaluable Patients Who Received Prior Doxorubicin (n = 20)
Response[b]		
Partial (PR)	27%	30%
Stable	29%	40%
Progression	44%	30%
Duration of PR (days)		
Median	73	89
Range	42+– 210+	42+– 210+
Time to PR (days)		
Median	43	53
Range	15–133	15–109

Indicator Lesion Assessment	All Evaluable Patients (n = 42)	Evaluable Patients Who Received Prior Doxorubicin (n = 23)
Response[b]		
Partial (PR)	48%	52%
Stable	26%	30%
Progression	26%	17%
Duration of PR (days)		
Median	71	79
Range	22+– 210+	35– 210+
Time to PR (days)		
Median	22	48
Range	15–109	15–109

a Patients with disease that progressed on prior combination chemotherapy or who were intolerant to such therapy.

b There were no complete responses in this population.

Clinical Benefit

Clinical benefit (e.g., decreased pain, disfigurement, pulmonary or gastrointestinal symptoms) was not well evaluated in the open studies carried out to date. A controlled trial with double-blinded assessment of clinical endpoints is ongoing.

INDICATIONS AND USAGE

DOXIL® (doxorubicin HCl liposome injection) is indicated for the treatment of AIDS-related Kaposi's sarcoma in patients with disease that has progressed on prior combination chemotherapy or in patients who are intolerant to such therapy.

CONTRAINDICATIONS

DOXIL® (doxorubicin HCl liposome injection) is contraindicated in patients who have a history of hypersensitivity reactions to a conventional formulation of doxorubicin HCl or the components of DOXIL®.

WARNINGS

Cardiac Toxicity

Experience with DOXIL® (doxorubicin HCl liposome injection) is limited in evaluating cardiac risk. Therefore, warnings related to the use of conventional formulation doxorubicin HCl should be observed.

Special attention must be given to the cardiac toxicity exhibited by doxorubicin HCl. Although uncommon, acute left ventricular failure has occurred, particularly in patients who have received total dosage of the drug exceeding the currently recommended limit of 550 mg/m². This limit appears to be lower (400 mg/m²) in patients who received radiotherapy to the mediastinal area or concomitant therapy with other potentially cardiotoxic agents such as cyclophosphamide.

Caution should be observed in patients who have received other anthracyclines. The total dose of doxorubicin HCl administered to the individual patient should also take into account any previous or concomitant therapy with related compounds such as daunorubicin. Congestive heart failure and/or cardiomyopathy may be encountered after discontinuation of therapy. Patients with a history of cardiovascular disease should be administered DOXIL® only when the potential benefit of treatment outweighs the risk.

The long-term cardiac effects of DOXIL® in patients relative to the conventional formulation of doxorubicin HCl have not been adequately evaluated.

Cardiac function should be carefully monitored in patients treated with DOXIL®. The most definitive test for anthracycline myocardial injury is endomyocardial biopsy. Other methods such as echocardiography or gated radionuclide scans have been used to monitor cardiac function during anthracycline therapy. Any of these methods should be employed to monitor potential cardiac toxicity during DOXIL® therapy. If these test results indicate possible cardiac injury associated with DOXIL® therapy, the benefit of continued therapy must be carefully weighed against the risk of myocardial injury. (See **ADVERSE REACTIONS—Cardiac Events.**)

Myelosuppression

The majority of experience with DOXIL® has been in AIDS-KS patients who present with baseline myelosuppression due to such factors as their HIV disease or numerous concomitant medications. In this population, myelosuppression appears to be the dose-limiting adverse event. Leukopenia is the most common adverse event (about 60%) experienced in this population; anemia (about 20%) and thrombocytopenia (about 10%) can also be expected.

Because of the potential for bone marrow suppression, careful hematologic monitoring is required during use of DOXIL®, including white blood cell and platelet counts and Hgb/Hct. With the recommended dosage schedule, leukopenia is usually transient. Hematologic toxicity may require dose reduction or suspension or delay of DOXIL® therapy. Persistent severe myelosuppression may result in superinfection or hemorrhage.

DOXIL® may potentiate the toxicity of other anticancer therapies. In particular, hematologic toxicity may be more severe when DOXIL® is administered in combination with other agents that cause bone marrow suppression. Patients treated with DOXIL® may require G-CSF (or GM-CSF) to support their blood counts. (See **ADVERSE REACTIONS—Hematologic.**)

Infusion Reactions

Acute infusion-associated reactions characterized by flushing, shortness of breath, facial swelling, headache, chills, back pain, tightness in the chest and throat, and/or hypotension have occurred in approximately 6.8% of patients

treated with DOXIL®. The reaction appears to occur with the first infusion and does not appear to occur with later infusions if not present initially. In most patients, these reactions resolve over the course of several hours to a day once the infusion is terminated. In some patients, the reaction resolves by slowing the rate of infusion. Similar reactions have not been reported with conventional doxorubicin and they presumably represent a reaction to the DOXIL® liposomes or one of its surface components.

Many patients were able to tolerate further infusions without complications, however, six patients were terminated from DOXIL® therapy because of an infusion reaction.

Palmar-Plantar Erythrodysesthesia

Among 705 patients with AIDS-related Kaposi's sarcoma treated with DOXIL®, 24 (3.4%) developed palmar-plantar skin eruptions characterized by swelling, pain, erythema and, for some patients, desquamation of the skin on the hands and the feet (palmar-plantar erythrodysesthesia). The syndrome was generally seen after six or more weeks of treatment but may occur earlier. The incidence of this reaction may be higher when DOXIL® is administered at doses that are higher or at intervals that are shorter than those recommended. In most patients, the reaction is mild and resolves in one to two weeks so that prolonged delay of therapy need not occur (See **DOSAGE AND ADMINISTRATION**). The reaction can be severe and debilitating in some patients, however, and may require discontinuation of treatment.

Pregnancy Category D

DOXIL® can cause fetal harm when administered to a pregnant woman. DOXIL® is embryotoxic at doses of 1 mg/kg/day (about $^1/_3$ the recommended human dose on a mg/m^2 basis) in rats. DOXIL® is embryotoxic and abortifacient at 0.5 mg/kg/day (about $^1/_4$ the recommended human dose on a mg/m^2 basis) in rabbits. Embryotoxicity was characterized by increased embryo-fetal deaths and reduced live litter sizes.

There are no adequate and well-controlled studies in pregnant women. If DOXIL® is to be used during pregnancy, or if the patient becomes pregnant during therapy, the patient should be apprised of the potential hazard to the fetus. Women of childbearing potential should be advised to avoid pregnancy.

Toxicity Potentiation

The doxorubicin in DOXIL® may potentiate the toxicity of other anticancer therapies. Exacerbation of cyclophosphamide-induced hemorrhagic cystitis and enhancement of the hepatotoxicity of 6-mercaptopurine have been reported with the conventional formulation of doxorubicin HCl. Radiation-induced toxicity to the myocardium, mucosae, skin and liver have been reported to be increased by the administration of doxorubicin HCl.

Injection Site Effects

DOXIL® should be considered an irritant and precautions should be taken to avoid extravasation. On intravenous administration of DOXIL®, extravasation may occur with or without an accompanying stinging or burning sensation and even if blood returns well on aspiration of the infusion needle (See **DOSAGE AND ADMINISTRATION**). If any signs or symptoms of extravasation have occurred, the infusion should be immediately terminated and restarted in another vein. The application of ice over the site of extravasation for approximately 30 minutes may be helpful in alleviating the local reaction. **DOXIL® must not be given by the intramuscular or subcutaneous route.**

In studies with rabbits, lesions that were induced by subcutaneous injection of DOXIL® were minor and reversible compared to more severe and irreversible lesions and tissue necrosis that were induced after subcutaneous injection of conventional doxorubicin HCl.

Hepatic Impairment

The pharmacokinetics of DOXIL® have not been studied in patients with hepatic impairment. Doxorubicin is known to be eliminated in large part by the liver. Thus DOXIL® dosage should be reduced in patients with impaired hepatic function. (See **DOSAGE AND ADMINISTRATION**.)

Prior to DOXIL® administration, evaluation of hepatic function is recommended using conventional clinical laboratory tests such as SGOT, SGPT, alkaline phosphatase and bilirubin. (See **DOSAGE AND ADMINISTRATION**.)

PRECAUTIONS

Laboratory Tests

Complete blood counts, including platelet counts, should be obtained frequently and at a minimum prior to each dose of DOXIL®.

Drug Interactions

No formal drug interaction studies have been conducted with DOXIL®. Until specific compatibility data are available, it is not recommended that DOXIL® be mixed with other drugs. DOXIL® may interact with drugs known to interact with the conventional formulation of doxorubicin HCl.

Carcinogenesis, Mutagenesis, Impairment of Fertility

Although no studies have been conducted with DOXIL®, doxorubicin HCl and related compounds have been shown to have mutagenic and carcinogenic properties when tested in experimental models.

STEALTH® liposomes without drug are negative when tested in Ames, mouse lymphoma and chromosomal aberration assays in vitro, and mammalian micronucleus assay in vivo.

The possible adverse effects on fertility in males and females in humans or experimental animals have not been adequately evaluated. However, DOXIL® resulted in mild to moderate ovarian and testicular atrophy in mice after a single dose of 36 mg/kg (about 5 times the recommended human dose on a mg/m^2 basis). Decreased testicular weights and hypospermia were present in rats after repeat doses of ≥ 0.25 mg/kg/day (about $^1/_{13}$ the recommended human dose on a mg/m^2 basis), and diffuse degeneration of the seminiferous tubules and a marked decrease in spermatogenesis were observed in dogs after repeat doses of 1 mg/kg/day (equivalent to the recommended human dose on a mg/m^2 basis).

Pregnancy

Pregnancy Category D: (See **WARNINGS**.)

Nursing Mothers

It is not known whether this drug is excreted in human milk. Because many drugs are excreted in human milk and because of the potential for serious adverse reactions in nursing infants from DOXIL®, mothers should discontinue nursing prior to taking this drug.

Pediatric Use

The safety and effectiveness of DOXIL® in pediatric patients have not been established.

Radiation Therapy

Recall of skin reaction due to prior radiotherapy has occurred with DOXIL® administration.

ADVERSE REACTIONS

Information on adverse events is based on the experience reported in 753 patients with AIDS-related KS enrolled in four studies. The majority of patients were treated with 20 mg/m^2 of DOXIL® (doxorubicin HCl liposome injection) every two to three weeks. The median time on study was 127 days and ranged from 1 to 811 days. The median cumulative dose was 120 mg/m^2 and ranged from 3.3 to 798.6 mg/m^2. Twenty-six patients (3.0%) received cumulative doses of greater than 450 mg/m^2.

Of these 753 patients, 61.2% were considered poor risk for KS tumor burden, 91.5% poor for immune system, and 46.9% for systemic illness; 36.2% were poor risk for all three categories. Patients' median CD4 count was 21.0 cells/mm^3, with 50.8% of patients having less than 50 cells/mm^3. The mean absolute neutrophil count at study entry was approximately 3000 cells/mm^3.

Patients received a variety of potentially myelotoxic drugs in combination with DOXIL®. Of the 693 patients with concomitant medication information, 58.7% were on one or more antiretroviral medications; 34.9% patients were on zidovudine (AZT), 20.8% on didanosine (ddI), 16.5% on zalcitabine (ddC), and 9.5% on stavudine (D4T). A total of 85.1% patients were on PCP prophylaxis, most (54.5%) on sulfamethoxazole/trimethoprim. Eighty-five percent of patients were receiving antifungal medications, primarily fluconazole (75.8%). Seventy-two percent of patients were receiving antivirals, 56.3% acyclovir, 29% ganciclovir, and 16% foscarnet. In addition, 47.8% patients received colony stimulating factors (sargramostim/filgrastim) sometime during their course of treatment.

Of the 753 patients enrolled in the DOXIL® clinical trials, adverse event information was available for 705 patients. In many instances it was difficult to determine whether adverse events resulted from DOXIL®, from concomitant therapy, or from the patients' underlying disease(s).

Hematologic

Neutropenia (<1000 neutrophils/mm^3) occurred in 49% of patients on study with 13% of patients having at least one episode of ANC < 500 cells/mm^3.

Sepsis occurred in 5% of patients; for 0.7% of patients the event was considered possibly or probably related to DOXIL®. Ten patients developed sepsis in the setting of neutropenia. Eleven patients (1.6%) discontinued study because of bone marrow suppression or neutropenia.

Opportunistic infections occurred in 355 patients (50.4%), most commonly candidiasis (23.5%), cytomegalovirus (20.1%), herpes simplex (10.5%), Pneumocystis carinii pneumonia (9.2%), and mycobacterium avium (8.4%). Four patients (0.6%) discontinued DOXIL® therapy because of opportunistic infection.

Infusion-Related Reactions (See WARNINGS)

Six patients (0.9%) discontinued DOXIL® therapy because of infusion reactions.

Palmar-Plantar Erythrodysesthesia

Three patients (0.4%) discontinued DOXIL® therapy because of palmar-plantar erythrodysesthesia. (See **WARNINGS**.)

Cardiac Events

Sixty-eight (9.6%) patients experienced cardiac-related adverse events. In 30 patients (4.3%), the event was thought to be possibly or probably related to DOXIL®. Nine cases of possibly or probably related cardiomyopathy and/or congestive heart failure were reported. Seven (1.0%) of the possibly or probably related cardiac events were severe. These severe events included arrhythmia (nonspecific), cardiomyopathy, heart failure, pericardial effusion, and tachycardia. Three patients discontinued study due to cardiac events.

Radiation Therapy

Recall of skin reaction due to prior radiotherapy has occurred with DOXIL® administration.

Eighty-three percent of the patients reported adverse events that were considered to be possibly or probably related to the treatment with DOXIL®. These adverse events are provided below. The table shows all events occurring at $\geq 5\%$ in the overall treated population that were considered by investigators at least possibly related to DOXIL®. Rates are also given for the subset of refractory/intolerant patients. Adverse reactions only infrequently (5%) led to discontinuation of treatment. Those that did so included bone marrow suppression, cardiac adverse events, infusion-related reactions, toxoplasmosis, palmar-plantar erythrodysesthesia, pneumonia, cough/dyspnea, fatigue, optic neuritis, progression of a non-KS tumor, allergy to penicillin, and unspecified reasons.

Probably and Possibly Drug-Related Adverse Events Reported in ≥ 5% of All Treated Patients

	Refractory or Intolerant AIDS-KS Patients	Total AIDS-KS Patients
Number of Patients	77	705
Number of Patients Reporting Adverse Events	57 (74.0%)	586 (83.1%)
Adverse Event		
Neutropenia (ANC <1000/mm^3)	34 (44.2%)	352 (49.9%)
Anemia	5 (6.5%)	137 (19.4%)
Nausea	14 (18.2%)	119 (16.9%)
Asthenia	5 (6.5%)	70 (9.9%)
Hypochromic Anemia	4 (5.2%)	69 (9.8%)
Thrombocytopenia	5 (6.5%)	65 (9.2%)
Fever	6 (7.8%)	64 (9.1%)
Alopecia	7 (9.1%)	63 (8.9%)
Alkaline Phosphatase Increase	1 (1.3%)	55 (7.8%)
Vomiting	6 (7.8%)	55 (7.8%)
Diarrhea	4 (5.2%)	55 (7.8%)
Stomatitis	4 (5.2%)	48 (6.8%)
Oral Moniliasis	1 (1.3%)	39 (5.5%)

Incidence 1% to 5% (Possibly or Probably Related)

Body as a Whole: headache, back pain, infection, allergic reaction, chills.

Cardiovascular: chest pain, hypotension, tachycardia.

Cutaneous: Herpes simplex, rash, itching.

Digestive System: mouth ulceration, glossitis, constipation, aphthous stomatitis, anorexia, dysphagia, abdominal pain.

Hematologic: hemolysis, increased prothrombin time.

Metabolic/Nutritional: SGPT increase, weight loss, hypocalcemia, hyperbilirubinemia, hyperglycemia.

Other: dyspnea, albuminuria, pneumonia, retinitis, emotional lability, dizziness, somnolence.

Incidence Less Than 1% (Possibly or Probably Related)

Body as a Whole: face edema, cellulitis, sepsis, abscess, radiation injury, flu syndrome, moniliasis, hypothermia, injection site hemorrhage, injection site pain, cryptococcosis, ascites.

Cardiovascular System: thrombophlebitis, cardiomyopathy, pericardial effusion, hemorrhage, palpitation, syncope, bundle branch block, congestive heart failure, cardiomegaly, heart arrest, migraine, thrombosis, ventricular arrhythmia.

Digestive System: dyspepsia, cholestatic jaundice, gastritis, gingivitis, ulcerative proctitis, colitis, esophageal ulcer, esophagitis, gastrointestinal hemorrhage, hepatic failure, leukoplakia of mouth, pancreatitis, ulcerative stomatitis, hepatitis, hepatosplenomegaly, increased appetite, jaundice, sclerosing cholangitis, tenesmus, fecal impaction.

Endocrine System: diabetes mellitus.

Hemic and Lymphatic System: eosinophilia, lymphadenopathy, lymphangitis, lymphedema, petechia, thromboplastin decrease.

Metabolic/Nutritional Disorders: lactic dehydrogenase increase, hypernatremia, creatinine increase, BUN increase, dehydration, edema, hypercalcemia, hyperkalemia, hyperlipemia, hyperuricemia, hypoglycemia, hypokalemia, hypolipemia, hypomagnesemia, hyponatremia, hypophosphatemia, hypoproteinemia, ketosis, weight gain.

Musculoskeletal System: myalgia, arthralgia, bone pain, myositis.

Nervous System: paresthesia, insomnia, peripheral neuritis, depression, neuropathy, anxiety, convulsion, hypotonia,

Continued on next page

Sequus—Cont.

acute brain syndrome, confusion, hemiplegia, hypertonia, hypokinesia, vertigo.

Respiratory System: pleural effusion, asthma, bronchitis, cough increase, hyperventilation, pharyngitis, pneumothorax, rhinitis, sinusitis.

Skin and Appendages: maculopapular rash, skin ulcer, exfoliative dermatitis, skin discoloration, herpes zoster, cutaneous moniliasis, erythema multiforme, erythema nodosum, furunculosis, psoriasis, pustular rash, skin necrosis, urticaria, vesiculobullous rash.

Special Senses: otitis media, taste perversion, abnormal vision, blindness, conjunctivitis, eye pain, optic neuritis, tinnitus, visual field defect.

Urogenital System: hematuria, balanitis, cystitis, dysuria, genital edema, glycosuria, kidney failure.

OVERDOSAGE

Acute overdosage with doxorubicin HCl causes increases in mucositis, leukopenia and thrombocytopenia.

Treatment of acute overdosage consists of treatment of the severely myelosuppressed patient with hospitalization, antibiotics, platelet and granulocyte transfusions and symptomatic treatment of mucositis.

DOSAGE AND ADMINISTRATION

AIDS-KS Patients

DOXIL® (doxorubicin HCl liposome injection) should be administered intravenously at a dose of 20 mg/m^2 (doxorubicin HCl equivalent) over 30 minutes, once every three weeks, for as long as patients respond satisfactorily and tolerate treatment.

Do not administer as a bolus injection or an undiluted solution. Rapid infusion may increase the risk of infusion-related reactions. (See **WARNINGS—Infusion Reactions.**)

Each vial contains 20 mg doxorubicin HCl at a concentration of 2 mg/mL.

DOXIL® should be considered an irritant and precautions should be taken to avoid extravasation. On intravenous administration of DOXIL®, extravasation may occur with or without an accompanying stinging or burning sensation and even if blood returns well on aspiration of the infusion needle. If any signs or symptoms of extravasation have occurred the infusion should be immediately terminated and restarted in another vein. The application of ice over the site of extravasation for approximately 30 minutes may be helpful in alleviating the local reaction. **DOXIL® must not be given by the intramuscular or subcutaneous route.**

Dose Modifications

The dose modifications shown in the tables below are recommended for managing possible adverse events.

[See table above.]

HEMATOLOGICAL TOXICITY

Grade	ANC (cells/mm³)	Platelets (cells/mm³)	Modification
1	1500–1900	75,000–150,000	None
2	1000–<1500	50,000–<75,000	None
3	500–999	25,000–<50,000	Wait until ANC ≥1,000 and/or platelets ≥50,000 then redose at 25% dose reduction
4	<500	<25,000	Wait until ANC ≥1,000 and/or platelets ≥50,000 then redose at 50% dose reduction

STOMATITIS

Grade	Symptoms	Modification
1	Painless ulcers, erythema or mild soreness	None
2	Painful erythema, edema or ulcers, but can eat	Wait one week and if symptoms improve redose at 100% dose
3	Painful erythema, edema or ulcers, and cannot eat	Wait one week and if symptoms improve redose at 25% dose reduction
4	Requires parenteral or enteral support	Wait one week and if symptoms improve redose at 50% dose reduction

Patients with Impaired Hepatic Function

Limited clinical experience exists in treating hepatically impaired patients with DOXIL®.

PALMAR-PLANTAR ERYTHRODYSESTHESIA

Toxicity Grade	Symptoms	Weeks Since Last Dose	
		3	4
0	no symptoms	Redose at 3-week interval	Redose at 3-week interval
1	mild erythema, swelling, or desquamation not interfering with daily activities	Redose unless patient has experienced a previous Grade 3 or 4 skin toxicity in which case wait an additional week	Redose at 25% dose reduction; return to 3-week interval
2	erythema, desquamation, or swelling interfering with, but not precluding normal physical activities; small blisters or ulcerations less than 2 cm in diameter	Wait an additional week	Redose at 50% dose reduction; return to 3-week interval
3	blistering, ulceration, or swelling interfering with walking or normal daily activities; cannot wear regular clothing	Wait an additional week	Discontinue DOXIL®
4	diffuse or local process causing infectious complications, or a bed ridden state or hospitalization	Wait an additional week	Discontinue DOXIL®

Therefore, based on experience with doxorubicin HCl, it is recommended that DOXIL® dosage be reduced if the bilirubin is elevated as follows: Serum bilirubin 1.2 to 3.0 mg/dL give $^1/_2$ normal dose, >3 mg/dL give $^1/_4$ normal dose.

Preparation for Intravenous Administration

The appropriate dose of DOXIL®, up to a maximum of 90 mg, must be diluted in 250 mL of 5% Dextrose Injection, USP prior to administration. Aseptic technique must be strictly observed since no preservative or bacteriostatic agent is present in DOXIL®. Diluted DOXIL® should be refrigerated at 2°C to 8°C (36°F to 46°F) and administered within 24 hours.

Do not use with in-line filters.

Do not mix with other drugs.

Do not use with any diluent other than 5% Dextrose Injection.

Do not use any bacteriostatic agent, such as benzyl alcohol.

DOXIL® is not a clear solution but a translucent, red liposomal dispersion. **Parenteral drug products should be inspected visually for particulate matter and discoloration prior to administration, whenever solution and container permit. Do not use if a precipitate or foreign matter is present.**

Storage and Stability

Refrigerate unopened vials of DOXIL® at 2°C to 8°C (36°F to 46°F). Avoid freezing. Prolonged freezing may adversely affect liposomal drug products; however, short-term freezing (less than 1 month) does not appear to have a deleterious effect on DOXIL®.

Procedure for Proper Handling and Disposal

Caution should be exercised in the handling and preparation of DOXIL®.

The use of gloves is required.

If DOXIL® comes into contact with skin or mucosa, immediately wash thoroughly with soap and water.

DOXIL® should be considered an irritant and precautions should be taken to avoid extravasation. On intravenous administration of DOXIL®, extravasation may occur with or without an accompanying stinging or burning sensation and even if blood returns well on aspiration of the infusion needle. If any signs or symptoms of extravasation have occurred, the infusion should be immediately terminated and restarted in another vein. DOXIL® must not be given by the intramuscular or subcutaneous route.

DOXIL® should be handled and disposed of in a manner consistent with other anticancer drugs. Several guidelines on this subject exist[2–8] although there is no general agreement that all of the procedures listed in these guidelines are appropriate or necessary.

HOW SUPPLIED

DOXIL® (doxorubicin HCl liposome injection) is supplied as a sterile, translucent, red liposomal dispersion in 10 mL glass, single use vials.

Each vial contains 20 mg doxorubicin HCl at a concentration of 2 mg/mL.

Refrigerate at 2-8°C. Avoid freezing. Prolonged freezing may adversely affect liposomal drug products: however, short-term freezing (less than 1 month) does not appear to have a deleterious affect on DOXIL®.

Available as individually cartoned vials in packages of six.

NDC #61471-295-12.

REFERENCES

1. Krown et al. Kaposi's sarcoma in the acquired immune deficiency syndrome: A proposal for uniform evaluation, response, and staging criteria. *J Clin Oncol.* 1989; 7(9):1201–1207.
2. Recommendations for the safe handling of cytotoxic drugs. NIH Publication No. 92–2621. US Government Printing Office, Washington, DC 20402.
3. OSHA Work-Practice guidelines for personnel dealing with cytotoxic (antineoplastic) drugs. *Am J Hosp Pharm.* 1986; 43:1193–1204.
4. American Society of Hospital Pharmacists Technical Assistance Bulletin on Handling Cytotoxic and Hazardous Drugs. *Am J Hosp Pharm.* 1985; 42:131–137.
5. National Study Commission on Cytotoxic Exposure—Recommendations for Handling Cytotoxic Agents. Available from Louis P. Jeffrey, Sc.D., Chairman, National Study Commission on Cytotoxic Exposure, Massachusetts College of Pharmacy and Allied Health Sciences, 179 Longwood Avenue, Boston, Massachusetts 02115.
6. AMA Council Report. Guidelines for handling parenteral antineoplastics. *JAMA* 1985; 253(11):1590–1592.
7. Clinical Oncologic Society of Australia: Guidelines and recommendation for safe handling of antineoplastic agents. *Med J Australia* 1983; 1:426–428.
8. Jones RB, et al. Safe handling of chemotherapeutic agents: a report from the Mount Sinai Medical Center. *Ca-A Cancer Journal for Clinicians.* 1983; Sept/Oct:258–263.

Manufactured by
Ben Venue Laboratories, Inc., Bedford, Ohio 44146
Distributed by:
SEQUUS Pharmaceuticals, Inc., Menlo Park, CA 94025 USA
Last Revised: November 28, 1995

Shown in Product Identification Guide, page 335

Serono Laboratories, Inc.
100 LONGWATER CIRCLE
NORWELL, MA 02061

Direct Inquiries to:
Customer Service, Sales and Ordering
(800) 283-8088 X 5141
(617) 982-9000 X 5141

For Medical Information or to report Adverse Drug Experiences Contact:
Drug Information and Surveillance Group
(800) 283-8088 X 5562
(617) 982-9000 X 5562

Serono Laboratories, Inc. will be pleased to answer inquiries about the following products:

METRODIN®
[me 'tro-den]
(urofollitropin for injection)
FOR INTRAMUSCULAR INJECTION

DESCRIPTION

Metrodin® (urofollitropin for injection) is a preparation of gonadotropin extracted from the urine of postmenopausal

women. Each ampule of Metrodin® contains 75 or 150 IU of follicle-stimulating hormone (FSH) activity, in not more than 0.83 mg (75 IU) or 1.66 mg (150 IU) of extract, plus 10 mg lactose in a sterile, lyophilized form. Metrodin® is administered by intramuscular injection.

Metrodin® contains an acidic, water soluble glycoprotein biologically standardized for FSH gonadotropin activity in terms of the Second International Reference Preparation for Human Menopausal Gonadotropins established in September, 1964 by the Expert Committee on Biological Standards of the World Health Organization. Negligible amounts (less than 1 IU per 75 IU FSH) of luteinizing hormone (LH) activity are contained in Metrodin®.

Therapeutic Class: Infertility.

CLINICAL PHARMACOLOGY

Metrodin® stimulates ovarian follicular growth in women who do not have primary ovarian failure. FSH, the active component of Metrodin®, is the primary hormone responsible for follicular recruitment and development. In order to effect final maturation of the follicle and ovulation in the absence of an endogenous LH surge, human chorionic gonadotropin (hCG) must be given following the administration of Metrodin® when monitoring of the patient indicates that sufficient follicular development has occurred. There may be a degree of interpatient variability in response to FSH administration.

INDICATIONS AND USAGE

Metrodin® and hCG given in a sequential manner are indicated for the stimulation of follicular development and the induction of ovulation in patients with polycystic ovary syndrome, and infertility, who have failed to respond or conceive following adequate clomiphene citrate therapy.

Metrodin® and hCG may also be used to stimulate the development of multiple follicles in ovulatory patients undergoing Assisted Reproductive Technologies (ART) such as in vitro fertilization.

Selection of Patients:

1. Before treatment with Metrodin® is instituted, a thorough gynecologic and endocrinologic evaluation must be performed. This should include an assessment of pelvic anatomy. Patients with tubal obstruction should receive Metrodin® only if enrolled in an in vitro fertilization program.
2. Primary ovarian failure should be excluded by the determination of gonadotropin levels.
3. Careful examination should be made to rule out the presence of early pregnancy.
4. Patients in late reproductive life have a greater predisposition to endometrial carcinoma as well as a higher incidence of anovulatory disorders. A thorough diagnostic examination should always be performed before starting Metrodin® therapy in such patients who demonstrate abnormal uterine bleeding or other signs of endometrial abnormalities.
5. Evaluation of the husband's fertility potential should be included in the workup.

CONTRAINDICATIONS

Metrodin® is contraindicated in women who exhibit:

1. High levels of FSH indicating primary ovarian failure.
2. Uncontrolled thyroid or adrenal dysfunction.
3. An organic intracranial lesion such as a pituitary tumor.
4. The presence of any cause of infertility other than anovulation, as stated in the "Indications" unless they are candidates for Assisted Reproductive Technologies.
5. Abnormal bleeding of undetermined origin (see "Selection of Patients").
6. Ovarian cysts or enlargement of undetermined origin.
7. Prior hypersensitivity to urofollitropin.

Metrodin® is also contraindicated in women who are pregnant and may cause fetal harm when administered to a pregnant woman. There are limited human data on the effects of Metrodin® when administered during pregnancy.

WARNINGS

Metrodin® should only be used by physicians who are thoroughly familiar with infertility problems and their management. It is a potent gonadotropic substance capable of causing mild to severe adverse reactions. Therefore, the lowest dose consistent with the expectation of good results should be used. Gonadotropin therapy requires a certain time commitment by physicians and supportive health professionals, and its use requires the availability of appropriate monitoring facilities (see "Precautions/Laboratory Tests"). Safe and effective use of Metrodin® requires monitoring of ovarian response with serum estradiol and vaginal ultrasound, on a regular basis.

Overstimulation of the Ovary During Metrodin® Therapy: Ovarian Enlargement: Mild to moderate uncomplicated ovarian enlargement which may be accompanied by abdominal distension and/or abdominal pain occurs in approximately 20% of those treated with Metrodin® and hCG, and generally regresses without treatment within two or three weeks. Careful monitoring of ovarian response can further minimize the risk of overstimulation.

If the ovaries are abnormally enlarged on the last day of Metrodin® therapy, hCG should not be administered in this course of therapy. This will reduce the chances of development of the Ovarian Hyperstimulation Syndrome.

The Ovarian Hyperstimulation Syndrome (OHSS): OHSS is a medical event distinct from uncomplicated ovarian enlargement. Severe OHSS may progress rapidly (within 24 hours to several days) to become a serious medical event. It is characterized by an apparent dramatic increase in vascular permeability which can result in a rapid accumulation of fluid in the peritoneal cavaity, thorax, and potentially, the pericardium. The early warning signs of development of OHSS are severe pelvic pain, nausea, vomiting, and weight gain. The following symptomatology has been seen with cases of OHSS: abdominal pain, abdominal distension, gastrointestinal symptoms including nausea, vomiting and diarrhea, severe ovarian enlargement, weight gain, dyspnea, and oliguria. Clinical evaluation may reveal hypovolemia, hemoconcentration, electrolyte imbalances, ascites, hemoperitoneum, pleural effusions, hydrothorax, acute pulmonary distress, and thromboembolic events (see "Pulmonary and Vascular Complications"). Transient liver function test abnormalities suggestive of hepatic dysfunction, which may be accompanied by morphologic changes on liver biopsy, have been reported in association with the Ovarian Hyperstimulation Syndrome (OHSS).

Severe OHSS occurred in approximately 6.0% of patients treated with Metrodin® therapy in the initial clinical trials, in patients treated for anovulation due to polycystic ovarian syndrome. In these studies, prospective monitoring of ovarian response using serum estradiol determination or ultrasonographic visualizations was not routinely employed. In more recent clinical trials in oligo-anovulatory and infertile women in which both estradiol and ultrasound measurements were utilized to monitor follicular development, the incidence of severe OHSS was 0.6% (see "Clinical Studies"). During studies for in vitro fertilization, four cases of OHSS were reported following 1,586 treatment cycles (0.25%). OHSS may be more severe and more protracted if pregnancy occurs. OHSS develops rapidly; therefore, patients should be followed for at least two weeks after hCG administration. Most often, OHSS occurs after treatment has been discontinued and reaches its maximum at about seven to ten days following treatment. Usually, OHSS resolves spontaneously with the onset of menses. If there is evidence that OHSS may be developing prior to hCG administration (see "Precautions/Laboratory Tests"), the hCG should be withheld.

If severe OHSS occurs, treatment should be stopped and the patient should be hospitalized. A physician experienced in the management of this syndrome, or who is experienced in the management in fluid and electrolyte imbalances should be consulted.

Pulmonary and Vascular Complications: The following paragraph describes serious medical events reported following gonadotropin therapy.

Serious pulmonary conditions (e.g., atelectasis, acute respiratory distress syndrome) have been reported. In addition, thromboembolic events both in association with, and separate from the Ovarian Hyperstimulation Syndrome have been reported. Intravascular thrombosis and embolism can result in reduced blood flow to critical organs or the extremities. Sequelae of such events have included venous thrombophlebitis, pulmonary embolism, pulmonary infarction, cerebral vascular occlusion (stroke), and arterial occlusion resulting in loss of limb. In rare cases, pulmonary complications and/or thromboembolic events have resulted in death.

Multiple Births: Reports of multiple births have been associated with Metrodin®-hCG treatment, including triplet and quintuplet gestations. In clinical studies with Metrodin®, **81.4%** of the pregnancies following ovulation induction therapy resulted in single births and 18.6% in multiple births. The risk of multiple births in patients undergoing ART procedures is related to the number of embryos replaced. The patient and her husband should be advised of the potential risk of multiple births before starting treatment.

PRECAUTIONS

General: Careful attention should be given to diagnosis in candidates for Metrodin® therapy (see "Indications and Usage/Selection of Patients").

Information for Patients: Prior to the therapy with Metrodin® patients should be informed of the duration of treatment and monitoring of their condition that will be required. Possible adverse reactions (see "Adverse Reactions") and the risk of multiple births should also be discussed.

Laboratory Tests: In most instances, treatment with Metrodin® results only in follicular recruitment and development. In order to effect ovulation in the absence of an endogenous LH surge, hCG must be given following the administration of Metrodin® when monitoring of the patient indicates that sufficient follicular development has occurred. This may be estimated by serum estradiol and vaginal ultrasound. The combination of ultrasound and estradiol is useful for monitoring the development of follicles, timing hCG administration, as well as for detecting ovarian enlargement and minimizing the risk of the Ovarian Hyperstimulation Syndrome and multiple gestation. It is recommended that the number of growing follicles be confirmed using ultrasonography because plasma estrogen alone does not give an indication of the size or number of follicles.

The clinical confirmation of ovulation, with the exception of pregnancy, is obtained by direct and indirect indices of progesterone production. The indices generally used are:

1. A rise in basal body temperature,
2. Increase in serum progesterone, and
3. Menstruation following the shift in basal body temperature.

When used in conjunction with indices of progesterone production, sonographic visualization of the ovaries will assist in determining if ovulation has occurred. Sonographic evidence of ovulation may include the following:

1. Fluid in the cul-de-sac,
2. Ovarian stigmata,
3. Collapsed follicle, and
4. Secretory endometrium.

Accurate interpretation of the indices of follicular development and maturation as well as the determination of ovulation require a physician who is experienced in the interpretation of these tests.

Drug Interactions: No clinically significant drug/drug or drug/food interactions have been reported during Metrodin® therapy.

Carcinogenesis and Mutagenesis: Carcinogenicity and mutagenicity studies have not been performed.

Pregnancy Category X: See "Contraindications".

Nursing Mothers: It is not known whether this drug is excreted in human milk. Because many drugs are excreted in human milk, caution should be exercised if Metrodin® is administered to a nursing woman.

ADVERSE REACTIONS

The following adverse reactions reported during Metrodin® therapy are listed in decreasing order of potential severity:

1. Pulmonary and vascular complications (see "Warnings"),
2. Ovarian Hyperstimulation Syndrome (see "Warnings"),
3. Adnexal torsion (as a complication of ovarian enlargement),
4. Mild to moderate ovarian enlargement,
5. Abdominal pain,
6. Sensitivity to Metrodin®,
   (Febrile reactions which may be accompanied by chills, musculoskeletal aches, joint pains, malaise, headache, and fatigue have occurred after the administration of Metrodin®. It is not clear whether or not these were pyrogenic responses or possible allergic reactions.)
7. Ovarian cysts,
8. Gastrointestinal symptoms (nausea, vomiting, diarrhea, abdominal cramps, bloating),
9. Pain, rash, swelling, and/or irritation at the site of injection,
10. Breast tenderness,
11. Headache,
12. Dermatological symptoms (dry skin, body rash, hair loss, hives),
13. Hemoperitoneum has been reported during menotropins therapy and, therefore, may also occur during Metrodin® therapy.
14. There have been infrequent reports of ovarian neoplasms, both benign and malignant, in women who have undergone multiple drug regimens for ovulation induction; however, a causal relationship has not been established.

The following medical events have been reported subsequent to pregnancies resulting from Metrodin® therapy:

1. Ectopic pregnancy
2. Congenital abnormalities
   (Three incidents of chromosomal abnormalities and four birth defects have been reported following Metrodin®-hCG or Metrodin®, Pergonal® (menotropins for injection, USP)-hCG therapy in clinical trials for stimulation prior to in vitro fertilization. The aborted pregnancies included one Trisomy 13, one Trisomy 18, and one fetus with multiple congenital anomalies (hydrocephaly, omphalocele, and meningocele). One meningocele, one external ear defect, one dislocated hip and ankle, and one dilated cardiomyopathy in presence of maternal Systemic Lupus Erythematosis were reported. None of these events was thought to be drug-related. The incidence does not exceed that found in the general population.)

DRUG ABUSE AND DEPENDENCE

There have been no reports of abuse or dependence with Metrodin®.

OVERDOSAGE

Aside from possible ovarian hyperstimulation and multiple gestations (see "WARNINGS"), little is known concerning the consequences of acute overdosage with Metrodin®.

Continued on next page

Serono Laboratories—Cont.

DOSAGE AND ADMINISTRATION

Dosage: Polycystic Ovary Syndrome: The dose of Metrodin® to stimulate development of the follicle must be individualized for each patient. The lowest dose consistent with the expectation of good results should be used. Over the course of treatment, doses of Metrodin® may range between 75 IU to 300 IU per day depending on the individual patient response. Metrodin® should be administered until adequate follicular development is indicated by serum estradiol and vaginal ultrasonography. A response is generally evident after 5 to 7 days. Subsequent monitoring intervals should be based on individual patient response.

It is recommended that the initial dose of the first cycle be 75 IU of Metrodin® per day, **ADMINISTERED INTRAMUSCULARLY.** An adjustment in dose may be considered after 5 to 7 days. An additional dose adjustment may also be considered based on individual patient response. The dose should not be increased more than twice in any cycle or by more than one ampule (75 IU) per adjustment. To complete follicular development and effect ovulation in the absense of an endogenous LH surge, hCG, 5,000 U to 10,000 U, should be given 1 day after the last dose of Metrodin®. HCG should be withheld if the serum estradiol is greater than 2,000 pg/mL. If the ovaries are abnormally enlarged or abdominal pain occurs, Metrodin® treatment should be discontinued, hCG should not be administered, and the patient should be advised not to have intercourse; this will reduce the chance of development of the Ovarian Hyperstimulation Syndrome and, should spontaneous ovulation occur, reduce the chance of multiple gestation. A follow-up visit should be conducted in the luteal phase.

The initial dose administered in the subsequent cycles should be individualized for each patient based on her response in the preceding cycle. Doses larger than 300 IU of FSH per day are not routinely recommended. As in the initial cycle, 5,000 U to 10,000 U of hCG must be given 1 day after the last dose of Metrodin® to complete follicular development and induce ovulation. The precautions described above should be followed to minimize the chance of development of the Ovarian Hyperstimulation Syndrome.

The couple should be encouraged to have intercourse daily, beginning on the day prior to the administration of hCG until ovulation becomes apparent from the indices employed for the determination of progestational activity. Care should be taken to ensure insemination. In light of the indices and parameters mentioned, it should become obvious that, unless a physician is willing to devote considerable time to these patients and be familiar with and conduct the necessary laboratory studies, he/she should not use Metrodin®.

Assisted Reproductive Technologies: As in the treatment of patients with polycystic ovary syndrome, the dose of Metrodin® to stimulate development of the follicle must be individualized for each patient. For Assisted Reproductive Technologies, therapy with Metrodin® should be initiated in the early follicular phase (cycle day 2 or 3) at a dose of 150 IU per day, until sufficient follicular development is attained. In most cases, therapy should not exceed ten days.

Administration: Dissolve the contents of one ampule of Metrodin® in one to two mL of sterile saline and **ADMINISTER INTRAMUSCULARLY** immediately. Any unused reconstituted material should be discarded.

Parenteral drug products should be inspected visually, for particulate matter and discoloration prior to administration, whenever solution and container permit.

HOW SUPPLIED

Metrodin® is supplied in a sterile, lyophilized form as a white to off-white powder or pellet in ampules containing 75 IU or 150 IU FSH activity. The following package combinations are available:

—1 ampule 75 IU Metrodin® and 1 ampule 2 mL Sodium Chloride Injection (USP), NDC 44087-6075-1
—1 ampule 150 IU Metrodin® and 1 ampule 2 mL Sodium Chloride Injection (USP), NDC 44087-6150-1
—10 ampules 75 IU Metrodin® and 10 ampules 2 mL Sodium Chloride Injection (USP), NDC 44087-6075-3
—100 ampules 75 IU Metrodin® and 100 ampules 2 mL Sodium Chloride Injection (USP), NDC 44087-6075-4

Lyophilized powder may be stored refrigerated or at room temperature (3°-25°C/37°-77°F). Protect from light. Use immediately after reconstitution. Discard unused material.

CLINICAL STUDIES

The results of the clinical experience and effectiveness of the administration of Metrodin® to 173 evaluable patients in 367 completed courses of therapy are summarized below. All patients received prior therapy with clomiphene citrate, without success.

	%
Patients ovulating	98
Patients pregnant	32
Patients aborting	11*
Multiple pregnancies	18.6
Hyperstimulation syndrome (% patients)	0.6**

* Based on total pregnancies.
**Based on 181 patients who received 446 courses of therapy.

Caution: Federal law prohibits dispensing without prescription.

Manufactured for:
SERONO LABORATORIES, INC.
Randolph, MA 02368 USA
by: Laboratoires Serono SA
Aubonne, Switzerland
© Serono Laboratories, Inc. 1986, 1994, 1995
Revised: July 1995
Code N0700101C   07/95

PERGONAL®   ℞
[per'go-nal]
(menotropins for injection, USP)
FOR INTRAMUSCULAR INJECTION

PRODUCT OVERVIEW

KEY FACTS

Pergonal® is a purified, lyophilized preparation of gonadotropins and contains equal amounts of follicle stimulating hormone and luteinizing hormone. Human Chorionic Gonadotropins (hCG), a naturally occurring hormone in postmenopausal urine, is detected in Pergonal®. Pergonal® is administered by intramuscular injection immediately after reconstitution with Sodium Chloride for Injection, USP.

MAJOR USES

Women: Pergonal® is used to stimulate follicular development in hypogonadotropic anovulatory women who do not have primary ovarian failure.

Men: Pergonal® is used concomitantly with Profasi® (hCG) to stimulate spermatogenesis in men with infertility due to primary or secondary hypogonadotropic hypogonadism.

SAFETY INFORMATION

Pergonal® is contraindicated in individuals who have previously demonstrated hypersensitivity to the drug. In rare instances, women may experience excessive ovarian enlargement, ascites, and pleural effusion requiring hospitalization. The risk can be minimized through careful patient monitoring. Multiple births, 75% of which are twins, have been reported in 20% of pregnancies resulting from Pergonal® therapy.

PRESCRIBING INFORMATION

PERGONAL®   ℞
[per'go-nal]
(menotropins for injection, USP)
FOR INTRAMUSCULAR INJECTION

DESCRIPTION

Pergonal® (menotropins for injection, USP) is a purified preparation of gonadotropins extracted from the urine of postmenopausal women. Each ampule of Pergonal® contains 75 IU or 150 IU of follicle-stimulating hormone (FSH) activity and 75 IU or 150 IU of luteinizing hormone (LH) activity, respectively, plus 10 mg lactose in a sterile, lyophilized form. Human Chorionic Gonadotropins (hCG), a naturally occurring hormone in post-menopausal urine, is detected in Pergonal®. Pergonal® is administered by intramuscular injection.

Pergonal® is biologically standardized for FSH and LH (ICSH) gonadotropin activities in terms of the Second International Reference Preparation for Human Menopausal Gonadotropins established in September, 1964 by the Expert Committee on Biological Standards of the World Health Organization.

Both FSH and LH are glycoproteins that are acidic and water soluble.

Therapeutic class: Infertility.

CLINICAL PHARMACOLOGY

Women:

Pergonal® administered for seven to twelve days produces ovarian follicular growth in women who do not have primary ovarian failure. Treatment with Pergonal® in most instances results only in follicular growth and maturation. In order to effect ovulation, human chorionic gonadotropin (hCG) must be given following the administration of Pergonal® when clinical assessment of the patient indicates that sufficient follicular maturation has occurred.

Men:

Pergonal® administered concomitantly with human chorionic gonadotropin (hCG) for at least three months induces spermatogenesis in men with primary or secondary pituitary hypofunction who have achieved adequate masculinization with prior hCG therapy.

INDICATIONS AND USAGE

Women:

Pergonal® and hCG given in a sequential manner are indicated for the induction of ovulation and pregnancy in the anovulatory infertile patient, in whom the cause of anovulation is functional and is not due to primary ovarian failure.

Pergonal® and hCG may also be used to stimulate the development of multiple follicles in ovulatory patients participating in an in vitro fertilization program.

Men:

Pergonal® with concomitant hCG is indicated for the stimulation of spermatogenesis in men who have primary or secondary hypogonadotropic hypogonadism.

Pergonal® with concomitant hCG has proven effective in inducing spermatogenesis in men with primary hypogonadotropic hypogonadism due to a congenital factor or prepubertal hypophysectomy and in men with secondary hypogonadotropic hypogonadism due to hypophysectomy, craniopharyngioma, cerebral aneurysm or chromophobe adenoma.

SELECTION OF PATIENTS

Women:

1. Before treatment with Pergonal® is instituted, a thorough gynecologic and endocrinologic evaluation must be performed. Except for those patients enrolled in an in vitro fertilization program, this should include a hysterosalpingogram (to rule out uterine and tubal pathology) and documentation of anovulation by means of basal body temperature, serial vaginal smears, examination of cervical mucus, determination of serum (or urinary) progesterone, urinary pregnanediol and endometrial biopsy. Patients with tubal pathology should receive Pergonal® only if enrolled in an in vitro fertilization program.
2. Primary ovarian failure should be excluded by the determination of gonadotropin levels.
3. Careful examination should be made to rule out the presence of an early pregnancy.
4. Patients in late reproductive life have a greater predilection to endometrial carcinoma as well as a higher incidence of anovulatory disorders. Cervical dilation and curettage should always be done for diagnosis before starting Pergonal® therapy in such patients who demonstrate abnormal uterine bleeding or other signs of endometrial abnormalities.
5. Evaluation of the husband's fertility potential should be included in the workup.

Men:

Patient selection should be made based on a documented lack of pituitary function. Prior to hormonal therapy, these patients will have low testosterone levels and low or absent gonadotropin levels. Patients with primary hypogonadotropic hypogonadism will have a subnormal development of masculinization, and those with secondary hypogonadotropic hypogonadism will have decreased masculinization.

CONTRAINDICATIONS

Women:

Pergonal® is contraindicated in women who have:
1. A high FSH level indicating primary ovarian failure.
2. Uncontrolled thyroid and adrenal dysfunction.
3. An organic intracranial lesion such as a pituitary tumor.
4. The presence of any cause of infertility other than anovulation, unless they are candidates for in vitro fertilization.
5. Abnormal bleeding of undetermined origin.
6. Ovarian cysts or enlargement not due to polycystic ovary syndrome.
7. Prior hypersensitivity to menotropins.
8. Pergonal® is contraindicated in women who are pregnant and may cause fetal harm when administered to a pregnant woman. There are limited human data on the effects of Pergonal® when administered during pregnancy.

Men:

Pergonal® is contraindicated in men who have:
1. Normal gonadotropin levels indicating normal pituitary function.
2. Elevated gonadotropin levels indicating primary testicular failure.
3. Infertility disorders other than hypogonadotropic hypogonadism.

WARNINGS

Pergonal® is a drug that should only be used by physicians who are thoroughly familiar with infertility problems. It is a potent gonadotropic substance capable of causing mild to severe adverse reactions in women. Gonadotropin therapy requires a certain time commitment by physicians and supportive health professionals, and its use requires the availability of appropriate monitoring facilities (see "Precautions—Laboratory Tests"). In female patients it must be used with a great deal of care.

Overstimulation of the Ovary During Pergonal® Therapy:
Ovarian Enlargement: Mild to moderate uncomplicated ovarian enlargement which may be accompanied by abdominal distension and/or abdominal pain occurs in approximately 20% of those treated with Pergonal® and hCG, and

generally regresses without treatment within two or three weeks.

In order to minimize the hazard associated with the occasional abnormal ovarian enlargement which may occur with Pergonal®-hCG therapy, the lowest dose consistent with expectation of good results should be used. Careful monitoring of ovarian response can further minimize the risk of overstimulation.

If the ovaries are abnormally enlarged on the last day of Pergonal® therapy, hCG should not be administered in this course of therapy; this will reduce the chances of development of the Ovarian Hyperstimulation Syndrome.

The Ovarian Hyperstimulation Syndrome (OHSS): OHSS is a medical event distinct from uncomplicated ovarian enlargement. OHSS may progress rapidly to become a serious medical event. It is characterized by an apparent dramatic increase in vascular permeability which can result in a rapid accumulation of fluid in the peritoneal cavity, thorax, and potentially, the pericardium. The early warning signs of development of OHSS are severe pelvic pain, nausea, vomiting, and weight gain. The following symptomatology has been seen with cases of OHSS: abdominal pain, abdominal distension, gastrointestinal symptoms including nausea, vomiting and diarrhea, severe ovarian enlargement, weight gain, dyspnea, and oliguria. Clinical evaluation may reveal hypovolemia, hemoconcentration, electrolyte imbalances, ascites, hemoperitoneum, pleural effusions, hydrothorax, acute pulmonary distress, and thromboembolic events (see "Pulmonary and Vascular Complications" below). Transient liver function test abnormalities suggestive of hepatic dysfunction, which may be accompanied by morphologic changes on liver biopsy, have been reported in association with the Ovarian Hyperstimulation Syndrome (OHSS).

OHSS occurs in approximately 0.4% of patients when the recommended dose is administered and in 1.3% of patients when higher than recommended doses are administered. Cases of OHSS are more common, more severe and more protracted if pregnancy occurs. OHSS develops rapidly; therefore patients should be followed for at least two weeks after hCG administration. Most often, OHSS occurs after treatment has been discontinued and reaches its maximum at about seven to ten days following treatment. Usually, OHSS resolves spontaneously with the onset of menses. If there is evidence that OHSS may be developing prior to hCG administration (see "Precautions—Laboratory Tests"), the hCG should be withheld.

If OHSS occurs, treatment should be stopped and the patient hospitalized. Treatment is primarily symptomatic, consisting of bed rest, fluid and electrolyte management, and analgesics if needed. The phenomenon of hemoconcentration associated with fluid loss into the peritoneal cavity, pleural cavity, and the pericardial cavity has been seen to occur and should be thoroughly assessed in the following manner: 1) fluid intake and output, 2) weight, 3) hematocrit, 4) serum and urinary electrolytes, 5) urine specific gravity, 6) BUN and creatinine, and 7) abdominal girth. These determinations are to be performed daily or more often if the need arises.

With OHSS there is an increased risk of injury to the ovary. The ascitic, pleural, and pericardial fluid should not be removed unless absolutely necessary to relieve symptoms such as pulmonary distress or cardiac tamponade. Pelvic examination may cause rupture of an ovarian cyst, which may result in hemoperitoneum, and should therefore be avoided. If this does occur, and if bleeding becomes such that surgery is required, the surgical treatment should be designed to control bleeding and to retain as much ovarian tissue as possible. Intercourse should be prohibited in those patients in whom significant ovarian enlargement occurs after ovulation because of the danger of hemoperitoneum resulting from ruptured ovarian cysts.

The management of OHSS may be divided into three phases: the acute, the chronic, and the resolution phases. Because the use of diuretics can accentuate the diminished intravascular volume, diuretics should be avoided except in the late phase of resolution as described below.

Acute Phase: Management during the acute phase should be designed to prevent hemoconcentration due to loss of intravascular volume to the third space and to minimize the risk of thromboembolic phenomena and kidney damage. Treatment is designed to normalize electrolytes while maintaining an acceptable but somewhat reduced intravascular volume. Full correction of the intravascular volume deficit may lead to an unacceptable increase in the amount of third space fluid accumulation. Management includes administration of limited intravenous fluids, electrolytes, and human serum albumin. Monitoring for the development of hyperkalemia is recommended.

Chronic Phase: After stabilizing the patient during the acute phase, excessive fluid accumulation in the third space should be limited by instituting severe potassium, sodium, and fluid restriction.

Resolution Phase: A fall in hematocrit and an increasing urinary output without an increased intake are observed due to the return of third space fluid to the intravascular compartment. Peripheral and/or pulmonary edema may result

if the kidneys are unable to excrete third space fluid as rapidly as it is mobilized. Diuretics may be indicated during the resolution phase if necessary to combat pulmonary edema.

Pulmonary and Vascular Complications: Serious pulmonary conditions (e.g., atelectasis, acute respiratory distress syndrome) have been reported. In addition, thromboembolic events both in association with, and separate from, the Ovarian Hyperstimulation Syndrome have been reported following Pergonal® therapy. Intravascular thrombosis and embolism, which may originate in venous or arterial vessels, can result in reduced blood flow to critical organs or the extremities. Sequelae of such events have included venous thrombophlebitis, pulmonary embolism, pulmonary infarction, cerebral vascular occlusion (stroke), and arterial occlusion resulting in loss of limb. In rare cases, pulmonary complications and/or thromboembolic events have resulted in death.

Multiple Births: Data from a clinical trial revealed the following results regarding multiple births: Of the pregnancies following therapy with Pergonal® and hCG, 80% resulted in single births, 15% in twins, and 5% of the total pregnancies resulted in three or more concepti. The patient and her husband should be advised of the frequency and potential hazards of multiple gestation before starting treatment.

Hypersensitivity/Anaphylactic Reactions: Hypersensitivity/anaphylactic reactions associated with Pergonal® administration have been reported in some patients. These reactions presented as generalized urticaria, facial edema, angioneurotic edema, and/or dyspnea suggestive of laryngeal edema. The relationship of these symptoms to uncharacterized urinary proteins is uncertain.

PRECAUTIONS

General: Careful attention should be given to diagnosis in the selection of candidates for Pergonal® therapy (see "Indications and Usage—Selection of Patients").

Information for Patients: Prior to therapy with Pergonal®, patients should be informed of the duration of treatment and the monitoring of their condition that will be required. Possible adverse reactions (see "Adverse Reactions" section) and the risk of multiple births should also be discussed.

Laboratory Tests:

Women:

Treatment for Induction of Ovulation

In most instances, treatment with Pergonal® results only in follicular growth and maturation. In order to effect ovulation, hCG must be given following the administration of Pergonal® when clinical assessment of the patient indicates that sufficient follicular maturation has occurred. This may be directly estimated by measuring serum (or urinary) estrogen levels and sonographic visualization of the ovaries. The combination of both estradiol levels and ultrasonography are useful for monitoring the growth and development of follicles, timing hCG administration, as well as minimizing the risk of the Ovarian Hyperstimulation Syndrome and multiple gestation.

Other clinical parameters which may have potential use for monitoring menotropins therapy include:

a) Changes in the vaginal cytology;
b) Appearance and volume of the cervical mucus;
c) Spinnbarkeit; and
d) Ferning of the cervical mucus.

The above clinical indices provide an indirect estimate of the estrogenic effect upon the target organs, and therefore should only be used adjunctively with more direct estimates of follicular development, i.e., serum estradiol and ultrasonography.

The clinical confirmation of ovulation, with the exception of pregnancy, is obtained by direct and indirect indices of progesterone production. The indices most generally used are as follows:

a) A rise in basal body temperature;
b) Increase in serum progesterone; and
c) Menstruation following the shift in basal body temperature.

When used in conjunction with indices of progesterone production, sonographic visualization of the ovaries will assist in determining if ovulation has occurred. Sonographic evidence of ovulation may include the following:

a) Fluid in the cul-de-sac;
b) Ovarian stigmata; and
c) Collapsed follicle.

Because of the subjectivity of the various tests for the determination of follicular maturation and ovulation, it cannot be overemphasized that the physician should choose tests with which he/she is thoroughly familiar.

Drug Interactions: No clinically significant drug/drug or drug/food adverse interactions have been reported during Pergonal® therapy.

Carcinogenesis and Mutagenesis: Long-term toxicity studies in animals have not been performed to evaluate the carcinogenic potential of Pergonal®.

Pregnancy: Pregnancy Category X. See "Contraindications" section.

Nursing Mothers: It is not known whether this drug is excreted in human milk. Because many drugs are excreted in human milk, caution should be exercised if Pergonal® is administered to a nursing woman.

ADVERSE REACTIONS

Women:

The following adverse reactions, reported during Pergonal® therapy, are listed in decreasing order of potential severity:

1. Pulmonary and vascular complications (see "Warnings")
2. Ovarian Hyperstimulation Syndrome (see "Warnings")
3. Hemoperitoneum
4. Adnexal torsion (as a complication of ovarian enlargement)
5. Mild to moderate ovarian enlargement
6. Ovarian cysts
7. Abdominal pain
8. Sensitivity to Pergonal®
   (Febrile reactions suggestive of allergic response have been reported following the administration of Pergonal®. Reports of flu-like symptoms including fever, chills, musculoskeletal aches, joint pains, nausea, headaches and malaise have also been reported).
9. Gastrointestinal symptoms (nausea, vomiting, diarrhea, abdominal cramps, bloating)
10. Pain, rash, swelling and/or irritation at the site of injection
11. Body rashes
12. Dizziness, tachycardia, dyspnea, tachypnea

The following medical events have been reported subsequent to pregnancies resulting from Pergonal® therapy:

1. Ectopic pregnancy
2. Congenital abnormalities
   From a study of 287 completed pregnancies following Pergonal®-hCG therapy five incidents of birth defects were reported (1.7%). One infant had multiple congenital anomalies consisting of imperforate anus, aplasia of the sigmoid colon, third degree hypospadias, cecovesicle fistula, bifid scrotum, meningocele, bilateral internal tibial torsion, and right metatarsus adductus. Another infant was born with an imperforate anus and possible congenital heart lesions; another had a supernumerary digit; another was born with hypospadias and exstrophy of the bladder; and the fifth child had Down's syndrome. None of the investigators felt that these defects were drug-related. Subsequently one report of an infant death due to hydrocephalus and cardiac anomalies has been received.

There have been infrequent reports of ovarian neoplasms, both benign and malignant, in women who have undergone multiple drug regimens for ovulation induction; however, a causal relationship has not been established.

Men:

1. Gynecomastia may occur occasionally during Pergonal®-hCG therapy. This is a known effect of hCG treatment.
2. Erythrocytosis (hct 50%, hgb 17.8 g%) was recorded in one patient.

DRUG ABUSE AND DEPENDENCE

There have been no reports of abuse or dependence with Pergonal®.

OVERDOSAGE

Aside from possible ovarian hyperstimulation (see "Warnings"), little is known concerning the consequences of acute overdosage with Pergonal®.

DOSAGE AND ADMINISTRATION

Women:

1. Dosage:

The dose of Pergonal® to produce maturation of the follicle must be individualized for each patient. It is recommended that the initial dose to any patient should be 75 IU of FSH/LH per day, **ADMINISTERED INTRAMUSCULARLY**, for seven to twelve days followed by hCG, 5,000 U to 10,000 U, one day after the last dose of Pergonal®. Administration of Pergonal® should not exceed 12 days in a single course of therapy. The patient should be treated until indices of estrogenic activity, as indicated under "Precautions" above, are equivalent to or greater than those of the normal individual. If serum or urinary estradiol determinations or ultrasonographic visualizations are available, they may be useful as a guide to therapy. If the ovaries are abnormally enlarged on the last day of Pergonal® therapy, hCG should not be administered in this course of therapy; this will reduce the chances of development of the Ovarian Hyperstimulation Syndrome. If there is evidence of ovulation but no pregnancy, repeat this dosage regime for at least two more courses before increasing the dose of Pergonal® to 150 IU of FSH/LH per day for seven to twelve days. As before, this dose should be followed by 5,000 U to 10,000 U of hCG one day after the last dose of Pergonal®. A Pergonal® dose of 150 IU of FSH/LH per day has proven to be the most effective dose espe-

Continued on next page

Serono Laboratories—Cont.

	% Pts. Ovul.	% Pts. Preg.	% Abort.	% Multi Preg.	% Twins	% 3 or More Concepti	% Hyperstim. Syndr.
Primary Amenorrhea	62	22	14	25	25	0	0
Secondary Amenorrhea	61	28	24	28	18	10	1.9
Secondary Amen. with Galactorrhea	77	42	21	41	31	10	1.2
Polycystic Ovaries	76	26	39	17	17	0	1.1
Anovulatory Cycles	77	24	15	14	9	5	2.0
Miscellaneous	83	20	36	2	2	0	0.1

cially for in vitro fertilization. If evidence of ovulation is present, but pregnancy does not ensue, repeat the same dose for two more courses. Doses larger than this are not routinely recommended.

During treatment with both Pergonal® and hCG and during a two-week post-treatment period, patients should be examined at least every other day for signs of excessive ovarian stimulation. It is recommended that Pergonal® administration be stopped if the ovaries become abnormally enlarged or abdominal pain occurs. Most of the Ovarian Hyperstimulation Syndrome occurs after treatment has been discontinued and reaches its maximum at about seven to ten days post-ovulation. Patients should be followed for at least two weeks after hCG administration.

The couple should be encouraged to have intercourse daily, beginning on the day prior to the administration of hCG until ovulation becomes apparent from the indices employed for the determination of progestational activity. Care should be taken to insure insemination. In the light of the foregoing indices and parameters mentioned, it should become obvious that, unless a physician is willing to devote considerable time to these patients and be familiar with and conduct the necessary laboratory studies, he/she should not use Pergonal®.

2. Administration:
Dissolve the contents of one ampule of Pergonal® in one to two ml of sterile saline and **ADMINISTER INTRAMUSCULARLY** immediately. Any unused reconstituted material should be discarded. Parenteral drug products should be inspected visually for particulate matter and discoloration prior to administration, whenever solution and container permit.

Men:

1. Dosage:
Prior to concomitant therapy with Pergonal® and hCG, pretreatment with hCG alone (5,000 U three times a week) is required. Treatment should continue for a period sufficient to achieve serum testosterone levels within the normal range and masculinization as judged by the appearance of secondary sex characteristics. Such pretreatment may require four to six months, then the recommended dose of Pergonal® is 75 IU FSH/LH **ADMINISTERED INTRAMUSCULARLY**, three times a week and the recommended dose of hCG is 2,000 U twice a week. Therapy should be carried on for a minimum of four more months to insure detecting spermatozoa in the ejaculate, as it takes 74± 4 days in the human male for germ cells to reach the spermatozoa stage.

If the patient has not responded with evidence of increased spermatogenesis at the end of four months of therapy, treatment may continue with 75 IU FSH/LH three times a week, or the dose can be increased to 150 IU FSH/LH three times a week, with the hCG dose unchanged.

2. Administration:
Dissolve the contents of one ampule of Pergonal® in one to two ml of sterile saline and **ADMINISTER INTRAMUSCULARLY** immediately. Any unused reconstituted material should be discarded. Parenteral drug products should be inspected visually for particulate matter and discoloration prior to administration, whenever solution and container permit.

HOW SUPPLIED
Pergonal® is supplied in a sterile lyophilized form as a white to off-white powder or pellet in ampules containing 75 IU or 150 IU FSH/LH activity. The following package combinations are available:
—1 ampule 75 IU Pergonal® and 1 ampule 2 ml Sodium Chloride Injection (USP), NDC 44087-0571-7.
—10 ampules 75 IU Pergonal® and 10 ampules 2 ml Sodium Chloride Injection (USP), NDC 44087-5075-3.
—1 ampule 150 IU Pergonal® and 1 ampule 2 ml Sodium Chloride Injection (USP), NDC 44087-5150-1.
By biological assay, one IU of LH for the Second International Reference Preparation (2nd-IRP) for hMG is biologically equivalent to approximately ½ U of hCG.
Lyophilized powder may be stored refrigerated or at room

temperature (3°–25°C/37°–77°F). Protect from light. Use immediately after reconstitution. Discard unused material.

CLINICAL STUDIES
Women:
The results of the clinical experience and effectiveness of the administration of Pergonal® to 1,286 patients in 3,002 courses of therapy were summarized below. The values include patients who were treated with other than the recommended dosage regime. The values for the presently recommended dosage regime are essentially the same.

	%
Patients ovulating	75
Patients pregnant	25
Patients aborting	25*
Multiple pregnancies	20†
Twins	15†
Three or more concepti	5†
Fetal abnormalities	1.7†
Hyperstimulation syndrome	1.3

* Based on total pregnancies
† Based on total deliveries
Results by diagnosis group are summarized below (these values include patients who were treated with other than the present recommended dosage regime):
[See table above.]
Men:
Clinical results of the treatment of men with primary or secondary hypogonadotropic hypogonadism are as follows:
In the Serono Cooperative study, with an adequate treatment period of 3 to 8 months, 60 of 70 men with primary hypogonadotropic hypogonadism and 8 of 11 men with secondary hypogonadotropic hypogonadism responded with mean increases in their sperm counts from less than 5 to 24 million spermatozoa per milliliter of ejaculate. Forty-one wives of 54 men with primary hypogonadotropic hypogonadism desiring offspring and 7 wives of men with secondary hypogonadotropic hypogonadism conceived. Patients treated with Pergonal® and hCG for less than 3 months or with Pergonal® alone did not respond to therapy.
A world-wide data search revealed that of 160 recorded pregnancies as the result of use of Pergonal®-hCG in men, there were 7 spontaneous abortions, one ectopic pregnancy and 3 congenital anomalies at birth (esophageal atresia in a female infant which was later corrected by surgery, unilateral cryptorchidism, inguinal hernia).
Caution: Federal law prohibits dispensing without prescription.

Manufactured for:
SERONO LABORATORIES, INC.
Randolph, MA 02368 USA
by: Laboratoires Serono, SA
Aubonne, Switzerland
© SERONO LABORATORIES, INC. 1969, 1994
Revised: November 1994

PROFASI® ℞
[pro 'fah-se]
(chorionic gonadotropin for injection, USP)

FOR INTRAMUSCULAR INJECTION

DESCRIPTION
Human chorionic gonadotropin (HCG), a polypeptide hormone produced by the human placenta, is composed of an alpha and a beta sub-unit. The alpha sub-unit is essentially identical to the alpha sub-units of the human pituitary gonadotropins, luteinizing hormone (LH) and follicle-stimulating hormone (FSH), as well as to the alpha sub-unit of human thyroid-stimulating hormone (TSH). The beta sub-units of these hormones differ in amino acid sequence.
Chorionic Gonadotropin is a water soluble glycoprotein derived from human pregnancy urine. The sterile lyophilized powder is stable. When reconstituted, the solution should be refrigerated and used within 30 days.
Each vial, when reconstituted with provided diluent, will contain:

Chorionic Gonadotropin 2,000, 5,000 or 10,000 USP Units, Mannitol 100 mg, Dibasic Sodium Phosphate 16 mg, Monobasic Sodium Phosphate 4 mg, with Benzyl Alcohol 0.9% as preservative, in Water for Injection.

CLINICAL PHARMACOLOGY
The action of HCG is virtually identical to that of pituitary LH, although HCG appears to have a small degree of FSH activity as well. It stimulates production of gonadal steroid hormones by stimulating the interstitial cells (Leydig cells) of the testis to produce androgens and the corpus luteum of the ovary to produce progesterone. Androgen stimulation in the male leads to the development of secondary sex characteristics and may stimulate testicular descent when no anatomical impediment to descent is present. This descent is usually reversible when HCG is discontinued. During the normal menstrual cycle, LH participates with FSH in the development and maturation of the normal ovarian follicle, and the mid-cycle LH surge triggers ovulation. HCG can substitute for LH in this function.
During a normal pregnancy, HCG secreted by the placenta maintains the corpus luteum after LH secretion decreases, supporting continued secretion of estrogen and progesterone, and preventing menstruation. HCG HAS NO KNOWN EFFECT ON FAT MOBILIZATION, APPETITE OR SENSE OF HUNGER, OR BODY FAT DISTRIBUTION.

INDICATIONS AND USAGE
HCG HAS NOT BEEN DEMONSTRATED TO BE EFFECTIVE ADJUNCTIVE THERAPY IN THE TREATMENT OF OBESITY. THERE IS NO SUBSTANTIAL EVIDENCE THAT IT INCREASES WEIGHT LOSS BEYOND THAT RESULTING FROM CALORIC RESTRICTION, THAT IT CAUSES A MORE ATTRACTIVE OR "NORMAL" DISTRIBUTION OF FAT, OR THAT IT DECREASES THE HUNGER AND DISCOMFORT ASSOCIATED WITH CALORIE-RESTRICTED DIETS.
1. Prepubertal cryptorchidism not due to anatomic obstruction. In general, HCG is thought to induce testicular descent in situations when descent would have occurred at puberty. HCG thus may help to predict whether or not orchiopexy will be needed in the future. Although, in some cases, descent following HCG administration is permanent, in most cases the response is temporary. Therapy is usually instituted between the ages of 4 and 9.
2. Selected cases of hypogonadotropic hypogonadism (hypogonadism secondary to a pituitary deficiency) in males.
3. Induction of ovulation and pregnancy in the anovulatory, infertile woman in whom the cause of anovulation is secondary and not due to primary ovarian failure, and who has been appropriately pretreated with human menotropins.

CONTRAINDICATIONS
Precocious puberty, prostatic carcinoma or other androgen-dependent neoplasm, prior allergic reaction to HCG. HCG may cause fetal harm when administered to a pregnant woman. Combined HCG/PMS (pregnant mare's serum) therapy has been noted to induce high incidences of external congenital anomalies in the offspring of mice, in a dose-dependent manner. The potential extrapolation to humans has not been determined.

WARNINGS
HCG should be used in conjunction with human menopausal gonadotropins only by physicians experienced with infertility problems who are familiar with the criteria for patient selection, contraindications, warnings, precautions, and adverse reactions described in the package insert for menotropins. The principal serious adverse reactions during this use are: (1) Ovarian hyperstimulation, a sydrome of sudden ovarian enlargement, ascites with or without pain, and/or pleural effusion; (2) Enlargement of preexisting ovarian cysts or rupture of ovarian cysts with resultant hemoperitoneum; (3) Multiple births, and (4) Arterial thromboembolism.
The diluent used for reconstitution contains benzyl alcohol. Benzyl alcohol has been reported to be associated with a fatal "Gasping Syndrome" in premature infants.

PRECAUTIONS
General: 1. Induction of androgen secretion by HCG may induce precocious puberty in patients treated for cryptorchidism. Therapy should be discontinued if signs of precocious puberty occur.
2. Since androgens may cause fluid retention, HCG should be used with caution in patients with cardiac or renal disease, epilepsy, migraine, or asthma.
Drug/Laboratory test: HCG can crossreact in the radioimmunoassay of gonadotropins, especially luteinizing hormone. Each individual laboratory should establish the degree of crossreactivity with their gonadotropin assay. Physicians should make the laboratory aware of patients on HCG if gonadotropin levels are requested.
Carcinogenesis, Mutagenesis, Impairment of Fertility: There have been sporadic reports of testicular tumors in otherwise healthy young men receiving HCG for secondary infertility. A causative relationship between HCG and tumor development in these men has not been established. Defects of fore-

limbs and of the central nervous system, as well as alterations in sex ratio, have been reported in mice on combined gonadotropin and HCG regimens. The dose of gonadotropin used was intended to induce superovulation. No mutagenic effect has been clearly established in humans. Fertility—see "Indications and Usage."

Pregnancy: Teratogenic effects- *Category X:* See "Contraindications" section. Combined HCG/PMS (pregnant mare's serum) therapy has been noted to induce high incidences of external congenital anomalies in the offspring of mice, in a dose-dependent manner. The potential extrapolation to humans has not been determined.

Nursing Mothers: It is not known whether this drug is excreted in human milk. Because many drugs are excreted in human milk, caution should be exercised when HCG is administered to a nursing woman.

Pediatric Use: Safety and effectiveness in children below the age of 4 have not been established.

ADVERSE REACTIONS (See WARNINGS)

Headache, irritability, restlessness, depression, fatigue, edema, precocious puberty, gynecomastia, pain at the site of injection. Hypersensitivity reactions both localized and systemic in nature, including erythema, urticaria, rash, angioedema, dyspnea and shortness of breath, have been reported. The relationship of these allergic-like events to the polypeptide hormone or the diluent containing benzyl alcohol is not clear.

DOSAGE AND ADMINISTRATION (Intramuscular Use Only):

The dosage regimen employed in any particular case will depend upon the indication for use, the age and weight of the patient, and the physician's preference. The following regimens have been advocated by various authorities.

Prepubertal cryptorchidism not due to anatomical obstruction:

(1) 4,000 USP Units three times weekly for three weeks.

(2) 5,000 USP Units every second day for four injections.

(3) 15 Injections of 500 to 1,000 USP Units over a period of six weeks.

(4) 500 USP Units three times weekly for four to six weeks. If this course of treatment is not successful, another is begun one month later, giving 1,000 USP Units per injection.

Selected cases of hypogonadotropic hypogonadism in males:

(1) 500 to 1,000 USP Units three times a week for three weeks, followed by the same dose twice a week for three weeks.

(2) 4,000 USP Units three times weekly for six to nine months, following which the dosage may be reduced to 2,000 USP Units three times weekly for an additional three months.

Induction of ovulation and pregnancy in the anovulatory, infertile woman in whom the cause of anovulation is secondary and not due to primary ovarian failure and who has been appropriately pre-treated with human menotropins (See prescribing information for menotropins for dosage and administration for that drug product).

5,000 to 10,000 USP Units one day following the last dose of menotropins. (A dosage of 10,000 USP Units is recommended in the labeling for menotropins).

Parenteral drug products should be inspected visually for particulate matter and discoloration prior to administration, whenever solution and container permit.

HOW SUPPLIED

Chorionic gonadotropin for injection, USP, is available in 10 mL lyophilized multiple dose vial sets containing either:
5,000 USP Units per Vial-NDC 44087-8005-3
10,000 USP Units per Vial-NDC 44087-8010-3 with 10 mL vial bacteriostatic water for injection, USP (containing benzyl alcohol 0.9% v/v).

Storage: Store dry product at controlled room temperature 15°-30° C (59°-86° F). AFTER RECONSTITUTION, REFRIGERATE THE PRODUCT AT 2°-8° C (36°-46° F) AND USE WITHIN 30 DAYS.

Caution: Federal law prohibits dispensing without prescription.

Manufactured for: SERONO LABORATORIES, INC.
Randolph, MA 02368 USA

Manufactured by: Steris Laboratories, Inc.
Phoenix, AZ 85043 USA
ST-12-90

®Serono Laboratories, Inc. 1984, 1992
Revised June 1993
1-1919-0692
6957012544087F1

SEROPHENE®   ℞
[*se'ro-fēn*]
(clomiphene citrate tablets, USP)

PRODUCT OVERVIEW

KEY FACTS

Serophene® is an orally administered, non-steroidal compound with some estrogenic activity. The exact mechanism of action is unknown, although it appears to involve the pituitary by stimulating release of pituitary gonadotropins to mediate ovulation.

MAJOR USES

Serophene® is effective in inducing ovulation in infertile women with physiological indications of normal estrogen production. Reduced estrogen levels, while less favorable, do not prevent successful therapy.

SAFETY INFORMATION

Serophene® is contraindicated in patients who have previously experienced hypersensitivity to clomiphene citrate. Visual disturbances, vasomotor flushes, and ovarian enlargement occasionally occur. Because the teratogenic potential of clomiphene citrate is unknown, it should not be administered during pregnancy. Multiple births occur in approximately 10% of pregnancies resulting from clomiphene citrate therapy; the vast majority of these are twins.

PRESCRIBING INFORMATION

SEROPHENE®   ℞
[*se'ro-fēn*]
(clomiphene citrate tablets, USP)

DESCRIPTION

Each scored white tablet contains: clomiphene citrate, USP 50 mg. Clomiphene citrate is designated chemically as 2-[p-(2-chloro-1,2-diphenylvinyl) phenoxy] triethylamine dihydrogen citrate and is represented structurally as:

$$(C_2H_5)_2NCH_2CH_2O \text{—} \bigcirc \text{—} O \text{—} C = C \text{—} \bigcirc \text{—} C_6H_6O_7$$

clomiphene citrate, USP (Serophene®)

As shown, one molecule of citric acid is chemically bound with one molecule of the organic base, clomiphene.

Clomiphene citrate is a chemical analog of other triarylethylene compounds such as chlorotrianisene and the cholesterol inhibitor, triparanol.

ACTIONS

Clomiphene citrate, an orally-administered, non-steroidal agent, may induce ovulation in selected anovulatory women. It is a drug of considerable pharmacologic potency. Careful evaluation and selection of the patient and close attention to the timing of the dose is mandatory prior to treatment with clomiphene citrate. Conservative selection and management of the patient contribute to successful therapy of anovulation. Clomiphene citrate induces ovulation in most selected anovulatory patients. The various criteria for ovulation include: an ovulation peak of estrogen excretion followed by a biphasic basal body temperature curve, urinary excretion of pregnanediol at post-ovulatory levels, and endometrial histologic findings characteristic of the luteal phase.

A review of eleven publications appearing between 1964 and 1978 showed that pregnancy occurred in 35% of 5154 patients with ovulatory dysfunction who received clomiphene citrate.

[See table below.]

Clomiphene citrate therapy appears to mediate ovulation through increased output of pituitary gonadotropins. These stimulate the maturation and endocrine activity of the ovarian follicle which is followed by the development and function of the corpus luteum. Increased urinary excretion of gonadotropins and estrogen suggests involvement of the pituitary.

Studies with ^{14}C labeled clomiphene citrate have shown that it is readily absorbed orally in humans and is excreted principally in the feces. An average of 51% of the administered

---

dose was excreted after 5 days. After intravenous administration, 37% was excreted in 5 days. The appearance of ^{14}C in the feces six weeks after administration suggests that the remaining drug and/or metabolites are slowly excreted from a sequestered enterohepatic recirculation pool.

INDICATIONS

Clomiphene citrate is indicated for the treatment of ovulatory failure in patients desiring pregnancy and whose husbands are fertile and potent. Impediments to this goal must be excluded or adequately treated before beginning therapy. Administration of clomiphene citrate is indicated only in patients with demonstrated ovulatory dysfunction and in whom the following conditions apply:

1. Normal liver function.

2. Physiologic indications of normal endogenous estrogen (as estimated from vaginal smears, endometrial biopsy, assay of serum [or urinary] estrogen, or from bleeding in response to progesterone). Reduced estrogen levels, while less favorable, do not prevent successful therapy.

3. Clomiphene citrate therapy is not effective for those patients with primary pituitary or ovarian failure. It cannot substitute for appropriate therapy of other disturbances leading to ovulatory dysfunction, e.g., diseases of the thyroid or adrenals.

4. Particularly careful evaluation prior to clomiphene citrate therapy should be done in patients with abnormal uterine bleeding. It is most important that neoplastic lesions are detected.

CONTRAINDICATIONS

Pregnancy:

Although no direct effect of clomiphene citrate therapy on the human fetus has been seen established, clomiphene citrate should not be administered in cases of suspected pregnancy as such effects have been reported in animals. To prevent inadvertent clomiphene citrate administration during early pregnancy, the basal body temperature should be recorded throughout all treatment cycles, and therapy should be discontinued if pregnancy is suspected. If the basal body temperature following clomiphene citrate is biphasic and is not followed by menses, the possibility of an ovarian cyst and/or pregnancy should be excluded. Until the correct diagnosis has been determined, the next course of therapy should be delayed.

Clomiphene citrate is also contraindicated in patients who have:

1. Uncontrolled thyroid or adrenal dysfunction.

2. An organic intracranial lesion such as a pituitary tumor.

3. Liver disease or a history of liver dysfunction.

4. Abnormal uterine bleeding of undetermined origin.

5. Ovarian cysts or enlargement not due to polycystic ovarian syndrome.

WARNINGS

Visual Symptoms:

Patients should be warned that blurring and/or other visual symptoms may occur occasionally with clomiphene citrate therapy. These may make activities such as driving or operating machinery more hazardous than usual, particularly under conditions of variable lighting. While their significance is not yet understood (see "Adverse Reactions"), patients having any visual symptoms should discontinue treatment and have a complete ophthalmologic evaluation.

Ovarian Hyperstimulation Syndrome:

The Ovarian Hyperstimulation Syndrome (OHSS) has been reported to occur in patients receiving drug therapy for ovulation induction, including in rare cases patients receiving clomiphene citrate therapy. OHSS is a medical event distinct from uncomplicated ovarian enlargement. OHSS may progress rapidly (within 24 hours to several days) to become a serious medical event. It is characterized by an apparent dramatic increase in vascular permeability which can result in a rapid accumulation of fluid in the peritoneal cavity, thorax, and potentially, the pericardium. The early warning signs of development of OHSS are severe pelvic pain, nausea, vomiting, and weight gain. The following symptomatology has been seen with cases of OHSS: abdominal pain, abdominal distension, gastrointestinal symptoms including nausea,

---

PREGNANCIES FOLLOWING CLOMIPHENE CITRATE, USP[a]		(Range)
Number of Patients	= 5154	
Percent of Patients Ovulating[b]	= 75	(50-94%)
Percent of Ovulatory Cycles	= 53	(33-69%)
Percent of Patients Pregnant	= 35	(11-52%)
Percent Patients Pregnant	= 46	(22-61%)
Percent Patients Ovulating		
Percent Live Births	= 86	(74-99.8%)
Percent Abortions	= 14	(0.2-26%)
Percent of Single Births	= 90	(67-100%)
Percent Surviving	= 99	(98.2-100%)
Percent of Multiple Births	= 10	(0-33%)
Percent Surviving	= 96	(82-100%)

a) includes patients receiving other than recommended dosage regimen.
b) average from studies.

Continued on next page

Serono Laboratories—Cont.

vomiting and diarrhea, severe ovarian enlargement, weight gain, dyspnea, and oliguria. Clinical evaluation may reveal hypovolemia, hemoconcentration, electrolyte imbalances, ascites, hemoperitoneum, pleural effusions, hydrothorax, acute pulmonary distress, and thromboembolic phenomena. Transient liver function test abnormalities, suggestive of hepatic dysfunction, which may be accompanied by morphologic changes on liver biopsy, have been reported in association with the Ovarian Hyperstimulation Syndrome (OHSS).

PRECAUTIONS

Diagnosis Prior to Clomiphene Citrate Therapy:
Careful evaluation should be given to candidates for clomiphene citrate therapy. A complete pelvic examination should be performed prior to treatment and repeated before each subsequent course. Clomiphene citrate should not be given to patients with an ovarian cyst, as further ovarian enlargement may result.

Since the incidence of endometrial carcinoma and of ovulatory disorders increases with age, endometrial biopsy should always exclude the former as causative in such patients. If abnormal uterine bleeding is present, full diagnostic measures are necessary.

Ovarian Overstimulation During Treatment with Clomiphene Citrate:
To minimize the hazard associated with the occasional abnormal ovarian enlargement during clomiphene citrate therapy (see "Adverse Reactions"), the lowest dose producing good results should be chosen. Some patients with polycystic ovarian syndrome are unusually sensitive to gonadotropins and may have an exaggerated response to usual doses of clomiphene citrate. Maximal enlargement of the ovary, whether abnormal or physiologic, does not occur until several days after discontinuation of clomiphene citrate. The patient complaining of pelvic pains after receiving clomiphene citrate should be examined carefully. If enlargement of the ovary occurs, clomiphene citrate therapy should be withheld until the ovaries have returned to pretreatment size, and the dosage or duration of the next course should be reduced. The ovarian enlargement and cyst formation following clomiphene citrate therapy regress spontaneously within a few days or weeks after discontinuing treatment. Therefore, unless a strong indication for laparoscopy (or laparotomy) exists, such cystic enlargement always should be managed conservatively.

Multiple Pregnancy:
In the reviewed publications, the incidence of multiple pregnancies was increased during those cycles in which clomiphene citrate was given. Among the 1,803 pregnancies on which the outcome was reported, 90% were single and 10% twins. Less than 1% of the reported deliveries resulted in triplets or more.

Of these multiple pregnancies, 96-99% resulted in the births of live infants. The patient and her husband should be advised of the frequency and potential hazards of multiple pregnancy before starting treatment.

Additional Precautions:
Prolonged use of clomiphene may increase the risk of a borderline or invasive ovarian tumor.

ADVERSE REACTIONS

At the recommended dosage of clomiphene citrate, side effects occur infrequently and generally do not interfere with treatment. Adverse reactions tend to occur more frequently at higher doses and in the longer treatment courses used in some early studies.

The most frequent adverse reactions to clomiphene citrate include ovarian enlargement (approximately 1 in 7 patients), vasomotor flushes resembling menopausal symptoms which are not usually severe and promptly disappear after treatment is discontinued (approximately 1 in 10 patients), and abdominal discomfort (approximately 1 in 15 patients). Adverse reactions which occur less frequently (approximately 1 in 50 patients or more) include breast tenderness, nausea and vomiting, nervousness, insomnia, and visual disturbances. Other side effects which occur in less than 1 in 100 patients include headache, dizziness and light-headedness, increased urination, depression, fatigue, urticaria and allergic dermatitis, abnormal uterine bleeding, weight gain, ovarian cysts (ovarian enlargement or cysts could, as such, be complicated by adnexal torsion), and reversible hair loss.

Thromboembolic events, such as pulmonary embolism, arterial occlusion, and phlebitis, have been reported rarely in patients treated with clomiphene citrate. It is not clear what, if any, relationship these events have to clomiphene citrate therapy.

When clomiphene citrate is administered at the recommended dose, abnormal ovarian enlargement (see "Precautions") is infrequent, although the usual cyclic variation in ovarian size may be exaggerated. Similarly, mid-cycle ovarian pain (mittelschmerz) may be accentuated.

With prolonged or higher dosage, ovarian enlargement and cyst formation (usually luteal) may occur more often, and the luteal phase of the cycle may be prolonged. Patients with polycystic ovarian syndrome may be unusually sensitive to clomiphene therapy. Rare occurrences of massive ovarian enlargement have been reported, for example, in a patient with polycystic ovarian syndrome whose clomiphene citrate therapy consisted of 100 mg daily for 14 days. Since abnormal ovarian enlargement usually regresses spontaneously, most of these patients should be treated conservatively. The Ovarian Hyperstimulation Syndrome has been reported to occur in rare cases in patients receiving clomiphene citrate therapy (see "Warnings").

The incidence of visual symptoms (see "Warnings" for further recommendations), usually described as "blurring" or spots or flashes (scintillating scotomata), correlates with increasing total dose. Other visual symptoms which may occur include diplopia, phosphenes, photophobia, decreased visual acuity, loss of peripheral vision, and spatial distortion. The symptoms disappear usually within a few days or weeks after clomiphene citrate is discontinued. This may be due to intensification and/or prolongation of after-images. Symptoms often appear first, or are accentuated, upon exposure to a more brightly lit environment.

While measured visual acuity generally has not been affected, in one patient taking 200 mg daily, visual blurring developed on the seventh day of treatment and progressed to severe diminution of visual acuity by the tenth day. No other abnormality was coincident, and the visual acuity was normal by the third day after treatment was stopped. Ophthalmologically definable scotomata and electroretinographic retinal function changes have also been reported.

BSP Laboratory Studies:
Greater than 5% retention of sulfobromophthalein (BSP) has been reported in approximately 10% to 20% of patients in whom it was measured. Retention was usually minimal but was elevated during prolonged clomiphene citrate administration or with apparently unrelated liver disease. In some patients, pre-existing BSP retention decreased even though clomiphene citrate therapy was continued. Other liver function tests were usually normal.

Other Laboratory Studies:
Clomiphene citrate has not been reported to cause a significant abnormality in hematologic or renal tests, in protein bound iodine, or in serum cholesterol levels.

Birth Defects:
The following medical events have been reported subsequent to pregnancies following ovulation induction therapy with clomiphene citrate: ectopic pregnancy and congenital abnormalities such as syndactyly, polydactyly, congenital heart defects, retinal aplasia, hypospadias, ovarian dysplasia, cleft lip/palate, microcephaly and neural tube defects, including anencephaly. Some medical literature reports have implied an increased occurrence of neural tube defects, while others indicate that an increased incidence over that found in the general population does not exist. One case of a congenital abnormality (adactyly) in an infant exposed to clomiphene citrate in utero has been reported.

Of 1,803 births following clomiphene citrate administration, 45 infants with birth defects were reported for a cumulative rate of 2.5%.

Six cases of Down's syndrome, one neonatal death with multiple malformations, and one case of each of the following were reported: club-foot, tibial torsion, blocked tear duct, and hemangioma. The other congenital abnormalities were not described. The investigators did not report that these were presumed to be due to therapy. The cumulative rate of congenital abnormalities does not exceed that reported in the general population.

Ovarian cancer has been reported in a very small number of infertile women who have been treated with clomiphene citrate. A causal relationship between treatment with clomiphene citrate and ovarian cancer has not been established.

DOSAGE AND ADMINISTRATION

General Considerations:
Physicians experienced in managing gynecologic or endocrine disorders should supervise the work-up and treatment of candidate patients for clomiphene citrate therapy. Patients should be chosen for clomiphene citrate therapy only after careful diagnostic evaluation (see "Indications"). The plan of therapy should be outlined in advance. Impediments to achieving the goal of therapy must be excluded or adequately treated before beginning clomiphene citrate.

In determining a starting dose schedule, efficacy must be balanced against potential side effects. For example, the available data so far suggest that ovulation and pregnancy are slightly more attainable with 100 mg/day for 5 days than with 50 mg/day for 5 days. As the dosage is increased, however, ovarian overstimulation and other side effects may be expected to increase. Although the data do not yet establish a relationship between dose level and multiple births, it is reasonable that such a correlation exists on pharmacologic grounds.

For these reasons, treatment of the usual patient should initiate with a 50 mg daily dose for 5 days. The dose may be increased only in those patients who do not respond to the first course (see "Recommended Dosage"). Special treatment with lower dosage over shorter duration is particularly recommended if unusual sensitivity to pituitary gonadotropin is suspected, including patients with polycystic ovarian syndrome (see "Precautions").

Recommended Dosage:
The recommended dosage for the first course of clomiphene citrate is 50 mg (1 tablet) daily for 5 days. Therapy may be started at any time if the patient has had no recent uterine bleeding. If progestin-induced bleeding is intended, or if spontaneous uterine bleeding occurs prior to therapy, the regimen of 50 mg daily for 5 days should be started on or about the fifth day of the cycle. When ovulation occurs at this dosage, there is no advantage to increasing the dose in subsequent cycles of treatment. If ovulation does not appear to have occurred after the first course of therapy, a second course of 100 mg daily (two 50 mg tablets given as a single daily dose) for 5 days may be started. This course may begin as early as 30 days after the previous one. It is recommended that the patient be examined for pregnancy, ovarian enlargement, or cyst formation between each treatment cycle. Increasing the dosage or duration of therapy beyond 100 mg/day for 5 days should not be undertaken.

The majority of patients who respond do so during the first course of therapy, and 3 courses constitute an adequate therapeutic trial. If ovulatory menses do not occur, the diagnosis should be re-evaluated. Treatment beyond this is not recommended in the patient who does not exhibit evidence of ovulation.

Pregnancy:
Properly timed coitus is very important for good results. For regularity of cyclic ovulatory response, it is also important that each course of clomiphene citrate be started on or about the fifth day of the cycle, once ovulation has been established. As with other therapeutic modalities, Serophene® therapy follows the rule of diminishing returns, such that the likelihood of conception diminishes with each succeeding course of therapy. If pregnancy has not been achieved after 3 ovulatory responses to Serophene®, further treatment generally is not recommended. Before starting treatment, patients should be advised of the possibility and potential hazards of multiple pregnancy if conception occurs following clomiphene citrate therapy.

Long-Term Cyclic Therapy —Not Recommended:
Since the relative safety of long-term cyclic therapy has not yet been demonstrated conclusively, and since the majority of patients will ovulate following 3 courses, long-term cyclic therapy is not recommended.

HOW SUPPLIED

Serophene® is available as 50 mg scored white tablets in the following package combinations:
- 1 carton 10 tablets, NDC 44087-8090-6

Each carton contains 2 strips of 5 tablets each.
- 1 carton 30 tablets, NDC 44087-8090-1

Each carton contains 3 strips of 10 tablets, each in a 2×5 arrangement.

Protect from light, moisture, and excessive heat. Dispense in well-closed, light resistant container as defined in the USP, with child resistant closure. Store at room temperature (15°–30°C/59°–86°F).

Caution: Federal law prohibits dispensing without prescription.

Manufactured for:
SERONO LABORATORIES, INC.
Randolph, MA 02368 USA
©SERONO LABORATORIES, INC. 1982, 1992
Revised: November 1994

For additional information, please contact:
Serono Laboratories, Inc.
Drug Information and Surveillance Group, x5562
Customer Service, Sales and Ordering, x5141
100 Longwater Circle
Norwell, MA 02061
800-283-8088 (Toll free)
617-982-9000

EDUCATIONAL MATERIAL

To obtain information about scientific, medical, nursing and consumer educational meetings and materials, please contact Serono Symposia USA, Inc.

Sigma-Tau Pharmaceuticals, Inc.
800 SOUTH FREDERICK AVENUE
GAITHERSBURG, MARYLAND 20877

Direct Inquiries to:
(301) 948-1041

CARNITOR® ℞
[car-nĭ-tor]
CARNITOR® (Levocarnitine) Injection 1 g per 5 mL and 500 mg per 2.5 mL
FOR INTRAVENOUS USE ONLY

DESCRIPTION

Levocarnitine is a carrier molecule in the transport of long chain fatty acids across the inner mitochondrial membrane. CARNITOR® (Levocarnitine) Injection is a sterile aqueous solution containing 1 gram of levocarnitine per 5 mL ampule and 500 mg of levocarnitine per 2.5 mL ampule. The pH is adjusted to 6.0–6.5 with hydrochloric acid. Chemically, levocarnitine is (R)-3-carboxy-2-hydroxy-N,N,N-trimethyl-1-propanaminium hydroxide, inner salt. It is a white powder with a melting point of 196–197°C and is readily soluble in water, hot alcohol, and insoluble in acetone. The pH of a solution (1 in 20) is between 6–8 and its pKa value is 3.8. Its chemical structure is:

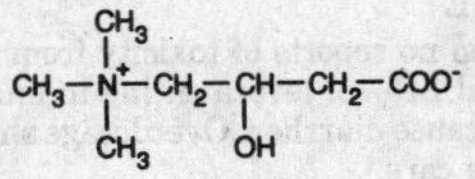

Empirical Formula: $C_7H_{15}NO_3$
Molecular Weight: 161.20

CLINICAL PHARMACOLOGY

CARNITOR® (Levocarnitine) is a naturally occurring substance required in mammalian energy metabolism. It has been shown to facilitate long-chain fatty acid entry into cellular mitochondria, therefore delivering substrate for oxidation and subsequent energy production. Fatty acids are utilized as an energy substrate in all tissues except the brain. In skeletal and cardiac muscle they serve as major fuel. Primary systemic carnitine deficiency is characterized by low plasma, RBC, and/or tissue levels. It has not been possible to determine which symptoms are due to carnitine deficiency and which are due to the underlying organic acidemia, as symptoms of both abnormalities may be expected to improve with carnitine. The literature reports that carnitine can promote the excretion of excess organic or fatty acids in patients with defects in fatty acid metabolism and/or specific organic acidopathies that bioaccumulate acyl CoA esters.[1–6]

Secondary levocarnitine deficiency can be a consequence of inborn errors of metabolism. CARNITOR® may alleviate the metabolic abnormalities of patients with inborn errors that result in accumulation of toxic organic acids. Conditions for which this effect was demonstrated are: glutaric aciduria II, methyl malonic aciduria, propionic acidemia, and medium chain fatty acyl CoA dehydrogenase deficiency.[7,8] Autointoxication occurs in these patients due to the accumulations of acyl CoA compounds that disrupt intermediary metabolism. The subsequent hydrolysis of the acyl CoA compound to its free acid results in acidosis that can be life threatening. Levocarnitine clears the acyl CoA compound by formation of acyl carnitine which is quickly excreted. Levocarnitine deficiency is defined biochemically as abnormally low plasma levels of free carnitine, less that 20 μM/L at age greater that one week post term and may be associated with low tissue and/or urine levels. Further, this condition may be associated with a ratio of plasma ester/free levocarnitine levels greater than 0.4 or abnormally elevated levels of esterified levocarnitine in the urine. In premature infants and newborns, secondary deficiency is defined as plasma free levocarnitine levels below age related normal levels.

BIOAVAILABILITY/PHARMACOKINETICS

In a relative bioavailability study in 15 healthy adult male volunteers CARNITOR® Tablets were found to be bioequivalent to CARNITOR® Oral Solution. Following the administration of 1980 mg b.i.d., the maximum plasma concentration level (C_{max}) was 80 nmol/mL and the time to maximum concentration (T_{max}) occurred at 3.3 hours. There were no significant differences for AUC and urinary excretion observed between these two formulations.

In the same bioavailability study of 15 healthy adult males, CARNITOR® (Levocarnitine) Injection administered as a slow 3 minute bolus intravenous injection at a dose of 20 mg/Kg showed that free levocarnitine plasma profiles are best fit by a two compartment model. Approximately 76% of free levocarnitine is eliminated in the urine. Using plasma levels uncorrected for endogenous levocarnitine, the mean distribution half life was 0.585 hours and the mean apparent terminal elimination half life was 17.4 hours following a single intravenous dose.

The absolute bioavailability of L-carnitine from CARNITOR® Tablets and Oral Solution was determined compared to the bioavailability of L-carnitine from CARNITOR® (Injection) Intravenous in 15 healthy male volunteers. After correction for circulating endogenous levels of L-carnitine in the plasma, absolute bioavailability was 15.1% ± 5.3% for L-carnitine from CARNITOR® Tablets and 15.9% ± 4.9% from the Oral Solution.

Total body clearance of L-carnitine (Dose/AUC including endogenous baseline levels) was a mean of 4.00 L/hr. Endogenous baseline levels were not subtracted since total body clearance of L-carnitine does not distinguish between exogenous sources of L-carnitine and endogenously synthesized L-carnitine. Volume of distribution of the intravenously administered dose above baseline endogenous levels was calculated to be a mean of 29.0 L ± 71.1 L (approximately 0.39 L/kg) which is an underestimate of the true volume of distribution since plasma L-carnitine is known to equilibrate slowly with, for instance, muscle L-carnitine.

L-carnitine was not bound to plasma protein or albumin when tested at any concentration or with any species including the human.[9]

METABOLISM AND EXCRETION

Five normal adult male volunteers, administered a dose of [^{3}H-methyl]-L-carnitine following 15 days of a high carnitine diet and additional carnitine supplement, excreted 58–65% of administered radioactive dose in 5 to 11 days in the urine and feces. Maximum concentration of [^{3}H-methyl]-L-carnitine in serum occurred from 2.0 to 4.5 hr after drug administration. Major metabolites found were trimethylamine N-oxide, primarily in urine (8% to 49% of the administered dose) and [^{3}H]-y-butyrobetaine, primarily in feces (0.44% to 45% of the administered dose). Urinary excretion of carnitine was 4% to 8% of the dose. Fecal excretion of total carnitine was less than 1% of total carnitine excretion.[10]

After attainment of steady state following 4 days of oral administration of L-carnitine with CARNITOR® Tablets (1980 mg q12h) or Oral Solution (2000 mg q12h) to 15 healthy male volunteers, urinary excretion of L-carnitine was a mean of 2107 and 2339 μmoles, respectively, equivalent to 8.6% and 9.4%, respectively, of the orally-administered doses (uncorrected for endogenous urinary excretion). After a single intravenous dose (20 mg/kg) prior to multiple oral doses, urinary excretion of L-carnitine was 6974 μmoles equivalent to 75.6% of the intravenously administered dose (uncorrected for endogenous urinary excretion).

INDICATIONS AND USAGE

For the acute treatment of patients with an inborn error of metabolism that results in secondary carnitine deficiency.

CONTRAINDICATIONS

None known.

WARNINGS

None.

PRECAUTIONS

Carcinogenesis, mutagenesis, impairment of fertility
Mutagenicity tests performed in *Salmonella typhimurium*, *Saccharomyces cerevisiae*, and *Schizosaccharomyces pombe* indicate that levocarnitine is not mutagenic. No long-term animal studies have been performed to evaluate the carcinogenic potential of levocarnitine.

Pregnancy
Pregnancy Category B.
Reproductive studies have been performed in rats and rabbits at doses up to 3.8 times the human dose on the basis of surface area and have revealed no evidence of impaired fertility or harm to the fetus due to CARNITOR®. There are, however, no adequate and well controlled studies in pregnant women.

Because animal reproduction studies are not always predictive of human response, this drug should be used during pregnancy only if clearly needed.

Nursing Mothers
It is not known whether this drug is excreted in human milk. Because many drugs are excreted in human milk, a decision should be made whether to discontinue nursing or to discontinue the drug, taking into account the importance of the drug to the mother.

Pediatric use
See Dosage and Administration.

ADVERSE REACTIONS

Transient nausea and vomiting have been observed. Less frequent adverse reactions are body odor, nausea, and gastritis. An incidence for these reactions is difficult to estimate due to the confounding effects of the underlying pathology.

OVERDOSAGE

There have been no reports of toxicity from levocarnitine overdosage. The oral LD_{50} of levocarnitine in mice is 19.2 g/kg. Large doses of levocarnitine may cause diarrhea.

DOSAGE AND ADMINISTRATION

CARNITOR® Injection is administered intravenously. The recommended dose is 50 mg/kg given as a slow 2–3 minute bolus injection or by infusion. Often a loading dose is given in patients with severe metabolic crisis followed by an equivalent dose over the following 24 hours. It should be administered q3h or q4h, and never less than q6h either by infusion or by intravenous injection. All subsequent daily doses are recommended to be in the range of 50 mg/kg or as therapy may require. The highest dose administered has been 300 mg/kg.

It is recommended that a plasma carnitine level be obtained prior to beginning this parenteral therapy. Weekly and monthly monitoring is recommended as well. This monitoring should include blood chemistries, vital signs, plasma carnitine concentrations (the plasma free carnitine level should be between 35 and 60 micromoles/liter) and overall clinical condition.

Parenteral drug products should be inspected visually for particulate matter and discoloration prior to administration, whenever solution and container permit.

COMPATIBILITY AND STABILITY

Carnitor® Injection is compatible and stable when mixed in parenteral solutions of Sodium Chloride 0.9% or Lactated Ringer's in concentrations ranging from 250 mg/500 mL (0.5 mg/mL) to 4200 mg/500 mL (8.0 mg/mL) and stored at room temperature (25°C) for up to 24 hours in PVC plastic bags.

HOW SUPPLIED

CARNITOR® (Levocarnitine) Injection, 200 mg per 1 mL, is available in 5 mL single dose ampoules packaged 5 ampoules per carton (NDC 54482-146-09) and in 2.5 mL single dose ampoules packaged 5 ampoules per carton (NDC 54482-146-10). Made in Italy.

Store ampoules at room temperature (25°C/77°F) in carton until their use to protect from light. Discard unused portion of an opened ampoule, as they contain no preservative.

CARNITOR® (Levocarnitine) is also available in the following dosage forms for oral administration:

CARNITOR® (Levocarnitine) Tablets are supplied as 330 mg (unit dose), individually foil wrapped tablets embossed with "CARNITOR-ST" in boxes of 90 (NDC 54482-144-07). Made in Italy.

CARNITOR® (Levocarnitine) Oral Solution, 118 mL (4 fl. oz.) supplied as a red, cherry flavored solution in a multiple-dose plastic bottle (NDC 54482-145-08). CARNITOR® (Levocarnitine) Oral Solution is manufactured for Sigma-Tau Pharmaceuticals, Inc. By: Barre-National, Inc. Baltimore, MD 21244-2654.

CAUTION

Federal (U.S.A.) law prohibits dispensing without prescription.

REFERENCES

1. Bohmer T, Rynding A, Solberg HE: Carnitine levels in human serum in health and disease. **Clin Chim Acta 57:** 55-61, 1974.
2. Brooks H, Goldberg L, Holland R et al: Carnitine-induced effects on cardiac and peripheral hemodynamics. **J Clin Pharmacol 17:** 561-578, 1977.
3. Christiansen R, Bremer J: Active transport of butyrobetaine and carnitine into isolated liver cells. **Biochem Biophys Acta 448:** 562-577, 1977.
4. Lindstedt S, Lindstedt G: Distribution and excretion of carnitine $^{14}CO_2$ in the rat. **Acta Chim Scand 15:** 701-701, 1961.
5. Rebouche CJ, Engel AG: Carnitine metabolism and deficiency syndromes. **Mayo Clin Proc 58:** 533-540.
6. Rebouche CJ, Paulson DJ: Carnitine metabolism and function in humans. **Ann Rev Nutr 6:** 41-68, 1986.
7. Scriver CR, Beaudet AL, Sly WS, Valle D: *The Metabolic Basis of Inherited Disease.* McGraw-Hill, New York, 1989.
8. Schaub J, Van Hoof F, Vis HL: *Inborn Errors of Metabolism.* Raven Press, New York, 1991.
9. Marzo A, Arrigoni Martelli E, Mancinelli A, Cardace G, Corbelletta C, Bassani E, Solbiati M: Protein binding of L-carnitine family components. **Eur J Drug Met Pharmacokin,** Special Issue III: 364-368, 1992.
10. Rebouche C: Quantitative estimation of absorption and degradation of a carnitine supplement by human adults. **Metabolism:** 1305-1310, 1991.

sigma-tau
Pharmaceuticals, Inc.
800 S. Frederick Avenue
Gaithersburg, MD 20877-4150
PREVIOUS EDITION IS OBSOLETE
ST-N20-182-10/95

Continued on next page

Sigma-Tau—Cont.

CARNITOR® ℞
[car-nĭ-tor]
(Levocarnitine) Tablets (330 mg)

CARNITOR®
(Levocarnitine) Oral Solution
1 g per 10 mL multidose)
For oral use only.
Not for parenteral use.

DESCRIPTION

CARNITOR® (Levocarnitine) is (R)-3-carboxy-2-hydroxy-N,N,N-trimethyl-1-propanaminium hydroxide, inner salt. Levocarnitine is a carrier molecule in the transport of long chain fatty acids across the inner mitochondrial membrane. As a bulk drug substance it is a white powder with a melting point of 196–197° C and is readily soluble in water, hot alcohol, and insoluble in acetone. The pH of a solution (1 in 20) is between 6–8 and its pKa value is 3.8. Its chemical structure is:

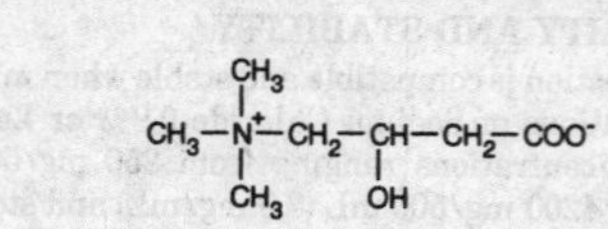

Each CARNITOR® (Levocarnitine) Tablet contains 330 mg of levocarnitine and the inactive ingredients magnesium stearate, microcrystalline cellulose and povidone.
Each 118 mL container of the CARNITOR® (Levocarnitine) Oral Solution contains 1 g of levocarnitine/10 mL. Also contains: Artificial Cherry Flavor, D&C Red No. 33, D,L-Malic Acid, FD&C Red No. 40, Purified Water, Sucrose Syrup. Methylparaben NF and Propylparaben NF are added as preservatives. The pH is approximately 5.

CLINICAL PHARMACOLOGY

CARNITOR® (Levocarnitine) is a naturally occurring substance required in mammalian energy metabolism. It has been shown to facilitate long-chain fatty acid entry into cellular mitochondria, therefore delivering substrate for oxidation and subsequent energy production. Fatty acids are utilized as an energy substrate in all tissues except the brain. In skeletal and cardiac muscle they serve as major fuel. Primary systemic carnitine deficiency is characterized by low plasma, RBC, and/or tissue levels. It has not been possible to determine which symptoms are due to carnitine deficiency and which are due to the underlying organic acidemia, as symptoms of both abnormalities may be expected to improve with carnitine. The literature reports that carnitine can promote the excretion of excess organic or fatty acids in patients with defects in fatty acid metabolism and/or specific organic acidopathies that bioaccumulate acyl CoA esters.[1–6]
Secondary levocarnitine deficiency can be a consequence of inborn errors of metabolism. CARNITOR® may alleviate the metabolic abnormalities of patients with inborn errors that result in accumulation of toxic organic acids. Conditions for which this effect was demonstrated are: glutaric aciduria II, methyl malonic aciduria, propionic acidemia, and medium chain fatty acyl CoA dehydrogenase deficiency.[7,8] Autointoxication occurs in these patients due to the accumulations of acyl CoA compounds that disrupt intermediary metabolism. The subsequent hydrolysis of the acyl CoA compound to its free acid results in acidosis that can be life threatening. Levocarnitine clears the acyl CoA compound by formation of acyl carnitine which is quickly excreted. Levocarnitine deficiency is defined biochemically as abnormally low plasma levels of free carnitine, less than 20 μM/L at age greater than one week post term and may be associated with low tissue and/or urine levels. Further, this condition may be associated with a ratio of plasma ester/free levocarnitine levels greater than 0.4 or abnormally elevated levels of esterified levocarnitine in the urine. In premature infants and newborns, secondary deficiency is defined as plasma free levocarnitine levels below age related normal levels.

BIOAVAILABILITY/PHARMACOKINETICS

In a relative bioavailability study in 15 healthy adult male volunteers CARNITOR® Tablets were found to be bio-equivalent to CARNITOR® Oral Solution. Following the administration of 1980 mg b.i.d., the maximum plasma concentration level (C_{max}) was 80 nmol/mL and the time to maximum concentration (T_{max}) occurred at 3.3 hours. There were no significant differences for AUC and urinary excretion observed between these two formulations.
In the same bioavailability study of 15 healthy adult males, CARNITOR® (Levocarnitine) Injection administered as a slow 3 minute bolus intravenous injection at a dose of 20 mg/kg showed that free levocarnitine plasma profiles are best fit by a two compartment model. Approximately 76% of free levocarnitine is eliminated in the urine. Using plasma levels uncorrected for endogenous levocarnitine, the mean distribution half life was 0.585 hours and the mean apparent terminal elimination half life was 17.4 hours following a single intravenous dose.
The absolute bioavailability of L-carnitine from CARNITOR® Tablets and Oral Solution was determined compared to the bioavailability of L-carnitine from CARNITOR® Injection Intravenous in 15 healthy male volunteers. After correction for circulating endogenous levels of L-carnitine in the plasma, absolute bioavailability was 15.1% $\pm$ 5.3% for L-carnitine from CARNITOR® Tablets and 15.9% $\pm$ 4.9% from the Oral Solution.
Total body clearance of L-carnitine (Dose/AUC including endogenous baseline levels) was a mean of 4.00 L/hr. Endogenous baseline levels were not subtracted since total body clearance of L-carnitine does not distinguish between exogenous sources of L-carnitine and endogenously synthesized L-carnitine. Volume of distribution of the intravenously administered dose above baseline endogenous levels was calculated to be a mean of 29.0 L $\pm$ 7.1 L (approximately 0.39 L/kg) which is an underestimate of the true volume of distribution since plasma L-carnitine is known to equilibrate slowly with, for instance, muscle L-carnitine.
L-carnitine was not bound to plasma protein or albumin when tested at any concentration or with any species including the human.[9]

METABOLISM AND EXCRETION

Five normal adult male volunteers, administered a dose of [^{3}H-methyl]-L-carnitine following 15 days of a high carnitine diet and additional carnitine supplement, excreted 58–65% of administered radioactive dose in 5 to 11 days in the urine and feces. Maximum concentration of [^{3}H-methyl]-L-carnitine in serum occurred from 2.0 to 4.5 hr after drug administration. Major metabolites found were trimethylamine N-oxide, primarily in urine (8% to 49% of the administered dose) and [^{3}H]-γ-butyrobetaine, primarily in feces (0.44% to 45% of the administered dose). Urinary excretion of carnitine was 4% to 8% of the dose. Fecal excretion of total carnitine was less than 1% of total carnitine excretion.[10]
After attainment of steady state following 4 days of oral administration of L-carnitine with CARNITOR® Tablets (1980 mg q12h) or Oral Solution (2000 mg q12h) to 15 healthy male volunteers, urinary excretion of L-carnitine was a mean of 2107 and 2339 μmoles, respectively, equivalent to 8.6% and 9.4%, respectively, of the orally administered doses (uncorrected for endogenous urinary excretion). After a single intravenous dose (20 mg/kg) prior to multiple oral doses, urinary excretion of L-carnitine was 6974 μmoles equivalent to 75.6% of the intravenously administered dose (uncorrected for endogenous urinary excretion).

INDICATIONS AND USAGE

CARNITOR® (Levocarnitine) is indicated in the treatment of primary systemic carnitine deficiency. In the reported cases, the clinical presentation consisted of recurrent episodes of Reye-like encephalopathy, hypoketotic hypoglycemia, and/or cardiomyopathy. Associated symptoms included hypotonia, muscle weakness and failure to thrive. A diagnosis of primary carnitine deficiency requires that serum, red cell and/or tissue carnitine levels be low and that the patient does not have a primary defect in fatty acid or organic acid oxidation (see Clinical Pharmacology). In some patients, particularly those presenting with cardiomyopathy, carnitine supplementation rapidly alleviated signs and symptoms. Treatment should include, in addition to carnitine, supportive and other therapy as indicated by the condition of the patient.
CARNITOR® (Levocarnitine) is also indicated for acute and chronic treatment of patients with an inborn error of metabolism that results in a secondary carnitine deficiency.

CONTRAINDICATIONS

None known.

WARNINGS

None.

PRECAUTIONS

General
CARNITOR® (Levocarnitine) Oral Solution is for oral/internal use only.
Not for parenteral use.
Gastrointestinal reactions may result from too rapid consumption of carnitine. CARNITOR® (Levocarnitine) Oral Solution may be consumed alone, or dissolved in drinks or other liquid foods to reduce taste fatigue. It should be consumed slowly and doses should be spaced evenly throughout the day to maximize tolerance.
Carcinogenesis, mutagenesis, impairment of fertility
Mutagenicity tests have been performed in *Salmonella typhimurium*, *Saccharomyces cerevisiae*, and *Schizosaccharomyces pombe* that do not indicate that CARNITOR® (Levocarnitine) is mutagenic. Long-term animal studies have not been conducted to evaluate the carcinogenicity of the compound.
Pregnancy
Pregnancy Category B.
Reproductive studies have been performed in rats and rabbits at doses up to 3.8 times the human dose on the basis of surface area and have revealed no evidence of impaired fertility or harm to the fetus due to CARNITOR®. There are, however, no adequate and well controlled studies in pregnant women. Because animal reproduction studies are not always predictive of human response, this drug should be used during pregnancy only if clearly needed.
Nursing mothers
It is not known whether this drug is excreted in human milk. Because many drugs are excreted in human milk, a decision should be made whether to discontinue nursing or to discontinue the drug, taking into account the importance of the drug to the mother.
Pediatric use
See Dosage and Administration.

ADVERSE REACTIONS

Various mild gastrointestinal complaints have been reported during the long-term administration of oral L- or D,L-carnitine; these include transient nausea and vomiting, abdominal cramps, and diarrhea. Mild myasthenia has been described only in uremic patients receiving D,L-carnitine. Gastrointestinal adverse reactions with CARNITOR® (Levocarnitine) Oral Solution dissolved in liquids might be avoided by a slow consumption of the solution or by a greater dilution. Decreasing the dosage often diminishes or eliminates drug-related patient body odor or gastrointestinal symptoms when present. Tolerance should be monitored very closely during the first week of administration, and after any dosage increases.

OVERDOSAGE

There have been no reports of toxicity from carnitine overdosage. The oral LD_{50} of levocarnitine in mice is 19.2 g/kg. Carnitine may cause diarrhea. Overdosage should be treated with supportive care.

DOSAGE AND ADMINISTRATION

CARNITOR® (Levocarnitine) Tablets.
Adults: The recommended oral dosage for adults is 990 mg two or three times a day using the 330 mg tablets, depending on clinical response.
Infants and children: The recommended oral dosage for infants and children is between 50 and 100 mg/kg/day in divided doses, with a maximum of 3 g/day. Dosage should begin at 50 mg/kg/day. The exact dosage will depend on clinical response.
Monitoring should include periodic blood chemistries, vital signs, plasma carnitine concentrations and overall clinical condition.
CARNITOR® (Levocarnitine) Oral Solution
For oral use only. **Not for parenteral use.**
Adults: The recommended dosage of levocarnitine is 1 to 3 g/day for a 50 kg subject which is equivalent to 10 to 30 mL/day of CARNITOR® (Levocarnitine) Oral Solution. Higher doses should be administered only with caution and only where clinical and biochemical considerations make it seem likely that higher doses will be of benefit. Dosage should start at 1 g/day, (10 mL/day), and be increased slowly while assessing tolerance and therapeutic response. Monitoring should include periodic blood chemistries, vital signs, plasma carnitine concentrations, and overall clinical condition.
Infants and children: The recommended dosage of levocarnitine is 50 to 100 mg/kg/day which is equivalent to 0.5 mL/kg/day CARNITOR® (Levocarnitine) Oral Solution. Higher doses should be administered only with caution and only where clinical and biochemical considerations make it seem likely that higher doses will be of benefit. Dosage should start at 50 mg/kg/day, and be increased slowly to a maximum of 3 g/day (30 mL/day) while assessing tolerance and therapeutic response. Monitoring should include periodic blood chemistries, vital signs, plasma carnitine concentrations, and overall clinical condition.
CARNITOR® (Levocarnitine) Oral Solution may be consumed alone or dissolved in drink or other liquid food. Doses should be spaced evenly throughout the day (every three or four hours) preferably during or following meals and should be consumed slowly in order to maximize tolerance.

HOW SUPPLIED

CARNITOR® (Levocarnitine) Tablets are supplied as 330 mg (unit dose) tablets embossed with "CARNITOR S-T" in individual blisters packaged in boxes of 90 (NDC 54482-144-07). Store at room temperature (25°C/77°F).
CARNITOR® (Levocarnitine) Oral Solution is supplied in 118 mL (4 FL. OZ.) multiple-unit plastic containers. The multiple-unit containers are packaged 24 per case (NDC 54482-145-08). Store at room temperature (25°C/77°F).
CARNITOR® (Levocarnitine) Oral Solution manufactured for: Sigma-Tau Pharmaceuticals, Inc. By: Barre-National, Inc. Baltimore, MD 21207-2642.
CARNITOR® (Levocarnitine) is also available in the following dosage form for intravenous injection: CARNITOR® (levocarnitine) Injection, 200 mg per 1 mL, is available in 5 mL single dose ampoules packaged 5 ampoules per carton (NDC 54482-146-09) and 2.5 mL single dose ampoules pack-

aged 5 ampoules per carton (NDC 54482-146-10). Made in Italy.

CAUTION

Federal (U.S.A.) law prohibits dispensing without prescription.

CARNITOR® (Levocarnitine) Oral Solution manufactured for: Sigma-Tau Pharmaceuticals, Inc. By: Barre-National, Inc. Baltimore, MD 21244-2654

REFERENCES

1. Bohmer T, Rynding A, Solberg HE: Carnitine levels in human serum in health and disease. **Clin Chim Acta 57**:55–61, 1974.
2. Brooks H, Goldberg L, Holland R et al: Carnitine-induced effects on cardiac and peripheral hemodynamics. **J Clin Pharmacol 17**:561–578, 1977.
3. Christiansen R, Bremer J: Active transport of butyrobetaine and carnitine into isolated liver cells. **Biochem Biophys Acta 448**:562–577, 1977.
4. Lindstedt S, Lindstedt G: Distribution and excretion of carnitine $^{14}CO_2$ in the rat. **Acta Chim Scand 15**:701–702, 1961.
5. Rebouche CJ, Engel AG: Carnitine metabolism and deficiency syndromes. **Mayo Clin Proc 58**:533–540, 1983.
6. Rebouche CJ, Paulson DJ: Carnitine metabolism and function in humans. **Ann Rev Nutr 6**:41–68, 1986.
7. Scriver CR, Beaudet AL, Sly WS, Valle D: The Metabolic Basis of Inherited Disease. McGraw-Hill, New York, 1989.
8. Schaub J, Van Hoof F, Vis HL: Inborn Errors of Metabolism. Raven Press, New York, 1991.
9. Marzo A, Arrigoni Martelli E, Mancinelli A, Cardace G, Corbelletta C, Bassani E, Solbiati M: Protein binding of L-carnitine family components. **Eur J Drug Met Pharmacokin**, Special Issue III: 364–368, 1992.
10. Rebouche C: Quantitative estimation of absorption and degradation of a carnitine supplement by human adults. **Metabolism**: 1305–1310, 1991.

sigma-tau
PHARMACEUTICALS, INC.
800 South Frederick Avenue,
Gaithersburg, MD 20877

PREVIOUS EDITION IS OBSOLETE
ST-N18-948-01/96

SmithKline Beecham Consumer Healthcare

Unit of SmithKline Beecham Inc.
POST OFFICE BOX 1467
PITTSBURGH, PA 15230

Direct Inquiries to:
1-800-245-1040 weekdays

CĒPASTAT® Lozenges — OTC

[sēp 'ă-stăt]

(See PDR For Nonprescription Drugs.)

DEBROX® Drops — OTC

[de 'brox]
Ear Wax Removal Aid

(See PDR For Nonprescription Drugs.)

ECOTRIN® — OTC

Enteric-Coated Aspirin
Antiarthritic, Antiplatelet

DESCRIPTION

'Ecotrin' is enteric-coated aspirin (acetylsalicylic acid, ASA) available in tablet form in 81 mg, 325 mg and 500 mg dosage units, and in caplet form in 500 mg dosage units.

The enteric coating covers a core of aspirin and is designed to resist disintegration in the stomach, dissolving in the more neutral-to-alkaline environment of the duodenum. Such action helps to protect the stomach from injury that may result from ingestion of plain, buffered or highly buffered aspirin (see SAFETY).

INDICATIONS

'Ecotrin' is indicated for:

- conditions requiring chronic or long-term aspirin therapy for pain and/or inflammation, e.g., rheumatoid arthritis, juvenile rheumatoid arthritis, systemic lupus erythematosus, osteoarthritis (degenerative joint disease), ankylosing spondylitis, psoriatic arthritis, Reiter's syndrome and fibrositis,
- antiplatelet indications of aspirin (see the ANTIPLATELET EFFECT section) and
- situations in which compliance with aspirin therapy may be affected because of the gastrointestinal side effects of plain, i.e., non-enteric-coated, or buffered aspirin.

DOSAGE

For analgesic or anti-inflammatory indications, the OTC maximum dosage for aspirin is 4000 mg per day in divided doses, i.e., up to 650 mg every 4 hours or 1000 mg every 6 hours.

For antiplatelet effect dosage: see the ANTIPLATELET EFFECT section.

Under a physician's direction, the dosage can be increased or otherwise modified as appropriate to the clinical situation. When 'Ecotrin' is used for anti-inflammatory effect, the physician should be attentive to plasma salicylate levels, and may also caution the patient to be alert to the development of tinnitus as an indicator of elevated salicylate levels. It should be noted that patients with a high frequency hearing loss (such as may occur in older individuals) may have difficulty perceiving the tinnitus. Tinnitus would then not be a reliable indicator in such individuals.

INACTIVE INGREDIENTS

81 mg: Carnauba Wax, D&C Yellow 10, FD&C Yellow 6, Hydroxypropyl Methylcellulose, Methacrylic Acid Copolymer, Microcrystalline Cellulose, Polyethylene Glycol, Polysorbate 80, Propylene Glycol, Silicon Dioxide, Starch, Stearic Acid, Talc, Titanium Dioxide, Triethyl Citrate.

325 mg and 500 mg: Carnauba wax, Colloidal Silicon Dioxide, FD&C Yellow #6, Hydroxypropyl Methylcellulose, Maltodextrin, Methacrylic Acid Copolymer, Microcrystalline Cellulose, Pregelatinized Starch, Propylene Glycol, Simethicone, Sodium Hydroxide, Sodium Starch Glycolate, Stearic Acid, Talc, Titanium Dioxide, Triethyl Citrate.

BIOAVAILABILITY

The bioavailability of aspirin from 'Ecotrin' has been demonstrated in a number of salicylate excretion studies. The studies show levels of salicylate (and metabolites) in urine excreted over 48 hours for 'Ecotrin' do not differ statistically from plain, i.e., non-enteric-coated, aspirin.

Plasma studies, in which 'Ecotrin' has been compared with plain aspirin in steady-state studies over eight days, also demonstrate that 'Ecotrin' provides plasma salicylate levels not statistically different from plain aspirin.

Information regarding salicylate levels over a range of doses was generated in a study in which 24 healthy volunteers (12 male and 12 female) took daily (divided) doses of either 2600 mg, 3900 mg, or 5200 mg of 'Ecotrin'. Plasma salicylate levels generally acknowledged to be anti-inflammatory (15 mg/dL) were attained at daily doses of 5200 mg, on Day 2 by females and Day 3 by males. At 3900 mg, anti-inflammatory levels were attained at Day 3 by females and Day 4 by males.

Dissolution of the enteric coating occurs at a neutral-to-basic pH and is therefore dependent on gastric emptying into the duodenum. With continued dosing, appropriate plasma levels are maintained.

SAFETY

The safety of 'Ecotrin' has been demonstrated in a number of endoscopic studies comparing 'Ecotrin', plain aspirin, buffered aspirin, and highly buffered aspirin preparations. In these studies, all forms of aspirin were dosed to the OTC maximum (3900–4000 mg per day) for up to 14 days. The normal healthy volunteers participating in these studies were gastroscoped before and after the courses of treatment and 14-day drug-free periods followed active drug. Compared to all the other preparations, there was less gastric damage at a statistically significant level during the 'Ecotrin' courses. There was also statistically less duodenal damage when compared with the plain i.e., non-enteric-coated aspirin.

Details of studies demonstrating the safety and bioavailability of 'Ecotrin' are available to health care professionals. Write: Professional Services Department, SmithKline Beecham Consumer Healthcare, P.O. Box 1467, Pittsburgh, Pa. 15230.

WARNINGS

Children and teenagers should not use this product for chicken pox or flu symptoms before a doctor is consulted about Reye Syndrome, a rare but serious illness reported to be associated with aspirin. Do not take this product for pain for more than 10 days or for fever for more than 3 days, or in conditions affecting children under 12 years of age, unless directed by a doctor. If pain or fever persists or gets worse, if new symptoms occur, or if redness or swelling is present, consult a doctor because these could be signs of a serious condition. Do not take this product if you are allergic to aspirin, have asthma, have stomach problems that persist or recur, or if you have ulcers or bleeding problems unless directed by a doctor. If ringing in the ears or a loss of hearing occurs, consult a doctor before taking any more of this product. **Keep this and all drugs out of the reach of children.** In case of accidental overdose, seek professional assistance or contact a poison control center immediately. As with any medicine, if you are pregnant or nursing a baby, seek the advice of a health professional before using this product. **IT IS ESPECIALLY IMPORTANT NOT TO USE ASPIRIN DURING THE LAST 3 MONTHS OF PREGNANCY UNLESS SPECIFICALLY DIRECTED TO DO SO BY A DOCTOR BECAUSE IT MAY CAUSE PROBLEMS IN THE UNBORN CHILD OR COMPLICATIONS DURING DELIVERY.**

Drug Interaction Precaution: Do not take this product if you are taking a prescription drug for anticoalgulation (thinning of the blood), diabetes, gout, or arthritis unless directed by a doctor.

Professional Warning: There have been occasional reports in the literature concerning individuals with impaired gastric emptying in whom there may be retention of one or more enteric coated aspirin tablets over time. This unusual phenomenon may occur as a result of outlet obstruction from ulcer disease alone or combined with hypotonic gastric peristalsis. Because of the integrity of the enteric coating in an acidic environment, these tablets may accumulate and form a bezoar in the stomach. Individuals with this condition may present with complaints of early satiety or of vague upper abdominal distress. Diagnosis may be made by endoscopy or by abdominal films which show opacities suggestive of a mass of small tablets *(Ref.: Bogacz, K. and Caldron, P.: Enteric-coated Aspirin Bezoar: Elevation of Serum Salicylate Level by Barium Study. Amer. J. Med. 1987:83, 783-6.)*. Management may vary according to the condition of the patient. Options include: gastrotomy and alternating slightly basic and neutral lavage *(Ref.: Baum, J.: Enteric-Coated Aspirin and the Problem of Gastric Retention. J. Rheum., 1984:11, 250-1.)*. While there have been no clinical reports, it has been suggested that such individuals may also be treated with parenteral cimetidine (to reduce acid secretion) and then given sips of slightly basic liquids to effect gradual dissolution of the enteric coating. Progress may be followed with plasma salicylate levels or via recognition of tinnitus by the patient.

It should be kept in mind that individuals with a history of partial or complete gastrectomy may produce reduced amounts of acid and therefore have less acidic gastric pH. Under these circumstances, the benefits offered by the acid-resistant enteric coating may not exist.

ANTIARTHRITIC AND ANTI-INFLAMMATORY INDICATIONS

For rheumatoid arthritis, juvenile rheumatoid arthritis, systemic lupus erythematosus, osteoarthritis (degenerative joint disease), ankylosing spondylitis, psoriatic arthritis, Reiter's syndrome, and fibrositis.

ANTIPLATELET EFFECT

Aspirin may be recommended to reduce the risk of death and/or nonfatal myocardial infarction (MI) in patients with a previous infarction or unstable angina pectoris and its use in reducing the risk of transient ischemic attacks in men.

Aspirin is also indicated to reduce the risk of vascular mortality in patients with suspected acute MI. Indications for these conditions follow:

ASPIRIN FOR MYOCARDIAL INFARCTION INDICATIONS

Recurrent Myocardial Infarction (MI) (Reinfarction) or Unstable Angina Pectoris: Aspirin is indicated to reduce the risk of death and/or nonfatal MI in patients with a previous MI or unstable angina pectoris.

Suspected Acute MI: Aspirin is indicated to reduce the risk of vascular mortality in patients with a suspected acute MI.

CLINICAL TRIALS

Recurrent MI (Reinfarction) and Unstable Angina Pectoris: The indication is supported by the results of six large, randomized multicenter, placebo-controlled studies involving 10,816, predominantly male, post-myocardial infarction (MI) patients and one randomized placebo-controlled study of 1,266 men with unstable angina (1–7). Therapy with aspirin was begun at intervals after the onset of acute MI varying from less than 3 days to more than 5 years and continued for periods of from less than 1 year to 4 years. In the unstable angina study, treatment was started within 1 month after the onset of unstable angina and continued for 12 weeks, and congestive heart failure were not included in the study.

Aspirin therapy in MI patients was associated with about a 20-percent reduction in the risk of subsequent death and/or non-fatal reinfarction, a median absolute decrease of 3 percent from the 12- to 22-percent event rates in the placebo groups. In aspirin-treated unstable angina patients the reduction in risk was about 50 percent, a reduction in event rate of 5 percent from the 10-percent rate in the placebo group over the 12-weeks of the study.

Daily dosage of aspirin in the post-myocardial infarction studies was 300 milligrams in one study and 900 to 1,500 milligrams in 5 studies. A dose of 325 milligrams was used in the study of unstable angina.

Continued on next page

SmithKline Beecham Consumer—Cont.

Suspected Acute MI: The use of aspirin in patients with a suspected acute MI is supported by the results of a large, multicenter 2 × 2 factorial study of 17,187 subjects with suspected acute MI (8). Subjects were randomized within 24 hours of the onset of symptoms so that 8,587 subjects received oral aspirin (162.5 milligrams, enteric-coated) daily for 1 month (the first dose crushed, sucked, or chewed) and 8,600 received oral placebo. Of the subjects, 8,592 were also randomized to receive a single dose of streptokinase (1.5 million units) infused intravenously for about 1 hour, and 8,595 received a placebo infusion. Thus, 4,295 subjects received aspirin plus placebo, 4,300 received streptokinase plus placebo, 4,292 received aspirin plus streptokinase, and 4,300 received double placebo.

Vascular mortality (attributed to cardiac, cerebral, hemorrhagic, other vascular, or unknown causes) occurred in 9.4 percent of the subjects in the aspirin group and in 11.8 percent of the subjects in the oral placebo group in the 35-day followup. This represents an absolute reduction of 2.4 percent in the mean 35-day vascular mortality attributable to aspirin and a 23 percent reduction in the odds of vascular death (2p <0.0001).

Significant absolute reductions in mortality and corresponding reductions in specific clinical events favoring aspirin were found for reinfarction (1.5 percent absolute reduction, 45 percent odds reduction, 2p <0.0001), cardiac arrest (1.2 percent absolute reduction, 14.2 percent odds reduction, 2p <0.01), and total stroke (0.4 percent absolute reduction, 41.5 percent odds reduction, 2p <0.01). The effect of aspirin over and above its effect on mortality was evidenced by small, but significant, reductions in vascular morbidity in those subjects who were discharged.

The beneficial effects of aspirin on mortality were present with or without streptokinase infusion. Aspirin reduced vascular mortality from 10.4 to 8.0 percent for days 0 to 35 in subjects given streptokinase and reduced vascular mortality from 13.2 to 10.7 percent in subjects given no streptokinase. The effects of aspirin and thrombolytic therapy with streptokinase in this study were approximately additive. subjects who received the combination of streptokinase infusion and daily aspirin had significantly lower vascular mortality at 35 days than those who received either active treatment alone (combination 8.0 percent, aspirin 10.7 percent, streptokinase 10.4 percent, and no treatment 13.2 percent). While this study demonstrated that aspirin has an additive benefit in patients given streptokinase, there is no reason to restrict its use to that specific thrombolytic.

ADVERSE REACTIONS

Gastrointestinal Reactions: Doses of 1,000 milligrams per day of aspirin caused gastrointestinal symptoms and bleeding that in some cases were clinically significant. In the largest post-infarction study (the Aspirin Myocardial Infarction Study (AMIS) with 4,500 people), the percentage incidences of gastrointestinal symptoms for the aspirin (1,000 milligrams of a standard, solid-tablet formulation) and placebo-treated subjects, respectively, were: stomach pain (14.5 percent; 4.4 percent); heartburn (11.9 percent; 4.8 percent); nausea and/or vomiting (7.6 percent; 2.1 percent); hospitalization for gastrointestinal disorder (4.8 percent; 3.5 percent). Symptoms and signs of gastrointestinal irritation were not significantly increased in subjects treated for unstable angina with 325 milligrams buffered aspirin in solution.

Bleeding: In the AMIS and other trials, aspirin-treated subjects had increased rates of gross gastrointestinal bleeding. In the ISIS-2 study (8), there was no significant difference in the incidence of major bleeding (bleeds requiring transfusion) between 8,587 subjects taking 162.5 milligrams aspirin daily and 8,600 subjects taking placebo (31 versus 33 subjects). There were five confirmed cerebral hemorrhages in the aspirin group compared with two in the placebo group, but the incidence of stroke of all causes was significantly reduced from 81 to 47 for the placebo versus aspirin group (0.4 percent absolute change). There was a small and statistically significant excess (0.6 percent) of minor bleeding in people taking aspirin (2.5 percent for aspirin, 1.9 percent for placebo). No other significant adverse effects were reported.

Cardiovascular and Biochemical: In the AMIS trial, the dosage of 1,000 milligrams per day of aspirin was associated with small increases in systolic blood pressure (BP) (average 1.5 to 2.1 millimeters), depending upon whether maximal or last available readings were used. Blood urea nitrogen and uric acid levels were also increased, but by less than 1.0 milligram percent.

Subjects with marked hypertension or renal insufficiency had been excluded from the trial so that the clinical importance of these observations for such subjects or for any subjects treated over more prolonged periods is not known. It is recommended that patients placed on long-term aspirin treatment, even at doses of 300 milligrams per day, be seen at regular intervals to assess changes in these measurements.

Sodium in Buffered Aspirin for Solution Formulations: One tablet daily of buffered aspirin in solutions adds 553 milligrams of sodium to that in the diet and may not be tolerated by patients with active sodium-retaining states such as congestive heart or renal failure. This amount of sodium adds about 30 percent to the 70- to 90-millieqivalents intake suggested as appropriate for dietary treatment of essential hypertension in the "1984 Report of the Joint National Committee on Detection, Evaluation, and Treatment of High Blood Pressure" (9).

DOSAGE AND ADMINISTRATION

Recurrent MI (Reinfarction) and Unstable Angina Pectoris:- Although most of the studies used dosages exceeding 300 milligrams, 2 trials used only 300 millgrams and pharmacologic data indicate that this dose inhibits platelet function fully. Therefore, 300 milligrams or a conventional 325 milligram aspirin dose is a reasonable, routine dose that would minimize gastrointestinal adverse reactions. This use of aspirin applies to both solid, oral dosage forms (buffered and plain aspirin) and buffered aspirin in solution.

Suspected Acute MI: The recommended dose of aspirin to treat suspected acute MI is 160 to 162.5 milligrams taken as soon as the infarct is suspected and then daily for at least 30 days. (One-half of a conventional 325-milligram aspirin tablet or two 80- or 81-milligram aspirin tablets may be taken.) This use of aspirin applies to both solid, oral dosage forms buffered, plain, and enteric-coated aspirin) and buffered aspirin in solution. If using a solid dosage form, the first dose should be crushed, sucked, or chewed. After the 30-day treatment, physicians should consider further therapy based on the labeling for dosage and administration of aspirin for prevention of recurrent MI (reinfarction).

REFERENCES

(1) Elwood, P.C. et al., "A Randomized Controlled Trial of Acetylsalicylic Acid in the Secondary Prevention of Mortality from Myocardial Infarction," British Medical Journal, 1:436–440, 1974.

(2) The Coronary Drug Project Research Group, "Aspirin in Coronary Heart Disease," Journal of Chronic Diseases, 29:625–642, 1976.

(3) Breddin, K. et al., "Secondary Prevention of Myocardial Infarction: A Comparison of Acetylsalicylic Acid, Phenprocoumon or Placebo," Homeostasis, 470:263–268, 1979.

(4) Aspirin Myocardial Infarction Study Research Group, "A Randomized, Controlled Trial of Aspirin in Persons Recovered from Myocardial Infarction," Journal of the American Medical Aassociation, 243:661–669, 1980.

(5) Elwood, P.C., and P.M. Sweetnam, "Aspirin and Secondary Mortality After Myocardial Infarction," Lancet, II:1313–1315, December 22–29, 1979.

(6) The Persantine-Aspirin Reinfarction Study Research Group, "Persantine and Aspirin in Coronary Heart Disease," Circulation, 62:449–461, 1980.

(7) Lewis, H.D. et al., "Protective Effects of Aspirin Against Acute Myocardial Infarction and Death in Men with Unstable Angina, Results of a Veterans Administration Cooperative Study," New England Journal of Medicine, 309:396–403, 1983.

(8) ISIS-2 (Second International Study of Infarct Survival) Collaborative Group, "Randomized Trial of Intravenous Streptokinase, Oral Aspirin, Both, or Neither Among 17,187 Cases of Suspected Acute Myocardial Infarction: ISIS-2," Lancet, 2:349-360, August 13, 1988.

(8) "1984 Report of the Joint National Committee on Detection, Evaluation, and Treatment of High Blood Pressure," United States Department of Health and Human Services and United States Public Health Service, National Institutes of Health, Publication No. NIH 84-1088, 1984.

"ASPIRIN FOR TRANSIENT ISCHEMIC ATTACKS"

Indication

For reducing the risk of recurrent Transient Ischemic Attacks (TIA's) or stroke in men who have had transient ischemia of the brain due to fibrin platelet emboli. There is inadequate evidence that aspirin or buffered aspirin is effective in reducing TIA's in women at the recommended dosage. There is no evidence that aspirin or buffered aspirin is of benefit in the treatment of completed strokes in men or women.

Clinical Trials

The indication is supported by the results of a Canadian study (1) in which 585 patients with threatened stroke were followed in a randomized clinical trial for an average of 26 months to determine whether aspirin or sulfinpyrazone, singly or in combination, was superior to placebo in preventing transient ischemic attacks, stroke or death. The study showed that, although sulfinpyrazone had no statistically significant effect, aspirin reduced the risk of continuing transient ischemic attacks, stroke or death by 19 percent and reduced the risk of stroke or death by 31 percent. Another aspirin study carried out in the United States with 178 patients, showed a statistically significant number of "favorable outcomes," including reduced transient ischemic attacks, stroke and death (2).

Precautions

Patients presenting with signs and/or symptoms of TIA's should have a complete medical and neurologic evaluation. Consideration should be given to other disorders that resemble TIA's. Attention should be given to risk factors: it is important to evaluate and treat, if appropriate, other diseases associated with TIA's and stroke, such as hypertension and diabetes.

Concurrent administration of absorbable antacids at therapeutic doses may increase the clearance of salicylates in some individuals. The concurrent administration of nonabsorbable antacids may alter the rate of absorption of aspirin, thereby resulting in a decreased acetylsalicylic acid/salicylate ratio in plasma. The clinical significance of these decreases in available aspirin is unknown.

Aspirin at dosages of 1,000 milligrams per day has been associated with small increases in blood pressure, blood urea nitrogen, and serum uric acid levels. It is recommended that patients placed on long-term aspirin treatment be seen at regular intervals to assess changes in these measurements.

Adverse Reactions:

At dosages of 1,000 milligrams or higher of aspirin per day, gastrointestinal side effects include stomach pain, heartburn, nausea and/or vomiting, as well as increased rates of gross gastrointestinal bleeding.

Dosage and Administration

Adult dosage for men is 1,300 mg a day, in divided doses of 650 mg twice a day or 325 mg four times a day.

References

(1) The Canadian Cooperative Study Group, "Randomized Trial of Aspirin and Sulfinpyrazone in Threatened Stroke," *New England Journal of Medicine,* 299:53–59, 1978.

(2) Fields, W. S., et al., "Controlled Trial of Aspirin in Cerebral Ischemia," *Stroke* 8:301–316, 1977."

HOW SUPPLIED

'Ecotrin' Tablets
- 81 mg in bottle of 36
- 325 mg in bottles of 100* and 250
- 500 mg in bottles of 60* and 150

'Ecotrin' Caplets
- 500 mg in bottles of 60.

*Without child-resistant caps.

TAMPER-RESISTANT PACKAGE FEATURES FOR YOUR PROTECTION:

- Bottle has imprinted seal under cap.
- The words ECOTRIN LOW or ECOTRIN REG or ECOTRIN MAX appear on each tablet or caplet (see product illustration printed on carton).
- **DO NOT USE THIS PRODUCT IF ANY OF THESE TAMPER-RESISTANT FEATURES ARE MISSING OR BROKEN.**

Comments or Questions? Call Toll-Free 800-245-1040 weekdays.

FEOSOL® Caplets **OTC**
Hematinic
Iron Supplement

DESCRIPTION

FEOSOL Caplets contain pure iron micro particles called carbonyl iron. Replacing FEOSOL Capsules, this advanced formula is specially designed to be well absorbed, gentle on the stomach and offers enhanced safety in the event of an accidental overdose. Each FEOSOL carbonyl iron caplet delivers 50 mg of pure elemental iron, the same amount of elemental iron contained in the 250 mg ferrous sulfate capsule. At equivalent doses, carbonyl iron and ferrous sulfate were shown to be equally efficacious in correcting hemoglobin, hematocrit and serum iron levels in iron-deficient patients[1].

SAFETY

According to the American Association of Poison Control Centers, iron containing supplements are the leading cause of pediatric poisoning deaths for children under six in the United States[2]. Widely used as a food additive, carbonyl iron must be gastrically solubilized before it can be absorbed, giving it lower toxicity and enhancing its safety versus any of the ferrous salts[3]. As a result, carbonyl iron presents less chance of harm from accidental overdose. In addition, at equivalent doses, carbonyl iron side effects are no greater than those experienced with ferrous sulfate[4].

WARNINGS

Do not exceed recommended dosage. The treatment of any anemic condition should be under the advice and supervision of a physician. Since oral iron products interfere with absorption of oral tetracycline antibiotics, these products should not be taken within two hours of each other. Occasional gastrointestinal discomfort (such as nausea) may be minimized by taking with meals. Iron containing medication may occasionally cause constipation or diarrhea.

Keep out of the reach of children. Contains iron, which can be harmful or fatal to children in large doses. In case of accidental overdose, seek professional assistance or contact a poison control center immediately. If you are pregnant or nursing a baby, seek the advice of a health professional before using this product.

NUTRITION FACTS
Serving Size: 1 Tablet

Amount per Tablet	% Daily Value
Iron 50 mg	280%

FORMULA
INGREDIENTS
Lactose, Sorbitol, Carbonyl Iron, Hydroxypropyl Methylcellulose, Polydextrose, Crospovidone, Polyethylene Glycol, Magnesium Stearate, Stearic Acid, Triacetin, Titanium Dioxide, Maltodextrin, FD&C Blue #2, FD&C Red #40, FD&C Yellow #6.

DIRECTIONS
Adults—one caplet daily or as directed by a physician. Children under 12 years: Consult a physician.

TAMPER-EVIDENT FEATURE
Each caplet is encased in a plastic cell with a foil back; do not use if cell or foil is broken.

REFERENCES
[1]Devasthali SD, Gordeuk VR, Brittenham GM, et al, "Bioavailability of Carbonyl Iron: A randomized, double-blind study." Eur J Haematology, 1991; 46:272–278.
[2]FDA Consumer; March 1996:7
[3]Heubers, JA, Brittenham GM, Csiba E and Finch CA. "Absorption of carbonyl iron." J Lab Clin Med 1986; 108:473–78.
[4]Devasthali SD, Gordeuk VR, Brittenham GM, et al, "Bioavailability of a Carbonyl Iron: A randomized, double-blind study." Eur J Haematology, 1991; 46:272–278.
Store at room temperature, avoid excessive heat (greater than 100°F) or humidity.

HOW SUPPLIED
Boxes of 30 and 60 caplets in blisters
Comments or Questions? Call Toll-Free 1-800-245-1040 Weekdays.
SmithKline Beecham Consumer Healthcare, L.P.
Pittsburgh, PA 15230   Made in USA

FEOSOL® ELIXIR   OTC
Hematinic
Iron Supplement

DESCRIPTION
'Feosol' Elixir, an unusually palatable iron elixir, provides the body with ferrous sulfate—iron in its most efficient form. The standard elixir for simple iron deficiency and iron-deficiency anemia when the need for such therapy has been determined by a physician.

NUTRITION FACTS
Serving Size: 1 teaspoonful
Servings per Container: 94

Amount per teaspoonful	% Daily Value
Iron 44 mg	244%

FORMULA
INGREDIENTS
Purified Water, Sucrose, Glucose, Alcohol 5%, Ferrous Sulfate, Citric Acid, Saccharin Sodium, FD&C Yellow #6, Flavors.

DIRECTIONS
Adults—1 teaspoonful daily or as directed by a doctor. Children under 12 years—Consult a physician. Mix with water or fruit juice to avoid temporary staining of teeth; do not mix with milk or wine-based vehicles.

TAMPER-RESISTANT PACKAGE FEATURE:
IMPRINTED SEAL AROUND BOTTLE CAP: DO NOT USE IF BROKEN.

WARNINGS
Do not exceed recommended dosage. The treatment of any anemic condition should be under the advice and supervision of a physician. Since oral iron products interfere with absorption of oral tetracycline antibiotics, these products should not be taken within two hours of each other. Occasional gastrointestinal discomfort (such as nausea) may be minimized by taking with meals. Iron containing medication may occasionally cause constipation or diarrhea and liquids may cause temporary staining of the teeth (this is less likely when diluted). **Keep away from children. Close tightly. Contains iron, which can be harmful or fatal to children in large doses. In case of accidental overdosage, seek professional** assistance or contact a poison control center immediately. If you are pregnant or nursing a baby, seek the advice of a health professional before using this product.
STORE AT ROOM TEMPERATURE (59–86 F), PROTECT FROM FREEZING.

HOW SUPPLIED
A clear orange liquid in 16 fl. oz. bottles.

ALSO AVAILABLE
'Feosol' Tablets, 'Feosol' Capsules.
NOTE: There are other Feosol products. Make sure this is the one you are interested in.

FEOSOL® TABLETS   OTC
Hematinic
Iron Supplement

DESCRIPTION
Feosol tablets provide the body with ferrous sulfate—iron in its most efficient form. An iron supplement for iron deficiency and iron deficiency anemia when the need for such therapy has been determined by a physician.

NUTRITION FACTS
Serving Size: 1 Tablet

Amount per Tablet	% Daily Value
Iron 65 mg	361%

FORMULA
INGREDIENTS
Dried ferrous sulfate 200 mg (65 mg of elemental iron) equivalent to 325 mg of ferrous sulfate USP per tablet. Calcium Sulfate, Starch, Glucose, Hydroxypropyl Methylcellulose, Talc, Stearic Acid, Polyethylene Glycol, Sodium Lauryl Sulfate, Mineral Oil, Titanium Dioxide, D&C Yellow 10, FD&C Blue 2.

DIRECTIONS
Adults and children 12 years and over—One tablet daily or as directed by a physician. Children under 12 years—Consult a physician.

TAMPER-RESISTANT PACKAGE FEATURES:
- Bottle has imprinted seal under cap. Do not use if missing or broken.
- FEOSOL Tablets are triangular shaped (see product illustration printed on carton).
CAUTION: DO NOT USE THIS PRODUCT IF ANY OF THESE TAMPER-RESISTANT FEATURES ARE MISSING OR BROKEN.

Comments or Questions?
Call toll-free 800-245-1040 weekdays.

WARNINGS
Do not exceed recommended dosage. The treatment of any anemic condition should be under the advice and supervision of a physician. Since oral iron products interfere with absorption of oral tetracycline antibiotics, these products should not be taken within two hours of each other. Occasional gastrointestinal discomfort (such as nausea) may be minimized by taking with meals. Iron containing medication may occasionally cause constipation or diarrhea. **Keep away from children. Close tightly. Contains iron, which can be harmful or fatal to children in large doses. In case of accidental overdose, seek professional assistance or contact a poison control center immediately. If you are pregnant or nursing a baby, seek the advice of a health professional before using this product.**
Store at room temperature (59–86 F).
Not USP for dissolution.

HOW SUPPLIED
Bottles of 100 tablets; in Single Unit Packages of 100 tablets (intended for institutional use only).
Also available in Capsules and Elixir.
NOTE: There are other FEOSOL Products. Make sure this is the one you are interested in.

GAVISCON® EXTRA STRENGTH   OTC
Antacid Tablets
[găv 'ĭs-kŏn]

(See PDR For Nonprescription Drugs.)

GAVISCON® EXTRA STRENGTH   OTC
Liquid Antacid
[găv 'ĭs-kŏn]

(See PDR For Nonprescription Drugs.)

GAVISCON® REGULAR STRENGTH   OTC
Antacid Tablets
[gav 'ĭs-kon]

(See PDR For Nonprescription Drugs.)

GAVISCON® REGULAR STRENGTH   OTC
Liquid Antacid
[gav 'ĭs-kon]

(See PDR For Nonprescription Drugs.)

GLY–OXIDE® Liquid   OTC
[gli 'ok-sĭd]

(See PDR For Nonprescription Drugs.)

MASSENGILL® Douches, Towelettes   OTC
and Cleansing Wash
[mas 'sen-gil]

PRODUCT OVERVIEW
KEY FACTS
Massengill is the brand name for a line of douches which are recommended for routine cleansing and for temporary relief of vaginal itching and irritation. Massengill disposable douches are available in two Vinegar & Water formulas (Extra Mild and Extra Cleansing), a Baking Soda formula, four Cosmetic solutions (Country Flowers, Fresh Baby Powder Scent, Mountain Breeze, and Spring Rain Freshness), and a Medicated formula (with povidone-iodine). Massengill is also available in a Non-Medicated liquid concentrate and powder form. Massengill also has products specially designed to safely and gently cleanse the external vaginal area: Massengill Soft Cloth Towelettes (Unscented and Baby Powder), Massengill Medicated Soft Cloth Towelettes and Massingill Feminine Cleansing Wash.

MAJOR USES
Massengill's Vinegar & Water, Baking Soda & Water, and Cosmetic douches are recommended for routine douching, or for cleansing following menstruation, prescribed use of vaginal medication or use of contraceptives. Massengill Medicated is recommended in a seven day regimen for the symptomatic relief of minor itching and irritation associated with vaginitis due to Candida albicans, Trichomonas vaginalis, and Gardnerella vaginalis. Massengill Feminine Cleansing Wash is a gentle soapfree way to clean the external vaginal area. Massengill Non-Medicated Soft Cloth Towelettes are a convenient and portable way to cleanse the external vaginal area and wash odor away. Massengill Medicated Soft Cloth Towelettes provide temporary relief of minor external itching associated with irritation or skin rashes.

SAFETY INFORMATION
Do not douche during pregnancy unless directed by a physician. Douching does not prevent pregnancy. Do not use this product and consult your physician if you are experiencing any of the following symptoms: unusual vaginal discharge, vaginal bleeding, painful and/or frequent urination, lower abdominal/pelvis pain, or you or your sex partner has genital sores or ulcers.
Massengill Vinegar & Water, Baking Soda & Water, and Cosmetic Douches—If vaginal dryness or irritation occurs, discontinue use.
Massengill Medicated — Women with iodine-sensitivity should not use this product. If symptoms persist after seven days, or if redness, swelling or pain develop, consult a physician. Do not use while nursing unless directed by a physician.

PRODUCT INFORMATION
MASSENGILL®
[mas 'sen-gil]
Disposable Douches
MASSENGILL®
Liquid Concentrate
MASSENGILL® Powder

INGREDIENTS
DISPOSABLES: Extra Mild Vinegar and Water—Purified Water and Vinegar.
Extra Cleansing Vinegar and Water—Purified Water, Vinegar, Puraclean™ (Cetylpyridinium Chloride), Diazolidinyl Urea, Disodium EDTA.
* Puraclean is a trademark for cetylpyridinium chloride, a safe, special cleansing ingredient not found in any other vinegar & water douche.
Baking Soda and Water—Sanitized Water, Sodium Bicarbonate (Baking Soda).

Continued on next page

SmithKline Beecham Consumer—Cont.

<u>Fresh Baby Powder Scent</u>—Water, SD Alcohol 40, Lactic Acid, Sodium Lactate, Octoxynol-9, Cetylpyridinium Chloride, Propylene Glycol (and) Diazolidinyl Urea (and) Methylparaben (and) Propylparaben, Disodium EDTA, Fragrance, FD&C Blue #1.

<u>Country Flowers</u>—Water, SD Alcohol 40, Lactic Acid, Sodium Lactate, Octoxynol-9, Cetylpyridinium Chloride, Propylene Glycol (and) Diazolidinyl Urea (and), Methylparaben (and) Propylparaben, Disodium EDTA, Fragrance, D&C Red #28, FD&C Blue #1.

<u>Mountain Breeze</u>—Water, SD Alcohol 40, Lactic Acid, Sodium Lactate, Octoxynol-9, Cetylpyridinium Chloride, Propylene Glycol (and) Diazolidinyl Urea (and) Methylparaben (and) Propylparaben, Disodium EDTA, Fragrance, D&C Yellow #10, FD&C Blue #1.

<u>Spring Rain Freshness</u>—Water, SD Alcohol 40, Lactic Acid, Sodium Lactate, Octoxynol-9, Cetylpyridinium Chloride, Propylene Glycol (and) Diazolidinyl Urea (and) Methylparaben (and) Propylparaben, Disodium EDTA, Fragrance.

LIQUID CONCENTRATE: Water, SD Alcohol 40, Lactic Acid, Sodium Bicarbonate, Octoxynol-9, Methyl Salicylate, Eucalyptol, Menthol, Thymol, D&C Yellow #10, FD&C Yellow #6 (Sunset Yellow).

POWDER: Sodium Chloride, Ammonium alum, PEG-8, Phenol, Methyl Salicylate, Eucalyptus Oil, Menthol, Thymol, D&C Yellow #10, FD&C Yellow #6 (Sunset Yellow).

INDICATIONS
Recommended for routine cleansing at the end of menstruation, after use of contraceptive creams or jellies (check the contraceptive package instructions first) or to rinse out the residue of prescribed vaginal medication (as directed by physician).

ACTIONS
The buffered acid solutions of Massengill Douches are valuable adjuncts to specific vaginal therapy following the prescribed use of vaginal medication or contraceptives and in feminine hygiene.

DIRECTIONS
DISPOSABLES: Twist off flat, wing-shaped tab from bottle containing premixed solution, attach nozzle supplied and use. The unit is completely disposable.
LIQUID CONCENTRATE: Fill cap ¾ full, to measuring line, and pour contents into douche bag containing 1 quart of warm water. Mix thoroughly.
POWDER: Packettes—Dissolve the contents of 1 packet in a quart of warm water. Mix thoroughly in a separate container or douche bag. Container—Dissolve two rounded teaspoonfuls in a douche bag containing 1 quart of warm water. Mix thoroughly.

WARNING
Douching does not prevent pregnancy. Do not use during pregnancy except under the advice and supervision of your physician. If vaginal dryness or irritation occurs, discontinue use. Use this product only as directed for routine cleansing. You should douche no more than twice a week except on the advice of your doctor.
An association has been reported between douching and pelvic inflammatory disease (PID), a serious infection of your reproductive system which can lead to sterility and/or ectopic (tubal) pregnancy. PID requires immediate medical attention.
PID's most common symptoms are pain and/or tenderness in the lower part of the abdomen and pelvis. You may also experience a vaginal discharge, vaginal bleeding, nausea or fever. Other sexually transmitted diseases (STDs) have similar symptoms and/or frequent urination, genital sores, or ulcers. Douches should not be used for the self treatment of any STDs or PID. If you suspect you have one of these infections or PID, stop using this product and see your doctor immediately.
See the enclosed insert for important health information concerning sexually transmitted diseases and PID.

HOW SUPPLIED
Disposable—6 oz. disposable plastic bottle.
Liquid Concentrate—4 oz. plastic bottles.
Powder—4 oz., Packettes—12's.

MASSENGILL® Medicated　　　　OTC
[mas'sen-gil]
Disposable Douche

ACTIVE INGREDIENT
Cepticin™ (povidone-iodine)

INDICATIONS
For symptomatic relief of minor vaginal irritation or itching associated with vaginitis due to Candida albicans, Trichomonas vaginalis, and Gardnerella vaginalis.

ACTION
Povidone-iodine is widely recognized as an effective broad spectrum microbicide against both gram negative and gram positive bacteria, fungi, yeasts and protozoa. While remaining active in the presence of blood, serum or bodily secretions, it possesses virtually none of the irritating properties of iodine.

WARNING
Douching does not prevent pregnancy. Do not use during pregnancy or while nursing except under the advice and supervision of your physician. If vaginal dryness or irritation occurs, discontinue use. Use this product only as directed. Do not use this product for routine cleansing.
An association has been reported between douching and pelvic inflammatory disease (PID), a serious infection of your reproductive system which can lead to sterility and/or ectopic (tubal) pregnancy. PID requires immediate medical attention.
PID's most common symptoms are pain and/or tenderness in the lower part of the abdomen and pelvis. You may also experience a vaginal discharge, vaginal bleeding, nausea or fever. Other sexually transmitted diseases (STDs) have similar symptoms and/or frequent urination, genital sores, or ulcers. Douches should not be used for the self treatment of any STDs or PID. If you suspect you have one of these infections or PID, stop using this product and see your doctor immediately.
See the enclosed insert for important health information concerning sexually transmitted diseases and PID.
Women with iodine sensitivity should not use this product. Keep out of the reach of children.
Avoid storing at high temperature (greater than 100°F). Protect from freezing.

DOSAGE AND ADMINISTRATION
Dosage is provided as a single unit concentrate to be added to 6 oz. of sanitized water supplied in a disposable bottle. A specially designed nozzle is provided. After use, the unit is discarded. Use one bottle a day for seven days. Although symptoms may be relieved earlier, for maximum relief, treatment should be continued for the full seven days.

HOW SUPPLIED
6 oz. bottle of sanitized water with 0.17 oz. vial of povidone-iodine and nozzle.

MASSENGILL® Feminine Cleansing Wash　　　OTC
[mas'sen-gil]

INGREDIENTS
Water, sodium laureth sulfate, magnesium laureth sulfate, sodium laureth-8 sulfate, magnesium laureth-8 sulfate, sodium oleth sulfate, magnesium oleth sulfate, lauramidopropyl betaine, myristamine oxide, lactic acid, PEG-120 methyl glucose dioleate, fragrance, sodium methylparaben, sodium ethylparaben, sodium propylparaben, methylchloroisothiazolinone, methylisothiazolinone, D&C Red #33.

INDICATIONS
For cleansing and refreshing of external vaginal area.

ACTIONS
Massengill feminine cleansing wash safely and gently cleanses the external vaginal area.

DIRECTIONS
Pour small amount into palm of hand or wash cloth and lather into wet skin. Rinse clean. Safe to use daily. For external use only.

HOW SUPPLIED
8 fl. oz plastic flip-top bottle.

MASSENGILL® Medicated　　　　OTC
[mas'sen-gil]
Soft Cloth Towelette

ACTIVE INGREDIENT
Hydrocortisone (0.5%).

INACTIVE INGREDIENTS
Diazolidinyl Urea, DMDM Hydantoin, Isopropyl Myristate, Methylparaben, Polysorbate 60, Propylene Glycol, Propylparaben, Sorbitan Stearate, Steareth-2, Steareth-21, Water.
Also available in non-medicated Baby Powder Scent and Unscented formulas to freshen and cleanse the external vaginal area.

INDICATIONS
For soothing relief of minor external feminine itching or other itching associated with minor skin irritations, and rashes. Other uses of this product should be only under the advice and supervision of a physician.

ACTION
Massengill Medicated Soft Cloth Towelettes contain hydrocortisone, a proven anti-inflammatory, anti-pruritic ingredient. The towelette delivery system makes the application soothing, soft, and gentle.

WARNINGS
For external use only. Avoid contact with eyes. If condition worsens, symptoms persist for more than seven days, or symptoms recur within a few days, do not use this or any other hydrocortisone product unless you have consulted a physician. If experiencing a vaginal discharge, see a physician. Do not use this product for the treatment of diaper rash.
Keep this and all drugs out of the reach of children. As with any drug, if pregnant or nursing a baby, seek the advice of a health professional before using this product. In case of accidental ingestion, seek professional assistance or contact a Poison Control Center immediately.

DIRECTIONS
Adults and Children two years of age and older—apply to the affected area not more than three to four times daily. Remove towelette from foil packet, gently wipe, and discard. Throw away towelette after it has been used once. Children under 2 years of age: DO NOT USE.

HOW SUPPLIED
Ten individually wrapped, disposable towelettes per carton.

MASSENGILL®　　　　OTC
[mas'sen-gil]
Fragrance-Free Soft Cloth Towelette and Baby Powder Scent

INGREDIENTS
Unscented
Water, Octoxynol-9, Lactic Acid, Sodium Lactate, Potassium Sorbate, Disodium EDTA, and Cetylpyridinium Chloride.
Baby Powder Scent
Water, Lactic Acid, Sodium Lactate, Potassium Sorbate, Octoxynol-9, Disodium EDTA, Cetylpyridinium Chloride, and Fragrance.

INDICATIONS
For cleansing and refreshing the external vaginal area.

ACTIONS
Massengill Baby Powder Scent and Fragrance-Free Soft Cloth Towelettes safely cleanse the external vaginal area. The towelette delivery system makes the application soft and gentle.

DIRECTIONS
Remove towelette from foil packet, unfold, and gently wipe. Throw away towelette after it has been used once.

HOW SUPPLIED
Sixteen individually wrapped, disposable towelettes per carton.

NICORETTE® 2 mg　　　　OTC
NICORETTE® 4 mg　　　　OTC
[nĭk'ŏ-rĕt"]
(nicotine polacrilex)

(See PDR For Nonprescription Drugs)

OS-CAL® 500 Tablets　　　　OTC
[ahs'kal]
calcium supplement

(See PDR For Nonprescription Drugs.)

OS-CAL® 500 Chewable Tablets　　　　OTC
[ahs'kal]
calcium supplement

(See PDR For Nonprescription Drugs.)

OS-CAL® 500+D Tablets　　　　OTC
[ahs'kal]
calcium supplement with vitamin D

(See PDR For Nonprescription Drugs.)

OS-CAL® 250+D Tablets　　　　　　　　OTC
[ahs'kal]
calcium supplement with vitamin D

(See PDR For Nonprescription Drugs.)

OS-CAL® FORTIFIED Tablets　　　　　OTC
[ahs'kal for'te-ftd]
multivitamin and minerals supplement
(Formerly marketed as Os-Cal Forte)

(See PDR For Nonprescription Drugs.)

SINGLET®　　　　　　　　　　　　　OTC
[sin'glet]
Pain Reliever-Fever Reducer/
Nasal Decongestant/Antihistamine

(See PDR For Nonprescription Drugs.)

TAGAMET® HB　　　　　　　　　　　OTC
Acid Reducer

(See PDR For Nonprescription Drugs)

TUMS®, TUMS EX®, & TUMS ULTRA®　OTC
Antacid/Calcium Supplement Tablets

TUMS® Anti-gas/Antacid　　　　　　OTC

(See PDR For Nonprescription Drugs.)

EDUCATIONAL MATERIAL

"The facts about Vaginal Infections and STDs"
A guide for women on vaginal infections and sexually transmitted diseases (STDs).
Free to physicians, pharmacists and patients in Limited quantities by writing SmithKline Beecham Consumer Healthcare, L.P. or calling 1-800-233-2426.
"A Personal Guide to Feminine Freshness"
A pamphlet on vaginal infections, feminine hygiene and douching. (BiLingual) free to physicians, pharmacists and patients in Limited quantities by writing SmithKline Beecham Consumer Healthcare, L.P. or calling 1-800-233-2426

SmithKline Beecham Pharmaceuticals
ONE FRANKLIN PLAZA
P.O. BOX 7929
PHILADELPHIA, PA 19101

For Medical Information Contact:
Medical Department
800-366-8900, ext. 5231

Questions should be directed to Product Information,
1-800-366-8900, ext. 5231.

PRODUCT CODE INDEX

Code	Product, Form and Strength
A55	Androderm Testosterone Transdermal System
189	Augmentin 125 mg Chewable Tablets
190	Augmentin 250 mg Chewable Tablets
185	Beepen-VK Tablets 250 mg
186	Beepen-VK Tablets 500 mg
C44	Compazine Spansule Capsules 10 mg
C46	Compazine Spansule Capsules 15 mg
C60	Compazine Suppositories 2½ mg
C61	Compazine Suppositories 5 mg
C62	Compazine Suppositories 25 mg
C66	Compazine Tablets 5 mg
C67	Compazine Tablets 10 mg

D14	Cytomel Tablets 5 mcg
D16	Cytomel Tablets 25 mcg
D17	Cytomel Tablets 50 mcg
E12	Dexedrine Spansule Capsules 5 mg
E13	Dexedrine Spansule Capsules 10 mg
E14	Dexedrine Spansule Capsules 15 mg
E19	Dexedrine Tablets 5 mg
E33	Dibenzyline Capsules 10 mg
165	Dycill Capsules 250 mg
166	Dycill Capsules 500 mg
J10	Eskalith Controlled Release Tablets 450 mg
125	Menest Tablets 0.3 mg
126	Menest Tablets 0.625 mg
127	Menest Tablets 1.25 mg
128	Menest Tablets 2.5 mg
S03	Stelazine Tablets 1 mg
S04	Stelazine Tablets 2 mg
S06	Stelazine Tablets 5 mg
S07	Stelazine Tablets 10 mg
T63	Thorazine Spansule Capsules 30 mg
T64	Thorazine Spansule Capsules 75 mg
T66	Thorazine Spansule Capsules 150 mg
T70	Thorazine Suppositories 25 mg
T71	Thorazine Suppositories 100 mg
T73	Thorazine Tablets 10 mg
T74	Thorazine Tablets 25 mg
T76	Thorazine Tablets 50 mg
T77	Thorazine Tablets 100 mg
T79	Thorazine Tablets 200 mg
140	Totacillin Capsules 250 mg
141	Totacillin Capsules 500 mg

ALBENZA™　　　　　　　　　　　　　℞
[al-ben'-za]
brand of
albendazole
Tablets

DESCRIPTION
Albenza (albendazole) is an orally administered broad-spectrum anthelmintic. Chemically it is Methyl 5-(propylthio)-2-benzimidazolecarbamate. Its molecular formula is $C_{12}H_{15}N_3O_2S$. Its molecular weight is 265.34. It has the following chemical structure:

albendazole

Albendazole is a white to off-white powder. It is soluble in dimethylsulfoxide, strong acids and strong bases. It is slightly soluble in methanol, chloroform, ethyl acetate and acetonitrile. Albendazole is practically insoluble in water. Each white to off-white, film-coated tablet contains 200 mg of albendazole.
Inactive ingredients consist of: carnauba wax, hydroxypropyl methylcellulose, lactose monohydrate, magnesium stearate, microcrystalline cellulose, povidone, sodium lauryl sulfate, sodium saccharin, sodium starch glycolate, and starch.

CLINICAL PHARMACOLOGY
Pharmacokinetics
Absorption and Metabolism
Albendazole is poorly absorbed from the gastrointestinal tract due to its low aqueous solubility. Albendazole concentrations are negligible or undetectable in plasma as it is rapidly converted to the sulfoxide metabolite prior to reaching the systemic circulation. The systemic anthelmintic activity has been attributed to the primary metabolite, albendazole sulfoxide. Oral bioavailability appears to be enhanced when albendazole is coadministered with a fatty meal (estimated fat content 40 g) as evidenced by higher (up to 5-fold on average) plasma concentrations of albendazole sulfoxide as compared to the fasted state.
Maximal plasma concentrations of albendazole sulfoxide are typically achieved 2 to 5 hours after dosing and are on average 1.31 mcg/mL (range 0.46 to 1.58 mcg/mL) following oral doses of albendazole (400 mg) in six hydatid disease patients, when administered with a fatty meal. Plasma concentrations of albendazole sulfoxide increase in a dose-proportional manner over the therapeutic dose range following ingestion of a fatty meal (fat content 43.1 g). The mean apparent terminal elimination half-life of albendazole sulfoxide typically ranges from 8 to 12 hours in twenty-five normal subjects, as well as in fourteen hydatid and eight neurocysticercosis patients.
Following 4 weeks of treatment with albendazole (200 mg three times daily), twelve patients' plasma concentrations of

albendazole sulfoxide were approximately 20% lower than those observed during the first half of the treatment period, suggesting that albendazole may induce its own metabolism.
Distribution
Albendazole sulfoxide is 70% bound to plasma protein and is widely distributed throughout the body; it has been detected in urine, bile, liver, cyst wall, cyst fluid, and cerebral spinal fluid (CSF). Concentrations in plasma were 3- to 10-fold and 2- to 4-fold higher than those simultaneously determined in cyst fluid and CSF, respectively. Limited in vitro and clinical data suggest that albendazole sulfoxide may be eliminated from cysts at a slower rate than observed in plasma.
Metabolism and Excretion
Albendazole is rapidly converted in the liver to the primary metabolite, albendazole sulfoxide, which is further metabolized to albendazole sulfone and other primary oxidative metabolites that have been identified in human urine. Following oral administration, albendazole has not been detected in human urine. Urinary excretion of albendazole sulfoxide is a minor elimination pathway with less than 1% of the dose recovered in the urine. Biliary elimination presumably accounts for a portion of the elimination as evidenced by biliary concentrations of albendazole sulfoxide similar to those achieved in plasma.
Special Populations
Patients with Impaired Renal Function: The pharmacokinetics of albendazole in patients with impaired renal function have not been studied. However, since renal elimination of albendazole and its primary metabolite, albendazole sulfoxide, is negligible, it is unlikely that clearance of these compounds would be altered in these patients.
Biliary Effects: In patients with evidence of extrahepatic obstruction (n=5), the systemic availability of albendazole sulfoxide was increased, as indicated by a 2-fold increase in maximum serum concentration and a 7-fold increase in area under the curve. The rate of absorption/conversion and elimination of albendazole sulfoxide appeared to be prolonged with mean T_{max} and serum elimination half-life values of 10 hours and 31.7 hours, respectively. Plasma concentrations of parent albendazole were measurable in only one of five patients.
Pediatrics: Following single-dose administration of 200 mg to 300 mg (approximately 10 mg/kg) albendazole to three fasted and two fed pediatric patients with hydatid cyst disease (age range 6 to 13 years), albendazole sulfoxide pharmacokinetics were similar to those observed in fed adults.
Elderly Patients: Although no studies have investigated the effect of age on albendazole sulfoxide pharmacokinetics, data in twenty-six hydatid cyst patients (up to 79 years) suggest pharmacokinetics similar to those in young healthy subjects.
Microbiology
The principal mode of action for albendazole is by its inhibitory effect on tubulin polymerization which results in the loss of cytoplasmic microtubules.
In the specified treatment indications albendazole appears to be active against the larval forms of the following organisms:
Echinococcus granulosus
Taenia solium

INDICATIONS AND USAGE
Albenza (albendazole) is indicated for the treatment of the following infections:
Neurocysticercosis. Albenza is indicated for the treatment of parenchymal neurocysticercosis due to active lesions caused by larval forms of the pork tapeworm, Taenia solium. Lesions considered responsive to albendazole therapy appear as nonenhancing cysts with no surrounding edema on contrast-enhanced computerized tomography. Clinical studies in patients with lesions of this type demonstrate a 74% to 88% reduction in number of cysts; 40% to 70% of albendazole-treated patients showed resolution of all active cysts.
Hydatid disease. Albenza is indicated for the treatment of cystic hydatid disease of the liver, lung, and peritoneum, caused by the larval form of the dog tapeworm, Echinococcus granulosus.
This indication is based on combined clinical studies which demonstrated non-infectious cyst contents in approximately 80-90% of patients given Albenza for 3 cycles of therapy of 28 days each. (See DOSAGE AND ADMINISTRATION.) Clinical cure (disappearance of cysts) was seen in approximately 30% of these patients, and improvement (reduction in cyst diameter of ≥25%) was seen in an additional 40%.
NOTE: When medically feasible, surgery is considered the treatment of choice for hydatid disease. When administering

Continued on next page

SmithKline Beecham—Cont.

Albenza in the pre- or post-surgical setting, optimal killing of cyst contents is achieved when three courses of therapy have been given.
NOTE: The efficacy of albendazole in the therapy of alveolar hydatid disease caused by *Echinococcus multilocularis* has not been clearly demonstrated in clinical studies.

CONTRAINDICATIONS

Albenza (albendazole) is contraindicated in patients with known hypersensitivity to the benzimidazole class of compounds or any components of *Albenza*.

WARNINGS

Rare fatalities associated with the use of *Albenza* have been reported due to granulocytopenia or pancytopenia. (See **PRECAUTIONS.**) Blood counts should be monitored at the beginning of each 28-day cycle of therapy, and every 2 weeks while on therapy with albendazole. Albendazole may be continued if the total white blood cell count and absolute neutrophil count decrease appear modest and do not progress. Albendazole should not be used in pregnant women except in clinical circumstances where no alternative management is appropriate. Patients should not become pregnant for at least 1 month following cessation of albendazole therapy. If a patient becomes pregnant while taking this drug, albendazole should be discontinued immediately. If pregnancy occurs while taking this drug, the patient should be apprised of the potential hazard to the fetus.

PRECAUTIONS

General: Patients being treated for neurocysticercosis should receive appropriate steroid and anticonvulsant therapy as required. Oral or intravenous corticosteroids should be considered to prevent cerebral hypertensive episodes during the first week of anticysticeral therapy.
Cysticercosis may, in rare cases, involve the retina. Before initiating therapy for neurocysticercosis, the patient should be examined for the presence of retinal lesions. If such lesions are visualized, the need for anticysticeral therapy should be weighed against the possibility of retinal damage caused by albendazole-induced changes to the retinal lesion.
Information for Patients
Patients should be advised that:
- Albendazole may cause fetal harm, therefore, women of childbearing age should begin treatment after a negative pregnancy test.
- Women of childbearing age should be cautioned against becoming pregnant while on albendazole or within 1 month of completing treatment.
- During albendazole therapy, because of the possibility of harm to the liver or bone marrow, routine (every 2 weeks) monitoring of blood counts and liver function tests should take place.
- Albendazole should be taken with food.
Laboratory Tests
White Blood Cell Count: Albendazole has been shown to cause occasional (less than 1% of treated patients) reversible reductions in total white blood cell count. Rarely, more significant reductions may be encountered including granulocytopenia, agranulocytosis, or pancytopenia. Blood counts should be performed at the start of each 28-day treatment cycle and every 2 weeks during each 28-day cycle. Albendazole may be continued if the total white blood cell count decrease appears modest and does not progress.
Liver Function: In clinical trials, treatment with albendazole has been associated with mild to moderate elevations of hepatic enzymes in approximately 16% of patients. These have returned to normal upon discontinuation of therapy.
Liver function tests (transaminases) should be performed before the start of each treatment cycle and at least every 2 weeks during treatment. If enzymes are significantly increased, albendazole therapy should be discontinued. Therapy can be reinstituted when liver enzymes have returned to pretreatment levels, but laboratory tests should be performed frequently during repeat therapy.
Patients with abnormal liver function test results prior to commencing albendazole therapy should be carefully evaluated, since the drug is metabolized by the liver and has been associated with hepatotoxicity in a few patients.
Theophylline: Although single doses of albendazole have been shown not to inhibit theophylline metabolism (see **Drug Interactions**), albendazole does induce cytochrome P450 1A in human hepatoma cells. Therefore, it is recommended that plasma concentrations of theophylline be monitored during and after treatment with Albenza (albendazole).
Drug Interactions
Dexamethasone: Steady-state trough concentrations of albendazole sulfoxide were about 56% higher when 8 mg dexamethasone was coadministered with each dose of albendazole (15 mg/kg/day) in eight neurocysticercosis patients.
Praziquantel: In the fed state, praziquantel (40 mg/kg) increased mean maximum plasma concentration and area under the curve of albendazole sulfoxide by about 50% in healthy subjects (n=10) compared with a separate group of

Indication	Patient Weight	Dose	Duration
Hydatid Disease	60 kg or greater	400 mg b.i.d., with meals	28-day cycle followed by a 14-day albendazole-free interval, for a total of 3 cycles
	less than 60 kg	15 mg/kg/day given in divided doses b.i.d. with meals (maximum total daily dose 800 mg)	

NOTE: When administering *Albenza* in the pre- or post-surgical setting, optimal killing of cyst contents is achieved when three courses of therapy have been given.

Neurocysticercosis	60 kg or greater	400 mg b.i.d., with meals	8–30 days
	less than 60 kg	15 mg/kg/day given in divided doses b.i.d. with meals (maximum total daily dose 800 mg)	

subjects (n=6) given albendazole alone. Mean T_{max} and mean plasma elimination half-life of albendazole sulfoxide were unchanged. The pharmacokinetics of praziquantel were unchanged following coadministration with albendazole (400 mg).
Cimetidine: Albendazole sulfoxide concentrations in bile and cystic fluid were increased (about 2-fold) in hydatid cyst patients treated with cimetidine (10 mg/kg/day) (n=7) compared with albendazole (20 mg/kg/day) alone (n=12). Albendazole sulfoxide plasma concentrations were unchanged 4 hours after dosing.
Theophylline: The pharmacokinetics of theophylline (aminophylline 5.8 mg/kg infused over 20 minutes) were unchanged following a single oral dose of albendazole (400 mg) in 6 healthy subjects.
Carcinogenesis, Mutagenesis, Impairment of Fertility
Long-term carcinogenicity studies were conducted in mice and rats. In the mouse study, albendazole was administered in the diet at doses of 25, 100 and 400 mg/kg/day (0.1, 0.5, and 2 times the recommended human dose based on body surface area in mg/m², respectively) for 108 weeks. In the rat study, albendazole was administered in the diet at doses of 3.5, 7, and 20 mg/kg/day (0.04, 0.08, and 0.21 times the recommended human dose based on body surface area in mg/m², respectively) for 117 weeks. There was no evidence of increased incidence of tumors in the treated mice and rats when compared to the control group.
In genotoxicity tests, albendazole was found negative in an Ames Salmonella/Microsome Plate mutation assay with and without metabolic activation or with and without pre-incubation, cell-mediated Chinese Hamster Ovary chromosomal aberration test and *in vivo* mouse micronucleus test. In the *in vitro* BALB/3T3 cells transformation assay, albendazole produced weak activity in the presence of metabolic activation while no activity was found in the absence of metabolic activation.
Albendazole did not adversely affect male or female fertility in the rat at an oral dose of 30 mg/kg/day (0.32 times the recommended human dose based on body surface area in mg/m²).
Pregnancy
Teratogenic Effects—Pregnancy Category C: Albendazole has been shown to be teratogenic (to cause embryotoxicity and skeletal malformations) in pregnant rats and rabbits. The teratogenic response in the rat was shown at oral doses of 10 and 30 mg/kg/day (0.10 times and 0.32 times the recommended human dose based on body surface area in mg/m², respectively) during gestation days 6 to 15 and in pregnant rabbits at oral doses of 30 mg/kg/day (0.60 times the recommended human dose based on body surface area in mg/m²) administered during gestation days 7 to 19. In the rabbit study, maternal toxicity (33% mortality) was noted at 30 mg/kg/day. In mice, no teratogenic effects were observed at oral doses up to 30 mg/kg/day (0.16 times the recommended human dose based on body surface area in mg/m²), administered during gestation days 6 to 15.
There are no adequate and well-controlled studies of albendazole administration in pregnant women. Albendazole should be used during pregnancy only if the potential benefit justifies the potential risk to the fetus. (See **WARNINGS.**)
Nursing Mothers: Albendazole is excreted in animal milk. It is not known whether it is excreted in human milk. Because many drugs are excreted in human milk, caution should be exercised when albendazole is administered to a nursing woman.
Pediatric Use: Experience in children under the age of 6 years is limited. In hydatid disease, infection in infants and young children is uncommon, but no problems have been

encountered in those who have been treated. In neurocysticercosis, infection is more frequently encountered. In five published studies involving pediatric patients as young as 1 year, no significant problems were encountered, and the efficacy appeared similar to the adult population.
Geriatric Use: Experience in patients 65 years of age or older is limited. The number of patients treated for either hydatid disease or neurocysticercosis is limited, but no problems associated with an older population have been observed.

ADVERSE REACTIONS

The adverse event profile of albendazole differs between hydatid disease and neurocysticercosis. Adverse events occurring with a frequency of ≥1% in either disease are described in the table below.
These symptoms were usually mild and resolved without treatment. Treatment discontinuations were predominantly due to leukopenia (0.7%) or hepatic abnormalities (3.8% in hydatid disease). The following incidence reflects events that were reported by investigators to be at least possibly or probably related to albendazole.

Adverse Event Incidence ≥1% in Hydatid Disease and Neurocysticercosis

Adverse Event	Hydatid Disease	Neurocysticercosis
Abnormal Liver Function Tests	15.6	<1.0
Abdominal Pain	6.0	0
Nausea/Vomiting	3.7	6.2
Headache	1.3	11.0
Dizziness/Vertigo	1.2	<1.0
Raised Intracranial Pressure	0	1.5
Meningeal Signs	0	1.0
Reversible Alopecia	1.6	<1.0
Fever	1.0	0

The following adverse events were observed at an incidence of <1%:
Hematologic: Leukopenia. There have been rare reports of granulocytopenia, pancytopenia, agranulocytosis, or thrombocytopenia. (See **WARNINGS**.)
Dermatologic: Rash, urticaria.
Hypersensitivity: Allergic reactions.
Renal: Acute renal failure related to albendazole therapy has been observed.

OVERDOSAGE

Significant toxicity and mortality were shown in male and female mice at doses exceeding 5,000 mg/kg; in rats, at estimated doses between 1,300 and 2,400 mg/kg; in hamsters, at doses exceeding 10,000 mg/kg; and in rabbits, at estimated doses between 500 and 1,250 mg/kg. In the animals, symptoms were demonstrated in a dose-response relationship and included diarrhea, vomiting, tachycardia, and respiratory distress.
One overdosage has been reported with Albenza (albendazole) in a patient who took at least 16 grams over 12 hours. No untoward effects were reported. In case of overdosage, symptomatic therapy (e.g., gastric lavage and activated charcoal) and general supportive measures are recommended.

DOSAGE AND ADMINISTRATION

Dosing of *Albenza* will vary, depending upon which of the following parasitic infections is being treated.

[See table at top of page.]

Patients being treated for neurocysticercosis should receive appropriate steroid and anticonvulsant therapy as required. Oral or intravenous corticosteroids should be considered to prevent cerebral hypertensive episodes during the first week of treatment.

HOW SUPPLIED

Albenza (albendazole) is supplied as 200 mg, white to off-white, circular, biconvex, bevel-edged, film-coated Tiltab® tablets in bottles of 112.
NDC 0007-5500-40 .... Bottles of 112
Store between 20° and 25°C (68° and 77°F).
AL:L1

AMOXIL® ℞

[ă-mŏx ′ĭl]
brand of amoxicillin
capsules, powder for oral suspension
and chewable tablets

DESCRIPTION

Amoxil (amoxicillin) is a semisynthetic antibiotic, an analog of ampicillin, with a broad spectrum of bactericidal activity against many gram-positive and gram-negative microorganisms. Chemically it is D-(-)-α-amino-p-hydroxybenzyl penicillin trihydrate.

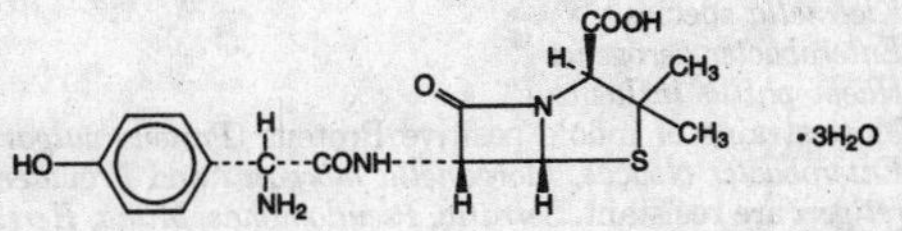

Amoxil capsules, tablets and powder for oral suspension are intended for oral administration.

Capsules: Each *Amoxil* capsule, with royal blue opaque cap and pink opaque body, contains 250 mg or 500 mg amoxicillin as the trihydrate. The cap and body of the 250 mg capsule is imprinted with the product name AMOXIL and 250; 500 mg—AMOXIL and 500. Inactive ingredients: D&C Red No. 28, FD&C Blue No. 1, FD&C Red No. 40, gelatin, magnesium stearate and titanium dioxide.

Tablets: Each oval, pink, cherry-banana-peppermint-flavored tablet contains 125 mg or 250 mg amoxicillin as the trihydrate. The tablets are imprinted with the product name AMOXIL on one side and 125 or 250 on the other side. Inactive ingredients: citric acid, corn starch, FD&C Red No. 40, flavorings, glycine, mannitol, magnesium stearate, saccharin sodium, silica gel and sucrose.

Oral Suspension: Each 5 mL of reconstituted suspension contains 125 mg or 250 mg amoxicillin as the trihydrate.

Pediatric Drops for Oral Suspension: Each mL of reconstituted suspension contains 50 mg amoxicillin as the trihydrate.

Amoxicillin trihydrate for oral suspension 125 mg/5 mL (reconstituted) is a strawberry-flavored pink suspension; the 250 mg/5 mL or 50 mg/mL is a bubble-gum-flavored pink suspension. Inactive ingredients: FD&C Red No. 3, flavorings, silica gel, sodium benzoate, sodium citrate, sucrose and xanthan gum.

ACTIONS

PHARMACOLOGY

Amoxicillin is stable in the presence of gastric acid and may be given without regard to meals. It is rapidly absorbed after oral administration. It diffuses readily into most body tissues and fluids, with the exception of brain and spinal fluid, except when meninges are inflamed. The half-life of amoxicillin is 61.3 minutes. Most of the amoxicillin is excreted unchanged in the urine; its excretion can be delayed by concurrent administration of probenecid. Amoxicillin is not highly protein-bound. In blood serum, amoxicillin is approximately 20% protein-bound as compared to 60% for penicillin G.

Orally administered doses of 250 mg and 500 mg amoxicillin capsules result in average peak blood levels 1 to 2 hours after administration in the range of 3.5 mcg/mL to 5.0 mcg/mL and 5.5 mcg/mL to 7.5 mcg/mL, respectively.

Orally administered doses of amoxicillin suspension 125 mg/5 mL and 250 mg/5 mL result in average peak blood levels 1 to 2 hours after administration in the range of 1.5 mcg/mL to 3.0 mcg/mL and 3.5 mcg/mL to 5.0 mcg/mL, respectively. Amoxicillin chewable tablets, 125 mg and 250 mg, produced blood levels similar to those achieved with the corresponding doses of amoxicillin oral suspensions.

Detectable serum levels are observed up to 8 hours after an orally administered dose of amoxicillin. Following a 1 gram dose and utilizing a special skin window technique to determine levels of the antibiotic, it was noted that therapeutic levels were found in the interstitial fluid. Approximately 60% of an orally administered dose of amoxicillin is excreted in the urine within 6 to 8 hours.

MICROBIOLOGY

Amoxil (amoxicillin) is similar to ampicillin in its bactericidal action against susceptible organisms during the stage of active multiplication. It acts through the inhibition of biosynthesis of cell wall mucopeptide. *In vitro* studies have demonstrated the susceptibility of most strains of the following gram-positive bacteria: alpha- and beta-hemolytic streptococci, *Diplococcus pneumoniae*, nonpenicillinase-producing staphylococci and *Streptococcus faecalis*. It is active *in vitro* against many strains of *Haemophilus influenzae*, *Neisseria gonorrhoeae*, *Escherichia coli* and *Proteus mirabilis*. Because it does not resist destruction by penicillinase, it is not effective against penicillinase-producing bacteria, particularly resistant staphylococci. All strains of *Pseudomonas* and most strains of *Klebsiella* and *Enterobacter* are resistant.

DISK SUSCEPTIBILITY TESTS: Quantitative methods that require measurement of zone diameters give the most precise estimates of antibiotic susceptibility. One such procedure* has been recommended for use with disks for testing susceptibility to ampicillin-class antibiotics. Interpretations correlate diameters of the disk test with MIC values for amoxicillin. With this procedure, a report from the laboratory of "susceptible" indicates that the infecting organism is likely to respond to therapy. A report of "resistant" indicates that the infecting organism is not likely to respond to therapy. A report of "intermediate susceptibility" suggests that the organism would be susceptible if high dosage is used, or if the infection is confined to tissues and fluids (e.g., urine), in which high antibiotic levels are attained.

*Bauer, A. W., Kirby, W. M. M., Sherris, J. C., and Turck, M.: Antibiotic Testing by a Standardized Single Disc Method, Am. J. Clin. Pathol. 45:493, 1966. Standardized Disc Susceptibility Test, Federal Register 37:20527–29, 1972.

INDICATIONS

Amoxil (amoxicillin) is indicated in the treatment of infections due to susceptible strains of the following:

Gram-negative organisms—*H. influenzae, E. coli, P. mirabilis* and *N. gonorrhoeae*.

Gram-positive organisms—Streptococci (including *Streptococcus faecalis*), *D. pneumoniae* and nonpenicillinase-producing staphylococci.

Therapy may be instituted prior to obtaining results from bacteriological and susceptibility studies to determine the causative organisms and their susceptibility to amoxicillin. Indicated surgical procedures should be performed.

CONTRAINDICATIONS

A history of allergic reaction to any of the penicillins is a contraindication.

WARNINGS

SERIOUS AND OCCASIONALLY FATAL HYPERSENSITIVITY (anaphylactic) REACTIONS HAVE BEEN REPORTED IN PATIENTS ON PENICILLIN THERAPY. THESE REACTIONS ARE MORE LIKELY TO OCCUR IN INDIVIDUALS WITH A HISTORY OF PENICILLIN HYPERSENSITIVITY AND/OR A HISTORY OF SENSITIVITY TO MULTIPLE ALLERGENS. BEFORE INITIATING THERAPY WITH *AMOXIL*, CAREFUL INQUIRY SHOULD BE MADE CONCERNING PREVIOUS HYPERSENSITIVITY REACTIONS TO PENICILLINS, CEPHALOSPORINS OR OTHER ALLERGENS. IF AN ALLERGIC REACTION OCCURS, *AMOXIL* SHOULD BE DISCONTINUED AND APPROPRIATE THERAPY INSTITUTED. **SERIOUS ANAPHYLACTIC REACTIONS REQUIRE IMMEDIATE EMERGENCY TREATMENT WITH EPINEPHRINE. OXYGEN, INTRAVENOUS STEROIDS AND AIRWAY MANAGEMENT, INCLUDING INTUBATION, SHOULD ALSO BE ADMINISTERED AS INDICATED.**

Pseudomembranous colitis has been reported with nearly all antibacterial agents, including amoxicillin, and may range in severity from mild to life-threatening. Therefore, it is important to consider this diagnosis in patients who present with diarrhea subsequent to the administration of antibacterial agents.

Treatment with antibacterial agents alters the normal flora of the colon and may permit overgrowth of clostridia. Studies indicate that a toxin produced by *Clostridium difficile* is a primary cause of "antibiotic-associated colitis."

After the diagnosis of pseudomembranous colitis has been established, therapeutic measures should be initiated. Mild cases of pseudomembranous colitis usually respond to drug discontinuation alone. In moderate to severe cases, consideration should be given to management with fluids and electrolytes, protein supplementation and treatment with an antibacterial drug clinically effective against *C. difficile* colitis.

USAGE IN PREGNANCY

Safety for use in pregnancy has not been established.

PRECAUTIONS

As with any potent drug, periodic assessment of renal, hepatic and hematopoietic function should be made during prolonged therapy. The possibility of superinfections with mycotic or bacterial pathogens should be kept in mind during therapy. If superinfections occur (usually involving *Enterobacter, Pseudomonas* or *Candida*), the drug should be discontinued and/or appropriate therapy instituted.

ADVERSE REACTIONS

As with other penicillins, it may be expected that untoward reactions will be essentially limited to sensitivity phenomena. They are more likely to occur in individuals who have previously demonstrated hypersensitivity to penicillins and in those with a history of allergy, asthma, hay fever or urticaria. The following adverse reactions have been reported as associated with the use of penicillins:

Gastrointestinal: Nausea, vomiting and diarrhea.

Hypersensitivity Reactions: Erythematous maculopapular rashes, erythema multiforme, Stevens-Johnson Syndrome, toxic epidermal necrolysis and urticaria have been reported.

NOTE: These hypersensitivity reactions may be controlled with antihistamines and, if necessary, systemic corticosteroids. Whenever such reactions occur, amoxicillin should be discontinued unless, in the opinion of the physician, the condition being treated is life-threatening and amenable only to amoxicillin therapy.

Liver: A moderate rise in serum glutamic oxaloacetic transaminase (SGOT) has been noted, but the significance of this finding is unknown.

Hemic and Lymphatic Systems: Anemia, thrombocytopenia, thrombocytopenic purpura, eosinophilia, leukopenia and agranulocytosis have been reported during therapy with penicillins. These reactions are usually reversible on discontinuation of therapy and are believed to be hypersensitivity phenomena.

Central Nervous System: Reversible hyperactivity, agitation, anxiety, insomnia, confusion, behavioral changes and/or dizziness have been reported rarely.

DOSAGE AND ADMINISTRATION

Infections of the ear, nose and throat due to streptococci, pneumococci, nonpenicillinase-producing staphylococci and *H. influenzae*;

Infections of the genitourinary tract due to *E. coli, Proteus mirabilis* and *Streptococcus faecalis*;

Infections of the skin and soft-tissues due to streptococci, susceptible staphylococci and *E. coli*:

USUAL DOSAGE:
Adults: 250 mg every 8 hours.
Children: 20 mg/kg/day in divided doses every 8 hours.
Children weighing 20 kg or more should be dosed according to the adult recommendations.

In severe infections or those caused by less susceptible organisms:
500 mg every 8 hours for adults and 40 mg/kg/day in divided doses every 8 hours for children may be needed.

Infections of the lower respiratory tract due to streptococci, pneumococci, nonpenicillinase-producing staphylococci and *H. influenzae*:

USUAL DOSAGE:
Adults: 500 mg every 8 hours.
Children: 40 mg/kg/day in divided doses every 8 hours.
Children weighing 20 kg or more should be dosed according to the adult recommendations.

Gonorrhea, acute uncomplicated ano-genital and urethral infections due to *N. gonorrhoeae* (males and females):

USUAL DOSAGE:
Adults: 3 grams as a single oral dose.
Prepubertal children: 50 mg/kg amoxicillin combined with 25 mg/kg probenecid as a single dose.

NOTE: SINCE PROBENECID IS CONTRAINDICATED IN CHILDREN UNDER 2 YEARS, THIS REGIMEN SHOULD NOT BE USED IN THESE CASES.

Cases of gonorrhea with a suspected lesion of syphilis should have dark-field examinations before receiving amoxicillin, and monthly serological tests for a minimum of 4 months. Larger doses may be required for stubborn or severe infections.

The children's dosage is intended for individuals whose weight will not cause a dosage to be calculated greater than that recommended for adults.

It should be recognized that in the treatment of chronic urinary tract infections, frequent bacteriological and clinical

Continued on next page

Information on the SmithKline Beecham Pharmaceuticals products appearing here is based on the labeling in effect on July 1, 1996. Further information on these and other products may be obtained from the Medical Department, SmithKline Beecham Pharmaceuticals, One Franklin Plaza, Philadelphia, PA 19101.

SmithKline Beecham—Cont.

appraisals are necessary. Smaller doses than those recommended above should not be used. Even higher doses may be needed at times. In stubborn infections, therapy may be required for several weeks. It may be necessary to continue clinical and/or bacteriological follow-up for several months after cessation of therapy. Except for gonorrhea, treatment should be continued for a minimum of 48 to 72 hours beyond the time that the patient becomes asymptomatic or evidence of bacterial eradication has been obtained. It is recommended that there be at least 10 days' treatment for any infection caused by hemolytic streptococci to prevent the occurrence of acute rheumatic fever or glomerulonephritis.

DOSAGE AND ADMINISTRATION OF PEDIATRIC DROPS

Usual dosage for all indications except infections of the lower respiratory tract:

Under 6 kg (13 lbs): 0.75 mL every 8 hours.
6 to 7 kg (13 to 15 lbs): 1.0 mL every 8 hours.
8 kg (16 to 18 lbs): 1.25 mL every 8 hours.

Infections of the lower respiratory tract:

Under 6 kg (13 lbs): 1.25 mL every 8 hours.
6 to 7 kg (13 to 15 lbs): 1.75 mL every 8 hours.
8 kg (16 to 18 lbs): 2.25 mL every 8 hours.

Children weighing more than 8 kg (18 lbs) should receive the appropriate dose of the Oral Suspension 125 mg or 250 mg/5 mL.

After reconstitution, the required amount of suspension should be placed directly on the child's tongue for swallowing. Alternate means of administration are to add the required amount of suspension to formula, milk, fruit juice, water, ginger ale or cold drinks. These preparations should then be taken immediately. To be certain the child is receiving full dosage, such preparations should be consumed in entirety.

DIRECTIONS FOR MIXING ORAL SUSPENSION

Prepare suspension at time of dispensing as follows: Tap bottle until all powder flows freely. Add approximately ¹/₃ of the total amount of water for reconstitution (see table below) and shake vigorously to wet powder. Add remainder of the water and again shake vigorously.

125 mg/5 mL

Bottle Size	Amount of Water Required for Reconstitution
80 mL	62 mL
100 mL	78 mL
150 mL	116 mL

Each teaspoonful (5 mL) will contain 125 mg amoxicillin.
125 mg unit dose .... 5 mL

250 mg/5 mL

Bottle Size	Amount of Water Required for Reconstitution
80 mL	59 mL
100 mL	74 mL
150 mL	111 mL

Each teaspoonful (5 mL) will contain 250 mg amoxicillin.
250 mg unit dose .... 5 mL

DIRECTIONS FOR MIXING PEDIATRIC DROPS

Prepare pediatric drops at time of dispensing as follows: Add the required amount of water (see table below) to the bottle and shake vigorously. Each mL of suspension will then contain amoxicillin trihydrate equivalent to 50 mg amoxicillin.

Bottle Size	Amount of Water Required for Reconstitution
15 mL	12 mL
30 mL	23 mL

NOTE: SHAKE BOTH ORAL SUSPENSION AND PEDIATRIC DROPS WELL BEFORE USING. Keep bottle tightly closed. Any unused portion of the reconstituted suspension must be discarded after 14 days. Refrigeration preferable, but not required.

HOW SUPPLIED

Amoxil (amoxicillin) Capsules. Each capsule contains 250 mg or 500 mg amoxicillin as the trihydrate.

250 mg Capsule

NDC 0029-6006-30 ....bottles of 100
NDC 0029-6006-32 ....bottles of 500

500 mg Capsule

NDC 0029-6007-30 ....bottles of 100
NDC 0029-6007-32 ....bottles of 500

Amoxil (amoxicillin) Chewable Tablets. Each cherry-banana-peppermint-flavored tablet contains 125 mg or 250 mg amoxicillin as the trihydrate.

125 mg Tablet

NDC 0029-6004-39 ....bottles of 60

250 mg Tablet

NDC 0029-6005-13 ....bottles of 30
NDC 0029-6005-30 ....bottles of 100

Amoxil (amoxicillin) for Oral Suspension.

125 mg/5 mL

NDC 0029-6008-21 ....80 mL bottle
NDC 0029-6008-23 ....100 mL bottle
NDC 0029-6008-22 ....150 mL bottle

250 mg/5 mL

NDC 0029-6009-21 ....80 mL bottle
NDC 0029-6009-23 ....100 mL bottle
NDC 0029-6009-22 ....150 mL bottle

Each 5 mL of reconstituted strawberry-flavored suspension contains 125 mg amoxicillin as the trihydrate.
Each 5 mL of reconstituted bubble-gum-flavored suspension contains 250 mg amoxicillin as the trihydrate.

NDC 0029-6008-18 ....125 mg unit dose bottle
NDC 0029-6009-18 ....250 mg unit dose bottle

Amoxil (amoxicillin) Pediatric Drops for Oral Suspension. Each mL of bubble-gum-flavored reconstituted suspension contains 50 mg amoxicillin as the trihydrate.

NDC 0029-6035-20 ....15 mL bottle
NDC 0029-6038-39 ....30 mL bottle

Veterans Administration/Military/PHS—Chewable Tablets, 125 mg, 60's 6505-01-159-9245; 250 mg, 100's, 6505-01-253-3834; Capsules, 250 mg, 100's, 6505-01-010-7953; 250 mg, 500's, 6505-01-116-6013; 500 mg, 100's, 6505-01-115-1474; 500 mg, 500's, 6505-01-250-8527; Oral Suspension, 125 mg, 10x5 mL SUP, 6505-01-197-2950; 125 mg/5 mL, 80 mL, 6505-01-412-9703; 125 mg/5 mL, 100 mL, 6505-01-153-3862; 125 mg/5 mL, 150 mL, 6505-01-011-1464; 250 mg, 10x5 mL SUP, 6505-01-160-6013; 250 mg/5 mL, 80 mL, 6505-01-153-3442; 250 mg/5 mL, 100 mL, 6505-01-156-2106; 250 mg/5 mL, 150 mL, 6505-01-066-4195.

AM:L10A

Shown in Product Identification Guide, page 335

ANCEF® ℞

[an-sef']

(brand of sterile cefazolin sodium and cefazolin sodium injection)

DESCRIPTION

Ancef (sterile cefazolin sodium) is a semi-synthetic cephalosporin for parenteral administration. It is the sodium salt of 3-[[(5-methyl-1, 3, 4-thiadiazol-2-yl) thio]-methyl]-8-oxo-7-[2-(1H-tetrazol-1-yl) acetamido]-5-thia-1-azabicyclo [4.2.0] oct-2-ene-2-carboxylic acid.

The sodium content is 46 mg per gram of cefazolin.

Ancef in lyophilized form is supplied in vials equivalent to 500 mg or 1 gram of cefazolin; in "Piggyback" Vials for intravenous admixture equivalent to 1 gram of cefazolin; and in Pharmacy Bulk Vials equivalent to 5 grams or 10 grams of cefazolin.

Ancef is also supplied as a frozen, sterile, nonpyrogenic solution of cefazolin sodium in an iso-osmotic diluent in plastic containers. After thawing, the solution is intended for intravenous use.

The plastic container is fabricated from a specially designed multilayer plastic, PL 2040. Solutions are in contact with the polyethylene layer of this container and can leach out certain of the chemical components of the plastic in very small amounts within the expiration period. However, the suitability of the plastic has been confirmed in tests in animals according to the USP biological tests for plastic containers as well as by tissue culture toxicity studies.

CLINICAL PHARMACOLOGY

Human Pharmacology: After intramuscular administration of Ancef to normal volunteers, the mean serum concentrations were 37 mcg/mL at 1 hour and 3 mcg/mL at 8 hours following a 500 mg dose, and 64 mcg/mL at 1 hour and 7 mcg/mL at 8 hours following a 1 gram dose.

Studies have shown that following intravenous administration of Ancef to normal volunteers, mean serum concentrations peaked at approximately 185 mcg/mL and were approximately 4 mcg/mL at 8 hours for a 1 gram dose.

The serum half-life for Ancef is approximately 1.8 hours following I.V. administration and approximately 2.0 hours following I.M. administration.

In a study (using normal volunteers) of constant intravenous infusion with dosages of 3.5 mg/kg for 1 hour (approximately 250 mg) and 1.5 mg/kg the next 2 hours (approximately 100 mg), Ancef produced a steady serum level at the third hour of approximately 28 mcg/mL.

Studies in patients hospitalized with infections indicate that Ancef (sterile cefazolin sodium) produces mean peak serum levels approximately equivalent to those seen in normal volunteers.

Bile levels in patients without obstructive biliary disease can reach or exceed serum levels by up to five times; however, in patients with obstructive biliary disease, bile levels of Ancef are considerably lower than serum levels (< 1.0 mcg/mL).

In synovial fluid, the Ancef level becomes comparable to that reached in serum at about 4 hours after drug administration.

Studies of cord blood show prompt transfer of Ancef across the placenta. Ancef is present in very low concentrations in the milk of nursing mothers.

Ancef is excreted unchanged in the urine. In the first 6 hours approximately 60% of the drug is excreted in the urine and this increases to 70% to 80% within 24 hours. Ancef achieves peak urine concentrations of approximately

2400 mcg/mL and 4000 mcg/mL respectively following 500 mg and 1 gram intramuscular doses.

In patients undergoing peritoneal dialysis (2 l/hr.), Ancef produced mean serum levels of approximately 10 and 30 mcg/mL after 24 hours' instillation of a dialyzing solution containing 50 mg/l and 150 mg/l, respectively. Mean peak levels were 29 mcg/mL (range 13–44 mcg/mL) with 50 mg/l (three patients), and 72 mcg/mL (range 26–142 mcg/mL) with 150 mg/l (six patients). Intraperitoneal administration of Ancef is usually well tolerated.

Controlled studies on adult normal volunteers, receiving 1 gram 4 times a day for 10 days, monitoring CBC, SGOT, SGPT, bilirubin, alkaline phosphatase, BUN, creatinine and urinalysis, indicated no clinically significant changes attributed to Ancef.

Microbiology: In vitro tests demonstrate that the bactericidal action of cephalosporins results from inhibition of cell wall synthesis. Ancef (sterile cefazolin sodium) is active against the following organisms in vitro and in clinical infections:

Staphylococcus aureus (including penicillinase-producing strains)
Staphylococcus epidermidis
Methicillin-resistant staphylococci are uniformly resistant to cefazolin
Group A beta-hemolytic streptococci and other strains of streptococci (many strains of enterococci are resistant)
Streptococcus pneumoniae
Escherichia coli
Proteus mirabilis
Klebsiella species
Enterobacter aerogenes
Haemophilus influenzae

Most strains of indole positive Proteus (Proteus vulgaris), Enterobacter cloacae, Morganella morganii and Providencia rettgeri are resistant. Serratia, Pseudomonas, Mima, Herellea species are almost uniformly resistant to cefazolin.

Disk Susceptibility Tests

Disk diffusion technique—Quantitative methods that require measurement of zone diameters give the most precise estimates of antibiotic susceptibility. One such procedure[1] has been recommended for use with disks to test susceptibility to cefazolin.

Reports from a laboratory using the standardized single-disk susceptibility test[1] with a 30 mcg cefazolin disk should be interpreted according to the following criteria:

Susceptible organisms produce zones of 18 mm or greater, indicating that the tested organism is likely to respond to therapy.

Organisms of intermediate susceptibility produce zones 15 to 17 mm, indicating that the tested organism would be susceptible if high dosage is used or if the infection is confined to tissues and fluids (e.g., urine), in which high antibiotic levels are attained.

Resistant organisms produce zones of 14 mm or less, indicating that other therapy should be selected.

---

1 Bauer, A.W.; Kirby, W.M.M.; Sherris, J.C., and Turck, M.: Antibiotic Testing by a Standardized Single Disc Method, Am. J. Clin. Path. 45:493, 1966. Standardized Disc Susceptibility Test, Federal Register 39:19182-19184, 1974.

For gram-positive isolates, a zone of 18 mm is indicative of a cefazolin-susceptible organism when tested with either the cephalosporin-class disk (30 mcg cephalothin) or the cefazolin disk (30 mcg cefazolin).

Gram-negative organisms should be tested with the cefazolin disk (using the above criteria), since cefazolin has been shown by in vitro tests to have activity against certain strains of Enterobacteriaceae found resistant when tested with the cephalothin disk. Gram-negative organisms having zones of less than 18 mm around the cephalothin disk may be susceptible to cefazolin.

Standardized procedures require use of control organisms. The 30 mcg cefazolin disk should give zone diameter between 23 and 29 mm for E. coli ATCC 25922 and between 29 and 35 mm for S. aureus ATCC 25923.

The cefazolin disk should not be used for testing susceptibility to other cephalosporins.

Dilution techniques—A bacterial isolate may be considered susceptible if the minimal inhibitory concentration (MIC) for cefazolin is not more than 16 mcg per mL. Organisms are considered resistant if the MIC is equal to or greater than 64 mcg per mL.

The range of MIC's for the control strains are as follows:

S. aureus ATCC 25923, 0.25 to 1.0 mcg/mL
E. coli ATCC 25922, 1.0 to 4.0 mcg/mL

INDICATIONS AND USAGE

Ancef (sterile cefazolin sodium) is indicated in the treatment of the following serious infections due to susceptible organisms:

RESPIRATORY TRACT INFECTIONS due to Streptococcus pneumoniae, Klebsiella species, Haemophilus influenzae, Staphylococcus aureus (penicillin-sensitive and penicillin-resistant) and group A beta-hemolytic streptococci.

Injectable benzathine penicillin is considered to be the drug of choice in treatment and prevention of streptococcal infections, including the prophylaxis of rheumatic fever.

Ancef is effective in the eradication of streptococci from the nasopharynx; however, data establishing the efficacy of *Ancef* in the subsequent prevention of rheumatic fever are not available at present.

URINARY TRACT INFECTIONS due to *Escherichia coli, Proteus mirabilis, Klebsiella* species and some strains of enterobacter and enterococci.

SKIN AND SKIN STRUCTURE INFECTIONS due to *Staphylococcus aureus* (penicillin-sensitive and penicillin-resistant), group A beta-hemolytic streptococci and other strains of streptococci.

BILIARY TRACT INFECTIONS due to *Escherichia coli,* various strains of streptococci, *Proteus mirabilis, Klebsiella* species and *Staphylococcus aureus.*

BONE AND JOINT INFECTIONS due to *Staphylococcus aureus.*

GENITAL INFECTIONS (i.e., prostatitis, epididymitis) due to *Escherichia coli, Proteus mirabilis, Klebsiella* species and some strains of enterococci.

SEPTICEMIA due to *Streptococcus pneumoniae, Staphylococcus aureus* (penicillin-sensitive and penicillin-resistant), *Proteus mirabilis, Escherichia coli* and *Klebsiella* species.

ENDOCARDITIS due to *Staphylococcus aureus* (penicillin-sensitive and penicillin-resistant) and group A beta-hemolytic streptococci.

Appropriate culture and susceptibility studies should be performed to determine susceptibility of the causative organism to *Ancef.*

PERIOPERATIVE PROPHYLAXIS: The prophylactic administration of *Ancef* preoperatively, intraoperatively and postoperatively may reduce the incidence of certain postoperative infections in patients undergoing surgical procedures which are classified as contaminated or potentially contaminated (e.g., vaginal hysterectomy, and cholecystectomy in high-risk patients such as those over 70 years of age, with acute cholecystitis, obstructive jaundice or common duct bile stones).

The perioperative use of *Ancef* may also be effective in surgical patients in whom infection at the operative site would present a serious risk (e.g., during open-heart surgery and prosthetic arthroplasty).

The prophylactic administration of *Ancef* should usually be discontinued within a 24-hour period after the surgical procedure. In surgery where the occurrence of infection may be particularly devastating (e.g., open-heart surgery and prosthetic arthroplasty), the prophylactic administration of *Ancef* may be continued for 3 to 5 days following the completion of surgery.

If there are signs of infection, specimens for cultures should be obtained for the identification of the causative organism so that appropriate therapy may be instituted. (See DOSAGE AND ADMINISTRATION.)

CONTRAINDICATIONS

ANCEF (STERILE CEFAZOLIN SODIUM) IS CONTRAINDICATED IN PATIENTS WITH KNOWN ALLERGY TO THE CEPHALOSPORIN GROUP OF ANTIBIOTICS.

WARNINGS

SERIOUS AND OCCASIONALLY FATAL HYPERSENSITIVITY (anaphylactic) REACTIONS HAVE BEEN REPORTED IN PATIENTS ON PENICILLIN THERAPY. THESE REACTIONS ARE MORE LIKELY TO OCCUR IN INDIVIDUALS WITH A HISTORY OF PENICILLIN HYPERSENSITIVITY AND/OR A HISTORY OF SENSITIVITY TO MULTIPLE ALLERGENS. THERE HAVE BEEN REPORTS OF INDIVIDUALS WITH A HISTORY OF PENICILLIN HYPERSENSITIVITY WHO HAVE EXPERIENCED SEVERE REACTIONS WHEN TREATED WITH CEPHALOSPORINS. BEFORE INITIATING THERAPY WITH *ANCEF,* CAREFUL INQUIRY SHOULD BE MADE CONCERNING PREVIOUS HYPERSENSITIVITY REACTIONS TO PENICILLINS, CEPHALOSPORINS OR OTHER ALLERGENS. IF AN ALLERGIC REACTION OCCURS, *ANCEF* SHOULD BE DISCONTINUED AND APPROPRIATE THERAPY SHOULD BE INSTITUTED. SERIOUS ANAPHYLACTIC REACTIONS REQUIRE IMMEDIATE EMERGENCY TREATMENT WITH EPINEPHRINE. OXYGEN, INTRAVENOUS STEROIDS AND AIRWAY MANAGEMENT, INCLUDING INTUBATION, SHOULD ALSO BE ADMINISTERED AS INDICATED.

Pseudomembranous colitis has been reported with nearly all antibacterial agents, including *Ancef,* and may range in severity from mild to life-threatening. Therefore, it is important to consider this diagnosis in patients who present with diarrhea subsequent to the administration of antibacterial agents.

Treatment with antibacterial agents alters the normal flora of the colon and may permit overgrowth of clostridia. Studies indicate that a toxin produced by *Clostridium difficile* is one primary cause of "antibiotic-associated colitis."

After the diagnosis of pseudomembranous colitis has been established, therapeutic measures should be initiated. Mild cases of pseudomembranous colitis usually respond to drug discontinuation alone. In moderate to severe cases, consideration should be given to management with fluids and electrolytes, protein supplementation and treatment with an antibacterial drug clinically effective against *C. difficile* colitis.

PRECAUTIONS

General—Prolonged use of Ancef (sterile cefazolin sodium) may result in the overgrowth of nonsusceptible organisms. Careful clinical observation of the patient is essential.

When *Ancef* is administered to patients with low urinary output because of impaired renal function, lower daily dosage is required (see DOSAGE AND ADMINISTRATION).

As with other beta-lactam antibiotics, seizures may occur if inappropriately high doses are administered to patients with impaired renal function (see DOSAGE AND ADMINISTRATION).

Ancef, as with all cephalosporins, should be prescribed with caution in individuals with a history of gastrointestinal disease, particularly colitis.

Drug Interactions—Probenecid may decrease renal tubular secretion of cephalosporins when used concurrently, resulting in increased and more prolonged cephalosporin blood levels.

Drug/Laboratory Test Interactions—A false positive reaction for glucose in the urine may occur with Benedict's solution, Fehling's solution or with Clinitest® tablets, but not with enzyme-based tests such as Clinistix® and Tes-Tape®. Positive direct and indirect antiglobulin (Coombs) tests have occurred; these may also occur in neonates whose mothers received cephalosporins before delivery.

Carcinogenesis/Mutagenesis — Mutagenicity studies and long-term studies in animals to determine the carcinogenic potential of Ancef (sterile cefazolin sodium) have not been performed.

Pregnancy — Teratogenic Effects — Pregnancy Category B. Reproduction studies have been performed in rats, mice and rabbits at doses up to 25 times the human dose and have revealed no evidence of impaired fertility or harm to the fetus due to *Ancef.* There are, however, no adequate and well-controlled studies in pregnant women. Because animal reproduction studies are not always predictive of human response, this drug should be used during pregnancy only if clearly needed.

Labor and Delivery—When cefazolin has been administered prior to caesarean section, drug levels in cord blood have been approximately one quarter to one third of maternal drug levels. The drug appears to have no adverse effect on the fetus.

Nursing Mothers—Ancef (sterile cefazolin sodium) is present in very low concentrations in the milk of nursing mothers. Caution should be exercised when *Ancef* is administered to a nursing woman.

Pediatric Use—Safety and effectiveness for use in prematures and infants under 1 month of age have not been established. See DOSAGE AND ADMINISTRATION for recommended dosage in children over 1 month.

The potential for the toxic effect in children from chemicals that may leach from the single-dose I.V. preparation in plastic has not been determined.

ADVERSE REACTIONS

The following reactions have been reported:

Gastrointestinal: Diarrhea, oral candidiasis (oral thrush), vomiting, nausea, stomach cramps, anorexia and pseudomembranous colitis. Onset of pseudomembranous colitis symptoms may occur during or after antibiotic treatment (see WARNINGS). Nausea and vomiting have been reported rarely.

Allergic: Anaphylaxis, eosinophilia, itching, drug fever, skin rash, Stevens-Johnson syndrome.

Hematologic: Neutropenia, leukopenia, thrombocytopenia, thrombocythemia.

Hepatic and Renal: Transient rise in SGOT, SGPT, BUN and alkaline phosphatase levels has been observed without clinical evidence of renal or hepatic impairment.

Local Reactions: Rare instances of phlebitis have been reported at site of injection. Pain at the site of injection after intramuscular administration has occurred infrequently. Some induration has occurred.

Other Reactions: Genital and anal pruritus (including vulvar pruritus, genital moniliasis and vaginitis).

DOSAGE AND ADMINISTRATION

Usual Adult Dosage

Type of Infection	Dose	Frequency
Moderate to severe infections	500 mg to 1 gram	every 6 to 8 hrs.
Mild infections caused by susceptible gram + cocci	250 mg to 500 mg	every 8 hours
Acute, uncomplicated urinary tract infections	1 gram	every 12 hours
Pneumococcal pneumonia	500 mg	every 12 hours
Severe, life-threatening infections (e.g., endocarditis, septicemia)*	1 gram to 1.5 grams	every 6 hours

* In rare instances, doses of up to 12 grams of *Ancef* per day have been used.

Perioperative Prophylactic Use

To prevent postoperative infection in contaminated or potentially contaminated surgery, recommended doses are:

a. 1 gram I.V. or I.M. administered 1/2 hour to 1 hour prior to the start of surgery.
b. For lengthy operative procedures (e.g., 2 hours or more), 500 mg to 1 gram I.V. or I.M. during surgery (administration modified depending on the duration of the operative procedure).
c. 500 mg to 1 gram I.V. or I.M. every 6 to 8 hours for 24 hours postoperatively.

It is important that (1) the preoperative dose be given just (1/2 to 1 hour) prior to the start of surgery so that adequate antibiotic levels are present in the serum and tissues at the time of initial surgical incision; and (2) *Ancef* be administered, if necessary, at appropriate intervals during surgery to provide sufficient levels of the antibiotic at the anticipated moments of greatest exposure to infective organisms.

In surgery where the occurrence of infection may be particularly devastating (e.g., open-heart surgery and prosthetic arthroplasty), the prophylactic administration of *Ancef* (sterile cefazolin sodium) may be continued for 3 to 5 days following the completion of surgery.

Dosage Adjustment for Patients with Reduced Renal Function

Ancef may be used in patients with reduced renal function with the following dosage adjustments: Patients with a creatinine clearance of 55 mL/min. or greater or a serum creatinine of 1.5 mg % or less can be given full doses. Patients with creatinine clearance rates of 35 to 54 mL/min. or serum creatinine of 1.6 to 3.0 mg % can also be given full doses but dosage should be restricted to at least 8 hour intervals. Patients with creatinine clearance rates of 11 to 34 mL/min. or serum creatinine of 3.1 to 4.5 mg % should be given 1/2 the usual dose every 12 hours. Patients with creatinine clearance rates of 10 mL/min. or less or serum creatinine of 4.6 mg % or greater should be given 1/2 the usual dose every 18 to 24 hours. All reduced dosage recommendations apply after an initial loading dose appropriate to the severity of the infection. Patients undergoing peritoneal dialysis: See Human Pharmacology.

Pediatric Dosage

In children, a total daily dosage of 25 to 50 mg per kg (approximately 10 to 20 mg per pound) of body weight, divided into three or four equal doses, is effective for most mild to moderately severe infections. Total daily dosage may be increased to 100 mg per kg (45 mg per pound) of body weight for severe infections. Since safety for use in premature infants and in infants under 1 month has not been established, the use of Ancef (sterile cefazolin sodium) in these patients is not recommended.

Pediatric Dosage Guide

Weight		25 mg/kg/Day Divided into 3 Doses		25 mg/kg/Day Divided into 4 Doses	
Lbs	Kg	Approximate Single Dose mg/q8h	Vol. (mL) needed with dilution of 125 mg/mL	Approximate Single Dose mg/q6h	Vol. (mL) needed with dilution of 125 mg/mL
10	4.5	40 mg	0.35 mL	30 mg	0.25 mL
20	9.0	75 mg	0.60 mL	55 mg	0.45 mL
30	13.6	115 mg	0.90 mL	85 mg	0.70 mL
40	18.1	150 mg	1.20 mL	115 mg	0.90 mL
50	22.7	190 mg	1.50 mL	140 mg	1.10 mL

Continued on next page

Information on the SmithKline Beecham Pharmaceuticals products appearing here is based on the labeling in effect on July 1, 1996. Further information on these and other products may be obtained from the Medical Department, SmithKline Beecham Pharmaceuticals, One Franklin Plaza, Philadelphia, PA 19101.

SmithKline Beecham—Cont.

Weight		50 mg/kg/Day Divided into 3 Doses		50 mg/kg/Day Divided into 4 Doses	
Lbs	Kg	Approximate Single Dose mg/q8h	Vol. (mL) needed with dilution of 225 mg/mL	Approximate Single Dose mg/q6h	Vol. (mL) needed with dilution of 225 mg/mL
10	4.5	75 mg	0.35 mL	55 mg	0.25 mL
20	9.0	150 mg	0.70 mL	110 mg	0.50 mL
30	13.6	225 mg	1.00 mL	170 mg	0.75 mL
40	18.1	300 mg	1.35 mL	225 mg	1.00 mL
50	22.7	375 mg	1.70 mL	285 mg	1.25 mL

In children with mild to moderate renal impairment (creatinine clearance of 70 to 40 mL/min.), 60 percent of the normal daily dose given in equally divided doses every 12 hours should be sufficient. In patients with moderate impairment (creatinine clearance of 40 to 20 mL/min.), 25 percent of the normal daily dose given in equally divided doses every 12 hours should be adequate. Children with severe renal impairment (creatinine clearance of 20 to 5 mL/min.) may be given 10 percent of the normal daily dose every 24 hours. All dosage recommendations apply after an initial loading dose.

RECONSTITUTION

Preparation of Parenteral Solution
Parenteral drug products should be SHAKEN WELL when reconstituted, and inspected visually for particulate matter prior to administration. If particulate matter is evident in reconstituted fluids, the drug solutions should be discarded. When reconstituted or diluted according to the instructions below, Ancef (sterile cefazolin sodium) is stable for 24 hours at room temperature or for 10 days if stored under refrigeration (5°C or 41°F). Reconstituted solutions may range in color from pale yellow to yellow without a change in potency.

Single-Dose Vials
For I.M. injection, I.V. direct (bolus) injection or I.V. infusion, reconstitute with Sterile Water for Injection according to the following table. SHAKE WELL.

Vial Size	Amount of Diluent	Approximate Concentration	Approximate Available Volume
500 mg	2.0 mL	225 mg/mL	2.2 mL
1 gram	2.5 mL	330 mg/mL	3.0 mL

Pharmacy Bulk Vials
Add Sterile Water for Injection, Bacteriostatic Water for Injection or Sodium Chloride Injection according to the table below. SHAKE WELL.

Vial Size	Amount of Diluent	Approximate Concentration	Approximate Available Volume
5 grams	23 mL	1 gram/5 mL	26 mL
	48 mL	1 gram/10 mL	51 mL
10 grams	45 mL	1 gram/5 mL	51 mL
	96 mL	1 gram/10 mL	102 mL

"Piggyback" Vials
Reconstitute with 50 to 100 mL of Sodium Chloride Injection or other I.V. solution listed under ADMINISTRATION. When adding diluent to vial, allow air to escape by using a small vent needle or by pumping the syringe. SHAKE WELL. Administer with primary I.V. fluids, as a single dose.

ADMINISTRATION
Intramuscular Administration—Reconstitute vials with Sterile Water for Injection according to the dilution table above. Shake well until dissolved. Ancef should be injected into a large muscle mass. Pain on injection is infrequent with Ancef.

Intravenous Administration—Direct (bolus) injection: Following reconstitution according to the above table, further dilute vials with approximately 5 mL Sterile Water for Injection. Inject the solution slowly over 3 to 5 minutes, directly or through tubing for patients receiving parenteral fluids (see list below).

Intermittent or continuous infusion: Dilute reconstituted Ancef in 50 to 100 mL of one of the following solutions:
Sodium Chloride Injection, USP
5% or 10% Dextrose Injection, USP
5% Dextrose in Lactated Ringer's Injection, USP
5% Dextrose and 0.9% Sodium Chloride Injection, USP
5% Dextrose and 0.45% Sodium Chloride Injection, USP
5% Dextrose and 0.2% Sodium Chloride Injection, USP
Lactated Ringer's Injection, USP
Invert Sugar 5% or 10% in Sterile Water for Injection

Ringer's Injection, USP
5% Sodium Bicarbonate Injection, USP

DIRECTIONS FOR USE OF ANCEF (CEFAZOLIN SODIUM INJECTION) GALAXY® CONTAINER (PL 2040 PLASTIC)
Ancef in Galaxy® Container (PL 2040 Plastic) is to be administered either as a continuous or intermittent infusion using sterile equipment.

Storage
Store in a freezer capable of maintaining a temperature of −20°C (−4°F).

Thawing of Plastic Container
Thaw frozen container at 25°C or 77°F or under refrigeration (5°C or 41°F). (DO NOT FORCE THAW BY IMMERSION IN WATER BATHS OR BY MICROWAVE IRRADIATION.)
Check for minute leaks by squeezing container firmly. If leaks are detected, discard solution as sterility may be impaired.
Do not add supplementary medication.
The container should be visually inspected. Components of the solution may precipitate in the frozen state and will dissolve upon reaching room temperature with little or no agitation. Potency is not affected. Agitate after solution has reached room temperature. If after visual inspection the solution remains cloudy or if an insoluble precipitate is noted or if any seals or outlet ports are not intact, the container should be discarded.
The thawed solution is stable for 30 days under refrigeration (5°C or 41°F) and 48 hours at 25°C or 77°F. Do not refreeze thawed antibiotics.
Use sterile equipment. It is recommended that the intravenous administration apparatus be replaced at least once every 48 hours.
CAUTION: Do not use plastic containers in series connections. Such use could result in air embolism due to residual air being drawn from the primary container before administration of the fluid from the secondary container is complete.

Preparation for administration:
1. Suspend container from eyelet support.
2. Remove plastic protector from outlet port at bottom of container.
3. Attach administration set. Refer to complete directions accompanying set.

HOW SUPPLIED
Ancef (sterile cefazolin sodium)—supplied in vials equivalent to 500 mg or 1 gram of cefazolin; in "Piggyback" Vials for intravenous admixture equivalent to 1 gram of cefazolin; and in Pharmacy Bulk Vials equivalent to 5 grams or 10 grams of cefazolin.
Ancef (cefazolin sodium injection) as a frozen, iso-osmotic, sterile, nonpyrogenic solution in plastic containers—supplied in 50 mL single-dose containers equivalent to 500 mg or 1 gram of cefazolin. Dextrose Hydrous, USP, has been added to the above dosages to adjust osmolality (approximately 2.4 grams and 2 grams, respectively). Store at or below −20°C (−4°F). (See DIRECTIONS FOR USE OF ANCEF [CEFAZOLIN SODIUM INJECTION] GALAXY® CONTAINER [PL 2040 PLASTIC].)
As with other cephalosporins, Ancef tends to darken depending on storage conditions; within the stated recommendations, however, product potency is not adversely affected. Before reconstitution protect from light and store between 15° and 30°C (59° and 86°F).
Ancef supplied as a frozen, iso-osmotic, sterile, nonpyrogenic solution in plastic containers is manufactured for SmithKline Beecham Pharmaceuticals by Baxter Healthcare Corporation, Deerfield, IL 60015.
Galaxy is a registered trademark of Baxter International Inc.
Veterans Administration /Military /PHS —500 mg/50 mL, frozen, 24's, 6505-01-274-9683; 1 gram/50 mL, frozen, 24's, 6505-01-237-8453

AF:L50

Shown in Product Identification Guide, page 336

ANDRODERM®
[an-drō-derm]
Testosterone Transdermal System
Controlled Delivery for Once-Daily Application

DESCRIPTION
Androderm (testosterone transdermal system) provides continuous delivery of testosterone (the primary endogenous androgen) for 24 hours following application to intact, non-scrotal skin (e.g., back, abdomen, thighs, upper arms).
Each Androderm system delivers in vivo 2.5 mg of testosterone per day across skin of average permeability.
Androderm has a 7.5 cm² central drug delivery reservoir surrounded by a peripheral adhesive area. The total contact surface area is 37 cm². Each system contains 12.2 mg testosterone USP, dissolved in an alcohol-based gel. Testosterone USP is a white, or creamy white crystalline powder or crystals chemically described as 17β-hydroxyandrost-4-en-3-one.

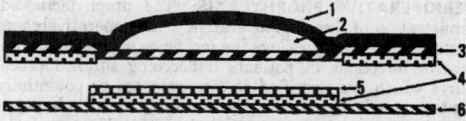

Testosterone
$C_{19}H_{28}O_2$ mw 288.43

The Androderm system has six components as shown in Figure 1. Proceeding from the top toward the surface attached to the skin, the system is composed of (1) a transparent ethylene vinyl acetate copolymer/polyester laminate backing film, (2) a drug reservoir of testosterone USP, alcohol USP, glycerin USP, glycerol monooleate, and methyl laurate gelled with an acrylic acid copolymer, (3) a permeable polyethylene microporous membrane, and (4) a peripheral layer of acrylic adhesive surrounding the central, active drug delivery area of the system. Prior to opening of the system and application to the skin, the central delivery surface of the system is sealed with a peelable laminate disc (5) composed of a five-layer laminate containing polyester/polyesterurethane adhesive/aluminum foil/polyesterurethane adhesive/polyethylene. The disc is attached to and removed with the release liner (6), a silicone-coated polyester film, which is removed before the system can be used.

1. Backing Film   3. Microporous Membrane   5. Disc
2. Drug Reservoir   4. Adhesive   6. Release Liner

Figure 1: System Schematic

The active ingredient in the system is testosterone. The remaining components of the system are pharmacologically inactive.

CLINICAL PHARMACOLOGY
Androderm (testosterone transdermal system) delivers physiologic amounts of testosterone producing circulating testosterone concentrations that approximate the normal circadian rhythm of healthy young men.

Testosterone
Androderm (testosterone transdermal system) delivers testosterone, the primary androgenic hormone. Testosterone is responsible for the normal growth and development of the male sex organs and for maintenance of secondary sex characteristics. These effects include the growth and maturation of the prostate, seminal vesicles, penis, and scrotum; development of male hair distribution, such as facial, pubic, chest, and axillary hair; laryngeal enlargement; vocal cord thickening; and alterations in body musculature and fat distribution.
Male hypogonadism results from insufficient secretion of testosterone and is characterized by low serum testosterone concentrations. Symptoms associated with male hypogonadism include the following: impotence and decreased sexual desire; fatigue and loss of energy; mood depression; and regression of secondary sexual characteristics.

General Androgen Effects
Androgens promote retention of nitrogen, sodium, potassium, and phosphorus, and decreased urinary excretion of calcium. Androgens have been reported to increase protein anabolism and decrease protein catabolism. Nitrogen balance is improved only when there is sufficient intake of calories and protein.
Androgens are also responsible for the growth spurt of adolescence and for the eventual termination of linear growth that is brought about by the fusion of the epiphyseal growth centers. In children, exogenous androgens accelerate linear growth rates but may cause disproportionate advancement in bone maturation. Use over long periods may result in fusion of the epiphyseal growth centers and termination of the growth process.
Androgens have been reported to stimulate the production of red blood cells by enhancing erythropoietin production.
During exogenous administration of androgens, endogenous testosterone release is inhibited through feedback inhibition of pituitary LH secretion. With large doses of exogenous androgens, spermatogenesis may also be suppressed through feedback inhibition of pituitary follicle stimulating hormone (FSH) secretion.
There is a lack of substantial evidence that androgens are effective in accelerating fracture healing or in shortening post-surgical convalescence.

Pharmacokinetics

Absorption

Following *Androderm* application to non-scrotal skin, testosterone is continuously absorbed during the 24-hour dosing period. Daily application of 2 systems at approximately 10 PM results in a serum testosterone concentration profile that mimics the normal circadian variation observed in healthy young men (Fig. 2 below). Maximum concentrations occur in the early morning hours with minimum concentrations in the evening (Table 1 below).

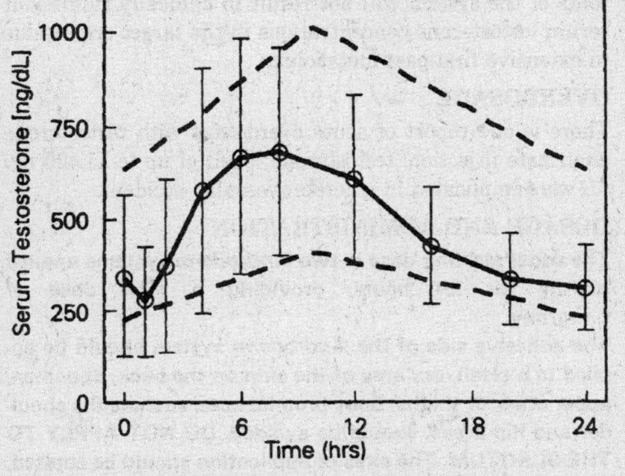

Figure 2: Mean (SD) steady state serum testosterone concentrations during nightly application of 2 systems in 29 hypogonadal male subjects. Area between the dashed lines shows the 95% confidence interval for the circadian variation observed in healthy young men.[1] System application (t=0) at approximately 10 PM.

Table 1: Steady-state serum testosterone pharmacokinetic parameters in hypogonadal men measured during continuous Androderm (testosterone transdermal system) treatment.

Parameter	Units	n	Mean	SD
C_{max}	ng/dL	56	753	276
C_{avg}	ng/dL	56	498	169
C_{min}	ng/dL	56	246	120
T_{max}	hr	56	7.9	2.2
$T_{1/2}$	min	29	71	32
CL	L/day	49	1304	464

C_{max}=maximum serum concentration
C_{avg}=average serum concentration (AUC/24 hr)
C_{min}=minimum serum concentration
T_{max}=time of maximum serum concentration
$T_{1/2}$=elimination half-life
CL=clearance

In a group of 34 hypogonadal men, application of two *Androderm* systems to the abdomen, back, thighs, or upper arms resulted in average testosterone absorption of 4 to 5 mg over 24 hours. The serum testosterone concentration profiles during application were similar for these sites (Table 2). Applications to the chest and shins resulted in greater inter-individual variability and average 24 hour absorption of 3 to 4 mg.

Table 2: Mean serum testosterone concentrations (ng/dL) measured during single-dose applications of 2 *Androderm* systems applied at night to different sites in 34 hypogonadal men.

Sample Time (hr)	Abdomen Mean	Abdomen SD	Back Mean	Back SD	Thigh Mean	Thigh SD	Upper Arm Mean	Upper Arm SD
0	90	82	80	74	85	76	81	69
3	286	201	429	252	271	201	308	226
6	476	236	608	250	489	254	468	245
9	570	234	613	214	592	251	534	204
12	575	244	588	233	594	247	527	199
24	352	164	403	174	367	161	332	124

In a steady-state study of 12 hypogonadal men, nightly application of 1, 2, or 3 *Androderm* systems resulted in increases in the mean morning serum testosterone concentrations. These concentrations averaged 424, 584, and 766 ng/dL with the application of 1, 2, and 3 systems, respectively. The mean baseline serum testosterone concentration was 76 ng/dL. Normal range morning serum testosterone concentrations are reached during the first day of dosing. There is no accumulation of testosterone during continuous treatment.

Distribution

In serum, testosterone is bound with high affinity to sex hormone binding globulin (SHBG) and with low affinity to albumin. The albumin bound portion easily dissociates and is presumed to be bioactive. The SHBG-bound portion is not considered to be bioactive. The amount of SHBG in serum and the total testosterone concentration determine the distribution of bioactive and non-bioactive androgen.

Bioactive serum testosterone concentrations (BT) measured during Androderm (testosterone transdermal system) treatment paralleled the serum testosterone profile (Figure 2) and remained within the normal reference range.

Metabolism

Inactivation of testosterone occurs primarily in the liver. Testosterone (T) is metabolized to various 17-keto steroids through two different pathways, and the major active metabolites are estradiol (E2) and dihydrotestosterone (DHT). DHT binds with greater affinity to SHBG than does testosterone. In reproductive tissues, DHT is further metabolized to 3-alpha and 3-beta androstanediol.

In many tissues, the activity of testosterone appears to depend on reduction to DHT, which binds to cytosol receptor proteins. The steroid-receptor complex is transported to the nucleus, where it initiates transcription events and cellular changes related to androgen action.

During steady-state pharmacokinetic studies in hypogonadal men treated with *Androderm*, the average DHT:T and E2:T ratios were comparable to those in normal men, approximately 1:10 and 1:200, respectively.

Upon removal of the *Androderm* systems, serum testosterone concentrations decrease with an apparent half-life of approximately 70 minutes. Hypogonadal concentrations are reached within 24 hours following system removal.

Androderm therapy suppresses endogenous testosterone secretion via the pituitary/gonadal axis, resulting in a reduction in baseline serum testosterone concentrations compared to the untreated state.

Excretion

Approximately 90% of a testosterone dose given intramuscularly is excreted in the urine as glucuronide and sulfate conjugates of testosterone and its metabolites; about 6% is excreted in the feces, mostly in unconjugated form.

Special Populations

Geriatric

No age related effects on testosterone pharmacokinetics were observed in clinical trials of *Androderm* in men up to 65 years of age. In a group of 9 elderly testosterone deficient men (65–79 years of age, average baseline testosterone level 184±50 ng/dL), a single application of 2 *Androderm* systems to the back resulted in an average testosterone level of 591±121 ng/dL with a T_{max} of 14.2±4.2 hours. The total testosterone delivered over the 24-hour application time was 3.8±0.6 mg, approximately 20% less than the average amount delivered in younger patients.

Race

There is insufficient information available from *Androderm* trials to compare testosterone pharmacokinetics in different racial groups.

Renal Insufficiency

There is no experience with use of *Androderm* in patients with renal insufficiency.

Hepatic Insufficiency

There is no experience with use of *Androderm* in patients with hepatic insufficiency.

Drug-Drug Interactions

See "Precautions" below

Clinical Studies

In clinical studies, 93% of patients were treated with two *Androderm* systems daily, 6% used three systems daily, and 1% used one system daily.

The hormonal effects of Androderm (testosterone transdermal system) as a treatment for male hypogonadism were demonstrated in four open-label trials that included 94 hypogonadal men, ages 15 to 65 years. In these trials, *Androderm* produced average morning serum testosterone concentrations within the normal reference range in 92% of patients. The mean (SD) serum hormone concentrations and percentage of patients who achieved average concentrations within the normal ranges are shown in Table 3 below.

Table 3: Individual morning serum hormone concentrations (ng/dL) and percent of patients with mean concentrations within the normal range during continuous *Androderm* treatment (n=94).

Normal Range	T (306–1031)	BT (93–420)	DHT (28–85)	E2 (0.9–3.6)
Mean	589	312	47	2.7
SD	209	127	18	1.2
% Normal	92	88	85	77
% High	1	12	2	22
% Low	7	0	13	1

A physiological suppression of the pituitary/gonadal axis occurs during continuous *Androderm* treatment leading to reduced serum LH concentrations. In clinical trials, 10 of 21 (48%) of men with primary (hypergonadotropic) hypogonadism achieved normal range LH concentrations within 6 to 12 months of treatment. LH concentrations may remain elevated in some patients despite serum testosterone concentrations within the normal range.

Twenty-nine patients, previously treated with testosterone, completed 12 months of *Androderm* treatment. Following an 8-week androgen withdrawal period, *Androderm* treatment produced positive effects on fatigue, mood and sexual function. The percent of patients complaining of fatigue decreased from 79% to 10% during treatment ($p<0.001$). The average patient depression score (Beck Depression Inventory) decreased from 6.9 to 3.9 ($p<0.001$). Nocturnal penile tumescence and rigidity monitoring showed an increase in mean duration of erections 0.23 to 0.39 hours per night ($p=0.01$) and an increase in penile tip rigidity from 18% to 50% ($p<0.001$). The total number of self-reported erections reported increased from 2.3 to 7.8 per week ($p<0.001$).

Comparison with intramuscular testosterone: Sixty-six patients, previously treated with testosterone injections, received *Androderm* or intramuscular testosterone enanthate (200 mg every 2 weeks) treatment for 6 months. The percent of time that serum concentrations measured throughout the dosing interval remained within the normal range were as follows:

	Androderm	IM	*p* value
T	82%	72%	0.05
BT	87%	39%	<0.001
DHT	76%	70%	0.06
E2	81%	35%	<0.001

Sexual function was comparable between groups.

Effect on plasma lipids: In 67 men treated for 6 to 12 months, the average (SE) serum total cholesterol and HDL concentrations were 199 (7.6) ng/dL and 46 (2.3) ng/dL.

Compared to baseline values during a hypogonadal state achieved by 8 weeks of androgen withdrawal in 29 patients, the following changes in lipids were observed during 1 year of *Androderm* treatment: Cholesterol decreased 1.2%; HDL decreased 8%; Cholesterol/HDL ratio increased 9%. In these patients, lipids measured during *Androderm* treatment were not significantly different from those measured during prior IM injection treatment.

Effects on the prostate: Prostate size and serum prostate specific antigen (PSA) concentrations during treatment were comparable to values reported for eugonadal men. One case of prostate carcinoma occurred during *Androderm* treatment; two cases were detected during IM treatment.

INDICATIONS AND USAGE

Androderm (testosterone transdermal system) is indicated for testosterone replacement therapy in men for conditions associated with a deficiency or absence of endogenous testosterone.

Primary hypogonadism (congenital or acquired)—Testicular failure due to cryptorchidism, bilateral torsion, orchitis, vanishing testis syndrome, or orchidectomy, Klinefelter's syndrome, chemotherapy, or toxic damage from alcohol or heavy metals. These men usually have low serum testosterone concentrations accompanied by gonadotropins (FSH, LH) above the normal range.

Secondary, i.e., hypogonadotropic hypogonadism (congenital or acquired)—idiopathic gonadotropin or luteinizing hormone-releasing hormone (LHRH) deficiency, or pituitary-hypothalamic injury from tumors, trauma, or radiation. These men have low serum testosterone concentrations without associated elevation in gonadotropins. Appropriate adrenal cortical and thyroid hormone replacement therapy may be necessary in patients with multiple pituitary or hypothalamic abnormalities.

CONTRAINDICATIONS

Androgens are contraindicated in men with carcinoma of the breast or known or suspected carcinoma of the prostate.

Androderm therapy has not been evaluated in women and must not be used in women. Testosterone may cause fetal harm.

Androderm is contraindicated in patients with known hypersensitivity to any of its components.

WARNINGS

Prolonged use of high doses of orally active 17-alpha-alkyl androgens (e.g., methyltestosterone) has been associated with the development of peliosis hepatis, cholestatic jaundice and hepatic neoplasms, including hepatocellular carcinoma (see PRECAUTIONS, Carcinogenesis). Peliosis hepatis can be a life-threatening or fatal complication. Testosterone is not known to produce these adverse effects.

Geriatric patients treated with androgens may be at an increased risk for the development of prostatic hyperplasia.

Geriatric patients and other patients with clinical or demographic characteristics that are recognized to be associated with an increased risk of prostate cancer should be evaluated for the presence of subclinical or clinical prostate cancer prior to initiation of testosterone replacement therapy, be-

Continued on next page

Information on the SmithKline Beecham Pharmaceuticals products appearing here is based on the labeling in effect on July 1, 1996. Further information on these and other products may be obtained from the Medical Department, SmithKline Beecham Pharmaceuticals, One Franklin Plaza, Philadelphia, PA 19101.

SmithKline Beecham—Cont.

cause testosterone therapy may promote the growth of existing subclinical foci of prostate cancer.[2]

In men receiving testosterone replacement therapy, surveillance for prostate cancer should be consistent with current practices for eugonadal men (see PRECAUTIONS, Carcinogenesis).

Edema, with or without congestive heart failure, may be a serious complication of androgen treatment in patients with preexisting cardiac, renal, or hepatic disease. In addition to discontinuation of the drug, diuretic therapy may be required.

Gynecomastia frequently develops and occasionally persists in patients being treated for hypogonadism.

PRECAUTIONS

General

The physician should instruct patients to report any of the following side effects of androgens:
- Too frequent or persistent erections of the penis
- Any nausea, vomiting, jaundice, or ankle swelling

Virilization of female sexual partners has been reported with male use of a topical testosterone solution. Topically applied creams leave as much as 90 mg residual testosterone on the skin. The occlusive backing film on Androderm (testosterone transdermal system) prevents the partner from coming in contact with the active material in the system. Transfer of the system to the partner is unlikely.

Changes in body hair distribution, significant increase in acne, or other signs of virilization of the female partner should be brought to the attention of a physician.

Information for Patients

An information brochure is available for patients concerning the use of Androderm.

Advise patients of the following:

Androderm should not be applied to the scrotum.

Androderm should not be applied over a bony prominence or on a part of the body that could be subject to prolonged pressure during sleep or sitting. Application to these sites has been associated with burn-like blister reactions.

Androderm does not have to be removed during sexual intercourse, nor while taking a shower or bath.

Androderm systems should be applied nightly.

Laboratory Tests

Hemoglobin and hematocrit should be checked periodically to detect polycythemia in patients who are receiving androgen therapy.

Liver function, prostate specific antigen, total cholesterol and HDL cholesterol should be checked periodically.

Drug Interactions

Anticoagulants: C-17 substituted derivatives of testosterone, such as methandrostenolone, have been reported to decrease the anticoagulant requirements of patients receiving oral anticoagulants. Patients receiving oral anticoagulants require close monitoring especially when androgens are started or stopped.

Oxyphenbutazone: Concurrent administration of oxyphenbutazone and androgens may result in elevated serum levels of oxyphenbutazone.

Insulin: In diabetic patients, the metabolic effects of androgens may decrease blood glucose and, therefore, insulin requirements.

Drug/Laboratory Test Interferences

Androgens may decrease levels of thyroxine-binding globulin, resulting in decreased total T_4 serum levels and increased resin uptake of T_3 and T_4. Free thyroid hormone levels remain unchanged, however, and there is no clinical evidence of thyroid dysfunction.

Carcinogenesis, Mutagenesis, Impairment of Fertility

Animal Data: Testosterone has been tested by subcutaneous injection and implantation in mice and rats. The implant induced cervical-uterine tumors in mice, which metastasized in some cases. There is suggestive evidence that injection of testosterone into some strains of female mice increases their susceptibility to hepatoma. Testosterone is also known to increase the number of tumors and decrease the degree of differentiation of chemically induced carcinomas of the liver in rats.

Human Data: There are rare reports of hepatocellular carcinoma in patients receiving long-term therapy with androgens in high doses. Withdrawal of drugs did not lead to regression of the tumors in all cases.

Geriatric patients treated with androgens may be at an increased risk for the development of prostatic hyperplasia.

Geriatric patients and other patients with clinical or demographic characteristics that are recognized to be associated with an increased risk of prostate cancer should be evaluated for the presence of subclinical or clinical prostate cancer prior to initiation of testosterone replacement therapy, because testosterone therapy may promote the growth of existing subclinical foci of prostate cancer.[2]

In men receiving testosterone replacement therapy, surveillance for prostate cancer should be consistent with current practices for eugonadal men.

Pregnancy Category X: (See Contraindications).

Teratogenic Effects: *Androderm* must not be used in women.

Nursing Mothers: *Androderm* must not be used in women.

Pediatric Use: *Androderm* has not been evaluated clinically in males under 15 years of age.

ADVERSE REACTIONS

Adverse Events Associated with Androderm (testosterone transdermal system)

In clinical studies of 122 patients treated with *Androderm*, the most common adverse events reported were skin reactions at the site of system application. Transient mild to moderate erythema was observed at the site of application in the majority of patients at some time during treatment.

The adverse reactions reported by more than 1% of patients are listed below shown in order of decreasing frequency.

Event	Percent of Patients
pruritus at application site	37%
burn-like blister reaction under system	12%
erythema at application site	7%
vesicles at application site	6%
prostate abnormalities	5%
headache	4%
allergic contact dermatitis to the system	4%
burning at application site	3%
induration at application site	3%
depression	3%
rash	2%
gastrointestinal bleeding	2%

The following reactions occurred in less than 1% of patients: fatigue; body pain; pelvic pain; hypertension; peripheral vascular disease; increased appetite; accelerated growth; anxiety; confusion; decreased libido; paresthesia; thinking abnormalities; vertigo; acne; bullae at application site; mechanical irritation at application site; rash at application site; contamination of application site; prostate carcinoma; dysuria; hematuria; impotence; urinary incontinence; urinary tract infection; testicular abnormalities.

Three types of application site reactions occurred: irritation which included mild to moderate erythema, induration or burning; allergic contact dermatitis; and burn-like blister reactions.

Chronic skin irritation caused 5% of patients to discontinue treatment. Mild skin irritation may be ameliorated by treatment of affected skin with over-the-counter topical hydrocortisone cream or topical antihistamine products.

Five patients (4%) developed allergic contact dermatitis after 3 to 8 weeks treatment that required discontinuation. These reactions were characterized by pruritus, erythema, induration and in some instances vesicles or bullae, which recurred with each system application. Rechallenge with components of the system showed ethanol sensitization in 4 patients. One patient's reaction was attributed to testosterone. None of these patients had adverse sequelae related to oral alcohol ingestion or to injectable testosterone use. Older patients may be more prone to develop allergic contact dermatitis.

Fourteen patients (12%) had burn-like blister reactions that involved bullae, epidermal necrosis or the development of ulcerated lesions. These reactions typically occurred once, at a single application site; 5 patients experienced a single recurrence. None withdrew from the clinical trials. These reactions occurred at a rate of approximately 1 in 6,500 system applications (1 in 3,250 treatment days). The majority of these lesions were associated with system application over bony prominences or on parts of the body that may have been subject to prolonged pressure during sleep or sitting (e.g., over the deltoid region of the upper arm, the greater trochanter of the femur, or the ischial tuberosity). The more severe lesions healed over several weeks with scarring in some cases. Such lesions should be treated as burns.

Adverse Events Associated with Injection or Oral Treatments

Skin and Appendages: Hirsutism, male pattern of baldness, seborrhea, and acne.

Endocrine and Urogenital: Gynecomastia and excessive frequency and duration of penile erections. Oligospermia may occur at high dosages (see CLINICAL PHARMACOLOGY).

Fluid and Electrolyte Disturbances: Retention of sodium, chloride, water, potassium, calcium, and inorganic phosphates.

Gastrointestinal: Nausea, cholestatic jaundice, alterations in liver function tests. Rare instances of hepatocellular neoplasms and peliosis hepatis have occurred (see WARNINGS).

Hematologic: Suppression of clotting factors II, V, VII, and X; bleeding in patients on concomitant anticoagulant therapy and polycythemia.

Nervous System: Increased or decreased libido, headache, anxiety, depression and generalized paresthesia.

Metabolic: Increased serum cholesterol.

Miscellaneous: Rarely, anaphylactoid reactions.

DRUG ABUSE AND DEPENDENCE

Androderm (testosterone transdermal system) is a Schedule III controlled substance under the Anabolic Steroids Control Act.

Oral consumption of the *Androderm* system or the gel contents of the system will not result in clinically significant serum testosterone concentrations in the target organs due to extensive first-pass metabolism.

OVERDOSAGE

There is one report of acute overdosage with testosterone enanthate injection: testosterone levels of up to 11,400 ng/dL were implicated in a cerebrovascular accident.

DOSAGE AND ADMINISTRATION

The usual starting dose is two *Androderm* systems applied nightly for 24 hours, providing a total dose of 5 mg/day.

The adhesive side of the *Androderm* system should be applied to a clean, dry area of the skin on the back, abdomen, upper arms, or thighs. Bony prominences, such as the shoulder and hip areas, should be avoided. DO NOT APPLY TO THE SCROTUM. The sites of application should be rotated, with an interval of 7 days between applications to the same site. The area selected should not be oily, damaged, or irritated. (See Table 2.)

The system should be applied immediately after opening the pouch and removing the protective release liner. The system should be pressed firmly in place, making sure there is good contact with the skin, especially around the edges.

To ensure proper dosing, the morning serum testosterone concentration may be measured following system application the previous evening. If the serum concentration is outside the normal range, sampling should be repeated with assurance of proper system adhesion as well as appropriate application time. Confirmed serum concentrations outside the normal range may require increasing the dosing regimen to 3 systems, or decreasing the regimen to 1 system, maintaining nightly application. Because of variability in analytical values among diagnostic laboratories, this laboratory work and any later analyses for assessing the effect of *Androderm* therapy, should be performed at the same laboratory so results can be more easily compared.

Androderm (testosterone transdermal system) therapy for non-virilized patients may be initiated with one system applied nightly.

HOW SUPPLIED

Each system contains 12.2 mg testosterone USP for delivery of 2.5 mg of testosterone per day (see DESCRIPTION).

Cartons of 60 systems NDC 0007-3155-18
Cartons of 30 systems NDC 0007-3155-13

Storage and Disposal

Store at room temperature, 15° to 30°C (59° to 86°F). Apply to skin immediately upon removal from the protective pouch. Do not store outside the pouch provided. Damaged systems should not be used. The drug reservoir may be burst by excessive pressure or heat. Discard systems in household trash in a manner that prevents accidental application or ingestion by children, pets or others.

REFERENCES

1. Mazer NA, et al. Mimicking the circadian pattern of testosterone and metabolite levels with an enhanced transdermal delivery system. In Gurney, Junjinger, Peppas, eds. *Pulsatile Drug Delivery: Current Applications and Future Trends.* Stuttgart: Wiss. Verl.-Ges.; 1993, 73-97.
2. Schroeder FH. Androgens and carcinoma of the prostate. In Neischlag E, Behre HM, eds. *Testosterone Action, Deficiency, Substitution.* Berlin/Heidelberg: Springer-Verlag; 1990, 245-260.

CAUTION: Federal law prohibits dispensing without prescription.

U.S. Patent Nos. 4,849,224, 4,855,294, 4,863,970, 4,983,395, 5,152,997, and 5,164,190.

Manufactured by:
TheraTech, Inc.
Salt Lake City, UT 84108
for SmithKline Beecham Pharmaceuticals
Philadelphia, PA

Veterans Administration/Military/PHS—
Testosterone Transdermal System,
2.5 mg, 60's 6505-01-423-4981.
AD:L3

Shown in Product Identification Guide, page 336

AUGMENTIN® ℞
[og'men-tin]
amoxicillin/clavulanate potassium
Powder for Oral Suspension and Chewable Tablets

Dose† (amoxicillin/clavulanate potassium)	AUC$_{0-\infty}$ (μg.hr./mL) amoxicillin (±S.D.)	clavulanate potassium (±S.D.)	C$_{max}$ (μg/mL)‡ amoxicillin (±S.D.)	clavulanate potassium (±S.D.)
400/57 mg (5 mL of suspension)	17.29 ±2.28	2.34 ±0.94	6.94 ±1.24	1.10 ±0.42
400/57 mg (one chewable tablet)	17.24 ±2.64	2.17 ±0.73	6.67 ±1.37	1.03 ±0.33

†Administered at the start of a light meal.
‡Mean values of 28 normal volunteers. Peak concentrations occurred approximately 1 hour after the dose.

DESCRIPTION

Augmentin is an oral antibacterial combination consisting of the semisynthetic antibiotic amoxicillin and the β-lactamase inhibitor, clavulanate potassium (the potassium salt of clavulanic acid). Amoxicillin is an analog of ampicillin, derived from the basic penicillin nucleus, 6-aminopenicillanic acid. The amoxicillin molecular formula is $C_{16}H_{19}N_3O_5S \bullet 3H_2O$ and the molecular weight is 419.46. Chemically, amoxicillin is (2S,5R,6R)-6-[(R)-(-)-2-Amino-2-(p-hydroxyphenyl)acetamido]-3,3-dimethyl-7-oxo-4-thia-1-azabicyclo[3.2.0]heptane-2- carboxylic acid trihydrate and may be represented structurally as:

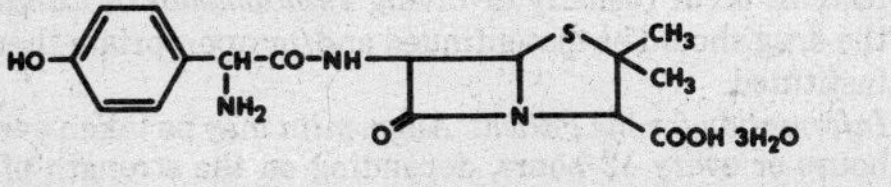

Clavulanic acid is produced by the fermentation of *Streptomyces clavuligerus*. It is a β-lactam structurally related to the penicillins and possesses the ability to inactivate a wide variety of β-lactamases by blocking the active sites of these enzymes. Clavulanic acid is particularly active against the clinically important plasmid mediated β-lactamases frequently responsible for transferred drug resistance to penicillins and cephalosporins. The clavulanate potassium molecular formula is $C_8H_8KNO_5$ and the molecular weight is 237.25. Chemically clavulanate potassium is potassium (Z)-(2R,5R)-3-(2-hydroxyethylidene)-7-oxo-4-oxa-1-azabicyclo [3.2.0]-heptane-2-carboxylate and may be represented structurally as:

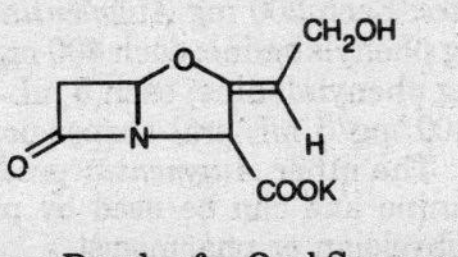

Inactive Ingredients: Powder for Oral Suspension—Colloidal silicon dioxide, flavorings (See HOW SUPPLIED), succinic acid, xanthan gum, and one or more of the following: aspartame*, hydroxypropyl methylcellulose, mannitol, silica gel, silicon dioxide and sodium saccharin. Chewable Tablets—Colloidal silicon dioxide, flavorings (See HOW SUPPLIED), magnesium stearate, mannitol and one or more of the following: aspartame*, D&C Yellow No. 10, FD&C Red No. 40, glycine, sodium saccharin and succinic acid.

*See PRECAUTIONS—Information for Patients.

Each 125 mg chewable tablet and each 5 mL of reconstituted *Augmentin* 125 mg/5 mL oral suspension contains 0.16 mEq potassium. Each 250 mg chewable tablet and each 5 mL of reconstituted *Augmentin* 250 mg/5 mL oral suspension contains 0.32 mEq potassium. Each 200 mg chewable tablet and each 5 mL of reconstituted *Augmentin* 200 mg/5 mL oral suspension contains 0.14 mEq potassium. Each 400 mg chewable tablet and each 5 mL of reconstituted *Augmentin* 400 mg/5 mL oral suspension contains 0.29 mEq of potassium.

CLINICAL PHARMACOLOGY

Amoxicillin and clavulanate potassium are well absorbed from the gastrointestinal tract after oral administration of *Augmentin*. Dosing in the fasted or fed state has minimal effect on the pharmacokinetics of amoxicillin. While *Augmentin* can be given without regard to meals, absorption of clavulanate potassium when taken with food is greater relative to the fasted state. In one study, the relative bioavailability of clavulanate was reduced when *Augmentin* was dosed at 30 and 150 minutes after the start of a high fat breakfast. The safety and efficacy of *Augmentin* have been established in clinical trials where *Augmentin* was taken without regard to meals.

Oral administration of single doses of 400 mg *Augmentin* chewable tablets and 400 mg/5 mL suspension to 28 adult volunteers yielded comparable pharmacokinetic data:

[See table above.]

Oral administration of 5 mL of *Augmentin* 250 mg/5 mL suspension or the equivalent dose of 10 mL *Augmentin* 125 mg/5 mL suspension provides average peak serum concentrations approximately 1 hour after dosing of 6.9 μg/mL for amoxicillin and 1.6 μg/mL for clavulanic acid. The areas under the serum concentration curves obtained during the first 4 hours after dosing were 12.6 μg.hr./mL for amoxicillin and 2.9 μg.hr./mL for clavulanic acid when 5 mL of *Augmentin* 250 mg/5 mL suspension or equivalent dose of 10 mL of *Augmentin* 125 mg/5 mL suspension was administered to adult volunteers. One *Augmentin* 250 mg chewable tablet or 2 *Augmentin* 125 mg chewable tablets are equivalent to 5 mL of *Augmentin* 250 mg/5 mL suspension and provide similar serum levels of amoxicillin and clavulanic acid.

Amoxicillin serum concentrations achieved with *Augmentin* are similar to those produced by the oral administration of equivalent doses of amoxicillin alone. The half-life of amoxicillin after the oral administration of *Augmentin* is 1.3 hours and that of clavulanic acid is 1.0 hour. Time above the minimum inhibitory concentration of 1.0 μg/mL for amoxicillin has been shown to be similar after corresponding q12h and q8h dosing regimens of *Augmentin* in adults and children. Approximately 50% to 70% of the amoxicillin and approximately 25% to 40% of the clavulanic acid are excreted unchanged in urine during the first 6 hours after administration of 10 mL of *Augmentin* 250 mg/5 mL suspension.

Concurrent administration of probenecid delays amoxicillin excretion but does not delay renal excretion of clavulanic acid.

Neither component in *Augmentin* is highly protein-bound; clavulanic acid has been found to be approximately 25% bound to human serum and amoxicillin approximately 18% bound.

Amoxicillin diffuses readily into most body tissues and fluids with the exception of the brain and spinal fluid. The results of experiments involving the administration of clavulanic acid to animals suggest that this compound, like amoxicillin, is well distributed in body tissues.

Two hours after oral administration of a single 35 mg/kg dose of *Augmentin* suspension to fasting children, average concentrations of 3.0 μg/mL of amoxicillin and 0.5 μg/mL of clavulanic acid were detected in middle ear effusions.

Microbiology: Amoxicillin is a semisynthetic antibiotic with a broad spectrum of bactericidal activity against many gram-positive and gram-negative microorganisms. Amoxicillin is, however, susceptible to degradation by β-lactamases and, therefore, the spectrum of activity does not include organisms which produce these enzymes. Clavulanic acid is a β-lactam, structurally related to the penicillins, which possesses the ability to inactivate a wide range of β-lactamase enzymes commonly found in microorganisms resistant to penicillins and cephalosporins. In particular, it has good activity against the clinically important plasmid mediated β-lactamases frequently responsible for transferred drug resistance.

The formulation of amoxicillin and clavulanic acid in *Augmentin* protects amoxicillin from degradation by β-lactamase enzymes and effectively extends the antibiotic spectrum of amoxicillin to include many bacteria normally resistant to amoxicillin and other β-lactam antibiotics. Thus, *Augmentin* possesses the distinctive properties of a broad-spectrum antibiotic and a β-lactamase inhibitor.

Amoxicillin/clavulanic acid has been shown to be active against most strains of the following microorganisms, both *in vitro* and in clinical infections as described in the INDICATIONS AND USAGE section.

GRAM-POSITIVE AEROBES
Staphylococcus aureus (β-lactamase and non-β-lactamase producing)§

§Staphylococci which are resistant to methicillin/oxacillin must be considered resistant to amoxicillin/clavulanic acid.

GRAM-NEGATIVE AEROBES
Enterobacter species (Although most strains of *Enterobacter* species are resistant *in vitro*, clinical efficacy has been demonstrated with *Augmentin* in urinary tract infections caused by these organisms.)
Escherichia coli (β-lactamase and non-β-lactamase producing)
Haemophilus influenzae (β-lactamase and non-β-lactamase producing)
Klebsiella species (All known strains are β-lactamase producing.)
Moraxella catarrhalis (β-lactamase and non-β-lactamase producing)

The following *in vitro* data are available, **but their clinical significance is unknown.**

Amoxicillin/clavulanic acid exhibits *in vitro* minimal inhibitory concentrations (MICs) of 0.5 μg/mL or less against most (≥90%) strains of *Streptococcus pneumoniae*[II]; MICs of 0.06 μg/mL or less against most (≥90%) strains of *Neisseria gonorrhoeae*; MICs of 4 μg/mL or less against most (≥90%) strains of staphylococci and anaerobic bacteria; and MICs of 8 μg/mL or less against most (≥90%) strains of other listed organisms. However, with the exception of organisms shown to respond to amoxicillin alone, the safety and effectiveness of amoxicillin/clavulanic acid in treating clinical infections due to these microorganisms have not been established in adequate and well-controlled clinical trials.

[II]Because amoxicillin has greater *in vitro* activity against *Streptococcus pneumoniae* than does ampicillin or penicillin, the majority of *S. pneumoniae* strains with intermediate susceptibility to ampicillin or penicillin are fully susceptible to amoxicillin.

GRAM-POSITIVE AEROBES
Enterococcus faecalis ¶
Staphylococcus epidermidis (β-lactamase and non-β-lactamase producing)
Staphylococcus saprophyticus (β-lactamase and non-β-lactamase producing)
Streptococcus pneumoniae ¶**
Streptococcus pyogenes ¶**
viridans group *Streptococcus* ¶**

GRAM-NEGATIVE AEROBES
Eikenella corrodens (β-lactamase and non-β-lactamase producing)
Neisseria gonorrhoeae ¶ (β-lactamase and non-β-lactamase producing)
Proteus mirabilis ¶ (β-lactamase and non-β-lactamase producing)

ANAEROBIC BACTERIA
Bacteroides species, including *Bacteroides fragilis* (β-lactamase and non-β-lactamase producing)
Fusobacterium species (β-lactamase and non-β-lactamase producing)
Peptostreptococcus species**

¶Adequate and well-controlled clinical trials have established the effectiveness of amoxicillin alone in treating certain clinical infections due to these organisms.

** These are non-β-lactamase-producing organisms and, therefore, are susceptible to amoxicillin alone.

SUSCEPTIBILITY TESTING

Dilution Techniques: Quantitative methods are used to determine antimicrobial minimal inhibitory concentrations (MICs). These MICs provide estimates of the susceptibility of bacteria to antimicrobial compounds. The MICs should be determined using a standardized procedure. Standardized procedures are based on a dilution method[1] (broth or agar) or equivalent with standardized inoculum concentrations and standardized concentrations of amoxicillin/clavulanate potassium powder.

The recommended dilution pattern utilizes a constant amoxicillin/clavulanate potassium ratio of 2 to 1 in all tubes with varying amounts of amoxicillin. MICs are expressed in terms of the amoxicillin concentration in the presence of clavulanic acid at a constant 2 parts amoxicillin to 1 part clavulanic acid. The MIC values should be interpreted according to the following criteria:

RECOMMENDED RANGES FOR AMOXICILLIN/CLAVULANIC ACID SUSCEPTIBILITY TESTING

For gram-negative enteric aerobes:

MIC (μg/mL)	Interpretation
≤8/4	Susceptible (S)
16/8	Intermediate (I)
≥32/16	Resistant (R)

For *Staphylococcus* †† and *Haemophilus* species:

MIC (μg/mL)	Interpretation
≤4/2	Susceptible (S)
≥8/4	Resistant (R)

†† Staphylococci which are susceptible to amoxicillin/clavulanic acid but resistant to methicillin/oxacillin must be considered as resistant.

Continued on next page

Information on the SmithKline Beecham Pharmaceuticals products appearing here is based on the labeling in effect on July 1, 1996. Further information on these and other products may be obtained from the Medical Department, SmithKline Beecham Pharmaceuticals, One Franklin Plaza, Philadelphia, PA 19101.

SmithKline Beecham—Cont.

For *Streptococcus pneumoniae:* Isolates should be tested using amoxicillin/clavulanic acid and the following criteria should be used:

MIC (µg/mL)	Interpretation
≤ 0.5/0.25	Susceptible (S)
1/0.5	Intermediate (I)
≥ 2/1	Resistant (R)

A report of "Susceptible" indicates that the pathogen is likely to be inhibited if the antimicrobial compound in the blood reaches the concentration usually achievable. A report of "Intermediate" indicates that the result should be considered equivocal, and, if the microorganism is not fully susceptible to alternative, clinically feasible drugs, the test should be repeated. This category implies possible clinical applicability in body sites where the drug is physiologically concentrated or in situations where high dosage of drug can be used. This category also provides a buffer zone that prevents small uncontrolled technical factors from causing major discrepancies in interpretation. A report of "Resistant" indicates that the pathogen is not likely to be inhibited if the antimicrobial compound in the blood reaches the concentrations usually achievable; other therapy should be selected.
Standardized susceptibility test procedures require the use of laboratory control microorganisms to control the technical aspects of the laboratory procedures. Standard amoxicillin/clavulanate potassium powder should provide the following MIC values:

Microorganism	MIC Range (µg/mL)‡‡
Escherichia coli ATCC 25922	2 to 8
Escherichia coli ATCC 35218	4 to 16
Enterococcus faecalis ATCC 29212	0.25 to 1.0
Haemophilus influenzae ATCC 49247	2 to 16
Staphylococcus aureus ATCC 29213	0.12 to 0.5
Streptococcus pneumoniae ATCC 49619	0.03 to 0.12

‡‡ Expressed as concentration of amoxicillin in the presence of clavulanic acid at a constant 2 parts amoxicillin to 1 part clavulanic acid.

Diffusion Techniques: Quantitative methods that require measurement of zone diameters also provide reproducible estimates of the susceptibility of bacteria to antimicrobial compounds. One such standardized procedure[2] requires the use of standardized inoculum concentrations. This procedure uses paper disks impregnated with 30 µg of amoxicillin/clavulanate potassium (20 µg amoxicillin plus 10 µg clavulanate potassium) to test the susceptibility of microorganisms to amoxicillin/clavulanic acid.
Reports from the laboratory providing results of the standard single-disk susceptibility test with a 30 µg amoxicillin/clavulanate potassium (20 µg amoxicillin plus 10 µg clavulanate potassium) disk should be interpreted according to the following criteria:
RECOMMENDED RANGES FOR AMOXICILLIN/CLAVULANIC ACID SUSCEPTIBILITY TESTING
For *Staphylococcus* §§ species and *H. influenzae* [a]:

Zone Diameter (mm)	Interpretation
≥ 20	Susceptible (S)
≤ 19	Resistant (R)

For other organisms except *S. pneumoniae* [b] and *N. gonorrhoeae* [c]:

Zone Diameter (mm)	Interpretation
≥ 18	Susceptible (S)
14 to 17	Intermediate (I)
≤ 13	Resistant (R)

§§ Staphylococci which are resistant to methicillin/oxacillin must be considered as resistant to amoxicillin/clavulanic acid.
[a] A broth microdilution method should be used for testing *H. influenzae*. Beta-lactamase negative, ampicillin-resistant strains must be considered resistant to amoxicillin/clavulanic acid.
[b] Susceptibility of *S. pneumoniae* should be determined using a 1 µg oxacillin disk. Isolates with oxacillin zone sizes of ≥ 20 mm are susceptible to amoxicillin/clavulanic acid. An amoxicillin/clavulanic acid MIC should be determined on isolates of *S. pneumoniae* with oxacillin zone sizes of ≤ 19 mm.
[c] A broth microdilution method should be used for testing *N. gonorrhoeae* and interpreted according to penicillin breakpoints.

Interpretation should be as stated above for results using dilution techniques. Interpretation involves correlation of the diameter obtained in the disk test with the MIC for amoxicillin/clavulanic acid.
As with standardized dilution techniques, diffusion methods require the use of laboratory control microorganisms that are used to control the technical aspects of the laboratory procedures. For the diffusion technique, the 30 µg amoxicillin/clavulanate potassium (20 µg amoxicillin plus 10 µg

clavulanate potassium) disk should provide the following zone diameters in these laboratory quality control strains:

Microorganism	Zone Diameter (mm)
Escherichia coli ATCC 25922	19 to 25 mm
Escherichia coli ATCC 35218	18 to 22 mm
Staphylococcus aureus ATCC 25923	28 to 36 mm

INDICATIONS AND USAGE

Augmentin is indicated in the treatment of infections caused by susceptible strains of the designated organisms in the conditions listed below:
Lower Respiratory Tract Infections—caused by β-lactamase-producing strains of *Haemophilus influenzae* and *Moraxella (Branhamella) catarrhalis.*
Otitis Media—caused by β-lactamase-producing strains of *Haemophilus influenzae* and *Moraxella (Branhamella) catarrhalis.*
Sinusitis—caused by β-lactamase-producing strains of *Haemophilus influenzae* and *Moraxella (Branhamella) catarrhalis.*
Skin and Skin Structure Infections—caused by β-lactamase-producing strains of *Staphylococcus aureus, Escherichia coli* and *Klebsiella* spp.
Urinary Tract Infections—caused by β-lactamase-producing strains of *Escherichia coli, Klebsiella* spp. and *Enterobacter* spp.
While *Augmentin* is indicated only for the conditions listed above, infections caused by ampicillin-susceptible organisms are also amenable to *Augmentin* treatment due to its amoxicillin content. Therefore, mixed infections caused by ampicillin-susceptible organisms and β-lactamase-producing organisms susceptible to *Augmentin* should not require the addition of another antibiotic. Because amoxicillin has greater *in vitro* activity against *Streptococcus pneumoniae* than does ampicillin or penicillin, the majority of *S. pneumoniae* strains with intermediate susceptibility to ampicillin or penicillin are fully susceptible to amoxicillin and *Augmentin.* (See Microbiology subsection.)
Bacteriological studies, to determine the causative organisms and their susceptibility to *Augmentin,* should be performed together with any indicated surgical procedures.
Therapy may be instituted prior to obtaining the results from bacteriological and susceptibility studies to determine the causative organisms and their susceptibility to *Augmentin* when there is reason to believe the infection may involve any of the β-lactamase-producing organisms listed above. Once the results are known, therapy should be adjusted, if appropriate.

CONTRAINDICATIONS

Augmentin is contraindicated in patients with a history of allergic reactions to any penicillin. It is also contraindicated in patients with a previous history of *Augmentin*-associated cholestatic jaundice/hepatic dysfunction.

WARNINGS

SERIOUS AND OCCASIONALLY FATAL HYPERSENSITIVITY (ANAPHYLACTIC) REACTIONS HAVE BEEN REPORTED IN PATIENTS ON PENICILLIN THERAPY. THESE REACTIONS ARE MORE LIKELY TO OCCUR IN INDIVIDUALS WITH A HISTORY OF PENICILLIN HYPERSENSITIVITY AND/OR A HISTORY OF SENSITIVITY TO MULTIPLE ALLERGENS. THERE HAVE BEEN REPORTS OF INDIVIDUALS WITH A HISTORY OF PENICILLIN HYPERSENSITIVITY WHO HAVE EXPERIENCED SEVERE REACTIONS WHEN TREATED WITH CEPHALOSPORINS. BEFORE INITIATING THERAPY WITH *AUGMENTIN,* CAREFUL INQUIRY SHOULD BE MADE CONCERNING PREVIOUS HYPERSENSITIVITY REACTIONS TO PENICILLINS, CEPHALOSPORINS OR OTHER ALLERGENS. IF AN ALLERGIC REACTION OCCURS, *AUGMENTIN* SHOULD BE DISCONTINUED AND THE APPROPRIATE THERAPY INSTITUTED. SERIOUS ANAPHYLACTIC REACTIONS REQUIRE IMMEDIATE EMERGENCY TREATMENT WITH EPINEPHRINE. OXYGEN, INTRAVENOUS STEROIDS AND AIRWAY MANAGEMENT, INCLUDING INTUBATION, SHOULD ALSO BE ADMINISTERED AS INDICATED.
Pseudomembranous colitis has been reported with nearly all antibacterial agents, including *Augmentin,* and has ranged in severity from mild to life-threatening. Therefore, it is important to consider this diagnosis in patients who present with diarrhea subsequent to the administration of antibacterial agents.
Treatment with antibacterial agents alters the normal flora of the colon and may permit overgrowth of clostridia. Studies indicate that a toxin produced by *Clostridium difficile* is one primary cause of "antibiotic associated colitis."
After the diagnosis of pseudomembranous colitis has been established, appropriate therapeutic measures should be initiated. Mild cases of pseudomembranous colitis usually respond to drug discontinuation alone. In moderate to severe cases, consideration should be given to management with fluids and electrolytes, protein supplementation and treatment with an antibacterial drug clinically effective against *Clostridium difficile* colitis.

Augmentin should be used with caution in patients with evidence of hepatic dysfunction. Hepatic toxicity associated with the use of *Augmentin* is usually reversible. On rare occasions, deaths have been reported (less than 1 death reported per estimated 4 million prescriptions worldwide). These have generally been cases associated with serious underlying diseases or concomitant medications. (See CONTRAINDICATIONS and ADVERSE REACTIONS—*Liver.*)

PRECAUTIONS

General: While *Augmentin* possesses the characteristic low toxicity of the penicillin group of antibiotics, periodic assessment of organ system functions, including renal, hepatic and hematopoietic function, is advisable during prolonged therapy. A high percentage of patients with mononucleosis who receive ampicillin develop an erythematous skin rash. Thus, ampicillin class antibiotics should not be administered to patients with mononucleosis.
The possibility of superinfections with mycotic or bacterial pathogens should be kept in mind during therapy. If superinfections occur (usually involving *Pseudomonas* or *Candida*), the drug should be discontinued and/or appropriate therapy instituted.
Information for the Patient: Augmentin may be taken every 8 hours or every 12 hours, depending on the strength of the product prescribed. Each dose should be taken with a meal or snack to reduce the possibility of gastrointestinal upset. Many antibiotics can cause diarrhea. If diarrhea is severe or lasts more than 2 or 3 days, call your doctor.
Make sure your child completes the entire prescribed course of treatment, even if he/she begins to feel better after a few days. Keep suspension refrigerated. Shake well before using. When dosing a child with *Augmentin* suspension (liquid), use a dosing spoon or medicine dropper. Be sure to rinse the spoon or dropper after each use. Bottles of *Augmentin* suspension may contain more liquid than required. Follow your doctor's instructions about the amount to use and the days of treatment your child requires. Discard any unused medicine.
Phenylketonurics: Each 200 mg *Augmentin* chewable tablet contains 2.1 mg phenylalanine; each 400 mg chewable tablet contains 4.2 mg phenylalanine; each 5 mL of either the 200 mg/5 mL or 400 mg/5 mL oral suspension contains 7 mg phenylalanine. The other *Augmentin* products do not contain phenylalanine and can be used by phenylketonurics. Contact your physician or pharmacist.
Drug Interactions: Probenecid decreases the renal tubular secretion of amoxicillin. Concurrent use with *Augmentin* may result in increased and prolonged blood levels of amoxicillin. Co-administration of probenecid cannot be recommended.
The concurrent administration of allopurinol and ampicillin increases substantially the incidence of rashes in patients receiving both drugs as compared to patients receiving ampicillin alone. It is not known whether this potentiation of ampicillin rashes is due to allopurinol or the hyperuricemia present in these patients. There are no data with *Augmentin* and allopurinol administered concurrently.
Drug/Laboratory Test Interactions: Oral administration of *Augmentin* will result in high urine concentrations of amoxicillin. High urine concentrations of ampicillin may result in false-positive reactions when testing for the presence of glucose in urine using Clinitest®, Benedict's Solution or Fehling's Solution. Since this effect may also occur with amoxicillin and therefore *Augmentin,* it is recommended that glucose tests based on enzymatic glucose oxidase reactions (such as Clinistix® or Tes-Tape®) be used.
Following administration of ampicillin to pregnant women a transient decrease in plasma concentration of total conjugated estriol, estriol-glucuronide, conjugated estrone and estradiol has been noted. This effect may also occur with amoxicillin and therefore *Augmentin.*
Carcinogenesis, Mutagenesis, Impairment of Fertility: Long-term studies in animals have not been performed to evaluate carcinogenic potential.
Mutagenesis: The mutagenic potential of *Augmentin* was investigated *in vitro* with an Ames test, a human lymphocyte cytogenetic assay, a yeast test and a mouse lymphoma forward mutation assay, and *in vivo* with mouse micronucleus tests and a dominant lethal test. All were negative apart from the *in vitro* mouse lymphoma assay where weak activity was found at very high, cytotoxic concentrations.
Impairment of Fertility: Augmentin at oral doses of up to 1200 mg/kg/day (5.7 times the maximum human dose, 1480 mg/m²/day, based on body surface area) was found to have no effect on fertility and reproductive performance in rats, dosed with a 2:1 ratio formulation of amoxicillin:clavulanate.
Teratogenic effects. Pregnancy (Category B): Reproduction studies performed in pregnant rats and mice given *Augmentin* at oral dosages up to 1200 mg/kg/day, equivalent to 7200 and 4080 mg/m²/day, respectively (4.9 and 2.8 times the maximum human oral dose based on body surface area), revealed no evidence of harm to the fetus due to *Augmentin.* There are, however, no adequate and well-controlled studies in pregnant women. Because animal reproduction studies

are not always predictive of human response, this drug should be used during pregnancy only if clearly needed.

Labor and Delivery: Oral ampicillin class antibiotics are generally poorly absorbed during labor. Studies in guinea pigs have shown that intravenous administration of ampicillin decreased the uterine tone, frequency of contractions, height of contractions and duration of contractions. However, it is not known whether the use of *Augmentin* in humans during labor or delivery has immediate or delayed adverse effects on the fetus, prolongs the duration of labor, or increases the likelihood that forceps delivery or other obstetrical intervention or resuscitation of the newborn will be necessary.

Nursing Mothers: Ampicillin class antibiotics are excreted in the milk; therefore, caution should be exercised when *Augmentin* is administered to a nursing woman.

Pediatric Use: Because of incompletely developed renal function in neonates and young infants, the elimination of amoxicillin may be delayed. Dosing of *Augmentin* should be modified in pediatric patients younger than 12 weeks (3 months). (See DOSAGE AND ADMINISTRATION–Pediatric.)

ADVERSE REACTIONS

Augmentin is generally well tolerated. The majority of side effects observed in clinical trials were of a mild and transient nature and less than 3% of patients discontinued therapy because of drug-related side effects. From the original premarketing studies, where both pediatric and adult patients were enrolled, the most frequently reported adverse effects were diarrhea/loose stools (9%), nausea (3%), skin rashes and urticaria (3%), vomiting (1%) and vaginitis (1%). The overall incidence of side effects, and in particular diarrhea, increased with the higher recommended dose. Other less frequently reported reactions include: abdominal discomfort, flatulence and headache.

In pediatric patients (aged 2 months to 12 years), one U.S./Canadian clinical trial was conducted which compared *Augmentin* 45/6.4 mg/kg/day (divided q12h) for 10 days versus *Augmentin* 40/10 mg/kg/day (divided q8h) for 10 days in the treatment of acute otitis media. A total of 575 patients were enrolled, and only the suspension formulations were used in this trial. Overall, the adverse event profile seen was comparable to that noted above. However, there were differences in the rates of diarrhea, skin rashes/urticaria, and diaper area rashes. (See CLINICAL STUDIES.)

The following adverse reactions have been reported for ampicillin class antibiotics:

Gastrointestinal: Diarrhea, nausea, vomiting, indigestion, gastritis, stomatitis, glossitis, black "hairy" tongue, enterocolitis, mucocutaneous candidiasis and pseudomembranous colitis. Onset of pseudomembranous colitis symptoms may occur during or after antibiotic treatment. (See WARNINGS.)

Hypersensitivity Reactions: Skin rashes, pruritus, urticaria, angioedema, serum sickness-like reactions (urticaria or skin rash accompanied by arthritis, arthralgia, myalgia and frequently fever), erythema multiforme (rarely Stevens-Johnson Syndrome) and an occasional case of exfoliative dermatitis (including toxic epidermal necrolysis) have been reported. These reactions may be controlled with antihistamines and, if necessary, systemic corticosteroids. Whenever such reactions occur, the drug should be discontinued, unless the opinion of the physician dictates otherwise. Serious and occasional fatal hypersensitivity (anaphylactic) reactions can occur with oral penicillin. (See WARNINGS.)

Liver: A moderate rise in AST (SGOT) and/or ALT (SGPT) has been noted in patients treated with ampicillin class antibiotics but the significance of these findings is unknown. Hepatic dysfunction, including increases in serum transaminases (AST and/or ALT), serum bilirubin and/or alkaline phosphatase, has been infrequently reported with *Augmentin*. The histologic findings on liver biopsy have consisted of predominantly cholestatic, hepatocellular, or mixed cholestatic-hepatocellular changes. The onset of signs/symptoms of hepatic dysfunction may occur during or several weeks after therapy has been discontinued. The hepatic dysfunction, which may be severe, is usually reversible. On rare occasions, deaths have been reported (less than 1 death reported per estimated 4 million prescriptions worldwide). These have generally been cases associated with serious underlying diseases or concomitant medications.

Renal: Interstitial nephritis and hematuria have been reported rarely.

Hemic and Lymphatic Systems: Anemia, thrombocytopenia, thrombocytopenic purpura, eosinophilia, leukopenia and agranulocytosis have been reported during therapy with penicillins. These reactions are usually reversible on discontinuation of therapy and are believed to be hypersensitivity phenomena. A slight thrombocytosis was noted in less than 1% of the patients treated with *Augmentin.*

Central Nervous System: Reversible hyperactivity, agitation, anxiety, insomnia, confusion, behavioral changes, and/or dizziness have been reported rarely.

OVERDOSAGE

Amoxicillin may be removed from circulation by hemodialysis. The molecular weight, degree of protein binding and pharmacokinetic profile of clavulanic acid together with information from a single patient with renal insufficiency all suggest that this compound may also be removed by hemodialysis.

DOSAGE AND ADMINISTRATION

Dosage:

Pediatric Patients: Based on the amoxicillin component, *Augmentin* should be dosed as follows:

Neonates and infants aged < 12 weeks (3 months)

Due to incompletely developed renal function affecting elimination of amoxicillin in this age group, the recommended dose of *Augmentin* is 30 mg/kg/day divided q12h, based on the amoxicillin component. Clavulanate elimination is unaltered in this age group. Experience with the 200 mg/5 mL formulation in this age group is limited and, thus, use of the 125 mg/5 mL oral suspension is recommended.

Patients aged 12 weeks (3 months) and older

INFECTIONS	DOSING REGIMEN	
	q12h‖	q8h
	200 mg/5 mL or 400 mg/5 mL oral suspension¶¶	125 mg/5 mL or 250 mg/5 mL oral suspension¶¶
Otitis media***, sinusitis, lower respiratory tract infections, and more severe infections	45 mg/kg/day q12h	40 mg/kg/day q8h
Less severe infections	25 mg/kg/day q12h	20 mg/kg/day q8h

‖ The q12h regimen is recommended as it is associated with significantly less diarrhea. (See CLINICAL STUDIES.) However, the q12h formulations (200 mg and 400 mg) contain aspartame and should not be used by phenylketonurics.

¶¶ Each strength of *Augmentin* suspension is available as a chewable tablet for use by older children.

*** Duration of therapy studied and recommended for acute otitis media is 10 days.

Pediatric patients weighing 40 kg and more should be dosed according to the following adult recommendations: The usual adult dose is 1 *Augmentin* 500 mg tablet every 12 hours or 1 *Augmentin* 250 mg tablet every 8 hours. For more severe infections and infections of the respiratory tract, the dose should be 1 *Augmentin* 875 mg tablet every 12 hours or 1 *Augmentin* 500 mg tablet every 8 hours. Among adults treated with 875 mg every 12 hours, significantly fewer experienced severe diarrhea or withdrawals with diarrhea vs. adults treated with 500 mg every 8 hours. For detailed adult dosage recommendations, please see complete prescribing information for *Augmentin* Tablets.

Hepatically impaired patients should be dosed with caution and hepatic function monitored at regular intervals. (See WARNINGS.)

Adults: Adults who have difficulty swallowing may be given the 125 mg/5 mL or 250 mg/5 mL suspension in place of the 500 mg tablet. The 200 mg/5 mL suspension or the 400 mg/5 mL suspension may be used in place of the 875 mg tablet. See dosage recommendations above for children weighing 40 kg or more.

The *Augmentin* 250 mg tablet and the 250 mg chewable tablet do *not* contain the same amount of clavulanic acid (as the potassium salt). The *Augmentin* 250 mg tablet contains 125 mg of clavulanic acid, whereas the 250 mg chewable tablet contains 62.5 mg of clavulanic acid. Therefore, the *Augmentin* 250 mg tablet and the 250 mg chewable tablet should *not* be substituted for each other, as they are not interchangeable.

Due to the different amoxicillin to clavulanic acid ratios in the *Augmentin* 250 mg tablet (250/125) versus the *Augmentin* 250 mg chewable tablet (250/62.5), the *Augmentin* 250 mg tablet should not be used until the child weighs at least 40 kg and more.

DIRECTIONS FOR MIXING ORAL SUSPENSION

Prepare a suspension at time of dispensing as follows: Tap bottle until all the powder flows freely. Add approximately $^{2}/_{3}$ of the total amount of water for reconstitution (see table below) and shake vigorously to suspend powder. Add remainder of the water and again shake vigorously.

***Augmentin* 125 mg/5 mL Suspension**

Bottle Size	Amount of Water Required for Reconstitution
75 mL	67 mL
100 mL	90 mL
150 mL	134 mL

Each teaspoonful (5 mL) will contain 125 mg amoxicillin and 31.25 mg of clavulanic acid as the potassium salt.

***Augmentin* 200 mg/5 mL Suspension**

Bottle Size	Amount of Water Required for Suspension
50 mL	47 mL
75 mL	69 mL
100 mL	91 mL

Each teaspoonful (5 mL) will contain 200 mg amoxicillin and 28.5 mg of clavulanic acid as the potassium salt.

***Augmentin* 250 mg/5 mL Suspension**

Bottle Size	Amount of Water Required for Reconstitution
75 mL	65 mL
100 mL	87 mL
150 mL	130 mL

Each teaspoonful (5 mL) will contain 250 mg amoxicillin and 62.5 mg of clavulanic acid as the potassium salt.

***Augmentin* 400 mg/5 mL Suspension**

Bottle Size	Amount of Water Required for Suspension
50 mL	44 mL
75 mL	66 mL
100 mL	87 mL

Each teaspoonful (5 mL) will contain 400 mg amoxicillin and 57.0 mg of clavulanic acid as the potassium salt.

Note: SHAKE ORAL SUSPENSION WELL BEFORE USING.

Reconstituted suspension must be stored under refrigeration and discarded after 10 days.

Administration: *Augmentin* may be taken without regard to meals; however, absorption of clavulanate potassium is enhanced when *Augmentin* is administered at the start of a meal. To minimize the potential for gastrointestinal intolerance, *Augmentin* should be taken at the start of a meal.

HOW SUPPLIED

***AUGMENTIN* 125 MG/5 ML FOR ORAL SUSPENSION:** Each 5 mL of reconstituted banana-flavored suspension contains 125 mg amoxicillin and 31.25 mg clavulanic acid as the potassium salt.

NDC 0029-6085-39 .... 75 mL bottle
NDC 0029-6085-23 .... 100 mL bottle
NDC 0029-6085-22 .... 150 mL bottle

***AUGMENTIN* 200 MG/5 ML FOR ORAL SUSPENSION:** Each 5 mL of reconstituted orange-raspberry-flavored suspension contains 200 mg amoxicillin and 28.5 mg clavulanic acid as the potassium salt.

NDC 0029-6087-29 .... 50 mL bottle
NDC 0029-6087-39 .... 75 mL bottle
NDC 0029-6087-51 .... 100 mL bottle

***AUGMENTIN* 250 MG/5 ML FOR ORAL SUSPENSION:** Each 5 mL of reconstituted orange-flavored suspension contains 250 mg amoxicillin and 62.5 mg clavulanic acid as the potassium salt.

NDC 0029-6090-39 .... 75 mL bottle
NDC 0029-6090-23 .... 100 mL bottle
NDC 0029-6090-22 .... 150 mL bottle

***AUGMENTIN* 400 MG/5 ML FOR ORAL SUSPENSION:** Each 5 mL of reconstituted orange-raspberry-flavored suspension contains 400 mg amoxicillin and 57 mg clavulanic acid as the potassium salt.

NDC 0029-6092-29 .... 50 mL bottle
NDC 0029-6092-39 .... 75 mL bottle
NDC 0029-6092-51 .... 100 mL bottle

***AUGMENTIN* 125 MG CHEWABLE TABLETS:** Each mottled yellow, round, lemon-lime-flavored tablet, debossed with BMP 189, contains 125 mg amoxicillin as the trihydrate and 31.25 mg clavulanic acid as the potassium salt.

NDC 0029-6073-47 .... carton of 30 tablets

***AUGMENTIN* 200 MG CHEWABLE TABLETS:** Each mottled pink, round, biconvex, cherry-banana-flavored tablet contains 200 mg amoxicillin as the trihydrate and 28.5 mg clavulanic acid as the potassium salt.

NDC 0029-6071-12 .... carton of 20 tablets

***AUGMENTIN* 250 MG CHEWABLE TABLETS:** Each mottled yellow, round, lemon-lime-flavored tablet, debossed with BMP 190, contains 250 mg amoxicillin as the trihydrate and 62.5 mg clavulanic acid as the potassium salt.

NDC 0029-6074-47 .... carton of 30 tablets

***AUGMENTIN* 400 MG CHEWABLE TABLETS:** Each mottled pink, round, biconvex, cherry-banana-flavored tablet contains 400 mg amoxicillin as the trihydrate and 57.0 mg clavulanic acid as the potassium salt.

NDC 0029-6072-12 .... carton of 20 tablets

Continued on next page

Information on the SmithKline Beecham Pharmaceuticals products appearing here is based on the labeling in effect on July 1, 1996. Further information on these and other products may be obtained from the Medical Department, SmithKline Beecham Pharmaceuticals, One Franklin Plaza, Philadelphia, PA 19101.

SmithKline Beecham—Cont.

AUGMENTIN is also supplied as:

***AUGMENTIN* 250 MG TABLETS** (250 mg amoxicillin/125 mg clavulanic acid):

NDC 0029-6075-27 .... bottles of 30
NDC 0029-6075-31 .... 100 Unit Dose tablets

***AUGMENTIN* 500 MG TABLETS** (500 mg amoxicillin/125 mg clavulanic acid):

NDC 0029-6080-12 .... bottles of 20
NDC 0029-6080-27 .... bottles of 30
NDC 0029-6080-31 .... 100 Unit Dose tablets

***AUGMENTIN* 875 MG TABLETS** (875 mg amoxicillin/125 mg clavulanic acid):

NDC 0029-6086-12 .... bottles of 20
NDC 0029-6086-21 .... 100 Unit Dose tablets

Store tablets and dry powder at or below 25°C (77°F). Dispense in tightly closed, moisture-proof containers. Store reconstituted suspension under refrigeration. Discard unused suspension after 10 days.

CLINICAL STUDIES

In pediatric patients (aged 2 months to 12 years), one U.S./Canadian clinical trial was conducted which compared *Augmentin* 45/6.4 mg/kg/day (divided q12h) for 10 days versus *Augmentin* 40/10 mg/kg/day (divided q8h) for 10 days in the treatment of acute otitis media. Only the suspension formulations were used in this trial. A total of 575 patients were enrolled, with an even distribution among the two treatment groups and a comparable number of patients were evaluable (i.e., ≥84%) per treatment group. Strict otitis media-specific criteria were required for eligibility and a strong correlation was found at the end of therapy and follow-up between these criteria and physician assessment of clinical response. The clinical efficacy rates at the end of therapy visit (defined as 2–4 days after the completion of therapy) and at the follow-up visit (defined as 22–28 days post-completion of therapy) were comparable for the two treatment groups, with the following cure rates obtained for the evaluable patients: At end of therapy, 87.2% (n=265) and 82.3% (n=260) for 45 mg/kg/day q12h and 40 mg/kg/day q8h, respectively. At follow-up, 67.1% (n=249) and 68.7% (n=243) for 45 mg/kg/day q12h and 40 mg/kg/day q8h, respectively.

The incidence of diarrhea††† was significantly lower in patients in the q12h treatment group compared to patients who received the q8h regimen (14.3% and 34.3%, respectively). In addition, the number of patients with either severe diarrhea or who were withdrawn with diarrhea was significantly lower in the q12h treatment group (3.1% and 7.6% for the q12h/10 day and q8h/10 day, respectively). In the q12h treatment group, 3 patients (1.0%) were withdrawn with an allergic reaction, while 1 patient (0.3%) in the q8h group was withdrawn for this reason. The number of patients with a candidal infection of the diaper area was 3.8% and 6.2% for the q12h and q8h groups, respectively.

It is not known if the finding of a statistically significant reduction in diarrhea with the oral suspensions dosed q12h, versus suspensions dosed q8h, can be extrapolated to the chewable tablets. The presence of mannitol in the chewable tablets may contribute to a different diarrhea profile. The q12h oral suspensions are sweetened with aspartame only.

††† Diarrhea was defined as either: (a) three or more watery or four or more loose/watery stools in one day; OR (b) two watery stools per day or three loose/watery stools per day for two consecutive days.

REFERENCES

1. National Committee for Clinical Laboratory Standards. Methods for Dilution Antimicrobial Susceptibility Tests for Bacteria That Grow Aerobically — Third Edition. Approved Standard NCCLS Document M7-A3, Vol. 13, No. 25. NCCLS, Villanova, PA, Dec. 1993.

2. National Committee for Clinical Laboratory Standards. Performance Standard for Antimicrobial Disk Susceptibility Tests — Fifth Edition. Approved Standard NCCLS Document M2-A5, Vol. 13, No. 24. NCCLS, Villanova, PA, Dec. 1993.

Veterans Administration/Military/PHS—Chewable Tablets, 125 mg, 30's 6505-01-282-6332; 250 mg, 30's 6505-01-264-2366; Tablets 250 mg, 30's 6505-01-203-6259; 250 mg, 100's SUP, 6505-01-339-6919; 500 mg, 30's 6505-01-206-6228; 500 mg, 100's SUP, 6505-01-303-8962; Oral Suspension, 125 mg/5 mL, 75 mL, 6505-01-340-0847; 125 mg/5 mL, 100 mL, 6505-01-408-8181; 125 mg/5 mL, 150 mL, 6505-01-204-5388; 250 mg/5 mL, 75 mL, 6505-01-207-8205; 250 mg/5 mL, 100 mL, 6505-01-408-8352; 250 mg/5 mL, 150 mL, 6506-01-207-0795.
AG:PL2A

Shown in Product Identification Guide, page 336

AUGMENTIN® ℞

[og' men-tin]
amoxicillin/clavulanate potassium
Tablets

DESCRIPTION

Augmentin is an oral antibacterial combination consisting of the semisynthetic antibiotic amoxicillin and the β-lactamase inhibitor, clavulanate potassium (the potassium salt of clavulanic acid). Amoxicillin is an analog of ampicillin, derived from the basic penicillin nucleus, 6-aminopenicillanic acid. The amoxicillin molecular formula is $C_{16}H_{19}N_3O_5S \cdot 3H_2O$ and the molecular weight is 419.46. Chemically, amoxicillin is (2*S*,5*R*,6*R*)-6-[(*R*)-(-)-2-Amino-2-(*p*-hydroxyphenyl)acetamido]-3,3-dimethyl-7-oxo-4-thia-1-azabicyclo[3.2.0]heptane-2-carboxylic acid trihydrate and may be represented structurally as:

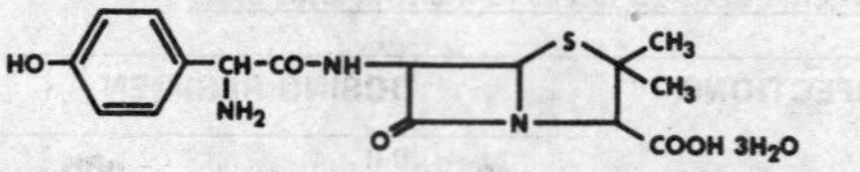

Clavulanic acid is produced by the fermentation of *Streptomyces clavuligerus*. It is a β-lactam structurally related to the penicillins and possesses the ability to inactivate a wide variety of β-lactamases by blocking the active sites of these enzymes. Clavulanic acid is particularly active against the clinically important plasmid mediated β-lactamases frequently responsible for transferred drug resistance to penicillins and cephalosporins. The clavulanate potassium molecular formula is $C_8H_8KNO_5$ and the molecular weight is 237.25. Chemically clavulanate potassium is potassium (*Z*)-(2*R*, 5*R*)-3-(2-hydroxyethylidene)-7-oxo-4-oxa-1-azabicyclo[3.2.0]-heptane-2-carboxylate, and may be represented structurally as:

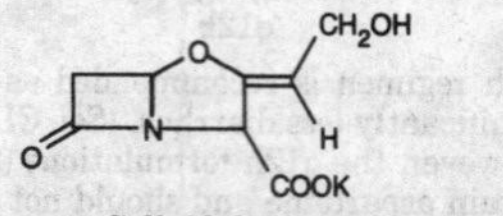

Inactive Ingredients: Colloidal silicon dioxide, hydroxypropyl methylcellulose, magnesium stearate, microcrystalline cellulose, polyethylene glycol, sodium starch glycolate and titanium dioxide.

Each *Augmentin* tablet contains 0.63 mEq potassium.

CLINICAL PHARMACOLOGY

Amoxicillin and clavulanate potassium are well absorbed from the gastrointestinal tract after oral administration of *Augmentin*. Dosing in the fasted or fed state has minimal effect on the pharmacokinetics of amoxicillin. While *Augmentin* can be given without regard to meals, absorption of clavulanate potassium when taken with food is greater relative to the fasted state. In one study, the relative bioavailability of clavulanate was reduced when *Augmentin* was dosed at 30 and 150 minutes after the start of a high fat breakfast. The safety and efficacy of *Augmentin* have been established in clinical trials where *Augmentin* was taken without regard to meals.

Mean* amoxicillin and clavulanate potassium pharmacokinetic parameters are shown in the table below:
[See table below.]

Amoxicillin serum concentrations achieved with *Augmentin* are similar to those produced by the oral administration of equivalent doses of amoxicillin alone. The half-life of amoxicillin after the oral administration of *Augmentin* is 1.3 hours and that of clavulanic acid is 1.0 hour.

Approximately 50% to 70% of the amoxicillin and approximately 25% to 40% of the clavulanic acid are excreted unchanged in urine during the first 6 hours after administration of a single *Augmentin* 250 mg or 500 mg tablet.

Concurrent administration of probenecid delays amoxicillin excretion but does not delay renal excretion of clavulanic acid.

Neither component in *Augmentin* is highly protein-bound; clavulanic acid has been found to be approximately 25% bound to human serum and amoxicillin approximately 18% bound.

Amoxicillin diffuses readily into most body tissues and fluids with the exception of the brain and spinal fluids. The results of experiments involving the administration of clavulanic acid to animals suggest that this compound, like amoxicillin, is well distributed in body tissues.

Microbiology: Amoxicillin is a semisynthetic antibiotic with a broad spectrum of bactericidal activity against many gram-positive and gram-negative microorganisms. Amoxicillin is, however, susceptible to degradation by β-lactamases and, therefore, the spectrum of activity does not include organisms which produce these enzymes. Clavulanic acid is a β-lactam, structurally related to the penicillins, which possesses the ability to inactivate a wide range of β-lactamase enzymes commonly found in microorganisms resistant to penicillins and cephalosporins. In particular, it has good activity against the clinically important plasmid mediated β-lactamases frequently responsible for transferred drug resistance.

The formulation of amoxicillin and clavulanic acid in *Augmentin* protects amoxicillin from degradation by β-lactamase enzymes and effectively extends the antibiotic spectrum of amoxicillin to include many bacteria normally resistant to amoxicillin and other β-lactam antibiotics. Thus *Augmentin* possesses the properties of a broad-spectrum antibiotic and a β-lactamase inhibitor.

Amoxicillin/clavulanic acid has been shown to be active against most strains of the following microorganisms, both *in vitro* and in clinical infections as described in the INDICATIONS AND USAGE section.

GRAM-POSITIVE AEROBES
Staphylococcus aureus (β-lactamase and non-β-lactamase producing)‡
‡Staphylococci which are resistant to methicillin/oxacillin must be considered resistant to amoxicillin/clavulanic acid.

GRAM-NEGATIVE AEROBES
Enterobacter species (Although most strains of *Enterobacter* species are resistant *in vitro*, clinical efficacy has been demonstrated with *Augmentin* in urinary tract infections caused by these organisms.)
Escherichia coli (β-lactamase and non-β-lactamase producing)
Haemophilus influenzae (β-lactamase and non-β-lactamase producing)
Klebsiella species (All known strains are β-lactamase producing.)
Moraxella catarrhalis (β-lactamase and non-β-lactamase producing)

The following *in vitro* data are available, **but their clinical significance is unknown.**

Amoxicillin/clavulanic acid exhibits *in vitro* minimal inhibitory concentrations (MICs) of 0.5 μg/mL or less against most (≥90%) strains of *Streptococcus pneumoniae* §; MICs of 0.06 μg/mL or less against most (≥90%) strains of *Neisseria gonorrhoeae*; MICs of 4 μg/mL or less against most (≥90%) strains of staphylococci and anaerobic bacteria; and MICs of 8 μg/mL or less against most (≥90%) strains of other listed organisms. However, with the exception of organisms shown to respond to amoxicillin alone, the safety and effectiveness of amoxicillin/clavulanic acid in treating clinical infections due to these microorganisms have not been established in adequate and well-controlled clinical trials.

§ Because amoxicillin has greater *in vitro* activity against *Streptococcus pneumoniae* than does ampicillin or penicillin, the majority of *S. pneumoniae* strains with intermediate susceptibility to amipicillin or penicillin are fully susceptible to amoxicillin.

GRAM-POSITIVE AEROBES
Enterococcus faecalis‖
Staphylococcus epidermidis (β-lactamase and non-β-lactamase producing)
Staphylococcus saprophyticus (β-lactamase and non-β-lactamase producing)
Streptococcus pneumoniae ‖ ¶
Streptococcus pyogenes ‖ ¶
viridans group *Streptococcus*‖ ¶

GRAM-NEGATIVE AEROBES
Eikenella corrodens (β-lactamase and non-β-lactamase producing)
Neisseria gonorrhoeae‖ (β-lactamase and non-β-lactamase producing)
Proteus mirabilis‖ (β-lactamase and non-β-lactamase producing)

ANAEROBIC BACTERIA
Bacteroides species, including *Bacteroides fragilis* (β-lactamase and non-β-lactamase producing)

Dose† and regimen amoxicillin/clavulanate potassium	AUC$_{0-24}$ (μg.hr/mL) amoxicillin (±S.D.)	AUC$_{0-24}$ (μg.hr/mL) clavulanate potassium (±S.D.)	C_{max} (μg/mL) amoxicillin (±S.D.)	C_{max} (μg/mL) clavulanate potassium (±S.D.)
250/125 mg q8h	26.7 ± 4.56	12.6 ± 3.25	3.3 ± 1.12	1.5 ± 0.70
500/125 mg q12h	33.4 ± 6.76	8.6 ± 1.95	6.5 ± 1.41	1.8 ± 0.61
500/125 mg q8h	53.4 ± 8.87	15.7 ± 3.86	7.2 ± 2.26	2.4 ± 0.83
875/125 mg q12h	53.5 ± 12.31	10.2 ± 3.04	11.6 ± 2.78	2.2 ± 0.99

* Mean values of 14 normal volunteers (n=15 for clavulanate potassium in the low-dose regimens). Peak concentrations occurred approximately 1.5 hours after the dose.
† Administered at the start of a light meal.

Fusobacterium species (β-lactamase and non-β-lactamase producing)
Peptostreptococcus species¶
ǁAdequate and well-controlled clinical trials have established the effectiveness of amoxicillin alone in treating certain clinical infections due to these organisms.
¶These are non-β-lactamase-producing organisms and, therefore, are susceptible to amoxicillin alone.

SUSCEPTIBILITY TESTING

Dilution Techniques: Quantitative methods are used to determine antimicrobial minimal inhibitory concentrations (MICs). These MICs provide estimates of the susceptibility of bacteria to antimicrobial compounds. The MICs should be determined using a standardized procedure. Standardized procedures are based on a dilution method[1] (broth or agar) or equivalent with standardized inoculum concentrations and standardized concentrations of amoxicillin/clavulanate potassium powder.
The recommended dilution pattern utilizes a constant amoxicillin/clavulanate potassium ratio of 2 to 1 in all tubes with varying amounts of amoxicillin. MICs are expressed in terms of the amoxicillin concentration in the presence of clavulanic acid at a constant 2 parts amoxicillin to 1 part clavulanic acid. The MIC values should be interpreted according to the following criteria:

RECOMMENDED RANGES FOR AMOXICILLIN/CLAVULANIC ACID SUSCEPTIBILITY TESTING

For gram-negative enteric aerobes:

MIC (μg/mL)	Interpretation
≤8/4	Susceptible (S)
16/8	Intermediate (I)
≥32/16	Resistant (R)

For *Staphylococcus*** and *Haemophilus* species:

MIC (μg/mL)	Interpretation
≤4/2	Susceptible (S)
≥8/4	Resistant (R)

** Staphylococci which are susceptible to amoxicillin/clavulanic acid but resistant to methicillin/oxacillin must be considered as resistant.

For *Streptococcus pneumoniae*: Isolates should be tested using amoxicillin/clavulanic acid and the following criteria should be used:

MIC (μg/mL)	Interpretation
≤0.5/0.25	Susceptible (S)
1/0.5	Intermediate (I)
≥2/1	Resistant (R)

A report of "Susceptible" indicates that the pathogen is likely to be inhibited if the antimicrobial compound in the blood reaches the concentration usually achievable. A report of "Intermediate" indicates that the result should be considered equivocal, and, if the microorganism is not fully susceptible to alternative, clinically feasible drugs, the test should be repeated. This category implies possible clinical applicability in body sites where the drug is physiologically concentrated or in situations where high dosage of drug can be used. This category also provides a buffer zone which prevents small uncontrolled technical factors from causing major discrepancies in interpretation. A report of "Resistant" indicates that the pathogen is not likely to be inhibited if the antimicrobial compound in the blood reaches the concentrations usually achievable; other therapy should be selected.
Standardized susceptibility test procedures require the use of laboratory control microorganisms to control the technical aspects of the laboratory procedures. Standard amoxicillin/clavulanate potassium powder should provide the following MIC values:

Microorganism	MIC Range (μg/mL)††
Escherichia coli ATCC 25922	2 to 8
Escherichia coli ATCC 35218	4 to 16
Enterococcus faecalis ATCC 29212	0.25 to 1.0
Haemophilus influenzae ATCC 49247	2 to 16
Staphylococcus aureus ATCC 29213	0.12 to 0.5
Streptococcus pneumoniae ATCC 49619	0.03 to 0.12

†† Expressed as concentration of amoxicillin in the presence of clavulanic acid at a constant 2 parts amoxicillin to 1 part clavulanic acid.

Diffusion Techniques: Quantitative methods that require measurement of zone diameters also provide reproducible estimates of the susceptibility of bacteria to antimicrobial compounds. One such standardized procedure[2] requires the use of standardized inoculum concentrations. This procedure uses paper disks impregnated with 30 μg of amoxicillin/clavulanate potassium (20 μg amoxicillin plus 10 μg clavulanate potassium) to test the susceptibility of microorganisms to amoxicillin/clavulanic acid.
Reports from the laboratory providing results of the standard single-disk susceptibility test with a 30 μg amoxicillin/clavulanate acid (20 μg amoxicillin plus 10 μg clavulanate potassium) disk should be interpreted according to the following criteria:

RECOMMENDED RANGES FOR AMOXICILLIN/CLAVULANIC ACID SUSCEPTIBILITY TESTING

For *Staphylococcus*‡‡ species and *H. influenzae*[a]:

Zone Diameter (mm)	Interpretation
≥20	Susceptible (S)
≤19	Resistant (R)

For other organisms except *S. pneumoniae*[b] and *N. gonorrhoeae*[c]:

Zone Diameter (mm)	Interpretation
≥18	Susceptible (S)
14 to 17	Intermediate (I)
≤13	Resistant (R)

‡‡ Staphylococci which are resistant to methicillin/oxacillin must be considered as resistant to amoxicillin/clavulanic acid.
[a] A broth microdilution method should be used for testing *H. influenzae*. Beta-lactamase negative, ampicillin-resistant strains must be considered resistant to amoxicillin/clavulanic acid.
[b] Susceptibility of *S. pneumoniae* should be determined using a 1 μg oxacillin disk. Isolates with oxacillin zone sizes of ≥20 mm are susceptible to amoxicillin/clavulanic acid. An amoxicillin/clavulanic acid MIC should be determined on isolates of *S. pneumoniae* with oxacillin zone sizes of ≤19 mm.
[c] A broth microdilution method should be used for testing *N. gonorrhoeae* and interpreted according to penicillin breakpoints.

Interpretation should be as stated above for results using dilution techniques. Interpretation involves correlation of the diameter obtained in the disk test with the MIC for amoxicillin/clavulanic acid.
As with standardized dilution techniques, diffusion methods require the use of laboratory control microorganisms that are used to control the technical aspects of the laboratory procedures. For the diffusion technique, the 30 μg amoxicillin/clavulanate potassium (20 μg amoxicillin plus 10 μg clavulanate potassium) disk should provide the following zone diameters in these laboratory quality control strains:

Microorganism	Zone Diameter (mm)
Escherichia coli ATCC 25922	19 to 25
Escherichia coli ATCC 35218	18 to 22
Staphylococcus aureus ATCC 25923	28 to 36

INDICATIONS AND USAGE

Augmentin is indicated in the treatment of infections caused by susceptible strains of the designated organisms in the conditions listed below:
Lower Respiratory Tract Infections—caused by β-lactamase-producing strains of *Haemophilus influenzae* and *Moraxella (Branhamella) catarrhalis*.
Otitis Media—caused by β-lactamase-producing strains of *Haemophilus influenzae* and *Moraxella (Branhamella) catarrhalis*.
Sinusitis—caused by β-lactamase-producing strains of *Haemophilus influenzae* and *Moraxella (Branhamella) catarrhalis*.
Skin and Skin Structure Infections—caused by β-lactamase-producing strains of *Staphylococcus aureus, Escherichia coli* and *Klebsiella* spp.
Urinary Tract Infections—caused by β-lactamase-producing strains of *Escherichia coli, Klebsiella* spp. and *Enterobacter* spp.
While *Augmentin* is indicated only for the conditions listed above, infections caused by ampicillin-susceptible organisms are also amenable to *Augmentin* treatment due to its amoxicillin content. Therefore, mixed infections caused by ampicillin-susceptible organisms and β-lactamase-producing organisms susceptible to *Augmentin* should not require the addition of another antibiotic. Because amoxicillin has greater *in vitro* activity against *Streptococcus pneumoniae* than does ampicillin or penicillin, the majority of *S. pneumoniae* strains with intermediate susceptibility to ampicillin or penicillin are fully susceptible to amoxicillin and *Augmentin*. (See Microbiology subsection.)
Bacteriological studies, to determine the causative organisms and their susceptibility to *Augmentin*, should be performed together with any indicated surgical procedures.
Therapy may be instituted prior to obtaining the results from bacteriological and susceptibility studies to determine the causative organisms and their susceptibility to *Augmentin* when there is reason to believe the infection may involve any of the β-lactamase-producing organisms listed above. Once the results are known, therapy should be adjusted, if appropriate.

CONTRAINDICATIONS

Augmentin is contraindicated in patients with a history of allergic reactions to any penicillin. It is also contraindicated in patients with a previous history of *Augmentin*-associated cholestatic jaundice/hepatic dysfunction.

WARNINGS

SERIOUS AND OCCASIONALLY FATAL HYPERSENSITIVITY (ANAPHYLACTIC) REACTIONS HAVE BEEN REPORTED IN PATIENTS ON PENICILLIN THERAPY. THESE REACTIONS ARE MORE LIKELY TO OCCUR IN INDIVIDUALS WITH A HISTORY OF PENICILLIN HYPERSENSITIVITY AND/OR A HISTORY OF SENSITIVITY TO MULTIPLE ALLERGENS. THERE HAVE BEEN REPORTS OF INDIVIDUALS WITH A HISTORY OF PENICILLIN HYPERSENSITIVITY WHO HAVE EXPERIENCED SEVERE REACTIONS WHEN TREATED WITH CEPHALOSPORINS. BEFORE INITIATING THERAPY WITH *AUGMENTIN*, CAREFUL INQUIRY SHOULD BE MADE CONCERNING PREVIOUS HYPERSENSITIVITY REACTIONS TO PENICILLINS, CEPHALOSPORINS OR OTHER ALLERGENS. IF AN ALLERGIC REACTION OCCURS, *AUGMENTIN* SHOULD BE DISCONTINUED AND THE APPROPRIATE THERAPY INSTITUTED. **SERIOUS ANAPHYLACTIC REACTIONS REQUIRE IMMEDIATE EMERGENCY TREATMENT WITH EPINEPHRINE. OXYGEN, INTRAVENOUS STEROIDS AND AIRWAY MANAGEMENT, INCLUDING INTUBATION, SHOULD ALSO BE ADMINISTERED AS INDICATED.**
Pseudomembranous colitis has been reported with nearly all antibacterial agents, including *Augmentin*, and has ranged in severity from mild to life-threatening. Therefore, it is important to consider this diagnosis in patients who present with diarrhea subsequent to the administration of antibacterial agents.
Treatment with antibacterial agents alters the normal flora of the colon and may permit overgrowth of clostridia. Studies indicate that a toxin produced by *Clostridium difficile* is one primary cause of "antibiotic associated colitis."
After the diagnosis of pseudomembranous colitis has been established, appropriate therapeutic measures should be initiated. Mild cases of pseudomembranous colitis usually respond to drug discontinuation alone. In moderate to severe cases, consideration should be given to management with fluids and electrolytes, protein supplementation and treatment with an antibacterial drug clinically effective against *Clostridium difficile* colitis.
Augmentin should be used with caution in patients with evidence of hepatic dysfunction. Hepatic toxicity associated with the use of *Augmentin* is usually reversible. On rare occasions, deaths have been reported (less than 1 death reported per estimated 4 million prescriptions worldwide). These have generally been cases associated with serious underlying diseases or concomitant medications. (See CONTRAINDICATIONS and ADVERSE REACTIONS—*Liver*.)

PRECAUTIONS

General: While *Augmentin* possesses the characteristic low toxicity of the penicillin group of antibiotics, periodic assessment of organ system functions, including renal, hepatic and hematopoietic function, is advisable during prolonged therapy.
A high percentage of patients with mononucleosis who receive ampicillin develop an erythematous skin rash. Thus, ampicillin class antibiotics should not be administered to patients with mononucleosis.
The possibility of superinfections with mycotic or bacterial pathogens should be kept in mind during therapy. If superinfections occur (usually involving *Pseudomonas* or *Candida*), the drug should be discontinued and/or appropriate therapy instituted.
Drug Interactions: Probenecid decreases the renal tubular secretion of amoxicillin. Concurrent use with *Augmentin* may result in increased and prolonged blood levels of amoxicillin. Co-administration of probenecid cannot be recommended.
The concurrent administration of allopurinol and ampicillin increases substantially the incidence of rashes in patients receiving both drugs as compared to patients receiving ampicillin alone. It is not known whether this potentiation of ampicillin rashes is due to allopurinol or the hyperuricemia present in these patients. There are no data with *Augmentin* and allopurinol administered concurrently.
Drug/Laboratory Test Interactions: Oral administration of *Augmentin* will result in high urine concentrations of amoxicillin. High urine concentrations of ampicillin may result in false-positive reactions when testing for the presence of glucose in urine using Clinitest®, Benedict's Solution or Fehling's Solution. Since this effect may also occur with amoxicillin and therefore *Augmentin*, it is recommended that glucose tests based on enzymatic glucose oxidase reactions (such as Clinistix® or Tes-Tape®) be used.
Following administration of ampicillin to pregnant women a transient decrease in plasma concentration of total conjugated estriol, estriol-glucuronide, conjugated estrone and estradiol has been noted. This effect may also occur with amoxicillin and therefore *Augmentin*.

Continued on next page

Information on the SmithKline Beecham Pharmaceuticals products appearing here is based on the labeling in effect on July 1, 1996. Further information on these and other products may be obtained from the Medical Department, SmithKline Beecham Pharmaceuticals, One Franklin Plaza, Philadelphia, PA 19101.

SmithKline Beecham—Cont.

Carcinogenesis, Mutagenesis, Impairment of Fertility: Long-term studies in animals have not been performed to evaluate carcinogenic potential.
Mutagenesis: The mutagenic potential of *Augmentin* was investigated *in vitro* with an Ames test, a human lymphocyte cytogenetic assay, a yeast test and a mouse lymphoma forward mutation assay, and *in vivo* with mouse micronucleus tests and a dominant lethal test. All were negative apart from the *in vitro* mouse lymphoma assay where weak activity was found at very high, cytotoxic concentrations.
Impairment of Fertility: *Augmentin* at oral doses of up to 1200 mg/kg/day (5.7 times the maximum human dose, 1480 mg/m^2/day, based on body surface area) was found to have no effect on fertility and reproductive performance in rats, dosed with a 2:1 ratio formulation of amoxicillin:clavulanate.
Teratogenic effects. Pregnancy (Category B): Reproduction studies performed in pregnant rats and mice given *Augmentin* at oral dosages up to 1200 mg/kg/day, equivalent to 7200 and 4080 mg/m^2/day, respectively (4.9 and 2.8 times the maximum human oral dose based on body surface area), revealed no evidence of harm to the fetus due to *Augmentin*. There are, however, no adequate and well-controlled studies in pregnant women. Because animal reproduction studies are not always predictive of human response, this drug should be used during pregnancy only if clearly needed.
Labor and Delivery: Oral ampicillin class antibiotics are generally poorly absorbed during labor. Studies in guinea pigs have shown that intravenous administration of ampicillin decreased the uterine tone, frequency of contractions, height of contractions and duration of contractions. However, it is not known whether the use of *Augmentin* in humans during labor or delivery has immediate or delayed adverse effects on the fetus, prolongs the duration of labor, or increases the likelihood that forceps delivery or other obstetrical intervention or resuscitation of the newborn will be necessary.
Nursing Mothers: Ampicillin class antibiotics are excreted in the milk; therefore, caution should be exercised when *Augmentin* is administered to a nursing woman.

ADVERSE REACTIONS

Augmentin is generally well tolerated. The majority of side effects observed in clinical trials were of a mild and transient nature and less than 3% of patients discontinued therapy because of drug-related side effects. The most frequently reported adverse effects were diarrhea/loose stools (9%), nausea (3%), skin rashes and urticaria (3%), vomiting (1%) and vaginitis (1%). The overall incidence of side effects, and in particular diarrhea, increased with the higher recommended dose. Other less frequently reported reactions include: abdominal discomfort, flatulence and headache.
The following adverse reactions have been reported for ampicillin class antibiotics:
Gastrointestinal: Diarrhea, nausea, vomiting, indigestion, gastritis, stomatitis, glossitis, black "hairy" tongue, enterocolitis, mucocutaneous candidiasis and pseudomembranous colitis. Onset of pseudomembranous colitis symptoms may occur during or after antibiotic treatment. (See WARNINGS.)
Hypersensitivity Reactions: Skin rashes, pruritus, urticaria, angioedema, serum sickness-like reactions (urticaria or skin rash accompanied by arthritis, arthralgia, myalgia and frequently fever), erythema multiforme (rarely Stevens-Johnson Syndrome) and an occasional case of exfoliative dermatitis (including toxic epidermal necrolysis) have been reported. These reactions may be controlled with antihistamines and, if necessary, systemic corticosteroids. Whenever such reactions occur, the drug should be discontinued, unless the opinion of the physician dictates otherwise. Serious and occasional fatal hypersensitivity (anaphylactic) reactions can occur with oral penicillin. (See WARNINGS.)
Liver: A moderate rise in AST (SGOT) and/or ALT (SGPT) has been noted in patients treated with ampicillin class antibiotics but the significance of these findings is unknown. Hepatic dysfunction, including increases in serum transaminases (AST and/or ALT), serum bilirubin and/or alkaline phosphatase, has been infrequently reported with *Augmentin*. The histologic findings on liver biopsy have consisted of predominantly cholestatic, hepatocellular, or mixed cholestatic-hepatocellular changes. The onset of signs/symptoms of hepatic dysfunction may occur during or several weeks after therapy has been discontinued. The hepatic dysfunction, which may be severe, is usually reversible. On rare occasions, deaths have been reported (less than 1 death reported per estimated 4 million prescriptions worldwide). These have generally been cases associated with serious underlying diseases or concomitant medications.
Renal: Interstitial nephritis and hematuria have been reported rarely.
Hemic and Lymphatic Systems: Anemia, thrombocytopenia, thrombocytopenic purpura, eosinophilia, leukopenia and agranulocytosis have been reported during therapy with penicillins. These reactions are usually reversible on discontinuation of therapy and are believed to be hypersensitivity phenomena. A slight thrombocytosis was noted in less than 1% of the patients treated with *Augmentin*.
Central Nervous System: Reversible hyperactivity, agitation, anxiety, insomnia, confusion, behavioral changes, and/or dizziness have been reported rarely.

OVERDOSAGE

Amoxicillin may be removed from circulation by hemodialysis.
The molecular weight, degree of protein binding and pharmacokinetic profile of clavulanic acid together with information from a single patient with renal insufficiency all suggest that this compound may also be removed by hemodialysis.

DOSAGE AND ADMINISTRATION

Since both the *Augmentin* 250 mg and 500 mg tablets contain the same amount of clavulanic acid (125 mg, as the potassium salt), 2 *Augmentin* 250 mg tablets are not equivalent to 1 *Augmentin* 500 mg tablet. Therefore, 2 *Augmentin* 250 mg tablets should not be substituted for 1 *Augmentin* 500 mg tablet.
Dosage:
Adults: The usual adult dose is 1 *Augmentin* 500 mg tablet every 12 hours or 1 *Augmentin* 250 mg tablet every 8 hours. For more severe infections and infections of the respiratory tract, the dose should be 1 *Augmentin* 875 mg tablet every 12 hours or 1 *Augmentin* 500 mg tablet every 8 hours.
Patients with impaired renal function do not generally require a reduction in dose unless the impairment is severe. Severely impaired patients with a glomerular filtration rate of <30 mL/minute should not receive the 875 mg tablet. Patients with a glomerular filtration rate of 10 to 30 mL/minute should receive 500 mg or 250 mg every 12 hours, depending on the severity of the infection. Patients with a less than 10 mL/minute glomerular filtration rate should receive 500 mg or 250 mg every 24 hours, depending on severity of the infection.
Hemodialysis patients should receive 500 mg or 250 mg every 24 hours, depending on the severity of the infection. They should receive an additional dose both during and at the end of dialysis.
Hepatically impaired patients should be dosed with caution and hepatic function monitored at regular intervals. (See WARNINGS.)
Pediatric Patients: Pediatric patients weighing 40 kg or more should be dosed according to the adult recommendations.
Due to the different amoxicillin to clavulanic acid ratios in the *Augmentin* 250 mg tablet (250/125) versus the *Augmentin* 250 mg chewable tablet (250/62.5), the *Augmentin* 250 mg tablet should not be used until the pediatric patient weighs at least 40 kg or more.
Administration: *Augmentin* may be taken without regard to meals; however, absorption of clavulanate potassium is enhanced when *Augmentin* is administered at the start of a meal. To minimize the potential for gastrointestinal intolerance, *Augmentin* should be taken at the start of a meal.

HOW SUPPLIED

***AUGMENTIN* 250 MG TABLETS:** Each white oval film-coated tablet, debossed with AUGMENTIN on 1 side and 250/125 on the other side, contains 250 mg amoxicillin as the trihydrate and 125 mg clavulanic acid as the potassium salt.
NDC 0029-6075-27 .... bottles of 30
NDC 0029-6075-31 .... Unit Dose (10×10) 100 tablets
***AUGMENTIN* 500 MG TABLETS:** Each white oval film-coated tablet, debossed with AUGMENTIN on 1 side and 500/125 on the other side, contains 500 mg amoxicillin as the trihydrate and 125 mg clavulanic acid as the potassium salt.
NDC 0029-6080-12 .... bottles of 20
NDC 0029-6080-27 .... bottles of 30
NDC 0029-6080-31 .... Unit Dose (10×10) 100 tablets
***AUGMENTIN* 875 MG TABLETS:** Each scored white capsule-shaped tablet, debossed with AUGMENTIN 875 on 1 side and *SB* on the other side, contains 875 mg amoxicillin as the trihydrate and 125 mg clavulanic acid as the potassium salt.
NDC 0029-6086-12 .... bottles of 20
NDC 0029-6086-21 .... Unit Dose (10×10) 100 tablets
***AUGMENTIN* is also supplied as:**
AUGMENTIN 125 MG/5 ML (125 mg amoxicillin/31.25 mg clavulanic acid) FOR ORAL SUSPENSION:
NDC 0029-6085-39 .... 75 mL bottle
NDC 0029-6085-23 .... 100 mL bottle
NDC 0029-6085-22 .... 150 mL bottle
AUGMENTIN 250 MG/5 ML (250 mg amoxicillin/62.5 mg clavulanic acid) FOR ORAL SUSPENSION:
NDC 0029-6090-39 .... 75 mL bottle
NDC 0029-6090-23 .... 100 mL bottle
NDC 0029-6090-22 .... 150 mL bottle
AUGMENTIN 125 MG (125 mg amoxicillin/31.25 mg clavulanic acid) CHEWABLE TABLETS:
NDC 0029-6073-47 .... carton of 30 (5×6) tablets
AUGMENTIN 250 MG (250 mg amoxicillin/62.5 mg clavulanic acid) CHEWABLE TABLETS:
NDC 0029-6074-47 .... carton of 30 (5×6) tablets
Store tablets and dry powder at or below 25°C (77°F). Dispense in tightly closed, moisture-proof containers.

CLINICAL STUDIES

Data from two pivotal studies in 1,191 patients treated for either lower respiratory tract infections or complicated urinary tract infections compared a regimen of 875 mg *Augmentin* tablets q12h to 500 mg *Augmentin* tablets dosed q8h (584 and 607 patients, respectively). Comparable efficacy was demonstrated between the q12h and q8h dosing regimens. There was no significant difference in the percentage of adverse events in each group. The most frequently reported adverse event was diarrhea; incidence rates were similar for the 875 mg q12h and 500 mg q8h dosing regimens (14.9% and 14.3%, respectively). However, there was a statistically significant difference ($p < 0.05$) in rates of severe diarrhea or withdrawals with diarrhea between the regimens: 1.0% for 875 mg q12h dosing versus 2.5% for the 500 mg q8h dosing.
In one of these pivotal studies, 629 patients with either pyelonephritis or a complicated urinary tract infection (i.e., patients with abnormalities of the urinary tract that predispose to relapse of bacteriuria following eradication) were randomized to receive either 875 mg *Augmentin* tablets q12h or 500 mg *Augmentin* tablets q8h in the following distribution:

	875 mg q12h	500 mg q8h
Pyelonephritis	173 patients	188 patients
Complicated UTI	135 patients	133 patients
Total patients	308	321

The number of bacteriologically evaluable patients was comparable between the two dosing regimens. *Augmentin* produced comparable bacteriological success rates in patients assessed 2 to 4 days immediately following end of therapy. The bacteriologic efficacy rates were comparable at one of the follow-up visits (5 to 9 days post-therapy) and at a late post-therapy visit (in the majority of cases, this was 2 to 4 weeks post-therapy), as seen in the table below:

	875 mg q12h	500 mg q8h
2 to 4 days	81%, n=58	80%, n=54
5 to 9 days	58.5%, n=41	51.9%, n=52
2 to 4 weeks	52.5%, n=101	54.8%, n=104

As noted before, though there was no significant difference in the percentage of adverse events in each group, there was a statistically significant difference in rates of severe diarrhea or withdrawals with diarrhea between the regimens.

REFERENCES

1. National Committee for Clinical Laboratory Standards. Methods for Dilution Antimicrobial Susceptibility Tests for Bacteria that Grow Aerobically—Third Edition. Approved Standard NCCLS Document M7-A3, Vol. 13, No. 25. NCCLS, Villanova, PA, December 1993.
2. National Committee for Clinical Laboratory Standards. Performance Standards for Antimicrobial Disk Susceptibility Tests—Fifth Edition. Approved Standard NCCLS Document M2-A5, Vol. 13, No. 24. NCCLS, Villanova, PA, December 1993.

Veterans Administration/Military/PHS—Chewable Tablets, 125 mg, 30's 6505-01-282-6332; 250 mg, 30's 6505-01-264-2366; Tablets 250 mg, 30's 6505-01-203-6259; 250 mg, 100's SUP, 6505-01-339-6919; 500 mg, 30's 6505-01-206-6228; 500 mg, 100's SUP, 6505-01-303-8962; Oral Suspension, 125 mg/5 mL, 75 mL, 6505-01-340-0847; 125 mg/5 mL, 100 mL, 6505-01-408-8181; 125 mg/5 mL, 150 mL, 6505-01-204-5388; 250 mg/5 mL, 75 mL, 6505-01-207-8205; 250 mg/5 mL, 100 mL, 6505-01-408-8352; 250 mg/5 mL, 150 mL, 6505-01-207-0795.
AG:AL2

Shown in Product Identification Guide, page 336

BACTROBAN® ℞

[back'tro-ban]
(mupirocin)
Ointment 2%
For Dermatologic Use

DESCRIPTION

Each gram of *Bactroban* Ointment 2% contains 20 mg mupirocin in a bland water miscible ointment base (polyethylene glycol ointment, N.F.) consisting of polyethylene glycol 400 and polyethylene glycol 3350. Mupirocin is a naturally occurring antibiotic. The chemical name is (*E*)-(2*S*,3*R*,4*R*,5*S*)-5-[(2*S*,3*S*,4*S*,5*S*)-2,3-Epoxy-5-hydroxy-4-methylhexyl] tetrahydro-3,4-dihydroxy-β-methyl-2*H*-pyran-2-crotonic acid, ester with 9-hydroxynonanoic acid. The chemical structure is:
[See chemical structure at top of next column.]

CLINICAL PHARMACOLOGY

Mupirocin is produced by fermentation of the organism *Pseudomonas fluorescens*. Mupirocin inhibits bacterial protein

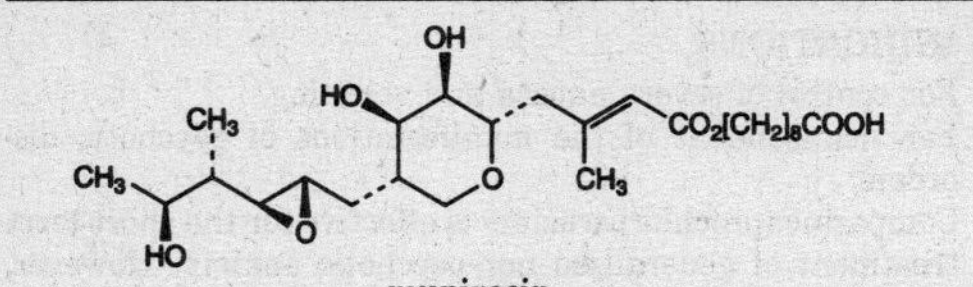

mupirocin

synthesis by reversibly and specifically binding to bacterial isoleucyl transfer-RNA synthetase. Due to this mode of action, mupirocin shows no cross resistance with chloramphenicol, erythromycin, fusidic acid, gentamicin, lincomycin, methicillin, neomycin, novobiocin, penicillin, streptomycin, and tetracycline.

Application of ^{14}C-labeled mupirocin ointment to the lower arm of normal male subjects followed by occlusion for 24 hours showed no measurable systemic absorption (<1.1 nanogram mupirocin per milliliter of whole blood). Measurable radioactivity was present in the stratum corneum of these subjects 72 hours after application.

Microbiology: The following bacteria are susceptible to the action of mupirocin *in vitro:* the aerobic isolates of *Staphylococcus aureus* (including methicillin-resistant and β-lactamase producing strains), *Staphylococcus epidermidis, Staphylococcus saprophyticus,* and *Streptococcus pyogenes.*

Only the organisms listed in the INDICATIONS AND USAGE section have been shown to be clinically susceptible to mupirocin.

INDICATIONS AND USAGE

Bactroban (mupirocin) Ointment is indicated for the topical treatment of impetigo due to: *Staphylococcus aureus,* beta-hemolytic *Streptococcus**, and *Streptococcus pyogenes.*

*Efficacy for this organism in this organ system was studied in fewer than ten infections.

CONTRAINDICATIONS

This drug is contraindicated in individuals with a history of sensitivity reactions to any of its components.

WARNINGS

Bactroban Ointment is not for ophthalmic use.

PRECAUTIONS

If a reaction suggesting sensitivity or chemical irritation should occur with the use of *Bactroban* Ointment, treatment should be discontinued and appropriate alternative therapy for the infection instituted.

As with other antibacterial products prolonged use may result in overgrowth of nonsusceptible organisms, including fungi.

Bactroban is not formulated for use on mucosal surfaces. Intranasal use has been associated with isolated reports of stinging and drying.

Polyethylene glycol can be absorbed from open wounds and damaged skin and is excreted by the kidneys. In common with other polyethylene glycol-based ointments, *Bactroban* should not be used in conditions where absorption of large quantities of polyethylene glycol is possible, especially if there is evidence of moderate or severe renal impairment.

Pregnancy Category B: Reproduction studies have been performed in rats and rabbits at systemic doses, i.e., orally, subcutaneously, and intramuscularly, up to 100 times the human topical dose and have revealed no evidence of impaired fertility or harm to the fetus due to mupirocin. There are, however, no adequate and well-controlled studies in pregnant women. Because animal studies are not always predictive of human response, this drug should be used during pregnancy only if clearly needed.

Nursing Mothers: It is not known whether *Bactroban* is present in breast milk. Nursing should be temporarily discontinued while using *Bactroban.*

ADVERSE REACTIONS

The following local adverse reactions have been reported in connection with the use of *Bactroban* Ointment: burning, stinging, or pain in 1.5% of patients; itching in 1% of patients; rash, nausea, erythema, dry skin, tenderness, swelling, contact dermatitis, and increased exudate in less than 1% of patients.

DOSAGE AND ADMINISTRATION

A small amount of *Bactroban* Ointment should be applied to the affected area three times daily. The area treated may be covered with a gauze dressing if desired. Patients not showing a clinical response within 3 to 5 days should be re-evaluated.

HOW SUPPLIED

Bactroban (mupirocin) Ointment 2% is supplied in 15 gram and 30 gram tubes.

NDC 0029-1525-22 (15 gram tube)

NDC 0029-1525-25 (30 gram tube)

Store between 15° and 30°C (59° and 86°F).

Veterans Administration/Military/PHS—15 gram, 6505-01-375-5686; 30 gram, 6505-01-352-3658.

BC:L6C

BACTROBAN® NASAL ℞

[back 'tro-ban]

brand of mupirocin calcium ointment, 2%
for intranasal use only

DESCRIPTION

Bactroban Nasal (mupirocin calcium ointment), 2% contains the dihydrate crystalline calcium hemi-salt of the antibiotic mupirocin. Chemically, it is (α *E*,2*S*,3*R*,4*R*,5*S*)-5-[(2*S*,3*S*,4*S*,5*S*)-2,3-epoxy-5-hydroxy-4-methylhexyl] tetrahydro-3,4-dihydroxy-β-methyl-2*H*-pyran-2-crotonic acid, ester with 9-hydroxynonanoic acid, calcium salt (2:1), dihydrate.

The molecular formula of mupirocin calcium is $(C_{52}H_{86}O_{18})_2Ca \cdot 2H_2O$, and the molecular weight is 1075.3. The molecular weight of mupirocin free acid is 500.6. The structural formula of mupirocin calcium is:

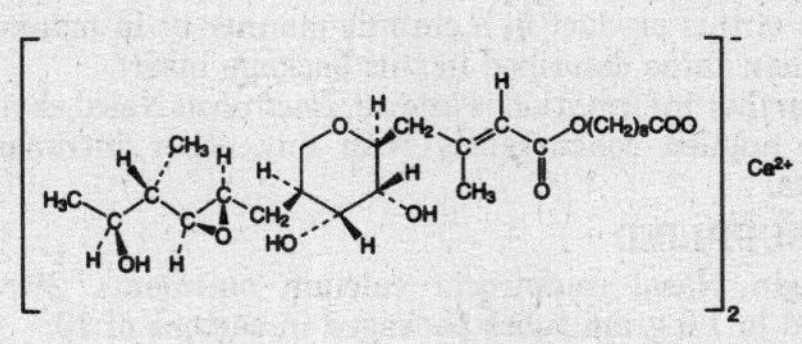

Bactroban Nasal is a white to off-white ointment that contains 2.15% w/w mupirocin calcium (equivalent to 2.0% pure mupirocin free acid) in a soft white ointment base. The inactive ingredients are paraffin and a mixture of glycerin esters (Softisan® 649).

CLINICAL PHARMACOLOGY

Pharmacokinetics

Following single or repeated intranasal applications of 0.2 gram of *Bactroban* Nasal t.i.d. for 3 days to five healthy adult male subjects, no evidence of systemic absorption of mupirocin was demonstrated. The dosage regimen used in this study was for pharmacokinetic characterization only. (See DOSAGE AND ADMINISTRATION for proper clinical dosing information.)

In this study, the concentrations of mupirocin in urine and of monic acid in urine and serum were below the limit of determination of the assay for up to 72 hours after the applications. The lowest levels of determination of the assay used were 50 ng/mL of mupirocin in urine, 75 ng/mL of monic acid in urine, and 10 ng/mL of monic acid in serum. Based on the detectable limit of the urine assay for monic acid, one can extrapolate that a mean of 3.3% (range: 1.2% to 5.1%) of the applied dose could be systemically absorbed from the nasal mucosa of **adults.**

Data from a report of a pharmacokinetic study in neonates and premature infants indicate that, unlike in adults, significant systemic absorption occurred following intranasal administration of *Bactroban* Nasal in this population. **At this time, the pharmacokinetic properties of mupirocin following intranasal application of *Bactroban* Nasal have not been adequately characterized in neonates or other children less than 12 years of age and, in addition, the safety of the product in children less than 12 years of age has not been established.**

The effect of the concurrent application of intranasal mupirocin calcium ointment, 2% with other intranasal products has not been studied. (See PRECAUTIONS, Drug Interactions.)

Following intravenous or oral administration, mupirocin is rapidly metabolized. The principal metabolite, monic acid, demonstrates no antibacterial activity. In a study conducted in seven healthy adult male subjects, the elimination half-life after intravenous administration of mupirocin was 20 to 40 minutes for mupirocin and 30 to 80 minutes for monic acid. Monic acid is predominantly eliminated by renal excretion. The pharmacokinetics of mupirocin has not been studied in individuals with renal insufficiency.

Microbiology

Mupirocin is an antibacterial agent produced by fermentation using the microorganism *Pseudomonas fluorescens.* Mupirocin inhibits bacterial protein synthesis by reversibly and specifically binding to bacterial isoleucyl transfer-RNA synthetase. Due to this mode of action, mupirocin demonstrates no *in vitro* cross-resistance with other classes of antimicrobial agents.

When mupirocin resistance does occur, it appears to result from the production of a modified isoleucyl-tRNA synthetase. High-level plasmid-mediated resistance (MIC >1024 mcg/mL) has been reported in some strains of *S. aureus* and coagulase-negative staphylococci.

Mupirocin is bactericidal at concentrations achieved topically by intranasal administration. However, the minimum bactericidal concentration (MBC) against relevant intranasal pathogens is generally eight-fold to thirty-fold higher than the minimum inhibitory concentration (MIC). In addition, mupirocin is highly protein bound (>97%), and the effect of nasal secretions on the MICs of intranasally applied mupirocin has not been determined.

Mupirocin has been shown to be active against most strains of methicillin-resistant *S. aureus,* both *in vitro* and in clinical studies of the eradication of nasal colonization. *Bactroban* Nasal has only established clinical utility in nasal eradication as part of a comprehensive program to curtail institutional outbreaks of infections with methicillin-resistant *S. aureus.* (See INDICATIONS AND USAGE.)

The following *in vitro* data are available, **but their clinical significance is unknown.** Mupirocin exhibits *in vitro* MICs of 1 mcg/mL or less against most (>90%) strains of methicillin-susceptible *S. aureus;* however, the safety and effectiveness of mupirocin calcium in eradicating nasal colonization and preventing subsequent infections due to methicillin-susceptible *S. aureus* have not been established.

INDICATIONS AND USAGE

Bactroban Nasal (mupirocin calcium ointment), 2% is indicated for the eradication of nasal colonization with methicillin-resistant *Staphylococcus aureus* in adult patients and health care workers as part of a comprehensive infection control program to reduce the risk of infection among patients at high risk of methicillin-resistant *S. aureus* infection during institutional outbreaks of infections with this pathogen.

NOTE:

(1) There are insufficient data at this time to establish that this product is safe and effective as part of an intervention program to prevent autoinfection of high-risk patients from their own nasal colonization with *S. aureus.*

(2) There are insufficient data at this time to recommend use of *Bactroban* Nasal for general prophylaxis of any infection in any patient population.

(3) Greater than 90% of subjects/patients in clinical trials had eradication of nasal colonization 2 to 4 days after therapy was completed. Approximately 30% recolonization was reported in one domestic study within 4 weeks after completion of therapy. These eradication rates were clinically and statistically superior to those reported in subjects/patients in the vehicle-treated arms of the adequate and well-controlled studies. Those treated with vehicle had eradication rates of 5% to 30% at 2 to 4 days post-therapy with 85% to 100% recolonization within 4 weeks.

All adequate and well-controlled trials of this product were vehicle-controlled; therefore, no data from direct, head-to-head comparisons with other products are available at this time.

CONTRAINDICATIONS

Bactroban Nasal is contraindicated in patients with known hypersensitivity to any of the constituents of the product.

WARNINGS

AVOID CONTACT WITH THE EYES. Application of *Bactroban* Nasal to the eye under testing conditions has caused severe symptoms such as burning and tearing. These symptoms resolved within days to weeks after discontinuation of the ointment.

In the event of a sensitization or severe local irritation from *Bactroban* Nasal, usage should be discontinued.

PRECAUTIONS

General

As with other antibacterial products, prolonged use may result in overgrowth of nonsusceptible microorganisms, including fungi. (See DOSAGE AND ADMINISTRATION.)

Information for Patients

Patients should be given the following instructions:

—Apply approximately one-half of the ointment from the single-use tube directly into one nostril and the other half into the other nostril;

—Avoid contact of the medication with the eyes;

—Discard the tube after using, do not re-use;

—Press the sides of the nose together and gently massage after application to spread the ointment throughout the inside of the nostrils; and

—Discontinue usage of the medication and call your health care practitioner if sensitization or severe local irritation occurs.

Drug Interactions

The effect of the concurrent application of intranasal mupirocin calcium and other intranasal products has not been studied. Until further information is known, mupirocin calcium ointment, 2% should not be applied concurrently with any other intranasal products.

Continued on next page

Information on the SmithKline Beecham Pharmaceuticals products appearing here is based on the labeling in effect on July 1, 1996. Further information on these and other products may be obtained from the Medical Department, SmithKline Beecham Pharmaceuticals, One Franklin Plaza, Philadelphia, PA 19101.

SmithKline Beecham—Cont.

Carcinogenesis, Mutagenesis, Impairment of Fertility
Long-term studies in animals to evaluate carcinogenic potential of mupirocin calcium have not been conducted.
Results of the following studies performed with mupirocin calcium or mupirocin sodium *in vitro* and *in vivo* did not indicate a potential for mutagenicity: rat primary hepatocyte unscheduled DNA synthesis, sediment analysis for DNA strand breaks, *Salmonella* reversion test (Ames), *Escherichia coli* mutation assay, metaphase analysis of human lymphocytes, mouse lymphoma assay, and bone marrow micronuclei assay in mice.
Reproduction studies were performed in rats with mupirocin administered subcutaneously at doses up to 40 times the human intranasal dose (approximately 20 mg mupirocin per day) on a mg/m² basis and revealed no evidence of impaired fertility from mupirocin sodium.

Pregnancy
Teratogenic Effects. Pregnancy Category B. Reproduction studies have been performed in rats and rabbits with mupirocin administered subcutaneously at doses up to 65 and 130 times, respectively, the human intranasal dose (approximately 20 mg mupirocin per day) on a mg/m² basis and revealed no evidence of harm to the fetus due to mupirocin. There are, however, no adequate and well-controlled studies in pregnant women. Because animal reproduction studies are not always predictive of human response, this drug should be used during pregnancy only if clearly needed.

Nursing Mothers
It is not known whether this drug is excreted in human milk. Because many drugs are excreted in human milk, caution should be exercised when *Bactroban* Nasal is administered to a nursing woman.

Pediatric Use
Safety in children under the age of 12 years has not been established. (See CLINICAL PHARMACOLOGY.)

ADVERSE REACTIONS

Clinical Trials
In clinical trials, 210 domestic and 2,130 foreign adult subjects/patients received *Bactroban* Nasal ointment. Less than 1% of domestic or foreign subjects and patients in clinical trials were withdrawn due to adverse events.
The most frequently reported adverse events in foreign clinical trials were as follows: rhinitis (1.0%), taste perversion (0.8%), pharyngitis (0.5%).
In domestic clinical trials, 17% (36/210) of adults treated with *Bactroban* Nasal ointment reported adverse events thought to be at least possibly drug-related. The incidence of adverse events thought to be at least possibly drug-related that were reported in at least 1% of adults enrolled in domestic clinical trials were as follows:

**ADVERSE EVENTS (≥ 1% INCIDENCE)-
ADULTS IN U.S. TRIALS**

	% of Subjects/Patients Experiencing Event *Bactroban* Nasal 2% (n=210)
Headache	9%
Rhinitis	6%
Respiratory disorder, including upper respiratory tract congestion	5%
Pharyngitis	4%
Taste perversion	3%
Burning/Stinging	2%
Cough	2%
Pruritus	1%

The following events thought possibly drug-related were reported in less than 1% of adults enrolled in domestic clinical trials: blepharitis, diarrhea, dry mouth, ear pain, epistaxis, nausea and rash.
All adequate and well-controlled clinical trials have been performed using *Bactroban* Nasal ointment, 2% in one arm and the vehicle ointment in the other arm of the study. No adequate and well-controlled safety data are available from direct, head-to-head comparative studies of this product and other products for this indication.

OVERDOSAGE

Following single or repeated intranasal applications of *Bactroban* Nasal to adults, no evidence for systemic absorption of mupirocin was obtained. Intravenous infusions of 252 mg, as well as single oral doses of 500 mg of mupirocin, have been well tolerated in healthy adult subjects. There is no information regarding local overdose of *Bactroban* Nasal or regarding oral ingestion of the nasal ointment formulation.

DOSAGE AND ADMINISTRATION
(See INDICATIONS AND USAGE.)
Adults (12 years of age and older): Approximately one-half of the ointment from the single-use tube should be applied into one nostril and the other half into the other nostril twice daily (morning and evening) for 5 days.
After application, the nostrils should be closed by pressing together and releasing the sides of the nose repetitively for approximately 1 minute. This will spread the ointment throughout the nares.
The single-use 1.0 gram tube will deliver a total of approximately 0.5 gram of the ointment (approximately 0.25 gram/nostril).
The tube should be discarded after usage; it should not be re-used.
The safety and effectiveness of applications of this medication for greater than 5 days have not been established. There are no human clinical or pre-clinical animal data to support the use of this product in a chronic manner or in manners other than those described in this package insert.
Until further information is known, *Bactroban* Nasal should not be applied concurrently with any other intranasal products.

HOW SUPPLIED
Bactroban Nasal (mupirocin calcium ointment), 2% is supplied in 1.0 gram tubes packaged in cartons of 10.
NDC 0029-1526-11 (1.0 gram tubes in packages of 10). Store at or below 25°C (77°F).

REFERENCE
1. National Committee for Clinical Laboratory Standards. Methods for Dilution Antimicrobial Susceptibility Tests for Bacteria That Grow Aerobically—Third Edition; Approved Standard NCCLS Document M7-A3. Vol. 12, No. 25, NCCLS, Villanova, PA, December 1993.
Manufactured by DPT Laboratories, Inc.
San Antonio, TX 78215
Distributed by SmithKline Beecham Pharmaceuticals
Philadelphia, PA 19101
BN:L1

COMPAZINE® ℞
[*komp'ah-zeen*]
(brand of prochlorperazine)

DESCRIPTION
Tablets—Each round, yellow-green, coated tablet contains prochlorperazine maleate equivalent to prochlorperazine as follows: 5 mg imprinted SKF and C66; 10 mg imprinted SKF and C67.
5 mg and 10 mg Tablets: Modified Formulation—Inactive ingredients consist of cellulose, lactose, magnesium stearate, polyethylene glycol, sodium croscarmellose, titanium dioxide, D&C Yellow No. 10, FD&C Blue No. 2, FD&C Yellow No. 6, FD&C Red No. 40, iron oxide, starch, stearic acid and trace amounts of other inactive ingredients.
NOTE: *Compazine* 5 mg and 10 mg tablets have been changed from yellow-green sugar-coated tablets to yellow-green film-coated tablets. The film-coated tablets are smaller in size than the sugar-coated tablets. The inactive ingredients have changed, but the drug content remains unchanged.
Spansule® sustained release capsules—Each Compazine® *Spansule* capsule is so prepared that an initial dose is released promptly and the remaining medication is released gradually over a prolonged period.
Each capsule, with black cap and natural body, contains prochlorperazine maleate equivalent to prochlorperazine as follows: 10 mg imprinted SKF and C44; 15 mg imprinted SKF and C46. Inactive ingredients consist of benzyl alcohol, cetylpyridinium chloride, D&C Green No. 5, D&C Yellow No. 10, FD&C Blue No. 1, FD&C Red No. 40, FD&C Yellow No. 6, gelatin, glyceryl monostearate, sodium lauryl sulfate, starch, sucrose, wax and trace amounts of other inactive ingredients.
Vials, 2 mL (5 mg/mL) and 10 mL (5 mg/mL)—Each mL contains, in aqueous solution, 5 mg prochlorperazine as the edisylate, 5 mg sodium biphosphate, 12 mg sodium tartrate, 0.9 mg sodium saccharin and 0.75% benzyl alcohol as preservative.
Disposable Syringes, 2 mL (5 mg/mL)—Each mL contains, in aqueous solution, 5 mg prochlorperazine as the edisylate, 5 mg sodium biphosphate, 12 mg sodium tartrate, 0.9 mg sodium saccharin and 0.75% benzyl alcohol as preservative.
Suppositories—Each suppository contains 2¹⁄₂ mg, 5 mg or 25 mg of prochlorperazine; with glycerin, glyceryl monopalmitate, glyceryl monostearate, hydrogenated cocoanut oil fatty acids and hydrogenated palm kernel oil fatty acids.
Syrup—Each 5 mL (1 teaspoonful) of clear, yellow-orange, fruit-flavored liquid contains 5 mg of prochlorperazine as the edisylate. Inactive ingredients consist of FD&C Yellow No. 6, flavors, polyoxyethylene polyoxypropylene glycol, sodium benzoate, sodium citrate, sucrose and water.

INDICATIONS
For control of severe nausea and vomiting.
For management of the manifestations of psychotic disorders.
Compazine (prochlorperazine) is effective for the short-term treatment of generalized non-psychotic anxiety. However, *Compazine* is not the first drug to be used in therapy for most patients with non-psychotic anxiety, because certain risks associated with its use are not shared by common alternative treatments (e.g., benzodiazepines).
When used in the treatment of non-psychotic anxiety, *Compazine* should not be administered at doses of more than 20 mg per day or for longer than 12 weeks, because the use of *Compazine* at higher doses or for longer intervals may cause persistent tardive dyskinesia that may prove irreversible (see Warnings).
The effectiveness of *Compazine* as treatment for non-psychotic anxiety was established in 4-week clinical studies of outpatients with generalized anxiety disorder. This evidence does not predict that *Compazine* will be useful in patients with other non-psychotic conditions in which anxiety, or signs that mimic anxiety, are found (e.g., physical illness, organic mental conditions, agitated depression, character pathologies, etc.).
Compazine has not been shown effective in the management of behavioral complications in patients with mental retardation.

CONTRAINDICATIONS
Do not use in patients with known hypersensitivity to phenothiazines.
Do not use in comatose states or in the presence of large amounts of central nervous system depressants (alcohol, barbiturates, narcotics, etc.).
Do not use in pediatric surgery.
Do not use in children under 2 years of age or under 20 lbs.
Do not use in children for conditions for which dosage has not been established.

WARNINGS
The extrapyramidal symptoms which can occur secondary to Compazine (prochlorperazine) may be confused with the central nervous system signs of an undiagnosed primary disease responsible for the vomiting, e.g., Reye's syndrome or other encephalopathy. The use of Compazine (prochlorperazine) and other potential hepatotoxins should be avoided in children and adolescents whose signs and symptoms suggest Reye's syndrome.
Tardive Dyskinesia: Tardive dyskinesia, a syndrome consisting of potentially irreversible, involuntary, dyskinetic movements, may develop in patients treated with neuroleptic (antipsychotic) drugs. Although the prevalence of the syndrome appears to be highest among the elderly, especially elderly women, it is impossible to rely upon prevalence estimates to predict, at the inception of neuroleptic treatment, which patients are likely to develop the syndrome. Whether neuroleptic drug products differ in their potential to cause tardive dyskinesia is unknown.
Both the risk of developing the syndrome and the likelihood that it will become irreversible are believed to increase as the duration of treatment and the total cumulative dose of neuroleptic drugs administered to the patient increase. However, the syndrome can develop, although much less commonly, after relatively brief treatment periods at low doses.
There is no known treatment for established cases of tardive dyskinesia, although the syndrome may remit, partially or completely, if neuroleptic treatment is withdrawn. Neuroleptic treatment itself, however, may suppress (or partially suppress) the signs and symptoms of the syndrome and thereby may possibly mask the underlying disease process. The effect that symptomatic suppression has upon the long-term course of the syndrome is unknown.
Given these considerations, neuroleptics should be prescribed in a manner that is most likely to minimize the occurrence of tardive dyskinesia. Chronic neuroleptic treatment should generally be reserved for patients who suffer from a chronic illness that, 1) is known to respond to neuroleptic drugs, and 2) for whom alternative, equally effective, but potentially less harmful treatments are *not* available or appropriate. In patients who do require chronic treatment, the smallest dose and the shortest duration of treatment producing a satisfactory clinical response should be sought. The need for continued treatment should be reassessed periodically.
If signs and symptoms of tardive dyskinesia appear in a patient on neuroleptics, drug discontinuation should be considered. However, some patients may require treatment despite the presence of the syndrome.
For further information about the description of tardive dyskinesia and its clinical detection, please refer to the sections on PRECAUTIONS and ADVERSE REACTIONS.
Neuroleptic Malignant Syndrome (NMS): A potentially fatal symptom complex sometimes referred to as Neuroleptic Malignant Syndrome (NMS) has been reported in association with antipsychotic drugs. Clinical manifestations of NMS are hyperpyrexia, muscle rigidity, altered mental sta-

tus and evidence of autonomic instability (irregular pulse or blood pressure, tachycardia, diaphoresis and cardiac dysrhythmias).

The diagnostic evaluation of patients with this syndrome is complicated. In arriving at a diagnosis, it is important to identify cases where the clinical presentation includes both serious medical illness (e.g., pneumonia, systemic infection, etc.) and untreated or inadequately treated extrapyramidal signs and symptoms (EPS). Other important considerations in the differential diagnosis include central anticholinergic toxicity, heat stroke, drug fever and primary central nervous system (CNS) pathology.

The management of NMS should include 1) immediate discontinuation of antipsychotic drugs and other drugs not essential to concurrent therapy, 2) intensive symptomatic treatment and medical monitoring, and 3) treatment of any concomitant serious medical problems for which specific treatments are available. There is no general agreement about specific pharmacological treatment regimens for uncomplicated NMS.

If a patient requires antipsychotic drug treatment after recovery from NMS, the potential reintroduction of drug therapy should be carefully considered. The patient should be carefully monitored, since recurrences of NMS have been reported.

An encephalopathic syndrome (characterized by weakness, lethargy, fever, tremulousness and confusion, extrapyramidal symptoms, leukocytosis, elevated serum enzymes, BUN and FBS) has occurred in a few patients treated with lithium plus a neuroleptic. In some instances, the syndrome was followed by irreversible brain damage. Because of a possible causal relationship between these events and the concomitant administration of lithium and neuroleptics, patients receiving such combined therapy should be monitored closely for early evidence of neurologic toxicity and treatment discontinued promptly if such signs appear. This encephalopathic syndrome may be similar to or the same as neuroleptic malignant syndrome (NMS).

Patients with bone marrow depression or who have previously demonstrated a hypersensitivity reaction (e.g., blood dyscrasias, jaundice) with a phenothiazine should not receive any phenothiazine, including *Compazine*, unless in the judgment of the physician the potential benefits of treatment outweigh the possible hazards.

Compazine (prochlorperazine) may impair mental and/or physical abilities, especially during the first few days of therapy. Therefore, caution patients about activities requiring alertness (e.g., operating vehicles or machinery).

Phenothiazines may intensify or prolong the action of central nervous system depressants (e.g., alcohol, anesthetics, narcotics).

Usage in Pregnancy: Safety for the use of *Compazine* during pregnancy has not been established. Therefore, *Compazine* is not recommended for use in pregnant patients except in cases of severe nausea and vomiting that are so serious and intractable that, in the judgment of the physician, drug intervention is required and potential benefits outweigh possible hazards.

There have been reported instances of prolonged jaundice, extrapyramidal signs, hyperreflexia or hyporeflexia in newborn infants whose mothers received phenothiazines.

Nursing Mothers: There is evidence that phenothiazines are excreted in the breast milk of nursing mothers. Caution should be exercised when *Compazine* is administered to a nursing woman.

PRECAUTIONS

The antiemetic action of Compazine (prochlorperazine) may mask the signs and symptoms of overdosage of other drugs and may obscure the diagnosis and treatment of other conditions such as intestinal obstruction, brain tumor and Reye's syndrome (see Warnings).

When *Compazine* is used with cancer chemotherapeutic drugs, vomiting as a sign of the toxicity of these agents may be obscured by the antiemetic effect of *Compazine*.

Because hypotension may occur, large doses and parenteral administration should be used cautiously in patients with impaired cardiovascular systems. To minimize the occurrence of hypotension after injection, keep patient lying down and observe for at least $^1/_2$ hour. If hypotension occurs after parenteral or oral dosing, place patient in head-low position with legs raised. If a vasoconstrictor is required, Levophed®* and Neo-Synephrine®† are suitable. Other pressor agents, including epinephrine, should not be used because they may cause a paradoxical further lowering of blood pressure.

Aspiration of vomitus has occurred in a few post-surgical patients who have received Compazine (prochlorperazine) as an antiemetic. Although no causal relationship has been established, this possibility should be borne in mind during surgical aftercare.

Deep sleep, from which patients can be aroused, and coma have been reported, usually with overdosage.

Neuroleptic drugs elevate prolactin levels; the elevation persists during chronic administration. Tissue culture experiments indicate that approximately one third of human

breast cancers are prolactin-dependent *in vitro*, a factor of potential importance if the prescribing of these drugs is contemplated in a patient with a previously detected breast cancer. Although disturbances such as galactorrhea, amenorrhea, gynecomastia and impotence have been reported, the clinical significance of elevated serum prolactin levels is unknown for most patients. An increase in mammary neoplasms has been found in rodents after chronic administration of neuroleptic drugs. Neither clinical nor epidemiologic studies conducted to date, however, have shown an association between chronic administration of these drugs and mammary tumorigenesis; the available evidence is considered too limited to be conclusive at this time.

Chromosomal aberrations in spermatocytes and abnormal sperm have been demonstrated in rodents treated with certain neuroleptics.

As with all drugs which exert an anticholinergic effect, and/or cause mydriasis, prochlorperazine should be used with caution in patients with glaucoma.

Because phenothiazines may interfere with thermoregulatory mechanisms, use with caution in persons who will be exposed to extreme heat.

Phenothiazines can diminish the effect of oral anticoagulants.

Phenothiazines can produce alpha-adrenergic blockade.

Thiazide diuretics may accentuate the orthostatic hypotension that may occur with phenothiazines.

Antihypertensive effects of guanethidine and related compounds may be counteracted when phenothiazines are used concomitantly.

Concomitant administration of propranolol with phenothiazines results in increased plasma levels of both drugs.

Phenothiazines may lower the convulsive threshold; dosage adjustments of anticonvulsants may be necessary. Potentiation of anticonvulsant effects does not occur. However, it has been reported that phenothiazines may interfere with the metabolism of Dilantin®‡ and thus precipitate *Dilantin* toxicity.

The presence of phenothiazines may produce false-positive phenylketonuria (PKU) test results.

Long-Term Therapy: Given the likelihood that some patients exposed chronically to neuroleptics will develop tardive dyskinesia, it is advised that all patients in whom chronic use is contemplated be given, if possible, full information about this risk. The decision to inform patients and/or their guardians must obviously take into account the clinical circumstances and the competency of the patient to understand the information provided.

To lessen the likelihood of adverse reactions related to cumulative drug effect, patients with a history of long-term therapy with Compazine (prochlorperazine) and/or other neuroleptics should be evaluated periodically to decide whether the maintenance dosage could be lowered or drug therapy discontinued.

Children with acute illnesses (e.g., chickenpox, CNS infections, measles, gastroenteritis) or dehydration seem to be much more susceptible to neuromuscular reactions, particularly dystonias, than are adults. In such patients, the drug should be used only under close supervision.

Drugs which lower the seizure threshold, including phenothiazine derivatives, should not be used with Amipaque®§. As with other phenothiazine derivatives, Compazine (prochlorperazine) should be discontinued at least 48 hours before myelography, should not be resumed for at least 24 hours postprocedure, and should not be used for the control of nausea and vomiting occurring either prior to myelography with *Amipaque*, or postprocedure.

ADVERSE REACTIONS

Drowsiness, dizziness, amenorrhea, blurred vision, skin reactions and hypotension may occur. Neuroleptic Malignant Syndrome (NMS) has been reported in association with antipsychotic drugs (see WARNINGS).

Cholestatic jaundice has occurred. If fever with grippe-like symptoms occurs, appropriate liver studies should be conducted. If tests indicate an abnormality, stop treatment. There have been a few observations of fatty changes in the livers of patients who have died while receiving the drug. No causal relationship has been established.

Leukopenia and agranulocytosis have occurred. Warn patients to report the sudden appearance of sore throat or other signs of infection. If white blood cell and differential counts indicate leukocyte depression, stop treatment and start antibiotic and other suitable therapy.

Neuromuscular (Extrapyramidal) Reactions

These symptoms are seen in a significant number of hospitalized mental patients. They may be characterized by motor restlessness, be of the dystonic type, or they may resemble parkinsonism.

Depending on the severity of symptoms, dosage should be reduced or discontinued. If therapy is reinstituted, it should be at a lower dosage. Should these symptoms occur in children or pregnant patients, the drug should be stopped and not reinstituted. In most cases barbiturates by suitable route of administration will suffice. (Or, injectable Benadryl®‖ may be useful.) In more severe cases, the administration of

an anti-parkinsonism agent, except levodopa, usually produces rapid reversal of symptoms. Suitable supportive measures such as maintaining a clear airway and adequate hydration should be employed.

Motor Restlessness: Symptoms may include agitation or jitteriness and sometimes insomnia. These symptoms often disappear spontaneously. At times these symptoms may be similar to the original neurotic or psychotic symptoms. Dosage should not be increased until these side effects have subsided.

If these symptoms become too troublesome, they can usually be controlled by a reduction of dosage or change of drug. Treatment with anti-parkinsonian agents, benzodiazepines or propranolol may be helpful.

Dystonias: Symptoms may include: spasm of the neck muscles, sometimes progressing to torticollis; extensor rigidity of back muscles, sometimes progressing to opisthotonos; carpopedal spasm, trismus, swallowing difficulty, oculogyric crisis and protrusion of the tongue.

These usually subside within a few hours, and almost always within 24 to 48 hours, after the drug has been discontinued. *In mild cases*, reassurance or a barbiturate is often sufficient. *In moderate cases*, barbiturates will usually bring rapid relief. *In more severe adult cases*, the administration of an anti-parkinsonism agent, except levodopa, usually produces rapid reversal of symptoms. *In children*, reassurance and barbiturates will usually control symptoms. (Or, injectable *Benadryl* may be useful. Note: See *Benadryl* prescribing information for appropriate *children's* dosage.) If appropriate treatment with anti-parkinsonism agents or *Benadryl* fails to reverse the signs and symptoms, the diagnosis should be reevaluated.

Pseudo-parkinsonism: Symptoms may include: mask-like facies; drooling; tremors; pillrolling motion; cogwheel rigidity; and shuffling gait. Reassurance and sedation are important. In most cases these symptoms are readily controlled when an anti-parkinsonism agent is administered concomitantly. Anti-parkinsonism agents should be used only when required. Generally, therapy of a few weeks to 2 or 3 months will suffice. After this time patients should be evaluated to determine their need for continued treatment. (Note: Levodopa has not been found effective in pseudo-parkinsonism.) Occasionally it is necessary to lower the dosage of Compazine (prochlorperazine) or to discontinue the drug.

Tardive Dyskinesia: As with all antipsychotic agents, tardive dyskinesia may appear in some patients on long-term therapy or may appear after drug therapy has been discontinued. The syndrome can also develop, although much less frequently, after relatively brief treatment periods at low doses. This syndrome appears in all age groups. Although its prevalence appears to be highest among elderly patients, especially elderly women, it is impossible to rely upon prevalence estimates to predict at the inception of neuroleptic treatment which patients are likely to develop the syndrome. The symptoms are persistent and in some patients appear to be irreversible. The syndrome is characterized by rhythmical involuntary movements of the tongue, face, mouth or jaw (e.g., protrusion of tongue, puffing of cheeks, puckering of mouth, chewing movements). Sometimes these may be accompanied by involuntary movements of extremities. In rare instances, these involuntary movements of the extremities are the only manifestations of tardive dyskinesia. A variant of tardive dyskinesia, tardive dystonia, has also been described.

There is no known effective treatment for tardive dyskinesia; anti-parkinsonism agents do not alleviate the symptoms of this syndrome. It is suggested that all antipsychotic agents be discontinued if these symptoms appear.

Should it be necessary to reinstitute treatment, or increase the dosage of the agent, or switch to a different antipsychotic agent, the syndrome may be masked.

It has been reported that fine vermicular movements of the tongue may be an early sign of the syndrome and if the medication is stopped at that time the syndrome may not develop.

Contact Dermatitis: Avoid getting the Injection solution on hands or clothing because of the possibility of contact dermatitis.

Adverse Reactions Reported with Compazine (prochlorperazine) or Other Phenothiazine Derivatives: Adverse reactions with different phenothiazines vary in type, frequency and mechanism of occurrence, i.e., some are dose-related, while others involve individual patient sensitivity. Some adverse reactions may be more likely to occur, or occur with greater intensity, in patients with special medical problems, e.g., patients with mitral insufficiency or pheochromocytoma

Continued on next page

Information on the SmithKline Beecham Pharmaceuticals products appearing here is based on the labeling in effect on July 1, 1996. Further information on these and other products may be obtained from the Medical Department, SmithKline Beecham Pharmaceuticals, One Franklin Plaza, Philadelphia, PA 19101.

SmithKline Beecham—Cont.

have experienced severe hypotension following recommended doses of certain phenothiazines.

Not all of the following adverse reactions have been observed with every phenothiazine derivative, but they have been reported with 1 or more and should be borne in mind when drugs of this class are administered: extrapyramidal symptoms (opisthotonos, oculogyric crisis, hyperreflexia, dystonia, akathisia, dyskinesia, parkinsonism) some of which have lasted months and even years—particularly in elderly patients with previous brain damage; grand mal and petit mal convulsions, particularly in patients with EEG abnormalities or history of such disorders; altered cerebrospinal fluid proteins; cerebral edema; intensification and prolongation of the action of central nervous system depressants (opiates, analgesics, antihistamines, barbiturates, alcohol), atropine, heat, organophosphorus insecticides; autonomic reactions (dryness of mouth, nasal congestion, headache, nausea, constipation, obstipation, adynamic ileus, ejaculatory disorders/impotence, priapism, atonic colon, urinary retention, miosis and mydriasis); reactivation of psychotic processes, catatonic-like states; hypotension (sometimes fatal); cardiac arrest; blood dyscrasias (pancytopenia, thrombocytopenic purpura, leukopenia, agranulocytosis, eosinophilia, hemolytic anemia, aplastic anemia); liver damage (jaundice, biliary stasis); endocrine disturbances (hyperglycemia, hypoglycemia, glycosuria, lactation, galactorrhea, gynecomastia, menstrual irregularities, false-positive pregnancy tests); skin disorders (photosensitivity, itching, erythema, urticaria, eczema up to exfoliative dermatitis); other allergic reactions (asthma, laryngeal edema, angioneurotic edema, anaphylactoid reactions); peripheral edema; reversed epinephrine effect; hyperpyrexia; mild fever after large I.M. doses; increased appetite; increased weight; a systemic lupus erythematosus-like syndrome; pigmentary retinopathy; with prolonged administration of substantial doses, skin pigmentation, epithelial keratopathy, and lenticular and corneal deposits.

EKG changes—particularly nonspecific, usually reversible Q and T wave distortions—have been observed in some patients receiving phenothiazine tranquilizers.

Although phenothiazines cause neither psychic nor physical dependence, sudden discontinuance in long-term psychiatric patients may cause temporary symptoms, e.g., nausea and vomiting, dizziness, tremulousness.

Note: There have been occasional reports of sudden death in patients receiving phenothiazines. In some cases, the cause appeared to be cardiac arrest or asphyxia due to failure of the cough reflex.

DOSAGE AND ADMINISTRATION

Notes on Injection: *Stability*—This solution should be protected from light. This is a clear, colorless to pale yellow solution; a slight yellowish discoloration will not alter potency. If markedly discolored, solution should be discarded.

Compatibility—It is recommended that Compazine (prochlorperazine) Injection not be mixed with other agents in the syringe.

DOSAGE AND ADMINISTRATION—ADULTS

(For children's dosage and administration, see below.) Dosage should be increased more gradually in debilitated or emaciated patients.

Elderly Patients: In general, dosages in the lower range are sufficient for most elderly patients. Since they appear to be more susceptible to hypotension and neuromuscular reactions, such patients should be observed closely. Dosage should be tailored to the individual, response carefully monitored and dosage adjusted accordingly. Dosage should be increased more gradually in elderly patients.

1. To Control Severe Nausea and Vomiting: Adjust dosage to the response of the individual. Begin with the lowest recommended dosage.

Oral Dosage—Tablets: Usually one 5 mg or 10 mg tablet 3 or 4 times daily. Daily dosages above 40 mg should be used only in resistant cases.

***Spansule* capsules:** Initially, usually one 15 mg capsule on arising or one 10 mg capsule q12h. Daily doses above 40 mg should be used only in resistant cases.

Rectal Dosage: 25 mg twice daily.

I.M. Dosage: Initially 5 to 10 mg (1 to 2 mL) injected *deeply* into the upper outer quadrant of the buttock. If necessary, repeat every 3 or 4 hours. Total I.M. dosage should not exceed 40 mg per day.

I.V. Dosage: $2^1/_2$ to 10 mg ($^1/_2$ to 2 mL) by slow I.V. injection or infusion at a rate not to exceed 5 mg per minute. *Compazine* Injection may be administered either undiluted or diluted in isotonic solution. A single dose of the drug should not exceed 10 mg; total I.V. dosage should not exceed 40 mg per day. When administered I.V., do not use bolus injection. Hypotension is a possibility if the drug is given by I.V. injection or infusion.

Subcutaneous administration is not advisable because of local irritation.

2. Adult Surgery (for severe nausea and vomiting): Total parenteral dosage should not exceed 40 mg per day. Hypotension is a possibility if the drug is given by I.V. injection or infusion.

I.M. Dosage: 5 to 10 mg (1 to 2 mL) 1 to 2 hours before induction of anesthesia (repeat once in 30 minutes, if necessary), or to control acute symptoms during and after surgery (repeat once if necessary).

I.V. Dosage: 5 to 10 mg (1 to 2 mL) as a slow I.V. injection or infusion 15 to 30 minutes before induction of anesthesia, or to control acute symptoms during or after surgery. Repeat once if necessary. Compazine (prochlorperazine) may be administered either undiluted or diluted in isotonic solution, but a single dose of the drug should not exceed 10 mg. The rate of administration should not exceed 5 mg per minute. When administered I.V., do not use bolus injection.

3. In Adult Psychiatric Disorders: Adjust dosage to the response of the individual and according to the severity of the condition. Begin with the lowest recommended dose. Although response ordinarily is seen within a day or 2, longer treatment is usually required before maximal improvement is seen.

Oral Dosage: *Non-Psychotic Anxiety*—Usual dosage is 5 mg 3 or 4 times daily; by *Spansule* capsule, usually one 15 mg capsule on arising or one 10 mg capsule q12h. Do not administer in doses of more than 20 mg per day or for longer than 12 weeks.

Psychotic Disorders—*In relatively mild conditions,* as seen in private psychiatric practice or in outpatient clinics, dosage is 5 or 10 mg 3 or 4 times daily.

In moderate to severe conditions, for hospitalized or adequately supervised patients, usual starting dosage is 10 mg 3 or 4 times daily. Increase dosage gradually until symptoms are controlled or side effects become bothersome. When dosage is increased by small increments every 2 or 3 days, side effects either do not occur or are easily controlled. Some patients respond satisfactorily on 50 to 75 mg daily.

In more severe disturbances, optimum dosage is usually 100 to 150 mg daily.

I.M. Dosage: For immediate control of severely disturbed adults, inject an initial dose of 10 to 20 mg (2 to 4 mL) *deeply* into the upper outer quadrant of the buttock. Many patients respond shortly after the first injection. If necessary, however, repeat the initial dose every 2 to 4 hours (or, in resistant cases, every hour) to gain control of the patient. More than three or four doses are seldom necessary. After control is achieved, switch patient to an oral form of the drug at the same dosage level or higher. If, in rare cases, parenteral therapy is needed for a prolonged period, give 10 to 20 mg (2 to 4 mL) every 4 to 6 hours. Pain and irritation at the site of injection have seldom occurred.

Subcutaneous administration is not advisable because of local irritation.

DOSAGE AND ADMINISTRATION—CHILDREN

Do not use in pediatric surgery.

Children seem more prone to develop extrapyramidal reactions, even on moderate doses. Therefore, use lowest effective dosage. Tell parents not to exceed prescribed dosage, since the possibility of adverse reactions increases as dosage rises. Occasionally the patient may react to the drug with signs of restlessness and excitement; if this occurs, do not administer additional doses. Take particular precaution in administering the drug to children with acute illnesses or dehydration (see under Dystonias).

When writing a prescription for the $2^1/_2$ mg size suppository, write "$2^1/_2$," not "2.5"; this will help avoid confusion with the 25 mg adult size.

1. Severe Nausea and Vomiting in Children: Compazine (prochlorperazine) should not be used in children under 20 pounds in weight or 2 years of age. It should not be used in conditions for which children's dosages have not been established. Dosage and frequency of administration should be adjusted according to the severity of the symptoms and the response of the patient. The duration of activity following intramuscular administration may last up to 12 hours. Subsequent doses may be given by the same route if necessary.

Oral or Rectal Dosage: More than 1 day's therapy is seldom necessary.

Weight	Usual Dosage	Not to Exceed
under 20 lbs not recommended		
20 to 29 lbs	$2^1/_2$ mg 1 or 2 times a day	7.5 mg per day
30 to 39 lbs	$2^1/_2$ mg 2 or 3 times a day	10 mg per day
40 to 85 lbs	$2^1/_2$ mg 3 times a day or 5 mg 2 times a day	15 mg per day

I.M. Dosage: Calculate each dose on the basis of 0.06 mg of the drug per lb of body weight; give by deep I.M. injection. Control is usually obtained with one dose.

2. In Psychotic Children:

Oral or Rectal Dosage: For children 2 to 12 years, starting dosage is $2^1/_2$ mg 2 or 3 times daily. Do not give more than 10 mg the first day. Then increase dosage according to patient's response.

FOR AGES 2 to 5, total daily dosage usually does not exceed 20 mg.

FOR AGES 6 to 12, total daily dosage usually does not exceed 25 mg.

I.M. Dosage: For ages under 12, calculate each dose on the basis of 0.06 mg of Compazine (prochlorperazine) per lb of body weight; give by deep I.M. injection. Control is usually obtained with one dose. After control is achieved, switch the patient to an oral form of the drug at the same dosage level or higher.

OVERDOSAGE

(See also Adverse Reactions.)

SYMPTOMS—Primarily involvement of the extrapyramidal mechanism producing some of the dystonic reactions described above.

Symptoms of central nervous system depression to the point of somnolence or coma. Agitation and restlessness may also occur. Other possible manifestations include convulsions, EKG changes and cardiac arrhythmias, fever and autonomic reactions such as hypotension, dry mouth and ileus.

TREATMENT—It is important to determine other medications taken by the patient since multiple-dose therapy is common in overdosage situations. Treatment is essentially symptomatic and supportive. Early gastric lavage is helpful. Keep patient under observation and maintain an open airway, since involvement of the extrapyramidal mechanism may produce dysphagia and respiratory difficulty in severe overdosage. **Do not attempt to induce emesis because a dystonic reaction of the head or neck may develop that could result in aspiration of vomitus.** Extrapyramidal symptoms may be treated with anti-parkinsonism drugs, barbiturates or *Benadryl*. See prescribing information for these products. Care should be taken to avoid increasing respiratory depression.

If administration of a stimulant is desirable, amphetamine, dextroamphetamine or caffeine with sodium benzoate is recommended.

Stimulants that may cause convulsions (e.g., picrotoxin or pentylenetetrazol) should be avoided.

If hypotension occurs, the standard measures for managing circulatory shock should be initiated. If it is desirable to administer a vasoconstrictor, *Levophed* and *Neo-Synephrine* are most suitable. Other pressor agents, including epinephrine, are not recommended because phenothiazine derivatives may reverse the usual elevating action of these agents and cause a further lowering of blood pressure.

Limited experience indicates that phenothiazines are *not* dialyzable.

Special note on Spansule *capsules*—Since much of the *Spansule* capsule medication is coated for gradual release, therapy directed at reversing the effects of the ingested drug and at supporting the patient should be continued for as long as overdosage symptoms remain. Saline cathartics are useful for hastening evacuation of pellets that have not already released medication.

HOW SUPPLIED

Tablets—5 and 10 mg, in bottles of 100; in Single Unit Packages of 100 (intended for institutional use only).
5 mg 100's: NDC 0007-3366-20
5 mg SUP 100's: NDC 0007-3366-21
10 mg 100's: NDC 0007-3367-20
10 mg SUP 100's: NDC 0007-3367-21

***Spansule* capsules**—10 and 15 mg, in bottles of 50.
10 mg 50's: NDC 0007-3344-15
15 mg 50's: NDC 0007-3346-15

Vials—2 mL (5 mg/mL), in boxes of 25 and 10 mL (5 mg/mL), in boxes of 1.
2 mL (5 mg/mL), in boxes of 25: NDC 0007-3352-16
10 mL (5 mg/mL), in boxes of 1: NDC 0007-3343-01

Disposable Syringes—2 mL (5 mg/mL), in individual cartons.
2 mL (5 mg/mL), in boxes of 1: NDC 0007-3351-01

Suppositories—$2^1/_2$ mg (for young children), 5 mg (for older children) and 25 mg (for adults), in boxes of 12.
$2^1/_2$ mg, in boxes of 12: NDC 0007-3360-03
5 mg, in boxes of 12: NDC 0007-3361-03
25 mg, in boxes of 12: NDC 0007-3362-03

Syrup—5 mg/5 mL (1 teaspoonful) in 4 fl oz bottles.
5 mg/5 mL, 4 fl oz: NDC 0007-3363-44

Store Compazine (prochlorperazine) vials and syringes below 86°F. Do not freeze.

Veterans Administration/Military/PHS—Vials, 2 mL, 25's, 6505-01-230-3931; 10 mL, 1's, 6505-00-684-9630; Suppositories, $2^1/_2$ mg, 12's, 6505-00-133-5213; 5 mg, 12's, 6505-01-153-2894; 25 mg, 12's, 6505-00-133-5214; Syrup, 5 mg/5 mL, 4 fl oz, 6505-01-039-5849; Tablets, 5 mg, 100's, 6505-00-761-5640;

5 mg, 100's (SUP), 6505-00-118-2563; 10 mg, 100's, 6505-01-354-1042; 10 mg, 100's (SUP), 6505-00-092-3139.

* norepinephrine bitartrate, Sanofi Winthrop Pharmaceuticals.
† phenylephrine hydrochloride, Sanofi Winthrop Pharmaceuticals.
‡ phenytoin, Parke-Davis.
§ metrizamide, Sanofi Winthrop Pharmaceuticals.
" diphenhydramine hydrochloride, Parke-Davis.
CZ:L85

Shown in Product Identification Guide, page 336

CYTOMEL®   ℞

[sigh "toe'mel]
**brand of liothyronine sodium
tablets**

DESCRIPTION

Thyroid hormone drugs are natural or synthetic preparations containing tetraiodothyronine (T_4, levothyroxine) sodium or triiodothyronine (T_3, liothyronine) sodium or both. T_4 and T_3 are produced in the human thyroid gland by the iodination and coupling of the amino acid tyrosine. T_4 contains four iodine atoms and is formed by the coupling of two molecules of diiodotyrosine (DIT). T_3 contains three atoms of iodine and is formed by the coupling of one molecule of DIT with one molecule of monoiodotyrosine (MIT). Both hormones are stored in the thyroid colloid as thyroglobulin.

Thyroid hormone preparations belong to two categories: (1) natural hormonal preparations derived from animal thyroid, and (2) synthetic preparations. Natural preparations include desiccated thyroid and thyroglobulin. Desiccated thyroid is derived from domesticated animals that are used for food by man (either beef or hog thyroid), and thyroglobulin is derived from thyroid glands of the hog. The United States Pharmacopeia (USP) has standardized the total iodine content of natural preparations. Thyroid USP contains not less than (NLT) 0.17 percent and not more than (NMT) 0.23 percent iodine, and thyroglobulin contains not less than (NLT) 0.7 percent of organically bound iodine. Iodine content is only an indirect indicator of true hormonal biologic activity.

Cytomel (liothyronine sodium) Tablets contain liothyronine (L-triiodothyronine or LT_3), a synthetic form of a natural thyroid hormone, and is available as the sodium salt.

Twenty-five mcg of liothyronine is equivalent to approximately 1 grain of desiccated thyroid or thyroglobulin and 0.1 mg of L-thyroxine.

Each round, white to off-white Cytomel (liothyronine sodium) tablet contains liothyronine sodium equivalent to liothyronine as follows: 5 mcg debossed SKF and D14; 25 mcg scored and debossed SKF and D16; 50 mcg scored and debossed SKF and D17. Inactive ingredients consist of calcium sulfate, gelatin, starch, stearic acid, sucrose and talc.

CLINICAL PHARMACOLOGY

The mechanisms by which thyroid hormones exert their physiologic action are not well understood. These hormones enhance oxygen consumption by most tissues of the body, increase the basal metabolic rate and the metabolism of carbohydrates, lipids and proteins. Thus, they exert a profound influence on every organ system in the body and are of particular importance in the development of the central nervous system.

Pharmacokinetics

Since liothyronine sodium (T_3) is not firmly bound to serum protein, it is readily available to body tissues. The onset of activity of liothyronine sodium is rapid, occurring within a few hours. Maximum pharmacologic response occurs within 2 or 3 days, providing early clinical response. The biological half-life is about $2\text{-}1/2$ days.

T_3 is almost totally absorbed, 95 percent in 4 hours. The hormones contained in the natural preparations are absorbed in a manner similar to the synthetic hormones.

Liothyronine sodium has a rapid cutoff of activity which permits quick dosage adjustment and facilitates control of the effects of overdosage, should they occur.

The higher affinity of levothyroxine (T_4) for both thyroid-binding globulin and thyroid-binding prealbumin as compared to triiodothyronine (T_3) partially explains the higher serum levels and longer half-life of the former hormone. Both protein-bound hormones exist in reverse equilibrium with minute amounts of free hormone, the latter accounting for the metabolic activity.

INDICATIONS AND USAGE

Thyroid hormone drugs are indicated:
1. As replacement or supplemental therapy in patients with hypothyroidism of any etiology, except transient hypothyroidism during the recovery phase of subacute thyroiditis. This category includes cretinism, myxedema and ordinary hypothyroidism in patients of any age (pediatric patients, adults, the elderly), or state (including pregnancy); primary hypothyroidism resulting from functional deficiency, primary atrophy, partial or total absence of thyroid gland, or the effects of surgery, radiation, or drugs, with or without the presence of goiter; and secondary (pituitary) or tertiary (hypothalamic) hypothyroidism (See WARNINGS).
2. As pituitary thyroid-stimulating hormone (TSH) suppressants, in the treatment or prevention of various types of euthyroid goiters, including thyroid nodules, subacute or chronic lymphocytic thyroiditis (Hashimoto's) and multinodular goiter.
3. As diagnostic agents in suppression tests to differentiate suspected mild hyperthyroidism or thyroid gland autonomy.

Cytomel (liothyronine sodium) Tablets can be used in patients allergic to desiccated thyroid or thyroid extract derived from pork or beef.

CONTRAINDICATIONS

Thyroid hormone preparations are generally contraindicated in patients with diagnosed but as yet uncorrected adrenal cortical insufficiency, untreated thyrotoxicosis and apparent hypersensitivity to any of their active or extraneous constituents. There is no well-documented evidence from the literature, however, of true allergic or idiosyncratic reactions to thyroid hormone.

WARNINGS

> Drugs with thyroid hormone activity, alone or together with other therapeutic agents, have been used for the treatment of obesity. In euthyroid patients, doses within the range of daily hormonal requirements are ineffective for weight reduction. Larger doses may produce serious or even life-threatening manifestations of toxicity, particularly when given in association with sympathomimetic amines such as those used for their anorectic effects.

The use of thyroid hormones in the therapy of obesity, alone or combined with other drugs, is unjustified and has been shown to be ineffective. Neither is their use justified for the treatment of male or female infertility unless this condition is accompanied by hypothyroidism.

Thyroid hormones should be used with great caution in a number of circumstances where the integrity of the cardiovascular system, particularly the coronary arteries, is suspected. These include patients with angina pectoris or the elderly, in whom there is a greater likelihood of occult cardiac disease. In these patients, liothyronine sodium therapy should be initiated with low doses, with due consideration for its relatively rapid onset of action. Starting dosage of Cytomel (liothyronine sodium) Tablets is 5 mcg daily, and should be increased by no more than 5 mcg increments at 2-week intervals. When, in such patients, a euthyroid state can only be reached at the expense of an aggravation of the cardiovascular disease, thyroid hormone dosage should be reduced.

Morphologic hypogonadism and nephrosis should be ruled out before the drug is administered. If hypopituitarism is present, the adrenal deficiency must be corrected prior to starting the drug.

Myxedematous patients are very sensitive to thyroid; dosage should be started at a very low level and increased gradually. Severe and prolonged hypothyroidism can lead to a decreased level of adrenocortical activity commensurate with the lowered metabolic state. When thyroid-replacement therapy is administered, the metabolism increases at a greater rate than adrenocortical activity. This can precipitate adrenocortical insufficiency. Therefore, in severe and prolonged hypothyroidism, supplemental adrenocortical steroids may be necessary.

In rare instances the administration of thyroid hormone may precipitate a hyperthyroid state or may aggravate existing hyperthyroidism.

PRECAUTIONS

General—Thyroid hormone therapy in patients with concomitant diabetes mellitus or insipidus or adrenal cortical insufficiency aggravates the intensity of their symptoms. Appropriate adjustments of the various therapeutic measures directed at these concomitant endocrine diseases are required.

The therapy of myxedema coma requires simultaneous administration of glucocorticoids.

Hypothyroidism decreases and hyperthyroidism increases the sensitivity to oral anticoagulants. Prothrombin time should be closely monitored in thyroid-treated patients on oral anticoagulants and dosage of the latter agents adjusted on the basis of frequent prothrombin time determinations. In infants, excessive doses of thyroid hormone preparations may produce craniosynostosis.

Information for the Patient—Patients on thyroid hormone preparations and parents of pediatric patients on thyroid therapy should be informed that:

1. Replacement therapy is to be taken essentially for life, with the exception of cases of transient hypothyroidism, usually associated with thyroiditis, and in those patients receiving a therapeutic trial of the drug.
2. They should immediately report during the course of therapy any signs or symptoms of thyroid hormone toxicity, e.g., chest pain, increased pulse rate, palpitations, excessive sweating, heat intolerance, nervousness, or any other unusual event.
3. In case of concomitant diabetes mellitus, the daily dosage of antidiabetic medication may need readjustment as thyroid hormone replacement is achieved. If thyroid medication is stopped, a downward readjustment of the dosage of insulin or oral hypoglycemic agent may be necessary to avoid hypoglycemia. At all times, close monitoring of urinary glucose levels is mandatory in such patients.
4. In case of concomitant oral anticoagulant therapy, the prothrombin time should be measured frequently to determine if the dosage of oral anticoagulants is to be readjusted.
5. Partial loss of hair may be experienced by pediatric patients in the first few months of thyroid therapy, but this is usually a transient phenomenon and later recovery is usually the rule.

Laboratory Tests—Treatment of patients with thyroid hormones requires the periodic assessment of thyroid status by means of appropriate laboratory tests besides the full clinical evaluation. The TSH suppression test can be used to test the effectiveness of any thyroid preparation, bearing in mind the relative insensitivity of the infant pituitary to the negative feedback effect of thyroid hormones. Serum T_4 levels can be used to test the effectiveness of all thyroid medications except products containing liothyronine sodium. When the total serum T_4 is low but TSH is normal, a test specific to assess unbound (free) T_4 levels is warranted. Specific measurements of T_4 and T_3 by competitive protein binding or radioimmunoassay are not influenced by blood levels of organic or inorganic iodine and have essentially replaced older tests of thyroid hormone measurements, i.e., PBI, BEI and T_4 by column.

Drug Interactions

Oral Anticoagulants—Thyroid hormones appear to increase catabolism of vitamin K-dependent clotting factors. If oral anticoagulants are also being given, compensatory increases in clotting factor synthesis are impaired. Patients stabilized on oral anticoagulants who are found to require thyroid replacement therapy should be watched very closely when thyroid is started. If a patient is truly hypothyroid, it is likely that a reduction in anticoagulant dosage will be required. No special precautions appear to be necessary when oral anticoagulant therapy is begun in a patient already stabilized on maintenance thyroid replacement therapy.

Insulin or Oral Hypoglycemics—Initiating thyroid replacement therapy may cause increases in insulin or oral hypoglycemic requirements. The effects seen are poorly understood and depend upon a variety of factors such as dose and type of thyroid preparations and endocrine status of the patient. Patients receiving insulin or oral hypoglycemics should be closely watched during initiation of thyroid replacement therapy.

Cholestyramine—Cholestyramine binds both T_4 and T_3 in the intestine, thus impairing absorption of these thyroid hormones. *In vitro* studies indicate that the binding is not easily removed. Therefore, 4 to 5 hours should elapse between administration of cholestyramine and thyroid hormones.

Estrogen, Oral Contraceptives—Estrogens tend to increase serum thyroxine-binding globulin (TBg). In a patient with a nonfunctioning thyroid gland who is receiving thyroid replacement therapy, free levothyroxine may be decreased when estrogens are started thus increasing thyroid requirements. However, if the patient's thyroid gland has sufficient function, the decreased free thyroxine will result in a compensatory increase in thyroxine output by the thyroid. Therefore, patients without a functioning thyroid gland who are on thyroid replacement therapy may need to increase their thyroid dose if estrogens or estrogen-containing oral contraceptives are given.

Tricyclic Antidepressants—Use of thyroid products with imipramine and other tricyclic antidepressants may increase receptor sensitivity and enhance antidepressant activity; transient cardiac arrhythmias have been observed. Thyroid hormone activity may also be enhanced.

Digitalis—Thyroid preparations may potentiate the toxic effects of digitalis. Thyroid hormonal replacement increases

Continued on next page

Information on the SmithKline Beecham Pharmaceuticals products appearing here is based on the labeling in effect on July 1, 1996. Further information on these and other products may be obtained from the Medical Department, SmithKline Beecham Pharmaceuticals, One Franklin Plaza, Philadelphia, PA 19101.

SmithKline Beecham—Cont.

metabolic rate, which requires an increase in digitalis dosage.

Ketamine—When administered to patients on a thyroid preparation, this parenteral anesthetic may cause hypertension and tachycardia. Use with caution and be prepared to treat hypertension, if necessary.

Vasopressors—Thyroxine increases the adrenergic effect of catecholamines such as epinephrine and norepinephrine. Therefore, injection of these agents into patients receiving thyroid preparations increases the risk of precipitating coronary insufficiency, especially in patients with coronary artery disease. Careful observation is required.

Drug/Laboratory Test Interactions—The following drugs or moieties are known to interfere with laboratory tests performed in patients on thyroid hormone therapy: androgens, corticosteroids, estrogens, oral contraceptives containing estrogens, iodine-containing preparations and the numerous preparations containing salicylates.

1. Changes in TBg concentration should be taken into consideration in the interpretation of T_4 and T_3 values. In such cases, the unbound (free) hormone should be measured. Pregnancy, estrogens and estrogen-containing oral contraceptives increase TBg concentrations. TBg may also be increased during infectious hepatitis. Decreases in TBg concentrations are observed in nephrosis, acromegaly and after androgen or corticosteroid therapy. Familial hyper- or hypo-thyroxine-binding-globulinemias have been described. The incidence of TBg deficiency approximates 1 in 9000. The binding of thyroxine by thyroxine-binding prealbumin (TBPA) is inhibited by salicylates.
2. Medicinal or dietary iodine interferes with all *in vivo* tests of radioiodine uptake, producing low uptakes which may not be reflective of a true decrease in hormone synthesis.
3. The persistence of clinical and laboratory evidence of hypothyroidism in spite of adequate dosage replacement indicates either poor patient compliance, poor absorption, excessive fecal loss, or inactivity of the preparation. Intracellular resistance to thyroid hormone is quite rare.

Carcinogenesis, Mutagenesis and Impairment of Fertility—A reportedly apparent association between prolonged thyroid therapy and breast cancer has not been confirmed and patients on thyroid for established indications should not discontinue therapy. No confirmatory long-term studies in animals have been performed to evaluate carcinogenic potential, mutagenicity, or impairment of fertility in either males or females.

Pregnancy—Category A. Thyroid hormones do not readily cross the placental barrier. The clinical experience to date does not indicate any adverse effect on fetuses when thyroid hormones are administered to pregnant women. On the basis of current knowledge, thyroid replacement therapy to hypothyroid women should not be discontinued during pregnancy.

Nursing Mothers—Minimal amounts of thyroid hormones are excreted in human milk. Thyroid is not associated with serious adverse reactions and does not have a known tumorigenic potential. However, caution should be exercised when thyroid is administered to a nursing woman.

Pediatric Use—Pregnant mothers provide little or no thyroid hormone to the fetus. The incidence of congenital hypothyroidism is relatively high (1:4000) and the hypothyroid fetus would not derive any benefit from the small amounts of hormone crossing the placental barrier. Routine determinations of serum T_4 and/or TSH is strongly advised in neonates in view of the deleterious effects of thyroid deficiency on growth and development.

Treatment should be initiated immediately upon diagnosis and maintained for life, unless transient hypothyroidism is suspected, in which case, therapy may be interrupted for 2 to 8 weeks after the age of 3 years to reassess the condition. Cessation of therapy is justified in patients who have maintained a normal TSH during those 2 to 8 weeks.

ADVERSE REACTIONS

Adverse reactions, other than those indicative of hyperthyroidism because of therapeutic overdosage, either initially or during the maintenance period are rare (See OVERDOSAGE).

In rare instances, allergic skin reactions have been reported with Cytomel (liothyronine sodium) Tablets.

OVERDOSAGE

Signs and Symptoms—Headache, irritability, nervousness, sweating, arrhythmia (including tachycardia), increased bowel motility and menstrual irregularities. Angina pectoris or congestive heart failure may be induced or aggravated. Shock may also develop. Massive overdosage may result in symptoms resembling thyroid storm. Chronic excessive dosage will produce the signs and symptoms of hyperthyroidism.

Treatment of Overdosage—Dosage should be reduced or therapy temporarily discontinued if signs and symptoms of overdosage appear. Treatment may be reinstituted at a

lower dosage. In normal individuals, normal hypothalamic-pituitary-thyroid axis function is restored in 6 to 8 weeks after thyroid suppression.

Treatment of acute massive thyroid hormone overdosage is aimed at reducing gastrointestinal absorption of the drugs and counteracting central and peripheral effects, mainly those of increased sympathetic activity. Vomiting may be induced initially if further gastrointestinal absorption can reasonably be prevented and barring contraindications such as coma, convulsions, or loss of the gagging reflex. Treatment is symptomatic and supportive. Oxygen may be administered and ventilation maintained. Cardiac glycosides may be indicated if congestive heart failure develops. Measures to control fever, hypoglycemia, or fluid loss should be instituted if needed. Antiadrenergic agents, particularly propranolol, have been used advantageously in the treatment of increased sympathetic activity. Propranolol may be administered intravenously at a dosage of 1 to 3 mg over a 10-minute period or orally, 80 to 160 mg/day, especially when no contraindications exist for its use.

DOSAGE AND ADMINISTRATION

The dosage of thyroid hormones is determined by the indication and must in every case be individualized according to patient response and laboratory findings.

Cytomel (liothyronine sodium) Tablets are intended for oral administration; once-a-day dosage is recommended. Although liothyronine sodium has a rapid cutoff, its metabolic effects persist for a few days following discontinuance.

Mild Hypothyroidism: Recommended starting dosage is 25 mcg daily. Daily dosage then may be increased by up to 25 mcg every 1 or 2 weeks. Usual maintenance dose is 25 to 75 mcg daily.

The rapid onset and dissipation of action of liothyronine sodium (T_3), as compared with levothyroxine sodium (T_4), has led some clinicians to prefer its use in patients who might be more susceptible to the untoward effects of thyroid medication. However, the wide swings in serum T_3 levels that follow its administration and the possibility of more pronounced cardiovascular side effects tend to counterbalance the stated advantages.

Cytomel (liothyronine sodium) Tablets may be used in preference to levothyroxine (T_4) during radioisotope scanning procedures, since induction of hypothyroidism in those cases is more abrupt and can be of short duration. It may also be preferred when impairment of peripheral conversion of T_4 to T_3 is suspected.

Myxedema: Recommended starting dosage is 5 mcg daily. This may be increased by 5 to 10 mcg every 1 or 2 weeks. When 25 mcg daily is reached, dosage may be increased by 5 to 25 mcg every 1 or 2 weeks until a satisfactory therapeutic response is attained. Usual maintenance dose is 50 to 100 mcg daily.

Myxedema Coma: Myxedema coma is usually precipitated in the hypothyroid patient of long standing by intercurrent illness or drugs such as sedatives and anesthetics and should be considered a medical emergency.

An intravenous preparation of liothyronine sodium is marketed by SmithKline Beecham Pharmaceuticals under the trade name Triostat™ for use in myxedema coma/precoma.

Congenital Hypothyroidism: Recommended starting dosage is 5 mcg daily, with a 5 mcg increment every 3 to 4 days until the desired response is achieved. Infants a few months old may require only 20 mcg daily for maintenance. At 1 year, 50 mcg daily may be required. Above 3 years, full adult dosage may be necessary (see PRECAUTIONS, Pediatric Use).

Simple (non-toxic) Goiter: Recommended starting dosage is 5 mcg daily. This dosage may be increased by 5 to 10 mcg daily every 1 or 2 weeks. When 25 mcg daily is reached, dosage may be increased every week or two by 12.5 or 25 mcg. Usual maintenance dosage is 75 mcg daily.

In the elderly or in pediatric patients, therapy should be started with 5 mcg daily and increased only by 5 mcg increments at the recommended intervals.

When switching a patient to Cytomel (liothyronine sodium) Tablets from thyroid, L-thyroxine or thyroglobulin, discontinue the other medication, initiate *Cytomel* at a low dosage, and increase gradually according to the patient's response. When selecting a starting dosage, bear in mind that this drug has a rapid onset of action, and that residual effects of the other thyroid preparation may persist for the first several weeks of therapy.

Thyroid Suppression Therapy: Administration of thyroid hormone in doses higher than those produced physiologically by the gland results in suppression of the production of endogenous hormone. This is the basis for the thyroid suppression test and is used as an aid in the diagnosis of patients with signs of mild hyperthyroidism in whom baseline laboratory tests appear normal or to demonstrate thyroid gland autonomy in patients with Graves' ophthalmopathy. ^{131}I uptake is determined before and after the administration of the exogenous hormone. A 50% or greater suppression of uptake indicates a normal thyroid-pituitary axis and thus rules out thyroid gland autonomy.

Cytomel (liothyronine sodium) Tablets are given in doses of 75 to 100 mcg/day for 7 days, and radioactive iodine uptake is determined before and after administration of the hormone. If thyroid function is under normal control, the radioiodine uptake will drop significantly after treatment. Cytomel (liothyronine sodium) Tablets should be administered cautiously to patients in whom there is a strong suspicion of thyroid gland autonomy, in view of the fact that the exogenous hormone effects will be additive to the endogenous source.

HOW SUPPLIED

Cytomel (liothyronine sodium) Tablets: 5 mcg in bottles of 100; 25 mcg in bottles of 100; and 50 mcg in bottles of 100.
5 mcg 100's: NDC 0007-3414-20
25 mcg 100's: NDC 0007-3416-20
50 mcg 100's: NDC 0007-3417-20
Store between 15° and 30°C (59° and 86°F).
Manufactured by
Schering Canada, Inc.
3535 Trans-Canada Highway
Pointe Claire, Quebec HqR 1B4 Canada for
SmithKline Beecham Pharmaceuticals
Philadelphia, Pa 19101
Veterans Administration/Military/PHS—
Tablets, 5 mcg, 100's, 6505-00-660-1609;
25 mcg, 100's, 6505-01-231-5697.
CY:L37

Shown in Product Identification Guide, page 336

DEXEDRINE®   Ⓒ

[dex 'eh-dreen]
(brand of dextroamphetamine sulfate)
SPANSULE® CAPSULES
brand of sustained release capsules
and TABLETS

WARNING

> AMPHETAMINES HAVE A HIGH POTENTIAL FOR ABUSE. THEY SHOULD THUS BE TRIED ONLY IN WEIGHT REDUCTION PROGRAMS FOR PATIENTS IN WHOM ALTERNATIVE THERAPY HAS BEEN INEFFECTIVE. ADMINISTRATION OF AMPHETAMINES FOR PROLONGED PERIODS OF TIME IN OBESITY MAY LEAD TO DRUG DEPENDENCE AND MUST BE AVOIDED. PARTICULAR ATTENTION SHOULD BE PAID TO THE POSSIBILITY OF SUBJECTS OBTAINING AMPHETAMINES FOR NON-THERAPEUTIC USE OR DISTRIBUTION TO OTHERS, AND THE DRUGS SHOULD BE PRESCRIBED OR DISPENSED SPARINGLY.

DESCRIPTION

Dexedrine (dextroamphetamine sulfate) is the dextro isomer of the compound d,l-amphetamine sulfate, a sympathomimetic amine of the amphetamine group. Chemically, dextroamphetamine is d-alpha-methylphenethylamine, and is present in all forms of *Dexedrine* as the neutral sulfate.

Spansule® capsules
Each *Spansule* sustained release capsule is so prepared that an initial dose is released promptly and the remaining medication is released gradually over a prolonged period.

Each capsule, with brown cap and clear body, contains dextroamphetamine sulfate. The 5 mg capsule is imprinted 5 mg and 3512 on the brown cap and is imprinted 5 mg and SB on the clear body. The 10 mg capsule is imprinted 10 mg and 3513 on the brown cap and is imprinted 10 mg and SB on the clear body. The 15 mg capsule is imprinted 15 mg and 3514 on the brown cap and is imprinted 15 mg and SB on the clear body. Inactive ingredients consist of acacia, benzyl alcohol, calcium sulfate, cetylpyridinium chloride, FD&C Blue No. 1, FD&C Red No. 40, FD&C Yellow No. 5 (tartrazine), FD&C Yellow No. 6, gelatin, glyceryl distearate, glyceryl monostearate, sodium lauryl sulfate, starch, sucrose, wax and trace amounts of other inactive ingredients.

Tablets
Each triangular, orange, scored tablet is debossed SKF and E19 and contains dextroamphetamine sulfate, 5 mg. Inactive ingredients consist of calcium sulfate, FD&C Yellow No. 5 (tartrazine), FD&C Yellow No. 6, gelatin, lactose, mineral oil, starch, stearic acid, sucrose, talc and trace amounts of other inactive ingredients.

CLINICAL PHARMACOLOGY

Amphetamines are non-catecholamine, sympathomimetic amines with CNS stimulant activity. Peripheral actions include elevations of systolic and diastolic blood pressures and weak bronchodilator and respiratory stimulant action. There is neither specific evidence which clearly establishes the mechanism whereby amphetamines produce mental and behavioral effects in children, nor conclusive evidence re-

garding how these effects relate to the condition of the central nervous system.

Drugs of this class used in obesity are commonly known as "anorectics" or "anorexigenics." It has not been established, however, that the action of such drugs in treating obesity is primarily one of appetite suppression. Other central nervous system actions, or metabolic effects, may be involved, for example.

Adult obese subjects instructed in dietary management and treated with "anorectic" drugs lose more weight on the average than those treated with placebo and diet, as determined in relatively short-term clinical trials.

The magnitude of increased weight loss of drug-treated patients over placebo-treated patients is only a fraction of a pound a week. The rate of weight loss is greatest in the first weeks of therapy for both drug and placebo subjects and tends to decrease in succeeding weeks. The origins of the increased weight loss due to the various possible drug effects are not established. The amount of weight loss associated with the use of an "anorectic" drug varies from trial to trial, and the increased weight loss appears to be related in part to variables other than the drug prescribed, such as the physician-investigator, the population treated and the diet prescribed. Studies do not permit conclusions as to the relative importance of the drug and nondrug factors on weight loss. The natural history of obesity is measured in years, whereas the studies cited are restricted to a few weeks' duration; thus, the total impact of drug-induced weight loss over that of diet alone must be considered clinically limited.

Dexedrine (dextroamphetamine sulfate) *Spansule* capsules are formulated to release the active drug substance *in vivo* in a more gradual fashion than the standard formulation, as demonstrated by blood levels. The formulation has not been shown superior in effectiveness over the same dosage of the standard, noncontrolled-release formulations given in divided doses.

Pharmacokinetics

Tablet—The single ingestion of two 5 mg tablets by healthy volunteers produced an average peak dextroamphetamine blood level of 29.2 ng/mL at 2 hours post-administration. The average half-life was 10.25 hours. The average urinary recovery was 45% in 48 hours.

Spansule capsule—Ingestion of a *Spansule* capsule containing 15 mg radiolabeled dextroamphetamine sulfate by healthy volunteers produced a peak blood level of radioactivity, on the average, at 8 to 10 hours post-administration with peak urinary recovery seen at 12 to 24 hours.

INDICATIONS AND USAGE

Dexedrine (dextroamphetamine sulfate) is indicated:

1. **In Narcolepsy.**
2. **In Attention Deficit Disorder with Hyperactivity,** as an integral part of a total treatment program which typically includes other remedial measures (psychological, educational, social) for a stabilizing effect in pediatric patients (ages 3 years to 16 years) with a behavioral syndrome characterized by the following group of developmentally inappropriate symptoms: moderate to severe distractibility, short attention span, hyperactivity, emotional lability, and impulsivity. The diagnosis of this syndrome should not be made with finality when these symptoms are only of comparatively recent origin. Nonlocalizing (soft) neurological signs, learning disability, and abnormal EEG may or may not be present, and a diagnosis of central nervous system dysfunction may or may not be warranted.

CONTRAINDICATIONS

Advanced arteriosclerosis, symptomatic cardiovascular disease, moderate to severe hypertension, hyperthyroidism, known hypersensitivity or idiosyncrasy to the sympathomimetic amines, glaucoma.

Agitated states.

Patients with a history of drug abuse.

During or within 14 days following the administration of monoamine oxidase inhibitors (hypertensive crises may result).

WARNING

When tolerance to the "anorectic" effect develops, the recommended dose should not be exceeded in an attempt to increase the effect; rather, the drug should be discontinued.

PRECAUTIONS

General: Caution is to be exercised in prescribing amphetamines for patients with even mild hypertension.

The least amount feasible should be prescribed or dispensed at one time in order to minimize the possibility of overdosage.

These products contain FD&C Yellow No. 5 (tartrazine), which may cause allergic-type reactions (including bronchial asthma) in certain susceptible individuals. Although the overall incidence of FD&C Yellow No. 5 (tartrazine) sensitivity in the general population is low, it is frequently seen in patients who also have aspirin hypersensitivity.

Information for Patients: Amphetamines may impair the ability of the patient to engage in potentially hazardous activities such as operating machinery or vehicles; the patient should therefore be cautioned accordingly.

Drug Interactions

Acidifying agents—Gastrointestinal acidifying agents (guanethidine, reserpine, glutamic acid HCl, ascorbic acid, fruit juices, etc.) lower absorption of amphetamines. Urinary acidifying agents (ammonium chloride, sodium acid phosphate, etc.) increase the concentration of the ionized species of the amphetamine molecule, thereby increasing urinary excretion. Both groups of agents lower blood levels and efficacy of amphetamines.

Adrenergic blockers—Adrenergic blockers are inhibited by amphetamines.

Alkalinizing agents—Gastrointestinal alkalinizing agents (sodium bicarbonate, etc.) increase absorption of amphetamines. Urinary alkalinizing agents (acetazolamide, some thiazides) increase the concentration of the non-ionized species of the amphetamine molecule, thereby decreasing urinary excretion. Both groups of agents increase blood levels and therefore potentiate the actions of amphetamines.

Antidepressants, tricyclic—Amphetamines may enhance the activity of tricyclic or sympathomimetic agents; d-amphetamine with desipramine or protriptyline and possibly other tricyclics cause striking and sustained increases in the concentration of d-amphetamine in the brain; cardiovascular effects can be potentiated.

MAO inhibitors—MAOI antidepressants, as well as a metabolite of furazolidone, slow amphetamine metabolism. This slowing potentiates amphetamines, increasing their effect on the release of norepinephrine and other monoamines from adrenergic nerve endings; this can cause headaches and other signs of hypertensive crisis. A variety of neurological toxic effects and malignant hyperpyrexia can occur, sometimes with fatal results.

Antihistamines—Amphetamines may counteract the sedative effect of antihistamines.

Antihypertensives—Amphetamines may antagonize the hypotensive effects of antihypertensives.

Chlorpromazine—Chlorpromazine blocks dopamine and norepinephrine reuptake, thus inhibiting the central stimulant effects of amphetamines, and can be used to treat amphetamine poisoning.

Ethosuximide—Amphetamines may delay intestinal absorption of ethosuximide.

Haloperidol—Haloperidol blocks dopamine and norepinephrine reuptake, thus inhibiting the central stimulant effects of amphetamines.

Lithium carbonate—The antiobesity and stimulatory effects of amphetamines may be inhibited by lithium carbonate.

Meperidine—Amphetamines potentiate the analgesic effect of meperidine.

Methenamine therapy—Urinary excretion of amphetamines is increased, and efficacy is reduced, by acidifying agents used in methenamine therapy.

Norepinephrine—Amphetamines enhance the adrenergic effect of norepinephrine.

Phenobarbital—Amphetamines may delay intestinal absorption of phenobarbital; co-administration of phenobarbital may produce a synergistic anticonvulsant action.

Phenytoin—Amphetamines may delay intestinal absorption of phenytoin; co-administration of phenytoin may produce a synergistic anticonvulsant action.

Propoxyphene—In cases of propoxyphene overdosage, amphetamine CNS stimulation is potentiated and fatal convulsions can occur.

Veratrum alkaloids—Amphetamines inhibit the hypotensive effect of veratrum alkaloids.

Drug/Laboratory Test Interactions

- Amphetamines can cause a significant elevation in plasma corticosteroid levels. This increase is greatest in the evening.
- Amphetamines may interfere with urinary steroid determinations.

Carcinogenesis/Mutagenesis: Mutagenicity studies and long-term studies in animals to determine the carcinogenic potential of Dexedrine (dextroamphetamine sulfate) have not been performed.

Pregnancy—Teratogenic Effects: Pregnancy Category C. *Dexedrine* has been shown to have embryotoxic and teratogenic effects when administered to A/Jax mice and C57BL mice in doses approximately 41 times the maximum human dose. Embryotoxic effects were not seen in New Zealand white rabbits given the drug in doses 7 times the human dose nor in rats given 12.5 times the maximum human dose. There are no adequate and well-controlled studies in pregnant women. *Dexedrine* should be used during pregnancy only if the potential benefit justifies the potential risk to the fetus.

Nonteratogenic Effects: Infants born to mothers dependent on amphetamines have an increased risk of premature delivery and low birth weight. Also, these infants may experience symptoms of withdrawal as demonstrated by dysphoria, including agitation, and significant lassitude.

Nursing Mothers: Amphetamines are excreted in human milk. Mothers taking amphetamines should be advised to refrain from nursing.

Pediatric Use: Long-term effects of amphetamines in pediatric patients have not been well established.

Amphetamines are not recommended for use as anorectic agents in pediatric patients under 12 years of age, or in pediatric patients under 3 years of age with Attention Deficit Disorder with Hyperactivity described under INDICATIONS AND USAGE.

Clinical experience suggests that in psychotic children, administration of amphetamines may exacerbate symptoms of behavior disturbance and thought disorder.

Amphetamines have been reported to exacerbate motor and phonic tics and Tourette's syndrome. Therefore, clinical evaluation for tics and Tourette's syndrome in children and their families should precede use of stimulant medications. Data are inadequate to determine whether chronic administration of amphetamines may be associated with growth inhibition; therefore, growth should be monitored during treatment.

Drug treatment is not indicated in all cases of Attention Deficit Disorder with Hyperactivity and should be considered only in light of the complete history and evaluation of the child. The decision to prescribe amphetamines should depend on the physician's assessment of the chronicity and severity of the child's symptoms and their appropriateness for his/her age. Prescription should not depend solely on the presence of one or more of the behavioral characteristics. When these symptoms are associated with acute stress reactions, treatment with amphetamines is usually not indicated.

ADVERSE REACTIONS

Cardiovascular: Palpitations, tachycardia, elevation of blood pressure. There have been isolated reports of cardiomyopathy associated with chronic amphetamine use.

Central Nervous System: Psychotic episodes at recommended doses (rare), overstimulation, restlessness, dizziness, insomnia, euphoria, dyskinesia, dysphoria, tremor, headache, exacerbation of motor and phonic tics and Tourette's syndrome.

Gastrointestinal: Dryness of the mouth, unpleasant taste, diarrhea, constipation, other gastrointestinal disturbances. Anorexia and weight loss may occur as undesirable effects when amphetamines are used for other than the anorectic effect.

Allergic: Urticaria.

Endocrine: Impotence, changes in libido.

DRUG ABUSE AND DEPENDENCE

Dextroamphetamine sulfate is a Schedule II controlled substance.

Amphetamines have been extensively abused. Tolerance, extreme psychological dependence and severe social disability have occurred. There are reports of patients who have increased the dosage to many times that recommended. Abrupt cessation following prolonged high dosage administration results in extreme fatigue and mental depression; changes are also noted on the sleep EEG.

Manifestations of chronic intoxication with amphetamines include severe dermatoses, marked insomnia, irritability, hyperactivity and personality changes. The most severe manifestation of chronic intoxication is psychosis, often clinically indistinguishable from schizophrenia. This is rare with oral amphetamines.

OVERDOSAGE

Individual patient response to amphetamines varies widely. While toxic symptoms occasionally occur as an idiosyncrasy at doses as low as 2 mg, they are rare with doses of less than 15 mg; 30 mg can produce severe reactions, yet doses of 400 to 500 mg are not necessarily fatal.

In rats, the oral LD_{50} of dextroamphetamine sulfate is 96.8 mg/kg.

Manifestations of acute overdosage with amphetamines include restlessness, tremor, hyperreflexia, rhabdomyolysis, rapid respiration, hyperpyrexia, confusion, assaultiveness, hallucinations, panic states.

Fatigue and depression usually follow the central stimulation.

Cardiovascular effects include arrhythmias, hypertension or hypotension and circulatory collapse. Gastrointestinal symptoms include nausea, vomiting, diarrhea and abdominal cramps. Fatal poisoning is usually preceded by convulsions and coma.

TREATMENT—Management of acute amphetamine intoxication is largely symptomatic and includes gastric lavage and sedation with a barbiturate. Experience with hemodialysis or peritoneal dialysis is inadequate to permit recommen-

Continued on next page

Information on the SmithKline Beecham Pharmaceuticals products appearing here is based on the labeling in effect on July 1, 1996. Further information on these and other products may be obtained from the Medical Department, SmithKline Beecham Pharmaceuticals, One Franklin Plaza, Philadelphia, PA 19101.

SmithKline Beecham—Cont.

dation in this regard. Acidification of the urine increases amphetamine excretion. If acute, severe hypertension complicates amphetamine overdosage, administration of intravenous phentolamine (Regitine®, CIBA) has been suggested. However, a gradual drop in blood pressure will usually result when sufficient sedation has been achieved. Chlorpromazine antagonizes the central stimulant effects of amphetamines and can be used to treat amphetamine intoxication.

Since much of the *Spansule* capsule medication is coated for gradual release, therapy directed at reversing the effects of the ingested drug and at supporting the patient should be continued for as long as overdosage symptoms remain. Saline cathartics are useful for hastening the evacuation of pellets that have not already released medication.

DOSAGE AND ADMINISTRATION

Regardless of indication, amphetamines should be administered at the lowest effective dosage and dosage should be individually adjusted. Late evening doses—particularly with the *Spansule* capsule form—should be avoided because of the resulting insomnia.

Narcolepsy: Usual dose 5 to 60 mg per day in divided doses, depending on the individual patient response.

Narcolepsy seldom occurs in children under 12 years of age; however, when it does, Dexedrine (dextroamphetamine sulfate) may be used. The suggested initial dose for patients aged 6–12 is 5 mg daily; daily dose may be raised in increments of 5 mg at weekly intervals until optimal response is obtained. In patients 12 years of age and older, start with 10 mg daily; daily dosage may be raised in increments of 10 mg at weekly intervals until optimal response is obtained. If bothersome adverse reactions appear (e.g., insomnia or anorexia), dosage should be reduced. *Spansule* capsules may be used for once-a-day dosage wherever appropriate. With tablets, give first dose on awakening; additional doses (1 or 2) at intervals of 4 to 6 hours.

Attention Deficit Disorder with Hyperactivity: Not recommended for pediatric patients under 3 years of age.

In pediatric patients from 3 to 5 years of age, start with 2.5 mg daily, by tablet; daily dosage may be raised in increments of 2.5 mg at weekly intervals until optimal response is obtained.

In pediatric patients 6 years of age and older, start with 5 mg once or twice daily; daily dosage may be raised in increments of 5 mg at weekly intervals until optimal response is obtained. Only in rare cases will it be necessary to exceed a total of 40 mg per day.

Spansule capsules may be used for once-a-day dosage wherever appropriate.

With tablets, give first dose on awakening; additional doses (1 or 2) at intervals of 4 to 6 hours.

Where possible, drug administration should be interrupted occasionally to determine if there is a recurrence of behavioral symptoms sufficient to require continued therapy.

HOW SUPPLIED

Dexedrine Spansule capsules: Each capsule, with brown cap and clear body, contains dextroamphetamine sulfate. The 5 mg capsule is imprinted 5 mg and 3512 on the brown cap and is imprinted 5 mg and SB on the clear body. The 10 mg capsule is imprinted 10 mg and 3513 on the brown cap and is imprinted 10 mg and SB on the clear body. The 15 mg capsule is imprinted 15 mg and 3514 on the brown cap and is imprinted 15 mg and SB on the clear body. Available: 5 mg, 10 mg, and 15 mg in bottles of 50.

Store between 15° and 30°C (59° and 86°F). Dispense in a tight, light-resistant container.

5 mg 50's: NDC 0007-3512-15
10 mg 50's: NDC 0007-3513-15
15 mg 50's: NDC 0007-3514-15

Dexedrine (dextroamphetamine sulfate) Tablets: Triangular, orange, scored, debossed SKF and E19. Available: 5 mg in bottles of 100.

5 mg 100's: NDC 0007-3519-20

Store between 15° and 30°C (59° and 86°F). Dispense in a tight, light-resistant container.

Veterans Administration/Military/PHS—Spansule Capsules, 5 mg, 50's, 6505-01-153-4029; 10 mg, 50's, 6505-01-153-3038; 15 mg, 50's, 6505-00-769-2090; Tablets, 5 mg, 100's, 6505-00-106-8715.

DX:L445A
Shown in Product Identification Guide, page 336

DIBENZYLINE® Capsules   ℞
[di-benz'eh-leen]
brand of phenoxybenzamine hydrochloride

DESCRIPTION

Each *Dibenzyline* capsule, with red cap and red body, is imprinted SKF and E33 and contains phenoxybenzamine hy-

drochloride, 10 mg. Inactive ingredients consist of benzyl alcohol, cetylpyridinium chloride, D&C Red No. 33, FD&C Red No. 3, FD&C Yellow No. 6, gelatin, lactose, sodium lauryl sulfate and trace amounts of other inactive ingredients.

Dibenzyline is N-(2-Chloroethyl)-N-(1-methyl-2-phenoxyethyl)benzylamine hydrochloride.

Phenoxybenzamine hydrochloride is a colorless, crystalline powder with a molecular weight of 340.3 which melts between 136° and 141°C. It is soluble in water, alcohol and chloroform; insoluble in ether.

CLINICAL PHARMACOLOGY

Dibenzyline (phenoxybenzamine hydrochloride) is a long-acting, adrenergic, *alpha* -receptor blocking agent which can produce and maintain "chemical sympathectomy" by oral administration. It increases blood flow to the skin, mucosa and abdominal viscera, and lowers both supine and erect blood pressures. It has no effect on the parasympathetic system.

Twenty to 30 percent of orally administered phenoxybenzamine appears to be absorbed in the active form.[1]

The half-life of orally administered phenoxybenzamine hydrochloride is not known; however, the half-life of intravenously administered drug is approximately 24 hours. Demonstrable effects with intravenous administration persist for at least 3 to 4 days, and the effects of daily administration are cumulative for nearly a week.[1]

INDICATION AND USAGE

Pheochromocytoma, to control episodes of hypertension and sweating. If tachycardia is excessive, it may be necessary to use a beta-blocking agent concomitantly.

CONTRAINDICATIONS

Conditions where a fall in blood pressure may be undesirable.

WARNING

Dibenzyline-induced *alpha* -adrenergic blockade leaves *beta* -adrenergic receptors unopposed. Compounds that stimulate both types of receptors may therefore produce an exaggerated hypotensive response and tachycardia.

PRECAUTIONS

General—Administer with caution in patients with marked cerebral or coronary arteriosclerosis or renal damage. Adrenergic blocking effect may aggravate symptoms of respiratory infections.

Drug Interactions[2]—Dibenzyline (phenoxybenzamine hydrochloride) may interact with compounds that stimulate both *alpha* - and *beta* -adrenergic receptors (i.e., epinephrine) to produce an exaggerated hypotensive response and tachycardia. (See WARNING.)

Dibenzyline blocks hyperthermia production by levarterenol, and blocks hypothermia production by reserpine.

Carcinogenesis, Mutagenesis, Impairment of Fertility—Phenoxybenzamine hydrochloride has shown *in vitro* mutagenic activity in the Ames test and in the mouse lymphoma assay; it has not shown mutagenic activity in the micronucleus test in mice. In rats and mice repeated intraperitoneal administration of phenoxybenzamine hydrochloride resulted in peritoneal sarcomas. Chronic oral dosing in rats has produced malignant tumors in the gastrointestinal tract. The majority of these tumors were found in the nonglandular stomach of the rats.

In chronic oral studies in rats, ulcerative and/or erosive gastritis of the glandular stomach occurred which was probably drug related.

Pregnancy-Teratogenic Effects—Pregnancy Category C. Adequate reproductive studies have not been performed with Dibenzyline (phenoxybenzamine hydrochloride). It is also not known whether *Dibenzyline* can cause fetal harm when administered to a pregnant woman. *Dibenzyline* should be given to a pregnant woman only if clearly needed.

Nursing Mothers—It is not known whether this drug is excreted in human milk. Because many drugs are excreted in human milk, and because of the potential for serious adverse reactions from phenoxybenzamine hydrochloride, a decision should be made whether to discontinue nursing or to discontinue the drug, taking into account the importance of the drug to the mother.

Pediatric Use—Safety and effectiveness in children have not been established.

ADVERSE REACTIONS

The following adverse reactions have been observed, but there are insufficient data to support an estimate of their frequency.

Autonomic Nervous System*: Postural hypotension, tachycardia, inhibition of ejaculation, nasal congestion, miosis.

Miscellaneous: Gastrointestinal irritation, drowsiness, fatigue.

---

*These so-called "side effects" are actually evidence of adrenergic blockade and vary according to the degree of blockade.

OVERDOSAGE

SYMPTOMS—These are largely the result of block of the sympathetic nervous system and of the circulating epinephrine. They may include postural hypotension resulting in dizziness or fainting; tachycardia, particularly postural; vomiting; lethargy; shock.

TREATMENT—When symptoms and signs of overdosage exist, discontinue the drug. Treatment of circulatory failure, if present, is a prime consideration. In cases of mild overdosage, recumbent position with legs elevated usually restores cerebral circulation. In the more severe cases, the usual measures to combat shock should be instituted. Usual pressor agents are *not* effective. Epinephrine is contraindicated because it stimulates both *alpha* and *beta* receptors; since *alpha* receptors are blocked, the net effect of epinephrine administration is vasodilation and a further drop in blood pressure (epinephrine reversal).

The patient may have to be kept flat for 24 hours or more in the case of overdose, as the effect of the drug is prolonged. Leg bandages and an abdominal binder may shorten the period of disability.

I.V. infusion of levarterenol bitartrate* may be used to combat severe hypotensive reactions, because it stimulates *alpha* receptors primarily. Although Dibenzyline (phenoxybenzamine hydrochloride) is an *alpha*-adrenergic blocking agent, a sufficient dose of levarterenol bitartrate will overcome this effect.

The oral LD_{50} for phenoxybenzamine hydrochloride is approximately 2000 mg/kg in rats and approximately 500 mg/kg in guinea pigs.

DOSAGE AND ADMINISTRATION

The dosage should be adjusted to fit the needs of each patient. Small initial doses should be *slowly* increased until the desired effect is obtained or the side effects from blockade become troublesome. *After each increase, the patient should be observed on that level before instituting another increase.* The dosage should be carried to a point where symptomatic relief and/or objective improvement are obtained, but not so high that the side effects from blockade become troublesome. Initially, 10 mg of Dibenzyline (phenoxybenzamine hydrochloride) twice a day. Dosage should be increased every other day, usually to 20 to 40 mg 2 or 3 times a day, until an optimal dosage is obtained, as judged by blood pressure control.

HOW SUPPLIED

Dibenzyline (phenoxybenzamine hydrochloride) capsules, 10 mg, in bottles of 100 (*NDC* 0007-3533-20).

Veterans Administration/Military/PHS—Capsules, 10 mg, 100's, 6505-00-890-1193.

REFERENCES

1. Weiner, N.: Drugs That Inhibit Adrenergic Nerves and Block Adrenergic Receptors, in Goodman, L., and Gilman, A., *The Pharmacological Basis of Therapeutics*, ed. 6, New York, Macmillan Publishing Co., 1980, p. 179; p. 182.
2. Martin, E.W.: *Drug Interactions Index 1978/1979*, Philadelphia, J.B. Lippincott Co., 1978, pp. 209–210.

*Available as Levophed® Bitartrate (brand of norepinephrine bitartrate) from Sanofi Winthrop Pharmaceuticals.
DI:L24
Shown in Product Identification Guide, page 336

DIPHTHERIA AND TETANUS TOXOIDS AND PERTUSSIS VACCINE ADSORBED   ℞

DESCRIPTION

Diphtheria and Tetanus Toxoids and Pertussis Vaccine Adsorbed (DTP) consists of a combination of purified tetanus and diphtheria toxoids, aluminum phosphate adsorbed, combined with a suspension of *Bordetella pertussis* organisms. Diphtheria toxin is produced by growing *Corynebacterium diphtheriae* in a medium composed chiefly of a porcine pancreatic hydrolysate of casein. Tetanus toxin is produced by growing *Clostridium tetani* in a medium composed of a porcine tryptic digest of casein. Both toxins are inactivated with formaldehyde, purified by fractionation with ammonium sulfate, adsorbed onto aluminum phosphate, and diluted with 0.85% saline containing thimerosal (mercury derivative) as a preservative.

Pertussis vaccine is prepared by growing Phase 1 *B. pertussis* organisms on Bordet-Gengou agar, which contains potato infusion, proteose peptone, agar, washed sheep red blood cells, glycerol and sodium chloride. The pertussis organisms are washed from the agar with 0.85% saline. Three strains of pertussis organisms are combined, inactivated at room temperature in the presence of thimerosal (mercury derivative), and diluted with 0.85% saline containing thimerosal as preservative.

Pertussis vaccine, diphtheria and tetanus toxoids are combined in physiological saline diluent containing thimerosal as a preservative.

Each single dose (0.5 mL) contains 0.2 to 0.6 mg of aluminum by assay as an adjuvant and less than 0.001% residual formaldehyde. It does not contain animal serum and is free of detectable sheep antigens. This product also contains 0.01% sodium ethylmercurithiosalicylate (thimerosal, a mercury derivative) as a preservative.

Each 0.5 mL dose of vaccine is formulated to contain 6.5 Lf of diphtheria toxoid and 5.5 Lf of tetanus toxoid. The pertussis component is formulated to contain not more than 16 opacity units per single human dose.

When appropriately tested in guinea pigs, the tetanus and diphtheria components stimulate *at least* 2 neutralizing units/mL of serum. The total human immunizing dose is 12 units of pertussis vaccine with an estimate of 4 protective units per single human dose.[1]

The vaccine is supplied as a sterile suspension for intramuscular administration that is ready to use without reconstitution. It contains 0.2 to 0.6 mg of aluminum as an adjuvant, 0.01% thimerosal as a preservative, less than 0.001% residual formaldehyde, sodium chloride, sodium phosphate and water. With thorough agitation, DTP is an opaque white suspension. The licensed name of the product is Diphtheria and Tetanus Toxoids and Pertussis Vaccine Adsorbed.

CLINICAL PHARMACOLOGY

Simultaneous immunization with diphtheria, tetanus and pertussis vaccine during infancy and childhood, a routine practice in the United States since the late 1940s, has played a major role in markedly reducing the incidence of cases and deaths from each of these diseases.

Diphtheria

Diphtheria is primarily a localized and generalized intoxication caused by diphtheria toxin, an extracellular protein metabolite of toxinogenic strains of *C. diphtheriae.* While the incidence of diphtheria in the United States has decreased from over 200,000 cases reported in 1921 to only 24 cases reported from 1980 to 1989, the ratio of fatalities to attack rate has remained constant at about 5% to 10%. The highest case fatality rates are in the very young and in the elderly. There is essentially no natural immunity to diphtheria toxin. Thus, universal primary immunization with diphtheria toxoid, with subsequent maintenance of adequate antitoxin levels by means of timed boosters, is necessary to protect all age groups.[1] Following adequate immunization with diphtheria toxoid, which induces antitoxin and neutralizing antibodies, it is thought that protection lasts for at least 10 years.[1] Serologic data demonstrate the ability of DTP vaccine to stimulate neutralizing antibody against diphtheria antigen in humans—the protective level is ≥0.01 units/mL. Following administration of three doses of diphtheria vaccine (having a potency of 2 to 4 antitoxin-inducing units per mL) geometric mean titers (GMTs) were 3.7 to 9.3 antitoxin units.[2,3] This significantly reduces both the risk of developing diphtheria and the severity of clinical illness. It does not, however, eliminate carriage of *C. diphtheriae* in the pharynx or nose, or on the skin.[1]

Tetanus

Tetanus is an intoxication manifested primarily by neuromuscular dysfunction caused by a potent exotoxin released by *C. tetani.* The incidence of tetanus in the United States has dropped dramatically with the routine use of tetanus toxoid to a record low of 48 cases in 1987. Spores of *C. tetani* are ubiquitous, and there is essentially no natural immunity to tetanus toxin. Thus, universal primary immunization with tetanus toxoid, with subsequent maintenance of adequate antitoxin levels by means of timed boosters, is necessary to protect all age groups.[1] Tetanus toxoid is a highly effective antigen and a completed primary series generally induces neutralizing antibodies and protective levels of serum antitoxin that persist for at least 10 years.[1] Serologic data demonstrate the ability of DTP vaccine to stimulate neutralizing antibody against tetanus antigen in humans. Following administration of three doses of tetanus vaccine (having a potency of 2 to 4 antitoxin-inducing units per mL) GMTs were 13.5 units to 29.1 antitoxin units.[2,3]

Pertussis

Pertussis ("whooping cough") is a disease of the respiratory tract caused by *B. pertussis.* This gram-negative coccobacillus produces a variety of active components including endotoxin and a number of other substances that have been defined primarily on the basis of their biological activity in animals. These active components have been associated with a number of effects, such as lymphocytosis, leukocytosis, sensitivity to histamine, changes in glucose and/or insulin levels, possible neurological effects and adjuvant activity.[4] The role of each of the different components in either the pathogenesis of, or immunity to, pertussis is not well understood.

Pertussis is a highly communicable disease which has an attack rate of over 90% in unimmunized household contacts.[1] Since pertussis vaccine has come into widespread use, the number of reported cases and associated mortality in the United States has declined from about 120,000 cases and 1,100 deaths in 1950,[5] to an average of about 2,300 cases annually in the 1970s. During the 1980s, the incidence increased to 4,157 cases in 1989, with about eight fatalities annually.[1] Accurate data do not exist, as bacteriological confirmation of pertussis can be obtained in less than half of the suspected cases. Most reported illnesses from *B. pertussis* occur in infants and young children; two thirds of reported deaths occur in children less than 1 year old. Older children and adults, in whom classic signs are often absent, may go undiagnosed and serve as reservoirs of disease.[1]

Potency of the pertussis component of the vaccine is measured and shown to be acceptable in the mouse potency test. Serum agglutinin titers of vaccinees were correlated with clinical protection in the Medical Research Council trials. In the second Medical Research Council Field Trial, which compared five pertussis vaccines (including the nonadsorbed component of the present vaccine) and involved more than 30,000 children aged 6 months to 3 years, attack rates in exposed vaccinated children ranged from 4% to 29%. In an earlier trial, the attack rate in unvaccinated exposed children was 87%. Efficacy of the present vaccine has been estimated at 80% to 85%.[6,7] All five vaccines were found to be efficacious. In this trial, protection was found to correlate with protection of mice against intracerebral infection, production of specific agglutinin in mice, and production of specific agglutinin in children.[6,7]

Because the severity of pertussis decreases with age, and the vaccine may cause side effects and adverse reactions, routine pertussis immunization is not recommended for persons 7 years of age or older.[1]

INDICATIONS AND USAGE

Diphtheria and Tetanus Toxoids and Pertussis Vaccine Adsorbed is recommended for active immunization of healthy children from 6 weeks to their seventh birthday against diphtheria, tetanus and pertussis. It should not be used for treatment of these illnesses. All vaccinated individuals may not be protected.

Infants and children under 7 years of age should be immunized with DTP. Individuals 7 years of age or older should not receive the vaccine.

In children 7 years of age and older and in adults, Tetanus and Diphtheria Toxoids Adsorbed for Adult Use (Td) is preferable to use of either tetanus or diphtheria vaccines alone.

If immunization with pertussis vaccine is contraindicated, Diphtheria and Tetanus Toxoids Adsorbed (DT) should be used in children under 7 years of age. Individuals recovering from confirmed pertussis do not need additional doses of DTP but should receive additional doses of diphtheria and tetanus toxoids in accordance with ACIP recommendations.[1] When confirmation is lacking, DTP vaccination should be completed.[1]

DTP may be used concomitantly with Tetanus Immune Globulin and Diphtheria Antitoxin (see DOSAGE AND ADMINISTRATION).

CONTRAINDICATIONS

DTP vaccine is contraindicated for (1) persons with allergic hypersensitivity to any component of the vaccine, including thimerosal; (2) persons who experienced an immediate anaphylactic reaction to a previous dose; (3) persons who developed an unacceptable adverse reaction to a previous dose, including anaphylactic reaction; (4) use during an outbreak of poliomyelitis; (5) persons with a febrile illness or acute infection (see below); (6) persons who experienced encephalopathy following a previous dose. Encephalopathy is defined as an acute, severe central nervous system disorder occurring within 7 days following vaccination; it generally consists of major alterations in consciousness, unresponsiveness, generalized or focal seizures that persist more than a few hours with failure to recover within 24 hours. Even though causation by DTP cannot be established, no subsequent doses of pertussis vaccine should be given.[1]

The decision to administer or delay DTP vaccination because of a current or recent febrile illness depends largely on the severity of the symptoms and their etiology. Although a moderate or severe febrile illness or acute infection is sufficient reason to postpone vaccination, minor illness such as mild upper respiratory infection with or without low-grade fever is not usually reason to defer immunization.

WARNINGS

If any of the following events occur in temporal relation to receipt of DTP, the decision to give subsequent doses of vaccine containing the pertussis component should be carefully considered. There may be circumstances, such as a high incidence of pertussis, when the potential benefits outweigh possible risks, particularly since these events are not associated with permanent sequelae.

- **Arthus-type reactions.** These are characterized by severe local reactions (generally starting 2 to 8 hours after an injection) and may follow receipt of tetanus toxoid, particularly in adults who have received frequent (e.g., annual) boosters of tetanus toxoid.
- **Temperature of ≥40.5°C (105°F) within 48 hours not due to another identifiable cause.** There is a likelihood of high fever following a subsequent dose of DTP vaccine. Because such febrile reactions are usually attributed to the pertussis component, vaccination with DT should not be discontinued.
- **Collapse or shock-like state (hypotonic-hyporesponsive episode) within 48 hours.** Although these uncommon events have not been recognized to cause death or to induce permanent neurologic sequelae, it is prudent to continue vaccination with DT, omitting the pertussis component.[8,9]
- **Persistent, inconsolable crying lasting ≥3 hours, occurring within 48 hours.** The evidence obtained from follow-up of infants who have cried inconsolably following DTP vaccination is insufficient to indicate whether DTP-associated inconsolable crying does or does not lead to chronic neurologic damage.[10] Inconsolable crying occurs most frequently following the first dose and is less frequently reported following subsequent doses of DTP vaccine.[11] However, crying for >30 minutes following DTP vaccination can be a predictor of increased likelihood of recurrence of persistent crying following subsequent doses.[1,12] Children with persistent crying have had a higher rate of substantial local reactions than children who had other DTP-associated reactions (including high fever, seizures and hypotonic-hyporesponsive episodes), suggesting that prolonged crying was really a pain reaction.[9]
- **Convulsions with or without fever occurring within 3 days.** If convulsions occur after a previous dose of DTP, it is desirable to delay subsequent doses until the patient's neurologic status is better defined. Short-lived convulsions, with or without fever, have not been shown to cause permanent sequelae. More prolonged seizures would require careful evaluation before administration of further doses of vaccine.[1]

Any of the following may increase the risk of DTP vaccination but do not preclude its use: thrombocytopenia, coagulation disorder, family history of convulsions, developing neurologic illness.

A family history of convulsions or other central nervous system disorders is not a contraindication to pertussis vaccination. Acetaminophen is useful in preventing the fever which may cause seizures among febrile-convulsion-prone children and should be given at the time of DTP vaccination and every 4 hours for 24 hours to reduce the possibility of post-vaccination fever.[1]

Infants and children with recognized possible or potential underlying neurologic conditions seem to be at enhanced risk for the appearance of manifestations of the underlying neurologic disorder within 2 or 3 days following vaccination. Whether to administer DTP to children with proven or suspected underlying neurologic disorders must be decided on an individual basis. Important considerations include the current local incidence of pertussis, the near absence of diphtheria in the United States and the low risk of infection with *C. tetani.*[1]

Partial doses of DTP should not be given.[1]

Deaths have been reported in temporal association with the administration of DTP vaccine (see ADVERSE REACTIONS section).

PRECAUTIONS

General

Care must be taken by the health care provider for the safe and effective use of DTP.

The customary precautions usually taken in administering vaccines, such as the immediate availability of epinephrine injection solution, 1:1000, are recommended because of the possibility of an allergic reaction to any vaccine.

The patient, parent or guardian should be questioned about previous reactions to a dose of this vaccine or similar products. They should also be questioned about the immunization history and current health status of the vaccinee.

DTP vaccine should not be injected into a blood vessel.

Immunosuppressed patients may not respond to the vaccine. Immunosuppressive therapies, including irradiation, antimetabolites, alkylating agents, cytotoxic drugs and corticosteroids (used in greater than physiologic doses), may reduce the immune response to vaccines. Short-term (less than 2 weeks) corticosteroid therapy or intra-articular, bursal or tendon injections with corticosteroids should not be immunosuppressive. If immunosuppressive therapy will be discontinued shortly, it would be reasonable to defer immunization until the patient has been off therapy for 1 month[13]; otherwise, the patient should be vaccinated while still on therapy.[1]

Administration of this vaccine is not contraindicated based on the presence of human immunodeficiency virus infection.[14]

Continued on next page

Information on the SmithKline Beecham Pharmaceuticals products appearing here is based on the labeling in effect on July 1, 1996. Further information on these and other products may be obtained from the Medical Department, SmithKline Beecham Pharmaceuticals, One Franklin Plaza, Philadelphia, PA 19101.

SmithKline Beecham—Cont.

An individual sterile needle and syringe should be used for each patient to avoid transmission of viral hepatitis and other infectious agents. Needles should be disposed of properly and should not be recapped.

Information for patients

Patients, parents or guardians should be informed of the benefits and risks of the vaccine, and of the importance of completing the immunization series. The adult accompanying the recipient should be told to report severe or unusual adverse reactions to the physician or clinic where the vaccine was administered. For further information call the Vaccine Adverse Events Reporting System at 1-800-822-7967.[15] The patient, parent or guardian should be given the Vaccine Information Pamphlets (VIPs), which are required to be given with each immunization.

Drug Interactions

Tetanus Immune Globulin or Diphtheria Antitoxin, if used, should be given in a separate site, with a separate needle and syringe.

As with other intramuscular injections, use with caution in patients on anticoagulant therapy.

See PRECAUTIONS, General, about use during immunosuppressive therapy.

Influenza Virus Vaccine should not be given within 3 days of immunization.

Carcinogenesis, Mutagenesis, Impairment of Fertility

Animal and human studies concerning possible carcinogenesis or teratogenic effects have not been done.

Pregnancy: Pregnancy Category C.

(Diphtheria and Tetanus Toxoids and Pertussis Vaccine Adsorbed).

DTP is not recommended for people 7 years of age or older. Animal reproduction studies have not been conducted with DTP. It is also not known whether DTP can cause fetal harm when administered to a pregnant woman or can affect reproductive capacity.

Pediatric Use

Safety and effectiveness in children below the age of 6 weeks have not been established.

Full protection is based on a full course of immunization of four doses. If the fourth dose is not given on or before the fourth birthday, a booster dose is recommended. (See DOSAGE AND ADMINISTRATION.) DTP should not be used in children 7 years of age or older.

If immunization with pertussis vaccine is contraindicated, Diphtheria and Tetanus Toxoids Adsorbed (For Pediatric Use) (DT) should be used. In children 7 years of age and older and in adults, Tetanus and Diphtheria Toxoids Adsorbed for Adult Use (Td), a multiple antigen vaccine, is preferable to use of either tetanus or diphtheria vaccines alone.

ADVERSE REACTIONS

Not all adverse events following administration of DTP are causally related to DTP vaccine. Table 1 indicates approximate rates of adverse events (regardless of dose number in the series).

Local reaction at injection site: edema; erythema; heat; induration with or without tenderness; sterile abscess (6 to 10 per million doses); subcutaneous atrophy; occasionally, temporary (few weeks) palpable nodule; pain. These events are usually self-limiting and require no therapy. If local redness of 2.5 cm or greater occurs, the likelihood of recurrence after another DTP dose increases significantly.[16]

Cardiovascular: rarely, hypotension or shock.

Body as a whole: drowsiness; fever (approximately 50% of DTP vaccinees develop temperatures >38°C [100.4°F] after one or more doses, approximately 6% >39°C [102.2°F] and approximately 0.3% ≥40.5°C [105°F]); fretfulness; persistent, inconsolable crying. These reactions are significantly more common following vaccination with DTP than with DT, are usually self-limiting and need no therapy other than, perhaps, systemic treatment (e.g., antipyretics). Some data suggest that febrile reactions are more likely to occur in those who have experienced such responses after prior doses.[16] However, these observations were not noted by Barkin RM, et al.[17]

Respiratory: respiratory difficulties, including apnea.

Gastrointestinal: anorexia, vomiting.

Lymphatic: cervical lymphadenopathy following injections in the arm.

Skin and appendages: arthralgias, erythema multiforme, rash, urticaria.

Central nervous system: bulging fontanel, collapse (hypotonic-hyporesponsive state), convulsions, encephalopathy, mono- and polyneuropathies including Guillain-Barré Syndrome.

Moderate to severe systemic events such as fever of 40.5°C (105°F) or higher, persistent inconsolable crying lasting 3 hours or more, unusual high-pitched crying, collapse or convulsion occur relatively infrequently. More severe neurologic complications, such as prolonged convulsion or encephalopathy, occasionally fatal, have been reported to be associated with DTP administration.[1]

In the National Childhood Encephalopathy Study (NCES), a large case-control study in England,[18] children 2 to 35 months of age with serious, acute neurologic disorders, such as encephalopathy or complicated convulsion(s), were more likely to have received DTP in the 7 days preceding onset than their age-, sex- and neighborhood-matched controls. Among children known to be neurologically normal before entering the study, the relative risk (estimated by odds ratio) of a neurologic illness occurring within the 7-day period following receipt of DTP dose, compared to children not receiving DTP vaccine in the 7-day period before onset of their illness, was 3.3 (p < 0.001). Within this 7-day period, the risk was significantly increased for immunized children only within 3 days of vaccination (relative risk 4.2, p < 0.001). The relative risk for illness occurring 4 to 7 days after vaccination was 2.1 (0.05 < p < 0.1). The attributable risk estimates for a serious acute neurologic disorder within 7 days after DTP vaccine (regardless of outcome) was one in 140,000 doses of DTP. The estimated risk for a permanent neurologic deficit was one in 330,000 doses with a wide confidence interval.[1] No specific clinical syndrome was identified. Overall, DTP vaccine accounted for only a small proportion of cases of serious neurologic disorders reported in the population studied.[1] Although there are uncertainties in the reported studies, recent data suggest that infants and young children who have had previous convulsions (whether febrile or nonfebrile) are more likely to have seizures following DTP than those without such histories.[1,19]

Sudden infant death syndrome (SIDS) has occurred in infants following administration of DTP. A large case-control study of SIDS in the United States showed that receipt of DTP was not causally related to SIDS.[20] It should be recognized that the first three primary immunizing doses of DTP are usually administered to infants 2 to 6 months old and that approximately 85% of SIDS cases occur at ages 1 to 6 months, with the peak incidence occurring at 6 weeks to 4 months of age. By chance alone, some SIDS victims can be expected to have recently received vaccine.[1]

Deaths due to causes other than SIDS, including deaths due to serious infections, have occurred in infants following the administration of DTP. A number of studies have evaluated the relative risk of death due to causes other than SIDS in temporal association with DTP vaccination and a causal relationship has neither been proved nor disproved.

Onset of infantile spasms has occurred in infants who have recently received DTP or DT. Analysis of data from the NCES on children with infantile spasms showed that receipt of DTP or DT was not causally related to infantile spasms.[21] The incidence of onset of infantile spasms increases at 3 to 9 months of age, the time period in which the second and third doses of DTP are generally given. Therefore, some cases of infantile spasms can be expected to be related by chance alone to recent receipt of DTP.[1] (See Table 1.)

Hypersensitivity: rarely, an anaphylactic reaction (i.e., hives, swelling of the mouth, difficulty breathing, hypotension or shock and death); Arthus-type hypersensitivity reaction. The latter, which is characterized by severe local reactions (generally starting 2 to 8 hours after an injection), may follow receipt of tetanus toxoid, particularly in adults who have received frequent (e.g., annual) boosters of tetanus toxoid. A few cases of peripheral neuropathy have been reported following tetanus toxoid administration, although a causal relationship has not been established.[1]

TABLE 1. Adverse events occurring within 48 hours of DTP immunizations[1]

Event	Frequency*
Local	
Redness	1/3 doses
Swelling	2/5 doses
Pain	1/2 doses
Systemic	
Fever >38°C (100.4°F)	1/2 doses
Drowsiness	1/3 doses
Fretfulness	1/2 doses
Vomiting	1/15 doses
Anorexia	1/5 doses
Persistent, inconsolable crying (duration ≥3 hours)	1/100 doses
Fever ≥40.5°C (≥105°F)	1/330 doses
Collapse (hypotonic-hyporesponsive episode)	1/1,750 doses
Convulsions (with or without fever)	1/1,750 doses

* Number of adverse events per total number of doses regardless of dose number in DTP series.

In a prospective study of serious reactions to Michigan Department of Public Health's DTP vaccine within 48 hours of vaccination, the following rates of adverse events were reported via mail-in questionnaires completed by parents followed by telephone contacts of positive responses: prolonged crying >3 hours 1:442; unusual crying 1:1,457; fever >40.5°C 1:1,770; hypotension/hyporesponsiveness 1:3,539 and seizure 1:24,776.[22]

Reporting of Adverse Reactions

Parents or guardians should report severe adverse reactions to their health care provider or to the clinic at which the vaccine was given. The National Childhood Vaccine Injury Act has established a procedure for compensation of children with certain injuries. Parents who believe that serious injury has been sustained should call the Vaccine Adverse Events Reporting System at 1-800-822-7967.

If serious adverse reactions are noted, report them promptly to the manufacturer: Michigan Department of Public Health, 517-335-8050 during working hours or 517-335-9030 at other times. Reports may also be submitted directly to the FDA on forms which may be obtained by calling 1-800-822-7967.

DOSAGE AND ADMINISTRATION

The primary series for children less than 7 years of age is four doses of 0.5 mL each given intramuscularly. The customary age for the first dose is 2 months but may be given as young as 6 weeks of age and up to the seventh birthday.

The first three doses should be given at 4 to 8 week intervals (preferably 8 weeks); the fourth dose should be given 6 to 12 months after the third dose.

Interruption of the recommended schedule with a delay between doses does not interfere with the final immunity achieved with DTP. There is no need to start the series over again, regardless of the time elapsed between doses.

The preferred sites are the anterolateral aspect of the thigh and the deltoid muscle of the upper arm.

The vaccine should not be injected into the gluteal area or areas where there may be a major nerve trunk.

The use of reduced volume (fractional doses) is not recommended. The effect of such practices on the frequency of serious adverse events and on protection against disease has not been determined.[1]

Preterm infants should be vaccinated according to their chronological age from birth.[1]

The concomitant administration of DTP, haemophilus b conjugate vaccine, inactivated poliovirus vaccine (IPV), hepatitis B vaccine, oral poliovirus vaccine (OPV) and/or measles-mumps-rubella vaccine (MMR) has resulted in seroconversion rates and rates of side effects similar to those observed when the vaccines are administered separately.[1,23-25] The ACIP recommends the concomitant administration of all vaccines appropriate to the age and previous vaccination status of the recipient, including the special circumstance of simultaneous administration of DTP, OPV, HbCV and MMR at ≥15 months of age.[1]

DTP may be used concomitantly with Tetanus Immune Globulin and Diphtheria Antitoxin.

Use a separate sterile needle and sterile syringe for each patient to avoid transmission of viral hepatitis and other infectious agents.

The bottle must be shaken thoroughly to ensure that the suspension is homogeneous during withdrawal. DO NOT USE IF RESUSPENSION DOES NOT OCCUR WITH VIGOROUS SHAKING.

After insertion of the needle and before injection of the vaccine, aspirate to avoid inadvertent intravenous injection of the preparation.

Parenteral drug products should be inspected visually for particulate matter and discoloration prior to administration, whenever solution and container permit.

Booster Doses

Children 4 to 6 years old (up to the seventh birthday), who received all required primary immunizing doses before the fourth birthday, should receive a single dose of DTP just before entering kindergarten or elementary school. This booster is not necessary if the fourth dose in the primary series was given on or after the fourth birthday.

For persons 7 years of age or older, Tetanus and Diphtheria Toxoids Adsorbed for Adult Use (Td) should be given for routine booster immunization against tetanus and diphtheria.

HOW SUPPLIED

Diphtheria and Tetanus Toxoids and Pertussis Vaccine Adsorbed is supplied in vials containing 5.0 mL (10 doses) of the product in packages of 1 and 10 vials.

Storage: DTP should be stored at 2° to 8°C (36° to 46°F). Do not freeze. Do not use after expiration date shown on the label.

Package of 1: NDC 0007-3555-01
Package of 10: NDC 0007-3555-53

REFERENCES

1. Centers for Disease Control. Diphtheria, tetanus and pertussis: Recommendations for vaccine use and other preventive measures: Recommendation of the Immunization Practices Advisory Committee. *MMWR.* 1991;40(No. RR-10):1-28.
2. Brown GC, Volk VK, Gottshall RY, et al: Responses of infants to DTP-P vaccine used in nine injection schedules. *Public Health Reports.* 1964;79:585-601.
3. Volk VK, Gottshall RY, Anderson HD, et al: Antibody response to booster dose of diphtheria and tetanus tox-

oids and pertussis vaccine. *Public Health Reports.* 1964;79:424-434.
4. Manclark CR, et al: Pertussis. In: Germanier R. (ed), *Bacterial Vaccines.* Academic Press Inc., New York. 1984, pp. 69-106.
5. Centers for Disease Control. Reported incidence of notifiable disease in the United States. *MMWR.* 1970;19(53):44.
6. *Federal Register.* December 13, 1985;50(240).
7. Whooping Cough Immunization Committee of the Medical Research Council: Vaccination against whooping cough. *Br Med J.* Aug 25, 1956;ii:454-462.
8. Baraff LJ, Shields WD, Beckwith L, et al: Infants and children with convulsions and hypotonic-hyporesponsive episodes following diphtheria-tetanus-pertussis immunization: follow-up evaluation. *Pediatrics.* 1988;81:789-794.
9. Blumberg DA, Mink CM, Lewis K, et al: Severe DTP-associated reactions (abstract). In: Manclark CR (ed). *The Sixth International Symposium on Pertussis, Abstracts.* Bethesda, Maryland: Department of Health and Human Services, 1990; DHHS publication no. (FDA) 90-1162, 223-224.
10. Howson CP, et al: A Report of the Committee to Review the Adverse Consequences of Pertussis and Rubella Vaccines. National Academy Press, Washington, DC, 1991.
11. Cody CL, Baraff LF, Cherry JD, et al: The nature and rate of adverse reactions associated with DTP and DT immunization in infants and children. *Pediatrics.* 1981; 68:650-660.
12. Long SS, Deforest A, Pennridget Pediatric Associates, Smith DG, et al: Longitudinal study of adverse reactions following diphtheria-tetanus-pertussis vaccine in infancy. *Pediatrics.* 1990;85:294.
13. Hirtz DG, et al: Seizures following childhood immunization. *J Pediatr.* 1983;102(1):14-18.
14. Centers for Disease Control. General recommendations on immunizations: Recommendation of the Immunization Practices Advisory Committee (ACIP). *MMWR.* 1989;38(13):205-227.
15. Centers for Disease Control. *MMWR.* October 19, 1990;39:730-733.
16. Baraff L, et al: DTP-associated reactions: An analysis by injection site, manufacturer, prior reactions and dose. *Pediatrics.* 1984;73:31.
17. Barkin RM, et al: Diphtheria-pertussis-tetanus vaccine: Reactogenicity of commercial products. *Pediatrics.* 1979;63:256.
18. Miller DL, et al: Pertussis immunization and serious acute neurological illness in children. *Br Med J* [*Clin Res*]. 1981;282:1595-1599.
19. Centers for Disease Control. Adverse events following immunization surveillance. Surveillance Report No. 1, 1979-1982 (August 1984).
20. Hoffman HJ: SIDS and DTP. 17th Immunization Conference Proceedings, Atlanta, GA: Centers for Disease Control: 79-88, 1982.
21 Bellman MH, et al: Infantile spasms and pertussis immunization. *Lancet.* 1983;i:1031-1034.
22. Murray D, Wilcok K, Berlin B and the Michigan DTP Study Group: Serious reactions to DTP vaccine: a Michigan survey. *Pediatr Res.* 1988;42(4 part 2):Abst. No. 1054.
23. Deforest A, Long SS, Lischner HW, et al: Simultaneous administration of measles-mumps-rubella vaccine with booster doses of diphtheria-tetanus-pertussis and poliovirus vaccines. *Pediatrics.* 1988;81:237-246.
24. Centers for Disease Control. *Haemophilus* b conjugate vaccines for prevention of *Haemophilus influenzae* type b disease among infants and children two months of age and older. Recommendation of the Immunization Practices Advisory Committee (ACIP). *MMWR.* 1991;40(No. RR-10):14.
25. Data on file. SmithKline Beecham Pharmaceuticals.

Manufactured by
Michigan Department of Public Health
Lansing, MI 48909
U.S. License No. 99
Distributed by
SmithKline Beecham Pharmaceuticals
Philadelphia, PA 19101
Veterans Administration/Military/PHS—Vial, 5 mL, 6505-01-378-3939.
DTP:L2SB

Shown in Product Identification Guide, page 336

DYAZIDE® ℞
[*dye-uh-zide'*]
capsules
diuretic • antihypertensive

DESCRIPTION

Each *Dyazide* capsule for oral use, with opaque red cap and opaque white body, contains hydrochlorothiazide 25 mg and triamterene 37.5 mg, and is imprinted with the product name DYAZIDE and SB. Hydrochlorothiazide is a diuretic/antihypertensive agent and triamterene is an antikaliuretic agent.

Hydrochlorothiazide is slightly soluble in water. It is soluble in dilute ammonia, dilute aqueous sodium hydroxide and dimethylformamide. It is sparingly soluble in methanol.

Hydrochlorothiazide is 6-chloro-3,4-dihydro-2H -1,2,4-benzothiadiazine-7-sulfonamide 1,1-dioxide and its structural formula is:

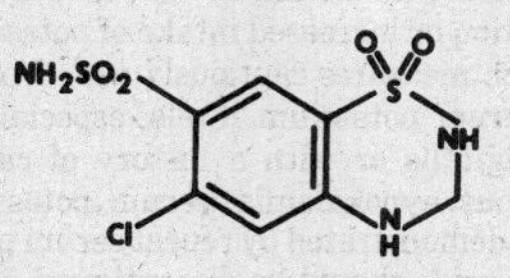

At 50°C, triamterene is practically insoluble in water (less than 0.1%). It is soluble in formic acid, sparingly soluble in methoxyethanol and very slightly soluble in alcohol.

Triamterene is 2,4,7-triamino-6-phenylpteridine and its structural formula is:

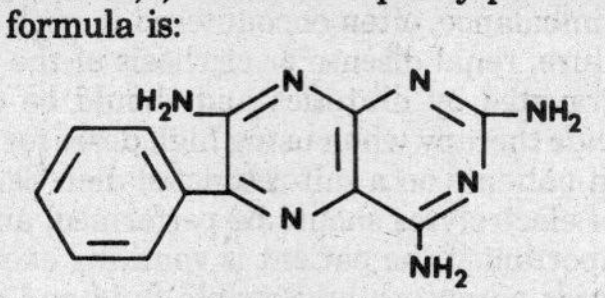

Inactive ingredients consist of benzyl alcohol, cetylpyridinium chloride, D&C Red No. 33, FD&C Yellow No. 6, gelatin, glycine, lactose, magnesium stearate, microcrystalline cellulose, povidone, polysorbate 80, sodium starch glycolate, titanium dioxide and trace amounts of other inactive ingredients.

CLINICAL PHARMACOLOGY

Dyazide is a diuretic/antihypertensive drug product that combines natriuretic and antikaliuretic effects. Each component complements the action of the other. The hydrochlorothiazide component blocks the reabsorption of sodium and chloride ions, and thereby increases the quantity of sodium traversing the distal tubule and the volume of water excreted. A portion of the additional sodium presented to the distal tubule is exchanged there for potassium and hydrogen ions. With continued use of hydrochlorothiazide and depletion of sodium, compensatory mechanisms tend to increase this exchange and may produce excessive loss of potassium, hydrogen and chloride ions. Hydrochlorothiazide also decreases the excretion of calcium and uric acid, may increase the excretion of iodide and may reduce glomerular filtration rate. The exact mechanism of the antihypertensive effect of hydrochlorothiazide is not known.

The triamterene component of *Dyazide* exerts its diuretic effect on the distal renal tubule to inhibit the reabsorption of sodium in exchange for potassium and hydrogen ions. Its natriuretic activity is limited by the amount of sodium reaching its site of action. Although it blocks the increase in this exchange that is stimulated by mineralocorticoids (chiefly aldosterone) it is not a competitive antagonist of aldosterone and its activity can be demonstrated in adrenalectomized rats and patients with Addison's disease. As a result, the dose of triamterene required is not proportionally related to the level of mineralocorticoid activity, but is dictated by the response of the individual patients, and the kaliuretic effect of concomitantly administered drugs. By inhibiting the distal tubular exchange mechanism, triamterene maintains or increases the sodium excretion and reduces the excess loss of potassium, hydrogen and chloride ions induced by hydrochlorothiazide. As with hydrochlorothiazide, triamterene may reduce glomerular filtration and renal plasma flow. Via this mechanism it may reduce uric acid excretion although it has no tubular effect on uric acid reabsorption or secretion. Triamterene does not affect calcium excretion. No predictable antihypertensive effect has been demonstrated for triamterene.

Duration of diuretic activity and effective dosage range of the hydrochlorothiazide and triamterene components of *Dyazide* are similar. Onset of diuresis with *Dyazide* takes place within 1 hour, peaks at 2 to 3 hours and tapers off during the subsequent 7 to 9 hours.

Dyazide capsule is well absorbed.

Upon administration of a single oral dose to fasted normal male volunteers, the following mean pharmacokinetic parameters were determined:

[See table above.]

	AUC(0–48) ng*hrs/mL (±SD)	Cmax ng/mL (±SD)	Median Tmax hrs	Ae mg (±SD)
triamterene	148.7 (87.9)	46.4 (29.4)	1.1	2.7 (1.4)
hydroxytriamterene sulfate	1865 (471)	720 (364)	1.3	19.7 (6.1)
hydrochlorothiazide	834 (177)	135.1 (35.7)	2.0	14.3 (3.8)

where AUC(0–48), Cmax, Tmax and Ae represent area under the plasma concentration versus time plot, maximum plasma concentration, time to reach Cmax and amount excreted in urine over 48 hours.

Dyazide capsule is bioequivalent to a single-entity 25 mg hydrochlorothiazide tablet and 37.5 mg triamterene capsule used in the double-blind clinical trial below. (See Clinical Trials.)

In a limited study involving 12 subjects, coadministration of *Dyazide* with a high-fat meal resulted in: (1) an increase in the mean bioavailability of triamterene by about 67% (90% confidence interval = 0.99, 1.90), p-hydroxytriamterene sulfate by about 50% (90% confidence interval = 1.06, 1.77), hydrochlorothiazide by about 17% (90% confidence interval = 0.90, 1.34); (2) increases in the peak concentrations of triamterene and p-hydroxytriamterene; and (3) a delay of up to 2 hours in the absorption of the active constituents.

Clinical Trials

A placebo-controlled, double-blind trial was conducted to evaluate the efficacy of *Dyazide* capsules. This trial demonstrated that *Dyazide* (25 mg hydrochlorothiazide/37.5 mg triamterene) was effective in controlling blood pressure while reducing the incidence of hydrochlorothiazide-induced hypokalemia. This trial involved 636 patients with mild to moderate hypertension controlled by hydrochlorothiazide 25 mg daily and who had hypokalemia (serum potassium < 3.5 mEq/L) secondary to the hydrochlorothiazide. Patients were randomly assigned to 4 weeks' treatment with once-daily regimens of 25 mg hydrochlorothiazide plus placebo, or 25 mg hydrochlorothiazide combined with one of the following doses of triamterene: 25 mg, 37.5 mg, 50 mg or 75 mg.

Blood pressure and serum potassium were monitored at baseline and throughout the trial. All five treatment groups had similar mean blood pressure and serum potassium concentrations at baseline (mean systolic blood pressure range: 137±14 mmHg to 140±16 mmHg; mean diastolic blood pressure range: 86±9 mmHg to 88±8 mmHg; mean serum potassium range: 2.3 to 3.4 mEq/L with the majority of patients having values between 3.1 and 3.4 mEq/L).

While all triamterene regimens reversed hypokalemia, at week 4 the 37.5 mg regimen proved optimal compared with the other tested regimens. On this regimen, 81% of the patients had a significant ($p < 0.05$) reversal of hypokalemia vs. 59% of patients on the placebo/hydrochlorothiazide regimen. The mean serum potassium concentration on 37.5 mg triamterene went from 3.2±0.2 mEq/L at baseline to 3.7±0.3 mEq/L at week 4, a significantly greater ($p < 0.05$) improvement than that achieved with placebo/hydrochlorothiazide (i.e., 3.2±0.2 mEq/L at baseline and 3.5±0.4 mEq/L at week 4). Also, 51% of patients in the 37.5 mg triamterene group had an increase in serum potassium of ≥0.5 mEq/L at week 4 vs. 33% in the placebo group. The 37.5 mg triamterene/25 mg hydrochlorothiazide regimen also maintained control of blood pressure; mean supine systolic blood pressure at week 4 was 138±21 mmHg while mean supine diastolic blood pressure was 87±13 mmHg.

INDICATIONS AND USAGE

This fixed combination drug is not indicated for the initial therapy of edema or hypertension except in individuals in whom the development of hypokalemia cannot be risked.

Dyazide is indicated for the treatment of hypertension or edema in patients who develop hypokalemia on hydrochlorothiazide alone.

Dyazide is also indicated for those patients who require a thiazide diuretic and in whom the development of hypokalemia cannot be risked.

Dyazide may be used alone or as an adjunct to other antihypertensive drugs, such as beta-blockers. Since *Dyazide* may enhance the action of these agents, dosage adjustments may be necessary.

Usage in Pregnancy: The routine use of diuretics in an otherwise healthy woman is inappropriate and exposes mother and fetus to unnecessary hazard. Diuretics do not prevent development of toxemia of pregnancy, and there is no satisfactory evidence that they are useful in the treatment of developed toxemia.

Continued on next page

Information on the SmithKline Beecham Pharmaceuticals products appearing here is based on the labeling in effect on July 1, 1996. Further information on these and other products may be obtained from the Medical Department, SmithKline Beecham Pharmaceuticals, One Franklin Plaza, Philadelphia, PA 19101.

Consult 1997 supplements and future editions for revisions

SmithKline Beecham—Cont.

Edema during pregnancy may arise from pathological causes or from the physiologic and mechanical consequences of pregnancy. Diuretics are indicated in pregnancy when edema is due to pathologic causes, just as they are in the absence of pregnancy. Dependent edema in pregnancy resulting from restriction of venous return by the expanded uterus is properly treated through elevation of the lower extremities and use of support hose; use of diuretics to lower intravascular volume in this case is illogical and unnecessary. There is hypervolemia during normal pregnancy which is harmful to neither the fetus nor the mother (in the absence of cardiovascular disease), but which is associated with edema, including generalized edema in the majority of pregnant women. If this edema produces discomfort, increased recumbency will often provide relief. In rare instances this edema may cause extreme discomfort which is not relieved by rest. In these cases a short course of diuretics may provide relief and may be appropriate.

CONTRAINDICATIONS

Antikaliuretic Therapy and Potassium Supplementation
Dyazide should not be given to patients receiving other potassium-sparing agents such as spironolactone, amiloride or other formulations containing triamterene. Concomitant potassium-containing salt substitutes should also not be used.

Potassium supplementation should not be used with *Dyazide* except in severe cases of hypokalemia. Such concomitant therapy can be associated with rapid increases in serum potassium levels. If potassium supplementation is used, careful monitoring of the serum potassium level is necessary.

Impaired Renal Function
Dyazide is contraindicated in patients with anuria, acute and chronic renal insufficiency or significant renal impairment.

Hypersensitivity
Hypersensitivity to either drug in the preparation or to other sulfonamide-derived drugs is a contraindication.

Hyperkalemia
Dyazide should not be used in patients with preexisting elevated serum potassium.

WARNINGS: Hyperkalemia

Abnormal elevation of serum potassium levels (greater than or equal to 5.5 mEq/liter) can occur with all potassium-sparing diuretic combinations, including *Dyazide*. Hyperkalemia is more likely to occur in patients with renal impairment and diabetes (even without evidence of renal impairment), and in the elderly or severely ill. Since uncorrected hyperkalemia may be fatal, serum potassium levels must be monitored at frequent intervals especially in patients first receiving *Dyazide*, when dosages are changed or with any illness that may influence renal function.

If hyperkalemia is suspected (warning signs include paresthesias, muscular weakness, fatigue, flaccid paralysis of the extremities, bradycardia and shock), an electrocardiogram (ECG) should be obtained. However, it is important to monitor serum potassium levels because hyperkalemia may not be associated with ECG changes.

If hyperkalemia is present, *Dyazide* should be discontinued immediately and a thiazide alone should be substituted. If the serum potassium exceeds 6.5 mEq/liter more vigorous therapy is required. The clinical situation dictates the procedures to be employed. These include the intravenous administration of calcium chloride solution, sodium bicarbonate solution and/or the oral or parenteral administration of glucose with a rapid-acting insulin preparation. Cationic exchange resins such as sodium polystyrene sulfonate may be orally or rectally administered. Persistent hyperkalemia may require dialysis.

The development of hyperkalemia associated with potassium-sparing diuretics is accentuated in the presence of renal impairment (see CONTRAINDICATIONS section). Patients with mild renal functional impairment should not receive this drug without frequent and continuing monitoring of serum electrolytes. Cumulative drug effects may be observed in patients with impaired renal function. The renal clearances of hydrochlorothiazide and the pharmacologically active metabolite of triamterene, the sulfate ester of hydroxytriamterene, have been shown to be reduced and the plasma levels increased following *Dyazide* administration to elderly patients and patients with impaired renal function. Hyperkalemia has been reported in diabetic patients with the use of potassium-sparing agents even in the absence of apparent renal impairment. Accordingly, serum electrolytes must be frequently monitored if *Dyazide* is used in diabetic patients.

Metabolic or Respiratory Acidosis
Potassium-sparing therapy should also be avoided in severely ill patients in whom respiratory or metabolic acidosis may occur. Acidosis may be associated with rapid elevations

in serum potassium levels. If *Dyazide* is employed, frequent evaluations of acid/base balance and serum electrolytes are necessary.

PRECAUTIONS

Impaired Hepatic Function
Thiazides should be used with caution in patients with impaired hepatic function. They can precipitate hepatic coma in patients with severe liver disease. Potassium depletion induced by the thiazide may be important in this connection. Administer *Dyazide* cautiously and be alert for such early signs of impending coma as confusion, drowsiness and tremor; if mental confusion increases discontinue *Dyazide* for a few days. Attention must be given to other factors that may precipitate hepatic coma, such as blood in the gastrointestinal tract or preexisting potassium depletion.

Hypokalemia
Hypokalemia is uncommon with *Dyazide*; but, should it develop, corrective measures should be taken such as potassium supplementation or increased intake of potassium-rich foods. Institute such measures cautiously with frequent determinations of serum potassium levels, especially in patients receiving digitalis or with a history of cardiac arrhythmias. If serious hypokalemia (serum potassium less than 3.0 mEq/L) is demonstrated by repeat serum potassium determinations, *Dyazide* should be discontinued and potassium chloride supplementation initiated. Less serious hypokalemia should be evaluated with regard to other coexisting conditions and treated accordingly.

Electrolyte Imbalance
Electrolyte imbalance, often encountered in such conditions as heart failure, renal disease or cirrhosis of the liver, may also be aggravated by diuretics and should be considered during *Dyazide* therapy when using high doses for prolonged periods or in patients on a salt-restricted diet. Serum determinations of electrolytes should be performed, and are particularly important if the patient is vomiting excessively or receiving fluids parenterally. Possible fluid and electrolyte imbalance may be indicated by such warning signs as: dry mouth, thirst, weakness, lethargy, drowsiness, restlessness, muscle pain or cramps, muscular fatigue, hypotension, oliguria, tachycardia and gastrointestinal symptoms.

Hypochloremia
Although any chloride deficit is generally mild and usually does not require specific treatment except under extraordinary circumstances (as in liver disease or renal disease), chloride replacement may be required in the treatment of metabolic alkalosis. Dilutional hyponatremia may occur in edematous patients in hot weather; appropriate therapy is water restriction, rather than administration of salt, except in rare instances when the hyponatremia is life threatening. In actual salt depletion, appropriate replacement is the therapy of choice.

Renal Stones
Triamterene has been found in renal stones in association with the other usual calculus components. *Dyazide* should be used with caution in patients with a history of renal stones.

Laboratory Tests
Serum Potassium: The normal adult range of serum potassium is 3.5 to 5.0 mEq per liter with 4.5 mEq often being used for a reference point. If hypokalemia should develop, corrective measures should be taken such as potassium supplementation or increased dietary intake of potassium-rich foods. Institute such measures cautiously with frequent determinations of serum potassium levels. Potassium levels persistently above 6 mEq per liter require careful observation and treatment. Serum potassium levels do not necessarily indicate true body potassium concentration. A rise in plasma pH may cause a decrease in plasma potassium concentration and an increase in the intracellular potassium concentration. Discontinue corrective measures for hypokalemia immediately if laboratory determinations reveal an abnormal elevation of serum potassium. Discontinue *Dyazide* and substitute a thiazide diuretic alone until potassium levels return to normal.

Serum Creatinine and BUN: *Dyazide* may produce an elevated blood urea nitrogen level, creatinine level or both. This apparently is secondary to a reversible reduction of glomerular filtration rate or a depletion of intravascular fluid volume (prerenal azotemia) rather than renal toxicity; levels usually return to normal when *Dyazide* is discontinued. If azotemia increases, discontinue *Dyazide*. Periodic BUN or serum creatinine determinations should be made, especially in elderly patients and in patients with suspected or confirmed renal insufficiency.

Serum PBI: Thiazide may decrease serum PBI levels without sign of thyroid disturbance.

Parathyroid Function: Thiazides should be discontinued before carrying out tests for parathyroid function. Calcium excretion is decreased by thiazides. Pathologic changes in the parathyroid glands with hypercalcemia and hypophosphatemia have been observed in a few patients on prolonged thiazide therapy. The common complications of hyperparathyroidism such as bone resorption and peptic ulceration have not been seen.

Drug Interactions
Angiotensin-converting enzyme inhibitors: Potassium-sparing agents should be used with caution in conjunction with angiotensin-converting enzyme (ACE) inhibitors due to an increased risk of hyperkalemia.

Oral hypoglycemic drugs: Concurrent use with chlorpropamide may increase the risk of severe hyponatremia.

Nonsteroidal anti-inflammatory drugs: A possible interaction resulting in acute renal failure has been reported in a few patients on *Dyazide* when treated with indomethacin, a nonsteroidal anti-inflammatory agent. Caution is advised in administering nonsteroidal anti-inflammatory agents with *Dyazide*.

Lithium: Lithium generally should not be given with diuretics because they reduce its renal clearance and increase the risk of lithium toxicity. Read circulars for lithium preparations before use of such concomitant therapy with *Dyazide*.

Surgical considerations: Thiazides have been shown to decrease arterial responsiveness to norepinephrine (an effect attributed to loss of sodium). This diminution is not sufficient to preclude effectiveness of the pressor agent for therapeutic use. Thiazides have also been shown to increase the paralyzing effect of nondepolarizing muscle relaxants such as tubocurarine (an effect attributed to potassium loss); consequently caution should be observed in patients undergoing surgery.

Other Considerations: Concurrent use of hydrochlorothiazide with amphotericin B or corticosteroids or corticotropin (ACTH) may intensify electrolyte imbalance, particularly hypokalemia, although the presence of triamterene minimizes the hypokalemic effect.

Thiazides may add to or potentiate the action of other antihypertensive drugs. See INDICATIONS AND USAGE for concomitant use with other antihypertensive drugs.

The effect of oral anticoagulants may be decreased when used concurrently with hydrochlorothiazide; dosage adjustments may be necessary.

Dyazide may raise the level of blood uric acid; dosage adjustments of antigout medication may be necessary to control hyperuricemia and gout.

The following agents given together with triamterene may promote serum potassium accumulation and possibly result in hyperkalemia because of the potassium-sparing nature of triamterene, especially in patients with renal insufficiency: blood from blood bank (may contain up to 30 mEq of potassium per liter of plasma or up to 65 mEq per liter of whole blood when stored for more than 10 days); low-salt milk (may contain up to 60 mEq of potassium per liter); potassium-containing medications (such as parenteral penicillin G potassium); salt substitutes (most contain substantial amounts of potassium).

Exchange resins, such as sodium polystyrene sulfonate, whether administered orally or rectally, reduce serum potassium levels by sodium replacement of the potassium; fluid retention may occur in some patients because of the increased sodium intake.

Chronic or overuse of laxatives may reduce serum potassium levels by promoting excessive potassium loss from the intestinal tract; laxatives may interfere with the potassium-retaining effects of triamterene.

The effectiveness of methenamine may be decreased when used concurrently with hydrochlorothiazide because of alkalinization of the urine.

Drug/Laboratory Test Interactions
Triamterene and quinidine have similar fluorescence spectra; thus, *Dyazide* will interfere with the fluorescent measurement of quinidine.

Carcinogenesis, Mutagenesis, Impairment of Fertility
Carcinogenesis
Long-term studies have not been conducted with *Dyazide* (the triamterene/hydrochlorothiazide combination), or with triamterene alone.

Hydrochlorothiazide: Two-year feeding studies in mice and rats, conducted under the auspices of the National Toxicology Program (NTP), treated mice and rats with doses of hydrochlorothiazide up to 600 and 100 mg/kg/day, respectively. On a body-weight basis, these doses are 600 times (in mice) and 100 times (in rats) the Maximum Recommended Human Dose (MRHD) for the hydrochlorothiazide component of *Dyazide* at 50 mg/day (or 1.0 mg/kg/day based on 50 kg individuals). On the basis of body-surface area, these doses are 56 times (in mice) and 21 times (in rats) the MRHD. These studies uncovered no evidence of carcinogenic potential of hydrochlorothiazide in rats or female mice, but there was equivocal evidence of hepatocarcinogenicity in male mice.

Mutagenesis
Studies of the mutagenic potential of *Dyazide* (the triamterene/hydrochlorothiazide combination), or of triamterene alone have not been performed.

Hydrochlorothiazide: Hydrochlorothiazide was not genotoxic in in vitro assays using strains TA 98, TA 100, TA 1535, TA 1537 and TA 1538 of *Salmonella typhimurium* (the Ames test); in the Chinese Hamster Ovary (CHO) test for chromosomal aberrations; or in in vivo assays using mouse germinal cell chromosomes, Chinese hamster bone marrow chromo-

somes, and the *Drosophila* sex-linked recessive lethal trait gene. Positive test results were obtained in the *in vitro* CHO Sister Chromatid Exchange (clastogenicity) test, and in the mouse Lymphoma Cell (mutagenicity) assays, using concentrations of hydrochlorothiazide of 43 to 1300 mcg/mL. Positive test results were also obtained in the *Aspergillus nidulans* nondisjunction assay, using an unspecified concentration of hydrochlorothiazide.

Impairment of Fertility
Studies of the effects of *Dyazide* (the triamterene/hydrochlorothiazide combination), or of triamterene alone on animal reproductive function have not been conducted.
Hydrochlorothiazide: Hydrochlorothiazide had no adverse effects on the fertility of mice and rats of either sex in studies wherein these species were exposed, via their diet, to doses of up to 100 and 4 mg/kg/day, respectively, prior to mating and throughout gestation. Corresponding multiples of the MRHD are 100 (mice) and 4 (rats) on the basis of body-weight and 9.4 (mice) and 0.8 (rats) on the basis of body-surface area.

Pregnancy: Category C
Teratogenic Effects
Dyazide: Animal reproduction studies to determine the potential for fetal harm by *Dyazide* have not been conducted. However, a One Generation Study in the rat approximated *Dyazide* composition by using a 1:1 ratio of triamterene to hydrochlorothiazide (30:30 mg/kg/day); there was no evidence of teratogenicity at those doses which were, on a body-weight basis, 15 and 30 times, respectively, the MRHD, and on the basis of body-surface area, 3.1 and 6.2 times, respectively, the MRHD.
The safe use of *Dyazide* in pregnancy has not been established since there are no adequate and well-controlled studies with *Dyazide* in pregnant women. *Dyazide* should be used during pregnancy only if the potential benefit justifies the risk to the fetus.
Triamterene: Reproduction studies have been performed in rats at doses as high as 20 times the MRHD on the basis of body-weight, and 6 times the human dose on the basis of body-surface area without evidence of harm to the fetus due to triamterene.
Because animal reproduction studies are not always predictive of human response, this drug should be used during pregnancy only if clearly needed.
Hydrochlorothiazide: Hydrochlorothiazide was orally administered to pregnant mice and rats during respective periods of major organogenesis at doses up to 3000 and 1000 mg/kg/day, respectively. At these doses, which are multiples of the MRHD equal to 3000 for mice and 1000 for rats, based on body-weight, and equal to 282 for mice and 206 for rats, based on body-surface area, there was no evidence of harm to the fetus.
There are, however, no adequate and well-controlled studies in pregnant women. Because animal reproduction studies are not always predictive of human response, this drug should be used during pregnancy only if clearly needed.
Nonteratogenic Effects—Thiazides and triamterene have been shown to cross the placental barrier and appear in cord blood. The use of thiazides and triamterene in pregnant women requires that the anticipated benefit be weighed against possible hazards to the fetus. These hazards include fetal or neonatal jaundice, pancreatitis, thrombocytopenia and possible other adverse reactions which have occurred in the adult.
Nursing Mothers—Thiazides and triamterene in combination have not been studied in nursing mothers. Triamterene appears in animal milk; this may occur in humans. Thiazides are excreted in human breast milk. If use of the combination drug product is deemed essential, the patient should stop nursing.
Pediatric Use—Safety and effectiveness in children have not been established.

ADVERSE REACTIONS
Adverse effects are listed in decreasing order of frequency; however, the most serious adverse effects are listed first regardless of frequency. The serious adverse effects associated with *Dyazide* have commonly occurred in less than 0.1% of patients treated with this product.
Hypersensitivity: anaphylaxis, rash, urticaria, photosensitivity.
Cardiovascular: arrhythmia, postural hypotension.
Metabolic: diabetes mellitus, hyperkalemia, hyperglycemia, glycosuria, hyperuricemia, hypokalemia, hyponatremia, acidosis, hypochloremia.
Gastrointestinal: jaundice and/or liver enzyme abnormalities, pancreatitis, nausea and vomiting, diarrhea, constipation, abdominal pain.
Renal: acute renal failure (one case of irreversible renal failure has been reported), interstitial nephritis, renal stones composed primarily of triamterene, elevated BUN and serum creatinine, abnormal urinary sediment.
Hematologic: leukopenia, thrombocytopenia and purpura, megaloblastic anemia.
Musculoskeletal: muscle cramps.
Central Nervous System: weakness, fatigue, dizziness, headache, dry mouth.

Miscellaneous: impotence, sialadenitis.
Thiazides alone have been shown to cause the following additional adverse reactions:
Central Nervous System: paresthesias, vertigo.
Ophthalmic: xanthopsia, transient blurred vision.
Respiratory: allergic pneumonitis, pulmonary edema, respiratory distress.
Other: necrotizing vasculitis, exacerbation of lupus.
Hematologic: aplastic anemia, agranulocytosis, hemolytic anemia.
Neonate and infancy: thrombocytopenia and pancreatitis—rarely, in newborns whose mothers have received thiazides during pregnancy.

DOSAGE AND ADMINISTRATION
The usual dose of *Dyazide* is one or two capsules given once daily, with appropriate monitoring of serum potassium and of the clinical effect. (See WARNINGS, Hyperkalemia.)

OVERDOSAGE
Electrolyte imbalance is the major concern (see WARNINGS section). Symptoms reported include: polyuria, nausea, vomiting, weakness, lassitude, fever, flushed face and hyperactive deep tendon reflexes. If hypotension occurs, it may be treated with pressor agents such as levarterenol to maintain blood pressure. Carefully evaluate the electrolyte pattern and fluid balance. Induce immediate evacuation of the stomach through emesis or gastric lavage. There is no specific antidote.
Reversible acute renal failure following ingestion of 50 tablets of a product containing a combination of 50 mg triamterene and 25 mg hydrochlorothiazide has been reported. Although triamterene is largely protein-bound (approximately 67%), there may be some benefit to dialysis in cases of overdosage.

HOW SUPPLIED
Capsules containing 25 mg hydrochlorothiazide and 37.5 mg triamterene, in bottles of 1000 capsules; in Single Unit Packages (unit-dose) of 100 (intended for institutional use only); in Patient-Pak™ unit-of-use bottles of 100.
They are supplied as follows:
NDC 0007-3650-21—Single Unit Packages (unit-dose) of 100 (intended for institutional use only).
NDC 0007-3650-22—in Patient-Pak™ unit-of-use bottles of 100.
NDC 0007-3650-30—bottles of 1000.
Store between 15° and 30°C (59° and 86°F). Protect from light. Dispense in a tight, light-resistant container.
Veterans Administration/Military/PHS—Capsules, 100's (SUP), 6505-01-390-0308; 100's, 6505-01-390-0348; 1000's, 6505-01-390-0358.
DZ:L65A
Shown in Product Identification Guide, page 336

DYRENIUM® ℞
[*di-ren'ee-um*]
brand of triamterene
Capsules
50 mg and 100 mg
potassium-sparing diuretic

DESCRIPTION
Dyrenium (triamterene) is a potassium-sparing diuretic. Triamterene is 2,4,7-triamino-6-phenyl-pteridine. Its molecular weight is 253.27. At 50°C, triamterene is slightly soluble in water. It is soluble in dilute ammonia, dilute aqueous sodium hydroxide and dimethylformamide. It is sparingly soluble in methanol.
Each capsule for oral use, with opaque red cap and body, contains triamterene, 50 or 100 mg, and is imprinted with the product name DYRENIUM, strength (50 or 100) and SKF. Inactive ingredients consist of benzyl alcohol, cetylpyridinium chloride, D&C Red No. 33, FD&C Yellow No. 6, gelatin, lactose, magnesium stearate, povidone, sodium lauryl sulfate, titanium dioxide and trace amounts of other inactive ingredients.

CLINICAL PHARMACOLOGY
Triamterene has a unique mode of action; it inhibits the reabsorption of sodium ions in exchange for potassium and hydrogen ions at that segment of the distal tubule under the control of adrenal mineralocorticoids (especially aldosterone). This activity is not directly related to aldosterone secretion or antagonism; it is a result of a direct effect on the renal tubule.
The fraction of filtered sodium reaching this distal tubular exchange site is relatively small, and the amount which is exchanged depends on the level of mineralocorticoid activity. Thus, the degree of natriuresis and diuresis produced by inhibition of the exchange mechanism is necessarily limited. Increasing the amount of available sodium and the level of mineralocorticoid activity by the use of more proximally acting diuretics will increase the degree of diuresis and potassium conservation.

Triamterene occasionally causes increases in serum potassium which can result in hyperkalemia. It does not produce alkalosis because it does not cause excessive excretion of titratable acid and ammonium.
Triamterene has been shown to cross the placental barrier and appear in the cord blood of animals.

Pharmacokinetics
Onset of action is 2 to 4 hours after ingestion. In normal volunteers the mean peak serum levels were 30 ng/mL at 3 hours. The average percent of drug recovered in the urine (0 to 48 hours) was 21%. Triamterene is primarily metabolized to the sulfate conjugate of hydroxytriamterene. Both the plasma and urine levels of this metabolite greatly exceed triamterene levels. Triamterene is rapidly absorbed, with somewhat less than 50% of the oral dose reaching the urine. Most patients will respond to Dyrenium (triamterene) during the first day of treatment. Maximum therapeutic effect, however, may not be seen for several days. Duration of diuresis depends on several factors, especially renal function, but it generally tapers off 7 to 9 hours after administration.

INDICATIONS AND USAGE
Dyrenium (triamterene) is indicated in the treatment of edema associated with congestive heart failure, cirrhosis of the liver, and the nephrotic syndrome; also in steroid-induced edema, idiopathic edema and edema due to secondary hyperaldosteronism.
Dyrenium may be used alone or with other diuretics either for its added diuretic effect or its potassium-sparing potential. It also promotes increased diuresis when patients prove resistant or only partially responsive to thiazides or other diuretics because of secondary hyperaldosteronism.
Usage in Pregnancy. The routine use of diuretics in an otherwise healthy woman is inappropriate and exposes mother and fetus to unnecessary hazard. Diuretics do not prevent development of toxemia of pregnancy, and there is no satisfactory evidence that they are useful in the treatment of developed toxemia.
Edema during pregnancy may arise from pathological causes or from the physiologic and mechanical consequences of pregnancy. Diuretics are indicated in pregnancy when edema is due to pathologic causes, just as they are in the absence of pregnancy (however, see PRECAUTIONS below). Dependent edema in pregnancy, resulting from restriction of venous return by the expanded uterus, is properly treated through elevation of the lower extremities and use of support hose; use of diuretics to lower intravascular volume in this case is illogical and unnecessary. There is hypervolemia during normal pregnancy which is harmful to neither the fetus nor the mother (in the absence of cardiovascular disease), but which is associated with edema, including generalized edema, in the majority of pregnant women. If this edema produces discomfort, increased recumbency will often provide relief. In rare instances, this edema may cause extreme discomfort which is not relieved by rest. In these cases, a short course of diuretics may provide relief and may be appropriate.

CONTRAINDICATIONS
Anuria. Severe or progressive kidney disease or dysfunction with the possible exception of nephrosis. Severe hepatic disease. Hypersensitivity to the drug.
Dyrenium (triamterene) should not be used in patients with pre-existing elevated serum potassium, as is sometimes seen in patients with impaired renal function or azotemia, or in patients who develop hyperkalemia while on the drug. Patients should not be placed on dietary potassium supplements, potassium salts or potassium-containing salt substitutes in conjunction with *Dyrenium*.
Dyrenium should not be given to patients receiving other potassium-sparing agents such as spironolactone, amiloride hydrochloride or other formulations containing triamterene. Two deaths have been reported in patients receiving concomitant spironolactone and *Dyrenium* or Dyazide®. Although dosage recommendations were exceeded in one case and in the other serum electrolytes were not properly monitored, these two drugs should not be given concomitantly.

WARNINGS

Abnormal elevation of serum potassium levels (greater than or equal to 5.5 mEq/liter) can occur with all potassium-sparing agents, including *Dyrenium*. Hyperkalemia is more likely to occur in patients with renal impairment and diabetes (even without evidence of renal impairment), and in the elderly or severely ill. Since

Continued on next page

Information on the SmithKline Beecham Pharmaceuticals products appearing here is based on the labeling in effect on July 1, 1996. Further information on these and other products may be obtained from the Medical Department, SmithKline Beecham Pharmaceuticals, One Franklin Plaza, Philadelphia, PA 19101.

SmithKline Beecham—Cont.

uncorrected hyperkalemia may be fatal, serum potassium levels must be monitored at frequent intervals especially in patients receiving *Dyrenium*, when dosages are changed or with any illness that may influence renal function.

There have been isolated reports of hypersensitivity reactions; therefore, patients should be observed regularly for the possible occurrence of blood dyscrasias, liver damage or other idiosyncratic reactions.

Periodic BUN and serum potassium determinations should be made to check kidney function, especially in patients with suspected or confirmed renal insufficiency. It is particularly important to make serum potassium determinations in elderly or diabetic patients receiving the drug; these patients should be observed carefully for possible serum potassium increases.

If hyperkalemia is present or suspected, an electrocardiogram should be obtained. If the ECG shows no widening of the QRS or arrhythmia in the presence of hyperkalemia, it is usually sufficient to discontinue Dyrenium (triamterene) and any potassium supplementation and substitute a thiazide alone. Sodium polystyrene sulfonate (Kayexalate®, Winthrop) may be administered to enhance the excretion of excess potassium. **The presence of a widened QRS complex or arrhythmia in association with hyperkalemia requires prompt additional therapy.** For tachyarrhythmia, infuse 44 mEq of sodium bicarbonate or 10 mL of 10% calcium gluconate or calcium chloride over several minutes. For asystole, bradycardia or A-V block transvenous pacing is also recommended.

The effect of calcium and sodium bicarbonate is transient and repeated administration may be required. When indicated by the clinical situation, excess K^+ may be removed by dialysis or oral or rectal administration of Kayexalate®. Infusion of glucose and insulin has also been used to treat hyperkalemia.

PRECAUTIONS
General
Dyrenium (triamterene) tends to conserve potassium rather than to promote the excretion as do many diuretics and, occasionally, can cause increases in serum potassium which, in some instances, can result in hyperkalemia. In rare instances, hyperkalemia has been associated with cardiac irregularities.

Electrolyte imbalance often encountered in such diseases as congestive heart failure, renal disease or cirrhosis may be aggravated or caused independently by any effective diuretic agent including *Dyrenium*. The use of full doses of a diuretic when salt intake is restricted can result in a low-salt syndrome.

Triamterene can cause mild nitrogen retention which is reversible upon withdrawal of the drug and is seldom observed with intermittent (every-other-day) therapy.

Triamterene may cause a decreasing alkali reserve with the possibility of metabolic acidosis.

By the very nature of their illness, cirrhotics with splenomegaly sometimes have marked variations in their blood pictures. Since triamterene is a weak folic acid antagonist, it may contribute to the appearance of megaloblastosis in cases where folic acid stores have been depleted. Therefore, periodic blood studies in these patients are recommended. They should also be observed for exacerbations of underlying liver disease.

Triamterene has elevated uric acid, especially in persons predisposed to gouty arthritis.

Triamterene has been reported in renal stones in association with other calculus components. *Dyrenium* should be used with caution in patients with histories of renal stones.

Information for Patients
To help avoid stomach upset, it is recommended that the drug be taken after meals.

If a single daily dose is prescribed, it may be preferable to take it in the morning to minimize the effect of increased frequency of urination on nighttime sleep.

If a dose is missed, the patient should not take more than the prescribed dose at the next dosing interval.

Laboratory Tests
Hyperkalemia will rarely occur in patients with adequate urinary output, but it is a possibility if large doses are used for considerable periods of time. If hyperkalemia is observed, Dyrenium (triamterene) should be withdrawn. The normal adult range of serum potassium is 3.5 to 5.0 mEq per liter with 4.5 mEq often being used for a reference point. Potassium levels persistently above 6 mEq per liter require careful observation and treatment. Normal potassium levels tend to be higher in neonates (7.7 mEq per liter) than in adults. Serum potassium levels do not necessarily indicate true body potassium concentration. A rise in plasma pH may cause a decrease in plasma potassium concentration and an increase in the intracellular potassium concentration. Because *Dyrenium* conserves potassium, it has been theorized that in

patients who have received intensive therapy or been given the drug for prolonged periods, a rebound kaliuresis could occur upon abrupt withdrawal. In such patients withdrawal of *Dyrenium* should be gradual.

Drug Interactions
Caution should be used when lithium and diuretics are used concomitantly because diuretic-induced sodium loss may reduce the renal clearance of lithium and increase serum lithium levels with risk of lithium toxicity. Patients receiving such combined therapy should have serum lithium levels monitored closely and the lithium dosage adjusted if necessary.

A possible interaction resulting in acute renal failure has been reported in a few subjects when indomethacin, a nonsteroidal anti-inflammatory agent, was given with triamterene. Caution is advised in administering nonsteroidal anti-inflammatory agents with triamterene.

The effects of the following drugs may be potentiated when given together with triamterene: antihypertensive medication, other diuretics, preanesthetic and anesthetic agents, skeletal muscle relaxants (nondepolarizing).

Potassium-sparing agents should be used with caution in conjunction with angiotensin-converting enzyme (ACE) inhibitors due to an increased risk of hyperkalemia.

The following agents, given together with triamterene, may promote serum potassium accumulation and possibly result in hyperkalemia because of the potassium-sparing nature of triamterene, especially in patients with renal insufficiency: blood from blood bank (may contain up to 30 mEq of potassium per liter of plasma or up to 65 mEq per liter of whole blood when stored for more than 10 days); low-salt milk (may contain up to 60 mEq of potassium per liter); potassium-containing medications (such as parenteral penicillin G potassium); salt substitutes (most contain substantial amounts of potassium).

Dyrenium (triamterene) may raise blood glucose levels; for adult-onset diabetes, dosage adjustments of hypoglycemic agents may be necessary during and after therapy; concurrent use with chlorpropamide may increase the risk of severe hyponatremia.

Drug/Laboratory Test Interactions
Triamterene and quinidine have similar fluorescence spectra; thus, triamterene will interfere with the fluorescent measurement of quinidine.

Carcinogenesis, Mutagenesis, Impairment of Fertility
Long-term studies to determine the carcinogenic potential of triamterene are not available. Studies to determine the mutagenic potential of triamterene are not available. Reproductive studies have been performed in rats at doses up to 30 times the human dose and have revealed no evidence of impaired fertility.

Pregnancy
Teratogenic Effects: Pregnancy Category B: Reproduction studies have been performed in rats at doses up to 30 times the human dose and have revealed no evidence of impaired fertility or harm to the fetus due to triamterene. There are, however, no adequate and well-controlled studies in pregnant women. Because animal reproductive studies are not always predictive of human response, this drug should be used during pregnancy only if clearly needed.

Nonteratogenic Effects: Triamterene has been shown to cross the placental barrier and appear in the cord blood of animals; this may occur in humans. The use of *Dyrenium* in pregnant women requires that the anticipated benefit be weighed against possible hazards to the fetus. These possible hazards include adverse reactions which have occurred in the adult.

Nursing Mothers: Triamterene appears in animal milk; this may occur in humans. If use of the drug is deemed essential, the patient should stop nursing.

Pediatric Use: Safety and effectiveness in children have not been established.

ADVERSE REACTIONS
Adverse effects are listed in decreasing order of frequency; however, the most serious adverse effects are listed first regardless of frequency. All adverse effects occur rarely (that is, 1 in 1000, or less).

Hypersensitivity: anaphylaxis, rash, photosensitivity.

Metabolic: hyperkalemia, hypokalemia.

Renal: azotemia, elevated BUN and creatinine, renal stones, acute interstitial nephritis (rare), acute renal failure (one case of irreversible renal failure has been reported).

Gastrointestinal: jaundice and/or liver enzyme abnormalities, nausea and vomiting, diarrhea.

Hematologic: thrombocytopenia, megaloblastic anemia.

Central Nervous System: weakness, fatigue, dizziness, headache, dry mouth.

OVERDOSAGE
In the event of overdosage it can be theorized that electrolyte imbalance would be the major concern, with particular attention to possible hyperkalemia. Other symptoms that might be seen would be nausea and vomiting, other G.I. disturbances and weakness. It is conceivable that some hypotension could occur. As with an overdose of any drug, imme-

diate evacuation of the stomach should be induced through emesis and gastric lavage. Careful evaluation of the electrolyte pattern and fluid balance should be made. There is no specific antidote.

Reversible acute renal failure following ingestion of 50 tablets of a product containing a combination of 50 mg triamterene and 25 mg hydrochlorothiazide has been reported. The oral LD_{50} in mice is 380 mg/kg. The amount of drug in a single dose ordinarily associated with symptoms of overdose or likely to be life-threatening is not known.

Although triamterene is 67% protein-bound, there may be some benefit to dialysis in cases of overdosage.

DOSAGE AND ADMINISTRATION
Adult Dosage
Dosage should be titrated to the needs of the individual patient. When used alone, the usual starting dose is 100 mg twice daily after meals. When combined with another diuretic or antihypertensive agent, the total daily dosage of each agent should usually be lowered initially and then adjusted to the patient's needs. The total daily dosage should not exceed 300 mg. Please refer to PRECAUTIONS-General. When Dyrenium (triamterene) is added to other diuretic therapy or when patients are switched to *Dyrenium* from other diuretics, all potassium supplementation should be discontinued.

HOW SUPPLIED
Capsules: 50 mg in bottles of 100 and 100 mg in bottles of 100. Store between 15° and 30°C (59° and 86°F).
Protect from light.
50 mg 100's: NDC 0108-3806-20
100 mg 100's: NDC 0108-3807-20
Veterans Administration/Military/PHS—Capsules, 50 mg, 100's, 6505-01-058-5726; 100 mg, 100's, 6505-00-982-9143.
DY:L42

Shown in Product Identification Guide, page 336

ENGERIX-B®
[en 'jur-ix bee]
Hepatitis B Vaccine (Recombinant)

℞

DESCRIPTION
Engerix-B [Hepatitis B Vaccine (Recombinant)] is a noninfectious recombinant DNA hepatitis B vaccine developed and manufactured by SmithKline Beecham Biologicals. It contains purified surface antigen of the virus obtained by culturing genetically engineered *Saccharomyces cerevisiae* cells, which carry the surface antigen gene of the hepatitis B virus. The surface antigen expressed in *Saccharomyces cerevisiae* cells is purified by several physicochemical steps and formulated as a suspension of the antigen adsorbed on aluminum hydroxide. The procedures used to manufacture *Engerix-B* result in a product that contains no more than 5% yeast protein. No substances of human origin are used in its manufacture.

Engerix-B is supplied as a sterile suspension for intramuscular administration. The vaccine is ready for use without reconstitution; it must be shaken before administration since a fine white deposit with a clear colorless supernatant may form on storage.

Each 1 mL of vaccine consists of 20 mcg of hepatitis B surface antigen adsorbed on 0.5 mg aluminum as aluminum hydroxide. Each 0.5 mL of vaccine consists of 10 mcg of hepatitis B surface antigen adsorbed on 0.25 mg aluminum as aluminum hydroxide. Both formulations contain 1:20,000 thimerosal (mercury derivative) as a preservative, sodium chloride (9 mg/mL) and phosphate buffers (disodium phosphate dihydrate, 0.98 mg/mL; sodium dihydrogen phosphate dihydrate, 0.71 mg/mL).

CLINICAL PHARMACOLOGY
Several hepatitis viruses are known to cause a systemic infection resulting in major pathologic changes in the liver (e.g., A, B, C, D, E). The estimated lifetime risk of HBV infection in the United States varies from almost 100% for the highest-risk groups to approximately 5% for the population as a whole.[1] Hepatitis B infection can have serious consequences including acute massive hepatic necrosis, chronic active hepatitis and cirrhosis of the liver. Sixty to 80% of neonates and 6 to 10% of adults who are infected in the United States will become hepatitis B virus carriers.[1] It has been estimated that more than 170 million people in the world today are persistently infected with hepatitis B virus.[2] The Centers for Disease Control (CDC) estimates that there are approximately 0.75 to 1.0 million chronic carriers of hepatitis B virus in the United States.[1] Those patients who become chronic carriers can infect others and are at increased risk of developing primary hepatocellular carcinoma. Among other factors, infection with hepatitis B may be the single most important factor for development of this carcinoma.[1,3] Considering the serious consequences of infection, immunization should be considered for all persons at potential risk of exposure to the hepatitis B virus. Mothers infected with hepatitis B virus can infect their infants at, or

shortly after, birth if they are carriers of the HBsAg antigen or develop an active infection during the third trimester of pregnancy. Infected infants usually become chronic carriers. Therefore, screening of pregnant women for hepatitis B is recommended.[1] Because a vaccination strategy limited to high-risk individuals has failed to substantially lower the overall incidence of hepatitis B infection, both the Immunization Practices Advisory Committee (ACIP) and the Committee on Infectious Diseases of the American Academy of Pediatrics (AAP) have endorsed universal infant immunization as part of a comprehensive strategy for the control of hepatitis B infection.[4,5] These advisory groups further recommend broad-based vaccination of adolescents. The ACIP encourages universal hepatitis B vaccination of adolescents in communities where use of illicit injectable drugs, pregnancy among teenagers, and/or sexually transmitted diseases are common.[4] Similarly, the AAP recommends that universal immunization of all adolescents should be implemented when resources permit with emphasis on those individuals in high-risk settings.[5] (See INDICATIONS AND USAGE.) There is no specific treatment for acute hepatitis B infection. However, those who develop anti-HBs antibodies after active infection are usually protected against subsequent infection. Antibody titers ≥10 mIU/mL against HBsAg are recognized as conferring protection against hepatitis B.[6] Seroconversion is defined as antibody titers ≥1 mIU/mL.

Immunogenicity in Healthy Adults and Adolescents: Clinical trials in healthy adult and adolescent subjects have shown that following a course of three doses of 20 mcg *Engerix-B* given according to the ACIP recommended schedule of injections at months 0, 1 and 6, the seroprotection (antibody titers ≥10 mIU/mL) rate for all individuals was 79% at month 6 and 96% at month 7; the geometric mean antibody titer (GMT) for seroconverters at month 7 was 2,204 mIU/mL. On an alternate schedule (injections at months 0, 1 and 2) designed for certain populations (e.g., neonates born of hepatitis B infected mothers, individuals who have or might have been recently exposed to the virus, and certain travelers to high-risk areas. See INDICATIONS AND USAGE.), 99% of all individuals were seroprotected at month 3 and remained protected through month 12. On the alternate schedule, an additional dose at 12 months produced a GMT for seroconverters at month 13 of 9,163 mIU/mL.

Immunogenicity in Adolescents: In clinical trials with healthy adolescent subjects 11 through 19 years of age, immunization with 10 mcg using a 0, 1, 6-month schedule produced a seroprotection rate of 97% at month 8 (N=119) with a GMT of 1,989 mIU/mL (N=118, 95% confidence intervals=1,318–3,020). Immunization with 20 mcg using a 0, 1, 6-month schedule produced a seroprotection rate of 99% at month 8 (N=122) with a GMT of 7,672 mIU/mL (N=122, 95% confidence intervals=5,248–10,965).

Immunogenicity in Neonates: Immunization with 10 mcg at 0, 1 and 2 months of age produced a seroprotection rate of 96% in infants by month 4, with a GMT among seroconverters of 210 mIU/mL (N=311); an additional dose at month 12 produced a GMT among seroconverters of 2,941 mIU/mL at month 13 (N=126).

Immunization with 10 mcg at 0, 1 and 6 months of age produced seroconversion in 100% of infants by month 7 with a GMT of 713 mIU/mL (N=52), and the seroprotection rate was 97%.

Clinical trials indicate that administration of hepatitis B immune globulin at birth does not alter the response to *Engerix-B.*

Immunogenicity in Children: In clinical trials with 242 children ages 6 months to, and including, 10 years given 10 mcg at months 0, 1 and 6, the seroprotection rate was 98% 1 to 2 months after the third dose; the GMT of seroconverters was 4,023 mIU/mL.

Immunogenicity in Older Subjects: Among older subjects given 20 mcg at months 0, 1 and 6, the seroprotection rate 1 month after the third dose was 88%. However, as with other hepatitis B vaccines, in adults over 40 years of age, *Engerix-B* vaccine produced anti-HBs titers that were lower than those in younger adults (GMT among seroconverters 1 month after the third 20 mcg dose with a 0, 1, 6-month schedule: 610 mIU/mL for individuals over 40 years of age, N=50).

Hemodialysis Patients: Hemodialysis patients given hepatitis B vaccines respond with lower titers,[7] which remain at protective levels for shorter durations than in normal subjects. In a study in which patients on chronic hemodialysis (mean time on dialysis was 24 months; N=562) received 40 mcg of the plasma-derived vaccine at months 0, 1 and 6, approximately 50% of patients achieved antibody titers ≥10 mIU/mL.[7] Since a fourth dose of *Engerix-B* given to healthy adults at month 12 following the 0, 1, 2-month schedule resulted in a substantial increase in the GMT (see above), a four-dose regimen was studied in hemodialysis patients. In a clinical trial of adults who had been on hemodialysis for a mean of 56 months (N=43), 67% of patients were seroprotected 2 months after the last dose of 40 mcg of *Engerix-B* (two × 20 mcg) given on a 0, 1, 2, 6-month schedule; the GMT among seroconverters was 93 mIU/mL.

Protective Efficacy: Protective efficacy with *Engerix-B* has been demonstrated in a clinical trial in neonates at high risk of hepatitis B infection.[8,9] Fifty-eight neonates born of mothers who were both HBsAg and HBeAg positive were given *Engerix-B* (10 mcg at 0, 1 and 2 months) without concomitant hepatitis B immune globulin. Two infants became chronic carriers in the 12-month follow-up period after initial inoculation. Assuming an expected carrier rate of 70%,[1] the protective efficacy rate against the chronic carrier state during the first 12 months of life was 95%.

Other Clinical Studies: In one study,[10] four of 244 (1.6%) adults (homosexual men) at high risk of contracting hepatitis B virus became infected during the period prior to completion of three doses of *Engerix-B* (20 mcg at 0, 1, 6 months). No additional patients became infected during the 18-month follow-up period after completion of the immunization course.

Interchangeability with Other Hepatitis B Vaccines: Recombinant DNA vaccines are produced in yeast by expression of a hepatitis B virus gene sequence that codes for the hepatitis B surface antigen. Like plasma-derived vaccine, the yeast-derived vaccines are protein particles visible by electron microscopy and have hepatitis B surface antigen epitopes as determined by monoclonal antibody analyses. Yeast-derived vaccines have been shown by *in vitro* analyses to induce antibodies (anti-HBs) which are immunologically comparable by epitope specificity and binding affinity to antibodies induced by plasma-derived vaccine.[11] In cross absorption studies, no differences were detected in the spectra of antibodies induced in man to plasma-derived or to yeast-derived hepatitis B vaccines.[11]

Additionally, patients immunized approximately 3 years previously with plasma-derived vaccine and whose antibody titers were <100 mIU/mL (GMT: 35 mIU/mL; range: 9–94) were given a 20 mcg dose of *Engerix-B.* All patients, including two who had not responded to the plasma-derived vaccine, showed a response to *Engerix-B* (GMT: 5,069 mIU/mL; range: 624–15,019). There have been no clinical studies in which a three-dose vaccine series was initiated with a plasma-derived hepatitis B vaccine and completed with *Engerix-B,* or vice versa. However, because the *in vitro* and *in vivo* studies described above indicate the comparability of the antibody produced in response to plasma-derived vaccine and *Engerix-B,* it should be possible to interchange the use of *Engerix-B* and plasma-derived vaccines (but see CONTRAINDICATIONS).

A controlled study (N=48) demonstrated that completion of a course of immunization with one dose of *Engerix-B* (20 mcg, month 6) following two doses of Recombivax HB®* (10 mcg, months 0 and 1) produced a similar GMT (4,077 mIU/mL) to immunization with three doses of *Recombivax HB* (10 mcg, months 0, 1 and 6; 2,654 mIU/mL). Thus, *Engerix-B* can be used to complete a vaccination course initiated with *Recombivax HB.*

INDICATIONS AND USAGE

Engerix-B is indicated for immunization against infection caused by all known subtypes of hepatitis B virus. As hepatitis D (caused by the delta virus) does not occur in the absence of hepatitis B infection, it can be expected that hepatitis D will also be prevented by *Engerix-B* vaccination.

Engerix-B will not prevent hepatitis caused by other agents, such as hepatitis A, C and E viruses, or other pathogens known to infect the liver.

Immunization is recommended in persons of all ages, especially those who are, or will be, at increased risk of exposure to hepatitis B virus,[1] for example:

Health Care Personnel: Dentists and oral surgeons. Dental, medical and nursing students. Physicians, surgeons and podiatrists. Nurses. Paramedical and ambulance personnel and custodial staff who may be exposed to the virus via blood or other patient specimens. Dental hygienists and dental nurses. Laboratory and blood-bank personnel handling blood, blood products, and other patient specimens. Hospital cleaning staff who handle waste.

Selected Patients and Patient Contacts: Patients and staff in hemodialysis units and hematology/oncology units. Patients requiring frequent and/or large volume blood transfusions or clotting factor concentrates (e.g., persons with hemophilia, thalassemia, sickle-cell anemia, cirrhosis). Clients (residents) and staff of institutions for the mentally handicapped. Classroom contacts of deinstitutionalized mentally handicapped persons who have persistent hepatitis B surface antigenemia and who show aggressive behavior. Household and other intimate contacts of persons with persistent hepatitis B surface antigenemia.

Infants, Including Those Born of HBsAG-Positive Mothers Whether HBeAg Positive or Negative (See DOSAGE AND ADMINISTRATION.)

Adolescents (See CLINICAL PHARMACOLOGY.)

Subpopulations with a Known High Incidence of the Disease, such as: Alaskan Eskimos. Pacific Islanders. Indochinese immigrants. Haitian immigrants. Refugees from other HBV endemic areas. All infants of women born in areas where the infection is highly endemic.

Persons Who May Be Exposed to the Hepatitis B Virus by Travel to High-Risk Areas (See ACIP Guidelines, 1990.)

Military Personnel Identified as Being at Increased Risk Morticians and Embalmers

Persons at Increased Risk of the Disease Due to Their Sexual Practices, such as: Persons with more than one sexual partner in a 6-month period. Persons who have contracted a sexually transmitted disease. Homosexually active males. Female prostitutes.

Prisoners

Users of Illicit Injectable Drugs

Others: Police and fire department personnel who render first aid or medical assistance, and any others who, through their work or personal life-style, may be exposed to the hepatitis B virus. Adoptees from countries of high HBV endemicity.

Use with Other Vaccines: The Immunization Practices Advisory Committee states that, in general, simultaneous administration of certain live and inactivated pediatric vaccines has not resulted in impaired antibody responses or increased rates of adverse reactions.[12] Separate sites and syringes should be used for simultaneous administration of injectable vaccines.

CONTRAINDICATIONS

Hypersensitivity to yeast or any other component of the vaccine is a contraindication for use of the vaccine.

WARNINGS

Patients experiencing hypersensitivity after an Engerix-B [Hepatitis B Vaccine (Recombinant)] injection should not receive further injections of *Engerix-B.* (See CONTRAINDICATIONS.)

Hepatitis B has a long incubation period. Hepatitis B vaccination may not prevent hepatitis B infection in individuals who had an unrecognized hepatitis B infection at the time of vaccine administration. Additionally, it may not prevent infection in individuals who do not achieve protective antibody titers.

PRECAUTIONS

General As with any percutaneous vaccine, epinephrine should be available for use in case of anaphylaxis or anaphylactoid reaction.

As with any vaccine, administration of *Engerix-B* should be delayed, if possible, in persons with any febrile illness or active infection.

Pregnancy Pregnancy Category C: Animal reproduction studies have not been conducted with *Engerix-B.* It is also not known whether *Engerix-B* can cause fetal harm when administered to a pregnant woman or can affect reproduction capacity. *Engerix-B* should be given to a pregnant woman only if clearly needed.

Nursing Mothers It is not known whether *Engerix-B* is excreted in human milk. Because many drugs are excreted in human milk, caution should be exercised when *Engerix-B* is administered to a nursing woman.

Pediatric Use *Engerix-B* has been shown to be well tolerated and highly immunogenic in infants and children of all ages. Newborns also respond well; maternally transferred antibodies do not interfere with the active immune response to the vaccine. (See CLINICAL PHARMACOLOGY for seroconversion rates and titers in neonates and children. See DOSAGE AND ADMINISTRATION for recommended pediatric dosage and for recommended dosage for infants born of HBsAg-positive mothers.)

ADVERSE REACTIONS

Engerix-B [Hepatitis B Vaccine (Recombinant)] is generally well tolerated. As with any vaccine, however, it is possible that expanded commercial use of the vaccine could reveal rare adverse reactions.

Ten double-blind studies involving 2,252 subjects showed no significant difference in the frequency or severity of adverse experiences between *Engerix-B* and plasma-derived vaccines. In 36 clinical studies a total of 13,495 doses of *Engerix-B* were administered to 5,071 healthy adults and children who were initially seronegative for hepatitis B markers, and healthy neonates. All subjects were monitored for 4 days post-administration. Frequency of adverse experiences tended to decrease with successive doses of *Engerix-B.* Using a symptom checklist,‡ the most frequently reported adverse reactions were injection site soreness (22%) and fatigue‡ (14%). Other reactions are listed below.

Continued on next page

Information on the SmithKline Beecham Pharmaceuticals products appearing here is based on the labeling in effect on July 1, 1996. Further information on these and other products may be obtained from the Medical Department, SmithKline Beecham Pharmaceuticals, One Franklin Plaza, Philadelphia, PA 19101.

Consult 1997 supplements and future editions for revisions

SmithKline Beecham—Cont.

Incidence 1% to 10% of Injections

Local reactions at injection site: Induration; erythema; swelling.
Body as a whole: Fever (> 37.5°C).
Nervous system: Headache[‡]; dizziness.[‡]
‡ Parent or guardian completed forms for children and neonates. Neonatal checklist did not include headache, fatigue or dizziness.

Incidence < 1% of Injections

Local reactions at injection site: Pain; pruritus; ecchymosis.
Body as a whole: Sweating; malaise; chills; weakness; flushing; tingling.
Cardiovascular system: Hypotension.
Respiratory system: Influenza-like symptoms; upper respiratory tract illnesses.
Gastrointestinal system: Nausea; anorexia; abdominal pain/cramps; vomiting; constipation; diarrhea.
Lymphatic system: Lymphadenopathy.
Musculoskeletal system: Pain/stiffness in arm, shoulder or neck; arthralgia; myalgia; back pain.
Skin and appendages: Rash; urticaria; petechiae; pruritus; erythema.
Nervous system: Somnolence; insomnia; irritability; agitation.

Additional adverse experiences have been reported with the commercial use of *Engerix-B*. Those listed below are to serve as alerting information to physicians.
Hypersensitivity: Anaphylaxis; erythema multiforme including Stevens-Johnson syndrome; angioedema; arthritis.
Cardiovascular system: Tachycardia/palpitations.
Respiratory system: Bronchospasm including asthma-like symptoms.
Gastrointestinal system: Abnormal liver function tests; dyspepsia.
Nervous system: Migraine; syncope; paresis; neuropathy including hypoesthesia, paresthesia, Guillain-Barré syndrome and Bell's palsy, transverse myelitis; optic neuritis; multiple sclerosis.
Hematologic: Thrombocytopenia.
Skin and appendages: Eczema; purpura; herpes zoster; erythema nodosum; alopecia.
Special senses: Conjunctivitis; keratitis; visual disturbances; vertigo; tinnitus; earache.
Potential Adverse Experiences: In addition, certain other adverse experiences not observed with *Engerix-B* have been reported with Heptavax-B®† and/or *Recombivax HB*. Those listed below are to serve as alerting information to physicians:
Urogenital system: Dysuria.

DOSAGE AND ADMINISTRATION

Injection: Engerix-B should be administered by intramuscular injection. *Do not inject intravenously or intradermally.* In adults, the injection should be given in the deltoid region but it may be preferable to inject in the anterolateral thigh in neonates and infants, who have smaller deltoid muscles. *Engerix-B* should not be administered in the gluteal region; such injections may result in suboptimal response. The attending physician should determine final selection of the injection site and needle size, depending upon the patient's age and the size of the target muscle. A 1-inch 23-gauge needle is sufficient to penetrate the anterolateral thigh in infants younger than 12 months of age. A 5/8-inch 25-gauge needle may be used to administer the vaccine in the deltoid region of toddlers and children up to, and including, 10 years of age. The 1-inch 23-gauge needle is appropriate for use in older children and adults.[13]
Engerix-B may be administered subcutaneously to persons at risk of hemorrhage (e.g., hemophiliacs). However, hepatitis B vaccines administered subcutaneously are known to result in lower GMTs. Additionally, when other aluminum-adsorbed vaccines have been administered subcutaneously, an increased incidence of local reactions including subcutaneous nodules has been observed. Therefore, subcutaneous administration should be used only in persons who are at risk of hemorrhage with intramuscular injections.
Preparation for Administration: Shake well before withdrawal and use. Parenteral drug products should be inspected visually for particulate matter or discoloration prior to administration. With thorough agitation, *Engerix-B* is a slightly opaque white suspension. Discard if it appears otherwise. The vaccine should be used as supplied; no dilution is necessary. The full recommended dose of the vaccine should be used.
Dosing Schedules: The usual immunization regimen (see Table 1) consists of three doses of vaccine given according to the following schedule: 1st dose: at elected date; 2nd dose: 1 month later; 3rd dose: 6 months after first dose.
There is an alternate schedule with injections at 0, 1 and 2 months designed for certain populations (e.g., neonates born of hepatitis B infected mothers, others who have or might have been recently exposed to the virus, certain travelers to high-risk areas. See INDICATIONS AND USAGE.). On this alternate schedule, an additional dose at 12 months is recommended for infants born of infected mothers and for others for whom prolonged maintenance of protective titers is desired.
In infants born of mothers who are not hepatitis B infected, *Engerix-B* may be administered at birth, 1 month of age and 6 months of age.

Table 1

Group	Dose	Schedule §
Infants born of:		
HBsAg-negative mothers	10 mcg/0.5 mL	Usual
HBsAg-positive mothers	10 mcg/0.5 mL	Either
Children:		
0 through 10 years of age	10 mcg/0.5 mL	Either
Adolescents:		
11 through 19 years of age	10 mcg/0.5 mL	Usual
	20 mcg/1.0 mL	Either
Adults (> 19 years)	20 mcg/1.0 mL	Either
Adult hemodialysis	40 mcg/2.0 mL[‖]	0, 1, 2, 6 months

§ Usual dosing schedule is 0, 1, 6 months; alternate dosing schedule is 0, 1, 2, 12 months. When the alternate schedule is used for adolescents, the 20 mcg/1.0 mL dose should be used.
‖ Two × 20 mcg in one or two injections.

For hemodialysis patients, in whom vaccine-induced protection is less complete and may persist only as long as antibody levels remain above 10 mIU/mL, the need for booster doses should be assessed by annual antibody testing. 40 mcg (two × 20 mcg) booster doses with *Engerix-B* should be given when antibody levels decline below 10 mIU/mL.[1] Data show individuals given a booster with *Engerix-B* achieve high antibody titers. (See CLINICAL PHARMACOLOGY.)
booster vaccinations: Whenever administration of a booster dose is appropriate, the dose of *Engerix-B* is 10 mcg for children 10 years of age and under; 20 mcg for adolescents 11 through 19 years of age and 20 mcg for adults. Studies have demonstrated a substantial increase in antibody titers after *Engerix-B* booster vaccination following an initial course with both plasma- and yeast-derived vaccines. (See CLINICAL PHARMACOLOGY.)
See previous section for discussion on booster vaccination for adult hemodialysis patients.
Known or presumed exposure to hepatitis B virus: Unprotected individuals with known or presumed exposure to the hepatitis B virus (e.g., neonates born of infected mothers, others experiencing percutaneous or permucosal exposure) should be given hepatitis B immune globulin (HBIG) in addition to *Engerix-B* in accordance with ACIP recommendations[1] and with the package insert for HBIG. *Engerix-B* can be given on either dosing schedule (see above).

STORAGE

Store between 2° and 8°C (35° to 46°F). *Do not freeze;* discard if product has been frozen. Do not dilute to administer.

HOW SUPPLIED

Adult Dose
20 mcg/mL in Single-Dose Vials in packages of 1 and 25 vials.
NDC 58160-860-01 (package of 1)
NDC 58160-860-16 (package of 25)
20 mcg/mL in Single-Dose Prefilled Disposable Syringes.
NDC 58160-861-05 (package of 5)
20 mcg/mL in 10 mL Multi-Dose Vials.
NDC 58160-862-01 (package of 1)
Adolescent/Pediatric Doses
10 mcg/0.5 mL in Single-Dose Vials in packages of 1 vial.
NDC 58160–859–01 (package of 1)
10 mcg/0.5 mL in Single-Dose Prefilled Disposable Syringes with 1-inch 23-gauge needles.
NDC 58160–859–05 (package of 5)
10 mcg/0.5 mL in Single-Dose Prefilled Disposable Syringes with 5/8-inch 25-gauge needles.
NDC 58160–859–06 (package of 5)

REFERENCES 1. Centers for Disease Control: Protection against viral hepatitis: recommendations of the Immunization Practices Advisory Committee (ACIP). *MMWR.* 39(No. RR-2), 1990. 2. Robinson, W.S.: Hepatitis B virus and the delta virus. In Mandell, G.L., Douglas, R.G., Bennett, J.E. (eds): *Principles and practice of infectious diseases,* vol. 3, New York, John Wiley & Sons, 1990, pp. 1204-1231. 3. Beasley, R.P., et al.: Efficacy of hepatitis B immune globulin for prevention of perinatal transmission of hepatitis B virus carrier state: final report of a randomized double-blind, placebo-controlled trial. *Hepatology* 3:135-141, 1983. 4. Centers for Disease Control: Hepatitis B virus: a comprehensive strategy for eliminating transmission in the United States through universal childhood vaccination: recommendations of the Immunization Practices Advisory Committee (ACIP). *MMWR.* 40(No. RR-13):1-25, 1991. 5. Committee on Infectious Diseases: Universal hepatitis B immunization. *Pediatrics.* 89(4):795-800, 1992. 6. Ambrosch, F.: Persistence of vaccine-induced antibodies to hepatitis B surface antigen–the need for booster vaccination in adult subjects. *Postgrad. Med. J.* 63(Suppl. 2):129-135, 1987. 7. Stevens, C.E., et al.: Hepatitis B vaccine in patients receiving hemodialysis. *N. Engl. J. Med.* 311:496-501, 1984. 8. Andre, F.E., and Safary, A.: Clinical experience with a yeast-derived hepatitis B vaccine. In Zuckerman, A.J.(ed): *Viral hepatitis and liver disease,* Alan R. Liss, Inc., 1988, pp. 1025-1030. 9. Poovorawan, Y., et al.: Protective efficacy of a recombinant DNA hepatitis B vaccine in neonates of HBe antigen-positive mothers. *JAMA.* 261(22):3278-3281, June 9, 1989. 10. Goilav, C., et al.: Immunization of homosexual men with a recombinant DNA vaccine against hepatitis B: immunogenicity and protection. In Zuckerman, A.J. (ed): *Viral hepatitis and liver disease,* Alan R. Liss, Inc., 1988, pp. 1057-1058. 11. Hauser, P., et al.: Immunological properties of recombinant HBsAg produced in yeast. *Postgrad. Med. J.* 63(Suppl. 2):83-91, 1987. 12. Centers for Disease Control: Recommendations of the Immunization Practices Advisory Committee (ACIP): General Recommendations on Immunization. *MMWR.* 38(13):April 7, 1989. 13. Centers for Disease Control and Prevention: General Recommendations on Immunization; Recommendations of the Advisory Committee on Immunization Practices (ACIP). *MMWR.* 1994; 43(RR-1):6.

* yeast-derived, Hepatitis B Vaccine, MSD.
† plasma-derived, Hepatitis B Vaccine, MSD.

Manufactured by **SmithKline Beecham Biologicals**
Rixensart, Belgium
Distributed by **SmithKline Beecham Pharmaceuticals**
Philadelphia, PA 19101
Engerix-B® is a registered trademark of SmithKline Beecham.
Veterans Administration/Military/PHS—Vial, 10 mcg/0.5 mL, 1's, 6505-01-311-5220; Prefilled Syringe, 10 mcg/0.5 mL, 6505-01-392-6766; Vial, 20 mcg/mL, 1's, 6505-01-311-5221; 20 mcg/mL, 25's, 6505-01-311-5222; Prefilled Syringe, 20 mcg/mL, 5's, 6505-1-392-6768; 10 mL Multi-Dose Vial, 20 mcg/mL, 6505-01-428-3900.

EB:L15B

Shown in Product Identification Guide, page 336

ESKALITH® ℞
[ess-kah 'lith]
(brand of lithium carbonate)
Capsules, 300 mg

ESKALITH CR® ℞
(brand of lithium carbonate)
Controlled Release Tablets, 450 mg

WARNING
Lithium toxicity is closely related to serum lithium levels, and can occur at doses close to therapeutic levels. Facilities for prompt and accurate serum lithium determinations should be available before initiating therapy (see DOSAGE AND ADMINISTRATION).

DESCRIPTION

Eskalith contains lithium carbonate, a white, light alkaline powder with molecular formula Li_2CO_3 and molecular weight 73.89. Lithium is an element of the alkali-metal group with atomic number 3, atomic weight 6.94 and an emission line at 671 nm on the flame photometer.
***Eskalith* Capsules:** Each capsule, with opaque gray cap and opaque yellow body, is imprinted with the product name ESKALITH and SB and contains lithium carbonate, 300 mg. Inactive ingredients consist of benzyl alcohol, cetylpyridinium chloride, D&C Yellow No. 10, FD&C Green No. 3, FD&C Red No. 40, FD&C Yellow No. 6, gelatin, lactose, magnesium stearate, povidone, sodium lauryl sulfate, titanium dioxide and trace amounts of other inactive ingredients.
***Eskalith CR* Controlled Release Tablets:** Each round, buff, scored tablet is debossed SKF and J10 and contains lithium carbonate, 450 mg. Inactive ingredients consist of alginic acid, gelatin, iron oxide, magnesium stearate and sodium starch glycolate.
Eskalith CR tablets 450 mg are designed to release a portion of the dose initially and the remainder gradually; the release pattern of the controlled release tablets reduces the variability in lithium blood levels seen with the immediate release dosage forms.

ACTIONS

Preclinical studies have shown that lithium alters sodium transport in nerve and muscle cells and effects a shift toward intraneuronal metabolism of catecholamines, but the spe-

cific biochemical mechanism of lithium action in mania is unknown.

INDICATIONS

Eskalith (lithium carbonate) is indicated in the treatment of manic episodes of manic-depressive illness. Maintenance therapy prevents or diminishes the intensity of subsequent episodes in those manic-depressive patients with a history of mania.

Typical symptoms of mania include pressure of speech, motor hyperactivity, reduced need for sleep, flight of ideas, grandiosity, elation, poor judgment, aggressiveness and possibly hostility. When given to a patient experiencing a manic episode, *Eskalith* may produce a normalization of symptomatology within 1 to 3 weeks.

WARNINGS

Lithium should generally not be given to patients with significant renal or cardiovascular disease, severe debilitation or dehydration, or sodium depletion, since the risk of lithium toxicity is very high in such patients. If the psychiatric indication is life-threatening, and if such a patient fails to respond to other measures, lithium treatment may be undertaken with extreme caution, including daily serum lithium determinations and adjustment to the usually low doses ordinarily tolerated by these individuals. In such instances, hospitalization is a necessity.

Chronic lithium therapy may be associated with diminution of renal concentrating ability, occasionally presenting as nephrogenic diabetes insipidus, with polyuria and polydipsia. Such patients should be carefully managed to avoid dehydration with resulting lithium retention and toxicity. This condition is usually reversible when lithium is discontinued.

Morphologic changes with glomerular and interstitial fibrosis and nephron atrophy have been reported in patients on chronic lithium therapy. Morphologic changes have also been seen in manic-depressive patients never exposed to lithium. The relationship between renal functional and morphologic changes and their association with lithium therapy have not been established.

When kidney function is assessed, for baseline data prior to starting lithium therapy or thereafter, routine urinalysis and other tests may be used to evaluate tubular function (e.g., urine specific gravity or osmolality following a period of water deprivation, or 24-hour urine volume) and glomerular function (e.g., serum creatinine or creatinine clearance). During lithium therapy, progressive or sudden changes in renal function, even within the normal range, indicate the need for reevaluation of treatment.

An encephalopathic syndrome (characterized by weakness, lethargy, fever, tremulousness and confusion, extrapyramidal symptoms, leukocytosis, elevated serum enzymes, BUN and FBS) has occurred in a few patients treated with lithium plus a neuroleptic. In some instances, the syndrome was followed by irreversible brain damage. Because of a possible causal relationship between these events and the concomitant administration of lithium and neuroleptics, patients receiving such combined therapy should be monitored closely for early evidence of neurologic toxicity and treatment discontinued promptly if such signs appear. This encephalopathic syndrome may be similar to or the same as neuroleptic malignant syndrome (NMS).

Lithium toxicity is closely related to serum lithium levels, and can occur at doses close to therapeutic levels (see DOSAGE AND ADMINISTRATION).

Outpatients and their families should be warned that the patient must discontinue lithium carbonate therapy and contact his physician if such clinical signs of lithium toxicity as diarrhea, vomiting, tremor, mild ataxia, drowsiness or muscular weakness occur.

Lithium carbonate may impair mental and/or physical abilities. Caution patients about activities requiring alertness (e.g., operating vehicles or machinery).

Lithium may prolong the effects of neuromuscular blocking agents. Therefore, neuromuscular blocking agents should be given with caution to patients receiving lithium.

Usage in Pregnancy: Adverse effects on implantation in rats, embryo viability in mice and metabolism *in vitro* of rat testes and human spermatozoa have been attributed to lithium, as have teratogenicity in submammalian species and cleft palates in mice.

In humans, lithium carbonate may cause fetal harm when administered to a pregnant woman. Data from lithium birth registries suggest an increase in cardiac and other anomalies, especially Ebstein's anomaly. If this drug is used in women of childbearing potential, or during pregnancy, or if a patient becomes pregnant while taking this drug, the patient should be apprised of the potential hazard to the fetus.

Usage in Nursing Mothers: Lithium is excreted in human milk. Nursing should not be undertaken during lithium therapy except in rare and unusual circumstances where, in the view of the physician, the potential benefits to the mother outweigh possible hazards to the child.

Usage in Pediatric Patients: Since information regarding the safety and effectiveness of lithium carbonate in children under 12 years of age is not available, its use in such patients is not recommended.

There has been a report of a transient syndrome of acute dystonia and hyperreflexia occurring in a 15 kg child who ingested 300 mg of lithium carbonate.

Usage in the Elderly: Elderly patients often require lower lithium dosages to achieve therapeutic serum levels. They may also exhibit adverse reactions at serum levels ordinarily tolerated by younger patients.

PRECAUTIONS

The ability to tolerate lithium is greater during the acute manic phase and decreases when manic symptoms subside (see DOSAGE AND ADMINISTRATION).

Caution should be used when lithium and diuretics are used concomitantly because diuretic-induced sodium loss may reduce the renal clearance of lithium and increase serum lithium levels with risk of lithium toxicity. Patients receiving such combined therapy should have serum lithium levels monitored closely and the lithium dosage adjusted if necessary.

The distribution space of lithium approximates that of total body water. Lithium is primarily excreted in urine with insignificant excretion in feces. Renal excretion of lithium is proportional to its plasma concentration. The half-life of elimination of lithium is approximately 24 hours. Lithium decreases sodium reabsorption by the renal tubules which could lead to sodium depletion. Therefore, it is essential for the patient to maintain a normal diet, including salt, and an adequate fluid intake (2500 to 3000 mL) at least during the initial stabilization period. Decreased tolerance to lithium has been reported to ensue from protracted sweating or diarrhea and, if such occur, supplemental fluid and salt should be administered under careful medical supervision and lithium intake reduced or suspended until the condition is resolved.

In addition to sweating and diarrhea, concomitant infection with elevated temperatures may also necessitate a temporary reduction or cessation of medication.

Previously existing underlying thyroid disorders do not necessarily constitute a contraindication to lithium treatment; where hypothyroidism exists, careful monitoring of thyroid function during lithium stabilization and maintenance allows for correction of changing thyroid parameters, if any; where hypothyroidism occurs during lithium stabilization and maintenance, supplemental thyroid treatment may be used.

Indomethacin and piroxicam have been reported to increase significantly, steady-state plasma lithium levels. In some cases, lithium toxicity has resulted from such interactions. There is also some evidence that other nonsteroidal anti-inflammatory agents may have a similar effect. When such combinations are used, increased plasma lithium level monitoring is recommended. Concurrent use of metronidazole with lithium may provoke lithium toxicity due to reduced renal clearance. Patients receiving such combined therapy should be monitored closely.

There is evidence that angiotensin-converting enzyme inhibitors, such as enalapril and captopril, may substantially increase steady-state plasma lithium levels, sometimes resulting in lithium toxicity. When such combinations are used, lithium dosage may need to be decreased, and plasma lithium levels should be measured more often.

Concurrent use of calcium channel blocking agents with lithium may increase the risk of neurotoxicity in the form of ataxia, tremors, nausea, vomiting, diarrhea and/or tinnitus. Caution is recommended.

The following drugs can lower serum lithium concentrations by increasing urinary lithium excretion: acetazolamide, urea, xanthine preparations and alkalinizing agents such as sodium bicarbonate.

ADVERSE REACTIONS

The occurrence and severity of adverse reactions are generally directly related to serum lithium concentrations as well as to individual patient sensitivity to lithium, and generally occur more frequently and with greater severity at higher concentrations.

Adverse reactions may be encountered at serum lithium levels below 1.5 mEq/L. Mild to moderate adverse reactions may occur at levels from 1.5 to 2.5 mEq/L, and moderate to severe reactions may be seen at levels of 2.0 mEq/L and above.

Fine hand tremor, polyuria and mild thirst may occur during initial therapy for the acute manic phase, and may persist throughout treatment. Transient and mild nausea and general discomfort may also appear during the first few days of lithium administration.

These side effects usually subside with continued treatment or a temporary reduction or cessation of dosage. If persistent, cessation of lithium therapy may be required.

Diarrhea, vomiting, drowsiness, muscular weakness and lack of coordination may be early signs of lithium intoxication, and can occur at lithium levels below 2.0 mEq/L. At higher levels, ataxia, giddiness, tinnitus, blurred vision and a large output of dilute urine may be seen. Serum lithium levels above 3.0 mEq/L may produce a complex clinical picture, involving multiple organs and organ systems. Serum lithium levels should not be permitted to exceed 2.0 mEq/L during the acute treatment phase.

The following reactions have been reported and appear to be related to serum lithium levels, including levels within the therapeutic range: **Neuromuscular/Central Nervous System**—tremor, muscle hyperirritability (fasciculations, twitching, clonic movements of whole limbs), hypertonicity, ataxia, choreo-athetotic movements, hyperactive deep tendon reflex, extrapyramidal symptoms including acute dystonia, cogwheel rigidity, blackout spells, epileptiform seizures, slurred speech, dizziness, vertigo, downbeat nystagmus, incontinence of urine or feces, somnolence, psychomotor retardation, restlessness, confusion, stupor, coma, tongue movements, tics, tinnitus, hallucinations, poor memory, slowed intellectual functioning, startled response, worsening of organic brain syndromes, myasthenia gravis (rarely); **Cardiovascular**—cardiac arrhythmia, hypotension, peripheral circulatory collapse, bradycardia, sinus node dysfunction with severe bradycardia (which may result in syncope); **Gastrointestinal**—anorexia, nausea, vomiting, diarrhea, gastritis, salivary gland swelling, abdominal pain, excessive salivation, flatulence, indigestion; **Genitourinary**—glycosuria, decreased creatinine clearance, albuminuria, oliguria, and symptoms of nephrogenic diabetes insipidus including polyuria, thirst and polydipsia; **Dermatologic**—drying and thinning of hair, alopecia, anesthesia of skin, acne, chronic folliculitis, xerosis cutis, psoriasis or its exacerbation, generalized pruritus with or without rash, cutaneous ulcers, angioedema; **Autonomic**—blurred vision, dry mouth, impotence/sexual dysfunction; **Thyroid Abnormalities**—euthyroid goiter and/or hypothyroidism (including myxedema) accompanied by lower T_3 and T_4. I^{131} uptake may be elevated. (See PRECAUTIONS.) Paradoxically, rare cases of hyperthyroidism have been reported; **EEG Changes**—diffuse slowing, widening of the frequency spectrum, potentiation and disorganization of background rhythm; **EKG Changes**—reversible flattening, isoelectricity or inversion of T-waves; **Miscellaneous**—fatigue, lethargy, transient scotomata, exophthalmos, dehydration, weight loss, leukocytosis, headache, transient hyperglycemia, hypercalcemia, hyperparathyroidism, excessive weight gain, edematous swelling of ankles or wrists, metallic taste, dysgeusia/taste distortion, salty taste, thirst, swollen lips, tightness in chest, swollen and/or painful joints, fever, polyarthralgia, dental caries.

Some reports of nephrogenic diabetes insipidus, hyperparathyroidism and hypothyroidism which persist after lithium discontinuation have been received.

A few reports have been received of the development of painful discoloration of fingers and toes and coldness of the extremities within one day of the starting of treatment with lithium. The mechanism through which these symptoms (resembling Raynaud's syndrome) developed is not known. Recovery followed discontinuance.

Cases of pseudotumor cerebri (increased intracranial pressure and papilledema) have been reported with lithium use. If undetected, this condition may result in enlargement of the blind spot, constriction of visual fields and eventual blindness due to optic atrophy.

Lithium should be discontinued, if clinically possible, if this syndrome occurs.

DOSAGE AND ADMINISTRATION

Immediate release capsules are usually given t.i.d. or q.i.d. Doses of controlled release tablets are usually given b.i.d. (approximately 12-hour intervals). When initiating therapy with immediate release or controlled release lithium, dosage must be individualized according to serum levels and clinical response.

When switching a patient from immediate release capsules to the Eskalith CR (lithium carbonate) Controlled Release Tablets, give the same total daily dose when possible. Most patients on maintenance therapy are stabilized on 900 mg daily, e.g., 450 mg *Eskalith CR* b.i.d. When the previous dosage of immediate release lithium is not a multiple of 450 mg, for example, 1500 mg, initiate *Eskalith CR* dosage at the multiple of 450 mg nearest to, but *below*, the original daily dose, i.e., 1350 mg. When the two doses are unequal, give the larger dose in the evening. In the above example, with a total daily dosage of 1350 mg, generally 450 mg *Eskalith CR* should be given in the morning and 900 mg *Eskalith CR* in the evening. If desired, the total daily dosage of 1350 mg can be given in three equal 450 mg *Eskalith CR* doses. These patients should be monitored at 1 to 2 week intervals, and dosage adjusted if necessary, until stable and satisfactory serum levels and clinical state are achieved.

Continued on next page

Information on the SmithKline Beecham Pharmaceuticals products appearing here is based on the labeling in effect on July 1, 1996. Further information on these and other products may be obtained from the Medical Department, SmithKline Beecham Pharmaceuticals, One Franklin Plaza, Philadelphia, PA 19101.

SmithKline Beecham—Cont.

When patients require closer titration than that available with *Eskalith CR* doses in increments of 450 mg, immediate release capsules should be used.

Acute Mania—Optimal patient response to Eskalith (lithium carbonate) can usually be established and maintained with 1800 mg per day in divided doses. Such doses will normally produce the desired serum lithium level ranging between 1.0 and 1.5 mEq/L.

Dosage must be individualized according to serum levels and clinical response. Regular monitoring of the patient's clinical state and serum lithium levels is necessary. Serum levels should be determined twice per week during the acute phase, and until the serum level and clinical condition of the patient have been stabilized.

Long-Term Control—The desirable serum lithium levels are 0.6 to 1.2 mEq/L. Dosage will vary from one individual to another, but usually 900 mg to 1200 mg per day in divided doses will maintain this level. Serum lithium levels in uncomplicated cases receiving maintenance therapy during remission should be monitored at least every two months.

Patients unusually sensitive to lithium may exhibit toxic signs at serum levels below 1.0 mEq/L.

N.B.: Blood samples for serum lithium determinations should be drawn immediately prior to the next dose when lithium concentrations are relatively stable (i.e., 8 to 12 hours after the previous dose). Total reliance must not be placed on serum levels alone. Accurate patient evaluation requires both clinical and laboratory analysis.

Elderly patients often respond to reduced dosage, and may exhibit signs of toxicity at serum levels ordinarily tolerated by younger patients.

OVERDOSAGE

The toxic levels for lithium are close to the therapeutic levels. It is therefore important that patients and their families be cautioned to watch for early toxic symptoms and to discontinue the drug and inform the physician should they occur. Toxic symptoms are listed in detail under ADVERSE REACTIONS.

Treatment

No specific antidote for lithium poisoning is known. Early symptoms of lithium toxicity can usually be treated by reduction or cessation of dosage of the drug and resumption of the treatment at a lower dose after 24 to 48 hours. In severe cases of lithium poisoning, the first and foremost goal of treatment consists of elimination of this ion from the patient. Treatment is essentially the same as that used in barbiturate poisoning: 1) gastric lavage, 2) correction of fluid and electrolyte imbalance, and 3) regulation of kidney function. Urea, mannitol and aminophylline all produce significant increases in lithium excretion. Hemodialysis is an effective and rapid means of removing the ion from the severely toxic patient. Infection prophylaxis, regular chest X-rays and preservation of adequate respiration are essential.

HOW SUPPLIED

Capsules: gray and yellow, imprinted with the product name ESKALITH and SB, in bottles of 100 and 500.

300 mg 100's: NDC 0007-4007-20
300 mg 500's: NDC 0007-4007-25

Controlled Release Tablets: round, buff, scored, debossed SKF and J10, in bottles of 100.

450 mg 100's: NDC 0007-4010-20

STORAGE CONDITIONS: Store between 15° and 30°C (59° and 86°F).

Veterans Administration/Military/PHS—Capsules, 300 mg, 100's, 6505-00-482-8058; 300 mg, 500's, 6505-01-016-7746; CR Tablets, 450 mg, 100's, 6505-01-170-2364.

EL:L41

Shown in Product Identification Guide, page 336

FAMVIR® ℞
brand of famciclovir Tablets

DESCRIPTION

Famvir contains famciclovir, an orally administered prodrug of the antiviral agent penciclovir. Chemically, famciclovir is known as 2-[2-(2-amino-9*H*-purin-9-yl)ethyl]-1,3-propanediol diacetate. Its molecular formula is $C_{14}H_{19}N_5O_4$; its molecular weight is 321.3. It is a synthetic acyclic guanine derivative and has the following structure:

[See structure at top of next column.]

Famciclovir is a white to pale yellow solid. It is freely soluble in acetone and methanol, and sparingly soluble in ethanol

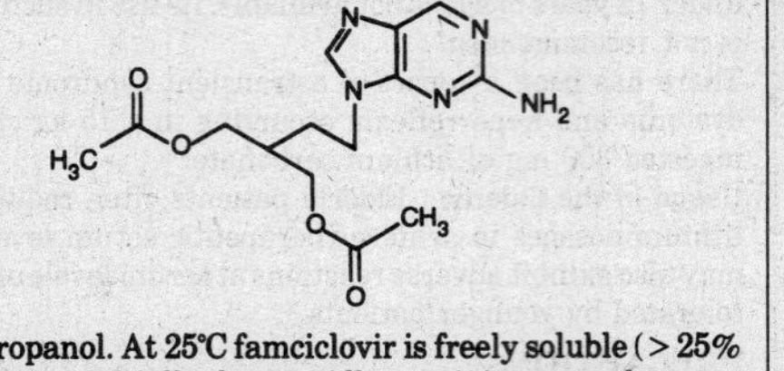

and isopropanol. At 25°C famciclovir is freely soluble (> 25% w/v) in water initially, but rapidly precipitates as the sparingly soluble (2-3% w/v) monohydrate. Famciclovir is not hygroscopic below 85% relative humidity. Partition coefficients are: octanol/water (pH 4.8) P=1.09 and octanol/phosphate buffer (pH 7.4) P=2.08.

Tablets for Oral Administration: Each white, film-coated tablet contains famciclovir. The 125 mg and 250 mg tablets are round; the 500 mg tablets are oval. Inactive ingredients consist of hydroxypropyl cellulose, hydroxypropyl methylcellulose, lactose, magnesium stearate, polyethylene glycols, sodium starch glycolate and titanium dioxide.

CLINICAL PHARMACOLOGY

Microbiology

Mechanism of Antiviral Activity: Famciclovir undergoes rapid biotransformation to the active antiviral compound penciclovir, which has inhibitory activity against herpes simplex virus types 1 (HSV-1) and 2 (HSV-2) and varicella zoster virus (VZV). In cells infected with HSV-1, HSV-2 or VZV, viral thymidine kinase phosphorylates penciclovir to a monophosphate form that, in turn, is converted to penciclovir triphosphate by cellular kinases. *In vitro* studies demonstrate that penciclovir triphosphate inhibits HSV-2 polymerase competitively with deoxyguanosine triphosphate. Consequently, herpes viral DNA synthesis and, therefore, replication are selectively inhibited.

Penciclovir triphosphate has an intracellular half-life of 10 hours in HSV-1-, 20 hours in HSV-2- and 7 hours in VZV-infected cells cultured *in vitro*; however, the clinical significance is unknown.

Antiviral Activity *In Vitro* and *In Vivo*: In cell culture studies, penciclovir has antiviral activity against the following herpesviruses (listed in decreasing order of potency): HSV-1, HSV-2 and VZV. Sensitivity test results expressed as the concentration of the drug required to inhibit the growth of the virus by 50% (IC_{50}) or 99% (IC_{99}) in cell culture vary greatly depending upon a number of factors. See Table 1.

[See table below.]

Drug Resistance: Penciclovir-resistant mutants of HSV and VZV can result from qualitative changes in viral thymidine kinase or DNA polymerase. The most commonly encountered acyclovir-resistant mutants that are deficient in viral thymidine kinase are also resistant to penciclovir. The possibility of viral resistance to penciclovir should be considered in patients who show poor clinical response during therapy.

Pharmacokinetics

Absorption and Bioavailability: Famciclovir is the diacetyl 6-deoxy analog of the active antiviral compound penciclovir. Following oral administration, little or no famciclovir is detected in plasma or urine.

The absolute bioavailability of famciclovir is 77±8% as determined following the administration of a 500 mg famciclovir oral dose and a 400 mg penciclovir intravenous dose to 12 healthy male subjects.

Following single oral-dose administration of 500 mg famciclovir to 124 healthy male volunteers across 10 studies, the mean ± SD area under the plasma concentration-time profile (AUC) was 8.6±1.9 mcg·hr/mL. The maximum concentration (C_{max}) was 3.3±0.8 mcg/mL and the time to C_{max} (T_{max}) was 0.9±0.5 hours.

Following single oral-dose administration of 500 mg famciclovir to seven patients with herpes zoster, the mean ± SD AUC, C_{max}, and T_{max} were 12.1±1.7 mcg·hr/mL, 4.0±0.7 mcg/mL, and 0.7±0.2 hours, respectively. The AUC of penciclovir was approximately 35% greater in patients with herpes zoster as compared to healthy volunteers. Some of this difference may be due to differences in renal function between the two groups.

There is no accumulation of penciclovir after the administration of 500 mg famciclovir t.i.d. for 7 days.

Penciclovir concentrations increased in proportion to dose over a famciclovir dose range of 125 mg to 750 mg administered as a single dose.

Penciclovir C_{max} decreased approximately 50% and T_{max} was delayed by 1.5 hours when a capsule formulation of famciclovir was administered with food (nutritional content was approximately 910 Kcal and 26% fat). There was no effect on the extent of availability (AUC) of penciclovir. There was an 18% decrease in C_{max} and a delay in T_{max} of about 1 hour when famciclovir was given 2 hours after a meal as compared to its administration 2 hours before a meal. Because there was no effect on the extent of systemic availability of penciclovir, it appears that *Famvir* can be taken without regard to meals.

Distribution: After a 1-hour intravenous infusion of penciclovir at doses of 5 mg/kg to 20 mg/kg, the volume of distribution (Vd_β) of penciclovir in 18 and 12 healthy male volunteers who received a dose of 5 mg/kg and 400 mg, respectively, was 83.1±7.7 L (1.13±0.11 L/kg) and 125±21.3 L (1.55±0.28 L/kg). Vd_{ss} was 72.6±11.5 L (0.98±0.13 L/kg) and 85.3±10.8 L (1.08±0.17 L/kg).

Penciclovir is < 20% bound to plasma proteins over the concentration range of 0.1 to 20 mcg/mL. The blood/plasma ratio of penciclovir is approximately 1.

Metabolism: Following oral administration, famciclovir is deacetylated and oxidized to form penciclovir. Metabolites that are inactive include 6-deoxy penciclovir, monoacetylated penciclovir, and 6-deoxy monoacetylated penciclovir (each < 0.5% of the dose). Little or no famciclovir is detected in plasma or urine.

An *in vitro* study using human liver microsomes demonstrated that cytochrome P450 does not play an important role in famciclovir metabolism. The conversion of 6-deoxy penciclovir to penciclovir is catalyzed by aldehyde oxidase.

Elimination: Approximately 94% of administered radioactivity was recovered in urine over 24 hours (83% of the dose was excreted in the first 6 hours) after the administration of 5 mg/kg radiolabeled penciclovir as a 1-hour infusion to three healthy male volunteers. Penciclovir accounted for 91% of the radioactivity excreted in the urine.

Following the oral administration of a single 500-mg dose of radiolabeled famciclovir to three healthy male volunteers, 73% and 27% of administered radioactivity were recovered in urine and feces over 72 hours, respectively. Penciclovir accounted for 82% and 6-deoxy penciclovir accounted for 7% of the radioactivity excreted in the urine. Approximately 60% of the administered radiolabeled dose was collected in urine in the first 6 hours.

After intravenous administration of penciclovir in 48 healthy male volunteers, mean ± SD total plasma clearance of penciclovir was 36.6±6.3 L/hr (0.48±0.09 L/hr/kg). Penciclovir renal clearance accounted for 74.5±8.8% of total plasma clearance.

Renal clearance of penciclovir following the oral administration of a single 500 mg dose of famciclovir to 109 healthy male volunteers was 27.7±7.6 L/hr.

The plasma elimination half-life of penciclovir was 2.0±0.3 hours after intravenous administration of penciclovir to 48 healthy male volunteers and 2.3±0.4 hours after oral administration of 500 mg famciclovir to 124 healthy male volunteers. The half-life in seven patients with herpes zoster was 3.0±1.1 hours.

Renal Insufficiency: Apparent plasma clearance, renal clearance, and the plasma-elimination rate constant of penciclovir decreased linearly with reductions in renal function. After the administration of a single 500 mg famciclovir oral dose (n=27) to healthy volunteers and to volunteers with varying degrees of renal insufficiency (CL_{CR} ranged from 6.4 to 138.8 mL/min.), the following results were obtained (Table 2):

[See table at top of next page.]

A dosage adjusment is recommended for patients with renal insufficiency (see DOSAGE AND ADMINISTRATION).

Table 1

Method of Assay	Virus Type	Cell Type	IC_{50} (mcg/mL)	IC_{99} (mcg/mL)
Plaque Reduction	VZV (c.i.)	MRC-5	5.0 ± 3.0	
	VZV (c.i.)	Hs68	0.9 ± 0.4	
	HSV-1 (c.i.)	MRC-5	0.2 – 0.6	
	HSV-1 (c.i.)	WISH	0.04 – 0.5	
	HSV-2 (c.i.)	MRC-5	0.9 – 2.1	
	HSV-2 (c.i.)	WISH	0.1 – 0.8	
Virus Yield Reduction	HSV-1 (c.i.)	MRC-5		0.4–0.5
	HSV-2 (c.i.)	MRC-5		0.6–0.7
DNA Synthesis Inhibition	VZV (Ellen)	MRC-5	0.1	
	HSV-1 (SC16)	MRC-5	0.04	
	HSV-2 (MS)	MRC-5	0.05	

(c.i.) = clinical isolates.

Hepatic Insufficiency: Well-compensated chronic liver disease (chronic hepatitis [n=6], chronic ethanol abuse [n=8], or primary biliary cirrhosis [n=1]) had no effect on the extent of availability (AUC) of penciclovir following a single dose of 500 mg famciclovir. However, there was a 44% decrease in penciclovir mean maximum plasma concentration and the time to maximum plasma concentration was increased by 0.75 hours in patients with hepatic insufficiency compared to normal volunteers. No dosage adjustment is recommended for patients with well-compensated hepatic impairment. The pharmacokinetics of penciclovir have not been evaluated in patients with severe uncompensated hepatic impairment.

Elderly Subjects: Based on cross-study comparisons, mean penciclovir AUC was 40% larger and penciclovir renal clearance was 22% lower after the oral administration of famciclovir in elderly volunteers (n=18, age 65 to 79 years) compared to younger volunteers. Some of this difference may be due to differences in renal function between the two groups.

Gender: The pharmacokinetics of penciclovir was evaluated in 18 healthy male and 18 healthy female volunteers after single-dose oral administration of 500 mg famciclovir. AUC of penciclovir was 9.3 ± 1.9 mcg·hr/mL and 11.1 ± 2.1 mcg·hr/mL in males and females, respectively. Penciclovir renal clearance was 28.5 ± 8.9 L/hr and 21.8 ± 4.3 L/hr, respectively. These differences were attributed to differences in renal function between the two groups. No famciclovir dosage adjustment based on gender is recommended.

Pediatric Patients: The pharmacokinetics of famciclovir or penciclovir have not been evaluated in patients <18 years of age.

Race: The pharmacokinetics of famciclovir or penciclovir with respect to race have not been evaluated.

Drug Interactions

No clinically significant alterations in penciclovir pharmacokinetics were observed following single-dose administration of 500 mg famciclovir after pre-treatment with multiple doses of cimetidine, allopurinol, or theophylline (see CLINICAL PHARMACOLOGY).

Cimetidine: Penciclovir AUC and urinary recovery increased $18 \pm 12\%$ (mean $\pm$ SD) and $12 \pm 16\%$, respectively, in 12 healthy volunteers following the administration of a single 500 mg famciclovir dose after pre-treatment with cimetidine 400 mg b.i.d. for 7 days. The magnitude of this effect is considered to be of no clinical importance.

Allopurinol: The pharmacokinetics of penciclovir were not altered following a single oral dose of 500 mg famciclovir in 12 healthy volunteers after pre-treatment with allopurinol 300 mg once daily for 7 days.

Theophylline: Penciclovir AUC and C_{max} increased $22 \pm 9\%$ and $26 \pm 27\%$, respectively, following a single oral dose of 500 mg famciclovir in 12 healthy volunteers who were pretreated with theophylline 300 mg b.i.d. for 7 days. Renal clearance of penciclovir decreased by $12 \pm 14\%$ (n=10). The magnitude of this effect is considered to be of no clinical importance.

Digoxin: After single-dose administration of digoxin and famciclovir in 12 healthy male volunteers, the C_{max} of digoxin increased $19 \pm 18\%$ as compared to digoxin administered alone. There was no change in digoxin AUC_{0-t} where t ranged from 10 to 72 hours.

CLINICAL TRIALS

Herpes Zoster

Placebo-Controlled Trial

Famvir (famciclovir) was studied in a placebo-controlled, double-blind trial of 419 otherwise healthy patients with uncomplicated herpes zoster who were treated with *Famvir* 500 mg t.i.d. (n=138), *Famvir* 750 mg t.i.d. (n=135) or placebo (n=146). Treatment was begun within 72 hours of initial lesion appearance and therapy was continued for 7 days.

Dermatology and Virology: The times to full crusting, loss of vesicles, loss of ulcers, and loss of crusts were shorter for *Famvir* 500 mg-treated patients than for placebo-treated patients in the overall study population. The median time to full crusting in *Famvir* 500 mg-treated patients was 5 days compared to 7 days in placebo-treated patients. No additional efficacy was demonstrated with the higher dose of famciclovir (750 mg t.i.d), when compared to *Famvir* 500 mg t.i.d. In the total population, 65.2% of patients had a positive viral culture at some time during their acute infection. Patients treated with *Famvir* 500 mg had a shorter median duration of viral shedding (time to last positive viral culture) than did placebo-treated patients (1 day and 2 days, respectively).

Acute Pain and Postherpetic Neuralgia: There were no overall differences in the duration of acute pain (i.e., pain before rash healing) between *Famvir* and placebo-treated groups. In addition, there was no difference in the incidence of postherpetic neuralgia (i.e., pain after rash healing) between the treatment groups. In the 186 patients (44.4% of total study population) who did develop postherpetic neuralgia, the median duration of postherpetic neuralgia was shorter in patients treated with *Famvir* 500 mg than in those treated with placebo (63 days and 119 days, respectively).

Table 2

Parameter (mean $\pm$ S.D.)	CL_{CR}* ≥ 60 (mL/min.)	CL_{CR} 40–59 (mL/min.)	CL_{CR} 20–39 (mL/min.)	CL_{CR} <20 (mL/min.)
CL_{CR} (mL/min)	88.1 ± 20.6	49.3 ± 5.9	26.5 ± 5.3	12.7 ± 5.9
CL_R (L/hr)	30.1 ± 10.6	13.0 ± 1.3**	4.2 ± 0.9	1.6 ± 1.0
CL/F*** (L/hr)	66.9 ± 27.5	27.3 ± 2.8	12.8 ± 1.3	5.8 ± 2.8
Half-life (hr)	2.3 ± 0.5	3.4 ± 0.7	6.2 ± 1.6	13.4 ± 10.2
n	15	5	4	3

* CL_{CR} is measured creatinine clearance.
** n=4.
*** CL/F consists of bioavailability factor and famciclovir to penciclovir conversion factor.

Active-Control Trial

A second double-blind controlled trial in 545 otherwise healthy patients with uncomplicated herpes zoster treated within 72 hours of initial lesion appearance compared *Famvir* 250 mg t.i.d. (n=134), *Famvir* 500 mg t.i.d. (n=134), *Famvir* 750 mg t.i.d. (n=138), and acyclovir 800 mg 5 times per day (n=139) for 7 days. In this study, patients treated with *Famvir* at each dose and acyclovir had comparable times to full lesion crusting and times to loss of acute pain. There were no statistically significant differences in the time to loss of postherpetic neuralgia between *Famvir* and acyclovir-treated groups.

Genital Herpes Infections

Recurrent Episodes: In two placebo-controlled trials, 626 otherwise healthy patients with a recurrence of genital herpes were treated with *Famvir* 125 mg b.i.d. (n=160), *Famvir* 250 mg b.i.d. (n=169), *Famvir* 500 mg b.i.d. (n=154) or placebo (n=143) for 5 days. Treatment was initiated within 6 hours of either symptom onset or lesion appearance. In the two studies combined, the median time to healing in *Famvir* 125 mg-treated patients was 4 days compared to 5 days in placebo-treated patients and the median time to cessation of viral shedding was 1.8 vs. 3.4 days in *Famvir* 125 mg and placebo recipients, respectively. The median time to loss of all symptoms was 3.2 days in *Famvir* 125 mg-treated patients vs. 3.8 days in placebo-treated patients. When used to treat acute recurrent genital herpes, no additional efficacy was demonstrated with higher doses of *Famvir* (250 mg b.i.d. or 500 mg b.i.d.) when compared to *Famvir* 125 mg b.i.d.

INDICATIONS AND USAGE

Herpes Zoster: *Famvir* is indicated for the management of acute herpes zoster (shingles).

Genital Herpes: *Famvir* is indicated for the treatment of recurrent episodes of genital herpes.

CONTRAINDICATIONS

Famvir (famciclovir) is contraindicated in patients with known hypersensitivity to the product.

PRECAUTIONS

General

The efficacy of *Famvir* has not been established for initial episode genital herpes infection, suppression of recurrent genital herpes, ophthalmic zoster, disseminated zoster, or in immunocompromised patients.

Dosage adjustment is recommended when administering *Famvir* to patients with creatinine clearance values <60 mL/min. (see DOSAGE AND ADMINISTRATION). There is no information from clinical trials about the safety of administering *Famvir* to patients with renal dysfunction.

Information for Patients

Patients should be informed that *Famvir* is not a cure for genital herpes. There are no data evaluating whether *Famvir* will prevent transmission of infection to others. As genital herpes is a sexually transmitted disease, patients should avoid contact with lesions or intercourse when lesions and/or symptoms are present to avoid infecting partners. Genital herpes can also be transmitted in the absence of symptoms through asymptomatic viral shedding.

Drug Interactions

No clinically significant alterations in penciclovir pharmacokinetics were observed following single-dose administration of 500 mg famciclovir after pre-treatment with multiple doses of cimetidine, allopurinol, or theophylline (see CLINICAL PHARMACOLOGY).

Concurrent use with probenecid or other drugs significantly eliminated by active renal tubular secretion may result in increased plasma concentrations of penciclovir.

The conversion of 6-deoxy penciclovir to penciclovir is catalyzed by aldehyde oxidase. Interactions with other drugs metabolized by this enzyme could potentially occur.

Carcinogenesis, Mutagenesis, Impairment of Fertility

Famciclovir was administered orally unless otherwise stated.

Carcinogenesis: Two-year dietary carcinogenicity studies on famciclovir were conducted in rats and mice. The high dose tested in rats and mice was lowered after 7 to 8 months of drug administration to ensure long-term survival (female rats and male/female mice from 750 to 600 mg/kg/day; male rats from 300 to 240 mg/kg/day). A significant increase in the incidence of mammary adenocarcinoma was seen in female rats receiving 600 mg/kg/day (1.5 to 9.0 times the human systemic exposure at the recommended oral dose of 500 mg t.i.d. or 125 mg b.i.d. based on area under the plasma concentration curve comparisons [24 hr AUC] for penciclovir). Marginal increases in the incidence of subcutaneous tissue fibrosarcomas or squamous cell carcinomas of the skin were seen in female rats (dosed at 600 mg/kg/day) and male mice (dosed at 600 mg/kg/day; 0.4 to 2.4x the human systemic exposure, based on 24 hr AUC for penciclovir), respectively. No increases in tumor incidence were reported for male rats treated at doses up to 240 mg/kg/day (0.9 to 5.4x the human AUC), or in female mice at doses up to 600 mg/kg/day (0.4 to 2.4x the human AUC).

Mutagenesis: Famciclovir and penciclovir (the active metabolite of famciclovir) were tested for genotoxic potential in a battery of in vitro and in vivo assays. Famciclovir and penciclovir were negative in in vitro tests for gene mutations in bacteria (S. typhimurium and E. coli) and unscheduled DNA synthesis in mammalian HeLa 83 cells (at doses up to 10,000 and 5000 mcg/plate, respectively). Famciclovir was also negative in the L5178Y mouse lymphoma assay (5000 mcg/mL), the in vivo mouse micronucleus test (4800 mg/kg), and rat dominant lethal study (5000 mg/kg). Famciclovir induced increases in polyploidy in human lymphocytes in vitro in the absence of chromosomal damage (1200 mcg/mL). Penciclovir was positive in the L5178Y mouse lymphoma assay for gene mutation/chromosomal aberrations, with and without metabolic activation (1000 mcg/mL). In human lymphocytes, penciclovir caused chromosomal aberrations in the absence of metabolic activation (250 mcg/mL). Penciclovir caused an increased incidence of micronuclei in mouse bone marrow in vivo when administered intravenously at doses highly toxic to bone marrow (500 mg/kg), but not when administered orally.

Impairment of Fertility: Testicular toxicity was observed in rats, mice, and dogs following repeated administration of famciclovir or penciclovir. Testicular changes included atrophy of the seminiferous tubules, reduction in sperm count, and/or increased incidence of sperm with abnormal morphology or reduced motility. The degree of toxicity to male reproduction was related to dose and duration of exposure. In male rats, decreased fertility was observed after 10 weeks of dosing at 500 mg/kg/day (1.9 to 11.4x the human AUC). The no observable effect level for sperm and testicular toxicity in rats following chronic administration (26 weeks) was 50 mg/kg/day (0.2 to 1.2x the human systemic exposure based on AUC comparisons). Testicular toxicity was observed following chronic administration to mice (104 weeks) and dogs (26 weeks) at doses of 600 mg/kg/day (0.4 to 2.4x the human AUC) and 150 mg/kg/day (1.7 to 10.2x the human AUC), respectively.

Famciclovir had no effect on general reproductive performance or fertility in female rats at doses up to 1000 mg/kg/day (3.6 to 21.6x the human AUC).

Pregnancy

Teratogenic Effects—Pregnancy Category B. Famciclovir was tested for effects on embryo-fetal development in rats and rabbits at oral doses up to 1000 mg/kg/day (approximately 3.6 to 21.6x and 1.8 to 10.8x the human systemic exposure to penciclovir based on AUC comparisons for the rat and rabbit, respectively) and intravenous doses of 360 mg/kg/day in rats (2 to 12x the human dose based on body surface area [BSA] comparisons) or 120 mg/kg/day in rabbits (1.5 to 9.0x the human dose [BSA]). No adverse effects were observed on embryo-fetal development. Similarly, no adverse effects were observed following intravenous administration of penciclovir to rats (80 mg/kg/day, 0.4 to 2.6x the human dose [BSA]) or rabbits (60 mg/kg/day, 0.7 to 4.2x the human dose [BSA]). There are, however, no adequate and

Continued on next page

Information on the SmithKline Beecham Pharmaceuticals products appearing here is based on the labeling in effect on July 1, 1996. Further information on these and other products may be obtained from the Medical Department, SmithKline Beecham Pharmaceuticals, One Franklin Plaza, Philadelphia, PA 19101.

SmithKline Beecham—Cont.

well-controlled studies in pregnant women. Because animal reproduction studies are not always predictive of human response, famciclovir should be used during pregnancy only if the benefit to the patient clearly exceeds the potential risk to the fetus.

Nursing Mothers
Following oral administration of famciclovir to lactating rats, penciclovir was excreted in breast milk at concentrations higher than those seen in the plasma. It is not known whether it is excreted in human milk. Because of the potential for tumorigenicity shown for famciclovir in rats, a decision should be made whether to discontinue nursing or to discontinue the drug, taking into account the importance of the drug to the mother.

Usage in Children
Safety and efficacy in children under the age of 18 years have not been established.

Geriatric Use
Of 816 patients with herpes zoster in clinical studies who were treated with *Famvir*, 248 (30.4%) were ≥ 65 years of age and 103 (13%) were ≥ 75 years of age. No overall differences were observed in the incidence or types of adverse events between younger and older patients.

ADVERSE REACTIONS

Herpes Zoster
In four clinical studies involving 816 *Famvir*-treated patients with herpes zoster (*Famvir*, 250 mg t.i.d. to 750 mg t.i.d.), the most frequent adverse events associated with *Famvir* were headache and nausea. Table 3 lists adverse events occurring on-therapy with an incidence of ≥ 2% per treatment group in *Famvir* clinical trials. The frequency and types of reported adverse events in trial 008 were representative of the safety experience in the active-controlled herpes zoster *Famvir* trials (007 and 094).

Recurrent Genital Herpes
In three placebo-controlled clinical trials involving 528 *Famvir*-treated patients with genital herpes (*Famvir*, 125 mg b.i.d. to 500 mg t.i.d.), the most frequent adverse events associated with *Famvir* were headache and nausea. Table 3 lists adverse events occurring on-therapy in *Famvir* clinical trials with an incidence of ≥ 2% per treatment group.

Table 3
Adverse Events Reported by ≥ 2% of Treatment Group in Patients in One Herpes Zoster and Three Placebo-controlled Recurrent Genital Herpes Famvir (famciclovir) Trials*

	Incidence			
	Herpes Zoster		**Genital Herpes**	
	Famvir	Placebo	*Famvir*	Placebo
Event	(n=273)	(n=146)	(n=640)	(n=225)
	%	%	%	%
Nervous System				
Headache	22.7	17.8	23.6	16.4
Dizziness	3.3	4.1	5.5	4.9
Insomnia	1.5	1.4	2.5	2.2
Somnolence	2.6	2.7	1.6	0.4
Paresthesia	2.6	0.0	1.3	0.0
Gastrointestinal				
Nausea	12.5	11.6	10.0	8.0
Diarrhea	7.7	4.8	4.5	7.6
Abdominal Pain	1.1	3.4	3.9	5.8
Dyspepsia	1.1	1.4	3.4	2.2
Flatulence	1.5	0.7	1.9	2.2
Constipation	4.4	4.8	1.4	0.9
Vomiting	4.8	3.4	1.3	0.9
Anorexia	2.6	4.1	1.1	0.9
Body as a Whole				
Fatigue	4.4	3.4	6.3	4.4
Pain	2.6	2.7	2.0	1.8
Injury	2.6	0.0	0.8	1.3
Fever	3.3	4.1	0.8	0.4
Rigors	1.5	2.7	0.5	0.4
Respiratory				
URI	0.7	0.7	3.3	2.7
Pharyngitis	2.6	4.8	2.7	2.2
Sinusitis	2.6	1.4	1.3	1.3
Musculoskeletal				
Back Pain	1.5	2.7	1.9	2.2
Arthralgia	1.5	2.1	1.3	0.0
Zoster/Genital Herpes-Related Signs/Symptoms/ Complications	2.9	3.4	1.7	2.2
Skin and Appendages				
Pruritus	3.7	2.7	0.9	0.0

*Patients may have entered into more than one clinical trial.

During clinical practice, confusion (including delirium, disorientation, confusional state) has been reported very rarely.

Most of these spontaneous reports have occurred in the elderly.

OVERDOSAGE
No acute overdosage has been reported. Appropriate symptomatic and supportive therapy should be given. Penciclovir is removed by hemodialysis.

DOSAGE AND ADMINISTRATION

Herpes Zoster
The recommended dosage is 500 mg every 8 hours for 7 days. Therapy should be initiated promptly as soon as herpes zoster is diagnosed. In clinical trials, the effect of *Famvir* on rash resolution was more pronounced in patients age 50 years and older. Treatment was begun within 72 hours of rash onset in these studies and was more useful if started within the first 48 hours. The efficacy of *Famvir* initiated more than 72 hours after rash onset has not been studied.

Genital Herpes
For recurrent episodes: The recommended dosage is 125 mg b.i.d. for 5 days. Initiate therapy at the first sign or symptom if medical management of a genital herpes recurrence is indicated. The efficacy of *Famvir* has not been established when treatment is initiated more than 6 hours after onset of symptoms or lesions.

In patients with reduced renal function, dosage reduction is recommended.

Table 4

Normal Dosage Regimen	Creatinine Clearance (mL/min.)	Adjusted Dosage Regimen	
		Dose (mg)	Dosing Interval
Herpes Zoster 500 mg every 8 hours	≥ 60	500	every 8 hours
	40–59	500	every 12 hours
	20–39	500	every 24 hours
	< 20	250	every 48 hours
Recurrent Genital Herpes 125 mg every 12 hours	≥ 40	125	every 12 hours
	20–39	125	every 24 hours
	< 20	125	every 48 hours

Hemodialysis patients: The recommended dose of *Famvir* is 250 mg (herpes zoster) or 125 mg (genital herpes) administered following each dialysis treatment.

Administration with Food
When famciclovir was administered with food, penciclovir C_{max} decreased approximately 50%. Because the systemic availability of penciclovir (AUC) was not altered, it appears that *Famvir* may be taken without regard to meals.

HOW SUPPLIED
Famvir is supplied as film-coated tablets as follows: 125 mg in bottles of 30 and Single Unit Packages of 100 (intended for institutional use only); 250 mg in bottles of 30; and 500 mg in bottles of 30 and Single Unit Packages of 50 (intended for institutional use only).

Famvir 125 mg tablets are white, round, debossed with FAMVIR on one side and 125 on the other.
125 mg 30's: NDC 0007-4115-13
125 mg SUP 100's: NDC 0007-4115-21
Famvir 250 mg tablets are white, round, debossed with FAMVIR on one side and 250 on the other.
250 mg 30's: NDC 0007-4116-13
Famvir 500 mg tablets are white, oval, debossed with FAMVIR on one side and 500 on the other.
500 mg 30's: NDC 0007-4117-13
500 mg SUP 50's: NDC 0007-4117-19
Store between 15° and 30°C (59° and 86°F).
Manufactured in Crawley, UK
by SmithKline Beecham Pharmaceuticals
for SmithKline Beecham Pharmaceuticals
Philadelphia, PA 19101
Veterans Administration/Military/PHS—
Tablets, 125 mg, 30's, 6505-01-425-3169;
125 mg, SUP, 100's, 6505-01-425-3170;
250 mg, 30's, 6505-01-425-3166.
FV:L5B

Shown in Product Identification Guide, page 336

FASTIN®   ℞
[făs 'tin]
(brand of phentermine hydrochloride)
Capsules

DESCRIPTION
Each Fastin (phentermine hydrochloride) capsule contains phentermine hydrochloride, 30 mg (equivalent to 24 mg phentermine).

Phentermine hydrochloride is a white crystalline powder, very soluble in water and alcohol. Chemically, the product is phenyl-tertiary-butylamine hydrochloride. **Inactive Ingredients:** FD&C Blue No. 1, invert sugar, methylcellulose, polyethylene glycol, starch, sucrose and titanium dioxide. The branding ink used on the gelatin capsules contains: aluminum lake, ethyl alcohol, FD&C Blue No. 1, isopropyl alcohol, n-butyl alcohol, pharmaceutical shellac (modified) or refined shellac (food grade) and propylene glycol.

ACTIONS
Fastin is a sympathomimetic amine with pharmacologic activity similar to the prototype drugs of this class used in obesity, the amphetamines. Actions include central nervous system stimulation and elevation of blood pressure. Tachyphylaxis and tolerance have been demonstrated with all drugs of this class in which these phenomena have been looked for.

Drugs of this class used in obesity are commonly known as "anorectics" or "anorexigenics." It has not been established that the action of such drugs in treating obesity is primarily one of appetite suppression. Other central nervous system actions, or metabolic effects, may be involved, for example. Adult obese subjects instructed in dietary management and treated with "anorectic" drugs lose more weight on the average than those treated with placebo and diet, as determined in relatively short-term clinical trials.

The magnitude of increased weight loss of drug-treated patients over placebo-treated patients is only a fraction of a pound a week. The rate of weight loss is greatest in the first weeks of therapy for both drug and placebo subjects and tends to decrease in succeeding weeks. The possible origins of the increased weight loss due to the various drug effects are not established. The amount of weight loss associated with the use of an "anorectic" drug varies from trial to trial, and the increased weight loss appears to be related in part to variables other than the drugs prescribed, such as the physician-investigator, the population treated and the diet prescribed. Studies do not permit conclusions as to the relative importance of the drug and non-drug factors on weight loss. The natural history of obesity is measured in years, whereas the studies cited are restricted to a few weeks' duration; thus, the total impact of drug-induced weight loss over that of diet alone must be considered clinically limited.

INDICATION
Fastin is indicated in the management of exogenous obesity as a short-term (a few weeks) adjunct in a regimen of weight reduction based on caloric restriction. The limited usefulness of agents of this class (see ACTIONS) should be measured against possible risk factors inherent in their use such as those described below.

CONTRAINDICATIONS
Advanced arteriosclerosis, symptomatic cardiovascular disease, moderate to severe hypertension, hyperthyroidism, known hypersensitivity or idiosyncrasy to the sympathomimetic amines, glaucoma.
Agitated states.
Patients with a history of drug abuse.
During or within 14 days following the administration of monoamine oxidase inhibitors (hypertensive crises may result).

WARNINGS
Tolerance to the anorectic effect usually develops within a few weeks. When this occurs, the recommended dose should not be exceeded in an attempt to increase the effect; rather, the drug should be discontinued.

Fastin may impair the ability of the patient to engage in potentially hazardous activities such as operating machinery or driving a motor vehicle; the patient should therefore be cautioned accordingly.

Drug Dependence: *Fastin* is related chemically and pharmacologically to the amphetamines. Amphetamines and related stimulant drugs have been extensively abused, and the possibility of abuse of *Fastin* should be kept in mind when evaluating the desirability of including a drug as part of a weight reduction program. Abuse of amphetamines and related drugs may be associated with intense psychological dependence and severe social dysfunction. There are reports of patients who have increased the dosage to many times that recommended. Abrupt cessation following prolonged high dosage administration results in extreme fatigue and mental depression; changes are also noted on the sleep EEG. Manifestations of chronic intoxication with anorectic drugs include severe dermatoses, marked insomnia, irritability, hyperactivity and personality changes. The most severe manifestation of chronic intoxications is psychosis, often clinically indistinguishable from schizophrenia.

Usage in Pregnancy: Safe use in pregnancy has not been established. Use of *Fastin* by women who are or who may become pregnant, and those in the first trimester of pregnancy, requires that the potential benefit be weighed against the possible hazard to mother and infant.
Usage in Children: *Fastin* is not recommended for use in children under 12 years of age.
Usage with Alcohol: Concomitant use of alcohol with *Fastin* may result in an adverse drug interaction.

PRECAUTIONS

Caution is to be exercised in prescribing Fastin (phentermine hydrochloride) for patients with even mild hypertension.
Insulin requirements in diabetes mellitus may be altered in association with the use of *Fastin* and the concomitant dietary regimen.
Fastin may decrease the hypotensive effect of guanethidine.
The least amount feasible should be prescribed or dispensed at one time in order to minimize the possibility of overdosage.

ADVERSE REACTIONS

Cardiovascular: Palpitation, tachycardia, elevation of blood pressure.
Central Nervous System: Overstimulation, restlessness, dizziness, insomnia, euphoria, dysphoria, tremor, headache; rarely psychotic episodes at recommended doses.
Gastrointestinal: Dryness of the mouth, unpleasant taste, diarrhea, constipation, other gastrointestinal disturbances.
Allergic: Urticaria.
Endocrine: Impotence, changes in libido.

DOSAGE AND ADMINISTRATION

Exogenous Obesity: One capsule at approximately 2 hours after breakfast for appetite control. Late evening medication should be avoided because of the possibility of resulting insomnia.
Administration of one capsule (30 mg) daily has been found to be adequate in depression of the appetite for 12 to 14 hours.
Fastin is not recommended for use in children under 12 years of age.

OVERDOSAGE

Manifestations of acute overdosage with phentermine include restlessness, tremor, hyperreflexia, rapid respiration, confusion, assaultiveness, hallucinations, panic states. Fatigue and depression usually follow the central stimulation. Cardiovascular effects include arrhythmias, hypertension or hypotension, and circulatory collapse. Gastrointestinal symptoms include nausea, vomiting, diarrhea and abdominal cramps. Fatal poisoning usually terminates in convulsions and coma.
Management of acute phentermine intoxication is largely symptomatic and includes lavage and sedation with a barbiturate. Experience with hemodialysis or peritoneal dialysis is inadequate to permit recommendations in this regard. Acidification of the urine increases phentermine excretion. Intravenous phentolamine (Regitine®, CIBA) has been suggested for possible acute, severe hypertension, if this complicates phentermine overdosage.

HOW SUPPLIED

Blue and clear capsules with blue and white beads containing 30 mg phentermine hydrochloride (equivalent to 24 mg phentermine) imprinted with BEECHAM on cap and product name FASTIN® on body.
NDC 0029-2205-30 ....bottles of 100
NDC 0029-2205-39 ....bottles of 450
Store at room temperature.
Manufactured by
King Pharmaceuticals, Inc.
Bristol, TN 37620 for
SmithKline Beecham Pharmaceuticals
Philadelphia, PA 19101

FA:L2

Shown in Product Identification Guide, page 336

HEPATITIS A VACCINE, INACTIVATED ℞

HAVRIX®
[*have'rix*]

DESCRIPTION

Havrix (Hepatitis A Vaccine, Inactivated) is a noninfectious hepatitis A vaccine developed and manufactured by SmithKline Beecham Biologicals. The virus (strain HM175) is propagated in MRC_5 human diploid cells. After removal of the cell culture medium, the cells are lysed to form a suspension. This suspension is purified through ultrafiltration and gel permeation chromatography procedures. Treatment of this lysate with formalin ensures viral inactivation. *Havrix* contains a sterile suspension of inactivated virus; viral antigen activity is referenced to a standard using an enzyme linked immunosorbent assay (ELISA), and is therefore expressed in terms of ELISA Units (EL.U.).
Havrix is supplied as a sterile suspension for intramuscular administration. The vaccine is ready for use without reconstitution; it must be shaken before administration to assure a uniform suspension.
Each 1 mL adult dose of vaccine consists of not less than 1440 EL.U. of viral antigen, adsorbed on 0.5 mg of aluminum, as aluminum hydroxide.
There are two pediatric dose formulations, each with its own dosing schedule (see DOSAGE AND ADMINISTRATION). The formulations are: not less than 360 EL.U. of viral antigen/0.5 mL; not less than 720 EL.U. of viral antigen/0.5 mL. Each dose is adsorbed onto 0.25 mg of aluminum, as aluminum hydroxide.
The vaccine preparations also contain 0.5% (w/v) of 2-phenoxyethanol as a preservative. Other excipients are: amino acid supplement (0.3% w/v) in a phosphate-buffered saline solution and polysorbate 20 (0.05 mg/mL). Residual MRC_5 cellular proteins (not more than 5 mcg/adult dose) and traces of formalin (not more than 0.1 mg/mL) are present.

CLINICAL PHARMACOLOGY

The hepatitis A virus (HAV) belongs to the picornavirus family. Only one serotype of HAV has been described.[1]
Hepatitis A is highly contagious with the predominant mode of transmission being person-to-person via the fecal-oral route. Infection has been shown to be spread (1) by contaminated water or food; (2) by infected food handlers[2]; (3) after breakdown in usual sanitary conditions or after floods or natural disasters; (4) by ingestion of raw or undercooked shellfish (oysters, clams, mussels) from contaminated waters[3]; (5) during travel to areas of the world with poor hygienic conditions[4,5]; (6) among institutionalized children and adults[6]; (7) in day-care centers where children have not been toilet trained[7]; (8) by parenteral transmission, either blood transfusions or sharing needles with infected people.[1]
The level of economic development influences the prevalence of hepatitis A and the age at which it is most likely to occur. In developing countries with poor hygiene and sanitation, about 90% of children are infected by age 5 years.[1] As conditions improve, the prevalence decreases and the age at which infection occurs increases. Hence it is more likely to occur in adulthood, when disease is generally more severe and more likely to be fatal.[1] In the United States, attack rates for hepatitis A infection are cyclical and vary by population. The rates have increased gradually from 9.2 per 100,000 in 1983 to 14.6 per 100,000 in 1989.[8]
The incubation period for hepatitis A averages 28 days (range: 15 to 50 days).[9] The course of hepatitis A infection is extremely variable, ranging from asymptomatic infection to icteric hepatitis. However, most adults (76% to 97%)[10] become symptomatic. Symptoms range from mild and transient to severe and prolonged and may include fever, nausea, vomiting and diarrhea in the prodromal phase, followed by jaundice in up to 88% of adults, as well as hepatomegaly and biochemical evidence of hepatocellular damage.[10] Recovery is generally complete and followed by protection against HAV infection. However, illness may be prolonged, and relapse of clinical illness and viral shedding have been described.[11]
Hepatitis A infection is often asymptomatic in children under 2 years of age, who nonetheless excrete the virus in their stool and thereby serve as a source of infection.[10] In older patients and persons with underlying liver disease,[1] it is generally much more severe. This is reflected in mortality rates. While an overall case fatality rate of 0.6% has been reported, a case fatality rate of 2.7% has been reported in patients ≥49 years of age.[1] Indeed, while 67% of cases occur in children, over 70% of deaths occur in those over the age of 49 years.[1]
There is no chronic carrier state. The virus replicates in the liver and is excreted in bile. The highest concentrations of HAV are found in stools of infected persons during the 2-week period immediately before the onset of jaundice and decline after jaundice appears.[12] Children and infants may shed HAV for longer periods than adults, possibly lasting as long as several weeks after the onset of clinical illness.[13] Chronic shedding of HAV in feces has not been demonstrated, but relapses of hepatitis A can occur in as many as 20% of patients[1,14] and fecal shedding of HAV may recur at this time.[11]
The presence of antibodies to HAV (anti-HAV) confers protection against hepatitis A infection. However, the lowest titer needed to confer protection has not been determined.
In a chimpanzee challenge study, the quality of protection afforded by immune globulin (IG) prepared from initially seronegative human volunteers vaccinated with *Havrix* was comparable to that afforded by commercial IG. In this experiment chimpanzees immunized with either preparation developed passive-active immunity, when challenged with wild-type HAV. No animal in either group developed clinical illness.
In vitro studies in a randomly selected subset of human subjects (n=80) showed anti-HAV induced by *Havrix* to have functional activity. This was demonstrated by a neutralization assay and a competitive inhibition assay using a panel of monoclonal antibodies known to have neutralizing activity.
Immunogenicity in Adults: In three clinical studies involving over 400 healthy adult volunteers given a single 1440 EL.U. dose of *Havrix*, specific humoral antibodies against HAV were elicited in more than 96% of subjects when measured 1 month after vaccination. By day 15, 80% to 98% of vaccinees had already seroconverted (anti-HAV ≥20 mIU/mL [the lower limit of antibody measurement by current assay]). Geometric mean titers (GMTs) of seroconverters ranged from 264 to 339 mIU/mL at day 15 and increased to a range of 335 to 637 mIU/mL by 1 month following vaccination.[15]
The GMTs obtained following a single dose of *Havrix* are at least several times higher than that expected following receipt of IG.
In a clinical study using 2.5 to 5 times the standard dose of IG (standard dose=0.02 to 0.06 mL/kg), the GMT in recipients was 146 mIU/mL at 5 days post-administration, 77 mIU/mL at month 1 and 63 mIU/mL at month 2.[15]
In two clinical trials in which a booster dose of 1440 EL.U. was given 6 months following the initial dose, 100% of vaccinees (n=269) were seropositive 1 month after the booster dose, with GMTs ranging from 3318 mIU/mL to 5925 mIU/mL. The titers obtained from this additional dose approximate those observed several years after natural infection.
In a subset of vaccinees (n=89), a single dose of *Havrix* 1440 EL.U. elicited specific anti-HAV neutralizing antibodies in more than 94% of vaccinees when measured 1 month after vaccination. These neutralizing antibodies persisted until month 6. One hundred percent of vaccinees had neutralizing antibodies when measured 1 month after a booster dose given at month 6.
Immunogenicity in Children and Adolescents: In six clinical studies involving pediatric vaccinees (n=762) ranging from 1 to 18 years of age, the GMT following two doses of *Havrix* 360 EL.U. given 1 month apart ranged from 197 to 660 mIU/mL. Ninety-nine percent of subjects seroconverted following two doses. When a booster (third) dose of *Havrix* 360 EL.U. was administered 6 months following the initial dose, all subjects were seropositive 1 month following the booster dose with GMTs rising to a range of 3388 to 4643 mIU/mL. In one study in which children were followed for an additional 6 months, all subjects remained seropositive. Solicited adverse effects were similar in frequency and nature to those seen following administration of Engerix-B® [Hepatitis B Vaccine (Recombinant)].
In four clinical studies, children and adolescents (n=314), ranging from 2 to 19 years of age, were immunized with two doses of *Havrix* 720 EL.U./0.5 mL given six months apart. One month after the first dose, seroconversion ranged from 96.8% to 100%, with GMTs of 194 mIU/mL to 305 mIU/mL. In studies in which sera were obtained 2 weeks following the initial dose, seroconversion ranged from 91.6% to 96.1%. One month following a booster dose at month 6, all subjects were seropositive with GMTs ranging from 2495 mIU/mL to 3644 mIU/mL.[15]
In one additional study in which the booster dose was delayed until 1 year following the initial dose, 95.2% of the subjects were seropositive just prior to administration of the booster dose. One month later, all subjects were seropositive with a GMT of 2657 mIU/mL.[15]
Also, *Havrix* has been found to be highly efficacious in a clinical study of children at high risk of HAV infection (see below).
At present, the duration of protection afforded by *Havrix* has not been established. Therefore it is unknown if the protection provided to immunized children will last until adulthood.
Protective Efficacy: Protective efficacy with *Havrix* has been demonstrated in a double-blind, randomized controlled study in school children (age 1 to 16 years) in Thailand who were at high risk of HAV infection. A total of 40,119 children were randomized to be vaccinated with either *Havrix* 360 EL.U. or *Engerix-B* at 0, 1, 12 months. 19,037 children received a primary course (0, 1 months) of *Havrix* and 19,120 children received a primary course (0, 1 months) of *Engerix-B*. 38,157 children entered surveillance at day 138 and were observed for an additional 8 months. Using the protocol-defined endpoint (≥2 days absence from school, ALT level >45 U/mL, and a positive result in the HAVAB-M test), 32 cases of clinical hepatitis A occurred in the control group; in the *Havrix* group, two cases were identified. These two cases were mild both in terms of biochemical and clinical indices of hepatitis A disease. Thus the calculated efficacy rate for prevention of clinical hepatitis A was 94% (95% confidence intervals 74% to 98%).[16]

Continued on next page

Information on the SmithKline Beecham Pharmaceuticals products appearing here is based on the labeling in effect on July 1, 1996. Further information on these and other products may be obtained from the Medical Department, SmithKline Beecham Pharmaceuticals, One Franklin Plaza, Philadelphia, PA 19101.

SmithKline Beecham—Cont.

In outbreak investigations occurring in the trial, 26 clinical cases of hepatitis A (of a total of 34 occurring in the trial) occurred. No cases occurred in *Havrix* vaccinees.

Using additional virological and serological analyses post hoc, the efficacy of *Havrix* was confirmed. Up to three additional cases of very mild clinical illness may have occurred in vaccinees. Using available testing, these illnesses could neither be proven nor disproven to have been caused by HAV. By including these as cases, the calculated efficacy rate for prevention of clinical hepatitis A would be 84% (95% confidence intervals 60% to 94%).

In a study designed to interrupt an epidemic of hepatitis A among Native Americans in Alaska, vaccination with a single dose of *Havrix* (1440 EL.U./mL in adults, 720 EL.U./0.5 mL in children and adolescents), appeared to be efficacious.[15]

INDICATIONS AND USAGE

Havrix is indicated for active immunization of persons ≥ 2 years of age against disease caused by hepatitis A virus (HAV).

Havrix will not prevent hepatitis caused by other agents such as hepatitis B virus, hepatitis C virus, hepatitis E virus or other pathogens known to infect the liver.

Immunization with *Havrix* is indicated for those people desiring protection against hepatitis A. Primary immunization should be completed at least 2 weeks prior to expected exposure to HAV. Individuals who are, or will be, at increased risk of infection by HAV include:

Travelers.
Persons traveling to areas of higher endemicity for hepatitis A. These areas include, but are not limited to, Africa, Asia (except Japan), the Mediterranean basin, eastern Europe, the Middle East, Central and South America, Mexico, and parts of the Caribbean. Current CDC advisories should be consulted with regard to specific locales.
Military personnel.
People living in, or relocating to, areas of high endemicity.
Certain ethnic and geographic populations that experience cyclic hepatitis A epidemics such as:
Native peoples of Alaska and the Americas.
Others.
—Persons engaging in high-risk sexual activity (such as men having sex with men)
—Residents of a community experiencing an outbreak of hepatitis A
—Users of illicit injectable drugs
Although the epidemiology of hepatitis A does not permit the identification of other specific populations at high risk of disease, outbreaks of hepatitis A or exposure to hepatitis A virus have been described in a variety of populations in which *Havrix* may be useful:
—Certain institutional workers (e.g., caretakers for the developmentally challenged)
—Employees of child day-care centers
—Laboratory workers who handle live hepatitis A virus
—Handlers of primate animals that may be harboring HAV
People exposed to hepatitis A.
For those requiring both immediate and long-term protection, *Havrix* may be administered concomitantly with IG.

CONTRAINDICATIONS

Havrix is contraindicated in people with known hypersensitivity to any component of the vaccine.

WARNINGS

There have been rare reports of anaphylaxis/anaphylactoid reactions following commercial use of the vaccine in other countries. Patients experiencing hypersensitivity reactions after a *Havrix* injection should not receive further *Havrix* injections. (See CONTRAINDICATIONS.)

Hepatitis A has a relatively long incubation period (15 to 50 days). Hepatitis A vaccine may not prevent hepatitis A infection in individuals who have an unrecognized hepatitis A infection at the time of vaccination. Additionally, it may not prevent infection in individuals who do not achieve protective antibody titers (although the lowest titer needed to confer protection has not been determined).

PRECAUTIONS

General
As with any parenteral vaccine, epinephrine should be available for use in case of anaphylaxis or anaphylactoid reaction. As with any vaccine, administration of *Havrix* should be delayed, if possible, in people with any febrile illness, except when, in the opinion of the physician, withholding vaccine entails the greater risk.

Havrix should be administered with caution to people with thrombocytopenia or a bleeding disorder since bleeding may occur following an intramuscular administration to these subjects.

As with any vaccine, if administered to immunosuppressed persons or persons receiving immunosuppressive therapy, the expected immune response may not be obtained.[17]

Care is to be taken by the health-care provider for the safe and effective use of *Havrix*.

Prior to an injection of any vaccine, all known precautions should be taken to prevent adverse reactions. This includes a review of the patient's history with respect to possible hypersensitivity to the vaccine or similar vaccines.

A separate sterile syringe and needle (for single-dose vial) or a sterile disposable unit (prefilled syringe) must be used for each patient to prevent the transmission of infectious agents from person to person. Needles should not be recapped and should be properly disposed.

Special care should be taken to ensure that *Havrix* is not injected into a blood vessel.

Information for Patients
Patients, parents or guardians should be fully informed of the benefits and risks of immunization with *Havrix*.

Havrix is indicated in a variety of situations (see INDICATIONS AND USAGE). For persons traveling to endemic or epidemic areas, current CDC advisories should be consulted with regard to specific locales.

Travelers should take all necessary precautions to avoid contact with or ingestion of contaminated food or water. The duration of immunity following a complete schedule of immunization with *Havrix* has not been established.

Drug Interactions
Preliminary results suggest that the concomitant administration of a wide variety of other vaccines is unlikely to interfere with the immune response to *Havrix*.

As with other intramuscular injections, *Havrix* should be given with caution to individuals on anticoagulant therapy. When concomitant administration of other vaccines or IG is required, they should be given with different syringes and at different injection sites.

Carcinogenesis, Mutagenesis, Impairment of Fertility
Havrix has not been evaluated for its carcinogenic potential, mutagenic potential or potential for impairment of fertility.

Pregnancy: Pregnancy Category C.
Animal reproduction studies have not been conducted with *Havrix*. It is also not known whether *Havrix* can cause fetal harm when administered to a pregnant woman or can affect reproduction capacity. *Havrix* should be given to a pregnant woman only if clearly needed.

Nursing Mothers
It is not known whether *Havrix* is excreted in human milk. Because many drugs are excreted in human milk, caution should be exercised when *Havrix* is administered to a nursing woman.

Pediatric Use
Havrix is well tolerated and highly immunogenic and effective in children ≥ 2 years of age. (See CLINICAL PHARMACOLOGY for immunogenicity and efficacy data. See DOSAGE AND ADMINISTRATION for recommended dosage.)

ADVERSE REACTIONS

During clinical trials involving more than 31,000 individuals receiving doses ranging from 360 EL.U. to 1440 EL.U. and during extensive postmarketing experience in Europe, Havrix (Hepatitis A Vaccine, Inactivated) has been generally well tolerated. As with all pharmaceuticals, however, it is possible that expanded commercial use of the vaccine could reveal rare adverse events not observed in clinical studies.

The frequency of solicited adverse events tended to decrease with successive doses of *Havrix*. Most events reported were considered by the subjects as mild and did not last for more than 24 hours.

Of solicited adverse events in clinical trials, the most frequently reported by volunteers was injection-site soreness (56% of adults and 21% of children); however, less than 0.5% of soreness was reported as severe. Headache was reported by 14% of adults and less than 9% of children. Other solicited and unsolicited events occurring during clinical trials are listed below:

Incidence 1% to 10% of Injections
Local reactions at injection site: induration, redness, swelling.
Body as a whole: fatigue, fever (> 37.5°C), malaise.
Gastrointestinal: anorexia, nausea.

Incidence < 1% of Injections
Local reaction at injection site: hematoma.
Dermatologic: pruritus, rash, urticaria.
Respiratory: pharyngitis, other upper respiratory tract infections.
Gastrointestinal: abdominal pain, diarrhea, dysgeusia, vomiting.
Musculoskeletal: arthralgia, elevation of creatine phosphokinase, myalgia.
Hematologic: lymphadenopathy.
Central nervous system: hypertonic episode, insomnia, photophobia, vertigo.

Additional Safety Data
Safety data were obtained from two additional sources in which large populations were vaccinated. In an outbreak setting in which 4,930 individuals were immunized with a single dose of either 720 EL.U. or 1440 EL.U. of *Havrix*, the vaccine was well-tolerated and no serious adverse events due

to vaccination were reported. Overall, less than 10% of vaccinees reported solicited general adverse events following the vaccine. The most common solicited local adverse event was pain at the injection site, reported in 22.3% of subjects at 24 hours and decreasing to 2.4% by 72 hours.

In a field efficacy trial, 19,037 children received the 360 EL.U. dose of *Havrix*. The most commonly reported adverse events following administration of *Havrix* were injection-site pain (9.5%) and tenderness (8.1%), which were reported following first doses of *Havrix*. Other adverse events were infrequent and comparable to the control vaccine *Engerix-B*. Additionally, no serious adverse events due to the vaccine were reported. The large trial further allowed for analysis of rare adverse events, including hospitalization and death. No significant differences were found between the cohorts.

Postmarketing Reports
Rare voluntary reports of adverse events in people receiving *Havrix* that have been reported since market introduction of the vaccine include the following:
Local: localized edema.
While no causal relationship has been established, the following rare events have been reported:
Body as a whole: anaphylaxis/anaphylactoid reactions, somnolence.
Cardiovascular: syncope.
Hepatobiliary: jaundice, hepatitis.
Dermatologic: erythema multiforme, hyperhydrosis, angioedema.
Respiratory: dyspnea.
Hematologic: lymphadenopathy.
Central nervous system: convulsions, encephalopathy, dizziness, neuropathy, myelitis, paresthesia, Guillain-Barré syndrome, multiple sclerosis.
Other: congenital abnormality.

Reporting of Adverse Events
The U.S. Department of Health and Human Services has established the Vaccine Adverse Events Reporting System (VAERS) to accept reports of suspected adverse events after the administration of any vaccine, including, but not limited to, the reporting of events required by the National Childhood Vaccine Injury Act of 1986. The toll-free number for VAERS forms and information is 1-800-822-7967.[18]

DOSAGE AND ADMINISTRATION

Havrix should be administered by intramuscular injection. *Do not inject intravenously, intradermally or subcutaneously.* In adults, the injection should be given in the deltoid region. *Havrix* should not be administered in the gluteal region; such injections may result in suboptimal response.

Havrix may be administered concomitantly with IG, although the ultimate antibody titer obtained is likely to be lower than when the vaccine is given alone. *Havrix* has been administered simultaneously with *Engerix-B* without interference with their respective immune responses.

When concomitant administration of other vaccines or IG is required, they should be given with different syringes and at different injection sites.

Preparation for Administration: Shake vial or syringe well before withdrawal and use. Parenteral drug products should be inspected visually for particulate matter or discoloration prior to administration. With thorough agitation, *Havrix* is a turbid white suspension. Discard if it appears otherwise.

The vaccine should be used as supplied; no dilution or reconstitution is necessary. The full recommended dose of the vaccine should be used. After removal of the appropriate volume from a single-dose vial, any vaccine remaining in the vial should be discarded.

Primary immunization for adults consists of a single dose of 1440 EL.U. in 1 mL. Primary immunization for children and adolescents (2 through 18 years of age) may follow either of these two schedules:

Group	Dose	Schedule
Children and adolescents (2 through 18 years of age)	Primary course: 360 EL.U./0.5 mL	two doses, given 1 month apart (month 0 and month 1)
	Booster: 360 EL.U./0.5 mL	6 to 12 months after primary course
	OR	
	Primary course: 720 EL.U./0.5 mL	one dose (month 0)
	Booster: 720 EL.U./0.5 mL	6 to 12 months after primary course

Individuals should not be alternated between the 360 EL.U. and 720 EL.U. doses. Those who receive an initial 360 EL.U. dose should continue on the 360 EL.U. dosing schedule. Like-

wise, those individuals who receive a single 720 EL.U. primary dose should receive a 720 EL.U. booster dose.
For all age groups, a booster dose is recommended anytime between 6 and 12 months after the initiation of the primary dose in order to ensure the highest antibody titers.
In those with an impaired immune system, adequate anti-HAV response may not be obtained after the primary immunization course. Such patients may therefore require administration of additional doses of vaccine.

STORAGE

Store between 2° and 8°C (36° and 47°F). Do not freeze; discard if product has been frozen. Do not dilute to administer.

HOW SUPPLIED

360 EL.U./0.5 mL in Single-Dose Vials.
NDC 58160-836-01 Package of 1
720 EL.U./0.5 mL in Single-Dose Vials and Prefilled Syringes.
NDC 58160-837-01 Package of 1 Single-Dose Vial
NDC 58160-837-02 Package of 1 Prefilled Syringe
1440 EL.U./mL in Single-Dose Vials and Prefilled Syringes.
NDC 58160-835-01 Package of 1 Single-Dose Vial
NDC 58160-835-02 Package of 1 Prefilled Syringe

REFERENCES

1. Hadler SC: Global impact of hepatitis A virus infection changing patterns. In Hollinger FB, Lemon SM, Margolis H (eds): *Viral Hepatitis and Liver Disease.* Baltimore, Williams & Wilkins, 1991, pp. 14-20. **2.** Dienstag JL, Routenberg JA, Purcell RH, et al: Foodhandler-associated outbreak of hepatitis type A. An immune electron microscopic study. *Ann Intern Med.* 1975;83:647. **3.** Mackowiak PA, Caraway CT, Portnoy BL: Oyster-associated hepatitis. Lessons from the Louisiana experience. *Am J Epidemiol.* 1976;103:181. **4.** Woodson RD, Clinton JJ: Hepatitis prophylaxis abroad. Effectiveness of immune serum globulin in protecting Peace Corps volunteers. *JAMA.* 1969;1009:1053. **5.** Krugman S, Giles JP: Viral hepatitis. New light on an old disease. *JAMA.* 1970;212:1019. **6.** Mosley JW: Hepatitis types B and non-B. Epidemiologic background. *JAMA.* 1975;233:967. **7.** Hadler SC, Erben JJ, Francis DP, et al: Risk factors for hepatitis A in daycare centers. *J Infect Dis.* 1982;145:255. **8.** Shapiro CN, Shaw SE, Mandel EJ, Hadler SC: Epidemiology of hepatitis A in the United States. In Hollinger FB, Lemon SM, Margolis H (eds): *Viral Hepatitis and Liver Disease.* Baltimore, Williams & Wilkins, 1991, pp. 71-76. **9.** Centers for Disease Control: Protection against viral hepatitis: Recommendations of the Immunization Practices Advisory Committee (ACIP). *MMWR.* 1990;39(No. RR-2):1-26. **10.** Lemon SM: Type A viral hepatitis: new developments in an old disease. *N Engl J Med.* Oct. 24, 1985;313(17):1059-1067. **11.** Sjogren MH, Tanno H, Fay O, et al: Hepatitis A virus in stool during clinical relapse. *Ann Intern Med.* 1987;106:221-226. **12.** Hollinger FB, Ticehurst J: Hepatitis A Virus. In Hollinger FB, Robinson WS, Purcell RH, et al (eds): *Viral Hepatitis.* New York, Raven Press, 1990, pp. 1-37. **13.** Tassopoulos NC, Papaevangelou GJ, Ticehurst JR, et al: Fecal excretion of Greek strains of hepatitis A virus in patients with hepatitis A and in experimentally infected chimpanzees. *J Infect Dis.* 1986; 154:231-237. **14.** Chiriaco P, Gaudalupi C, Armigliato MK, et al: Polyphasic course of hepatitis type A in children. *J Infect Dis.* 1986; 153:378. **15.** Data on file, SmithKline Beecham Pharmaceuticals. **16.** Innis BL, Snitbhan R, Kunasol P, et al: Protection against hepatitis A by an inactivated vaccine. *JAMA.* 1994;271(17):1328-1364. **17.** ACIP: Use of vaccines and immune globulins in persons with altered immunocompetence. *MMWR.* 1993;42 (No. RR-4). **18.** Centers for Disease Control: Vaccine Adverse Event Reporting System-United States. *MMWR.* 1990;39:730-733.

U.S. License No. 1090
Manufactured by **SmithKline Beecham Biologicals**
Rixensart, Belgium
Distributed by **SmithKline Beecham Pharmaceuticals**
Philadelphia, PA 19101
Havrix is a registered trademark of SmithKline Beecham.
Veterans Administration/Military/PHS—1440 EL.U./mL. single dose, 1's, 6505-01-398-3325: 1440 EL.U./mL. prefilled syringe, 1's, 6505-01-397-6045.
360 EL.U./0.5 mL, single dose, 1's, 6505-01-413-1330; 720 EL.U./0.5 mL, prefilled syringe, 1's, 6505-01-431-9401.
HA:L5A

Shown in Product Identification Guide, page 336

HYCAMTIN™ ℞

[hī-kam'-tin]
brand of topotecan hydrochloride for Injection (for intravenous use)

WARNING

Hycamtin (topotecan hydrochloride) for Injection should be administered under the supervision of a physician experienced in the use of cancer chemotherapeutic agents. Appropriate management of complications is possible only when adequate diagnostic and treatment facilities are readily available.
Therapy with *Hycamtin* should not be given to patients with baseline neutrophil counts of less than 1500 cells/mm^3. In order to monitor the occurrence of bone marrow suppression, primarily neutropenia, which may be severe and result in infection and death, frequent peripheral blood cell counts should be performed on all patients receiving *Hycamtin.*

DESCRIPTION

Hycamtin (topotecan hydrochloride) is a semi-synthetic derivative of camptothecin and is an anti-tumor drug with topoisomerase I-inhibitory activity.
Hycamtin (topotecan hydrochloride) for Injection is supplied as a sterile lyophilized, buffered, light yellow to greenish powder available in single-dose vials. Each vial contains topotecan hydrochloride equivalent to 4 mg of topotecan as free base. The reconstituted solution ranges in color from yellow to yellow-green and is intended for administration by intravenous infusion.
Inactive ingredients are mannitol, 48 mg, and tartaric acid, 20 mg. Hydrochloric acid and sodium hydroxide may be used to adjust the pH. The solution pH ranges from 2.5 to 3.5. The chemical name for topotecan hydrochloride is (*S*)-10-[(dimethylamino)methyl]-4-ethyl-4,9-dihydroxy-1*H*-pyrano [3′, 4′:6,7]indolizino[1,2-*b*]quinoline-3,14-(4*H*,12*H*)-dione monohydrochloride. It has the molecular formula $C_{23}H_{23}N_3O_5{\bullet}HCl$ and a molecular weight of 457.9.
Topotecan hydrochloride has the following structural formula:

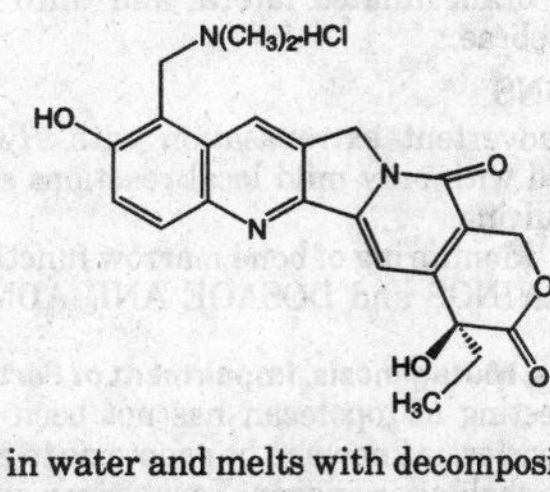

It is soluble in water and melts with decomposition at 213° to 218°C.

CLINICAL PHARMACOLOGY

Mechanism of Action

Topoisomerase I relieves torsional strain in DNA by inducing reversible single strand breaks. Topotecan binds to the topoisomerase I-DNA complex and prevents religation of these single strand breaks. The cytotoxicity of topotecan is thought to be due to double strand DNA damage produced during DNA synthesis when replication enzymes interact with the ternary complex formed by topotecan, topoisomerase I and DNA. Mammalian cells cannot efficiently repair these double strand breaks.

Pharmacokinetics

The pharmacokinetics of topotecan have been evaluated in cancer patients following doses of 0.5 to 1.5 mg/m^2 administered as a 30-minute infusion. Topotecan exhibits multiexponential pharmacokinetics with a terminal half-life of 2 to 3 hours. Total exposure (AUC) is approximately dose-proportional. Binding of topotecan to plasma proteins is about 35%.
Metabolism and Elimination: Topotecan undergoes a reversible pH dependent hydrolysis of its lactone moiety; it is the lactone form that is pharmacologically active. At pH$\leq$4 the lactone is exclusively present whereas the ring-opened hydroxy-acid form predominates at physiologic pH. *In vitro* studies in human liver microsomes indicate that metabolism of topotecan to an N-demethylated metabolite represents a minor metabolic pathway.
In humans, about 30% of the dose is excreted in the urine and renal clearance is an important determinant of topotecan elimination (see Special Populations).

Special Populations

Gender: The overall mean topotecan plasma clearance in male patients was approximately 24% higher than in female patients, largely reflecting difference in body size.
Geriatrics: Topotecan pharmacokinetics have not been specifically studied in an elderly population, but population pharmacokinetic analysis in female patients did not identify age as a significant factor. Decreased renal clearance, common in the elderly, is a more important determinant of topotecan clearance.
Race: The effect of race on topotecan pharmacokinetics has not been studied.
Renal Impairment: In patients with mild renal impairment (creatinine clearance of 40 to 60 mL/min.), topotecan plasma clearance was decreased to about 67% of the value in patients with normal renal function. In patients with moderate renal impairment (Cl_{cr} of 20 to 39 mL/min.), topotecan plasma clearance was reduced to about 34% of the value in control patients, with an increase in half-life. Mean half-life, estimated in three renally impaired patients, was about 5.0 hours. Dosage adjustment is recommended for these patients (see DOSAGE AND ADMINISTRATION).
Hepatic Impairment: Plasma clearance in patients with hepatic impairment (serum bilirubin levels between 1.7 and 15.0 mg/dL) was decreased to about 67% of the value in patients without hepatic impairment. Topotecan half-life increased slightly, from 2.0 hours to 2.5 hours, but these hepatically impaired patients tolerated the usual recommended topotecan dosage regimen (see DOSAGE AND ADMINISTRATION).
Drug Interactions: Pharmacokinetic studies of the interaction of topotecan with concomitantly administered medications have not been formally investigated. *In vitro* inhibition studies using marker substrates known to be metabolized by human P450 CYP1A2, CYP2A6, CYP2C8/9, CYP2C19, CYP2D6, CYP2E, CYP3A or CYP4A or dihydropyrimidine dehydrogenase indicate that the activities of these enzymes were not altered by topotecan. Enzyme inhibition by topotecan has not been evaluated *in vivo.*
Pharmacodynamics: The dose-limiting toxicity of topotecan is leukopenia. White blood cell count decreases with increasing topotecan dose or topotecan AUC. When topotecan is administered at a dose of 1.5 mg/m^2/day for 5 days, an 80 to 90% decrease in white blood cell count at nadir is typically observed after the first cycle of therapy.

CLINICAL STUDIES

Hycamtin (topotecan hydrochloride) was studied in four clinical trials of 452 patients with metastatic ovarian carcinoma. All patients had disease that had recurred on, or was unresponsive to, a platinum-containing regimen. Patients in these four studies received an initial dose of 1.5 mg/m^2 given by intravenous infusion over 30 minutes for 5 consecutive days, starting on day one of a 21-day course.
Two of the studies, involving 223 patients given topotecan, are mature enough for evaluation (although survival results are incomplete). *Hycamtin* was compared with paclitaxel in a randomized trial involving 112 patients treated with *Hycamtin* (1.5 mg/m^2/day x 5 days starting on day one of a 21-day course) and 114 patients treated with paclitaxel (175 mg/m^2 over 3 hours on day 1 of a 21-day course). All patients had recurrent ovarian cancer after a platinum-containing regimen or had not responded to at least one prior platinum-containing regimen. Patients who did not respond to the study therapy, or who progressed, could be given the alternative treatment.
Response rates, response duration and time to progression are shown in Table 1.

Table 1. Efficacy of *Hycamtin* vs. Paclitaxel in Ovarian Cancer

Parameter	*Hycamtin* (n=112)	Paclitaxel (n=114)
Complete Response Rate	5.4%	3.5%
Partial Response Rate	14.3%	8.8%
Overall Response Rate	19.6%	12.3%
95% Confidence Interval	12.8 to 28.2%	6.9 to 19.7%
(p-value)	(0.092)	
Response Duration (weeks) Median	32.1	23.1
95% Confidence Interval	24.1† to ∞	23.1† to 24.4†
hazard-ratio (*Hycamtin*:paclitaxel)	0.424	
(p-value)	(0.224)	
Time to Progression (weeks) Median	23.1	14.0
95% Confidence Interval	17.1† to 29.6†	11.9† to 18.3†
hazard-ratio (*Hycamtin*:paclitaxel)	0.578	
(p-value)	(0.002)	

The calculation for duration of response was based on the interval between first response and time to progression.
† Value corresponds to a censored event; i.e., patient had not yet progressed.

Continued on next page

Information on the SmithKline Beecham Pharmaceuticals products appearing here is based on the labeling in effect on July 1, 1996. Further information on these and other products may be obtained from the Medical Department, SmithKline Beecham Pharmaceuticals, One Franklin Plaza, Philadelphia, PA 19101.

SmithKline Beecham—Cont.

The time to response was longer with *Hycamtin* compared to paclitaxel with a mean of 10 weeks (range 3.1 to 24.1) vs 7 weeks (range 2.4 to 12.3). Consequently, the efficacy of *Hycamtin* may not be achieved if patients are withdrawn from treatment prematurely.

In the crossover phase, 5 of 53 (9.4%) patients who received *Hycamtin* after paclitaxel had a partial response and 1 of 37 (2.7%) patients who received paclitaxel after *Hycamtin* had a complete response.

Hycamtin was active in patients who had developed resistance to platinum-containing therapy, defined as tumor progression while on, or tumor relapse within 6 months after completion of, a platinum-containing regimen. One complete and seven partial responses were seen in 60 patients, for a response rate of 13%. In the same study, there were no complete responders and four partial responders on the paclitaxel arm, for a response rate of 7%.

The adverse reaction profile for paclitaxel in this study was consistent with the product's approved labeling; the adverse reaction profile for *Hycamtin* in this study was consistent with that observed in all 452 patients from the four ovarian cancer clinical trials (see ADVERSE REACTIONS).

Hycamtin was also studied in an open-label, non-comparative trial in 111 patients with recurrent ovarian cancer after treatment with a platinum-containing regimen, or who had not responded to one prior platinum-containing regimen. The response rate was 14% (95% CI=7.9% to 20.9%). The median duration of response was 18 weeks (range 5 to 42 weeks). The time to progression was 8.4 weeks (range: 0.7 to 72.1 weeks).

INDICATIONS AND USAGE

Hycamtin (topotecan hydrochloride) is indicated for the treatment of patients with metastatic carcinoma of the ovary after failure of initial or subsequent chemotherapy.

CONTRAINDICATIONS

Hycamtin is contraindicated in patients who have a history of hypersensitivity reactions to topotecan or to any of its ingredients. *Hycamtin* should not be used in patients who are pregnant or breast-feeding, or those with severe bone marrow depression.

WARNINGS

Bone marrow suppression (primarily neutropenia) is the dose-limiting toxicity of topotecan. Neutropenia is not cumulative over time.

Neutropenia: Severe (grade 4, <500 cells/mm^3) neutropenia was most common during course 1 of treatment (60% of patients) and occurred in 40% of all courses, with a median duration of 7 days. The nadir neutrophil count occurred at a median of 11 days. Prophylactic G-CSF was given in 27% of courses after the first cycle. Therapy-related sepsis or febrile neutropenia occurred in 26% of patients and sepsis was fatal in 0.7%.

Thrombocytopenia: Grade 4 thrombocytopenia (<25,000/mm^3) occurred in 26% of patients and in 9% of courses, with a median duration of 5 days and platelet nadir at a median of 15 days. There were no episodes of serious bleeding. Platelet transfusions were given to 13% of patients and in 4% of courses.

Anemia: Severe anemia (grade 3/4, <8 gm/dL) occurred in 40% of patients and in 16% of courses. Median nadir was at Day 15. Transfusions were needed in 56% of patients and in 23% of courses.

Monitoring of Bone Marrow Function: *Hycamtin* should only be administered in patients with adequate bone marrow reserves, including baseline neutrophil counts of at least 1,500 cells/mm^3 and platelet count at least 100,000/mm^3. Frequent monitoring of peripheral blood cell counts should be instituted during treatment with *Hycamtin*. Patients should not be treated with subsequent courses of *Hycamtin* until neutrophils recover to >1,000 cells/mm^3, platelets recover to >100,000 cells/mm^3 and hemoglobin levels recover to 9.0 mg/dL, (with transfusion if necessary). Severe myelotoxicity has been reported when *Hycamtin* is used in combination with cisplatin (see Drug Interactions).

Pregnancy: *Hycamtin* may cause fetal harm when administered to a pregnant woman. The effects of topotecan on pregnant women have not been studied. If topotecan is used during a patient's pregnancy, or if a patient becomes pregnant while taking topotecan, she should be warned of the potential hazard to the fetus. Fecund women should be warned to avoid becoming pregnant. In rabbits, a dose of 0.10 mg/kg/day (about equal to the clinical dose on a mg/m^2 basis) given on days 6 through 20 of gestation caused maternal toxicity, embryolethality, and reduced fetal body weight. In the rat, a dose of 0.23 mg/kg/day (about equal to the clinical dose on a mg/m^2 basis) given for 14 days before mating through gestation day six caused fetal resorption, microphthalmia, preimplant loss, and mild maternal toxicity. A dose of 0.10 mg/kg/day (about half the clinical dose on a mg/m^2 basis) given to rats on days six through 17 of gestation caused an increase in post-implantation mortality. This dose also caused an increase in total fetal malformations. The most frequent malformations were of the eye (microphthalmia, anophthalmia, rosette formation of the retina, coloboma of the retina, ectopic orbit), brain (dilated lateral and third ventricles), skull and vertebrae.

PRECAUTIONS

General: Inadvertent extravasation with *Hycamtin* has been associated with only mild local reactions such as erythema and bruising.

Hematology: Monitoring of bone marrow function is essential (see WARNINGS and DOSAGE AND ADMINISTRATION).

Carcinogenesis, Mutagenesis, Impairment of Fertility: Carcinogenicity testing of topotecan has not been performed. Topotecan, however, is known to be genotoxic to mammalian cells and is a probable carcinogen. Topotecan was mutagenic to L5178Y mouse lymphoma cells and clastogenic to cultured human lymphocytes with and without metabolic activation. It was also clastogenic to mouse bone marrow. Topotecan did not cause mutations in bacterial cells.

Drug Interactions: Concomitant administration of G-CSF can prolong the duration of neutropenia, so if G-CSF is to be used, it should not be initiated until day 6 of the course of therapy, 24 hours after completion of treatment with *Hycamtin*.[1]

Myelosuppression was more severe when *Hycamtin* was given in combination with cisplatin in Phase I studies. In a reported study on concomitant administration of cisplatin 50 mg/m^2 and *Hycamtin* at a dose of 1.25 mg/m^2/day ×5 days, one of three patients had neutropenia for 12 days and a second patient died with neutropenic sepsis. There are no adequate data to define a safe and effective regimen for *Hycamtin* and cisplatin in combination.

Pregnancy: Pregnancy Category D. (See WARNINGS section.)

Nursing Mothers: It is not known whether the drug is excreted in human milk. Breast-feeding should be discontinued when women are receiving *Hycamtin* (see CONTRAINDICATIONS).

Pediatric Use: Safety and effectiveness in pediatric patients have not been established.

ADVERSE REACTIONS

Data in the following section are based on the experience of 452 patients with metastatic ovarian carcinoma treated with *Hycamtin*. Table 2 lists the principal hematologic toxicities and Table 3 lists non-hematologic toxicities occurring in at least 19% of patients.

Table 2. Summary of Hematologic Adverse Events in Patients Receiving *Hycamtin*

Hematologic Adverse Events	Patients n=452 % Incidence	Courses n=2375 % Incidence
Neutropenia		
<1,500 cells/mm^3	98	78
<500 cells/mm^3	81	40
Leukopenia		
<3,000 cells/mm^3	98	77
<1,000 cells/mm^3	32	11
Thrombocytopenia		
<75,000/mm^3	63	39
<25,000/mm^3	26	9
Anemia		
<10 g/dL	95	76
<8 g/dL	40	16
Sepsis or fever/infection with Grade 4 neutropenia	26	7
Platelet transfusions	13	4
RBC transfusions	56	23

[See Table 3 below.]

Premedications were not routinely used in these clinical studies.

Hematologic: (See WARNINGS)

Gastrointestinal: The incidence of nausea was 77% (10% grade 3/4) and vomiting occurred in 58% (9% grade 3/4) of patients (See Table 3). The prophylactic use of antiemetics was not routine in patients treated with *Hycamtin*. Forty-two percent of patients had diarrhea (5% grade 3/4), 39% constipation (3% grade 3/4) and 33% had abdominal pain (6% grade 3/4).

Skin/Appendages: Total alopecia (Grade 2) occurred in 42% of patients.

Central and Peripheral Nervous System: Headache (21%) was the most frequently reported neurologic toxicity. Paresthesia occurred in 9% of patients but was generally Grade 1.

Liver/Biliary: Grade 1 transient elevations in SGOT/AST and SGPT/ALT occurred in 5% of patients. Greater elevations, grade 3/4, occurred in <1%. Grade 3/4 elevated bilirubin occurred in <3% of patients.

Respiratory: Dyspnea (20%); Grade 3/4 dyspnea (4%).

Table 4 shows the grade 3/4 hematologic and major non-hematologic adverse events in the topotecan/paclitaxel comparator trial.

Table 4. Comparative Toxicity Profiles for Ovarian Cancer Patients Randomized to Receive *Hycamtin* or Paclitaxel

Adverse Event	Hycamtin		Paclitaxel	
	Pts	Courses	Pts	Courses
	n=112	n=555	n=114	n=550
Hematologic Grade 3/4	%	%	%	%
Grade 4 neutropenia (<500 cells/mL)	79.5	36.7	21.9	8.5
Grade 3/4 Anemia (Hgb <8 g/dL)	40.5	16.0	6.3	2.0
Grade 4 Thrombocytopenia (<25,000 plts/mL)	25.3	9.6	1.8	0.4
Fever/Grade 4 neutropenia	23.2	5.4	2.6	0.5
Documented Sepsis	5.4	1.1	1.8	0.4
Death related to Sepsis	1.8	0.4	0.0	0.0
Non-hematologic Grade 3/4				
Gastrointestinal				
Abdominal pain	5.4	1.1	3.5	0.9
Constipation	5.4	1.1	0.0	0.0
Diarrhea	6.3	1.6	0.9	0.2
Intestinal Obstruction	4.5	1.1	4.4	0.9
Nausea	8.9	3.1	1.8	0.4
Stomatitis	0.9	0.2	0.9	0.2
Vomiting	9.8	2.0	2.6	0.5

Table 3. Summary of Non-hematologic Adverse Events in Patients Receiving *Hycamtin*

Non-hematologic Adverse Events	All Grades %Incidence		Grade 3 %Incidence		Grade 4 %Incidence	
	n=452 Patients	n=2375 Courses	n=452 Patients	n=2375 Courses	n=452 Patients	n=2375 Courses
Gastrointestinal						
Nausea	77	50	10	3	<1	<1
Vomiting	58	26	6	3	3	<1
Diarrhea	42	19	4	1	<1	<1
Constipation	39	18	2	<1	1	<1
Abdominal Pain	33	13	4	<1	<1	<1
Stomatitis	24	9	2	<1	<1	<1
Anorexia	19	8	2	<1	0	0
Body as a Whole						
Fatigue	37	25	6	2	0	0
Fever	34	13	1	<1	<1	<1
Asthenia	21	10	3	<1	1	<1
Skin/Appendages						
Alopecia	59	62	NA	NA	NA	NA

Constitutional				
Anorexia	3.6	0.2	0.0	0.0
Dyspnea	6.3	1.8	5.3	1.3
Fatigue	8.0	2.2	5.3	2.0
Malaise	1.8	0.5	1.8	0.4
Neuromuscular				
Arthralgia	0.9	0.2	3.5	0.5
Asthenia	5.4	1.8	3.5	1.3
Headache	0.9	0.2	1.8	0.9
Myalgia	0.0	0.0	2.6	1.6
Pain	5.4	1.1	10.5	2.2

Premedications were not routinely used in patients randomized to *Hycamtin*, while patients receiving paclitaxel received routine pretreatment with corticosteroids, diphenhydramine, and histamine receptor type 2 blockers.

OVERDOSAGE

There is no known antidote for overdosage with *Hycamtin*. The primary anticipated complication of overdosage would consist of bone marrow suppression.

The LD_{10} in mice receiving single intravenous infusions of *Hycamtin* was 75 mg/m^2 (CI 95%: 47 to 97).

DOSAGE AND ADMINISTRATION

Prior to administration of the first course of *Hycamtin*, patients must have a baseline neutrophil count of >1500 cells/mm^3 and a platelet count of >100,000 cells/mm^3. The recommended dose of Hycamtin (topotecan hydrochloride) is 1.5 mg/m^2 by intravenous infusion over 30 minutes daily for 5 consecutive days, starting on day one of a 21-day course. A minimum of four courses is recommended because median time to response in three clinical trials was 9 to 12 weeks. In the event of severe neutropenia during any course, the dose should be reduced by 0.25 mg/m^2 for subsequent courses. Alternatively, in the event of severe neutropenia, G-CSF may be administered following the subsequent course (before resorting to dose reduction) starting from Day 6 of the course (24 hours after completion of topotecan administration).

Adjustment of Dose in Special Populations

Hepatic Impairment: No dosage adjustment appears to be required for treating patients with impaired hepatic function (plasma bilirubin >1.5 to <10 mg/dL).

Renal Functional Impairment: No dosage adjustment appears to be required for treating patients with mild renal impairment (Cl_{cr} 40 to 60 mL/min). Dosage adjustment to 0.75 mg/m^2 is recommended for patients with moderate renal impairment (20 to 39 mL/min). Insufficient data are available in patients with severe renal impairment to provide a dosage recommendation.

Elderly Patients: No dosage adjustment appears to be needed in the elderly, other than adjustments related to renal function.

PREPARATION FOR ADMINISTRATION

Precautions: *Hycamtin* is a cytotoxic anticancer drug. As with other potentially toxic compounds, *Hycamtin* should be prepared under a vertical laminar flow hood while wearing gloves and protective clothing. If *Hycamtin* solution contacts the skin, wash the skin immediately and thoroughly with soap and water. If *Hycamtin* contacts mucous membranes, flush thoroughly with water.

Preparation for Intravenous Administration: Each *Hycamtin* 4 mg vial is reconstituted with 4 mL Sterile Water for Injection. Then the appropriate volume of the reconstituted solution is diluted in either 0.9% Sodium Chloride Intravenous Infusion or 5% Dextrose Intravenous Infusion prior to administration.

Because the lyophilized dosage form contains no antibacterial preservative, the reconstituted product should be used immediately.

STABILITY

Unopened vials of Hycamtin (topotecan hydrochloride) are stable until the date indicated on the package when stored between 20° and 25°C (68° and 77°F) [see USP] and protected from light in the original package. Because the vials contain no preservative, contents should be used immediately after reconstitution.

Reconstituted vials of *Hycamtin* diluted for infusion are stable at approximately 20° to 25°C (68° to 77°F) and ambient lighting conditions for 24 hours.

HOW SUPPLIED

NDC 0007-4201-05: Hycamtin (topotecan hydrochloride) for Injection is supplied in 4 mg (free base) single-dose vials, in packages of 5 vials.

Storage: Store the vials protected from light in the original cartons at controlled room temperature between 20° and 25°C (68° and 77°F) [see USP].

Handling and Disposal: Procedures for proper handling and disposal of anticancer drugs should be used. Several guidelines on this subject have been published.[2-8] There is no general agreement that all of the procedures recommended in the guidelines are necessary or appropriate.

REFERENCES

1. Rowinsky, et al. Phase 1 and pharmacologic study of high doses of the topoisomerase I inhibitor topotecan with granulocyte colony-stimulating factor in patients with solid tumors. J Clin Oncol. 1996;14:1224-1235.
2. Recommendations for the safe handling of parenteral antineoplastic drugs. NIH Publication No. 83-2621. For sale by the Superintendent of Documents, US Government Printing Office, Washington, DC 20402.
3. AMA Council Report. Guidelines for handling parenteral antineoplastics. JAMA 1985;253(11):1590-1592.
4. National Study Commission on Cytotoxic Exposure-recommendations for handling cytotoxic agents. Available from Louis P. Jeffry, Chairman, National Study Commission on Cytotoxic Exposure. Massachusetts College of Pharmacy and Allied Health Sciences, 179 Longwood Avenue, Boston, Massachusetts, 02115.
5. Clinical Oncological Society of Australia. Guidelines and recommendations for safe handling of antineoplastic agents. Med J Austr. 1983;1:426-428.
6. Jones RB, et al. Safe handling of chemotherapeutic agents: A report from the Mount Sinai Medical Center. CA-A Cancer Journal for Clinicians 1983;Sept./Oct.:258-263.
7. American Society of Hospital Pharmacists Technical Assistance Bulletin on Handling Cytotoxic and Hazardous Drugs. Am J Hos Pharm 1990;47:1033-1049.
8. OSHA Work-Practice guidelines for personnel dealing with cytotoxic (antineoplastic) drugs. Am J Hosp Pharm 1986;43:1193-1204.

HY:L2

Shown in Product Identification Guide, page 336

KYTRIL® ℞
[ki'-tril]
granisetron hydrochloride Injection

DESCRIPTION

Kytril (granisetron hydrochloride) Injection is an antinauseant and antiemetic agent. Chemically it is *endo*-N-(9-methyl-9-azabicyclo [3.3.1] non-3-yl)-1-methyl-1H-indazole-3-carboxamide hydrochloride with a molecular weight of 348.9 (312.4 free base). Its empirical formula is $C_{18}H_{24}N_4O \cdot HCl$ while its chemical structure is:

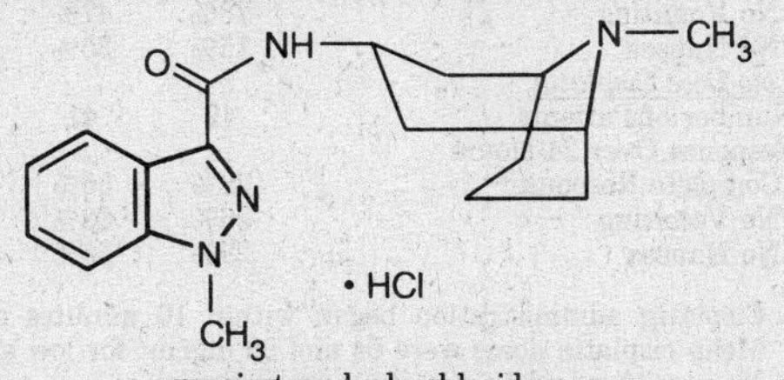

granisetron hydrochloride

Granisetron hydrochloride is a white to off-white solid that is readily soluble in water and normal saline at 20°C. *Kytril* Injection is a clear, colorless, sterile, nonpyrogenic, aqueous solution for intravenous administration.

Each 1 mL of preservative-free aqueous solution contains 1.12 mg granisetron hydrochloride equivalent to granisetron, 1.0 mg and sodium chloride, 9.0 mg. The solution's pH ranges from 4.7 to 7.3.

CLINICAL PHARMACOLOGY

Granisetron is a selective 5-hydroxytryptamine$_3$ (5-HT_3) receptor antagonist with little or no affinity for other serotonin receptors, including 5-HT_1; 5-HT_{1A}; 5-$HT_{1B/C}$; 5-HT_2; for alpha$_1$-, alpha$_2$- or beta-adrenoreceptors; for dopamine-D_2; or for histamine-H_1; benzodiazepine; picrotoxin, or opioid receptors.

Serotonin receptors of the 5-HT_3 type are located peripherally on vagal nerve terminals and centrally in the chemoreceptor trigger zone of the area postrema. During chemotherapy-induced vomiting, mucosal enterochromaffin cells release serotonin, which stimulates 5-HT_3 receptors. This evokes vagal afferent discharge, inducing vomiting. Animal studies demonstrate that, in binding to 5-HT_3 receptors, granisetron blocks serotonin stimulation and subsequent vomiting after emetogenic stimuli such as cisplatin. In the ferret animal model, a single granisetron injection prevented vomiting due to high-dose cisplatin or arrested vomiting within 5 to 30 seconds.

In most human studies, granisetron has had little effect on blood pressure, heart rate or ECG. No evidence of an effect on plasma prolactin or aldosterone concentrations has been found in other studies.

Kytril Injection exhibited no effect on oro-cecal transit time in normal volunteers given a single intravenous infusion of 50 mcg/kg or 200 mcg/kg. Single and multiple oral doses slowed colonic transit in normal volunteers.

Pharmacokinetics

In adult cancer patients undergoing chemotherapy and in volunteers, infusion of a single 40 mcg/kg dose of *Kytril* Injection produced the following mean pharmacokinetic data:

[See Table 1 on top of next page.]

There was high inter and intrasubject variability noted in these studies. No difference in mean AUC was found between males and females, although males had a higher C_{max} generally.

Granisetron metabolism involves N-demethylation and aromatic ring oxidation followed by conjugation. Animal studies suggest that some of the metabolites may also have 5-HT_3 receptor antagonist activity.

Clearance is predominantly by hepatic metabolism. In normal volunteers, approximately 12% of the administered dose is eliminated unchanged in the urine in 48 hours. The remainder of the dose is excreted as metabolites, 49% in the urine and 34% in the feces.

In vitro liver microsomal studies show that granisetron's major route of metabolism is inhibited by ketoconazole, suggestive of metabolism mediated by the cytochrome P-450 3A subfamily.

Plasma protein binding is approximately 65% and granisetron distributes freely between plasma and red blood cells.

Elderly: The ranges of the pharmacokinetic parameters in elderly volunteers (mean age 71 years), given a single 40 mcg/kg intravenous dose of *Kytril* Injection, were generally similar to those in younger healthy volunteers; mean values were lower for clearance and longer for half-life in the elderly (see Table 1).

Pediatrics: The pharmacokinetics of granisetron has not been adequately studied in children.

Renal Failure Patients: Total clearance of granisetron was not affected in patients with severe renal failure who received a single 40 mcg/kg intravenous dose of *Kytril* Injection.

Hepatically Impaired Patients: A pharmacokinetic study in patients with hepatic impairment due to neoplastic liver involvement showed that total clearance was approximately halved compared to patients without hepatic impairment. Given the wide variability in pharmacokinetic parameters noted in patients and the good tolerance of doses well above the recommended 10 mcg/kg dose, dosage adjustment in patients with possible hepatic functional impairment is not necessary.

CLINICAL TRIALS

Kytril Injection has been shown to prevent nausea and vomiting associated with single-day and repeat cycle cancer chemotherapy.

Single-Day Chemotherapy

Cisplatin-Based Chemotherapy: In a double-blind, placebo-controlled study in 28 cancer patients, *Kytril* Injection, administered as a single intravenous infusion of 40 mcg/kg, was significantly more effective than placebo in preventing nausea and vomiting induced by cisplatin chemotherapy. See Table 2.

Table 2. Prevention of Chemotherapy-Induced Nausea and Vomiting—Single-Day Cisplatin Therapy[1]

	***Kytril* Injection**	**Placebo**	***P*-Value**
Number of Patients	14	14	
Response Over 24 Hours			
Complete Response[2]	93%	7%	<0.001
No Vomiting	93%	14%	<0.001
No More Than Mild Nausea	93%	7%	<0.001

1. Cisplatin administration began within 10 minutes of *Kytril* Injection infusion and continued for 1.5 to 3.0 hours. Mean cisplatin dose was 86 mg/m^2 in the *Kytril* Injection group and 80 mg/m^2 in the placebo group.
2. No vomiting and no moderate or severe nausea.

Kytril Injection was also evaluated in a randomized dose response study of cancer patients receiving cisplatin ≥75 mg/m^2. Additional chemotherapeutic agents included: anthracyclines, carboplatin, cytostatic antibiotics, folic acid derivatives, methylhydrazine, nitrogen mustard analogs, podophyllotoxin derivatives, pyrimidine analogs and vinca alkaloids. *Kytril* Injection doses of 10 and 40 mcg/kg were superior to 2 mcg/kg in preventing cisplatin-induced nausea and vomiting, but 40 mcg/kg was not significantly superior to 10 mcg/kg. See Table 3.

[See Table 3 on next page.]

Continued on next page

Information on the SmithKline Beecham Pharmaceuticals products appearing here is based on the labeling in effect on July 1, 1996. Further information on these and other products may be obtained from the Medical Department, SmithKline Beecham Pharmaceuticals, One Franklin Plaza, Philadelphia, PA 19101.

SmithKline Beecham—Cont.

Kytril (granisetron hydrochloride) Injection was also evaluated in a double-blind, randomized dose response study of 353 patients stratified for high ($\geq$ 80 to 120 mg/m²) or low (50 to 79 mg/m²) cisplatin dose. Response rates of patients for both cisplatin strata are given in Table 4.

[See Table 4 at right.]

For both the low and high cisplatin strata, the 10, 20 and 40 mcg/kg doses were more effective than the 5 mcg/kg dose in preventing nausea and vomiting within 24 hours of chemotherapy administration. The 10 mcg/kg dose was at least as effective as the higher doses.

Moderately Emetogenic Chemotherapy: Kytril Injection, 40 mcg/kg, was compared with the combination of chlorpromazine (50 to 200 mg/24 hours) and dexamethasone (12 mg) in patients treated with moderately emetogenic chemotherapy, including primarily carboplatin > 300 mg/m², cisplatin 20 to 50 mg/m² and cyclophosphamide > 600 mg/m². Kytril Injection was superior to the chlorpromazine regimen in preventing nausea and vomiting. See Table 5.

Table 5. Prevention of Chemotherapy-Induced Nausea and Vomiting—Single-Day Moderately Emetogenic Chemotherapy

	Kytril Injection 133	Chlor-promazine[1] 133	P-Value
Number of Patients	133	133	
Response Over 24 Hours			
Complete Response[2]	68%	47%	< 0.001
No Vomiting	73%	53%	< 0.001
No More Than Mild Nausea	77%	59%	< 0.001

1. Patients also received dexamethasone, 12 mg.
2. No vomiting and no moderate or severe nausea.

In other studies of moderately emetogenic chemotherapy, no significant difference in efficacy was found between Kytril doses of 40 mcg/kg and 160 mcg/kg doses.

Repeat-Cycle Chemotherapy

In an uncontrolled trial, 512 cancer patients received Kytril Injection, 40 mcg/kg, prophylactically, for two cycles of chemotherapy, 224 patients received it for at least four cycles and 108 patients received it for at least six cycles. Kytril Injection efficacy remained relatively constant over the first six repeat cycles, with complete response rates (no vomiting and no moderate or severe nausea in 24 hours) of 60% to 69%. No patients were studied for more than 15 cycles.

Pediatric Studies

A randomized double-blind study evaluated the 24-hour response of 80 pediatric cancer patients (age 2 to 16 years) to Kytril Injection 10, 20 or 40 mcg/kg. Patients were treated with cisplatin $\geq$ 60 mg/m², cytarabine $\geq$ 3 g/m², cyclophosphamide $\geq$ 1 g/m² or nitrogen mustard $\geq$ 6 mg/m². See Table 6.

Table 6. Prevention of Chemotherapy-Induced Nausea and Vomiting in Pediatric Patients

	Kytril Injection 10	Dose 20	(mcg/kg) 40
Number of Patients	29	26	25
Median Number of Vomiting Episodes	2	3	1
Complete Response Over 24 Hours[1]	21%	31%	32%

1. No vomiting and no moderate or severe nausea.

A second pediatric study compared Kytril Injection 20 mcg/kg to chlorpromazine plus dexamethasone in 88 patients treated with ifosfamide $\geq$ 3 g/m²/day for two or three days. Kytril Injection was administered on each day of ifosfamide treatment. At 24 hours, 22% of Kytril Injection patients achieved complete response (no vomiting and no moderate or severe nausea in 24 hours) compared with 10% on the chlorpromazine regimen. The median number of vomiting episodes with Kytril Injection was 1.5; with chlorpromazine it was 7.0.

INDICATIONS AND USAGE

Kytril (granisetron hydrochloride) Injection is indicated for the prevention of nausea and vomiting associated with initial and repeat courses of emetogenic cancer therapy, including high-dose cisplatin.

CONTRAINDICATIONS

Kytril Injection is contraindicated in patients with known hypersensitivity to the drug.

PRECAUTIONS

Drug Interactions

Granisetron does not induce or inhibit the cytochrome P-450 drug-metabolizing enzyme system. There have been no definitive drug-drug interaction studies to examine pharmacokinetic or pharmacodynamic interaction with other drugs, but

Table 1. Pharmacokinetic Parameters in Adult Cancer Patients Undergoing Chemotherapy and in Volunteers, Following a Single Intravenous 40 mcg/kg Dose of Kytril (granisetron hydrochloride) Injection

	Peak Plasma Concentration (ng/mL)	Terminal Phase Plasma Half-Life (h)	Total Clearance (L/h/kg)	Volume of Distribution (L/kg)
Cancer Patients				
Mean	63.8*	8.95*	0.38*	3.07*
Range	18.0 to 176	0.90 to 31.1	0.14 to 1.54	0.85 to 10.4
Volunteers				
21 to 42 years				
Mean	64.3†	4.91†	0.79†	3.04†
Range	11.2 to 182	0.88 to 15.2	0.20 to 2.56	1.68 to 6.13
65 to 81 years				
Mean	57.0†	7.69†	0.44†	3.97†
Range	14.6 to 153	2.65 to 17.7	0.17 to 1.06	1.75 to 7.01

* 5-minute infusion.
† 3-minute infusion.

Table 3. Prevention of Chemotherapy-Induced Nausea and Vomiting—Single-Day High-Dose Cisplatin Therapy[1]

	Kytril Injection (mcg/kg) 2	10	40	P-Value (vs. 2 mcg/kg) 10	40
Number of Patients	52	52	53		
Response Over 24 Hours					
Complete Response[2]	31%	62%	68%	< 0.002	< 0.001
No Vomiting	38%	65%	74%	< 0.001	< 0.001
No More Than Mild Nausea	58%	75%	79%	NS	0.007

1. Cisplatin administration began within 10 minutes of Kytril Injection infusion and continued for 2.6 hours (mean). Mean cisplatin doses were 96 to 99 mg/m².
2. No vomiting and no moderate or severe nausea.

Table 4. Prevention of Chemotherapy-Induced Nausea and Vomiting—Single-Day High-Dose and Low-Dose Cisplatin Therapy[1]

	Kytril Injection (mcg/kg) 5	10	20	40	P-Value (vs. 5 mcg/kg) 10	20	40
High-Dose Cisplatin							
Number of Patients	40	49	48	47			
Response Over 24 Hours							
Complete Response[2]	18%	41%	40%	47%	0.018	0.025	0.004
No Vomiting	28%	47%	44%	53%	NS	NS	0.016
No Nausea	15%	35%	38%	43%	0.036	0.019	0.005
Low-Dose Cisplatin							
Number of Patients	42	41	40	46			
Response Over 24 Hours							
Complete Response[2]	29%	56%	58%	41%	0.012	0.009	NS
No Vomiting	36%	63%	65%	43%	0.012	0.008	NS
No Nausea	29%	56%	38%	33%	0.012	NS	NS

1. Cisplatin administration began within 10 minutes of Kytril Injection infusion and continued for 2 hours (mean). Mean cisplatin doses were 64 and 98 mg/m² for low and high strata.
2. No vomiting and no use of rescue antiemetic.

in humans, Kytril Injection has been safely administered with drugs representing benzodiazepines, neuroleptics and anti-ulcer medications commonly prescribed with antiemetic treatments. Kytril Injection also does not appear to interact with emetogenic cancer chemotherapies. Because granisetron is metabolized by hepatic cytochrome P-450 drug-metabolizing enzymes, inducers or inhibitors of these enzymes may change the clearance and, hence, the half-life of granisetron.

Carcinogenesis, Mutagenesis, Impairment of Fertility

In a 24-month carcinogenicity study, rats were treated orally with granisetron 1, 5 or 50 mg/kg/day (6, 30 or 300 mg/m²/day). The 50 mg/kg/day dose was reduced to 25 mg/kg/day (150 mg/m²/day) during week 59 due to toxicity. For a 50 kg person of average height (1.46m² body surface area), these doses represent 16, 81 and 405 times the recommended clinical dose (0.37 mg/m², i.v.) on a body surface area basis. There was a statistically significant increase in the incidence of hepatocellular carcinomas and adenomas in males treated with 5 mg/kg/day (30 mg/m²/day, 81 times the recommended human dose based on body surface area) and above, and in females treated with 25 mg/kg/day (150 mg/m²/day, 405 times the recommended human dose based on body surface area). No increase in liver tumors was observed at a dose of 1 mg/kg/day (6 mg/m²/day, 16 times the recommended human dose based on body surface area) in males and 5 mg/kg/day (30 mg/m²/day, 81 times the recommended human dose based on body surface area) in females. In a 12-month oral toxicity study, treatment with granisetron 100 mg/kg/day (600 mg/m²/day, 1622 times the recommended human dose based on body surface area) produced hepatocellular adenomas in male and female rats while no such tumors were found in the control rats. A 24-month mouse carcinogenicity study of granisetron did not show a statistically significant increase in tumor incidence, but the study was not conclusive.

Because of the tumor findings in rat studies, Kytril (granisetron hydrochloride) Injection should be prescribed only at the dose and for the indication recommended (see INDICATIONS AND USAGE, and DOSAGE AND ADMINISTRATION).

Granisetron was not mutagenic in *in vitro* Ames test and mouse lymphoma cell forward mutation assay, and *in vivo* mouse micronucleus test and *in vitro* and *ex vivo* rat hepatocyte UDS assays. It, however, produced a significant increase in UDS in HeLa cells *in vitro* and a significant increased incidence of cells with polyploidy in an *in vitro* human lymphocyte chromosomal aberration test.

Granisetron at subcutaneous doses up to 6 mg/kg/day (36 mg/m²/day, 97 times the recommended human dose based on body surface area) was found to have no effect on fertility and reproductive performance of male and female rats.

Pregnancy

Teratogenic Effects. Pregnancy Category B. Reproduction studies have been performed in pregnant rats at intravenous doses up to 9 mg/kg/day (54 mg/m²/day, 146 times the recommended human dose based on body surface area) and pregnant rabbits at intravenous doses up to 3 mg/kg/day (35.4 mg/m²/day, 96 times the recommended human dose based on body surface area) and have revealed no evidence of impaired fertility or harm to the fetus due to granisetron. There are, however, no adequate and well-controlled studies in pregnant women. Because animal reproduction studies are not always predictive of human response, this drug should be used during pregnancy only if clearly needed.

Nursing Mothers

It is not known whether granisetron is excreted in human milk. Because many drugs are excreted in human milk, caution should be exercised when Kytril Injection is administered to a nursing woman.

Pediatric Use

See DOSAGE AND ADMINISTRATION for use in children 2 to 16 years of age. Safety and effectiveness in children under 2 years of age have not been established.

Geriatric Use

During clinical trials, 713 patients 65 years of age or older received Kytril (granisetron HCl) Injection. Effectiveness and safety were similar in patients of various ages.

ADVERSE REACTIONS

The following have been reported during controlled clinical trials or in the routine management of patients. The percentage figures are based on clinical trial experience only. Table 7 gives the comparative frequencies of the five most commonly reported adverse events (≥3%) in patients receiving *Kytril* Injection, in single-day chemotherapy trials. These patients received chemotherapy, primarily cisplatin, and intravenous fluids during the 24-hour period following *Kytril* Injection administration. Events were generally recorded over seven days post-*Kytril* Injection administration. In the absence of a placebo group, there is uncertainty as to how many of these events should be attributed to *Kytril*, except for headache, which was clearly more frequent than in comparison groups.

Table 7. Principal Adverse Events in Clinical Trials—Single-Day Chemotherapy

	Percent of Patients with Event	
	Kytril Injection 40 mcg/kg (n=1,268)	Comparator[1] (n=422)
Headache	14%	6%
Asthenia	5%	6%
Somnolence	4%	15%
Diarrhea	4%	6%
Constipation	3%	3%

1. Metoclopramide/dexamethasone and phenothiazines/dexamethasone.

In over 3,000 patients receiving *Kytril* Injection (2 to 160 mcg/kg) in single-day and multiple-day clinical trials with emetogenic cancer therapies, adverse events, other than those in Table 7, were observed; attribution of many of these events to *Kytril* is uncertain.

Hepatic: In comparative trials, mainly with cisplatin regimens, elevations of AST and ALT (>2 times the upper limit of normal) following administration of *Kytril* Injection occurred in 2.8% and 3.3% of patients, respectively. These frequencies were not significantly different from those seen with comparators (AST: 2.1%; ALT: 2.4%).

Cardiovascular: Hypertension (2%); hypotension, arrhythmias such as sinus bradycardia, atrial fibrillation, varying degrees of A-V block, ventricular ectopy including non-sustained tachycardia, and ECG abnormalities have been observed rarely.

Central Nervous System: Agitation, anxiety, CNS stimulation and insomnia were seen in less than 2% of patients. Extrapyramidal syndrome occurred rarely and only in the presence of other drugs associated with this syndrome.

Hypersensitivity: Rare cases of hypersensitivity reactions, sometimes severe (e.g., anaphylaxis, shortness of breath, hypotension, urticaria) have been reported.

Other: Fever (3%), taste disorder(2%), skin rashes (1%). In multiple-day comparative studies, fever occurred more frequently with *Kytril* Injection (8.6%) than with comparative drugs (3.4%, $P<0.014$), which usually included dexamethasone.

OVERDOSAGE

There is no specific antidote for Kytril (granisetron hydrochloride) Injection overdosage. In case of overdosage, symptomatic treatment should be given. Overdosage of up to 38.5 mg of granisetron hydrochloride injection has been reported without symptoms or only the occurrence of a slight headache.

DOSAGE AND ADMINISTRATION

The recommended dosage for *Kytril* Injection is 10 mcg/kg infused intravenously over 5 minutes, beginning within 30 minutes before initiation of chemotherapy, and only on the day(s) chemotherapy is given.

Pediatric Use: The recommended dose in children 2 to 16 years of age is 10 mcg/kg (see CLINICAL TRIALS). Children under 2 years of age have not been studied.

Use in the Elderly, Renal Failure Patients or Hepatically Impaired Patients: No dosage adjustment is recommended. (See CLINICAL PHARMACOLOGY, Pharmacokinetics.)

Infusion Preparation

Kytril Injection should be diluted in 0.9% Sodium Chloride or 5% Dextrose to a total volume of 20 to 50 mL.

Stability

Intravenous infusion of *Kytril* Injection should be prepared at the time of administration. However, *Kytril* Injection has been shown to be stable for at least 24 hours when diluted in 0.9% Sodium Chloride or 5% Dextrose and stored at room temperature under normal lighting conditions.

As a general precaution, *Kytril* Injection should not be mixed in solution with other drugs. Parenteral drug products should be inspected visually for particulate matter and discoloration before administration whenever solution and container permit.

HOW SUPPLIED

Kytril (granisetron hydrochloride) Injection, 1 mg/mL (free base), is supplied in 1 mL Single-Use Vials, in packages of 1.
NDC 0029-4149-01 (package of 1)

Store vials at 30°C (86°F) or below. Do not freeze. Protect from light.

Veterans Administration/Military/PHS—vial, 1 mg/mL, 1's (multiples of 6), 6505-01-391-6108; Tablets, 1 mg, 2's, 6505-01-412-0329; 1 mg, 20's, 6505-01-412-0324.

KY:L5

Shown in Product Identification Guide, page 337

KYTRIL® ℞

[*kī'-tril*]

granisetron hydrochloride
Tablets

DESCRIPTION

Kytril Tablets contain granisetron hydrochloride, an antinauseant and antiemetic agent. Chemically it is *endo*-N-(9-methyl-9-azabicyclo [3.3.1] non-3-yl)-1-methyl-1H-indazole-3-carboxamide hydrochloride with a molecular weight of 348.9 (312.4 free base). Its empirical formula is $C_{18}H_{24}N_4O \cdot HCl$, while its chemical structure is:

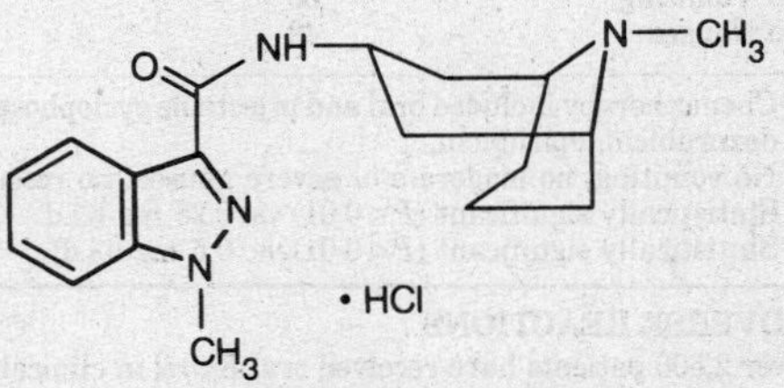

granisetron hydrochloride

Granisetron hydrochloride is a white to off-white solid that is readily soluble in water and normal saline at 20°C.

Tablets for Oral Administration: Each white, triangular, biconvex, film-coated *Kytril* Tablet contains 1.12 mg granisetron hydrochloride equivalent to granisetron, 1 mg. Inactive ingredients are: hydroxypropyl methylcellulose, lactose, magnesium stearate, microcrystalline cellulose, polyethylene glycol, polysorbate 80, sodium starch glycolate and titanium dioxide.

CLINICAL PHARMACOLOGY

Granisetron is a selective 5-hydroxytryptamine$_3$ (5-HT_3) receptor antagonist with little or no affinity for other serotonin receptors, including 5-HT_1; 5-HT_{1A}; 5-$HT_{1B/C}$; 5-HT_2; for alpha$_1$-, alpha$_2$-, or beta-adrenoreceptors; for dopamine-D_2; or for histamine-H_1; benzodiazepine; picrotoxin, or opioid receptors.

Serotonin receptors of the 5-HT_3 type are located peripherally on vagal nerve terminals and centrally in the chemoreceptor trigger zone of the area postrema. During chemotherapy that induces vomiting, mucosal enterochromaffin cells release serotonin, which stimulates 5-HT_3 receptors. This evokes vagal afferent discharge, inducing vomiting. Animal studies demonstrate that, in binding to 5-HT_3 receptors, granisetron blocks serotonin stimulation and subsequent vomiting after emetogenic stimuli such as cisplatin. In the ferret animal model, a single granisetron injection prevented vomiting due to high-dose cisplatin or arrested vomiting within 5 to 30 seconds.

In most human studies, granisetron has had little effect on blood pressure, heart rate or ECG. No evidence of an effect on plasma prolactin or aldosterone concentrations has been found in other studies.

Following single and multiple oral doses, *Kytril* slowed colonic transit in normal volunteers. However, *Kytril* had no effect on oro-cecal transit time in normal volunteers when given as a single intravenous (IV) infusion of 50 mcg/kg or 200 mcg/kg.

Pharmacokinetics

In healthy volunteers and adult cancer patients undergoing chemotherapy, administration of oral *Kytril* produced the following mean pharmacokinetic data:

[See Table 1 on top of next page.]

The effects of gender on the pharmacokinetics of oral *Kytril* have not been studied. However, after intravenous infusion of *Kytril*, no difference in mean AUC was found between males and females, although males had a higher C_{max} generally.

When oral *Kytril* was administered with food, AUC was decreased by 5% and C_{max} increased by 30% in non-fasted healthy volunteers who received a single dose of 10 mg.

Granisetron metabolism involves N-demethylation and aromatic ring oxidation followed by conjugation. Animal studies suggest that some of the metabolites may also have 5-HT_3 receptor antagonist activity.

Clearance is predominantly by hepatic metabolism. In normal volunteers, approximately 11% of the orally administered dose is eliminated unchanged in the urine in 48 hours. The remainder of the dose is excreted as metabolites, 48% in the urine and 38% in the feces.

In vitro liver microsomal studies show that granisetron's major route of metabolism is inhibited by ketoconazole, suggestive of metabolism mediated by the cytochrome P-450 3A subfamily.

Plasma protein binding is approximately 65% and granisetron distributes freely between plasma and red blood cells.

In the elderly and in patients with renal failure or hepatic impairment, the pharmacokinetics of granisetron was determined following administration of intravenous *Kytril:*

Elderly: The ranges of the pharmacokinetic parameters in elderly volunteers (mean age 71 years), given a single 40 mcg/kg intravenous dose of *Kytril* Injection, were generally similar to those in younger healthy volunteers; mean values were lower for clearance and longer for half-life in the elderly.

Renal Failure Patients: Total clearance of granisetron was not affected in patients with severe renal failure who received a single 40 mcg/kg intravenous dose of *Kytril* Injection.

Hepatically Impaired Patients: A pharmacokinetic study with intravenous *Kytril* in patients with hepatic impairment due to neoplastic liver involvement showed that total clearance was approximately halved compared to patients without hepatic impairment. Given the wide variability in pharmacokinetic parameters noted in patients and the good tolerance of doses well above the recommended 1.0 mg b.i.d. dose, dosage adjustment in patients with possible hepatic functional impairment is not necessary.

Pediatrics: The pharmacokinetics of granisetron has not been adequately studied in children.

CLINICAL TRIALS

Oral *Kytril* prevents nausea and vomiting associated with emetogenic cancer therapy as shown by 24-hour efficacy data from three double-blind studies. The first trial compared oral *Kytril* doses of 0.25 to 2.0 mg b.i.d., in 930 cancer patients receiving, principally, cyclophosphamide, carboplatin and cisplatin (20 mg/m^2 to 50 mg/m^2). Efficacy was based on: complete response (i.e., no vomiting, no moderate or severe nausea, no rescue medication), no vomiting and no nausea. Table 2 summarizes the results of this study.

[See Table 2 on top of next page.]

A second double-blind, randomized trial compared oral *Kytril* 1.0 mg b.i.d. with prochlorperazine sustained release capsules 10.0 mg b.i.d., in 230 cancer patients receiving moderately emetogenic chemotherapeutic agents. Oral *Kytril* was significantly better than prochlorperazine in preventing nausea and vomiting (see Table 3).

Table 3. Prevention of Nausea and Vomiting 24 Hours Post-Chemotherapy[1]

	Percentages of Patients Antiemetic Regimen	
	Kytril **1.0 mg b.i.d. (n=119)**	**Prochlorperazine 10.0 mg b.i.d. (n=111)**
Efficacy Measures	**%**	**%**
Complete Response[2]	74*	41
No Vomiting	82*	48
No Nausea	58*	35

1. Chemotherapy included injectable cyclophosphamide, carboplatin, cisplatin (20 mg/m^2 to 50 mg/m^2), dacarbazine, doxorubicin, epirubicin.
2. No vomiting, no moderate or severe nausea, no rescue medication.

* Statistically significant ($P<0.001$) vs. prochlorperazine.

A third double-blind trial compared oral *Kytril* 1.0 mg b.i.d., relative to placebo (historical control), in 119 cancer patients receiving high-dose cisplatin (mean dose 80 mg/m^2). At 24 hours, oral *Kytril* 1.0 mg b.i.d. was significantly ($P<0.001$) superior to placebo (historical control) in all efficacy parameters: complete response (52%), no vomiting (56%) and no nausea (45%). The placebo rates were 7%, 14% and 7%, respectively, for the three efficacy parameters.

No controlled study comparing granisetron injection with the oral formulation to prevent chemotherapy-induced nausea and vomiting has been performed.

Continued on next page

Information on the SmithKline Beecham Pharmaceuticals products appearing here is based on the labeling in effect on July 1, 1996. Further information on these and other products may be obtained from the Medical Department, SmithKline Beecham Pharmaceuticals, One Franklin Plaza, Philadelphia, PA 19101.

SmithKline Beecham—Cont.

INDICATIONS AND USAGE

Kytril (granisetron hydrochloride) is indicated for the prevention of nausea and vomiting associated with initial and repeat courses of emetogenic cancer therapy, including high-dose cisplatin.

CONTRAINDICATIONS

Kytril is contraindicated in patients with known hypersensitivity to the drug or any of its components.

PRECAUTIONS

Drug Interactions

Granisetron does not induce or inhibit the cytochrome P-450 drug-metabolizing enzyme system. There have been no definitive drug-drug interaction studies to examine pharmacokinetic or pharmacodynamic interaction with other drugs but, in humans, Kytril Injection has been safely administered with drugs representing benzodiazepines, neuroleptics and anti-ulcer medications commonly prescribed with antiemetic treatments. Kytril Injection also does not appear to interact with emetogenic cancer chemotherapies. Because granisetron is metabolized by hepatic cytochrome P-450 drug-metabolizing enzymes, inducers or inhibitors of these enzymes may change the clearance and, hence, the half-life of granisetron.

Carcinogenesis, Mutagenesis, Impairment of Fertility

In a 24-month carcinogenicity study, rats were treated orally with granisetron 1, 5 or 50 mg/kg/day (6, 30 or 300 mg/m^2/day). The 50 mg/kg/day dose was reduced to 25 mg/kg/day (150 mg/m^2/day) during week 59 due to toxicity. For a 50 kg person of average height (1.46m^2 body surface area), these doses represent 4, 20 and 101 times the recommended clinical dose (1.48 mg/m^2, oral) on a body surface area basis. There was a statistically significant increase in the incidence of hepatocellular carcinomas and adenomas in males treated with 5 mg/kg/day (30 mg/m^2/day, 20 times the recommended human dose based on body surface area) and above, and in females treated with 25 mg/kg/day (150 mg/m^2/day, 101 times the recommended human dose based on body surface area). No increase in liver tumors was observed at a dose of 1 mg/kg/day (6 mg/m^2/day, 4 times the recommended human dose based on body surface area) in males and 5 mg/kg/day (30 mg/m^2/day, 20 times the recommended human dose based on body surface area) in females. In a 12-month oral toxicity study, treatment with granisetron 100 mg/kg/day (600 mg/m^2/day, 405 times the recommended human dose based on body surface area) produced hepatocellular adenomas in male and female rats while no such tumors were found in the control rats. A 24-month mouse carcinogenicity study of granisetron did not show a statistically significant increase in tumor incidence, but the study was not conclusive.

Because of the tumor findings in rat studies, Kytril (granisetron hydrochloride) Tablets should be prescribed only at the dose and for the indication recommended (see INDICATIONS AND USAGE, and DOSAGE AND ADMINISTRATION).

Granisetron was not mutagenic in in vitro Ames test and mouse lymphoma cell forward mutation assay, and in vivo mouse micronucleus test and in vitro and ex vivo rat hepatocyte UDS assays. It, however, produced a significant increase in UDS in HeLa cells in vitro and a significant increased incidence of cells with polyploidy in an in vitro human lymphocyte chromosomal aberration test.

Granisetron at oral doses up to 100 mg/kg/day (600 mg/m^2/day, 405 times the recommended human dose based on body surface area) was found to have no effect on fertility and reproductive performance of male and female rats.

Pregnancy

Teratogenic Effects. Pregnancy Category B. Reproduction studies have been performed in pregnant rats at oral doses up to 125 mg/kg/day (750 mg/m^2/day, 507 times the recommended human dose based on body surface area) and pregnant rabbits at oral doses up to 32 mg/kg/day (378 mg/m^2/day, 255 times the recommended human dose based on body surface area) and have revealed no evidence of impaired fertility or harm to the fetus due to granisetron. There are, however, no adequate and well-controlled studies in pregnant women. Because animal reproduction studies are not always predictive of human response, this drug should be used during pregnancy only if clearly needed.

Nursing Mothers

It is not known whether granisetron is excreted in human milk. Because many drugs are excreted in human milk, caution should be exercised when Kytril is administered to a nursing woman.

Pediatric Use

Safety and effectiveness in children have not been established.

Geriatric Use

During clinical trials, 325 patients 65 years of age or older received oral Kytril; 298 were 65 to 74 years of age and 27 were 75 years of age or older. Efficacy and safety were maintained with increasing age.

Table 1. Pharmacokinetic Parameters (Median [range]) Following Oral Kytril (granisetron hydrochloride)

	Peak Plasma Concentration (ng/mL)	Terminal Phase Plasma Half-Life (h)	Volume of Distribution (L/kg)	Total Clearance (L/h/kg)
Cancer Patients 1.0 mg b.i.d., 7 days (n=27)	5.99 [0.63 to 30.9]	N.D.*	N.D.	0.52 [0.09 to 7.37]
Volunteers single 1.0 mg dose (n=39)	3.63 [0.27 to 9.14]	6.23 [0.96 to 19.9]	3.94 [1.89 to 39.4]	0.41 [0.11 to 24.6]

* Not determined after oral administration; following a single intravenous dose of 40 mcg/kg, terminal phase half-life was determined to be 8.95 hours.
N.D. Not determined

Table 2. Prevention of Nausea and Vomiting 24 Hours Post-Chemotherapy[1]

Efficacy Measures	Percentages of Patients Oral Kytril Dose			
	0.25 mg b.i.d. (n=229) %	0.5 mg b.i.d. (n=235) %	1.0 mg b.i.d. (n=233) %	2.0 mg b.i.d. (n=233) %
Complete Response[2]	61	70*	81*†	72*
No Vomiting	66	77*	88*	79*
No Nausea	48	57	63*	54

1. Chemotherapy included oral and injectable cyclophosphamide, carboplatin, cisplatin (20 mg/m^2 to 50 mg/m^2), dacarbazine, doxorubicin, epirubicin.
2. No vomiting, no moderate or severe nausea, no rescue medication.
* Statistically significant ($P < 0.01$) vs. 0.25 mg b.i.d.
† Statistically significant ($P < 0.01$) vs. 0.5 mg b.i.d.

ADVERSE REACTIONS

Over 2,600 patients have received oral Kytril in clinical trials with emetogenic cancer therapies consisting primarily of cyclophosphamide or cisplatin regimens.

In patients receiving oral Kytril 1 mg b.i.d. for 1, 7 or 14 days, the following table lists adverse experiences reported in more than 5% of the patients with comparator and placebo incidences.

Table 4. Principal Adverse Events in Clinical Trials

	Percent of Patients with Event		
	Oral Kytril[1] 1 mg b.i.d. (n=978)	Comparator[2] (n=599)	Placebo (n=185)
Headache[3]	21%	13%	12%
Constipation	18%	16%	9%
Asthenia	14%	10%	4%
Diarrhea	8%	10%	4%
Abdominal pain	6%	6%	3%

1. Adverse events were recorded for 7 days when oral Kytril was given on a single day and for up to 28 days when oral Kytril was administered for 7 or 14 days.
2. Metoclopramide/dexamethasone; phenothiazines/dexamethasone; dexamethasone alone; prochlorperazine.
3. Usually mild to moderate in severity.

Other adverse events reported in clinical trials were:

Gastrointestinal: In single-day dosing studies in which adverse events were collected for 7 days, nausea (15%) and vomiting (9%) were recorded as adverse events after the 24-hour efficacy assessment period.

Hepatic: In comparative trials, elevation of AST and ALT (> 2 times the upper limit of normal) following the administration of oral Kytril occurred in 5% and 6% of patients, respectively. These frequencies were not significantly different from those seen with comparators (AST: 2%; ALT: 9%).

Cardiovascular: Hypertension (1%); hypotension, angina pectoris, atrial fibrillation and syncope have been observed rarely.

Central Nervous System: Dizziness (3%), insomnia (3%), anxiety (2%), somnolence (1%). One case compatible with but not diagnostic of extrapyramidal symptoms has been reported in a patient treated with oral Kytril.

Hypersensitivity: Rare cases of hypersensitivity reactions, sometimes severe (e.g., anaphylaxis, shortness of breath, hypotension, urticaria) have been reported.

Other: Fever (5%). Events often associated with chemotherapy also have been reported: leukopenia (11%), decreased appetite (5%), anemia (4%), alopecia (3%), thrombocytopenia (3%).

Over 5,000 patients have received injectable Kytril in clinical trials.

Table 5 gives the comparative frequencies of the five commonly reported adverse events (≥ 3%) in patients receiving

---

Kytril Injection, 40 mcg/kg, in single-day chemotherapy trials. These patients received chemotherapy, primarily cisplatin, and intravenous fluids during the 24-hour period following Kytril Injection administration.

Table 5. Principal Adverse Events in Clinical Trials—Single-Day Chemotherapy

	Percent of Patients with Event	
	Kytril Injection[1] 40 mcg/kg (n=1,268)	Comparator[2] (n=422)
Headache	14%	6%
Asthenia	5%	6%
Somnolence	4%	15%
Diarrhea	4%	6%
Constipation	3%	3%

1. Adverse events were generally recorded over 7 days post-Kytril Injection administration.
2. Metoclopramide/dexamethasone and phenothiazines/dexamethasone.

In the absence of a placebo group, there is uncertainty as to how many of these events should be attributed to Kytril, except for headache, which was clearly more frequent than in comparison groups.

OVERDOSAGE

There is no specific treatment for granisetron hydrochloride overdosage. In case of overdosage, symptomatic treatment should be given. Overdosage of up to 38.5 mg of granisetron hydrochloride injection has been reported without symptoms or only the occurrence of a slight headache.

DOSAGE AND ADMINISTRATION

The recommended adult dosage of oral Kytril (granisetron hydrochloride) is 1 mg twice daily. The first 1 mg tablet is given up to 1 hour before chemotherapy, and the second tablet, 12 hours after the first, only on the day(s) chemotherapy is given. Continued treatment, while not on chemotherapy, has not been found to be useful.

Use in the Elderly, Renal Failure Patients or Hepatically Impaired Patients: No dosage adjustment is recommended. (See CLINICAL PHARMACOLOGY, Pharmacokinetics.)

Pediatric Use: Data on oral Kytril are not available.

HOW SUPPLIED

Tablets: White, triangular, biconvex, film-coated tablets debossed K1 on one face: 1 mg in Unit-of-Use Packages of 2; in Single Unit Packages of 20 (intended for institutional use only).

1 mg Unit-of-Use 2's: NDC 0029-4151-39
1 mg SUP 20's: NDC 0029-4151-05
Store between 15° and 30°C (59° and 86°F). Protect from light.
Manufactured in Crawley, UK, by
SmithKline Beecham Pharmaceuticals
for **SmithKline Beecham Pharmaceuticals**
Philadelphia, PA 19101

Veterans Administration/Military/PHS—Tablets, 1 mg, 2's, 6505-01-412-0329; 1 mg, 20's, 6505-01-412-0324. KY:L2T

Shown in Product Identification Guide, page 337

MENEST™

℞

[men-est']
brand of esterified estrogens tablets, USP

WARNINGS

1. ESTROGENS HAVE BEEN REPORTED TO INCREASE THE RISK OF ENDOMETRIAL CARCINOMA.

Three independent case control studies have shown an increased risk of endometrial cancer in postmenopausal women exposed to exogenous estrogens for prolonged periods.[1–3] This risk was independent of the other known risk factors for endometrial cancer. These studies are further supported by the finding that incidence rates of endometrial cancer have increased sharply since 1969 in eight different areas of the United States with population-based cancer reporting systems, an increase which may be related to the rapidly expanding use of estrogens during the last decade.[4]

The three case control studies reported that the risk of endometrial cancer in estrogen users was about 4.5 to 13.9 times greater than in nonusers. The risk appears to depend on both duration of treatment[1] and on estrogen dose.[3] In view of these findings, when estrogens are used for the treatment of menopausal symptoms, the lowest dose that will control symptoms should be utilized and medication should be discontinued as soon as possible. When prolonged treatment is medically indicated, the patient should be reassessed on at least a semiannual basis to determine the need for continued therapy. Although the evidence must be considered preliminary, one study suggests that cyclic administration of low doses of estrogen may carry less risk than continuous administration[3]; it therefore appears prudent to utilize such a regimen.

Close clinical surveillance of all women taking estrogens is important. In all cases of undiagnosed persistent or recurring abnormal vaginal bleeding, adequate diagnostic measures should be undertaken to rule out malignancy.

There is no evidence at present that "natural" estrogens are more or less hazardous than "synthetic" estrogens at equiestrogenic doses.

2. ESTROGENS SHOULD NOT BE USED DURING PREGNANCY.

The use of female sex hormones, both estrogens and progestagens, during early pregnancy may seriously damage the offspring. It has been shown that females exposed in utero to diethylstilbestrol, a nonsteroidal estrogen, have an increased risk of developing in later life a form of vaginal or cervical cancer that is ordinarily extremely rare.[5,6] The risk has been estimated as not greater than 4 per 1000 exposures.[7] Furthermore, a high percentage of such exposed women (from 30 to 90 percent) have been found to have vaginal adenosis,[8–12] epithelial changes of the vagina and cervix. Although these changes are histologically benign, it is not known whether they are precursors of malignancy. Although similar data are not available with the use of other estrogens, it cannot be presumed they would not induce similar changes. Several reports suggest an association between intrauterine exposure to female sex hormones and congenital anomalies, including congenital heart defects and limb reduction defects.[13–16] One case control study[16] estimated a 4.7-fold increased risk of limb reduction defects in infants exposed in utero to sex hormones (oral contraceptives, hormone withdrawal tests for pregnancy, or attempted treatment for threatened abortion). Some of these exposures were very short and involved only a few days of treatment. The data suggest that the risk of limb reduction defects in exposed fetuses is somewhat less than 1 per 1000. In the past, female sex hormones have been used during pregnancy in an attempt to treat threatened or habitual abortion. There is considerable evidence that estrogens are ineffective for these indications, and there is no evidence from well-controlled studies that progestagens are effective for these uses. If Menest (esterified estrogens tablets) is used during pregnancy, or if the patient becomes pregnant while taking this drug, she should be apprised of the potential risks to the fetus, and the advisability of pregnancy continuation.

DESCRIPTION

Esterified estrogens is a mixture of the sodium salts of the sulfate esters of the estrogenic substances, principally estrone, that are of the type excreted by pregnant mares. The content of total esterified estrogens is not less than 90 percent and not more than 110 percent of the labeled amount. Esterified estrogens contain not less than 75 percent and not more than 85 percent of sodium estrone sulfate, and not less than 6 percent and not more than 15 percent of sodium equilin sulfate, in such proportion that the total of these two components is not less than 90 percent, all percentages being calculated on the basis of the total esterified estrogens content.

Inactive Ingredients: Ethyl cellulose, fragrances, hydroxypropyl cellulose, hydroxypropyl methylcellulose 2910, lactose, magnesium stearate, methylcellulose, polyethylene glycol, sodium bicarbonate, shellac, starch, stearic acid, titanium dioxide, and vanillin. Dyes in the form of aluminum lakes are contained in each tablet strength as follows: **0.3 mg Tablet:** FD&C Yellow No. 6, D&C Yellow No. 10. **0.625 mg Tablet:** FD&C Yellow No. 6, D&C Yellow No. 10. **1.25 mg Tablet:** FD&C Yellow No. 6, D&C Yellow No. 10, FD&C Blue No. 1. **2.5 mg Tablet:** D&C Red No. 30.

CLINICAL PHARMACOLOGY

Estrogens are important in the development and maintenance of the female reproductive system and secondary sex characteristics. They promote growth and development of the vagina, uterus, and fallopian tubes, and enlargement of the breasts. Indirectly, they contribute to the shaping of the skeleton, maintenance of tone and elasticity of urogenital structures, changes in the epiphyses of the long bones that allow for the pubertal growth spurt and its termination, growth of axillary and pubic hair, and pigmentation of the nipples and genitals. Decline of estrogenic activity at the end of the menstrual cycle can bring on menstruation, although the cessation of progesterone secretion is the most important factor in the mature ovulatory cycle. However, in the preovulatory or nonovulatory cycle, estrogen is the primary determinant in the onset of menstruation. Estrogens also affect the release of pituitary gonadotropins. The pharmacologic effects of esterified estrogens are similar to those of endogenous estrogens. They are soluble in water and are well absorbed from the gastrointestinal tract.

In responsive tissues (female genital organs, breasts, hypothalamus, pituitary) estrogens enter the cell and are transported into the nucleus. As a result of estrogen action, specific RNA and protein synthesis occurs. Metabolism and inactivation occur primarily in the liver. Some estrogens are excreted into the bile; however, they are reabsorbed from the intestine and returned to the liver through the portal venous system. Water soluble estrogen conjugates are strongly acidic and are ionized in body fluids, which favor excretion through the kidneys since tubular reabsorption is minimal.

INDICATIONS AND USAGE

Menest (esterified estrogens tablets) is indicated in the treatment of:

1. Moderate to severe *vasomotor* symptoms associated with the menopause. (There is no evidence that estrogens are effective for nervous symptoms or depression which might occur during menopause, and they should not be used to treat these conditions.)
2. Atrophic vaginitis.
3. Kraurosis vulvae.
4. Female hypogonadism.
5. Female castration.
6. Primary ovarian failure.
7. Breast cancer (for palliation only) in appropriately selected women and men with metastatic disease.
8. Prostatic carcinoma—palliative therapy of advanced disease.

MENEST (esterified estrogens tablets) HAS NOT BEEN SHOWN TO BE EFFECTIVE FOR ANY PURPOSE DURING PREGNANCY AND ITS USE MAY CAUSE SEVERE HARM TO THE FETUS (SEE BOXED WARNING).

CONTRAINDICATIONS

Estrogens should not be used in women (or men) with any of the following conditions:

1. Known or suspected cancer of the breast except in appropriately selected patients being treated for metastatic disease.
2. Known or suspected estrogen-dependent neoplasia.
3. Known or suspected pregnancy (See Boxed Warning).
4. Undiagnosed abnormal genital bleeding.
5. Active thrombophlebitis or thromboembolic disorders.
6. A past history of thrombophlebitis, thrombosis or thromboembolic disorders associated with previous estrogen use (except when used in treatment of breast or prostatic malignancy).

WARNINGS

1. *Induction of malignant neoplasms.* Long-term continuous administration of natural and synthetic estrogens in certain animal species increases the frequency of carcinomas of the breast, cervix, vagina, and liver. There is now evidence that estrogens increase the risk of carcinoma of the endometrium in humans. (See Boxed Warning.) At the present time there is no satisfactory evidence that estrogens given to postmenopausal women increase the risk of cancer of the breast[18] although a recent long-term followup of a single physician's practice has raised this possibility.[18a] Because of the animal data, there is a need for caution in prescribing estrogens for women with a strong family history of breast cancer or who have breast nodules, fibrocystic disease, or abnormal mammograms.

2. *Gall bladder disease.* A recent study has reported a 2- to 3-fold increase in the risk of surgically confirmed gall bladder disease in women receiving postmenopausal estrogens,[18] similar to the 2-fold increase previously noted in users of oral contraceptives.[19–24] In the case of oral contraceptives the increased risk appeared after 2 years of use.[24]

3. *Effects similar to those caused by estrogen-progestagen oral contraceptives.* There are several serious adverse effects of oral contraceptives, most of which have not, up to now, been documented as consequences of postmenopausal estrogen therapy. This may reflect the comparatively low doses of estrogen used in post-menopausal women. It would be expected that the larger doses of estrogen used to treat prostatic or breast cancer or postpartum breast engorgement are more likely to result in these adverse effects and, in fact, it has been shown that there is an increased risk of thrombosis in men receiving estrogens for prostatic cancer and women for postpartum breast engorgement.[20–23]

a. *Thromboembolic disease.* It is now well established that users of oral contraceptives have an increased risk of various thromboembolic and thrombotic vascular diseases, such as thrombophlebitis, pulmonary embolism, stroke, and myocardial infarction.[24–31] Cases of retinal thrombosis, mesenteric thrombosis, and optic neuritis have been reported in oral contraceptive users. There is evidence that the risk of several of these adverse reactions is related to the dose of the drug.[32, 33] An increased risk of post-surgery thromboembolic complications has also been reported in users of oral contraceptives.[34,35] If feasible, estrogen should be discontinued at least 4 weeks before surgery of the type associated with an increased risk of thromboembolism, or during periods of prolonged immobilization.

While an increased rate of thromboembolic and thrombotic disease in postmenopausal users of estrogens has not been found,[18–36] this does not rule out the possibility that such an increase may be present or that subgroups of women who have underlying risk factors or who are receiving relatively large doses of estrogens may have increased risk.

Therefore estrogens should not be used in persons with active thrombophlebitis or thromboembolic disorders, and they should not be used (except in treatment of malignancy) in persons with a history of such disorders in association with estrogen use. They should be used with caution in patients with cerebral vascular or coronary artery disease and only for those in whom estrogens are clearly needed.

Large doses of estrogen (5 mg esterified estrogens per day), comparable to those used to treat cancer of the prostate and breast, have been shown in a large prospective clinical trial in men[37] to increase the risk of nonfatal myocardial infarction, pulmonary embolism and thrombophlebitis. When estrogen doses of this size are used, any of the thromboembolic and thrombotic adverse effects associated with oral contraceptive use should be considered a clear risk.

b. *Hepatic adenoma.* Benign hepatic adenomas appear to be associated with the use of oral contraceptives.[38–40] Although benign, and rare, these may rupture and may cause death through intra-abdominal hemorrhage. Such lesions have not yet been reported in association with other estrogen or progestagen preparations but should be considered in estrogen users having abdominal pain and tenderness, abdominal mass, or hypovolemic shock. Hepatocellular carcinoma has also been reported in women taking estrogen-containing oral contraceptives.[39] The relationship of this malignancy to these drugs is not known at this time.

c. *Elevated blood pressure.* Increased blood pressure is not uncommon in women using oral contraceptives. There is now a report that this may occur with use of estrogens in

Continued on next page

Information on the SmithKline Beecham Pharmaceuticals products appearing here is based on the labeling in effect on July 1, 1996. Further information on these and other products may be obtained from the Medical Department, SmithKline Beecham Pharmaceuticals, One Franklin Plaza, Philadelphia, PA 19101.

SmithKline Beecham—Cont.

the menopause[41] and blood pressure should be monitored with estrogen use, especially if high doses are used.

d. *Glucose tolerance.* A worsening of glucose tolerance has been observed in a significant percentage of patients on estrogen-containing oral contraceptives. For this reason, diabetic patients should be carefully observed while receiving estrogen.

4. *Hypercalcemia.* Administration of estrogens may lead to severe hypercalcemia in patients with breast cancer and bone metastases. If this occurs, the drug should be stopped and appropriate measures taken to reduce the serum calcium level.

See footnotes at end of article.

PRECAUTIONS

A. *General Precautions:*

1. A complete medical and family history should be taken prior to the initiation of any estrogen therapy. The pretreatment and periodic physical examinations should include special reference to blood pressure, breast, abdomen, and pelvic organs, and should include a Papanicolau smear. As a general rule, estrogen should not be prescribed for longer than 1 year without another physical examination being performed.

2. Fluid retention—Because estrogens may cause some degree of fluid retention, conditions which might be influenced by this factor, such as epilepsy, migraine, and cardiac or renal dysfunction, require careful observation.

3. Certain patients may develop undesirable manifestations of excessive estrogenic stimulation, such as abnormal or excessive uterine bleeding, mastodynia, etc.

4. Oral contraceptives appear to be associated with an increased incidence of mental depression.[24] Although it is not clear whether this is due to the estrogenic or progestagenic component of the contraceptive, patients with a history of depression should be carefully observed.

5. Pre-existing uterine leiomyomata may increase in size during estrogen use.

6. The pathologist should be advised of estrogen therapy when relevant specimens are submitted.

7. Patients with a past history of jaundice during pregnancy have an increased risk of recurrence of jaundice while receiving estrogen-containing oral contraceptive therapy. If jaundice develops in any patient receiving estrogen, the medication should be discontinued while the cause is investigated.

8. Estrogens may be poorly metabolized in patients with impaired liver function and they should be administered with caution in such patients.

9. Because estrogens influence the metabolism of calcium and phosphorus, they should be used with caution in patients with metabolic bone diseases that are associated with hypercalcemia or in patients with renal insufficiency.

10. Because of the effects of estrogens on epiphyseal closure, they should be used judiciously in young patients in whom bone growth is not complete.

11. The lowest effective dose appropriate for the specific indication should be utilized. Studies of the addition of a progestin for 7 or more days of a cycle of estrogen administration have reported a lowered incidence of endometrial hyperplasia. Morphological and biochemical studies of endometrium suggest that 10 to 13 days of progestin are needed to provide maximal maturation of the endometrium and to eliminate any hyperplastic changes. Whether this will provide protection from endometrial carcinoma has not been clearly established. There are possible additional risks which may be associated with the inclusion of progestin in estrogen replacement regimens. The potential risks include adverse effects on carbohydrate and lipid metabolism. The choice of progestin and dosage may be important in minimizing these adverse effects.

12. Certain endocrine and liver function tests may be affected by estrogen-containing oral contraceptives. The following similar changes may be expected with larger doses of estrogen:

a. Increased sulfobromophthalein retention.

b. Increased prothrombin and factors VII, VIII, IX, and X; decreased antithrombin 3; increased norepinephrine-induced platelet aggregability.

c. Increased thyroid binding globulin (TBG) leading to increased circulating total thyroid hormone, as measured by PBI, T4 by column or T4 by radioimmunoassay. Free T3 resin uptake is decreased, reflecting the elevated TBG; free T4 concentration is unaltered.

d. Impaired glucose tolerance.

e. Decreased pregnanediol excretion.

f. Reduced response to metyrapone test.

g. Reduced serum folate concentration.

h. Increased serum triglyceride and phospholipid concentration.

B. *Information for patients:* See text which appears after PHYSICIAN REFERENCES.

C. *Pregnancy Category X*—See Contraindications and Boxed Warning.

D. *Nursing Mothers.* As a general principle, the administration of any drug to nursing mothers should be done only when clearly necessary since many drugs are excreted in human milk.

ADVERSE REACTIONS

(See Warnings regarding induction of neoplasia, adverse effects on the fetus, increased incidence of gall bladder disease, and adverse effects similar to those of oral contraceptives, including thromboembolism.) The following additional adverse reactions have been reported with estrogenic therapy, including oral contraceptives:

1. *Genitourinary system.*
Breakthrough bleeding, spotting, change in menstrual flow.
Dysmenorrhea.
Premenstrual-like syndrome.
Amenorrhea during and after treatment.
Increase in size of uterine fibromyomata.
Vaginal candidiasis.
Change in cervical eversion and in degree of cervical secretion.
Cystitis-like syndrome.

2. *Breasts.*
Tenderness, enlargement, secretion.

3. *Gastrointestinal.*
Nausea, vomiting.
Abdominal cramps, bloating.
Cholestatic jaundice.

4. *Skin.*
Chloasma or melasma which may persist when drug is discontinued.
Erythema multiforme.
Erythema nodosum.
Hemorrhagic eruption.
Loss of scalp hair.
Hirsutism.

5. *Eyes.*
Steepening of corneal curvature.
Intolerance to contact lenses.

6. *CNS.*
Headache, migraine, dizziness.
Mental depression.
Chorea.

7. *Miscellaneous.*
Increase or decrease in weight.
Reduced carbohydrate tolerance.
Aggravation of porphyria.
Edema.
Changes in libido.

ACUTE OVERDOSAGE

Numerous reports of ingestion of large doses of estrogen-containing oral contraceptives by young children indicate that serious ill effects do not occur. Overdosage of estrogen may cause nausea, and withdrawal bleeding may occur in females.

DOSAGE AND ADMINISTRATION

1. *Given cyclically for short term use only:*
For treatment of moderate to severe *vasomotor symptoms, atrophic vaginitis* or *kraurosis vulvae* associated with the menopause.
The lowest dose that will control symptoms should be chosen and medication should be discontinued as promptly as possible.
Administration should be cyclic (e.g., 3 weeks on and 1 week off).
Attempts to discontinue or taper medication should be made at 3 to 6 month intervals.

USUAL DOSAGE RANGES:

Vasomotor symptoms—1.25 mg daily. If the patient has not menstruated within the last 2 months or more, cyclic administration is started arbitrarily. If the patient is menstruating, cyclic administration is started on day 5 of bleeding.

Atrophic vaginitis and kraurosis vulvae—0.3 mg to 1.25 mg or more daily, depending upon the tissue response of the individual patient. Administer cyclically.

2. *Given cyclically:* Female hypogonadism; female castration; primary ovarian failure.

USUAL DOSAGE RANGES:

Female hypogonadism—2.5 to 7.5 mg daily, in divided doses for 20 days, followed by a rest period of 10 days' duration. If bleeding does not occur by the end of this period, the same dosage schedule is repeated. The number of courses of estrogen therapy necessary to produce bleeding may vary depending on responsiveness of the endometrium.
If bleeding occurs before the end of the 10 day period, begin a 20 day estrogen-progestin cyclic regimen with Menest (esterified estrogens tablets), 2.5 to 7.5 mg daily in divided doses, for 20 days. During the last 5 days of estrogen therapy, give an oral progestin. If bleeding occurs before this regimen is

concluded, therapy is discontinued and may be resumed on the fifth day of bleeding.

Female castration and primary ovarian failure—1.25 mg daily, cyclically. Adjust dosage upward or downward according to severity of symptoms and response of the patient. For maintenance, adjust dosage to lowest level that will provide effective control.

3. *Given chronically:* Inoperable progressing prostatic cancer—1.25 to 2.5 mg three times daily. The effectiveness of therapy can be judged by phosphatase determinations as well as by symptomatic improvement of the patient.
Inoperable progressing breast cancer in appropriately selected men and postmenopausal women. (See INDICATIONS AND USAGE)—Suggested dosage is 10 mg three times daily for a period of at least 3 months.
Treated patients with an intact uterus should be monitored closely for signs of endometrial cancer and appropriate diagnostic measures should be taken to rule out malignancy in the event of persistent or recurring abnormal vaginal bleeding.

HOW SUPPLIED

Tablets:
0.3 mg yellow, film-coated oblong tablet imprinted with BMP 125 100's: NDC 0029-2800-30
0.625 mg orange, film-coated oblong tablet imprinted with BMP 126 100's: NDC 0029-2810-30
1.25 mg green, film-coated oblong tablet imprinted with BMP 127 100's: NDC 0029-2820-30
2.5 mg pink, film-coated oblong tablet imprinted with BMP 128 50's: NDC 0029-2830-29

PHYSICIAN REFERENCES

1. Ziel HK, Finkel WD: Increased Risk of Endometrial Carcinoma Among Users of Conjugated Estrogens, *New England Journal of Medicine* 293:1167–1170, 1975.

2. Smith DC, Prentic R, Thompson DJ, Hermann WL: Association of Exogenous Estrogen and Endometrial Carcinoma, *New England Journal of Medicine* 293:1164–1167, 1975.

3. Mack TM, Pike MC, Henderson BE, et al: Estrogens and Endometrial Cancer in a Retirement Community, *New England Journal of Medicine* 294:1262–1267, 1976.

4. Weiss NS, Szekely DR, Austin DF: Increasing Incidence of Endometrial Cancer in the United States, *New England Journal of Medicine* 294:1259–1262, 1976.

5. Herbst AL, Ulfelder H, Poskanzer DC: Adenocarcinoma of Vagina, *New England Journal of Medicine* 284:878–881, 1971.

6. Greenwald P, Barlow J, Nasca P, Burnett W: Vaginal Cancer After Maternal Treatment with Synthetic Estrogens, *New England Journal of Medicine* 285:390–392, 1971.

7. Lanier A, Noller K, Decker D, et al: Cancer and Stilbestrol. A Follow-up of 1719 Persons Exposed to Estrogens in Utero and Born 1943–1959, *Mayo Clinic Proceedings* 48:793–799, 1973.

8. Herbst A, Kurman R, Scully R: Vaginal and Cervical Abnormalities After Exposure to Stilbestrol In Utero, *Obstetrics and Gynecology* 40:287–298, 1972.

9. Herbst A, Robboy S, Macdonald G, Scully R: The Effects of Local Progesterone on Stilbestrol-Associated Vaginal Adenosis, *American Journal of Obstetrics and Gynecology* 118:607–615, 1974.

10. Herbst A, Poskanzer D, Robboy S, et al: Prenatal Exposure to Stilbestrol, A Prospective Comparison of Exposed Female Offspring with Unexposed Controls, *New England Journal of Medicine* 292:334–339, 1975.

11. Stafl A, Mattingly R, Foley D, Fetherston W: Clinical Diagnosis of Vaginal Adenosis, *Obstetrics and Gynecology* 43:118–128, 1974.

12. Sherman AI, Goldrath M, Berlin A, et al: Cervical-Vaginal Adenosis After In Utero Exposure to Synthetic Estrogens, *Obstetrics and Gynecology* 44:531–545, 1974.

13. Gal I, Kirman B, Stern J: Hormone Pregnancy Tests and Congenital Malformation, *Nature* 216:83, 1967.

14. Levy EP, Cohen A, Fraser FC: Hormone Treatment During Pregnancy and Congenital Heart Defects, *Lancet* 1:611, 1973.

15. Nora J, Nora A: Birth Defects and Oral Contraceptives, *Lancet* 1:941–942, 1973.

16. Janerich DT, Piper JM, Glebatis, DM: Oral Contraceptives and Congenital Limb-Reduction Defects, *New England Journal of Medicine* 291:697–700, 1974.

17. Estrogens for Oral or Parenteral Use, *Federal Register* 40:8212, 1975.

18. Boston Collaborative Drug Surveillance Program: Surgically Confirmed Gall Bladder Disease, Venous Thromboembolism and Breast Tumors in Relations to Post-Menopausal Estrogen Therapy, *New England Journal of Medicine* 290:15–19, 1974.

18a. Hoover R, Gray LA Sr, Cole P, MacMahon B: Menopausal Estrogens and Breast Cancer, *New England Journal of Medicine* 295:401–405, 1976.

19. Boston Collaborative Drug Surveillance Program: Oral Contraceptives and Venous Thromboembolic Disease,

Surgically Confirmed Gall Bladder Disease, and Breast Tumors, *Lancet* 1:1399–1404, 1973.

20. Daniel DG, Campbell H, Turnbull AC: Puerperal Thromboembolism and Suppression of Lactation, *Lancet* 2:287–289, 1967.

21. The Veterans Administration Cooperative Urological Research Group: Carcinoma of the Prostate: Treatment Comparisons, *Journal of Urology* 98:516–522, 1967.

22. Bailar JC: Thromboembolism and Oestrogen Therapy, *Lancet* 2:560, 1967.

23. Blackard C, Doe R, Mellinger G, Byar D: Incidence of Cardiovascular Disease and Death in Patients Receiving Diethylstilbestrol for Carcinoma of the Prostate, *Cancer* 26:249–256, 1970.

24. Royal College of General Practitioners: Oral Contraception and Thromboembolic Disease, *Journal of the Royal College of General Practitioners* 13:267–279, 1967.

25. Inman WHW, Vessey MP: Investigation of Deaths from Pulmonary, Coronary and Cerebral Thrombosis and Embolism in Women of Child-Bearing Age, *British Medical Journal* 2:193–199, 1968.

26. Vessey MP, Doll R: Investigation of Relation Between Use of Oral Contraceptives and Thromboembolic Disease. A Further Report, *British Medical Journal* 2:651–657, 1969.

27. Sartwell PE, Masi AT, Arthes FG, et al: Thromboembolism and Oral Contraceptives: An Epidemiological Case Control Study, *American Journal of Epidemiology* 90:365–380, 1969.

28. Collaborative Group for the Study of Stroke in Young Women: Oral Contraception and Increased Risk of Cerebral Ischemia or Thrombosis, *New England Journal of Medicine* 288:871–878, 1973.

29. Collaborative Group for the Study of Stroke in Young Women: Oral Contraceptives and Stroke in Young Women: Associated Risk Factors, *Journal of the American Medical Association* 231:718–722, 1975.

30. Mann JI, Inman WHW: Oral Contraceptives and Death from Myocardial Infarction, *British Medical Journal* 2:245–248, 1975.

31. Mann JI, Vessey MP, Thorogood M, Doll R: Myocardial Infarction in Young Women with Special Reference to Oral Contraceptive Practice, *British Medical Journal* 2:241–245, 1975.

32. Inman WHW, Vessey VP, Westerholm B, Engelund A: Thromboembolic Disease and the Steroidal Content of Oral Contraceptives, *British Medical Journal* 2:203–209, 1970.

33. Stolley PD, Tonascia JA, Tockman MS, et al: Thrombosis with Low-Estrogen Oral Contraceptives, *American Journal of Epidemiology* 102:197–208, 1975.

34. Vessey MP, Doll R, Fairbairn AS, Glober G: Post-Operative Thromboembolism and the Use of the Oral Contraceptives, *British Medical Journal* 3:123–126, 1970.

35. Greene GR, Sartwell PE: Oral Contraceptive Use in Patients with Thromboembolism Following Surgery, Trauma or Infection, *American Journal of Public Health* 62:680–685, 1972.

36. Rosenberg L, Armstrong MB, Jick H: Myocardial Infarction and Estrogen Therapy in Postmenopausal Women, *New England Journal of Medicine* 294:1256–1259, 1976.

37. Coronary Drug Project Research Group: The Coronary Drug Project: Initial Findings Leading to Modification of Its Research Protocol, *Journal of the American Medical Association* 214:1303–1313, 1970.

38. Baum J, Holtz F, Bookstein JJ, Klein EW: Possible Association Between Benign Hepatomas and Oral Contraceptives, *Lancet* 2:926–928, 1973.

39. Mays ET, Christopherson WM, Mahr MM, Williams HC: Hepatic Changes in Young Women Ingesting Contraceptive Steroids, Hepatic Hemorrhage and Primary Hepatic Tumors, *Journal of the American Medical Association* 235:730–782, 1976.

40. Edmondson HA, Henderson B, Benton B: Liver Cell Adenomas Associated with the Use of Oral Contraceptives, *New England Journal of Medicine* 294:470–472, 1976.

41. Pfeffer RI, Van Den Noort S: Estrogen Use and Stroke Risk in Postmenopausal Women, *American Journal of Epidemiology* 103:445–456, 1976.

PATIENT INFORMATION

WHAT YOU SHOULD KNOW ABOUT ESTROGENS

Estrogens are female hormones produced by the ovaries. The ovaries make several different kinds of estrogens. In addition, scientists have been able to make a variety of synthetic estrogens. As far as we know, all these estrogens have similar properties and therefore much the same usefulness, side effects, and risks. This leaflet is intended to help you understand what estrogens are used for, the risks involved in their use, and how to use them as safely as possible.

This leaflet includes the most important information about estrogens, but not all the information. If you want to know more, you can ask your doctor or pharmacist to let you read the package insert prepared for the doctor.

USES OF ESTROGEN

Estrogens are prescribed by doctors for a number of purposes, including:

1. To provide estrogen during a period of adjustment when a woman's ovaries no longer produce it, in order to prevent certain uncomfortable symptoms of estrogen deficiency. (All women normally stop producing estrogens, generally between the ages of 45 and 55; this is called the menopause.)
2. To prevent symptoms of estrogen deficiency when a woman's ovaries have been removed surgically before the natural menopause.
3. To prevent pregnancy. (Estrogens are given along with a progestagen, another female hormone; these combinations are called oral contraceptives or birth control pills. Patient labeling is available to women taking oral contraceptives, and they will not be discussed in this leaflet.)
4. To treat certain cancers in women and men.

THERE IS NO PROPER USE OF ESTROGENS IN A PREGNANT WOMAN.

ESTROGENS IN THE MENOPAUSE

In the natural course of their lives, all women eventually experience a decrease in estrogen production. This usually occurs between ages 45 and 55, but may occur earlier or later. Sometimes the ovaries may need to be removed before natural menopause by an operation, producing a "surgical menopause."

When the amount of estrogen in the blood begins to decrease, many women may develop typical symptoms: Feelings of warmth in the face, neck, and chest or sudden intense episodes of heat and sweating throughout the body (called "hot flashes" or "hot flushes"). These symptoms are sometimes very uncomfortable. A few women eventually develop changes in the vagina (called "atrophic vaginitis") which cause discomfort, especially during and after intercourse. Estrogens can be prescribed to treat these symptoms of the menopause. It is estimated that considerably more than half of all women undergoing the menopause have only mild symptoms or no symptoms at all and therefore do not need estrogens. Other women may need estrogens for a few months, while their bodies adjust to lower estrogen levels. Sometimes the need will be for periods longer than 6 months. In an attempt to avoid overstimulation of the uterus (womb), estrogens are usually given cyclically during each month of use, that is 3 weeks of pills followed by 1 week without pills. Sometimes women experience nervous symptoms or depression during menopause. There is no evidence that estrogens are effective for such symptoms and they should not be used to treat them, although other treatments may be needed.

You may have heard that taking estrogens for long periods (years) after menopause will keep your skin soft and supple and keep you feeling young. There is no evidence that this is so, however, and such long-term treatment carries important risks.

THE DANGERS OF ESTROGENS

1. *Cancer of the uterus.* If estrogens are used in the post-menopausal period for more than a year, there is an increased risk of *endometrial cancer* (cancer of the uterus). Women taking estrogens have roughly 5 to 10 times as great a chance of getting this cancer as women who take no estrogens. To put this another way, while a postmenopausal woman not taking estrogens has 1 chance in 1,000 each year of getting cancer of the uterus, a woman taking estrogens has 5 to 10 chances in 1,000 each year. For this reason *it is important to take estrogens only when you really need them.*

   The risk of this cancer is greater the longer estrogens are used and also seems to be greater when larger doses are taken. For this reason *it is important to take the lowest dose of estrogen that will control symptoms and to take it only as long as it is needed.* If estrogens are needed for longer periods of time, your doctor will want to re-evaluate your need for estrogens at least every 6 months.

   Women using estrogens should report any irregular vaginal bleeding to their doctors; such bleeding may be of no importance, but it can be an early warning of cancer of the uterus. If you have undiagnosed vaginal bleeding, you should not use estrogens until a diagnosis is made and you are certain there is no cancer of the uterus. If you have had your uterus completely removed (total hysterectomy) there is no danger of developing cancer of the uterus.
2. *Other possible cancers.* Estrogens can cause development of other tumors in animals, such as tumors of the breast, cervix, vagina, or liver, when given for a long time. At present there is no good evidence that women using estrogen in the menopause have an increased risk of such tumors, but there is no way yet to be sure they do not; and one study raises the possibility that use of estrogens in the menopause may increase risk of breast cancer many years later. This is a further reason to use estrogens only when clearly needed. While you are taking estrogens, it is important that you go to your doctor at least once a year for a physical examination. Also, if members of your family have had breast cancer or if you have breast nodules or abnormal mammograms (breast x-rays), your doctor may wish to carry out more frequent examinations of your breasts.
3. *Gall bladder disease.* Women who use estrogens after menopause are more likely to develop gall bladder disease needing surgery than women who do not use estrogens. Birth control pills have a similar effect.
4. *Abnormal blood clotting.* Oral contraceptives increase the risk of blood clotting in various parts of the body. This can result in a stroke (if the clot is in the brain), a heart attack (clot in a blood vessel of the heart), or a pulmonary embolus (a clot which forms in the legs or pelvis, then breaks off and travels to the lungs). Any of these can be fatal.

   At this time use of estrogens in the menopause is not known to cause such blood clotting, but this has not been fully studied and there could still prove to be such a risk. It is recommended that if you have had clotting in the legs or lungs or a heart attack or stroke while you were using estrogens or birth control pills, you should not use estrogens (unless they are being used to treat cancer of the breast or prostate). If you have had a stroke or heart attack or if you have angina pectoris, estrogens should be used with great caution and only if clearly needed (for example, if you have severe symptoms of the menopause).

SPECIAL WARNING ABOUT PREGNANCY

You should not receive estrogen if you are pregnant. If this should occur there is a greater than usual chance that the developing child will be born with a birth defect, although the possibility remains fairly small. A female child may have an increased risk of developing cancer of the vagina or cervix later in life (in the teens or twenties). Every possible effort should be made to avoid exposure to estrogens during pregnancy. If exposure occurs, see your doctor.

OTHER EFFECTS OF ESTROGENS

In addition to the serious known risks of estrogens described above, estrogens have the following side effects and potential risks:

1. *Nausea and vomiting.* The most common side effect of estrogen therapy is nausea. Vomiting is less common.
2. *Effects on breasts.* Estrogens may cause breast tenderness or enlargement and may cause the breasts to secrete a liquid. These effects are not dangerous.
3. *Effects on the uterus.* Estrogens may cause benign fibroid tumors of the uterus to get larger. Some women will have menstrual bleeding when estrogens are stopped. But if the bleeding occurs on days you are still taking estrogens you should report this to your doctor.
4. *Effects on liver.* Women taking oral contraceptives develop on rare occasions a tumor of the liver which can rupture and bleed into the abdomen. So far, these tumors have not been reported in women using estrogens in the menopause, but you should report any swelling or unusual pain or tenderness in the abdomen to your doctor immediately. Women with a past history of jaundice (yellowing of the skin and white parts of the eyes) may get jaundice again during estrogen use. If this occurs, stop taking estrogen and see your doctor.
5. *Other effects.* Estrogens may cause excess fluid to be retained in the body. This may make some conditions worse, such as epilepsy, migraine, heart disease, or kidney disease.

SUMMARY

Estrogens have important uses, but they have serious risks as well. You must decide, with your doctor, whether the risks are acceptable to you in view of the benefits of treatment. Except where your doctor has prescribed estrogens for use in special cases of cancer of the breast or prostate, you should not use estrogens if you have cancer of the breast or uterus, are pregnant, have undiagnosed abnormal vaginal bleeding, clotting in the legs or lungs, or have had a stroke, heart attack or angina, or clotting in the legs or lungs in the past while you were taking estrogens.

You can use estrogens as safely as possible by understanding that your doctor will require regular physical examinations while you are taking them and will try to discontinue the drug as soon as possible and use the smallest dose possible. Be alert for signs of trouble including:

1. Abnormal bleeding from the vagina.
2. Pains in the calves or chest or sudden shortness of breath, or coughing blood (indicating possible clots in the legs, heart, or lungs).

Continued on next page

Information on the SmithKline Beecham Pharmaceuticals products appearing here is based on the labeling in effect on July 1, 1996. Further information on these and other products may be obtained from the Medical Department, SmithKline Beecham Pharmaceuticals, One Franklin Plaza, Philadelphia, PA 19101.

SmithKline Beecham—Cont.

3. Severe headache, dizziness, faintness, or changes in vision (indicating possible developing clots in the brain or eye).
4. Breast lumps (you should ask your doctor how to examine your own breasts).
5. Jaundice (yellowing of the skin).
6. Mental depression.

Based on his or her assessment of your medical needs, your doctor has prescribed this drug for you. Do not give the drug to anyone else.

CAUTION
Federal law prohibits dispensing without prescription.
Manufactured by King Pharmaceuticals, Inc.
Bristol, TN 37620 for
SmithKline Beecham Pharmaceuticals
Philadelphia, PA 19101
ME:L6

Shown in Product Identification Guide, page 337

MONOCID®
[*mon 'oh-sid*]
brand of sterile cefonicid sodium
(lyophilized)

℞

DESCRIPTION
Monocid (sterile cefonicid sodium), a sterile, lyophilized, semi-synthetic, broad-spectrum cephalosporin antibiotic for intravenous and intramuscular administration, is 5–Thia-1-azabicyclo[4.2.0]oct-2-ene-2-carboxylic acid, 7-[(hydroxyphenyl - acetyl) - amino] -8- oxo -3- [[[1-(sulfomethyl)-1*H* - tetrazol -5- yl] thio] methyl] -disodium salt, [6*R* - [6α, 7β(*R**)]].
Cefonicid sodium contains 85 mg (3.7 mEq) sodium per gram of cefonicid activity.

CLINICAL PHARMACOLOGY
Human Pharmacology
The table below demonstrates the levels and duration of Monocid (sterile cefonicid sodium) in serum following intravenous and intramuscular administration of 1 gram to normal volunteers.
[See table below.]
Serum half-life is approximately 4.5 hours with intravenous and intramuscular administration. *Monocid* is highly (greater than 90%) and reversibly protein bound.
Monocid is not metabolized; 99% is excreted unchanged in the urine in 24 hours. A 500 mg IM dose provides a high (384 mcg/mL) urinary concentration at 6 to 8 hours. Probenecid, given concurrently with *Monocid*, slows renal excretion, produces higher peak serum levels and significantly increases the serum half-life of the drug (8.2 hours).
Monocid reaches therapeutic levels in the following tissues and fluids:
[See table above.]
Note: Although *Monocid* reaches therapeutic levels in bile, those levels are lower than those seen with other cephalosporins, and amounts of *Monocid* released into the gastrointestinal tract are minute. This small amount of *Monocid* in the gastrointestinal tract is thought to be the reason for the low incidence of gastrointestinal reactions following therapy with *Monocid*.
No disulfiram-like reactions were reported in a crossover study conducted in healthy volunteers receiving *Monocid* and alcohol.
Microbiology
The bactericidal action of Monocid (sterile cefonicid sodium) results from inhibition of cell-wall synthesis. *Monocid* is highly resistant to beta-lactamases produced by *Staphylococcus aureus, Haemophilus influenzae, Neisseria gonorrhoeae* and Richmond type I beta-lactamases. *Monocid* is resistant to degradation by beta-lactamases from certain members of *Enterobacteriaceae*. Active against a wide range of gram-positive and gram-negative organisms, *Monocid* is usually active against the following organisms *in vitro* and in clinical situations:
Gram-Positive Aerobes: *Staphylococcus aureus* (beta-lactamase producing and non-beta-lactamase producing) and *S. epidermidis* (Note: Methicillin-resistant staphylococci are resistant to cephalosporins, including cefonicid.); *Streptococcus pneumoniae, S. pyogenes* (Group A beta-hemolytic *Streptococcus*), and *S. agalactiae* (Group B *Streptococcus*).
Gram-Negative Aerobes: *Escherichia coli; Klebsiella pneumoniae; Providencia rettgeri* (formerly *Proteus rettgeri*);

Proteus vulgaris; Morganella morganii (formerly *Proteus morganii*); *Proteus mirabilis;* and *Haemophilus influenzae* (ampicillin-sensitive and -resistant).
The following *in vitro* data are available but their clinical significance is unknown. *Monocid* is usually active against the following organisms *in vitro*:
Gram-Negative Aerobes: *Moraxella* (formerly *Branhamella*) *catarrhalis; Klebsiella oxytoca; Enterobacter aerogenes; Neisseria gonorrhoeae* (penicillin-sensitive and -resistant); *Citrobacter freundii* and *C. diversus.*
Gram-Positive Anaerobes: *Clostridium perfringens; Peptostreptococcus anaerobius; Peptococcus magnus; P. prevotii;* and *Propionibacterium acnes.*
Gram-Negative Anaerobes: *Fusobacterium nucleatum.*
Monocid (sterile cefonicid sodium) is usually inactive *in vitro* against most strains of *Pseudomonas, Serratia, Enterococcus* and *Acinetobacter.* Most strains of *B. fragilis* are resistant.
Susceptibility Testing
Results from standardized single-disk susceptibility tests using a 30 mcg *Monocid* disk should be interpreted according to the following criteria:
Zones of 18 mm or greater indicate that the tested organism is susceptible to *Monocid* and is likely to respond to therapy.
Zones from 15 to 17 mm indicate that the tested organism is of intermediate (moderate) susceptibility, and is likely to respond to therapy if a higher dosage is used or if the infection is confined to tissues and fluids in which high antibiotic levels are attained.
Zones of 14 mm or less indicate that the organism is resistant.
Only the *Monocid* disk should be used to determine susceptibility, since *in vitro* tests show that *Monocid* has activity against certain strains not susceptible to other cephalosporins. The *Monocid* disk should not be used for testing susceptibility to other cephalosporins.
A bacterial isolate may be considered susceptible if the MIC value for *Monocid* is equal to or less than 8 mcg/mL in accordance with the National Committee for Clinical Laboratory Standards (NCCLS) guidelines. Organisms are considered resistant if the MIC is equal to or greater than 32 mcg/mL. For most organisms the MBC value for *Monocid* is the same as the MIC value.
The standardized quality control procedure requires use of control organisms. The 30 mcg *Monocid* disk should give the zone diameters listed below for the quality control strains.

Organism	ATCC	Zone Size Range
E. coli	25922	25 to 29 mm
S. aureus	25923	22 to 28 mm

INDICATIONS AND USAGE
Due to the long half-life of *Monocid*, a 1 gram dose results in therapeutic serum levels which provide coverage against susceptible organisms (listed below) for 24 hours.
Studies on specimens obtained prior to therapy should be used to determine the susceptibility of the causative organisms to *Monocid*. Therapy with *Monocid* may be initiated pending results of the studies; however, treatment should be adjusted according to study findings.
Treatment
Monocid (sterile cefonicid sodium) is indicated in the treatment of infections due to susceptible strains of the microorganisms listed below:
LOWER RESPIRATORY TRACT INFECTIONS, due to *Streptococcus pneumoniae; Klebsiella pneumoniae**; *Escherichia coli;* and *Haemophilus influenzae* (ampicillin-resistant and ampicillin-sensitive).

URINARY TRACT INFECTIONS, due to *Escherichia coli; Proteus mirabilis* and *Proteus* spp. (which may include the organisms now called *Proteus vulgaris,** *Providencia rettgeri* and *Morganella morganii*); and *Klebsiella pneumoniae.**
SKIN AND SKIN STRUCTURE INFECTIONS, due to *Staphylococcus aureus* and *S. epidermidis; Streptococcus pyogenes* (Group A *Streptococcus*) and *S. agalactiae* (Group B *Streptococcus*).
SEPTICEMIA, due to *Streptococcus pneumoniae* and *Escherichia coli.**
BONE AND JOINT INFECTIONS, due to *Staphylococcus aureus.*
*Efficacy for this organism in this organ system has been demonstrated in fewer than 10 infections.
Surgical Prophylaxis
Administration of a single 1 gram dose of *Monocid* before surgery may reduce the incidence of postoperative infections in patients undergoing surgical procedures classified as contaminated or potentially contaminated (e.g., colorectal surgery, vaginal hysterectomy, or cholecystectomy in high-risk patients), or in patients in whom infection at the operative site would present a serious risk (e.g., prosthetic arthroplasty, open heart surgery). Although cefonicid has been shown to be as effective as cefazolin in prevention of infection following coronary artery bypass surgery, no placebo-controlled trials have been conducted to evaluate any cephalosporin antibiotic in the prevention of infection following coronary artery bypass surgery or prosthetic heart valve replacement.
In cesarean section, the use of *Monocid* (after the umbilical cord has been clamped) may reduce the incidence of certain postoperative infections.
When administered 1 hour prior to surgical procedures for which it is indicated, a single 1 gram dose of *Monocid* provides protection from most infections due to susceptible organisms throughout the course of the procedure. Intraoperative and/or postoperative administrations of *Monocid* are not necessary. Daily doses of *Monocid* may be administered for 2 additional days in patients undergoing prosthetic arthroplasty or open heart surgery.
If there are signs of infection, the causative organisms should be identified and appropriate therapy determined through susceptibility testing.
Before using *Monocid* concomitantly with other antibiotics, the prescribing information for those agents should be reviewed for contraindications, warnings, precautions and adverse reactions. Renal function should be carefully monitored.

CONTRAINDICATIONS
Monocid (sterile cefonicid sodium) is contraindicated in persons who have shown hypersensitivity to cephalosporin antibiotics.

WARNINGS
BEFORE THERAPY WITH MONOCID (STERILE CEFONICID SODIUM) IS INSTITUTED, CAREFUL INQUIRY SHOULD BE MADE TO DETERMINE WHETHER THE PATIENT HAS HAD PREVIOUS HYPERSENSITIVITY REACTIONS TO CEPHALOSPORINS, PENICILLINS OR OTHER DRUGS. THIS PRODUCT SHOULD BE GIVEN CAUTIOUSLY TO PENICILLIN-SENSITIVE PATIENTS. ANTIBIOTICS SHOULD BE ADMINISTERED WITH CAUTION TO ANY PATIENT WHO HAS DEMONSTRATED SOME FORM OF ALLERGY, PARTICULARLY TO DRUGS. SERIOUS ACUTE HYPERSENSITIVITY REACTIONS MAY REQUIRE EPINEPHRINE AND OTHER EMERGENCY MEASURES.
Pseudomembranous colitis has been reported with nearly all antibacterial agents, including *Monocid,* and has ranged in severity from mild to life-threatening. Therefore, it is important to consider this diagnosis in patients who present with diarrhea subsequent to the administration of antibacterial agents.
Treatment with antibacterial agents alters the normal flora of the colon and may permit overgrowth of clostridia. Studies

Tissue and Body Fluid Levels

Tissue or Body Fluid	Dosage and Route (No. of Patients Sampled)		Time of Sampling After Dose	Average Tissue or Fluid Levels (mcg/g or/mL)
Bone	1 g IM	(7)	60 to 90 min.	6.8
	1 g IV	(10)	44 to 99 min.	14.0
Gallbladder	1 g IM	(10)	60 to 70 min.	15.5
Bile	1 g IM	(10)	60 to 70 min.	7.5
Prostate	1 g IM	(10)	50 to 115 min.	13.0
Uterine Tissue	1 g IM	(6)	60 to 90 min.	17.5
Wound Fluid	1 g IM	(10)	60 to 75 min.	37.7
Purulent Wound	1 g IM	(9)	60 min.	11.5
Adipose Tissue	1 g IM	(5)	60 min.	4.0
Atrial Appendage	1 g IM	(7)	77 to 170 min.	7.5
	2 g IM	(7)	105 to 170 min.	8.7
	15 mg/kg IV	(10)	53 to 160 min.	15.4

Serum Concentrations After 1 Gram Administration
(mcg/mL)

Interval	5 min.	15 min.	30 min.	1 hr.	2 hr.	4 hr.	6 hr.	8 hr.	10 hr.	12 hr.	24 hr.
IV	221.3	176.4	147.6	124.2	88.9	61.4	40.0	29.3	20.6	15.2	2.6
IM	13.5	45.9	73.1	98.6	97.1	77.8	54.9	38.5	28.9	20.6	4.5

indicate that a toxin produced by *Clostridium difficile* is one primary cause of "antibiotic-associated colitis."

Mild cases of pseudomembranous colitis usually respond to drug discontinuation alone. In moderate to severe cases, consideration should be given to management with fluids and electrolytes, protein supplementation and treatment with an antibacterial drug clinically effective against *C. difficile* colitis.

PRECAUTIONS

General: With any antibiotic, prolonged use may result in overgrowth of nonsusceptible organisms. Careful observation is essential, and appropriate measures should be taken if superinfection occurs.

Drug Interactions: Nephrotoxicity has been reported following concomitant administration of other cephalosporins and aminoglycosides.

Carcinogenesis, Mutagenesis, Impairment of Fertility: Beta-lactam antibiotics with methyl-thio-tetrazole side chains have been shown to cause testicular atrophy in prepubertal rats, which persisted into adulthood and resulted in decreased spermatogenesis and decreased fertility. Cefonicid, which contains a methylsulfonic-thio-tetrazole moiety, has no adverse effect on the male reproductive system of prepubertal, juvenile or adult rats when given under identical conditions.

Carcinogenicity studies of cefonicid have not been conducted; however, results of mutagenicity studies (i.e., Ames/Salmonella/microsome plate assay and the micronucleus test in mice) were negative.

Pregnancy: (Category B.) Reproduction studies have been performed in mice, rabbits and rats at doses up to an equivalent of 40 times the usual adult human dose and have revealed no evidence of impaired fertility or harm to the fetus due to Monocid (sterile cefonicid sodium). There are, however, no adequate and well-controlled studies in pregnant women. Because animal reproduction studies are not always predictive of human response, this drug should be used in pregnancy only if clearly needed.

Labor and Delivery: In cesarean section, *Monocid* should be administered only after the umbilical cord has been clamped.

Nursing Mothers: *Monocid* is excreted in human milk in low concentrations. Caution should be exercised when *Monocid* is administered to a nursing woman.

Pediatric Use: Safety and effectiveness in children have not been established.

ADVERSE REACTIONS

Monocid (sterile cefonicid sodium) is generally well tolerated and adverse reactions have occurred infrequently. The most common adverse reaction has been pain on IM injection. On-therapy conditions occurring in greater than 1% of Monocid-treated patients were:

Injection Site Phenomena (5.7%): Pain and/or discomfort on injection; less often, burning, phlebitis at IV site.

Increased Platelets (1.7%).

Increased Eosinophils (2.9%).

Liver Function Test Alterations (1.6%): Increased alkaline phosphatase, increased SGOT, increased SGPT, increased GGTP, increased LDH.

Less frequent on-therapy conditions occurring in less than 1% of Monocid-treated patients were:

Hypersensitivity Reactions: Fever, rash, pruritus, erythema, myalgia and anaphylactoid-type reactions have been reported.

Hematology: Decreased WBC, neutropenia, thrombocytopenia, positive Coombs' test.

Renal: Increased BUN and creatinine levels have occasionally been seen. Rare reports of acute renal failure associated with interstitial nephritis, observed with other beta-lactam antibiotics, have also occurred with *Monocid.*

Gastrointestinal: Diarrhea and pseudomembranous colitis. Onset of pseudomembranous colitis symptoms may occur during or after antibiotic treatment (see WARNINGS).

DOSAGE AND ADMINISTRATION

General

The usual adult dosage is 1 gram of Monocid (sterile cefonicid sodium) given once every 24 hours, intravenously or by deep intramuscular injection. Doses in excess of 1 gram daily are rarely necessary; however, in exceptional cases dosage of up to 2 grams given once daily have been well tolerated. When administering 2 gram IM doses once daily, ½ the dose should be administered in different large muscle masses.

Outpatient Use

Monocid has been used (once daily IM or IV) on an outpatient basis. Individuals responsible for outpatient administration of *Monocid* should be instructed thoroughly in appropriate procedures for storage, reconstitution and administration.

Surgical Prophylaxis

When administered 1 hour prior to appropriate surgical procedures (see INDICATIONS AND USAGE), a 1 gram dose of *Monocid* provides protection from most infections due to

Dosage of Monocid® in Adults with Reduced Renal Function

(Monitor renal function and adjust accordingly.)

Creatinine Clearance (mL/min per 1.73 M²)	Dosage Regimen	
	Mild to Moderate Infections	Severe Infections
79 to 60	10 mg/kg (every 24 hours)	25 mg/kg (every 24 hours)
59 to 40	8 mg/kg (every 24 hours)	20 mg/kg (every 24 hours)
39 to 20	4 mg/kg (every 24 hours)	15 mg/kg (every 24 hours)
19 to 10	4 mg/kg (every 48 hours)	15 mg/kg (every 48 hours)
9 to 5	4 mg/kg (every 3 to 5 days)	15 mg/kg (every 3 to 5 days)
<5	3 mg/kg (every 3 to 5 days)	4 mg/kg (every 3 to 5 days)

susceptible organisms throughout the course of the procedure. Intraoperative and/or postoperative administrations of *Monocid* are not necessary. Daily doses of *Monocid* may be administered for 2 additional days in patients undergoing prosthetic arthroplasty or open heart surgery.

In cesarean section *Monocid* should be administered only after the umbilical cord has been clamped.

General Guidelines for Dosage of Monocid®, IV or IM

Type of Infection	Daily Dose (grams)	Frequency
Uncomplicated Urinary Tract	0.5	once every 24 hours
Mild to Moderate	1	once every 24 hours
Severe or Life-Threatening	2*	once every 24 hours
Surgical Prophylaxis	1	1 hour preoperatively

* When administering 2 gram IM doses once daily, ½ the dose should be administered in different large muscle masses.

Impaired Renal Function

Modification of Monocid (sterile cefonicid sodium) dosage is necessary in patients with impaired renal function. Following an initial loading dosage of 7.5 mg/kg IM or IV, the maintenance dosing schedule shown below should be followed. Further dosing should be determined by severity of the infection and susceptibility of the causative organism. [See table on top of page.]

Note: It is not necessary to administer additional dosage following dialysis.

Preparation of Parenteral Solution

Parenteral drug products should be SHAKEN WELL when reconstituted, and inspected visually for particulate matter prior to administration. If particulate matter is evident in reconstituted fluids, the drug solutions should be discarded.

RECONSTITUTION

Single-Dose Vials

For IM injection, IV direct (bolus) injection or IV infusion, reconstitute with Sterile Water for Injection according to the following table. SHAKE WELL.

Vial Size	Diluent to Be Added	Approx. Avail. Volume	Approx. Avg. Concentration
500 mg	2.0 mL	2.2 mL	225 mg/mL
1 gram	2.5 mL	3.1 mL	325 mg/mL

These solutions of Monocid (sterile cefonicid sodium) are stable 24 hours at room temperature or 72 hours if refrigerated (5°C). Slight yellowing does not affect potency.

For IV infusion, dilute reconstituted solution in 50 to 100 mL of the parenteral fluids listed under ADMINISTRATION.

Pharmacy Bulk Vials (10 grams)

For IM injection, IV direct (bolus) injection or IV infusion, reconstitute with Sterile Water for Injection, Bacteriostatic Water for Injection or Sodium Chloride Injection according to the following table:

Amount of Diluent	Approx. Concentration	Approx. Avail. Volume
25 mL	1 gram/3 mL	31 mL
45 mL	1 gram/5 mL	51 mL

These solutions of *Monocid* are stable 24 hours at room temperature or 72 hours if refrigerated (5°C). Slight yellowing does not affect potency.

For IV infusion add to parenteral fluids listed under ADMINISTRATION.

"Piggyback" Vials

Reconstitute with 50 to 100 mL of Sodium Chloride Injection or other IV solution listed under ADMINISTRATION. Administer with primary IV fluids, as a single dose. These solutions of *Monocid* are stable 24 hours at room temperature or 72 hours if refrigerated (5°C). Slight yellowing does not affect potency.

A solution of 1 gram of *Monocid* in 18 mL of Sterile Water for Injection is isotonic.

ADMINISTRATION

IM Injection: Inject well within the body of a relatively large muscle. Aspiration is necessary to avoid inadvertent injection into a blood vessel. When administering 2 gram IM doses once daily, ½ the dose should be given in different large muscle masses.

IV Administration: For direct (bolus) injection, administer reconstituted *Monocid* slowly over 3 to 5 minutes, directly or through tubing for patients receiving parenteral fluids (see list below). For infusion, dilute reconstituted *Monocid* in 50 to 100 mL of 1 of the following solutions:

 0.9% Sodium Chloride Injection, USP
 5% Dextrose Injection, USP
 5% Dextrose and 0.9% Sodium Chloride Injection, USP
 5% Dextrose and 0.45% Sodium Chloride Injection, USP
 5% Dextrose and 0.2% Sodium Chloride Injection, USP
 10% Dextrose Injection, USP
 Ringer's Injection, USP
 Lactated Ringer's Injection, USP
 5% Dextrose and Lactated Ringer's Injection
 10% Invert Sugar in Sterile Water for Injection
 5% Dextrose and 0.15% Potassium Chloride Injection
 Sodium Lactate Injection, USP

In these fluids *Monocid* is stable 24 hours at room temperature or 72 hours if refrigerated (5°C). Slight yellowing does not affect potency.

HOW SUPPLIED

Monocid (sterile cefonicid sodium) is supplied in vials equivalent to 1 gram of cefonicid and in "Piggyback" Vials for IV admixture equivalent to 1 gram of cefonicid.

1 gram vial: NDC 0007-4353-01
1 gram "Piggyback" Vial (pack of 10): NDC 0007-4354-11

As with other cephalosporins, *Monocid* may darken on storage. However, if stored as recommended, this color change does not affect potency.

Before reconstitution, *Monocid* should be protected from light and refrigerated (2° to 8°C).

Veterans Administration/Military/PHS—Vial, 1 gram/10 mL, 1's, 6505-01-189-4698.

MC:L27

Shown in Product Identification Guide, page 337

Continued on next page

Information on the SmithKline Beecham Pharmaceuticals products appearing here is based on the labeling in effect on July 1, 1996. Further information on these and other products may be obtained from the Medical Department, SmithKline Beecham Pharmaceuticals, One Franklin Plaza, Philadelphia, PA 19101.

SmithKline Beecham—Cont.

OmniHIB™ ℞

[ahm-nee-hib]

Haemophilus b Conjugate Vaccine
(Tetanus Toxoid Conjugate)

Caution: Federal (U.S.A.) law prohibits dispensing without prescription.

NOTE: Haemophilus b Conjugate Vaccine (Tetanus Toxoid Conjugate)—OmniHIB™ (distributed by SmithKline Beecham Pharmaceuticals) is identical to Haemophilus b Conjugate Vaccine (Tetanus Toxoid Conjugate)—ActHIB™; both products are manufactured by Pasteur Mérieux Sérums & Vaccins S.A.

DESCRIPTION

OmniHIB™, Haemophilus b Conjugate Vaccine (Tetanus Toxoid Conjugate), produced by Pasteur Mérieux Sérums & Vaccins S.A., for intramuscular use, is a sterile, lyophilized powder which is reconstituted at the time of use with saline diluent (0.4% Sodium Chloride). The vaccine consists of the Haemophilus b polysaccharide, a high molecular weight polymer prepared from the *Haemophilus influenzae* type b strain 1482 grown in a semi-synthetic medium, covalently bound to tetanus toxoid.[1] The lyophilized powder and saline diluent contain no preservatives. Each single dose of 0.5 mL is formulated to contain 10 μg of purified capsular polysaccharide, 24 μg of tetanus toxoid and 8.5% of sucrose. The tetanus toxoid is prepared by extraction, ammonium sulfate purification, and formalin inactivation of the toxin from cultures of *Clostridium tetani* (Harvard strain) grown in a modified Mueller and Miller medium.[2] The toxoid is filter sterilized prior to the conjugation process. Potency of OmniHIB is specified on each lot by limits on the content of PRP polysaccharide and protein in each dose and the proportion of polysaccharide and protein in the vaccine which is characterized as high molecular weight conjugate. The reconstituted vaccine is clear and colorless.

CLINICAL PHARMACOLOGY

NOTE: Haemophilus b Conjugate Vaccine (Tetanus Toxoid Conjugate)—OmniHIB (distributed by SmithKline Beecham Pharmaceuticals) is identical to Haemophilus b Conjugate Vaccine (Tetanus Toxoid Conjugate)—ActHIB; both products are manufactured by Pasteur Mérieux Sérums & Vaccins S.A.

H influenzae type b was the leading cause of invasive bacterial disease among children in the United States prior to licensing of Haemophilus b conjugate vaccines. Based on its active surveillance areas, the Centers for Disease Control and Prevention (CDC) now estimate that *H influenzae* type b disease in children under the age of 5 years has been reduced by 95%.[3] Before effective vaccines were introduced, it was estimated that one in 200 children developed invasive *H influenzae* type b disease by the age of 5 years. In children less than 5 years of age, the mortality rate for invasive *H influenzae* type b disease ranged between 3% and 6%.[3] In more than 60% of these children, meningitis was the clinical syndrome and permanent sequelae ranging from mild hearing loss to mental retardation affecting 20% to 30% of all survivors.[3] Ninety-five percent of the cases of invasive *H influenzae* disease among children <5 years of age were caused by organisms with the type b polysaccharide capsule. Approximately two-thirds of all cases of invasive *H influenzae* type b disease affected infants and children <15 months of age, a group for which a vaccine was not available until late 1990.[4,5]

Incidence rates of invasive *H influenzae* type b disease have been shown to be increased in certain high-risk groups, such as native Americans (both American Indians and Eskimos), blacks, individuals of lower socioeconomic status, and patients with asplenia, sickle cell disease, Hodgkin's disease, and antibody deficiency syndromes.[5,6] Studies also have suggested that the risk of acquiring primary invasive *H influenzae* type b disease for children under 5 years of age appears to be greater for those who attend day-care facilities.[7,8,9,10]

The potential for person to person transmission of the organism among susceptible individuals has been recognized. Studies of secondary spread of disease in household contacts of index patients have shown a substantially increased risk among exposed household contacts under 4 years of age.[11] Adults can be colonized with *H influenzae* type b from children infected with the organism.[12]

The response to OmniHIB is typical of a T-dependent immune response to antigen. The predominant isotype of anticapsular polysaccharide (polyribosyl-ribitol-phosphate or PRP) antibody induced by OmniHIB is IgG.[13] A substantial booster response has been demonstrated in children 12 months of age or older who previously received two or three doses. Bactericidal activity against *H influenzae* type b is demonstrated in serum after immunization and statistically correlates with the anti-PRP antibody response induced by OmniHIB.[14]

Antibody to *H influenzae* capsular polysaccharide (anti-PRP) titers of >1.0 μg/mL following vaccination with unconjugated PRP vaccine correlated with long-term protection against invasive *H influenzae* type b disease in children older than 24 months of age.[15] Although the relevance of this threshold to clinical protection after immunization with conjugate vaccines is not known, particularly in light of the induced, immunologic memory, this level continues to be considered as indicative of long-term protection.[4] The immu-

nogenicity and safety of OmniHIB has been demonstrated in the United States and worldwide. OmniHIB induced, on average anti-PRP levels ≥1.0 μg/mL in 90% of infants after the primary series and in more than 98% of infants after a booster dose.[14]

Two clinical trials supported by the National Institutes of Health (NIH) have compared the anti-PRP antibody responses to three Haemophilus b conjugate vaccines in a racially mixed population of children. These studies were done in Tennessee[16] (Table 1) and in Minnesota, Missouri and Texas[17] (Table 2) in infants immunized with OmniHIB and other Haemophilus b conjugate vaccines at 2, 4 and 6 months of age. All Haemophilus b conjugate vaccines were administered concomitantly with Poliovirus Vaccine Live Oral and DTP vaccines at separate sites.

[See Tables 1 and 2 below.]

N/A Not applicable in this comparison trial although third dose data have been published.[16,17]

Native American populations have high rates of *H influenzae* type b disease and have been observed to have low immune responses to Haemophilus b conjugate vaccines. Following three doses of OmniHIB at six weeks, four and six months of age, 75% of Native Americans in Alaska showed an anti-PRP antibody titer of ≥1.0 μg/mL.[18]

In three U.S. trials in 12- to 15-month-old children and one trial in 17- to 24-month-old children who had not previously received Haemophilus b conjugate vaccination, a single dose of OmniHIB produced an anti-PRP antibody response comparable to those seen after three doses were administered in infants (Table 3).[18]

TABLE 3[18] ANTI-PRP ANTIBODY RESPONSES IN 12- TO 24-MONTH-OLD CHILDREN IMMUNIZED WITH A SINGLE DOSE OF OmniHIB

AGE GROUP	N	GMT (μg/mL)		% SUBJECTS RESPONDING WITH ≥1.0 μg/mL	
		Pre	Post	Pre	Post
12 to 15 months	256	0.06	5.12	1.6	90.2
17 to 24 months	81	0.10	4.4	3.7	81.5

These trials demonstrated that OmniHIB consistently conferred an anti-PRP antibody response previously shown to correlate with protection, when administered either as a regimen of three doses at least four to eight weeks apart in infants 2 to 6 months of age or as a single dose in children 12 months of age and older.[18]

OmniHIB has been found to be immunogenic in children with sickle cell anemia, a condition which may cause increased susceptibility to Haemophilus b disease. Two doses of OmniHIB given at two month intervals induced anti-PRP antibody titers of >1.0 μg/mL in 89% of these children with a mean age of 11 months. This is comparable to anti-PRP antibody levels demonstrated in normal children of similar age following two doses of OmniHIB.[19]

Although OmniHIB produces an antibody response to tetanus toxoid, data do not exist to substantiate the correlation of this response with protection against tetanus. IMMUNIZATION WITH OmniHIB ALONE DOES NOT SUBSTITUTE FOR ROUTINE TETANUS IMMUNIZATION.

INDICATIONS AND USAGE

NOTE: Haemophilus b Conjugate Vaccine (Tetanus Toxoid Conjugate)—OmniHIB (distributed by SmithKline Beecham Pharmaceuticals) is identical to Haemophilus b Conjugate Vaccine (Tetanus Toxoid Conjugate)—ActHIB; both products are manufactured by Pasteur Mérieux Sérums & Vaccins S.A.

OmniHIB is indicated for the active immunization of infants and children 2 months through 5 years of age for the prevention of invasive disease caused by *H influenzae* type b. Antibody levels associated with protection may not be achieved earlier than two weeks following the last recommended dose.

As with any vaccine, vaccination with OmniHIB may not protect 100% of susceptible individuals.

CONTRAINDICATIONS

OmniHIB IS CONTRAINDICATED IN CHILDREN WITH A HISTORY OF HYPERSENSITIVITY TO ANY COMPONENT OF THIS VACCINE, INCLUDING TETANUS TOXOID.

WARNINGS

If OmniHIB is administered to immunosuppressed persons or persons receiving immunosuppressive therapy, the expected antibody response may not be obtained. This includes patients with asymptomatic or symptomatic HIV-infection,[20] severe combined immunodeficiency, hypogammaglobulinemia, or agammaglobulinemia; altered immune

TABLE 1[16] ANTI-PRP ANTIBODY RESPONSES IN 2-MONTH-OLD INFANTS NIH TRIAL IN TENNESSEE

VACCINE	N*	GEOMETRIC MEAN TITER (GMT) (μg/mL)			POST THIRD IMMUNIZATION
		Pre-Immunization	Post Second Immunization	Post Third Immunization	% ≥1.0 μg/mL
PRP-T† (OmniHIB™)	65	0.10	0.30	3.64	83%
PRP-OMPΔ (PedvaxHIB®)	64	0.11	0.84	N/A	50%**
HbOC‡ (HibTITER®)	61	0.07	0.13	3.08	75%

TABLE 2[17] ANTI-PRP ANTIBODY RESPONSES IN 2-MONTH-OLD INFANTS NIH TRIAL IN MINNESOTA, MISSOURI AND TEXAS

VACCINE	N*	GEOMETRIC MEAN TITER (GMT) (μg/mL)			POST THIRD§ IMMUNIZATION
		Pre-Immunization	Post Second Immunization	Post Third§ Immunization	% ≥1.0 μg/mL
PRP-T† (OmniHIB™)	142	0.25	1.25	6.37	97%
PRP-OMPΔ (PedvaxHIB®)	149	0.18	4.00	N/A	85%**
HbOC‡ (HibTITER®)	167	0.17	0.45	6.31	90%

* N = Number of Children
§ Sera were obtained after the third dose from 86 and 110 infants, in PRP-T and HbOC vaccine groups, respectively.
† Haemophilus b Conjugate Vaccine (Tetanus Toxoid Conjugate)
Δ Haemophilus b Conjugate Vaccine (Meningococcal Protein Conjugate)
** Seroconversion after the recommended 2-dose primary immunization series is shown.
‡ Haemophilus b Conjugate Vaccine (Diphtheria CRM₁₉₇ Protein Conjugate)

states due to diseases such as leukemia, lymphoma, or generalized malignancy; or an immune system compromised by treatment with corticosteroids, alkylating drugs, antimetabolites or radiation.[21]

IMMUNIZATION WITH OmniHIB ALONE DOES NOT SUBSTITUTE FOR ROUTINE TETANUS IMMUNIZATION.

PRECAUTIONS

GENERAL

EPINEPHRINE INJECTION (1:1000) MUST BE IMMEDIATELY AVAILABLE SHOULD AN ANAPHYLACTIC OR OTHER ALLERGIC REACTION OCCUR DUE TO ANY COMPONENT OF THE VACCINE.

Prior to an injection of any vaccine, all known precautions should be taken to prevent adverse reactions. This includes a review of the patient's history with respect to possible hypersensitivity to this vaccine or similar vaccines. The health-care provider should ask the parent or guardian about the recent health status of the infant or child to be immunized including the infant's or child's previous immunization history prior to administration of OmniHIB.

Any acute infection or febrile illness is reason for delaying use of OmniHIB except when in the opinion of the physician, withholding the vaccine entails a greater risk.

As reported with Haemophilus b polysaccharide vaccines,[22] cases of *H influenzae* type b disease may occur subsequent to vaccination and prior to the onset of protective effects of the vaccine.[18] (See INDICATIONS AND USAGE section)

Antigenuria has been detected in some instances following receipt of OmniHIB; therefore, urine antigen detection may not have definitive diagnostic value in suspected *H influenzae* type b disease within one week of immunization.[23]

Special care should be taken to ensure that OminHIB is not injected into a blood vessel.

Administration of OmniHIB is not contraindicated in individuals with an HIV infection.[21]

A separate, sterile syringe and needle or a sterile disposable unit should be used for each patient to prevent transmission of hepatitis or other infectious agents from person to person. Needles should not be recapped and should be properly disposed.

INFORMATION FOR PATIENT

The health-care provider should inform the parent or guardian of the benefits and risks of the vaccine.

The physician should inform the parent or guardian about the significant adverse reactions that have been temporally associated with OmniHIB administration. The parent or guardian should be instructed to report any serious adverse reactions to the health-care provider.

As part of the child's immunization record, the date, lot number and manufacturer of the vaccine administered should be recorded.[24,25,26]

The U.S. Department of Health and Human Services has established a new Vaccine Adverse Event Reporting System (VAERS) to accept all reports of suspected adverse events after the administration of any vaccine, including but not limited to the reporting of events required by the National Childhood Vaccine Injury Act of 1986.[24] The toll-free number for VAERS forms and information is 1-800-822-7967.

The National Vaccine Injury Compensation Program, established by the National Childhood Vaccine Injury Act of 1986, requires physicians and other health-care providers who administer vaccines to maintain permanent vaccination records and to report occurrences of certain adverse events to the U.S. Department of Health and Human Services. Reportable events include those listed in the Act for each vaccine and events specified in the package insert as contraindications to further doses of the vaccine.[25,26]

The health-care provider should inform the parent or guardian of the importance of completing the immunization series.

The health-care provider should provide the Vaccine Information Materials (VIMs) which are required to be given with each immunization.

DRUG INTERACTIONS

There are no known interactions of OmniHIB with drugs or foods.

In clinical trials, OmniHIB was routinely administered, at separate sites, concomitantly with one or more of the following vaccines: DTP vaccine, Poliovirus Vaccine Live Oral, Measles, Mumps and Rubella vaccine (MMR), Hepatitis B vaccine and occasionally Inactivated Polio Vaccine (IPV). No significant impairment of the antibody response to any antigen was observed in three clinical trials when Connaught Laboratories, Inc. (CLI) DTP vaccine was given concurrently with OmniHIB at separate sites.[18] Interference with the antibody response to the pertussis component has been suggested with a DTP vaccine unlicensed in the U.S.[27] No impairment of the antibody response to the individual antigens was demonstrated when OmniHIB was given at the same time, at separate sites, with Inactivated Polio Vaccine (IPV) or Measles, Mumps and Rubella vaccine (MMR).[18] In addition, more than 47,000 infants in Finland have received a third dose of OmniHIB concomitantly with MMR vaccine.[18] No data are available on the antibody response to OPV or Hepatitis B vaccines when given concurrently with OmniHIB.

TABLE 5[14] PERCENTAGE OF INFANTS PRESENTING WITH LOCAL OR SYSTEMIC REACTIONS AT 6, 24, AND 48 HOURS OF IMMUNIZATION WITH OmniHIB ADMINISTERED SIMULTANEOUSLY, AT SEPARATE SITES, WITH CLI DTP VACCINE

	AGE AT IMMUNIZATION								
REACTION	2 Months (n=365)			4 Months (n=364)			6 Months (n=365)		
	6 Hrs.	24 Hrs.	48 Hrs.	6 Hrs.	24 Hrs.	48 Hrs.	6 Hrs.	24 Hrs.	48 Hrs.
Local§									
Tenderness	46.3%	11.5%	2.2%	23.4%	7.4%	1.1%	19.2%	6.0%	1.1%
Erythema	14.3%	4.1%	0.3%	8.8%	5.8%	0.6%	11.5%	6.9%	1.6%
Induration	22.5%	6.3%	1.9%	12.4%	4.7%	0.8%	9.6%	3.8%	1.1%
Systemic*									
Fever > 100.8°F†	20.1%	1.3%	0.6%	14.6%	6.6%	1.4%	15.7%	8.8%	0.8%
Irritability	72.6%	21.9%	12.6%	48.4%	25.0%	13.2%	44.1%	25.2%	10.1%
Drowsiness	57.5%	29.9%	10.4%	44.2%	18.1%	7.4%	32.6%	13.4%	2.5%
Anorexia	15.3%	5.8%	4.9%	8.0%	5.0%	3.0%	5.5%	4.9%	2.2%
Diarrhea	4.4%	6.6%	5.2%	5.0%	4.7%	4.7%	4.7%	6.3%	3.6%
Vomiting	2.7%	4.1%	2.7%	2.5%	3.3%	2.8%	2.2%	2.7%	1.9%
Persistent Crying	Percentage of infants within 72 hours after immunization was 1.6% after dose one, 0.6% after dose two, and 0.3% after dose three.								

§Local reactions were evaluated at the OmniHIB injection site.
*The adverse reaction profile is defined by the concomitant use of CLI DTP vaccine.
†The number of individuals observed at each time point for fever varied from 357 to 363.

CARCINOGENESIS, MUTAGENESIS, IMPAIRMENT OF FERTILITY

OmniHIB has not been evaluated for its carcinogenic, mutagenic potential or impairment of fertility.

PREGNANCY

REPRODUCTIVE STUDIES–PREGNANCY CATEGORY C

Animal reproduction studies have not been conducted with OmniHIB. It is also not known whether OmniHIB can cause fetal harm when administered to a pregnant woman or can affect reproduction capacity. OmniHIB is NOT recommended for use in a pregnant woman.

PEDIATRIC USE

SAFETY AND EFFECTIVENESS OF OmniHIB IN INFANTS BELOW THE AGE OF SIX WEEKS HAVE NOT BEEN ESTABLISHED. (See DOSAGE AND ADMINISTRATION section.)

ADVERSE REACTIONS

NOTE: Haemophilus b Conjugate Vaccine (Tetanus Toxoid Conjugate)—OmniHIB (distributed by SmithKline Beecham Pharmaceuticals) is identical to Haemophilus b Conjugate Vaccine (Tetanus Toxoid Conjugate)—ActHIB; both products are manufactured by Pasteur Mérieux Sérums & Vaccins S.A.

More than 7,000 infants and young children (≤2 years of age) have received at least one dose of OmniHIB during U.S. clinical trials. Of these, 1,064 subjects 12 to 24 months of age who received OmniHIB alone reported no serious or life threatening adverse reactions.

Summarized in Table 4 are adverse reactions temporally associated with OmniHIB immunization in 188 subjects 12 to 15 months of age.[18]

TABLE 4[18] PERCENTAGE OF 12- TO 15-MONTH-OLD CHILDREN PRESENTING WITH LOCAL OR SYSTEMIC REACTIONS WITHIN THE FIRST 24 HOURS OF IMMUNIZATION WITH OmniHIB (n=188)

REACTIONS	DOSE 1*	DOSE 2*
Local		
Pain	9.0%	6.4%
Erythema (1 to 5 cm)	24.0%	18.6%
Induration	9.6%	9.0%
Systemic		
Fever (> 100.6°F)	7.4%	6.4%
Irritability	30.9%	28.2%
Lethargy	18.6%	17.0%
Anorexia	9.0%	8.5%
Rhinorrhea	24.5%	21.3%
Diarrhea	5.8%	8.5%
Vomiting	4.3%	3.7%
Cough	9.6%	4.3%

*DTP was not administered concomitantly with OmniHIB.

When OmniHIB was administered to infants at 2, 4, and 6 months of age concomitantly, at separate sites, with CLI DTP vaccine, the systemic adverse experience profile was not different from that seen when CLI DTP vaccine was administered alone.[18] ***Refer to product insert for CLI whole-cell DTP.***

Adverse reactions from a U.S. multicenter trial in 2-, 4- and 6-month-old infants are summarized in Table 5. Systemic adverse reactions listed in Table 5 are more prominent than those in Table 4 because infants also received concomitant immunization with DTP.[14,18]

[See Table 5 above.]

In general, the rates of minor systemic reactions after OmniHIB and DTP immunization were comparable to those usually reported after DTP vaccine alone.[28,29,30,31]

Adverse reactions associated with OmniHIB generally subsided after 24 hours and usually do not persist beyond 48 hours after immunization.

In a randomized, double-blind U.S. clinical trial, OmniHIB was given concomitantly with DTP to more than 5,000 infants and hepatitis B vaccine was given with DTP to a similar number. In this large study, deaths due to sudden infant death syndrome (SIDS) and other causes were observed but were not different in the two groups. In the first 48 hours following immunization, two definite and three possible seizures were observed after OmniHIB and DTP in comparison with none after hepatitis B vaccine and DTP.[18] This rate of seizures following OmniHIB and DTP was not greater than previously reported in infants receiving DTP alone. Other adverse reactions reported with administration of other Haemophilus b conjugate vaccines include urticaria, seizures, hives, renal failure and Guillain-Barré syndrome (GBS).[18,32]

A cause and effect relationship among any of these events and the vaccination has not been established.

When OmniHIB was given with DTP and inactivated poliovirus vaccine to more than 100,000 Finnish infants, the rate and extent of serious adverse reactions were not different from those seen when other Haemophilus b conjugate vaccines were evaluated in Finland (i.e. HibTITER®, ProHIBiT®).[18]

Reporting of Adverse Events

Reporting by the parent or guardian of all adverse events occurring after vaccine administration should be encouraged. Adverse events following immunization with vaccine should be reported by the health-care provider to the U.S. Department of Health and Human Services (DHHS) Vaccine Adverse Event Reporting System (VAERS). Reporting forms and information about reporting requirements or completion of the form can be obtained from VAERS through a toll-free number 1-800-822-7967.[24,25,26]

Health-care providers also should report these events to the Director of Medical Affairs, Connaught Laboratories, Inc., Route 611, P.O. Box 187, Swiftwater, PA 18370 or call 1-800-822-2463.

DOSAGE AND ADMINISTRATION

NOTE: Haemophilus b Conjugate Vaccine (Tetanus Toxoid Conjugate)—OmniHIB (distributed by SmithKline Beecham Pharmaceuticals) is identical to Haemophilus b Conjugate Vaccine (Tetanus Toxoid Conjugate)—ActHIB; both products are manufactured by Pasteur Mérieux Sérums & Vaccins S.A.

Parenteral drug products should be inspected visually for particulate matter and/or discoloration prior to administration, whenever solution and container permit. If these conditions exist, the vaccine should not be administered.

Continued on next page

Information on the SmithKline Beecham Pharmaceuticals products appearing here is based on the labeling in effect on July 1, 1996. Further information on these and other products may be obtained from the Medical Department, SmithKline Beecham Pharmaceuticals, One Franklin Plaza, Philadelphia, PA 19101.

SmithKline Beecham—Cont.

RECONSTITUTION:

WITH DILUENT SUPPLIED: Prior to reconstitution, cleanse the vaccine vial rubber barrier with a suitable germicide and inject the entire volume of diluent contained in the syringe into the vial of lyophilized vaccine. Thorough agitation is advised to ensure complete rehydration. The entire volume of reconstituted vaccine is then drawn back into a new syringe before injection of one 0.5 mL dose. The vaccine will appear clear and colorless.

Reconstitution instructions for diluent supplied: see Figures 1, 2, and 3 below.

Administer OmniHIB intramuscularly after reconstitution with diluent supplied. (In the event of coagulation disorders, OmniHIB may be given subcutaneously in the mid-lateral aspect of the thigh.[14]) **Vaccine should be used immediately after reconstitution.**

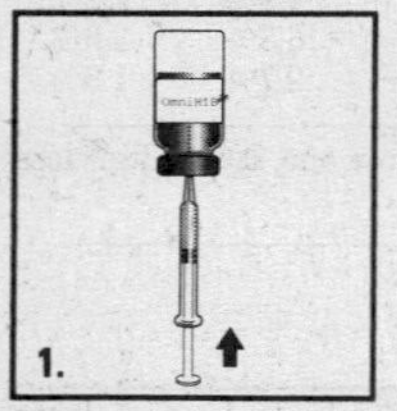

Figure 1. Insert syringe needle through the rubber barrier into the OmniHIB vial and inject 0.6 mL of diluent supplied.

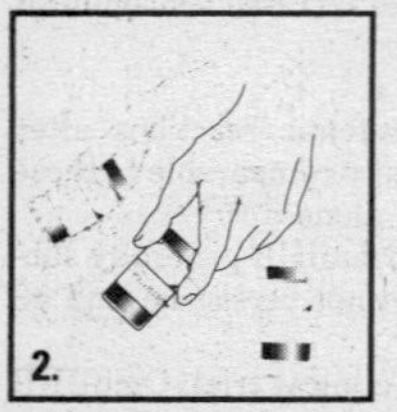

Figure 2. Agitate vial thoroughly to ensure complete reconstitution.

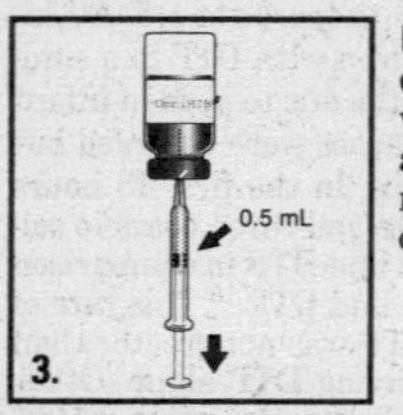

Figure 3. After reconstitution, discard syringe and withdraw total volume of reconstituted vaccine in a new syringe and administer 0.5 mL intramuscularly (or subcutaneously if coagulation disorders exist).

Each 0.5 mL dose is formulated to contain 10 μg of purified capsular polysaccharide conjugated to 24 μg of inactivated tetanus toxoid and 8.5% of sucrose.

Before injection, the skin over the site to be injected should be cleansed with a suitable germicide. After insertion of the needle, aspirate to ensure that the needle has not entered a blood vessel.

DO NOT INJECT INTRAVENOUSLY.

Each dose of OmniHIB is administered intramuscularly in the outer aspect of the vastus lateralis (mid-thigh) or deltoid. The vaccine should not be injected into the gluteal area or areas where there may be a nerve trunk. During the course of primary immunizations, injections should not be made more than once at the same site.

OmniHIB is indicated for infants and children 2 months through 5 years of age for intramuscular administration in accordance with the schedule indicated in Table 6.[14,16]

Infants between 2 and 6 months of age should receive three 0.5 mL doses at eight week intervals, followed by a booster dose at 15 to 18 months of age. Infants 7 to 11 months of age who have not been previously immunized should receive two 0.5 mL doses at eight week intervals, followed by a booster dose at 15 to 18 months of age; children 12 to 14 months of age who have not been previously immunized should receive one 0.5 mL dose, followed by a booster dose at 15 to 18 months of age; and children 15 to 60 months of age who have not been previously immunized should receive a single 0.5 mL dose.

TABLE 6[14,16,33]

IMMUNIZATION SCHEDULE

AGE AT FIRST DOSE	PRIMARY SERIES	BOOSTER
2 to 6 months	3 Doses, 8 weeks apart	1 Dose, 15 to 18 months
7 to 11 months	2 Doses, 8 weeks apart	1 Dose, 15 to 18 months
12 to 14 months	1 Dose	1 Dose, 15 to 18 months*
15 to 60 months	1 Dose	None

*Administer vaccine not earlier than 2 months after the previous dose.

Preterm infants should be vaccinated according to their chronological age from birth.[33]

Interruption of the recommended schedule with a delay between doses should not interfere with the final immunity achieved with OmniHIB. There is no need to start the series over again, regardless of the time elapsed between doses.

No data are available to support the interchangeably of OmniHIB and ActHIB with other Haemophilus b conjugate vaccines. Therefore, it is recommended that the same conjugate vaccine be used throughout each immunization schedule, consistent with the data supporting approval and licensure of the vaccine. Since OmniHIB and ActHIB are the same vaccine these may be used interchangeably.

HOW SUPPLIED

Vial, 1 Dose, lyophilized vaccine (5 × 1 Dose vials per package), packaged with prefilled 0.6 mL Syringe containing diluent (5 × 0.6 mL syringes per package)–Product No. 0007-4408-05

Administer vaccine immediately after reconstitution.

STORAGE

Store lyophilized vaccine and prefilled syringe containing diluent between 2°-8°C (35°-46°F). DO NOT FREEZE.

REFERENCES

1. Chu CY, et al. Further studies on the immunogenicity of *Haemophilus influenzae* type b and pneumococcal type 6A polysaccharide-protein conjugate. Infect Immun 40: 245-246, 1983
2. Mueller JH, et al. Production of diphtheria toxin of high potency (100 Lf) on a reproducible medium. J Immunol 40:21-32, 1941
3. Adams WG, et al. Decline of Childhood *Haemophilus influenzae* Type b (Hib) Disease in the Hib Vaccine Era. JAMA 269: 221-226, 1993
4. Recommendations of the Immunization Practices Advisory Committee (ACIP). Haemophilus b conjugate vaccines for prevention of *Haemophilus influenzae* type b disease among infants and children two months of age and older. MMWR 40: No. RR-1, 1991
5. Broome CV. Epidemiology of *Haemophilus influenzae* type b infections in the United States. Pediatr Infect Dis J 6: 779-782, 1987
6. ACIP. Polysaccharide vaccine for prevention of *Haemophilus influenzae* type b disease. MMWR 34:201-205, 1985
7. Istre GR, et al. Risk factors for primary invasive *Haemophilus influenzae* disease: Increased risk from day care attendance and school-aged household members. J Pediatr 106:190-195, 1985
8. Redmond SR, et al. *Haemophilus influenzae* type b disease. An epidemiologic study with special reference to day-care centers. JAMA 252: 2581-2584, 1984
9. Murphy TV, et al. County-wide surveillance of invasive Haemophilus infections: Risk of associated cases in Child Care Programs (CCPs). Twenty-third Interscience Conference on Antimicrobial Agents and Chemotherapy (Abstract #788) 229, 1983
10. Fleming D, et al. *Haemophilus influenzae* b (Hib) disease-secondary spread in day care. Twenty-fourth Interscience Conference on Antimicrobial Agents and Chemotherapy (Abstract #967) 261, 1984
11. CDC. Prevention of secondary cases of *Haemophilus influenzae* type b disease. MMWR 31: 672-680, 1982
12. Michaels RH, et al. Pharyngeal colonization with *Haemophilus influenzae* type b: A longitudinal study of families with a child with meningitis or epiglottitis due to *H. influenzae* type b. J Infec Dis 136: 222-227, 1977
13. Holmes SJ, et al. Immunogenicity of four *Haemophilus influenzae* type b conjugate vaccines in 17- to 19-month-old children. J Pediatr 118: 364-371, 1991
14. Data on file, Pasteur Mérieux Sérums & Vaccins S.A.
15. Peltola H, et al. Prevention of *Haemophilus influenzae* type b bacteremic infections with the capsular polysaccharide vaccine. N Engl J Med 310: 1561-1566, 1984
16. Decker MD, et al. Comparative trial in infants of four conjugate *Haemophilus influenzae* type b vaccines. J Pediatr 120:184-189, 1992
17. Granoff DM, et al. Differences in the immunogenicity of three *Haemophilus influenzae* type b conjugate vaccines in infants. J Pediatr 121:187-194, 1992
18. Data on file, Connaught Laboratories, Inc.
19. Kaplan SL, et al. Immunogenicity of *Haemophilus influenzae* type b, polysaccharide-tetanus protein conjugate vaccine in children with sickle hemoglobinopathy or malignancies, and after systemic *Haemophilus influenzae* type b infection. J Pediatr 120:367-370, 1992
20. Steinhoff MC, et al. Antibody responses to *Haemophilus influenzae* type b vaccines in men with human immunodeficiency virus infection. N Engl J Med 325 (26): 1837-1842, 1991
21. ACIP. General recommendations on immunization. MMWR 38: 205-227, 1989
22. FDA Workshop on Haemophilus b Polysaccharide Vaccine-A Preliminary Report. MMWR 36: 529-531, 1987
23. Rothstein EP, et al. Comparison of antigenuria after immunization with three *Haemophilus influenzae* type b conjugate vaccines. Pediatr Infect Dis J 10: 311-314, 1991
24. Vaccine Adverse Event Reporting System-United States. MMWR 39: 730-733, 1990
25. CDC. National Childhood Vaccine Injury Act: Requirements for permanent vaccination records and for reporting of selected events after vaccination. MMWR 37: 197-200, 1988
26. National Childhood Vaccine Injury Act of 1986 (Amended 1987)
27. Clemens JD, et al. Impact of *Haemophilus influenzae* Type b Polysaccharide-Tetanus Protein Conjugate Vaccine on responses to concurrently administered Diphtheria-Tetanus-Pertussis Vaccine. JAMA 267: 673-678, 1992
28. Cody CL, et al. Nature and rates of adverse reactions associated with DTP and DT immunizations in infants and children. Pediatr 68: 650-660, 1981
29. Barkin RM, et al. Diphtheria-tetanus-pertussis vaccine: reactogenicity of commercial products. Pediatr 63: 256-260, 1979
30. Baraff LJ, et al. DTP-associated reactions: an analysis by injection site, manufacturer, prior reactions and dose. Pediatr 73: 31-39, 1984
31. Long SS, et al. Longitudinal study of adverse reactions following diphtheria-tetanus-pertussis vaccine in infancy. Pediatr 85: 294-302, 1990
32. D'Cruz OF, et al. Acute inflammatory demyelinating polyradiculoneuropathy (Guillain-Barré Syndrome) after immunization with *Haemophilus influenzae* type b conjugate vaccine. J Pediatr 115: 743-746, 1989
33. Report on the Committee on Infectious Diseases. American Academy of Pediatrics. Twenty-second Edition, 1991

A.H.F.S. Category 80:12

Manufactured by

PASTEUR MÉRIEUX Sérums & Vaccins S.A.

Lyon, France U.S. License No. 384

Distributed by

SmithKline Beecham Pharmaceuticals

Philadelphia, PA 19101

Veterans Administration/Military/PHS—Vial, 0.5 mL, 5's, 6505-01-371-1161.

OM:L1

Shown in Product Identification Guide, page 337

ORNADE® SPANSULE® CAPSULES ℞

[or 'naid]

brand of sustained release capsules

DESCRIPTION

Ornade is a combination of an oral nasal decongestant and an antihistamine.

Each *Ornade* Spansule capsule contains phenylpropanolamine hydrochloride, 75 mg and chlorpheniramine maleate, 12 mg. Inactive ingredients consist of benzyl alcohol, cetylpyridinium chloride, FD&C Blue No. 1, FD&C Red No. 3, FD&C Yellow No. 6, D&C Red No. 27, D&C Red No. 30, gelatin, glyceryl distearate, iron oxide, polyethylene glycol, povidone, silicon dioxide, sodium lauryl sulfate, starch, sucrose, titanium dioxide, wax and trace amounts of other inactive ingredients.

Each *Ornade* Spansule capsule is so prepared that an initial dose is released promptly and the remaining medication is released gradually over a prolonged period.

CLINICAL PHARMACOLOGY

Phenylpropanolamine Hydrochloride

Phenylpropanolamine hydrochloride is a sympathomimetic agent which is closely related to ephedrine in chemical structure and pharmacologic action, but produces less central nervous system stimulation than ephedrine. It is a vasoconstrictor with decongestant action on nasal and upper respiratory tract mucosal membranes.

Chlorpheniramine Maleate

Chlorpheniramine maleate is an antihistamine with anticholinergic (drying) and sedative side effects. Antihistamines appear to compete with histamine for H_1 cell receptor sites on effector cells.

Pharmacokinetics

A single *Ornade* Spansule capsule produces blood levels comparable to those produced by administration of three 25 mg doses of phenylpropanolamine hydrochloride and three 4 mg doses of chlorpheniramine maleate in conventional release form given at 4-hour intervals. At steady-state conditions, the following peak levels are reached after the oral administration of an *Ornade* Spansule capsule: 21 ng/mL chlorpheniramine maleate in 7.7 hours; 173 ng/mL phenylpropanolamine hydrochloride in 6.1 hours; under these circumstances, the half-lives are approximately 21 and 7 hours, respectively.

INDICATIONS AND USAGE

For the treatment of the symptoms of seasonal and perennial allergic rhinitis and vasomotor rhinitis, including nasal obstruction (congestion); also for the treatment of runny nose, sneezing and nasal congestion associated with the common cold.

CONTRAINDICATIONS

Hypersensitivity to either phenylpropanolamine hydrochloride or chlorpheniramine maleate and other antihistamines of similar chemical structure; severe hypertension; coronary artery disease.

This drug should NOT be used in newborn or premature infants.

Because of the higher risk of antihistamines for infants generally, and for newborns and prematures in particular, antihistamine therapy is contraindicated in nursing mothers.

As with any product containing a sympathomimetic, *Ornade* Spansule capsules should NOT be used in patients taking monoamine oxidase (MAO) inhibitors.

WARNINGS

Ornade Spansule capsules may potentiate the effects of alcohol and other CNS depressants. Also, this product should not be taken simultaneously with other products containing phenylpropanolamine hydrochloride or amphetamines.

Ornade Spansule capsules should be used with considerable caution in patients with narrow-angle glaucoma, stenosing peptic ulcer, pyloroduodenal obstruction, symptomatic prostatic hypertrophy, or bladder neck obstruction.

Use in Children: In infants and children, especially, antihistamines in *overdosage* may cause hallucinations, convulsions, or death. As in adults, antihistamines may diminish mental alertness in children. In the young child, particularly, they may produce excitation.

Use in the Elderly (approximately 60 years or older): Antihistamines are more likely to cause dizziness, sedation and hypotension in elderly patients.

PRECAUTIONS

General: Use with caution in patients with lower respiratory disease including asthma, hypertension, cardiovascular disease, hyperthyroidism, increased intraocular pressure, or diabetes.

Information for Patients: Caution patients about activities requiring alertness (e.g., operating vehicles or machinery). Also caution patients about the possible additive effects of alcohol and other CNS depressants (hypnotics, sedatives, tranquilizers, etc.), and not to take simultaneously other products containing phenylpropanolamine hydrochloride or amphetamines. Patients should not take *Ornade* Spansule capsules in conjunction with a monoamine oxidase inhibitor or an oral anticoagulant.

Drug Interactions: *Ornade* Spansule capsules may interact with alcohol and other CNS depressants to potentiate their effects.

This product may have additive effects when taken simultaneously with other products containing phenylpropanolamine hydrochloride or amphetamines.

MAO inhibitors prolong and intensify the anticholinergic (drying) effects of antihistamines and potentiate the pressor effects of sympathomimetics such as phenylpropanolamine hydrochloride (see CONTRAINDICATIONS).

Phenylpropanolamine hydrochloride should not be used with ganglionic blocking drugs—such as mecamylamine—which potentiate reactions of sympathomimetics. It also should not be used with adrenergic blocking drugs, such as guanethidine sulfate or bethanidine, since it antagonizes the hypotensive action of these drugs.

The action of oral anticoagulants may be inhibited by antihistamines.

The CNS depressant and atropine-like effects of anticholinergics may be potentiated by concomitant administration of antihistamines. Concomitant administration of anticholinergics such as trihexyphenidyl, and other drugs with anticholinergic action (such as imipramine), with antihistamines may result in xerostomia.

β-adrenergic blockers may be antagonized by antihistamines.

Concomitant administration of corticosteroids and antihistamines may decrease the effects of the corticosteroids by enzyme induction.

Antihistamines inhibit norepinephrine reuptake by tissues and therefore potentiate the cardiovascular effects of norepinephrine.

Concomitant use of antihistamines with phenothiazines may produce an additive CNS depressant effect; concomitant use also may cause urinary retention or glaucoma.

Carcinogenesis, Mutagenesis, Impairment of Fertility: A long-term oncogenic study in rats with the chlorpheniramine maleate component of *Ornade* Spansule capsules did not produce an increase in the incidence of tumors in the drug-treated groups, as compared with the controls. No evidence of mutagenicity was found when chlorpheniramine maleate was evaluated in a battery of mutagenic studies, including the Ames test.

In an early study in rats with chlorpheniramine maleate a reduction in fertility was observed in female rats at doses approximately 67 times the human dose. More recent studies in rabbits and rats, using more appropriate methodology and doses up to approximately 50 and 85 times the human dose, showed no reduction in fertility.

There are no studies available which indicate whether phenylpropanolamine hydrochloride has carcinogenic or mutagenic effects or impairs fertility.

Pregnancy, Teratogenic Effects, Pregnancy Category B: Reproduction studies have been performed with the components of *Ornade* Spansule capsules. Studies with chlorpheniramine maleate in rabbits and rats at doses up to 50 times and 85 times the human dose, respectively, revealed no evidence of harm to the fetus. A study with phenylpropanolamine hydrochloride in rats at doses up to 7 times the human dose revealed no evidence of harm to the fetus. There are, however, no adequate and well-controlled studies in pregnant women. Because animal reproduction studies are not always predictive of human response, *Ornade* Spansule capsules should be used during pregnancy only if clearly needed.

Nonteratogenic Effects: Studies of chlorpheniramine maleate in rats showed a decrease in the postnatal survival rate of offspring of animals dosed with 33 and 67 times the human dose.

Nursing Mothers: Small amounts of antihistamines are excreted in breast milk. Because of the higher risk with antihistamines in infants generally, and for newborns and prematures in particular, *Ornade* Spansule capsules should not be administered to a nursing mother (see CONTRAINDICATIONS).

Pediatric Use: The safety and effectiveness of *Ornade* Spansule capsules in children under 12 years of age have not been established.

In infants and children, especially, antihistamines in *overdosage* may cause hallucinations, convulsions, or death. As in adults, antihistamines may diminish mental alertness in children. In the young child, particularly, they may produce excitation. (See WARNINGS.)

ADVERSE REACTIONS

The following adverse reactions have been reported following the use of antihistamines and/or sympathomimetic amines:

General: Anaphylactic shock; chills; drug rash; excessive dryness of mouth, nose and throat; increased intraocular pressure; excessive perspiration; photosensitivity; urticaria; weakness.

Cardiovascular System: Angina pain; extrasystoles; headache; hypertension; hypotension; palpitations; tachycardia.

Hematologic: Agranulocytosis; hemolytic anemia; leukopenia; thrombocytopenia.

Nervous System: Blurred vision; confusion; convulsions; diplopia; disturbed coordination; dizziness; drowsiness; euphoria; excitation; fatigue; hysteria; insomnia; irritability; acute labyrinthitis; nervousness; neuritis; paresthesia; restlessness; sedation; tinnitus; tremor; vertigo.

GI System: Abdominal pain; anorexia; constipation; diarrhea; epigastric distress; nausea; vomiting.

GU System: Dysuria; early menses; urinary frequency; urinary retention.

Respiratory System: Thickening of bronchial secretions; tightness of chest and wheezing; nasal stuffiness.

OVERDOSAGE

In the event of overdosage, emergency treatment should be started immediately.

Symptoms: Effects of antihistamine overdosage may vary from central nervous system depression (sedation, apnea, diminished mental alertness, cardiovascular collapse) to stimulation (insomnia, hallucinations, tremors, or convulsions) to death.

Other signs and symptoms may be dizziness, tinnitus, ataxia, blurred vision and hypotension. Stimulation is particularly likely in children, as are atropine-like signs and symptoms (dry mouth; fixed, dilated pupils; flushing; hyperthermia; and gastrointestinal symptoms). In large doses, sympathomimetics may cause giddiness, headache, nausea, vomiting, sweating, thirst, tachycardia, precordial pain, palpitations, difficulty in micturition, muscular weakness and tenseness, anxiety, restlessness and insomnia. Many patients can present a toxic psychosis with delusions and hallucinations. Some may develop cardiac arrhythmias, circulatory collapse, convulsions, coma and respiratory failure.

Toxicity: In acute oral toxicity tests in rats, the LD_{50} for the ratio of 75 mg phenylpropanolamine hydrochloride and 12 mg chlorpheniramine maleate was 774.2 mg/kg; in mice, the LD_{50} for the formulation was 757.4 mg/kg.

Treatment: The patient should be induced to vomit even if emesis has occurred spontaneously. Pharmacologically induced vomiting by the administration of ipecac syrup is a preferred method. But vomiting should not be induced in patients with impaired consciousness. The action of ipecac is facilitated by physical activity and by the administration of 8 to 12 fluid ounces of water. If emesis does not occur within 15

minutes, the dose of ipecac should be repeated. Precautions against aspiration must be taken, especially in infants and children.

Following emesis, any drug remaining in the stomach may be adsorbed by activated charcoal administered as a slurry with water. If vomiting is unsuccessful or contraindicated, gastric lavage should be performed. Isotonic and one-half isotonic saline are the lavage solutions of choice. Since much of the *Spansule* capsule medication is coated for gradual release, saline cathartics should be administered to hasten evacuation of pellets that have not already released medication. Saline cathartics, such as milk of magnesia, draw water into the bowel by osmosis and therefore may be valuable for their action in rapid dilution of bowel content. Dialysis has not been reported to be effective in the treatment of phenylpropanolamine hydrochloride and chlorpheniramine maleate overdosage. After emergency treatment, the patient should continue to be medically monitored.

Treatment of the signs and symptoms of overdosage is symptomatic and supportive. *Stimulants* (analeptic agents) should *not* be used. Vasopressors may be used to treat hypotension. Short-acting barbiturates, diazepam, or paraldehyde may be administered to control seizures. Hyperpyrexia, especially in children, may require treatment with tepid water sponge baths or a hypothermic blanket. Apnea is treated with ventilatory support.

DOSAGE AND ADMINISTRATION

Adults and children 12 years of age and over—one capsule every 12 hours.

Ornade Spansule capsules are not recommended in children under 12.

HOW SUPPLIED

In gelatin capsules with opaque red cap and natural body. Each capsule is imprinted with the product name ORNADE and SB, and filled with small red, white and gray pellets; in bottles of 50 and 500 capsules, and in Single Unit Packages of 100 capsules (intended for institutional use only). Each capsule contains 75 mg phenylpropanolamine hydrochloride and 12 mg chlorpheniramine maleate. Capsules should be stored between 15° and 30°C (59° and 86°F).

NDC 0007-4421-15 50's
NDC 0007-4421-25 500's

WARNING: Manufactured with carbon tetrachloride and methyl chloroform, substances which harm public health and environment by destroying ozone in the upper atmosphere.

Veterans Administration/Military/PHS—*Spansule* capsules, 500's, 6505-01-108-9574.

OR:L42

Shown in Product Identification Guide, page 337

PARNATE® ℞
[*pahr'naight*]
(brand of tranylcypromine sulfate)
Tablets 10 mg

Before prescribing, the physician should be familiar with the entire contents of this prescribing information.

DESCRIPTION

Chemically, tranylcypromine sulfate is (±)-*trans*-2-phenylcyclopropylamine sulfate (2:1).

Each round, rose-red, coated tablet is imprinted with the product name PARNATE and SKF and contains tranylcypromine sulfate equivalent to 10 mg of tranylcypromine. Inactive ingredients consist of gelatin, lactose, cellulose, citric acid, croscarmellose sodium, talc, magnesium stearate, iron oxide, D&C Red No. 7, FD&C Blue No. 2, FD&C Yellow No. 6, FD&C Red No. 40, titanium dioxide and trace amounts of other inactive ingredients.

NOTE: Parnate (tranylcypromine sulfate) tablets have been changed from rose-red sugar-coated tablets to rose-red film-coated tablets. The film-coated tablets differ in size from the sugar-coated tablets, but the drug content remains unchanged.

ACTION

Tranylcypromine is a non-hydrazine monoamine oxidase inhibitor with a rapid onset of activity. It increases the concentration of epinephrine, norepinephrine, and serotonin in storage sites throughout the nervous system and, in theory, this increased concentration of monoamines in the brain stem is the basis for its antidepressant activity. When tranylcypromine is withdrawn, monoamine oxidase activity is re-

Continued on next page

Information on the SmithKline Beecham Pharmaceuticals products appearing here is based on the labeling in effect on July 1, 1996. Further information on these and other products may be obtained from the Medical Department, SmithKline Beecham Pharmaceuticals, One Franklin Plaza, Philadelphia, PA 19101.

SmithKline Beecham—Cont.

covered in 3 to 5 days, although the drug is excreted in 24 hours.

INDICATIONS

For the treatment of Major Depressive Episode Without Melancholia.

Parnate (tranylcypromine sulfate) should be used in adult patients who can be closely supervised. It should rarely be the first antidepressant drug given. Rather, the drug is suited for patients who have failed to respond to the drugs more commonly administered for depression.

The effectiveness of *Parnate* has been established in adult outpatients, most of whom had a depressive illness which would correspond to a diagnosis of Major Depressive Episode Without Melancholia. As described in the American Psychiatric Association's Diagnostic and Statistical Manual, third edition (DSM III), Major Depressive Episode implies a prominent and relatively persistent (nearly every day for at least 2 weeks) depressed or dysphoric mood that usually interferes with daily functioning and includes at least 4 of the following 8 symptoms: change in appetite, change in sleep, psychomotor agitation or retardation, loss of interest in usual activities or decrease in sexual drive, increased fatigability, feelings of guilt or worthlessness, slowed thinking or impaired concentration and suicidal ideation or attempts.

The effectiveness of *Parnate* in patients who meet the criteria for Major Depressive Episode with Melancholia (endogenous features) has not been established.

SUMMARY OF CONTRAINDICATIONS

Parnate (tranylcypromine sulfate) should not be administered in combination with any of the following: MAO inhibitors or dibenzazepine derivatives; sympathomimetics (including amphetamines); some central nervous system depressants (including narcotics and alcohol); antihypertensive, diuretic, antihistaminic, sedative or anesthetic drugs; bupropion HCl; buspirone HCl; dextromethorphan; cheese or other foods with a high tyramine content; or excessive quantities of caffeine.

Parnate (tranylcypromine sulfate) should not be administered to any patient with a confirmed or suspected cerebrovascular defect or to any patient with cardiovascular disease, hypertension or history of headache.

(For complete discussion of contraindications and warnings, see below.)

CONTRAINDICATIONS

Parnate (tranylcypromine sulfate) is contraindicated:

1. In patients with cerebrovascular defects or cardiovascular disorders

Parnate should not be administered to any patient with a confirmed or suspected cerebrovascular defect or to any patient with cardiovascular disease or hypertension.

2. In the presence of pheochromocytoma

Parnate should not be used in the presence of pheochromocytoma since such tumors secrete pressor substances.

3. In combination with MAO inhibitors or with dibenzazepine-related entities

Parnate (tranylcypromine sulfate) should not be administered together or in rapid succession with other MAO inhibitors or with dibenzazepine-related entities. Hypertensive crises or severe convulsive seizures may occur in patients receiving such combinations.

In patients being transferred to *Parnate* from another MAO inhibitor or from a dibenzazepine-related entity, allow a medication-free interval of at least a week, then initiate *Parnate* using half the normal starting dosage for at least the first week of therapy. Similarly, at least a week should elapse between the discontinuance of *Parnate* and the administration of another MAO inhibitor or a dibenzazepine-related entity, or the readministration of *Parnate*.

The following list includes some other MAO inhibitors, dibenzazepine-related entities and tricyclic antidepressants.

Other MAO Inhibitors

Generic Name	Trademark
Furazolidone	Furoxone® (Roberts Laboratories)
Isocarboxazid	Marplan® (Roche Laboratories)
Pargyline HCl	Eutonyl® (Abbott Laboratories)
Pargyline HCl and methyclothiazide	Eutron® (Abbott Laboratories)
Phenelzine sulfate	Nardil® (Parke-Davis)
Procarbazine HCl	Matulane® (Roche Laboratories)

Dibenzazepine-Related and Other Tricyclics

Generic Name	Trademark
Amitriptyline HCl	Elavil® (Merck Sharp & Dohme)
	Endep® (Roche Products)
Perphenazine and amitriptyline HCl	Etrafon® (Schering)
	Triavil® (Merck Sharp & Dohme)
Clomipramine hydrochloride	Anafranil® (CIBA-GEIGY)
Desipramine HCl	Norpramin® (Marion Merrell Dow)
	Pertofrane® (Rhône-Poulenc Rorer Pharmaceuticals)
Imipramine HCl	Janimine® (Abbott Laboratories)
	Tofranil® (GEIGY Pharmaceuticals)
Nortriptyline HCl	Aventyl® (Eli Lilly & Co.)
	Pamelor® (Sandoz)
Protriptyline HCl	Vivactil® (Merck Sharp & Dohme)
Doxepin HCl	Adapin® (Fisons)
	Sinequan® (Roerig)
Carbamazepine	Tegretol® (GEIGY Pharmaceuticals)
Cyclobenzaprine HCl	Flexeril® (Merck Sharp & Dohme)
Amoxapine	Asendin® (Lederle)
Maprotiline HCl	Ludiomil® (CIBA)
Trimipramine maleate	Surmontil® (Wyeth-Ayerst Laboratories)

4. In combination with bupropion

The concurrent administration of a MAO inhibitor and bupropion hydrochloride (Wellbutrin®, Burroughs Wellcome) is contraindicated. At least 14 days should elapse between discontinuation of a MAO inhibitor and initiation of treatment with bupropion hydrochloride.

5. In combination with selective serotonin reuptake inhibitors (SSRIs)

As a general rule, *Parnate* should not be administered in combination with any SSRI. There have been reports of serious, sometimes fatal, reactions (including hyperthermia, rigidity, myoclonus, autonomic instability with possible rapid fluctuations of vital signs, and mental status changes that include extreme agitation progressing to delirium and coma) in patients receiving fluoxetine (Prozac®, Lilly) in combination with a monoamine oxidase inhibitor (MAOI), and in patients who have recently discontinued fluoxetine and are then started on a MAOI. Some cases presented with features resembling neuroleptic malignant syndrome. Therefore, fluoxetine and other SSRIs should not be used in combination with a MAOI, or within 14 days of discontinuing therapy with a MAOI. Since fluoxetine and its major metabolite have very long elimination half-lives, at least 5 weeks should be allowed after stopping fluoxetine before starting a MAOI.

At least 2 weeks should be allowed after stopping sertraline (Zoloft®, Roerig) or paroxetine (Paxil®, SmithKline Beecham Pharmaceuticals) before starting a MAOI.

6. In combination with buspirone

Parnate (tranylcypromine sulfate) should not be used in combination with buspirone HCl (Buspar®, Mead Johnson), since several cases of elevated blood pressure have been reported in patients taking MAO inhibitors who were then given buspirone HCl. At least 10 days should elapse between the discontinuation of *Parnate* and the institution of buspirone HCl.

7. In combination with sympathomimetics

Parnate (tranylcypromine sulfate) should not be administered in combination with sympathomimetics, including amphetamines, and over-the-counter drugs such as cold, hay fever or weight-reducing preparations that contain vasoconstrictors.

During *Parnate* therapy, it appears that certain patients are particularly vulnerable to the effects of sympathomimetics when the activity of certain enzymes is inhibited. Use of sympathomimetics and compounds such as guanethidine, methyldopa, reserpine, dopamine, levodopa and tryptophan with *Parnate* may precipitate hypertension, headache and related symptoms. In addition, use with tryptophan may precipitate disorientation, memory impairment and other neurologic and behavioral signs.

8. In combination with meperidine

Do not use meperidine concomitantly with MAO inhibitors or within 2 or 3 weeks following MAOI therapy. Serious reactions have been precipitated with concomitant use, including coma, severe hypertension or hypotension, severe respiratory depression, convulsions, malignant hyperpyrexia, excitation, peripheral vascular collapse and death. It is thought that these reactions may be mediated by accumulation of 5-HT (serotonin) consequent to MAO inhibition.

9. In combination with dextromethorphan

The combination of MAO inhibitors and dextromethorphan has been reported to cause brief episodes of psychosis or bizarre behavior.

10. In combination with cheese or other foods with a high tyramine content

Hypertensive crises have sometimes occurred during *Parnate* therapy after ingestion of foods with a high tyramine content. In general, the patient should avoid protein foods in which aging or protein breakdown is used to increase flavor. In particular, patients should be instructed not to take foods such as cheese (particularly strong or aged varieties), sour cream, Chianti wine, sherry, beer (including nonalcoholic beer), liqueurs, pickled herring, anchovies, caviar, liver, canned figs, raisins, bananas or avocados (particularly if overripe), chocolate, soy sauce, sauerkraut, the pods of broad beans (fava beans), yeast extracts, yogurt, meat extracts or meat prepared with tenderizers.

11. In patients undergoing elective surgery

Patients taking *Parnate* should not undergo elective surgery requiring general anesthesia. Also, they should not be given cocaine or local anesthesia containing sympathomimetic vasoconstrictors. The possible combined hypotensive effects of *Parnate* and spinal anesthesia should be kept in mind. *Parnate* should be discontinued at least 10 days prior to elective surgery.

ADDITIONAL CONTRAINDICATIONS

In general, the physician should bear in mind the possibility of a lowered margin of safety when Parnate (tranylcypromine sulfate) is administered in combination with potent drugs.

1. *Parnate* should not be used in combination with some central nervous system depressants such as narcotics and alcohol, or with hypotensive agents. A marked potentiating effect on these classes of drugs has been reported.
2. Anti-parkinsonism drugs should be used with caution in patients receiving *Parnate* since severe reactions have been reported.
3. *Parnate* should not be used in patients with a history of liver disease or in those with abnormal liver function tests.
4. Excessive use of caffeine in any form should be avoided in patients receiving *Parnate*.

WARNING TO PHYSICIANS

Parnate (tranylcypromine sulfate) is a potent agent with the capability of producing serious side effects. *Parnate* is not recommended in those depressive reactions where other antidepressant drugs may be effective. **It should be reserved for patients who can be closely supervised and who have not responded satisfactorily to the drugs more commonly administered for depression.**

Before prescribing, the physician should be completely familiar with the full material on dosage, side effects and contraindications on these pages, with the principles of MAO inhibitor therapy and the side effects of this class of drugs. Also, the physician should be familiar with the symptomatology of mental depressions and alternate methods of treatment to aid in the careful selection of patients for *Parnate* therapy. In depressed patients, the possibility of suicide should always be considered and adequate precautions taken.

Pregnancy Warning: Use of any drug in pregnancy, during lactation or in women of childbearing age requires that the potential benefits of the drug be weighed against its possible hazards to mother and child.

Animal reproductive studies show that *Parnate* passes through the placental barrier into the fetus of the rat, and into the milk of the lactating dog. The absence of a harmful action of *Parnate* on fertility or on postnatal development by either prenatal treatment or from the milk of treated animals has not been demonstrated. Tranylcypromine is excreted in human milk.

WARNING TO THE PATIENT

Patients should be instructed to report promptly the occurrence of headache or other unusual symptoms, i.e., palpitation and/or tachycardia, a sense of constriction in the throat or chest, sweating, dizziness, neck stiffness, nausea or vomiting.

Patients should be warned against eating the foods listed in Section 9 under Contraindications while on Parnate (tranylcypromine sulfate) therapy. Also, they should be told not to drink alcoholic beverages. The patient should also be warned about the possibility of hypotension and faintness, as well as drowsiness sufficient to impair performance of potentially hazardous tasks such as driving a car or operating machinery.

Patients should also be cautioned not to take concomitant medications, whether prescription or over-the-counter drugs such as cold, hay fever or weight-reducing preparations, without the advice of a physician. They should be advised not to consume excessive amounts of caffeine in any form. Likewise, they should inform other physicians, and their dentist, about their use of *Parnate*.

WARNINGS

HYPERTENSIVE CRISES: The most important reaction associated with Parnate (tranylcypromine sulfate) is the occurrence of hypertensive crises which have sometimes been fatal.

These crises are characterized by some or all of the following symptoms: occipital headache which may radiate frontally, palpitation, neck stiffness or soreness, nausea or vomiting, sweating (sometimes with fever and sometimes with cold, clammy skin) and photophobia. Either tachycardia or bradycardia may be present, and associated constricting chest pain and dilated pupils may occur. **Intracranial bleeding, sometimes fatal in outcome, has been reported in association with the paradoxical increase in blood pressure.**

In all patients taking *Parnate* blood pressure should be followed closely to detect evidence of any pressor response. It is emphasized that full reliance should not be placed on blood pressure readings, but that the patient should also be observed frequently.

Therapy should be discontinued immediately upon the occurrence of palpitation or frequent headaches during *Parnate* therapy. These signs may be prodromal of a hypertensive crisis.

Important:
Recommended treatment in
hypertensive crises

If a hypertensive crisis occurs, Parnate (tranylcypromine sulfate) should be discontinued and therapy to lower blood pressure should be instituted immediately. Headache tends to abate as blood pressure is lowered. On the basis of present evidence, phentolamine (available as Regitine®*) is recommended. (The dosage reported for phentolamine is 5 mg I.V.) Care should be taken to administer this drug slowly in order to avoid producing an excessive hypotensive effect. Fever should be managed by means of external cooling. Other symptomatic and supportive measures may be desirable in particular cases. Do not use parenteral reserpine.

PRECAUTIONS

Hypotension

Hypotension has been observed during Parnate (tranylcypromine sulfate) therapy. Symptoms of postural hypotension are seen most commonly but not exclusively in patients with pre-existent hypertension; blood pressure usually returns rapidly to pretreatment levels upon discontinuation of the drug. At doses above 30 mg daily, postural hypotension is a major side effect and may result in syncope. Dosage increases should be made more gradually in patients showing a tendency toward hypotension at the beginning of therapy. Postural hypotension may be relieved by having the patient lie down until blood pressure returns to normal.

Also, when *Parnate* is combined with those phenothiazine derivatives or other compounds known to cause hypotension, the possibility of additive hypotensive effects should be considered.

OTHER PRECAUTIONS

There have been reports of drug dependency in patients using doses of tranylcypromine significantly in excess of the therapeutic range. Some of these patients had a history of previous substance abuse. The following withdrawal symptoms have been reported: restlessness, anxiety, depression, confusion, hallucinations, headache, weakness and diarrhea. Drugs which lower the seizure threshold, including MAO inhibitors, should not be used with Amipaque®†. As with other MAO inhibitors, Parnate (tranylcypromine sulfate) should be discontinued at least 48 hours before myelography and should not be resumed for at least 24 hours postprocedure.

In depressed patients, the possibility of suicide should always be considered and adequate precautions taken. Exclusive reliance on drug therapy to prevent suicidal attempts is unwarranted, as there may be a delay in the onset of therapeutic effect or an increase in anxiety and agitation. Also, some patients fail to respond to drug therapy or may respond only temporarily.

MAO inhibitors may have the capacity to suppress anginal pain that would otherwise serve as a warning of myocardial ischemia.

The usual precautions should be observed in patients with impaired renal function since there is a possibility of cumulative effects in such patients.

Older patients may suffer more morbidity than younger patients during and following an episode of hypertension or malignant hyperthermia. Older patients have less compensatory reserve to cope with any serious adverse reaction. Therefore, *Parnate* should be used with caution in the elderly population.

Although excretion of *Parnate* is rapid, inhibition of MAO may persist up to 10 days following discontinuation.

Because the influence of *Parnate* on the convulsive threshold is variable in animal experiments, suitable precautions should be taken if epileptic patients are treated.

Some MAO inhibitors have contributed to hypoglycemic episodes in diabetic patients receiving insulin or oral hypoglycemic agents. Therefore, *Parnate* should be used with caution in diabetics using these drugs.

Parnate may aggravate coexisting symptoms in depression, such as anxiety and agitation.

Use Parnate (tranylcypromine sulfate) with caution in hyperthyroid patients because of their increased sensitivity to pressor amines.

Parnate should be administered with caution to patients receiving Antabuse®‡. In a single study, rats given high intraperitoneal doses of *d* or *l* isomers of tranylcypromine sulfate plus disulfiram experienced severe toxicity including convulsions and death. Additional studies in rats given high oral doses of racemic tranylcypromine sulfate (*Parnate*) and disulfiram produced no adverse interaction.

ADVERSE REACTIONS

Overstimulation which may include increased anxiety, agitation and manic symptoms is usually evidence of excessive therapeutic action. Dosage should be reduced, or a phenothiazine tranquilizer should be administered concomitantly. Patients may experience restlessness or insomnia; may notice some weakness, drowsiness, episodes of dizziness or dry mouth; or may report nausea, diarrhea, abdominal pain or constipation. Most of these effects can be relieved by lowering the dosage or by giving suitable concomitant medication. Tachycardia, significant anorexia, edema, palpitation, blurred vision, chills and impotence have each been reported.

Headaches without blood pressure elevation have occurred. Rare instances of hepatitis and skin rash have been reported. Impaired water excretion compatible with the syndrome of inappropriate secretion of antidiuretic hormone (SIADH) has been reported.

Tinnitus, muscle spasm, tremors, myoclonic jerks, numbness, paresthesia, urinary retention and retarded ejaculation have been reported.

Hematologic disorders including anemia, leukopenia, agranulocytosis and thrombocytopenia have been reported.

Post-Introduction Reports

The following are spontaneously reported adverse events temporally associated with *Parnate* therapy. No clear relationship between *Parnate* and these events has been established. Localized scleroderma, flare-up of cystic acne, ataxia, confusion, disorientation, memory loss, urinary frequency, urinary incontinence, urticaria, fissuring in corner of mouth, akinesia.

DOSAGE AND ADMINISTRATION

Dosage should be adjusted to the requirements of the individual patient. Improvement should be seen within 48 hours to 3 weeks after starting therapy.

The usual effective dosage is 30 mg per day, usually given in divided doses. If there are no signs of improvement after a reasonable period (up to 2 weeks), then the dosage may be increased in 10 mg per day increments at intervals of 1 to 3 weeks; the dosage range may be extended to a maximum of 60 mg per day from the usual 30 mg per day.

OVERDOSAGE

SYMPTOMS: The characteristic symptoms that may be caused by overdosage are usually those described above. However, an intensification of these symptoms and sometimes severe additional manifestations may be seen, depending on the degree of overdosage and on individual susceptibility. Some patients exhibit insomnia, restlessness and anxiety, progressing in severe cases to agitation, mental confusion and incoherence. Hypotension, dizziness, weakness and drowsiness may occur, progressing in severe cases to extreme dizziness and shock. A few patients have displayed hypertension with severe headache and other symptoms. Rare instances have been reported in which hypertension was accompanied by twitching or myoclonic fibrillation of skeletal muscles with hyperpyrexia, sometimes progressing to generalized rigidity and coma.

TREATMENT: Gastric lavage is helpful if performed early. Treatment should normally consist of general supportive measures, close observation of vital signs and steps to counteract specific symptoms as they occur, since MAO inhibition may persist. The management of hypertensive crises is described under WARNINGS in the HYPERTENSIVE CRISES section.

External cooling is recommended if hyperpyrexia occurs. Barbiturates have been reported to help relieve myoclonic reactions, but frequency of administration should be controlled carefully because Parnate (tranylcypromine sulfate) may prolong barbiturate activity. When hypotension requires treatment, the standard measures for managing circulatory shock should be initiated. If pressor agents are used, the rate of infusion should be regulated by careful observation of the patient because an exaggerated pressor response sometimes occurs in the presence of MAO inhibition. Remember that the toxic effect of *Parnate* may be delayed or prolonged following the last dose of the drug. Therefore, the patient should be closely observed for at least a week. It is not known if tranylcypromine is dialyzable.

HOW SUPPLIED

Parnate is supplied as round, rose-red, film-coated tablets imprinted with the product name PARNATE and SKF and contains tranylcypromine sulfate equivalent to 10 mg of tranylcypromine, in bottles of 100 with a desiccant.
10 mg 100's: NDC 0007-4471-20
Store between 15° and 30°C (59° to 86°F).

* phentolamine mesylate USP, CIBA.
†metrizamide, Sanofi Winthrop Pharmaceuticals.
‡disulfiram, Wyeth-Ayerst Laboratories.
Veterans Administration/Military/PHS—Tablets, 10 mg, 100's, 6505-01-211-9008.
PT:L60
Shown in Product Identification Guide, page 337

PAXIL® ℞
[*packs 'ill*]
brand of
paroxetine
hydrochloride
tablets

DESCRIPTION

Paxil (paroxetine hydrochloride) is an orally administered antidepressant with a chemical structure unrelated to other selective serotonin reuptake inhibitors or to tricyclic, tetracyclic or other available antidepressant agents. It is the hydrochloride salt of a phenylpiperidine compound identified chemically as (-)-*trans*-4R-(4'-fluorophenyl)-3S-[(3',4'-methylenedioxyphenoxy) methyl] piperidine hydrochloride hemihydrate and has the empirical formula of $C_{19}H_{20}FNO_3 \cdot HCl \cdot 1/2H_2O$. The molecular weight is 374.8 (329.4 as free base). The structural formula is:

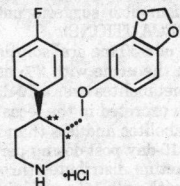

paroxetine hydrochloride

Paroxetine hydrochloride is an odorless, off-white powder, having a melting point range of 120° to 138°C and a solubility of 5.4 mg/mL in water.

Each film-coated tablet contains paroxetine hydrochloride equivalent to paroxetine as follows: 10 mg-yellow; 20 mg-pink (scored); 30 mg-blue, 40 mg-green. Inactive ingredients consist of dibasic calcium phosphate dihydrate, hydroxypropyl methylcellulose, magnesium stearate, polyethylene glycols, polysorbate 80, sodium starch glycolate, titanium dioxide and one or more of the following: D&C Red No. 30, D&C Yellow No. 10, FD&C Blue No. 2, FD&C Yellow No. 6.

CLINICAL PHARMACOLOGY

Pharmacodynamics

The antidepressant action of paroxetine and its efficacy in the treatment of obsessive compulsive disorder (OCD) and panic disorder (PD) is presumed to be linked to potentiation of serotonergic activity in the central nervous system resulting from inhibition of neuronal reuptake of serotonin (5-hydroxy-tryptamine, 5-HT). Studies at clinically relevant doses in humans have demonstrated that paroxetine blocks the uptake of serotonin into human platelets. *In vitro* studies in animals also suggest that paroxetine is a potent and highly selective inhibitor of neuronal serotonin reuptake and has only very weak effects on norepinephrine and dopamine neuronal reuptake. *In vitro* radioligand binding studies indicate that paroxetine has little affinity for muscarinic, alpha$_1$-, alpha$_2$-, beta-adrenergic-, dopamine (D$_2$)-, 5-HT$_1$-, 5-HT$_2$- and histamine (H$_1$)-receptors; antagonism of muscarinic, histaminergic and alpha$_1$-adrenergic receptors has been associated with various anticholinergic, sedative and cardiovascular effects for other psychotropic drugs.

Because the relative potencies of paroxetine's major metabolites are at most 1/50 of the parent compound, they are essentially inactive.

Pharmacokinetics

Paroxetine hydrochloride is completely absorbed after oral dosing of a solution of the hydrochloride salt. In a study in which normal male subjects (n=15) received 30 mg tablets

Continued on next page

Information on the SmithKline Beecham Pharmaceuticals products appearing here is based on the labeling in effect on July 1, 1996. Further information on these and other products may be obtained from the Medical Department, SmithKline Beecham Pharmaceuticals, One Franklin Plaza, Philadelphia, PA 19101.

SmithKline Beecham—Cont.

daily for 30 days, steady-state paroxetine concentrations were achieved by approximately 10 days for most subjects, although it may take substantially longer in an occasional patient. At steady state, mean values of C_{max}, T_{max}, C_{min} and $T_{1/2}$ were 61.7 ng/mL (CV 45%), 5.2 hr. (CV 10%), 30.7 ng/mL (CV 67%) and 21.0 hr. (CV 32%), respectively. The steady-state C_{max} and C_{min} values were about 6 and 14 times what would be predicted from single-dose studies. Steady-state drug exposure based on AUC_{0-24} was about 8 times greater than would have been predicted from single-dose data in these subjects. The excess accumulation is a consequence of the fact that one of the enzymes that metabolizes paroxetine is readily saturable.

In steady-state dose proportionality studies involving elderly and nonelderly patients, at doses of 20 to 40 mg daily for the elderly and 20 to 50 mg daily for the nonelderly, some nonlinearity was observed in both populations, again reflecting a saturable metabolic pathway. In comparison to C_{min} values after 20 mg daily, values after 40 mg daily were only about 2 to 3 times greater than doubled.

Paroxetine is extensively metabolized after oral administration. The principal metabolites are polar and conjugated products of oxidation and methylation, which are readily cleared. Conjugates with glucuronic acid and sulfate predominate, and major metabolites have been isolated and identified. Data indicate that the metabolites have no more than 1/50 the potency of the parent compound at inhibiting serotonin uptake. The metabolism of paroxetine is accomplished in part by cytochrome $P_{450}IID_6$. Saturation of this enzyme at clinical doses appears to account for the nonlinearity of paroxetine kinetics with increasing dose and increasing duration of treatment. The role of this enzyme in paroxetine metabolism also suggests potential drug-drug interactions (see PRECAUTIONS).

Approximately 64% of a 30 mg oral solution dose of paroxetine was excreted in the urine with 2% as the parent compound and 62% as metabolites over a 10-day post-dosing period. About 36% was excreted in the feces (probably via the bile), mostly as metabolites and less than 1% as the parent compound over the 10-day post-dosing period.

Distribution: Paroxetine distributes throughout the body, including the CNS, with only 1% remaining in the plasma.

Protein Binding: Approximately 95% and 93% of paroxetine is bound to plasma protein at 100 ng/mL and 400 ng/mL, respectively. Under clinical conditions, paroxetine concentrations would normally be less than 400 ng/mL. Paroxetine does not alter the *in vitro* protein binding of phenytoin or warfarin.

Renal and Liver Disease: Increased plasma concentrations of paroxetine occur in subjects with renal and hepatic impairment. The mean plasma concentrations in patients with creatinine clearance below 30 mL/min was approximately 4 times greater than seen in normal volunteers. Patients with creatinine clearance of 30 to 60 mL/min and patients with hepatic functional impairment had about a 2-fold increase in plasma concentrations (AUC, C_{max}).

The initial dosage should therefore be reduced in patients with severe renal or hepatic impairment, and upward titration, if necessary, should be at increased intervals (see DOSAGE AND ADMINISTRATION).

Elderly Patients: In a multiple-dose study in the elderly at daily paroxetine doses of 20, 30 and 40 mg, C_{min} concentrations were about 70% to 80% greater than the respective C_{min} concentrations in nonelderly subjects. Therefore the initial dosage in the elderly should be reduced. (See DOSAGE AND ADMINISTRATION.)

Clinical Trials
Depression
The efficacy of *Paxil* as a treatment for depression has been established in 6 placebo-controlled studies of patients with depression (ages 18 to 73). In these studies *Paxil* was shown to be significantly more effective than placebo in treating depression by at least 2 of the following measures: Hamilton Depression Rating Scale (HDRS), the Hamilton depressed mood item, and the Clinical Global Impression (CGI)-Severity of Illness. *Paxil* was significantly better than placebo in improvement of the HDRS sub-factor scores, including the depressed mood item, sleep disturbance factor and anxiety factor.

A study of depressed outpatients who had responded to *Paxil* (HDRS total score <8) during an initial 8-week open-treatment phase and were then randomized to continuation on *Paxil* or placebo for 1 year demonstrated a significantly lower relapse rate for patients taking *Paxil* (15%) compared to those on placebo (39%). Effectiveness was similar for male and female patients.

Obsessive Compulsive Disorder
The effectiveness of *Paxil* in the treatment of obsessive compulsive disorder (OCD) was demonstrated in two 12-week multicenter placebo-controlled studies of adult outpatients (Studies 1 and 2). Patients in all studies had moderate to severe OCD (DSM-IIIR) with mean baseline ratings on the Yale Brown Obsessive Compulsive Scale (YBOCS) total score ranging from 23 to 26. Study 1, a dose-range finding study where patients were treated with fixed doses of 20, 40 or 60 mg of paroxetine/day demonstrated that daily doses of paroxetine 40 and 60 mg are effective in the treatment of OCD. Patients receiving doses of 40 and 60 mg paroxetine experienced a mean reduction of approximately 6 and 7 points respectively on the YBOCS total score which was significantly greater than the approximate 4 point reduction at 20 mg and a 3 point reduction in the placebo-treated patients. Study 2 was a flexible dose study comparing paroxetine (20 to 60 mg daily) with clomipramine (25 to 250 mg daily). In this study, patients receiving paroxetine experienced a mean reduction of approximately 7 points on the YBOCS total score which was significantly greater than the mean reduction of approximately 4 points in placebo-treated patients.

The following table provides the outcome classification by treatment group on Global Improvement items of the Clinical Global Impressions (CGI) scale for Study 1.

Outcome Classification (%) on CGI-Global Improvement Item for Completers in Study 1			
Outcome Classification	Placebo (N=74)	Paxil 20 mg (N=75)	Paxil 40 mg (N=66)	Paxil 60 mg (N=66)
---	---	---	---	---
Worse	14%	7%	7%	3%
No Change	44%	35%	22%	19%
Minimally Improved	24%	33%	29%	34%
Much Improved	11%	18%	22%	24%
Very Much Improved	7%	7%	20%	20%

Subgroup analyses did not indicate that there were any differences in treatment outcomes as a function of age or gender.

The long-term maintenance effects of *Paxil* in OCD were demonstrated in a long-term extension to Study 1. Patients who were responders on paroxetine during the 3-month double-blind phase and a 6-month extension on open-label paroxetine (20 to 60 mg/day) were randomized to either paroxetine or placebo in a 6-month double-blind relapse prevention phase. Patients randomized to paroxetine were significantly less likely to relapse than comparably treated patients who were randomized to placebo.

Panic Disorder
The effectiveness of *Paxil* in the treatment of panic disorder was demonstrated in three 10 to 12 week multicenter, placebo-controlled studies of adult outpatients (Studies 1-3). Patients in all studies had panic disorder (DSM-IIIR), with or without agoraphobia. In these studies, *Paxil* was shown to be significantly more effective than placebo in treating panic disorder by at least 2 out of 3 measures of panic attack frequency and on the Clinical Global Impression Severity of Illness score.

Study 1 was a 10-week dose-range finding study: patients were treated with fixed paroxetine doses of 10, 20, or 40 mg/day or placebo. A significant difference from placebo was observed only for the 40 mg/day group. At endpoint, 76% of patients receiving paroxetine 40 mg/day were free of panic attacks, compared to 44% of placebo-treated patients.

Study 2 was a 12-week flexible-dose study comparing paroxetine (10 to 60 mg daily) and placebo. At endpoint, 51% of paroxetine patients were free of panic attacks compared to 32% of placebo-treated patients.

Study 3 was a 12-week flexible-dose study comparing paroxetine (10 to 60 mg daily) to placebo in patients concurrently receiving standardized cognitive behavioral therapy. At endpoint, 33% of the paroxetine-treated patients showed a reduction to 0 or 1 panic attacks compared to 14% of placebo patients.

In both Studies 2 and 3, the mean paroxetine dose for completers at endpoint was approximately 40 mg/day of paroxetine.

Long-term maintenance effects of *Paxil* in panic disorder were demonstrated in an extension to Study 1. Patients who were responders during the 10-week double-blind phase and during a 3-month double-blind extension phase were randomized to either paroxetine (10, 20, or 40 mg/day) or placebo in a 3-month double-blind relapse prevention phase. Patients randomized to paroxetine were significantly less likely to relapse than comparably treated patients who were randomized to placebo.

Subgroup analyses did not indicate that there were any differences in treatment outcomes as a function of age or gender.

INDICATIONS AND USAGE
Depression
Paxil (paroxetine hydrochloride) is indicated for the treatment of depression.

The efficacy of *Paxil* in the treatment of a major depressive episode was established in 6 week controlled trials of outpatients whose diagnoses corresponded most closely to the DSM-III category of major depressive disorder (see CLINI-CAL PHARMACOLOGY). A major depressive episode implies a prominent and relatively persistent depressed or dysphoric mood that usually interferes with daily functioning (nearly every day for at least 2 weeks); it should include at least 4 of the following 8 symptoms: change in appetite, change in sleep, psychomotor agitation or retardation, loss of interest in usual activities or decrease in sexual drive, increased fatigue, feelings of guilt or worthlessness, slowed thinking or impaired concentration, and a suicide attempt or suicidal ideation.

The antidepressant action of *Paxil* in hospitalized depressed patients has not been adequately studied.

The efficacy of *Paxil* in maintaining an antidepressant response for up to 1 year was demonstrated in a placebo-controlled trial (see CLINICAL PHARMACOLOGY). Nevertheless, the physician who elects to use *Paxil* for extended periods should periodically re-evaluate the long-term usefulness of the drug for the individual patient.

Obsessive Compulsive Disorder
Paxil is indicated for the treatment of obsessions and compulsions in patients with obsessive compulsive disorder (OCD) as defined in the DSM-IV. The obsessions or compulsions cause marked distress, are time-consuming, or significantly interfere with social or occupational functioning.

The efficacy of *Paxil* was established in two 12 week trials with obsessive compulsive outpatients whose diagnoses corresponded most closely to the DSM-IIIR category of obsessive compulsive disorder (see CLINICAL PHARMACOLOGY—Clinical Trials).

Obsessive compulsive disorder is characterized by recurrent and persistent ideas, thoughts, impulses or images (obsessions) that are ego-dystonic and/or repetitive, purposeful and intentional behaviors (compulsions) that are recognized by the person as excessive or unreasonable.

Long-term maintenance of efficacy was demonstrated in a 6-month relapse prevention trial. In this trial, patients assigned to paroxetine showed a lower relapse rate compared to patients on placebo (see Clinical Pharmacology). Nevertheless, the physician who elects to use *Paxil* for extended periods should periodically reevaluate the long-term usefulness of the drug for the individual patient (see DOSAGE AND ADMINISTRATION).

Panic Disorder
Paxil is indicated for the treatment of panic disorder, with or without agoraphobia, as defined in DSM-IV. Panic disorder is characterized by the occurrence of unexpected panic attacks and associated concern about having additional attacks, worry about the implications or consequences of the attacks, and/or a significant change in behavior related to the attacks.

The efficacy of *Paxil* was established in three 10 to 12 week trials in panic disorder patients whose diagnoses corresponded to the DSM-IIIR category of panic disorder (see Clinical Pharmacology—Clinical Trials).

Panic disorder (DSM-IV) is characterized by recurrent unexpected panic attacks, i.e., a discrete period of intense fear or discomfort in which four (or more) of the following symptoms develop abruptly and reach a peak within 10 minutes: [(1) palpitations, pounding heart, or accelerated heart rate; (2) sweating; (3) trembling or shaking; (4) sensations of shortness of breath or smothering; (5) feeling of choking; (6) chest pain or discomfort; (7) nausea or abdominal distress; (8) feeling dizzy, unsteady, lightheaded, or faint; (9) derealization (feelings of unreality) or depersonalization (being detached from oneself); (10) fear of losing control; (11) fear of dying; (12) paresthesias (numbness or tingling sensations); (13) chills or hot flushes.]

Long-term maintenance of efficacy was demonstrated in a 3-month relapse prevention trial. In this trial, patients with panic disorder assigned to paroxetine demonstrated a lower relapse rate compared to patients on placebo (see CLINICAL PHARMACOLOGY). Nevertheless, the physician who prescribes *Paxil* for extended periods should periodically reevaluate the long-term usefulness of the drug for the individual patient.

CONTRAINDICATIONS
Concomitant use in patients taking monoamine oxidase inhibitors (MAOIs) is contraindicated (see WARNINGS and PRECAUTIONS).

WARNINGS
Potential for Interaction with Monoamine Oxidase Inhibitors
In patients receiving another serotonin reuptake inhibitor drug in combination with a monoamine oxidase inhibitor (MAOI), there have been reports of serious, sometimes fatal, reactions including hyperthermia, rigidity, myoclonus, autonomic instability with possible rapid fluctuations of vital signs, and mental status changes that include extreme agitation progressing to delirium and coma. These reactions have also been reported in patients who have recently discontinued that drug and have been started on a MAOI. Some cases presented with features resembling neuroleptic malignant syndrome. While there are no human data showing such an interaction with *Paxil*, limited animal data on the effects of

combined use of paroxetine and MAOIs suggest that these drugs may act synergistically to elevate blood pressure and evoke behavioral excitation. Therefore, it is recommended that Paxil (paroxetine hydrochloride) not be used in combination with a MAOI, or within 14 days of discontinuing treatment with a MAOI. At least 2 weeks should be allowed after stopping Paxil before starting a MAOI.

PRECAUTIONS

General

Activation of Mania/Hypomania: During premarketing testing, hypomania or mania occurred in approximately 1.0% of Paxil-treated unipolar patients compared to 1.1% of active-control and 0.3% of placebo-treated unipolar patients. In a subset of patients classified as bipolar, the rate of manic episodes was 2.2% for Paxil and 11.6% for the combined active-control groups. As with all antidepressants, Paxil should be used cautiously in patients with a history of mania.

Seizures: During premarketing testing, seizures occurred in 0.1% of Paxil-treated patients, a rate similar to that associated with other antidepressants. Paxil should be used cautiously in patients with a history of seizures. It should be discontinued in any patient who develops seizures.

Suicide: The possibility of a suicide attempt is inherent in depression and may persist until significant remission occurs. Close supervision of high-risk patients should accompany initial drug therapy. Prescriptions for Paxil should be written for the smallest quantity of tablets consistent with good patient management, in order to reduce the risk of overdose.

Hyponatremia: Several cases of hyponatremia have been reported. The hyponatremia appeared to be reversible when Paxil was discontinued. The majority of these occurrences have been in elderly individuals, some in patients taking diuretics or who were otherwise volume depleted.

Abnormal Bleeding: There have been several reports of abnormal bleeding (mostly ecchymosis and purpura) associated with paroxetine treatment, including a report of impaired platelet aggregation. While a causal relationship to paroxetine is unclear, impaired platelet aggregation may result from platelet serotonin depletion and contribute to such occurrences.

Use in Patients with Concomitant Illness: Clinical experience with Paxil in patients with certain concomitant systemic illness is limited. Caution is advisable in using Paxil in patients with diseases or conditions that could affect metabolism or hemodynamic responses.

Paxil has not been evaluated or used to any appreciable extent in patients with a recent history of myocardial infarction or unstable heart disease. Patients with these diagnoses were excluded from clinical studies during the product's premarket testing. Evaluation of electrocardiograms of 682 patients who received Paxil in double-blind, placebo-controlled trials, however, did not indicate that Paxil is associated with the development of significant ECG abnormalities. Similarly, Paxil (paroxetine hydrochloride) does not cause any clinically important changes in heart rate or blood pressure.

Increased plasma concentrations of paroxetine occur in patients with severe renal impairment (creatinine clearance < 30 mL/min.) or severe hepatic impairment. A lower starting dose should be used in such patients (see DOSAGE AND ADMINISTRATION).

Information for Patients

Physicians are advised to discuss the following issues with patients for whom they prescribe Paxil:

Interference with Cognitive and Motor Performance: Any psychoactive drug may impair judgment, thinking or motor skills. Although in controlled studies Paxil has not been shown to impair psychomotor performance, patients should be cautioned about operating hazardous machinery, including automobiles, until they are reasonably certain that Paxil therapy does not affect their ability to engage in such activities.

Completing Course of Therapy: While patients may notice improvement with Paxil therapy in 1 to 4 weeks, they should be advised to continue therapy as directed.

Concomitant Medication: Patients should be advised to inform their physician if they are taking, or plan to take, any prescription or over-the-counter drugs, since there is a potential for interactions.

Alcohol: Although Paxil has not been shown to increase the impairment of mental and motor skills caused by alcohol, patients should be advised to avoid alcohol while taking Paxil.

Pregnancy: Patients should be advised to notify their physician if they become pregnant or intend to become pregnant during therapy.

Nursing: Patients should be advised to notify their physician if they are breast-feeding an infant. (See PRECAUTIONS-Nursing Mothers.)

Laboratory Tests

There are no specific laboratory tests recommended.

Drug Interactions

Tryptophan: As with other serotonin reuptake inhibitors, an interaction between paroxetine and tryptophan may occur when they are co-administered. Adverse experiences, consisting primarily of headache, nausea, sweating and dizziness, have been reported when tryptophan was administered to patients taking Paxil (paroxetine hydrochloride). Consequently, concomitant use of Paxil with tryptophan is not recommended.

Monoamine Oxidase Inhibitors: See CONTRAINDICATIONS and WARNINGS.

Warfarin: Preliminary data suggest that there may be a pharmacodynamic interaction (that causes an increased bleeding diathesis in the face of unaltered prothrombin time) between paroxetine and warfarin. Since there is little clinical experience, the concomitant administration of Paxil and warfarin should be undertaken with caution.

Drugs Affecting Hepatic Metabolism: The metabolism and pharmacokinetics of paroxetine may be affected by the induction or inhibition of drug-metabolizing enzymes.

Cimetidine—Cimetidine inhibits many cytochrome P_{450} (oxidative) enzymes. In a study where Paxil (30 mg q.d.) was dosed orally for 4 weeks, steady-state plasma concentrations of paroxetine were increased by approximately 50% during co-administration with oral cimetidine (300 mg t.i.d.) for the final week. Therefore, when these drugs are administered concurrently, dosage adjustment of Paxil after the 20 mg starting dose should be guided by clinical effect. The effect of paroxetine on cimetidine's pharmacokinetics was not studied.

Phenobarbital—Phenobarbital induces many cytochrome P_{450} (oxidative) enzymes. When a single oral 30 mg dose of Paxil was administered at phenobarbital steady state (100 mg q.d. for 14 days), paroxetine AUC and $T_{1/2}$ were reduced (by an average of 25% and 38%, respectively) compared to paroxetine administered alone. The effect of paroxetine on phenobarbital pharmacokinetics was not studied. Since Paxil exhibits nonlinear pharmacokinetics, the results of this study may not address the case where the 2 drugs are both being chronically dosed. No initial Paxil dosage adjustment is considered necessary when co-administered with phenobarbital; any subsequent adjustment should be guided by clinical effect.

Phenytoin—When a single oral 30 mg dose of Paxil was administered at phenytoin steady state (300 mg q.d. for 14 days), paroxetine AUC and $T_{1/2}$ were reduced (by an average of 50% and 35%, respectively) compared to Paxil administered alone. In a separate study, when a single oral 300 mg dose of phenytoin was administered at paroxetine steady state (30 mg q.d. for 14 days), phenytoin AUC was slightly reduced (12% on average) compared to phenytoin administered alone. Since both drugs exhibit nonlinear pharmacokinetics, the above studies may not address the case where the 2 drugs are both being chronically dosed. No initial dosage adjustments are considered necessary when these drugs are co-administered; any subsequent adjustments should be guided by clinical effect. (see ADVERSE REACTIONS-Postmarketing Reports).

Drugs Metabolized by Cytochrome $P_{450}IID_6$: Many drugs, including most antidepressants (paroxetine, other SSRIs and many tricyclics), are metabolized by the cytochrome P_{450} isozyme $P_{450}IID_6$. Like other agents that are metabolized by $P_{450}IID_6$, paroxetine may significantly inhibit the activity of this isozyme. In most patients (> 90%), this $P_{450}IID_6$ isozyme is saturated early during Paxil dosing. In one study, daily dosing of Paxil (20 mg q.d.) under steady-state conditions increased single dose desipramine (100 mg) C_{max}, AUC and $T_{1/2}$ by an average of approximately two-, five- and threefold, respectively. Concomitant use of Paxil with other drugs metabolized by cytochrome $P_{450}IID_6$ has not been formally studied but may require lower doses than usually prescribed for either Paxil or the other drug.

Therefore, co-administration of Paxil with other drugs that are metabolized by this isozyme, including certain antidepressants (e.g., nortriptyline, amitriptyline, imipramine, desipramine and fluoxetine), phenothiazines (e.g., thioridazine) and Type 1C antiarrhythmics (e.g., propafenone, flecainide and encainide), or that inhibit this enzyme (e.g., quinidine), should be approached with caution.

At steady state, when the $P_{450}IID_6$ pathway is essentially saturated, paroxetine clearance is governed by alternative P_{450} isozymes which, unlike $P_{450}IID_6$, show no evidence of saturation. (see PRECAUTIONS-Tricyclic Antidepressants).

Drugs Metabolized by Cytochrome $P_{450}IIIA_4$: An in vivo interaction study involving the co-administration under steady-state conditions of paroxetine and terfenadine, a substrate for cytochrome $P_{450}IIIA_4$, revealed no effect of paroxetine on terfenadine pharmacokinetics. In addition, in vitro studies have shown ketoconazole, a potent inhibitor of $P_{450}IIIA_4$ activity, to be at least 100 times more potent than paroxetine as an inhibitor of the metabolism of several substrates for this enzyme, including terfenadine, astemizole, cisapride, triazolam, and cyclosporin. Based on the assumption that the relationship between paroxetine's in vitro K_i

and its lack of effect on terfenadine's in vivo clearance predicts its effect on other $IIIA_4$ substrates, paroxetine's extent of inhibition of $IIIA_4$ activity is not likely to be of clinical significance.

Tricyclic Antidepressants (TCA): Caution is indicated in the co-administration of tricyclic antidepressants (TCAs) with Paxil, because paroxetine may inhibit TCA metabolism. Plasma TCA concentrations may need to be monitored, and the dose of TCA may need to be reduced, if a TCA is co-administered with Paxil (see PRECAUTIONS-Drugs Metabolized by Cytochrome $P_{450}IID_6$).

Drugs Highly Bound to Plasma Protein: Because paroxetine is highly bound to plasma protein, administration of Paxil to a patient taking another drug that is highly protein bound may cause increased free concentrations of the other drug, potentially resulting in adverse events. Conversely, adverse effects could result from displacement of paroxetine by other highly bound drugs.

Alcohol: Although Paxil does not increase the impairment of mental and motor skills caused by alcohol, patients should be advised to avoid alcohol while taking Paxil (paroxetine hydrochloride).

Lithium: A multiple-dose study has shown that there is no pharmacokinetic interaction between Paxil and lithium carbonate. However, since there is little clinical experience, the concurrent administration of paroxetine and lithium should be undertaken with caution.

Digoxin: The steady-state pharmacokinetics of paroxetine was not altered when administered with digoxin at steady state. Mean digoxin AUC at steady state decreased by 15% in the presence of paroxetine. Since there is little clinical experience, the concurrent administration of paroxetine and digoxin should be undertaken with caution.

Diazepam: Under steady-state conditions, diazepam does not appear to affect paroxetine kinetics. The effects of paroxetine on diazepam were not evaluated.

Procyclidine: Daily oral dosing of Paxil (30 mg q.d.) increased steady-state AUC_{0-24}, C_{max} and C_{min} values of procyclidine (5 mg oral q.d.) by 35%, 37% and 67%, respectively, compared to procyclidine alone at steady state. If anticholinergic effects are seen, the dose of procyclidine should be reduced.

Beta-Blockers: In a study where propranolol (80 mg b.i.d.) was dosed orally for 18 days, the established steady-state plasma concentrations of propranolol were unaltered during co-administration with Paxil (30 mg q.d.) for the final 10 days. The effects of propranolol on paroxetine have not been evaluated. (See ADVERSE REACTIONS-Postmarketing Reports).

Theophylline: Reports of elevated theophylline levels associated with Paxil treatment have been reported. While this interaction has not been formally studied, it is recommended that theophylline levels be monitored when these drugs are concurrently administered.

Electroconvulsive Therapy (ECT): There are no clinical studies of the combined use of ECT and Paxil.

Carcinogenesis, Mutagenesis, Impairment of Fertility

Carcinogenesis: Two-year carcinogenicity studies were conducted in rodents given paroxetine in the diet at 1, 5, and 25 mg/kg/day (mice) and 1, 5, and 20 mg/kg/day (rats). These doses are up to 2.4 (mouse) and 3.9 (rat) times the maximum recommended human dose (MRHD) for depression on a mg/m² basis. Because the MRHD for depression is slightly less than that for OCD (50 mg vs. 60 mg), the doses used in these carcinogenicity studies were only 2.0 (mouse) and 3.2 (rat) times the MRHD for OCD. There was a significantly greater number of male rats in the high-dose group with reticulum cell sarcomas (1/100, 0/50, 0/50 and 4/50 for control, low-, middle- and high-dose groups, respectively) and a significantly increased linear trend across dose groups for the occurrence of lymphoreticular tumors in male rats. Female rats were not affected. Although there was a dose-related increase in the number of tumors in mice, there was no drug-related increase in the number of mice with tumors. The relevance of these findings to humans is unknown.

Mutagenesis: Paroxetine produced no genotoxic effects in a battery of 5 in vitro and 2 in vivo assays that included the following: bacterial mutation assay, mouse lymphoma mutation assay, unscheduled DNA synthesis assay, and tests for cytogenetic aberrations in vivo in mouse bone marrow and in vitro in human lymphocytes and in a dominant lethal test in rats.

Impairment of Fertility: A reduced pregnancy rate was found in reproduction studies in rats at a dose of paroxetine of 15 mg/kg/day which is 2.9 times the MRHD for depression

Continued on next page

Information on the SmithKline Beecham Pharmaceuticals products appearing here is based on the labeling in effect on July 1, 1996. Further information on these and other products may be obtained from the Medical Department, SmithKline Beecham Pharmaceuticals, One Franklin Plaza, Philadelphia, PA 19101.

SmithKline Beecham—Cont.

or 2.4 times the MRHD for OCD on a mg/m² basis. Irreversible lesions occurred in the reproductive tract of male rats after dosing in toxicity studies for 2 to 52 weeks. These lesions consisted of vacuolation of epididymal tubular epithelium at 50 mg/kg/day and atrophic changes in the seminiferous tubules of the testes with arrested spermatogenesis at 25 mg/kg/day (9.8 and 4.9 times the MRHD for depression; 8.2 and 4.1 times the MRHD for OCD and PD on a mg/m² basis).

Pregnancy

Teratogenic Effects–Pregnancy Category C

Reproduction studies were performed at doses up to 50 mg/kg/day in rats and 6 mg/kg/day in rabbits administered during organogenesis. These doses are equivalent to 9.7 (rat) and 2.2 (rabbit) times the maximum recommended human dose (MRHD) for depression (50 mg) and 8.1 (rat) and 1.9 (rabbit) times the MRHD for OCD, on a mg/m² basis. These studies have revealed no evidence of teratogenic effects. However, in rats, there was an increase in pup deaths during the first 4 days of lactation when dosing occurred during the last trimester of gestation and continued throughout lactation. This effect occurred at a dose of 1 mg/kg/day or 0.19 times (mg/m²) the MRHD for depression and at 0.16 times (mg/m²) the MRHD for OCD. The no-effect dose for rat pup mortality was not determined. The cause of these deaths is not known. There are no adequate and well-controlled studies in pregnant women. Because animal reproduction studies are not always predictive of human response, this drug should be used during pregnancy only if the potential benefit justifies the potential risk to the fetus.

Labor and Delivery

The effect of paroxetine on labor and delivery in humans is unknown.

Nursing Mothers

Like many other drugs, paroxetine is secreted in human milk, and caution should be exercised when Paxil (paroxetine hydrochloride) is administered to a nursing woman.

Pediatric Use

Safety and effectiveness in the pediatric population have not been established.

Geriatric Use

In worldwide premarketing Paxil clinical trials, 17% of Paxil-treated patients (approximately 700) were 65 years of age or older. Pharmacokinetic studies revealed a decreased clearance in the elderly, and a lower starting dose is recommended; there were, however, no overall differences in the adverse event profile between elderly and younger patients, and effectiveness was similar in younger and older patients. (See CLINICAL PHARMACOLOGY and DOSAGE AND ADMINISTRATION).

ADVERSE REACTIONS

Associated with Discontinuation of Treatment

Twenty percent of (1,199/6,145) of Paxil patients in worldwide clinical trials in depression and 11.8% (64/542) and 9.4% (44/469) of Paxil patients in worldwide trials in OCD and panic disorder, respectively, discontinued treatment due to an adverse event. The most common events (≥1%) associated with discontinuation and considered to be drug related (i.e., those events associated with dropout at a rate approximately twice or greater for Paxil compared to placebo) included the following:

[See table on top of page.]

Where numbers are not provided the incidence of the adverse events in Paxil patients was not >1% or was greater than or equal to two times the incidence of placebo.

1. Incidence corrected for gender.

Commonly Observed Adverse Events

Depression

The most commonly observed adverse events associated with the use of paroxetine (incidence of 5% or greater and incidence for Paxil at least twice that for placebo, derived from Table 1 below) were: asthenia, sweating, nausea, decreased appetite, somnolence, dizziness, insomnia, tremor, nervousness, ejaculatory disturbance and other male genital disorders.

Obsessive Compulsive Disorder

The most commonly observed adverse events associated with the use of paroxetine (incidence of 5% or greater and incidence for Paxil at least twice that for placebo, derived from Table 2 below) were: nausea, dry mouth, decreased appetite, constipation, dizziness, somnolence, tremor, sweating, impotence and abnormal ejaculation.

Panic Disorder

The most commonly observed adverse events associated with the use of paroxetine (incidence of 5% or greater and incidence for Paxil at least twice that for placebo, derived from Table 2 below were: asthenia, sweating, decreased appetite,

	Depression		OCD		Panic Disorder	
	Paxil	Placebo	Paxil	Placebo	Paxil	Placebo
CNS						
Somnolence	2.3%	0.7%	—		1.9%	0.3%
Insomnia	—		1.7%	0%	1.3%	0.3%
Agitation	1.1%	0.5%	—			
Tremor	1.1%	0.3%	—			
Anxiety	—		—			
Dizziness	—		1.5%	0%		
Gastrointestinal						
Constipation			1.1%	0%		
Nausea	3.2%	1.1%	1.9%	0%	3.2%	1.2%
Diarrhea	1.0%	0.3%				
Dry mouth	1.0%	0.3%				
Vomiting	1.0%	0.3%				
Other						
Asthenia	1.6%	0.4%	1.9%	0.4%		
Abnormal ejaculation[1]	1.6%	0%	2.1%	0%		
Sweating	1.0%	0.3%				
Impotence[1]	—		1.5%	0%		

Table 1. Treatment-Emergent Adverse Experience Incidence in Placebo-Controlled Clinical Trials for Depression[1]

Body System	Preferred Term	Paxil (n=421)	Placebo (n=421)
Body as a Whole	Headache	18%	17%
	Asthenia	15%	6%
Cardiovascular	Palpitation	3%	1%
	Vasodilation	3%	1%
Dermatologic	Sweating	11%	2%
	Rash	2%	1%
Gastrointestinal	Nausea	26%	9%
	Dry Mouth	18%	12%
	Constipation	14%	9%
	Diarrhea	12%	8%
	Decreased Appetite	6%	2%
	Flatulence	4%	2%
	Oropharynx Disorder[2]	2%	0%
	Dyspepsia	2%	1%
Musculoskeletal	Myopathy	2%	1%
	Myalgia	2%	1%
	Myasthenia	1%	0%
Nervous System	Somnolence	23%	9%
	Dizziness	13%	6%
	Insomnia	13%	6%
	Tremor	8%	2%
	Nervousness	5%	3%
	Anxiety	5%	3%
	Paresthesia	4%	2%
	Libido Decreased	3%	0%
	Drugged Feeling	2%	1%
	Confusion	1%	0%
Respiration	Yawn	4%	0%
Special Senses	Blurred Vision	4%	1%
	Taste Perversion	2%	0%
Urogenital System	Ejaculatory Disturbance[3,4]	13%	0%
	Other Male Genital Disorders[3,5]	10%	0%
	Urinary Frequency	3%	1%
	Urination Disorder[6]	3%	0%
	Female Genital Disorders[3,7]	2%	0%

1. Events reported by at least 1% of patients treated with Paxil (paroxetine hydrochloride) are included, except the following: events which had an incidence on placebo ≥ Paxil: abdominal pain, agitation, back pain, chest pain, CNS stimulation, fever, increased appetite, myoclonus, pharyngitis, postural hypotension, respiratory disorder (includes mostly "cold symptoms" or "URI"), trauma and vomiting.
2. Includes mostly "lump in throat" and "tightness in throat."
3. Percentage corrected for gender.
4. Mostly "ejaculatory delay."
5. Includes "anorgasmia," "erectile difficulties," "delayed ejaculation/orgasm," and "sexual dysfunction," and "impotence."
6. Includes mostly "difficulty with micturition" and "urinary hesitancy."
7. Includes mostly "anorgasmia" and "difficulty reaching climax/orgasm."

libido decreased, tremor, abnormal ejaculation, female genital disorders and impotence.

Incidence in Controlled Clinical Trials

Depression

Table 1 enumerates adverse events that occurred at an incidence of 1% or more among paroxetine-treated patients who participated in short term (6-week) placebo-controlled trials in which patients were dosed in a range of 20 to 50 mg/day. Reported adverse events were classified using a standard COSTART-based Dictionary terminology.

The prescriber should be aware that these figures cannot be used to predict the incidence of side effects in the course of usual medical practice where patient characteristics and other factors differ from those which prevailed in the clinical trials. Similarly, the cited frequencies cannot be compared with figures obtained from other clinical investigations involving different treatments, uses and investigators. The

cited figures, however, do provide the prescribing physician with some basis for estimating the relative contribution of drug and nondrug factors to the side effect incidence rate in the population studied.

[See Table 1 above.]

Obsessive Compulsive Disorder and Panic Disorder

Table 2 enumerates adverse events that occurred at a frequency of 2% or more among OCD patients on Paxil who participated in placebo-controlled trials of 12-weeks duration in which patients were dosed in a range of 20 to 60 mg/day or among patients with panic disorder on Paxil who participated in placebo-controlled trials of 10 to 12 weeks duration in which patients were dosed in a range of 10 to 60 mg/day.

[See Table 2 at top of next page.]

Dose Dependency of Adverse Events: A comparison of adverse event rates in a fixed-dose study comparing Paxil 10, 20, 30 and 40 mg/day with placebo in the treatment of de-

pression revealed a clear dose dependency for some of the more common adverse events associated with *Paxil* use, as shown in the following table:

Table 3. Treatment-Emergent Adverse Experience Incidence in a Depression Dose-Comparison Trial*

Body System/ Preferred Term	Placebo n=51	Paxil 10 mg n=102	20 mg n=104	30 mg n=101	40 mg n=102
Body as a Whole					
Asthenia	0.0%	2.9%	10.6%	13.9%	12.7%
Dermatology					
Sweating	2.0%	1.0%	6.7%	8.9%	11.8%
Gastrointestinal					
Constipation	5.9%	4.9%	7.7%	9.9%	12.7%
Decreased Appetite	2.0%	2.0%	5.8%	4.0%	4.9%
Diarrhea	7.8%	9.8%	19.2%	7.9%	14.7%
Dry Mouth	2.0%	10.8%	18.3%	15.8%	20.6%
Nausea	13.7%	14.7%	26.9%	34.7%	36.3%
Nervous System					
Anxiety	0.0%	2.0%	5.8%	5.9%	5.9%
Dizziness	3.9%	6.9%	6.7%	8.9%	12.7%
Nervousness	0.0%	5.9%	5.8%	4.0%	2.9%
Paresthesia	0.0%	2.9%	1.0%	5.0%	5.9%
Somnolence	7.8%	12.7%	18.3%	20.8%	21.6%
Tremor	0.0%	0.0%	7.7%	7.9%	14.7%
Special Senses					
Blurred Vision	2.0%	2.9%	2.9%	2.0%	7.8%
Urogenital System					
Abnormal Ejaculation	0.0%	5.8%	6.5%	10.6%	13.0%
Impotence	0.0%	1.9%	4.3%	6.4%	1.9%
Male Genital Disorders	0.0%	3.8%	8.7%	6.4%	3.7%

*Rule for including adverse events in table: incidence at least 5% for one of paroxetine groups and ≥ twice the placebo incidence for at least one paroxetine group.

In a fixed-dose study comparing placebo and *Paxil* 20, 40 and 60 mg in the treatment of OCD, there was no clear relationship between adverse events and the dose of *Paxil* to which patients were assigned. No new adverse events were observed in the *Paxil* 60 mg dose group compared to any of the other treatment groups.

In a fixed-dose study comparing placebo and *Paxil* 10, 20 and 40 mg in the treatment of panic disorder, there was no clear relationship between adverse events and the dose of *Paxil* to which patients were assigned, except for asthenia, dry mouth, anxiety, libido decreased, tremor and abnormal ejaculation. In flexible dose studies, no new adverse events were observed in patients receiving *Paxil* 60 mg compared to any of the other treatment groups.

Adaptation to Certain Adverse Events: Over a 4- to 6-week period, there was evidence of adaptation to some adverse events with continued therapy (e.g., nausea and dizziness), but less to other effects (e.g., dry mouth, somnolence and asthenia).

Weight and Vital Sign Changes: Significant weight loss may be an undesirable result of treatment with *Paxil* for some patients but, on average, patients in controlled trials had minimal (about 1 pound) weight loss vs. smaller changes on placebo and active control. No significant changes in vital signs (systolic and diastolic blood pressure, pulse and temperature) were observed in patients treated with *Paxil* in controlled clinical trials.

ECG Changes: In an analysis of ECGs obtained in 682 patients treated with *Paxil* and 415 patients treated with placebo in controlled clinical trials, no clinically significant changes were seen in the ECGs of either group.

Liver Function Tests: In placebo-controlled clinical trials, patients treated with *Paxil* exhibited abnormal values on liver function tests at no greater rate than that seen in placebo-treated patients. In particular, the *Paxil*-vs.-placebo comparisons for alkaline phosphatase, SGOT, SGPT and bilirubin revealed no differences in the percentage of patients with marked abnormalities.

Other Events Observed During the Premarketing Evaluation of Paxil (paroxetine hydrochloride)

During its premarketing assessment in depression, multiple doses of *Paxil* were administered to 6,145 patients in phase 2 and 3 studies. The conditions and duration of exposure to *Paxil* varied greatly and included (in overlapping categories) open and double-blind studies, uncontrolled and controlled studies, inpatient and outpatient studies, and fixed-dose and titration studies. During premarketing clinical trials in OCD and panic disorder, 542 and 469 patients, respectively, received multiple doses of *Paxil*. Untoward events associated with this exposure were recorded by clinical investigators using terminology of their own choosing. Consequently, it is not possible to provide a meaningful estimate of the proportion of individuals experiencing adverse events without first

Table 2. Treatment Emergent Adverse Experience Incidence in Placebo-Controlled Clinical Trials for Obsessive Compulsive Disorder and Panic Disorder[1]

Body System	Preferred Term	Obsessive Compulsive Disorder Paxil (n=542)	Placebo (n=265)	Panic Disorder Paxil (n=469)	Placebo (n=324)
Body as a Whole	Asthenia	22%	14%	14%	5%
	Abdominal Pain	—	—	4%	3%
	Chest Pain	3%	2%	—	—
	Back Pain	—	—	3%	2%
	Chills	2%	1%	2%	1%
Cardiovascular	Vasodilation	4%	1%	—	—
	Palpitation	2%	0%	—	—
Dermatologic	Sweating	9%	3%	14%	6%
	Rash	3%	2%	—	—
Gastrointestinal	Nausea	23%	10%	23%	17%
	Dry Mouth	18%	9%	18%	11%
	Constipation	16%	6%	8%	5%
	Diarrhea	10%	10%	12%	7%
	Decreased Appetite	9%	3%	7%	3%
	Increased Appetite	4%	3%	2%	1%
Nervous System	Insomnia	24%	13%	18%	10%
	Somnolence	24%	7%	19%	11%
	Dizziness	12%	6%	14%	10%
	Tremor	11%	1%	9%	1%
	Nervousness	9%	8%	—	—
	Libido Decreased	7%	4%	9%	1%
	Agitation	—	—	5%	4%
	Anxiety	—	—	5%	4%
	Abnormal Dreams	4%	1%	—	—
	Concentration Impaired	3%	2%	—	—
	Depersonalization	3%	0%	—	—
	Myoclonus	3%	0%	3%	2%
	Amnesia	2%	1%	—	—
Respiratory System	Rhinitis	—	—	3%	0%
Special Senses	Abnormal Vision	4%	2%	—	—
	Taste Perversion	2%	0%	—	—
Urogenital System	Abnormal Ejaculation[2]	23%	1%	21%	1%
	Female Genital Disorder[2]	3%	0%	9%	1%
	Impotence[2]	8%	1%	5%	0%
	Urinary Frequency	3%	1%	2%	0%
	Urination Impaired	3%	0%	—	—
	Urinary Tract Infection	2%	1%	2%	1%

1. Events reported by at least 2% of OCD or panic disorder *Paxil*-treated patients are included, except the following events which had an incidence on placebo ≥ *Paxil*: [OCD]: abdominal pain, agitation, anxiety, back pain, cough increased, depression, headache, hyperkinesia, infection, paresthesia, pharyngitis, respiratory disorder, rhinitis and sinusitis. [panic disorder]: abnormal dreams, abnormal vision, chest pain, cough increased, depersonalization, depressions, dysmenorrhea, dyspepsia, flu syndrome, headache, infection, myalgia, nervousness, palpitation, paresthesia, pharyngitis, rash, respiratory disorder, sinusitis, taste perversion, trauma, urination impaired and vasodilation.
2. Percentage corrected for gender.

grouping similar types of untoward events into a smaller number of standardized event categories.

In the tabulations that follow, reported adverse events were classified using a standard COSTART-based Dictionary terminology. The frequencies presented, therefore, represent the proportion of the 7,156 patients exposed to multiple doses of Paxil (paroxetine hydrochloride) who experienced an event of the type cited on at least one occasion while receiving *Paxil*. All reported events are included except those already listed in Tables 1 and 2, those reported in terms so general as to be uninformative and those events where a drug cause was remote. It is important to emphasize that although the events reported occurred during treatment with paroxetine, they were not necessarily caused by it.

Events are further categorized by body system and listed in order of decreasing frequency according to the following definitions: frequent adverse events are those occurring in one or more occasions in at least 1/100 patients (only those not already listed in the tabulated results from placebo-controlled trials appear in this listing); infrequent adverse events are those occurring in 1/100 to 1/1000 patients; rare events are those occurring in fewer than 1/1000 patients. Events of major clinical importance are also described in the PRECAUTIONS section.

Body as a Whole: *frequent:* chills, malaise; *infrequent:* allergic reaction, carcinoma, face edema, moniliasis, neck pain; *rare:* abscess, adrenergic syndrome, cellulitis, neck rigidity, pelvic pain, peritonitis, ulcer.

Cardiovascular System: *frequent:* hypertension, syncope, tachycardia; *infrequent:* bradycardia, conduction abnormalities, electrocardiogram abnormal, hematoma, hypotension, migraine, peripheral vascular disorder; *rare:* angina pectoris, arrhythmia, atrial fibrillation, bundle branch block, cerebral ischemia, cerebrovascular accident, congestive heart failure, heart block, low cardiac output, myocardial infarct, myocardial ischemia, pallor, phlebitis, pulmonary embolus, supraventricular extrasystoles, thrombophlebitis, thrombosis, varicose vein, vascular headache, ventricular extrasystoles.

Digestive System: *infrequent:* bruxism, colitis, dysphagia, eructation, gastroenteritis, gingivitis, glossitis, increased salivation, liver function tests abnormal, mouth ulceration, rectal hemorrhage, ulcerative stomatitis; *rare:* aphthous stomatitis, bloody diarrhea, bulimia, choleithiasis, duodenitis, enteritis, esophagitis, fecal impactions, fecal incontinence, gastritis, gum hemorrhage, hematemesis, hepatitis, ileus, intestinal obstruction, jaundice, melena, peptic ulcer, salivary gland enlargement, stomach ulcer, stomatitis, tongue discoloration, tongue edema, tooth caries, tooth malformation.

Endocrine System: *rare:* diabetes mellitus, hyperthyroidism, hypothyroidism, thyroiditis.

Hemic and Lymphatic Systems: *infrequent:* anemia, leukopenia, lymphadenopathy, purpura; *rare:* abnormal erythrocytes, basophilia, eosinophilia, hypochromic anemia, iron deficiency anemia, leukocytosis, lymphedema, abnormal lymphocytes, lymphocytosis, microcytic anemia, monocytosis, normocytic anemia, thrombocythemia.

Metabolic and Nutritional: *frequent:* edema, weight gain, weight loss; *infrequent:* hyperglycemia, peripheral edema, SGOT increased, SGPT increased, thirst; *rare:* alkaline phosphatase increased, bilirubinemia, BUN increased, creatinine phosphokinase increased, dehydration, gamma globulins increased, gout, hypercalcemia, hypercholesteremia, hyperkalemia, hyperphosphatemia, hypocalcemia, hypoglycemia, hypokalemia, hyponatremia, ketosis, lactic dehydrogenase increased.

Musculoskeletal System: *frequent:* arthralgia; *infrequent:* arthritis; *rare:* arthrosis, bursitis, myositis, osteoporosis, generalized spasm, tenosynovitis, tetany.

Nervous System: *frequent:* amnesia, CNS stimulation, concentration impaired, depression, emotional lability, vertigo; *infrequent:* abnormal thinking, akinesia, alcohol abuse, ataxia, convulsion, depersonalization, dystonia, hallucina-

Continued on next page

Information on the SmithKline Beecham Pharmaceuticals products appearing here is based on the labeling in effect on July 1, 1996. Further information on these and other products may be obtained from the Medical Department, SmithKline Beecham Pharmaceuticals, One Franklin Plaza, Philadelphia, PA 19101.

SmithKline Beecham—Cont.

tions, hostility, hyperkinesia, hypertonia, hypesthesia, incoordination, lack of emotion, manic reaction, neurosis, paralysis, paranoid reaction; *rare:* abnormal electroencephalogram, abnormal gait, antisocial reaction, aphasia, choreoathetosis, circumoral paresthesias, delirium, delusions, diplopia, drug dependence, dysarthria, dyskinesia, euphoria, extrapyramidal syndrome, fasciculations, grand mal convulsion, hyperalgesia, hypokinesia, hysteria, libido increased, manic-depressive reaction, meningitis, myelitis, neuralgia, neuropathy, nystagmus, peripheral neuritis, psychosis, psychotic depression, reflexes decreased, reflexes increased, stupor, trismus, withdrawal syndrome.

Respiratory System: frequent: cough increased, rhinitis; *infrequent:* asthma, bronchitis, dyspnea, epistaxis, hyperventilation, pneumonia, respiratory flu, sinusitis, voice alteration; *rare:* emphysema, hemoptysis, hiccups, lung fibrosis, pulmonary edema, sputum increased.

Skin and Appendages: frequent: pruritus; *infrequent:* acne, alopecia, dry skin, ecchymosis, eczema, furunculosis, urticaria; *rare:* angioedema, contact dermatitis, erythema nodosum, erythema multiforme, fungal dermatitis, herpes simplex, herpes zoster, hirsutism, maculopapular rash, photosensitivity, seborrhea, skin discoloration, skin hypertrophy, skin ulcer, vesiculobullous rash.

Special Senses: frequent: tinnitus; *infrequent:* abnormality of accommodation, conjunctivitis, ear pain, eye pain, mydriasis, otitis media, taste loss, visual field defect; *rare:* amblyopia, aniso croia, blepharitis, cataract, conjunctival edema, corneal ulcer, deafness, exophthalmos, eye hemorrhage, glaucoma, hyperacusis, keratoconjunctivitis, night blindness, otitis externa, parosmia, photophobia, ptosis, retinal hemorrhage.

Urogenital System: infrequent: abortion, amenorrhea, breast pain, cystitis, dysmenorrhea, dysuria, hematuria, menorrhagia, nocturia, polyuria, urethritis, urinary incontinence, urinary retention, urinary urgency, vaginitis; *rare:* breast atrophy, breast carcinoma, breast enlargement, breast neoplasm, epididymitis, female lactation, fibrocystic breast, kidney calculus, kidney function abnormal, kidney pain, leukorrhea, mastitis, metrorrhagia, nephritis, oliguria, prostatic carcinoma, pyuria, urethritis, uterine spasm, urolith, vaginal moniliasis, vaginal hemorrhage.

Postmarketing Reports

Voluntary reports of adverse events in patients taking *Paxil* that have been received since market introduction and not listed above that may have no causal relationship with the drug include acute pancreatitis, elevated liver function tests (the most severe cases were deaths due to liver necrosis, and grossly elevated transaminases associated with severe liver dysfunction), Guillain-Barré syndrome, toxic epidermal necrolysis, priapism, thrombocytopenia, syndrome of inappropriate ADH secretion, symptoms suggestive of prolactinemia and galactorrhea, neuroleptic malignant syndrome-like events; extrapyramidal symptoms which have included akathisia, bradykinesia, cogwheel rigidity, dystonia, hypertonia, oculogyric crisis which has been associated with concomitant use of pimozide, tremor and trismus; and serotonin syndrome, associated in some cases with concomitant use of serotonergic drugs and with drugs which may have impaired *Paxil* metabolism (symptoms have included agitation, confusion, diaphoresis, hallucinations, hyperreflexia, myoclonus, shivering, tachycardia and tremor). There have been spontaneous reports that abrupt discontinuation may lead to symptoms such as dizziness, sensory disturbances, agitation or anxiety, nausea and sweating; these events are generally self-limiting. There has been a case report of an elevated phenytoin level after 4 weeks of *Paxil* and phenytoin co-administration. There has been a case report of severe hypotension when *Paxil* was added to chronic metoprolol treatment.

DRUG ABUSE AND DEPENDENCE

Controlled Substance Class: Paxil (paroxetine hydrochloride) is not a controlled substance.

Physical and Psychologic Dependence: Paxil has not been systematically studied in animals or humans for its potential for abuse, tolerance or physical dependence. While the clinical trials did not reveal any tendency for any drug-seeking behavior, these observations were not systematic and it is not possible to predict on the basis of this limited experience the extent to which a CNS-active drug will be misused, diverted and/or abused once marketed. Consequently, patients should be evaluated carefully for history of drug abuse, and such patients should be observed closely for signs of *Paxil* misuse or abuse (e.g., development of tolerance, incrementations of dose, drug-seeking behavior).

OVERDOSAGE

Human Experience: No deaths were reported following acute overdose with *Paxil* alone or in combination with other drugs and/or alcohol (18 cases, with doses up to 850 mg) during premarketing clinical trials in depression, OCD, and panic disorder. Signs and symptoms of overdose with *Paxil* included: nausea, vomiting, drowsiness, sinus tachycardia

and dilated pupils. There were no reports of ECG abnormalities, coma or convulsions following overdosage with *Paxil* alone.

Overdosage Management: Treatment should consist of those general measures employed in the management of overdosage with any antidepressant. There are no specific antidotes for *Paxil.* Establish and maintain an airway; ensure adequate oxygenation and ventilation. Gastric evacuation either by the induction of emesis or lavage or both should be performed. In most cases, following evacuation, 20 to 30 grams of activated charcoal may be administered every 4 to 6 hours during the first 24 to 48 hours after ingestion. An ECG should be taken and monitoring of cardiac function instituted if there is any evidence of abnormality. Supportive care with frequent monitoring of vital signs and careful observation is indicated. Due to the large volume of distribution of *Paxil,* forced diuresis, dialysis, hemoperfusion and exchange transfusion are unlikely to be of benefit.

A specific caution involves patients taking or recently having taken paroxetine who might ingest by accident or intent excessive quantities of a tricyclic antidepressant. In such a case, accumulation of the parent tricyclic and its active metabolite may increase the possibility of clinically significant sequelae and extend the time needed for close medical observation.

In managing overdosage, consider the possibility of multiple-drug involvement. The physician should consider contacting a poison control center for additional information on the treatment of any overdose. Telephone numbers for certified poison control centers are listed in the *Physicians' Desk Reference* (PDR).

DOSAGE AND ADMINISTRATION

Depression

Usual Initial Dosage: Paxil (paroxetine hydrochloride) should be administered as a single daily dose, usually in the morning. The recommended initial dose is 20 mg/day. Patients were dosed in a range of 20 to 50 mg/day in the clinical trials demonstrating the antidepressant effectiveness of *Paxil.* As with all antidepressants, the full antidepressant effect may be delayed. Some patients not responding to a 20 mg dose may benefit from dose increases, in 10 mg/day increments, up to a maximum of 50 mg/day. Dose changes should occur at intervals of at least 1 week.

Maintenance Therapy: There is no body of evidence available to answer the question of how long the patient treated with *Paxil* should remain on it. It is generally agreed that acute episodes of depression require several months or longer of sustained pharmacologic therapy. Whether the dose of an antidepressant needed to induce remission is identical to the dose needed to maintain and/or sustain euthymia is unknown.

Systematic evaluation of the efficacy of *Paxil* (paroxetine hydrochloride) has shown that efficacy is maintained for periods of up to 1 year with doses that averaged about 30 mg.

Obsessive Compulsive Disorder

Usual Initial Dosage: Paxil should be administered as a single daily dose, usually in the morning. The recommended dose of *Paxil* in the treatment of OCD is 40 mg daily. Patients should be started on 20 mg/day and the dose can be increased in 10 mg/day increments. Dose changes should occur at intervals of at least 1 week. Patients were dosed in a range of 20 to 60 mg/day in the clinical trials demonstrating the effectiveness of *Paxil* in the treatment of OCD. The maximum dosage should not exceed 60 mg/day.

Maintenance Therapy: Long-term maintenance of efficacy was demonstrated in a 6-month relapse prevention trial. In this trial, patients with OCD assigned to paroxetine demonstrated a lower relapse rate compared to patients on placebo (see Clinical Pharmacology). OCD is a chronic condition, and it is reasonable to consider continuation for a responding patient. Dosage adjustments should be made to maintain the patient on the lowest effective dosage, and patients should be periodically reassessed to determine the need for continued treatment.

Panic Disorder

Usual Initial Dosage: Paxil should be administered as a single daily dose, usually in the morning. The target dose of *Paxil* in the treatment of panic disorder is 40 mg/day. Patients should be started on 10 mg/day. Dose changes should occur in 10 mg/week increments and at intervals of at least 1 week. Patients were dosed in a range of 10 to 60 mg/day in the clinical trials demonstrating the effectiveness of *Paxil.* The maximum dosage should not exceed 60 mg/day.

Maintenance Therapy: Long-term maintenance of efficacy was demonstrated in a 3-month relapse prevention trial. In this trial, patients with panic disorder assigned to paroxetine demonstrated a lower relapse rate compared to patients on placebo (see CLINICAL PHARMACOLOGY). Panic disorder is a chronic condition, and it is reasonable to consider continuation for a responding patient. Dosage adjustments should be made to maintain the patient on the lowest effective dosage, and patients should be periodically reassessed to determine the need for continued treatment.

Dosage for Elderly or Debilitated, and Patients with Severe Renal or Hepatic Impairment: The recommended initial dose is 10 mg/day for elderly patients, debilitated patients, and/or patients with severe renal or hepatic impairment. Increases may be made if indicated. Dosage should not exceed 40 mg/day.

Switching Patients to or from a Monoamine Oxidase Inhibitor: At least 14 days should elapse between discontinuation of a MAOI and initiation of *Paxil* therapy. Similarly, at least 14 days should be allowed after stopping *Paxil* before starting a MAOI.

HOW SUPPLIED

Paxil is supplied as film-coated, modified-oval tablets as follows:

10 mg yellow tablets engraved on the front with PAXIL and on the back with 10.

    NDC 0029-3210-13 Bottles of 30

20 mg pink, scored tablets engraved on the front with PAXIL and on the back with 20.

    NDC 0029-3211-13 Bottles of 30
    NDC 0029-3211-20 Bottles of 100
    NDC 0029-3211-21 SUP 100's (intended for institutional use only)

30 mg blue tablets engraved on the front with PAXIL and on the back with 30.

    NDC 0029-3212-13 Bottles of 30

40 mg green tablets engraved on the front with PAXIL and on the back with 40.

    NDC 0029-3213-13 Bottles of 30

Store between (15° and 30°C; 59° and 86°F).

Veterans Administration/Military/PHS—Tablets, 20 mg, 30's 6505-01-371-8323; 20 mg, 100's, 6505-01-371-8322; 20 mg, SUP, 100's 6505-01-371-8321; 30 mg, 30's, 6505-01-371-8320.
PX:L10

Shown in Product Identification Guide, page 337

RABIES VACCINE ADSORBED   ℞

DESCRIPTION

Rabies Vaccine Adsorbed is a sterile, cell-culture derived rabies vaccine for pre- and post-exposure prophylaxis in humans. It is prepared with the CVS Kissling/MDPH strain of rabies virus. The virus is propagated in a diploid cell line derived from fetal rhesus lung cells (FRhL-2 cell line) in a serum-free, chemically defined, antibiotic-free medium. The virus harvest, which is clarified by centrifugation and filtration, is inactivated with betapropiolactone. After inactivation, the virus is adsorbed to aluminum phosphate.

The final vaccine is a suspension containing 2.5 international units or more of rabies antigen per 1.0 mL dose. It contains no more than 2.0 mg aluminum phosphate per mL and also contains 0.01% sodium ethylmercurithiosalicylate (thimerosal) as a preservative. The solution is a light pink color due to the presence of phenol red.

Rabies Vaccine Adsorbed is intended for intramuscular (IM) injection. CAUTION: THIS VACCINE IS NOT FOR USE BY THE INTRADERMAL (ID) ROUTE.

CLINICAL PHARMACOLOGY

The immune response to rabies vaccines can be ascertained by measuring antibody directed against rabies virus by means of the rapid fluorescent focus inhibition test (RFFIT). Serum antibody levels against rabies virus are usually expressed in terms of international units or serum titers. The definition of a minimally acceptable antibody titer in vaccinees varies among laboratories and is dependent on the type of test performed. The Centers for Disease Control considers complete virus neutralization at a 1:5 serum dilution by the RFFIT a minimally acceptable response to pre-exposure vaccination. The World Health Organization specifies that a minimum titer of 0.5 international units is an adequate response to vaccination.

In field trials of Rabies Vaccine Adsorbed, 99% or greater of 1,567 persons who had not been immunized previously against rabies responded with serum titers of 0.5 international units (a dilution titer of approximately 1:25) or greater by 2 weeks after the last of 3 IM injections of Rabies Vaccine Adsorbed given over a 3- or 4-week period. At 9 to 12 months post-immunization, 97% of 605 persons had antibody titers at or above a level of 0.1 international units (a 1:5 dilution of serum). In addition, 97% or more of 2,148 persons previously immunized with Duck Embryo Rabies Vaccine, Human Diploid Rabies Vaccine or Rabies Vaccine Adsorbed showed 4-fold increased antibody titers following a single booster injection of Rabies Vaccine Adsorbed.

In post-exposure field trials and clinical simulations of post-exposure prophylaxis, 5 doses of Rabies Vaccine Adsorbed, in conjunction with Rabies Immune Globulin, induced active antibody production in all previously unvaccinated persons between the seventh and fourteenth day following initiation of treatment. In post-exposure rabies prophylaxis, Rabies Immune Globulin is given concomitantly with the first injection of rabies vaccine to provide immediate passive immunoprophylaxis. If not given when vaccination was begun, Ra-

bies Immune Globulin may be given up to 7 days after administration of the first dose of vaccine.

Rabies Vaccine Adsorbed has been used successfully to immunize both adults and children 6 years of age and older. There have been reports of possible vaccine failures when human diploid cell rabies vaccine (HDCV) has been administered in the gluteal area. Subcutaneous fat in the gluteal area may interfere with the immunogenicity of HDCV.[1-3] It is not known if an adequate response would be obtained after gluteal administration of Rabies Vaccine Adsorbed. Therefore, adults and older children should receive this vaccine in the deltoid muscle. For younger children the anterolateral aspect of the thigh is also acceptable.

INDICATIONS AND USAGE

Rabies Vaccine Adsorbed is indicated for immunization against rabies in the following circumstances: primary pre-exposure immunization which is intended to induce immunity before exposure to the virus; pre-exposure booster immunization which is intended to augment or reinforce the level of immunity induced by previous immunization against rabies; or post-exposure prophylaxis which is given to persons who, in the judgment of the treating physician, may have been exposed to rabies virus. Each circumstance requires a different schedule of injections.

A. **Primary Pre-Exposure Vaccination** (see Table 1): Pre-exposure vaccination is given to persons who are at greater than usual risk of possible rabies exposure by reason of occupation or avocation. The list of such persons includes, but is not limited to, veterinarians and staff, certain laboratory workers, animal handlers and persons spending time (e.g., 1 month or more) in foreign countries where canine rabies is enzootic. Persons whose vocational or avocational pursuits bring them into contact with potentially rabid dogs, cats, foxes, skunks, raccoons, bats or other species at risk of having rabies should also be considered for pre-exposure prophylaxis.

Pre-exposure vaccination is given as a series of 3 individual injections of Rabies Vaccine Adsorbed with the second and third injections being given 7 and 21 or 28 days after the first injection, respectively. Pre-exposure vaccination does not eliminate the need for prompt post-exposure prophylaxis following an exposure; it only eliminates the need for Rabies Immune Globulin and reduces the number of injections of rabies vaccine needed for post-exposure prophylaxis. Criteria for pre-exposure vaccination are summarized in Table 1.

B. **Pre-Exposure Booster Vaccination** (see Table 1): Pre-exposure booster vaccination is given to persons who have received previous rabies vaccination and remain at increased risk of rabies exposure by reasons of occupation or avocation. Persons who work with live rabies virus in research laboratories or vaccine production facilities (continuous-risk category; see Table 1) should have a serum sample tested for rabies antibody every 6 months. Booster doses of vaccine should be given to maintain a serum titer corresponding to at least complete neutralization at a 1:5 serum dilution by the RFFIT. The frequent-risk category includes other laboratory workers, such as those doing rabies diagnostic testing, spelunkers, veterinarians and staff, animal-control and wildlife officers in areas where animal rabies is epizootic, and international travelers living or visiting (for > 30 days) in areas where canine rabies is endemic. Persons among this group should have a serum sample tested for rabies antibody every 2 years and, if the titer is less than complete neutralization at a 1:5 serum dilution by the RFFIT, should have a booster dose of vaccine. Alternatively, a booster can be administered in lieu of a titer determination. Veterinarians and animal-control and wildlife officers working in areas of low rabies enzooticity (infrequent-exposure group) do not require routine pre-exposure booster doses of Rabies Vaccine Adsorbed after completion of primary pre-exposure vaccination (Table 1).

A single booster injection of Rabies Vaccine Adsorbed has been shown to increase antibody titers in persons who have previously been immunized with Rabies Vaccine Adsorbed or Human Diploid Cell Rabies Vaccine. Persons who have been shown to have developed antibody responses to a previous series of injections of Duck Embryo Rabies Vaccine also respond to a single booster dose of Rabies Vaccine Adsorbed.

[See Tables 1 and 2 above.]

C. **Post-Exposure Prophylaxis:** Factors to be considered for appropriate post-exposure antirabies treatment are given in Table 2.[4,5] These include the species of animal with which the person has had contact, the circumstances of the biting incident and vaccination status of the exposing animal, the type of exposure and the previous rabies immunization history of the person exposed. Carnivorous wild animals (especially skunks, raccoons and foxes) and bats are the animals most commonly infected with rabies and the cause of most of the indigenous cases of human rabies in the United States since 1960. In contrast, with the exception of woodchucks, rodents (such

PRE-EXPOSURE VACCINATION. Primary pre-exposure vaccination consists of 3 doses of Rabies Vaccine Adsorbed, 1.0 mL, IM (i.e., deltoid area), 1 each on days 0, 7 and 21 or 28. Administration of routine booster doses of vaccine depends on exposure risk category as noted below.

Table 1. Pre-Exposure Vaccination Criteria*

Criteria for Pre-Exposure Vaccination

Risk Category	Nature of Risk	Typical Populations	Pre-Exposure Regimen
Continuous	Virus present continuously, often in high concentrations. Aerosol, mucous membrane, bite or non-bite exposure possible. Exposure may go unrecognized.	Rabies research laboratory workers†; rabies biologics production workers.	Primary course. Serology every 6 months; booster vaccination when antibody level falls below acceptable level.‡
Frequent	Exposure usually episodic, with source recognized, but exposure may also be unrecognized. Aerosol, mucous membrane, bite or non-bite exposure.	Rabies diagnostic laboratory workers,† spelunkers, veterinarians and staff, and animal-control and wildlife workers in rabies enzootic areas; travelers visiting foreign areas of enzootic rabies for more than 30 days.	Primary course. Serologic testing or booster vaccination every 2 years.‡
Infrequent (greater than population at large)	Exposure nearly always episodic with source recognized. Mucous membrane, bite or non-bite exposure.	Veterinarians and animal-control and wildlife workers in areas of low rabies enzooticity. Veterinary students.	Primary course. No serologic testing or booster vaccination.
Rare (population at large)	Exposure always episodic. Mucous membrane or bite with source recognized.	U.S. population at large, including individuals in rabies enzootic areas.	No vaccination necessary.

* References 4 and 5.
†Judgment of relative risk and extra monitoring of immunization status is the responsibility of the laboratory supervisor (see U.S. Department of Health and Human Services' Biosafety in *Microbiological and Biomedical Laboratories*, 1984).
‡Pre-exposure booster vaccination consists of 1 dose of Rabies Vaccine Adsorbed, 1.0 mL dose intramuscular (deltoid muscle). Minimum acceptable antibody level is complete virus neutralization at a 1:5 serum dilution by RFFIT. Administer booster dose if titer falls below 1:5.

Table 2. Rabies Post-Exposure Prophylaxis Guide*

Animal Type	Evaluation and Disposition of Animal	Post-Exposure Prophylaxis Recommendations
Dogs and cats	Healthy and available for 10 days' observation	Should not begin prophylaxis unless animal develops symptoms of rabies†
	Rabid or suspected rabid	Immediate vaccination
	Unknown (escaped)	Consult public health officials
Skunks, raccoons, bats, foxes and most other carnivores; woodchucks	Regarded as rabid unless geographic area is known to be free of rabies or until animal proven negative by laboratory tests‡	Immediate vaccination
Livestock, rodents and lagomorphs (rabbits and hares)	Consider individually	Consult public health officials. Bites of squirrels, hamsters, guinea pigs, gerbils, chipmunks, rats, mice, other rodents, rabbits and hares almost never require antirabies treatment.

* References 4 and 5.
†During the 10-day holding period, begin treatment with Rabies Vaccine Adsorbed with or without Rabies Immune Globulin (Human) at first sign of rabies in a dog or cat that has bitten someone (see Post-Exposure Prophylaxis below). The symptomatic animal should be killed immediately and tested.
‡The animal should be killed and tested as soon as possible. Holding for observation is not recommended. Discontinue vaccine if immunofluorescence test results of the animal are negative.

as squirrels, hamsters, guinea pigs, gerbils, chipmunks, rats and mice) and lagomorphs (including rabbits and hares) are rarely found to be infected with rabies and have not been known to cause human rabies in the United States. The likelihood that a domestic dog or cat is infected with rabies varies from region to region and depends, in part, on the vaccination history of the animal. In addition, an unprovoked attack is more likely than a provoked attack to indicate that an animal is rabid. Moreover, rabies is transmitted by introducing the virus into open wounds or mucous membranes. Thus, the likelihood of rabies infection depends, in part, on whether the exposure occurred by penetrating the skin or by contamination of mucous membranes by saliva or other potentially infectious material. Physicians should evaluate each possible exposure to rabies and, if necessary, consult with their state or local public health officials regarding the need for rabies prophylaxis.

1. Local Treatment of Wounds: Immediate and thorough washing of all bite wounds and scratches with soap and water is perhaps the most effective measure for preventing rabies. In experimental animals, simple local wound cleaning has been shown to reduce markedly the likelihood of rabies. Tetanus prophylaxis and measures to control bacterial infection should be given as indicated.

2. Specific Treatment: RABIES VACCINE ADSORBED IS NOT INTENDED FOR USE IN PATIENTS KNOWN TO HAVE CLINICAL MANIFESTATION OF RABIES. The injection schedule for post-exposure prophylaxis depends on whether the patient has had or has not had previous vaccination against rabies. For persons who have not previously been vaccinated against rabies, the schedule consists of an initial injection IM of Rabies Immune Globulin (Human) (HRIG), 20 international units per kilogram body weight in total. If anatomically feasible, up to half the dose of HRIG should be thoroughly infiltrated around the wound(s) and the remainder should be administered IM in the gluteal region (for specific instructions for HRIG use, see the product package insert). The HRIG injection is followed by a series of 5 individual injections

Continued on next page

Information on the SmithKline Beecham Pharmaceuticals products appearing here is based on the labeling in effect on July 1, 1996. Further information on these and other products may be obtained from the Medical Department, SmithKline Beecham Pharmaceuticals, One Franklin Plaza, Philadelphia, PA 19101.

SmithKline Beecham—Cont.

of Rabies Vaccine Adsorbed given IM on days 0, 3, 7, 14 and 28. The HRIG and Rabies Vaccine Adsorbed should be given at separate sites using separate syringes. Post-exposure rabies prophylaxis should begin the same day exposure occurred or as soon after exposure as possible. The combined use of HRIG and Rabies Vaccine Adsorbed is recommended for both bite and non-bite exposures, regardless of the interval between exposure and initiation of treatment. The sooner treatment is begun after exposure, the better. However, there have been instances in which the decision to begin treatment was made as late as 6 months or longer after exposure due to delay in recognition that an exposure had occurred. Post-exposure antirabies vaccine should always include administration of both passive antibody and vaccination with the exception of persons who have previously received complete vaccination regimens (pre-exposure or post-exposure) with a cell culture vaccine, or persons who have been vaccinated with other types of vaccines and have had documented rabies antibody titers. Persons who have previously received rabies vaccination are given 2 IM doses of Rabies Vaccine Adsorbed: 1 on day 0 and another on day 3. They should not be given HRIG.

3. Treatment Outside the United States: If post-exposure prophylaxis is begun outside the United States with locally produced biologics, it may be desirable to provide additional treatment when the patient reaches the United States. State health departments should be contacted for specific advice in each case.[4]

CONTRAINDICATIONS

Rabies Vaccine Adsorbed is contraindicated in persons who have had life-threatening allergic reactions to previous injections of this vaccine or to components of this vaccine, including thimerosal. No such reactions have been seen to date but are theoretically possible since less severe allergic reactions have been observed. Persons who have experienced non-life-threatening allergic reactions to Rabies Vaccine Adsorbed may receive additional injections under appropriate medical supervision, if the indications for vaccination justify the risk and vaccines are not available to which the patient has not had a reaction.

WARNINGS

Pre-exposure immunization should be delayed in persons with an acute intercurrent illness.

Rabies Vaccine Adsorbed should be injected into the deltoid muscle unless the use of that muscle is contraindicated. As is the case in giving any adsorbed vaccine, care should be taken to avoid accidently depositing Rabies Vaccine Adsorbed in close approximation to a peripheral nerve or in adipose and subcutaneous tissue.

PRECAUTIONS

General: In adults and children, the vaccine should be injected into the deltoid muscle. In small children, the mid-lateral aspect of the thigh area may be preferable.

As with the injection of any biologic material that may induce an allergic reaction, epinephrine injection (1:1,000) should be available for immediate use should an anaphylactic reaction occur.

This vaccine should be given with caution to persons who are known to be sensitive to or allergic to monkey proteins. If a patient known to be allergic to monkey proteins has been exposed to a known rabid animal, and if no other rabies vaccine is available, then administration of Rabies Vaccine Adsorbed to the allergic patient should be done under the supervision of a physician qualified in the management of allergic reactions. Local or mild post-vaccination reactions are not a contraindication to continuing immunization.

Drug Interactions: Immunosuppressive agents, antimalarials and immunosuppressive diseases can interfere with development of active immunity after vaccination and may reduce the effectiveness of rabies vaccine. Immunosuppressive agents should not be given during post-exposure therapy unless essential for treatment of other conditions. When post-exposure prophylaxis is given to immunosuppressed persons, it is important that serum be tested for rabies antibody to ensure that an adequate response occurred.

Laboratory Tests: Routine testing for rabies antibody response to vaccination is not necessary. Experience from clinical trials documented that antibodies can be detected consistently in serum samples obtained approximately 2 weeks after the last injection. For immunosuppressed persons see Drug Interactions.

Pregnancy Category C: Animal reproduction studies have not been conducted with Rabies Vaccine Adsorbed. It is also not known whether Rabies Vaccine Adsorbed can cause fetal harm when administered to a pregnant woman or can affect reproductive capacity. Rabies Vaccine Adsorbed should be given to a pregnant woman only if clearly needed.

Pediatric Use: Rabies Vaccine Adsorbed has been administered to children as young as 6 years old without noticeable difference in effects from its administration to adults. All children from whom post-vaccination serum was obtained showed rabies antibody titers greater than 1:5. However, because of the limited experience with this vaccine in children, special precautions should be taken for unexpected adverse events.

ADVERSE REACTIONS

Once initiated, rabies prophylaxis should not be interrupted due to mild local or systemic reactions.

Local: Approximately 65% to 70% of persons given IM injections of Rabies Vaccine Adsorbed reported subjective mild, transient discomfort localized to the injection site. In a few, aching of the injected muscle and a mild local inflammatory reaction consisting of swelling, induration or erythema were present for 48 hours. These local complaints can usually be successfully treated with simple analgesics.

Systemic: Mild, transient constitutional reactions have been reported by 8% to 10% of Rabies Vaccine Adsorbed recipients. These consisted chiefly of headache, nausea, slight fever or fatigue. Also, serum-sickness-like reactions, some with arthralgia, suggestive of hypersensitivity to Rabies Vaccine Adsorbed, have been reported in less than 1% of vaccinees between 7 and 14 days after vaccination. These hypersensitivity reactions have occurred after booster vaccination, but have not been seen following primary immunization with Rabies Vaccine Adsorbed.

The occurrence of allergic reactions in patients receiving either Rabies Vaccine Adsorbed or Human Diploid Cell Rabies Vaccine raises special difficulties for the managing physician. The use of pre-exposure booster doses of Human Diploid Cell Rabies Vaccine has been limited by the observation of serum-sickness-like allergic reactions that occur in approximately 6% of individuals who receive boosters with that vaccine.[5] These reactions are thought to be due to small amounts of human serum albumin that have been rendered allergenic by betapropiolactone. Human serum albumin is not used in the medium used to grow the rabies virus for Rabies Vaccine Adsorbed and therefore is not present when betapropiolactone is added to inactivate the virus. Nevertheless, systemic allergic reactions have also occurred in some individuals following booster doses of Rabies Vaccine Adsorbed at a rate of less than 1%. However, it is not known whether patients who are allergic to Rabies Vaccine Adsorbed are also allergic to Human Diploid Cell Rabies Vaccine and vice versa. Thus, judgments must be made regarding whether or not to continue the vaccination schedule and whether or not to change the vaccines.

Other: Neurologic reactions such as those reported to be temporally associated with the administration of other viral vaccines, including Human Diploid Cell Rabies Vaccine, for example, allergic peripheral neuritis, encephalomyelitis or transverse myelitis, have not been reported in recipients of Rabies Vaccine Adsorbed.

If serious adverse reactions are noted, report them promptly to the manufacturer: Michigan Department of Public Health, 517-335-8050 during working hours or 517-335-9030 at other times. Reports may also be submitted directly to the FDA on form FDA-1639, single copies of which may be obtained from the Division of Epidemiology and Surveillance (HFN-730), 5600 Fishers Lane, Rockville, MD 20857.

DOSAGE AND ADMINISTRATION

Each vial of Rabies Vaccine Adsorbed contains a sufficient volume of vaccine to enable withdrawing a full dose of 1.0 mL. The vial should be shaken gently before withdrawing the vaccine to ensure complete suspension of the aluminum phosphate adjuvant. The vaccine should be given IM. THIS VACCINE IS NOT FOR USE BY THE ID ROUTE. Before injecting the vaccine, the syringe barrel should be retracted sufficiently to create a back-pressure to ascertain whether the needle is in the lumen of a blood vessel.

In adults and children, the site of the injection is the deltoid muscle. Administration into the buttock is not recommended since experience with other vaccines has shown that acceptable antibody titers may not be obtained.[3] In small children, who may have insufficient deltoid muscle mass, the anterolateral aspect of the thigh is an acceptable injection site.

Pre-Exposure Vaccination: Pre-exposure vaccination consists of three 1.0 mL IM injections of rabies vaccine, 1 each given at 0, 7 and 21 or 28 days. (Also see Table 1.)

Booster Vaccination: Booster vaccination consists of a single 1.0 mL IM injection of vaccine.

Post-Exposure Prophylaxis: Post-exposure prophylaxis for persons not previously vaccinated against rabies consists of an injection of HRIG, 20 international units per kilogram body weight, and five 1.0 mL injections of Rabies Vaccine Adsorbed, intramuscularly, 1 each to be given on days 0, 3, 7, 14 and 28. The amount of HRIG administered should not exceed the recommended amount. Post-exposure prophylaxis for persons who have been previously vaccinated against rabies consists of two 1.0 mL IM injections of Rabies Vaccine Adsorbed: 1 at day 0 and the second on day 3. HRIG should not be given. Persons should be considered to have been immunized previously if they received pre- or post-exposure prophylaxis with Rabies Vaccine Adsorbed or Human Diploid Cell Rabies Vaccine or have been documented to have had an adequate antibody response to Duck Embryo Rabies Vaccine. (Also see Table 2.)

Parenteral drug products should be inspected for particulate matter and discoloration prior to administration, whenever solution and container permit. This vaccine should have a light pink color due to the presence of phenol red in a neutral solution. Do not use vials that are discolored or contain particulate matter.

HOW SUPPLIED

Rabies Vaccine Adsorbed is supplied in a single-dose, rubber-stoppered vial which contains sufficient volume to enable withdrawing a full 1.0 mL dose.

Package of 1: NDC 0007-4840-01

STORAGE

Rabies Vaccine Adsorbed should be stored at 2° to 8°C (35° to 46°F). Do not freeze; discard if product has been frozen.

REFERENCES

1. Shill, M., Baynes, R.D., and Miller, S.D.: Fatal Rabies Encephalitis Despite Appropriate Post-Exposure Prophylaxis. *N. Engl. J. Med.* 316:1257–1258, 1987.
2. Baer, G.M., and Fishbein, D.B.: Rabies Post-Exposure Prophylaxis. *N. Engl. J. Med.* 316:1270–1272, 1987.
3. Centers for Disease Control: Human Rabies Despite Treatment with Rabies Immune Globulin and Human Diploid Cell Rabies Vaccine—Thailand. *MMWR.* 36:(November 27) 757–760, 765, 1987.
4. Centers for Disease Control: Rabies Prevention—United States, 1991: Recommendations of the Immunization Practices Advisory Committee (ACIP). *MMWR.* 40 (No. RR-3): 1–19, 1991.
5. Centers for Disease Control: Rabies Vaccine Adsorbed: A New Rabies Vaccine for Use in Humans. *MMWR.* April 1988.

Additional References

6. Corey, L., and Hattwick, M.A.W.: Treatment of Persons Exposed to Rabies. *JAMA.* 232:272–276, 1975.
7. Burgoyne, G.H., Kajiya, K.D., Brown, D.W., and Mitchell, J.R.: Rhesus Diploid Rabies Vaccine (Adsorbed): A New Rabies Vaccine Using FRhL-2 Cells. *J. Infect. Dis.* 152:204–210, 1985.
8. Berlin, B.S., Mitchell, J.R., Burgoyne, G.H., et al.: Rhesus Diploid Rabies Vaccine (Adsorbed), A New Rabies Vaccine: Results of Initial Clinical Studies of Pre-Exposure Vaccination. *JAMA.* 247:1726–1728, 1982.
9. Berlin, B.S., Mitchell, J.R., Burgoyne, G.H., et al.: Rhesus Diploid Rabies Vaccine (Adsorbed), A New Rabies Vaccine II. Results of Clinical Studies Simulating Prophylactic Therapy for Rabies Exposure. *JAMA.* 249:2663–2665, 1983.
10. Bahmanyar, M., Fayaz, A., Nour-Salehi, S., et al.: Successful Protection of Humans Exposed to Rabies Infection. *JAMA.* 236:2751–2754, 1976.

Manufactured by
Michigan Department of Public Health
Lansing, MI 48909
U.S. License No. 99
Distributed by
SmithKline Beecham Pharmaceuticals
Philadelphia, PA 19101
Veterans Administration/Military/PHS—Vial, 1 mL, 1's, 6505-01-378-0232.
RV:L3

Shown in Product Identification Guide, page 337

RELAFEN® ℞

[rel 'ah-fen]
brand of nabumetone
tablets

DESCRIPTION

Relafen (nabumetone) is a naphthylalkanone designated chemically as 4-(6-methoxy-2-naphthalenyl)-2-butanone. It has the following structure:

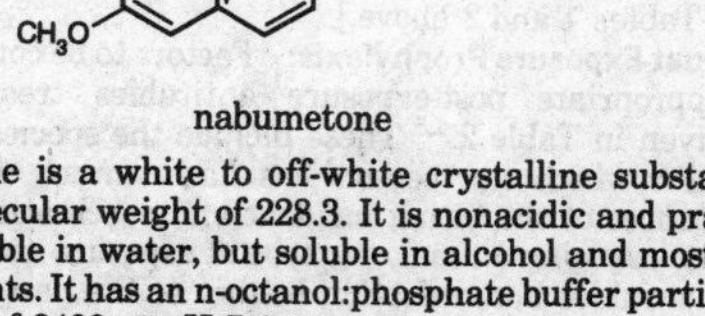

nabumetone

Nabumetone is a white to off-white crystalline substance with a molecular weight of 228.3. It is nonacidic and practically insoluble in water, but soluble in alcohol and most organic solvents. It has an n-octanol:phosphate buffer partition coefficient of 2400 at pH 7.4.

Tablets for Oral Administration: Each oval-shaped, film-coated tablet contains 500 mg or 750 mg of nabumetone. Inactive ingredients consist of hydroxypropyl methylcellulose, microcrystalline cellulose, polyethylene glycol, polysorbate

Table 1. Mean pharmacokinetic parameters of nabumetone active metabolite (6MNA) at steady state following oral administration of 1000 mg or 2000 mg doses of Relafen (nabumetone)

Abbreviation (units)	Young Adults Mean ± SD 1000 mg n=31	Young Adults Mean ± SD 2000 mg n=12	Elderly Mean ± SD 1000 mg n=27
t_{max} (hours)	3.0 (1.0 to 12.0)	2.5 (1.0 to 8.0)	4.0 (1.0 to 10.0)
$t_{1/2}$ (hours)	22.5 ± 3.7	26.2 ± 3.7	29.8 ± 8.1
CL_{SS}/F (mL/min.)	26.1 ± 17.3	21.0 ± 4.0	18.6 ± 13.4
Vd_{SS}/F (L)	55.4 ± 26.4	53.4 ± 11.3	50.2 ± 25.3

80, sodium lauryl sulfate, sodium starch glycolate and titanium dioxide. The 750 mg tablets also contain iron oxides.

CLINICAL PHARMACOLOGY

Relafen is a nonsteroidal anti-inflammatory drug (NSAID) that exhibits anti-inflammatory, analgesic and antipyretic properties in pharmacologic studies. As with other nonsteroidal anti-inflammatory agents, its mode of action is not known. However, the ability to inhibit prostaglandin synthesis may be involved in the anti-inflammatory effect.

The parent compound is a prodrug, which undergoes hepatic biotransformation to the active component, 6-methoxy-2-naphthylacetic acid (6MNA), that is a potent inhibitor of prostaglandin synthesis.

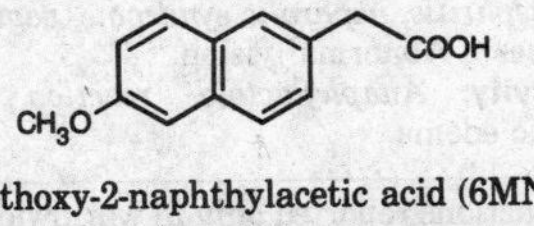

6-methoxy-2-naphthylacetic acid (6MNA)

It is acidic and has an n-octanol:phosphate buffer partition coefficient of 0.5 at pH 7.4.

Pharmacokinetics

After oral administration, approximately 80% of a radiolabelled dose of nabumetone is found in the urine, indicating that nabumetone is well absorbed from the gastrointestinal tract. Nabumetone itself is not detected in the plasma because, after absorption, it undergoes rapid biotransformation to the principal active metabolite, 6-methoxy-2-naphthylacetic acid (6MNA). Approximately 35% of a 1000 mg oral dose of nabumetone is converted to 6MNA and 50% is converted into unidentified metabolites which are subsequently excreted in the urine. Following oral administration of *Relafen,* 6MNA exhibits pharmacokinetic characteristics that generally follow a one-compartment model with first order input and first order elimination.

6MNA is more than 99% bound to plasma proteins. The free fraction is dependent on total concentration of 6MNA and is proportional to dose over the range of 1000 mg to 2000 mg. It is 0.2% to 0.3% at concentrations typically achieved following administration of *Relafen* 1000 mg and is approximately 0.6% to 0.8% of the total concentrations at steady state following daily administration of 2000 mg.

Steady-state plasma concentrations of 6MNA are slightly lower than predicted from single-dose data. This may result from the higher fraction of unbound 6MNA which undergoes greater hepatic clearance.

Coadministration of food increases the rate of absorption and subsequent appearance of 6MNA in the plasma but does not affect the extent of conversion of nabumetone into 6MNA. Peak plasma concentrations of 6MNA are increased by approximately one third.

Coadministration with an aluminum-containing antacid had no significant effect on the bioavailability of 6MNA.

[See Table 1 above.]

The simulated curves in the graph below illustrate the range of active metabolite plasma concentrations that would be expected from 95% of patients following 1000 mg to 2000 mg doses to steady state. The cross-hatched area represents the expected overlap in plasma concentrations due to intersubject variation following oral administration of 1000 mg to 2000 mg of *Relafen.*

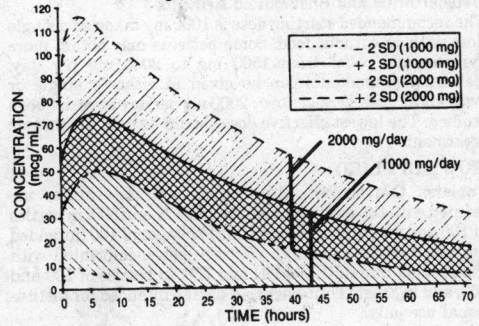

Nabumetone Active Metabolite (6MNA) Plasma Concentrations at Steady State Following Once-Daily Dosing of Nabumetone
1000 mg (n=31) 2000 mg (n=12)

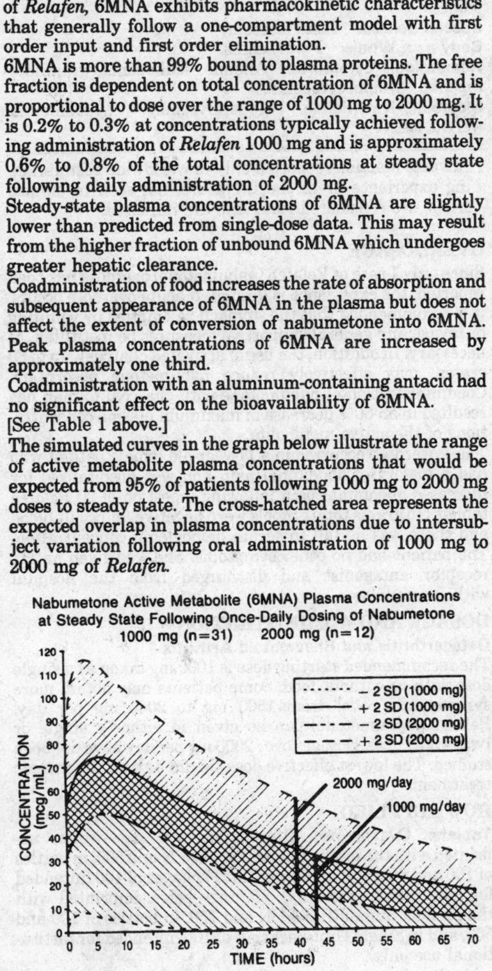

6MNA undergoes biotransformation in the liver, producing inactive metabolites that are eliminated as both free metabolites and conjugates. None of the known metabolites of 6MNA has been detected in plasma. Preliminary *in vivo* and *in vitro* studies suggest that unlike other NSAIDs, there is no evidence of enterohepatic recirculation of the active metabolite. Approximately 75% of a radiolabelled dose was recovered in urine in 48 hours. Approximately 80% was recovered in 168 hours. A further 9% appeared in the feces. In the first 48 hours, metabolites consisted of:

—nabumetone, unchanged	not detectable
—6-methoxy-2-naphthylacetic acid (6MNA), unchanged	<1%
—6MNA, conjugated	11%
—6-hydroxy-2-naphthylacetic acid (6HNA), unchanged	5%
—6HNA, conjugated	7%
—4-(6-hydroxy-2-naphthyl)-butan-2-ol, conjugated	9%
—*O*-desmethyl-nabumetone, conjugated	7%
—unidentified minor metabolites	34%
Total % Dose:	73%

Following oral administration of dosages of 1000 mg to 2000 mg to steady state, the mean plasma clearance of 6MNA is 20 to 30 mL/min. and the elimination half-life is approximately 24 hours.

Elderly Patients: Steady-state plasma concentrations in elderly patients were generally higher than in young healthy subjects. (See Table 1 for summary of pharmacokinetic parameters.)

Renal Insufficiency: In studies of patients with renal insufficiency, the mean terminal half-life of 6MNA was increased in patients with severe renal dysfunction (creatinine clearance <30 mL/min./1.73 m^2). In patients undergoing hemodialysis, steady-state plasma concentrations of the active metabolite were similar to those observed in healthy subjects. Due to extensive protein-binding, 6MNA is not dialyzable.

Hepatic Impairment: Data in patients with severe hepatic impairment are limited. Biotransformation of nabumetone to 6MNA and the further metabolism of 6MNA to inactive metabolites is dependent on hepatic function and could be reduced in patients with severe hepatic impairment (history of or biopsy-proven cirrhosis).

Special Studies

Gastrointestinal: Relafen (nabumetone) was compared to aspirin in inducing gastrointestinal blood loss. Food intake was not monitored. Studies utilizing ^{51}Cr-tagged red blood cells in healthy males showed no difference in fecal blood loss after 3 or 4 weeks' administration of *Relafen* 1000 mg or 2000 mg daily when compared to either placebo-treated or nontreated subjects. In contrast, aspirin 3600 mg daily produced an increase in fecal blood loss when compared to the *Relafen*-treated, placebo-treated or nontreated subjects. The clinical relevance of the data is unknown.

The following endoscopy trials entered patients who had been previously treated with NSAIDs. These patients had varying baseline scores and different courses of treatment. The trials were not designed to correlate symptoms and endoscopy scores. The clinical relevance of these endoscopy trials, i.e., either G.I. symptoms or serious G.I. events, is not known.

Ten endoscopy studies were conducted in 488 patients who had baseline and post-treatment endoscopy. In 5 clinical trials that compared a total of 194 patients on *Relafen* 1000 mg daily or naproxen 250 mg or 500 mg twice daily for 3 to 12 weeks, *Relafen* treatment resulted in fewer patients with endoscopically detected lesions (>3 mm). In 2 trials a total of 101 patients on *Relafen* 1000 mg or 2000 mg daily or piroxicam 10 mg to 20 mg for 7 to 10 days, there were fewer *Relafen* patients with endoscopically detected lesions. In 3 trials of a total of 47 patients on *Relafen* 1000 mg daily or indomethacin 100 mg to 150 mg daily for 3 to 4 weeks, the endoscopy scores were higher with indomethacin. Another 12-week trial in a total of 171 patients compared the results of treatment with *Relafen* 1000 mg/day to ibuprofen 2400 mg/day and ibuprofen 2400 mg/day plus misoprostol 800 mcg/day. The results showed that patients treated with *Relafen* had a lower number of endoscopically detected lesions (>5 mm) than patients treated with ibuprofen alone but comparable to the combination of ibuprofen plus misoprostol. The results did not correlate with abdominal pain.

Other: In 1-week repeat-dose studies in healthy volunteers, *Relafen* 1000 mg daily had little effect on collagen-induced platelet aggregation and no effect on bleeding time. In comparison, naproxen 500 mg daily suppressed collagen-induced platelet aggregation and significantly increased bleeding time.

CLINICAL TRIALS

Osteoarthritis: The use of *Relafen* in relieving the signs and symptoms of osteoarthritis was assessed in double-blind controlled trials in which 1,047 patients were treated for 6 weeks to 6 months. In these trials, *Relafen* in a dose of 1000 mg/day administered at night was comparable to naproxen 500 mg/day and to aspirin 3600 mg/day.

Rheumatoid Arthritis: The use of *Relafen* in relieving the signs and symptoms of rheumatoid arthritis was assessed in double-blind, randomized, controlled trials in which 770 patients were treated for 3 weeks to 6 months. *Relafen,* in a dose of 1000 mg/day administered at night was comparable to naproxen 500 mg/day and to aspirin 3600 mg/day.

In controlled clinical trials of rheumatoid arthritis patients, *Relafen* has been used in combination with gold, d-penicillamine and corticosteroids.

INDIVIDUALIZATION OF DOSING

There is considerable interpatient variation in response to *Relafen.* Therapy is usually initiated at a *Relafen* dose of 1000 mg daily, then adjusted, if needed, based on clinical response.

In clinical trials with osteoarthritis and rheumatoid arthritis patients, most patients responded to *Relafen* in doses of 1000 mg/day administered nightly; total daily dosages up to 2000 mg were used. In open-labelled studies, 1,490 patients were permitted dosage increases and were followed for approximately 1 year (mode). Twenty percent of patients (n=294) were withdrawn for lack of effectiveness during the first year of these open-labelled studies. The following table provides patient-exposure to doses used in the U.S. clinical trials:

Table 2. Clinical double-blind and open-labelled trials of Relafen (nabumetone) in osteoarthritis and rheumatoid arthritis

Relafen Dose	Number of Patients OA	Number of Patients RA	Mean/Mode Duration of Treatment (yrs.) OA	Mean/Mode Duration of Treatment (yrs.) RA
500 mg	17	6	0.4/–	0.2/–
1000 mg	917	701	1.2/1	1.4/1
1500 mg	645	224	2.3/1	1.7/1
2000 mg	15	100	0.6/1	1.3/1

As with other NSAIDs, the lowest dose should be sought for each patient. Patients weighing under 50 kg may be less likely to require dosages beyond 1000 mg. Therefore, after observing the response to initial therapy, the dose should be adjusted to meet individual patients' requirements.

INDICATIONS AND USAGE

Relafen is indicated for acute and chronic treatment of signs and symptoms of osteoarthritis and rheumatoid arthritis.

CONTRAINDICATIONS

Relafen is contraindicated in patients who have previously exhibited hypersensitivity to it.

Relafen is contraindicated in patients in whom *Relafen,* aspirin or other NSAIDs induce asthma, urticaria or other allergic-type reactions. Fatal asthmatic reactions have been reported in such patients receiving NSAIDs.

WARNINGS

Risk of G.I. Ulceration, Bleeding and Perforation with NSAID Therapy: Serious gastrointestinal toxicity such as bleeding, ulceration and perforation can occur at any time, with or without warning symptoms, in patients treated chronically with NSAID therapy. Although minor upper gastrointestinal problems, such as dyspepsia, are common, usually developing early in therapy, physicians should remain alert for ulceration and bleeding in patients treated chronically with NSAIDs even in the absence of previous G.I. tract symptoms. In controlled clinical trials involving 1,677 patients treated with *Relafen* (1,140 followed for 1 year and 927 for 2 years),

Continued on next page

Information on the SmithKline Beecham Pharmaceuticals products appearing here is based on the labeling in effect on July 1, 1996. Further information on these and other products may be obtained from the Medical Department, SmithKline Beecham Pharmaceuticals, One Franklin Plaza, Philadelphia, PA 19101.

SmithKline Beecham—Cont.

the cumulative incidence of peptic ulcers was 0.3% (95% Cl; 0%, 0.6%) at 3 to 6 months, 0.5% (95% Cl; 0.1%, 0.9%) at 1 year and 0.8% (95% Cl; 0.3%, 1.3%) at 2 years. Physicians should inform patients about the signs and symptoms of serious G.I. toxicity and what steps to take if they occur. In patients with active peptic ulcer, physicians must weigh the benefits of Relafen (nabumetone) therapy against possible hazards, institute an appropriate ulcer treatment regimen and monitor the patients' progress carefully.

Studies to date have not identified any subset of patients not at risk of developing peptic ulceration and bleeding. Except for a prior history of serious G.I. events and other risk factors known to be associated with peptic ulcer disease, such as alcoholism, smoking, etc., no risk factors (e.g., age, sex) have been associated with increased risk. Elderly or debilitated patients seem to tolerate ulceration or bleeding less well than other individuals and most spontaneous reports of fatal G.I. events are in this population.

High doses of any NSAID probably carry a greater risk of these reactions, although controlled clinical trials showing this do not exist in most cases. In considering the use of relatively large doses (within the recommended dosage range), sufficient benefit should be anticipated to offset the potential increased risk of G.I. toxicity.

PRECAUTIONS

General

Renal Effects: As a class, NSAIDs have been associated with renal papillary necrosis and other abnormal renal pathology during long-term administration to animals.

A second form of renal toxicity often associated with NSAIDs is seen in patients with conditions leading to a reduction in renal blood flow or blood volume, where renal prostaglandins have a supportive role in the maintenance of renal perfusion. In these patients, administration of an NSAID results in a dose-dependent decrease in prostaglandin synthesis and, secondarily, in a reduction of renal blood flow, which may precipitate overt renal decompensation. Patients at greatest risk of this reaction are those with impaired renal function, heart failure, liver dysfunction, those taking diuretics, and the elderly. Discontinuation of NSAID therapy is typically followed by recovery to the pretreatment state.

Because nabumetone undergoes extensive hepatic metabolism, no adjustment of *Relafen* dosage is generally necessary in patients with renal insufficiency. However, as with all NSAIDs, patients with impaired renal function should be monitored more closely than patients with normal renal function (see CLINICAL PHARMACOLOGY, Special Studies). The oxidized and conjugated metabolites of 6MNA are eliminated primarily by the kidneys. The extent to which these largely inactive metabolites may accumulate in patients with renal failure has not been studied. As with other drugs whose metabolites are excreted by the kidneys, the possibility that adverse reactions (not listed in ADVERSE REACTIONS) may be attributable to these metabolites should be considered.

Hepatic Function: As with other NSAIDs, borderline elevations of one or more liver function tests may occur in up to 15% of patients. These abnormalities may progress, may remain essentially unchanged, or may return to normal with continued therapy. The ALT (SGPT) test is probably the most sensitive indicator of liver dysfunction. Meaningful (3 times the upper limit of normal) elevations of ALT (SGPT) or AST (SGOT) have occurred in controlled clinical trials of Relafen (nabumetone) in less than 1% of patients. A patient with symptoms and/or signs suggesting liver dysfunction, or in whom an abnormal liver test has occurred, should be evaluated for evidence of the development of a more severe hepatic reaction while on *Relafen* therapy. Severe hepatic reactions, including jaundice and fatal hepatitis, have been reported with other NSAIDs. Although such reactions are rare, if abnormal liver tests persist or worsen, if clinical signs and symptoms consistent with liver disease develop, or if systemic manifestations occur (e.g., eosinophilia, rash, etc.), *Relafen* should be discontinued. Because nabumetone's biotransformation to 6MNA is dependent upon hepatic function, the biotransformation could be decreased in patients with severe hepatic dysfunction. Therefore, *Relafen* should be used with caution in patients with severe hepatic impairment (see Pharmacokinetics, *Hepatic Impairment*).

Fluid Retention and Edema: Fluid retention and edema have been observed in some patients taking *Relafen*. Therefore, as with other NSAIDs, *Relafen* should be used cautiously in patients with a history of congestive heart failure, hypertension or other conditions predisposing to fluid retention.

Photosensitivity: Based on U.V. light photosensitivity testing, *Relafen* may be associated with more reactions to sun exposure than might be expected based on skin tanning types.

Information for Patients: *Relafen*, like other drugs of its class, is not free of side effects. The side effects of these drugs can cause discomfort and, rarely, there are more serious side effects, such as gastrointestinal bleeding, which may result in hospitalization and even fatal outcome.

NSAIDs are often essential agents in the management of arthritis, but they also may be commonly employed for conditions which are less serious. Physicians may wish to discuss with their patients the potential risks (see WARNINGS, PRECAUTIONS and ADVERSE REACTIONS) and likely benefits of NSAID treatment, particularly when the drugs are used for less serious conditions where treatment without NSAIDs may represent an acceptable alternative to both the patient and the physician.

Laboratory Tests: Because severe G.I. tract ulceration and bleeding can occur without warning symptoms, physicians should follow chronically treated patients for signs and symptoms of ulceration and bleeding, and should inform them of the importance of this follow-up (see WARNINGS, Risk of G.I. Ulceration, Bleeding and Perforation with NSAID Therapy).

Drug Interactions: *In vitro* studies have shown that, because of its affinity for protein, 6MNA may displace other protein-bound drugs from their binding site. Caution should be exercised when administering *Relafen* with warfarin since interactions have been seen with other NSAIDs. Concomitant administration of an aluminum-containing antacid had no significant effect on the bioavailability of 6MNA. When administered with food or milk, there is more rapid absorption; however, the total amount of 6MNA in the plasma is unchanged (see Pharmacokinetics).

Carcinogenesis, Mutagenesis: In two-year studies conducted in mice and rats, nabumetone had no statistically significant tumorigenic effect. Nabumetone did not show mutagenic potential in the Ames test and mouse micronucleus test *in vivo*. However, nabumetone- and 6MNA-treated lymphocytes in culture showed chromosomal aberrations at 80 mcg/mL and higher concentrations (equal to the average human exposure to *Relafen* at the maximum recommended dose).

Impairment of Fertility: Nabumetone did not impair fertility of male or female rats treated orally at doses of 320 mg/kg/day (1888 mg/m^2) before mating.

Pregnancy: Teratogenic Effects. Pregnancy Category C. Nabumetone did not cause any teratogenic effect in rats given up to 400 mg/kg (2360 mg/m^2) and in rabbits up to 300 mg/kg (3540 mg/m^2) orally. However, increased post-implantation loss was observed in rats at 100 mg/kg (590 mg/m^2) orally and at higher doses (equal to the average human exposure to 6MNA at the maximum recommended human dose). There are no adequate, well-controlled studies in pregnant women. This drug should be used during pregnancy only if clearly needed.

Because of the known effect of prostaglandin-synthesis-inhibiting drugs on the human fetal cardiovascular system (closure of ductus arteriosus), use of Relafen (nabumetone) during the third trimester of pregnancy is not recommended.

Labor and Delivery: The effects of *Relafen* on labor and delivery in women are not known. As with other drugs known to inhibit prostaglandin synthesis, an increased incidence of dystocia and delayed parturition occurred in rats treated throughout pregnancy.

Nursing Mothers: *Relafen* is not recommended for use in nursing mothers because of the possible adverse effects of prostaglandin-synthesis-inhibiting drugs on neonates. It is not known whether nabumetone or its metabolites are excreted in human milk; however, 6MNA is excreted in the milk of lactating rats.

Pediatric Use: *Relafen* is not recommended for use in children because the safety and efficacy in children have not been established.

Geriatric Use: Of the 1,677 patients in U.S. clinical studies who were treated with *Relafen*, 411 patients (24%) were 65 years of age or older; 22 patients (1%) were 75 years of age or older. No overall differences in efficacy or safety were observed between these older patients and younger ones. Similar results were observed in a 1-year, non-U.S. postmarketing surveillance study of 10,800 *Relafen* patients, of whom 4,577 patients (42%) were 65 years of age or older.

ADVERSE REACTIONS

Adverse reaction information was derived from blinded-controlled and open-labelled clinical trials and from worldwide marketing experience. In the description below, rates of the more common events (greater than 1%) and many of the less common events (less than 1%) represent results of U.S. clinical studies.

Of the 1,677 patients who received *Relafen* during U.S. clinical trials, 1,524 were treated for at least 1 month, 1,327 for at least 3 months, 929 for at least a year and 750 for at least 2 years. Over 300 patients have been treated for 5 years or longer.

The most frequently reported adverse reactions were related to the gastrointestinal tract. They were diarrhea, dyspepsia and abdominal pain.

Incidence ≥ 1% — Probably Causally Related
Gastrointestinal: Diarrhea (14%), dyspepsia (13%), abdominal pain (12%), constipation*, flatulence*, nausea*, positive stool guaiac*, dry mouth, gastritis, stomatitis, vomiting.
Central Nervous System: Dizziness*, headache*, fatigue, increased sweating, insomnia, nervousness, somnolence.
Dermatologic: Pruritus*, rash*.
Special Senses: Tinnitus*.
Miscellaneous: Edema*.

---

* Incidence of reported reaction between 3% and 9%. Reactions occurring in 1% to 3% of the patients are unmarked.

Incidence < 1% — Probably Causally Related†
Gastrointestinal: Anorexia, cholestatic jaundice, duodenal ulcer, dysphagia, gastric ulcer, gastroenteritis, gastrointestinal bleeding, increased appetite, liver function abnormalities, melena.
Central Nervous System: Asthenia, agitation, anxiety, confusion, depression, malaise, paresthesia, tremor, vertigo.
Dermatologic: Bullous eruptions, photosensitivity, urticaria, pseudoporphyria cutanea tarda, *toxic epidermal necrolysis*.
Cardiovascular: Vasculitis.
Metabolic: Weight gain.
Respiratory: Dyspnea, *eosinophilic pneumonia, hypersensitivity pneumonitis*.
Genitourinary: Albuminuria, azotemia, *hyperuricemia, interstitial nephritis, nephrotic syndrome, vaginal bleeding*.
Special Senses: Abnormal vision.
Hypersensitivity: *Anaphylactoid reaction, anaphylaxis*, angioneurotic edema.

---

† Adverse reactions reported only in worldwide postmarketing experience or in the literature, not seen in clinical trials, are considered rarer and are italicized.

Incidence < 1% — Causal Relationship Unknown‡
Gastrointestinal: Bilirubinuria, duodenitis, eructation, gallstones, gingivitis, glossitis, pancreatitis, rectal bleeding.
Central Nervous System: Nightmares.
Dermatologic: Acne, alopecia, *erythema multiforme, Stevens-Johnson Syndrome.*
Cardiovascular: Angina, arrhythmia, hypertension, myocardial infarction, palpitations, syncope, thrombophlebitis.
Respiratory: Asthma, cough.
Genitourinary: Dysuria, hematuria, impotence, renal stones.
Special Senses: Taste disorder.
Body as a Whole: Fever, chills.
Hematologic/Lymphatic: Anemia, leukopenia, granulocytopenia, thrombocytopenia.
Metabolic/Nutritional: Hyperglycemia, hypokalemia, weight loss.

---

‡ Adverse reactions reported only in worldwide postmarketing experience or in the literature, not seen in clinical trials, are considered rarer and are italicized.

OVERDOSAGE

Since only 1 case of Relafen (nabumetone) overdose has been reported, the experience is limited. If acute overdose occurs, it is recommended that the stomach be emptied by vomiting or lavage and general supportive measures be instituted, as necessary. In addition, the use of activated charcoal, up to 60 grams, may effectively reduce nabumetone absorption. Coadministration of nabumetone with charcoal to man has resulted in an 80% decrease in maximum plasma concentrations of the active metabolite.

The 1 overdose occurred in a 17-year-old female patient who had a history of abdominal pain and was hospitalized for increased abdominal pain following ingestion of 30 *Relafen* tablets (15 grams total). Stools were negative for occult blood and there was no fall in serum hemoglobin concentration. The patient had no other symptoms. She was given an H$_2$-receptor antagonist and discharged from the hospital without sequelae.

DOSAGE AND ADMINISTRATION

Osteoarthritis and Rheumatoid Arthritis

The recommended starting dose is 1000 mg taken as a single dose with or without food. Some patients may obtain more symptomatic relief from 1500 mg to 2000 mg per day. Relafen (nabumetone) can be given in either a single or twice-daily dose. Dosages over 2000 mg per day have not been studied. The lowest effective dose should be used for chronic treatment.

HOW SUPPLIED

Tablets: Oval-shaped, film-coated: 500 mg—white, imprinted with the product name RELAFEN and 500, in bottles of 100 and 500, and in Single Unit Packages of 100 (intended for institutional use only). 750 mg—beige, imprinted with the product name RELAFEN and 750, in bottles of 100 and 500, and in Single Unit Packages of 100 (intended for institutional use only).

Store at controlled room temperature (59° to 86°F) in well-closed container; dispense in light-resistant container.

500 mg 100's: NDC 0029-4851-20
500 mg 500's: NDC 0029-4851-25
500 mg SUP 100's: NDC 0029-4851-21

750 mg 100's: NDC 0029-4852-20
750 mg 500's: NDC 0029-4852-25
750 mg SUP 100's: NDC 0029-4852-21

Veterans Administration/Military/PHS—Tablets, 500 mg, 100's, 6505-01-352-9299; 500 mg, 100's (SUP), 6505-01-352-9300; 750 mg, 100's, 6505-01-377-1644.

RL:L7

Shown in Product Identification Guide, page 337

RIDAURA® ℞
[ri-door 'ah]
(brand of auranofin)
Capsules

> Ridaura (auranofin) contains gold and, like other gold-containing drugs, can cause gold toxicity, signs of which include: fall in hemoglobin, leukopenia below 4,000 WBC/cu mm, granulocytes below 1,500/cu mm, decrease in platelets below 150,000/cu mm, proteinuria, hematuria, pruritus, rash, stomatitis or persistent diarrhea. Therefore, the results of recommended laboratory work (See PRECAUTIONS) should be reviewed before writing each *Ridaura* prescription. Like other gold preparations, *Ridaura* is only indicated for use in selected patients with active rheumatoid arthritis. Physicians planning to use *Ridaura* should be experienced with chrysotherapy and should thoroughly familiarize themselves with the toxicity and benefits of *Ridaura*.
>
> In addition, the following precautions should be routinely employed:
>
> 1. The possibility of adverse reactions should be explained to patients before starting therapy.
> 2. Patients should be advised to report promptly any symptoms suggesting toxicity. (See PRECAUTIONS—Information for Patients.)

DESCRIPTION

Ridaura (auranofin) is available in oral form as capsules containing 3 mg auranofin.

Auranofin is (2,3,4,6-tetra-O-acetyl-1-thio-β-D-glucopyranosato-S-) (triethylphosphine) gold.

Auranofin contains 29% gold and has the following chemical structure:

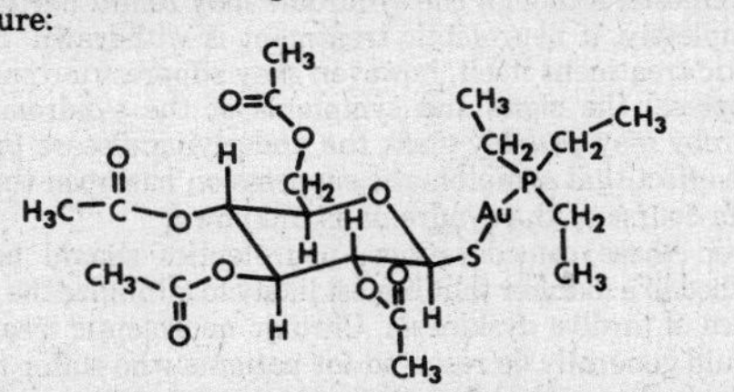

Each *Ridaura* capsule, with opaque brown cap and opaque tan body, contains auranofin, 3 mg, and is imprinted with the product name RIDAURA and SKF. Inactive ingredients consist of benzyl alcohol, cellulose, cetylpyridinium chloride, D&C Red No. 33, FD&C Blue No. 1, FD&C Red No. 40, FD&C Yellow No. 6, gelatin, lactose, magnesium stearate, povidone, sodium lauryl sulfate, sodium starch glycolate, starch, titanium dioxide and trace amounts of other inactive ingredients.

CLINICAL PHARMACOLOGY

The mechanism of action of Ridaura (auranofin) is not understood. In patients with adult rheumatoid arthritis, *Ridaura* may modify disease activity as manifested by synovitis and associated symptoms, and reflected by laboratory parameters such as ESR. There is no substantial evidence, however, that gold-containing compounds induce remission of rheumatoid arthritis.

Pharmacokinetics: Pharmacokinetic studies were performed in rheumatoid arthritis patients, not in normal volunteers. Auranofin is rapidly metabolized and intact auranofin has never been detected in the blood. Thus, studies of the pharmacokinetics of auranofin have involved measurement of gold concentrations. Approximately 25% of the gold in auranofin is absorbed.

The mean terminal plasma half-life of auranofin gold at steady state was 26 days (range 21 to 31 days; n=5). The mean terminal body half-life was 80 days (range 42 to 128; n=5). Approximately 60% of the absorbed gold (15% of the administered dose) from a single dose of auranofin is excreted in urine; the remainder is excreted in the feces.

In clinical studies, steady state blood-gold concentrations are achieved in about three months. In patients on 6 mg auranofin/day, mean steady state blood-gold concentrations were 0.68 ± 0.45 mcg/mL (n=63 patients). In blood, approximately 40% of auranofin gold is associated with red cells, and 60% associated with serum proteins. In contrast, 99% of injectable gold is associated with serum proteins.

Mean blood-gold concentrations are proportional to dose; however, no correlation between blood-gold concentrations and safety or efficacy has been established.

INDICATIONS AND USAGE

Ridaura (auranofin) is indicated in the management of adults with active classical or definite rheumatoid arthritis (ARA criteria) who have had an insufficient therapeutic response to, or are intolerant of, an adequate trial of full doses of one or more nonsteroidal anti-inflammatory drugs. *Ridaura* should be added to a comprehensive baseline program, including non-drug therapies.

Unlike anti-inflammatory drugs, *Ridaura* does not produce an immediate response. Therapeutic effects may be seen after three to four months of treatment, although improvement has not been seen in some patients before six months.

When cartilage and bone damage has already occurred, gold cannot reverse structural damage to joints caused by previous disease. The greatest potential benefit occurs in patients with active synovitis, particularly in its early stage.

In controlled clinical trials comparing *Ridaura* with injectable gold, *Ridaura* was associated with fewer dropouts due to adverse reactions, while injectable gold was associated with fewer dropouts for inadequate or poor therapeutic effect. Physicians should consider these findings when deciding on the use of *Ridaura* in patients who are candidates for chrysotherapy.

CONTRAINDICATIONS

Ridaura (auranofin) is contraindicated in patients with a history of any of the following gold-induced disorders: anaphylactic reactions, necrotizing enterocolitis, pulmonary fibrosis, exfoliative dermatitis, bone marrow aplasia or other severe hematologic disorders.

WARNINGS

Danger signs of possible gold toxicity include fall in hemoglobin, leukopenia below 4,000 WBC/cu mm, granulocytes below 1,500/cu mm, decrease in platelets below 150,000/cu mm, proteinuria, hematuria, pruritus, rash, stomatitis or persistent diarrhea.

Thrombocytopenia has occurred in 1–3% of patients (See ADVERSE REACTIONS) treated with Ridaura (auranofin), some of whom developed bleeding. The thrombocytopenia usually appears to be peripheral in origin and is usually reversible upon withdrawal of *Ridaura*. Its onset bears no relationship to the duration of *Ridaura* therapy and its course may be rapid. While patients' platelet counts should normally be monitored at least monthly (See PRECAUTIONS—Laboratory Tests), the occurrence of a precipitous decline in platelets or a platelet count less than 100,000/cu mm or signs and symptoms (e.g., purpura, ecchymoses or petechiae) suggestive of thrombocytopenia indicates a need to immediately withdraw *Ridaura* and other therapies with the potential to cause thrombocytopenia, and to obtain additional platelet counts. No additional *Ridaura* should be given unless the thrombocytopenia resolves and further studies show it was not due to gold therapy.

Proteinuria has developed in 3–9% of patients (See ADVERSE REACTIONS) treated with *Ridaura*. If clinically significant proteinuria or microscopic hematuria is found (See PRECAUTIONS—Laboratory Tests), *Ridaura* and other therapies with the potential to cause proteinuria or microscopic hematuria should be stopped immediately.

PRECAUTIONS

General: The safety of concomitant use of Ridaura (auranofin) with injectable gold, hydroxychloroquine, penicillamine, immunosuppressive agents (e.g., cyclophosphamide, azathioprine, or methotrexate) or high doses of corticosteroids has not been established.

Medical problems that might affect the signs or symptoms used to detect *Ridaura* toxicity should be under control before starting Ridaura (auranofin).

The potential benefits of using *Ridaura* in patients with progressive renal disease, significant hepatocellular disease, inflammatory bowel disease, skin rash or history of bone marrow depression should be weighed against 1) the potential risks of gold toxicity on organ systems previously compromised or with decreased reserve, and 2) the difficulty in quickly detecting and correctly attributing the toxic effect.

The following adverse reactions have been reported with the use of gold preparations and require modification of *Ridaura* treatment or additional monitoring. See ADVERSE REACTIONS for the approximate incidence of those reactions specifically reported with *Ridaura*.

Gastrointestinal Reactions: Gastrointestinal reactions reported with gold therapy include diarrhea/loose stools, nausea, vomiting, anorexia and abdominal cramps. The most common reaction to *Ridaura* is diarrhea/loose stools reported in approximately 50% of the patients. This is generally manageable by reducing the dosage (e.g., from 6 mg daily to 3 mg) and in only 6% of the patients is it necessary to discontinue Ridaura (auranofin) permanently.

Ulcerative enterocolitis is a rare serious gold reaction. Therefore, patients with gastrointestinal symptoms should be monitored for the appearance of gastrointestinal bleeding.

Cutaneous Reactions: Dermatitis is the most common reaction to injectable gold therapy and the second most common reaction to *Ridaura*. *Any eruption, especially if pruritic, that develops during treatment should be considered a gold reaction until proven otherwise.* Pruritus often exists before dermatitis becomes apparent, and therefore should be considered to be a warning signal of a cutaneous reaction. Gold dermatitis may be aggravated by exposure to sunlight or an actinic rash may develop. The most serious form of cutaneous reaction reported with injectable gold is generalized exfoliative dermatitis.

Mucous Membrane Reactions: Stomatitis, another common gold reaction, may be manifested by shallow ulcers on the buccal membranes, on the borders of the tongue, and on the palate or in the pharynx. Stomatitis may occur as the only adverse reaction or with a dermatitis. Sometimes diffuse glossitis or gingivitis develops. A metallic taste may precede these oral mucous membrane reactions and should be considered a warning signal.

Renal Reactions: Gold can produce a nephrotic syndrome or glomerulitis with proteinuria and hematuria. These renal reactions are usually relatively mild and subside completely if recognized early and treatment is discontinued. They may become severe and chronic if treatment is continued after the onset of the reaction. *Therefore it is important to perform urinalyses regularly* and to discontinue treatment promptly if proteinuria or hematuria develops.

Hematologic Reactions: Blood dyscrasias including leukopenia, granulocytopenia, thrombocytopenia and aplastic anemia have all been reported as reactions to injectable gold and *Ridaura*. These reactions may occur separately or in combination at anytime during treatment. Because they have potentially serious consequences, *blood dyscrasias should be constantly watched for through regular monitoring (at least monthly) of the formed elements of the blood throughout treatment.*

Miscellaneous Reactions: Rare reactions attributed to gold include cholestatic jaundice; gold bronchitis and interstitial pneumonitis and fibrosis; peripheral neuropathy; partial or complete hair loss; fever.

Information for Patients: Patients should be advised of the possibility of toxicity from *Ridaura* and of the signs and symptoms that they should report promptly. (Patient information sheets are available.)

Women of childbearing potential should be warned of the potential risks of *Ridaura* therapy during pregnancy (See PRECAUTIONS—Pregnancy).

Laboratory Tests: CBC with differential, platelet count, urinalysis, and renal and liver function tests should be performed prior to Ridaura (auranofin) therapy to establish a baseline and to identify any preexisting conditions.

CBC with differential, platelet count and urinalysis should then be monitored at least monthly; other parameters should be monitored as appropriate.

Drug Interactions: In a single patient-report, there is the suggestion that concurrent administration of *Ridaura* and phenytoin may have increased phenytoin blood levels.

Carcinogenesis/Mutagenesis: In a 24-month study in rats, animals treated with auranofin at 0.4, 1.0 or 2.5 mg/kg/day orally (3, 8 or 21 times the human dose) or gold sodium thiomalate at 2 or 6 mg/kg injected twice weekly (4 or 12 times the human dose) were compared to untreated control animals.

There was a significant increase in the frequency of renal tubular cell karyomegaly and cytomegaly and renal adenoma in the animals treated with 1.0 or 2.5 mg/kg/day of auranofin and 2 or 6 mg/kg twice weekly of gold sodium thiomalate. Malignant renal epithelial tumors were seen in the 1.0 mg/kg/day and the 2.5 mg/kg/day auranofin and in the 6 mg/kg twice weekly gold sodium thiomalate-treated animals.

In a 12-month study, rats treated with auranofin at 23 mg/kg/day (192 times the human dose) developed tumors of the renal tubular epithelium, whereas those treated with 3.6 mg/kg/day (30 times the human dose) did not.

In an 18-month study in mice given oral auranofin at doses of 1, 3 and 9 mg/kg/day (8, 24 and 72 times the human dose), there was no statistically significant increase above controls in the instances of tumors.

Continued on next page

Information on the SmithKline Beecham Pharmaceuticals products appearing here is based on the labeling in effect on July 1, 1996. Further information on these and other products may be obtained from the Medical Department, SmithKline Beecham Pharmaceuticals, One Franklin Plaza, Philadelphia, PA 19101.

SmithKline Beecham—Cont.

In the mouse lymphoma forward mutation assay, auranofin at high concentrations (313 to 700 ng/mL) induced increases in the mutation frequencies in the presence of a rat liver microsomal preparation. Auranofin produced no mutation effects in the Ames test (Salmonella), in the in vitro assay (Forward and Reverse Mutation Inducement Assay with Saccharomyces), in the in vitro transformation of BALB/T3 cell mouse assay or in the Dominant Lethal Assay.

Pregnancy: Teratogenic Effects—Pregnancy Category C. Use of Ridaura (auranofin) by pregnant women is not recommended. Furthermore, women of childbearing potential should be warned of the potential risks of Ridaura therapy during pregnancy. (See below.)

Pregnant rabbits given auranofin at doses of 0.5, 3 or 6 mg/kg/day (4.2 to 50 times the human dose) had impaired food intake, decreased maternal weights, decreased fetal weights and an increase above controls in the incidence of resorptions, abortions and congenital abnormalities, mainly abdominal defects such as gastroschisis and umbilical hernia.

Pregnant rats given auranofin at a dose of 5 mg/kg/day (42 times the human dose) had an increase above controls in the incidence of resorptions and a decrease in litter size and weight linked to maternal toxicity. No such effects were found in rats given 2.5 mg/kg/day (21 times the human dose).

Pregnant mice given auranofin at a dose of 5 mg/kg/day (42 times the human dose) had no teratogenic effects.

There are no adequate and well-controlled Ridaura studies in pregnant women.

Nursing Mothers: Nursing during Ridaura therapy is not recommended. Following auranofin administration to rats and mice, gold is excreted in milk. Following the administration of injectable gold, gold appears in the milk of nursing women; human data on auranofin are not available.

Pediatric Use: Ridaura (auranofin) is not recommended for use in children because its safety and effectiveness have not been established.

ADVERSE REACTIONS

The adverse reactions incidences listed below are based on observations of 1) 4,784 Ridaura-treated patients in clinical trials (2,474 U.S., 2,310 foreign), of whom 2,729 were treated more than one year and 573 for more than three years; and 2) postmarketing experience. The highest incidence is during the first six months of treatment; however, reactions can occur after many months of therapy. With rare exceptions, all patients were on concomitant nonsteroidal anti-inflammatory therapy; some of them were also taking low dosages of corticosteroids.

Reactions occurring in more than 1% of Ridaura-treated patients

Gastrointestinal: loose stools or diarrhea (47%); abdominal pain (14%); nausea with or without vomiting (10%); constipation; anorexia*; flatulence*; dyspepsia*; dysgeusia.
Dermatological: rash (24%); pruritus (17%); hair loss; urticaria.
Mucous Membrane: stomatitis (13%); conjunctivitis*; glossitis.
Hematological: anemia; leukopenia; thrombocytopenia; eosinophilia.
Renal: proteinuria*; hematuria.
Hepatic: elevated liver enzymes.

---

* Reactions marked with an asterisk occurred in 3–9% of the patients. The other reactions listed occurred in 1–3%.

Reactions occurring in less than 1% of Ridaura-treated patients

Gastrointestinal: dysphagia; gastrointestinal bleeding†; melena†; positive stool for occult blood†; ulcerative enterocolitis.
Dermatological: angioedema.
Mucous Membrane: gingivitis†.
Hematological: aplastic anemia; neutropenia†; agranulocytosis; pure red cell aplasia; pancytopenia.
Hepatic: jaundice.
Respiratory: interstitial pneumonitis.
Neurological: peripheral neuropathy.
Ocular: gold deposits in the lens or cornea unassociated clinically with eye disorders or visual impairment.

---

† Reactions marked with a dagger occurred in 0.1–1% of the patients. The other reactions listed occurred in less than 0.1%.

Reactions reported with injectable gold preparations, but not with Ridaura (auranofin) (based on clinical trials and on postmarketing experience)
Cutaneous Reactions: generalized exfoliative dermatitis.

Incidence of Adverse Reactions for Specific Categories— 18 Comparative Trials

	Ridaura (445 patients)	Injectable Gold (445 patients)
Proteinuria	0.9%	5.4%
Rash	26 %	39 %
Diarrhea	42.5%	13 %
Stomatitis	13 %	18 %
Anemia	3.1%	2.7%
Leukopenia	1.3%	2.2%
Thrombocytopenia	0.9%	2.2%
Elevated liver function tests	1.9%	1.7%
Pulmonary	0.2%	0.2%

OVERDOSAGE

The acute oral LD$_{50}$ for auranofin is 310 mg/kg in adult mice and 265 mg/kg in adult rats. The minimum lethal dose in rats is 30 mg/kg.

In case of acute overdosage, immediate induction of emesis or gastric lavage and appropriate supportive therapy are recommended.

Ridaura overdosage experience is limited. A 50-year-old female, previously on 6 mg Ridaura daily, took 27 mg (9 capsules) daily for 10 days and developed an encephalopathy and peripheral neuropathy. Ridaura was discontinued and she eventually recovered.

There has been no experience with treating Ridaura overdosage with modalities such as chelating agents. However, they have been used with injectable gold and may be considered for Ridaura overdosage.

DOSAGE AND ADMINISTRATION

Usual Adult Dosage: The usual adult dosage of Ridaura (auranofin) is 6 mg daily, given either as 3 mg twice daily or 6 mg once daily. Initiation of therapy at dosages exceeding 6 mg daily is not recommended because it is associated with an increased incidence of diarrhea. If response is inadequate after six months, an increase to 9 mg (3 mg three times daily) may be tolerated. If response remains inadequate after a three-month trial of 9 mg daily, Ridaura therapy should be discontinued. Safety at dosages exceeding 9 mg daily has not been studied.

Transferring from Injectable Gold: In controlled clinical studies, patients on injectable gold have been transferred to Ridaura (auranofin) by discontinuing the injectable agent and starting oral therapy with Ridaura, 6 mg daily. When patients are transferred to Ridaura, they should be informed of its adverse reaction profile, in particular the gastrointestinal reactions. (See PRECAUTIONS—Information for Patients.) At six months, control of disease activity of patients transferred to Ridaura and those maintained on the injectable agent was not different. Data beyond six months are not available.

HOW SUPPLIED

Capsules, containing 3 mg auranofin, in bottles of 60.
STORAGE AND HANDLING
Store at controlled room temperature (59°–86°F). Dispense in a tight, light-resistant container.
Veterans Administration/Military/PHS—Capsules, 3 mg, 60's, 6505-01-226-9907.

RI:L31

Shown in Product Identification Guide, page 337

STELAZINE® ℞
[stel'ah-zeen]
brand of trifluoperazine hydrochloride
Antianxiety/Antipsychotic

DESCRIPTION

Tablets: Each round, blue, film-coated tablet contains trifluoperazine hydrochloride equivalent to trifluoperazine as follows: 1 mg imprinted SKF and S03; 2 mg imprinted SKF and S04; 5 mg imprinted SKF and S06; 10 mg imprinted SKF and S07. Inactive ingredients consist of cellulose, croscarmellose sodium, FD&C Blue No. 2, FD&C Yellow No. 6, FD&C Red No. 40, gelatin, iron oxide, lactose, magnesium stearate, talc, titanium dioxide and trace amounts of other inactive ingredients.

Multi-Dose Vials, 10 mL (2 mg/mL)—Each mL contains, in aqueous solution, trifluoperazine, 2 mg, as the hydrochloride; sodium tartrate, 4.75 mg; sodium biphosphate, 11.6 mg; sodium saccharin, 0.3 mg; benzyl alcohol, 0.75%, as preservative.

Concentrate—Each mL of clear, yellow, banana-vanilla-flavored liquid contains 10 mg of trifluoperazine as the hydrochloride. Inactive ingredients consist of D&C Yellow No. 10, FD&C Yellow No. 6, flavor, sodium benzoate, sodium bisulfite, sucrose and water.

N.B.: The Concentrate is for use in severe neuropsychiatric conditions when oral medication is preferred and other oral forms are considered impractical.

INDICATIONS

For the management of the manifestations of psychotic disorders.

Stelazine (trifluoperazine HCl) is effective for the short-term treatment of generalized non-psychotic anxiety. However, Stelazine is not the first drug to be used in therapy for most patients with non-psychotic anxiety because certain risks associated with its use are not shared by common alternative treatments (i.e., benzodiazepines).

When used in the treatment of non-psychotic anxiety, Stelazine should not be administered at doses of more than 6 mg per day or for longer than 12 weeks because the use of Stelazine at higher doses or for longer intervals may cause persistent tardive dyskinesia that may prove irreversible (see WARNINGS).

The effectiveness of Stelazine as a treatment for non-psychotic anxiety was established in a 4-week clinical multicenter study of outpatients with generalized anxiety disorder (DSM-III). This evidence does not predict that Stelazine will be useful in patients with other non-psychotic conditions in which anxiety, or signs that mimic anxiety, are found (i.e., physical illness, organic mental conditions, agitated depression, character pathologies, etc.).

Stelazine (trifluoperazine HCl) has not been shown effective in the management of behavioral complications in patients with mental retardation.

CONTRAINDICATIONS

A known hypersensitivity to phenothiazines, comatose or greatly depressed states due to central nervous system depressants and, in cases of existing blood dyscrasias, bone marrow depression and pre-existing liver damage.

WARNINGS

Tardive Dyskinesia: Tardive dyskinesia, a syndrome consisting of potentially irreversible, involuntary, dyskinetic movements, may develop in patients treated with neuroleptic (antipsychotic) drugs. Although the prevalence of the syndrome appears to be highest among the elderly, especially elderly women, it is impossible to rely upon prevalence estimates to predict, at the inception of neuroleptic treatment, which patients are likely to develop the syndrome. Whether neuroleptic drug products differ in their potential to cause tardive dyskinesia is unknown.

Both the risk of developing the syndrome and the likelihood that it will become irreversible are believed to increase as the duration of treatment and the total cumulative dose of neuroleptic drugs administered to the patient increase. However, the syndrome can develop, although much less commonly, after relatively brief treatment periods at low doses. There is no known treatment for established cases of tardive dyskinesia, although the syndrome may remit, partially or completely, if neuroleptic treatment is withdrawn. Neuroleptic treatment itself, however, may suppress (or partially suppress) the signs and symptoms of the syndrome and thereby may possibly mask the underlying disease process. The effect that symptomatic suppression has upon the long-term course of the syndrome is unknown.

Given these considerations, neuroleptics should be prescribed in a manner that is most likely to minimize the occurrence of tardive dyskinesia. Chronic neuroleptic treatment should generally be reserved for patients who suffer from a chronic illness that 1) is known to respond to neuroleptic drugs, and, 2) for whom alternative, equally effective, but potentially less harmful treatments are *not* available or appropriate. In patients who do require chronic treatment, the smallest dose and the shortest duration of treatment producing a satisfactory clinical response should be sought. The need for continued treatment should be reassessed periodically.

If signs and symptoms of tardive dyskinesia appear in a patient on neuroleptics, drug discontinuation should be considered. However, some patients may require treatment despite the presence of the syndrome.

For further information about the description of tardive dyskinesia and its clinical detection, please refer to the sections on PRECAUTIONS and ADVERSE REACTIONS.

Neuroleptic Malignant Syndrome (NMS)
A potentially fatal symptom complex sometimes referred to as Neuroleptic Malignant Syndrome (NMS) has been reported in association with antipsychotic drugs. Clinical manifestations of NMS are hyperpyrexia, muscle rigidity, altered mental status and evidence of autonomic instability (irregular pulse or blood pressure, tachycardia, diaphoresis, and cardiac dysrhythmias).

The diagnostic evaluation of patients with this syndrome is complicated. In arriving at a diagnosis, it is important to identify cases where the clinical presentation includes both serious medical illness (e.g., pneumonia, systemic infection, etc.) and untreated or inadequately treated extrapyramidal signs and symptoms (EPS). Other important considerations in the differential diagnosis include central anticholinergic toxicity, heat stroke, drug fever and primary central nervous system (CNS) pathology.

The management of NMS should include 1) immediate discontinuation of antipsychotic drugs and other drugs not es-

sential to concurrent therapy, 2) intensive symptomatic treatment and medical monitoring, and 3) treatment of any concomitant serious medical problems for which specific treatments are available. There is no general agreement about specific pharmacological treatment regimens for uncomplicated NMS.

If a patient requires antipsychotic drug treatment after recovery from NMS, the potential reintroduction of drug therapy should be carefully considered. The patient should be carefully monitored, since recurrences of NMS have been reported.

An encephalopathic syndrome (characterized by weakness, lethargy, fever, tremulousness and confusion, extrapyramidal symptoms, leukocytosis, elevated serum enzymes, BUN and FBS) has occurred in a few patients treated with lithium plus a neuroleptic. In some instances, the syndrome was followed by irreversible brain damage. Because of a possible causal relationship between these events and the concomitant administration of lithium and neuroleptics, patients receiving such combined therapy should be monitored closely for early evidence of neurologic toxicity and treatment discontinued promptly if such signs appear. This encephalopathic syndrome may be similar to or the same as neuroleptic malignant syndrome (NMS).

Patients who have demonstrated a hypersensitivity reaction (e.g., blood dyscrasias, jaundice) with a phenothiazine should not be re-exposed to any phenothiazine, including Stelazine (trifluoperazine HCl), unless in the judgment of the physician the potential benefits of treatment outweigh the possible hazard.

Stelazine Concentrate contains sodium bisulfite, a sulfite that may cause allergic-type reactions including anaphylactic symptoms and life-threatening or less severe asthmatic episodes in certain susceptible people. The overall prevalence of sulfite sensitivity in the general population is unknown and probably low. Sulfite sensitivity is seen more frequently in asthmatic than in non-asthmatic people.

Stelazine (trifluoperazine HCl) may impair mental and/or physical abilities, especially during the first few days of therapy. Therefore, caution patients about activities requiring alertness (e.g., operating vehicles or machinery).

If agents such as sedatives, narcotics, anesthetics, tranquilizers or alcohol are used either simultaneously or successively with the drug, the possibility of an undesirable additive depressant effect should be considered.

Usage in Pregnancy: Safety for the use of *Stelazine* during pregnancy has not been established. Therefore, it is not recommended that the drug be given to pregnant patients except when, in the judgment of the physician, it is essential. The potential benefits should clearly outweigh possible hazards. There are reported instances of prolonged jaundice, extrapyramidal signs, hyperreflexia or hyporeflexia in newborn infants whose mothers received phenothiazines.

Reproductive studies in rats given over 600 times the human dose showed an increased incidence of malformations above controls and reduced litter size and weight linked to maternal toxicity. These effects were not observed at half this dosage. No adverse effect on fetal development was observed in rabbits given 700 times the human dose nor in monkeys given 25 times the human dose.

Nursing Mothers: There is evidence that phenothiazines are excreted in the breast milk of nursing mothers. Because of the potential for serious adverse reactions in nursing infants from trifluoperazine, a decision should be made whether to discontinue nursing or to discontinue the drug, taking into account the importance of the drug to the mother.

PRECAUTIONS

General

Given the likelihood that some patients exposed chronically to neuroleptics will develop tardive dyskinesia, it is advised that all patients in whom chronic use is contemplated be given, if possible, full information about this risk. The decision to inform patients and/or their guardians must obviously take into account the clinical circumstances and the competency of the patient to understand the information provided.

Thrombocytopenia and anemia have been reported in patients receiving the drug. Agranulocytosis and pancytopenia have also been reported—warn patients to report the sudden appearance of sore throat or other signs of infection. If white blood cell and differential counts indicate cellular depression, stop treatment and start antibiotic and other suitable therapy.

Jaundice of the cholestatic type of hepatitis or liver damage has been reported. If fever with grippe-like symptoms occurs, appropriate liver studies should be conducted. If tests indicate an abnormality, stop treatment.

One result of therapy may be an increase in mental and physical activity. For example, a few patients with angina pectoris have complained of increased pain while taking the drug. Therefore, angina patients should be observed carefully and, if an unfavorable response is noted, the drug should be withdrawn.

Because hypotension has occurred, large doses and parenteral administration should be avoided in patients with impaired cardiovascular systems. To minimize the occurrence of hypotension after injection, keep patient lying down and observe for at least ½ hour. If hypotension occurs from parenteral or oral dosing, place patient in head-low position with legs raised. If a vasoconstrictor is required, Levophed®* and Neo-Synephrine®† are suitable. Other pressor agents, including epinephrine, should not be used as they may cause a paradoxical further lowering of blood pressure.

Since certain phenothiazines have been reported to produce retinopathy, the drug should be discontinued if ophthalmoscopic examination or visual field studies should demonstrate retinal changes.

An antiemetic action of Stelazine (trifluoperazine HCl) may mask the signs and symptoms of toxicity or overdosage of other drugs and may obscure the diagnosis and treatment of other conditions such as intestinal obstruction, brain tumor and Reye's syndrome.

With prolonged administration at high dosages, the possibility of cumulative effects, with sudden onset of severe central nervous system or vasomotor symptoms, should be kept in mind.

Neuroleptic drugs elevate prolactin levels; the elevation persists during chronic administration. Tissue culture experiments indicate that approximately ⅓ of human breast cancers are prolactin-dependent in vitro, a factor of potential importance if the prescribing of these drugs is contemplated in a patient with a previously detected breast cancer. Although disturbances such as galactorrhea, amenorrhea, gynecomastia and impotence have been reported, the clinical significance of elevated serum prolactin levels is unknown for most patients. An increase in mammary neoplasms has been found in rodents after chronic administration of neuroleptic drugs. Neither clinical nor epidemiologic studies conducted to date, however, have shown an association between chronic administration of these drugs and mammary tumorigenesis; the available evidence is considered too limited to be conclusive at this time.

Chromosomal aberrations in spermatocytes and abnormal sperm have been demonstrated in rodents treated with certain neuroleptics.

Because phenothiazines may interfere with thermoregulatory mechanisms, use with caution in persons who will be exposed to extreme heat.

As with all drugs which exert an anticholinergic effect, and/or cause mydriasis, trifluoperazine should be used with caution in patients with glaucoma.

Phenothiazines may diminish the effect of oral anticoagulants.

Phenothiazines can produce alpha-adrenergic blockade.

Concomitant administration of propranolol with phenothiazines results in increased plasma levels of both drugs.

Antihypertensive effects of guanethidine and related compounds may be counteracted when phenothiazines are used concurrently.

Thiazide diuretics may accentuate the orthostatic hypotension that may occur with phenothiazines.

Phenothiazines may lower the convulsive threshold; dosage adjustments of anticonvulsants may be necessary. Potentiation of anticonvulsant effects does not occur. However, it has been reported that phenothiazines may interfere with the metabolism of Dilantin®‡ and thus precipitate *Dilantin* toxicity.

Drugs which lower the seizure threshold, including phenothiazine derivatives, should not be used with Amipaque®§.

As with other phenothiazine derivatives, *Stelazine* should be discontinued at least 48 hours before myelography, should not be resumed for at least 24 hours postprocedure and should not be used for the control of nausea and vomiting occurring either prior to myelography or postprocedure with *Amipaque.*

The presence of phenothiazines may produce false-positive phenylketonuria (PKU) test results.

Long-Term Therapy: To lessen the likelihood of adverse reactions related to cumulative drug effect, patients with a history of long-term therapy with Stelazine (trifluoperazine HCl) and/or other neuroleptics should be evaluated periodically to decide whether the maintenance dosage could be lowered or drug therapy discontinued.

ADVERSE REACTIONS

Drowsiness, dizziness, skin reactions, rash, dry mouth, insomnia, amenorrhea, fatigue, muscular weakness, anorexia, lactation, blurred vision and neuromuscular (extrapyramidal) reactions.

Neuromuscular (Extrapyramidal) Reactions

These symptoms are seen in a significant number of hospitalized mental patients. They may be characterized by motor restlessness, be of the dystonic type, or they may resemble parkinsonism.

Depending on the severity of symptoms, dosage should be reduced or discontinued. If therapy is reinstituted, it should be at a lower dosage. Should these symptoms occur in children or pregnant patients, the drug should be stopped and not reinstituted. In most cases barbiturates by suitable route of administration will suffice. (Or, injectable Benadryl®‖ may be useful.) In more severe cases, the administration of an anti-parkinsonism agent, except levodopa, usually produces rapid reversal of symptoms. Suitable supportive measures such as maintaining a clear airway and adequate hydration should be employed.

Motor Restlessness: Symptoms may include agitation or jitteriness and sometimes insomnia. These symptoms often disappear spontaneously. At times these symptoms may be similar to the original neurotic or psychotic symptoms. Dosage should not be increased until these side effects have subsided.

If this phase becomes too troublesome, the symptoms can usually be controlled by a reduction of dosage or change of drug. Treatment with anti-parkinsonian agents, benzodiazepines or propranolol may be helpful.

Dystonias: Symptoms may include: spasm of the neck muscles, sometimes progressing to torticollis; extensor rigidity of back muscles, sometimes progressing to opisthotonos; carpopedal spasm, trismus, swallowing difficulty, oculogyric crisis and protrusion of the tongue.

These usually subside within a few hours, and almost always within 24 to 48 hours, after the drug has been discontinued.

In mild cases, reassurance or a barbiturate is often sufficient. *In moderate cases,* barbiturates will usually bring rapid relief. *In more severe adult cases,* the administration of an anti-parkinsonism agent, except levodopa, usually produces rapid reversal of symptoms. Also, intravenous caffeine with sodium benzoate seems to be effective. *In children,* reassurance and barbiturates will usually control symptoms. (Or, injectable *Benadryl* may be useful.) Note: See *Benadryl* prescribing information for appropriate children's dosage. If appropriate treatment with anti-parkinsonism agents or *Benadryl* fails to reverse the signs and symptoms, the diagnosis should be reevaluated.

Pseudo-parkinsonism: Symptoms may include: mask-like facies; drooling; tremors; pill-rolling motion; cogwheel rigidity; and shuffling gait. Reassurance and sedation are important. In most cases these symptoms are readily controlled when an anti-parkinsonism agent is administered concomitantly. Anti-parkinsonism agents should be used only when required. Generally, therapy of a few weeks to 2 to 3 months will suffice. After this time patients should be evaluated to determine their need for continued treatment. (Note: Levodopa has not been found effective in pseudo-parkinsonism.) Occasionally it is necessary to lower the dosage of Stelazine (trifluoperazine HCl) or to discontinue the drug.

Tardive Dyskinesia: As with all antipsychotic agents, tardive dyskinesia may appear in some patients on long-term therapy or may appear after drug therapy has been discontinued. The syndrome can also develop, although much less frequently, after relatively brief treatment periods at low doses. This syndrome appears in all age groups. Although its prevalence appears to be highest among elderly patients, especially elderly women, it is impossible to rely upon prevalence estimates to predict at the inception of neuroleptic treatment which patients are likely to develop the syndrome. The symptoms are persistent and in some patients appear to be irreversible. The syndrome is characterized by rhythmical involuntary movements of the tongue, face, mouth or jaw (e.g., protrusion of tongue, puffing of cheeks, puckering of mouth, chewing movements). Sometimes these may be accompanied by involuntary movements of extremities. In rare instances, these involuntary movements of the extremities are the only manifestations of tardive dyskinesia. A variant of tardive dyskinesia, tardive dystonia, has also been described.

There is no known effective treatment for tardive dyskinesia; anti-parkinsonism agents do not alleviate the symptoms of this syndrome. If clinically feasible, it is suggested that all antipsychotic agents be discontinued if these symptoms appear. Should it be necessary to reinstitute treatment, or increase the dosage of the agent, or switch to a different antipsychotic agent, the syndrome may be masked.

It has been reported that fine vermicular movements of the tongue may be an early sign of the syndrome and if the medication is stopped at that time the syndrome may not develop.

Adverse Reactions Reported with Stelazine (trifluoperazine HCl) or Other Phenothiazine Derivatives: Adverse effects with different phenothiazines vary in type, frequency, and mechanism of occurrence, i.e., some are dose-related, while others involve individual patient sensitivity. Some adverse effects may be more likely to occur, or occur with greater intensity, in patients with special medical problems, e.g.,

Continued on next page

Information on the SmithKline Beecham Pharmaceuticals products appearing here is based on the labeling in effect on July 1, 1996. Further information on these and other products may be obtained from the Medical Department, SmithKline Beecham Pharmaceuticals, One Franklin Plaza, Philadelphia, PA 19101.

SmithKline Beecham—Cont.

patients with mitral insufficiency or pheochromocytoma have experienced severe hypotension following recommended doses of certain phenothiazines.

Neuroleptic Malignant Syndrome (NMS) has been reported in association with antipsychotic drugs. (See WARNINGS.) Not all of the following adverse reactions have been observed with every phenothiazine derivative, but they have been reported with one or more and should be borne in mind when drugs of this class are administered: extrapyramidal symptoms (opisthotonos, oculogyric crisis, hyperreflexia, dystonia, akathisia, dyskinesia, parkinsonism) some of which have lasted months and even years—particularly in elderly patients with previous brain damage; grand mal and petit mal convulsions, particularly in patients with EEG abnormalities or history of such disorders; altered cerebrospinal fluid proteins; cerebral edema; intensification and prolongation of the action of central nervous system depressants (opiates, analgesics, antihistamines, barbiturates, alcohol), atropine, heat, organophosphorus insecticides; autonomic reactions (dryness of mouth, nasal congestion, headache, nausea, constipation, obstipation, adynamic ileus, ejaculatory disorders/impotence, priapism, atonic colon, urinary retention, miosis and mydriasis); reactivation of psychotic processes, catatonic-like states; hypotension (sometimes fatal); cardiac arrest; blood dyscrasias (pancytopenia, thrombocytopenic purpura, leukopenia, agranulocytosis, eosinophilia, hemolytic anemia, aplastic anemia); liver damage (jaundice, biliary stasis); endocrine disturbances (hyperglycemia, hypoglycemia, glycosuria, lactation, galactorrhea, gynecomastia, menstrual irregularities, false-positive pregnancy tests); skin disorders (photosensitivity, itching, erythema, urticaria, eczema up to exfoliative dermatitis); other allergic reactions (asthma, laryngeal edema, angioneurotic edema, anaphylactoid reactions); peripheral edema; reversed epinephrine effect; hyperpyrexia; mild fever after large I.M. doses; increased appetite; increased weight; a systemic lupus erythematosus-like syndrome; pigmentary retinopathy; with prolonged administration of substantial doses, skin pigmentation, epithelial keratopathy, and lenticular and corneal deposits.

EKG changes—particularly nonspecific, usually reversible Q and T wave distortions—have been observed in some patients receiving phenothiazine tranquilizers. Although phenothiazines cause neither psychic nor physical dependence, sudden discontinuance in long-term psychiatric patients may cause temporary symptoms, e.g., nausea and vomiting, dizziness, tremulousness.

Note: There have been occasional reports of sudden death in patients receiving phenothiazines. In some cases, the cause appeared to be cardiac arrest or asphyxia due to failure of the cough reflex.

DOSAGE AND ADMINISTRATION—ADULTS

Dosage should be adjusted to the needs of the individual. The lowest effective dosage should always be used. Dosage should be increased more gradually in debilitated or emaciated patients. When maximum response is achieved, dosage may be reduced gradually to a maintenance level. Because of the inherent long action of the drug, patients may be controlled on convenient b.i.d. administration; some patients may be maintained on once-a-day administration.

When Stelazine (trifluoperazine HCl) is administered by intramuscular injection, equivalent oral dosage may be substituted once symptoms have been controlled.

Note: Although there is little likelihood of contact dermatitis due to the drug, persons with known sensitivity to phenothiazine drugs should avoid direct contact.

Elderly Patients: In general, dosages in the lower range are sufficient for most elderly patients. Since they appear to be more susceptible to hypotension and neuromuscular reactions, such patients should be observed closely. Dosage should be tailored to the individual, response carefully monitored, and dosage adjusted accordingly. Dosage should be increased more gradually in elderly patients.

Non-psychotic Anxiety
Usual dosage is 1 or 2 mg twice daily. Do not administer at doses of more than 6 mg per day or for longer than 12 weeks.

Psychotic Disorders
Oral: Usual starting dosage is 2 mg to 5 mg b.i.d. (Small or emaciated patients should always be started on the lower dosage.)

Most patients will show optimum response on 15 mg or 20 mg daily, although a few may require 40 mg a day or more. Optimum therapeutic dosage levels should be reached within 2 or 3 weeks.

When the Concentrate dosage form is to be used, it should be added to 60 mL (2 fl oz) or more of diluent *just prior to administration* to insure palatability and stability. Vehicles suggested for dilution are: tomato or fruit juice, milk, simple syrup, orange syrup, carbonated beverages, coffee, tea or water. Semisolid foods (soup, puddings, etc.) may also be used.

Intramuscular (for prompt control of severe symptoms): Usual dosage is 1 mg to 2 mg (½ to 1 mL) by deep intramuscular injection q4 to 6h, p.r.n. More than 6 mg within 24 hours is rarely necessary.

Only in very exceptional cases should intramuscular dosage exceed 10 mg within 24 hours. Injections should not be given at intervals of less than 4 hours because of a possible cumulative effect.

Note: Stelazine (trifluoperazine HCl) Injection has been usually well tolerated and there is little, if any, pain and irritation at the site of injection.

This solution should be protected from light. This is a clear, colorless to pale yellow solution; a slight yellowish discoloration will not alter potency. If markedly discolored, solution should be discarded.

DOSAGE AND ADMINISTRATION—PSYCHOTIC CHILDREN

Dosage should be adjusted to the weight of the child and severity of the symptoms. These dosages are for children, ages 6 to 12, who are hospitalized or under close supervision.

Oral: The starting dosage is 1 mg administered once a day or b.i.d. Dosage may be increased gradually until symptoms are controlled or until side effects become troublesome.

While it is usually not necessary to exceed dosages of 15 mg daily, some older children with severe symptoms may require higher dosages.

Intramuscular: There has been little experience with the use of Stelazine (trifluoperazine HCl) Injection in children. However, if it is necessary to achieve rapid control of severe symptoms, 1 mg (½ mL) of the drug may be administered intramuscularly once or twice a day.

OVERDOSAGE

(See also under ADVERSE REACTIONS.) SYMPTOMS— Primarily involvement of the extrapyramidal mechanism producing some of the dystonic reactions described above. Symptoms of central nervous system depression to the point of somnolence or coma. Agitation and restlessness may also occur. Other possible manifestations include convulsions, EKG changes and cardiac arrhythmias, fever and autonomic reactions such as hypotension, dry mouth and ileus.

TREATMENT—It is important to determine other medications taken by the patient since multiple dose therapy is common in overdosage situations. Treatment is essentially symptomatic and supportive. Early gastric lavage is helpful. Keep patient under observation and maintain an open airway, since involvement of the extrapyramidal mechanism may produce dysphagia and respiratory difficulty in severe overdosage. **Do not attempt to induce emesis because a dystonic reaction of the head or neck may develop that could result in aspiration of vomitus.** Extrapyramidal symptoms may be treated with anti-parkinsonism drugs, barbiturates, or *Benadryl*. See prescribing information for these products. Care should be taken to avoid increasing respiratory depression. If administration of a stimulant is desirable, amphetamine, dextroamphetamine or caffeine with sodium benzoate is recommended. Stimulants that may cause convulsions (e.g., picrotoxin or pentylenetetrazol) should be avoided.

If hypotension occurs, the standard measures for managing circulatory shock should be initiated. If it is desirable to administer a vasoconstrictor, *Levophed* and *Neo-Synephrine* are most suitable. Other pressor agents, including epinephrine, are not recommended because phenothiazine derivatives may reverse the usual elevating action of these agents and cause a further lowering of blood pressure.

Limited experience indicates that phenothiazines are *not* dialyzable.

HOW SUPPLIED

Tablets, 1 mg, 2 mg, 5 mg and 10 mg in bottles of 100.
1 mg 100's: NDC 0108-4903-20
2 mg 100's: NDC 0108-4904-20
5 mg 100's: NDC 0108-4906-20
10 mg 100's: NDC 0108-4907-20
Multi-Dose Vials, 10 mL (2 mg/mL), in 1's:
NDC 0108-4902-01
Concentrate (for institutional use), 10 mg/mL, in 2 fl oz bottles and in cartons of 12 bottles.
The Concentrate form is light-sensitive. For this reason, it should be protected from light and dispensed in amber bottles. *Refrigeration is not required.*
10 mg/mL 2 fl oz (carton of 12): NDC 0108-4901-42
Store all Stelazine (trifluoperazine HCl) formulations between 15° and 30°C (59° and 86°F).

---

* norepinephrine bitartrate, Sanofi Winthrop Pharmaceuticals.
† phenylephrine hydrochloride, Sanofi Winthrop Pharmaceuticals.
‡ phenytoin, Parke-Davis.
§ metrizamide, Sanofi Winthrop Pharmaceuticals.
‖ diphenhydramine hydrochloride, Parke-Davis.
Veterans Administration/Military/PHS—Injection, 10 mL, 1's, 6505-01-220-1479; Tablets, 1 mg, 100's, 6505-00-761-5658;

---

2 mg, 100's, 6505-01-361-5235; 5 mg, 100's, 6505-01-311-3784; 10 mg, 100's, 6505-01-246-1918.

SZ:L70

Shown in Product Identification Guide, page 337

TAGAMET® ℞

[*tag'ah-met*]
brand of cimetidine tablets
cimetidine hydrochloride liquid and
cimetidine hydrochloride injection

DESCRIPTION

Tagamet (cimetidine) is a histamine H_2-receptor antagonist. Chemically it is N''-cyano- N-methyl-N'-[2-[[(5-methyl-1 H-imidazol-4-yl) methyl] thio]-ethyl]-guanidine.

The empirical formula for cimetidine is $C_{10}H_{16}N_6S$ and for cimetidine hydrochloride, $C_{10}H_{16}N_6S$HCl; these represent molecular weights of 252.34 and 288.80, respectively.

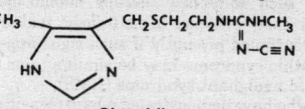

Cimetidine

Cimetidine contains an imidazole ring, and is chemically related to histamine.

(The liquid and injection dosage forms contain cimetidine as the hydrochloride.)

Cimetidine has a bitter taste and characteristic odor.

Solubility Characteristics: Cimetidine is soluble in alcohol, slightly soluble in water, very slightly soluble in chloroform and insoluble in ether. Cimetidine hydrochloride is freely soluble in water, soluble in alcohol, very slightly soluble in chloroform and practically insoluble in ether.

Tablets for Oral Administration: Each light green, film-coated tablet contains cimetidine as follows: 200 mg—round, imprinted with the product name TAGAMET, SKF and 200; 300 mg—round, debossed with the product name TAGAMET, SB and 300; 400 mg—oval Tiltab® tablets, debossed with the product name TAGAMET, SB and 400; 800 mg—oval Tiltab® tablets, debossed with the product name TAGAMET, SB and 800. Inactive ingredients consist of cellulose, D&C Yellow No. 10, FD&C Blue No. 2, FD&C Red No. 40, FD&C Yellow No. 6, hydroxypropyl methylcellulose, iron oxides, magnesium stearate, povidone, propylene glycol, sodium lauryl sulfate, sodium starch glycolate, starch, titanium dioxide and trace amounts of other inactive ingredients.

Liquid for Oral Administration: Each 5 mL (1 teaspoonful) of clear, light orange, mint-peach flavored liquid contains cimetidine hydrochloride equivalent to cimetidine, 300 mg; alcohol, 2.8%. Inactive ingredients consist of FD&C Yellow No. 6, flavors, methylparaben, polyoxyethylene polyoxypropylene glycol, propylene glycol, propylparaben, saccharin sodium, sodium chloride, sodium phosphate, sorbitol and water.

Injection:
Single-Dose Vials for Intramuscular or Intravenous Administration: Each 2 mL contains, in sterile aqueous solution (pH range 3.8 to 6), cimetidine hydrochloride equivalent to cimetidine, 300 mg; phenol, 10 mg.
Multi-Dose Vials for Intramuscular or Intravenous Administration: 8 mL (300 mg/2 mL): Each 2 mL contains, in sterile aqueous solution (pH range 3.8 to 6), cimetidine hydrochloride equivalent to cimetidine, 300 mg; phenol, 10 mg.
Single-Dose Premixed Plastic Containers for Intravenous Administration: Each 50 mL of sterile aqueous solution (pH range 5 to 7) contains cimetidine hydrochloride equivalent to 300 mg cimetidine and 0.45 grams sodium chloride. No preservative has been added.
The plastic container is fabricated from specially formulated polyvinyl chloride. The amount of water that can permeate from inside the container into the overwrap is insufficient to affect the solution significantly. Solutions in contact with the plastic container can leach out certain of its chemical components in very small amounts within the expiration period, e.g., di 2-ethylhexyl phthalate (DEHP), up to 5 parts per million. However, the safety of the plastic has been confirmed in tests in animals according to the USP biological tests for plastic containers as well as by tissue culture toxicity studies.
ADD-Vantage®* Vials for Intravenous Administration: Each 2 mL contains, in sterile aqueous solution (pH range 3.8 to 6), cimetidine hydrochloride equivalent to cimetidine, 300 mg; phenol, 10 mg.
All of the above injection formulations are pyrogen free, and sodium hydroxide N.F. is used as an ingredient to adjust the pH.

CLINICAL PHARMACOLOGY

Tagamet (cimetidine) competitively inhibits the action of histamine at the histamine H_2 receptors of the parietal cells and thus is a histamine H_2-receptor antagonist.

Tagamet is not an anticholinergic agent. Studies have shown that *Tagamet* inhibits both daytime and nocturnal basal gastric acid secretion. *Tagamet* also inhibits gastric acid secretion stimulated by food, histamine, pentagastrin, caffeine and insulin.

Antisecretory Activity

1) **Acid Secretion:** *Nocturnal: Tagamet* 800 mg orally at bedtime reduces mean hourly H^+ activity by greater than 85% over an 8-hour period in duodenal ulcer patients, with no effect on daytime acid secretion. *Tagamet* 1600 mg orally h.s. produces 100% inhibition of mean hourly H^+ activity over an 8-hour period in duodenal ulcer patients, but also reduces H^+ activity by 35% for an additional 5 hours into the following morning. *Tagamet* 400 mg b.i.d. and 300 mg q.i.d. decrease nocturnal acid secretion in a dose-related manner, i.e., 47% to 83% over a 6- to 8-hour period and 54% over a 9-hour period, respectively.

Food Stimulated: During the first hour after a standard experimental meal, oral *Tagamet* 300 mg inhibited gastric acid secretion in duodenal ulcer patients by at least 50%. During the subsequent 2 hours *Tagamet* inhibited gastric acid secretion by at least 75%.

The effect of a 300 mg breakfast dose of *Tagamet* continued for at least 4 hours and there was partial suppression of the rise in gastric acid secretion following the luncheon meal in duodenal ulcer patients. This suppression of gastric acid output was enhanced and could be maintained by another 300 mg dose of *Tagamet* given with lunch.

In another study, *Tagamet* 300 mg given with the meal increased gastric pH as compared with placebo.

	Mean Gastric pH	
	Tagamet	Placebo
1 hour	3.5	2.6
2 hours	3.1	1.6
3 hours	3.8	1.9
4 hours	6.1	2.2

24-Hour Mean H^+ Activity: *Tagamet* 800 mg h.s., 400 mg b.i.d. and 300 mg q.i.d. all provide a similar, moderate (less than 60%) level of 24-hour acid suppression. However, the 800 mg h.s. regimen exerts its entire effect on nocturnal acid, and does not affect daytime gastric physiology.

Chemically Stimulated: Oral Tagamet (cimetidine) significantly inhibited gastric acid secretion stimulated by betazole (an isomer of histamine), pentagastrin, caffeine and insulin as follows:

Stimulant	Stimulant Dose	*Tagamet*	% Inhibition
Betazole	1.5mg/kg (sc)	300mg (po)	85% at 2½ hours
Pentagastrin	6mcg/kg/hr (iv)	100mg/hr (iv)	60% at 1 hour
Caffeine	5mg/kg/hr (iv)	300mg (po)	100% at 1 hour
Insulin	0.03 units/kg/hr (iv)	100mg/hr (iv)	82% at 1 hour

When food and betazole were used to stimulate secretion, inhibition of hydrogen ion concentration usually ranged from 45% to 75% and the inhibition of volume ranged from 30% to 65%.

Parenteral administration also significantly inhibits gastric acid secretion. In a crossover study involving patients with active or healed duodenal or gastric ulcers, either continuous I.V. infusion of *Tagamet* 37.5 mg/hour (900 mg/day) or intermittent injection of *Tagamet* 300 mg q6h (1200 mg/day) maintained gastric pH above 4.0 for more than 50% of the time under steady-state conditions.

2) **Pepsin:** Oral *Tagamet* 300 mg reduced total pepsin output as a result of the decrease in volume of gastric juice.

3) **Intrinsic Factor:** Intrinsic factor secretion was studied with betazole as a stimulant. Oral *Tagamet* 300 mg inhibited the rise in intrinsic factor concentration produced by betazole, but some intrinsic factor was secreted at all times.

*ADD-Vantage® is a trademark of Abbott Laboratories.

Other

Lower Esophageal Sphincter Pressure and Gastric Emptying

Tagamet has no effect on lower esophageal sphincter (LES) pressure or the rate of gastric emptying.

Pharmacokinetics

Tagamet is rapidly absorbed after oral administration and peak levels occur in 45 to 90 minutes. The half-life of *Tagamet* is approximately 2 hours. Both oral and parenteral (I.V. or I.M.) administration provide comparable periods of therapeutically effective blood levels; blood concentrations remain above that required to provide 80% inhibition of basal gastric acid secretion for 4 to 5 hours following a dose of 300 mg.

Steady-state blood concentrations of cimetidine with continuous infusion of *Tagamet* are determined by the infusion rate and clearance of the drug in the individual patient. In a study of peptic ulcer patients with normal renal function, an infusion rate of 37.5 mg/hour produced average steady-state plasma cimetidine concentrations of about 0.9 mcg/mL. Blood levels with other infusion rates will vary in direct proportion to the infusion rate.

The principal route of excretion of *Tagamet* is the urine. Following parenteral administration, most of the drug is excreted as the parent compound; following oral administration, the drug is more extensively metabolized, the sulfoxide being the major metabolite. Following a single oral dose, 48% of the drug is recovered from the urine after 24 hours as the parent compound. Following I.V. or I.M. administration, approximately 75% of the drug is recovered from the urine after 24 hours as the parent compound.

CLINICAL TRIALS

Duodenal Ulcer

Tagamet (cimetidine) has been shown to be effective in the treatment of active duodenal ulcer and, at reduced dosage, in maintenance therapy following healing of active ulcers.

Active Duodenal Ulcer: *Tagamet* accelerates the rate of duodenal ulcer healing. Healing rates reported in U.S. and foreign controlled trials with *Tagamet* are summarized below, beginning with the regimen providing the lowest nocturnal dose.

Duodenal Ulcer Healing Rates with Various *Tagamet* Dosage Regimens*

Regimen	300 mg q.i.d.	400 mg b.i.d.	800 mg h.s.	1600 mg h.s.
week 4	68%	73%	80%	86%
week 6	80%	80%	89%	
week 8	—	92%	94%	

*Averages from controlled clinical trials.

A U.S., double-blind, placebo-controlled, dose-ranging study demonstrated that all once-daily at bedtime (h.s.) *Tagamet* regimens were superior to placebo in ulcer healing and that *Tagamet* 800 mg h.s. healed 75% of patients at 4 weeks. The healing rate with 800 mg h.s. was significantly superior to 400 mg h.s. (66%) and not significantly different from 1600 mg h.s. (81%).

In the U.S. dose-ranging trial, over 80% of patients receiving *Tagamet* 800 mg h.s. experienced nocturnal pain relief after 1 day. Relief from daytime pain was reported in approximately 70% of patients after 2 days. As with ulcer healing, the 800 mg h.s. dose was superior to 400 mg h.s. and not different from 1600 mg h.s.

In foreign, double-blind studies with *Tagamet* 800 mg h.s., 79% to 85% of patients were healed at 4 weeks.

While short-term treatment with Tagamet (cimetidine) can result in complete healing of the duodenal ulcer, acute therapy will not prevent ulcer recurrence after *Tagamet* has been discontinued. Some follow-up studies have reported that the rate of recurrence once therapy was discontinued was slightly higher for patients healed on *Tagamet* than for patients healed on other forms of therapy; however, the *Tagamet*-treated patients generally had more severe disease.

Maintenance Therapy in Duodenal Ulcer: Treatment with a reduced dose of *Tagamet* has been proven effective as maintenance therapy following healing of active duodenal ulcers.

In numerous placebo-controlled studies conducted worldwide, the percent of patients with observed ulcers at the end of 1 year's therapy with *Tagamet* 400 mg h.s. was significantly lower (10% to 45%) than in patients receiving placebo (44% to 70%). Thus, from 55% to 90% of patients were maintained free of observed ulcers at the end of 1 year with *Tagamet* 400 mg h.s.

Factors such as smoking, duration and severity of disease, gender, and genetic traits may contribute to variations in actual percentages.

Trials of other anti-ulcer therapy, whether placebo-controlled, positive-controlled or open, have demonstrated a range of results similar to that seen with *Tagamet*.

Active Benign Gastric Ulcer

Tagamet has been shown to be effective in the short-term treatment of active benign gastric ulcer.

In a multicenter, double-blind U.S. study, patients with endoscopically confirmed benign gastric ulcer were treated with *Tagamet* 300 mg four times a day or with placebo for 6 weeks. Patients were limited to those with ulcers ranging from 0.5 to 2.5 cm in size. Endoscopically confirmed healing at 6 weeks was seen in significantly* more *Tagamet*-treated patients than in patients receiving placebo, as shown below:

	Tagamet	Placebo
week 2	14/63 (22%)	7/63 (11%)
total at week 6	43/65 (66%)*	30/67 (45%)

*$p < 0.05$

In a similar multicenter U.S. study of the 800 mg h.s. oral regimen, the endoscopically confirmed healing rates were:

	Tagamet	Placebo
total at week 6	63/83 (76%)*	44/80 (55%)

*$p = 0.005$

Similarly, in worldwide double-blind clinical studies, endoscopically evaluated benign gastric ulcer healing rates were consistently higher with *Tagamet* than with placebo.

Gastroesophageal Reflux Disease

In two multicenter, double-blind, placebo-controlled studies in patients with gastroesophageal reflux disease (GERD) and endoscopically proven erosions and/or ulcers, *Tagamet* was significantly more effective than placebo in healing lesions. The endoscopically confirmed healing rates were:

Trial	*Tagamet* (800 mg b.i.d.)	*Tagamet* (400 mg q.i.d.)	Placebo	p-Value (800 mg b.i.d. vs. placebo)
1 Week 6	45%	52%	26%	0.02
Week 12	60%	66%	42%	0.02
2 Week 6	50%		20%	<0.01
Week 12	67%		36%	<0.01

In these trials *Tagamet* was superior to placebo by most measures in improving symptoms of day- and night-time heartburn, with many of the differences statistically significant. The q.i.d. regimen was generally somewhat better than the b.i.d. regimen where these were compared.

Prevention of Upper Gastrointestinal Bleeding in Critically Ill Patients

A double-blind, placebo-controlled randomized study of continuous infusion cimetidine was performed in 131 critically ill patients (mean APACHE II score = 15.99) to compare the incidence of upper gastrointestinal bleeding, manifested as hematemesis or bright red blood which did not clear after adjustment of the nasogastric tube and a 5 to 10 minute lavage, persistent Gastroccult® positive coffee grounds for 8 consecutive hours which did not clear with 100 cc lavage and/or which were accompanied by a drop in hematocrit of 5 percentage points, or melena, with an endoscopically documented upper gastrointestinal source of bleed. 14% (9/65) of patients treated with cimetidine continuous infusion developed bleeding compared to 33% (22/66) of the placebo group. Coffee grounds was the manifestation of bleeding that accounted for the difference between groups. Another randomized, double-blind placebo-controlled study confirmed these results for an end point of upper gastrointestinal bleeding with a confirmed upper gastrointestinal source noted on endoscopy, and by post hoc analyses of bleeding episodes between groups.

Pathological Hypersecretory Conditions
(such as Zollinger-Ellison Syndrome)

Tagamet significantly inhibited gastric acid secretion and reduced occurrence of diarrhea, anorexia and pain in patients with pathological hypersecretion associated with Zollinger-Ellison Syndrome, systemic mastocytosis and multiple endocrine adenomas. Use of *Tagamet* was also followed by healing of intractable ulcers.

INDICATIONS AND USAGE

Tagamet (cimetidine) is indicated in:

(1) Short-term treatment of active duodenal ulcer. Most patients heal within 4 weeks and there is rarely reason to use *Tagamet* at full dosage for longer than 6 to 8 weeks (see Dosage and Administration–Duodenal Ulcer). Concomitant antacids should be given as needed for relief of pain. However, simultaneous administration of *Tagamet* and antacids is not recommended, since antacids have been reported to interfere with the absorption of *Tagamet*.

(2) Maintenance therapy for duodenal ulcer patients at reduced dosage after healing of active ulcer. Patients have been maintained on continued treatment with *Tagamet* 400 mg h.s. for periods of up to 5 years.

(3) Short-term treatment of active benign gastric ulcer. There is no information concerning usefulness of treatment periods of longer than 8 weeks.

(4) Erosive gastroesophageal reflux disease (GERD). Erosive esophagitis diagnosed by endoscopy. Treatment is indicated for 12 weeks for healing of lesions and control of symptoms. The use of *Tagamet* beyond 12 weeks has not been established (see Dosage and Administration—GERD).

(5) Prevention of upper gastrointestinal bleeding in critically ill patients.

Continued on next page

Information on the SmithKline Beecham Pharmaceuticals products appearing here is based on the labeling in effect on July 1, 1996. Further information on these and other products may be obtained from the Medical Department, SmithKline Beecham Pharmaceuticals, One Franklin Plaza, Philadelphia, PA 19101.

SmithKline Beecham—Cont.

(6) The treatment of pathological hypersecretory conditions (i.e., Zollinger-Ellison Syndrome, systemic mastocytosis, multiple endocrine adenomas).

CONTRAINDICATIONS

Tagamet is contraindicated for patients known to have hypersensitivity to the product.

PRECAUTIONS

General: Rare instances of cardiac arrhythmias and hypotension have been reported following the rapid administration of Tagamet (cimetidine hydrochloride) Injection by intravenous bolus.

Symptomatic response to *Tagamet* therapy does not preclude the presence of a gastric malignancy. There have been rare reports of transient healing of gastric ulcers despite subsequently documented malignancy.

Reversible confusional states (see Adverse Reactions) have been observed on occasion, predominantly, but not exclusively, in severely ill patients. Advancing age (50 or more years) and preexisting liver and/or renal disease appear to be contributing factors. In some patients these confusional states have been mild and have not required discontinuation of *Tagamet* therapy. In cases where discontinuation was judged necessary, the condition usually cleared within 3 to 4 days of drug withdrawal.

Drug Interactions: *Tagamet,* apparently through an effect on certain microsomal enzyme systems, has been reported to reduce the hepatic metabolism of warfarin-type anticoagulants, phenytoin, propranolol, nifedipine, chlordiazepoxide, diazepam, certain tricyclic antidepressants, lidocaine, theophylline and metronidazole, thereby delaying elimination and increasing blood levels of these drugs.

Clinically significant effects have been reported with the warfarin anticoagulants; therefore, close monitoring of prothrombin time is recommended, and adjustment of the anticoagulant dose may be necessary when *Tagamet* is administered concomitantly. Interaction with phenytoin, lidocaine and theophylline has also been reported to produce adverse clinical effects.

However, a crossover study in healthy subjects receiving either *Tagamet* 300 mg q.i.d. or 800 mg h.s. concomitantly with a 300 mg b.i.d. dosage of theophylline (Theo-Dur®, Key Pharmaceuticals, Inc.) demonstrated less alteration in steady-state theophylline peak serum levels with the 800 mg h.s. regimen, particularly in subjects aged 54 years and older. Data beyond 10 days are not available. (Note: All patients receiving theophylline should be monitored appropriately, regardless of concomitant drug therapy.)

Dosage of the drugs mentioned above and other similarly metabolized drugs, particularly those of low therapeutic ratio or in patients with renal and/or hepatic impairment, may require adjustment when starting or stopping concomitantly administered *Tagamet* to maintain optimum therapeutic blood levels.

Alteration of pH may affect absorption of certain drugs (e.g., ketoconazole). If these products are needed, they should be given at least 2 hours before cimetidine administration.

Additional clinical experience may reveal other drugs affected by the concomitant administration of *Tagamet.*

Carcinogenesis, Mutagenesis, Impairment of Fertility: In a 24-month toxicity study conducted in rats, at dose levels of 150, 378 and 950 mg/kg/day (approximately 8 to 48 times the recommended human dose), there was a small increase in the incidence of benign Leydig cell tumors in each dose group; when the combined drug-treated groups and control groups were compared, this increase reached statistical significance. In a subsequent 24-month study, there were no differences between the rats receiving 150 mg/kg/day and the untreated controls. However, a statistically significant increase in benign Leydig cell tumor incidence was seen in the rats that received 378 and 950 mg/kg/day. These tumors were common in control groups as well as treated groups and the difference became apparent only in aged rats.

Tagamet (cimetidine) has demonstrated a weak antiandrogenic effect. In animal studies this was manifested as reduced prostate and seminal vesicle weights. However, there was no impairment of mating performance or fertility, nor any harm to the fetus in these animals at doses 8 to 48 times the full therapeutic dose of *Tagamet,* as compared with controls. The cases of gynecomastia seen in patients treated for 1 month or longer may be related to this effect.

In human studies, *Tagamet* has been shown to have no effect on spermatogenesis, sperm count, motility, morphology or *in vitro* fertilizing capacity.

Pregnancy: Teratogenic Effects. Pregnancy Category B: Reproduction studies have been performed in rats, rabbits and mice at doses up to 40 times the normal human dose and have revealed no evidence of impaired fertility or harm to the fetus due to *Tagamet.* There are, however, no adequate and well-controlled studies in pregnant women. Because animal reproductive studies are not always predictive of human response, this drug should be used during pregnancy only if clearly needed.

Nursing Mothers: Cimetidine is secreted in human milk and, as a general rule, nursing should not be undertaken while a patient is on a drug.

Pediatric Use: Clinical experience in children is limited. Therefore, *Tagamet* therapy cannot be recommended for children under 16, unless, in the judgment of the physician, anticipated benefits outweigh the potential risks. In very limited experience, doses of 20 to 40 mg/kg per day have been used.

Immunocompromised Patients: In immunocompromised patients, decreased gastric acidity, including that produced by acid-suppressing agents such as cimetidine, may increase the possibility of a hyperinfection of strongyloidiasis.

ADVERSE REACTIONS

Adverse effects reported in patients taking *Tagamet* are described below by body system. Incidence figures of 1 in 100 and greater are generally derived from controlled clinical studies.

Gastrointestinal: Diarrhea (usually mild) has been reported in approximately 1 in 100 patients.

CNS: Headaches, ranging from mild to severe, have been reported in 3.5% of 924 patients taking 1600 mg/day, 2.1% of 2,225 patients taking 800 mg/day and 2.3% of 1,897 patients taking placebo. Dizziness and somnolence (usually mild) have been reported in approximately 1 in 100 patients on either 1600 mg/day or 800 mg/day.

Reversible confusional states, e.g., mental confusion, agitation, psychosis, depression, anxiety, hallucinations, disorientation, have been reported predominantly, but not exclusively, in severely ill patients. They have usually developed within 2 to 3 days of initiation of *Tagamet* therapy and have cleared within 3 to 4 days of discontinuation of the drug.

Endocrine: Gynecomastia has been reported in patients treated for 1 month or longer. In patients being treated for pathological hypersecretory states, this occurred in about 4% of cases while in all others the incidence was 0.3% to 1% in various studies. No evidence of induced endocrine dysfunction was found, and the condition remained unchanged or returned toward normal with continuing Tagamet (cimetidine) treatment.

Reversible impotence has been reported in patients with pathological hypersecretory disorders, e.g., Zollinger-Ellison Syndrome, receiving *Tagamet,* particularly in high doses, for at least 12 months (range 12 to 79 months, mean 38 months). However, in large-scale surveillance studies at regular dosage, the incidence has not exceeded that commonly reported in the general population.

Hematologic: Decreased white blood cell counts in *Tagamet*-treated patients (approximately 1 per 100,000 patients), including agranulocytosis (approximately 3 per million patients), have been reported, including a few reports of recurrence on rechallenge. Most of these reports were in patients who had serious concomitant illnesses and received drugs and/or treatment known to produce neutropenia. Thrombocytopenia (approximately 3 per million patients) and, very rarely, cases of pancytopenia or aplastic anemia have also been reported. As with some other H₂-receptor antagonists, there have been extremely rare reports of immune hemolytic anemia.

Hepatobiliary: Dose-related increases in serum transaminase have been reported. In most cases they did not progress with continued therapy and returned to normal at the end of therapy. There have been rare reports of cholestatic or mixed cholestatic-hepatocellular effects. These were usually reversible. Because of the predominance of cholestatic features, severe parenchymal injury is considered highly unlikely. However, as in the occasional liver injury with other H₂-receptor antagonists, in exceedingly rare circumstances fatal outcomes have been reported.

There has been reported a single case of biopsy-proven periportal hepatic fibrosis in a patient receiving *Tagamet.* Rare cases of pancreatitis, which cleared on withdrawal of the drug, have been reported.

Hypersensitivity: Rare cases of fever and allergic reactions including anaphylaxis and hypersensitivity vasculitis, which cleared on withdrawal of the drug, have been reported.

Renal: Small, possibly dose-related increases in plasma creatinine, presumably due to competition for renal tubular secretion, are not uncommon and do not signify deteriorating renal function. Rare cases of interstitial nephritis and urinary retention, which cleared on withdrawal of the drug, have been reported.

Cardiovascular: Rare cases of bradycardia, tachycardia and A-V heart block have been reported with H₂-receptor antagonists.

Musculoskeletal: There have been rare reports of reversible arthralgia and myalgia; exacerbation of joint symptoms in patients with preexisting arthritis has also been reported. Such symptoms have usually been alleviated by a reduction in Tagamet (cimetidine) dosage. Rare cases of polymyositis have been reported, but no causal relationship has been established.

Integumental: Mild rash and, very rarely, cases of severe generalized skin reactions including Stevens-Johnson syndrome, epidermal necrolysis, erythema multiforme, exfoliative dermatitis and generalized exfoliative erythroderma have been reported with H₂-receptor antagonists. Reversible alopecia has been reported very rarely.

Immune Function: There have been extremely rare reports of strongyloidiasis hyperinfection in immunocompromised patients.

OVERDOSAGE

Studies in animals indicate that toxic doses are associated with respiratory failure and tachycardia that may be controlled by assisted respiration and the administration of a beta-blocker.

Reported acute ingestions orally of up to 20 grams have been associated with transient adverse effects similar to those encountered in normal clinical experience. The usual measures to remove unabsorbed material from the gastrointestinal tract, clinical monitoring and supportive therapy should be employed.

There have been reports of severe CNS symptoms, including unresponsiveness, following ingestion of between 20 and 40 grams of cimetidine, and extremely rare reports following concomitant use of multiple CNS-active medications and ingestion of cimetidine at doses less than 20 grams. An elderly, terminally ill dehydrated patient with organic brain syndrome receiving concomitant antipsychotic agents and *Tagamet* 4800 mg intravenously over a 24-hour period experienced mental deterioration with reversal on *Tagamet* discontinuation.

There have been two deaths in adults who were reported to have ingested over 40 grams orally on a single occasion.

DOSAGE AND ADMINISTRATION

Duodenal Ulcer

Active Duodenal Ulcer: Clinical studies have indicated that suppression of nocturnal acid is the most important factor in duodenal ulcer healing (see Clinical Pharmacology—Acid Secretion). This is supported by recent clinical trials (see Clinical Trials—Active Duodenal Ulcer). Therefore, there is no apparent rationale, except for familiarity with use, for treating with anything other than a once-daily at bedtime dosage regimen (h.s.).

In a U.S. dose-ranging study of 400 mg h.s., 800 mg h.s. and 1600 mg h.s., a continuous dose response relationship for ulcer healing was demonstrated.

However, 800 mg h.s. is the dose of choice for most patients, as it provides a high healing rate (the difference between 800 mg h.s. and 1600 mg h.s. being small), maximal pain relief, a decreased potential for drug interactions (see Precautions—Drug Interactions) and maximal patient convenience. Patients unhealed at 4 weeks, or those with persistent symptoms, have been shown to benefit from 2 to 4 weeks of continued therapy.

It has been shown that patients who both have an endoscopically demonstrated ulcer larger than 1.0 cm and are also heavy smokers (i.e., smoke one pack of cigarettes or more per day) are more difficult to heal. There is some evidence which suggests that more rapid healing can be achieved in this subpopulation with *Tagamet* 1600 mg at bedtime. While early pain relief with either 800 mg h.s. or 1600 mg h.s. is equivalent in all patients, 1600 mg h.s. provides an appropriate alternative when it is important to ensure healing within 4 weeks for this subpopulation. Alternatively, approximately 94% of all patients will also heal in 8 weeks with *Tagamet* 800 mg h.s.

Other *Tagamet* regimens in the U.S. which have been shown to be effective are: 300 mg four times daily, with meals and at bedtime, the original regimen with which U.S. physicians have the most experience, and 400 mg twice daily, in the morning and at bedtime (see Clinical Trials—Active Duodenal Ulcer).

Concomitant antacids should be given as needed for relief of pain. However, simultaneous administration of *Tagamet* and antacids is not recommended, since antacids have been reported to interfere with the absorption of Tagamet (cimetidine).

While healing with *Tagamet* often occurs during the first week or two, treatment should be continued for 4 to 6 weeks unless healing has been demonstrated by endoscopic examination.

Maintenance Therapy for Duodenal Ulcer: In those patients requiring maintenance therapy, the recommended adult oral dose is 400 mg at bedtime.

Active Benign Gastric Ulcer

The recommended adult oral dosage for short-term treatment of active benign gastric ulcer is 800 mg h.s., or 300 mg four times a day with meals and at bedtime. Controlled clinical studies were limited to 6 weeks of treatment (see Clinical Trials). 800 mg h.s. is the preferred regimen for most patients based upon convenience and reduced potential for drug interactions. Symptomatic response to *Tagamet* does not preclude the presence of a gastric malignancy. It is important to follow gastric ulcer patients to assure rapid progress to complete healing.

Erosive Gastroesophageal Reflux Disease (GERD)
The recommended adult oral dosage for the treatment of erosive esophagitis that has been diagnosed by endoscopy is 1600 mg daily in divided doses (800 mg b.i.d. or 400 mg q.i.d.) for 12 weeks. The use of *Tagamet* beyond 12 weeks has not been established.

Prevention of Upper Gastrointestinal Bleeding
The recommended adult dosing regimen is continuous I.V. infusion of 50 mg/hour. Patients with creatinine clearance less than 30 cc/min. should receive half the recommended dose. Treatment beyond 7 days has not been studied.

Pathological Hypersecretory Conditions
(such as Zollinger-Ellison Syndrome)
Recommended adult oral dosage: 300 mg four times a day with meals and at bedtime. In some patients it may be necessary to administer higher doses more frequently. Doses should be adjusted to individual patient needs, but should not usually exceed 2400 mg per day and should continue as long as clinically indicated.

Parenteral Administration
In hospitalized patients with pathological hypersecretory conditions or intractable ulcers, or in patients who are unable to take oral medication, *Tagamet* may be administered parenterally.
The doses and regimen for parenteral administration in patients with GERD have not been established.
All parenteral drug products should be inspected visually for particulate matter and discoloration prior to administration.

Recommendations for parenteral administration:
Intramuscular injection: 300 mg q 6 to 8 hours (no dilution necessary). Transient pain at the site of injection has been reported.
Intravenous injection: 300 mg q 6 to 8 hours. In some patients it may be necessary to increase dosage. When this is necessary, the increases should be made by more frequent administration of a 300 mg dose, but should not exceed 2400 mg per day. Dilute Tagamet (cimetidine hydrochloride) Injection, 300 mg, in Sodium Chloride Injection (0.9%) or another compatible I.V. solution (see Stability of *Tagamet* Injection) to a total volume of 20 mL and inject over a period of not less than 5 minutes (see Precautions).
Intermittent intravenous infusion: 300 mg q 6 to 8 hours, infused over 15 to 20 minutes. In some patients it may be necessary to increase dosage. When this is necessary, the increases should be made by more frequent administration of a 300 mg dose, but should not exceed 2400 mg per day. **Vials:** Dilute *Tagamet* Injection, 300 mg, in at least 50 mL of 5% Dextrose Injection, or another compatible I.V. solution (see Stability of *Tagamet* Injection). **Plastic containers:** Use premixed *Tagamet* Injection, 300 mg, in 0.9% Sodium Chloride in 50 mL plastic containers. **ADD-Vantage® Vials:** Dilute contents of one vial in an ADD-Vantage® Diluent Container, available in 50 mL and 100 mL sizes of 0.9% Sodium Chloride Injection, and 5% Dextrose Injection.
Continuous intravenous infusion: 37.5 mg/hour (900 mg/day). For patients requiring a more rapid elevation of gastric pH, continuous infusion may be preceded by a 150 mg loading dose administered by I.V. infusion as described above. Dilute 900 mg *Tagamet* Injection in a compatible I.V. fluid (see Stability of *Tagamet* Injection) for constant rate infusion over a 24-hour period. Note: *Tagamet* may be diluted in 100 to 1000 mL; however, a volumetric pump is recommended if the volume for 24-hour infusion is less than 250 mL. In one study in patients with pathological hypersecretory states, the mean infused dose of cimetidine was 160 mg/hour with a range of 40 to 600 mg/hour.
These doses maintained the intragastric acid secretory rate at 10 mEq/hour or less. The infusion rate should be adjusted to individual patient requirements.

DIRECTIONS FOR USE OF TAGAMET (cimetidine hydrochloride) INJECTION IN PLASTIC CONTAINERS
To open: Tear overwrap down side at slit and remove solution containers.
Some opacity of the plastic due to moisture absorption during the sterilization process may be observed. This is normal and does not affect solution quality or safety. The opacity will diminish gradually.
Do not add other drugs to premixed *Tagamet* Injection in plastic containers.
CAUTION: Check for minute leaks by squeezing inner bag firmly. If leaks are found, discard solution as sterility may be impaired. Additives should not be introduced into this solution. Do not use if the solution is cloudy or precipitated or if the seal is not intact.
Do not use plastic containers in series connections. Such use could result in air embolism due to residual air being drawn from the primary container before administration of the fluid from the secondary container is complete.
Use sterile equipment.
Preparation for administration:
1. Suspend container from eyelet support.
2. Remove plastic protector from outlet port at bottom of container.
3. Attach administration set. Refer to complete directions accompanying set.

DIRECTIONS FOR USE OF TAGAMET® INJECTION IN ADD-VANTAGE® VIALS are enclosed in ADD-Vantage® Vial packaging.

Stability of *Tagamet* Injection
When added to or diluted with most commonly used intravenous solutions, e.g., Sodium Chloride Injection (0.9%), Dextrose Injection (5% or 10%), Lactated Ringer's Solution, 5% Sodium Bicarbonate Injection, Tagamet (cimetidine hydrochloride) Injection should not be used after more than 48 hours of storage at room temperature.
Tagamet Injection premixed in plastic containers is stable through the labeled expiration date when stored under the recommended conditions.

Dosage Adjustment for Patients with Impaired Renal Function
Patients with severely impaired renal function have been treated with *Tagamet*. However, such usage has been very limited. On the basis of this experience the recommended dosage is 300 mg q 12 hours orally or by intravenous injection. Should the patient's condition require, the frequency of dosing may be increased to q 8 hours or even further with caution. In severe renal failure, accumulation may occur and the lowest frequency of dosing compatible with an adequate patient response should be used. When liver impairment is also present, further reductions in dosage may be necessary. Hemodialysis reduces the level of circulating *Tagamet*. Ideally, the dosage schedule should be adjusted so that the timing of a scheduled dose coincides with the end of hemodialysis.
Patients with creatinine clearance less than 30 cc/min. who are being treated for prevention of upper gastrointestinal bleeding should receive half the recommended dose.

HOW SUPPLIED
Tablets: Light green, film-coated as follows: 200 mg—round, imprinted with the product name TAGAMET, SKF and 200—tablets in bottles of 100; 300 mg—round, debossed with the product name TAGAMET, SB and 300—tablets in bottles of 100 and Single Unit Packages of 100 (intended for institutional use only); 400 mg—oval-shaped Tiltab®, debossed with the product name, TAGAMET, SB and 400—tablets in bottles of 60 and Single Unit Packages of 100 (intended for institutional use only); 800 mg—oval-shaped Tiltab®, debossed with the product name TAGAMET, SB and 800—tablets in bottles of 30 and Single Unit Packages of 100 (intended for institutional use only).
Store between 15° and 30°C (59° and 86°F); dispense in a tight light-resistant container.
200 mg 100's: NDC 0108-5012-20
300 mg 100's: NDC 0108-5013-20
300 mg SUP 100's: NDC 0108-5013-21
400 mg 60's: NDC 0108-5026-18
400 mg SUP 100's: NDC 0108-5026-21
800 mg 30's: NDC 0108-5027-13
800 mg SUP 100's: NDC 0108-5027-21
Liquid: Clear, light orange, mint-peach flavored, as follows: 300 mg/5 mL in 8 fl oz (237 mL) amber glass bottles; 300 mg/5 mL in single-dose units in packages of 10 (intended for institutional use only).
Store between 15° and 30°C (59° and 86°F); dispense in a tight light-resistant container.
300 mg/5 mL 8 fl oz: NDC 0108-5014-48
300 mg/5 mL SUP 10's: NDC 0108-5014-10
Injection:
Vials: 300 mg/2 mL in single-dose vials, in packages of 25, and in 8 mL multi-dose vials, in packages of 10 and 25.
Store between 15° and 30°C (59° and 86°F); do not refrigerate.
300 mg/2 mL Single-Dose Vials: NDC 0108-5017-16 (package of 25 vials)
300 mg/2 mL in 8 mL Multi-Dose Vials:
NDC 0108-5022-11 (package of 10 vials)
NDC 0108-5022-16 (package of 25 vials)
Single-Dose Premixed Plastic Containers: 300 mg in 50 mL of 0.9% Sodium Chloride in single-dose plastic containers, in packages of 4 units. No preservative has been added.
Exposure of the premixed product to excessive heat should be avoided. It is recommended the product be stored between 15° and 30°C (59° and 86°F). Brief exposure up to 40°C does not adversely affect the premixed product.
300 mg/50 mL SUP's: NDC 0108-5029-04
ADD-Vantage® Vials: 300 mg/2 mL in single-dose ADD-Vantage® Vials, in packages of 25.
Store between 15° and 30°C (59° and 86°F); do not refrigerate.
300 mg/2 mL: NDC 0108-5031-16 (package of 25 vials)
Tagamet (cimetidine hydrochloride) Injection premixed in single-dose plastic containers is manufactured for SmithKline Beecham Pharmaceuticals by Baxter Healthcare Corporation, Deerfield, IL 60015.
Veterans Administration/Military/PHS—Tablets, 200 mg, 100's, 6505-01-103-6335; 300 mg, SUP, 100's, 6505-01-050-3546; 300 mg, 100's, 6505-01-050-3547; 300 mg, 500's × 12 Bulk, 6505-01-323-5256; 300 mg, 5000's, 6505-01-388-1904; 400 mg, 60's, 6505-01-176-0712; 400 mg, SUP, 100's, 6505-01-207-3113; 400 mg, 500's × 12 Bulk, 6505-01-323-5255; 400 mg, 5000's, 6505-01-388-1901; 800 mg, 30's, 6505-01-291-8374; 800 mg, SUP, 100's, 6505-01-339-1872; 800 mg, 500's, 6505-01-388-1022; Injection, 300 mg/2 mL, 25's, 6505-01-351-9271; 8 mL, 300 mg/2 mL, 10's, 6505-01-069-1661; 8 mL, 300 mg/2 mL, 6505-01-282-2970; 300 mg/50 mL, MINI-BAG, 48's, 6505-01-242-8865; 300 mg/2 mL, ADD-Vantage, 25's, 6505-01-307-8201. Liquid, 300 mg/5 mL, 8 fl oz, 6505-01-119-0616; 300 mg/5 mL, SUP, 10's, 6505-01-222-3560.

TG:L91A

Shown in Product Identification Guide, page 337

TAZICEF® ℞
[taz 'i-sef]
brand of ceftazidime for injection for intravenous or intramuscular use

DESCRIPTION
Ceftazidime is a semisynthetic, broad-spectrum, beta-lactam antibiotic for intravenous or intramuscular administration. It is the pentahydrate of Pyridinium, 1-[[7- [[(2- amino-4-thiazolyl) [(1-carboxy-1-methylethoxy) imino]acetyl]amino]-2-carboxy -8- oxo -5- thia-1-azabicyclo (4.2.0.) oct -2- en -3- yl] methyl]-,hydroxide,inner salt, [6R-[6α,7β(Z)]].
Its molecular formula is $C_{22}H_{22}N_6O_7S_2 \cdot 5H_20$ and the molecular weight is 636.65.
Tazicef (ceftazidime for injection) is a sterile, dry, powdered mixture of ceftazidime pentahydrate and sodium carbonate. The sodium carbonate at a concentration of 118 mg/gram of ceftazidime activity has been admixed to facilitate dissolution. The total sodium content of the mixture is approximately 54 mg (2.3 mEq)/gram of ceftazidime activity.
Tazicef in sterile crystalline form is supplied in vials equivalent to 1 gram or 2 grams of anhydrous ceftazidime, in piggyback vials equivalent to 1 gram or 2 grams of anhydrous ceftazidime and ADD-Vantage® vials equivalent to 1 gram or 2 grams of anhydrous ceftazidime. Solutions of *Tazicef* range in color from light yellow to amber, depending upon the diluent and volume used. The pH of freshly reconstituted solutions usually ranges from 5.0 to 8.0.

CLINICAL PHARMACOLOGY
After intravenous administration of 500 mg and 1 gram doses of ceftazidime over 5 minutes to normal adult male volunteers, mean peak serum concentrations of 45 mcg/mL and 90 mcg/mL, respectively, were achieved. After intravenous infusion of 500 mg, 1 gram and 2 gram doses of ceftazidime over 20 to 30 minutes to normal adult male volunteers, mean peak serum concentrations of 42 mcg/mL, 69 mcg/mL and 170 mcg/mL, respectively, were achieved. The average serum concentrations following intravenous infusion of 500 mg, 1 gram and 2 gram doses to these volunteers over an 8-hour interval are given in Table 1.

Table 1

Ceftazidime IV Dosage	Serum Concentrations (mcg/mL)				
	0.5 hr.	1 hr.	2 hr.	4 hr.	8 hr.
500 mg	42	25	12	6	2
1 gram	60	39	23	11	3
2 grams	129	75	42	13	5

The absorption and elimination of ceftazidime were directly proportional to the size of the dose. The half-life following intravenous administration was approximately 1.9 hours. Less than 10% of ceftazidime was protein bound. The degree of protein binding was independent of concentration. There was no evidence of accumulation of ceftazidime in the serum in individuals with normal renal function following multiple intravenous doses of 1 gram and 2 grams every 8 hours for 10 days.
Following intramuscular administration of 500 mg and 1 gram doses of ceftazidime to normal adult volunteers, the mean peak serum concentrations were 17 mcg/mL and 39 mcg/mL, respectively, at approximately 1 hour. Serum concentrations remained above 4 mcg/mL for 6 and 8 hours after the intramuscular administration of 500 mg and 1 gram doses, respectively. The half-life of ceftazidime in these volunteers was approximately 2 hours.
The presence of hepatic dysfunction had no effect on the pharmacokinetics of ceftazidime in individuals administered 2 grams intravenously every 8 hours for 5 days. Therefore, a

Continued on next page

Information on the SmithKline Beecham Pharmaceuticals products appearing here is based on the labeling in effect on July 1, 1996. Further information on these and other products may be obtained from the Medical Department, SmithKline Beecham Pharmaceuticals, One Franklin Plaza, Philadelphia, PA 19101.

SmithKline Beecham—Cont.

dosage adjustment from the normal recommended dosage is not required for patients with hepatic dysfunction, provided renal function is not impaired.

Approximately 80% to 90% of an intramuscular or intravenous dose of ceftazidime is excreted unchanged by the kidneys over a 24-hour period. After the intravenous administration of single 500 mg or 1 gram doses, approximately 50% of the dose appeared in the urine in the first 2 hours. An additional 20% was excreted between 2 and 4 hours after dosing, and approximately another 12% of the dose appeared in the urine between 4 and 8 hours later. The elimination of ceftazidime by the kidneys resulted in high therapeutic concentrations in the urine.

The mean renal clearance of ceftazidime was approximately 100 mL/min. The calculated plasma clearance of approximately 115 mL/min. indicated nearly complete elimination of ceftazidime by the renal route. Administration of probenecid prior to dosing had no effect on the elimination kinetics of ceftazidime. This suggests that ceftazidime is eliminated by glomerular filtration and is not actively secreted by renal tubular mechanisms.

Since ceftazidime is eliminated almost solely by the kidneys, its serum half-life is significantly prolonged in patients with impaired renal function. Consequently, dosage adjustments in such patients as described in the DOSAGE AND ADMINISTRATION section are suggested.

Therapeutic concentrations of ceftazidime are achieved in the following body tissues and fluid.

[See Table 2 below.]

Microbiology

Ceftazidime is bactericidal in action, exerting its effect by inhibition of enzymes responsible for cell-wall synthesis. A wide range of gram-negative organisms is susceptible to ceftazidime *in vitro*, including strains resistant to gentamicin and other aminoglycosides. In addition, ceftazidime has been shown to be active against gram-positive organisms. It is highly stable to most clinically important beta-lactamases, plasmid or chromosomal, which are produced by both gram-negative and gram-positive organisms and, consequently, is active against many strains resistant to ampicillin and other cephalosporins.

Ceftazidime has been shown to be active against the following organisms both *in vitro* and in clinical infections (see INDICATIONS AND USAGE).

Aerobes, Gram-Negative: *Citrobacter* species (including *Citrobacter freundii* and *Citrobacter diversus*); *Enterobacter* species (including *Enterobacter cloacae* and *Enterobacter aerogenes*); *Escherichia coli; Haemophilus influenzae,* including ampicillin-resistant strains; *Klebsiella* species (including *Klebsiella pneumoniae*); *Neisseria meningitidis; Proteus mirabilis; Proteus vulgaris; Pseudomonas* species (including *Pseudomonas aeruginosa*); and *Serratia* species.

Aerobes, Gram-Positive: *Staphylococcus aureus,* including penicillinase- and non-penicillinase-producing strains; *Streptococcus agalactiae* (group B streptococci); and *Streptococcus pneumoniae;* and *Streptococcus pyogenes* (group A beta-hemolytic streptococci).

Anaerobes: *Bacteroides* species (NOTE: Many strains of *Bacteroides fragilis* are resistant).

Ceftazidime has been shown to be active *in vitro* against most strains of the following organisms; however, the clinical significance of these data is unknown: *Acinetobacter* species; *Clostridium* species (not including *Clostridium difficile*); *Haemophilus parainfluenzae; Morganella morganii* (formerly *Proteus morganii*); *Neisseria gonorrhoeae; Peptococcus* species; *Peptostreptococcus* species; *Providencia* species (including *Providencia rettgeri,* formerly *Proteus rettgeri*); *Salmonella* species; *Shigella* species; *Staphylococcus epidermidis*; and *Yersinia enterocolitica.*

Ceftazidime and the aminoglycosides have been shown to be synergistic *in vitro* against Enterobacteriaceae and *Pseudomonas aeruginosa.* Ceftazidime and carbenicillin have also been shown to be synergistic *in vitro* against *P. aeruginosa.*

Ceftazidime is not active *in vitro* against: *Campylobacter* species; *Clostridium difficile; Listeria monocytogenes;* methicillin-resistant staphylococci; or *Streptococcus faecalis* and many other enterococci.

Susceptibility Tests

Diffusion Techniques

Quantitative methods that require measurement of zone diameters give an estimate of antibiotic susceptibility. One such procedure[1–3] has been recommended for use with disks to test susceptibility to ceftazidime.

Reports from the laboratory giving results of the standard single-disk susceptibility test with a 30 mcg ceftazidime disk should be interpreted according to the following criteria:

Susceptible organisms produce zones of 18 mm or greater, indicating that the test organism is likely to respond to therapy.

Organisms that produce zones of 15 mm to 17 mm are expected to be susceptible if high dosage is used or if the infection is confined to tissues and fluids (e.g., urine) in which high antibiotic levels are attained.

Resistant organisms produce zones of 14 mm or less, indicating that other therapy should be selected.

Organisms should be tested with the ceftazidime disk, since ceftazidime has been shown by *in vitro* tests to be active against certain strains found resistant when other beta-lactam disks are used.

Standardized procedures require the use of laboratory control organisms. The 30 mcg ceftazidime disk should give zone diameters between 25 mm and 32 mm for *E. coli* ATCC 25922. For *P. aeruginosa* ATCC 27853, the zone diameters should be between 22 mm and 29 mm. For *S. aureus* ATCC 25923, the zone diameters should be between 16 mm and 20 mm.

Dilution Techniques

In other susceptibility testing procedures, e.g., ICS agar dilution or the equivalent, a bacterial isolate may be considered susceptible if the MIC value for ceftazidime is not more than 16 mcg/mL. Organisms are considered resistant to ceftazidime if the MIC is equal to or greater than 64 mcg/mL. Organisms having an MIC value of less than 64 mcg/mL but greater than 16 mcg/mL are expected to be susceptible if high dosage is used or if the infection is confined to tissues and fluids (e.g., urine) in which high antibiotic levels are attained.

As with standard diffusion methods, dilution procedures require the use of laboratory control organisms. Standard ceftazidime powder should give MIC values in the range of 4 mcg/mL and 16 mcg/mL for *S. aureus* ATCC 25923. For *E. coli* ATCC 25922, the MIC range should be between 0.125 mcg/mL and 0.5 mcg/mL. For *P. aeruginosa* ATCC 27853, the MIC range should be between 0.5 mcg/mL and 2 mcg/mL.

INDICATIONS AND USAGE

Tazicef (ceftazidime for injection) is indicated for the treatment of patients with infections caused by susceptible strains of the designated organisms in the diseases listed below:

LOWER RESPIRATORY TRACT INFECTIONS, including pneumonia, caused by *P. aeruginosa* and other *Pseudomonas* species; *H. influenzae,* including ampicillin-resistant strains; *Klebsiella* species; *Enterobacter* species, *P. mirabilis; E. coli; Serratia* species; *Citrobacter* species; *S. pneumoniae;* and *S. aureus* (methicillin-susceptible strains).

Table 2. Ceftazidime Concentrations in Body Tissues and Fluids

Tissue or Fluid	Dose/ Route	No. Patients	Time of Sample Post-Dose	Average Tissue or Fluid Level (mcg/mL or mcg/g)
Urine	500 mg IM	6	0 to 2 hours	2,100
	2 grams IV	6	0 to 2 hours	12,000
Bile	2 grams IV	3	90 min.	36.4
Synovial fluid	2 grams IV	13	2 hours	25.6
Peritoneal fluid	2 grams IV	8	2 hours	48.6
Sputum	1 gram IV	8	1 hour	9
Cerebrospinal fluid	2 grams q8h IV	5	120 min.	9.8
(inflamed meninges)	2 grams q8h IV	6	180 min.	9.4
Aqueous humor	2 grams IV	13	1 to 3 hours	11
Blister fluid	1 gram IV	7	2 to 3 hours	19.7
Lymphatic fluid	1 gram IV	7	2 to 3 hours	23.4
Bone	2 grams IV	8	0.67 hour	31.1
Heart muscle	2 grams IV	35	30 to 280 min.	12.7
Skin	2 grams IV	22	30 to 180 min.	6.6
Skeletal muscle	2 grams IV	35	30 to 280 min.	9.4
Myometrium	2 grams IV	31	1 to 2 hours	18.7

SKIN AND SKIN STRUCTURE INFECTIONS, caused by *P. aeruginosa, Klebsiella* species; *E. coli; Proteus* species including *P. mirabilis* and indole-positive *Proteus, Enterobacter* species; *Serratia* species; *S. aureus* (methicillin-susceptible strains) and *S. pyogenes* (group A beta-hemolytic streptococci).

URINARY TRACT INFECTIONS, both complicated and uncomplicated, caused by *P. aeruginosa; Enterobacter* species; *Proteus* species, including *P. mirabilis* and indole-positive *Proteus; Klebsiella* species and *E. coli.*

BACTERIAL SEPTICEMIA, caused by *P. aeruginosa, Klebsiella* species; *H. influenzae; E. coli, Serratia* species, *S. pneumoniae* and *S. aureus* (methicillin-susceptible strains).

BONE AND JOINT INFECTIONS, caused by *P. aeruginosa; Klebsiella* species; *Enterobacter* species; and *S. aureus* (methicillin-susceptible strains).

GYNECOLOGIC INFECTIONS, including endometritis, pelvic cellulitis and other infections of the female genital tract caused by *E. coli.*

INTRA-ABDOMINAL INFECTIONS, including peritonitis caused by *E. coli, Klebsiella* species; *S. aureus* (methicillin-susceptible strains), and polymicrobial infections caused by aerobic and anaerobic organisms, and *Bacteroides* species (many strains of *B. fragilis* are resistant).

CENTRAL NERVOUS SYSTEM INFECTIONS, including meningitis caused by *H. influenzae* and *Neisseria meningitidis.* Ceftazidime has also been used successfully in a limited number of cases of meningitis due to *P. aeruginosa* and *S. pneumoniae.*

Specimens for bacterial cultures should be obtained prior to therapy in order to isolate and identify causative organisms and to determine their susceptibility to ceftazidime. Therapy may be instituted before results of susceptibility studies are known; however, once these results become available, the antibiotic treatment should be adjusted accordingly.

Tazicef (ceftazidime for injection) may be used alone in cases of confirmed or suspected sepsis. Ceftazidime has been used successfully in clinical trials as empiric therapy in cases where various concomitant therapies with other antibiotics have been used.

Tazicef may also be used concomitantly with other antibiotics, such as aminoglycosides, vancomycin and clindamycin, in severe and life-threatening infections and in the immunocompromised patient. When such concomitant treatment is appropriate, prescribing information in the labeling for the other antibiotics should be followed. The dose depends on the severity of the infection and the patient's condition.

CONTRAINDICATIONS

Tazicef is contraindicated in patients who have shown hypersensitivity to ceftazidime or the cephalosporin group of antibiotics.

WARNINGS

SERIOUS AND OCCASIONALLY FATAL HYPERSENSITIVITY (anaphylactic) REACTIONS HAVE BEEN REPORTED IN PATIENTS ON PENICILLIN THERAPY. THESE REACTIONS ARE MORE LIKELY TO OCCUR IN INDIVIDUALS WITH A HISTORY OF PENICILLIN HYPERSENSITIVITY AND/OR A HISTORY OF SENSITIVITY TO MULTIPLE ALLERGENS. THERE HAVE BEEN REPORTS OF INDIVIDUALS WITH A HISTORY OF PENICILLIN HYPERSENSITIVITY WHO HAVE EXPERIENCED SEVERE REACTIONS WHEN TREATED WITH CEPHALOSPORINS. BEFORE INITIATING THERAPY WITH *TAZICEF*, CAREFUL INQUIRY SHOULD BE MADE CONCERNING PREVIOUS HYPERSENSITIVITY REACTIONS TO PENICILLINS, CEPHALOSPORINS OR OTHER ALLERGENS. IF AN ALLERGIC REACTION OCCURS, *TAZICEF* SHOULD BE DISCONTINUED AND APPROPRIATE THERAPY SHOULD BE INSTITUTED. SERIOUS ANAPHYLACTIC REACTIONS REQUIRE IMMEDIATE EMERGENCY TREATMENT WITH EPINEPHRINE. OXYGEN, INTRAVENOUS STEROIDS AND AIRWAY MANAGEMENT, INCLUDING INTUBATION, SHOULD ALSO BE ADMINISTERED AS INDICATED.

Pseudomembranous colitis has been reported with nearly all antibacterial agents, including *Tazicef,* and may range in severity from mild to life-threatening. Therefore, it is important to consider this diagnosis in patients who present with diarrhea subsequent to the administration of antibacterial agents.

Treatment with antibacterial agents alters the normal flora of the colon and may permit overgrowth of clostridia. Studies indicate that a toxin produced by *Clostridium difficile* is one primary cause of "antibiotic-associated colitis."

After the diagnosis of pseudomembranous colitis has been established, therapeutic measures should be initiated. Mild cases of pseudomembranous colitis usually respond to drug discontinuation alone. In moderate to severe cases, consideration should be given to management with fluids and electrolytes, protein supplementation and treatment with an antibacterial drug clinically effective against *C. difficile* colitis.

Elevated levels of ceftazidime in patients with renal insufficiency can lead to seizures, encephalopathy, asterixis and neuromuscular excitability (see PRECAUTIONS).

Table 3. Recommended Dosage Schedule

	Dose	Frequency
Adults		
Usual recommended dose	1 gram IV or IM	q8 to 12h
Uncomplicated urinary tract infections	250 mg IV or IM	q12h
Bone and joint infections	2 grams IV	q12h
Complicated urinary tract infections	500 mg IV or IM	q8 to 12h
Uncomplicated pneumonia; mild skin and skin structure infections	500 mg to 1 gram IV or IM	q8h
Serious gynecological and intra-abdominal infections	2 grams IV	q8h
Meningitis	2 grams IV	q8h
Very severe life-threatening infections, especially in immunocompromised patients	2 grams IV	q8h
Lung infections caused by *Pseudomonas* species in patients with cystic fibrosis with normal renal function*	30 to 50 mg/kg IV to a maximum of 6 grams/day	q8h
Neonates (0 to 4 weeks)	30 mg/kg IV	q12h
Infants and children (1 month to 12 years)	30 to 50 mg/kg IV to a maximum of 6 grams/day†	q8h

* Although clinical improvement has been shown, bacteriological cures cannot be expected in patients with chronic respiratory disease and cystic fibrosis.

† The higher dose should be reserved for immunocompromised children or children with cystic fibrosis or meningitis.

PRECAUTIONS

General: Ceftazidime has not been shown to be nephrotoxic; however, high and prolonged serum antibiotic concentrations can occur from usual doses in patients with transient or persistent reduction of urinary output because of renal insufficiency. The total daily dosage should be reduced when ceftazidime is administered to patients with renal insufficiency (see DOSAGE AND ADMINISTRATION). In these patients, elevated levels of ceftazidime can lead to seizures, encephalopathy, asterixis and neuromuscular excitability. Continued dosage should be determined by degree of renal impairment, severity of infection and susceptibility of the causative organisms.

As with other antibiotics, prolonged use of Tazicef (ceftazidime for injection) may result in overgrowth of nonsusceptible organisms. Repeated evaluation of the patient's condition is essential. If superinfection occurs during therapy, appropriate measures should be taken.

Cephalosporins may be associated with a fall in prothrombin activity. Those at risk include patients with renal or hepatic impairment, or poor nutritional state, as well as patients receiving a protracted course of antimicrobial therapy. Prothrombin time should be monitored in patients at risk and exogenous vitamin K administered as indicated.

Tazicef should be prescribed with caution in individuals with a history of gastrointestinal disease, particularly colitis.

Drug Interactions: Nephrotoxicity has been reported following concomitant administration of cephalosporins with aminoglycoside antibiotics or potent diuretics, such as furosemide. Renal function should be carefully monitored, especially if higher dosages of the aminoglycosides are to be administered or if therapy is prolonged, because of the potential nephrotoxicity and ototoxicity of aminoglycoside antibiotics. Nephrotoxicity and ototoxicity were not noted when ceftazidime was given alone in clinical trials.

Chloramphenicol in combination with cephalosporins, including ceftazidime, has been shown to be antagonistic *in vitro*. Due to the possibility of antagonism *in vivo*, this combination should be avoided.

Drug/Laboratory Test Interactions: The administration of ceftazidime may result in a false-positive reaction for glucose in the urine when using Clinitest® tablets, Benedict's solution or Fehling's solution. It is recommended that glucose tests based on enzymatic glucose oxidase reactions (such as Clinistix® or Tes-Tape® [Glucose Enzymatic Test Strip USP]) be used.

Carcinogenesis, Mutagenesis, Impairment of Fertility: Long-term studies in animals have not been performed to evaluate carcinogenic potential. However, a mouse micronucleus test and an Ames test were both negative for mutagenic effects.

Pregnancy: Teratogenic Effects: Pregnancy Category B. Reproduction studies have been performed in mice and rats at doses up to 40 times the human dose and have revealed no evidence of impaired fertility or harm to the fetus due to *Tazicef*. There are, however, no adequate and well-controlled studies in pregnant women. Because animal reproduction studies are not always predictive of human response, this drug should be used during pregnancy only if clearly needed.

Nursing Mothers: Ceftazidime is excreted in human milk in low concentrations. Caution should be exercised when *Tazicef* is administered to a nursing woman.

Pediatric Use: See DOSAGE AND ADMINISTRATION.

ADVERSE REACTIONS

Ceftazidime is generally well-tolerated. The incidence of adverse reactions associated with the administration of ceftazidime was low in clinical trials. The most common were local reactions following IV injection and allergic and gastrointestinal reactions. Other adverse reactions were encountered infrequently. No disulfiram-like reactions were reported.

The following adverse effects from clinical trials were considered to be either related to ceftazidime therapy or were of uncertain etiology:

Local Effects, reported in less than 2% of patients, were phlebitis and inflammation at the site of injection (1 in 69 patients).

Hypersensitivity Reactions, reported in 2% of patients, were pruritus, rash and fever. Immediate reactions, generally manifested by rash and/or pruritus, occurred in 1 in 285 patients. Angioedema and anaphylaxis (bronchospasm and/or hypotension) have been reported very rarely.

Gastrointestinal Symptoms, reported in less than 2% of patients, were diarrhea (1 in 78), nausea (1 in 156), vomiting (1 in 500) and abdominal pain (1 in 416). The onset of pseudomembranous colitis symptoms may occur during or after treatment (see WARNINGS).

Central Nervous System Reactions (fewer than 1%) include headache, dizziness and paresthesia. Seizures have been reported with several cephalosporins, including ceftazidime. In addition, encephalopathy, asterixis and neuromuscular excitability have been reported in renally impaired patients treated with unadjusted dosage regimens of ceftazidime (see PRECAUTIONS: General).

Less Frequent Adverse Events (less than 1%) were candidiasis (including oral thrush) and vaginitis.

Laboratory Test Changes noted during Tazicef (ceftazidime for injection) clinical trials were transient and included: eosinophilia (1 in 13), positive Coombs' test without hemolysis (1 in 23), thrombocytosis (1 in 45), and slight elevations in one or more of the hepatic enzymes, aspartate aminotransferase (AST, SGOT) (1 in 16), alanine aminotransferase (ALT, SGPT) (1 in 15), LDH (1 in 18), GGT (1 in 19) and alkaline phosphatase (1 in 23). As with some other cephalosporins, transient elevations of blood urea, blood urea nitrogen and/or serum creatinine were observed occasionally. Transient leukopenia, neutropenia, agranulocytosis, thrombocytopenia and lymphocytosis were seen very rarely.

In addition to the adverse reactions listed above that have been observed with ceftazidime, the following adverse reactions and altered laboratory tests have been reported for cephalosporin-class antibiotics:

Adverse Reactions: Urticaria, Stevens-Johnson syndrome, erythema multiforme, toxic epidermal necrolysis, colitis, renal dysfunction, toxic nephropathy, hepatic dysfunction including cholestasis, aplastic anemia, hemolytic anemia, hemorrhage.

Altered Laboratory Tests: Prolonged prothrombin time, false-positive test for urinary glucose, elevated bilirubin, pancytopenia.

OVERDOSAGE

Ceftazidime overdosage has occurred in patients with renal failure. Reactions have included seizure activity, encephalopathy, asterixis and neuromuscular excitability. Patients who receive an acute overdosage should be carefully observed and given supportive treatment. In the presence of renal insufficiency, hemodialysis or peritoneal dialysis may aid in the removal of ceftazidime from the body.

DOSAGE AND ADMINISTRATION

Dosage: The usual adult dosage is 1 gram administered intravenously or intramuscularly every 8 or 12 hours. The dosage and route should be determined by the susceptibility of the causative organisms, the severity of infection and the condition and renal function of the patient.

The guidelines for dosage of *Tazicef* are listed in Table 3. The following dosage schedule is recommended.
[See table at left.]

Impaired Hepatic Function: No adjustment in dosage is required for patients with hepatic dysfunction.

Impaired Renal Function: Ceftazidime is excreted by the kidneys, almost exclusively by glomerular filtration. Therefore, in patients with impaired renal function (GFR <50 mL/min.), it is recommended that the dosage of ceftazidime be reduced to compensate for its slower excretion. In patients with suspected renal insufficiency, an initial loading dose of 1 gram of ceftazidime may be given. An estimate of GFR should be made to determine the appropriate maintenance dose. The recommended dosage is presented in Table 4.

Table 4. Recommended Maintenance Doses of Tazicef (ceftazidime for injection) in Renal Insufficiency

NOTE: IF THE DOSE RECOMMENDED IN TABLE 3 ABOVE IS LOWER THAN THAT RECOMMENDED FOR PATIENTS WITH RENAL INSUFFICIENCY AS OUTLINED IN TABLE 4, THE LOWER DOSE SHOULD BE USED.

Creatinine Clearance (mL/min.)	Recommended Unit Dose of Ceftazidime	Frequency of Dosing
50 to 31	1 gram	q12h
30 to 16	1 gram	q24h
15 to 6	500 mg	q24h
<5	500 mg	q48h

When only serum creatinine is available, the following formula (Cockcroft's equation)[4] may be used to estimate creatinine clearance. The serum creatinine should represent a steady state of renal function:

Males:

$$\text{Creatinine clearance (mL/min.)} = \frac{\text{Weight (kg)} \times (140 - \text{age})}{72 \times \text{serum creatinine (mg/dL)}}$$

Females:

$0.85 \times$ male value

In patients with severe infections who would normally receive 6 grams of ceftazidime daily were it not for renal insufficiency, the unit dose given in the table above may be increased by 50% or the dosing frequency increased appropriately. Further dosing should be determined by therapeutic monitoring, severity of the infection and susceptibility of the causative organism.

In children as for adults, the creatinine clearance should be adjusted for body surface area or lean body mass and the dosing frequency reduced in cases of renal insufficiency.

In patients undergoing hemodialysis, a loading dose of 1 gram is recommended, followed by 1 gram after each hemodialysis period.

Tazicef (ceftazidime for injection) can also be used in patients undergoing intra-peritoneal dialysis (IPD) and continuous ambulatory peritoneal dialysis (CAPD). In such patients, a loading dose of *Tazicef* 1 gram may be given, followed by 500 mg every 24 hours. In addition to intravenous use, *Tazicef* can be incorporated in the dialysis fluid at a concentration of 250 mg for 2 liters of dialysis fluid.

NOTE: Generally, *Tazicef* should be continued for 2 days after the signs and symptoms of infection have disappeared, but in complicated infections longer therapy may be required.

Administration: *Tazicef* may be given intravenously or by deep intramuscular injection into a large muscle mass such as the upper outer quadrant of the gluteus maximus or lateral part of the thigh.

NOTE: Ceftazidime for injection in ADD-Vantage® vials is not intended for direct intravenous or intramuscular injection.

Continued on next page

Information on the SmithKline Beecham Pharmaceuticals products appearing here is based on the labeling in effect on July 1, 1996. Further information on these and other products may be obtained from the Medical Department, SmithKline Beecham Pharmaceuticals, One Franklin Plaza, Philadelphia, PA 19101.

SmithKline Beecham—Cont.

Intramuscular Administration: For intramuscular administration, *Tazicef* should be reconstituted with Sterile Water for Injection. Refer to Table 5.

Intravenous Administration: The IV route is preferable for patients with bacterial septicemia, bacterial meningitis, peritonitis, or other severe or life-threatening infections, or for patients who may be poor risks because of lowered resistance resulting from such debilitating conditions as malnutrition, trauma, surgery, diabetes, heart failure or malignancy, particularly if shock is present or pending.

For direct intermittent intravenous administration, reconstitute *Tazicef* as directed in Table 5 with Sterile Water for Injection. Slowly inject directly into the vein over a period of 3 to 5 minutes or give through the tubing of an administration set while the patient is also receiving one of the compatible intravenous fluids (see COMPATIBILITY AND STABILITY).

For intravenous infusion, reconstitute the 1 or 2 gram piggyback vial with 100 mL of Sodium Chloride Injection or one of the compatible intravenous fluids listed under the COMPATIBILITY AND STABILITY section. Alternatively, reconstitute the 1 gram or 2 gram vial and add an appropriate quantity of the resulting solution to an IV container with one of the compatible intravenous fluids.

Intermittent intravenous infusion with a Y-type administration set can be accomplished with compatible solutions. However, during infusion of a solution containing *Tazicef* it is advisable to discontinue the other solution.

All vials of *Tazicef* as supplied are under reduced pressure. When *Tazicef* is dissolved, carbon dioxide is released and a positive pressure develops. See RECONSTITUTION.

Solutions of *Tazicef*, like those of most beta-lactam antibiotics, should not be added to solutions of aminoglycoside antibiotics because of potential interaction.

However, if concurrent therapy with *Tazicef* and an aminoglycoside is indicated, each of these antibiotics can be administered separately to the same patient.

***TAZICEF* INJECTION IN ADD-VANTAGE® VIALS**

NOTE: Tazicef (ceftazidime for injection) in the ADD-Vantage® vial is intended to be administered as a single-dose intravenous infusion with the ADD-Vantage® flexible diluent container.

Tazicef in single-dose ADD-Vantage® vials should be prepared as directed (see RECONSTITUTION, for ADD-Vantage® Vials) with either 0.9% Sodium Chloride Injection in the 50 mL or 100 mL flexible diluent containers, 0.45% Sodium Chloride Injection in the 50 mL container or 5% Dextrose Injection in the 50 mL or 100 mL containers.

RECONSTITUTION

Single-Dose Vials:
For IM injection, IV direct (bolus) injection or IV infusion, reconstitute with Sterile Water for Injection according to the following table. The vacuum may assist entry of the diluent. SHAKE WELL.

Table 5

Vial Size	Diluent to Be Added	Approx. Avail. Volume	Average Concentration
Intramuscular or Intravenous Direct (bolus) Injection			
1 gram	3.0 mL	3.6 mL	280 mg/mL
Intravenous Infusion			
1 gram	10 mL	10.6 mL	95 mg/mL
2 gram	10 mL	11.2 mL	180 mg/mL

Withdraw the total volume of solution into the syringe (the pressure in the vial may aid withdrawal). The withdrawn solution may contain some bubbles of carbon dioxide.

NOTE: As with the administration of all parenteral products, accumulated gases should be expressed from the syringe immediately before injection of *Tazicef*.

These solutions of *Tazicef* are stable for 24 hours at room temperature or 7 days if refrigerated (5°C). Slight yellowing does not affect potency.

For IV infusion, dilute reconstituted solution in 50 to 100 mL of one of the parenteral fluids listed under COMPATIBILITY AND STABILITY.

"Piggyback" Vials:
For IV infusion, reconstitute with 10 mL of Sodium Chloride Injection according to the following table. The vacuum may assist entry of the diluent. SHAKE WELL.

Table 6

Vial Size	Diluent to Be Added	Approx. Avail. Volume	Approx. Avg. Concentration
1 gram	100 mL*	100 mL	10 mg/mL
2 gram	100 mL*	100 mL	20 mg/mL

* Addition should be in two stages.

Insert a gas relief needle through the vial closure to relieve the internal pressure. With the gas relief needle in position, add the remaining 90 mL of Sodium Chloride Injection. Remove the gas relief needle and syringe needle; shake the vial and set up for infusion in the normal way.

NOTE: To preserve product sterility, it is important that a gas relief needle is not inserted through the vial closure before the product has dissolved.

These solutions of Tazicef (ceftazidime for injection) are stable for 24 hours at room temperature or 7 days if refrigerated (5°C). Slight yellowing does not affect potency.

ADD-Vantage® Vials: ADD-Vantage® vials of Tazicef (ceftazidime for injection) are to be reconstituted only with 0.9% Sodium Chloride Injection or 5% Dextrose Injection in the 50 mL or 100 mL flexible diluent containers, or with 0.45% Sodium Chloride Injection in the 50 mL container.

DIRECTIONS FOR USE OF TAZICEF® INJECTION IN ADD-VANTAGE® VIALS

To Open Diluent Container:
Peel overwrap at corner and remove solution container. Some opacity of the plastic due to moisture absorption during the sterilization process may be observed. This is normal and does not affect the solution quality or safety. The opacity will diminish gradually.

To Assemble Vial and Flexible Diluent Container:
(Use Aseptic Technique)
1. Remove the protective covers from the top of the vial and the vial port on the diluent container as follows:
   a. To remove the breakaway vial cap, swing the pull ring over the top of the vial and pull down far enough to start the opening (SEE FIGURE 1), then pull straight up to remove the cap. (SEE FIGURE 2.)
   NOTE: Do not access vial with syringe.

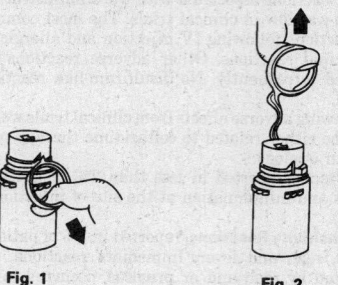

Fig. 1   **Fig. 2**

   b. To remove the vial port cover, grasp the tab on the pull ring, pull up to break the three tie strings, then pull back to remove the cover. (SEE FIGURE 3.)
2. Screw the vial into the vial port until it will go no further. THE VIAL MUST BE SCREWED IN TIGHTLY TO ASSURE A SEAL. This occurs approximately ½ turn (180°) after the first audible click. (SEE FIGURE 4.) The clicking sound does not assure a seal; the vial must be turned as far as it will go.
   NOTE: Once vial is sealed, do not attempt to remove. (SEE FIGURE 4.)
3. Recheck the vial to assure that it is tight by trying to turn it further in the direction of assembly.
4. Label appropriately.

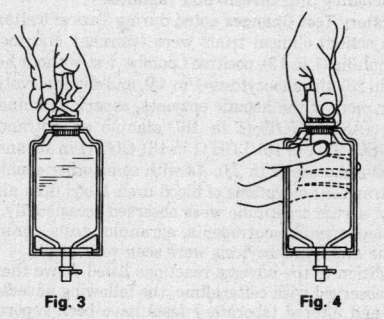

Fig. 3   **Fig. 4**

To Reconstitute the Drug:
1. Squeeze the bottom of the diluent container gently to inflate the portion of the container surrounding the end of the drug vial.
2. With the other hand, push the drug vial down into the container telescoping the walls of the container. Grasp the inner cap of the vial through the walls of the container. (SEE FIGURE 5.)
3. Pull the inner cap from the drug vial. (SEE FIGURE 6.) Verify that the rubber stopper has been pulled out, allowing the drug and diluent to mix.
4. Mix container contents thoroughly and use within the specified time.

[See Figures at top of next column.]

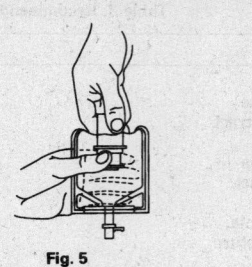
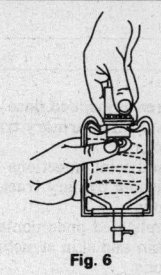

Fig. 5   **Fig. 6**

Preparation for Administration:
(Use Aseptic Technique)
1. Confirm the activation and admixture of vial contents.
2. Check for leaks by squeezing container firmly. If leaks are found discard unit as sterility may be impaired.
3. Close flow control clamp of administration set.
4. Remove cover from outlet port at bottom of container.
5. Insert piercing pin of administration set into port with a twisting motion until the pin is firmly seated. **NOTE:** See full directions on administration set carton.
6. Lift the free end of the hanger loop on the bottom of the vial, breaking the two tie strings. Bend the loop outward to lock it in the upright position, then suspend container from hanger.
7. Squeeze and release drip chamber to establish proper fluid level in chamber.
8. Open flow control clamp and clear air from set. Close clamp.
9. Attach set to venipuncture device. If device is not indwelling, prime and make venipuncture.
10. Regulate rate of administration with flow control clamp.
WARNING: Do not use flexible container in series connections.

COMPATIBILITY AND STABILITY

Intramuscular: Tazicef (ceftazidime for injection) when reconstituted as directed with Sterile Water for Injection, maintains satisfactory potency for 24 hours at room temperature or for 7 days under refrigeration (5°C). Solutions in Sterile Water for Injection that are frozen immediately after reconstitution in the original container are stable for 3 months when stored at −20°C. Once thawed, solutions should not be refrozen. Thawed solutions may be stored for up to 8 hours at room temperature or for 4 days in a refrigerator (5°C).

Intravenous: Tazicef (ceftazidime for injection) when reconstituted as directed with Sterile Water for Injection, maintains satisfactory potency for 24 hours at room temperature or for 7 days under refrigeration (5°C). Solutions in Sterile Water for Injection in the original container or in 0.9% Sodium Chloride Injection in Viaflex® small volume containers that are frozen immediately after reconstitution are stable for 3 months when stored at −20°C. For larger volumes where it may be necessary to warm the frozen product (to a maximum of 40°C), care should be taken to avoid heating after thawing is complete. Once thawed, solutions should not be refrozen. Thawed solutions may be stored for up to 8 hours at room temperature or for 4 days in a refrigerator (5°C).

Tazicef is compatible with the more commonly used intravenous infusion fluids. Solutions at concentrations between 1 mg/mL and 40 mg/mL in the following infusion fluids may be stored for up to 18 hours at room temperature or 7 days if refrigerated: 0.9% Sodium Chloride Injection; Ringer's Injection USP; Lactated Ringer's Injection USP; 5% Dextrose Injection; 5% Dextrose and 0.225% Sodium Chloride Injection; 5% Dextrose and 0.45% Sodium Chloride Injection; 5% Dextrose and 0.9% Sodium Chloride Injection; 10% Dextrose Injection.

Tazicef is less stable in Sodium Bicarbonate Injection than in other intravenous fluids. It is not recommended as a diluent. Solutions of *Tazicef* in 5% Dextrose and 0.9% Sodium Chloride Injection are stable for at least 6 hours at room temperature in plastic tubing, drip chambers and volume control devices of common intravenous infusion sets.

Ceftazidime at a concentration of 20 mg/mL has been found physically compatible for 18 hours at room temperature or 7 days under refrigeration in Sterile Water for Injection when admixed with: cefazolin sodium (Ancef®) 330 mg/mL; heparin 1000 units/mL; and cimetidine HCl (Tagamet®) 150 mg/mL.

Ceftazidime at a concentration of 20 mg/mL has been found physically compatible for 18 hours at room temperature or 7 days under refrigeration in 5% Dextrose Injection when admixed with potassium chloride 40 mEq/L.

Vancomycin solution exhibits a physical incompatibility when mixed with a number of drugs, including ceftazidime. The likelihood of precipitation with ceftazidime is dependent on the concentrations of vancomycin and ceftazidime present. It is therefore recommended, when both drugs are to be administered by intermittent IV infusion, that they be given

separately, flushing the IV lines (with one of the compatible IV fluids) between the administration of these two agents.
ADD-Vantage®* Vials: Ordinarily, ADD-Advantage® vials should be reconstituted only when it is certain that the patient is ready to receive the drug. However, *Tazicef* in ADD-Vantage® vials is stable for 24 hours at room temperature when reconstituted as directed (see RECONSTITUTION, ADD-Vantage® Vials and DIRECTIONS FOR USE OF TAZICEF® INJECTION IN ADD-VANTAGE® VIALS).
Note: Parenteral drug products should be inspected visually for particulate matter prior to administration wherever solution and container permit.
As with other cephalosporins, *Tazicef* powder, as well as solutions, tends to darken depending on storage conditions; within the stated recommendations, however, product potency is not adversely affected.

HOW SUPPLIED

Tazicef in the dry state should be stored between 15° and 30°C (59° and 86°F) and protected from light. Tazicef (ceftazidime for injection) is a dry, white to off-white powder supplied in vials as follows:
Vials: equivalent to 1 gram and 2 grams of ceftazidime.
1 gram (tray of 25): NDC 0007-5082-16
2 gram (tray of 10): NDC 0007-5084-11
"Piggyback" Vials for IV admixture: equivalent to 1 gram and 2 grams of ceftazidime.
1 gram (tray of 10): NDC 0007-5083-11
2 gram (tray of 10): NDC 0007-5085-11
ADD-Vantage® Vials: equivalent to 1 gram and 2 grams of ceftazidime.
1 gram: NDC 0007-5090-16
2 gram: NDC 0007-5091-11
Also available as:
Pharmacy Bulk Vials: equivalent to 6 grams of ceftazidime.
6 gram (tray of 10): NDC 0007-5086-11
Galaxy® Containers (PL 2040 Plastic): equivalent to 1 gram and 2 grams of ceftazidime.
1 gram 1's: NDC 0007-5088-04
2 gram 1's: NDC 0007-5089-04
* ADD-Vantage® is a trademark of Abbott Laboratories.

REFERENCES

1. Bauer, A.W.; Kirby, W.M.M., and Sherris, J.C., et al.: Antibiotic susceptibility testing by a standardized single disc method, Am. J. Clin. Pathol. 45:493, 1966.
2. National Committee for Clinical Laboratory Standards, Approved Standard: Performance Standards for Antimicrobial Disc Susceptibility Tests (M2-A3), December, 1984.
3. Standardized disc susceptibility test, Federal Register 39:19182–19184, 1974.
4. Cockcroft, D.W., and Gault, M.H.: Prediction of creatinine clearance from serum creatinine, Nephron 16:31–41, 1976.

Jointly manufactured by
SmithKline Beecham Pharmaceuticals
Philadelphia, PA 19101 and
Bristol-Myers Squibb Co.
New York, NY 10154
Veterans Administration/Military/PHS—
Injection, 1 gram/50 mL in Galaxy container, 24's, 6505-01-393-5864; 2 gram/50 mL in Galaxy container, 24's, 6505-01-393-5862.
TF:L15

THORAZINE® ℞

[thor'ah-zeen]
(brand of chlorpromazine)tranquilizer · antiemetic

DESCRIPTION

Thorazine (chlorpromazine) is 10-(3-dimethylaminopropyl)-2-chlorphenothiazine, a dimethylamine derivative of phenothiazine. It is present in oral and injectable forms as the hydrochloride salt, and in the suppositories as the base.
Tablets—Each round, orange, coated tablet contains chlorpromazine hydrochloride as follows: 10 mg imprinted SKF and T73; 25 mg imprinted SKF and T74; 50 mg imprinted SKF and T76; 100 mg imprinted SKF and T77; 200 mg imprinted SKF and T79. Inactive ingredients consist of benzoic acid, croscarmellose sodium, D&C Yellow No. 10, FD&C Blue No. 2, FD&C Yellow No. 6, gelatin, hydroxypropyl methylcellulose, lactose, magnesium stearate, methylparaben, polyethylene glycol, propylparaben, talc, titanium dioxide and trace amounts of other inactive ingredients.
Spansule® sustained release capsules—Each *Thorazine* Spansule® capsule is so prepared that an initial dose is released promptly and the remaining medication is released gradually over a prolonged period.
Each capsule, with opaque orange cap and natural body, contains chlorpromazine hydrochloride as follows: 30 mg imprinted SKF and T63; 75 mg imprinted SKF and T64; 150 mg imprinted SKF and T66. Inactive ingredients consist of benzyl alcohol, calcium sulfate, cetylpyridinium chloride, FD&C Yellow No. 6, gelatin, glyceryl distearate, glyceryl monostearate, iron oxide, povidone, silicon dioxide, sodium lauryl sulfate, starch, sucrose, titanium dioxide, wax and trace amounts of other inactive ingredients.
Ampuls—Each mL contains, in aqueous solution, chlorpromazine hydrochloride, 25 mg; ascorbic acid, 2 mg; sodium bisulfite, 1 mg; sodium chloride, 6 mg; sodium sulfite, 1 mg.
Multi-Dose Vials—Each mL contains, in aqueous solution, chlorpromazine hydrochloride, 25 mg; ascorbic acid, 2 mg; sodium bisulfite, 1 mg; sodium chloride, 1 mg; sodium sulfite, 1 mg; benzyl alcohol, 2%, as a preservative.
Syrup—Each 5 mL (1 teaspoonful) of clear, orange-custard flavored liquid contains chlorpromazine hydrochloride, 10 mg. Inactive ingredients consist of citric acid, flavors, sodium benzoate, sodium citrate, sucrose and water.
Suppositories—Each suppository contains chlorpromazine, 25 or 100 mg, glycerin, glyceryl monopalmitate, glyceryl monostearate, hydrogenated coconut oil fatty acids and hydrogenated palm kernel oil fatty acids.
Concentrate—Each mL of clear, custard flavored liquid contains chlorpromazine hydrochloride, 30 or 100 mg. Inactive ingredients consist of calcium disodium edetate, citric acid, flavors, hydroxypropyl methylcellulose, propylene glycol, saccharin sodium, sodium benzoate, water and trace amounts of other inactive ingredients.

ACTIONS

The precise mechanism whereby the therapeutic effects of chlorpromazine are produced is not known. The principal pharmacological actions are psychotropic. It also exerts sedative and antiemetic activity. Chlorpromazine has actions at all levels of the central nervous system—primarily at subcortical levels—as well as on multiple organ systems. Chlorpromazine has strong antiadrenergic and weaker peripheral anticholinergic activity; ganglionic blocking action is relatively slight. It also possesses slight antihistaminic and antiserotonin activity.

INDICATIONS

For the management of manifestations of psychotic disorders.
To control nausea and vomiting.
For relief of restlessness and apprehension before surgery.
For acute intermittent porphyria.
As an adjunct in the treatment of tetanus.
To control the manifestations of the manic type of manic-depressive illness.
For relief of intractable hiccups.
For the treatment of severe behavioral problems in children marked by combativeness and/or explosive hyperexcitable behavior (out of proportion to immediate provocations), and in the short-term treatment of hyperactive children who show excessive motor activity with accompanying conduct disorders consisting of some or all of the following symptoms: impulsivity, difficulty sustaining attention, aggressivity, mood lability and poor frustration tolerance.

CONTRAINDICATIONS

Do not use in patients with known hypersensitivity to phenothiazines.
Do not use in comatose states or in the presence of large amounts of central nervous system depressants (alcohol, barbiturates, narcotics, etc.).

WARNINGS

The extrapyramidal symptoms which can occur secondary to Thorazine (chlorpromazine) may be confused with the central nervous system signs of an undiagnosed primary disease responsible for the vomiting, e.g., Reye's syndrome or other encephalopathy. The use of *Thorazine* and other potential hepatotoxins should be avoided in children and adolescents whose signs and symptoms suggest Reye's syndrome.
Tardive Dyskinesia: Tardive dyskinesia, a syndrome consisting of potentially irreversible, involuntary, dyskinetic movements, may develop in patients treated with neuroleptic (antipsychotic) drugs. Although the prevalence of the syndrome appears to be highest among the elderly, especially elderly women, it is impossible to rely upon prevalence estimates to predict, at the inception of neuroleptic treatment, which patients are likely to develop the syndrome. Whether neuroleptic drug products differ in their potential to cause tardive dyskinesia is unknown.
Both the risk of developing the syndrome and the likelihood that it will become irreversible are believed to increase as the duration of treatment and the total cumulative dose of neuroleptic drugs administered to the patient increase. However, the syndrome can develop, although much less commonly, after relatively brief treatment periods at low doses.
There is no known treatment for established cases of tardive dyskinesia, although the syndrome may remit, partially or completely, if neuroleptic treatment is withdrawn. Neuroleptic treatment itself, however, may suppress (or partially suppress) the signs and symptoms of the syndrome and thereby may possibly mask the underlying disease process. The effect that symptomatic suppression has upon the long-term course of the syndrome is unknown.
Given these considerations, neuroleptics should be prescribed in a manner that is most likely to minimize the occurrence of tardive dyskinesia. Chronic neuroleptic treatment should generally be reserved for patients who suffer from a chronic illness that, 1) is known to respond to neuroleptic drugs, and, 2) for whom alternative, equally effective, but potentially less harmful treatments are *not* available or appropriate. In patients who do require chronic treatment, the smallest dose and the shortest duration of treatment producing a satisfactory clinical response should be sought. The need for continued treatment should be reassessed periodically.
If signs and symptoms of tardive dyskinesia appear in a patient on neuroleptics, drug discontinuation should be considered. However, some patients may require treatment despite the presence of the syndrome.
For further information about the description of tardive dyskinesia and its clinical detection, please refer to the sections on PRECAUTIONS and ADVERSE REACTIONS.
Neuroleptic Malignant Syndrome (NMS): A potentially fatal symptom complex sometimes referred to as Neuroleptic Malignant Syndrome (NMS) has been reported in association with antipsychotic drugs. Clinical manifestations of NMS are hyperpyrexia, muscle rigidity, altered mental status and evidence of autonomic instability (irregular pulse or blood pressure, tachycardia, diaphoresis and cardiac dysrhythmias).
The diagnostic evaluation of patients with this syndrome is complicated. In arriving at a diagnosis, it is important to identify cases where the clinical presentation includes both serious medical illness (e.g., pneumonia, systemic infection, etc.) and untreated or inadequately treated extrapyramidal signs and symptoms (EPS). Other important considerations in the differential diagnosis include central anticholinergic toxicity, heat stroke, drug fever and primary central nervous system (CNS) pathology.
The management of NMS should include 1) immediate discontinuation of antipsychotic drugs and other drugs not essential to concurrent therapy, 2) intensive symptomatic treatment and medical monitoring, and 3) treatment of any concomitant serious medical problems for which specific treatments are available. There is no general agreement about specific pharmacological treatment regimens for uncomplicated NMS.
If a patient requires antipsychotic drug treatment after recovery from NMS, the potential reintroduction of drug therapy should be carefully considered. The patient should be carefully monitored, since recurrences of NMS have been reported.
An encephalopathic syndrome (characterized by weakness, lethargy, fever, tremulousness and confusion, extrapyramidal symptoms, leukocytosis, elevated serum enzymes, BUN and FBS) has occurred in a few patients treated with lithium plus a neuroleptic. In some instances, the syndrome was followed by irreversible brain damage. Because of a possible causal relationship between these events and the concomitant administration of lithium and neuroleptics, patients receiving such combined therapy should be monitored closely for early evidence of neurologic toxicity and treatment discontinued promptly if such signs appear. This encephalopathic syndrome may be similar to or the same as neuroleptic malignant syndrome (NMS).
Thorazine (chlorpromazine) ampuls and multi-dose vials contain sodium bisulfite and sodium sulfite, sulfites that may cause allergic-type reactions including anaphylactic symptoms and life-threatening or less severe asthmatic episodes in certain susceptible people. The overall prevalence of sulfite sensitivity in the general population is unknown and probably low. Sulfite sensitivity is seen more frequently in asthmatic than in nonasthmatic people.
Patients with bone marrow depression or who have previously demonstrated a hypersensitivity reaction (e.g., blood dyscrasias, jaundice) with a phenothiazine should not receive any phenothiazine, including *Thorazine,* unless in the judgment of the physician the potential benefits of treatment outweigh the possible hazard.
Thorazine may impair mental and/or physical abilities, especially during the first few days of therapy. Therefore, caution patients about activities requiring alertness (e.g., operating vehicles or machinery).
The use of alcohol with this drug should be avoided due to possible additive effects and hypotension.
Thorazine may counteract the antihypertensive effect of guanethidine and related compounds.
Usage in Pregnancy: Safety for the use of Thorazine (chlorpromazine) during pregnancy has not been established. Therefore, it is not recommended that the drug be given to

Continued on next page

Information on the SmithKline Beecham Pharmaceuticals products appearing here is based on the labeling in effect on July 1, 1996. Further information on these and other products may be obtained from the Medical Department, SmithKline Beecham Pharmaceuticals, One Franklin Plaza, Philadelphia, PA 19101.

SmithKline Beecham—Cont.

pregnant patients except when, in the judgment of the physician, it is essential. The potential benefits should clearly outweigh possible hazards. There are reported instances of prolonged jaundice, extrapyramidal signs, hyperreflexia or hyporeflexia in newborn infants whose mothers received phenothiazines.

Reproductive studies in rodents have demonstrated potential for embryotoxicity, increased neonatal mortality and nursing transfer of the drug. Tests in the offspring of the drug-treated rodents demonstrate decreased performance. The possibility of permanent neurological damage cannot be excluded.

Nursing Mothers: There is evidence that chlorpromazine is excreted in the breast milk of nursing mothers. Because of the potential for serious adverse reactions in nursing infants from chlorpromazine, a decision should be made whether to discontinue nursing or to discontinue the drug, taking into account the importance of the drug to the mother.

PRECAUTIONS

General

Given the likelihood that some patients exposed chronically to neuroleptics will develop tardive dyskinesia, it is advised that all patients in whom chronic use is contemplated be given, if possible, full information about this risk. The decision to inform patients and/or their guardians must obviously take into account the clinical circumstances and the competency of the patient to understand the information provided.

Thorazine (chlorpromazine) should be administered cautiously to persons with cardiovascular, liver or renal disease. There is evidence that patients with a history of hepatic encephalopathy due to cirrhosis have increased sensitivity to the CNS effects of Thorazine (i.e., impaired cerebration and abnormal slowing of the EEG).

Because of its CNS depressant effect, Thorazine should be used with caution in patients with chronic respiratory disorders such as severe asthma, emphysema and acute respiratory infections, particularly in children.

Because Thorazine can suppress the cough reflex, aspiration of vomitus is possible.

Thorazine (chlorpromazine) prolongs and intensifies the action of CNS depressants such as anesthetics, barbiturates and narcotics. When Thorazine is administered concomitantly, about $1/4$ to $1/2$ the usual dosage of such agents is required. When Thorazine is not being administered to reduce requirements of CNS depressants, it is best to stop such depressants before starting Thorazine treatment. These agents may subsequently be reinstated at low doses and increased as needed.

Note: Thorazine does not intensify the anticonvulsant action of barbiturates. Therefore, dosage of anticonvulsants, including barbiturates, should not be reduced if Thorazine is started. Instead, start Thorazine at low doses and increase as needed.

Use with caution in persons who will be exposed to extreme heat, organophosphorus insecticides, and in persons receiving atropine or related drugs.

Neuroleptic drugs elevate prolactin levels; the elevation persists during chronic administration. Tissue culture experiments indicate that approximately $1/3$ of human breast cancers are prolactin-dependent in vitro, a factor of potential importance if the prescribing of these drugs is contemplated in a patient with a previously detected breast cancer. Although disturbances such as galactorrhea, amenorrhea, gynecomastia and impotence have been reported, the clinical significance of elevated serum prolactin levels is unknown for most patients. An increase in mammary neoplasms has been found in rodents after chronic administration of neuroleptic drugs. Neither clinical nor epidemiologic studies conducted to date, however, have shown an association between chronic administration of these drugs and mammary tumorigenesis; the available evidence is considered too limited to be conclusive at this time.

Chromosomal aberrations in spermatocytes and abnormal sperm have been demonstrated in rodents treated with certain neuroleptics.

As with all drugs which exert an anticholinergic effect, and/or cause mydriasis, chlorpromazine should be used with caution in patients with glaucoma.

Chlorpromazine diminishes the effect of oral anticoagulants. Phenothiazines can produce alpha-adrenergic blockade.

Chlorpromazine may lower the convulsive threshold; dosage adjustments of anticonvulsants may be necessary. Potentiation of anticonvulsant effects does not occur. However, it has been reported that chlorpromazine may interfere with the metabolism of Dilantin®* and thus precipitate Dilantin toxicity.

Concomitant administration with propranolol results in increased plasma levels of both drugs.

Thiazide diuretics may accentuate the orthostatic hypotension that may occur with phenothiazines.

The presence of phenothiazines may produce false-positive phenylketonuria (PKU) test results.

Drugs which lower the seizure threshold, including phenothiazine derivatives, should not be used with Amipaque®†. As with other phenothiazine derivatives, Thorazine should be discontinued at least 48 hours before myelography, should not be resumed for at least 24 hours postprocedure, and should not be used for the control of nausea and vomiting occurring either prior to myelography or postprocedure with Amipaque.

Long-Term Therapy: To lessen the likelihood of adverse reactions related to cumulative drug effect, patients with a history of long-term therapy with Thorazine and/or other neuroleptics should be evaluated periodically to decide whether the maintenance dosage could be lowered or drug therapy discontinued.

Antiemetic Effect: The antiemetic action of Thorazine may mask the signs and symptoms of overdosage of other drugs and may obscure the diagnosis and treatment of other conditions such as intestinal obstruction, brain tumor and Reye's syndrome. (See WARNINGS.)

When Thorazine is used with cancer chemotherapeutic drugs, vomiting as a sign of the toxicity of these agents may be obscured by the antiemetic effect of Thorazine.

Abrupt Withdrawal: Like other phenothiazines, Thorazine (chlorpromazine) is not known to cause psychic dependence and does not produce tolerance or addiction. There may be, however, following abrupt withdrawal of high-dose therapy, some symptoms resembling those of physical dependence such as gastritis, nausea and vomiting, dizziness and tremulousness. These symptoms can usually be avoided or reduced by gradual reduction of the dosage or by continuing concomitant anti-parkinsonism agents for several weeks after Thorazine is withdrawn.

ADVERSE REACTIONS

Note: Some adverse effects of Thorazine may be more likely to occur, or occur with greater intensity, in patients with special medical problems, e.g., patients with mitral insufficiency or pheochromocytoma have experienced severe hypotension following recommended doses.

Drowsiness, usually mild to moderate, may occur, particularly during the first or second week, after which it generally disappears. If troublesome, dosage may be lowered.

Jaundice: Overall incidence has been low, regardless of indication or dosage. Most investigators conclude it is a sensitivity reaction. Most cases occur between the second and fourth weeks of therapy. The clinical picture resembles infectious hepatitis, with laboratory features of obstructive jaundice, rather than those of parenchymal damage. It is usually promptly reversible on withdrawal of the medication; however, chronic jaundice has been reported.

There is no conclusive evidence that preexisting liver disease makes patients more susceptible to jaundice. Alcoholics with cirrhosis have been successfully treated with Thorazine (chlorpromazine) without complications. Nevertheless, the medication should be used cautiously in patients with liver disease. Patients who have experienced jaundice with a phenothiazine should not, if possible, be reexposed to Thorazine or other phenothiazines.

If fever with grippe-like symptoms occurs, appropriate liver studies should be conducted. If tests indicate an abnormality, stop treatment.

Liver function tests in jaundice induced by the drug may mimic extrahepatic obstruction; withhold exploratory laparotomy until extrahepatic obstruction is confirmed.

Hematological Disorders, including agranulocytosis, eosinophilia, leukopenia, hemolytic anemia, aplastic anemia, thrombocytopenic purpura and pancytopenia have been reported.

Agranulocytosis—Warn patients to report the sudden appearance of sore throat or other signs of infection. If white blood cell and differential counts indicate cellular depression, stop treatment and start antibiotic and other suitable therapy.

Most cases have occurred between the fourth and tenth weeks of therapy; patients should be watched closely during that period.

Moderate suppression of white blood cells is not an indication for stopping treatment unless accompanied by the symptoms described above.

Cardiovascular:

Hypotensive Effects—Postural hypotension, simple tachycardia, momentary fainting and dizziness may occur after the first injection; occasionally after subsequent injections; rarely, after the first oral dose. Usually recovery is spontaneous and symptoms disappear within $1/2$ to 2 hours. Occasionally, these effects may be more severe and prolonged, producing a shock-like condition.

To minimize hypotension after injection, keep patient lying down and observe for at least $1/2$ hour. To control hypotension, place patient in head-low position with legs raised. If a vasoconstrictor is required, Levophed®‡ and Neo-Synephrine®§ are the most suitable. Other pressor agents, including epinephrine, should not be used as they may cause a paradoxical further lowering of blood pressure.

EKG Changes—particularly nonspecific, usually reversible Q and T wave distortions—have been observed in some patients receiving phenothiazine tranquilizers, including Thorazine (chlorpromazine).

Note: Sudden death, apparently due to cardiac arrest, has been reported.

CNS Reactions:

Neuromuscular (Extrapyramidal) Reactions—Neuromuscular reactions include dystonias, motor restlessness, pseudoparkinsonism and tardive dyskinesia, and appear to be dose-related. They are discussed in the following paragraphs:

Dystonias: Symptoms may include spasm of the neck muscles, sometimes progressing to acute, reversible torticollis; extensor rigidity of back muscles, sometimes progressing to opisthotonos; carpopedal spasm, trismus, swallowing difficulty, oculogyric crisis and protrusion of the tongue.

These usually subside within a few hours, and almost always within 24 to 48 hours after the drug has been discontinued.

In mild cases, reassurance or a barbiturate is often sufficient. In moderate cases, barbiturates will usually bring rapid relief. In more severe adult cases, the administration of an anti-parkinsonism agent, except levodopa, usually produces rapid reversal of symptoms. In children, reassurance and barbiturates will usually control symptoms. (Or, parenteral Benadryl®ll may be useful. See Benadryl prescribing information for appropriate children's dosage.) If appropriate treatment with anti-parkinsonism agents or Benadryl fails to reverse the signs and symptoms, the diagnosis should be reevaluated.

Suitable supportive measures such as maintaining a clear airway and adequate hydration should be employed when needed. If therapy is reinstituted, it should be at a lower dosage. Should these symptoms occur in children or pregnant patients, the drug should not be reinstituted.

Motor Restlessness: Symptoms may include agitation or jitteriness and sometimes insomnia. These symptoms often disappear spontaneously. At times these symptoms may be similar to the original neurotic or psychotic symptoms. Dosage should not be increased until these side effects have subsided.

If these symptoms become too troublesome, they can usually be controlled by a reduction of dosage or change of drug. Treatment with anti-parkinsonian agents, benzodiazepines or propranolol may be helpful.

Pseudo-parkinsonism: Symptoms may include: mask-like facies, drooling, tremors, pillrolling motion, cogwheel rigidity and shuffling gait. In most cases these symptoms are readily controlled when an anti-parkinsonism agent is administered concomitantly. Anti-parkinsonism agents should be used only when required. Generally, therapy of a few weeks to 2 or 3 months will suffice. After this time patients should be evaluated to determine their need for continued treatment. (Note: Levodopa has not been found effective in neuroleptic-induced pseudo-parkinsonism.) Occasionally it is necessary to lower the dosage of Thorazine (chlorpromazine) or to discontinue the drug.

Tardive Dyskinesia: As with all antipsychotic agents, tardive dyskinesia may appear in some patients on long-term therapy or may appear after drug therapy has been discontinued. The syndrome can also develop, although much less frequently, after relatively brief treatment periods at low doses. This syndrome appears in all age groups. Although its prevalence appears to be highest among elderly patients, especially elderly women, it is impossible to rely upon prevalence estimates to predict at the inception of neuroleptic treatment which patients are likely to develop the syndrome. The symptoms are persistent and in some patients appear to be irreversible. The syndrome is characterized by rhythmical involuntary movements of the tongue, face, mouth or jaw (e.g., protrusion of tongue, puffing of cheeks, puckering of mouth, chewing movements). Sometimes these may be accompanied by involuntary movements of extremities. In rare instances, these involuntary movements of the extremities are the only manifestations of tardive dyskinesia. A variant of tardive dyskinesia, tardive dystonia, has also been described.

There is no known effective treatment for tardive dyskinesia; anti-parkinsonism agents do not alleviate the symptoms of this syndrome. If clinically feasible, it is suggested that all antipsychotic agents be discontinued if these symptoms appear. Should it be necessary to reinstitute treatment, or increase the dosage of the agent, or switch to a different antipsychotic agent, the syndrome may be masked.

It has been reported that fine vermicular movements of the tongue may be an early sign of the syndrome and if the medication is stopped at that time the syndrome may not develop.

Adverse Behavioral Effects—Psychotic symptoms and catatonic-like states have been reported rarely.

Other CNS Effects—Neuroleptic Malignant Syndrome (NMS) has been reported in association with antipsychotic drugs. (See WARNINGS.)

Cerebral edema has been reported.

Convulsive seizures (petit mal and grand mal) have been reported, particularly in patients with EEG abnormalities or history of such disorders.

Abnormality of the cerebrospinal fluid proteins has also been reported.

Allergic Reactions of a mild urticarial type or photosensitivity are seen. Avoid undue exposure to sun. More severe reactions, including exfoliative dermatitis, have been reported occasionally.

Contact dermatitis has been reported in nursing personnel; accordingly, the use of rubber gloves when administering *Thorazine* liquid or injectable is recommended.

In addition, asthma, laryngeal edema, angioneurotic edema and anaphylactoid reactions have been reported.

Endocrine Disorders: Lactation and moderate breast engorgement may occur in females on large doses. If persistent, lower dosage or withdraw drug. False-positive pregnancy tests have been reported, but are less likely to occur when a serum test is used. Amenorrhea and gynecomastia have also been reported. Hyperglycemia, hypoglycemia and glycosuria have been reported.

Autonomic Reactions: Occasional dry mouth; nasal congestion; nausea; obstipation; constipation; adynamic ileus; urinary retention; priapism; miosis and mydriasis, atonic colon, ejaculatory disorders/impotence.

Special Considerations in Long-Term Therapy: Skin pigmentation and ocular changes have occurred in some patients taking substantial doses of Thorazine (chlorpromazine) for prolonged periods.

Skin Pigmentation—Rare instances of skin pigmentation have been observed in hospitalized mental patients, primarily females who have received the drug usually for 3 years or more in dosages ranging from 500 mg to 1500 mg daily. The pigmentary changes, restricted to exposed areas of the body, range from an almost imperceptible darkening of the skin to a slate gray color, sometimes with a violet hue. Histological examination reveals a pigment, chiefly in the dermis, which is probably a melanin-like complex. The pigmentation may fade following discontinuance of the drug.

Ocular Changes—Ocular changes have occurred more frequently than skin pigmentation and have been observed both in pigmented and nonpigmented patients receiving Thorazine (chlorpromazine) usually for 2 years or more in dosages of 300 mg daily and higher. Eye changes are characterized by deposition of fine particulate matter in the lens and cornea. In more advanced cases, star-shaped opacities have also been observed in the anterior portion of the lens. The nature of the eye deposits has not yet been determined. A small number of patients with more severe ocular changes have had some visual impairment. In addition to these corneal and lenticular changes, epithelial keratopathy and pigmentary retinopathy have been reported. Reports suggest that the eye lesions may regress after withdrawal of the drug.

Since the occurrence of eye changes seems to be related to dosage levels and/or duration of therapy, it is suggested that long-term patients on moderate to high dosage levels have periodic ocular examinations.

Etiology—The etiology of both of these reactions is not clear, but exposure to light, along with dosage/duration of therapy, appears to be the most significant factor. If either of these reactions is observed, the physician should weigh the benefits of continued therapy against the possible risks and, on the merits of the individual case, determine whether or not to continue present therapy, lower the dosage, or withdraw the drug.

Other Adverse Reactions: Mild fever may occur after large I.M. doses. Hyperpyrexia has been reported. Increases in appetite and weight sometimes occur. Peripheral edema and a systemic lupus erythematosus-like syndrome have been reported.

Note: There have been occasional reports of sudden death in patients receiving phenothiazines. In some cases, the cause appeared to be cardiac arrest or asphyxia due to failure of the cough reflex.

DOSAGE AND ADMINISTRATION—ADULTS

Adjust dosage to individual and the severity of his condition, recognizing that the milligram for milligram potency relationship among all dosage forms has not been precisely established clinically. It is important to increase dosage until symptoms are controlled. Dosage should be increased more gradually in debilitated or emaciated patients. In continued therapy, gradually reduce dosage to the lowest effective maintenance level, after symptoms have been controlled for a reasonable period.

In general, dosage recommendations for other oral forms of the drug may be applied to Spansule® brand sustained release capsules on the basis of total daily dosage in milligrams.

The 100 mg and 200 mg tablets are for use in severe neuropsychiatric conditions.

Increase parenteral dosage only if hypotension has not occurred. Before using I.M., see IMPORTANT NOTES ON INJECTION.

Elderly Patients—In general, dosages in the lower range are sufficient for most elderly patients. Since they appear to be more susceptible to hypotension and neuromuscular reactions, such patients should be observed closely. Dosage

should be tailored to the individual, response carefully monitored, and dosage adjusted accordingly. Dosage should be increased more gradually in elderly patients.

Psychotic Disorders—Increase dosage gradually until symptoms are controlled. Maximum improvement may not be seen for weeks or even months. Continue optimum dosage for 2 weeks; then gradually reduce dosage to the lowest effective maintenance level. Daily dosage of 200 mg is not unusual. Some patients require higher dosages (e.g., 800 mg daily is not uncommon in discharged mental patients).

HOSPITALIZED PATIENTS: ACUTELY DISTURBED OR MANIC—*I.M.:* 25 mg (1 mL). If necessary, give additional 25 to 50 mg injection in 1 hour. Increase subsequent I.M. doses gradually over several days—up to 400 mg q4 to 6h in exceptionally severe cases—until patient is controlled. Usually patient becomes quiet and cooperative within 24 to 48 hours and oral doses may be substituted and increased until the patient is calm. 500 mg a day is generally sufficient. While gradual increases to 2,000 mg a day or more may be necessary, there is usually little therapeutic gain to be achieved by exceeding 1,000 mg a day for extended periods. In general, dosage levels should be lower in the elderly, the emaciated and the debilitated. LESS ACUTELY DISTURBED—*Oral:* 25 mg t.i.d. Increase gradually until effective dose is reached—usually 400 mg daily. OUTPATIENTS—*Oral:* 10 mg t.i.d. or q.i.d., or 25 mg b.i.d. or t.i.d. MORE SEVERE CASES—*Oral:* 25 mg t.i.d. After 1 or 2 days, daily dosage may be increased by 20 to 50 mg at semiweekly intervals until patient becomes calm and cooperative. PROMPT CONTROL OF SEVERE SYMPTOMS—*I.M.:* 25 mg (1 mL). If necessary, repeat in 1 hour. Subsequent doses should be oral, 25 to 50 mg t.i.d.

Nausea and Vomiting—*Oral:* 10 to 25 mg q4 to 6h, p.r.n., increased, if necessary. *I.M.:* 25 mg (1 mL). If no hypotension occurs, give 25 to 50 mg q3 to 4h, p.r.n., until vomiting stops. Then switch to oral dosage. *Rectal:* One 100 mg suppository q6 to 8h, p.r.n. In some patients, half this dose will do. DURING SURGERY—*I.M.:* 12.5 mg (0.5 mL). Repeat in 1/2 hour if necessary and if no hypotension occurs. *I.V.:* 2 mg per fractional injection, at 2-minute intervals. Do not exceed 25 mg. Dilute to 1 mg/mL, i.e., 1 mL (25 mg) mixed with 24 mL of saline.

Presurgical Apprehension—*Oral:* 25 to 50 mg, 2 to 3 hours before the operation. *I.M.:* 12.5 to 25 mg (0.5 to 1 mL), 1 to 2 hours before operation.

Intractable Hiccups—*Oral:* 25 to 50 mg t.i.d. or q.i.d. If symptoms persist for 2 to 3 days, give 25 to 50 mg (1 to 2 mL) I.M. Should symptoms persist, use *slow* I.V. infusion with patient flat in bed: 25 to 50 mg (1 to 2 mL) in 500 to 1,000 mL of saline. Follow blood pressure closely.

Acute Intermittent Porphyria—*Oral:* 25 to 50 mg t.i.d. or q.i.d. Can usually be discontinued after several weeks, but maintenance therapy may be necessary for some patients. *I.M.:* 25 mg (1 mL) t.i.d. or q.i.d. until patient can take oral therapy.

Tetanus—*I.M.:* 25 to 50 mg (1 to 2 mL) given 3 or 4 times daily, usually in conjunction with barbiturates. Total doses and frequency of administration must be determined by the patient's response, starting with low doses and increasing gradually. *I.V.:* 25 to 50 mg (1 to 2 mL). Dilute to at least 1 mg per mL and administer at a rate of 1 mg per minute.

DOSAGE AND ADMINISTRATION—CHILDREN

Thorazine (chlorpromazine) should generally not be used in children under 6 months of age except where potentially lifesaving. It should not be used in conditions for which specific children's dosages have not been established.

Severe Behavioral Problems—OUTPATIENTS—Select route of administration according to severity of patient's condition and increase dosage gradually as required. *Oral:* 1/4 mg/lb body weight q4 to 6h, p.r.n. (e.g., for 40 lb child—10 mg q4 to 6h). *Rectal:* 1/2 mg/lb body weight q6 to 8h, p.r.n. (e.g., for 20 to 30 lb child—half a 25 mg suppository q6 to 8h). *I.M.:* 1/4 mg/lb body weight q6 to 8h, p.r.n.

HOSPITALIZED PATIENTS—As with outpatients, start with low doses and increase dosage gradually. In severe behavior disorders or psychotic conditions, higher dosages (50 to 100 mg daily, and in older children, 200 mg daily or more) may be necessary. There is little evidence that behavior improvement in severely disturbed mentally retarded patients is further enhanced by doses beyond 500 mg per day. *Maximum I.M. Dosage:* Children up to 5 years (or 50 lbs), not over 40 mg/day; 5 to 12 years (or 50 to 100 lbs), not over 75 mg/day except in unmanageable cases.

Nausea and Vomiting—Dosage and frequency of administration should be adjusted according to the severity of the symptoms and response of the patient. The duration of activity following intramuscular administration may last up to 12 hours. Subsequent doses may be given by the same route if necessary. *Oral:* 1/4 mg/lb body weight (e.g., 40 lb child—10 mg q4 to 6h). *Rectal:* 1/2 mg/lb body weight q6 to 8h, p.r.n. (e.g., 20 to 30 lb child—half of a 25 mg suppository q6 to 8h). *I.M.:* 1/4 mg/lb body weight q6 to 8h, p.r.n. *Maximum I.M. Dosage:* Children up to 5 yrs. (or 50 lbs), not over 40 mg/day; 5 to 12 yrs. (or 50 to 100 lbs), not over 75 mg/day except in severe cases. DURING SURGERY—*I.M.:* 1/8 mg/lb body

weight. Repeat in 1/2 hour if necessary and if no hypotension occurs. *I.V.:* 1 mg per fractional injection at 2-minute intervals and not exceeding recommended I.M. dosage. Always dilute to 1 mg/mL, i.e., 1 mL (25 mg) mixed with 24 mL of saline.

Presurgical Apprehension—1/4 mg/lb body weight, either *orally* 2 to 3 hours before operation, or *I.M.* 1 to 2 hours before.

Tetanus—*I.M.* or *I.V.:* 1/4 mg/lb body weight q6 to 8h. When given I.V., dilute to at least 1 mg/mL and administer at rate of 1 mg per 2 minutes. In children up to 50 lbs, do not exceed 40 mg daily; 50 to 100 lbs, do not exceed 75 mg, except in severe cases.

IMPORTANT NOTES ON INJECTION

Inject slowly, deep into upper outer quadrant of buttock. Because of possible hypotensive effects, reserve parenteral administration for bedfast patients or for acute ambulatory cases, and keep patient lying down for at least 1/2 hour after injection. If irritation is a problem, dilute Injection with saline or 2% procaine; mixing with other agents in the syringe is not recommended. Subcutaneous injection is not advised. Avoid injecting undiluted Thorazine (chlorpromazine) into vein. I.V. route is only for severe hiccups, surgery and tetanus.

Because of the possibility of contact dermatitis, avoid getting solution on hands or clothing. This solution should be protected from light. This is a clear, colorless to pale yellow solution; a slight yellowish discoloration will not alter potency. If markedly discolored, solution should be discarded. For information on sulfite sensitivity, see the WARNINGS section of this labeling.

Note on Concentrate: When the Concentrate is to be used, add the desired dosage of Concentrate to 60 mL (2 fl oz) or more of diluent *just prior to administration.* This will insure palatability and stability. Vehicles suggested for dilution are: tomato or fruit juice, milk, simple syrup, orange syrup, carbonated beverages, coffee, tea or water. Semisolid foods (soups, puddings, etc.) may also be used. The Concentrate is light sensitive; it should be protected from light and dispensed in amber glass bottles. *Refrigeration is not required.*

OVERDOSAGE

(See also ADVERSE REACTIONS.)

SYMPTOMS—Primarily symptoms of central nervous system depression to the point of somnolence or coma. Hypotension and extrapyramidal symptoms.

Other possible manifestations include agitation and restlessness, convulsions, fever, autonomic reactions such as dry mouth and ileus, EKG changes and cardiac arrhythmias.

TREATMENT—It is important to determine other medications taken by the patient since multiple drug therapy is common in overdosage situations. Treatment is essentially symptomatic and supportive. Early gastric lavage is helpful. Keep patient under observation and maintain an open airway, since involvement of the extrapyramidal mechanism may produce dysphagia and respiratory difficulty in severe overdosage. **Do not attempt to induce emesis because a dystonic reaction of the head or neck may develop that could result in aspiration of vomitus.** Extrapyramidal symptoms may be treated with anti-parkinsonism drugs, barbiturates, or *Benadryl.* See prescribing information for these products. Care should be taken to avoid increasing respiratory depression.

If administration of a stimulant is desirable, amphetamine, dextroamphetamine, or caffeine with sodium benzoate is recommended. Stimulants that may cause convulsions (e.g., picrotoxin or pentylenetetrazol) should be avoided.

If hypotension occurs, the standard measures for managing circulatory shock should be initiated. If it is desirable to administer a vasoconstrictor, *Levophed* and *Neo-Synephrine* are most suitable. Other pressor agents, including epinephrine, are not recommended because phenothiazine derivatives may reverse the usual elevating action of these agents and cause a further lowering of blood pressure.

Limited experience indicates that phenothiazines are *not* dialyzable.

Special note on Spansule® capsules—Since much of the Spansule capsule medication is coated for gradual release, therapy directed at reversing the effects of the ingested drug and at supporting the patient should be continued for as long as overdosage symptoms remain. Saline cathartics are useful for hastening evacuation of pellets that have not already released medication.

Continued on next page

Information on the SmithKline Beecham Pharmaceuticals products appearing here is based on the labeling in effect on July 1, 1996. Further information on these and other products may be obtained from the Medical Department, SmithKline Beecham Pharmaceuticals, One Franklin Plaza, Philadelphia, PA 19101.

SmithKline Beecham—Cont.

HOW SUPPLIED

Tablets: 10 mg, in bottles of 100; 25 mg or 50 mg, in bottles of 100 and 1000. For use in severe neuropsychiatric conditions, 100 mg and 200 mg, in bottles of 100 and 1000.

NDC 0007-5073-20 10 mg 100's
NDC 0007-5074-20 25 mg 100's
NDC 0007-5074-30 25 mg 1000's
NDC 0007-5076-20 50 mg 100's
NDC 0007-5076-30 50 mg 1000's
NDC 0007-5077-20 100 mg 100's
NDC 0007-5077-30 100 mg 1000's
NDC 0007-5079-20 200 mg 100's
NDC 0007-5079-30 200 mg 1000's

Spansule® brand of sustained release capsules: 30 mg, 75 mg or 150 mg, in bottles of 50.

NDC 0007-5063-15 30 mg 50's
NDC 0007-5064-15 75 mg 50's
NDC 0007-5066-15 150 mg 50's

Ampuls: 1 mL and 2 mL (25 mg/mL), in boxes of 10.

NDC 0007-5060-11 25 mg/mL in 1 mL Ampuls (box of 10)
NDC 0007-5061-11 25 mg/mL in 2 mL Ampuls (box of 10)

Multi-Dose Vials: 10 mL (25 mg/mL), in boxes of 1.

NDC 0007-5062-01 25 mg/mL in 10 mL Multi-Dose Vials (box of 1)

Syrup: 10 mg/5 mL, in 4 fl oz bottles.

NDC 0007-5072-44 10 mg/5 mL 4 fl oz

Suppositories: 25 mg or 100 mg, in boxes of 12.

NDC 0007-5070-03 25 mg (box of 12)
NDC 0007-5071-03 100 mg (box of 12)

Concentrate: Intended for institutional use. 30 mg/mL, in 4 fl oz bottles, and 100 mg/mL, in 8 fl oz bottles, in cartons of 12.

The Concentrate form is light-sensitive. For this reason, it should be protected from light and dispensed in amber bottles. *Refrigeration is not required.*

NDC 0007-5047-44 30 mg/mL 4 fl oz (carton of 12)
NDC 0007-5049-48 100 mg/mL 8 fl oz (carton of 12)

---

* phenytoin, Parke-Davis.

† metrizamide, Sanofi Winthrop Pharmaceuticals.

‡ norepinephrine bitartrate, Sanofi Winthrop Pharmaceuticals.

§ phenylephrine hydrochloride, Sanofi Winthrop Pharmaceuticals.

″ diphenhydramine hydrochloride, Parke-Davis.

WARNING: Thorazine® *Spansule* capsules are manufactured with carbon tetrachloride and methyl chloroform, substances which harm public health and environment by destroying ozone in the upper atmosphere.

Veterans Administration/Military/PHS—Concentrate, 30 mg/mL, 4 oz, 6505-00-660-1664; 100 mg/mL, 8 oz, 6505-00-126-2044; Ampuls, 25 mg/mL, 1 mL, 10's, 6505-01-196-6216; 25 mg/mL, 2 mL, 10's, 6505-00-129-6709; *Spansule* capsules, 30 mg, 50's, 6505-01-343-3074; 75 mg, 50's, 6505-00-684-8672; Suppositories, 25 mg, 12's, 6505-01-153-3217; 100 mg, 12's, 6505-01-142-6379; Syrup, 10 mg/5 mL, 4 oz, 6505-01-156-1640; Tablets, 10 mg, 100's, 6505-00-763-5750; 25 mg, 1000's, 6505-00-022-1326; 50 mg, 1000's, 6505-00-022-1327; 100 mg, 100's, 6505-00-763-5748; 100 mg, 1000's, 6505-00-014-1182; 200 mg, 100's, 6505-00-014-1183; 200 mg, 1000's, 6505-00-014-1186.

TZ:L80

Shown in Product Identification Guide, page 337

TICAR®

[ti'kar]

**brand of sterile ticarcillin disodium
for Intramuscular or Intravenous Administration**

DESCRIPTION

Ticar is a semisynthetic injectable penicillin derived from the penicillin nucleus, 6-aminopenicillanic acid. Chemically, it is *N*-(2-Carboxy-3,3-dimethyl-7-oxo-4-thia-1-azabicyclo [3.2.0]hept-6-yl)-3-thiophenemalonamic acid disodium salt.

TICARCILLIN SERUM LEVELS
mcg/mL

Dosage	Route	¼ hr.	½ hr.	1 hr.	2 hr.	3 hr.	4 hr.	6 hr.
Adults:								
500 mg	I.M.	—	7.7	8.6	6.0	4.0	—	2.9
1 gram	I.M.	—	31.0	18.7	15.7	9.7	—	3.4
2 grams	I.M.	—	63.6	39.7	32.3	18.9	—	3.4
3 grams	I.V.	190.0	140.0	107.0	52.2	31.3	13.8	4.2
5 grams	I.V.	327.0	280.0	175.0	106.0	63.0	28.5	9.6
3 grams + 1 gram probenecid	I.V. Oral	223.0	166.0	123.0	78.0	54.0	35.4	17.1

Neonates:		½ hr.	1 hr.	1½ hr.	2 hr.	4 hr.	8 hr.
50 mg/kg	I.M.	64.0	70.7	63.7	60.1	33.2	11.6

Culture	Susceptible	Intermediate	Resistant
P. aeruginosa and *Enterobacteriaceae*	≥ 15 mm	12 to 14 mm	≤ 11 mm

The MIC correlates are: Resistant > 128 mcg/mL
Susceptible ≤ 64 mcg/mL

It is supplied as a white to pale yellow powder for reconstitution. The reconstituted solution is clear, colorless or pale yellow, having a pH of 6.0 to 8.0. Ticarcillin is very soluble in water; its solubility is greater than 600 mg/mL.

ACTIONS

Pharmacology

Ticarcillin is not absorbed orally; therefore, it must be given intravenously or intramuscularly. Following intramuscular administration, peak serum concentrations occur within ½ to 1 hour. Somewhat higher and more prolonged serum levels can be achieved with the concurrent administration of probenecid.

The minimum inhibitory concentrations (MICs) for many strains of *Pseudomonas* are relatively high by usual standards; serum levels of 60 mcg/mL or greater are required. However, the low degree of toxicity of ticarcillin permits the use of doses large enough to achieve inhibitory levels for these strains in serum or tissues. Other susceptible organisms usually require serum levels in the 10 to 25 mcg/mL range.

[See first table above.]

As with other penicillins, ticarcillin is eliminated by glomerular filtration and tubular secretion. It is not highly bound to serum protein (approximately 45%) and is excreted unchanged in the urine. After the administration of a 1 to 2 gram I.M. dose, a urine concentration of 2000 to 4000 mcg/mL may be obtained in patients with normal renal function. The serum half-life of ticarcillin in normal individuals is approximately 70 minutes.

An inverse relationship exists between serum half-life and creatinine clearance, but the dosage of *Ticar* need only be adjusted in cases of severe renal impairment (see DOSAGE AND ADMINISTRATION). The administered ticarcillin may be removed from patients undergoing dialysis; the actual amount removed depends on the duration and type of dialysis.

Ticarcillin can be detected in tissues and interstitial fluid following parenteral administration. Penetration into the cerebrospinal fluid, bile and pleural fluid has been demonstrated.

Microbiology

Ticarcillin is bactericidal and demonstrates substantial *in vitro* activity against both gram-positive and gram-negative organisms. Many strains of the following organisms were found to be susceptible to ticarcillin *in vitro*:

Pseudomonas aeruginosa (and other species)
Escherichia coli
Proteus mirabilis
Morganella morganii (formerly *Proteus morganii*)
Providencia rettgeri (formerly *Proteus rettgeri*)
Proteus vulgaris
Enterobacter species
Haemophilus influenzae
Neisseria species
Salmonella species
Staphylococcus aureus (non-penicillinase producing)
Staphylococcus epidermidis
Beta-hemolytic streptococci (Group A)
Streptococcus faecalis (*Enterococcus*)
Streptococcus pneumoniae
Anaerobic bacteria, including:
Bacteroides species including *B. fragilis*
Fusobacterium species
Veillonella species
Clostridium species
Eubacterium species
Peptococcus species
Peptostreptococcus species

In vitro synergism between ticarcillin and gentamicin sulfate, tobramycin sulfate or amikacin sulfate against certain strains of *Pseudomonas aeruginosa* has been demonstrated. Some strains of such microorganisms as *Mima-Herellea* (*Acinetobacter*), *Citrobacter* and *Serratia* have shown susceptibility.

Ticarcillin is not stable in the presence of penicillinase.

Some strains of *Pseudomonas* have developed resistance fairly rapidly.

DISK SUSCEPTIBILITY TESTS

Susceptibility Tests: Ticarcillin disks or powders should be used for testing susceptibility to ticarcillin. However, organisms reportedly susceptible to carbenicillin are susceptible to ticarcillin.

Diffusion Techniques: For the disk diffusion method of susceptibility testing a 75 mcg *Ticar* disk should be used. The method for this test is the one outlined in NCCLS publication M2-A3* with the following interpretative criteria:

[See second table above.]

Dilution Techniques: Dilution techniques for determining the MIC (minimum inhibitory concentration) are published by NCCLS for the broth and agar dilution procedures. The MIC data should be interpreted in light of the concentrations present in serum, tissue and body fluids. Organisms with MIC ≤ 64 are considered susceptible when they are in tissue but organisms with MIC ≤ 128 would be susceptible in urine where the *Ticar* concentrations are much greater. At present, only dilution methods can be recommended for testing antibiotic susceptibility of obligate anaerobes. Susceptibility testing methods require the use of control organisms. The 75 mcg ticarcillin disk should give zone diameters between 22 and 28 mm for *P. aeruginosa* ATCC 27853 and 24 and 30 mm for *E. coli* ATCC 25922. Reference strains are available for dilution testing of ticarcillin. 95% of the MICs should fall within the following MIC ranges and the majority of MICs should be at values close to the center of the pertinent range (reference NCCLS publication M7-A†).

S. aureus ATCC 29213, 2.0 to 8.0 mcg/mL; *S. faecalis* ATCC 29212, 16 to 64 mcg/mL; *E. coli* ATCC 25922, 2.0 to 8.0 mcg/mL; *P. aeruginosa* ATCC 27853, 8.0 to 32 mcg/mL.

*Performance Standards for Antimicrobial Disc Susceptibility Tests, National Committee for Clinical Laboratory Standards, Vol. 4, No. 16, pp. 369–402, 1984.

†Methods for Dilution Antimicrobial Susceptibility Tests for Bacteria That Grow Aerobically, Vol. 5, No. 22, pp. 579–618, 1985.

INDICATIONS

Ticar is indicated for the treatment of the following infections:

Bacterial septicemia†
Skin and soft-tissue infections‡
Acute and chronic respiratory tract infections‡§
‡Caused by susceptible strains of *Pseudomonas aeruginosa*, *Proteus* species (both indole-positive and indole-negative) and *Escherichia coli*.
§Though clinical improvement has been shown, bacteriological cures cannot be expected in patients with chronic respiratory disease or cystic fibrosis.

Genitourinary tract infections (complicated and uncomplicated) due to susceptible strains of *Pseudomonas aeruginosa*, *Proteus* species (both indole-positive and indole-negative), *Escherichia coli*, *Enterobacter* and *Streptococcus faecalis* (enterococcus).

Ticarcillin is also indicated in the treatment of the following infections due to susceptible anaerobic bacteria:
1. Bacterial septicemia.
2. Lower respiratory tract infections such as empyema, anaerobic pneumonitis and lung abscess.

Adults:

Bacterial septicemia Respiratory tract infections Skin and soft-tissue infections Intra-abdominal infections Infections of the female pelvis and genital tract	200 to 300 mg/kg/day by I.V. infusion in divided doses every 4 or 6 hours. (The usual dose is 3 grams given every 4 hours [18 grams/day] or 4 grams given every 6 hours [16 grams/day] depending on weight and the severity of the infection.)

Urinary tract infections
    Complicated: 150 to 200 mg/kg/day by I.V. infusion in divided doses every 4 or 6 hours.
                                         (Usual recommended dosage for average [70 kg] adults: 3 grams q.i.d.)
    Uncomplicated: 1 gram I.M. or direct I.V. every 6 hours.

Infections complicated by renal insufficiency*:

Initial loading dose of 3 grams I.V. followed by I.V. doses, based on creatinine clearance and type of dialysis, as indicated below:

Creatinine clearance mL/min.:	
over 60	3 grams every 4 hours
30 to 60	2 grams every 4 hours
10 to 30	2 grams every 8 hours
less than 10	2 grams every 12 hours (or 1 gram I.M. every 6 hours)
less than 10 with hepatic dysfunction	2 grams every 24 hours (or 1 gram I.M. every 12 hours)
patients on peritoneal dialysis	3 grams every 12 hours
patients on hemodialysis	2 grams every 12 hours supplemented with 3 grams after each dialysis

To calculate creatinine clearance† from a serum creatinine value use the following formula:

$$C_{cr} = \frac{(140 - Age)\ (wt.\ in\ kg)}{72 \times S_{cr}(mg/100\ mL)}$$

This is the calculated creatinine clearance for adult males; for females it is 15% less.

†Cockcroft, D.W., et al: Prediction of Creatinine Clearance from Serum Creatinine. <u>Nephron</u> 16:31–41, 1976.

*The half-life of ticarcillin in patients with renal failure is approximately 13 hours.

Children under 40 kg (88 lbs):

The daily dose for children should not exceed the adult dosage.

Bacterial septicemia Respiratory tract infections Skin and soft-tissue infections Intra-abdominal infections Infections of the female pelvis and genital tract	200 to 300 mg/kg/day by I.V. infusion in divided doses every 4 or 6 hours.

Urinary tract infections
    Complicated: 150 to 200 mg/kg/day by I.V. infusion in divided doses every 4 or 6 hours.
    Uncomplicated: 50 to 100 mg/kg/day I.M. or direct I.V. in divided doses every 6 or 8 hours.

Infections complicated by renal insufficiency: Clinical data are insufficient to recommend an optimum dose.

Children weighing more than 40 kg (88 lbs) should receive adult dosages.

Neonates: In the neonate, for severe infections (sepsis) due to susceptible strains of *Pseudomonas, Proteus* and *E. coli*, the following ticarcillin dosages may be given I.M. or by 10 to 20 minute I.V. infusion:

Infants under 2000 grams body weight:	Infants over 2000 grams body weight:
Aged 0 to 7 days 75 mg/kg/12 hours (150 mg/kg/day)	Aged 0 to 7 days 75 mg/kg/8 hours (225 mg/kg/day)
Aged over 7 days 75 mg/kg/8 hours (225 mg/kg/day)	Aged over 7 days 100 mg/kg/8 hours (300 mg/kg/day)

This dosage schedule is intended to produce peak serum concentrations of 125 to 150 mcg/mL 1 hour after a dose of ticarcillin and trough concentrations of 25 to 50 mcg/mL immediately before the next dose.

3. Intra-abdominal infections such as peritonitis and intra-abdominal abscess (typically resulting from anaerobic organisms resident in the normal gastrointestinal tract).

4. Infections of the female pelvis and genital tract, such as endometritis, pelvic inflammatory disease, pelvic abscess and salpingitis.

5. Skin and soft-tissue infections.

Although ticarcillin is primarily indicated in gram-negative infections, its *in vitro* activity against gram-positive organisms should be considered in treating infections caused by both gram-negative and gram-positive organisms (see Microbiology).

Based on the *in vitro* synergism between ticarcillin and gentamicin sulfate, tobramycin sulfate or amikacin sulfate against certain strains of *Pseudomonas aeruginosa*, combined therapy has been successful, using full therapeutic dosages. (For additional prescribing information, see the gentamicin sulfate, tobramycin sulfate and amikacin sulfate package inserts.)

NOTE: Culturing and susceptibility testing should be performed initially and during treatment to monitor the effectiveness of therapy and the susceptibility of the bacteria.

CONTRAINDICATIONS

A history of allergic reaction to any of the penicillins is a contraindication.

WARNINGS

Serious and occasionally fatal hypersensitivity (anaphylactoid) reactions have been reported in patients receiving penicillin. These reactions are more likely to occur in persons with a history of sensitivity to multiple allergens.

There are reports of patients with a history of penicillin hypersensitivity reactions who experience severe hypersensitivity reactions when treated with a cephalosporin. Before therapy with a penicillin, careful inquiry should be made about previous hypersensitivity reactions to penicillins, cephalosporins and other allergens. If a reaction occurs, the drug should be discontinued unless, in the opinion of the physician, the condition being treated is life-threatening and amenable only to ticarcillin therapy. **Serious anaphylactoid reactions require immediate emergency treatment with epi-**

nephrine. Oxygen, intravenous steroids and airway management, including intubation, should also be administered as indicated.

Some patients receiving high doses of ticarcillin may develop hemorrhagic manifestations associated with abnormalities of coagulation tests, such as bleeding time and platelet aggregation. On withdrawal of the drug, the bleeding cease and coagulation abnormalities revert to normal. Other causes of abnormal bleeding should also be considered. Patients with renal impairment, in whom excretion of ticarcillin is delayed, should be observed for bleeding manifestations. Such patients should be dosed strictly according to recommendations (see DOSAGE AND ADMINISTRATION). If bleeding manifestations appear, ticarcillin treatment should be discontinued and appropriate therapy instituted. **Pseudomembranous colitis has been reported with nearly all antibacterial agents, including *Ticar*, and has ranged in severity from mild to life-threatening. Therefore, it is important to consider this diagnosis in patients who present with diarrhea subsequent to the administration of antibacterial agents.**

Treatment with antibacterial agents alters the normal flora of the colon and may permit overgrowth of clostridia. Studies indicate that a toxin produced by *Clostridium difficile* is 1 primary cause of "antibiotic-associated colitis."

Mild cases of pseudomembranous colitis usually respond to drug discontinuation alone. In moderate to severe cases, consideration should be given to management with fluids and electrolytes, protein supplementation and treatment with an antibacterial drug effective against *C. difficile*.

PRECAUTIONS

Although *Ticar* exhibits the characteristic low toxicity of the penicillins, as with any other potent agent, it is advisable to check periodically for organ system dysfunction (including renal, hepatic and hematopoietic) during prolonged treatment. If overgrowth of resistant organisms occurs, the appropriate therapy should be initiated.

Since the theoretical sodium content is 5.2 mEq (120 mg) per gram of ticarcillin, and the actual vial content can be as high as 6.5 mEq/gram, electrolyte and cardiac status should be monitored carefully.

In a few patients receiving intravenous ticarcillin, hypokalemia has been reported. Serum potassium should be measured periodically, and, if necessary, corrective therapy should be implemented.

As with any penicillin, the possibility of an allergic response, including anaphylaxis, exists, particularly in hypersensitive patients.

Usage During Pregnancy

Reproduction studies have been performed in mice and rats and have revealed no evidence of impaired fertility or harm to the fetus due to ticarcillin. There are no well-controlled studies in pregnant women, but investigational experience does not include any positive evidence of adverse effects on the fetus. Although there is no clearly defined risk, such experience cannot exclude the possibility of infrequent or subtle damage to the fetus. Ticarcillin should be used in pregnant women only when clearly needed.

ADVERSE REACTIONS

The following adverse reactions may occur:

Hypersensitivity Reactions: Skin rashes, pruritus, urticaria, drug fever.

Gastrointestinal Disturbances: Nausea and vomiting, pseudomembranous colitis. Onset of pseudomembranous colitis symptoms may occur during or after antibiotic treatment. (See WARNINGS.)

Hemic and Lymphatic Systems: As with other penicillins, anemia, thrombocytopenia, leukopenia, neutropenia and eosinophilia.

Abnormalities of Blood, Hepatic and Renal Laboratory Studies: As with other semisynthetic penicillins, SGOT and SGPT

Continued on next page

Information on the SmithKline Beecham Pharmaceuticals products appearing here is based on the labeling in effect on July 1, 1996. Further information on these and other products may be obtained from the Medical Department, SmithKline Beecham Pharmaceuticals, One Franklin Plaza, Philadelphia, PA 19101.

SmithKline Beecham—Cont.

Intravenous Solution (concentration of 10 mg/mL to 100 mg/mL)	STABILITY PERIOD Room Temperature 21° to 24°C (70° to 75°F)	Refrigeration 4°C (40°F)
Sodium Chloride Injection, USP	72 hours	14 days
Dextrose Injection 5%	72 hours	14 days
Lactated Ringer's Injection	48 hours	14 days

elevations have been reported. To date, clinical manifestations of hepatic or renal disorders have not been observed which could be ascribed solely to ticarcillin.
CNS: Patients, especially those with impaired renal function, may experience convulsions or neuromuscular excitability when very high doses of the drug are administered.
Other: Local reactions such as pain (rarely accompanied by induration) at the site of the injection have been reported. Vein irritation and phlebitis can occur, particularly when undiluted solution is directly injected into the vein.

DOSAGE AND ADMINISTRATION

Clinical experience indicates that in serious urinary tract and systemic infections, intravenous therapy in the higher doses should be used. Intramuscular injections should not exceed 2 grams per injection.
[See table on preceding page.]
NOTE: Gentamicin, tobramycin or amikacin may be used concurrently with ticarcillin for initial therapy until results of culture and susceptibility studies are known.
Seriously ill patients should receive the higher doses. *Ticar* has proved to be useful in infections in which protective mechanisms are impaired, such as in acute leukemia and during therapy with immunosuppressive or oncolytic drugs.

DIRECTIONS FOR USE

1 gram, 3 gram and 6 gram Standard Vials

Intramuscular Use (concentration of approximately 385 mg/mL): For initial reconstitution use Sterile Water for Injection, USP, Sodium Chloride Injection, USP, or 1% Lidocaine Hydrochloride solution‡ (without epinephrine).
Each gram of ticarcillin should be reconstituted with 2 mL of Sterile Water for Injection, USP, Sodium Chloride Injection, USP, or 1% Lidocaine Hydrochloride solution‡ (without epinephrine) and **used promptly.** Each 2.6 mL of the resulting solution will then contain 1 gram of ticarcillin.
‡For full product information, refer to manufacturer's package insert for Lidocaine Hydrochloride.
Only the 1 gram vial should be used for intramuscular administration. As with all intramuscular preparations, Ticar (ticarcillin disodium) should be injected well within the body of a relatively large muscle using usual techniques and precautions.
Intravenous Administration (concentration of approximately 200 mg/mL): For initial reconstitution use Sodium Chloride Injection, Dextrose Injection 5% or Lactated Ringer's Injection.
Reconstitute each gram of ticarcillin with 4 mL of the appropriate diluent. After the addition of 4 mL of diluent per gram of ticarcillin, each 1.0 mL of the resulting solution will have an approximate concentration of 200 mg. Once dissolved, further dilute if desired.
Direct Intravenous Injection: In order to avoid vein irritation, administer solution as slowly as possible.
Intravenous Infusion: Administer by continuous or intermittent intravenous drip. Intermittent infusion should be administered over a 30 minute to 2-hour period in equally divided doses.

3 gram Piggyback Bottle

Intravenous Infusion (concentrations of approximately 29 mg/mL to 100 mg/mL): The 3 gram bottle should be reconstituted with a minimum of 30 mL of the desired intravenous solution listed below.

Amount of Diluent	Concentration of Solution
100 mL	1 gram/34 mL (~29 mg/mL)
60 mL	1 gram/20 mL (50 mg/mL)
30 mL	1 gram/10 mL (100 mg/mL)

In order to avoid vein irritation, the solution should be administered as slowly as possible. A dilution of approximately 50 mg/mL or more will further reduce the incidence of vein irritation.
Intravenous Infusion: Stability studies in the intravenous solutions listed below indicate that ticarcillin disodium will provide sufficient activity between 21° and 24°C (70° and 75°F) within the stated time periods at concentrations between 10 mg/mL and 50 mg/mL — see Stability Period section below.
After reconstitution and prior to administration *Ticar* as with other parenteral drugs should be inspected visually for particulate matter and discoloration.
[See table at top of page.]
Refrigerated solutions stored longer than 72 hours should not be used for multidose purposes.
After reconstitution and dilution to a concentration of 10 mg/mL to 100 mg/mL, this solution can be frozen −18°C (0°F) and stored for up to 30 days. The thawed solution must be used within 24 hours.
Unused solutions should be discarded after the time periods mentioned above.
It is recommended that *Ticar* and gentamicin sulfate, tobramycin sulfate or amikacin sulfate not be mixed together in the same I.V. solution due to the gradual inactivation of gentamicin sulfate, tobramycin sulfate or amikacin sulfate under these circumstances. The therapeutic effect of *Ticar* and these aminoglycoside drugs remains unimpaired when administered separately.

HOW SUPPLIED

Ticar (sterile ticarcillin disodium). Each vial contains ticarcillin disodium equivalent to 1 gram, 3 grams, 6 grams of ticarcillin.
NDC 0029-6550-22 .... 1 gram Vial
NDC 0029-6552-26 .... 3 gram Vial
NDC 0029-6555-26 .... 6 gram Vial
NDC 0029-6552-21 .... 3 gram Piggyback Bottle
Ticar is also supplied as:
NDC 0029-6558-21 .... 20 gram Pharmacy Bulk Package
NDC 0029-6559-21 .... 30 gram Pharmacy Bulk Package
NDC 0029-6552-40 .... 3 gram ADD-Vantage®§ Antibiotic Vial
Ticar (sterile ticarcillin disodium). Each vial contains ticarcillin disodium equivalent to 20 grams, 30 grams, 3 grams of ticarcillin.
Store dry powder at room temperature or below.
§ADD-Vantage® is a trademark of Abbott Laboratories.
TR:L4IV

TIMENTIN® ℞

[*tī'mĕn-tĭn*]
brand of sterile ticarcillin disodium and clavulanate potassium for Intravenous Administration

DESCRIPTION

Timentin is an injectable antibacterial combination consisting of the semisynthetic antibiotic, ticarcillin disodium, and the β-lactamase inhibitor, clavulanate potassium (the potassium salt of clavulanic acid), for intravenous administration. Ticarcillin is derived from the basic penicillin nucleus, 6-amino-penicillanic acid.
Chemically, it is 4-Thia-1-azabicyclo[3.2.0]heptane-2-carboxylic acid, 6-[(carboxy-3-thienylacetyl)amino]-3,3-dimethyl-7-oxo-, disodium salt, [2*S*-[2α, 5α, 6β(*S**)]]- and may be represented as:

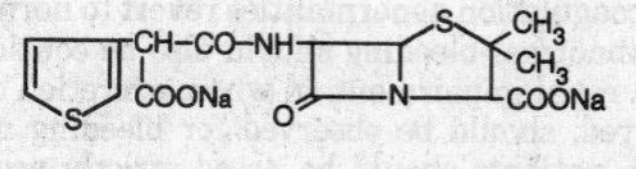

Clavulanic acid is produced by the fermentation of *Streptomyces clavuligerus.* It is a β-lactam structurally related to the penicillins and possesses the ability to inactivate a wide variety of β-lactamases by blocking the active sites of these enzymes. Clavulanic acid is particularly active against the clinically important plasmid-mediated β-lactamases frequently responsible for transferred drug resistance to penicillins and cephalosporins.
Chemically, clavulanate potassium is potassium 4-Oxa-1-azabicyclo[3.2.0]heptane-2-carboxylic acid, 3-(2-hydroxyethylidene)-7-oxo-, monopotassium salt [2*R*-(2α, 3*Z*,5α)]- and may be represented structurally as:

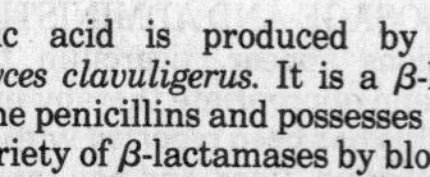

Timentin is supplied as a white to pale yellow powder for reconstitution. *Timentin* is very soluble in water, its solubility being greater than 600 mg/mL. The reconstituted solution is clear, colorless or pale yellow, having a pH of 5.5 to 7.5.
For the *Timentin* 3.1 gram and 3.2 gram dosages, the theoretical sodium content is 4.75 mEq (109 mg) per gram of *Timentin.* The theoretical potassium content is 0.15 mEq (6 mg) and 0.3 mEq (11.9 mg) per gram of *Timentin* for the 3.1 gram and 3.2 gram dosages, respectively.

CLINICAL PHARMACOLOGY

After an intravenous infusion (30 min.) of 3.1 grams or 3.2 grams *Timentin*, peak serum concentrations of both ticarcillin and clavulanic acid are attained immediately after completion of infusion. Ticarcillin serum levels are similar to those produced by the administration of equivalent amounts of ticarcillin alone with a mean peak serum level of 330 mcg/mL for the 3.1 gram and 3.2 gram formulations. The corresponding mean peak serum levels for clavulanic acid were 8 mcg/mL and 16 mcg/mL for the 3.1 gram and 3.2 gram formulations, respectively. (See following table.)
[See table at top of next page.]
The mean area under the serum concentration curves for ticarcillin was 485 mcg/mL.hr. for the *Timentin* 3.1 gram and 3.2 gram formulations. The corresponding areas under the serum concentration curves for clavulanic acid were 8.2 mcg/mL.hr. and 15.6 mcg/mL.hr. for the *Timentin* 3.1 gram and 3.2 gram formulations, respectively.
The mean serum half-lives of ticarcillin and clavulanic acid in healthy volunteers are 68 minutes and 64 minutes, respectively, following administration of 3.1 grams or 3.2 grams of *Timentin.*
Approximately 60% to 70% of ticarcillin and approximately 35% to 45% of clavulanic acid are excreted unchanged in urine during the first 6 hours after administration of a single dose of *Timentin* to normal volunteers with normal renal function. Two hours after an intravenous injection of 3.1 grams or 3.2 grams *Timentin*, concentrations of ticarcillin in urine generally exceed 1500 mcg/mL. The corresponding concentrations of clavulanic acid in urine generally exceed 40 mcg/mL and 70 mcg/mL following administration of the 3.1 gram and 3.2 gram doses, respectively. By 4 to 6 hours after injection, the urine concentrations of ticarcillin and clavulanic acid usually decline to approximately 190 mcg/mL and 2 mcg/mL, respectively, for both doses. Neither component of *Timentin* is highly protein bound; ticarcillin has been found to be approximately 45% bound to human serum protein and clavulanic acid approximately 9% bound.
Somewhat higher and more prolonged serum levels of ticarcillin can be achieved with the concurrent administration of probenecid; however, probenecid does not enhance the serum levels of clavulanic acid.
Ticarcillin can be detected in tissues and interstitial fluid following parenteral administration.
Penetration of ticarcillin into the bile, pleural fluid and cerebrospinal fluid with inflamed meninges has been demonstrated. The results of experiments involving the administration of clavulanic acid to animals suggest that this compound, like ticarcillin, is well distributed in body tissues.
An inverse relationship exists between the serum half-life of ticarcillin and creatinine clearance. The dosage of *Timentin* need only be adjusted in cases of severe renal impairment (see DOSAGE AND ADMINISTRATION).
Ticarcillin may be removed from patients undergoing dialysis; the actual amount removed depends on the duration and type of dialysis.
MICROBIOLOGY: Ticarcillin is a semisynthetic antibiotic with a broad spectrum of bactericidal activity against many gram-positive and gram-negative aerobic and anaerobic bacteria.
Ticarcillin is, however, susceptible to degradation by β-lactamases and therefore the spectrum of activity does not normally include organisms which produce these enzymes.
Clavulanic acid is a β-lactam, structurally related to the penicillins, which possesses the ability to inactivate a wide range of β-lactamase enzymes commonly found in microorganisms resistant to penicillins and cephalosporins. In particular, it has good activity against the clinically important plasmid-mediated β-lactamases frequently responsible for transferred drug resistance.
The formulation of ticarcillin with clavulanic acid in *Timentin* protects ticarcillin from degradation by β-lactamase enzymes and effectively extends the antibiotic spectrum of ticarcillin to include many bacteria normally resistant to ticarcillin and other β-lactam antibiotics. Thus *Timentin* possesses the distinctive properties of a broad-spectrum antibiotic and a β-lactamase inhibitor.
While *in vitro* studies have demonstrated the susceptibility of most strains of the following organisms, clinical efficacy for infections other than those included in the INDICATIONS AND USAGE section has not been documented:
GRAM-NEGATIVE BACTERIA: *Pseudomonas aeruginosa* (β-lactamase and non-β-lactamase producing), *Pseudomonas* species including *P. maltophilia* (β-lactamase and non-β-lactamase producing), *Escherichia coli* (β-lactamase and non-β-lactamase producing), *Proteus mirabilis* (β-lactamase and non-β-lactamase producing), *Proteus vulgaris* (β-lactamase and non-β-lactamase producing), *Providencia rettgeri* (formerly *Proteus rettgeri*) (β-lactamase and non-β-lactamase producing), *Providencia stuartii* (β-lactamase and non-β-lactamase producing), *Morganella morganii* (formerly *Proteus morganii*) (β-lactamase and non-β-lactamase producing), *Enterobacter* species (Although most strains of *Enterobacter* species are resistant *in vitro*, clinical efficacy has been demonstrated with *Timentin* in urinary tract infections

caused by these organisms.), *Acinetobacter* species (β-lactamase and non-β-lactamase producing), *Hemophilus influenzae* (β-lactamase and non-β-lactamase producing), *Branhamella catarrhalis* (β-lactamase and non-β-lactamase producing), *Serratia* species including *S. marcescens* (β-lactamase and non-β-lactamase producing), *Neisseria gonorrhoeae* (β-lactamase and non-β-lactamase producing), *Neisseria meningitidis**, *Salmonella* species (β-lactamase and non-β-lactamase producing), *Klebsiella* species including *K. pneumoniae* (β-lactamase and non-β-lactamase producing), *Citrobacter* species including *C. freundii, C. diversus* and *C. amalonaticus* (β-lactamase and non-β-lactamase producing).

GRAM-POSITIVE BACTERIA: *Staphylococcus aureus* (β-lactamase and non-β-lactamase producing), *Staphylococcus saprophyticus, Staphylococcus epidermidis* (coagulase-negative staphylococci) (β-lactamase and non-β-lactamase producing), *Streptococcus pneumoniae* * (*D. pneumoniae*), *Streptococcus bovis* *, *Streptococcus agalactiae* * (Group B), *Streptococcus faecalis* * (*Enterococcus*), *Streptococcus pyogenes* * (Group A, β-hemolytic), Viridans group streptococci *.

ANAEROBIC BACTERIA: *Bacteroides* species, including *B. fragilis* group (*B. fragilis, B. vulgatus*) (β-lactamase and non-β-lactamase producing), non-*B. fragilis* (*B. melaninogenicus*) (β-lactamase and non-β-lactamase producing), *B. thetaiotaomicron, B. ovatus, B. distasonis* (β-lactamase and non-β-lactamase producing), *Clostridium* species including *C. perfringens, C. difficile, C. sporogenes, C. ramosum* and *C. bifermentans* *, *Eubacterium* species, *Fusobacterium* species including *F. nucleatum* and *F. necrophorum* *, *Peptococcus* species*, *Peptostreptococcus* species*, *Veillonella* species.

* These are non-β-lactamase-producing strains and therefore are susceptible to ticarcillin alone. Some of the β-lactamase-producing strains are also susceptible to ticarcillin alone.

In vitro synergism between *Timentin* and gentamicin, tobramycin or amikacin against multiresistant strains of *Pseudomonas aeruginosa* has been demonstrated.

SUSCEPTIBILITY TESTING:

Diffusion Technique: An 85 mcg *Timentin* (75 mcg ticarcillin plus 10 mcg clavulanic acid) diffusion disk is available for use with the Kirby-Bauer method. Based on the zone sizes given below, a report of "Susceptible" indicates that the infecting organism is likely to respond to *Timentin* therapy, while a report of "Resistant" indicates that the organism is not likely to respond to therapy with this antibiotic. A report of "Intermediate" susceptibility indicates that the organism would be susceptible to *Timentin* at a higher dosage or if the infection is confined to tissues or fluids (e.g., urine) in which high antibiotic levels are attained.

Dilution Technique: Broth or agar dilution methods may be used to determine the minimal inhibitory concentration (MIC) values for bacterial isolates to *Timentin*. Tubes should be inoculated with the test culture containing 10^4 to 10^5 CFU/mL or plates spotted with a test solution containing 10^3 to 10^4 CFU/mL.

The recommended dilution pattern utilizes a constant level of clavulanic acid, 2 mcg/mL, in all tubes together with varying amounts of ticarcillin. MICs are expressed in terms of the ticarcillin concentration in the presence of 2 mcg/mL clavulanic acid.

RECOMMENDED RANGES FOR *TIMENTIN* SUSCEPTIBILITY TESTING[1–3]

Diffusion Method
Disk Zone Size, mm

Res.	Inter.	Susc.
≤11	12 to 14	≥15

Dilution Method
MIC Correlates[4], mcg/mL

Res.	Susc.
≥128	≤64

[1] The non-β-lactamase-producing organisms which are normally susceptible to ticarcillin will have similar zone sizes as for ticarcillin.

[2] Staphylococci which are susceptible to *Timentin* but resistant to methicillin, oxacillin or nafcillin must be considered as resistant.

[3] The quality control cultures should have the following assigned daily ranges for *Timentin*:

		Disks	MIC Range (mcg/mL)
E. coli	(ATCC 25922)	24 to 30 mm	2/2 to 8/2
S. aureus	(ATCC 25923)	32 to 40 mm	—
Ps. aeruginosa	(ATCC 27853)	20 to 28 mm	8/2 to 32/2
E. coli	(ATCC 35218)	21 to 25 mm	4/2 to 16/2
S. aureus	(ATCC 29213)	—	0.5/2 to 2/2

[4] Expressed as concentration of ticarcillin in the presence of a constant 2.0 mcg/mL concentration of clavulanic acid.

INDICATIONS AND USAGE

Timentin is indicated in the treatment of infections caused by susceptible strains of the designated organisms in the conditions listed below:

Septicemia: including bacteremia, caused by β-lactamase-producing strains of *Klebsiella* spp.*, *E. coli**, *Staphylococcus aureus** or *Pseudomonas aeruginosa** (or other *Pseudomonas* species*).

SERUM LEVELS IN ADULTS
AFTER A 30-MINUTE I.V. INFUSION OF TIMENTIN®

TICARCILLIN SERUM LEVELS (mcg/mL)

Dose	0	15 min.	30 min.	1 hr.	1.5 hr.	3.5 hr.	5.5 hr.
3.1 gram	324 (293 to 388)	223 (184 to 293)	176 (135 to 235)	131 (102 to 195)	90 (65 to 119)	27 (19 to 37)	6 (5 to 7)
3.2 gram	336 (301 to 386)	214 (180 to 258)	186 (160 to 218)	122 (108 to 136)	78 (33 to 113)	29 (19 to 44)	10 (5 to 15)

CLAVULANIC ACID SERUM LEVELS (mcg/mL)

Dose	0	15 min.	30 min.	1 hr.	1.5 hr.	3.5 hr.	5.5 hr.
3.1 gram	8.0 (5.3 to 10.3)	4.6 (3.0 to 7.6)	2.6 (1.8 to 3.4)	1.8 (1.6 to 2.2)	1.2 (0.8 to 1.6)	0.3 (0.2 to 0.3)	0
3.2 gram	15.8 (11.7 to 21.0)	8.3 (6.4 to 10.0)	5.2 (3.5 to 6.3)	3.4 (1.9 to 4.0)	2.5 (1.3 to 3.4)	0.5 (0.2 to 0.8)	0

Lower Respiratory Infections: caused by β-lactamase-producing strains of *Staphylococcus aureus, Hemophilus influenzae** or *Klebsiella* spp.*

Bone and Joint Infections: caused by β-lactamase-producing strains of *Staphylococcus aureus.*

Skin and Skin Structure Infections: caused by β-lactamase-producing strains of *Staphylococcus aureus, Klebsiella* spp.* or *E. coli**.

Urinary Tract Infections (complicated and uncomplicated): caused by β-lactamase-producing strains of *E. coli, Klebsiella* spp., *Pseudomonas aeruginosa** (or other *Pseudomonas* spp.*), *Citrobacter* spp.*, *Enterobacter cloacae**, *Serratia marcescens** or *Staphylococcus aureus**.

Gynecologic Infections: endometritis caused by β-lactamase-producing strains of *B. melaninogenicus**, *Enterobacter* spp. (including *E. cloacae**), *Escherichia coli, Klebsiella pneumoniae**, *Staphylococcus aureus* or *Staphylococcus epidermidis.*

Intra-abdominal Infections: peritonitis caused by β-lactamase-producing strains of *Escherichia coli, Klebsiella pneumoniae* or *Bacteroides fragilis** group.

*Efficacy for this organism in this organ system was studied in fewer than 10 infections.

While *Timentin* is indicated only for the conditions listed above, infections caused by ticarcillin-susceptible organisms are also amenable to *Timentin* treatment due to its ticarcillin content. Therefore, mixed infections caused by ticarcillin-susceptible organisms and β-lactamase-producing organisms susceptible to *Timentin* should not require the addition of another antibiotic.

Appropriate culture and susceptibility tests should be performed before treatment in order to isolate and identify organisms causing infection and to determine their susceptibility to *Timentin*. Because of its broad spectrum of bactericidal activity against gram-positive and gram-negative bacteria, *Timentin* is particularly useful for the treatment of mixed infections and for presumptive therapy prior to the identification of the causative organisms. *Timentin* has been shown to be effective as single drug therapy in the treatment of some serious infections where normally combination antibiotic therapy might be employed. Therapy with *Timentin* may be initiated before results of such tests are known when there is reason to believe the infection may involve any of the β-lactamase-producing organisms listed above; however, once these results become available, appropriate therapy should be continued.

Based on the *in vitro* synergism between *Timentin* and aminoglycosides against certain strains of *Pseudomonas aeruginosa*, combined therapy has been successful, especially in patients with impaired host defenses. Both drugs should be used in full therapeutic doses. As soon as results of culture and susceptibility tests become available, antimicrobial therapy should be adjusted as indicated.

CONTRAINDICATIONS

Timentin is contraindicated in patients with a history of hypersensitivity reactions to any of the penicillins.

WARNINGS

SERIOUS AND OCCASIONALLY FATAL HYPERSENSITIVITY (ANAPHYLACTIC) REACTIONS HAVE BEEN REPORTED IN PATIENTS ON PENICILLIN THERAPY. THESE REACTIONS ARE MORE LIKELY TO OCCUR IN INDIVIDUALS WITH A HISTORY OF PENICILLIN HYPERSENSITIVITY AND/OR A HISTORY OF SENSITIVITY TO MULTIPLE ALLERGENS. THERE HAVE BEEN REPORTS OF INDIVIDUALS WITH A HISTORY OF PENICILLIN HYPERSENSITIVITY WHO HAVE EXPERIENCED SEVERE REACTIONS WHEN TREATED WITH CEPHALOSPORINS. BEFORE INITIATING THERAPY WITH *TIMENTIN*, CAREFUL INQUIRY SHOULD BE MADE CONCERNING PREVIOUS HYPERSENSITIVITY REACTIONS TO PENICILLINS, CEPHALOSPORINS OR OTHER ALLERGENS. IF AN ALLERGIC REACTION OCCURS. *TIMENTIN* SHOULD BE DISCONTINUED AND THE APPROPRIATE THERAPY INSTITUTED. **SERIOUS ANAPHYLACTIC REACTIONS REQUIRE IMMEDIATE EMERGENCY TREATMENT WITH EPINEPHRINE. OXYGEN, INTRAVENOUS STEROIDS AND AIRWAY MANAGEMENT, INCLUDING INTUBATION, SHOULD ALSO BE PROVIDED AS INDICATED.**

Pseudomembranous colitis has been reported with nearly all antibacterial agents, including *Timentin*, and may range in severity from mild to life-threatening. Therefore, it is important to consider this diagnosis in patients who present with diarrhea subsequent to the administration of antibacterial agents.

Treatment with antibacterial agents alters the normal flora of the colon and may permit overgrowth of clostridia. Studies indicate that a toxin produced by *Clostridium difficile* is one primary cause of "antibiotic-associated colitis."

After the diagnosis of pseudomembranous colitis has been established, therapeutic measures should be initiated. Mild cases of pseudomembranous colitis usually respond to drug discontinuation alone. In moderate to severe cases, consideration should be given to management with fluids and electrolytes, protein supplementation and treatment with an antibacterial drug clinically effective against *C. difficile* colitis.

PRECAUTIONS

General: While *Timentin* possesses the characteristic low toxicity of the penicillin group of antibiotics, periodic assessment of organ system functions, including renal, hepatic and hematopoietic function, is advisable during prolonged therapy.

Bleeding manifestations have occurred in some patients receiving β-lactam antibiotics. These reactions have been associated with abnormalities of coagulation tests such as clotting time, platelet aggregation and prothrombin time and are more likely to occur in patients with renal impairment.

If bleeding manifestations appear, *Timentin* treatment should be discontinued and appropriate therapy instituted.

Timentin has only rarely been reported to cause hypokalemia; however, the possibility of this occurring should be kept in mind particularly when treating patients with fluid and electrolyte imbalance. Periodic monitoring of serum potassium may be advisable in patients receiving prolonged therapy.

The theoretical sodium content is 4.75 mEq (109 mg) per gram of *Timentin*. This should be considered when treating patients requiring restricted salt intake.

As with any penicillin, an allergic reaction, including anaphylaxis, may occur during *Timentin* administration, particularly in a hypersensitive individual.

The possibility of superinfections with mycotic or bacterial pathogens should be kept in mind, particularly during prolonged treatment. If superinfections occur, appropriate measures should be taken.

Drug/Laboratory Test Interactions: As with other penicillins, the mixing of *Timentin* with an aminoglycoside in solutions for parenteral administration can result in substantial inactivation of the aminoglycoside.

Probenecid interferes with the renal tubular secretion of ticarcillin, thereby increasing serum concentrations and prolonging serum half-life of the antibiotic.

High urine concentrations of ticarcillin may produce false-positive protein reactions (pseudoproteinuria) with the following methods: sulfosalicylic acid and boiling test, acetic acid test, biuret reaction and nitric acid test. The bromphenol blue (Multi-stix®) reagent strip test has been reported to be reliable.

Continued on next page

Information on the SmithKline Beecham Pharmaceuticals products appearing here is based on the labeling in effect on July 1, 1996. Further information on these and other products may be obtained from the Medical Department, SmithKline Beecham Pharmaceuticals, One Franklin Plaza, Philadelphia, PA 19101.

SmithKline Beecham—Cont.

The presence of clavulanic acid in *Timentin* may cause a nonspecific binding of IgG and albumin by red cell membranes leading to a false-positive Coombs test.

Carcinogenesis, Mutagenesis, Impairment of Fertility: Long-term studies in animals have not been performed to evaluate carcinogenic potential. Results of studies performed with *Timentin in vitro* and *in vivo* did not indicate a potential for mutagenicity.

Pregnancy (Category B): Reproduction studies have been performed in rats given doses up to 1050 mg/kg/day and have revealed no evidence of impaired fertility or harm to the fetus due to *Timentin*. There are, however, no adequate and well-controlled studies in pregnant women. Because animal reproduction studies are not always predictive of human response, this drug should be used during pregnancy only if clearly needed.

Nursing Mothers: Caution should be exercised when *Timentin* is administered to a nursing woman.

Pediatric Use: The efficacy and safety of *Timentin* have not been established in infants and children under the age of 12.

ADVERSE REACTIONS

As with other penicillins, the following adverse reactions may occur:

Hypersensitivity reactions: skin rash, pruritus, urticaria, arthralgia, myalgia, drug fever, chills, chest discomfort and anaphylactic reactions.

Central nervous system: headache, giddiness, neuromuscular hyperirritability or convulsive seizures.

Gastrointestinal disturbances: disturbances of taste and smell, stomatitis, flatulence, nausea, vomiting and diarrhea, epigastric pain and pseudomembranous colitis. Onset of pseudomembranous colitis symptoms may occur during or after antibiotic treatment (see WARNINGS).

Hemic and lymphatic systems: thrombocytopenia, leukopenia, neutropenia, eosinophilia and reduction of hemoglobin or hematocrit. Prolongation of prothrombin time and bleeding time.

Abnormalities of hepatic and renal function tests: elevation of serum aspartate aminotransferase (SGOT), serum alanine aminotransferase (SGPT), serum alkaline phosphatase, serum LDH, serum bilirubin. Rarely, transient hepatitis and cholestatic jaundice—as with some other penicillins and some cephalosporins. Elevation of serum creatinine and/or BUN, hypernatremia. Reduction in serum potassium and uric acid.

Local reactions: pain, burning, swelling and induration at the injection site and thrombophlebitis with intravenous administration.

DRUG ABUSE AND DEPENDENCE

Neither *Timentin* abuse nor *Timentin* dependence has been reported.

OVERDOSAGE

As with other penicillins, *Timentin* in overdosage has the potential to cause neuromuscular hyperirritability or convulsive seizures. Ticarcillin may be removed from circulation by hemodialysis. The molecular weight, degree of protein binding and pharmacokinetic profile of clavulanic acid together with information from a single patient with renal insufficiency all suggest that this compound may also be removed by hemodialysis.

DOSAGE AND ADMINISTRATION

Timentin should be administered by intravenous infusion (30 min.).

Adults: The usual recommended dosage for systemic and urinary tract infections for average (60 kg) adults is 3.1 grams *Timentin* (3.1 gram vial containing 3 grams ticarcillin and 100 mg clavulanic acid) given every 4 to 6 hours. For gynecologic infections, *Timentin* should be administered as follows: Moderate infections 200 mg/kg/day in divided doses every 6 hours and for severe infections 300 mg/kg/day in divided doses every 4 hours. For patients weighing less than 60 kg, the recommended dosage is 200 to 300 mg/kg/day, based on ticarcillin content, given in divided doses every 4 to 6 hours.

In urinary tract infections, a dosage of 3.2 grams *Timentin* (3.2 gram vial containing 3 grams ticarcillin and 200 mg clavulanic acid) given every 8 hours is adequate.

For infections complicated by renal insufficiency[1], an initial loading dose of 3.1 grams should be followed by doses based on creatinine clearance and type of dialysis as indicated below:

Creatinine clearance mL/min.	Dosage
over 60	3.1 grams every 4 hrs.
30 to 60	2 grams every 4 hrs.
10 to 30	2 grams every 8 hrs.
less than 10	2 grams every 12 hrs.

less than 10 with hepatic dysfunction	2 grams every 24 hrs.
patients on peritoneal dialysis	3.1 grams every 12 hrs.
patients on hemodialysis	2 grams every 12 hrs. supplemented with 3.1 grams after each dialysis

To calculate creatinine clearance* from a serum creatinine value use the following formula.

$$C_{cr} = \frac{(140 - Age)\,(wt.\,in\,kg)}{72 \times S_{cr}(mg/100\,mL)}$$

This is the calculated creatinine clearance for adult males; for females it is 15% less.

*Cockcroft, D. W., et al: Prediction of Creatinine Clearance from Serum Creatinine. Nephron 16:31-41, 1976.

[1] The half-life of ticarcillin in patients with renal failure is approximately 13 hours.

Dosage for any individual patient must take into consideration the site and severity of infection, the susceptibility of the organisms causing infection and the status of the patient's host defense mechanisms.

The duration of therapy depends upon the severity of infection. Generally, *Timentin* should be continued for at least 2 days after the signs and symptoms of infection have disappeared. The usual duration is 10 to 14 days; however, in difficult and complicated infections, more prolonged therapy may be required.

Frequent bacteriologic and clinical appraisal is necessary during therapy of chronic urinary tract infection and may be required for several months after therapy has been completed; persistent infections may require treatment for several weeks and doses smaller than those indicated above should not be used.

In certain infections, involving abscess formation, appropriate surgical drainage should be performed in conjunction with antimicrobial therapy.

INTRAVENOUS ADMINISTRATION

DIRECTIONS FOR USE

3.1 gram and 3.2 gram Vials and Piggyback Bottles

The 3.1 gram or 3.2 gram vial should be reconstituted by adding approximately 13 mL of Sterile Water for Injection, USP, or Sodium Chloride Injection, USP, and shaking well. When dissolved, the concentration of ticarcillin will be approximately 200 mg/mL with corresponding concentrations of 6.7 mg/mL and 13.4 mg/mL clavulanic acid for the 3.1 gram and 3.2 gram respective doses. Conversely, each 5.0 mL of the 3.1 gram dose reconstituted with approximately 13 mL of diluent will contain approximately 1 gram of ticarcillin and 33 mg of clavulanic acid. For the 3.2 gram dose reconstituted with 13 mL of diluent, each 5.0 mL will contain 1 gram of ticarcillin and 66 mg of clavulanic acid.

INTRAVENOUS INFUSION: The dissolved drug should be further diluted to desired volume using the recommended solution listed in the COMPATIBILITY AND STABILITY SECTION (STABILITY PERIOD) to a concentration between 10 mg/mL to 100 mg/mL. The solution of reconstituted drug may then be administered over a period of 30 minutes by direct infusion or through a Y-type intravenous infusion set. If this method or the "piggyback" method of administration is used, it is advisable to discontinue temporarily the administration of any other solutions during the infusion of *Timentin*.

Stability—For I.V. solutions, see STABILITY PERIOD below.

When *Timentin* is given in combination with another antimicrobial, such as an aminoglycoside, each drug should be given separately in accordance with the recommended dosage and routes of administration for each drug.

After reconstitution and prior to administration, *Timentin*, as with other parenteral drugs, should be inspected visually for particulate matter. If this condition is evident, the solution should be discarded.

The color of reconstituted solutions of *Timentin* normally ranges from light to dark yellow depending on concentration, duration and temperature of storage while maintaining label claim characteristics.

COMPATIBILITY AND STABILITY

3.1 gram and 3.2 gram Vials and Piggyback Bottles (Dilutions derived from a stock solution of 200 mg/mL)

The concentrated stock solution at 200 mg/mL is stable for up to 6 hours at room temperature 21° to 24°C (70° to 75°F) or up to 72 hours under refrigeration 4°C (40°F).

If the concentrated stock solution (200 mg/mL) is held for up to 6 hours at room temperature 21° to 24°C (70° to 75°F) or up to 72 hours under refrigeration 4°C (40°F) and further diluted to a concentration between 10 mg/mL and 100 mg/mL with any of the diluents listed below, then the following stability periods apply.

[See table on top of next column.]

STABILITY PERIOD
(3.1 gram and 3.2 gram Vials and Piggyback Bottles)

Intravenous Solution (ticarcillin concentrations of 10 mg/mL to 100 mg/mL)	Room Temperature 21° to 24°C (70° to 75°F)	Refrigerated 4°C (40°F)
Dextrose Injection 5%, USP	24 hours	3 days
Sodium Chloride Injection, USP	24 hours	7 days
Lactated Ringer's Injection, USP	24 hours	7 days

If the concentrated stock solution (200 mg/mL) is stored for up to 6 hours at room temperature and then further diluted to a concentration between 10 mg/mL and 100 mg/mL, solutions of Sodium Chloride Injection, USP, and Lactated Ringer's Injection, USP, may be stored frozen –18°C (0°F) for up to 30 days. Solutions prepared with Dextrose Injection 5%, USP, may be stored frozen –18°C (0°F) for up to 7 days. All thawed solutions should be used within 8 hours or discarded. Once thawed, solutions should not be refrozen.

NOTE: *Timentin* is incompatible with Sodium Bicarbonate.

Unused solutions must be discarded after the time periods listed above.

HOW SUPPLIED

Timentin (sterile ticarcillin disodium and clavulanate potassium).

Each 3.1 gram vial contains sterile ticarcillin disodium equivalent to 3 grams ticarcillin and sterile clavulanate potassium equivalent to 0.1 gram clavulanic acid.
NDC 0029-6571-26 ....3.1 gram Vial
NDC 0029-6571-21 ....3.1 gram Piggyback Bottle

Timentin is also supplied as:
NDC 0029-6571-40 ....3.1 gram ADD-Vantage® *Antibiotic Vial

Each 31 gram Pharmacy Bulk Package contains sterile ticarcillin disodium equivalent to 30 grams ticarcillin and sterile clavulanate potassium equivalent to 1 gram clavulanic acid.
NDC 0029-6579-21 ....31 gram Pharmacy Bulk Package
Timentin vials should be stored at or below 24°C (75°F).
NDC 0029-6571-31 .... *Timentin* as an iso-osmotic, sterile, nonpyrogenic, frozen solution in Galaxy® † (PL 2040) Plastic Containers—supplied in 100 mL single-dose containers equivalent to 3 grams ticarcillin and clavulanate potassium equivalent to 0.1 gram clavulanic acid.

* ADD-Vantage® is a trademark of Abbott Laboratories.
†Galaxy® is a trademark of Baxter International Inc.

Veterans Administration/Military/PHS—Injection, 3.1 gram, 50 mL, 1's, 6505-01-312-9086; 3.1 gram, 100 mL Pharmacy Bulk, 1's, 6505-01-231-9930; 3.1 gram, ADD-Vantage, 1's, 6505-01-283-0066; 31.0 gram, 100 mL Bulk, 1's, 6505-01-267-7965; 3.1 gram, frozen bag, 12's, 6505-01-344-1132.
TI:L5IV

Shown in Product Identification Guide, page 338

TRIOSTAT™   ℞
[*try'o-stat*]
brand of
liothyronine sodium
injection
(T₃)

DESCRIPTION

Thyroid hormone drugs are natural or synthetic preparations containing tetraiodothyronine (T_4, levothyroxine) sodium or triiodothyronine (T_3, liothyronine) sodium or both. T_4 and T_3 are produced in the human thyroid gland by the iodination and coupling of the amino acid tyrosine. T_4 contains four iodine atoms and is formed by the coupling of two molecules of diiodotyrosine (DIT). T_3 contains three atoms of iodine and is formed by the coupling of one molecule of DIT with one molecule of monoiodotyrosine (MIT). Both hormones are stored in the thyroid colloid as thyroglobulin and released into the circulation. The major source of T_3 has been shown to be peripheral deiodination of T_4. T_3 is bound less firmly than T_4 in the serum, enters peripheral tissues more readily, and binds to specific nuclear receptor(s) to initiate hormonal, metabolic effects. T_4 is the prohormone which is deiodinated to T_3 for hormone activity.

Thyroid hormone preparations belong to two categories: (1) natural hormonal preparations derived from animal thyroid, and (2) synthetic preparations. Natural preparations include desiccated thyroid and thyroglobulin. Desiccated thyroid is derived from domesticated animals that are used for food by man (either beef or hog thyroid), and thyroglobulin is derived from thyroid glands of the hog.

Triostat (liothyronine sodium injection) (T_3) contains liothyronine (L-triiodothyronine or L-T_3), a synthetic form of a natural thyroid hormone, as the sodium salt.

The structural and empirical formulas and molecular weight of liothyronine sodium are given below.

Liothyronine Sodium

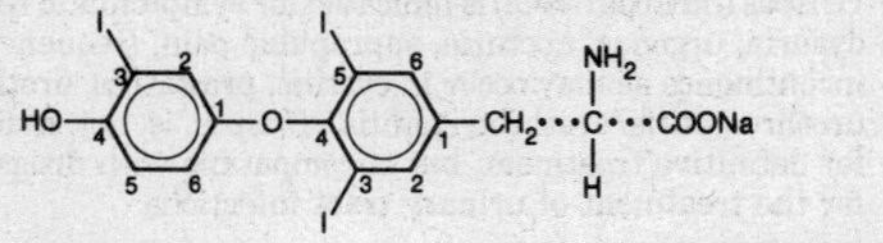

$C_{15}H_{11}I_3NNaO_4$ **M.W. 672.96**

L-Tyrosine, *O*-(4-hydroxy -3- iodophenyl) -3,5-diiodo-, monosodium salt

In euthyroid patients, 25 mcg of liothyronine is equivalent to approximately 1 grain of desiccated thyroid or thyroglobulin and 0.1 mg of L-thyroxine.

Each mL of *Triostat* in amber-glass vials contains, in sterile non-pyrogenic aqueous solution, sodium liothyronine equivalent to 10 mcg of liothyronine; alcohol, 6.8% by volume; anhydrous citric acid, 0.175 mg; ammonia, 2.19 mg, as ammonium hydroxide.

CLINICAL PHARMACOLOGY

Thyroid hormones enhance oxygen consumption by most tissues of the body and increase the basal metabolic rate and the metabolism of carbohydrates, lipids and proteins. In vitro studies indicate that T_3 increases aerobic mitochondrial function, thereby increasing the rates of synthesis and utilization of myocardial high-energy phosphates. This, in turn, stimulates myosin ATPase and reduces tissue lactic acidosis. Thus, thyroid hormones exert a profound influence on virtually every organ system in the body and are of particular importance in the development of the central nervous system.

While the source of levothyroxine (T_4) and some triiodothyronine (T_3) is via secretion from the thyroid gland, it is now well-established that approximately 80% of circulating T_3 arises predominantly by way of the extrathyroidal conversion of T_4. The membrane-bound enzyme responsible for this reaction is iodothyronine 5′-deiodinase. Activity of the enzyme is greatest in the liver and kidney. A second pathway of T_4 to T_3 conversion occurs via a PTU-insensitive 5′-deiodinase located primarily in the pituitary and central nervous system.

The prohormone T_4 must be converted to T_3 in the body before it can exert biological effects. During periods of illness or stress, this conversion is often inhibited and can be diverted to the inactive reverse T_3 (rT_3) moiety. Therefore, correction of the hypothyroid condition in patients with myxedema coma is facilitated by the parenteral administration of triiodothyronine (T_3). T_3 is bound much less firmly to serum binding proteins and therefore penetrates into the cells much more rapidly than T_4. Also, the binding of T_3 to a nuclear thyroid hormone receptor seems to initiate most of the effects of thyroid hormone in tissues. Although most thyroid hormone analogs, both natural and synthetic, will bind to this protein, the affinity of T_3 for this receptor is roughly 10-fold higher than that of T_4. Thus, T_3 is the biologically active thyroid hormone.

Pharmacodynamics

The clinical features of myxedema coma include depression of the cardiovascular, respiratory, gastrointestinal and central nervous systems, impaired diuresis, and hypothermia. Administration of thyroid hormones reverses or attenuates these conditions. Thyroid hormones increase heart rate, ventricular contractility and cardiac output, as well as decrease total systemic vascular resistance. They also increase the rate and depth of respiration, motility of the gastrointestinal tract, rapidity of cerebration, and vasodilatation. Thyroid hormones correct hypothermia by markedly increasing the basal metabolic rate, as well as the number and activity of mitochondria in almost all cells of the body.

Pharmacokinetics

Since liothyronine sodium (T_3) is not firmly bound to serum protein, it is readily available to body tissues.

Liothyronine sodium has a rapid cutoff of activity which permits quick dosage adjustment and facilitates control of the effects of overdosage, should they occur.

The higher affinity of levothyroxine (T_4) as compared to triiodothyronine (T_3) for both thyroid-binding globulin and thyroid-binding prealbumin partially explains the higher serum levels and longer half-life of the former hormone. Both protein-bound hormones exist in reverse equilibrium with minute amounts of free hormone, the latter accounting for the metabolic activity. T_4 is deiodinated to T_3.

A single dose of liothyronine sodium administered intravenously produces a detectable metabolic response in as little as two to four hours and a maximum therapeutic response within two days. However, no pharmacokinetic studies have been performed with intravenous liothyronine (T_3) in myxedema coma or precoma patients.

INDICATIONS AND USAGE

Triostat (liothyronine sodium injection) (T_3) is indicated in the treatment of myxedema coma/precoma.

Triostat can be used in patients allergic to desiccated thyroid or thyroid extract derived from pork or beef.

CONTRAINDICATIONS

Thyroid hormone preparations are generally contraindicated in patients with diagnosed but as yet uncorrected adrenal cortical insufficiency or untreated thyrotoxicosis. Thyroid hormone preparations are also generally contraindicated in patients with hypersensitivity to any of the active or extraneous constituents of these preparations; however, there is no well-documented evidence in the literature of true allergic or idiosyncratic reactions to thyroid hormone.

Concomitant use of *Triostat* and artificial rewarming of patients is contraindicated. (See PRECAUTIONS.)

WARNINGS

> Drugs with thyroid hormone activity, alone or together with other therapeutic agents, have been used for the treatment of obesity. In euthyroid patients, doses within the range of daily hormonal requirements are ineffective for weight reduction. Larger doses may produce serious or even life-threatening manifestations of toxicity, particularly when given in association with sympathomimetic amines such as those used for their anorectic effects.

The use of thyroid hormones in the therapy of obesity, alone or combined with other drugs, is unjustified and has been shown to be ineffective. Neither is their use justified for the treatment of male or female infertility unless this condition is accompanied by hypothyroidism.

Thyroid hormones should be used with great caution in a number of circumstances where the integrity of the cardiovascular system, particularly the coronary arteries, is suspect. These include patients with angina pectoris or the elderly, in whom there is a greater likelihood of occult cardiac disease. Therefore, in patients with compromised cardiac function, use thyroid hormones in conjunction with careful cardiac monitoring. Although the specific dosage of *Triostat* depends upon individual circumstances, in patients with known or suspected cardiovascular disease the extremely rapid onset of action of *Triostat* may warrant initiating therapy at a dose of 10 mcg to 20 mcg. (See DOSAGE AND ADMINISTRATION.)

Myxedematous patients are very sensitive to thyroid hormones; dosage should be started at a low level and increased gradually as acute changes may precipitate adverse cardiovascular events.

Severe and prolonged hypothyroidism can lead to a decreased level of adrenocortical activity commensurate with the lowered metabolic state. When thyroid-replacement therapy is administered, the metabolism increases at a greater rate than adrenocortical activity. This can precipitate adrenocortical insufficiency. Therefore, in severe and prolonged hypothyroidism, supplemental adrenocortical steroids may be necessary.

In rare instances, the administration of thyroid hormone may precipitate a hyperthyroid state or may aggravate existing hyperthyroidism.

Extreme caution is advised when administering thyroid hormones with digitalis or vasopressors. (See PRECAUTIONS—Drug Interactions.)

Fluid therapy should be administered with great care to prevent cardiac decompensation. (See PRECAUTIONS—Adjunctive Therapy.)

PRECAUTIONS

General

Thyroid hormone therapy in patients with concomitant diabetes mellitus (see PRECAUTIONS—Drug Interactions, Insulin or Oral Hypoglycemics regarding interaction and dose adjustment with insulin) or insipidus or adrenal cortical insufficiency may aggravate the intensity of their symptoms. Appropriate adjustments of the various therapeutic measures directed at these concomitant endocrine diseases are required.

The therapy of myxedema coma requires simultaneous administration of glucocorticoids. (See PRECAUTIONS—Adjunctive Therapy.)

Hypothyroidism decreases and hyperthyroidism increases the sensitivity to anticoagulants. Prothrombin time should be closely monitored in thyroid-treated patients on anticoagulants and dosage of the latter agents adjusted on the basis of frequent prothrombin time determinations.

Oral therapy should be resumed as soon as the clinical situation has been stabilized and the patient is able to take oral medication. If L-thyroxine rather than liothyronine sodium is used in initiating oral therapy, the physician should bear in mind that there is a delay of several days in the onset of L-thyroxine activity and that intravenous therapy should be discontinued gradually.

Adjunctive Therapy

Many investigators recommend that corticosteroids be administered routinely in the initial emergency treatment of all patients with myxedema coma. Patients with pituitary myxedema should receive adrenocortical hormone replacement therapy at or before the start of *Triostat* therapy. Similarly, patients with primary myxedema may also require adrenocortical hormone replacement therapy since a rapid return to normal body metabolism from a severely hypothyroid state may result in acute adrenocortical insufficiency and shock.

In considering the need to elevate blood pressure, it should be kept in mind that tissue metabolic requirements are markedly reduced in the hypothyroid patient. Because arrhythmias and circulatory collapse have infrequently occurred following the concomitant administration of thyroid hormones and vasopressor therapies, use caution when administering these therapies concomitantly. (See PRECAUTIONS—Drug Interactions, Vasopressors.)

Hyponatremia is frequently present in myxedema coma, but usually resolves without specific therapy as the metabolic status of the patient is improved with thyroid hormone treatment. Fluid therapy should be administered with great care to prevent cardiac decompensation. In addition, some patients with myxedema have inappropriate secretion of ADH and are susceptible to water intoxication.

In some patients, respiratory depression has been a significant factor in the development or persistence of the comatose state. Decreased oxygen saturation and elevated CO_2 levels respond quickly to artificial respiration.

Infection is often present in myxedema coma and should be looked for and treated appropriately.

Concomitant use of *Triostat* and artificial rewarming of patients is contraindicated. Although patients in myxedema coma are often hypothermic, most investigators believe that artificial rewarming is of little value or may be harmful. The peripheral vasodilation produced by external heat serves to further decrease circulation to vital internal organs and to increase shock if present. It has been reported that the administration of liothyronine sodium will restore a normal body temperature in 24 to 48 hours if heat loss is prevented by keeping the patient covered with blankets in a warm room.

Laboratory Tests

Treatment of patients with thyroid hormones requires the periodic assessment of thyroid status by means of appropriate laboratory tests besides the full clinical evaluation. Serum T_3 and TSH levels should be monitored to assess dosage adequacy and biologic effectiveness.

Drug Interactions

Oral Anticoagulants: Thyroid hormones appear to increase catabolism of vitamin K-dependent clotting factors. If oral anticoagulants are also being given, compensatory increases in clotting factor synthesis are impaired. Patients stabilized on oral anticoagulants who are found to require thyroid replacement therapy should be watched very closely when thyroid is started. If a patient is truly hypothyroid, it is likely that a reduction in anticoagulant dosage will be required. No special precautions appear to be necessary when oral anticoagulant therapy is begun in a patient already stabilized on maintenance thyroid replacement therapy.

Insulin or Oral Hypoglycemics: Initiating thyroid replacement therapy may cause increases in insulin or oral hypoglycemic requirements. The effects seen are poorly understood and depend upon a variety of factors such as dose and type of thyroid preparations and endocrine status of the patient. Patients receiving insulin or oral hypoglycemics should be closely watched during initiation of thyroid replacement therapy.

Estrogen, Oral Contraceptives: Estrogens tend to increase serum thyroxine-binding globulin (TBG). In a patient with a nonfunctioning thyroid gland who is receiving thyroid replacement therapy, free levothyroxine may be decreased when estrogens are started thus increasing thyroid requirements. However, if the patient's thyroid gland has sufficient function, the decreased free thyroxine will result in a compensatory increase in thyroxine output by the thyroid. Therefore, patients without a functioning thyroid gland who are on thyroid replacement therapy may need to increase their thyroid dose if estrogens or estrogen-containing oral contraceptives are given.

Tricyclic Antidepressants: Use of thyroid products with imipramine and other tricyclic antidepressants may increase receptor sensitivity and enhance antidepressant activity; transient cardiac arrhythmias have been observed. Thyroid hormone activity may also be enhanced.

Digitalis: Thyroid preparations may potentiate the toxic effects of digitalis. Thyroid hormonal replacement increases metabolic rate, which requires an increase in digitalis dosage.

Ketamine: When administered to patients on a thyroid preparation, this parenteral anesthetic may cause hypertension and tachycardia. Use with caution and be prepared to treat hypertension, if necessary.

Continued on next page

Information on the SmithKline Beecham Pharmaceuticals products appearing here is based on the labeling in effect on July 1, 1996. Further information on these and other products may be obtained from the Medical Department, SmithKline Beecham Pharmaceuticals, One Franklin Plaza, Philadelphia, PA 19101.

SmithKline Beecham—Cont.

Vasopressors: Thyroid hormones increase the adrenergic effect of catecholamines such as epinephrine and norepinephrine. Therefore, use of vasopressors in patients receiving thyroid hormone preparations may increase the risk of precipitating coronary insufficiency, especially in patients with coronary artery disease. Therefore, use caution when administering vasopressors with liothyronine (T_3).

Drug/Laboratory Test Interactions

The following drugs or moieties are known to interfere with laboratory tests performed in patients on thyroid hormone therapy: androgens, corticosteroids, estrogens, oral contraceptives containing estrogens, iodine-containing preparations and the numerous preparations containing salicylates.

1. Changes in TBG concentration should be taken into consideration in the interpretation of T_4 and T_3 values. In such cases, the unbound (free) hormone should be measured. Pregnancy, estrogens and estrogen-containing oral contraceptives increase TBG concentrations. TBG may also be increased during infectious hepatitis. Decreases in TBG concentrations are observed in nephrosis, acromegaly and after androgen or corticosteroid therapy. Familial hyper- or hypothyroxine-binding globulinemias have been described. The incidence of TBG deficiency approximates 1 in 9000. The binding of thyroxine by thyroxine-binding prealbumin (TBPA) is inhibited by salicylates.

2. Medicinal or dietary iodine interferes with all *in vivo* tests of radioiodine uptake, producing low uptakes which may not be reflective of a true decrease in hormone synthesis.

Carcinogenesis, Mutagenesis and Impairment of Fertility

A reportedly apparent association between prolonged thyroid therapy and breast cancer has not been confirmed and patients on thyroid for established indications should not discontinue therapy. No confirmatory long-term studies in animals have been performed to evaluate carcinogenic potential, mutagenicity, or impairment of fertility in either males or females.

Pregnancy

Pregnancy Category A: Thyroid hormones do not readily cross the placental barrier. The clinical experience to date does not indicate any adverse effect on fetuses when thyroid hormones are administered to pregnant women. On the basis of current knowledge, thyroid replacement therapy to hypothyroid women should not be discontinued during pregnancy.

Nursing Mothers

Minimal amounts of thyroid hormones are excreted in human milk. Thyroid hormones are not associated with serious adverse reactions and do not have a known tumorigenic potential. However, caution should be exercised when thyroid hormones are administered to a nursing woman.

Pediatric Use

There is limited experience with *Triostat* in children. Safety and effectiveness have not been established.

ADVERSE REACTIONS

The most frequently reported adverse events were arrhythmia (6% of patients) and tachycardia (3%). Cardiopulmonary arrest, hypotension and myocardial infarction occurred in approximately 2% of patients. The following events occurred in approximately 1% or fewer of patients: angina, congestive heart failure, fever, hypertension, phlebitis and twitching. In rare instances, allergic skin reactions have been reported with liothyronine sodium tablets.

OVERDOSAGE

Signs and Symptoms: Headache, irritability, nervousness, tremor, sweating, increased bowel motility and menstrual irregularities. Angina pectoris, arrhythmia, tachycardia, acute myocardial infarction or congestive heart failure may be induced or aggravated. Shock may also develop if there is untreated pituitary or adrenocortical failure. Massive overdosage may result in symptoms resembling thyroid storm.

Treatment of Overdosage: Dosage should be reduced or therapy temporarily discontinued if signs and symptoms of overdosage appear. Treatment may be reinstituted at a lower dosage. In normal individuals, normal hypothalamic-pituitary-thyroid axis function is restored in six to eight weeks after cessation of therapy following thyroid suppression.

Treatment is symptomatic and supportive. Oxygen may be administered and ventilation maintained. Cardiac glycosides may be indicated if congestive heart failure develops. Beta-adrenergic antagonists have been used advantageously in the treatment of increased sympathetic activity. Measures to control fever, hypoglycemia or fluid loss should be instituted if needed.

DOSAGE AND ADMINISTRATION

Adults

Myxedema coma is usually precipitated in the hypothyroid patient of long standing by intercurrent illness or drugs such as sedatives and anesthetics and should be considered a medical emergency. Therapy should be directed at the correction of electrolyte disturbances, possible infection, or other inter-

current illness in addition to the administration of intravenous liothyronine (T_3). Simultaneous glucocorticosteroids are required.

Triostat (liothyronine sodium injection) (T_3) is for intravenous administration only. It should not be given intramuscularly or subcutaneously.

- Prompt administration of an adequate dose of intravenous liothyronine (T_3) is important in determining clinical outcome.
- Initial and subsequent doses of *Triostat* should be based on continuous monitoring of the patient's clinical status and response to therapy.
- *Triostat* doses should normally be administered at least four hours—and not more than 12 hours—apart.
- Administration of at least 65 mcg/day of intravenous liothyronine (T_3) in the initial days of therapy was associated with lower mortality.
- There is limited clinical experience with intravenous liothyronine (T_3) at total daily doses exceeding 100 mcg/day.

No controlled clinical studies have been done with *Triostat*. The following dosing guidelines have been derived from data analysis of myxedema coma/precoma case reports collected by SmithKline Beecham Pharmaceuticals since 1963 and from scientific literature since 1956.

An initial intravenous *Triostat* dose ranging from 25 mcg to 50 mcg is recommended in the emergency treatment of myxedema coma/precoma in adults. In patients with known or suspected cardiovascular disease, an initial dose of 10 mcg to 20 mcg is suggested (see WARNINGS). However, both the initial dose and subsequent doses should be determined on the basis of continuous monitoring of the patient's clinical condition and response to *Triostat* therapy. Normally at least four hours should be allowed between doses to adequately assess therapeutic response and no more than 12 hours should elapse between doses to avoid fluctuations in hormone levels. Caution should be exercised in adjusting the dose due to the potential of large changes to precipitate adverse cardiovascular events. Review of the myxedema case reports indicates decreased mortality in patients receiving at least 65 mcg/day in the initial days of treatment. However, there is limited clinical experience at total daily doses above 100 mcg. See PRECAUTIONS—Drug Interactions for potential interactions between thyroid hormones and digitalis and vasopressors.

Pediatric Use

There is limited experience with *Triostat* in children. Safety and effectiveness have not been established.

Switching to Oral Therapy

Oral therapy should be resumed as soon as the clinical situation has been stabilized and the patient is able to take oral medication. When switching a patient to liothyronine sodium tablets from *Triostat*, discontinue *Triostat*, initiate oral therapy at a low dosage, and increase gradually according to the patient's response.

If L-thyroxine rather than liothyronine sodium is used in initiating oral therapy, the physician should bear in mind that there is a delay of several days in the onset of L-thyroxine activity and that intravenous therapy should be discontinued gradually.

HOW SUPPLIED

In packages of six 1 mL vials at a concentration of 10 mcg/mL.
NDC 0007-5210-06
Store between 2° and 8°C.
TS:L3

Shown in Product Identification Guide, page 338

URISPAS®

[yore 'eh-spaz]
brand of flavoxate HCl
100 mg tablets

℞

DESCRIPTION

Urispas (flavoxate HCl) tablets contain flavoxate hydrochloride, a synthetic urinary tract spasmolytic.

Chemically, flavoxate hydrochloride is 2-piperidinoethyl 3-methyl -4- oxo-2- phenyl -4H- 1-benzopyran -8- carboxylate hydrochloride. The empirical formula of flavoxate hydrochloride is $C_{24}H_{25}NO_4 \cdot HCl$. The molecular weight is 427.94. *Urispas* is supplied in tablets for oral administration. Each round, white, film-coated *Urispas* tablet is debossed URISPAS SKF and contains flavoxate hydrochloride, 100 mg. Inactive ingredients consist of calcium phosphate, castor oil, cellulose acetate phthalate, magnesium stearate, polyethylene glycol, starch and talc.

CLINICAL PHARMACOLOGY

Flavoxate hydrochloride counteracts smooth muscle spasm of the urinary tract and exerts its effect directly on the muscle.

In a single study of 11 normal male subjects, the time to onset of action was 55 minutes. The peak effect was observed at 112 minutes. 57% of the flavoxate HCl was excreted in the urine within 24 hours.

INDICATIONS AND USAGE

Urispas (flavoxate HCl) is indicated for symptomatic relief of dysuria, urgency, nocturia, suprapubic pain, frequency and incontinence as may occur in cystitis, prostatitis, urethritis, urethrocystitis/urethrotrigonitis. *Urispas* is not indicated for definitive treatment, but is compatible with drugs used for the treatment of urinary tract infections.

CONTRAINDICATIONS

Urispas (flavoxate HCl) is contraindicated in patients who have any of the following obstructive conditions: pyloric or duodenal obstruction, obstructive intestinal lesions or ileus, achalasia, gastrointestinal hemorrhage and obstructive uropathies of the lower urinary tract.

WARNINGS

Urispas (flavoxate HCl) should be given cautiously in patients with suspected glaucoma.

PRECAUTIONS

Information for Patients: Patients should be informed that if drowsiness and blurred vision occur, they should not operate a motor vehicle or machinery or participate in activities where alertness is required.

Carcinogenesis, Mutagenesis, Impairment of Fertility: Mutagenicity studies and long-term studies in animals to determine the carcinogenic potential of Urispas (flavoxate HCl) have not been performed.

Pregnancy: Teratogenic Effects—Pregnancy Category B. Reproduction studies have been performed in rats and rabbits at doses up to 34 times the human dose and revealed no evidence of impaired fertility or harm to the fetus due to flavoxate HCl. There are, however, no well-controlled studies in pregnant women. Because animal reproduction studies are not always predictive of human response, this drug should be used during pregnancy only if clearly needed.

Nursing Mothers: It is not known whether this drug is excreted in human milk. Because many drugs are excreted in human milk, caution should be exercised when *Urispas* is administered to a nursing woman.

Pediatric Use: Safety and effectiveness in children below the age of 12 years have not been established.

ADVERSE REACTIONS

The following adverse reactions have been observed, but there are not enough data to support an estimate of their frequency.

Gastrointestinal: Nausea, vomiting, dry mouth.

CNS: Vertigo, headache, mental confusion, especially in the elderly, drowsiness, nervousness.

Hematologic: Leukopenia (one case which was reversible upon discontinuation of the drug).

Cardiovascular: Tachycardia and palpitation.

Allergic: Urticaria and other dermatoses, eosinophilia and hyperpyrexia.

Ophthalmic: Increased ocular tension, blurred vision, disturbance in eye accommodation.

Renal: Dysuria.

OVERDOSAGE

The oral LD_{50} for flavoxate HCl in rats is 4273 mg/kg. The oral LD_{50} for flavoxate HCl in mice is 1837 mg/kg. It is not known whether flavoxate HCl is dialyzable.

DOSAGE AND ADMINISTRATION

Adults and children over 12 years of age: One or two 100 mg tablets 3 or 4 times a day. With improvement of symptoms, the dose may be reduced. This drug cannot be recommended for infants and children under 12 years of age because safety and efficacy have not been demonstrated in this age group.

HOW SUPPLIED

Urispas (flavoxate HCl), 100 mg, is supplied as round, white, film-coated tablets debossed with the product name URISPAS and SKF, in bottles of 100 and in Single Unit Packages of 100 (intended for institutional use only).
100 mg 100's: NDC 0007-5290-20
100 mg SUP 100's: NDC 0007-5290-21
Store between 15° and 30°C (59° and 86°F).
Veterans Administration/Military/PHS—Tablets, 100 mg, 100's, 6505-00-172-3420; 100 mg, 100's SUP, 6505-01-156-1935.
UR:L18

Shown in Product Identification Guide, page 338

For information on over-the-counter drugs, consult **PDR For Nonprescription Drugs**

SoloPak Laboratories Inc.
6001 BROKEN SOUND PKWY
BOCA RATON, FL 33487

Direct Inquiries to:
(800) 276-5672
FAX: (561) 998-3059

GANITE® ℞
(gallium nitrate injection)

WARNING

Concurrent use of gallium nitrate with other potentially nephrotoxic drugs (e.g., aminoglycosides, amphotericin B) may increase the risk for developing severe renal insufficiency in patients with cancer-related hypercalcemia. If use of a potentially nephrotoxic drug is indicated during gallium nitrate therapy, gallium nitrate administration should be discontinued and it is recommended that hydration be continued for several days after administration of the potentially nephrotoxic drug. Serum creatinine and urine output should be closely monitored during and subsequent to this period. Ganite therapy should be discontinued if the serum creatinine level exceeds 2.5 mg/dL.

DESCRIPTION

Gallium nitrate injection is a clear, colorless, odorless, sterile solution of gallium nitrate, a hydrated nitrate salt of the group IIIa element, gallium. Gallium nitrate is formed by the reaction of elemental gallium with nitric acid, followed by crystallization of the drug from the solution. The stable, nonahydrate, $Ga(NO_3)_3 \cdot 9H_2O$ is a white, slightly hygroscopic, crystalline powder of molecular weight 417.87, that is readily soluble in water. Each mL of Ganite (gallium nitrate injection) contains gallium nitrate 25 mg (on an anhydrous basis and sodium citrate dihydrate 28.75 mg. The solution may contain sodium hydroxide for pH adjustment to 6.0–7.0.

CLINICAL PHARMACOLOGY

Mechanism of Action

Ganite exerts a hypocalcemic effect by inhibiting calcium resorption from bone, possibly by reducing increased bone turnover. Although *in vitro* and animal studies have been performed to investigate the mechanism of action of gallium nitrate, the precise mechanism for inhibiting calcium resorption has not been determined. No cytotoxic effects were observed on bone cells in drug-treated animals.

Pharmacokinetics

Gallium nitrate was infused at a daily dose of 200 mg/m^2 for 5 (n=2) or 7 (n=10) consecutive days to 12 cancer patients. In most patients apparent steady-state is achieved by 24 to 48 hours. The range of average steady-state plasma levels of gallium observed among 7 fully evaluable patients was between 1134 and 2399 ng/mL. The average plasma clearance of gallium (n=7) following daily infusion of gallium nitrate at a dose of 200 mg/m^2 for 5 or 7 days was 0.15 L/hr/kg (range: 0.12 to 0.20 L/hr/kg). In one patient who received daily infusion doses of 100, 150 and 200 mg/m^2 the apparent steady-state levels of gallium did not increase proportionally with an increase in dose. Gallium nitrate is not metabolized either by the liver or the kidney and appears to be significantly excreted via the kidney. Urinary excretion data for a dose of 200 mg/m^2 has not been determined.

Cancer-Related Hypercalcemia

Hypercalcemia is a common problem in hospitalized patients with malignancy. It may affect 10–20% of patients with cancer. Different types of malignancy seem to vary in their propensity to cause hypercalcemia. A higher incidence of hypercalcemia has been observed in patients with non-small cell lung cancer, breast cancer, multiple myeloma, kidney cancer, and cancer of head and neck. Hypercalcemia of malignancy seems to result from an imbalance between the net resorption of bone and urinary excretion of calcium. Patients with extensive osteolytic bone metastases frequently develop hypercalcemia; this type of hypercalcemia is common with primary breast cancer. Some of these patients have been reported to have increased renal tubular calcium resorption. Breast cancer cells have been reported to produce several potential bone-resorbing factors which stimulate the local osteoclast activity. Humoral hypercalcemia is common with the solid tumors of the lung, head and neck, kidney, and ovaries. Systemic factors (e.g., PTH-rP) produced either by the tumor or host cells have been implicated for the altered calcium fluxes between the extracellular fluid, the kidney, and the skeleton. About 30% of patients with myeloma develop hypercalcemia associated with extensive osteolytic lesions and impaired glomerular filtration. Myeloma cells have been reported to produce local factors that stimulate adjacent osteoclasts.

Hypercalcemia may produce a spectrum of signs and symptoms including: anorexia, lethargy, fatigue, nausea, vomiting, constipation, dehydration, renal insufficiency, impaired mental status, coma and cardiac arrest. A rapid rise in serum calcium may cause more severe symptoms for a given level of hypercalcemia. Since calcium is bound to serum proteins, which may fluctuate in concentration as a response to changes in blood volume, changes in total serum calcium (especially during rehydration) may not accurately reflect changes in the concentration of free-ionized calcium. In the absence of a direct measurement of free-ionized calcium, measurement of the serum albumin concentration and correction of the total serum calcium concentration may help in assessing the severity of hypercalcemia. The patient's acid-base status should also be taken into consideration while assessing the degree of hypercalcemia. Mild or asymptomatic hypercalcemia may be treated with conservative measures (i.e., saline hydration, with or without diuretics). The patient's cardiovascular status should be taken into consideration in the use of saline. In patients who have an underlying cancer type that may be sensitive to corticosteroids (e.g., hematologic cancers), the use or addition of corticosteroid therapy may be indicated.

Hypocalcemic Activity

A randomized double-blind clinical study comparing Ganite with calcitonin was conducted in patients with a serum calcium concentration (corrected for albumin) ≥12.0 mg/dL following 2 days of hydration. Ganite was given as a continuous intravenous infusion at a dose of 200 mg/m^2/day for 5 days and calcitonin was given intramuscularly at a dose of 8 I.U./kg every 6 hours for 5 days. Elevated serum calcium (corrected for albumin) was normalized in 75% (18 to 24) of the patients receiving Ganite and in 27% (7 of 26) of the patients receiving calcitonin (p=0.0016). The time-course of effect on serum calcium (corrected for albumin) is summarized in the following table.

Change in Corrected Serum Calcium by Time From Initiation of Treatment

Time Period[1] (hours)	Mean Change in Serum Calcium (mg/dL)[2] GANITE	Calcitonin
24	−0.4	−1.6*
48	−0.9	−1.4
72	−1.5	−1.1
96	−2.9*	−1.1
120	−3.3*	−1.3

[1] Time after initiation of therapy in hours.
[2] Change from baseline in serum calcium (corrected for albumin).
* Comparison between treatment groups (p<0.01).

The median duration of normocalcemia/hypocalcemia was 7.5 days for patients treated with Ganite and 1 day for patients treated with calcitonin. A total of 92% of patients treated with Ganite had a decrease in serum calcium (corrected for albumin) ≥2.0 mg/dL as compared to 54% of the patients treated with calcitonin (p=0.004).

An open-label, non-randomized study was conducted to examine a range of doses and dosing schedules of Ganite for control of cancer-related hypercalcemia. The principal dosing regimens were 100 and 200 mg/m^2/day, administered as continuous intravenous infusions for 5 days. Ganite, at a dose of 200 mg/m^2/day for 5 days was found to normalize elevated serum calcium levels (corrected for albumin) in 83% of patients as compared to 50% of patients receiving a dose of 100 mg/m^2/day for 5 days. A decrease in serum calcium (corrected for albumin) ≥2.0 mg/dL was observed in 83% and 94% of patients treated with Ganite at dosages of 100 and 200 mg/m^2/day for 5 days, respectively. There were no significant differences in the proportion of patients responding to Ganite when considering either the presence or absence of bone metastasis, or whether the tumor histology was epidermoid or nonepidermoid.

INDICATIONS AND USAGE

Ganite is indicated for the treatment of clearly symptomatic cancer-related hypercalcemia that has not responded to adequate hydration. In general, patients with a serum calcium (corrected for albumin) <12 mg/dL would not be expected to be symptomatic. Mild or asymptomatic hypercalcemia may be treated with conservative measures (i.e., saline hydration, with or without diuretics). In the treatment of cancer-related hypercalcemia, it is important first to establish adequate hydration, preferably with intravenous saline, in order to increase the renal excretion of calcium and correct dehydration caused by hypercalcemia.

CONTRAINDICATIONS

Ganite should not be administered to patients with severe renal impairment (serum creatinine >2.5 mg/dL).

WARNINGS

(See boxed **WARNING**.) The hypercalcemic state in cancer patients is commonly associated with impaired renal function. Abnormalities in renal function (elevated BUN and/or serum creatinine) have been observed in clinical trials with Ganite. **It is strongly recommended that serum creatinine be monitored during Ganite therapy.** Since patients with cancer-related hypercalcemia are frequently dehydrated, it is important that such patients be adequately hydrated with oral and/or intravenous fluids (preferably saline) and that a satisfactory urine output (a urine output of 2 L/day is recommended) be established before therapy with Ganite is started. Adequate hydration should be maintained throughout the treatment period, with careful attention to avoid overhydration in patients with compromised cardiovascular status. Diuretic therapy should not be employed prior to correction of hypovolemia. Ganite therapy should be discontinued if the serum creatinine level exceeds 2.5 mg/dL.

The use of Ganite in patients with marked renal insufficiency (serum creatinine >2.5 mg/dL) has not been systematically examined. If therapy is undertaken in patients with moderately impaired renal function (serum creatinine 2.0 to 2.5 mg/dL), frequent monitoring of the patient's renal status is recommended. Treatment should be discontinued if the serum creatinine level exceeds 2.5 mg/dL.

Combined use of Ganite with other potentially nephrotoxic drugs (e.g., aminoglycosides, amphotericin B) may increase the risk of developing renal insufficiency in patients with cancer-related hypercalcemia (see boxed **WARNING**).

PRECAUTIONS

General

Asymptomatic or mild to moderate hypocalcemia (6.5–8.0 mg/dL, corrected for serum albumin) occurred in approximately 38% of patients treated with Ganite in the controlled clinical trial. One patient exhibited a positive Chvostek's sign. If hypocalcemia occurs, Ganite therapy should be stopped and short-term calcium therapy may be necessary.

Laboratory Tests

Renal function (serum creatinine and BUN) and serum calcium must be closely monitored during Ganite therapy. In addition to baseline assessment, the suggested frequency of calcium and phosphorus determinations is daily and twice weekly, respectively. Ganite should be discontinued if the serum creatinine exceeds 2.5 mg/dL.

Drug Interactions

The concomitant use of highly nephrotoxic drugs in combination with Ganite may increase the risk for development of renal insufficiency (see **WARNINGS**). Available information does not indicate any adverse interaction with diuretics such as furosemide.

Carcinogenesis, Mutagenesis, Impairment of Fertility

Long-term studies in animals have not been performed to evaluate the carcinogenic potential of gallium nitrate. Gallium nitrate is not mutagenic in standard tests (i.e., Ames test and chromosomal aberration studies on human lymphocytes).

Usage in Pregnancy

Pregnancy Category C. Animal reproduction studies have not been conducted with gallium nitrate. It is also not known whether gallium nitrate can cause fetal harm when administered to a pregnant woman or can affect reproductive capacity. Ganite should be administered to a pregnant woman only if clearly needed.

Nursing Mothers

It is not known whether gallium nitrate is excreted in human milk. Because of the potential for serious adverse reactions in nursing infants from gallium nitrate, a decision should be made whether to discontinue nursing or discontinue the drug, taking into account the importance of the drug to the mother.

Pediatric Use

The safety and effectiveness of Ganite in children have not been established.

ADVERSE REACTIONS

Kidney

Adverse renal effects, as demonstrated by rising BUN and creatinine, have been reported in about 12.5% of patients treated with Ganite. In a controlled clinical trial of patients with cancer-related hypercalcemia, two patients receiving Ganite and one patient receiving calcitonin developed acute renal failure. Due to the serious nature of the patients' underlying conditions, the relationship of these events to the drug was unclear. Ganite should not be administered to patients with serum creatinine >2.5 mg/dL (see **CONTRAINDICATIONS** and **WARNINGS**).

Metabolic

Hypocalcemia may occur after Ganite treatment (see **PRECAUTIONS**).

Transient hypophosphatemia of mild-to-moderate degree may occur in up to 79% of hypercalcemic patients following treatment with Ganite. In a controlled clinical trial, 33% of patients had at least 1 serum phosphorus measurement be-

Continued on next page

SoloPak—Cont.

tween 1.5–2.4 mg/dL, while 46% of patients had at least 1 serum phosphorus value < 1.5 mg/dL. Patients who develop hypophosphatemia may require oral phosphorus therapy.

Decreased serum bicarbonate, possibly secondary to mild respiratory alkalosis was reported in 40–50% of cancer patients treated with Ganite. The cause for this effect is not clear. This effect has been asymptomatic and has not required specific treatment.

Hematologic

The use of very high doses of gallium nitrate (up to 1400 mg/m^2) in treating patients for advanced cancer has been associated with anemia, and several patients have received red blood cell transfusions. Due to the serious nature of the underlying illness, it is uncertain that the anemia was caused by gallium nitrate.

Blood Pressure

A decrease in mean systolic and diastolic blood pressure was observed several days after treatment with gallium nitrate in a controlled clinical trial. The decrease in blood pressure was asymptomatic and did not require specific treatment.

Visual and Auditory

In cancer chemotherapy trials, a small proportion (< 1%) of patients treated with multiple high doses of gallium nitrate combined with other investigational anticancer drugs, have developed acute optic neuritis. While these patients were critically ill and had received multiple drugs, a reaction to high-dose gallium nitrate is possible. Most patients had full recovery; however, at least one case of permanent blindness has been reported. One patient with cancer-related hypercalcemia was reported to develop decreased hearing following gallium nitrate administration. Due to the patient's underlying condition and concurrent therapies, the relationship of this event to gallium nitrate administration is unclear. Tinnitus and partial loss of auditory acuity have been reported rarely (< 1%) in patients who received high-dose gallium nitrate as anticancer treatment.

Miscellaneous

Other clinical events reported in association with gallium nitrate treatment for cancer as well as cancer-related hypercalcemia include: nausea and/or vomiting, tachycardia, lethargy, confusion, dreams and hallucinations, diarrhea, constipation, lower extremity edema, hypothermia, fever, dyspnea, rales and rhonchi, anemia, leukopenia, paresthesia, skin rash, pleural effusion, and pulmonary infiltrates. Due to the serious nature of the underlying condition of these patients, the relationship of these events to therapy with gallium nitrate is unknown.

OVERDOSAGE

Rapid intravenous infusion of gallium nitrate or use of doses higher than recommended (200 mg/m^2) may cause nausea and vomiting and a substantially increased risk of renal insufficiency. In the event of overdosage, further drug administration should be discontinued, serum calcium should be monitored, and the patient should receive vigorous intravenous hydration, with or without diuretics, for 2-3 days. During this time period, renal function and urinary output should be carefully monitored so that fluid intake and output are balanced.

DOSAGE AND ADMINISTRATION

The usual recommended dose of Ganite is 200 mg per square meter of body surface area (200 mg/m^2) daily for 5 consecutive days. In patients with mild hypercalcemia and few symptoms, a lower dosage of 100 mg/m^2/day for 5 days may be considered. If serum calcium levels are lowered into the normal range in less than 5 days, treatment may be discontinued early. The daily dose must be administered as an intravenous infusion over 24 hours. The daily dose should be diluted, preferably in 1,000 mL of 0.9% Sodium Chloride Injection USP, or 5% Dextrose Injection USP, for administration as an intravenous infusion over 24 hours. Adequate hydration must be maintained throughout the treatment period, with careful attention to avoid overhydration in patients with compromised cardiovascular status. Controlled studies have not been undertaken to evaluate the safety and effectiveness of retreatment with gallium nitrate.

When Ganite is added to either 0.9% Sodium Chloride Injection USP, or 5% Dextrose Injection USP, it is stable for 48 hours at room temperature (15°-30°C) and for seven (7) days if stored under refrigeration (2°-8°C). Parenteral drug products should be inspected visually for particulate matter and discoloration prior to administration whenever solution and container permit.

HOW SUPPLIED

Ganite* (gallium nitrate injection)
Cat. 34220, NDC 39769-342-20
500 mg (25 mg/mL) in 20 mL single-dose, flip-top vials, individually packaged.
Store at controlled room temperature 15°-30°C (59°-86°F).
Contains no preservative. Discard unused portion.
CAUTION: Federal law prohibits dispensing without prescription.

Manufactured by:
Fujisawa USA, Inc.
Deerfield, IL 60015
for: **SoloPak Laboratories Inc.**
1845 Tonne Road
Elk Grove Village, IL 60007-5125 USA
Telephone: 847/806-0080
45524F/Revised: May 1996

Shown in Product Identification Guide, page 338

HYDRALAZINE HYDROCHLORIDE INJECTION USP ℞

DESCRIPTION

Hydralazine Hydrochloride Injection USP is an antihypertensive available in 1 mL vials for intravenous and intramuscular administration. Each milliliter of the sterile, colorless solution contains 20 mg hydralazine hydrochloride USP, 103.6 mg propylene glycol USP, and 0.65 mg methylparaben NF and 0.35 mg propylparaben NF as preservatives, in water for injection. The pH of the solution is 3.4 to 4.0.

Hydralazine hydrochloride is a white to off-white, odorless crystalline powder. It is soluble in water, slightly soluble in alcohol, and very slightly soluble in ether. It melts at about 275°C, with decomposition. Its chemical formula is $C_8H_8N_4 \cdot HC$ and its molecular weight is 196.64. Hydralazine hydrochloride is 1-hydrazinophthalazine monohydrochloride, and its structural formula is:

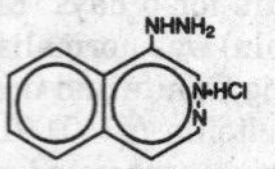

CLINICAL PHARMACOLOGY

Although the precise mechanism of action of hydralazine is not fully understood, the major effects are on the cardiovascular system. Hydralazine apparently lowers blood pressure by exerting a peripheral vasodilating effect through a direct relaxation of vascular smooth muscle. Hydralazine, by altering cellular calcium metabolism, interferes with the calcium movements within the vascular smooth muscle that are responsible for initiating or maintaining the contractile state.

The peripheral vasodilating effect of hydralazine results in decreased arterial blood pressure (diastolic more than systolic); decreased peripheral vascular resistance; and an increased heart rate, stroke volume, and cardiac output. The preferential dilatation of arterioles, as compared to veins, minimizes postural hypotension and promotes the increase in cardiac output. Hydralazine usually increases renin activity in plasma, presumably as a result of increased secretion of renin by the renal juxtaglomerular cells in response to reflex sympathetic discharge. This increase in renin activity leads to the production of angiotensin II, which then causes stimulation of aldosterone and consequent sodium reabsorption. Hydralazine also maintains or increases renal and cerebral blood flow.

The average maximal decrease in blood pressure usually occurs 10-80 minutes after administration of hydralazine hydrochloride injection. No other pharmacokinetic data on hydralazine hydrochloride injection are available.

INDICATIONS AND USAGE

Severe essential hypertension when the drug cannot be given orally or when there is an urgent need to lower blood pressure.

CONTRAINDICATIONS

Hypersensitivity to hydralazine; coronary artery disease; mitral valvular rheumatic heart disease.

WARNING

In a few patients, hydralazine may produce a clinical picture simulating systemic lupus erythematosus including glomerulonephritis. In such patients hydralazine should be discontinued unless the benefit-to-risk determination requires continued antihypertensive therapy with this drug. Symptoms and signs usually regress when the drug is discontinued but residua have been detected many years later. Long-term treatment with steroids may be necessary. **(See PRECAUTIONS, Laboratory Tests.)**

PRECAUTIONS

General: Myocardial stimulation produced by hydralazine can cause anginal attacks and ECG changes of myocardial ischemia. The drug has been implicated in the production of myocardial infarction. It must, therefore, be used with caution in patients with suspected coronary artery disease.

The "hyperdynamic" circulation caused by hydralazine may accentuate specific cardiovascular inadequacies. For example, hydralazine may increase pulmonary artery pressure in patients with mitral valvular disease. The drug may reduce the pressor responses to epinephrine. Postural hypotension may result from hydralazine but is less common than with ganglionic blocking agents. It should be used with caution in patients with cerebral vascular accidents.

In hypertensive patients with normal kidneys who are treated with hydralazine, there is evidence of increased renal blood flow and a maintenance of glomerular filtration rate. In some instances where control values were below normal, improved renal function has been noted after administration of hydralazine. However, as with any antihypertensive agent, hydralazine should be used with caution in patients with advanced renal damage.

Peripheral neuritis, evidenced by paresthesia, numbness and tingling, has been observed. Published evidence suggests an antipyridoxine effect, and that pyridoxine should be added to the regimen if symptoms develop.

Laboratory Tests: Complete blood counts and antinuclear antibody titer determinations are indicated before and periodically during prolonged therapy with hydralazine even though the patient is asymptomatic. These studies are also indicated if the patient develops arthralgia, fever, chest pain, continued malaise, or other unexplained signs or symptoms.

A positive antinuclear antibody titer requires that the physician carefully weigh the implications of the test results against the benefits to be derived from antihypertensive therapy with hydralazine.

Blood dyscrasias, consisting of reduction in hemoglobin and red cell count, leukopenia, agranulocytosis, and purpura, have been reported. If such abnormalities develop, therapy should be discontinued.

Drug/Drug Interactions: MAO inhibitors should be used with caution in patients receiving hydralazine.

When other potent parenteral antihypertensive drugs, such as diazoxide, are used in combination with hydralazine, patients should be continuously observed for several hours for any excessive fall in blood pressure. Profound hypotensive episodes may occur when diazoxide injection and hydralazine are used concomitantly.

Carcinogenesis, Mutagenesis, Impairment of Fertility: In a life-time study in Swiss albino mice, there was a statistically significant increase in the incidence of lung tumors (adenomas and adenocarcinomas) of both male and female mice given hydralazine continuously in their drinking water at a dosage of about 250 mg/kg per day (about 80 times the maximum recommended human dose). In a 2-year carcinogenicity study of rats given hydralazine by gavage at dose levels of 15, 30, and 60 mg/kg/day (approximately 5 to 20 times the recommended human daily dosage), microscopic examination of the liver revealed a small, but statistically significant, increase in benign neoplastic nodules in male and female rats from the high-dose group and in female rats from the intermediate-dose group. Benign interstitial cell tumors of the testes were also significantly increased in male rats from the high-dose group. The tumors observed are common in aged rats and a significantly increased incidence was not observed until 18 months of treatment. Hydralazine was shown to be mutagenic in bacterial systems (Gene Mutation and DNA Repair) and in one of two rat and one rabbit hepatocyte *in vitro* DNA repair studies. Additional *in vivo* and *in vitro* studies using lymphoma cells, germinal cells, and fibroblasts from mice, bone marrow cells from chinese hamsters and fibroblasts from human cell lines did not demonstrate any mutagenic potential for hydralazine.

The extent to which these findings indicate a risk to man is uncertain. While long-term clinical observation has not suggested that human cancer is associated with hydralazine use, epidemiologic studies have so far been insufficient to arrive at any conclusions.

Pregnancy Category C: Animal studies indicate that hydralazine is teratogenic in mice at 20–30 times the maximum daily human dose of 200–300 mg and possibly in rabbits at 10–15 times the maximum daily human dose, but that it is non-teratogenic in rats. Teratogenic effects observed were cleft palate and malformations of facial and cranial bones. There are no adequate and well-controlled studies in pregnant women. Although clinical experience does not include any positive evidence of adverse effects on the human fetus, hydralazine should be used during pregnancy only if the expected benefit justifies the potential risk to the fetus.

Nursing Mothers: It is not known whether this drug is excreted in human milk. Because many drugs are excreted in human milk, caution should be exercised when hydralazine is administered to a nursing woman.

Pediatric Use: Safety and effectiveness in children have not been established in controlled clinical trials, although there is experience with the use of hydralazine hydrochloride in children. The usual recommended parenteral dosage, administered intramuscularly or intravenously, is 1.7–3.5 mg/kg of body weight daily, divided into four to six doses.

ADVERSE REACTIONS

Adverse reactions with hydralazine hydrochloride are usually reversible when dosage is reduced. However, in some cases it may be necessary to discontinue the drug.

The following adverse reactions have been observed, but there has not been enough systematic collection of data to support an estimate to their frequency.
Common: headache, anorexia, nausea, vomiting, diarrhea, palpitations, tachycardia, angina pectoris.
Less Frequent: Digestive: constipation, paralytic ileus.
Cardiovascular: hypotension, paradoxical pressor response, edema.
Respiratory: dyspnea.
Neurologic: peripheral neuritis, evidenced by paresthesia, numbness, and tingling; dizziness; tremors; muscle cramps; psychotic reactions characterized by depression, disorientation, or anxiety.
Genitourinary: difficulty in urination.
Hematologic: blood dyscrasias, consisting of reduction in hemoglobin and red cell count, leukopenia, agranulocytosis, purpura; lymphadenopathy; splenomegaly.
Hypersensitive Reactions: rash, urticaria, pruritus, fever, chills, arthralgia, eosinophilia, and, rarely, hepatitis.
Other: nasal congestion, flushing, lacrimation, conjunctivitis.

OVERDOSAGE

Acute Toxicity: No deaths due to acute poisoning have been reported.
Highest known dose survived: adults, 10 g orally. Oral LD_{50} in rats: 173 and 187 mg/kg
Signs and Symptoms: Signs and symptoms of overdosage include hypotension, tachycardia, headache, and generalized skin flushing. Complications can include myocardial ischemia and subsequent myocardial infarction, cardiac arrhythmia, and profound shock.
Treatment: There is no specific antidote.
Support of the cadiovascular system is of primary importance. Shock should be treated with plasma expanders. If possible, vasopressors should not be given, but if a vasopressor is required, care should be taken not to precipitate or aggravate cardiac arrhythmia. Tachycardia responds to beta blockers. Digitalization may be necessary, and renal function should be monitored and supported as required.
No experience has been reported with extracorporeal or peritoneal dialysis.

DOSAGE AND ADMINISTRATION

When there is urgent need, therapy in the hospitalized patient may be initiated intramuscularly or as a rapid intravenous bolus injection directly into the vein. Hydralazine hydrochloride injection should be used only when the drug cannot be given orally. The usual dose is 20–40 mg, repeated as necessary. Certain patients (especially those with marked renal damage) may require a lower dose. Blood pressure should be checked frequently. It may begin to fall within a few minutes after injection, with the average maximum decrease occurring in 10–80 minutes. In cases where there has been increased intracranial pressure, lowering the blood pressure may increase cerebral ischemia. Most patients can be transferred to oral hydralazine within 24–48 hours.
The product should be used immediately after the stopper is punctured. It should not be added to infusion solutions. Hydralazine hydrochloride injection may discolor upon contact with metal; discolored solutions should be discarded. Parenteral drug products should be inspected visually for particulate matter and discoloration prior to administration, whenever solution and container permit.

HOW SUPPLIED

Hydralazine Hydrochloride Injection USP (20 mg/mL)
Cat. 02101—1 mL fill in 2 mL vial—25/tray
NDC 39769-021-01
Store at controlled room temperature 15°-30°C (59°-86°F)
Caution: Federal (USA) law prohibits dispensing without prescription.
SoloPak Laboratories, Inc.
1845 Tonne Rd
Elk Grove Village, IL 60007-5125 USA
Telephone: 847-806-0080

Shown in Product Identification Guide, page 338

Solvay Pharmaceuticals, Inc.

**901 SAWYER ROAD
MARIETTA, GA 30062**

For Medical Information Contact:
Generally:
Medical Services Department
(770) 578-9000
FAX: (770) 578-5586
In Emergencies:
(800) 241-1643

Sales and Ordering:
Orders may be placed by calling this toll free number:
(800) 241-1643
Mail orders should be sent to:
Solvay Pharmaceuticals
Order Entry Department
901 Sawyer Road
Marietta, GA 30062

CORTENEMA® ℞

(Hydrocortisone Retention Enema)
Disposable Unit for Rectal Use Only

Each disposable unit (60 mL) contains:
Hydrocortisone, 100 mg in an aqueous solution containing carboxypolymethylene, polysorbate 80, and methylparaben, 0.18% as a preservative.

DESCRIPTION

CORTENEMA® is a convenient disposable single-dose hydrocortisone enema designed for ease of self-administration. Hydrocortisone is a naturally occurring glucocorticoid (adrenal corticosteroid) which, similarly as its acetate and sodium hemisuccinate derivatives, is partially absorbed following rectal administration. Absorption studies in ulcerative colitis patients have shown up to 50% absorption of hydrocortisone administered as CORTENEMA® and up to 30% of hydrocortisone acetate administered in an identical vehicle.

ACTIONS

CORTENEMA® provides the potent anti-inflammatory effect of hydrocortisone. Because this drug is absorbed from the colon, it acts both topically and systemically. Although rectal hydrocortisone, used as recommended for CORTENEMA®, has a low incidence of reported adverse reactions, prolonged use presumably may cause systemic reactions associated with oral dosage forms.

INDICATIONS

CORTENEMA® is indicated as adjunctive therapy in the treatment of ulcerative colitis, especially distal forms, including ulcerative proctitis, ulcerative proctosigmoiditis, and left-sided ulcerative colitis. It has proved useful also in some cases involving the transverse and ascending colons.

CONTRAINDICATIONS

Systemic fungal infections; and ileocolostomy during the immediate or early post-operative period.

WARNINGS

In severe ulcerative colitis, it is hazardous to delay needed surgery while awaiting response to medical treatment.
Damage to the rectal wall can result from careless or improper insertion of an enema tip.
In patients on corticosteroid therapy subjected to unusual stress, increased dosage of rapidly acting corticosteroids before, during, and after the stressful situation is indicated.
Corticosteroids may mask some signs of infection, and new infections may appear during their use. There may be decreased resistance and inability to localize infection when corticosteroids are used.
Prolonged use of corticosteroids may produce posterior subcapsular cataracts, glaucoma with possible damage to the optic nerves, and may enhance the establishment of secondary ocular infections due to fungi or viruses.
Usage in pregnancy: Since adequate human reproduction studies have not been done with corticosteroids, the use of these drugs in pregnancy, nursing mothers or women of childbearing potential requires that the possible benefits of the drug be weighed against the potential hazards to the mother and embryo or fetus. Infants born of mothers who have received substantial doses of corticosteroids during pregnancy should be carefully observed for signs of hypoadrenalism.
Average and large doses of hydrocortisone or cortisone can cause elevation of blood pressure, salt and water retention, and increased excretion of potassium. These effects are less likely to occur with the synthetic derivatives except when used in large doses. Dietary salt restriction and potassium supplementation may be necessary. All corticosteroids increase calcium excretion.
While on corticosteroid therapy patients should not be vaccinated against smallpox. Other immunization procedures should not be undertaken in patients who are on corticosteroids, especially on high dose, because of possible hazards of neurological complications and a lack of antibody response.
If corticosteroids are indicated in patients with latent tuberculosis or tuberculin reactivity, close observation is necessary as reactivation of the disease may occur. During prolonged corticosteroid therapy, these patients should receive chemoprophylaxis.

PRECAUTIONS

CORTENEMA® hydrocortisone retention enema should be used with caution where there is a probability of impending perforation, abscess or other pyogenic infection; fresh intestinal anastomoses; obstruction; or extensive fistulas and sinus tracts. Use with caution in presence of active or latent peptic ulcer; diverticulitis; renal insufficiency; hypertension; osteoporosis; and myasthenia gravis.
Steroid therapy might impair prognosis in surgery by increasing the hazard of infection. If infection is suspected, appropriate antibiotic therapy must be administered, usually in larger than ordinary doses.
Drug-induced secondary adrenocortical insufficiency may occur with prolonged CORTENEMA® therapy. This is minimized by gradual reduction of dosage. This type of relative insufficiency may persist for months after discontinuation of therapy; therefore, in any situation of stress occurring during that period, hormone therapy should be reinstituted.
Since mineralocorticoid secretion may be impaired, salt and/or a mineralocorticoid should be administered concurrently.
There is an enhanced effect of corticosteroids on patients with hypothyroidism and in those with cirrhosis.
Corticosteroid should be used cautiously in patients with ocular herpes simplex because of possible corneal perforation.
The lowest possible dose of corticosteroid should be used to control the conditions under treatment, and when reduction in dosage is possible, the reduction should be gradual.
Psychic derangement may appear when corticosteroids are used, ranging from euphoria, insomnia, mood swings, personality changes, and severe depression, to frank psychotic manifestations. Also, existing emotional instability or psychotic tendencies may be aggravated by corticosteroids.
Aspirin should be used cautiously in conjunction with corticosteroids in hypoprothrombinemia.
Growth and development of infants and children on prolonged corticosteroid therapy should be carefully observed.

ADVERSE REACTIONS

Local pain or burning, and rectal bleeding attributed to CORTENEMA® have been reported rarely. Apparent exacerbations or sensitivity reactions also occur rarely. The following adverse reactions should be kept in mind whenever corticosteroids are given by rectal administration.
Fluid and Electrolyte Disturbances: Sodium retention; fluid retention; congestive heart failure in susceptible patients; potassium loss; hypokalemic alkalosis; hypertension. **Musculoskeletal:** Muscle weakness; steroid myopathy; loss of muscle mass; osteoporosis; vertebral compression fractures; asceptic necrosis of femoral and humeral heads; pathologic fracture of long bones. **Gastrointestinal:** Peptic ulcer with possible perforation and hemorrhage; pancreatitis; abdominal distention; ulcerative esophagitis. **Dermatologic:** Impaired wound healing; thin fragile skin; petechiae and ecchymoses; facial erythema; increased sweating; may suppress reactions to skin tests. **Neurological:** Convulsions; increased intracranial pressure with papilledema (pseudo-tumor cerebri) usually after treatment; vertigo; headache. **Endocrine:** Menstrual irregularities; development of Cushingoid state; suppression of growth in children; secondary adrenocortical and pituitary unresponsiveness, particularly in times of stress, as in trauma, surgery or illness; decreased carbohydrate tolerance; manifestations of latent diabetes requirements for insulin or oral hypoglycemic agents in diabetics. **Ophthalmic:** Posterior subcapsular cataracts; increased intraocular pressure; glaucoma; exophthalmos. **Metabolic:** Negative nitrogen balance due to protein catabolism.

DOSAGE AND ADMINISTRATION

The use of CORTENEMA® hydrocortisone retention enema is predicated upon the concomitant use of modern supportive measures such as rational dietary control, sedatives, antidiarrheal agents, antibacterial therapy, blood replacement if necessary, etc.
The usual course of therapy is one CORTENEMA® nightly for 21 days, or until the patient comes into remission both clinically and proctologically. Clinical symptoms usually subside promptly within 3 to 5 days. Improvement in the appearance of the mucosa, as seen by sigmoidoscopic examination, may lag somewhat behind clinical improvement. Difficult cases may require as long as 2 or 3 months of CORTENEMA® treatment. Where the course of therapy extends beyond 21 days, CORTENEMA® should be discon-

Continued on next page

Solvay—Cont.

tinued gradually by reducing administration to every other night for 2 or 3 weeks.

If clinical or proctologic improvement fails to occur within 2 or 3 weeks after starting CORTENEMA® discontinue its use.

Symptomatic improvement, evidenced by decreased diarrhea and bleeding; weight gain; improved appetite; lessened fever; and decreased leukocytosis, may be misleading and should not be used as the sole criterion in judging efficacy. Sigmoidoscopic examination and X-ray visualization are essential for adequate monitoring of ulcerative colitis. Biopsy is useful for differential diagnosis.

Patient instructions for administering CORTENEMA® are enclosed in each box of seven units. We recommend that the patient lie on his left side during administration and for 30 minutes thereafter, so that the fluid will distribute throughout the left colon. Every effort should be made to retain the enema for at least an hour and preferably, all night. This may be facilitated by prior sedation and/or antidiarrheal medication, especially early in therapy, when the urge to evacuate is great.

HOW SUPPLIED

CORTENEMA®, hydrocortisone 100 mg retention enema is supplied as disposable single-dose bottles with lubricated rectal applicator tips, in boxes of seven × 60 mL (NDC 0032-1904-82) and boxes of one × 60 mL (NDC 0032-1904-73). Store at controlled room temperature, 15°–30°C (59°–86°F).

CAUTION: Federal law prohibits dispensing without prescription.

5E Rev. 4/93

SOLVAY
PHARMACEUTICALS, INC.
Marietta, GA 30062

CREON® 5
CREON® 10
CREON® 20
(Pancrelipase)
Delayed-Release
MINIMICROSPHERES™
CAPSULES

℞

PRESCRIBING INFORMATION

DESCRIPTION

CREON® 5, CREON® 10, and CREON® 20 Capsules are orally administered and contain delayed-release MINIMICROSPHERES™ of pancrelipase, which is of porcine pancreatic origin. Each CREON 5 Capsule contains lipase 5,000 USP Units, protease 18,750 USP Units and amylase 16,600 USP Units. Each capsule of CREON 10 contains lipase 10,000 USP Units, protease 37,500 USP Units and amylase 33,200 USP Units. Each capsule of CREON 20 contains lipase 20,000 USP Units, protease 75,000 USP Units and amylase 66,400 USP Units.

Inactive ingredients include dibutyl phthalate, dimethicone, hydroxypropylmethylcellulose phthalate, light mineral oil and polyethylene glycol. The capsule shells contain gelatin, red iron oxide, titanium dioxide, yellow iron oxide. The CREON 5 capsule shell contains FD & C blue No. 2. In addition, the CREON 10 capsule shell contains black iron oxide and the CREON 20 capsule contains black iron oxide, D & C yellow No. 10 and FD & C red No. 40.

CLINICAL PHARMACOLOGY

The pancreatic enzymes in CREON 5, CREON 10, and CREON 20 Capsules are enteric-coated to resist gastric destruction or inactivation. The pancreatic enzymes catalyze the hydrolysis of fats to glycerol and fatty acids, protein into proteoses and derived substances and starch into dextrins and short chain sugars.

INDICATIONS

CREON 5, CREON 10, and CREON 20 Capsules are indicated for patients with pancreatic exocrine insufficiency as is often associated with:
- cystic fibrosis
- chronic pancreatitis
- post-pancreatectomy
- post-gastrointestinal bypass surgery (e.g., Billroth II gastroenterostomy)
- ductal obstruction from neoplasm (e.g., of the pancreas or common bile duct)

CONTRAINDICATIONS

CREON 5, CREON 10, and CREON 20 Capsules are contraindicated in the early stages of acute pancreatitis or in patients who are known to be hypersensitive to pork protein.

WARNINGS

Should symptoms of hypersensitivity appear, discontinue medication and initiate symptomatic and supportive therapy if necessary.

Strictures in the ileo-cecal region and/or ascending colon have been reported in cystic fibrosis patients treated with high doses of high-potency pancreatic enzyme supplements containing 20,000 or greater USP units of lipase per capsule. The underlying mechanism is unknown, but caution should be exercised when doses in excess of 6,000 USP units per kg per meal fail to resolve symptoms, especially in patients with a history of intestinal complications such as meconium ileus equivalent, short bowel syndrome, surgery or Crohn's disease. If symptoms suggestive of gastrointestinal obstruction occur, the possibility of bowel stricture should be investigated including evaluation of pancreatic enzyme therapy.

PRECAUTIONS

CREON 5, CREON 10, and CREON 20 Capsules MINIMICROSPHERES™ SHOULD NOT BE CRUSHED OR CHEWED or placed on foods having a pH greater than 5.5. These can dissolve the protective enteric coating resulting in early release of enzymes, irritation of oral mucosa, and/or loss of enzyme activity.

Information for Patients: CREON 5, CREON 10, and CREON 20 Capsules are a pancreatic enzyme product prescribed to promote improved digestion of foods, especially fat. The prescribed dosage should be taken with each meal and snack or as directed by the physician. The capsules can be swallowed whole, or the contents poured on soft, bland food. Care should be taken to avoid chewing or crushing of the capsule contents, which can result in early release of enzymes, irritation of oral mucosa, and/or loss of enzyme activity. Patients should maintain adequate fluid intake. The prescribed dose range should not be exceeded without calling your doctor.

The most common adverse reactions involve the stomach and intestine including diarrhea, nausea, vomiting, bloating, constipation, stomach cramps or pain. If these symptoms are persistent, contact your doctor.

Carcinogenesis, Mutagenesis, Impairment of Fertility: Long-term studies in animals have not been performed to evaluate carcinogenic potential.

Pregnancy, Category C: Animal reproduction studies have not been conducted with pancrelipase. It is also not known whether pancrelipase can cause fetal harm when administered to a pregnant woman or can affect reproduction capacity. CREON 5, CREON 10, and CREON 20 Capsules should be given to a pregnant woman only if clearly needed.

Nursing Mothers: It is not known whether this drug is excreted in human milk. Because many drugs are excreted in human milk, caution should be exercised when CREON 5, CREON 10, and CREON 20 Capsules are administered to a nursing mother.

ADVERSE REACTIONS

The most frequently reported adverse reactions to pancreatic enzyme-containing products are gastrointestinal in nature which may include nausea, vomiting, bloating, cramping, constipation or diarrhea. Less frequently, allergic-type reactions have also been observed. Very high doses of pancreatin have been associated with hyperuricosuria and hyperuricemia.

DOSAGE AND ADMINISTRATION

Clinical experience should dictate initial starting dose. Doses should be taken during meals or snacks, not before or after. Do not take without food.

Adults and Children Over 6 Years Old:

CREON 5: Usual initial starting dosage is two to four CREON 5 Capsules per meal or snack.

CREON 10: Usual initial starting dosage is one to two CREON 10 Capsules per meal or snack.

CREON 20: Usual initial starting dosage is one CREON 20 capsule per meal or snack.

Children Under 6 Years Old:

CREON 5: The exact dosage of CREON 5 Capsules should be selected based on clinical experience for this age group. Patients can be started on one to two capsules per meal or snack.

CREON 10: Usual initial starting dosage is up to one CREON 10 Capsule per meal or snack.

CREON 20: The exact dosage of CREON 20 should be selected based on clinical experience for this age group.

For cystic fibrosis patients typical doses are 1,500–3,000 USP lipase units/kg/meal.

Dosage should be adjusted according to the severity of the disease, control of steatorrhea and maintenance of good nutritional status. Doses in excess of 6,000 USP lipase units/kg/meal are not recommended.

Dose increases, if required, should occur with careful monitoring of body weight and stool fat content. When changing strengths of pancreatic enzyme products, care should be taken to maintain equivalent lipase units for each divided dosage.

It is important to ensure adequate hydration of patients at all times while taking pancreatic enzymes.

Where swallowing of capsules is difficult, the capsules may be carefully opened and the MINIMICROSPHERES™ added to a small amount of soft food, with a pH less than 5.5. The soft food should be swallowed immediately without

chewing and followed with a glass of water or juice to insure swallowing.

HOW SUPPLIED

CREON® 5 (pancrelipase) Capsules are available in a two-piece gelatin capsule (orange opaque top half, blue opaque bottom half) imprinted in white with "SOLVAY" and "1205". Each capsule contains tan-colored delayed-release MINIMICROSPHERES™ of pancrelipase supplied in bottles of:

100	NDC 0032-1205-01
250	NDC 0032-1205-07

CREON® 10 (pancrelipase) Delayed-Release MINIMICROSPHERES™ are available in a two-piece gelatin capsule (brown opaque top half, natural transparent bottom half) imprinted in white with "SOLVAY" and "1210". Each capsule contains tan-colored enteric-coated MINIMICROSPHERES™ of pancrelipase supplied in bottles of:

100	NDC 0032-1210-01
250	NDC 0032-1210-07

CREON® 20 (pancrelipase) Capsules are available in a two-piece gelatin capsule (orange opaque top half, natural transparent bottom half) imprinted in white with "SOLVAY" and "1220". Each capsule contains tan-colored delayed release MINIMICROSPHERES™ of pancrelipase supplied in bottles of:

100	NDC 0032-1220-01
250	NDC 0032-1220-07

CREON 5, CREON 10, and CREON 20 Capsules must be stored at controlled room temperature, 15°–30°C (59°–86°F). PROTECT FROM MOISTURE. Dispense in tight, light-resistant containers. For human consumption only.

CAUTION: Federal law prohibits dispensing without prescription.

Manufactured By:
Kali-Chemie Pharma GmbH,
Hannover, Germany

Marketed by:
SOLVAY
PHARMACEUTICALS
MARIETTA, GA 30062

Rev 8/94
©1995
SOLVAY PHARMACEUTICALS, INC.

Shown in Product Identification Guide, page 338

DUPHALAC®
(Lactulose Solution, USP)
10 g/15 mL

℞

DESCRIPTION

DUPHALAC® (lactulose solution, USP) is a synthetic disaccharide in solution form for oral administration.

Each 15 mL of DUPHALAC Solution contains: 10 g lactulose (and less than 1.6 g galactose less than 1.2 g lactose, and 1.2 g or less of other sugars).

DUPHALAC Solution is a colonic acidifier which promotes laxation.

The chemical name for lactulose is 4-O-β-D-galactopyranosyl-D-fructofuranose. It has the following structural formula:

Its empirical formula is $C_{12}H_{22}O_{11}$ and its molecular weight is 342.30. It is freely soluble in water.

CLINICAL PHARMACOLOGY

DUPHALAC Solution is poorly absorbed from the gastrointestinal tract and no enzyme capable of hydrolysis of this disaccharide is present in human gastrointestinal tissue. As a result, oral doses of DUPHALAC Solution reach the colon virtually unchanged. In the colon, DUPHALAC Solution is broken down primarily to lactic acid, and also to small amounts of formic and acetic acids, by the action of colonic bacteria, which results in an increase in osmotic pressure and slight acidification of the colonic contents. This in turn causes an increase in stool water content and softens the stool.

Since DUPHALAC Solution does not exert its effect until it reaches the colon, and since transit time through the colon may be slow, 24 to 48 hours may be required to produce the desired bowel movement.

DUPHALAC Solution given orally to man and experimental animals resulted in only small amounts reaching the blood.

Urinary excretion has been determined to be 3% or less and is essentially complete within 24 hours.

INDICATIONS AND USAGE

For the treatment of constipation. In patients with a history of chronic constipation, DUPHALAC (lactulose solution) therapy increases the number of bowel movements per day and the number of days on which bowel movements occur.

CONTRAINDICATIONS

Since DUPHALAC Solution contains galactose (less than 1.6 g/15 mL), it is contraindicated in patients who require a low galactose diet.

WARNINGS

A theoretical hazard may exist for patients being treated with lactulose solution who may be required to undergo electrocautery procedures during proctoscopy or colon-oscopy. Accumulation of H_2 gas in significant concentration in the presence of an electrical spark may result in an explosive reaction. Although this complication has not been reported with lactulose, patients on lactulose therapy undergoing such procedures should have a thorough bowel cleansing with a non-fermentable solution. Insufflation of CO_2 as an additional safeguard may be pursued but is considered to be a redundant measure.

PRECAUTIONS

General: Since DUPHALAC Solution contains galactose (less than 1.6 g/15 mL and lactose (less than 1.2 g/15 mL), it should be used with caution in diabetics.

Information for Patients: In the event that an unusual diarrheal condition occurs, contact your physician.

Laboratory Tests: Elderly, debilitated patients who receive DUPHALAC Solution for more than six months should have serum electrolytes (potassium, chloride, carbon dioxide) measured periodically.

Drug Interaction: Results of preliminary studies in humans and rats suggest that nonabsorbable antacids given concurrently with lactulose may inhibit the desired lactulose-induced drop in colonic pH. Therefore, a possible lack of desired effect of treatment should be taken into consideration before such drugs are given concomitantly with DUPHALAC Solution.

Carcinogenesis, Mutagenesis, Impairment of Fertility: There are no known human data on long-term potential for carcinogenicity, mutagenicity, or impairment of fertility.
There are no known animal data on long-term potential for mutagenicity.
Administration of lactulose solution in the diet of mice for 18 months in concentrations of 3 and 10 percent (V/W) did not produce any evidence of carcinogenicity.
In studies in mice, rats and rabbits doses of lactulose solution up to 6 or 12 mL/kg/day produced no deleterious effects in breeding, conception, or parturition.

Pregnancy:

Teratogenic Effects:

Pregnancy Category B: Reproduction studies have been performed in mice, rats, and rabbits at doses up to 3 or 6 times the usual human oral dose and have revealed no evidence of impaired fertility or harm to the fetus due to lactulose. There are, however, no adequate and well-controlled studies in pregnant women. Because animal reproduction studies are not always predictive of human response, this drug should be used during pregnancy only if clearly needed.

Nursing Mothers: It is not known whether this drug is excreted in human milk. Because many drugs are excreted in human milk, caution should be exercised when DUPHALAC® (Lactulose Solution) is administered to a nursing woman.

Pediatric Use: Safety and effectiveness in children have not been established.

ADVERSE REACTIONS

Precise frequency data are not available.
Initial dosing may produce flatulence and intestinal cramps, which are usually transient. Excessive dosage can lead to diarrhea with potential complications such as loss of fluids, hypokalemia and hypernatremia.
Nausea and vomiting have been reported.

OVERDOSAGE

Signs and Symptoms: There have been no reports of accidental overdosage. In the event of overdosage, it is expected that diarrhea and abdominal cramps would be the major symptoms. Medication should be terminated.

Oral LD_{50}: The acute oral LD_{50} of the drug is 48.8 mL/kg in mice and greater than 30 mL/kg in rats.

Dialysis: Dialysis data are not available for lactulose. Its molecular similarity to sucrose, however, would suggest that it should be dialyzable.

DOSAGE AND ADMINISTRATION

The usual dose is 1 to 2 tablespoonfuls (15 to 30 mL. containing 10 g to 20 g of lactulose) daily. The dose may be increased to 60 mL daily if necessary. Twenty-four to 48 hours may be required to produce a normal bowel movement.
Note: Some patients have found that DUPHALAC Solution may be more acceptable when mixed with fruit juice, water or milk.

HOW SUPPLIED

DUPHALAC (lactulose solution) is a colorless to yellow color + solution that may darken on standing, for oral administration, containing 10 g/15 mL lactulose (667 mg/mL). It is available as:
NDC 0032-1602-08
8 fl oz bottles
NDC 0032-1602-78
16 fl oz bottles
NDC 0032-1602-80
32 fl oz bottles
NDC 0032-1602-84
30 mL unit dose cups in trays of 10 cups.
Store at controlled room temperature, 15°–30°C (59°–86°F). Do not freeze.
+Under recommended storage conditions, a normal darkening of color may occur. Such darkening is characteristic of sugar solutions and does not affect therapeutic action. Prolonged exposure to temperatures above 30°C (86°F) or to direct light may cause extreme darkening and turbidity which may be pharmaceutically objectionable. If this condition develops, do not use.
Prolonged exposure to freezing temperatures may cause change to a semisolid, too viscous to pour. Viscosity will return to normal upon warming to room temperature.
CAUTION: Federal law prohibits dispensing without prescription.
DUPHALAC is a registered trademark of Solvay Duphar B.V.
Manufactured By:
Solvay Duphar B.V.
Weesp, The Netherlands
Marketed by:
SOLVAY PHARMACEUTICALS
MARIETTA, GA 30062
6E1379 Rev 11/94
©1994
SOLVAY PHARMACEUTICALS, INC.

Physician Labeling
ESTRATAB® ℞
Esterified Estrogens Tablets, USP
0.3 mg; 0.625 mg; 1.25 mg; 2.5 mg.

WARNING:

1. ESTROGENS HAVE BEEN REPORTED TO INCREASE THE RISK OF ENDOMETRIAL CARCINOMA.
Three independent case control stuides have reported an increased risk of endomentrial cancer in postmenopausal women exposed to exogenous estrogens for prolonged periods.[1–3] This risk was independent of the other known risk factors for endometrial cancer. These studies are further supported by the finding that incidence rates of endometrial cancer have increased sharply since 1969 in eight different areas of the United States with population-based cancer reporting systems, an increase which may be related to the rapidly expanding use of estrogens during the last decade.[4]
The three case control studies reported that the risk of endometrial cancer in estrogen users was about 4.5 to 13.9 times greater than in nonusers. The risk appears to depend on both duration of treatment[1] and on estrogen dose.[3] In view of these findings, when estrogens are used for the treatment of menopausal symptoms, the lowest dose that will control symptoms should be utilitzed and medication should be discontinued as soon as possible. When prolonged treatment is medically indicated, the patient should be reassessed on at least a semiannual basis to determine the need for continued therapy. Although the evidence must be considered preliminary, one study suggests that cyclic administration of low doses of estrogen may carry less risk than continuous administration,[3] it therefore appears prudent to utilize such a regimen.
Close clinical surveillance of all women taking estrogens is important. In all cases of undiagnosed persistent or recurring abnormal vaginal bleeding, adequate diagnostic measures should be undertaken to rule out malignancy.
There is no evidence at present that "natural" estrogens are more or less hazardous than "synthetic" estrogens at equiestrogenic doses.
2. ESTROGENS SHOULD NOT BE USED DURING PREGNANCY. The use of female sex hormones, both estrogens and progestogens, during early pregnancy may seriously damage the off-spring. It has been shown that females exposed in utero to diethylstilbestrol, a non-steroidal estrogen, have an increased risk of developing in later life a form of vaginal or cervical cancer that is ordinarily extremely rare.[5–6] This risk has been estimated as not greater than 4 per 1000 exposures.[7] Furthermore a high percentage of such exposed women (from 30 to 90 percent) have been found to have vaginal adenosis,[8–12] epithelial changes of the vagina and cervix. Although these changes are histologically benign, it is not known whether they are precursors of malignancy. Although similar data are not available with the use of other estrogens, it cannot be presumed they would not induce similar changes.
Several reports suggest an association between intrauterine exposure to female sex hormones and congenital anomalies, including congenital heart defects and limb reduction defects.[13–16] One case control study[16] estimated a 4.7 fold increased risk of limb reduction defects in infants exposed in utero to sex hormones (oral contraceptives, hormone withdrawal tests for pregnancy, or attempted treatment for threatened abortion). Some of these exposures were very short and involved only a few days of treatment. The data suggest that the risk of limb reduction defects in exposed fetuses is somewhat less than 1 per 1000.
In the past, female sex hormones have been used during pregnancy in an attempt to treat threatened or habitual abortion. There is considerable evidence that estrogens are ineffective for these indications, and there is no evidence from well controlled studies that progestogens are effective for these uses.
If ESTRATAB® is used during pregnancy, or if the patient becomes pregnant while taking this drug, she should be apprised of the potential risks to the fetus, and the advisability of pregnancy continuation.

DESCRIPTION

ESTRATAB® (Esterified Estrogens Tablets). Each blue, sugar coated tablet contains 0.3 mg. Each yellow, sugar coated tablet contains 0.625 mg. Each orange-red, sugar coated tablet contains 1.25 mg. Each light purple, sugar coated tablet contains 2.5 mg.

Inactive Ingredients: Acacia, calcium carbonate, carnauba wax, carboxymethylcellulose sodium, citric acid, colloidal silicon dioxide, diacetylated monoglyceride, gelatin, lactose, magnesium stearate, methylparaben, microcrystalline cellulose, pharmaceutical glaze, povidone, propylparaben, shellac, sodium benzoate, sodium bicarbonate, sorbic acid, sucrose, corn starch, talc, titanium dioxide and tribasic calcium phosphate. The 0.3 mg tablet coating contains FD&C Blue #1 Lake; the 0.625 mg tablet coating contains D&C Yellow #10 Lake, FD&C Yellow #6 Lake and FD&C Blue #2 Lake; the 1.25 mg tablet coating contains FD&C Yellow #6 Lake and 2.5 mg tablet coating contains FD&C Red #40 Lake and FD&C Blue #2 Lake. In addition the tablet imprinting ink for the 0.3 mg, 0.625 mg and the 1.25 mg tablets contain black iron oxide, FD&C Blue #2 Lake, FD&C Red #40 Lake and FD&C Yellow #6 Lake. The 2.5 mg imprinting ink contains Soya lecithin, Dimethyl Polysiloxane, pharmaceutical Shellac and Titanium dioxide.

ESTRATAB® (Esterified Estrogens Tablets) for oral administration is a mixture of the sodium salts of the sulfate esters of the estrogenic substances, principally estrone, that are of the type excreted by pregnant mares. Esterified Estrogens contain not less than 75.0 percent and not more than 85.0 percent of sodium estrone sulfate, and not less than 6.0 percent and not more than 15.0 percent of sodium equilin sulfate, in such proportion that the total of these two components is not less than 90.0 percent.

CLINICAL PHARMACOLOGY

Estrogens are important in the development and maintenance of the female reproductive system and secondary sex characteristics. They promote growth and development of the vagina, uterus, and fallopian tubes, and enlargement of the breasts. Indirectly, they contribute to the shaping of the skeleton, maintenance of tone and elasticity of urogenital structures, changes in the epiphyses of the long bones that allow for the pubertal growth spurt and its termination, growth of axillary and pubic hair, and pigmentation of the nipples and genitals. Decline of estrogenic activity at the end of the menstrual cycle can bring on menstruation, although the cessation of progesterone secretion is the most important factor in the mature ovulatory cycle. However, in the preovulatory or nonovulatory cycle, estrogen is the primary determinant in the onset of menstruation. Estrogens also affect the release of pituitary gonadotropins.
The pharmacologic effects of conjugated estrogens are similar to those of endogenous estrogens. They are soluble in water and are well absorbed from the gastrointestinal tract.

Continued on next page

Solvay—Cont.

In responsive tissues (female genital organs, breasts, hypothalamus, pituitary) estrogens enter the cell and are transported into the nucleus. As a result of estrogen action, specific RNA and protein synthesis occurs.
Metabolism and inactivation occur primarily in the liver. Some estrogens are excreted into the bile; however they are reabsorbed from the intestine and returned to the liver through the portal venous system. Water soluble estrogen conjugates are strongly acidic and are ionized in body fluids, which favor excretion through the kidneys since tubular reabsorption is minimal.

INDICATIONS AND USAGE

ESTRATAB® is indicated in the treatment of:
1. Moderate to severe *vasomotor* symptoms associated with the menopause. (There is no evidence that estrogens are effective for nervous symptoms or depression which might occur during menopause and they should not be used to treat these conditions).
2. Atrophic vaginitis.
3. Kraurosis vulvae.
4. Female hypogonadism.
5. Female castration.
6. Primary ovarian failure.
7. Breast cancer (for palliation only) in appropriately selected women and men with metastatic disease.
8. Prostatic carcinoma—palliative therapy of advanced disease.

ESTRATAB® HAS NOT BEEN SHOWN TO BE EFFECTIVE FOR ANY PURPOSE DURING PREGNANCY AND ITS USE MAY CAUSE SEVERE HARM TO THE FETUS (SEE BOXED WARNING).

CONTRAINDICATIONS

Estrogens should not be used in women (or men) with any of the following conditions:
1. Known or suspected cancer of the breast except in appropriately selected patients being treated for metastatic disease.
2. Known or suspected estrogen-dependent neoplasia.
3. Known or suspected pregnancy (See Boxed Warning).
4. Undiagnosed abnormal genital bleeding.
5. Active thrombophlebitis or thromboembolic disorders.
6. A past history of thrombophlebitis, thrombosis, or thromboembolic disorders associated with previous estrogen use (except when used in treatment of breast or prostatic malignancy).

WARNINGS

1. **Induction of malignant neoplasms.** Long term continuous administration of natural and synthetic estrogens in certain animal species increases the frequency of carcinomas of the breast, cervix, vagina, and liver. There is now evidence that estrogens increase the risk of carcinoma of the endometrium in humans (See Boxed Warning).
   At the present time there is no satisfactory evidence that estrogens given to postmenopausal women increase the risk of cancer of the breast,[18] although a recent long-term follow up of a single physician's practice has raised this possibility.[18a] Because of the animal data, there is need for caution in prescribing estrogens for women with a strong family history of breast cancer or who have breast nodules, fibrocytic disease, or abnormal mammograms.
2. **Gall bladder disease.** A recent study has reported a 2 to 3-fold increase in the risk of surgically confirmed gall bladder disease in women receiving postmenopausal estrogens,[18] similar to the 2-fold increase previously noted in users of oral contraceptives.[19–24] In the case of oral contraceptives the increase risk appeared after two years of use.[24]
3. **Effects similar to these caused by estrogen-progestogen oral contraceptives.** There are several serious adverse effects of oral contraceptives, most of which have not, up to now, been documented as consequences of postmenopausal estrogen therapy. This may reflect the comparatively low doses of estrogen used in postmenopausal women. It would be expected that the larger doses of estrogen used to treat prostatic or breast cancer or postpartum breast engorgement are more likely to result in these adverse effects, and, in fact, it has been shown that there is an increased risk of thrombosis in men receiving estrogens for prostatic cancer and women for postpartum breast engorgement.[20–23]
   a. **Thromboembolic disease.** It is now well established that users of oral contraceptives have an increased risk of various thromboembolic and thrombotic vascular diseases, such as thrombophlebitis, pulmonary embolism, stroke, and myocardial infarction.[24–31] Cases of retinal thrombosis, mesenteric thrombosis, and optic neuritis have been reported in oral contraceptive users. There is evidence that the risk of several of these adverse reactions is related to the dose of the drug.[32–33]
   An increased risk of postsurgery thromboembolic complications has also been reported in users of oral contraceptives.[34–35] If feasible, estrogen should be discontinued at least 4 weeks before surgery of the type associated with an increased risk of thromboembolism, or during periods of prolonged immobilization.
   While an increased rate of thromboembolic and thrombotic disease in postmenopausal users of estrogen has not been found,[18–36] this does not rule out the possibility that such an increase may be present or that subgroups of women who have underlying risk factors or who are receiving relatively large doses of estrogens may have increased risk. Therefore estrogens should not be used in persons with active thrombophlebitis or thromboemblic disorders, and they should not be used (except in treatment of malignancy) in persons with a history of such disorders in association with estrogen use. They should be used with caution in patients with cerebral vascular or coronary artery disease and only for those in whom estrogens are clearly needed. Large doses of estrogen (5 mg esterified estrogens per day) comparable to those used to treat cancer of the prostate and breast, have been shown in a large prospective clinical trial in men[37] to increase the risk of nonfatal myocardial infarction, pulmonary embolism and thrombophlebitis. When estrogen doses of this size are used, any of the thromboembolic and thrombotic adverse effects associated with oral contraceptive use should be considered a clear risk.
   b. **Hepatic adenoma.** Benign hepatic adenomas appear to be associated with the use of oral contraceptives.[38–40] Although benign and rare, these may rupture and may cause death through intraabdominal hemorrhage. Such lesions have not yet been reported in association with other estrogen or progestogen preparations but should be considered in estrogen users having abdominal pain and tenderness, abdominal mass, or hypovolemic shock. Hepatocellular carcinoma has also been reported in women taking estrogen-containing oral contraceptives.[39] The relationship of this malignancy to these drugs is not known at this time.
   c. **Elevated blood pressure.** Increased blood pressure is not uncommon in women using oral contraceptives. There is now a report that this may occur with use of estrogens in the menopause[41] and blood pressure, should be monitored with estrogen use, especially if high doses are used.
   d. **Glucose tolerance.** A worsening of glucose tolerance has been observed in a significant percentage of patients on estrogen-containing oral contraceptives. For this reason, diabetic patients should be carefully observed while receiving estrogens.
4. **Hypercalcemia.** Administration of estrogens may lead to severe hypercalcemia in patients with breast cancer and bone metastases. If this occurs, the drug should be stopped and appropriate measures taken to reduce the serum calcium level.

PRECAUTIONS

A. General Precautions

1. A complete medical and family history should be taken prior to the initiation of any estrogen therapy. The pretreatment and periodic physical examinations should include special reference to blood pressure, abdomen, and pelvic organs, and should include a Papanicolaou smear. As a general rule, estrogen should not be prescribed for longer than one year without another physical examination being performed.
2. Fluid-retention—Because estrogen may cause some degree of fluid retention, conditions which might be influenced by this factor such as epilepsy, migraine, and cardiac or renal dysfunction, require careful observation.
3. Certain patients may develop undesirable manifestations of excessive estrogenic stimulation, such as abnormal or excessive uterine bleeding, mastodynia, etc.
4. Oral contraceptives appear to be associated with an increased incidence of mental depression.[24] Although it is not clear whether this is due to the estrogenic or progestogenic component of the contraceptive, patients with a history of depression should be carefully observed.
5. Preexisting uterine leiomyomata may increase in size during estrogen use.
6. The pathologist should be advised of estrogen therapy when relevant specimens are submitted.
7. Patients with a past history of jaundice during pregnancy have an increased risk of recurrence of jaundice while receiving estrogen-containing oral contraceptive therapy. If jaundice develops in any patient receiving estrogen, the medication should be discontinued while the cause is investigated.
8. Estrogens may be poorly metabolized in patients with impaired liver functions and they should be administered with caution in such patients.
9. Because estrogens influence the metabolism of calcium and phosphorus, they should be used with caution in patients with metabolic bone diseases that are associated with hypercalcemia or in patients with renal insufficiency.
10. Because of the effects of estrogens on epiphyseal closure, they should be used judiciously in young patients in whom bone growth is not complete.
11. Certain endocrine and liver function tests may be affected by estrogen-containing oral contraceptives. The following similar changes may be expected with larger doses of estrogen:
    a. Increased sulfobromophthalein retention.
    b. Increased prothrombin and factors VII, VIII, IX, and X; decreased antitrombin 3, increased norepinephrine-induced platelet aggregability.
    c. Increased thyroid binding globulin (TBG) leading to increased circulating total thyroid hormone, as measured by PBI, T4 by column, or T4 by radioimmunoassay. Free T3 resin uptake is decreased, reflecting the elevated TBG; free T4 concentration is unaltered.
    d. Impaired glucose tolerance.
    e. Decreased pregnanediol excretion.
    f. Reduced response to metyrapone test.
    g. Reduced serum folate concentration.
    h. Increased serum triglyceride and phospholipid concentration.
12. The lowest effective dose appropriate for the specific indication should be utilized. Studies of the addition of a progestin for seven or more days of a cycle of estrogen administration have reported a lowered incidence of endometrial hyperplasia. Morphological and biochemical studies of endometrium suggest that 10 to 13 days of progestin are needed to provide maximal maturation of the endometrium and to eliminate any hyperplastic changes. Whether this will provide protection from endometrial carcinoma has not been clearly established. There are possible additional risks which may be associated with the inclusion of progestin in estrogen replacement regimens. The potential risks include adverse effects on carbohydrate and lipid metabolism. The choice of progestin and dosage may be important in minimizing these adverse effects.

B. Information for the Patient. See text of Patient Package Insert which appears after the REFERENCES.

C. Pregnancy Category X. See CONTRAINDICATIONS and Boxed WARNING.

D. Nursing Mothers. As a general principle, the administration of any drug to nursing mothers should be done only when clearly necessary since many drugs are excreted in human milk.

ADVERSE REACTIONS

(See Warnings regarding induction of neoplasia, adverse effects on the fetus, increased incidence of gall bladder disease, and adverse effects similar to those of oral contraceptives, including thromboembolism). The following additional adverse reactions have been reported with estrogenic therapy, including oral contraceptives:

1. **Genitourinary system.**
   Breakthrough bleeding, spotting, change in menstrual flow.
   Dysmenorrhea.
   Premenstrual-like syndrome.
   Increase in size of uterine fibromyomata.
   Vaginal candidiasis.
   Change in cervical erosion and in degree of cervical secretion.
   Cystitis-like syndrome.
2. **Breasts.**
   Tenderness, enlargement, secretion.
3. **Gastrointestinal.**
   Nausea, vomiting.
   Abdominal cramps, bloating.
   Cholestatic jaundice.
4. **Skin.**
   Chloasma or melasma which may persist when drug is discontinued.
   Erythema multiforme.
   Erythema nodosum.
   Hemorrhagic eruption.
   Loss of scalp hair.
   Hirsutism.
5. **Eyes.**
   Steepening of corneal curvature.
   Intolerance to contact lens.
6. **CNS.**
   Headache, migraine, dizziness.
   Mental depression.
   Chorea.
7. **Miscellaneous.**
   Increase or decrease in weight.
   Reduced carbohydrate tolerance.
   Aggravation of porphyria.
   Edema.
   Changes in libido.

OVERDOSAGE

Numerous reports of ingestion of large doses of estrogen-containing oral contraceptives by young children indicate that serious ill effects do not occur. Overdosage of estrogen

may cause nausea, and withdrawal bleeding may occur in females.

DOSAGE AND ADMINISTRATION

1. Given cyclically for short term use only:

For treatment of moderate to severe *vasomotor* symptoms, atrophic vaginitis, or kraurosis vulvae associated with the menopause. The lowest dose that will control symptoms should be chosen and medication should be discontinued as promptly as possible. Administration should by cyclic (e.g., three weeks on and one week off). Attempts to discontinue or taper medication should be made at three to six month intervals.

Usual dosage ranges.

Vasomotor symptoms—1.25 mg daily. If the patient has not menstruated within the last two months or more, cyclic administration is started arbitrarily. If the patient is menstruating, cyclic administration is started on day 5 of bleeding.

Atrophic vaginitis and kraurosis vulvae—0.3 mg to 1.25 mg or more daily, depending upon the tissue response of the individual patient. Administer cyclically.

2. Given cyclically: Female hypogonadism; female castration; primary ovarian failure.

Usual dosage ranges:

Female hypogonadism—2.5 to 7.5 mg daily, in divided doses for 20 days, followed by a rest period of 10 days' duration. If bleeding does not occur by the end of this period, the same dosage schedule is repeated. The number of courses of estrogen therapy necessary to produce bleeding may vary depending on the responsiveness of the endometrium.

If bleeding occurs before the end of the 10 day period, begin a 20 day estrogen-progestin cyclic regimen with ESTRATAB® (Esterified Estrogens Tablets, USP), 2.5 to 7.5 mg daily in divided doses, for 20 days. During the last five days of estrogen therapy, give an oral progestin. If bleeding occurs before this regimen is concluded, therapy is discontinued and may be resumed on the fifth day of bleeding.

Female castration, and primary ovarian failure—1.25 mg daily, cyclically. Adjust dosage upward or downward according to severity of symptoms and response of the patient. For maintenance, adjust dosage to lowest level that will provide effective control.

3. Given chronically: Inoperable progressing prostatic cancer —1.25 to 2.5 mg three times daily. The effectiveness of therapy can be judged by phosphatase determinations as well as by symptomatic improvement of the patient. Inoperable progressing breast cancer in appropriately selected men and postmenopausal women (See INDICATIONS)—Suggested dosage is 10 mg three times daily for a period of at least three months.

Treated patients with an intact uterus should be monitored closely for signs of endometrial cancer and appropriate diagnosis measures should be taken to rule out malignancy in the event of persistent or recurring abnormal vaginal bleeding.

HOW SUPPLIED

ESTRATAB® (Esterified Estrogens Tablets, USP): Each blue tablet contains 0.3 mg in bottles of 100 (NDC 0032-1014-01) imprinted "SOLVAY 1014" in black.

Each yellow tablet contains 0.625 mg in bottles of 100 (NDC 0032-1022-01) and 1000 (NDC 0032-1022-10) imprinted "SOLVAY 1022" in black.

Each orange-red tablet contains 1.25 mg in bottles of 100 (NDC 0032-1024-01) and 1000 (NDC 0032-1024-10) imprinted "SOLVAY 1024" in black.

Each light purple tablet contains 2.5 mg in bottles of 100 (NDC 0032-1025-01) imprinted "SOLVAY 1025" in white.

STORAGE: Store and dispense in tight, light-resistant containers as defined in the USP. Store below 30°C (86°F). Protect from moisture.

REFERENCES

1. Ziel, H.K. and W.D. Finkel, "Increased Risk of Endometrial Carcinoma Among Users of Conjugated Estrogens," **New England Journal of Medicine**, 293:1167–1170, 1975.
2. Smith, D.C., R. Prentic, D.J. Thompson, and W.L. Hermann, "Association of Exogenous Estrogen and Endometrial Carcinoma," **New England Journal of Medicine**, 293:1164–1167, 1975.
3. Mack, T.M., M.C. Pike, B.E. Henderson, R.I. Pfeffer, V.R. Gerkins, M. Arthur, and S.E. Brown, "Estrogens, and Endometrial Cancer in a Retirement Community," **New England Journal of Medicine**, 284:1262–1267, 1976.
4. Weiss, N.S., D.R. Szekely and D.F. Austin, "Increasing Incidence of Endometrial Cancer in the United States," **New England Journal of Medicine**, 294:1259–1262, 1976.
5. Herbst, A.L., H. Ulfelder and D.C. Poskanzer, "Adenocarcinoma of Vagina," **New England Journal of Medicine**, 284:878–881, 1971.
6. Greenwald, P., J. Barlow, P. Nasca, and W. Burnett, "Vaginal Cancer after Maternal Treatment with Synthetic Estrogens," **New England Journal of Medicine**, 285:390–392, 1971.
7. Lanier, A., K. Noller, D. Decker, L. Elveback, and L. Kurland, "Cancer and Stilbestrol. A Followup of 1791 Persons Exposed to Estrogens in Utero and Born 1943–1959," **Mayo Clinic Proceedings**, 48:793–799, 1973.
8. Herbst, A., R. Kurman, and R. Scully, "Vaginal and Cervical Abnormalities After Exposure to Stilbestrol in Utero," **Obstetrics and Gynecology**, 40:287–298, 1972.
9. Herbst, A., S. Robboy, G. Macdonald, and R. Scully, "The Effects of Local Progesterone on Stilbestrol-Associated Vaginal Adenosis," **American Journal of Obstetrics and Gynecology**. 118:607–615, 1974.
10. Herbst, A., D. Poskanzer, S. Robboy, L. Friedlander, and R. Scully, "Prenatal Exposure to Stilbestrol, A Prospective Comparison of Exposed Female Offspring with Unexposed Controls," **New England Journal of Medicine**, 292:334–339. 1975
11. Stafl, A., R. Mattingly, D. Foley, and W. Fetherston, "Clinical Diagnosis of Vaginal Adenosis," **Obstetrics and Gynecology**, 43:118–128, 1974.
12. Sherman, A.I., M. Goldrath, A. Berlin, V. Vakhariya, F. Banooni, W. Michaels, P. Goodman, S. Brown, "Cervical-Vaginal Adenosis After In Utero Exposure to Synthetic Estrogens," **Obstetrics and Gynecology**, 44:531–545, 1974.
13. Gal, I., B. Kirman, and J. Stern, "Hormone Pregnancy Tests and Congenital and Malformation," **Nature**, 216:83, 1967.
14. Levy, E.P., A. Cohen, and F.C. Fraser, "Hormone Treatment During Pregnancy and Congenital Heart Defects," **Lancet**, 1:611, 1973.
15. Nora, J., and A. Nora, "Birth Defects and Oral Contraceptives," **Lancet**, 1:941–942, 1973.
16. Janerich, D.T., J.M. Piper, and D.M. Glebatis, "Oral Contraceptives and Congenital Limb-Reduction Defects," **New England Journal of Medicine**, 291:697–700, 1974.
17. "Estrogens for Oral or Parental Use," **Federal Register**, 40:8212, 1975.
18. Boston Collaborative Drug Surveillance Program "Surgically Confirmed Gall Bladder Disease, Venous Thromboembolism and Breast Tumors in Relation to Post-Menopausal Estrogen Therapy," **New England Journal of Medicine**, 290:15–19, 1974.
18a.Hoover, R., L.A. Gray, Sr., P. Cole, and B. MacMahon, "Menopausal Estrogens and Breast Cancer," **New England Journal of Medicine**, 295:401–405, 1976.
19. Boston Collaborative Drug Surveillance Program, "Oral Contraceptives and Venous Thromboembolic Disease, Surgically Confirmed Gall Bladder Disease, and Breast Tumors," **Lancet**, 1:1399–1404, 1973.
20. Daniel, D., G.H. Campbell, and A.C. Turnbull, "Puerperal Thromboembolism and Suppression of Lactation," **Lancet**, 2:287–289, 1967.
21. The Veterans Administration Cooperative Urological Research Group, "Carcinoma of the Prostate: Treatment Comparisons," **Journal of Urology**, 98:516–522, 1967.
22. Ballar, J.C., "Thromboembolism and Oestrogen Therapy," **Lancet**, 2:560, 1967.
23. Blackard, C., R. Doe, G. Mellinger, and D. Byar, "Incidence of Cardiovascular Disease and Death in Patients Receiving Diethyistilbestrol for Carcinoma of the Prostate," **Cancer**, 26:249–256, 1970.
24. Royal College of General Practitioners, "Oral Contraception and Thromboembolic Disease," **Journal of the Royal College of General Practitioners**, 13:267–279, 1967.
25. Inman, W.H.W., and M.P. Veseey, "Investigation of Deaths from Pulmonary, Coronary, and Cerebral Thrombosis, and Embolism in Women of Child-Bearing Age," **British Medical Journal**, 2:193–199, 1968.
26. Vessey, M.P., and R. Doll, "Investigation of Relation Between Use of Oral Contraceptives and Thromboembolic Disease, A Further Report," **British Medical Journal**, 2:651–657, 1969.
27. Sartwell, P.E., A.T. Masi, F.G. Arthes, G.R. Greene, and H.E. Smith, "Thromboembolism and Oral Contraceptives: An Epidemiological Case Control Study," **American Journal of Epidemiology**, 90:365–380, 1969.
28. Collaborative Group for the Study of Stroke in Young Women, "Oral Contraception and Increased Risk of Cerebral Ischemia of Thrombosis," **New England Journal of Medicine**, 288:871–878, 1973.
29. Collaborative Group for the Study of Stroke in Young Women, "Oral Contraceptives and Stroke in Young Women: Associated Risk Factors," **Journal of American Medical Association**, 231:718–722, 1975.
30. Mann, J.I., and W.H.W. Inman, "Oral Contraceptives and Death from Myocardial Infarction," **British Medical Journal, 2:245–248, 1975.**
31. Mann, J.I., M.P. Vessey, M. Thorogood, and R. Doll, "Myocardial Infarction in Young Women with Special Reference to Oral Contraceptive Practice," **British Medical Journal**, 2:241–245, 1975.
32. Inman, W.H.W., V.P. Vessey, B. Westerholm, and A. Engelund, "Thromboembolic Disease and the Steroidal Content of Oral Contraceptives," **British Medical Journal**, 2:203–209, 1970.
33. Stolley, P.D., J.A. Tonascia, M.S. Tockman, P.E. Sartwell, A.H. Rutledge, and M.P. Jacobs, "Thrombosis with Low-Estrogen Oral Contraceptives," **American Journal of Epidemiology**, 102:197–208, 1975.
34. Vessey, M.P., R. Doll, A.S. Fairbairn, and G. Golber, "Post-Operative Thromboembolism and the Use of the Oral Contraceptives," **British Medical Journal**, 3:123–126, 1970.
35. Greene, G.R., and P.E. Sartwell, "Oral Contraceptives Use in Patients with Thromboembolism Following Surgery, Trauma or Infection," **American Journal of Public Health**, 62:680–685, 1972.
36. Rosenberg, L., M.B. Armstrong, and H. Jick, "Myocardial Infarction and Estrogen Therapy in Postmenopausal Women," **New England Journal of Medicine**, 294:1256–1259, 1976.
37. Coronary Drug Project Research Group. The Coronary Drug Project: Initial Findings Leading to Modifications of its Research Protocol, **Journal of the American Medical Association**, 214:1303–1313, 1970.
38. Baum, J., F. Holtz, J.J. Bookstein, and E.W. Klein, "Possible Association between Benign Hepatomas and Oral Contraceptives," **Lancet**, 2:926–928, 1973.
39. Mays, E.T., W.M. Christopherson, M.M. Mahr, and H.C. Williams, "Hepatic Changes in Young Women Ingesting Contraceptive Steroids, Hepatic Hemorrhage and Primary Hepatic Tumors," **Journal of the American Medical Association**, 235:730–782, 1976.
40. Edmondson, H.A., B. Henderson, and B. Benton, "Liver Cell Adenomas Associated with the Use of Oral Contraceptives," **New England Journal of Medicine**, 294:470–472, 1976.
41. Pfeffer, R.I., and S. Van Den Noore, "Estrogen Use and Stroke Risk in Postmenopausal Women," **American Journal of Epidemiolgy**, 103:445–456, 1976.

INFORMATION FOR THE PATIENT

WHAT YOU SHOULD KNOW ABOUT ESTROGENS

Estrogens are female hormones produced by the ovaries. The ovaries make several different kinds of estrogens. In addition, scientists have been able to make a variety of synthetic estrogens. As far as we know, all these estrogens have similar properties and therefore much the same usefulness, side effects, and risks. This leaflet is intended to help you understand what estrogens are used for the risks involved in their use, and how to use them as safely as possible.

This leaflet includes the most important information about estrogens, but not all the information. If you want to know more, you can ask your doctor or pharmacist to let you read the package insert prepared for the doctor.

USES OF ESTROGEN

Estrogens are prescribed by doctors for a number of purposes, including:

1. To provide estrogen during a period of adjustment when a woman's ovaries no longer produce it, in order to prevent certain uncomfortable symptoms of estrogen deficiency. (All women normally stop producing estrogens, generally between the ages of 45 and 55; this is called the menopause).
2. To prevent symptoms of estrogen deficiency when a woman's ovaries have been removed surgically before the natural menopause.
3. To prevent pregnancy. (Estrogens are given along with a progestogen, another female hormone; these combinations are called oral contraceptives or birth controll pills. Patient labeling is available to women taking oral contraceptives and they will not be discussed in this leaflet).
4. To treat certain cancers in women and men.

THERE IS NO PROPER USE OF ESTROGENS IN A PREGNANT WOMAN.

ESTROGEN IN THE MENOPAUSE

In the natural course of their lives, all women eventually experience a decrease in estrogen production. This usually occurs between ages 45 and 55 but may occur earlier or later. Sometimes the ovaries may need to be removed before natural menopause by an operation, producing a "surgical menopause."

When the amount of estrogen in the blood begins to decrease, many women may develop typical symptoms: Feelings of warmth in the face, neck, and chest or sudden intense episodes of heat and sweating throughout the body (called "hot flashes" or "hot flushes"). These symptoms are sometimes very uncomfortable. A few women eventually develop changes in the vagina (called "atrophic vaginitis") which cause discomfort, especially during and after intercourse. Estrogens can be prescribed to treat these symptoms of the menopause. It is estimated that considerably more than half of all women undergoing the menopause have only mild symptoms or no symptoms at all and therefore do not need estrogens. Other women may need estrogens for a few months, while their bodies adjust to lower estrogen levels. Sometimes the need will be for periods longer than six months. In an attempt to avoid overstimulation of the uterus (womb), estrogens are usually given cyclically during each

Continued on next page

Solvay—Cont.

month of use, that is three weeks of pills followed by one week without pills.

Sometimes women experience nervous symptoms or depression during menopause. There is no evidence that estrogens are effective for such symptoms and they should not be used to treat them, although other treatment may be needed. You may have heard that taking estrogens for long periods (years) after the menopause will keep your skin soft and supple and keep you feeling young. There is no evidence that this is so, however, and such long-term treatment carries important risks.

THE DANGERS OF ESTROGENS

1. **Cancer of the uterus.** If estrogens are used in the postmenopausal period for more than a year, there is an increased risk of endometrial cancer (cancer of the uterus). Women taking estrogens have roughly 5 to 10 times as great a chance of getting this cancer as women who take no estrogens. To put this another way, while a postmenopausal woman not taking estrogens has 1 chance in 1,000 each year of getting cancer of the uterus, a woman taking estrogens has 5 to 10 chances in 1,000 each year. For this reason **it is important to take estrogens only when you really need them.**

The risk of this cancer is greater the longer estrogens are used and also seems to be greater when larger doses are taken. For this reason, **it is important to take the lowest dose of estrogen that will control symptoms and to take it only as long as it is needed.** If estrogens are needed for longer periods of time, your doctor will want to reevaluate your need for estrogens at least every six months.

Women using estrogens should report any irregular vaginal bleeding to their doctors; such bleeding may be of no importance, but it can be an early warning of cancer of the uterus. If you have undiagnosed vaginal bleeding, you should not use estrogens until a diagnosis is made and you are certain there is no cancer of the uterus.

2. **Other possible cancers.** Estrogens can cause development of other tumors in animals, such as tumors of the breast, cervix, vagina, or liver, when given for a long time. At present there is no good evidence that women using estrogen in the menopause have an increased risk of such tumors, but there is no way yet to be sure they do not; and one study raises the possibility that use of estrogens in the menopause may increase the risk of breast cancer many years later. This is a further reason to use estrogens only when clearly needed. While you are taking estrogens, it is important that you go to your doctor at least once a year for a physical examination. Also, if members of your family have had breast cancer or if you have had breast nodules or abnormal mammograms (breast x-rays), your doctor may wish to carry out more frequent examinations of your breasts.

3. **Gall bladder disease.** Women who use estrogens after menopause are more likely to develop gall bladder disease needing surgery as women who do not use estrogens. Birth control pills have a similar effect.

4. **Abnormal blood clotting.** Oral contraceptives increase the risk of blood clotting in various parts of the body. This can result in a stroke (if the clot is in the brain), a heart attack (clot in a blood vessel of the heart), or pulmonary embolus (a clot which forms in the legs or pelvis, then breaks off and travels to the lungs). Any of these can be fatal. At this time use of estrogens in the menopause is not known to cause such blood clotting, but this has not been fully studied and there could still prove to be such a risk. It is recommended that if you have had clotting in the legs or lungs or a heart attack or stroke while you were using estrogens or birth control pills, you should not use estrogens (unless they are being used to treat cancer of the breast or prostate). If you have had a stroke or heart attack or if you have angina pectoris, estrogens should be used with great caution and only if clearly needed (for example, if you have severe symptoms of the menopause). The larger doses of estrogen used to prevent swelling of the breasts after pregnancy have been reported to cause clotting in the legs and lungs.

SPECIAL WARNING ABOUT PREGNANCY: You should not receive estrogen if you are pregnant. If this should occur, there is a greater than usual chance that the developing child will be born with a birth defect, although the possibility remains fairly small. A female child may have an increased risk of developing cancer of the vagina or cervix later in life (in the teens or twenties). Every possible effort should be made to avoid exposure to estrogens during pregnancy. If exposure occurs, see your doctor.

OTHER EFFECTS OF ESTROGENS: In addition to the serious known risks of estrogens described above, estrogens have the following side effects and potential risks:

1. **Nausea and vomiting.** The most common side effect of estrogen therapy is nausea. Vomiting is less common.

2. **Effects on breasts.** Estrogens may cause breast tenderness or enlargement and may cause the breasts to secrete a liquid. These effects are not dangerous.

3. **Effects on the uterus.** Estrogens may cause benign fibroid tumors of the uterus to get larger.
Some women will have menstrual bleeding when estrogens are stopped. But if the bleeding occurs on days you are still taking estrogens you should report this to your doctor.

4. **Effect on liver.** Women taking oral contraceptives develop on rare occasions a benign tumor of the liver which can rupture and bleed into the abdomen. So far, these tumors have not been reported in women using estrogens in the menopause, but you should report any swelling or unusual pain or tenderness in the abdomen to your doctor immediately.
Women with a past history of jaundice (yellowing of the skin and white parts of the eyes) may get jaundice again during estrogen use. If this occurs, stop taking estrogens and see your doctor.

5. **Other effects.** Estrogens may cause excess fluid to be retained in the body. This may make some conditions worse, such as epilepsy, migraine, heart disease, or kidney disease.

SUMMARY

Estrogens have important uses, but they have serious risks as well. You must decide, with your doctor, whether the risks are acceptable to you in view of the benefits of treatment. Except where your doctor has prescribed estrogens for use in special cases of cancer of the breast or prostate, you should not use estrogens if you have cancer of the breast or uterus, are pregnant, have undiagnosed abnormal vaginal bleeding, or have had a stroke, heart attack or angina, or clotting in the legs or lungs in the past while you were taking estrogens. You can use estrogens as safely as possible by understanding that your doctor will require regular physical examinations while you are taking them and will try to discontinue the drug as soon as possible and use the smallest dose possible. Be alert for signs of trouble including:

1. Abnormal bleeding from the vagina.
2. Pains in the calves or chest or sudden shortness of breath, or coughing blood (indicating possible clots in the legs, heart, or lungs).
3. Severe headaches, dizziness, faintness, or changes in vision (indicating possible developing clots in the brain or eye).
4. Breast lumps (you should ask your doctor how to examine your own breasts).
5. Jaundice (yellowing of the skin).
6. Mental depression.

Based on his or her assessment of your medical needs, your doctor has prescribed this drug for you. Do not give the drug to anyone else.

HOW SUPPLIED

ESTRATAB® (Esterified Estrogen Tablets, USP)—Tablets for oral administration.
0.3 mg/Tablet (Blue); 0.625 mg/Tablet (Yellow); 1.25 mg/Tablet (Orange-Red); and 2.5 mg/Tablet (Light Purple).

4E Rev. 2/92

SOLVAY PHARMACEUTICALS
MARIETTA, GA 30062
Shown in Product Identification Guide, page 338

ESTRATEST®
[es 'trah-test]
ESTRATEST® H.S.
(Esterified Estrogens and Methyltestosterone) Tablets

℞
℞

WARNING

1. ESTROGENS HAVE BEEN REPORTED TO INCREASE THE RISK OF ENDOMETRIAL CARCINOMA.

Three independent case control studies have reported an increased risk of endometrial cancer in postmenopausal women exposed to exogenous estrogens for prolonged periods.[1-3] This risk was independent of the other known risk factors for endometrial cancer. These studies are further supported by the finding that incidence rates of endometrial cancer have increased sharply since 1969 in eight different areas of the United States with population-based cancer reporting systems, an increase which may be related to the rapidly expanding use of estrogens during the last decade.[4]

The three case control studies reported that the risk of endometrial cancer in estrogen users was about 4.5 to 13.9 times greater than in nonusers. The risk appears to depend on both duration of treatment[1] and on estrogen dose.[3] In view of these findings, when estrogens are used for the treatment of menopausal symptoms, the lowest dose that will control symptoms should be utilized and medication should be discontinued as soon as possible. When prolonged treatment is medically indicated, the patient should be reassessed on at least a semiannual basis to determine the need for continued therapy. Although the evidence must be considered preliminary, one study suggests that cyclic administration of low doses of estrogen may carry less risk than continuous administration;[3] it therefore appears prudent to utilize such a regimen.

Close clinical surveillance of all women taking estrogens is important. In all cases of undiagnosed persistent or recurring abnormal vaginal bleeding, adequate diagnostic measures should be undertaken to rule out malignancy.

There is no evidence at present that "natural" estrogens are more or less hazardous than "synthetic" estrogens at equiestrogenic doses.

2. ESTROGENS SHOULD NOT BE USED DURING PREGNANCY.

The use of female sex hormones, both estrogens and progestogens, during early pregnancy may seriously damage the offspring. It has been shown that females exposed in utero to diethylstilbestrol, a non-steroidal estrogen, have an increased risk of developing in later life a form of vaginal or cervical cancer that is ordinarily extremely rare.[5,6] This risk has been estimated as not greater than 4 per 1000 exposures.[7] Furthermore, a high percentage of such exposed women (from 30 to 90 percent) have been found to have vaginal adenosis,[8-12] epithelial changes of the vagina and cervix. Although these changes are histologically benign, it is not known whether they are precursors of malignancy. Although similar data are not available with the use of other estrogens, it cannot be presumed they would not induce similar changes.

Several reports suggest an association between intrauterine exposure to female sex hormones and congenital anomalies, including congenital heart defects and limb reduction defects.[13-16] One case control study[16] estimated a 4.7 fold increased risk of limb reduction defects in infants exposed in utero to sex hormones (oral contraceptives, hormone withdrawal tests for pregnancy, or attempted treatment for threatened abortion). Some of these exposures were very short and involved only a few days of treatment. The data suggest that the risk of limb reduction defects in exposed fetuses is somewhat less than 1 per 1000.

In the past, female sex hormones have been used during pregnancy in an attempt to treat threatened or habitual abortion. There is considerable evidence that estrogens are ineffective for these indications, and there is no evidence from well controlled studies that progestogens are effective for these uses.

If ESTRATEST® or ESTRATEST® H.S. is used during pregnancy, or if the patient becomes pregnant while taking this drug, she should be apprised of the potential risks to the fetus, and the advisability of pregnancy continuation.

DESCRIPTION

ESTRATEST®: Each dark green, capsule shaped, sugar-coated oral tablet contains: 1.25 mg of Esterified Estrogens, USP and 2.5 mg of Methyltestosterone.
ESTRATEST® H.S. (Half-Strength): Each light green, capsule shaped, sugar-coated oral tablet contains: 0.625 mg of Esterified Estrogens, USP and 1.25 mg of Methyltestosterone.
ESTERIFIED ESTROGENS: Esterified Estrogens, USP is a mixture of the sodium salts of the sulfate esters of the estrogenic substances, principally estrone, that are of the type excreted by pregnant mares. Esterified Estrogens contain not less than 75.0 percent and not more than 85.0 percent of sodium estrone sulfate, and not less than 6.0 percent and not more than 15.0 percent of sodium equilin sulfate, in such proportion that the total of these two components is not less than 90.0 percent.
Category: Estrogens
METHYLTESTOSTERONE: Methyltestosterone is an androgen.
Androgens are derivatives of cyclopentano-perhydrophenanthrene. Endogenous androgens are C-19 steroids with a side chain at C-17, and with two angular methyl groups. Testosterone is the primary endogenous androgen. Fluoxymesterone and methyltestosterone are synthetic derivatives of testosterone.
Methyltestosterone is a white to light yellow crystalline substance that is virtually insoluble in water but soluble in organic solvents. It is stable in air but decomposes in light.

Methyltestosterone structural formula:

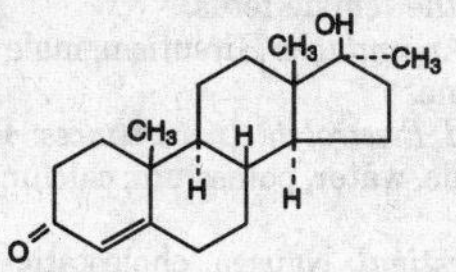

$C_{20}H_{30}O_2$, 302.46
Androst-4-en-3-one, 17-hydroxy-17-methyl-, (17B)-
Category: Androgen.

ESTRATEST® and ESTRATEST® H.S. Tablets contain the following inactive ingredients: acacia, calcium carbonate, citric acid, gelatin, lactose (anhydrous), magnesium stearate, methylparaben, microcrystalline cellulose, pharmaceutical glaze, povidone, propylparaben, sodium benzoate, sodium bicarbonate, sodium carboxymethylcellulose, sorbic acid, sucrose, starch (corn), talc, titanium dioxide, tribasic calcium phosphate, and other minor ingredients.
ESTRATEST® Tablets also contain: FD&C Blue No. 1 Lake, FD&C Yellow No. 6 Lake, and FD&C Yellow No. 10 Lake.
ESTRATEST® H.S. Tablets also contain: FD&C Yellow No. 10 Lake, FD&C Blue No. 1 Lake, and FD&C Blue No. 2 Lake.

CLINICAL PHARMACOLOGY

Estrogens: Estrogens are important in the development and maintenance of the female reproductive system and secondary sex characteristics. They promote growth and development of the vagina, uterus, and fallopian tubes, and enlargement of the breasts. Indirectly, they contribute to the shaping of the skeleton, maintenance of tone and elasticity of urogenital structures, changes in the epiphyses of the long bones that allow for the pubertal growth spurt and its termination, growth of axillary and pubic hair, and pigmentation of the nipples and genitals. Decline of estrogenic activity at the end of the menstrual cycle can bring on menstruation, although the cessation of progesterone secretion is the most important factor in the mature ovulatory cycle. However, in the preovulatory or nonovulatory cycle, estrogen is the primary determinant in the onset of menstruation. Estrogens also affect the release of pituitary gonadotropins.
The pharmacologic effects of esterified estrogens are similar to those of endogenous estrogens. They are soluble in water and are well absorbed from the gastrointestinal tract.
In responsive tissues (female genital organs, breasts, hypothalamus, pituitary) estrogens enter the cell and are transported into the nucleus. As a result of estrogen action, specific RNA and protein synthesis occurs.

Estrogen Pharmacokinetics
Metabolism and inactivation occur primarily in the liver. Some estrogens are excreted into the bile; however they are reabsorbed from the intestine and returned to the liver through the portal venous system. Water soluble esterified estrogens are strongly acidic and are ionized in body fluids, which favor excretion through the kidneys since tubular reabsorption is minimal.

Androgens Endogenous androgens are responsible for the normal growth and development of the male sex organs and for maintenance of secondary sex characteristics. These effects include the growth and maturation of prostate, seminal vesicles, penis, and scrotum; the development of male hair distribution, such as beard, pubic, chest, and axillary hair, laryngeal enlargement, vocal cord thickening, alterations in body musculature, and fat distribution. Drugs in this class also cause retention of nitrogen, sodium, potassium, phosphorus, and decreased urinary excretion of calcium. Androgens have been reported to increase protein anabolism and decrease protein catabolism. Nitrogen balance is improved only when there is sufficient intake of calories and protein. Androgens are responsible for the growth spurt of adolescence and for the eventual termination of linear growth which is brought about by fusion of the epiphyseal growth centers. In children, exogenous androgens accelerate linear growth rates, but may cause a disproportionate advancement in bone maturation. Use over long periods may result in fusion of the epiphyseal growth centers and termination of growth process. Androgens have been reported to stimulate the production of red blood cells by enhancing the production of erythropoietic stimulating factor.

Androgen Pharmacokinetics
Testosterone given orally is metabolized by the gut and 44 percent is cleared by the liver in the first pass. Oral doses as high as 400 mg per day are needed to achieve clinically effective blood levels for full replacement therapy. The synthetic androgens (methyltestosterone and fluoxymesterone) are less extensively metabolized by the liver and have longer half-lives. They are more suitable than testosterone for oral administration.
Testosterone in plasma is 98 percent bound to a specific testosterone-estradiol binding globulin, and about 2 percent is free. Generally, the amount of this sex-hormone binding globulin in the plasma will determine the distribution of testosterone between free and bound forms, and the free testosterone concentration will determine its half-life.
About 90 percent of a dose of testosterone is excreted in the urine as glucuronic and sulfuric acid conjugates of testosterone and its metabolites; about 6 percent of a dose is excreted in the feces, mostly in the unconjugated form. Inactivation of testosterone occurs primarily in the liver. Testosterone is metabolized to various 17-keto steroids through two different pathways. There are considerable variations of the half-life of testosterone as reported in the literature, ranging from 10 to 100 minutes.
In many tissues the activity of testosterone appears to depend on reduction to dihydrotestosterone, which binds to cytosol receptor proteins. The steroid-receptor complex is transported to the nucleus where it initiates transcription events and cellular changes related to androgen action.

INDICATIONS AND USAGE

ESTRATEST® and ESTRATEST® H.S. are indicated in the treatment of:
Moderate to severe *vasomotor* symptoms associated with the menopause in those patients not improved by estrogens alone. (There is no evidence that estrogens are effective for nervous symptoms or depression without associated vasomotor symptoms, and they should not be used to treat such conditions.)
ESTRATEST® AND ESTRATEST® H.S. HAVE NOT BEEN SHOWN TO BE EFFECTIVE FOR ANY PURPOSE DURING PREGNANCY AND ITS USE MAY CAUSE SEVERE HARM TO THE FETUS (SEE BOXED WARNING).

CONTRAINDICATIONS

Estrogens should not be used in women with any of the following conditions:
1. Known or suspected cancer of the breast except in appropriately selected patients being treated for metastatic disease.
2. Known or suspected estrogen-dependent neoplasia.
3. Known or suspected pregnancy (See Boxed Warning).
4. Undiagnosed abnormal genital bleeding.
5. Active thrombophlebitis or thromboembolic disorders.
6. A past history of thrombophlebitis, thrombosis, or thromboembolic disorders associated with previous estrogen use (except when used in treatment of breast malignancy).

Methyltestosterone should not be used in:
1. The presence of severe liver damage.
2. Pregnancy and in breast-feeding mothers because of the possibility of masculinization of the female fetus or breast-fed infant.

WARNINGS

Associated with Estrogens:
1. **Induction of malignant neoplasms.** Long term continuous administration of natural and synthetic estrogens in certain animal species increases the frequency of carcinomas of the breast, cervix, vagina, and liver. There is now evidence that estrogens increase the risk of carcinoma of the endometrium in humans (See Boxed Warning).
   At the present time there is no satisfactory evidence that estrogens given to postmenopausal women increase the risk of cancer of the breast,[18] although a recent long-term follow-up of a single physician's practice has raised this possibility.[18a] Because of the animal data, there is a need for caution in prescribing estrogens for women with a strong family history of breast cancer or who have breast nodules, fibrocystic disease, or abnormal mammograms.
2. **Gallbladder disease.** A recent study has reported a 2 to 3-fold increase in the risk of surgically confirmed gallbladder disease in women receiving postmenopausal estrogens,[18] similar to the 2-fold increase previously noted in users of oral contraceptives.[19–24a] In the case of oral contraceptives the increased risk appeared after two years of use.[24]
3. **Effects similar to those caused by estrogen-progestogen oral contraceptives.** There are several serious adverse effects of oral contraceptives, most of which have not, up to now, been documented as consequences of postmenopausal estrogen therapy. This may reflect the comparatively low doses of estrogen used in postmenopausal women. It would be expected that the larger doses of estrogen used to treat prostatic or breast cancer or postpartum breast engorgement are more likely to result in these adverse effects, and, in fact, it has been shown that there is an increased risk of thrombosis in men receiving estrogens for prostatic cancer and women for postpartum breast engorgement.[20–23]
   a. **Thromboembolic disease.** It is now well established that users of oral contraceptives have an increased risk of various thromboembolic and thrombotic vascular diseases, such as thrombophlebitis, pulmonary embolism, stroke, and myocardial infarction.[24–31] Cases of retinal thrombosis, mesenteric thrombosis, and optic neuritis have been reported in oral contraceptive users. There is evidence that the risk of several of these adverse reactions is related to the dose of the drug.[32,33] An increased risk of postsurgery thromboembolic complications has also been reported in users of oral contraceptives.[34,35] If feasible, estrogen should be discontinued at least 4 weeks before surgery of the type associated with an increased risk of thromboembolism, or during periods of prolonged immobilization.
   While an increased rate of thromboembolic and thrombotic disease in postmenopausal users of estrogens has not been found,[18–36] this does not rule out the possibility that such an increase may be present or that subgroups of women who have underlying risk factors or who are receiving relatively large doses of estrogens may have increased risk. Therefore estrogens should not be used in persons with active thrombophlebitis or thromboembolic disorders, and they should not be used (except in treatment of malignancy) in persons with a history of such disorders in association with estrogen use. They should be used with caution in patients with cerebral vascular or coronary artery disease and only for those in whom estrogens are clearly needed.
   Large doses of estrogen (5 mg esterified estrogens per day), comparable to those used to treat cancer of the prostate and breast, have been shown in a large prospective clinical trial in men[37] to increase the risk of nonfatal myocardial infarction, pulmonary embolism and thrombophlebitis. When estrogen doses of this size are used, any of the thromboembolic and thrombotic adverse effects associated with oral contraceptive use should be considered a clear risk.
   b. **Hepatic adenoma.** Benign hepatic adenomas appear to be associated with the use of oral contraceptives.[38–40] Although benign and rare, these may rupture and may cause death through intra-abdominal hemorrhage. Such lesions have not yet been reported in association with other estrogen or progestogen preparations but should be considered in estrogen users having abdominal pain and tenderness, abdominal mass, or hypovolemic shock. Hepatocellular carcinoma has also been reported in women taking estrogen-containing oral contraceptives.[39] The relationship of this malignancy to these drugs is not known at this time.
   c. **Elevated blood pressure.** Increased blood pressure is not uncommon in women using oral contraceptives. There is now a report that this may occur with use of estrogens in the menopause[41] and blood pressure should be monitored with estrogen use, especially if high doses are used.
   d. **Glucose tolerance.** A worsening of glucose tolerance has been observed in a significant percentage of patients on estrogen-containing oral contraceptives. For this reason, diabetic patients should be carefully observed while receiving estrogens.
4. **Hypercalcemia.** Administration of estrogens may lead to severe hypercalcemia in patients with breast cancer and bone metastases. If this occurs, the drug should be stopped and appropriate measures taken to reduce the serum calcium level.

Associated with Methyltestosterone
In patients with breast cancer, androgen therapy may cause hypercalcemia by stimulating osteolysis. In this case, the drug should be discontinued.
Prolonged use of high doses of androgens has been associated with the development of peliosis hepatis and hepatic neoplasms including hepatocellular carcinoma. (See PRECAUTIONS—*Carcinogenesis*). Peliosis hepatis can be a life-threatening or fatal complication.
Cholestatic hepatitis and jaundice occur with 17-alpha-alkylandrogens at a relatively low dose. If cholestatic hepatitis with jaundice appears or if liver function tests become abnormal, the androgen should be discontinued and the etiology should be determined. Drug-induced jaundice is reversible when the medication is discontinued.
Edema with or without heart failure may be a serious complication in patients with preexisting cardiac, renal, or hepatic disease. In addition to discontinuation of the drug, diuretic therapy may be required.

PRECAUTIONS

Associated with Estrogens
A. General Precautions.
1. A complete medical and family history should be taken prior to the initiation of any estrogen therapy. The pretreatment and periodic physical examinations should include special reference to blood pressure, breasts, abdomen, and pelvic organs, and should include a Papanicolaou smear. As a general rule, estrogen should not be prescribed for longer than one year without another physical examination being performed.
2. Fluid retention—Because estrogens may cause some degree of fluid retention, conditions which might be influenced by this factor such as asthma, epilepsy, migraine, and cardiac or renal dysfunction, require careful observation.
3. Certain patients may develop undesirable manifestations of excessive estrogenic stimulation, such as abnormal or excessive uterine bleeding, mastodynia, etc.
4. Oral contraceptives appear to be associated with an increased incidence of mental depression.[24] Although it is

Continued on next page

Solvay—Cont.

not clear whether this is due to the estrogenic or progestogenic component of the contraceptive, patients with a history of depression should be carefully observed.

5. Preexisting uterine leiomyomata may increase in size during estrogen use.

6. The pathologist should be advised of estrogen therapy when relevant specimens are submitted.

7. Patients with a past history of jaundice during pregnancy have an increased risk of recurrence of jaundice while receiving estrogen-containing oral contraceptive therapy. If jaundice develops in any patient receiving estrogen, the medication should be discontinued while the cause is investigated.

8. Estrogens may be poorly metabolized in patients with impaired liver function and they should be administered with caution in such patients.

9. Because estrogens influence the metabolism of calcium and phosphorus, they should be used with caution in patients with metabolic bone diseases that are associated with hypercalcemia or in patients with renal insufficiency.

10. Because of the effects of estrogens on epiphyseal closure, they should be used judiciously in young patients in whom bone growth is not complete.

11. Certain endocrine and liver function tests may be affected by estrogen-containing oral contraceptives. The following similar changes may be expected with larger doses of estrogen:

a. Increased sulfobromophthalein retention.

b. Increased prothrombin and factors VII, VIII, IX and X; decreased antithrombin 3; increased norepinephrine-induced platelet aggregability.

c. Increased thyroid binding globulin (TBG) leading to increased circulating total thyroid hormone, as measured by PBI, T_4 by column, or T_4 by radioimmunoassay. Free T_3 resin uptake is decreased, reflecting the elevated TBG; free T_4 concentration is unaltered.

d. Impaired glucose tolerance.

e. Decreased pregnanediol excretion.

f. Reduced response to metyrapone test.

g. Reduced serum folate concentration.

h. Increased serum triglyceride and phospholipid concentration.

B. Information for the Patient. See text of Patient Package Insert which appears after the REFERENCES.

C. Pregnancy Category X. See CONTRAINDICATIONS and Boxed WARNING.

D. Nursing Mothers. As a general principle, the administration of any drug to nursing mothers should be done only when clearly necessary since many drugs are excreted in human milk.

Associated with Methyltestosterone:

A. General Precautions

1. Women should be observed for signs of virilization (deepening of the voice, hirsutism, acne, clitoromegaly, and menstrual irregularities). Discontinuation of drug therapy at the time of evidence of mild virilism is necessary to prevent irreversible virilization. Such virilization is usual following androgen use at high doses.

2. Prolonged dosage of androgen may result in sodium and fluid retention. This may present a problem, especially in patients with compromised cardiac reserve or renal disease.

3. Hypersensitivity may occur rarely.

4. PBI may be decreased in patients taking androgens.

5. Hypercalcemia may occur. If this does occur, the drug should be discontinued.

B. Information for the Patient

The physician should instruct patients to report any of the following side effects of androgens:

Women: Hoarseness, acne, changes in menstrual periods, or more hair on the face.

All Patients: Any nausea, vomiting, changes in skin color or ankle swelling.

C. Laboratory tests

1. Women with disseminated breast carcinoma should have frequent determination of urine and serum calcium levels during the course of androgen therapy (See WARNINGS).

2. Because of the hepatotoxicity associated with the use of 17-alpha-alkylated androgens, liver function tests should be obtained periodically.

3. Hemoglobin and hematocrit should be checked periodically for polycythemia in patients who are receiving high doses of androgens.

D. Drug Interactions

1. *Anticoagulants* C-17 substituted derivatives of testosterone, such as methandrostenolone, have been reported to decrease the anticoagulant requirements of patients receiving oral anticoagulants. Patients receiving oral anticoagulant therapy require close monitoring, especially when androgens are started or stopped.

2. *Oxyphenbutazone.* Concurrent administration of oxyphenbutazone and androgens may result in elevated serum levels of oxyphenbutazone.

3. *Insulin.* In diabetic patients the metabolic effects of androgens may decrease blood glucose and insulin requirements.

E. Drug/Laboratory Test Interferences

Androgens may decrease levels of thyroxine-binding globulin, resulting in decreased T_4 serum levels and increased resin uptake of T_3 and T_4. Free thyroid hormone levels remain unchanged, however, and there is no clinical evidence of thyroid dysfunction.

F. Carcinogenesis

Animal Data. Testosterone has been tested by subcutaneous injection and implantation in mice and rats. The implant induced cervical-uterine tumors in mice, which metastasized in some cases. There is suggestive evidence that injection of testosterone into some strains of female mice increases their susceptibility to hepatoma. Testosterone is also known to increase the number of tumors and decrease the degree of differentiation of chemically induced carcinomas of the liver in rats.

Human Data. There are rare reports of hepatocellular carcinoma in patients receiving long-term therapy with androgens in high doses. Withdrawal of the drugs did not lead to regression of the tumors in all cases.

Geriatric patients treated with androgens may be at an increased risk for the development of prostatic hypertrophy and prostatic carcinoma.

G. Pregnancy

Teratogenic Effects. Pregnancy Category X (see CONTRAINDICATIONS).

H. Nursing Mothers

It is not known whether androgens are excreted in human milk. Because many drugs are excreted in human milk and because of the potential for serious adverse reactions in nursing infants from androgens, a decision should be made whether to discontinue nursing or to discontinue the drug, taking into account the importance of the drug to the mother.

ADVERSE REACTIONS

Associated with Estrogens (See Warnings regarding induction of neoplasia, adverse effects on the fetus, increased incidence of gallbladder disease, and adverse effects similar to those of oral contraceptives, including thromboembolism). The following additional adverse reactions have been reported with estrogenic therapy, including oral contraceptives:

1. Genitourinary system.

Breakthrough bleeding, spotting, change in menstrual flow.

Dysmenorrhea.

Premenstrual-like syndrome.

Amenorrhea during and after treatment.

Increase in size of uterine fibromyomata.

Vaginal candidiasis.

Change in cervical erosion and in degree of cervical secretion.

Cystitis-like syndrome.

2. Breasts.

Tenderness, enlargement, secretion.

3. Gastrointestinal.

Nausea, vomiting.

Abdominal cramps, bloating.

Cholestatic jaundice.

4. Skin.

Chloasma or melasma which may persist when drug is discontinued.

Erythema multiforme.

Erythema nodosum.

Hemorrhagic eruption.

Loss of scalp hair.

Hirsutism.

5. Eyes.

Steepening of corneal curvature.

Intolerance to contact lenses.

6. CNS.

Headache, migraine, dizziness.

Mental depression.

Chorea.

7. Miscellaneous.

Increase or decrease in weight.

Reduced carbohydrate tolerance.

Aggravation of porphyria.

Edema.

Changes in libido.

Associated with Methyltestosterone

A. Endocrine and Urogenital

1. *Female:* The most common side effects of androgen therapy are amenorrhea and other menstrual irregularities, inhibition of gonadotropin secretion, and virilization, including deepening of the voice and clitoral enlargement. The latter usually is not reversible after androgens are discontinued. When administered to a preg-

nant woman androgens cause virilization of external genitalia of the female fetus.

2. *Skin and Appendages:* Hirsutism, male pattern of baldness, and acne.

3. *Fluid and Electrolyte Disturbances:* Retention of sodium, chloride, water, potassium, calcium, and inorganic phosphates.

4. *Gastrointestinal:* Nausea, cholestatic jaundice, alterations in liver function test, rarely hepatocellular neoplasms, and peliosis hepatis (see WARNINGS).

5. *Hematologic:* Suppression of clotting factors II, V, VII, and X, bleeding in patients on concomitant anticoagulant therapy, and polycythemia.

6. *Nervous System:* Increased or decreased libido, headache, anxiety, depression, and generalized paresthesia.

7. *Metabolic:* Increased serum cholesterol.

8. *Miscellaneous:* Inflammation and pain at the site of intramuscular injection or subcutaneous implantation of testosterone containing pellets, stomatitis with buccal preparations, and rarely anaphylactoid reactions.

OVERDOSAGE

Numerous reports of ingestion of large doses of estrogen-containing oral contraceptives by young children indicate that serious ill effects do not occur. Overdosage of estrogen may cause nausea, and withdrawal bleeding may occur in females.

There have been no reports of acute overdosage with the androgens.

DOSAGE AND ADMINISTRATION

1. *Given cyclically for short-term use only:*

For treatment of moderate to severe *vasomotor* symptoms associated with the menopause in patients not improved by estrogen alone.

The lowest dose that will control symptoms should be chosen and medication should be discontinued as promptly as possible.

Administration should be cyclic (e.g., three weeks on and one week off).

Attempts to discontinue or taper medication should be made at three to six month intervals.

Usual Dosage Range: 1 tablet of ESTRATEST or 1 to 2 tablets of ESTRATEST H.S. daily as recommended by the physician.

Treated patients with an intact uterus should be monitored closely for signs of endometrial cancer and appropriate diagnostic measures should be taken to rule out malignancy in the event of persistent or recurring abnormal vaginal bleeding.

HOW SUPPLIED

ESTRATEST® (Imprinted "SOLVAY 1026") in bottles of 100—NDC 0032-1026-01 and 1000—NDC 0032-1026-10.

ESTRATEST® (Dark green, capsule shaped, sugar-coated oral tablets) contains: 1.25 mg of Esterified Estrogens, USP and 2.5 mg of Methyltestosterone, USP.

ESTRATEST® H.S. (Imprinted "SOLVAY 1023") in bottles of 100—NDC 0032-1023-01.

ESTRATEST® H.S. "Half-Strength" (Light green, capsule shaped, sugar-coated oral tablets) contains: 0.625 mg of Esterified Estrogens, USP and 1.25 mg of Methyltestosterone, USP.

Store at controlled room temperature, 15°–30°C (59°–86°F).

REFERENCES

1. Ziel, H.K., *et al.:* N. Engl. J. Med. *293* :1167–1170, 1975.
2. Smith, D.C., *et al.:* N. Engl. J. Med. *293* :1164–1167, 1975.
3. Mack, T.M., *et al.:* N. Engl. J. Med. *294* :1262–1267, 1976.
4. Weiss, N.S., *et al.:* N. Engl. J. Med. *294* :1259–1262, 1976.
5. Herbst, A.L., *et al.:* N. Engl. J. Med. *284* :878–881, 1971.
6. Greenwald, P., *et al.:* N. Engl. J. Med. *285* :390–392, 1971.
7. Lanier, A., *et al.:* Mayo Clin. Proc. *48* :793–799, 1973.
8. Herbst, A., *et al.:* Obstet. Gynecol. *40* :287–298, 1972.
9. Herbst, A., *et al.:* Am. J. Obstet. Gynecol. *118* :607–615, 1974.
10. Herbst, A., *et al.:* N. Engl. J. Med. *292* :334–339, 1975.
11. Stafl, A., *et al.:* Obstet. Gynecol. *43* –128, 1974.
12. Sherman, A.I., *et al.:* Obstet. Gynecol. *44* :531–545, 1974.
13. Gal, I., *et al.:* Nature *216* :83, 1967.
14. Levy, E.P., *et al.:* Lancet *1* :611, 1973.
15. Nora, J., *et al.:* Lancet *1* :941–942, 1973.
16. Janerich, D.T., *et al.:* N. Engl. J. Med. *291* :697–700, 1974.
17. Estrogens for Oral or Parenteral Use: Federal Register *40* :8212, 1975.
18. Boston Collaborative Drug Surveillance Program: N. Engl. J. Med. *290* :15–19, 1974.
18a. Hoover, R., *et al.:* N. Engl. J. Med. *295* :401–405, 1976.
19. Boston Collaborative Drug Surveillance Program: Lancet *1* :1399–1404, 1973.
20. Daniel, D.G., *et al.:* Lancet *2* :287–289, 1967.
21. The Veterans Administration Cooperative Urological Research Group: J. Urol. *98* :516–522, 1967.
22. Bailar, J. C.: Lancet *2* :560, 1967.
23. Blackard, C., *et al.:* Cancer *26* :249–256, 1970.
24. Royal College of General Practitioners: J.R. Coll, Gen. Pract. *13* :267–279, 1967.

25. Inman, W.H.W., *et al.:* Br. Med. J. *2*:193–199, 1968.
26. Vessey, M.P., *et al.:* Br. Med. J. *2*:651–657, 1969.
27. Sartwell, P.E., *et al.:* Am. J. Epidemiol, *90*:365–380, 1969.
28. Collaborative Group for the Study of Stroke in Young Women: N. Engl. J. Med. *288*:871–878, 1973.
29. Collaborative Group for the Study of Stroke in Young Women: J.A.M.A. *231*:718–722, 1975.
30. Mann, J.I., *et al.:* Br. Med. J. *2*:245–248, 1975.
31. Mann, J.I., *et al.:* Br. Med. J. *2*:241–245, 1975.
32. Inman, W.H.W., *et al.:* Br. Med. J. *2*:203–209, 1970.
33. Stolley, P.D., *et al.:* Am. J. Epidemiol, *102*:197–208, 1975.
34. Vessey, M.P., *et al.:* Br. Med. J. *3*:123–126, 1970.
35. Greene, G.R., *et al.:* Am. J. Public Health *62*:680–685, 1972.
36. Rosenberg, L., *et al.:* N. Engl. J. Med. *294*:1256–1259, 1976.
37. Coronary Drug Project Research Group: J.A.M.A. *214*:1303–1313, 1970.
38. Baum, J., *et al.:* Lancet *2*:926–928, 1973.
39. Mays, E.T., *et al.:* J.A.M.A. *235*:730–732, 1976.
40. Edmondson, H.A., *et al.:* N. Engl. J. Med. *294*:470–472, 1976.
41. Pfeffer, R.I., *et al.:* Am. J. Epidemiol, *103*:445–456, 1976.

INFORMATION FOR THE PATIENT:

WHAT YOU SHOULD KNOW ABOUT ESTROGENS: Estrogens are female hormones produced by the ovaries. The ovaries make several different kinds of estrogens. In addition, scientists have been able to make a variety of synthetic estrogens. As far as we know, all these estrogens have similar properties and therefore much the same usefulness, side effects, and risks. This leaflet is intended to help you understand what estrogens are used for, the risks involved in their use, and how to use them as safely as possible.

This leaflet includes the most important information about estrogens, but not all the information. If you want to know more, you can ask your doctor or pharmacist to let you read the package insert prepared for the doctor.

USES OF ESTROGEN:

Estrogens are prescribed by doctors for a number of purposes, including:

1. To provide estrogen during a period of adjustment when a woman's ovaries no longer produce it, in order to prevent certain uncomfortable symptoms of estrogen deficiency. (All women normally stop producing estrogens, generally between the ages of 45 and 55; this is called the menopause).
2. To prevent symptoms of estrogen deficiency when a woman's ovaries have been removed surgically before the natural menopause.
3. To prevent pregnancy. (Estrogens are given along with a progestogen, another female hormone; these combinations are called oral contraceptives or birth controll pills. Patient labeling is available to women taking oral contraceptives and they will not be discussed in this leaflet).
4. To treat certain cancers in women and men.

THERE IS NO PROPER USE OF ESTROGENS IN A PREGNANT WOMAN.

ESTROGENS IN THE MENOPAUSE: In the natural course of their lives, all women eventually experience a decrease in estrogen production. This usually occurs between ages 45 and 55 but may occur earlier or later. Sometimes the ovaries may need to be removed before natural menopause by an operation, producing a "surgical menopause."

When the amount of estrogen in the blood begins to decrease, many women may develop typical symptoms: Feelings of warmth in the face, neck, and chest or sudden intense episodes of heat and sweating throughout the body (called "hot flashes" or "hot flushes"). These symptoms are sometimes very uncomfortable. A few women eventually develop changes in the vagina (called "atrophic vaginitis") which cause discomfort, especially during and after intercourse.

Estrogens can be prescribed to treat these symptoms of the menopause. It is estimated that considerably more than half of all women undergoing the menopause have only mild symptoms or no symptoms at all and therefore do not need estrogens. Other women may need estrogens for a few months, while their bodies adjust to lower estrogen levels. Sometimes the need will be for periods longer than six months. In an attempt to avoid overstimulation of the uterus (womb), estrogens are usually given cyclically during each month of use, that is three weeks of pills followed by one week without pills.

Sometimes women experience nervous symptoms or depression during menopause. There is no evidence that estrogens are effective for such symptoms and they should not be used to treat them, although other treatment may be needed.

You may have heard that taking estrogens for long periods (years) after the menopause will keep your skin soft and supple and keep you feeling young. There is no evidence that this is so, however, and such long-term treatment carries important risks.

THE DANGERS OF ESTROGENS:

1. **Cancer of the uterus.** If estrogens are used in the postmenopausal period for more than a year, there is an increased risk of **endometrial cancer** (cancer of the uterus). Women taking estrogens have roughly 5 to 10 times as great a chance of getting this cancer as women who take no estrogens. To put this another way, while a postmenopausal woman not taking estrogens has 1 chance in 1,000 each year of getting cancer of the uterus, a woman taking estrogens has 5 to 10 chances in 1,000 each year. For this reason **it is important to take estrogens only when you really need them.**

   The risk of this cancer is greater the longer estrogens are used and also seems to be greater when larger doses are taken. For this reason, **it is important to take the lowest dose of estrogen that will control symptoms and to take it only as long as it is needed.** If estrogens are needed for longer periods of time, your doctor will want to reevaluate your need for estrogens at least every six months.

   Women using estrogens should report any irregular vaginal bleeding to their doctors; such bleeding may be of no importance, but it can be an early warning of cancer of the uterus. If you have undiagnosed vaginal bleeding, you should not use estrogens until a diagnosis is made and you are certain there is no cancer of the uterus.
2. **Other possible cancers.** Estrogens can cause development of other tumors in animals, such as tumors of the breast, cervix, vagina, or liver, when given for a long time. At present there is no good evidence that women using estrogen in the menopause have an increased risk of such tumors, but there is no way yet to be sure they do not; and one study raises the possibility that use of estrogens in the menopause may increase the risk of breast cancer many years later. This is a further reason to use estrogens only when clearly needed. While you are taking estrogens, it is important that you go to your doctor at least once a year for a physical examination. Also, if members of your family have had breast cancer or if you have had breast nodules or abnormal mammograms (breast x-rays), your doctor may wish to carry out more frequent examinations of your breasts.
3. **Gallbladder disease.** Women who use estrogens after menopause are more likely to develop gallbladder disease needing surgery as women who do not use estrogens. Birth control pills have a similar effect.
4. **Abnormal blood clotting.** Oral contraceptives increase the risk of blood clotting in various parts of the body. This can result in a stroke (if the clot is in the brain), a heart attack (clot in a blood vessel of the heart), or pulmonary embolus (a clot which forms in the legs or pelvis, then breaks off and travels to the lungs). Any of these can be fatal.

   At this time use of estrogens in the menopause is not known to cause such blood clotting, but this has not been fully studied and there could still prove to be such a risk. It is recommended that if you have had clotting in the legs or lungs or a heart attack or stroke while you were using estrogens or birth control pills, you should not use estrogens (unless they are being used to treat cancer of the breast or prostate). If you have had a stroke or heart attack or if you have angina pectoris, estrogens should be used with great caution and only if clearly needed (for example, if you have severe symptoms of the menopause).

   The larger doses of estrogen used to prevent swelling of the breasts after pregnancy have been reported to cause clotting in the legs and lungs.

SPECIAL WARNING ABOUT PREGNANCY: You should not receive estrogen if you are pregnant. If this should occur, there is a greater than usual chance that the developing child will be born with a birth defect, although the possibility remains fairly small. A female child may have an increased risk of developing cancer of the vagina or cervix later in life (in the teens or twenties). Every possible effort should be made to avoid exposure to estrogens during pregnancy. If exposure occurs, see your doctor.

OTHER EFFECTS OF ESTROGENS: In addition to the serious known risks of estrogens described above, estrogens have the following side effects and potential risks:

1. **Nausea and vomiting.** The most common side effect of estrogen therapy is nausea. Vomiting is less common.
2. **Effects on breasts.** Estrogens may cause breast tenderness or enlargement and may cause the breasts to secrete a liquid. These effects are not dangerous.
3. **Effects on the uterus.** Estrogens may cause benign fibroid tumors of the uterus to get larger.

   Some women will have menstrual bleeding when estrogens are stopped. But if the bleeding occurs on days you are still taking estrogens you should report this to your doctor.
4. **Effect on liver.** Women taking oral contraceptives develop on rare occasions a benign tumor of the liver which can rupture and bleed into the abdomen. So far, these tumors have not been reported in women using estrogens in the menopause, but you should report any swelling or unusual pain or tenderness in the abdomen to your doctor immediately.

   Women with a past history of jaundice (yellowing of the skin and white parts of the eyes) may get jaundice again during estrogen use. If this occurs, stop taking estrogens and see your doctor.
5. **Other effects.** Estrogens may cause excess fluid to be retained in the body. This may make some conditions worse, such as epilepsy, migraine, heart disease, or kidney disease.

SUMMARY: Estrogens have important uses, but they have serious risks as well. You must decide, with your doctor, whether the risks are acceptable to you in view of the benefits of treatment. Except where your doctor has prescribed estrogens for use in special cases of cancer of the breast or prostate, you should not use estrogens if you have cancer of the breast or uterus, are pregnant, have undiagnosed abnormal vaginal bleeding, or have had a stroke, heart attack or angina, or clotting in the legs or lungs in the past while you were taking estrogens.

You can use estrogens as safely as possible by understanding that your doctor will require regular physical examinations while you are taking them and will try to discontinue the drug as soon as possible and use the smallest dose possible. Be alert for signs of trouble including:

1. Abnormal bleeding from the vagina.
2. Pains in the calves or chest or sudden shortness of breath, or coughing blood (indicating possible clots in the legs, heart, or lungs).
3. Severe headaches, dizziness, faintness, or changes in vision (indicating possible developing clots in the brain or eye).
4. Breast lumps (you should ask your doctor how to examine your own breasts).
5. Jaundice (yellowing of the skin).
6. Mental depression.

Based on his or her assessment of your medical needs, your doctor has prescribed this drug for you. Do not give the drug to anyone else.

HOW SUPPLIED

ESTRATEST® H.S. a combination of Esterified Estrogens and Methyltestosterone. Each capsule-shaped Light Green sugar coated Tablet contains: 0.625 mg of Esterified Estrogens, USP and 1.25 mg of Methyltestosterone, USP.

ESTRATEST® a combination of Esterified Estrogens and Methyltestosterone. Each capsule-shaped Dark Green Sugar Coated Tablet contains: 1.25 mg of Esterified Estrogens, USP and 2.5 mg of Methyltestosterone, USP.

SOLVAY PHARMACEUTICALS, INC.
Marietta, GA 30062 4E 0978 Rev 7/94

Shown in Product Identification Guide, page 338

LITHOBID® ℞
(Lithium Carbonate, USP)
Slow-Release Tablets
300 mg

LITHONATE® ℞
(Lithium Carbonate
Capsules, USP)
300 mg

LITHOTABS™ ℞
(Lithium Carbonate
Tablets, USP)
300 mg

> **WARNING**
> Lithium toxicity is closely related to serum lithium levels, and can occur at doses close to therapeutic levels. Facilities for prompt and accurate serum lithium determinations should be available before initiating therapy (see DOSAGE AND ADMINISTRATION).

DESCRIPTION

LITHOBID® Tablets, LITHONATE® Capsules and LITHOTABS™ Tablets contain lithium carbonate, a white, odorless alkaline powder with molecular formula Li_2CO_3 and molecular weight 73.89. Lithium is an element of the alkali-metal group with atomic number 3, atomic weight 6.94 and an emission line at 671 nm on the flame photometer.

LITHOBID® Slow-Release Tablets: Each peach-colored, film-coated, slow-release tablet contains 300 mg of lithium carbonate. This slowly dissolving, film-coated tablet is designed to give lower serum lithium peak concentrations than obtained with conventional oral lithium dosage forms. Inactive ingredients consist of calcium stearate, carnauba wax, cellulose compounds, FD&C Blue No. 2 Aluminum Lake, FD&C Red No. 40 Aluminum Lake, FD&C Yellow No. 6 Aluminum Lake, povidone, propylene glycol, sodium chloride, sodium lauryl sulfate, sodium starch glycolate, sorbitol and titanium dioxide.

Continued on next page

Solvay—Cont.

LITHONATE® Capsules: Each peach-colored capsule contains 300 mg of lithium carbonate. Inactive ingredients consist of FD&C Red No. 40, gelatin, polyethylene glycol, talc and titanium dioxide. Capsule imprinting ink contains red ferric oxide.

LITHOTABS™ Tablets: Each scored, white, film-coated tablet contains 300 mg of lithium carbonate. Inactive ingredients consist of calcium stearate, carnauba wax, cellulose, povidone, propylene glycol, sodium lauryl sulfate and sodium starch glycolate.

ACTIONS
Preclinical studies have shown that lithium alters sodium transport in nerve and muscle cells and effects a shift toward intraneuronal metabolism of catecholamines, but the specific biochemical mechanism of lithium action in mania is unknown.

INDICATIONS
Lithium is indicated in the treatment of manic episodes of manic-depressive illness. Maintenance therapy prevents or diminishes the intensity of subsequent episodes in those manic-depressive patients with a history of mania.

Typical symptoms: of mania include pressure of speech, motor hyperactivity, reduced need for sleep, flight of ideas, grandiosity, elation, poor judgment, aggressiveness, and possibly hostility. When given to a patient experiencing a manic episode, lithium may produce a normalization of symptomatology within 1 to 3 weeks.

WARNINGS
Lithium should generally not be given to patients with significant renal or cardiovascular disease, severe debilitation, dehydration, sodium depletion, and to patients receiving diuretics, or angiotensin converting enzyme (ACE) inhibitors, since the risk of lithium toxicity is very high in such patients. If the psychiatric indication is life threatening, and if such a patient fails to respond to other measures, lithium treatment may be undertaken with extreme caution, including daily serum lithium determinations and adjustment to the usually low doses ordinarily tolerated by these individuals. In such instances, hospitalization is a necessity.

Chronic lithium therapy may be associated with diminution of renal concentrating ability, occasionally presenting as nephrogenic diabetes insipidus, with polyuria and polydipsia. Such patients should be carefully managed to avoid dehydration with resulting lithium retention and toxicity. This condition is usually reversible when lithium is discontinued.

Morphologic changes with glomerular and interstitial fibrosis and nephron atrophy have been reported in patients on chronic lithium therapy. Morphologic changes have also been seen in manic-depressive patients never exposed to lithium. The relationship between renal function and morphologic changes and their association with lithium therapy have not been established.

Kidney function should be assessed, prior to and during lithium therapy. Routine urinalysis and other tests may be used to evaluate tubular function (e.g., urine specific gravity or osmolality following a period of water deprivation, or 24-hour urine volume) and glomerular function (e.g., serum creatinine or creatinine clearance). During lithium therapy, progressive or sudden changes in renal function, even within the normal range, indicate the need for reevaluation of treatment.

An encephalopathic syndrome (characterized by weakness, lethargy, fever, tremulousness and confusion, extrapyramidal symptoms, leukocytosis, elevated serum enzymes, BUN and FBS) has occurred in a few patients treated with lithium plus a neuroleptic, most notably haloperidol. In some instances, the syndrome was followed by irreversible brain damage. Because of possible causal relationship between these events and the concomitant administration of lithium and neuroleptic drugs, patients receiving such combined therapy or patients with organic brain syndrome or other CNS impairment should be monitored closely for early evidence of neurologic toxicity and treatment discontinued promptly if such signs appear. This encephalopathic syndrome may be similar to or the same as Neuroleptic Malignant Syndrome (NMS).

Lithium toxicity is closely related to serum lithium concentrations and can occur at doses close to the therapeutic concentrations (see DOSAGE AND ADMINISTRATION).

Outpatients and their families should be warned that the patient must discontinue lithium therapy and contact his physician if such clinical signs of lithium toxicity as diarrhea, vomiting, tremor, mild ataxia, drowsiness, or muscular weakness occur.

Lithium may prolong the effects of neuromuscular blocking agents. Therefore, neuromuscular blocking agents should be given with caution to patients receiving lithium.

Usage in Pregnancy: Adverse effects on nidation in rats, embryo viability in mice, and metabolism in vitro of rat testis and human spermatozoa have been attributed to lithium, as have teratogenicity in submammalian species and cleft palate in mice.

In humans, lithium may cause fetal harm when administered to a pregnant woman. Data from lithium birth registries suggest an increase in cardiac and other anomalies especially Ebstein's anomaly. If this drug is used in women of childbearing potential, or during pregnancy, or if a patient becomes pregnant while taking this drug, the patient should be apprised by their physician of the potential hazard to the fetus.

Usage in Nursing Mothers: Lithium is excreted in human milk. Nursing should not be undertaken during lithium therapy except in rare and unusual circumstances where, in the view of the physician, the potential benefits to the mother outweigh possible hazard to the child. Signs and symptoms of lithium toxicity such as hypertonia, hypothermia, cyanosis and ECG changes have been reported in some infants.

Usage in Children: Since the safety and effectiveness of lithium in children under 12 years of age has not been established, its use in such patients is not recommended at this time.

There has been a report of transient syndrome of acute dystonia and hyperreflexia occurring in a 15 kg child who ingested 300 mg of lithium carbonate.

PRECAUTIONS
The ability to tolerate lithium is greater during the acute manic phase and decreases when manic symptoms subside (see DOSAGE AND ADMINISTRATION.)

The distribution space of lithium approximates that of total body water. Lithium is primarily excreted in urine with insignificant excretion in feces. Renal excretion of lithium is proportional to its plasma concentration. The elimination half-life of lithium is approximately 24 hours. Lithium decreases sodium reabsorption by the renal tubules which could lead to sodium depletion. Therefore, it is essential for the patient to maintain a normal diet, including salt, and an adequate fluid intake (2500–3500 mL) at least during the initial stabilization period. Decreased tolerance to lithium has been reported to ensue from protracted sweating or diarrhea and, if such occur, supplemental fluid and salt should be administered under careful medical supervision and lithium intake reduced or suspended until the condition is resolved. In addition to sweating and diarrhea, concomitant infection with elevated temperatures may also necessitate a temporary reduction or cessation of medication.

Previously existing underlying thyroid disorders do not necessarily constitute a contraindication to lithium treatment. Where hypothyroidism preexists, careful monitoring of thyroid function during lithium stabilization and maintenance allows for correction of changing thyroid parameters and/or adjustment of lithium doses, if any. If hypothyroidism occurs during lithium stabilization and maintenance, supplemental thyroid treatment may be used.

In general the concomitant use of diuretics or angiotensin converting enzyme (ACE) inhibitors with lithium carbonate should be avoided. In those cases where concomitant use is necessary, extreme caution is advised since sodium loss from these drugs may reduce the renal clearance of lithium resulting in increased serum lithium concentrations with the risk of lithium toxicity. When such combinations are used, the lithium dosage may need to be decreased, and more frequent monitoring of lithium serum concentrations is recommended. See WARNINGS for additional caution information.

Concomitant administration of carbamazepine and lithium may increase the risk of neurotoxic side effects.

The following drugs can lower serum lithium concentrations by increasing urinary lithium excretion: acetazolamide, urea, xanthine preparations and alkalinizing agents such as sodium bicarbonate.

Concomitant extended use of iodide preparations, especially potassium iodide, with lithium may produce hypothyroidism. Indomethacin and piroxicam have been reported to significantly increase steady state serum lithium concentrations. In some cases, lithium toxicity has resulted from such interactions. There is also some evidence that other nonsteroidal, anti-inflammatory agents may have a similar effect. When such combinations are used, increased serum lithium concentrations monitoring is recommended.

Concurrent use of calcium channel blocking agents with lithium may increase the risk of neurotoxicity in the form of ataxia, tremors, nausea, vomiting, diarrhea and/or tinnitus.

Concurrent use of metronidazole with lithium may provoke lithium toxicity due to reduced renal clearance. Patients receiving such combined therapy should be monitored closely.

Concurrent use of fluoxetine with lithium has resulted in both increased and decreased serum lithium concentrations. Patients receiving such combined therapy should be monitored closely.

Lithium may impair mental and/or physical abilities. Patients should be cautioned about activities requiring alertness (e.g., operating vehicles or machinery).

Usage in Pregnancy:
Pregnancy Category D. (see WARNINGS).

Usage in Nursing Mothers: Because of the potential for serious adverse reactions in nursing infants from lithium, a decision should be made whether to discontinue nursing or to discontinue the drug, taking into account the importance of the drug to the mother (see WARNINGS).

Usage in Children: Safety and effectiveness in children below the age of 12 have not been established (see WARNINGS).

Usage in the Elderly:
Elderly patients often require lower lithium dosages to achieve therapeutic serum concentrations. They may also exhibit adverse reactions at serum concentrations ordinarily tolerated by younger patients. Additionally, patients with renal impairment may also require lower lithium doses (see WARNINGS).

ADVERSE REACTIONS
The occurrence and severity of adverse reactions are generally directly related to serum lithium concentrations and to individual patient sensitivity to lithium. They generally occur more frequently and with greater severity at higher concentrations.

Adverse reactions may be encountered at serum lithium concentrations below 1.5 mEq/L. Mild to moderate adverse reactions may occur at concentrations from 1.5–2.5 mEq/L, and moderate to severe reactions may be seen at concentrations from 2.0 mEq/L and above.

Fine hand tremor, polyuria and mild thirst may occur during initial therapy for the acute manic phase, and may persist throughout treatment. Transient and mild nausea and general discomfort may also appear during the first few days of lithium administration.

These side effects usually subside with continued treatment or with a temporary reduction or cessation of dosage. If persistent, a cessation of lithium therapy may be required. Diarrhea, vomiting, drowsiness, muscular weakness and lack of coordination may be early signs of lithium intoxication, and can occur at lithium concentrations below 2.0 mEq/L. At higher concentrations giddiness, ataxia, blurred vision, tinnitus and a large output of dilute urine may be seen. Serum lithium concentrations above 3.0 mEq/L may produce a complex clinical picture involving multiple organs and organ systems. Serum lithium concentrations should not be permitted to exceed 2.0 mEq/L during the acute treatment phase.

The following reactions have been reported and appear to be related to serum lithium concentrations, including concentrations within the therapeutic range:

Central Nervous System: tremor, muscle hyperirritability (fasiculations, twitching, clonic movements of whole limbs), hypertonicity, ataxia, choreoathetotic movements, hyperactive deep tendon reflex, extrapyramidal symptoms including acute dystonia, cogwheel rigidity, blackout spells, epileptiform seizures, slurred speech, dizziness, vertigo, downbeat nystagmus, incontinence of urine or feces, somnolence, psychomotor retardation, restlessness, confusion, stupor, coma, tongue movements, tics, tinnitus, hallucinations, poor memory, slowed intellectual functioning, startled response, worsening of organic brain syndromes. Cases of Pseudotumor Cerebri (increased intracranial pressure and papilledema) have been reported with lithium use. If undetected, this condition may result in enlargement of the blind spot, constriction of visual fields and eventual blindness due to optic atrophy. Lithium should be discontinued, if clinically possible, if this syndrome occurs. **Cardiovascular:** cardiac arrhythmia, hypotension, peripheral circulatory collapse, bradycardia, sinus node dysfunction with severe bradycardia (which may result in syncope); **Gastrointestinal:** anorexia, nausea, vomiting, diarrhea, gastritis, salivary gland swelling, abdominal pain, excessive salivation, flatulence, indigestion; **Genitourinary:** glycosuria, decreased creatinine clearance, albuminuria, oliguria, and symptoms of nephrogenic diabetes insipidus including polyuria, thirst and polydipsia; **Dermatologic:** drying and thinning of hair, alopecia, anesthesia of skin, acne, chronic folliculitis, xerosis cutis, psoriasis or its exacerbation, generalized pruritus with or without rash, cutaneous ulcers, angioedema; **Autonomic Nervous System:** blurred vision, dry mouth, impotence/sexual dysfunction; **Thyroid Abnormalities:** euthyroid goiter and/or hypothyroidism (including myxedema) accompanied by lower T_3 and T_4. [131]Iodine uptake may be elevated (see PRECAUTIONS). Paradoxically, rare cases of hyperthyroidism have been reported.

EEG Changes: diffuse slowing, widening of frequency spectrum, potentiation and disorganization of background rhythm. **EKG Changes:** reversible flattening, isoelectricity or inversion of T-waves. **Miscellaneous:** fatigue, lethargy, transient scotomata, exophthalmos, dehydration, weight loss, leucocytosis, headache, transient hyperglycemia, hypercalcemia, hyperparathyroidism, albuminuria, excessive weight gain, edematous swelling of ankles or wrists, metallic taste, dysgeusia/taste distortion, salty taste, thirst, swollen lips, tightness in chest, swollen and/or painful joints, fever, polyarthralgia, and dental caries.

Some reports of nephrogenic diabetes insipidus, hyperparathyroidism and hypothyroidism which persist after lithium discontinuation have been received.

A few reports have been received of the development of painful discoloration of fingers and toes and coldness of the extremities within one day of starting lithium treatment. The mechanism through which these symptoms (resembling Raynaud's Syndrome) developed is not known. Recovery followed discontinuance.

DOSAGE AND ADMINISTRATION

Acute Mania: Optimal patient response can usually be established with 1800 mg/day in the following dosages:

ACUTE MANIA

	Morning	Afternoon	Nighttime
LITHOBID® Slow-Release Tablets[1]	3 tabs (900 mg)		3 tabs (900 mg)
LITHONATE® Capsules	2 caps (600 mg)	2 caps (600 mg)	2 caps (600 mg)
LITHOTABS™ Tablets	2 tabs (600 mg)	2 tabs (600 mg)	2 tabs (600 mg)

[1]Can also be administered on 600mg t.i.d. recommended dosing interval.

Such doses will normally produce an effective serum lithium concentration ranging between 1.0 and 1.5 mEq/L. Dosage must be individualized according to serum concentrations and clinical response. Regular monitoring of the patient's clinical state and of serum lithium concentrations is necessary. Serum concentrations should be determined twice per week during the acute phase, and until the serum concentrations and clinical condition of the patient have been stabilized.

Long-Term Control: Desirable serum lithium concentrations are 0.6 to 1.2 mEq/L which can usually be achieved with 900–1200 mg/day. Dosage will vary from one individual to another, but generally the following dosages will maintain this concentration.

LONG TERM

	Morning	Afternoon	Nighttime
LITHOBID® Slow-Release Tablets[1]	2 tabs (600 mg)		2 tabs (600 mg)
LITHONATE® Capsules[2]	1 cap (300 mg)	1 cap (300 mg)	1 cap (300 mg)
LITHOTABS™ Tablets[2]	1 tab (300 mg)	1 tab (300 mg)	1 tab (300 mg)

[1]Can be administered on t.i.d. recommended dosing interval up to 1200mg/day
[2]Can be administered on 300mg q.i.d. recommended dosing interval.

Serum lithium concentrations in uncomplicated cases receiving maintenance therapy during remission should be monitored at least every two months. Patients abnormally sensitive to lithium may exhibit toxic signs at serum concentrations of 1.0 to 1.5 mEq/L. Elderly patients often respond to reduced dosage, and may exhibit signs of toxicity at serum concentrations ordinarily tolerated by other patients.

N.B.: Blood samples for serum lithium determinations should be drawn immediately prior to the next dose when lithium concentrations are relatively stable (i.e., 8–12 hours after previous dose). Total reliance must not be placed on serum concentrations alone. Accurate patient evaluation requires both clinical and laboratory analysis. LITHOBID® Slow-Release Tablets must be swallowed whole and never chewed or crushed.

OVERDOSAGE

The toxic concentrations for lithium (≥ 1.5 mEq/L) are close to the therapeutic concentrations (0.6–1.2 mEq/L). It is therefore important that patients and their families be cautioned to watch for early toxic symptoms and to discontinue the drug and inform the physician should they occur.(Toxic symptoms are listed in detail under ADVERSE REACTIONS.)

Treatment: No specific antidote for lithium poisoning is known. Treatment is supportive. Early symptoms of lithium toxicity can usually be treated by reduction or cessation of dosage of the drug and resumption of the treatment at a lower dose after 24 to 48 hours. In severe cases of lithium poisoning, the first and foremost goal of treatment consists of elimination of this ion from the patient.
Treatment is essentially the same as that used in barbiturate poisoning: 1) gastric lavage, 2) correction of fluid and electro-

lyte imbalance and, 3) regulation of kidney functioning. Urea, mannitol, and aminophylline all produce significant increases in lithium excretion. Hemodialysis is an effective and rapid means of removing the ion from the severely toxic patient. However, patient recovery may be slow.
Infection prophylaxis, regular chest X-rays, and preservation of adequate respiration are essential.

HOW SUPPLIED

LITHOBID® (Lithium Carbonate, USP) Slow-Release Tablets, 300 mg, peach-colored debossed "SOLVAY 4492"
Bottles of 100
NDC 0032-4492-01
Bottles of 1000
NDC 0032-4492-10
Unit Dose Box of 100
NDC 0032-4492-11
Store between 59°–86°F (15°–30°C). Protect from moisture. Dispense in tight, child-resistant container (USP).
LITHONATE® (Lithium Carbonate Capsules, USP) 300 mg, peach-colored, No. 3 capsules, imprinted "SOLVAY 7512" in red.
Bottles of 100
NDC 0032-7512-01
Bottles of 1000
NDC 0032-7512-10
Unit Dose Boxes of 100
NDC 0032-7512-11
Store at controlled room temperature 59°–86°F (15°–30°C). Dispense in tight, child-resistant container (USP).
LITHOTABS™ (Lithium Carbonate Tablets, USP) 300 mg, scored, white film-coated tablets debossed "SOLVAY 7516."
Bottles of 100
NDC 0032-7516-01
Bottles of 1000
NDC 0032-7516-10
Unit Dose Box of 100
NDC 0032-7516-11
Store at controlled room temperature 59°–86°F (15°–30°C). Dispense in tight, child-resistant container (USP).
Caution: Federal law prohibits dispensing without prescription.
SOLVAY PHARMACEUTICALS
MARIETTA, GA 30062
22E0803 Rev 2/95
©1995 SOLVAY PHARMACEUTICALS, INC.
Shown in Product Identification Guide, page 338

LUVOX® ℞
(Fluvoxamine Maleate) Tablets
50 mg and 100 mg

DESCRIPTION

Fluvoxamine maleate is a selective serotonin (5-HT) reuptake inhibitor (SSRI) belonging to a new chemical series, the 2-aminoethyl oxime ethers of aralkylketones. It is chemically unrelated to other SSRIs and clomipramine. It is chemically designated as 5-methoxy-4'-(trifluoromethyl)valerophenone-(E)-O-(2-aminoethyl)oxime maleate (1:1) and has the empirical formula $C_{15}H_{21}O_2N_2F_3 \cdot C_4H_4O_4$. Its molecular weight is 434.4.
The structural formula is:

Fluvoxamine maleate is a white or off white, ordorless, crystalline powder which is sparingly soluble in water, freely soluble in ethanol and chloroform and practically insoluble in diethyl ether.
LUVOX® (fluvoxamine maleate) Tablets are available in 50 mg and 100 mg strengths for oral administration. In addition to the active ingredient, fluvoxamine maleate, each tablet contains the following inactive ingredients: carnauba wax, hydroxypropyl methylcellulose, mannitol, polyethylene glycol, polysorbate 80, pregelatinized starch, silicon dioxide, sodium stearyl fumarate, starch, synthetic iron oxides, and titanium dioxide.

CLINICAL PHARMACOLOGY
Pharmacodynamics

The mechanism of action of fluvoxamine maleate in Obsessive Compulsive Disorder is presumed to be linked to its specific serotonin reuptake inhibition in brain neurons. In preclinical studies, it was found that fluvoxamine inhibited neuronal uptake of serotonin.
In *in vitro* studies fluvoxamine maleate had no significant affinity for histaminergic, alpha or beta adrenergic, muscarinic, or dopaminergic receptors. Antagonism of some of these receptors is thought to be associated with various sedative, cardiovascular, anticholinergic, and extrapyramidal effects of some psychotropic drugs.

Pharmacokinetics

Bioavailability: The absolute bioavailability of fluvoxamine maleate is 53%. Oral bioavailability is not significantly affected by food.
In a dose proportionality study involving fluvoxamine maleate at 100, 200 and 300 mg/day for 10 consecutive days in 30 normal volunteers, steady state was achieved after about a week of dosing. Maximum plasma concentrations at steady state occurred within 3–8 hours of dosing and reached concentrations averaging 88, 283 and 546 ng/mL, respectively. Thus, fluvoxamine had nonlinear pharmacokinetics over this dose range, i.e., higher doses of fluvoxamine maleate produced disproportionately higher concentrations than predicted from the lower dose.
Distribution/Protein Binding: The mean apparent volume of distribution for fluvoxamine is approximately 25 L/kg, suggesting extensive tissue distribution.
Approximately 80% of fluvoxamine is bound to plasma protein, mostly albumin, over a concentration range of 20 to 2000 ng/mL.
Metabolism: Fluvoxamine maleate is extensively metabolized by the liver; the main metabolic routes are oxidative demethylation and deamination. Nine metabolites were identified following a 5 mg radiolabelled dose of fluvoxamine maleate, constituting approximately 85% of the urinary excretion products of fluvoxamine. The main human metabolite was fluvoxamine acid which, together with its N-acetylated analog, accounted for about 60% of the urinary excretion products. A third metabolite, fluvoxethanol, formed by oxidative deamination, accounted for about 10%. Fluvoxamine acid and fluvoxethanol were tested in an *in vitro* assay of serotonin and norepinephrine reuptake inhibition in rats; they were inactive except for a weak effect of the former metabolite on inhibition of serotonin uptake (1–2 orders of magnitude less potent than the parent compound). Approximately 2% of fluvoxamine was excreted in urine unchanged. (See PRECAUTIONS—Drug Interactions)
Elimination: Following a ^{14}C-labelled oral dose of fluvoxamine maleate (5 mg), an average of 94% of drug-related products was recovered in the urine within 71 hours.
The mean plasma half-life of fluvoxamine at steady state after multiple oral doses of 100 mg/day in healthy, young volunteers was 15.6 hours.
Elderly Subjects: In a study of LUVOX Tablets at 50 and 100 mg comparing elderly (aged 66–73) and young subjects (aged 19–35), mean maximum plasma concentrations in the elderly were 40% higher. The multiple dose elimination half-life of fluvoxamine was 17.4 and 25.9 hours in the elderly compared to 13.6 and 15.6 hours in the young subjects at steady state for 50 and 100 mg doses, respectively.
In elderly patients, the clearance of fluvoxamine was reduced by about 50% and, therefore, LUVOX Tablets should be slowly titrated during initiation of therapy.
Hepatic and Renal Disease: A cross study comparison (healthy subjects vs. patients with hepatic dysfunction) suggested a 30% decrease in fluvoxamine clearance in association with hepatic dysfunction. The mean minimum plasma concentrations in renally impaired patients (creatinine clearance of 5 to 45 mL/min) after 4 and 6 weeks of treatment (50 mg bid, N=13) were comparable to each other, suggesting no accumulation of fluvoxamine in these patients. (See PRECAUTIONS—*Use in Patients with Concomitant Illness*)
Clinical Trials
The effectiveness of LUVOX Tablets for the treatment of Obsessive Compulsive Disorder (OCD) was demonstrated in two 10-week multicenter, parallel group studies of adult outpatients. Patients in these trials were titrated to a total daily fluvoxamine maleate dose of 150 mg/day over the first two weeks of the trial, following which the dose was adjusted within a range of 100–300 mg/day (on a bid schedule), on the basis of response and tolerance. Patients in these studies had moderate to severe OCD (DSM-III-R), with mean baseline ratings on the Yale-Brown Obsessive Compulsive Scale (Y-BOCS), total score of 23. Patients receiving fluvoxamine maleate experienced mean reductions of approximately 4 to 5 units on the Y-BOCS total score, compared to a 2 unit reduction for placebo patients.
The following table provides the outcome classification by treatment group on the Global Improvement item of the Clinical Global Impressions (CGI) scale for both studies combined.

OUTCOME CLASSIFICATION (%) ON CGI-GLOBAL IMPROVEMENT ITEM FOR COMPLETERS IN POOL OF TWO OCD STUDIES

Outcome Classification	Fluvoxamine (N=120)	Placebo (N=134)
Worse	4%	6%
No Change	31%	51%

Continued on next page

Solvay—Cont.

Minimally Improved	22%	32%
Much Improved	30%	10%
Very Much Improved	13%	2%

Exploratory analyses for age and gender effects on outcomes did not suggest any differential responsiveness on the basis of age or sex.

INDICATIONS AND USAGE

LUVOX Tablets are indicated for the treatment of obsessions and compulsions in patients with Obsessive Compulsive Disorder (OCD), as defined in the DSM-III-R. The obsessions or compulsions cause marked distress, are time-consuming, or significantly interfere with social or occupational functioning.

The efficacy of LUVOX Tablets was established in two 10-week trials with obsessive compulsive outpatients with the diagnosis of Obsessive Compulsive Disorder as defined in DSM-III-R. (See Clinical Trials under CLINICAL PHARMACOLOGY.)

Obsessive Compulsive Disorder is characterized by recurrent and persistent ideas, thoughts, impulses or images (obsessions) that are ego-dystonic and/or repetitive, purposeful, and intentional behaviors (compulsions) that are recognized by the person as excessive or unreasonable.

The effectiveness of LUVOX Tablets for long-term use, i.e., for more than 10 weeks, has not been systematically evaluated in placebo-controlled trials. Therefore, the physician who elects to use LUVOX Tablets for extended periods should periodically re-evaluate the long-term usefulness of the drug for the individual patient. (See DOSAGE AND ADMINISTRATION)

CONTRAINDICATIONS

Co-administration of terfenadine, astemizole, or cisapride with LUVOX Tablets is contraindicated (see WARNINGS and PRECAUTIONS).

LUVOX Tablets are contraindicated in patients with a history of hypersensitivity to fluvoxamine maleate.

WARNINGS

Potential for Interaction with Monoamine Oxidase Inhibitors

In patients receiving another serotonin reuptake inhibitor drug in combination with monoamine oxidase inhibitors (MAOI), there have been reports of serious, sometimes fatal, reactions including hyperthermia, rigidity, myoclonus, autonomic instability with possible rapid fluctuations of vital signs, and mental status changes that include extreme agitation progressing to delirium and coma. These reactions have also been reported in patients who have discontinued that drug and have been started on a MAOI. Some cases presented with features resembling neuroleptic malignant syndrome. Therefore, it is recommended that LUVOX Tablets not be used in combination with a MAOI, or within 14 days of discontinuing treatment with a MAOI. After stopping LUVOX Tablets, at least 2 weeks should be allowed before starting a MAOI.

Potential Terfenadine, Astemizole, and Cisapride Interactions

Terfenadine, astemizole, and cisapride are all metabolized by the cytochrome P450IIIA4 isozyme, and it has been demonstrated that ketoconazole, a potent inhibitor of IIIA4, blocks the metabolism of these drugs, resulting in increased plasma concentrations of parent drug. Increased plasma concentrations of terfenadine, astemizole, and cisapride cause QT prolongation and have been associated with torsades de pointes-type ventricular tachycardia, sometimes fatal. As noted below, a substantial pharmacokinetic interaction has been observed for fluvoxamine in combination with alprazolam, a drug that is known to be metabolized by the IIIA4 isozyme. Although it has not been definitively demonstrated that fluvoxamine is a potent IIIA4 inhibitor, it is likely to be, given the substantial interaction of fluvoxamine with alprazolam. Consequently, it is recommended that fluvoxamine not be used in combination with either terfenadine, astemizole, or cisapride (see CONTRAINDICATIONS and PRECAUTIONS).

Other Potentially Important Drug Interactions

(Also see PRECAUTIONS—Drug Interactions)

Benzodiazepines: Benzodiazepines metabolized by hepatic oxidation (e.g., alprazolam, midazolam, triazolam, etc.) should be used with caution because the clearance of these drugs is likely to be reduced by fluvoxamine. The clearance of benzodiazepines metabolized by glucuronidation (e.g., lorazepam, oxazepam, temazepam) is unlikely to be affected by fluvoxamine.

Alprazolam—When fluvoxamine maleate (100 mg qd) and alprazolam (1 mg qid) were co-administered to steady state, plasma concentrations and other pharmacokinetic parameters (AUC, C_{max}, $T_{1/2}$) of alprazolam were approximately twice those observed when alprazolam was administered alone; oral clearance was reduced by about 50%. The elevated plasma alprazolam concentrations resulted in decreased psychomotor performance and memory. This interaction, which has not been investigated using higher doses of fluvoxamine, may be more pronounced if a 300 mg daily dose is co-administered, particularly since fluvoxamine exhibits non-linear pharmacokinetics over the dosage range 100–300 mg. If alprazolam is co-administered with LUVOX Tablets, the initial alprazolam dosage should be at least halved and titration to the lowest effective dose is recommended. No dosage adjustment is required for LUVOX Tablets.

Diazepam—The co-administration of LUVOX Tablets and diazepam is generally not advisable. Because fluvoxamine reduces the clearance of both diazepam and its active metabolite, N-desmethyldiazepam, there is a strong likelihood of substantial accumulation of both species during chronic co-administration.

Evidence supporting the conclusion that it is inadvisable to co-administer fluvoxamine and diazepam is derived from a study in which healthy volunteers taking 150 mg/day of fluvoxamine were administered a single oral dose of 10 mg of diazepam. In these subjects (N=8), the clearance of diazepam was reduced by 65% and that of N-desmethyldiazepam to a level that was too low to measure over the course of the 2 week long study.

It is likely that this experience significantly underestimates the degree of accumulation that might occur with repeated diazepam administration. Moreover, as noted with alprazolam, the effect of fluvoxamine may even be more pronounced when it is administered at higher doses.

Accordingly, diazepam and fluvoxamine should not ordinarily be co-administered.

Theophylline: The effect of steady-state fluvoxamine (50 mg bid) on the pharmacokinetics of a single dose of theophylline (375 mg as 442 mg aminophylline) was evaluated in 12 healthy non-smoking, male volunteers. The clearance of theophylline was decreased approximately 3-fold. Therefore, if theophylline is co-administered with fluvoxamine maleate, its dose should be reduced to one third of the usual daily maintenance dose and plasma concentrations of theophylline should be monitored. No dosage adjustment is required for LUVOX Tablets.

Warfarin: When fluvoxamine maleate (50 mg tid) was administered concomitantly with warfarin for two weeks, warfarin plasma concentrations increased by 98% and prothrombin times were prolonged. Thus patients receiving oral anticoagulants and LUVOX Tablets should have their prothrombin time monitored and their anticoagulant dose adjusted accordingly. No dosage adjustment is required for LUVOX Tablets.

PRECAUTIONS

General

Activation of Mania/Hypomania: During premarketing studies involving primarily depressed patients, hypomania or mania occurred in approximately 1% of patients treated with fluvoxamine. Activation of mania/hypomania has also been reported in a small proportion of patients with major affective disorder who were treated with other marketed antidepressants. As with all antidepressants, LUVOX Tablets should be used cautiously in patients with a history of mania.

Seizures: During premarketing studies, seizures were reported in 0.2% of fluvoxamine-treated patients. LUVOX Tablets should be used cautiously in patients with a history of seizures. It should be discontinued in any patient who develops seizures.

Suicide: The possibility of a suicide attempt is inherent in patients with depressive symptoms, whether these occur in primary depression or in association with another primary disorder such as OCD. Close supervision of high risk patients should accompany initial drug therapy. Prescriptions for LUVOX Tablets should be written for the smallest quantity of tablets consistent with good patient management in order to reduce the risk of overdose.

Use in Patients with Concomitant Illness: Closely monitored clinical experience with LUVOX Tablets in patients with concomitant systemic illness is limited. Caution is advised in administering LUVOX Tablets to patients with diseases or conditions that could affect hemodynamic responses or metabolism.

LUVOX Tablets have not been evaluated or used to any appreciable extent in patients with a recent history of myocardial infarction or unstable heart disease. Patients with these diagnoses were systematically excluded from many clinical studies during the product's premarketing testing. Evaluation of the electrocardiograms for patients with depression or OCD who participated in premarketing studies revealed no differences between fluvoxamine and placebo in the emergence of clinically important ECG changes.

In patients with liver dysfunction, fluvoxamine clearance was decreased by approximately 30%. LUVOX Tablets should be slowly titrated in patients with liver dysfunction during the initiation of treatment.

Information for Patients

Physicians are advised to discuss the following issues with patients for whom they prescribe LUVOX Tablets:

Interference with Cognitive or Motor Performance: Since any psychoactive drug may impair judgement, thinking , or motor skills, patients should be cautioned about operating hazardous machinery, including automobiles, until they are certain that LUVOX Tablets therapy does not adversely affect their ability to engage in such activities.

Pregnancy: Patients should be advised to notify their physicians if they become pregnant or intend to become pregnant during therapy with LUVOX Tablets.

Nursing: Patients receiving LUVOX Tablets should be advised to notify their physicians if they are breast feeding an infant. (See PRECAUTIONS—Nursing Mothers)

Concomitant Medication: Patients should be advised to notify their physicians if they are taking, or plan to take, any prescription or over-the-counter drugs, since there is a potential for clinically important interactions with LUVOX Tablets.

Alcohol: As with other psychotropic medications, patients should be advised to avoid alcohol while taking LUVOX Tablets.

Allergic Reactions: Patients should be advised to notify their physicians if they develop a rash, hives, or a related allergic phenomenon during therapy with LUVOX Tablets.

Laboratory Tests

There are no specific laboratory tests recommended.

Drug Interactions

Potential Interactions with Drugs that Inhibit or are Metabolized by Cytochrome P450 Isozymes: Multiple hepatic cytochrome P450 (CYP450) enzymes are involved in the oxidative biotransformation of a large number of structurally different drugs and endogenous compounds. The available knowledge concerning the relationship of fluvoxamine and the CYP450 enzyme system has been obtained mostly from pharmacokinetic interaction studies conducted in healthy volunteers, but some preliminary *in vitro* data are also available. Based on a finding of substantial interactions of fluvoxamine with certain of these drugs (see later parts of this section and also WARNINGS for details) and limited *in vitro* data for the IIIA4 isozyme, it appears that fluvoxamine inhibits the following isozymes that are known to be involved in the metabolism of the listed drugs:

IA2	IIC9	IIIA4
Warfarin	Warfarin	Alprazolam
Theophylline		
Propranolol		

In vitro data suggest that fluvoxamine is a relatively weak inhibitor of the IID6 isozyme.

Approximately 7% of the normal population has a genetic defect that leads to reduced levels of activity of cytochrome P450IID6 isozyme. Such individuals have been referred to as "poor metabolizers" (PM) of drugs such as debrisoquin, dextromethorphan, and tricyclic antidepressants. While none of the drugs studied for drug interactions significantly affected the pharmacokinetics of fluvoxamine, an *in vivo* study of fluvoxamine single-dose pharmacokinetics in 13 PM subjects demonstrated altered pharmacokinetic properties compared to 16 "extensive metabolizers" (EM): mean Cmax, AUC, and half-life were increased by 52%, 200%, and 62%, respectively, in the PM compared to the EM group. This suggests that fluvoxamine is metabolized, at least in part, by IID6 isozyme. Caution is indicated in patients known to have reduced levels of P450IID6 activity and those receiving concomitant drugs known to inhibit this isozyme (e.g. quinidine).

The metabolism of fluvoxamine has not been fully characterized and the effects of potent P450 isozyme inhibition, such as the ketoconazole inhibition of IIIA4, on fluvoxamine metabolism have not been studied.

A clinically significant fluvoxamine interaction is possible with drugs having a narrow therapeutic ratio such as terfenadine, astemizole, or cisapride, warfarin, theophylline, certain benzodiazepines and phenytoin. If LUVOX Tablets are to be administered together with a drug that is eliminated via oxidative metabolism and has a narrow therapeutic window, plasma levels and/or pharmacodynamic effects of the latter drug should be monitored closely, at least until steady-state conditions are reached (See CONTRAINDICATIONS and WARNINGS).

CNS Active Drugs:

Monoamine Oxidase Inhibitors: See WARNINGS

Alprazolam: See WARNINGS

Diazepam: See WARNINGS

Lorazepam: A study of multiple doses of fluvoxamine maleate (50 mg bid) in healthy male volunteers (N=12) and a single dose of lorazepam (4 mg single dose) indicated no significant pharmacokinetic interaction. On average, both lorazepam alone and lorazepam with fluvoxamine produced substantial decrements in cognitive functioning; however,

the co-administration of fluvoxamine and lorazepam did not produce larger mean decrements compared to lorazepam alone.

Lithium: As with other serotonergic drugs, lithium may enhance the serotonergic effects of fluvoxamine and, therefore, the combination should be used with caution. Seizures have been reported with the co-administration of fluvoxamine maleate and lithium.

Tryptophan: Tryptophan may enhance the serotonergic effects of fluvoxamine, and the combination should, therefore, be used with caution. Severe vomiting has been reported with the co-administration of fluvoxamine maleate and tryptophan.

Clozapine: Elevated serum levels of clozapine have been reported in patients taking fluvoxamine maleate and clozapine. Since clozapine related seizures and orthostatic hypotension appear to be dose related, the risk of these adverse events may be higher when fluvoxamine and clozapine are co-administered. Patients should be closely monitored when fluvoxamine maleate and clozapine are used concurrently.

Alcohol: Studies involving single 40 g doses of ethanol (oral administration in one study and intravenous in the other) and multiple dosing with fluvoxamine maleate (50 mg bid) revealed no effect of either drug on the pharmacokinetics or pharmacodynamics of the other.

Tricyclic Antidepressants (TCAs): Significantly increased plasma TCA levels have been reported with the co-administration of fluvoxamine maleate and amitriptyline, clomipramine or imipramine. Caution is indicated with the co-administration of LUVOX Tablets and TCAs; plasma TCA concentrations may need to be monitored, and the dose of TCA may need to be reduced.

Carbamazepine: Elevated carbamazepine levels and symptoms of toxicity have been reported with the co-administration of fluvoxamine maleate and carbamazepine.

Methadone: Significantly increased methadone (plasma level:dose) ratios have been reported when fluvoxamine maleate was administered to patients receiving maintenance methadone treatment, with symptoms of opioid intoxication in one patient. Opioid withdrawal symptoms were reported following fluvoxamine maleate discontinuation in another patient.

Other Drugs:

Theophylline: See WARNINGS

Propranolol and Other Beta-Blockers: Co-administration of fluvoxamine maleate 100 mg per day and propranolol 160 mg per day in normal volunteers resulted in a mean five-fold increase (range 2 to 17) in minimum propranolol plasma concentrations. In this study, there was a slight potentiation of the propranolol-induced reduction in heart rate and reduction in the exercise diastolic pressure.

One case of bradycardia and hypotension and a second case of orthostatic hypotension have been reported with the co-administration of fluvoxamine and metoprolol.

If propranolol or metoprolol is co-administered with LUVOX Tablets, a reduction in the initial beta-blocker dose and more cautious dose titration is recommended. No dosage adjustment is required for LUVOX Tablets.

Co-administration of fluvoxamine maleate 100 mg per day with atenolol 100 mg per day (N=6) did not affect the plasma concentrations of atenolol. Unlike propranolol and metoprolol which undergo hepatic metabolism, atenolol is eliminated primarily by renal excretion.

Warfarin: See WARNINGS

Digoxin: Administration of fluvoxamine maleate 100 mg daily for 18 days (N=8) did not significantly affect the pharmacokinetics of a 1.25 mg single intravenous dose of digoxin.

Diltiazem: Bradycardia has been reported with the co-administration of fluvoxamine maleate and diltiazem.

Effects of Smoking on Fluvoxamine Metabolism: Smokers had a 25% increase in the metabolism of fluvoxamine compared to nonsmokers.

Electroconvulsive Therapy (ECT): There are no clinical studies establishing the benefits or risks of combined use of ECT and fluvoxamine maleate.

Carcinogenesis, Mutagenesis, Impairment of Fertility

Carcinogenesis: There is no evidence of carcinogenicity, mutagenicity or impairment of fertility with fluvoxamine maleate.

There was no evidence of carcinogenicity in rats treated orally with fluvoxamine maleate for 30 months or hamsters treated orally with fluvoxamine maleate for 20 (females) or 26 (males) months. The daily doses in the high dose groups in these studies were increased over the course of the study from a minimum of 160 mg/kg to a maximum of 240 mg/kg in rats, and from a minimum of 135 mg/kg to a maximum of 240 mg/kg in hamsters. The maximum dose of 240 mg/kg is approximately 6 times the maximum human daily dose on a mg/m² basis.

Mutagenesis: No evidence of mutagenic potential was observed in a mouse micronucleus test, an *in vitro* chromosome aberration test, or the Ames microbial mutagen test with or without metabolic activation.

Impairment of Fertility: In fertility studies of male and female rats, up to 80 mg/kg/day orally of fluvoxamine maleate, (approximately 2 times the maximum human daily dose

on a mg/m² basis) had no effect on mating performance, duration of gestation, or pregnancy rate.

Pregnancy

Teratogenic Effects—Pregnancy Category C: In teratology studies in rats and rabbits, daily oral doses of fluvoxamine maleate of up to 80 and 40 mg/kg, respectively (approximately 2 times the maximum human daily dose on a mg/m² basis) caused no fetal malformations. However, in other reproduction studies in which pregnant rats were dosed through weaning there was (1) an increase in pup mortality at birth (seen at 80 mg/kg and above but not at 20 mg/kg, and (2) decreases in postnatal pup weights (seen at 160 but not at 80 mg/kg) and survival (seen at all doses; lowest dose tested = 5 mg/kg). (Doses of 5, 20, 80, and 160 mg/kg are approximately 0.1, 0.5, 2, and 4 times the maximum human daily dose on a mg/m² basis.) While the results of a cross-fostering study implied that at least some of these results likely occurred secondarily to maternal toxicity, the role of a direct drug effect on the fetuses or pups could not be ruled out. There are no adequate and well-controlled studies in pregnant women. Fluvoxamine maleate should be used during pregnancy only if the potential benefit justifies the potential risk to the fetus.

Labor and Delivery

The effect of fluvoxamine on labor and delivery in humans is unknown.

Nursing Mothers

As for many other drugs, fluvoxamine is secreted in human breast milk. The decision of whether to discontinue nursing or to discontinue the drug should take into account the potential for serious adverse effects from exposure to fluvoxamine in the nursing infant as well as the potential benefits of LUVOX® (fluvoxamine maleate) Tablets therapy to the mother.

Pediatric Use

Safety and effectiveness of LUVOX Tablets in individuals below 18 years of age have not been established.

Geriatric Use

Approximately 230 patients participating in controlled premarketing studies with LUVOX Tablets were 65 years of age or over. No overall differences in safety were observed between these patients and younger patients. Other reported clinical experience has not identified differences in response between the elderly and younger patients. However, the clearance of fluvoxamine is decreased by about 50% in elderly compared to younger patients (see Pharmacokinetics under CLINICAL PHARMACOLOGY), and greater sensitivity of some older individuals also cannot be ruled out. Consequently, LUVOX Tablets should be slowly titrated during initiation of therapy.

ADVERSE REACTIONS

Associated with Discontinuation of Treatment

Of the 1087 OCD and depressed patients treated with fluvoxamine maleate in controlled clinical trials conducted in North America, 22% discontinued treatment due to an adverse event. The most common events (≥1%) associated with discontinuation and considered to be drug related (i.e., those events associated with dropout at a rate at least twice that of placebo) included:

Table 1

ADVERSE EVENTS ASSOCIATED WITH DISCONTINUATION OF TREATMENT IN OCD AND DEPRESSION POPULATIONS

BODY SYSTEM/ ADVERSE EVENT	PERCENTAGE OF PATIENTS FLUVOXAMINE	PLACEBO
BODY AS A WHOLE		
Headache	3%	1%
Asthenia	2%	<1%
Abdominal Pain	1%	0%
DIGESTIVE		
Nausea	9%	1%
Diarrhea	1%	<1%
Vomiting	2%	<1%
Anorexia	1%	<1%
Dyspepsia	1%	<1%
NERVOUS SYSTEM		
Insomnia	4%	1%
Somnolence	4%	<1%
Nervousness	2%	<1%
Agitation	2%	<1%
Dizziness	2%	<1%
Anxiety	1%	<1%
Dry Mouth	1%	<1%

Incidence in Controlled Trials

Commonly Observed Adverse Events in Controlled Clinical Trials:

LUVOX Tablets have been studied in controlled trials of OCD (N=320) and depression (N=1350). In general, adverse event rates were similar in the two data sets. The most commonly observed adverse events associated with the use of LUVOX Tablets and likely to be drug-related (incidence of

5% or greater and at least twice that for placebo) derived from Table 2 were: *somnolence, insomnia, nervousness, tremor, nausea, dyspepsia, anorexia, vomiting, abnormal ejaculation, asthenia, and sweating.* In a pool of two studies involving only patients with OCD, the following additional events were identified using the above rule: *dry mouth, decreased libido, urinary frequency, anorgasmia, rhinitis and taste perversion.*

Adverse Events Occurring at an Incidence of 1%: Table 2 enumerates adverse events that occurred at a frequency of 1% or more, and were more frequent than in the placebo group, among patients treated with LUVOX Tablets in two short-term placebo controlled OCD trials (10 week) and depression trials (6 week) in which patients were dosed in a range of generally 100 to 300 mg/day. This table shows the percentage of patients in each group who had at least one occurrence of an event at some time during their treatment. Reported adverse events were classified using a standard COSTART-based Dictionary terminology.

The prescriber should be aware that these figures cannot be used to predict the incidence of side effects in the course of usual medical practice where patient characteristics and other factors may differ from those that prevailed in the clinical trials. Similarly, the cited frequencies cannot be compared with figures obtained from other clinical investigations involving different treatments, uses, and investigators. The cited figures, however, do provide the prescribing physician with some basis for estimating the relative contribution of drug and non-drug factors to the side-effect incidence rate in the population studied.

Adverse Events in OCD Placebo Controlled Studies Which are Markedly Different (defined as at least a two-fold difference) in Rate from the Pooled Event Rates in OCD and Depression Placebo Controlled Studies: The events in OCD studies with a two-fold decrease in rate compared to event rates in OCD and depression studies were dysphagia and amblyopia (mostly blurred vision). Additionally, there was an approximate 25% decrease in nausea.

The events in OCD studies with a two-fold increase in rate compared to event rates in OCD and depression studies were: *asthenia, abnormal ejaculation (mostly delayed ejaculation), anxiety, infection, rhinitis, anorgasmia (in males), depression, libido decreased, pharyngitis, agitation, impotence, myoclonus/twitch, thirst, weight loss, leg cramps, myalgia and urinary retention.* These events are listed in order of decreasing rates in the OCD trials.

Vital Sign Changes

Comparisons of fluvoxamine maleate and placebo groups in separate pools of short-term OCD and depression trials on (1) median change from baseline on various vital signs variables and on (2) incidence of patients meeting criteria for potentially important changes from baseline on various vital signs variables revealed no important differences between fluvoxamine maleate and placebo.

Laboratory Changes

Comparisons of fluvoxamine maleate and placebo groups in separate pools of short-term OCD and depression trials on (1) median change from baseline on various serum chemistry, hematology, and urinalysis variables and on (2) incidence of patients meeting criteria for potentially important changes from baseline on various serum chemistry, hematology, and urinalysis variables revealed no important differences between fluvoxamine maleate and placebo.

ECG Changes

Comparisons of fluvoxamine maleate and placebo groups in separate pools of short-term OCD and depression trials on (1) mean change from baseline on various ECG variables and on (2) incidence of patients meeting criteria for potentially important changes from baseline on various ECG variables revealed no important differences between fluvoxamine maleate and placebo.

Table 2

TREATMENT-EMERGENT ADVERSE EVENT INCIDENCE RATES BY BODY SYSTEM IN OCD AND DEPRESSION POPULATIONS COMBINED[1]

BODY SYSTEM/ ADVERSE EVENT	Percentage of Patients Reporting Event FLUVOXAMINE N = 892	PLACEBO N = 778
BODY AS WHOLE		
Headache	22	20
Asthenia	14	6
Flu Syndrome	3	2
Chills	2	1
CARDIOVASCULAR		
Palpitations	3	2
DIGESTIVE SYSTEM		
Nausea	40	14
Diarrhea	11	7
Constipation	10	8

Continued on next page

Solvay—Cont.

Dyspepsia	10	5
Anorexia	6	2
Vomiting	5	2
Flatulence	4	3
Tooth Disorder[2]	3	1
Dysphagia	2	1
NERVOUS SYSTEM		
Somnolence	22	8
Insomnia	21	10
Dry Mouth	14	10
Nervousness	12	5
Dizziness	11	6
Tremor	5	1
Anxiety	5	3
Vasodilatation[3]	3	1
Hypertonia	2	1
Agitation	2	1
Decreased Libido	2	1
Depression	2	1
CNS Stimulation	2	1
RESPIRATORY SYSTEM		
Upper Respiratory Infection	9	5
Dyspnea	2	1
Yawn	2	0
SKIN		
Sweating	7	3
SPECIAL SENSES		
Taste Perversion	3	1
Amblyopia[4]	3	2
UROGENITAL		
Abnormal Ejaculation[5,6]	8	1
Urinary Frequency	3	2
Impotence[6]	2	1
Anorgasmia	2	0
Urinary Retention	1	0

[1] Events for which fluvoxamine maleate incidence was equal to or less than placebo are not listed in the table above, but include the following: abdominal pain, abnormal dreams, appetite increase, back pain, chest pain, confusion, dysmenorrhea, fever, infection, leg cramps, migraine, myalgia, pain, paresthesia, pharyngitis, postural hypotension, pruritus, rash, rhinitis, thirst and tinnitus.

[2] Includes "toothache," "tooth extraction and abscess," and "caries."

[3] Mostly feeling warm, hot, or flushed.

[4] Mostly "blurred vision."

[5] Mostly "delayed ejaculation."

[6] Incidence based on number of male patients.

Other Events Observed During the Premarketing Evaluation of LUVOX Tablets

During premarketing clinical trials conducted in North America and Europe, multiple doses of fluvoxamine maleate were administered for a combined total of 2737 patient exposures in patients suffering OCD or Major Depressive Disorder. Untoward events associated with this exposure were recorded by clinical investigators using descriptive terminology of their own choosing. Consequently, it is not possible to provide a meaningful estimate of the proportion of individuals experiencing adverse events without first grouping similar types of untoward events into a limited (i.e., reduced) number of standard event categories.

In the tabulations which follow, a standard COSTART-based Dictionary terminology has been used to classify reported adverse events. If the COSTART term for an event was so general as to be uninformative, it was replaced with a more informative term. The frequencies presented, therefore, represent the proportion of the 2737 patient exposures to multiple doses of fluvoxamine maleate who experienced an event of the type cited on at least one occasion while receiving fluvoxamine maleate. All reported events are included in the list below, with the following exceptions: 1) those events already listed in Table 2, which tabulates incidence rates of common adverse experiences in placebo-controlled OCD and depression clinical trials, are excluded; 2) those events for which a drug cause was considered remote (i.e., neoplasia, gastrointestinal carcinoma, herpes simplex, herpes zoster, application site reaction, and unintended pregnancy) are omitted; and 3) events which were reported in only one patient and judged to not be potentially serious are not included. It is important to emphasize that, although the events reported did occur during treatment with fluvoxamine maleate, a causal relationship to fluvoxamine maleate has not been established.

Events are further classified within body system categories and enumerated in order of decreasing frequency using the following definitions: frequent adverse events are defined as those occurring on one or more occasions in at least 1/100 patients; infrequent adverse events are those occurring between 1/100 and 1/1000 patients; and rare adverse events are those occurring in less than 1/1000 patients.

Body as a Whole: *Frequent:* accidental injury, malaise; *Infrequent:* allergic reaction, neck pain, neck rigidity, overdose, photosensitivity reaction, suicide attempt; *Rare:* cyst, pelvic pain, sudden death.

Cardiovascular System: *Frequent:* hypertension, hypotension, syncope, tachycardia; *Infrequent:* angina pectoris, bradycardia, cardiomyopathy, cardiovascular disease, cold extremities, conduction delay, heart failure, myocardial infarction, pallor, pulse irregular, ST segment changes; *Rare:* AV block, cerebrovascular accident, coronary artery disease, embolus, pericarditis, phlebitis, pulmonary infarction, supraventricular extrasystoles.

Digestive System: *Frequent:* elevated liver transaminases; *Infrequent:* colitis, eructation, esophagitis, gastritis, gastroenteritis, gastrointestinal hemorrhage, gastrointestinal ulcer, gingivitis, glossitis, hemorrhoids, melena, rectal hemorrhage, stomatitis; *Rare:* biliary pain, cholecystitis, cholelithiasis, fecal incontinence, hematemesis, intestinal obstruction, jaundice.

Endocrine System: *Infrequent:* hypothyroidism; *Rare:* goiter.

Hemic and Lymphatic Systems: *Infrequent:* anemia, ecchymosis, leukocytosis, lymphadenopathy, thrombocytopenia; *Rare:* leukopenia, purpura.

Metabolic and Nutritional Systems: *Frequent:* edema, weight gain, weight loss; *Infrequent:* dehydration, hypercholesterolemia; *Rare:* diabetes mellitus, hyperglycemia, hyperlipidemia, hypoglycemia, hypokalemia, lactate dehydrogenase increased.

Musculoskeletal System: *Infrequent:* arthralgia, arthritis, bursitis, generalized muscle spasm, myasthenia, tendinous contracture, tenosynovitis; *Rare:* arthrosis, myopathy, pathological fracture.

Nervous System: *Frequent:* amnesia, apathy, hyperkinesia, hypokinesia, manic reaction, myoclonus, psychotic reaction; *Infrequent:* agoraphobia, akathisia, ataxia, CNS depression, convulsion, delirium, delusion, depersonalization, drug dependence, dyskinesia, dystonia, emotional lability, euphoria, extrapyramidal syndrome, gait unsteady, hallucinations, hemiplegia, hostility, hypersomnia, hypochondriasis, hypotonia, hysteria, incoordination, increased salivation, increased libido, neuralgia, paralysis, paranoid reaction, phobia, psychosis, sleep disorder, stupor, twitching, vertigo; *Rare:* akinesia, coma, fibrillations, mutism, obsessions, reflexes decreased, slurred speech, tardive dyskinesia, torticollis, trismus, withdrawal syndrome.

Respiratory System: *Frequent:* cough increased, sinusitis; *Infrequent:* asthma, bronchitis, epistaxis, hoarseness, hyperventilation; *Rare:* apnea, congestion of upper airway, hemoptysis, hiccups, laryngismus, obstructive pulmonary disease, pneumonia.

Skin: *Infrequent:* acne, alopecia, dry skin, eczema, exfoliative dermatitis, furunculosis, seborrhea, skin discoloration, urticaria.

Special Senses: *Infrequent:* accommodation abnormal, conjunctivitis, deafness, diplopia, dry eyes, ear pain, eye pain, mydriasis, otitis media, parosmia, photophobia, taste loss, visual field defect; *Rare:* corneal ulcer, retinal detachment.

Urogenital System: *Infrequent:* anuria, breast pain, cystitis, delayed menstruation[1], dysuria, female lactation[1], hematuria, menopause[1], menorrhagia[1], metrorrhagia[1], nocturia, polyuria, premenstrual syndrome[1], urinary incontinence, urinary tract infection, urinary urgency, urination impaired, vaginal hemorrhage[1], vaginitis[1]; *Rare:* kidney calculus, hematospermia[2], oliguria.

[1] Based on the number of females.

[2] Based on the number of males.

Non-US Postmarketing Reports

Voluntary reports of adverse events in patients taking LUVOX Tablets that have been received since market introduction and are of unknown causal relationship to LUVOX Tablets use include: toxic epidermal necrolysis, Stevens-Johnson syndrome, Henoch-Schoenlein purpura, bullous eruption, priapism, agranulocytosis, neuropathy, aplastic anemia, anaphylactic reaction, hyponatremia, acute renal failure, hepatitis, and severe akinesia with fever when fluvoxamine was co-administered with antipsychotic medication.

DRUG ABUSE AND DEPENDENCE

Controlled Substance Class

LUVOX Tablets are not controlled substances.

Physical and Psychological Dependence

The potential for abuse, tolerance and physical dependence with fluvoxamine maleate has been studied in a nonhuman primate model. No evidence of dependency phenomena was found. The discontinuation effects of LUVOX Tablets were not systematically evaluated in controlled clinical trials. LUVOX Tablets were not systematically studied in clinical trials for potential for abuse, but there was no indication of drug-seeking behavior in clinical trials. It should be noted, however, that patients at risk for drug dependency were systematically excluded from investigational studies of fluvoxamine maleate. Generally, it is not possible to predict on the basis of preclinical or premarketing clinical experience the extent to which a CNS active drug will be misused, diverted, and/or abused once marketed. Consequently, physicians should carefully evaluate patients for a history of drug abuse and follow such patients closely, observing them for signs of fluvoxamine maleate misuse or abuse (i.e., development of tolerance, incrementation of dose, drug-seeking behavior).

OVERDOSAGE

Human Experience

Worldwide exposure to fluvoxamine maleate includes over 37,000 patients treated in clinical trials and an estimated exposure of 4,500,000 patients treated during foreign marketing experience (circa 1992). Of the 354 cases of deliberate or accidental overdose involving fluvoxamine maleate reported from this population, there were 19 deaths. Of the 19 deaths, 2 were in patients taking fluvoxamine maleate alone and the remaining 17 were in patients taking fluvoxamine maleate along with other drugs. In the remaining 335 patients, 309 had complete recovery after gastric lavage or symptomatic treatment. One patient had persistent mydriasis after the event, and a second patient had a bowel infarction requiring a hemicolectomy. In the remaining 24 patients the outcome was unknown. The highest reported overdose of fluvoxamine maleate involved a non-lethal ingestion of 10,000 mg (equivalent of 1–3 months' dosage). The patient fully recovered with no sequelae.

Commonly observed adverse events associated with fluvoxamine maleate overdose included drowsiness, vomiting, diarrhea, and dizziness. Other notable signs and symptoms seen with fluvoxamine maleate overdose (single or mixed drugs) included coma, tachycardia, bradycardia, hypotension, ECG abnormalities, liver function abnormalities, convulsions, and symptoms such as aspiration pneumonitis, respiratory difficulties or hypokalemia that may occur secondary to loss of consciousness or vomiting.

Management of Overdose

1. An unobstructed airway should be established with maintenance of respiration as required. Vital signs and ECG should be monitored.
2. Administration of activated charcoal may be as effective as emesis or lavage and should be considered in treating overdose. Since absorption with overdose may be delayed, measures to minimize absorption may be necessary for up to 24 hours post-ingestion.
3. Maintain close observation as clinically indicated.
4. There are no specific antidotes for LUVOX Tablets.
5. In managing overdosage, consider the possibility of multiple drug involvement. The physician should consider contacting a poison control center for additional information on the treatment of any overdosage.
6. Dialysis is not believed to be beneficial.

DOSAGE AND ADMINISTRATION

The recommended starting dose for LUVOX Tablets is 50 mg, administered as a single daily dose at bedtime. In the controlled clinical trials establishing the effectiveness of LUVOX Tablets in OCD, patients were titrated within a dose range of 100 to 300 mg/day. Consequently, the dose should be increased in 50 mg increments every 4 to 7 days, as tolerated, until maximum therapeutic benefit is achieved, not to exceed 300 mg per day. It is advisable that a total daily dose of more than 100 mg should be given in two divided doses. If the doses are not equal, the larger dose should be given at bedtime.

Dosage for Elderly or Hepatically Impaired Patients

Elderly patients and those with hepatic impairment have been observed to have a decreased clearance of fluvoxamine maleate. Consequently, it may be appropriate to modify the initial dose and the subsequent dose titration for these patient groups.

Maintenance/Continuation Extended Treatment

Although the efficacy of LUVOX Tablets beyond 10 weeks of dosing for OCD has not been documented in controlled trials, OCD is a chronic condition, and it is reasonable to consider continuation for a responding patient. Dosage adjustments should be made to maintain the patient on the lowest effective dosage, and patients should be periodically reassessed to determine the need for continued treatment.

HOW SUPPLIED

Tablets 50 mg: scored, yellow, elliptical, film-coated (debossed "SOLVAY" and "4205" on one side and scored on the other)

Bottles of 100	NDC 0032-4205-01
Bottles of 1000	NDC 0032-4205-10
Unit dose pack of 100	NDC 0032-4205-11

Tablets 100 mg: scored, beige, elliptical, film-coated (debossed "SOLVAY" and "4210" on one side and scored on the other)

Bottles of 100	NDC 0032-4210-01
Bottles of 1000	NDC 0032-4210-10
Unit dose pack of 100	NDC 0032-4210-11

LUVOX Tablets should be protected from high humidity and stored at controlled room temperature, 15°–30°C (59°–86°F). Dispense in tight containers.

CAUTION: Federal law prohibits dispensing without prescription.

SOLVAY PHARMACEUTICALS
MARIETTA, GA 30062
5E1252 Rev 8/96

Shown in Product Identification Guide, page 338

ROWASA® ℞

[*rō -ā 'să*]
(mesalamine)
Rectal Suspension Enema 4.0 grams/unit (60 mL)
Rectal Suppositories 500 mg

DESCRIPTION

The active ingredient in ROWASA® is mesalamine, also known as 5-aminosalicylic acid (5-ASA). Chemically, mesalamine is 5-amino-2-hydroxybenzoic acid, and is classified as an anti-inflammatory drug.
The empirical formula is $C_7H_7NO_3$, representing a molecular weight of 153.14. The structural formula is:

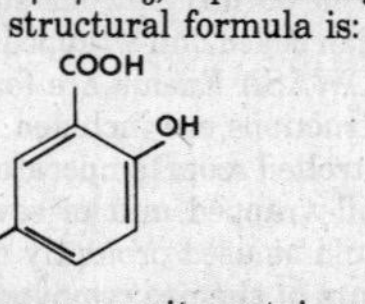

Each rectal suspension enema unit contains 4 grams of mesalamine. In addition to mesalamine the preparation contains the inactive ingredients potassium metabisulfite, carbomer 934P. edetate disodium, potassium acetate, water and xanthan gum. Sodium benzoate is added as a preservative. The disposable unit consists of an applicator tip protected by a polyethylene cover and lubricated with USP white petrolatum. The unit has a one-way valve to prevent back flow of the dispensed product.
Each ROWASA® suppository contains 500 mg of mesalamine in a base of Hard Fat, NF. Each suppository is individually wrapped in foil.

CLINICAL PHARMACOLOGY

Sulfasalazine is split by bacterial action in the colon into sulfapyridine (SP) and mesalamine (5-ASA). It is thought that the mesalamine component is therapeutically active in ulcerative colitis [A.K. Azad Khan et al, **Lancet** 2:892–895 (1977)]. The usual oral dose of sulfasalazine for active ulcerative colitis in adults is two to four grams per day in divided doses. Four grams of sulfasalazine provide 1.6 g of free mesalamine to the colon. Each ROWASA® suspension enema delivers up to 4 g of mesalamine to the left side of the colon. Each ROWASA® suppository delivers 500 mg of mesalamine to the rectum.
The mechanism of action of mesalamine (and sulfasalazine) is unknown, but appears to be topical rather than systemic. Mucosal production of arachidonic acid (AA) metabolites, both through the cyclooxygenase pathways, i.e., prostanoids, and through the lipoxygenase pathways, i.e., leukotrienes (LTs) and hydroxyeicosatetraenoic acids (HETEs) is increased in patients with chronic inflammatory bowel disease, and it is possible that mesalamine diminishes inflammation by blocking cyclooxygenase and inhibiting prostaglandin (PG) production in the colon.

Preclinical Toxicology

Preclinical studies have shown the kidney to be the major target organ for mesalamine toxicity. Adverse renal function changes were observed in rats after a single 600 mg/kg oral dose, but not after a 200 mg/kg dose. Gross kidney lesions, including papillary necrosis, were observed after a single oral > 900 mg/kg dose, and after i.v. doses of > 214 mg/kg. Mice responded similarly. In a 13-week oral (gavage) dose study in rats, the high dose of 640 mg/kg/day mesalamine caused deaths, probably due to renal failure, and dose-related renal lesions (papillary necrosis and/or multifocal tubular injury) were seen in most rats given the high dose (males and females) as well as in males receiving lower doses 160 mg/kg/day. Renal lesions were not observed in the 160 mg/kg/day female rats. Minimal tubular epithelial damage was seen in the 40 mg/kg/day males and was reversible. In a six-month oral study in dogs, the no-observable dose level of mesalamine was 40 mg/kg/day and doses of 80 mg/kg/day and higher caused renal pathology similar to that described for the rat. In a combined 52-week toxicity and 127-week carcinogenicity study in rats, degeneration in kidneys was observed at doses of 100 mg/kg/day and above admixed with diet for 52 weeks, and at 127 weeks increased incidence of kidney degeneration and hyalinization of basement membranes and Bowman's capsules was seen at 100 mg/kg/day and above. In the 12 month eye toxicity study in dogs, Keratoconjunctivitis Sicca (KCS) occurred at oral doses of 40 mg/kg/day and above. The oral preclinical studies were done with a highly bioavailable suspension where absorption throughout the gastrointestinal tract occurred. The human dose of 4 grams represents approximately 80 mg/kg but when mesalamine is given rectally as a suspension, absorption is poor and limited to the distal colon (see **Pharmacokinetics**). Overt renal toxicity has not been observed (see **ADVERSE REACTIONS** and **PRECAUTIONS**), but the potential must be considered.

EFFECT OF TREATMENT ON SEVERITY OF DISEASE
DATA FROM U.S.-CANADA TRIAL
COMBINED RESULTS OF EIGHT CENTERS
Activity Indices, mean

		N	Baseline	Day 22	End-Point	Change Baseline to End-Point†
Overall DAI	ROWASA®	76	7.42	4.05**	3.37***	−55.07%***
	Placebo	77	7.40	6.03	5.83	−21.58%
Stool Frequency	ROWASA®		1.58	1.11*	1.01**	−0.57*
	Placebo		1.92	1.47	1.50	−0.41
Rectal Bleeding	ROWASA®		1.82	0.59***	0.51***	−1.30***
	Placebo		1.73	1.21	1.11	−0.61
Mucosal inflammation	ROWASA®		2.17	1.22**	0.96***	−1.21**
	Placebo		2.18	1.74	1.61	−0.56
Physician's Assessment of Disease Severity	ROWASA®		1.86	1.13***	0.88***	−0.97***
	Placebo		1.87	1.62	1.55	−0.30

Each parameter has a 4-point scale with a numerical rating:
0 = normal, 1 = mild, 2 = moderate, 3 = severe. The four parameters are added together to produce a maximum overall DAI of 12.
† Percent change for overall DAI only (calculated by taking the average of the change for each individual patient).
* Significant ROWASA®/placebo difference. $p < 0.05$
** Significant ROWASA®/placebo difference. $p < 0.01$
*** Significant ROWASA®/placebo difference. $p < 0.001$

Pharmacokinetics

Mesalamine administered rectally as ROWASA® suspension enema is poorly absorbed from the colon and is excreted principally in the feces during subsequent bowel movements. The extent of absorption is dependent upon the retention time of the drug product, and there is considerable individual variation. At steady state, approximatey 10 to 30% of the daily 4-gram dose can be recovered in cumulative 24-hour urine collections. Other than the kidney, the organ distribution and other bioavailability characteristics of absorbed mesalamine in man are not known. It is known that the compound undergoes acetylation but whether this process takes place at colonic or systemic sites has not been elucidated. Whatever the metabolic site, most of the absorbed mesalamine is excreted in the urine as the N-acetyl-5-ASA metabolite. The poor colonic absorption of rectally administered mesalamine is substantiated by the low serum concentration of 5-ASA and N-acetyl-5-ASA seen in ulcerative colitis patients after dosage with mesalamine. Under clinical conditions patients demonstrated plasma levels 10 to 12 hours post mesalamine administration of 2 μg/mL, about two-thirds of which was the N-acetyl metabolite. While the elimination half-life of mesalamine is short (0.5 to 1.5 h), the acetylated metabolite exhibits a half-life of 5 to 10 hours [U. Klotz, **Clin. Pharmacokin.** 10:285–302 (1985)]. In addition, steady state plasma levels demonstrated a lack of accumulation of either free or metabolized drug during repeated daily administrations. Following single doses of ROWASA® 500 mg suppository in normal volunteers, 24-hr urines contained (only) N-acetyl-mesalamine equivalent to 15 to 38% (avg. 24%) of the administered dose. This is commensurate with the finding of 3 to 36% (avg. 10%) in urine in a study of ROWASA 4 g enema in normals. In that study, 40 to 107% (avg. 75%) of the administered dose was recovered in feces. At steady state in ulcerative colitis patients (N=38) being treated with ROWASA® Rectal Suspension, 24-hr urines contained 0 to 41% (avg. 8%) of the 4 g daily dose and plasma levels 10 to 12 hr post administration ranged from 0 to 2.1 mcg/mL (avg. 0.37 mcg/mL) of mesalamine equivalent (84% as N-acetyl metabolite). Multiple dose pharmacokinetic studies have not been conducted with ROWASA Suppository nor have plasma levels been reported from single dose studies.

Efficacy

ROWASA® Suspension Enema: In a placebo-controlled, international, multicenter trial of 153 patients with active distal ulcerative colitis, proctosigmoiditis or proctitis, ROWASA® suspension enema reduced the overall disease activity index (DAI) and individual components as follows: [See table above.]
Differences between ROWASA® and placebo were also statistically different in subgroups of patients on concurrent sulfasalazine and in those having an upper disease boundary between 5 and 20 or 20 and 40 cm. Significant differences between ROWASA® and placebo were not achieved in those subgroups of patients on concurrent prednisone or with an upper disease boundary between 40 and 50 cm.

ROWASA® Suppositories: Two double-blind placebo-controlled, multicenter studies were conducted in North America in patients with active ulcerative proctitis. The primary measures of efficacy were the same in both trials. The main difference between the two studies was the dosage regimen: 500 mg three times daily (1.5 g/d) in Study 1 and 500 mg twice daily (1.0 g/d) in Study 2. A total of 173 patients were studied (Study 1, N=79; Study 2, N=94) Patients were evaluated clinically and sigmoidoscopically after three and six weeks of suppository treatment.
Compared to placebo, ROWASA® (mesalamine) Suppository treatment was statistically ($p < .01$) superior in both trials with respect to stool frequency, rectal bleeding, mucosal appearance, disease severity and overall disease activity after both three and six weeks of treatment. Daily diary records indicated significant improvement in rectal bleeding in the first week of therapy while tenesmus and diarrhea improved significantly within two weeks. Investigators rated patients much improved in 84% and 79% with mesalamine in Studies 1 and 2, respectively compared to 41% and 26% with placebo ($p < .001$, $p < .001$).
Normalization of rectal mucosa was achieved by 62% and 60% of mesalamine treated patients in Studies 1 and 2 compared to 25% and 10% of placebo-treated patients ($p < .001$, $p < .001$). The effectiveness of ROWASA® Suppositories was statistically significant irrespective of sex, extent of proctitis, duration of current episode or duration of disease. Overall the efficacy demonstrated with the twice daily regimen (Study 2) was comparable to that observed with three times daily dosing (Study 1).

INDICATIONS AND USAGE

ROWASA® suspension enema is indicated for the treatment of active mild to moderate distal ulcerative colitis, proctosigmoiditis or proctitis.
ROWASA® Suppositories are indicated for the treatment of active ulcerative proctitis.

CONTRAINDICATIONS

ROWASA® suspension enema is contraindicated for patients known to have hypersensitivity to the drug or any component of this medication.
ROWASA® Suppositories are contraindicated for patients known to have hypersensitivity to mesalamine (5-aminosalicylic acid) or to the suppository vehicle [saturated vegetable fatty acid esters (Hard Fat, NF)].

WARNING

ROWASA® suspension enema contains potassium metabisulfite, a sulfite that may cause allergic-type reactions including anaphylactic symptoms and life-threatening or less severe asthmatic episodes in certain susceptible people. The overall prevalence of sulfite sensitivity in the general population is unknown but probably low. Sulfite sensitivity is seen more frequently in asthmatic or in atopic nonasthmatic persons. Epinephrine is the preferred treatment for serious allergic or emergency situations even though epinephrine injection contains sodium or potassium metabisulfite with the above-mentioned potential liabilities. The alternatives to using epinephrine in a life-threatening situation may not be satisfactory. The presence of a sulfite(s) in epinephrine injection should not deter the administration of the drug for treatment of serious allergic or other emergency situations.

PRECAUTIONS

Mesalamine has been implicated in the production of an acute intolerance syndrome characterized by cramping,

Continued on next page

Solvay—Cont.

acute abdominal pain and bloody diarrhea, sometimes fever, headache and a rash; in such cases prompt withdrawal is required. The patient's history of sulfasalazine intolerance, if any, should be re-evaluated. If a rechallenge is performed later in order to validate the hypersensitivity it should be carried out under close supervision and only if clearly needed, giving consideration to reduced dosage. In the literature one patient previously sensitive to sulfasalazine was rechallenged with 400 mg oral mesalamine, within eight hours she experienced headache, fever, intensive abdominal colic, profuse diarrhea and was readmitted as an emergency. She responded poorly to steroid therapy and two weeks later a pancolectomy was required.

Although renal abnormalities were not noted in the clinical trials with ROWASA® suspension enema, the possibility of increased absorption of mesalamine and concomitant renal tubular damage as noted in the preclinical studies must be kept in mind. Patients on ROWASA®, especially those on concurrent oral products which liberate mesalamine and those with preexisting renal disease, should be carefully monitored with urinalysis, BUN and creatinine studies.

In a clinical trial most patients who were hypersensitive to sulfasalazine were able to take mesalamine rectally without evidence of any allergic reaction. Nevertheless, caution should be exercised when mesalamine is initially used in patients known to be allergic to sulfasalazine. These patients should be instructed to discontinue therapy if signs of rash or fever become apparent.

While using ROWASA® some patients have developed pancolitis. However, extension of upper disease boundary and/or flare-ups occurred less often in the ROWASA-treated group than in the placebo-treated group.

Rare instances of pericarditis have been reported with mesalamine containing products including sulfasalazine. Cases of pericarditis have also been reported as manifestations of inflammatory bowel disease. In the cases reported with ROWASA® Rectal Suspension Enema there have been positive rechallenges with mesalamine or mesalamine containing products. In one of these cases, however, a second rechallenge with sulfasalazine was negative throughout a 2 month follow-up. Chest pain or dypsnea in patients treated with ROWASA® should be investigated with this information in mind. Discontinuation of ROWASA® may be warranted in some cases, but rechallenge with mesalamine can be performed under careful clinical observation should the continued therapeutic need for mesalamine be present.

Carcinogenesis, Mutagenesis, Impairment of Fertility

Mesalamine caused no increase in the incidence of neoplastic lesions over controls in a two-year study of Wistar rats fed up to 320 mg/kg/day of mesalamine admixed with diet. Mesalamine is not mutagenic to Salmonella typhimurium tester strains TA98, TA100, TA1535, TA1537, TA1538. There were no reverse mutations in an assay using E. coli strain WP2UVRA. There were no effects in an in vivo mouse micronucleus assay at 600 mg/kg and in an in vivo sister chromatid exchange at I.P. doses up to 610 mg/kg. No effects on fertility were observed in rats receiving oral doses up to 320 mg/kg/day. The oligospermia and infertility in men associated with sulfasalazine have not been reported with mesalamine.

Pregnancy (Category B)

Teratologic studies have been performed in rats and rabbits at oral doses of up to ten and sixteen times respectively, the maximum recommended human rectal suppository dose, and have revealed no evidence of harm to the embryo or the fetus. There are, however, no adequate and well controlled studies in pregnant women for either sulfasalazine or mesalamine. Because animal reproduction studies are not always predictive of human response, mesalamine should be used during pregnancy only if clearly needed.

Nursing Mothers

It is not known whether mesalamine or its metabolite(s) are excreted in human milk. As a general rule, nursing should not be undertaken while a patient is on a drug since many drugs are excreted in human milk.

Pediatric Use

Safety and effectiveness in pediatric patients have not been established.

ADVERSE REACTIONS

Clinical Adverse Experience

ROWASA Suspension Enema is usually well tolerated. Most adverse effects have been mild and transient.

ADVERSE REACTIONS OCCURRING IN MORE THAN 0.1% OF ROWASA® SUSPENSION ENEMA TREATED PATIENTS (COMPARISON TO PLACEBO)

	ROWASA (N=815)		PLACEBO (N=128)	
SYMPTOM	N	%	N	%
Abdominal Pain/Cramps/Discomfort	66	8.10	10	7.81
Headache	53	6.50	16	12.50
Gas/Flatulence	50	6.13	5	3.91
Nausea	47	5.77	12	9.38
Flu	43	5.28	1	0.78
Tired/Weak/Malaise/Fatigue	28	3.44	8	6.25
Fever	26	3.19	0	0.00
Rash/Spots	23	2.82	4	3.12
Cold/Sore Throat	19	2.33	9	7.03
Diarrhea	17	2.09	5	3.91
Leg/Joint Pain	17	2.09	1	0.78
Dizziness	15	1.84	3	2.34
Bloating	12	1.47	2	1.56
Back Pain	11	1.35	1	0.78
Pain on Insertion of Enema Tip	11	1.35	1	0.78
Hemorrhoids	11	1.35	0	0.00
Itching	10	1.23	1	0.78
Rectal Pain	10	1.23	0	0.00
Constipation	8	0.98	4	3.12
Hair Loss	7	0.86	0	0.00
Peripheral Edema	5	0.61	11	8.59
UTI/Urinary Burning	5	0.61	4	3.12
Rectal Pain/Soreness/Burning	5	0.61	3	2.34
Asthenia	1	0.12	4	3.12
Insomnia	1	0.12	3	2.34

ADVERSE REACTIONS OCCURRING IN MORE THAN 1% OF ROWASA SUPPOSITORY-TREATED PATIENTS (COMPARISON TO PLACEBO)

	ROWASA (N=168)		PLACEBO (N=84)	
SYMPTOM	N	%	N	%
Headache	11	6.5	10	11.9
Flatulence	6	3.6	6	7.1
Abdominal Pain	5	3.0	7	8.3
Diarrhea	5	3.0	5	6.0
Dizziness	5	3.0	2	2.4
Rectal Pain	3	1.8	0	0.0
Upper Resp. Infection	3	1.8	2	2.4
Acne	2	1.2	0	0.0
Asthenia	2	1.2	4	4.8
Colitis	2	1.2	0	0.0
Fever	2	1.2	0	0.0
Generalized Edema	2	1.2	1	1.2
Nausea	2	1.2	6	7.1
Rash	2	1.2	0	0.0

In addition, the following adverse events have been associated with ROWASA and other mesalamine containing products: nephrotoxicity, pancreatitis, fibrosing alveolitis and elevated liver enzymes. Cases of pancreatitis and fibrosing alveolitis have been reported as manifestations of inflammatory bowel disease as well.

Hair Loss

Mild hair loss characterized by "more hair in the comb" but no withdrawal from clinical trials has been observed in seven of 815 mesalamine patients but none of the placebo-treated patients. In the literature there are at least six additional patients with mild hair loss who received either mesalamine or sulfasalazine. Retreatment is not always associated with repeated hair loss.

OVERDOSAGE

There have been no documented reports of serious toxicity in man resulting from massive overdosing with mesalamine. Under ordinary circumstances, mesalamine absorption from the colon is limited.

DOSAGE AND ADMINISTRATION

ROWASA® Suspension Enema: The usual dosage of ROWASA® (mesalamine) suspension enema in 60 mL units is one rectal instillation (4 grams) once a day, preferably at bedtime, and retained for approximately eight hours. While the effect of ROWASA® (mesalamine) may be seen within three to twenty-one days, the usual course of therapy would be from three to six weeks depending on symptoms and sigmoidoscopic findings. Studies available to date have not assessed if ROWASA® suspension enema will modify relapse rates after the 6-week short-term treatment.

Patients should be instructed to shake the bottle well to make sure the suspension is homogeneous. The patient should remove the protective sheath from the applicator tip. Holding the bottle at the neck will not cause any of the medication to be discharged. The position most often used is obtained by lying on the left side (to facilitate migration into the sigmoid colon); with the lower leg extended and the upper right leg flexed forward for balance. An alternative is the knee-chest position. The applicator tip should be gently inserted in the rectum pointing toward the umbilicus. A steady squeezing of the bottle will discharge most of the preparation. The preparation should be taken at bedtime with the objective of retaining it all night. Patient instructions are included with every seven units.

ROWASA® Suppositories: The usual dosage of ROWASA® Suppositories 500 mg is one rectal suppository 2 times daily. The suppository should be retained for one to three hours or longer, if possible, to achieve the maximum benefit. While the effect of ROWASA® Suppositories may be seen within three to twenty-one days, the usual course of therapy would be from three to six weeks depending on symptoms and sigmoidoscopic findings. Studies available to date have not assessed if ROWASA® Suppositories will modify relapse rates after the six-week short-term treatment.

Patient Instructions:

1. Detach one suppository from strip of suppositories.
2. Hold suppository upright and carefully remove the foil wrapper.
3. Avoid excessive handling of suppository, which is designed to melt at body temperature.
4. Insert suppository completely into rectum with gentle pressure, pointed end first.

HOW SUPPLIED

ROWASA® Suspension Enema: ROWASA® suspension for rectal administration is an off-white to tan colored suspension. Each disposable enema bottle contains 4.0 grams of mesalamine in 60 mL aqueous suspension. Enema bottles are supplied in boxed, foil-wrapped trays of seven (NDC 0032-1924-82). ROWASA Enema are for rectal use only.

Patient instructions are included.

Store at controlled room temperature 15° to 30°C (59° to 86°F). Once the foil-wrapped unit of seven bottles is opened, all enemas should be used promptly as directed by your physician. **Contents of enemas removed from the foil pouch may darken with time. Slight darkening will not affect potency, however enemas with dark brown contents should be discarded.**

ROWASA® Suppositories: ROWASA® Suppositories for rectal administration are available as bullet-shaped, light tan suppositories containing 500 mg mesalamine supplied in boxes of 12 (NDC 0032-1928-46) or boxes of 24 (NDC 0032-1928-24) individually foil-wrapped suppositories. Patient instructions are on back of boxes. Store at 19° to 26°C (66°–79°F).

NOTE: ROWASA® will cause staining of direct contact surfaces, including but not limited to fabrics, flooring, painted surfaces, marble, granite, vinyl, and enamel. Take care in choosing a suitable location for administration of this product.

CAUTION: Federal law prohibits dispensing without prescription.

ROWASA® Suspension Enema
Manufactured and Marketed By:
Solvay Pharmaceuticals, Inc.
Marietta, GA 30062
ROWASA® Suppository
Manufactured By:
G & W Laboratories Inc.
South Plainfield, NJ 07080
Marketed By:
Solvay Pharmaceuticals, Inc
Marietta, GA 30062

REV 9/95

Shown in Product Identification Guide, page 338

Advanced Formula ZENATE® ℞
[*ze 'nāt*]
Prenatal Multivitamin/Mineral Supplement Tablets

DESCRIPTION

Each film-coated tablet contains:

Vitamins:

A*	3,000 I.U.
D (as cholecalciferol)	400 I.U.
E (as dl-alpha tocopheryl acetate)	10 I.U.
C (ascorbic acid)	70 mg
Folic Acid	1 mg
B_1 (as thiamine mononitrate)	1.5 mg
B_2 (riboflavin)	1.6 mg
Niacin (as niacinamide)	17 mg
B_6 (as pyridoxine hydrochloride)	2.2 mg
B_{12} (cyanocobalamin)	2.2 mcg

Minerals:

Calcium (from calcium carbonate)	200 mg
Iodine (from potassium iodide)	175 mcg
Iron (from ferrous fumarate)	65 mg
Magnesium (from magnesium oxide)	100 mg
Zinc (from zinc oxide)	15 mg

*Input as rentinylpalmitate and beta-carotene

Inactive Ingredients: Amorphous Precipitated Silica, Aqueous Shellac, Croscarmellose Sodium, Crospovidone, Hydrogenated Soybean Oil, Hydrogenated Castor Oil, Hydroxypropyl Cellulose, Hydroxypropyl Methylcellulose, Magnesium Stearate, Polyethylene Glycol, Polysorbate 80, Powdered Cellulose, Pregelatinized Starch, and Titanium Dioxide.

INDICATIONS AND USAGE

As a dietary adjunct in nutritional stress associated with periconception, pregnancy and lactation.

CONTRAINDICATIONS

This product is contraindicated in patients with a known hypersensitivity to any of the ingredients.

WARNINGS

As with all medications, keep out of the reach of children. Contains iron, which can be harmful or fatal to children if taken in large doses. In case of accidental overdose, seek professional assistance or contact a Poison Control Center immediately.

PRECAUTIONS

Folic Acid may obscure pernicious anemia, in that hematologic remission can occur while neurologic manifestations remain progressive.

Pediatric Use: Safety and effectiveness in pediatric patients have not been established.

ADVERSE REACTIONS

Allergic sensitization has been reported following both oral and parenteral administration of folic acid.

DOSAGE AND ADMINISTRATION

One tablet daily or as directed by physician.

HOW SUPPLIED

Advanced Formula ZENATE® Tablets are white, film-coated, scored, capsule-shaped tablets debossed SOLVAY on one side and 1472 on the other and supplied in bottles of 100 tablets (NDC 0032-1472-01).

Store at controlled room temperature, 15°–30°C (59°–86°F). Dispense in tight, light-resistant container with child resistant closure.

CAUTION: Federal law prohibits dispensing without prescription.

SOLVAY PHARMACEUTICALS
MARIETTA, GA 30062
2E1030 Rev 5/96

Shown in Product Identification Guide, page 338

Somerset Pharmaceuticals, Inc.

5215 WEST LAUREL STREET
TAMPA, FLORIDA 33607

For Medical Information Contact:
Generally:
Professional Services Department
(813) 288-0040
FAX: (813) 282-0085
In Emergencies:
Cheryl D. Blume, Ph.D.
(800) 892-8889
FAX: (813) 282-0085

ELDEPRYL® ℞
(SELEGILINE HYDROCHLORIDE)
CAPSULES

DESCRIPTION

ELDEPRYL (selegiline hydrochloride) is a levorotatory acetylenic derivative of phenethylamine. It is commonly referred to in the clinical and pharmacological literature as l-deprenyl.

The chemical name is: (R)-(-)-N,2-dimethyl-N-2-propynylphenethylamine hydrochloride. It is a white to near white crystalline powder, freely soluble in water, chloroform, and methanol, and has a molecular weight of 223.75. The structural formula is as follows:

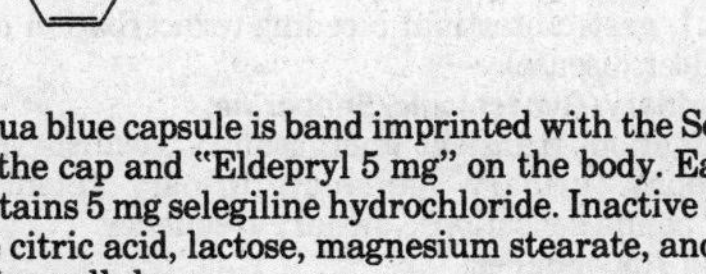

Each aqua blue capsule is band imprinted with the Somerset logo on the cap and "Eldepryl 5 mg" on the body. Each capsule contains 5 mg selegiline hydrochloride. Inactive ingredients are citric acid, lactose, magnesium stearate, and microcrystalline cellulose.

CLINICAL PHARMACOLOGY

The mechanisms accounting for selegiline's beneficial adjunctive action in the treatment of Parkinson's disease are not fully understood. Inhibition of monoamine oxidase, type B, activity is generally considered to be of primary importance; in addition, there is evidence that selegiline may act through other mechanisms to increase dopaminergic activity.

Selegiline is best known as an irreversible inhibitor of monoamine oxidase (MAO), an intracellular enzyme associated with the outer membrane of mitochondria. Selegiline inhibits MAO by acting as a 'suicide' substrate for the enzyme; that is, it is converted by MAO to an active moiety which combines irreversibly with the active site and/or the enzyme's essential FAD cofactor. Because selegiline has greater affinity for type B rather than for type A active sites, it can serve as a selective inhibitor of MAO type B if it is administered at the recommended dose.

MAOs are widely distributed throughout the body; their concentration is especially high in liver, kidney, stomach, intestinal wall, and brain. MAOs are currently subclassified into two types, A and B, which differ in their substrate specificity and tissue distribution. In humans, intestinal MAO is predominantly type A, while most of that in brain is type B. In CNS neurons, MAO plays an important role in the catabolism of catecholamines (dopamine, norepinephrine and epinephrine) and serotonin. MAOs are also important in the catabolism of various exogenous amines found in a variety of foods and drugs. MAO in the GI tract and liver (primarily type A), for example, is thought to provide vital protection from exogenous amines (e.g., tyramine) that have the capacity, if absorbed intact, to cause a 'hypertensive crisis', the so-called 'cheese reaction.' (If large amounts of certain exogenous amines gain access to the systemic circulation —e.g., from fermented cheese, red wine, herring, over-the-counter cough/cold medications, etc.—they are taken up by adrenergic neurons and displace norepinephrine from storage sites within membrane bound vesicles. Subsequent release of the displaced norepinephrine causes the rise in systemic blood pressure, etc.)

In theory, since MAO A of the gut is not inhibited, patients treated with selegiline at a dose of 10 mg a day should be able to take medications containing pharmacologically active amines and consume tyramine-containing foods without risk of uncontrolled hypertension. However, one case of hypertensive crisis has been reported in a patient taking the recommended dose of selegiline and a sympathomimetic medication (ephedrine). The pathophysiology of the 'cheese reaction' is complicated and, in addition to its ability to inhibit MAO B selectively, selegiline's relative freedom from this reaction has been attributed to an ability to prevent tyramine and other indirect acting sympathomimetics from displacing norepinephrine from adrenergic neurons. However, until the pathophysiology of the cheese reaction is more completely understood, it seems prudent to assume that selegiline can ordinarily only be used safely without dietary restrictions at doses where it presumably selectively inhibits MAO B (e.g., 10 mg/day).

In short, attention to the dose dependent nature of selegiline's selectivity is critical if it is to be used without elaborate restrictions being placed on diet and concomitant drug use although, as noted above, a case of hypertensive crisis has been reported at the recommended dose. (See WARNINGS and PRECAUTIONS.)

It is important to be aware that selegiline may have pharmacological effects unrelated to MAO B inhibition. As noted above, there is some evidence that it may increase dopaminergic activity by other mechanisms, including interfering with dopamine re-uptake at the synapse. Effects resulting from selegiline administration may also be mediated through its metabolites. Two of its three principal metabolites, amphetamine and methamphetamine, have pharmacological actions of their own; they interfere with neuronal uptake and enhance release of several neurotransmitters (e.g., norepinephrine, dopamine, serotonin). However, the extent to which these metabolites contribute to the effects of selegiline are unknown.

Rationale for the Use of a Selective Monoamine Oxidase Type B Inhibitor in Parkinson's Disease: Many of the prominent symptoms of Parkinson's disease are due to a deficiency of striatal dopamine that is the consequence of a progressive degeneration and loss of a population of dopaminergic neurons which originate in the substantia nigra of the midbrain and project to the basal ganglia or striatum. Early in the course of Parkinson's Disease, the deficit in the capacity of these neurons to synthesize dopamine can be overcome by administration of exogenous levodopa, usually given in combination with a peripheral decarboxylase inhibitor (carbidopa).

With the passage of time, due to the progression of the disease and/or the effect of sustained treatment, the efficacy and quality of the therapeutic response to levodopa diminishes. Thus, after several years of levodopa treatment, the response, for a given dose of levodopa, is shorter, has less predictable onset and offset (i.e., there is 'wearing off'), and is often accompanied by side effects (e.g., dyskinesia, akinesias, on-off phenomena, freezing, etc.).

This deteriorating response is currently interpreted as a manifestation of the inability of the ever decreasing population of intact nigrostriatal neurons to synthesize and release adequate amounts of dopamine.

MAO B inhibition may be useful in this setting because, by blocking the catabolism of dopamine, it would increase the net amount of dopamine available (i.e., it would increase the pool of dopamine). Whether or not this mechanism or an alternative one actually accounts for the observed beneficial effects of adjunctive selegiline is unknown.

Selegiline's benefit in Parkinson's disease has only been documented as an adjunct to levodopa/carbidopa. Whether or not it might be effective as a sole treatment is unknown, but past attempts to treat Parkinson's disease with non-selective MAOI monotherapy are reported to have been unsuccessful. It is important to note that attempts to treat Parkinsonian patients with combinations of levodopa and currently marketed non-selective MAO inhibitors were abandoned because of multiple side effects including hypertension, increase in involuntary movement, and toxic delirium.

Pharmacokinetic Information (Absorption, Distribution, Metabolism and Elimination—ADME):

The absolute bioavailability of selegiline following oral dosing is not known; however, selegiline undergoes extensive metabolism (presumably attributable to presystemic clearance in gut and liver). The major plasma metabolites are N-desmethylselegiline, L-amphetamine and L-methamphetamine. Only N-desmethylselegiline has MAO-B inhibiting activity. The peak plasma levels of these metabolites following a single oral dose of 10 mg are from 4 to almost 20 times greater than that of the maximum plasma concentration of selegiline [1 ng/mL]. The maximum concentrations of amphetamine and methamphetamine, however, are far below those ordinarily expected to produce clinically important effects.

Single oral dose studies do not predict multiple dose kinetics, however. At steady state the peak plasma level of selegiline is 4 fold that obtained following a single dose. Metabolite concentrations increase to a lesser extent, averaging 2 fold that seen after a single dose.

The bioavailability of selegiline is increased 3 to 4 fold when it is taken with food.

The extent of systemic exposure to selegiline at a given dose varies considerably among individuals. Estimates of systemic clearance of selegiline are not available. Following a single oral dose, the mean elimination half-life of selegiline is two hours. Under steady state conditions the elimination half-life increases to ten hours.

Because selegiline's inhibition of MAO-B is irreversible, it is impossible to predict the extent of MAO-B inhibition from steady state plasma levels. For the same reason, it is not possible to predict the rate of recovery of MAO-B activity as a function of plasma levels. The recovery of MAO-B activity is a function of de novo protein synthesis; however, information about the rate of de novo protein synthesis is not yet available. Although platelet MAO-B activity returns to the normal range within 5 to 7 days of selegiline discontinuation, the linkage between platelet and brain MAO-B inhibition is not fully understood nor is the relationship of MAO-B inhibition to the clinical effect established (see Clinical Pharmacology).

Special Populations:

Renal Impairment:
No pharmacokinetic information is available on selegiline or its metabolites in renally impaired subjects.

Hepatic Impairment:
No pharmacokinetic information is available on selegiline or its metabolites in hepatically impaired subjects.

Age:
Although a general conclusion about the effects of age on the pharmacokinetics of selegiline is not warranted because of the size of the sample evaluated (12 subjects greater than 60 years of age, 12 subjects between the ages of 18 to 30), systemic exposure was about twice as great in older as compared to a younger population given a single oral dose of 10 mg.

Gender:
No information is available on the effects of gender on the pharmacokinetics of selegiline.

INDICATIONS AND USAGE

ELDEPRYL is indicated as an adjunct in the management of Parkinsonian patients being treated with levodopa/carbidopa who exhibit deterioration in the quality of their response to this therapy. There is no evidence from controlled studies that selegiline has any beneficial effect in the absence of concurrent levodopa therapy.

Evidence supporting this claim was obtained in randomized controlled clinical investigations that compared the effects of added selegiline or placebo in patients receiving levodopa/carbidopa. Selegiline was significantly superior to placebo on all three principal outcome measures employed: change from baseline in daily levodopa/carbidopa dose, the amount of 'off' time, and patient self-rating of treatment success. Beneficial effects were also observed on other measures of treatment success (e.g., measures of reduced end of dose akinesia, decreased tremor and sialorrhea, improved speech

Continued on next page

Somerset—Cont.

and dressing ability and improved overall disability as assessed by walking and comparison to previous state).

CONTRAINDICATIONS

ELDEPRYL is contraindicated in patients with a known hypersensitivity to this drug.
ELDEPRYL is contraindicated for use with meperidine (DEMEROL & other trade names). This contraindication is often extended to other opioids. (See Drug Interactions.)

WARNINGS

Selegiline should not be used at daily doses exceeding those recommended (10 mg/day) because of the risks associated with non-selective inhibition of MAO. (See CLINICAL PHARMACOLOGY.)
The selectivity of selegiline for MAO B may not be absolute even at the recommended daily dose of 10 mg a day and selectivity is further diminished with increasing daily doses. The precise dose at which selegiline becomes a non-selective inhibitor of all MAO is unknown, but may be in the range of 30 to 40 mg a day.
Severe CNS toxicity associated with hyperpyrexia and death have been reported with the combination of tricyclic antidepressants and non-selective MAOIs (NARDIL, PARNATE). A similar reaction has been reported for a patient on amitriptyline and ELDEPRYL. Another patient receiving protriptyline and ELDEPRYL developed tremors, agitation, and restlessness followed by unresponsiveness and death two weeks after ELDEPRYL was added. Related adverse events including hypertension, syncope, asystole, diaphoresis, seizures, changes in behavioral and mental status, and muscular rigidity have also been reported in some patients receiving ELDEPRYL and various tricyclic antidepressants.
Serious, sometimes fatal, reactions with signs and symptoms that may include hyperthermia, rigidity, myoclonus, autonomic instability with rapid fluctuations of the vital signs, and mental status changes that include extreme agitation progressing to delirium and coma have been reported with patients receiving a combination of fluoxetine hydrochloride (PROZAC) and non-selective MAOIs. Similar signs have been reported in some patients on the combination of ELDEPRYL (10 mg a day) and selective serotonin reuptake inhibitors including fluoxetine, sertraline and paroxetine.
Since the mechanisms of these reactions are not fully understood, it seems prudent, in general, to avoid this combination of ELDEPRYL and tricyclic antidepressants as well as ELDEPRYL and selective serotonin reuptake inhibitors. At least 14 days should elapse between discontinuation of ELDEPRYL and initiation of treatment with a tricyclic antidepressant or selective serotonin reuptake inhibitors. Because of the long half-lives of fluoxetine and its active metabolite, at least five weeks (perhaps longer, especially if fluoxetine has been prescribed chronically and/or at higher doses) should elapse between discontinuation of fluoxetine and initiation of treatment with ELDEPRYL.

PRECAUTIONS

General:
Some patients given selegiline may experience an exacerbation of levodopa associated side effects, presumably due to the increased amounts of dopamine reaction with super sensitive, post-synaptic receptors. These effects may often be mitigated by reducing the dose of levodopa/carbidopa by approximately 10 to 30%.
The decision to prescribe selegiline should take into consideration that the MAO system of enzymes is complex and incompletely understood and there is only a limited amount of carefully documented clinical experience with selegiline. Consequently, the full spectrum of possible responses to selegiline may not have been observed in pre-marketing evaluation of the drug. It is advisable, therefore, to observe patients closely for atypical responses.
Information for Patients:
Patients should be advised of the possible need to reduce levodopa dosage after the initiation of ELDEPRYL therapy.
Patients (or their families if the patient is incompetent) should be advised not to exceed the daily recommended dose of 10 mg. The risk of using higher daily doses of selegiline should be explained, and a brief description of the 'cheese reaction' provided. While hypertensive reactions with selegiline associated with dietary influences have not been reported, documented experience is limited.
Consequently, it may be useful to inform patients (or their families) about the signs and symptoms associated with MAOI induced hypertensive reactions. In particular, patients should be urged to report, immediately, any severe headache or other atypical or unusual symptoms not previously experienced.
Laboratory Tests:
No specific laboratory tests are deemed essential for the management of patients on ELDEPRYL. Periodic routine evaluation of all patients, however, is appropriate.
Drug Interactions:
The occurrence of stupor, muscular rigidity, severe agitation, and elevated temperature has been reported in some patients receiving the combination of selegiline and meperidine. Symptoms usually resolve over days when the combination is discontinued. This is typical of the interaction of meperidine and MAOIs. Other serious reactions (including severe agitation, hallucinations, and death) have been reported in patients receiving this combination (see **CONTRAINDICATIONS**). Severe toxicity has also been reported in patients receiving the combination of tricyclic antidepressants and ELDEPRYL and selective serotonin reuptake inhibitors and ELDEPRYL. (See **WARNINGS** for details.) One case of hypertensive crisis has been reported in a patient taking the recommended doses of selegiline and a sympathomimetic medication (ephedrine).
Carcinogenesis, Mutagenesis, and Impairment of Fertility:
Assessment of the carcinogenic potential of selegiline in mice and rats is ongoing. Selegiline did not induce mutations or chromosomal damage when tested in the bacterial mutation assay in Salmonella typhimurium and in an in vivo chromosomal aberration assay. While these studies provide some reassurance that selegiline is not mutagenic or clastogenic, they are not definitive because of methodological limitations. No definitive in vitro chromosomal aberration or in vitro mammalian gene mutation assays have been performed.
The effect of selegiline on fertility has not been adequately assessed.
Pregnancy:
Pregnancy Category C: No teratogenic effects were observed in a study of embryo-fetal development in Sprague-Dawley rats at oral doses of 4, 12, and 36 mg/kg or 4, 12 and 35 times the human therapeutic dose on a mg/m2 basis. No teratogenic effects were observed in a study of embryo-fetal development in New Zealand White rabbits at oral doses of 5, 25, and 50 mg/kg or 10, 48, and 95 times the human therapeutic dose on a mg/m2 basis; however, in this study, the number of litters produced at the two higher doses was less than reccmmended for assessing teratogenic potential. In the rat study, there was a decrease in fetal body weight at the highest dose tested. In the rabbit study, increases in total resorptions and % post-implantation loss, and a decrease in the number of live fetuses per dam occurred at the highest dose tested. In a peri- and postnatal development study in Sprague-Dawley rats (oral doses of 4, 16, and 64 mg/kg or 4, 15, and 62 times the human therapeutic dose on a mg/m2 basis), an increase in the number of stillbirths and decreases in the number of pups per dam, pup survival, and pup body weight (at birth and throughout the lactation period) were observed at the two highest doses. At the highest dose tested, no pups born alive survived to Day 4 postpartum. Postnatal development at the highest dose tested in dams could not be evaluated because of the lack of surviving pups. The reproductive performance of the untreated offspring was not assessed. There are no adequate and well-controlled studies in pregnant women. Selegiline should be used during pregnancy only if the potential benefit justifies the potential risk to the fetus.
Nursing Mothers:
It is not known whether selegiline hydrochloride is excreted in human milk. Because many drugs are excreted in human milk, consideration should be given to discontinuing the use of all but absolutely essential drug treatments in nursing women.
Pediatric Use:
The effects of selegiline hydrochloride in children have not been evaluated.

ADVERSE REACTIONS

Introduction:
The number of patients who received selegiline in prospectively monitored pre-marketing studies is limited. While other sources of information about the use of selegiline are available (e.g., literature reports, foreign post-marketing reports, etc.) they do not provide the kind of information necessary to estimate the incidence of adverse events. Thus, overall incidence figures for adverse reactions associated with the use of selegiline cannot be provided. Many of the adverse reactions seen have also been reported as symptoms of dopamine excess.
Moreover, the importance and severity of various reactions reported often cannot be ascertained. One index of relative importance, however, is whether or not a reaction caused treatment discontinuation. In prospective pre-marketing studies, the following events led, in decreasing order of frequency, to discontinuation of treatment with selegiline: nausea, hallucinations, confusion, depression, loss of balance, insomnia, orthostatic hypotension, increased akinetic involuntary movements, agitation, arrhythmia, bradykinesia, chorea, delusions, hypertension, new or increased angina pectoris, and syncope. Events reported only once as a cause of discontinuation are ankle edema, anxiety, burning lips/mouth, constipation, drowsiness/lethargy, dystonia, excess perspiration, increased freezing, gastrointestinal bleeding, hair loss, increased tremor, nervousness, weakness, and weight loss.
Experience with ELDEPRYL obtained in parallel, placebo controlled, randomized studies provides only a limited basis for estimates of adverse reaction rates. The following reactions that occurred with greater frequency among the 49 patients assigned to selegiline as compared to the 50 patients assigned to placebo in the only parallel, placebo controlled trial performed in patients with Parkinson's disease are shown in the following Table. None of these adverse reactions led to a discontinuation of treatment.

INCIDENCE OF TREATMENT-EMERGENT ADVERSE EXPERIENCES IN THE PLACEBO-CONTROLLED CLINICAL TRIAL

Adverse Event	Number of Patients Reporting Events selegiline hydrochloride N=49	placebo N=50
Nausea	10	3
Dizziness/Lighthead/Fainting	7	1
Abdominal Pain	4	2
Confusion	3	0
Hallucinations	3	1
Dry mouth	3	1
Vivid Dreams	2	0
Dyskinesias	2	5
Headache	2	1
The following events were reported once in either or both groups		
Ache, generalized	1	0
Anxiety/Tension	1	1
Anemia	0	1
Diarrhea	1	0
Hair Loss	0	1
Insomnia	1	1
Lethargy	1	0
Leg pain	1	0
Low back pain	1	0
Malaise	0	1
Palpitations	1	0
Urinary Retention	1	0
Weight Loss	1	0

In all prospectively monitored clinical investigations, enrolling approximately 920 patients, the following adverse events, classified by body system, were reported.
Central Nervous System:
Motor/Coordination/Extrapyramidal:
increased tremor, chorea, loss of balance, restlessness, blepharospasm, increased bradykinesia, facial grimace, falling down, heavy leg, muscle twitch*, myoclonic jerks*, stiff neck, tardive dyskinesia, dystonic symptoms, dyskinesia, involuntary movements, freezing, festination, increased apraxia, muscle cramps.
Mental Status/Behavioral/Psychiatric:
hallucinations, dizziness, confusion, anxiety, depression, drowsiness, behavior/mood change, dreams/nightmares, tiredness, delusions, disorientation, lightheadedness, impaired memory*, increased energy*, transient high*, hollow feeling, lethargy/malaise, apathy, overstimulation, vertigo, personality change, sleep disturbance, restlessness, weakness, transient irritability.
Pain/Altered Sensation:
headache, back pain, leg pain, tinnitus, migraine, supraorbital pain, throat burning, generalized ache, chills, numbness of toes/fingers, taste disturbance.
Autonomic Nervous System:
dry mouth, blurred vision, sexual dysfunction.
Cardiovascular:
orthostatic hypotension, hypertension, arrhythmia, palpitations, new or increased angina pectoris, hypotension, tachycardia, peripheral edema, sinus bradycardia, syncope.
Gastrointestinal:
nausea/vomiting, constipation, weight loss, anorexia, poor appetite, dysphagia, diarrhea, heartburn, rectal bleeding, bruxism*, gastrointestinal bleeding (exacerbation of preexisting ulcer disease).
Genitourinary/Gynecologic/Endocrine:
slow urination, transient anorgasmia*, nocturia, prostatic hypertrophy, urinary hesitancy, urinary retention, decreased penile sensation*, urinary frequency.
Skin and Appendages:
increased sweating, diaphoresis, facial hair, hair loss, hematoma, rash, photosensitivity.
Miscellaneous:
asthma, diplopia, shortness of breath, speech affected.
Postmarketing Reports:
The following experiences were described in spontaneous post-marketing reports. These reports do not provide suffi-

cient information to establish a clear causal relationship with the use of ELDEPRYL.

CNS:

Seizure in dialyzed chronic renal failure patient on concomitant medications.

* indicates events reported only at doses greater than 10 mg/day.

OVERDOSAGE

Selegiline:

No specific information is available about clinically significant overdoses with ELDEPRYL. However, experience gained during selegiline's development reveals that some individuals exposed to doses of 600 mg of d,l-selegiline suffered severe hypotension and psychomotor agitation.

Since the selective inhibition of MAO B by selegiline hydrochloride is achieved only at doses in the range recommended for the treatment of Parkinson's disease (e.g., 10 mg/day), overdoses are likely to cause significant inhibition of both MAO A and MAO B. Consequently, the signs and symptoms of overdose may resemble those observed with marketed non-selective MAO inhibitors [e.g., tranylcypromine (PARNATE), isocarboxazide (MARPLAN), and phenelzine (NARDIL)].

Overdose with Non-Selective MAO Inhibition:

NOTE: This section is provided for reference; it does not describe events that have actually been observed with selegiline in overdose.

Characteristically, signs and symptoms of non-selective MAOI overdose may not appear immediately. Delays of up to 12 hours between ingestion of drug and the appearance of signs may occur. Importantly, the peak intensity of the syndrome may not be reached for upwards of a day following the overdose. Death has been reported following overdosage. Therefore, immediate hospitalization, with continuous patient observation and monitoring for a period of at least two days following the ingestion of such drugs in overdose, is strongly recommended.

The clinical picture of MAOI overdose varies considerably; its severity may be a function of the amount of drug consumed. The central nervous and cardiovascular systems are prominently involved.

Signs and symptoms of overdosage may include, alone or in combination, any of the following: drowsiness, dizziness, faintness, irritability, hyperactivity, agitation, severe headache, hallucinations, trismus, opisthotonos, convulsions, and coma; rapid and irregular pulse, hypertension, hypotension and vascular collapse; precordial pain, respiratory depression and failure, hyperpyrexia, diaphoresis, and cool, clammy skin.

Treatment Suggestions For Overdose:

NOTE: Because there is no recorded experience with selegiline overdose, the following suggestions are offered based upon the assumption that selegiline overdose may be modeled by non-selective MAOI poisoning. In any case, up-to-date information about the treatment of overdose can often be obtained from a certified Regional Poison Control Center. Telephone numbers of certified Poison Control Centers are listed in the Physicians' Desk Reference (PDR).

Treatment of overdose with non-selective MAOIs is symptomatic and supportive. Induction of emesis or gastric lavage with instillation of charcoal slurry may be helpful in early poisoning, provided the airway has been protected against aspiration. Signs and symptoms of central nervous system stimulation, including convulsions, should be treated with diazepam, given slowly intravenously. Phenothiazine derivatives and central nervous system stimulants should be avoided. Hypotension and vascular collapse should be treated with intravenous fluids and, if necessary, blood pressure titration with an intravenous infusion of a dilute pressor agent. It should be noted that adrenergic agents may produce a markedly increased pressor response.

Respiration should be supported by appropriate measures, including management of the airway, use of supplemental oxygen, and mechanical ventilatory assistance, as required. Body temperature should be monitored closely. Intensive management of hyperpyrexia may be required. Maintenance of fluid and electrolyte balance is essential.

DOSAGE AND ADMINISTRATION

ELDEPRYL is intended for administration to Parkinsonian patients receiving levodopa/carbidopa therapy who demonstrate a deteriorating response to this treatment. The recommended regimen for the administration of ELDEPRYL is 10 mg per day administered as divided doses of 5 mg each taken at breakfast and lunch. There is no evidence that additional benefit will be obtained from the administration of higher doses. Moreover, higher doses should ordinarily be avoided because of the increased risk of side effects.

After two to three days of selegiline treatment, an attempt may be made to reduce the dose of levodopa/carbidopa. A reduction of 10 to 30% was achieved with the typical participant in the domestic placebo controlled trials who was assigned to selegiline treatment. Further reductions of

levodopa/carbidopa may be possible during continued selegiline therapy.

HOW SUPPLIED

ELDEPRYL capsules are available containing 5 mg of selegiline hydrochloride. Each aqua blue capsule is band imprinted with the Somerset logo on the cap and "Eldepryl 5 mg" on the body.

They are available as:
NDC 39506-022-60 bottles of 60 capsules.
NDC 39506-022-30 bottles of 300 capsules.

Store at controlled room temperature, 59° to 86°F (15° to 30°C).

CAUTION—Federal (USA) law prohibits dispensing without prescription.

Tampa, FL 33607

Literature issued May 1996

ELD:R9

Shown in Product Identification Guide, page 338

Speywood Pharmaceuticals, Inc.
27 MAPLE STREET
MILFORD, MA 01757-3650

Direct Inquiries to:
Customer Service:
(508) 478-8900
Educational Information:
(508) 478-8900
For Medical Information Contact:
In Emergencies:
(800) 456-7322
Sales and Ordering:
(800) 456-7322
Reimbursement Services:
(800) 334-1142

HYATE:C® ℞
Antihemophilic Factor (Porcine)

DESCRIPTION

Antihemophilic Factor (Porcine)—HYATE:C® is a highly purified sterile freeze-dried concentrate of porcine antihemophilic factor (Factor VIII:C) in the form of a white lyophilized powder for reconstitution.

HOW SUPPLIED

Antihemophilic Factor (Porcine)—HYATE:C® is supplied in vials containing between 400–700 porcine units of Factor VIII:C, to be reconstituted with 20mL Sterile Water for Injection U.S.P. (not supplied).

1 Vial   NDC 55688-106-02

Manufactured by:
Speywood Biopharm Ltd.
Ash Road, Wrexham Industrial Estate
Wrexham, Clwyd LL13 9UF
United Kingdom
Tel. 978 661181
US License #1014

Distributed by:
Speywood Pharmaceuticals, Inc.
27 Maple Street
Milford, MA 01757-3650
Tel: (508) 478-8900
FAX (508) 478-1883

For customer service or medical emergency contact:
(508) 478-8900
For HYATE: C Reimbursement Services contact (800) 334-1142

EDUCATIONAL MATERIAL

Educational Information concerning Factor VIII Inhibitors or Acquired Hemophilia is available free of charge. Please call or write Speywood Pharmaceuticals, Inc.

Star Pharmaceuticals, Inc.
1990 N.W. 44TH STREET
POMPANO BEACH, FL 33064-8712

Direct Inquiries to:
Scott L. Davidson, President
(954) 971-9704
For Medical Information Contact:
Scott L. Davidson
(800) 845-7827
Sales and Ordering:
(800) 845-7827
FAX: (954) 971-7718

APHRODYNE® ℞
[af"ro-din']
brand of yohimbine hydrochloride

Each scored aqua caplet contains 5.4 mg yohimbine hydrochloride.

HOW SUPPLIED

Bottles of 100 and 1000.
NDC 0076-0401-03 and 04

PROSED®/DS ℞
Tablets/Double Strength

Each dark blue, round sugar-coated tablet contains:

Methenamine	81.6 mg.
Phenyl Salicylate	36.2 mg.
Methylene Blue	10.8 mg.
Benzoic Acid	9.0 mg.
Atropine Sulfate	0.06 mg.
Hyoscyamine Sulfate	0.06 mg.

HOW SUPPLIED

Bottles of 100 and 1000
NDC 0076-0108-03 & 04

URO–KP–NEUTRAL® ℞
[ū'ro-kp-nū'tral]
Phosphorus Supplement

Each peach capsule-shaped, film coated tablet contains:

Phosphorus	258 mg.
Potassium	49.4 mg.
Sodium	262.4 mg.

Derived from Sodium Phosphate Monobasic Anhydrous, Dipotassium Phosphate Anhydrous, and Disodium Phosphate Anhydrous.

HOW SUPPLIED

Bottles of 100.
NDC 0076-0109-03

UROLENE BLUE® ℞
[ū'ro-lene blue]
Methylene Blue Tablets

Each blue coated tablet contains Methylene blue USP 65 mg.

HOW SUPPLIED

Bottles of 100 and 1000.
NDC 0076-0501-03 & 04

VIRILON® ℗ ℞
[vir'i-lon]
Methyltestosterone Macro-Beads Capsules
Oral Androgen Macro-Beads

Each capsule contains Methyltestosterone.........USP 10 mg. In a special base. Look for the grey and white seeds in the black and transparent capsule, available only from Star Pharmaceuticals.

HOW SUPPLIED

Bottles of 100 and 1000.
NDC 0076-0301-03 & 04

Continued on next page

Star—Cont.

VIRILON® IM
brand of testosterone cypionate
injection sterile solution
200 mg/ml
For Intramuscular Use Only

HOW SUPPLIED
Multiple dose vials of 10 ml containing 200 mg/ml.
NDC 0076-0302-10

Write for complete prescribing information for all Star products.

Stiefel Laboratories, Inc.
255 ALHAMBRA CIRCLE
CORAL GABLES, FL 33134

Direct Inquiries to:
Professional Services Department
(305) 443-3800

BREVOXYL®-4
[brĕv-ăhx-il]
(benzoyl peroxide 4%)
BREVOXYL®-8
(benzoyl peroxide 8%)

DESCRIPTION
Brevoxyl-4 and Brevoxyl-8 are topical preparations containing benzoyl peroxide 4% and 8%, respectively, as the active ingredient in a gel vehicle containing purified water, cetyl alcohol, dimethyl isosorbide, fragrance, simethicone, stearyl alcohol and ceteareth-20. The structural formula of benzoyl peroxide is:

CLINICAL PHARMACOLOGY
The exact method of action of benzoyl peroxide in acne vulgaris is not known. Benzoyl peroxide is an antibacterial agent with demonstrated activity against *Propionibacterium acnes*. This action, combined with the mild keratolytic effect of benzoyl peroxide is believed to be responsible for its usefulness in acne.
Benzoyl peroxide is absorbed by the skin where it is metabolized to benzoic acid and excreted as benzoate in the urine.

INDICATIONS AND USAGE
Brevoxyl-4 and Brevoxyl-8 are indicated for use in the topical treatment of mild to moderate acne vulgaris. Brevoxyl may be used as an adjunct in acne treatment regimens including antibiotics, retinoic acid products, and sulfur/salicylic acid containing preparations.

CONTRAINDICATIONS
Brevoxyl-4 and Brevoxyl-8 should not be used in patients who have shown hypersensitivity to benzoyl peroxide or to any of the other ingredients in the product.

PRECAUTIONS
General—For external use only. Avoid contact with eyes and mucous membranes. AVOID CONTACT WITH HAIR, FABRICS OR CARPETING AS BENZOYL PEROXIDE WILL CAUSE BLEACHING.
Carcinogenesis, Mutagenesis, Impairment of Fertility—Based upon all available evidence, benzoyl peroxide is not considered to be a carcinogen. However, data from a study using mice known to be highly susceptible to cancer suggest that benzoyl peroxide acts as a tumor promoter. The clinical significance of the findings is not known.
Pregnancy: Category C—Animal reproduction studies have not been conducted with benzoyl peroxide. It is also not known whether benzoyl peroxide can cause fetal harm when administered to a pregnant woman or can affect reproduction capacity. Benzoyl peroxide should be used by a pregnant woman only if clearly needed.
Nursing Mothers—It is not known whether this drug is excreted in human milk. Because many drugs are excreted in human milk, caution should be exercised when benzoyl peroxide is administered to a nursing woman.
Pediatric Use—Safety and effectiveness in children below the age of 12 have not been established.

ADVERSE REACTIONS
Contact sensitization reactions are associated with the use of topical benzoyl peroxide products and may be expected to occur in 10 to 25 of 1000 patients. The most frequent adverse reactions associated with benzoyl peroxide use are excessive erythema and peeling which may be expected to occur in 5 of 100 patients. Excessive erythema and peeling most frequently appear during the initial phase of drug use and may normally be controlled by reducing frequency of use.

DOSAGE AND ADMINISTRATION
Therapy may be initiated with either Brevoxyl-4 or Brevoxyl-8. The medication should be applied once or twice daily to affected areas. Frequency of use should be adjusted to obtain the desired clinical response. Gentle cleansing of the affected areas prior to application of Brevoxyl-4 or Brevoxyl-8 may be beneficial. Clinically visible improvement will normally occur by the third week of therapy. Maximum lesion reduction may be expected after approximately eight to twelve weeks of drug use. Continuing use of the drug is normally required to maintain a satisfactory clinical response.

HOW SUPPLIED
Brevoxyl-4 and Brevoxyl-8 are supplied in 42.5 g (1.5 oz) and 90 g (3.1 oz) tubes.
Brevoxyl-4
42.5 g tube NDC 0145-2374-06
90 g tube NDC 0145-2374-08
Brevoxyl-8
42.5 g tube NDC 0145-2384-06
90 g tube NDC 0145-2384-08
Store at controlled room temperature 15°–30°C (59°–86°F).
U.S. Patent No. 4,923,900

BREVOXYL® CLEANSING LOTION
[brev-ăhx-il]
(benzoyl peroxide 4%)

DESCRIPTION
Brevoxyl Cleansing Lotion is a topical preparation containing benzoyl peroxide as the active ingredient.
Brevoxyl Cleansing Lotion contains benzoyl peroxide 4% in a lathering vehicle containing purified water, cetyl alcohol, citric acid, dimethyl isosorbide, docusate sodium, hydroxypropyl methylcellulose, laureth-12, magnesium aluminum silicate, propylene glycol, sodium hydroxide, sodium lauryl sulfoacetate, and sodium octoxynol-2 ethane sulfonate.
The structural formula of benzoyl peroxide is:

CLINICAL PHARMACOLOGY
The exact method of action of benzoyl peroxide in acne vulgaris is not known. Benzoyl peroxide is an antibacterial agent with demonstrated activity against *Propionibacterium acnes*. This action, combined with the mild keratolytic effect of benzoyl peroxide is believed to be responsible for its usefulness in acne.
Benzoyl peroxide is absorbed by the skin where it is metabolized to benzoic acid and excreted as benzoate in the urine.

INDICATIONS AND USAGE
Brevoxyl Cleansing Lotion is indicated for use in the topical treatment of mild to moderate acne vulgaris. Brevoxyl Cleansing Lotion may be used as an adjunct in acne treatment regimens including antibiotics, retinoic acid products, and sulfur/salicylic acid containing preparations.

CONTRAINDICATIONS
Brevoxyl Cleansing Lotion should not be used in patients who have shown hypersensitivity to benzoyl peroxide or to any of the other ingredients in the product.

PRECAUTIONS
General—For external use only. Avoid contact with eyes and mucous membranes. AVOID CONTACT WITH HAIR, FABRICS OR CARPETING AS BENZOYL PEROXIDE WILL CAUSE BLEACHING.
Carcinogenesis, Mutagenesis, Impairment of Fertility—Based upon all available evidence, benzoyl peroxide is not considered to be a carcinogen. However, data from a study using mice known to be highly susceptible to cancer suggest that benzoyl peroxide acts as a tumor promoter. The clinical significance of the findings is not known.
Pregnancy: Category C—Animal reproduction studies have not been conducted with benzoyl peroxide. It is also not known whether benzoyl peroxide can cause fetal harm when administered to a pregnant woman or can affect reproduction capacity. Benzoyl peroxide should be used by a pregnant woman only if clearly needed.
Nursing Mothers—It is not known whether this drug is excreted in human milk. Because many drugs are excreted in human milk, caution should be exercised when benzoyl peroxide is administered to a nursing woman.
Pediatric Use—Safety and effectiveness in children below the age of 12 have not been established.

ADVERSE REACTIONS
Contact sensitization reactions are associated with the use of topical benzoyl peroxide products and may be expected to occur in 10 to 25 of 1000 patients. The most frequent adverse reactions associated with benzoyl peroxide use are excessive erythema and peeling which may be expected to occur in 5 of 100 patients. Excessive erythema and peeling most frequently appear during the initial phase of drug use and may normally be controlled by reducing frequency of use.

DOSAGE AND ADMINISTRATION
Shake well before using. Wash the affected areas once a day during the first week, and twice a day thereafter as tolerated. Wet skin areas to be treated; apply Brevoxyl Cleansing Lotion, work to a full lather, rinse thoroughly and pat dry. Frequency of use should be adjusted to obtain the desired clinical response. Clinically visible improvement will normally occur by the third week of therapy. Maximum lesion reduction may be expected after approximately eight to twelve weeks of drug use. Continuing use of the drug is normally required to maintain a satisfactory clinical response.

HOW SUPPLIED
Brevoxyl Cleansing Lotion is supplied in 297 g (10.5 oz) plastic bottles NDC 0145-2310-05.
Store at controlled room temperature 15°–30°C (59°–86°F).

LACTICARE®–HC Lotion 1%, 2½%
[lăk 'tĭ-kār ']
(hydrocortisone lotion, USP)

CONTAINS
Each ml of LactiCare-HC Lotion 1% and 2½% (hydrocortisone lotion, USP) contains 10 mg and 25 mg respectively of hydrocortisone in a vehicle consisting of carbomer 940, sodium PCA, lactic acid, sodium hydroxide, stearyl alcohol (and) ceteareth-20, glyceryl stearate (and) PEG-100 stearate, cetyl alcohol, isopropyl palmitate, light mineral oil, myristyl lactate, DMDM hydantoin, dehydroacetic acid, fragrance and purified water.

HOW SUPPLIED
Lacticare®-HC Lotion 1% (hydrocortisone lotion, USP) is available in the following size:
118 mL (4 fl oz) bottle NDC 0145-2537-04
Lacticare®-HC Lotion 2½% (hydrocortisone lotion, USP) is available in the following sizes:
59 mL (2 fl oz) bottle NDC 0145-2538-02
118 mL (4 fl oz) bottle NDC 0145-2538-04

PANOXYL® 5
[pan 'ăhx-il]
(benzoyl peroxide 5%)
PANOXYL® 10
(benzoyl peroxide 10%)

HOW SUPPLIED
PanOxyl 5 and PanOxyl 10 are supplied in 56.7 gram and 113.4 gram tubes.
PanOxyl 5
56.7 g (2.0 oz) tube NDC 0145-2372-06
113.4 g (4.0 oz) tube NDC 0145-2372-08
PanOxyl 10
56.7 g (2.0 oz) tube NDC 0145-2373-06
113.4 g (4.0 oz) tube NDC 0145-2373-08
U.S. Patent 4056611

PANOXYL® AQ 2½
[pan 'ăhx-il]
(benzoyl peroxide 2½%)
PANOXYL® AQ 5
(benzoyl peroxide 5%)
PANOXYL® AQ 10
(benzoyl peroxide 10%)

HOW SUPPLIED
PanOxyl AQ 2½, PanOxyl AQ 5, and PanOxyl AQ 10 are supplied in 56.7 gram and 113.4 gram tubes.
PanOxyl AQ 2½
56.7 g (2.0 oz) tube NDC 0145-2375-06
113.4 g (4.0 oz) tube NDC 0145-2375-08
PanOxyl AQ 5
56.7 g (2.0 oz) tube NDC 0145-2376-06
113.4 g (4.0 oz) tube NDC 0145-2376-08

PanOxyl AQ 10
56.7 g (2.0 oz) tube NDC 0145-2377-06
113.4 g (4.0 oz) tube NDC 0145-2377-08

SULFOXYL® Lotion Regular
SULFOXYL® Lotion Strong
[sul'fox-ul]

HOW SUPPLIED
Sulfoxyl Lotion Regular and Sulfoxyl Lotion Strong are supplied in 59 milliliter (2 fluid ounce) plastic bottles.

Sulfoxyl Lotion Regular   **Sulfoxyl Lotion Strong**
NDC 0145-3518-07   NDC 0145-3519-07

Summit Pharmaceuticals
Ciba-Geigy Corporation
556 MORRIS AVENUE
SUMMIT, NJ 07901

For Information Contact:
Consumer Affairs Department:
(800) 742-2422
Medical Services Department:
556 Morris Avenue
Summit, NJ, 07901

PLEASE NOTE:
Due to the alliance between Ciba Pharmaceuticals (which includes Basel Pharmaceuticals, Ciba Pharmaceutical Company, Geigy Pharmaceuticals, and Summit Pharmaceuticals) and Geneva Pharmaceuticals, Inc, please refer to **CibaGeneva** for product information.

To provide a convenient and accurate means of identifying CibaGeneva Pharmaceuticals' solid dosage form products, a code number has been imprinted on all tablets and capsules. To help you quickly identify a CibaGeneva tablet or capsule by its code number, an alphabetical listing of products (with corresponding codes and identification numbers) has been compiled below.

See CibaGeneva Pharmaceuticals for information on the following products:
Actigall®
Slow-K®
Transderm-Nitro®

Supergen, Inc.
6450 HOLLIS STREET
EMERYVILLE, CA 94608

For Customer Service and Placing Orders Contact:
800-905-5474
FAX: 800-903-5474
For Medical or Drug Information Contact:
Generally:
Professional Services Department:
888-43-SUPER
888-437-8737
FAX: 510-655-1098
In Emergencies:
415-749-7897

ETOPOSIDE INJECTION

DESCRIPTION
Etoposide is a semisynthetic derivative of podophyllotoxin used in the treatment of certain neoplastic diseases. It is 4'-demethylepipodophyllotoxin 9-[4,6-O-(R)-ethylidene-b-O-glucopyranoside]. It is very soluble in methanol and chloroform, slightly soluble in ethanol, and sparingly soluble in water and ether. It is made more miscible with water by means of organic solvents. It has a molecular weight of 588.56 and a molecular formula of $C_{29}H_{32}O_{13}$.

Etoposide injection is available for intravenous use as a 20 mg/mL sterile solution in 5 mL (100 mg) and 12.5 mL (250 mg) multiple dose vials. The pH of the clear yellow solution is 3 to 4. Each mL contains 20 mg etoposide, 2 mg citric acid, 30 mg benzyl alcohol, 80 mg polysorbate 80/tween 80, 650 mg polyethylene glycol 300, and 30.5 percent (v/v) alcohol.

HOW SUPPLIED
Etoposide Injection is available as 20 mg/mL and is supplied as follows:
5 mL Multiple Dose Vial (100 mg):
NDC 62701-110-01
12.5 mL Multiple Dose Vial (250 mg):
NDC 62701-113-01
Store between 15°–30°C (59°–86°F).
0218-00   Rev. October 1995

LEUCOVORIN CALCIUM TABLETS

DESCRIPTION
Leucovorin is one of several active, chemically reduced derivatives of folic acid. It is useful as an antidote to drugs which act as folic acid antagonists. Also known as folinic acid, Citrovorum factor, or 5-formyl-5,6,7,8-tetrahydro folic acid, this compound has the chemical designation of: L-Glutamic acid, N-[4-[[(2-amino-5-formyl-1,4,5,6,7,8-hexahydro-4-oxo-6-pteridinyl)- methyl]amino]benzoyl]-, calcium salt (1:1).
Each tablet for oral administration contains leucovorin calcium, equivalent to 5 mg or 25 mg of leucovorin.
Inactive Ingredients: Colloidal silicon dioxide, croscarmellose sodium type A, lactose, magnesium stearate, and microcrystalline cellulose.
The 25 mg tablet also contains D&C yellow no. 10 and FD&C blue no. 1.

HOW SUPPLIED
Leucovorin Calcium Tablets are available as:
5 mg: White, round, unscored, biconvex tablets. Debossed with **b** on one side and 484 on the other side. Available in bottles of:
    30   **NDC 62701-900-30**
    100 **NDC 62701-900-99**
25 mg: Pale green, round, unscored, biconvex tablets. Debossed with **b** on one side and 485 on the other side. Available in bottles of:
    25   **NDC 62701-901-25**
PROTECT FROM LIGHT.
Dispense with child-resistant closure in a tight, light-resistant container as defined in the USP/NF.
Store at controlled room temperature 15°–30°C (59°–86°F).
BR-484, 485   Rev. March 1996

MEGESTROL ACETATE
TABLETS, USP

DESCRIPTION
Megestrol acetate is a synthetic, anti-neoplastic and progestational drug. Megestrol acetate is a white, crystalline solid chemically designated as 17α-acetyloxy-6-methylpregna-4,6-diene-3,20-dione. Solubility at 37° C in water is 2 mcg per mL, solubility in plasma is 24 mcg per mL.
Megestrol acetate is supplied as tablets for oral administration containing 20 mg and 40 mg megestrol acetate.
Inactive Ingredients: Anhydrous lactose, dibasic calcium phosphate, magnesium stearate, microcrystalline cellulose, and sodium starch glycolate.

HOW SUPPLIED
Megestrol Acetate Tablets, USP are available as:
20 mg: White, round, flat-faced, beveledged, scored tablet. Debossed with 555/606 on one side and **barr** on the other side. Available in bottles of:
    100 **NDC 62701-920-99**
40 mg: White, round, flat-faced, beveledged, scored tablet. Debossed with 555/607 on one side and **barr** on the other side. Available in bottles of:
    100 **NDC 62701-921-99**
    250 **NDC 62701-921-51**
    500 **NDC 62701-921-52**
Dispense with a child-resistant closure in a well-closed container as defined in the USP.
Store at controlled room temperature 15°–30°C (59°–86°F).
BR-607   Rev. Nov, 1995

METHOTREXATE
TABLETS, USP

DESCRIPTION
Methotrexate is an antimetabolite used in the treatment of certain neoplastic diseases, severe psoriasis, and adult rheumatoid arthritis. Chemically methotrexate is N-[4-[[2,4-diamino-6-pteridinyl] methyl] methyl-amino]benzoyl]-L-glutamic acid.
Methotrexate Tablets for oral administration are available in bottles of 36 and 100. Methotrexate tablets contain an amount of methotrexate sodium equivalent to 2.5 mg of methotrexate.
Inactive Ingredients: Hydroxypropyl methylcellulose, lactose anhydrous, magnesium stearate, microcrystalline cellulose, polyethylene glycol, pregelatinized starch, propylene glycol, sodium carbonate monohydrate and talc.

HOW SUPPLIED
Methotrexate Tablets, USP contain an amount of methotrexate sodium equivalent to 2.5 mg of methotrexate.
2.5 mg: Yellow, oval shaped, scored tablet. Debossed with **b**/ 572 on one side. Available in bottles of:
    36   **NDC 62701-940-36**
    100 **NDC 62701-940-99**
Dispense with child-resistant closure in a well-closed container as defined in the USP.
Store at controlled room temperature 15°–30°C (59°–86°F).
Protect from light.
BR-572   Rev. Nov, 1995

NIPENT®
(pentostatin for injection)

> **WARNING**
> NIPENT should be administered under the supervision of a physician qualified and experienced in the use of cancer chemotherapeutic agents. The use of higher doses than those specified (see **DOSAGE AND ADMINISTRATION**) is not recommended. Dose-limiting severe renal, liver, pulmonary, and CNS toxicities occurred in Phase 1 studies that used NIPENT at higher doses (20–50 mg/m^2 in divided doses over 5 days) than recommended.
> In a clinical investigation in patients with refractory chronic lymphocytic leukemia using NIPENT at the recommended dose in combination with fludarabine phosphate, 4 of 6 patients entered in the study had severe or fatal pulmonary toxicity. The use of NIPENT in combination with fludarabine phosphate is not recommended.

DESCRIPTION
NIPENT® (pentostatin for injection) is supplied as a sterile, apyrogenic, lyophilized powder in single-dose vials for intravenous administration. Each vial contains 10 mg of pentostatin and 50 mg of mannitol USP. The pH of the final product is maintained between 7.0 and 8.5 by addition of sodium hydroxide or hydrochloric acid.
Pentostatin, also known as 2'-deoxycoformycin (DCF), is a potent inhibitor of the enzyme adenosine deaminase and is isolated from fermentation cultures of *Streptomyces antibioticus*. Pentostatin is known chemically as (R)-3-(2-deoxy-β-D-*erythro*-pentofuranosyl) -3.6.7,8- tetrahydroimidazo[4,5-d] [1,3]diazepin-8-ol with a molecular formula of $C_{11}H_{16}N_4O_4$ and a molecular weight of 268.27.
Pentostain is a white to off-white solid, freely soluble in distilled water.
The molecular structure of pentostatin is:

CLINICAL PHARMACOLOGY
Mechanism of Action
Pentostatin is a potent transition state inhibitor of the enzyme adenosine deaminase (ADA). The greatest activity of ADA is found in cells of the lymphoid system with T-cells having higher activity than B-cells and T-cell malignancies higher ADA activity than B-cell malignancies. Pentostatin inhibition of ADA, particularly in the presence of adenosine or deoxyadenosine, leads to cytotoxicity, and this is believed to be due to elevated intracellular levels of dATP which can block DNA synthesis through inhibition of ribonucleotide reductase. Pentostatin can also inhibit RNA synthesis as well as cause increased DNA damage. In addition to elevated

Continued on next page

Supergen—Cont.

dATP, these mechanisms may also contribute to the overall cytotoxic effect of pentostatin. The precise mechanism of pentostain's antitumor effect, however, in hairy cell leukemia is not known.

Pharmacokinetics/Drug Metabolism

A tissue distribution and whole-body autoradiography study in the rat revealed that radioactivity concentrations were highest in the kidneys with very little central nervous system penetration.

In man, following a single dose of 4 mg/m^2 of pentostain infused over 5 minutes, the distribution half-life was 11 minutes, the mean terminal half-life was 5.7 hours, the mean plasma clearance was 68 mL/min/m^2, and approximately 90% of the dose was excreted in the urine as unchanged pentostatin and/or metabolites as measured by adenosine deaminase inhibitory activity. The plasma protein binding of pentostain is low, approximately 4%.

A positive correlation was observed between pentostatin clearance and creatinine clearance (CrCl) in patients with creatinine clearance values ranging from 60 mL/min to 130 mL/min.[1] Pentostatin half-life in patients with renal impairment (CrCl <50 mL/min, n=2) was 18 hours, which was much longer than that observed in patients with normal renal function (CrCl >60 mL/min, n=14), about 6 hours.

CLINICAL STUDIES

The following table provides efficacy results for 4 groups (columns) of patients with hairy cell leukemia: patients who initially received NIPENT, patients who initially received alpha-interferon (IFN), and 2 different groups of patients who received NIPENT after proving to be refractory to, or intolerant of IFN therapy. The first 2 groups represent treatment results from the SWOG 8691 study, a large multicenter study comparing NIPENT and IFN in untreated (frontline) patients with confirmed hairy cell leukemia. The third group represents evaluable patients from the SWOG study who crossed over to NIPENT after initially receiving IFN. The fourth group, labeled NCI Phase 2 studies, displays pooled results of 2 noncomparative studies (MD Anderson and CALGB), in which NIPENT was used to treat patients with confirmed IFN-refractory disease.

In the SWOG 8691 study, NIPENT was administered at a dose of 4 mg/m^2 every 2 weeks. After 6 months of treatment, patients were evaluated for response. If a complete response was achieved, 2 additional doses of NIPENT were administered and then discontinued. If a partial response was achieved. NIPENT was continued for up to an additional 6 months. NIPENT was discontinued for stable disease after 6 months or progressive disease after 2 months of therapy. IFN was administered 3 million units subcutaneously 3 times per week. Patients who achieved a complete or partial response after 6 months of treatment continued on IFN for another 6 months. IFN was discontinued if patients did not achieve a complete or partial response after 6 months of initial treatment or progressed after 2 months. This study allowed crossover of patients intolerant of, or refractory to, initial treatment.

Interferon-refractory patients enrolled into the MD Anderson study received NIPENT at a dose of 4 mg/m^2 every other week for 3 months and responding patients received 3 additional months. CALGB patients received 4 mg/m^2 of NIPENT every other week for 3 months and responding patients were treated monthly for up to 9 additional months. Almost all patients had a PS of 0 to 2 in the Phase 2 and 3 studies.

For each study, a complete response (CR) required clearing of the peripheral blood and bone marrow of all hairy cells, normalization of organomegaly and lymphadenopathy by physical examination, and recovery of hemoglobin to at least 12 g/dL, platelet count to at least 100,000/mm^3, and granulocyte count to at least 1500/mm^3. A partial response (PR) required that the percentage of hairy cells in the blood and bone marrow decrease by more than 50%, enlarged organs and lymph nodes decrease by more than 50% by physical examination, and hematologic parameters had to meet the same criteria as for complete response. The table below reports the response rate for 2 groups of patients: (1) Evaluable, ie, patients who could be evaluated for response and (2) Intent-to-Treat, ie, patients diagnosed with hairy cell leukemia.

[See table below.]

The results show that frontline patients treated with NIPENT achieved a significantly higher rate of response than those treated with IFN. The time to recovery of neutrophil and platelet counts was shorter with NIPENT treatment and the estimated duration of response was longer. The response rate in IFN-refractory patients treated with NIPENT was similar to that in NIPENT-treated frontline patients. At a median follow-up duration of 46 months, there was no statistically significant difference in survival between hairy cell leukemia patients initially treated with NIPENT and those initially treated with IFN. However, no definite conclusions regarding survival can be made from these results because they are complicated by the fact that the majority of IFN patients crossed over to NIPENT treatment.

In the Phase 3 SWOG study, 25 patients with hairy cell leukemia died during treatment or follow-up: 18 patients had last received NIPENT (3 of whom had crossed over from IFN), and 7 patients had last received IFN (1 of whom crossed over from NIPENT). Eleven of the 25 deaths occurred within 60 days of the last dose of treatment. Of these, hairy cell leukemia was cited by the investigators as a contributory cause for 1 death in the NIPENT group and 3 deaths in the IFN group. Additionally, infection contributed to the deaths of 3 patients in the NIPENT group and 2 patients in the IFN group. Approximately 4% of hairy cell leukemia patients, in each arm, died more than 60 days after the last dose of either treatment and there was no outstanding cause of death among these patients.

INDICATIONS AND USAGE

NIPENT is indicated as single-agent treatment for both untreated and alpha-interferon-refractory hairy cell leukemia patients with active disease as defined by clinically significant anemia, neutropenia, thrombocytopenia, or disease-related symptoms.

CONTRAINDICATIONS

NIPENT is contraindicated in patients who have demonstrated hypersensitivity to NIPENT.

WARNINGS

See Boxed Warning.

Patients with hairy cell leukemia may experience myelosuppression primarily during the first few courses of treatment. Patients with infections prior to NIPENT treatment have in some cases developed worsening of their condition leading to death, whereas others have achieved complete response. Patients with infection should be treated only when the potential benefit of treatment justifies the potential risk to the patient. Efforts should be made to control the infection before treatment is initiated or resumed.

In patients with progressive hairy cell leukemia, the initial courses of NIPENT treatment were associated with worsening of neutropenia. Therefore, frequent monitoring of complete blood counts during this time is necessary. If severe neutropenia continues beyond the initial cycles, patients should be evaluated for disease status, including a bone marrow examination.

Elevations in liver function tests occurred during treatment with NIPENT and were generally reversible.

Renal toxicity was observed at higher doses in early studies; however, in patients treated at the recommended dose, elevations in serum creatinine were usually minor and reversible. There were some patients who began treatment with normal renal function who had evidence of mild to moderate toxicity at a final assessment. (See **DOSAGE AND ADMINISTRATION.**)

Rashes, occasionally severe, were commonly reported and may worsen with continued treatment. Withholding of treatment may be required (See **DOSAGE AND ADMINISTRATION.**)

Acute pulmonary edema and hypotension, leading to death, have been reported in the literature in patients treated with pentostatin in combination with carmustine, etoposide and high dose cyclophosphamide as part of the ablative regimen for bone marrow transplant.

Pregnancy Category D

Pentostatin can cause fetal harm when administered to a pregnant woman. Pentostatin was administered intravenously at doses of 0, 0.01, 0.1, or 0.75 mg/kg/day (0, 0.06, 0.6, and 4.5 mg/m^2) to pregnant rats on days 6 through 15 of gestation. Drug-related maternal toxicity occurred at doses of 0.1 and 0.75 mg/kg/day (0.6 and 4.5 mg/m^2). Teratogenic effects were observed at 0.75 mg/kg/day (4.5 mg/m^2) manifested by increased incidence of various skeletal malformations. In a dose range-finding study, pentostatin was administered intravenously to rats at doses of 0, 0.05, 0.1, 0.5, 0.75, or 1 mg/kg/day (0, 0.3, 0.6, 3, 4.5, 6 mg/m^2) on days 6 through 15 of gestation. Fetal malformations that were observed were an omphalocele at 0.05 mg/kg (0.3 mg/m^2), gastroschisis at 0.75 mg/kg and 1 mg/kg (4.5 and 6 mg/m^2), and a flexure defect of the hindlimbs at 0.75 mg/kg (4.5 mg/m^2). Pentostatin was also shown to be teratogenic in mice when administered as a single 2 mg/kg (6 mg/m^2) intraperitoneal injection on day 7 of gestation. Pentostatin was not teratogenic in rabbits when administered intravenously on days 6 through 18 of gestation at doses of 0, 0.005, 0.01, or 0.02 mg/kg/day (0, 0.015, 0.03, or 0.06 mg/m^2); however maternal toxicity, abortions, early deliveries, and deaths occurred in all drug-treated groups. There are no adequate and well-controlled studies in pregnant women. If NIPENT is used during pregnancy, or if the patient becomes pregnant while taking (receiving) this drug, the patient should be apprised of the potential hazard to the fetus. Women of childbearing potential receiving NIPENT should be advised to avoid becoming pregnant.

PRECAUTIONS

General

Therapy with NIPENT requires regular patient observation and monitoring of hematologic parameters and blood chemistry values. If severe adverse reactions occur, the drug should be withheld (see **DOSAGE AND ADMINISTRATION**), and appropriate corrective measures should be taken according to the clinical judgment of the physician. NIPENT treatment should be withheld or discontinued in patients showing evidence of nervous system toxicity.

Information for Patients

Patients should be advised of the signs and symptoms of adverse events associated with NIPENT therapy. (See **ADVERSE REACTIONS.**)

Laboratory Tests

Prior to initiating therapy witn NIPENT, renal function should be assessed with a serum creatinine and/or a creatinine clearance assay. (See **CLINICAL PHARMACOLOGY** and **DOSAGE AND ADMINISTRATION.**) Complete blood counts and serum creatinine should be performed before each dose of NIPENT and at other appropriate periods during therapy (see **DOSAGE AND ADMINISTRATION**). Severe neutropenia has been observed following the early courses of treatment with NIPENT and therefore frequent monitoring of complete blood counts is recommended during this time. If hematologic parameters do not improve with subsequent courses, patients should be evaluated for disease status, including a bone marrow examination. Periodic monitoring of the peripheral blood for hairy cells should be performed to assess the response to treatment.

In addition, bone marrow aspirates and biopsies may be required at 2 to 3 month intervals to assess the response to treatment.

Parameter	FRONTLINE: Evaluable NIPENT N=138	FRONTLINE: Evaluable IFN N=130	IFN-REFRACTORY[a]: SWOG 8691[b] Crossover N=79	IFN-REFRACTORY[a]: NCI Phase 2 Studies N=44
Response Rates (%)				
Evaluable CR	84	18	85	58
PR	6	24	4	28
Intent-to-Treat	*N=170*	*N=170*		
CR	*68*	*14*		
PR	*5*	*18*		
Median Time to Response (months)				
CR	6.6	11.5	6.0	4.2
PR	4.0	6.2	5.8	—
Median Duration of Response (months)				
CR	NR	8.3	NR	>7.7[c] (CALGB) >15.2[c] (MDA)
PR	NR	15.2	NR	—
% Estimated to be in Response After 24 Months				
CR	76	16	85	—
PR	50	21	—	—
Median Time to Recovery (days)				
ANC (1500/m^3)	70	106	—	—
Platelets (100,000/m^3)	22	36	—	—

NR = Not reached by Kaplan-Meier method; ANC = Absolute neutrophil count.
[a] Evaluable patients
[b] Patients either refractory to, or intolerant of, IFN
[c] Kaplan-Meier estimate

Drug Interactions

Allopurinol and NIPENT are both associated with skin rashes. Based on clinical studies in 25 refractory patients who received both NIPENT and allopurinol, the combined use of NIPENT and allopurinol did not appear to produce a higher incidence of skin rashes than observed with NIPENT alone. There has been a report of one patient who received both drugs and experienced a hypersensitivity vasculitis that resulted in death. It was unclear whether this adverse event and subsequent death resulted from the drug combination.

Biochemical studies have demonstrated that pentostatin enhances the effects of vidarabine, a purine nucleoside with antiviral activity. The combined use of vidarabine and NIPENT may result in an increase in adverse reactions associated with each drug. The therapeutic benefit of the drug combination has not been established.

The combined use of NIPENT and fludarabine phosphate is not recommended because it may be associated with an increased risk of fatal pulmonary toxicity (see WARNINGS). Acute pulmonary edema and hypotension, leading to death, have been reported in the literature in patients treated with pentostatin in combination with carmustine, etoposide and high dose cyclophosphamide as part of the ablative regimen for bone marrow transplant.

Carcinogenesis, Mutagenesis, Impairment of Fertility

Carcinogenesis: No animal carcinogenicity studies have been conducted with pentostatin.

Mutagenesis: Pentostatin was nonmutagenic when tested in *Salmonella typhimurium* strains TA-98, TA-1535, TA-1537, and TA-1538. When tested with strain TA-100, a repeatable statistically significant response trend was observed with and without metabolic activation. The response was 2.1 to 2.2 fold higher than the background at 10 mg/plate, the maximum possible drug concentration. Formulated pentostatin was clastogenic in the *in vivo* mouse bone marrow micronucleus assay at 20, 120, and 240 mg/kg. Pentostatin was not mutagenic to V79 Chinese hamster lung cells at the HGPRT locus exposed 3 hours to concentrations of 1 to 3 mg/mL, with or without metabolic activation. Pentostatin did not significantly increase chromosomal aberrations in V79 Chinese hamster lung cells exposed 3 hours to 1 to 3 mg/mL in the presence or absence of metabolic activation.

Impairment of Fertility: No fertility studies have been conducted in animals; however, in a 5-day intravenous toxicity study in dogs, mild seminiferous tubular degeneration was observed with doses of 1 and 4 mg/kg. The possible adverse effects on fertility in humans have not been determined.

Pregnancy

Pregnancy Category D: (See WARNINGS)

Nursing Mothers

It is not known whether NIPENT is excreted in human milk. Because many drugs are excreted in human milk, and because of the potential for serious adverse reactions in nursing infants from pentostatin, a decision should be made whether to discontinue nursing or discontinue the drug, taking into account the importance of NIPENT to the mother.

Pediatric Use

Safety and effectiveness in children or adolescents have not been established.

ADVERSE REACTIONS

Most patients treated for hairy cell leukemia in the five NCI-sponsored Phase 2 and the Phase 3 SWOG study experienced an adverse event. The following table lists the most frequently occurring adverse events in patients treated with NIPENT (both frontline and IFN-refractory patients) compared with IFN (frontline only), regardless of drug association. The drug association of some adverse events is uncertain as they may be associated with the disease itself (eg, infection, hematologic suppression), but other events, such as the gastrointestinal symptoms, rashes, and abnormal liver function tests, can in many cases be attributed to the drug. Most adverse events that were assessed for severity were either mild or moderate, and diminished in frequency with continued therapy.

All Adverse Events[a]	Percent of Patients		
	Frontline, Treated With NIPENT N=180	Frontline, Treated With IFN N=176	IFN-Refractory Treated With NIPENT N=197
Nausea and/or Vomiting	63	22	53[b]
Fever	46	59	42
Rash	43	30	26
Fatigue	42	55	29
Leukopenia	22	15	60
Pruritus	21	6	10
Coughing/Increased Cough	20	15	17
Myalgia	19	36	11
Chills	19	34	11
Headache	17	29	13
Diarrhea	17	17	15
Abdominal Pain	16	15	4
Anorexia	13	10	16
Upper Respiratory Infection	13	8	16
Asthenia	12	13	10
Stomatitis	12	7	5
Rhinitis	11	15	10
Dyspnea	11	13	8
Anemia	8	5	35
Pain	8	19	20
Pharyngitis	8	11	10
Sweating Increased/ Sweating	8	21	10
Viral Infection	8	17	NR
Infection	7	2[c]	36
Arthralgia	6	14	3
Thrombocytopenia	6	6	32
Skin Disorder	4	5	17
Allergic Reaction	2	1	11
Hepatic Disorder/ Elevated Liver Function Tests[d]	2	2	19
Neurologic Disorder, CNS/CNS Toxicity	1	NR	11
Lung Disorder/ Disease	NR	1	12
Nausea	NR	NR	22
Genitourinary Disorder	NR	NR	15

NR = Not Reported
a Occurring in more than 10% of patients, in any group, regardless of drug association
b Includes only nausea with vomiting
c These figures represent only unspecified infections. Refer to infection table.
d Elevated liver enzymes and liver disorder for SWOG

The total incidence for all types of infections is considerably higher for both treatment groups in the SWOG 8691 study than is listed in the table above. An intent-to-treat analysis of infections found that 38% of patients treated with NIPENT and 34% of patients treated with IFN averaged 2.4 and 1.9 documented infections during treatment, respectively. The following table lists the different types of infections that were reported as adverse events during the initial phase of the SWOG study. There were no apparent differences in the types of infection between the 2 treatment groups, with the possible exception of herpes zoster which was reported more frequently for NIPENT (8%) than for IFN (1%).

Type of Infection	Percent of Patients	
	Frontline, Treated With NIPENT N=180	Frontline, Treated With IFN N=176
Upper Respiratory Infection	13	8
Rhinitis	11	15
Herpes Zoster	8	1
Pharyngitis	8	11
Viral Infection	8	17
Infection (Unspecified)	7	2
Sinusitis	6	4
Cellulitis	6	3
Bacterial Infection	5	4
Pneumonia	5	7
Conjunctivitis	4	2
Furunculosis	4	<1
Herpes Simplex	4	1
Bronchitis	3	2
Sepsis	3	2
Urinary Tract Infection	3	3
Abscess, Skin	2	4
Moniliasis, Oral	2	<1
Mycotic Infection, Skin	<1	3
Osteomyelitis	1	0

The drug relatedness of the adverse events listed below cannot be excluded. The following adverse events occurred in 3% to 10% of NIPENT-treated patients in the initial phase of the SWOG study:

Body as a Whole—Chest Pain, Death, Face Edema, Peripheral Edema
Cardiovascular System—Hemorrhage, Hypotension
Digestive System—Dental Abnormalities, Dyspepsia, Flatulence, Gingivitis
Hemic and Lymphatic System—Agranulocytosis
Laboratory Deviations—Elevated Creatinine
Musculoskeletal System—Arthralgia
Nervous System—Confusion, Dizziness, Insomnia, Paresthesia, Somnolence
Psychobiologic Function—Anxiety, Depression, Nervousness
Respiratory System—Asthma
Skin & Appendages—Skin Dry, Urticaria

The remaining adverse events which occurred in less than 3% of NIPENT-treated patients during the initial phase of the SWOG study:

Body as a Whole—Flu-like Symptoms, Hangover Effect, Neoplasm
Cardiovascular System—Angina Pectoris, Arrhythmia, A-V Block, Bradycardia, Extrasystoles Ventricular, Heart Arrest, Heart Failure, Hypertension, Pericardial Effusion, Phlebitis, Pulmonary Embolus, Sinus Arrest, Tachycardia, Thrombophlebitis Deep, Vasculitis
Digestive System—Constipation, Dysphagia, Glossitis, Ileus
Hemic and Lymphatic System—Acute Leukemia, Anemia-Hemolytic, Aplastic Anemia
Laboratory Deviations—Hypercalcemia, Hyponatremia
Musculoskeletal System—Arthritis, Gout
Nervous System—Amnesia, Ataxia, Convulsions, Dreaming Abnormal, Dysarthria, Encephalitis, Hyperkinesia, Meningism, Neuralgia, Neuritis, Neuropathy, Paralysis, Syncope, Twitching, Vertigo
Psychobiologic Function—Decrease/Loss Libido, Emotional Liability, Hallucination, Hostility, Neurosis, Thinking Abnormal
Respiratory System—Bronchospasm, Larynx Edema
Skin and Appendages—Acne, Alopecia, Eczema, Petechial Rash, Photosensitivity Reaction
Special Senses—Amblyopia, Deafness, Earache, Eyes Dry, Labyrinthitis, Lacrimation Disorder, Nonreactive Eye, Photophobia, Retinopathy, Tinnitus, Unusual Taste, Vision Abnormal, Watery Eyes
Urogenital System—Amenorrhea, Breast Lump, Impotence, Kidney Function Abnormal, Nephropathy, Renal Failure, Renal Insufficiency, Renal Stone

One patient with hairy cell leukemia treated with NIPENT during another clinical study developed unilateral uveitis with vision loss.

Nineteen (5%) patients withdrew from the Phase 3 SWOG 8691 study because of adverse events; 9 during initial NIPENT treatment, 4 during NIPENT crossover, 5 during initial IFN treatment, and 1 during both initial IFN treatment and NIPENT crossover. In the Phase 2 studies in IFN-refractory hairy cell leukemia, 11% of patients withdrew from treatment with NIPENT due to an adverse event.

OVERDOSAGE

No specific antidote for NIPENT overdose is known. NIPENT administered at higher doses (20-50 mg/m² in divided doses over 5 days) than recommended was associated with deaths due to severe renal, hepatic, pulmonary, and CNS toxicity. In case of overdose, management would include general supportive measures through any period of toxicity that occurs.

DOSAGE AND ADMINISTRATION

It is recommended that patients receive hydration with 500 to 1,000 mL of 5% Dextrose in 0.5 Normal Saline or equivalent before NIPENT administration. An additional 500 mL of 5% Dextrose or equivalent should be administered after NIPENT is given.

The recommended dosage of NIPENT for the treatment of hairy cell leukemia is 4 mg/m² every other week. NIPENT may be administered intravenously by bolus injection or diluted in a larger volume and given over 20 to 30 minutes. (See **Preparation of Intravenous Solution.**)

Higher doses are not recommended.

No extravasation injuries were reported in clinical studies. The optimal duration of treatment has not been determined. In the absence of major toxicity and with observed continuing improvement, the patient should be treated until a complete response has been achieved. Although not established as required, the administration of two additional doses has been recommended following the achievement of a complete response.

All patients receiving NIPENT at 6 months should be assessed for response to treatment. If the patient has not achieved a complete or partial response, treatment with NIPENT should be discontinued.

If the patient has achieved a partial response, NIPENT treatment should be continued in an effort to achieve a complete response. At any time thereafter that a complete response is achieved, two additional doses of NIPENT are recommended. NIPENT treatment should then be stopped. If the best response to treatment at the end of 12 months is a partial response, it is recommended that treatment with NIPENT be stopped.

Continued on next page

Supergen—Cont.

Withholding or discontinuation of individual doses may be needed when severe adverse reactions occur. Drug treatment should be withheld in patients with severe rash, and withheld or discontinued in patients showing evidence of nervous system toxicity.

NIPENT treatment should be withheld in patients with active infection occurring during the treatment but may be resumed when the infection is controlled.

Patients who have elevated serum creatinine should have their dose withheld and a creatinine clearance determined. There are insufficient data to recommend a starting or a subsequent dose for patients with impaired renal function (creatinine clearance < 60 mL/min).

Patients with impaired renal function should be treated only when the potential benefit justifies the potential risk. Two patients with impaired renal function (creatinine clearances 50 to 60 mL/min) achieved complete response without unusual adverse events when treated with 2 mg/m^2.

No dosage reduction is recommended at the start of therapy with NIPENT in patients with anemia, neutropenia, or thrombocytopenia. In addition, dosage reductions are not recommended during treatment in patients with anemia and thrombocytopenia if patients can be otherwise supported hematologically. NIPENT should be temporarily withheld if the absolute neutrophil count falls during treatment below 200 cells/mm^3 in a patient who had an initial neutrophil count greater than 500 cells/mm^3 and may be resumed when the count returns to predose levels.

Preparation of Intravenous Solution

1. Procedures for proper handling and disposal of anticancer drugs should be followed. Several guidelines on this subject have been published.[2-7] There is no general agreement that all of the procedures recommended in the guidelines are necessary or appropriate. Spills and wastes should be treated with a 5% sodium hypochlorite solution prior to disposal.
2. Protective clothing including polyethylene gloves must be worn.
3. Transfer 5 mL of Sterile Water for Injection USP to the vial containing NIPENT and mix thoroughly to obtain complete dissolution of a solution yielding 2 mg/mL. Parenteral drug products should be inspected visually for particulate matter and discoloration prior to administration.
4. NIPENT may be given intravenously by bolus injection or diluted in a larger volume (25 to 50 mL) with 5% Dextrose Injection USP or 0.9% Sodium Chloride Injection USP. Dilution of the entire contents of a reconstituted vial with 25 mL or 50 mL provides a pentostatin concentration of 0.33 mg/mL or 0.18 mg/mL, respectively, for the diluted solutions.
5. NIPENT solution when diluted for infusion with 5% Dextrose Injection USP or 0.9% Sodium Chloride Injection USP does not interact with PVC infusion containers or administration sets at concentrations of 0.18 mg/mL to 0.33 mg/mL.

Stability

NIPENT vials are stable at refrigerated storage temperature 2° to 8°C) (36° to 46°F) for the period stated on the package. Vials reconstituted or reconstituted and further diluted as directed may be stored at room temperature and ambient light but should be used within 8 hours because NIPENT contains no preservatives.

HOW SUPPLIED

NIPENT (pentostatin for injection) is supplied as a sterile lyophilized white to off-white powder in single-dose vials containing 10 mg of pentostatin. The vials are packed in individual cartons. NDC 62701-800-01
Storage: Store NIPENT vials under refrigerated storage conditions 2° to 8°C (36° to 46°F).
Caution—Federal law prohibits dispensing without prescription.

REFERENCES

1. Malspeis L, et al. Clinical Pharmacokinetics of 2'-Deoxycoformycin. Cancer Treatment Symposia 2:7–15, 1984.
2. Recommendations for the safe handling of parenteral antineoplastic drugs. NIH publication 83-2621. For sale by the Superintendent of Documents, US Government Printing Office, Washington, NC 20402.
3. AMA council report. Guidelines for handling parenteral antineoplastics. JAMA 253:590–2, 1985.
4. National Study Commission on Cytotoxic Exposure–Recommendations for handling cytotoxic agents. Director of Pharmacy Services. Rhode Island Hospital, 593 Eddy Street, Providence, RI 02902.
5. Clinical Oncology Society of Australia: Guidelines and recommendations for safe handling of antineoplastic agents. Med J Australia 1:426–8, 1983.
6. Jones RB, et al. Safe handling of chemotherapeutic agents: A report from the Mount Sinai Medical Center. CA: A Cancer Journal for Clinicians 33:258–63, 1983.
7. American Society of Hospital Pharmacists technical assistance bulletin on handling cytotoxic and hazardous drugs. Am J Hosp Pharm 47:1033–49, 1990.

4243G034   Rev. September, 1994

Syntex (F.P.) Inc.
HUMACAO, PUERTO RICO 00791

Syntex Laboratories, Inc
3401 HILLVIEW AVE.
P.O. BOX 10850
PALO ALTO, CA 94303

Syntex Puerto Rico, Inc.
HUMACAO, PUERTO RICO 00791

For Medical Information Contact:
Roche Laboratories
(800) 526-6367

For Customer Service (Distribution) contact:
Roche Laboratories
(800) 526-0625

For Product Information:
See Roche Laboratories

TAP Pharmaceuticals Inc.
DEERFIELD, IL 60015

For Medical Information Contact:
Generally:
Medical Department
(800) 622-2011 (LUPRON)
(800) 478-9526 (PREVACID)
In Emergencies:
Medical Department
(800) 622-2011 (LUPRON)
(800) 478-9526 (PREVACID)

LUPRON®   ℞
(leuprolide acetate) Injection

DESCRIPTION

LUPRON (leuprolide acetate) Injection is a synthetic nonapeptide analog of naturally occurring gonadotropin releasing hormone (GnRH or LH-RH). The analog possesses greater potency than the natural hormone. The chemical name is 5-Oxo-L-prolyl-L-histidyl-L-tryptophyl-L-seryl-L-tyrosyl-D-leucyl-L-leucyl-L-arginyl -N- ethyl-L - prolinamide acetate (salt) with the following structural formula:

[See structure below.]

LUPRON is a sterile, aqueous solution intended for subcutaneous injection. It is available in a 2.8 mL multiple-dose vial containing 5 mg/mL of leuprolide acetate, sodium chloride for tonicity adjustment, 9 mg/mL of benzyl alcohol as a preservative and water for injection. The pH may have been adjusted with sodium hydroxide and/or acetic acid.

CLINICAL PHARMACOLOGY

Leuprolide acetate, an LH-RH agonist, acts as a potent inhibitor of gonadotropin secretion when given continuously and in therapeutic doses. Animal and human studies indicate that following an initial stimulation, chronic administration of leuprolide acetate results in suppression of ovarian and testicular steroidogenesis. This effect is reversible upon discontinuation of drug therapy. Administration of leuprolide acetate has resulted in inhibition of the growth of certain hormone dependent tumors (prostatic tumors in Noble and Dunning male rats and DMBA-induced mammary tumors in female rats) as well as atrophy of the reproductive organs. In humans, subcutaneous administration of single daily doses of leuprolide acetate results in an initial increase in

---

circulation levels of luteinizing hormone (LH) and follicle stimulating hormone (FSH), leading to a transient increase in levels of the gonadal steroids (testosterone and dihydrotestosterone in males, and estrone and estradiol in pre-menopausal females). However, continuous daily administration of leuprolide acetate results in decreased levels of LH and FSH in all patients. In males, testosterone is reduced to castrate levels. In pre-menopausal females, estrogens are reduced to post-menopausal levels. These decreases occur within two to four weeks after initiation of treatment, and castrate levels of testosterone in prostatic cancer patients have been demonstrated for periods of up to five years. Leuprolide acetate is not active when given orally. Bioavailability by subcutaneous administration is comparable to that by intravenous administration. Leuprolide acetate has a plasma half-life of approximately three hours. The metabolism, distribution and excretion of leuprolide acetate in man have not been determined.

INDICATIONS AND USAGE

LUPRON (leuprolide acetate) Injection is indicated in the palliative treatment of advanced prostatic cancer. It offers an alternative treatment of prostatic cancer when orchiectomy or estrogen administration are either not indicated or unacceptable to the patient. In a controlled study comparing LUPRON 1 mg/day given subcutaneously to DES (diethylstilbestrol), 3 mg/day, the survival rate for the two groups was comparable after two years treatment. The objective response to treatment was also similar for the two groups.

CONTRAINDICATIONS

A report of an anaphylactic reaction to synthetic GnRH (Factrel) has been reported in the medical literature.[1]

LUPRON is contraindicated in women who are or may become pregnant while receiving the drug. When administered on day 6 of pregnancy at test dosages of 0.00024, 0.0024, and 0.024 mg/kg (1/600 to 1/6 the human dose) to rabbits, LUPRON produced a dose-related increase in major fetal abnormalities. Similar studies in rats failed to demonstrate an increase in fetal malformations. There was increased fetal mortality and decreased fetal weights with the two higher doses of LUPRON in rabbits and with the highest dose in rats. The effects on fetal mortality are logical consequences of the alterations in hormonal levels brought about by this drug. Therefore, the possibility exists that spontaneous abortion may occur if the drug is administered during pregnancy.

WARNINGS

Isolated cases of worsening of signs and symptoms during the first weeks of treatment have been reported. Worsening of symptoms may contribute to paralysis with or without fatal complications.

PRECAUTIONS

Patients with metastatic vertebral lesions and/or with urinary tract obstruction should be closely observed during the first few weeks of therapy (see "ADVERSE REACTIONS" section).

Patients with known allergies to benzyl alcohol, an ingredient of the drug's vehicle, may present symptoms of hypersensitivity, usually local, in the form of erythema and induration at the injection site.

Information for Patients: See Information for Patients which appears after the "HOW SUPPLIED" section.

Laboratory Tests: Response to leuprolide acetate should be monitored by measuring serum levels of testosterone and acid phosphatase. In the majority of patients, testosterone levels increased above baseline during the first week, declining thereafter to baseline levels or below by the end of the second week of treatment. Castrate levels were reached within two to four weeks and once attained were maintained for as long as drug administration continued. Transient increases in acid phosphatase levels occurred sometimes early in treatment. However, by the fourth week, the elevated levels usually decreased to values at or near baseline.

Drug Interactions: None have been reported.

Carcinogenesis, Mutagenesis, Impairment of Fertility: Two-year carcinogenicity studies were conducted in rats and mice. In rats, a dose-related increase of benign pituitary hyperplasia and benign pituitary adenomas was noted at 24

months when the drug was administered subcutaneously at high daily doses (0.6 to 4 mg/kg). In mice no pituitary abnormalities were observed at a dose as high as 60 mg/kg for two years. Patients have been treated with leuprolide acetate for up to three years with doses as high as 10 mg/day and for two years with doses as high as 20 mg/day without demonstrable pituitary abnormalities.

Mutagenicity studies have been performed with leuprolide acetate using bacterial and mammalian systems. These studies provided no evidence of a mutagenic potential.

Clinical and pharmacologic studies with leuprolide acetate and similar analogs have shown full reversibility of fertility suppression when the drug is discontinued after continuous administration for periods of up to 24 weeks. However, no clinical studies have been conducted with leuprolide acetate to assess the reversibility of fertility suppression.

Pregnancy Category X. See CONTRAINDICATIONS section.

ADVERSE REACTIONS

In the majority of patients testosterone levels increased above baseline during the first week, declining thereafter to baseline levels or below by the end of the second week of treatment. This transient increase was occasionally associated with a temporary worsening of signs and symptoms, usually manifested by an increase in bone pain (See "WARNINGS" section). In a few cases a temporary worsening of existing hematuria and urinary tract obstruction occurred during the first week. Temporary weakness and paresthesia of the lower limbs have been reported in a few cases.

Potential exacerbations of signs and symptoms during the first few weeks of treatment is a concern in patients with vertebral metastases and/or urinary obstruction which, if aggravated, may lead to neurological problems or increase the obstruction.

In a comparative trial of LUPRON (leuprolide acetate) Injection versus DES, in 5% or more of the patients receiving either drug, the following adverse reactions were reported to have a possible or probable relationship to drug as ascribed by the treating physician. Often, causality is difficult to assess in patients with metastatic prostate cancer. Reactions considered not drug related are excluded.

	LUPRON (N=98)	DES (N=101)
	Number of Reports	
Cardiovascular System		
Congestive heart failure	1	5
ECG changes/ischemia	19	22
High blood pressure	8	5
Murmur	3	8
Peripheral edema	12	30
Phlebitis/thrombosis	2	10
Gastrointestinal System		
Anorexia	6	5
Constipation	7	9
Nausea/vomiting	5	17
Endocrine System		
*Decreased testicular size	7	11
*Gynecomastia/breast tenderness or pain	7	63
*Hot flashes	55	12
*Impotence	4	12
Hemic and Lymphatic System		
Anemia	5	5
Musculoskeletal System		
Bone pain	5	2
Myalgia	3	9
Central/Peripheral Nervous System		
Dizziness/lightheadedness	5	7
General pain	13	13
Headache	7	4
Insomnia/sleep disorders	7	5
Respiratory System		
Dyspnea	2	8
Sinus congestion	5	6
Integumentary System		
Dermatitis	5	8
Urogenital System		
Frequency/urgency	6	8
Hematuria	6	4
Urinary tract infection	3	7
Miscellaneous		
Asthenia	10	10

*Physiologic effect of decreased testosterone.

In this same study, the following adverse reactions were reported in less than 5% of the patients on LUPRON.

Cardiovascular System- Angina, Cardiac arrhythmias, Myocardial infarction, Pulmonary emboli; *Gastrointestinal System* - Diarrhea, Dysphagia, Gastrointestinal bleeding, Gastrointestinal disturbance, Peptic ulcer, Rectal polyps; *Endocrine System* - Libido decrease, Thyroid enlargement; *Musculoskeletal System* - Joint pain; *Central/Peripheral Nervous System* - Anxiety, Blurred vision, Lethargy, Memory disorder, Mood swings, Nervousness, Numbness, Paresthesia, Peripheral neuropathy, Syncope/blackouts, Taste disorders; *Respiratory System* - Cough, Pleural rub, Pneumonia, Pulmonary fibrosis; *Integumentary System* - Carcinoma of skin/ear, Dry skin, Ecchymosis, Hair loss, Itching, Local skin reactions, Pigmentation, Skin lesions; *Urogenital System* - Bladder spasms, Dysuria, Incontinence, Testicular pain, Urinary obstruction; *Miscellaneous* - Depression, Diabetes, Fatigue, Fever/chills, Hypoglycemia, Increased BUN, Increased calcium, Increased creatinine, Infection/inflammation, Ophthalmologic disorders, Swelling (temporal bone).

The following additional adverse reactions have been reported with LUPRON or LUPRON DEPOT (leuprolide acetate for depot suspension) during other clinical trials and/or during postmarketing surveillance. Reactions considered as nondrug related by the treating physician are excluded.

Cardiovascular System - Hypotension, Transient ischemic attack/stroke; *Gastrointestinal System* - Hepatic dysfunction; *Endocrine System* - Libido increase; *Hemic and Lymphatic System* - Decreased WBC, Hemoptysis; *Musculoskeletal System* - Ankylosing spondylosis, Pelvic fibrosis; *Central/Peripheral Nervous System* - Hearing disorder, Peripheral neuropathy, Spinal fracture/paralysis; *Respiratory System* - Pulmonary infiltrate, Respiratory disorders; *Integumentary System* - Hair growth; *Urogenital System* - Penile swelling, Prostate pain; *Miscellaneous* - Hypoproteinemia, Hard nodule in throat, Weight gain, Increased uric acid.

OVERDOSAGE

In rats subcutaneous administration of 250 to 500 times the recommended human dose, expressed on a per body weight basis, resulted in dyspnea, decreased activity, and local irritation at the injection site. There is no evidence at present that there is a clinical counterpart of this phenomenon. In early clinical trials with leuprolide acetate doses as high as 20 mg/day for up to two years caused no adverse effects differing from those observed with the 1 mg/day dose.

DOSAGE AND ADMINISTRATION

The recommended dose is 1 mg (0.2 mL) administered as a single daily subcutaneous injection. As with other drugs administered chronically by subcutaneous injection, the injection site should be varied periodically.

NOTE: As with all parenteral products, inspect container's solution for discoloration and particulate matter before each use.

HOW SUPPLIED

LUPRON (leuprolide acetate) Injection is a sterile solution supplied in a 2.8 mL multiple-dose vial, **NDC** 0300-3626-28. Store below 77°F (25°C). Do not freeze. Protect from light—store vial in carton until use.

Each 0.2 mL contains 1 mg of leuprolide acetate, sodium chloride for tonicity adjustment, 1.8 mg of benzyl alcohol as preservative and water for injection. The pH may have been adjusted with sodium hydroxide and/or acetic acid.

Caution: Federal (U.S.A.) law prohibits dispensing without a prescription.

U.S. Patent Nos. 4,005,063 and 4,005,194.

REFERENCE

1. MacLeod TL, Eisen A, Sussman GL, et al: Anaphylactic reaction to synthetic luteinizing hormone-releasing hormone. *Fertil Steril* 1987 Sept;48(3):500-502.

INFORMATION FOR PATIENTS

NOTE: Be sure to consult your physician with any questions you may have or for information about LUPRON (leuprolide acetate) Injection and its use.

WHAT IS LUPRON?

LUPRON (leuprolide acetate) Injection is chemically similar to gonadotropin releasing hormone (GnRH or LH-RH) a hormone which occurs naturally in your body.

Normally, your body releases small amounts of LH-RH and this leads to events which stimulate the production of sex hormones.

However, when you inject LUPRON (leuprolide acetate) Injection, the normal events that lead to sex hormone production are interrupted and testosterone is no longer produced by the testes.

LUPRON must be injected because, like insulin which is injected by diabetics, LUPRON is inactive when taken by mouth.

If you were to discontinue the drug for any reason, your body would begin making testosterone again.

DIRECTIONS FOR USING LUPRON

1. Wash hands thoroughly with soap and water.
2. If using a new bottle for the first time, flip off the plastic cover to expose the gray rubber stopper. Wipe metal ring and rubber stopper with an alcohol wipe each time you use LUPRON. Check the liquid in the container. If it is not clear or has particles in it, DO NOT USE IT. Exchange it at your pharmacy for another container.
3. Remove outer wrapping from one syringe. Pull plunger back until the tip of the plunger is at the .2 or 20 unit mark.
4. Take cover off needle. Push the needle through the center of the rubber stopper on the LUPRON bottle.
5. Push the plunger all the way in to inject air into the bottle.
6. Keep the needle in the bottle and turn the bottle upside down. Check to make sure the tip of the needle is in the liquid. Slowly pull back on the plunger, until the syringe fills to the .2 or 20 unit mark.
7. Toward the end of a two-week period, the amount of LUPRON left in the bottle will be small. Take special care to hold the bottle straight and to keep the needle tip in liquid while pulling back on the plunger.
8. Keeping the needle in the bottle and the bottle upside down, check for air bubbles in the syringe. If you see any, push the plunger *slowly* in to push the air bubble back into the bottle. Keep the tip of the needle in the liquid and pull the plunger back again to fill to the .2 or 20 unit mark.
9. Do this again if necessary to eliminate air bubbles. Remove needle from bottle and lay syringe down. DO NOT TOUCH THE NEEDLE OR ALLOW THE NEEDLE TO TOUCH ANY SURFACE.
10. To protect your skin, inject each daily dose at a different body spot.
11. Choose an injection spot. Cleanse the injection spot with another alcohol wipe.
12. Hold the syringe in one hand. Hold the skin taut, or pull up a little flesh with the other hand, as you were instructed.
13. Holding the syringe as you would a pencil, thrust the needle all the way into the skin at a 90° angle.
14. Hold an alcohol wipe down on your skin where the needle is inserted and withdraw the needle at the same angle it was inserted.
15. Use the disposable syringe only once and dispose of it properly as you were instructed. Needles thrown into a garbage bag could accidentally stick someone. NEVER LEAVE SYRINGES, NEEDLES OR DRUGS WHERE CHILDREN CAN REACH THEM.

SOME SPECIAL ADVICE

- You may experience hot flashes when using LUPRON (leuprolide acetate) Injection. During the first few weeks of treatment you may experience increased bone pain, increased difficulty in urinating, and less commonly but most importantly, you may experience the onset or aggravation of nerve symptoms. In any of these events, discuss the symptoms with your doctor.
- You may experience some irritation at the injection site, such as burning, itching or swelling. These reactions are usually mild and go away. If they do not, tell your doctor.
- Do not stop taking your injections because you feel better. You need an injection every day to make sure LUPRON keeps working for you.
- If you need to use an alternate to the syringe supplied with LUPRON, insulin syringes should be utilized.
- When the drug level gets low, take special care to hold the bottle straight up and down and to keep the needle tip in liquid while pulling back on the plunger.
- Do not try to get every last drop out of the bottle. This will increase the possibility of drawing air into the syringe and getting an incomplete dose. Some extra drug has been provided so that you can withdraw the recommended number of doses.
- Tell your pharmacist when you will need LUPRON so it will be at the pharmacy when you need it.
- Store below 77°F (25°C). Do not store near a radiator or other very warm place. Do not freeze. Protect from light - store vial in carton until use.
- Do not leave your drug or hypodermic syringes where anyone can pick them up.
- Keep this and all other medications out of reach of children.

TAP Pharmaceuticals Inc.
Deerfield, IL 60015, U.S.A.
Lupron Injection
manufactured by
Abbott Laboratories,
North Chicago, IL 60064
® – Registered
Revised: April, 1996

For Pediatric Use
LUPRON®
(leuprolide acetate) Injection ℞

DESCRIPTION

Leuprolide acetate is a synthetic nonapeptide analog of naturally occurring gonadotropin releasing hormone (GnRH or LH-RH). The analog possesses greater potency than the natural hormone. The chemical name is 5-Oxo-L-prolyl

Continued on next page

TAP—Cont.

-L-histidyl -L-tryptophyl-L-seryl -L- tyrosyl-D-leucyl-L-leucyl -L-arginyl-N-ethyl-L-prolinamide acetate (salt) with the following structural formula:
[See structure below.]
LUPRON Injection is a sterile, aqueous solution intended for daily subcutaneous injection.

- A 2.8 mL multiple dose vial contains leuprolide acetate (5 mg/mL), sodium chloride (6.3 mg/mL) for tonicity adjustment, benzyl alcohol as a preservative (9 mg/mL), and water for injection. The pH may have been adjusted with sodium hydroxide and/or acetic acid.

CLINICAL PHARMACOLOGY

Leuprolide acetate, a GnRH agonist, acts as a potent inhibitor of gonadotropin secretion when given continuously and in therapeutic doses. Human studies indicate that following an initial stimulation of gonadotropins, chronic stimulation with leuprolide acetate results in suppression or "downregulation" of these hormones and consequent suppression of ovarian and testicular steroidogenesis. These effects are reversible on discontinuation of drug therapy.
Leuprolide acetate is not active when given orally. In adults, bioavailability by subcutaneous administration is comparable to that by intravenous administration; and leuprolide acetate has a plasma half-life of approximately three hours. The metabolism, distribution and excretion of leuprolide acetate in humans have not been determined. A pharmacokinetic study of leuprolide acetate in children has not been performed.
In children with central precocious puberty (CPP), stimulated and basal gonadotropins are reduced to prepubertal levels. Testosterone and estradiol are reduced to prepubertal levels in males and females respectively. Reduction of gonadotropins will allow for normal physical and psychological growth and development. Natural maturation occurs when gonadotropins return to pubertal levels following discontinuation of leuprolide acetate.
The following physiologic effects have been noted with the chronic administration of leuprolide acetate in this patient population.

1. **Skeletal Growth.** A measurable increase in body length can be noted since the epiphyseal plates will not close prematurely.
2. **Organ growth.** Reproductive organs will return to a prepubertal state.
3. **Menses.** Menses, if present, will cease.

INDICATIONS AND USAGE

LUPRON Injection is indicated in the treatment of children with central precocious puberty. Children should be selected using the following criteria:

1. Clinical diagnosis of CPP (idiopathic or neurogenic) with onset of secondary sexual characteristics earlier than 8 years in females and 9 years in males.
2. Clinical diagnosis should be confirmed prior to initiation of therapy:
   - Confirmation of diagnosis by a pubertal response to a GnRH stimulation test. The sensitivity and methodology of this assay must be understood.
   - Bone age advanced one year beyond the chronological age.
3. Baseline evaluation should also include:
   - Height and weight measurements.
   - Sex steroid levels.
   - Adrenal steroid level to exclude congenital adrenal hyperplasia.
   - Beta human chorionic gonadotropin level to rule out a chorionic gonadotropin secreting tumor.
   - Pelvic/adrenal/testicular ultrasound to rule out a steroid secreting tumor.
   - Computerized tomography of the head to rule out intracranial tumor.

CONTRAINDICATIONS

LUPRON Injection is contraindicated in women who are or may become pregnant while receiving the drug. When administered on day 6 of pregnancy at test dosages of 0.00024, 0.0024, and 0.024 mg/kg (1/1200 to 1/12 the human pediatric dose) to rabbits, LUPRON produced a dose-related increase in major fetal abnormalities. Similar studies in rats failed to demonstrate an increase in fetal malformations. There was increased fetal mortality and decreased fetal weights with the two higher doses of LUPRON in rabbits and with the highest dose in rats. The effects on fetal mortality are logical consequences of the alterations in hormonal levels brought about by this drug. Therefore, the possibility exists that spontaneous abortion may occur if the drug is administered during pregnancy.
Leuprolide acetate is contraindicated in children demonstrating hypersensitivity to GnRH, GnRH agonist analogs, or any of the excipients.
A report of an anaphylactic reaction to synthetic GnRH (Factrel) has been reported in the medical literature.[1]

WARNINGS

During the early phase of therapy, gonadotropins and sex steroids rise above baseline because of the natural stimulatory effect of the drug. Therefore, an increase in clinical signs and symptoms may be observed (see "Clinical Pharmacology" section).
Noncompliance with drug regimen or inadequate dosing may result in inadequate control of the pubertal process. The consequences of poor control include the return of pubertal signs such as menses, breast development, and testicular growth. The long-term consequences of inadequate control of gonadal steroid secretion are unknown, but may include a further compromise of adult stature.

PRECAUTIONS

Patients with known allergies to benzyl alcohol, an ingredient of the vehicle of Lupron Injection, may present symptoms of hypersensitivity, usually local, in the form of erythema and induration at the injection site.
Laboratory Tests: Response to leuprolide acetate should be monitored 1-2 months after the start of therapy with a GnRH stimulation test and sex steroid levels. Measurement of bone age for advancement should be done every 6-12 months.
Sex steroids may increase or rise above prepubertal levels if the dose is inadequate (see "WARNINGS" section). Once a therapeutic dose has been established, gonadotropin and sex steroid levels will decline to prepubertal levels.
Drug Interactions: No pharmacokinetic-based drug-drug interaction studies have been conducted. However, because leuprolide acetate is a peptide that is primarily degraded by peptidase and not by cytochrome P-450 enzymes as noted in specific studies, and the drug is only about 46% bound to plasma proteins, drug interactions would not be expected to occur.
Drug/Laboratory Test Interactions: Administration of leuprolide acetate in therapeutic doses results in suppression of the pituitary-gonadal system. Normal function is usually restored within 4 to 12 weeks after treatment is discontinued.
Information for Parents: Prior to starting therapy with LUPRON Injection, the parent or guardian must be aware of the importance of continuous therapy. Adherence to daily drug administration schedules must be accepted if therapy is to be successful.

- During the first 2 months of therapy, a female may experience menses or spotting. If bleeding continues beyond the second month, notify the physician.
- Any irritation at the injection site should be reported to the physician immediately.
- Report any unusual signs or symptoms to the physician.

Carcinogenesis, Mutagenesis, Impairment of Fertility: A two-year carcinogenicity study was conducted in rats and mice. In rats, a dose-related increase of benign pituitary hyperplasia and benign pituitary adenomas was noted at 24 months when the drug was administered subcutaneously at high daily doses (0.6 to 4 mg/kg). There was a significant but not dose-related increase of pancreatic islet-cell adenomas in females and of testes interstitial cell adenomas in males (highest incidence in the low dose group). In mice, no leuprolide acetate-induced tumors or pituitary abnormalities were observed at a dose as high as 60 mg/kg for two years. Adult patients have been treated with leuprolide acetate for up to three years with doses as high as 10 mg/day and for two years with doses as high as 20 mg/day without demonstrable pituitary abnormalities.
Although no clinical studies have been completed in children to assess the full reversibility of fertility suppression, animal studies (prepubertal and adult rats and monkeys) with leuprolide acetate and other GnRH analogs have shown functional recovery. However, following a study with leuprolide acetate, immature male rats demonstrated tubular degeneration in the testes even after a recovery period. In spite of the failure to recover histologically, the treated males proved to be as fertile as the controls. Also, no histologic changes were observed in the female rats following the same protocol. In both sexes, the offspring of the treated animals appeared normal. The effect of the treatment of the parents on the reproductive performance of the F1 generation was not tested. The clinical significance of these findings is unknown.
Pregnancy Category X. See "CONTRAINDICATIONS" section.
Nursing Mothers: It is not known whether leuprolide acetate is excreted in human milk. LUPRON should not be used by nursing mothers.

ADVERSE REACTIONS

Potential exacerbation of signs and symptoms during the first few weeks of treatment (See "PRECAUTIONS" section) is a concern in patients with rapidly advancing central precocious puberty.
In two studies of children with central precocious puberty, in 2% or more of the patients receiving the drug, the following adverse reactions were reported to have a possible or probable relationship to drug as ascribed by the treating physician. Reactions considered not drug related are excluded.

	Number of Patients N = 395	(Percent)
Body as a Whole		
General Pain	7	(2)
Integumentary System		
Acne/Seborrhea	7	(2)
Injection Site Reactions Including Abscess	21	(5)
Rash Including Erythema Multiforme	8	(2)
Urogenital System		
Vaginitis/Bleeding/ Discharge	7	(2)

In those same studies, the following adverse reactions were reported in less than 2% of the patients.
Body as a Whole - Body Odor, Fever, Headache, Infection; *Cardiovascular System* - Syncope, Vasodilation; *Digestive System* - Dysphagia, Gingivitis, Nausea/Vomiting; *Endocrine System* - Accelerated Sexual Maturity; *Metabolic and Nutritional Disorders* - Peripheral Edema, Weight Gain; *Nervous System* - Nervousness, Personality Disorder, Somnolence, Emotional Lability; *Respiratory System* - Epistaxis; *Integumentary System* - Alopecia, Skin Striae; *Urogenital System* - Cervix Disorder, Gynecomastia/Breast Disorders, Urinary Incontinence.
See other package inserts for adverse events reported in other patient populations.

OVERDOSAGE

In rats, subcutaneous administration of 125 to 250 times the recommended human pediatric dose, expressed on a per body weight basis, resulted in dyspnea, decreased activity, and local irritation at the injection site. There is no evidence at present that there is a clinical counterpart of this phenomenon. In early clinical trials using leuprolide acetate in adult patients, doses as high as 20 mg/day for up to two years caused no adverse effects differing from those observed with the 1 mg/day dose.

DOSAGE AND ADMINISTRATION

LUPRON INJECTION can be administered by a patient/ parent or health care professional.
The dose of LUPRON Injection must be individualized for each child. The dose is based on a mg/kg ratio of drug to body weight. Younger children require higher doses on a mg/kg ratio.
For either dosage form, after 1-2 months of initiating therapy or changing doses, the child must be monitored with a GnRH stimulation test, sex steroids, and Tanner staging to confirm downregulation. Measurements of bone age for advancement should be monitored every 6-12 months. The dose should be titrated upward until no progression of the condition is noted either clinically and/or by laboratory parameters.
The first dose found to result in adequate downregulation can probably be maintained for the duration of therapy in most children. However, there are insufficient data to guide dosage adjustment as patients move into higher weight categories after beginning therapy at very young ages and low dosages. It is recommended that adequate downregulation be verified in such patients whose weight has increased significantly while on therapy.

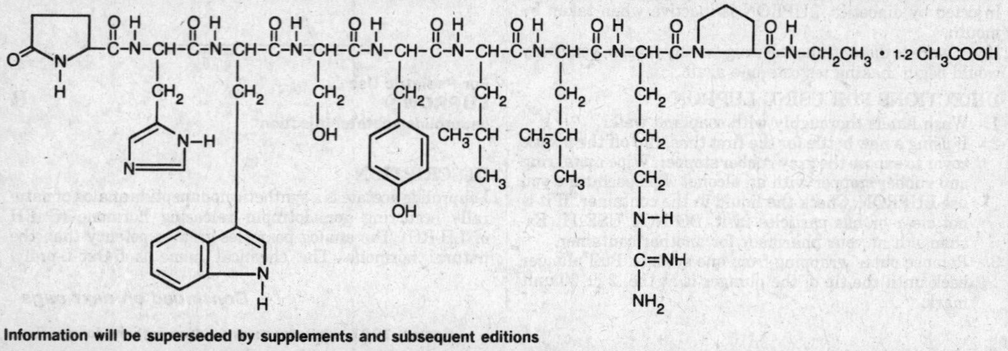

As with other drugs administered by injection, the injection site should be varied periodically.

Discontinuation of LUPRON Injection should be considered before age 11 for females and age 12 for males.

The recommended starting dose is 50 mcg/kg/day administered as a single subcutaneous injection. If total downregulation is not achieved, the dose should be titrated upward by 10 mcg/kg/day. This dose will be considered the maintenance dose.

NOTE: As with other parenteral products, inspect container's solution for discoloration and particulate matter before each use.

HOW SUPPLIED

LUPRON (leuprolide acetate) Injection is a sterile solution.

- A 2.8 mL multiple dose vial (NDC 0300-3626-28) contains leuprolide acetate (5 mg/mL), sodium chloride (6.3 mg/mL) for tonicity adjustment, benzyl alcohol as a preservative (9 mg/mL), and water for injection. The pH may have been adjusted with sodium hydroxide and/or acetic acid.
- Store below 77°F (25°C). Do not freeze. Protect from light - store vial in carton until use.
- Use the syringes supplied with LUPRON Injection. Insulin syringes may be substituted for use with Lupron Injection. The volume of drug for the dose will vary depending on the syringe used and the concentration of drug.

Caution: Federal (U.S.A.) law prohibits dispensing without a prescription.

U.S. Patent Nos. 4,005,063; 4,005,194.

REFERENCE

1. MacLeod TL, et al. Anaphylactic reaction to synthetic luteinizing hormone-releasing hormone. *Fertil Steril* 1987 Sept;48(3):500-502.

TAP Pharmaceuticals Inc.
Deerfield, IL 60015, U.S.A.
Lupron Injection
manufactured by
Abbott Laboratories,
North Chicago, IL 60064
® – Registered
Revised: April, 1996

This is combined labeling. Examples of different fonts appear below.
- General information
- Information on endometrosis
- Information on uterine fibroids

LUPRON DEPOT® 3.75 mg ℞
(leuprolide acetate for depot suspension)

DESCRIPTION

Leuprolide acetate is a synthetic nonapeptide analog of naturally occurring gonadotropin-releasing hormone (GnRH or LH-RH). The analog possesses greater potency than the natural hormone. The chemical name is 5-oxo-L-prolyl-L-his-

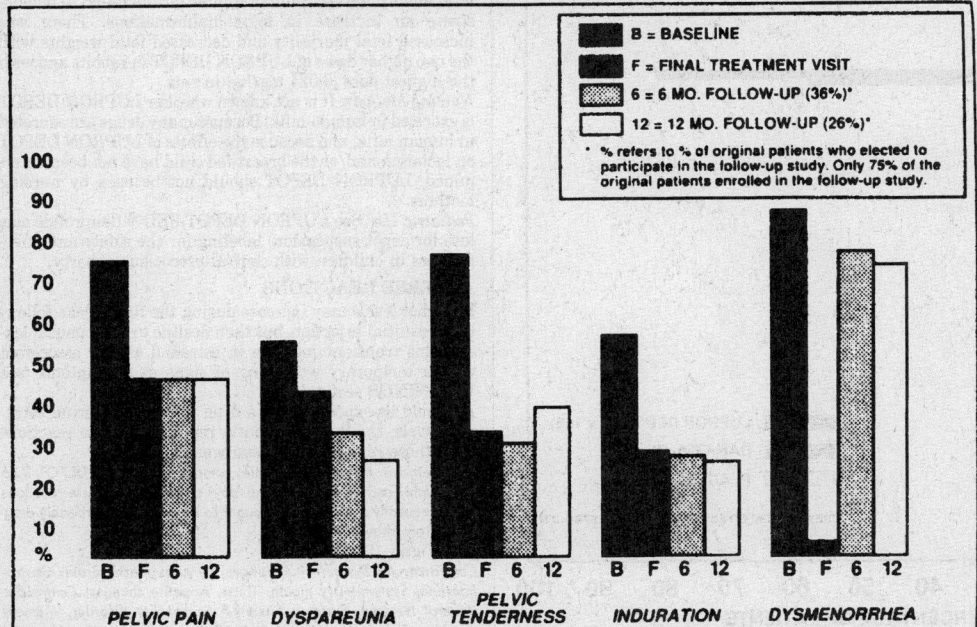

tidyl -L-tryptophyl-L-seryl-L-tyrosyl-D-leucyl -L- leucyl-L-arginyl-N-ethyl-L-prolinamide acetate (salt) with the following structural formula:

[See structure above.]

LUPRON DEPOT is available in a vial containing sterile lyophilized microspheres, which when mixed with diluent, become a suspension which is intended as a monthly intramuscular injection.

The single-dose vial contains leuprolide acetate (3.75 mg), purified gelatin (0.65 mg), DL-lactic and glycolic acids copolymer (33.1 mg), and D-mannitol (6.6 mg). The accompanying ampule of diluent contains carboxymethylcellulose sodium (10 mg), D-mannitol (100 mg), polysorbate 80 (2 mg), water for injection, USP, and glacial acetic acid, USP to control pH.

During the manufacture of LUPRON DEPOT 3.75 mg, acetic acid is lost, leaving the peptide.

CLINICAL PHARMACOLOGY

Leuprolide acetate is a long-acting GnRH analog. A single monthly injection of LUPRON DEPOT 3.75 mg results in an initial stimulation followed by a prolonged suppression of pituitary gonadotropins. Repeated dosing at monthly intervals results in decreased secretion of gonadal steroids; consequently, tissues and functions that depend on gonadal steroids for their maintenance become quiescent. This effect is reversible on discontinuation of drug therapy.

Leuprolide acetate is not active when given orally. Intramuscular injection of the depot formulation provides plasma concentrations of leuprolide over a period of one month.

PHARMACOKINETICS

Absorption: A single dose of LUPRON DEPOT 3.75 mg was administered by intramuscular injection to healthy female volunteers. The absorption of leuprolide was characterized by an initial increase in plasma concentration, with peak concentration ranging from 4.6 to 10.2 ng/mL at four hours postdosing. However, intact leuprolide and an inactive metabolite could not be distinguished by the assay used in the study. Following the initial rise, leuprolide concentrations started to plateau within two days after dosing and remained relatively stable for about four to five weeks with plasma concentrations of about 0.30 ng/mL.

Distribution: The mean steady-state volume of distribution of leuprolide following intravenous bolus administration to

healthy male volunteers was 27 L. In vitro binding to human plasma proteins ranged from 43% to 49%.

Metabolism: In healthy male volunteers, a 1 mg bolus of leuprolide administered intravenously revealed that the mean systemic clearance was 7.6 L/h, with a terminal elimination half-life of approximately 3 hours based on a two compartment model.

In rats and dogs, administration of ^{14}C-labeled leuprolide was shown to be metabolized to smaller inactive peptides, a pentapeptide (Metabolite I), tripeptides (Metabolites II and III) and a dipeptide (Metabolite IV). These fragments may be further catabolized.

The major metabolite (M-I) plasma concentrations measured in 5 prostate cancer patients reached maximum concentration 2 to 6 hours after dosing and were approximately 6% of the peak parent drug concentration. One week after dosing, mean plasma M-I concentrations were approximately 20% of mean leuprolide concentrations.

Excretion: Following administration of LUPRON DEPOT 3.75 mg to 3 patients, less than 5% of the dose was recovered as parent and M-I metabolite in the urine.

Special Populations: The pharmacokinetics of the drug in hepatically and renally impaired patients have not been determined.

CLINICAL STUDIES

Endometriosis: In controlled clinical studies, LUPRON DEPOT 3.75 mg monthly for six months was shown to be comparable to danazol 800 mg/day in relieving the clinical sign/symptoms of endometriosis (pelvic pain, dysmenorrhea, dyspareunia, pelvic tenderness, and induration) and in reducing the size of endometrial implants as evidenced by laparoscopy. The clinical significance of a decrease in endometriotic lesions is not known at this time, and in addition laparoscopic staging of endometriosis does not necessarily correlate with the severity of symptoms.

[See Figure 1 below.]

LUPRON DEPOT 3.75 mg monthly induced amenorrhea in 74% and 98% of the patients after the first and second treatment months respectively. Most of the remaining patients reported episodes of only light bleeding or spotting. In the first, second and third post-treatment months, normal menstrual cycles resumed in 7%, 71% and 95% respectively, of those patients who did not become pregnant.

Figure 1 illustrates the percent of patients with symptoms at baseline, final treatment visit and sustained relief at six and 12 months following discontinuation of treatment for the various symptoms evaluated during the study. This included all patients at end of treatment and those who elected to participate at the follow-up periods. This might provide a slight bias in the results at follow-up as 75% of the original patients entered the follow-up study, and 36% were evaluated at six months and 26% at 12 months respectively.

Uterine Leiomyomata (Fibroids): In controlled clinical trials, administration of LUPRON DEPOT 3.75 mg for a period of three or six months was shown to decrease uterine and fibroid volume, thus allowing for relief of clinical symptoms (abdominal bloating, pelvic pain, and pressure). Excessive vaginal bleeding (menorrhagia and menometrorrhagia) decreased, resulting in improvement in hematologic parameters. In three clinical trials, enrollment was not based on hematologic status. Mean uterine volume decreased by 41% and myoma volume decreased by 37% at final visit as evidenced by ultrasound or MRI. These patients also experienced a decrease in symptoms including excessive vaginal bleeding and pelvic discomfort. Benefit occurred by three months of therapy, but additional gain was observed with an additional three months of LUPRON DEPOT 3.75 mg. Ninety-five percent of these patients became amenorrheic with 61%, 25%, and 4% experiencing amenorrhea during the first, second, and third treatment months respectively.

Post-treatment follow-up was carried out for a small percentage of LUPRON DEPOT 3.75 mg patients among the 77% who demonstrated a ≥ 25% decrease in uterine volume while on therapy. Menses usually returned within two months of cessation of therapy. Mean time to return to pretreatment uterine size was 8.3 months. Regrowth did not appear to be related to pretreatment uterine volume.

In another controlled clinical study, enrollment was based on hematocrit ≤ 30% and/or hemoglobin ≤ 10.2 g/dL. Administration of LUPRON DEPOT 3.75 mg, concomitantly with

FIGURE 1

PERCENT OF PATIENTS WITH SYMPTOMS AT BASELINE, FINAL TREATMENT VISIT, AND AFTER 6 AND 12 MONTHS OF FOLLOW–UP

Legend:
- B = BASELINE
- F = FINAL TREATMENT VISIT
- 6 = 6 MO. FOLLOW-UP (36%)*
- 12 = 12 MO. FOLLOW-UP (26%)*

* % refers to % of original patients who elected to participate in the follow-up study. Only 75% of the original patients enrolled in the follow-up study.

Symptoms (x-axis): PELVIC PAIN, DYSPAREUNIA, PELVIC TENDERNESS, INDURATION, DYSMENORRHEA

Continued on next page

TAP—Cont.

iron, produced an increase of ≥ 6% hematocrit and ≥ 2 g/dL hemoglobin in 77% of patients at three months of therapy. The mean change in hematocrit was 10.1% and the mean change in hemoglobin was 4.2 g/dL. Clinical response was judged to be a hematocrit of ≥ 36% and hemoglobin of ≥ 12 g/dL, thus allowing for autologous blood donation prior to surgery. At three months, 75% of patients met this criterion.

At three months, 80% of patients experienced relief from either menorrhagia or menometrorrhagia. As with the previous studies, episodes of spotting and menstrual-like bleeding were noted in some patients.

In this same study, a decrease of ≥ 25% was seen in uterine and myoma volumes in 60% and 54% of patients respectively. LUPRON DEPOT 3.75 mg was found to relieve symptoms of bloating, pelvic pain, and pressure.

There is no evidence that pregnancy rates are enhanced or adversely affected by the use of LUPRON DEPOT 3.75 mg.

INDICATIONS AND USAGE

Endometriosis:
LUPRON DEPOT 3.75 mg is indicated for management of endometriosis, including pain relief and reduction of endometriotic lesions.
Experience with LUPRON DEPOT 3.75 mg in females has been limited to women 18 years of age and older treated for 6 months.
Uterine Leiomyomata (Fibroids):
LUPRON DEPOT 3.75 mg concomitantly with iron therapy is indicated for the preoperative hematologic improvement of patients with anemia caused by uterine leiomyomata. The clinician may wish to consider a one-month trial period on iron alone inasmuch as some of the patients will respond to iron alone (see clinical trial results below). LUPRON may be added if the response to iron alone is considered inadequate. Recommended duration of therapy with LUPRON DEPOT 3.75 mg is **up to three** months.
Experience with LUPRON DEPOT in females has been limited to women 18 years of age and older.

PERCENT OF PATIENTS ACHIEVING HEMOGLOBIN ≥ 12 GM/DL

Treatment Group	Week 4	Week 8	Week 12
LUPRON DEPOT 3.75 mg with Iron	41*	71**	79*
Iron Alone	17	40	56

* P-Value < 0.01
** P-Value < 0.001

CONTRAINDICATIONS

1. Hypersensitivity to GnRH, GnRH agonist analogs or any of the excipients in LUPRON DEPOT.
2. Undiagnosed abnormal vaginal bleeding.
3. LUPRON DEPOT is contraindicated in women who are or may become pregnant while receiving the drug. LUPRON DEPOT may cause fetal harm when administered to a pregnant woman. Major fetal abnormalities were observed in rabbits but not in rats after administration of LUPRON DEPOT throughout gestation. There was increased fetal mortality and decreased fetal weights in rats and rabbits (see *Pregnancy* section). The effects on fetal mortality are expected consequences of the alterations in hormonal levels brought about by the drug. If this drug is used during pregnancy or if the patient becomes pregnant while taking this drug, she should be apprised of the potential hazard to the fetus.
4. Use in women who are breast feeding (see *Nursing Mothers* section).
5. A report of an anaphylactic reaction to synthetic GnRH (Factrel) has been reported in the medical literature.[1]

WARNINGS

Safe use of leuprolide acetate in pregnancy has not been established clinically. Before starting treatment with LUPRON DEPOT, pregnancy must be excluded.

When used monthly at the recommended dose, LUPRON DEPOT usually inhibits ovulation and stops menstruation. Contraception is not insured, however, by taking LUPRON DEPOT. Therefore, patients should use nonhormonal methods of contraception. Patients should be advised to see their physician if they believe they may be pregnant. If a patient becomes pregnant during treatment, the drug must be discontinued and the patient must be apprised of the potential risk to the fetus.

During the early phase of therapy, sex steroids temporarily rise above baseline because of the physiologic effect of the drug. Therefore, an increase in clinical signs and symptoms may be observed during the initial days of therapy, but these will dissipate with continued therapy.

PRECAUTIONS

Information for Patients: An information pamphlet for patients is included with the product. Patients should be aware of the following information:
1. Since menstruation should stop with effective doses of LUPRON DEPOT, the patient should notify her physician if regular menstruation persists. Patients missing successive doses of LUPRON DEPOT may experience breakthrough bleeding.
2. Patients should not use LUPRON DEPOT if they are pregnant, breast feeding, have undiagnosed abnormal vaginal bleeding, or are allergic to any of the ingredients in LUPRON DEPOT.
3. Safe use of the drug in pregnancy has not been established clinically. Therefore, a nonhormonal method of contraception should be used during treatment. Patients should be advised that if they miss successive doses of LUPRON DEPOT, breakthrough bleeding or ovulation may occur with the potential for conception. If a patient becomes pregnant during treatment, she should discontinue treatment and consult her physician.
4. Adverse events occurring in clinical studies with LUPRON DEPOT that are associated with hypoestrogenism include: hot flashes, headaches, emotional lability, decreased libido, acne, myalgia, reduction in breast size, and vaginal dryness. Estrogen levels returned to normal after treatment was discontinued.
5. The induced hypoestrogenic state **also** results in a small loss in bone density over the course of treatment, some of which may not be reversible. For a period up to six months, this bone loss should not be important. In patients with major risk factors for decreased bone mineral content such as chronic alcohol and/or tobacco use, strong family history of osteoporosis, or chronic use of drugs that can reduce bone mass such as anticonvulsants or corticosteroids, LUPRON DEPOT therapy may pose an additional risk. In these patients, the risks and benefits must be weighed carefully before therapy with LUPRON DEPOT is instituted. Repeated courses of therapy with gonadotropin-releasing hormone analogs beyond six months are not advisable in patients with major risk factors for loss of bone mineral content.
6. Retreatment cannot be recommended since safety data beyond six months are not available.

Drug Interactions: No pharmacokinetic-based drug-drug interaction studies have been conducted with LUPRON DEPOT. However, because leuprolide acetate is a peptide that is primarily degraded by peptidase and not by cytochrome P-450 enzymes as noted in specific studies, and the drug is only about 46% bound to plasma proteins, drug interactions would not be expected to occur.

Drug/Laboratory Test Interactions: Administration of LUPRON DEPOT in therapeutic doses results in suppression of the pituitary-gonadal system. Normal function is usually restored within three months after treatment is discontinued. Therefore, diagnostic tests of pituitary gonadotropic and gonadal functions conducted during treatment and for up to three months after discontinuation of LUPRON DEPOT may be misleading.

Carcinogenesis, Mutagenesis, Impairment of Fertility: A two-year carcinogenicity study was conducted in rats and mice. In rats, a dose-related increase of benign pituitary hyperplasia and benign pituitary adenomas was noted at 24 months when the drug was administered subcutaneously at high daily doses (0.6 to 4 mg/kg). There was a significant but not dose-related increase of pancreatic islet-cell adenomas in females and of testicular interstitial cell adenomas in males (highest incidence in the low dose group). In mice, no leuprolide acetate-induced tumors or pituitary abnormalities were observed at a dose as high as 60 mg/kg for two years. Patients have been treated with leuprolide acetate for up to three years with doses as high as 10 mg/day and for two years with doses as high as 20 mg/day without demonstrable pituitary abnormalities.

Mutagenicity studies have been performed with leuprolide acetate using bacterial and mammalian systems. These studies provided no evidence of a mutagenic potential.

Clinical and pharmacologic studies in adults (> 18 years) with leuprolide acetate and similar analogs have shown reversibility of fertility suppression when the drug is discontinued after continuous administration for periods of up to 24 weeks. Although no clinical studies have been completed in children to assess the full reversibility of fertility suppression, animal studies (prepubertal and adult rats and monkeys) with leuprolide acetate and other GnRH analogs have shown functional recovery.

Pregnancy, Teratogenic Effects: Pregnancy Category X. (See **CONTRAINDICATIONS** section.) When administered on day 6 of pregnancy at test dosages of 0.00024, 0.0024, and 0.024 mg/kg (1/300 to 1/3 the human dose) to rabbits, LUPRON DEPOT produced a dose-related increase in major fetal abnormalities. Similar studies in rats failed to demonstrate an increase in fetal malformations. There was increased fetal mortality and decreased fetal weights with the two higher doses of LUPRON DEPOT in rabbits and with the highest dose (0.024 mg/kg) in rats.

Nursing Mothers: It is not known whether LUPRON DEPOT is excreted in human milk. Because many drugs are excreted in human milk, and because the effects of LUPRON DEPOT on lactation and/or the breast-fed child have not been determined, LUPRON DEPOT should not be used by nursing mothers.

Pediatric Use: See LUPRON DEPOT-PED® (leuprolide acetate for depot suspension) labeling for the safety and effectiveness in children with central precocious puberty.

ADVERSE REACTIONS

Estradiol levels may increase during the first weeks following the initial injection, but then decline to menopausal levels. This transient increase in estradiol can be associated with a temporary worsening of signs and symptoms (see **WARNINGS** section).

As would be expected with a drug that lowers serum estradiol levels, the most frequently reported adverse reactions were those related to hypoestrogenism.

Endometriosis: In controlled studies comparing LUPRON DEPOT 3.75 mg monthly and danazol (800 mg/day) or placebo, adverse reactions most frequently reported and thought to be possibly or probably drug-related are shown in Figure 2.
[See Figure 2 at left.]

Cardiovascular System—Palpitations, Syncope, Tachycardia; *Gastrointestinal System*—Dry mouth, Thirst, Appetite changes; *Central/Peripheral Nervous System*—Anxiety,* Personality disorder, Memory disorder, Delusions; *Integumentary System*—Ecchymosis, Alopecia,

FIGURE 2—ADVERSE EVENTS REPORTED DURING 6 MONTHS OF TREATMENT WITH LUPRON DEPOT 3.75 MG

COSTART CATEGORIES (vertical axis):
EDEMA; NAUSEA/VOMITING; GI DISTURBANCES*; HOT FLASHES/SWEATS*; BREAST CHANGES, TENDERNESS/PAIN*; DECREASED LIBIDO*; ANDROGEN-LIKE EFFECTS; MYALGIA*; JOINT DISORDER*; DEPRESSION EMOTIONAL LABILITY*; HEADACHES*; DIZZINESS; INSOMNIA/SLEEP DISORDERS*; GENERAL PAIN; NEUROMUSCULAR DISORDERS*; NERVOUSNESS*; PARESTHESIAS; SKIN REACTIONS; VAGINITIS*; ASTHENIA; WEIGHT GAIN/LOSS

Legend:
- LUPRON DEPOT (N = 166)
- DANAZOL (N = 136)
- PLACEBO (N = 31)

*PHYSIOLOGIC EFFECT OF DECREASED ESTROGEN

PERCENTAGE OF PATIENTS (horizontal axis): 0 10 20 30 40 50 60 70 80 90 100

Hair disorder; *Urogenital System*—Dysuria,* Lactation;*Miscellaneous*—Ophthalmologic disorders,* Lymphadenopathy.

Uterine Leiomyomata (Fibroids): In controlled clinical trials comparing LUPRON DEPOT 3.75 mg and placebo, adverse events reported in >5% of patients and thought to be potentially related to drug are noted in the following table.

	Lupron Depot 3.75 mg N=166 (%)	**Placebo N=163 (%)**
Body as a Whole		
Asthenia	14 (8.4)	8 (4.9)
General pain	14 (8.4)	10 (6.1)
Headache*	43 (25.9)	29 (17.8)
Cardiovascular System		
Hot flashes/sweats*	121 (72.9)	29 (17.8)
Metabolic and Nutritional Disorders		
Edema	9 (5.4)	2 (1.2)
Musculoskeletal System		
Joint disorder*	13 (7.8)	5 (3.1)
Nervous System		
Depression/emotional lability*	18 (10.8)	7 (4.3)
Urogenital System		
Vaginitis*	19 (11.4)	3 (1.8)

Symptoms reported in <5% of patients included: *Body as Whole*—Body odor, Flu syndrome, Injection site reactions; *Cardiovascular System*—Tachycardia; *Digestive System*—Appetite changes, Dry mouth, GI disturbances, Nausea/vomiting; *Metabolic and Nutritional Disorders*—Weight changes; *Musculoskeletal System*—Myalgia; *Nervous System*—Anxiety, Decreased libido,* Dizziness, Insomnia, Nervousness,* Neuromuscular disorders,* Paresthesias; *Respiratory System*—Rhinitis; *Integumentary System*—Androgen-like effects, Nail disorder, Skin reactions; *Special Senses*—Conjunctivitis, Taste perversion; *Urogenital System*—Breast changes,* Menstrual disorders.

* = Physiologic effect of the drug.

In one controlled clinical trial, patients received a higher dose (7.5 mg) of LUPRON DEPOT. Events seen with this dose that were thought to be potentially related to drug and were not seen at the lower dose included palpitations, syncope, glossitis, ecchymosis, hypesthesia, confusion, lactation, pyelonephritis, and urinary disorders. Generally, a higher incidence of hypoestrogenic effects was observed at the higher dose.

Postmarketing

During postmarketing surveillance, the following adverse events were reported. Like other drugs in this class, mood swings, including depression, have been reported as a physiologic effect of decreased sex steroids. There have been very rare reports of suicidal ideation and attempt. Many, but not all, of these patients had a history of depression or other psychiatric illness. Patients should be counseled on the possibility of worsening of depression.

Symptoms consistent with an anaphylactoid or asthmatic process have been rarely reported. Rash, urticaria, and photosensitivity reactions have also been reported.

Localized reactions including induration and abscess have been reported at the site of injection.

Cardiovascular System - Hypotension; *Hemic and Lymphatic System* - Decreased WBC; *Central/Peripheral Nervous System* - Peripheral neuropathy, Spinal fracture/paralysis; *Musculoskeletal System* - Tenosynovitis-like symptoms; *Urogenital System* - Prostate pain.

See other LUPRON DEPOT and LUPRON Injection package inserts for other events reported in different patient populations.

Changes in Bone Density:

Endometriosis: A controlled study in endometriosis patients showed that vertebral bone density as measured by dual energy x-ray absorptiometry (DEXA) decreased by an average of 3.9% at six months compared with the pretreatment value. For those patients who were tested at six or twelve months after discontinuation of therapy, mean bone density returned to within 2% of pretreatment. Use of LUPRON DEPOT 3.75 mg for longer than six months or in the presence of other known risk factors for decreased bone mineral content may cause additional bone loss.

Uterine Leiomyomata (Fibroids): In one study, vertebral trabecular bone mineral density as assessed by quantitative digital radiography (QDR) revealed a mean decrease of 2.7% at three months compared with the pretreatment value. Six months after discontinuation of therapy a trend toward recovery was observed. Use of LUPRON DEPOT 3.75 mg for uterine leiomyomata for longer than three months or in the presence of other known risk factors for decreased bone mineral content may cause additional bone loss **and is not recommended.**

Changes in Laboratory Values During Treatment:

Plasma Enzymes

Endometriosis: During clinical trials with LUPRON DEPOT 3.75 mg, regular laboratory monitoring revealed that AST levels were more than twice the upper limit of normal in only one patient. There was no clinical or other laboratory evidence of abnormal liver function.

Uterine Leiomyomata (Fibroids): In clinical trials with LUPRON DEPOT 3.75 mg, five (3%) patients had a post-treatment transaminase value that was at least twice the baseline value and above the upper limit of the normal range. None of the laboratory increases were associated with clinical symptoms.

Lipids

Endometriosis: At enrollment, 4% of the LUPRON DEPOT 3.75 mg patients and 1% of the danazol patients had total cholesterol values above the normal range. These patients also had cholesterol values above the normal range at the end of treatment.

Of those patients whose pretreatment cholesterol values were in the normal range, 7% of the LUPRON DEPOT 3.75 mg patients and 9% of the danazol patients had post-treatment values above the normal range.

The mean (±SEM) pretreatment values for total cholesterol from all patients were 178.8 (2.9) mg/dL in the LUPRON DEPOT 3.75 mg groups and 175.3 (3.0) mg/dL in the danazol group. At the end of treatment, the mean values for total cholesterol from all patients were 193.3 mg/dL in the LUPRON DEPOT 3.75 mg group and 194.4 mg/dL in the danazol group. These increases from the pretreatment values were statistically significant ($p < 0.03$) in both groups.

Triglycerides were increased above the upper limit of normal in 12% of the patients who received LUPRON DEPOT 3.75 mg and in 6% of the patients who received danazol.

At the end of treatment, HDL cholesterol fractions decreased below the lower limit of the normal range in 2% of the LUPRON DEPOT 3.75 mg patients compared with 54% of those receiving danazol. LDL cholesterol fractions increased above the upper limit of the normal range in 6% of the patients receiving LUPRON DEPOT 3.75 mg compared with 23% of those receiving danazol. There was no increase in the LDL/HDL ratio in patients receiving LUPRON DEPOT 3.75 mg but there was approximately a two-fold increase in the LDL/HDL ratio in patients receiving danazol.

Uterine Leiomyomata (Fibroids): In patients receiving LUPRON DEPOT 3.75 mg, mean changes in cholesterol (+11 mg/dL to +29 mg/dL), LDL cholesterol (+8 mg/dL to +22 mg/dL), HDL cholesterol (0 to +6 mg/dL), and the LDL/HDL ratio (−0.1 to +0.5) were observed across studies. In the one study in which triglycerides were determined, the mean increase from baseline was 32 mg/dL.

Other Changes

Endometriosis: In comparative studies, the following changes were seen in approximately 5% to 8% of patients. LUPRON DEPOT 3.75 mg was associated with elevations of LDH and phosphorus, and deceases in WBC counts. Danazol therapy was associated with increases in hematocrit, platelet count, and LDH.

Uterine Leiomyomata (Fibroids):

Hematology: (See Clinical Studies section.) In LUPRON DEPOT 3.75 mg treated patients, although there were statistically significant mean decreases in platelet counts from baseline to final visit, the last mean platelet counts were within the normal range. Decreases in total WBC count and neutrophils were observed, but were not clinically significant.

Chemistry: Slight to moderate mean increases were noted for glucose, uric acid, BUN, creatinine, total protein, albumin, bilirubin, alkaline phosphatase, LDH, calcium, and phosphorus. None of these increases were clinically significant.

OVERDOSAGE

In rats subcutaneous administration of 250 to 500 times the recommended human dose, expressed on a per body weight basis, resulted in dyspnea, decreased activity, and local irritation at the injection site. There is no evidence that there is a clinical counterpart of this phenomenon. In early clinical trials using daily subcutaneous leuprolide acetate in patients with prostate cancer, doses as high as 20 mg/day for up to two years caused no adverse effects differing from those observed with the 1 mg/day dose.

DOSAGE AND ADMINISTRATION

LUPRON DEPOT Must Be Administered Under The Supervision Of A Physician.

The recommended dose of LUPRON DEPOT is 3.75 mg, incorporated in a depot formulation. The lyophilized microspheres are to be reconstituted and administered monthly as a single intramuscular injection, in accord with the following directions:

1. Using a syringe with a 23 gauge needle, withdraw 1 mL of diluent from the ampule, and inject it into the vial. (Extra diluent is provided; any remaining should be discarded.)
2. Shake well to thoroughly disperse particles to obtain a uniform suspension. The suspension will appear milky.
3. Withdraw the entire contents of the vial into the syringe and inject it at the time of reconstitution.

Although the potency of the reconstituted suspension has been shown to be stable for 24 hours, since the product does not contain a preservative, the suspension should be discarded if not used immediately.

Endometriosis: The recommended duration of administration is six months. Retreatment cannot be recommended since safety data for retreatment are not available. If the symptoms of endometriosis recur after a course of therapy, and further treatment with LUPRON DEPOT 3.75 mg is contemplated, it is recommended that bone density be assessed before retreatment begins to ensure that values are within normal limits.

Uterine Leiomyomata (Fibroids): Recommended duration of therapy with LUPRON DEPOT 3.75 mg is up to 3 months. The symptoms associated with uterine leiomyomata will recur following discontinuation of therapy. If additional treatment with LUPRON DEPOT 3.75 mg is contemplated, bone density should be assessed prior to initiation of therapy to ensure that values are within normal limits.

As with other drugs administered by injection, the injection site should be varied periodically.

The vial of LUPRON DEPOT and the ampule of diluent may be stored at room temperature.

HOW SUPPLIED

LUPRON DEPOT 3.75 mg is available in a single use kit (NDC 0300-3639-01) and in a six pack of drug only (NDC 0300-3639-06). Each vial contains sterile lyophilized microspheres which is leuprolide incorporated in a biodegradable copolymer of lactic and glycolic acids. When mixed with 1 mL of diluent, LUPRON DEPOT 3.75 mg is administered as a single monthly IM injection.

No refrigeration necessary. Protect from freezing.

Caution: Federal (U.S.A.) law prohibits dispensing without a prescription.

REFERENCE

1. MacLeod TL, et al. Anaphylactic reaction to synthetic luteinizing hormone-releasing hormone. *Fertil Steril* 1987 Sept; 48(3):500-502.

U.S. Patent Nos. 4,652,441; 4,677,191; 4,728,721; 4,849,228; 4,917,893; 4,954,298; 5,330,767; and 5,476,663.

(No. 3639)

03-4638-R5-Rev. May, 1996

TAP Pharmaceuticals Inc.
Deerfield, Illinois 60015-1595, U.S.A.

LUPRON DEPOT 3.75 mg
manufactured by Takeda Chemical Industries, Ltd.
Osaka, JAPAN 541

®—Registered trademark

Shown in Product Identification Guide, page 338

LUPRON DEPOT® 7.5 mg ℞
(leuprolide acetate for depot suspension)

DESCRIPTION

Leuprolide acetate is a synthetic nonapeptide analog of naturally occurring gonadotropin-releasing hormone (GnRH or LH-RH). The analog possesses greater potency than the natural hormone. The chemical name is 5-oxo-L-prolyl-L-histidyl-L-tryptophyl-L-seryl-L-tyrosyl-D-leucyl-L-leucyl-L-arginyl-N-ethyl-L-prolinamide acetate (salt) with the following structural formula:

[See structure on top of next page.]

LUPRON DEPOT is available in a vial containing sterile lyophilized microspheres, which when mixed with diluent, become a suspension which is intended as a monthly intramuscular injection.

The single-dose vial of LUPRON DEPOT 7.5 mg contains leuprolide acetate (7.5 mg), purified gelatin (1.3 mg), DL-lactic and glycolic acids copolymer (66.2 mg), and D-mannitol (13.2 mg). The accompanying ampule of diluent contains carboxymethylcellulose sodium (10 mg), D-mannitol (100 mg), polysorbate 80 (2 mg), water for injection, USP, and glacial acetic acid, USP to control pH.

During the manufacture of LUPRON DEPOT 7.5 mg, acetic acid is lost, leaving the peptide.

CLINICAL PHARMACOLOGY

Leuprolide acetate, an LH-RH agonist, acts as a potent inhibitor of gonadotropin secretion when given continuously and in therapeutic doses. Animal and human studies indicate that following an initial stimulation, chronic administration of leuprolide acetate results in suppression of ovarian and testicular steroidogenesis. This effect is reversible upon discontinuation of drug therapy. Administration of leuprolide acetate has resulted in inhibition of the growth of certain hormone dependent tumors (prostatic tumors in Noble and Dunning male rats and DMBA-induced mammary tumors in female rats) as well as atrophy of the reproductive organs.

In humans, administration of leuprolide acetate results in an initial increase in circulating levels of luteinizing hormone (LH) and follicle stimulating hormone (FSH), leading to a transient increase in levels of the gonadal steroids (testosterone and dihydrotestosterone in males, and estrone and estradiol in premenopausal females). However, continuous administration of leuprolide acetate results in decreased levels of LH and FSH. In males, testosterone is reduced to castrate levels. In premenopausal females, estrogens are reduced to postmenopausal levels. These decreases occur within two to four weeks after initiation of treatment, and castrate levels of testosterone in prostate cancer patients have been demonstrated for more than five years.

Leuprolide acetate is not active when given orally.

Continued on next page

TAP—Cont.

PHARMACOKINETICS

Absorption: Following a single LUPRON DEPOT 7.5 mg injection to patients, mean peak leuprolide plasma concentration was almost 20 ng/mL at 4 hours and 0.36 ng/mL at 4 weeks. However, intact leuprolide and an inactive major metabolite could not be distinguished by the assay which was employed in the study. Nondetectable leuprolide plasma concentrations have been observed during chronic LUPRON DEPOT 7.5 mg administration, but testosterone levels appear to be maintained at castrate levels.
Distribution: The mean steady-state volume of distribution of leuprolide following intravenous bolus administration to healthy male volunteers was 27 L. In vitro binding to human plasma proteins ranged from 43% to 49%.
Metabolism: In healthy male volunteers, a 1 mg bolus of leuprolide administered intravenously revealed that the mean systemic clearance was 7.6 L/h, with a terminal elimination half-life of approximately 3 hours based on a two compartment model.
In rats and dogs, administration of ^{14}C-labeled leuprolide was shown to be metabolized to smaller inactive peptides, a pentapeptide (Metabolite I), tripeptides (Metabolites II and III) and a dipeptide (Metabolite IV). These fragments may be further catabolized.
The major metabolite (M-I) plasma concentrations measured in 5 prostate cancer patients reached maximum concentration 2 to 6 hours after dosing and were approximately 6% of the peak parent drug concentration.
One week after dosing, mean plasma M-I concentrations were approximately 20% of mean leuprolide concentrations.
Excretion: Following administration of LUPRON DEPOT 3.75 mg to 3 patients, less than 5% of the dose was recovered as parent and M-I metabolite in the urine.
Special Populations: The pharmacokinetics of the drug in hepatically and renally impaired patients have not been determined.

INDICATIONS AND USAGE

LUPRON DEPOT 7.5 mg is indicated in the palliative treatment of advanced prostatic cancer. It offers an alternative treatment of prostatic cancer when orchiectomy or estrogen administration are either not indicated or unacceptable to the patient. In clinical trials, the safety and efficacy of LUPRON DEPOT 7.5 mg does not differ from that of the original daily subcutaneous injection.

CONTRAINDICATIONS

A report of an anaphylactic reaction to synthetic GnRH (Factrel) has been reported in the medical literature.[1]
LUPRON DEPOT is contraindicated in women who are or may become pregnant while receiving the drug. When administered on day 6 of pregnancy at test dosages of 0.00024, 0.0024, and 0.024 mg/kg (1/600 to 1/6 the human dose) to rabbits, LUPRON DEPOT produced a dose-related increase in major fetal abnormalities. Similar studies in rats failed to demonstrate an increase in fetal malformations. There was increased fetal mortality and decreased fetal weights with the two higher doses of LUPRON DEPOT in rabbits and with the highest dose in rats. The effects on fetal mortality are logical consequences of the alterations in hormonal levels brought about by this drug. Therefore, the possibility exists that spontaneous abortion may occur if the drug is administered during pregnancy.

WARNINGS

Isolated cases of worsening of signs and symptoms during the first weeks of treatment have been reported with LH-RH analogs. Worsening of symptoms may contribute to paralysis with or without fatal complications. For patients at risk, the physician may consider initiating therapy with daily LUPRON® (leuprolide acetate) Injection for the first two weeks to facilitate withdrawal of treatment if that is considered necessary.

PRECAUTIONS

Patients with metastatic vertebral lesions and/or with urinary tract obstruction should be closely observed during the first few weeks of therapy (see **WARNINGS** section).
Laboratory Tests: Response to LUPRON DEPOT 7.5 mg should be monitored by measuring serum levels of testosterone, as well as prostate-specific antigen and prostatic acid phosphatase. In the majority of patients, testosterone levels increased above baseline during the first week, declining thereafter to baseline levels or below by the end of the second week. Castrate levels were reached within two to four weeks and once achieved were maintained for as long as the patients received their injections. Transient increases in prostatic acid phosphatase levels may occur sometime early in treatment. However, by the fourth week, the elevated levels can be expected to decrease to values at or near baseline.
Drug Interactions: No pharmacokinetic-based drug-drug interaction studies have been conducted with LUPRON DEPOT. However, because leuprolide acetate is a peptide that is primarily degraded by peptidase and not by cyto-

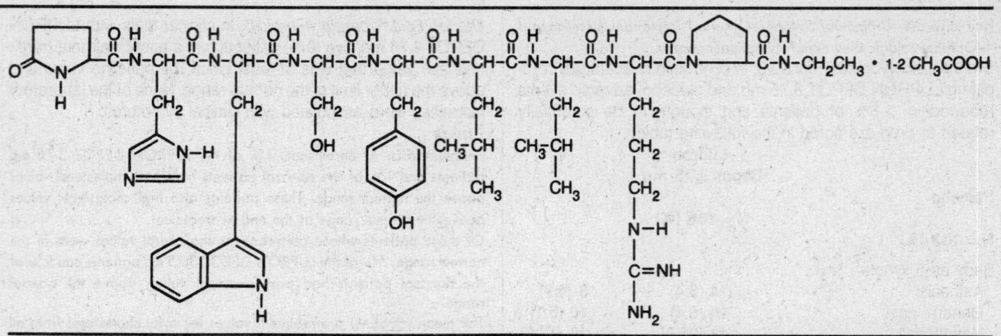

chrome P-450 enzymes as noted in specific studies, and the drug is only about 46% bound to plasma proteins, drug interactions would not be expected to occur.
Drug/Laboratory Test Interactions: Administration of LUPRON DEPOT in therapeutic doses results in suppression of the pituitary-gonadal system. Normal function is usually restored within one to three months after treatment is discontinued. Therefore, diagnostic tests of pituitary gonadotropic and gonadal functions conducted during treatment and up to one to two months after discontinuation of LUPRON DEPOT therapy may be misleading.
Carcinogenesis, Mutagenesis, Impairment of Fertility: Two-year carcinogenicity studies were conducted in rats and mice. In rats, a dose-related increase of benign pituitary hyperplasia and benign pituitary adenomas was noted at 24 months when the drug was administered subcutaneously at high daily doses (0.6 to 4 mg/kg). There was a significant but not dose-related increase of pancreatic islet-cell adenomas in females and of testicular interstitial cell adenomas in males (highest incidence in the low dose group). In mice, no leuprolide acetate-induced tumors or pituitary abnormalities were observed at a dose as high as 60 mg/kg for two years. Patients have been treated with leuprolide acetate for up to three years with doses as high as 10 mg/day and for two years with doses as high as 20 mg/day without demonstrable pituitary abnormalities.
Mutagenicity studies have been performed with leuprolide acetate using bacterial and mammalian systems. These studies provided no evidence of a mutagenic potential.
Clinical and pharmacologic studies in adults (≥18 years) with leuprolide acetate and similar analogs have shown reversibility of fertility suppression when the drug is discontinued after continuous administration for periods of up to 24 weeks.
Pregnancy Category X. (See **CONTRAINDICATIONS** section.)
Pediatric Use: See LUPRON DEPOT-PED® (leuprolide acetate for depot suspension) labeling for the safety and effectiveness of the monthly formulation in children with central precocious puberty.

ADVERSE REACTIONS

In the majority of patients testosterone levels increased above baseline during the first week, declining thereafter to baseline levels or below by the end of the second week of treatment.
Potential exacerbations of signs and symptoms during the first few weeks of treatment is a concern in patients with vertebral metastases and/or urinary obstruction or hematuria which, if aggravated, may lead to neurological problems such as temporary weakness and/or paresthesia of the lower limbs or worsening of urinary symptoms (see **WARNINGS** section).
In a clinical trial of LUPRON DEPOT 7.5 mg, the following adverse reactions were reported to have a possible or probable relationship to drug as ascribed by the treating physician in 5% or more of the patients receiving the drug. **Often, causality is difficult to assess in patients with metastatic prostate cancer.** Reactions considered not drug-related are excluded.

	LUPRON DEPOT 7.5 mg N=56	(Percent)
Cardiovascular System		
Edema	7	(12.5%)
Gastrointestinal System		
Nausea/vomiting	3	(5.4%)
Endocrine System		
*Decreased testicular size	3	(5.4%)
*Hot flashes/sweats	33	(58.9%)
*Impotence	3	(5.4%)
Central/Peripheral Nervous System		
General pain	4	(7.1%)
Respiratory System		
Dyspnea	3	(5.4%)
Miscellaneous		
Asthenia	3	(5.4%)

*Physiologic effect of decreased testosterone.

Laboratory: Elevations of certain parameters were observed, but it is difficult to assess these abnormalities in this population.

SGOT (>2N)	4	(7.1%)
LDH (>2N)	11	(19.6%)
Alkaline phos (>1.5N)	4	(7.1%)

In this same study, the following adverse reactions were reported in less than 5% of the patients on LUPRON DEPOT 7.5 mg.
Cardiovascular System—Angina, Cardiac arrhythmia; *Gastrointestinal System*—Anorexia, Diarrhea; *Endocrine System*—Gynecomastia, Libido decrease; *Musculoskeletal System*—Bone pain, Myalgia; *Central/Peripheral Nervous System*—Paresthesia, Insomnia; *Respiratory System*—Hemoptysis; *Integumentary System*—Dermatitis, Local skin reactions, Hair growth; *Urogenital System*—Dysuria, Frequency/urgency, Hematuria, Testicular pain; *Miscellaneous—Diabetes,* Fever/chills, Hard nodule in throat, Increased calcium, Weight gain, Increased uric acid.
Postmarketing
During postmarketing surveillance, which includes other dosage forms, the following adverse events were reported.
Symptoms consistent with an anaphylactoid or asthmatic process have been rarely reported with GnRH analogs. Rash, urticaria, and photosensitivity reactions have also been reported.
Localized reactions including induration and abscess have been reported at the site of injection.
Cardiovascular System—Hypotension; *Hemic and Lymphatic System*— Decreased WBC; *Central/Peripheral Nervous System*—Peripheral neuropathy, Spinal fracture/paralysis; *Musculoskeletal System*—Tenosynovitis-like symptoms; *Urogenital System*—Prostate pain.
See other LUPRON DEPOT and LUPRON Injection package inserts for other events reported in different patient populations.

OVERDOSAGE

In rats subcutaneous administration of 250 to 500 times the recommended human dose, expressed on a per body weight basis, resulted in dyspnea, decreased activity, and local irritation at the injection site. There is no evidence that there is a clinical counterpart of this phenomenon. In early clinical trials with daily subcutaneous leuprolide acetate, doses as high as 20 mg/day for up to two years caused no adverse effects differing from those observed with the 1 mg/day dose.

DOSAGE AND ADMINISTRATION

LUPRON DEPOT Must Be Administered Under The Supervision Of A Physician.
The recommended dose of LUPRON DEPOT is 7.5 mg, incorporated in a depot formulation. The lyophilized microspheres are to be reconstituted and administered monthly as a single intramuscular injection, in accord with the following directions:
1. Using a syringe with a 23 gauge needle, withdraw 1 mL of diluent from the ampule, and inject it into the vial. (Extra diluent is provided; any remaining should be discarded.)
2. Shake well to thoroughly disperse particles to obtain a uniform suspension. The suspension will appear milky.
3. Withdraw the entire contents of the vial into the syringe and inject it at the time of reconstitution.

Although the potency of the reconstituted suspension has been shown to be stable for 24 hours, since the product does not contain a preservative, the suspension should be discarded if not used immediately.
As with other drugs administered by injection, the injection site should be varied periodically.
The vial of LUPRON DEPOT 7.5 mg and the ampule of diluent may be stored at room temperature.

HOW SUPPLIED

LUPRON DEPOT 7.5 mg is available in a single use kit (NDC 0300-3629-01) and in a six pack of drug only (NDC 0300-3629-06). Each vial contains sterile lyophilized microspheres which is leuprolide incorporated in a biodegradable copolymer of lactic and glycolic acids. When mixed with 1 mL of diluent, LUPRON DEPOT 7.5 mg is administered as a single monthly IM injection.
An information pamphlet for patients is included with the kit.

No refrigeration necessary. Protect from freezing.
Caution: Federal (U.S.A.) law prohibits dispensing without a prescription.

REFERENCE

1. MacLeod TL, et al. Anaphylactic reaction to synthetic luteinizing hormone-releasing hormone. Fertil Steril 1987 Sept; 48(3):500–502.

U.S. Patent Nos. 4,652,441; 4,677,191; 4,728,721; 4,849,228; 4,917,893; 4,954,298; 5,330,767; and 5,476,663.
TAP Pharmaceuticals Inc.
Deerfield, Illinois 60015-1595, U.S.A.
LUPRON DEPOT 7.5 mg manufactured by
Takeda Chemical Industries, Ltd.
Osaka, JAPAN 541
®—Registered trademark
(No. 3629)
03-4639-R5–Rev. Feb., 1996

Shown in Product Identification Guide, page 338

LUPRON DEPOT®-3 Month 22.5 mg ℞
(leuprolide acetate for depot suspension)

3-MONTH FORMULATION

DESCRIPTION

Leuprolide acetate is a synthetic nonapeptide analog of naturally occurring gonadotropin-releasing hormone (GnRH or LH-RH). The analog possesses greater potency than the natural hormone. The chemical name is 5-oxo-L-prolyl-L-histidyl-L-tryptophyl -L- seryl-L-tyrosyl-D-leucyl-L- leucyl-L-arginyl-N-ethyl-L-prolinamide acetate (salt) with the following structural formula:
[See structure above.]

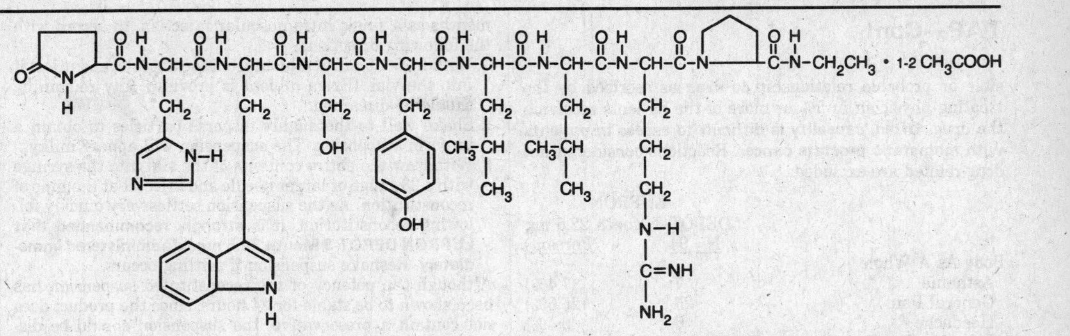

LUPRON DEPOT-3 Month 22.5 mg is available in a vial containing sterile lyophilized microspheres, which when mixed with diluent, become a suspension which is intended as an intramuscular injection to be given **ONCE EVERY THREE MONTHS (84 days).**
The single-dose vial of LUPRON DEPOT-3 Month 22.5 mg contains leuprolide acetate (22.5 mg), polylactic acid (198.6 mg), and D-mannitol (38.9 mg). The accompanying ampule of diluent contains carboxymethylcellulose sodium (10 mg), D-mannitol (100 mg), polysorbate 80 (2 mg), water for injection, USP, and glacial acetic acid, USP to control pH.
During the manufacture of LUPRON DEPOT-3 Month 22.5 mg, acetic acid is lost, leaving the peptide.

CLINICAL PHARMACOLOGY

Leuprolide acetate, an LH-RH agonist, acts as a potent inhibitor of gonadotropin secretion when given continuously and in therapeutic doses. Animal and human studies indicate that following an initial stimulation, chronic administration of leuprolide acetate results in suppression of ovarian and testicular steroidogenesis. This effect is reversible upon discontinuation of drug therapy. Administration of leuprolide acetate has resulted in inhibition of the growth of certain hormone dependent tumors (prostatic tumors in Noble and Dunning male rats and DMBA-induced mammary tumors in female rats) as well as atrophy of the reproductive organs.
In humans, administration of leuprolide acetate results in an initial increase in circulating levels of luteinizing hormone (LH) and follicle stimulating hormone (FSH), leading to a transient increase in levels of the gonadal steroids (testosterone and dihydrotestosterone in males, and estrone and estradiol in premenopausal females). However, continuous administration of leuprolide acetate results in decreased levels of LH and FSH. In males, testosterone is reduced to castrate levels. In premenopausal females, estrogens are reduced to postmenopausal levels. These decreases occur within two to four weeks after initiation of treatment, and castrate levels of testosterone in prostatic cancer patients have been demonstrated for more than five years.
Leuprolide acetate is not active when given orally.

PHARMACOKINETICS

Absorption: Following a single injection of the three month formulation of LUPRON DEPOT-3 Month 22.5 mg in patients, mean peak plasma leuprolide concentration of 48.9 ng/mL was observed at 4 hours and then declined to 0.67 ng/mL at 12 weeks. Leuprolide appeared to be released at a constant rate following the onset of steady-state levels during the third week after dosing, providing steady plasma concentrations through the 12-week dosing interval. However, intact leuprolide and an inactive major metabolite could not be distinguished by the assay which was employed in the study. Detectable levels of leuprolide were present at all measurement points in all patients. The initial burst, followed by the rapid decline to a steady-state level, was similar to the release pattern seen with the monthly formulation.
Distribution: The mean steady-state volume of distribution of leuprolide following intravenous bolus administration to healthy male volunteers was 27 L. In vitro binding to human plasma proteins ranged from 43% to 49%.
Metabolism: In healthy male volunteers, a 1 mg bolus of leuprolide administered intravenously revealed that the mean systemic clearance was 7.6 L/h, with a terminal elimination half-life of approximately 3 hours based on a two compartment model.
In rats and dogs, administration of ^{14}C-labeled leuprolide was shown to be metabolized to smaller inactive peptides, a pentapeptide (Metabolite I), tripeptides (Metabolites II and III) and a dipeptide (Metabolite IV). These fragments may be further catabolized.
The major metabolite (M-I) plasma concentrations measured in 5 prostate cancer patients reached maximum concentration 2 to 6 hours after dosing and were approximately 6% of the peak parent drug concentration. One week after dosing, mean plasma M-I concentrations were approximately 20% of mean leuprolide concentrations.
Excretion: Following administration of LUPRON DEPOT 3.75 mg to 3 patients, less than 5% of the dose was recovered as parent and M-I metabolite in the urine.
Special Populations: The pharmacokinetics of the drug in hepatically and renally impaired patients have not been determined.

CLINICAL STUDIES

In clinical studies, serum testosterone was suppressed to castrate within 30 days in 87 of 92 (95%) patients and within an additional two weeks in three patients. Two patients did not suppress for 15 and 28 weeks, respectively. Suppression was maintained in all of these patients with the exception of transient minimal testosterone elevations in one of them, and in another an increase in serum testosterone to above the castrate range was recorded during the 12 hour observation period after a subsequent injection. This represents stimulation of gonadotropin secretion.
An 85% rate of "no progression" was achieved during the initial 24 weeks of treatment. A decrease from baseline in serum PSA of ≥90% was reported in 71% of the patients and a change to within the normal range (≤3.99 ng/mL) in 63% of the patients.
Periodic monitoring of serum testosterone and PSA levels is recommended, especially if the anticipated clinical or biochemical response to treatment has not been achieved. It should be noted that results of testosterone determinations are dependent on assay methodology. It is advisable to be aware of the type and precision of the assay methodology to make appropriate clinical and therapeutic decisions.

INDICATIONS AND USAGE

LUPRON DEPOT-3 Month 22.5 mg is indicated in the palliative treatment of advanced prostatic cancer. It offers an alternative treatment of prostatic cancer when orchiectomy or estrogen administration are either not indicated or unacceptable to the patient. In clinical trials, the safety and efficacy of LUPRON DEPOT-3 Month 22.5 mg were similar to that of the original daily subcutaneous injection and the monthly depot formulation.

CONTRAINDICATIONS

A report of an anaphylactic reaction to synthetic GnRH (Factrel) has been reported in the medical literature.[1]
LUPRON DEPOT is contraindicated in women who are or may become pregnant while receiving the drug. When administered on day 6 of pregnancy at test dosages of 0.00024, 0.0024, and 0.024 mg/kg (1/600 to 1/6 the human dose) to rabbits, the monthly formulation of LUPRON DEPOT produced a dose-related increase in major fetal abnormalities. Similar studies in rats failed to demonstrate an increase in fetal malformations. There was increased fetal mortality and decreased fetal weights with the two higher doses of the monthly formulation of LUPRON DEPOT in rabbits and with the highest dose in rats. The effects on fetal mortality are logical consequences of the alterations in hormonal levels brought about by this drug. Therefore, the possibility exists that spontaneous abortion may occur if the drug is administered during pregnancy.

WARNINGS

Isolated cases of worsening of signs and symptoms during the first weeks of treatment have been reported with LH-RH analogs. Worsening of symptoms may contribute to paralysis with or without fatal complications. For patients at risk, the physician may consider initiating therapy with daily LUPRON® (leuprolide acetate) Injection for the first two weeks to facilitate withdrawal of treatment if that is considered necessary.

PRECAUTIONS

Patients with metastatic vertebral lesions and/or with urinary tract obstruction should be closely observed during the first few weeks of therapy (see **WARNINGS** section).
Laboratory Tests: Response to LUPRON DEPOT-3 Month 22.5 mg should be monitored by measuring serum levels of testosterone, as well as prostate-specific antigen and prostatic acid phosphatase. In the majority of patients, testosterone levels increased above baseline during the first week, declining thereafter to baseline levels or below by the end of the second week. Castrate levels were reached within two to four weeks and once achieved were maintained for as long as the patients received their injections.
Drug Interactions: No pharmacokinetic-based drug-drug interaction studies have been conducted with LUPRON DEPOT. However, because leuprolide acetate is a peptide that is primarily degraded by peptidase and not by cytochrome P-450 enzymes as noted in specific studies, and the drug is only about 46% bound to plasma proteins, drug interactions would not be expected to occur.
Drug/Laboratory Test Interactions: Administration of LUPRON DEPOT 3.75 mg in women results in suppression of the pituitary-gonadal system. Normal function is usually restored within one to three months after treatment is discontinued. Therefore, diagnostic tests of pituitary gonadotropic and gonadal functions conducted during treatment and up to three months after discontinuation of LUPRON DEPOT 3.75 mg therapy may be misleading.
Carcinogenesis, Mutagenesis, Impairment of Fertility: Two-year carcinogenicity studies were conducted in rats and mice. In rats, a dose-related increase of benign pituitary hyperplasia and benign pituitary adenomas was noted at 24 months when the drug was administered subcutaneously at high daily doses (0.6 to 4 mg/kg). There was a significant but not dose-related increase of pancreatic islet-cell adenomas in females and of testicular interstitial cell adenomas in males (highest incidence in the low dose group). In mice no pituitary abnormalities were observed at a dose as high as 60 mg/kg for two years. Patients have been treated with leuprolide acetate for up to three years with doses as high as 10 mg/day and for two years with doses as high as 20 mg/day without demonstrable pituitary abnormalities.
Mutagenicity studies have been performed with leuprolide acetate using bacterial and mammalian systems. These studies provided no evidence of a mutagenic potential.
Clinical and pharmacologic studies in adults (≥18 years) with leuprolide acetate and similar analogs have shown reversibility of fertility suppression when the drug is discontinued after continuous administration for periods of up to 24 weeks.
Pregnancy Category X. (See **CONTRAINDICATIONS** section.)
Pediatric Use: See LUPRON DEPOT-PED® (leuprolide acetate for depot suspension) labeling for the safety and effectiveness of the monthly formulation in children with central precocious puberty.

ADVERSE REACTIONS

In the majority of patients testosterone levels increased above baseline during the first week, declining thereafter to baseline levels or below by the end of the second week of treatment.
Potential exacerbations of signs and symptoms during the first few weeks of treatment is a concern in patients with vertebral metastases and/or urinary obstruction or hematuria which, if aggravated, may lead to neurological problems such as temporary weakness and/or paresthesia of the lower limbs or worsening of urinary symptoms (see **WARNINGS** section).
In two clinical trials of LUPRON DEPOT-3 Month 22.5 mg, the following adverse reactions were reported to have a pos-

Continued on next page

TAP—Cont.

sible or probable relationship to drug as ascribed by the treating physician in 5% or more of the patients receiving the drug. **Often, causality is difficult to assess in patients with metastatic prostate cancer. Reactions considered not drug-related are excluded.**

	LUPRON DEPOT-3 Month 22.5 mg N = 94	(Percent)
Body As A Whole		
Asthenia	7	(7.4%)
General Pain	25	(26.6%)
Headache	6	(6.4%)
Injection Site Reaction	13	(13.8%)
Cardiovascular System		
Hot flashes/Sweats*	55	(58.5%)
Digestive System		
GI Disorders	15	(16.0%)
Musculoskeletal System		
Joint Disorders	11	(11.7%)
Central/Peripheral Nervous System		
Dizziness/Vertigo	6	(6.4%)
Insomnia/Sleep Disorders	8	(8.5%)
Neuromuscular Disorders	9	(9.6%)
Respiratory System		
Respiratory Disorders	6	(6.4%)
Skin and Appendages		
Skin Reaction	8	(8.5%)
Urogenital System		
Testicular Atrophy*	19	(20.2%)
Urinary Disorders	14	(14.9%)

In these same studies, the following adverse reactions were reported in less than 5% of the patients on LUPRON DEPOT-3 Month 22.5 mg.
Body As A Whole— Enlarged abdomen, Fever; *Cardiovascular System*—Arrhythmia, Bradycardia, Heart failure, Hypertension, Hypotension, Varicose vein; *Digestive System* — Anorexia, Duodenal ulcer, Increased appetite, Thirst/dry mouth; *Hemic and Lymphatic System*— Anemia, Lymphedema; *Metabolic and Nutritional Disorders*— Dehydration, Edema; *Central/Peripheral Nervous System*— Anxiety, Delusions, Depression, Hypesthesia, Libido decreased*, Nervousness, Paresthesia; *Respiratory System*— Epistaxis, Pharyngitis, Pleural effusion, Pneumonia; *Special Senses*— Abnormal vision, Amblyopia, Dry eyes, Tinnitus; *Urogenital System*— Gynecomastia, Impotence*, Penis disorders, Testis disorders. *Laboratory:* Abnormalities of certain parameters were observed, but are difficult to assess in this population. The following were recorded in ≥5% of patients: Increased BUN, Hyperglycemia, Hyperlipidemia (total cholesterol, LDL-cholesterol, triglycerides), Hyperphosphatemia, Abnormal liver function tests, Increased PT, Increased PTT. Additional laboratory abnormalities reported were: Decreased platelets, Decreased potassium and Increased WBC.
*Physiologic effect of decreased testosterone.
Postmarketing
During postmarketing surveillance, which includes other dosage forms, the following adverse events were reported. Symptoms consistent with an anaphylactoid or asthmatic process have been rarely reported. Rash, urticaria, and photosensitivity reactions have also been reported.
Localized reactions including induration and abscess have been reported at the site of injection.
Hemic and Lymphatic System—Decreased WBC; *Central/ Peripheral Nervous System*—Peripheral neuropathy, Spinal fracture/paralysis; *Musculoskeletal System*—Tenosynovitis-like symptoms; *Urogenital System*—Prostate pain.
See other LUPRON DEPOT and LUPRON Injection package inserts for other events reported in different patient populations.

OVERDOSAGE

In rats subcutaneous administration of 250 to 500 times the recommended human dose, expressed on a per body weight basis, resulted in dyspnea, decreased activity, and local irritation at the injection site. There is no evidence at present that there is a clinical counterpart of this phenomenon. In early clinical trials with daily subcutaneous leuprolide acetate, doses as high as 20 mg/day for up to two years caused no adverse effects differing from those observed with the 1 mg/day dose.

DOSAGE AND ADMINISTRATION

LUPRON DEPOT Must Be Administered Under The Supervision Of A Physician.

The recommended dose of LUPRON DEPOT-3 Month 22.5 mg to be administered is one injection every three months **(84 days).** Due to different release characteristics, a fractional dose of this 3-month depot formulation is not equivalent to the same dose of the monthly formulation and should not be given.

Incorporated in a depot formulation, the lyophilized microspheres are to be reconstituted and administered every three

months as a single intramuscular injection, in accord with the following directions:
1. Withdraw 1.5 mL of diluent from the ampule, and inject it into the vial. (Extra diluent is provided; any remaining should be discarded.)
2. Shake well to thoroughly disperse particles to obtain a uniform suspension. The suspension will appear milky.
3. Withdraw the entire contents of the vial into the syringe with a 23 gauge or larger needle and inject it at the time of reconstitution. As the suspension settles very quickly following reconstitution, **it is strongly recommended that LUPRON DEPOT-3 Month 22.5 mg be administered immediately.** Reshake suspension if settling occurs.
Although the potency of the reconstituted suspension has been shown to be stable for 24 hours, since the product does not contain a preservative, the suspension should be discarded if not used immediately.
As with other drugs administered by injection, the injection site should be varied periodically.
The vial of LUPRON DEPOT-3 Month 22.5 mg and the ampule of diluent may be stored at room temperature.

HOW SUPPLIED

LUPRON DEPOT — 3 Month 22.5 mg (NDC 0300-3336-01) is available in a single use kit. Each kit contains a vial of sterile lyophilized microspheres which is leuprolide incorporated in a biodegradable polymer of polylactic acid. When mixed with 1.5 mL of accompanying diluent, LUPRON DEPOT-3 Months 22.5 mg is administered as a single IM injection **EVERY THREE MONTHS (84 days).**
An information pamphlet for patients is included with the kit.
No refrigeration necessary. Protect from freezing.
Caution: Federal (U.S.A.) law prohibits dispensing without a prescription.

REFERENCE

1. MacLeod TL, et al. Anaphylactic reaction to synthetic luteinizing hormone-releasing hormone. *Fertil Steril* 1987 Sept; 48(3):500-502.
U.S. Patent Nos. 4,652,441; 4,677,191 4,728,721; 4,849,228; 4,917,893; 4,954,298; 5,330,767; and 5,476,663.
TAP Pharmaceuticals Inc.
Deerfield, Illinois 60015-1595, U.S.A.
LUPRON DEPOT-3 Month 22.5 mg
manufactured by
Takeda Chemical Industries, LTD.
Osaka, JAPAN 541
®—Registered Trademark
(No. 3336)
03-4673-R2-Revised: April, 1996
Shown in Product Identification Guide, page 338

LUPRON DEPOT-PED®
(leuprolide acetate for depot suspension)
7.5 mg, 11.25 mg and 15 mg

℞

DESCRIPTION

Leuprolide acetate is a synthetic nonapeptide analog of naturally occurring gonadotropin-releasing hormone (GnRH or LH-RH). The analog possesses greater potency than the natural hormone. The chemical name is 5-oxo-L-prolyl-L-histidyl -L- tryptophyl-L-seryl-L-tyrosyl-D-leucyl-L-leucyl-L-arginyl-N-ethyl-L-prolinamide acetate (salt) with the following structural formula:
[See structure below.]
LUPRON DEPOT-PED is available in a vial containing sterile lyophilized microspheres, which when mixed with diluent, become a suspension which is intended as a single intramuscular injection.
The single-dose vial contains, respectively for each dosage strength, leuprolide acetate (7.5/11.25/15 mg), purified gelatin (1.3/1.95/2.6 mg), DL-lactic and glycolic acids copolymer (66.2/99.3/132.4 mg), and D-mannitol (13.2/19.8/26.4 mg). The accompanying ampule of diluent contains carboxymethylcellulose sodium (10 mg), D-mannitol (100 mg), polysorbate 80 (2 mg), water for injection, USP, and glacial acetic acid, USP to control pH.

During the manufacture of LUPRON DEPOT-PED, acetic acid is lost, leaving the peptide.

CLINICAL PHARMACOLOGY

Leuprolide acetate, a GnRH agonist, acts as a potent inhibitor of gonadotropin secretion when given continuously and in therapeutic doses. Human studies indicate that following an initial stimulation of gonadotropins, chronic stimulation with leuprolide acetate results in suppression or "downregulation" of these hormones and consequent suppression of ovarian and testicular steroidogenesis. These effects are reversible on discontinuation of drug therapy.
Leuprolide acetate is not active when given orally.

PHARMACOKINETICS

Absorption: Following a single LUPRON DEPOT 7.5 mg injection to adult patients, mean peak leuprolide plasma concentration was almost 20 ng/mL at 4 hours and then declined to 0.36 ng/mL at 4 weeks. However, intact leuprolide and an inactive major metabolite could not be distinguished by the assay which was employed in the study. Nondetectable leuprolide plasma concentrations have been observed during chronic LUPRON DEPOT 7.5 mg administration, but testosterone levels appear to be maintained at castrate levels.
Distribution: The mean steady-state volume of distribution of leuprolide following intravenous bolus administration to healthy male volunteers was 27 L. In vitro binding to human plasma proteins ranged from 43% to 49%.
Metabolism: In healthy male volunteers, a 1 mg bolus of leuprolide administered intravenously revealed that the mean systemic clearance was 7.6 L/h, with a terminal elimination half-life of approximately 3 hours based on a two compartment model.
In rats and dogs, administration of ^{14}C-labeled leuprolide was shown to be metabolized to smaller inactive peptides, a pentapeptide (Metabolite I), tripeptides (Metabolites II and III) and a dipeptide (Metabolite IV). These fragments may be further catabolized.
The major metabolite (M-I) plasma concentrations measured in 5 prostate cancer patients reached maximum concentration 2 to 6 hours after dosing and were approximately 6% of the peak parent drug concentration. One week after dosing, mean plasma M-I concentrations were approximately 20% of mean leuprolide concentrations.
Excretion: Following administration of LUPRON DEPOT 3.75 mg to 3 patients, less than 5% of the dose was recovered as parent and M-I metabolite in the urine.
Special Populations: The pharmacokinetics of the drug in hepatically and renally impaired patients have not been determined.

CLINICAL STUDIES

In children with central precocious puberty (CPP), stimulated and basal gonadotropins are reduced to prepubertal levels. Testosterone and estradiol are reduced to prepubertal levels in males and females respectively. Reduction of gonadotropins will allow for normal physical and psychological growth and development. Natural maturation occurs when gonadotropins return to pubertal levels following discontinuation of leuprolide acetate.
The following physiologic effects have been noted with the chronic administration of leuprolide acetate in this patient population.
1. **Skeletal Growth.** A measurable increase in body length can be noted since the epiphyseal plates will not close prematurely.
2. **Organ growth.** Reproductive organs will return to a prepubertal state.
3. **Menses.** Menses, if present, will cease.

In a study of 22 children with central precocious puberty, doses of LUPRON DEPOT were given every 4 weeks and plasma levels were determined according to weight categories as summarized below:
[See table at top of next page.]

INDICATIONS AND USAGE

LUPRON DEPOT-PED is indicated in the treatment of children with central precocious puberty. Children should be selected using the following criteria:

1. Clinical diagnosis of CPP (idiopathic or neurogenic) with onset of secondary sexual characteristics earlier than 8 years in females and 9 years in males.
2. Clinical diagnosis should be confirmed prior to initiation of therapy:
   - Confirmation of diagnosis by a pubertal response to a GnRH stimulation test. The sensitivity and methodology of this assay must be understood.
   - Bone age advanced one year beyond the chronological age.
3. Baseline evaluation should also include:
   - Height and weight measurements.
   - Sex steroid levels.
   - Adrenal steroid level to exclude congenital adrenal hyperplasia.
   - Beta human chorionic gonadotropin level to rule out a chorionic gonadotropin secreting tumor.
   - Pelvic/adrenal/testicular ultrasound to rule out a steroid secreting tumor.
   - Computerized tomography of the head to rule out intracranial tumor.

CONTRAINDICATIONS

LUPRON DEPOT-PED is contraindicated in women who are or may become pregnant while receiving the drug. When administered on day 6 of pregnancy at test dosages of 0.00024, 0.0024, and 0.024 mg/kg (1/1200 to 1/12 the human pediatric dose) to rabbits, LUPRON DEPOT produced a dose-related increase in major fetal abnormalities. Similar studies in rats failed to demonstrate an increase in fetal malformations. There was increased fetal mortality and decreased fetal weights with the two higher doses of LUPRON DEPOT in rabbits and with the highest dose in rats. The effects on fetal mortality are logical consequences of the alterations in hormonal levels brought about by this drug. Therefore, the possibility exists that spontaneous abortion may occur if the drug is administered during pregnancy.

Leuprolide acetate is contraindicated in children demonstrating hypersensitivity to GnRH, GnRH agonist analogs, or any of the excipients.

A report of an anaphylactic reaction to synthetic GnRH (Factrel) has been reported in the medical literature.[1]

WARNINGS

During the early phase of therapy, gonadotropins and sex steroids rise above baseline because of the natural stimulatory effect of the drug. Therefore, an increase in clinical signs and symptoms may be observed (see **CLINICAL PHARMACOLOGY** section).

Noncompliance with drug regimen or inadequate dosing may result in inadequate control of the pubertal process. The consequences of poor control include the return of pubertal signs such as menses, breast development, and testicular growth. The long-term consequences of inadequate control of gonadal steroid secretion are unknown, but may include a further compromise of adult stature.

PRECAUTIONS

Laboratory Tests: Response to LUPRON DEPOT-PED should be monitored 1–2 months after the start of therapy with a GnRH stimulation test and sex steroid levels. Measurement of bone age for advancement should be done every 6–12 months.

Sex steroids may increase or rise above prepubertal levels if the dose is inadequate (see **WARNINGS** section). Once a therapeutic dose has been established, gonadotropin and sex steroid levels will decline to prepubertal levels.

Drug Interactions: No pharmacokinetic-based drug-drug interaction studies have been conducted. However, because leuprolide acetate is a peptide that is primarily degraded by peptidase and not by cytochrome P-450 enzymes as noted in specific studies, and the drug is only about 46% bound to plasma proteins, drug interactions would not be expected to occur.

Drug/Laboratory Test Interactions: Administration of LUPRON DEPOT in therapeutic doses results in suppression of the pituitary-gonadal system. Normal function is usually restored within 4 to 12 weeks after treatment is discontinued. Therefore, diagnostic tests of pituitary gonadotropic and gonadal functions conducted during treatment and up to one to two months after discontinuation of LUPRON DEPOT therapy may be misleading.

Information for Parents: Prior to starting therapy with LUPRON DEPOT-PED, the parent or guardian must be aware of the importance of continuous therapy. Adherence to 4 week drug administration schedules must be accepted if therapy is to be successful.

- During the first 2 months of therapy, a female may experience menses or spotting. If bleeding continues beyond the second month, notify the physician.
- Any irritation at the injection site should be reported to the physician immediately.
- Report any unusual signs or symptoms to the physician.

Carcinogenesis, Mutagenesis, Impairment of Fertility: A two-year carcinogenicity study was conducted in rats and mice. In rats, a dose-related increase of benign pituitary hyperplasia and benign pituitary adenomas was noted at 24 months when the drug was administered subcutaneously at high daily doses (0.6 to 4 mg/kg). There was a significant but not dose-related increase of pancreatic islet-cell adenomas in females and of testicular interstitial cell adenomas in males (highest incidence in the low dose group). In mice, no leuprolide acetate-induced tumors or pituitary abnormalities were observed at a dose as high as 60 mg/kg for two years. Adult patients have been treated with leuprolide acetate for up to three years with doses as high as 10 mg/day and for two years with doses as high as 20 mg/day without demonstrable pituitary abnormalities.

Patient Weight Range (kg)	Group Weight Average (kg)	Dose (mg)	Trough Plasma Leuprolide Level Mean ± SD (ng/mL)*
20.2–27.0	22.7	7.5	0.77±0.033
28.4–36.8	32.5	11.25	1.25±1.06
39.3–57.5	44.2	15.0	1.59±0.65

* Group average values determined at Week 4 immediately prior to leuprolide injection. Drug levels at 12 and 24 weeks were similar to respective 4 week levels.

Although no clinical studies have been completed in children to assess the full reversibility of fertility suppression, animal studies (prepubertal and adult rats and monkeys) with leuprolide acetate and other GnRH analogs have shown functional recovery. However, following a study with leuprolide acetate, immature male rats demonstrated tubular degeneration in the testes even after a recovery period. In spite of the failure to recover histologically, the treated males proved to be as fertile as the controls. Also, no histologic changes were observed in the female rats following the same protocol. In both sexes, the offspring of the treated animals appeared normal. The effect of the treatment of the parents on the reproductive performance of the F1 generation was not tested. The clinical significance of these findings is unknown.

Pregnancy Category X. See **CONTRAINDICATIONS** section.

Nursing Mothers: It is not known whether leuprolide acetate is excreted in human milk. LUPRON should not be used by nursing mothers.

ADVERSE REACTIONS

Potential exacerbation of signs and symptoms during the first few weeks of treatment (See **PRECAUTIONS** section) is a concern in patients with rapidly advancing central precocious puberty.

In two studies of children with central precocious puberty, in 2% or more of the patients receiving the drug, the following adverse reactions were reported to have a possible or probable relationship to drug as ascribed by the treating physician. Reactions considered not drug related are excluded.

	Number of Patients N=395	(Percent)
Body as a Whole		
General Pain	7	(2)
Integumentary System		
Acne/Seborrhea	7	(2)
Injection Site Reactions Including Abscess	21	(5)
Rash Including Erythema Multiforme	8	(2)
Urogenital System		
Vaginitis/Bleeding/Discharge	7	(2)

In those same studies, the following adverse reactions were reported in less than 2% of the patients.

Body as a Whole—Body Odor, Fever, Headache, Infection; *Cardiovascular System*—Syncope, Vasodilation; *Digestive System*—Dysphagia, Gingivitis, Nausea/Vomiting; *Endocrine System*—Accelerated Sexual Maturity; *Metabolic and Nutritional Disorders*—Peripheral Edema, Weight Gain; *Nervous System*—Emotional Lability, Nervousness, Personality Disorder, Somnolence; *Respiratory System*—Epistaxis; *Integumentary System*—Alopecia, Skin Striae; *Urogenital System*—Cervix Disorder, Gynecomastia/Breast Disorders, Urinary Incontinence.

Postmarketing

During postmarketing surveillance, which includes other dosage forms, the following adverse events were reported.

Symptoms consistent with an anaphylactoid or asthmatic process have been rarely reported. Rash, urticaria, and photosensitivity reactions have also been reported.

Localized reactions including induration and abscess have been reported at the site of injection.

Cardiovascular System—Hypotension; *Hemic and Lymphatic System*—Decreased WBC; *Central/Peripheral Nervous System*—Peripheral neuropathy, Spinal fracture/paralysis; *Musculoskeletal System*—Tenosynovitis-like symptoms; *Urogenital System*—Prostate pain.

See other LUPRON DEPOT and LUPRON Injection package inserts for other events reported in different patient populations.

OVERDOSAGE

In rats, subcutaneous administration of 125 to 250 times the recommended human pediatric dose, expressed on a per body weight basis, resulted in dyspnea, decreased activity, and local irritation at the injection site. There is no evidence at present that there is a clinical counterpart of this phenomenon. In early clinical trials using leuprolide acetate in adult patients, doses as high as 20 mg/day for up to two years caused no adverse effects differing from those observed with the 1 mg/day dose.

DOSAGE AND ADMINISTRATION

LUPRON DEPOT-PED must be administered under the supervision of a physician.

The dose of LUPRON DEPOT-PED must be individualized for each child. The dose is based on a mg/kg ratio of drug to body weight. Younger children require higher doses on a mg/kg ratio.

For each dosage form, after 1-2 months of initiating therapy or changing doses, the child must be monitored with a GnRH stimulation test, sex steroids, and Tanner staging to confirm downregulation. Measurements of bone age for advancement should be monitored every 6-12 months. The dose should be titrated upward until no progression of the condition is noted either clinically and/or by laboratory parameters.

The first dose found to result in adequate downregulation can probably be maintained for the duration of therapy in most children. However, there are insufficient data to guide dosage adjustment as patients move into higher weight categories after beginning therapy at very young ages and low dosages. It is recommended that adequate downregulation be verified in such patients whose weight has increased significantly while on therapy.

Discontinuation of LUPRON DEPOT-PED should be considered before age 11 for females and age 12 for males.

The recommended starting dose is 0.3 mg/kg/4 weeks (minimum 7.5 mg) administered as a single intramuscular injection. The starting dose will be dictated by the child's weight.

≤ 25 kg	7.5 mg
> 25–37.5 kg	11.25 mg
> 37.5 kg	15 mg

If total downregulation is not achieved, the dose should be titrated upward in increments of 3.75 mg every 4 weeks. This dose will be considered the maintenance dose.

The lyophilized microspheres are to be reconstituted and administered as a single intramuscular injection, in accord with the following directions:

1. Using a syringe with a 23 gauge needle, withdraw 1 mL of diluent from the ampule, and inject it into the vial. (Extra diluent is provided; any remaining should be discarded.)
2. Shake well to thoroughly disperse particles to obtain a uniform suspension. The suspension will appear milky.
3. Withdraw the entire contents of the vial into the syringe and inject it at the time of reconstitution.

Although the potency of the reconstituted suspension has been shown to be stable for 24 hours, since the product does not contain a preservative, the suspension should be discarded if not used immediately.

As with other drugs administered by injection, the injection site should be varied periodically.

The vial of LUPRON DEPOT-PED and the ampule of diluent may be stored at room temperature.

HOW SUPPLIED

LUPRON DEPOT-PED is available in three single use kits providing a dose of 7.5 mg (NDC 0300-2106-01), 11.25 mg (NDC 0300-2270-01) or 15 mg (NDC 0300-2437-01). Each vial contains sterile lyophilized microspheres which is leuprolide incorporated in a biodegradable copolymer of lactic and glycolic acids. When mixed with 1 mL of diluent, LUPRON DEPOT-PED is administered as a single IM injection.

An information pamphlet for parents is included with the kit.

No refrigeration necessary. Protect from freezing.

Caution: Federal (U.S.A.) law prohibits dispensing without a prescription.

REFERENCE

1. MacLeod TL, et al. Anaphylactic reaction to synthetic luteinizing hormone-releasing hormone. *Fertil Steril* 1987 Sept;48(3):500–502.

Continued on next page

TAP—Cont.

U.S. Patent Nos. 4,652,441; 4,677,191; 4,728,721; 4,849,228; 4,917,893; 4,954,298; 5,330,767; and 5,476,663.
TAP Pharmaceuticals Inc.
Deerfield, IL 60015, U.S.A.
LUPRON DEPOT-PED manufactured by
Takeda Chemical
Industries, Ltd.
Osaka, JAPAN 541
®—Registered trademark
(Nos. 2106, 2270, 2437)
03-4637-R5-Revised: April, 1996

PREVACID® ℞

[prĕ′-va-sĭd]
(lansoprazole)
Delayed-Release Capsules

DESCRIPTION

The active ingredient in PREVACID (lansoprazole) Delayed-Release Capsules is a substituted benzimidazole, 2-[[[3-methyl -4- (2,2,2-trifluroethoxy) -2- pyridyl]methyl]sulfinyl] benzimidazole, a compound that inhibits gastric acid secretion. Its empirical formula is $C_{16}H_{14}F_3N_3O_2S$ with a molecular weight of 369.37. The structural formula is:

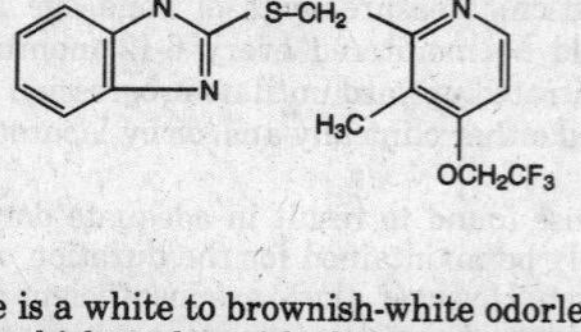

Lansoprazole is a white to brownish-white odorless, crystalline powder which melts with decomposition at approximately 166°C. Lansoprazole is freely soluble in dimethylformamide; soluble in methanol; sparingly soluble in ethanol; slightly soluble in ethyl acetate, dichloromethane and acetonitrile; very slightly soluble in ether; and practically insoluble in hexane and water.
Lansoprazole is stable when exposed to light for up to two months. The compound degrades in aqueous solution, the rate of degradation increasing with decreasing pH. At 25°C the $t_{1/2}$ is approximately 0.5 hour at pH 5.0 and approximately 18 hours at pH 7.0.
PREVACID is supplied in delayed-release capsules for oral administration. The delayed-release capsules contain the active ingredient, lansoprazole, in the form of enteric-coated granules and are available in two dosage strengths; 15 mg and 30 mg of lansoprazole per capsule. Each delayed-release capsule contains enteric-coated granules consisting of lansoprazole, hydroxypropyl cellulose, low substituted hydroxypropyl cellulose, colloidal silicon dioxide, magnesium carbonate, methacrylic acid copolymer, starch, talc, sugar sphere, sucrose, polyethylene glycol, polysorbate 80, and titanium dioxide. Components of the gelatin capsule include gelatin, titanium dioxide, D&C Red No. 28, FD&C Blue No. 1, FD&C Green No. 3*, and FD&C Red No. 40.
*PREVACID 15 mg capsules only.

CLINICAL PHARMACOLOGY

Pharmacokinetics and Metabolism
PREVACID Delayed-Release Capsules contain an enteric-coated granule formulation of lansoprazole. Absorption of lansoprazole begins only after the granules leave the stomach. Absorption is rapid, with mean peak plasma levels of lansoprazole occurring after approximately 1.7 hours. Peak plasma concentrations of lansoprazole (C_{max}) and the area under the plasma concentration curve (AUC) of lansoprazole are approximately proportional in doses from 15 mg to 60 mg after single-oral administration. Lansoprazole does not accumulate and its pharmacokinetics are unaltered by multiple dosing.

Absorption
The absorption of lansoprazole is rapid, with mean C_{max} occurring approximately 1.7 hours after oral dosing, and relatively complete with absolute bioavailability over 80%. In healthy subjects, the mean (± SD) plasma half-life was 1.5 (± 1.0) hours. Both C_{max} and AUC are diminished by about 50% if the drug is given 30 minutes after food as opposed to the fasting condition. There is no significant food effect if the drug is given before meals.

Distribution
Lansoprazole is 97% bound to plasma proteins. Plasma protein binding is constant over the concentration range of 0.05 to 5.0 mcg/mL.

Metabolism
Lansoprazole is extensively metabolized in the liver. Two metabolites have been identified in measurable quantities in plasma (the hydroxylated sulfinyl and sulfone derivatives of lansoprazole). These metabolites have very little or no antisecretory activity. Lansoprazole is thought to be transformed into two active species which inhibit acid secretion by (H^+, K^+)-ATPase within the parietal cell canaliculus, but are not present in the system circulation. The plasma elimination half-life of lansoprazole does not reflect its duration of suppression of gastric acid secretion. Thus, the plasma elimination half-life is less than two hours while the acid inhibitory effect lasts more than 24 hours.

Elimination
Following single-dose oral administration of lansoprazole, virtually no unchanged lansoprazole was excreted in the urine. In one study, after a single oral dose of ^{14}C-lansoprazole, approximately one-third of the administered radiation was excreted in the urine and two-thirds was recovered in the feces. This implies a significant biliary excretion of the metabolites of lansoprazole.

Special Populations

Geriatric
The clearance of lansoprazole is decreased in the elderly, with elimination half-life increased approximately 50% to 100%. Because the mean half-life in the elderly remains between 1.9 to 2.9 hours, repeated once daily dosing does not result in accumulation of lansoprazole. Peak plasma levels were not increased in the elderly.

Pediatric
The pharmacokinetics of lansoprazole has not been investigated in patients < 18 years of age.

Gender
In a study comparing 12 male and six female human subjects, no gender differences were found in pharmacokinetics and intragastric pH results (also see Use in Women).

Renal Insufficiency
In patients with severe renal insufficiency, plasma protein binding decreased by 1.0%–1.5% after administration of 60 mg of lansoprazole. Patients with renal insufficiency had a shortened elimination half-life and decreased total AUC (free and bound). AUC for free lansoprazole in plasma, however, was not related to the degree of renal impairment, and C_{max} and T_{max} were not different from subjects with healthy kidneys.

Hepatic Insufficiency
In patients with various degrees of chronic hepatic disease, the mean plasma half-life of the drug was prolonged from 1.5 hours to 3.2–7.2 hours. An increase in mean AUC of up to 500% was observed at steady state in hepatically-impaired patients compared to healthy subjects. Dose reduction in patients with severe hepatic disease should be considered.

Race
The pooled pharmacokinetic parameters of lansoprazole from twelve U.S. Phase I studies (N=513) were compared to the mean pharmacokinetic parameters from two Asian studies (N=20). The mean AUCs of lansoprazole in Asian subjects are approximately twice that seen in pooled U.S. data, however the inter-individual variability is high. The C_{max} values are comparable.

Mean Antisecretory Effects after Single and Multiple Daily Dosing

Parameter	Baseline Value	PREVACID 15 mg Day 1		PREVACID 30 mg Day 1		Omeprazole 20 mg Day 1	
		Day 1	Day 5	Day 1	Day 5	Day 1	Day 5
Mean 24-Hour pH	2.1	2.7+	4.0+	3.6*	4.9*	2.5	4.2+
Mean Nighttime pH	1.9	2.4	3.0+	2.6	3.8*	2.2	3.0+
% Time Gastric pH > 3	18	33+	59+	51*	72*	30+	61+
% Time Gastric pH > 4	12	22+	49+	41*	66*	19	51+

NOTE: An intragastric pH of > 4 reflects a reduction in gastric acid by 99%.
*(p < 0.05) versus baseline, lansoprazole 15 mg and omeprazole 20 mg.
+(p < 0.05) versus baseline only.

PHARMACODYNAMICS

Mechanism of action
Lansoprazole belongs to a class of antisecretory compounds, the substituted benzimidazoles, that do not exhibit anticholinergic or histamine H_2-receptor antagonist properties, but that suppress gastric acid secretion by specific inhibition of the (H^+, K^+)-ATPase enzyme system at the secretory surface of the gastric parietal cell. Because this enzyme system is regarded as the acid (proton) pump within the parietal cell, lansoprazole has been characterized as a gastric acid-pump inhibitor, in that it blocks the final step of acid production. This effect is dose-related and leads to inhibition of both basal and stimulated gastric acid secretion irrespective of the stimulus.

Antisecretory activity
After oral administration, lansoprazole was shown to significantly decrease the basal acid output and significantly increase the mean gastric pH and percent of time the gastric pH was > 3 and > 4. Lansoprazole also significantly reduced meal-stimulated gastric acid output and secretion volume, as well as pentagastrin-stimulated acid output. In patients with hypersecretion of acid, lansoprazole significantly reduced basal and pentagastrin-stimulated gastric acid secretion. Lansoprazole inhibited the normal increases in secretion volume, acidity and acid output induced by insulin.
In a crossover study comparing lansoprazole 15 and 30 mg with omeprazole 20 mg for five days, the following effects on intragastric pH were noted:
[See table below.]
After the initial dose in this study, increased gastric pH was seen within 1–2 hours with lansoprazole 30 mg, 2–3 hours with lansoprazole 15 mg, and 3–4 hours with omeprazole 20 mg. After multiple daily dosing, increased gastric pH was seen within the first hour postdosing with lansoprazole 30 mg and within 1–2 hours postdosing with lansoprazole 15 mg and omeprazole 20 mg.
The inhibition of gastric acid secretion as measured by intragastric pH returns gradually to normal over two to four days after multiple doses. There is no indication of rebound gastric acidity.

Enterochromaffin-like (ECL) cell effects
During lifetime exposure of rats with up to 150 mg/kg/day of lansoprazole dosed seven days per week, marked hypergastrinemia was observed followed by ECL cell proliferation and formation of carcinoid tumors, especially in female rats (see PRECAUTIONS, Carcinogenesis, Mutagenesis, and Fertility).
Gastric biopsy specimens from the body of the stomach from approximately 150 patients treated continuously with lansoprazole for at least one year have not shown evidence of ECL cell effects similar to those seen in rat studies. Longer term data are needed to rule out the possibility of an increased risk of the development of gastric tumors in patients receiving long-term therapy with lansoprazole.

Other gastric effects in humans
Lansoprazole did not significantly affect mucosal blood flow in the fundus of the stomach. Due to the normal, physiologic effect caused by the inhibition of gastric acid secretion, a decrease of about 17% in blood flow in the antrum, pylorus and duodenal bulb was seen. Lansoprazole significantly slowed the gastric emptying of digestible solids. Lansoprazole increased serum pepsinogen levels and decreased pepsin activity under basal conditions and in response to meal stimulation or insulin injection. As with other agents that elevate intragastric pH, increases in gastric pH were associated with increases in nitrate-reducing bacteria and elevation of nitrite concentration in gastric juice in patients with gastric ulcer. No significant increase in nitrosamine concentrations was observed.

Serum gastrin effects
In over 2100 patients, median fasting serum gastrin levels increased 50% to 100% from baseline, but remained within normal range after treatment with lansoprazole given orally in doses of 15 mg to 60 mg. These elevations reached a plateau within two months of therapy and returned to pretreatment levels within four weeks after discontinuation of therapy.

Endocrine effects
Human studies for up to eight weeks have not detected any clinically significant effects on the endocrine system. Hormones studied include testosterone, luteinizing hormone (LH), follicle stimulating hormone (FSH), sex hormone binding globulin (SHBG), dehydroepiandrosterone sulfate (DHEA-S), prolactin, cortisol, estradiol, insulin, aldosterone, parathormone, glucagon, thyroid stimulating hormone (TSH), triiodothyronine (T_3), thyroxine (T_4), and somatotropic hormone (STH). Lansoprazole in oral doses of 15 to 60 mg for up to one year, had no clinically significant effect on sexual function. In addition, lansoprazole in oral doses of 15 to 60 mg for two to eight weeks had no clinically significant effect on thyroid function.
In 24-month carcinogenicity studies in Sprague-Dawley rats with daily dosages up to 150 mg/kg, proliferative changes in the Leydig cells of the testes, including benign neoplasm, were increased compared to control rates.

Other effects

No systemic effects of lansoprazole on the central nervous system, lymphoid, hematopoietic, renal hepatic, cardiovascular or respiratory systems have been found in humans. No visual toxicity was observed among 56 patients who had extensive baseline eye evaluations, were treated with up to 180 mg/day of lansoprazole and were observed for up to 58 months. Other rat-specific findings after lifetime exposure included focal pancreatic atrophy, diffuse lymphoid hyperplasia in the thymus, and spontaneous retinal atrophy.

CLINICAL STUDIES

Duodenal Ulcer

In a U.S. multicenter, double-blind, placebo-controlled, dose-response (15, 30, and 60 mg of PREVACID once daily) study of 284 patients with endoscopically documented duodenal ulcer, the percentage of patients healed after two and four weeks was significantly higher with all doses of PREVACID than with placebo. There was no evidence of a greater or earlier response with the two higher doses compared with PREVACID 15 mg. Based on this study and the second study described below, the recommended dose of PREVACID in duodenal ulcer is 15 mg per day.

Duodenal Ulcer Healing Rates

Week	PREVACID 15 mg qd (N=68)	PREVACID 30 mg qd (N=74)	PREVACID 60 mg qd (N=70)	Placebo (N=72)
2	42.4%*	35.6%*	39.1%*	11.3%
4	89.4%*	91.7%*	89.9%*	46.1%

* (p ≤ 0.001) versus placebo.

PREVACID 15 mg was significantly more effective than placebo in relieving day and nighttime abdominal pain and in decreasing the amount of antacid taken per day.

In a second U.S. multicenter study, also double-blind, placebo-, dose-comparison (15 and 30 mg of PREVACID once daily), and including a comparison with ranitidine, in 280 patients with endoscopically documented duodenal ulcer, the percentage of patients healed after four weeks was significantly higher with both doses of PREVACID than with placebo. There was no evidence of a greater or earlier response with the higher dose of PREVACID. Although the 15 mg dose of PREVACID was superior to ranitidine at 4 weeks, the lack of significant difference at 2 weeks and the absence of a difference between 30 mg of PREVACID and ranitidine leaves the comparative effectiveness of the two agents undetermined.

Duodenal Ulcer Healing Rates

Week	PREVACID 15 mg qd (N=80)	PREVACID 30 mg qd (N=77)	Ranitidine 300 mg hs (N=82)	Placebo (N=41)
2	35.0%	44.2%	30.5%	34.2%
4	92.3%**	80.3%*	70.5%*	47.5%

* (p ≤ 0.05) versus placebo.
**(p ≤ 0.05) versus placebo and ranitidine.

Erosive Esophagitis

In a U.S. multicenter, double-blind, placebo-controlled study of 269 patients entering with an endoscopic diagnosis of esophagitis with mucosal grading of 2 or more and grades 3 and 4 signifying erosive disease, the percentages of patients with healing were as follows:

Erosive Esophagitis Healing Rates

Week	PREVACID 15 mg qd (N=69)	PREVACID 30 mg qd (N=65)	PREVACID 60 mg qd (N=72)	Placebo (N=63)
4	67.6%*	81.3%**	80.6%**	32.8%
6	87.7%*	95.4%*	94.3%*	52.5%
8	90.9%*	95.4%*	94.4%*	52.5%

* (p ≤ 0.001) versus placebo.
**(p ≤ 0.05) versus PREVACID 15 mg and placebo.

In this study, all PREVACID groups reported significantly greater relief of heartburn and less day and night abdominal pain along with fewer days of antacid use and fewer antacid tablets taken per day than the placebo group.

Although all doses were effective, the earlier healing in the higher two doses suggest 30 mg qd as the recommended dose. PREVACID was also compared in a U.S. multicenter, double-blind study to a low dose of ranitidine in 242 patients with erosive reflux esophagitis. PREVACID at a dose of 30 mg was significantly more effective than ranitidine 150 mg bid as shown below.

Endoscopic Remission Rates

Trial	Drug	No of Pts.	Percent in Endoscopic Remission 0–3 mo.	0–6 mo	0–12 mo.
#1	PREVACID 15 mg qd	59	83%*	81%*	79%*
	PREVACID 30 mg qd	56	93%*	93%*	90%*
	Placebo	55	31%	27%	24%
#2	PREVACID 15 mg qd	50	74%*	72%*	67%*
	PREVACID 30 mg qd	49	75%*	72%*	55%*
	Placebo	47	16%	13%	13%

% =Life Table estimate
* (p ≤ 0.001) versus placebo

Erosive Esophagitis Healing Rates

Week	PREVACID 30 mg qd (N=115)	Ranitidine 150 mg bid (N=127)
2	66.7%*	38.7%
4	82.5%*	52.0%
6	93.0%*	67.8%
8	92.1%*	69.9%

*(p ≤ 0.001) versus ranitidine.

In addition, patients treated with PREVACID reported less day and nighttime heartburn and took less antacid tablets for fewer days than patients taking ranitidine 150 mg bid. Although this study demonstrates effectiveness of PREVACID in healing erosive esophagitis, it does not represent an adequate comparison with ranitidine because the recommended ranitidine dose for esophagitis is 150 mg qid, twice the dose used in this study.

In the two trials described and in several smaller studies involving patients with moderate to severe erosive esophagitis, PREVACID produced healing rates similar to those shown above.

In a U.S. multicenter, double-blind, active-controlled study, 30 mg of PREVACID was compared with ranitidine 150 mg bid in 151 patients with erosive reflux esophagitis that was poorly responsive to a minimum of 12 weeks of treatment with at least one H$_2$-receptor antagonist given at the dose indicated for symptom relief or greater, namely cimetidine 800 mg/day, ranitidine 300 mg/day, famotidine 40 mg/day or nizatidine 300 mg/day. PREVACID 30 mg was more effective than ranitidine 150 mg bid in healing reflux esophagitis and the percentage of patients with healing were as follows. This study does not constitute a comparison of the effectiveness of histamine H$_2$-receptor antagonists with PREVACID as all patients had demonstrated unresponsiveness to the histamine H$_2$-receptor antagonist mode of treatment. It does indicate, however, that PREVACID may be useful in patients failing on a histamine H$_2$-receptor antagonist.

Reflux Esophagitis Healing Rates in Patients Poorly Responsive to Histamine H$_2$-Receptor Antagonist Therapy

Week	PREVACID 30 mg qd (N=100)	Ranitidine 150 mg bid (N=51)
4	74.7%*	42.6%
8	83.7%*	32.0%

*(p ≤ 0.001) versus ranitidine.

Long-Term Maintenance Treatment of Erosive Esophagitis

Two independent, double-blind, multicenter, controlled trials were conducted in patients with endoscopically confirmed healed esophagitis. Patients remained in remission significantly longer and the number of recurrences of erosive esophagitis was significantly less in patients treated with PREVACID than in patients treated with placebo over a 12-month period.

[See table on top of page.]

Regardless of initial grade of erosive esophagitis, PREVACID 15 mg and 30 mg were similar in maintaining remission.

Pathological Hypersecretory Conditions Including Zollinger-Ellison Syndrome

In open studies of 57 patients with pathological hypersecretory conditions, such as Zollinger-Ellison (ZE) syndrome with or without multiple endocrine adenomas, PREVACID significantly inhibited gastric acid secretion and controlled associated symptoms of diarrhea, anorexia and pain. Doses ranging from 15 mg every other day to 180 mg per day maintained basal acid secretion below 10 mEq/hr in patients without prior gastric surgery, and below 5 mEq/hr in patients with prior gastric surgery.

Initial doses were titrated to the individual patient need, and adjustments were necessary with time in some patients (see DOSAGE AND ADMINISTRATION). PREVACID was well tolerated at these high dose levels for prolonged periods (greater than four years in some patients). In most ZE patients, serum gastrin levels were not modified by PREVACID. However, in some patients serum gastrin increased to levels greater than those present prior to initiation of lansoprazole therapy.

INDICATIONS AND USAGE

Short-Term Treatment of Active Duodenal Ulcer

PREVACID Delayed-Release Capsules are indicated for short-term treatment (up to 4 weeks) for healing and symptom relief of active duodenal ulcer.

Short-Term Treatment of Erosive Esophagitis

PREVACID Delayed-Release Capsules are indicated for short-term treatment (up to 8 weeks) for healing and symptom relief of all grades of erosive esophagitis.

For patients who do not heal with PREVACID for 8 weeks (5–10%) it may be helpful to give an additional 8 weeks of treatment.

If there is a recurrence of erosive esophagitis an additional 8 week course of PREVACID may be considered.

Maintenance of Healing of Erosive Esophagitis

PREVACID Delayed-Release Capsules are indicated to maintain healing of erosive esophagitis. Controlled studies do not extend beyond 12 months.

Pathological Hypersecretory Conditions Including Zollinger-Ellison Syndrome

PREVACID Delayed-Release Capsules are indicated for the long-term treatment of pathological hypersecretory conditions, including Zollinger-Ellison syndrome.

CONTRAINDICATIONS

PREVACID Delayed-Release Capsules are contraindicated in patients with known hypersensitivity to any component of the formulation.

PRECAUTIONS

General

Symptomatic response to therapy with lansoprazole does not preclude the presence of gastric malignancy.

Information for Patients

PREVACID Delayed-Release Capsules should be taken before eating.

Patients should be cautioned that PREVACID Delayed-Release Capsules should be swallowed whole. However, for patients who have difficulty swallowing capsules, PREVACID Delayed-Release Capsules can be opened, and the intact granules contained within can be sprinkled on one tablespoon of applesauce and swallowed immediately. The granules should not be chewed or crushed.

Drug Interactions

Lansoprazole is metabolized through the cytochrome P$_{450}$ system, specifically through the CYP3A and CYP2C19 isozymes. Studies have shown that lansoprazole does not have clinically significant interactions with other drugs metabolized by the cytochrome P$_{450}$ system, such as warfarin, antipyrine, indomethacin, ibuprofen, phenytoin, propranolol, prednisone, or diazepam in healthy subjects. These compounds are metabolized through various cytochrome P$_{450}$ isozymes including CYP1A2, CYP2C9, CYP2C19, CYP2D6, and CYP3A. When lansoprazole was administered concomitantly with theophylline (CYP1A2, CYP3A), a minor increase (10%) in the clearance of theophylline was seen. Because of the small magnitude and the direction of the effect on theophylline clearance, this interaction is unlikely to be of clinical concern. Nonetheless, individual patients may require additional titration of their theophylline dosage when lansoprazole is started or stopped to ensure clinically effective blood levels.

Coadministration of lansoprazole with sucralfate delayed absorption and reduced lansoprazole bioavailability by approximately 30%. Therefore, lansoprazole should be taken at least 30 minutes prior to sucralfate. In clinical trials, antacids were administered concomitantly with PREVACID Delayed-Release Capsules; this did not interfere with its effect.

Lansoprazole causes a profound and long lasting inhibition of gastric acid secretion; therefore, it is theoretically possible that lansoprazole may interfere with the absorption of drugs where gastric pH is an important determinant of bioavailability (e.g., ketoconazole, ampicillin esters, iron salts, digoxin).

Continued on next page

TAP—Cont.

Carcinogenesis, Mutagenesis, and Fertility

In two 24-month carcinogenicity studies, Sprague-Dawley rats were treated orally with doses of 5 to 150 mg/kg/day, about 1 to 40 times the exposure on a body surface (mg/m^2) basis, of a 50 kg person of average height (1.46 m^2 body surface area) given the recommended human dose of 30 mg/day (22.2 mg/m^2). Lansoprazole produced dose-related gastric enterochromaffin like (ECL) cell hyperplasia and ECL cell carcinoids in both male and female rats. It also increased the incidence of intestinal metaplasia of the gastric epithelium in both sexes. In male rats, lansoprazole produced a dose-related increase of testicular interstitial cell adenomas. The incidence of these adenomas in rats receiving doses of 15 to 150 mg/kg/day (4 to 40 times the recommended human dose based on body surface area) exceeded the low background incidence (range = 1.4 to 10%) for this strain of rat. Testicular interstitial cell adenoma also occurred in 1 of 30 rats treated with 50 mg/kg/day (13 times the recommended human dose based on body surface area) in a 1-year toxicity study.

In a 24-month carcinogenicity study, CD-1 mice were treated orally with doses of 15 to 600 mg/kg/day, 2 to 80 times the recommended human dose based on body surface area. Lansoprazole produced a dose related increased incidence of gastric ECL cell hyperplasia. It also produced an increased incidence of liver tumors (hepatocellular adenoma plus carcinoma). The tumor incidences in male mice treated with 300 and 600 mg/kg/day (40 to 80 times the recommended human dose based on body surface area) and female mice treated with 150 to 600 mg/kg/day (20 to 80 times the recommended human dose based on body surface area) exceeded the ranges of background incidences in historical controls for this strain of mice. Lansoprazole treatment produced adenoma of rete testis in male mice receiving 75 to 600 mg/kg/day (10 to 80 times the recommended human dose based on body surface area).

Lansoprazole was not genotoxic in the Ames test, the *ex vivo* rat hepatocyte unscheduled DNA synthetics (UDS) test, the *in vivo* mouse micronucleus test or the rat bone marrow cell chromosomal aberration test. It was positive in *in vitro* human lymphocyte chromosomal aberration assays.

Lansoprazole at oral doses up to 150 mg/kg/day (40 times the recommended human dose based on body surface area) was found to have no effect on fertility and reproductive performance of male and female rats.

Pregnancy

Teratogenic Effects. Pregnancy Category B

Teratology studies have been performed in pregnant rats at oral doses up to 150 mg/kg/day (40 times the recommended human dose based on body surface area) and pregnant rabbits at oral doses up to 30 mg/kg/day (16 times the recommended human dose based on body surface area) and have revealed no evidence of impaired fertility or harm to the fetus due to lansoprazole.

There are, however, no adequate or well-controlled studies in pregnant women. Because animal reproduction studies are not always predictive of human response, this drug should be used during pregnancy only if clearly needed.

Nursing Mothers

Lansoprazole or its metabolites are excreted in the milk of rats. It is not known whether lansoprazole is excreted in human milk. Because many drugs are excreted in human milk, because of the potential for serious adverse reactions in nursing infants from lansoprazole, and because of the potential for tumorigenicity shown for lansoprazole in rat carcinogenicity studies, a decision should be made whether to discontinue nursing or to discontinue the drug, taking into account the importance of the drug to the mother.

Pediatric Use

Safety and effectiveness in children have not been established.

Use in Women

Over 800 women were treated with lansoprazole. Ulcer healing rates in females are similar to those in males. The incidence rates of adverse events are also similar to those seen in males.

Use in Elderly Patients

Ulcer healing rates in elderly patients are similar to those in a younger age group. The incidence rates of adverse events and laboratory test abnormalities are also similar to those seen in younger patients. The initial dosing regimen need not be altered for elderly patients, but subsequent doses higher than 30 mg per day should not be administered unless additional gastric acid suppression is necessary.

ADVERSE REACTIONS

Worldwide, over 6100 patients have been treated with lansoprazole in Phase II-III clinical trials involving various dosages and duration of treatment. In general, lansoprazole treatment has been well tolerated in both short-term and long-term trials.

Incidence in Clinical Trials

The following adverse events were reported by the treating physician to have a possible or probable relationship to drug in 1% or more of PREVACID-treated patients and occurred at a greater rate in PREVACID-treated patients than placebo-treated patients:

Incidence of Possibly or Probably Treatment-Related Adverse Events in Short-term, Placebo-Controlled Studies

Body System/Adverse Event	PREVACID (N=1457) %	Placebo (N=467) %
Body as a Whole		
Abdominal Pain	1.8	1.3
Digestive System		
Diarrhea	3.6	2.6
Nausea	1.4	1.3

Headache was also seen at greater than 1% incidence but was more common on placebo. The incidence of diarrhea is similar between placebo and lansoprazole 15 mg and 30 mg patients, but higher in the lansoprazole 60 mg patients (2.9%, 1.4%, 4.2%, and 7.4%, respectively).

The most commonly reported possibly or probably treatment-related adverse event during maintenance therapy was diarrhea.

In short-term and long-term studies, the following adverse events were reported in <1% of the lansoprazole-treated patients:

Body as a Whole — asthenia, candidiasis, chest pain (not otherwise specified), edema, fever, flu syndrome, halitosis, infection (not otherwise specified), malaise; *Cardiovascular System* — angina, cereborvascular accident, hypertension/hypotension, myocardial infarction, palpitations, shock (circulatory failure), vasodilation; *Digestive System* — melena, anorexia, bezoar, cardiospasm, cholelithiasis, constipation, dry mouth/thirst, dyspepsia, dysphagia, eructation, esophageal stenosis, esophageal ulcer, esophagitis, fecal discoloration, flatulence, gastric nodules/fundic gland polyps, gastroenteritis, gastrointestinal hemorrhage, hematemesis, increased appetite, increased salivation, rectal hemorrhage, stomatitis, tenesmus, ulcerative colitis vomiting; *Endocrine System* — diabetes mellitus, goiter, hyperglycemia/hypoglycemia; *Hematologic and Lymphatis System* — anemia, hemolysis; *Metabolic and Nutritional Disorders* — gout, weight gain/loss; *Musculoskeletal System* — arthritis/arthralgia, musculoskeletal pain, myalgia; *Nervous System* — agitation, amnesia, anxiety, apathy, confusion, depression, dizziness/syncope, hallucinations, hemiplegia, hostility aggravated, libido decreased, nervousness, paresthesia, thinking abnormality; *Respiratory System* — asthma, bronchitis, cough increased, dyspnea, epistaxis, hemoptysis, hiccup, pneumonia, upper respiratory inflammation/infection; *Skin and Appendages* — acne, alopecia, pruritis, rash, urticaria; *Special Senses* — amblyopia, deafness, eye pain, visual field defect, otitis media, taste perversion, tinnitus; *Urogenital System* — abnormal menses, albuminuria, breast enlargement/gynecomastia, breast tenderness, glycosuria, hematuria, impotence, kidney calculus.

Laboratory Values

The following changes in laboratory parameters were reported as adverse events.

Abnormal liver function tests, increased SGOT (AST), increased SGPT (ALT), increased creatinine, increased alkaline phosphatase, increased globulins, increased GGTP, increased/decreased/abnormal WBC, abnormal AG ratio, abnormal RBC, bilirubinemia, eosinophilia, hyperlipemia, increased/decreased electrolytes, increased/decreased cholesterol, increased glucocorticoids, increased LDH, increased/decreased/abnormal platelets, and increased gastrin levels. Additional isolated laboratory abnormalities were reported.

In the placebo controlled studies, when SGOT (AST) and SGPT (ALT) were evaluated, 0.4% (1/250) placebo patients and 0.3% (2/795) lansoprazole patients had enzyme elevations greater than three times the upper limit of normal range at the final treatment visit. None of these patients reported jaundice at any time during the study.

OVERDOSAGE

Oral doses up to 5000 mg/kg in rats (approximately 1300 times the recommended human dose based on body surface area) and mice (about 675.7 times the recommended human dose based on body surface area) did not produce deaths or any clinical signs.

Lansoprazole is not removed from the circulation by hemodialysis. In one reported case of overdose, the patient consumed 600 mg of lansoprazole with no adverse reaction.

DOSAGE AND ADMINISTRATION

Treatment of Duodenal Ulcer

The recommended adult oral dose is 15 mg once daily for 4 weeks. (See INDICATIONS AND USAGE).

Treatment of Erosive Esophagitis

The recommended adult oral dose is 30 mg daily for up to 8 weeks. For patients who do not heal with PREVACID for 8 weeks (5-10%) it may be helpful to give an additional 8 weeks of treatment. (See INDICATIONS AND USAGE).

If there is a recurrence of erosive esophagitis, an additional 8 weeks course of PREVACID may be considered.

Maintenance of Healing of Erosive Esophagitis

The recommended adult oral dose is 15 mg once daily (See CLINICAL STUDIES).

Pathological Hypersecretory Conditions Including Zollinger-Ellison Syndrome

The dosage of PREVACID in patients with pathologic hypersecretory conditions varies with the individual patient. The recommended adult oral starting dose is 60 mg once a day. Doses should be adjusted to individual patient needs and should continue for as long as clinically indicated. Dosages up to 90 mg bid have been administered. Daily dosages of greater than 120 mg should be administered in divided doses. Some patients with Zollinger-Ellison syndrome have been treated continuously with PREVACID for more than four years.

No dosage adjustment is necessary in patients with renal insufficiency or the elderly. For patients with severe liver disease, dosage adjustment should be considered.

PREVACID Delayed-Release Capsules should be taken before eating. In the clinical trials, antacids were used concomitantly with PREVACID.

HOW SUPPLIED

PREVACID Delayed-Release Capsules, 15 mg, are opaque, hard gelatin, colored pink and green. The 30 mg are opaque, hard gelatin, pink and black colored capsules. They are available as follows:

NDC 0300-1541-30
Unit of use bottles of 30: 15 mg capsules
NDC 0300-1541-13
Bottles of 100: 15 mg capsules
NDC 0300-1541-11
Unit dose package of 100: 15 mg capsules
NDC 0300-3046-30
Unit of use bottles of 30: 30 mg capsules
NDC 0300-3046-13
Bottles of 100: 30 mg capsules
NDC 0300-3046-11
Unit dose package of 100: 30 mg capsules

Storage: PREVACID capsules should be stored in a tight container protected from moisture.

Store between 59°F and 86°F.

Caution: Federal (USA) law prohibits dispensing without a prescription.

U.S. Patent Nos. 4,628,098; 4,689,333; 5,013,743; 5,026,560 and 5,045,321.

Manufactured for
TAP Pharmaceuticals Inc.
Deerfield, Illinois 60015-1595, U.S.A.
by Takeda Chemical Industries Limited,
Osaka, Japan 541
®—Registered Trademark
Ref. 03-4662-R4-Rev. February, 1996

Shown in Product Identification Guide, page 338

TEVA Pharmaceuticals USA
650 Cathill Road
Sellersville, PA 18960

Direct Inquiries to:
650 Cathill Road
Sellersville, PA 18960
(888) TEVA-USA

Product
Acetaminophen and Codeine Phosphate Tablets 300 mg/15 mg CIII
Acetaminophen and Codeine Phosphate Tablets 300 mg/30 mg CIII
Acetaminophen and Codeine Phosphate Tablets 300 mg/60 mg CIII
Albuterol Sulfate Syrup 2 mg/5 mL
Albuterol Tablets 2 mg
Albuterol Tablets 4 mg
Amitriptyline HCl Tablets 10 mg
Amitriptyline HCl Tablets 25 mg
Amitriptyline HCl Tablets 50 mg
Amitriptyline HCl Tablets 75 mg
Amitriptyline HCl Tablets 100 mg
Amoxicillin Capsules 250 mg
Amoxicillin Capsules 500 mg

Amoxicillin Chewable Tablets 125 mg
Amoxicillin Chewable Tablets 250 mg
Amoxicillin for Oral Suspension 125 mg/5 mL
Amoxicillin for Oral Suspension 250 mg/5 mL
Ampicillin Capsules 250 mg
Ampicillin Capsules 500 mg
Atenolol Tablets 50 mg
Atenolol Tablets 100 mg
Baclofen Tablets 10 mg
Baclofen Tablets 20 mg
Benzonatate Capsules 100 mg
Betamethasone Dipropionate Lotion 0.05%
Beta-Val™ Cream 0.1% (Betamethasone Valerate-equivalent to 0.1% Betamethasone)
Beta-Val™ Lotion 0.1% (Betamethasone Valerate-equivalent to 0.1% Betamethasone)
Butalbital, Acetaminophen and Caffeine Tablets 50 mg/325 mg/40 mg
Captopril Tablets 12.5 mg
Captopril Tablets 25 mg
Captopril Tablets 50 mg
Captopril Tablets 100 mg
Carbamazepine Chewable Tablets 100 mg
Carbamazepine Tablets 200 mg
Carbidopa and Levodopa Tablets 10 mg/100 mg
Carbidopa and Levodopa Tablets 25 mg/100 mg
Carbidopa and Levodopa Tablets 25 mg/250 mg
Cephalexin Capsules 250 mg
Cephalexin Capsules 500 mg
Cephalexin for Oral Suspension 125 mg/5 mL
Cephalexin for Oral Suspension 250 mg/5 mL
Cephalexin Tablets 250 mg
Cephalexin Tablets 500 mg
Cephradine Capsules 250 mg
Cephradine Capsules 500 mg
Cephradine for Oral Suspension 125 mg/5 mL
Cephradine for Oral Suspension 250 mg/5 mL
Chlorhexidine Gluconate Oral Rinse 0.12%
Chlorzoxazone Tablets 500 mg
Cimetidine Tablets 200 mg
Cimetidine Tablets 300 mg
Cimetidine Tablets 400 mg
Cimetidine Tablets 800 mg
Cinoxacin Capsules 500 mg
Clemastine Fumarate Syrup 0.5 mg/5 mL
Clemastine Fumarate Tablets 2.68 mg
Clindamycin HCl Capsules 150 mg
Clomiphene Citrate Tablets 50 mg
Clotrimazole Topical Solution 1%
Cloxacillin Sodium for Oral Solution 125 mg/5 mL
Cloxacillin Sodium Capsules 250 mg
Cloxacillin Sodium Capsules 500 mg
Cotrim D.S. Tablets (Sulfamethoxazole 800 mg, Trimethoprim 160 mg)
Cotrim Pediatric Suspension (Sulfamethoxazole 200 mg/5 mL, Trimethoprim 40 mg/5 mL)
Cotrim Tablets (Sulfamethoxazole 400 mg, Trimethoprim 80 mg)
Dicloxacillin Sodium Capsules 250 mg
Dicloxacillin Sodium Capsules 500 mg
Diflunisal Tablets 500 mg
Diltiazem HCl Extended-Release Capsules 60 mg
Diltiazem HCl Extended-Release Capsules 90 mg
Diltiazem HCl Extended-Release Capsules 120 mg
Diltiazem HCl Tablets 30mg
Diltiazem HCl Tablets 60mg
Diltiazem HCl Tablets 90mg
Diltiazem HCl Tablets 120mg
Disopyramide Phosphate Capsules 100 mg
Disopyramide Phosphate Capsules 150 mg
Doxycycline Hyclate Capsules 50 mg
Doxycycline Hyclate Capsules 100 mg
Doxycycline Hyclate Tablets 100 mg
Epitol Tablets (Carbamazepine 200 mg)
Fluocinonide Cream 0.05%
Fluocinonide Cream 0.05% (Emulsified Base)
Fluocinonide Gel 0.05%
Fluocinonide Ointment 0.05%
Fluocinonide Topical Solution 0.05%
Flurbiprofen Tablets 100 mg
Gemfibrozil Tablets 600 mg
Haloperidol Oral Solution (Concentrate) 2 mg/mL
Hydrocodone Bitartrate and Acetaminophen Tablets 5 mg/500 mg CIII
Hydrocodone Bitartrate and Acetaminophen Tablets 7.5 mg/650 mg CIII
Hydrocodone Bitartrate and Acetaminophen Tablets 7.5 mg/750 mg CIII
Imipramine HCl Tablets 10 mg
Imipramine HCl Tablets 25 mg
Imipramine HCl Tablets 50 mg
Indomethacin Extended-Release Capsules 75 mg
Ketoprofen Capsules 25 mg
Ketoprofen Capsules 50 mg
Ketoprofen Capsules 75 mg
Loperamide HCl Capsules 2 mg

Megestrol Acetate Tablets 40 mg
Metaproterenol Sulfate Tablets 10 mg
Metaproterenol Sulfate Tablets 20 mg
Metaproterenol Sulfate Syrup 10 mg/5 mL
Metoclopramide Oral Solution 5 mg/5 mL
Metoclopramide Tablets 5 mg
Metoclopramide Tablets 10 mg
Metoprolol Tartrate Tablets 50 mg
Metoprolol Tartrate Tablets 100 mg
Metronidazole Tablets 250 mg
Metronidazole Tablets 500 mg
Minocycline HCl Capsules 50 mg
Minocycline HCl Capsules 100 mg
Minoxidil Topical Solution 2%
Myco-Triacet® II Cream (Nystatin 100,000 units/gm, Triamcinolone Acetonide 1 mg/gm)
Myco-Triacet® II Ointment (Nystatin 100,000 units/gm, Triamcinolone Acetonide 1 mg/gm)
Naproxen Sodium Tablets 275 mg
Naproxen Sodium Tablets 550 mg
Naproxen Tablets 250 mg
Naproxen Tablets 375 mg
Naproxen Tablets 500 mg
Neomycin Sulfate Tablets 500 mg
Nortriptyline Hydrochloride Capsules 10 mg
Nortriptyline Hydrochloride Capsules 25 mg
Nortriptyline Hydrochloride Capsules 50 mg
Nortriptyline Hydrochloride Capsules 75 mg
Nystatin Oral Suspension (Nystatin 100,000 units/mL)
Nystatin Oral Tablets (Nystatin 500,000 units)
Otocort® Sterile Solution - Each mL contains: Neomycin Sulfate equivalent to 3.5 mg Neomycin Base, Polymyxin B Sulfate 10,000 Units, Hydrocortisone 10 mg (1%)
Otocort® Sterile Suspension - Each mL contains: Neomycin Sulfate equivalent to 3.5 mg Neomycin Base, Polymyxin B Sulfate 10,000 Units, Hydrocortisone 10 mg (1%)
Oxacillin Sodium Capsules 250 mg
Oxacillin Sodium Capsules 500 mg
Oxacillin Sodium for Oral Solution 250 mg/5 mL
Penicillin V Potassium for Oral Solution 125 mg/5 mL
Penicillin V Potassium for Oral Solution 250 mg/5 mL
Penicillin V Potassium Tablets 250 mg
Penicillin V Potassium Tablets 500 mg
Piroxicam Capsules 10 mg
Piroxicam Capsules 20 mg
Propacet™ 100 Tablets CIV (Propoxyphene Napsylate 100 mg, Acetaminophen 650 mg)
Propoxyphene Compound 65 CIV Capsules (Propoxyphene Hydrochloride 65 mg, Aspirin 389 mg, Caffeine 32.4 mg)
Propoxyphene HCl Capsules 65 mg CIV
Propoxyphene Napsylate and Acetaminophen Tablets 100 mg/650 mg (Pink) CIV
Propoxyphene Napsylate and Acetaminophen Tablets 100 mg/650 mg (White) CIV
Propranolol HCl Extended-Release Capsules 60 mg
Propranolol HCl Extended-Release Capsules 80 mg
Propranolol HCl Extended-Release Capsules 120 mg
Propranolol HCl Extended-Release Capsules 160 mg
Sucralfate Tablets 1 gm
Sulfamethoxazole and Trimethoprim Oral Suspension (Sulfamethoxazole 200 mg/5 mL, Trimethoprim 40 mg/5 mL)
Sulfamethoxazole and Trimethoprim Tablets (Sulfamethoxazole 400 mg, Trimethoprim 80 mg)
Sulfamethoxazole and Trimethoprim Tablets (Sulfamethoxazole 800 mg, Trimethoprim 160 mg)
Sulfanilamide Vaginal Cream 15%
Theochron Extended-Release Tablets 100 mg (Theophylline Anhydrous 100 mg)
Theochron Extended-Release Tablets 200 mg (Theophylline Anhydrous 200 mg)
Theochron Extended-Release Tablets 300 mg (Theophylline Anhydrous 300 mg)
Theophylline Extended-Release Capsules 100 mg
Theophylline Extended-Release Capsules 125 mg
Theophylline Extended-Release Capsules 200 mg
Theophylline Extended-Release Capsules 300 mg
Trazodone HCl Tablets 50 mg
Trazodone HCl Tablets 100 mg
Triacet™ Cream 0.1% (Triamcinolone Acetonide 0.1%)
Trimethoprim Tablets 100 mg
Trimethoprim Tablets 200 mg

For EMERGENCY telephone numbers,
consult the **Manufacturers' Index.**

Tyson & Associates, Inc.
12832 CHADRON AVENUE
HAWTHORNE, CA 90250

Direct Inquiries to:
Customer Service Department
(310) 675-1080
(800) 318-9766

AMINOMINE™ (Excitatory neurotransmitters)	OTC 700mg/cap
ARGININE HCl	OTC 700mg/cap
NUTROX	OTC
(Encapsulated Anti-oxidant)	
AMINOSTASIS® (Branched Chain formula)	OTC 700mg/cap
MVM (High potency multivitamin/mineral)	OTC
AMINOVIROX™ (Arginine-free formula)	OTC 700mg/cap
AMINOXIN (Enteric Pyridoxal 5'– Phosphate)	OTC 20mg/tab
ATP (Enteric Adenosine Triphosphate)	OTC 20mg/tab
L-CARNITINE (Fatty Acid Combustion)	OTC 250mg/cap
ENDORPHENYL® (Enkephalinase inhibitor D-Phenylalanine)	OTC 500mg/cap
RIBO-2™ (Enteric Riboflavin 5' = Phosphate)	OTC 5mg/tab
Co-Q-10	OTC 10mg/cap
THIAMILATE® (Enteric Thiamine Pyrophosphate)	OTC 20mg/tab
THREOSTAT™ (L-Threonine USP)	OTC 500mg/cap

AMINOPLEX®   OTC

DESCRIPTION
U.S.P. crystalline amino acid formulation. Formula contains 740 mg Anhydrous of 18 crystalline L-amino acids including neurotransmitter precursors and sulfur amino acids, and supplies 130 mg Nitrogen per capsule. Balanced formulation replacement based on quantitative Amino Acid Fractionation.

COMPOSITION
L-Lysine, L-Arginine, L-Isoleucine, L-Leucine, L-Alanine, L-Threonine, L-Histidine, L-Cystine, L-Methionine, L-Glutamine, L-Tyrosine, L-Aspartic Acid, L-Valine, L-Glutamic Acid, L-Phenylalanine, Glycine, L-Serine, L-Cysteine HCl.

DOSAGE AND ADMINISTRATION
1–3 capsules half an hour before meals.

HOW SUPPLIED
Bottles of 100 capsules—NDC 53335-701-14

AMINOTATE®   OTC
(Glucogenic formula)

DESCRIPTION
Isolated, singular, L-crystalline amino acid supplement for adults and children 4 or more years of age. Capsules contain 700 mg of 15 isolated singular amino acids without fillers, binders, preservatives or sugars. Contains 102 milligrams of Nitrogen per capsule. Formula rich source of glucogenic amino acids.

COMPOSITION
Glycine, L-Alanine, L-Leucine, L-Lysine, L-Valine, L-Isoleucine, L-Arginine, L-Phenylalanine, Proline, L-Glutamine, L-Tyrosine.

DOSAGE AND ADMINISTRATION
Initially it is recommended 2–4 capsules b.i.d. in between meals.

HOW SUPPLIED
700 mg capsule; Bottles of 100 capsules.

Continued on next page

Tyson—Cont.

CATEMINE®   OTC
(Catecholamine Precursor)

DESCRIPTION
Enterically coated preparation of 800 mg L-Tyrosine and 10 mg pyridoxal-5'-phosphate.

ACTIONS AND USES
Biochemical precursor of dopamine and norepinephrine.

DOSAGE AND ADMINISTRATION
2 tablets b.i.d. in between meals.

HOW SUPPLIED
Bottles of 60—NDC 53335-056-12

UAD Laboratories
Division of Forest Pharmaceuticals, Inc.
13622 LAKEFRONT DRIVE
ST. LOUIS, MO 63045

Address Inquiries to:
Professional Services Department
13622 Lakefront Drive
St. Louis, MO 63045
(314) 344-8870

See Forest Pharmaceuticals, Inc.

UCB Pharma, Inc.
1950 LAKE PARK DRIVE
P.O. BOX 723308
SMYRNA (ATLANTA), GA 31139

Direct Inquiries to:
UCB Pharma, Inc.
1950 Lake Park Drive
Smyrna (Atlanta), GA 30080
(800) 477-7877

For Medical Information Contact:
Suzan E. Leake
Manager, Med. Affairs
770-437-5558
In Emergencies:
Medical Affairs
(800) 477-7877

DURATUSS™ Tablets   ℞
120 mg pseudoephedrine hydrochloride and 600 mg guaifenesin

DESCRIPTION
Each long-acting, film-coated, dye-free Duratuss™ Tablet contains:
Pseudoephedrine Hydrochloride .... 120 mg
Guaifenesin .... 600 mg
Also contains colloidal silicon dioxide, magnesium stearate, microcrystalline cellulose, stearic acid and other ingredients. Film coating composed of hydroxypropyl methylcellulose and polyethylene glycol.
Pseudoephedrine hydrochloride is a nasal decongestant. Chemically it is [S-(R*,R*)]-α-[1-(methylamino)ethyl] benzenemethanol hydrochloride with the following structure:

Guaifenesin is an expectorant. Chemically it is 3-(O-methoxyphenoxy)-1,2 propanediol with the following structure:

CLINICAL PHARMACOLOGY
Pseudoephedrine hydrochloride is an orally effective nasal decongestant that acts on alpha-adrenergic receptors in the mucosa of the respiratory tract producing vasoconstriction. Pseudoephedrine shrinks swollen nasal mucous membranes, reduces tissue hyperemia, edema and nasal congestion and increases nasal airway patency. Drainage of sinus secretions is increased and obstructed Eustachian ostia may be opened. Pseudoephedrine produces little, if any, rebound congestion. Guaifenesin is an expectorant which enhances the flow of respiratory tract secretions. The enhanced flow of less viscid secretions lubricates irritated respiratory tract membranes, promotes ciliary action and facilitates the removal of inspissated mucus. As a result, sinus and bronchial drainage is improved and nonproductive coughs become more productive and less frequent.

INDICATIONS
Duratuss Tablets are indicated for the relief of nasal congestion due to the common cold, hay fever or other upper respiratory allergies and nasal congestion associated with sinusitis. To promote nasal or sinus drainage; for the relief of Eustachian tube congestion; for adjunctive therapy in serous otitis media; for the symptomatic relief of respiratory conditions characterized by dry, nonproductive cough and in the presence of tenacious mucus and/or mucus plugs in the respiratory tract.

CONTRAINDICATIONS
Duratuss Tablets are contraindicated in individuals with known hypersensitivity to sympathomimetics, severe hypertension or in patients receiving MAO inhibitors.

PRECAUTIONS
DO NOT CRUSH OR CHEW DURATUSS TABLETS BEFORE INGESTION TO PRESERVE THE LONG-ACTING EFFECT.
Information for Patients: As with other sympathomimetic drugs, Duratuss Tablets should be used with caution in the presence of hypertension, hyperthyroidism, diabetes, heart disease, peripheral vascular disease, glaucoma and prostatic hypertrophy.
Laboratory Test Interactions: Guaifenesin interferes with the colorimetric determination of 5-hydroxyindoleacetic acid (5-HIAA) and vanillylmandelic acid (VMA).
Pregnancy Category C.: Animal reproduction studies have not been conducted with pseudoephedrine or guaifenesin. It is also not known whether pseudoephedrine or guaifenesin can cause fetal harm when administered to a pregnant woman or can affect reproduction capacity. Pseudoephedrine and guaifenesin may be given to a pregnant woman only if clearly needed.
Nursing Mothers: Because of potential serious adverse reactions in nursing infants from sympathomimetic amines, pseudoephedrine is contraindicated in nursing mothers.

ADVERSE REACTIONS
Possible adverse reactions include nervousness, insomnia, restlessness or headache. These reactions seldom, if ever, require discontinuation of therapy. Urinary retention may occur in patients with prostatic hypertrophy.

OVERDOSAGE
Since the effects of Duratuss Tablets may last up to 12 hours, treatment of overdosage directed towards supporting the patient and reversing the effects of the drug should be continued for at least that length of time.
Saline cathartics may be useful in hastening the evacuation of unreleased medication.

DOSAGE AND ADMINISTRATION
Adults: 1 tablet every 12 hours. Children 6—12 years of age: one half (½) tablet every 12 hours. Tablet may be broken in half without affecting release of medication but not crushed or chewed.

HOW SUPPLIED
Duratuss Tablets (120 mg pseudoephedrine hydrochloride and 600 mg guaifenesin) are supplied as white, film-coated, dye-free, oval-shaped tablets debossed "ucb" on one side and scored and debossed "612" on the other side in bottles of 100 (NDC 50474-612-01), and 500 tablets (NCD 50474-612-50).
CAUTION: Federal Law prohibits dispensing without prescription.
Manufactured for
UCB Pharma, Inc.,
Smyrna (Atlanta), GA 30080
by Mikart, Inc.,
Atlanta, GA 30318

Rev. 4/96
Shown in Product Identification Guide, page 338

DURATUSS™ HD Elixir
2.5 mg hydrocodone bitartrate
(Warning: May be habit forming),
30 mg pseudoephedrine hydrochloride, and
100 mg guaifenesin per 5 mL

DESCRIPTION
Each 5 mL (one teaspoonful) of Duratuss™ HD Elixir contains:
Hydrocodone* Bitartrate .... 2.5 mg
  ***WARNING:** May be habit forming
Pseudoephedrine Hydrochloride .... 30 mg
Guaifenesin .... 100 mg
Alcohol 5%
Also contains citric acid anhydrous, glucose liquid, methylparaben, propylene glycol, propylparaben, purified water, saccharin sodium, sorbitol solution, sucrose, FD&C Red #40, natural and artificial flavoring.
Hydrocodone bitartrate is an antitussive. Chemically it is 4,5 α-epoxy-3-methoxy-17-methylmorphinan-6-one-tartrate (1:1) hydrate (2:5) with the following structure:

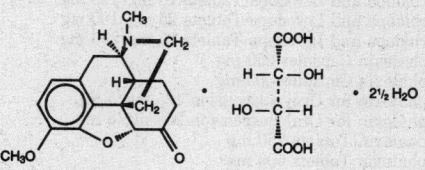

Pseudoephedrine hydrochloride is a nasal decongestant. Chemically it is [S-(R*,R*)]-α-[1-(methylamino)ethyl] benzenemethanol hydrochloride with the following structure:

Guaifenesin is an expectorant. Chemically it is 3-(2-methoxyphenoxy)-1,2 propanediol with the following structure:

CLINICAL PHARMACOLOGY
Hydrocodone is a semisynthetic narcotic analgesic and antitussive with multiple actions qualitatively similar to those of codeine. Most of these involve the central nervous system and smooth muscle. Hydrocodone suppresses the cough reflex by depressing the medullary cough center. The precise mechanism of action of hydrocodone and other opiates is not known, although it is believed to relate to the existence of opiate receptors in the central nervous system.
Pseudoephedrine hydrochloride is an orally effective nasal decongestant that acts on alpha-adrenergic receptors in the mucosa of the respiratory tract producing vasoconstriction. Pseudoephedrine shrinks swollen nasal mucous membranes, reduces tissue hyperemia, edema and nasal congestion and increases nasal airway patency. Drainage of sinus secretions is increased and obstructed Eustachian ostia may be opened. Pseudoephedrine produces little if any rebound congestion. Guaifenesin is an expectorant which enhances the flow of respiratory tract secretions. The enhanced flow of less viscid secretions lubricates irritated respiratory tract membranes, promotes cilliary action and facilitates the removal of inspissated mucus. As as result, sinus and bronchial drainage is improved and nonproductive coughs become more productive and less frequent.

INDICATIONS AND USAGE
For exhausting, nonproductive cough accompanying respiratory tract congestion associated with the common cold, influenza, sinusitis, and bronchitis.

CONTRAINDICATIONS
Duratuss HD Elixir (2.5 mg hydrocodone bitartrate [Warning: May be habit forming]. 30 mg pseudoephedrine hydrochloride, and 100 mg guaifenesin per teaspoonful) is contraindicated in patients with severe hypertension, severe coronary artery disease, and in patients on MAO inhibitor therapy.
Hypersensitivity: Contraindicated in patients with hypersensitivity or idiosyncracy to sympathomimetic amines, phenanthrene derivatives, or to any other formula ingredients.
Nursing Mothers: Contraindicated because of the higher than usual risk for infants for sympathomimetic amines.

WARNINGS

Hydrocodone should be prescribed and administered with the same degree of caution as all oral medications containing a narcotic analgesic. Extreme caution should be exercised in the use of hydrocodone in patients with severe respiratory impairment or patients with impaired respiratory drive. If sympathomimetic amines are used in patients with hypertension, diabetes mellitus, ischemic heart disease, hyperthyroidism, increased intraocular pressure or prostatic hypertrophy, judicious caution should be exercised (see CONTRAINDICATIONS).

Use in Elderly: The elderly (60 years and older) are more likely to have adverse reactions to sympathomimetics. Overdosage of sympathomimetics in this age group may cause hallucinations, convulsions, CNS depression and death.

PRECAUTIONS

General: Caution should be exercised if used in patients with diabetes, hypertension, cardiovascular diseases, hyperreactivity to ephedrine or decreased respiratory drive (see CONTRAINDICATIONS).

Information for Patients: Hydrocodone may produce drowsiness. Persons who perform hazardous tasks requiring mental alertness or physical coordination should be cautioned accordingly. Concomitant use of hydrocodone with tranquilizers, alcohol or other depressants may produce additive depressant effects. Do not exceed the prescribed dosage.

Drug Interactions: Hydrocodone may potentiate the effects of other narcotics, general anesthetics, tranquilizers, sedatives and hypnotics, tricyclic antidepressants, MAO inhibitors, alcohol, and other CNS depressants. Beta-adrenergic blockers and MAO inhibitors potentiate the sympathomimetic effects of pseudoephedrine. Sympathomimetics may reduce the antihypertensive effects of methyldopa, mecamylamine, reserpine and veratrum alkaloids.

Laboratory Test Interactions: Guaifenesin interferes with the colorimetric determination of 5-hydroxyindoleacetic acid (5-HIAA) and vanillylmandelic acid (VMA).

Pregnancy Category C: Animal reproduction studies have not been conducted with pseudoephedrine, guaifenesin, or hydrocodone. It is also not known whether pseudoephedrine, guaifenesin or hydrocodone can cause fetal harm when administered to a pregnant woman or can affect reproduction capacity. Pseudoephedrine, guaifenesin or hydrocodone may be given to a pregnant woman only if clearly needed.

Nursing Mothers: Because of the potential for serious adverse reactions in nursing infants from sympathomimetic amines, pseudoephedrine is contraindicated in nursing mothers.

ADVERSE REACTIONS

Gastrointestinal upset, nausea, drowsiness and constipation. A slight elevation in serum transaminase levels has been noted.

Individuals hyperreactive to pseudoephedrine may display ephedrine-like reactions such as tachycardia, palpitations, headache, dizziness or nausea. Sympathomimetic drugs have been associated with certain untoward reactions including fear, anxiety, tenseness, restlessness, tremor, weakness, pallor, respiratory difficulty, dysuria, insomnia, hallucinations, convulsions, CNS depression, arrhythmias, and cardiovascular collapse with hypotension. Patient idiosyncrasy to adrenergic agents may be manifested by insomnia, dizziness, weakness, tremor or arrhythmias.

DRUG ABUSE AND DEPENDENCE

Controlled Substance: Hydrocodone in Duratuss HD Elixir is controlled by the Drug Enforcement Administration. Duratuss HD Elixir is a Schedule III controlled substance.

Abuse: Hydrocodone is a narcotic drug related to codeine with similar abuse potential.

Dependence: Hydrocodone can produce drug dependence of the morphine type. Psychic dependence, physical dependence and tolerance may develop if dosage recommendations are greatly exceeded over a prolonged period of time.

OVERDOSAGE

Acute overdosage with Duratuss HD Elixir may produce variable clinical signs as hydrocodone produces CNS depression and cardiovascular depression while pseudoephedrine produces CNS stimulation and variable cardiovascular effects. Hydrocodone is likely to be responsible for most of the severe reactions from overdosage. Pressor amines should be used with great caution when taking pseudoephedrine. Patients with signs of stimulation should be treated conservatively and depressant medications should be avoided if possible because of potential drug interaction with hydrocodone.

DOSAGE AND ADMINISTRATION

Adults: 2 teaspoonfuls (10 mL) every 4–6 hours. Children 6–12 years of age: 1 teaspoonful (5 mL) every 4–6 hours. May be given four times a day as needed. May be taken with meals.

HOW SUPPLIED

Duratuss HD Elixir is a red-colored, fruit punch-flavored liquid containing 2.5 mg hydrocodone bitartrate (Warning: May be habit forming), 30 mg pseudoephedrine hydrochloride, and 100 mg guaifenesin per 5 mL, with 5% alcohol. It is supplied in containers of 1 pint (473 mL), NDC 50474-610-16, and 1 gallon (3785 mL), NDC 50474-610-28.

CAUTION

Federal law prohibits dispensing without prescription.
Manufactured for
UCB Pharma, Inc.,
Smyrna (Atlanta), GA 30080
by Mikart, Inc.,
Atlanta, GA 30318
Rev. 1/96

Shown in Product Identification Guide, page 338

Fe50™ Caplets   OTC
Extended release iron caplet

Each off-white caplet debossed with the symbol ⊗ contains:
Elemental Iron (ferrous sulfate) .... 50 mg

HOW SUPPLIED

Bottles of 100; NDC 58436-072-01

LORTAB® 2.5/500 TABLETS   Ⓒ
HYDROCODONE* BITARTRATE AND ACETAMINOPHEN TABLETS, USP
2.5 mg/500 mg
*Warning: May be habit forming

LORTAB® 5/500 TABLETS   Ⓒ
HYDROCODONE* BITARTRATE AND ACETAMINOPHEN TABLETS, USP
5 mg/500 mg
*Warning: May be habit forming

LORTAB® 7.5/500 TABLETS   Ⓒ
HYDROCODONE* BITARTRATE AND ACETAMINOPHEN TABLETS, USP
7.5 mg/500 mg
*Warning: May be habit forming

LORTAB® 10/500 TABLETS   Ⓒ
HYDROCODONE* BITARTRATE AND ACETAMINOPHEN TABLETS, USP
10 mg/500 mg
*Warning: May be habit forming

LORTAB® Elixir   Ⓒ
HYDROCODONE* BITARTRATE AND ACETAMINOPHEN ELIXIR
7.5 mg/500 mg PER 15 mL
*Warning: May be habit forming

DESCRIPTION

Hydrocodone bitartrate and acetaminophen is supplied in tablet and liquid form for oral administration.

Hydrocodone bitartrate is an opioid analgesic and antitussive and occurs as fine, white crystals or as a crystalline powder. It is affected by light. The chemical name is 4,5α-epoxy-3-methoxy-17-methylmorphinan-6-one tartrate (1:1) hydrate (2:5). It has the following structural formula:

$C_{18}H_{21}NO_3 \cdot C_4H_6O_6 \cdot 2\frac{1}{2}H_2O$ MW = 494.50

Acetaminophen, 4'-hydroxyacetanilide, a slightly bitter, white, odorless, crystalline powder, is a non-opiate, non-salicylate analgesic and antipyretic. It has the following structural formula:

$C_8H_9NO_2$ MW = 151.16

Each Lortab 2.5/500 contains:
Hydrocodone Bitartrate .... 2.5 mg
(Warning: May be habit forming)
Acetaminophen .... 500 mg

In addition each tablet contains the following inactive ingredients: colloidal silicon dioxide, croscarmellose sodium, crospovidone, microcrystalline cellulose, povidone, pregelatinized starch, stearic acid and sugar spheres which are composed of starch derived from corn, sucrose, FD&C Red #3.

Each Lortab 5/500 contains:
Hydrocodone Bitartrate .... 5 mg
(Warning: May be habit forming)
Acetaminophen .... 500 mg

In addition each tablet contains the following inactive ingredients: corn starch, FD&C Blue #1 lake, gelatin, magnesium stearate, microcrystalline cellulose, sugar spheres, povidone, pregelatinized starch, sodium starch glycolate.

Each Lortab 7.5/500 contains:
Hydrocodone Bitartrate .... 7.5 mg
(Warning: May be habit forming)
Acetaminophen .... 500 mg

In addition each tablet contains the following inactive ingredients: colloidal silicon dioxide, croscarmellose sodium, crospovidone, microcrystalline cellulose, povidone, pregelatinized starch, stearic acid, and sugar spheres which are composed of starch derived from corn, sucrose, FD&C Blue #1 and D&C Yellow #10.

Each Lortab 10/500 tablet contains:
Hydrocodone Bitartrate .... 10 mg
(Warning: May be habit forming)
Acetaminophen .... 500 mg

In addition each tablet contains the following inactive ingredients: D&C Red No. 27 Aluminum Lake, D&C Red No. 30 Aluminum Lake, croscarmellose sodium, microcrystalline cellulose, colloidal silicon dioxide, starch (corn), stearic acid, pregelatinized starch, povidone, and crospovidone.

Lortab Elixir contains:	Per 5 mL	Per 15 mL
Hydrocodone Bitartrate	2.5 mg	7.5 mg
(Warning: May be habit forming)		
Acetaminophen	167 mg	500 mg
Alcohol	7%	7%

In addition the liquid contains the following inactive ingredients: Citric acid anhydrous, ethyl maltol, glycerin, methyl paraben, propylene glycol, propylparaben, purified water, saccharin sodium, sorbitol solution, sucrose, with D&C Yellow #10 and FD&C Yellow #6 as coloring and natural and artificial flavoring.

CLINICAL PHARMACOLOGY

Hydrocodone is a semisynthetic narcotic analgesic and antitussive with multiple actions qualitatively similar to those of codeine. Most of these involve the central nervous system and smooth muscle. The precise mechanism of action of hydrocodone and other opiates is not known, although it is believed to relate to the existence of opiate receptors in the central nervous system. In addition to analgesia, narcotics may produce drowsiness, changes in mood and mental clouding. The analgesic action of acetaminophen involves peripheral influences, but the specific mechanism is as yet undetermined. Antipyretic activity is mediated through hypothalamic heat regulating centers. Acetaminophen inhibits prostaglandin synthetase. Therapeutic doses of acetaminophen have negligible effects on the cardiovascular or respiratory systems; however, toxic doses may cause circulatory failure and rapid, shallow breathing.

Pharmacokinetics: The behavior of the individual components is described below.

Hydrocodone: Following a 10 mg oral dose of hydrocodone administered to five adult male subjects, the mean peak concentration was 23.6 ± 5.2 ng/mL. Maximum serum levels were achieved at 1.3 ± 0.3 hours and the half-life was determined to be 3.8 ± 0.3 hours. Hydrocodone exhibits a complex pattern of metabolism including O-demethylation, N-demethylation and 6-keto reduction to the corresponding 6-α- and 6-β- hydroxymetabolites.
See OVERDOSAGE for toxicity information.

Acetaminophen: Acetaminophen is rapidly absorbed from the gastrointestinal tract and is distributed throughout most body tissues. The plasma half-life is 1.25 to 3 hours, but may be increased by liver damage and following overdosage. Elimination of acetaminophen is principally by liver metabolism (conjugation) and subsequent renal excretion of metabolites. Approximately 85% of an oral dose appears in the urine within 24 hours of administration, most as the glucuronide conjugate, with small amounts of other conjugates and unchanged drug.
See OVERDOSAGE for toxicity information.

INDICATIONS AND USAGE

Lortab Tablets & Elixir are indicated for the relief of moderate to moderately severe pain.

CONTRAINDICATIONS

This product should not be administered to patients who have previously exhibited hypersensitivity to hydrocodone or acetaminophen.

WARNINGS

Respiratory Depression: At high doses or in sensitive patients, hydrocodone may produce dose-related respiratory depression by acting directly on the brain stem respiratory center. Hydrocodone also affects the center that controls

Continued on next page

UCB—Cont.

respiratory rhythm, and may produce irregular and periodic breathing.

Head Injury and Increased Intracranial Pressure: The respiratory depressant effects of narcotics and their capacity to elevate cerebrospinal fluid pressure may be markedly exaggerated in the presence of head injury, other intracranial lesions or a preexisting increase in intracranial pressure. Furthermore, narcotics produce adverse reactions which may obscure the clinical course of patients with head injuries.

Acute Abdominal Conditions: The administration of narcotics may obscure the diagnosis or clinical course of patients with acute abdominal conditions.

PRECAUTIONS

General: Special Risk Patients: As with any narcotic analgesic agent, Lortab Tablets & Elixir should be used with caution in elderly or debilitated patients, and those with severe impairment of hepatic or renal function, hypothyroidism, Addison's disease, prostatic hypertrophy or urethral stricture. The usual precautions should be observed and the possibility of respiratory depression should be kept in mind.

Cough Reflex: Hydrocodone suppresses the cough reflex; as with all narcotics, caution should be exercised when Lortab Tablets or Elixir are used postoperatively and in patients with pulmonary disease.

Information for Patients: Hydrocodone, like all narcotics, may impair the mental and/or physical abilities required for the performance of potentially hazardous tasks such as driving a car or operating machinery; patients should be cautioned accordingly.

Alcohol and other CNS depressants may produce an additive CNS depression, when taken with this combination product, and should be avoided.

Hydrocodone may be habit-forming. Patients should take the drug only for as long as it is prescribed, in the amounts prescribed, and no more frequently than prescribed.

Laboratory Tests: In patients with severe hepatic or renal disease, effects of therapy should be monitored with serial liver and/or renal function tests.

Drug Interactions: Patients receiving narcotics, antihistamines, antipsychotics, antianxiety agents, or other CNS depressants (including alcohol) concomitantly with hydrocodone bitartrate and acetaminophen tablets or elixir may exhibit an additive CNS depression. When combined therapy is contemplated, the dose of one or both agents should be reduced.

The use of MAO inhibitors or tricyclic antidepressants with hydrocodone preparations may increase the effect of either the antidepressant or hydrocodone.

Drug/Laboratory Test Interactions: Acetaminophen may produce false-positive test results for urinary 5-hydroxyindoleacetic acid.

Carcinogenesis, Mutagenesis, Impairment of Fertility: No adequate studies have been conducted in animals to determine whether hydrocodone or acetaminophen have a potential for carcinogenesis, mutagenesis, or impairment of fertility.

Pregnancy:

Teratogenic Effects: Pregnancy Category C: There are no adequate and well-controlled studies in pregnant women. Lortab Tablets or Elixir should be used during pregnancy only if the potential benefit justifies the potential risk to the fetus.

Nonteratogenic Effects: Babies born to mothers who have been taking opioids regularly prior to delivery will be physically dependent. The withdrawal signs include irritability and excessive crying, tremors, hyperactive reflexes, increased respiratory rate, increased stools, sneezing, yawning, vomiting, and fever. The intensity of the syndrome does not always correlate with the duration of maternal opioid use or dose. There is no consensus on the best method of managing withdrawal.

Labor and Delivery: As with all narcotics, administration of this product to the mother shortly before delivery may result in some degree of respiratory depression in the newborn, especially if higher doses are used.

Nursing Mothers: Acetaminophen is excreted in breast milk in small amounts, but the significance of its effects on nursing infants is not known. It is not known whether hydrocodone is excreted in human milk. Because many drugs are excreted in human milk and because of the potential for serious adverse reactions in nursing infants from hydrocodone and acetaminophen, a decision should be made whether to discontinue nursing or to discontinue the drug, taking into account the importance of the drug to the mother.

Pediatric Use: Safety and effectiveness in the pediatric population have not been established.

ADVERSE REACTIONS

The most frequently reported adverse reactions are lightheadedness, dizziness, sedation, nausea and vomiting. These effects seem to be more prominent in ambulatory than in non-ambulatory patients, and some of these adverse reactions may be alleviated if the patient lies down.

Other adverse reactions include:

Central Nervous System: Drowsiness, mental clouding, lethargy, impairment of mental and physical performance, anxiety, fear, dysphoria, psychic dependence, mood changes.

Gastrointestinal System: Prolonged administration of Lortab Tablets or Elixir may produce constipation.

Genitourinary System: Ureteral spasm, spasm of vesical sphincters and urinary retention have been reported with opiates.

Respiratory Depression: Hydrocodone bitartrate may produce dose-related respiratory depression by acting directly on brain stem respiratory center (see OVERDOSAGE).

Dermatological: Skin rash, pruritus.

The following adverse drug events may be borne in mind as potential effects of acetaminophen: allergic reactions, rash, thrombocytopenia, agranulocytosis.

Potential effects of high dosage are listed in the OVERDOSAGE section.

DRUG ABUSE AND DEPENDENCE

Controlled Substance: Lortab Tablets & Elixir are classified as Schedule III controlled substances.

Abuse and Dependence: Psychic dependence, physical dependence, and tolerance may develop upon repeated administration of narcotics; therefore, this product should be prescribed and administered with caution. However, psychic dependence is unlikely to develop when hydrocodone bitartrate and acetaminophen tablets or elixir are used for a short time for the treatment of pain.

Physical dependence, the condition in which continued administration of the drug is required to prevent the appearance of a withdrawal syndrome, assumes clinically significant proportions only after several weeks of continued narcotic use, although some mild degree of physical dependence may develop after a few days of narcotic therapy. Tolerance, in which increasingly large doses are required in order to produce the same degree of analgesia, is manifested initially by a shortened duration of analgesic effect, and subsequently by decreases in the intensity of analgesia. The rate of development of tolerance varies among patients.

OVERDOSAGE

Following an acute overdosage, toxicity may result from hydrocodone or acetaminophen.

Signs and Symptoms:

Hydrocodone: Serious overdose with hydrocodone is characterized by respiratory depression (a decrease in respiratory rate and/or tidal volume, Cheyne-Stokes respiration, cyanosis), extreme somnolence progressing to stupor or coma, skeletal muscle flaccidity, cold and clammy skin, and sometimes bradycardia and hypotension. In severe overdosage, apnea, circulatory collapse, cardiac arrest and death may occur.

Acetaminophen: In acetaminophen overdosage: dose-dependent, potentially fatal hepatic necrosis is the most serious adverse effect. Renal tubular necrosis, hypoglycemic coma, and thrombocytopenia may also occur.

Early symptoms following a potentially hepatotoxic overdose may include: nausea, vomiting, diaphoresis and general malaise. Clinical and laboratory evidence of hepatic toxicity may not be apparent until 48 to 72 hours post-ingestion.

In adults, hepatic toxicity has rarely been reported with acute overdose of less than 10 grams or fatalities with less than 15 grams.

Treatment: A single or multiple overdose with hydrocodone and acetaminophen is a potentially lethal polydrug overdose, and consultation with a regional poison control center is recommended.

Immediate treatment includes support of cardiorespiratory function and measures to reduce drug absorption. Vomiting should be induced mechanically, or with syrup of ipecac, if the patient is alert (adequate pharyngeal and laryngeal reflexes). Oral activated charcoal (1 g/kg) should follow gastric emptying. The first dose should be accompanied by an appropriate cathartic. If repeated doses are used, the cathartic might be included with alternate doses as required. Hypotension is usually hypovolemic and should respond to fluids. Vasopressors and other supportive measures should be employed as indicated. A cuffed endo-tracheal tube should be inserted before gastric lavage of the unconscious patient and, when necessary, to provide assisted respiration.

Meticulous attention should be given to maintaining adequate pulmonary ventilation. In severe cases of intoxication, peritoneal dialysis, or preferably hemodialysis may be considered. If hypoprothrombinemia occurs due to acetaminophen overdose, vitamin K should be administered intravenously.

Naloxone, a narcotic antagonist, can reverse respiratory depression and coma associated with opioid overdose. Naloxone hydrochloride 0.4 mg to 2 mg is given parenterally. Since the duration of action of hydrocodone may exceed that of naloxone, the patient should be kept under continuous surveillance and repeated doses of the antagonist should be administered as needed to maintain adequate respiration. A narcotic antagonist should not be administered in the absence of clinically significant respiratory or cardiovascular depression.

If the dose of acetaminophen may have exceeded 140 mg/kg, acetylcysteine should be administered as early as possible. Serum acetaminophen levels should be obtained, since levels four or more hours following ingestion help predict acetaminophen toxicity. Do not await acetaminophen assay results before initiating treatment. Hepatic enzymes should be obtained initially, and repeated at 24-hour intervals.

Methemoglobinemia over 30% should be treated with methylene blue by slow intravenous administration.

The toxic dose for adults for acetaminophen is 10 g.

DOSAGE AND ADMINISTRATION

Dosage should be adjusted according to severity of pain and response of the patient. However, it should be kept in mind that tolerance to hydrocodone can develop with continued use and that the incidence of untoward effects is dose related.

The usual adult dosage for LORTAB® 2.5/500 tablets is one or two tablets every four to six hours as needed for pain. The total daily dosage should not exceed 8 tablets.

The usual adult dosage for LORTAB® 5/500 tablets is one or two tablets every four to six hours as needed for pain. The total daily dosage should not exceed 8 tablets.

The usual adult dosage for LORTAB® 7.5/500 tablets is one tablet every four to six hours as needed for pain. The total daily dosage should not exceed 6 tablets.

The usual adult dosage for LORTAB® 10/500 tablets is one tablet every four to six hours as needed for pain. The total daily dosage should not exceed 6 tablets.

The usual adult dosage for LORTAB® ELIXIR is one tablespoonful (15 mL) every four to six hours as needed for pain. The total daily dosage should not exceed 6 tablespoonfuls.

HOW SUPPLIED

LORTAB® 2.5/500 (Hydrocodone Bitartrate and Acetaminophen Tablets, USP) contain hydrocodone* bitartrate 2.5 mg *(Warning: May be habit forming) and acetaminophen 500 mg. They are supplied as white with pink specks, capsule-shaped, bisected tablets, debossed "ucb/901" in containers of 100 tablets NDC 50474-925-01.

LORTAB® 5/500 (Hydrocodone Bitartrate and Acetaminophen Tablets, USP) contain hydrocodone* bitartrate 5 mg *(Warning: May be habit forming) and acetaminophen 500 mg. They are supplied as white with blue specks, capsule-shaped, bisected tablets, debossed "ucb/902" in containers of 100 tablets NDC 50474-902-01, in containers of 500 tablets NDC 50474-902-50, and in hospital unit-dose packages of 100 tablets [4×25] NDC 50474-902-60.

LORTAB® 7.5/500 (Hydrocodone Bitartrate and Acetaminophen Tablets, USP) contain hydrocodone* bitartrate 7.5 mg *(Warning: May be habit forming) and acetaminophen 500 mg. They are supplied as white with green specks, capsule-shaped, bisected tablets, debossed "ucb/903" in containers of 100 tablets NDC 50474-907-01 and in containers of 500 tablets NDC 50474-907-50, and in hospital unit-dose packages of 100 tablets [4×25] NDC 50474-907-60.

Lortab® 10/500 (Hydrocodone Bitartrate and Acetaminophen Tablets, USP) contain hydrocodone bitartrate 10 mg (Warning: May be habit forming) and acetaminophen 500 mg. They are supplied as pink capsule-shaped tablets debossed "ucb/910," in containers of 100 tablets NDC 50474–910–01, 500 tablets NDC 50474–910–50, and in hospital unit-dose packages of 100 tablets [4×25] NDC 50474–910–60.

LORTAB® Elixir (Hydrocodone Bitartrate and Acetaminophen Elixir, 7.5mg/500 mg per 15 mL) is a yellow-colored, tropical fruit punch flavored liquid containing 7.5 mg hydrocodone* bitartrate (*Warning: May be habit forming) and 500 mg acetaminophen per 15 mL, with 7% alcohol. It is supplied in containers of 1 pint (473 mL) NDC 50474-909-16 and 1 gallon (3785 mL) NDC 50474-909-28.

Storage: Store at controlled room temperature, 15°–30°C (59°–86°F).

Dispense in a tight, light-resistant container with a child-resistant closure.

CAUTION: Federal law prohibits dispensing without prescription.

A Schedule CIII Narcotic

Manufactured for:

UCB PHARMA, INC.

Smyrna (Atlanta), GA 30080

Lortab® 2.5/500, Lortab® 7.5/500, Lortab® Elixir

Manufactured by:

Mikart, Inc.

Atlanta, GA 30318

Lortab® 5/500, Lortab® 10/500

Manufactured by:

D.M. Graham Laboratories, Inc.

Hobart, NY 13788

Rev. 5/96

Shown in Product Identification Guide, page 338

LORTAB® ASA Ⓒ
Hydrocodone* Bitartrate and Aspirin Tablets
5 mg/500 mg

Each tablet contains:

Hydrocodone bitartrate	5 mg
Warning: May be habit forming	
Aspirin	500 mg

HOW SUPPLIED

Bottles of 100; NDC 50474-500-01

Shown in Product Identification Guide, page 338

PRECARE® ℞
PRENATAL
MULTI-VITAMIN/MINERAL
FILM COATED CAPLET

DESCRIPTION

Each peach film-coated caplet contains:

Vitamin C (ascorbic acid)	50 mg
Calcium (as calcium carbonate)	250 mg
Iron (as ferrous fumarate)	40 mg
Vitmain D (cholecalciferol)	6 mcg
Vitamin E (dl-α-tocopherol acetate)	3.5 mg
Vitamin B_6 (pyridoxine hydrochloride)	2 mg
Folic Acid (folate)	1 mg
Magnesium (as magnesium oxide)	50 mg
Zinc (as zinc sulfate)	15 mg
Copper (as cupric sulfate)	2 mg

INACTIVE INGREDIENTS

Castor Oil, Corn Starch, Ethyl Cellulose, FD&C Yellow #6 Lake, Gelatin Hydroxypropyl Cellulose, Hydroxypropyl Methylcellulose, Magnesium Stearate, Pharmaceutical Glaze, Polyethylene Glycol, Povidone, Propylene Glycol, Silicon Dioxide, Sodium Benzoate, Sodium Lauryl Sulfate, Sodium Starch Glycolate, Sorbic Acid, Titanium Dioxide.

INDICATIONS

Precare is indicated to provide vitamin and mineral supplementation throughout pregnancy and during the postnatal period—for both lactating and non-lactating mothers. It is also useful for improving nutritional status prior to conception.

CONTRAINDICATIONS

This product is contraindicated in patients with a known hypersensitivity to any of the ingredients.

WARNINGS

Folic acid alone is improper therapy in the treatment of pernicious anemia and other megaloblastic anemias where Vitamin B_{12} is deficient.

WARNING—Close tightly and keep out of reach of children. Contains iron, which can be harmful or fatal to children in large doses. In case of accidental overdose, seek professional assistance or contact a Poison Control Center immediately.

PRECAUTIONS

Folic acid, in doses above 0.1 mg daily may obscure pernicious anemia, in that hematologic remission can occur while neurological manifestations remain progressive.

ADVERSE REACTIONS

Allergic sensitization has been reported following both oral and parenteral administration of folic acid.

DOSAGE AND ADMINISTRATION

One caplet daily between meals or at bedtime, or as prescribed by a physician.

HOW SUPPLIED

Precare caplets for oral administration are supplied as peach film-coated caplets, debossed "nmi" on one side and scored on the other side in bottles of 100 caplets (NDC 58436-071-01) with child-resistant closures.

DISPENSE IN A TIGHT, LIGHT-RESISTANT CONTAINER AS DEFINED IN THE USP/NF WITH A CHILD-RESISTANT CLOSURE.

STORE AT CONTROLLED ROOM TEMPERATURE 15°–30°C (59°–86°F).

CAUTION

Federal law prohibits dispensing without prescription.

Manufactured for:
northampton medical, inc.
Smyrna (Atlanta), GA 30080
Manufactured by:
Central Pharmaceuticals, Inc.
Seymour, IN 47274

Rev. 12/94

THEO-24® ℞
(theophylline anhydrous)
Extended-release capsules 100, 200, 300, & 400 mg

DESCRIPTION

Theophylline

Theophylline is structurally classified as a methylxanthine. It occurs as a white, odorless, crystalline powder with a bitter taste. Anhydrous theophylline has the chemical name 1H-Purine-2,6-dione,3,7-dihydro-1,3-dimethyl-, and is represented by the following structural formula:

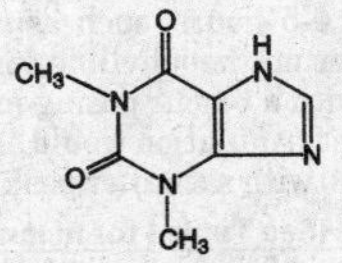

The molecular formula of anhydrous theophylline is $C_7H_8N_4O_2$ with a molecular weight of 180.17.

Theo-24® is available as capsules intended for oral administration, containing 100 mg, 200 mg, 300 mg, or 400 mg of anhydrous theophylline per capsule, in an extended-release formulation which allows a 24-hour dosing interval for appropriate patients.

Inactive ingredients are edible ink (which contains synthetic black iron oxide, FD&C Blue No. 1, FD&C Blue No. 2, FD&C Yellow No. 6, FD&C Yellow No. 10, FD&C Red No. 40), ethylcellulose, gelatin, pharmaceutical glaze, colloidal silicon dioxide, starch, sucrose, talc, titanium dioxide, and coloring agents: 100-mg—includes FD&C Yellow No. 6; 200-mg—FD&C Red No. 3 and D&C Yellow No. 10; 300-mg—FD&C Blue No.1 and FD&C Red No. 40; 400-mg—FD&C Red No. 40 and D&C Red No. 28.

Theo-24® Extended-release capsules meet Drug Release Test 6 as published in the USP 23 monograph for Theophylline Extended-release Capsules.

CLINICAL PHARMACOLOGY

Mechanism of Action;

Theophylline has two distinct actions in the airways of patients with reversible obstruction; smooth muscle relaxation (i.e., bronchodilation) and suppression of the response of the airways to stimuli (i.e., non-bronchodilator prophylactic effects). While the mechanisms of action of theophylline are not known with certainty, studies in animals suggest that bronchodilation is mediated by the inhibition of two isozymes of phosphodiesterase (PDE III and, to a lesser extent, PDE IV) while non-bronchodilator prophylactic actions are probably mediated through one or more different molecular mechanisms, that do not involve inhibition of PDE III or antagonism of adenosine receptors. Some of the adverse effects associated with theophylline appear to be mediated by inhibition of PDE III (e.g., hypotension, tachycardia, headache, and emesis) and adenosine receptor antagonism (e.g., alterations in cerebral blood flow).

Theophylline increases the force of contraction of diaphragmatic muscles. This action appears to be due to enhancement of calcium uptake through an adenosine-mediated channel.

Serum Concentration-Effect Relationship:

Bronchodilation occurs over the serum theophylline concentration range of 5–20 mcg/mL. Clinically important improvement in symptom control has been found in most studies to require peak serum theophylline concentrations >10 mcg/mL, but patients with mild disease may benefit from lower concentrations. At serum theophylline concentrations >20 mcg/mL, both the frequency and severity of adverse reactions increase. In general, maintaining peak serum theophylline concentrations between 10 and 15 mcg/mL will achieve most of the drug's potential therapeutic benefit while minimizing the risk of serious adverse events.

Pharmacokinetics:

Overview Theophylline is rapidly and completely absorbed after oral administration in solution or immediate-release solid oral dose form. Theophylline does not undergo any appreciable pre-systemic elimination, distributes freely into fat-free tissues and is extensively metabolized in the liver.

The pharmacokinetics of theophylline vary widely among similar patients and cannot be predicted by age, sex, body weight or other demographic characteristics. In addition, certain concurrent illnesses and alterations in normal physiology (see Table I) and co-administration of other drugs (see Table II) can significantly alter the pharmacokinetic characteristics of theophylline. Within-subject variability in metabolism has also been reported in some studies, especially in acutely ill patients. It is, therefore, recommended that serum theophylline concentrations be measured frequently in acutely ill patients (e.g., at 24-hr intervals) and periodically in patients receiving long-term therapy, e.g., at 6–12 month intervals. More frequent measurements should be made in the presence of any condition that may significantly alter theophylline clearance (see PRECAUTIONS, Laboratory tests).

[See Table 1 at bottom of next page.]

Absorption Theophylline is rapidly and completely absorbed after oral administration in solution or immediate-release solid oral dosage form. After a single immediate-release dose of 5 mg/kg in adults, a mean peak serum concentration of about 10 mcg/mL (range 5–15 mcg/mL) can be expected 1–2 hr after dose. Co-administration of theophylline with food or antacids does not cause clinically significant changes in the absorption of theophylline from immediate-release dosage forms.

Theo-24 capsules contain hundreds of coated beads of theophylline. Each bead is an individual extended-release delivery system. After dissolution of the capsules these beads are released and distributed in the gastrointestinal tract, thus minimizing the probability of high local concentrations of theophylline at any particular site.

In a 6–day multiple-dose study involving 18 subjects (with theophylline clearance rates between 0.57 and 1.02 mL/kg/min) who had fasted overnight and 2 hours after morning dosing, Theo-24 given once daily in a dose of 1500 mg produced serum theophylline levels that ranged between 5.7 mcg/mL and 22 mcg/mL. The mean minimum and maximum values were 11.6 mcg/mL and 18.1 mcg/mL, respectively, with an average peak-trough difference of 6.5 mcg/mL. The mean percent fluctuation [(Cmax-Cmin/Cmin)×100] equals 80%. A 24-hour single-dose study demonstrated an approximately proportional increase in serum levels as the dose was increased from 600 to 1500 mg.

Taking Theo-24 with a high-fat-content meal may result in a significant increase in the peak serum level and in the extent of absorption of theophylline as compared to administration in the fasted state (see Precautions: Drug/Food interactions).

Following the single-dose administration (8 mg/kg) of Theo-24 to 20 normal subjects who had fasted overnight and 2 hours after morning dosing, peak serum theophylline concentrations of 4.8 ± 1.5 (SD) mcg/mL were obtained at 13.3 ± 4.7 (SD) hours. The amount of the dose absorbed was approximately 13% at 3 hours, 31% at 6 hours, 55% at 12 hours, 70% at 16 hours, and 88% at 24 hours. The extent of theophylline bioavailability from Theo-24 was comparable to the most widely used 12-hour extended-release product when both products were administered every 12 hours.

Distribution Once theophylline enters the systemic circulation, about 40% is bound to plasma protein, primarily albumin. Unbound theophylline distributes throughout body water, but distributes poorly into body fat. The apparent volume of distribution of theophylline is approximately 0.45 L/kg (range 0.3–0.7 L/kg) based on ideal body weight. Theophylline passes freely across the placenta, into breast milk and into the cerebrospinal fluid (CSF). Saliva theophylline concentrations approximate unbound serum concentrations, but are not reliable for routine or therapeutic monitoring unless special techniques are used. An increase in the volume of distribution of theophylline, primarily due to reduction in plasma protein binding, occurs in premature neonates, patients with hepatic cirrhosis, uncorrected acidemia, the elderly and in women during the third trimester of pregnancy. In such cases, the patient may show signs of toxicity at total (bound + unbound) serum concentrations of theophylline in the therapeutic range (10–20 mcg/mL) due to elevated concentrations of the pharmacologically active unbound drug. Similarly, a patient with decreased theophylline binding may have a sub-therapeutic total drug concentration while the pharmacologically active unbound concentration is in the therapeutic range. If only total serum theophylline concentration is measured, this may lead to an unnecessary and potentially dangerous dose increase. In patients with reduced protein binding, measurement of unbound serum theophylline concentration provides a more reliable means of dosage adjustment than measurement of total serum theophylline concentration. Generally, concentrations of unbound theophylline should be maintained in the range of 6–12 mcg/mL.

Metabolism Following oral dosing, theophylline does not undergo any measurable first-pass elimination. In adults and children beyond one year of age, approximately 90% of the dose is metabolized in the liver. Biotransformation takes place through demethylation to 1-methylxanthine and 3-methylxanthine and hydroxylation to 1,3-dimethyluric acid. 1-methylxanthine is further hydroxylated, by xanthine oxidase, to 1-methyluric acid. About 6% of a theophylline dose is N-methylated to caffeine. Theophylline demethylation to 3-methylxanthine is catalyzed by cytochrome P-450 1A2, while cytochromes P-450 2E1 and P-450 3A3 catalyze the hydroxylation to 1,3-dimethyluric acid. Demethylation to 1-methylxanthine appears to be catalyzed either by cytochrome P-450 1A2 or a closely related cytochrome. In neonates, the N-demethylation pathway is absent while the function of the hydroxylation pathway is markedly deficient. The activity of these pathways slowly increases to maximal levels by one year of age.

Continued on next page

UCB—Cont.

Caffeine and 3-methylxanthine are the only theophylline metabolites with pharmacologic activity. 3-methylxanthine has approximately one tenth the pharmacologic activity of theophylline and serum concentrations in adults with normal renal function are < 1 mcg/mL. In patients with end-stage renal disease, 3-methylxanthine may accumulate to concentrations that approximate the unmetabolized theophylline concentration. Caffeine concentrations are usually undetectable in adults regardless of renal function. In neonates, caffeine may accumulate to concentrations that approximate the unmetabolized theophylline concentration and thus, exert a pharmacologic effect.

Both the N-demethylation and hydroxylation pathways of theophylline biotransformation are capacity-limited. Due to the wide intersubject variability of the rate of theophylline metabolism, non-linearity of elimination may begin in some patients at serum theophylline concentrations < 10 mcg/mL. Since this non-linearity results in more than proportional changes in serum theophylline concentrations with changes in dose, it is advisable to make increases or decreases in dose in small increments in order to achieve desired changes in serum theophylline concentrations (see DOSAGE AND ADMINISTRATION, Table VI). Accurate prediction of dose-dependency of theophylline metabolism in patients *a priori* is not possible, but patients with very high initial clearance rates (i.e., low steady state serum theophylline concentrations at above average doses) have the greatest likelihood of experiencing large changes in serum theophylline concentration in response to dosage changes.

Excretion In neonates, approximately 50% of the theophylline dose is excreted unchanged in the urine. Beyond the first three months of life, approximately 10% of the theophylline dose is excreted unchanged in the urine. The remainder is excreted in the urine mainly as 1,3-dimethyluric acid (35-40%), 1-methyluric acid (20-25%) and 3-methylxanthine (15-20%). Since little theophylline is excreted unchanged in the urine and since active metabolites of theophylline (i.e., caffeine, 3-methylxanthine) do not accumulate to clinically significant levels even in the face of end-stage renal disease, no dosage adjustment for renal insufficiency is necessary in adults and children > 3 months of age. In contrast, the large fraction of the theophylline dose excreted in the urine as unchanged theophylline and caffeine in neonates requires careful attention to dose reduction and frequent monitoring of serum theophylline concentrations in neonates with reduced renal function (See WARNINGS).

Serum concentrations at Steady State After multiple doses of theophylline, steady state is reached in 30–65 hours (average 40 hours) in adults. At steady state, on a dosage regimen with 6-hour intervals, the expected mean trough concentration is approximately 60% of the mean peak concentration, assuming a mean theophylline half-life of 8 hours. The difference between peak and trough concentrations is larger in patients with more rapid theophylline clearance. In patients with high theophylline clearance and half-lives of about 4–5 hours, such as children age 1 to 9 years, the trough serum theophylline concentration may be only 30% of peak with a 6-hour dosing interval. In these patients a slow release formulation would allow a longer dosing interval (8–12 hours) with a smaller peak/trough difference.

Special Populations (See Table I for mean clearance and half-life values) Geriatric The clearance of theophylline is decreased by an average of 30% in healthy elderly adults (> 60 years) compared to healthy young adults. Careful attention to dose reduction and frequent monitoring of serum theophylline concentrations are required in elderly patients (see WARNINGS).

Pediatrics The clearance of theophylline is very low in neonates (see WARNINGS). Theophylline clearance reaches maximal values by one year of age, remains relatively constant until about 9 years of age and then slowly decreases by approximately 50% to adult values at about age 16. Renal excretion of unchanged theophylline in neonates amounts to about 50% of the dose, compared to about 10% in children older than three months and in adults. Careful attention to dosage selection and monitoring of serum theophylline concentrations are required in pediatric patients (see WARNINGS and DOSAGE AND ADMINISTRATION).

Gender Gender differences in theophylline clearance are relatively small and unlikely to be of clinical significance. Significant reduction in theophylline clearance, however, has been reported in women on the 20th day of the menstrual cycle and during the third trimester of pregnancy.

Table I. Mean and range of total body clearance and half-life of theophylline related to age and altered physiological states.¶

Population characteristics	Total body clearance* mean (range)†† (mL/kg/min)	Half-life mean (range)††, (hr)
Age		
Premature neonates		
postnatal age 3–15 days	0.29 (0.09–0.49)	30 (17–43)
postnatal age 25–57 days	0.64 (0.04–1.2)	20 (9.4–30.6)
Term infants		
postnatal age 1–2 days	NR†	25.7 (25–26.5)
postnatal age 3–30 weeks	NR†	11 (6–29)
Children		
1–4 years	1.7 (0.5–2.9)	3.4 (1.2–5.6)
4–12 years	1.6 (0.8–2.4)	NR†
13–15 years	0.9 (0.48–1.3)	NR†
6–17 years	1.4 (0.2–2.6)	3.7 (1.5–5.9)
Adults (16–60 years) otherwise healthy non-smoking asthmatics	0.65 (0.27–1.03)	8.7 (6.1–12.8)
Elderly (> 60 years) non-smokers with normal cardiac, liver, and renal function	0.41 (0.21–0.61)	9.8 (1.6–18)
Concurrent illness or altered physiological state		
Acute pulmonary edema	0.33** (0.07–2.45)	19** (3.1–82)
COPD- > 60 years, stable non-smoker > 1 year	0.54 (0.44–0.64)	11 (9.4–12.6)
COPD with cor pulmonale	0.48 (0.08–0.88)	NR†
Cystic fibrosis (14–28 years)	1.25 (0.31–2.2)	6.0 (1.8–10.2)
Fever associated with acute viral respiratory illness (children 9–15 years)	NR†	7.0 (1.0–13)
Liver disease - cirrhosis	0.31 ** (0.1–0.7)	32** (10–56)
acute hepatitis	0.35 (0.25–0.45)	19.2 (16.6–21.8)
cholestasis	0.65 (0.25–1.45)	14.4 (5.7–31.8)
Pregnancy - 1st trimester	NR†	8.5 (3.1–13.9)
2nd trimester	NR†	8.8 (3.8–13.8)
3rd trimester	NR†	13.0 (8.4–17.6)
Sepsis with multi-organ failure	0.47 (0.19–1.9)	18.8 (6.3–24.1)
Thyroid disease - hypothyroid	0.38 (0.13–0.57)	11.6 (8.2–25)
hyperthyroid	0.8 (0.68–0.97)	4.5 (3.7–5.6)

¶ For various North American patient populations from literature reports. Different rates of elimination and consequent dosage requirements have been observed among other peoples.

* Clearance represents the volume of blood completely cleared of theophylline by the liver in one minute. Values listed were generally determined at serum theophylline concentrations < 20 mcg/mL; clearance may decrease and half-life may increase at higher serum concentrations due to non-linear pharmacokinetics.

†† Reported range or estimated range (mean ± 2 SD) where actual range not reported.

† NR = not reported or not reported in a comparable format.

** Median

Note: In addition to the factors listed above, theophylline clearance is increased and half-life decreased by low carbohydrate/high protein diets, parenteral nutrition, and daily consumption of charcoal-broiled beef. A high carbohydrate/low protein diet can decrease the clearance and prolong the half-life of theophylline.

Race Pharmacokinetic differences in theophylline clearance due to race have not been studied.

Renal Insufficiency Only a small fraction, e.g., about 10% of the administered theophylline dose is excreted unchanged in the urine of children greater than three months of age and adults. Since little theophylline is excreted unchanged in the urine and since active metabolites of theophylline (i.e., caffeine, 3-methylxanthine) do not accumulate to clinically significant levels even in the face of end-stage renal disease, no dosage adjustment for renal insufficiency is necessary in adults and children > 3 months of age. In contrast, approximately 50% of the administered theophylline dose is excreted unchanged in the urine in neonates. Careful attention to dose reduction and frequent monitoring of serum theophylline concentrations are required in neonates with decreased renal function (see WARNINGS).

Hepatic Insufficiency Theophylline clearance is decreased by 50% or more in patients with hepatic insufficiency (e.g., cirrhosis, acute hepatitis, cholestasis). Careful attention to dose reduction and frequent monitoring of serum theophylline concentrations are required in patients with reduced hepatic function (see WARNINGS).

Congestive Heart Failure (CHF) Theophylline clearance is decreased by 50% or more in patients with CHF. The extent of reduction in theophylline clearance in patients with CHF appears to be directly correlated to the severity of the cardiac disease. Since theophylline clearance is independent of liver blood flow, the reduction in clearance appears to be due to impaired hepatocyte function rather than reduced perfusion. Careful attention to dose reduction and frequent monitoring of serum theophylline concentrations are required in patients with CHF (see WARNINGS).

Smokers Tobacco and marijuana smoking appears to increase the clearance of theophylline by induction of metabolic pathways. Theophylline clearance has been shown to increase by approximately 50% in young adult tobacco smokers and by approximately 80% in elderly tobacco smokers compared to non-smoking subjects. Passive smoke exposure has also been shown to increase theophylline clearance by up to 50%. Abstinence from tobacco smoking for one week causes a reduction of approximately 40% in theophylline clearance. Careful attention to dose reduction and frequent monitoring of serum theophylline concentrations are required in patients who stop smoking (see WARNINGS). Use of nicotine gum has been shown to have no effect on theophylline clearance.

Fever Fever, regardless of its underlying cause, can decrease the clearance of theophylline. The magnitude and duration of the fever appear to be directly correlated to the degree of decrease of theophylline clearance. Precise data are lacking, but a temperature of 39°C (102°F) for at least 24 hours is probably required to produce a clinically significant increase in serum theophylline concentrations. Children with rapid rates of theophylline clearance (i.e., those who require a dose that is substantially larger than average [e.g., > 22 mg/kg/day] to achieve a therapeutic peak serum theophylline concentration when afebrile) may be at greater risk of toxic effects from decreased clearance during sustained fever. Careful attention to dose reduction and frequent monitoring of serum theophylline concentrations are required in patients with sustained fever (see WARNINGS).

Miscellaneous

Other factors associated with decreased theophylline clearance include the third trimester of pregnancy, sepsis with multiple organ failure, and hypothyroidism. Careful attention to dose reduction and frequent monitoring of serum theophylline concentrations are required in patients with any of these conditions (see WARNINGS). Other factors associated with increased theophylline clearance include hyperthyroidism and cystic fibrosis.

Clinical Studies:

In patients with chronic asthma, including patients with severe asthma requiring inhaled corticosteroids or alternate-day oral corticosteroids, many clinical studies have shown that theophylline decreases the frequency and severity of symptoms, including nocturnal exacerbations, and decreases the "as needed" use of inhaled beta-2 agonists. Theophylline has also been shown to reduce the need for short courses of daily oral prednisone to relieve exacerbations of airway obstruction that are unresponsive to bronchodilators in asthmatics.

In patients with chronic obstructive pulmonary disease (COPD), clinical studies have shown that theophylline decreases dyspnea, air trapping, the work of breathing, and improves contractility of diaphragmatic muscles with little or no improvement in pulmonary function measurements.

INDICATIONS AND USAGE

Theophylline is indicated for the treatment of the symptoms and reversible airflow obstruction associated with chronic asthma and other chronic lung diseases, e.g., emphysema and chronic bronchitis.

CONTRAINDICATIONS

Theo-24 is contraindicated in patients with a history of hypersensitivity to theophylline or other components in the product.

WARNINGS

Concurrent Illness:
Theophylline should be used with extreme caution in patients with the following clinical conditions due to the increased risk of exacerbation of the concurrent condition:
- Active peptic ulcer disease
- Seizure disorders
- Cardiac arrhythmias (not including bradyarrhythmias)

Conditions That Reduce Theophylline Clearance:
There are several readily indentifiable causes of reduced theophylline clearance. ***If the total daily dose is not appropriately reduced in the presence of these risk factors, severe and potentially fatal theophylline toxicity can occur.*** Careful consideration must be given to the benefits and risks of theophylline use and the need for more intensive monitoring of serum theophylline concentrations in patients with the following risk factors:

Age
- Neonates (term and premature)
- Children <1 year
- Elderly (>60 years)

Concurrent Diseases
- Acute pulmonary edema
- Congestive heart failure
- Cor-pulmonale
- Fever; ≥102° for 24 hours or more; or lesser temperature elevations for longer periods
- Hypothyroidism
- Liver disease; cirrhosis, acute hepatitis
- Reduced renal function in infants <3 months of age
- Sepsis with multi-organ failure
- Shock

Cessation of Smoking

Drug Interactions Adding a drug that inhibits theophylline metabolism (e.g., cimetidine, erythromycin, tacrine) or stopping a concurrently administered drug that enhances theophylline metabolism (e.g., carbamazepine, rifampin). (see PRECAUTIONS, Drug Interactions, Table II).

When Signs or Symptoms of Theophylline Toxicity Are Present:
Whenever a patient receiving theophylline develops nausea or vomiting, particularly repetitive vomiting, or other signs or symptoms consistent with theophylline toxicity (even if another cause may be suspected), additional doses of theophylline should be withheld and a serum theophylline concentration measured immediately. Patients should be instructed not to continue any dosage that causes adverse effects and to withhold subsequent doses until the symptoms have resolved, at which time the clinician may instruct the patient to resume the drug at a lower dosage (see DOSAGE AND ADMINISTRATION, Dosing Guidelines, Table VI).

Dosage Increases:
Increases in the dose of theophylline should not be made in response to an acute exacerbation of symptoms of chronic lung disease since theophylline provides little added benefit to inhaled beta$_2$-selective agonists and systemically administered corticosteroids in this circumstance and increases the risk of adverse effects. A peak steady-state serum theophylline concentration should be measured before increasing the dose in response to persistent chronic symptoms to ascertain whether an increase in dose is safe. Before increasing the theophylline dose on the basis of a low serum concentration, the clinician should consider whether the blood sample was obtained at an appropriate time in relationship to the dose and whether the patient has adhered to the prescribed regimen (see PRECAUTIONS, Laboratory Tests).
As the rate of theophylline clearance may be dose-dependent (i.e., steady-state serum concentrations may increase disproportionately to the increase in dose), an increase in dose based upon a sub-therapeutic serum concentration measurement should be conservative. In general, limiting dose increases to about 25% of the previous total daily dose will reduce the risk of unintended excessive increases in serum theophylline concentration (see DOSAGE AND ADMINISTRATION, Table VI).

PRECAUTIONS

General:
Careful consideration of the various interacting drugs and physiologic conditions that can alter theophylline clearance and require dosage adjustment should occur prior to initiation of theophylline therapy, prior to increases in theophylline dose, and during follow up (see WARNINGS). The dose of theophylline selected for initiation of therapy should be low and, ***if tolerated***, increased slowly over a period of a week or longer with the final dose guided by monitoring serum theophylline concentrations and the patient's clinical response (see DOSAGE AND ADMINISTRATION, Table V).

Monitoring Serum Theophylline Concentrations:
Serum theophylline concentration measurements are readily available and should be used to determine whether the dosage is appropriate. Specifically, the serum theophylline concentration should be measured as follows:

1. When initiating therapy to guide final dosage adjustment after titration.
2. Before making a dose increase to determine whether the serum concentration is sub-therapeutic in a patient who continues to be symptomatic.
3. Whenever signs or symptoms of theophylline toxicity are present.
4. Whenever there is a new illness, worsening of a chronic illness or a change in the patient's treatment regimen that may alter theophylline clearance (e.g., fever >102°F sustained for ≥24 hours, hepatitis, or drugs listed in Table II are added or discontinued).

To guide a dose increase, the blood sample should be obtained at the time of the expected peak serum theophylline concentration; 12 hours after a dose at steady-state (expected peak serum theophylline concentration range is between 5–15 mcg/mL). For most patients, steady-state will be reached after 3 days of dosing when no doses have been missed, no extra doses have been added, and none of the doses have been taken at unequal intervals. A trough concentration (i.e., at the end of the dosing interval) provides no additional useful information and may lead to an inappropriate dose increase since the peak serum theophylline concentration can be two or more times greater than the trough concentration with an extended-release formulation. If the serum sample is drawn more or less than twelve (12) hours after the dose, the results must be interpreted with caution since the concentration may not be reflective of the peak concentration. In contrast, when signs or symptoms of theophylline toxicity are present, the serum sample should be obtained as soon as possible, analyzed immediately, and the result reported to the clinician without delay. In patients in whom decreased serum protein binding is suspected (e.g., cirrhosis, women during the third trimester of pregnancy), the concentration of unbound theophylline should be measured and the dosage adjusted to achieve an unbound concentration of 6-12 mcg/mL.
Saliva concentrations of theophylline cannot be used reliably to adjust dosage without special techniques.

Effects on Laboratory Tests:
As a result of its pharmacological effects, theophylline at serum concentrations within the 10–20 mcg/mL range modestly increases plasma glucose (from a mean of 88 mg% to 98 mg%), uric acid (from a mean of 4 mg/dL to 6 mg/dL), free fatty acids (from a mean of 451 μEq/L to 800 μEq/L, total cholesterol (from a mean of 140 vs 160 mg/dL), HDL (from a mean of 36 to 50 mg/dL), HDL/LDL ratio (from a mean of 0.5 to 0.7), and urinary free cortisol excretion (from a mean of 44 to 63 mcg/24 hr). Theophylline at serum concentrations within the 10–20 mcg/mL range may also transiently decrease serum concentrations of triiodothyronine (144 before, 131 after one week and 142 ng/dL after 4 weeks of theophylline). The clinical importance of these changes should be weighed against the potential therapeutic benefit of theophylline in individual patients.

Information for Patients:
The patient (or parent/care giver) should be instructed to seek medical advice whenever nausea, vomiting, persistent headache, insomnia or rapid heart beat occurs during treatment with theophylline, even if another cause is suspected. The patient should be instructed to contact their clinician if they develop a new illness, especially if accompanied by a persistent fever, if they experience worsening of a chronic illness, if they start or stop smoking cigarettes or marijuana, or if another clinician adds a new medication or discontinues a previously prescribed medication. Patients should be instructed to inform all clinicians involved in their care that they are taking theophylline, especially when a medication is being added or deleted from their treatment. Patients should be instructed to not alter the dose, timing of the dose, or frequency of administration without first consulting their clinician. If a dose is missed, the patient should be instructed to take the next dose at the usually scheduled time and to not attempt to make up for the missed dose.
Patients should be instructed to take this medication each morning at approximately the same time and not to exceed the prescribed dose.
Patients who require a relatively high dose of theophylline should be informed of important considerations relating to time of drug administration and meal content (see Precautions: Drug/Food interactions; and Dosage and Administration).

Drug Interactions:
Drug/Drug Interactions Theophylline interacts with a wide variety of drugs. The interaction may be pharmacodynamic, i.e., alterations in the therapeutic response to theophylline or another drug or occurrence of adverse effects without a change in serum theophylline concentration. More frequently, however, the interaction is pharmacokinetic, i.e., the rate of theophylline clearance is altered by another drug resulting in increased or decreased serum theophylline concentrations. Theophylline only rarely alters the pharmacokinetics of other drugs.
The drugs listed in Table II have the potential to produce clinically significant pharmacodynamic or pharmacokinetic interactions with theophylline. The information in the "Effect" column of Table II assumes that the interacting drug is being added to a steady-state theophylline regimen. If theophylline is being initiated in a patient who is already taking a drug that inhibits theophylline clearance (e.g., cimetidine, erythromycin), the dose of theophylline required to achieve a therapeutic serum theophylline concentration will be smaller. Conversely, if theophylline is being initiated in a patient who is already taking a drug that enhances theophylline clearance (e.g., rifampin), the dose of theophylline required to achieve a therapeutic serum theophylline concentration will be larger. Discontinuation of a concomitant drug that increases theophylline clearance will result in accumulation of theophylline to potentially toxic levels, unless the theophylline dose is appropriately reduced.
Discontinuation of a concomitant drug that inhibits theophylline clearance will result in decreased serum theophylline concentrations, unless the theophylline dose is appropriately increased.
The drugs listed in Table III have either been documented not to interact with theophylline or do not produce a clinically significant interaction (i.e., <15% change in theophylline clearance).
The listing of drugs in Tables II and III are current as of January 2, 1996. New interactions are continuously being reported for theophylline, especially with new chemical entities. **The clinician should not assume that a drug does not interact with theophylline if it is not listed in Table II.** Before addition of a newly available drug in a patient receiving theophylline, the package insert of the new drug and/or the medical literature should be consulted to determine if an interaction between the new drug and theophylline has been reported.
[See Table 2 on next page and at top of page 2757.]

Table III. Drugs that have been documented not to interact with theophylline or drugs that produce no clinically significant interaction with theophylline.*

albuterol, systemic and inhaled	lomefloxacin
amoxicillin	mebendazole
ampicillin, with or without sulbactam	medroxyprogesterone
atenolol	methylprednisolone
azithromycin	metronidazole
caffeine, dietary ingestion	metoprolol
cefaclor	nadolol
co-trimoxazole (trimethoprim and sulfamethoxazole)	nifedipine
diltiazem	nizatidine
dirithomycin	norfloxacin
enflurane	ofloxacin
famotidine	omeprazole
felodipine	prednisone, prednisolone
finasteride	ranitidine
hydrocortisone	rifabutin
isoflurane	roxithromycin
isoniazid	sorbitol (purgative doses do not inhibit theophylline absorption)
isradipine	sucralfate
influenza vaccine	terbutaline, systemic
ketoconazole	terfenadine
	tetracycline
	tocainide

***Refer to PRECAUTIONS, Drug Interactions for information regarding table.**

Drug/Food Interactions Taking Theo-24 less than one hour before a high-fat-content meal, such as 8 oz whole milk, 2 fried eggs, 2 bacon strips, 2 oz hashed brown potatoes, and 2 slices of buttered toast (about 985 calories, including approximately 71g of fat) may result in a significant increase in peak serum level and in the extent of absorption of theophylline as compared to administration in the fasted state. In some cases (especially with doses of 900 mg or more taken less than one hour before a high-fat-content meal) serum theophylline levels may exceed the 20 mcg/mL level, above which theophylline toxicity is more likely to occur.

The Effect of Other Drugs on Theophylline Serum Concentration Measurements:
Most serum theophylline assays in clinical use are immunoassays which are specific for theophylline. Other xanthines such as caffeine, dyphylline, and pentoxifylline are not detected by these assays. Some drugs (e.g., cefazolin, cephalothin), however, may interfere with certain HPLC techniques. Caffeine and xanthine metabolites in neonates or patients with renal dysfunction may cause the reading from some dry reagent office methods to be higher than the actual serum theophylline concentration.

Carcinogenesis, Mutagenesis, and Impairment of Fertility:
Long term carcinogenicity studies have been carried out in mice (oral doses 30–150 mg/kg) and rats (oral doses 5–75 mg/kg). Results are pending.

Continued on next page

UCB—Cont.

Theophylline has been studied in Ames salmonella, *in vivo* and *in vitro* cytogenetics, micronucleus and Chinese hamster ovary test systems and has not been shown to be genotoxic. In a 14 week continuous breeding study, theophylline, administered to mating pairs of B6C3F$_1$ mice at oral doses of 120, 270 and 500 mg/kg (approximately 1.0–3.0 times the human dose on a mg/m^2 basis) impaired fertility, as evidenced by decreases in the number of live pups per litter, decreases in the mean number of litters per fertile pair, and increases in the gestation period at the high dose as well as decreases in the proportion of pups born alive at the mid and high dose. In 13 week toxicity studies, theophylline was administered to F344 rats and B6C3F$_1$ mice at oral doses of 40–300 mg/kg (approximately 2.0 times the human dose on a mg/m^2 basis). At the high dose, systemic toxicity was observed in both species including decreases in testicular weight.

Pregnancy:

CATEGORY C: There are no adequate and well controlled studies in pregnant women. Additionally, there are no teratogenicity studies in non-rodents (e.g., rabbits). Theophylline was not shown to be teratogenic in CD-1 mice at oral doses up to 400 mg/kg, approximately 2.0 times the human dose on a mg/m^2 basis or in CD-1 rats at oral doses up to 260 mg/kg, approximately 3.0 times the recommended human dose on a mg/m^2 basis. At a dose of 220 mg/kg, embryotoxicity was observed in rats in the absence of maternal toxicity.

Nursing Mothers:

Theophylline is excreted into breast milk and may cause irritability or other signs of mild toxicity in nursing human infants. The concentration of theophylline in breast milk is about equivalent to the maternal serum concentration. An infant ingesting a liter of breast milk containing 10–20 mcg/mL of theophylline day is likely to receive 10–20 mg of theophylline per day. Serious adverse effects in the infant are unlikely unless the mother has toxic serum theophylline concentrations.

Pediatric Use:

Theophylline is safe and effective for the approved indications in pediatric patients (See, INDICATIONS AND USAGE). The maintenance dose of theophylline must be selected with caution in pediatric patients since the rate of theophylline clearance is highly variable across the age range of neonates to adolescents (see CLINICAL PHARMACOLOGY, Table I, WARNINGS, and DOSAGE AND ADMINISTRATION, Table V). Due to the immaturity of theophylline metabolic pathways in infants under the age of one year, particular attention to dosage selection and frequent monitoring of serum theophylline concentrations are required when theophylline is prescribed to pediatric patients in this group.

Geriatric Use:

Elderly patients are at significantly greater risk of experiencing serious toxicity from theophylline than younger patients due to pharmacokinetic and pharmacodynamic changes associated with aging. Theophylline clearance is reduced in patients greater than 60 years of age, resulting in increased serum theophylline concentrations in response to a given theophylline dose. Protein binding may be decreased in the elderly resulting in a larger proportion of the total serum theophylline concentration in the pharmacologically active unbound form. Elderly patients also appear to be more sensitive to the toxic effects of theophylline after chronic overdosage than younger patients. For these reasons, the maximum daily dose of theophylline in patients greater than 60 years of age ordinarily should not exceed 400 mg/day unless the patient continues to be symptomatic and the peak steady state serum theophylline concentration is < 10 mcg/mL (see DOSAGE AND ADMINISTRATION). Theophylline doses greater than 400 mg/d should be prescribed with caution in elderly patients.

ADVERSE REACTIONS

Adverse reactions associated with theophylline are generally mild when peak serum theophylline concentrations are < 20 mcg/mL and mainly consist of transient caffeine-like adverse effects such as nausea, vomiting, headache, and insomnia. When peak serum theophylline concentrations exceed 20 mcg/mL, however, theophylline produces a wide range of adverse reactions including persistent vomiting, cardiac arrhythmias, and intractable seizures which can be lethal (see OVERDOSE). The transient caffeine-like adverse reactions occur in about 50% of patients when theophylline therapy is initiated at doses higher than recommended initial doses (e.g., > 300 mg/day in adults and > 12 mg/kg/day in children beyond > 1 year of age). During the initiation of theophylline therapy, caffeine-like adverse effects may transiently alter patient behavior, especially in school age children, but this response rarely persists. Initiation of theophylline therapy at a low dose with subsequent slow titration to a predetermined age-related maximum dose will significantly reduce the frequency of these transient adverse effects (see DOSAGE AND ADMINISTRATION, Table V). In a small percentage of patients (< 3% of children and < 10% of adults) the caffeine-like adverse effects persist during maintenance therapy, even at peak serum theophylline concentrations within the therapeutic range (i.e., 10–20 mcg/mL). Dosage reduction may alleviate the caffeine-like adverse effects in these patients, however, persistent adverse effects should result in a reevaluation of the need for continued theophylline therapy and the potential therapeutic benefit of alternative treatment.

Other adverse reactions that have been reported at serum theophylline concentrations < 20 mcg/mL include diarrhea, irritability, restlessness, fine skeletal muscle tremors, and transient diuresis. In patients with hypoxia secondary to COPD, multifocal atrial tachycardia and flutter have been reported at serum theophylline concentrations ≥ 15 mcg/mL. There have been a few isolated reports of seizures at serum theophylline concentrations < 20 mcg/mL in patients with an underlying neurological disease or in elderly patients. The occurrence of seizures in elderly patients with serum theophylline concentrations < 20 mcg/mL may be secondary to decreased protein binding resulting in a larger proportion of the total serum theophylline concentration in the pharmacologically active unbound form. The clinical characteristics of the seizures reported in patients with serum theophylline concentrations < 20 mcg/mL have generally been milder than seizures associated with excessive serum theophylline concentrations resulting from an overdose (i.e., they have generally been transient, often stopped without anticonvulsant therapy, and did not result in neurological residua).

Table II. Clinically significant drug interactions with theophylline*.

Drug	Type of Interaction	Effect**
Adenosine	Theophylline blocks adenosine receptors.	Higher doses of adenosine may be required to achieve desired effect.
Alcohol	A single large dose of alcohol (3 mL/kg of whiskey) decreases theophylline clearance for up to 24 hours.	30% increase
Allopurinol	Decreases theophylline clearance at allopurinol doses ≥ 600 mg/day.	25% increase
Aminoglutethimide	Increases theophylline clearance by induction of microsomal enzyme activity.	25% decrease
Carbamazepine	Similar to aminoglutethimide.	30% decrease
Cimetidine	Decreases theophylline clearance by inhibiting cytochrome P450 1A2.	70% increase
Ciprofloxacin	Similar to cimetidine.	40% increase
Clarithomycin	Similar to erythromycin.	25% increase
Diazepam	Benzodiazepines increase CNS concentrations of adenosine, a potent CNS depressant, while theophylline blocks adenosine receptors.	Larger diazepam doses may be required to produce desired level of sedation. Discontinuation of theophylline without reduction of diazepam dose may result in respiratory depression.
Disulfiram	Decreases theophylline clearance by inhibiting hydroxylation and demethylation.	50% increase
Enoxacin	Similar to cimetidine.	300% increase
Ephedrine	Synergistic CNS effects	Increased frequency of nausea, nervousness, and insomnia.
Erythromycin	Erythromycin metabolite decreases theophylline clearance by inhibiting cytochrome P450 3A3.	35% increase. Erythromycin steady-state serum concentrations decrease by a similar amount.
Estrogen	Estrogen containing oral contraceptives decrease theophylline clearance in a dose-dependent fashion. The effect of progesterone on theophylline clearance is unknown.	30% increase
Flurazepam	Similar to diazepam.	Similar to diazepam.
Fluvoxamine	Similar to cimetidine	Similar to cimetidine
Halothane	Halothane sensitizes the myocardium to catecholamines, theophylline increases release of endogenous catecholamines.	Increased risk of ventricular arrhythmias.
Interferon, human recombinant alpha-A	Decreases theophylline clearance.	100% increase
Isoproterenol (IV)	Increases theophylline clearance.	20% decrease

Table IV. Manifestations of theophylline toxicity.*

	Percentage of patients reported with sign or symptom			
	Acute Overdose (Large Single Ingestion)		Chronic Overdosage (Multiple Excessive Doses)	
Sign/Symptom	Study 1 (n=157)	Study 2 (n=14)	Study 1 (n=92)	Study 2 (n=102)
Asymptomatic	NR**	0	NR**	6
Gastrointestinal				
Vomiting	73	93	30	61
Abdominal Pain	NR**	21	NR**	12
Diarrhea	NR**	0	NR**	14
Hematemesis	NR**	0	NR**	2
Metabolic/Other				
Hypokalemia	85	79	44	43
Hyperglycemia	98	NR**	18	NR**
Acid/base disturbance	34	21	9	5
Rhabdomyolysis	NR**	7	NR**	0
Cardiovascular				
Sinus tachycardia	100	86	100	62
Other supraventricular tachycardias	2	21	12	14
Ventricular premature beats	3	21	10	19
Atrial fibrillation or flutter	1	NR**	12	NR**
Multifocal atrial tachycardia	0	NR**	2	NR**
Ventricular arrhythmias with hemodynamic instability	7	14	40	0
Hypotension/shock	NR**	21	NR**	8
Neurologic				
Nervousness	NR**	64	NR**	21
Tremors	38	29	16	14

Disorientation	NR**	7	NR**	11
Seizures	5	14	14	5
Death	3	21	10	4

* These data are derived from two studies in patients with serum theophylline concentrations >30 mcg/mL. In the first study (Study #1—Shanon, Ann Intern Med 1993; 119:1161–67), data were prospectively collected from 249 consecutive cases of theophylline toxicity referred to a regional poison center for consultation. In the second study (Study #2—Sessler, Am J Med 1990;88:567–76), data were retrospectively collected from 116 cases with serum theophylline concentrations >30 mcg/mL among 6000 blood samples obtained for measurement of serum theophylline concentrations in three emergency departments. Differences in the incidence of manifestations of theophylline toxicity between the two studies may reflect sample selection as a result of study design (e.g., in Study #1, 48% of the patients had acute intoxications versus only 10% in Study #2) and different methods of reporting results.

** NR = Not reported in a comparable manner.

OVERDOSAGE

General:

The chronicity and pattern of theophylline overdosage significantly influences clinical manifestations of toxicity, management and outcome. There are two common presentations: (1) acute overdose, i.e., ingestion of a single large excessive dose (>10 mg/kg) as occurs in the context of an attempted suicide or isolated medication error, and (2) chronic overdosage, i.e., ingestion of repeated doses that are excessive for the patient's rate of theophylline clearance. The most common causes of chronic theophylline overdosage include patient or care giver error in dosing, clinician prescribing of an excessive dose or a normal dose in the presence of factors known to decrease the rate of theophylline clearance, and increasing the dose in response to an exacerbation of symptoms without first measuring the serum theophylline concentration to determine whether a dose increase is safe.

Severe toxicity from theophylline overdose is a relatively rare event. In one health maintenance organization, the frequency of hospital admissions for chronic overdosage of theophylline was about 1 per 1000 person-years exposure. In another study, among 6000 blood samples obtained for measurement of serum theophylline concentration, for any reason, from patients treated in an emergency department, 7% were in the 20-30 mcg/mL range and 3% were >30 mcg/mL. Approximately two-thirds of the patients with serum theophylline concentrations in the 20-30 mcg/mL range had one or more manifestations of toxicity while >90% of patients with serum theophylline concentrations >30 mcg/mL were clinically intoxicated. Similarly, in other reports, serious toxicity from theophylline is seen principally at serum concentrations >30 mcg/mL.

Several studies have described the clinical manifestations of theophylline overdose and attempted to determine the factors that predict life-threatening toxicity. In general, patients who experience an acute overdose are less likely to experience seizures than patients who have experienced a chronic overdosage, unless the peak serum theophylline concentration is >100 mcg/mL. After a chronic overdosage, generalized seizures, life-threatening cardiac arrhythmias, and death may occur at serum theophylline concentrations >30 mcg/mL. The severity of toxicity after chronic overdosage is more strongly correlated with the patient's age than the peak serum theophylline concentration; patients >60 years are at the greatest risk for severe toxicity and mortality after a chronic overdosage. Pre-existing or concurrent disease may also significantly increase the susceptibility of a patient to a particular toxic manifestation, e.g., patients with neurologic disorders have an increased risk of seizures and patients with cardiac disease have an increased risk of cardiac arrhythmias for a given serum theophylline concentration compared to patients without the underlying disease. The frequency of various reported manifestations of theophylline overdose according to the mode of overdose are listed in Table IV.

Other manifestations of theophylline toxicity include increases in serum calcium, creatine kinase, myoglobin and leukocyte count, decreases in serum phosphate and magnesium, acute myocardial infarction, and urinary retention in men with obstructive uropathy.

Seizures associated with serum theophylline concentrations >30 mcg/mL are often resistant to anticonvulsant therapy and may result in irreversible brain injury if not rapidly controlled. Death from theophylline toxicity is most often secondary to cardiorespiratory arrest and/or hypoxic encephalopathy following prolonged generalized seizures or intractable cardiac arrhythmias causing hemodynamic compromise.

Overdose Management:

General Recommendations for Patients with Symptoms of Theophylline Overdose or Serum Theophylline Concentrations >30 mcg/mL (Note: Serum theophylline concentra-

Table II. Clinically significant drug interactions with theophylline*. (Continued)

Drug	Type of Interaction	Effect**
Ketamine	Pharmacologic	May lower theophylline seizure threshold.
Lithium	Theophylline increases renal lithium clearance.	Lithium dose required to achieve a therapeutic serum concentration increased an average of 60%.
Lorazepam	Similar to diazepam.	Similar to diazepam.
Methotrexate (MTX)	Decreases theophylline clearance.	20% increase after low dose MTX, higher dose MTX may have a greater effect.
Mexiletine	Similar to disulfiram.	80% increase
Midazolam	Similar to diazepam.	Similar to diazepam.
Moricizine	Increases theophylline clearance.	25% decrease
Pancuronium	Theophylline may antagonize non-depolarizing neuromuscular blocking effects; possibly due to phosphodiesterase inhibition.	Larger dose of pancuronium may be required to achieve neuromuscular blockade.
Pentoxifylline	Decreases theophylline clearance.	30% increase
Phenobarbital (PB)	Similar to aminoglutethimide.	25% decrease after two weeks of concurrent PB.
Phenytoin	Phenytoin increases theophylline clearance by increasing microsomal enzyme activity. Theophylline decreases phenytoin absorption.	Serum theophylline and phenytoin concentrations decrease about 40%.
Propafenone	Decreases theophylline clearance and pharmacologic interaction.	40% increase. Beta-2 blocking effect may decrease efficacy of theophylline.
Propranolol	Similar to cimetidine and pharmacologic interaction.	100% increase. Beta-2 blocking effect may decrease efficacy of theophylline.
Rifampin	Increases theophylline clearance by increasing cytochrome P450 1A2 and 3A3 activity.	20–40% decrease
Sulfinpyrazone	Increases theophylline clearance by increasing demethylation and hydroxylation. Decreases renal clearance of theophylline.	20% decrease
Tacrine	Similar to cimetidine, also increases renal clearance of theophylline.	90% increase
Thiabendazole	Decreases theophylline clearance.	190% increase
Ticlopidine	Decreases theophylline clearance.	60% increase
Troleandomycin	Similar to erythromycin.	33–100% increase depending on troleandomycin dose.
Verapamil	Similar to disulfiram.	20% increase

*   Refer to PRECAUTIONS, Drug Interactions for further information regarding table.
** Average effect on steady-state theophylline concentration or other clinical effect for pharmacologic interactions. Individual patients may experience larger changes in serum theophylline concentration than the value listed.

tions may continue to increase after presentation of the patient for medical care.

1. While simultaneously instituting treatment, contact a regional poison center to obtain updated information and advice on individualizing the recommendations that follow.

2. Institute supportive care, including establishment of intravenous access, maintenance of the airway, and electrocardiographic monitoring.

3. Treatment of seizures Because of the high morbidity and mortality associated with theophylline-induced seizures, treatment should be rapid and aggressive. Anticonvulsant therapy should be initiated with an intravenous benzodiazepine, e.g., diazepam, in increments of 0.1-0.2 mg/kg every 1-3 minutes until seizures are terminated. Repetitive seizures should be treated with a loading dose of phenobarbital (20 mg/kg infused over 30-60 minutes). Case reports of theophylline overdose in humans and animal studies suggest that phenytoin is ineffective in terminating theophylline-induced seizures. The doses of benzodiazepines and phenobarbital required to terminate theophylline-induced seizures are close to the doses that may cause severe respiratory depression or respiratory arrest; the clinician should therefore be prepared to provide assisted ventilation. Elderly patients and patients with COPD may be more susceptible to the respiratory depressant effects of anticonvulsants. Barbiturate-induced coma or administration of general anesthesia may be required to terminate repetitive seizures or status epilepticus. General anesthesia should be used with caution in patients with theophylline overdose because fluorinated volatile anesthetics may sensitize the myocardium to endogenous catecholamines released by theophylline. Enflurane appears less likely to be associated with this effect than halothane and may, therefore, be safer. Neuromuscular blocking agents alone should not be used to terminate seizures since they abolish the musculoskeletal

manifestations without terminating seizure activity in the brain.

4. Anticipate Need for Anticonvulsants In patients with theophylline overdose who are at a high risk for theophylline-induced seizures, e.g., patients with acute overdoses and serum theophylline concentrations >100 mcg/mL or chronic overdosage in patients >60 years of age with serum theophylline concentrations >30 mcg/mL, the need for anticonvulsant therapy should be anticipated. A benzodiazepine such as diazepam should be drawn into a syringe and kept at the patient's bedside and medical personnel qualified to treat seizures should be immediately available. In selected patients at high risk for theophylline-induced seizures, consideration should be given to the administration of prophylactic anticonvulsant therapy. Situations where prophylactic anticonvulsant therapy should be considered in high risk patients include anticipated delays in instituting methods for extracorporeal removal of theophylline (e.g., transfer of a high risk patient from one health care facility to another for extracorporeal removal) and clinical circumstances that significantly interfere with efforts to enhance theophylline clearance (e.g., a neonate where dialysis may not be technically feasible or a patient with vomiting unresponsive to antiemetics who is unable to tolerate multiple-dose oral activated charcoal). In animal studies, prophylactic administration of phenobarbital, but not phenytoin, has been shown to delay the onset of theophylline-induced generalized seizures and to increase the dose of theophylline required to induce seizures (i.e., markedly increases the LD50). Although there are no controlled studies in humans, a loading dose of intravenous phenobarbital (20 mg/kg infused over 60 minutes) may delay or prevent life-threatening seizures in high risk patients while efforts to enhance theophylline clearance are continued. Phenobarbital may cause respiratory depression, particularly in elderly patients and patients with COPD.

Continued on next page

UCB—Cont.

5. Treatment of cardiac arrhythmias Sinus tachycardia and simple ventricular premature beats are not harbingers of life-threatening arrhythmias, they do not require treatment in the absence of hemodynamic compromise, and they resolve with declining serum theophylline concentrations. Other arrhythmias, especially those associated with hemodynamic compromise, should be treated with antiarrhythmic therapy appropriate for the type of arrhythmia.

6. Gastrointestinal decontamination Oral activated charcoal (0.5 g/kg up to 20 g and repeat at least once 1-2 hours after the first dose) is extremely effective in blocking the absorption of theophylline throughout the gastrointestinal tract, even when administered several hours after ingestion. If the patient is vomiting, the charcoal should be administered through a nasogastric tube or after administration of an antiemetic. Phenothiazine antiemetics such as prochlorperazine or perphenazine should be avoided since they can lower the seizure threshold and frequently cause dystonic reactions. A single dose of sorbitol may be used to promote stooling to facilitate removal of theophylline bound to charcoal from the gastrointestinal tract. Sorbitol, however, should be dosed with caution since it is a potent purgative which can cause profound fluid and electrolyte abnormalities, particularly after multiple doses. Commercially available fixed combinations of liquid charcoal and sorbitol should be avoided in young children and after the first dose in adolescents and adults since they do not allow for individualization of charcoal and sorbitol dosing. Ipecac syrup should be avoided in theophylline overdoses. Although ipecac induces emesis, it does not reduce the absorption of theophylline unless administered within 5 minutes of ingestion and even then is less effective than oral activated charcoal. Moreover, ipecac-induced emesis may persist for several hours after a single dose and significantly decrease the retention and the effectiveness of oral activated charcoal.

7. Serum Theophylline Concentration Monitoring The serum theophylline concentration should be measured immediately upon presentation, 2-4 hours later, and then at sufficient intervals, e.g., every 4 hours, to guide treatment decisions and to assess the effectiveness of therapy. Serum theophylline concentrations may continue to increase after presentation of the patient for medical care as a result of continued absorption of theophylline from the gastrointestinal tract. Serial monitoring of serum theophylline serum concentrations should be continued until it is clear that the concentration is no longer rising and has returned to non-toxic levels.

8. General Monitoring Procedures Electrocardiographic monitoring should be initiated on presentation and continued until the serum theophylline level has returned to a non-toxic level. Serum electrolytes and glucose should be measured on presentation and at appropriate intervals indicated by clinical circumstances. Fluid and electrolyte abnormalities should be promptly corrected. **Monitoring and treatment should be continued until the serum concentration decreases below 20 mcg/mL.**

9. Enhance clearance of theophylline Multiple-dose oral activated charcoal (e.g., 0.5 mg/kg up to 20 g, every two hours) increases the clearance of theophylline at least twofold by adsorption of theophylline secreted into gastrointestinal fluids. Charcoal must be retained in, and pass through, the gastrointestinal tract to be effective; emesis should therefore be controlled by administration of appropriate antiemetics. Alternatively, the charcoal can be administered continuously through a nasogastric tube in conjunction with appropriate antiemetics. A single dose of sorbitol may be administered with the activated charcoal to promote stooling to facilitate clearance of the adsorbed theophylline from the gastrointestinal tract. Sorbitol alone does not enhance clearance of theophylline and should be dosed with caution to prevent excessive stooling which can result in severe fluid and electrolyte imbalances. Commercially available fixed combinations of liquid charcoal and sorbitol should be avoided in young children and after the first dose in adolescents and adults since they do not allow for individualization of charcoal and sorbitol dosing. In patients with intractable vomiting, extracorporeal methods of theophylline removal should be instituted (see OVERDOSAGE, Extracorporeal Removal).

Specific Recommendations:
Acute Overdose
A. Serum Concentration >20 <30 mcg/mL
1. Administer a single dose of oral activated charcoal.
2. Monitor the patient and obtain a serum theophylline concentration in 2-4 hours to insure that the concentration is not increasing.

B. Serum Concentration >30 <100 mcg/mL
1. Administer multiple dose oral activated charcoal and measures to control emesis.
2. Monitor the patient and obtain serial theophylline concentrations every 2-4 hours to gauge the effectiveness of therapy and to guide further treatment decisions.

3. Institute extracorporeal removal if emesis, seizures, or cardiac arrhythmias cannot be adequately controlled (see OVERDOSAGE, Extracorporeal Removal).
C. Serum Concentration >100 mcg/mL
1. Consider prophylactic anticonvulsant therapy.
2. Administer multiple-dose oral activated charcoal and measures to control emesis.
3. Consider extracorporeal removal, even if the patient has not experienced a seizure (see OVERDOSAGE, Extracorporeal Removal).
4. Monitor the patient and obtain serial theophylline concentrations every 2-4 hours to gauge the effectiveness of therapy and to guide further treatment decisions.

Chronic Overdosage
A. Serum Concentration >20 <30 mcg/mL (with manifestations of theophylline toxicity)
1. Administer a single dose of oral activated charcoal.
2. Monitor the patient and obtain a serum theophylline concentration in 2-4 hours to insure that the concentration is not increasing.
B. Serum Concentration >30 mcg/mL in patients <60 years of age
1. Administer multiple-dose oral activated charcoal and measures to control emesis.
2. Monitor the patient and obtain serial theophylline concentrations every 2-4 hours to gauge the effectiveness of therapy and to guide further treatment decisions.
3. Institute extracorporeal removal if emesis, seizures, or cardiac arrhythmias cannot be adequately controlled (see OVERDOSAGE, Extracorporeal Removal).
C. Serum Concentration >30 mcg/mL in patients ≥60 years of age.
1. Consider prophylactic anticonvulsant therapy.
2. Administer multiple-dose oral activated charcoal and measures to control emesis.
3. Consider extracorporeal removal even if the patient has not experienced a seizure (see OVERDOSAGE, Extracorporeal Removal).
4. Monitor the patient and obtain serial theophylline concentrations every 2-4 hours to gauge the effectiveness of therapy and to guide further treatment decisions.

Extracorporeal Removal:
Increasing the rate of theophylline clearance by extracorporeal methods may rapidly decrease serum concentrations, but the risks of the procedure must be weighed against the potential benefit. Charcoal hemoperfusion is the most effective method of extracorporeal removal, increasing theophylline clearance up to six fold, but serious complications, including hypotension, hypocalcemia, platelet consumption and bleeding diatheses may occur. Hemodialysis is about as efficient as multiple-dose oral activated charcoal and has a lower risk of serious complications than charcoal hemoperfusion. Hemodialysis should be considered as an alternative when charcoal hemoperfusion is not feasible and multiple-dose oral charcoal is ineffective because of intractable emesis. Serum theophylline concentrations may rebound 5-10 mcg/mL after discontinuation of charcoal hemoperfusion or hemodialysis due to redistribution of theophylline from the tissue compartment. Peritoneal dialysis is ineffective for theophylline removal; exchange transfusions in neonates have been minimally effective.

DOSAGE AND ADMINISTRATION
General Considerations:
Theo-24, like other extended-release theophylline products, is intended for patients with relatively continuous or recurring symptoms who have a need to maintain therapeutic serum levels of theophylline. It is not intended for patients experiencing an acute episode of bronchospasm (associated with asthma, chronic bronchitis, or emphysema). Such patients require rapid relief of symptoms and should be treated with an immediate-release or intravenous theophylline preparation (or other bronchodilators) and not with extended-release products.
Patients who metabolize theophylline at a normal or slow rate are reasonable candidates for once-daily dosing with Theo-24. Patients who metabolize theophylline rapidly (e.g., the young, smokers, and some nonsmoking adults) and who have symptoms repeatedly at the end of a dosing interval, will require either increased doses given once a day or preferably, are likely to be better controlled by a schedule of twice-daily dosing. Those patients who require increased daily doses are more likely to experience relatively wide peak-trough differences and may be candidates for twice-a-day dosing with Theo-24.
Patients should be instructed to take this medication each morning at approximately the same time and not to exceed the prescribed dose.
Recent studies suggest that dosing of extended-release theophylline products at night (after the evening meal) results in serum concentrations of theophylline which are not identical to those recorded during waking hours and may be characterized by early trough and delayed peak levels. This appears to occur whether the drug is given as an immediate-release, extended-release, or intravenous product. To avoid

this phenomenon when two doses per day are prescribed, it is recommended that the second dose be given 10 to 12 hours after the morning dose and before the evening meal.
Food and posture, along with changes associated with circadian rhythm, may influence the rate of absorption and/or clearance rates of theophylline from extended-release dosage forms administered at night. The exact relationship of these and other factors to nighttime serum concentrations and the clinical significance of such findings require additional study. Therefore, it is not recommended that Theo-24 (when used as a once-a-day product) be administered at night.
Patients who require a relatively high dose of theophylline (i.e., a dose equal to or greater than 900 mg or 13 mg/kg, whichever is less) should not take Theo-24 less than 1 hour before a high-fat-content meal since this may result in a significant increase in peak serum level and in the extent of absorption of theophylline as compared to administration in the fasted state (see PRECAUTIONS: Drug/Food interactions).
The steady-state peak serum theophylline concentration is a function of the dose, the dosing interval, and the rate of theophylline absorption and clearance in the individual patient. Because of marked individual differences in the rate of theophylline clearance the dose required to achieve a peak serum theophylline concentration in the 10-20 mcg/mL range varies fourfold among otherwise similar patients in the absence of factors known to alter theophylline clearance (e.g., 400-1600 mg/day in adults <60 years old and 10-36 mg/kg/day in children 1-9 years old). For a given population there is no single theophylline dose that will provide both safe and effective serum concentrations for all patients. Administration of the median theophylline dose required to achieve a therapeutic serum theophylline concentration in a given population may result in either sub-therapeutic or potentially toxic serum theophylline concentrations in individual patients. For example, at a dose of 900 mg/d in adults <60 years or 22 mg/kg/d in children 1-9 years, the steady-state peak serum theophylline concentration will be <10 mcg/mL in about 30% of patients, 10-20 mcg/mL in about 50% and 20-30 mcg/mL in about 20% of patients. The dose of theophylline must be individualized on the basis of peak serum theophylline concentration measurements in order to achieve a dose that will provide maximum potential benefit with minimal risk of adverse effects.
Transient caffeine-like adverse effects and excessive serum concentrations in slow metabolizers can be avoided in most patients by starting with a sufficiently low dose and slowly increasing the dose, if judged to be clinically indicated, in small increments (See Table V). Dose increases should only be made if the previous dosage is well tolerated and at intervals of no less than 3 days to allow serum theophylline concentrations to reach the new steady state. Dosage adjustment should be guided by serum theophylline concentration measurement (see PRECAUTIONS, Laboratory Tests and DOSAGE AND ADMINISTRATION, Table VI). Health care providers should instruct patients and care givers to discontinue any dosage that causes adverse effects, to withhold the medication until these symptoms are gone and to then resume therapy at a lower, previously tolerated dosage (see WARNINGS).
If the patient's symptoms are well controlled, there are no apparent adverse effects, and no intervening factors that might alter dosage requirements (see WARNINGS and PRECAUTIONS), serum theophylline concentrations should be monitored at 6 month intervals for rapidly growing children and at yearly intervals for all others. In acutely ill patients, serum theophylline concentrations should be monitored at frequent intervals, e.g., every 24 hours.
Theophylline distributes poorly into body fat, therefore, mg/kg dose should be calculated on the basis of ideal body weight.
Table V contains theophylline dosing titration schema recommended for patients in various age groups and clinical circumstances. Table VI contains recommendations for theophylline dosage adjustment based upon serum theophylline concentrations. Application of these general dosing recommendations to individual patients must take into account the unique clinical characteristics of each patient. In general, these recommendations should serve as the upper limit for dosage adjustments in order to decrease the risk of potentially serious adverse events associated with unexpected large increases in serum theophylline concentration.

Table V.   Dosing initiation and titration
(as anhydrous theophylline).*

A. **Children (12–15 years) and adults (16–60 years) without risk factors for impaired clearance.**

Titration Step	Children <45 kg	Children >45 kg and adults
1. Starting Dosage	12–14 mg/kg/day up to a maximum of 300 mg/day divided Q 24 hrs*	300–400 mg/day[1] divided Q 24 hrs*

2. After 3 days, *if tolerated,* increase dose to: | 16 mg/kg/day up to a maximum of 400 mg/day divided Q 24 hrs* | 400–600 mg/day[1] divided Q 24 hrs*

3. After 3 more days, *if tolerated* and *if needed,* increase dose to: | 20 mg/kg/day up to a maximum of 600 mg/day divided Q 24 hrs* | As with all theophylline products, doses greater than 600 mg should be titrated according to blood level (see Table VI)

[1] If caffeine-like effects occur, then consideration should be given to a lower dose and titrating the dose more slowly (see ADVERSE REACTIONS).

B. **Patients With Risk Factors For Impaired Clearance, The Elderly (> 60 Years), And Those In Whom It Is Not Feasible To Monitor Serum Theophylline Concentrations:**

In children 1–15 years of age, the final theophylline dose should not exceed 16 mg/kg/day up to a maximum of 400 mg/day in the presence of risk factors for reduced theophylline clearance (see WARNINGS) or if it is not feasible to monitor serum theophylline concentrations.

In adolescents ≥ 16 years and adults, including the elderly, the final theophylline dose should not exceed 400 mg/day in the presence of risk factors for reduced theophylline clearance (see WARNINGS) or if it is not feasible to monitor serum theophylline concentrations.

* Patients with more rapid metabolism, clinically identified by higher than average dose requirements, should receive a smaller dose more frequently to prevent breakthrough symptoms resulting from low trough concentrations before the next dose. A reliably absorbed slow-release formulation will decrease fluctuations and permit longer dosing intervals.

Table VI. Dosage adjustment guided by serum theophylline concentration.

Peak Serum Concentration	Dosage Adjustment
<9.9 mcg/mL	If symptoms are not controlled and current dosage is tolerated, increase dose about 25%. Recheck serum concentration after three days for further dosage adjustment.
10–14.9 mcg/mL	If symptoms are controlled and current dosage is tolerated, maintain dose and recheck serum concentration at 6–12 month intervals.¶ If symptoms are not controlled and current dosage is tolerated consider adding additional medication(s) to treatment regimen.
15–19.9 mcg/mL	Consider 10% decrease in dose to provide greater margin of safety even if current dosage is tolerated.¶
20–24.9 mcg/mL	Decrease dose by 25% even if no adverse effects are present. Recheck serum concentration after 3 days to guide further dosage adjustment.
25–30 mcg/mL	Skip next dose and decrease subsequent doses at least 25% even if no adverse effects are present. Recheck serum concentration after 3 days to guide further dosage adjustment. If symptomatic, consider whether overdose treatment is indicated (see recommendations for chronic overdosage).
>30 mcg/mL	Treat overdose as indicated (see recommendations for chronic overdosage). If theophylline is subsequently resumed, decrease dose by at least 50% and recheck serum concentration after 3 days to guide further dosage adjustment.

¶ Dose reduction and/or serum theophylline concentration measurement is indicated whenever adverse effects are present, physiologic abnormalities that can reduce theophylline clearance occur (e.g., sustained fever), or a drug that interacts with theophylline is added or discontinued (see WARNINGS).

HOW SUPPLIED

Theo-24 (theophylline anhydrous) is supplied in extended-release capsules containing 100, 200, 300 or 400 mg of anhydrous theophylline.

Theo-24 100-mg capsules are yellow-orange and clear, with markings Theo-24, 100 mg, ucb, and 2832, supplied as:

NDC Number	Size
50474-100-01	bottle of 100

Theo-24 200-mg capsules are red-orange and clear, with markings Theo-24, 200 mg, ucb, and 2842, supplied as:

NDC Number	Size
50474-200-01	bottle of 100
50474-200-50	bottle of 500
50474-200-60	carton of 100 unit dose

Theo-24 300-mg capsules are red and clear, with markings Theo-24, 300 mg, ucb, and 2852, supplied as:

NDC Number	Size
50474-300-01	bottle of 100
50474-300-50	bottle of 500
50474-300-60	carton of 100 unit dose

Theo-24 400-mg capsules are pink and clear, with markings Theo-24, 400 mg, ucb, and 2902, supplied as:

NDC Number	Size
50474-400-01	bottle of 100
50474-400-50	bottle of 500

Store below 77° F (25° C).

Caution: Federal law prohibits dispensing without prescription.

Manufactured for: Revised: 3/96
UCB Pharma, Inc.
Smyrna (Atlanta), GA 30080
by: **G. D. Searle & Co.,**
Chicago, IL 60680

Shown in Product Identification Guide, page 338

TRINSICON®   ℞
[tren 'sa-kon]
Hematinic Concentrate
With Intrinsic Factor
A Highly Potent Oral Antianemia Preparation

DESCRIPTION

Each TRINSICON® capsule contains:

Special liver-stomach concentrate (containing intrinsic factor)	240 mg
Vitamin B_{12} (activity equivalent)	15 mcg
Iron elemental (as ferrous fumarate)	110 mg
Ascorbic acid (vitamin C)	75 mg
Folic acid	0.5 mg

with other factors of vitamin B complex present in the liver-stomach concentrate.

Each capsule also contains the inactive ingredients corn starch, edible ink, FD&C Blue No. 1, D&C Red No. 28, FD&C Red No. 40, D&C Yellow No. 10, gelatin, silicon dioxide, silicon fluid, sodium lauryl sulfate and titanium dioxide.

CLINICAL PHARMACOLOGY

Vitamin B_{12} with Intrinsic Factor: When secretion of intrinsic factor in gastric juice is inadequate or absent (eg, in Addisonian pernicious anemia or after gastrectomy), vitamin B_{12} in physiologic doses is absorbed poorly, if at all. The resulting deficiency of vitamin B_{12} leads to the clinical manifestations of pernicious anemia. Similar megaloblastic anemias may develop in fish tapeworm (*Diphyllobothrium latum*) infection or after a surgically created small-bowel blind loop; in these situations, treatment requires freeing the host of the parasites or bacteria that appear to compete for the available vitamin B_{12}. Strict vegetarianism and malabsorption syndromes may also lead to vitamin B_{12} deficiency. In the latter case, parenteral therapy, or oral therapy with so-called massive doses of vitamin B_{12}, may be necessary for adequate treatment of the patient.

Potency of intrinsic factor concentrates is determined physiologically, ie, by their use in patients with pernicious anemia. The liver-stomach concentrate with intrinsic factor and the vitamin B_{12} contained in two TRINSICON® capsules provide 1½ times the minimum amount of therapeutic agent, which, when given daily in an uncomplicated case of pernicious anemia, will produce a satisfactory reticulocyte response and relief of anemia and symptoms.

Concentrates of intrinsic factor derived from hog gastric, pyloric, and duodenal mucosa have been used successfully in patients who lack intrinsic factor. For example, Fouts et al maintained patients with pernicious anemia in clinical remission with oral therapy (liver extracts or intrinsic factor concentrate with vitamin B_{12}) for as long as 29 years.

After total gastrectomy, Ficarra found multifactor preparations taken orally to be "just as effective in maintaining blood levels as any medication that has to be administered parenterally." His study was based on 24 patients who had survived for five years after total gastrectomy for cancer and who had been taking two TRINSICON capsules daily.

Folic Acid: Folic acid deficiency is the immediate cause of most, if not all, cases of nutritional megaloblastic anemia and of the megaloblastic anemias of pregnancy and infancy; usually, it is also at least partially responsible for the megaloblastic anemias of malabsorption syndromes, eg, tropical and nontropical sprue.

It is apparent that in vitamin B_{12} deficiency (eg, pernicious anemia), lack of this vitamin results in impaired utilization of folic acid. There are other evidences of the close folic acid-

vitamin B_{12} interrelationship: (1) B_{12} influences the storage, absorption, and utilization of folic acid, and (2) as a deficiency of B_{12} progresses, the requirement for folic acid increases. However, folic acid does not change the requirement for vitamin B_{12}.

Iron: A very common anemia is that due to iron deficiency. In most cases, the response to iron salts is prompt, safe, and predictable. Within limits, the response is quicker and more certain to large doses of iron than to small doses.

Each TRINSICON capsule furnishes 110 mg of elemental iron (as ferrous fumarate) to provide a maximum response.

Ascorbic Acid: Vitamin C plays a role in anemia therapy. It augments the conversion of folic acid to its active form, folinic acid. In addition, ascorbic acid promotes the reduction of ferric iron in food to the more readily absorbed ferrous form. Severe and prolonged vitamin C deficiency is associated with an anemia that is usually hypochromic but occasionally megaloblastic in type.

INDICATIONS AND USAGE

TRINSICON® (hematinic concentrate with intrinsic factor) is a multifactor preparation effective in the treatment of anemias that respond to oral hematinics, including pernicious anemia and other megaloblastic anemias and also iron-deficiency anemia. Therapeutic quantities of hematopoietic factors that are known to be important are present in the recommended daily dose.

CONTRAINDICATIONS

Hemochromatosis and hemosiderosis are contraindications to iron therapy.

PRECAUTIONS

General: Anemia is a manifestation that requires appropriate investigation to determine its cause or causes. Folic acid *alone* is unwarranted in the treatment of pure vitamin B_{12} deficiency states, such as pernicious anemia.

Folic acid may obscure pernicious anemia in that the blood picture may revert to normal while neurolological manifestations remain progressive.

As with all preparations containing intrinsic factor, resistance may develop in some cases of pernicious anemia to the potentiation of absorption of physiologic doses of vitamin B_{12}. If resistance occurs, parenteral therapy or oral therapy with so-called massive doses of vitamin B_{12} may be necessary for adequate treatment of the patient. No single regimen fits all cases, and the status of the patient observed in follow-up is the final criterion for adequacy of therapy. Periodic clinical and laboratory studies are considered essential and are recommended.

Pregnancy:
Teratogenic Effects: *Pregnancy Category C:* Animal reproduction studies have not been conducted with TRINSICON®. It is also not known whether TRINSICON can cause fetal harm when administered to a pregnant woman or can affect reproduction capacity. TRINSICON should be given to a pregnant woman only if clearly needed.

Nursing Mothers: It is not known whether this drug is excreted in human milk. Because many drugs are excreted in human milk, caution should be exercised when TRINSICON is administered to a nursing woman.

Pediatric Use: Safety and effectiveness in children below the age of 10 have not been established.

ADVERSE REACTIONS

Rarely, iron in therapeutic doses produces gastrointestinal reactions, such as diarrhea or constipation. Reducing the dose and administering it with meals will minimize these effects in the iron-sensitive patient.

In extremely rare instances, skin rash suggesting allergy has been noted following the oral administration of liver-stomach material. Allergic sensitization has been reported following both oral and parenteral administration of folic acid.

OVERDOSAGE

Symptoms: Those of iron intoxication, which may include pallor and cyanosis, vomiting, hematemesis, diarrhea, melena, shock, drowsiness, and coma.

Treatment: For specific therapy, exchange transfusion and chelating agents. For general management, gastric and rectal lavage with sodium bicarbonate solution or milk, administration of intravenous fluids and electrolytes, and use of oxygen.

DOSAGE AND ADMINISTRATION

One capsule twice a day. (Two capsules daily produce a standard response in the average uncomplicated case of pernicious anemia.)

HOW SUPPLIED

Dark pink and dark red capsules imprinted 'UCB/364' in bottles of 60 (NDC 50474-364-22) and 500 (NDC 50474-364-24) and unit dose packages of 100 (NDC 50474-364-27).

CAUTION: Federal law prohibits dispensing without prescription.

Continued on next page

UCB—Cont.

Manufactured for
UCB Pharma, Inc.
Smyrna (Atlanta), GA 30080
By D.M. Graham Laboratories, Inc.
Hobart, NY 13788
Revised 5/95
Shown in Product Identification Guide, page 338

VICON FORTE® Capsules
[vī'kon for'tā]
(Therapeutic Vitamins-Minerals)

DESCRIPTION
Each black and orange VICON FORTE® capsule for oral administration contains:

Vitamin A	8,000 IU
Vitamin E	50 IU
Ascorbic acid	150 mg
Zinc sulfate, USP*	80 mg
Magnesium sulfate, USP†	70 mg
Niacinamide	25 mg
Thiamine mononitrate	10 mg
d-Calcium pantothenate	10 mg
Riboflavin	5 mg
Manganese chloride	4 mg
Pyridoxine hydrochloride	2 mg
Folic acid	1 mg
Vitamin B$_{12}$ (Cyanocobalamin)	10 mcg

* As 50 mg dried zinc sulfate.
† As 50 mg dried magnesium sulfate.
Each capsule also contains edible ink, FD&C Blue No. 1, FD&C Red No. 40, FD&C Yellow No. 6, gelatin, lactose, magnesium stearate, silicon dioxide, sodium lauryl sulfate, and titanium dioxide.

INDICATIONS AND USAGE
VICON FORTE® is indicated for the treatment and/or prevention of vitamin and mineral deficiencies associated with restricted diets, improper food intake, alcoholism, and decreased absorption. VICON FORTE is also indicated in patients with increased requirements for vitamins and minerals due to chronic disease, infection, and burns and in persons using alcohol to excess. Preoperative and postoperative use of VICON FORTE can provide the increased amounts of vitamins and minerals necessary for optimal recovery from the stress of surgery.

CONTRAINDICATIONS
None known.

PRECAUTIONS
General: Folic acid in doses above 0.1 mg daily may obscure pernicious anemia in that hematologic remission can occur while neurological manifestations remain progressive.

DOSAGE AND ADMINISTRATION
One capsule daily or as directed by physician.

HOW SUPPLIED
Orange and black capsules imprinted with 'UCB' and "316" in bottles of 60 (NDC 50474-316-22) and 500 (NDC 50474-316-24) and unit dose packs of 100 (NDC 50474-316-27).
Dispense in tight, light-resistant container with a child resistant closure.
CAUTION: Federal law prohibits dispensing without prescription.

Manufactured for
UCB Pharma, Inc.,
Smyrna (Atlanta), GA 30080
by D.M. Graham Laboratories, Inc.,
Hobart, NY 13788
Revised 5/95
Shown in Product Identification Guide, page 338

NOTICE
Before prescribing or administering
any product described in
PHYSICIANS' DESK REFERENCE,
check the **PDR Supplements**
for revised information.

U.S. Bioscience, Inc.
ONE TOWER BRIDGE
100 FRONT STREET
WEST CONSHOHOCKEN, PA 19428

Direct Inquiries to:
US Bioscience
(610) 832-0570

For Medical Information or Emergencies Contact:
1-800-872-4672

Ethyol® (amifostine), see Listing under ALZA Pharmaceuticals

HEXALEN®   ℞
[hex'a-len]
(ALTRETAMINE)
CAPSULES
50 mg

> **WARNINGS**
> 1. HEXALEN® should only be given under the supervision of a physician experienced in the use of antineoplastic agents.
> 2. Peripheral blood counts should be monitored at least monthly, prior to the initiation of each course of HEXALEN, and as clinically indicated (see Adverse Reactions).
> 3. Because of the possibility of HEXALEN-related neurotoxicity, neurologic examination should be performed regularly during HEXALEN administration (see Adverse Reactions).

DESCRIPTION
HEXALEN (altretamine) is a synthetic cytotoxic antineoplastic s-triazine derivative. HEXALEN capsules contain 50 mg of altretamine for oral administration. Inert ingredients include lactose, anhydrous and calcium stearate. Altretamine, known chemically as N,N,N',N',N'',N''-hexamethyl-1,3,5-triazine-2,4,6-triamine, has the following structural formula:

Its empirical formula is $C_9H_{18}N_6$ with a molecular weight of 210.28. Altretamine is a white crystalline powder, melting at 172° ± 1°C. Altretamine is practically insoluble in water but is increasingly soluble at pH 3 and below.

CLINICAL PHARMACOLOGY
The precise mechanism by which HEXALEN exerts its cytotoxic effect is unknown, although a number of theoretical possibilities have been studied. Structurally, HEXALEN resembles the alkylating agent triethylenemelamine, yet *in vitro* tests for alkylating activity of HEXALEN and its metabolites have been negative. HEXALEN has been demonstrated to be efficacious for certain ovarian tumors resistant to classical alkylating agents. Metabolism of altretamine is a requirement for cytotoxicity. Synthetic monohydroxymethylmelamines, and products of altretamine metabolism, *in vitro* and *in vivo*, can form covalent adducts with tissue macromolecules including DNA, but the relevance of these reactions to antitumor activity is unknown.
HEXALEN is well-absorbed following oral administration in humans, but undergoes rapid and extensive demethylation in the liver, producing variation in altretamine plasma levels. The principal metabolites are pentamethylmelamine and tetramethylmelamine.
Pharmacokinetic studies were performed in a limited number of patients and should be considered preliminary. After oral administration of HEXALEN to 11 patients with advanced ovarian cancer in doses of 120–300 mg/m², peak plasma levels (as measured by gas-chromatographic assay) were reached between 0.5 and 3 hours, varying from 0.2 to 20.8 mg/l. Half-life of the β-phase of elimination ranged from 4.7 to 10.2 hours. Altretamine and metabolites show binding to plasma proteins. The free fractions of altretamine, pentamethylmelamine and tetramethylmelamine are 6%, 25% and 50%, respectively.
Following oral administration of ¹⁴C-ring-labeled altretamine (4 mg/kg), urinary recovery of radioactivity was 61% at 24 hours and 90% at 72 hours. Human urinary metabolites were N-demethylated homologues of altretamine with <1% unmetabolized altretamine excreted at 24 hours.
After intraperitoneal administration of ¹⁴C-ring-labeled altretamine to mice, tissue distribution was rapid in all organs, reaching a maximum at 30 minutes. The excretory organs (liver and kidney) and the small intestine showed high concentrations of radioactivity, whereas relatively low concentrations were found in other organs, including the brain.
There have been no formal pharmacokinetic studies in patients with compromised hepatic and/or renal function, though HEXALEN has been administered both concurrently and following nephrotoxic drugs such as cisplatin. HEXALEN has been administered in 4 divided doses, with meals and at bedtime, though there is no pharmacokinetic data on this schedule nor information from formal interaction studies about the effect of food on its bioavailability or pharmacokinetics.
In two studies in patients with persistent or recurrent ovarian cancer following first-line treatment with cisplatin and/or alkylating agent-based combinations, HEXALEN was administered as a single agent for 14 or 21 days of a 28 day cycle. In the 51 patients with measurable or evaluable disease, there were 6 clinical complete responses, 1 pathologic complete response, and 2 partial responses for an overall response rate of 18%. The duration of these responses ranged from 2 months in a patient with a palpable pelvic mass to 36 months in a patient who achieved a pathologic complete response. In some patients, tumor regression was associated with improvement in symptoms and performance status.

INDICATIONS AND USAGE
HEXALEN (altretamine) is indicated for use as a single agent in the palliative treatment of patients with persistent or recurrent ovarian cancer following first-line therapy with a cisplatin and/or alkylating agent-based combination.

CONTRAINDICATIONS
HEXALEN is contraindicated in patients who have shown hypersensitivity to it. HEXALEN should not be employed in patients with preexisting severe bone marrow depression or severe neurologic toxicity. HEXALEN has been administered safely, however, to patients heavily pretreated with cisplatin and/or alkylating agents, including patients with preexisting cisplatin neuropathies. Careful monitoring of neurologic function in these patients is essential.

WARNINGS
See boxed Warnings.
Concurrent administration of HEXALEN and antidepressants of the monoamine oxidase (MAO) inhibitor class may cause severe orthostatic hypotension. Four patients, all over 60 years of age, were reported to have experienced symptomatic hypotension after 4 to 7 days of concomitant therapy with HEXALEN and MAO inhibitors.
HEXALEN causes mild to moderate myelosuppression and neurotoxicity. Blood counts and a neurologic examination should be performed prior to the initiation of each course of therapy and the dose of HEXALEN adjusted as clinically indicated (see Dosage and Administration).
Pregnancy: Category D
HEXALEN has been shown to be embryotoxic and teratogenic in rats and rabbits when given at doses 2 and 10 times the human dose. HEXALEN may cause fetal damage when administered to a pregnant woman. If HEXALEN is used during pregnancy, or if the patient becomes pregnant while taking the drug, the patient should be appraised of the potential hazard to the fetus. Women of childbearing potential should be advised to avoid becoming pregnant.

PRECAUTIONS
General
Neurologic examination should be performed regularly (see Adverse Reactions).
Laboratory Tests
Peripheral blood counts should be monitored at least monthly, prior to the initiation of each course of HEXALEN, and as clinically indicated (see Adverse Reactions).
Drug Interactions
Concurrent administration of HEXALEN and antidepressants of the MAO inhibitor class may cause severe orthostatic hypotension (see Warnings section). Cimetidine, an inhibitor of microsomal drug metabolism, increased altretamine's half-life and toxicity in a rat model.
Data from a randomized trial of HEXALEN and cisplatin plus or minus pyridoxine in ovarian cancer indicated that pyridoxine significantly reduced neurotoxicity; however, it adversely affected response duration suggesting that pyridoxine should not be administered with HEXALEN and/or cisplatin (1).
Carcinogenesis, Mutagenesis and Impairment of Fertility
The carcinogenic potential of HEXALEN has not been studied in animals, but drugs with similar mechanisms of action have been shown to be carcinogenic. HEXALEN was weakly mutagenic when tested in strain TA100 of *Salmonella typhimurium*. HEXALEN administered to female rats 14 days

prior to breeding through the gestation period had no adverse effect on fertility, but decreased post-natal survival at 120 mg/m^2/day and was embryocidal at 240 mg/m^2/day. Administration of 120 mg/m^2/day HEXALEN to male rats for 60 days prior to mating resulted in testicular atrophy, reduced fertility and a possible dominant lethal mutagenic effect. Male rats treated with HEXALEN at 450 mg/m^2/day for 10 days had decreased spermatogenesis, atrophy of testes, seminal vesicles and ventral prostate.

Pregnancy
Pregnancy Category D: see Warnings section.

Nursing Mothers
It is not known whether altretamine is excreted in human milk. Because there is a possibility of toxicity in nursing infants secondary to HEXALEN treatment of the mother, it is recommended that breast feeding be discontinued if the mother is treated with HEXALEN.

Pediatric Use
The safety and effectiveness of HEXALEN in children have not been established.

ADVERSE REACTIONS

Gastrointestinal
With continuous high-dose daily HEXALEN, nausea and vomiting of gradual onset occur frequently. Although in most instances these symptoms are controllable with antiemetics, at times the severity requires HEXALEN dose reduction or, rarely, discontinuation of HEXALEN therapy. In some instances, a tolerance of these symptoms develops after several weeks of therapy. The incidence and severity of nausea and vomiting are reduced with moderate-dose administration of HEXALEN. In 2 clinical studies of single-agent HEXALEN utilizing a moderate, intermittent dose and schedule, only 1 patient (1%) discontinued HEXALEN due to severe nausea and vomiting.

Neurotoxicity
Peripheral neuropathy and central nervous system symptoms (mood disorders, disorders of consciousness, ataxia, dizziness, vertigo) have been reported. They are more likely to occur in patients receiving continuous high-dose daily HEXALEN than moderate-dose HEXALEN administered on an intermittent schedule. Neurologic toxicity has been reported to be reversible when therapy is discontinued. Data from a randomized trial of HEXALEN and cisplatin plus or minus pyridoxine in ovarian cancer indicated that pyridoxine significantly reduced neurotoxicity; however, it adversely affected response duration suggesting that pyridoxine should not be administered with HEXALEN and/or cisplatin (1).

Hematologic
HEXALEN (altretamine) causes mild to moderate dose-related myelosuppression. Leukopenia below 3000 WBC/mm^3 occurred in <15% of patients on a variety of intermittent or continuous dose regimens. Less than 1% had leukopenia below 1000 WBC/mm^3. Thrombocytopenia below 50,000 platelets/mm^3 was seen in <10% of patients. When given in doses of 8–12 mg/kg/day over a 21 day course, nadirs of leukocyte and platelet counts were reached by 3–4 weeks, and normal counts were regained by 6 weeks. With continuous administration at doses of 6–8 mg/kg/day, nadirs are reached in 6–8 weeks (median).

Data in the following table are based on the experience of 76 patients with ovarian cancer previously treated with a cisplatin-based combination regimen who received single-agent HEXALEN. In one study, HEXALEN, 260 mg/m^2/day, was administered for 14 days of a 28 day cycle. In another study, HEXALEN, 6–8 mg/kg/day, was administered for 21 days of a 28 day cycle.

[See table on top of next column.]

Additional adverse reaction information is available from 13 single-agent altretamine studies (total of 1014 patients) conducted under the auspices of the National Cancer Institute. The treated patients had a variety of tumors and many were heavily pretreated with other chemotherapies; most of these trials utilized high, continuous daily doses of altretamine (6–12 mg/kg/day). In general, adverse reaction experiences were similar in the two trials described above. Additional toxicities, not reported in the above table, included hepatic toxicity, skin rash, pruritus and alopecia, each occurring in <1% of patients.

OVERDOSAGE
No case of acute overdosage in humans has been described. The oral LD50 dose in rats was 1050 mg/kg and 437 mg/kg in mice.

DOSAGE AND ADMINISTRATION
HEXALEN is administered orally. Doses are calculated on the basis of body surface area.

HEXALEN may be administered either for 14 or 21 consecutive days in a 28 day cycle at a dose of 260 mg/m^2/day. The total daily dose should be given as 4 divided oral doses after meals and at bedtime. There is no pharmacokinetic information supporting this dosing regimen and the effect of food on

ADVERSE EXPERIENCES IN 76 PREVIOUSLY TREATED OVARIAN CANCER PATIENTS RECEIVING SINGLE-AGENT HEXALEN

Adverse Experiences	% Patients
Gastrointestinal	
Nausea and Vomiting	33
Mild to Moderate	32
Severe	1
Increased Alkaline Phosphatase	9
Neurologic	
Peripheral Sensory Neuropathy	31
Mild	22
Moderate to Severe	9
Anorexia and Fatigue	1
Seizures	1
Hematologic	
Leukopenia	5
WBC 2000–2999/mm^3	4
WBC <2000/mm^3	1
Thrombocytopenia	9
Platelets 75,000–99,000/mm^3	6
Platelets <75,000/mm^3	3
Anemia	33
Mild	20
Moderate to Severe	13
Renal	
Serum Creatinine 1.6–3.75 mg/dl	7
BUN	9
25–40 mg%	5
41–60 mg%	3
>60 mg%	1

HEXALEN bioavailability or pharmacokinetics has not been evaluated.

HEXALEN should be temporarily discontinued (for 14 days or longer) and subsequently restarted at 200 mg/m^2/day for any of the following situations:

1) Gastrointestinal intolerance unresponsive to symptomatic measures;
2) White blood count <2000/mm^3 or granulocyte count <1000/mm^3;
3) Platelet count <75,000/mm^3;
4) Progressive neurotoxicity.

If neurologic symptoms fail to stabilize on the reduced dose schedule, HEXALEN should be discontinued indefinitely. Procedures for proper handling and disposal of anticancer drugs should be considered. Several guidelines on this subject have been published (2–8). There is no general agreement that all of the procedures recommended in the guidelines are necessary or appropriate.

HOW SUPPLIED
HEXALEN (altretamine) is available in 50 mg clear, hard gelatin capsules in bottles of 100 (**NDC** 58178-001-70). The capsules are imprinted with the following inscription: USB001 HEXALEN 50 mg. Store at controlled room temperature 15°–30°C (59°–86°F).

REFERENCES
1. Wiernik PH, et al. Hexamethylmelamine and Low or Moderate Dose Cisplatin With or Without Pyridoxine for Treatment of Advanced Ovarian Carcinoma: A Study of the Eastern Cooperative Oncology Group. *Cancer Investigation* 10(1): 1–9, 1992.
2. Recommendations for the Safe Handling of Parenteral Antineoplastic Drugs. NIH Publication No. 83-2621. For sale by the Superintendent of Documents, U.S. Government Printing Office, Washington, D.C. 20402.
3. AMA Council Report. Guidelines for Handling Parenteral Antineoplastics. *Journal of the American Medical Association* March 15, 1985.
4. National Study Commission on Cytotoxic Exposure—Recommendation for Handling Cytotoxic Agents. Available from Louis P. Jeffrey, Sc.D., Director of Pharmacy Services, Rhode Island Hospital, 593 Eddy Street, Providence, Rhode Island 02902.
5. Clinical Oncological Society of Australia: Guidelines and Recommendations for Safe Handling of Antineoplastic Agents. *Medical Journal of Australia* 1:426–428, 1983.
6. Jones, RB, et al. Safe Handling of Chemotherapeutic Agents: A Report from the Mount Sinai Medical Center. *CA—A Cancer Journal for Clinicians* Sept/Oct, 258–263, 1983.
7. American Society of Hospital Pharmacists Technical Assistance Bulletin on Handling Cytotoxic Drugs in Hospitals. *American Journal of Hospital Pharmacy* 42:131–137, 1985.
8. OSHA Work Practice Guidelines for Personnel Dealing with Cytotoxic (Antineoplastic) Drugs. *American Journal of Hospital Pharmacy* 43:1193–1204, 1986.

Manufactured by:
Applied Analytical Industries, Inc.
Wilmington, NC 28405
For: **U.S. Bioscience**
One Tower Bridge
100 Front Street
West Conshohocken, PA 19428
Revision Date 7/95　　　　　　　　　　　PE
Shown in Product Identification Guide, page 338

NEUTREXIN®　　　　　　　　　　　℞
[n(y)ü-trex ′in]
(trimetrexate glucuronate for injection)

> **WARNINGS**
> NEUTREXIN (TRIMETREXATE GLUCURONATE FOR INJECTION) MUST BE USED WITH CONCURRENT LEUCOVORIN (LEUCOVORIN PROTECTION) TO AVOID POTENTIALLY SERIOUS OR LIFE-THREATENING TOXICITIES (SEE PRECAUTIONS AND DOSAGE AND ADMINISTRATION).

DESCRIPTION
Neutrexin is the brand name for trimetrexate glucuronate. Trimetrexate, a 2,4-diaminoquinazoline, non-classical folate antagonist, is a synthetic inhibitor of the enzyme dihydrofolate reductase (DHFR). Neutrexin is available as a sterile lyophilized powder in single-dose vials, each containing trimetrexate glucuronate equivalent to 25 mg of trimetrexate without any preservatives or excipients. The powder is reconstituted prior to intravenous infusion (see **DOSAGE AND ADMINISTRATION, RECONSTITUTION AND DILUTION**.

Trimetrexate glucuronate is chemically known as 2, 4-diamino-5-methyl-6- [(3, 4, 5-trimethoxyanilino) methyl] quinazoline mono-D-glucuronate, and has the following structure:

The empirical formula for trimetrexate glucuronate is $C_{19}H_{23}N_5O_3 \cdot C_6H_{10}O_7$ with a molecular weight of 563.56. The active ingredient, trimetrexate free base, has an empirical formula of $C_{19}H_{23}N_5O_3$ with a molecular weight of 369.42. Trimetrexate glucuronate for injection is a pale greenish-yellow powder or cake. Trimetrexate glucuronate is soluble in water (>50 mg/mL), whereas trimetrexate free base is practically insoluble in water (<0.1 mg/mL). The pKa of trimetrexate free base in 50% methanol/water is 8.0. The logarithm$_{10}$ of the partition coefficient of trimetrexate free base between octanol and water is 1.63.

CLINICAL PHARMACOLOGY
Mechanism of Action
In vitro studies have shown that trimetrexate is a competitive inhibitor of dihydrofolate reductase (DHFR) from bacterial, protozoan, and mammalian sources. DHFR catalyzes the reduction of intracellular dihydrofolate to the active coenzyme tetrahydrofolate. Inhibition of DHFR results in the depletion of this coenzyme, leading directly to interference with thymidylate biosynthesis, as well as inhibition of folate-dependent formyltransferases, and indirectly to inhibition of purine biosynthesis. The end result is disruption of DNA, RNA, and protein synthesis, with consequent cell death.

Leucovorin (folinic acid) is readily transported into mammalian cells by an active, carrier-mediated process and can be assimilated into cellular folate pools following its metabolism. *In vitro* studies have shown that leucovorin provides a source of reduced folates necessary for normal cellular biosynthetic processes. Because the *Pneumocystis carinii* organism lacks the reduced folate carrier-mediated transport system, leucovorin is prevented from entering the organism. Therefore, at concentrations achieved with therapeutic doses of trimetrexate plus leucovorin, the selective transport of trimetrexate, but not leucovorin, into the *Pneumocystis carinii* organism allows the concurrent administration of leucovorin to protect normal host cells from the cytotoxicity of trimetrexate without inhibiting the antifolate's inhibition of *Pneumocystis carinii*. It is not known if considerably

Continued on next page

U.S. Bioscience—Cont.

higher doses of leucovorin would affect trimetrexate's effect on *Pneumocystis carinii*.

Microbiology

Trimetrexate inhibits, in a dose-related manner, *in vitro* growth of the trophozoite stage of rat *Pneumocystis carinii* cultured on human embryonic lung fibroblast cells. Trimetrexate concentrations between 3 and 54.1 μM were shown to inhibit the growth of trophozoites. Leucovorin alone at a concentration of 10 μM did not alter either the growth of the trophozoites or the anti-pneumocystis activity of trimetrexate. Resistance to trimetrexate's antimicrobial activity against *Pneumocystis carinii* has not been studied.

Pharmacokinetics

Trimetrexate pharmacokinetics were assessed in six patients with acquired immunodeficiency syndrome (AIDS) who had *Pneumocystis carinii* pneumonia (4 patients) or toxoplasmosis (2 patients). Trimetrexate was administered intravenously as a bolus injection at a dose of 30 mg/m^2/day along with leucovorin 20 mg/m^2 every 6 hours for 21 days. Trimetrexate clearance (mean $\pm$ SD) was 38 ± 15 mL/min/m^2 and volume of distribution at steady state (Vd_{ss}) was 20 ± 8 L/m^2. The plasma concentration time profile declined in a biphasic manner over 24 hours with a terminal half-life of 11 ± 4 hours.

The pharmacokinetics of trimetrexate without the concomitant administration of leucovorin have been evaluated in cancer patients with advanced solid tumors using various dosage regimens. The decline in plasma concentrations over time has been described by either biexponential or triexponential equations. Following the single-dose administration of 10 to 130 mg/m^2 to 37 patients, plasma concentrations were obtained for 72 hours. Nine plasma concentration time profiles were described as biexponential. The alpha phase half-life was 57 ± 28 minutes, followed by a terminal phase with a half-life of 16 ± 3 hours. The plasma concentrations in the remaining patients exhibited a triphasic decline with half-lives of 8.6 ± 6.5 minutes, 2.4 ± 1.3 hours, and 17.8 ± 8.2 hours.

Trimetrexate clearance in cancer patients has been reported as 53 ± 41 mL/min (14 patients) and 32 ± 18 mL/min/m^2 (23 patients) following single-dose administration. After a five-day infusion of trimetrexate to 16 patients, plasma clearance was 30 ± 8 mL/min/m^2.

Renal clearance of trimetrexate in cancer patients has varied from about 4 ± 2 mL/min/m^2 to 10 ± 6 mL/min/m^2. Ten to 30% of the administered dose is excreted unchanged in the urine. Considering the free fraction of trimetrexate, active tubular secretion may possibly contribute to the renal clearance of trimetrexate. Renal clearance has been associated with urine flow, suggesting the possibility of tubular reabsorption as well.

The Vd_{ss} of trimetrexate in cancer patients after single-dose administration and for whom plasma concentrations were obtained for 72 hours was 36.9 ± 17.6 L/m^2 (n=23) and 0.62 ± 0.24 L/kg (n=14). Following a constant infusion of trimetrexate for five days, Vd_{ss} was 32.8 ± 16.6 L/m^2. The volume of the central compartment has been estimated as 0.17 ± 0.08 L/kg and 4.0 ± 2.9 L/m^2.

There have been inconsistencies in the reporting of trimetrexate protein binding. The *in vitro* plasma protein binding of trimetrexate using ultrafiltration is approximately 95% over the concentration range of 18.75 to 1000 ng/mL. There is a suggestion of capacity limited binding (saturable binding) at concentrations greater than about 1000 ng/mL, with free fraction progressively increasing to about 9.3% as concentration is increased to 15 μg/mL. Other reports have declared trimetrexate to be greater than 98% bound at concentrations of 0.1 to 10 μg/mL; however, specific free fractions were not stated. The free fraction of trimetrexate also has been reported to be about 15 to 16% at a concentration of 60 ng/mL, increasing to about 20% at a trimetrexate concentration of 6 μg/mL.

Trimetrexate metabolism in man has not been characterized. Preclinical data strongly suggest that the major metabolic pathway is oxidative O-demethylation, followed by conjugation to either glucuronide or the sulfate. N-demethylation and oxidation is a related minor pathway. Preliminary findings in humans indicate the presence of a glucuronide conjugate with DHFR inhibition and a demethylated metabolite in urine.

The presence of metabolite(s) in human plasma following the administration of trimetrexate is suggested by the differences seen in trimetrexate plasma concentrations when measured by HPLC and a nonspecific DHFR inhibition assay. The profiles are similar initially, but diverge with time; concentrations determined by DHFR being higher than those determined by HPLC. This suggests the presence of one or more metabolites with DHFR inhibition activity. After intravenous administration of trimetrexate to humans, urinary recovery averaged about 40%, using a DHFR assay, in comparison to 10% urinary recovery as determined by HPLC, suggesting the presence of one or more metabolites that retain inhibitory activity against DHFR. Fecal recovery of trimetrexate over 48 hours after intravenous administration ranged from 0.09 to 7.6% of the dose as determined by DHFR inhibition and 0.02 to 5.2% of the dose as determined by HPLC.

The pharmacokinetics of trimetrexate have not been determined in patients with renal insufficiency or hepatic dysfunction.

TABLE 1
TREATMENT IND
Baseline Characteristics

	IST (n = 227)	RIST (n = 146)	RST (n = 204)	TOTAL (n = 577)
Ventilatory Support Required n (%)	39 (17)	50 (34)	129 (63)	218 (38)
Median Days on Standard Therapy	10	12	16	14
First Episode of PCP n (%)	104 (46)	103 (71)	190 (93)	397 (69)

TABLE 2
TREATMENT IND
Survival Rate One Month After Completion of Neutrexin Therapy

	IST		RIST		RST	
All Patients	153/227	(67%)	73/146	(50%)	50/204	(25%)
Baseline Ventilatory Support	9/39	(23%)	15/50	(30%)	18/129	(14%)
No Baseline Ventilatory Support	144/188	(77%)	58/96	(60%)	32/75	(43%)

INDICATIONS AND USAGE

Neutrexin (trimetrexate glucuronate for injection) with concurrent leucovorin administration (leucovorin protection) is indicated as an alternative therapy for the treatment of moderate-to-severe *Pneumocystis carinii* pneumonia (PCP) in immunocompromised patients, including patients with the acquired immunodeficiency syndrome (AIDS), who are intolerate of, or are refractory to, trimethoprim-sulfamethoxazole therapy or for whom trimethoprim-sulfamethoxazole is contraindicated.

This indication is based on the results of a randomized, controlled double-blind trial comparing Neutrexin with concurrent leucovorin protection (TMTX/LV) to trimethoprim-sulfamethoxazole (TMP/SMX) in patients with moderate-to-severe *Pneumocystis carinii* pneumonia, as well as results of a Treatment IND. These studies are summarized below:

Neutrexin Comparative Study with TMP/SMX: This double-blind, randomized trial initiated by the AIDS Clinical Trials Group (ACTG) in 1988 was designed to compare the safety and efficacy of TMTX/LV to that of TMP/SMX for the treatment of histologically confirmed, moderate-to-severe PCP, defined as (A-a) baseline gradient >30 mmHg, in patients with AIDS.

Of the 220 patients with histologically confirmed PCP, 109 were randomized to receive TMTX/LV and 111 to TMP/SMX. Study patients randomized to TMTX/LV treatment were to receive 45 mg/m^2 of TMTX daily for 21 days plus 20 mg/m^2 of LV every 6 hours for 24 days. Those randomized to TMP/SMX were to receive 5 mg/kg TMP plus 25 mg/kg SMX four times daily for 21 days.

Response to therapy, defined as alive and off ventilatory support at completion of therapy, with no change in antipneumocystis therapy, or addition of supraphysiologic doses of steroids, occurred in fifty percent of patients in each treatment group.

The observed mortality in the TMTX/LV treatment group was approximately twice that in the TMP/SMX treatment group (95% CI: 0.99–4.11). Thirty of 109 (27%) patients treated with TMTX/LV and 18 of 111 (16%) patients receiving TMP/SMX died during the 21-day treatment course or 4-week follow-up period. Twenty-seven of 30 deaths in the TMTX/LV arm were attributed to PCP; all 18 deaths in the TMP/SMX arm were attributed to PCP.

A significantly smaller proportion of patients who received TMTX/LV compared to TMP/SMX failed therapy due to toxicity (10% vs. 25%), and a significantly greater proportion of patients failed due to lack of efficacy (40% vs. 24%). Six patients (12%) who responded to TMTX/LV relapsed during the one-month follow-up period; no patient responding to TMP/SMX relapsed during this period. Information is not available as to whether these patients received prophylaxis therapy for PCP.

Treatment IND: The FDA granted a Treatment IND for Neutrexin with leucovorin protection in February 1988 to make Neutrexin therapy available to HIV-infected patients with histologically confirmed PCP who had disease refractory to or who are intolerant of TMP/SMX and/or intravenous pentamidine.

Over 500 physicians in the United States participated in the Treatment IND. Of the first 753 patients enrolled, 577 were evaluable for efficacy. Of these, 227 patients were intolerant of both TMP/SMX and pentamidine (IST—patients intolerant of both standard therapies), 146 were intolerant of one therapy and refractory to the other (RIST=patients refractory to one therapy and intolerant of the other) and 204 were refractory to both therapies (RST=refractory to both standard therapies). This was a very ill patient population; 38% required ventilatory support at entry (Table 1). These studies did not have concurrent control groups.

[See Table 1 above.]

The overall survival rate one month after completion of TMTX/LV as salvage therapy was 48%. Patients who had not responded to treatment with both TMP/SMX and pentamidine, of whom 63% required mechanical ventilation at entry, achieved a survival rate of 25% following treatment with TMTX/LV. Survival was 67% in patients who were intolerant to both TMP/SMX and pentamidine (Table 2).

[See Table 2 above.]

In the Treatment IND, 12% of the patients discontinued Neutrexin therapy (with leucovorin protection) for toxicity.

CONTRAINDICATIONS

Neutrexin (trimetrexate glucuronate for injection) is contraindicated in patients with clinically significant sensitivity to trimetrexate, leucovorin, or methotrexate.

WARNINGS

Neutrexin (trimetrexate glucuronate for injection) must be used with concurrent leucovorin to avoid potentially serious or life-threatening complications including bone marrow suppression, oral and gastrointestinal mucosal ulceration, and renal and hepatic dysfunction. Leucovorin therapy must extend for 72 hours past the last dose of Neutrexin. Patients should be informed that failure to take the recommended dose and duration of leucovorin can lead to fatal toxicity. Patients should be closely monitored for the development of serious hematologic adverse reactions (see **PRECAUTIONS** and **DOSAGE AND ADMINISTRATION**).

Neutrexin can cause fetal harm when administered to a pregnant woman. Trimetrexate has been shown to be fetotoxic and teratogenic in rats and rabbits. Rats administered 1.5 and 2.5 mg/kg/day intravenously on gestational days 6–15 showed substantial postimplantation loss and severe inhibition of maternal weight gain. Trimetrexate administered intravenously to rats at 0.5 and 1.0 mg/kg/day on gestational days 6–15 retarded normal fetal development and was teratogenic. Rabbits administered trimetrexate intravenously at daily doses of 2.5 and 5.0 mg/kg/day on gestational days 6–18 resulted in significant maternal and fetal toxicity. In rabbits, trimetrexate at 0.1 mg/kg/day was teratogenic in the absence of significant maternal toxicity. These effects were observed using doses 1/20 to 1/2 the equivalent human therapeutic dose based on a mg/m^2 basis. Teratogenic effects included skeletal, visceral, ocular, and cardiovascular abnormalities. If Neutrexin is used during pregnancy, or if the patient becomes pregnant while taking this drug, the patient should be apprised of the potential hazard to the fetus. Women of childbearing potential should be advised to avoid becoming pregnant.

PRECAUTIONS

General

Patients receiving Neutrexin (trimetrexate glucuronate for injection) may experience severe hematologic, hepatic, renal, and gastrointestinal toxicities. Caution should be used in treating patients with impaired hematologic, renal, or hepatic function. Patients who require concomitant therapy with nephrotoxic, myelosuppressive, or hepatotoxic drugs should be treated with Neutrexin at the discretion of the physician and monitored carefully. To allow for full therapeutic doses of Neutrexin, treatment with zidovudine should be discontinued during Neutrexin therapy.

Neutrexin-associated myelosuppression, stomatitis, and gastrointestinal toxicities generally can be ameliorated by adjusting the dose of leucovorin. Mild elevations in transaminases and alkaline phosphatase have been observed with Neutrexin administration and are usually not cause for

modification of Neutrexin therapy (see **DOSAGE AND ADMINISTRATION**). Seizures have been reported rarely (<1%) in AIDS patients receiving Neutrexin; however, a causal relationship has not been established. An anaphylactoid reaction has been reported in a cancer patient receiving Neutrexin as a bolus injection.

Neutrexin has not been evaluated clinically for the treatment of concurrent pulmonary conditions such as bacterial, viral, or fungal pneumonia or mycobacterial diseases. *In vitro* activity has been observed against *Toxoplasma gondii, Mycobacterium avium* complex, gram positive cocci, and gram negative rods. If clinical deterioration is observed in patients, they should be carefully evaluated for other possible causes of pulmonary disease and treated with additional agents as appropriate.

Laboratory Tests
Patients receiving Neutrexin and leucovorin protection should be seen frequently by a physician. Blood tests to assess the following parameters should be performed at least twice a week during therapy: hematology (absolute neutrophil counts [ANC], platelets), renal function (serum creatinine, BUN), and hepatic function (AST, ALT, alkaline phosphatase).

Drug Interactions
Since trimetrexate is metabolized by a P450 enzyme system, drugs that induce or inhibit this drug metabolizing enzyme system may elicit important drug-drug interactions that may alter trimetrexate plasma concentrations. Agents that might be coadministered with trimetrexate in AIDS patients for other indications that could elicit this activity include erythromycin, rifampin, rifabutin, ketoconazole, and fluconazole. *In vitro* perfusion of isolated rat liver has shown that cimetidine caused a significant reduction in trimetrexate metabolism and that acetaminophen altered the relative concentration of trimetrexate metabolites possibly by competing for sulfate metabolities. Based on an *in vitro* rat liver model, nitrogen substituted imidazole drugs (clotrimazole, ketoconazole, miconazole) were potent, non-competitive inhibitors of trimetrexate metabolism. Patients medicated with these drugs and trimetrexate should be carefully monitored.

Carcinogenesis, Mutagenesis, Impairment of Fertility
Carcinogenesis: Long term studies in animals to evaluate the carcinogenic potential of trimetrexate have not been performed.
Mutagenesis: Trimetrexate was not mutagenic when tested using the standard Ames *Salmonella* mutagenicity assay with and without metabolic activation. Trimetrexate did not induce mutations in Chinese hamster lung cells or sister-chromatid exchange in Chinese hamster ovary cells. Trimetrexate did induce an increase in the chromosomal aberration frequency of cultured Chinese hamster lung cells; however, trimetrexate showed no clastogenic activity in a mouse micronucleus assay.
Impairment of fertility: No studies have been conducted to evaluate the potential of trimetrexate to impair fertility. However, during standard toxicity studies conducted in mice and rats, degeneration of the testes and spermatocytes including the arrest of spermatogenesis was observed.

Pregnancy, Teratogenic Effects—See WARNINGS.
Pregnancy Category D
Nursing Mothers
It is not known if trimetrexate is excreted in human milk. Because many drugs are excreted in human milk and because of the potential for serious adverse reactions in nursing infants from trimetrexate, it is recommended that breast feeding be discontinued if the mother is treated with Neutrexin.

Pediatric Use
The safety and effectiveness of Neutrexin for the treatment of histologically confirmed PCP has not been established for patients under 18 years of age. Two children, ages 15 months and 9 months, were treated with trimetrexate and leucovorin using a dose of 45 mg/m^2 of trimetrexate per day for 21 days and 20 mg/m^2 of leucovorin every 6 hours for 24 days. There were no serious or unexpected adverse effects.

ADVERSE REACTIONS
Because many patients who participated in clinical trials of Neutrexin (trimetrexate glucuronate for injection) had complications of advanced HIV disease, it is difficult to distinguish adverse events caused by Neutrexin from those resulting from underlying medical conditions.
Table 3 lists the adverse events that occurred in ≥1% of the patients who participated in the Comparative Study of Neutrexin plus leucovorin versus TMP/SMX.
[See Table 3 above.]
Laboratory toxicities were generally manageable with dose modification of trimetrexate/leucovorin (see **DOSAGE AND ADMINISTRATION**).
Table 4 lists the adverse events resulting in discontinuation of study therapy in the Neutrexin Comparative Study with TMP/SMX. Twenty-nine percent of the patients on the

TABLE 3
NEUTREXIN COMPARATIVE TRIAL
Comparison of Adverse Events Reported for ≥ 1% of Patients

Adverse Events	Number and Percent (%) of Patients with Adverse Events			
	TMTX/LV (n = 109)		TMP/SMX (n = 111)	
Non-Laboratory Adverse Events:				
Fever	9	(8.3)	14	(12.6)
Rash/Pruritus	6	(5.5)	14	(12.6)
Nausea/Vomiting	5	(4.6)[a]	15	(13.5)[a]
Confusion	3	(2.8)	3	(2.7)
Fatigue	2	(1.8)	0	(0.0)
Hematologic Toxicity:				
Neutropenia (≤1000/mm^3)	33	(30.3)	37	(33.3)
Thrombocytopenia (≤75,000/mm^3)	11	(10.1)	17	(15.3)
Anemia (Hgb <8 g/dL)	8	(7.3)	10	(9.0)
Hepatotoxicity:				
Increased AST (>5 × ULN[b])	15	(13.8)	10	(9.0)
Increased ALT (>5 × ULN)	12	(11.0)	13	(11.7)
Increased Alkaline Phosphatase (>5 × ULN)	5	(4.6)	3	(2.7)
Increased Bilirubin (2.5 × ULN)	2	(1.8)	1	(0.9)
Renal:				
Increased Serum Creatinine (>3 × ULN)	1	(0.9)	2	(1.8)
Electrolyte Imbalance:				
Hyponatremia	5	(4.6)	10	(9.0)
Hypocalcemia	2	(1.8)	0	(0.0)
No. of Patients With at least one Adverse Event[c]	**58**	**(53.2)**	**60**	**(54.1)**

a Statistically significant difference between treatment groups (Chi-square: p = 0.022)
b ULN = Upper limit of normal range
c Patients could have reported more than one adverse event; therefore, the sum of adverse events exceeds the number of patients

TABLE 4
NEUTREXIN COMPARATIVE TRIAL
Adverse Events Resulting in Discontinuation of Therapy

Adverse Events	Number and Percent (%) of Patients Discontinued for Adverse Events[b]			
	TMTX/LV (n = 109)		TMP/SMX (n = 111)	
Non-Laboratory Adverse Events:				
Rash/Pruritus	3	(2.8)	5	(4.5)
Fever	2	(1.8)	4	(3.6)
Nausea/Vomiting	1	(0.9)	8	(7.2)
Neurologic Toxicity	1	(0.9)[c]	2	(1.8)
Hematologic Toxicity:				
Neutropenia (≤1000/mm^3)	4	(3.7)	6	(5.4)
Thrombocytopenia (≤75,000/mm^3)	0	(0.0)	4	(3.6)
Anemia (Hgb <8 g/dL)	0	(0.0)	4	(3.6)
Hepatotoxicity:				
Increased AST (>5 × ULN[a])	3	(2.8)	9	(8.1)
Increased ALT (>5 × ULN)	1	(0.9)	4	(3.6)
Increased Alkaline Phosphatase (>5 × ULN)	0	(0.0)	1	(0.9)
Electrolyte Imbalance:				
Hyponatremia	0	(0.0)	3	(2.7)
No. of Patients Discontinuing Therapy Due to an Adverse Event[b]	**11**	**(10.1)[d]**	**32**	**(28.8)[d]**

a ULN = Upper limit of normal range
b Patients could discontinue therapy due to more than one toxicity; therefore the sum exceeds number of patients who discontinued due to toxicity
c Patient discontinued TMTX/LV due to seizure, though causal relationship could not be established
d Statistically significant difference between treatment groups (Chi-square: p < 0.001)

TMP/SMX arm discontinued therapy due to adverse events compared to 10% of the patients treated with TMTX/LV (p <0.001).
[See Table 4 above.]
Hematologic toxicity was the principal dose-limiting side effect. One case of anaphylactoid reaction was reported in a cancer patient receiving Neutrexin as a bolus injection.

OVERDOSAGE
Neutrexin (trimetrexate glucuronate for injection) administered without concurrent leucovorin can cause lethal complications. There has been no extensive experience in humans receiving single intravenous doses of trimetrexate greater than 90 mg/m^2/day with concurrent leucovorin. The toxicit-

ies seen at this dose were primarily hematologic. In the event of overdose, Neutrexin should be stopped and leucovorin should be administered at a dose of 40 mg/m^2 every 6 hours for 3 days. The LD$_{50}$ of intravenous trimetrexate in mice is 62 mg/kg (186 mg/m^2).

DOSAGE AND ADMINISTRATION
Caution: Neutrexin (trimetrexate glucuronate for injection) must be administered with concurrent leucovorin (leucovorin protection) to avoid potentially serious or life-threatening toxicities. Leucovorin therapy must extend for 72 hours past the last dose of Neutrexin.

Continued on next page

U.S. Bioscience—Cont.

TABLE 5
DOSE MODIFICATIONS FOR HEMATOLOGIC TOXICITY

Toxicity Grade	Neutrophils (Polys and Bands)	Platelets	Recommended Dosages of Neutrexin	Recommended Dosages of Leucovorin
1	$>1000/mm^3$	$>75,000/mm^3$	$45\ mg/m^2$ once daily	$20\ mg/m^2$ every 6 hours
2	$750–1000/mm^3$	$50,000–75,000/mm^3$	$45\ mg/m^2$ once daily	$40\ mg/m^2$ every 6 hours
3	$500–749/mm^3$	$25,000–49,999/mm^3$	$22\ mg/m^2$ once daily	$40\ mg/m^2$ every 6 hours
4	$<500/mm^3$	$<25,000/mm^3$	Day 1–9 Discontinue Day 10–21 Interrupt up to 96 hours[a]	$40\ mg/m^2$ every 6 hours

a If Grade 4 hematologic toxicity occurs prior to Day 10, Neutrexin should be discontinued. Leucovorin $(40\ mg/m^2,\ q6h)$ should be administered for an additional 72 hours. If Grade 4 hematologic toxicity occurs at Day 10 or later, Neutrexin may be held up to 96 hours to allow counts to recover. If counts recover to Grade 3 within 96 hours, Neutrexin should be administered at a dose of $22\ mg/m^2$ and leucovorin maintained at $40\ mg/m^2$, q6h. When counts recover to Grade 2 toxicity, Neutrexin dose may be increased to $45\ mg/m^2$, but the leucovorin dose should be maintained at $40\ mg/m^2$ for the duration of treatment. If counts do not improve to $\leq$ Grade 3 toxicity within 96 hours, Neutrexin should be discontinued. Leucovorin at a dose of $40\ mg/m^2$, q6h should be administered for 72 hours following the last dose of Neutrexin.

Neutrexin (trimetrexate glucuronate for injection) is administered at a dose of $45\ mg/m^2$ once daily by intravenous infusion over 60–90 minutes. Leucovorin must be administered daily during treatment with Neutrexin and for 72 hours past the last dose of Neutrexin. Leucovorin may be administered intravenously at a dose of $20\ mg/m^2$ over 5 to 10 minutes every 6 hours for a total daily dose of $80\ mg/m^2$, or orally as 4 doses of $20\ mg/m^2$ spaced equally throughout the day. The oral dose should be rounded up to the next higher 25 mg increment. The recommended course of therapy is 21 days of Neutrexin and 24 days of leucovorin.
Dosage Modifications
Hematologic toxicity: Neutrexin (trimetrexate glucuronate for injection) and leucovorin doses should be modified based on the worst hematologic toxicity according to the following table. If leucovorin is given orally, doses should be rounded up to the next higher 25 mg increment.
[See Table 5 above.]
Hepatic toxicity: Transient elevation of transaminases and alkaline phosphatase have been observed in patients treated with Neutrexin. Interruption of treatment is advisable if transaminase levels or alkaline phosphatase levels increase to >5 times the upper limit of normal range.
Renal toxicity: Interruption of Neutrexin is advisable if serum creatinine levels increase to >2.5 mg/dL and the elevation is considered to be secondary to Neutrexin.
Other toxicities: Interruption of treatment is advisable in patients who experience severe mucosal toxicity that interferes with oral intake. Treatment should be discontinued for fever (oral temperature $\geq$ 105°F/40.5°C) that cannot be controlled with antipyretics.
Leucovorin therapy must extend for 72 hours past the last dose of Neutrexin.
RECONSTITUTION AND DILUTION
Neutrexin (trimetrexate glucuronate for injection) should be reconstituted with 2 mL of 5% Dextrose Injection, USP, or Sterile Water for Injection, USP, to yield a concentration of 12.5 mg of trimetrexate per mL (complete dissolution should occur within 30 seconds). The reconstituted product will appear as a pale greenish-yellow solution and must be inspected visually for particulate matter prior to dilution. **Do not use if cloudiness or precipitate is observed, but even if the solution appears clear, it should be filtered (0.22μm) prior to dilution.** Neutrexin should not be reconstituted with solutions containing either chloride ion or leucovorin, since precipitation occurs instantly.
After reconstitution, the solution is stable under refrigeration or at room temperature for up to 24 hours. Do not freeze reconstituted solution. Discard any unused portion after 24 hours.
Reconstituted solution should be further diluted with 5% Dextrose Injection, USP, to yield a final concentration of 0.25 to 2 mg of trimetrexate per mL. The diluted solution should be administered by intravenous infusion over 60 minutes. Neutrexin should not be mixed with solutions containing either chloride ion or leucovorin, since precipitation occurs instantly. It is stable under refrigeration or at room temperature for up to 24 hours. Do not freeze. Discard any unused portion after 24 hours after initial reconstitution. The intravenous line must be flushed thoroughly with at least 10 mL of 5% Dextrose Injection, USP, before and after administering Neutrexin.
Leucovorin protection may be administered prior to or following Neutrexin. In either case, the intravenous line must be flushed thoroughly with at least 10 mL of 5% Dextrose Injection, USP. Leucovorin calcium for injection should be diluted according to the instructions in the leucovorin package insert, and administered over 5 to 10 minutes every 6 hours.

Caution: Parenteral products should be inspected visually for particulate matter and discoloration prior to administration, whenever solution and container permit. Neutrexin forms a precipitate instantly upon contact with chloride ion or leucovorin, therefore it should not be added to solutions containing sodium chloride or other anions. Neutrexin and leucovorin solutions must be administered separately. Intravenous lines should be flushed with at least 10 mL of 5% Dextrose Injection, USP, between Neutrexin and leucovorin infusions.

HANDLING AND DISPOSAL
If Neutrexin (trimetrexate glucuronate for injection) contacts the skin or mucosa, immediately wash thoroughly with soap and water. Procedures for proper disposal of cytotoxic drugs should be considered. Several guidelines on this subject have been published (1–5).

HOW SUPPLIED
Neutrexin (trimetrexate glucuronate for injection) (NDC 58178-020-01) is supplied as a sterile lyophilized powder in 5 mL, single-dose vials. Each 5 mL vial contains trimetrexate glucuronate equivalent to 25 mg of trimetrexate. The vials are packaged and available in five market presentations as listed below:
Bulk Pack—4 trays of 25 vials per shrink-wrapped tray (NDC 58178-020-70)
10 Pack—10 vials in a white chip-board carton (NDC 58178-020-10)
25 Pack—25 vials per shrink-wrapped tray (NDC 58178-020-25)
50 Pack—2 trays of 25 vials per shrink-wrapped tray (NDC 58178-020-50)
Starter Pack—21 vials per shrink-wrapped tray (NDC 58178-020-21) presented in combination with 28 vials of Leucovorin Calcium for Injection in a shrink-wrapped tray each vial of which contains 50 mg of leucovorin as the calcium salt.
Store at controlled room temperature 15° to 30°C (59° to 86°F).
Protect from exposure to light.
• **CAUTION:** Federal (U.S.A.) law prohibits dispensing without prescription. U.S. Patents 4,376,858; 4,694,007

REFERENCES
1. AMA Council Report. Guidelines for Handling Parenteral Antineoplastics. *Journal of the American Medical Association* March 15, 1985.
2. Clinical Oncological Society of Australia: Guidelines and Recommendations for Safe Handling of Antineoplastic Agents. *Medical Journal of Australia* 1:426–428, 1983.
3. Jones RB, et al. Safe Handling of Chemotherapeutic Agents: A Report from the Mount Sinai Medical Center. *CA-A Cancer Journal for Clinicians* Sept/Oct, 258–263, 1983.
4. American Society of Hospital Pharmacists Technical Assistance Bulletin on Handling Cytotoxic Drugs in Hospitals. *American Journal of Hospital Pharmacy* 42: 131–137, 1985.
5. OSHA Work Practice Guidelines for Personnel Dealing with Cytotoxic (Antineoplastic) Drugs. *American Journal of Hospital Pharmacy* 43: 1193–1204, 1986.

Manufactured by: For:
Ben Venue Laboratories, Inc.   U.S. Bioscience, Inc.
Bedford, Ohio 44146   West Conshohocken, PA 19428
or
USB PHARMA B.V.
Nijmegen, The Netherlands
© 1994, U.S. Bioscience, Inc.   1-800-USBIOSC
Revision Date 7/95   (1-800-872-4672)

Shown in Product Identification Guide, page 339

U.S. Pharmaceutical Corporation
2401-C MELLON COURT
DECATUR, GA 30035

Direct Inquiries to:
Raymond F. Meyer, R.Ph.,
Marketing Director
(800) 330-3040

HEMOCYTE™ Tablets   OTC
(ferrous fumarate 324 mg.)

HOW SUPPLIED
Bottles of 100 NDC 52747-307-60

HEMOCYTE PLUS™ Tabules   ℞
Iron-Vitamin-Mineral Complex

DESCRIPTION
Each tabule contains:

Ferrous Fumarate (anhydrous)	324	mg.
[Equivalent to about 106 mg. of Elemental Iron]		
Sodium Ascorbate (Vit. C)	200	mg.
Vit. B-1—Thiamine Mononitrate	10	mg.
Vit. B-2—Riboflavin	6	mg.
Vit. B-6—Pyridoxine HCl	5	mg.
Vit. B-12—Cyanocobalamin Concentrate	15	mcg.
Folic Acid	1	mg.
Niacinamide	30	mg.
Calcium Pantothenate	10	mg.
Zinc (as Zinc Sulfate)	18.2	mg.
Magnesium (as Magnesium Sulfate)	6.9	mg.
Manganese (as Manganese Sulfate)	1.3	mg.
Copper (as Copper Sulfate)	0.8	mg.

HOW SUPPLIED
Bottles of 100 NDC 52747-308-60

HEMOCYTE–C Tablets   OTC
(Chewable Iron/Vitamin C)

DESCRIPTION
Each tablet contains:

Iron (elemental) (as Ferrous Fumarate)	50 mg
Ascorbic Acid (as Ascorbic Acid and Sodium Ascorbate)	250 mg

HOW SUPPLIED
Tablets: Bottles of 50 NDC 52747-303-50

HEMOCYTE–F ELIXIR   ℞
Iron, Folic Acid, and Vitamin B12 Complex

DESCRIPTION
Each Teaspoon Contains:

Elemental Iron (As a polysaccharide-iron complex)	100 mg
Folic Acid	1 mg
Vitamin B12	25 mcg
Alcohol	10%
(Sugar Free)	

HOW SUPPLIED
Bottles of 16 oz. and 2 oz.

HEMOCYTE–F TABLETS   ℞

DESCRIPTION
Each tablet contains:

Ferrous Fumarate (anhydrous)	324 mg.
Folic Acid	1 mg.

HOW SUPPLIED
Bottles of 100 NDC 52747-306-60

MAGSAL™ TABLETS   ℞

DESCRIPTION
Each tablet contains:
Magnesium Salicylate .... 600 mg.
Phenyltoloxamine Dihydrogen Citrate .... 25 mg.

HOW SUPPLIED
Bottles of 100 NDC 52747-321-60

MEDIGESIC® Capsules   ℞

DESCRIPTION
Each capsule or tablet contains:
Butalbital* .... 50 mg
    *WARNING: May be habit forming.
Acetaminophen .... 325 mg
Caffeine .... 40 mg

HOW SUPPLIED
Capsules: Bottles of 100 NDC 52747-600-60

MEDIPLEX™   OTC
Vitamin-Mineral Complex

DESCRIPTION: Each tabule contains:
Vitamin E—dl-alpha Tocopherol Acetete .... 60 I.U.
Vitamin C—Ascorbic Acid .... 300 mg.
Vitamin B¹²—Cyanocabalmin
    Concentrate .... 25 mcg.
Vitamin B¹—Thiamine .... 25 mg.
Niacinamide .... 100 mg.
Vitamin B⁶—Pyridoxine .... 10 mg.
Vitamin B²—Riboflavin .... 10 mg.
Calcium Pantothenate .... 25 mg.
Zinc (as Zinc Sulfate) .... 18 mg.
Magnesium (as Magnesium Sulfate) .... 7 mg.
Manganese (as Manganese Sulfate) .... 1.3 mg.
Copper .... 0.8 mg.

HOW SUPPLIED
Bottles of 100 NDC 52747-142-60

NOREL   ℞
Decongestant/Expectorant

DESCRIPTION:
Each capsule contains:
Guaifenesin .... 200 mg
Phenylpropanolamine .... 45 mg
Phenylephrine .... 5 mg

HOW SUPPLIED:
Bottles of 100 NDC 52747-610-60

NOREL PLUS   ℞
Decongestant–Analgesic–Antihistaminic

DESCRIPTION
Each yellow and white capsule for oral administration
contains:
Acetaminophen .... 325 mg
Phenyltoloxamine Dihydrogen Citrate .... 25 mg
Phenylpropanolamine Hydrochloride .... 25 mg
Chlorpheniramine Maleate .... 4 mg

HOW SUPPLIED
Bottles of 100 NDC 52747-128-60

IDENTIFICATION PROBLEM?
Turn to the **Product Identification** Guide,
where you'll find more than
1600 products pictured in actual
size and full color.

Upsher-Smith Laboratories, Inc.
14905 23RD AVE. NORTH
MINNEAPOLIS, MN 55447

For Medical Information Contact:
Write: Professional Services Department
or call: (800) 654-2299
(during business hours-8:00 am to 5:00 pm CST)

KLOR–CON® POWDER   ℞
[klōr 'kon]
Potassium Chloride for Oral Solution, USP
20 mEq (1.5 g) per packet

DESCRIPTION
Each packet contains 1.5 g potassium chloride providing
potassium 20 mEq and chloride 20 mEq. Fruit-flavored with
artificial color and sweetener (saccharin) added.

HOW SUPPLIED
KLOR-CON® Powder 20 mEq (1.5 g Potassium Chloride). In
cartons of 30 and 100 packets.
30's NDC 0245-0035-30, 100's NDC 0245-0035-01

KLOR–CON®/25 POWDER   ℞
[klōr 'kon]
Potassium Chloride for Oral Solution, USP
25 mEq (1.875 g) per packet

DESCRIPTION
Each packet contains 1.875 g potassium chloride providing
potassium 25 mEq and chloride 25 mEq. Fruit-flavored with
artificial color and sweetener (saccharin) added.

HOW SUPPLIED
KLOR-CON®/25 Powder 25 mEq:
Cartons of 30, 100 and 250 packets.
30's NDC 0245-0037-30, 100's NDC 0245-0037-01
250's NDC 0245-0037-25

KLOR–CON® 8/KLOR–CON® 10   ℞
[klōr 'kon]
Potassium Chloride
Extended–release Tablets, USP
8 mEq and 10 mEq

DESCRIPTION
KLOR-CON® Extended-release Tablets, USP are a solid
oral dosage form of potassium chloride. Each contains 600
mg or 750 mg of potassium chloride equivalent to 8 mEq or
10 mEq of potassium in a wax matrix tablet. This formulation is intended to slow the release of potassium so that the
likelihood of a high localized concentration of potassium
chloride within the gastrointestinal tract is reduced.
Klor-Con® Extended-release Tablets are an electrolyte replenisher. The chemical name is potassium chloride, and the
structural formula is KCl. Potassium chloride USP occurs as
a white, granular powder or as colorless crystals. It is odorless and has a saline taste. Its solutions are neutral to litmus.
It is freely soluble in water and insoluble in alcohol.
Inactive Ingredients: Castor oil, hydroxypropyl methylcellulose 2910, magnesium stearate, polyethylene glycol 3350,
propylene glycol, synthetic iron oxide, titanium dioxide, and
other ingredients. Yellow tablets also contain FD& C Yellow
No. 10 aluminum lake and FD & C Yellow No. 6 aluminum
lake. Blue tablets also contain FD & C Blue No. 1 aluminum
lake.

HOW SUPPLIED
Film coated, Klor-Con® 8 (blue), Klor-Con® 10 (yellow),
imprinted round tablets containing:
    600 mg potassium chloride (equivalent to 8 mEq) in bottles
    of 100 (NDC 0245-0040-11), bottles of 500 (NDC 0245-0040-
    15), and unit-dose packages of 100 (NDC 0245-0040-01);
    750 mg potassium chloride (equivalent to 10 mEq) in bot-
    tles of 100 (NDC 0245-0041-11), bottles of 500 (NDC 0245-
    0041-15), and unit-dose packages of 100 (NDC 0245-
    0041-01).
Protect from light and moisture. Store at controlled room
temperature 59°–86°F (15°–30°C). Dispense in container with
child resistant closure.
CAUTION: Federal law prohibits dispensing without prescription.
Shown in Product Identification Guide, page 339

KLOR-CON®/EF 25mEq   ℞
[klōr 'kon]
Potassium Bicarbonate Effervescent Tablets for Oral
Solution, USP

DESCRIPTION
Each effervescent tablet in solution provides 25 mEq (978
mg) potassium as bicarbonate and citrate. KLOR-CON®/EF
tablets are sugar-free.

HOW SUPPLIED
KLOR-CON®/EF 25 mEq effervescent tablets in cartons of
30 and 100 individually wrapped tablets.
30's NDC 0245-0039-30, 100's NDC 0245-0039-01

NIACOR®   ℞
[nī 'ă-kōr]
NIACIN TABLETS, USP
500 mg

DESCRIPTION
Niacin or nicotinic acid, a water-soluble B complex vitamin
and antihyperlipidemic agent, is 3-pyridinecarboxylic acid.
It is a white, crystalline powder, sparingly soluble in water.
It has the following structural formula:

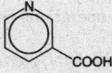

MW = 123.11 $C_6H_5NO_2$

Each NIACOR® tablet for oral administration, contains
500 mg of nicotinic acid. In addition, each tablet contains the
following inactive ingredients: colloidal silicon dioxide, corn
starch, lactose, microcrystalline cellulose, povidone (K-25),
purified stearic acid.

HOW SUPPLIED
Each tablet is circular, biconvex, white tablet, debossed
W 901 on one side and scored on other side.
NIACOR® is available in bottles of 100 tablets (NDC 0245-
0067-11).
Dispense in a tight, light-resistant container as defined in the
USP, with a child-resistant closure.
Store at controlled room temperature 15–30°C (59–86°F).
CAUTION: Federal law prohibits dispensing without
prescription.

OMS® Concentrate   Ⓒ ℞
Morphine Sulfate Immediate-release Concentrated Oral
Solution

DESCRIPTION
Each ml of OMS® Concentrate contains:
Morphine Sulfate .... 20 mg
            (WARNING: May be habit forming)

HOW SUPPLIED
OMS® Concentrate
Immediate Release (Morphine Sulfate Concentrated Oral
Solution)
20 mg per ml
NDC 0245-0167-31: Bottle of 30 ml with calibrated
dropper.
NDC 0245-0167-04: Bottle of 120 ml with calibrated
dropper.
DEA ORDER FORM REQUIRED
Caution: Federal law prohibits dispensing without pre-
scription.

PREVALITE®   ℞
[prĕ 'vă līt]
(Cholestyramine for Oral Suspension, USP)

DESCRIPTION
Prevalite®, the chloride salt of a basic anion exchange resin,
a cholesterol-lowering agent, is intended for oral administration. Cholestyramine resin is quite hydrophilic, but insoluble
in water. The cholestyramine resin in Prevalite® is not absorbed from the digestive tract. 5.5 grams of Prevalite® contain 4 grams of anhydrous cholestyramine resin. It is represented by the following structural formula:
[See chemical structure at top of next column.]

Continued on next page

Upsher-Smith Laboratories—Cont.

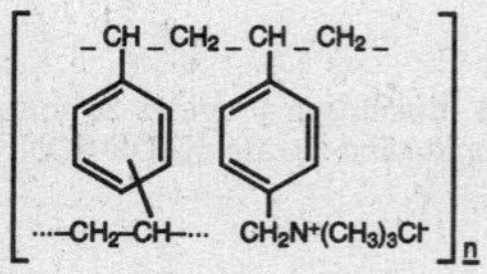

Representation of structure of main polymeric groups

This product contains the following inactive ingredients: aspartame, FD&C Yellow No. 6, malic acid, polysorbate 80, propylene glycol alginate, and natural orange flavor.

HOW SUPPLIED

Prevalite® (Cholestyramine for Oral Suspension, USP) available in cartons of sixty 5.5 gram single dose packets. Each 5.5 gram packet of Prevalite® contains 4 grams of anhydrous cholestyramine resin.

NDC 0245-0036-60   Cartons of 60, 5.5 g packets

Store at controlled room temperature 15°–30°C (59°–86°F).

CAUTION: FEDERAL LAW PROHIBITS DISPENSING WITHOUT PRESCRIPTION.

Manufactured by
UPSHER-SMITH LABORATORIES, INC.
Minneapolis, MN 55447

Certain manufacturing operations have been performed by other firms.

Please refer to the *PDR for Generics* for full prescribing information.

RMS® Suppositories Ⓒ ℞

(Rectal Morphine Sulfate)
WARNING—MAY BE HABIT FORMING

DESCRIPTION

Suppositories contain 5, 10, 20, or 30 mg of morphine sulfate. Morphine sulfate occurs as white, feathery, silky crystals, cubical masses of crystals or white crystalline powder. The chemical name of morphine sulfate is morphinan-3. 6-diol, 7, 8-didehydro-4, 5-epoxy-17-methyl, (5α, 6α)-, sulfate (2:1) (salt), pentahydrate.

The empirical formula is $(C_{17}H_{19}NO_3)2 \cdot H_2SO_4 \cdot 5H_2O$.

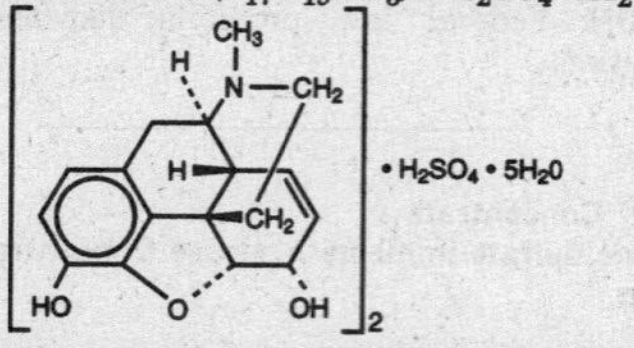

Morphine sulfate belongs to the pharmacological class of the narcotic analgesics. Morphine sulfate suppositories are prepared from a bland hydrogenated vegetable oil base and other ingredients (contains BHA and BHT as preservatives), and are suitable for rectal administration.

CLINICAL PHARMACOLOGY

Morphine sulfate is a potent analgesic, with major effects on the central nervous system and organs containing smooth muscle. Opioids act as agonists, interacting with stereospecific and saturable binding sites on receptors in the brain and other tissues. Pharmacological effects include analgesia, drowsiness, alteration in mood (euphoria), reduction in body temperature (at low doses), dose-related depression of respiration, interference with adrenocortical response to stress (at high doses), reduction in peripheral resistance with little or no effect on cardiac index and miosis.

Morphine sulfate given as a rectal suppository can produce analgesic effects and duration similar to that of oral adminstration at similar dose levels. Analgesic effects are commonly seen 20 to 60 minutes after administration.

INDICATIONS AND USAGE

Morphine is a potent analgesic indicated for the relief of severe acute and severe chronic pain.

CONTRAINDICATIONS

Hypersensitivity to morphine; respiratory insufficiency or depression; severe CNS depression; attack of bronchial asthma; heart failure secondary to chronic lung disease; cardiac arrhythmias; increased intracranial or cerebrospinal pressure; head injuries; brain tumor; acute alcoholism; delerium tremens; convulsive disorders; after biliary tract surgery, suspected surgical abdomen; surgical abdomen; surgical anastomosis; concomitantly with MAO inhibitors or within 14 days of such treatment.

WARNINGS

Morphine can cause tolerance, psychological and physical dependence. Withdrawal will occur on abrupt discontinuation or administration of a narcotic antagonist.

Interaction with Other Central Nervous System Depressants—Morphine should be used with caution and in reduced dosage with patients who are concurrently receiving other narcotic analgesics, general anesthetics, phenothiazines, other tranquilizers, sedative-hypnotics, tricyclic antidepressants, and other CNS depressants (including alcohol). Respiratory depression, hypotension, and profound sedation or coma may result.

PRECAUTIONS

General: *Head Injury and Intracranial Pressure*—The respiratory depressant effects of morphine and its capacity to elevate cerebrospinal fluid pressure may be markedly exaggerated in the presence of increased intracranial pressure. Furthermore, narcotics produce side effects that may obscure the clinical course of patients with head injuries. In such patients, morphine must be used with caution and only if it is deemed essential. *Asthma and Other Respiratory Conditions*—Morphine should be used with caution in patients having acute asthmatic attack, in those with chronic obstructive pulmonary disease or cor pulmonale, and in individuals with a substantially decreased respiratory reserve, preexisting respiratory depression, hypoxia, or hypercapnia. In such patients, even usual therapeutic doses of narcotics may decrease respiratory drive while simultaneously increasing airway resistance to the point of apnea.

Acute Abdominal Condition—The administration of morphine or other narcotics may obscure the diagnosis or clinical course in patients with acute abdominal conditions. *Special Risk Patients*—Morphine should be given with caution to certain patients, such as the elderly or debilitated and those with severe impairment of hepatic or renal function, hypothyroidism, Addison's disease, and prostatic hypertrophy or urethral structure. Morphine sulfate should be used with extreme caution in patients with disorders characterized by hypoxia, since even usual therapeutic doses of narcotics may decrease respiratory drive to the point of apnea while simultaneously increasing airway resistance.

Hypotensive Effect—The adminstration of morphine sulfate may result in severe hypotension in the postoperative patient or any individual whose ability to maintain blood pressure has been compromised by a depleted blood volume or the administration of such drugs as the phenothiazines or certain anesthetics. *Supraventricular Tachycardias*—Because of possible vagolytic action may produce a significant increase in the ventricular response rate, morphine sulfate should be used with caution in patients with atrial flutter and other supraventricular tachycardias. *Convulsions*—Morphine sulfate may aggravate preexisting convulsions in patients with convulsive disorders. If dosage is escalated substantially above recommended levels because of tolerance development, convulsions may occur in individuals without a history of convulsive disorders. *Kidney or Liver Dysfunction*—Morphine sulfate may have a prolonged duration and cumulative effect in patients with kidney or liver dysfunction.

Information for Patients—Morphine may impair the mental and/or physical abilities required for the performance of potentially hazardous tasks, such as driving a car or operating machinery. Morphine in combination with other narcotic analgesics, phenothiazines, sedative/hypnotics, and alcohol has additive depressant effects. The patient should be cautioned accordingly.

Drug Interactions—Morphine in combination with other narcotic analgesics, general anesthetics, antihistamines, phenothiazines, barbiturates, other tranquilizers, sedative/hypnotics, tricyclic antidepressants, or other CNS depressants (including alcohol) has additive depressant effects. When such combination therapy is contemplated, the dosage of one or both agents should be reduced.

Carcinogenesis, Mutagenesis, Impairment of Fertility—Morphine has no known carcinogenic or mutagenic potential. However, no long-term animal studies are available to support this observation.

Usage in Pregnancy: Category C—Animal reproduction studies have not been conducted with morphine sulfate. It is not known whether morphine sulfate can cause fetal harm when administered to a pregnant woman or can affect reproduction capacity. On the basis of the historical use of morphine sulfate during all stages of pregnancy, there is no known risk of fetal abnormality. However, infants born from mothers who have been taking morphine chronically may exhibit withdrawal symptoms. Morphine sulfate should be given to a pregnant woman only if clearly needed.

Labor and Delivery—The use of morphine sulfate in obstetrics may prolong labor. It crosses the placental barrier and may produce depression of respiration in the newborn. Resuscitation and, in the case of severe depression, the administration of a narcotic antagonist such as naloxone may be required.

Nursing Mothers—Morphine sulfate appears in the milk of nursing mothers. Caution should be exercised when it is administered to a nursing mother.

Pediatric Usage—Safety and effectiveness in children have not been established.

ADVERSE REACTIONS

As with other narcotic analgesics, the major hazards of morphine are respiratory depression, and to a lesser degree, circulatory depression, respiratory arrest, shock, and cardiac arrest. The most frequently observed adverse reactions include lightheadedness, dizziness, sedation, nausea, vomiting, and sweating. These effects seem to be more prominent in ambulatory patients and in those who are not suffering severe pain. In such individuals, lower doses are advisable. Some adverse reactions may be alleviated in the ambulatory patient if he lies down. Other adverse reactions include the following: *Central Nervous System*—Euphoria, dysphoria, weakness, headache, insomnia, agitation, disorientation, and visual disturbances. *Gastrointestinal*—Dry mouth, anorexia, constipation, and biliary tract spasms. *Cardiovascular*—Flushing of the face, bradycardia, palpitation, faintness, and syncope. *Genitourinary*—Urinary retention or hesitancy, anti-diuretic effect and reduced libido and/or potency. *Allergic*—Pruritus, urticaria, other skin rashes, edema, and rarely hemorrhagic urticaria.

Treatment of the most frequent adverse reactions: *Constipation*—Ample intake of water or other liquids should be encouraged. Concomitant administration of a stool softener and a peristaltic stimulant with the narcotic analgesic can be effective preventive measure for those patients in need of therapeutics. If elimination does not occur for two days, an enema should be administered to prevent impaction.

In the event diarrhea occurs, seepage around a fecal impaction is a possible cause to consider before antidiarrheal measures are employed.

Nausea and Vomiting—Phenothiazines and antihistamines can be effective treatments for nausea of the medullary and vestibular sources, respectively. However, these drugs may potentiate the side effects of the narcotics or the antinauseant.

Drowsiness (sedation)—Once pain control is achieved, undesirable sedation can be minimized by titrating the dosage to a level that just maintains a tolerable pain or pain free state.

DRUG ABUSE AND DEPENDENCE

Controlled Substance—Morphine sulfate is a Schedule II narcotic. *Dependence*—Morphine can produce drug dependence and, therefore, has the potential for being abused. Patients receiving therapeutic dosage regimens of 10 mg every 4 hours for 1 to 2 weeks have exhibited mild withdrawal symptoms. Development of the dependent state is recognizable by an increased tolerance to the analgesic effect and the appearance of purposive phenomena (complaints, pleas, demands or manipulative actions) shortly before the time of the next scheduled dose. A patient in withdrawal should be treated in a hospital environment. Usually, it is necessary only to provide supportive care with administration of a tranquilizer to suppress anxiety. Severe symptoms of withdrawal may require administration of a replacement narcotic.

In treating the terminally ill patient, the benefit of pain relief may outweigh the possibility of drug dependence. The chance of drug dependence is substantially reduced when the patient is placed on scheduled narcotic programs instead of a "pain to relief-of-pain" cycle typical of a PRN regimen.

OVERDOSAGE

Signs and Symptoms—serious overdosage of morphine is characterized by respiratory depression (a decrease in respiratory rate and/or tidal volume, Cheyne-Stokes respiration, cyanosis), extreme somnolence progressing to stupor or coma, skeletal muscle flaccidity, cold and clammy skin, and sometimes, bradycardia and hypotension. In severe overdosage, apnea, circulatory collapse, cardiac arrest, and death may occur. *Treatment*—Primary attention should be given to the re-establishment of adequate respiratory exchange through provision of a patent airway and institution of assisted or controlled ventilation. The narcotic antagonists naloxone and levallorphan are specific antidotes against the respiratory depression that may result from overdosage or unusual sensitivity to narcotics. Therefore, an appropriate dose of one of these antagonists should be administered, preferably by the intravenous route, simultaneously with efforts at respiratory resuscitation. Since the duration of action of morphine may exceed that of the antagonist, the patient should be kept under continued surveillance, and repeated doses of the antagonist should be administered as needed to maintain adequate respiration. An antagonist should not be administered in the absence of clinically significant respiratory or cardiovascular depression. Oxygen, intravenous fluids, vasopressors, and other supportive measures should be employed as indicated.

DOSAGE AND ADMINISTRATION

Dosage should be adjusted according to the severity of the pain and the response of the patient. RMS® Suppositories

are to be administered rectally. *For Analgesia*—Usual Adult Dose: 10 to 30 mg every 4 hours or as directed by physician: Dosage is a patient dependent variable, and increased dosage may be required for adequate analgesia. For control of chronic, agonizing pain in patients with certain terminal disease, this drug should be administered on a regularly scheduled basis, every 4 hours, at the lowest dosage level that will achieve adequate analgesia. **Note:** Medication may suppress respiration in the elderly, the very ill, and those patients with respiratory problems, therefore lower doses may be required.

MORPHINE DOSAGE REDUCTION

During the first two to three days of effective pain relief, the patient may sleep for many hours. This can be misinterpreted as the effect of excessive analgesic dosing rather than the first sign of relief in a pain exhausted patient. The dose, therefore, should be maintained for at least three days before reduction, if respiratory activity and other vital signs are adequate. Following successful relief of severe pain, periodic attempts to reduce the narcotic dose should be made. Smaller doses or complete discontinuation of the narcotic analgesic may become feasible due to a physiologic change or the improved mental state of the patient.

HOW SUPPLIED

RMS® Suppositories are individually sealed in color-coded wrappers to aid in identification. 5 mg suppositories (white wrapper/blue type), NDC 0245-0160-12, 12 per carton. 10 mg suppositories (white wrapper/green type), NDC 0245-0161-12, 12 per carton. 20 mg suppositories (white wrapper/red type), NDC 0245-0162-12, 12 per carton. 30 mg suppositories (white wrapper/gold type), NDC 0245-0163-12, 12 per carton.

DEA ORDER FORM REQUIRED—

Caution: Federal law prohibits dispensing without prescription.

SSKI®
**Potassium Iodide Oral Solution, USP
(Saturated) 1 g/ml**

℞

DESCRIPTION

SSKI® (potassium iodide oral solution, USP) is a saturated solution of potassium iodide containing 1 g of potassium iodide per ml.

CLINICAL PHARMACOLOGY

Potassium iodide is thought to act as an expectorant by increasing respiratory tract secretions and thereby decreasing the viscosity of mucus.

INDICATIONS AND USAGE

For use as an expectorant in the symptomatic treatment of chronic pulmonary diseases where tenacious mucus complicates the problem, including bronchial asthma, bronchitis and pulmonary emphysema.

CONTRAINDICATIONS

Contraindicated in patients with a known sensitivity to iodides.

WARNINGS

Potassium iodide can cause fetal harm, abnormal thyroid function, and goiter when administered to a pregnant woman. Because of the possible development of fetal goiter, if the drug is used during pregnancy or if the patient becomes pregnant during therapy, apprise the patient of the potential hazard.

PRECAUTIONS

General: In some patients, prolonged use of iodides can lead to hypothyroidism. Iodides should be used with caution in patients having Addison's disease, cardiac disease, hyperthyroidism, myotonia congenita, tuberculosis, acute bronchitis, or renal function impairment.

Drug Interactions: Concurrent use with lithium and other antithyroid drugs may potentiate the hypothyroid and goitrogenic effects of these medications. Concurrent use with potassium-containing medications, potassium-sparing diuretics and angiotensin-converting enzyme inhibitors (ACE inhibitors) may result in hyperkalemia and cardiac arrhythmias or cardiac arrest.

Drug/Laboratory Test Interactions: Thyroid function tests may be altered by iodide.

Pregnancy: Category D—see "Warnings" section.

Nursing Mothers: Potassium iodide is excreted in breast milk. Use by nursing mothers may cause skin rash and thyroid suppression in the infant.

Pediatric Use: Safety and effectiveness in children have not been established.

ADVERSE REACTIONS

The most frequent adverse reactions to potassium iodide are stomach upset, diarrhea, nausea, vomiting, stomach pain, skin rash, and salivary gland swelling or tenderness. Less frequent adverse reactions include gastrointestinal bleeding, confusion, irregular heartbeat, numbness, tingling, pain or weakness in hands or feet, unusual tiredness, weakness or heaviness of legs, fever, and swelling of neck or throat. Thyroid adenoma, goiter, and myxedema are possible side effects.

Iodism or chronic iodine poisoning may occur during prolonged treatment or with the use of high doses. The symptoms of iodism include burning of mouth or throat, severe headache, metallic taste, soreness of teeth and gums, symptoms of head cold, irritation of the eyes with swelling of the eyelids, unusual increase in salivation, acneform skin lesions in the seborrheic areas, and rarely, severe skin eruptions. If symptoms of iodism appear, the drug should be withdrawn and the patient given appropriate supportive therapy. Hypersensitivity to iodides may occur and may be manifested by angioedema, cutaneous and mucosal hemorrhage, and signs and symptoms resembling serum sickness, such as fever, arthralgia, lymph node enlargement, and eosinophilia.

OVERDOSAGE

Acute toxicity from potassium iodide is relatively rare. An occasional individual may show marked sensitivity and the onset of acute poisoning can occur immediately or hours after administration. Angioedema, laryngeal edema and cutaneous hemorrhages may occur.

Iodism or chronic iodine poisoning may occur during prolonged treatment or with the use of high doses. Symptoms of iodism typically disappear soon after discontinuation of the drug. Abundant fluid and salt intake aids in iodide elimination.

DOSAGE AND ADMINISTRATION

Adults—0.3 ml (300 mg) or 0.6 ml (600 mg) diluted in one glassful of water, fruit juice or milk 3 to 4 times daily. To minimize gastric irritation, take with food or milk.

The medication should be used no longer than is necessary to produce the desired effect.

HOW SUPPLIED

SSKI® (potassium iodide oral solution, USP) is supplied in 1 fluid ounce (30 ml) bottles (NDC 0245-0003-31) with a calibrated dropper marked to deliver 0.3 ml (300 mg) and 0.6 ml (600 mg); and 8 fluid ounce (237 ml) bottles (NDC 0245-0003-08). Inactive ingredient: Sodium thiosulfate as a preservative.

Caution: Federal law prohibits dispensing without prescription.

Store at controlled room temperature 59°–86° F (15°–30°C). Keep tightly closed and protect from light.

Dispense in tight, light resistant containers with child resistant closures.

Notice: When exposed to cold temperatures, crystallization may occur, but on warming and shaking, the crystals will redissolve. If the solution turns brownish yellow in color, it should be discarded.

SALSITAB®
[*sal'si"tab*]
**Salsalate
Tablets**

℞

DESCRIPTION

Salsitab® (salsalate) is a nonsteroidal anti-inflammatory agent for oral administration.

Each round, blue, film coated Salsitab® Tablet contains 500 mg salsalate. Each capsule-shaped, blue, scored, film coated Salsitab® Tablet contains 750 mg salsalate.

HOW SUPPLIED

500 mg tablets in bottles of 100 (NDC 0245-0153-11)
500 mg tablets in bottles of 500 (NDC 0245-0153-15)
500 mg tablets in cartons of 100 unit dose (NDC 0245-0153-01)
750 mg tablets in bottles of 100 (NDC 0245-0154-11)
750 mg tablets in bottles of 500 (NDC 0245-0154-15)
750 mg tablets in cartons of 100 unit dose (NDC 0245-0154-01)

SLO-NIACIN® Tablets
**(polygel® controlled-release niacin)
Dietary Supplement**

OTC

DESCRIPTION

Slo-Niacin® Tablets are manufactured utilizing a unique, patented polygel® controlled-release delivery system. This exclusive technology assures the gradual and measured release of niacin (nicotinic acid) and is designed to reduce the incidence of flushing and itching commonly associated with niacin use. Slo-Niacin® Tablets are available in 250 mg, 500 mg, and 750 mg strengths.

SUGGESTED USE

Slo-Niacin® is a member of the vitamin B-complex group (nicotinic acid, vitamin B_3) and is suggested as a dietary supplement. This product has the advantage of a slower release of niacin than conventional dosage forms. This may permit its use by those who do not tolerate immediate-release tablets.

DIRECTIONS

250 mg: Adults—One Slo-Niacin® Tablet morning or evening, or as directed by a physician.
500 mg: Adults—One Slo-Niacin® Tablet morning or evening, or as directed by a physician.
750 mg: Adults—One-half Slo-Niacin® Tablet morning or evening, or as directed by a physician.
Before using more than 500 mg daily, consult a physician.
Note: Slo-Niacin® Tablets may be broken on the score line, but should not be crushed or chewed. The inactive matrix of the tablet is not absorbed and may be excreted intact in the stool.
Store at room temperature, 59°–86°F.
Keep tightly closed.

CAUTION

Niacin may cause temporary flushing, itching and tingling, feelings of warmth and headache, particularly when beginning, increasing amount or changing brand of niacin. These effects seldom require discontinuing niacin use. Skin rash, upset stomach, and low blood pressure when standing are less common symptoms; if they persist, contact a physician.

WARNINGS

Slo-Niacin® Tablets should not be used by persons with a known sensitivity or allergy to niacin. Persons with heart disease, particularly those who have recurrent chest pain (angina) or who recently suffered a heart attack, should take niacin only under the supervision of a physician. Persons taking high blood pressure or cholesterol-lowering drugs should contact a physician before taking niacin because of possible interactions. Do not take niacin unless recommended by and taken under the supervision of a physician if you have any of the following conditions; gallbladder disease, gout, arterial bleeding, glaucoma, diabetes, impaired liver function, peptic ulcer, pregnancy or lactating women. Increased uric acid and glucose levels and abnormal liver function tests have been reported in persons taking daily doses of 500 mg or more of niacin.

Discontinue use and consult a physician immediately if any of the following symptoms occur: persistent flu-like symptoms (nausea, vomiting, a general "not well" feeling); loss of appetite; a decrease in urine output associated with dark-colored urine; muscle discomfort such as tender, swollen muscles or muscle weakness; irregular heartbeat; or cloudy or blurry vision.

Keep out of the reach of children.

INGREDIENTS

250 mg niacin (nicotinic acid), supplying 1,250% of the Reference Daily Intake (RDI) for niacin.
500 mg niacin (nicotinic acid), supplying 2,500% of the Reference Daily Intake (RDI) for niacin.
750 mg niacin (nicotinic acid), supplying 3,750% of the Reference Daily Intake (RDI) for niacin.
Each tablet also contains: cellulose polymer derivative, vegetable stearine, magnesium stearate, silicon dioxide, glyceryl behenate, and FD&C Red # 40.

HOW SUPPLIED

250 mg tablets in bottles of 100: List No. 0245-0062-11
500 mg tablets in bottles of 100: List No. 0245-0063-11
750 mg tablets in bottles of 100: List No. 0245-0064-11
U.S. Patent No. 5,126,145 and other patents pending.
Shown in Product Identification Guide, page 339

Vitaline Corporation
**385 WILLIAMSON WAY
ASHLAND, OR 97520**

Direct Inquiries to:
Jed D. Meese, Technical Director
(541) 482-9231
FAX: (541) 482-9112

L–CARNITINE USP
**250mg Tablets, 500mg Scored Caplets and 500mg
Chewable Wafers
Renal Patient L-Carnitine
Dietary Supplement**

OTC

DESCRIPTION

Carnitine is a naturally occurring substance, and is essential for fatty acid oxidation and energy production. Without it, long-chain fatty acids cannot cross from cellular cytoplasm

Continued on next page

Vitaline—Cont.

into the mitochondria and out again, resulting in loss of energy and toxic accumulations of free fatty acids. Ninety-five percent of the body's carnitine is found in cardiac and skeletal tissue; these muscles rely upon fatty acid oxidation for most of their energy.

INDICATIONS

Dietary supplementation of L-Carnitine for renal patients. Because of dietary restrictions and other factors renal dialysis patients have a limited intake of this essential nutrient.

WARNINGS

None reported.

SUGGESTED USE

As a dietary supplement: Adults, 500mg–1500mg daily or as directed by physician, registered dietitian or nutritionist. Children, as directed by physician.

HOW SUPPLIED

250mg tablets in bottles of 90 NDC 54022-2100-01
500mg scored caplets in bottles of 30 NDC 54022-2120-01
500mg chewable wafers in bottles of 30 NDC 54022-2700-01

REFERENCES

1)Effect of Oral L-Carnitine on Serum Myoglobin in Hemodialysis Patients. *Renal Failure. 18(1):91-96, 1996.*
2)Effects of Nutritional Status and Oral Essential Amino Acid Replacement on Serum L-Carnitine Levels of Chronically Hemodialyzed Patients. *Nephron, 72(2):341-342, February 1996.*
3)A Randomised, Double-Blind, Placebo-Controlled Trial of L-Carnitine in Suspected Acute Myocardial Infarction. *Postgraduate Medical Journal, 72(843):45-50, January 1996.*

COENZYME Q$_{10}$ (Ubiquinone) OTC
200mg, 100mg & 60mg Chewable Wafers, and 200mg, 60mg & 25mg Tablets

DESCRIPTION

Coenzyme Q$_{10}$(CoQ$_{10}$) is an essential nutrient that is a cofactor in the mitochondrial electron transport chain, the biochemical pathway in cellular respiration from which ATP and metabolic energy are derived. Since nearly all cellular functions are dependent on energy, CoQ$_{10}$ is essential for the health of all human tissues and organs. The involvement of CoQ$_{10}$ as a redox carrier of the respiratory chain is well established on the basis of both reconstitution studies and kinetic evidence.
CoQ$_{10}$ is a naturally occurring antioxidant nutrient that retards free radical formation in biological systems.

> Unlike drugs, which pharmacologically act within minutes or hours, CoQ$_{10}$ is a vitamin which acts by natural biochemical and intrinsic mechanisms in the human body over a period of time up to three months.

SUGGESTED USE

As a dietary supplement: Adults, 60mg–200mg daily or as directed by physician or registered dietitian. Children, as directed by physician.

ADVERSE REACTIONS

None reported.

HOW SUPPLIED

200mg with 400 I.U. Vitamin E chewable wafers in bottles of 30; 100mg with 300 I.U. Vitamin E chewable wafers in bottles of 30; 60mg chewable wafers in bottles of 30; 200mg tablets in bottles of 30; 60mg tablets in bottles of 30 & 60; 25mg tablets in bottles of 60

REFERENCES

1) Introduction to Coenzyme Q$_{10}$.Langsjoen, Peter H., M.D., F.A.C.C., 1996. Tyler, TX 75701.
2) Energy and Defense, Facts and Perspectives on Coenzyme Q$_{10}$ in Biology and Medicine. *Littarru, G.P Pub: CESI, Rome, Italy, 1995; ISBN 88-86062-24-9.*
3) Neuroprotective Strategies for Treatment of Lesions Produced by Mitochondrial Toxins: Implications for Neurodegenerative Diseases. *Beal, M.F., et al. Neuroscience, 71(4):1043-1048,1996.*

Wakefield Pharmaceuticals, Inc.
**1050 CAMBRIDGE SQUARE, SUITE C
ALPHARETTA, GA 30201**

WAKEFIELD PHARMACEUTICALS, INC.

1050 Cambridge Square, Suite C
Alpharetta, GA 30201
   Phone (770) 664-1661
   Fax (770) 664-1126
Products Described
● Biohist®-LA Tablets
● Muco-Fen®-LA Tablets
● Muco-Fen® DM Tablets
● Profen-LA® Tablets
● Profen II® Tablets
Other Products

BIOHIST®-LA Tablets ℞
Antihistamine, Decongestant

DESCRIPTION

Each dye-free, timed-released, scored tablet contains:
Carbinoxamine Maleate .... 8 mg
Pseudoephedrine HCl .... 120 mg

HOW SUPPLIED

Bottles of 100 (NDC 59310-101-10)

MUCO-FEN® DM ℞
[mūco-fin]
Dextromethorphan HBR/Guaifenesin

DESCRIPTION

Each dye free, timed release, scored tablet contains:
Dextromethorphan Hydrobromide 30 mg
Guaifemesin 600 mg

HOW SUPPLIED

Bottle of 100 (NDC 59310-108-10)

MUCO-FEN®-LA Tablets ℞
[mūco-fin]
Guaifenesin

DESCRIPTION

Each dye-free, timed-release, scored tablet contains:
Guaifenesin .... 600 mg

HOW SUPPLIED

Bottle of 100 (NDC 59310-102-10)

PROFEN-LA®Tablets ℞
[Pro-fin]
Phenylpropanolamine HCl, Guaifenesin

DESCRIPTION

Each dye-free, timed-release, scored tablet contains:
Phenylpropanolamine HCl .... 75 mg
Guaifenesin .... 600 mg

HOW SUPPLIED

Bottle of 100 (NDC 59310-104-10)

PROFEN II® ℞
[Pro-fin]
Phenylpropanolamine HCl, Guaifenesin

DESCRIPTION

Each dye-free, timed-release, scored tablet contains:
Phenylpropanolamine HCl .... 37.5 mg
Guaifenesin .... 600 mg

HOW SUPPLIED

Bottle of 100 (NDC 59310-107-10)

Wallace Laboratories
**P.O. BOX 1001
CRANBURY, NJ 08512**

**For Medical Information Contact:
Generally:**
Professional Services
(609) 655-6000
After Hours and Weekend Emergencies:
(609) 655-6474

Sales and Ordering:
Wallace Laboratories
Div. of Carter-Wallace, Inc
P.O. Box 1001
Cranbury, NJ 08512

AQUATENSEN® ℞
**(methyclothiazide tablets, USP 5 mg)
Tablets**

BUTISOL SODIUM® ℞ (℃Ⅲ)
**(Butabarbital Sodium Tablets, USP
and Butabarbital Sodium Elixir, USP)
Tablets & Elixir**

DESCRIPTION

BUTISOL SODIUM (butabarbital sodium tablets and butabarbital sodium elixir) is a non-selective central nervous system depressant which is used as a sedative or hypnotic (**WARNING:** May be habit-forming). It is available for oral administration as *Tablets* containing 15 mg, 30 mg, 50 mg, or 100 mg butabarbital sodium; and as *Elixir* containing 30 mg/5 mL, with alcohol (by volume) 7%. Other ingredients in the Tablets are: calcium stearate, corn starch, dibasic calcium phosphate, FD&C Blue No. 1 (15 mg and 30 mg only), FD&C Blue No. 2 (100 mg only), FD&C Red No. 3 (15 mg and 100 mg only), FD&C Yellow No. 5 (30 mg and 50 mg only — see Precautions), FD&C Yellow No. 6 (50 mg only). Other ingredients in the Elixir are: D&C Green No. 5, edetate disodium, FD&C Yellow No. 5 (see Precautions), flavors (natural and artificial), propylene glycol, purified water, saccharin sodium, sodium benzoate. Butabarbital sodium occurs as a white, bitter powder which is freely soluble in water and alcohol, but practically insoluble in benzene and ether.
The structural formula for butabarbital sodium is:

Sodium 5-*sec*-butyl-5-ethylbarbiturate

CLINICAL PHARMACOLOGY

BUTISOL SODIUM (butbarbital sodium tablets and butabarbital sodium elixir), like other barbiturates, is capable of producing all levels of CNS mood alteration from excitation to mild sedation, to hypnosis, and deep coma. Overdosage can produce death. Barbiturates depress the sensory cortex, decrease motor activity, alter cerebellar function, and produce drowsiness, sedation, and hypnosis.
Barbiturate-induced sleep differs from physiological sleep. Sleep laboratory studies have demonstrated that barbiturates reduce the amount of time spent in the rapid eye movement (REM) phase of sleep or dreaming stage. Also, Stages III and IV sleep are decreased. Following abrupt cessation of barbiturates used regularly, patients may experience markedly increased dreaming, nightmares, and/or insomnia. Therefore, withdrawal of a single therapeutic dose over 5 or 6 days has been recommended to lessen the REM rebound and disturbed sleep which contribute to drug withdrawal syndrome (for example, decrease the dose from 3 to 2 doses a day for 1 week).
In studies, secobarbital sodium and pentobarbital sodium have been found to lose most of their effectiveness for both inducing and maintaining sleep by the end of 2 weeks of continued drug administration even with the use of multiple doses. As with secobarbital sodium and pentobarbital sodium, other barbiturates might be expected to lose their effectiveness for inducing and maintaining sleep after about 2 weeks. The short-, intermediate-, and, to a lesser degree, long-acting barbiturates have been widely prescribed for treating insomnia. Although the clinical literature abounds with claims that the short-acting barbiturates are superior for producing sleep while the intermediate-acting compounds are more effective in maintaining sleep, controlled

studies have failed to demonstrate these differential effects. Therefore as sleep medications, the barbiturates are of limited value beyond short-term use.

Barbiturates are respiratory depressants. The degree of respiratory depression is dependent upon dose. With hypnotic doses, respiratory depression produced by barbiturates is similar to that which occurs during physiologic sleep with slight decrease in blood pressure and heart rate.

Barbiturates do not impair normal hepatic function, but have been shown to induce liver microsomal enzymes, thus increasing and/or altering the metabolism of barbiturates and other drugs (see Precautions-*Drug interactions*).

Pharmacokinetics: BUTISOL SODIUM (butabarbital sodium tablets and butabarbital sodium elixir) is the sodium salt of a weak acid. Barbiturates are weak acids that are absorbed and rapidly distributed to all tissues and fluids with high concentrations in the brain, liver, and kidneys. Barbiturates are bound to plasma and tissue proteins. The rate of absorption is increased if it is ingested as a dilute solution or taken on an empty stomach.

Barbiturates are metabolized primarily by the hepatic microsomal enzyme system, and most metabolic products are excreted in the urine. The excretion of unchanged butabarbital in the urine is negligible. BUTISOL SODIUM (butabarbital sodium tablets and butabarbital sodium elixir) is classified as an intermediate-acting barbiturate. The average plasma half-life for butabarbital is 100 hours in the adult. Although variable from patient to patient, butabarbital has an onset of action of about $^3/_4$ to 1 hour, and a duration of action of about 6 to 8 hours.

INDICATIONS AND USAGE

BUTISOL SODIUM (butabarbital sodium tablets and butabarbital sodium elixir) is indicated for use **as a sedative or hypnotic**.

Since barbiturates appear to lose their effectiveness for sleep induction and sleep maintenance after 2 weeks, use of BUTISOL SODIUM in treating insomnia should be limited to this time (see Clinical Pharmacology above).

CONTRAINDICATIONS

Barbiturates are contraindicated in patients with known barbiturate sensitivity. Barbiturates are also contraindicated in patients with a history of manifest or latent porphyria.

WARNINGS

Habit-forming: Barbiturates may be habit-forming. Tolerance, psychological and physical dependence may occur with continued use (see **Drug Abuse and Dependence** below). Patients who have psychological dependence on barbiturates may increase the dosage or decrease the dosage interval without consulting a physician and may subsequently develop a physical dependence on barbiturates. To minimize the possibility of overdosage or the development of dependence, the prescribing and dispensing of sedative-hypnotic barbiturates should be limited to the amount required for the interval until the next appointment. Abrupt cessation after prolonged use in the dependent person may result in withdrawal symptoms, including delirium, convulsions, and possibly death. Barbiturates should be withdrawn gradually from any patient known to be taking excessive dosage over long periods of time. (See **Drug Abuse and Dependence** below.)

Acute or chronic pain: Caution should be exercised when barbiturates are administered to patients with acute or chronic pain, because paradoxical excitement could be induced, or important symptoms could be masked. However, the use of barbiturates as sedatives in the postoperative surgical period, and as adjuncts to cancer chemotherapy, is well established.

Use in pregnancy: Barbiturates can cause fetal damage when administered to a pregnant woman. Retrospective, case-controlled studies have suggested a connection between the maternal consumption of barbiturates and a higher than expected incidence of fetal abnormalities. Following oral administration, barbiturates readily cross the placental barrier and are distributed throughout fetal tissues with highest concentrations found in the placenta, fetal liver, and brain. Withdrawal symptoms occur in infants born to mothers who receive barbiturates throughout the last trimester of pregnancy (see **Drug Abuse and Dependence**). If this drug is used during pregnancy, or if the patient becomes pregnant while taking this drug, the patient should be apprised of the potential hazard to the fetus.

PRECAUTIONS

General: Barbiturates should be administered with caution, if at all, to patients who are mentally depressed, have suicidal tendencies, or a history of drug abuse.

Elderly or debilitated patients may react to barbiturates with marked excitement, depression, and confusion. In some persons, barbiturates repeatedly produce excitement rather than depression.

In patients with hepatic damage, barbiturates should be administered with caution and initially in reduced doses.

Barbiturates should not be administered to patients showing the premonitory signs of hepatic coma.

BUTISOL SODIUM (butabarbital sodium tablets and butabarbital sodium elixir) Tablets, 30 mg and 50 mg, and Elixir contain FD&C Yellow No. 5 (tartrazine) which may cause allergic-type reactions (including bronchial asthma) in certain susceptible individuals. Although the overall incidence of FD&C Yellow No. 5 (tartrazine) sensitivity in the general population is low, it is frequently seen in patients who also have aspirin hypersensitivity.

Information for patients: Practitioners should give the following information and instructions to patients receiving barbiturates.

The use of barbiturates carries with it an associated risk of psychological and/or physical dependence. The patient should be warned against increasing the dose of the drug without consulting a physician.

Barbiturates may impair mental and/or physical abilities required for the performance of potentially hazardous tasks, such as driving or operating machinery.

Alcohol should not be consumed while taking barbiturates. Concurrent use of the barbiturates with other CNS depressants, including other sedatives or hypnotics, alcohol, narcotics, tranquilizers, and antihistamines, may result in additional CNS depressant effects.

Laboratory tests: Prolonged therapy with barbiturates should be accompanied by periodic laboratory evaluation of organ systems, including hematopoietic, renal, and hepatic systems (see **Precautions**—*General* and **Adverse Reactions**).

Drug interactions: Most reports of clinically significant drug interactions occurring with the barbiturates have involved phenobarbital. However, the application of these data to other barbiturates appears valid and warrants serial blood level determinations of the relevant drugs when there are multiple therapies.

1. *Anticoagulants.* Phenobarbital lowers the plasma levels of dicumarol and causes a decrease in anticoagulant activity as measured by the prothrombin time. Barbiturates can induce hepatic microsomal enzymes resulting in increased metabolism and decreased anticoagulant response of oral anticoagulants (e.g., warfarin, acenocoumarol, dicumarol, and phenprocoumon). Patients stabilized on anticoagulant therapy may require dosage adjustments if barbiturates are added to or withdrawn from their dosage regimen.

2. *Corticosteroids.* Barbiturates appear to enhance the metabolism of exogenous corticosteroids probably through the induction of hepatic microsomal enzymes. Patients stabilized on corticosteroid therapy may require dosage adjustments if barbiturates are added to or withdrawn from their dosage regimen.

3. *Griseofulvin.* Phenobarbital appears to interfere with the absorption of orally administered griseofulvin, thus decreasing its blood level. The effect of the resultant decreased blood levels of griseofulvin on therapeutic response has not been established. However, it would be preferable to avoid concomitant administration of these drugs.

4. *Doxycycline.* Phenobarbital has been shown to shorten the half-life of doxycycline for as long as 2 weeks after barbiturate therapy is discontinued. This mechanism is probably through the induction of hepatic microsomal enzymes that metabolize the antibiotic. If phenobarbital and doxycycline are administered concurrently, the clinical response to doxycycline should be monitored closely.

PRECAUTIONS

5. *Phenytoin, sodium valproate, valproic acid.* The effect of barbiturates on the metabolism of phenytoin appears to be variable. Some investigators report an accelerating effect, while others report no effect. Because the effect of barbiturates on the metabolism of phenytoin is not predictable, phenytoin and barbiturate blood levels should be monitored more frequently if these drugs are given concurrently. Sodium valproate and valproic acid appear to decrease barbiturate metabolism; therefore, barbiturate blood levels should be monitored and appropriate dosage adjustments made as indicated.

6. *Central nervous system.* The concomitant use of other central nervous system depressants, including other sedatives or hypnotics, antihistamines, tranquilizers, or alcohol, may produce additive depressant effects.

7. *Monoamine oxidase inhibitors (MAOI).* MAOI prolong the effects of barbiturates probably because metabolism of the barbiturate is inhibited.

8. *Estradiol, estrone, progesterone, and other steroid hormones.* Pretreatment with or concurrent administration of phenobarbital may decrease the effect of estradiol by increasing its metabolism. There have been reports of patients treated with antiepileptic drugs (e.g., phenobarbital) who become pregnant while taking oral contraceptives. An alternate contraceptive method might be suggested to women taking phenobarbital.

Carcinogenesis, mutagenesis, impairment of fertility: No long-term studies in animals have been performed with butabarbital sodium to determine carcinogenic and mutagenic potential, or effects on fertility.

Pregnancy: Teratogenic effects - Pregnancy Category D (see Warnings - *Use in pregnancy* above).

Nonteratogenic effects - Infants suffering from long-term barbiturate exposure *in utero* may have an acute withdrawal syndrome of seizures and hyperirritability from birth to a delayed onset of up to 14 days (see Drug Abuse and Dependence).

Labor and delivery: Hypnotic doses of barbiturates do not appear to significantly impair uterine activity during labor. Administration of sedative-hypnotic barbiturates to the mother during labor may result in respiratory depression in the newborn. Premature infants are particularly susceptible to the depressant effects of barbiturates. If barbiturates are used during labor and delivery, resuscitation equipment should be available.

Nursing mothers: Caution should be exercised when a barbiturate is administered to a nursing woman since small amounts of some barbiturates are excreted in the milk.

ADVERSE REACTIONS

The following adverse reactions have been observed with the use of barbiturates in hospitalized patients. Because such patients may be less aware of certain of the milder adverse effects of barbiturates, the incidence of these reactions may be somewhat higher in fully ambulatory patients.

More than 1 in 100 patients. The most common adverse reaction, somnolence, is estimated to occur at a rate of 1 to 3 patients per 100.

Less than 1 in 100 patients. The most common adverse reactions estimated to occur at a rate of less than 1 in 100 patients listed below, grouped by organ system, and by decreasing order of occurrence are:

Central nervous system/psychiatric: Agitation, confusion, hyperkinesia, ataxia, CNS depression, nightmares, nervousness, psychiatric disturbance, hallucinations, insomnia, anxiety, dizziness, thinking abnormality.
Respiratory: Hypoventilation, apnea.
Cardiovascular: Bradycardia, hypotension, syncope.
Gastrointestinal: Nausea, vomiting, constipation.
Other reported reactions: Headache, hypersensitivity (angioedema, skin rashes, exfoliative dermatitis), fever, liver damage.

DRUG ABUSE AND DEPENDENCE

Controlled substance: Schedule III.

Abuse and dependence: Barbiturates may be habit-forming. Tolerance, psychological dependence, and physical dependence may occur especially following prolonged use of high doses of barbiturates. Daily administration in excess of 400 milligrams (mg) of pentobarbital or secobarbitol for approximately 90 days is likely to produce some degree of physical dependence. A dosage of from 600 to 800 mg taken for at least 35 days is sufficient to produce withdrawal seizures. The average daily dose for the barbiturate addict is usually about 1.5 grams. As tolerance to barbiturates develops, the amount needed to maintain the same level of intoxication increases; tolerance to a fatal dosage, however, does not increase more than two-fold. As this occurs, the margin between an intoxicating dosage and a fatal dosage becomes smaller.

Symptoms of acute intoxication with barbiturates include unsteady gait, slurred speech, and sustained nystagmus. Mental signs of chronic intoxication include confusion, poor judgment, irritability, insomnia, and somatic complaints. Symptoms of barbiturate dependence are similar to those of chronic alcoholism.

If an individual appears to be intoxicated with alcohol to a degree that is radically disproportionate to the amount of alcohol in his or her blood, the use of barbiturates should be suspected. The lethal dose of a barbiturate is far less if alcohol is also ingested.

The symptoms of barbiturate withdrawal can be severe and may cause death. Minor withdrawal symptoms may appear 8 to 12 hours after the last dose of a barbiturate. These symptoms usually appear in the following order: anxiety, muscle twitching, tremor of hands and fingers, progressive weakness, dizziness, distortion in visual perception, nausea, vomiting, insomnia, and orthostatic hypotension. Major withdrawal symptoms (convulsions and delirium) may occur within 16 hours and last up to 5 days after abrupt cessation of these drugs. Intensity of withdrawal symptoms gradually declines over a period of approximately 15 days.

Drug dependence to barbiturates arises from repeated administration of a barbiturate or agent with barbiturate-like effect on a continuous basis, generally in amounts exceeding therapeutic dose levels. The characteristics of drug dependence to barbiturates include: (a) a strong desire or need to continue taking the drug; (b) a tendency to increase the dose; (c) a psychic dependence on the effects of the drug related to subjective and individual appreciation for those effects; and (d) a physical dependence on the effects of the drug requiring its presence for maintenance of homeostasis and resulting in a definite, characteristic, and self-limited abstinence syndrome when the drug is withdrawn.

Continued on next page

Wallace Laboratories—Cont.

Treatment of barbiturate dependence consists of cautious and gradual withdrawal of the drug. Barbiturate-dependent patients can be withdrawn by using a number of different withdrawal regimens. In all cases, withdrawal takes an extended period of time. One method involves initiating treatment at the patient's regular dosage level, in 3 to 4 divided doses, and decreasing the daily dose by 10 percent if tolerated by the patient.

Infants physically dependent on barbiturates may be given phenobarbital 3 to 10 mg/kg/day. After withdrawal symptoms (hyperactivity, disturbed sleep, tremors, hyperreflexia) are relieved, the dosage of phenobarbital should be gradually decreased and completely withdrawn over a 2-week period.

OVERDOSAGE

Signs and symptoms: The toxic dose of barbiturates varies considerably. In general, an oral dose of 1 gram of most barbiturates produces serious poisoning in an adult. Death commonly occurs after 2 to 10 grams of ingested barbiturates. Symptoms of acute intoxication with barbiturates include unsteady gait, slurred speech, and sustained nystagmus. Mental signs of chronic intoxication include confusion, poor judgment, irritability, insomnia, and somatic complaints. Barbiturate intoxication may be confused with alcoholism, bromide intoxication, and with various neurological disorders.

Acute overdosage with barbiturates is manifested by CNS and respiratory depression which may progress to Cheyne-Stokes respiration, areflexia, constriction of the pupils to a slight degree (though in severe poisoning they may show paralytic dilation), oliguria, tachycardia, hypotension, lowered body temperature, and coma. Typical shock syndrome (apnea, circulatory collapse, respiratory arrest, and death) may occur.

In extreme overdose, all electrical activity in the brain may cease, in which case a "flat" EEG normally equated with clinical death cannot be accepted. This effect is fully reversible unless hypoxic damage occurs. Consideration should be given to the possibility of barbiturate intoxication even in situations that appear to involve trauma.

Complications: Pneumonia, pulmonary edema, cardiac arrhythmias, congestive heart failure, and renal failure may occur. Uremia may increase CNS sensitivity to barbiturates if renal function is impaired. Differential diagnosis should include hypoglycemia, head trauma, cerebrovascular accidents, convulsive states, and diabetic coma.

Treatment: Treatment of overdosage is mainly supportive and consists of the following:

1. Maintenance of an adequate airway, with assisted respiration and oxygen administration as necessary.
2. Monitoring of vital signs and fluid balance.
3. If the patient is conscious and has not lost the gag reflex, emesis may be induced with ipecac. Care should be taken to prevent pulmonary aspiration of vomitus. After completion of vomiting, 30 grams activated charcoal in a glass of water may be administered.
4. If emesis is contraindicated, gastric lavage may be performed with a cuffed endotracheal tube in place with the patient in the face down position. Activated charcoal may be left in the emptied stomach and a saline cathartic administered.
5. Fluid therapy and other standard treatment for shock, if needed.
6. If renal function is normal, forced diuresis may aid in the elimination of the barbiturate.
7. Although not recommended as a routine procedure, hemodialysis may be used in severe barbiturate intoxications or if the patient is anuric or in shock.
8. Appropriate nursing care, including rolling patients from side-to-side every 30 minutes, to prevent hypostatic pneumonia, decubiti, aspiration, and other complications of patients with altered states of consciousness.
9. Antibiotics should be given if pneumonia is suspected.

DOSAGE AND ADMINISTRATION

Usual adult dosage:
Daytime sedative—15 to 30 mg, 3 or 4 times daily.
Bedtime hypnotic—50 to 100 mg.
Preoperative sedative—50 to 100 mg, 60 to 90 minutes before surgery.
Usual pediatric dosage:
Preoperative sedative—2 to 6 mg/kg maximum 100 mg.
Special patient population:
Dosage should be reduced in the elderly or debilitated because these patients may be more sensitive to barbiturates. Dosage should be reduced for patients with impaired renal function or hepatic disease (see **Precautions**).

HOW SUPPLIED

BUTISOL SODIUM® (butabarbital sodium tablets and butabarbital sodium elixir) Tablets:

15 mg— colored lavender, scored, imprinted "BUTISOL SODIUM"

and $\frac{37}{112}$ in bottles of 100

(NDC 0037-0112-60) and 1000 (NDC 0037-0112-80).

30 mg*— colored green, scored, imprinted "BUTISOL SODIUM"

and $\frac{37}{113}$ in bottles of 100

(NDC 0037-0113-60) and 1000 (NDC 0037-0113-80).

50 mg*— colored orange, scored, imprinted "BUTISOL SODIUM"

and $\frac{37}{114}$ in bottles of 100

(NDC 0037-0114-60).

100 mg— colored pink, scored, imprinted "BUTISOL SODIUM"

and $\frac{37}{115}$ in bottles of 100

(NDC 0037-0115-60).

BUTISOL SODIUM® (butabarbital sodium tablets and butabarbital sodium elixir) Elixir*: 30 mg/5 mL, alcohol (by volume) 7%-colored green, in bottles of one pint (NDC 0037-0110-16) and one gallon (NDC 0037-0110-28).

*Contains FD&C Yellow No. 5 (see Precautions).

Storage: Store at controlled room temperature 15°–30°C (59°–86°F).

Dispense in a tight container.

WALLACE LABORATORIES
Division of
CARTER-WALLACE, INC.
Cranbury, New Jersey 08512
IN-0110-05   Rev. 11/94

DEPEN®   ℞
(penicillamine tablets, USP)
Titratable Tablets

> Physicians planning to use penicillamine should thoroughly familiarize themselves with its toxicity, special dosage considerations, and therapeutic benefits. Penicillamine should never be used casually. Each patient should remain constantly under the close supervision of the physician. Patients should be warned to report promptly any symptoms suggesting toxicity.

DESCRIPTION

Penicillamine is 3-mercapto-D-valine, a disease modifying antirheumatic drug. It is a white or practically white, crystalline powder, freely soluble in water, slightly soluble in alcohol, and insoluble in ether, acetone, benzene, and carbon tetrachloride. Although its configuration is D, it is levorotatory as usually measured:

$$[\alpha]\,^{25°}_D = -62.5° \pm 2.0° \ (C = 1, 1N \ NaOH)$$

The empirical formula is $C_5H_{11}NO_2S$, giving it a molecular weight of 149.21. The structural formula is:

$$HS-\underset{\underset{CH_3}{|}}{\overset{\overset{CH_3}{|}}{C}}-\underset{\underset{NH_2}{|}}{\overset{\overset{H}{|}}{C}}-COOH$$

It reacts readily with formaldehyde or acetone to form a thiazolidine-carboxylic acid.

Depen® (penicillamine tablets, USP) Titratable Tablets for oral administration contain 250 mg of penicillamine.

Other ingredients (inactive): edetate disodium, hydroxypropyl methylcellulose, lactose, magnesium stearate, magnesium trisilicate, polyethylene glycol, povidone, simethicone emulsion, starch, and stearic acid.

CLINICAL PHARMACOLOGY

Penicillamine is a chelating agent recommended for the removal of excess copper in patients with Wilson's disease. From *in vitro* studies which indicate that one atom of copper combines with two molecules of penicillamine, it would appear that one gram of penicillamine should be followed by the excretion of about 200 milligrams of copper; however, the actual amount excreted is about one percent of this. Penicillamine also reduces excess cystine excretion in cystinuria. This is done, at least in part, by disulfide interchange between penicillamine and cystine, resulting in formation of penicillamine-cysteine disulfide, a substance that is much more soluble than cystine and is excreted readily.

Penicillamine interferes with the formation of cross-links between tropocollagen molecules and cleaves them when newly formed.

The mechanism of action of penicillamine in rheumatoid arthritis is unknown, although it appears to suppress disease activity. Unlike cytotoxic immunosuppressants, penicillamine markedly lowers IgM rheumatoid factor but produces no significant depression in absolute levels of serum immunoglobulins. Also unlike cytotoxic immunosuppressants, which act on both, penicillamine *in vitro* depresses T-cell activity but not B-cell activity.

In vitro, penicillamine dissociates macroglobulins (rheumatoid factor) although the relationship of the activity to its effect in rheumatoid arthritis is not known.

In rheumatoid arthritis, the onset of therapeutic response to DEPEN may not be seen for two or three months. In those patients who respond, however, the first evidence of suppression of symptoms such as pain, tenderness, and swelling usually is generally apparent within three months. The optimum duration of therapy has not been determined. If remissions occur, they may last from months to years but usually require continued treatment (see DOSAGE AND ADMINISTRATION).

In all patients receiving penicillamine, it is important that DEPEN be given on an empty stomach, at least one hour before meals or two hours after meals, and at least one hour apart from any other drug, food or milk. This permits maximum absorption and reduces the likelihood of inactivation by metal binding in the gastrointestinal tract.

Methodology for determining the bioavailability of penicillamine is not available; however, penicillamine is known to be a very soluble substance.

INDICATIONS

DEPEN is indicated in the treatment of Wilson's disease, cystinuria, and in patients with severe, active rheumatoid arthritis who have failed to respond to an adequate trial of conventional therapy. Available evidence suggests that DEPEN is not of value in ankylosing spondylitis.

Wilson's disease—Wilson's disease (hepatolenticular degeneration) results from the interaction of an inherited defect and an abnormality in copper metabolism. The metabolic defect, which is the consequence of the autosomal inheritance of one abnormal gene from each parent, manifests itself in a greater positive copper balance than normal. As a result, copper is deposited in several organs and appears eventually to produce pathologic effects most prominently seen in the brain, where degeneration is widespread; in the liver, where fatty infiltration, inflammation, and hepatocellular damage progress to postnecrotic cirrhosis; in the kidney, where tubular and glomerular dysfunction results; and in the eye, where characteristic corneal copper deposits are known as Kayser-Fleischer rings.

Two types of patients require treatment for Wilson's disease: (1) the symptomatic, and (2) the asymptomatic in whom it can be assumed the disease will develop in the future if the patient is not treated.

Diagnosis, suspected on the basis of family or individual history, physical examination, or a low serum concentration of ceruloplasmin,* is confirmed by the demonstration of Kayser-Fleischer rings or, particularly in the asymptomatic patient, by the quantitative demonstration in a liver biopsy specimen of a concentration of copper in excess of 250 mcg/g dry weight.

* For quantitative test for serum ceruloplasmin see: Morell, A. G.; Windsor, J.; Sternlieb, I.; Scheinberg, I. H.: Measurement of the concentration of ceruloplasmin in serum by determination of its oxidase activity, in "Laboratory Diagnosis of Liver Disease," F. W. Sunderman; F. W Sunderman, Jr. (eds.), St. Louis, Warren H. Green, Inc., 1968, pp. 193–195.

Treatment has two objectives:
(1) to minimize dietary intake and absorption of copper.
(2) to promote excretion of copper deposited in tissues.

The first objective is attained by a daily diet that contains no more than one or two milligrams of copper. Such a diet should exclude, most importantly, chocolate, nuts, shellfish, mushrooms, liver, molasses, broccoli, and cereals enriched with copper, and be composed to as great an extent as possible of foods with a low copper content. Distilled or demineralized water should be used if the patient's drinking water contains more than 0.1 mg of copper per liter.

For the second objective, a copper chelating agent is used. In symptomatic patients, this treatment usually produces marked neurologic improvement, fading of Kayser-Fleischer rings, and gradual amelioration of hepatic dysfunction and psychic disturbances.

Clinical experience to date suggests that life is prolonged with the above regimen.

Noticeable improvement may not occur for one to three months. Occasionally, neurologic symptoms become worse during initiation of therapy with DEPEN. Despite this, the drug should not be discontinued permanently. Although temporary interruption may result in clinical improvement of the neurological symptoms, it carries an increased risk of

developing a sensitivity reaction upon resumption of therapy (See WARNINGS).

Treatment of asymptomatic patients has been carried out for over ten years. Symptoms and signs of the disease appear to be prevented indefinitely if daily treatment with DEPEN can be continued.

Cystinuria—Cystinuria is characterized by excessive urinary excretion of the dibasic amino acids, arginine, lysine, ornithine, and cystine, and the mixed disulfide of cysteine and homocysteine. The metabolic defect that leads to cystinuria is inherited as an autosomal, recessive trait. Metabolism of the affected amino acids is influenced by at least two abnormal factors: (1) defective gastrointestinal absorption and (2) renal tubular dysfunction.

Arginine, lysine, ornithine, and cysteine are soluble substances, readily excreted. There is no apparent pathology connected with their excretion in excessive quantities.

Cystine, however, is so slightly soluble at the usual range of urinary pH that it is not excreted readily, and so crystallizes and forms stones in the urinary tract. Stone formation is the only known pathology in cystinuria. Normal daily output of cystine is 40 to 80 mg. In cystinuria, output is greatly increased and may exceed 1 g/day. At 500 to 600 mg/day, stone formation is almost certain. When it is more than 300 mg/day, treatment is indicated.

Conventional treatment is directed at keeping urinary cystine diluted enough to prevent stone formation, keeping the urine alkaline enough to dissolve as much cystine as possible, and minimizing cystine production by a diet low in methionine (the major dietary precursor of cystine). Patients must drink enough fluid to keep urine specific gravity below 1.010, take enough alkali to keep urinary pH at 7.5 to 8, and maintain a diet low in methionine. This diet is not recommended in growing children and probably is contraindicated in pregnancy because of its low protein content (see PRECAUTIONS).

When these measures are inadequate to control recurrent stone formation, DEPEN may be used as additional therapy. When patients refuse to adhere to conventional treatment, DEPEN may be a useful substitute. It is capable of keeping cystine excretion to near normal values, thereby hindering stone formation and the serious consequences of pyelonephritis and impaired renal function that develop in some patients.

Bartter and colleagues depict the process by which penicillamine interacts with cystine to form penicillamine-cysteine mixed disulfide as:

$$\text{CSSC} + \text{PS}' \rightleftarrows \text{CS}' + \text{CSSP}$$
$$\text{PSSP} + \text{CS}' \rightleftarrows \text{PS}' + \text{CSSP}$$
$$\text{CSSC} + \text{PSSP} \rightleftarrows 2\,\text{CSSP}$$

CSSC = cystine
CS′ = deprotonated cysteine
PSSP = penicillamine
PS′ = deprotonated penicillamine sulfhydryl
CSSP = penicillamine-cysteine mixed disulfide

In this process, it is assumed that the deprotonated form of penicillamine, PS′, is the active factor in bringing about the disulfide interchange.

Rheumatoid Arthritis—Because DEPEN can cause severe adverse reactions, its use in rheumatoid arthritis should be restricted to patients who have severe, active disease and who have failed to respond to an adequate trial of conventional therapy. Even then, benefit-to-risk ratio should be carefully considered. Other measures, such as rest, physiotherapy, salicylates, and corticosteroids should be used, when indicated, in conjunction with DEPEN (see PRECAUTIONS).

CONTRAINDICATIONS

Except for treatment of Wilson's disease or certain cases of cystinuria, use of penicillamine during pregnancy is contraindicated (see WARNINGS).

Although breast milk studies have not been reported in animals or humans, mothers on therapy with penicillamine should not nurse their infants.

Patients with a history of penicillamine-related aplastic anemia or agranulocytosis should not be restarted on penicillamine (see WARNINGS and ADVERSE REACTIONS).

Because of its potential for causing renal damage, penicillamine should not be administered to rheumatoid arthritis patients with a history or other evidence of renal insufficiency.

WARNINGS

The use of penicillamine has been associated with fatalities due to certain diseases, such as aplastic anemia, agranulocytosis, thrombocytopenia, Goodpasture's syndrome, and myasthenia gravis.

Because of the potential for serious hematological and renal adverse reactions to occur at any time, routine urinalysis, white and differential blood cell count, hemoglobin determination, and direct platelet count must be done every two weeks for at least the first six months of penicillamine therapy and monthly thereafter. Patients should be instructed to report promptly the development of signs and symptoms of granulocytopenia and/or thrombocytopenia such as fever, sore throat, chills, bruising, or bleeding. The above laboratory studies should then be promptly repeated.

Leukopenia and thrombocytopenia have been reported to occur in up to five percent of patients during penicillamine therapy. Leukopenia is of the granulocytic series and may or may not be associated with an increase in eosinophils. A confirmed reduction in WBC below 3500 per cubic mL mandates discontinuance of penicillamine therapy. Thrombocytopenia may be on an idiosyncratic basis with decreased or absent megakaryocytes in the marrow, when it is part of an aplastic anemia. In other cases the thrombocytopenia is presumably on an immune basis since the number of megakaryocytes in the marrow has been reported to be normal or sometimes increased. The development of a platelet count below 100,000 per cubic mL, even in the absence of clinical bleeding, requires at least temporary cessation of penicillamine therapy. A progressive fall in either platelet count or WBC in three successive determinations, even though values are still within the normal range, likewise requires at least temporary cessation.

Proteinuria and/or hematuria may develop during therapy and may be warning signs of membranous glomerulopathy which can progress to a nephrotic syndrome. Close observation of these patients is essential. In some patients the proteinuria disappears with continued therapy; in others penicillamine must be discontinued. When a patient develops proteinuria or hematuria the physician must ascertain whether it is a sign of drug-induced glomerulopathy or is unrelated to penicillamine.

Rheumatoid arthritis patients who develop moderate degrees of proteinuria may be continued cautiously on penicillamine therapy, provided that quantitative 24-hour urinary protein determinations are obtained at intervals of one to two weeks. Penicillamine dosage should not be increased under these circumstances. Proteinuria which exceeds 1 g/24 hours, or proteinuria which is progressively increasing requires either discontinuance of the drug or a reduction in the dosage. In some patients, proteinuria has been reported to clear following reduction in dosage.

In rheumatoid arthritis patients, penicillamine should be discontinued if unexplained gross hematuria or persistent microscopic hematuria develops.

In patients with Wilson's disease or cystinuria the risks of continued penicillamine therapy in patients manifesting potentially serious urinary abnormalities must be weighed against the expected therapeutic benefits.

When penicillamine is used in cystinuria, an annual x-ray for renal stones is advised. Cystine stones form rapidly, sometimes in six months.

Up to one year or more may be required for any urinary abnormalities to disappear after penicillamine has been discontinued.

Because of rare reports of intrahepatic cholestasis and toxic hepatitis, liver function tests are recommended every six months for the duration of therapy.

Goodpasture's syndrome has occurred rarely. The development of abnormal urinary findings associated with hemoptysis and pulmonary infiltrates on x-ray requires immediate cessation of penicillamine.

Obliterative bronchiolitis has been reported rarely. The patient should be cautioned to report immediately pulmonary symptoms such as exertional dyspnea, unexplained cough, or wheezing. Pulmonary function studies should be considered at that time.

Myasthenic syndrome sometimes progressing to myasthenia gravis has been reported. Ptosis and diplopia, with weakness of the extraocular muscles, are often early signs of myasthenia. In the majority of cases, symptoms of myasthenia have receded after withdrawal of penicillamine.

Most of the various forms of pemphigus have occurred during treatment with penicillamine. Pemphigus vulgaris and pemphigus foliaceus are reported most frequently, usually as a late complication of therapy. The seborrhea-like characteristics of pemphigus foliaceus may obscure an early diagnosis. When pemphigus is suspected, DEPEN should be discontinued. Treatment has consisted of high doses of corticosteroids alone or, in some cases, concomitantly with an immunosuppressant. Treatment may be required for only a few weeks or months, but may need to be continued for more than a year.

Once instituted for Wilson's disease or cystinuria, treatment with penicillamine should, as a rule, be continued on a daily basis. Interruptions for even a few days have been followed by sensitivity reactions after reinstitution of therapy.

Use in Pregnancy—Penicillamine has been shown to be teratogenic in rats when given in doses 6 times higher than the highest dose recommended for human use (based on a standard weight of 50 kg). Skeletal defects, cleft palates, and fetal toxicity (resorptions) have been reported.

There are no controlled studies on the use of penicillamine in pregnant women. Although normal outcomes have been reported, characteristic congenital cutis laxa and associated birth defects have been reported in infants born of mothers who received therapy with penicillamine during pregnancy. Penicillamine should be used in women of childbearing potential only when the expected benefits outweigh the possible hazards. Women on therapy with penicillamine who are of childbearing potential should be apprised of this risk, advised to report promptly any missed menstrual periods or other indications of possible pregnancy, and followed closely for early recognition of pregnancy.

Wilson's Disease—Reported experience* shows that continued treatment with penicillamine throughout pregnancy protects the mother against relapse of the Wilson's disease, and that discontinuation of penicillamine has deleterious effects on the mother.

* Scheinberg, I. H., Sternlieb, I.: *N Engl J Med 293:* 1300–1302, December 18, 1975.

If penicillamine is administered during pregnancy to patients with Wilson's disease, it is recommended that the daily dosage be limited to 1 g. If cesarean section is planned, the daily dosage should be limited to 250 mg during the last six weeks of pregnancy and postoperatively until wound healing is complete.

Cystinuria—If possible, penicillamine should not be given during pregnancy to women with cystinuria (see CONTRAINDICATIONS). There are reports of women with cystinuria on therapy with penicillamine who gave birth to infants with generalized connective tissue defects who died following abdominal surgery. If stones continue to form in these patients, the benefits of therapy to the mother must be evaluated against the risk to the fetus.

Rheumatoid Arthritis—Penicillamine should not be administered to rheumatoid arthritis patients who are pregnant (see CONTRAINDICATIONS) and should be discontinued promptly in patients in whom pregnancy is suspected or diagnosed.

There is a report that a woman with rheumatoid arthritis treated with less than one gram a day of penicillamine during pregnancy gave birth (cesarean delivery) to an infant with growth retardation, flattened face with broad nasal bridge, low set ears, short neck with loose skin folds, and unusually lax body skin.

PRECAUTIONS

Some patients may experience drug fever, a marked febrile response to penicillamine, usually in the second or third week following initiation of therapy. Drug fever may sometimes be accompanied by a macular cutaneous eruption.

In the case of drug fever in patients with Wilson's disease or cystinuria, penicillamine should be temporarily discontinued until the reaction subsides. Then penicillamine should be reinstituted with a small dose that is gradually increased until the desired dosage is attained. Systemic steroid therapy may be necessary, and is usually helpful, in such patients in whom toxic reactions develop a second or third time.

In the case of drug fever in rheumatoid arthritis patients, because other treatments are available, penicillamine should be discontinued and another therapeutic alternative tried, since experience indicates that the febrile reaction will recur in a very high percentage of patients upon readministration of penicillamine.

The skin and mucous membranes should be observed for allergic reactions. Early and late rashes have occurred. Early rash occurs during the first few months of treatment and is more common. It is usually a generalized pruritic, erythematous, maculopapular, or morbilliform rash and resembles the allergic rash seen with other drugs. Early rash usually disappears within days after stopping penicillamine and seldom recurs when the drug is restarted at a lower dosage. Pruritus and early rash may often be controlled by the concomitant administration of antihistamines. Less commonly, a late rash may be seen, usually after six months or more of treatment, and requires discontinuation of penicillamine. It is usually on the trunk, is accompanied by intense pruritus, and is usually unresponsive to topical corticosteroid therapy. Late rash may take weeks to disappear after penicillamine is stopped and usually recurs if the drug is restarted.

The appearance of a drug eruption accompanied by fever, arthralgia, lymphadenopathy, or other allergic manifestations usually requires discontinuation of penicillamine.

Certain patients will develop a positive antinuclear antibody (ANA) test and some of these may show a lupus erythematosus-like syndrome similar to drug-induced lupus associated with other drugs. The lupus erythematosus-like syndrome is not associated with hypocomplementemia and may be present without nephropathy. The development of a positive ANA test does not mandate discontinuance of the drug; however, the physician should be alerted to the possibility that a lupus erythematosus-like syndrome may develop in the future.

Some patients may develop oral ulcerations which in some cases have the appearance of aphthous stomatitis. The stomatitis usually recurs on rechallenge but often clears on a lower dosage. Although rare, cheilosis, glossitis, and gingivostomatitis have also been reported. These oral lesions are frequently dose-related and may preclude further increase

Continued on next page

Wallace Laboratories—Cont.

in penicillamine dosage or require discontinuation of the drug.

Hypogeusia (a blunting or diminution in taste perception) has occurred in some patients. This may last two to three months or more and may develop into a total loss of taste; however, it is usually self-limited, despite continued penicillamine treatment. Such taste impairment is rare in patients with Wilson's disease.

Penicillamine should not be used in patients who are receiving concurrently gold therapy, antimalarial or cytotoxic drugs, oxyphenbutazone, or phenylbutazone because these drugs are also associated with similar serious hematologic and renal adverse reactions. Patients who have had gold salt therapy discontinued due to a major toxic reaction may be at greater risk of serious adverse reactions with penicillamine, but not necessarily of the same type.

Patients who are allergic to penicillin may theoretically have cross-sensitivity to penicillamine. The possibility of reactions from contamination of penicillamine by trace amounts of penicillin has been eliminated now that penicillamine is being produced synthetically rather than as a degradation product of penicillin.

Because of their dietary restrictions, patients with Wilson's disease and cystinuria should be given 25 mg/day of pyridoxine during therapy, since penicillamine increases the requirement for this vitamin. Patients also may receive benefit from a multivitamin preparation, although there is no evidence that deficiency of any vitamin other than pyridoxine is associated with penicillamine. In Wilson's disease, multivitamin preparations must be copper-free.

Rheumatoid arthritis patients whose nutrition is impaired should also be given a daily supplement of pyridoxine. Mineral supplements should not be given, since they may block the response to penicillamine.

Iron deficiency may develop, especially in children and in menstruating women. In Wilson's disease, this may be a result of adding the effects of the low copper diet, which is probably also low in iron, and the penicillamine to the effects of blood loss or growth. In cystinuria, a low methionine diet may contribute to iron deficiency, since it is necessarily low in protein. If necessary, iron may be given in short courses, but a period of two hours should elapse between administration of penicillamine and iron, since orally administered iron has been shown to reduce the effects of penicillamine.

Penicillamine causes an increase in the amount of soluble collagen. In the rat this results in inhibition of normal healing and also a decrease in tensile strength of intact skin. In man this may be the cause of increased skin friability at sites especially subject to pressure or trauma, such as shoulders, elbows, knees, toes, and buttocks. Extravasations of blood may occur and may appear as purpuric areas, with external bleeding if the skin is broken, or as vesicles containing dark blood. Neither type is progressive. There is no apparent association with bleeding elsewhere in the body and no associated coagulation defect has been found. Therapy with penicillamine may be continued in the presence of these lesions. They may not recur if dosage is reduced. Other reported effects probably due to the action of penicillamine on collagen are excessive wrinkling of the skin and development of small, white papules at venipuncture and surgical sites.

The effects of penicillamine on collagen and elastin make it advisable to consider a reduction in dosage to 250 mg/day when surgery is contemplated. Reinstitution of full therapy should be delayed until wound healing is complete.

Carcinogenesis—Long-term animal carcinogenicity studies have not been done with penicillamine. There is a report that five of ten autoimmune disease-prone NZB hybrid mice developed lymphocytic leukemia after 6 months' intraperitoneal treatment with a dose of 400 mg/kg penicillamine 5 days per week.

Nursing Mothers—See CONTRAINDICATIONS.

Usage in Children—The efficacy of DEPEN in juvenile rheumatoid arthritis has not been established.

ADVERSE REACTIONS

Penicillamine is a drug with a high incidence of untoward reactions, some of which are potentially fatal. Therefore, it is mandatory that patients receiving penicillamine therapy remain under close medical supervision throughout the period of drug administration (see WARNINGS and PRECAUTIONS).

Reported incidences (%) for the most commonly occurring adverse reactions in rheumatoid arthritis patients are noted, based on 17 representative clinical trials reported in the literature (1270 patients).

Allergic—Generalized pruritus, early and late rashes (5%), pemphigus (see WARNINGS), and drug eruptions which may be accompanied by fever, arthralgia, or lymphadenopathy have occurred (see WARNINGS and PRECAUTIONS). Some patients may show a lupus erythematosus-like syndrome similar to drug-induced lupus produced by other pharmacological agents (see PRECAUTIONS).

Urticaria and exfoliative dermatitis have occurred. Thyroiditis has been reported; hypoglycemia in association with anti-insulin antibodies has been reported. These reactions are extremely rare.

Some patients may develop a migratory polyarthralgia, often with objective synovitis (see DOSAGE AND ADMINISTRATION).

Gastrointestinal—Anorexia, epigastric pain, nausea, vomiting, or occasional diarrhea may occur (17%).

Isolated cases of reactivated peptic ulcer have occurred, as have hepatic dysfunction and pancreatitis. Intrahepatic cholestasis and toxic hepatitis have been reported rarely. There have been a few reports of increased serum alkaline phosphatase, lactic dehydrogenase, and positive cephalin flocculation and thymol turbidity tests.

Some patients may report a blunting, diminution, or total loss of taste perception (12%); or may develop oral ulcerations. Although rare, cheilosis, glossitis, and gingivostomatitis have been reported (see PRECAUTIONS).

Gastrointestinal side effects are usually reversible following cessation of therapy.

Hematological—Penicillamine can cause bone marrow depression (see WARNINGS). Leukopenia (2%) and thrombocytopenia (4%) have occurred. Fatalities have been reported as a result of thrombocytopenia, agranulocytosis, aplastic anemia, and sideroblastic anemia.

Thrombotic thrombocytopenic purpura, hemolytic anemia, red cell aplasia, monocytosis, leukocytosis, eosinophilia, and thrombocytosis have also been reported.

Renal—Patients on penicillamine therapy may develop proteinuria (6%) and/or hematuria which, in some, may progress to the development of the nephrotic syndrome as a result of an immune complex membranous glomerulopathy (see WARNINGS).

Central Nervous System—Tinnitus, optic neuritis, and peripheral sensory and motor neuropathies (including polyradiculoneuropathy, i.e., Guillain-Barre Syndrome) have been reported. Muscular weakness may or may not occur with the peripheral neuropathies.

Neuromuscular—Myasthenia gravis (see WARNINGS).

Other—Adverse reactions that have been reported rarely include thrombophlebitis; hyperpyrexia (see PRECAUTIONS); falling hair or alopecia; lichen planus; polymyositis; dermatomyositis; mammary hyperplasia; elastosis perforans serpiginosa; toxic epidermal necrolysis; anetoderma (cutaneous macular atrophy); and Goodpasture's syndrome, a severe and ultimately fatal glomerulonephritis associated with intra-alveolar hemorrhage (see WARNINGS). Fatal renal vasculitis has also been reported. Allergic alveolitis, obliterative bronchiolitis, interstitial pneumonitis, and pulmonary fibrosis have been reported in patients with severe rheumatoid arthritis, some of whom were receiving penicillamine. Bronchial asthma has also been reported.

Increased skin friability, excessive wrinkling of skin, and development of small, white papules at venipuncture and surgical sites have been reported (see PRECAUTIONS).

The chelating action of the drug may cause increased excretion of other heavy metals such as zinc, mercury and lead. There have been reports associating penicillamine with leukemia. However, circumstances involved in these reports are such that a cause and effect relationship to the drug has not been established.

DOSAGE AND ADMINISTRATION

In all patients receiving penicillamine, it is important that DEPEN be given on an empty stomach, at least one hour before meals or two hours after meals, and at least one hour apart from any other drug, food, or milk. Because penicillamine increases the requirement for pyridoxine, patients may require a daily supplement of pyridoxine (see PRECAUTIONS).

Wilson's Disease—Optimal dosage can be determined by measurement of urinary copper excretion and the determination of free copper in the serum. The urine must be collected in copper-free glassware, and should be quantitatively analyzed for copper before and soon after initiation of therapy with DEPEN.

Determination of 24-hour urinary copper excretions is of greatest value in the first week of therapy with penicillamine. In the absence of any drug reaction, a dose between 0.75 and 1.5 g that results in an initial 24-hour cupriuresis of over 2 mg should be continued for about three months, by which time the most reliable method of monitoring maintenance treatment is the determination of free copper in the serum. This equals the difference between quantitatively determined total copper and ceruloplasmin-copper. Adequately treated patients will usually have less than 10 mcg free copper/dL of serum. It is seldom necessary to exceed a dosage of 2 g/day. If the patient is intolerant to therapy with DEPEN, alternative treatment is trientine hydrochloride.

In patients who cannot tolerate as much as 1 g/day initially, initiating dosage with 250 mg/day, and increasing gradually to the requisite amount, gives closer control of the effects of the drug and may help to reduce the incidence of adverse reactions.

Cystinuria—It is recommended that DEPEN be used along with conventional therapy. By reducing urinary cystine, it decreases crystalluria and stone formation. In some instances, it has been reported to decrease the size of, and even to dissolve, stones already formed.

The usual dosage of DEPEN in the treatment of cystinuria is 2 g/day for adults, with a range of 1 to 4 g/day. For children, dosage can be based on 30 mg/kg/day. The total daily amount should be divided into four doses. If four equal doses are not feasible, give the larger portion at bedtime. If adverse reactions necessitate a reduction in dosage, it is important to retain the bedtime dose.

Initiating dosage with 250 mg/day, and increasing gradually to the requisite amount, gives closer control of the effects of the drug and may help to reduce the incidence of adverse reactions.

In addition to taking DEPEN, patients should drink copiously. It is especially important to drink about a pint of fluid at bedtime and another pint once during the night when urine is more concentrated and more acid than during the day. The greater the fluid intake, the lower the required dosage of DEPEN.

Dosage must be individualized to an amount that limits cystine excretion to 100–200 mg/day in those with no history of stones, and below 100 mg/day in those who have had stone formation and/or pain. Thus, in determining dosage, the inherent tubular defect, the patient's size, age, and rate of growth, and his diet and water intake all must be taken into consideration.

The standard nitroprusside cyanide test has been reported useful as a qualitative measure of the effective dose[*]: Add 2 mL of freshly prepared 5 percent sodium cyanide to 5 mL of a 24-hour aliquot of protein-free urine and let stand ten minutes. Add 5 drops of freshly prepared 5 percent sodium nitroprusside and mix. Cystine will turn the mixture magenta. If the result is negative, it can be assumed that cystine excretion is less than 100 mg/g creatinine.

[*] Lotz, M., Potts, J. T. and Bartter, F. C.: *Brit Med J 2* :521, August 28, 1965 (in Medical Memoranda).

Although penicillamine is rarely excreted unchanged, it also will turn the mixture magenta. If there is any question as to which substance is causing the reaction, a ferric chloride test can be done to eliminate doubt: Add 3 percent ferric chloride dropwise to the urine. Penicillamine will turn the urine an immediate and quickly fading blue. Cystine will not produce any change in appearance.

Rheumatoid Arthritis—The principal rule of treatment with DEPEN in rheumatoid arthritis is patience. The onset of therapeutic response is typically delayed. Two or three months may be required before the first evidence of a clinical response is noted (see CLINICAL PHARMACOLOGY).

When treatment with DEPEN has been interrupted because of adverse reactions or other reasons, the drug should be reintroduced cautiously by starting with a lower dosage and increasing slowly.

Initial Therapy—The currently recommended dosage regimen in rheumatoid arthritis begins with a single daily dose of 125 mg or 250 mg which is thereafter increased at one to three month intervals, by 125 mg or 250 mg/day, as patient response and tolerance indicate. If a satisfactory remission of symptoms is achieved, the dose associated with the remission should be continued (see Maintenance Therapy). If there is no improvement and there are no signs of potentially serious toxicity after two to three months of treatment with doses of 500–750 mg/day, increases of 250 mg/day at two to three month intervals may be continued until a satisfactory remission occurs (see Maintenance Therapy) or signs of toxicity develop (see WARNINGS and PRECAUTIONS). If there is no discernible improvement after three to four months of treatment with 1000 to 1500 mg of penicillamine/day, it may be assumed the patient will not respond and DEPEN should be discontinued.

Maintenance Therapy—The maintenance dosage of DEPEN must be individualized, and may require adjustment during the course of treatment. Many patients respond satisfactorily to a dosage within the 500–750 mg/day range. Some need less.

Changes in maintenance dosage levels may not be reflected clinically or in the erythrocyte sedimentation rate for two to three months after each dosage adjustment.

Some patients will subsequently require an increase in the maintenance dosage to achieve maximal disease suppression. In those patients who do respond, but who evidence incomplete suppression of their disease after the first six to nine months of treatment, the daily dosage of DEPEN may be increased by 125 mg or 250 mg/day at three-month intervals. It is unusual in current practice to employ a dosage in excess of 1 g/day, but up to 1.5 g/day has sometimes been required.

Management of Exacerbations—During the course of treatment some patients may experience an exacerbation of disease activity following an initial good response. These may be self-limited and can subside within twelve weeks. They are usually controlled by the addition of nonsteroidal anti-inflammatory drugs, and only if the patient has demon-

strated a true "escape" phenomenon (as evidenced by failure of the flare to subside within this time period) should an increase in the maintenance dose ordinarily be considered.

In the rheumatoid patient, migratory polyarthralgia due to penicillamine is extremely difficult to differentiate from an exacerbation of the rheumatoid arthritis. Discontinuance or a substantial reduction in the dosage of DEPEN for up to several weeks will usually determine which of these processes is responsible for the arthralgia.

Duration of Therapy—The optimum duration of DEPEN therapy in rheumatoid arthritis has not been determined. If the patient has been in remission for six months or more, a gradual, stepwise dosage reduction in decrements of 125 mg or 250 mg/day at approximately three month intervals may be attempted.

Concomitant Drug Therapy—DEPEN should not be used in patients who are receiving gold therapy, antimalarial or cytotoxic drugs, oxyphenbutazone, or phenylbutazone (see PRECAUTIONS). Other measures, such as salicylates, other nonsteroidal anti-inflammatory drugs or systemic corticosteroids may be continued when DEPEN is initiated. After improvement commences, analgesic and anti-inflammatory drugs may be slowly discontinued as symptoms permit. Steroid withdrawal must be done gradually, and many months of DEPEN treatment may be required before steroids can be completely eliminated.

Dosage Frequency—Based on clinical experience, dosages up to 500 mg/day can be given as a single daily dose. Dosages in excess of 500 mg/day should be administered in divided doses.

HOW SUPPLIED

DEPEN® (penicillamine tablets, USP) Titratable Tablets: 250 mg scored, oval, white tablets coded with 37-4401 and Wallace; available in bottles of 100 (NDC 0037-4401-01).

Storage: Store at controlled room temperature 15°–30°C (59°–86°F). Protect from moisture.

Dispense in a tight container.

WALLACE LABORATORIES
Division of
CARTER-WALLACE, INC.
Cranbury, New Jersey 08512
Manufactured under license from ASTA Medica AG,
Frankfurt, Federal Republic of Germany
IN-030F2-09 Rev. 8/92

DIUTENSEN®-R ℞

(methyclothiazide and reserpine)
Tablets

DORAL Ⓒ ℞

(quazepam)
Tablets

DESCRIPTION

DORAL (brand of quazepam) Tablets contain quazepam, a trifluoroethyl benzodiazepine hypnotic agent, having the chemical name 7-chloro-5-(o-fluoro-phenyl)-1,3-dihydro-1-(2,2,2-trifluoroethyl)-2*H*-1,4-benzodiazepine-2-thione and the following structural formula:

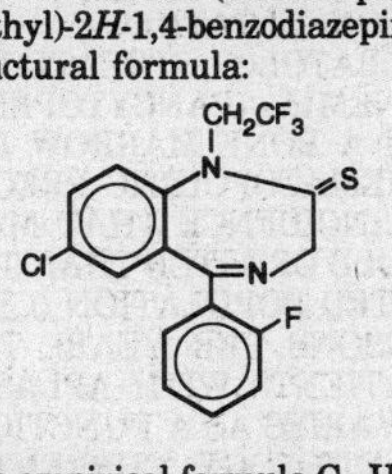

Quazepam has the empirical formula $C_{17}H_{11}ClF_4N_2S$, and a molecular weight of 386.8. It is a white crystalline compound, soluble in ethanol and insoluble in water. Each DORAL Tablet contains either 7.5 or 15 mg of quazepam. The inactive ingredients for DORAL Tablets 7.5 or 15 mg include cellulose, corn starch, FD&C Yellow No. 6 Al Lake, lactose, magnesium stearate, silicon dioxide, and sodium lauryl sulfate.

CLINICAL PHARMACOLOGY

Central nervous system agents of the 1,4-benzodiazepine class presumably exert their effects by binding to stereospecific receptors at several sites within the central nervous system (CNS). Their exact mechanism of action is unknown.

In a sleep laboratory study, DORAL Tablets significantly decreased sleep latency and total wake time, and significantly increased total sleep time and percent sleep time, for one or more nights. Quazepam 15 mg was effective on the first night of administration. Sleep latency, total wake time, and wake time after sleep onset were still decreased and percent sleep time was still increased for several nights after the drug was discontinued. Percent slow wave sleep was decreased, and REM sleep was essentially unchanged. No transient sleep disturbance, such as "rebound insomnia," was observed after withdrawal of the drug in sleep laboratory studies in 12 patients using 15 mg doses.

In outpatient studies, DORAL Tablets improved all subjective measures of sleep including sleep induction time, duration of sleep, number of nocturnal awakenings, occurrence of early morning awakening, and sleep quality. Some effects were evident on the first night of administration of DORAL Tablets (sleep induction time, number of nocturnal awakenings, and duration of sleep). Residual medication effects ("hangover") were minimal.

Quazepam is rapidly (absorption half-life of about 30 minutes) and well absorbed from the gastrointestinal tract. The peak plasma concentration of quazepam is approximately 20 ng/mL after a 15 mg dose and is obtained at about 2 hours. Quazepam, the active parent compound, is extensively metabolized in the liver; two of the plasma metabolites are 2-oxoquazepam and N-desalkyl-2-oxoquazepam. All three compounds show pharmacological central nervous system activity in animals.

Following administration of ^{14}C-quazepam, approximately 31% of the dose appears in the urine and 23% in the feces over a five-day period; only trace amounts of unchanged drug are present in the urine.

The mean elimination half-life of quazepam and 2-oxoquazepam is 39 hours and that of N-desalkyl-2-oxoquazepam is 73 hours. Steady-state levels of quazepam and 2-oxoquazepam are attained by the seventh daily dose and that of N-desalkyl-2-oxoquazepam by the thirteenth daily dose.

The pharmacokinetics of quazepam and 2-oxoquazepam in geriatric subjects are comparable to those seen in young adults; as with desalkyl metabolites of other benzodiazepines, the elimination half-life of N-desalkyl-2-oxoquazepam in geriatric patients is about twice that of young adults.

The degree of plasma protein binding for quazepam and its two major metabolites is greater than 95%. The absorption, distribution, metabolism, and excretion of benzodiazepines may be altered in various disease states including alcoholism, impaired hepatic function, and impaired renal function.

The type and duration of hypnotic effects and the profile of unwanted effects during administration of benzodiazepine drugs may be influenced by the biologic half-life of administered drug and any active metabolites formed. When half-lives are long, drug or metabolites may accumulate during periods of nightly adminstration and be associated with impairments of cognitive and/or motor performance during waking hours; the possibility of interaction with other psychoactive drugs or alcohol will be enhanced. In contrast, if half-lives are short, drug and metabolites will be cleared before the next dose is ingested, and carry-over effects related to excessive sedation or CNS depression should be minimal or absent. However, during nightly use for an extended period, pharmacodynamic tolerance or adaptation to some effects of benzodiazepine hypnotics may develop. If the drug has a short half-life of elimination, it is possible that a relative deficiency of the drug or its active metabolites (i.e., in relationship to the receptor site) may occur at some point in the interval between each night's use. This sequence of events may account for two clinical findings reported to occur after several weeks of nightly use of rapidly eliminated benzodiazepine hypnotics, namely, increased wakefulness during the last third of the night, and the appearance of increased signs of daytime anxiety in selected patients.

Quazepam crosses the placental barrier of mice. Quazepam, 2-oxoquazepam and N-desalkyl-2-oxoquazepam are present in breast milk of lactating women, but the total amount found in the milk represents only about 0.1% of the administered dose.

INDICATIONS AND USAGE

DORAL Tablets are indicated for the treatment of insomnia characterized by difficulty in falling asleep, frequent nocturnal awakenings, and/or early morning awakenings. The effectiveness of DORAL has been established in placebo-controlled clinical studies of 5 nights duration in acute and chronic insomnia. The sustained effectiveness of DORAL has been established in chronic insomnia in a sleep lab (polysomnographic) study of 28 nights duration.

Because insomnia is often transient and intermittent, the prolonged administration of DORAL Tablets is generally not necessary or recommended. Since insomnia may be a symptom of several other disorders, the possibility that the complaint may be related to a condition for which there is a more specific treatment should be considered.

CONTRAINDICATIONS

DORAL Tablets are contraindicated in patients with known hypersensitivity to this drug or other benzodiazepines, and in patients with established or suspected sleep apnea.

Usage in Pregnancy: Benzodiazepines may cause fetal damage when administered during pregnancy. An increased risk of congenital malformations associated with the use of diazepam and chlordiazepoxide during the first trimester of pregnancy has been suggested in several studies. Transplacental distribution has resulted in neonatal CNS depression following the ingestion of therapeutic doses of a benzodiazepine hypnotic during the last weeks of pregnancy.

DORAL Tablets are contraindicated in pregnancy because the potential risks outweigh the possible advantages of their use during this period. If there is a likelihood of the patient becoming pregnant while receiving DORAL, she should be warned of the potential risk to the fetus. Patients should be instructed to discontinue the drug prior to becoming pregnant. The possibility that a woman of childbearing potential may be pregnant at the time of institution of therapy should be considered. (see **Pregnancy, Teratogenic Effects: Pregnancy Category X**).

WARNINGS

Patients receiving benzodiazepines should be cautioned about possible combined effects with alcohol and other CNS depressants. Also, caution patients that an additive effect may occur if alcoholic beverages are consumed during the day following the use of benzodiazepines for nighttime sedation. The potential for this interaction continues for several days following their discontinuance until serum levels of psychoactive metabolites have declined.

Patients should also be cautioned about engaging in hazardous occupations requiring complete mental alertness, such as operating machinery or driving a motor vehicle, after ingesting benzodiazepines, including potential impairment of the performance of such activities which may occur the day following ingestion.

Withdrawal symptoms of the type associated with sedatives/hypnotics (e.g., barbiturates, bromides, etc.) and alcohol have been reported after the discontinuation of benzodiazepines. While these symptoms have been more frequently reported after the discontinuation of excessive benzodiazepine doses, there have also been controlled studies demonstrating the occurrence of such symptoms after discontinuation of therapeutic doses of benzodiazepines, generally following prolonged use (but in some instances after periods as brief as six weeks). It is generally believed that the gradual reduction of dosage will diminish the occurrence of such symptoms (see **Drug Abuse and Dependence**).

PRECAUTIONS

General: Impaired motor and/or cognitive performance attributable to the accumulation of benzodiazepines and their active metabolites following several days of repeated use at their recommended doses is a concern in certain vulnerable patients (e.g., those especially sensitive to the effects of benzodiazepines or those with a reduced capacity to metabolize and eliminate them). Consequently, elderly or debilitated patients and those with impaired renal or hepatic function should be cautioned about the risk and advised to monitor themselves for signs of excessive sedation or impaired coordination.

The possibility of respiratory depression in patients with chronic pulmonary insufficiency should be considered.

When benzodiazepines are administered to depressed patients, there is a risk that the signs and symptoms of depression may be intensified. Consequently, appropriate precautions (e.g., limiting the total prescription size and increased monitoring for suicidal ideation) should be considered.

Information for Patients: It is suggested that physicians discuss the following information with patients. This information is intended to aid in the safe and effective use of this medication. It is not a disclosure of all possible adverse or intended effects.

1. Inform your physician about any alcohol consumption and medicine you are taking now, including drugs you may buy without a prescription. Alcohol should generally not be used during treatment with hypnotics.
2. Inform your physician if you are planning to become pregnant, if you are pregnant, or if you become pregnant while you are taking this medicine.
3. Inform your physician if you are nursing.
4. Until you experience how this medicine affects you, do not drive a car or operate potentially dangerous machinery, etc.
5. Benzodiazepines may cause daytime sedation, which may persist for several days following drug discontinuation.
6. Patients should be told not to increase the dose on their own and should inform their physician if they believe the drug "does not work anymore".
7. If benzodiazepines are taken on a prolonged and regular basis (even for periods as brief as six weeks), patients should be advised not to stop taking them abruptly or to decrease the dose without consulting their physician, because withdrawal symptoms may occur.

Laboratory Tests: Laboratory tests are not ordinarily required in otherwise healthy patients when quazepam is used as recommended.

Drug Interactions: The benzodiazepines, including DORAL Tablets, produce additive CNS depressant effects when co-administered with psychotropic medications, anticonvul-

Continued on next page

Wallace Laboratories—Cont.

sants, antihistaminics, ethanol, and other drugs which produce CNS depression.

Carcinogenesis, Mutagenesis, Impairment of Fertility: Quazepam showed no evidence of carcinogenicity or other significant pathology in oral oncogenicity studies in mice and hamsters.

Quazepam was tested for mutagenicity using the L5178Y TK +/-Mouse Lymphoma Mutagenesis Assay and Ames Test. The L5178Y TK +/-Assay was equivocal and the Ames Test did not show mutagenic activity.

Reproduction studies in mice conducted with quazepam at doses equal to 60 and 180 times the human dose of 15 mg, and with diazepam at 67 times the human dose, produced slight reductions in the pregnancy rate. Similar reduction in pregnancy rates have been reported in mice dosed with other benzodiazepines, and is believed to be related to the sedative effects of these drugs at high doses.

Pregnancy: Teratogenic Effects: Pregnancy Category X (See **CONTRAINDICATIONS, Usage in Pregnancy** section.) Reproduction studies of quazepam in mice at doses up to 400 times the human dose revealed no major drug-related malformations. Minor developmental variations that occurred were delayed ossification of the sternum, vertebrae, distal phalanges and suprooccipital bones, at doses of 66 and 400 times the human dose. Studies with diazepam at 200 times the human dose showed a similar or greater incidence than quazepam. A reproduction study of quazepam in New Zealand rabbits at doses up to 134 times the human dose demonstrated no effect on fetal morphology or development of offspring.

Nonteratogenic Effects: The child born of a mother who is taking benzodiazepines may be at some risk of withdrawal symptoms from the drug during the postnatal period. Neonatal flaccidity has been reported in children born of mothers who had been receiving benzodiazepines.

Labor and Delivery: DORAL Tablets have no established use in labor or delivery.

Nursing Mothers: Quazepam and its metabolites are excreted in milk of lactating women. Therefore, administration of DORAL Tablets to nursing women is not recommended.

Pediatric Use: Safety and effectiveness in children below the age of 18 years have not been established.

ADVERSE REACTIONS

Adverse events most frequently encountered in patients treated with quazepam are drowsiness and headache.

Accurate estimates of the incidence of adverse events associated with the use of any drug are difficult to obtain. Estimates are influenced by drug dose, detection technique, setting, physician judgments, etc. Consequently, the table below is presented solely to indicate the relative frequency of adverse events reported in representative controlled clinical studies conducted to evaluate the safety and efficacy of quazepam. The figures cited cannot be used to predict precisely the incidence of such events in the course of usual medical practice. These figures, also, cannot be compared with those obtained from other clinical studies involving related drug products and placebo.

The figures cited below are estimates of untoward clinical event incidences of 1% or greater among subjects who participated in the relatively short duration placebo-controlled clinical trials of quazepam.

	DORAL*	PLACEBO
NUMBER OF PATIENTS	267	268
% OF PATIENTS REPORTING		
Central Nervous System		
Daytime Drowsiness	12.0	3.3
Headache	4.5	2.2
Fatigue	1.9	0
Dizziness	1.5	<1
Autonomic Nervous System		
Dry Mouth	1.5	<1
Gastrointestinal System		
Dyspepsia	1.1	<1

*Doral 15 mg

The following incidences of laboratory abnormalities occurred at a rate of 1% or greater in patients receiving quazepam and the corresponding placebo group. None of these changes were considered to be of physiological significance.

	DORAL		PLACEBO	
NUMBER OF PATIENTS	234		244	
% of Patients Reporting	Low	High	Low	High
Hematology				
Hemoglobin	1.4	0	1.2	0
Hematocrit	1.5	0	1.7	0
Lymphocyte	1.3	1.6	1.2	1.9
Eosinophil	*	1.5	*	1.3
SEG	1.1	*	1.6	*
Monocyte	*	1.1	*	*
Blood Chemistry				
Glucose	*	*	*	1.2
SGOT	*	1.3	*	1.1
Urinalysis				
Specific Gravity	*	*	*	1.1
WBC	0	2.6	0	3.0
RBC	0	*	0	1.1
Epithelial Cells	0	2.5	0	3.2
Crystals	0	*	0	1.0

*These laboratory abnormalities occurred in less than 1% of patients. In addition, abnormalities in the following laboratory tests were observed in less than 1% of the patients evaluated: WBC count, platelet count, total protein, albumin, BUN, creatinine, total bilirubin, alkaline phosphatase, and SGPT.

The following additional events occurred among individuals receiving quazepam at doses equivalent to or greater than those recommended during its clinical testing and development. There is no way to establish whether or not the administration of DORAL caused these events.

Hypokinesia, ataxia, confusion, incoordination, hyperkinesia, speech disorder, and tremor were reported.

Also, depression, nervousness, agitation, amnesia, anorexia, anxiety, apathy, euphoria, impotence, decreased libido, paranoid reaction, nightmares, abnormal thinking, abnormal taste perception, abnormal vision, and cataract were reported.

Also reported were urinary incontinence, palpitations, nausea, constipation, diarrhea, abdominal pain, pruritus, rash, asthenia, and malaise.

The following list provides an overview of adverse experiences that have been reported and are considered to be reasonably related to the administration of benzodiazepines: incontinence, slurred speech, urinary retention, jaundice, dysarthria, dystonia, changes in libido, irritability, and menstrual irregularities.

As with all benzodiazepines, paradoxical reactions such as stimulation, agitation, increased muscle spasticity, sleep disturbances, hallucinations, and other adverse behavioral effects may occur in rare instances and in a random fashion. Should these occur, use of the drug should be discontinued.

There have been reports of withdrawal signs and symptoms of the type associated with withdrawal from CNS depressant drugs following the rapid decrease or the abrupt discontinuation of benzodiazepines (see **Drug Abuse and Dependence** section).

DRUG ABUSE AND DEPENDENCE

Controlled Substance: DORAL is a controlled substance under the Controlled Substance Act and has been assigned by the Drug Enforcement Administration to Schedule IV.

Abuse and Dependence: Withdrawal symptoms, similar in character to those noted with barbiturates and alcohol (e.g., convulsions, tremor, abdominal and muscle cramps, vomiting and sweating), have occurred following abrupt discontinuance of benzodiazepines. The more severe withdrawal symptoms have usually been limited to those patients who received excessive doses over an extended period of time. Generally milder withdrawal symptoms (e.g., dysphoria and insomnia) have been reported following abrupt discontinuance of benzodiazepines taken continuously at therapeutic levels for several months. Consequently, after extended therapy, abrupt discontinuation should generally be avoided and a gradual dosage tapering schedule followed. Addiction-prone individuals (such as drug addicts or alcoholics) should be under careful surveillance when receiving quazepam or other psychotropic agents because of the predisposition of such patients to habituation and dependence.

OVERDOSAGE Manifestations of overdosage seen with other benzodiazepines include somnolence, confusion, and coma. In the event that an overdose occurs, the following is the recommended treatment. Respiration, pulse, and blood pressure should be monitored, as in all cases of drug overdosage. General supportive measures should be employed, along with immediate gastric lavage. Intravenous fluids should be administered and an adequate airway maintained. Hypotension may be treated with the use of norepinephrine bitartrate or metaraminol bitartrate. Dialysis is of limited value. Animal experiments suggest that forced diuresis or hemodialysis are probably of little value in treating overdosage. As with the management of intentional overdosing with any drug, it should be borne in mind that multiple agents may have been ingested.

The oral LD_{50} in mice was greater that 5,000 mg/kg.

DOSAGE AND ADMINISTRATION *Adults:* Initiate therapy at 15 mg until individual responses are determined. In some patients, the dose may then be reduced to 7.5 mg.

Elderly and debilitated patients: Because the elderly and debilitated may be more sensitive to benzodiazepines, attempts to reduce the nightly dosage after the first one or two nights of therapy are suggested.

HOW SUPPLIED

DORAL Tablets, 7.5 mg, unscored, capsule-shaped, light orange, slightly white speckled tablets, impressed with the product identification number 7.5 on one side of the tablet, and the product name (DORAL) on the other.

7.5 mg	Bottles of 100	NDC 0037-9000-01
	Unit-dose package (10 strips of 10)	NDC 0037-9000-02

DORAL Tablets, 15 mg, unscored, capsule-shaped, light orange, slightly white speckled tablets, impressed with the product identification number 15 on one side of the tablet, and the product name (DORAL) on the other.

15 mg	Bottles of 100	NDC 0037-9002-01
	Unit-dose package (10 strips of 10)	NDC 0037-9002-02

Store DORAL Tablets between 2° and 30°C (36° and 86°F). Protect unit doses from excessive moisture.

CAUTION: Federal law prohibits dispensing without prescription.

Distributed by
WALLACE LABORATORIES
Division of
CARTER-WALLACE, INC.
Cranbury, NJ 08512
Under license from Baker Norton Pharmaceuticals, Inc.
Manufactured by Schering Corporation
Kenilworth, NJ 07033
©1989, 1990 Carter-Wallace, Inc.
IN9000-03 Rev. 7/94

Shown in Product Identification Guide, page 339

FELBATOL® ℞

(felbamate)
Tablets 400 mg and 600 mg,
Oral Suspension 600 mg/5 mL

Before Prescribing FELBATOL® (felbamate), the physician should be thoroughly familiar with the details of this prescribing information.

FELBATOL® SHOULD NOT BE USED BY PATIENTS UNTIL THERE HAS BEEN A COMPLETE DISCUSSION OF THE RISKS AND THE PATIENT, PARENT, OR GUARDIAN HAS PROVIDED WRITTEN INFORMED CONSENT (SEE PATIENT INFORMATION/CONSENT SECTION).

WARNING

1. **APLASTIC ANEMIA**

THE USE OF FELBATOL® (felbamate) IS ASSOCIATED WITH A MARKED INCREASE IN THE INCIDENCE OF APLASTIC ANEMIA. ACCORDINGLY, FELBATOL® SHOULD ONLY BE USED IN PATIENTS WHOSE EPILEPSY IS SO SEVERE THAT THE RISK OF APLASTIC ANEMIA IS DEEMED ACCEPTABLE IN LIGHT OF THE BENEFITS CONFERRED BY ITS USE (SEE **INDICATIONS**). ORDINARILY, A PATIENT SHOULD NOT BE PLACED ON AND/OR CONTINUED ON FELBATOL® WITHOUT CONSIDERATION OF APPROPRIATE EXPERT HEMATOLOGIC CONSULTATION.

AMONG FELBATOL® TREATED PATIENTS, APLASTIC ANEMIA (PANCYTOPENIA IN THE PRESENCE OF A BONE MARROW LARGELY DEPLETED OF HEMATOPOIETIC PRECURSORS) OCCURS AT AN INCIDENCE THAT MAY BE MORE THAN A 100 FOLD GREATER THAN THAT SEEN IN THE UNTREATED POPULATION (I.E., 2 TO 5 PER MILLION PERSONS PER YEAR). THE RISK OF DEATH IN PATIENTS WITH APLASTIC ANEMIA GENERALLY VARIES AS A FUNCTION OF ITS SEVERITY AND ETIOLOGY; CURRENT ESTIMATES OF THE OVERALL CASE FATALITY RATE ARE IN THE RANGE OF 20 TO 30%, BUT RATES AS HIGH AS 70% HAVE BEEN REPORTED IN THE PAST.

THERE ARE TOO FEW FELBATOL® ASSOCIATED CASES, AND TOO LITTLE KNOWN ABOUT THEM TO PROVIDE A RELIABLE ESTIMATE OF THE SYNDROME'S INCIDENCE OR ITS CASE FATALITY RATE OR TO IDENTIFY THE FACTORS, IF ANY, THAT MIGHT CONCEIVABLY BE USED TO PREDICT WHO IS AT GREATER OR LESSER RISK.

IN MANAGING PATIENTS ON FELBATOL®, IT SHOULD BE BORNE IN MIND THAT THE CLINICAL MANIFESTATION OF APLASTIC ANEMIA MAY NOT BE SEEN UNTIL AFTER A PATIENT HAS BEEN ON FELBATOL® FOR SEVERAL MONTHS (E.G., ONSET OF APLASTIC ANEMIA AMONG FELBATOL® EXPOSED PATIENTS FOR WHOM DATA ARE AVAILABLE HAS RANGED FROM 5 TO 30 WEEKS). HOWEVER, THE INJURY TO BONE MARROW STEM CELLS THAT IS HELD TO BE ULTI-

MATELY RESPONSIBLE FOR THE ANEMIA MAY OCCUR WEEKS TO MONTHS EARLIER. ACCORDINGLY, PATIENTS WHO ARE DISCONTINUED FROM FELBATOL® REMAIN AT RISK FOR DEVELOPING ANEMIA FOR A VARIABLE, AND UNKNOWN, PERIOD AFTERWARDS.

IT IS NOT KNOWN WHETHER OR NOT THE RISK OF DEVELOPING APLASTIC ANEMIA CHANGES WITH DURATION OF EXPOSURE. CONSEQUENTLY, IT IS NOT SAFE TO ASSUME THAT A PATIENT WHO HAS BEEN ON FELBATOL® WITHOUT SIGNS OF HEMATOLOGIC ABNORMALITY FOR LONG PERIODS OF TIME IS WITHOUT RISK.

IT IS NOT KNOWN WHETHER OR NOT THE DOSE OF FELBATOL® AFFECTS THE INCIDENCE OF APLASTIC ANEMIA.

IT IS NOT KNOWN WHETHER OR NOT CONCOMITANT USE OF ANTIEPILEPTIC DRUGS AND/OR OTHER DRUGS AFFECTS THE INCIDENCE OF APLASTIC ANEMIA.

APLASTIC ANEMIA TYPICALLY DEVELOPS WITHOUT PREMONITORY CLINICAL OR LABORATORY SIGNS, THE FULL BLOWN SYNDROME PRESENTING WITH SIGNS OF INFECTION, BLEEDING, OR ANEMIA. ACCORDINGLY, ROUTINE BLOOD TESTING CANNOT BE RELIABLY USED TO REDUCE THE INCIDENCE OF APLASTIC ANEMIA, BUT, IT WILL, IN SOME CASES, ALLOW THE DETECTION OF THE HEMATOLOGIC CHANGES BEFORE THE SYNDROME DECLARES ITSELF CLINICALLY.

FELBATOL® SHOULD BE DISCONTINUED IF ANY EVIDENCE OF BONE MARROW DEPRESSION OCCURS.

2. HEPATIC FAILURE

HEPATIC FAILURE RESULTING IN FATALITIES HAS BEEN REPORTED WITH A MARKED INCREASE IN THE FREQUENCY IN PATIENTS RECEIVING FELBATOL® (felbamate). ACCORDINGLY, FELBATOL SHOULD ONLY BE USED IN PATIENTS WHOSE EPILEPSY IS SO SEVERE THAT THE RISK OF LIVER FAILURE IS OUTWEIGHED BY THE POTENTIAL BENEFITS OF SEIZURE CONTROL.

ALTHOUGH FULL INFORMATION IS NOT YET AVAILABLE, THE NUMBER OF CASES REPORTED GREATLY EXCEEDS THE NUMBER THAT IS EXPECTED BASED ON THE ANNUAL INCIDENCE OF ACUTE LIVER FAILURE IN THE UNITED STATES (I.E., ABOUT 2,000 CASES PER YEAR).

THERE ARE TOO FEW FELBATOL® ASSOCIATED CASES OF HEPATIC FAILURE AND TOO LITTLE KNOWN ABOUT THEM TO PROVIDE EITHER A RELIABLE ESTIMATE OF ITS INCIDENCE OR TO IDENTIFY THE FACTORS, IF ANY, THAT MIGHT BE USED TO PREDICT WHICH PATIENT IS AT GREATER OR LESSER RISK.

IT IS NOT KNOWN WHETHER OR NOT THE RISK OF DEVELOPING HEPATIC FAILURE CHANGES WITH DURATION OF EXPOSURE.

IT IS NOT KNOWN WHETHER OR NOT THE DOSAGE OF FELBATOL® AFFECTS THE INCIDENCE OF HEPATIC FAILURE.

IT IS NOT KNOWN WHETHER CONCOMITANT USE OF OTHER ANTIEPILEPTIC DRUGS AND/OR OTHER DRUGS AFFECTS THE INCIDENCE OF HEPATIC FAILURE.

FELBATOL® SHOULD NOT BE PRESCRIBED FOR ANYONE WITH A HISTORY OF HEPATIC DYSFUNCTION.

PATIENTS PRESCRIBED FELBATOL® SHOULD HAVE LIVER FUNCTION TESTS (AST, ALT, BILIRUBIN) PERFORMED BEFORE INITIATING FELBATOL® AND AT 1- TO 2-WEEK INTERVALS WHILE TREATMENT CONTINUES. A PATIENT WHO DEVELOPS ABNORMAL LIVER FUNCTION TESTS SHOULD BE IMMEDIATELY WITHDRAWN FROM FELBATOL® TREATMENT.

DESCRIPTION

FELBATOL® (felbamate) is an antiepileptic available as 400 mg and 600 mg tablets and as a 600 mg/5 mL suspension for oral administration. Its chemical name is 2-phenyl-1,3-propanediol dicarbamate.

Felbamate is a white to off-white crystalline powder with a characteristic odor. It is very slightly soluble in water, slightly soluble in ethanol, sparingly soluble in methanol, and freely soluble in dimethyl sulfoxide. The molecular weight is 238.24; felbamate's molecular formula is $C_{11}H_{14}N_2O_4$; its structural formula is:

[See chemical structure at top of next column.]

The inactive ingredients for FELBATOL® (felbamate) tablets 400 mg and 600 mg are starch, microcrystalline cellulose, croscarmellose sodium, lactose, magnesium stearate, FD&C Yellow No. 6, D&C Yellow No. 10, and FD&C Red No. 40 (600 mg tablets only). The inactive ingredients for FELBATOL® (felbamate) suspension 600 mg/5 mL are sor-

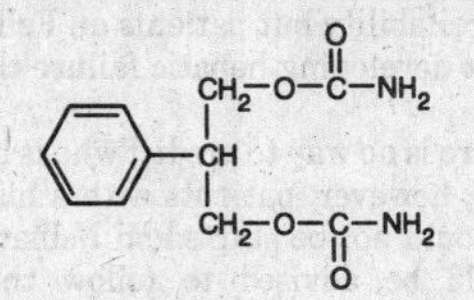

bitol, glycerin, microcrystalline cellulose, carboxymethylcellulose sodium, simethicone, polysorbate 80, methylparaben, saccharin sodium, propylparaben, FD&C Yellow No. 6, FD&C Red No. 40, flavorings, and purified water.

CLINICAL PHARMACOLOGY

Mechanism of Action:

The mechanism by which felbamate exerts its anticonvulsant activity is unknown, but in animal test systems designed to detect anticonvulsant activity, felbamate has properties in common with other marketed anticonvulsants. Felbamate is effective in mice and rats in the maximal electroshock test, the subcutaneous pentylenetetrazol seizure test, and the subcutaneous picrotoxin seizure test. Felbamate also exhibits anticonvulsant activity against seizures induced by intracerebroventricular administration of glutamate in rats and N-methyl-D,L-aspartic acid in mice. Protection against maximal electroshock-induced seizures suggests that felbamate may reduce seizure spread, an effect possibly predictive of efficacy in generalized tonic-clonic or partial seizures. Protection against pentylenetetrazol-induced seizures suggests that felbamate may increase seizure threshold, an effect considered to be predictive of potential efficacy in absence seizures.

Receptor-binding studies *in vitro* indicate that felbamate has weak inhibitory effects on GABA-receptor binding, benzodiazepine receptor binding, and is devoid of activity at the MK-801 receptor binding site of the NMDA receptor-ionophore complex. However, felbamate does interact as an antagonist at the strychnine-insensitive glycine recognition site of the NMDA receptor-ionophore complex. Felbamate is not effective in protecting chick embryo retina tissue against the neurotoxic effects of the excitatory amino acid agonists NMDA, kainate, or quisqualate *in vitro*.

The monocarbamate, p-hydroxy, and 2-hydroxy metabolites were inactive in the maximal electroshock-induced seizure test in mice. The monocarbamate and p-hydroxy metabolites had only weak (0.2 to 0.6) activity compared with felbamate in the subcutaneous pentylenetetrazol seizure test. These metabolites did not contribute significantly to the anticonvulsant action of felbamate.

Pharmacokinetics:

The numbers in the pharmacokinetic section are mean ± standard deviation.

Felbamate is well-absorbed after oral administration. Over 90% of the radioactivity after a dose of 1000 mg ^{14}C felbamate was found in the urine. Absolute bioavailability (oral vs. parenteral) has not been measured. The tablet and suspension were each shown to be bioequivalent to the capsule used in clinical trials, and pharmacokinetic parameters of the tablet and suspension are similar. There was no effect of food on absorption of the tablet; the effect of food on absorption of the suspension has not been evaluated.

Following oral administration, felbamate is the predominant plasma species (about 90% of plasma radioactivity). About 40–50% of absorbed dose appears unchanged in urine, and an additional 40% is present as unidentified metabolites and conjugates. About 15% is present as parahydroxyfelbamate, 2-hydroxyfelbamate, and felbamate monocarbamate, none of which have significant anticonvulsant activity.

Binding of felbamate to human plasma protein was independent of felbamate concentrations between 10 and 310 micrograms/mL. Binding ranged from 22% to 25%, mostly to albumin, and was dependent on the albumin concentration.

Felbamate is excreted with a terminal half-life of 20–23 hours, which is unaltered after multiple doses. Clearance after a single 1200 mg dose is 26±3 mL/hr/kg, and after multiple daily doses of 3600 mg is 30±8 mL/hr/kg. The apparent volume of distribution was 756±82 mL/kg after a 1200 mg dose. Felbamate Cmax and AUC are proportionate to dose after single and multiple doses over a range of 100–800 mg single doses and 1200–3600 mg daily doses. Cmin (trough) blood levels are also dose proportional. Multiple daily doses of 1200, 2400, and 3600 mg gave Cmin values of 30±5, 55±8, and 83±21 micrograms/mL (N=10 patients). Felbamate gave dose proportional steady-state peak plasma concentrations in children age 4–12 over a range of 15, 30, and 45 mg/kg/day with peak concentrations of 17, 32, and 49 micrograms/mL.

The effects of race and gender on felbamate pharmacokinetics have not been systematically evaluated, but plasma concentrations in males (N=5) and females (N=4) given felbamate have been similar. The effects of felbamate kinetics on renal and hepatic functional impairment have not been evaluated.

Pharmacodynamics:

Typical Physiologic Responses:

1. Cardiovascular:

In adults, there is no effect of felbamate on blood pressure. Small but statistically significant mean increases in heart rate were seen during adjunctive therapy and monotherapy; however, these mean increases of up to 5 bpm were not clinically significant. In children, no clinically relevant changes in blood pressure or heart rate were seen during adjunctive therapy or monotherapy with felbamate.

2. Other Physiologic Effects:

The only other change in vital signs was a mean decrease of approximately 1 respiration per minute in respiratory rate during adjunctive therapy in children. In adults, statistically significant mean reductions in body weight were observed during felbamate monotherapy and adjunctive therapy. In children, there were mean decreases in body weight during adjunctive therapy and monotherapy; however, these mean changes were not statistically significant. These mean reductions in adults and children were approximately 5% of the mean weights at baseline.

CLINICAL STUDIES

The results of controlled clinical trials established the efficacy of FELBATOL® (felbamate) as monotherapy and adjunctive therapy in adults with partial-onset seizures with or without secondary generalization and in partial and generalized seizures associated with Lennox-Gastaut syndrome in children.

FELBATOL® Monotherapy Trials in Adults

FELBATOL® (3600 mg/day given QID) and low-dose valproate (15 mg/kg/day) were compared as monotherapy during a 112-day treatment period in a multicenter and a single-center double-blind efficacy trial. Both trials were conducted according to an identical study design. During a 56-day baseline period, all patients had at least four partial-onset seizures per 28 days and were receiving one antiepileptic drug at a therapeutic level, the most common being carbamazepine. In the multicenter trial, baseline seizure frequencies were 12.4 per 28 days in the FELBATOL® group and 21.3 per 28 days in the low-dose valproate group. In the single-center trial, baseline seizure frequencies were 18.1 per 28 days in the FELBATOL® group and 15.9 per 28 days in the low-dose valproate group. Patients were converted to monotherapy with FELBATOL® or low-dose valproic acid during the first 28 days of the 112-day treatment period. Study endpoints were completion of 112 study days or fulfilling an escape criterion. Criteria for escape relative to baseline were: (1) twofold increase in monthly seizure frequency, (2) twofold increase in highest 2-day seizure frequency, (3) single generalized tonic-clonic seizure (GTC) if none occurred during baseline, or (4) significant prolongation of GTCs. The primary efficacy variable was the number of patients in each treatment group who met escape criteria.

In the multicenter trial, the percentage of patients who met escape criteria was 40% (18/45) in the Felbatol® group and 78% (39/50) in the low-dose valproate group. In the single-center trial, the percentage of patients who met escape criteria was 14% (3/21) in the Felbatol® group and 90% (19/21) in the low-dose valproate group. In both trials, the difference in the percentage of patients meeting escape criteria was statistically significant (P<.001) in favor of Felbatol®. These two studies by design were intended to demonstrate the effectiveness of Felbatol® monotherapy. The studies were not designed or intended to demonstrate comparative efficacy of the two drugs. For example, valproate was not used at the maximally effective dose.

Felbatol® Adjunctive Therapy Trials in Adults

A double-blind, placebo-controlled crossover trial consisted of two 10-week outpatient treatment periods. Patients with refractory partial-onset seizures who were receiving phenytoin and carbamazepine at therapeutic levels were administered Felbatol® (felbamate) as add-on therapy at a starting dosage of 1400 mg/day in three divided doses, which was increased to 2600 mg/day in three divided doses. Among the 56 patients who completed the study, the baseline seizure frequency was 20 per month. Patients treated with Felbatol® had fewer seizures than patients treated with placebo for each treatment sequence. There was a 23% (P=.018) difference in percentage seizure frequency reduction in favor of Felbatol®.

Felbatol® 3600 mg/day given QID and placebo were compared in a 28-day double-blind add-on trial in patients who had their standard antiepileptic drugs reduced while undergoing evaluations for surgery of intractable epilepsy. All patients had confirmed partial-onset seizures with or without generalization, seizure frequency during surgical evaluation not exceeding an average of four partial seizures per day or more than one generalized seizure per day, and a minimum average of one partial or generalized tonic-clonic seizure per day for the last 3 days of the surgical evaluation. The primary efficacy variable was time to fourth seizure after randomization to treatment with Felbatol® or placebo. Thirteen (46%) of 28 patients in the Felbatol® group

Continued on next page

Wallace Laboratories—Cont.

versus 29 (88%) of 33 patients in the placebo group experienced a fourth seizure. The median times to fourth seizure were greater than 28 days in the Felbatol® group and 5 days in the placebo group. The difference between Felbatol® and placebo in time to fourth seizure was statistically significant (P=.002) in favor of Felbatol®.

Felbatol® Adjunctive Therapy Trial in Children with Lennox-Gastaut Syndrome

In a 70-day double-blind, placebo-controlled add-on trial in the Lennox-Gastaut syndrome, Felbatol® 45 mg/kg/day given QID was superior to placebo in controlling the multiple seizure types associated with this condition. Patients had at least 90 atonic and/or atypical absence seizures per month while receiving therapeutic dosages of one or two other antiepileptic drugs. Patients had a past history of using an average of eight antiepileptic drugs. The most commonly used antiepileptic drug during the baseline period was valproic acid. The frequency of all types of seizures during the baseline period was 1617 per month in the Felbatol® group and 716 per month in the placebo group. Statistically significant differences in the effect on seizure frequency favored Felbatol® over placebo for total seizures (26% reduction vs 5% increase, P<.001), atonic seizures (44% reduction vs 7% reduction, P=.002), and generalized tonic-clonic seizures (40% reduction vs 12% increase, P=.017). Parent/guardian global evaluations based on impressions of quality of life with respect to alertness, verbal responsiveness, general well-being, and seizure control significantly (P<.001) favored Felbatol® over placebo.

When efficacy was analyzed by gender in four well-controlled trials of felbamate as adjunctive and monotherapy for partial-onset seizures and Lennox-Gastaut syndrome, a similar response was seen in 122 males and 142 females.

INDICATIONS AND USAGE

Felbatol® is not indicated as a first line antiepileptic treatment (see **Warnings**). Felbatol® is recommended for use only in those patients who respond inadequately to alternative treatments and whose epilepsy is so severe that a substantial risk of aplastic anemia and/or liver failure is deemed acceptable in light of the benefits conferred by its use.

If these criteria are met and the patient has been fully advised of the risk and has provided written, informed consent, Felbatol® can be considered for either monotherapy or adjunctive therapy in the treatment of partial seizures, with and without generalization, in adults with epilepsy and as adjunctive therapy in the treatment of partial and generalized seizures associated with Lennox-Gastaut syndrome in children.

CONTRAINDICATIONS

Felbatol® is contraindicated in patients with known hypersensitivity to Felbatol®, its ingredients, or known sensitivity to other carbamates. It should not be used in patients with a history of any blood dyscrasia or hepatic dysfunction.

WARNINGS

See Boxed Warning regarding aplastic anemia and hepatic failure.

Antiepileptic drugs should not be suddenly discontinued because of the possibility of increasing seizure frequency.

PRECAUTIONS

Information for Patients: Patients should be informed that the use of Felbatol® is associated with aplastic anemia and hepatic failure, potentially fatal conditions acutely or over a long term.

The physician should obtain written, informed consent prior to initiation of Felbatol® therapy (see **PATIENT INFORMATION/CONSENT** section).

Aplastic anemia in the general population is relatively rare. The absolute risk for the individual patient is not known with any degree of reliability, but patients on Felbatol® may be at more than a 100 fold greater risk for developing the syndrome than the general population.

The long term outlook for patients with aplastic anemia is variable. Although many patients are apparently cured, others require repeated transfusions and other treatments for relapses, and some, although surviving for years, ultimately develop serious complications that sometimes prove fatal (e.g., leukemia).

At present there is no way to predict who is likely to get aplastic anemia, nor is there a documented effective means to monitor the patient so as to avoid and/or reduce the risk. Patients with a history of any blood dyscrasia should not receive Felbatol®.

Patients should be advised to be alert for signs of infection, bleeding, easy bruising, or signs of anemia (fatigue, weakness, lassitude, etc.), and should be advised to report to the physician immediately if any such signs or symptoms appear.

Hepatic failure in the general population is relatively rare. The absolute risk for an individual patient is not known with

any degree of reliability but patients on Felbatol® are at a greater risk for developing hepatic failure than the general population.

At present, there is no way to predict who is likely to develop hepatic failure, however, patients with a history of hepatic dysfunction should not be started on Felbatol®.

Patients should be advised to follow their physician's directives for liver function testing both before starting Felbatol® (felbamate) and at frequent intervals while taking Felbatol®.

Laboratory Tests: Full hematologic evaluations should be performed before Felbatol® therapy, frequently during therapy, and for a significant period of time after discontinuation of Felbatol® therapy. While it might appear prudent to perform frequent CBCs in patients continuing on Felbatol®, there is no evidence that such monitoring will allow early detection of marrow suppression before aplastic anemia occurs. (See **Boxed Warnings**). Complete pretreatment blood counts, including platelets and reticulocytes should be obtained as a baseline. If any hematologic abnormalities are detected during the course of treatment, immediate consultation with a hematologist is advised. Felbatol® should be discontinued if any evidence of bone marrow depression occurs.

Liver function testing (AST, ALT, bilirubin) should be done before Felbatol® is started and at 1- to 2-week intervals while the patient is taking Felbatol®. If any liver abnormalities are detected during the course of treatment, Felbatol® should be discontinued immediately. (see **PATIENT INFORMATION/CONSENT**).

Drug Interactions:

The drug interaction data described in this section were obtained from controlled clinical trials and studies involving otherwise healthy adults with epilepsy.

Use in Conjunction with Other Antiepileptic Drugs (See DOSAGE AND ADMINISTRATION):

The addition of Felbatol® to antiepileptic drugs (AEDs) affects the steady-state plasma concentrations of AEDs. The net effect of these interactions is summarized in the following table:

AED Coadministered	AED Concentration	Felbatol® Concentration
Phenytoin	↑	↓
Valproate	↑	↔**
Carbamazepine (CBZ)	↓	↓
*CBZ epoxide	↑	

* Not administered, but an active metabolite of carbamazepine.
** No significant effect.

Specific Effects of Felbatol® on Other Antiepileptic Drugs:

Phenytoin: Felbatol® causes an increase in steady-state phenytoin plasma concentrations. In 10 otherwise healthy subjects with epilepsy ingesting phenytoin, the steady-state trough (Cmin) phenytoin plasma concentration was 17±5 micrograms/mL. The steady-state Cmin increased to 21±5 micrograms/mL when 1200 mg/day of felbamate was coadministered. Increasing the felbamate dose to 1800 mg/day in six of these subjects increased the steady-state phenytoin Cmin to 25±7 micrograms/mL. In order to maintain phenytoin levels, limit adverse experiences, and achieve the felbamate dose of 3600 mg/day, a phenytoin dose reduction of approximately 40% was necessary for eight of these 10 subjects.

In a controlled clinical trial, a 20% reduction of the phenytoin dose at the initiation of Felbatol® therapy resulted in phenytoin levels comparable to those prior to Felbatol® administration.

Carbamazepine: Felbatol® causes a decrease in the steady-state carbamazepine plasma concentrations and an increase in the steady-state carbamazepine epoxide plasma concentration. In nine otherwise healthy subjects with epilepsy ingesting carbamazepine, the steady-state trough (Cmin) carbamazepine concentration was 8±2 micrograms/mL. The carbamazepine steady-state Cmin decreased 31% to 5±1 micrograms/mL when felbamate (3000 mg/day, divided into three doses) was coadministered. Carbamazepine epoxide steady-state Cmin concentrations increased 57% from 1.0±0.3 to 1.6±0.4 micrograms/mL with the addition of felbamate.

In clinical trials, similar changes in carbamazepine and carbamazepine epoxide were seen.

Valproate: Felbatol® causes an increase in steady-state valproate concentrations. In four subjects with epilepsy ingesting valproate, the steady-state trough (Cmin) valproate plasma concentration was 63±16 micrograms/mL. The steady-state Cmin increased to 78±14 micrograms/mL when 1200 mg/day of felbamate was coadministered. Increasing the felbamate dose to 2400 mg/day increased the

steady-state valproate Cmin to 96±25 micrograms/mL. Corresponding values for free valproate Cmin concentrations were 7±3, 9±4, and 11±6 micrograms/mL for 0, 1200, and 2400 mg/day Felbatol®, respectively. The ratios of the AUCs of unbound valproate to the AUCs of the total valproate were 11.1%, 13.0%, and 11.5%, with coadministration of 0, 1200, and 2400 mg/day of Felbatol®, respectively. This indicates that the protein binding of valproate did not change appreciably with increasing doses of Felbatol®.

Effects of Other Antiepileptic Drugs on Felbatol®:

Phenytoin: Phenytoin causes an approximate doubling of the clearance of Felbatol® (felbamate) at steady state and, therefore, the addition of phenytoin causes an approximate 45% decrease in the steady-state trough concentrations of Felbatol® as compared to the same dose of Felbatol® given as monotherapy.

Carbamazepine: Carbamazepine causes an approximate 50% increase in the clearance of Felbatol® at steady state and, therefore, the addition of carbamazepine results in an approximate 40% decrease in the steady-state trough concentrations of Felbatol® as compared to the same dose of Felbatol® given as monotherapy.

Valproate: Available data suggest that there is no significant effect of valproate on the clearance of Felbatol® at steady state. Therefore, the addition of valproate is not expected to cause a clinically important effect on Felbatol® (felbamate) plasma concentrations.

Effects of Antacids on Felbatol®:

The rate and extent of absorption of a 2400 mg dose of Felbatol® as monotherapy given as tablets was not affected when coadministered with antacids.

Drug/Laboratory Test Interactions: There are no known interactions of Felbatol® with commonly used laboratory tests.

Carcinogenesis, Mutagenesis, Impairment of Fertility: Carcinogenicity studies were conducted in mice and rats. Mice received felbamate as a feed admixture for 92 weeks at doses of 300, 600, and 1200 mg/kg and rats were also dosed by feed admixture for 104 weeks at doses of 30, 100, and 300 (males) or 10, 30, and 100 (females) mg/kg. The maximum doses in these studies produced steady-state plasma concentrations that were equal to or less than the steady-state plasma concentrations in epileptic patients receiving 3600 mg/day. There was a statistically significant increase in hepatic cell adenomas in high-dose male and female mice and in high-dose female rats. Hepatic hypertrophy was significantly increased in a dose-related manner in mice, primarily males, but also in females. Hepatic hypertrophy was not found in female rats. The relationship between the occurrence of benign hepatocellular adenomas and the finding of liver hypertrophy resulting from liver enzyme induction has not been examined. There was a statistically significant increase in benign interstitial cell tumors of the testes in high-dose male rats receiving felbamate. The relevance of these findings to humans is unknown.

As a result of the synthesis process, felbamate could contain small amounts of two known animal carcinogens, the genotoxic compound ethyl carbamate (urethane) and the nongenotoxic compound methyl carbamate. It is theoretically possible that a 50 kg patient receiving 3600 mg of felbamate could be exposed to up to 0.72 micrograms of urethane and 1800 micrograms of methyl carbamate. These daily doses are approximately 1/35,000 (urethane) and 1/5,500 (methyl carbamate) on a mg/kg basis, and 1/10,000 (urethane) and 1/1,600 (methyl carbamate) on a mg/m^2 basis, of the dose levels shown to be carcinogenic in rodents. Any presence of these two compounds in felbamate used in the lifetime carcinogenicity studies was inadequate to cause tumors.

Microbial and mammalian cell assays revealed no evidence of mutagenesis in the Ames *Salmonella*/microsome plate test, CHO/HGPRT mammalian cell forward gene mutation assay, sister chromatid exchange assay in CHO cells, and bone marrow cytogenetics assay.

Reproduction and fertility studies in rats showed no effects on male or female fertility at oral doses of up to 13.9 times the human total daily dose of 3600 mg on a mg/kg basis, or up to 3 times the human total daily dose on a mg/m^2 basis.

Pregnancy: Pregnancy Category C. The incidence of malformations was not increased compared to control in offspring of rats or rabbits given doses up to 13.9 times (rat) and 4.2 times (rabbit) the human daily dose on a mg/kg basis, or 3 times (rat) and less than 2 times (rabbit) the human daily dose on a mg/m^2 basis. However, in rats, there was a decrease in pup weight and an increase in pup deaths during lactation. The cause for these deaths is not known. The no effect dose for rat pup mortality was 6.9 times the human dose on a mg/kg basis or 1.5 times the human dose on a mg/m^2 basis.

Placental transfer of felbamate occurs in rat pups. There are, however, no studies in pregnant women. Because animal reproduction studies are not always predictive of human response, this drug should be used during pregnancy only if clearly needed.

Labor and Delivery: The effect of felbamate on labor and delivery in humans is unknown.

Nursing Mothers: Felbamate has been detected in human milk. The effect on the nursing infant is unknown (see **Pregnancy** section).

Pediatric Use: The safety and effectiveness of Felbatol® in children other than those with Lennox-Gastaut syndrome has not been established.

Geriatric Use: No systematic studies in geriatric patients have been conducted. Clinical studies of Felbatol® did not include sufficient numbers of patients aged 65 and over to determine whether they respond differently from younger patients. Other reported clinical experience has not identified differences in responses between the elderly and younger patients. In general, dosage selection for an elderly patient should be cautious, usually starting at the low end of the dosing range, reflecting the greater frequency of decreased hepatic, renal, or cardiac function, and of concomitant disease or other drug therapy.

ADVERSE REACTIONS

The most common adverse reactions seen in association with Felbatol® (felbamate) in adults during monotherapy are anorexia, vomiting, insomnia, nausea, and headache. The most common adverse reactions seen in association with Felbatol® in adults during adjunctive therapy are anorexia, vomiting, insomnia, nausea, dizziness, somnolence and headache.

The most common adverse reactions seen in association with Felbatol® in children during adjunctive therapy are anorexia, vomiting, insomnia, headache, and somnolence.

The dropout rate because of adverse experiences or intercurrent illnesses among adult felbamate patients was 12 percent (120/977). The dropout rate because of adverse experiences or intercurrent illnesses among pediatric felbamate patients was six percent (22/357). In adults, the body systems associated with causing these withdrawals in order of frequency were: digestive (4.3%), psychological (2.2%), whole body (1.7%), neurological (1.5%), and dermatological (1.5%). In children, the body systems associated with causing these withdrawals in order of frequency were: digestive (1.7%), neurological (1.4%), dermatological (1.4%), psychological (1.1%), and whole body (1.0%). In adults, specific events with an incidence of 1% or greater associated with causing these withdrawals, in order of frequency were: anorexia (1.6%), nausea (1.4%), rash (1.2%), and weight decrease (1.1%). In children, specific events with an incidence of 1% or greater associated with causing these withdrawals, in order of frequency was rash (1.1%).

Incidence in Clinical Trials:

The prescriber should be aware that the figures cited in the following table cannot be used to predict the incidence of side effects in the course of usual medical practice where patient characteristics and other factors differ from those which prevailed in the clinical trials. Similarly, the cited frequencies cannot be compared with figures obtained from other clinical investigations involving different investigators, treatments, and uses including the use of Felbatol® (felbamate) as adjunctive therapy where the incidence of adverse events may be higher due to drug interactions. The cited figures, however, do provide the prescribing physician with some basis for estimating the relative contribution of drug and nondrug factors to the side effect incidence rate in the population studied.

Adults

Incidence in Controlled Clinical Trials—Monotherapy Studies in Adults:

The table that follows enumerates adverse events that occurred at an incidence of 2% or more among 58 adult patients who received Felbatol® monotherapy at dosages of 3600 mg/day in double-blind controlled trials. Reported adverse events were classified using standard WHO-based dictionary terminology.

Adults
Treatment-Emergent Adverse Event
Incidence in Controlled Monotherapy Trials

Body System/Event	Felbatol®* (N=58) %	Low Dose Valproate** (N=50) %
Body as a Whole		
Fatigue	6.9	4.0
Weight Decrease	3.4	0
Face Edema	3.4	0
Central Nervous System		
Insomnia	8.6	4.0
Headache	6.9	18.0
Anxiety	5.2	2.0
Dermatological		
Acne	3.4	0
Rash	3.4	0
Digestive		
Dyspepsia	8.6	2.0
Vomiting	8.6	2.0
Constipation	6.9	2.0
Diarrhea	5.2	0
SGPT Increased	5.2	2.0
Metabolic/Nutritional		
Hypophosphatemia	3.4	0
Respiratory		
Upper Respiratory Tract Infection	8.6	4.0
Rhinitis	6.9	0
Special Senses		
Diplopia	3.4	4.0
Otitis Media	3.4	0
Urogenital		
Intramenstrual Bleeding	3.4	0
Urinary Tract Infection	3.4	2.0

* 3600 mg/day; **15 mg/kg/day

Incidence in Controlled Add-On Clinical Studies in Adults:

The table that follows enumerates adverse events that occurred at an incidence of 2% or more among 114 adult patients who received Felbatol® adjunctive therapy in add-on controlled trials at dosages up to 3600 mg/day. Reported adverse events were classified using standard WHO-based dictionary terminology.

Many adverse experiences that occurred during adjunctive therapy may be a result of drug interactions. Adverse experiences during adjunctive therapy typically resolved with conversion to monotherapy, or with adjustment of the dosage of other antiepileptic drugs.

Adults
Treatment-Emergent Adverse Event
Incidence in Controlled Add-On Trials

Body System/Event	Felbatol® (N=114) %	Placebo (N=43) %
Body as a Whole		
Fatigue	16.8	7.0
Fever	2.6	4.7
Chest Pain	2.6	0
Central Nervous System		
Headache	36.8	9.3
Somnolence	19.3	7.0
Dizziness	18.4	14.0
Insomnia	17.5	7.0
Nervousness	7.0	2.3
Tremor	6.1	2.3
Anxiety	5.3	4.7
Gait Abnormal	5.3	0
Depression	5.3	0
Paraesthesia	3.5	2.3
Ataxia	3.5	0
Mouth Dry	2.6	0
Stupor	2.6	0
Dermatological		
Rash	3.5	4.7
Digestive		
Nausea	34.2	2.3
Anorexia	19.3	2.3
Vomiting	16.7	4.7
Dyspepsia	12.3	7.0
Constipation	11.4	2.3
Diarrhea	5.3	2.3
Abdominal Pain	5.3	0
SGPT Increased	3.5	0
Musculoskeletal		
Myalgia	2.6	0
Respiratory		
Upper Respiratory Tract Infection	5.3	7.0
Sinusitis	3.5	0
Pharyngitis	2.6	0
Special Senses		
Diplopia	6.1	0
Taste Perversion	6.1	0
Vision Abnormal	5.3	2.3

Children

Incidence in a Controlled Add-On Trial in Children with Lennox-Gastaut Syndrome:

The table that follows enumerates adverse events that occurred more than once among 31 pediatric patients who received Felbatol® up to 45 mg/kg/day or a maximum of 3600 mg/day. Reported adverse events were classified using standard WHO-based dictionary terminology.

Children
Treatment-Emergent Adverse Event
Incidence in a Controlled Add-On Lennox-Gastaut Trial

Body System/Event	Felbatol® (N=31) %	Placebo (N=27) %
Body as a Whole		
Fever	22.6	11.1
Fatigue	9.7	3.7
Weight Decrease	6.5	0
Pain	6.5	0
Central Nervous System		
Somnolence	48.4	11.1
Insomnia	16.1	14.8
Nervousness	16.1	18.5
Gait Abnormal	9.7	0
Headache	6.5	18.5
Thinking Abnormal	6.5	3.7
Ataxia	6.5	3.7
Urinary Incontinence	6.5	7.4
Emotional Lability	6.5	0
Miosis	6.5	0
Dermatological		
Rash	9.7	7.4
Digestive		
Anorexia	54.8	14.8
Vomiting	38.7	14.8
Constipation	12.9	0
Hiccup	9.7	3.7
Nausea	6.5	0
Dyspepsia	6.5	3.7
Hematologic		
Purpura	12.9	7.4
Leukopenia	6.5	0
Respiratory		
Upper Respiratory Tract Infection	45.2	25.9
Pharyngitis	9.7	3.7
Coughing	6.5	0
Special Senses		
Otitis Media	9.7	0

Other Events Observed in Association with the Administration of Felbatol® (felbamate):

In the paragraphs that follow, the adverse clinical events, other than those in the preceding tables, that occurred in a total of 977 adults and 357 children exposed to Felbatol® (felbamate) and that are reasonably associated with its use are presented. They are listed in order of decreasing frequency. Because the reports cite events observed in open-label and uncontrolled studies, the role of Felbatol® in their causation cannot be reliably determined.

Events are classified within body system categories and enumerated in order of decreasing frequency using the following definitions: frequent adverse events are defined as those occurring on one or more occasions in at least 1/100 patients; infrequent adverse events are those occurring in 1/100–1/1000 patients; and rare events are those occurring in fewer than 1/1000 patients.

Event frequencies are calculated as the number of patients reporting an event divided by the total number of patients (N = 1334) exposed to Felbatol®.

Body as a Whole: *Frequent:* Weight increase, asthenia, malaise, influenza-like symptoms; *Rare:* anaphylactoid reaction, chest pain substernal.

Cardiovascular: *Frequent:* Palpitation, tachycardia; *Rare:* supraventricular tachycardia.

Central Nervous System: *Frequent:* Agitation, psychological disturbance, aggressive reaction; *Infrequent:* hallucination, euphoria, suicide attempt, migraine.

Digestive: *Frequent:* SGOT increased; *Infrequent:* esophagitis, appetite increased; *Rare:* GGT elevated.

Hematologic: *Infrequent:* Lymphadenopathy, leukopenia, leukocytosis, thrombocytopenia, granulocytopenia; *Rare:* antinuclear factor test positive, qualitative platelet disorder, agranulocytosis.

Metabolic/Nutritional: *Infrequent:* Hypokalemia, hyponatremia, LDH increased, alkaline phosphatase increased, hypophosphatemia; *Rare:* creatinine phosphokinase increased.

Musculoskeletal: *Infrequent:* Dystonia.

Dermatological: *Frequent:* Pruritus; *Infrequent:* urticaria, bullous eruption; *Rare:* buccal mucous membrane swelling, Stevens-Johnson Syndrome.

Special Senses: *Rare:* Photosensitivity allergic reaction.

Postmarketing Adverse Event Reports:

Voluntary reports of adverse events in patients taking Felbatol® (usually in conjunction with other drugs) have been received since market introduction and may have no causal relationship with the drug(s). These include the following by body system:

Body as a Whole: neoplasm, sepsis, L.E. syndrome, SIDS, sudden death, edema, hypothermia, rigors, hyperpyrexia.

Cardiovascular: atrial fibrillation, atrial arrhythmia, cardiac arrest, torsade de pointes, cardiac failure, hypotension, hypertension, flushing, thrombophlebitis, ischemic necrosis, gangrene, peripheral ischemia, bradycardia, Henoch-Schönlein purpura (vasculitis).

Central & Peripheral Nervous System: delusion, paralysis, mononeuritis, cerebrovascular disorder, cerebral edema,

Continued on next page

Wallace Laboratories—Cont.

coma, manic reaction, encephalopathy, paranoid reaction, nystagmus, choreoathetosis, extrapyramidal disorder, confusion, psychosis, status epilepticus, dyskinesia, dysarthria, respiratory depression, apathy, concentration impaired.

Dermatological: abnormal body odor, sweating, lichen planus, livedo reticularis, alopecia, toxic epidermal necrolysis.

Digestive: (Refer to **WARNINGS**) hepatitis, hepatic failure, G.I. hemorrhage, hyperammonemia, pancreatitis, hematemesis, gastritis, rectal hemorrhage, flatulence, gingival bleeding, acquired megacolon, ileus, intestinal obstruction, enteritis, ulcerative stomatitis, glossitis, dysphagia, jaundice, gastric ulcer, gastric dilatation, gastroesophageal reflux.

Fetal Disorders: fetal death, microcephaly, genital malformation, anencephaly, encephalocele.

Hematologic: (Refer to **WARNINGS**) increased and decreased prothrombin time, anemia, hypochromic anemia, aplastic anemia, pancytopenia, hemolytic uremic syndrome, increased mean corpuscular volume (MCV), with and without anemia, coagulation disorder, embolism-limb, disseminated intravascular coagulation, eosinophilia, hemolytic anemia.

Metabolic/Nutritional: hypernatremia, hypoglycemia, SIADH, hypomagnesemia, dehydration, hyperglycemia, hypocalcemia.

Musculoskeletal: arthralgia, muscle weakness, involuntary muscle contraction, rhabdomyolysis.

Respiratory: dyspnea, pneumonia, pneumonitis, hypoxia, epistaxis, pleural effusion, respiratory insufficiency, pulmonary hemorrhage, asthma.

Special Senses: hemianopsia, decreased hearing, conjunctivitis.

Urogenital: menstrual disorder, acute renal failure, hepatorenal syndrome, hematuria, urinary retention, nephrosis, vaginal hemorrhage, abnormal renal function, dysuria, placental disorder.

DRUG ABUSE AND DEPENDENCE

Abuse: Abuse potential was not evaluated in human studies.

Dependence: Rats administered felbamate orally at doses 8.3 times the recommended human dose 6 days each week for 5 consecutive weeks demonstrated no signs of physical dependence as measured by weight loss following drug withdrawal on day 7 of each week.

OVERDOSAGE

Four subjects inadvertently received Felbatol® (felbamate) as adjunctive therapy in dosages ranging from 5400 to 7200 mg/day for durations between 6 and 51 days. One subject who received 5400 mg/day as monotherapy for 1 week reported no adverse experiences. Another subject attempted suicide by ingesting 12,000 mg of Felbatol® in a 12-hour period. The only adverse experiences reported were mild gastric distress and a resting heart rate of 100 bpm. No serious adverse reactions have been reported.

General supportive measures should be employed if overdosage occurs. It is not known if felbamate is dialyzable.

DOSAGE AND ADMINISTRATION

Felbatol® (felbamate) has been studied as monotherapy and adjunctive therapy in adults and as adjunctive therapy in children with seizures associated with Lennox-Gastaut syndrome. As Felbatol® is added to or substituted for existing AEDs, it is strongly recommended to reduce the dosage of those AEDs in the range of 20–33% to minimize side effects (see **Drug Interactions** subsection).

Adults (14 years of age and over)
The majority of patients received 3600 mg/day in clinical trials evaluating its use as both monotherapy and adjunctive therapy.

Monotherapy: (Initial therapy) Felbatol® (felbamate) has not been systematically evaluated as initial monotherapy. Initiate Felbatol® at 1200 mg/day in divided doses three or four times daily. The prescriber is advised to titrate previously untreated patients under close clinical supervision, increasing the dosage in 600-mg increments every 2 weeks to 2400 mg/day based on clinical response and thereafter to 3600 mg/day if clinically indicated.

Conversion to Monotherapy: Initiate Felbatol® at 1200 mg/day in divided doses three or four times daily. Reduce the dosage of concomitant AEDs by one-third at initiation of Felbatol® therapy. At week 2, increase the Felbatol® dosage to 2400 mg/day while reducing the dosage of other AEDs up to an additional one-third of their original dosage. At week 3, increase the Felbatol® dosage up to 3600 mg/day and continue to reduce the dosage of other AEDs as clinically indicated.

Adjunctive Therapy: Felbatol® should be added at 1200 mg/day in divided doses three or four times daily while reducing present AEDs by 20% in order to control plasma concentrations of concurrent phenytoin, valproic acid, and carbamazepine and its metabolites. Further reductions of the concomitant AEDs dosage may be necessary to minimize side effects due to drug interactions. Increase the dosage of

Felbatol® by 1200 mg/day increments at weekly intervals to 3600 mg/day. Most side effects seen during Felbatol® adjunctive therapy resolve as the dosage of concomitant AEDs is decreased.

Dosage Table (adults)			
	WEEK 1	**WEEK 2**	**WEEK 3**
Dosage reduction of concomitant AEDs	REDUCE original dose by 20–33%*	REDUCE original dose by up to an additional ⅓*	REDUCE as clinically indicated
Felbatol® Dosage	1200 mg/day Initial dose	2400 mg/day Therapeutic dosage range	3600 mg/day Therapeutic dosage range

*See **Adjunctive** and **Conversion to Monotherapy** sections.

While the above Felbatol® conversion guidelines may result in a Felbatol® 3600 mg/day dose within 3 weeks, in some patients titration to a 3600 mg/day Felbatol® dose has been achieved in as little as 3 days with appropriate adjustment of other AEDs.

Children with Lennox-Gastaut Syndrome (Ages 2–14 years)
Adjunctive Therapy: Felbatol® should be added at 15 mg/kg/day in divided doses three or four times daily while reducing present AEDs by 20% in order to control plasma levels of concurrent phenytoin, valproic acid, and carbamazepine and its metabolites. Further reductions of the concomitant AED dosage may be necessary to minimize side effects due to drug interactions. Increase the dosage of Felbatol® by 15 mg/kg/day increments at weekly intervals to 45 mg/kg/day. Most side effects seen during Felbatol® adjunctive therapy resolve as the dosage of concomitant AEDs is decreased.

HOW SUPPLIED

Felbatol® (felbamate) Tablets, 400 mg, are yellow, scored, capsule-shaped tablets, debossed "0430" on one side and "WALLACE" on the other; available in:

Bottles of 100 .... NDC 0037-0430-01
Unit Dose 100's .... NDC 0037-0430-11

Felbatol® (felbamate) Tablets, 600 mg, are peach-colored, scored, capsule-shaped tablets, debossed "0431" on one side and "WALLACE" on the other; available in:

Bottles of 100 .... NDC 0037-0431-01
Unit Dose 100's .... NDC 0037-0431-11

Felbatol® (felbamate) Oral Suspension, 600 mg/5 mL, is peach-colored; available in:

8 oz bottles .... NDC 0037-0442-67
32 oz bottles .... NDC 0037-0442-17

Shake suspension well before using.
Store at controlled room temperature 15°–30°C (59°–86°F).
Dispense in tight container.

PATIENT INFORMATION/CONSENT

FELBATOL® (felbamate) SHOULD NOT BE USED BY PATIENTS UNTIL THERE HAS BEEN A COMPLETE DISCUSSION OF THE RISKS AND WRITTEN INFORMED CONSENT HAS BEEN OBTAINED.

IMPORTANT INFORMATION AND WARNING:
Felbatol®, taken by itself or with other prescription and/or non-prescription drugs, can result in severe, potentially fatal blood abnormality ("aplastic anemia") and/or severe, potentially fatal liver damage.

PATIENT CONSENT:
My [My son, daughter, ward, _____
_____ 's]
treatment with Felbatol® has been personally/
explained to me by Dr. _____ .
The following points of information, among others, have been specifically discussed and made clear and I have had the opportunity to ask any questions concerning this information.

1. I, _____
_____ (Patient's Name), understand that Felbatol® is used to treat certain types of seizures and my physician has told me that I have this type(s) of seizures:
INITIALS: _____

2. I understand that Felbatol® is being used since my seizures have not been satisfactorily treated with other antiepileptic drugs;
INITIALS: _____

3. I understand there is a serious risk that I could develop aplastic anemia and/or liver failure, both of which are potentially fatal, by using Felbatol®;
INITIALS: _____

4. I understand that there are no laboratory tests which will predict if I am at an increased risk for one of the potentially fatal conditions;
INITIALS: _____

5. I understand that I should have the recommended blood work before my treatment with Felbatol® is begun or continued and then every 1–2 weeks while taking Felbatol®. I understand that although this blood work may help detect if I develop one of these conditions, it may do so only after significant, irreversible and potentially fatal damage has already occurred;
INITIALS: _____

6. If I am currently taking another antiepileptic drug, I understand that the manufacturer of Felbatol® recommends that the dosage of these other drugs be decreased by a certain amount when Felbatol® is started; if my physician determines that this should not be done in my case, he/she has explained the reason(s) for this decision;
INITIALS: _____

7. I understand that I must immediately report any unusual symptoms to Dr. _____
and be especially aware of any rashes, easy bruising, bleeding, sore throats, fever, and/or dark urine;
INITIALS: _____

I now authorize Dr. _____
to begin my treatment with Felbatol®; OR, if my treatment has already begun with Felbatol®, to continue such treatment.

_____
Patient, Parent, or Guardian

_____
Address

_____
Telephone

PHYSICIAN STATEMENT:
I have fully explained to the patient, _____,
the nature and purpose of the treatment with Felbatol® (felbamate) and the potential risks associated with that treatment. I have asked the patient if he/she has any questions regarding this treatment or the risks and have answered those questions to the best of my ability. I also acknowledge that I have read and understand the prescribing information listed above.

_____
Physician   Date

NOTE TO PHYSICIAN: It is strongly recommended that you retain a signed copy of the informed consent with the patient's medical records.

SUPPLY OF PATIENT INFORMATION/CONSENT FORMS:
A supply of "Patient Information/Consent" forms as printed above is available, free of charge, from your local Wallace representative, or may be obtained by calling 609-655-6147. Permission to use the above Patient Information/Consent by photocopy reproduction is also hereby granted by Carter-Wallace, Inc.

CAUTION: Federal law prohibits dispensing without prescription.

WALLACE LABORATORIES
Division of Carter-Wallace, Inc.
Cranbury, New Jersey 08512
Rev. 11/95   IN-00431-07 PP
Shown in Product Identification Guide, page 339

LUFYLLIN®
(dyphylline)
Elixir   ℞

LUFYLLIN® Tablets
(dyphylline tablets, USP, 200 mg)   ℞
LUFYLLIN®–400 Tablets
(dyphylline tablets, USP, 400 mg)   ℞

DESCRIPTION

LUFYLLIN (dyphylline), a xanthine derivative, is a bronchodilator available for oral administration as tablets containing 200 mg and 400 mg of dyphylline. Other ingredients: magnesium stearate, microcrystalline cellulose.

Chemically, dyphylline is 7-(2,3-dihydroxypropyl)-theophylline, a white, extremely bitter, amorphous powder that is freely soluble in water and soluble in alcohol to the extent of

2 g/100 mL. Dyphylline forms a neutral solution that is stable in gastrointestinal fluids over a wide range of pH.
The molecular formula for dyphylline is $C_{10}H_{14}N_4O_4$ with a molecular weight of 254.25. Its structural formula is:

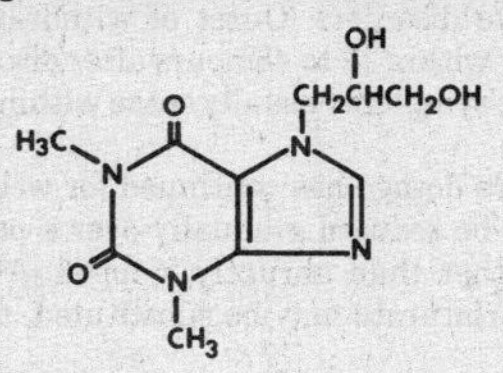

CLINICAL PHARMACOLOGY

Dyphylline is a xanthine derivative with pharmacologic actions similar to theophylline and other members of this class of drugs. Its primary action is that of bronchodilation, but it also exhibits peripheral vasodilatory and other smooth muscle relaxant activity to a lesser degree. The bronchodilatory action of dyphylline, as with other xanthines, is thought to be mediated through competitive inhibition of phosphodiesterase with a resulting increase in cyclic AMP producing relaxation of bronchial smooth muscle.
LUFYLLIN is well tolerated and produces less nausea than aminophylline and other alkaline theophylline compounds when administered orally. Unlike the hydrolyzable salts of theophylline, dyphylline is not converted to free theophylline *in vivo.* It is absorbed rapidly in therapeutically active form and in healthy volunteers reaches a mean peak plasma concentration of 17.1 mcg/mL in approximately 45 minutes following a single oral dose of 1000 mg of LUFYLLIN.
Dyphylline exerts its bronchodilatory effects directly and, unlike theophylline, is excreted unchanged by the kidneys without being metabolized by the liver. Because of this, dyphylline pharmacokinetics and plasma levels are not influenced by various factors that affect liver function and hepatic enzyme activity, such as smoking, age, congestive heart failure, or concomitant use of drugs which affect liver function.
The elimination half-life of dyphylline is approximately two hours (1.8–2.1 hr) and approximately 88% of a single oral dose can be recovered from the urine unchanged. The renal clearance would be correspondingly reduced in patients with impaired renal function. In anuric patients, the half-life may be increased 3 to 4 times normal.
Dyphylline plasma levels are dose-related and generally predictable. The range of plasma levels within which dyphylline can be expected to produce effective bronchodilation has not been determined.
Dyphylline plasma concentrations can be accurately determined using high pressure liquid chromatography (HPLC)* or gas-liquid chromatography (GLC).

INDICATIONS AND USAGE

For relief of acute bronchial asthma and for reversible bronchospasm associated with chronic bronchitits and emphysema.

CONTRAINDICATIONS

Hypersensitivity to dyphylline or related xanthine compounds.

WARNINGS

LUFYLLIN is not indicated in the management of status asthmaticus, which is a serious medical emergency.
Although the relationship between plasma levels of dyphylline and appearance of toxicity is unknown, excessive doses may be expected to be associated with an increased risk of adverse effects.

PRECAUTIONS

General: Use LUFYLLIN with caution in patients with severe cardiac disease, hypertension, hyperthyroidism, acute myocardial injury, or peptic ulcer.
Drug interactions: Synergism between xanthine bronchodilators (e.g., theophylline), ephedrine, and other sympathomimetic bronchodilators has been reported. This should be considered whenever these agents are prescribed concomitantly.
Concurrent administration of dyphylline and probenecid, which competes for tubular secretion, has been shown to increase the plasma half-life of dyphylline (see Clinical Pharmacology).
Carcinogenesis, mutagenesis, impairment of fertility: No long-term animal studies have been performed with LUFYLLIN.
Pregnancy: Teratogenic effects—Pregnancy Category C. Animal reproduction studies have not been conducted with LUFYLLIN. It is also not known if LUFYLLIN can cause fetal harm when administered to a pregnant woman or can affect reproduction capacity. LUFYLLIN should be given to a pregnant woman only if clearly needed.
Nursing mothers: Dyphylline is present in human milk at approximately twice the maternal plasma concentration. Caution should be exercised when LUFYLLIN is administered to a nursing woman.
Pediatric use: Safety and effectiveness in children have not been established.

*See Valia, *et al. J. Chromatogr.* **221**: 170 (1980). Small quantities of pure dyphylline powder may be obtained from Wallace Laboratories, Cranbury, N.J. The internal standard, β-hydroxyethyl-theophylline, may be obtained from companies supplying analytical chemicals.

ADVERSE REACTIONS

Adverse reactions with the use of LUFYLLIN have been infrequent, relatively mild, and rarely required reduction in dosage or withdrawal of therapy.
The following adverse reactions which have been reported with other xanthine bronchodilators, and which have most often been related to excessive drug plasma levels, should be considered as potential adverse effects when dyphylline is administered:
Gastrointestinal: nausea, vomiting, epigastric pain, hematemesis, diarrhea.
Central nervous system: headache, irritability, restlessness, insomnia, hyperexcitability, agitation, muscle twitching, generalized clonic and tonic convulsions.
Cardiovascular: palpitation, tachycardia, extrasystoles, flushing, hypotension, circulatory failure, ventricular arrhythmias.
Respiratory: tachypnea.
Renal: albuminuria, gross and microscopic hematuria, diuresis.
Other: hyperglycemia, inappropriate ADH syndrome.

OVERDOSAGE

There have been no reports, in the literature, of overdosage with LUFYLLIN. However, the following information based on reports of theophylline overdosage are considered typical of the xanthine class of drugs and should be kept in mind.
Signs and symptoms: Restlessness, anorexia, nausea, vomiting, diarrhea, insomnia, irritability, and headache. Marked overdosage with resulting severe toxicity has produced agitation, severe vomiting, dehydration, excessive thirst, tinnitus, cardiac arrhythmias, hyperthermia, diaphoresis, and generalized clonic and tonic convulsions. Cardiovascular collapse has also occcurred, with some fatalities. Seizures have occurred in some cases associated with very high theophylline plasma concentrations, without any premonitory symptoms of toxicity.
Treatment: There is no specific antidote for overdosage with drugs of the xanthine class. Symptomatic treatment and general supportive measures should be instituted with careful monitoring and maintenance of vital signs, fluids, and electrolytes. The stomach should be emptied by inducing emesis if the patient is conscious and responsive, or by gastric lavage, taking care to protect against aspiration, especially in stuporous or comatose patients. Maintenance of an adequate airway is essential in case oxygen or assisted respiration is needed. Sympathomimetic agents should be avoided but sedatives such as short-acting barbiturates may be useful.
Dyphylline is dialyzable and, although not recommended as a routine procedure in overdosage cases, hemodialysis may be of some benefit when severe intoxication is present or when the patient has not responded to general supportive and symptomatic treatment.

DOSAGE AND ADMINISTRATION

Dosage should be individually titrated according to the severity of the condition and the response of the patient.
Usual adult dosage: Up to 15 mg/kg every six hours.
Appropriate dosage adjustments should be made in patients with impaired renal function (see Clinical Pharmacology).

HOW SUPPLIED

LUFYLLIN Tablets contain 200 mg dyphylline and are white, rectangular, scored on one side and imprinted WALLACE 521 on the other side.
The tablets are available in bottles of 100 (NDC 0037-0521-92), 1000 (NDC 0037-0521-97), and 5000 (NDC 0037-0521-98), and individually film-sealed in unit-dose boxes of 100 (NDC 0037-0521-85).
LUFYLLIN-400 Tablets contain 400 mg dyphylline and are white, capsule-shaped, scored on one side and imprinted WALLACE 731 on the other side. The tablets are available in bottles of 100 (NDC 0037-0731-92), 1000 (NDC 0037-0731-97), and 2500 (NDC 0037-0731-99.
Storage: Store at controlled room temperature 15°–30°C (59°–86°F).
Dispense in a tight container.
CAUTION: Federal law prohibits dispensing without prescription.

WALLACE LABORATORIES
Division of
CARTER-WALLACE, INC.
Cranbury, New Jersey 08512
IN05 Rev. 5/94

LUFYLLIN®–GG ℞

(dyphylline and guaifenesin tablets and elixir, USP)
Tablets and Elixir

DESCRIPTION

LUFYLLIN®-GG is a bronchodilator/expectorant combination available for oral administration as *Tablets* and *Elixir.*
Each Tablet contains:

Dyphylline	200 mg
Guaifenesin	200 mg

Other ingredients: corn starch, D&C Yellow No. 10, magnesium aluminium silicate, magnesium stearate, microcrystalline cellulose.
Each 15 mL (one tablespoonful) of Elixir contains:

Dyphylline	100 mg
Guaifenesin	100 mg
Alcohol (by volume)	17%

Other ingredients: citric acid, FD&C Yellow No. 6, flavor (artificial), purified water, saccharin sodium, sodium citrate, sucrose.
Dyphylline is 7-(2,3-dihydroxypropyl)-theophylline, a white, extremely bitter, amorphous powder that is fully soluble in water and soluble in alcohol to the extent of 2 g/100 mL. Dyphylline forms a neutral solution that is stable in gastrointestinal fluids over a wide range of pH.

CLINICAL PHARMACOLOGY

Dyphylline is a xanthine derivative with pharmacologic actions similar to theophylline and other members of this class of drugs. Its primary action is that of bronchodilation, but it also exhibits peripheral vasodilatory and other smooth muscle relaxant activity to a lesser degree. The bronchodilatory action of dyphylline, as with as other xanthines, is thought to be mediated through competitive inhibition of phosphodiesterase with a resulting increase in cyclic AMP producing relaxation of bronchial smooth muscle.
Dyphylline in LUFYLLIN-GG is well tolerated and produces less nausea than aminophylline and other alkaline theophylline compounds when administered orally. Unlike the hydrolyzable salts of theophylline, dyphylline is not converted to free theophylline *in vivo.* It is absorbed rapidly in therapeutically active form and in healthy volunteers reaches a mean peak plasma concentration of 17.1 mcg/mL in approximately 45 minutes following a single oral dose of 1000 mg of dyphylline.
Dyphylline exerts its bronchodilatory effects directly and, unlike theophylline, is excreted unchanged by the kidneys without being metabolized by the liver. Because of this, dyphylline pharmacokinetics and plasma levels are not influenced by various factors that affect liver function and hepatic enzyme activity, such as smoking, age, or concomitant use of drugs which affect liver function.
The elimination half-life of dyphylline is approximately two hours (1.8–2.1 hr) and approximately 88% of a single oral dose can be recovered from the urine unchanged. The renal clearance would be correspondingly reduced in patients with impaired renal function. In anuric patients, the half-life may be increased 3 to 4 times normal.
Dyphylline plasma levels are dose-related and generally predictable. The therapeutic range of plasma levels within which dyphylline can be expected to produce effective bronchodilation has not been determined.
Dyphylline plasma concentrations can be accurately determined using high pressure liquid chromatography (HPLC)* or gas-liquid chromatography (GLC).
Guaifenesin is an expectorant whose action helps increase the output of thin respiratory tract fluid to facilitate mucociliary clearance and removal of inspissated mucus.

*See Valia, *et al, J Chromatogr.* **221**: 170 (1980). Small quantities of pure dyphylline powder may be obtained from Wallace Laboratories, Cranbury, N.J. The internal standard, β-hydroxyethyl-theophylline may be obtained from companies supplying analytical chemicals.

INDICATIONS AND USAGE

For relief of acute bronchial asthma and for reversible bronchospasm associated with chronic bronchitis and emphysema.

CONTRAINDICATIONS

Hypersensitivity to any of the ingredients or related compounds.

WARNINGS

LUFYLLIN-GG is not indicated in the management of status asthmaticus, which is a serious medical emergency.
Although the relationship between plasma levels of dyphylline and appearance of toxicity is unknown, excessive doses may be expected to be associated with an increased risk of adverse effects.

PRECAUTIONS

General: Use LUFYLLIN-GG with caution in patients with severe cardiac disease, hypertension, hyperthyroidism, acute myocardial injury or peptic ulcer.

Continued on next page

Wallace Laboratories—Cont.

Drug interactions: Synergism between xanthine bronchodilators (e.g., theophylline), ephedrine and other sympathomimetic bronchodilators has been reported. This should be considered whenever these agents are prescribed concomitantly. Concurrent administration of dyphylline and probenecid, which competes for tubular secretion, has been shown to increase plasma half-life of dyphylline (see Clinical Pharmacology).

Carcinogenesis, mutagenesis, impairment of fertility: No long-term animal studies have been performed with LUFYLLIN-GG.

Pregnancy: Teratogenic effects—Pregnancy Category C. Animal reproduction studies have not been conducted with LUFYLLIN-GG. It is also not known whether the product can cause fetal harm when administered to a pregnant woman or can affect reproduction capacity. LUFYLLIN-GG should be given to a pregnant woman only if clearly needed.

Nursing mothers: Dyphylline is present in human milk at approximately twice the maternal plasma concentration. Caution should be exercised when LUFYLLIN-GG is administered to a nursing woman.

Pediatric use: Safety and effectiveness in children below the age of six have not been established. Use caution when administering to children six years of age or older.

ADVERSE REACTIONS

LUFYLLIN-GG may cause nausea, headache, cardiac palpitation and CNS stimulation. Postprandial administration may help avoid gastric discomfort.

The following adverse reactions which have been reported with other xanthine bronchodilators, and which have most often been related to excessive drug plasma levels, should be considered as potential adverse effects when dyphylline is administered:

Gastrointestinal: nausea, vomiting, epigastric pain, hematemesis, diarrhea.

Central nervous system: headache, irritability, restlessness, insomnia, hyperexcitability, agitation, muscle twitching, generalized clonic and tonic convulsions.

Cardiovascular: palpitation, tachycardia, extrasystoles, flushing, hypotension, circulatory failure, ventricular arrhythmias.

Respiratory: tachypnea.

Renal: albuminuria, gross and microscopic hematuria, diuresis.

Other: hyperglycemia, inappropriate ADH syndrome.

OVERDOSAGE

There have been no reports, in the literature, of overdosage with LUFYLLIN-GG. However, the following information based on reports of theophylline overdosage are considered typical of the xanthine class of drugs and should be kept in mind.

Signs & symptoms: Restlessness, anorexia, nausea, vomiting, diarrhea, insomnia, irritability, and headache. Marked overdosage with resulting severe toxicity has produced agitation, severe vomiting, dehydration, excessive thirst, tinnitus, cardiac arrhythmias, hyperthermia, diaphoresis, and generalized clonic and tonic convulsions. Cardiovascular collapse has also occurred, with some fatalities. Seizures have occurred in some cases associated with very high theophylline plasma concentrations, without any premonitory symptoms of toxicity.

Treatment: There is no specific antidote for overdosage with drugs of the xanthine class. Symptomatic treatment and general supportive measures should be instituted with careful monitoring and maintenance of vital signs, fluids and electrolytes. The stomach should be emptied by inducing emesis if the patient is conscious and responsive, or by gastric lavage, taking care to protect against aspiration, especially in stuporous or comatose patients. Maintenance of an adequate airway is essential in case oxygen or assisted respiration is needed. Sympathomimetic agents should be avoided but sedatives such as short-acting barbiturates may be useful.

Dyphylline is dialyzable and, although not recommended as a routine procedure in overdosage cases, hemodialysis may be of some benefit when severe intoxication is present or when the patient has not responded to general supportive and symptomatic treatment.

DOSAGE AND ADMINISTRATION

Dosage should be individually titrated according to the severity of the condition and the response of the patient.

Usual adult dosage:
One tablet or 30 mL (two tablespoonfuls) elixir, four times daily.

Children above age six:
One-half to one tablet or 15 to 30 mL (one to two tablespoonfuls) elixir, three or four times daily.

Not recommended for use in children below age six: (see Precautions).

HOW SUPPLIED

LUFYLLIN-GG Tablets (dyphylline 200 mg and guaifenesin 200 mg) are round, convex, light yellow, scored on one side and imprinted on the other side with WALLACE 541. The tablets are available in bottles of 100 (NDC 0037-0541-92), 1000 (NDC 0037-0541-97), and 3000 (NDC 0037-0541-96), and in boxes of 100 unit-dose (NDC 0037-0541-85).

LUFYLLIN-GG Elixir (dyphylline 100 mg, quaifenesin 100 mg and alcohol 17% by volume per 15 mL) is a clear, light yellow-orange liquid with a mild wine-like odor and taste. The elixir is available in bottles of one pint (NDC 0037-0545-68) and one gallon (NDC 0037-0545-69).

Storage:
Tablets and Elixir—Store at controlled room temperature 15°–30°C (59°–86°F).

Dispense in a tight container.

CAUTION: Federal law prohibits dispensing without prescription.

WALLACE LABORATORIES
Division of
CARTER-WALLACE, INC.
Cranbury, New Jersey 08512
IN-0541-06   Rev. 2/95

MALTSUPEX®   OTC
(malt soup extract)
Powder, Liquid, Tablets

(See PDR For Nonprescription Drugs.)

MILTOWN®   © ℞
(meprobamate tablets, USP)

DESCRIPTION

Meprobamate is a white powder with a *characteristic odor* and a bitter taste. It is slightly soluble in water, freely soluble in acetone and alcohol, and sparingly soluble in ether. The structural formula of meprobamate is:

$$NH_2COOCH_2 - \overset{\overset{\displaystyle CH_3}{|}}{\underset{\underset{\displaystyle CH_2CH_2CH_3}{|}}{C}} - CH_2OOCNH_2$$

MILTOWN-200 contains 200 mg meprobamate per tablet. Other ingredients: acacia, carnauba wax, corn starch, gelatin, magnesium carbonate, magnesium stearate, methylcellulose, shellac, sugar, talc, titanium dioxide, white wax and other ingredients.

MILTOWN-400 contains 400 mg meprobamate per tablet. Other ingredients: corn starch, magnesium stearate, methylcellulose.

MILTOWN-600 contains 600 mg meprobamate per tablet. Other ingredients: alginic acid, corn starch, ethylcellulose, magnesium stearate, purified stearic acid.

ACTIONS

Meprobamate is a carbamate derivative which has been shown in animal studies to have effects at multiple sites in the central nervous system, including the thalamus and limbic system.

INDICATIONS

MILTOWN (meprobamate) is indicated for the management of anxiety disorders or for the short-term relief of the symptoms of anxiety. Anxiety or tension associated with the stress of everyday life usually do not require treatment with an anxiolytic.

The effectiveness of MILTOWN in long-term use, that is, more than 4 months, has not been assessed by systematic clinical studies. The physician should periodically reassess the usefulness of the drug for the individual patient.

CONTRAINDICATIONS

Acute intermittent porphyria as well as allergic or idiosyncratic reactions to meprobamate or related compounds such as carisoprodol, mebutamate, tybamate or carbromal.

WARNINGS

Drug Dependence
Physical dependence, psychological dependence, and abuse have occurred. When chronic intoxication from prolonged use occurs, it usually involves ingestion of greater than recommended doses and is manifested by ataxia, slurred speech, and vertigo. Therefore, careful supervision of dose and amounts prescribed is advised, as well as avoidance of prolonged administration, especially for alcoholics and other patients with a known propensity for taking excessive quantities of drugs.

Sudden withdrawal of the drug after prolonged and excessive use may precipitate recurrence of pre-existing symptoms, such as anxiety, anorexia, or insomnia, or withdrawal

reactions, such as vomiting, ataxia, tremors, muscle twitching, confusional states, hallucinosis, and, rarely, convulsive seizures. Such seizures are more likely to occur in persons with central nervous system damage or pre-existent or latent convulsive disorders. Onset of withdrawal symptoms occurs usually within 12 to 48 hours after discontinuation of meprobamate; symptoms usually cease within the next 12 to 48 hours.

When excessive dosage has continued for weeks or months, dosage should be reduced gradually over a period of one or two weeks rather than abruptly stopped. Alternatively, a long-acting barbiturate may be substituted, then gradually withdrawn.

Potentially Hazardous Tasks
Patients should be warned that this drug may impair the mental and/or physical abilities required for the performance of potentially hazardous tasks such as driving a motor vehicle or operating machinery.

Additive Effects
Since the effects of meprobamate and alcohol or meprobamate and other CNS depressants or psychotropic drugs may be additive, appropriate caution should be exercised with patients who take more than one of these agents simultaneously.

Usage in Pregnancy and Lactation
An increased risk of congenital malformations associated with the use of minor tranquilizers (meprobamate, chlordiazepoxide, and diazepam) during the first trimester of pregnancy has been suggested in several studies. Because use of these drugs is rarely a matter of urgency, their use during this period should almost always be avoided. The possibility that a woman of childbearing potential may be pregnant at the time of institution of therapy should be considered. Patients should be advised that if they become pregnant during therapy or intend to become pregnant they should communicate with their physician about the desirability of discontinuing the drug.

Meprobamate passes the placental barrier. It is present both in umbilical cord blood at or near maternal plasma levels and in breast milk of lactating mothers at concentrations two to four times that of maternal plasma. When use of meprobamate is contemplated in breast-feeding patients, the drug's higher concentration in breast milk as compared to maternal plasma levels should be considered.

Usage in Children
MILTOWN-200 and MILTOWN-400 should not be administered to children under age six, since there is a lack of documented evidence for safety and effectiveness in this age group.

MILTOWN-600 is not intended for use in children.

PRECAUTIONS

The lowest effective dose should be administered, particularly to elderly and/or debilitated patients, in order to preclude oversedation.

The possibility of suicide attempts should be considered and the least amount of drug feasible should be dispensed at any one time.

Meprobamate is metabolized in the liver and excreted by the kidney; to avoid its excess accumulation, caution should be exercised in administration to patients with compromised liver or kidney function.

Meprobamate occasionally may precipitate seizures in epileptic patients.

ADVERSE REACTIONS

Central Nervous System
Drowsiness, ataxia, dizziness, slurred speech, headache, vertigo, weakness, paresthesias, impairment of visual accomodation, euphoria, overstimulation, paradoxical excitement, fast EEG activity.

Gastrointestinal
Nausea, vomiting, diarrhea.

Cardiovascular
Palpitations, tachycardia, various forms of arrhythmia, transient ECG changes, syncope; also, hypotensive crises (including one fatal case).

Allergic or Idiosyncratic
Allergic or idiosyncratic reactions are usually seen within the period of the first to fourth dose in patients having had no previous contact with the drug. Milder reactions are characterized by an itchy, urticarial, or erythematous maculopapular rash which may be generalized or confined to the groin. Other reactions have included leukopenia, acute nonthrombocytopenic purpura, petechiae, ecchymoses, eosinophilia, peripheral edema, adenopathy, fever, fixed drug eruption with cross reaction to carisoprodol, and cross sensitivity between meprobamate/mebutamate and meprobamate/carbromal.

More severe hypersensitivity reactions, rarely reported, include hyperpyrexia, chills, angioneurotic edema, bronchospasm, oliguria, and anuria. Also, anaphylaxis, erythema multiforme, exfoliative dermatitis, stomatitis, proctitis, Stevens-Johnson syndrome, and bullous dermatitis, including one fatal case of the latter following administration of meprobamate in combination with prednisolone.

In case of allergic or idiosyncratic reactions to meprobamate, discontinue the drug and initiate appropriate symptomatic therapy, which may include epinephrine, antihistamines, and in severe cases corticosteroids. In evaluating possible allergic reactions, also consider allergy to excipients.

Hematologic

(See also **Allergic or Idiosyncratic**.) Agranulocytosis and aplastic anemia have been reported. These cases rarely were fatal. Rare cases of thrombocytopenic purpura have been reported.

Other

Exacerbation of porphyric symptoms.

DOSAGE AND ADMINISTRATION

MILTOWN-200 and 400:

The usual adult dosage is 1200 mg to 1600 mg, in three or four divided doses; a daily dosage above 2400 mg is not recommended. The usual daily dosage for children ages six to twelve is 200 mg to 600 mg, in two or three divided doses.

Not recommended for children under age 6 (see **Usage in Children**).

MILTOWN-600:

Adults—One tablet twice a day. Doses of meprobamate above 2400 mg daily are not recommended.

Not recommended for use in children (see **Usage in Children**).

OVERDOSAGE

Suicidal attempts with meprobamate have resulted in drowsiness, lethargy, stupor, ataxia, coma, shock, vasomotor and respiratory collapse. Some suicidal attempts have been fatal. The following data on meprobamate tablets have been reported in the literature and from other sources. These data are not expected to correlate with each case (considering factors such as individual susceptibility and length of time from ingestion to treatment), but represent the **usual ranges** reported.

Acute simple overdose (meprobamate alone): Death has been reported with ingestion of as little as 12 g meprobamate and survival with as much as 40 g.

Blood Levels:

0.5–2.0 mg% represents the usual blood level range of meprobamate after therapeutic doses. The level may occasionally be as high as 3.0 mg%.

3–10 mg% usually corresponds to findings of mild to moderate symptoms of overdosage, such as stupor or light coma.

10–20 mg% usually corresponds to deeper coma, requiring more intensive treatment. Some fatalities occur.

At levels greater than 20%, more fatalities than survivals can be expected.

Acute combined overdose (meprobamate with alcohol or other CNS depressants or psychotropic drugs): Since effects can be additive, a history of ingestion of a low dose of meprobamate plus any of these compounds (or of a relative low blood or tissue level) cannot be used as a prognostic indicator. In cases where excessive doses have been taken, sleep ensues rapidly and blood pressure, pulse, and respiratory rates are reduced to basal levels. Any drug remaining in the stomach should be removed and symptomatic therapy given. Should respiration or blood pressure become compromised, respiratory assistance, central nervous system stimulants, and pressor agents should be administered cautiously as indicated. Meprobamate is metabolized in the liver and excreted by the kidney. Diuresis, osmotic (mannitol) diuresis, peritoneal dialysis, and hemodialysis have been used successfully. Careful monitoring of urinary output is necessary and caution should be taken to avoid overhydration. Relapse and death, after initial recovery, have been attributed to incomplete gastric emptying and delayed absorption. Meprobamate can be measured in biological fluids by two methods: colorimetric (Hoffman, A.J. and Ludwig, B.J.: *J Amer Pharm Assn 48:* 740, 1959) and gas chromatographic (Douglas, J.F. et al.: *Anal Chem 39* : 956, 1967).

HOW SUPPLIED

MILTOWN-200: 200 mg white, sugar-coated tablets coded 37-1101 and Wallace; available in bottles of 100 (NDC 0037-1101-01).

MILTOWN-400: 400 mg white, scored tablets coded 37-1001 and Wallace: available in bottles of 100 (NDC 0037-1001-01), 500 (NDC 0037-1001-03), and 1000 (NDC 0037-1001-02).

MILTOWN-600: 600 mg white, capsule-shaped tablets coded 37-1601 and Wallace on one side and 600 on the other side; available in bottles of 100 (NDC 0037-1601-01).

Storage: Store at controlled room temperature 15°–30°C (59°–86°F). Dispense in a tight container.

WALLACE LABORATORIES
Division of CARTER-WALLACE, INC.
Cranbury, New Jersey 08512
IN-070J2-07   Rev. 6/92

ORGANIDIN® NR*   ℞
(*Newly Reformulated)
(guaifenesin)
Tablets and Liquid

Professional Labeling Information and Directions for Use
This product labeled for sale on prescription only.

DESCRIPTION

ORGANIDIN® NR* (*Newly Reformulated) (guaifenesin) is an expectorant available for oral administration as tablets and liquid.

Each tablet contains 200 mg guaifenesin, USP.

Other ingredients: Microcrystalline cellulose, corn starch, croscarmellose sodium, magnesium stearate, FD&C Red No. 40.

Each teaspoonful (5 mL) of liquid contains 100 mg guaifenesin, USP.

Other ingredients: Citric acid, caramel, glycerin, sorbitol solution, propylene glycol, saccharin sodium, sodium benzoate, flavor compound (raspberry), purified water.

Guaifenesin (glycerol guaiacolate) has the chemical name 3-(2-methoxyphenoxy)-1,2-propanediol. Its molecular formula is $C_{10}H_{14}O_4$, with a molecular weight of 198.21. It is a white, colorless crystalline substance with a slightly bitter aromatic taste. One gram dissolves in 20 mL water at 25°C; freely soluble in ethanol. Guaifenesin is readily absorbed from the GI tract and is rapidly metabolized and excreted in the urine. Guaifenesin has a plasma half-life of one hour. The major urinary metabolite is beta-(2-methoxyphenoxy) lactic acid.

CLINICAL PHARMACOLOGY

Guaifenesin is an expectorant the action of which promotes or facilitates the removal of secretions from the respiratory tract. By increasing sputum volume and making sputum less viscous, guaifenesin facilitates expectoration of retained secretions.

INDICATIONS AND USAGE

Helps loosen phlegm (mucus) and thin bronchial secretions to rid the bronchial passageways of bothersome mucus, drain bronchial tubes, and make coughs more productive. Helps loosen phlegm and thin bronchial secretions in patients with stable chronic bronchitis.

CONTRAINDICATIONS

ORGANIDIN® NR* (*Newly Reformulated) is contraindicated in patients hypersensitive to any of the ingredients.

PRECAUTIONS

Carcinogenesis, Mutagenesis, Impairment of Fertility. Animal studies to assess the long-term carcinogenic and mutagenic potential or the effect of fertility in animals or humans have not been performed.

Pregnancy

Teratogenic Effects—Pregnancy Category C: Animal reproduction studies have not been conducted. Safe use in pregnancy has not been established relative to possible adverse effects on fetal development. Therefore, this product should not be used in pregnant patients, unless in the judgment of the physician, the potential benefits outweigh possible hazards.

Nursing Mothers: It is not known whether guaifenesin is excreted in human milk. Because many drugs are excreted in human milk, caution should be exercised when these products are administered to a nursing woman and a decision should be made whether to discontinue nursing or to discontinue the drug, taking into account the importance of the drug to the mother.

Laboratory Test Interactions: Guaifenesin or its metabolites may cause color interference with the VMA (vanillylmandelic acid) test for catechols. It may also falsely elevate the level of urinary 5-HIAA (5-hydroxyindoleacetic acid) in certain serotonin metabolite chemical tests because of color interference.

ADVERSE REACTIONS

Guaifenesin is well tolerated and has a wide margin of safety. Side effects have been generally mild and infrequent. Nausea and vomiting are the side effects that occur most commonly. Dizziness, headache, and rash (including urticaria) have been reported rarely.

OVERDOSAGE

The acute toxicity of guaifenesin is low and overdosage is unlikely to produce serious toxic effects. In laboratory animals no toxicity resulted when guaifenesin was administered by stomach tube in doses up to 5 grams/kg.

In massive overdosage the stomach should be emptied (emesis and/or gastric lavage) and further absorption prevented. Treatment is symptomatic and supportive.

DOSAGE AND ADMINISTRATION

Tablets—Adults and children 12 years of age and older: One to 2 tablets (200 mg to 400 mg) every four hours, not to exceed 2400 mg (12 tablets) in 24 hours.

Liquid—Adults and children 12 years of age and older: Two to four teaspoonfuls (200 mg to 400 mg) every four hours, not to exceed 2400 mg (24 teaspoonfuls) in 24 hours.

Children 6 years to under 12 years of age: One to two teaspoonfuls (100 mg to 200 mg) every four hours, not to exceed 1200 mg (12 teaspoonfuls) in 24 hours.

Children 2 years to under 6 years of age: ½ to 1 teaspoonful (50 mg to 100 mg) every four hours, not to exceed 600 mg (6 teaspoonfuls) in 24 hours.

Children 6 mo. to under 2 years of age: A common dosage is ¼ to ½ teaspoonful (25 to 50 mg) every four hours, not to exceed 300 mg (3 teaspoonfuls) in 24 hours. Individualized dosage should be determined by evaluation of patient.

HOW SUPPLIED

Tablet—Each round scored rose-colored tablet contains 200 mg guaifenesin USP—available in bottles of 100 (NDC 0037-4312-01)

Liquid—Each teaspoonful (5 mL) contains 100 mg guaifenesin—available as a clear amber liquid in bottles of 1 pint (NDC 0037-4214-10) and 1 gallon (NDC 0037-4214-20)

Storage—Store at controlled room temperature—15°–30°C (59°–86°F). Protect from light. Keep bottle tightly closed.

ORGANIDIN® NR* (*Newly Reformulated) (guaifenesin) Tablets are Manufactured and Distributed by:
WALLACE LABORATORIES
Division of CARTER-WALLACE, Inc.
Cranbury, NJ 08512

ORGANIDIN® NR* (*Newly Reformulated) (guaifenesin) Liquid is distributed by:
WALLACE LABORATORIES
Division of CARTER-WALLACE, Inc.
Cranbury, NJ 08512

Manufactured by:
Denver Chemical (Puerto Rico) Inc.
Subsidiary of Carter-Wallace, Inc.
Humacao, Puerto Rico 00791
IN-046F8-01   Rev. 7/94

Shown in Product Identification Guide, page 339

RYNA® (Liquid)   ©
RYNA-C®
(Liquid)
RYNA-CX®   ©
(Liquid)

(See PDR For Nonprescription Drugs.)

RYNATAN®   ℞
Tablets
Pediatric Suspension

RYNATAN®-S*
Pediatric Suspension

DESCRIPTION

RYNATAN® is an antihistamine/nasal decongestant combination available for oral administration as *Tablets* and as *Pediatric Suspension*. Each tablet contains:

Phenylephrine Tannate	25 mg
Chlorpheniramine Tannate	8 mg
Pyrilamine Tannate	25 mg

Other ingredients: corn starch, dibasic calcium phosphate, magnesium stearate, methylcellulose, polygalacturonic acid, talc.

Each 5 mL (one teaspoonful) of the Pediatric Suspension contains:

Phenylephrine Tannate	5 mg
Chlorpheniramine Tannate	2 mg
Pyrilamine Tannate	12.5 mg

Other ingredients: benzoic acid, FD&C Red No. 3, flavors (natural and artificial), glycerin, kaolin, magnesium aluminum silicate, methylparaben, pectin, purified water, saccharin sodium, sucrose.

CLINICAL PHARMACOLOGY

RYNATAN combines the sympathomimetic decongestant effect of phenylephrine with the antihistaminic actions of chlorpheniramine and pyrilamine.

INDICATIONS AND USAGE

RYNATAN is indicated for symptomatic relief of the coryza and nasal congestion associated with the common cold, sinusitis, allergic rhinitis and other upper respiratory tract conditions. Appropriate therapy should be provided for the primary disease.

CONTRAINDICATIONS

RYNATAN is contraindicated for newborns, nursing mothers and patients sensitive to any of the ingredients or related compounds.

Continued on next page

Wallace Laboratories—Cont.

WARNINGS

Use with caution in patients with hypertension, cardiovascular disease, hyperthyroidism, diabetes, narrow angle glaucoma or prostatic hypertrophy. Use with caution or avoid use in patients taking monoamine oxidase (MAO) inhibitors, or within 14 days of stopping such treatment. This product contains antihistamines which may cause drowsiness and may have additive central nervous system (CNS) effects with alcohol or other CNS depressants (e.g., hypnotics, sedatives, tranquilizers).

PRECAUTIONS

General: Antihistamines are more likely to cause dizziness, sedation and hypotension in elderly patients. Antihistamines may cause excitation, particularly in children, but their combination with sympathomimetics may cause either mild stimulation or mild sedation.

Information for patients: Caution patients against drinking alcoholic beverages or engaging in potentially hazardous activities requiring alertness, such as driving a car or operating machinery while using this product. Patients should be warned not to use this product if they are now taking a prescription monoamine oxidase inhibitor (MAOI) (certain drugs for depression, psychiatric or emotional conditions, or Parkinson's disease), or for 2 weeks after stopping the MAOI drug. If patients are uncertain whether a prescription drug contains an MAOI, they should be instructed to consult a health professional before taking such a product.

Drug Interactions: MAO inhibitors may prolong and intensify the anticholinergic effects of antihistamines and the overall effects of sympathomimetic agents.

Carcinogenesis, mutagenesis, impairment of fertility: No long term animal studies have been performed with RYNATAN®.

Pregnancy: Teratogenic effects: Pregnancy Category C. Animal reproduction studies have not been conducted with RYNATAN. It is also not known whether RYNATAN can cause fetal harm when administered to a pregnant woman or can affect reproduction capacity. RYNATAN should be given to a pregnant woman only if clearly needed.

Nursing mothers: RYNATAN should not be administered to a nursing woman.

ADVERSE REACTIONS

Adverse effects associated with RYNATAN at recommended doses have been minimal. The most common have been drowsiness, sedation, dryness of mucous membranes, and gastrointestinal effects. Serious side effects with oral antihistamines or sympathomimetics have been rare.

OVERDOSAGE

Signs & Symptoms: May vary from CNS depression to stimulation (restlessness to convulsions). Antihistamine overdosage in young children may lead to convulsions and death. Atropine-like signs and symptoms may be prominent.

Treatment: Induce vomiting if it has not occurred spontaneously. Precautions must be taken against aspiration especially in infants, children and comatose patients. If gastric lavage is indicated, isotonic or half-isotonic saline solution is preferred. Stimulants should not be used. If hypotension is a problem, vasopressor agents may be considered.

DOSAGE AND ADMINISTRATION

Administer the recommended dose every 12 hours.

RYNATAN Tablets: Adults—1 or 2 tablets.

RYNATAN Pediatric Suspension: Children over six years of age —5 to 10 mL (1 to 2 teaspoonfuls); Children two to six years of age —2.5 to 5 mL (1/2 to 1 teaspoonful); *Children under two years of age* —Titrate dose individually.

HOW SUPPLIED

RYNATAN® Tablets (phenylephrine tannate 25 mg, chlorpheniramine tannate 8 mg, and pyrilamine tannate 25 mg): buff-colored, capsule-shaped, scored on one side and imprinted WALLACE 713 on the other side. The tablets are available in bottles of 100 (NDC 0037-0713-92), 500 (NDC 0037-0713-96), and 2000 (NDC 0037-0713-95).

RYNATAN® Pediatric Suspension (phenylephrine tannate 5 mg, chlorpheniramine tannate 2 mg, and pyrilamine tannate 12.5 mg per 5 mL): pink with strawberry-currant flavor in 4 fl oz **unit of use** container with a 10 mL graduated oral syringe and fitment (NDC 0037-0715-67, labeled RYNATAN®-S*) and in pint bottles (NDC 0037-0715-68).

Storage: RYNATAN Tablets—Store at controlled room temperature 15°-30°C (59°-86°F).

RYNATAN Pediatric Suspension—Store at controlled room temperature 15°-30°C (59°-86°F).

Dispense in a tight container.

CAUTION: Federal law prohibits dispensing without prescription.

*RYNATAN®-S is RYNATAN Pediatric Suspension either in a 4 fl oz **unit of use** container with a 10 mL graduated oral syringe and fitment or in a 15 mL sample container.

WALLACE LABORATORIES
Division of
CARTER-WALLACE, INC.
Cranbury, New Jersey 08512
IN-0713-08 Rev. 4/95

Shown in Product Identification Guide, page 339

RYNATUSS® ℞
Tablets
Pediatric Suspension

DESCRIPTION

RYNATUSS® is an antitussive/antihistamine/nasal decongestant/bronchodilator combination available for oral administration as *Tablets* and as *Pediatric Suspension*

Each tablet contains:

Carbetapentane Tannate	60 mg
Chlorpheniramine Tannate	5 mg
Ephedrine Tannate	10 mg
Phenylephrine Tannate	10 mg

Other ingredients: corn starch, dibasic calcium phosphate, FD&C Blue No. 1, FD&C Red No. 40, magnesium stearate, methylcellulose, polygalacturonic acid, povidone, talc.

Each 5 mL (one teaspoonful) of the Pediatric Suspension contains:

Carbetapentane Tannate	30 mg
Chlorpheniramine Tannate	4 mg
Ephedrine Tannate	5 mg
Phenylephrine Tannate	5 mg

Other ingredients: benzoic acid, FD&C Blue No. 1, FD&C Red No. 3, FD&C Red No. 40, FD&C Yellow No. 5 (see Precautions), flavors (natural and artificial), glycerin, Kaolin, magnesium aluminum silicate, methylparaben, pectin, purified water, saccharin sodium, sucrose.

CLINICAL PHARMACOLOGY

RYNATUSS combines the antitussive action of carbetapentane, the sympathomimetic decongestant effect of phenylephrine, the antihistaminic action of chlorpheniramine, and the bronchodilator action of ephedrine.

INDICATIONS AND USAGE

RYNATUSS is indicated for the symptomatic relief of cough associated with respiratory tract conditions such as the common cold, bronchial asthma, acute and chronic bronchitis. Appropriate therapy should be provided for the primary disease.

CONTRAINDICATIONS

RYNATUSS is contraindicated for newborns, nursing mothers, and patients who are sensitive to any of the ingredients or related compounds.

WARNINGS

Use with caution in patients with hypertension, cardiovascular disease, hyperthyroidism, diabetes, narrow angle glaucoma, or prostatic, hypertrophy. Do not use in patients taking monoamine oxidase (MAO) inhibitors, or for 14 days after stopping treatment with an MAOI.

This product contains antihistamines which may cause drowsiness and may have additive central nervous system (CNS) effects with alcohol or other CNS depressants (e.g., hypnotics, sedatives, tranquilizers).

PRECAUTIONS

For RYNATUSS Pediatric Suspension only: This product contains FD&C Yellow No. 5 (tartrazine) which may cause allergic-type reactions (including bronchial asthma) in certain susceptible individuals. Although the overall incidence of FD&C Yellow No. 5 (tartrazine) sensitivity in the general population is low, it is frequently seen in patients who also have aspirin hypersensitivity.

General: Antihistamines are more likely to cause dizziness, sedation, and hypotension in elderly patients. Antihistamines may cause excitation, particularly in children, but their combination with sympathomimetics may cause either mild stimulation or mild sedation.

Information for patients: Caution patients against drinking alcoholic beverages or engaging in potentially hazardous activities requiring alertness, such as driving a car or operating machinery while using this product. Patients should be warned not to use this product if they are now taking a prescription monoamine oxidase inhibitor (MAOI) (certain drugs for depression, psychiatric or emotional conditions, or Parkinson's disease), or for 2 weeks after stopping the MAOI drug. If patients are uncertain whether a prescription drug contains an MAOI, they should be instructed to consult a health professional before taking such a product.

Drug Interactions: MAO inhibitors may prolong and intensify the anticholinergic effects of antihistamines and the overall effects of sympathomimetic agents.

Carcinogenesis, mutagenesis, impairment of fertility: No long term animal studies have been performed with RYNATUSS.

Pregnancy: Teratogenic effects: Pregnancy Category C. Animal reproduction studies have not been conducted with RYNATUSS. It is also not known whether RYNATUSS can cause fetal harm when administered to a pregnant woman or can affect reproduction capacity. RYNATUSS should be given to a pregnant woman only if clearly needed.

Nursing mothers: RYNATUSS should not be administered to a nursing woman.

ADVERSE REACTIONS

Adverse effects associated with RYNATUSS at recommended doses have been minimal. The most common have been drowsiness, sedation, dryness of mucous membranes, and gastrointestinal effects. Serious side effects with oral antihistamines or sympathomimetics have been rare.

OVERDOSAGE

Signs and symptoms: May vary from CNS depression to stimulation (restlessness to convulsions). Antihistamine overdosage in young children may lead to convulsions and death. Atropine-like signs and symptoms may be prominent.

Treatment: Induce vomiting if it has not occurred spontaneously. Precautions must be taken against aspiration especially in infants, children, and comatose patients. If gastric lavage is indicated, isotonic or half-isotonic saline solution is preferred. Stimulants should not be used. If hypotension is a problem, vasopressor agents may be considered.

DOSAGE AND ADMINISTRATION

Administer the recommended dose every 12 hours.

RYNATUSS Tablets: Adults – 1 to 2 tablets.

RYNATUSS Pediatric Suspension: Children over six years of age– 5 to 10 mL (1 to 2 teaspoonfuls); *Children two to six years of age*– 2.5 to 5 mL (1/2 to 1 teaspoonful); *Children under two years of age*– Titrate dose individually.

HOW SUPPLIED

RYNATUSS® Tablets are mauve, capsule-shaped, scored on one side and imprinted WALLACE 717 on the other side, containing in each tablet: carbetapentane tannate 60 mg, chlorpheniramine tannate 5 mg, ephedrine tannate 10 mg, phenylephrine tannate 10 mg, available in bottles of 100 (NDC 0037-0717-92), 500 (NDC 0037-0717-96), and 2000 (NDC 0037-0717-95).

RYNATUSS® Pediatric Suspension is pink with strawberry-currant flavor, containing in each 5 mL (one teaspoonful): carbetapentane tannate 30 mg, chlorpheniramine tannate 4 mg, ephedrine tannate 5 mg, phenylephrine tannate 5 mg, available in bottles of 8 fl oz (NDC 0037-0718-67) and one pint (NDC 0037-0718-68).

Storage: RYNATUSS Tablets and RYNATUSS Pediatric Suspension: Store at controlled room temperature 15°-30°C (59°-86°F).

Dispense in a tight container.

WALLACE LABORATORIES
Division of
CARTER-WALLACE, INC.
Cranbury, New Jersey 08512
IN-0717-05 Rev: 1/95

Shown in Product Identification Guide, page 339

SOMA® ℞
(carisoprodol)
Tablets, USP

DESCRIPTION

'SOMA' (carisoprodol) Tablets, USP is available as 350 mg round, white tablets. Chemically, carisoprodol is N-isopropyl-2-methyl-2-propyl-1,3-propanediol dicarbamate. Carisoprodol is a white, crystalline powder, having a mild, characteristic odor and a bitter taste. It is very slightly soluble in water; freely soluble in alcohol, in chloroform, and in acetone; its solubility is practically independent of pH. Carisoprodol is present as a racemic mixture. The molecular formula is $C_{12}H_{24}N_2O_4$, with a molecular weight of 260.33. The structural formula is:

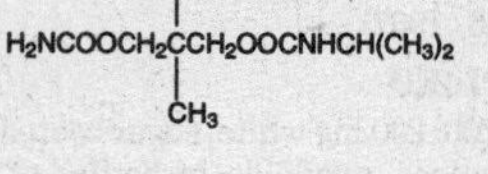
CH2CH2CH3
H2NCOOCH2CCH2OOCNHCH(CH3)2
CH3

Other ingredients: alginic acid, magnesium stearate, potassium sorbate, starch, tribasic calcium phosphate.

ACTIONS

Carisoprodol produces muscle relaxation in animals by blocking interneuronal activity in the descending reticular formation and spinal cord. The onset of action is rapid and effects last four to six hours.

INDICATIONS

Carisoprodol is indicated as an adjunct to rest, physical therapy, and other measures for the relief of discomfort associated with acute, painful musculoskeletal conditions. The mode of action of this drug has not been clearly identified,

but may be related to its sedative properties. Carisoprodol does not directly relax tense skeletal muscles in man.

CONTRAINDICATIONS

Acute intermittent porphyria as well as allergic or idiosyncratic reactions to carisoprodol or related compounds.

WARNINGS

Idiosyncratic Reactions—On very rare occasions, the first dose of carisoprodol has been followed by idiosyncratic symptoms appearing within minutes or hours. Symptoms reported include: extreme weakness, transient quadriplegia, dizziness, ataxia, temporary loss of vision, diplopia, mydriasis, dysarthria, agitation, euphoria, confusion, and disorientation. Symptoms usually subside over the course of the next several hours. Supportive and symptomatic therapy, including hospitalization, may be necessary.

Usage in Pregnancy and Lactation—Safe usage of this drug in pregnancy or lactation has not been established. Therefore, use of this drug in pregnancy, in nursing mothers, or in women of childbearing potential requires that the potential benefits of the drug be weighed against the potential hazards to mother and child. Carisoprodol is present in breast milk of lactating mothers at concentrations two to four times that of maternal plasma. This factor should be taken into account when use of the drug is contemplated in breast-feeding patients.

Usage in Children—Because of limited clinical experience, 'SOMA' is not recommended for use in patients under 12 years of age.

Potentially Hazardous Tasks—Patients should be warned that this drug may impair the mental and/or physical abilities required for the performance of potentially hazardous tasks such as driving a motor vehicle or operating machinery.

Additive Effects—Since the effects of carisoprodol and alcohol or carisoprodol and other CNS depressants or psychotropic drugs may be additive, appropriate caution should be exercised with patients who take more than one of these agents simultaneously.

Drug Dependence—In dogs, no withdrawal symptoms occurred after abrupt cessation of carisoprodol from dosages as high as 1 gm/kg/day. In a study in man, abrupt cessation of 100 mg/kg/day (about five times the recommended daily adult dosage) was followed in some subjects by mild withdrawal symptoms such as abdominal cramps, insomnia, chilliness, headache, and nausea. Delirium and convulsions did not occur. In clinical use, psychological dependence and abuse have been rare, and there have been no reports of significant abstinence signs. Nevertheless, the drug should be used with caution in addiction-prone individuals.

PRECAUTIONS

Carisoprodol is metabolized in the liver and excreted by the kidney; to avoid its excess accumulation, caution should be exercised in administration to patients with compromised liver or kidney function.

ADVERSE REACTIONS

Central Nervous System—Drowsiness and other CNS effects may require dosage reduction. Also observed: dizziness, vertigo, ataxia, tremor, agitation, irritability, headache, depressive reactions, syncope, and insomnia. (See also Idiosyncratic Reactions under "Warnings.")

Allergic or Idiosyncratic—Allergic or idiosyncratic reactions occasionally develop. They are usually seen within the period of the first to fourth dose in patients having had no previous contact with the drug. Skin rash, erythema multiforme, pruritus, eosinophilia, and fixed drug eruption with cross reaction to meprobamate have been reported with carisoprodol. Severe reactions have been manifested by asthmatic episodes, fever, weakness, dizziness, angioneurotic edema, smarting eyes, hypotension, and anaphylactoid shock. (See also Idiosyncratic Reactions under "Warnings.") In case of allergic or idiosyncratic reactions to carisoprodol, discontinue the drug and initiate appropriate symptomatic therapy, which may include epinephrine, antihistamines, and in severe cases corticosteroids. In evaluating possible allergic reactions, also consider allergy to excipients (information on excipients is available to physicians on request).

Cardiovascular—Tachycardia, postural hypotension, and facial flushing.

Gastrointestinal—Nausea, vomiting, hiccup, and epigastric distress.

Hematologic—Leukopenia, in which other drugs or viral infection may have been responsible, and pancytopenia, attributed to phenylbutazone, have been reported. No serious blood dyscrasias have been attributed to carisoprodol.

DOSAGE AND ADMINISTRATION

The usual adult dosage of 'SOMA' (carisoprodol) Tablets, USP is one 350 mg tablet, three times daily and at bedtime. Usage in patients under age 12 is not recommended.

OVERDOSAGE

Overdosage of carisoprodol has produced stupor, coma, shock, respiratory depression, and, very rarely, death. The effects of an overdosage of carisoprodol and alcohol or other CNS depressants or psychotropic agents can be additive even when one of the drugs has been taken in the usual recommended dosage. Any drug remaining in the stomach should be removed and symptomatic therapy given. Should respiration or blood pressure become compromised, respiratory assistance, central nervous system stimulants, and pressor agents should be administered cautiously as indicated. Carisoprodol is metabolized in the liver and excreted by the kidney. Although carisoprodol overdosage experience is limited, the following types of treatment have been used successfully with the related drug meprobamate: diuresis, osmotic (mannitol) diuresis, peritoneal dialysis, and hemodialysis (carisoprodol is dialyzable). Careful monitoring of urinary output is necessary and caution should be taken to avoid overhydration. Observe for possible relapse due to incomplete gastric emptying and delayed absorption. Carisoprodol can be measured in biological fluids by gas chromatography (Douglas, J. F. et al.: *J Pharm Sci 58*: 145, 1969).

HOW SUPPLIED

'SOMA' (carisoprodol) Tablets, USP 350 mg: Round, convex, white tablets, inscribed with 'SOMA' on one side and 37-WALLACE 2001 on the other side, are available in bottles of 100 (NDC 0037-2001-01) and 500 (NDC 0037-2001-03), and unit-dose packages of 100 (NDC 0037-2001-85).

Storage: Store at controlled room temperature 15°–30°C (59°–86°F).

Dispense in a tight container.

WALLACE LABORATORIES
Division of
CARTER-WALLACE, INC.
Cranbury, New Jersey 08512
IN-090H2-10   Rev. 9/94
Shown in Product Identification Guide, page 339

SOMA® COMPOUND†   ℞
(carisoprodol and aspirin tablets, USP)
carisoprodol 200 mg + aspirin 325 mg
TABLETS

DESCRIPTION

SOMA Compound is a combination product containing carisoprodol, a centrally-acting muscle relaxant, plus aspirin, an analgesic with antipyretic and anti-inflammatory properties. It is available as a two-layered, white and orange, round tablet for oral administration. Each tablet contains carisoprodol, USP 200 mg and aspirin 325 mg. Chemically, carisoprodol is N-isopropyl-2-methyl-2-propyl-1,3-propanediol dicarbamate. Its empirical formula is $C_{12}H_{24}N_2O_4$, with a molecular weight of 260.33. The structural formula is:

$$CH_2CH_2CH_3$$
$$|$$
$$H_2NCOOCH_2CCH_2OOCNHCH(CH_3)_2$$
$$|$$
$$CH_3$$

Other ingredients: croscarmellose sodium, FD&C Red #40, FD&C Yellow #6, hydroxypropyl methylcellulose, magnesium stearate, microcrystalline cellulose, povidone, starch, stearic acid.

CLINICAL PHARMACOLOGY

Carisoprodol: Carisoprodol is a centrally-acting muscle relaxant that does not directly relax tense skeletal muscles in man. The mode of action of carisoprodol in relieving acute muscle spasm of local origin has not been clearly identified, but may be related to its sedative properties. In animals, carisoprodol has been shown to produce muscle relaxation by blocking interneuronal activity and depressing transmission of polysynaptic neurons in the spinal cord and in the descending reticular formation of the brain. The onset of action is rapid and lasts four to six hours.

Carisoprodol is metabolized in the liver and is excreted by the kidneys. It is dialyzable by peritoneal and hemodialysis.

Aspirin: Aspirin is a nonnarcotic analgesic with anti-inflammatory and antipyretic activity. Inhibition of prostaglandin biosynthesis appears to account for most of its anti-inflammatory and for at least part of its analgesic and antipyretic properties.

Aspirin is rapidly absorbed and almost totally hydrolyzed to salicylic acid following oral administration. Although aspirin has a half-life of only about 15 minutes, the apparent biologic half-life of salicylic acid in the therapeutic plasma concentration range is between 6 and 12 hours. Salicylic acid is eliminated by renal excretion and by biotransformation to inactive metabolites. Clearance of salicylic acid in the high-dose range is sensitive to urinary pH (see *Drug Interactions*) and is reduced by renal dysfunction.

INDICATIONS AND USAGE

SOMA Compound is indicated as an adjunct to rest, physical therapy, and other measures for the relief of pain, muscle spasm, and limited mobility associated with acute, painful musculoskeletal conditions.

Patent No. 4534973

CONTRAINDICATIONS

Acute intermittent porphyria; bleeding disorders; allergic or idiosyncratic reactions to carisoprodol, aspirin or related compounds.

WARNINGS

On very rare occasions, the first dose of carisoprodol has been followed by an idiosyncratic reaction with symptoms appearing within minutes or hours. These may include extreme weakness, transient quadriplegia, dizziness, ataxia, temporary loss of vision, diplopia, mydriasis, dysarthria, agitation, euphoria, confusion, and disorientation. Although symptoms usually subside over the course of the next several hours, discontinue SOMA Compound and initiate appropriate supportive and symptomatic therapy, which may include epinephrine and/or antihistamines. In severe cases, corticosteroids may be necessary. Severe reactions have been manifested by asthmatic episodes, fever, weakness, dizziness, angioneurotic edema, smarting eyes, hypotension, and anaphylactoid shock.

The effects of carisoprodol with agents such as alcohol, other CNS depressants, or psychotropic drugs may be additive. Appropriate caution should be exercised with patients who may take one or more of these agents simultaneously with SOMA Compound.

PRECAUTIONS

General: To avoid excessive accumulation of carisoprodol, aspirin, or their metabolites, use SOMA Compound with caution in patients with compromised liver or kidney function, or in elderly or debilitated patients (see CLINICAL PHARMACOLOGY).

Use with caution in patients with history of gastritis or peptic ulcer, in patients on anticoagulant therapy, and in addiction-prone individuals.

Information for Patients: Caution patients that this drug may impair the mental and/or physical abilities required for the performance of potentially hazardous tasks such as driving a motor vehicle or operating machinery.

Caution patients with a predisposition for gastrointestinal bleeding that concomitant use of aspirin and alcohol may have an additive effect in this regard.

Caution patients that dosage of medications used for gout, arthritis, or diabetes may have to be adjusted when aspirin is administered or discontinued (see *Drug Interactions*).

Drug Interactions: Clinically important interactions may occur when certain drugs are administered concomitantly with aspirin or aspirin-containing drugs.

1. *Oral Anticoagulants*—By interfering with platelet function or decreasing plasma prothrombin concentration, aspirin enhances the potential for bleeding in patients on anticoagulants.

2. *Methotrexate*—aspirin enhances the toxic effects of this drug.

3. *Probenecid and Sulfinpyrazone*—large doses of aspirin reduce the uricosuric effect of both drugs. Renal excretion of salicylate may also be reduced.

4. *Oral Antidiabetic Drugs*—enhancement of hypoglycemia may occur.

5. *Antacids*—to the extent that they raise urinary pH, antacids may substantially decrease plasma salicylate concentrations; conversely, their withdrawal can result in a substantial increase.

6. *Ammonium Chloride*—this and other drugs that acidify a relatively alkaline urine can elevate plasma salicylate concentrations.

7. *Ethyl Alcohol*—enhanced aspirin-induced fecal blood loss has been reported.

8. *Corticosteroids*—salicylate plasma levels may be decreased when adrenal corticosteroids are given, and may be increased substantially when they are discontinued.

Carcinogenesis, Mutagenesis, Impairment of Fertility: No long-term studies have been done with SOMA Compound.

Pregnancy—Teratogenic Effects: **Pregnancy Category C.** Adequate animal reproduction studies have not been conducted with SOMA Compound. It is also not known whether SOMA Compound can cause fetal harm when administered to a pregnant woman or can affect reproduction capacity. SOMA Compound should be given to a pregnant woman only if clearly needed.

Studies in rodents have shown salicylates to be teratogenic when given in early gestation, and embryocidal when given in later gestation in doses considerably greater than usual therapeutic doses in humans. Studies in women who took aspirin during pregnancy have not demonstrated an increased incidence of congenital abnormalities in the offspring.

Labor and Delivery: Ingestion of aspirin near term or prior to delivery may prolong delivery or lead to bleeding in mother, fetus, or neonate.

Nursing Mothers: Carisoprodol is excreted in human milk in concentrations two-to-four times that in maternal plasma. Aspirin is excreted in human milk in moderate amounts and

Continued on next page

Wallace Laboratories—Cont.

can produce a bleeding tendency in nursing infants. Because of the potential for serious adverse reactions in nursing infants, a decision should be made whether to discontinue nursing or the drug, taking into account the importance of the drug to the mother.

Pediatric Use: Safety and effectiveness in children below the age of twelve have not been established.

ADVERSE REACTIONS

If severe reactions occur, discontinue SOMA Compound and initiate appropriate symptomatic and supportive therapy. The following side effects which have occurred with the administration of the individual ingredients alone may also occur with the combination.

Carisoprodol: Central Nervous System—Drowsiness is the most frequent complaint and along with other CNS effects may require dosage reduction. Observed less frequently are dizziness, vertigo and ataxia. Tremor, agitation, irritability, headache, depressive reactions, syncope, and insomnia have been infrequent or rare.

Idiosyncratic—Idiosyncratic reactions are very rare. They are usually seen within the period of the first to fourth dose in patients having had no previous contact with the drug (see WARNINGS).

Allergic—Skin rash, erythema multiforme, pruritus, eosinophilia, and fixed drug eruptions with cross-reaction to meprobamate have been reported. If allergic reactions occur, discontinue SOMA Compound and treat symptomatically. In evaluating possible allergic reactions, also consider allergy to excipients (information on excipients is available to physicians on request).

Cardiovascular—Tachycardia, postural hypotension, and facial flushing.

Gastrointestinal—Nausea, vomiting, epigastric distress, and hiccup.

Hematologic—No serious blood dyscrasias have been attributed to carisoprodol alone. Leukopenia and pancytopenia have been reported, very rarely, in situations in which other drugs or viral infections may have been responsible.

Aspirin: The most common adverse reactions associated with the use of aspirin have been gastrointestinal, including nausea, vomiting, gastritis, occult bleeding, constipation, and diarrhea. Gastric erosion, angioedema, asthma, rash, pruritus and urticaria have been reported less commonly. Tinnitus is a sign of high serum salicylate levels (see OVERDOSAGE).

Aspirin Intolerance—Allergic type reactions in aspirin-sensitive individuals may involve the respiratory tract or the skin. Symptoms of the former range from rhinorrhea and shortness of breath to severe asthma, and the latter may consist of urticaria, edema, rash, or angioedema (giant hives). These may occur independently or in combination.

DRUG ABUSE AND DEPENDENCE

Abuse: In clinical use, abuse has been rare.

Dependence: In clinical use, dependence with SOMA Compound has been rare, and there have been no reports of significant abstinence signs. Nevertheless, the following information on the individual ingredients should be kept in mind.

Carisoprodol—In dogs, no withdrawal symptoms occurred after abrupt cessation of carisoprodol from dosages as high as 1 gm/kg/day. In a study in man, abrupt cessation of 100 mg/kg/day (about five times the recommended daily adult dosage) was followed in some subjects by mild withdrawal symptoms such as abdominal cramps, insomnia, chills, headache, and nausea. Delirium and convulsions did not occur (see PRECAUTIONS).

OVERDOSAGE

Signs and Symptoms: Any of the following which have been reported with the individual ingredients may occur and may be modified to a varying degree by the effects of the other ingredients present in SOMA Compound.

Carisoprodol—Stupor, coma, shock, respiratory depression, and, very rarely, death. Overdosage with carisoprodol in combination with alcohol, other CNS depressants, or psychotropic agents can have additive effects, even when one of the agents has been taken in the usually recommended dosage.

Aspirin—Headache, tinnitus, hearing difficulty, dim vision, dizziness, lassitude, hyperpnea, rapid breathing, thirst, nausea, vomiting, sweating and occasionally diarrhea are characteristic of mild to moderate salicylate poisoning. Salicylate poisoning should be considered in children with symptoms of vomiting, hyperpnea, and hyperthermia.

Hyperpnea is an early sign of salicylate poisoning, but dyspnea supervenes at plasma levels above 50 mg/dL. These respiratory changes eventually lead to serious acid-base disturbances. Metabolic acidosis is a constant finding in infants but occurs in older children only with severe poisoning; adults usually exhibit respiratory alkalosis initially and acidosis terminally.

Other symptoms of severe salicylate poisoning include hyperthermia, dehydration, delirium, and mental distur-

bances. Skin eruptions, GI hemorrhage, or pulmonary edema are less common. Early CNS stimulation is replaced by increasing depression, stupor, and coma. Death is usually due to respiratory failure or cardiovascular collapse.

Treatment: General: Provide symptomatic and supportive treatment, as indicated. Any drug remaining in the stomach should be removed using appropriate procedures and caution to protect the airway and prevent aspiration, especially in the stuporous or comatose patient. Incomplete gastric emptying with delayed absorption of carisoprodol has been reported as a cause for relapse. Should respiration or blood pressure become compromised, respiratory assistance, central nervous system stimulants, and pressor agents should be administered cautiously, as indicated.

Carisoprodol: The following have been used successfully in overdosage with the related drug meprobamate: diuretics, osmotic (mannitol) diuresis, peritoneal dialysis, and hemodialysis (see CLINICAL PHARMACOLOGY). Careful monitoring of urinary output is necessary and caution should be taken to avoid overhydration. Carisoprodol can be measured in biological fluid by gas chromatography (Douglas, J. F., et al: *J Pharm Sci 58:* 145, 1969).

Aspirin—Since there are no specific antidotes for salicylate poisoning, the aim of treatment is to enhance elimination of salicylate and prevent or reduce further absorption; to correct any fluid, electrolyte or metabolic imbalance; and to provide general and cardiorespiratory support. If acidosis is present, intravenous sodium bicarbonate must be given, along with adequate hydration, until salicylate levels decrease to within the therapeutic range. To enhance elimination, forced diuresis and alkalinization of the urine may be beneficial. The need for hemoperfusion or hemodialysis is rare and should be used only when other measures have failed.

DOSAGE AND ADMINISTRATION

Usual Adult Dosage: 1 or 2 tablets, four times daily. Not recommended for use in children under age twelve (see PRECAUTIONS).

HOW SUPPLIED

SOMA Compound Tablets (carisoprodol, USP 200 mg and aspirin 325 mg) are round, convex, two-layered and inscribed on the white layer with SOMA C and on the light orange layer with WALLACE 2103. The tablets are available in bottles of 100 (NDC 0037-2103-01) and 500 (NDC 0037-2103-03) and unit-dose packages of 100 (NDC 0037-2103-85).

Storage: Store at controlled room temperature 15°–30°C (59°–86°F). Protect from moisture.
Dispense in a tight container.

WALLACE LABORATORIES
Division of CARTER-WALLACE, INC.
Cranbury, New Jersey 08512

Rev. 9/93

Shown in Product Identification Guide, page 339

SOMA® COMPOUND with CODEINE† ℃ ℞
(carisoprodol, aspirin and codeine phosphate tablets, USP)
carisoprodol 200 mg †
aspirin 325 mg †
codeine phosphate 16 mg·
Warning: May be habit-forming.
TABLETS

DESCRIPTION

'Soma' Compound with Codeine is a combination product containing carisoprodol, a centrally-acting muscle relaxant, plus aspirin, an analgesic with antipyretic and anti-inflammatory properties and codeine phosphate, a centrally-acting narcotic analgesic. It is available as a two-layered, white and yellow, oval-shaped tablet for oral administration. Each tablet contains carisoprodol 200 mg, aspirin 325 mg, and codeine phosphate 16 mg. Chemically, carisoprodol is N-isopropyl-2-methyl-2-propyl-1,3-propanediol dicarbamate. Its empirical formula is $C_{12}H_{24}N_2O_4$, with a molecular weight of 260.33. The structural formula is:

$$CH_2CH_2CH_3$$
$$|$$
$$H_2NCOOCH_2CCH_2OOCNHCH(CH_3)_2$$
$$|$$
$$CH_3$$

Other ingredients: croscarmellose sodium, D&C Yellow #10, hydroxypropyl methylcellulose, magnesium stearate, microcrystalline cellulose, povidone, sodium metabisulfite, starch, stearic acid.

CLINICAL PHARMACOLOGY

Carisoprodol: Carisoprodol is a centrally-acting muscle relaxant that does not directly relax tense skeletal muscles in man. The mode of action of carisoprodol in relieving acute muscle spasm of local origin has not been clearly identified, but may be related to its sedative properties. In animals,

carisoprodol has been shown to produce muscle relaxation by blocking interneuronal activity and depressing transmission of polysynaptic neurons in the spinal cord and in the descending reticular formation of the brain. The onset of action is rapid and lasts four to six hours.

Carisoprodol is metabolized in the liver and is excreted by the kidneys. It is dialyzable by peritoneal and hemodialysis.

Aspirin: Aspirin is a non-narcotic analgesic with anti-inflammatory and antipyretic activity. Inhibition of prostaglandin biosynthesis appears to account for most of its anti-inflammatory and for at least part of its analgesic and antipyretic properties.

Aspirin is rapidly absorbed and almost totally hydrolyzed to salicylic acid following oral administration. Although aspirin has a half-life of only about 15 minutes, the apparent biologic half-life of salicylic acid in the therapeutic plasma concentration range is between 6 and 12 hours. Salicylic acid is eliminated by renal excretion and by biotransformation to inactive metabolites. Clearance of salicylic acid in the high-dose range is sensitive to urinary pH (see *Drug Interactions*) and is reduced by renal dysfunction.

Codeine Phosphate: Codeine phosphate is a centrally-acting narcotic-analgesic. Its actions are qualitatively similar to morphine, but its potency is substantially less.

Clinical studies have shown that combining aspirin and codeine produces a significant additive effect in analgesic efficacy.

INDICATIONS AND USAGE

'Soma' Compound with Codeine is indicated as an adjunct to rest, physical therapy, and other measures for the relief of pain, muscle spasm, and limited mobility associated with acute, painful musculoskeletal conditions when the additional action of codeine is desired.

CONTRAINDICATIONS

Acute intermittent porphyria; bleeding disorders; allergic or idiosyncratic reactions to carisoprodol, aspirin, codeine, or related compounds.

WARNINGS

On very rare occasions, the first dose of carisoprodol has been followed by idiosyncratic reactions, with symptoms appearing within minutes or hours. These may include extreme weakness, transient quadriplegia, dizziness, ataxia, temporary loss of vision, diplopia, mydriasis, dysarthria, agitation, euphoria, confusion, and disorientation. Although symptoms usually subside over the course of the next several hours, discontinue 'Soma' Compound with Codeine and initiate appropriate supportive and symptomatic therapy, which may include epinephrine and/or antihistamines. In severe cases, corticosteroids may be necessary. Severe reactions have been manifested by asthmatic episodes, fever, weakness, dizziness, angioneurotic edema, smarting eyes, hypotension, and anaphylactoid shock.

The effects of carisoprodol with agents such as alcohol, other CNS depressants, or psychotropic drugs may be additive. Appropriate caution should be exercised with patients who take one or more of these agents simultaneously with Soma Compound with Codeine.

Contains sodium metabisulfite, a sulfite that may cause allergic-type reactions including anaphylactic symptoms and life-threatening or less severe asthmatic episodes in certain susceptible people. The overall prevalence of sulfite sensitivity in the general population is unknown and probably low. Sulfite sensitivity is seen more frequently in asthmatic than in nonasthmatic people.

PRECAUTIONS

General: To avoid excessive accumulation of carisoprodol, aspirin, or their metabolites, use 'Soma' Compound with Codeine with caution in patients with compromised liver or kidney function, or in elderly or debilitated patients (see CLINICAL PHARMACOLOGY).

Use with caution in patients with history of gastritis or peptic ulcer, in patients on anticoagulant therapy, and in addiction-prone individuals.

Information for Patients: Caution patients that this drug may impair the mental and/or physical abilities required for the performance of potentially hazardous tasks such as driving a motor vehicle or operating machinery.

Caution patients with a predisposition for gastrointestinal bleeding that concomitant use of aspirin and alcohol may have an additive effect in this regard.

Caution patients that dosage of medications used for gout, arthritis, or diabetes may have to be adjusted when aspirin is administered or discontinued (see *Drug Interactions*).

Drug Interactions: Clinically important interactions may occur when certain drugs are administered concomitantly with aspirin or aspirin-containing drugs.

1. *Oral Anticoagulants*—By interfering with platelet function or decreasing plasma prothrombin concentration, aspirin enhances the potential for bleeding in patients on anticoagulants.

2. *Methotrexate*—aspirin enhances the toxic effects of this drug.

3. *Probenecid and Sulfinpyrazone*—large doses of aspirin reduce the uricosuric effect of both drugs. Renal excretion of salicylate may also be reduced.

4. *Oral Antidiabetic Drugs*—enhancement of hypoglycemia may occur.

5. *Antacids*—to the extent that they raise urinary pH, antacids may substantially decrease plasma salicylate concentrations; conversely, their withdrawal can result in a substantial increase.

6. *Ammonium Chloride*—this and other drugs that acidify a relatively alkaline urine can elevate plasma salicylate concentrations.

7. *Ethyl Alcohol*—enhanced aspirin-induced fecal blood loss has been reported.

8. *Corticosteroids*—salicylate plasma levels may be decreased when adrenal corticosteroids are given, and may be increased substantially when they are discontinued.

Carcinogenesis, Mutagenesis, Impairment of Fertility: No long-term studies have been done with 'Soma' Compound with Codeine.

Pregnancy—Teratogenic Effects: Pregnancy Category C. Adequate animal reproduction studies have not been conducted with 'Soma' Compound with Codeine. It is also not known whether 'Soma' Compound with Codeine can cause fetal harm when administered to a pregnant woman or can affect reproduction capacity. 'Soma' Compound with Codeine should be given to a pregnant woman only if clearly needed. Studies in rodents have shown salicylates to be teratogenic when given in early gestation, and embryocidal when given in later gestation in doses considerably greater than usual therapeutic doses in humans. Studies in women who took aspirin during pregnancy have not demonstrated an increased incidence of congenital abnormalities in the offspring.

Labor and Delivery: Ingestion of aspirin near term or prior to delivery may prolong delivery or lead to bleeding in mother, fetus, or neonate.

Nursing Mothers: Carisoprodol is excreted in human milk in concentrations two-to-four times that in maternal plasma. Aspirin is excreted in human milk in moderate amounts and can produce a bleeding tendency in nursing infants. Because of the potential for serious adverse reactions in nursing infants, a decision should be made whether to discontinue nursing or the drug, taking into account the importance of the drug to the mother.

Pediatric Use: Safety and effectiveness in children below the age of twelve have not been established.

ADVERSE REACTIONS

If severe reactions occur, discontinue 'Soma' Compound with Codeine and initiate appropriate symptomatic and supportive therapy.

The following side effects which have occurred with the administration of the individual ingredients alone may also occur with the combination.

Carisoprodol: Central Nervous System—Drowsiness is the most frequent complaint and along with other CNS effects may require dosage reduction. Observed less frequently are dizziness, vertigo and ataxia. Tremor, agitation, irritability, headache, depressive reactions, syncope, and insomnia have been infrequent or rare.

Idiosyncratic—Idiosyncratic reactions are very rare. They are usually seen within the period of the first to fourth dose in patients having had no previous contact with the drug (see WARNINGS).

Allergic—Skin rash, erythema multiforme, pruritus, eosinophilia, and fixed drug eruptions with cross-reaction to meprobamate have been reported. If allergic reactions occur, discontinue 'Soma' Compound with Codeine and treat symptomatically. In evaluating possible allergic reactions, also consider allergy to excipients (information on excipients is available to physicians on request).

Cardiovascular—Tachycardia, postural hypotension, and facial flushing.

Gastrointestinal—Nausea, vomiting, epigastric distress and hiccup.

Hematologic—No serious blood dyscrasias have been attributed to carisoprodol alone. Leukopenia and pancytopenia have been reported, very rarely, in situations in which other drugs or viral infections may have been responsible.

Aspirin: The most common adverse reactions associated with the use of aspirin have been gastrointestinal, including nausea, vomiting, gastritis, occult bleeding, constipation and diarrhea. Gastric erosion, angioedema, asthma, rash, pruritus and urticaria have been reported less commonly. Tinnitus is a sign of high serum salicylate levels (see OVERDOSAGE).

Aspirin Intolerance—Allergic type reactions in aspirin-sensitive individuals may involve the respiratory tract or the skin. Symptoms of the former range from rhinorrhea and shortness of breath to severe asthma, and the latter may consist of urticaria, edema, rash, or angioedema (giant hives). These may occur independently or in combination.

Codeine Phosphate: Nausea, vomiting, constipation, miosis, sedation, and dizziness have been reported.

DRUG ABUSE AND DEPENDENCE

Controlled Substance: Schedule C-III (see PRECAUTIONS).

Abuse: In clinical use, abuse has been rare.

Dependence: In clinical use, dependence with 'Soma' Compound with Codeine has been rare and there have been no reports of significant abstinence signs. Nevertheless, the following information on the individual ingredients should be kept in mind.

Carisoprodol—In dogs, no withdrawal symptoms occurred after abrupt cessation of carisoprodol from dosages as high as 1 gm/kg/day. In a study in man, abrupt cessation of 100 mg/kg/day (about five times the recommended daily adult dosage) was followed in some subjects by mild withdrawal symptoms such as abdominal cramps, insomnia, chills, headache, and nausea. Delirium and convulsions did not occur (see PRECAUTIONS).

Codeine Phosphate—Drug dependence of the morphine type may result.

OVERDOSAGE

Signs and Symptoms: Any of the following which have been reported with the individual ingredients may occur and may be modified to a varying degree by the effects of the other ingredients present in 'Soma' Compound with Codeine.

Carisoprodol—Stupor, coma, shock, respiratory depression and, very rarely, death. Overdosage with carisoprodol in combination with alcohol, other CNS depressants, or psychotropic agents can have additive effects, even when one of the agents has been taken in the usually recommended dosage.

Aspirin—Headache, tinnitus, hearing difficulty, dim vision, dizziness, lassitude, hyperpnea, rapid breathing, thirst, nausea, vomiting, sweating and occasionally diarrhea are characteristic of mild to moderate salicylate poisoning. Salicylate poisoning should be considered in children with symptoms of vomiting, hyperpnea, and hyperthermia.

Hyperpnea is an early sign of salicylate poisoning, but dyspnea supervenes at plasma levels above 50 mg/dl. These respiratory changes eventually lead to serious acid-base disturbances. Metabolic acidosis is a constant finding in infants but occurs in older children only with severe poisoning; adults usually exhibit respiratory alkalosis initially and acidosis terminally.

Other symptoms of severe salicylate poisoning include hyperthermia, dehydration, delirium, and mental disturbances. Skin eruptions, GI hemorrhage, or pulmonary edema are less common. Early CNS stimulation is replaced by increasing depression, stupor, and coma. Death is usually due to respiratory failure or cardiovascular collapse.

Codeine Phosphate—pinpoint pupils, CNS depression, coma, respiratory depression, and shock.

Treatment: General—Provide symptomatic and supportive treatment, as indicated. Any drug remaining in the stomach should be removed using appropriate procedures and caution to protect the airway and prevent aspiration, especially in the stuporous or comatose patient. Incomplete gastric emptying with delayed absorption of carisoprodol has been reported as a cause for relapse. Should respiration or blood pressure become compromised, respiratory assistance, central nervous system stimulants, and pressor agents should be administered cautiously, as indicated.

Carisoprodol—The following have been used successfully in overdosage with the related drug meprobamate: diuretics, osmotic (mannitol) diuresis, peritoneal dialysis, and hemodialysis (see CLINICAL PHARMACOLOGY). Careful monitoring of urinary output is necessary and caution should be taken to avoid overhydration. Carisoprodol can be measured in biological fluid by gas chromatography (Douglas, J. F., et al: *J Pharm Sci 58*: 145, 1969).

Aspirin—Since there are no specific antidotes for salicylate poisoning, the aim of treatment is to enhance elimination of salicylate and prevent or reduce further absorption; to correct any fluid, electrolyte or metabolic imbalance; and to provide general and cardiorespiratory support. If acidosis is present, intravenous sodium bicarbonate must be given, along with adequate hydration, until salicylate levels decrease to within the therapeutic range. To enhance elimination, forced diuresis and alkalinization of the urine may be beneficial. The need for hemoperfusion or hemodialysis is rare and should be used only when other measures have failed.

Codeine Phosphate—Narcotic antagonists, such as nalorphine and levallorphan, may be indicated.

DOSAGE AND ADMINISTRATION

Usual Adult Dosage: 1 or 2 tablets, four times daily. Not recommended for use in children under age twelve.

HOW SUPPLIED

'Soma' Compound with Codeine Tablets (carisoprodol, USP 200 mg, aspirin 325 mg, and codeine phosphate, USP 16 mg) are oval, convex, two-layered and inscribed on the white layer with SOMA CC and on the yellow layer with WALLACE 2403. The tablets are available in bottles of 100 (NDC 0037-2403-01).

Storage: Store at controlled room temperature 15°–30°C (59°–86°F). Protect from moisture.

Dispense in a tight container.

WALLACE LABORATORIES
Division of CARTER-WALLACE, INC.
Cranbury, New Jersey 08512

Rev. 9/93

Shown in Product Identification Guide, page 339

THYRO-BLOCK®   OTC
TABLETS
(POTASSIUM IODIDE TABLETS, USP)
(pronounced poe-TASS-e-um EYE-oh-dyed)
(abbreviated: KI)

TAKE POTASSIUM IODIDE ONLY WHEN PUBLIC HEALTH OFFICIALS TELL YOU. IN A RADIATION EMERGENCY, RADIOACTIVE IODINE COULD BE RELEASED INTO THE AIR. POTASSIUM IODIDE (A FORM OF IODINE) CAN HELP PROTECT YOU.
IF YOU ARE TOLD TO TAKE THIS MEDICINE, TAKE IT ONE TIME EVERY 24 HOURS. DO NOT TAKE IT MORE OFTEN. MORE WILL NOT HELP YOU AND MAY INCREASE THE RISK OF SIDE EFFECTS. *DO NOT TAKE THIS DRUG IF YOU KNOW YOU ARE ALLERGIC TO IODIDE.* (SEE SIDE EFFECTS BELOW.)

INDICATIONS

THYROID BLOCKING IN A RADIATION EMERGENCY ONLY.

DIRECTIONS FOR USE

Use only as directed by State or local public health authorities in the event of a radiation emergency.

DOSE

Tablets: ADULTS AND CHILDREN 1 YEAR OF AGE OR OLDER: One (1) tablet once a day. Crush for small children.
BABIES UNDER 1 YEAR OF AGE:
One-half (1/2) tablet once a day. Crush first.

Take for 10 days unless directed otherwise by State or local public health authorities.

Store at controlled room temperatures between 15° and 30°C (59° to 86°F). Keep container tightly closed and protect from light.

WARNING

Potassium iodide should not be used by people allergic to iodide. Keep out of the reach of children. In case of overdose or allergic reaction, contact a physician or the public health authority.

DESCRIPTION

Each white, round, scored, monogrammed THYRO-BLOCK® Tablet contains 130 mg of potassium iodide. Other ingredients: magnesium stearate, microcrystalline cellulose, silica gel, and sodium thiosulfate.

HOW POTASSIUM IODIDE WORKS

Certain forms of iodine help your thyroid gland work right. Most people get the iodine they need from foods, like iodized salt or fish. The thyroid can "store" or hold only a certain amount of iodine.

In a radiation emergency, radioactive iodine may be released in the air. This material may be breathed or swallowed. It may enter the thyroid gland and damage it. The damage would probably not show itself for years. Children are most likely to have thyroid damage.

If you take potassium iodide, it will fill up your thyroid gland. This reduces the chance that harmful radioactive iodine will enter the thyroid gland.

WHO SHOULD NOT TAKE POTASSIUM IODIDE

The only people who should not take potassium iodide are people who know they are allergic to iodide. You may take potassium iodide even if you are taking medicines for a thyroid problem (for example, a thyroid hormone or antithyroid drug). Pregnant and nursing women and babies and children may also take this drug.

HOW AND WHEN TO TAKE POTASSIUM IODIDE

Potassium iodide should be taken as soon as possible after public health officials tell you. You should take one dose every 24 hours. More will not help you because the thyroid can "hold" only limited amounts of iodine. Larger doses will increase the risk of side effects. You will probably be told not to take the drug for more than 10 days.

SIDE EFFECTS

Usually, side effects of potassium iodide happen when people take higher doses for a long time. You should be careful not to take more than the recommended dose or take it for longer than you are told. Side effects are unlikely because of the low dose and the short time you will be taking the drug.

Continued on next page

Wallace Laboratories—Cont.

Possible side effects include skin rashes, swelling of the salivary glands, and "iodism" (metallic taste, burning mouth and throat, sore teeth and gums, symptoms of a head cold, and sometimes stomach upset and diarrhea).

A few people have an allergic reaction with more serious symptoms. These could be fever and joint pains, or swelling of parts of the face and body and at times severe shortness of breath requiring immediate medical attention.

Taking iodide may rarely cause overactivity of the thyroid gland, underactivity of the thyroid gland, or enlargement of the thyroid gland (goiter).

WHAT TO DO IF SIDE EFFECTS OCCUR

If the side effects are severe or if you have an allergic reaction, stop taking potassium iodide. Then, if possible, call a doctor or public health authority for instructions.

HOW SUPPLIED

THYRO-BLOCK® Tablets (Potassium Iodide Tablets, USP) are white, round tablets, one side scored, other side debossed 472 WALLACE, each containing 130 mg potassium iodide. Available in bottles of 14 tablets (NDC 0037-0472-20).

WALLACE LABORATORIES
Division of
CARTER-WALLACE, INC.
Cranbury, New Jersey 08512
IN-0472-03   Rev. 5/94

TUSSI-ORGANIDIN® DM NR* ℞
(*Newly Reformulated) Liquid
TUSSI-ORGANIDIN® DM-S† NR* ℞
(*Newly Reformulated) Liquid
(guaifenesin, dextromethorphan hydrobromide)

Professional Labeling Information and Directions for Use
This product labeled for sale on prescription only.

DESCRIPTION

TUSSI-ORGANIDIN® DM NR* (*Newly Reformulated) Liquid is a clear yellow liquid with a raspberry flavor.
Each 5 mL (1 teaspoon) contains:
Guaifenesin, USP .... 100 mg
Dextromethorphan Hydrobromide, USP .... 10 mg
Other ingredients: Citric acid, D&C Yellow No. 10, FD&C Red No. 40, flavor (artificial), glycerin, propylene glycol, purified water, saccharin sodium, sodium benzoate, sorbitol.
Guaifenesin (glyceryl guaiacolate) has the chemical name 3-(2-methoxyphenoxy)-1,2-propanediol. Its molecular formula is $C_{10}H_{14}O_4$, with a molecular weight of 198.21. It is a white, colorless crystalline substance with a slightly bitter aromatic taste. One gram dissolves in 20 mL water at 25°C; freely soluble in ethanol. Guaifenesin is readily absorbed from the GI tract and is rapidly metabolized and excreted in the urine. Guaifenesin has a plasma half-life of one hour. The major urinary metabolite is beta-(2-methoxyphenoxy) lactic acid.

CLINICAL PHARMACOLOGY

TUSSI-ORGANIDIN® DM NR* (*Newly Reformulated) combines the expectorant, guaifenesin and the cough suppressant, dextromethorphan hydrobromide. Guaifenesin is an expectorant the action of which promotes or facilitates the removal of secretions from the respiratory tract. By increasing sputum volume and making sputum less viscous, guaifenesin facilitates expectoration of retained secretions. Dextromethorphan is a synthetic nonopioid cough suppressant, the dextro isomer of the codeine analogue of levorphanol. Dextromethorphan acts centrally to elevate the threshold for coughing, but does not have addictive, analgesic or sedative actions and does not produce respiratory depression with usual doses.

INDICATIONS AND USAGE

Temporarily relieves cough due to minor throat and bronchial irritation as may occur with the common cold or inhaled irritants. Calms the cough control center and relieves coughing. Helps loosen phlegm (mucus) and thin bronchial secretions to rid the bronchial passageways of bothersome mucus, drain bronchial tubes, and make coughs more productive.

CONTRAINDICATIONS

Hypersensitivity to any of the ingredients. The use of dextromethorphan-containing products is contraindicated in patients receiving monoamine oxidase inhibitors (MAOIs).

PRECAUTIONS

Carcinogenesis, Mutagenesis, Impairment of Fertility: Animal studies to assess the long-term carcinogenic and mutagenic potential or the effect on fertility in animals or humans of TUSSI-ORGANIDIN DM NR* (*Newly Reformulated) Liquid have not been performed.
Pregnancy.
Teratogenic Effects—Pregnancy Category C: Animal reproduction studies have not been conducted. Safe use in pregnancy

has not been established relative to possible adverse effects on fetal development. Therefore, this product should not be used in pregnant patients, unless in the judgment of the physician, the potential benefits outweigh possible hazards.
Nursing Mothers: It is not known whether guaifenesin or dextromethorphan is excreted in human milk. Because many drugs are excreted in human milk, caution should be exercised when these products are administered to a nursing woman and a decision should be made whether to discontinue nursing or to discontinue the drug, taking into account the importance of the drug to the mother.
Laboratory Test Interactions: Guaifenesin or its metabolites may cause color interference with the VMA (vanillylmandelic acid) test for catechols. It may also falsely elevate the level of urinary 5-HIAA (5-hydroxyindoleacetic acid) in certain serotonin metabolite chemical tests because of color interference.
Drug Interactions: Serious toxicity may result if dextromethorphan is coadministered with monoamine oxidase inhibitors (MAOIs). The use of dextromethorphan hydrobromide may result in additive CNS depressant effects when coadministered with alcohol, antihistamines, psychotropics or other drugs which produce CNS depression.
Information for Patients: Patients should be warned not to use this product if they are now taking a prescription monoamine oxidase inhibitor (MAOI) (certain drugs for depression, psychiatric or emotional conditions, or Parkinson's disease), or for 2 weeks after stopping the MAOI drug. If patients are uncertain whether a prescription drug contains an MAOI, they should be instructed to consult a health professional before taking such a product.

ADVERSE REACTIONS

Guaifenesin is well tolerated and has a wide margin of safety. Nausea and vomiting are the side effects that occur most commonly. Other reported adverse reactions have included dizziness, headache and rash (including urticaria). Rare drowsiness or mild gastrointestinal disturbances are the only side effects associated with dextromethorphan in clinical use. (see also Drug Interactions)

OVERDOSAGE

Overdosage with guaifenesin is unlikely to produce toxic effects since its toxicity is low. Guaifenesin, when administered by stomach tube to test animals in doses up to 5 grams/kg, produced no signs of toxicity. In severe cases of overdosage, treatment should be aimed at reducing further absorption of the drug. Gastric emptying (emesis and/or gastric lavage) is recommended as soon as possible after ingestion. Overdosage with dextromethorphan may produce excitement and mental confusion. Very high doses may produce respiratory depression. One case of toxic psychosis (hyperactivity, marked visual and auditory hallucinations) after ingestion of a single 300 mg dose of dextromethorphan has been reported.

DOSAGE AND ADMINISTRATION

Adults and children 12 years of age and older: 2 teaspoonfuls (10 mL) every four hours not to exceed 12 teaspoonfuls (60 mL) in 24 hours.
Children 6 years to under 12 years of age: 1 teaspoonful (5 mL) every four hours not to exceed 6 teaspoonfuls (30 mL) in 24 hours.
Children 2 to under 6 years of age: ½ teaspoonful (2.5 mL) every four hours not to exceed 3 teaspoonfuls (15 mL) in 24 hours.
Children 6 mo. to under 2 years of age: A common dosage is ⅛ teaspoonful to ¼ teaspoonful (0.6 mL to 1.25 mL) every 4 hours or ½ teaspoonful (2.5 mL) every 6–8 hours, not to exceed 1.5 teaspoonfuls (7.5 mL) in 24 hours. Individualized dosage should be determined by evaluation of patient.

HOW SUPPLIED

Guaifenesin 100 mg and dextromethorphan hydrobromide 10 mg per 5 mL of clear yellow liquid in bottles of one pint (NDC 0037-4714-10) and one gallon (NDC 0037-4714-20), and 4 fl oz (NDC 0037-4714-01) labeled TUSSI-ORGANIDIN® DM-S† NR.*
Storage—Store at controlled room temperature—15°–30°C (59°–86°F). Protect from light. Keep bottle tightly closed.
†TUSSI-ORGANIDIN® DM-S NR* is TUSSI-ORGANIDIN® DM NR* Liquid either in a 4 fl oz unit of use container with a 10 mL graduated oral syringe and fitment or in a 30 mL sample container.
TUSSI-ORGANIDIN® DM NR* (*Newly Reformulated) Liquid is distributed by:
WALLACE LABORATORIES
Division of CARTER-WALLACE, Inc.
Cranbury, NJ 08512
Manufactured by:
Denver Chemical (Puerto Rico) Inc.
Subsidiary of Carter-Wallace, Inc.
Humacao, Puerto Rico 00791
IN-053J8-01   Rev. 7/94
Shown in Product Identification Guide, page 339

VASCOR® ℞
brand of bepridil hydrochloride
Tablets

Marketed jointly by McNeil Pharmaceutical and Wallace Laboratories. See McNeil Pharmaceutical for product information.

VōSoL® ℞
OTIC SOLUTION
(acetic acid otic solution, USP)

VōSoL® HC ℞
OTIC SOLUTION
(hydrocortisone and acetic acid otic solution, USP)

DESCRIPTION

VōSoL (acetic acid otic solution, USP) is a solution of acetic acid (2%), in a propylene glycol vehicle containing propylene glycol diacetate (3%), benzethonium chloride (0.02%), and sodium acetate (0.015%). The empirical formula for acetic acid is CH_3COOH, with a molecular weight of 60.05. The structural formula is:

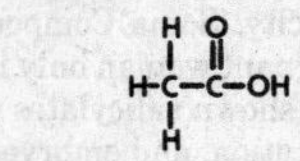

VōSoL is available as a nonaqueous otic solution buffered at pH 3 for use in the external ear canal.
VōSoL HC (hydrocortisone and acetic acid otic solution, USP) is a solution containing hydrocortisone (1%) and acetic acid (2%), in a propylene glycol vehicle containing propylene glycol diacetate (3%), benzethonium chloride (0.02%), sodium acetate (0.015%) and citric acid (0.05%). The empirical formulas for acetic acid and hydrocortisone are CH_3COOH and $C_{21}H_{30}O_5$, with a molecular weight of 60.05 and 362.46, respectively. The structural formulas are:

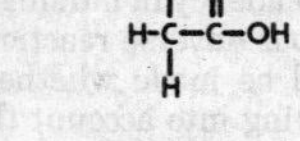

Acetic Acid

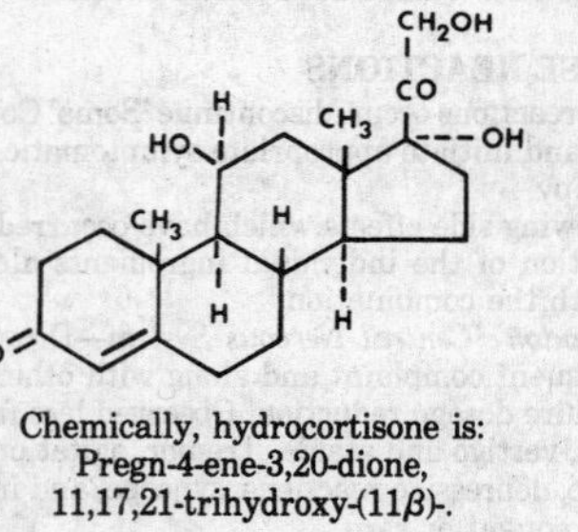

Chemically, hydrocortisone is:
Pregn-4-ene-3,20-dione,
11,17,21-trihydroxy-(11β)-.

VōSoL HC is available as a nonaqueous otic solution buffered at pH 3 for use in the external ear canal.

CLINICAL PHARMACOLOGY

VōSoL—Acetic acid is antibacterial and antifungal; propylene glycol is hydrophilic and provides a low surface tension; benzethonium chloride is a surface active agent that promotes contact of the solution with tissues.
VōSoL HC—Acetic acid is antibacterial and antifungal; hydrocortisone is anti-inflammatory, antiallergic, and antipruritic; propylene glycol is hydrophilic and provides a low surface tension; benzethonium chloride is a surface active agent that promotes contact of the solution with tissues.

INDICATIONS AND USAGE

VōSoL—For the treatment of superficial infections of the external auditory canal caused by organisms susceptible to the action of the antimicrobial.
VōSoL HC—For the treatment of superficial infections of the external auditory canal caused by organisms susceptible to the action of the antimicrobial, complicated by inflammation.

CONTRAINDICATIONS

VōSoL—Hypersensitivity to VōSoL or any of the ingredients. Perforated tympanic membrane is considered a contraindication to the use of any medication in the external ear canal.
VōSoL HC—Hypersensitivity to VōSoL HC or any of the ingredients; herpes simplex, vaccinia and varicella. Perfo-

rated tympanic membrane is considered a contraindication to the use of any medication in the external ear canal.

WARNINGS

VōSoL—Discontinue promptly if sensitization or irritation occurs.

VōSoL HC—Discontinue promptly if sensitization or irritation occurs.

PRECAUTIONS

VōSoL—Transient stinging or burning may be noted occasionally when the solution is first instilled into the acutely inflamed ear.

VōSoL HC—Transient stinging or burning may be noted occasionally when the solution is first instilled into the acutely inflamed ear.

ADVERSE REACTIONS

VōSoL—Stinging or burning may be noted occasionally; local irritation has occurred very rarely.

VōSoL HC—Stinging or burning may be noted occasionally; local irritation has occurred very rarely.

DOSAGE AND ADMINISTRATION

VōSoL—Carefully remove all cerumen and debris to allow VōSoL to contact infected surfaces directly. To promote continuous contact, insert a wick of cotton saturated with VōSoL into the ear canal; the wick may also be saturated after insertion. Instruct the patient to keep the wick in for at least 24 hours and to keep it moist by adding 3 to 5 drops of VōSoL every 4 to 6 hours. The wick may be removed after 24 hours but the patient should continue to instill 5 drops of VōSoL 3 or 4 times daily thereafter, for as long as indicated.

VōSoL HC—Carefully remove all cerumen and debris to allow VōSoL HC to contact infected surfaces directly. To promote continuous contact, insert a wick of cotton saturated with VōSoL HC into the ear canal; the wick may also be saturated after insertion. Instruct the patient to keep the wick in for at least 24 hours and to keep it moist by adding 3 to 5 drops of VōSoL HC every 4 to 6 hours. The wick may be removed after 24 hours but the patient should continue to instill 5 drops of VōSoL HC 3 or 4 times daily thereafter, for as long as indicated.

HOW SUPPLIED

VōSoL (acetic acid otic solution, USP), containing 2% acetic acid, is available in 15 mL (NDC 0037-3611-10) and 30 mL (NDC 0037-3611-30) measured-drop, safety-tip plastic bottles.

VōSoL HC (hydrocortisone and acetic acid otic solution, USP), containing hydrocortisone (1%) and acetic acid (2%), is available in 10 mL, measured-drop, safety-tip plastic bottles (NDC 0037-3811-12).

STORAGE

VōSoL—Store at controlled room temperature, 20°–25°C (68°–77°F). Keep container tightly closed.

VōSoL HC—Store at controlled room temperature, 20°–25°C (68°–77°F). Keep container tightly closed.

WALLACE LABORATORIES
Division of
CARTER-WALLACE, INC.
Cranbury, New Jersey 08512
VōSoL: IN-056S3–02D
VōSoL HC: IN-056H9–02D   Rev. 3/96

Warner Chilcott, Inc.
182 TABOR ROAD
MORRIS PLAINS, NJ 07950

Direct Inquiries to:
800-521-8813
Product/Medical Information
800-521-8813
201-540-7181
After Hours and Weekend Medical Emergencies:
303-739-1110

NDC #	PRODUCT	
0956	Albuterol Sulfate Tablets, 2 mg	℞
0957	Albuterol Sulfate Tablets, 4 mg	℞
0515	Allopurinol Tablets, 100 mg	℞
0787	Alprazolam Tablets .25 mg	ℂ/℞
0786	Alprazolam Tablets .5 mg	ℂ/℞
0785	Alprazolam Tablets 1.0 mg	ℂ/℞
0853	Amantadine HCl Capsules, USP 100 mg	℞
0730	Amoxicillin Capsules, USP 250 mg	℞
0731	Amoxicillin Capsules, USP 500 mg	℞
2500	Amoxicillin for Oral Suspension, USP 125 mg/5 mL	℞
2501	Amoxicillin for Oral Suspension, USP 250 mg/5 mL	℞

0402	Ampicillin Capsules, USP 250 mg	℞
0404	Ampicillin Capsules, USP 500 mg	℞
2301	Ampicillin for Oral Suspension, USP 125 mg/5 mL	℞
2302	Ampicillin for Oral Suspension, USP 250 mg/5 mL	℞
0048	Benzonatate Capsules USP 100 mg	℞
0106	Butalbital, Acetaminophen, and Caffeine Tablets, USP 50mg/325 mg/40 mg	℞
0114	Butalbital, Aspirin, Caffeine and Codeine Phosphate Capsules, USP 50 mg/325 mg/40 mg/30 mg	ℂ/℞
0242	Carbamazepine Chewable Tablets, 100 mg	℞
0559	Captopril Tablets, USP 12.5 mg	℞
0522	Captopril Tablets, USP 25 mg	℞
0542	Captopril Tablets, USP 50 mg	℞
0543	Captopril Tablets, USP 100 mg	℞
0938	Cephalexin Capsules, USP 250 mg	℞
0939	Cephalexin Capsules, USP 500 mg	℞
2375	Cephalexin for Oral Suspension, USP 125 mg/5 mL	℞
2376	Cephalexin for Oral Suspension, USP 250 mg/5 mL	℞
0768	Cimetidine Tablets 300 mg	℞
0765	Cimetidine Tablets 400 mg	℞
0508	Cimetidine Tablets 800 mg	℞
0451	Clorazepate Dipotassium Tablets 3.75 mg	℞
0452	Clorazepate Dipotassium Tablets 7.5 mg	℞
0453	Clorazepate Dipotassium Tablets 15 mg	℞
0057	Cyclobenzaprine Tablets 10 mg	℞
0594	Desipramine Tablets 25 mg	℞
0595	Desipramine Tablets 50 mg	℞
0596	Desipramine Tablets 75 mg	℞
0945	Dicloxacillin Sodium Capsules, USP 250 mg	℞
0946	Dicloxacillin Sodium Capsules, USP 500 mg	℞
2623	Doxepin HCl Oral Solution 10 mg/mL	℞
0829	Doxycycline Hyclate Capsules, USP 50 mg	℞
0830	Doxycycline Hyclate Capsules, USP 100 mg	℞
0091	Doxycycline HYC Capsules (coated Pellets) 100 mg	℞
0813	Doxycycline Hyclate Tablets, USP 100 mg	℞
2545	Erythromycin Ethlsuccinate w/Sulfisoxazole	℞
0124	Estropipate Tablets .75 mg	
0126	Estropipate Tablets 1.5 mg	
0128	Estropipate Tablets 3 mg	
0988	Flurazepam HCl Capsules, USP 15 mg	ℂ/℞
0989	Flurazepam HCl Capsules, USP 30 mg	ℂ/℞
0084	Gemfibrozil Tablets 600 mg	
0463	Glipizide Tablets 5 mg	℞
0464	Glipizide Tablets 10 mg	℞
0560	Guanabenz Acetate Tablets 4 mg	℞
0561	Guanabenz Acetate Tablets 8 mg	℞
0312	Guanfacine Hydrochloride Tablets 1 mg	℞
0313	Guanfacine Hydrochloride Tablets 2 mg	℞
0448	Hydrocodone w/APAP Tablets 5/500 mg	ℂ/℞
0318	Hydrocodone Bitartrate and Acetaminophen Tablets 2.5 mg/500 mg	ℂ/℞
0355	Hydrocodone Bitartrate and Acetaminophen Tablets, USP 7.5 mg/650 mg	ℂ/℞
0164	Hydrocodone Bitartrate and Acetaminophen Tablets, USP 10 mg/650 mg	ℂ/℞
0319	Hydrocodone Bitartrate w/APAP Tablets 7.5/500 mg	ℂ/℞
0486	Hydrocodone Bitartrate w/APAP Tablets 7.5/750 mg	ℂ/℞
0516	Ibuprofen Tablets, 400 mg	℞
0922	Ibuprofen Tablets, 600 mg	℞
0914	Ibuprofen Tablets, 800 mg	℞
0887	Indomethacin Capsules, USP 25 mg	℞
0888	Indomethacin Capsules, USP 50 mg	℞
0875	Indomethacin Extended-Release Capsules, USP 75 mg	℞
0528	Ketoprofen Capsules 50 mg	℞
0566	Ketoprofen Capsules 75 mg	℞
0334	Levothyroxine Sodium Tablets .025 mg	
0336	Levothyroxine Sodium Tablets .05 mg	
0338	Levothyroxine Sodium Tablets .075 mg	
0341	Levothyrozine Sodium Tablets .1 mg	
0343	Levothyrozine Sodium Tablets .125 mg	
0344	Levothyrozine Sodium Tablets .15 mg	
0347	Levothyrozine Sodium Tablets .2 mg	
0348	Levothyrozine Sodium Tablets .3 mg	
0431	Lorazepam Tablets 0.5 mg	ℂ/℞
0432	Lorazepam Tablets 1 mg	ℂ/℞
0433	Lorazepam Tablets 2 mg	ℂ/℞
0621	Loxapine Succinate Capsules 5 mg	
0632	Loxapine Succinate Capsules 10 mg	

0650	Loxapine Succinate Capsules 25 mg	℞
0651	Loxapine Succinate Capsules 50 mg	℞
0874	Medroxyprogesterone Tablets 10 mg	℞
0108	Megestrol Acetate Tablets, USP 40 mg	℞
0615	Minocycline HCl Capsules 50 mg	℞
0616	Minocycline HCl Capsules 100 mg	℞
0930/ 0927	Nelova™ 1/35E (norethindrone 1 mg and ethinyl estradiol 35 mcg)	℞
0929/ 0926	Nelova™ 0.5/35E (norethindrone 0.5 mg and ethinyl estradiol 35 mcg)	℞
0941/ 0942/ 0947	Nelova™ 10/11 (norethindrone 0.5 mg and ethinyl estradiol 35 mcg)	℞
0942/ 0947	Nelova™ 1/50M (norethindrone 1 mg and mestranol 50 mcg)	℞
0690	Oxazepam Capsules 10 mg	ℂ/℞
0665	Oxazepam Capsules 15 mg	ℂ/℞
0667	Oxazepam Capsules 30 mg	ℂ/℞
0648	Penicillin V Potassium Tablets, USP 250 mg	℞
0673	Penicillin V Potassium Tablets, USP 500 mg	℞
2449	Penicillin VK for Oral Solution, USP 125 mg/5 mL	℞
2506	Penicillin VK for Oral Solution, USP 250 mg/5 mL	℞
0951	Potassium Chloride Extended-Release Tablets, USP 8 mEq (600 mg)	℞
0784	Potassium Chloride ER Tablets 750 mg (10 MEq)	℞
0070	Propranolol HCl Tablets, USP 10 mg	℞
0071	Propranolol HCl Tablets, USP 20 mg	℞
0072	Propranolol HCl Tablets, USP 40 mg	℞
0073	Propranolol HCl Tablets, USP 60 mg	℞
0074	Propranolol HCl Tablets, USP 80 mg	℞
2885	R-Tannate Pediatric Suspension	℞
0940	R-Tannate Tablets phenylephrine tannate 25 mg chlorpheniramine tannate 8 mg pyrilamine tannate 25 mg	℞
0773	Sulindac Tablets, USP 150 mg	℞
0774	Sulindac Tablets, USP 200 mg	℞
0407	Tetracycline HCl Capsules, USP 250 mg	℞
0697	Tetracycline HCl Capsules, USP 500 mg	℞
0657	Theophylline Controlled-Release Tablets 100 mg	℞
0659	Theophylline Controlled-Release Tablets 200 mg	℞
0592	Theophylline Controlled-Release Tablets 300 mg	℞
0593	Theophylline Extended–Release Tablets 450 mg	℞
0835	Transdermal-NTG (nitroglycerin transdermal system) 0.2 mg/hour	℞
0837	Transdermal-NTG (nitroglycerin transdermal system) 0.4 mg/hour	℞
0839	Transdermal-NTG (nitroglycerin transdermal system) 0.6 mg/hour	℞
0577	Trazodone HCl Tablets 50 mg	℞
0578	Trazodone HCl Tablets 100 mg	℞
0716	Trazodone HCl Tablets 150 mg	℞
0833	Triamterene and Hydrochlorothiazide Tablets, 75 mg/50 mg	℞
3122	Unibase	OTC
0328	Verapamil HCl Tablets 80 mg	℞
0329	Verapamil HCl Tablets 120 mg	℞
0472	Verapamil SR Tablets 180 mg	℞
0474	Verapamil SR Tablets 240 mg	℞

NOTICE
Before prescribing or administering any product described in PHYSICIANS' DESK REFERENCE, check the **PDR Supplements** for revised information.

Warner Wellcome
Consumer Healthcare
201 TABOR ROAD
MORRIS PLAINS, NJ 07950

Direct Inquiries and For Medical Information Contact:
Consumer Affairs
1-(800) 524-2624
1-(800) 223-0182
(See PDR For Nonprescription Drugs)

ACTIFED® ALLERGY   OTC
Daytime/Nighttime Caplets
[ăk'-tĭ-fĕd]

Daytime
Pseudoephedrine HCl (30 mg)
Nasal Decongestant
Nighttime:
Diphenhydramine HCl (25 mg)
Pseudoephedrine HCl (30 mg)
Nasal Decongestant /Antihistamine

ACTIFED COLD & ALLERGY® Tablets   OTC
[ăk'-tĭ-fĕd]

Pseudoephedrine HCl (60 mg)
Triprolidine HCl (2.5 mg)
Antihistamine/Nasal Decongestant

ACTIFED® COLD & SINUS   OTC
Tablets and Caplets
[ăk'tĭ-fĕd]

Acetaminophen (500 mg)
Pseudoephedrine HCl (30 mg)
Triprolidine HCl (1.25 mg)
Antihistamine/Nasal Decongestant
Pain Reliever-Fever Reducer

ACTIFED® SINUS Daytime/Nighttime   OTC
Caplets & Tablets
[ăk'-tĭ-fĕd]

Daytime:
Acetaminophen (500 mg)
Pseudoephedrine HCl (30 mg)
Pain Reliever/Nasal Decongestant
Nighttime:
Acetaminophen (500 mg)
Diphenhydramine HCl (25 mg)
Pseudoephedrine HCl (30 mg)
Pain Reliever/Nasal Decongestant/Antihistamine

AGORAL®   OTC
[ăg'-a-rŏl]

Phenolphthalein (0.2 gm)
Lubricant/Stimulant Laxative

ALOPHEN® Pills   OTC
[al'-ō-fen]

Phenolphthalein (60 mg)
Stimulant Laxative

ANUSOL® HC-1 Ointment   OTC
[an'-ū-sol]

Hydrocortisone Acetate (equivalent to 1% Hydrocortisone)
Anti-Itch Hydrocortisone Ointment

ANUSOL® Hemorrhoidal Ointment   OTC
[an'-ū-sol]

Pramoxine HCl (1%)
Zinc Oxide (12.5%)
Mineral Oil

ANUSOL® Hemorrhoidal Suppositories   OTC
[ăn"-ū'-sŏl]

Topical Starch (51%)
Hemorrhoidal Suppositories

BENADRYL® ALLERGY CHEWABLES   OTC
[bĕ'-nă-drĭl]

Diphenhydramine HCl (12.5 mg)
Antihistamine

BENADRYL® ALLERGY/COLD Tablets   OTC
[bĕ'-nă-drĭl]

Diphenhydramine HCl (12.5 mg)
Pseudoephedrine HCl (30 mg)
Acetaminophen (500 mg)
Antihistamine/Nasal Decongestant/Pain
Reliever-Fever Reducer

BENADRYL® ALLERGY DECONGESTANT   OTC
Liquid
[bĕ'-nă-drĭl]

Diphenhydramine HCl (12.5 mg)
Pseudoephedrine HCl (30 mg)
Antihistamine/Nasal Decongestant

BENADRYL® ALLERGY DECONGESTANT   OTC
Tablets
[bĕ'-nă-drĭl]

Diphenhydramine HCl (25 mg)
Pseudoephedrine HCl (60 mg)
Antihistamine/Nasal Decongestant 4

BENADRYL® ALLERGY Kapseals   OTC
[bĕ'-nă-drĭl]

Diphenhydramine HCl (25 mg)
Antihistamine

BENADRYL® ALLERGY Liquid   OTC
[bĕ'-nă-drĭl]

Diphenhydramine HCl (12.5 mg)
Antihistamine

BENADRYL® ALLERGY Tablets   OTC
[bĕ'-nă-drĭl]

Diphenhydramine HCl (25 mg)
Antihistamine

BENADRYL® ALLERGY/SINUS Headache   OTC
Caplets
[bĕ'-nă-drĭl]

Diphenhydramine HCl (12.5 mg)
Pseudoephedrine HCl (30 mg)
Acetaminophen (500 mg)
Antihistamine/Nasal Decongestant Pain Reliever

BENADRYL® DYE-FREE ALLERGY Liqui-gels®   OTC
[bĕ'-nă-drĭl]

Diphenhydramine HCl (25 mg)
Antihistamine

BENADRYL® DYE-FREE ALLERGY Liquid   OTC
[bĕ'-nă-drĭl]

Diphenhydramine HCl (6.25 mg)
Antihistamine

BENADRYL® Itch Relief Stick   OTC
Extra Strength
[bĕ'-nă-drĭl]

Diphenhydramine HCl (2%)
Zinc Acetate (0.1%)
Topical Analgesic/Skin Protectant

BENADRYL® Itch Stopping Cream   OTC
Original Strength
[bĕ'-nă-drĭl]

Diphenhydramine HCl (1%)
Zinc Acetate (0.1%)
Topical Analgesic/Skin Protectant

BENADRYL® Itch Stopping Cream   OTC
Extra Strength
[bĕ'-nă-drĭl]

Diphenhydramine HCl (2%)
Zinc Acetate (0.1%)
Topical Analgesic/Skin Protectant

BENADRYL® Itch Stopping Gel   OTC
Original Strength
[bĕ'-nă-drĭl]

Diphenhydramine HCl (1%)
Zinc Acetate (1%)
Topical Analgesic/Skin Protectant

BENADRYL® Itch Stopping Gel   OTC
Extra Strength
[bĕ'-nă-drĭl]

Diphenhydramine HCl (2%)
Zinc Acetate (1%)
Topical Analgesic/Skin Protectant

BENADRYL® Itch Stopping Spray   OTC
Original Strength
[bĕ'-nă-drĭl]

Diphenhydramine HCl (1%)
Zinc Acetate (0.1%)
Topical Analgesic/Skin Protectant

BENADRYL® Itch Stopping Spray   OTC
Extra Strength
[bĕ'-nă-drĭl]

Diphenhydramine HCl (2%)
Zinc Acetate (0.1%)
Topical Analgesic/Skin Protectant

BENYLIN® ADULT Formula   OTC
[bĕ'-nă-lĭn]

Dextromethorphan HBr (15 mg)
Cough Suppressant

BENYLIN® EXPECTORANT   OTC
[bĕ'-nă-lĭn]

Dextromethorphan HBr (5 mg)
Guaifenesin (100 mg)
Cough Suppressant

BENYLIN® MULTI-SYMPTOM   OTC
[bĕ'-nă-lĭn]

Dextromethorphan HBr (5 mg)
Pseudoephedrine HCl (15 mg)
Guaifenesin (100 mg)
Cough Suppressant/Expectorant/Nasal Decongestant

BENYLIN® PEDIATRIC OTC
[bĕ'-nă-lĭn]

Dextromethorphan HBr (7.5 mg)
Cough Suppressant

BOROFAX® Ointment OTC
[bōr'-ō-făks]

Zinc Oxide (15%)
White Petrolatum (68.6%)
Skin Protectant

CALADRYL® CLEAR Lotion OTC
[kăl'-ă-drĭl]

Pramoxine HCl (1%)
Zinc Acetate (0.1%)
External Analgesic/Skin Protectant

CALADRYL® Cream for Kids OTC
[kăl'-ă-drĭl]

Calamine (8%)
Pramoxine HCl (1%)
External Analgesic/Skin Protectant

CALADRYL® Lotion OTC
[kăl'-ă-drĭl]

Calamine (8%)
Pramoxine HCl (1%)
External Analgesic/Skin Protectant

GELUSIL® Tablets OTC
[jĕl'ū-sĭl]

Aluminum Hydroxide Dried Gel (200 mg)
Magnesium Hydroxide (200 mg)
Simethicone (25 mg)
Antacid/Anti-Gas

LAVACOL® OTC
[lav'a kol]

Ethyl Alcohol Solution (denatured) (70%)
Rubbing Alcohol/1st Aid Antiseptic

COOL MINT LISTERINE® OTC
[lĭs'tərēn]

Thymol (0.064%)
Eucalyptol (0.092%)
Methyl Salicylate (0.060%)
Menthol (0.042%)
Antiseptic

FRESHBURSH LISTERINE® OTC
[lĭs'tərēn]

Thymol (0.064%)
Eucalyptol (0.092%)
Methyl Salicylate (0.060%)
Menthol (0.042%)
Antiseptic

LISTERINE® Antiseptic OTC
[lĭs'tərēn]

Thymol (0.064%)
Eucalyptol (0.092%)
Methyl Salicylate (0.060%)
Menthol (0.042%)
Antiseptic

LISTERMINT® OTC
Alcohol-Free Mouthwash
[lĭs'tər mĭnt]

NEOSPORIN® ORIGINAL Ointment OTC
[nē"ō-spōr'ĭn]

Polymyxin B Sulfate (5000 units)
Bacitracin Zinc (400 units)
Neomycin (3.5 mg)
First Aid Antibiotic Ointment

NEOSPORIN® PLUS OTC
Maximum Strength Cream
[nē"ō-spor'ĭn]

Polymyxin B Sulfate (10,000 units)
Neomycin (3.5 mg)
Pramoxine HCl (10 mg)
First Aid Antibiotic/Pain Relieving Cream

NEOSPORIN® PLUS OTC
Maximum Strength Ointment
[nē"ō-spor'ĭn]

Polymyxin B Sulfate (10,000 units)
Bacitracin Zinc (500 units)
Neomycin (3.5 mg)
Pramoxine HCl (10 mg)
First Aid Antibiotic/Pain Relieving Ointment

NIX® Creme Rinse OTC
[nĭks]

Permethrin 280 mg (1%)
Lice Treatment

POLYSPORIN® Ointment OTC
[pah"lē-spor'ĭn]

Polymyxin B. Sulfate (10,000 Units)
Bacitracin Zinc (500 Units)
First Aid Antibiotic Ointment

POLYSPORIN® Powder OTC
[pah"lēspor'ĭn]

Polymyxin B Sulfate (10,000 units)
Bacitracin Zinc (500 units)
First Aid Antibiotic Powder

PROXACOL™ OTC
[prŏks'a kŏl]

Hydrogen Peroxide, (3%)
First Aid Antiseptic

REPLENS® OTC
[ree'plenz]

Vaginal Moisturizer

SINUTAB® Non Drying Liquid Caps OTC
[sĭn'ū tăb]

Pseudoephedrine HCl (30 mg)
Guaifenesin (200 mg)
Nasal Decongestant/Expectorant

SINUTAB® SINUS ALLERGY OTC
Maximum Strength
Caplets & Tablets
[sĭn'ū tăb]

Acetaminophen (500 mg)
Pseudoephedrine HCl (30 mg)
Chlorpheniramine Maleate (2 mg)
Pain Reliever/Nasal Decongestant/Antihistamine

SINUTAB® SINUS Regular Strength OTC
Without Drowsiness Tablets
[sĭn'ū tăb]

Acetaminophen (325 mg)
Pseudoephedrine HCl (30 mg)
Analgesic/Decongestant

SINUTAB® SINUS Maximum Strength OTC
Without Drowsiness Caplets & Tablets
[sĭn'ū tăb]

Acetaminophen (500 mg)
Pseudoephedrine HCl (30 mg)
Pain Reliever/Nasal Decongestant

SUDAFED® 30 mg Tablets OTC
[sū'dah-fĕd"]

Pseudoephedrine HCl (30 mg)
Nasal Decongestant

SUDAFED® 60 mg Tablets OTC
[sū'dah-fĕd"]

Pseudoephedrine HCl (60 mg)
Nasal Decongestant

SUDAFED® 12 Hour Caplets OTC
[sū'dah-fĕd"]

Pseudoephedrine HCl (120 mg)
Long-Acting Nasal Decongestant

SUDAFED® COLD & ALLERGY Tablets OTC
[sū'dah-fĕd"]

Pseudoephedrine HCl (60 mg)
Chlorpheniramine Maleate (4 mg)
Nasal Decongestant, Antihistamine

SUDAFED® Cold & Cough Liquid Caps OTC
[sū'dah-fĕd"]

Acetaminophen (250 mg)
Dextromethorphan HBr (10 mg)
Guaifenesin (100 mg)
Pseudoephedrine HCl (30 mg)
Nasal Decongestant/Pain Reliever/Fever
Reducer/Cough Suppressant/Expectorant

SUDAFED® Severe Cold Formula OTC
Maximum Strength
Caplets & Tablets
[sū'dah-fĕd"]

Acetaminophen (500 mg)
Dextromethorphan Hydrobromide (15 mg)
Pseudoephedrine HCl (30 mg)
Nasal Decongestant/Cough Suppressant/
Pain Reliever/Fever Reducer

SUDAFED® NON-DRYING SINUS OTC
Liquid Caps
[sū'dah-fĕd"]

Guaifenesin (200 mg)
Pseudoephedrine HCl (30 mg)
Nasal Decongestant, Expectorant

Continued on next page

Warner Wellcome—Cont.

SUDAFED® SINUS OTC
Maximum Strength
Caplets and Tablets
[sū'dah-fĕd"]

Acetaminophen (500 mg)
Pseudoephedrine HCl (30 mg)
Pain Reliever/Nasal Decongestant

**PEDIATRIC SUDAFED® NASAL
DECONGESTANT** OTC
[sū'dah-fĕd"]

Pseudoephedrine HCl (7.5 mg)
Nasal Decongestant

CHILDREN'S SUDAFED® COLD & COUGH OTC
[sū'dah-fĕd"]

Pseudoephedrine HCl (15 mg)
Dextromethorphan Hydrobromide (5 mg)
Guaifenesin (100 mg)
Nasal Decongestant, Cough
Suppressant, Expectorant

**CHILDREN'S SUDAFED® NASAL
DECONGESTANT** OTC
[sū'dah-fĕd"]

Pseudoephedrine HCl (15 mg)
Nasal Decongestant

TUCKS® Clear Gel OTC
[tŭks]

Witch Hazel (50%)
Glycerin (10%)
Hemorrhoidal Gel

TUCKS® Hemorrhoidal Pads OTC
[tŭks]

Witch Hazel (50%),
Hemorrhoidal Pads

TUCKS® Take Alongs OTC
[tŭks]

Witch Hazel (50%)
Hemorrhoidal Pads

ZANTAC® 75 OTC
[zan'tak]

Ranitidine Hydrochloride (84 mg)
(equivalent to 75 mg ranitidine)
Acid Reducer

IDENTIFICATION PROBLEM?
Turn to the **Product Identification** Guide,
where you'll find more than
1600 products pictured in actual
size and full color.

Watson Laboratories, Inc.
**311 BONNIE CIRCLE
CORONA, CA 91720**

Address Inquiries to:
Customer Service Department
Telephone: 800/272-5525
FAX: 909/270-1096

The following list of Watson Laboratories products is
provided to facilitate identification. It includes the color(s)
and identification codes for all tablets and capsules.

PRODUCT	IDENTIFICATION CODE
GENERIC NAME	(Front/Back*)
Description	
Color(s), Shape	
ACEBUTOLOL HYDROCHLORIDE	WATSON 437/200 mg
Capsules, 200 mg ℞	
Red/Gray	
ACEBUTOLOL HYDROCHLORIDE	WATSON 438/400 mg
Capsules, 400 mg ℞	
Maroon/Green	
ALBUTEROL SULFATE	
Syrup, 2 mg/5 ml ℞	
Clear, yellow	
AMOXAPINE	WATSON 379/Bisected
Tablets, USP, 25 mg ℞	
White, Round	
AMOXAPINE	WATSON 380/Bisected
Tablets, USP, 50 mg ℞	
Salmon, Round	
AMOXAPINE	WATSON 381/Bisected
Tablets, USP, 100 mg ℞	
Blue, Round	
AMOXAPINE	WATSON 382/Bisected
Tablets, USP, 150 mg ℞	
Peach, Round	
BUTALBITAL, ASPIRIN, CAFFEINE, and CODEINE PHOSPHATE	WATSON/425
Capsules, USP 50 mg/325 mg/40 mg/30 mg ℃ ℞	
Blue/Yellow	
CARBIDOPA and LEVODOPA	WATSON 430/Scored
Tablets, USP, 10 mg/100 mg ℞	
Blue, Round	
CARBIDOPA and LEVODOPA	WATSON 431/Scored
Tablets, USP, 25 mg/100 mg ℞	
Tan, Round	
CARBIDOPA and LEVODOPA	WATSON 432/Scored
Tablets, USP, 25 mg/250 mg ℞	
Blue, Round	
CLORAZEPATE DIPOTASSIUM	WATSON 363/3.75 Scored
Tablets, 3.75 mg ℃ ℞	
Light Blue, Round	
CLORAZEPATE DIPOTASSIUM	WATSON 364/7.5 Scored
Tablets, 7.5 mg ℃ ℞	
Light beige, Round	
CLORAZEPATE DIPOTASSIUM	WATSON 365/15 Scored
Tablets, 15 mg ℃ ℞	
Pink, Round	
CYCLOBENZAPRINE HYDRO-CHLORIDE ℞	WATSON/418
Tablets, USP, 10 mg	
White, Film Coated, Round	
ESTRADIOL	WATSON 528/Scored
Tablets, USP, 0.5 mg ℞	
White, Round	
ESTRADIOL	WATSON 487/Scored
Tablets, USP, 1 mg ℞	
Gray, Round	
ESTRADIOL	WATSON 488/Scored
Tablets, USP, 2 mg ℞	
Light Green, Round	
ESTROPIPATE	WATSON 414/Scored
Tablets, USP, 0.75 mg ℞	
(calculated as sodium estrone sulfate 0.625 mg)	
Yellow, Round	
ESTROPIPATE	WATSON 415/Scored
Tablets, USP, 1.5 mg ℞	
(calculated as sodium estrone sulfate 1.25 mg)	
Peach, Round	
ESTROPIPATE	WATSON 416/Scored
Tablets, USP, 3 mg ℞	
(calculated as sodium estrone sulfate 2.5 mg)	
Blue, Round	

PRODUCT	IDENTIFICATION CODE
FUROSEMIDE	WATSON 300/Blank
Tablets, USP, 20 mg ℞	
White, Round	
FUROSEMIDE	WATSON/311
Tablets, USP, 20 mg ℞	
White, Oval	
FUROSEMIDE	WATSON 301/Scored
Tablets, USP, 40 mg ℞	
White, Round	
FUROSEMIDE	WATSON 302/Scored
Tablets, USP, 80 mg ℞	
White, Round	
GEMFIBROZIL	WATSON 454/Bisected
Tablets, USP, 600 mg ℞	
White, Film-coated Oval	
GLIPIZIDE	WATSON 460/Scored
Tablets, USP, 5 mg ℞	
White, Round	
GLIPIZIDE	WATSON 461/Scored
Tablets, USP, 10 mg ℞	
White, Round	
GUANABENZ ACETATE	WATSON 451/Blank
Tablets, USP, 4 mg ℞	
Orange, Round	
GUANABENZ ACETATE	WATSON 452/Scored
Tablets, USP, 8 mg ℞	
Grey, Round	
GUANFACINE HYDROCHLORIDE	WATSON 444/Blank
Tablets, 1 mg ℞	
Pink, Round	
GUANFACINE HYDROCHLORIDE	WATSON 453/Blank
Tablets, 2 mg ℞	
Peach, Round	
HYDROCODONE BITARTRATE and APAP	WATSON 388/Bisected
Tablets, 2.5 mg/500 mg ℃ ℞	
White, Oblong	
HYDROCODONE BITARTRATE and APAP	WATSON 385/Bisected
Tablets, 7.5 mg/500 mg ℃ ℞	
White, Capsule-shaped	
HYDROCODONE BITARTRATE and APAP	WATSON 349/Bisected
Tablets, 5 mg/ 500 mg ℃ ℞	
White, Capsule-shaped	
HYDROCODONE BITARTRATE and APAP	WATSON 502/Bisected
Tablets, USP, 7.5 mg/650 mg ℃ ℞	
Pink, Capsule-shaped	
HYDROCODONE BITARTRATE and APAP	WATSON 387/Bisected
Tablets, 7.5 mg/ 750 mg ℃ ℞	
White, Oblong	
HYDROCODONE BITARTRATE and APAP	WATSON 503/Bisected
Tablets, 10 mg/650mg ℃ ℞	
Light Green, Capsule-Shaped	
LORAZEPAM	WATSON/332 Scored 0.5
Tablets, USP, 0.5 mg ℃ ℞	
White, Round	
LORAZEPAM	WATSON/333 Scored 1.0
Tablets, USP, 1 mg ℃ ℞	
White, Round	
LORAZEPAM	WATSON/334 Scored 2.0
Tablets, USP, 2 mg ℃ ℞	
White, Round	
LOXAPINE SUCCINATE	WATSON 369/5 mg
Capsules, 5 mg ℞	
White/white	
LOXAPINE SUCCINATE	WATSON 370/10 mg
Capsules, 10 mg ℞	
Yellow/white	
LOXAPINE SUCCINATE	WATSON 371/25 mg
Capsules, 25 mg ℞	
Green/white	
LOXAPINE SUCCINATE	WATSON 372/50 mg
Capsules, 50 mg ℞	
Blue/white	
MAPROTILINE HYDROCHLORIDE	WATSON/373 (Partial Bisect)
Tablets, USP, 25 mg ℞	
Peach, Film Coated, Oval	
MAPROTILINE HYDROCHLORIDE	WATSON 374/Scored
Tablets, USP, 50 mg ℞	
Peach, Film Coated, Round	
MAPROTILINE HYDROCHLORIDE	WATSON/375 (Partial Bisect)
Tablets, USP, 75 mg ℞	
White, Film Coated, Oval	
METOCLOPRAMIDE HYDROCHLORIDE	WATSON 312/Scored
Tablets, 10 mg ℞	
White, Round	
METOPROLOL TARTRATE	WATSON 462/Scored
Tablets, USP, 50 mg ℞	
Pink, Film Coated, Round	
METOPROLOL TARTRATE	WATSON 463/Scored
Tablets, USP, 100 mg ℞	
Light Blue, Film Coated, Round	
PROPRANOLOL HYDROCHLORIDE	WATSON 305/Scored
Tablets, USP, 10 mg ℞	
Orange, Round	
PROPRANOLOL HYDROCHLORIDE	WATSON 306/Scored
Tablets, USP, 20 mg ℞	
Blue, Round	

PROPRANOLOL HYDROCHLORIDE — WATSON 307/
Tablets, USP, 40 mg ℞ — Scored
Green, Round
PROPRANOLOL HYDROCHLORIDE — WATSON 352/
Tablets, USP, 60 mg ℞ — Scored
Pink, Round
PROPRANOLOL HYDROCHLORIDE — WATSON 308/
Tablets, USP, 80 mg ℞ — Scored
Yellow, Round
TRIAMTERENE and
HYDROCHLOROTHIAZIDE — WATSON 424/Scored
Tablets, USP, 37.5 mg/25 mg ℞
Light green, Round
TRIAMTERENE and
HYDROCHLOROTHIAZIDE — WATSON 348/Scored
Tablets, USP, 75 mg/50 mg ℞
Yellow, Round
VERAPAMIL HYDROCHLORIDE — WATSON 404/Blank
Tablets, 40 mg ℞
Light Peach, Film Coated, Round
VERAPAMIL HYDROCHLORIDE — WATSON 343/Scored
Tablets, 80 mg ℞
White, Film Coated, Round
VERAPAMIL HYDROCHLORIDE — WATSON 344/Scored
Tablets, 80 mg ℞
Light peach, Film Coated, Round
VERAPAMIL HYDROCHLORIDE — WATSON 345/Scored
Tablets, 120 mg ℞
White, Film Coated, Round
VERAPAMIL HYDROCHLORIDE — WATSON 346/Scored
Tablets, 120 mg ℞
Peach, Film Coated, Round

ORAL CONTRACEPTIVE PRODUCTS:
(available in 21 day and 28 day packs)

NORETHINDRONE AND ETHINYL ℞
ESTRADIOL TABLETS USP:
NECON® 0.5/35 — WATSON/507
(0.5 mg norethindrone and
35 mcg ethinyl estradiol)
NECON® 1/35 — WATSON/508
(1 mg norethindrone and
35 mcg ethinyl estradiol)
NECON® 10/11 — 10 tablets of
(10 tablets—each contains — WATSON/507
0.5 mg norethindrone and — and 11 tablets of
35 mcg ethinyl estradiol; — WATSON/508
11 tablets—each contains
1 mg norethindrone and
35 mcg ethinyl estradiol.)

NORETHINDRONE AND MESTRANOL ℞
TABLETS USP:
NECON® 1/50 — WATSON/510
(1 mg norethindrone and
50 mcg mestranol)

ETHYNODIOL DIACETATE AND ℞
ETHINYL ESTRADIOL TABLETS USP:
ZOVIA® 1/35E — WATSON 383/Blank
(1 mg ethynodiol diacetate
and 35 mcg ethinyl estradiol)
ZOVIA® 1/50E — WATSON 384/Blank
(1 mg ethynodiol diacetate
and 50 mcg ethinyl estradiol)

WE Pharmaceuticals, Inc.
P.O. BOX 1142
RAMONA, CA, 92065

Direct Inquiries to:
(619) 788-9155
For Medical Emergencies Contact:
(619) 788-9155

AH-CHEW® Chewable Tablets ℞

Each tablet contains chlorpheniramine maleate 2mg. phenylephrine HCl 10mg. methscopolamine nitrate 1.25mg.
DOSAGE
12 yrs. & Older 1 or 2 Tabs (Q.I.D.), 6–12 yrs. 1 Tab (Q.I.D.).
HOW SUPPLIED
Bottles of 100, NDC# 59196-003-01

AH-CHEW®D Chewable Tablets ℞

Each tablet contains phenylephrine HCl 10mg.
DOSAGE
12 yrs. & Older 1 or 2 Tabs (Q.I.D.), 6–12 yrs. 1 Tab (Q.I.D.)
HOW SUPPLIED
Bottles of 100, NDC# 59196-007-01

D-FEDA™ II Tablets ℞

East tablet contains pseudoephedrine HCl 60mg, guaifenesin 600mg.

DOSAGE
12 yrs. & Older 1 or 2 Tabs (B.I.D.), 6–12 yrs. 1 Tab (B.I.D.),
2–6 Yrs. ½ Tab (B.I.D.).
HOW SUPPLIED
Bottles of 100, NDC #59196-005-01

E-Z SPACER® ℞
Portable Drug Delivery System for
use with metered dose inhalers.

HOW SUPPLIED
One Unit plus Instructions for Single Patient Use.
NDC #59196-009-01

HUMAVENT™ L.A. Tablets ℞
600 mg Guaifenesin

HOW SUPPLIED
NDC # 59196-008-01 — Bottles of 100
59196-008-05 — Bottles of 500

OMNIHIST® L.A. Tablets ℞

Each tablet contains chlorpheniramine maleate 8 mg, phenylephrine HCl 20 mg, methscopolamine nitrate 2.5 mg.
DOSAGE
12 yrs. & Older 1 Tab (B.I.D.), 6–12 yrs. ½ Tab (B.I.D.)
HOW SUPPLIED
Bottles of 100, NDC #59196-002-01

SINUVENT® Tablets ℞

Each tablet contains phenylpropanolamine HCl 75mg, guaifenesin 600mg.
DOSAGE
12 yrs. & Older 1 Tab (B.I.D.), 6–12 yrs. ½ Tab (B.I.D.)
HOW SUPPLIED
Bottles of 100, NDC# 59196-001-01

ULTRABROM® Capsules ℞

Each capsule contains brompheniramine maleate 12mg. pseudoephedrine HCl 120mg.
DOSAGE
12 yrs. and Older 1 Cap (B.I.D.)
HOW SUPPLIED
Bottles of 100, NDC# 59196-006-01

ULTRABROM® PD Capsules ℞

Each capsule contains brompheniramine maleate 6mg, pseudoephedrine HCl 60mg.
DOSAGE
12 yrs. & Older 1 or 2 Caps B.I.D., 6–12 yrs. 1 Cap B.I.D.
HOW SUPPLIED
Bottles of 100, NDC# 59196-004-01

Westwood-Squibb Pharmaceuticals, Inc.
100 FOREST AVENUE
BUFFALO, NY 14213

For Medical Information Contact:
Generally:
Consumer Affairs Department:
(716) 887-7667
Adverse Drug Experiences
and Product Defects Reporting call during business hours only:
(716) 887-7667

CAPITROL® ℞
(chloroxine 2%)
Shampoo

CAUTION
Federal law prohibits dispensing without a prescription.

DESCRIPTION
CAPITROL is an antibacterial shampoo containing 2% (w/w) chloroxine (each gram contains 20 mg chloroxine) suspended in a base of sodium octoxynol-2 ethane sulfonate, water, PEG-6 lauramide, dextrin, sodium lauryl sulfoacetate, sodium dioctyl sulfosuccinate, 1% benzyl alcohol, PEG-14M, magnesium aluminum silicate, fragrance, EDTA, and color. May contain citric acid to adjust pH.
Chloroxine is a synthetic antibacterial compound that is effective in the treatment of dandruff and seborrheic dermatitis when incorporated in a shampoo.
The chemical name of chloroxine is 5,7-dichloro-8-hydroxyquinoline. The chemical structure of chloroxine is:

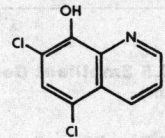

CLINICAL PHARMACOLOGY
Well controlled studies demonstrate Capitrol effectively reduces the excess scaling in patients with dandruff or seborrheic dermatitis. Though the cause of dandruff is not known, it is thought to be the result of accelerated mitotic activity in the epidermis. The presumed mechanism of action to reduce scaling would be to slow down the mitotic activity.
The role of microbes in seborrheic dermatitis is not known; however, *Staphylococcus aureus* and *Pityrosporon* species are often present in increased numbers during the course of the disease. Chloroxine is antibacterial, inhibiting the growth of Gram-positive as well as some Gram-negative organisms. Antifungal activity against some dermatophytes and yeasts also has been shown.
The absorption, metabolism and pharmacokinetics of Capitrol in humans have not been studied.

INDICATIONS AND USAGE
Capitrol is indicated in the treatment of dandruff and mild-to-moderately severe seborrheic dermatitis of the scalp. Clinical studies indicate that improvement may be observed after 14 days of therapy.

CONTRAINDICATIONS
Capitrol is contraindicated in those patients with a history of hypersensitivity to any of the listed ingredients.

WARNINGS
Capitrol should not be used on acutely inflamed (exudative) lesions of the scalp.

PRECAUTIONS
Information for patients: Exercise care to prevent Capitrol from entering the eyes. If contact occurs, the patient should flush eyes with cool water. Discoloration of light-colored hair (e.g. blond, gray or bleached) may follow use of this preparation.
Irritation and a burning sensation on the scalp and adjacent areas have been reported.
Drug/Laboratory Test Interactions: There is no known interference of Capitrol with laboratory tests.
Carcinogenesis, Mutagenesis: No long term studies in animals have been performed to evaluate the carcinogenic potential of Capitrol.
Results of the *in vitro* Ames Salmonella/Microsome Plate test show that Capitrol does not demonstrate genetic activity and is considered non-mutagenic.

Continued on next page

Westwood-Squibb—Cont.

Pregnancy Category C: Animal reproduction studies have not been conducted with Capitrol. It is also not known whether Capitrol can cause fetal harm when administered to a pregnant woman or can affect reproduction capacity. Capitrol should be given to a pregnant woman only if clearly needed.

Nursing Mothers: It is not known whether this drug is excreted in human milk. Because many drugs are excreted in human milk, caution should be exercised when Capitrol is administered to a nursing woman.

Pediatric Use: Specific studies to demonstrate the safety and effectiveness for use of Capitrol in children have not been conducted.

ADVERSE REACTION

One patient out of 225 in clinical studies was reported to have contact dermatitis.

OVERDOSAGE

The acute oral LD_{50} in mice was found to be 200 mg/kg and in rats 450 mg/kg. On the basis of these animal studies, Capitrol may be considered practically non-toxic.

DOSAGE AND ADMINISTRATION

Shake well. Capitrol should be massaged thoroughly onto the wet scalp, avoiding contact with the eyes. Lather should remain on the scalp for approximately three minutes, then rinsed. The application should be repeated and the scalp rinsed thoroughly. Two treatments per week are usually sufficient.

HOW SUPPLIED

Capitrol shampoo contains 2% (w/w) chloroxine (20 mg chloroxine per gram) and is supplied in 110g plastic bottles (NDC 0072-6850-04).
Store at room temperature.

WATER BASE
DESQUAM-E™ 2.5 Emollient Gel ℞
(2.5% benzoyl peroxide)

WATER BASE
DESQUAM-E™ 5 Emollient Gel ℞
(5% benzoyl peroxide)

WATER BASE
DESQUAM-E™ 10 Emollient Gel ℞
(10% benzoyl peroxide)

WATER BASE
DESQUAM-X® 5 Gel ℞
(5% Benzoyl Peroxide)

WATER BASE
DESQUAM-X® 10 Gel ℞
(10% Benzoyl Peroxide)

WATER BASE
DESQUAM-X® 5 Wash ℞
(5% benzoyl peroxide)

WATER BASE
DESQUAM-X 10 ® Wash ℞
(10% benzoyl peroxide)

DESQUAM-X® 10 Bar ℞
(10% benzoyl peroxide)

CAUTION

Federal law prohibits dispensing without prescription.

DESCRIPTION

DESQUAM-E 2.5, DESQUAM-E 5 and DESQUAM-E 10 brand topical anti-acne gels contain benzoyl peroxide (2.5, 5 and 10%) in a water-base vehicle of carbomer 940, diisopropanolamine, disodium edetate, docusate sodium, methyl gluceth-20 and polyquaternium-7.

DESQUAM-X 5 and DESQUAM-X 10 brand topical anti-acne gels contain benzoyl peroxide (5 and 10%), in a water-base vehicle of carbomer 940, disodium edetate and laureth-4. May contain diisopropanolamine or triethanolamine to adjust pH.

DESQUAM-X^5 and DESQUAM-X^{10} brand topical therapeutic anti-acne cleansers contain benzoyl peroxide (5% and 10%) in a lathering water base of sodium octoxynol-3 sulfonate, dioctyl sodium sulfosuccinate, magnesium aluminum silicate, methylcellulose and EDTA.

DESQUAM-X 10 brand therapeutic anti-acne BAR contains 10% benzoyl peroxide, boric acid, cellulose gum, dextrin (may contain wheat starch), disodium EDTA, docusate sodium, lactic acid, PEG-14M, sodium lauryl sulfoacetate (or sodium dodecyl benzene sulfonate and trisodium sulfosuccinate), sorbitol, urea and water.

[See chemical structure at top of next column.]

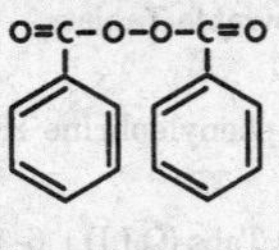

Benzoyl Peroxide

CLINICAL PHARMACOLOGY

The effectiveness of benzoyl peroxide in the treatment of acne vulgaris is primarily attributable to its antibacterial activity, especially with respect to *Propionibacterium acnes*, the predominant organism in sebaceous follicles and comedones. The antibacterial activity of this compound is presumably due to the release of active or free-radical oxygen capable of oxidizing bacterial proteins. In acne patients treated topically with benzoyl peroxide, resolution of the acne usually coincides with reduction in the level of *P. acnes* and free fatty acids (FFA). Mild desquamation is another observed action of topically applied benzoyl peroxide and may also play a role in the drug's effectiveness in acne. Studies also indicate that topical benzoyl peroxide may exert a sebostatic effect with a resultant reduction of skin surface lipids.

Benzoyl peroxide has been shown to be absorbed by the skin, where it is metabolized to benzoic acid and then excreted as benzoate in the urine.

INDICATIONS AND USAGE

DESQUAM-E (5 or 10) EMOLLIENT GEL is indicated for the topical treatment of mild to moderate acne vulgaris and as an adjunct in therapeutic regimens including antibiotics, retinoic acid products and sulfur or salicylic acid-containing preparations. DESQUAM-E EMOLLIENT GEL has been shown effective in the treatment of the following acne lesion types: papules, pustules, open and closed comedones. Clinical studies have demonstrated therapeutic response after two to three weeks.

DESQUAM-X (5 or 10) GEL is indicated for the topical treatment of mild to moderate acne vulgaris and as an adjunct in therapeutic regimens including antibiotics, retinoic acid products and sulfur or salicylic acid-containing preparations. DESQUAM-X GEL has been shown effective in the treatment of the following acne lesion types: papules, pustules, open and closed comedones. Clinical studies have demonstrated therapeutic response after two to three weeks.

DESQUAM-X GEL may also be used as adjunctive treatment for nodulo-cystic acne (acne conglobata), although its effectiveness for this condition has not been proven.

DESQUAM-X (5 or 10) WASH is indicated for the topical treatment of mild to moderate acne. In more severe cases, it may be used as an adjunct in therapeutic regimens including benzoyl peroxide gels, antibiotics, retinoic acid products and sulfur/salicylic acid-containing preparations. The improvement of the treated condition is dependent on the degree and type of acne, the frequency of use of DESQUAM-X WASH and the nature of other therapies employed.

DESQUAM-X 10 BAR is indicated for the topical treatment of acne. It may be used as an adjunct in therapeutic regimens including benzoyl peroxide gels, antibiotics, retinoic acid products and sulfur/salicylic acid-containing preparations. The improvement of the treated condition is dependent on the degree and type of acne, the frequency of use of DESQUAM-X 10 BAR and the nature of other therapies employed.

CONTRAINDICATIONS

This product should not be used in patients known to be sensitive to benzoyl peroxide or any of the other listed ingredients.

PRECAUTIONS

General: Avoid contact with eyes and other mucous membranes. For external use only. In patients known to be sensitive to the following substances, there is a possibility of cross-sensitization: benzoic acid derivatives (including certain topical anesthetics) and cinnamon.

Information for Patients: This product may bleach colored fabric or hair. Concurrent use with PABA-containing sunscreens may result in transient discoloration of the skin.

Carcinogenesis, Mutagenesis, Impairment of Fertility: Based upon considerable evidence, benzoyl peroxide is not considered to be a carcinogen. However, in one study, using mice known to be highly susceptible to cancer, there was evidence for benzoyl peroxide as a tumor promoter. Benzoyl peroxide has been found to be inactive as a mutagen in the *Ames Salmonella* and other assays, including the mouse dominant lethal assay. This assay is frequently used to assess the effect of substances on spermatogenesis.

Pregnancy (Category C): Animal reproduction studies have not been conducted with benzoyl peroxide. It is also not known whether benzoyl peroxide can cause fetal harm when administered to a pregnant woman or can affect reproductive capacity. Benzoyl peroxide should be given to a pregnant woman only if clearly needed.

Nursing Mothers: It is not known whether this drug is excreted in human milk. Caution should be exercised when benzoyl peroxide is administered to a nursing woman.

Pediatric Use: Safety and effectiveness in children below the age of 12 have not been established.

ADVERSE REACTIONS

Adverse reactions which may be encountered with topical benzoyl peroxide include excessive drying (manifested by marked peeling, erythema and possible edema), and allergic contact sensitization.

Excessive dryness would appear to occur in approximately 2 patients in 50.

Pertinent literature indicates that allergic sensitization to benzoyl peroxide may occur in 10 to 25 patients in 1,000. There is one reference that reports an occurrence of sensitization in 5 of 100 patients.

OVERDOSAGE

In the event that excessive scaling, erythema or edema occur, the use of this preparation should be discontinued. If the reaction is judged to be due to excessive use and not allergenicity, after symptoms and signs subside, a reduced dosage schedule may be cautiously tried.

To hasten resolution of the adverse effects, emollients, cool compresses and/or topical corticosteroid preparations may be used.

DOSAGE AND ADMINISTRATION

DESQUAM-E EMOLLIENT GEL should be gently rubbed into all affected areas once or twice daily. Suitable cleansing of the affected area should precede application. In fair-skinned individuals or under excessively drying conditions, it is suggested that therapy be initiated with one application daily. The degree of drying or peeling may be controlled by modification of dose frequency or drug concentration. The use of DESQUAM-E EMOLLIENT GEL may be continued as long as deemed necessary.

DESQUAM-X GEL should be gently rubbed into all affected areas once or twice daily. Suitable cleansing of the affected area should precede application. In fair-skinned individuals or under excessively drying conditions, it is suggested that therapy be initiated with one application daily. The degree of drying or peeling may be controlled by modification of dose frequency or drug concentration. The use of DESQUAM-X GEL may be continued as long as deemed necessary.

DESQUAM-X (5 or 10) WASH—
Shake well before use. Wash affected areas once or twice daily, avoiding contact with eyes or mucous membranes. Wet skin areas to be treated prior to administration; apply DESQUAM-X WASH, work to a full lather, rinse thoroughly and pat dry. The amount of drying or peeling may be controlled by modification of dose frequency or drug concentration.

DESQUAM-X 10 BAR—
Wash entire area gently with fingertips for 1 to 2 minutes 2 or 3 times daily or as physician directs. Rinse well. The desired degree of dryness and peeling may be obtained by regulating frequency of use.

HOW SUPPLIED

DESQUAM-E 2.5 EMOLLIENT GEL		
1.5 oz. (42.5g)	Plastic Tubes	NDC 0072-6003-45
DESQUAM-E 5 EMOLLIENT GEL		
1.5 oz. (42.5g)	Plastic Tubes	NDC 0072-6103-45
DESQUAM-E 10 EMOLLIENT GEL		
1.5 oz. (42.5g)	Plastic Tubes	NDC 0072-6203-45

Store at controlled room temperature (59°–86°F).

DESQUAM-X 5 GEL		
1.5 oz. (42.5 g)	Plastic Tubes	NDC 0072-6621-01
3 oz. (85 g)	Plastic Tubes	NDC 0072-6621-03
DESQUAM-X 10 GEL		
1.5 oz. (42.5 g)	Plastic Tubes	NDC 0072-6721-01
3 oz. (85 g)	Plastic Tubes	NDC 0072-6721-03

Store at controlled room temperature (59°–86° F).

DESQUAM-X WASH (5%)		
5 oz.	Plastic Bottle	NDC 0072-6905-05
DESQUAM-X WASH (10%)		
5 oz.	Plastic Bottle	NDC 0072-7000-05

Store at controlled room temperature (59°–86°F; 15°–30°C).

DESQUAM-X BAR (10%):		
3.75 oz.	carton	NDC 0072-2000-04

Store at controlled room temperature (59°–86°F).

DOVONEX® ℞
[*dōvă-nex*]
(calcipotriene cream)
Cream, 0.005%
FOR TOPICAL DERMATOLOGIC USE ONLY.
Not for ophthalmic, oral or intravaginal use.

DESCRIPTION

DOVONEX (calcipotriene cream) Cream contains calcipotriene monohydrate, a synthetic vitamin D_3 derivative, for topical dermatological use.

Chemically, calcipotriene monohydrate is (5Z,7E,22E,24S)-24-cyclopropyl-9, 10-secochola-5,7,10(19), 22-tetraene-

1α,3β,24-triol monohydrate, with empirical formula $C_{27}H_{40}O_3 \cdot H_2O$, a molecular weight of 430.6, and the following structural formula:

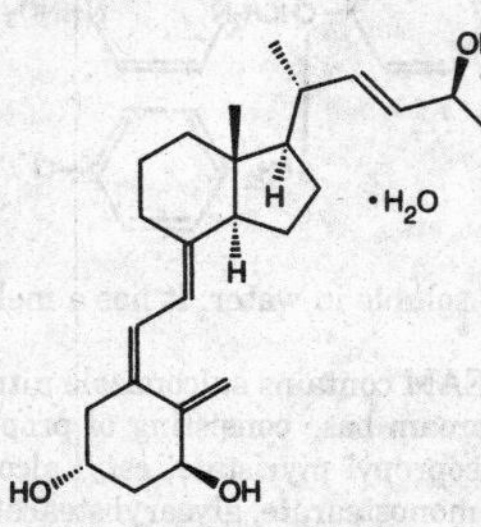

Calcipotriene monohydrate is a white or off-white crystalline substance. DOVONEX Cream contains calcipotriene monohydrate equivalent to 50 μg/g anhydrous calcipotriene in a cream base of cetearyl alcohol, ceteth-20, diazolidinyl urea, dichlorobenzyl alcohol, dibasic sodium phosphate, edetate disodium, glycerin, mineral oil, petrolatum, and water.

CLINICAL PHARMACOLOGY

In humans, the natural supply of vitamin D depends mainly on exposure to the ultraviolet rays of the sun for conversion of 7-dehydrocholesterol to vitamin D_3 (cholecalciferol) in the skin. Calcipotriene is a synthetic analog of vitamin D_3.

Clinical studies with radiolabelled calcipotriene ointment indicate that approximately 6% (±3%, SD) of the applied dose of calcipotriene is absorbed systemically when the ointment is applied topically to psoriasis plaques or 5% (±2.6%, SD) when applied to normal skin, and much of the absorbed active is converted to inactive metabolites within 24 hours of application. Systemic absorption of the cream has not been studied.

Vitamin D and its metabolites are transported in the blood, bound to specific plasma proteins. The active form of the vitamin, 1,25-dihydroxy vitamin D_3 (calcitriol) is known to be recycled via the liver and excreted in the bile. Calcipotriene metabolism following systemic uptake is rapid and occurs via a similar pathway to the natural hormone.

CLINICAL STUDIES

Adequate and well-controlled trials of patients treated with DOVONEX Cream have demonstrated improvement usually beginning after 2 weeks of therapy. This improvement continued with approximately 50% of patients showing at least marked improvement in the signs and symptoms of psoriasis after 8 weeks of therapy, but only approximately 4% showed complete clearing.

INDICATIONS AND USAGE

DOVONEX (calcipotriene cream) Cream, 0.005%, is indicated for the treatment of plaque psoriasis. The safety and effectiveness of topical calcipotriene in dermatoses other than psoriasis have not been established.

CONTRAINDICATIONS

DOVONEX Cream is contraindicated in those patients with a history of hypersensitivity to any of the components of the preparation. It should not be used by patients with demonstrated hypercalcemia or evidence of vitamin D toxicity. DOVONEX Cream should not be used on the face.

PRECAUTIONS

General: Use of DOVONEX Cream may cause transient irritation of both lesions and surrounding uninvolved skin. If irritation develops, DOVONEX Cream should be discontinued.

Reversible elevation of serum calcium has occurred with use of topical calcipotriene. If elevation in serum calcium outside the normal range should occur, discontinue treatment until normal calcium levels are restored.

Information for Patients: Patients using DOVONEX Cream should receive the following information and instructions:

1. This medication is to be used only as directed by the physician. It is for external use only. Avoid contact with the face or eyes. As with any topical medication, patients should wash their hands after application.
2. This medication should not be used for any disorder other than that for which it was prescribed.
3. Patients should report to their physician any signs of adverse reactions.

Carcinogenesis, Mutagenesis, Impairment of Fertility: Animal studies have not been conducted to evaluate the carcinogenic potential of calcipotriene. Studies in rats at doses up to 54 μg/kg/day (318 μg/m²/day) of calcipotriene indicated no impairment of fertility or general reproductive performance.

Calcipotriene did not elicit any mutagenic effects in the Ames mutagenicity assay, the mouse lymphoma TK locus assay, the human lymphocyte chromosome aberration test, or the mouse micronucleus test.

Pregnancy: Teratogenic Effects: Pregnancy Category C. Studies of teratogenicity were done by the oral route where bioavailability is expected to be approximately 40–60% of the administered dose. Increased rabbit maternal and fetal toxicity was noted at 12 μg/kg/day (132 μg/m²/day). Rabbits administered 36 μg/kg/day (396 μg/m²/day) resulted in fetuses with a significant increase in the incidence of pubic bones, forelimb phalanges, and incomplete bone ossification. In a rat study, oral doses of 54 μg/kg/day (318 μg/m²/day) resulted in a significantly higher incidence of skeletal abnormalities consisting primarily of enlarged fontanelles and extra ribs. The enlarged fontanelles are most likely due to calcipotriene's effect upon calcium metabolism. The maternal and fetal calculated no-effect exposures in the rat (43.2 μg/m²/day) and rabbit (17.6 μg/m²/day) studies are approximately equal to the expected human systemic exposure level (18.5 μg/m²/day) from dermal applicatioin. There are no adequate and well-controlled studies in pregnant women. Therefore, DOVONEX Cream should be used during pregnancy only if the potential benefit justifies the potential risk to the fetus.

Nursing Mothers: There is evidence that maternal 1,25-dihydroxy vitamin D_3 (calcitriol) may enter the fetal circulation, but it is not known whether it is excreted in human milk. The systemic disposition of calcipotriene is expected to be similar to that of the naturally occurring vitamin. Because many drugs are excreted in human milk, caution should be exercised when DOVONEX Cream is administered to a nursing woman.

Pediatric Use: Safety and effectiveness of DOVONEX Cream in pediatric patients have not been established. Because of a higher ratio of skin surface area to body mass, pediatric patients are at greater risk than adults of systemic adverse effects when they are treated with topical medication.

ADVERSE REACTIONS

In controlled clinical trials, the most frequent adverse experiences reported for DOVONEX Cream were cases of skin irritation which occurred in approximately 10–15% of patients. Rash, pruritus, dermatitis, and worsening of psoriasis were reported in 1 to 10% of patients.

OVERDOSAGE

Topically applied calcipotriene can be absorbed in sufficient amounts to produce systemic effects. Elevated serum calcium has been observed with excessive use of topical calcipotriene. If elevation in serum calcium should occur, discontinue treatment until normal calcium levels are restored (See PRECAUTIONS).

DOSAGE AND ADMINISTRATION

Apply a thin layer of DOVONEX Cream to the affected skin twice daily and rub in gently and completely. The safety and efficacy of DOVONEX Cream have been demonstrated in patients treated for eight weeks.

HOW SUPPLIED

DOVONEX Cream is available in 30 g, 60 g, and 100 g aluminum tubes. Store at controlled room temperature 15°–25°C (59°–77°F). Do not freeze.

CAUTION: Federal Law prohibits dispensing without a prescription.

Manufactured by
Leo Laboratories Ltd.,
Dublin, Ireland
©1994 Distributed by
Westwood-Squibb Pharmaceuticals Inc.,
Buffalo, NY, USA 14213
1996 03-6012-0

DOVONEX® ℞

[*dō vă-nex*]
(calcipotriene ointment), 0.005%
For topical dermatologic use only. Not for ophthalmic, oral or intravaginal use.

DESCRIPTION

DOVONEX (calcipotriene ointment) contains the compound calcipotriene, a synthetic vitamin D_3 derivative for topical dermatological use.

Chemically, calcipotriene is (5Z, 7E, 22E, 24S)-24-cyclopropyl-9,10-secochola-5,7,10(19),22-tetraene-1α, 3β, 24-triol-, with the empirical formula $C_{27}H_{40}O_3$, a molecular weight of 412.6, and the following structural formula:

[See chemical structure at top of next column.]

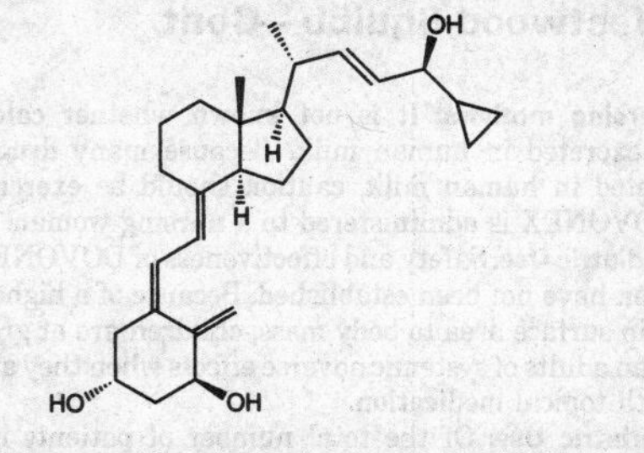

Calcipotriene is a white or off-white crystalline substance. DOVONEX contains calcipotriene 50 μg/g in an ointment base of dibasic sodium phosphate, edetate disodium, mineral oil, petrolatum, propylene glycol, tocopherol, steareth-2 and water.

CLINICAL PHARMACOLOGY

In humans, the natural supply of vitamin D depends mainly on exposure to the ultraviolet rays of the sun for conversion of 7-dehydrocholesterol to vitamin D_3 (cholecalciferol) in the skin. Calcipotriene is a synthetic analog of vitamin D_3.

Clinical studies with radiolabelled ointment indicate that approximately 6% (±3%, SD) of the applied dose of calcipotriene is absorbed systemically when the ointment is applied topically to psoriasis plaques or 5% (±2.6%, SD) when applied to normal skin, and much of the absorbed active is converted to inactive metabolites within 24 hours of application.

Vitamin D and its metabolites are transported in the blood, bound to specific plasma proteins. The active form of the vitamin, 1,25-dihydroxy vitamin D_3 (calcitriol), is known to be recycled via the liver and excreted in the bile. Calcipotriene metabolism following systemic uptake is rapid, and occurs via a similar pathway to the natural hormone. The primary metabolites are much less potent than the parent compound.

There is evidence that maternal 1,25-dihydroxy vitamin D_3 (calcitriol) may enter the fetal circulation, but it is not known whether it is excreted in human milk. The systemic disposition of calcipotriene is expected to be similar to that of the naturally occurring vitamin.

CLINICAL STUDIES

Adequate and well-controlled trials of patients treated with DOVONEX have demonstrated improvement usually beginning after two weeks of therapy. This improvement continued with approximately 70% of patients showing at least marked improvement after 8 weeks of therapy, but only approximately 10% showing complete clearing.

INDICATIONS AND USAGE

DOVONEX (calcipotriene ointment), 0.005%, is indicated for the treatment of moderate plaque psoriasis. The safety and effectiveness of topical calcipotriene in dermatoses other than psoriasis have not been established.

CONTRAINDICATIONS

DOVONEX is contraindicated in those patients with a history of hypersensitivity to any of the components of the preparation. It should not be used by patients with demonstrated hypercalcemia or evidence of vitamin D toxicity. DOVONEX should not be used on the face.

PRECAUTIONS

General

Use of DOVONEX may cause irritation of lesions and surrounding uninvolved skin. If irritation develops, DOVONEX should be discontinued.

Transient, rapidly reversible elevation of serum calcium has occurred with use of DOVONEX. If elevation in serum calcium outside the normal range should occur, discontinue treatment until normal calcium levels are restored.

Information for patients: Patients using DOVONEX should receive the following information and instructions:

1. This medication is to be used as directed by the physician. It is for external use only. Avoid contact with the face or eyes. As with any topical medication, patients should wash hands after application.
2. This medication should not be used for any disorder other than that for which it was prescribed.
3. Patients should report to their physician any signs of local adverse reactions.

Carcinogenesis, Mutagenesis, Impairment of fertility: Long-term animal studies have not been conducted to evaluate the carcinogenic potential of calcipotriene. Studies in rats at doses up to 54 μg/kg/day (318 μg/m²/day) of calcipotriene indicated no impairment of fertility or general reproductive performance.

Calcipotriene did not elicit any mutagenic effects in the Ames mutagenicity assay, the mouse lymphoma TK locus assay, the human lymphocyte chromosome aberration test or the mouse micronucleus test.

Pregnancy; Teratogenic Effects; Pregnancy Category C. Doses of calcipotriene up to 36 μg/kg/day (396 μg/m²/day) in the rabbit did not result in teratogenic effects; however, increased maternal and fetal toxicity was observed at 12 μg/kg/day (132 μg/m²/day) and higher. In the rat oral doses of 54 μg/kg/day (318 μg/m²/day) resulted in a significantly higher incidence of skeletal abnormalities consisting primarily of enlarged fontanelles and extra ribs. The enlarged fontanelles is most likely due to calcipotriene's effect upon calcium metabolism. There are no adequate and well-controlled studies in pregnant women. Therefore, DOVONEX should be used during pregnancy only if the potential benefit justifies the potential risk to the fetus.

Continued on next page

Westwood-Squibb—Cont.

Nursing mothers: It is not known whether calcipotriene is excreted in human milk. Because many drugs are excreted in human milk, caution should be exercised when DOVONEX is administered to a nursing woman.

Pediatric Use: Safety and effectiveness of DOVONEX in children have not been established. Because of a higher ratio of skin surface area to body mass, children are at greater risk than adults of systemic adverse effects when they are treated with topical medication.

Geriatric Use: Of the total number of patients in clinical studies of calcipotriene ointment, approximately 12% were 65 or older, while approximately 4% were 75 and over. The results of an analysis of severity of skin-related adverse events showed a statistically significant difference for subjects over 65 years (more severe) compared to those under 65 years (less severe).

ADVERSE REACTIONS

In controlled clinical trials, the most frequent adverse experiences reported for DOVONEX were burning, itching, and skin irritation, which occurred in approximately 10–15% of patients. Erythema, dry skin, peeling, rash, dermatitis, worsening of psoriasis including development of facial/scalp psoriasis were reported in 1 to 10% of patients. Other experiences reported in less than 1% of patients included skin atrophy, hyperpigmentation, hypercalcemia, and folliculitis.

OVERDOSAGE

Topically applied DOVONEX can be absorbed in sufficient amounts to produce systemic effects. Elevated serum calcium has been observed with excessive use of DOVONEX.

DOSAGE AND ADMINISTRATION

Apply a thin layer of DOVONEX to the affected skin twice daily and rub in gently and completely. The safety and efficacy of DOVONEX have been demonstrated in patients treated for eight weeks.

HOW SUPPLIED

DOVONEX Ointment is available in 30 g, 60 g, and 100 g aluminum tubes. Store at controlled room temperature 15°–25°C (59°–77°F). Do not freeze.

CAUTION: Federal Law prohibits dispensing without a prescription.

Manufactured by Leo Laboratories Ltd.,
Dublin, Ireland   12/93
©1993 Distributed by Westwood-Squibb Pharmaceuticals Inc., Buffalo, N.Y., U.S.A. 14213

EURAX®
(crotamiton USP)
Lotion/Cream
Scabicide/Antipruritic   ℞

For topical use only. Not for opthalmic use.

CAUTION

Federal law prohibits dispensing without prescription.

DESCRIPTION

EURAX, crotamiton USP, is a scabicidal and antipruritic agent available as a cream or lotion for topical use only. EURAX provides 10% (w/w) of the synthetic, crotamiton USP, in a vanishing-cream or emollient-lotion base containing: water, petrolatum, propylene glycol, steareth-2, cetyl alcohol, dimethicone, laureth-23, fragrance, magnesium aluminum silicate, carbomer-934, sodium hydroxide, diazolidinyl urea, methylchloroisothiazolinone, methylisothiazolinone and magnesium nitrate. In addition, the cream contains glyceryl stearate. Crotamiton is N-ethyl-N-(o-methylphenyl)-2-butenamide and its structural formula is:

$$CH_3 \ CH = CHCONCH_2 \ CH_3$$

Crotamiton USP is a colorless to slightly yellowish oil, having a faint amine-like odor. It is miscible with alcohol and with methanol. Crotamiton is a mixture of the *cis* and *trans* isomers. Its molecular weight is 203.28.

CLINICAL PHARMACOLOGY

EURAX has scabicidal and antipruritic actions. The mechanisms of these actions are not known.

INDICATIONS AND USAGE

For eradication of scabies (*Sarcoptes scabiei*) and for symptomatic treatment of pruritic skin.

CONTRAINDICATIONS

EURAX should not be applied topically to patients who develop a sensitivity or are allergic to it or who manifest a primary irritation response to topical medications.

WARNINGS

If severe irritation or sensitization develops, treatment with this product should be discontinued and appropriate therapy instituted.

PRECAUTIONS

General: EURAX should not be applied in the eyes or mouth because it may cause irritation. It should not be applied to acutely inflamed skin or raw or weeping surfaces until the acute inflammation has subsided.

Information for Patients: See "Directions for patients with scabies".

Drug Interactions: None known.

Carcinogenesis, Mutagenesis, Impairment of Fertility: Long-term carcinogenicity studies in animals have not been conducted.

Pregnancy (Category C): Animal reproduction studies have not been conducted with EURAX. It is also not known whether EURAX can cause fetal harm when applied topically to a pregnant woman or can affect reproduction capacity. EURAX should be given to a pregnant woman only if clearly needed.

Pediatric Use: Safety and effectiveness in children have not been established.

ADVERSE REACTIONS

Allergic sensitivity or primary irritation reactions may occur in some patients.

OVERDOSAGE

There is no specific information on the effect of overtreatment with repeated topical applications in humans. Acute toxicity (after accidental oral administration in children): Highest known doses ingested: Cream: children—2g (age 1½ years); Lotion: 1 ounce (age 2 years). A death was reported but cause was not confirmed.

Oral LD$_{50}$ in animals (mg/kg): rats, 2212; mice, 2011.

Signs and symptoms (of oral ingestion): Burning sensation in the mouth, irritation of the buccal, esophageal and gastric mucosa, nausea, vomiting, abdominal pain.

Treatment: There is no specific antidote if taken orally. General measures to eliminate the drug and reduce its absorption, combined with symptomatic treatment, are recommended.

DOSAGE AND ADMINISTRATION

LOTION: Shake well before using—*In Scabies:* Thoroughly massage into the skin of the whole body from the chin down, paying particular attention to all folds and creases. A second application is advisable 24 hours later. Clothing and bed linen should be changed the next morning. A cleansing bath should be taken 48 hours after the last application. *In Pruritus:* Massage gently into affected areas until medication is completely absorbed. Repeat as needed.

DIRECTIONS FOR PATIENTS WITH SCABIES

1. Take a routine bath or shower. Thoroughly massage EURAX cream or lotion into the skin from the chin to the toes including folds and creases.
2. A second application is advisable 24 hours later.
3. This 60 gram tube or bottle is sufficient for two applications.
4. Clothing and bed linen should be changed the next day. Contaminated clothing and bed linen may be dry-cleaned, or washed in the hot cycle of the washing machine.
5. A cleansing bath should be taken 48 hours after the last application.

HOW SUPPLIED

Cream: 60g tubes (NDC 0072-2103-60; NSN 6505-00-116-0200).

Lotion: 60g (2 oz.) bottles (NDC 0072-2203-60, NSN 6505-01-153-4423). 454g (16 oz.) bottles (NDC 0072-2203-16).

Store at room temperature.

EXELDERM®
(sulconazole nitrate)
Cream, 1.0%
For topical use only. Not for ophthalmic use.   ℞

CAUTION

Federal law prohibits dispensing without prescription.

DESCRIPTION

EXELDERM (sulconazole nitrate) CREAM, 1.0% is a broad-spectrum antifungal agent intended for topical application. Sulconazole nitrate, the active ingredient in EXELDERM CREAM, is an imidazole derivative with in vitro antifungal and antiyeast activity. Its chemical name is (±)-1-[2.4-dichloro-β-[(p-chlorobenzyl)-thio]-phenethyl] imidazole mononitrate and it has the following chemical structure:
[See chemical structure at top of next column.]
Sulconazole nitrate is a white to off-white crystalline powder with a molecular weight of 460.77. It is freely soluble in pyridine; slightly soluble in ethanol, acetone, and chloroform;

and very slightly soluble in water. It has a melting point of about 130°C.

EXELDERM CREAM contains sulconazole nitrate 10 mg/g in an emollient cream base consisting of propylene glycol, stearyl alcohol, isopropyl myristate, cetyl alcohol, polysorbate 60, sorbitan monostearate, glyceryl stearate (and) PEG-100 stearate, ascorbyl palmitate, and purified water, with sodium hydroxide and/or nitric acid added to adjust the pH.

CLINICAL PHARMACOLOGY

Sulconazole nitrate is an imidazole derivative with broad-spectrum antifungal activity that inhibits the growth in vitro of the common pathogenic dermatophytes including *Trichophyton rubrum*, *Trichophyton mentagrophytes*, *Epidermophyton floccosum* and *Microsporum canis*. It also inhibits (*in vitro*) the organism responsible for tinea versicolor, *Malassezia furfur*. Sulconazole nitrate has been shown to be active in vitro against the following microorganisms, although clinical efficacy has not been established: *Candida albicans* and certain gram positive bacteria.

A modified Draize test showed no allergic contact dermatitis and a phototoxicity study showed no phototoxic or photoallergic reaction to sulconazole nitrate cream. Maximization tests with sulconazole nitrate cream showed no evidence of contact sensitization or irritation.

INDICATIONS AND USAGE

EXELDERM (sulconazole nitrate) CREAM, 1.0% is an antifungal agent indicated for the treatment of tinea pedis (athlete's foot), tinea cruris, and tinea corporis caused by *Trichophyton rubrum*, *Trichophyton mentagrophytes*, *Epidermophyton floccosum*, and *Microsporum canis*,* and for the treatment of tinea versicolor.

* Efficacy for this organism in the organ system was studied in fewer than ten infections.

CONTRAINDICATIONS

EXELDERM (sulconazole nitrate) CREAM, 1.0% is contraindicated in patients who have a history of hypersensitivity to any of its ingredients.

PRECAUTIONS

General: EXELDERM (sulconazole nitrate) CREAM, 1.0% is for external use only. Avoid contact with the eyes. If irritation develops, the cream should be discontinued and appropriate therapy instituted.

Information for Patients: Patients should be told to use EXELDERM CREAM as directed by the physician, to use it externally only, and to avoid contact with the eyes.

Carcinogenesis, Mutagenesis, Impairment of Fertility: Long-term animal studies to determine carcinogenic potential have not been performed. In vitro studies have shown no mutagenic activity.

Pregnancy (Category C): There are no adequate and well controlled studies in pregnant women. Sulconazole nitrate should be used during pregnancy only if clearly needed. Sulconazole nitrate has been shown to be embryotoxic in rats when given in doses of 125 times the adult human dose (in mg/kg). The drug was not teratogenic in rats or rabbits at oral doses of 50 mg/kg/day.

Sulconazole nitrate given orally to rats at a dose 125 times the human dose resulted in prolonged gestation and dystocia. Several females died during the prenatal period, most likely due to labor complications.

Nursing Mothers: It is not known whether sulconazole nitrate is excreted in human milk. Caution should be exercised when sulconazole nitrate is administered to a nursing woman.

Pediatric Use: Safety and effectiveness in children have not been established.

ADVERSE REACTIONS

There were no systemic effects and only infrequent cutaneous adverse reactions in 1185 patients treated with sulconazole nitrate cream in controlled clinical trials. Approximately 3% of these patients reported itching, 3% burning or stinging, and 1% redness. These complaints did not usually interfere with treatment.

CLINICAL STUDIES

In a vehicle-controlled study for the treatment of tinea pedis (moccasin type) due to *T. rubrum*, after 4–6 weeks of treatment 69% of patients on the active drug and 19% of patients on the drug vehicle had become KOH and culture negative. In addition, 68% of patients on the active drug and 20% of patients on the drug vehicle showed a good or excellent clinical response.

DOSAGE AND ADMINISTRATION

A small amount of cream should be gently massaged into the affected and surrounding skin areas once or twice daily, except in tinea pedis, where administration should be twice daily.

Early relief of symptoms is experienced by the majority of patients and clinical improvement may be seen fairly soon after treatment is begun; however, tinea corporis/cruris and tinea versicolor should be treated for 3 weeks and tinea pedis for 4 weeks to reduce the possibility of recurrence.

If significant clinical improvement is not seen after 4 to 6 weeks of treatment, an alternate diagnosis should be considered.

HOW SUPPLIED

EXELDERM (sulconazole nitrate) CREAM, 1.0%:
15 g tube—NDC 0072-8200-15
30 g tube—NDC 0072-8200-30
60 g tube—NDC 0072-8200-60
Avoid excessive heat, above 40°C (104°F).

EXELDERM®

(sulconazole nitrate)
Solution, 1.0%
For topical use only. Not for ophthalmic use.

℞

CAUTION

Federal law prohibits dispensing without prescription.

DESCRIPTION

EXELDERM (sulconazole nitrate) SOLUTION, 1.0% is a broad-spectrum antifungal agent intended for topical application. Sulconazole nitrate, the active ingredient in EXELDERM SOLUTION, is an imidazole derivative with antifungal and antiyeast activity. Its chemical name is $(\pm)$-1-[2,4-dichloro-β-[(p-chlorobenzyl)-thio]-phenethyl] imidazole mononitrate and it has the following chemical structure:

Sulconazole nitrate is a white to off-white crystalline powder with a molecular weight of 460.77. It is freely soluble in pyridine; slightly soluble in ethanol, acetone, and chloroform; and very slightly soluble in water. It has a melting point of about 130°C.

EXELDERM SOLUTION contains sulconazole nitrate 10 mg/mL in a solution of propylene glycol, poloxamer 407, polysorbate 20, butylated hydroxyanisole, and purified water, with sodium hydroxide and, if necessary, nitric acid added to adjust the pH.

CLINICAL PHARMACOLOGY

Sulconazole nitrate is an imidazole derivative that inhibits the growth of the common pathogenic dermatophytes including *Trichophyton rubrum*, *Trichophyton mentagrophytes*, *Epidermophyton floccosum*, and *Microsporum canis*. It also inhibits the organism responsible for tinea versicolor, *Malassezia furfur*, and certain gram positive bacteria.

A maximization test with sulconazole nitrate solution showed no evidence of irritation or contact sensitization.

INDICATIONS AND USAGE

EXELDERM (sulconazole nitrate) SOLUTION, 1.0% is a broad-spectrum antifungal agent indicated for the treatment of tinea cruris and tinea corporis caused by *Trichophyton rubrum*, *Trichophyton mentagrophytes*, *Epidermophyton floccosum*, and *Microsporum canis;* and for the treatment of tinea versicolor. Effectiveness has not been proven in tinea pedis (athlete's foot).

Symptomatic relief usually occurs within a few days after starting EXELDERM SOLUTION and clinical improvement usually occurs within one week.

CONTRAINDICATIONS

EXELDERM (sulconazole nitrate) SOLUTION, 1.0% is contraindicated in patients who have a history of hypersensitivity to any of the ingredients.

PRECAUTIONS

General: EXELDERM (sulconazole nitrate) SOLUTION, 1.0% is for external use only. Avoid contact with the eyes. If irritation develops, the solution should be discontinued and appropriate therapy instituted.

Information for Patients: Patients should be told to use EXELDERM SOLUTION as directed by the physician, to use it externally only, and to avoid contact with the eyes.

Carcinogenesis, Mutagenesis, Impairment of Fertility: Long-term animal studies to determine carcinogenic poten-

tial have not been performed. In vitro studies have shown no mutagenic activity.

Pregnancy: Pregnancy Category C: Sulconazole nitrate has been shown to be embryotoxic in rats when given in doses 125 times the human dose (in mg/kg). The drug at this dose given orally to rats also resulted in prolonged gestation and dystocia. Several females died during the perinatal period, most likely due to labor complications. Sulconazole nitrate was not teratogenic in rats or rabbits at oral doses of 50 mg/kg/day.

There are no adequate and well-controlled studies in pregnant women. Sulconazole nitrate should be used during pregnancy only if the potential benefit justifies the potential risk to the fetus.

Nursing Mothers: It is not known whether this drug is excreted in human milk. Because many drugs are excreted in human milk, caution should be exercised when sulconazole nitrate is administered to a nursing woman.

Pediatric Use: Safety and effectiveness in children have not been established.

ADVERSE REACTIONS

There were no systemic effects and only infrequent cutaneous adverse reactions in 370 patients treated with sulconazole nitrate solution in controlled clinical trials. Approximately 1% of these patients reported itching and 1% burning or stinging. These complaints did not usually interfere with treatment.

DOSAGE AND ADMINISTRATION

A small amount of the solution should be gently massaged into the affected and surrounding skin areas once or twice daily.

Symptomatic relief usually occurs within a few days after starting EXELDERM (sulconazole nitrate) SOLUTION, 1.0%, and clinical improvement usually occurs within one week. To reduce the possibility of recurrence, tinea cruris, tinea corporis, and tinea versicolor should be treated for 3 weeks.

If significant clinical improvement is not seen after 4 weeks of treatment, an alternate diagnosis should be considered.

HOW SUPPLIED

EXELDERM SOLUTION, 1.0%
30 mL   Plastic Bottle   NDC 0072-8400-30
Avoid excessive heat, above 40°C (104°F), and protect from light.

HALOG CREAM

Halcinonide Cream USP 0.1%   ℞
HALOG Ointment
Halcinonide Ointment USP 0.1%   ℞
HALOG Solution
Halcinonide Topical Solution USP 0.1% ℞
HALOG-E Cream
Halcinonide Cream USP 0.1%   ℞
For dermatologic use only.
Not for ophthalmic use.

DESCRIPTION

The topical corticosteroids constitute a class of primarily synthetic steroids used as anti-inflammatory and antipruritic agents. The steroids in this class include halcinonide. Halcinonide is designated chemically as 21-Chloro-9-fluoro-11β, 16α, 17-trihydroxypregn-4-ene-3,20-dione cyclic 16,17-acetal with acetone.

$C_{24}H_{32}ClFO_5$, MW 454.96, CAS-3093-35-4

Each gram of 0.1% HALOG Cream (Halcinonide Cream) contains 1 mg halcinonide in a specially formulated cream base consisting of glyceryl monostearate NF XII, cetyl alcohol, isopropyl palmitate, dimethicone 350, polysorbate 60, titanium dioxide, propylene glycol, and purified water.

Each gram of 0.1% **HALOG Ointment (Halcinonide Ointment)** contains 1 mg halcinonide in Plastibase® (Plasticized Hydrocarbon Gel), a polyethylene and mineral oil gel base with polyethylene glycol 400, polyethylene glycol 6000 distearate, polyethylene glycol 300, polyethylene glycol 1450, and butylated hydroxytoluene as an antioxidant.

Each mL of 0.1% **HALOG Solution (Halcinonide Topical Solution)** contains 1 mg halcinonide with edetate disodium, polyethylene glycol 300, purified water, and butylated hydroxytoluene as an antioxidant.

Each gram of 0.1% **HALOG-E Cream (Halcinonide Cream)** contains 1 mg halcinonide in a hydrophilic vanishing cream base consisting of propylene glycol, dimethicone 350, castor oil, cetearyl alcohol (and) ceteareth-20, propylene glycol stearate, white petrolatum, and purified water. This formulation is water-washable, greaseless, and nonstaining, with moisturizing and emollient properties.

CLINICAL PHARMACOLOGY

Topical corticosteroids share anti-inflammatory, antipruritic and vasoconstrictive actions.

The mechanism of anti-inflammatory activity of the topical corticosteroids is unclear. Various laboratory methods, including vasoconstrictor assays, are used to compare and predict potencies and/or clinical efficacies of the topical corticosteroids. There is some evidence to suggest that a recognizable correlation exists between vasoconstrictor potency and therapeutic efficacy in man.

PHARMACOKINETICS

The extent of percutaneous absorption of topical corticosteroids is determined by many factors including the vehicle, the integrity of the epidermal barrier, and the use of occlusive dressings.

Topical corticosteroids can be absorbed from normal intact skin. Inflammation and/or other disease processes in the skin increase percutaneous absorption. Occlusive dressings substantially increase the percutaneous absorption of topical corticosteroids. Thus, occlusive dressings may be a valuable therapeutic adjunct for treatment of resistant dermatoses (see DOSAGE AND ADMINISTRATION).

Once absorbed through the skin, topical corticosteroids are handled through pharmacokinetic pathways similar to systemically administered corticosteroids. Corticosteroids are bound to plasma proteins in varying degrees. Corticosteroids are metabolized primarily in the liver and are then excreted by the kidneys. Some of the topical corticosteroids and their metabolites are also excreted into the bile.

INDICATIONS AND USAGE

HALOG (Halcinonide) preparations are indicated for the relief of the inflammatory and pruritic manifestations of corticosteroid-responsive dermatoses.

CONTRAINDICATIONS

Topical corticosteroids are contraindicated in those patients with a history of hypersensitivity to any of the components of the preparations.

PRECAUTIONS

General
Systemic absorption of topical corticosteroids has produced reversible hypothalamic-pituitary-adrenal (HPA) axis suppression, manifestations of Cushing's syndrome, hyperglycemia, and glucosuria in some patients.

Conditions which augment systemic absorption include the application of the more potent steroids, use over large surface areas, prolonged use, and the addition of occlusive dressings.

Therefore, patients receiving a large dose of any potent topical steroid applied to a large surface area or under an occlusive dressing should be evaluated periodically for evidence of HPA axis suppression by using the urinary free cortisol and ACTH stimulation tests, and for impairment of thermal homeostasis. If HPA axis suppression or elevation of the body temperature occurs, an attempt should be made to withdraw the drug, to reduce the frequency of application, substitute a less potent steroid, or use a sequential approach when utilizing the occlusive technique.

Recovery of HPA axis function and thermal homeostasis are generally prompt and complete upon discontinuation of the drug. Infrequently, signs and symptoms of steroid withdrawal may occur, requiring supplemental systemic corticosteroids. Occasionally, a patient may develop a sensitivity reaction to a particular occlusive dressing material or adhesive and a substitute material may be necessary.

Children may absorb proportionally larger amounts of topical corticosteroids and thus be more susceptible to systemic toxicity (see PRECAUTIONS, Pediatric Use).

If irritation develops, topical corticosteroids should be discontinued and appropriate therapy instituted.

In the presence of dermatological infections, the use of an appropriate antifungal or antibacterial agent should be instituted. If a favorable response does not occur promptly, the corticosteroid should be discontinued until the infection has been adequately controlled.

These preparations are not for ophthalmic use.

Information for the Patient
Patients using topical corticosteroids should receive the following information and instructions:

1. These medications are to be used as directed by the physician. They are for dermatologic use only. Avoid contact with the eyes.
2. Patients should be advised not to use these medications for any disorder other than for which it was prescribed.

Continued on next page

Westwood-Squibb—Cont.

3. The treated skin area should not be bandaged or otherwise covered or wrapped as to be occlusive unless directed by the physician.
4. Patients should report any signs of local adverse reactions especially under occlusive dressing.
5. Parents of pediatric patients should be advised not to use tight-fitting diapers or plastic pants on a child being treated in the diaper area, as these garments may constitute occlusive dressings.

Laboratory Tests
A urinary free cortisol test and ACTH stimulation test may be helpful in evaluating HPA axis suppression.

Carcinogenesis, Mutagenesis, and Impairment of Fertility
Long-term animal studies have not been performed to evaluate the carcinogenic potential or the effect on fertility of topical corticosteroids. Studies to determine mutagenicity with prednisolone and hydrocortisone showed negative results.

Pregnancy: Teratogenic Effects
Category C. Corticosteroids are generally teratogenic in laboratory animals when administered systemically at relatively low dosage levels. The more potent corticosteroids have been shown to be teratogenic after dermal application in laboratory animals. There are no adequate and well-controlled studies in pregnant women on teratogenic effects from topically applied corticosteroids. Therefore, topical corticosteroids should be used during pregnancy only if the potential benefit justifies the potential risk to the fetus. Drugs of this class should not be used extensively on pregnant patients, in large amounts, or for prolonged periods of time.

Nursing Mothers
It is not known whether topical administration of corticosteroids could result in sufficient systemic absorption to produce detectable quantities in breast milk. Systemically administered corticosteroids are secreted into breast milk in quantities not likely to have a deleterious effect on the infant. Nevertheless, caution should be exercised when topical corticosteroids are administered to a nursing woman.

Pediatric Use
Pediatric patients may demonstrate greater susceptibility to topical corticosteroid-induced HPA axis suppression and Cushing's syndrome than mature patients because of a larger skin surface area to body weight ratio.
HPA axis suppression, Cushing's syndrome, and intracranial hypertension have been reported in children receiving topical corticosteroids. Manifestations of adrenal suppression in children include linear growth retardation, delayed weight gain, low plasma cortisol levels, and absence of response to ACTH stimulation. Manifestations of intracranial hypertension include bulging fontanelles, headaches, and bilateral papilledema.
Administration of topical corticosteroids to children should be limited to the least amount compatible with an effective therapeutic regimen. Chronic corticosteroid therapy may interfere with the growth and development of children.

ADVERSE REACTIONS
The following local adverse reactions are reported infrequently with topical corticosteroids, but may occur more frequently with the use of occlusive dressings (reactions are listed in an approximate decreasing order of occurrence): burning, itching, irritation, dryness, folliculitis, hypertrichosis, acneiform eruptions, hypopigmentation, perioral dermatitis, allergic contact dermatitis, maceration of the skin, secondary infection, skin atrophy, striae, and miliaria.

OVERDOSAGE
Topically applied corticosteroids can be absorbed in sufficient amounts to produce systemic effects (see PRECAUTIONS, General).

DOSAGE AND ADMINISTRATION
HALOG Creams (Halcinonide Cream): Apply the 0.1% HALOG Cream (Halcinonide Cream) to the affected area two to three times daily. Rub in gently.
HALOG Ointment (Halcinonide Ointment): Apply a thin film of 0.1% HALOG Ointment (Halcinonide Ointment) to the affected area two to three times daily.
HALOG Solution (Halcinonide Topical Solution): Apply HALOG Solution (Halcinonide Topical Solution) 0.1% to the affected area two to three times daily.
HALOG-E Cream (Halcinonide Cream): Apply HALOG-E Cream (Halcinonide Cream) 0.1% to the affected area one to three times daily. Rub in gently.

Occlusive Dressing Technique
Occlusive dressings may be used for the management of psoriasis or other recalcitrant conditions.
HALOG Cream (Halcinonide Cream) 0.1% and HALOG-E Cream (Halcinonide Cream) 0.1%: Gently rub a small amount of the cream into the lesion until it disappears. Reapply the preparation leaving a thin coating on the lesion, cover with a pliable nonporous film, and seal the edges. If needed, additional moisture may be provided by covering the lesion with a dampened clean cotton cloth before the nonporous film is applied or by briefly wetting the affected area with water immediately prior to applying the medication.

The frequency of changing dressings is best determined on an individual basis. It may be convenient to apply HALOG/HALOG-E Cream under an occlusive dressing in the evening and to remove the dressing in the morning (i.e., 12-hour occlusion). When utilizing the 12-hour occlusion regimen, additional cream should be applied, without occlusion, during the day. Reapplication is essential at each dressing change.
If an infection develops, the use of occlusive dressings should be discontinued and appropriate antimicrobial therapy instituted.
HALOG Ointment (Halcinonide Ointment) 0.1%: Apply a thin film of the ointment to the lesion, cover with a pliable nonporous film, and seal the edges. If needed, additional moisture may be provided by covering the lesion with a dampened clean cotton cloth before the nonporous film is applied or by briefly wetting the affected area with water immediately prior to applying the medication. The frequency of changing dressings is best determined on an individual basis. It may be convenient to apply HALOG Ointment under an occlusive dressing in the evening and to remove the dressing in the morning (i.e., 12-hour occlusion). When utilizing the 12-hour occlusion regimen, additional ointment should be applied, without occlusion, during the day. Reapplication is essential at each dressing change.
If an infection develops, the use of occlusive dressings should be discontinued and appropriate antimicrobial therapy instituted.
HALOG Solution (Halcinonide Topical Solution) 0.1%: Apply the solution to the lesion, cover with a pliable nonporous film, and seal the edges. If needed, additional moisture may be provided by covering the lesion with a dampened clean cotton cloth before the nonporous film is applied or by briefly wetting the affected area with water immediately prior to applying the medication. The frequency of changing dressings is best determined on an individual basis. It may be convenient to apply HALOG solution under an occlusive dressing in the evening and to remove the dressing in the morning (i.e., 12-hour occlusion). When utilizing the 12-hour occlusion regimen, additional solution should be applied, without occlusion, during the day. Reapplication is essential at each dressing change.
If an infection develops, the use of occlusive dressings should be discontinued and appropriate antimicrobial therapy instituted.

HOW SUPPLIED
HALOG Cream (Halcinonide Cream USP)
0.1%: tubes containing 15 g (NDC 0003-1482-15), 30 g (NDC 0003-1482-20), 60 g (NDC 0003-1482-30); and jars containing 240 g (NDC 0003-1482-40) of cream.
HALOG Ointment (Halcinonide Ointment USP)
0.1%: tubes containing 15 g (NDC 0003-0248-15), 30 g (NDC 0003-0248-20), and 60 g (NDC 0003-0248-30); and jars containing 240 g (NDC 0003-0248-40) of ointment.
HALOG Solution (Halcinonide Topical Solution USP)
0.1%: plastic squeeze bottles containing 20 mL (NDC 0003-0249-15) and 60 mL (NDC 0003-0249-20) of solution.
HALOG-E Cream (Halcinonide Cream USP)
0.1%: 30 g (NDC 0003-1494-21), and 60 g (NDC 0003-1494-31) of cream.
Storage
HALOG Cream (Halcinonide Cream USP)
Store at room temperature; avoid excessive heat (104°F).
HALOG Ointment (Halcinonide Ointment USP)
Store at room temperature; avoid excessive heat (104°F).
HALOG Solution (Halcinonide Topical Solution USP)
Store at room temperature; avoid freezing and temperatures above 104°F.
HALOG-E Cream (Halcinonide Cream USP)
Store at room temperature; avoid freezing and refrigeration.

LAC–HYDRIN® 12%* ℞
(ammonium lactate)
Lotion
For topical use only. Not for ophthalmic use.

CAUTION
Federal law prohibits dispensing without a prescription.

DESCRIPTION*
LAC-HYDRIN, specially formulates 12% lactic acid neutralized with ammonium hydroxide, as ammonium lactate to provide a lotion pH of 4.5–5.5. LAC-HYDRIN also contains light mineral oil, glyceryl stearate, PEG-100 stearate, propylene glycol, polyoxyl 40 stearate, glycerin, magnesium aluminum silicate, laureth-4, cetyl alcohol, methyl and propylparabens, methylcellulose, fragrance, and water. Lactic acid is a racemic mixture of 2-hydroxypropanoic acid and has the following structural formula:

$$\begin{array}{c} COOH \\ | \\ CHOH \\ | \\ CH_3 \end{array}$$

CLINICAL PHARMACOLOGY
It is generally accepted that the water content of the stratum corneum is a controlling factor in maintaining skin flexibility. When the stratum corneum contains more than 10% water it remains soft and pliable; however, when the water content drops below 10% the stratum corneum becomes less flexible and rough, and may exhibit scaling and cracking and the underlying skin may become irritated.
Symptomatic relief of dry skin is provided by skin protectants containing hygroscopic substances (humectants) which increase skin moisture. Lactic acid, an α-hydroxy acid, is reported to be one of the most effective naturally occurring humectants in the skin. The α-hydroxy acids (and their salts), in addition to having beneficial effects on dry skin, have also been shown to reduce excessive epidermal keratinization in patients with hyperkeratotic conditions (e.g., ichthyosis).
Pharmacokinetics: The mechanism of action of topically applied neutralized lactic acid is not yet known.

INDICATIONS AND USAGE
LAC-HYDRIN is indicated for the treatment of dry, scaly skin (xerosis) and ichthyosis vulgaris and for temporary relief of itching associated with these conditions.

CONTRAINDICATIONS
Known hypersensitivity to any of the label ingredients.

PRECAUTIONS
General: For external use only. Avoid contact with eyes, lips or mucous membranes. Caution is advised when used on the face of fair-skinned individuals since irritation may occur. A mild, transient stinging may occur on application to abraded or inflamed areas or in individuals with sensitive skin.
Carcinogenesis, Mutagenesis, Impairment of Fertility: LAC-HYDRIN was nonmutagenic in the Ames/Salmonella/Microsome Plate Assay. Reproductive studies in rats given lactic acid orally showed no effect on the sex ratio of the offspring.
Pregnancy (Category C): Animal reproduction studies have not been conducted with LAC-HYDRIN. It is also not known whether LAC-HYDRIN can cause fetal harm when administered to a pregnant woman or can affect reproduction capacity. LAC-HYDRIN should be given to a pregnant woman only if clearly needed.
Nursing Mothers: Although lactic acid is a normal constituent of blood and tissues, it is not known to what extent this drug affects normal lactic acid levels in human milk. Because many drugs are excreted in human milk, caution should be exercised when LAC-HYDRIN is administered to a nursing woman.
Pediatric Use: Safety and effectiveness of LAC-HYDRIN have been demonstrated in infants and children. No unusual toxic effects were reported.

ADVERSE REACTIONS
The most frequent adverse experiences in patients with xerosis are transient stinging (1 in 30 patients), burning (1 in 30 patients), erythema (1 in 50 patients) and peeling (1 in 60 patients). Other adverse reactions which occur less frequently are irritation, eczema, petechiae, dryness and hyperpigmentation.
Due to the more severe initial skin conditions associated with ichthyosis, there was a higher incidence of transient stinging, burning and erythema (each occurring in 1 in 10 patients).

OVERDOSAGE
The oral administration of LAC-HYDRIN to rats and mice showed this drug to be practically non-toxic ($LD_{50} >$ 15 ml/kg).

DOSAGE AND ADMINISTRATION
Shake well. Apply to the affected areas and rub in thoroughly. Use twice daily or as directed by a physician.

HOW SUPPLIED
225g (NDC 0072-5712-08; NSN 6505-01-216-6274) plastic bottle and 400g (NDC 0072-5712-14) plastic bottle.
Store at controlled room temperature (15°–30°C; 59°–86°F).

MOISTUREL® CREAM OTC
Fragrance Free Skin Protectant—Moisturizer

COMPOSITION
Active Ingredients: Dimethicone 1%, petrolatum 30%. Also contains: Water, glycerin, PG dioctanoate, cetyl alcohol, steareth-2, PVP/hexadecene copolymer, laureth-23, magnesium aluminum silicate, diazolidinyl urea, carbomer-934, sodium hydroxide, methylchloroisothiazolinone and methylisothiazolinone.

ACTIONS AND USES
A highly effective, concentrated formula clinically proven to relieve dry skin and designed not to cause acne or blemishes. Ideal for sensitive skin. Free of lanolins, fragrances, and parabens that can sensitize or irritate skin.

Helps prevent and temporarily protects chafed, chapped, cracked or windburned skin. For temporary protection of minor cuts, scrapes, burns and sunburn. Helps treat and prevent minor skin irritation due to diaper rash and helps seal out wetness.

WARNINGS
For external use only. Avoid contact with the eyes. Not to be applied over puncture wounds or infections.

ADMINISTRATION AND DOSAGE
Apply liberally as often as needed. If used for diaper rash, change wet diapers promptly, cleanse the diaper area and allow to dry. Apply cream liberally with each changing.

HOW SUPPLIED
4 oz. (113g) (NDC 0072-9500-04) and 16 oz. (453g) (NDC 0072-9500-16) plastic jars.

MOISTUREL® LOTION   OTC
Skin Protectant—Moisturizer

COMPOSITION
Active Ingredient: Dimethicone 3%. Also contains: Water, petrolatum, glycerin, steareth-2, cetyl alcohol, benzyl alcohol, laureth-23, magnesium aluminum silicate, carbomer-934, sodium hydroxide, quaternium-15.

ACTION AND USES
Quick absorbing, long lasting formula that leaves the skin feeling smooth and soft. Clinically proven to relieve dry skin and designed not to cause acne. Free of lanolins and parabens that can irritate sensitive skin. Generalized dry skin. Helps prevent and temporarily protects chafed, chapped, cracked or windburned skin. Helps treat and prevent minor skin irritation due to diaper rash and helps seal out wetness.

WARNINGS
For external use only. Avoid contact with the eyes. Not to be applied over puncture wounds or infections.

ADMINISTRATION AND DOSAGE
Apply liberally as often as needed to soothe and soften sensitive skin. If used for diaper rash, change wet diapers promptly, cleanse the diaper area and allow to dry. Apply lotion liberally with each changing.

HOW SUPPLIED
8 oz. (226g) (NDC 0072-9100-08) and 14 oz. (397g) (NDC 0072-9100-14) plastic bottles.

MYCOSTATIN® CREAM   ℞
[*mtk´ō-stat"in*]
Nystatin Cream USP
MYCOSTATIN® TOPICAL POWDER   ℞
Nystatin Topical Powder USP
For topical use only.
Not for ophthalmic use.

DESCRIPTION
MYCOSTATIN Cream (Nystatin Cream), and MYCOSTATIN Topical Powder (Nystatin Topical Powder) are for dermatologic use.
MYCOSTATIN Cream contains the antifungal antibiotic nystatin with the following chemical structure:

Nystatin

Each gram of MYCOSTATIN Cream contains 100,000 USP nystatin units in an aqueous, perfumed vanishing cream base containing aluminum hydroxide concentrated wet gel, titanium dioxide, propylene glycol, cetearyl alcohol (and) ceteareth-20, white petrolatum, sorbitol solution, glyceryl monostearate, polyethylene glycol monostearate, sorbic acid and simethicone.
MYCOSTATIN Topical Powder provides, in each gram, 100,000 USP nystatin units dispersed in talc.

CLINICAL PHARMACOLOGY
Nystatin is an antifungal antibiotic which is both fungistatic and fungicidal *in vitro* against a wide variety of yeasts and yeast-like fungi. It probably acts by binding to sterols in the cell membrane of the fungus with a resultant change in membrane permeability allowing leakage of intracellular components. Nystatin is a polyene antibiotic of undetermined structural formula that is obtained from *Streptomyces noursei*, and is the first well tolerated antifungal antibiotic of dependable efficacy for the treatment of cutaneous, oral and intestinal infections caused by *Candida* (Monilia) *albicans* and other Candida species. It exhibits no appreciable activity against bacteria.
Nystatin provides specific therapy for all localized forms of candidiasis. Symptomatic relief is rapid, often occurring within 24 to 72 hours after the initiation of treatment. Cure is effected both clinically and mycologically in most cases of localized candidiasis.

INDICATIONS AND USAGE
MYCOSTATIN (nystatin) topical preparations are indicated in the treatment of cutaneous or mucocutaneous mycotic infections caused by *Candida* (Monilia) *albicans* and other Candida species.

CONTRAINDICATIONS
MYCOSTATIN topical preparations are contraindicated in patients with a history of hypersensitivity to any of their components.

PRECAUTIONS
Should a reaction of hypersensitivity occur the drug should be immediately withdrawn and appropriate measures taken. These preparations are not for ophthalmic use.

ADVERSE REACTIONS
Nystatin is virtually nontoxic and nonsensitizing and is well tolerated by all age groups including debilitated infants, even on prolonged administration. If irritation on topical application should occur, discontinue medication.

DOSAGE AND ADMINISTRATION
The cream should be applied liberally to affected areas twice daily or as indicated until healing is complete. The powder should be applied to candidal lesions two or three times daily until lesions have healed. For fungal infection of the feet caused by Candida species, the powder should be dusted freely on the feet as well as in shoes and socks. The cream is usually preferred in candidiasis involving intertriginous areas; very moist lesions, however, are best treated with the topical dusting powder.
The preparations do not stain skin or mucous membranes and they provide a simple, convenient means of treatment.

HOW SUPPLIED
MYCOSTATIN Cream (Nystatin Cream USP) is supplied in 30g (NDC 0003-0579-31) tubes providing 100,000 USP nystatin units per gram in an aqueous, perfumed vanishing cream base.
MYCOSTATIN Topical Powder (Nystatin Topical Powder USP) is supplied in 15g (NDC 0003-0593-20) plastic squeeze bottles providing, in each gram, 100,000 USP nystatin units.
Storage
MYCOSTATIN Cream (Nystatin Cream USP)
Store at room temperature; avoid freezing.
MYCOSTATIN Topical Powder (Nystatin Topical Powder USP)
Store at room temperature; avoid excessive heat (40°C; 104°F).
Keep tightly closed.

T-STAT®   ℞
(erythromycin) 2.0% Topical Solution and Pads
For topical use only. Not for ophthalmic use.

CAUTION
Federal law prohibits dispensing without prescription.

DESCRIPTION
Erythromycin is an antibiotic produced from a strain of Streptomyces erythraeus. It is basic and readily forms salts with acids. Each ml of T-STAT (erythromycin). 2.0% Topical Solution contains 20 mg of erythromycin base in a vehicle consisting of alcohol (71.2%), propylene glycol and fragrance. It may contain citric acid to adjust pH.

ACTIONS
Although the mechanism by which T-STAT Solution acts in reducing inflammatory lesions of acne vulgaris is unknown, it is presumably due to its antibiotic action.

INDICATIONS
T-STAT Solution is indicated for the topical control of acne vulgaris.

CONTRAINDICATIONS
T-STAT Solution is contraindicated in persons who have shown hypersensitivity to any of its ingredients.

WARNING
The safe use of T-STAT (erythromycin) 2.0% Solution during pregnancy or lactation has not been established.

PRECAUTIONS
General—The use of antibiotic agents may be associated with the overgrowth of antibiotic-resistant organisms. If this occurs, administration of this drug should be discontinued and appropriate measures taken.
Information for Patients—T-STAT Solution is for external use only and should be kept away from the eyes, nose, mouth, and other mucous membranes. Concomitant topical acne therapy should be used with caution because a cumulative irritant effect may occur, especially with the use of peeling, desquamating, or abrasive agents.
Carcinogensis, Mutagenesis, Impairment of Fertility—Long-term animal studies to evaluate carcinogenic potential, mutagenicity, or the effect on fertility of erythromycin have not been performed.
Pregnancy: Pregnancy Category C.—Animal reproduction studies have not been conducted with erythromycin. It is also not known whether erythromycin can cause fetal harm when administered to a pregnant woman or can affect reproduction capacity. Erythromycin should be given to a pregnant woman only if clearly needed.
Nursing Mothers—Erythromycin is excreted in breast milk. Caution should be exercised when erythromycin is administered to a nursing woman.

ADVERSE REACTIONS
Adverse conditions reported include dryness, tenderness, pruritus, desquamation, erythema, oiliness, and burning sensation. Irritation of the eyes has also been reported. A case of generalized urticarial reaction, possibly related to the drug, which required the use of systemic steroid therapy has been reported.

DOSAGE AND ADMINISTRATION
T-STAT Solution or Pads should be applied over the affected area twice a day after the skin is thoroughly washed with warm water and soap and patted dry. Acne lesions on the face, neck, shoulder, chest, and back may be treated in this manner. Additional pads may be used, if needed.
This medication should be applied with applicator top or the disposable applicator pads. If fingertips or pads are used, wash hands after application. Drying and peeling may be controlled by reducing the frequency of applications.

HOW SUPPLIED
T-STAT Solution, 60 ml plastic bottle with optional applicator, NDC 0072-8300-60. T-STAT Pads, 60 disposable premoistened applicator pads in a plastic jar. NDC 0072-8303-60. Store in a dry place at temperatures between 15°C and 25°C (59°F and 77°F).

ULTRAVATE®   ℞
(halobetasol propionate cream)
Cream, 0.05%
For Dermatological Use Only. Not for Ophthalmic Use.
Caution: Federal law prohibits dispensing without a prescription.

DESCRIPTION
ULTRAVATE (halobetasol propionate cream) Cream contains halobetasol propionate, a synthetic corticosteroid for topical dermatological use. The corticosteroids constitute a class of primarily synthetic steroids used topically as an anti-inflammatory and antipruritic agent.
Chemically halobetasol propionate is 21-chloro-6α, 9-difluoro-11β, 17-dihydroxy-16β-methylpregna-1, 4-diene-3-20-dione, 17 propionate, $C_{25}H_{31}ClF_2O_5$. It has the following structural formula:

Halobetasol propionate has the molecular weight of 485. It is a white crystalline powder insoluble in water.
Each gram of ULTRAVATE Cream contains 0.5 mg/g of halobetasol propionate in a cream base of cetyl alcohol, glycerin, isopropyl isostearate, isopropyl palmitate, steareth-21, diazolidinyl urea, methylchloroisothiazolinone, methylisothiazolinone and water.

CLINICAL PHARMACOLOGY
Like other topical corticosteroids, halobetasol propionate has anti-inflammatory, antipruritic and vasoconstrictive actions. The mechanism of the anti-inflammatory activity of the topical corticosteroids, in general, is unclear. However, corticosteroids are thought to act by the induction of phospholipase A_2 inhibitory proteins, collectively called lipocor-

Continued on next page

Westwood-Squibb—Cont.

tins. It is postulated that these proteins control the biosynthesis of potent mediators of inflammation such as prostaglandins and leukotrienes by inhibiting the release of their common precursor arachidonic acid. Arachidonic acid is released from membrane phospholipids by phospholipase A_2.

Pharmacokinetics—The extent of percutaneous absorption of topical corticosteroids is determined by many factors including the vehicle and the integrity of the epidermal barrier. Occlusive dressings with hydrocortisone for up to 24 hours have not been demonstrated to increase penetration; however, occlusion of hydrocortisone for 96 hours markedly enhances penetration. Topical corticosteroids can be absorbed from normal intact skin. Inflammation and/or other disease processes in the skin may increase percutaneous absorption.

Human and animal studies indicate that less than 6% of the applied dose of halobetasol propionate enters the circulation with 96 hours following topical administration of the cream. Studies performed with ULTRAVATE (halobetasol propionate cream) Cream indicate that it is in the super-high range of potency as compared with other topical corticosteroids.

INDICATIONS AND USAGE

ULTRAVATE (halobetasol propionate cream) Cream 0.05% is a super-high potency corticosteroid indicated for the relief of the inflammatory and pruritic manifestations of corticosteroid-responsive dermatoses. Treatment beyond two consecutive weeks is not recommended, and the total dosage should not exceed 50 g/week because of the potential for the drug to suppress the hypothalamic-pituitary-adrenal (HPA) axis.

CONTRAINDICATIONS

ULTRAVATE (halobetasol propionate cream) Cream is contraindicated in those patients with a history of hypersensitivity to any of the components of the preparation.

PRECAUTIONS

General: Systemic absorption of topical corticosteroids can produce reversible hypothalamic-pituitary-adrenal (HPA) axis suppression with the potential for glucocorticosteroid insufficiency after withdrawal of treatment. Manifestations of Cushing's syndrome, hyperglycemia, and glucosuria can also be produced in some patients by systemic absorption of topical corticosteroids while on treatment.

Patients applying a topical steroid to a large surface area or to areas under occlusion should be evaluated periodically for evidence of HPA axis suppression. This may be done by using the ACTH stimulation, A.M. plasma cortisol, and urinary free-cortisol tests. Patients receiving super potent corticosteroids should not be treated for more than 2 weeks at a time and only small areas should be treated at any one time due to increased risk of HPA suppression.

ULTRAVATE (halobetasol propionate cream) Cream produced HPA axis suppression when used in divided doses at 7 grams per day for one week in patients with psoriasis. These effects were reversible upon discontinuation of treatment.

If HPA axis suppression is noted, an attempt should be made to withdraw the drug, to reduce the frequency of application, or to substitute a less potent corticosteroid. Recovery of HPA axis function is generally prompt upon discontinuation of topical corticosteroids. Infrequently, signs and symptoms of glucocorticosteroids insufficiency may occur requiring supplemental systemic corticosteroids. For information on systemic supplementation, see prescribing information for those products.

Pediatric patients may be more susceptible to systemic toxicity from equivalent doses due to their larger skin surface to body mass ratios (See PRECAUTIONS: Pediatric Use).

If irritation develops, ULTRAVATE (halobetasol propionate cream) Cream should be discontinued and appropriate therapy instituted. Allergic contact dermatitis with corticosteroids is usually diagnosed by observing failure to heal rather than noting a clinical exacerbation as with most topical products not containing corticosteroids. Such an observation should be corroborated with appropriate diagnostic patch testing.

If concomitant skin infections are present or develop, an appropriate antifungal or antibacterial agent should be used. If a favorable response does not occur promptly, use of ULTRAVATE (halobetasol propionate cream) Cream should be discontinued until the infection has been adequately controlled.

ULTRAVATE (halobetasol propionate cream) Cream should not be used in the treatment of rosacea or perioral dermatitis, and it should not be used on the face, groin, or in the axillae.

Information for Patients: Patients using topical corticosteroids should receive the following information and instructions:

1. The medication is to be used as directed by the physician. It is for external use only. Avoid contact with the eyes.
2. The medication should not be used for any disorder other than that for which it was prescribed.

3. The treated skin area should not be bandaged, otherwise covered or wrapped, so as to be occlusive unless directed by the physician.
4. Patients should report to the their physician any signs of local adverse reactions.
5. Parents of pediatric patients should be advised not to use tight-fitting diapers or plastic pants on a child being treated in the diaper area, as these garments may constitute occlusive dressing.

Laboratory Tests: The following tests may be helpful in evaluating patients for HPA axis suppression: ACTH-stimulation test; A.M. plasma cortisol test; Urinary free-cortisol test.

Carcinogenesis, mutagenesis, and Impairment of fertility: Long-term animal studies have not been performed to evaluate the carcinogenic potential of halobetasol propionate.

Positive mutagenicity effects were observed in two genotoxicity assays. Halobetasol propionate was positive in a Chinese hamster micronucleus test, and in a mouse lymphoma gene mutation assay in vitro.

Studies in the rat following oral administration at dose levels up to 50 μg/kg/day indicated no impairment of fertility or general reproductive performance.

In other genotoxicity testing, halobetasol propionate was not found to be genotoxic in the Ames/Salmonella assay, in the sister chromatid exchange test in somatic cells of the Chinese hamster, in chromosome aberration studies of germinal and somatic cells of rodents, and in a mammalian spot test to determine point mutations.

Pregnancy: *Teratogenic effects: Pregnancy Category C:* Corticosteroids have been shown to be teratogenic in laboratory animals when administered systemically at relatively low dosage levels. Some corticosteroids have been shown to be teratogenic after dermal application in laboratory animals. Halobetasol propionate has been shown to be teratogenic in SPF rats and chinchilla-type rabbits when given systemically during gestation at doses of 0.04 to 0.1 mg/kg in rats and 0.01 mg/kg in rabbits. These doses are approximately 13.33 and 3 times, respectively, the human topical dose of ULTRAVATE (halobetasol propionate cream) Cream. Halobetasol propionate was embryotoxic in rabbits but not in rats.

Cleft palate was observed in both rats and rabbits. Omphalocele was seen in rats, but not in rabbits.

There are no adequate and well-controlled studies of the teratogenic potential of halobetasol propionate in pregnant women. ULTRAVATE (halobetasol propionate cream) Cream should be used during pregnancy only if the potential benefit justifies the potential risk to the fetus.

Nursing Mothers: Systemically administered corticosteroids appear in human milk and could suppress growth, interfere with endogenous corticosteroid production, or cause other untoward effects. It is not known whether topical administration of corticosteroids could result in sufficient systemic absorption to produce detectable quantities in human milk. Because many drugs are excreted in human milk, caution should be exercised when ULTRAVATE (halobetasol propionate cream) Cream is administered to a nursing woman.

Pediatric Use: Safety and effectiveness of ULTRAVATE (halobetasol propionate cream) Cream in pediatric patients have not been established and use in pediatric patients under 12 is not recommended. Because of a higher ratio of skin surface area to body mass, pediatric patients are at a greater risk than adults of HPA axis suppression and Cushing's syndrome when they are treated with topical corticosteroids. They are therefore also at greater risk of adrenal insufficiency during or after withdrawal of treatment. Adverse effects including striae have been reported with inappropriate use of topical corticosteroids in infants and children.

HPA axis suppression, Cushing's syndrome, linear growth retardation, delayed weight gain and intracranial hypertension have been reported in children receiving topical corticosteroids. Manifestations of adrenal suppression in children include low plasma cortisol levels and an absence of response to ACTH stimulation. Manifestations of intracranial hypertension include bulging fontanelles, headaches, and bilateral papilledema.

ADVERSE REACTIONS

In controlled clinical trials, the most frequent adverse events reported for ULTRAVATE (halobetasol propionate cream) Cream included stinging, burning or itching in 4.4% of the patients. Less frequently reported adverse reactions were dry skin, erythema, skin atrophy, leukoderma, vesicles and rash.

The following additional local adverse reactions are reported infrequently with topical corticosteroids, and they may occur more frequently with high potency corticosteroids, such as ULTRAVATE (halobetasol propionate cream) Cream. These reactions are listed in an approximate decreasing order of occurrence: folliculitis, hypertrichosis, acneiform eruptions, hypopigmentation, perioral dermatitis, allergic contact dermatitis, secondary infection, striae and miliaria.

OVERDOSAGE

Topically applied ULTRAVATE (halobetasol propionate cream) Cream can be absorbed in sufficient amounts to produce systemic effects (see PRECAUTIONS).

DOSAGE AND ADMINISTRATION

Apply a thin layer of ULTRAVATE (halobetasol propionate cream) Cream to the affected skin once or twice daily, as directed by your physician, and rub in gently and completely. ULTRAVATE (halobetasol propionate cream) Cream is a high potency topical corticosteroids; therefore, treatment should be limited to two weeks, and amounts greater than 50 g/wk should not be used. As with other corticosteroids, therapy should be discontinued when control is achieved. If no improvement is seen within 2 weeks, reassessment of diagnosis may be necessary.

ULTRAVATE (halobetasol propionate cream) Cream should not be used with occlusive dressings.

HOW SUPPLIED

ULTRAVATE CREAM, 0.05% is supplied in the following tube sizes:
15 g (NDC 0072-1400-15)
50 g (NDC 0072-1400-50)
Store between 15° and 30°C (59° and 86°F).

WESTWOOD SQUIBB™
© 1995 Westwood-Squibb Pharmaceuticals Inc.
A Bristol-Myers Squibb Company
Buffalo, New York U.S.A. 14213   03-5994-0

ULTRAVATE®   ℞
(halobetasol propionate ointment)
Ointment, 0.05%
For Dermatological Use Only. Not for Ophthalmic Use.
Caution: Federal law prohibits dispensing without a prescription.

DESCRIPTION

ULTRAVATE (halobetasol propionate ointment) Ointment contains halobetasol propionate, a synthetic corticosteroid for topical dermatological use. The corticosteroids constitute a class of primarily synthetic steroids used topically as an anti-inflammatory and antipruritic agent.

Chemically halobetasol propionate is 21-chloro-6α, 9-difluoro-11β, 17-dihydroxy-16β-methylpregna-1, 4-diene-3-20-dione, 17-propionate, $C_{25}H_{31}CIF_2O_5$. It has the following structural formula:

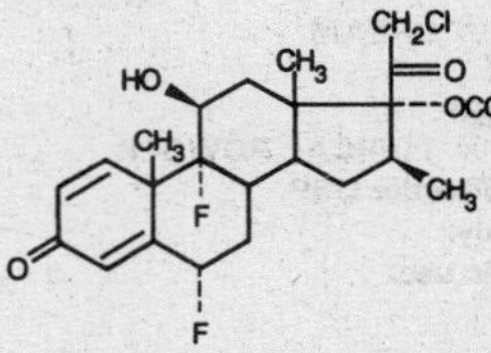

Halobetasol propionate has the molecular weight of 485. It is a white crystalline powder insoluble in water.

Each gram of ULTRAVATE Ointment contains 0.5 mg/g of halobetasol propionate in a base of aluminum stearate, beeswax, pentaerythritol cocoate, petrolatum, propylene glycol, sorbitan sesquioleate, and stearyl citrate.

CLINICAL PHARMACOLOGY

Like other topical corticosteroids, halobetasol propionate has anti-inflammatory, antipruritic and vasoconstrictive actions. The mechanism of the anti-inflammatory activity of the topical corticosteroids, in general, is unclear. However, corticosteroids are thought to act by the induction of phospholipase A_2 inhibitory proteins, collectively called lipocortins. It is postulated that these proteins control the biosynthesis of potent mediators of inflammation such as prostaglandins and leukotrienes by inhibiting the release of their common precursor arachidonic acid. Arachidonic acid is released from membrane phospholipids by phospholipase A_2.

Pharmacokinetics
The extent of percutaneous absorption of topical corticosteroids is determined by many factors including the vehicle and the integrity of the epidermal barrier. Occlusive dressings with hydrocortisone for up to 24 hours have not been demonstrated to increase penetration; however, occlusion of hydrocortisone for 96 hours markedly enhances penetration. Topical corticosteroids can be absorbed from normal intact skin. Inflammation and/or other disease processes in the skin may increase percutaneous absorption.

Human and animal studies indicate that less than 6% of the applied dose of halobetasol propionate enters the circulation within 96 hours following topical administration of the ointment.

Studies performed with ULTRAVATE (halobetasol propionate ointment) Ointment indicate that it is in the super-high

range of potency as compared with other topical corticosteroids.

INDICATIONS AND USAGE

ULTRAVATE (halobetasol propionate ointment) Ointment 0.05% is a super-high potency corticosteroid indicated for the relief of the inflammatory and pruritic manifestations of corticosteroid-responsive dermatoses. Treatment beyond two consecutive weeks is not recommended, and the total dosage should not exceed 50 g/week because of the potential for the drug to suppress the hypothalamic-pituitary-adrenal (HPA) axis.

CONTRAINDICATIONS

ULTRAVATE (halobetasol propionate ointment) Ointment is contraindicated in those patients with a history of hypersensitivity to any of the components of the preparation.

PRECAUTIONS

General: Systemic absorption of topical corticosteroids can produce reversible hypothalamic-pituitary-adrenal (HPA) axis suppression with the potential for glucocorticosteroid insufficiency after withdrawal of treatment. Manifestations of Cushing's syndrome, hyperglycemia, and glucosuria can also be produced in some patients by systemic absorption of topical corticosteroids while on treatment.

Patients applying a topical steroid to a large surface area or to areas under occlusion should be evaluated periodically for evidence of HPA axis suppression. This may be done by using the ACTH stimulation, A.M. plasma cortisol, and urinary free-cortisol tests. Patients receiving super potent corticosteroids should not be treated for more than 2 weeks at a time and only small areas should be treated at any one time due to the increased risk of HPA suppression.

ULTRAVATE (halobetasol propionate ointment) Ointment produced HPA axis suppression when used in divided doses at 7 grams per day for one week in patients with psoriasis. These effects were reversible upon discontinuation of treatment.

If HPA axis suppression is noted, an attempt should be made to withdraw the drug, to reduce the frequency of application, or to substitute a less potent corticosteroid. Recovery of HPA axis function is generally prompt upon discontinuation of topical corticosteroids. Infrequently, signs and symptoms of glucocorticosteroid insufficiency may occur requiring supplemental systemic corticosteroids. For information on systemic supplementation, see prescribing information for those products.

Pediatric patients may be more susceptible to systemic toxicity from equivalent doses due to their larger skin surface to body mass ratios (See PRECAUTIONS: Pediatric Use).

If irritation develops, ULTRAVATE (halobetasol propionate ointment) Ointment should be discontinued and appropriate therapy instituted. Allergic contact dermatitis with corticosteroids is usually diagnosed by observing failure to heal rather than noting a clinical exacerbation as with most topical products not containing corticosteroids. Such an observation should be corroborated with appropriate diagnostic patch testing.

If concomitant skin infections are present or develop, an appropriate antifungal or antibacterial agent should be used. If a favorable response does not occur promptly, use of ULTRAVATE (halobetasol propionate ointment) Ointment should be discontinued until the infection has been adequately controlled.

ULTRAVATE (halobetasol propionate ointment) Ointment should not be used in the treatment of rosacea or perioral dermatitis, and it should not be used on the face, groin, or in the axillae.

Information for Patients

Patients using topical corticosteroids should receive the following information and instructions:

1. The medication is to be used as directed by the physician. It is for external use only. Avoid contact with the eyes.
2. The medication should not be used for any disorder other than that for which it was prescribed.
3. The treated skin area should not be bandaged, otherwise covered or wrapped, so as to be occlusive unless directed by the physician.
4. Patients should report to their physician any signs of local adverse reactions.
5. Parents of pediatric patients should be advised not to use tight-fitting diapers or plastic pants on a child being treated in the diaper area, as these garments may constitute occlusive dressing.

Laboratory Tests

The following tests may be helpful in evaluating patients for HPA axis suppression: ACTH-stimulation test; A.M. plasma cortisol test; Urinary free-cortisol test.

Carcinogenesis, mutagenesis, and Impairment of fertility

Long-term animal studies have not been performed to evaluate the carcinogenic potential of halobetasol propionate.

Positive mutagenicity effects were observed in two genotoxicity assays. Halobetasol propionate was positive in a Chinese hamster micronucleus test, and in a mouse lymphoma gene mutation assay *in vitro*.

Studies in the rat following oral administration at dose levels up to 50 μg/kg/day indicated no impairment of fertility or general reproductive performance.

In other genotoxicity testing, halobetasol propionate was not found to be genotoxic in the Ames/Salmonella assay, in the sister chromatid exchange test in somatic cells of the Chinese hamster, in chromosome aberration studies of germinal and somatic cells of rodents, and in a mammalian spot test to determine point mutations.

Pregnancy

Teratogenic effects: Pregnancy Category C: Corticosteroids have been shown to be teratogenic in laboratory animals when administered systemically at relatively low dosage levels. Some corticosteroids have been shown to be teratogenic after dermal application in laboratory animals.

Halobetasol propionate has been shown to be teratogenic in SPF rats and chinchilla-type rabbits when given systematically during gestation at doses of 0.04 to 0.1 mg/kg in rats and 0.01 mg/kg in rabbits. These doses are approximately 13, 33 and 3 times, respectively, the human topical dose of ULTRAVATE (halobetasol propionate ointment) Ointment. Halobetasol propionate was embryotoxic in rabbits but not in rats.

Cleft palate was observed in both rats and rabbits. Omphalocele was seen in rats, but not in rabbits.

There are no adequate and well-controlled studies of the teratogenic potential of halobetasol propionate in pregnant women. ULTRAVATE (halobetasol propionate ointment) Ointment should be used during pregnancy only if the potential benefit justifies the potential risk to the fetus.

Nursing Mothers

Systematically administered corticosteroids appear in human milk and could suppress growth, interfere with endogenous corticosteroid production, or cause other untoward effects. It is not known whether topical administration of corticosteroids could result in sufficient systemic absorption to produce detectable quantities in human milk. Because many drugs are excreted in human milk, caution should be exercised when ULTRAVATE (halobetasol propionate ointment) Ointment is administered to a nursing woman.

Pediatric Use

Safety and effectiveness of ULTRAVATE (halobetasol propionate ointment) Ointment in pediatric patients have not been established and use in pediatric patients under 12 is not recommended. Because of a higher ratio of skin surface area to body mass, pediatric patients are at a greater risk than adults of HPA axis suppression and Cushing's syndrome when they are treated with topical corticosteroids. They are therefore also at greater risk of adrenal insufficiency during or after withdrawal of treatment. Adverse effects including striae have been reported with inappropriate use of topical corticosteroids in infants and children.

HPA axis suppression, Cushing's syndrome, linear growth retardation, delayed weight gain and intracranial hypertension have been reported in children receiving topical corticosteroids. Manifestations of adrenal suppression in children include low plasma cortisol levels and an absence of response to ACTH stimulation. Manifestations of intracranial hypertension include bulging fontanelles, headaches, and bilateral papilledema.

ADVERSE REACTIONS

In controlled clinical trials, the most frequent adverse events reported for ULTRAVATE (halobetasol propionate ointment) Ointment included stinging or burning in 1.6% of the patients. Less frequently reported adverse reactions were pustulation, erythema, skin atrophy, leukoderma, acne, itching, secondary infection, telangiectasia, urticaria, dry skin, miliaria, paresthesia, and rash.

The following additional local adverse reactions are reported infrequently with topical corticosteroids, and they may occur more frequently with high potency corticosteroids, such as ULTRAVATE (halobetasol propionate ointment) Ointment. These reactions are listed in an approximate decreasing order of occurrence: folliculitis, hypertrichosis, acneiform eruptions, hypopigmentation, perioral dermatitis, allergic contact dermatitis, secondary infection, striae and miliaria.

OVERDOSAGE

Topically applied ULTRAVATE (halobetasol propionate ointment) Ointment can be absorbed in sufficient amounts to produce systemic effects (see **PRECAUTIONS**).

DOSAGE AND ADMINISTRATION

Apply a thin layer of ULTRAVATE (halobetasol propionate ointment) Ointment to the affected skin once or twice daily, as directed by your physician, and rub in gently and completely.

ULTRAVATE (halobetasol propionate ointment) Ointment is a high potency topical corticosteroid; therefore, treatment should be limited to two weeks, and amounts greater than 50 g/wk should not be used. As with other corticosteroids, therapy should be discontinued when control is achieved. If no improvement is seen within 2 weeks, reassessment of diagnosis may be necessary.

ULTRAVATE (halobetasol propionate ointment) Ointment should not be used with occlusive dressings.

HOW SUPPLIED

ULTRAVATE OINTMENT, 0.05% is supplied in the following tube sizes:

15 g (NDC 0072-1450-15)
50 g (NDC 0072-1450-50)

Store between 15° and 30°C (59° and 86°F).

WESTWOOD SQUIBB™
© 1995 Westwood-Squibb Pharmaceuticals Inc.
A Bristol-Myers Squibb Company
Buffalo, New York U.S.A. 14213 03-5995-1

WESTCORT®

(hydrocortisone valerate)
Cream, 0.2%

℞

For topical use only. Not for use in eyes.

CAUTION: Federal law prohibits dispensing without a prescription.

DESCRIPTION

WESTCORT CREAM is a topical formulation containing hydrocortisone valerate, a non-fluorinated steroid. It has the chemical name Pregn-4-ene-3,20-dione. 11, 21-dihydroxy-17-[(1-oxopentyl) oxy]-, (11β)-; the empirical formula is: $C_{26}H_{38}O_6$; the molecular weight is 446.58, and the CAS registry number is: 57524-89-7. The structural formula is:

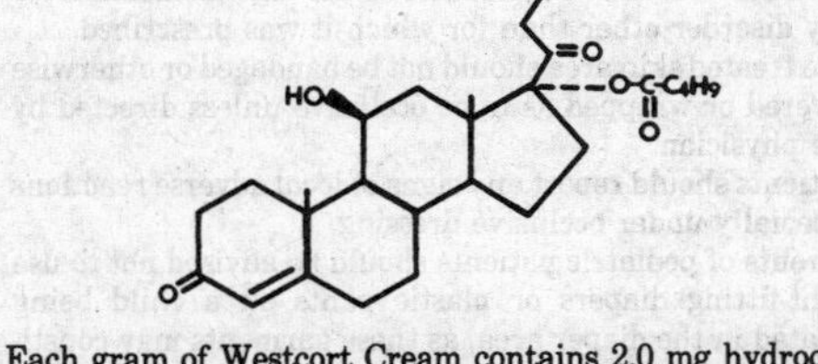

Each gram of Westcort Cream contains 2.0 mg hydrocortisone valerate in a hydrophilic base composed of white petrolatum, stearyl alcohol, propylene glycol, amphoteric-9, carbomer 940, dried sodium phosphate, sodium lauryl sulfate, sorbic acid and water.

CLINICAL PHARMACOLOGY

Topical corticosteroids share anti-inflammatory, anti-pruritic and vasoconstrictive actions.

The mechanism of anti-inflammatory activity of the topical corticosteroids is unclear.[1] Various laboratory methods, including vasoconstrictor assays, are used to compare and predict potencies and/or clinical efficacies of the topical corticosteroids.[2] There is some evidence to suggest that a recognizable correlation exists between vasoconstrictor potency and therapeutic efficacy in man.[3]

Pharmacokinetics—The extent of percutaneous absorption of topical corticosteroids is determined by many factors including the vehicle, the integrity of the epidermal barrier, and the use of occlusive dressings.[4,5,6]

Topical corticosteroids can be absorbed from normal intact skin.[5,6,7] Inflammation and/or other disease processes in the skin increase percutaneous absorption.[8] Occlusive dressings substantially increase the percutaneous absorption of topical corticosteroids.[4,7] Thus, occlusive dressings may be valuable therapeutic adjunct for treatment of resistant dermatoses (see DOSAGE AND ADMINISTRATION).

Once absorbed through the skin, topical corticosteroids are handled through pharmacokinetic pathways similar to systemically administered corticosteroids. Corticosteroids are bound to plasma proteins in varying degrees. Corticosteroids are metabolized primarily in the liver and are then excreted by the kidneys. Some of the topical corticosteroids and their metabolites are also excreted into the bile.

INDICATIONS AND USAGE

Westcort Cream is indicated for the relief of the inflammatory and pruritic manifestations of the corticosteroid-responsive dermatoses.

CONTRAINDICATIONS

Topical corticosteroids are contraindicated in those patients with a history of hypersensitivity to any of the components of the preparation.

PRECAUTIONS

General—Systemic absorption of topical corticosteroids has produced reversible hypothalamic-pituitary-adrenal (HPA) axis suppression, manifestations of Cushing's syndrome, hyperglycemia, and glucosuria in some patients.[9]

Conditions which augment systemic absorption include the application of the more potent steroids, use over large surface areas, prolonged use, and the addition of occlusive dressings.[10]

Therefore, patients receiving a large dose of a potent topical steroid applied to a large surface area or under an occlusive dressing should be evaluated periodically for evidence of

Continued on next page

Westwood-Squibb—Cont.

HPA axis suppression by using the urinary free cortisol and ACTH stimulation tests. If HPA axis suppression is noted, an attempt should be made to withdraw the drug, to reduce the frequency of application, or to substitute a less potent steroid.

Recovery of HPA axis function is generally prompt and complete upon discontinuation of the drug.[10] Infrequently, signs and symptoms of steroid withdrawal may occur, requiring supplemental systemic corticosteroids.[11,12]

Children may absorb proportionally larger amounts of topical corticosteroids and thus be more susceptible to systemic toxicity.[13,14] (see PRECAUTIONS—*Pediatric Use*).

If irritation develops, topical corticosteroids should be discontinued and appropriate therapy instituted.

In the presence of dermatological infections, the use of an appropriate antifungal or antibacterial agent should be instituted. If a favorable response does not occur promptly, the corticosteroid should be discontinued until the infection has been adequately controlled.

Information for the Patient—Patients using topical corticosteroids should receive the following information and instructions:

1. This medication is to be used as directed by the physician. It is for external use only. Avoid contact with the eyes.
2. Patients should be advised not to use this medication for any disorder other than for which it was prescribed.
3. The treated skin area should not be bandaged or otherwise covered or wrapped as to be occlusive unless directed by the physician.
4. Patients should report any signs of local adverse reactions especially under occlusive dressing.
5. Parents of pediatric patients should be advised not to use tight-fitting diapers or plastic pants on a child being treated in the diaper area, as these garments may constitute occlusive dressing.

Laboratory Tests—The following tests may be helpful in evaluating the HPA axis suppression:

Urinary free cortisol test
ACTH stimulation test

Carcinogenesis, Mutagenesis, and Impairment of Fertility—Long-term animal studies have not been performed to evaluate the carcinogenic potential or the effect on fertility of topical corticosteroids.

Studies to determine mutagenicity with prednisolone and hydrocortisone have revealed negative results.[15,16]

Pregnancy (Category C)—Corticosteroids are generally teratogenic in laboratory animals when administered systemically at relatively low dosage levels. The more potent corticosteroids have been shown to be teratogenic after dermal application in laboratory animals. There are no adequate and well-controlled studies in pregnant women on teratogenic effects from topically applied corticosteroids. Therefore, topical corticosteroids should be used during pregnancy only if the potential benefit justifies the potential risk to the fetus. Drugs of this class should not be used extensively on pregnant patients, in large amounts, or for prolonged periods of time.

Nursing Mothers—It is not known whether topical administration of corticosteroids could result in sufficient systemic absorption to produce detectable quantities in breast milk. Systemically administered corticosteroids are secreted into breast milk in quantities *not* likely to have a deleterious effect on the infant.[17,18] Nevertheless, caution should be exercised when topical corticosteroids are administered to a nursing woman.

Pediatric Use—*Pediatric patients may demonstrate greater susceptibility to topical corticosteroid-induced HPA axis suppression and Cushing's syndrome than mature patients because of a larger skin surface area to body weight ratio.*

Hypothalamic-pituitary-adrenal (HPA) axis suppression. Cushing's syndrome, and intracranial hypertension have been reported in children receiving topical corticosteroids. Manifestations of adrenal suppression in children include linear growth retardation, delayed weight gain, low plasma cortisol levels, and absence of response to ACTH stimulation. Manifestations of intracranial hypertension include bulging fontanelles, headaches, and bilateral papilledema.

Administration of topical corticosteroids to children should be limited to the least amount compatible with an effective therapeutic regimen. Chronic corticosteroid therapy may interfere with the growth and development of children.

ADVERSE REACTIONS

The following local adverse reactions are reported infrequently with topical corticosteroids, but may occur more frequently with the use of occlusive dressings. These reactions are listed in an approximate decreasing order of occurrence: burning, itching, irritation, dryness, folliculitis, hypertrichosis, acneiform eruptions, hypopigmentation, perioral dermatitis, allergic contact dermatitis, maceration of the skin, secondary infection, skin atrophy, striae, miliaria.

OVERDOSAGE

Topically applied corticosteroids can be absorbed in sufficient amounts to produce systemic effects (see PRECAUTIONS).

DOSAGE AND ADMINISTRATION

Westcort Cream should be applied to the affected area as a thin film two or three times daily depending on the severity of the condition.

Occlusive dressings may be used for the management of psoriasis or recalcitrant conditions.

If an infection develops, the use of occlusive dressings should be discontinued and appropriate antimicrobial therapy instituted.

HOW SUPPLIED

WESTCORT CREAM, 0.2% is supplied in the following tube sizes:

15 g NDC 0072-8100-15; NSN 6505-01-093-9901
45 g NDC 0072-8100-45; NSN 6505-01-083-9901
60 g NDC 0072-8100-60
Store below 78°F (26°C).

©1982, 1990 WESTWOOD-SQUIBB PHARMACEUTICALS, INC.
Buffalo, N.Y., U.S.A. 14213   03-5971-0

WESTCORT®   ℞
(hydrocortisone valerate ointment)
Ointment, 0.2%
For Dermatologic Use Only. Not for Ophthalmic Use.
Caution: Federal law prohibits dispensing without a prescription.

DESCRIPTION

Ointment contains hydrocortisone valerate, 11, 21-dihydroxy-17-[(1-oxopentyl)oxy]-,(11β)-pregn-4-ene-3, 20-dione, a synthetic corticosteroid for topical dermatologic use. The corticosteroids constitute a class of primarily synthetic steroids used topically as anti-inflammatory and antipruritic agents.

Chemically, hydrocortisone valerate is $C_{26}H_{38}O_6$. It has the following structural formula:

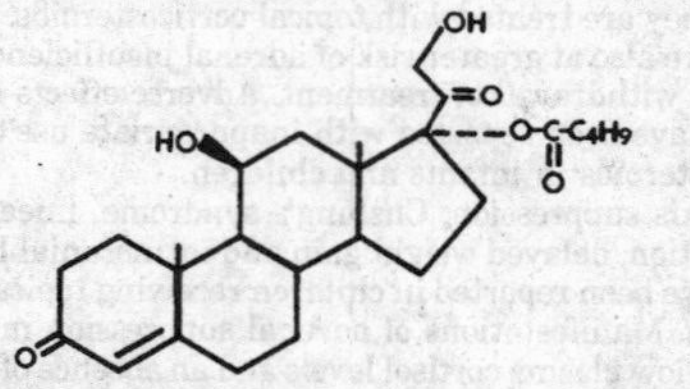

Hydrocortisone valerate has a molecular weight of 446.58. It is a white, crystalline solid, soluble in ethanol and methanol, sparingly soluble in propylene glycol and insoluble in water. Each gram of WESTCORT Ointment contains 2 mg hydrocortisone valerate in a hydrophilic base composed of white petrolatum, stearyl alcohol, propylene glycol, sorbic acid, sodium lauryl sulfate, carbomer 934, dried sodium phosphate, mineral oil, steareth-2, steareth-100, and water.

CLINICAL PHARMACOLOGY

Like other topical corticosteroids, hydrocortisone valerate has anti-inflammatory, anti-pruritic and vasoconstrictive properties. The mechanism of the anti-inflammatory activity of the topical steroids, in general, is unclear. However, corticosteroids are thought to act by the induction of phospholipase A₂ inhibitory proteins, collectively called lipocortins. It is postulated that these proteins control the biosynthesis of potent mediators of inflammation such as prostaglandins and leukotrienes by inhibiting the release of their common precursor arachidonic acid. Arachidonic acid is released from membrane phospholipids by phospholipase A₂.

Pharmacokinetics: The extent of percutaneous absorption of topical corticosteroids is determined by many factors including the vehicle and the integrity of the epidermal barrier. Occlusive dressings with hydrocortisone for up to 24 hours have not been demonstrated to increase penetration; however, occlusion of hydrocortisone for 96 hours markedly enhances penetration. Topical corticosteroids can be absorbed from normal intact skin. Inflammation and/or other disease processes in the skin may increase percutaneous absorption.

Studies performed with WESTCORT Ointment indicate that it is in the medium range of potency as compared with other topical corticosteroids.

INDICATIONS AND USAGE

WESTCORT Ointment is a medium potency corticosteroid indicated for the relief of the inflammatory and pruritic manifestations of corticosteroid responsive dermatoses.

CONTRAINDICATIONS

WESTCORT Ointment is contraindicated in those patients with a history of hypersensitivity to any of the components of the preparation.

PRECAUTIONS

General: Systemic absorption of topical corticosteroids can produce reversible hypothalamic-pituitary-adrenal (HPA) axis suppression with the potential for glucocorticosteroid insufficiency after withdrawal of treatment. Manifestations of Cushing's syndrome, hyperglycemia, and glucosuria can also be produced in some patients by systemic absorption of topical corticosteroids while on treatment.

Patients applying a topical steroid to a large surface area or to areas under occlusion should be evaluated periodically for evidence of HPA axis suppression. This may be done by using the ACTH stimulation, A.M. plasma cortisol, and urinary free cortisol tests.

WESTCORT Ointment has produced mild, reversible adrenal suppression when used under occlusion for 5 days or on extensive areas of psoriasis for 3–4 weeks.

If HPA axis suppression is noted, an attempt should be made to withdraw the drug, to reduce the frequency of application, or to substitute a less potent corticosteroid. Recovery of HPA axis function is generally prompt upon discontinuation of topical corticosteroids. Infrequently, signs and symptoms of glucocorticosteroid insufficiency may occur, requiring supplemental systemic corticosteroids. For information on systemic supplementation, see prescribing information for these products.

Pediatric patients may be more susceptible to systemic toxicity from equivalent doses due to their larger skin surface to body mass ratios. (See PRECAUTIONS—Pediatric Use)

If irritation develops, WESTCORT Ointment should be discontinued and appropriate therapy instituted. Allergic contact dermatitis with corticosteroids is usually diagnosed by observing a failure to heal rather than noting a clinical exacerbation, as with most topical products not containing corticosteroids. Such an observation should be corroborated with appropriate diagnostic patch testing.

If concomitant skin infections are present or develop, an appropriate antifungal or antibacterial agent should be used. If a favorable response does not occur promptly, use of WESTCORT Ointment should be discontinued until the infection has been adequately controlled.

Information for Patients: Patients using topical corticosteroids should receive the following information and instructions:

1. This medication is to be used as directed by the physician. It is for external use only. Avoid contact with the eyes.
2. This medication should not be used for any disorder other than that for which it was prescribed.
3. The treated skin area should not be bandaged, otherwise covered or wrapped, so as to be occlusive unless directed by the physician.
4. Patients should report to their physician any signs of local adverse reactions.
5. This medication should not be used on the face, underarms, or groin areas unless directed by the physician.
6. As with other corticosteroids, therapy should be discontinued when control is achieved. If no improvement is seen within 2 weeks, contact the physician.

Laboratory Tests: The following tests may be helpful in evaluating patients for HPA axis suppression:
ACTH stimulation test
A.M. plasma cortisol test
Urinary free cortisol test

Carcinogenesis, mutagenesis, and impairment of fertility: Long-term animal studies have not been performed to evaluate the carcinogenic potential of hydrocortisone valerate. WESTCORT Ointment was shown to be non-mutagenic in the Ames-Salmonella/Microsome Plate Test.

There are no studies which assess the effects of hydrocortisone valerate on fertility and general reproductive performance.

Pregnancy: Teratogenic Effects: Pregnancy Category C: Corticosteroids have been shown to be teratogenic in laboratory animals when administered systematically at relatively low dosage levels. Some corticosteroids have been shown to be teratogenic after dermal application in laboratory animals. Hydrocortisone valerate was found to be teratogenic in rabbits treated topically with a daily dose 5 times the estimated average human dose. However, there was no evidence of teratogenicity in rats treated topically with 22 times the estimated average human dose.

There are no adequate and well-controlled studies in pregnant women. WESTCORT Ointment should be used during pregnancy only if the potential benefit justifies the potential risk to the fetus.

Nursing Mothers: Systematically administered corticosteroids appear in human milk and could suppress growth, interfere with endogenous corticosteroid production, or cause other untoward effects. It is not known whether topical administration of corticosteroids could result in sufficient systemic absorption to produce detectable quantities in human

milk. Because many drugs are excreted in human milk, caution should be exercised when WESTCORT Ointment is administered to a nursing woman.

Pediatric Use: Safety and effectiveness in pediatric patients have not been established. Because of a higher ratio of skin surface area to body mass, pediatric patients are at a greater risk than adults of HPA axis suppression and Cushing's syndrome when they are treated with topical corticosteroids. They are therefore also at a greater risk of adrenal insufficiency during and/or after withdrawal of treatment. Adverse effects including striae have been reported with inappropriate use of topical corticosteroids in infants and children. (See PRECAUTIONS)

HPA axis suppression, Cushing's syndrome, linear growth retardation, delayed weight gain, and intracranial hypertension have been reported in children receiving topical corticosteroids. Manifestations of adrenal suppression in children include low plasma cortisol levels, and an absence of response to ACTH stimulation. Manifestations of intracranial hypertension include bulging fontanelles, headaches, and bilateral papilledema.

ADVERSE REACTIONS

In controlled clinical trials, the total incidence of adverse reactions associated with the use of WESTCORT Ointment was approximately 12%. These include worsening of condition (2%), transient itching (2%), irritation (1%) and redness (1%).

The following additional local adverse reactions have been reported with topical corticosteroids, and they may occur more frequently with the use of occlusive dressings. These reactions are listed in an approximate decreasing order of occurrence: burning, dryness, folliculitis, acneiform eruptions, hypopigmentation, perioral dermatitis, allergic contact dermatitis, secondary infection, skin atrophy, striae, and miliaria.

OVERDOSAGE

Topically applied WESTCORT Ointment can be absorbed in sufficient amounts to produce systemic effects (see PRECAUTIONS).

DOSAGE AND ADMINISTRATION

WESTCORT Ointment should be applied to the affected area as a thin film two or three times daily depending on the severity of the condition.

As with other corticosteroids, therapy should be discontinued when control is achieved. If no improvement is seen within 2 weeks, reassessment of the diagnosis may be necessary.

WESTCORT Ointment should not be used with occlusive dressings unless directed by a physician. WESTCORT Ointment should not be applied in the diaper area if the patient requires diapers or plastic pants as these garments may constitute occlusive dressing.

HOW SUPPLIED

WESTCORT OINTMENT, 0.2% is supplied in the following tube sizes:
15 g NDC 0072-7800-15
45 g NDC 0072-7800-45
60 g NDC 0072-7800-60
Store between 59°–78°F (15°–26°C)

WESTWOOD SQUIBB™

©1995 Westwood-Squibb Pharmaceuticals Inc., Buffalo, NY, USA 14213   03-5996-0
A Bristol-Myers Squibb Company

Whitby Pharmaceuticals, Inc.

The following products previously marketed by Whitby Pharmaceuticals are now marketed by UCB Pharma, Inc. Please see UCB Pharma, Inc.

Duratuss™   ℞
Duratuss™HD Elixir   Ⓒ℞, ℞
Lortab® Tablets   Ⓒ℞, ℞
Lortab® Elixir   Ⓒ℞, ℞
Lortab® ASA   Ⓒ℞, ℞
Theo-24®   ℞
Trinsicon®   ℞
Vicon®Forte   ℞

Wyeth-Ayerst Laboratories
Division of American Home
Products Corporation
P.O. BOX 8299
PHILADELPHIA, PA 19101

Direct General Inquiries to:
(610) 688-4400

For Medical Information Contact:
Medical Affairs
Day: (800) 934-5556
8:30 AM to 4:30 PM (Eastern Standard Time), Weekdays only
In Emergencies:
Day: (800) 934-5556
Night: (610) 688-4400
(Emergencies only;
non-emergencies should wait until the next day)

For prescribing information for products of Elkins-Sinn Incorporated, see page 980 of the 1997 PDR; ESI Lederle Inc. see page 990; Lederle Laboratories, see page 1414; and page 2232 for products of A.H. Robins Company. Information for these products can also be obtained by writing to Professional Service, Wyeth-Ayerst Laboratories, P.O. Box 8299, Philadelphia, PA 19101, or by contacting your local Wyeth-Ayerst representative.

Product Identification Codes
The following is a numerical list of National Drug Code (NDC) numbers with their corresponding product names for all oral solid dosage forms manufactured by Wyeth-Ayerst Laboratories.

Numerical Listing
Wyeth-Labeled Products

Product Ident. Code	Product
1	Equanil® (meprobamate) Tablet 400 mg. Ⓒ℣
2	Equanil® (meprobamate) Tablet 200 mg. Ⓒ℣
6	Serax® (oxazepam) Capsule 15 mg. Ⓒ℣
13	Amphojel® [dried aluminum hydroxide gel (hydrated alumina)] Tablet 0.6 Gm. (10 gr.)
19	Phenergan® (promethazine HCl) Tablet 12.5 mg.
27	Phenergan® (promethazine HCl) Tablet 25 mg.
28	Sparine® (promazine HCl) Tablet 50 mg.
29	Sparine® (promazine HCl) Tablet 25 mg.
51	Serax® (oxazepam) Capsule 10 mg. Ⓒ℣
52	Serax® (oxazepam) Capsule 30 mg. Ⓒ℣
53	Omnipen® (ampicillin) Capsule 250 mg.
56	Ovral® (each tablet contains 0.5 mg. norgestrel with 0.05 mg. ethinyl estradiol) Tablet, white
57	Unipen® [(nafcillin sodium) as the monohydrate] Capsule 250 mg.
59	Pen·Vee® K (penicillin V potassium) Tablet 250 mg. (400,000 units)
62	Ovrette® (norgestrel) Tablet
64	Ativan® (lorazepam) Tablet 1 mg. Ⓒ℣
65	Ativan® (lorazepam) Tablet 2 mg. Ⓒ℣
71	Mazanor® (mazindol) Tablet 1 mg. Ⓒ℣
73	Wytensin® (guanabenz acetate) Tablet 4 mg.
74	Wytensin® (guanabenz acetate) Tablet 8 mg.
75	Nordette-21® (each tablet contains 0.15 mg. levonorgestrel with 0.03 mg. ethinyl estradiol) Tablet
78	Lo/Ovral® (each tablet contains 0.3 mg. norgestrel with 0.03 mg. ethinyl estradiol) Tablet, white
81	Ativan® (lorazepam) Tablet 0.5 mg. Ⓒ℣
85	Wygesic® (each tablet contains 65 mg. propoxyphene HCl, U.S.P., and 650 mg. acetaminophen, U.S.P.) Tablet Ⓒ℣
91	Equagesic® (meprobamate with aspirin) Tablet
119	Amphojel® [dried aluminum hydroxide gel (hydrated alumina)] Tablet 0.3 Gm. (5 gr.)
227	Phenergan® (promethazine HCl) Tablet 50 mg.
261	Mepergan® Fortis (meperidine HCl and promethazine HCl) Capsule Ⓒ℣
308	Meperidine HCl Tablet USP 50 mg. Ⓒ℣
309	Omnipen® (ampicillin) Capsule 500 mg.
317	Serax® (oxazepam) Capsule 15 mg. Ⓒ℣
390	Pen·Vee® K (penicillin V potassium) Tablet 500 mg. (800,000 units)
445	Ovral®-28 pink inert tablet
472	Basaljel® (dried basic aluminum carbonate gel) Capsule
486	Nordette®-28, Lo/Ovral®-28 pink inert tablet

559	Wymox® (amoxicillin) Capsule 250 mg.
560	Wymox® (amoxicillin) Capsule 500 mg.
690	Oruvail® (ketoprofen) Extended-Release Capsules 200 mg.
701	Effexor® (venlafaxine HCl) Tablet 25 mg.
703	Effexor® (venlafaxine HCl) Tablet 50 mg.
704	Effexor® (venlafaxine HCl) Tablet 75 mg.
705	Effexor® (venlafaxine HCl) Tablet 100 mg.
750	Basaljel® (dried basic aluminum carbonate gel) Tablet
771	Ismo® (isosorbide dinitrate) Tablet 20 mg.
781	Effexor® (venlafaxine HCl) Tablet 37.5 mg.
821	Oruvail® (ketoprofen) Extended-Release Capsules 100 mg.
822	Oruvail® (ketoprofen) Extended-Release Capsules 150 mg.
901	Naprelan® (naproxen sodium) Controlled Release Tablet 375 mg.
902	Naprelan® (naproxen sodium) Controlled Release Tablet 500 mg.
904	Redux™(dexfenfluramine HCl) Capsule 15 mg. Ⓒ℣
2511	Ovral®-28 Pilpak® (21 white tablets each containing 0.5 mg. norgestrel with 0.05 mg. ethinyl estradiol and 7 pink inert tablets)
2514	Lo/Ovral®-28 Pilpak® (21 white tablets each containing 0.3 mg. norgestrel with 0.03 mg. ethinyl estradiol and 7 pink inert tablets)
2533	Nordette®-28 Pilpak® (21 light-orange tablets each containing 0.15 mg. levonorgestrel with 0.03 mg ethinyl estradiol and 7 pink inert tablets)
2535	Triphasil®-21 Tablets (levonorgestrel and ethinyl estradiol tablets—triphasic regimen)
2536	Triphasil®-28 Tablets (levonorgestrel and ethinyl estradiol tablets—triphasic regimen)
4124	Cyclospasmol® (cyclandelate) Capsule 200 mg.
4125	Isordil® Tembids® Tablet 40 mg.
4126	Isordil® Sublingual Tablet 5 mg.
4130	Trecator®-SC (ethionamide) Tablet 250 mg.
4132	Surmontil® (trimipramine) Capsule 25 mg.
4133	Surmontil® (trimipramine) Capsule 50 mg.
4139	Isordil® (isosorbide dinitrate) Sublingual Tablet 2.5 mg.
4140	Isordil® (isosorbide dinitrate) Tembids® Capsule 40 mg.
4148	Cyclospasmol® (cyclandelate) Capsule 400 mg.
4152	Isordil® (isosorbide dinitrate) 5 Titradose Tablet 5 mg.
4153	Isordil® (isosorbide dinitrate) 10 Titradose Tablet 10 mg.
4154	Isordil® (isosorbide dinitrate) 20 Titradose Tablet 20 mg.
4158	Surmontil® (trimipramine) Capsule 100 mg.
4159	Isordil® (isosorbide dinitrate) 30 Titradose Tablet 30 mg.
4161	Isordil® (isosorbide dinitrate) Sublingual Tablet 10 mg.
4177	Sectral® (acebutolol) Capsule 200 mg.
4179	Sectral® (acebutolol) Capsule 400 mg.
4181	Orudis® (ketoprofen) Capsule 50 mg.
4186	Orudis® (ketoprofen) Capsule 25 mg.
4187	Orudis® (ketoprofen) Capsule 75 mg.
4188	Cordarone® (amiodarone) Tablet 200 mg.
4191	Synalgos®-DC (each capsule contains 16 mg. dihydrocodeine bitartrate, 356.4 mg. aspirin, and 30 mg. caffeine) Capsule
4192	Isordil® (isosorbide dinitrate) 40 Titradose Tablet 40 mg.

Ayerst-Labeled Products

243	Atromid-S® (clofibrate) Capsule 500 mg.
421	Inderal® (propranolol HCl) Tablet 10 mg.
422	Inderal® (propranolol HCl) Tablet 20 mg.
424	Inderal® (propranolol HCl) Tablet 40 mg.
426	Inderal® (propranolol HCl) Tablet 60 mg.
428	Inderal® (propranolol HCl) Tablet 80 mg.
430	Mysoline® (primidone) Tablet 250 mg.
431	Mysoline® (primidone) Tablet 50 mg.
443	Grisactin® 250 (griseofulvin, microsize) Capsule 250 mg.
444	Grisactin® 500 (griseofulvin, microsize) Tablet 500 mg.
455	Inderide® LA (each capsule contains 80 mg. Inderal® LA [propranolol HCl] and 50 mg. hydrochlorothiazide) Capsule
457	Inderide® LA (each capsule contains 120 mg. Inderal® LA [propranolol HCl] and 50 mg. hydrochlorothiazide) Capsule
459	Inderide® LA (each capsule contains 160 mg. Inderal® LA [propranolol HCl] and 50 mg. hydrochlorothiazide) Capsule
470	Inderal® LA (propranolol HCl) Capsule 60 mg.
471	Inderal® LA (propranolol HCl) Capsule 80 mg.
473	Inderal® LA (propranolol HCl) Capsule 120 mg.

Continued on next page

Consult 1997 supplements and future editions for revisions

Wyeth-Ayerst Laboratories—Cont.

479 Inderal® LA (propranolol HCl) Capsule 160 mg.
484 Inderide® (each tablet contains 40 mg. Inderal® [propranolol HCl] and 25 mg. hydrochlorothiazide) Tablet
488 Inderide® (each tablet contains 80 mg. Inderal® [propranolol HCl] and 25 mg. hydrochlorothiazide) Tablet
702 Diucardin® (hydroflumethiazide) Tablet 50 mg.
738 Lodine® (etodolac) Capsule 200 mg.
739 Lodine® (etodolac) Capsule 300 mg.
755 Plegine® (phendimetrazine tartrate) Tablet 35 mg. CIII
761 Lodine® (etodolac) Tablet 400 mg.
787 Lodine® (etodolac) Tablet 500 mg.
809 Antabuse® (disulfiram) Tablet 250 mg.
810 Antabuse® (disulfiram) Tablet 500 mg.
864 Premarin® (conjugated estrogens tablets, USP) Tablet 0.9 mg.
865 Premarin® (conjugated estrogens tablets, USP) Tablet 2.5 mg.
866 Premarin® (conjugated estrogens tablets, USP) Tablet 1.25 mg.
867 Premarin® (conjugated estrogens tablets, USP) Tablet 0.625 mg.
868 Premarin® (conjugated estrogens tablets, USP) Tablet 0.3 mg.
875 Prempro™ (conjugated estrogens/medroxyprogesterone acetate 0.625 mg./2.5 mg. [continuous regimen] Tablets)
880 PMB® 200 (each tablet contains 0.45 mg. Premarin® [conjugated estrogens, USP] and 200 mg. meprobamate) Tablet
881 PMB® 400 (each tablet contains 0.45 mg. Premarin® [conjugated estrogens, USP] and 400 mg. meprobamate) Tablet
2573 Premphase® (conjugated estrogens/medroxyprogesterone acetate 0.625 mg./5 mg. [sequential regimen] Tablets)

AMPHOJEL® OTC

[am 'fo-jel]
(aluminum hydroxide gel)
ORAL SUSPENSION • TABLETS

COMPOSITION

Suspension—Peppermint flavored—Each teaspoonful (5 ml) contains 320 mg of aluminum hydroxide [$Al(OH)_3$] as a gel, and not more than 0.10 mEq of sodium. The inactive ingredients present are calcium benzoate, glycerin, hydroxypropyl methylcellulose, menthol, peppermint oil, potassium butylparaben, potassium propylparaben, saccharin, simethicone, sorbitol solution, and water.
Suspension—Without flavor—Each teaspoonful (5 ml) contains 320 mg of aluminum hydroxide [$Al(OH)_3$] as a gel. The inactive ingredients present are butylparaben, calcium benzoate, glycerin, hydroxypropyl methylcellulose, methylparaben, propylparaben, saccharin, simethicone, sorbitol solution, and water.
Tablets available in 0.3 Gm and 0.6 Gm strengths. Each contains, respectively, the equivalent of 300 mg and 600 mg aluminum hydroxide as a dried gel. The inactive ingredients present are artificial and natural flavors, cellulose, hydrogenated vegetable oil, magnesium stearate, polacrilin potassium, saccharin, starch, and talc. The 0.3 Gm (5 grain) strength is equivalent to about 1 teaspoonful of the suspension and the 0.6 Gm (10 grain) strength is equivalent to about 2 teaspoonfuls. Each 0.3 Gm tablet contains 0.08 mEq of sodium and each 0.6 Gm tablet contains 0.13 mEq of sodium.

INDICATIONS

For the symptomatic relief of hyperacidity associated with the diagnosis of peptic ulcer, gastritis, peptic esophagitis, gastric hyperacidity, and hiatal hernia.

DOSAGE

Suspension—two teaspoonfuls followed by a sip of water if desired, five or six times daily, between meals and on retiring. Two teaspoonfuls have the capacity to neutralize 20 mEq of acid. *Tablets*—Two tablets of the 0.3 Gm. strength, or one tablet of the 0.6 Gm. strength, five or six times daily between meals and on retiring. Two tablets have the capacity to neutralize 16 mEq of acid.
It is unnecessary to chew the 0.3 Gm tablet before swallowing with water. After chewing the 0.6 Gm tablet, one-half glass of water should be sipped.

WARNINGS

Patients are advised not to take more than 1 teaspoonfuls (60 ml) or twelve (12) 0.3 Gm tablets or six (6) 0.6 Gm tablets in a 24-hour period or use this maximum dosage for more than two weeks except under the advice and supervision of a physician. Prolonged use of aluminum-containing antacids in patients with renal failure may result in or worsen dialysis osteomalacia. Elevated tissue aluminum levels contribute to the development of dialysis encephalopathy and osteomalacia syndromes. Also, a number of cases of dialysis encephalopathy have been associated with elevated aluminum levels in the dialysate water. Small amounts of aluminum are absorbed from the gastrointestinal tract and reneal excretion of aluminum is impaired in renal failure. Prolonged use of aluminum-containing antacids in such patients may contribute to increased plasma levels of aluminum. Aluminum is not well removed by dialysis because it is bound to albumin and transferrin, which do not cross dialysis membranes. As a result, aluminum is deposited in bone, and dialysis osteomalacia may develop when large amounts of aluminum are ingested orally by patients with impaired renal function. Pregnant women and nursing mothers are advised to seek the advice of a health professional before using this product.

PRECAUTION

May cause constipation.

DRUG INTERACTION PRECAUTIONS

Antacids may interact with certain prescription drugs.
This product must not be taken if the patient is presently taking a prescription antibiotic drug containing any form of tetracycline.
If patients are presently taking a prescription drug, they are advised to check with their physicians before taking this product.

HOW SUPPLIED

Suspension—Peppermint flavored; without flavor—bottles of 12 fluidounces. *Tablets*—a convenient auxiliary dosage form—0.3 Gm. (5 gr.), bottles of 100; 0.6 Gm. (10 gr.), boxes of 100.

ANTABUSE® ℞

[an 'tah-būse]
(disulfiram)
IN ALCOHOLISM

Caution: Federal law prohibits dispensing without prescription.

> **WARNING**
> Antabuse should *never* be administered to a patient when he is in a state of alcohol intoxication, or without his full knowledge.
> The physician should instruct relatives accordingly.

DESCRIPTION

CHEMICAL NAME: bis(diethylthiocarbamoyl) disulfide
STRUCTURAL FORMULA:

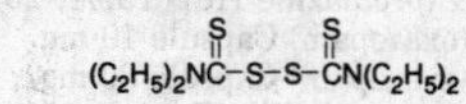

Antabuse occurs as a white to off-white, odorless, and almost tasteless powder, soluble in water to the extent of about 20 mg in 100 mL, and in alcohol to the extent of about 3.8 g in 100 mL.
Antabuse contains these inactive ingredients: magnesium aluminum silicate; magnesium stearate, NF; povidone, USP; starch, NF.

ACTION

Antabuse produces a sensitivity to alcohol which results in a highly unpleasant reaction when the patient under treatment ingests even small amounts of alcohol.
Antabuse blocks the oxidation of alcohol at the acetaldehyde stage. During alcohol metabolism following Antabuse intake, the concentration of acetaldehyde occurring in the blood may be 5- to 10-times higher than that found during metabolism of the same amount of alcohol alone.
Accumulation of acetaldehyde in the blood produces a complex of highly unpleasant symptoms referred to hereinafter as the Antabase-alcohol reaction. This reaction, which is proportional to the dosage of both Antabuse and alcohol, will persist as long as alcohol is being metabolized. Antabuse does not appear to influence the rate of alcohol elimination from the body.
Antabuse is absorbed slowly from the gastrointestinal tract and eliminated slowly from the body. One (or even two) weeks after a patient has taken his last dose of Antabuse, ingestion of alcohol may produce unpleasant symptoms.
Prolonged administration of Antabuse does not produce tolerance; the longer a patient remains on therapy, the more exquisitely sensitive he becomes to alcohol.

INDICATION

Antabuse is an aid in the management of selected chronic alcoholic patients who *want* to remain in a state of enforced sobriety so that supportive and psychotherapeutic treatment may be applied to best advantage.
Antabuse is not a cure for alcoholism. When used alone, without proper motivation and supportive therapy, it is unlikely that it will have any substantive effect on the drinking pattern of the chronic alcoholic.

CONTRAINDICATIONS

Patients who are receiving or have recently received metronidazole, paraldehyde, alcohol, or alcohol-containing preparations, e.g., cough syrups, tonics and the like, should not be given Antabuse.
Antabuse is contraindicated in the presence of severe myocardial disease or coronary occlusion, psychoses, and hypersensitivity to disulfiram or to other thiuram derivatives used in pesticides and rubber vulcanization.

WARNINGS

> Antabuse should *never* be administered to a patient when he is in a state of alcohol intoxication, or without his full knowledge.
> The physician should instruct relatives accordingly.

The patient must be fully informed of the Antabuse-alcohol reaction. He must be strongly cautioned against surreptitious drinking while taking the drug, and he must be fully aware of possible consequences. He should be warned to avoid alcohol in disguised form, i.e., in sauces, vinegars, cough mixtures, and even aftershave lotions and back rubs. He should also be warned that reactions may occur with alcohol up to 14 days after ingesting Antabuse.
THE ANTABUSE-ALCOHOL REACTION:
Antabuse plus alcohol, even small amounts, produces flushing, throbbing in head and neck, throbbing headache, respiratory difficulty, nausea, copious vomiting, sweating, thirst, chest pain, palpitation, dyspnea, hyperventilation, tachycardia, hypotension, syncope, marked uneasiness, weakness, vertigo, blurred vision, and confusion. In severe reactions there may be respiratory depression, cardiovascular collapse, arrhythmias, myocardial infarction, acute congestive heart failure, unconsciousness, convulsions, and death.
The intensity of the reaction varies with each individual but is generally proportional to the amounts of Antabuse and alcohol ingested. Mild reactions may occur in the sensitive individual when the blood alcohol concentration is increased to as little as 5 to 10 mg per 100 mL. Symptoms are fully developed at 50 mg per 100 mL, and unconsciousness usually results when the blood alcohol level reaches 125 to 150 mg.
The duration of the reaction varies from 30 to 60 minutes, to several hours in the more severe cases, or as long as there is alcohol in the blood.
DRUG INTERACTIONS
Disulfiram appears to decrease the rate at which certain drugs are metabolized and therefore may increase the blood levels and the possibility of clinical toxicity of drugs given concomitantly.
DISULFIRAM SHOULD BE USED WITH CAUTION IN THOSE PATIENTS RECEIVING PHENYTOIN AND ITS CONGENERS, SINCE THE CONCOMITANT ADMINISTRATION OF THESE TWO DRUGS CAN LEAD TO PHENYTOIN INTOXICATION. PRIOR TO ADMINISTERING DISULFIRAM TO A PATIENT ON PHENYTOIN THERAPY, A BASELINE PHENYTOIN SERUM LEVEL SHOULD BE OBTAINED. SUBSEQUENT TO INITIATION OF DISULFIRAM THERAPY, SERUM LEVELS OF PHENYTOIN SHOULD BE DETERMINED ON DIFFERENT DAYS FOR EVIDENCE OF AN INCREASE OR FOR A CONTINUING RISE IN LEVELS. INCREASED PHENYTOIN LEVELS SHOULD BE TREATED WITH APPROPRIATE DOSAGE ADJUSTMENT.
It may be necessary to adjust the dosage of oral anticoagulants upon beginning or stopping disulfiram, since disulfiram may prolong prothrombin time.
Patients taking isoniazid when disulfiram is given should be observed for the appearance of unsteady gait or marked changes in mental status; the disulfiram should be discontinued if such signs appear.
In rats, simultaneous ingestion of disulfiram and nitrite in the diet for 78 weeks has been reported to cause tumors, and it has been suggested that disulfiram may react with nitrites in the rat stomach to form a nitrosamine, which is tumorigenic. Disulfiram alone in the rats' diet did not lead to such tumors. The relevance of this finding to humans is not known at this time.
CONCOMITANT CONDITIONS
Because of the possibility of an accidental Antabuse-alcohol reaction, Antabuse should be used with extreme caution in patients with any of the following conditions: diabetes mellitus, hypothyroidism, epilepsy, cerebral damage, chronic and acute nephritis, hepatic cirrhosis or insufficiency.
USAGE IN PREGNANCY
The safe use of this drug in pregnancy has not been established. Therefore, Antabuse should be used during pregnancy only when, in the judgment of the physician, the probable benefits outweigh the possible risks.

PRECAUTIONS

Patients with a history of rubber contact dermatitis should be evaluated for hypersensitivity to thiuram derivatives before receiving Antabuse (see "Contraindications").

It is suggested that every patient under treatment carry an *Identification Card*, stating that he is receiving Antabuse and describing the symptoms most likely to occur as a result of the Antabuse-alcohol reaction. In addition, this card should indicate the physician or institution to be contacted in an emergency. (Cards may be obtained from Wyeth-Ayerst Laboratories upon request.)

Alcoholism may accompany or be followed by dependence on narcotics or sedatives. Barbiturates and Antabuse have been administered concurrently without untoward effects; the possibility of initiating a new abuse should be considered.

Baseline and follow-up transaminase tests (10 to 14 days) are suggested to detect any hepatic dysfunction that may result with Antabuse therapy. In addition, a complete blood count and a sequential multiple analysis-12 (SMA-12) test should be made every six months.

Patients taking Antabuse Tablets should not be exposed to ethylene dibromide or its vapors. This precaution is based on preliminary results of animal research currently in progress that suggest a toxic interaction between inhaled ethylene dibromide and ingested disulfiram resulting in a higher incidence of tumors and mortality in rats. A correlation between this finding and humans, however, has not been demonstrated.

ADVERSE REACTIONS

(See "Contraindications," "Warnings," and "Precautions.")

OPTIC NEURITIS, PERIPHERAL NEURITIS, POLYNEURITIS, AND PERIPHERAL NEUROPATHY MAY OCCUR FOLLOWING ADMINISTRATION OF ANTABUSE.

Multiple cases of hepatitis, including both cholestatic and fulminant hepatitis, have been reported to be associated with administration of Antabuse.

Occasional skin eruptions are, as a rule, readily controlled by concomitant administration of an antihistaminic drug.

In a small number of patients, a transient mild drowsiness, fatigability, impotence, headache, acneform eruptions, allergic dermatitis, or a metallic or garlic-like aftertaste may be experienced during the first two weeks of therapy. These complaints usually disappear spontaneously with the continuation of therapy, or with reduced dosage.

Psychotic reactions have been noted, attributable in most cases to high dosage, combined toxicity (with metronidazole or isoniazid), or to the unmasking of underlying psychoses in patients stressed by the withdrawal of alcohol.

DOSAGE AND ADMINISTRATION

Antabuse should never be administered until the patient has abstained from alcohol for at least 12 hours.

INITIAL DOSAGE SCHEDULE

In the first phase of treatment, a *maximum* of 500 mg daily is given in a single dose for one to two weeks. Although usually taken in the morning, Antabuse may be taken on retiring by patients who experience a sedative effect. Alternatively, to minimize, or eliminate, the sedative effect, dosage may be adjusted downward.

MAINTENANCE REGIMEN

The average maintenance dose is 250 mg daily (range, 125 to 500 mg); it should not exceed 500 mg daily.

Note: Occasionally patients, while seemingly on adequate maintenance doses of Antabuse, report that they are able to drink alcoholic beverages with impunity and without any symptomatology. All appearances to the contrary, such patients must be presumed to be disposing of their tablets in some manner without actually taking them. Until such patients have been observed reliably taking their daily Antabuse Tablets (preferably crushed and well mixed with liquid), it cannot be concluded that Antabuse is ineffective.

DURATION OF THERAPY

The daily, uninterrupted administration of Antabuse must be continued until the patient is fully recovered socially and a basis for permanent self-control is established. Depending on the individual patient, maintenance therapy may be required for months, or even years.

TRIAL WITH ALCOHOL

During early experience with Antabuse, it was thought advisable for each patient to have at least one supervised alcohol-drug reaction. More recently, the test reaction has been largely abandoned. Furthermore, such a test reaction should never be administered to a patient over 50 years of age. A clear, detailed, and convincing description of the reaction is felt to be sufficient in most cases.

However, where a test reaction is deemed necessary, the suggested procedure is as follows:

After the first one to two weeks' therapy with 500 mg daily, a drink of 15 mL (½ oz) of 100 proof whiskey, or equivalent, is taken slowly. This test dose of alcoholic beverage may be repeated once only, so that the total dose does not exceed 30 mL (1 oz) of whiskey. Once a reaction develops, no more alcohol should be consumed. Such tests should be carried out only when the patient is hospitalized, or comparable supervision and facilities, including oxygen, are available.

MANAGEMENT OF ANTABUSE-ALCOHOL REACTION:

In severe reactions, whether caused by an excessive test dose or by the patient's unsupervised ingestion of alcohol, supportive measures to restore blood pressure and treat shock should be instituted. Other recommendations include: oxygen, carbogen (95% oxygen and 5% carbon dioxide), vitamin C intravenously in massive doses (1 g), and ephedrine sulfate. Antihistamines have also been used intravenously. Potassium levels should be monitored, particularly in patients on digitalis, since hypokalemia has been reported.

HOW SUPPLIED

Antabuse® (disulfiram) Tablets are available in the following dosage strengths:

250 mg, NDC 0046-0809-81, white-to-off-white, octagonal-shaped, scored, compressed tablet, embossed with a stylized "A" on one side and imprinted with "ANTABUSE" and "250" on the scored reverse side, in bottles of 100 tablets.

500 mg, NDC 0046-0810-50, white-to-off-white, octagonal-shaped, scored compressed tablet, embossed with a stylized "A" on one side and imprinted with "ANTABUSE" and "500" on the scored reverse side, in bottles of 50 tablets.

Store at room temperature, approximately 25°C.

Dispense in a tight, light-resistant container as defined in the USP

Shown in Product Identification Guide, page 339

ANTIVENIN (CROTALIDAE) ℞

[an "te ven 'in]

POLYVALENT

(equine origin)

IMPORTANT

Pit viper bites may cause severe tissue damage or fatal envenomation, or both. The physician responsible for treatment of an envenomated patient should be familiar with the contents of this brochure and the pertinent medical literature concerning current concepts of first-aid and general supportive therapy as presented in the references listed at the end of this pamphlet.

COMPOSITION

Antivenin (Crotalidae) Polyvalent, Wyeth, is a refined and concentrated preparation of serum globulins obtained by fractionating blood from healthy horses immunized with the following venoms: *Crotalus adamanteus* (Eastern diamond rattlesnake), *C. atrox* (Western diamond rattlesnake), *C. durissus terrificus* (tropical rattlesnake, Cascabel), and *Bothrops atrox* ("Fer-de-lance"). Phenol, 0.25%, and thimerosal, 0.005%, are added as preservatives. The product is standardized by its ability to neutralize the lethal action of standard venoms by intravenous injection in mice.[1] Dried from the frozen state, the lyophilized serum has a moisture content of less than 1% and is soluble on addition of the diluent contained in each package (Bacteriostatic Water for Injection, USP, with preservative: 0.001% phenylmercuric nitrate).

Antivenin (Crotalidae) Polyvalent, Wyeth (hereinafter referred to as Antivenin) contains protective substances capable of neutralizing the toxic effects of venoms of crotalids (pit vipers) native to North, Central, and South America, including rattlesnakes *(Crotalus, Sistrurus);* copperhead and cottonmouth moccasins *(Agkistrodon),* including *A. halys* of Korea and Japan; the Fer-de-lance and other species of *Bothrops;* the tropical rattler *(Crotalus durissus* and similar species); the Cantil *(A. bilineatus);* and bushmaster *(Lachesis mutus)* of South and Central America.

INDICATION

Antivenin is indicated only for the treatment of envenomation caused by bites of those crotalids (pit vipers) specified in the immediately preceding paragraph.

PIT VIPER BITES AND ENVENOMATION

The symptoms, signs, and severity of snake-venom poisoning resulting from pit viper bites depend on many factors, including, but not limited to, the following variables: species, age, and size of the biting snake; the number and location of bite(s); the depth of venom deposit by the snake's fangs; the condition of the snake's fangs and venom glands; the length of time the snake "hangs on"; the age, general health, and size of the victim; the type and efficacy of any first-aid treatment rendered in an attempt to remove venom and how soon such treatment was applied. In any venomous snake bite, the actual amount of venom introduced into the victim is always an unknown. Even the type of clothing or leg-footwear through which the snake's fangs pass may affect the amount of venom delivered by the bite. Although most North American pit vipers tend to bite and introduce venom superficially, their fangs may get hung-up in the subcutaneous tissues during the biting act and can penetrate deeper tissues during the attempt to release the bitten part. In some bites the fangs may penetrate into muscle. In such cases, the usual local superficial manifestations of envenomation may not appear early in the course of poisoning. In bites by some species, systemic evidence of envenomation may be present in the absence of significant local manifestations. It may be difficult to determine the severity of envenomation during the first several hours after a pit viper bite and estimates of severity may need to be revised as poisoning progresses. It must be remembered, too, that not all pit viper bites result in envenomation. In approximately 20% of rattlesnake bites, the snake may not inject any venom. The local and systemic symptoms and signs of envenomation include the following:

LOCAL:

Fang puncture(s).

Swelling—edema is usually seen around the site of bite within five minutes. It may progress rapidly and involve the entire extremity within an hour. More than 95% of all snakebites are inflicted on extremities.[2] Generally, however, edema spreads more slowly, usually over a period of 8 or more hours. Swelling is usually most severe following envenomation by the Eastern diamondback; less severe after bites by the Western diamondback, prairie, timber, red, Pacific, Mojave, and blacktailed rattlers, the sidewinder and cottonmouth moccasins; least severe after bites by copperheads, massasaugas, and pygmy rattlers.

Ecchymosis and discoloration of the skin—often appear in the area of the bite within a few hours. Vesicules may form within a few hours and are usually present at 24 hours. Hemorrhagic blebs and petechiae are common. Necrosis may develop, necessitating amputation of an extremity or a portion thereof.

Pain—frequently a complaint of the victim beginning shortly after the bite by most pit vipers. Pain may be absent after bites by Mojave rattlers.

SYSTEMIC:

Weakness; faintness; nausea; sweating; numbness or tingling around the mouth, tongue, scalp, fingers, toes, site of bite; muscle fasciculations; hypotension; prolongation of bleeding and clotting times; hemoconcentration, early followed by a decrease in erythrocytes; thrombocytopenia; hematuria; proteinuria; vomiting, including hematemesis; melena; hemoptysis; epistaxis. In fatal poisoning, a frequent cause of death is associated with destruction of erythrocytes and changes in capillary permeability, especially of the pulmonary vascular system, leading to pulmonary edema; hemoconcentration usually occurs early, probably as a result of plasma loss secondary to vascular permeability; the hemoglobin may fall, and bleeding may occur throughout the body as early as 6 hours after the bite. Renal involvement is not uncommon. Mojave rattler venom may cause neuromuscular changes leading to respiratory failure.

An estimate of the severity of envenomation should be made as soon as possible and before any Antivenin is administered. The amount (volume) of the first dose of Antivenin is determined on this estimate of severity. Every symptom, sign, laboratory-test result, and any other pertinent information should be considered in estimating severity—local manifestations; systemic manifestations, including abnormal laboratory findings; species and size of the biting snake, if known; number and location of bite(s); size and health of the patient; type of first-aid treatment rendered; and interval between bite and arrival for treatment. Russell et al,[3] and Wingert and Wainschel[4] grade severity as follows:

No envenomation—no local or systemic manifestations.

Minimal envenomation—local swelling and other local changes; no systemic manifestations; normal laboratory findings.

Moderate envenomation—swelling progressing beyond the site of bite and one or more systemic manifestations; abnormal laboratory findings, for example, a fall in hematocrit or platelets.

Severe envenomation—marked local response, severe systemic manifestations and significant alteration in laboratory findings.

Parrish and Hayes,[5] McCollough and Gennaro,[6] and Watt and Gennaro[7] have used a Grade 0 (no envenomation) through Grade IV (very severe) classification of severity which was developed for the most part in treatment of envenomation by the Eastern diamondback and timber rattlers. This classification is more dependent on local manifestations, or the absence thereof, as the venoms of these species seem to be more consistent in inducing local tissue damage.

Any suspected envenomation should be treated as a medical emergency, and until careful observation provides clear evidence that envenomation has not occurred or is minimal, the following procedures are recommended:

Monitor vital signs at frequent intervals: Blood pressure, pulse, respiration.

Draw sufficient blood as soon as possible for baseline laboratory studies, including type and cross-match, CBC, hematocrit, platelet count, prothrombin time, clot retraction, bleeding and coagulation times, BUN, electrolytes, bilirubin. Some of these studies may need to be repeated at daily intervals, or less, depending on the severity of envenomation and the response to treatment. During the first 4 or 5 days of se-

Continued on next page

Wyeth-Ayerst Laboratories—Cont.

vere envenomations, hemoglobin, hematocrit, and platelet counts should be carried out several times a day.
Obtain urine samples at frequent intervals for analysis, with special attention to microscopic examination for presence of erythrocytes.
Chart fluid intake and urine output.
Measure and record the circumference of the bitten extremity just proximal to the bite and at one or more additional points each several inches closer to the trunk. Repeat measurements every 15-30 minutes to obtain information about progression of edema.
Have available and ready for immediate use: oxygen, resuscitation equipment including airway, tourniquet, epinephrine, injectable antihistaminic agents and corticosteroids.
Start an intravenous infusion in one or two extremities: one line to be used for supportive therapy, if needed, such as whole blood, plasma, packed red cells, specific clotting factors, platelet transfusion, plasma expanders; the other line to be used for administration of Antivenin and electrolytes.
Carry out and interpret a skin test for horse-serum sensitivity. (See "Precautions" section below.)

DOSAGE AND ADMINISTRATION

Before administration, read "Precautions" and "Systemic Reactions" sections below. Since the possibility of a severe immediate reaction (anaphylaxis) exists whenever a horse-serum-containing product is administered, appropriate therapeutic agents, including a tourniquet, airway, oxygen, epinephrine, an injectable pressor amine, and corticosteroid, must be available and ready for immediate use. Constant attendance and observation of the patient for untoward reactions are mandatory when Antivenin is administered. Should any systemic reaction occur, administration should be discontinued immediately and appropriate treatment initiated.
The intravenous route of administration is preferred, and probably should always be used for moderate or severe envenomation. Intravenous administration is mandatory if venom-induced shock is present. To be most effective, Antivenin should be administered within 4 hours of the bite; it is less effective when given after 8 hours and may be of questionable value after 12 hours. However, it is recommended that Antivenin therapy be given in severe poisonings, even if 24 hours have elapsed since the time of the bite. It should be kept in mind that maximum blood levels of Antivenin may not be obtained for 8 or more hours after intramuscular administration.
For intravenous-drip use, prepare a 1:1 to 1:10 dilution of reconstituted Antivenin in Sodium Chloride Injection, USP, or 5% Dextrose Injection, USP. To avoid foaming, mix by gently swirling rather than shaking. Allow the initial 5 to 10 mL to infuse over a 3- to 5-minute period, with careful observation of the patient for evidence of untoward reaction. If no symptoms or signs of an immediate systemic reaction appear, continue the infusion with delivery at the maximum safe rate for intravenous fluid administration. The dilution of Antivenin to be used, the type of electrolyte solution used for dilution, and the rate of intravenous delivery of the diluted Antivenin must take into consideration the age, weight, and cardiac status of the patient; the severity of envenomation; the total amount and type of parenteral fluids it is anticipated will be given or are needed; and the interval between bite and initiation of specific therapy.
It is important to give as soon as possible the entire initial dose of Antivenin as based on the best estimate of the severity of envenomation at the time treatment is begun. The following initial doses are recommended:[3,4,8]
no envenomation—none
minimal envenomation—20-40 mL (contents of 2 to 4 vials)
moderate envenomation—50-90 mL (contents of 5 to 9 vials)
severe envenomation—100-150 mL or more (contents of 10 to 15 or more vials)
These recommended initial-dosage volumes are in general accord with those of others.[5-7,9]
The need for additional Antivenin must be based on the clinical response to the initial dose and continuing assessment of the severity of poisoning. If swelling continues to progress or if systemic symptoms or signs of envenomation increase in severity or if new manifestations appear, for example, fall in hematocrit or hypotension, administer an additional 10 to 50 mL (contents of 1 to 5 vials) intravenously.
Envenomation by large snakes in children or small adults requires larger doses of Antivenin. The amount administered to a child is not based on weight.
If Antivenin is given intramuscularly, it should be given into a large muscle mass, preferably the gluteal area, with care to avoid nerve trunks. Antivenin should never be injected into a finger or toe.
The effectiveness of corticosteroids in treatment of envenomation per se or venom shock is not resolved. Russell[3] and others[9,10] believe corticosteroids may mask the seriousness of hypovolemia in moderate or severe poisoning and have little, if any, effect on the local-tissue response to rattler venoms. Corticosteroids should not be given simultaneously with Antivenin on a routine basis or during the acute state of envenomation; however, their use may be necessary to treat immediate allergic reactions to Antivenin, and corticosteroids are the agents of choice for treating serious delayed reactions to Antivenin.
Snakes' mouths do not harbor *Clostridium tetani*. However, appropriate tetanus prophylaxis is indicated, since tetanus spores may be carried into the fang puncture wounds by dirt present on skin at time of bite or by nonsterile first-aid procedures.
A broad-spectrum antibiotic in adequate dosage is indicated if local tissue damage is evident.
Shock following envenomation is treated like shock resulting from hypovolemia from any cause, including administration of whole blood, plasma, albumin, or other plasma expanders, as indicated.
Aspirin or codeine is usually adequate for relieving pain. Sedation with phenobarbital or mild tranquilizers may be used if indicated, but not in the presence of respiratory failure.
The bitten extremity should not be packed in ice, and so-called "cryotherapy" is contraindicated.
Compartment syndromes may complicate pit viper envenomations, especially those caused by bites on the lower extremities. Prompt surgical consultation is indicated whenever a closed-compartment syndrome is suspected.[3,12]
Defibrination and disseminated intravascular coagulation (DIC) syndromes have been associated with envenomation caused by some pit vipers native to the United States, and appropriate therapy may be indicated.[3,9,10,13–17]

TECHNIC FOR RECONSTITUTING THE DRIED ANTIVENIN

Pry off the small metal disc in the cap over the diaphragms of the vials of Antivenin and diluent. Swab the exposed surface of the rubber diaphragms of both vials with an appropriate germicide. With a sterile 10 mL syringe and needle, withdraw the diluent (Bacteriostatic Water for Injection, USP, containing phenylmercuric nitrate 1:100,000) from the vial of diluent and inject it into the vial of Antivenin. Gentle agitation will hasten complete dissolution of the lyophilized Antivenin.

PRECAUTIONS

Before administration of any product prepared from horse serum, appropriate measures must be taken in an effort to detect the presence of dangerous sensitivity: (1) A careful review of the patient's history, including any report of (a) asthma, hay fever, urticaria, or other allergic manifestations; (b) allergic reactions upon exposure to horses; and (c) prior injections of horse serum. (2) A suitable test for detection of sensitivity. A skin test should be performed in every patient prior to administration, regardless of clinical history.
Skin test—Inject intracutaneously 0.02 to 0.03 mL of a 1:10 dilution of Normal Horse Serum or Antivenin. A control test on the opposite extremity, using Sodium Chloride Injection, USP, facilitates interpretation. Use of larger amounts for the skin-test dose increases the likelihood of false-positive reactions, and in the exquisitely sensitive patient, increases the risk of a systemic reaction from the skin-test dose. A 1:100 or greater dilution should be used for preliminary skin testing if the history suggests sensitivity. A positive reaction to a skin test occurs within five to thirty minutes and is manifested by a wheal with or without pseudopodia and surrounding erythema. In general, the shorter the interval between injection and the beginning of the skin reaction, the greater the sensitivity.
If the history is negative for allergy and the result of a skin test is negative, proceed with administration of Antivenin as outlined above. If the history is positive and a skin test is strongly positive, administration may be dangerous, especially if the positive sensitivity test is accompanied by systemic allergic manifestations. In such instances, the risk of administering Antivenin must be weighed against the risk of withholding it, keeping in mind that severe envenomation can be fatal. (See last paragraph of this section.)
A negative allergic history and absence of reaction to a properly applied skin test do not rule out the possibility of an immediate reaction. Also, a negative skin test has no bearing on whether or not delayed serum reactions (serum sickness) will occur after administration of the full dose.
If the history is negative, and the skin test is mildly or questionably positive, administer as follows to reduce the risk of a severe immediate systemic reaction: (a) Prepare, in separate sterile vials or syringes, 1:100 and 1:10 dilutions of Antivenin. (b) Allow at least 15 minutes between injections and proceed with the next dose if no reaction follows the previous dose. (c) Inject subcutaneously, using a tuberculin-type syringe, 0.1, 0.2, and 0.5 mL of the 1:100 dilution at 15-minute intervals; repeat with the 1:10 dilution, and finally undiluted Antivenin. (d) If a systemic reaction occurs after any injection, place a tourniquet proximal to the site of injections and administer an appropriate dose of epinephrine, 1:1000, proximal to the tourniquet or into another extremity. Wait at least 30 minutes before injecting another dose. The amount of the next dose should be the same as the last that did not evoke a reaction. (e) If no reaction occurs after 0.5 mL of undiluted Antivenin has been administered, switch to the intramuscular route and continue doubling the dose at 15-minute intervals until the entire dose has been injected intramuscularly or proceed to the intravenous route as described above under "Dosage and Administration."
Obviously, if the just-described schedule is used, 3 to 5 or more hours would be required to administer the initial dose suggested for a moderate or severe envenomation, and time is an important factor in neutralization of venom in a critically ill patient. Wingert and Wainschel[4] have described a procedure based on the experience of their group which they have used in some severely envenomated patients who have positive sensitivity tests: 50 to 100 mg of diphenhydramine hydrochloride is given intravenously, followed by slow intravenous infusion of diluted Antivenin for 15 to 20 minutes while carefully observing the patient for symptoms and signs of anaphylaxis; if anaphylaxis does not occur, Antivenin is continued, maintaining close observation of the patient. Patients who require Antivenin but develop signs of impending anaphylaxis in spite of this or the procedure described earlier present a difficult problem, and consultation should be sought.

SYSTEMIC REACTIONS

A. The immediate reaction (shock, anaphylaxis) usually occurs within 30 minutes. Symptoms and signs may develop before the needle is withdrawn and may include apprehension, flushing, itching, urticaria; edema of the face, tongue, and throat; cough, dyspnea, cyanosis, vomiting, and collapse.
B. Serum sickness usually occurs 5 to 24 days after administration. The incubation period may be less than 5 days, especially in those who have received horse-serum-containing preparations in the past. The usual symptoms and signs are malaise, fever, urticaria, lymphadenopathy, edema, arthralgia, nausea, and vomiting. Occasionally, neurological manifestations develop, such as meningismus or peripheral neuritis. Peripheral neuritis usually involves the shoulders and arms. Pain and muscle weakness are frequently present, and permanent atrophy may develop.

REFERENCES

1. GINGRICH, W. & HOHENADEL, J.: Standardization of polyvalent antivenin. "Venoms", edited by E. Buckley and N. Porges. Publication No. 44, Amer. Assoc. for the Advancement of Science, Washington, D.C., 1956, Pages 337–80.
2. PARRISH, H.: Incidence of treated snakebite in the United States. Pub. Hlth. Rep. *81*:269, 1966.
3. RUSSELL, F., et al.: Snake venom poisoning in the United States. Experiences with 550 cases. JAMA *233*:341, 1975. RUSSELL, F.: Venomous bites and stings: Poisonous snakes. In The Merck Manual of Diagnosis and Therapy, pp. 2450–2456, 14th Ed., 1982.
4. WINGERT, W. and WAINSCHEL, J.: Diagnosis and management of envenomation by poisonous snakes. South. Med. J. *68*:1015, 1975.
5. PARRISH, H. & HAYES, R.: Hospital management of pit viper venenations. Clinical Toxicol. *3*:501, 1970.
6. McCOLLOUGH, N. & GENNARO, J.: Diagnosis, symptoms, treatment and sequelae of envenomation by *Crotalus adamanteus* and Genus *Agkistrodon*. J. Florida Med. Assoc. *55*:327, 1968.
7. WATT, C. & GENNARO, J.: Pit viper bites in South Georgia and North Florida. Tr. South. Surg. Assoc. *77*:378, 1966.
8. MINTON, S.: Venom Diseases: Snakebite. In Textbook of Medicine, P. Beeson and W. McDermott (Eds.), pp. 88–92; Saunders, Philadelphia, 1975.
9. VAN MIEROP, L.: Snakebite symposium. J. Florida Med. Assoc. *63*:101, 1976.
10. ARNOLD, R.: Treatment of snakebite. JAMA *236*:1843, 1976; Controversies and hazards in the treatment of pit viper bites. South Med. J. *72*:902, 1979.
11. Poisonous Snakes of the World. U.S. Government Printing Office, Washington, D.C., NAVMED, 1965.
12. GARFIN, S. et al.: Rattlesnake bites: Current concepts. Clin. Orthop. *140*:50, 1979; Role of surgical decompression in treatment of rattlesnake bites. Surg. Forum *30*:502, 1979.
13. VAN MIEROP, L. & KITCHENS, C.: Defibrination syndrome following bites by the Eastern diamondback rattlesnake. J. Florida Med. Assoc. *67*:21, 1980.
14. HASIBA, U. et al.: DIC-like syndrome after envenomation by the snake, *Crotalus horridus horridus*. New Eng. J. Med. *292*:505, 1975.
15. WEISS, H. et al.: Afibrinogenemia in man following the bite of a rattlesnake *(Crotalus adamanteus)*. Am. J. Med. *47*:625, 1969.
16. SIVAPRASAD, R. & CANTINI, E.: Western diamondback rattlesnake *(Crotalus atrox)* poisoning. Postgrad. Med. *71*:223, 1982.
17. SABBACK, M. et al.: A study of the treatment of pit viper envenomization in 45 patients. J. Trauma *17*:569, 1977.

HOW SUPPLIED

Each combination package contains one vacuum vial to yield 10 mL of serum—to be used immediately after reconstitu-

tion—(with preservatives: phenol 0.25% and thimerosal [mercury derivative] 0.005%). One vial containing 10 mL of Bacteriostatic Water for Injection, USP (with preservative: phenylmercuric nitrate 0.001%). One 1 mL vial of normal horse serum (diluted 1:10) as sensitivity testing material with preservatives: thimerosal (mercury derivative) 0.005% and phenol 0.35%. Not returnable.
Manufactured by: Wyeth Laboratories Inc., Marietta, PA 17547.

ANTIVENIN (Micrurus fulvius) ℞
[an "te ven 'in]
(equine origin)
North American Coral Snake Antivenin

COMPOSITION
Each combination package contains one vial of lyophilized Antivenin (Micrurus fulvius) with 0.25% phenol and 0.005% thimerosal (mercury derivative) as preservatives (before lyophilization); one vial of diluent containing 10 ml. of Bacteriostatic Water for Injection, U.S.P., with phenylmercuric nitrate (1:100,000) as preservative.

HOW SUPPLIED
Combination packages as described (not returnable).
Manufactured by Wyeth Laboratories Inc., Marietta, PA 17547.
For prescribing information write to Professional Service, Wyeth-Ayerst Laboratories, P.O. Box 8299, Philadelphia, PA 19101, or contact your local Wyeth-Ayerst representative.

A.P.L.® ℞
(chorionic gonadotropin for injection, USP)
For Intramuscular Injection Only

Caution: Federal law prohibits dispensing without prescription.

DESCRIPTION
Human chorionic gonadotropin (HCG), a polypeptide hormone produced by the human placenta, is composed of an alpha and a beta subunit. The alpha subunit is essentially identical to the alpha subunits of the human pituitary gonadotropins, luteinizing hormone (LH) and follicle-stimulating hormone (FSH), as well as to the alpha subunit of human thyroid stimulating hormone (TSH). The beta subunits of these hormones differ in amino acid sequence.
A.P.L. (chorionic gonadotropin, USP) is a gonad-stimulating principle obtained from the urine of pregnant women. It is a sterile, amorphous powder prepared by cryodesiccation, and is freely soluble in water.
When reconstituted with the accompanying 10 mL of sterile diluent water, each SECULE® vial contains:
5,000 USP units of chorionic gonadotropin, 2.0% benzyl alcohol, 0.9% lactose, and not more than 0.2% phenol;
10,000 USP units of chorionic gonadotropin, 2.0% benzyl alcohol, 1.8% lactose, and not more than 0.2% phenol;
20,000 USP units of chorionic gonadotropin, 2.0% benzyl alcohol, 3.6% lactose, and not more than 0.2% phenol.
The pH is adjusted with sodium hydroxide or hydrochloric acid.
After reconstitution, store refrigerated and use within 30 days.
THIS PRODUCT IS FOR INTRAMUSCULAR INJECTION ONLY.

HOW SUPPLIED
A.P.L. (chorionic gonadotropin for injection, USP)
NDC 0046-0970-10 — Each package provides:
(1) One vial containing 5,000 USP units chorionic gonadotropin in dry form, and
(2) One 10 mL ampul sterile diluent.
NDC 0046-0971-10 — Each package provides:
(1) One vial containing 10,000 USP units chorionic gonadotropin in dry form, and
(2) One 10 mL ampul sterile diluent.
NDC 0046-0972-10 — Each package provides:
(1) One vial containing 20,000 USP units chorionic gonadotropin in dry form, and
(2) One 10 mL ampul sterile diluent.
The product is assayed in accord with USP method; USP potency units are defined in terms of the USP Chorionic Gonadotropin Reference Standard.
When reconstituted with 10 mL of accompanying sterile diluent, the resulting solutions also contain 2.0% benzyl alcohol, not more than 0.2% phenol, and the following concentrations of lactose: No. 970, 0.9%; No. 971, 1.8%; No. 972, 3.6%. The pH is adjusted with sodium hydroxide or hydrochloric acid.
DIRECTIONS FOR RECONSTITUTION
Withdraw sterile air from lyophilized vial and inject into sterile diluent vial. Remove 10 mL from diluent vial and add to lyophilized vial; agitate gently until powder is completely dissolved.
MAY BE STORED FOR 30 DAYS IN A REFRIGERATOR AFTER RECONSTITUTION.
For prescribing information write to Professional Service, Wyeth-Ayerst Laboratories, P.O. Box 8299, Philadelphia, PA 19101, or contact your local Wyeth-Ayerst representative.

ATIVAN® Ⓒ ℞
[at 'i-van]
(lorazepam)
Injection

DESCRIPTION
Ativan (lorazepam) Injection, a benzodiazepine with antianxiety and sedative effects, is intended for intramuscular or intravenous routes of administration. It has the chemical formula: 7-chloro-5-(o-chlorophenyl)-1,3-dihydro-3-hydroxy-2*H*-1,4-benzodiazepin-2-one. The molecular weight is 321.2, and the C.A.S. No. is [846-49-1].
Lorazepam is a nearly white powder almost insoluble in water. Each mL of sterile injection contains either 2.0 or 4.0 mg of lorazepam, 0.18 mL polyethylene glycol 400 in propylene glycol with 2.0% benzyl alcohol as preservative.

CLINICAL PHARMACOLOGY
Intravenous or intramuscular administration of the recommended dose of 2 mg to 4 mg of Ativan (lorazepam) Injection to adult patients is followed by dose-related effects of sedation (sleepiness or drowsiness), relief of preoperative anxiety, and lack of recall of events related to the day of surgery in the majority of patients. The clinical sedation (sleepiness or drowsiness) thus noted is such that the majority of patients are able to respond to simple instructions whether they give the appearance of being awake or asleep. The lack of recall is relative rather than absolute, as determined under conditions of careful patient questioning and testing, using props designed to enhance recall. The majority of patients under these reinforced conditions had difficulty recalling perioperative events or recognizing props from before surgery. The lack of recall and recognition was optimum within 2 hours following intramuscular administration and 15 to 20 minutes after intravenous injection.
The intended effects of the recommended adult dose of lorazepam injection usually last 6 to 8 hours. In rare instances and where patients received greater than the recommended dose, excessive sleepiness and prolonged lack of recall were noted. As with other benzodiazepines, unsteadiness, enhanced sensitivity to CNS-depressant effects of ethyl alcohol and other drugs were noted in isolated and rare cases for greater than 24 hours.
Studies in healthy adult volunteers reveal that intravenous lorazepam in doses up to 3.5 mg/70 kg does not alter sensitivity to the respiratory stimulating effect of carbon dioxide and does not enhance the respiratory depressant effects of doses of meperidine up to 100 mg/70 kg (also determined by carbon dioxide challenge) as long as patients remain sufficiently awake to undergo testing. Upper airway obstruction has been observed in rare instances where the patient received greater than the recommended dose and was excessively sleepy and difficult to arouse. (See "**Warnings**" and "**Adverse Reactions**.")
Clinically employed doses of lorazepam injectable do not greatly affect the circulatory system in the supine position or employing a 70-degree tilt test. Doses of 8 mg to 10 mg of intravenous lorazepam (2 to 2½ times the maximum recommended dosage) will produce loss of lid reflexes within 15 minutes.
Studies in six (6) healthy young adults who received lorazepam injection and no other drugs revealed that visual tracking (the ability to keep a moving line centered) was impaired for a mean of eight (8) hours following administration of 4 mg of intramuscular lorazepam and four (4) hours following administration of 2 mg intramuscularly with considerable subject variation. Similar findings were noted with pentobarbital, 150 and 75 mg. Although this study showed that both lorazepam and pentobarbital interfered with eye-hand coordination, the data are insufficient to predict when it would be safe to operate a motor vehicle or engage in a hazardous occupation or sport.
PHARMACOKINETICS
Injectable Ativan (lorazepam) is readily absorbed when given intramuscularly. Peak plasma concentrations occur approximately 60 to 90 minutes following administration and appear to be dose-related, e.g., a 2.0 mg dose provides a level of approximately 20 ng/mL and a 4.0 mg dose approximately 40 ng/mL in plasma. The mean half-life of lorazepam is about 16 hours when given intravenously or intramuscularly. Ativan (lorazepam) is rapidly conjugated at the 3-hydroxyl group into its major metabolite, lorazepam glucuronide, which is then excreted in the urine. Lorazepam glucuronide has no demonstrable CNS activity in animals. When 5 mg of intravenous lorazepam was administered to volunteers once a day for four consecutive days, a steady state of free lorazepam was achieved by the second day (approximately 52 ng/mL of plasma three hours after the first dose and approximately 62 ng/mL three hours after each subsequent dose, one day apart). At clinically relevant concentrations, lorazepam is bound 85% to plasma proteins.

INDICATIONS AND USAGE
Ativan (lorazepam) Injection is indicated in adult patients for preanesthetic medication, producing sedation (sleepiness or drowsiness), relief of anxiety, and a decreased ability to recall events related to the day of surgery. It is most useful in those patients who are anxious about their surgical procedure and who would prefer to have diminished recall of the events of the day of surgery (see "**Precautions**—INFORMATION FOR PATIENTS").

CONTRAINDICATIONS
Ativan (lorazepam) Injection is contraindicated in patients with a known sensitivity to benzodiazepines or its vehicle (polyethylene glycol, propylene glycol, and benzyl alcohol) and in patients with acute narrow-angle glaucoma. The use of Ativan (lorazepam) Injection intra-arterially is contraindicated because, as with other injectable benzodiazepines, inadvertent intra-arterial injection may produce arteriospasm resulting in gangrene which may require amputation (see "**Warnings**").

WARNINGS
PRIOR TO INTRAVENOUS USE, ATIVAN INJECTION MUST BE DILUTED WITH AN EQUAL AMOUNT OF COMPATIBLE DILUENT (SEE "**DOSAGE AND ADMINISTRATION**"). INTRAVENOUS INJECTION SHOULD BE MADE SLOWLY AND WITH REPEATED ASPIRATION. CARE SHOULD BE TAKEN TO DETERMINE THAT ANY INJECTION WILL NOT BE INTRA-ARTERIAL AND THAT PERIVASCULAR EXTRAVASATION WILL NOT TAKE PLACE.
PARTIAL AIRWAY OBSTRUCTION MAY OCCUR IN HEAVILY SEDATED PATIENTS. INTRAVENOUS LORAZEPAM, WHEN GIVEN ALONE IN GREATER THAN THE RECOMMENDED DOSE, OR AT THE RECOMMENDED DOSE AND ACCOMPANIED BY OTHER DRUGS USED DURING THE ADMINISTRATION OF ANESTHESIA, MAY PRODUCE HEAVY SEDATION; THEREFORE, EQUIPMENT NECESSARY TO MAINTAIN A PATENT AIRWAY AND TO SUPPORT RESPIRATION/VENTILATION SHOULD BE AVAILABLE.
There is no evidence to support the use of lorazepam injection in coma, shock, or acute alcohol intoxication at this time. Since the liver is the most likely site of conjugation of lorazepam and since excretion of conjugated lorazepam (glucuronide) is a renal function, this drug is not recommended for use in patients with hepatic and/or renal *failure*. This does not preclude use of the drug in patients with mild-to-moderate hepatic or renal disease. When injectable lorazepam is selected for use in patients with mild-to-moderate hepatic or renal disease, the lowest effective dose should be considered since drug effect may be prolonged. Experience with other benzodiazepines and limited experience with parenteral lorazepam has demonstrated that tolerance to alcoholic beverages and other central-nervous-system depressants is diminished when used concomitantly.
As is true of similar CNS-acting drugs, patients receiving injectable lorazepam should not operate machinery or engage in hazardous occupations or drive a motor vehicle for a period of 24 to 48 hours. Impairment of performance may persist for greater intervals because of extremes of age, concomitant use of other drugs, stress of surgery, or the general condition of the patient.
Clinical trials have shown that patients over the age of 50 years may have a more profound and prolonged sedation with intravenous lorazepam. Ordinarily, an initial dose of 2 mg may be adequate unless a greater degree of lack of recall is desired.
As with all central-nervous-system depressant drugs, care should be exercised in patients given injectable lorazepam as premature ambulation may result in injury from falling.
There is no added beneficial effect to the addition of scopolamine to injectable lorazepam, and their combined effect may result in an increased incidence of sedation, hallucination, and irrational behavior.
PREGNANCY
ATIVAN (LORAZEPAM) MAY CAUSE FETAL DAMAGE WHEN ADMINISTERED TO PREGNANT WOMEN. An increased risk of congenital malformations associated with the use of minor tranquilizers (chlordiazepoxide, diazepam, and meprobamate) during the first trimester of pregnancy has been suggested in several studies. In humans, blood levels obtained from umbilical cord blood indicate placental transfer of lorazepam and lorazepam glucuronide.
Ativan Injection should not be used during pregnancy. There are insufficient data regarding obstetrical safety of parenteral lorazepam, including use in cesarean section. Such use, therefore, is not recommended.

Continued on next page

Wyeth-Ayerst Laboratories—Cont.

Reproductive studies in animals were performed in mice, rats, and two strains of rabbits. Occasional anomalies (reduction of tarsals, tibia, metatarsals, malrotated limbs, gastroschisis, malformed skull, and microphthalmia) were seen in drug-treated rabbits without relationship to dosage. Although all of these anomalies were not present in the concurrent control group, they have been reported to occur randomly in historical controls. At doses of 40 mg/kg orally or 4 mg/kg intravenously and higher, there was evidence of fetal resorption and increased fetal loss in rabbits which was not seen at lower doses.

ENDOSCOPIC PROCEDURES

There are insufficient data to support the use of Ativan (lorazepam) Injection for outpatient endoscopic procedures. Inpatient endoscopic procedures require adequate recovery room observations.

Pharyngeal reflexes are not impaired when Ativan Injection is used for peroral endoscopic procedures; therefore, adequate topical or regional anesthesia is recommended to minimize reflex activity associated with such procedures.

PRECAUTIONS

GENERAL

The additive central-nervous-system effects of other drugs such as phenothiazines, narcotic analgesics, barbiturates, antidepressants, scopolamine, and monoamine-oxidase inhibitors, should be borne in mind when these other drugs are used concomitantly with or during the period of recovery from Ativan (lorazepam) Injection. (See "**Clinical Pharmacology**" and "**Warnings**".)

Extreme care must be used in administering Ativan Injection to elderly patients, very ill patients, and to patients with limited pulmonary reserve because of the possibility that underventilation and/or hypoxic cardiac arrest may occur. Resuscitative equipment for ventilatory support should be readily available. (See "**Warnings**" and "**Dosage and Administration**".)

When lorazepam injection is used IV as the premedicant prior to regional or local anesthesia, the possibility of excessive sleepiness or drowsiness may interfere with patient cooperation to determine levels of anesthesia. This is most likely to occur when greater than 0.05 mg/kg is given and when narcotic analgesics are used concomitantly with the recommended dose. (See "**Adverse Reactions**".)

INFORMATION FOR PATIENTS

As appropriate, the patient should be informed of the pharmacological effects of the drug, such as sedation, relief of anxiety, and lack of recall, and the duration of these effects (about 8 hours), so that they may adequately perceive the risks as well as the benefits to be derived from its use.

Patients who receive Ativan Injection as a premedicant should be cautioned that driving an automobile or operating hazardous machinery, or engaging in a hazardous sport, should be delayed for 24 to 48 hours following the injection. Sedatives, tranquilizers, and narcotic analgesics may produce a more prolonged and profound effect when administered along with injectable Ativan. This effect may take the form of excessive sleepiness or drowsiness and, on rare occasions, interfere with recall and recognition of events of the day of surgery and the day after.

Getting out of bed unassisted may result in falling and injury if undertaken within 8 hours of receiving lorazepam injection. Alcoholic beverages should not be consumed for at least 24 to 48 hours after receiving lorazepam injectable due to the additive effects on central-nervous-system depression seen with benzodiazepines in general. Elderly patients should be told that Ativan (lorazepam) Injection may make them very sleepy for a period longer than six (6) to eight (8) hours following surgery.

LABORATORY TESTS

In clinical trials no laboratory test abnormalities were identified with either single or multiple doses of Ativan (lorazepam) Injection. These tests included: CBC, urinalysis, SGOT, SGPT, bilirubin, alkaline phosphatase, LDH, cholesterol, uric acid, BUN, glucose, calcium, phosphorus, and total proteins.

DRUG INTERACTIONS

Ativan (lorazepam) Injection, like other injectable benzodiazepines, produces depression of the central nervous system when administered with ethyl alcohol, phenothiazines, barbiturates, MAO inhibitors, and other antidepressants. When scopolamine is used concomitantly with injectable lorazepam, an increased incidence of sedation, hallucinations, and irrational behavior has been observed.

DRUG/LABORATORY TEST INTERACTIONS

No laboratory test abnormalities were identified when lorazepam was given alone or concomitantly with another drug, such as narcotic analgesics, inhalation anesthetics, scopolamine, atropine, and a variety of tranquilizing agents.

CARCINOGENESIS, MUTAGENESIS, IMPAIRMENT OF FERTILITY

No evidence of carcinogenic potential emerged in rats and mice during an 18-month study with oral lorazepam. No studies regarding mutagenesis have been performed. Preimplantation study in rats was performed with oral lorazepam at a 20 mg/kg dose and showed no impairment of fertility.

PREGNANCY

Pregnancy Category D; See "**Warnings**."

LABOR AND DELIVERY

There are insufficient data to support the use of Ativan (lorazepam) Injection during labor and delivery, including cesarean section; therefore, its use in this situation is not recommended.

NURSING MOTHERS

Injectable lorazepam should not be administered to nursing mothers, because, like other benzodiazepines, the possibility exists that lorazepam may be excreted in human milk and sedate the infant.

PEDIATRIC USE

There are insufficient data to support efficacy or make dosage recommendations for injectable lorazepam in patients less than 18 years of age; therefore, such use is not recommended.

ADVERSE REACTIONS

CENTRAL NERVOUS SYSTEM

The most frequent adverse effects seen with injectable lorazepam are an extension of the central-nervous-system-depressant effects of the drug. The incidence varied from one study to another, depending on the dosage, route of administration, use of other central-nervous-system depressants, and the investigator's opinion concerning the degree and duration of desired sedation. Excessive sleepiness and drowsiness were the main side effects. This interfered with patient cooperation in approximately 6% (25/446) of patients undergoing regional anesthesia in that they were unable to assess levels of anesthesia in regional blocks or with caudal anesthesia. Patients over 50 years of age had a higher incidence of excessive sleepiness or drowsiness when compared with those under 50 (21/106 vs 24/245) when lorazepam was given intravenously (see "**Dosage and Administration**"). On rare occasion (3/1580) the patient was unable to give personal identification in the operating room on arrival, and one patient fell when attempting premature ambulation in the postoperative period.

Symptoms such as restlessness, confusion, depression, crying, sobbing, and delirium occurred in about 1.3% (20/1580). One patient injured himself by picking at his incision during the immediate postoperative period.

Hallucinations were present in about 1% (14/1580) of patients and were visual and self-limiting.

An occasional patient complained of dizziness, diplopia, and/or blurred vision. Depressed hearing was infrequently reported during the peak-effect period.

An occasional patient had a prolonged recovery room stay, either because of excessive sleepiness or because of some form of inappropriate behavior. The latter was seen most commonly when scopolamine was given concomitantly as a premedicant.

Limited information derived from patients who were discharged the day after receiving injectable lorazepam showed one patient complained of some unsteadiness of gait and a reduced ability to perform complex mental functions. Enhanced sensitivity to alcoholic beverages has been reported more than 24 hours after receiving injectable lorazepam, similar to experience with other benzodiazepines.

LOCAL EFFECTS

Intramuscular injection of lorazepam has resulted in pain at the injection site, a sensation of burning, or observed redness in the same area in a very variable incidence from one study to another. The overall incidence of pain and burning was about 17% (146/859) in the immediate postinjection period and about 1.4% (12/859) at the 24-hour observation time. Reactions at the injection site (redness) occurred in approximately 2% (17/859) in the immediate postinjection period and were present 24 hours later in about 0.8% (7/859).

Intravenous administration of lorazepam resulted in painful responses in 13/771 patients or approximately 1.6% in the immediate postinjection period, and 24 hours later 4/771 patients or about 0.5% still complained of pain. Redness did not occur immediately following intravenous injection but was noted in 19/771 patients at the 24-hour observation period. This incidence is similar to that observed with an intravenous infusion before lorazepam is given.

CARDIOVASCULAR SYSTEM

Hypertension (0.1%) and hypotension (0.1%) have occasionally been observed after patients have received injectable lorazepam.

RESPIRATORY SYSTEM

Five patients (5/446) who underwent regional anesthesia were observed to have partial airway obstruction. This was believed due to excessive sleepiness at the time of the procedure and resulted in temporary underventilation. Immediate attention to the airway, employing the usual countermeasures, will usually suffice to manage this condition (see also "**Clinical Pharmacology**," "**Warnings**," and "**Precautions**").

OTHER ADVERSE EXPERIENCES

Skin rash, nausea, and vomiting have occasionally been noted in patients who have received injectable lorazepam combined with other drugs during anesthesia and surgery.

DRUG ABUSE AND DEPENDENCE

As with other benzodiazepines, Ativan (lorazepam) Injection has a low potential for abuse and may lead to limited dependence. Although there are no clinical data available for injectable lorazepam in this respect, physicians should be aware that repeated doses over a prolonged period of time may result in limited physical and psychological dependence.

OVERDOSAGE

Overdosage of benzodiazepines is usually manifested by varying degrees of central-nervous-system depression, ranging from drowsiness to coma. In mild cases symptoms include drowsiness, mental confusion, and lethargy. In more serious examples, symptoms may include ataxia, hypotonia, hypotension, hypnosis, stages one (1) to three (3) coma, and very rarely death.

Treatment of overdosage is mainly supportive until the drug is eliminated from the body. Vital signs and fluid balance should be carefully monitored. An adequate airway should be maintained and assisted respiration used as needed. With normally functioning kidneys, forced diuresis with intravenous fluids and electrolytes may accelerate elimination of benzodiazepines from the body. In addition, osmotic diuretics, such as mannitol, may be effective as adjunctive measures. In more critical situations, renal dialysis and exchange blood transfusions may be indicated.

The benzodiazepine antagonist flumazenil may be used in hospitalized patients as an adjunct to, not as a substitute for, proper management of benzodiazepine overdose. **The prescriber should be aware of a risk of seizure in association with flumazenil treatment, particularly in long-term benzodiazepine users and in cyclic antidepressant overdose.** The complete flumazenil package insert including "**Contraindications**," "**Warnings**," and "**Precautions**" should be consulted prior to use.

DOSAGE AND ADMINISTRATION

INTRAMUSCULAR INJECTION

For the designated indications as a premedicant, the usual recommended dose of lorazepam for intramuscular injection is 0.05 mg/kg up to a maximum of 4 mg. As with all premedicant drugs, the dose should be individualized. (See also "**Clinical Pharmacology**," "**Warnings**," "**Precautions**," and "**Adverse Reactions**.") Doses of other central-nervous-system depressant drugs should be ordinarily reduced (See "**Precautions**"). *For optimum effect, measured as lack of recall, intramuscular lorazepam should be administered at least 2 hours before the anticipated operative procedure.* Narcotic analgesics should be administered at their usual preoperative time. There are insufficient data to support efficacy to make dosage recommendations for intramuscular lorazepam in patients less than 18 years of age; therefore, such use is not recommended.

INTRAVENOUS INJECTION

For the primary purpose of sedation and relief of anxiety, the usual recommended initial dose of lorazepam for intravenous injection is 2 mg total, or 0.02 mg/lb (0.044 mg/kg), whichever is smaller. This dose will suffice for sedating most adult patients and should not ordinarily be exceeded in patients over 50 years of age. In those patients in whom a greater likelihood of lack of recall for perioperative events would be beneficial, larger doses as high as 0.05 mg/kg up to a total of 4 mg may be administered. (See "**Clinical Pharmacology**," "**Warnings**," "**Precautions**," and "**Adverse Reactions**.") Doses of other injectable central-nervous-system depressant drugs should ordinarily be reduced (see "**Precautions**"). *For optimum effect, measured as lack of recall, intravenous lorazepam should be administered 15 to 20 minutes before the anticipated operative procedure.*

EQUIPMENT NECESSARY TO MAINTAIN A PATENT AIRWAY SHOULD BE IMMEDIATELY AVAILABLE PRIOR TO INTRAVENOUS ADMINISTRATION OF LORAZEPAM (see "**Warnings**").

There are insufficient data to support efficacy or make dosage recommendations for intravenous lorazepam in patients less than 18 years of age; therefore, such use is not recommended.

ADMINISTRATION

The TUBEX® BLUNT POINTE™ Sterile Cartridge Unit is suitable for substances to be administered intravenously only. It is intended for use with injection sets specifically manufactured as "needle-less" injection systems. TUBEX® BLUNT POINTE™ is compatible with Abbott's Life-Shield® prepierced reseal injection site, Baxter's Inter-Link® Injection Site, and B. Braun Medical's SafSite® Reflux Valve. Consult manufacturer's recommendations regarding "Directions for Use" of the "needle-less" system. It is also intended for admixture with, and convenient administration of, various medicaments when using Drug Vial Adapters for "needle-less" injection systems.

The TUBEX® Sterile Cartridge-Needle Unit is suitable for substances to be administered intravenously or intramuscularly.
When given intramuscularly, Ativan Injection, undiluted, should be injected deep in the muscle mass.
Injectable Ativan (lorazepam) can be used with atropine sulfate, narcotic analgesics, other parenterally used analgesics, commonly used anesthetics, and muscle relaxants.
Immediately prior to intravenous use, Ativan (lorazepam) Injection must be diluted with an equal volume of compatible solution. When properly diluted the drug may be injected directly into a vein or into the tubing of an existing intravenous infusion (see above for tubing products compatible with the BLUNT POINTE™ Sterile Cartridge Unit). The rate of injection should not exceed 2.0 mg per minute.
Parenteral drug products should be inspected visually for particulate matter and discoloration prior to administration, whenever solution and container permit. Do not use if solution is discolored or contains a precipitate.
Ativan (lorazepam) Injection is compatible for dilution purposes with the following solutions: Sterile Water for Injection, USP; Sodium Chloride Injection, USP; 5% Dextrose Injection, USP.

HOW SUPPLIED

Ativan® (lorazepam) Injection is available in TUBEX® BLUNT POINTE™ Sterile Cartridge Units and Sterile Cartridge-Needle Units (22 gauge × 1¼ inch needle), in boxes of 10 TUBEX as follows:
1 mg per TUBEX, NDC 0008-0581-50, 0.5 mL fill in 1 mL size Blunt Pointe™
1 mg per TUBEX, NDC 0008-0581-07, 0.5 mL fill in 1 mL size
2 mg per mL, NDC 0008-0581-52, 1 mL fill in 2 mL size Blunt Pointe™
2 mg per mL, NDC 0008-0581-02, 1 mL fill in 2 mL size
4 mg per mL, NDC 0008-0570-50, 1 mL fill in 2 mL size Blunt Pointe™
4 mg per mL, NDC 0008-0570-02, 1 mL fill in 2 mL size
For IM or IV injection.
Protect from light.
Store in a refrigerator.
Use carton to protect contents from light.

ALSO AVAILABLE

TUBEX® BLUNT POINTE™ Sterile Cartridge Units and Sterile Cartridge-Needle Units (22 gauge × 1¼ inch needle), packaged in boxes of 10 TUBEX in TAMP-R-TEL® tamper-resistant packages as follows:
1 mg per TUBEX, NDC 0008-0581-51, 0.5 mL fill in 1 mL size Blunt Pointe™
1 mg per TUBEX, NDC 0008-0581-05, 0.5 mL fill in 1 mL size
2 mg per mL, NDC 0008-0581-53, 1 mL fill in 2 mL size Blunt Pointe™
2 mg per mL, NDC 0008-0581-06, 1 mL fill in 2 mL size
4 mg per mL, NDC 0008-0570-51, 1 mL fill in 2 mL size Blunt Pointe™
4 mg per mL, NDC 0008-0570-05, 1 mL fill in 2 mL size
Single-dose and multiple-dose vials are available as follows:
2 mg per mL, NDC 0008-0581-04, 1 mL vial and NDC 0008-0581-01, 10 mL vial
4 mg per mL, NDC 0008-0570-04, 1 mL vial and NDC 0008-0570-01, 10 mL vial

DIRECTIONS FOR DILUTION FOR IV USE

To dilute, adhere to the following procedure:
For TUBEX—
1. Extrude the entire amount of air in the half-filled TUBEX.
2. Slowly aspirate the desired volume of diluent.
3. Pull back slightly on the plunger to provide additional mixing space.
4. Immediately mix contents thoroughly by gently inverting TUBEX repeatedly until a homogenous solution results. Do not shake vigorously, as this will result in air entrapment.

For Vial—
Aspirate the desired amount of Ativan Injection into the syringe. Then proceed as described under TUBEX.

ATIVAN® ℂ ℞

[at'i-van]
(lorazepam)
Tablets

DESCRIPTION

Ativan (lorazepam), an antianxiety agent, has the chemical formula, 7-chloro-5-(*o*-chlorophenyl)-1,3-dihydro-3-hydroxy-2*H*-1,4-benzodiazepin-2-one.
It is a nearly white powder almost insoluble in water. Each Ativan (lorazepam) tablet, to be taken orally, contains 0.5 mg, 1 mg, or 2 mg of lorazepam. The inactive ingredients present are lactose and other ingredients.

CLINICAL PHARMACOLOGY

Studies in healthy volunteers show that in single high doses Ativan (lorazepam) has a tranquilizing action on the central nervous system with no appreciable effect on the respiratory or cardiovascular systems.
Ativan (lorazepam) is readily absorbed with an absolute bioavailability of 90 percent. Peak concentrations in plasma occur approximately 2 hours following administration. The peak plasma level of lorazepam from a 2 mg dose is approximately 20 ng/mL.
The mean half-life of unconjugated lorazepam in human plasma is about 12 hours and for its major metabolite, lorazepam glucuronide, about 18 hours. At clinically relevant concentrations, lorazepam is approximately 85% bound to plasma proteins. Ativan (lorazepam) is rapidly conjugated at its 3-hydroxy group into lorazepam glucuronide which is then excreted in the urine. Lorazepam glucuronide has no demonstrable CNS activity in animals.
The plasma levels of lorazepam are proportional to the dose given. There is no evidence of accumulation of lorazepam on administration up to six months.
Studies comparing young and elderly subjects have shown that the pharmacokinetics of lorazepam remain unaltered with advancing age.

INDICATIONS AND USAGE

Ativan (lorazepam) is indicated for the management of anxiety disorders or for the short-term relief of the symptoms of anxiety or anxiety associated with depressive symptoms. Anxiety or tension associated with the stress of everyday life usually does not require treatment with an anxiolytic.
The effectiveness of Ativan (lorazepam) in long-term use, that is, more than 4 months, has not been assessed by systematic clinical studies. The physician should periodically reassess the usefulness of the drug for the individual patient.

CONTRAINDICATIONS

Ativan (lorazepam) is contraindicated in patients with known sensitivity to the benzodiazepines or with acute narrow-angle glaucoma.

WARNINGS

Ativan (lorazepam) is not recommended for use in patients with a primary depressive disorder or psychosis. As with all patients on CNS-acting drugs, patients receiving lorazepam should be warned not to operate dangerous machinery or motor vehicles and that their tolerance for alcohol and other CNS depressants will be diminished.

PHYSICAL AND PSYCHOLOGICAL DEPENDENCE
Withdrawal symptoms, similar in character to those noted with barbiturates and alcohol (convulsions, tremor, abdominal and muscle cramps, vomiting, and sweating), have occurred following abrupt discontinuance of lorazepam. The more severe withdrawal symptoms have usually been limited to those patients who received excessive doses over an extended period of time. Generally milder withdrawal symptoms (e.g., dysphoria and insomnia) have been reported following abrupt discontinuance of benzodiazepines taken continuously at therapeutic levels for several months. Consequently, after extended therapy, abrupt discontinuation should generally be avoided and a gradual dosage-tapering schedule followed. Addiction-prone individuals (such as drug addicts or alcoholics) should be under careful surveillance when receiving lorazepam or other psychotropic agents because of the predisposition of such patients to habituation and dependence.

PRECAUTIONS

In patients with depression accompanying anxiety, a possibility for suicide should be borne in mind.
For elderly or debilitated patients, the initial daily dosage should not exceed 2 mg in order to avoid oversedation.
The usual precautions for treating patients with impaired renal or hepatic function should be observed.
In patients where gastrointestinal or cardiovascular disorders coexist with anxiety, it should be noted that lorazepam has not been shown to be of significant benefit in treating the gastrointestinal or cardiovascular component.
Esophageal dilation occurred in rats treated with lorazepam for more than one year at 6 mg/kg/day. The no-effect dose was 1.25 mg/kg/day (approximately 6 times the maximum human therapeutic dose of 10 mg per day). The effect was reversible only when the treatment was withdrawn within two months of first observation of the phenomenon. The clinical significance of this is unknown. However, use of lorazepam for prolonged periods and in geriatric patients requires caution, and there should be frequent monitoring for symptoms of upper G.I. disease.
Safety and effectiveness of Ativan (lorazepam) in children of less than 12 years have not been established.

INFORMATION FOR PATIENTS
To assure the safe and effective use of Ativan (lorazepam), patients should be informed that, since benzodiazepines may produce psychological and physical dependence, it is advisable that they consult with their physician before either increasing the dose or abruptly discontinuing this drug.

ESSENTIAL LABORATORY TESTS
Some patients on Ativan (lorazepam) have developed leukopenia, and some have had elevations of LDH. As with other benzodiazepines, periodic blood counts and liver-function tests are recommended for patients on long-term therapy.

CLINICALLY SIGNIFICANT DRUG INTERACTIONS
The benzodiazepines, including Ativan (lorazepam), produce CNS-depressant effects when administered with such medications as barbiturates or alcohol.

CARCINOGENESIS AND MUTAGENESIS
No evidence of carcinogenic potential emerged in rats during an 18-month study with Ativan (lorazepam). No studies regarding mutagenesis have been performed.

PREGNANCY
Reproductive studies in animals were performed in mice, rats, and two strains of rabbits. Occasional anomalies (reduction of tarsals, tibia, metatarsals, malrotated limbs, gastroschisis, malformed skull, and microphthalmia) were seen in drug-treated rabbits without relationship to dosage. Although all of these anomalies were not present in the concurrent control group, they have been reported to occur randomly in historical controls. At doses of 40 mg/kg and higher, there was evidence of fetal resorption and increased fetal loss in rabbits which was not seen at lower doses.
The clinical significance of the above findings is not known. However, an increased risk of congenital malformations associated with the use of minor tranquilizers (chlordiazepoxide, diazepam, and meprobamate) during the first trimester of pregnancy has been suggested in several studies. Because the use of these drugs is rarely a matter of urgency, the use of lorazepam during this period should almost always be avoided. The possibility that a woman of childbearing potential may be pregnant at the time of institution of therapy should be considered. Patients should be advised that if they become pregnant, they should communicate with their physician about the desirability of discontinuing the drug.
In humans, blood levels obtained from umbilical cord blood indicate placental transfer of lorazepam and lorazepam glucuronide.

NURSING MOTHERS
It is not known whether oral lorazepam is excreted in human milk like the other benzodiazepine tranquilizers. As a general rule, nursing should not be undertaken while a patient is on a drug, since many drugs are excreted in human milk.

ADVERSE REACTIONS

Adverse reactions, if they occur, are usually observed at the beginning of therapy and generally disappear on continued medication or upon decreasing the dose. In a sample of about 3,500 anxious patients, the most frequent adverse reaction to Ativan (lorazepam) is sedation (15.9%), followed by dizziness (6.9%), weakness (4.2%), and unsteadiness (3.4%). Less frequent adverse reactions are disorientation, depression, nausea, change in appetite, headache, sleep disturbance, agitation, dermatological symptoms, eye-function disturbance, together with various gastrointestinal symptoms and autonomic manifestations. The incidence of sedation and unsteadiness increased with age.
Small decreases in blood pressure have been noted but are not clinally significant, probably being related to the relief of anxiety produced by Ativan (lorazepam).
Transient amnesia or memory impairment has been reported in association with the use of benzodiazepines.

OVERDOSAGE

In the management of overdosage with any drug, it should be borne in mind that multiple agents may have been taken.

SYMPTOMS
Overdosage of benzodiazepines is usually manifested by varying degrees of central nervous system depression ranging from drowsiness to coma. In mild cases, symptoms include drowsiness, mental confusion and lethary. In more serious cases, and especially when other drugs or alcohol were ingested, symptoms may include ataxia, hypotonia, hypotension, hypnotic state, stage one (1) to three (3) coma, and very rarely, death.

MANAGEMENT
Induced vomiting and/or gastric lavage should be undertaken, followed by general supportive care, monitoring of vital signs, and close observation of the patient.
Hypotension, though unlikely, usually may be controlled with norepinephrine bitartrate injection. The value of dialysis has not been adequately determined for lorazepam. The benzodiazepine antagonist flumazenil may be used in hospitalized patients as an adjunct to, not as a substitute for, proper management of benzodiazepine overdose.
The prescriber should be aware of a risk of seizure in association with flumazenil treatment, particularly in long-term benzodiazepine users and in cyclic antidepressant overdose. The complete flumazenil package insert including "**Contraindications**," "**Warnings**," and "**Precautions**" should be consulted prior to use.

Continued on next page

Wyeth-Ayerst Laboratories—Cont.

DOSAGE AND ADMINISTRATION

Ativan (lorazepam) is administered orally. For optimal results, dose, frequency of administration, and duration of therapy should be individualized according to patient response. To facilitate this, 0.5 mg, 1 mg, and 2 mg tablets are available.
The usual range is 2 to 6 mg/day given in divided doses, the largest dose being taken before bedtime, but the daily dosage may vary from 1 to 10 mg/day.
For anxiety, most patients require an initial dose of 2 to 3 mg/day given b.i.d. or t.i.d.
For insomnia due to anxiety or transient situational stress, a single daily dose of 2 to 4 mg may be given, usually at bedtime.
For elderly or debilitated patients, an initial dosage of 1 to 2 mg/day in divided doses is recommended, to be adjusted as needed and tolerated.
The dosage of Ativan (lorazepam) should be increased gradually when needed to help avoid adverse effects. When higher dosage is indicated, the evening dose should be increased before the daytime doses.

HOW SUPPLIED

Ativan® (lorazepam) Tablets are available in the following dosage strengths:
0.5 mg, NDC 0008-0081, white, five-sided tablet with a raised "A" on one side and "WYETH" and "81" on reverse side, in bottles of 100 and 500 tablets, in Redipak® cartons of 250 tablets (10 blister folders of 25), and in Redipak cartons of 100 tablets (10 blister strips of 10).
1 mg, NDC 0008-0064, white, five-sided tablet with a raised "A" on one side and "WYETH" and "64" on scored reverse side, in bottles of 100, 500, and 1000 tablets, in Redipak cartons of 250 tablets (10 blister folders of 25), and in Redipak cartons of 100 tablets (10 blister strips of 10).
2 mg, NDC 0008-0065, white, five-sided tablet with a raised "A" on one side and "WYETH" and "65" on scored reverse side, in bottles of 100, 500, and 1000 tablets, in Redipak cartons of 250 tablets (10 blister folders of 25), and in Redipak cartons of 100 tablets (10 blister strips of 10).

BOTTLES:
Keep tightly closed.
Store at controlled room temperature.
Dispense in tight container.
BLISTER PACKAGES:
Store at controlled room temperature.
Protect from light.
Use carton to protect contents from light.

The appearance of ATIVAN tablets is a registered trademark of Wyeth-Ayerst Laboratories.

Shown in Product Identification Guide, page 339

ATROMID-S® ℞

[*ă'trō-mid*]
Capsules
(clofibrate capsules)
Antilipidemic agent for reduction of elevated serum lipids

Caution: Federal law prohibits dispensing without prescription.

DESCRIPTION

Atromid-S Capsules (clofibrate capsules) is ethyl 2-(p-chlorophenoxy)-2-methyl-propionate, an antilipidemic agent.

structural formula

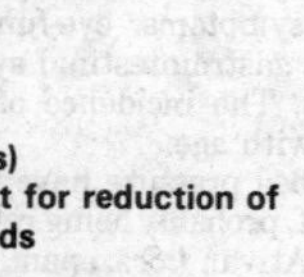

CH3
CH3CCOOCH2CH3
O
Cl

Its molecular formula is $C_{12}H_{15}O_3Cl$, molecular weight 242.7, and boiling point 148–150°C at 25 mm Hg. It is a stable, colorless to pale-yellow liquid with a faint odor and characteristic taste, soluble in common solvents but not in water. Each Atromid-S Capsule contains 500 mg clofibrate for oral administration.
Atromid-S Capsules contain the following inactive ingredients: D&C Red No. 28, D&C Red No. 30, D&C Yellow No. 10, FD&C Blue No. 1, FD&C Red No. 28, FD&C Red No. 40, FD&C Yellow No. 6, gelatin.

CLINICAL PHARMACOLOGY

Atromid-S is an antilipidemic agent. It acts to lower elevated serum lipids by reducing the very low-density lipoprotein fraction (S_f20–400) rich in triglycerides. Serum cholesterol may be decreased, particularly in those patients whose cholesterol elevation is due to the presence of IDL as a result of Type III hyperlipoproteinemia.
The mechanism of action has not been established definitively. Clofibrate may inhibit the hepatic release of lipoproteins (particularly VLDL), potentiate the action of lipoprotein lipase, and increase the fecal excretion of neutral sterols.
Between 95% and 99% of an oral dose of clofibrate is excreted in the urine as free and conjugated clofibric acid; thus, the absorption of clofibrate is virtually complete. The half-life of clofibric acid in normal volunteers averages 18 to 22 hours (range 14 to 35 hours) but can vary by up to 7 hours in the same subject at different times. Clofibric acid is highly protein-bound (95% to 97%). In subjects undergoing continuous clofibrate treatment, 1 g q12h, plasma concentrations of clofibric acid range from 120 to 125 mcg/mL to an approximate peak of 200 mcg/mL.
Several investigators have observed in their studies that clofibrate may produce a decrease in cholesterol linoleate but an increase in palmitoleate and oleate, the latter being considered atherogenic in experimental animals. The significance of this finding is unknown at this time.
Reduction of triglycerides in some patients treated with clofibrate or certain of its chemically and clinically similar analogs may be associated with an increase in LDL cholesterol. Increase in LDL cholesterol has been observed in patients whose cholesterol is initially normal.
Animal studies suggest that clofibrate interrupts cholesterol biosynthesis prior to mevalonate formation.

INDICATIONS AND USAGE

The initial treatment of choice for hyperlipidemia is dietary therapy specific for the type of hyperlipidemia.[1]
Excess body weight and alcoholic intake may be important factors in hypertriglyceridemia and should be addressed prior to any drug therapy. Physical exercise can be an important ancillary measure. Estrogen therapy, some beta-blockers, and thiazide diuretics may also be associated with increases in plasma triglycerides. Discontinuation of such products may obviate the need for specific antilipidemic therapy. Contributory diseases such as hypothyroidism or diabetes mellitus should be looked for and adequately treated. The use of drugs should be considered only when reasonable attempts have been made to obtain satisfactory results with nondrug methods. If the decision ultimately is to use drugs, the patient should be instructed that this does not reduce the importance of adhering to diet.
Because Atromid-S is associated with certain serious adverse findings reported in two large clinical trials (see "**Warnings**"), agents other than clofibrate may be more suitable for a particular patient.
Atromid-S is indicated for Primary Dysbetalipoproteinemia (Type III hyperlipidemia) that does not respond adequately to diet.
Atromid-S may be considered for the treatment of adult patients with very high serum-triglyceride levels (Type IV and V hyperlipidemia) who present a risk of abdominal pain and pancreatitis and who do not respond adequately to a determined dietary effort to control them. Patients who present such risk typically have serum triglycerides over 2000 mg/dl and have elevations of VLDL-cholesterol as well as fasting chylomicrons (Type V hyperlipidemia). Subjects who consistently have total serum or plasma triglycerides below 1000 mg/dl are unlikely to present a risk of pancreatitis. Atromid-S therapy may be considered for those subjects with triglyceride elevations between 1000 and 2000 mg/dl who have a history of pancreatitis or of recurrent abdominal pain typical of pancreatitis. It is recognized that some Type IV patients with triglycerides under 1000 mg/dl may, through dietary or alcoholic indiscretion, convert to a Type V pattern with massive triglyceride elevations accompanying fasting chylomicronemia, but the influence of Atromid-S therapy on the risk of pancreatitis in such situations has not been adequately studied.
Atromid-S is not useful for the hypertriglyceridemia of Type I hyperlipidemia, where elevations of chylomicrons and plasma triglycerides are accompanied by normal levels of very low-density lipoprotein (VLDL). Inspection of plasma refrigerated for 12 to 14 hours is helpful in distinguishing Types I, IV, and V hyperlipoproteinemia.[2]
Atromid-S has not been shown to be effective for prevention of coronary heart disease.
The biochemical response to Atromid-S is variable, and it is not always possible to predict from the lipoprotein type or other factors which patients will obtain favorable results. LDL cholesterol, as well as triglycerides, should be rechecked during the first several months of therapy in order to detect rises in LDL cholesterol that often accompany fibric-acid-type drug-induced reductions in elevated triglycerides. It is essential that lipid levels be reassessed periodically and that the drug be discontinued in any patient in whom lipids do not show significant improvement.

CONTRAINDICATIONS

Clofibrate is contraindicated in pregnant women. While teratogenic studies have not demonstrated any effect attributable to clofibrate, it is known that serum of the rabbit fetus accumulates a higher concentration of clofibrate than that found in maternal serum, and it is possible that the fetus may not have developed the enzyme system required for the excretion of clofibrate.
It is contraindicated in patients with clinically significant hepatic or renal dysfunction. Rhabdomyolysis and severe hyperkalemia have been reported in association with preexisting renal insufficiency.
It is contraindicated in patients with primary biliary cirrhosis, since it may raise the already elevated cholesterol in these cases.
It is contraindicated in patients with a known hypersensitivity to clofibrate.
It is contraindicated in nursing women (see "**Precautions**").

WARNINGS

In a large study involving 5,000 patients in a clofibrate-treated group and 5,000 in a placebo-treated group followed for an average of five years on drug or placebo and one year beyond (the WHO study), there was a statistically significant 44% higher age-adjusted total mortality in the clofibrate-treated group than in a comparable placebo group. The excess deaths were due to non-cardiovascular causes; half of this difference was due to malignancy; other causes of death included postcholecystectomy complications and pancreatitis.[3] In another prospective study involving 1,000 clofibrate- and 3,000 placebo-treated patients followed for an average of six years on drug or placebo (the Coronary Drug Project study), the noncardiovascular mortality rate, including that of malignancy, was not significantly different in the clofibrate- and placebo-treated groups.[4] This should not be interpreted to mean that clofibrate is not associated with an increased risk of noncardiovascular death, because the patients in the Coronary Drug Project were much older than those in the WHO study and they all had had a previous myocardial infarction, so that the deaths in the Coronary Drug Project were overwhelmingly due to cardiovascular causes, and it would have been very difficult to discern a clofibrate-associated risk of death due to noncardiovascular causes if it existed. Both studies demonstrated that clofibrate users have twice the risk of developing cholelithiasis and cholecystitis requiring surgery as do nonusers.

A potential benefit of clofibrate was, however, reported in the WHO study which involved patients with hypercholesterolemia and no history of myocardial infarction or angina pectoris. In this study, there was a statistically significant 25% decrease in subsequent nonfatal myocardial infarctions in the clofibrate-treated group when compared with the placebo group. There was no difference in incidence of fatal myocardial infarction in the two groups. In the Coronary Drug Project study, which involved patients with or without hypercholesterolemia and/or hypertriglyceridemia and with a history of previous myocardial infarction, there was no significant difference in incidence of either nonfatal or fatal myocardial infarction between the clofibrate- and placebo-treated groups.[3]

As a result of these and other studies, the following can be stated:

1. Clofibrate, in general, causes a relatively modest reduction of serum cholesterol and a somewhat greater reduction of serum triglycerides. In Type III hyperlipidemia, however, substantial reductions of both cholesterol and triglycerides can occur with clofibrate use.
2. No study to date has shown a convincing reduction in incidence of *fatal* myocardial infarction.
3. A significantly increased incidence of cholelithiasis has been demonstrated consistently in clofibrate-treated groups, and an increase in morbidity from this complication and mortality from cholecystectomy must be anticipated during clofibrate treatment.
4. Several types of other undesirable events have been associated in a statistically significant way with clofibrate administration in the WHO and the Coronary Drug Project studies. There was an increase in incidence of noncardiovascular deaths reported in the WHO study. There was an increase in cardiac arrhythmias, intermittent claudication, and definite or suspected thromboembolic events, and angina reported in the Coronary Drug Project, which was not, however, reported in the WHO study.
5. Administration of clofibrate to mice and rats in long-term studies at 1 to 2 times the maximum recommended human dose (based on surface area,

mg/m²), resulted in a higher incidence of benign and malignant liver tumors than in controls.

There was an increase in benign Leydig cell tumors in male rats treated at 400 mg/kg/day or 2 times the human dose in one study.

A comparative carcinogenicity study was also done in rats comparing three drugs in this class: fenofibrate (10 and 60 mg/kg; 0.3 and 1.6 times the human dose), clofibrate (400 mg/kg; 1.6 times the human dose), and gemfibrozil (250 mg/kg; 1.7 times the human dose). Pancreatic acinar adenomas were increased in males and females on fenofibrate; hepatocellular carcinoma and pancreatic acinar adenomas were increased in males and hepatic neoplastic nodules in females treated with clofibrate; hepatic neoplastic nodules were increased in males and females treated with gemfibrozil while testicular interstitial cell tumors were increased in males on all three drugs.

6. Administration of clofibrate to male monkeys at dosages of 1 to 2 times the maximum recommended human dose resulted in increases in mortality of 2- to 5-fold. As in the case of men in the WHO study, no single cause of death was identified.

BECAUSE OF THE TUMORIGENICITY OF CLOFIBRATE IN RODENTS AND THE POSSIBLE INCREASED RISK OF MALIGNANCY ASSOCIATED WITH CLOFIBRATE IN THE HUMAN, AS WELL AS THE INCREASED RISK OF CHOLELITHIASIS, AND BECAUSE THERE IS NOT, TO DATE, SUBSTANTIAL EVIDENCE OF A BENEFICIAL EFFECT ON CARDIOVASCULAR MORTALITY FROM CLOFIBRATE, THIS DRUG SHOULD BE UTILIZED ONLY FOR THOSE PATIENTS DESCRIBED IN THE "INDICATIONS AND USAGE" SECTION, AND SHOULD BE DISCONTINUED IF SIGNIFICANT LIPID RESPONSE IS NOT OBTAINED.

CONCOMITANT ANTICOAGULANTS
CAUTION SHOULD BE EXERCISED WHEN ANTICOAGULANTS ARE GIVEN IN CONJUNCTION WITH ATROMID-S. THE DOSAGE OF THE ANTICOAGULANT SHOULD BE REDUCED USUALLY BY ONE-HALF (DEPENDING ON THE INDIVIDUAL CASE) TO MAINTAIN THE PROTHROMBIN TIME AT THE DESIRED LEVEL TO PREVENT BLEEDING COMPLICATIONS. FREQUENT PROTHROMBIN DETERMINATIONS ARE ADVISABLE UNTIL IT HAS BEEN DEFINITELY DETERMINED THAT THE PROTHROMBIN LEVEL HAS BEEN STABILIZED.

SKELETAL MUSCLE
Myalgia, myositis, myopathy, and rhabdomyolysis with or without elevation of CPK have been associated with Atromid-S therapy. Consideration should be given to withholding or discontinuing drug therapy in any patient with a risk factor predisposing to the development of renal failure secondary to rhabdomyolysis, including: severe acute infection; hypotension; major surgery; trauma; severe metabolic, endocrine, or electrolyte disorders; and uncontrolled seizures. Atromid-S therapy should be discontinued if markedly elevated CPK levels occur or myositis is diagnosed.

AVOIDANCE OF PREGNANCY
Strict birth control procedures must be exercised by women of child-bearing potential. In patients who plan to become pregnant, clofibrate should be withdrawn several months before conception. Because of the possibility of pregnancy occurring despite birth-control precautions in patients taking clofibrate, the possible benefits of the drug to the patient must be weighed against possible hazards to the fetus. (See "PREGNANCY" section.)

PRECAUTIONS
GENERAL
Before instituting therapy with clofibrate, attempts should be made to control serum lipids with appropriate dietary regimens, weight loss in obese patients, control of diabetes mellitus, etc.

Because of the long-term administration of a drug of this nature, adequate baseline studies should be performed to determine that the patient has significantly elevated serum lipid levels. Frequent determinations of serum lipids should be obtained during the first few months of Atromid-S administration, and periodic determinations made thereafter. The drug should be withdrawn after three months if response is inadequate. However, in the case of xanthoma tuberosum, the drug should be employed for longer periods (even up to one year) provided that there is a reduction in the size and/or number of the xanthomata.

Since cholelithiasis is a possible side effect of clofibrate therapy, appropriate diagnostic procedures should be performed if signs and symptoms related to disease of the biliary system should occur.

Clofibrate may produce "flu-like" symptoms (muscular aching, soreness, cramping) associated with increased creatine kinase levels indicative of drug-induced myopathy. The physician should differentiate this from actual viral and/or bacterial disease.

Use with caution in patients with peptic ulcer, since reactivation has been reported. Whether this is drug related is unknown.

Various cardiac arrhythmias have been reported with the use of clofibrate.

LABORATORY TESTS
Subsequent serum lipid determinations should be done to detect a paradoxical rise in serum cholesterol or triglyceride levels. Clofibrate will not alter the seasonal variations of serum cholesterol: peak elevations in midwinter and late summer and decreases in fall and spring. If the drug is discontinued, the patient should be continued on an appropriate hypolipidemic diet, and serum lipids should be monitored until stabilized, as a rise in these values to or above the original baseline may occur.

During clofibrate therapy, frequent serum-transaminase determinations and other liver-function tests should be performed, since the drug may produce abnormalities in these parameters. These effects are usually reversible when the drug is discontinued. Hepatic biopsies are usually within normal limits. If the hepatic-function tests steadily rise or show excessive abnormalities, the drug should be withdrawn. Therefore, use with caution in those patients with a past history of jaundice or hepatic disease.

Complete blood counts should be done periodically since anemia, and more frequently, leukopenia have been reported in patients who have been taking clofibrate.

DRUG INTERACTIONS
Caution should be exercised when anticoagulants are given in conjunction with Atromid-S. Usually, the dosage of the anticoagulant should be reduced by one-half (depending on the individual case) to maintain the prothrombin time at the desired level to prevent bleeding complications. Frequent prothrombin determinations are advisable until it has been determined definitely that the prothrombin level has been stabilized.

Atromid-S may displace acidic drugs such as phenytoin or tolbutamide from their binding sites. Caution should be exercised when treating patients with either of these drugs or other highly protein-bound drugs and Atromid-S. The hypoglycemic effect of tolbutamide has been reported to increase when Atromid-S is given concurrently.

Fulminant rhabdomyolysis has been seen as early as three weeks after initiation of combined therapy with another fibrate and lovastatin but may be seen after several months. For these reasons, it is felt that, in most subjects who have had an unsatisfactory lipid response to either drug alone, the possible benefits of combined therapy with lovastatin and a fibrate do not outweigh the risks of severe myopathy, rhabdomyolysis, and acute renal failure. While it is not known whether this interaction occurs with fibrates other than gemfibrozil, myopathy and rhabdomyolysis have occasionally been associated with the use of fibrates alone, including clofibrate. Therefore, the combined use of lovastatin with fibrates should generally be avoided.

CARCINOGENESIS, MUTAGENESIS, IMPAIRMENT OF FERTILITY
See "Warnings" section for information on carcinogenesis and mutagenesis.

Arrest of spermatogenesis has been seen in both dogs and monkeys at doses approximately 2 times the maximum recommended human dose (based on surface area).

Electron microscopy studies have demonstrated peroxisomal proliferation following clofibrate administration to the rat. Changes in peroxisome morphology and numbers have been observed in humans after treatment with several members of the fibrate class, including clofibrate, when liver biopsies were compared before and after treatment in the same individual.

PREGNANCY
Teratogenic effects
Pregnancy Category C. Animal reproduction studies have not been conducted with Atromid-S. It is also not known whether Atromid-S can cause fetal harm when administered to a pregnant woman or can affect reproductive capacity. However, animal reproduction studies with clofibrate plus androsterone showed increases in neonatal deaths and pup mortality during lactation.

NURSING MOTHERS
Atromid-S is contraindicated in lactating women, since an active metabolite (CPIB) has been measured in breast milk.

PEDIATRIC USE
Safety and efficacy in pediatric patients have not been established.

ADVERSE REACTIONS
The most common is nausea. Less frequently encountered gastrointestinal reactions are vomiting, loose stools, dyspepsia, flatulence, and abdominal distress. Reactions reported less often than gastrointestinal ones are headache, dizziness, and fatigue; muscle cramping, aching, and weakness; skin rash, urticaria, and pruritus; dry brittle hair, and alopecia. The following reported adverse reactions are listed alphabetically by systems:

CARDIOVASCULAR
Increased or decreased angina.
Cardiac arrhythmias.
Both swelling and phlebitis at site of xanthomas.

DERMATOLOGIC
Allergic reactions including urticaria.
Skin rash.
Pruritus.
Dry skin and dry, brittle hair.
Alopecia.
Toxic epidermal necrolysis.
Erythema multiforme.
Stevens-Johnson syndrome.

GASTROINTESTINAL
Gallstones.
Nausea.
Vomiting.
Diarrhea.
Gastrointestinal upset (bloating, flatulence, abdominal distress).
Hepatomegaly (not associated with hepatotoxicity).
Stomatitis and gastritis.

GENITOURINARY
Findings consistent with renal dysfunction as evidenced by dysuria, hematuria, proteinuria, decreased urine output. One patient's renal biopsy suggested "allergic reaction."
Impotence and decreased libido.

HEMATOLOGIC
Leukopenia.
Potentiation of anticoagulant effect.
Anemia.
Eosinophilia.
Agranulocytosis.

MUSCULOSKELETAL
Myalgia (muscle cramping, aching, weakness).
"Flu-like" symptoms.
Myositis.
Myopathy.
Rhabdomyolysis in the setting of preexisting renal insufficiency.
Arthralgia.

NEUROLOGIC
Fatigue, weakness, drowsiness.
Dizziness.
Headache.

MISCELLANEOUS
Weight gain.
Polyphagia.

LABORATORY FINDINGS
Abnormal liver-function tests as evidenced by increased transaminase (SGOT and SGPT), BSP retention, and increased thymol turbidity
Proteinuria
Increased creatine phosphokinase
Hyperkalemia in association with renal insufficiency and continuous ambulatory peritoneal dialysis treatment
Reported adverse reactions whose direct relationship with the drug has not been established: peptic ulcer, gastrointestinal hemorrhage, rheumatoid arthritis, tremors, increased perspiration, systemic lupus erythematosus, blurred vision, gynecomastia, thrombocytopenic purpura.

OVERDOSAGE
While there has been no reported case of overdosage, should it occur, symptomatic supportive measures should be taken.

DOSAGE AND ADMINISTRATION
INITIAL: The recommended dosage for adults is 2 g daily in divided doses. Some patients may respond to a lower dosage.
MAINTENANCE: Same as for initial dosage.

HOW SUPPLIED
Atromid-S Capsules (clofibrate capsules)—Each orange, oblong, soft gelatin capsule contains 500 mg clofibrate, in bottles of 100 (NDC 0046-0243-81).
The appearance of these orange, oblong, soft-gelatin capsules is a trademark of Wyeth-Ayerst Laboratories.
Store at room temperature, approximately 25° C.
Dispense in a well-closed, light-resistant container as defined in the USP.
Avoid freezing and excessive heat.

REFERENCES
1. Coronary Risk Handbook (1973). American Heart Association.
2. Nikkila, EA: Familial lipoprotein lipase deficiency and related disorders of chylomicron metabolism. In Stanbury JB et al (eds): The Metabolic Basis of Inherited Disease, 5th ed., McGraw-Hill, 1983, Chap. 30. p.622–642.
3. Report from the Committee of Principal Investigators: A cooperative trial in the primary prevention of ischaemic heart disease using clofibrate. Br Heart J 40:1069, 1978.

Continued on next page

Wyeth-Ayerst Laboratories—Cont.

4. The Coronary Drug Project Research Group: Clofibrate and niacin in coronary heart disease. JAMA *231*:360, 1975.

Shown in Product Identification Guide, page 339

AURALGAN® ℞

[aw-răl 'gan]

Otic Solution

Caution: Federal law prohibits dispensing without prescription.

DESCRIPTION

Each mL contains:

Antipyrine	54.0 mg
Benzocaine	14.0 mg
Glycerin dehydrated q.s. to	1.0 mL

(contains not more than 0.6% moisture)
(also contains oxyquinoline sulfate)

TOPICAL DECONGESTANT AND ANALGESIC

Auralgan is an otic solution containing antipyrine, benzocaine, and dehydrated glycerin. The solution congeals at 0° C (32° F), but returns to normal consistency, unchanged, at room temperature.

The structures of the components are:

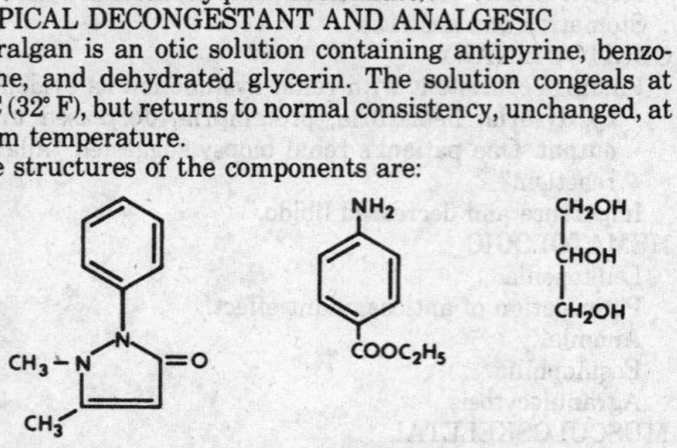

antipyrine benzocaine glycerin

CLINICAL PHARMACOLOGY

Auralgan combines the hygroscopic property of dehydrated glycerin with the analgesic action of antipyrine and benzocaine to relieve pressure, reduce inflammation and congestion, and alleviate pain and discomfort in acute otitis media. Auralgan does not blanch the tympanic membrane or mask the landmarks and, therefore, does not distort the otoscopic picture.

INDICATIONS AND USAGE

ACUTE OTITIS MEDIA OF VARIOUS ETIOLOGIES

— prompt relief of pain and reduction of inflammation in the congestive and serous stages

— adjuvant therapy during systemic antibiotic administration for resolution of the infection

Because of the close anatomical relationship of the eustachian tube to the nasal cavity, otitis media is a frequent problem, especially in children in whom the tube is shorter, wider, and more horizontal than in adults.

REMOVAL OF CERUMEN

—facilitates the removal of excessive or impacted cerumen

CONTRAINDICATIONS

Hypersensitivity to any of the components or substances related to them.

Perforated tympanic membrane is considered a contraindication to the use of any medication in the external ear canal.

WARNINGS

Discontinue promptly if sensitization or irritation occurs.

PRECAUTIONS

CARCINOGENESIS, MUTAGENESIS, IMPAIRMENT OF FERTILITY

No long-term studies in animals or humans have been conducted

PREGNANCY CATEGORY C

Animal reproduction studies have not been conducted with Auralgan. It is also not known whether Auralgan can cause fetal harm when administered to a pregnant woman, or can affect reproduction capacity. Auralgan should be given to a pregnant woman only if clearly needed.

NURSING MOTHERS

It is not known whether this drug is excreted in human milk. Because many drugs are excreted in human milk, caution should be exercised when Auralgan is administered to a nursing woman.

DOSAGE AND ADMINISTRATION

ACUTE OTITIS MEDIA

Instill Auralgan permitting the solution to run along the wall of the canal until it is filled. Avoid touching the ear with dropper. Then moisten a cotton pledget with Auralgan and insert into meatus. Repeat every one to two hours until pain and congestion are relieved.

REMOVAL OF CERUMEN

Before: Instill Auralgan three times daily for two or three days to help detach cerumen from wall of canal and facilitate removal.

After: Auralgan is useful for drying out the canal or relieving discomfort.

Before and after removal of cerumen, a cotton pledget moistened with Auralgan should be inserted into the meatus following instillation.

Note: Do not rinse dropper after use.

Replace dropper in bottle after each use. Hold dropper assembly by screw cap and, without compressing the rubber bulb, insert into drug container and screw down tightly.

Protect the solution from light and heat, and do not use if it is brown or contains a precipitate.

DISCARD THIS PRODUCT SIX MONTHS AFTER DROPPER IS FIRST PLACED IN THE DRUG SOLUTION.

HOW SUPPLIED

Auralgan® Otic Solution, in package containing 10 mL bottle with separate dropper-screw cap attachment (NDC 0046-1000-10).

Store at room temperature (approximately 25° C).

BASALJEL® OTC

[bā 'sel-jel]

(basic aluminum carbonate gel)

SUSPENSION • CAPSULES • TABLETS

COMPOSITION

Suspension—each 5 mL teaspoonful contains basic aluminum carbonate gel equivalent to 400 mg aluminum hydroxide. Inactive ingredients are artificial and natural flavors, butylparaben, calcium benzoate, glycerin, hydroxypropyl methylcellulose, methylparaben, mineral oil, propylparaben, saccharin, simethicone, sorbitol solution, and water. Capsule contains dried basic aluminum carbonate gel equivalent to 608 mg of dried aluminum hydroxide gel or 500 mg aluminum hydroxide. Inactive ingredients are D&C Yellow 10, FD&C Blue 1, FD&C Red 40, FD&C Yellow 6, gelatin, polacrilin potassium, polyethylene glycol, talc, and titanium dioxide. Tablet contains dried basic aluminum carbonate gel equivalent to 608 mg of dried aluminum hydroxide gel or 500 mg aluminum hydroxide. Inactive ingredients are cellulose, hydrogenated vegetable oil, magnesium stearate, polacrilin potassium, starch, and talc.

INDICATIONS

Symptomatic relief of hyperacidity associated with peptic ulcer, gastritis, peptic esophagitis, gastric hyperacidity, and hiatal hernia. For the treatment, control, or management of hyperphosphatemia, or for use with a low phosphate diet to prevent formation of phosphate urinary stones, through the reduction of phosphates in the serum and urine.

WARNINGS

No more than 24 tablets/capsules/teaspoonfuls of BASALJEL should be taken in a 24-hour period. Aluminum forms insoluble complexes with phosphate in the gastrointestinal tract, thus decreasing phosphate absorption. Prolonged use of aluminum-containing antacids by normophosphatemic patients may result in hypophosphatemia if phosphate intake is not adequate. In its more severe forms, hypophosphatemia can lead to anorexia, malaise, muscle weakness, and osteomalacia. A usually transient hypercalciuria of mild degree may be associated with the early weeks of therapy. Prolonged use of aluminum-containing antacids in patients with renal failure may result in or worsen dialysis osteomalacia. Elevated tissue aluminum levels contribute to the development of dialysis encephalopathy and osteomalacia syndromes. Also, a number of cases of dialysis encephalopathy have been associated with elevated aluminum levels in the dialysate water. Small amounts of aluminum are absorbed from the gastrointestinal tract and renal excretion of aluminum is impaired in renal failure. Prolonged use of aluminum-containing antacids in such patients may contribute to increased plasma levels of aluminum. Aluminum is not well removed by dialysis because it is bound to albumin and transferrin, which do not cross dialysis membranes. As a result, aluminum is deposited in bone, and dialysis osteomalacia may develop when large amounts of aluminum are ingested orally by patients with impaired renal function. Pregnant women and nursing mothers are advised to seek the advice of a health professional before using this product.

PRECAUTIONS

May cause constipation. Adequate fluid intake should be maintained in addition to the specific medical or surgical management indicated by the patient's condition.

DRUG INTERACTIONS

Alumina-containing antacids should not be used concomitantly with any form of tetracycline therapy.

DOSAGE AND ADMINISTRATION

Suspension—2 teaspoonfuls (10 mL) in water or fruit juice taken as often as every 2 hours up to 12 times daily. Two teaspoonfuls have the capacity to neutralize 23 mEq of acid. Capsules—2 capsules as often as every 2 hours up to 12 times daily. Two capsules have the capacity to neutralize 24 mEq of acid. Tablets—2 tablets as often as every 2 hours up to 12 times daily. Two tablets have the capacity to neutralize 25 mEq of acid.

Hyperphosphatemia: An initial dose of Basaljel equivalent to 1.0 gm aluminum hydroxide—2 capsules, 2 tablets, or 2.5 teaspoonfuls (12 mL) suspension—taken 3 to 4 times per day with meals (total daily dose 3–4 gm) is recommended. After therapy is initiated, Basaljel dosage should be adjusted to the minimum required amount by carefully monitoring dietary phosphate intake (patients should be instructed on maintaining a low phosphate diet) and measurement of serum phosphorus levels on a regular basis. Sodium content is: 0.13 mEq/5 mL for the suspension, 0.12 mEq per capsule, and 0.12 mEq per tablet.

HOW SUPPLIED

Suspension—bottles of 12 fluidounces; Capsules—bottles of 100 and 500; Tablets (scored)—bottles of 100.

BICILLIN® C-R ℞

[bī-sil 'in]

(penicillin G benzathine and penicillin G procaine suspension)

INJECTION

FOR DEEP INTRAMUSCULAR INJECTION ONLY

DESCRIPTION

Bicillin C-R (penicillin G benzathine and penicillin G procaine suspension), contains equal amounts of the benzathine and procaine salts of penicillin G. It is available for deep intramuscular injection.

Penicillin G benzathine is prepared by the reaction of dibenzylethylene diamine with two molecules of penicillin G. It is chemically designated as 3,3-dimethyl-7-oxo-6-(2-phenylacetamido)-4-thia-1-azabicyclo [3.2.0] heptane-2-carboxylic acid compound with *N,N'* -dibenzylethylenediamine (2:1), tetrahydrate. It occurs as a white, crystalline powder and is very slightly soluble in water and sparingly soluble in alcohol.

Penicillin G procaine, 3,3-dimethyl-7-oxo-6-(2-phenylacetamido)-4-thia-1-azabicyclo [3.2.0] heptane-2-carboxylic acid 2-(diethylamino)ethyl p-aminobenzoate compound(1:1) monohydrate, is an equimolar salt of procaine and penicillin G. It occurs as white crystals or a white, microcrystalline powder and is slightly soluble in water.

Bicillin C-R (penicillin G benzathine and penicillin G procaine suspension) contains in each mL the equivalent of 150,000 units of penicillin G as the benzathine salt and 150,000 units of penicillin G as the procaine salt in a stabilized aqueous suspension with sodium citrate buffer; and as w/v, approximately 0.5% lecithin, 0.55% carboxymethylcellulose, 0.55% povidone, 0.1% methylparaben, and 0.01% propylparaben.

Each disposable syringe (4 mL size) contains the equivalent of 2,400,000 units of penicillin G comprising: the equivalent of 1,200,000 units of penicillin G as the benzathine salt and the equivalent of 1,200,000 units of penicillin G as the procaine salt in a stabilized aqueous suspension with sodium citrate buffer; and as w/v, approximately 0.5% lecithin, 0.55% carboxymethylcellulose, 0.55% povidone, 0.1% methylparaben, and 0.01% propylparaben.

Each TUBEX cartridge (1 mL size) contains the equivalent of 600,000 units of penicillin G comprising: the equivalent of 300,000 units penicillin G as the benzathine salt and the equivalent of 300,000 units penicillin G as the procaine salt in a stabilized aqueous suspension with sodium citrate buffer; and as w/v, approximately 0.5% lecithin, 0.55% carboxymethylcellulose, 0.55% povidone, 0.1% methylparaben, and 0.01% propylparaben.

Each TUBEX cartridge (2 mL size) contains the equivalent of 1,200,000 units of penicillin G comprising: the equivalent of 600,000 units of penicillin G as the benzathine salt and the equivalent of 600,000 units of penicillin G as the procaine salt in a stabilized aqueous suspension with sodium citrate buffer; and as w/v, approximately 0.5% lecithin, 0.55% carboxymethylcellulose, 0.55% povidone, 0.1% methylparaben, and 0.01% propylparaben.

Bicillin C-R suspension in the multiple-dose-vial formulation, disposable-syringe formulation, and the TUBEX formulation is viscous and opaque. Read **"Contraindications," "Warnings," "Precautions,"** and **"Dosage and Administration"** sections prior to use.

CLINICAL PHARMACOLOGY

GENERAL

Penicillin G benzathine and penicillin G procaine have a low solubility and, thus, the drugs are slowly released from intramuscular injection sites. The drugs are hydrolyzed to penicillin G. This combination of hydrolysis and slow absorption results in blood serum levels much lower but more prolonged than other parenteral penicillins.

Intramuscular administration of 600,000 units of Bicillin C-R in adults usually produces peak blood levels of 1.0 to 1.3 units per mL within 3 hours; this level falls to an average concentration of 0.32 units per mL at 12 hours, 0.19 units per mL at 24 hours, and 0.03 units per mL at seven days.
Intramuscular administration of 1,200,000 units of Bicillin C-R in adults usually produces peak blood levels of 2.1 to 2.6 units per mL within 3 hours; this level falls to an average concentration of 0.75 units per mL at 12 hours, 0.28 units per mL at 24 hours, and 0.04 units per mL at seven days.
Approximately 60% of penicillin G is bound to serum protein. The drug is distributed throughout the body tissues in widely varying amounts. Highest levels are found in the kidneys with lesser amounts in the liver, skin, and intestines. Penicillin G penetrates into all other tissues and the spinal fluid to a lesser degree. With normal kidney function, the drug is excreted rapidly by tubular excretion. In neonates and young infants and in individuals with impaired kidney function, excretion is considerably delayed.

MICROBIOLOGY

Penicillin G exerts a bactericidal action against penicillin-susceptible microorganisms during the stage of active multiplication. It acts through the inhibition of biosynthesis of cell-wall mucopeptide. It is not active against the penicillinase-producing bacteria, which include many strains of staphylococci. The following *in vitro* data are available, but their clinical significance is unknown. Penicillin G exerts high *in vitro* activity against staphylococci (except penicillinase-producing strains), streptococci (Groups A, C, G, H, L, and M), and pneumococci. Other organisms susceptible to penicillin G are *Neisseria gonorrhoeae, Corynebacterium diphtheriae, Bacillus anthracis,* Clostridia species, *Actinomyces bovis, Streptobacillus moniliformis, Listeria monocytogenes,* and Leptospira species. *Treponema pallidum* is extremely susceptible to the bactericidal action of penicillin G.
Susceptibility Test: If the Kirby-Bauer method of disc susceptibility is used, a 10-unit penicillin disc should give a zone greater than 28 mm when tested against a penicillin-sensitive bacterial strain.

INDICATIONS AND USAGE

This drug is indicated in the treatment of moderately severe infections due to penicillin-G-susceptible microorganisms that are susceptible to serum levels common to this particular dosage form. Therapy should be guided by bacteriological studies (including susceptibility testing) and by clinical response.
Bicillin C-R is indicated in the treatment of the following in children of all ages:
Moderately severe to severe infections of the upper-respiratory tract, scarlet fever, erysipelas, and skin and soft-tissue infections due to susceptible streptococci.
NOTE: Streptococci in Groups A, C, G, H, L, and M are very sensitive to penicillin G. Other groups, including Group D (enterococci), are resistant. Penicillin G sodium or potassium is recommended for streptococcal infections with bacteremia.
Moderately severe pneumonia and otitis media due to susceptible pneumococci.
NOTE: Severe pneumonia, empyema, bacteremia, pericarditis, meningitis, peritonitis, and arthritis of pneumococcal etiology are better treated with penicillin G sodium or potassium during the acute stage.
When high, sustained serum levels are required, penicillin G sodium or potassium, either IM or IV, should be used. This drug should not be used in the treatment of venereal diseases, including syphilis, gonorrhea, yaws, bejel, and pinta.

CONTRAINDICATIONS

A previous hypersensitivity reaction to any penicillin or to procaine is a contraindication.
Do not inject into or near an artery or nerve.

WARNINGS

The combination of penicillin G benzathine and penicillin G procaine should only be prescribed for the indications listed in this insert.
Serious and occasionally fatal hypersensitivity (anaphylactoid) reactions have been reported in patients receiving penicillin. Although anaphylaxis is more frequent following parenteral therapy, it has occurred in patients on oral penicillins. These reactions are more apt to occur in individuals with a history of sensitivity to multiple allergens.
There are reports of patients with a history of penicillin hypersensitivity reactions who experienced severe hypersensitivity reactions when treated with a cephalosporin. Before therapy with a penicillin, careful inquiry should be made about previous hypersensitivity reactions to penicillins, cephalosporins, and other allergens. If an allergic reaction occurs, the drug should be discontinued and appropriate therapy should be instituted. Serious anaphylactoid reactions require immediate emergency treatment with epinephrine. Oxygen, intravenous steroids, airway management, including intubation, should also be administered as indicated.
Inadvertent intravascular administration, including inadvertent direct intra-arterial injection or injection immediately adjacent to arteries, of Bicillin C-R and other penicillin preparations has resulted in severe neurovascular damage, including transverse myelitis with permanent paralysis, gangrene requiring amputation of digits and more proximal portions of extremities, and necrosis and sloughing at and surrounding the injection site. Such severe effects have been reported following injections into the buttock, thigh, and deltoid areas. Other serious complications of suspected intravascular administration which have been reported include immediate pallor, mottling or cyanosis of the extremity both distal and proximal to the injection site followed by bleb formation; severe edema requiring anterior and/or posterior compartment fasciotomy in the lower extremity. The above-described severe effects and complications have most often occurred in infants and small children. Prompt consultation with an appropriate specialist is indicated if any evidence of compromise of the blood supply occurs at, proximal to, or distal to the site of injection.[1–9] See "**Contraindications,**" "**Precautions,**" and "**Dosage and Administration**" sections.
Quadriceps femoris fibrosis and atrophy have been reported following repeated intramuscular injections of penicillin preparations into the anterolateral thigh.
Injection into or near a nerve may result in permanent neurological damage.

PRECAUTIONS

GENERAL

Penicillin should be used with caution in individuals with histories of significant allergies and/or asthma.
Care should be taken to avoid intravenous or intra-arterial administration, or injection into or near major peripheral nerves or blood vessels, since such injections may produce neurovascular damage. See "**Contraindications,**" "**Warnings,**" and "**Dosage and Administration**" sections.
A small percentage of patients are sensitive to procaine. If there is a history of sensitivity, make the usual test: Inject intradermally 0.1 mL of a 1 to 2 percent procaine solution. Development of an erythema, wheal, flare, or eruption indicates procaine sensitivity. Sensitivity should be treated by the usual methods, including barbiturates, and procaine penicillin preparations should not be used. Antihistaminics appear beneficial in treatment of procaine reactions.
The use of antibiotics may result in overgrowth of nonsusceptible organisms. Constant observation of the patient is essential. If new infections due to bacteria or fungi appear during therapy, the drug should be discontinued and appropriate measures taken.
Whenever allergic reactions occur, penicillin should be withdrawn unless, in the opinion of the physician, the condition being treated is life-threatening and amenable only to penicillin therapy.
In prolonged therapy with penicillin, and particularly with high-dosage schedules, periodic evaluation of the renal and hematopoietic systems is recommended.

LABORATORY TESTS

In streptococcal infections, therapy must be sufficient to eliminate the organism; otherwise, the sequelae of streptococcal disease may occur. Cultures should be taken following completion of treatment to determine whether streptococci have been eradicated.

DRUG INTERACTIONS

Tetracycline, a bacteriostatic antibiotic, may antagonize the bactericidal effect of penicillin, and concurrent use of these drugs should be avoided.
Concurrent administration of penicillin and probenecid increases and prolongs serum penicillin levels by decreasing the apparent volume of distribution and slowing the rate of excretion by competitively inhibiting renal tubular secretion of penicillin.

PREGNANCY CATEGORY B

Reproduction studies performed in the mouse, rat, and rabbit have revealed no evidence of impaired fertility or harm to the fetus due to penicillin G. Human experience with the penicillins during pregnancy has not shown any positive evidence of adverse effects on the fetus. There are, however, no adequate and well-controlled studies in pregnant women showing conclusively that harmful effects of these drugs on the fetus can be excluded. Because animal reproduction studies are not always predictive of human response, this drug should be used during pregnancy only if clearly needed.

NURSING MOTHERS

Soluble penicillin G is excreted in breast milk. Caution should be exercised when penicillin G benzathine and penicillin G procaine are administered to a nursing woman.

CARCINOGENESIS, MUTAGENESIS, IMPAIRMENT OF FERTILITY

No long-term animal studies have been conducted with these drugs.

PEDIATRIC USE

See "**Indications and Usage**" and "**Dosage and Administration.**"

ADVERSE REACTIONS

As with other penicillins, untoward reactions of the sensitivity phenomena are likely to occur, particularly in individuals who have previously demonstrated hypersensitivity to penicillins or in those with a history of allergy, asthma, hay fever, or urticaria.
The following have been reported with parenteral penicillin G:
General: Hypersensitivity reactions including the following: skin eruptions (maculopapular to exfoliative dermatitis), urticaria, laryngeal edema, fever, eosinophilia; other serum-sicknesslike reactions (including chills, fever, edema, arthralgia, and prostration); anaphylaxis. Note: Urticaria, other skin rashes, and serum-sicknesslike reactions may be controlled with antihistamines and, if necessary, systemic corticosteriods. Whenever such reactions occur, penicillin G should be discontinued unless, in the opinion of the physician, the condition being treated is life-threatening and amenable only to therapy with penicillin G. Serious anaphylactic reactions require the immediate use of epinephrine, oxygen, and intravenous steroids.
Hematologic: Hemolytic anemia, leukopenia, thrombocytopenia.
Neurologic: Neuropathy.
Urogenital: Nephropathy.

OVERDOSAGE

Penicillin in overdosage has the potential to cause neuromuscular hyperirritability or convulsive seizures.

DOSAGE AND ADMINISTRATION

Administer by DEEP, INTRAMUSCULAR INJECTION in the upper, outer quadrant of the buttock. In infants and small children, the midlateral aspect of the thigh may be preferable. When doses are repeated, vary the injection site.
When using the multiple-dose vial:
Shake multiple-dose vial vigorously before withdrawing the desired dose.
Due to the viscous nature of this medication, a 23 gauge or larger bore needle should be used to withdraw medication from the vial and for patient administration. A smaller bore needle, such as a 24 or 25 gauge, is not recommended.
After selection of the proper site and insertion of the needle into the selected muscle, aspirate by pulling back on the plunger. While maintaining negative pressure for 2 to 3 seconds, carefully observe the neck of the syringe immediately proximal to the needle hub for appearance of blood or any discoloration. Blood or "typical blood color" may *not* be seen if a blood vessel has been entered—only a mixture of blood and Bicillin C-R. The appearance of any discoloration is reason to withdraw the needle and discard the syringe. If it is elected to inject at another site, a new syringe and needle should be used. If no blood or discoloration appears, inject the contents of the syringe slowly. Discontinue delivery of the dose if the subject complains of severe immediate pain at the injection site or if in infants and young children symptoms or signs occur suggesting onset of severe pain.
When using the TUBEX cartridge:
The Wyeth-Ayerst TUBEX cartridge for this product incorporates several features that are designed to facilitate the visualization of blood on aspiration if a blood vessel is inadvertently entered.

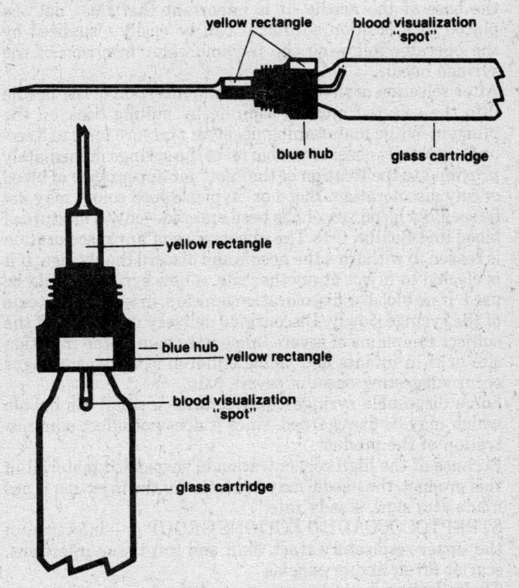

yellow rectangle
blood visualization "spot"
blue hub
glass cartridge
yellow rectangle
blue hub
yellow rectangle
blood visualization "spot"
glass cartridge

The design of this cartridge is such that blood which enters its needle will be quickly visualized as a red or dark-colored "spot." This "spot" will appear on the barrel of the glass cartridge immediately proximal to the blue hub. The TUBEX is designed with two orientation marks, in order to determine where the "spot" can be seen. First insert and secure the

Continued on next page

Wyeth-Ayerst Laboratories—Cont.

cartridge in the TUBEX injector in the usual fashion. Locate the yellow rectangle at the base of the blue hub. This yellow rectangle is aligned with the blood visualization "spot." An imaginary straight line, drawn from this yellow rectangle to the shoulder of the glass cartridge, will point to the area on the cartridge where the "spot" can be visualized. When the needle cover is removed, a second yellow rectangle will be visible. The second yellow rectangle is also aligned with the blood visualization "spot" to assist the operator in locating this "spot." If the 2 mL metal or plastic syringe is used, the glass cartridge should be rotated by turning the plunger of the syringe clockwise until the yellow rectangle is visualized. If the 1 mL metal syringe is used, it will not be possible to continue to rotate the glass cartridge clockwise once it is properly engaged and fully threaded; it can, however, then be rotated counterclockwise as far as necessary to properly orient the yellow rectangles and locate the observation area. (In this same area in some cartridges, a dark spot may sometimes be visualized prior to injection. This is the proximal end of the needle and does not represent a foreign body in, or other abnormality of, the suspension.)

Thus, before the needle is inserted into the selected muscle, it is important for the operator to orient the yellow rectangle so that any blood which may enter after needle insertion and during aspiration can be visualized in the area on the cartridge where it will appear and not be obscured by any obstructions.

After selection of the proper site and insertion of the needle into the selected muscle, aspirate by pulling back on the plunger. While maintaining negative pressure for 2 to 3 seconds, carefully observe the neck of the glass TUBEX cartridge immediately proximal to the blue plastic needle hub for appearance of blood or any discoloration.

Blood or "typical blood color" may *not* be seen if a blood vessel has been entered—only a mixture of blood and Bicillin C-R. The appearance of any discoloration is reason to withdraw the needle and discard the TUBEX. If it is elected to inject at another site, a new TUBEX cartridge should be used. If no blood or discoloration appears, inject the contents of the TUBEX slowly. Discontinue delivery of the dose if the subject complains of severe immediate pain at the injection site or if in infants and young children symptoms or signs occur suggesting onset of severe pain.

Some TUBEX cartridges may contain a small air bubble which may be disregarded since it does not affect administration of the product.

Because of the high concentration of suspended material in this product, the needle may be blocked if the injection is not made at a slow, steady rate.

When using the disposable syringe:

The Wyeth-Ayerst disposable syringe for this product incorporates several new features that are designed to facilitate its use.

A single small indentation, or "dot," has been punched into the metal ring that surrounds the neck of the syringe near the base of the needle. It is important that this "dot" be placed in a position so that it can be easily visualized by the operator following the intramuscular insertion of the syringe needle.

After selection of the proper site and insertion of the needle into the selected muscle, aspirate by pulling back on the plunger. While maintaining negative pressure for 2 to 3 seconds, carefully observe the barrel of the syringe immediately proximal to the location of the "dot" for appearance of blood or any discoloration. Blood or "typical blood color" may *not* be seen if a blood vessel has been entered—only a mixture of blood and Bicillin C-R. The appearance of any discoloration is reason to withdraw the needle and discard the syringe. If it is elected to inject at another site, a new syringe should be used. If no blood or discoloration appears, inject the contents of the syringe slowly. Discontinue delivery of the dose if the subject complains of severe immediate pain at the injection site or if in infants and young children symptoms or signs occur suggesting onset of severe pain.

Some disposable syringes may contain a small air bubble which may be disregarded, since it does not affect administration of the product.

Because of the high concentration of suspended material in this product, the needle may be blocked if the injection is not made at a slow, steady rate.

STREPTOCOCCAL INFECTIONS GROUP A —Infections of the upper-respiratory tract, skin and soft-tissue infections, scarlet fever, and erysipelas.

The following doses are recommended:

Adults and children over 60 lbs. in weight: 2,400,000 units.
Children from 30 to 60 lbs.: 900,000 units to 1,200,000 units.
Infants and children under 30 lbs.: 600,000 units.

NOTE: Treatment with the recommended dosage is usually given at a single session using multiple IM sites when indicated. An alternative dosage schedule may be used, giving one-half ($^1/_2$) the total dose on day 1 and one-half ($^1/_2$) on day 3. This will also insure the penicillinemia required over a 10-day period; however, this alternate schedule should be used only when the physician can be assured of the patient's cooperation.

PNEUMOCOCCAL INFECTIONS (except pneumococcal meningitis)

600,000 units in children and 1,200,000 units in adults, repeated every 2 or 3 days until the temperature is normal for 48 hours. Other forms of penicillin may be necessary for severe cases.

Parenteral drug products should be inspected visually for particulate matter and discoloration prior to administration whenever solution and container permit.

HOW SUPPLIED

Bicillin® C-R (penicillin G benzathine and penicillin G procaine suspension) is supplied in packages of 10 TUBEX® Sterile Cartridge-Needle Units (20 gauge × $1^1/_4$ inch needle) as follows:

1 mL size, containing 600,000 units per TUBEX, NDC 0008-0026-17.

2 mL size, containing 1,200,000 units per TUBEX, NDC 0008-0026-16.

Store in a refrigerator.
Keep from freezing.

ALSO AVAILABLE

Bicillin C-R (penicillin G benzathine and penicillin G procaine suspension) is also available in packages of 10 disposable syringes as follows:

4 mL size, 2,400,000 units per syringe (18 gauge × 2 inch needle), NDC 0008-0026-22.

Bicillin C-R (penicillin G benzathine and penicillin G procaine suspension) is also available in packages of single multiple-dose vials as follows:

10 mL size, 300,000 units per mL, NDC 0008-0176-01.

Store in a refrigerator.
Keep from freezing.
Shake multiple-dose vials well before using.

REFERENCES

1. SHAW, E.: Transverse myelitis from injection of penicillin. *Am. J. Dis. Child., 111*:548, 1966.
2. KNOWLES, J.: Accidental intra-arterial injection of penicillin. *Am. J. Dis. Child., 111*:552, 1966.
3. DARBY, C., et al: Ischemia following an intragluteal injection of benzathine-procaine penicillin G mixture in a one-year-old boy. *Clin. Pediatrics, 12*:485, 1973.
4. BROWN, L. & NELSON, A.: Postinfectious intravascular thrombosis with gangrene. *Arch. Surg., 94*:652, 1967.
5. BORENSTINE, J.: Transverse myelitis and penicillin (Correspondence). *Am. J. Dis. Child., 112*:166, 1966.
6. ATKINSON, J.: Transverse myelopathy secondary to penicillin injection. *J. Pediatrics, 75*:867, 1969.
7. TALBERT, J. et al: Gangrene of the foot following intramuscular injection in the lateral thigh: A case report with recommendations for prevention. *J. Pediatrics, 70*:110, 1967.
8. FISHER, T.: Medicolegal affairs. *Canad. Med. Assoc. J., 112*:395, 1975.
9. SCHANZER, H. et al: Accidental intraarterial injection of penicillin G. *JAMA, 242*:1289, 1979.

BICILLIN® C-R 900/300 ℞

[*bī-sil'in*]
(penicillin G benzathine and penicillin G procaine suspension)
INJECTION

FOR DEEP INTRAMUSCULAR INJECTION ONLY

DESCRIPTION

Bicillin C-R 900/300 (penicillin G benzathine and penicillin G procaine suspension) contains the equivalent of 900,000 units of penicillin G as the benzathine and 300,000 units of penicillin G as the procaine salts. It is available for deep intramuscular injection.

Penicillin G benzathine is prepared by the reaction of dibenzylethylene diamine with two molecules of penicillin G. It is chemically designated as 3,3-dimethyl-7-oxo-6-(2-phenylacetamido)-4-thia-1-azabicyclo[3.2.0]heptane-2-carboxylic acid compound with *N,N'*-dibenzylethylenediamine (2:1), tetrahydrate. It occurs as a white, crystalline powder and is very slightly soluble in water and sparingly soluble in alcohol.

Penicillin G procaine, 3,3-dimethyl-7-oxo-6-(2-phenylacetamido)-4-thia-1-azabicyclo[3.2.0] heptane-2- carboxylic acid compound with 2-(diethylamino)ethyl *p*-aminobenzoate compound (1:1) monohydrate, is an equimolar salt of procaine and penicillin G. It occurs as white crystals or a white, microcrystalline powder and is slightly soluble in water.

Each TUBEX® cartridge (2 mL size) contains the equivalent to 1,200,000 units of penicillin G as follows: penicillin G benzathine equivalent to 900,000 units of penicillin G and penicillin G procaine equivalent to 300,000 units of penicillin G in a stabilized aqueous suspension with sodium citrate buffer; and as w/v, approximately 0.5% lecithin, 0.55% carboxymethylcellulose, 0.55% povidone, 0.1% methylparaben, and 0.01% propylparaben.

Bicillin C-R 900/300 suspension in TUBEX formulation is viscous and opaque. Read "**Contraindications**," "**Warnings**," "**Precautions**," and "**Dosage and Administration**" sections prior to use.

CLINICAL PHARMACOLOGY

GENERAL

Penicillin G benzathine and penicillin G procaine have a low solubility and, thus, the drugs are slowly released from intramuscular injection sites. The drugs are hydrolyzed to penicillin G. This combination of hydrolysis and slow absorption results in blood serum levels much lower but more prolonged than other parenteral penicillins. Intramuscular administration of 1,200,000 units of Bicillin C-R 900/300 in patients weighing 100 to 140 lbs. usually produces average blood levels of 0.24 units/mL at 24 hours, 0.039 units/mL at 7 days, and 0.024 units/mL at 10 days.

Approximately 60% of penicillin G is bound to serum protein. The drug is distributed throughout the body tissues in widely varying amounts. Highest levels are found in the kidneys with lesser amounts in the liver, skin, and intestines. Penicillin G penetrates into all other tissues and the spinal fluid to a lesser degree. With normal kidney function, the drug is excreted rapidly by tubular excretion. In neonates and young infants and in individuals with impaired kidney function, excretion is considerably delayed.

MICROBIOLOGY

Penicillin G exerts a bactericidal action against penicillin-susceptible microorganisms during the stage of active multiplication. It acts through the inhibition of biosynthesis of cell-wall mucopeptide. It is not active against the penicillinase-producing bacteria, which include many strains of staphylococci.

The following *in vitro* data are available, but their clinical significance is unknown. Penicillin G exerts high *in vitro* activity against staphylococci (except penicillinase-producing strains), streptococci (Groups A, C, G, H, L, and M), and pneumococci. Other organisms susceptible to penicillin G are *Neisseria gonorrhoeae, Corynebacterium diphtheriae, Bacillus anthracis,* Clostridia species, *Actinomyces bovis, Streptobacillus moniliformis, Listeria monocytogenes,* and Leptospira species. *Treponema pallidum* is extremely susceptible to the bactericidal action of penicillin G.

Susceptibility Test: If the Kirby-Bauer method of disc susceptibility is used, a 10-unit penicillin disc should give a zone greater than 28 mm when tested against a penicillin-susceptible bacterial strain.

INDICATIONS AND USAGE

Bicillin C-R 900/300 is indicated in the treatment of infections as described below that are susceptible to serum levels characteristic of this particular dosage form. Therapy should be guided by bacteriological studies (including susceptibility testing) and by clinical response.

Bicillin C-R 900/300 is indicated in the treatment of the following in children of all ages:

Moderately severe to severe infections of the upper-respiratory tract, scarlet fever, erysipelas, and skin and soft-tissue infections due to susceptible streptococci.

NOTE: Streptococci in Groups A, C, G, H, L, and M are very susceptible to penicillin G. Other groups, including Group D (enterococci), are resistant. Penicillin G sodium or potassium is recommended for streptococcal infections with bacteremia.

Moderately severe pneumonia and otitis media due to susceptible pneumococci.

NOTE: Severe pneumonia, empyema, bacteremia, pericarditis, meningitis, peritonitis, and arthritis of pneumococcal etiology are better treated with penicillin G sodium or potassium during the acute stage.

When high, sustained serum levels are required, penicillin G sodium or potassium, either IM or IV, should be used. This drug should not be used in the treatment of venereal diseases, including syphilis, gonorrhea, yaws, bejel, and pinta.

CONTRAINDICATIONS

A previous hypersensitivity reaction to any penicillin or to procaine is a contraindication.

Do not inject into or near an artery or nerve.

WARNINGS

The combination of penicillin G benzathine and penicillin G procaine should only be prescribed for the indications listed in this insert.

Serious and occasionally fatal hypersensitivity (anaphylactoid) reactions have been reported in patients on penicillin therapy. Although anaphylaxis is more frequent following parenteral administration, it has occurred in patients on oral penicillins. These reactions are more apt to occur in individuals with a history of sensitivity to multiple allergens.

There are reports of patients with a history of penicillin hypersensitivity reactions who experienced severe hypersensitivity reactions when treated with a cephalosporin. Before therapy with a penicillin, careful inquiry should be made

about previous hypersensitivity reactions to penicillins, cephalosporins, and other allergens. If an allergic reaction occurs, the drug should be discontinued and appropriate therapy should be instituted. Serious anaphylactoid reactions require immediate emergency treatment with epinephrine. Oxygen, intravenous steroids, airway management, including intubation, should also be administered as indicated.

Inadvertent intravascular administration, including inadvertent direct intra-arterial injection or injection immediately adjacent to arteries, of Bicillin C-R 900/300 and other penicillin preparations has resulted in severe neurovascular damage, including transverse myelitis with permanent paralysis, gangrene requiring amputation of digits and more proximal portions of extremities, and necrosis and sloughing at and surrounding the injection site. Such severe effects have been reported following injections into the buttock, thigh, and deltoid areas. Other serious complications of suspected intravascular administration which have been reported include immediate pallor, mottling or cyanosis of the extremity both distal and proximal to the injection site followed by bleb formation; severe edema requiring anterior and/or posterior compartment fasciotomy in the lower extremity. The above-described severe effects and complications have most often occurred in infants and small children. Prompt consultation with an appropriate specialist is indicated if any evidence of compromise of the blood supply occurs at, proximal to, or distal to the site of injection.[1–9] See "**Contraindications**," "**Precautions**," and "**Dosage and Administration**" sections.

Quadriceps femoris fibrosis and atrophy have been reported following repeated intramuscular injections of penicillin preparations into the anterolateral thigh.

Injection into or near a nerve may result in permanent neurological damage.

PRECAUTIONS

GENERAL

Penicillin should be used with caution in individuals with histories of significant allergies and/or asthma.

Care should be taken to avoid intravenous or intra-arterial administration, or injection into or near major peripheral nerves or blood vessels, since such injections may produce neurovascular damage. See "**Contraindications**," "**Warnings**," and "**Dosage and Administration**" sections.

A small percentage of patients are sensitive to procaine. If there is a history of sensitivity, make the usual test: Inject intradermally 0.1 mL of a 1 to 2 percent procaine solution. Development of an erythema, wheal, flare, or eruption indicates procaine sensitivity. Sensitivity should be treated by the usual methods, including barbiturates, and procaine penicillin preparations should not be used. Antihistaminics appear beneficial in treatment of procaine reactions.

The use of antibiotics may result in overgrowth of nonsusceptible organisms. Constant observation of the patient is essential. If new infections due to bacteria or fungi appear during therapy, the drug should be discontinued and appropriate measures taken.

Whenever allergic reactions occur, penicillin should be withdrawn unless, in the opinion of the physician, the condition being treated is life-threatening and amenable only to penicillin therapy.

In prolonged therapy with penicillin, and particularly with high-dosage schedules, periodic evaluation of the renal and hematopoietic systems is recommended.

LABORATORY TESTS

In streptococcal infections, therapy must be sufficient to eliminate the organism; otherwise, the sequelae of streptococcal disease may occur. Cultures should be taken following completion of treatment to determine whether streptococci have been eradicated.

DRUG INTERACTIONS

Tetracycline, a bacteriostatic antibiotic, may antagonize the bactericidal effect of penicillin, and concurrent use of these drugs should be avoided.

Concurrent administration of penicillin and probenecid increases and prolongs serum penicillin levels by decreasing the apparent volume of distribution and slowing the rate of excretion by competitively inhibiting renal tubular secretion of penicillin.

PREGNANCY CATEGORY B

Reproduction studies performed in the mouse, rat, and rabbit have revealed no evidence of impaired fertility or harm to the fetus due to penicillin G. Human experience with the penicillins during pregnancy has not shown any positive evidence of adverse effects on the fetus. There are, however, no adequate and well-controlled studies in pregnant women showing conclusively that harmful effects of these drugs on the fetus can be excluded. Because animal reproduction studies are not always predictive of human response, this drug should be used during pregnancy only if clearly needed.

NURSING MOTHERS

Soluble penicillin G is excreted in breast milk. Caution should be exercised when penicillin G benzathine and penicillin G procaine are administered to a nursing woman.

CARCINOGENESES, MUTAGENESIS, IMPAIRMENT OF FERTILITY

No long-term animal studies have been conducted with these drugs.

PEDIATRIC USE

See "**Indications and Usage**" and "**Dosage and Administration.**"

ADVERSE REACTIONS

As with other penicillins, untoward reactions of the sensitivity phenomena are likely to occur, particularly in individuals who have previously demonstrated hypersensitivity to penicillins or in those with a history of allergy, asthma, hay fever, or urticaria.

The following have been reported with parenteral penicillin G:

General: Hypersensitivity reactions including the following: skin eruptions (maculopapular to exfoliative dermatitis), urticaria, laryngeal edema, fever, eosinophilia; other serum-sicknesslike reactions (including chills, fever, edema, arthralgia, and prostration); anaphylaxis. Note: Urticaria, other skin rashes, and serum-sicknesslike reactions may be controlled with antihistamines and, if necessary, systemic corticosteroids.

Whenever such reactions occur, penicillin G should be discontinued unless, in the opinion of the physician, the condition being treated is life-threatening and amenable only to therapy with penicillin G. Serious anaphylactic reactions require the immediate use of epinephrine, oxygen, and intravenous steroids.

Hematologic: Hemolytic anemia, leukopenia, thrombocytopenia.

Neurologic: Neuropathy.

Urogenital: Nephropathy.

OVERDOSAGE

Penicillin in overdosage has the potential to cause neuromuscular hyperirritability or convulsive seizures.

DOSAGE AND ADMINISTRATION

Administer by DEEP, INTRAMUSCULAR INJECTION in the upper, outer quadrant of the buttock. In infants and small children, the midlateral aspect of the thigh may be preferable. When doses are repeated, vary the injection site.

The Wyeth-Ayerst TUBEX cartridge for this product incorporates several features that are designed to facilitate the visualization of blood on aspiration if a blood vessel is inadvertently entered.

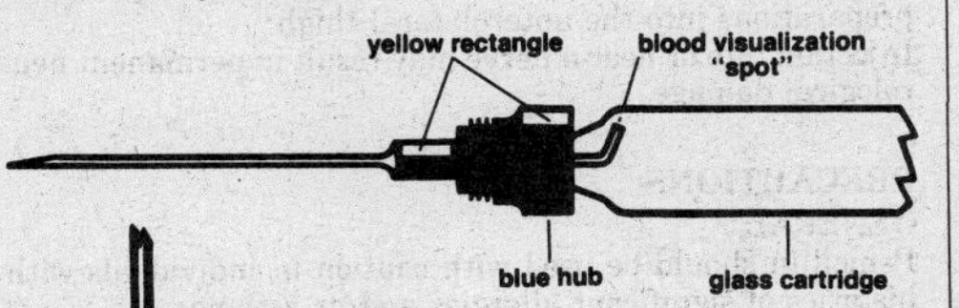

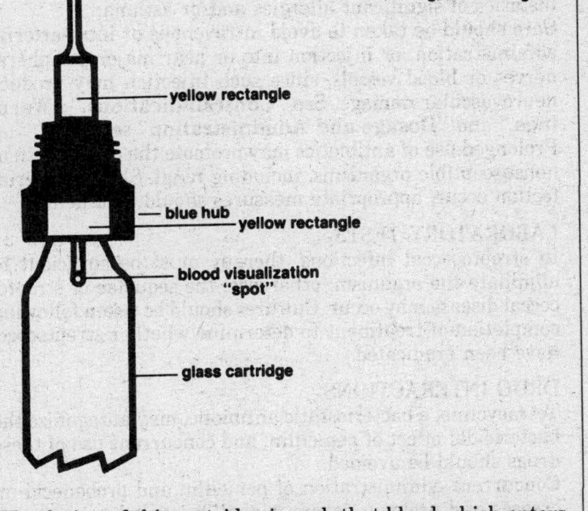

The design of this cartridge is such that blood which enters its needle will be quickly visualized as a red or dark-colored "spot." This "spot" will appear on the barrel of the glass cartridge immediately proximal to the blue hub. The TUBEX is designed with two orientation marks, in order to determine where the "spot" can be seen. First insert and secure the cartridge in the TUBEX injector in the usual fashion. Locate the yellow rectangle at the base of the blue hub. This yellow rectangle is aligned with the blood visualization "spot." An imaginary straight line, drawn from this yellow rectangle to the shoulder of the glass cartridge, will point to the area on the cartridge where the "spot" can be visualized. When the needle cover is removed, a second yellow rectangle will be visible. The second yellow rectangle is also aligned with the blood visualization "spot" to assist the operator in locating the "spot." If the 2 mL metal or plastic syringe is used, the glass cartridge should be rotated by turning the plunger of the syringe clockwise until the yellow rectangle is visualized. If the 1 mL metal syringe is used, it will not be possible to continue to rotate the glass cartridge clockwise once it is properly engaged and fully threaded; it can, however, then be rotated counterclockwise as far as necessary to properly orient the yellow rectangles and locate the observation area. (In this same area in some cartridges, a dark spot may sometimes be visualized prior to injection. This is the proximal end of the needle and does not represent a foreign body in, or other abnormality of, the suspension.)

Thus, before the needle is inserted into the selected muscle, it is important for the operator to orient the yellow rectangle so that any blood which may enter after needle insertion and during aspiration can be visualized in the area on the cartridge where it will appear and not be obscured by any obstructions.

After selection of the proper site and insertion of the needle into the selected muscle, aspirate by pulling back on the plunger. While maintaining negative pressure for 2 to 3 seconds, carefully observe the neck of the glass TUBEX cartridge immediately proximal to the blue plastic needle hub for appearance of blood or any discoloration.

Blood or "typical blood color" may *not* be seen if a blood vessel has been entered—only a mixture of blood and Bicillin C-R 900/300. The appearance of any discoloration is reason to withdraw the needle and discard the TUBEX. If it is elected to inject at another site, a new TUBEX cartridge should be used. If no blood or discoloration appears, inject the contents of the TUBEX slowly. Discontinue delivery of the dose if the subject complains of severe immediate pain at the injection site or if in infants and young children symptoms or signs occur suggesting onset of severe pain.

Some TUBEX cartridges may contain a small air bubble which may be disregarded since it does not affect administration of the product. Because of the high concentration of suspended material in this product, the needle may be blocked if the injection is not made at a slow, steady rate.

STREPTOCOCCAL INFECTIONS

Group A Infections of the upper-respiratory tract, skin and soft-tissue infections, scarlet fever, and erysipelas: A single injection of Bicillin C-R 900/300 is usually sufficient for the treatment of Group A streptococcal infections in children of all ages.

PNEUMOCOCCAL INFECTIONS (except pneumococcal meningitis)

One TUBEX Bicillin C-R 900/300 repeated at 2- or 3-day intervals until the temperature is normal for 48 hours. Other forms of penicillin may be necessary for severe cases.

Parenteral drug products should be inspected visually for particulate matter and discoloration prior to administration, whenever solution and container permit.

HOW SUPPLIED

Bicillin® C-R 900/300 (penicillin G benzathine and penicillin G procaine suspension) is supplied in 2 mL size TUBEX® Sterile Cartridge-Needle Units (20 gauge × 1¼ inch needle) in packages of 10 TUBEX, as follows:

1,200,000 units per TUBEX, NDC 0008-0079-01.

Store in a refrigerator.

Keep from freezing.

REFERENCES

1. SHAW, E.: Transverse myelitis from injection of penicillin. *Am. J. Dis. Child., 111:* 548, 1966.
2. KNOWLES, J.: Accidental intra-arterial injection of penicillin. *Am. J. Dis. Child., 111:* 552, 1966.
3. DARBY, C., et al: Ischemia following an intragluteal injection of benzathine-procaine penicillin G mixture in a one-year-old boy. *Clin. Pediatrics, 12:* 485, 1973.
4. BROWN, L. & NELSON, A.: Postinfectious intravascular thrombosis with gangrene. *Arch. Surg., 94:* 652, 1967.
5. BORENSTINE, J.: Transverse myelitis and penicillin (Correspondence). *Am. J. Dis. Child., 112:* 166, 1966.
6. ATKINSON, J.: Transverse myelopathy secondary to penicillin injection. *J. Pediatrics, 75:* 867, 1969.
7. TALBERT, J. et al: Gangrene of the foot following intramuscular injection in the lateral thigh: A case report with recommendations for prevention. *J. Pediatrics, 70:* 110, 1967.
8. FISHER, T.: Medicolegal affairs. *Canad. Med. Assoc. J., 112:* 395, 1975.
9. SCHANZER, H. et al: Accidental intra-arterial injection of penicillin G. *JAMA, 242:* 1289, 1979.

BICILLIN® L-A ℞

[*bī-sil 'in*]

(penicillin G benzathine suspension)

INJECTION

FOR DEEP INTRAMUSCULAR INJECTION ONLY

DESCRIPTION

Bicillin L-A (penicillin G benzathine suspension) is prepared by the reaction of dibenzylethylene diamine with two molecules of penicillin G. It is chemically designated as 3,3-dimethyl-7-oxo -6- (2-phenylacetamido) -4-thia-1-azabicy-

Continued on next page

Wyeth-Ayerst Laboratories—Cont.

clo[3.2.0]heptane-2-carboxylic acid compound with N,N'-dibenzylethylenediamine (2:1), tetrahydrate.

It is available for deep, intramuscular injection. It contains penicillin G benzathine in aqueous suspension with sodium citrate buffer and, as w/v, approximately 0.5% lecithin, 0.6% carboxymethylcellulose, 0.6% povidone, 0.1% methylparaben, and 0.01% propylparaben. It occurs as a white, crystalline powder and is very slightly soluble in water and sparingly soluble in alcohol.

Bicillin L-A suspension in the multiple-dose vial formulation, disposable syringe formulation and TUBEX formulation is viscous and opaque. The multiple-dose vial formulation contains the equivalent of 300,000 units per mL of penicillin G as the benzathine salt. The disposable syringe formulation is available in a 4 mL size containing the equivalent of 2,400,000 units of penicillin G as the benzathine salt. The TUBEX formulation is available in 1 mL and 2 mL TUBEX Sterile Cartridge-Needle Units containing the equivalent of 600,000 units and 1,200,000 units respectively of penicillin G as the benzathine salt. Read "**Contraindications**," "**Warnings**," "**Precautions**," and "**Dosage and Administration**" sections prior to use.

CLINICAL PHARMACOLOGY
GENERAL
Penicillin G benzathine has an extremely low solubility and, thus, the drug is slowly released from intramuscular injection sites. The drug is hydrolyzed to penicillin G. This combination of hydrolysis and slow absorption results in blood serum levels much lower but much more prolonged than other parenteral penicillins.

Intramuscular administration of 300,000 units of penicillin G benzathine in adults results in blood levels of 0.03 to 0.05 units per mL, which are maintained for 4 to 5 days. Similar blood levels may persist for 10 days following administration of 600,000 units and for 14 days following administration of 1,200,000 units. Blood concentrations of 0.003 units per mL may still be detectable 4 weeks following administration of 1,200,000 units.

Approximately 60% of penicillin G is bound to serum protein. The drug is distributed throughout the body tissues in widely varying amounts. Highest levels are found in the kidneys with lesser amounts in the liver, skin, and intestines. Penicillin G penetrates into all other tissues and the spinal fluid to a lesser degree. With normal kidney function, the drug is excreted rapidly by tubular excretion. In neonates and young infants and in individuals with impaired kidney function, excretion is considerably delayed.

MICROBIOLOGY
Penicillin G exerts a bactericidal action against penicillin-susceptible microorganisms during the stage of active multiplication. It acts through the inhibition of biosynthesis of cell-wall mucopeptide. It is not active against the penicillinase-producing bacteria, which include many strains of staphylococci.

The following *in vitro* data are available, but their clinical significance is unknown. Penicillin G exerts high *in vitro* activity against staphylococci (except penicillinase-producing strains), streptococci (Groups A, C, G, H, L, and M), and pneumococci. Other organisms susceptible to penicillin G are *Neisseria gonorrhoeae*, *Corynebacterium diphtheriae*, *Bacillus anthracis*, Clostridia species, *Actinomyces bovis*, *Streptobacillus moniliformis*, *Listeria monocytogenes*, and Leptospira species. *Treponema pallidum* is extremely susceptible to the bactericidal action of penicillin G.

Susceptibility Test: If the Kirby-Bauer method of disc susceptibility is used, a 20-unit penicillin disc should give a zone greater than 28 mm when tested against a penicillin-susceptible bacterial strain.

INDICATIONS AND USAGE
Intramuscular penicillin G benzathine is indicated in the treatment of infections due to penicillin-G-sensitive microorganisms that are susceptible to the low and very prolonged serum levels common to this particular dosage form. Therapy should be guided by bacteriological studies (including sensitivity tests) and by clinical response.

The following infections will usually respond to adequate dosage of intramuscular penicillin G benzathine:
Mild-to-moderate infections of the upper respiratory tract due to susceptible streptococci.
Venereal infections—Syphilis, yaws, bejel, and pinta.
Medical Conditions in which Penicillin G Benzathine Therapy is Indicated as Prophylaxis:
Rheumatic fever and/or chorea—Prophylaxis with penicillin G benzathine has proven effective in preventing recurrence of these conditions. It has also been used as follow-up prophylactic therapy for rheumatic heart disease and acute glomerulonephritis.

CONTRAINDICATIONS
A history of a previous hypersensitivity reaction to any of the penicillins is a contraindication.
Do not inject into or near an artery or nerve.

WARNINGS
Penicillin G benzathine should only be prescribed for the indications listed in this insert.
Serious and occasionally fatal hypersensitivity (anaphylactoid) reactions have been reported in patients receiving penicillin. Although anaphylaxis is more frequent following parenteral administration, it has occurred in patients on oral penicillins. These reactions are more apt to occur in individuals with a history of sensitivity to multiple allergens.
There are reports of patients with a history of penicillin hypersensitivity reactions who experienced severe hypersensitivity reactions when treated with a cephalosporin. Before therapy with a penicillin, careful inquiry should be made about previous hypersensitivity reactions to penicillins, cephalosporins, and other allergens. If an allergic reaction occurs, the drug should be discontinued and appropriate therapy should be instituted. Serious anaphylactoid reactions require immediate emergency treatment with epinephrine. Oxygen, intravenous steroids, airway management, including intubation, should also be administered as indicated.
Inadvertent intravascular administration, including inadvertent direct intra-arterial injection or injection immediately adjacent to arteries, of Bicillin L-A and other penicillin preparations has resulted in severe neurovascular damage, including transverse myelitis with permanent paralysis, gangrene requiring amputation of digits and more proximal portions of extremities, and necrosis and sloughing at and surrounding the injection site. Such severe effects have been reported following injections into the buttock, thigh, and deltoid areas. Other serious complications of suspected intravascular administration which have been reported include immediate pallor, mottling, or cyanosis of the extremity both distal and proximal to the injection site, followed by bleb formation; severe edema requiring anterior and/or posterior compartment fasciotomy in the lower extremity. The above-described severe effects and complications have most often occurred in infants and small children. Prompt consultation with an appropriate specialist is indicated if any evidence of compromise of the blood supply occurs at, proximal to, or distal to the site of injection.[1-9] See "**Contraindications**," "**Precautions**," and "**Dosage and Administration**" sections.
Quadriceps femoris fibrosis and atrophy have been reported following repeated intramuscular injections of penicillin preparations into the anterolateral thigh.
Injection into or near a nerve may result in permanent neurological damage.

PRECAUTIONS
GENERAL
Penicillin should be used with caution in individuals with histories of significant allergies and/or asthma.
Care should be taken to avoid intravenous or intra-arterial administration, or injection into or near major peripheral nerves or blood vessels, since such injection may produce neurovascular damage. See "**Contraindications**," "**Warnings**," and "**Dosage and Administration**" sections.
Prolonged use of antibiotics may promote the overgrowth of nonsusceptible organisms, including fungi. Should superinfection occur, appropriate measures should be taken.

LABORATORY TESTS
In streptococcal infections, therapy must be sufficient to eliminate the organism; otherwise, the sequelae of streptococcal disease may occur. Cultures should be taken following completion of treatment to determine whether streptococci have been eradicated.

DRUG INTERACTIONS
Tetracycline, a bacteriostatic antibiotic, may antagonize the bactericidal effect of penicillin, and concurrent use of these drugs should be avoided.
Concurrent administration of penicillin and probenecid increases and prolongs serum penicillin levels by decreasing the apparent volume of distribution and slowing the rate of excretion by competitively inhibiting renal tubular secretion of penicillin.

PREGNANCY CATEGORY B
Reproduction studies performed in the mouse, rat, and rabbit have revealed no evidence of impaired fertility or harm to the fetus due to penicillin G. Human experience with the penicillins during pregnancy has not shown any positive evidence of adverse effects on the fetus. There are, however, no adequate and well-controlled studies in pregnant women showing conclusively that harmful effects of these drugs on the fetus can be excluded. Because animal reproduction studies are not always predictive of human response, this drug should be used during pregnancy only if clearly needed.

NURSING MOTHERS
Soluble penicillin G is excreted in breast milk. Caution should be exercised when penicillin G benzathine is administered to a nursing woman.

CARCINOGENESIS, MUTAGENESIS, IMPAIRMENT OF FERTILITY
No long-term animal studies have been conducted with this drug.
PEDIATRIC USE
See "**Indications and Usage**" and "**Dosage and Administration**."

ADVERSE REACTIONS
As with other penicillins, untoward reactions of the sensitivity phenomena are likely to occur, particularly in individuals who have previously demonstrated hypersensitivity to penicillins or in those with a history of allergy, asthma, hay fever, or urticaria.
As with other treatments for syphilis, the Jarisch-Herxheimer reaction has been reported.
The following have been reported with parenteral penicillin G:
General: Hypersensitivity reactions including the following: skin eruptions (maculopapular to exfoliative dermatitis), urticaria, laryngeal edema, fever, eosinophilia; other serum-sicknesslike reactions (including chills, fever, edema, arthralgia, and prostration); anaphylaxis. Note: Urticaria, other skin rashes, and serum-sicknesslike reactions may be controlled with antihistamines and, if necessary, systemic corticosteroids.
Whenever such reactions occur, penicillin G should be discontinued unless, in the opinion of the physician, the condition being treated is life-threatening and amenable only to therapy with penicillin G. Serious anaphylactic reactions require the immediate use of epinephrine, oxygen, and intravenous steroids.
Hematologic: Hemolytic anemia, leukopenia, thrombocytopenia.
Neurologic: Neuropathy.
Urogenital: Nephropathy.

OVERDOSAGE
Penicillin in overdosage has the potential to cause neuromuscular hyperirritability or convulsive seizures.

DOSAGE AND ADMINISTRATION
Due to the viscous nature of this medication, a 23 gauge or larger bore needle should be used to withdraw medication from the vial and for patient administration. A smaller bore needle, such as a 24 or 25 gauge, is not recommended.
STREPTOCOCCAL (GROUP A) UPPER-RESPIRATORY INFECTIONS (for example, pharyngitis)
Adults—a single injection of 1,200,000 units; older children—a single injection of 900,000 units; infants and children (under 60 lbs.)—300,000 to 600,000 units.
SYPHILIS
Primary, secondary, and latent—2,400,000 units (1 dose). Late (tertiary and neurosyphilis)—2,400,000 units at 7-day intervals for three doses.
Congenital—under 2 years of age: 50,000 units/kg/body weight; ages 2–12 years: adjust dosage based on adult dosage schedule.
YAWS, BEJEL, and PINTA—1,200,000 units (1 injection).
PROPHYLAXIS—for rheumatic fever and glomerulonephritis.
Following an acute attack, penicillin G benzathine (parenteral) may be given in doses of 1,200,000 units once a month or 600,000 units every 2 weeks.
Administer by DEEP INTRAMUSCULAR INJECTION in the upper, outer quadrant of the buttock. In infants and small children, the midlateral aspect of the thigh may be preferable. When doses are repeated, vary the injection site.
When using the multiple-dose vial:
After selection of the proper site and insertion of the needle into the selected muscle, aspirate by pulling back on the plunger. While maintaining negative pressure for 2 to 3 seconds, carefully observe the barrel of the syringe immediately proximal to the needle hub for appearance of blood or any discoloration. Blood or "typical blood color" may *not* be seen if a blood vessel has been entered—only a mixture of blood and Bicillin L-A. The appearance of any discoloration is reason to withdraw the needle and discard the syringe. If it is elected to inject at another site, a new syringe and needle should be used. If no blood or discoloration appears, inject the contents of the syringe slowly. Discontinue delivery of the dose if the subject complains of severe immediate pain at the injection site or if in infants and young children symptoms or signs occur suggesting onset of severe pain.
Because of the high concentration of suspended material in this product, the needle may be blocked if the injection is not made at a slow, steady rate.
When using the TUBEX cartridge:
The Wyeth-Ayerst TUBEX® cartridge for this product incorporates several features that are designed to facilitate the visualization of blood on aspiration if a blood vessel is inadvertently entered.

[See figure at top of next page.]

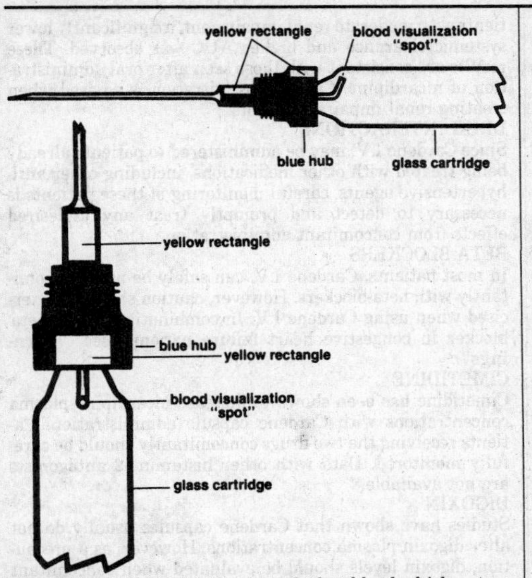

The design of this cartridge is such that blood which enters its needle will be quickly visualized as a red or dark-colored "spot." This "spot" will appear on the barrel of the glass cartridge immediately proximal to the blue hub. The TUBEX is designed with two orientation marks, in order to determine where the "spot" can be seen. First insert and secure the cartridge in the TUBEX injector in the usual fashion. Locate the yellow rectangle at the base of the blue hub. This yellow rectangle is aligned with the blood visualization "spot." An imaginary straight line, drawn from this yellow rectangle to the shoulder of the glass cartridge, will point to the area on the cartridge where the "spot" can be visualized. When the needle cover is removed, a second yellow rectangle will be visible. The second yellow rectangle is also aligned with the blood visualization "spot" to assist the operator in locating this "spot." If the 2 mL metal or plastic syringe is used, the glass cartridge should be rotated by turning the plunger of the syringe clockwise until the yellow rectangle is visualized. If the 1 mL metal syringe is used, it will not be possible to continue to rotate the glass cartridge clockwise once it is properly engaged and fully threaded; it can, however, then be rotated counterclockwise as far as necessary to properly orient the yellow rectangles and locate the observation area. (In this same area in some cartridges, a dark spot may sometimes be visualized prior to injection. This is the proximal end of the needle and does not represent a foreign body in, or other abnormality of, the suspension.)

Thus, before the needle is inserted into the selected muscle, it is important for the operator to orient the yellow rectangle so that any blood which may enter after needle insertion and during aspiration can be visualized in the area on the cartridge where it will appear and not be obscured by any obstructions.

After selection of the proper site and insertion of the needle into the selected muscle, aspirate by pulling back on the plunger. While maintaining negative pressure for 2 to 3 seconds, carefully observe the barrel of the cartridge in the area previously identified (see above) for the appearance of a red or dark-colored "spot."

Blood or "typical blood color" may *not* be seen if a blood vessel has been entered—only a mixture of blood and Bicillin L-A. The appearance of any discoloration is reason to withdraw the needle and discard the glass TUBEX cartridge. If it is elected to inject at another site, a new cartridge should be used. If no blood or discoloration appears, inject the contents of the cartridge slowly. Discontinue delivery of the dose if the subject complains of severe immediate pain at the injection site or if, especially in infants and young children, symptoms or signs occur suggesting onset of severe pain.

Some TUBEX cartridges may contain a small air bubble which may be disregarded, since it does not affect administration of the product.

Because of the high concentration of suspended material in this product, the needle may be blocked if the injection is not made at a slow, steady rate.

When using the disposable syringe:

The Wyeth-Ayerst disposable syringe for this product incorporates several new features that are designed to facilitate its use.

A single small indentation, or "dot," has been punched into the metal or plastic ring that surrounds the neck of the syringe near the base of the needle. It is important that this "dot" be placed in a position so that it can be easily visualized by the operator following the intramuscular insertion of the syringe needle.

After selection of the proper site and insertion of the needle into the selected muscle, aspirate by pulling back on the plunger. While maintaining negative pressure for 2 to 3 seconds, carefully observe the barrel of the syringe immediately proximal to the location of the "dot" for appearance of blood or any discoloration. Blood or "typical blood color" may *not* be seen if a blood vessel has been entered—only a mixture of blood and Bicillin L-A. The appearance of any discoloration is reason to withdraw the needle and discard the syringe. If it is elected to inject at another site, a new syringe should be used. If no blood or discoloration appears, inject the contents of the syringe slowly. Discontinue delivery of the dose if the subject complains of severe immediate pain at the injection site or if in infants and young children symptoms or signs occur suggesting onset of severe pain.

Some disposable syringes may contain a small air bubble which may be disregarded, since it does not affect administration of the product.

Because of the high concentration of suspended material in this product, the needle may be blocked if the injection is not made at a slow, steady rate.

Parenteral drug products should be inspected visually for particulate matter and discoloration prior to administration whenever solution and container permit.

HOW SUPPLIED

Bicillin® L-A (penicillin G benzathine suspension) is supplied in packages of 10 TUBEX® Sterile Cartridge-Needle Units (20 gauge × 1¼ inch needle) as follows:

1 mL size, containing 600,000 units per TUBEX, NDC 0008-0021-08.

2 mL size, containing 1,200,000 units per TUBEX, NDC 0008-0021-07.

Store in a refrigerator.

Keep from freezing.

ALSO AVAILABLE

Bicillin L-A (penicillin G benzathine suspension) is also available in packages of 10 disposable syringes as follows:

4 mL size, containing 2,400,000 units per syringe (18 gauge × 2 inch needle), NDC 0008-0021-12

Bicillin L-A (penicillin G benzathine suspension) is also available in packages of single multiple-dose vials as follows:

10 mL size, 300,000 units per mL, NDC 0008-0163-01.

Store in a refrigerator.

Keep from freezing.

Shake multiple-dose vials well before using.

REFERENCES

1. SHAW, E.: Transverse myelitis from injection of penicillin. *Am. J. Dis. Child., 111:* 548, 1966.

2. KNOWLES, J.: Accidental intra-arterial injection of penicillin. *Am. J. Dis. Child., 111:* 552, 1966.

3. DARBY, C., et al: Ischemia following an intragluteal injection of benzathine-procaine penicillin G mixture in a one-year-old boy. *Clin. Pediatrics, 12:* 485, 1973.

4. BROWN, L. & NELSON, A.: Postinfectious intravascular thrombosis with gangrene. *Arch. Surg., 94:* 652, 1967.

5. BORENSTINE, J.: Transverse myelitis and penicillin (Correspondence). *Am. J. Dis. Child., 112:* 166, 1966.

6. ATKINSON, J.: Transverse myelopathy secondary to penicillin injection. *J. Pediatrics, 75:* 867, 1969.

7. TALBERT, J. et al: Gangrene of the foot following intramuscular injection in the lateral thigh: A case report with recommendations for prevention. *J. Pediatrics, 70:* 110, 1967.

8. FISHER, T.: Medicolegal affairs. *Canad. Med. Assoc. J., 112:* 395, 1975.

9. SCHANZER, H. et al: Accidental intra-arterial injection of penicillin G. *JAMA, 242:* 1289, 1979.

BIOLOGICALS

Each of Wyeth-Ayerst's biological products is listed separately in alphabetical order in Wyeth-Ayerst's Product Information Section.

For prescribing information on the products listed—and for which information is not provided—write to Professional Service, Wyeth-Ayerst Laboratories, P.O. Box 8299, Philadelphia, PA 19101, or contact your local Wyeth-Ayerst representative.

CARDENE® I.V. ℞

[*kar 'deen*]

(nicardipine hydrochloride)

DESCRIPTION

Cardene (nicardipine HCl) is a calcium ion influx inhibitor (slow channel blocker or calcium channel blocker). Cardene I.V. for intravenous administration contains 2.5 mg/mL of nicardipine hydrochloride.

Nicardipine hydrochloride is a dihydropyridine derivative with IUPAC (International Union of Pure and Applied Chemistry) chemical name (±)-2-(benzyl-methyl amino) ethyl methyl 1,4-dihydro-2,6-dimethyl-4-(*m*-nitrophenyl)-3,5-pyridinedicarboxylate monohydrochloride and has the following structure:

[See chemical structure at top of next column.]

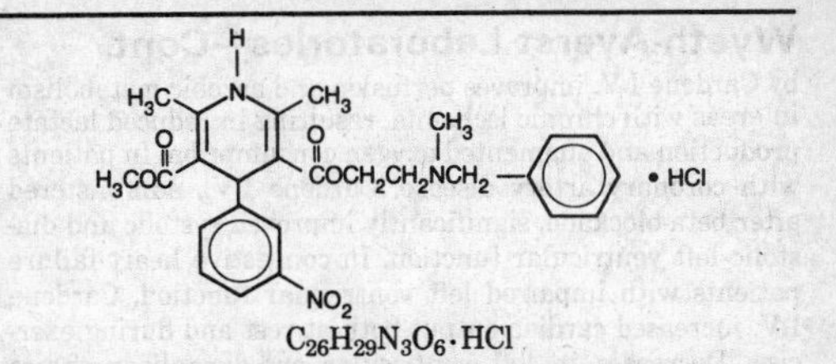

$C_{26}H_{29}N_3O_6 \cdot HCl$

Nicardipine hydrochloride is a greenish-yellow, odorless, crystalline powder that melts at about 169°C. It is freely soluble in chloroform, methanol, and glacial acetic acid, sparingly soluble in anhydrous ethanol, slightly soluble in n-butanol, water, 0.01 M potassium dihydrogen phosphate, acetone, and dioxane, very slightly soluble in ethyl acetate, and practically insoluble in benzene, ether, and hexane. It has a molecular weight of 515.99.

Cardene I.V. is available as a sterile, non-pyrogenic, clear, yellow solution in 10 mL ampuls for intravenous infusion after dilution. Each mL contains 2.5 mg nicardipine hydrochloride in Water for Injection, USP, with 48.00 mg Sorbitol, NF, buffered to pH 3.5 with 0.525 mg citric acid monohydrate, USP, and 0.09 mg sodium hydroxide, NF. Additional citric acid and/or sodium hydroxide may have been added to adjust pH.

CLINICAL PHARMACOLOGY

MECHANISM OF ACTION

Nicardipine inhibits the transmembrane influx of calcium ions into cardiac muscle and smooth muscle without changing serum calcium concentrations. The contractile processes of cardiac muscle and vascular smooth muscle are dependent upon the movement of extracellular calcium ions into these cells through specific ion channels. The effects of nicardipine are more selective to vascular smooth muscle than cardiac muscle. In animal models, nicardipine produced relaxation of coronary vascular smooth muscle at drug levels which cause little or no negative inotropic effect.

PHARMACOKINETICS AND METABOLISM

Following infusion, nicardipine plasma concentrations decline tri-exponentially, with a rapid early distribution phase (α-half-life of 2.7 minutes), an intermediate phase (β-half-life of 44.8 minutes), and a slow terminal phase (γ-half-life of 14.4 hours) that can only be detected after long-term infusions. Total plasma clearance (Cl) is 0.4 L/hr·kg, and the apparent volume of distribution (V_d) using a non-compartment model is 8.3 L/kg. The pharmacokinetics of Cardene I.V. are linear over the dosage range of 0.5 to 40.0 mg/hr.

Rapid dose-related increases in nicardipine plasma concentrations are seen during the first two hours after the start of an infusion of Cardene I.V. Plasma concentrations increase at a much slower rate after the first few hours, and approach steady state at 24 to 48 hours. On termination of the infusion, nicardipine concentrations decrease rapidly, with at least a 50% decrease during the first two hours post-infusion. The effects of nicardipine on blood pressure significantly correlate with plasma concentrations.

Nicardipine is highly protein bound (>95%) in human plasma over a wide concentration range.

Cardene I.V. has been shown to be rapidly and extensively metabolized by the liver. After coadministration of a radioactive intravenous dose of Cardene I.V. with an oral 30 mg dose given every 8 hours, 49% of the radioactivity was recovered in the urine and 43% in the feces within 96 hours. None of the dose was recovered as unchanged nicardipine.

Nicardipine does not induce or inhibit its own metabolism and does not induce or inhibit hepatic microsomal enzymes.

The steady-state pharmacokinetics of nicardipine are similar in elderly hypertensive patients (>65 years) and young healthy adults.

HEMODYNAMICS

Cardene I.V. produces significant decreases in systemic vascular resistance. In a study of intra-arterially administered Cardene I.V., the degree of vasodilation and the resultant decrease in blood pressure were more prominent in hypertensive patients than in normotensive volunteers. Administration of Cardene I.V. to normotensive volunteers at dosages of 0.25 to 3.0 mg/hr for eight hours produced changes of <5 mmHg in systolic blood pressure and <3 mmHg in diastolic blood pressure.

An increase in heart rate is a normal response to vasodilation and decrease in blood pressure; in some patients these increases in heart rate may be pronounced. In placebo-controlled trials, the mean increases in heart rate were 7±1 bpm in postoperative patients and 8±1 bpm in patients with severe hypertension at the end of the maintenance period.

Hemodynamic studies following intravenous dosing in patients with coronary artery disease and normal or moderately abnormal left ventricular function have shown significant increases in ejection fraction and cardiac output with no significant change, or a small decrease, in left ventricular end-diastolic pressure (LVEDP). There is evidence that Cardene increases blood flow. Coronary dilatation induced

Continued on next page

Wyeth-Ayerst Laboratories—Cont.

by Cardene I.V. improves perfusion and aerobic metabolism in areas with chronic ischemia, resulting in reduced lactate production and augmented oxygen consumption. In patients with coronary artery disease, Cardene I.V., administered after beta-blockade, significantly improved systolic and diastolic left ventricular function. In congestive heart failure patients with impaired left ventricular function, Cardene I.V. increased cardiac output both at rest and during exercise. Decreases in left ventricular end-diastolic pressure were also observed. However, in some patients with severe left ventricular dysfunction, it may have a negative inotropic effect and could lead to worsened failure.

"Coronary steal" has not been observed during treatment with Cardene I.V. (Coronary steal is the detrimental redistribution of coronary blood flow in patients with coronary artery disease from underperfused areas toward better perfused areas.) Cardene I.V. has been shown to improve systolic shortening in both normal and hypokinetic segments of myocardial muscle. Radionuclide angiography has confirmed that wall motion remained improved during increased oxygen demand. (Occasional patients have developed increased angina upon receiving Cardene capules. Whether this represents coronary steal in these patients, or is the result of increased heart rate and decreased diastolic pressure, is not clear.)

In patients with coronary artery disease, Cardene I.V. improves left ventricular diastolic distensibility during the early filling phase, probably due to a faster rate of myocardial relaxation in previously underperfused areas. There is little or no effect on normal myocardium, suggesting the improvement is mainly by indirect mechanisms such as afterload reduction and reduced ischemia. Cardene I.V. has no negative effect on myocardial relaxation at therapeutic doses. The clinical benefits of these properties have not yet been demonstrated.

ELECTROPHYSIOLOGIC EFFECTS

In general, no detrimental effects on the cardiac conduction system have been seen with Cardene I.V. During acute electrophysiologic studies, it increased heart rate and prolonged the corrected QT interval to a minor degree. It did not affect sinus node recovery or SA conduction times. The PA, AH, and HV intervals* or the functional and effective refractory periods of the atrium were not prolonged. The relative and effective refractory periods of the His-Purkinje system were slightly shortened.

*PA=conduction time from high to low right atrium; AH=conduction time from low right atrium to His bundle deflection, or AV nodal conduction time; HV=conduction time through the His bundle and the bundle branch-Purkinje system.

HEPATIC FUNCTION

Because nicardipine is extensively metabolized by the liver, plasma concentrations are influenced by changes in hepatic function. In a clincial study with Cardene capsules in patients with severe liver disease, plasma concentrations were elevated and the half-life was prolonged (see "Precautions"). Similar results were obtained in patients with hepatic disease when Cardene I.V. (nicardipine hydrochloride) was administered for 24 hours at 0.6 mg/hr.

RENAL FUNCTION

When Cardene I.V. was given to mild to moderate hypertensive patients with moderate degrees of renal impairment, significant reduction in glomerular filtration rate (GFR) and effective renal plasma flow (RPF) was observed. No significant differences in liver blood flow were observed in these patients. A significantly lower systemic clearance and higher area under the curve (AUC) were observed.

When Cardene capsules (20 mg or 30 mg TID) were given to hypertensive patients with impaired renal function, mean plasma concentrations, AUC, and C_{max} were approximately two-fold higher than in healthy controls. There is a transient increase in electrolyte excretion, including sodium (see "Precautions").

Acute bolus administration of Cardene I.V. (2.5 mg) in healthy volunteers decreased mean arterial pressure and renal vascular resistance; glomerular filtration rate (GFR), renal plasma flow (RPF), and the filtration fraction were unchanged. In healthy patients undergoing abdominal surgery, Cardene I.V. (10 mg over 20 minutes) increased GFR with no change in RPF when compared with placebo. In hypertensive Type II diabetic patients with nephropathy, Cardene capsules (20 mg TID) did not change RPF and GFR, but reduced renal vascular resistance.

PULMONARY FUNCTION

In two well-controlled studies of patients with obstructive airway disease treated with Cardene capsules, no evidence of increased bronchospasm was seen. In one of the studies, Cardene capsules improved forced expiratory volume 1 second (FEV 1) and forced vital capacity (FVC) in comparison with metoprolol. Adverse experiences reported in a limited number of patients with asthma, reactive airway disease, or obstructive airway disease are similar to all patients treated with Cardene capsules.

EFFECTS IN HYPERTENSION

In patients with mild to moderate chronic stable essential hypertension, Cardene I.V. (0.5. to 4.0 mg/hr) produced dose-dependent decreases in blood pressure, although only the decreases at 4.0 mg/hr were statistically different from placebo. At the end of a 48-hour infusion at 4.0 mg/hr, the decreases were 26.0 mmHg (17%) in systolic blood pressure and 20.7 mmHg (20%) in diastolic blood pressure.

In other settings (e.g., patients with severe or postoperative hypertension), Cardene I.V. (5 to 15 mg/hr) produced dose-dependent decreases in blood pressure. Higher infusion rates produced therapeutic responses more rapidly. The mean time to therapeutic response for severe hypertension, defined as diastolic blood pressure ≤ 95 mmHg or ≥ 25 mmHg decrease and systolic blood pressure ≤ 160 mmHg, was 77 ± 5.2 minutes. The average maintenance dose was 8.0 mg/hr. The mean time to therapeutic response for postoperative hypertension, defined as $\geq 15\%$ reduction in diastolic or systolic blood pressure, was 11.5 ± 0.8 minutes. The average maintenance dose was 3.0 mg/hr.

INDICATION AND USAGE

Cardene I.V. is indicated for the short-term treatment of hypertension when oral therapy is not feasible or not desirable.

For prolonged control of blood pressure, patients should be transferred to oral medication as soon as their clinical condition permits (see "Dosage and Administration").

CONTRAINDICATIONS

Cardene I.V. is contraindicated in patients with known hypersensitivity to the drug.

Cardene I.V. is also contraindicated in patients with advanced aortic stenosis because part of the effect of Cardene I.V. is secondary to reduced afterload.

Reduction of diastolic pressure in these patients may worsen rather than improve myocardial oxygen balance.

WARNINGS

BETA-BLOCKER WITHDRAWAL

Nicardipine is not a beta-blocker and therefore gives no protection against the dangers of abrupt beta-blocker withdrawal; any such withdrawal should be by gradual reduction of dose of beta-blocker.

RAPID DECREASES IN BLOOD PRESSURE

No clincial events have been reported suggestive of a too rapid decrease in blood pressure with Cardene I.V. However, as with any antihypertensive agent, blood pressure lowering should be accomplished over as long a time as is compatible with the patient's clincial status.

USE IN PATIENTS WITH ANGINA

Increases in frequency, duration, or severity of angina have been seen in chronic oral therapy with Cardene capsules. Induction or exacerbation of angina has been seen in less than 1% of coronary artery disease patients treated with Cardene I.V. The mechanism of this effect has not been established.

USE IN PATIENTS WITH CONGESTIVE HEART FAILURE

Cardene I.V. reduced afterload without impairing myocardial contractility in preliminary hemodynamic studies of CHF patients. However, *in vitro* and in some patients, a negative inotropic effect has been observed. Therefore, caution should be exercised when using Cardene I.V., particularly in combination with a beta-blocker, in patients with CHF or significant left ventricular dysfunction.

USE IN PATIENTS WITH PHEOCHROMOCYTOMA

Only limited clinical experience exists in use of Cardene I.V. for patients with hypertension associated with pheochromocytoma. Caution should therefore be exercised when using the drug in these patients.

PERIPHERAL VEIN INFUSION SITE

To minimize the risk of peripheral venous irritation, it is recommended that the site of infusion of Cardene I.V. be changed every 12 hours.

PRECAUTIONS

GENERAL

Blood Pressure: Because Cardene I.V. decreases peripheral resistance, monitoring of blood pressure during administration is required. Cardene I.V., like other calcium channel blockers, may occasionally produce symptomatic hypotension. Caution is advised to avoid systemic hypotension when administering the drug to patients who have sustained an acute cerebral infarction or hemorrhage.

Use in Patients with Impaired Hepatic Function: Since nicardipine is metabolized in the liver, the drug should be used with caution in patients with impaired liver function or reduced hepatic blood flow. The use of lower dosages should be considered.

Nicardipine administered intravenously has been reported to increase hepatic venous pressure gradient by 4 mmHg in cirrhotic patients at high doses (5 mg/20 min). Cardene I.V. should therefore be used with caution in patients with portal hypertension.

Use in Patients with Impaired Renal Function: When Cardene I.V. was given to mild to moderate hypertensive patients with moderate renal impairment, a significantly lower systemic clearance and higher AUC was observed. These results are consistent with those seen after oral administration of nicardipine. Careful dose titration is advised when treating renal impaired patients.

DRUG INTERACTIONS

Since Cardene I.V. may be administered to patients already being treated with other medications, including other antihypertensive agents, careful monitoring of these patients is necessary to detect and promptly treat any undesired effects from concomitant administration.

BETA-BLOCKERS

In most patients, Cardene I.V. can safely be used concomitantly with beta-blockers. However, caution should be exercised when using Cardene I.V. In combination with a beta-blocker in congestive heart failure patients (see "**Warnings**").

CIMETIDINE

Cimetidine has been shown to increase nicardipine plasma concentrations with Cardene capsule administration. Patients receiving the two drugs concomitantly should be carefully monitored. Data with other histamine-2 antagonists are not available.

DIGOXIN

Studies have shown that Cardene capsules usually do not alter digoxin plasma concentrations. However, as a precaution, digoxin levels should be evaluated when concomitant therapy with Cardene I.V. is initiated.

FENTANYL ANESTHESIA

Hypotension has been reported during fentanyl anesthesia with concomitant use of a beta-blocker and a calcium channel blocker. Even though such interactions were not seen during clinical studies with Cardene I.V. (nicardipine hydrochloride), an increased volume of circulating fluids might be required if such an interaction were to occur.

CYCLOSPORINE

Concomitant administration of Cardene capsules and cyclosporine results in elevated plasma cyclosporine levels. Plasma concentrations of cyclosporine should therefore be closely monitored during Cardene I.V. administration, and the dose of cyclosporine reduced accordingly.

IN VITRO INTERACTION

The plasma protein binding of nicardipine was not altered when therapeutic concentrations of furosemide, propranolol, dipyridamole, warfarin, quinidine, or naproxen were added to human plasma *in vitro*.

CARCINOGENESIS, MUTAGENESIS, IMPAIRMENT OF FERTILITY

Rats treated with nicardipine in the diet (at concentrations calculated to provide daily dosage levels of 5, 15, or 45 mg/kg/day) for two years showed a dose-dependent increase in thyroid hyperplasia and neoplasia (follicular adenoma/carcinoma). One- and three-month studies in the rat have suggested that these results are linked to a nicardipine-induced reduction in plasma thyroxine (T4) levels with a consequent increase in plasma levels of thyroid stimulating hormone (TSH). Chronic elevation of TSH is known to cause hyperstimulation of the thyroid. In rats on an iodine deficient diet, nicardipine administration for one month was associated with thyroid hyperplasia that was prevented by T4 supplementation. Mice treated with nicardipine in the diet (at concentrations calculated to provide daily dosage levels of up to 100 mg/kg/day) for up to 18 months showed no evidence of neoplasia of any tissue and no evidence of thyroid changes. There was no evidence of thyroid pathology in dogs treated with up to 25 mg nicardipine/kg/day for one year and no evidence of effects of nicardipine on thyroid function (plasma T4 and TSH) in man. There was no evidence of a mutagenic potential of nicardipine in a battery of genotoxicity tests conducted on microbial indicator organisms, in micronucleus tests in mice and hamsters, or in a sister chromatid exchange study in hamsters. No impairment of fertility was seen in male or female rats administered nicardipine at oral doses as high as 100 mg/kg/day (50 times the 40 mg TID maximum recommended dose in man, assuming a patient weight of 60 kg).

Pregnancy Category C: Cardene I.V. at doses up to 5 mg/kg/day to pregnant rats and up to 0.5 mg/kg/day to pregnant rabbits produced no embryotoxicity or teratogenicity. Embryotoxicity was seen at 10 mg/kg/day in rats and at 1 mg/kg/day in rabbits, but no teratogenicity was observed at these doses.

Nicardipine was embryocidal when administered orally to pregnant Japanese White rabbits, during organogenesis, at 150 mg/kg/day (a dose associated with marked body weight gain suppression in the treated doe), but not at 50 mg/kg/day (25 times the maximum recommended dose in man). No adverse effects on the fetus were observed when New Zealand albino rabbits were treated, during organogenesis, with up to 100 mg nicardipine/kg/day (a dose associated with significant mortality in the treated doe). In pregnant rats administered nicardipine orally at up to 100 mg/kg/day (50 times the maximum recommended human dose) there was no evidence of embryolethality or teratogenicity. However, dystocia, reduced birth weights, reduced neonatal survival, and reduced neonatal weight gain were noted. There

are no adequate and well-controlled studies in pregnant women. Cardene should be used during pregnancy only if the potential benefit justifies the potential risk to the fetus.

NURSING MOTHERS
Studies in rats have shown significant concentrations of nicardipine in maternal milk. For this reason, it is recommended that women who wish to breastfeed should not be given this drug.

PEDIATRIC USE
Safety and efficacy in patients under the age of 18 have not been established.

USE IN THE ELDERLY
No significant difference has been observed in the antihypertensive effect of Cardene I.V. in elderly patients (≥ 65 years) compared with other adult patients in clinical studies.

ADVERSE EXPERIENCES
Two hundred forty-four patients participated in two multicenter, double-blind, placebo controlled trials of Cardene I.V. Adverse experiences were generally not serious and most were expected consequences of vasodilation. Adverse experiences occasionally required dosage adjustment. Therapy was discontinued in approximately 12% of patients, mainly due to hypotension, headache, and tachycardia.
[See table at right.]

RARE EVENTS
The following rare events have been reported in clinical trials or in the literature in association with the use of intravenously administered nicardipine.
Body as a Whole: fever, neck pain
Cardiovascular: angina pectoris, atrioventricular block, ST segment depression, inverted T wave, deep-vein thrombophlebitis
Digestive: dyspepsia
Hemic and Lymphatic: thrombocytopenia
Metabolic and Nutritional: hypophosphatemia, peripheral edema
Nervous: confusion, hypertonia
Respiratory: respiratory disorder
Special Senses: conjunctivitis, ear disorder, tinnitus
Urogenital: urinary frequency
Sinus node dysfunction and myocardial infarction, which may be due to disease progression, have been seen in patients on chronic therapy with orally administered nicardipine.

OVERDOSAGE
Several overdosages with orally administered nicardipine have been reported. One adult patient allegedly ingested 600 mg of nicardipine [standard (immediate release) capsules], and another patient, 2160 mg of the sustained release formulation of nicardipine. Symptoms included marked hypotension, bradycardia, palpitations, flushing, drowsiness, confusion and slurred speech. All symptoms resolved without sequelae. An overdosage occurred in a one year old child who ingested half of the powder in a 30 mg nicardipine standard capsule. The child remained asymptomatic. Based on results obtained in laboratory animals, lethal overdose may cause systemic hypotension, bradycardia (following initial tachycardia) and progressive atrioventricular conduction block. Reversible hepatic function abnormalities and sporadic focal hepatic necrosis were noted in some animal species receiving very large doses of nicardipine.
For treatment of overdosage, standard measures including monitoring of cardiac and respiratory functions should be implemented. The patient should be positioned so as to avoid cerebral anoxia. Frequent blood pressure determinations are essential. Vasopressors are clinically indicated for patients exhibiting profound hypotension. Intravenous calcium gluconate may help reverse the effects of calcium entry blockade.

DOSAGE AND ADMINISTRATION
Cardene I.V. (nicardipine hydrochloride) is intended for intravenous use. DOSAGE MUST BE INDIVIDUALIZED depending upon the severity of hypertension and the response of the patient during dosing.
Blood pressure should be monitored both during and after the infusion; too rapid or excessive reduction in either systolic or diastolic blood pressure during parenteral treatment should be avoided.

PREPARATION
WARNING: AMPULS MUST BE DILUTED BEFORE INFUSION
Dilution: Cardene I.V. is administered by slow continuous infusion at a CONCENTRATION OF 0.1 MG/ML. Each ampul (25 mg) should be diluted with 240 mL of compatible intravenous fluid (see below), resulting in 250 mL of solution at a concentration of 0.1 mg/mL.
Cardene I.V. has been found to be compatible and stable in glass or polyvinyl chloride containers for 24 hours at controlled room temperature with:
Dextrose (5%) Injection, USP
Dextrose (5%) and Sodium Chloride (0.45%) Injection, USP
Dextrose (5%) and Sodium Chloride (0.9%) Injection, USP
Dextrose (5%) with 40 mEq Potassium, USP

Sodium Chloride (0.45%) Injection, USP
Sodium Chloride (0.9%) Injection, USP
Cardene I.V. is NOT compatible with Sodium Bicarbonate (5%) Injection, USP, or Lactated Ringer's Injection, USP.
THE DILUTED SOLUTION IS STABLE FOR 24 HOURS AT ROOM TEMPERATURE.
Inspection: As with all parenteral drugs, Cardene I.V. should be inspected visually for particulate matter and discoloration prior to administration, whenever solution and container permit. Cardene I.V. is normally light yellow in color.

DOSAGE
As a Substitute for Oral Nicardipine Therapy
The intravenous infusion rate required to produce an average plasma concentration equivalent to a given oral dose at steady state is shown in the following table:

Oral Cardene Dose	Equivalent I.V. Infusion Rate
20 mg q8h	0.5 mg/hr
30 mg q8h	1.2 mg/hr
40 mg q8h	2.2 mg/hr

For Initiation of Therapy in a Drug Free Patient
The time course of blood pressure decrease is dependent on the initial rate of infusion and the frequency of dosage adjustment.
Cardene I.V. is administered by slow continuous infusion at a CONCENTRATION OF 0.1 MG/ML. With constant infusion, blood pressure begins to fall within minutes. It reaches about 50% of its ultimate decrease in about 45 minutes and does not reach final steady state for about 50 hours.
When treating acute hypertensive episodes in patients with chronic hypertension, discontinuation of infusion is followed by a 50% offset of action in 30±7 minutes but plasma levels of drug and gradually decreasing antihypertensive effects exist for about 50 hours.
Titration: For gradual reduction in blood pressure, initiate therapy at 50 mL/hr (5.0 mg/hr). If desired blood pressure reduction is not achieved at this dose, the infusion rate may be increased by 25 mL/hr (2.5 mg/hr) every 15 minutes up to a maximum of 150 mL/hr (15.0 mg/hr), until desired blood pressure reduction is achieved. For more rapid blood pressure reduction, initiate therapy at 50 mL/hr (5.0 mg/hr). If desired blood pressure reduction is not achieved at this dose, the infusion rate may be increased by 25 mL/hr (2.5 mg/hr) every 5 minutes up to a maximum of 150 mL/hr (15.0 mg/hr), until desired blood pressure reduction is achieved. Following achievement of the blood pressure goal, the infusion rate should be decreased to 30 mL/hr (3 mg/hr).
Maintenance: The rate of infusion should be adjusted as needed to maintain desired response.

CONDITIONS REQUIRING INFUSION ADJUSTMENT
Hypotension or Tachycardia: If there is concern of impending hypotension or tachycardia, the infusion should be dicontinued. When blood pressure has stabilized, infusion of Cardene I.V. may be restarted at low doses such as 30–50 mL/hr (3.0–5.0 mg/hr) and adjusted to maintain desired blood pressure.
Infusion Site Changes: Cardene I.V. should be continued as long as blood pressure control is needed. The infusion site should be changed every 12 hours if administered via peripheral vein.
Impaired Cardiac, Hepatic, or Renal Function: Caution is advised when titrating Cardene I.V. in patients with congestive heart failure or impaired hepatic or renal function (see "Precautions").

TRANSFER TO ORAL ANTIHYPERTENSIVE AGENTS
If treatment includes transfer to an oral antihypertensive agent other than Cardene capsules, therapy should generally be initiated upon discontinuation of Cardene I.V. If Cardene capsules are to be used, the first dose of a TID regimen should be administered 1 hour prior to discontinuation of the infusion.

HOW SUPPLIED
Cardene I.V. (nicardipine hydrochloride) is available in packages of 10 ampuls of 10 mL as follows:
25 mg (2.5 mg/mL), NDC 0008-0812.
Store at controlled room temperature, 15°–30° C (59°–86° F).
Freezing does not adversely affect the product, but exposure to elevated temperatures should be avoided.
Protect from light. Store ampuls in carton until used.
Caution: Federal law prohibits dispensing without prescription.
U.S. Patent No. 3,985,758
Cardene® is a registered trademark of Syntex (U.S.A.) Inc.
Manufactured under license
from Syntex (U.S.A.) Inc. for
Wyeth Laboratories, Inc.
A Wyeth-Ayerst Company
Philadelphia, PA 19101
by Berk Pharmaceuticals
Eastbourne, East Sussex BN22 9AG
U.K.

CEROSE®-DM   OTC
[se-rōs′ DM]

(See PDR For Nonprescription Drugs.)

Percent of Patients with Adverse Experiences During the Double-Blind Portion of Controlled Trials

Adverse Experience	Cardene (n = 144)	Placebo (n = 100)
Body as a Whole		
Headache	14.6	2.0
Asthenia	0.7	0.0
Abdominal pain	0.7	0.0
Chest pain	0.7	0.0
Cardiovascular		
Hypotension	5.6	1.0
Tachycardia	3.5	0.0
ECG abnormality	1.4	0.0
Postural hypotension	1.4	0.0
Ventricular extrasystoles	1.4	0.0
Extrasystoles	0.7	0.0
Hemopericardium	0.7	0.0
Hypertension	0.7	0.0
Supraventricular tachycardia	0.7	0.0
Syncope	0.7	0.0
Vasodilation	0.7	0.0
Ventricular tachycardia	0.7	0.0
Digestive		
Nausea/vomiting	4.9	1.0
Injection Site		
Injection site reaction	1.4	0.0
Injection site pain	0.7	0.0
Metabolic and Nutritional		
Hypokalemia	0.7	0.0
Nervous		
Dizziness	1.4	0.0
Hypesthesia	0.7	0.0
Intracranial hemorrhage	0.7	0.0
Paresthesia	0.7	0.0
Respiratory		
Dyspnea	0.7	0.0
Skin and Appendages		
Sweating	1.4	0.0
Urogenital		
Polyuria	1.4	0.0
Hematuria	0.7	0.0

Continued on next page

Consult 1997 supplements and future editions for revisions

Wyeth-Ayerst Laboratories—Cont.

CHOLERA VACCINE ℞
USP

DESCRIPTION

Cholera Vaccine, USP is a sterile suspension of equal parts of Ogawa and Inaba serotypes of killed *Vibrio cholerae (V. comma)* in buffered sodium chloride injection. The Inaba and Ogawa strains of *V. cholerae* are grown on trypticase soy agar medium, removed from the medium with buffered sodium chloride injection and killed by the addition of 0.5 percent phenol. Phenol in a concentration of 0.5 percent is also used as the preservative in the finished vaccine. The vaccine contains 8 units of each serotype antigen (Ogawa and Inaba) per milliliter.

Cholera vaccine may be injected intracutaneously (intradermally), subcutaneously or intramuscularly.

CLINICAL PHARMACOLOGY

Cholera vaccine is used for active immunization against cholera. Field studies carried out in endemic cholera areas have shown cholera vaccines to be approximately 50% effective in reducing incidence of disease and for only 3 to 6 months. Use of cholera vaccine does not prevent transmission of infection.

INDICATION AND USAGE

Active immunization against cholera is indicated only for individuals traveling to or residing in countries where cholera is endemic or epidemic.

CONTRAINDICATIONS

Use of cholera vaccine should be postponed in the presence of any acute illness.

A history of severe systemic reaction or allergic response following a prior dose of cholera vaccine is a contraindication to further use.

WARNINGS

DO NOT INJECT INTRAVENOUSLY.

Cholera vaccine should not be administered intramuscularly to persons with thrombocytopenia or any coagulation disorder that would contraindicate intramuscular injection.

PRECAUTIONS

GENERAL

A separate, sterilized syringe and needle should be used for each patient to prevent transmission of hepatitis B virus and other infectious agents from one person to another.

Before delivering the dose intramuscularly or subcutaneously, aspirate to help avoid inadvertent injection into a blood vessel.

Before the injection of any biological, the physician should take all precautions known for prevention of allergic or other side reactions. This should include: a review of the patient's history regarding possible sensitivity; and a knowledge of the recent literature pertaining to the use of the biological concerned.

Epinephrine (1:1000) should be available for immediate use when this product is injected.

DRUG INTERACTIONS

Some data suggest that administration of cholera and yellow fever vaccines within three weeks of each other may result in decreased levels of antibody response to both vaccines as compared with administration at longer intervals. However, there is no evidence that protection to either disease is diminished following simultaneous administration.[1] It is currently recommended that, when feasible, cholera and yellow fever vaccines should be administered at a minimal interval of three weeks, unless time constraints preclude this. If the vaccines cannot be administered at least three weeks apart, they should be given simultaneously.[2]

PREGNANCY

Pregnancy Category C

Animal reproduction studies have not been conducted with cholera vaccine. It is also not known whether cholera vaccine can cause fetal harm when administered to a pregnant woman or can affect reproductive capacity. However, as with other inactivated bacterial vaccines, its use is not contraindicated during pregnancy unless the intended recipient has manifested significant systemic or allergic reaction following administration of prior doses. Use of cholera vaccine during pregnancy should be individualized to reflect actual need.[1,3]

ADVERSE REACTIONS

Local reactions manifested by erythema, induration, pain, and tenderness at the site of injection occur in most recipients, and such local reactions may persist for a few days.

Recipients frequently develop malaise, headache, and mild-to-moderate temperature elevations which may persist for 1 to 2 days.[1,4]

DOSAGE AND ADMINISTRATION

Shake vial vigorously before withdrawing each dose.

Parenteral drug products should be inspected visually for presence of particulate matter and discoloration prior to use.

The primary immunizing course consists of two doses administered one week to one month or more apart. The table below summarizes the recommended doses for both primary and booster immunizations by age, volume (mL), and route of administration.[3,5] The intracutaneous (intradermal) route is satisfactory for persons 5 years of age and older, but higher levels of antibody may be achieved in children less than 5 years old by the subcutaneous or intramuscular routes.

	Route & Age			
Dose number	Intra-dermal	Subcutaneous or Intramuscular		
	5 years and over	6 mos-4 years	5–10 years	Over 10 years
1 & 2	0.2 mL	0.2 mL	0.3 mL	0.5 mL
Boosters	0.2 mL	0.2 mL	0.3 mL	0.5 mL

In areas where cholera is epidemic or endemic, booster doses should be given every six months.

The primary immunizing series need never be repeated for booster doses to be effective.

Before injection, the rubber diaphragm of the vial and the skin over the site to be injected should be cleansed and prepared with a suitable germicide.

HOW SUPPLIED

Cholera Vaccine, USP, is supplied as 1.5 and 20 mL vials.

STORAGE

Keep between 2° and 8°C (35° and 46°F).

Keep from freezing.

REFERENCES

1. Recommendation of the Immunization Practices Advisory Committee (ACIP). General recommendations on immunization. MMWR 32(1):1, 1983.
2. Recommendations of the Immunization Practices Advisory Committee (ACIP). Yellow fever vaccine. MMWR 32(52):679, 1984.
3. Recommendation of the Public Health Service Advisory Committee on Immunization Practices—Cholera Vaccine. MMWR 27(20):173, 1978.
4. GANGAROSA, E. and FAICH, G.: Cholera: The risk to American travelers. Ann. Int. Med. 74:412, 1971.
5. Report of the Committee on Infectious Diseases, American Academy of Pediatrics, 1982 (Red Book).

Manufactured by Wyeth Laboratories Inc.,
Marietta, PA 17547.

CORDARONE® ℞
[*kŏr'dă-rōn*]
(amiodarone HCl)
Tablets

DESCRIPTION

Cordarone is a member of a new class of antiarrhythmic drugs with predominantly Class III (Vaughan Williams' classification) effects, available for oral administration as pink, scored tablets containing 200 mg of amiodarone hydrochloride. The inactive ingredients present are colloidal silicon dioxide, lactose, magnesium stearate, povidone, starch, and FD&C Red 40. Cordarone is a benzofuran derivative: 2-butyl-3-benzofuranyl 4-[2-(diethylamino)-ethoxy]-3,5-diiodophenyl ketone, hydrochloride. It is not chemically related to any other available antiarrhythmic drug.

The structural formula is as follows:

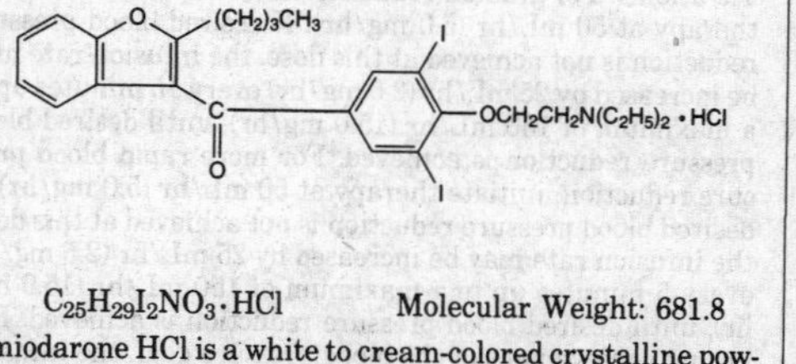

$C_{25}H_{29}I_2NO_3 \cdot HCl$ Molecular Weight: 681.8

Amiodarone HCl is a white to cream-colored crystalline powder. It is slightly soluble in water, soluble in alcohol, and freely soluble in chloroform. It contains 37.3% iodine by weight.

CLINICAL PHARMACOLOGY

ELECTROPHYSIOLOGY/MECHANISMS OF ACTION

In animals, Cordarone is effective in the prevention or suppression of experimentally induced arrhythmias. The antiarrhythmic effect of Cordarone may be due to at least two major properties: 1) a prolongation of the myocardial cell-action potential duration and refractory period and 2) noncompetitive α- and β-adrenergic inhibition.

Cordarone prolongs the duration of the action potential of all cardiac fibers while causing minimal reduction of dV/dt (maximal upstroke velocity of the action potential). The refractory period is prolonged in all cardiac tissues. Cordarone increases the cardiac refractory period without influencing resting membrane potential, except in automatic cells where the slope of the prepotential is reduced, generally reducing automaticity. These electrophysiologic effects are reflected in a decreased sinus rate of 15 to 20%, increased PR and QT intervals of about 10%, the development of U-waves, and changes in T-wave contour. These changes should not require discontinuation of Cordarone as they are evidence of its pharmacological action, although Cordarone can cause marked sinus bradycardia or sinus arrest and heart block. On rare occasions, QT prolongation has been associated with worsening of arrhythmia (see "**Warnings**").

HEMODYNAMICS

In animal studies and after intravenous administration in man, Cordarone relaxes vascular smooth muscle, reduces peripheral vascular resistance (afterload), and slightly increases cardiac index. After oral dosing, however, Cordarone produces no significant change in left ventricular ejection fraction (LVEF), even in patients with depressed LVEF. After acute intravenous dosing in man, Cordarone may have a mild negative inotropic effect.

PHARMACOKINETICS

Following oral administration in man, Cordarone is slowly and variably absorbed. The bioavailability of Cordarone is approximately 50%, but has varied between 35 and 65% in various studies. Maximum plasma concentrations are attained 3 to 7 hours after a single dose. Despite this, the onset of action may occur in 2 to 3 days, but more commonly takes 1 to 3 weeks, even with loading doses. Plasma concentrations with chronic dosing at 100 to 600 mg/day are approximately dose proportional, with a mean 0.5 mg/L increase for each 100 mg/day. These means, however, include considerable individual variability.

Cordarone has a very large but variable volume of distribution, averaging about 60 L/kg, because of extensive accumulation in various sites, especially adipose tissue and highly perfused organs, such as the liver, lung, and spleen. One major metabolite of Cordarone, desethylamiodarone, has been identified in man; it accumulates to an even greater extent in almost all tissues. The pharmacological activity of this metabolite, however, is not known. During chronic treatment, the plasma ratio of metabolite to parent compound is approximately one.

The main route of elimination is via hepatic excretion into bile, and some enterohepatic recirculation may occur. However, its kinetics in patients with hepatic insufficiency have not been elucidated. Cordarone has a very low plasma clearance with negligible renal excretion, so that it does not appear necessary to modify the dose in patients with renal failure. In patients with renal impairment, the plasma concentration of Cordarone is not elevated. Neither Cordarone nor its metabolite is dialyzable.

In patients, following discontinuation of chronic oral therapy, Cordarone has been shown to have a biphasic elimination with an initial one-half reduction of plasma levels after 2.5 to 10 days. A much slower terminal plasma-elimination phase shows a half-life of the parent compound ranging from 26 to 107 days, with a mean of approximately 53 days and most patients in the 40- to 55-day range. In the absence of a loading-dose period, steady-state plasma concentrations, at constant oral dosing, would therefore be reached between 130 and 535 days, with an average of 265 days. For the metabolite, the mean plasma-elimination half-life was approximately 61 days. These data probably reflect an initial elimination of the drug from well-perfused tissue (the 2.5- to 10-day half-life phase), followed by a terminal phase representing extremely slow elimination from poorly perfused tissue compartments such as fat.

The considerable intersubject variation in both phases of elimination, as well as uncertainty as to what compartment is critical to drug effect, requires attention to individual responses once arrhythmia control is achieved with loading doses because the correct maintenance dose is determined, in part, by the elimination rates. Daily maintenance doses of Cordarone should be based on individual patient requirements (see "**Dosage and Administration**").

Cordarone and its metabolite have a limited transplacental transfer of approximately 10 to 50%. The parent drug and its metabolite have been detected in breast milk.

Cordarone is highly protein-bound (approximately 96%).

Although electrophysiologic effects, such as prolongation of QTc, can be seen within hours after a parenteral dose of Cordarone, effects on abnormal rhythms are not seen before

2 to 3 days and usually require 1 to 3 weeks, even when a loading dose is used. There may be a continued increase in effect for longer periods still. There is evidence that the time to effect is shorter when a loading-dose regimen is used. Consistent with the slow rate of elimination, antiarrhythmic effects persist for weeks or months after Cordarone is discontinued, but the time of recurrence is variable and unpredictable. In general, when the drug is resumed after recurrence of the arrhythmia, control is established relatively rapidly compared to the initial response, presumably because tissue stores were not wholly depleted at the time of recurrence.

PHARMACODYNAMICS

There is no well-established relationship of plasma concentration to effectiveness, but it does appear that concentrations much below 1 mg/L are often ineffective and that levels above 2.5 mg/L are generally not needed. Within individuals dose reductions and ensuing decreased plasma concentrations can result in loss of arrhythmia control. Plasma-concentration measurements can be used to identify patients whose levels are unusually low, and who might benefit from a dose increase, or unusually high, and who might have dosage reduction in the hope of minimizing side effects. Some observations have suggested a plasma concentration, dose, or dose/duration relationship for side effects such as pulmonary fibrosis, liver-enzyme elevations, corneal deposits and facial pigmentation, peripheral neuropathy, gastrointestinal and central nervous system effects.

MONITORING EFFECTIVENESS

Predicting the effectiveness of any antiarrhythmic agent in long-term prevention of recurrent ventricular tachycardia and ventricular fibrillation is difficult and controversial, with highly qualified investigators recommending use of ambulatory monitoring, programmed electrical stimulation with various stimulation regimens, or a combination of these, to assess response. There is no present consensus on many aspects of how best to assess effectiveness, but there is a reasonable consensus on some aspects:

1. If a patient with a history of cardiac arrest does not manifest a hemodynamically unstable arrhythmia during electrocardiographic monitoring prior to treatment, assessment of the effectiveness of Cordarone requires some provocative approach, either exercise or programmed electrical stimulation (PES).
2. Whether provocation is also needed in patients who do manifest their life-threatening arrhythmia spontaneously is not settled, but there are reasons to consider PES or other provocation in such patients. In the fraction of patients whose PES-inducible arrhythmia can be made noninducible by Cordarone (a fraction that has varied widely in various series from less than 10% to almost 40%, perhaps due to different stimulation criteria), the prognosis has been almost uniformly excellent, with very low recurrence (ventricular tachycardia or sudden death) rates. More controversial is the meaning of continued inducibility. There has been an impression that continued inducibility in Cordarone patients may not foretell a poor prognosis but, in fact, many observers have found greater recurrence rates in patients who remain inducible than in those who do not. A number of criteria have been proposed, however, for identifying patients who remain inducible but who seem likely nonetheless to do well on Cordarone. These criteria include increased difficulty of Induction (more stimuli or more rapid stimuli), which has been reported to predict a lower rate of recurrence, and ability to tolerate the induced ventricular tachycardia without severe symptoms, a finding that has been reported to correlate with better survival but not with lower recurrence rates. While these criteria require confirmation and further study in general, *easier* inducibility or *poorer* tolerance of the induced arrhythmia should suggest consideration of a need to revise treatment.

Several predictors of success not based on PES have also been suggested, including complete elimination of all nonsustained ventricular tachycardia on ambulatory monitoring and very low premature ventricular-beat rates (less than 1 VPB/1,000 normal beats).

While these issues remain unsettled for Cordarone, as for other agents, the prescriber of Cordarone should have access to (direct or through referral), and familiarity with, the full range of evaluatory procedures used in the care of patients with life-threatening arrhythmias.

It is difficult to describe the effectiveness rates of Cordarone, as these depend on the specific arrhythmia treated, the success criteria used, the underlying cardiac disease of the patient, the number of drugs tried before resorting to Cordarone, the duration of follow-up, the dose of Cordarone, the use of additional antiarrhythmic agents, and many other factors. As Cordarone has been studied principally in patients with refractory life-threatening ventricular arrhythmias, in whom drug therapy must be selected on the basis of response and cannot be assigned arbitrarily, randomized comparisons with other agents or placebo have not been possible. Reports of series of treated patients with a history of cardiac arrest and mean follow-up of one year or more have given mortality (due to arrhythmia) rates that were highly variable, ranging from less than 5% to over

30%, with most series in the range of 10 to 15%. Overall arrhythmia-recurrence rates (fatal and nonfatal) also were highly variable (and, as noted above, depended on response to PES and other measures), and depend on whether patients who do not seem to respond initially are included. In most cases, considering only patients who seemed to respond well enough to be placed on long-term treatment, recurrence rates have ranged from 20 to 40% in series with a mean follow-up of a year or more.

INDICATIONS AND USAGE

Because of its life-threatening side effects and the substantial management difficulties associated with its use (see **"Warnings"** below), Cordarone is indicated only for the treatment of the following documented, life-threatening recurrent ventricular arrhythmias when these have not responded to documented adequate doses of other available antiarrhythmics or when alternative agents could not be tolerated.

1. Recurrent ventricular fibrillation.
2. Recurrent hemodynamically unstable ventricular tachycardia.

As is the case for other antiarrhythmic agents, there is no evidence from controlled trials that the use of Cordarone favorably affects survival.

Cordarone should be used only by physicians familiar with and with access to (directly or through referral) the use of all available modalities for treating recurrent life-threatening ventricular arrhythmias, and who have access to appropriate monitoring facilities, including in-hospital and ambulatory continuous electrocardiographic monitoring and electrophysiologic techniques. Because of the life-threatening nature of the arrhythmias treated, potential interactions with prior therapy, and potential exacerbation of the arrhythmia, initiation of therapy with Cordarone should be carried out in the hospital.

CONTRAINDICATIONS

Cordarone is contraindicated in severe sinus-node dysfunction, causing marked sinus bradycardia; second- and third-degree atrioventricular block; and when episodes of bradycardia have caused syncope (except when used in conjunction with a pacemaker).

Cordarone is contraindicated in patients with a known hypersensitivity to the drug.

WARNINGS

> Cordarone is intended for use only in patients with the indicated life-threatening arrhythmias because its use is accompanied by substantial toxicity.
>
> Cordarone has several potentially fatal toxicities, the most important of which is pulmonary toxicity (hypersensitivity pneumonitis or interstitial/alveolar pneumonitis) that has resulted in clinically manifest disease at rates as high as 10 to 17% in some series of patients with ventricular arrhythmias given doses around 400 mg/day, and as abnormal diffusion capacity without symptoms in a much higher percentage of patients. Pulmonary toxicity has been fatal about 10% of the time. Liver injury is common with Cordarone, but is usually mild and evidenced only by abnormal liver enzymes. Overt liver disease can occur, however, and has been fatal in a few cases. Like other antiarrhythmics, Cordarone can exacerbate the arrhythmia, e.g., by making the arrhythmia less well tolerated or more difficult to reverse. This has occurred in 2 to 5% of patients in various series, and significant heart block or sinus bradycardia has been seen in 2 to 5%. All of these events should be manageable in the proper clinical setting in most cases. Although the frequency of such proarrhythmic events does not appear greater with Cordarone than with many other agents used in this population, the effects are prolonged when they occur. Even in patients at high risk of arrhythmic death, in whom the toxicity of Cordarone is an acceptable risk, Cordarone poses major management problems that could be life-threatening in a population at risk of sudden death, so that every effort should be made to utilize alternative agents first.
>
> The difficulty of using Cordarone effectively and safely itself poses a significant risk to patients. Patients with the indicated arrhythmias must be hospitalized while the loading dose of Cordarone is given, and a response generally requires at least one week, usually two or more. Because absorption and elimination are variable, maintenance-dose selection is difficult, and it is not unusual to require dosage decrease or discontinuation of treatment. In a retrospective survey of 192 patients with ventricular tachyarrhythmias, 84 required dose reduction and 18 required at least temporary discontinuation because of adverse effects, and several series have reported 15 to 20% overall frequencies of discontinuation due to adverse reactions. The time at which a previously controlled life-threatening arrhythmia will recur after discontinuation or dose adjustment is unpredictable, ranging from weeks to months. The patient is obviously at great risk during this time and may need prolonged hospitalization. Attempts to substitute other antiarrhythmic agents when Cordarone must be stopped will be made difficult by the gradually, but unpredictably, changing amiodarone body burden. A similar problem exists when Cordarone is not effective; it still poses the risk of an interaction with whatever subsequent treatment is tried.

MORTALITY

In the National Heart, Lung and Blood Institute's Cardiac Arrhythmia Suppression Trial (CAST), a long-term, multi-centered, randomized, double-blind study in patients with asymptomatic non-life-threatening ventricular arrhythmias who had had myocardial infarctions more than six days but less than two years previously, an excessive mortality or non-fatal cardiac arrest rate was seen in patients treated with encainide or flecainide (56/730) compared with that seen in patients assigned to matched placebo-treated groups (22/725). The average duration of treatment with encainide or flecainide in this study was ten months.

The applicability of these results to other populations (e.g., those without recent myocardial infarctions) or to Cordarone-treated patients is uncertain. While definitive controlled trials with Cordarone are in progress, pooled analysis of small controlled studies in patients with structural heart disease (including post-mycardial infarction) have not shown excess mortality in the Cordarone-treated population.

PULMONARY TOXICITY

Cordarone may cause a clinical syndrome of cough and progressive dyspnea accompanied by functional, radiographic, gallium-scan, and pathological data consistent with pulmonary toxicity, the frequency of which varies from 2 to 7% in most published reports, but is as high as 10 to 17% in some reports. Therefore, when Cordarone therapy is initiated, a baseline chest X ray and pulmonary-function tests, including diffusion capacity, should be performed. The patient should return for a history, physical exam, and chest X ray every 3 to 6 months.

Preexisting pulmonary disease does not appear to increase the risk of developing pulmonary toxicity; however, these patients have a poorer prognosis if pulmonary toxicity does develop.

Pulmonary toxicity secondary to Cordarone seems to result from either indirect or direct toxicity as represented by hypersensitivity pneumonitis or interstitial/alveolar pneumonitis, respectively.

Hypersensitivity pneumonitis usually appears earlier in the course of therapy, and rechallenging these patients with Cordarone results in a more rapid recurrence of greater severity. Bronchoalveolar lavage is the procedure of choice to confirm this diagnosis, which can be made when a T suppressor/cytotoxic (CD8-positive) lymphocytosis is noted. Steroid therapy should be instituted and Cordarone therapy discontinued in these patients.

Interstitial/alveolar pneumonitis may result from the release of oxygen radicals and/or phospholipidosis and is characterized by findings of diffuse alveolar damage, interstitial pneumonitis or fibrosis in lung biopsy specimens. Phospholipidosis (foamy cells, foamy macrophages), due to inhibition of phospholipase, will be present in most cases of Cordarone-induced pulmonary toxicity; however, these changes also are present in approximately 50% of all patients on Cordarone therapy. These cells should be used as markers of therapy, but not as evidence of toxicity. A diagnosis of Cordarone-induced interstitial/alveolar pneumonitis should lead, at a minimum, to dose reduction or, preferably, to withdrawal of the Cordarone to establish reversibility, especially if other acceptable antiarrhythmic therapies are available. Where these measures have been instituted, a reduction in symptoms of amiodarone-induced pulmonary toxicity was usually noted within the first week, and a clinical improvement was greatest in the first two to three weeks. Chest X ray changes usually resolve within two to four months. According to some experts, steroids may prove beneficial. Prednisone in doses of 40 to 60 mg/day or equivalent doses of other steroids have been given and tapered over the course of several weeks depending upon the condition of the patient. In some cases rechallenge with Cordarone at a lower dose has not resulted in return of toxicity. Recent reports suggest that the use of lower loading and maintenance doses of Cordarone are associated with a decreased incidence of Cordarone-induced pulmonary toxicity.

In a patient receiving Cordarone, any new respiratory symptoms should suggest the possibility of pulmonary toxicity, and the history, physical exam, chest X ray, and pulmonary-function tests (with diffusion capacity) should be repeated and evaluated. A 15% decrease in diffusion capacity has a high sensitivity but only a moderate specificity for pulmonary toxicity; as the decrease in diffusion capacity approaches 30%, the sensitivity decreases but the specificity in-

Continued on next page

Wyeth-Ayerst Laboratories—Cont.

creases. A gallium scan also may be performed as part of the diagnostic workup.

Fatalities, secondary to pulmonary toxicity, have occurred in approximately 10% of cases. However, in patients with life-threatening arrhythmias, discontinuation of Cordarone therapy due to suspected drug-induced pulmonary toxicity should be undertaken with caution, as the most common cause of death in these patients is sudden cardiac death. Therefore, every effort should be made to rule out other causes of respiratory impairment (i.e., congestive heart failure with Swan-Ganz catheterization if necessary, respiratory infection, pulmonary embolism, malignancy, etc.) before discontinuing Cordarone in these patients. In addition, bronchoalveolar lavage, transbronchial lung biopsy and/or open lung biopsy may be necessary to confirm the diagnosis, especially in those cases where no acceptable alternative therapy is available.

If a diagnosis of Cordarone-induced hypersensitivity pneumonitis is made, Cordarone should be discontinued, and treatment with steroids should be instituted. If a diagnosis of Cordarone-induced interstitial/alveolar pneumonitis is made, steroid therapy should be instituted and, preferably, Cordarone discontinued or, at a minimum, reduced in dosage. Some cases of Cordarone-induced interstitial/alveolar pneumonitis may resolve following a reduction in Cordarone dosage in conjunction with the administration of steroids. In some patients, rechallenge at a lower dose has not resulted in return of interstitial/alveolar pneumonitis; however, in some patients (perhaps because of severe alveolar damage) the pulmonary lesions have not been reversible.

WORSENED ARRHYTHMIA

Cordarone, like other antiarrhythmics, can cause serious exacerbation of the presenting arrhythmia, a risk that may be enhanced by the presence of concomitant antiarrhythmics. Exacerbation has been reported in about 2 to 5% in most series, and has included new ventricular fibrillation, incessant ventricular tachycardia, increased resistance to cardioversion, and polymorphic ventricular tachycardia associated with QT prolongation (Torsade de Pointes). In addition, Cordarone has caused symptomatic bradycardia or sinus arrest with suppression of escape foci in 2 to 4% of patients.

LIVER INJURY

Elevations of hepatic enzyme levels are seen frequently in patients exposed to Cordarone and in most cases are asymptomatic. If the increase exceeds three times normal, or doubles in a patient with an elevated baseline, discontinuation of Cordarone or dosage reduction should be considered. In a few cases in which biopsy has been done, the histology has resembled that of alcoholic hepatitis or cirrhosis. Hepatic failure has been a rare cause of death in patients treated with Cordarone.

PREGNANCY: PREGNANCY CATEGORY D

Cordarone has been shown to be embryotoxic (increased fetal resorption and growth retardation) in the rat when given orally at a dose of 200 mg/kg/day (18 times the maximum recommended maintenance dose). Similar findings have been noted in one strain of mice at a dose of 5 mg/kg/day (approximately $^1/_2$ the maximum recommended maintenance dose) and higher, but not in a second strain nor in the rabbit at doses up to 100 mg/kg/day (9 times the maximum recommended maintenance dose).

Neonatal hypo- or hyperthyroidism

Cordarone can cause fetal harm when administered to a pregnant woman. Although Cordarone use during pregnancy is uncommon, there have been a small number of published reports of congenital goiter/hypothyroidism and hyperthyroidism. If Cordarone is used during pregnancy, or if the patient becomes pregnant while taking Cordarone, the patient should be apprised of the potential hazard to the fetus.

In general, Cordarone should be used during pregnancy only if the potential benefit to the mother justifies the unknown risk to the fetus.

PRECAUTIONS

CORNEAL MICRODEPOSITS; IMPAIRMENT OF VISION

Corneal microdeposits appear in the majority of adults treated with Cordarone®. They are usually discernible only by slit-lamp examination, but give rise to symptoms such as visual halos or blurred vision in as many as 10% of patients. Corneal microdeposits are reversible upon reduction of dose or termination of treatment. Asymptomatic microdeposits are not a reason to reduce dose or discontinue treatment.

PHOTOSENSITIVITY

Cordarone has induced photosensitization in about 10% of patients; some protection may be afforded by the use of sun-barrier creams or protective clothing. During long-term treatment, a blue-gray discoloration of the exposed skin may occur. The risk may be increased in patients of fair complexion or those with excessive sun exposure, and may be related to cumulative dose and duration of therapy.

THYROID ABNORMALITIES

Cordarone inhibits peripheral conversion of thyroxine (T_4) to triiodothyronine (T_3) and may cause increased thyroxine levels, decreased T_3 levels, and increased levels of inactive reverse T_3 (rT_3) in clinically euthyroid patients. It is also a potential source of large amounts of inorganic iodine. Because of its release of inorganic iodine, or perhaps for other reasons, Cordarone can cause either hypothyroidism or hyperthyroidism. Thyroid function should be monitored prior to treatment and periodically thereafter, particularly in elderly patients, and in any patient with a history of thyroid nodules, goiter, or other thyroid dysfunction. Because of the slow elimination of Cordarone and its metabolites, high plasma iodide levels, altered thyroid function, and abnormal thyroid-function tests may persist for several weeks or even months following Cordarone withdrawal.

Hypothyroidism has been reported in 2 to 4% of patients in most series, but in 8 to 10% in some series. This condition may be identified by relevant clinical symptoms and particularly by elevated serum TSH levels. In some clinically hypothyroid amiodarone-treated patients, free thyroxine index values may be normal. Hypothyroidism is best managed by Cordarone dose reduction and/or thyroid hormone supplement. However, therapy must be individualized, and it may be necessary to discontinue Cordarone in some patients.

Hyperthyroidism occurs in about 2% of patients receiving Cordarone, but the incidence may be higher among patients with prior inadequate dietary iodine intake. Cordarone-induced hyperthyroidism usually poses a greater hazard to the patient than hypothyroidism because of the possibility of arrhythmia breakthrough or aggravation. In fact, IF ANY NEW SIGNS OF ARRHYTHMIA APPEAR, THE POSSIBILITY OF HYPERTHYROIDISM SHOULD BE CONSIDERED. Hyperthyroidism is best identified by relevant clinical symptoms and signs, accompanied usually by abnormally elevated levels of serum T_3 RIA, and further elevations of serum T_4, and a subnormal serum TSH level (using a sufficiently sensitive TSH assay). The finding of a flat TSH response to TRH is confirmatory of hyperthyroidism and may be sought in equivocal cases. Since arrhythmia breakthroughs may accompany Cordarone-induced hyperthyroidism, aggressive medical treatment is indicated, including, if possible, dose reduction or withdrawal of Cordarone. The institution of antithyroid drugs, β-adrenergic blockers and/or temporary corticosteroid therapy may be necessary. The action of antithyroid drugs may be especially delayed in amiodarone-induced thyrotoxicosis because of substantial quantities of preformed thyroid hormones stored in the gland. Radioactive iodine therapy is contraindicated because of the low radioiodine uptake associated with amiodarone-induced hyperthyroidism. Experience with thyroid surgery in this setting is extremely limited, and this form of therapy runs the theoretical risk of inducing thyroid storm. Cordarone-induced hyperthyroidism may be followed by a transient period of hypothyroidism.

SURGERY

Hypotension Postbypass: Rare occurrences of hypotension upon discontinuation of cardiopulmonary bypass during open-heart surgery in patients receiving Cordarone have been reported. The relationship of this event to Cordarone therapy is unknown.

Adult Respiratory Distress Syndrome (ARDS): Postoperatively, rare occurrences of ARDS have been reported in patients receiving Cordarone therapy who have undergone either cardiac or noncardiac surgery. Although patients usually respond well to vigorous respiratory therapy, in rare instances the outcome has been fatal. One possible mechanism of this deleterious effect may be the generation of superoxide radicals during oxygenation; therefore, the operative FiO_2 should be kept as close to room air as possible.

LABORATORY TESTS

Elevations in liver enzymes (SGOT and SGPT) can occur. Liver enzymes in patients on relatively high maintenance doses should be monitored on a regular basis. Persistent significant elevations in the liver enzymes or hepatomegaly should alert the physician to consider reducing the maintenance dose of Cordarone or discontinuing therapy.

Cordarone alters the results of thyroid-function tests, causing an increase in serum T_4 and serum reverse T_3, and a decline in serum T_3 levels. Despite these biochemical changes, most patients remain clinically euthyroid.

DRUG INTERACTIONS

Although only a small number of drug-drug interactions with Cordarone have been explored formally, most of these have shown such an interaction. The potential for other interactions should be anticipated, particularly for drugs with potentially serious toxicity, such as other antiarrhythmics. If such drugs are needed, their dose should be reassessed and, where appropriate, plasma concentration measured.

In view of the long and variable half-life of Cordarone, potential for drug interactions exists not only with concomitant medication but also with drugs administered after discontinuation of Cordarone.

Cyclosporine

Concomitant use of amiodarone and cyclosporine has been reported to produce persistently elevated plasma concentrations of cyclosporine resulting in elevated creatinine, despite reduction in dose of cyclosporine.

Digitalis

Administration of Cordarone to patients receiving digoxin therapy regularly results in an increase in the serum digoxin concentration that may reach toxic levels with resultant clinical toxicity. **On initiation of Cordarone, the need for digitalis therapy should be reviewed and the dose reduced by approximately 50% or discontinued.** If digitalis treatment is continued, serum levels should be closely monitored and patients observed for clinical evidence of toxicity. These precautions probably should apply to digitoxin administration as well.

Anticoagulants

Potentiation of warfarin-type anticoagulant response is almost always seen in patients receiving Cordarone and can result in serious or fatal bleeding. **The dose of the anticoagulant should be reduced by one-third to one-half, and prothrombin times should be monitored closely.**

Antiarrhythmic Agents

Other antiarrhythmic drugs, such as quinidine, procainamide, disopyramide, and phenytoin, have been used concurrently with Cordarone.

There have been case reports of increased steady-state levels of quinidine, procainamide, and phenytoin during concomitant therapy with Cordarone. In general, any added antiarrhythmic drug should be initiated at a lower than usual dose with careful monitoring.

In general, combination of Cordarone with other antiarrhythmic therapy should be reserved for patients with life-threatening ventricular arrhythmias who are incompletely responsive to a single agent or incompletely responsive to Cordarone. During transfer to Cordarone the dose levels of previously administered agents should be reduced by 30 to 50% several days after the addition of Cordarone, when arrhythmia suppression should be beginning. The continued need for the other antiarrhythmic agent should be reviewed after the effects of Cordarone have been established, and discontinuation ordinarily should be attempted. If the treatment is continued, these patients should be particularly carefully monitored for adverse effects, especially conduction disturbances and exacerbation of tachyarrhythmias, as Cordarone is continued. In Cordarone-treated patients who require additional antiarrhythmic therapy, the initial dose of such agents should be approximately half of the usual recommended dose.

Cordarone should be used with caution in patients receiving β-blocking agents or calcium antagonists because of the possible potentiation of bradycardia, sinus arrest, and AV block; if necessary, Cordarone can continue to be used after insertion of a pacemaker in patients with severe bradycardia or sinus arrest.

[See table at left.]

ELECTROLYTE DISTURBANCES

Since antiarrhythmic drugs may be ineffective or may be arrhythmogenic in patients with hypokalemia, any potassium or magnesium deficiency should be corrected before instituting Cordarone therapy.

CARCINOGENESIS, MUTAGENESIS, IMPAIRMENT OF FERTILITY

Cordarone reduced fertility of male and female rats at a dose level of 90 mg/kg/day (8 × highest recommended human maintenance dose).

SUMMARY OF DRUG INTERACTIONS WITH CORDARONE

Concomitant Drug	Interaction: Onset (days)	Interaction: Magnitude	Recommended Dose Reduction of Concomitant Drug
Warfarin	3 to 4	Increases prothrombin time by 100%	↓ $^1/_3$ to $^1/_2$
Digoxin	1	Increases serum concentration by 70%	↓ $^1/_2$
Quinidine	2	Increases serum concentration by 33%	↓ $^1/_3$ to $^1/_2$ (or discontinue)
Procainamide	<7	Increases plasma concentration by 55%, NAPA* concentration by 33%	↓ $^1/_3$ (or discontinue)

*NAPA = n-acetyl procainamide.

Cordarone caused a statistically significant, dose-related increase in the incidence of thyroid tumors (follicular adenoma and/or carcinoma) in rats. The incidence of thyroid tumors was greater than control even at the lowest dose level of Cordarone tested, i.e., 5 mg/kg/day or approximately equal to $^1/_2$ the highest recommended human maintenance dose. Mutagenicity studies (Ames, micronucleus, and lysogenic tests) with Cordarone were negative.

PREGNANCY: PREGNANCY CATEGORY D

See "**Warnings**."

LABOR AND DELIVERY

It is not known whether the use of Cordarone during labor or delivery has any immediate or delayed adverse effects. Preclinical studies in rodents have not shown any effect of Cordarone on the duration of gestation or on parturition.

NURSING MOTHERS

Cordarone is excreted in human milk, suggesting that breast-feeding could expose the nursing infant to a significant dose of the drug. Nursing offspring of lactating rats administered Cordarone have been shown to be less viable and have reduced body-weight gains. Therefore, when Cordarone therapy is indicated, the mother should be advised to discontinue nursing.

PEDIATRIC USE

The safety and effectiveness of Cordarone in pediatric patients have not been established.

ADVERSE REACTIONS

Adverse reactions have been very common in virtually all series of patients treated with Cordarone for ventricular arrhythmias with relatively large doses of drug (400 mg/day and above), occurring in about three-fourths of all patients and causing discontinuation in 7 to 18%. The most serious reactions are pulmonary toxicity, exacerbation of arrhythmia, and rare serious liver injury (see "**Warnings**"), but other adverse effects constitute important problems. They are often reversible with dose reduction and virtually always reversible with cessation of Cordarone treatment. Most of the adverse effects appear to become more frequent with continued treatment beyond six months, although rates appear to remain relatively constant beyond one year. The time and dose relationships of adverse effects are under continued study.

Neurologic problems are extremely common, occurring in 20 to 40% of patients and including malaise and fatigue, tremor and involuntary movements, poor coordination and gait, and peripheral neuropathy; they are rarely a reason to stop therapy and may respond to dose reductions.

Gastrointestinal complaints, most commonly nausea, vomiting, constipation, and anorexia, occur in about 25% of patients but rarely require discontinuation of drug. These commonly occur during high-dose administration (i.e., loading dose) and usually respond to dose reduction or divided doses.

Asymptomatic corneal microdeposits are present in virtually all adult patients who have been on drug for more than 6 months. Some patients develop eye symptoms of halos, photophobia, and dry eyes. Vision is rarely affected and drug discontinuation is rarely needed.

Dermatological adverse reactions occur in about 15% of patients, with photosensitivity being most common (about 10%). Sunscreen and protection from sun exposure may be helpful, and drug discontinuation is not usually necessary. Prolonged exposure to Cordarone occasionally results in a blue-gray pigmentation. This is slowly and occasionally incompletely reversible on discontinuation of drug but is of cosmetic importance only.

Cardiovascular adverse reactions, other than exacerbation of the arrhythmias, include the uncommon occurrence of congestive heart failure (3%) and bradycardia. Bradycardia usually responds to dosage reduction but may require a pacemaker for control. CHF rarely requires drug discontinuation. Cardiac conduction abnormalities occur infrequently and are reversible on discontinuation of drug.

The following side-effect rates are based on a retrospective study of 241 patients treated for 2 to 1,515 days (mean 441.3 days).

The following side effects were reported in 10 to 33% of patients:

Gastrointestinal: Nausea and vomiting.

The following side effects were each reported in 4 to 9% of patients:

Dermatologic: Solar dermatitis/photosensitivity.

Neurologic: Malaise and fatigue, tremor/abnormal involuntary movements, lack of coordination, abnormal gait/ataxia, dizziness, paresthesias.

Gastrointestinal: Constipation, anorexia.

Ophthalmologic: Visual disturbances.

Hepatic: Abnormal liver-function tests.

Respiratory: Pulmonary inflammation or fibrosis.

The following side effects were each reported in 1 to 3% of patients:

Thyroid: Hypothyroidism, hyperthyroidism.

Neurologic: Decreased libido, insomnia, headache, sleep disturbances.

Cardiovascular: Congestive heart failure, cardiac arrhythmias, SA node dysfunction.

	Loading Dose (Daily)	Adjustment and Maintenance Dose (Daily)	
Ventricular Arrhythmias	1 to 3 weeks	~1 month	usual maintenance
	800 to 1,600 mg	600 to 800 mg	400 mg

Gastrointestinal: Abdominal pain.

Hepatic: Nonspecific hepatic disorders.

Other: Flushing, abnormal taste and smell, edema, abnormal salivation, coagulation abnormalities.

The following side effects were each reported in less than 1% of patients:

Blue skin discoloration, rash, spontaneous ecchymosis, alopecia, hypotension, and cardiac conduction abnormalities.

Rare occurrences of hepatitis, cholestatic hepatitis, cirrhosis, optic neuritis, epididymitis, vasculitis, pseudotumor cerebri, and thrombocytopenia have been reported in patients receiving Cordarone.

In surveys of almost 5,000 patients treated in open U.S. studies and in published reports of treatment with Cordarone, the adverse reactions most frequently requiring discontinuation of Cordarone included pulmonary infiltrates or fibrosis, paroxysmal ventricular tachycardia, congestive heart failure, and elevation of liver enzymes. Other symptoms causing discontinuations less often included visual disturbances, solar dermatitis, blue skin discoloration, hyperthyroidism and hypothyroidism.

OVERDOSAGE

There have been a few reported cases of Cordarone overdose in which 3 to 8 grams were taken. There were no deaths or permanent sequelae. Animal studies indicate that Cordarone has a high oral LD_{50} (> 3,000 mg/kg).

In addition to general supportive measures, the patient's cardiac rhythm and blood pressure should be monitored, and if bradycardia ensues, a β-adrenergic agonist or a pacemaker may be used. Hypotension with inadequate tissue perfusion should be treated with positive inotropic and/or vasopressor agents. Neither Cordarone nor its metabolite is dialyzable.

DOSAGE AND ADMINISTRATION

BECAUSE OF THE UNIQUE PHARMACOKINETIC PROPERTIES, DIFFICULT DOSING SCHEDULE, AND SEVERITY OF THE SIDE EFFECTS IF PATIENTS ARE IMPROPERLY MONITORED, CORDARONE SHOULD BE ADMINISTERED ONLY BY PHYSICIANS WHO ARE EXPERIENCED IN THE TREATMENT OF LIFE-THREATENING ARRHYTHMIAS WHO ARE THOROUGHLY FAMILIAR WITH THE RISKS AND BENEFITS OF CORDARONE THERAPY, AND WHO HAVE ACCESS TO LABORATORY FACILITIES CAPABLE OF ADEQUATELY MONITORING THE EFFECTIVENESS AND SIDE EFFECTS OF TREATMENT.

In order to insure that an antiarrhythmic effect will be observed without waiting several months, loading doses are required. A uniform, optimal dosage schedule for administration of Cordarone has not been determined. Individual patient titration is suggested according to the following guidelines.

For life-threatening ventricular arrhythmias, such as ventricular fibrillation or hemodynamically unstable ventricular tachycardia: Close monitoring of the patients is indicated during the loading phase, particularly until risk of recurrent ventricular tachycardia or fibrillation has abated. Because of the serious nature of the arrhythmia and the lack of predictable time course of effect, loading should be performed in a hospital setting. Loading doses of 800 to 1,600 mg/day are required for 1 to 3 weeks (occasionally longer) until initial therapeutic response occurs. (Administration of Cordarone in divided doses with meals is suggested for total daily doses of 1,000 mg or higher, or when gastrointestinal intolerance occurs.) If side effects become excessive, the dose should be reduced. Elimination of recurrence of ventricular fibrillation and tachycardia usually occurs within 1 to 3 weeks, along with reduction in complex and total ventricular ectopic beats.

Upon starting Cordarone therapy, an attempt should be made to gradually discontinue prior antiarrhythmic drugs (see section on "DRUG INTERACTIONS"). When adequate arrhythmia control is achieved, or if side effects become prominent, Cordarone dose should be reduced to 600 to 800 mg/day for one month and then to the maintenance dose, usually 400 mg/day (see "**Clinical Pharmacology**"—"MONITORING EFFECTIVENESS"). Some patients may require larger maintenance doses, up to 600 mg/day, and some can be controlled on lower doses. Cordarone may be administered as a single daily dose, or in patients with severe gastrointestinal intolerance, as a b.i.d. dose. In each patient, the chronic maintenance dose should be determined according to antiarrhythmic effect as assessed by symptoms, Holter recordings, and/or programmed electrical stimulation and by patient tolerance. Plasma concentrations may be helpful in evaluating nonresponsiveness or unexpectedly severe toxicity (see "**Clinical Pharmacology**").

The lowest effective dose should be used to prevent the occurrence of side effects. In all instances, the physician must be guided by the severity of the individual patient's arrhythmia and response to therapy.

When dosage adjustments are necessary, the patient should be closely monitored for an extended period of time because of the long and variable half-life of Cordarone and the difficulty in predicting the time required to attain a new steady-state level of drug. Dosage suggestions are summarized below:

[See table above.]

HOW SUPPLIED

Cordarone® (amiodarone HCl) Tablets are available in bottles of 60 tablets and in Redipak® cartons containing 100 tablets (10 blister strips of 10) as follows:

200 mg, NDC 0008-4188, round, convex-faced, pink tablets with a raised "C" and marked "200" on one side, with reverse side scored and marked "Wyeth" and "4188."

Keep tightly closed.

Store at Room Temperature, approximately 25° C (77° F).

Protect from light

Dispense in a light-resistant, tight container.

Use carton to protect contents from light.

Caution: Federal law prohibits dispensing without prescription.

Manufactured for
Wyeth Laboratories Inc.
A Wyeth-Ayerst Company
Philadelphia, PA 19101
by Sanofi Winthrop Industrie
1, rue de la Vierge
33440 Ambares, France

Shown in Product Identification Guide, page 339

CORDARONE® INTRAVENOUS ℞

(amiodarone hydrochloride)

DESCRIPTION

Cordarone Intravenous (Cordarone I.V.) contains amiodarone HCl ($C_{25}H_{29}I_2NO_3 \cdot HCl$), a class III antiarrhythmic drug. Amiodarone HCl is (2-butyl-3-benzofuranyl)[4-[2-(diethylamino)ethoxy]-3,5-diiodophenyl]methanone hydrochloride. Amiodarone HCl has the following structural formula:

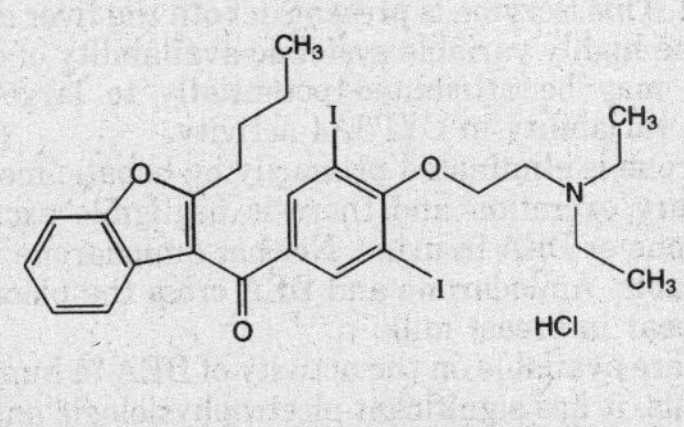

Amiodarone HCl is a white to slightly yellow crystalline powder, and is very slightly soluble in water. It has a molecular weight of 681.78 and contains 37.3% iodine by weight. Cordarone I.V. is a sterile clear, pale-yellow solution visually free from particulates. Each milliliter of the Cordarone I.V. formulation contains 50 mg of amiodarone HCl, 20.2 mg of benzyl alcohol, 100 mg of polysorbate 80, and water for injection.

CLINICAL PHARMACOLOGY

MECHANISMS OF ACTION

Amiodarone is generally considered a class III antiarrhythmic drug, but it possesses electrophysiologic characteristics of all four Vaughan Williams classes. Like class I drugs, amiodarone blocks sodium channels at rapid pacing frequencies, and like class II drugs, it exerts a noncompetitive antisympathetic action. One of its main effects, with prolonged administration, is to lengthen the cardiac action potential, a class III effect. The negative chronotropic effect of amiodarone in nodal tissues is similar to the effect of class IV drugs. In addition to blocking sodium channels, amiodarone blocks myocardial potassium channels, which contributes to slowing of conduction and prolongation of refractoriness. The antisympathetic action and the block of calcium and potassium channels are responsible for the negative dromotropic effects on the sinus node and for the slowing of conduction and prolongation of refractoriness in the atrioventricular (AV) node. Its vasodilatory action can decrease cardiac workload and consequently myocardial oxygen consumption.

Cordarone I.V. administration prolongs intranodal conduction (Atrial-His, AH) and refractoriness of the atrioventricu-

Continued on next page

Wyeth-Ayerst Laboratories—Cont.

lar node (ERP AVN), but has little or no effect on sinus cycle length (SCL), refractoriness of the right atrium and right ventricle (ERP RA and ERP RV), repolarization (QTc), intraventricular conduction (QRS), and infranodal conduction (His-ventricular, HV). A comparison of the electrophysiologic effects of Cordarone I.V. and oral Cordarone is shown in the table below.

EFFECTS OF INTRAVENOUS AND ORAL CORDARONE ON ELECTROPHYSIOLOGIC PARAMETERS

Formulation	SCL	QRS	QTc	AH	HV	ERP RA	ERP RV	ERP AVN
I.V.	↔	↔	↔	↑	↔	↔	↔	↑
Oral	↑	↔	↑	↑	↔	↑	↑	↑

↔No change

At higher doses (> 10 mg/kg) of Cordarone I.V., prolongation of the ERP RV and modest prolongation of the QRS have been seen. These differences between oral and intravenous administration suggest that the initial acute effects of Cordarone I.V. may be predominantly focused on the AV node, causing an intranodal conduction delay and increased nodal refractoriness due to slow channel blockade (class IV activity) and noncompetitive adrenergic antagonism (class II activity).

PHARMACOKINETICS AND METABOLISM

Amiodarone exhibits complex disposition characteristics after intravenous administration. Peak serum concentrations after single 5 mg/kg 15-minute intravenous infusions in healthy subjects range between 5 and 41 mg/L. Peak concentrations after 10-minute infusions of 150 mg Cordarone I.V. in patients with ventricular fibrillation (VF) or hemodynamically unstable ventricular tachycardia (VT) range between 7 and 26 mg/L. Due to rapid distribution, serum concentrations decline to 10% of peak values within 30 to 45 minutes after the end of the infusion. In clinical trials, after 48 hours of continued infusions (125, 500, or 1000 mg/day) plus supplemental (150 mg) infusions (for recurrent arrhythmias), amiodarone mean serum concentrations between 0.7 to 1.4 mg/L were observed (n=260).

N-desethylamiodarone (DEA) is the major active metabolite of amiodarone in humans. DEA serum concentrations above 0.05 mg/L are not usually seen until after several days of continuous infusion but with prolonged therapy reach approximately the same concentration as amiodarone. The enzymes responsible for the N-deethylation are believed to be the cytochrome P-450 3A (CYP3A) subfamily, principally CYP3A4. This isozyme is present in both the liver and intestines. The highly variable systemic availability of oral amiodarone may be attributed potentially to large interindividual variability in CYP3A4 activity.

Amiodarone is eliminated primarily by hepatic metabolism and biliary excretion and there is negligible excretion of amiodarone or DEA in urine. Neither amiodarone nor DEA is dialyzable. Amiodarone and DEA cross the placenta and both appear in breast milk.

No data are available on the activity of DEA in humans, but in animals, it has significant electrophysiologic and antiarrhythmic effects generally similar to amiodarone itself. DEA's precise role and contribution to the antiarrhythmic activity of oral amiodarone are not certain. The development of maximal ventricular class III effects after oral Cordarone administration in humans correlates more closely with DEA accumulation over time than with amiodarone accumulation. On the other hand (see CLINICAL TRIALS), after Cordarone I.V. administration, there is evidence of activity well before significant concentrations of DEA are attained.

The following table summarizes the mean ranges of pharmacokinetic parameters of amiodarone reported in single dose i.v. (5 mg/kg over 15 min) studies of healthy subjects.

PHARMACOKINETIC PROFILE AFTER I.V. AMIODARONE ADMINISTRATION

Drug	Clearance (mL/h/kg)	V_c (L/kg)	V_{ss} (L/kg)	$t_{1/2}$ (days)
Amiodarone	90–158	0.2	40–84	20–47
Desethylamiodarone	197–290	—	68–168	≥AMI $t_{1/2}$

Notes: V_c and V_{ss} denote the central and steady-state volumes of distribution from i.v. studies.

"—" denotes not available.

Desethylamiodarone clearance and volume involve an unknown biotransformation factor.

The systemic availability of ***oral*** amiodarone in healthy subjects ranges between 33% and 65%.

From *in vitro* studies, the protein binding of amiodarone is >96%.

In clinical studies of 2 to 7 days, clearance of amiodarone after intravenous administration in patients with VT and VF ranged between 220 and 440 mL/h/kg. Age, sex, renal disease, and hepatic disease (cirrhosis) do not have marked effects on the disposition of amiodarone or DEA. Renal impairment does not influence the pharmacokinetics of amiodarone. After a single dose of Cordarone I.V. in cirrhotic patients, significantly lower C_{max} and average concentration values are seen for DEA, but mean amiodarone levels are unchanged. Normal subjects over 65 years of age show lower clearances (about 100 mL/hr/kg) than younger subjects (about 150 mL/hr/kg) and an increase in $t_{1/2}$ from about 20 to 47 days. In patients with severe left ventricular dysfunction, the pharmacokinetics of amiodarone are not significantly altered but the terminal disposition $t_{1/2}$ of DEA is prolonged. Although no dosage adjustment for patients with renal, hepatic, or cardiac abnormalities has been defined during chronic treatment with ***oral*** Cordarone, close clinical monitoring is prudent for elderly patients and those with severe left ventricular dysfunction.

There is no established relationship between drug concentration and therapeutic response for short-term intravenous use. Steady-state amiodarone concentrations of 1 to 2.5 mg/L have been associated with antiarrhythmic effects and acceptable toxicity following chronic ***oral*** Cordarone therapy.

PHARMCODYNAMICS

Cordarone I.V. has been reported to produce negative inotropic and vasodilatory effects in animals and humans. In clinical studies of patients with refractory VF or hemodynamically unstable VT, treatment-emergent, drug-related hypotension occurred in 288 of 1836 patients (16%) treated with Cordarone I.V. No correlations were seen between the baseline ejection fraction and the occurrence of clinically significant hypotension during infusion of Cordarone I.V.

CLINICAL TRIALS

Apart from studies in patients with VT or VF, described below, there are two other studies of amiodarone showing an antiarrhythmic effect before significant levels of DEA could have accumulated. A placebo-controlled study of i.v. amiodarone (300 mg over 2 hours followed by 1200 mg/day) in post-coronary artery bypass graft patients with supraventricular and 2- to 3-consecutive-beat ventricular arrhythmias showed a reduction in arrhythmias from 12 hours on. A baseline-controlled study using a similar i.v. regimen in patients with recurrent, refractory VT/VF also showed rapid onset of antiarrhythmic activity; amiodarone therapy reduced episodes of VT by 85% compared to baseline.

The acute effectiveness of Cordarone I.V. in suppressing recurrent VF or hemodynamically unstable VT is supported by two randomized, parallel, dose-response studies of approximately 300 patients each. In these studies, patients with at least two episodes of VF or hemodynamically unstable VT in the preceding 24 hours were randomly assigned to receive doses of approximately 125 or 1000 mg over the first 24 hours, an 8-fold difference. In one study, a middle dose of approximately 500 mg was evaluated. The dose regimen consisted of an initial rapid loading infusion, followed by a slower 6-hour loading infusion, and then an 18-hour maintenance infusion. The maintenance infusion was continued up to hour 48. Additional 10-minute infusions of 150 mg Cordarone I.V. were given for "breakthrough" VT/VF more frequently to the 125-mg dose group, thereby considerably reducing the planned 8-fold differences in total dose to 1.8- and 2.6- fold, respectively, in the two studies.

The prospectively defined primary efficacy end point was the rate of VT/VF episodes per hour. For both studies, the median rate was 0.02 episodes per hour in patients receiving the high dose and 0.07 episodes per hour in patients receiving the low dose, or approximately 0.5 versus 1.7 episodes per day ($p = 0.07$, 2-sided, in both studies). In one study, the time to first episode of VT/VF was significantly prolonged (approximately 10 hours in patients receiving the low dose and 14 hours in patients receiving the high dose). In both studies, significantly fewer supplemental infusions were given to patients in the high-dose group. Mortality was not affected in these studies; at the end of double-blind therapy or after 48 hours, all patients were given open access to whatever treatment (including Cordarone I.V.) was deemed necessary.

INDICATIONS AND USAGE

Cordarone I.V. is indicated for initiation of treatment and prophylaxis of frequently recurring ventricular fibrillation and hemodynamically unstable ventricular tachycardia in patients refractory to other therapy. Cordarone I.V. also can be used to treat patients with VT/VF for whom oral Cordarone is indicated, but who are unable to take oral medication. During or after treatment with Cordarone I.V., patients may be transferred to oral Cordarone theray (see **DOSAGE AND ADMINISTRATION**).

Cordarone I.V. should be used for acute treatment until the patient's ventricular arrhythmias are stabilized. Most patients will require this therapy for 48 to 96 hours, but Cordarone I.V. may be safely administered for longer periods if necessary.

CONTRAINDICATIONS

Cordarone I.V. is contraindicated in patients with known hypersensitivity to any of the components of Cordarone I.V., or in patients with cardiogenic shock, marked sinus bradycardia, and second- or third-degree AV block unless a functioning pacemaker is available.

WARNINGS

HYPOTENSION

Hypotension is the most common adverse effect seen with Cordarone I.V. In clinical trials, treatment-emergent, drug-related hypotension was reported as an adverse effect in 288 (16%) of 1836 patients treated with Cordarone I.V. Clinically significant hypotension during infusions was seen most often in the first several hours of treatment and was not dose related, but appeared to be related to the rate of infusion. Hypotension necessitating alterations in Cordarone I.V. therapy was reported in 3% of patients, with permanent discontinuation required in less than 2% of patients. Hypotension should be treated initially by slowing the infusion; additional standard therapy may be needed, including the following; vasopressor drugs, positive inotropic agents, and volume expansion. ***The initial rate of infusion should be monitored closely and should not exceed that prescribed in*** **DOSAGE AND ADMINISTRATION.**

BRADYCARDIA AND AV BLOCK

Drug-related bradycardia occurred in 90 (4.9%) of 1836 patients in clinical trials while they were receiving Cordarone I.V. for life-threatening VT/VF; it was not dose-related. Bradycardia should be treated by slowing the infusion rate or discontinuing Cordarone I.V. In some patients, inserting a pacemaker is required. Despite such measures, bradycardia was progressive and terminal in 1 patient during the controlled trials. Patients with a known predisposition to bradycardia or AV block should be treated with Cordarone I.V. in a setting where a temporary pacemaker is available.

LONG-TERM USE

See labeling for oral Cordarone. There has been limited experience in patients receiving Cordarone I.V. for longer than 3 weeks.

NEONATAL HYPO- OR HYPERTHYROIDISM

Although ***oral*** Cordarone use during pregnancy is uncommon, there have been a small number of published reports of congenital goiter/hypothyroidism and hyperthyroidism. If Cordarone I.V. is administered during pregnancy, the patient should be apprised of the potential hazard to the fetus.

PRECAUTIONS

Cordarone I.V. should be administered only by physicians who are experienced in the treatment of life-threatening arrhythmias, who are thoroughly familiar with the risks and benefits of Cordarone therapy, and who have access to facilities adequate for monitoring the effectiveness and side effects of treatment.

LIVER ENZYME ELEVATIONS

Elevations of blood hepatic enzyme values—alanine aminotransferase (ALT), aspartate aminotransferase (AST), and gamma-glutamyl transferase (GGT)—are seen commonly in patients with immediately life-threatening VT/VF. Interpreting elevated AST activity can be difficult because the values may be elevated in patients who have had recent myocardial infarction, congestive heart failure, or multiple electrical defibrillations. Approximately 54% of patients receiving Cordarone I.V. in clinical studies had baseline liver enzyme elevations, and 13% had clinically significant elevations. In 81% of patients with both baseline and on-therapy data available, the liver enzyme elevations either improved during therapy or remained at baseline levels. Baseline abnormalities in hepatic enzymes are not a contraindication to treatment.

Two (2) cases of fatal hepatocellular necrosis after treatment with Cordarone I.V. have been reported. The patients, one 28 years of age and the other 60 years of age, were treated for atrial arrhythmias with an initial infusion of 1500 mg over 5 hours, a rate much higher than recommended. Both patients developed hepatic and renal failure within 24 hours after the start of Cordarone I.V. treatment and died on day 14 and day 4, respectively. Because these episodes of hepatic necrosis may have been due to the rapid rate of infusion with possible rate-related hypotension, ***the initial rate of infusion should be monitored closely and should not exceed that prescribed in*** **DOSAGE AND ADMINISTRATION.**

In patients with life-threatening arrhythmias, the potential risk of hepatic injury should be weighed against the potential benefit of Cordarone I.V. therapy, but patients receiving Cordarone I.V. should be monitored carefully for evidence of progressive hepatic injury. Consideration should be given to reducing the rate of administration or withdrawing Cordarone I.V. in such cases.

PROARRHYTHMIA

Like all antiarrhythmic agents, Cordarone I.V. may cause a worsening of existing arrhythmias or precipitate a new arrhythmia. Proarrhythmia, primarily torsades de pointes, has been associated with prolongation by Cordarone I.V. of the QTc interval to 500 ms or greater. Although QTc prolongation occurred frequently in patients receiving Cordarone

I.V., torsades de pointes or new-onset VF occurred infrequently (less than 2%). Patients should be monitored for QTc prolongation during infusion with Cordarone I.V.

PULMONARY DISORDERS

ARDS

Two percent (2%) of patients were reported to have adult respiratory distress syndrome (ARDS) during clinical studies. ARDS is a disorder characterized by bilateral, diffuse pulmonary infiltrates with pulmonary edema and varying degrees of respiratory insufficiency. The clinical and radiographic picture can arise after a variety of lung injuries, such as those resulting from trauma, shock, prolonged cardiopulmonary resuscitation, and aspiration pneumonia, conditions present in many of the patients enrolled in the clinical studies. It is not possible to determine what role, if any, Cordarone I.V. played in causing or exacerbating the pulmonary disorder in those patients.

Pulmonary fibrosis

Only 1 of more than 1000 patients treated with Cordarone I.V. in clinical studies developed pulmonary fibrosis. In that patient, the condition was diagnosed 3 months after treatment with Cordarone I.V., during which time she received ***oral*** Cordarone. Pulmonary toxicity is a well-recognized complication of long-term Cordarone use (see labeling for oral Cordarone).

DRUG INTERACTIONS

Amiodarone can inhibit metabolism mediated by cytochrome P-450 enzymes, probably accounting for the significant effects of oral Cordarone (and presumably Cordarone I.V.) on the pharmacokinetics of various therapeutic agents including digoxin, quinidine, procainamide, warfarin (CYP2C9), dextromethorphan (CYP2D6), and cyclosporine (CYP3A4). Hemodynamic and electrophysiologic interactions have also been observed after concomitant administration with propranolol, diltiazem, and verapamil. Conversely, agents producing a significant effect on amiodarone pharmacokinetics include phenytoin, cimetidine, and cholestyramine. Because of the long half-life of amiodarone, drug interactions may persist long after discontinuation of drug administration. Few data are available on drug interactions with Cordarone I.V. Except as noted, the following tables summarize the important interactions between ***oral*** Cordarone and other therapeutic agents.

SUMMARY OF DRUG INTERACTIONS WITH CORDARONE

Drugs Whose Effects May Be Increased by Cordarone

Concomitant Drug	Interaction
Warfarin	Increases prothrombin time.
Digoxin	Increases serum concentration.
Quinidine	Increases serum concentration.
Procainamide	Increases serum concentration, NAPA concentration.
Disopyramide	Increases QT prolongation which could cause arrhythmia.
Fentanyl	May cause hypotension, bradycardia, decreased cardiac output.
Flecainide	Reduces the dose of flecainide needed to maintain therapeutic plasma concentrations.
Lidocaine	**Oral:** Sinus bradycardia was observed in a patient receiving oral Cordarone who was given lidocaine for local anesthesia. **I.V.:** Seizure associated with increased lidocaine concentrations was observed in one patient.
Cyclosporine	Produces persistently elevated plasma concentrations of cyclosporine resulting in elevated creatinine, despite reduction in dose of cyclosporine.

SUMMARY OF DRUG INTERACTIONS WITH CORDARONE

Drugs that May Interfere with the Actions of Cordarone

Concomitant Drug	Interaction
Cholestyramine	Increases enterohepatic elimination of amiodarone and may reduce serum levels and $t_{1/2}$.
Cimetidine	Increases serum amiodarone levels.
Phenytoin	Decreases serum amiodarone levels.

Potential drug class interactions with Cordarone

Beta Blockers: Since Cordarone has weak beta blocking activity, use with beta blocking agents could increase risk of hypotension and bradycardia.

Calcium Channel Blockers: Cordarone inhibits atrioventricular conduction and decreases myocardial contractility, increasing the risk of AV block with verapamil or diltiazem or of hypotension with any calcium channel blocker.

In addition to the interactions noted above, chronic (>2 weeks) ***oral*** Cordarone administration impairs metabolism of phenytoin, dextromethorphan, and methotrexate.

SUMMARY TABULATION OF TREATMENT-EMERGENT DRUG-RELATED STUDY EVENTS IN PATIENTS RECEIVING CORDARONE I.V. IN CONTROLLED AND OPEN-LABEL STUDIES (≥2% INCIDENCE)

Study Event	Controlled Studies (n=814)	Open-Label Studies (n=1022)	Total (n=1836)
Body as a Whole			
Fever	24 (2.9%)	13 (1.2%)	37 (2.0%)
Cardiovascular System			
Bradycardia	49 (6.0%)	41 (4.0%)	90 (4.9%)
Congestive heart failure	18 (2.2%)	21 (2.0%)	39 (2.1%)
Heart arrest	29 (3.5%)	26 (2.5%)	55 (2.9%)
Hypotension	165 (20.2%)	123 (12.0%)	288 (15.6%)
Ventricular tachycardia	15 (1.8%)	30 (2.9%)	45 (2.4%)
Digestive System			
Liver function test abnormal	35 (4.2%)	29 (2.8%)	64 (3.4%)
Nausea	29 (3.5%)	43 (4.2%)	72 (3.9%)

ELECTROLYTE DISTURBANCES

Patients with hypokalemia or hypomagnesemia should have the condition corrected whenever possible before being treated with Cordarone I.V., as these disorders can exaggerate the degree of QTc prolongation and increase the potential for torsades de pointes. Special attention should be given to electrolyte and acid-base balance in patients experiencing severe or prolonged diarrhea or in patients receiving concomitant diuretics.

CARCINOGENESIS, MUTAGENESIS, IMPAIRMENT OF FERTILITY

No carcinogenicity studies were conducted with Cordarone I.V. However, ***oral*** Cordarone caused a statistically significant, dose-related increase in the incidence of thyroid adenomas in rats. The incidence of thyroid adenomas in rats was greater than the incidence in controls even at the lowest tested dose of 5 mg/kg/day (about 0.1 times the maximum recommended oral human maintenance dose in mg/m^2).

Mutagenicity studies conducted with amiodarone HCl (Ames, micronucleus, and lysogenic induction tests) were negative.

No fertility studies were conducted with Cordarone I.V. However, ***oral*** Cordarone administration resulted in reduced fertility of rats at a dose of 90 mg/kg/day (about 1.3 times the maximum recommended oral human maintenance dose in mg/m^2). No significant effects on fertility occurred at 30 mg/kg/day.

PREGNANCY

Category D. See **WARNINGS** and NEONATAL HYPO- OR HYPERTHYROIDISM.

In addition to causing infrequent congenital goiter/hypothyroidism and hyperthyroidism, amiodarone has caused a variety of adverse effects in animals.

In a reproductive study in which amiodarone was given intravenously to rabbits at dosages of 5, 10, or 25 mg/kg per day (about 0.1, 0.3, and 0.7 times the maximum recommended human dose [MRHD] on a body surface area basis), maternal deaths occurred in all groups, including controls. Embryotoxicity (as manifested by fewer full-term fetuses and increased resorptions with concomitantly lower litter weights) occurred at dosages of 10 mg/kg and above. No evidence of embryotoxicity was observed at 5 mg/kg and no teratogenicity was observed at any dosages.

In a teratology study in which amiodarone was administered by continuous i.v. infusion to rats at dosages of 25, 50, or 100 mg/kg per day (about 0.4, 0.7, and 1.4 times the MRHD when compared on a body surface area basis), maternal toxicity (as evidenced by reduced weight gain and food consumption) and embryotoxicity (as evidenced by increased resorptions, decreased live litter size, reduced body weights, and retarded sternum and metacarpal ossification) were observed in the 100 mg/kg group.

Cordarone I.V. should be used during pregnancy only if the potential benefit to the mother justifies the risk to the fetus.

NURSING MOTHERS

Amiodarone is excreted in human milk, suggesting that breast-feeding could expose the nursing infant to a significant dose of the drug. Nursing offspring of lactating rats administered amiodarone have demonstrated reduced viability and reduced body weight gains. The risk of exposing the infant to amiodarone should be weighed against the potential benefit of arrhythmia suppression in the mother. The mother should be advised to discontinue nursing.

LABOR AND DELIVERY

It is not known whether the use of Cordarone during labor or delivery has any immediate or delayed adverse effects. Preclinical studies in rodents have not shown any effect on the duration of gestation or on parturition.

PEDIATRIC USAGE

The safety and efficacy of Cordarone in the pediatric population have not been established; therefore, its use in pediatric patients is not recommended.

ADVERSE REACTIONS

In a total of 1836 patients in controlled and uncontrolled clinical trials, 14% of patients received Cordarone I.V. for at least 1 week, 5% received it for at least 2 weeks, 2% received it for at least 3 weeks, and 1% received it for more than 3 weeks, without an increased incidence of severe adverse reactions. The mean duration of therapy in these studies was 5.6 days; median exposure was 3.7 days.

The most important treatment-emergent adverse effects were hypotension, asystole/cardiac arrest/electromechanical dissociation (EMD), cardiogenic shock, congestive heart failure, bradycardia, liver function test abnormalities, VT, and AV block. Overall, treatment was discontinued for about 9% of the patients because of adverse effects. The most common adverse effects leading to discontinuation of Cordarone I.V. therapy were hypotension (1.6%), asystole/cardiac arrest/EMD (1.2%), VT (1.1%), and cardiogenic shock (1%).

The following table lists the most common (incidence ≥2%) treatment-emergent adverse events during Cordarone I.V. therapy considered at least possibly drug-related. These data were collected from the Wyeth-Ayerst clinical trials involving 1836 patients with life-threatening VT/VF. Data from all assigned treatment groups are pooled because none of the adverse events appeared to be dose-related.

[See table above.]

Other treatment-emergent possibly drug-related adverse events reported in less than 2% of patients receiving Cordarone I.V. in Wyeth-Ayerst controlled and uncontrolled studies included the following: abnormal kidney function, atrial fibrillation, diarrhea, increased ALT, increased AST, lung edema, nodal arrhythmia, prolonged QT interval, respiratory disorder, shock, sinus bradycardia, Stevens-Johnson syndrome, thrombocytopenia, VF, and vomiting.

OVERDOSAGE

The most likely effects of an inadvertent overdose of Cordarone I.V. are hypotension, cardiogenic shock, bradycardia, AV block, and hepatotoxicity. Hypotension and cardiogenic shock should be treated by slowing the infusion rate or with standard therapy: vasopressor drugs, positive inotropic agents, and volume expansion. Bradycardia and AV block may require temporary pacing. Hepatic enzyme concentrations should be monitored closely.

Amiodarone is not dialyzable.

DOSAGE AND ADMINISTRATION

Amiodarone shows considerable interindividual variation in response. Thus, although a starting dose adequate to suppress life-threatening arrhythmias is needed, close monitoring with adjustment of dose as needed is essential. The recommended starting dose of Cordarone I.V. is about 1000 mg over the first 24 hours of therapy, delivered by the following infusion regimen:

CORDARONE I.V. DOSE RECOMMENDATIONS — FIRST 24 HOURS —

Loading infusions	
***First* Rapid:**	**150 mg over the FIRST 10 minutes (15 mg/min).** Add 3 mL of Cordarone I.V. (150 mg) to 100 mL D_5W (concentration = 1.5 mg/mL). Infuse 100 mL over 10 minutes.
***Followed by* Slow:**	**360 mg over the NEXT 6 hours (1 mg/min).** Add 18 mL of Cordarone I.V. (900 mg) to 500 mL D_5W (concentration = 1.8 mg/mL).
Maintenance infusion	**540 mg over the REMAINING 18 hours (0.5 mg/min).** Decrease the rate of the slow loading infusion to 0.5 mg/min.

Continued on next page

Wyeth-Ayerst Laboratories—Cont.

AMIODARONE HCl SOLUTION STABILITY

Solution	Concentration (mg/mL)	Container	Comments
5% Dextrose in Water (D₅W)	1.0–6.0	PVC	Physically compatible, with amiodarone loss <10% at 2 hours.
5% Dextrose in Water (D₅W)	1.0–6.0	Polyolefin, Glass	Physically compatible, with no amiodarone loss at 24 hours.

Y-SITE INJECTION INCOMPATIBILITY

Drug	Vehicle	Amiodarone Concentration	Comments
Aminophylline	D₅W	4 mg/mL	Precipitate
Cefamandole Nafate	D₅W	4 mg/mL	Precipitate
Cefazolin Sodium	D₅W	4 mg/mL	Precipitate
Mezlocillin Sodium	D₅W	4 mg/mL	Precipitate
Heparin Sodium	D₅W	—	Precipitate
Sodium Bicarbonate	D₅W	3 mg/mL	Precipitate

After the first 24 hours, the maintenance infusion rate of 0.5 mg/min (720 mg/24 hours) should be continued utilizing a concentration of 1 to 6 mg/mL (Cordarone I.V. concentrations greater than 2 mg/mL should be administered via a central venous catheter). In the event of breakthrough episodes of VF or hemodynamically unstable VT, 150-mg supplemental infusions of Cordarone I.V. mixed in 100 mL of D₅W may be administered. Such infusions should be administered over 10 minutes to minimize the potential for hypotension. The rate of the maintenance infusion may be increased to achieve effective arrhythmia suppression.

The first 24-hour dose may be individualized for each patient; however, in controlled clinical trials, mean daily doses above 2100 mg were associated with an increased risk of hypotension. The initial infusion rate should not exceed 30 mg/min.

Based on the experience from clinical studies of Cordarone I.V., a maintenance infusion of up to 0.5 mg/min can be cautiously continued for 2 to 3 weeks regardless of the patient's age, renal function, or left ventricular function. There has been limited experience in patients receiving Cordarone I.V. for longer than 3 weeks.

The surface properties of solutions containing injectable amiodarone are altered such that the drop size may be reduced. This reduction may lead to underdosage of the patient by up to 30% if drop counter infusion sets are used. Cordarone I.V. must be delivered by a volumetric infusion pump.

Cordarone I.V. should, whenever possible, be administered through a central venous catheter dedicated to that purpose. An in-line filter should be used during administration.

Cordarone I.V. concentrations greater than 3 mg/mL in D₅W have been associated with a high incidence of peripheral vein phlebitis; however, concentrations of 2.5 mg/mL or less appear to be less irritating. Therefore, for infusions longer than 1 hour, Cordarone I.V. concentrations should not exceed 2 mg/mL unless a central venous catheter is used. Cordarone I.V. infusions exceeding 2 hours must be administered in glass or polyolefin bottles containing D₅W.

It is well known that amiodarone adsorbs to polyvinyl chloride (PVC) tubing and the clinical trial dose administration schedule was designed to account for this adsorption. All of the clinical trials were conducted using PVC tubing and its use is therefore recommended. The concentrations and rates of infusion provided in **DOSAGE AND ADMINISTRATION** reflect doses identified in these studies. It is important that the recommended infusion regimen be followed closely. Cordarone I.V. does not need to be protected from light during administration.

[See first table above.]

ADMIXTURE INCOMPATIBILITY

Cordarone I.V. in D₅W is incompatible with the drugs shown below.

[See second table above.]

INTRAVENOUS TO ORAL TRANSITION

Patients whose arrhythmias have been suppressed by Cordarone I.V. may be switched to oral Cordarone. The optimal dose for changing from intravenous to oral administration of Cordarone will depend on the dose of Cordarone I.V. already administered, as well as the bioavailability of oral Cordarone. When changing to oral Cordarone therapy, clinical monitoring is recommended, particularly for elderly patients.

The following table provides suggested doses of oral Cordarone to be initiated after varying durations of Cordarone I.V. administration. These recommendations are made on the basis of a comparable total body amount of amiodarone delivered by the intravenous and oral routes, based on 50% bioavailability of oral amiodarone.

RECOMMENDATIONS FOR ORAL DOSAGE AFTER I.V. INFUSION

Duration of Cordarone I.V. Infusion#	Initial Daily Dose of Oral Cordarone
<1 week	800–1600 mg
1—3 weeks	600–800 mg
>3 weeks*	400 mg

#Assuming a 720 mg/day infusion (0.5 mg/min).
* Cordarone I.V is not intended for maintenance treatment.

HOW SUPPLIED

Cordarone I.V. (amiodarone HCl) is available in packages of 10 ampuls (2 cartons each containing 5 ampuls), 3 mL each, as follows:

50 mg per mL, NDC 0008-0814-01.

Store at room temperature, 15° to 25°C (59° to 77°F).
Protect from light and excessive heat.
Use carton to protect contents from light until used.

DIUCARDIN®
[dī″ū-car′din]
(hydroflumethiazide tablets, USP)

℞

DESCRIPTION

Diucardin (hydroflumethiazide) is an oral thiazide (benzothiadiazine) diuretic-antihypertensive agent.

Diucardin is available as 50 mg tablets for oral administration.

Chemical name: 3,4-Dihydro-6-(trifluoromethyl)-2H-1,2,4-benzothiadiazine-7-sulfonamide 1,1-dioxide.

Structural formula:

Hydroflumethiazide is an odorless white to cream-colored, finely divided, crystalline powder. It has a melting point between 270° and 275° C. Hydroflumethiazide is freely soluble in acetone, soluble in alcohol, and very slightly soluble in water.

The inactive ingredients contained in Diucardin tablets are: lactose, magnesium stearate, microcrystalline cellulose, povidone, and starch.

CLINICAL PHARMACOLOGY

Hydroflumethiazide is incompletely but fairly rapidly absorbed from the gastrointestinal tract. It appears to have a biphasic biological half-life with an estimated alpha-phase of about 2 hours and an estimated beta-phase of about 17 hours; it has a metabolite with a longer half-life, which is extensively bound to the red blood cells. Hydroflumethiazide is excreted in the urine; its metabolite has also been detected in the urine.

The mechanism of action results in an interference with the renal tubular mechanism of electrolyte reabsorption. At maximal therapeutic dosage, all thiazides are approximately equal in their diuretic potency. The mechanism whereby thiazides function in the control of hypertension is unknown.

INDICATIONS AND USAGE

Diucardin is indicated as adjunctive therapy in edema associated with congestive heart failure, hepatic cirrhosis, and corticosteroid and estrogen therapy.

Diucardin has also been found useful in edema due to various forms of renal dysfunction such as: nephrotic syndrome; acute glomerulonephritis; and chronic renal failure.

Diucardin is indicated in the management of hypertension either as the sole therapeutic agent or to enhance the effect of other antihypertensive drugs in the more severe forms of hypertension.

USAGE IN PREGNANCY

The routine use of diuretics in an otherwise healthy woman is inappropriate and exposes mother and fetus to unnecessary hazard. Diuretics do not prevent development of toxemia of pregnancy, and there is no satisfactory evidence that they are useful in the treatment of developed toxemia.

Edema during pregnancy may arise from pathological causes or from the physiologic and mechanical consequences of pregnancy. Thiazides are indicated in pregnancy when edema is due to pathologic causes just as they are in the absence of pregnancy (however, see "Precautions—PREGNANCY" below).

Dependent edema in pregnancy, resulting from restriction of venous return by the expanded uterus, is properly treated through elevation of the lower extremities and use of support hose. Use of diuretics to lower intravascular volume in this case is illogical and unnecessary. There is hypervolemia during normal pregnancy which is harmful to neither the fetus nor the mother (in absence of cardiovascular disease), but which is associated with, including generalized edema, in the majority of pregnant women. If this edema produces discomfort, increased recumbency will often provide relief. In rare instances, this edema may cause extreme discomfort which is not relieved by rest. In these cases, a short course of diuretics may provide relief and may be appropriate.

CONTRAINDICATIONS

Anuria.
Hypersensitivity to this or other sulfonamide-derived drugs.

WARNINGS

Diucardin should be used with caution in severe renal disease. In patients with renal disease, thiazides may precipitate azotemia. Cumulative effects of the drug may develop in patients with impaired renal function.

Thiazides should be used with caution in patients with impaired hepatic function or progressive liver disease, since minor alterations of fluid and electrolyte balance may precipitate hepatic coma.

Thiazides may add to or potentiate the action of other antihypertensive drugs. Potentiation occurs with ganglionic or peripheral adrenergic blocking drugs.

Sensitivity reactions may occur in patients with a history of allergy or bronchial asthma.

The possibility of exacerbation or activation of systemic lupus erythematosus has been reported.

PRECAUTIONS

GENERAL

All patients receiving thiazide therapy should be observed for clinical signs of fluid or electrolyte imbalance; namely, hyponatremia, hypochloremic alkalosis, and hypokalemia. Serum and urine electrolyte determinations are particularly important when the patient is vomiting excessively or receiving parenteral fluids. Medication such as digitalis may also influence serum electrolytes. Warning signs, irrespective of cause, are: dryness of mouth, thirst, weakness, lethargy, drowsiness, restlessness, muscle pains or cramps, muscular fatigue, hypotension, oliguria, tachycardia, and gastrointestinal disturbances such as nausea and vomiting.

Hypokalemia may develop with thiazides as with any other potent diuretic, especially with brisk diuresis, when severe cirrhosis is present, or during concomitant use of corticosteroids or ACTH.

Interference with adequate oral electrolyte intake will also contribute to hypokalemia. Digitalis therapy may exaggerate metabolic effects of hypokalemia, especially with reference to myocardial activity.

Any chloride deficit is generally mild and usually does not require specific treatment except under extraordinary circumstances (as in liver disease or renal disease). Dilutional hyponatremia may occur in edematous patients in hot weather; appropriate therapy is water restriction, rather than administration of salt, except in rare instances when the hyponatremia is life-threatening. In actual salt depletion, appropriate replacement is the therapy of choice.

Hyperuricemia may occur or frank gout may be precipitated in certain patients receiving thiazide therapy.

Insulin requirements in diabetic patients may be increased, decreased, or unchanged. Latent diabetes mellitus may become manifested during thiazide administration.

The antihypertensive effects of the drug may be enhanced in the post-sympathectomy patient.

If progressive renal impairment becomes evident, as indicated by a rising creatinine or blood urea nitrogen, a careful reappraisal of therapy is necessary with consideration given to withholding or discontinuing diuretic therapy.

Thiazides may decrease serum PBI levels without signs of thyroid disturbance.

Lithium generally should not be given with diuretics because they reduce its renal clearance and increase the risk of lithium toxicity. Read circulars for lithium preparations before use of such concomitant therapy with Diucardin.

Thiazides have been shown to increase the urinary excretion of magnesium; this may result in hypomagnesemia.

Calcium excretion is decreased by thiazides. Pathological changes in the parathyroid gland with hypercalcemia and hypophosphatemia have been observed in a few patients on prolonged thiazide therapy. The common complications of hyperparathyroidism, such as renal lithiasis, bone resorption, and peptic ulceration, have not been seen.

LABORATORY TESTS
Periodic determination of serum electrolytes to detect possible electrolyte imbalance should be performed at appropriate intervals.

DRUG INTERACTIONS
Anticoagulants, oral
(Effects may be decreased when used concurrently with thiazide diuretics; dosage adjustments may be necessary.)

Antigout medications
(Thiazide diuretics may raise the level of blood uric acid; dosage adjustment of antigout medications may be necessary to control hyperuricemia and gout.)

Antihypertensive medications, other, especially diazoxide, or preanesthetic and anesthetic agents used in surgery or skeletal-muscle relaxants, nondepolarizing, used in surgery
(Effects may be potentiated when used concurrently with thiazide diuretics; dosage adjustments may be necessary.)

Amphotericin B or Corticosteroids or Corticotropin (ACTH)
(Concurrent use with thiazide diuretics may intensify electrolyte imbalance, particularly hypokalemia.)

Cardiac glycosides
(Concurrent use with thiazide diuretics may enhance the possibility of digitalis toxicity associated with hypokalemia.)

Colestipol
(May inhibit gastrointestinal absorption of the thiazide diuretics; administration 1 hour before or 4 hours after colestipol is recommended.)

Hypoglycemics
(Thiazide diuretics may raise blood glucose levels; for adult-onset diabetics, dosage adjustment of hypoglycemic medications may be necessary during and after thiazide diuretic therapy; insulin requirements may be increased, decreased, or unchanged.)

Lithium salts
(Concurrent use with thiazide diuretics is not recommended, as they may provoke lithium toxicity because of reduced renal clearance.)

Methenamine
(Effectiveness may be decreased when used concurrently with thiazide diuretics because of alkalinization of the urine.)

Nonsteroidal anti-inflammatory agents
(In some patients, the steroidal anti-inflammatory agent can reduce the diuretic, natriuretic, and antihypertensive effects of loop, potassium sparing, and thiazide diuretics. Therefore, when hydroflumethiazide and nonsteroidal anti-inflammatory agents are used concomitantly, the patient should be observed closely to determine if the desired effect of the diuretic is obtained.)

Norepinephrine
(Thiazides may decrease arterial responsiveness to norepinephrine. This diminution is not sufficient to preclude effectiveness of the pressor agent for therapeutic use.)

Tubocurarine
(Thiazide drugs may increase the responsiveness to tubocurarine.)

DIAGNOSTIC INTERFERENCE—With expected physiologic effects:
Blood and urine glucose levels (usually only in patients with a predisposition for glucose intolerance) and
Serum bilirubin levels (by displacement from albumin binding) and
Serum calcium levels (thiazide diuretics should be discontinued before parathyroid-function tests are carried out) and
Serum uric acid levels (may be increased)
Serum magnesium, potassium, and sodium levels (may be decreased; serum magnesium levels may increase in uremic patients)
Serum protein-bound iodine (PBI) levels (may be decreased)
Thiazides should be discontinued before carrying out tests for parathyroid function (see "Precautions—GENERAL, Calcium excretion.)

CARCINOGENESIS, MUTAGENESIS, IMPAIRMENT OF FERTILITY
No studies have been performed to evaluate carcinogenic or mutagenic potential of Diucardin or the potential of Diucardin to impair fertility.

PREGNANCY
Teratogenic Effects—Pregnancy Category C
Animal reproduction studies have not been conducted with Diucardin. It is also not known whether Diucardin can cause fetal harm when administered to a pregnant woman or can affect reproduction capacity. Diucardin should be given to a pregnant woman only if clearly needed.
Nonteratogenic Effects
Fetal or neonatal jaundice, thrombocytopenia, and possibly other adverse reactions which have occurred in the adult.

NURSING MOTHERS
Thiazides appear in breast milk. If use of the drug is deemed essential, the patient may consider stopping nursing.

PEDIATRIC USE
Safety and effectiveness in children have not been established.

ADVERSE REACTIONS
The following adverse reactions have been observed, but there is not enough systematic collection of data to support an estimate of their frequency.

GASTROINTESTINAL SYSTEMS
Anorexia, gastric irritation, nausea, vomiting, cramping, diarrhea, constipation, jaundice (intrahepatic cholestatic jaundice), pancreatitis, sialadenitis.

CENTRAL NERVOUS SYSTEM
Dizziness, vertigo, paresthesias, headache, xanthopsia.

HEMATOLOGIC
Leukopenia, agranulocytosis, thrombocytopenia, aplastic anemia, hemolytic anemia.

CARDIOVASCULAR
Orthostatic hypotension (may be aggravated by alcohol, barbiturates, or narcotics).

DERMATOLOGIC—HYPERSENSITIVITY
Purpura, photosensitivity, rash, urticaria, necrotizing angiitis (vasculitis, cutaneous vasculitis), fever, respiratory distress including pneumonitis, anaphylactic reactions.

OTHER
Hyperglycemia, glycosuria, hyperuricemia, muscle spasm, weakness, restlessness, transient blurred vision.
Whenever adverse reactions are moderate or severe, thiazide dosage should be reduced or therapy withdrawn.

OVERDOSAGE
SIGNS AND SYMPTOMS
Diuresis, lethargy progressing to coma, with minimal cardiorespiratory depression and with or without significant serum electrolyte changes or dehydration; GI irritation; hypermotility; transient elevation in BUN level.

TREATMENT
Empty stomach by gastric lavage, taking care to avoid aspiration. Monitor serum electrolyte levels and renal function, and institute supportive measures, as required to maintain hydration, electrolyte balance, respiration, and cardiovascular and renal function. Treat GI effects symptomatically.

DOSAGE AND ADMINISTRATION
The average adult dose is 25 to 200 mg per day. The average adult antihypertensive dose is 50 to 100 mg per day.
Therapy should be individualized according to patient response. This therapy should be titrated to gain maximal response as well as the minimal dose possible to maintain that therapeutic response.

HOW SUPPLIED
Diucardin®—Each scored, white oval compressed tablet, inscribed "DIUCARDIN 50," contains 50 mg hydroflumethiazide, in bottles of 100 (NDC 0046-0702-81).
Store at room temperature (approximately 25° C)
Dispense in a well-closed container as defined in the USP
Caution: Federal law prohibits dispensing without prescription.
Shown in Product Identification Guide, page 339

EFFEXOR®
(venlafaxine hydrochloride)
Tablets

℞

DESCRIPTION
Effexor (venlafaxine hydrochloride) is a structurally novel antidepressant for oral administration. It is chemically unrelated to tricyclic, tetracyclic, or other available antidepressant agents. It is designated (R/S)-1-[2-(dimethylamino)-1-(4-methoxyphenyl)ethyl] cyclohexanol hydrochloride or (±)-1-[α-[(dimethylamino)methyl]-p-methoxybenzyl] cyclohexanol hydrochloride and has the empirical formula of $C_{17}H_{27}NO_2HCl$. Its molecular weight is 313.87. The structural formula is shown below.
[See chemical structure at top of next column.]

Venlafaxine hydrochloride is a white to off-white crystalline solid with a solubility of 572 mg/mL in water (adjusted to ionic strength of 0.2 M with sodium chloride). Its octanol: water (0.2 M sodium chloride) partition coefficient is 0.43.

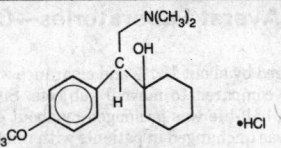
venlafaxine hydrochloride

Compressed tablets contain venlafaxine hydrochloride equivalent to 25 mg, 37.5 mg, 50 mg, 75 mg, or 100 mg venlafaxine. Inactive ingredients consist of cellulose, iron oxides, lactose, magnesium stearate, and sodium starch glycolate.

CLINICAL PHARMACOLOGY
PHARMACODYNAMICS
The mechanism of the antidepressant action of venlafaxine in humans is believed to be associated with its potentiation of neurotransmitter activity in the CNS. Preclinical studies have shown that venlafaxine and its active metabolite, O-desmethylvenlafaxine (ODV), are potent inhibitors of neuronal serotonin and norepinephrine reuptake and weak inhibitors of dopamine reuptake. Venlafaxine and ODV have no significant affinity for muscarinic, histaminergic, or α-1 adrenergic receptors *in vitro*. Pharmacologic activity at these receptors is hypothesized to be associated with the various anticholinergic, sedative, and cardiovascular effects seen with other psychotropic drugs. Venlafaxine and ODV do not possess monoamine oxidase (MAO) inhibitory activity.

PHARMACOKINETICS
Venlafaxine is well absorbed and extensively metabolized in the liver. O-desmethylvenlafaxine (ODV) is the only major active metabolite. On the basis of mass balance studies, at least 92% of a single dose of venlafaxine is absorbed. Approximately 87% of a venlafaxine dose is recovered in the urine within 48 hours as either unchanged venlafaxine (5%), unconjugated ODV (29%), conjugated ODV (26%), or other minor inactive metabolites (27%). Renal elimination of venlafaxine and its metabolites is the primary route of excretion. The relative bioavailability of venlafaxine from a tablet was 100% when compared to an oral solution. Food has no significant effect on the absorption of venlafaxine or on the formation of ODV.

The degree of binding of venlafaxine to human plasma is 27%±2% at concentrations ranging from 2.5 to 2215 ng/mL. The degree of ODV binding to human plasma is 30%±12% at concentrations ranging from 100 to 500 ng/mL. Protein-binding-induced drug interactions with venlafaxine are not expected.

Steady-state concentrations of both venlafaxine and ODV in plasma were attained within 3 days of multiple-dose therapy. Venlafaxine and ODV exhibited linear kinetics over the dose range of 75 to 450 mg total dose per day (administered on a q8h schedule). Plasma clearance, elimination half-life and steady-state volume of distribution were unaltered for both venlafaxine and ODV after multiple-dosing. Mean±SD steady-state plasma clearance of venlafaxine and ODV is 1.3±0.6 and 0.4±0.2 L/h/kg, respectively; elimination half-life is 5±2 and 11±2 hours, respectively; and steady-state volume of distribution is 7.5±3.7 L/kg and 5.7±1.8 L/kg, respectively. When equal daily doses of venlafaxine were administered as either b.i.d. or t.i.d. regimens, the drug exposure (AUC) and fluctuation in plasma levels of venlafaxine and ODV were comparable following both regimens.

Age and Gender
A pharmacokinetic analysis of 404 venlafaxine-treated patients from two studies involving both b.i.d. and t.i.d. regimens showed that dose-normalized trough plasma levels of either venlafaxine or ODV were unaltered due to age or gender differences. Dosage adjustment based upon the age or gender of a patient is generally not necessary (see "**Dosage and Administration**").

Liver Disease
In 9 patients with hepatic cirrhosis, the pharmacokinetic disposition of both venlafaxine and ODV was significantly altered after oral administration of venlafaxine. Venlafaxine elimination half-life was prolonged by about 30%, and clearance decreased by about 50% in cirrhotic patients compared to normal subjects. ODV elimination half-life was prolonged by about 60% and clearance decreased by about 30% in cirrhotic patients compared to normal subjects. A large degree of intersubject variability was noted. Three patients with more severe cirrhosis had a more substantial decrease in venlafaxine clearance (about 90%) compared to normal subjects.
Dosage adjustment is necessary in these patients (see "**Dosage and Administration**").

Renal Disease
In a renal impairment study, venlafaxine elimination half-life after oral administration was prolonged by about 50% and clearance was reduced by about 24% in renally impaired patients (GFR =10-70 mL/min), compared to normal subjects. In dialysis patients, venlafaxine elimination half-life

Continued on next page

Wyeth-Ayerst Laboratories—Cont.

was prolonged by about 180% and clearance was reduced by about 57% compared to normal subjects. Similarly, ODV elimination half-life was prolonged by about 40% although clearance was unchanged in patients with renal impairment (GFR = 10-70 mL/min) compared to normal subjects. In dialysis patients, ODV elimination half-life was prolonged by about 142% and clearance was reduced by about 56%, compared to normal subjects. A large degree of intersubject variability was noted.

Dosage adjustment is necessary in these patients (see "**Dosage and Administration**").

CLINICAL TRIALS

The efficacy of Effexor (venlafaxine hydrochloride) as a treatment for depression was established in 5 placebo-controlled, short-term trials. Four of these were 6-week trials in outpatients meeting DSM-III or DSM-III-R criteria for major depression: two involving dose titration with Effexor in a range of 75 to 225 mg/day (t.i.d. schedule), the third involving fixed Effexor doses of 75, 225, and 375 mg/day (t.i.d. schedule), and the fourth involving doses of 25, 75, and 200 mg/day (b.i.d. schedule). The fifth was a 4-week study of inpatients meeting DSM-III-R criteria for major depression with melancholia whose Effexor doses were titrated in a range of 150 to 375 mg/day (t.i.d schedule). In these 5 studies, Effexor was shown to be significantly superior to placebo on at least 2 of the following 3 measures: Hamilton Depression Rating Scale (total score), Hamilton depressed mood item, and Clinical Global Impression—Severity of Illness rating. Doses from 75 to 225 mg/day were superior to placebo in outpatient studies and a mean dose of about 350 mg/day was effective in inpatients. Data from the 2 fixed-dose outpatient studies were suggestive of a dose-response relationship in the range of 75 to 225 mg/day. There was no suggestion of increased response with doses greater than 225 mg/day.

While there were no efficacy studies focusing specifically on an elderly population, elderly patients were included among the patients studied. Overall, approximately $^2/_3$ of all patients in these trials were women. Exploratory analyses for age and gender effects on outcome did not suggest any differential responsiveness on the basis of age or sex.

INDICATIONS AND USAGE

Effexor (venlafaxine hydrochloride) is indicated for the treatment of depression.

The efficacy of Effexor in the treatment of depression was established in 6-week controlled trials of outpatients whose diagnoses corresponded most closely to the DSM-III or DSM-III-R category of major depressive disorder and in a 4-week controlled trial of inpatients meeting diagnostic criteria for major depressive disorder with melancholia (see "**Clinical Pharmacology**").

A major depressive episode implies a prominent and relatively persistent depressed or dysphoric mood that usually interferes with daily functioning (nearly every day for at least 2 weeks); it should include at least 4 of the following 8 symptoms: change in appetite, change in sleep, psychomotor agitation or retardation, loss of interest in usual activities or decrease in sexual drive, increased fatigue, feelings of guilt or worthlessness, slowed thinking or impaired concentration, and a suicide attempt or suicidal ideation.

The effectiveness of Effexor in long-term use, that is, for more than 4 to 6 weeks, has not been systematically evaluated in controlled trials. Therefore, the physician who elects to use Effexor for extended periods should periodically re-evaluate the long-term usefulness of the drug for the individual patient.

CONTRAINDICATIONS

Effexor (venlafaxine hydrochloride) is contraindicated in patients known to be hypersensitive to it.

Concomitant use in patients taking monoamine oxidase inhibitors (MAOIs) is contraindicated (see "**Warnings**").

WARNINGS

POTENTIAL FOR INTERACTION WITH MONOAMINE OXIDASE INHIBITORS

Adverse reactions, some of which were serious, have been reported in patients who have recently been discontinued from a monoamine oxidase inhibitor (MAOI) and started on Effexor, or who have recently had Effexor therapy discontinued prior to initiation of an MAOI. These reactions have included tremor, myoclonus, diaphoresis, nausea, vomiting, flushing, dizziness, hyperthermia with features resembling neuroleptic malignant syndrome, seizures, and death. In patients receiving antidepressants with pharmacological properties similar to venlafaxine in combination with a monoamine oxidase inhibitor, there have also been reports of serious, sometimes fatal, reactions. For a selective serotonin reuptake inhibitor, these reactions have included hyperthermia, rigidity, myoclonus, autonomic instability with possible rapid fluctuations of vital signs, and mental status changes that include extreme agitation progressing to delirium and coma. Some cases presented with features resembling neuroleptic malignant syndrome. Severe hyperthermia and seizures, sometimes fatal, have been reported in association with the combined use of tricyclic antidepressants and MAOIs. These reactions have also been reported in patients who have recently discontinued these drugs and have been started on an MAOI. Therefore, it is recommended that Effexor not be used in combination with an MAOI, or within at least 14 days of discontinuing treatment with an MAOI. Based on the half-life of Effexor, at least 7 days should be allowed after stopping Effexor before starting an MAOI.

SUSTAINED HYPERTENSION

Venlafaxine treatment is associated with sustained increases in blood pressure. (1) In a premarketing study comparing three fixed doses of venlafaxine (75, 225, and 375 mg/day) and placebo, a mean increase in supine diastolic blood pressure (SDBP) of 7.2 mm Hg was seen in the 375 mg/day group at week 6 compared to essentially no changes in the 75 and 225 mg/day groups and a mean decrease in SDBP of 2.2 mm Hg in the placebo group. (2) An analysis for patients meeting criteria for sustained hypertension (defined as treatment-emergent SDBP ≥ 90 mm Hg *and* ≥ 10 mm Hg above baseline for 3 consecutive visits) revealed a dose-dependent increase in the incidence of sustained hypertension for venlafaxine:

Probability of Sustained Elevation in SDBP (Pool of Premarketing Venlafaxine Studies)

Treatment Group	Incidence of Sustained Elevation in SDBP
Venlafaxine	
< 100 mg/day	3%
101–200 mg/day	5%
201–300 mg/day	7%
> 300 mg/day	13%
Placebo	2%

An analysis of the patients with sustained hypertension and the 19 venlafaxine patients who were discontinued from treatment because of hypertension (< 1% of total venlafaxine-treated group) revealed that most of the blood pressure increases were in a modest range (10–15 mm Hg, SDBP). Nevertheless, sustained increases of this magnitude could have adverse consequences. Therefore, it is recommended that patients receiving venlafaxine have regular monitoring of blood pressure. For patients who experience a sustained increase in blood pressure while receiving venlafaxine, either dose reduction or discontinuation should be considered.

PRECAUTIONS

GENERAL

Anxiety and Insomnia

Treatment-emergent anxiety, nervousness, and insomnia were more commonly reported for venlafaxine-treated patients compared to placebo-treated patients in a pooled analysis of short-term, double-blind, placebo-controlled depression studies:

Symptom	Venlafaxine n = 1033	Placebo n = 609
Anxiety	6%	3%
Nervousness	13%	6%
Insomnia	18%	10%

Anxiety, nervousness, and insomnia led to drug discontinuation in 2%, 2%, and 3%, respectively, of the patients treated with venlafaxine in the phase 2–3 depression studies.

Changes in Appetite and Weight

Treatment-emergent anorexia was more commonly reported for venlafaxine-treated (11%) than placebo-treated patients (2%) in the pool of short-term, double-blind, placebo-controlled depression studies. A dose-dependent weight loss was often noted in patients treated with venlafaxine for several weeks. Significant weight loss, especially in underweight depressed patients, may be an undesirable result of venlafaxine treatment. A loss of 5% or more of body weight occurred in 6% of patients treated with venlafaxine compared with 1% of patients treated with placebo and 3% of patients treated with another antidepressant. However, discontinuation for weight loss associated with venlafaxine was uncommon (0.1% of venlafaxine-treated patients in the phase 2–3 depression trials).

Activation of Mania/Hypomania

During phase 2–3 trials, hypomania or mania occurred in 0.5% of patients treated with venlafaxine. Activation of mania/hypomania has also been reported in a small proportion of patients with major affective disorder who were treated with other marketed antidepressants. As with all antidepressants, Effexor (venlafaxine hydrochloride) should be used cautiously in patients with a history of mania.

Seizures

During premarketing testing, seizures were reported in 0.26% (8/3082) of venlafaxine-treated patients. Most seizures (5 of 8) occurred in patients receiving doses of 150 mg/day or less. Effexor should be used cautiously in patients with a history of seizures. It should be discontinued in any patient who develops seizures.

Suicide

The possibility of a suicide attempt is inherent in depression and may persist until significant remission occurs. Close supervision of high-risk patients should accompany initial drug therapy. Prescriptions for Effexor should be written for the smallest quantity of tablets consistent with good patient management in order to reduce the risk of overdose.

Use in Patients with Concomitant Illness

Clinical experience with Effexor in patients with concomitant systemic illness is limited. Caution is advised in administering Effexor to patients with diseases or conditions that could affect hemodynamic responses or metabolism.

Effexor has not been evaluated or used to any appreciable extent in patients with a recent history of myocardial infarction or unstable heart disease. Patients with these diagnoses were sytematically excluded from many clinical studies during the product's premarketing testing. Evaluation of the electrocardiograms for 769 patients who received Effexor in 4- to 6-week double-blind placebo-controlled trials, however, showed that the incidence of trial-emergent conduction abnormalities did not differ from that with placebo. The mean heart rate in Effexor-treated patients was increased relative to baseline by about 4 beats per minute.

In patients with renal impairment (GFR = 10-70 mL/min) or cirrhosis of the liver, the clearances of venlafaxine and its active metabolite were decreased, thus prolonging the elimination half-lives of these substances. A lower dose may be necessary (see "**Dosage and Administration**"). Effexor (venlafaxine hydrochloride), like all antidepressants, should be used with caution in such patients.

INFORMATION FOR PATIENTS

Physicians are advised to discuss the following issues with patients for whom they prescribe Effexor:

Interference with Cognitive and Motor Performance

Clinical studies were performed to examine the effects of venlafaxine on behavioral performance of healthy individuals. The results revealed no clinically significant impairment of psychomotor, cognitive, or complex behavior performance. However, since any psychoactive drug may impair judgment, thinking, or motor skills, patients should be cautioned about operating hazardous machinery, including automobiles, until they are reasonably certain that Effexor therapy does not adversely affect their ability to engage in such activities.

Pregnancy

Patients should be advised to notify their physician if they become pregnant or intend to become pregnant during therapy.

Nursing

Patients should be advised to notify their physician if they are breast-feeding an infant.

Concomitant Medication

Patients should be advised to inform their physicians if they are taking, or plan to take, any prescription or over-the-counter drugs, since there is a potential for interactions.

Alcohol

Although Effexor has not been shown to increase the impairment of mental and motor skills caused by alcohol, patients should be advised to avoid alcohol while taking Effexor.

Allergic Reactions

Patients should be advised to notify their physician if they develop a rash, hives, or a related allergic phenomenon.

LABORATORY TESTS

There are no specific laboratory tests recommended.

DRUG INTERACTIONS

As with all drugs, the potential for interaction by a variety of mechanisms is a possibility.

Drugs Highly Bound to Plasma Protein

Venlafaxine is not highly bound to plasma proteins; therefore, administration of Effexor to a patient taking another drug that is highly protein bound should not cause increased free concentrations of the other drug.

Lithium

The steady-state pharmacokinetics of venlafaxine administered as 50 mg every 8 hours were not affected when a single 600 mg oral dose of lithium was administered to 12 healthy male subjects. O-desmethylvenlafaxine (ODV) was also unaffected. Venlafaxine had no effect on the pharmacokinetics of lithium.

Diazepam

Under steady-state conditions for venlafaxine administered as 50 mg every 8 hours, a single 10 mg dose of diazepam did not appear to affect the pharmacokinetics of either venlafaxine or ODV in 18 healthy male subjects. Venlafaxine also did

not have any effect on the pharmacokinetics of diazepam or its active metabolite, desmethyldiazepam.

Administration of Effexor did not affect the psychomotor and psychometric effects induced by diazepam.

Cimetidine

Concomitant administration of cimetidine and Effexor in a steady-state study for both drugs resulted in inhibition of first-pass metabolism of venlafaxine in 18 healthy subjects. The oral clearance of venlafaxine was reduced by about 43%, and the exposure (AUC) and maximum concentration (C_{max}) of the drug were increased by about 60%. However, co-administration of cimetidine had no apparent effect on the pharmacokinetics of ODV, which is present in much greater quantity in the circulation than is venlafaxine. Consequently, the overall pharmacological activity of venlafaxine plus ODV is expected to increase only slightly, and no dosage adjustment should be necessary for most normal adults. However, for patients with pre-existing hypertension, and for elderly patients or patients with hepatic dysfunction, the interaction associated with the concomitant use of Effexor (venlafaxine hydrochloride) and cimetidine is not known and potentially could be more pronounced. Therefore, caution is advised with such patients.

Alcohol

A single dose of ethanol (0.5 g/kg) had no effect on the pharmacokinetics of venlafaxine or ODV when venlafaxine was administered as a 50 mg dose every 8 hours in 15 healthy male subjects. The administration of Effexor in a stable regimen did not exaggerate the psychomotor and psychometric effects induced by ethanol in these same subjects when they were not receiving Effexor.

Drugs that Inhibit Cytochrome $P_{450}IID_6$ Metabolism

In vitro studies indicate that venlafaxine is metabolized to its active metabolite, ODV, by cytochrome $P_{450}IID_6$, the isoenzyme that is responsible for the genetic polymorphism seen in the metabolism of many antidepressants. Therefore, the potential exists for a drug interaction between Effexor and drugs that inhibit cytochrome $P_{450}IID_6$ metabolism. Drug interactions that reduce the metabolism of venlafaxine to ODV could potentially increase the plasma concentrations of venlafaxine and lower the concentrations of the active metabolite.

Drugs Metabolized by Cytochrome $P_{450}IID_6$

In vitro studies indicate that venlafaxine is a relatively weak inhibitor of cytochrome $P_{450}IID_6$. However, the clinical significance of this finding is unknown.

Monoamine Oxidase Inhibitors

See "**Contraindications**" and "**Warnings**."

CNS-Active Drugs

The risk of using venlafaxine in combination with other CNS-active drugs has not been systematically evaluated (except in the case of lithium and diazepam, as noted above). Consequently, caution is advised if the concomitant administration of venlafaxine and such drugs is required.

Electroconvulsive Therapy

There are no clinical data establishing the benefit of electroconvulsive therapy combined with Effexor treatment.

CARCINOGENESIS, MUTAGENESIS, IMPAIRMENT OF FERTILITY

Carcinogenesis

Venlafaxine was given by oral gavage to mice for 18 months at doses up to 120 mg/kg per day, which was 16 times, on a mg/kg basis, and 1.7 times on a mg/m² basis, the maximum recommended human dose. Venlafaxine was also given to rats by oral gavage for 24 months at doses up to 120 mg/kg per day. In rats receiving the 120 mg/kg dose, plasma levels of venlafaxine were 1 times (male rats) and 6 times (female rats) the plasma levels of patients receiving the maximum recommended human dose. Plasma levels of the O-desmethyl metabolite were lower in rats than in patients receiving the maximum recommended dose. Tumors were not increased by venlafaxine treatment in mice or rats.

Mutagenicity

Venlafaxine and the major human metabolite, O-desmethylvenlafaxine (ODV), were not mutagenic in the Ames reverse mutation assay in Salmonella bacteria or the CHO/HGPRT mammalian cell forward gene mutation assay. Venlafaxine was also not mutagenic in the *in vitro* BALB/c-3T3 mouse cell transformation assay, the sister chromatid exchange assay in cultured CHO cells, or the *in vivo* chromosomal aberration assay in rat bone marrow. ODV was not mutagenic in the *in vitro* CHO cell chromosomal aberration assay. There was a clastogenic response in the *in vivo* chromosomal aberration assay in rat bone marrow in male rats receiving 200 times, on a mg/kg basis, or 50 times, on a mg/m² basis, the maximum human daily dose. The no effect dose was 67 times (mg/kg) or 17 times (mg/m²) the human dose.

Impairment of Fertility

Reproduction and fertility studies in rats showed no effects on male or female fertility at oral doses of up to 8 times the maximum recommended human daily dose on a mg/kg basis, or up to 2 times on a mg/m² basis.

PREGNANCY

Teratogenic Effects—Pregnancy Category C

Venlafaxine did not cause malformations in offspring of rats or rabbits given doses up to 11 times (rat) or 12 times (rabbit) the maximum recommended human daily dose on a mg/kg basis, or 2.5 times (rat) and 4 times (rabbit) the human daily dose on a mg/m² basis. However, in rats, there was a decrease in pup weight, an increase in stillborn pups, and an increase in pup deaths during the first 5 days of lactation, when dosing began during pregnancy and continued until weaning. The cause of these deaths is not known. These effects occurred at 10 times (mg/kg) or 2.5 times (mg/m²) the maximum human daily dose. The no effect dose for rat pup mortality was 1.4 times the human dose on a mg/kg basis or 0.25 times the human dose on a mg/m² basis. There are no adequate and well-controlled studies in pregnant women. Because animal reproduction studies are not always predictive of human response, this drug should be used during pregnancy only if clearly needed.

LABOR AND DELIVERY

The effect of Effexor (venlafaxine hydrochloride) on labor and delivery in humans is unknown.

NURSING MOTHERS

It is not known whether venlafaxine hydrochloride or its metabolites are excreted in human milk. Because many drugs are excreted in human milk, caution should be exercised when Effexor is administered to a nursing woman.

USAGE IN CHILDREN

Safety and effectiveness in individuals below 18 years of age have not been established.

GERIATRIC USE

Of the 2,897 patients in phase 2-3 depression studies with Effexor, 12% (357) were 65 years of age or over. No overall differences in effectiveness or safety were observed between these patients and younger patients, and other reported clinical experience has not identified differences in response between the elderly and younger patients. However, greater sensitivity of some older individuals cannot be ruled out.

ADVERSE REACTIONS

ASSOCIATED WITH DISCONTINUATION OF TREATMENT

Nineteen percent (537/2897) of venlafaxine patients in phase 2-3 depression studies discontinued treatment due to an adverse event. The more common events (≥1%) associated with discontinuation and considered to be drug-related (i.e., those events associated with dropout at a rate approximately twice or greater for venlafaxine compared to placebo) included:

CNS	Venlafaxine	Placebo
Somnolence	3%	1%
Insomnia	3%	1%
Dizziness	3%	—
Nervousness	2%	—
Dry mouth	2%	—
Anxiety	2%	1%
Gastrointestinal		
Nausea	6%	1%
Urogenital		
Abnormal ejaculation*	3%	—
Other		
Headache	3%	1%
Asthenia	2%	—
Sweating	2%	—

* Percentages based on the number of males.
— Less than 1%

INCIDENCE IN CONTROLLED TRIALS

Commonly Observed Adverse Events in Controlled Clinical Trials

The most commonly observed adverse events associated with the use of Effexor (incidence of 5% or greater) and not seen at an equivalent incidence among placebo-treated patients (i.e., incidence for Effexor at least twice that for placebo), derived from the 1% incidence table below, were asthenia, sweating, nausea, constipation, anorexia, vomiting, somnolence, dry mouth, dizziness, nervousness, anxiety, tremor, and blurred vision as well as abnormal ejaculation/orgasm and impotence in men.

Adverse Events Occurring at an Incidence of 1% or More Among Effexor-Treated Patients

The table that follows enumerates adverse events that occurred at an incidence of 1% or more, and were more frequent than in the placebo group, among Effexor-treated patients who participated in short-term (4- to 8-week) placebo-controlled trials in which patients were administered doses in a range of 75 to 375 mg/day. This table shows the percentage of patients in each group who had at least one episode of an event at some time during their treatment. Reported adverse events were classified using a standard COSTART-based Dictionary terminology.

The prescriber should be aware that these figures cannot be used to predict the incidence of side effects in the course of usual medical practice where patient characteristics and other factors differ from those which prevailed in the clinical trials. Similarly, the cited frequencies cannot be compared with figures obtained from other clinical investigations involving different treatments, uses and investigators. The cited figures, however, do provide the prescribing physician with some basis for estimating the relative contribution of drug and nondrug factors to the side effect incidence rate in the population studied.

[See Table 1 at bottom of next page.]

Dose Dependency of Adverse Events

A comparison of adverse event rates in a fixed-dose study comparing Effexor (venlafaxine hydrochloride) 75, 225, and 375 mg/day with placebo revealed a dose dependency for some of the more common adverse events associated with Effexor use, as shown in the table that follows. The rule for including events was to enumerate those that occurred at an incidence of 5% or more for at least one of the venlafaxine groups and for which the incidence was at least twice the placebo incidence for at least one Effexor group. Tests for potential dose relationships for these events (Cochran-Armitage Test, with a criterion of exact 2-sided p-value ≤ 0.05) suggested a dose-dependency for several adverse events in this list, including chills, hypertension, anorexia, nausea, agitation, dizziness, somnolence, tremor, yawning, sweating, and abnormal ejaculation.

[See Table 2 at top of page 2829.]

Adaptation to Certain Adverse Events

Over a 6-week period, there was evidence of adaptation to some adverse events with continued therapy (e.g., dizziness and nausea), but less to other effects (e.g., abnormal ejaculation and dry mouth).

Vital Sign Changes

Effexor (venlafaxine hydrochloride) treatment (averaged over all dose groups) in clinical trials was associated with a mean increase in pulse rate of approximately 3 beats per minute, compared to no change for placebo. It was associated with mean increases in diastolic blood pressure ranging from 0.7 to 2.5 mm Hg averaged over all dose groups, compared to mean decreases ranging from 0.9 to 3.8 mm Hg for placebo. However, there is a dose dependency for blood pressure increase (see "**Warnings**").

Laboratory Changes

Of the serum chemistry and hematology parameters monitored during clinical trials with Effexor, a statistically significant difference with placebo was seen only for serum cholesterol, i.e., patients treated with Effexor had mean increases from baseline of 3 mg/dL, a change of unknown clinical significance.

ECG Changes

In an analysis of ECGs obtained in 769 patients treated with Effexor and 450 patients treated with placebo in controlled clinical trials, the only statistically significant difference observed was for heart rate, i.e., a mean increase from baseline of 4 beats per minute for Effexor.

OTHER EVENTS OBSERVED DURING THE PREMARKETING EVALUATION OF VENLAFAXINE

During its premarketing assessment, multiple doses of Effexor were administered to 2181 patients in phase 2 and 3 studies. The conditions and duration of exposure to Effexor varied greatly, and included (in overlapping categories) open and double-blind studies, uncontrolled and controlled studies, inpatient and outpatient studies, fixed-dose and titration studies. Untoward events associated with this exposure were recorded by clinical investigators using terminology of their own choosing. Consequently, it is not possible to provide a meaningful estimate of the proportion of individuals experiencing adverse events without first grouping similar types of untoward events into a smaller number of standardized event categories.

In the tabulations that follow, reported adverse events were classified using a standard COSTART-based Dictionary terminology. The frequencies presented, therefore, represent the proportion of the 2181 patients exposed to multiple doses of Effexor who experienced an event of the type cited on at least one occasion while receiving Effexor. All reported events are included except those already listed in Table 1 and those events for which a drug cause was remote. If the COSTART term for an event was so general as to be uninformative, it was replaced with a more informative term. It is important to emphasize that, although the events reported occurred during treatment with Effexor, they were not necessarily caused by it.

Events are further categorized by body system and listed in order of decreasing frequency according to the following definitions: frequent adverse events are those occurring on one or more occasions in at least 1/100 patients (only those not already listed in the tabulated results from placebo-controlled trials appear in this listing); infrequent adverse events are those occurring in 1/100 to 1/1000 patients; rare events are those occurring in fewer than 1/1000 patients.

Body as a whole—Frequent: accidental injury, malaise, neck pain; Infrequent: abdomen enlarged, allergic reaction, cyst, face edema, generalized edema, hangover effect, hernia, intentional injury, moniliasis, neck rigidity, overdose, chest

Continued on next page

Wyeth-Ayerst Laboratories—Cont.

pain substernal, pelvic pain, photosensitivity reaction, suicide attempt; Rare: appendicitis, body odor, carcinoma, cellulitis, halitosis, ulcer, withdrawal syndrome.

Cardiovascular system—Frequent: migraine; Infrequent: angina pectoris, extrasystoles, hypotension, peripheral vascular disorder (mainly cold feet and/or cold hands), syncope, thrombophlebitis; Rare: arrhythmia, first-degree atrioventricular block, bradycardia, bundle branch block, mitral valve disorder, mucocutaneous hemorrhage, sinus bradycardia, varicose vein.

Digestive system—Frequent: dysphagia, eructation; Infrequent: colitis, tongue edema, esophagitis, gastritis, gastroenteritis, gingivitis, glossitis, rectal hemorrhage, hemorrhoids, melena, stomatitis, stomach ulcer, mouth ulceration; Rare: cheilitis, cholecystitis, cholelithiasis, hematemesis, gum hemorrhage, hepatitis, ileitis, jaundice, oral moniliasis, intestinal obstruction, proctitis, increased salivation, soft stools, tongue discoloration, esophageal ulcer, peptic ulcer syndrome.

Endocrine system—Rare: goiter, hyperthyroidism, hypothyroidism.

Hemic and lymphatic system—Frequent: ecchymosis; Infrequent: anemia, leukocytosis, leukopenia, lymphadenopathy, lymphocytosis, thrombocythemia, thrombocytopenia, WBC abnormal; Rare: basophilia, cyanosis, eosinophilia, erythrocytes abnormal.

Metabolic and nutritional—Frequent: peripheral edema, weight gain; Infrequent: alkaline phosphatase increased, creatinine increased, diabetes mellitus, edema, glycosuria, hypercholesteremia, hyperglycemia, hyperlipemia, hyperuricemia, hypoglycemia, hypokalemia, SGOT increased, thirst; Rare: alcohol intolerance, bilirubinemia, BUN increased, gout, hemochromatosis, hyperkalemia, hyperphosphatemia, hypoglycemic reaction, hyponatremia, hypophosphatemia, hypoproteinemia, SGPT increased, uremia.

Musculoskeletal system—Infrequent: arthritis, arthrosis, bone pain, bone spurs, bursitis, joint disorder, myasthenia, tenosynovitis; Rare: osteoporosis.

Nervous system—Frequent: emotional lability, trismus, vertigo; Infrequent: apathy, ataxia, circumoral paresthesia, CNS stimulation, euphoria, hallucinations, hostility, hyperesthesia, hyperkinesia, hypertonia, hypotonia, incoordination, libido increased, manic reaction, myoclonus, neuralgia, neuropathy, paranoid reaction, psychosis, psychotic depression, sleep disturbance, abnormal speech, stupor, torticollis;

Rare: akathisia, akinesia, alcohol abuse, aphasia, bradykinesia, cerebrovascular accident, loss of consciousness, delusions, dementia, dystonia, hypokinesia, neuritis, nystagmus, reflexes increased, seizures.

Respiratory system—Frequent: bronchitis, dyspnea; Infrequent: asthma, chest congestion, epistaxis, hyperventilation, laryngismus, laryngitis, pneumonia, voice alteration; Rare: atelectasis, hemoptysis, hypoxia, pleurisy, pulmonary embolus, sleep apnea, sputum increased.

Skin and appendages—Infrequent: acne, alopecia, brittle nails, contact dermatitis, dry skin, herpes simplex, herpes zoster, maculopapular rash, urticaria; Rare: skin atrophy, exfoliative dermatitis, fungal dermatitis, lichenoid dermatitis, hair discoloration, eczema, furunculosis, hirsutism, skin hypertrophy, leukoderma, psoriasis, pustular rash, vesiculobullous rash.

Special senses—Frequent: abnormal vision, ear pain; Infrequent: cataract, conjunctivitis, corneal lesion, diplopia, dry eyes, exophthalmos, eye pain, otitis media, parosmia, photophobia, subconjunctival hemorrhage, taste loss, visual field defect; Rare: blepharitis, chromatopsia, conjunctival edema, deafness, glaucoma, hyperacusis, keratitis, labyrinthitis, miosis, papilledema, decreased pupillary reflex, scleritis.

Urogenital system—Frequent: anorgasmia, dysuria, hematuria, metrorrhagia*, urination impaired, vaginitis*; Infrequent: albuminuria, amenorrhea*, kidney calculus, cystitis, leukorrhea, menorrhagia*, nocturia, bladder pain, breast pain, kidney pain, polyuria, prostatitis*, pyelonephritis, pyuria, urinary incontinence, urinary urgency, uterine fibroids enlarged*, uterine hemorrhage*, vaginal hemorrhage*, vaginal moniliasis*, Rare: abortion*, breast engorgement, breast enlargement, calcium crystalluria, female lactation*, hypomenorrhea*, menopause*, prolonged erection*, uterine spasm*.

* Based on the number of male or female patients as appropriate.

DRUG ABUSE AND DEPENDENCE
CONTROLLED SUBSTANCE CLASS
Effexor (venlafaxine hydrochloride) is not a controlled substance.

PHYSICAL AND PSYCHOLOGICAL DEPENDENCE
In vitro studies revealed that venlafaxine has virtually no affinity for opiate, benzodiazepine, phencyclidine (PCP), or N-methyl-D-aspartic acid (NMDA) receptors.

Venlafaxine was not found to have any significant CNS stimulant activity in rodents. In primate drug discrimination studies, venlafaxine showed no significant stimulant or depressant abuse liability.

While the discontinuation effects of Effexor have not been systematically evaluated in controlled clinical trials, a retrospective survey of new events occurring during taper or following discontinuation revealed the following six events that occurred at an incidence of at least 5% and for which the incidence for Effexor was at least twice the placebo incidence: asthenia, dizziness, headache, insomnia, nausea, and nervousness. Therefore, it is recommended that the dosage be tapered gradually and the patient monitored (see "Dosage and Administration").

While Effexor has not been systematically studied in clinical trials for its potential for abuse, there was no indication of drug-seeking behavior in the clinical trials. However, it is not possible to predict on the basis of premarketing experience the extent to which a CNS active drug will be misused, diverted, and/or abused once marketed. Consequently, physicians should carefully evaluate patients for history of drug abuse and follow such patients closely, observing them for signs of misuse or abuse of Effexor (e.g., development of tolerance, incrementation of dose, drug-seeking behavior).

OVERDOSAGE
HUMAN EXPERIENCE
There were 14 reports of acute overdose with Effexor (venlafaxine hydrochloride), either alone or in combination with other drugs and/or alcohol, among the patients included in the premarketing evaluation. The majority of the reports involved ingestions in which the total dose of Effexor taken was estimated to be no more than several-fold higher than the usual therapeutic dose. The 3 patients who took the highest doses were estimated to have ingested approximately 6.75 g, 2.75 g, and 2.5 g. The resultant peak plasma levels of venlafaxine for the latter 2 patients were 6.24 and 2.35 μg/mL, respectively, and the peak plasma levels of O-desmethylvenlafaxine were 3.37 and 1.30 μg/mL, respectively. Plasma venlafaxine levels were not obtained for the patient who ingested 6.75 g of venlafaxine. All 14 patients recovered without sequelae. Most patients reported no symptoms. Among the remaining patients, somnolence was the most commonly reported symptom. The patient who ingested 2.75 g of venlafaxine was observed to have 2 generalized convulsions and a prolongation of QTc to 500 msec, compared with 405 msec at baseline. Mild sinus tachycardia was reported in 2 of the other patients.

In postmarketing experience, venlafaxine, taken alone, has not been clearly associated with lethal overdose. However,

TABLE 1
Treatment-Emergent Adverse Experience Incidence in 4- to 8-Week Placebo-Controlled Clinical Trials[1]

Body System	Preferred Term	Effexor (n = 1033)	Placebo (n = 609)
Body as a Whole	Headache	25%	24%
	Asthenia	12%	6%
	Infection	6%	5%
	Chills	3%	—
	Chest pain	2%	1%
	Trauma	2%	1%
Cardiovascular	Vasodilatation	4%	3%
	Increased blood pressure/hypertension	2%	—
	Tachycardia	2%	—
	Postural hypotension	1%	—
Dermatological	Sweating	12%	3%
	Rash	3%	2%
	Pruritus	1%	—
Gastrointestinal	Nausea	37%	11%
	Constipation	15%	7%
	Anorexia	11%	2%
	Diarrhea	8%	7%
	Vomiting	6%	2%
	Dyspepsia	5%	4%
	Flatulence	3%	2%
Metabolic	Weight loss	1%	—
Nervous System	Somnolence	23%	9%
	Dry mouth	22%	11%
	Dizziness	19%	7%
	Insomnia	18%	10%
	Nervousness	13%	6%
	Anxiety	6%	3%
	Tremor	5%	1%
	Abnormal dreams	4%	3%
	Hypertonia	3%	2%
	Paresthesia	3%	2%
	Libido decreased	2%	—
	Agitation	2%	—
	Confusion	2%	1%
	Thinking abnormal	2%	1%
	Depersonalization	1%	—
	Depression	1%	—
	Urinary retention	1%	—
	Twitching	1%	—
Respiration	Yawn	3%	—
Special Senses	Blurred vision	6%	2%
	Taste perversion	2%	—
	Tinnitus	2%	—
	Mydriasis	2%	—
Urogenital System	Abnormal ejaculation/orgasm	12%[2]	—[2]
	Impotence	6%[2]	—[2]
	Urinary frequency	3%	2%
	Urination impaired	2%	—
	Orgasm disturbance	2%[3]	—[3]
	Menstrual disorder	1%[3]	—[3]

[1] Events reported by at least 1% of patients treated with Effexor® (venlafaxine hydrochloride) are included, and are rounded to the nearest %. Events for which the Effexor incidence was equal to or less than placebo are not listed in the table, but included the following: abdominal pain, pain, back pain, flu syndrome, fever, palpitation, increased appetite, myalgia, arthralgia, amnesia, hypesthesia, rhinitis, pharyngitis, sinusitis, cough increased, urinary tract infection, and dysmenorrhea[3].
— Incidence less than 1%.
[2] Incidence based on number of male patients.
[3] Incidence based on number of female patients.

TABLE 2
Treatment-Emergent Adverse Experience Incidence in a
Dose Comparison Trial

Body System/ Preferred Term	Placebo (n=92)	Effexor (mg/day)		
		75 (n=89)	225 (n=89)	375 (n=88)
Body as a Whole				
Abdominal pain	3.3%	3.4%	2.2%	8.0%
Asthenia	3.3%	16.9%	14.6%	14.8%
Chills	1.1%	2.2%	5.6%	6.8%
Infection	2.2%	2.2%	5.6%	2.3%
Cardiovascular System				
Hypertension	1.1%	1.1%	2.2%	4.5%
Vasodilatation	0.0%	4.5%	5.6%	2.3%
Digestive System				
Anorexia	2.2%	14.6%	13.5%	17.0%
Dyspepsia	2.2%	6.7%	6.7%	4.5%
Nausea	14.1%	32.6%	38.2%	58.0%
Vomiting	1.1%	7.9%	3.4%	6.8%
Nervous System				
Agitation	0.0%	1.1%	2.2%	4.5%
Anxiety	4.3%	11.2%	4.5%	2.3%
Dizziness	4.3%	19.1%	22.5%	23.9%
Insomnia	9.8%	22.5%	20.2%	13.6%
Libido decreased	1.1%	2.2%	1.1%	5.7%
Nervousness	4.3%	21.3%	13.5%	12.5%
Somnolence	4.3%	16.9%	18.0%	26.1%
Tremor	0.0%	1.1%	2.2%	10.2%
Respiratory System				
Yawn	0.0%	4.5%	5.6%	8.0%
Skin and Appendages				
Sweating	5.4%	6.7%	12.4%	19.3%
Special Senses				
Abnormality of accommodation	0.0%	9.1%	7.9%	5.6%
Urogenital System				
Abnormal ejaculation/orgasm	0.0%	4.5%	2.2%	12.5%
Impotence	0.0%	5.8%	2.1%	3.6%
(Number of men)	(n=63)	(n=52)	(n=48)	(n=56)

fatal reactions have been reported in patients taking overdoses of venlafaxine in combination with alcohol and/or other drugs.

OVERDOSAGE MANAGEMENT
Treatment should consist of those general measures employed in the management of overdosage with any antidepressant. Ensure an adequate airway, oxygenation, and ventilation. Monitoring of cardiac rhythm and vital signs is recommended. General supportive and symptomatic measures are also recommended. Use of activated charcoal, induction of emesis, or gastric lavage should be considered. Due to the large volume of distribution of venlafaxine hydrochloride, forced diuresis, dialysis, hemoperfusion and exchange transfusion are unlikely to be of benefit. No specific antidotes for Effexor are known.
In managing overdosage, consider the possibility of multiple drug involvement. The physician should consider contacting a poison control center on the treatment of any overdose.

DOSAGE AND ADMINISTRATION
INITIAL TREATMENT
The recommended starting dose for Effexor is 75 mg/day, administered in two or three divided doses, taken with food. Depending on tolerability and the need for further clinical effect, the dose may be increased to 150 mg/day. If needed, the dose should be further increased up to 225 mg/day. When increasing the dose, increments of up to 75 mg/day should be made at intervals of no less than 4 days. In outpatient settings there was no evidence of usefulness of doses greater than 225 mg/day for moderately depressed patients, but more severely depressed inpatients responded to a mean dose of 350 mg/day. Certain patients, including more severely depressed patients, may therefore respond more to higher doses, up to a maximum of 375 mg/day, generally in three divided doses.
DOSAGE FOR PATIENTS WITH HEPATIC IMPAIRMENT
Given the decrease in clearance and increase in elimination half-life for both venlafaxine and ODV that is observed in patients with hepatic cirrhosis compared to normal subjects (see "**Clinical Pharmacology**"), it is recommended that the total daily dose be reduced by 50% in patients with moderate hepatic impairment. Since there was much individual variability in clearance between patients with cirrhosis, it may be necessary to reduce the dose even more than 50%, and individualization of dosing may be desirable in some patients.
DOSAGE FOR PATIENTS WITH RENAL IMPAIRMENT
Given the decrease in clearance for venlafaxine and the increase in elimination half-life for both venlafaxine and ODV

that is observed in patients with renal impairment (GFR = 10-70 mL/min) compared to normals (see "**Clinical Pharmacology**"), it is recommended that the total daily dose be reduced by 25% in patients with mild to moderate renal impairment. It is recommended that the total daily dose be reduced by 50% and the dose be withheld until the dialysis treatment is completed (4 hrs) in patients undergoing hemodialysis. Since there was much individual variability in clearance between patients with renal impairment, individualization of dosing may be desirable in some patients.
DOSAGE FOR ELDERLY PATIENTS
No dose adjustment is recommended for elderly patients on the basis of age. As with any antidepressant, however, caution should be exercised in treating the elderly. When individualizing the dosage, extra care should be taken when increasing the dose.
MAINTENANCE/CONTINUATION/EXTENDED TREATMENT
There is no body of evidence available to answer the question of how long a patient should continue to be treated with Effexor. It is generally agreed that acute episodes of major depression require several months or longer of sustained pharmacologic therapy. Whether the dose of antidepressant needed to induce remission is identical to the dose needed to maintain and/or sustain euthymia is unknown.
DISCONTINUING EFFEXOR (venlafaxine hydrochloride)
When discontinuing Effexor after more than 1 week of therapy, it is generally recommended that the dose be tapered to minimize the risk of discontinuation symptoms. Patients who have received Effexor for 6 weeks or more should have their dose tapered gradually over a 2-week period.
SWITCHING PATIENTS TO OR FROM A MONOAMINE OXIDASE INHIBITOR
At least 14 days should elapse between discontinuation of an MAOI and initiation of therapy with Effexor. In addition, at least 7 days should be allowed after stopping Effexor before starting an MAOI (see "**Contraindications**" and "**Warnings**").
HOW SUPPLIED
Effexor® (venlafaxine HCl tablets) is available in bottles of 100 tablets and in Redipak® cartons of 100 tablets (10 blister strips of 10) in the following dosage strengths (expressed in equivalent amounts of venlafaxine):
25 mg, NDC 0008-0701, peach, shield-shaped tablet with "25" and a "**W**" on one side and "701" on scored reverse side.
37.5 mg, NDC 0008-0781, peach, shield-shaped tablet with "37.5" and a "**W**" on one side and "781" on scored reverse side.

50 mg, NDC 0008-0703, peach, shield-shaped tablet with "50" and a "**W**" on one side and "703" on scored reverse side.
75 mg, NDC 0008-0704, peach, shield-shaped tablet with "75" and a "**W**" on one side and "704" on scored reverse side.
100 mg, NDC 0008-0705, peach, shield-shaped tablet with "100" and a "**W**" on one side and "705" on scored reverse side.
The appearance of these tablets is a trademark of Wyeth-Ayerst Laboratories.
Store at controlled room temperature, 20°C to 25°C (68°F to 77°F), in a dry place.
Dispense in a well-closed container as defined in the USP.
Shown in Product Identification Guide, page 339

EQUAGESIC®　　　　　　　　　　Ⓒ Ⓡ
[ek "wa-je 'zik]
(meprobamate with aspirin)

DESCRIPTION
Each tablet of Equagesic contains 200 mg meprobamate and 325 mg aspirin. The inactive ingredients present are cellulose, D&C Yellow 10, FD&C Red 3, FD&C Yellow 6, hydrogenated vegetable oil, magnesium stearate, polacrilin potassium, and starch.
HOW SUPPLIED
Equagesic® (meprobamate with aspirin) Tablets, 200 mg meprobamate and 325 mg aspirin, are available as follows: NDC 0008-0091, pink and yellow, double-layer, round, scored tablet marked "WYETH" and "91", in bottles of 100 tablets.
Store at room temperature, approx. 25°C (77°F).
Keep tightly closed.
Protect from light.
Dispense in light-resistant, tight container.
The appearance of EQUAGESIC tablets is a registered trademark of Wyeth-Ayerst Laboratories.
For full prescribing information write to Professional Service, Wyeth-Ayerst Laboratories, P.O. Box 8299, Philadelphia, PA 19101, or contact your local Wyeth-Ayerst representative.

EQUANIL®　　　　　　　　　　Ⓒ Ⓡ
[ek 'wah-nil]
(meprobamate)
Tablets

DESCRIPTION
Meprobamate is a white powder with a characteristic odor and a bitter taste. It is slightly soluble in water, freely soluble in acetone and alcohol, and sparingly soluble in ether. Equanil tablets contain 200 mg or 400 mg meprobamate. The inactive ingredients present are lactose, methylcellulose, polacrilin potassium, and stearic acid.
HOW SUPPLIED
Equanil® (meprobamate) Tablets are available in the following dosage strengths:
200 mg, NDC 0008-0002, white, five-sided tablet marked "WYETH" and "2", in bottles of 100 tablets.
400 mg, NDC 0008-0001, white, round, scored tablet marked "WYETH" and "1", in bottles of 100 and 500 tablets.
Keep tightly closed.
Dispense in tight container.
Store at room temperature, approximately 25°C (77°F).
For prescribing information write to Professional Service, Wyeth-Ayerst Laboratories, P.O. Box 8299, Philadelphia, PA 19101, or contact your local Wyeth-Ayerst representative.

FACTREL®　　　　　　　　　　Ⓡ
[făc-trĕl ']
(gonadorelin hydrochloride)
Synthetic Luteinizing Hormone Releasing Hormone (LH-RH)
DIAGNOSTIC USE ONLY

HOW SUPPLIED
LYOPHILIZED POWDER
in single-dose Secule® vials containing 100 mcg (NDC 0046-0507-05) and 500 mcg (NDC 0046-0509-05) gonadorelin as the hydrochloride with 100 mg lactose, USP. Each Secule® vial is accompanied by one ampul containing 2 mL sterile diluent of 2% benzyl alcohol in sterile water.
Secule® —Registered trademark to designate a vial containing an injectable preparation in dry form.
For full prescribing information turn to the Diagnostic Product Information section of this edition of the PDR.

Continued on next page

Wyeth-Ayerst Laboratories—Cont.

FLUOTHANE® ℞
[*flū'o-thān*]
(halothane, USP)
Inhalation

Caution: Federal law prohibits dispensing without prescription.

DESCRIPTION
Fluothane (halothane, USP) is supplied as a liquid and is vaporized for use as an inhalation anesthetic. It is 2-bromo-2-chloro-1, 1, 1-trifluoro-ethane and has the following structural formula:

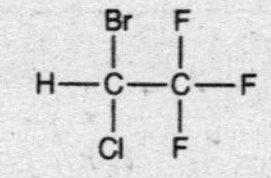

$C_2HBrClF_3$

The molecular weight is 197.38. The drug substance halothane molecule has an asymmetric carbon atom; the commercial product is a racemic mixture. Resolution of the mixture has not been reported.*

*Klaus Florey, editor, Analytical Profiles of Drug Substances, Vol. 1, page 127, (1972).

Halothane is miscible with alcohol, chloroform, ether, and other fat solvents.
The specific gravity is 1.872–1.877 at 20°C, and the boiling point (range) is 49°C–51°C at 760 mm Hg. The vapor pressure is 243 mm Hg at 20°C. The blood/gas coefficient is 2.5 at 37°C, and the olive oil/water coefficient is 220 at 37°C. Vapor concentrations within anesthetic range are nonirritating and have a pleasant odor.
Fluothane is nonflammable, and its vapors mixed with oxygen in proportions from 0.5 to 50% (v/v) are not explosive.
Fluothane does not decompose in contact with warm soda lime. When moisture is present, the vapor attacks aluminum, brass, and lead, but not copper. Rubber, some plastics, and similar materials are soluble in Fluothane; such materials will deteriorate rapidly in contact with Fluothane vapor or liquid. Stability of Fluothane is maintained by the addition of 0.01% thymol (w/w), up to 0.00025% ammonia (w/w).

CLINICAL PHARMACOLOGY
Fluothane is an inhalation anesthetic. Induction and recovery are rapid, and depth of anesthesia can be rapidly altered. Fluothane progressively depresses respiration. There may be tachypnea with reduced tidal volume and alveolar ventilation. Fluothane is not an irritant to the respiratory tract, and no increase in salivary or bronchial secretions ordinarily occurs. Pharyngeal and laryngeal reflexes are rapidly obtunded. It causes bronchodilation. Hypoxia, acidosis, or apnea may develop during deep anesthesia.
Fluothane reduces the blood pressure and frequently decreases the pulse rate. The greater the concentration of the drug, the more evident these changes become. Atropine may reverse the bradycardia. Fluothane does not cause the release of catecholamines from adrenergic stores. Fluothane also causes dilation of the vessels of the skin and skeletal muscles.
Cardiac arrhythmias may occur during Fluothane anesthesia. These include nodal rhythm, AV dissociation, ventricular extrasystoles, and asystole. Fluothane sensitizes the myocardial conduction system to the action of epinephrine and norepinephrine, and the combination may cause serious cardiac arrhythmias. Fluothane increases cerebrospinal-fluid pressure. Fluothane produces moderate muscular relaxation. Muscle relaxants are used as adjuncts in order to maintain lighter levels of anesthesia. Fluothane augments the action of nondepolarizing relaxants and ganglionic-blocking agents. Fluothane is a potent uterine relaxant.
The mechanism(s) whereby Fluothane and other substances induce general anesthesia is unknown. Fluothane is a very potent anesthetic in humans, with a minimum alveolar concentration (MAC) determined to be 0.64%. The MAC has been found to decrease with age (see MAC table in "Dosage and Administration").

INDICATIONS AND USAGE
Fluothane (halothane, USP) is indicated for the induction and maintenance of general anesthesia.

CONTRAINDICATIONS
Fluothane is not recommended for obstetrical anesthesia except when uterine relaxation is required.

WARNINGS
When previous exposure to Fluothane was followed by unexplained hepatic dysfunction and/or jaundice, consideration should be given to the use of other agents.

PRECAUTIONS
GENERAL
Fluothane should be used in vaporizers that permit a reasonable approximation of output, and preferably of the calibrated type. The vaporizer should be placed out of circuit in closed-circuit rebreathing systems; otherwise, overdosage is difficult to avoid. The patient should be closely observed for signs of overdosage, i.e., depression of blood pressure, pulse rate, and ventilation, particularly during assisted or controlled ventilation.
Fluothane increases cerebrospinal-fluid pressure. Therefore, in patients with markedly raised intracranial pressure, if Fluothane is indicated, administration should be preceded by measures ordinarily used to reduce cerebrospinal-fluid pressure. Ventilation should be carefully assessed, and it may be necessary to assist or control ventilation to ensure adequate oxygenation and carbon dioxide removal.
In susceptible individuals, halothane anesthesia may trigger a skeletal-muscle hypermetabolic state leading to a high oxygen demand and the clinical syndrome known as malignant hyperthermia. The syndrome includes nonspecific features such as muscle rigidity, tachycardia, tachypnea, cyanosis, arrhythmias, and unstable blood pressure. (It should also be noted that many of these nonspecific signs may appear with light anesthesia, acute hypoxia, etc.) An increase in overall metabolism may be reflected in an elevated temperature (which may rise rapidly, early or late in the case, but usually is not the first sign of augmented metabolism) and an increased usage of the CO_2 absorption system (hot canister). PaO_2 and pH may decrease, and hyperkalemia and a base deficit may appear. Treatment includes discontinuance of triggering agents (e.g., halothane), administration of intravenous dantrolene, and application of supportive therapy. Such therapy includes vigorous efforts to restore body temperature to normal, respiratory and circulatory support as indicated, and management of electrolyte-fluid-acid-base derangements. Renal failure may appear later, and urine flow should be sustained if possible. It should be noted that the syndrome of malignant hyperthermia secondary to halothane appears to be rare.
INFORMATION FOR PATIENTS
When appropriate, as in some cases where discharge is anticipated soon after general anesthesia, patients should be cautioned not to drive automobiles, operate hazardous machinery, or engage in hazardous sports for 24 hours or more (depending on the total dose of Fluothane, condition of the patient, and consideration given to other drugs administered after anesthesia).
DRUG INTERACTIONS
Epinephrine or norepinephrine should be employed cautiously, if at all, during Fluothane (halothane, USP) anesthesia since their simultaneous use may induce ventricular tachycardia or fibrillation.
Nondepolarizing relaxants and ganglionic-blocking agents should be administered cautiously, since their actions are augmented by Fluothane (halothane, USP).
Clinical experience and animal experiments suggest that pancuronium should be given with caution to patients receiving chronic tricyclic antidepressant therapy who are anesthetized with halothane, because severe ventricular arrhythmias may result from such usage.
CARCINOGENESIS, MUTAGENESIS, IMPAIRMENT OF FERTILITY
An 18-month inhalational carcinogenicity study of halothane at 0.05% in the mouse revealed no evidence of anesthetic-related carcinogenicity. This concentration is equivalent to 24 hours of 1% halothane.
Mutagenesis testing of halothane revealed both positive and negative results. In the rat, one-year exposure to trace concentrations of halothane (1 and 10 ppm) and nitrous oxide produced chromosomal damage to spermatogonia cells and bone marrow cells. Negative mutagenesis tests included: Ames bacterial assay, Chinese hamster lung fibroblast assay, sister chromatid exchange in Chinese hamster ovary cells, and human leukocyte culture assay.
Reproduction studies of halothane (10 ppm) and nitrous oxide in the rat caused decreased fertility. This trace concentration corresponds to 1/1000 the human maintenance dose.
PREGNANCY
Teratogenic Effects: Pregnancy Category C. Some studies have shown Fluothane to be teratogenic, embryotoxic, and fetotoxic in the mouse, rat, hamster, and rabbit at subanesthetic and/or anesthetic concentrations. There are no adequate and well-controlled studies in pregnant women. Fluothane should be used during pregnancy only if the potential benefit justifies the potential risk to the fetus.
LABOR AND DELIVERY
The uterine relaxation obtained with Fluothane, unless carefully controlled, may fail to respond to ergot derivatives and oxytocic posterior pituitary extract.
NURSING MOTHERS
It is not known whether this drug is excreted in human milk. Because many drugs are excreted in human milk, caution should be exercised when Fluothane is administered to a nursing woman.
PEDIATRIC USE
Extensive clinical experience reveals that maintenance concentrations of halothane are generally higher in infants and children, and that maintenance requirements decrease with age. See MAC table, based upon age, in "Dosage and Administration."

ADVERSE REACTIONS
The following adverse reactions have been reported: mild, moderate, and severe hepatic dysfunction (including hepatic necrosis); cardiac arrest; hypotension; respiratory arrest; cardiac arrhythmias; hyperpyrexia; shivering; nausea; and emesis.

OVERDOSAGE
In the event of overdosage, or what may appear to be overdosage, drug administration should be stopped, and assisted or controlled ventilation with pure oxygen initiated.

DOSAGE AND ADMINISTRATION
Fluothane may be administered by the nonrebreathing technique, partial rebreathing, or closed technique. The induction dose varies from patient to patient but is usually within the range of 0.5% to 3%. The maintenance dose varies from 0.5% to 1.5%.
Fluothane may be administered with either oxygen or a mixture of oxygen and nitrous oxide.
Fluothane should not be kept indefinitely in vaporizer bottles not specifically designed for its use. Thymol does not volatilize along with Fluothane and, therefore, accumulates in the vaporizer and may, in time, impart a yellow color to the remaining liquid or to wicks in vaporizers. The development of such discoloration may be used as an indicator that the vaporizer should be drained and cleaned, and the discolored Fluothane (halothane, USP) discarded. Accumulation of thymol may be removed by washing with diethyl ether. After cleaning a wick or vaporizer, make certain all the diethyl ether has been removed before reusing the equipment to avoid introducing ether into the system.
Because of the more rapid uptake of Fluothane and the increased blood concentration required for anesthesia in younger patients, the minimum alveolar concentration (MAC)[1] values will decrease with age as follows:

Age	MAC %
Infants	1.08
3 yrs.	0.91
10 yrs.	0.87
15 yrs.	0.92
24 yrs.	0.84
42 yrs.	0.76
81 yrs.	0.64

HOW SUPPLIED
Fluothane® (halothane, USP) is available in unit packages of 125 mL (NDC 0046-3125-81) and 250 mL (NDC 0046-3125-82) of halothane, USP, stabilized with 0.01% thymol (w/w) and up to 0.00025% ammonia (w/w).
HANDLING AND STORAGE
Store at room temperature (approximately 25°C) in a tight, closed container.
Protect from light.
Use carton to protect contents from light.

PHYSICIAN REFERENCE
1. Gregory, GA et al: *Anesthesiology* 1969; *30*(5):488–491.

GRISACTIN® ℞
[*grĭz-ăc'tĭn*]
(griseofulvin) microsize

Caution: Federal law prohibits dispensing without prescription.

DESCRIPTION
Griseofulvin is an oral fungistatic antibiotic for the treatment of superficial mycoses. It is derived from a species of *Penicillium*.
Grisactin is produced by a special process that fractures griseofulvin particles into minute crystals of irregular shape offering a greater and more effective surface area for increased gastrointestinal absorption.
Grisactin Capsules and Tablets contain the following inactive ingredients:
—250 mg capsules: black iron oxide, D&C Yellow No. 10, FD&C Blue No. 2, FD&C Red No. 40, FD&C Yellow No. 6, gelatin, lactose, magnesium stearate, titanium dioxide, water.
—500 mg tablets: calcium carboxymethylcellulose, D&C Red No. 36, gelatin, magnesium stearate, starch.

HOW SUPPLIED

GRISACTIN (griseofulvin) microsize—

GRISACTIN 250, each capsule contains 250 mg, in bottles of 100 (NDC 0046-0443-81) and 500 (NDC 0046-0443-85).

GRISACTIN 500, each tablet (scored) contains 500 mg, in bottles of 60 (NDC 0046-0444-60).

Store at room temperature (approximately 25°C)

Dispense in a well-closed container as defined in the USP

For prescribing information write to Professional Service, Wyeth-Ayerst Laboratories, P.O. Box 8299, Philadelphia, PA 19101, or contact your local Wyeth-Ayerst representative.

Shown in Product Identification Guide, page 339

HEPARIN ℞

[hep'ah-rin]

Lock Flush Solution, USP

Heparin Flush Kits

Heparin Lock Flush Solution is intended for maintenance of patency of intravenous injection devices only, and is not to be used for anticoagulant therapy.

DESCRIPTION

Wyeth-Ayerst's TUBEX® Heparin Lock Flush Solution, USP, is a sterile solution. Each mL contains either 10 or 100 USP units heparin sodium derived from porcine intestinal mucosa (standardized for use as an anticoagulant) in normal saline solution, and not more than 10 mg benzyl alcohol as a preservative.

The potency is determined by biological assay, using a USP reference standard based upon units of heparin activity per milligram.

Heparin is a heterogenous group of straight-chain anionic mucopolysaccharides, called glycosaminoglycans, having anticoagulant properties. Although others may be present, the main sugars occurring in heparin are: (1) α-L-iduronic acid 2-sulfate, (2) 2-deoxy-2-sulfamino-α-D-glucose 6-sulfate, (3) β-D-glucuronic acid, (4) 2-acetamido-2-deoxy-α-D-glucose, and (5) α-L-iduronic acid. These sugars are present in decreasing amounts, usually in the order (2) > (1) > (4) > (3) > (5), and are joined by glycosidic linkages, forming polymers of varying sizes. Heparin is strongly acidic because of its content of covalently linked sulfate and carboxylic acid groups. In heparin sodium, the acidic protons of the sulfate units are partially replaced by sodium ions.

STRUCTURE OF HEPARIN SODIUM (representative subunits):

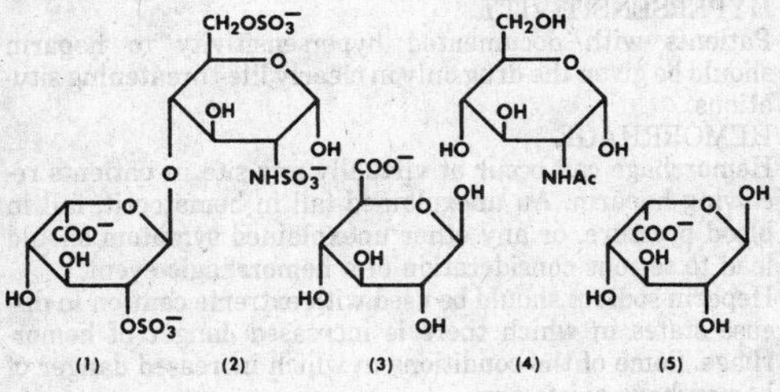

(1) (2) (3) (4) (5)

CLINICAL PHARMACOLOGY

Heparin inhibits reactions that lead to the clotting of blood and the formation of fibrin clots both *in vitro* and *in vivo.* Heparin acts at multiple sites in the normal coagulation system. Small amounts of heparin in combination with antithrombin III (heparin cofactor) can inhibit thrombosis by inactivating activated Factor X and inhibiting the conversion of prothrombin to thrombin. Once active thrombosis has developed, larger amounts of heparin can inhibit further coagulation by inactivating thrombin and preventing the conversion of fibrinogen to fibrin. Heparin also prevents the formation of a stable fibrin clot by inhibiting the activation of the fibrin stabilizing factor.

Bleeding time is usually unaffected by heparin. Clotting time is prolonged by full therapeutic doses of heparin; in most cases, it is not measurably affected by low doses of heparin. Peak plasma levels of heparin are achieved 2 to 4 hours following subcutaneous administration, although there are considerable individual variations. Loglinear plots of heparin plasma concentrations with time, for a wide range of dose levels, are linear which suggests the absence of zero order processes. Liver and the reticulo-endothelial system are the sites of biotransformation. The biphasic elimination curve, a rapidly declining alpha phase ($t_{1/2}$ = 10 min.), and after the age of 40 a slower beta phase, indicates uptake in organs. The absence of a relationship between anticoagulant half-life and concentration half-life may reflect factors such as protein binding of heparin.

Heparin does not have fibrinolytic activity; therefore, it will not lyse existing clots.

INDICATIONS AND USAGE

Heparin Lock Flush Solution, USP, is intended to maintain patency of an indwelling venipuncture device designed for intermittent injection or infusion therapy, or blood sampling. Heparin Lock Flush Solution, USP, may be used following initial placement of the device in the vein, after each injection of a medication, or after withdrawal of blood for laboratory tests.

Heparin Lock Flush Solution, USP, is not to be used for anticoagulant therapy.

CONTRAINDICATIONS

Heparin sodium should not be used in patients with the following conditions:

Severe thrombocytopenia; An uncontrollable active bleeding state (see "**Warnings**"), except when this is due to disseminated intravascular coagulation.

WARNINGS

Heparin is not intended for intramuscular use.

HYPERSENSITIVITY

Patients with documented hypersensitivity to heparin should be given the drug only in clearly life-threatening situations.

HEMORRHAGE

Hemorrhage can occur at virtually any site in patients receiving heparin. An unexplained fall in hematocrit, fall in blood pressure, or any other unexplained symptom should lead to serious consideration of a hemorrhagic event.

Heparin sodium should be used with extreme caution in disease states in which there is increased danger of hemorrhage. Some of the conditions in which increased danger of hemorrhage exists are:

Cardiovascular—Subacute bacterial endocarditis. Severe hypertension.

Surgical—During and immediately following (a) spinal tap or spinal anesthesia or (b) major surgery, especially involving the brain, spinal cord, or eye.

Hematologic—Conditions associated with increased bleeding tendencies, such as hemophilia, thrombocytopenia, and some vascular purpuras.

Gastrointestinal—Ulcerative lesions and continuous tube drainage of the stomach or small intestine.

Other—Menstruation, liver disease with impaired hemostasis.

THROMBOCYTOPENIA

Thrombocytopenia has been reported to occur in patients receiving heparin with a reported incidence of 0 to 30%. Mild thrombocytopenia (count greater than 100,000/mm^3) may remain stable or reverse even if heparin is continued. However, thrombocytopenia of any degree should be monitored closely. If the count falls below 100,000/mm^3 or if recurrent thrombosis develops (see "*White-clot Syndrome,*" "**Precautions**"), the heparin product should be discontinued. If continued heparin therapy is essential, administration of heparin from a different organ source can be reinstituted with caution.

MISCELLANEOUS

This product contains benzyl alcohol as preservative. Benzyl alcohol has been reported to be associated with a fatal "Gasping Syndrome" in premature infants.

PRECAUTIONS

GENERAL

White-clot Syndrome

It has been reported that patients on heparin may develop new thrombus formation in association with thrombocytopenia, resulting from irreversible aggregation of platelets induced by heparin, the so-called "white-clot syndrome." The process may lead to severe thromboembolic complications like skin necrosis, gangrene of the extremities that may lead to amputation, myocardial infarction, pulmonary embolism, stroke, and possibly death. Therefore, heparin administration should be promptly discontinued if a patient develops new thrombosis in association with thrombocytopenia.

Heparin Resistance

Increased resistance to heparin is frequently encountered in fever, thrombosis, thrombophlebitis, infections with thrombosing tendencies, myocardial infarction, cancer, and in postsurgical patients.

Increased Risk in Older Women

A higher incidence of bleeding has been reported in women over 60 years of age.

LABORATORY TESTS

Periodic platelet counts, hematocrits, and tests for occult blood in stool are recommended during the entire course of heparin therapy, regardless of the route of administration (see "**Dosage and Administration**").

DRUG INTERACTIONS

Platelet Inhibitors

Drugs such as acetylsalicylic acid, dextran, phenylbutazone, ibuprofen, indomethacin, dipyridamole, hydroxychloroquine, and others that interfere with platelet-aggregation reactions (the main hemostatic defense of heparinized patients) may induce bleeding and should be used with caution in patients receiving heparin sodium.

Other Interactions

Digitalis, tetracyclines, nicotine, or antihistamines may partially counteract the anticoagulant action of heparin sodium.

CARCINOGENESIS, MUTAGENESIS, IMPAIRMENT OF FERTILITY

No long-term studies in animals have been performed to evaluate carcinogenic potential of heparin. Also, no reproduction studies in animals have been performed concerning mutagenesis or impairment of fertility.

PREGNANCY

Teratogenic Effects—Pregnancy Category C

Animal reproduction studies have not been conducted with heparin sodium. It is also not known whether heparin sodium can cause fetal harm when administered to a pregnant woman or can affect reproduction capacity. Heparin sodium should be given to a pregnant woman only if clearly needed.

Nonteratogenic Effects

Heparin does not cross the placental barrier.

NURSING MOTHERS

Heparin is not excreted in human milk.

ADVERSE REACTIONS

HEMORRHAGE

Hemorrhage is the chief complication that may result from heparin therapy (see "**Warnings**"). An overly prolonged clotting time or minor bleeding during therapy can usually be controlled by withdrawing the drug (see "**Overdosage**"). It should be appreciated that gastrointestinal- or urinary-tract bleeding during anticoagulant therapy may indicate the presence of an underlying occult lesion. Bleeding can occur at any site but certain specific hemorrhagic complications may be difficult to detect:

a. Adrenal hemorrhage, with resultant acute adrenal insufficiency, has occurred during anticoagulant therapy. Therefore, such treatment should be discontinued in patients who develop signs and symptoms of acute adrenal hemorrhage and insufficiency. Initiation of corrective therapy should not depend on laboratory confirmation of the diagnosis, since any delay in an acute situation may result in the patient's death.
b. Ovarian (corpus luteum) hemorrhage developed in a number of women of reproductive age receiving short- or long-term anticoagulant therapy. This complication, if unrecognized, may be fatal.
c. Retroperitoneal hemorrhage.

LOCAL IRRITATION

Local irritation, erythema, mild pain, hematoma, or ulceration may follow deep, subcutaneous (intrafat) injection of heparin sodium. These complications are much more common after intramuscular use, and such use is not recommended.

HYPERSENSITIVITY

Generalized hypersensitivity reactions have been reported, with chills, fever, and urticaria as the most usual manifestations, and asthma, rhinitis, lacrimation, headache, nausea and vomiting, and anaphylactoid reactions, including shock, occurring more rarely. Itching and burning, especially on the plantar side of the feet, may occur.

Thrombocytopenia has been reported to occur in patients receiving heparin with a reported incidence of 0 to 30%. While often mild and of no obvious clinical significance, such thrombocytopenia can be accompanied by severe thromboembolic complications, such as skin necrosis, gangrene of the extremities that may lead to amputation, myocardial infarction, pulmonary embolism, stroke, and possibly death. (See "**Warnings,**" "**Precautions.**")

Certain episodes of painful, ischemic and cyanosed limbs have in the past been attributed to allergic vasospastic reactions. Whether these are, in fact, identical to the thrombocytopenia-associated complications remains to be determined.

MISCELLANEOUS

Osteoporosis following long-term administration of high doses of heparin, cutaneous necrosis after systemic administration, suppression of aldosterone synthesis, delayed transient alopecia, priapism, and rebound hyperlipemia on discontinuation of heparin sodium have also been reported.

Significant elevations of aminotransferase (SGOT [S-AST] and SGPT [S-ALT]) levels have occurred in a high percentage of patients (and healthy subjects) who have received heparin.

OVERDOSAGE

SYMPTOMS

Bleeding is the chief sign of heparin overdosage. Nosebleeds, blood in urine, or tarry stools may be noted as the first sign of bleeding. Easy bruising or petechial formations may precede frank bleeding.

TREATMENT—Neutralization of Heparin Effect

When clinical circumstances (bleeding) require reversal of heparinization, protamine sulfate (1% solution) by slow infusion will neutralize heparin sodium. No more than 50 mg should be administered, very slowly, in any 10-minute period. Each mg of protamine sulfate neutralizes approximately 100 USP heparin units. The amount of protamine required decreases over time as heparin is metabolized. Although the metabolism of heparin is complex, it may, for the

Continued on next page

Wyeth-Ayerst Laboratories—Cont.

purpose of choosing a protamine dose, be assumed to have a half-life of about ½ hour after intravenous injection.
Administration of protamine sulfate can cause severe hypotensive and anaphylactoid reactions. Because fatal reactions, often resembling anaphylaxis, have been reported, the drug should be given only when resuscitation techniques and treatment of anaphylactoid shock are readily available.
For additional information consult the labeling of Protamine Sulfate Injection, USP, products.

DOSAGE AND ADMINISTRATION

Parenteral drug products should be inspected visually for particulate matter and discoloration prior to administration, whenever solution and container permit. Slight discoloration does not alter potency.
MAINTENANCE OF PATENCY OF INTRAVENOUS DEVICES
To prevent clot formation in a heparin lock set or central venous catheter following its proper insertion, Heparin Lock Flush Solution, USP, is injected via the injection hub in a quantity sufficient to fill the entire device. This solution should be replaced each time the device is used. Aspirate before administering any solution via the device in order to confirm patency and location of needle or catheter tip. If the drug to be administered is incompatible with heparin, the entire device should be flushed with normal saline before and after the medication is administered; following the second saline flush, Heparin Lock Flush Solution, USP, may be reinstilled into the device. The device manufacturer's instructions should be consulted for specifics concerning its use. Usually this dilute heparin solution will maintain anticoagulation within the device for up to 4 hours.
NOTE: Since repeated injections of small doses of heparin can alter tests for activated partial thromboplastin time (APTT), a baseline value for APTT should be obtained prior to insertion of an intravenous device.
WITHDRAWAL OF BLOOD SAMPLES
Heparin Lock Flush Solution, USP, may also be used after each withdrawal of blood for laboratory tests. When heparin (or sodium chloride) would interfere with or alter the results of blood tests, the heparin solution should be cleared from the device by aspirating and discarding it before withdrawing the blood sample.
The TUBEX® BLUNT POINTE™ Sterile Cartridge Unit is suitable for substances to be administered intravenously only. It is intended for use with injection sets specifically manufactured as "needle-less" injection systems. TUBEX® BLUNT POINTE™ is compatible with Abbott's LifeShield® prepierced reseal injection site. Baxter's Interlink® Injection Site and B. Braun Medical's SafSite® Reflux Valve. Consult manufacturer's recommendations regarding "Directions for Use" of the "needle-less" system. It is also intended for admixture with, and convenient administration of, various medicaments when using Drug Vial Adapters for "needle-less" injection systems.

HOW SUPPLIED

Heparin Lock Flush Solution, USP, is available in TUBEX® BLUNT POINTE™ Sterile Cartridge Units and in TUBEX® Sterile Cartridge-Needle Units.
Each 1 mL size TUBEX contains one of the following concentrations of heparin sodium, in packages of 50 TUBEX:
10 USP Units per mL:
NDC 0008-0523-50, BLUNT POINTE™.
NDC 0008-0523-01, (25 gauge × ⅝ inch needle).
100 USP Units per mL:
NDC 0008-0487-50, BLUNT POINTE™.
NDC 0008-0487-01, (25 gauge × ⅝ inch needle).
Each 2.5 mL size TUBEX contains one of the following concentrations of heparin sodium, in packages of 50 TUBEX:
25 USP Units per TUBEX (10 USP Units per mL):
NDC 0008-0523-51, BLUNT POINTE™.
NDC 0008-0523-02, (25 gauge × ⅝ inch needle).
250 USP Units per TUBEX (100 USP Units per mL):
NDC 0008-0487-51, BLUNT POINTE™.
NDC 0008-0487-03, (25 gauge × ⅝ inch needle).
Do not use if solution is discolored or contains a precipitate
Store at room temperature, 15°-25°C (59°-77°F)
Do not freeze
HEPARIN FLUSH KITS
NOTE: There are two package inserts associated with the use of Heparin Flush Kits (Heparin Lock Flush Solution, USP, and Bacteriostatic Sodium Chloride Injection, USP).
Heparin Flush Kits are available in packages of TUBEX® BLUNT POINTE™ Sterile Cartridge Units and in TUBEX® Sterile Cartridge-Needle Units as follows:
10 USP UNITS HEPARIN SODIUM PER ML
Each Unit of Use Kit contains:
One TUBEX (1 mL) Heparin Lock Flush Solution, USP; two TUBEX (2.5 mL each) Bacteriostatic Sodium Chloride Injection, USP; in packages of 50 Kits.
NDC 0008-2528-50, BLUNT POINTE™.
NDC 0008-2528-01, (25 gauge × ⅝ inch needle).
One TUBEX (2.5 mL) Heparin Lock Flush Solution, USP (25 USP Units heparin sodium per TUBEX); two TUBEX (2.5 mL each) Bacteriostatic Sodium Chloride Injection, USP; in packages of 30 Kits.
NDC 0008-2528-51, BLUNT POINTE™.
NDC 0008-2528-02, (25 gauge × ⅝ inch needle).
One TUBEX (1 mL) Heparin Lock Flush Solution, USP; two TUBEX (1 mL each) Bacteriostatic Sodium Chloride Injection, USP; in packages of 50 Kits.
NDC 0008-2528-52, BLUNT POINTE™.
NDC 0008-2528-03, (25 gauge × ⅝ inch needle).
100 USP UNITS HEPARIN SODIUM PER ML
Each Unit of Use Kit contains:
One TUBEX (1 mL) Heparin Lock Flush Solution, USP; two TUBEX (2.5 mL each) Bacteriostatic Sodium Chloride Injection, USP; in packages of 50 Kits.
NDC 0008-2529-50, BLUNT POINTE™.
NDC 0008-2529-01, (25 gauge × ⅝ inch needle).
One TUBEX (2.5 mL) Heparin Lock Flush Solution, USP (250 USP Units heparin sodium per TUBEX); two TUBEX (2.5 mL each) Bacteriostatic Sodium Chloride Injection, USP; in packages of 30 Kits.
NDC 0008-2529-51, BLUNT POINTE™.
NDC 0008-2529-02, (25 gauge × ⅝ inch needle).
One TUBEX (1 mL) Heparin Lock Flush Solution, USP; two TUBEX (1 mL each) Bacteriostatic Sodium Chloride Injection, USP; in packages of 50 Kits.
NDC 0008-2529-52, BLUNT POINTE™.
NDC 0008-2529-03, (25 gauge × ⅝ inch needle).
Do not use if solution is discolored or contains a precipitate
Store at room temperature, 15°-25°C (59°-77°F)
Do not freeze

HEPARIN ℞

[hep'ah-rin]
Sodium Injection, USP

DESCRIPTION

Wyeth-Ayerst's TUBEX® Heparin Sodium Injection, USP, is a sterile solution. Each mL contains 1,000, 2,500, 5,000, 7,500, 10,000, 15,000, or 20,000 USP units heparin sodium, derived from porcine intestinal mucosa (standardized for use as an anticoagulant), in water for injection, and not more than 10 mg benzyl alcohol as a preservative.
The potency is determined by biological assay, using a USP reference standard based upon units of heparin activity per milligram. The pH range is 5.0 to 7.5.
Heparin is a heterogenous group of straight-chain anionic mucopolysaccharides, called glycosaminoglycans, having anticoagulant properties. Although others may be present, the main sugars occurring in heparin are: (1) α-L-iduronic acid 2-sulfate, (2) 2-deoxy-2-sulfamino-α-D-glucose 6-sulfate, (3) β-D-glucuronic acid, (4) 2-acetamido-2-deoxy-α-D-glucose, and (5) α-L-iduronic acid. These sugars are present in decreasing amounts, usually in the order (2) > (1) > (4) > (3) > (5), and are joined by glycosidic linkages, forming polymers of varying sizes. Heparin is strongly acidic because of its content of covalently linked sulfate and carboxylic acid groups. In heparin sodium, the acidic protons of the sulfate units are partially replaced by sodium ions.
STRUCTURE OF HEPARIN SODIUM (representative subunits):

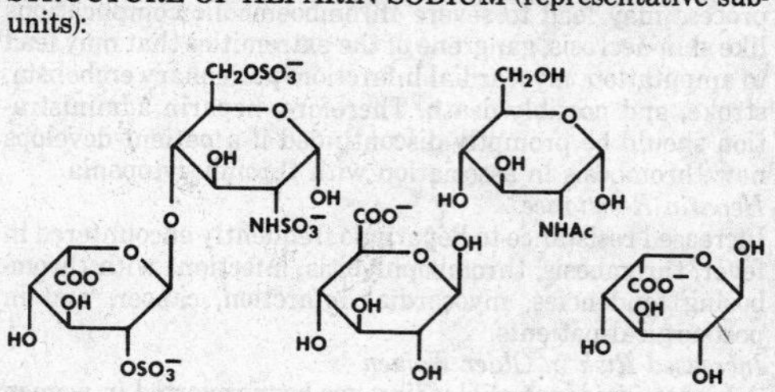

(1) (2) (3) (4) (5)

CLINICAL PHARMACOLOGY

Heparin inhibits reactions that lead to the clotting of blood and the formation of fibrin clots both *in vitro* and *in vivo.* Heparin acts at multiple sites in the normal coagulation system. Small amounts of heparin in combination with antithrombin III (heparin cofactor) can inhibit thrombosis by inactivating activated Factor X and inhibiting the conversion of prothrombin to thrombin. Once active thrombosis has developed, larger amounts of heparin can inhibit further coagulation by inactivating thrombin and preventing the conversion of fibrinogen to fibrin. Heparin also prevents the formation of a stable fibrin clot by inhibiting the activation of the fibrin stabilizing factor.
Bleeding time is usually unaffected by heparin. Clotting time is prolonged by full therapeutic doses of heparin; in most cases it is not measurably affected by low doses of heparin.
Peak plasma levels of heparin are achieved 2 to 4 hours following subcutaneous administration, although there are considerable individual variations. Loglinear plots of heparin plasma concentrations with time, for a wide range of dose levels, are linear which suggests the absence of zero order processes. Liver and the reticulo-endothelial system are the sites of biotransformation. The biphasic elimination curve, a rapidly declining alpha phase ($t_{1/2}$ = 10 min.), and after the age of 40 a slower beta phase, indicates uptake in organs. The absence of a relationship between anticoagulant half-life and concentration half-life may reflect factors such as protein binding of heparin.
Heparin does not have fibrinolytic activity; therefore, it will not lyse existing clots.

INDICATIONS AND USAGE

Heparin sodium injection is indicated for anticoagulant therapy in prophylaxis and treatment of venous thrombosis and its extension; in low-dose regimen for prevention of postoperative deep venous thrombosis and pulmonary embolism in patients undergoing major abdominothoracic surgery who are at risk of developing thromboembolic disease (see "Dosage and Administration"); for prophylaxis and treatment of pulmonary embolism; in atrial fibrillation with embolization; for diagnosis and treatment of acute and chronic consumptive coagulopathies (disseminated intravascular coagulation); for prevention of clotting in arterial and cardiac surgery; and for prophylaxis and treatment of peripheral arterial embolism.
Heparin may also be employed as an anticoagulant in blood transfusions, extracorporeal circulation, dialysis procedures, and in blood samples for laboratory purposes.

CONTRAINDICATIONS

Heparin sodium should not be used in patients:
with severe thrombocytopenia;
in whom suitable blood-coagulation tests—e.g., the whole-blood clotting time, partial thromboplastin time, etc.—cannot be performed at appropriate intervals (this contraindication refers to full-dose heparin; there is usually no need to monitor coagulation parameters in patients receiving low-dose heparin);
with an uncontrollable active bleeding state (see "Warnings"), except when this is due to disseminated intravascular coagulation.

WARNINGS

Heparin is not intended for intramuscular use.
HYPERSENSITIVITY
Patients with documented hypersensitivity to heparin should be given the drug only in clearly life-threatening situations.
HEMORRHAGE
Hemorrhage can occur at virtually any site in patients receiving heparin. An unexplained fall in hematocrit, fall in blood pressure, or any other unexplained symptom should lead to serious consideration of a hemorrhagic event.
Heparin sodium should be used with extreme caution in disease states in which there is increased danger of hemorrhage. Some of the conditions in which increased danger of hemorrhage exists are:
Cardiovascular—Subacute bacterial endocarditis. Severe hypertension.
Surgical—During and immediately following (a) spinal tap or spinal anesthesia or (b) major surgery, especially involving the brain, spinal cord, or eye.
Hematologic—Conditions associated with increased bleeding tendencies, such as hemophilia, thrombocytopenia, and some vascular purpuras.
Gastrointestinal—Ulcerative lesions and continuous tube drainage of the stomach or small intestine.
Other—Menstruation, liver disease with impaired hemostasis.
COAGULATION TESTING
When heparin sodium is administered in therapeutic amounts, its dosage should be regulated by frequent blood coagulation tests. If the coagulation test is unduly prolonged or if hemorrhage occurs, heparin sodium should be discontinued promptly (see "Overdosage").
THROMBOCYTOPENIA
Thrombocytopenia has been reported to occur in patients receiving heparin with a reported incidence of 0 to 30%. Mild thrombocytopenia (count greater than 100,000/mm³) may remain stable or reverse even if heparin is continued. However, thrombocytopenia of any degree should be monitored closely. If the count falls below 100,000/mm³ or if recurrent thrombosis develops (see "White-clot Syndrome," "Precautions"), the heparin product should be discontinued. If continued heparin therapy is essential, administration of heparin from a different organ source can be reinstituted with caution.
MISCELLANEOUS
This product contains benzyl alcohol as preservative. Benzyl alcohol has been reported to be associated with a fatal "Gasping Syndrome" in premature infants.

PRECAUTIONS

GENERAL

White-clot Syndrome

It has been reported that patients on heparin may develop new thrombus formation in association with thrombocytopenia, resulting from irreversible aggregation of platelets induced by heparin, the so-called "white-clot syndrome." The process may lead to severe thromboembolic complications like skin necrosis, gangrene of the extremities that may lead to amputation, myocardial infarction, pulmonary embolism, stroke, and possibly death. Therefore, heparin administration should be promptly discontinued if a patient develops new thrombosis in association with thrombocytopenia.

Heparin Resistance

Increased resistance to heparin is frequently encountered in fever, thrombosis, thrombophlebitis, infections with thrombosing tendencies, myocardial infarction, cancer, and in postsurgical patients.

Increased Risk in Older Women

A higher incidence of bleeding has been reported in women over 60 years of age.

LABORATORY TESTS

Periodic platelet counts, hematocrits, and tests for occult blood in stool are recommended during the entire course of heparin therapy, regardless of the route of administration (see "Dosage and Administration").

DRUG INTERACTIONS

Oral Anticoagulants

Heparin sodium may prolong the one-stage prothrombin time. Therefore, when heparin sodium is given with dicumarol or warfarin sodium, a period of at least 5 hours after the last intravenous dose or 24 hours after the last subcutaneous dose should elapse before blood is drawn if a valid prothrombin time is to be obtained.

Platelet Inhibitors

Drugs such as acetylsalicylic acid, dextran, phenylbutazone, ibuprofen, indomethacin, dipyridamole, hydroxychloroquine, and others that interfere with platelet-aggregation reactions (the main hemostatic defense of heparinized patients) may induce bleeding and should be used with caution in patients receiving heparin sodium.

Other Interactions

Digitalis, tetracyclines, nicotine, or antihistamines may partially counteract the anticoagulant action of heparin sodium.

DRUG/LABORATORY TEST INTERACTIONS

Hyperaminotransferasemia

Significant elevations of aminotransferase (SGOT [S-AST] and SGPT [S-ALT]) levels have occurred in a high percentage of patients (and healthy subjects) who have received heparin. Since aminotransferase determinations are important in the differential diagnosis of myocardial infarction, liver disease, and pulmonary emboli, rises that might be caused by drugs (like heparin) should be interpreted with caution.

CARCINOGENESIS, MUTAGENESIS, IMPAIRMENT OF FERTILITY

No long-term studies in animals have been performed to evaluate carcinogenic potential of heparin. Also, no reproduction studies in animals have been performed concerning mutagenesis or impairment of fertility.

PREGNANCY

Teratogenic Effects—Pregnancy Category C

Animal reproduction studies have not been conducted with heparin sodium. It is also not known whether heparin sodium can cause fetal harm when administered to a pregnant woman or can affect reproduction capacity. Heparin sodium should be given to a pregnant woman only if clearly needed.

Nonteratogenic Effects

Heparin does not cross the placental barrier.

NURSING MOTHERS

Heparin is not excreted in human milk.

PEDIATRIC USE

See "Dosage and Administration."

ADVERSE REACTIONS

HEMORRHAGE

Hemorrhage is the chief complication that may result from heparin therapy (see "Warnings").

An overly prolonged clotting time or minor bleeding during therapy can usually be controlled by withdrawing the drug (see "Overdosage"). It should be appreciated that gastrointestinal- or urinary-tract bleeding during anticoagulant therapy may indicate the presence of an underlying occult lesion. Bleeding can occur at any site but certain specific hemorrhagic complications may be difficult to detect:

a. Adrenal hemorrhage, with resultant acute adrenal insufficiency, has occurred during anticoagulant therapy. Therefore, such treatment should be discontinued in patients who develop signs and symptoms of acute adrenal hemorrhage and insufficiency. Initiation of corrective therapy should not depend on laboratory confirmation of the diagnosis, since any delay in an acute situation may result in the patient's death.

b. Ovarian (corpus luteum) hemorrhage developed in a number of women of reproductive age receiving short- or long-term anticoagulant therapy. This complication, if unrecognized, may be fatal.

c. Retroperitoneal hemorrhage.

LOCAL IRRITATION

Local irritation, erythema, mild pain, hematoma, or ulceration may follow deep, subcutaneous (intrafat) injection of heparin sodium. These complications are much more common after intramuscular use, and such use is not recommended.

HYPERSENSITIVITY

Generalized hypersensitivity reactions have been reported, with chills, fever, and urticaria as the most usual manifestations, and asthma, rhinitis, lacrimation, headache, nausea and vomiting, and anaphylactoid reactions, including shock, occurring more rarely. Itching and burning, especially on the plantar side of the feet, may occur.

Thrombocytopenia has been reported to occur in patients receiving heparin with a reported incidence of 0 to 30%. While often mild and of no obvious clinical significance, such thrombocytopenia can be accompanied by severe thromboembolic complications, such as skin necrosis, gangrene of the extremities that may lead to amputation, myocardial infarction, pulmonary embolism, stroke, and possibly death. (See "Warnings," "Precautions.")

Certain episodes of painful, ischemic and cyanosed limbs have in the past been attributed to allergic vasospastic reactions. Whether these are, in fact, identical to the thrombocytopenia-associated complications remains to be determined.

MISCELLANEOUS

Osteoporosis following long-term administration of high doses of heparin, cutaneous necrosis after systemic administration, suppression of aldosterone synthesis, delayed transient alopecia, priapism, and rebound hyperlipemia on discontinuation of heparin sodium have also been reported.

Significant elevations of aminotransferase (SGOT [S-AST] and SGPT [S-ALT]) levels have occurred in a high percentage of patients (and healthy subjects) who have received heparin.

OVERDOSAGE

SYMPTOMS

Bleeding is the chief sign of heparin overdosage. Nosebleeds, blood in urine, or tarry stools may be noted as the first sign of bleeding. Easy bruising or petechial formations may precede frank bleeding.

TREATMENT—Neutralization of Heparin Effect

When clinical circumstances (bleeding) require reversal of heparinization, protamine sulfate (1% solution) by slow infusion will neutralize heparin sodium. No more than 50 mg should be administered, very slowly, in any 10-minute period. Each mg of protamine sulfate neutralizes approximately 100 USP heparin units. The amount of protamine required decreases over time as heparin is metabolized. Although the metabolism of heparin is complex, it may, for the purpose of choosing a protamine dose, be assumed to have a half-life of about ½ hour after intravenous injection.

Administration of protamine sulfate can cause severe hypotensive and anaphylactoid reactions. Because fatal reactions, often resembling anaphylaxis, have been reported, the drug should be given only when resuscitation techniques and treatment of anaphylactoid shock are readily available.

For additional information consult the labeling of Protamine Sulfate Injection, USP, products.

DOSAGE AND ADMINISTRATION

Parenteral drug products should be inspected visually for particulate matter and discoloration prior to administration, whenever solution and container permit. Slight discoloration does not alter potency.

When heparin is added to an infusion solution for continuous intravenous administration, the container should be inverted at least six times to insure adequate mixing and prevent pooling of the heparin in the solution.

Heparin sodium is not effective by oral administration and should be given by intermittent intravenous injection, intravenous infusion, or deep, subcutaneous (intrafat, i.e., above the iliac crest or abdominal fat layer) injection. *The intramuscular route of administration should be avoided because of the frequent occurrence of hematoma at the injection site.*

The TUBEX® BLUNT POINTE™ Sterile Cartridge Unit is suitable for substances to be administered intravenously only. It is intended for use with injection sets specifically manufactured as "needle-less" injection systems. TUBEX® BLUNT POINTE™ is compatible with Abbott's LifeShield® prepierced reseal injection site, Baxter's InterLink® Injection Site and B. Braun Medical's SafSite® Reflux Valve. Consult manufacturer's recommendations regarding "Directions for Use" of the "needle-less" system. It is also intended for admixture with, and convenient administration of, various medicaments when using Drug Vial Adapters for "needle-less" injection systems.

The dosage of heparin sodium should be adjusted according to the patient's coagulation-test results. When heparin is given by continuous intravenous infusion, the coagulation time should be determined approximately every 4 hours in the early stages of treatment. When the drug is administered intermittently by intravenous injection, coagulation tests should be performed before each injection during the early stages of treatment and at appropriate intervals thereafter. Dosage is considered adequate when the activated partial thromboplastin time (APTT) is 1.5 to 2 times normal or when the whole-blood clotting time is elevated approximately 2.5 to 3 times the control value. After deep subcutaneous (intrafat) injections, tests for adequacy of dosage are best performed on samples drawn 4 to 6 hours after the injections.

Periodic platelet counts, hematocrits, and tests for occult blood in stool are recommended during the entire course of heparin therapy, regardless of the route of administration.

CONVERTING TO ORAL ANTICOAGULANT

When an oral anticoagulant of the coumarin or similar type is to be begun in patients already receiving heparin sodium, baseline and subsequent tests of prothrombin activity must be determined at a time when heparin activity is too low to affect the prothrombin time. This is about 5 hours after the last IV bolus and 24 hours after the last subcutaneous dose. If continuous IV heparin infusion is used, prothrombin time can usually be measured at any time.

In converting from heparin to an oral anticoagulant, the dose of the oral anticoagulant should be the usual initial amount, and thereafter prothrombin time should be determined at the usual intervals. To ensure continuous anticoagulation, it is advisable to continue full heparin therapy for several days after the prothrombin time has reached the therapeutic range. Heparin therapy may then be discontinued without tapering.

THERAPEUTIC ANTICOAGULANT EFFECT WITH FULL-DOSE HEPARIN

Although dosage must be adjusted for the individual patient according to the results of suitable laboratory tests, the following dosage schedules may be used as guidelines:

[See table above.]

Method of Administration	Frequency	Recommended Dose [based on 150 lb (68 kg) patient]
Deep, Subcutaneous (Intrafat) Injection	Initial Dose	5,000 units by IV injection followed by 10,000–20,000 units of a concentrated solution, subcutaneously
A different site should be used for each injection to prevent the development of massive hematoma.	Every 8 hours	8,000–10,000 units of a concentrated solution
	(or) Every 12 hours	15,000–20,000 units of a concentrated solution
Intermittent, Intravenous Injection	Initial Dose	10,000 units, either undiluted or in 50–100 ml isotonic sodium chloride injection
	Every 4 to 6 hours	5,000–10,000 units, either undiluted or in 50–100 mL isotonic sodium chloride injection
Intravenous Infusion	Initial Dose	5,000 units by IV injection
	Continuous	20,000–40,000 units in 1,000 mL of isotonic sodium chloride solution for infusion/day

PEDIATRIC USE

Follow recommendations of appropriate pediatric reference texts. In general, the following dosage schedule may be used as a guideline.

Initial Dose: 50 units/kg (IV, drip).

Maintenance Dose: 100 units/kg (IV, drip) every four hours, or 20,000 units/M^2/24 hours continuously.

Continued on next page

Wyeth-Ayerst Laboratories—Cont.

SURGERY OF THE HEART AND BLOOD VESSELS

Patients undergoing total body perfusion for open-heart surgery should receive an initial dose of not less than 150 units of heparin sodium per kilogram of body weight. Frequently, a dose of 300 units of heparin sodium per kilogram of body weight is used for procedures estimated to last less than 60 minutes; or 400 units per kilogram for those estimated to last longer than 60 minutes.

LOW-DOSE PROPHYLAXIS OF POSTOPERATIVE THROMBOEMBOLISM

A number of well-controlled clinical trials have demonstrated that low-dose heparin prophylaxis, given just prior to and after surgery, will reduce the incidence of postoperative deep-vein thrombosis in the legs, as measured by the l-125 fibrinogen technique and venography, and of clinical pulmonary embolism. The most widely used dosage has been 5,000 units 2 hours before surgery and 5,000 units every 8 to 12 hours thereafter for 7 days or until the patient is fully ambulatory, whichever is longer. The heparin is given by deep, subcutaneous injection in the arm or abdomen with a fine needle (25 to 26 gauge) to minimize tissue trauma. A concentrated solution of heparin sodium is recommended. Such prophylaxis should be reserved for patients over 40 undergoing major surgery. Patients with bleeding disorders, those having neurosurgery, spinal anesthesia, eye surgery, or potentially sanguineous operations should be excluded, as well as patients receiving oral anticoagulants or platelet-active drugs (see "Warnings"). The value of such prophylaxis in hip surgery has not been established. The possibility of increased bleeding during surgery or postoperatively should be borne in mind. If such bleeding occurs, discontinuance of heparin and neutralization with protamine sulfate is advisable. If clinical evidence of thromboembolism develops despite low-dose prophylaxis, full therapeutic doses of anticoagulants should be given unless contraindicated. All patients should be screened prior to heparinization to rule out bleeding disorders, and monitoring should be performed with appropriate coagulation tests just prior to surgery. Coagulation-test values should be normal or only slightly elevated. There is usually no need for daily monitoring of the effect of low-dose heparin in patients with normal coagulation parameters.

EXTRACORPOREAL DIALYSIS USE

Follow equipment manufacturer's operating directions carefully.

BLOOD TRANSFUSION

Addition of 400 to 600 USP units per 100 ml of whole blood. Usually, 7,500 USP units of heparin sodium are added to 100 mL of Sterile Sodium Chloride Injection (or 75,000 USP units per 1,000 mL of Sterile Sodium Chloride Injection) and mixed, and from this sterile solution, 6 to 8 mL is added per 100 mL of whole blood.

LABORATORY SAMPLES

Addition of 70 to 150 units of heparin sodium per 10 to 20 mL sample of whole blood is usually employed to prevent coagulation of the sample. Leukocyte counts should be performed on heparinized blood within two hours after addition of the heparin. Heparinized blood should not be used for isoagglutinin, complement, erythrocyte fragility tests, or platelet counts.

HOW SUPPLIED

Heparin Sodium Injection, USP, is available in TUBEX® Sterile Cartridge-Needle Units.
Each 1 mL size TUBEX contains one of the following concentrations of heparin sodium:
1,000 USP Units per mL
NDC 0008-0275-01, (22 gauge × 1¼ inch needle), in packages of 10 TUBEX.
2,500 USP Units per mL
NDC 0008-0482-01, (25 gauge × ⅝ inch needle), in packages of 10 TUBEX.
5,000 USP Units per 0.5 mL (10,000 USP Units per mL)
NDC 0008-0277-02, (25 gauge ×⅝ inch needle), in packages of 10 TUBEX.
NDC 0008-0277-03, (25 gauge × ⅝ inch needle), in packages of 50 TUBEX.
5,000 USP Units per mL
NDC 0008-0278-02, (25 gauge × ⅝ inch needle), in packages of 10 TUBEX.
7,500 USP Units per mL
NDC 0008-0293-01, (25 gauge × ⅝ inch needle), in packages of 10 TUBEX.
10,000 USP Units per mL
NDC 0008-0277-01, (25 gauge × ⅝ inch needle), in packages of 10 TUBEX.
20,000 USP Units per mL
NDC 0008-0276-01, (25 gauge × ⅝ inch needle), in packages of 10 TUBEX.
Heparin Sodium Injection, USP, 1,000 USP Units per mL, is also available in packages of 10 TUBEX® BLUNT POINTE™ Sterile Cartridge Units, NDC 0008-0275-50.

Store at room temperature, 15°–25°C (59°–77°F).
Do not freeze
Do not use if solution is discolored or contains a precipitate

---

INDERAL®   ℞
[ĭn 'der-al]
(propranolol hydrochloride)
TABLETS

Caution: Federal law prohibits dispensing without prescription.

DESCRIPTION

Inderal (propranolol hydrochloride) is a synthetic beta-adrenergic receptor blocking agent chemically described as 1-(Isopropylamino)-3-(1-naphthyloxy)-2-propanol hydrochloride. Its structural formula is

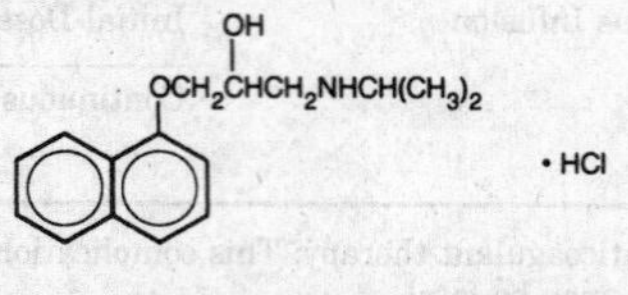

$$OH$$
$$OCH_2CHCH_2NHCH(CH_3)_2$$
$$\cdot HCl$$

Propranolol hydrochloride is a stable, white, crystalline solid which is readily soluble in water and ethanol. Its molecular weight is 295.81.
Inderal is available as 10 mg, 20 mg, 40 mg, 60 mg, and 80 mg tablets for oral administration and as a 1 mg/mL sterile injectable solution for intravenous administration.
The inactive ingredients contained in Inderal Tablets are: lactose, magnesium stearate, microcrystalline cellulose, and stearic acid. In addition, Inderal 10 mg and 80 mg Tablets contain FD&C Yellow No. 6 and D&C Yellow No. 10; Inderal 20 mg Tablets contain FD&C Blue No. 1; Inderal 40 mg Tablets contain FD&C Blue No. 1, FD&C Yellow No. 6, and D&C Yellow No. 10; Inderal 60 mg Tablets contain D&C Red No. 30.

CLINICAL PHARMACOLOGY

Inderal is a nonselective beta-adrenergic receptor blocking agent possessing no other autonomic nervous system activity. It specifically competes with beta-adrenergic receptor stimulating agents for available receptor sites. When access to beta-receptor sites is blocked by Inderal, the chronotropic, inotropic, and vasodilator responses to beta-adrenergic stimulation are decreased proportionately.
Propranolol is almost completely absorbed from the gastrointestinal tract, but a portion is immediately bound by the liver. Peak effect occurs in one to one and one-half hours. The biologic half-life is approximately four hours.
There is no simple correlation between dose or plasma level and therapeutic effect, and the dose-sensitivity range as observed in clinical practice is wide. The principal reason for this is that sympathetic tone varies widely between individuals. Since there is no reliable test to estimate sympathetic tone or to determine whether total beta blockade has been achieved, proper dosage requires titration.
The mechanism of the antihypertensive effect of Inderal has not been established. Among the factors that may be involved in contributing to the antihypertensive action are (1) decreased cardiac output, (2) inhibition of renin release by the kidneys, and (3) diminution of tonic sympathetic nerve outflow from vasomotor centers in the brain. Although total peripheral resistance may increase initially, it readjusts to or below the pretreatment level with chronic use. Effects on plasma volume appear to be minor and somewhat variable. Inderal has been shown to cause a small increase in serum potassium concentration when used in the treatment of hypertensive patients.
In angina pectoris, propranolol generally reduces the oxygen requirement of the heart at any given level of effort by blocking the catecholamine-induced increases in the heart rate, systolic blood pressure, and the velocity and extent of myocardial contraction. Propranolol may increase oxygen requirements by increasing left ventricular fiber length, end diastolic pressure, and systolic ejection period. The net physiologic effect of beta-adrenergic blockade is usually advantageous and is manifested during exercise by delayed onset of pain and increased work capacity. Propranolol exerts its antiarrhythmic effects in concentrations associated with beta-adrenergic blockade, and this appears to be its principal antiarrhythmic mechanism of action. In dosages greater than required for beta blockade, Inderal also exerts a quinidine-like or anesthetic-like membrane action, which affects the cardiac action potential. The significance of the membrane action in the treatment of arrhythmias is uncertain.
The mechanism of the antimigraine effect of propranolol has not been established. Beta-adrenergic receptors have been demonstrated in the pial vessels of the brain.
The specific mechanism of Inderal's antitremor effects has not been established, but beta-2 (noncardiac) receptors may be involved. A central effect is also possible. Clinical studies

---

have demonstrated that Inderal is of benefit in exaggerated physiological and essential (familial) tremor.
Beta-receptor blockade can be useful in conditions in which, because of pathologic or functional changes, sympathetic activity is detrimental to the patient. But there are also situations in which sympathetic stimulation is vital. For example, in patients with severely damaged hearts, adequate ventricular function is maintained by virtue of sympathetic drive, which should be preserved. In the presence of AV block greater than first degree, beta blockade may prevent the necessary facilitating effect of sympathetic activity on conduction. Beta blockade results in bronchial constriction by interfering with adrenergic bronchodilator activity, which should be preserved in patients subject to bronchospasm.
Propranolol is not significantly dialyzable.
The Beta-Blocker Heart Attack Trial (BHAT) was a National Heart, Lung and Blood Institute-sponsored multicenter, randomized, double-blind, placebo-controlled trial conducted in 31 U.S. centers (plus one in Canada) in 3,837 persons without history of severe congestive heart failure or presence of recent heart failure; certain conduction defects; angina since infarction, who had survived the acute phase of myocardial infarction. Propranolol was administered at either 60 or 80 mg t.i.d. based on blood levels achieved during an initial trial of 40 mg t.i.d. Therapy with Inderal, begun 5 to 21 days following infarction, was shown to reduce overall mortality up to 39 months, the longest period of follow-up. This was primarily attributable to a reduction in cardiovascular mortality. The protective effect of Inderal was consistent regardless of age, sex, or site of infarction. Compared with placebo, total mortality was reduced 39% at 12 months and 26% over an average follow-up period of 25 months. The Norwegian Multicenter Trial in which propranolol was administered at 40 mg q.i.d. gave overall results which support the findings in the BHAT.
Although the clinical trials used either t.i.d. or q.i.d. dosing, clinical, pharmacologic, and pharmacokinetic data provide a reasonable basis for concluding that b.i.d. dosing with propranolol should be adequate in the treatment of postinfarction patients.

CLINICAL

In the BHAT, patients on Inderal were prescribed either 180 mg/day (82% of patients) or 240 mg/day (18% of patients). Patients were instructed to take the medication 3 times a day at mealtimes. This dosing schedule would result in an overnight dosing interval of 12 to 14 hours which is similar to the dosing interval for a b.i.d regimen. In addition, blood samples were drawn at various times and analyzed for propranolol. When the patients were grouped into tertiles based on the blood levels observed and the mortality in the upper and lower tertiles was compared, there was no evidence that blood levels affected mortality.

PHARMACOLOGIC

Studies in normal volunteers have shown that a 90 mg b.i.d. regimen maintains beta blockade at, or above, the minimum for 60 mg t.i.d. dosing for 24 hours even though differences occurred at two time intervals. At 10 to 12 hours after the first dose of the day, t.i.d. dosing gave more beta blockade than b.i.d. dosing; at 20 to 24 hours the trend of the relationship was reversed. These relationships were similar in direction to those observed for plasma propranolol levels. (See "PHARMACOKINETIC".)

PHARMACOKINETIC

A bioavailability study in normal volunteers showed that the blood levels produced by 180 mg/day given b.i.d. are below those provided by the same daily dosage given t.i.d. at 10 to 12 hours after the first dose of the day, but above those of a t.i.d. regimen at 20 to 24 hours. However, the blood levels produced by b.i.d. dosing were always equivalent to or above the minimum for t.i.d. dosing throughout the 24 hours. In addition, the mean AUC on the fourth day for the b.i.d. regimen was about 17% greater than for the t.i.d. regimen (1,194 vs. 1,024 ng/mL·hr).

INDICATIONS AND USAGE

HYPERTENSION

Inderal is indicated in the management of hypertension. It may be used alone or used in combination with other antihypertensive agents, particularly a thiazide diuretic. Inderal is not indicated in the management of hypertensive emergencies.

ANGINA PECTORIS DUE TO CORONARY ATHEROSCLEROSIS

Inderal is indicated for the long-term management of patients with angina pectoris.

CARDIAC ARRHYTHMIAS

1.) Supraventricular arrhythmias
   a) Paroxysmal atrial tachycardias, particularly those arrhythmias induced by catecholamines or digitalis or associated with the Wolff-Parkinson-White syndrome. (See W-P-W under "Warnings".)
   b) Persistent sinus tachycardia which is noncompensatory and impairs the well-being of the patient.
   c) Tachycardias and arrhythmias due to thyrotoxicosis when causing distress or increased hazard and when

immediate effect is necessary as adjunctive, short-term (2 to 4 weeks) therapy. May be used with, but not in place of, specific therapy. (See THYROTOXICOSIS under "Warnings".)

d) Persistent atrial extrasystoles which impair the well-being of the patient and do not respond to conventional measures.

e) Atrial flutter and fibrillation when ventricular rate cannot be controlled by digitalis alone, or when digitalis is contraindicated.

2.) Ventricular tachycardias.
Ventricular arrhythmias do not respond to propranolol as predictably as do the supraventricular arrhythmias.

a) Ventricular tachycardias
With the exception of those induced by catecholamines or digitalis, Inderal is not the drug of first choice. In critical situations when cardioversion techniques or other drugs are not indicated or are not effective, Inderal may be considered. If, after consideration of the risks involved, Inderal is used, it should be given intravenously in low dosage and very slowly. (See "Dosage and Administration".) *Care in the administration of Inderal with constant electrocardiographic monitoring is essential as the failing heart requires some sympathetic drive for maintenance of myocardial tone.*

b) Persistent premature ventricular extrasystoles which do not respond to conventional measures and impair the well-being of the patient.

3.) Tachyarrhythmias of digitalis intoxication
If digitalis-induced tachyarrhythmias persist following discontinuance of digitalis and correction of electrolyte abnormalities, they are usually reversible with *oral* Inderal. Severe bradycardia may occur. (See "OVERDOSAGE.")

Intravenous propranolol hydrochloride is reserved for life-threatening arrhythmias. Temporary maintenance with oral therapy may be indicated. (See "Dosage and Administration.")

4.) Resistant tachyarrhythmias due to excessive catecholamine action during anesthesia
Tachyarrhythmias due to excessive catecholamine action during anesthesia may sometimes arise because of release of endogenous catecholamines or administration of catecholamines. When usual measures fail in such arrhythmias, Inderal may be given intravenously to abolish them. All general inhalation anesthetics produce some degree of myocardial depression. Therefore, when Inderal is used to treat arrhythmias during anesthesia, it should be used with extreme caution and constant ECG and central venous pressure monitoring. (See "Warnings.")

MYOCARDIAL INFARCTION
Inderal is indicated to reduce cardiovascular mortality in patients who have survived the acute phase of myocardial infarction and are clinically stable.

MIGRAINE
Inderal is indicated for the prophylaxis of common migraine headache. The efficacy of propranolol in the treatment of a migraine attack that has started has not been established, and propranolol is not indicated for such use.

ESSENTIAL TREMOR
Inderal is indicated in the management of familial or hereditary essential tremor. Familial or essential tremor consists of involuntary, rhythmic, oscillatory movements, usually limited to the upper limbs. It is absent at rest but occurs when the limb is held in a fixed posture or position against gravity and during active movement. Inderal causes a reduction in the tremor amplitude but not in the tremor frequency. Inderal is not indicated for the treatment of tremor associated with Parkinsonism.

HYPERTROPHIC SUBAORTIC STENOSIS
Inderal is useful in the management of hypertrophic subaortic stenosis, especially for treatment of exertional or other stress-induced angina, palpitations, and syncope. Inderal also improves exercise performance. The effectiveness of propranolol hydrochloride in this disease appears to be due to a reduction of the elevated outflow pressure gradient, which is exacerbated by beta-receptor stimulation. Clinical improvement may be temporary.

PHEOCHROMOCYTOMA
After primary treatment with an alpha-adrenergic blocking agent has been instituted, Inderal may be useful as *adjunctive* therapy if the control of tachycardia becomes necessary before or during surgery. It is hazardous to use Inderal unless alpha-adrenergic blocking drugs are already in use, since this would predispose to serious blood pressure elevation. Blocking only the peripheral dilator (beta) action of epinephrine leaves its constrictor (alpha) action unopposed. In the event of hemorrhage or shock, there is a disadvantage in having both beta and alpha blockade since the combination prevents the increase in heart rate and peripheral vasoconstriction needed to maintain blood pressure.
With inoperable or metastatic pheochromocytoma, Inderal may be useful as an adjunct to the management of symptoms due to excessive beta-receptor stimulation.

CONTRAINDICATIONS
Inderal is contraindicated in 1) cardiogenic shock, 2) sinus bradycardia and greater than first degree block, 3) bronchial asthma, 4) congestive heart failure (see "Warnings") unless the failure is secondary to a tachyarrhythmia treatable with Inderal.

WARNINGS
CARDIAC FAILURE
Sympathetic stimulation may be a vital component supporting circulatory function in patients with congestive heart failure, and its inhibition by beta blockade may precipitate more severe failure. Although beta blockers should be avoided in overt congestive heart failure, if necessary, they can be used with close follow-up in patients with a history of failure who are well compensated and are receiving digitalis and diuretics. Beta-adrenergic blocking agents do not abolish the inotropic action of digitalis on heart muscle. IN PATIENTS WITHOUT A HISTORY OF HEART FAILURE, continued use of beta blockers can, in some cases, lead to cardiac failure. Therefore, at the first sign or symptom of heart failure, the patient should be digitalized and/or treated with diuretics, and the response observed closely, or Inderal should be discontinued (gradually, if possible).

> IN PATIENTS WITH ANGINA PECTORIS, there have been reports of exacerbation of angina and, in some cases, myocardial infarction, following *abrupt* discontinuance of Inderal therapy. Therefore, when discontinuance of Inderal is planned, the dosage should be gradually reduced over at least a few weeks and the patient should be cautioned against interruption or cessation of therapy without the physician's advice. If Inderal therapy is interrupted and exacerbation of angina occurs, it usually is advisable to reinstitute Inderal therapy and take other measures appropriate for the management of unstable angina pectoris. Since coronary artery disease may be unrecognized, it may be prudent to follow the above advice in patients considered at risk of having occult atherosclerotic heart disease who are given propranolol for other indications.

Nonallergic Bronchospasm (e.g., chronic bronchitis, emphysema)
PATIENTS WITH BRONCHOSPASTIC DISEASES SHOULD IN GENERAL NOT RECEIVE BETA BLOCKERS. Inderal should be administered with caution since it may block bronchodilation produced by endogenous and exogenous catecholamine stimulation of beta receptors.

MAJOR SURGERY
The necessity or desirability of withdrawal of beta-blocking therapy prior to major surgery is controversial. It should be noted, however, that the impaired ability of the heart to respond to reflex adrenergic stimuli may augment the risks of general anesthesia and surgical procedures.
Inderal, like other beta blockers, is a competitive inhibitor of beta-receptor agonists and its effects can be reversed by administration of such agents, e.g., dobutamine or isoproterenol. However, such patients may be subject to protracted severe hypotension. Difficulty in starting and maintaining the heartbeat has also been reported with beta blockers.

DIABETES AND HYPOGLYCEMIA
Beta blockers should be used with caution in diabetic patients if a beta-blocking agent is required. Beta blockers may mask tachycardia occurring with hypoglycemia, but other manifestations such as dizziness and sweating may not be significantly affected. Following insulin-induced hypoglycemia, propranolol may cause a delay in the recovery of blood glucose to normal levels.

THYROTOXICOSIS
Beta blockade may mask certain clinical signs of hyperthyroidism. Therefore, abrupt withdrawal of propranolol may be followed by an exacerbation of symptoms of hyperthyroidism, including thyroid storm. Propranolol may change thyroid-function tests, increasing T_4 and reverse T_3 and decreasing T_3.

IN PATIENTS WITH WOLFF-PARKINSON-WHITE SYNDROME, several cases have been reported in which, after propranolol, the tachycardia was replaced by a severe bradycardia requiring a demand pacemaker. In one case this resulted after an initial dose of 5 mg propranolol.

PRECAUTIONS
GENERAL
Propranolol should be used with caution in patients with impaired hepatic or renal function. Inderal is not indicated for the treatment of hypertensive emergencies.
Beta-adrenoreceptor blockade can cause reduction of intraocular pressure. Patients should be told that Inderal may interfere with the glaucoma screening test. Withdrawal may lead to a return of increased intraocular pressure.

CLINICAL LABORATORY TESTS
Elevated blood urea levels in patients with severe heart disease, elevated serum transaminase, alkaline phosphatase, lactate dehydrogenase.

DRUG INTERACTIONS
Patients receiving catecholamine-depleting drugs such as reserpine should be closely observed if Inderal is administered. The added catecholamine-blocking action may produce an excessive reduction of resting sympathetic nervous activity, which may result in hypotension, marked bradycardia, vertigo, syncopal attacks, or orthostatic hypotension. Caution should be exercised when patients receiving a beta blocker are administered a calcium-channel blocking drug, especially intravenous verapamil, for both agents may depress myocardial contractility or atrioventricular conduction. On rare occasions, the concomitant intravenous use of a beta blocker and verapamil has resulted in serious adverse reactions, especially in patients with severe cardiomyopathy, congestive heart failure or recent myocardial infarction. Blunting of the antihypertensive effect of beta-adrenoceptor blocking agents by nonsteroidal anti-inflammatory drugs has been reported.
Hypotension and cardiac arrest have been reported with the concomitant use of propranolol and haloperidol.
Aluminum hydroxide gel greatly reduces intestinal absorption of propranolol.
Ethanol slows the rate of absorption of propranolol.
Phenytoin, phenobarbitone, and *rifampin* accelerate propranolol clearance.
Chlorpromazine, when used concomitantly with propranolol, results in increased plasma levels of both drugs.
Antipyrine and *lidocaine* have reduced clearance when used concomitantly with propranolol.
Thyroxine may result in a lower than expected T_3 concentration when used concomitantly with propranolol.
Cimetidine decreases the hepatic metabolism of propranolol, delaying elimination and increasing blood levels.
Theophylline clearance is reduced when used concomitantly with propranolol.

CARCINOGENESIS, MUTAGENESIS, IMPAIRMENT OF FERTILITY
Long-term studies in animals have been conducted to evaluate toxic effects and carcinogenic potential. In 18-month studies, in both rats and mice, employing doses up to 150 mg/kg/day, there was no evidence of significant drug-induced toxicity. There were no drug-related tumorigenic effects at any of the dosage levels. Reproductive studies in animals did not show any impairment of fertility that was attributable to the drug.

PREGNANCY: PREGNANCY CATEGORY C
In a series of reproduction and developmental toxicology studies, propranolol was given to rats at dosages up to 150 mg/kg/day by gavage or in the diet throughout pregnancy and through lactation. In rats given 150 mg/kg/day (about 10 times the maximum recommended human dose) propranolol was embryotoxic (reduced litter sizes and increased resorption sites). In addition, an unexplained increase in neonatal toxicity (death) was noted at all dosage groups in some of the studies. Maternal toxicity (decreased body weight) was evident at 150 mg/kg/day. Propranolol also was given to rabbits at dosages up to 250 mg/kg/day (approximately 20 times the maximum recommended human dose) throughout pregnancy. No evidence of embryotoxicity was noted. Teratogenicity was not noted in either species.
There are no adequate and well-controlled studies in pregnant women. Intrauterine growth retardation has been reported in neonates whose mothers received propranolol during pregnancy. Neonates whose mothers are receiving propranolol at parturition have exhibited bradycardia, hypoglycemia and respiratory depression. Adequate facilities for monitoring these infants at birth should be available. Inderal should be used during pregnancy only if the potential benefit justifies the potential risk to the fetus.

NURSING MOTHERS
Inderal is excreted in human milk. Caution should be exercised when Inderal is administered to a nursing woman.

PEDIATRIC USE
High serum propranolol levels have been noted in patients with Down's syndrome (trisomy 21), suggesting that the bioavailability of propranolol may be increased in patients with this condition.
Evaluation of the effects of propranolol in children, relative to the drug's efficacy and safety, has not been as systematically performed as in adults. Information is available in the medical literature to allow fair estimates, and specific dosing information has been reasonably studied.
Cardiovascular diseases that are common to adults and children are generally as responsive to propranolol intervention in children as they are in adults.
Adverse reactions are also similar: for example, bronchospasm and congestive heart failure related to propranolol therapy have been reported in children and occur through the same mechanisms as previously described in adults.
The normal echocardiogram evolves through a series of changes as the heart matures during growth and development in children. Should echocardiography be used to moni-

Continued on next page

Wyeth-Ayerst Laboratories—Cont.

tor propranolol therapy in children, the age-related changes in the echocardiogram need to be borne in mind.

ADVERSE REACTIONS

Most adverse effects have been mild and transient and have rarely required the withdrawal of therapy.

CARDIOVASCULAR: Bradycardia; congestive heart failure; intensification of AV block; hypotension; paresthesia of hands; thrombocytopenic purpura; arterial insufficiency, usually of the Raynaud type.

CENTRAL NERVOUS SYSTEM: Light-headedness; mental depression manifested by insomnia, lassitude, weakness, fatigue; reversible mental depression progressing to catatonia; visual disturbances; hallucinations, vivid dreams, an acute reversible syndrome characterized by disorientation for time and place, short-term memory loss, emotional lability, slightly clouded sensorium, and decreased performance on neuropsychometrics. Total daily doses above 160 mg (when administered as divided doses of greater than 80 mg each) may be associated with an increased incidence of fatigue, lethargy, and vivid dreams.

GASTROINTESTINAL: Nausea, vomiting, epigastric distress, abdominal cramping, diarrhea, constipation, mesenteric arterial thrombosis, ischemic colitis.

ALLERGIC: Pharyngitis and agranulocytosis, erythematous rash, fever combined with aching and sore throat, laryngospasm, and respiratory distress.

RESPIRATORY: Bronchospasm.

HEMATOLOGIC: Agranulocytosis, nonthrombocytopenic purpura, thrombocytopenic purpura.

AUTOIMMUNE: In extremely rare instances, systemic lupus erythematosus has been reported.

MISCELLANEOUS: Alopecia, LE-like reactions, psoriasiform rashes, dry eyes, male impotence, and Peyronie's disease have been reported rarely. Oculomucocutaneous reactions involving the skin, serous membranes and conjunctivae reported for a beta blocker (practolol) have not been associated with propranolol.

DOSAGE AND ADMINISTRATION

The dosage range for Inderal is different for each indication.

ORAL

HYPERTENSION—*Dosage must be individualized.*

The usual initial dosage is 40 mg Inderal twice daily, whether used alone or added to a diuretic. Dosage may be increased gradually until adequate blood pressure control is achieved. The usual maintenance dosage is 120 mg to 240 mg per day. In some instances a dosage of 640 mg a day may be required. The time needed for full antihypertensive response to a given dosage is variable and may range from a few days to several weeks.

While twice-daily dosing is effective and can maintain a reduction in blood pressure throughout the day, some patients, especially when lower doses are used, may experience a modest rise in blood pressure toward the end of the 12-hour dosing interval. This can be evaluated by measuring blood pressure near the end of the dosing interval to determine whether satisfactory control is being maintained throughout the day. If control is not adequate, a larger dose, or 3-times-daily therapy may achieve better control.

ANGINA PECTORIS—*Dosage must be individualized.*

Total daily doses of 80 mg to 320 mg, when administered orally, twice a day, three times a day, or four times a day, have been shown to increase exercise tolerance and to reduce ischemic changes in the ECG. If treatment is to be discontinued, reduce dosage gradually over a period of several weeks. (See "Warnings".)

ARRHYTHMIAS—10 mg to 30 mg three or four times daily, before meals and at bedtime.

MYOCARDIAL INFARCTION—The recommended daily dosage is 180 mg to 240 mg per day in divided doses. Although a t.i.d. regimen was used in the Beta-Blocker Heart Attack Trial and a q.i.d. regimen in the Norwegian Multicenter Trial, there is a reasonable basis for the use of either a t.i.d. or b.i.d. regimen (see "Clinical Pharmacology"). The effectiveness and safety of daily dosages greater than 240 mg for prevention of cardiac mortality have not been established. However, higher dosages may be needed to effectively treat coexisting diseases such as angina or hypertension (see above).

MIGRAINE—*Dosage must be individualized.*

The initial oral dose is 80 mg Inderal daily in divided doses. The usual effective dose range is 160 mg to 240 mg per day. The dosage may be increased gradually to achieve optimum migraine prophylaxis. If a satisfactory response is not obtained within four to six weeks after reaching the maximum dose, Inderal therapy should be discontinued. It may be advisable to withdraw the drug gradually over a period of several weeks.

ESSENTIAL TREMOR—*Dosage must be individualized.*

The initial dosage is 40 mg Inderal twice daily. Optimum reduction of essential tremor is usually achieved with a dose

of 120 mg per day. Occasionally, it may be necessary to administer 240 mg to 320 mg per day.

HYPERTROPHIC SUBAORTIC STENOSIS—20 mg to 40 mg three or four times daily, before meals and at bedtime.

PHEOCHROMOCYTOMA—*Preoperatively*—60 mg daily in divided doses for three days prior to surgery, concomitantly with an alpha-adrenergic blocking agent.

—*Management of inoperable tumor*—30 mg daily in divided doses.

USE IN CHILDREN: Intravenous administration of Inderal is not recommended in children. Oral dosage for treating hypertension requires individual titration, beginning with a 1.0 mg per kg (body weight) per day dosage regimen (i.e., 0.5 mg per kg b.i.d.).

The usual pediatric dosage range is 2 mg to 4 mg per kg per day in two equally divided doses (i.e., 1.0 mg per kg b.i.d. to 2.0 mg per kg b.i.d.). Pediatric dosage calculated by weight (recommended) generally produces propranolol plasma levels in a therapeutic range similar to that in adults. On the other hand, pediatric doses calculated on the basis of body surface area (*not* recommended) usually result in plasma levels above the mean adult therapeutic range. Doses above 16 mg per kg per day should not be used in children. If treatment with Inderal is to be discontinued, a gradually decreasing dose titration over a 7- to 14-day period is necessary.

INTRAVENOUS

Parenteral drug products should be inspected visually for particulate matter and discoloration prior to administration, whenever solution and container permit.

Intravenous administration is reserved for life-threatening arrhythmias or those occurring under anesthesia. The usual dose is from 1 mg to 3 mg administered under careful monitoring, e.g., electrocardiographic, central venous pressure. The rate of administration should not exceed 1 mg (1 mL) per minute to diminish the possibility of lowering blood pressure and causing cardiac standstill. Sufficient time should be allowed for the drug to reach the site of action even when a slow circulation is present. If necessary, a second dose may be given after two minutes. Thereafter, additional drug should not be given in less than four hours. Additional Inderal should not be given when the desired alteration in rate and/or rhythm is achieved.

Transference to oral therapy should be made as soon as possible.

The intravenous administration of Inderal has not been evaluated adequately in the management of hypertensive emergencies.

OVERDOSAGE

Inderal is not significantly dialyzable. In the event of overdosage or exaggerated response, the following measures should be employed:

General—If ingestion is or may have been recent, evacuate gastric contents, taking care to prevent pulmonary aspiration.

BRADYCARDIA—ADMINISTER ATROPINE (0.25 mg to 1.0 mg); IF THERE IS NO RESPONSE TO VAGAL BLOCKADE, ADMINISTER ISOPROTERENOL CAUTIOUSLY.

CARDIAC FAILURE—DIGITALIZATION AND DIURETICS.

HYPOTENSION — VASOPRESSORS, *e.g.*, LEVARTERENOL OR EPINEPHRINE (THERE IS EVIDENCE THAT EPINEPHRINE IS THE DRUG OF CHOICE).

BRONCHOSPASM — ADMINISTER ISOPROTERENOL AND AMINOPHYLLINE.

HOW SUPPLIED

Inderal®
(propranolol hydrochloride)
TABLETS

INDERAL 10—Each hexagonal-shaped, orange, scored tablet, embossed with an "I" and imprinted with "INDERAL 10," contains 10 mg propranolol hydrochloride, in bottles of 100 (NDC 0046-0421-81); 1,000 (NDC 0046-0421-91); and 5,000 (NDC 0046-0421-95). Also in Unit Dose packages of 100 (NDC 0046-0421-99).

Store at room temperature (approximately 25° C).
Dispense in a well-closed container as defined in the USP.

INDERAL 20—Each hexagonal-shaped, blue, scored tablet, embossed with an "I" and imprinted with "INDERAL 20", contains 20 mg propranolol hydrochloride, in bottles of 100 (NDC 0046-0422-81); 1,000 (NDC 0046-0422-91); and 5,000 (NDC 0046-0422-95). Also in Unit Dose packages of 100 (NDC 0046-0422-99).

Store at room temperature (approximately 25° C).
Dispense in a well-closed, light-resistant container as defined in the USP.
Protect from light.
Use carton to protect contents from light.

INDERAL 40—Each hexagonal-shaped, green, scored tablet, embossed with an "I" and imprinted with "INDERAL 40," contains 40 mg propranolol hydrochloride, in bottles of 100 (NDC 0046-0424-81); 1,000 (NDC 0046-0424-91); and 5,000 (NDC 0046-0424-95). Also in Unit Dose packages of 100 (NDC 0046-0424-99).

Store at room temperature (approximately 25° C).
Dispense in a well-closed, light-resistant container as defined in the USP.
Protect from light.
Use carton to protect contents from light.

INDERAL 60—Each hexagonal-shaped, pink, scored tablet, embossed with an "I" and imprinted with "INDERAL 60," contains 60 mg propranolol hydrochloride, in bottles of 100 (NDC 0046-0426-81), and 1,000 (NDC 0046-0426-91).

Store at room temperature (approximately 25° C).
Dispense in a well-closed container as defined in the USP.

INDERAL 80—Each hexagonal-shaped, yellow, scored tablet, embossed with an "I" and imprinted with "INDERAL 80", contains 80 mg propranolol hydrochloride, in bottles of 100 (NDC 0046-0428-81); 1,000 (NDC 0046-0428-91); and 5,000 (NDC 0046-0428-95).

Store at room temperature (approximately 25° C).
Dispense in a well-closed container as defined in the USP.

The appearance of these tablets is a registered trademark of Wyeth-Ayerst Laboratories.

INJECTABLE

—Each mL contains 1 mg of propranolol hydrochloride in Water for Injection. The pH is adjusted with citric acid. Supplied as: 1 mL ampuls in boxes of 10 (NDC 0046-3265-10).

Store at room temperature (approximately 25°C).
Protect from freezing or excessive heat.

Shown in Product Identification Guide, page 339

INDERAL® LA ℞
[in'der-al]
(propranolol hydrochloride)
Long-Acting Capsules

Caution: Federal law prohibits dispensing without prescription.

DESCRIPTION

Inderal (propranolol hydrochloride) is a synthetic beta-adrenergic receptor-blocking agent chemically described as 1-(Isopropylamino)-3-(1-naphthyloxy)-2-propanol hydrochloride. Its structural formula is

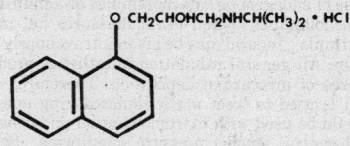

Propranolol hydrochloride is a stable, white, crystalline solid which is readily soluble in water and ethanol. Its molecular weight is 295.81.

Inderal LA is formulated to provide a sustained release of propranolol hydrochloride. Inderal LA is available as 60 mg, 80 mg, 120 mg, and 160 mg capsules.

Inderal LA capsules contain the following inactive ingredients: cellulose, ethylcellulose, gelatin capsules, hydroxypropyl methylcellulose, and titanium dioxide. In addition, Inderal LA 60 mg, 80 mg, and 120 mg capsules contain D&C Red No. 28 and FD&C Blue No. 1; Inderal LA 160 mg capsules contain FD&C Blue No. 1.

These capsules comply with USP Drug Release Test 1.

CLINICAL PHARMACOLOGY

Inderal is a nonselective, beta-adrenergic receptor-blocking agent possessing no other autonomic nervous system activity. It specifically competes with beta-adrenergic receptor-stimulating agents for available receptor sites. When access to beta-receptor sites is blocked by Inderal, the chronotropic, inotropic, and vasodilator responses to beta-adrenergic stimulation are decreased proportionately.

Inderal LA Capsules (60, 80, 120, and 160 mg) release propranolol HCl at a controlled and predictable rate. Peak blood levels following dosing with Inderal LA occur at about 6 hours, and the apparent plasma half-life is about 10 hours. When measured at steady state over a 24-hour period the areas under the propranolol plasma concentration-time curve (AUCs) for the capsules are approximately 60% to 65% of the AUCs for a comparable divided daily dose of Inderal Tablets. The lower AUCs for the capsules are due to greater hepatic metabolism of propranolol, resulting from the slower rate of absorption of propranolol. Over a twenty-four (24) hour period, blood levels are fairly constant for about twelve (12) hours, then decline exponentially.

Inderal LA should not be considered a simple mg-for-mg substitute for conventional propranolol and the blood levels achieved do not match (are lower than) those of two to four times daily dosing with the same dose. When changing to Inderal LA from conventional propranolol, a possible need for retitration upwards should be considered, especially to maintain effectiveness at the end of the dosing interval. In most clinical settings, however, such as hypertension or angina where there is little correlation between plasma levels and clinical effect, Inderal LA has been therapeutically

equivalent to the same mg dose of conventional Inderal as assessed by 24-hour effects on blood pressure and on 24-hour exercise responses of heart rate, systolic pressure, and rate pressure product. Inderal LA can provide effective beta blockade for a 24-hour period.

The mechanism of the antihypertensive effect of Inderal has not been established. Among the factors that may be involved in contributing to the antihypertensive action are: (1) decreased cardiac output, (2) inhibition of renin release by the kidneys, and (3) diminution of tonic sympathetic nerve outflow from vasomotor centers in the brain. Although total peripheral resistance may increase initially, it readjusts to or below the pretreatment level with chronic use. Effects on plasma volume appear to be minor and somewhat variable. Inderal has been shown to cause a small increase in serum potassium concentration when used in the treatment of hypertensive patients.

In angina pectoris, propranolol generally reduces the oxygen requirement of the heart at any given level of effort by blocking the catecholamine-induced increases in the heart rate, systolic blood pressure, and the velocity and extent of myocardial contraction. Propranolol may increase oxygen requirements by increasing left ventricular fiber length, end diastolic pressure, and systolic ejection period. The net physiologic effect of beta-adrenergic blockade is usually advantageous and is manifested during exercise by delayed onset of pain and increased work capacity.

In dosages greater than required for beta blockade, Inderal also exerts a quinidine-like or anesthetic-like membrane action which affects the cardiac action potential. The significance of the membrane action in the treatment of arrhythmias is uncertain.

The mechanism of the antimigraine effect of propranolol has not been established. Beta-adrenergic receptors have been demonstrated in the pial vessels of the brain.

Beta-receptor blockade can be useful in conditions in which, because of pathologic or functional changes, sympathetic activity is detrimental to the patient. But there are also situations in which sympathetic stimulation is vital. For example, in patients with severely damaged hearts, adequate ventricular function is maintained by virtue of sympathetic drive, which should be preserved. In the presence of AV block, greater than first degree, beta blockade may prevent the necessary facilitating effect of sympathetic activity on conduction. Beta blockade results in bronchial constriction by interfering with adrenergic bronchodilator activity, which should be preserved in patients subject to bronchospasm.

Propranolol is not significantly dialyzable.

INDICATIONS AND USAGE
HYPERTENSION
Inderal LA is indicated in the management of hypertension; it may be used alone or used in combination with other antihypertensive agents, particularly a thiazide diuretic. Inderal LA is not indicated in the management of hypertensive emergencies.
ANGINA PECTORIS DUE TO CORONARY ATHEROSCLEROSIS
Inderal LA is indicated for the long-term management of patients with angina pectoris.
MIGRAINE
Inderal LA is indicated for the prophylaxis of common migraine headache. The efficacy of propranolol in the treatment of a migraine attack that has started has not been established and propranolol is not indicated for such use.
HYPERTROPHIC SUBAORTIC STENOSIS
Inderal LA is useful in the management of hypertrophic subaortic stenosis, especially for treatment of exertional or other stress-induced angina, palpitations, and syncope. Inderal LA also improves exercise performance. The effectiveness of propranolol hydrochloride in this disease appears to be due to a reduction of the elevated outflow pressure gradient which is exacerbated by beta-receptor stimulation. Clinical improvement may be temporary.

CONTRAINDICATIONS
Inderal is contraindicated in 1) cardiogenic shock; 2) sinus bradycardia and greater than first-degree block; 3) bronchial asthma; 4) congestive heart failure (see WARNINGS) unless the failure is secondary to a tachyarrhythmia treatable with Inderal.

WARNINGS
CARDIAC FAILURE: Sympathetic stimulation may be a vital component supporting circulatory function in patients with congestive heart failure, and its inhibition by beta blockade may precipitate more severe failure. Although beta blockers should be avoided in overt congestive heart failure, if necessary, they can be used with close follow-up in patients with a history of failure who are well compensated and are receiving digitalis and diuretics. Beta-adrenergic blocking agents do not abolish the inotropic action of digitalis on heart muscle.

IN PATIENTS WITHOUT A HISTORY OF HEART FAILURE, continued use of beta blockers can, in some cases, lead to cardiac failure. Therefore, at the first sign or symptom of heart failure, the patient should be digitalized and/or treated with diuretics, and the response observed closely, or Inderal should be discontinued (gradually, if possible).

IN PATIENTS WITH ANGINA PECTORIS, there have been reports of exacerbation of angina and, in some cases, myocardial infarction, following *abrupt* discontinuance of Inderal therapy. Therefore, when discontinuance of Inderal is planned, the dosage should be gradually reduced over at least a few weeks, and the patient should be cautioned against interruption or cessation of therapy without the physician's advice. If Inderal therapy is interrupted and exacerbation of angina occurs, it usually is advisable to reinstitute Inderal therapy and take other measures appropriate for the management of unstable angina pectoris. Since coronary artery disease may be unrecognized, it may be prudent to follow the above advice in patients considered at risk of having occult atherosclerotic heart disease who are given propranolol for other indications.

NONALLERGIC BRONCHOSPASM (e.g., CHRONIC BRONCHITIS, EMPHYSEMA)—PATIENTS WITH BRONCHOSPASTIC DISEASES SHOULD IN GENERAL NOT RECEIVE BETA BLOCKERS. INDERAL should be administered with caution since it may block bronchodilation produced by endogenous and exogenous catecholamine stimulation of beta receptors.

MAJOR SURGERY: The necessity or desirability of withdrawal of beta-blocking therapy prior to major surgery is controversial. It should be noted, however, that the impaired ability of the heart to respond to reflex adrenergic stimuli may augment the risks of general anesthesia and surgical procedures.

Inderal, like other beta blockers, is a competitive inhibitor of beta-receptor agonists and its effects can be reversed by administration of such agents, e.g., dobutamine or isoproterenol. However, such patients may be subject to protracted severe hypotension. Difficulty in starting and maintaining the heartbeat has also been reported with beta blockers.

DIABETES AND HYPOGLYCEMIA: Beta blockers should be used with caution in diabetic patients if a beta-blocking agent is required. Beta blockers may mask tachycardia occurring with hypoglycemia, but other manifestations such as dizziness and sweating may not be significantly affected. Following insulin-induced hypoglycemia, propranolol may cause a delay in the recovery of blood glucose to normal levels.

THYROTOXICOSIS: Beta blockade may mask certain clinical signs of hyperthyroidism. Therefore, abrupt withdrawal of propranolol may be followed by an exacerbation of symptoms of hyperthyroidism, including thyroid storm. Propranolol may change thyroid-function tests, increasing T_4 and reverse T_3, and decreasing T_3.

IN PATIENTS WITH WOLFF-PARKINSON-WHITE SYNDROME, several cases have been reported in which, after propranolol, the tachycardia was replaced by a severe bradycardia requiring a demand pacemaker. In one case this resulted after an initial dose of 5 mg propranolol.

PRECAUTIONS
GENERAL
Propranolol should be used with caution in patients with impaired hepatic or renal function. Inderal is not indicated for the treatment of hypertensive emergencies.

Beta-adrenoreceptor blockade can cause reduction of intraocular pressure. Patients should be told that Inderal may interfere with the glaucoma screening test. Withdrawal may lead to a return of increased intraocular pressure.

CLINICAL LABORATORY TESTS
Elevated blood urea levels in patients with severe heart disease, elevated serum transaminase, alkaline phosphatase, lactate dehydrogenase.

DRUG INTERACTIONS
Patients receiving catecholamine-depleting drugs such as reserpine should be closely observed if Inderal is administered. The added catecholamine-blocking action may produce an excessive reduction of resting sympathetic nervous activity, which may result in hypotension, marked bradycardia, vertigo, syncopal attacks, or orthostatic hypotension.

Caution should be exercised when patients receiving a beta blocker are administered a calcium-channel-blocking drug, especially intravenous verapamil, for both agents may depress myocardial contractility or atrioventricular conduction. On rare occasions, the concomitant intravenous use of a beta blocker and verapamil has resulted in serious adverse reactions, especially in patients with severe cardiomyopathy, congestive heart failure or recent myocardial infarction.

Blunting of the antihypertensive effect of beta-adrenoceptor blocking agents by nonsteroidal anti-inflammatory drugs has been reported.

Hypotension and cardiac arrest have been reported with the concomitant use of propranolol and haloperidol.

Aluminum hydroxide gel greatly reduces intestinal absorption of propranolol.

Ethanol slows the rate of absorption of propranolol.

Phenytoin, phenobarbitone, and *rifampin* accelerate propranolol clearance.

Chlorpromazine, when used concomitantly with propranolol, results in increased plasma levels of both drugs.

Antipyrine and *lidocaine* have reduced clearance when used concomitantly with propranolol.

Thyroxine may result in a lower than expected T_3 concentration when used concomitantly with propranolol.

Cimetidine decreases the hepatic metabolism of propranolol, delaying elimination and increasing blood levels.

Theophylline clearance is reduced when used concomitantly with propranolol.

CARCINOGENESIS, MUTAGENESIS, IMPAIRMENT OF FERTILITY
Long-term studies in animals have been conducted to evaluate toxic effects and carcinogenic potential. In 18-month studies, in both rats and mice, employing doses up to 150 mg/kg/day, there was no evidence of significant drug-induced toxicity. There were no drug-related tumorigenic effects at any of the dosage levels. Reproductive studies in animals did not show any impairment of fertility that was attributable to the drug.

PREGNANCY: PREGNANCY CATEGORY C
In a series of reproduction and developmental toxicology studies, propranolol was given to rats at dosages up to 150 mg/kg/day by gavage or in the diet throughout pregnancy and through lactation. In rats given 150 mg/kg/day (about 10 times the maximum recommended human dose) propranolol was embryotoxic (reduced litter sizes and increased resorption sites). In addition, an unexplained increase in neonatal toxicity (death) was noted at all dosage groups in some of the studies. Maternal toxicity (decreased body weight) was evident at 150 mg/kg/day. Propranolol also was given to rabbits at dosages up to 250 mg/kg/day (approximately 20 times the maximum recommended human dose) throughout pregnancy. No evidence of embryotoxicity was noted. Teratogenicity was not noted in either species.

There are no adequate and well-controlled studies in pregnant women. Intrauterine growth retardation has been reported in neonates whose mothers received propranolol during pregnancy. Neonates whose mothers are receiving propranolol at parturition have exhibited bradycardia, hypoglycemia and respiratory depression. Adequate facilities for monitoring these infants at birth should be available. Inderal should be used during pregnancy only if the potential benefit justifies the potential risk to the fetus.

NURSING MOTHERS
Inderal is excreted in human milk. Caution should be exercised when Inderal is administered to a nursing woman.

PEDIATRIC USE
Safety and effectiveness in pediatric patients have not been established.

ADVERSE REACTIONS
Most adverse effects have been mild and transient and have rarely required the withdrawal of therapy.

CARDIOVASCULAR: Bradycardia; congestive heart failure; intensification of AV block; hypotension; paresthesia of hands; thrombocytopenic purpura; arterial insufficiency, usually of the Raynaud type.

CENTRAL NERVOUS SYSTEM: Light-headedness, mental depression manifested by insomnia, lassitude, weakness, fatigue; reversible mental depression progressing to catatonia; visual disturbances; hallucinations; vivid dreams; an acute reversible syndrome characterized by disorientation for time and place, short-term memory loss, emotional lability, slightly clouded sensorium, and decreased performance on neuropsychometrics. For immediate formulations, fatigue, lethargy, and vivid dreams appear dose related.

GASTROINTESTINAL: Nausea, vomiting, epigastric distress, abdominal cramping, diarrhea, constipation, mesenteric arterial thrombosis, ischemic colitis.

ALLERGIC: Pharyngitis and agranulocytosis; erythematous rash, fever combined with aching and sore throat; laryngospasm, and respiratory distress.

RESPIRATORY: Bronchospasm.

HEMATOLOGIC: Agranulocytosis, nonthrombocytopenic purpura, thrombocytopenic purpura.

AUTOIMMUNE: In extremely rare instances, systemic lupus erythematosus has been reported.

MISCELLANEOUS: Alopecia; LE-like reactions; psoriasiform rashes; dry eyes; male impotence; and Peyronie's disease have been reported rarely. Oculomucocutaneous reactions involving the skin, serous membranes and conjunctivae reported for a beta blocker (practolol) have not been associated with propranolol.

DOSAGE AND ADMINISTRATION
Inderal LA provides propranolol hydrochloride in a sustained-release capsule for administration once daily. If patients are switched from Inderal Tablets to Inderal LA Capsules, care should be taken to assure that the desired therapeutic effect is maintained. Inderal LA should not be consid-

Continued on next page

Wyeth-Ayerst Laboratories—Cont.

ered a simple mg-for-mg substitute for Inderal. Inderal LA has different kinetics and produces lower blood levels. Retitration may be necessary, especially to maintain effectiveness at the end of the 24-hour dosing interval.

HYPERTENSION

Dosage must be individualized. The usual initial dosage is 80 mg Inderal LA once daily, whether used alone or added to a diuretic. The dosage may be increased to 120 mg once daily or higher until adequate blood pressure control is achieved. The usual maintenance dosage is 120 to 160 mg once daily. In some instances a dosage of 640 mg may be required. The time needed for full hypertensive response to a given dosage is variable and may range from a few days to several weeks.

ANGINA PECTORIS

Dosage must be individualized. Starting with 80 mg Inderal LA once daily, dosage should be gradually increased at three- to seven-day intervals until optimal response is obtained. Although individual patients may respond at any dosage level, the average optimal dosage appears to be 160 mg once daily. In angina pectoris, the value and safety of dosage exceeding 320 mg per day have not been established.

If treatment is to be discontinued, reduce dosage gradually over a period of a few weeks (see WARNINGS).

MIGRAINE

Dosage must be individualized. The initial oral dose is 80 mg Inderal LA once daily. The usual effective dose range is 160 to 240 mg once daily. The dosage may be increased gradually to achieve optimal migraine prophylaxis. If a satisfactory response is not obtained within four to six weeks after reaching the maximal dose, Inderal LA therapy should be discontinued. It may be advisable to withdraw the drug gradually over a period of several weeks.

HYPERTROPHIC SUBAORTIC STENOSIS

80 to 160 mg Inderal LA once daily.

PEDIATRIC DOSAGE

At this time the data on the use of the drug in this age group are too limited to permit adequate directions for use.

Overdosage

Inderal is not significantly dialyzable. In the event of overdosage or exaggerated response, the following measures should be employed:

GENERAL

If ingestion is, or may have been, recent, evacuate gastric contents, taking care to prevent pulmonary aspiration.

BRADYCARDIA

ADMINISTER ATROPINE (0.25 to 1.0 mg); IF THERE IS NO RESPONSE TO VAGAL BLOCKADE, ADMINISTER ISOPROTERENOL CAUTIOUSLY.

CARDIAC FAILURE

DIGITALIZATION AND DIURETICS.

HYPOTENSION

VASOPRESSORS, e.g., LEVARTERENOL OR EPINEPHRINE (THERE IS EVIDENCE THAT EPINEPHRINE IS THE DRUG OF CHOICE).

BRONCHOSPASM

ADMINISTER ISOPROTERENOL AND AMINOPHYLLINE.

HOW SUPPLIED

Inderal® LA Capsules (propranolol hydrochloride)

Each white/light-blue capsule, identified by 3 narrow bands, 1 wide band, and "INDERAL LA 60," contains 60 mg of propranolol hydrochloride in bottles of 100 (NDC 0046-0470-81) and in bottles of 1,000 (NDC 0046-0470-91).

Each light-blue capsule, identified by 3 narrow bands, 1 wide band, and "INDERAL LA 80," contains 80 mg of propranolol hydrochloride in bottles of 100 (NDC 0046-0471-81) and in bottles of 1,000 (NDC 0046-0471-91). Also available in a Unit Dose package of 100 (NDC 0046-0471-99).

Each light-blue/dark-blue capsule, identified by 3 narrow bands, 1 wide band, and "INDERAL LA 120," contains 120 mg of propranolol hydrochloride in bottles of 100 (NDC 0046-0473-81) and in bottles of 1,000 (NDC 0046-0473-91). Also available in a Unit Dose package of 100 (NDC 0046-0473-99).

Each dark-blue capsule, identified by 3 narrow bands, 1 wide band, and "INDERAL LA 160," contains 160 mg of propranolol hydrochloride in bottles of 100 (NDC 0046-0479-81) and in bottles of 1,000 (NDC 0046-0479-91). Also available in a Unit Dose package of 100 (NDC 0046-0479-99).

The appearance of these capsules is a registered trademark of Wyeth-Ayerst Laboratories.

Store at room temperature (approximately 25° C).

Protect from light, moisture, freezing, and excessive heat.

Dispense in a tight, light-resistant container as defined in the USP.

Use carton to protect contents from light.

Shown in Product Identification Guide, page 339

INDERIDE® ℞

[*in 'de-rīde*]

(propranolol hydrochloride [INDERAL®] and hydrochlorothiazide)

Caution: Federal law prohibits dispensing without prescription.

DESCRIPTION

Inderide Tablets for oral administration combine two antihypertensive agents: Inderal (propranolol hydrochloride), a beta-adrenergic blocking agent, and hydrochlorothiazide, a thiazide diuretic-antihypertensive. Inderide 40/25 Tablets contain 40 mg propranolol hydrochloride and 25 mg hydrochlorothiazide; Inderide 80/25 Tablets contain 80 mg propranolol hydrochloride and 25 mg hydrochlorothiazide.

Inderal (propranolol hydrochloride) is a synthetic beta-adrenergic receptor-blocking agent chemically described as 1-(Isopropylamino)-3-(1-naphthyloxy)-2-propanol hydrochloride. Its structural formula is:

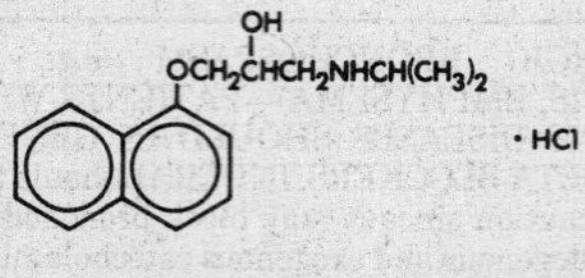

OH
OCH2CHCH2NHCH(CH3)2
· HCl

Propranolol hydrochloride is a stable, white, crystalline solid which is readily soluble in water and ethanol. Its molecular weight is 295.81.

Hydrochlorothiazide is a white, or practically white, practically odorless, crystalline powder. It is slightly soluble in water; freely soluble in sodum hydroxide solution; sparingly soluble in methanol; insoluble in ether, chloroform, benzene, and dilute mineral acids. Its chemical name is: 6-Chloro-3,4-dihydro-2H-1,2,4-benzothiadiazine-7-sulfonamide 1,1-dioxide. Its structural formula is:

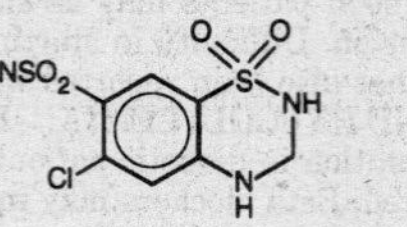

H2NSO2
Cl
NH
N
H

The inactive ingredients contained in Inderide Tablets are lactose, magnesium stearate, microcrystalline cellulose, stearic acid, and yellow ferric oxide.

CLINICAL PHARMACOLOGY

Propranolol hydrochloride (Inderal®)

Propranolol hydrochloride is a nonselective beta-adrenergic receptor blocking agent possessing no other autonomic nervous system activity. It specifically competes with beta-adrenergic receptor stimulating agents for available receptor sites. When access to beta-receptor sites is blocked by propranolol, the chronotropic, inotropic, and vasodilator responses to beta-adrenergic stimulation are decreased proportionately.

Propranolol is almost completely absorbed from the gastrointestinal tract, but a portion is immediately metabolized by the liver on its first pass through the portal circulation.

Peak effect occurs in one to one-and-one-half hours. The biologic half-life is approximately four hours. Propranolol is not significantly dialyzable. There is no simple correlation between dose or plasma level and therapeutic effect, and the dose-sensitivity range, as observed in clinical practice, is wide. The principal reason for this is that sympathetic tone varies widely between individuals. Since there is no reliable test to estimate sympathetic tone or to determine whether total beta blockade has been achieved, proper dosage requires titration.

The mechanism of the antihypertensive effects of propranolol has not been established. Among the factors that may be involved in contributing to the antihypertensive action are (1) decreased cardiac output, (2) inhibition of renin release by the kidneys, and (3) diminution of tonic sympathetic nerve outflow from vasomotor centers in the brain. Although total peripheral resistance may increase initially, it readjusts to, or below, the pretreatment level with chronic use. Effects on plasma volume appear to be minor and somewhat variable.

Propranolol has been shown to cause a small increase in serum potassium concentration when used in the treatment of hypertensive patients. Propranolol hydrochloride decreases heart rate, cardiac output, and blood pressure.

Beta-receptor blockade can be useful in conditions in which, because of pathologic or functional changes, sympathetic activity is detrimental to the patient. But there are also situations in which sympathetic stimulation is vital. For example, in patients with severely damaged hearts, adequate ventricular function is maintained by virtue of sympathetic drive, which should be preserved. In the presence of AV block greater than first degree, beta blockade may prevent the necessary facilitating effect of sympathetic activity on conduction. Beta blockade results in bronchial constriction by interfering with adrenergic bronchodilator activity, which should be preserved in patients subject to bronchospasm.

The proper objective of beta-blockade therapy is to decrease adverse sympathetic stimulation, but not to the degree that may impair necessary sympathetic support.

Hydrochlorothiazide

Hydrochlorothiazide is a benzothiadiazine (thiazide) diuretic closely related to chlorothiazide. The mechanism of the antihypertensive effect of the thiazides is unknown. Thiazides do not affect normal blood pressure.

Thiazides affect the renal tubular mechanism of electrolyte reabsorption. At maximal therapeutic dosage, all thiazides are approximately equal in their diuretic potency.

Thiazides increase excretion of sodium and chloride in approximately equivalent amounts. Natriuresis causes a secondary loss of potassium and bicarbonate. Onset of diuretic action of hydrochlorothiazide occurs in two hours, and the peak effect in about four hours. Its action persists for approximately six to 12 hours. Thiazides are eliminated rapidly by the kidney.

INDICATIONS AND USAGE

Inderide is indicated in the management of hypertension.

This fixed combination is not indicated for initial therapy of hypertension. Hypertension requires therapy titrated to the individual patient. If the fixed combination represents the dosage so determined, its use may be more convenient in patient management.

CONTRAINDICATIONS

Propranolol hydrochloride (Inderal®)

Propranolol is contraindicated in: 1) cardiogenic shock; 2) sinus bradycardia and greater than first-degree block; 3) bronchial asthma; 4) congestive heart failure (see WARNINGS) unless the failure is secondary to a tachyarrhythmia treatable with propranolol.

Hydrochlorothiazide

Hydrochlorothiazide is contraindicated in patients with anuria or hypersensitivity to this or other sulfonamide-derived drugs.

WARNINGS

Propranolol hydrochloride (Inderal®)

CARDIAC FAILURE: Sympathetic stimulation is a vital component supporting circulatory function in congestive heart failure, and inhibition with beta blockade always carries the potential hazard of further depressing myocardial contractility and precipitating cardiac failure. Propranolol acts selectively without abolishing the inotropic action of digitalis on the heart muscle (i.e., that of supporting the strength of myocardial contractions). In patients already receiving digitalis, the positive inotropic action of digitalis may be reduced by propranolol's negative inotropic effect. The effects of propranolol and digitalis are additive in depressing AV conduction.

PATIENTS WITHOUT A HISTORY OF HEART FAILURE: Continued depression of the myocardium over a period of time can, in some cases, lead to cardiac failure. In rare instances, this has been observed during propranolol therapy. Therefore, at the first sign or symptom of impending cardiac failure, patients should be fully digitalized and/or given additional diuretic, and the response observed closely: a) if cardiac failure continues, despite adequate digitalization and diuretic therapy, propranolol therapy should be withdrawn (gradually, if possible); b) if tachyarrhythmia is being controlled, patients should be maintained on combined therapy and the patient closely followed until threat of cardiac failure is over.

ANGINA PECTORIS: There have been reports of exacerbation of angina and, in some cases, myocardial infarction following *abrupt* discontinuation of propranolol therapy. Therefore, when discontinuance of propranolol is planned, the dosage should be gradually reduced and the patient should be carefully monitored. In addition, when propranolol is prescribed for angina pectoris, the patient should be cautioned against interruption or cessation of therapy without the physician's advice. If propranolol therapy is interrupted and exacerbation of angina occurs, it usually is advisable to reinstitute propranolol therapy and take other measures appropriate for the management of unstable angina pectoris. Since coronary artery disease may be unrecognized, it may be prudent to follow the above advice in patients considered at risk of having occult atherosclerotic heart disease, who are given propranolol for other indications.

NONALLERGIC BRONCHOSPASM (e.g., chronic bronchitis, emphysema): PATIENTS WITH BRONCHOSPASTIC DISEASES SHOULD, IN GENERAL, NOT RECEIVE BETA BLOCKERS. Propranolol should be administered with caution since it may block bronchodilation produced by endogenous and exogenous catecholamine stimulation of beta receptors.

MAJOR SURGERY: The necessity or desirability of withdrawal of beta-blocking therapy prior to major surgery is

controversial. It should be noted, however, that the impaired ability of the heart to respond to reflex adrenergic stimuli may augment the risks of general anesthesia and surgical procedures.

Propranolol, like other beta blockers, is a competitive inhibitor of beta-receptor agonists, and its effects can be reversed by administration of such agents, e.g., dobutamine or isoproterenol. However, such patients may be subject to protracted severe hypotension. Difficulty in starting and maintaining the heartbeat has also been reported with beta blockers.

DIABETES AND HYPOGLYCEMIA: Beta blockers should be used with caution in diabetic patients if a beta-blocking agent is required. Beta blockers may mask tachycardia occurring with hypoglycemia, but other manifestations such as dizziness and sweating may not be significantly affected. Following insulin-induced hypoglycemia, propranolol may cause a delay in the recovery of blood glucose to normal levels.

THYROTOXICOSIS: Beta blockade may mask certain clinical signs of hyperthyroidism. Therefore, abrupt withdrawal of propranolol may be followed by an exacerbation of symptoms of hyperthyroidism, including thyroid storm. Propranolol may change thyroid-function tests, increasing T_4 and reverse T_3, and decreasing T_3.

WOLFF-PARKINSON-WHITE SYNDROME: Several cases have been reported in which, after propranolol, the tachycardia was replaced by a severe bradycardia requiring a demand pacemaker. In one case this resulted after an initial dose of 5 mg propranolol.

Hydrochlorothiazide

Thiazides should be used with caution in severe renal disease. In patients with renal disease, thiazides may precipitate azotemia. In patients with impaired renal function, cumulative effects of the drug may develop.

Thiazides should also be used with caution in patients with impaired hepatic function or progressive liver disease, since minor alterations of fluid and electrolyte balance may precipitate hepatic coma.

Thiazides may add to or potentiate the action of other antihypertensive drugs. Potentiation occurs with ganglionic or peripheral adrenergic-blocking drugs.

Sensitivity reactions may occur in patients with a history of allergy or bronchial asthma. The possibility of exacerbation or activation of systemic lupus erythematosus has been reported.

PRECAUTIONS
GENERAL
Propranolol hydrochloride (Inderal®)

Propranolol should be used with caution in patients with impaired hepatic or renal function. Inderide is not indicated for the treatment of hypertensive emergencies.

Hydrochlorothiazide

All patients receiving thiazide therapy should be observed for clinical signs of fluid or electrolyte imbalance, namely hyponatremia, hypochloremic alkalosis, and hypokalemia. Serum and urine electrolyte determinations are particularly important when the patient is vomiting excessively or receiving parenteral fluids. Medication such as digitalis may also influence serum electrolytes. Warning signs, irrespective of cause, are: dryness of mouth, thirst, weakness, lethargy, drowsiness, restlessness, muscle pains or cramps, muscular fatigue, hypotension, oliguria, tachycardia, and gastrointestinal disturbances such as nausea and vomiting.

Hypokalemia may develop, especially with brisk diuresis or when severe cirrhosis is present.

Interference with adequate oral electrolyte intake will also contribute to hypokalemia. Hypokalemia can sensitize or exaggerate the response of the heart to the toxic effects of digitalis (e.g., increased ventricular irritability).

Hypokalemia may be avoided or treated by use of potassium supplements or foods with a high potassium content.

Any chloride deficit is generally mild, and usually does not require specific treatment except under extraordinary circumstances (as in liver or renal disease). Dilutional hyponatremia may occur in edematous patients in hot weather; appropriate therapy is water restriction rather than administration of salt, except in rare instances when the hyponatremia is life-threatening. In actual salt depletion, appropriate replacement is the therapy of choice.

Hyperuricemia may occur or frank gout may be precipitated in certain patients receiving thiazide therapy.

Diabetes mellitus which has been latent may become manifest during thiazide administration.

The antihypertensive effects of the drug may be enhanced in the postsympathectomy patient.

If progressive renal impairment becomes evident, consider withholding or discontinuing diuretic therapy.

Calcium excretion is decreased by thiazides. Pathologic changes in the parathyroid gland with hypercalcemia and hypophosphatemia have been observed in a few patients on prolonged thiazide therapy. The common complications of hyperparathyroidism, such as renal lithiasis, bone resorption, and peptic ulceration, have not been seen.

INFORMATION FOR PATIENTS

Beta-adrenoreceptor blockade can cause reduction of intraocular pressure. Patients should be told that Inderide may interfere with the glaucoma screening test. Withdrawal may lead to a return of increased intraocular pressure.

LABORATORY TESTS
Propranolol hydrochloride (Inderal®)

Elevated blood urea levels in patients with severe heart disease, elevated serum transaminase, alkaline phosphatase, lactate dehydrogenase.

Hydrochlorothiazide

Periodic determination of serum electrolytes to detect possible electrolyte imbalance should be performed at appropriate intervals.

DRUG/DRUG INTERACTIONS
Propranolol hydrochloride (Inderal®)

Patients receiving catecholamine-depleting drugs such as reserpine should be closely observed if Inderide is administered. The added catecholamine-blocking action may produce an excessive reduction of resting sympathetic nervous activity, which may result in hypotension, marked bradycardia, vertigo, syncopal attacks, or orthostatic hypotension. Caution should be exercised when patients receiving a beta blocker are administered a calcium-channel blocking drug, especially intravenous verapamil, for both agents may depress myocardial contractility or atrioventricular conduction. On rare occasions, the concomitant intravenous use of a beta blocker and verapamil has resulted in serious adverse reactions, especially in patients with severe cardiomyopathy, congestive heart failure, or recent myocardial infarction.

Blunting of the antihypertensive effect of beta-adrenoceptor blocking agents by nonsteroidal anti-inflammatory drugs has been reported.

Hypotension and coronary arrest have been reported with the concomitant use of propranolol and haloperidol.

Aluminum hydroxide gel greatly reduces intestinal absorption of propranolol.

Ethanol slows the rate of absorption of propranolol.

Phenytoin, phenobarbitone, and rifampin accelerate propranolol clearance.

Chlorpromazine, when used concomitantly with propranolol, results in increased plasma levels of both drugs.

Antipyrine and *lidocaine* have reduced clearance when used concomitantly with propranolol.

Thyroxine may result in a lower than expected T_3 concentration when used concomitantly with propranolol.

Cimetidine decreases the hepatic metabolism of propranolol, delaying elimination and increasing blood levels.

Theophylline clearance is reduced when used concomitantly with propranolol.

Hydrochlorothiazide

Thiazide drugs may increase the responsiveness to tubocurarine.

Thiazides may decrease arterial responsiveness to norepinephrine. This diminution is not sufficient to preclude effectiveness of the pressor agent for therapeutic use.

Insulin requirements in diabetic patients may be increased, decreased, or unchanged.

Hypokalemia may develop during concomitant use of corticosteroids or ACTH.

DRUG/LABORATORY TEST INTERACTIONS
Hydrochlorothiazide

Thiazides may decrease serum PBI levels without signs of thyroid disturbance.

Thiazides should be discontinued before carrying out tests for parathyroid function (see "PRECAUTIONS—GENERAL").

CARCINOGENESIS, MUTAGENESIS, IMPAIRMENT OF FERTILITY
Propranolol hydrochloride (Inderal®)

Long-term studies in animals have been conducted to evaluate toxic effects and carcinogenic potential. In 18-month studies in both rats and mice, employing doses up to 150 mg/kg/day, there was no evidence of significant drug-induced toxicity. There were no drug-related tumorigenic effects at any of the dosage levels. Reproductive studies in animals did not show any impairment of fertility that was attributable to the drug. Long-term studies in animals have not been conducted to evaluate the toxic effects and carcinogenic potential of Inderide.

Hydrochlorothiazide

Hydrochlorothiazide is presently under study for carcinogenesis in rats and mice in the National Toxicology Research and Testing Program.

Hydrochlorothiazide was not mutagenic in *in vitro* Ames mutagenicity assays of *Salmonella typhimurium* strains TA 98, TA 100, TA 1535, TA 1537, and TA 1538 or in *in vivo* mutagenicity assays of mouse germinal-cell chromosomes and Chinese hamster bone-marrow-cell chromosomes. It was, however, mutagenic in inducing nondisjunction (96% frequency) in diploid strains of *Aspergillus nidulans.*

Hydrochlorothiazide had no adverse effect on fertility in rats at a dose 4 times the Maximum Recommended Human Dose (MRHD) and in mice at a dose equivalent to 100 times the MRHD (1 mg/kg, assumed body weight of 50 kg).

PREGNANCY: PREGNANCY CATEGORY C
Propranolol hydrochloride (Inderal®)

In a series of reproduction and developmental toxicology studies, propranolol was given to rats at dosages up to 150 mg/kg/day by gavage or in the diet throughout pregnancy and through lactation. In rats given 150 mg/kg/day (about 10 times the maximum recommended human dose of propranolol alone or about 30 times the maximum recommended human dose of the combined propranolol/hydrochlorothiazide product) propranolol was embryotoxic (reduced litter sizes and increased resorption sites). In addition, an unexplained increase in neonatal toxicity (death) was noted in all dosage groups in some of the studies. Maternal toxicity (decreased body weight) was evident at 150 mg/kg/day. Propranolol also was given to rabbits at dosages up to 250 mg/kg/day (approximately 20 times the maximum recommended human dose of propranolol) throughout pregnancy. No evidence of embryotoxicity was noted. Teratogenicity was not noted in either species. There are no adequate and well-controlled studies in pregnant women. Intrauterine growth retardation has been reported in neonates whose mothers received propranolol during pregnancy. Neonates whose mothers are receiving propranolol at parturition have exhibited bradycardia, hypoglycemia and respiratory depression. Adequate facilities for monitoring these infants at birth should be available. Propranolol should be used during pregnancy only if the potential benefit justifies the potential risk to the fetus.

Hydrochlorothiazide

Thiazides cross the placental barrier and appear in cord blood. The use of thiazides in pregnant women requires that the anticipated benefit be weighed against possible hazards to the fetus. These hazards include fetal or neonatal jaundice, thrombocytopenia, and possibly other adverse reactions which have occurred in the adult.

Available information indicates that hydrochlorothiazide at doses as high as 1320 times the MRHD was not teratogenic in pregnant rats.

NURSING MOTHERS
Propranolol hydrochloride (Inderal®)

Propranolol is excreted in human milk. Caution should be exercised when Inderide is administered to a nursing woman.

Hydrochlorothiazide

Thiazides appear in breast milk. If the use of drug is deemed essential, the patient should stop nursing.

PEDIATRIC USE

Safety and effectiveness in pediatric patients have not been established.

ADVERSE REACTIONS

The following adverse reactions have been observed, but there is not enough systematic collection of data to support an estimate of their frequency. Within each category, adverse reactions are listed in decreasing order of severity. Although many side effects are mild and transient, some require discontinuation of therapy.

Propranolol hydrochloride (Inderal®)

Cardiovascular: Congestive heart failure; hypotension; intensification of AV block; bradycardia; thrombocytopenic purpura; arterial insufficiency, usually of the Raynaud type; paresthesia of hands.

Central Nervous System: Reversible mental depression progressing to catatonia; mental depression manifested by insomnia, lassitude, weakness, fatigue; an acute reversible syndrome characterized by disorientation for time and place, short-term memory loss, emotional lability, slightly clouded sensorium, decreased performance on neuropsychometrics; hallucinations; visual disturbances; vivid dreams; lightheadedness. Total daily doses above 160 mg (when administered as divided doses of greater than 80 mg each) may be associated with an increased incidence of fatigue, lethargy, and vivid dreams.

Gastrointestinal: Mesenteric arterial thrombosis; ischemic colitis; nausea, vomiting, epigastric distress, abdominal cramping, diarrhea, constipation.

Allergic: Laryngospasm and respiratory distress; pharyngitis and agranulocytosis; fever combined with aching and sore throat; erythematous rash.

Respiratory: Bronchospasm.

Hematologic: Agranulocytosis; nonthrombocytopenic purpura; thrombocytopenic purpura.

Autoimmune: In extremely rare instances, systemic lupus erythematosus has been reported.

Miscellaneous: Male impotence. Alopecia, LE-like reactions, psoriasiform rashes, dry eyes, and Peyronie's disease have been reported rarely. Oculomucocutaneous reactions involving the skin, serous membranes, and conjunctivae reported for a beta blocker (practolol) have not been associated with propranolol.

Hydrochlorothiazide

Cardiovascular: Orthostatic hypotension (may be aggravated by alcohol, barbiturates or narcotics).

Continued on next page

Wyeth-Ayerst Laboratories—Cont.

Central Nervous System: Dizziness, vertigo, headache, xanthopsia, paresthesias.
Gastrointestinal: Pancreatitis; jaundice (intrahepatic cholestatic jaundice); sialadenitis; anorexia, nausea, vomiting, gastric irritation, cramping, diarrhea, constipation.
Hypersensitivity: Anaphylactic reactions; necrotizing angiitis (vasculitis, cutaneous vasculitis); respiratory distress including pneumonitis; fever; urticaria, rash, purpura, photosensitivity.
Hematologic: Aplastic anemia, agranulocytosis, leukopenia, thrombocytopenia.
Miscellaneous: Hyperglycemia, glycosuria; hyperuricemia; muscle spasm; weakness; restlessness; transient blurred vision.
Whenever adverse reactions are moderate or severe, thiazide dosage should be reduced or therapy withdrawn.

OVERDOSAGE

The propranolol hydrochloride component may cause bradycardia, cardiac failure, hypotension, or bronchospasm. Propranolol is not significantly dialyzable.
The hydrochlorothiazide component can be expected to cause diuresis. Lethargy of varying degree may appear and may progress to coma within a few hours, with minimal depression of respiration and cardiovascular function, and in the absence of significant serum electrolyte changes or dehydration. The mechanism of central nervous system depression with thiazide overdosage is unknown. Gastrointestinal irritation and hypermotility can occur, temporary elevation of BUN has been reported, and serum electrolyte changes could occur, especially in patients with impairment of renal function.
The oral LD_{50} dosages in rats and mice for propranolol, hydrochlorothiazide, and combined propranolol/hydrochlorothiazide (40/25, 80/25) are 364 to 533 mg/kg, greater than 2,750 to 5,000 mg/kg, and 538 to 845 mg/kg, respectively.

TREATMENT
The following measures should be employed:
General—If ingestion is, or may have been, recent, evacuate gastric contents, taking care to prevent pulmonary aspiration.
Bradycardia—Administer atropine (0.25 to 1.0 mg). If there is no response to vagal blockade, administer isoproterenol cautiously.
Cardiac Failure—Digitalization and diuretics.
Hypotension—Vasopressors, e.g., levarterenol or epinephrine.
Bronchospasm—Administer isoproterenol and aminophylline.
Stupor or Coma—Administer supportive therapy as clinically warranted.
Gastrointestinal Effects—Though usually of short duration, these may require symptomatic treatment.
Abnormalities in BUN and/or Serum Electrolytes—Monitor serum electrolyte levels and renal function; institute supportive measures as required individually to maintain hydration, electrolyte balance, respiration, and cardiovascular-renal function.

DOSAGE AND ADMINISTRATION

The dosage must be determined by individual titration.
Hydrochlorothiazide can be given at doses of 25 to 100 mg per day when used alone, but in most patients, 50 mg exerts a maximal effect. The initial dose of propranolol is 80 mg daily, and it may be increased gradually until optimal blood pressure control is achieved. The usual effective dose when used alone is 160 to 480 mg per day.
One Inderide Tablet twice daily can be used to administer up to 160 mg of propranolol and 50 mg of hydrochlorothiazide. For doses of propranolol greater than 160 mg the combination products are not appropriate, because their use would lead to an excessive dose of the thiazide component.
When necessary, another antihypertensive agent may be added gradually beginning with 50 percent of the usual recommended starting dose to avoid an excessive fall in blood pressure.

HOW SUPPLIED

Inderide 40/25
 Each hexagonal-shaped, off-white, scored tablet, embossed with an "I" and imprinted with "INDERIDE 40/25," contains 40 mg propranolol hydrochloride (Inderal®) and 25 mg hydrochlorothiazide, in bottles of 100 (NDC 0046-0484-81) and 1,000 (NDC 0046-0484-91).
Inderide 80/25
 Each hexagonal-shaped, off-white, scored tablet, embossed with an "I" and imprinted with "INDERIDE 80/25," contains 80 mg propranolol hydrochloride (Inderal®) and 25 mg hydrochlorothiazide, in bottles of 100 (NDC 0046-0488-81).

Store at room temperature (approximately 25° C).
Protect from moisture, freezing, and excessive heat.
Dispense in a well-closed container as defined in the USP.
The appearance of these tablets is a registered trademark of Wyeth-Ayerst Laboratories.
Shown in Product Identification Guide, page 339

INDERIDE® LA ℞
[ĭn 'de-rīde]
(propranolol hydrochloride and hydrochlorothiazide)
Long-Acting Capsules

No. 455—Each Inderide® LA 80/50 Capsule contains:
Propranolol hydrochloride
 (Inderal® LA) .... 80 mg
Hydrochlorothiazide .... 50 mg
No. 457—Each Inderide® LA 120/50
Capsule contains:
Propranolol hydrochloride
 (Inderal® LA) .... 120 mg
Hydrochlorothiazide .... 50 mg
No. 459—Each Inderide® LA 160/50
Capsule contains:
Propranolol hydrochloride
 (Inderal® LA) .... 160 mg
Hydrochlorothiazide .... 50 mg
Caution: Federal law prohibits dispensing without prescription.

DESCRIPTION

Inderide LA is indicated in the once-daily management of hypertension.
Inderide LA combines two antihypertensive agents: Inderal (propranolol hydrochloride), a beta-adrenergic receptor-blocking agent, and hydrochlorothiazide, a thiazide diuretic-antihypertensive. Inderide LA is formulated to provide a sustained release of propranolol hydrochloride. Hydrochlorothiazide in Inderide LA exists in a conventional (not sustained-release) formulation.
Inderal (propranolol hydrochloride) is a synthetic beta-adrenergic receptor-blocking agent chemically described as 1-(Isopropylamino)-3-(1-naphthyloxy)-2-propanol hydrochloride. Its structural formula is:

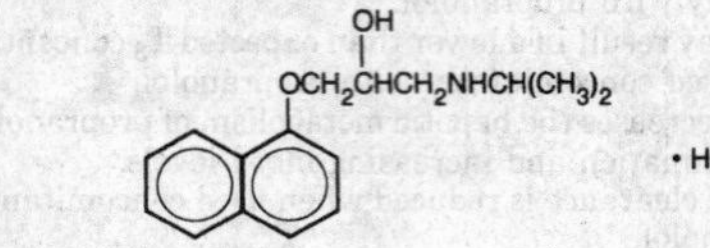

$$OCH_2CHCH_2NHCH(CH_3)_2$$
$$OH$$
$$\cdot HCl$$

Propranolol hydrochloride is a stable, white, crystalline solid which is readily soluble in water and ethanol. Its molecular weight is 295.81.
Hydrochlorothiazide is a white, or practically white, practically odorless, crystalline powder. It is slightly soluble in water; freely soluble in sodium hydroxide solution; sparingly soluble in methanol; insoluble in ether, chloroform, benzene, and dilute mineral acids. Its chemical name is 6-Chloro-3,4-dihydro-2H-1,2,4-benzothiadiazine-7-sulfonamide 1,1-dioxide. Its structural formula is:

$$H_2NSO_2 \quad \begin{array}{c} O \;\; O \\ S \\ NH \end{array}$$
$$Cl \qquad N$$
$$H$$

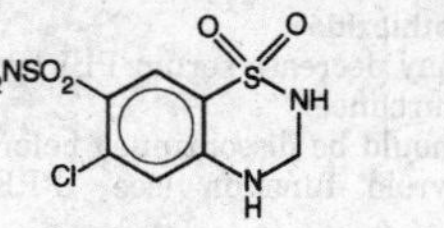

Inderide LA contains the following inactive ingredients: calcium carbonate, ethylcellulose, gelatin capsules, hydroxypropyl methylcellulose, lactose, magnesium stearate, microcrystalline cellulose, sodium lauryl sulfate, sodium starch glycolate, titanium dioxide, and D&C Yellow No. 10. In addition, Inderide LA 80/50 mg and 120/50 mg Capsules contain D&C Red No. 33; Inderide LA 120/50 mg and 160/50 mg Capsules contain FD&C Blue No. 1 and FD&C Red No. 40.

CLINICAL PHARMACOLOGY

PROPRANOLOL HYDROCHLORIDE (INDERAL®)
Inderal is a nonselective, beta-adrenergic receptor-blocking agent possessing no other autonomic nervous system activity. It specifically competes with beta-adrenergic receptor-stimulating agents for available receptor sites. When access to beta-receptor sites is blocked by Inderal, the chronotropic, inotropic, and vasodilator responses to beta-adrenergic stimulation are decreased proportionately.
Inderide LA Capsules (80/50, 120/50, and 160/50 mg) release propranolol hydrochloride at a controlled and predictable rate. Peak propranolol blood levels following dosing with Inderide LA occur at about 6 hours, and the apparent plasma half-life is about 10 hours. Over a 24-hour period, propranolol blood levels are fairly constant for about 12 hours, then decline exponentially. When measured at steady state over a 24-hour period, the areas under the propranolol plasma concentration-time curve (AUCs) for the capsules are approxi-

mately 60% to 65% of the AUCs for a comparable divided daily dose of Inderal Tablets. The lower AUCs for the capsules are due to greater hepatic metabolism of propranolol resulting from the slower rate of absorption of propranolol. Inderide LA should not be considered a simple mg-for-mg substitute for conventional Inderide Tablets, and the propranolol blood levels achieved do not match (are lower than) those of twice-daily dosing of Inderide Tablets with the same dose. When changing to Inderide LA from conventional Inderide Tablets, a possible need for retitration upwards should be considered.
The mechanism of the antihypertensive effect of propranolol has not been established. Among the factors that may be involved in contributing to the antihypertensive action are: (1) decreased cardiac output, (2) inhibition of renin release by the kidneys, and (3) diminution of tonic sympathetic nerve outflow from vasomotor centers in the brain.
Propranolol hydrochloride decreases heart rate, cardiac output, and blood pressure. Although total peripheral vascular resistance may increase initially, it readjusts to or below the pretreatment level with chronic usage. Effects on plasma volume appear to be minor and somewhat variable. Inderal has been shown to cause a small increase in serum potassium concentration when used in the treatment of hypertensive patients.
Beta-receptor blockade is useful in conditions in which, because of pathologic or functional changes, sympathetic activity is excessive or inappropriate, and detrimental to the patient. But there are also situations in which sympathetic stimulation is vital. For example, in patients with severely damaged hearts, adequate ventricular function is maintained by virtue of sympathetic drive, which should be preserved. In the presence of AV block, beta blockade may prevent the necessary facilitating effect of sympathetic activity on conduction. Beta blockade results in bronchial constriction by interfering with adrenergic bronchodilator activity, which should be preserved in patients subject to bronchospasm.
The proper objective of beta-blockade therapy is to decrease adverse sympathetic stimulation, but not to the degree that may impair necessary sympathetic support.

HYDROCHLOROTHIAZIDE
Hydrochlorothiazide is a benzothiadiazine (thiazide) diuretic closely related to chlorothiazide. The mechanism of the antihypertensive effect of the thiazides is unknown. Thiazides usually do not affect normal blood pressure.
Thiazides affect the renal tubular mechanism of electrolyte reabsorption. At maximal therapeutic dosage, all thiazides are approximately equal in their diuretic efficacy.
Thiazides increase excretion of sodium and chloride in approximately equivalent amounts. Natriuresis causes a secondary loss of potassium and bicarbonate.
Onset of diuretic action of thiazides occurs in 2 hours, and the peak effect in about 4 hours. Its action persists for approximately 6 to 12 hours. Thiazides are eliminated rapidly by the kidney. The hydrochlorothiazide in Inderide LA is a conventional (not sustained-release) formulation.

INDICATIONS AND USAGE

Inderide LA is indicated in the management of hypertension.
This fixed-combination drug is not indicated for initial therapy of hypertension. Hypertension requires therapy titrated to the individual patient. If the fixed combination represents the dosage so determined, its use may be more convenient in patient management. The treatment of hypertension is not static, but must be reevaluated as conditions in each patient warrant.

CONTRAINDICATIONS

PROPRANOLOL HYDROCHLORIDE (INDERAL®)
Propranolol is contraindicated in: 1) cardiogenic shock; 2) sinus bradycardia and greater than first-degree block; 3) bronchial asthma; 4) congestive heart failure (see **WARNINGS**), unless the failure is secondary to a tachyarrhythmia treatable with propranolol.
HYDROCHLOROTHIAZIDE
Hydrochlorothiazide is contraindicated in patients with anuria or hypersensitivity to this or other sulfonamide-derived drugs.

WARNINGS

PROPRANOLOL HYDROCHLORIDE (INDERAL®)
Cardiac Failure: Sympathetic stimulation may be a vital component supporting circulatory function in patients with congestive heart failure, and its inhibition by beta blockade may precipitate more severe failure. Although beta blockers should be avoided in overt congestive heart failure, if necessary, they can be used with close follow-up in patients with a history of failure who are well compensated and are receiving digitalis and diuretics. Beta-adrenergic blocking agents do not abolish the inotropic action of digitalis on heart muscle.
In Patients Without a History of Heart Failure, continued use of beta blockers can, in some cases, lead to cardiac failure. Therefore, at the first sign or symptom of heart failure, the patient should be digitalized and/or treated with diuretics,

and the response observed closely, or propranolol should be discontinued (gradually, if possible).

In Patients with Angina Pectoris, there have been reports of exacerbation of angina and, in some cases, myocardial infarction, following *abrupt* discontinuance of propranolol therapy. Therefore, when discontinuance of propranolol is planned, the dosage should be gradually reduced and the patient carefully monitored. In addition, when propranolol is prescribed for angina pectoris, the patient should be cautioned against interruption or cessation of therapy without the physician's advice. If propranolol therapy is interrupted and exacerbation of angina occurs, it usually is advisable to reinstitute propranolol therapy and take other measures appropriate for the management of unstable angina pectoris. Since coronary artery disease may be unrecognized, it may be prudent to follow the above advice in patients considered at risk of having occult atherosclerotic heart disease who are given propranolol for other indications.

Thyrotoxicosis: Beta blockade may mask certain clinical signs of hyperthyroidism. Therefore, abrupt withdrawal of propranolol may be followed by an exacerbation of symptoms of hyperthyroidism, including thyroid storm. Propranolol does not distort thyroid function tests.

In Patients With Wolff-Parkinson-White Syndrome, several cases have been reported in which, after propranolol, the tachycardia was replaced by a severe bradycardia requiring a demand pacemaker. In one case this resulted after an initial dose of 5 mg propranolol.

Major Surgery: The necessity or desirability of withdrawal of beta-blocking therapy prior to major surgery is controversial. It should be noted, however, that the impaired ability of the heart to respond to reflex adrenergic stimuli may augment the risks of general anesthesia and surgical procedures.

Nonallergic Bronchospasm (e.g., chronic bronchitis, emphysema): PATIENTS WITH BRONCHOSPASTIC DISEASES SHOULD, IN GENERAL, NOT RECEIVE BETA BLOCKERS. Inderal should be administered with caution since it may block bronchodilation produced by endogenous and exogenous catecholamine stimulation of beta receptors.

Diabetes and Hypoglycemia: Beta-adrenergic blockade may prevent the appearance of certain premonitory signs and symptoms (pulse rate and pressure changes) of acute hypoglycemia in labile insulin-dependent diabetes. In these patients, it may be more difficult to adjust the dosage of insulin. Hypoglycemic attacks may be accompanied by a precipitous elevation of blood pressure.

HYDROCHLOROTHIAZIDE

Thiazides should be used with caution in severe renal disease. In patients with renal disease, thiazides may precipitate azotemia. In patients with impaired renal function, cumulative effects of the drug may develop.

Thiazides should also be used with caution in patients with impaired hepatic function or progressive liver disease, since minor alterations of fluid and electrolyte balance may precipitate hepatic coma.

Thiazides may add to or potentiate the action of other antihypertensive drugs. Potentiation occurs with ganglionic or peripheral adrenergic-blocking drugs.

Sensitivity reactions may occur in patients with a history of allergy or bronchial asthma. The possibility of exacerbation or activation of systemic lupus erythematosus has been reported.

PRECAUTIONS

PROPRANOLOL HYDROCHLORIDE (INDERAL®)

General: Propranolol should be used with caution in patients with impaired hepatic or renal function. Propranolol is not indicated for the treatment of hypertensive emergencies.

Beta-adrenoreceptor blockade can cause reduction of intraocular pressure. Patients should be told that propranolol may interfere with the glaucoma screening test. Withdrawal may lead to a return of increased intraocular pressure.

Clinical Laboratory Tests: Elevated blood urea levels in patients with severe heart disease, elevated serum transaminase, alkaline phosphatase, lactate dehydrogenase.

Drug Interactions: Patients receiving catecholamine-depleting drugs, such as reserpine, should be closely observed if propranolol is administered. The added catecholamine-blocking action may produce an excessive reduction of resting sympathetic nervous activity, which may result in hypotension, marked bradycardia, vertigo, syncopal attacks, or orthostatic hypotension.

Blunting of the antihypertensive effect of beta-adrenoceptor blocking agents by nonsteroidal anti-inflammatory drugs has been reported.

Hypotension and cardiac arrest have been reported with the concomitant use of propranolol and haloperidol.

Carcinogenesis, Mutagenesis, Impairment of Fertility: Long-term studies in animals have been conducted to evaluate toxic effects and carcinogenic potential. In 18-month studies, in both rats and mice, employing doses up to 150 mg/kg/day there was no evidence of significant drug-induced toxicity. There were no drug-related tumorigenic effects at any of the dosage levels. Reproductive studies in animals did not show any impairment of fertility that was attributable to the drug.

Pregnancy: Pregnancy Category C. In a series of reproduction and developmental toxicology studies, propranolol was given to rats at dosages up to 150 mg/kg/day by gavage or in the diet throughout pregnancy and through lactation. In rats given 150 mg/kg/day (about 10 times the maximum recommended human dose of propranolol alone or about 30 times the maximum recommended human dose of the combined propranolol/hydrochlorothiazide product) propranolol was embryotoxic (reduced litter sizes and increased resorption sites). In addition, an unexplained increase in neonatal toxicity (death) was noted in all dosage groups in some of the studies. Maternal toxicity (decreased body weight) was evident at 150 mg/kg/day. Propranolol also was given to rabbits at dosages up to 250 mg/kg/day (approximately 20 times the maximum recommended human dose of propranolol) throughout pregnancy. No evidence of embryotoxicity was noted. Teratogenicity was not noted in either species. There are no adequate and well-controlled studies in pregnant women. Intrauterine growth retardation has been reported in neonates whose mothers received propranolol during pregnancy. Neonates whose mothers are receiving propranolol at parturition have exhibited bradycardia, hypoglycemia and respiratory depression. Adequate facilities for monitoring these infants at birth should be available. Propranolol should be used during pregnancy only if the potential benefit justifies the potential risk to the fetus.

Nursing Mothers: Propranolol is excreted in human milk. Caution should be exercised when propranolol is administered to a nursing mother.

Pediatric Use: Safety and effectiveness in pediatric patients have not been established.

HYDROCHLOROTHIAZIDE

General: Periodic determination of serum electrolytes to detect possible electrolyte imbalance should be performed at appropriate intervals.

All patients receiving thiazide therapy should be observed for clinical signs of fluid or electrolyte imbalance, namely: Hyponatremia, hypochloremic alkalosis, and hypokalemia. Serum and urine electrolyte determinations are particularly important when the patient is vomiting excessively or receiving parenteral fluids. Medication such as digitalis may also influence serum electrolytes. Warning signs irrespective of cause are: Dryness of mouth, thirst, weakness, lethargy, drowsiness, restlessness, muscle pains or cramps, muscular fatigue, hypotension, oliguria, tachycardia, and gastrointestinal disturbances such as nausea and vomiting.

Hypokalemia may develop, especially with brisk diuresis, when severe cirrhosis is present or during concomitant use of corticosteroids or ACTH.

Interference with adequate oral electrolyte intake will also contribute to hypokalemia. Hypokalemia can sensitize or exaggerate the response of the heart to the toxic effect of digitalis (e.g., increased ventricular irritability). Hypokalemia may be avoided or treated by use of potassium supplements, such as foods with a high potassium content.

Any chloride deficit is generally mild and usually does not require specific treatment, except under extraordinary circumstances (as in liver or renal disease). Dilutional hyponatremia may occur in edematous patients in hot weather; appropriate therapy is water restriction, rather than administration of salt, except in rare instances when the hyponatremia is life-threatening. In actual salt depletion, appropriate replacement is the therapy of choice.

Hyperuricemia may occur or frank gout may be precipitated in certain patients receiving thiazide therapy.

Insulin requirements in diabetic patients may be increased, decreased, or unchanged. Diabetes mellitus which has been latent may become manifest during thiazide administration.

If progressive renal impairment becomes evident, consider withholding or discontinuing diuretic therapy.

Thiazides may decrease serum PBI levels without signs of thyroid disturbance.

Calcium excretion is decreased by thiazides. Pathologic changes in the parathyroid gland with hypercalcemia and hypophosphatemia have been observed in a few patients on prolonged thiazide therapy. The common complications of hyperparathyroidism, such as renal lithiasis, bone resorption, and peptic ulceration have not been seen. Thiazides should be discontinued before carrying out tests for parathyroid function.

Drug Interactions: Thiazide drugs may increase the responsiveness to tubocurarine.

The antihypertensive effects of thiazides may be enhanced in the postsympathectomy patient. Thiazides may decrease arterial responsiveness to norepinephrine. This diminution is not sufficient to preclude effectiveness of the pressor agent for therapeutic use.

Hydrochlorothiazide had no adverse effect on fertility in rats at a dose 4 times the Maximum Recommended Human Dose (MRHD) and in mice at a dose equivalent to 100 times the MRHD (1 mg/kg, assumed body weight of 50 kg).

Pregnancy: Pregnancy Category C. Thiazides cross the placental barrier and appear in cord blood. The use of thiazides in pregnancy requires that the anticipated benefit be weighed against possible hazards to the fetus. These hazards include fetal or neonatal jaundice, thrombocytopenia, and possibly other adverse reactions which have occurred in the adult.

Available information indicates that hydrochlorothiazide at doses as high as 1320 times the MRHD was not teratogenic in pregnant rats.

Nursing Mothers: Thiazides appear in human milk. If use of the drug is deemed essential, the patient should stop nursing.

Pediatric Use: Safety and effectiveness in pediatric patients have not been established.

ADVERSE REACTIONS

PROPRANOLOL HYDROCHLORIDE (INDERAL®)

Most adverse effects have been mild and transient and have rarely required the withdrawal of therapy.

Cardiovascular: Bradycardia; congestive heart failure; intensification of AV block; hypotension; paresthesia of hands; thrombocytopenic purpura; arterial insufficiency, usually of the Raynaud type.

Central Nervous System: Light-headedness; mental depression manifested by insomnia, lassitude, weakness, fatigue; reversible mental depression progressing to catatonia; visual disturbances; hallucinations; an acute reversible syndrome characterized by disorientation for time and place, short-term memory loss, emotional lability, slightly clouded sensorium, and decreased performance on neuropsychometrics.

Gastrointestinal: Nausea, vomiting, epigastric distress, abdominal cramping, diarrhea, constipation, mesenteric arterial thrombosis, ischemic colitis.

Allergic: Pharyngitis and agranulocytosis; erythematous rash; fever combined with aching and sore throat; laryngospasm and respiratory distress.

Respiratory: Bronchospasm.

Hematologic: Agranulocytosis; nonthrombocytopenic purpura, thrombocytopenic purpura.

Autoimmune: In extremely rare instances, systemic lupus erythematosus has been reported.

Miscellaneous: Alopecia, LE-like reactions; psoriasiform rashes; dry eyes; male impotence; and Peyronie's disease have been reported rarely. Oculomucocutaneous reactions involving the skin, serous membranes, and conjunctivae reported for a beta blocker (practolol) have not been associated with propranolol.

HYDROCHLOROTHIAZIDE

Gastrointestinal: Anorexia, gastric irritation, nausea, vomiting, cramping; diarrhea; constipation; jaundice (intrahepatic cholestatic jaundice); pancreatitis; sialadenitis.

Central Nervous System: Dizziness, vertigo; paresthesias; headache; xanthopsia.

Hematologic: Leukopenia; agranulocytosis; thrombocytopenia; aplastic anemia.

Cardiovascular: Orthostatic hypotension (may be aggravated by alcohol, barbiturates, or narcotics).

Hypersensitivity: Purpura; photosensitivity; rash; urticaria; necrotizing angiitis (vasculitis, cutaneous vasculitis); fever; respiratory distress, including pneumonitis; anaphylactic reactions.

Other: Hyperglycemia; glycosuria; hyperuricemia; muscle spasm; weakness; restlessness; transient blurred vision.

Whenever adverse reactions are moderate or severe, thiazide dosage should be reduced or therapy withdrawn.

DOSAGE AND ADMINISTRATION

The dosage must be determined by individual titration.

Hydrochlorothiazide can be given at doses of 25 to 100 mg per day when used alone, but in most patients, 50 mg exerts a maximal effect. The initial dose of propranolol is 80 mg daily, and it may be increased gradually until optimal blood pressure control is achieved. The usual effective dose, when used alone, is 160 to 480 mg per day.

One Inderide LA Capsule once a day can be used to administer up to 160 mg of propranolol and 50 mg of hydrochlorothiazide. For doses of propranolol greater than 160 mg, the combination products are not appropriate because their use would lead to an excessive dose of the thiazide component.

Inderide LA provides propranolol hydrochloride in a sustained-release form and hydrochlorothiazide in conventional formulation, for once-daily administration. If patients are switched from Inderide Tablets (or Inderal plus hydrochlorothiazide) to Inderide LA, care should be taken to ensure that the desired therapeutic effect is maintained. Inderide LA should not be considered a mg-for-mg substitute for Inderide or Inderal plus hydrochlorothiazide. Inderide LA has different kinetics and produces lower blood levels. Retitration may be necessary, especially to maintain effectiveness at the end of the 24-hour dosing interval.

When necessary, another antihypertensive agent may be added gradually, beginning with 50% of the usual recom-

Continued on next page

Wyeth-Ayerst Laboratories—Cont.

mended starting dose, to avoid an excessive fall in blood pressure.

OVERDOSAGE OR EXAGGERATED RESPONSE

The propranolol hydrochloride (Inderal) component may cause bradycardia, cardiac failure, hypotension, or bronchospasm.

The hydrochlorothiazide component can be expected to cause diuresis. Lethargy of varying degree may appear and may progress to coma within a few hours, with minimal depression of respiration and cardiovascular function, and in the absence of significant serum electrolyte changes or dehydration. The mechanism of central nervous system depression with thiazide overdosage is unknown. Gastrointestinal irritation and hypermotility can occur; temporary elevation of BUN has been reported and serum electrolyte changes could occur, especially in patients with impairment of renal function.

TREATMENT

The following measures should be employed:

General: If ingestion is, or may have been, recent, evacuate gastric contents, taking care to prevent pulmonary aspiration.

Bradycardia: Administer atropine (0.25 to 1.0 mg). If there is no response to vagal blockade, administer isoproterenol cautiously.

Cardiac Failure: Digitalization and diuretics.

Hypotension: Vasopressors, e.g., levarterenol or epinephrine.

Bronchospasm: Administer isoproterenol and aminophylline.

Stupor or Coma: Administer supportive therapy as clinically warranted.

Gastrointestinal Effects: Though usually of short duration, these may require symptomatic treatment.

Abnormalities in BUN and/or Serum Electrolytes: Monitor serum electrolyte levels and renal function; institute supportive measures, as required individually, to maintain hydration, electrolyte balance, respiration, and cardiovascular function.

HOW SUPPLIED

Each beige capsule, identified by one wide band and 3 narrow bands, all in gold, and "Inderide LA 80/50," contains 80 mg of propranolol hydrochloride (Inderal® LA) and 50 mg of hydrochlorothiazide, in bottles of 100 (NDC 0046-0455-81).

Each beige/brown capsule, identified by one wide band and 3 narrow bands, all in gold, and "Inderide LA 120/50," contains 120 mg of propranolol hydrochloride (Inderal® LA) and 50 mg of hydrochlorothiazide, in bottles of 100 (NDC 0046-0457-81).

Each brown capsule, identified by one wide band and 3 narrow bands, all in gold, and "Inderide LA 160/50", contains 160 mg of propranolol hydrochloride (Inderal® LA) and 50 mg of hydrochlorothiazide, in bottles of 100 (NDC 0046-0459-81).

Store at room temperature (approximately 25° C).
Protect from light, moisture, freezing, and excessive heat.
Dispense in a tight, light-resistant container as defined in the USP.

The appearance of these capsules is a registered trademark of Wyeth-Ayerst Laboratories.

Shown in Product Identification Guide, page 339

INFLUENZA VIRUS VACCINE, ℞
TRIVALENT, TYPES A AND B
(chromatograph- and filter-purified subvirion antigen)

FluShield®
1996-97 formula
DO NOT INJECT INTRAVENOUSLY

DESCRIPTION

FluShield® (Influenza Virus Vaccine, Trivalent, Types A and B [Purified Subvirion]) is a sterile injectable for administration intramuscularly.

FluShield is prepared from the allantoic fluids of chick embryos inoculated with a specific type of influenza virus. During processing, not more than 5 μg of gentamicin sulfate per mL is added. The harvested virus is concentrated, purified, then inactivated with formaldehyde.

FluShield, Trivalent (chromatograph- and filter-purified subvirion antigen), is concentrated and refined by a column-chromatographic procedure. At the same time, addition of tri(n)butylphosphate and Polysorbate 80, USP to the column-eluting fluids effects inactivation and disruption of a significant proportion of the virus to smaller subunit particles. The recovered subvirion (split-virus) suspension is freed of substantial portions of the disrupting agents by dialysis and of other undesirable materials by selective filtration through membranes of controlled pore size.

The viral antigen content has been standardized by immunodiffusion tests, according to current U.S. Public Health Service requirements. Each dose (0.5 mL) contains the proportions and not less than the microgram amounts of hemagglutinin antigens (μg HA) representative of the specific components recommended for the 1996-1997 season: 15 μg HA of A/Texas/36/91-like (H1N1), 15 μg HA of A/Nanchang/933/95 (H3N2) (A/Wuhan/359/95-like [H3N2]), and 15 μg HA of B/Harbin/07/94 (B/Beijing/184/93-like).

The vaccine contains 1:10,000 thimerosal (mercury derivative) as a preservative. Gentamicin sulfate is used during manufacturing but is not detectable in the final product by current assay procedures.

CLINICAL PHARMACOLOGY

The administration of inactivated influenza vaccine to high-risk persons each year before the influenza season is the single most important influenza-control measure.[1]

The injection of antigens prepared from inactivated influenza virus stimulates the production of specific antibodies. Any protection afforded is only against those strains of virus from which the vaccine is prepared or closely related strains. With the passing of time, there may be major antigenic changes in the prevalent strains, or there may be continuous and progressive antigenic variation within a given virus subtype over time (antigenic drift), so that infection or immunization with one strain may not induce immunity to distantly related strains. Field studies of influenza vaccines conducted on many occasions since the 1940's have shown marked variation in efficacy, as measured by protection from disease, ranging from undemonstrable to 70-80%. The PHS regularly reviews the antigenic characteristics of circulating strains in order to select those to be included in the contemporary vaccine.

Based upon the epidemiological data available through the early months of 1996, the Federal Government determined, after consultation with advisory groups, that the influenza vaccines to be distributed in 1996-1997 will be trivalent, including 15 μg HA each of strains that are antigenically similar to A/Texas/36/91, A/Wuhan/359/95, and B/Beijing/184/93.

INDICATIONS AND USAGE

FluShield is recommended for 1) high-risk persons 6 months of age or older and for their medical-care providers or household contacts; 2) for children and teenagers receiving long-term aspirin therapy who, therefore, may be at increased risk of developing Reye's syndrome after an influenza virus infection; and 3) for other persons who wish to reduce their chances of acquiring influenza.

Guidelines for the use of vaccine among different groups are given below.

TARGET GROUPS FOR VACCINATION

Groups at increased risk for influenza-related complications:
1. Otherwise healthy persons 65 years of age or older.
2. Residents of nursing homes and other chronic-care facilities housing patients of any age with chronic medical conditions.
3. Adults and children with chronic disorders of the pulmonary or cardiovascular systems requiring regular medical follow-up or hospitalization during the preceding year, including children with asthma.
4. Adults and children who have required regular medical follow-up or hospitalization during the preceding year because of chronic metabolic diseases (including diabetes mellitus), renal dysfunction, hemoglobinopathies, or immunosuppression (including immunosuppression caused by medications).[1]
5. Children and teenagers (aged 6 months to 18 years) who are receiving long-term aspirin therapy and, therefore, may be at risk of developing Reye's syndrome after influenza infection.

Elderly persons and persons with certain chronic diseases may develop lower postvaccination antibody titers than healthy young adults and thus may remain susceptible to influenza-related upper-respiratory-tract infections. However, even if such persons develop influenza illness despite vaccination, the vaccine has been shown to be effective in helping to prevent lower-respiratory-tract involvement or other secondary complications, thereby reducing the risk of hospitalization and death.[1]

Groups potentially capable of nosocomial transmission of influenza to high-risk-persons:
Individuals attending high-risk persons can transmit influenza infections to them while they are themselves incubating infection, undergoing subclinical infection, or working despite the existence of symptoms. Some high-risk-persons, e.g., the elderly, transplant recipients, and persons with acquired immunodeficiency syndrome (AIDS), can have relatively low antibody responses to influenza vaccine. Efforts to help protect these members of high-risk groups against influenza may be improved by reducing the likelihood of influenza exposure from their caregivers. Therefore, the following groups should be vaccinated:
1. Physicians, nurses, and other personnel in both hospital and outpatient settings.

2. Employees of nursing homes and chronic-care facilities who have contact with patients or residents.
3. Providers of home care to high-risk persons (e.g., visiting nurses, volunteer workers).
4. Household members (including children) of high-risk groups, whether or not they provide care.[1]

VACCINATION OF OTHER GROUPS

General population:
Physicians should administer influenza vaccine to any person who wishes to reduce his/her chances of acquiring influenza infection. Persons who provide essential community services should be considered for vaccination to minimize disruption of essential activities during influenza outbreaks. Students or other healthy individuals in institutional settings (e.g., those who reside in dormitories) should be encouraged to receive vaccine to minimize the disruption of routine activities during outbreaks.[1]

Pregnant women:
Although animal reproductive studies have not been conducted (see "**Precautions**—PREGNANCY" section below), the prescribing health-care provider should be aware of the recommendations of the Advisory Committee on Immunization Practices (ACIP), which are incorporated below. Influenza-associated excess mortality among pregnant women has not been documented, except in the largest pandemics of 1918-19 and 1957-58. However, additional case reports and limited studies suggest that women in the third trimester of pregnancy and early puerperium, including those women without underlying risk factors, might be at increased risk for serious complications from influenza. The ACIP recommends: "Health-care workers who provide care for pregnant women should consider administering influenza vaccine to all women who would be in the third trimester of pregnancy or early puerperium during the influenza season. Pregnant women who have medical conditions that increase their risk for complications from influenza should be vaccinated before the influenza season, regardless of the stage of pregnancy."[1] The benefits of preventing influenza-related complications versus the theoretical risk of fetal harm should be considered, and discussed with the patient before administering influenza vaccine to a pregnant woman (see "**Precautions—PREGNANCY**").

Persons infected with human immunodeficiency virus (HIV):
Limited information exists regarding the frequency and severity of influenza illness among HIV-infected persons, but reports suggest that symptoms might be prolonged and the risk of complications increased for some HIV-infected persons. Influenza vaccine has produced protective antibody titers against influenza in vaccinated HIV-infected persons who have minimal AIDS-related symptoms and high CD4+ T-lymphocyte cell counts. In patients who have advanced HIV disease and low CD4+ T-lymphocyte cell counts, however influenza vaccine may not induce protective antibody titers; a second dose of vaccine does not improve the immune response for these persons. Because influenza may result in serious illness and complications and because influenza vaccination may result in protective antibody levels, vaccination will benefit many HIV-infected patients.[1]

Foreign travelers:
The risk of exposure to influenza during foreign travel varies, depending on, among other factors, season of travel and destination. Influenza can occur throughout the year in the tropics; the season of greatest influenza activity in the Southern Hemisphere is April through September. Because of the short incubation period for influenza, exposure to the virus during travel will often result in clinical illness that begins during travel, an inconvenience or potential danger, especially for persons at increased risk for complications. Persons preparing to travel to the tropics at any time of year or to the Southern Hemisphere from April through September should review their vaccination histories. If they were not vaccinated the previous fall or winter, they should be considered for influenza vaccination prior to travel. Persons in the high-risk categories especially should be encouraged to receive the most current vaccine. Persons at high risk who received the previous season's vaccine prior to travel should be revaccinated in the fall or winter with the current vaccine.[1]

Immunization programs:
If this product is to be used in an immunization program sponsored by an organization WHERE A TRADITIONAL PHYSICIAN/PATIENT RELATIONSHIP DOES NOT EXIST, each participant (or legal guardian) should be made aware of the possible risks that have been associated with the use of influenza virus vaccines, including the possible risk of a form of paralysis sometimes known as Guillain-Barré syndrome. Information about possible side effects and adverse reactions is presented below, and consent, preferably written, should be obtained from the intended recipient (or legal guardian) before vaccine administration. FluShield is a prescription product and shall only be administered upon prescription by a health-care provider who is licensed to prescribe biologicals. The prescribing health-care provider should be familiar with the text of this insert, including the "**Contraindications**," "**Precautions**," and "**Adverse Reactions**" sections.

SIMULTANEOUS ADMINISTRATION OF PNEUMOCOCCAL OR PEDIATRIC VACCINES
The target groups for influenza and pneumococcal vaccination overlap considerably. For persons at high risk who have not previously been vaccinated with pneumococcal vaccine, health-care providers should strongly consider administering pneumococcal and influenza vaccine concurrently. These vaccines can be administered at the same time at different sites without increasing side effects. However, it should be emphasized that whereas influenza vaccine is given annually, pneumococcal vaccine is generally given only once to all but those at highest risk of fatal pneumococcal disease.[2]
It may be desirable to simultaneously administer influenza vaccine, if indicated, with routine pediatric vaccines, but at different sites. Although studies have not been done, no diminution of immunogenicity or enhancement of adverse reactions should be expected. Because influenza vaccine can cause fever when administered to young children, it should generally not be given within 3 days of vaccination with pertussis vaccine. The ACIP permits immunization of children at high risk for influenza-related complications with influenza and pertussis vaccines at the same visit, but that DTaP may be preferable to DTP (for children ≥ 15 months of age who are receiving the fourth or fifth dose of pertussis vaccine).[1]

CONTRAINDICATIONS
INFLUENZA VIRUS VACCINE SHOULD NOT BE ADMINISTERED TO INDIVIDUALS WITH A HISTORY OF HYPERSENSITIVITY (ALLERGY) TO CHICKEN EGG OR TO ANY COMPONENT(S) OF INFLUENZA VIRUS VACCINE, INCLUDING THIMEROSAL, WITHOUT FIRST CONSULTING A PHYSICIAN (see "**Adverse Reactions**").
Before being vaccinated, persons known to be hypersensitive to egg protein or other components should be given a skin test or other allergy-evaluating test, using the influenza virus vaccine as the antigen. Persons with adverse reactions to such testing should not be vaccinated. Chemoprophylaxis may be indicated for prevention of influenza A in such persons. However, persons with a history of anaphylactic hypersensitivity to vaccine components but who are also at highest risk for complications of influenza infections may benefit from vaccine after appropriate evaluation and desensitization.[1]
Persons with a past history of Guillain-Barré syndrome (GBS) should not be given influenza virus vaccine. (See "**Adverse Reactions**.")
Persons with acute febrile illnesses usually should not be vaccinated until their symptoms have abated. However, minor illnesses with or without fever should not contraindicate the use of influenza vaccine, particularly in children with a mild upper-respiratory-tract infection or allergic rhinitis.[1,3]

WARNING
Patients with impaired immune responsiveness, whether due to the use of immunosuppressive therapy (including irradiation, large amounts of corticosteroids, antimetabolites, alkylating agents, and cytotoxic agents), a genetic defect, human immunodeficiency virus (HIV) infection, leukemia, lymphoma, generalized malignancy, or other causes, may have a reduced antibody response to active immunization procedures.[4] Short-term (less than 2 weeks) corticosteroid therapy or intra-articular, bursal, or tendon injections with corticosteroids should not be immunosuppressive. Inactivated vaccines are not a risk to immunocompromised individuals, although their efficacy may be substantially reduced. Because patients with immunodeficiencies may not have an adequate response to immunizing agents, they may remain susceptible despite having received an appropriate vaccine. If feasible, specific serum antibody titers or other immunologic responses may be determined after immunization to assess immunity.[3] Chemoprophylaxis may be indicated for high-risk persons who are expected to have a poor antibody response to influenza vaccine.[1]

PRECAUTIONS
GENERAL
Influenza virus is remarkably capricious antigenically, and significant changes may occur from time to time. *It is known definitely that FluShield, as now constituted, is not effective against all possible strains of influenza virus. Any protection afforded is only against those strains of virus from which the vaccine is prepared or against closely related strains.*
Influenza vaccine often contains one or more antigens used in previous years. However, immunity declines during the year following immunization. Therefore, revaccination on a yearly basis is necessary to provide optimal protection for the current season. REMAINING 1995-1996 VACCINE SHOULD NOT BE USED.
Epinephrine injection (1:1000) must be immediately available should an acute anaphylactoid reaction occur due to any component of the vaccine.
A separate sterile syringe and needle should be used for each patient to prevent transmission of hepatitis B or other infectious agents from one person to another. Reusable glass syringes and needles should be heat-sterilized.

DRUG INTERACTIONS
There have been conflicting reports[5–15] on the effects of influenza virus vaccine on the elimination of some drugs metabolized by the hepatic cytochrome P-450 system. Hypoprothrombinemia in patients receiving warfarin and elevated theophylline serum concentrations have occurred. Most studies have failed to show any adverse effects of influenza vaccine in patients receiving these drugs. Nevertheless, monitoring for possible enhanced drug effect or toxicity is indicated for those persons taking theophylline preparations or warfarin sodium.
Individuals receiving therapy with immunosuppressive agents (large amounts of corticosteroids, antimetabolites, alkylating agents, cytotoxic agents) may not respond optimally to active immunization procedures (see "**Warning**").

PREGNANCY
Pregnancy Category C:
Animal reproduction studies have not been conducted with influenza virus vaccine. It is also not known whether influenza virus vaccine can cause fetal harm when administered to a pregnant woman or can affect reproduction capacity. Influenza virus vaccine should be given to a pregnant woman only if clearly needed (see also "**Indications and Usage**").

ADVERSE REACTIONS
Side effects of influenza vaccination are generally inconsequential in adults and occur at low frequency, but at younger ages side effects may be more common.
BECAUSE INFLUENZA VACCINE CONTAINS ONLY NONINFECTIOUS VIRUSES, IT CANNOT CAUSE INFLUENZA. Occasional cases of respiratory disease following vaccination represent coincidental illnesses unrelated to influenza vaccination.
The most frequent side effect of vaccination is soreness around the vaccination site for up to 2 days; this occurs in less than one-third of vaccinees.
In addition, the following types of systemic reactions have occurred:
Fever, malaise, myalgia, and other systemic symptoms occur infrequently and most often affect persons who have had no exposure to the influenza virus antigens in the vaccine (e.g., young children). These reactions begin 6 to 12 hours after vaccination and can persist for 1 or 2 days.
Immediate, presumably allergic, reactions such as hives, angioedema, allergic asthma, or systemic anaphylaxis occur rarely after influenza vaccination. These reactions probably result from hypersensitivity to some vaccine component—the majority of reactions are most likely related to residual egg protein. Although current influenza vaccines contain only a small quantity of egg protein, this protein can induce immediate hypersensitivity reactions among persons who have severe egg allergy. Persons who have developed hives, have had swelling of the lips or tongue, or experienced acute respiratory distress or collapse after eating eggs should consult a physician for appropriate evaluation to help determine if vaccine should be administered. Persons who have documented immunoglobulin E (IgE)-mediated hypersensitivity to eggs, including those who have had occupational asthma or other allergic responses due to exposure to egg protein, might also be at increased risk for reactions from influenza vaccine and similar consultation should be considered. The protocol for influenza vaccination developed by Murphy and Strunk may be considered for patients who have egg allergies and medical conditions that place them at increased risk for influenza-associated complications.[16] Hypersensitivity reactions to any vaccine component can occur. Although exposure to vaccines containing thimerosal can lead to induction of hypersensitivity, most patients do not develop reactions to thimerosal when administered as a component of vaccines even when patch or intradermal tests for thimerosal indicate hypersensitivity. When reported, hypersensitivity to thimerosal has usually consisted of local, delayed-type hypersensitivity reactions.[1]
There have been rare reports of Guillain-Barré syndrome (GBS) following receipt of influenza virus vaccine. GBS is an uncommon illness characterized by ascending paralysis which is usually self-limited and reversible. Though most persons with GBS recover without residual weakness, approximately 5% of cases are fatal. Before 1976, no association of GBS with influenza vaccine use was recognized.
Except for the 1976–77 swine influenza vaccine, subsequent vaccines prepared from other virus strains have not been clearly associated with an increased frequency of Guillain-Barré syndrome.[1,17–20] However, a precise estimate of risk is difficult to determine for a rare condition such as GBS which has an annual background incidence of only one to two cases per 100,000 adult population. Among persons who received the swine influenza vaccine, the rate of GBS that exceeded the background rate was slightly less than one case per 100,000 vaccinations.[1]
Although, in 1990–91, there may have been a small increase in GBS cases in vaccinated persons 18 to 64 years of age, the epidemiologic features of the possible association of the 1990–91 vaccine with GBS were not as convincing as those found with the swine influenza vaccine. The rate of GBS cases after vaccination that was passively reported to the Vaccine Adverse Event Reporting System (VAERS) during 1993–94 was estimated to be approximately twice the average rate reported during other recent seasons (i.e., 1990–91, 1991–92, 1992–93, and 1994–95). The data currently available are not sufficient to determine whether this represents an actual risk.[1]
Whereas the incidence of GBS in the general population is very low, persons with a history of GBS have a substantially greater likelihood of subsequently developing GBS than persons without such a history. Thus, the likelihood of coincidentally developing GBS after influenza vaccination is expected to be greater among persons with a history of GBS than among persons with no history of this syndrome. Whether influenza vaccination might be causally associated with this risk for recurrence is not known.[1] Therefore, candidates for influenza virus vaccine should be made aware of the possible risks, including GBS, and the benefits of administration.
Other neurologic disorders, including encephalopathies not defined as GBS, have been temporally associated with influenza vaccination.[21]

DOSAGE AND ADMINISTRATION
Although influenza virus vaccine often contains one or more antigens used in previous years, immunity declines during the year following vaccination. Therefore, a history of vaccination in any previous year with a vaccine containing one or more antigens included in the current vaccine does NOT preclude the need for revaccination for the 1996–1997 influenza season to help provide optimal protection. REMAINING 1995–1996 VACCINE SHOULD NOT BE USED.
Influenza vaccine may be offered to high-risk persons presenting for routine care or hospitalization beginning in September, but not until new vaccine is available (see above for foreign-travel-related exceptions). Opportunities to vaccinate persons at high risk for complications of influenza should not be missed. In the United States, influenza activity generally peaks between late December and early March, and high levels of influenza activity infrequently occur in the contiguous 48 states before December. Therefore, the optimal time for organized vaccination campaigns for high-risk persons usually is the period between the beginning of October and mid-November. In facilities such as nursing homes it is particularly important to avoid administering vaccine too far in advance of the influenza season because antibody may begin to decline within a few months. Such vaccination programs may be undertaken as soon as current vaccine is available in September or October if regional influenza activity is expected to begin earlier than normal.
Children less than 9 years of age who have not been vaccinated previously should receive two doses with at least 1 month between doses to maximize the chance of a satisfactory antibody response to all three vaccine antigens. The second dose should be given before December, if possible. Vaccine should continue to be offered to both children and adults up to and even after influenza virus activity is documented in a community.
Parenteral drug products should be inspected visually for particulate matter and discoloration prior to administration, whenever solution and container permit.
DO NOT INJECT INTRAVENOUSLY. Injections of FluShield® are recommended to be given intramuscularly. The recommended site is the deltoid muscle for adults and older children. The preferred site for infants and young children is the anterolateral aspect of the thigh musculature. Because of lack of adequate evaluation of other routes in high-risk persons, the preferred route of vaccination is intramuscularly whenever possible. Before injection, the skin over the site to be injected should be cleansed with a suitable germicide. After insertion of the needle, aspirate to help avoid inadvertent injection into a blood vessel.

AGE GROUP	DOSAGE SCHEDULE
9 years and older	0.5 mL (one dose)
3 to 8 years	0.5 mL (1 or 2 doses)*
6 to 35 months	0.25 mL (1 or 2 doses)*

For those under 13 years, only split-virus (subvirion) vaccine is recommended.
*A single dose is considered sufficient for those under 9 years who have received at least 1 dose of influenza virus vaccine. With the 2-dose regimen, allow 4 weeks or more between doses. Both doses are recommended for maximum protection.
Immunogenicity and reactogenicity of split- and whole-virus vaccines are similar in adults when used according to the recommended dosage.[1]

HOW SUPPLIED
Influenza Virus Vaccine, Trivalent, Types A and B, (Purified Subvirion), FluShield®, is available in vials of 5 mL as follows:

Continued on next page

Wyeth-Ayerst Laboratories—Cont.

NDC 0009-0849-01
NDC 0009-0849-35 (Non-returnable)
ALSO AVAILABLE
TUBEX® Sterile Cartridge-Needle Units, 0.5 mL fill in 1 mL size (25 gauge × 5/8 inch needle), in packages of 10 TUBEX as follows:
NDC 0009-0849-02
NDC 0009-0849-45 (Non-returnable)

Storage
Store between 2°–8°C (35°–46°F). Potency is destroyed by freezing; do not use FluShield that has been frozen.

REFERENCES

1. Prevention and control of influenza: Recommendations of the Advisory Committee on Immunization Practices (ACIP). Morbidity and Mortality Weekly Report—May 3, 1996; *45 (No. RR-5)*.
2. ACIP. Pneumococcal polysaccharide vaccine. MMWR 1989; *38*: 64–8, 73–6.
3. American Academy of Pediatrics: Report of the Committee on Infectious Diseases. 23rd ed. Elk Grove Village, IL, American Academy of Pediatrics, 1994.
4. Recommendations of the Advisory Committee on Immunization Practices (ACIP): Use of vaccines and immune globulins in persons with altered immunocompetence. MMWR 1993: *42 (No. RR-4)*.
5. KRAMER, P. and McCLAIN, C.: Depression of aminopyrine metabolism by influenza vaccination. NEJM 1981; *305*: 1262.
6. RENTON, K. et al: Decreased elimination of theophylline after influenza vaccination. Can Med Assoc J 1980; *123*: 288.
7. GOLDSTEIN, R.S. et al: Decreased elimination of theophylline after influenza vaccination. Can Med Assoc J 1982; *126*: 470.
8. BRITTON, L. and RUBEN, F.L.: Serum and theophylline levels after influenza vaccination. Can Med Assoc J 1982; *126*: 1375.
9. FISCHER, R.G. et al: Influence of trivalent influenza vaccine on serum theophylline levels. Can Med Assoc J 1982; *126*: 1312–13.
10. SAN JOAQUIN, V.H., REYES, S., AND MARKS, M.I.: Influenza vaccination in asthmatic children on maintenance theophylline therapy. Clin Pediatrics 1982; *21*: 724–6.
11. STULTS, B. AND HASISAKI, P.: Influenza vaccination and theophylline pharmacokinetics in patients with chronic obstructive lung disease. West J Med 1983; *139*: 651–4.
12. PATRIARCA, P.A. et al: Influenza vaccination and warfarin or theophylline toxicity in nursing-home residents. NEJM 1983; *308*: 1601.
13. MEREDITH, C.G. et al: Effects of influenza virus vaccine on hepatic drug metabolism. Clin Pharm Ther 1985; *37*: 396–401.
14. LIPSKY, B.A. et al: Influenza vaccination and warfarin anticoagulation. Ann Int Med 1984; *100*: 835–7.
15. KRAMER, P. et al: Effect of influenza vaccine on warfarin anticoagulation. Clin Pharmacol Ther 1984; *35*: 416.
16. MURPHY, K.R. and STRUNK, R.L.: Safe administration of influenza vaccine in asthmatic children hypersensitive to egg proteins. J Pediatr 1985; *106*: 931–3.
17. SCHONBERGER, L. et al: Guillian-Barré syndrome following vaccination in the National Immunization Program, United States 1976–1977. Am J Epidemiol 1979; *110*: 105.
18. SCHONBERGER, L. et al: Guillian-Barré syndrome: Its epidemiology and associations with influenza vaccination. Ann Neurol 1981; *9 (suppl)*: 31.
19. HURWITZ, E. et al: Guillain-Barré syndrome and the 1978–1979 influenza vaccine. NEJM 1981; *304*: 1557.
20. KAPLAN, J. et al: Guillain-Barré syndrome in the United States, 1979–1980 and 1980–1981. Lack of association with influenza vaccination. JAMA 1982; *248*: 698.
21. RETAILLIAU, H. et al: Illness after influenza vaccination reported through a nation-wide surveillance system, 1976–1977. Am J Epidemiol 1980; *111*: 170.

Manufactured by Wyeth Laboratories Inc.,
A Wyeth-Ayerst Company
Marietta, PA 17547.

ISMO® ℞

[*ĭs'mō*]
(isosorbide mononitrate)
20 mg tablets

DESCRIPTION

Isosorbide mononitrate is 1,4:3,6-dianhydro-D-glucitol,5-nitrate, an organic nitrate whose structural formula is
[See chemical structure at top of next column.]
and whose molecular weight is 191.14. The organic nitrates are vasodilators, active on both arteries and veins.

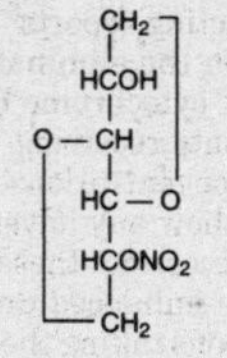

Each Ismo® tablet contains 20 mg of isosorbide mononitrate. The inactive ingredients in each tablet are D&C Yellow 10 Aluminum Lake, FD&C Yellow 6 Aluminum Lake, hydroxypropyl methylcellulose, lactose, magnesium stearate, microcrystalline cellulose, polyethylene glycol, polysorbate 20, povidone, silicon dioxide, sodium starch glycolate, titanium dioxide and hydroxypropyl cellulose.

CLINICAL PHARMACOLOGY

Isosorbide mononitrate is the major active metabolite of isosorbide dinitrate (ISDN), and most of the clinical activity of the dinitrate is attributable to the mononitrate.
The principal pharmacological action of isosorbide mononitrate is relaxation of vascular smooth muscle and consequent dilatation of peripheral arteries and veins, especially the latter. Dilation of the veins promotes peripheral pooling of blood and decreases venous return to the heart, thereby reducing left ventricular end-diastolic pressure and pulmonary capillary wedge pressure (preload). Arteriolar relaxation reduces systemic vascular resistance, systolic arterial pressure, and mean arterial pressure (afterload). Dilatation of the coronary arteries also occurs. The relative importance of preload reduction, afterload reduction, and coronary dilatation remains undefined.

PHARMACODYNAMICS
Dosing regimens for most chronically used drugs are designed to provide plasma concentrations that are continuously greater than a minimally effective concentration. This strategy is inappropriate for organic nitrates. Several well-controlled clinical trials have used exercise testing to assess the antianginal efficacy of continuously delivered nitrates. In the large majority of these trials, active agents were indistinguishable from placebo after 24 hours (or less) of continuous therapy. Attempts to overcome tolerance by dose escalation, even to doses far in excess of those used acutely, have consistently failed. Only after nitrates have been absent from the body for several hours has their antianginal efficacy been restored.
The drug-free interval sufficient to avoid tolerance to isosorbide mononitrate has not been completely defined. In the only regimen of twice-daily isosorbide mononitrate that has been shown to avoid development of tolerance, the two doses of Ismo tablets are given 7 hours apart, so there is a gap of 17 hours between the second dose of each day and the first dose of the next day. Taking account of the relatively long half-life of isosorbide mononitrate this result is consistent with those obtained for other organic nitrates.
The same twice-daily regimen of Ismo tablets successfully avoided significant rebound/withdrawal effects. The incidence and magnitude of such phenomena have appeared, in studies of other nitrates, to be highly dependent upon the schedule of nitrate administration.

PHARMACOKINETICS
In humans, isosorbide mononitrate is not subject to first pass metabolism in the liver. The absolute bioavailability of isosorbide mononitrate from Ismo tablets is nearly 100%. Maximum serum concentrations of isosorbide mononitrate are achieved 30 to 60 minutes after ingestion of Ismo.
The volume of distribution of isosorbide mononitrate is approximately 0.6 L/kg, and less than 4% is bound to plasma proteins. It is cleared from the serum by denitration to isosorbide; glucuronidation to the mononitrate glucuronide; and denitration/hydration to sorbitol. None of these metabolites is vasoactive. Less than 1% of administered isosorbide mononitrate is eliminated in the urine.
The overall elimination half-life of isosorbide mononitrate is about 5 hours; the rate of clearance is the same in healthy young adults, in patients with various degrees of renal, hepatic, or cardiac dysfunction, and in the elderly. In a single-dose study, the pharmacokinetics of isosorbide mononitrate were dose-proportional up to at least 60 mg.

CLINICAL TRIALS
Controlled trials of single doses of Ismo tablets have demonstrated that antianginal activity is present about 1 hour after dosing, with peak effect seen from 1–4 hours after dosing.
In placebo-controlled trials lasting 2–3 weeks, Ismo tablets were administered twice daily, in asymmetric regimens (with interdosing intervals of 7 and 17 hours) designed to avoid tolerance. One trial tested doses of 10 mg and 20 mg; one trial tested doses of 20 mg, 40 mg, and 60 mg; and three trials tested only doses of 20 mg. In each trial, the subjects were persons with known chronic stable angina, and the primary measure of efficacy was exercise tolerance on a standardized treadmill test. After initial dosing and for at least 3 weeks, exercise tolerance in patients treated with Ismo 20 mg tablets was significantly greater than that seen in patients treated with placebo, although there was some attenuation of effect with time. Treatment with Ismo tablets was superior to placebo for at least 12 hours after the first dose (i.e., 5 hours after the second dose) of each day. Significant tolerance and rebound phenomena were not observed.
The 10-mg dose was not unequivocally superior to placebo, while the effect of the 40-mg dose was similar to that of the 20-mg dose. The 60-mg dose appeared to be less effective, and it was associated with a rebound phenomenon (early-morning worsening).

INDICATIONS AND USAGE

Ismo tablets are indicated for the prevention of angina pectoris due to coronary artery disease. The onset of action of oral isosorbide mononitrate is not sufficiently rapid for this product to be useful in aborting an acute anginal episode.

CONTRAINDICATIONS

Allergic reactions to organic nitrates are extremely rare, but they do occur. Isosorbide mononitrate is contraindicated in patients who are allergic to it.

WARNINGS

The benefits of isosorbide mononitrate in patients with acute myocardial infarction or congestive heart failure have not been established. Because the effects of isosorbide mononitrate are difficult to terminate rapidly, this drug is not recommended in these settings.
If isosorbide mononitrate is used in these conditions, careful clinical or hemodynamic monitoring must be used to avoid the hazards of hypotension and tachycardia.

PRECAUTIONS

GENERAL
Severe hypotension, particularly with upright posture, may occur with even small doses of isosorbide mononitrate. This drug should therefore be used with caution in patients who may be volume depleted or who, for whatever reason, are already hypotensive. Hypotension induced by isosorbide mononitrate may be accompanied by paradoxical bradycardia and increased angina pectoris.
Nitrate therapy may aggravate the angina caused by hypertrophic cardiomyopathy.
In industrial workers who have had long-term exposure to unknown (presumably high) doses of organic nitrates, tolerance clearly occurs. Chest pain, acute myocardial infarction, and even sudden death have occurred during temporary withdrawal of nitrates from these workers, demonstrating the existence of true physical dependence. The importance of these observations to the routine, clinical use of oral isosorbide mononitrate is not known.

INFORMATION FOR PATIENTS
Patients should be told that the antianginal efficacy of Ismo tablets can be maintained by carefully following the prescribed schedule of dosing (two doses taken 7 hours apart). For most patients, this can be accomplished by taking the first dose on awakening and the second dose 7 hours later.
As with other nitrates, daily headaches sometimes accompany treatment with isosorbide mononitrate. In patients who get these headaches, the headaches are a marker of the activity of the drug. Patients should resist the temptation to avoid headaches by altering the schedule of their treatment with isosorbide mononitrate, since loss of headache may be associated with simultaneous loss of antianginal efficacy. Aspirin and/or acetaminophen, on the other hand, often successfully relieve isosorbide mononitrate-induced headaches with no deleterious effect on isosorbide mononitrate's antianginal efficacy.
Treatment with isosorbide mononitrate may be associated with light-headedness on standing, especially just after rising from a recumbent or seated position. This effect may be more frequent in patients who have also consumed alcohol.

DRUG INTERACTIONS
The vasodilating effects of isosorbide mononitrate may be additive with those of other vasodilators. Alcohol, in particular, has been found to exhibit additive effects of this variety.
Marked symptomatic orthostatic hypotension has been reported when calcium channel blockers and organic nitrates were used in combination. Dose adjustments of either class of agents may be necessary.

CARCINOGENESIS, MUTAGENESIS, AND IMPAIRMENT OF FERTILITY
No carcinogenic effects were observed in mice exposed to oral isosorbide mononitrate for 104 weeks at doses of up to 900 mg/kg/day (102 × the human exposure comparing body surface area). Rats treated with 900 mg/kg/day for 26 weeks (225 × the human exposure comparing body surface area) and 500 mg/kg/day for the remaining 95–111 weeks (males and females, respectively) showed no evidence of tumors.
No mutagenic activity was seen in a variety of *in vitro* and *in vivo* assays.
No adverse effects on fertility were observed when isosorbide mononitrate was administered to male and female rats at doses up to 500 mg/kg/day (125 × the human exposure comparing body surface area).

PREGNANCY CATEGORY C
Isosorbide mononitrate has been shown to be associated with stillbirths and neonatal death in rats receiving 500 mg/kg/day of isosorbide mononitrate (125 × the human exposure comparing body surface area). At 250 mg/kg/day, no adverse effects on reproduction and development were reported.
In rats and rabbits receiving isosorbide mononitrate at up to 250 mg/kg/day, no developmental abnormalities, fetal abnormalities, or other effects upon reproductive performance were detected; these doses are larger than the maximum recommended human dose by factors between 70 (body-surface-area basis in rabbits) and 310 (body-weight basis, either species). In rats receiving 500 mg/kg/day, there were small but statistically significant increases in the rates of prolonged gestation, prolonged parturition, stillbirth, and neonatal death; and there were small but statistically significant decreases in birth weight, live litter size, and pup survival.
There are no adequate and well-controlled studies in pregnant women. Isosorbide mononitrate should be used during pregnancy only if the potential benefit justifies the potential risk to the fetus.
NURSING MOTHERS
It is not known whether isosorbide mononitrate is excreted in human milk. Because many drugs are excreted in human milk, caution should be exercised when isosorbide mononitrate is administered to a nursing woman.
PEDIATRIC USE
Safety and effectiveness of isosorbide mononitrate in pediatric patients have not been established.

ADVERSE REACTIONS

The table below shows the frequencies of the adverse reactions observed in more than 1% of the subjects (a) in 6 placebo-controlled domestic studies in which patients in the active-treatment arm received 20 mg of isosorbide mononitrate twice daily, and (b) in all studies in which patients received isosorbide mononitrate in a variety of regimens. In parentheses, the same table shows the frequencies with which these adverse reactions led to discontinuation of treatment. Overall, 11% of the patients who received isosorbide mononitrate in the six controlled U.S. studies discontinued treatment because of adverse reactions. Most of these discontinued because of headache.
"Dizziness" and nausea were also frequently associated with withdrawal from these studies.

Frequency of Adverse Reactions (Discontinuations)*

	6 Controlled Studies		92 Clinical Studies
Dose	Placebo	20 mg	(varied)
Patients	204	219	3344
Headache	9% (0%)	38% (9%)	19% (4.3%)
Dizziness	1% (0%)	5% (1%)	3% (0.2%)
Nausea, Vomiting	<1% (0%)	4% (3%)	2% (0.2%)

* Some individuals discontinued for multiple reasons.

Other adverse reactions, each reported by fewer than 1% of exposed patients, and in many cases of uncertain relation to drug treatment, were:
Cardiovascular: angina pectoris, arrhythmias, atrial fibrillation, hypotension, palpitations, postural hypotension, premature ventricular contractions, supraventricular tachycardia, syncope.
Dermatologic: pruritus, rash.
Gastrointestinal: abdominal pain, diarrhea, dyspepsia, tenesmus, tooth disorder, vomiting.
Genitourinary: dysuria, impotence, urinary frequency.
Miscellaneous: asthenia, blurred vision, cold sweat, diplopia, edema, malaise, neck stiffness, rigors.
Musculoskeletal: arthralgia.
Neurologic: agitation, anxiety, confusion, dyscoordination, hypoesthesia, hypokinesia, increased appetite, insomnia, nervousness, nightmares.
Respiratory: bronchitis, pneumonia, upper respiratory tract infection.
Extremely rarely, ordinary doses of organic nitrates have caused methemoglobinemia in normal-seeming patients; for further discussion of its diagnosis and treatment see under **OVERDOSAGE.**

OVERDOSAGE

HEMODYNAMIC EFFECTS
The ill effects of isosorbide mononitrate overdose are generally the results of isosorbide mononitrate's capacity to induce vasodilatation, venous pooling, reduced cardiac output, and hypotension. These hemodynamic changes may have protean manifestations, including increased intracranial pressure, with any or all of persistent throbbing headache, confusion, and moderate fever; vertigo; palpitations; visual disturbances; nausea and vomiting (possibly with colic and even bloody diarrhea); syncope (especially in the upright posture); air hunger and dyspnea, later followed by reduced ventilatory effort; diaphoresis, with the skin either flushed or cold and clammy; heart block and bradycardia; paralysis; coma; seizures and death.
Laboratory determinations of serum levels of isosorbide mononitrate and its metabolites are not widely available, and such determinations have, in any event, no established role in the management of isosorbide mononitrate overdose.
There are no data suggesting what dose of isosorbide mononitrate is likely to be life-threatening in humans. In rats and mice, there is significant lethality at doses of 2000 mg/kg and 3000 mg/kg, respectively.
No data are available to suggest physiological maneuvers (e.g., maneuvers to change the pH of the urine) that might accelerate elimination of isosorbide mononitrate. In particular, dialysis is known to be ineffective in removing isosorbide mononitrate from the body.
No specific antagonist to the vasodilator effects of isosorbide mononitrate is known, and no intervention has been subject to controlled study as a therapy of isosorbide mononitrate overdose. Because the hypotension associated with isosorbide mononitrate overdose is the result of venodilatation and arterial hypovolemia, prudent therapy in this situation should be directed toward an increase in central fluid volume. Passive elevation of the patient's legs may be sufficient, but intravenous infusion of normal saline or similar fluid may also be necessary.
The use of epinephrine or other arterial vasoconstrictors in this setting is likely to do more harm than good.
In patients with renal disease or congestive heart failure, therapy resulting in central volume expansion is not without hazard. Treatment of isosorbide mononitrate overdose in these patients may be subtle and difficult, and invasive monitoring may be required.
METHEMOGLOBINEMIA
Methemoglobinemia has been reported in patients receiving other organic nitrates, and it probably could also occur as a side effect of isosorbide mononitrate. Certainly nitrate ions liberated during metabolism of isosorbide mononitrate can oxidize hemoglobin into methemoglobin. Even in patients totally without cytochrome b_5 reductase activity, however, and even assuming that the nitrate moiety of isosorbide mononitrate is quantitatively applied to oxidation of hemoglobin, about 2 mg/kg of isosorbide mononitrate should be required before any of these patients manifests clinically significant (≥ 10%) methemoglobinemia. In patients with normal reductase function, significant production of methemoglobin should require even larger doses of isosorbide mononitrate. In one study in which 36 patients received 2–4 weeks of continuous nitroglycerin therapy at 3.1 to 4.4 mg/hr (equivalent, in total administered dose of nitrate ions, to 7.8–11.1 mg of isosorbide mononitrate per hour), the average methemoglobin level measured was 0.2%; this was comparable to that observed in parallel patients who received placebo.
Not withstanding these observations, there are case reports of significant methemoglobinemia in association with moderate overdoses of organic nitrates. None of the affected patients had been thought to be unusually susceptible.
Methemoglobin levels are available from most clinical laboratories. The diagnosis should be suspected in patients who exhibit signs of impaired oxygen delivery despite adequate cardiac output and adequate arterial pO_2. Classically, methemoglobinemic blood is described as chocolate brown, without color change on exposure to air.
When methemoglobinemia is diagnosed, the treatment of choice is methylene blue, 1–2 mg/kg intravenously.

DOSAGE AND ADMINISTRATION

The recommended regimen of Ismo tablets is 20 mg (one tablet) twice daily, with the two doses given 7 hours apart. For most patients, this can be accomplished by taking the first dose on awakening and the second dose 7 hours later. Dosage adjustments are not necessary for elderly patients or patients with altered renal or hepatic function.
As noted above (**CLINICAL PHARMACOLOGY**), multiple studies of organic nitrates have shown that maintenance of continuous 24-hour plasma levels results in refractory tolerance. The dosing regimen for Ismo tablets provides a daily nitrate-free interval to avoid the development of this tolerance.
As also noted under **CLINICAL PHARMACOLOGY,** well-controlled studies have shown that tolerance to Ismo tablets is avoided when using the twice-daily regimen in which the two doses are given 7 hours apart. This regimen has been shown to have antianginal efficacy beginning 1 hour after the first dose and lasting at least 5 hours after the second dose. The duration (if any) of antianginal activity beyond 12 hours has not been studied; large controlled studies with other nitrates suggest that no dosing regimen should be expected to provide more than about 12 hours of continuous antianginal efficacy per day.
In clinical trials, Ismo tablets have been administered in a variety of regimens. Single doses less than 20 mg have not been adequately studied, while single doses greater than 20 mg have demonstrated no greater efficacy than doses of 20 mg.

HOW SUPPLIED

Ismo® (isosorbide mononitrate) tablets, 20 mg, are available in bottles of 100 (NDC 0008-0771-01) and in unit dose packages of 10 blister strips of 10 tablets (NDC 0008-0771-02). Each orange, round, film-coated tablet is engraved "ISMO 20" on one side and scored on the reverse side.
Store at controlled room temperature between 20°C and 25°C (68°F and 77°F).
Dispense in tight container.
Shown in Product Identification Guide, page 340

ISORDIL® ℞
(isosorbide dinitrate)
Sublingual Tablets

DESCRIPTION

Isosorbide dinitrate (ISDN) is 1,4:3,6-dianhydro-D-glucitol 2,5-dinitrate, an organic nitrate whose structural formula is

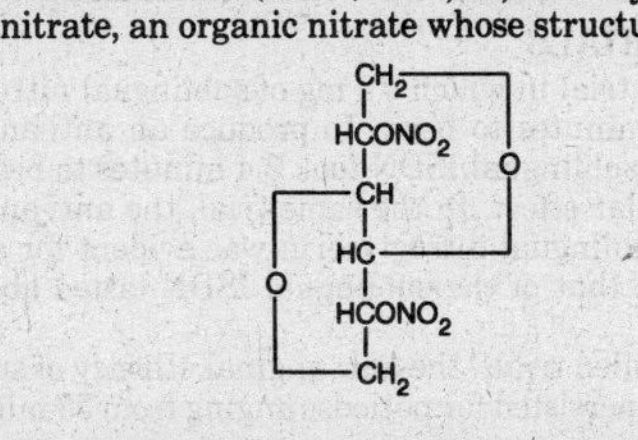

and whose molecular weight is 236.14. The organic nitrates are vasodilators, active on both arteries and veins.
Isosorbide dinitrate is a white, crystalline, odorless compound which is stable in air and in solution, has a melting point of 70°C and has an optical rotation of +134° (c=1.0, alcohol, 20°C). Isosorbide dinitrate is freely soluble in organic solvents such as acetone, alcohol, and ether, but is only sparingly soluble in water.
Each Isordil® Sublingual tablet contains 2.5, 5, or 10 mg of isosorbide dinitrate. The inactive ingredients in each tablet are cellulose, lactose, magnesium stearate, and starch. The 2.5 mg dosage strength also contains D&C Yellow 10 and FD&C Yellow 6, and the 5 mg dosage strength also contains FD&C Red 40.

CLINICAL PHARMACOLOGY

The principal pharmacological action of isosorbide dinitrate is relaxation of vascular smooth muscle and consequent dilatation of peripheral arteries and veins, especially the latter. Dilatation of the veins promotes peripheral pooling of blood and decreases venous return to the heart, thereby reducing left ventricular end-diastolic pressure and pulmonary capillary wedge pressure (preload). Arteriolar relaxation reduces systemic vascular resistance, systolic arterial pressure, and mean arterial pressure (afterload). Dilatation of the coronary arteries also occurs. The relative importance of preload reduction, afterload reduction, and coronary dilatation remains undefined.
Dosing regimens for most chronically used drugs are designed to provide plasma concentrations that are continuously greater than a minimally effective concentration. This strategy is inappropriate for organic nitrates. Several well-controlled clinical trials have used exercise testing to assess the anti-anginal efficacy of continuously-delivered nitrates. In the large majority of these trials, active agents were no more effective than placebo after 24 hours (or less) of continuous therapy. Attempts to overcome nitrate tolerance by dose escalation, even to doses far in excess of those used acutely, have consistently failed. Only after nitrates have been absent from the body for several hours has their antianginal efficacy been restored.
PHARMACOKINETICS
Bioavailability of ISDN after single sublingual doses is 40 to 50%. Multiple-dose studies of sublingual ISDN pharmacokinetics have not been reported; multiple-dose studies of ingested ISDN have observed progressive increases in bioavailability during chronic therapy. Serum levels of ISDN reach their maxima 10 to 15 minutes after sublingual dosing.
Once absorbed, the volume of distribution of isosorbide dinitrate is 2 to 4 L/kg, and this volume is cleared at the rate of 2 to 4 L/min, so ISDN's half-life in serum is about an hour. Since the clearance exceeds hepatic blood flow, considerable extrahepatic metabolism must also occur. Clearance is affected primarily by denitration to the 2-mononitrate (15 to 25%) and the 5-mononitrate (75 to 85%).
Both metabolites have biological activity, especially the 5-mononitrate. With an overall half-life of about 5 hours, the 5-mononitrate is cleared from the serum by denitration to isosorbide, glucuronidation to the 5-mononitrate glucuronide, and denitration/hydration to sorbitol. The 2-mononitrate has been less well studied, but it appears to participate

Continued on next page

Wyeth-Ayerst Laboratories—Cont.

in the same metabolic pathways, with a half-life of about 2 hours.

The daily dose-free interval sufficient to avoid tolerance to organic nitrates has not been well defined. Studies of nitroglycerin (an organic nitrate with a very short half-life) have shown that daily dose-free intervals of 10 to 12 hours are usually sufficient to minimize tolerance. Daily dose-free intervals that have succeeded in avoiding tolerance during trials of moderate doses (*e.g.,* 30 mg) of immediate-release ISDN have generally been somewhat longer (at least 14 hours), but this is consistent with the longer half-lives of ISDN and its active metabolites.

Few well-controlled clinical trials of organic nitrates have been designed to detect rebound or withdrawal effects. In one such trial, however, subjects receiving nitroglycerin had *less* exercise tolerance at the end of the daily dose-free interval than the parallel group receiving placebo. The incidence, magnitude, and clinical significance of similar phenomena in patients receiving ISDN have not been studied.

CLINICAL TRIALS

In a controlled trial in which 0.4 mg of sublingual nitroglycerin took 1.9 minutes to begin to produce an anti-anginal effect, 5 mg of sublingual ISDN took 3.4 minutes to begin to produce a similar effect. In the same trial, the anti-anginal effect of the sublingual nitroglycerin was evident for about an hour, while that of the sublingual ISDN lasted about 2 hours.

In other controlled trials, the anti-anginal efficacy of sublingual ISDN has persisted for periods ranging from 30 minutes up to 4 hours.

Multiple-dose trials of sublingual ISDN have not been reported. Multiple-dose trials of ingested formulations of ISDN have shown that ISDN's anti-anginal efficacy is substantially attenuated by tolerance unless the daily regimen includes a dose-free interval of at least 14 hours. The daily dose-free interval necessary in any chronic regimen using sublingual ISDN is not known.

From large, well-controlled studies of other nitrates, it is reasonable to believe that the maximal achievable daily duration of anti-anginal effect from isosorbide dinitrate is about 12 hours. No dosing regimen for isosorbide dinitrate has, however, ever actually been shown to achieve this duration of effect. In the absence of data from multiple-dose trials, and considering the capacity of organic nitrates to induce tolerance, it is not reasonable to assume that multiple sublingual ISDN tablets taken during the course of a day will all have similar effects.

INDICATIONS AND USAGE

Isordil Sublingual tablets are indicated for the prevention and treatment of angina pectoris due to coronary artery disease. However, because the onset of action of sublingual ISDN is significantly slower than that of sublingual nitroglycerin, sublingual ISDN is not the drug of first choice for abortion of an acute anginal episode.

CONTRAINDICATIONS

Allergic reactions to organic nitrates are extremely rare, but they do occur. Isordil is contraindicated in patients who are allergic to isosorbide dinitrate or any of its other ingredients.

WARNINGS

The benefits of sublingual isosorbide dinitrate in patients with acute myocardial infarction or congestive heart failure have not been established. If one elects to use isosorbide dinitrate in these conditions, careful clinical or hemodynamic monitoring must be used to avoid the hazards of hypotension and tachycardia.

PRECAUTIONS

GENERAL

Severe hypotension, particularly with upright posture, may occur with even small doses of isosorbide dinitrate. This drug should therefore be used with caution in patients who may be volume depleted or who, for whatever reason, are already hypotensive. Hypotension induced by isosorbide dinitrate may be accompanied by paradoxical bradycardia and increased angina pectoris.

Nitrate therapy may aggravate the angina caused by hypertrophic cardiomyopathy.

As tolerance to isosorbide dinitrate develops, the effect of sublingual nitroglycerin on exercise tolerance, although still observable, is somewhat blunted.

Some clinical trials in angina patients have provided nitroglycerin for about 12 continuous hours of every 24-hour day. During the daily dose-free interval in some of these trials, anginal attacks have been more easily provoked than before treatment, and patients have demonstrated hemodynamic rebound and *decreased* exercise tolerance. The importance of these observations to the routine, clinical use of sublingual isosorbide dinitrate is not known.

In industrial workers who have had long-term exposure to unknown (presumably high) doses of organic nitrates, tolerance clearly occurs. Chest pain, acute myocardial infarction, and even sudden death have occurred during temporary withdrawal of nitrates from these workers, demonstrating the existence of true physical dependence.

INFORMATION FOR PATIENTS

Patients should be told that the anti-anginal efficacy of isosorbide dinitrate is strongly related to its dosing regimen, so the prescribed schedule of dosing should be followed carefully. In particular, daily headaches sometimes accompany treatment with isosorbide dinitrate. In patients who get these headaches, the headaches are a marker of the activity of the drug. Patients should resist the temptation to avoid headaches by altering the schedule of their treatment with isosorbide dinitrate, since loss of headache may be associated with simultaneous loss of anti-anginal efficacy. Aspirin and/or acetaminophen, on the other hand, often successfully relieve isosorbide dinitrate-induced headaches with no deleterious effect on isosorbide dinitrate's anti-anginal efficacy.

Treatment with isosorbide dinitrate may be associated with lightheadedness on standing, especially just after rising from a recumbent or seated position. This effect may be more frequent in patients who have also consumed alcohol.

DRUG INTERACTIONS

The vasodilating effects of isosorbide dinitrate may be additive with those of other vasodilators. Alcohol, in particular, has been found to exhibit additive effects of this variety.

CARCINOGENESIS, MUTAGENESIS, IMPAIRMENT OF FERTILITY

No long-term studies in animals have been performed to evaluate the carcinogenic potential of isosorbide dinitrate. In a modified two-litter reproduction study, there was no remarkable gross pathology and no altered fertility or gestation among rats fed isosorbide dinitrate at 25 or 100 mg/kg/day.

PREGNANCY CATEGORY C

At oral doses 35 and 150 times the maximum recommended human daily dose, isosorbide dinitrate has been shown to cause a dose-related increase in embryotoxicity (increase in mummified pups) in rabbits. There are no adequate, well-controlled studies in pregnant women. Isosorbide dinitrate should be used during pregnancy only if the potential benefit justifies the potential risk to the fetus.

NURSING MOTHERS

It is not known whether isosorbide dinitrate is excreted in human milk. Because many drugs are excreted in human milk, caution should be exercised when isosorbide dinitrate is administered to a nursing woman.

PEDIATRIC USE

Safety and effectiveness in pediatric patients have not been established.

ADVERSE REACTIONS

Adverse reactions to isosorbide dinitrate are generally dose-related, and almost all of these reactions are the result of isosorbide dinitrate's activity as a vasodilator. Headache, which may be severe, is the most commonly reported side effect. Headache may be recurrent with each daily dose, especially at higher doses. Transient episodes of lightheadedness, occasionally related to blood pressure changes, may also occur. Hypotension occurs infrequently, but in some patients it may be severe enough to warrant discontinuation of therapy. Syncope, crescendo angina, and rebound hypertension have been reported but are uncommon.

Extremely rarely, ordinary doses of organic nitrates have caused methemoglobinemia in normal-seeming patients. Methemoglobinemia is so infrequent at these doses that further discussion of its diagnosis and treatment is deferred (see **"Overdosage"**).

Data are not available to allow estimation of the frequency of adverse reactions during treatment with Isordil® Sublingual tablets.

OVERDOSAGE

HEMODYNAMIC EFFECTS

The ill effects of isosorbide dinitrate overdose are generally the results of isosorbide dinitrate's capacity to induce vasodilatation, venous pooling, reduced cardiac output, and hypotension. These hemodynamic changes may have protean manifestations, including increased intracranial pressure, with any or all of persistent throbbing headache, confusion, and moderate fever; vertigo; palpitations; visual disturbances; nausea and vomiting (possibly with colic and even bloody diarrhea); syncope (especially in the upright posture); air hunger and dyspnea, later followed by reduced ventilatory effort; diaphoresis, with the skin either flushed or cold and clammy; heart block and bradycardia; paralysis; coma; seizures; and death.

Laboratory determinations of serum levels of isosorbide dinitrate and its metabolites are not widely available, and such determinations have, in any event, no established role in the management of isosorbide dinitrate overdose.

There are no data suggesting what dose of isosorbide dinitrate is likely to be life-threatening in humans. In rats, the median acute lethal dose (LD_{50}) was found to be 1100 mg/kg.

No data are available to suggest physiological maneuvers (*e.g.,* maneuvers to change the pH of the urine) that might accelerate elimination of isosorbide dinitrate and its active metabolites. Similarly, it is not known which, if any, of these substances can usefully be removed from the body by hemodialysis.

No specific antagonist to the vasodilator effects of isosorbide dinitrate is known, and no intervention has been subject to controlled studies as a therapy for isosorbide dinitrate overdose. Because the hypotension associated with isosorbide dinitrate overdose is the result of venodilatation and arterial hypovolemia, prudent therapy in this situation should be directed toward increase in central fluid volume. Passive elevation of the patient's legs may be sufficient, but intravenous infusion of normal saline or similar fluid may also be necessary.

The use of epinephrine or other arterial vasoconstrictors in this setting is likely to do more harm than good.

In patients with renal disease or congestive heart failure, therapy resulting in central volume expansion is not without hazard. Treatment of isosorbide dinitrate overdose in these patients may be subtle and difficult, and invasive monitoring may be required.

METHEMOGLOBINEMIA

Nitrate ions liberated during metabolism of isosorbide dinitrate can oxidize hemoglobin into methemoglobin. Even in patients totally without cytochrome b_5 reductase activity, however, and even assuming that the nitrate moieties of isosorbide dinitrate are quantitatively applied to oxidation of hemoglobin, about 1 mg/kg of isosorbide dinitrate should be required before any of these patients manifests clinically significant ($\geq 10\%$) methemoglobinemia. In patients with normal reductase function, significant production of methemoglobin should require even larger doses of isosorbide dinitrate. In one study in which 36 patients received 2 to 4 weeks of continuous nitroglycerin therapy at 3.1 to 4.4 mg/hr (equivalent, in total administered dose of nitrate ions, to 4.8 to 6.9 mg of bioavailable isosorbide dinitrate per hour), the average methemoglobin level measured was 0.2%; this was comparable to that observed in parallel patients who received placebo.

Notwithstanding these observations, there are case reports of significant methemoglobinemia in association with moderate overdoses of organic nitrates. None of the affected patients had been thought to be unusually susceptible.

Methemoglobin levels are available from most clinical laboratories. The diagnosis should be suspected in patients who exhibit signs of impaired oxygen delivery despite adequate cardiac output and adequate arterial pO_2. Classically, methemoglobinemic blood is described as chocolate brown, without color change on exposure to air.

When methemoglobinemia is diagnosed, the treatment of choice is methylene blue, 1 to 2 mg/kg intravenously.

DOSAGE AND ADMINISTRATION

As noted under **"Clinical Pharmacology,"** multiple-dose studies with ISDN and other nitrates have shown that maintenance of continuous 24-hour plasma levels results in refractory tolerance. Every dosing regimen for ISDN must provide a daily dose-free interval to minimize the development of this tolerance. In the case of sublingual tablets, it is probably true that one of the daily dose-free intervals must be somewhat longer than 14 hours.

As also noted under **"Clinical Pharmacology,"** the efficacy of daily doses after the first dose has never been demonstrated.

Large controlled studies with other nitrates suggest that no dosing regimen with Isordil Sublingual tablets should be expected to provide more than about 12 hours of continuous anti-anginal efficacy per day.

A patient anticipating activity likely to cause angina should take one Isordil Sublingual tablet (2.5 to 5 mg) about 15 minutes before the activity is expected to begin. Isordil Sublingual tablets may be used to abort an acute anginal episode, but its use is recommended only in patients who fail to respond to sublingual nitroglycerin.

HOW SUPPLIED

Isordil® (isosorbide dinitrate) Sublingual Tablets are available as follows:

2.5 mg, round, yellow tablets imprinted "2.5" on one side and "W" on reverse side:

NDC 0008-4139-01, bottles of 100.
NDC 0008-4139-03, bottles of 500.
NDC 0008-4139-05, Redipak® cartons of 100 (10 blister strips of 10).

5 mg, round, pink tablets imprinted "5" on one side and "W" on reverse side:

NDC 0008-4126-01, bottles of 100.
NDC 0008-4126-03, bottles of 500.
NDC 0008-4126-07, Redipak cartons of 100 (10 blister strips of 10).

Store at room temperature, approximately 25°C (77°F)
Protect from light
Keep bottles tightly closed
Dispense in a light-resistant, tight container
Use carton to protect blisters from light

10 mg, round, white tablets imprinted "10" on one side and "Wyeth" on reverse side:
NDC 0008-4161-01, bottles of 100.
Store at room temperature, approximately 25°C (77°F)
Keep tightly closed
Dispense in a tight container
ALSO AVAILABLE
Oral Titradose® Tablets in the following dosage strengths:
5 mg, NDC 0008-4152, in bottles of 100, 500 or 1,000 and in Redipak cartons of 100 (10 blister strips of 10).
10 mg, NDC 0008-4153, in bottles of 100, 500 or 1,000 and in Redipak cartons of 100 (10 blister strips of 10).
20 mg, NDC 0008-4154, in bottles of 100 or 500 and in Redipak cartons of 100 (10 blister strips of 10).
30 mg, NDC 0008-4159, in bottles of 100 or 500 and in Redipak cartons of 100 (10 blister strips of 10).
40 mg, NDC 0008-4192, in bottles of 100 and in Redipak cartons of 100 (10 blister strips of 10).
Tembids® Tablets, 40 mg, controlled-release tablets, NDC 0008-4125, in bottles of 100, 500 or 1,000.
Tembids® Capsules, 40 mg, controlled-release capsules, NDC 0008-4140, in bottles of 100 or 500.
Shown in Product Identification Guide, page 340

ISORDIL® TEMBIDS® ℞
(isosorbide dinitrate)
Controlled-Release Tablets and Capsules

DESCRIPTION
Isosorbide dinitrate (ISDN) is 1,4:3,6-dianhydro-D-glucitol 2,5-dinitrate, an organic nitrate whose structural formula is

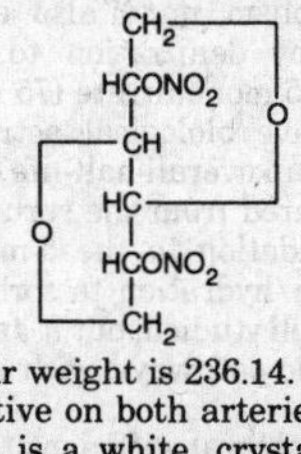

and whose molecular weight is 236.14. The organic nitrates are vasodilators, active on both arteries and veins.
Isosorbide dinitrate is a white, crystalline, odorless compound which is stable in air and in solution, has a melting point of 70°C and has an optical rotation of +134° (c=1.0, alcohol, 20°C). Isosorbide dinitrate is freely soluble in organic solvents such as acetone, alcohol, and ether, but is only sparingly soluble in water.
Each Isordil® Tembids® controlled-release tablet and capsule contains 40 mg of isosorbide dinitrate, in a matrix that causes the active drug to be released over a sustained period. The inactive ingredients contained in Isordil Tembids tablets are: D&C Yellow 10, FD&C Blue 1, FD&C Yellow 6, lactose, magnesium stearate, sodium silicoaluminate, talc, aluminum stearate, methylcellulose, and polacrilin potassium. The inactive ingredients contained in Isordil Tembids capsules are: confectioners' sugar, starch, gelatin capsule, and other ingredients.

CLINICAL PHARMACOLOGY
The principal pharmacological action of isosorbide dinitrate is relaxation of vascular smooth muscle and consequent dilatation of peripheral arteries and veins, especially the latter. Dilatation of the veins promotes peripheral pooling of blood and decreases venous return to the heart, thereby reducing left ventricular end-diastolic pressure and pulmonary capillary wedge pressure (preload). Arteriolar relaxation reduces systemic vascular resistance, systolic arterial pressure, and mean arterial pressure (afterload). Dilatation of the coronary arteries also occurs. The relative importance of preload reduction, afterload reduction, and coronary dilatation remains undefined.
Dosing regimens for most chronically used drugs are designed to provide plasma concentrations that are continuously greater than a minimally effective concentration. This strategy is inappropriate for organic nitrates. Several well-controlled clinical trials have used exercise testing to assess the anti-anginal efficacy of continuously-delivered nitrates. In the large majority of these trials, active agents were no more effective than placebo after 24 hours (or less) of continuous therapy. Attempts to overcome nitrate tolerance by dose escalation, even to doses far in excess of those used acutely, have consistently failed. Only after nitrates have been absent from the body for several hours has their anti-anginal efficacy been restored.
PHARMACOKINETICS
The kinetics of absorption of isosorbide dinitrate from Isordil Tembids controlled-release tablets and capsules have not been well studied. Studies of immediate-release formulations of ISDN have found highly variable bioavailability (10% to 90%) with extensive first-pass metabolism in the liver. Most such studies have observed progressive increases in bioavailability during chronic therapy; it is not known whether similar increases in bioavailability appear during the course of chronic therapy with Isordil Tembids controlled-release tablets and capsules.
Once absorbed, the volume of distribution of isosorbide dinitrate is 2 to 4 L/kg, and this volume is cleared at the rate of 2 to 4 L/min, so ISDN's half-life in serum is about an hour. Since the clearance exceeds hepatic blood flow, considerable extrahepatic metabolism must also occur. Clearance is effected primarily by denitration to the 2-mononitrate (15 to 25%) and the 5-mononitrate (75 to 85%).
Both metabolites have biological activity, especially the 5-mononitrate. With an overall half-life of about 5 hours, the 5-mononitrate is cleared from the serum by denitration to isosorbide, glucuronidation to the 5-mononitrate glucuronide, and denitration/hydration to sorbitol. The 2-mononitrate has been less well studied, but it appears to participate in the same metabolic pathways, with a half-life of about 2 hours.
The daily dose-free interval sufficient to avoid tolerance to ISDN has not been well defined. Studies of nitroglycerin (an organic nitrate with a very short half-life) have shown that daily dose-free intervals of 10 to 12 hours are usually sufficient to minimize tolerance. Daily dose-free intervals that have succeeded in avoiding tolerance during trials of moderate doses (*e.g.,* 30 mg) of immediate-release ISDN have generally been somewhat longer (at least 14 hours), but this is consistent with the longer half-lives of ISDN and its active metabolites. A dose-free interval sufficient to avoid tolerance with Isordil Tembids has not been demonstrated. Clinical trials using Isordil Tembids in a regimen designed to avoid tolerance have not been conducted, but in a multiple-dose study of another controlled-release isosorbide dinitrate product, 40 mg capsules were administered at 0800 and 1400 hours. After two weeks of this regimen, the controlled-release isosorbide dinitrate product was statistically indistinguishable from placebo. For the formulation of controlled-release isosorbide dinitrate that was tested, the necessary dose-free interval must therefore be greater than 18 hours; the necessary interval for Isordil Tembids remains unknown.
Few well-controlled clinical trials of organic nitrates have been designed to detect rebound or withdrawal effects. In one such trial, however, subjects receiving nitroglycerin had *less* exercise tolerance at the end of the daily dose-free interval than the parallel group receiving placebo. The incidence, magnitude, and clinical significance of similar phenomena in patients receiving ISDN have not been studied.

CLINICAL TRIALS
In clinical trials, immediate-release oral isosorbide dinitrate has been administered in a variety of regimens, with total daily doses ranging from 30 mg to 480 mg. Controlled trials of single doses of controlled-release isosorbide dinitrate have demonstrated effective reductions in exercise-related angina for up to 8 hours. Anti-anginal activity is present about 1 hour after dosing.
Adequate multiple-dose trials of Isordil Tembids controlled-release tablets and capsules have not been reported.
Most controlled trials of multiple-dose immediate-release oral ISDN taken every 12 hours (or more frequently) for several weeks have shown statistically significant anti-anginal efficacy for only 2 hours after dosing. Once-daily regimens, and regimens with one daily dose-free interval of at least 14 hours (*e.g.,* a regimen providing doses at 0800, 1400, and 1800 hours), have shown efficacy after the first dose of each day that was similar to that shown in the single-dose studies cited above. The efficacy of subsequent doses has not been demonstrated. From large, well-controlled studies of other nitrates, it is reasonable to believe that the maximal achievable daily duration of anti-anginal effect from isosorbide dinitrate is about 12 hours. No dosing regimen for Isordil Tembids controlled-release tablets and capsules has, however, ever actually been shown to achieve this duration of effect.

INDICATIONS AND USAGE
Isordil Tembids controlled-release tablets and capsules are indicated for the prevention of angina pectoris due to coronary artery disease. The onset of action of controlled-release oral isosorbide dinitrate is not sufficiently rapid for this product to be useful in aborting an acute anginal episode.

CONTRAINDICATIONS
Allergic reactions to organic nitrates are extremely rare, but they do occur. Isordil Tembids are contraindicated in patients who are allergic to isosorbide dinitrate or any of its ingredients.

WARNINGS
The benefits of controlled-release oral isosorbide dinitrate in patients with acute myocardial infarction or congestive heart failure have not been established. If one elects to use isosorbide dinitrate in these conditions, careful clinical or hemodynamic monitoring must be used to avoid the hazards of hypotension and tachycardia. Because the effects of controlled-release oral isosorbide dinitrate are so difficult to terminate rapidly, this formulation is not recommended in these settings.

PRECAUTIONS
GENERAL
Severe hypotension, particularly with upright posture, may occur with even small doses of isosorbide dinitrate. This drug should therefore be used with caution in patients who may be volume depleted or who, for whatever reason, are already hypotensive. Hypotension induced by isosorbide dinitrate may be accompanied by paradoxical bradycardia and increased angina pectoris.
Nitrate therapy may aggravate the angina caused by hypertrophic cardiomyopathy.
As tolerance to isosorbide dinitrate develops, the effect of sublingual nitroglycerin on exercise tolerance, although still observable, is somewhat blunted.
Some clinical trials in angina patients have provided nitroglycerin for about 12 continuous hours of every 24-hour day. During the daily dose-free intervals in some of these trials, anginal attacks have been more easily provoked than before treatment, and patients have demonstrated hemodynamic rebound and *decreased* exercise tolerance. The importance of these observations to the routine, clinical use of controlled-release oral isosorbide dinitrate is not known.
In industrial workers who have had long-term exposure to unknown (presumably high) doses of organic nitrates, tolerance clearly occurs. Chest pain, acute myocardial infarction, and even sudden death have occurred during temporary withdrawal of nitrates from these workers, demonstrating the existence of true physical dependence.
INFORMATION FOR PATIENTS
Patients should be told that the anti-anginal efficacy of isosorbide dinitrate is strongly related to its dosing regimen, so the prescribed schedule of dosing should be followed carefully. In particular, daily headaches sometimes accompany treatment with isosorbide dinitrate. In patients who get these headaches, the headaches are a marker of the activity of the drug. Patients should resist the temptation to avoid headaches by altering the schedule of their treatment with isosorbide dinitrate, since loss of headache may be associated with simultaneous loss of anti-anginal efficacy. Aspirin and/or acetaminophen, on the other hand, often successfully relieve isosorbide dinitrate-induced headaches with no deleterious effect on isosorbide dinitrate's anti-anginal efficacy.
Treatment with isosorbide dinitrate may be associated with lightheadedness on standing, especially just after rising from a recumbent or seated position. This effect may be more frequent in patients who have also consumed alcohol.
DRUG INTERACTIONS
The vasodilating effects of isosorbide dinitrate may be additive with those of other vasodilators. Alcohol, in particular, has been found to exhibit additive effects of this variety.
CARCINOGENESIS, MUTAGENESIS, IMPAIRMENT OF FERTILITY
No long-term studies in animals have been performed to evaluate the carcinogenic potential of isosorbide dinitrate. In a modified two-litter reproduction study, there was no remarkable gross pathology and no altered fertility or gestation among rats fed isosorbide dinitrate at 25 or 100 mg/kg/day.
PREGNANCY CATEGORY C
At oral doses 35 and 150 times the maximum recommended human daily dose, isosorbide dinitrate has been shown to cause a dose-related increase in embryotoxicity (increase in mummified pups) in rabbits. There are no adequate, well-controlled studies in pregnant women. Isosorbide dinitrate should be used during pregnancy only if the potential benefit justifies the potential risk to the fetus.
NURSING MOTHERS
It is not known whether isosorbide dinitrate is excreted in human milk. Because many drugs are excreted in human milk, caution should be exercised when isosorbide dinitrate is administered to a nursing woman.
PEDIATRIC USE
Safety and effectiveness in pediatric patients have not been established.

ADVERSE REACTIONS
Adverse reactions to isosorbide dinitrate are generally dose-related, and almost all of these reactions are the result of isosorbide dinitrate's activity as a vasodilator. Headache, which may be severe, is the most commonly reported side effect. Headache may be recurrent with each daily dose, especially at higher doses. Transient episodes of lightheadedness, occasionally related to blood pressure changes, may also occur. Hypotension occurs infrequently, but in some patients it may be severe enough to warrant discontinuation of therapy. Syncope, crescendo angina, and rebound hypertension have been reported but are uncommon.
Extremely rarely, ordinary doses of organic nitrates have caused methemoglobinemia in normal-seeming patients. Methemoglobinemia is so infrequent at these doses that further discussion of its diagnosis and treatment is deferred (see "**Overdosage**").

Continued on next page

Wyeth-Ayerst Laboratories—Cont.

Data are not available to allow estimation of the frequency of adverse reactions during treatment with Isordil® Tembids® controlled-release tablets and capsules.

OVERDOSAGE

HEMODYNAMIC EFFECTS

The ill effects of isosorbide dinitrate overdose are generally the results of isosorbide dinitrate's capacity to induce vasodilatation, venous pooling, reduced cardiac output, and hypotension. These hemodynamic changes may have protean manifestations, including increased intracranial pressure, with any or all of persistent throbbing headache, confusion, and moderate fever; vertigo; palpitations; visual disturbances; nausea and vomiting (possibly with colic and even bloody diarrhea); syncope (especially in the upright posture); air hunger and dyspnea, later followed by reduced ventilatory effort; diaphoresis, with the skin either flushed or cold and clammy; heart block and bradycardia; paralysis; coma; seizures; and death.

Laboratory determinations of serum levels of isosorbide dinitrate and its metabolites are not widely available, and such determinations have, in any event, no established role in the management of isosorbide dinitrate overdose.

There are no data suggesting what dose of isosorbide dinitrate is likely to be life-threatening in humans. In rats, the median acute lethal dose (LD_{50}) was found to be 1100 mg/kg.

No data are available to suggest physiological maneuvers (*e.g.,* maneuvers to change the pH of the urine) that might accelerate elimination of isosorbide dinitrate and its active metabolites. Similarly, it is not known which, if any, of these substances can usefully be removed from the body by hemodialysis.

No specific antagonist to the vasodilator effects of isosorbide dinitrate is known, and no intervention has been subject to controlled studies as a therapy for isosorbide dinitrate overdose. Because the hypotension associated with isosorbide dinitrate overdose is the result of venodilatation and arterial hypovolemia, prudent therapy in this situation should be directed toward increase in central fluid volume. Passive elevation of the patient's legs may be sufficient, but intravenous infusion of normal saline or similar fluid may also be necessary.

The use of epinephrine or other arterial vasoconstrictors in this setting is likely to do more harm than good.

In patients with renal disease or congestive heart failure, therapy resulting in central volume expansion is not without hazard. Treatment of isosorbide dinitrate overdose in these patients may be subtle and difficult, and invasive monitoring may be required.

METHEMOGLOBINEMIA

Nitrate ions liberated during metabolism of isosorbide dinitrate can oxidize hemoglobin into methemoglobin. Even in patients totally without cytochrome b_5 reductase activity, however, and even assuming that the nitrate moieties of isosorbide dinitrate are quantitatively applied to oxidation of hemoglobin, about 1 mg/kg of isosorbide dinitrate should be required before any of these patients manifests clinically significant ($\geq 10\%$) methemoglobinemia. In patients with normal reductase function, significant production of methemoglobin should require even larger doses of isosorbide dinitrate. In one study in which 36 patients received 2 to 4 weeks of continuous nitroglycerin therapy at 3.1 to 4.4 mg/hr (equivalent, in total administered dose of nitrate ions, to 4.8 to 6.9 mg of bioavailable isosorbide dinitrate per hour), the average methemoglobin level measured was 0.2%; this was comparable to that observed in parallel patients who received placebo.

Notwithstanding these observations, there are case reports of significant methemoglobinemia in association with moderate overdoses of organic nitrates. None of the affected patients had been thought to be unusually susceptible.

Methemoglobin levels are available from most clinical laboratories. The diagnosis should be suspected in patients who exhibit signs of impaired oxygen delivery despite adequate cardiac output and adequate arterial pO_2. Classically, methemoglobinemic blood is described as chocolate brown, without color change on exposure to air.

When methemoglobinemia is diagnosed, the treatment of choice is methylene blue, 1 to 2 mg/kg intravenously.

DOSAGE AND ADMINISTRATION

As noted under "**Clinical Pharmacology**," multiple-dose studies with ISDN and other nitrates have shown that maintenance of continuous 24-hour plasma levels results in refractory tolerance. Every dosing regimen for Isordil Tembids controlled-release tablets and capsules must provide a daily dose-free interval to minimize the development of this tolerance. With immediate-release ISDN, it appears that one daily dose-free interval must be at least 14 hours long. The necessary dose-free interval for Isordil Tembids controlled-release tablets and capsules has not been clearly identified, but is presumably somewhat longer. As also noted under "**Clinical Pharmacology**," only one trial has ever studied the use of controlled-release isosorbide dinitrate for more than one dose. In that trial, 40 mg of a different formulation of controlled-release ISDN was administered twice daily in doses given 6 hours apart. After 4 weeks, active treatment could not be distinguished from placebo.

Large controlled studies with other nitrates suggest that no dosing regimen with Isordil Tembids should be expected to provide more than about 12 hours of continuous anti-anginal efficacy per day.

In clinical trials, immediate-release oral isosorbide dinitrate has been administered in a variety of regimens, with total daily doses ranging from 30 mg to 480 mg.

HOW SUPPLIED

Isordil® (isosorbide dinitrate) Tembids® Controlled-Release Tablets and Capsules are available as follows:

40 mg, round, canary-colored (slight greenish tinge) controlled-release tablets imprinted "Wyeth" on one side and "4125" on scored reverse side:

NDC 0008-4125-01, bottles of 100.
NDC 0008-4125-02, bottles of 500.
NDC 0008-4125-03, bottles of 1,000.

40 mg, controlled-release capsules with a transparent colorless body and opaque blue cap, marked "Wyeth 4140" in black ink:

NDC 0008-4140-01, bottles of 100.
NDC 0008-4140-02, bottles of 500.

Store at room temperature, approximately 25°C (77°F)
Protect from light
Keep tightly closed
Dispense in a light-resistant, tight container

The appearances of Tembids® Tablets and Capsules are trademarks of Wyeth-Ayerst Laboratories.

ALSO AVAILABLE

Sublingual Tablets, 2.5 mg, NDC 0008-4139, in bottles of 100 or 500 and in Redipak® cartons of 100 (10 blister strips of 10).

Sublingual Tablets, 5 mg, NDC 0008-4126, in bottles of 100 or 500 and in Redipak cartons of 100 (10 blister strips of 10).

Sublingual Tablets, 10 mg, NDC 0008-4161, in bottles of 100.

Oral Titradose® Tablets in the following dosage strengths:
5 mg, NDC 0008-4152, in bottles of 100, 500 or 1,000 and in Redipak cartons of 100 (10 blister strips of 10).
10 mg, NDC 0008-4153, in bottles of 100, 500 or 1,000 and in Redipak cartons of 100 (10 blister strips of 10).
20 mg, NDC 0008-4154, in bottles of 100 or 500 and in Redipak cartons of 100 (10 blister strips of 10).
30 mg, NDC 0008-4159, in bottles of 100 or 500 and in Redipak cartons of 100 (10 blister strips of 10).
40 mg, NDC 0008-4192, in bottles of 100 and in Redipak cartons of 100 (10 blister strips of 10).

Only Isordil Tembids Capsules manufactured by
K-V Pharmaceutical Co., St. Louis, MO 63144

Shown in Product Identification Guide, page 340

ISORDIL® TITRADOSE® ℞
(isosorbide dinitrate)
Tablets

DESCRIPTION

Isosorbide dinitrate (ISDN) is 1,4:3,6-dianhydro-D-glucitol 2,5-dinitrate, an organic nitrate whose structural formula is

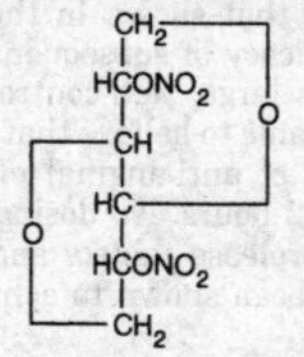

and whose molecular weight is 236.14. The organic nitrates are vasodilators, active on both arteries and veins.

Isosorbide dinitrate is a white, crystalline, odorless compound which is stable in air and in solution, has a melting point of 70°C and has an optical rotation of +134° (c=1.0, alcohol, 20°C). Isosorbide dinitrate is freely soluble in organic solvents such as acetone, alcohol, and ether, but is only sparingly soluble in water.

Each Isordil® Titradose® tablet contains 5, 10, 20, 30, or 40 mg of isosorbide dinitrate. The inactive ingredients in each tablet are lactose, cellulose, and magnesium stearate. The 5 mg, 20 mg, 30 mg, and 40 mg dosage strengths also contain the following: 5 mg—FD&C Red 40; 20 mg and 40 mg—D&C Yellow 10, FD&C Blue 1, and FD&C Yellow 6; 30 mg—FD&C Blue 1.

CLINICAL PHARMACOLOGY

The principal pharmacological action of isosorbide dinitrate is relaxation of vascular smooth muscle and consequent dilatation of peripheral arteries and veins, especially the latter. Dilatation of the veins promotes peripheral pooling of blood and decreases venous return to the heart, thereby reducing left ventricular end-diastolic pressure and pulmonary capillary wedge pressure (preload). Arteriolar relaxation reduces systemic vascular resistance, systolic arterial pressure, and mean arterial pressure (afterload). Dilatation of the coronary arteries also occurs. The relative importance of preload reduction, afterload reduction, and coronary dilatation remains undefined.

Dosing regimens for most chronically used drugs are designed to provide plasma concentrations that are continuously greater than a minimally effective concentration. This strategy is inappropriate for organic nitrates. Several well-controlled clinical trials have used exercise testing to assess the anti-anginal efficacy of continuously-delivered nitrates. In the large majority of these trials, active agents were no more effective than placebo after 24 hours (or less) of continuous therapy. Attempts to overcome nitrate tolerance by dose escalation, even to doses far in excess of those used acutely, have consistently failed. Only after nitrates have been absent from the body for several hours has their anti-anginal efficacy been restored.

PHARMACOKINETICS

Absorption of isosorbide dinitrate after oral dosing is nearly complete, but bioavailability is highly variable (10% to 90%), with extensive first-pass metabolism in the liver. Serum levels reach their maxima about an hour after ingestion. The average bioavailability of ISDN is about 25%; most studies have observed progressive increases in bioavailability during chronic therapy.

Once absorbed, the volume of distribution of isosorbide dinitrate is 2 to 4 L/kg, and this volume is cleared at the rate of 2 to 4 L/min, so ISDN's half-life in serum is about an hour. Since the clearance exceeds hepatic blood flow, considerable extrahepatic metabolism must also occur. Clearance is affected primarily by denitration to the 2-mononitrate (15 to 25%) and the 5-mononitrate (75 to 85%).

Both metabolites have biological activity, especially the 5-mononitrate. With an overall half-life of about 5 hours, the 5-mononitrate is cleared from the serum by denitration to isosorbide, glucuronidation to the 5-mononitrate glucuronide, and denitration/hydration to sorbitol. The 2-mononitrate has been less well studied, but it appears to participate in the same metabolic pathways, with a half-life of about 2 hours.

The daily dose-free interval sufficient to avoid tolerance to organic nitrates has not been well defined. Studies of nitroglycerin (an organic nitrate with a very short half-life) have shown that daily dose-free intervals of 10 to 12 hours are usually sufficient to minimize tolerance. Daily dose-free intervals that have succeeded in avoiding tolerance during trials of moderate doses (*e.g.,* 30 mg) of immediate-release ISDN have generally been somewhat longer (at least 14 hours), but this is consistent with the longer half-lives of ISDN and its active metabolites.

Few well-controlled clinical trials of organic nitrates have been designed to detect rebound or withdrawal effects. In one such trial, however, subjects receiving nitroglycerin had *less* exercise tolerance at the end of the daily dose-free interval than the parallel group receiving placebo. The incidence, magnitude, and clinical significance of similar phenomena in patients receiving ISDN have not been studied.

CLINICAL TRIALS

In clinical trials, immediate-release oral isosorbide dinitrate has been administered in a variety of regimens, with total daily doses ranging from 30 mg to 480 mg. Controlled trials of single oral doses of isosorbide dinitrate have demonstrated effective reductions in exercise-related angina for up to 8 hours. Anti-anginal activity is present about 1 hour after dosing.

Most controlled trials of multiple-dose oral ISDN taken every 12 hours (or more frequently) for several weeks have shown statistically significant anti-anginal efficacy for only 2 hours after dosing. Once-daily regimens, and regimens with one daily dose-free interval of at least 14 hours (*e.g.,* a regimen providing doses at 0800, 1400, and 1800 hours), have shown efficacy after the first dose of each day that was similar to that shown in the single-dose studies cited above. The effects of the second and later doses have been smaller and shorter-lasting than the effect of the first.

From large, well-controlled studies of other nitrates, it is reasonable to believe that the maximum achievable daily duration of anti-anginal effect from isosorbide dinitrate is about 12 hours. No dosing regimen for isosorbide dinitrate has, however, ever actually been shown to achieve this duration of effect. One study of 8 patients, who were administered a pretitrated dose (average 27.5 mg) of immediate-release ISDN at 0800, 1300, and 1800 hours for 2 weeks, revealed that significant anti-anginal effectiveness was discontinuous and totaled about 6 hours in a 24 hour period.

INDICATIONS AND USAGE

Isordil Titradose tablets are indicated for the prevention of angina pectoris due to coronary artery disease. The onset of action of immediate-release oral isosorbide dinitrate is not sufficiently rapid for this product to be useful in aborting an acute anginal episode.

CONTRAINDICATIONS

Allergic reactions to organic nitrates are extremely rare, but they do occur. Isordil Titradose is contraindicated in patients who are allergic to isosorbide dinitrate or any of its other ingredients.

WARNINGS

The benefits of immediate-release oral isosorbide dinitrate in patients with acute myocardial infarction or congestive heart failure have not been established. If one elects to use isosorbide dinitrate in these conditions, careful clinical or hemodynamic monitoring must be used to avoid the hazards of hypotension and tachycardia. Because the effects of oral isosorbide dinitrate are so difficult to terminate rapidly, this formulation is not recommended in these settings.

PRECAUTIONS
GENERAL

Severe hypotension, particularly with upright posture, may occur with even small doses of isosorbide dinitrate. This drug should therefore be used with caution in patients who may be volume depleted or who, for whatever reason, are already hypotensive. Hypotension induced by isosorbide dinitrate may be accompanied by paradoxical bradycardia and increased angina pectoris.

Nitrate therapy may aggravate the angina caused by hypertrophic cardiomyopathy.

As tolerance to isosorbide dinitrate develops, the effect of sublingual nitroglycerin on exercise tolerance, although still observable, is somewhat blunted.

Some clinical trials in angina patients have provided nitroglycerin for about 12 continuous hours of every 24-hour day. During the daily dose-free interval in some of these trials, anginal attacks have been more easily provoked than before treatment, and patients have demonstrated hemodynamic rebound and *decreased* exercise tolerance. The importance of these observations to the routine, clinical use of immediate-release oral isosorbide dinitrate is not known.

In industrial workers who have had long-term exposure to unknown (presumably high) doses of organic nitrates, tolerance clearly occurs. Chest pain, acute myocardial infarction, and even sudden death have occurred during temporary withdrawal of nitrates from these workers, demonstrating the existence of true physical dependence.

INFORMATION FOR PATIENTS

Patients should be told that the anti-anginal efficacy of isosorbide dinitrate is strongly related to its dosing regimen, so the prescribed schedule of dosing should be followed carefully. In particular, daily headaches sometimes accompany treatment with isosorbide dinitrate. In patients who get these headaches, the headaches are a marker of the activity of the drug. Patients should resist the temptation to avoid headaches by altering the schedule of their treatment with isosorbide dinitrate, since loss of headache may be associated with simultaneous loss of anti-anginal efficacy. Aspirin and/or acetaminophen, on the other hand, often successfully relieve isosorbide dinitrate-induced headaches with no deleterious effect on isosorbide dinitrate's anti-anginal efficacy.

Treatment with isosorbide dinitrate may be associated with lightheadedness on standing, especially just after rising from a recumbent or seated position. This effect may be more frequent in patients who have also consumed alcohol.

DRUG INTERACTIONS

The vasodilating effects of isosorbide dinitrate may be additive with those of other vasodilators. Alcohol, in particular, has been found to exhibit additive effects of this variety.

CARCINOGENESIS, MUTAGENESIS, IMPAIRMENT OF FERTILITY

No long-term studies in animals have been performed to evaluate the carcinogenic potential of isosorbide dinitrate. In a modified two-litter reproduction study, there was no remarkable gross pathology and no altered fertility or gestation among rats fed isosorbide dinitrate at 25 or 100 mg/kg/day.

PREGNANCY CATEGORY C

At oral doses 35 and 150 times the maximum recommended human daily dose, isosorbide dinitrate has been shown to cause a dose-related increase in embryotoxicity (increase in mummified pups) in rabbits. There are no adequate, well-controlled studies in pregnant women. Isosorbide dinitrate should be used during pregnancy only if the potential benefit justifies the potential risk to the fetus.

NURSING MOTHERS

It is not known whether isosorbide dinitrate is excreted in human milk. Because many drugs are excreted in human milk, caution should be exercised when isosorbide dinitrate is administered to a nursing woman.

PEDIATRIC USE

Safety and effectiveness in pediatric patients have not been established.

ADVERSE REACTIONS

Adverse reactions to isosorbide dinitrate are generally dose-related, and almost all of these reactions are the result of isosorbide dinitrate's activity as a vasodilator. Headache, which may be severe, is the most commonly reported side

effect. Headache may be recurrent with each daily dose, especially at higher doses. Transient episodes of lightheadedness, occasionally related to blood pressure changes, may also occur. Hypotension occurs infrequently, but in some patients it may be severe enough to warrant discontinuation of therapy. Syncope, crescendo angina, and rebound hypertension have been reported but are uncommon.

Extremely rarely, ordinary doses of organic nitrates have caused methemoglobinemia in normal-seeming patient. Methemoglobinemia is so infrequent at these doses that further discussion of its diagnosis and treatment is deferred (see "**Overdosage**").

Data are not available to allow estimation of the frequency of adverse reactions during treatment with Isordil® Titradose® tablets.

OVERDOSAGE
HEMODYNAMIC EFFECTS

The ill effects of isosorbide dinitrate overdose are generally the results of isosorbide dinitrate's capacity to induce vasodilatation, venous pooling, reduced cardiac output, and hypotension. These hemodynamic changes may have protean manifestations, including increased intracranial pressure, with any or all of persistent throbbing headache, confusion, and moderate fever; vertigo; palpitations; visual disturbances; nausea and vomiting (possibly with colic and even bloody diarrhea); syncope (especially in the upright posture); air hunger and dyspnea, later followed by reduced ventilatory effort; diaphoresis, with the skin either flushed or cold and clammy; heart block and bradycardia; paralysis; coma; seizures; and death.

Laboratory determinations of serum levels of isosorbide dinitrate and its metabolites are not widely available, and such determinations have, in any event, no established role in the management of isosorbide dinitrate overdose.

There are no data suggesting what dose of isosorbide dinitrate is likely to be life-threatening in humans. In rats, the median acute lethal dose (LD_{50}) was found to be 1100 mg/kg.

No data are available to suggest physiological maneuvers (*e.g.*, maneuvers to change the pH of the urine) that might accelerate elimination of isosorbide dinitrate and its active metabolites. Similarly, it is not known which, if any, of these substances can usefully be removed from the body by hemodialysis.

No specific antagonist to the vasodilator effects of isosorbide dinitrate is known, and no intervention has been subject to controlled studies as a therapy for isosorbide dinitrate overdose. Because the hypotension associated with isosorbide dinitrate overdose is the result of venodilatation and arterial hypovolemia, prudent therapy in this situation should be directed toward increase in central fluid volume. Passive elevation of the patient's legs may be sufficient, but intravenous infusion of normal saline or similar fluid may also be necessary.

The use of epinephrine or other arterial vasoconstrictors in this setting is likely to do more harm than good.

In patients with renal disease or congestive heart failure, therapy resulting in central volume expansion is not without hazard. Treatment of isosorbide dinitrate overdose in these patients may be subtle and difficult, and invasive monitoring may be required.

METHEMOGLOBINEMIA

Nitrate ions liberated during metabolism of isosorbide dinitrate can oxidize hemoglobin into methemoglobin. Even in patients totally without cytochrome b_5 reductase activity, however, and even assuming that the nitrate moieties of isosorbide dinitrate are quantitatively applied to oxidation of hemoglobin, about 1 mg/kg of isosorbide dinitrate should be required before any of these patients manifests clinically significant ($\geq 10\%$) methemoglobinemia. In patients with normal reductase function, significant production of methemoglobin should require even larger doses of isosorbide dinitrate. In one study in which 36 patients received 2 to 4 weeks of continuous nitroglycerin therapy at 3.1 to 4.4 mg/hr (equivalent, in total administered dose of nitrate ions, to 4.8 to 6.9 mg of bioavailable isosorbide dinitrate per hour), the average methemoglobin level measured was 0.2%; this was comparable to that observed in parallel patients who received placebo.

Notwithstanding these observations, there are case reports of significant methemoglobinemia in association with moderate overdoses of organic nitrates. None of the affected patients had been thought to be unusually susceptible.

Methemoglobin levels are available from most clinical laboratories. The diagnosis should be suspected in patients who exhibit signs of impaired oxygen delivery despite adequate cardiac output and adequate arterial pO_2. Classically, methemoglobinemic blood is described as chocolate brown, without color change on exposure to air.

When methemoglobinemia is diagnosed, the treatment of choice is methylene blue, 1 to 2 mg/kg intravenously.

DOSAGE AND ADMINISTRATION

As noted under "**Clinical Pharmacology**," multiple-dose studies with ISDN and other nitrates have shown that maintenance of continuous 24-hour plasma levels results in

refractory tolerance. Every dosing regimen for Isordil Titradose tablets must provide a daily dose-free interval to minimize the development of this tolerance. With immediate-release ISDN, it appears that one daily dose-free interval must be at least 14 hours long.

As also noted under "**Clinical Pharmacology**," the effects of the second and later doses have been smaller and shorter-lasting than the effects of the first.

Large controlled studies with other nitrates suggest that no dosing regimen with Isordil Titradose tablets should be expected to provide more than about 12 hours of continuous anti-anginal efficacy per day.

As with all titratable drugs, it is important to administer the minimum dose which produces the desired clinical effect. The usual starting dose of Isordil Titradose is 5 mg to 20 mg, two or three times daily. For maintenance therapy, 10 mg to 40 mg, two or three times daily is recommended. Some patients may require higher doses. A daily dose-free interval of at least 14 hours is advisable to minimize tolerance. The optimal interval will vary with the individual patient, dose and regimen.

HOW SUPPLIED

Isordil® (isosorbide dinitrate) Oral Titradose® Tablets are available as follows:

5 mg, round, pink tablets imprinted "WYETH 4152" on one side and deeply scored on reverse side:
NDC 0008-4152-01, bottles of 100.
NDC 0008-4152-02, bottles of 500.
NDC 0008-4152-03, bottles of 1,000.
NDC 0008-4152-05, Redipak® cartons of 100 (10 blister strips of 10).
Store at room temperature, approximately 25°C (77°F)
Protect from light
Keep bottles tightly closed
Dispense in a light-resistant, tight container
Use carton to protect blisters from light
10 mg, round, white tablets imprinted "WYETH 4153" on one side and deeply scored on reverse side:
NDC 0008-4153-01, bottles of 100.
NDC 0008-4152-02, bottles of 500.
NDC 0008-4153-03, bottles of 1,000.
NDC 0008-4153-05, Redipak cartons of 100 (10 blister strips of 10).
Store at room temperature, approximately 25°C (77°F)
Keep bottles tightly closed
Dispense in a tight container
20 mg, round, green tablets imprinted "WYETH 4154" on one side and deeply scored on reverse side:
NDC 0008-4154-01, bottles of 100.
NDC 0008-4154-02, bottles of 500.
NDC 0008-4154-05, Redipak cartons of 100 (10 blister strips of 10).
30 mg, round, blue tablets imprinted "WYETH 4159" on one side and deeply scored on reverse side:
NDC 0008-4159-01, bottles of 100.
NDC 0008-4159-02, bottles of 500.
NDC 0008-4159-04, Redipak cartons of 100 (10 blister strips of 10).
40 mg, round, light green tablets imprinted "WYETH 4192" on one side and deeply scored on reverse side:
NDC 0008-4192-01, bottles of 100.
NDC 0008-4192-04, Redipak cartons of 100 (10 blister strips of 10).
Store at room temperature, approximately 25°C (77°F)
Protect from light
Keep bottles tightly closed
Dispense in a light-resistant, tight container
Use carton to protect blisters from light
US Pat No. Re. 29077
The appearances of these tablets are trademarks of Wyeth-Ayerst Laboratories.
ALSO AVAILABLE
Sublingual Tablets, 2.5 mg, NDC 0008-4139, in bottles of 100 or 500 and in Redipak cartons of 100 (10 blister strips of 10).
Sublingual Tablets, 5 mg, NDC 0008-4126, in bottles of 100 or 500 and in Redipak cartons of 100 (10 blister strips of 10).
Sublingual Tablets, 10 mg, NDC 0008-4161, in bottles of 100.
Tembids® Tablets, 40 mg, controlled-release tablets, NDC 0008-4125, in bottles of 100, 500 or 1,000.
Tembids® Capsules, 40 mg, controlled-release capsules, NDC 0008-4140, in bottles of 100 or 500.
Shown in Product Identification Guide, page 340

LODINE®
[lō 'deen]
(etodolac capsules and tablets)

℞

DESCRIPTION

Lodine® (etodolac capsules and tablets) is a pyranocarboxylic acid chemically designated as (±) 1,8-diethyl-

Continued on next page

Wyeth-Ayerst Laboratories—Cont.

1,3,4,9-tetrahydropyrano-[3,4-b]indole-1-acetic acid. The structural formula for etodolac is shown below:

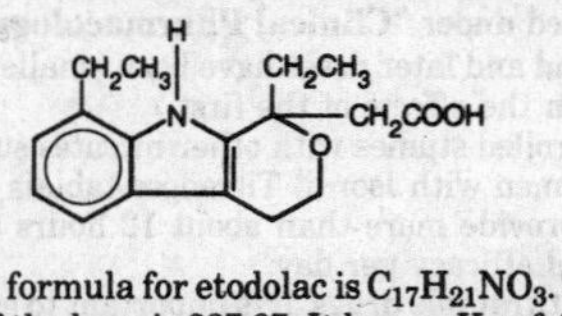

The empirical formula for etodolac is $C_{17}H_{21}NO_3$. The molecular weight of the base is 287.37. It has a pKa of 4.65 and an n-octanol:water partition coefficient of 11.4 at pH 7.4. Etodolac is a white crystalline compound, insoluble in water but soluble in alcohols, chloroform, dimethyl sulfoxide, and aqueous polyethylene glycol.

Inactive ingredients are:

—*in capsules:* cellulose, gelatin, iron oxides, lactose, magnesium stearate, povidone, sodium lauryl sulfate, sodium starch glycolate, and titanium dioxide.

—*in tablets:* cellulose, hydroxypropyl methylcellulose, lactose, magnesium stearate, polyethylene glycol, polysorbate 80, povidone, sodium starch glycolate, and titanium dioxide. The 400 mg tablets contain D&C Yellow #10, FD&C Blue #2, and FD&C Yellow #6 as color additives. The 500 mg tablets contain FD&C Blue #2 only.

Lodine is available in 200 and 300 mg capsules, and 400 and 500 mg tablets, for oral administration.

CLINICAL PHARMACOLOGY

PHARMACOLOGY

Etodolac is a nonsteroidal anti-inflammatory drug (NSAID) that exhibits anti-inflammatory, analgesic, and antipyretic activities in animal models. The mechanism of action of etodolac, like that of other NSAIDs, is not known but is believed to be associated with the inhibition of prostaglandin biosynthesis.

Lodine is a racemic mixture of [-]R- and [+]S-etodolac. As with other NSAIDs, it has been demonstrated in animals that the [+]S-form is biologically active. Both enantiomers are stable and there is no [-]R to [+]S conversion *in vivo*.

PHARMACODYNAMICS

Analgesia was demonstrable $^1/_2$ hour following single doses of 200 to 400 mg Lodine, with the peak effect occurring in 1 to 2 hours. The analgesic effect generally lasted for 4 to 6 hours (see **Clinical Trials**).

PHARMACOKINETICS

The pharmacokinetics of etodolac have been evaluated in 267 normal subjects, 44 elderly patients (>65 years old), 19 patients with renal failure (creatinine clearance 37 to 88 mL/min), 9 patients on hemodialysis, and 10 patients with compensated hepatic cirrhosis.

Etodolac, when administered orally, exhibits kinetics that are well described by a two-compartment model with first-order absorption.

Lodine has no apparent pharmacokinetic interaction when administered with phenytoin, glyburide, furosemide or hydrochlorothiazide.

ABSORPTION

Etodolac is well absorbed and had a relative bioavailability of 100% when 200 mg capsules were compared with a solution of etodolac. Based on mass balance studies, the systemic availability of etodolac from either the tablet or capsule formulation, is at least 80%. Etodolac does not undergo significant first-pass metabolism following oral administration. Mean (± 1 SD) peak plasma concentrations range from approximately 14 ± 4 to 37 ± 9 μg/mL after 200 to 600 mg single doses and are reached in 80 ± 30 minutes (see Table 1 for summary of pharmacokinetic parameters). The dose-proportionality based on AUC (the area under the plasma concentration-time curve) is linear following doses up to 600 mg every 12 hours. Peak concentrations are dose proportional for both total and free etodolac following doses up to 400 mg every 12 hours, but following a 600 mg dose, the peak is about 20% higher than predicted on the basis of lower doses.

Table 1. Etodolac Steady-State Pharmacokinetic Parameters (N=267)

Kinetic Parameters	Mean ± SD
Extent of oral absorption (bioavailability) [F]	≥80%
Oral-dose clearance [CL/F]	47 ± 16 mL/h/kg
Steady-state volume [V_{ss}/F]	362 ± 129 mL/kg
Distribution half-life [$t_{1/2,}$ α]	0.71 ± 0.50 h
Terminal half-life [$t_{1/2,}$ β]	7.3 ± 4.0 h

Antacid Effects

The extent of absorption of etodolac is not affected when Lodine is administered with an antacid. Coadministration with an antacid decreases the peak concentration reached by about 15 to 20%, with no measurable effect on time-to-peak.

Food Effects

The extent of absorption of etodolac is not affected when Lodine is administered after a meal. Food intake, however, reduces the peak concentration reached by approximately one half and increases the time-to-peak concentration by 1.4 to 3.8 hours.

Distribution

Etodolac has an apparent steady-state volume of distribution about 0.362 L/kg. Within the therapeutic dose range, etodolac is more than 99% bound to plasma proteins. The free fraction is less than 1% and is independent of etodolac total concentration over the dose range studied.

Metabolism

Etodolac is extensively metabolized in the liver, with renal elimination of etodolac and its metabolites being the primary route of excretion. The intersubject variability of etodolac plasma levels, achieved after recommended doses, is substantial.

Protein Binding

Data from *in vitro* studies, using peak serum concentrations at reported therapeutic doses in humans, show that the etodolac free fraction is not significantly altered by acetaminophen, ibuprofen, indomethacin, naproxen, piroxicam, chlorpropamide, glipizide, glyburide, phenytoin, and probenecid.

Elimination

The mean plasma clearance of etodolac, following oral dosing is 47 (± 16) mL/h/kg, and terminal disposition half-life is 7.3 (± 4.0) hours. Approximately 72% of the administered dose is recovered in the urine as the following, indicated as % of the administered dose:

— etodolac, unchanged	1%
— etodolac glucuronide	13%
— hydroxylated metabolites (6-, 7-, and 8-OH)	5%
— hydroxylated metabolite glucuronides	20%
— unidentified metabolites	33%

Fecal excretion accounted for 16% of the dose.

SPECIAL POPULATIONS

Elderly Patients

In clinical studies, etodolac clearance was reduced by about 15% in older patients (>65 years of age). In these studies, age was shown not to have any effect on etodolac half-life or protein binding, and there was no change in expected drug accumulation. No dosage adjustment is generally necessary in the elderly on the basis of pharmacokinetics. The elderly may need dosage adjustment, however, on the basis of body size (see **Precautions**—GERIATRIC POPULATION), as they may be more sensitive to antiprostaglandin effects than younger patients (see **Precautions**—GERIATRIC POPULATION).

Renal Impairment

Studies in patients with mild-to-moderate renal impairment (creatinine clearance 37 to 88 mL/min) showed no significant differences in the disposition of total and free etodolac. In patients undergoing hemodialysis, there was a 50% greater apparent clearance of total etodolac, due to a 50% greater unbound fraction. Free etodolac clearance was not altered, indicating the importance of protein binding in etodolac's disposition. Nevertheless, etodolac is not dialyzable.

Hepatic Impairment

In patients with compensated hepatic cirrhosis, the disposition of total and free etodolac is not altered. Although no dosage adjustment is generally required in this patient population, etodolac clearance is dependent on hepatic function and could be reduced in patients with severe hepatic failure.

CLINICAL TRIALS

ANALGESIA

Controlled clinical trials in analgesia were single-dose, randomized, double-blind, parallel studies in three pain models, including dental extractions. The analgesic effective dose for Lodine established in these acute pain models was 200 to 400 mg. The onset of analgesia occurred approximately 30 minutes after oral administration. Lodine 200 mg provided efficacy comparable to that obtained with aspirin (650 mg). Lodine 400 mg provided efficacy comparable to that obtained with acetaminophen with codeine (600 mg + 60 mg). The peak analgesic effect was between 1 to 2 hours. Duration of relief averaged 4 to 5 hours for 200 mg of Lodine and 5 to 6 hours for 400 mg of Lodine as measured by when approximately half of the patients required remedication.

OSTEOARTHRITIS

The use of Lodine in managing the signs and symptoms of osteoarthritis of the hip or knee was assessed in double-blind, randomized, controlled clinical trials in 341 patients. In patients with osteoarthritis of the knee, Lodine, in doses of 600 to 1000 mg/day, was better than placebo in two studies. The clinical trials in osteoarthritis used b.i.d. dosage regimens.

RHEUMATOID ARTHRITIS

In a 3-month study with 426 patients, Lodine 300 mg b.i.d. was effective in management of rheumatoid arthritis and comparable in efficacy to piroxicam 20 mg/day. In a long-term study with 1,446 patients in which 60% of patients completed 6 months of therapy and 20% completed 3 years of therapy, Lodine in a dose of 500 mg b.i.d. provided efficacy comparable to that obtained with ibuprofen 600 mg q.i.d. In clinical trials of rheumatoid arthritis patients, Lodine has been used in combination with gold, d-penicillamine, chloroquine, corticosteroids, and methotrexate.

INDICATIONS AND USAGE

Lodine is indicated for acute and long-term use in the management of signs and symptoms of osteoarthritis and rheumatoid arthritis. Lodine is also indicated for the management of pain.

CONTRAINDICATIONS

Lodine is contraindicated in patients with known hypersensitivity to etodolac. Lodine should not be given to patients who have experienced asthma, urticaria, or other allergic-type reactions after taking aspirin or other NSAIDs. Severe, rarely fatal, anaphylactic-like reactions to Lodine have been reported in such patients (see **Warnings**—ANAPHYLACTOID REACTIONS).

WARNINGS

RISK OF GASTROINTESTINAL (GI) ULCERATION, BLEEDING, AND PERFORATION WITH NONSTEROIDAL ANTI-INFLAMMATORY DRUG (NSAID) THERAPY

Serious GI toxicity, such as bleeding, ulceration, and perforation, can occur at any time, with or without warning symptoms, in patients treated chronically with NSAIDs. Although minor upper GI problems, such as dyspepsia, are common, usually developing early in therapy, physicians should remain alert for ulceration and bleeding in patients treated chronically with NSAIDs, even in the absence of previous GI-tract symptoms. In patients observed in clinical trials of such agents for several months' to 2 years' duration, symptomatic upper GI ulcers, gross bleeding, or perforation appears to occur in approximately 1% of patients treated for 3 to 6 months and in about 2% to 4% of patients treated for 1 year. Physicians should inform patients about the signs and/or symptoms of serious GI toxicity and what steps to take if they occur.

Studies to date have not identified any subset of patients not at risk of developing peptic ulceration and bleeding. Except for a prior history of serious GI events and other risk factors known to be associated with peptic ulcer disease, such as alcoholism, smoking, etc., no risk factors (e.g., age, sex) have been associated with increased risk. Elderly or debilitated patients seem to tolerate ulceration or bleeding less well than other individuals, and most spontaneous reports of fatal GI events are in this population. Studies to date are inconclusive concerning the relative risk of various NSAIDs in causing such reactions. High doses of any NSAID probably carry a greater risk of these reactions, although controlled clinical trials showing this do not exist in most cases. In considering the use of relatively large doses (within the recommended dosage range), sufficient benefit should be anticipated to offset the potential increased risk of GI toxicity.

ANAPHYLACTOID REACTIONS

Anaphylactoid reactions may occur in patients without prior exposure to etodolac. Lodine should not be given to patients with the aspirin triad. The triad typically occurs in asthmatic patients who experience rhinitis with or without nasal polyps, or who exhibit severe, potentially fatal bronchospasm after taking aspirin or other nonsteroidal anti-inflammatory drugs. Fatal reactions have been reported in such patients (see **Contraindications** and **Precautions**—*Preexisting Asthma*). Emergency help should be sought in cases where an anaphylactoid reaction occurs.

ADVANCED RENAL DISEASE

In cases with advanced kidney disease, as with other NSAIDs, treatment with Lodine should only be initiated with close monitoring of the patient's kidney function (see **Precautions**—*Renal Effects*).

PREGNANCY

In late pregnancy, as with other NSAIDs, Lodine should be avoided because it may cause premature closure of the ductus arteriosus (see **Precautions**—*Teratogenic Effects—Pregnancy Category C*).

PRECAUTIONS

GENERAL PRECAUTIONS

Renal Effects

As with other NSAIDs, long-term administration of etodolac to rats has resulted in renal papillary necrosis and other renal medullary changes. Renal pelvic transitional epithelial hyperplasia, a spontaneous change occurring with variable frequency, was observed with increased frequency in treated male rats in a 2-year chronic study.

A second form of renal toxicity encountered with Lodine, as with other NSAIDs, is seen in patients with conditions in which renal prostaglandins have a supportive role in the maintenance of renal perfusion. In these patients, administration of a nonsteroidal anti-inflammatory drug may cause a dose-dependent reduction in prostaglandin formation and, secondarily, in renal blood flow, which may precipitate overt renal decompensation. Patients at greatest risk of this reaction are those with impaired renal function, heart failure, or

liver dysfunction; those taking diuretics; and the elderly. Discontinuation of nonsteroidal anti-inflammatory drug therapy is usually followed by recovery to the pretreatment state.

Etodolac metabolites are eliminated primarily by the kidneys. The extent to which the inactive glucuronide metabolites may accumulate in patients with renal failure has not been studied. As with other drugs whose metabolites are excreted by the kidney, the possibility that adverse reactions (not listed in **Adverse Reactions**) may be attributable to these metabolites should be considered.

Hepatic Effects

Borderline elevations of one or more liver tests may occur in up to 15% of patients taking NSAIDs, including Lodine. These abnormalities may disappear, remain essentially unchanged, or progress with continued therapy. Meaningful elevations of ALT or AST (approximately three or more times the upper limit of normal) have been reported in approximately 1% of patients in clinical trials with Lodine. A patient with symptoms and/or signs suggesting liver dysfunction, or in whom an abnormal liver test has occurred, should be evaluated for evidence of the development of a more severe hepatic reaction while on therapy with Lodine. Rare cases of liver necrosis and hepatic failure, some of them with fatal outcomes have been reported. If clinical signs and symptoms consistent with liver disease develop, or if systemic manifestations occur (e.g. eosinophilia, rash, etc.), Lodine should be discontinued.

Hematological Effects

Anemia is sometimes seen in patients receiving NSAIDs including Lodine. This may be due to fluid retention, GI blood loss, or an incompletely described effect upon erythropoiesis. Patients on long-term treatment with NSAIDs, including Lodine, should have their hemoglobin or hematocrit checked if they exhibit any signs or symptoms of anemia. All drugs which inhibit the biosynthesis of prostaglandins may interfere to some extent with platelet function and vascular responses to bleeding.

Fluid Retention and Edema

Fluid retention and edema have been observed in some patients taking NSAIDs, including Lodine. Therefore, Lodine should be used with caution in patients with fluid retention, hypertension, or heart failure.

Pre-existing Asthma

About 10% of patients with asthma may have aspirin-sensitive asthma. The use of aspirin in patients with aspirin-sensitive asthmas has been associated with severe bronchospasm which can be fatal. Since cross reactivity, including bronchospasm, between aspirin and other nonsteroidal anti-inflammatory drugs has been reported in such aspirin-sensitive patients, etodolac should not be administered to patients with this form of aspirin sensitivity and should be used with caution in all patients with pre-existing asthma.

INFORMATION FOR PATIENTS

Lodine, like other drugs of its class, can cause discomfort and, rarely, more serious side effects, such as gastrointestinal bleeding, which may result in hospitalization and even fatal outcomes.

Physicians may wish to discuss with their patients the potential risks (see **Warnings, Precautions, Adverse Reactions**) and likely benefits of nonsteroidal anti-inflammatory drug treatment.

Patients on Lodine should report to their physicians signs or symptoms of gastrointestinal ulceration or bleeding, blurred vision or other eye symptoms, skin rash, weight gain, or edema.

Because serious gastrointestinal tract ulcerations and bleeding can occur without warning symptoms, physicians should follow chronically treated patients for the signs and symptoms of ulcerations and bleeding and should inform them of the importance of this follow-up (see **Warnings**—RISK OF GI ULCERATION, BLEEDING AND PERFORATION WITH NONSTEROIDAL ANTI-INFLAMMATORY THERAPY).

Patients should also be instructed to seek medical emergency help in case of an occurrence of anaphylactoid reactions (see **Warnings**).

LABORATORY TESTS

Patients on long-term treatment with Lodine, as with other NSAIDs, should have their hemoglobin or hematocrit checked periodically for signs or symptoms of anemia. Appropriate measures should be taken in case such signs of anemia occur.

If clinical signs and symptoms consistent with liver disease develop or if systematic manifestations occur (e.g., eosinophilia, rash, etc.) and if abnormal liver tests are detected, persist or worsen, Lodine should be discontinued.

DRUG INTERACTIONS

Antacids

The concomitant administration of antacids has no apparent effect on the extent of absorption of Lodine. However, antacids can decrease the peak concentration reached by 15% to 20% but have no detectable effect on the time-to-peak.

Aspirin

When Lodine is administered with aspirin, its protein binding is reduced, although the clearance of free etodolac is not altered. The clinical significance of this interaction is not known; however, as with other NSAIDs, concomitant administration of Lodine and aspirin is not generally recommended because of the potential of increased adverse effects.

Warfarin

Short-term pharmacokinetic studies have demonstrated that concomitant administration of warfarin and Lodine results in reduced protein binding of warfarin, but there was no change in the clearance of free warfarin. There was no significant difference in the pharmacodynamic effect of warfarin administered alone and warfarin administered with Lodine as measured by prothrombin time. Thus, concomitant therapy with warfarin and Lodine should not require dosage adjustment of either drug. However, there have been a few spontaneous reports of prolonged prothrombin times in Lodine-treated patients receiving concomitant warfarin therapy. Caution should be exercised because interactions have been seen with other NSAIDs.

Cyclosporin, Digoxin, Lithium, Methotrexate

Lodine, like other NSAIDs, through effects on renal prostaglandins, may cause changes in the elimination of these drugs leading to elevated serum levels of digoxin, lithium, and methotrexate and increased toxicity. Nephrotoxicity associated with cyclosporine may also be enhanced. Patients receiving these drugs who are given Lodine, or any other NSAID, and particularly those patients with altered renal function, should be observed for the development of the specific toxicities of these drugs.

Phenylbutazone

Phenylbutazone causes increase (by about 80%) in the free fraction of etodolac. Although *in vivo* studies have not been done to see if etodolac clearance is changed by coadministration of phenylbutazone, it is not recommended that they be coadministered.

DRUG/LABORATORY TEST INTERACTIONS

The urine of patients who take Lodine can give a false-positive reaction for urinary bilirubin (urobilin) due to the presence of phenolic metabolites of etodolac. Diagnostic dip-stick methodology, used to detect ketone bodies in urine, has resulted in false-positive findings in some patients treated with Lodine. Generally, this phenomenon has not been associated with other clinically significant events. No dose relationship has been observed.

Lodine treatment is associated with a small decrease in serum uric acid levels. In clinical trials, mean decreases of 1 to 2 mg/dL were observed in arthritic patients receiving etodolac (600 mg to 1000 mg/day) after 4 weeks of therapy. These levels then remained stable for up to 1 year of therapy.

CARCINOGENESIS, MUTAGENESIS, AND IMPAIRMENT OF FERTILITY

No carcinogenic effect of etodolac was observed in mice or rats receiving oral doses of 15 mg/kg/day (45 to 89 mg/m², respectively) or less for periods of 2 years or 18 months, respectively. Etodolac was not mutagenic in *in vitro* tests performed with *S. typhimurium* and mouse lymphoma cells as well as in an *in vivo* mouse micronucleus test. However, data from the *in vitro* human peripheral lymphocyte test showed an increase in the number of gaps (3.0 to 5.3% unstained regions in the chromatid without dislocation) among the Lodine-treated cultures (50 to 200 µg/mL) compared to negative controls (2.0%); no other difference was noted between the controls and drug-treated groups. Etodolac showed no impairment of fertility in male and female rats up to oral doses of 16 mg/kg (94 mg/m²). However, reduced implantation of fertilized eggs occurred in the 8 mg/kg group.

PREGNANCY

Teratogenic Effects—Pregnancy Category C

In teratology studies, isolated occurrences of alterations in limb development were found and included polydactyly, oligodactyly, syndactyly, and unossified phalanges in rats and oligodactyly and synostosis of metatarsals in rabbits. These were observed at dose levels (2 to 14 mg/kg/day) close to human clinical doses. However, the frequency and the dosage group distribution of these findings in initial or repeated studies did not establish a clear drug or dose-response relationship.

There are no adequate or well-controlled studies in pregnant women. Lodine should be used during pregnancy only if the potential benefits justify the potential risk to the fetus. Because of the known effects of NSAIDs on parturition and on the human fetal cardiovascular system with respect to closure of the ductus arteriosus, use during late pregnancy should be avoided.

LABOR AND DELIVERY

In rat studies with etodolac, as with other drugs known to inhibit prostaglandin synthesis, an increased incidence of dystocia, delayed parturition, and decreased pup survival occurred. The effects of Lodine on labor and delivery in pregnant women are unknown.

NURSING MOTHERS

It is not known whether etodolac is excreted in human milk. Because many drugs are excreted in human milk and because of the potential for serious adverse reactions in nursing infants from etodolac, a decision should be made whether to discontinue nursing or to discontinue the drug taking into account the importance of the drug to the mother.

PEDIATRIC USE

Safety and effectiveness in pediatric patients have not been established.

GERIATRIC POPULATION

As with any NSAID, however, caution should be exercised in treating the elderly, and when individualizing their dosage, extra care should be taken when increasing the dose because the elderly seem to tolerate NSAID side effects less well than younger patients. In patients 65 years and older, no substantial differences in the side effect profile of Lodine were seen compared with the general population (see **Clinical Pharmacology**—PHARMACOKINETICS.)

ADVERSE REACTIONS

Adverse-reaction information for Lodine was derived from 2,629 arthritic patients treated with Lodine in double-blind and open-label clinical trials of 4 to 320 weeks in duration and worldwide postmarketing surveillance studies. In clinical trials, most adverse reactions were mild and transient. The discontinuation rate in controlled clinical trials, because of adverse events, was up to 10% for patients treated with Lodine.

New patient complaints (with an incidence greater than or equal to 1%) are listed below by body system. The incidences were determined from clinical trials involving 465 patients with osteoarthritis treated with 300 to 500 mg of Lodine b.i.d. (i.e., 600 to 1000 mg/day).

INCIDENCE GREATER THAN OR EQUAL TO 1%—PROBABLY CAUSALLY RELATED

Body as a whole—Chills and fever.

Digestive system—Dyspepsia (10%), abdominal pain*, diarrhea*, flatulence*, nausea*, constipation, gastritis, melena, vomiting.

Nervous system—Asthenia/malaise*, dizziness*, depression, nervousness.

Skin and appendages—Pruritus, rash.

Special senses—Blurred vision, tinnitus.

Urogenital system—Dysuria, urinary frequency.

*Drug-related patient complaints occurring in 3 to 9% of patients treated with Lodine.

Drug-related patient-complaints occurring in fewer than 3%, but more than 1%, are unmarked.

INCIDENCE LESS THAN 1%—PROBABLY CAUSALLY RELATED

(Adverse reactions reported only in worldwide postmarketing experience, not seen in clinical trials, are considered rarer and are italicized)

Body as a whole—*Allergic reaction, anaphylactoid reaction.*

Cardiovascular system—Hypertension, congestive heart failure, flushing, palpitations, syncope, *vasculitis (including necrotizing and allergic).*

Digestive system—Thirst, dry mouth, ulcerative stomatitis, anorexia, eructation, elevated liver enzymes, *cholestatic hepatitis,* hepatitis, *cholestatic jaundice, duodenitis, jaundice, hepatic failure, liver necrosis,* peptic ulcer with or without bleeding and/or perforation, *intestinal ulceration, pancreatitis.*

Hemic and lymphatic system—Ecchymosis, anemia, thrombocytopenia, bleeding time increased, *agranulocytosis, hemolytic anemia, leukopenia, neutropenia, pancytopenia.*

Metabolic and nutritional—Edema, serum creatinine increase, *hyperglycemia in previously controlled diabetic patients.*

Nervous system—Insomnia, somnolence.

Respiratory system—Asthma.

Skin and appendages—Angioedema, sweating, urticaria, vesiculobullous rash, *cutaneous vasculitis with purpura, Stevens-Johnson Syndrome,* hyperpigmentation, *erythema multiforme.*

Special senses—Photophobia, transient visual disturbances.

Urogenital system—*Elevated BUN, renal failure, renal insufficiency, renal papillary necrosis.*

INCIDENCE LESS THAN 1%—CAUSAL RELATIONSHIP UNKNOWN (Medical events occurring under circumstances where causal relationship to Lodine is uncertain. These reactions are listed as alerting information for physicians)

Body as a whole—Infection, headache.

Cardiovascular system—Arrhythmias, myocardial infarction, cerebrovascular accident.

Digestive system—Esophagitis with or without stricture or cardiospasm, colitis.

Metabolic and nutritional—Change in weight.

Nervous system—Paresthesia, confusion.

Respiratory system—Bronchitis, dyspnea, pharyngitis, rhinitis, sinusitis.

Skin and appendages—Alopecia, maculopapular rash, photosensitivity, skin peeling.

Special senses—Conjunctivitis, deafness, taste perversion.

Urogenital system—Cystitis, hematuria, leukorrhea, renal calculus, interstitial nephritis, uterine bleeding irregularities.

Continued on next page

Wyeth-Ayerst Laboratories—Cont.

OVERDOSAGE

Symptoms following acute NSAID overdose are usually limited to lethargy, drowsiness, nausea, vomiting, and epigastric pain, which are generally reversible with supportive care. Gastrointestinal bleeding can occur and coma has occurred following massive ibuprofen or mefenamic-acid overdose. Hypertension, acute renal failure, and respiratory depression may occur but are rare. Anaphylactoid reactions have been reported with therapeutic ingestion of NSAIDs, and may occur following overdose.

Patients should be managed by symptomatic and supportive care following an NSAID overdose. There are no specific antidotes. Gut decontamination may be indicated in patients seen within 4 hours of ingestion with symptoms or following a large overdose (5 to 10 times the usual dose). This should be accomplished via emesis and/or activated charcoal (60 to 100 g in adults, 1 to 2 g/kg in children) with an osmotic cathartic. Forced diuresis, alkalinization of the urine, hemodialysis, or hemoperfusion would probably not be useful due to etodolac's high protein binding.

DOSAGE AND ADMINISTRATION

As with other NSAIDs, the lowest dose and longest dosing interval should be sought for each patient. Therefore, after observing the response to initial therapy with Lodine, the dose and frequency should be adjusted to suit an individual patient's needs.

Dosage adjustment of Lodine is generally not required in patients with mild to moderate renal impairment. Etodolac should be used with caution in such patients, because, as with other NSAIDs, it may further decrease renal function in some patients with impaired renal function. (see **Precautions**—GENERAL PRECAUTIONS, *Renal Effects*).

ANALGESIA

The recommended total daily dose of Lodine for acute pain is up to 1000 mg, given as 200–400 mg every 6 to 8 hours. In some patients, if the potential benefits outweigh the risks; the dose may be increased to 1200 mg/day in order to achieve a therapeutic benefit that might not have been achieved with 1000 mg/day. Doses of etodolac greater than 1000 mg/day have not been adequately evaluated in well-controlled clinical trials.

OSTEOARTHRITIS AND RHEUMATOID ARTHRITIS

The recommended starting dose of Lodine for the management of the signs and symptoms of osteoarthritis or rheumatoid arthritis is: 300 mg b.i.d., t.i.d., or 400 mg b.i.d., or 500 mg b.i.d. During long-term administration, the dose of Lodine may be adjusted up or down depending on the clinical response of the patient. A lower dose of 600 mg/day may suffice for long-term administration. In patients who tolerate 1000 mg/day, the dose may be increased to 1200 mg/day when a higher level of therapeutic activity is required. When treating patients with higher doses, the physician should observe sufficient increased clinical benefit to justify the higher dose. Physicians should be aware that doses above 1000 mg/day have not been adequately evaluated in well-controlled clinical trials.

In chronic conditions, a therapeutic response to therapy with Lodine is sometimes seen within one week of therapy, but most often is observed by two weeks. After a satisfactory response has been achieved, the patient's dose should be reviewed and adjusted as required.

HOW SUPPLIED

Lodine (etodolac capsules and tablets) is available as:
Lodine® (etodolac capsules) Capsules
200 mg capsules (light gray with one wide red band with LODINE 200/white with two narrow red bands)
—in bottles of 100, NDC 0046-0738-81
—in unit-dose packages of 100, NDC 0046-0738-99
300 mg capsules (light gray with one red band with LODINE 300/light gray with two narrow red bands)
—in bottles of 100, NDC 0046-0739-81
—in unit-dose packages of 100, NDC 0046-0739-99
Store at controlled room temperature 20°–25°C (68°–77°F), protected from moisture.
Lodine® (etodolac tablets) Tablets
400 mg tablets (yellow-orange, oval, film-coated tablet, debossed LODINE 400 on one side)
—in bottles of 100, NDC 0046-0761-81
—in unit-dose packages of 100, NDC 0046-0761-99
Store at controlled room temperature 20°–25°C (68°–77°F). Store tablets in original container until ready to use. Dispense in light-resistant container.
500 mg tablets (blue, oval, film-coated tablet, branded LODINE 500 on one side)
—in bottles of 100, NDC 0046-0787-81
—in unit-dose packages of 100, NDC 0046-0787-99
Store at controlled room temperature 20°–25°C (68°–77°F). Store tablets in original container until ready to use. Dispense in light-resistant container.

The appearance of these capsules is a registered trademark of Wyeth-Ayerst Laboratories and the appearance of these tablets is a trademark of Wyeth-Ayerst Laboratories.
Caution: Federal law prohibits dispensing without prescription.

Shown in Product Identification Guide, page 340

LO/OVRAL®   ℞
[*lōh-ōh 'vral*]
Tablets
(norgestrel and ethinyl estradiol tablets)

Patients should be counseled that this product does not protect against HIV infection (AIDS) and other sexually transmitted diseases.

DESCRIPTION

Each LO/OVRAL tablet contains 0.3 mg of norgestrel (*dl* -13-beta-ethyl -17- alpha-ethinyl -17- beta - hydroxygon - 4- en -3-one), a totally synthetic progestogen, and 0.03 mg of ethinyl estradiol (19-nor-17α-pregna-1,3,5 (10)-trien-20-yne-3,17-diol). The inactive ingredients present are cellulose, lactose, magnesium stearate, and polacrilin potassium.

CLINICAL PHARMACOLOGY

Combination oral contraceptives act by suppression of gonadotropins. Although the primary mechanism of this action is inhibition of ovulation, other alterations include changes in the cervical mucus (which increase the difficulty of sperm entry into the uterus) and the endometrium (which reduce the likelihood of implantation).

INDICATIONS AND USAGE

Oral contraceptives are indicated for the prevention of pregnancy in women who elect to use this product as a method of contraception.

Oral contraceptives are highly effective. Table I lists the typical accidental pregnancy rates for users of combination oral contraceptives and other methods of contraception. The efficacy of these contraceptive methods, except sterilization and the IUD, depends upon the reliability with which they are used. Correct and consistent use of methods can result in lower failure rates.

TABLE I: LOWEST EXPECTED AND TYPICAL FAILURE RATES DURING THE FIRST YEAR OF CONTINUOUS USE OF A METHOD
% of Women Experiencing an Accidental Pregnancy in the First Year of Continuous Use

Method	Lowest Expected*	Typical**
(No Contraception)	(85)	(85)
Oral contraceptives		3
combined	0.1	N/A***
progestin only	0.5	N/A***
Diaphragm with spermicidal cream or jelly	6	18
Spermicides alone (foams and vaginal suppositories)	3	21
Vaginal Sponge		
nulliparous	6	18
multiparous	9	28
DEPO-PROVERA® (injectable progestogen)	0.3	0.3
NORPLANT® SYSTEM (implants)	0.2#	0.2#
IUD		3
progesterone	2	N/A***
copper T 380A	0.8	N/A***
Condom without spermicides	2	12
Periodic abstinence (all methods)	1–9	20
Female sterilization	0.2	0.4
Male sterilization	0.1	0.15

Adapted from J. Trussell et al., Table 1, Studies in Family Planning, 21(1). Jan.–Feb. 1990.

* The authors' best guess of the percentage of women expected to experience an accidental pregnancy among couples who initiate a method (not necessarily for the first time) and who use it consistently and correctly during the first year if they do not stop for any other reason.
** This term represents "typical" couples who initiate use of a method (not necessarily for the first time), who experience an accidental pregnancy during the first year if they do not stop use for any other reason.
*** N/A—Data not available.
# This data is based on NORPLANT® SYSTEM clinical trials.

CONTRAINDICATIONS

Oral contraceptives should not be used in women with any of the following conditions:

Thrombophlebitis or thromboembolic disorders.
A past history of deep-vein thrombophlebitis or thromboembolic disorders.
Cerebral-vascular or coronary-artery disease.
Known or suspected carcinoma of the breast.
Carcinoma of the endometrium or other known or suspected estrogen-dependent neoplasia.
Undiagnosed abnormal genital bleeding.
Cholestatic jaundice of pregnancy or jaundice with prior pill use.
Hepatic adenomas or carcinomas.
Known or suspected pregnancy.

WARNINGS

Cigarette smoking increases the risk of serious cardiovascular side effects from oral-contraceptive use. This risk increases with age and with heavy smoking (15 or more cigarettes per day) and is quite marked in women over 35 years of age. Women who use oral contraceptives should be strongly advised not to smoke.

The use of oral contraceptives is associated with increased risks of several serious conditions including myocardial infarction, thromboembolism, stroke, hepatic neoplasia, gallbladder disease, and hypertension, although the risk of serious morbidity or mortality is very small in healthy women without underlying factors. The risk of morbidity and mortality increases significantly in the presence of other underlying risk factors such as hypertension, hyperlipidemias, obesity, and diabetes.

Practitioners prescribing oral contraceptives should be familiar with the following information relating to these risks. The information contained in this package insert is based principally on studies carried out in patients who used oral contraceptives with higher formulations of estrogens and progestogens than those in common use today. The effect of long-term use of the oral contraceptives with lower formulations of both estrogens and progestogens remains to be determined.

Throughout this labeling, epidemiological studies reported are of two types: retrospective or case control studies and prospective or cohort studies. Case control studies provide a measure of the relative risk of disease, namely, a ratio of the incidence of a disease among oral-contraceptive users to that among nonusers. The relative risk does not provide information on the actual clinical occurrence of a disease. Cohort studies provide a measure of attributable risk, which is the difference in the incidence of disease between oral-contraceptive users and nonusers. The attributable risk does provide information about the actual occurrence of a disease in the population. For further information, the reader is referred to a text on epidemiological methods.

1. THROMBOEMBOLIC DISORDERS AND OTHER VASCULAR PROBLEMS

a. *Myocardial infarction*

An increased risk of myocardial infarction has been attributed to oral-contraceptive use. This risk is primarily in smokers or women with other underlying risk factors for coronary-artery disease such as hypertension, hypercholesterolemia, morbid obesity, and diabetes. The relative risk of heart attack for current oral-contraceptive users has been estimated to be two to six. The risk is very low under the age of 30.

Smoking in combination with oral-contraceptive use has been shown to contribute substantially to the incidence of myocardial infarctions in women in their mid-thirties or older with smoking accounting for the majority of excess cases. Mortality rates associated with circulatory disease have been shown to increase substantially in smokers over the age of 35 and nonsmokers over the age of 40 (Table II) among women who use oral contraceptives.
[See graph on top of next page.]
Oral contraceptives may compound the effects of well-known risk factors, such as hypertension, diabetes, hyperlipidemias, age, and obesity. In particular, some progestogens are known to decrease HDL cholesterol and cause glucose intolerance, while estrogens may create a state of hyperinsulinism. Oral contraceptives have been shown to increase blood pressure among users (see section 9 in "Warnings"). Similar effects on risk factors have been associated with an increased risk of heart disease. Oral contraceptives must be used with caution in women with cardiovascular disease risk factors.

b. *Thromboembolism*

An increased risk of thromboembolic and thrombotic disease associated with the use of oral contraceptives is well estab-

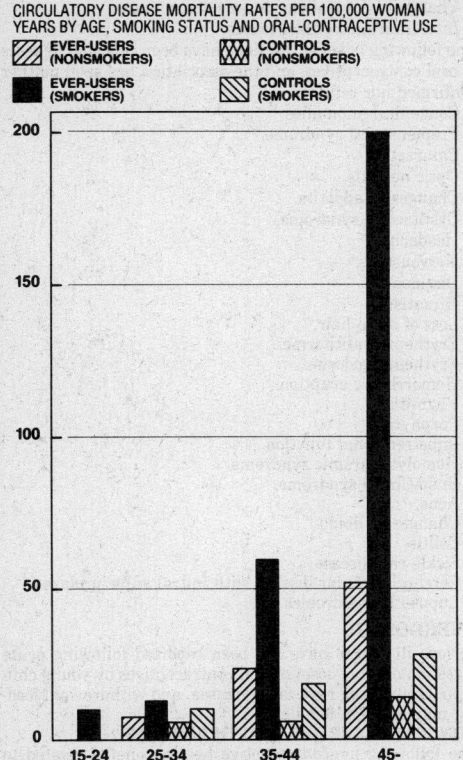

CIRCULATORY DISEASE MORTALITY RATES PER 100,000 WOMAN YEARS BY AGE, SMOKING STATUS AND ORAL-CONTRACEPTIVE USE

- EVER-USERS (NONSMOKERS)
- CONTROLS (NONSMOKERS)
- EVER-USERS (SMOKERS)
- CONTROLS (SMOKERS)

TABLE II. (Adapted from P.M. Layde and V. Beral, Lancet. 1:541–546, 1981.)

TABLE III—ANNUAL NUMBER OF BIRTH-RELATED OR METHOD-RELATED DEATHS ASSOCIATED WITH CONTROL OF FERTILITY PER 100,000 NONSTERILE WOMEN, BY FERTILITY-CONTROL METHOD ACCORDING TO AGE

Method of control and outcome	15–19	20–24	25–29	30–34	35–39	40–44
No fertility-control methods*	7.0	7.4	9.1	14.8	25.7	28.2
Oral contraceptives non-smoker**	0.3	0.5	0.9	1.9	13.8	31.6
Oral contraceptives smoker**	2.2	3.4	6.6	13.5	51.1	117.2
IUD**	0.8	0.8	1.0	1.0	1.4	1.4
Condom*	1.1	1.6	0.7	0.2	0.3	0.4
Diaphragm/spermicide*	1.9	1.2	1.2	1.3	2.2	2.8
Periodic abstinence*	2.5	1.6	1.6	1.7	2.9	3.6

* Deaths are birth related
** Deaths are method related

Adapted from H.W. Ory, Family Planning Perspectives, 15:57–63, 1983.

lished. Case control studies have found the relative risk of users compared to nonusers to be 3 for the first episode of superficial venous thrombosis, 4 to 11 for deep vein thrombosis or pulmonary embolism, and 1.5 to 6 for women with predisposing conditions for venous thromboembolic disease. Cohort studies have shown the relative risk to be somewhat lower, about 3 for new cases and about 4.5 for new cases requiring hospitalization. The risk of thromboembolic disease due to oral contraceptives is not related to length of use and disappears after pill use is stopped.

A two- to four-fold increase in relative risk of postoperative thromboembolic complications has been reported with the use of oral contraceptives. The relative risk of venous thrombosis in women who have predisposing conditions is twice that of women without such medical conditions. If feasible, oral contraceptives should be discontinued at least four weeks prior to and for two weeks after elective surgery of a type associated with an increase in risk of thromboembolism and during and following prolonged immobilization. Since the immediate postpartum period is also associated with an increased risk of thromboembolism, oral contraceptives should be started no earlier than four to six weeks after delivery in women who elect not to breast-feed, or a midtrimester pregnancy termination.

c. Cerebrovascular diseases

Oral contraceptives have been shown to increase both the relative and attributable risks of cerebrovascular events (thrombotic and hemorrhagic strokes), although, in general, the risk is greatest among older (> 35 years), hypertensive women who also smoke. Hypertension was found to be a risk factor for both users and nonusers, for both types of strokes, while smoking interacted to increase the risk for hemorrhagic strokes.

In a large study, the relative risk of thrombotic strokes has been shown to range from 3 for normotensive users to 14 for users with severe hypertension. The relative risk of hemorrhagic stroke is reported to be 1.2 for nonsmokers who used oral contraceptives, 2.6 for smokers who did not use oral contraceptives, 7.6 for smokers who used oral contraceptives, 1.8 for normotensive users, and 25.7 for users with severe hypertension. The attributable risk is also greater in older women.

d. Dose-related risk of vascular disease from oral contraceptives

A positive association has been observed between the amount of estrogen and progestogen in oral contraceptives and the risk of vascular disease. A decline in serum high-density lipoproteins (HDL) has been reported with many progestational agents. A decline in serum high-density lipoproteins has been associated with an increased incidence of ischemic heart disease. Because estrogens increase HDL cholesterol, the net effect of an oral contraceptive depends on a balance achieved between doses of estrogen and progestogen and the nature and absolute amount of progestogen used

in the contraceptive. The amount of both hormones should be considered in the choice of an oral contraceptive.

Minimizing exposure to estrogen and progestogen is in keeping with good principles of therapeutics. For any particular estrogen/progestogen combination, the dosage regimen prescribed should be one which contains the least amount of estrogen and progestogen that is compatible with a low failure rate and the needs of the individual patient. New acceptors of oral-contraceptive agents should be started on preparations containing less than 50 mcg of estrogen.

e. Persistence of risk of vascular disease

There are two studies which have shown persistence of risk of vascular disease for ever-users of oral contraceptives. In a study in the United States, the risk of developing myocardial infarction after discontinuing oral contraceptives persists for at least 9 years for women 40 to 49 years who had used oral contraceptives for five or more years, but this increased risk was not demonstrated in other age groups. In another study in Great Britain, the risk of developing cerebrovascular disease persisted for at least 6 years after discontinuation of oral contraceptives, although excess risk was very small. However, both studies were performed with oral-contraceptive formulations containing 50 micrograms or higher of estrogens.

2. ESTIMATES OF MORTALITY FROM CONTRACEPTIVE USE

One study gathered data from a variety of sources which have estimated the mortality rate associated with different methods of contraception at different ages (Table III). These estimates include the combined risk of death associated with contraceptive methods plus the risk attributable to pregnancy in the event of method failure. Each method of contraception has its specific benefits and risks. The study concluded that with the exception of oral-contraceptive users 35 and older who smoke and 40 and older who do not smoke, mortality associated with all methods of birth control is less than that associated with childbirth. The observation of a possible increase in risk of mortality with age for oral-contraceptive users is based on data gathered in the 1970's—but not reported until 1983. However, current clinical practice involves the use of lower estrogen dose formulations combined with careful restriction of oral contraceptive use to women who do not have the various risk factors listed in this labeling.

Because of these changes in practice and, also, because of some limited new data which suggest that the risk of cardiovascular disease with the use of oral contraceptives may now be less than previously observed, the Fertility and Maternal Health Drugs Advisory Committee was asked to review the topic in 1989. The Committee concluded that although cardiovascular disease risks may be increased with oral-contraceptive use after age 40 in healthy nonsmoking women (even with the newer low-dose formulations), there are greater potential health risks associated with pregnancy in older women and with the alternative surgical and medical procedures which may be necessary if such women do not have access to effective and acceptable means of contraception. Therefore, the Committee recommended that the benefits of oral-contraceptive use by healthy nonsmoking women over 40 may outweigh the possible risks. Of course, older women, as all women who take oral contraceptives, should take the lowest possible dose formulation that is effective.

[See Table III above.]

3. CARCINOMA OF THE REPRODUCTIVE ORGANS

Numerous epidemiological studies have been performed on the incidence of breast, endometrial, ovarian, and cervical cancer in women using oral contraceptives. The overwhelming evidence in the literature suggests that use of oral contraceptives is not associated with an increase in the risk of developing breast cancer, regardless of the age and parity of first use or with most of the marketed brands and doses. The Cancer and Steroid Hormone (CASH) study also showed no

latent effect on the risk of breast cancer for at least a decade following long-term use. A few studies have shown a slightly increased relative risk of developing breast cancer, although the methodology of these studies, which included differences in examination of users and nonusers and differences in age at start of use, has been questioned.

Some studies suggest that oral-contraceptive use has been associated with an increase in the risk of cervical intraepithelial neoplasia in some populations of women. However, there continues to be controversy about the extent to which such findings may be due to differences in sexual behavior and other factors.

In spite of many studies of the relationship between oral-contraceptive use and breast and cervical cancers, a cause-and-effect relationship has not been established.

4. HEPATIC NEOPLASIA

Benign hepatic adenomas are associated with oral-contraceptive use, although the incidence of benign tumors is rare in the United States. Indirect calculations have estimated the attributable risk to be in the range of 3.3 cases/100,000 for users, a risk that increases after four or more years of use. Rupture of rare, benign, hepatic adenomas may cause death through intra-abdominal hemorrhage.

Studies from Britain have shown an increased risk of developing hepatocellular carcinoma in long-term (> 8 years) oral-contraceptive users. However, these cancers are extremely rare in the U.S., and the attributable risk (the excess incidence) of liver cancers in oral contraceptive users approaches less than one per million users.

5. OCULAR LESIONS

There have been clinical case reports of retinal thrombosis associated with the use of oral contraceptives. Oral contraceptives should be discontinued if there is unexplained partial or complete loss of vision; onset of proptosis or diplopia; papilledema; or retinal vascular lesions. Appropriate diagnostic and therapeutic measures should be undertaken immediately.

6. ORAL-CONTRACEPTIVE USE BEFORE OR DURING EARLY PREGNANCY

Extensive epidemiological studies have revealed no increased risk of birth defects in women who have used oral contraceptives prior to pregnancy. Studies also do not suggest a teratogenic effect, particularly insofar as cardiac anomalies and limb reduction defects are concerned, when taken inadvertently during early pregnancy.

The administration of oral contraceptives to induce withdrawal bleeding should not be used as a test for pregnancy. Oral contraceptives should not be used during pregnancy to treat threatened or habitual abortion.

It is recommended that for any patient who has missed two consecutive periods, pregnancy should be ruled out before continuing oral contraceptive use. If the patient has not adhered to the prescribed schedule, the possibility of pregnancy should be considered at the time of the first missed period. Oral contraceptive use should be discontinued if pregnancy is confirmed.

7. GALLBLADDER DISEASE

Earlier studies have reported an increased lifetime relative risk of gallbladder surgery in users of oral contraceptives and estrogens. More recent studies, however, have shown that the relative risk of developing gallbladder disease among oral-contraceptive users may be minimal. The recent findings of minimal risk may be related to the use of oral-contraceptive formulations containing lower hormonal doses of estrogens and progestogens.

8. CARBOHYDRATE AND LIPID METABOLIC EFFECTS

Oral contraceptives have been shown to cause glucose intolerance in a significant percentage of users. Oral contraceptives containing greater than 75 micrograms of estrogens

Continued on next page

Wyeth-Ayerst Laboratories—Cont.

cause hyperinsulinism, while lower doses of estrogen cause less glucose intolerance. Progestogens increase insulin secretion and create insulin resistance, this effect varying with different progestational agents. However, in the nondiabetic woman, oral contraceptives appear to have no effect on fasting blood glucose. Because of these demonstrated effects, prediabetic and diabetic women should be carefully observed while taking oral contraceptives.

A small proportion of women will have persistent hypertriglyceridemia while on the pill. As discussed earlier (see "Warnings", 1a and 1d), changes in serum triglycerides and lipoprotein levels have been reported in oral-contraceptive users.

9. ELEVATED BLOOD PRESSURE

An increase in blood pressure has been reported in women taking oral contraceptives, and this increase is more likely in older oral-contraceptive users and with continued use. Data from the Royal College of General Practitioners and subsequent randomized trials have shown that the incidence of hypertension increases with increasing quantities of progestogens.

Women with a history of hypertension or hypertension-related diseases, or renal disease, should be encouraged to use another method of contraception. If women with hypertension elect to use oral contraceptives, they should be monitored closely, and if significant elevation of blood pressure occurs, oral contraceptives should be discontinued. For most women, elevated blood pressure will return to normal after stopping oral contraceptives, and there is no difference in the occurrence of hypertension among ever- and never-users.

10. HEADACHE

The onset or exacerbation of migraine or development of headache with a new pattern that is recurrent, persistent, or severe requires discontinuation of oral contraceptives and evaluation of the cause.

11. BLEEDING IRREGULARITIES

Breakthrough bleeding and spotting are sometimes encountered in patients on oral contraceptives, especially during the first three months of use. The type and dose of progestogen may be important. Non-hormonal causes should be considered and adequate diagnostic measures taken to rule out malignancy or pregnancy in the event of breakthrough bleeding, as in the case of any abnormal vaginal bleeding. If pathology has been excluded, time or a change to another formulation may solve the problem. In the event of amenorrhea, pregnancy should be ruled out.

Some women may encounter post-pill amenorrhea or oligomenorrhea, especially when such a condition was preexistent.

PRECAUTIONS

Patients should be counseled that this product does not protect against HIV infection (AIDS) and other sexually transmitted diseases.

1. PHYSICAL EXAMINATION AND FOLLOW-UP

A periodic history and physical examination is appropriate for all women, including women using oral contraceptives. The physical examination, however, may be deferred until after initiation of oral contraceptives if requested by the woman and judged appropriate by the clinician. The physical examination should include special reference to blood pressure, breasts, abdomen and pelvic organs, including cervical cytology, and relevant laboratory tests. In case of undiagnosed, persistent or recurrent abnormal vaginal bleeding, appropriate measures should be conducted to rule out malignancy. Women with a strong family history of breast cancer or who have breast nodules should be monitored with particular care.

2. LIPID DISORDERS

Women who are being treated for hyperlipidemias should be followed closely if they elect to use oral contraceptives. Some progestogens may elevate LDL levels and may render the control of hyperlipidemias more difficult. (See Warnings, 1d.)

3. LIVER FUNCTION

If jaundice develops in any woman receiving such drugs, the medication should be discontinued. Steroid hormones may be poorly metabolized in patients with impaired liver function.

4. FLUID RETENTION

Oral contraceptives may cause some degree of fluid retention. They should be prescribed with caution, and only with careful monitoring, in patients with conditions which might be aggravated by fluid retention.

5. EMOTIONAL DISORDERS

Patients becoming significantly depressed while taking oral contraceptives should stop the medication and use an alternate method of contraception in an attempt to determine whether the symptom is drug related. Women with a history of depression should be carefully observed and the drug discontinued if depression recurs to a serious degree.

6. CONTACT LENSES

Contact-lens wearers who develop visual changes or changes in lens tolerance should be assessed by an ophthalmologist.

7. DRUG INTERACTIONS

Reduced efficacy and increased incidence of breakthrough bleeding and menstrual irregularities have been associated with concomitant use of rifampin. A similar association, though less marked, has been suggested with barbiturates, phenylbutazone, phenytoin sodium, and possibly with griseofulvin, ampicillin, and tetracyclines.

8. INTERACTIONS WITH LABORATORY TESTS

Certain endocrine- and liver-function tests and blood components may be affected by oral contraceptives:

a. Increased prothrombin and factors VII, VIII, IX, and X; decreased antithrombin 3; increased norepinephrine-induced platelet aggregability.

b. Increased thyroid-binding globulin (TBG) leading to increased circulating total thyroid hormone, as measured by protein-bound iodine (PBI), T4 by column or by radioimmunoassay. Free T3 resin uptake is decreased, reflecting the elevated TBG; free T4 concentration is unaltered.

c. Other binding proteins may be elevated in serum.

d. Sex-binding globulins are increased and result in elevated levels of total circulating sex steroids and corticoids; however, free or biologically active levels remain unchanged.

e. Triglycerides may be increased.

f. Glucose tolerance may be decreased.

g. Serum folate levels may be depressed by oral-contraceptive therapy. This may be of clinical significance if a woman becomes pregnant shortly after discontinuing oral contraceptives.

9. CARCINOGENESIS

See "Warnings" section.

10. PREGNANCY

Pregnancy Category X. See "Contraindications" and "Warnings" sections.

11. NURSING MOTHERS

Small amounts of oral-contraceptive steroids have been identified in the milk of nursing mothers, and a few adverse effects on the child have been reported, including jaundice and breast enlargement. In addition, oral contraceptives given in the postpartum period may interfere with lactation by decreasing the quantity and quality of breast milk. If possible, the nursing mother should be advised not to use oral contraceptives but to use other forms of contraception until she has completely weaned her child.

INFORMATION FOR THE PATIENT

See Patient Labeling Printed Below.

ADVERSE REACTIONS

An increased risk of the following serious adverse reactions has been associated with the use of oral contraceptives (see "Warnings"section):

Thrombophlebitis.
Arterial thromboembolism.
Pulmonary embolism.
Myocardial infarction.
Cerebral hemorrhage.
Cerebral thrombosis.
Hypertension.
Gallbladder disease.
Hepatic adenomas or benign liver tumors.

There is evidence of an association between the following conditions and the use of oral contraceptives, although additional confirmatory studies are needed:

Mesenteric thrombosis.
Retinal thrombosis.

The following adverse reactions have been reported in patients receiving oral contraceptives and are believed to be drug related:

Nausea.
Vomiting.
Gastrointestinal symptoms (such as abdominal cramps and bloating).
Breakthrough bleeding.
Spotting.
Change in menstrual flow.
Amenorrhea.
Temporary infertility after discontinuation of treatment.
Edema.
Melasma which may persist.
Breast changes: tenderness, enlargement, secretion.
Change in weight (increase or decrease).
Change in cervical erosion and secretion.
Diminution in lactation when given immediately postpartum.
Cholestatic jaundice.
Migraine.
Rash (allergic).
Mental depression.
Reduced tolerance to carbohydrates.
Vaginal candidiasis.

Change in corneal curvature (steepening).
Intolerance to contact lenses.

The following adverse reactions have been reported in users of oral contraceptives, and the association has been neither confirmed nor refuted:

Congenital anomalies.
Premenstrual syndrome.
Cataracts.
Optic neuritis.
Changes in appetite.
Cystitis-like syndrome.
Headache.
Nervousness.
Dizziness.
Hirsutism.
Loss of scalp hair.
Erythema multiforme.
Erythema nodosum.
Hemorrhagic eruption.
Vaginitis.
Porphyria.
Impaired renal function.
Hemolytic uremic syndrome.
Budd-Chiari syndrome.
Acne.
Changes in libido.
Colitis.
Sickle cell disease.
Cerebral-vascular disease with mitral valve prolapse.
Lupus-like syndromes.

OVERDOSAGE

Serious ill effects have not been reported following acute ingestion of large doses of oral contraceptives by young children. Overdosage may cause nausea, and withdrawal bleeding may occur in females.

NONCONTRACEPTIVE HEALTH BENEFITS

The following noncontraceptive health benefits related to the use of oral contraceptives are supported by epidemiological studies which largely utilized oral contraceptive formulations containing doses exceeding 0.035 mg of ethinyl estradiol or 0.05 mg of mestranol.

Effects on menses:
Increased menstrual cycle regularity.
Decreased blood loss and decreased incidence of iron-deficiency anemia.
Decreased incidence of dysmenorrhea.

Effects related to inhibition of ovulation:
Decreased incidence of functional ovarian cysts.
Decreased incidence of ectopic pregnancies.

Effects from long-term use:
Decreased incidence of fibroadenomas and fibrocystic disease of the breast.
Decreased incidence of acute pelvic inflammatory disease.
Decreased incidence of endometrial cancer.
Decreased incidence of ovarian cancer.

DOSAGE AND ADMINISTRATION

To achieve maximum contraceptive effectiveness, LO/OVRAL must be taken exactly as directed and at intervals not exceeding 24 hours.

The dosage of LO/OVRAL is one tablet daily for 21 consecutive days per menstrual cycle according to prescribed schedule. Tablets are then discontinued for 7 days (three weeks on, one week off).

It is recommended that LO/OVRAL tablets be taken at the same time each day, preferably after the evening meal or at bedtime.

During the first cycle of medication, the patient is instructed to take one LO/OVRAL tablet daily for twenty-one consecutive days, beginning on the first day (Day 1 Start) of her menstrual cycle or on the Sunday after her period begins (Sunday Start). (The first day of menstruation is day one.) The tablets are then discontinued for one week (7 days). Withdrawal bleeding should usually occur within 3 days following discontinuation of LO/OVRAL. (For Day 1 Start: If LO/OVRAL is first taken later than the first day of the first menstrual cycle of medication or postpartum, contraceptive reliance should not be placed on LO/OVRAL until after the first seven consecutive days of administration. For Sunday Start: Contraceptive reliance should not be placed on LO/OVRAL until after the first seven consecutive days of administration. The possibility of ovulation and conception prior to initiation of medication should be considered.)

The patient begins her next and all subsequent 21-day courses of LO/OVRAL tablets on the same day of the week that she began her first course, following the same schedule: 21 days on—7 days off. She begins taking her tablets on the 8th day after discontinuance, regardless of whether or not a menstrual period has occurred or is still in progress. Any time a new cycle of LO/OVRAL is started later than the 8th day, the patient should be protected by another means of contraception until she has taken a tablet daily for seven consecutive days.

If spotting or breakthrough bleeding occurs, the patient is instructed to continue on the same regimen. This type of

bleeding is usually transient and without significance; however, if the bleeding is persistent or prolonged, the patient is advised to consult her physician. Although the occurrence of pregnancy is highly unlikely if LO/OVRAL is taken according to directions, if withdrawal bleeding does not occur, the possibility of pregnancy must be considered. If the patient has not adhered to the prescribed schedule (missed one or more tablets or started taking them on a day later than she should have), the probability of pregnancy should be considered at the time of the first missed period and appropriate diagnostic measures taken before the medication is resumed. If the patient has adhered to the prescribed regimen and misses two consecutive periods, pregnancy should be ruled out before continuing the contraceptive regimen.

For additional patient instructions regarding missed pills, see the "WHAT TO DO IF YOU MISS PILLS" section in the **DETAILED PATIENT LABELING** below.

Any time a patient misses two or more tablets, she should also use another method of contraception until she has taken a tablet daily for seven consecutive days. If breakthrough bleeding occurs following missed tablets, it will usually be transient and of no consequence. While there is little likelihood of ovulation occurring if only one or two tablets are missed, the possibility of ovulation increases with each successive day that scheduled tablets are missed.

In the nonlactating mother, LO/OVRAL may be initiated postpartum, for contraception. When the tablets are administered in the postpartum period, the increased risk of thromboembolic disease associated with the postpartum period must be considered (see "Contraindications," "Warnings", and "Precautions" concerning thromboembolic disease). It is to be noted that early resumption of ovulation may occur if Parlodel® (bromocriptine mesylate) has been used for the prevention of lactation.

HOW SUPPLIED

LO/OVRAL® Tablets (0.3 mg norgestrel and 0.03 mg ethinyl estradiol) are available in packages of 6 PILPAK® dispensers with 21 tablets each as follows:
NDC 0008-0078, white, round tablet marked "WYETH" and "78".

REFERENCES

Available Upon Request.
Brief Summary Patient Package Insert
This product (like all oral contraceptives) is intended to prevent pregnancy. It does not protect against HIV infection (AIDS) and other sexually transmitted diseases.

Oral contraceptives, also known as "birth-control pills" or "the pill", are taken to prevent pregnancy, and when taken correctly, have a failure rate of less than 1.0% per year when used without missing any pills. The typical failure rate of large numbers of pill users is less than 3.0% per year when women who miss pills are included. For most women oral contraceptives are also free of serious or unpleasant side effects. However, forgetting to take pills considerably increases the chances of pregnancy.

For the majority of women, oral contraceptives can be taken safely. But there are some women who are at high risk of developing certain serious diseases that can be life-threatening or may cause temporary or permanent disability or death. The risks associated with taking oral contraceptives increase significantly if you:
- smoke
- have high blood pressure, diabetes, high cholesterol
- have or have had clotting disorders, heart attack, stroke, angina pectoris, cancer of the breast or sex organs, jaundice, or malignant or benign liver tumors.
You should not take the pill if you suspect you are pregnant or have unexplained vaginal bleeding.

> Cigarette smoking increases the risk of serious cardiovascular side effects on the heart and blood vessels from oral contraceptive use. This risk increases with age and with heavy smoking (15 or more cigarettes per day) and is quite marked in women over 35 years of age. Women who use oral contraceptives should not smoke.

Most side effects of the pill are not serious. The most common such effects are nausea, vomiting, bleeding between menstrual periods, weight gain, breast tenderness, and difficulty wearing contact lenses. These side effects, especially nausea and vomiting, may subside within the first three months of use.

The serious side effects of the pill occur very infrequently, especially if you are in good health and do not smoke. However, you should know that the following medical conditions have been associated with or made worse by the pill:
1. Blood clots in the legs (thrombophlebitis), lungs (pulmonary embolism), stoppage or rupture of a blood vessel in the brain (stroke), blockage of blood vessels in the heart (heart attack or angina pectoris) or other organs of the body. As mentioned above, smoking increases the risk of heart attacks and strokes and subsequent serious medical consequences.
2. Liver tumors, which may rupture and cause severe bleeding. A possible but not definite association has been found

with the pill and liver cancer. However, liver cancers are extremely rare. The chance of developing liver cancer from using the pill is thus even rarer.
3. High blood pressure, although blood pressure usually returns to normal when the pill is stopped.
The symptoms associated with these serious side effects are discussed in the detailed leaflet given to you with your supply of pills. Notify your doctor or health-care provider if you notice any unusual physical disturbances while taking the pill. In addition, drugs such as rifampin, as well as some anticonvulsants and some antibiotics, may decrease oral contraceptive effectiveness.

Studies to date of women taking the pill have not shown an increase in the incidence of cancer of the breast or cervix. There is, however, insufficient evidence to rule out the possibility that pills may cause such cancers.

Taking the pill provides some important noncontraceptive benefits. These include less painful menstruation, less menstrual blood loss and anemia, fewer pelvic infections, and fewer cancers of the ovary and the lining of the uterus.

Be sure to discuss any medical condition you may have with your health-care provider. Your health-care provider will take a medical and family history before prescribing oral contraceptives and will examine you. The physical examination may be delayed to another time if you request it and the health-care provider believes that it is appropriate to postpone it. You should be reexamined at least once a year while taking oral contraceptives. The detailed patient information leaflet gives you further information which you should read and discuss with your health-care provider.

DETAILED PATIENT LABELING

This product (like all oral contraceptives) is intended to prevent pregnancy. It does not protect against HIV infection (AIDS) and other sexually transmitted diseases.

INTRODUCTION

Any woman who considers using oral contraceptives (the birth-control pill or the pill) should understand the benefits and risks of using this form of birth control. This leaflet will give you much of the information you will need to make this decision and will also help you determine if you are at risk of developing any of the serious side effects of the pill. It will tell you how to use the pill properly so that it will be as effective as possible. However, this leaflet is not a replacement for a careful discussion between you and your health-care provider. You should discuss the information provided in this leaflet with him or her, both when you first start taking the pill and during your revisits. You should also follow your health-care provider's advice with regard to regular checkups while you are on the pill.

EFFECTIVENESS OF ORAL CONTRACEPTIVES

Oral contraceptives or "birth-control pills" or "the pill" are used to prevent pregnancy and are more effective than other nonsurgical methods of birth control. When they are taken correctly, the chance of becoming pregnant is less than 1.0% when used perfectly, without missing any pills. Typical failure rates are less than 3.0% per year. The chance of becoming pregnant increases with each missed pill during the menstrual cycle.

In comparison, typical failure rates for other nonsurgical methods of birth control during the first year of use are as follows:
IUD: 3%
DEPO-PROVERA® (injectable progestogen): 0.3%
NORPLANT® SYSTEM (implants): 0.2%
Diaphragm with spermicides: 18%
Spermicides alone: 21%
Vaginal sponge: 18% to 28%
Condom alone: 12%
Periodic abstinence: 20%
No methods: 85%

WHO SHOULD NOT TAKE ORAL CONTRACEPTIVES

> Cigarette smoking increases the risk of serious adverse effects on the heart and blood vessels from oral-contraceptive use. This risk increases with age and with heavy smoking (15 or more cigarettes per day) and is quite marked in women over 35 years of age. Women who use oral contraceptives should not smoke.

Some women should not use the pill. For example, you should not take the pill if you are pregnant or think you may be pregnant. You should also not use the pill if you have had any of the following conditions:
- Heart attack or stroke.
- Blood clots in the legs (thrombophlebitis), lungs (pulmonary embolism), or eyes.
- Blood clots in the deep veins of your legs.
- Known or suspected breast cancer or cancer of the lining of the uterus, cervix, or vagina.
- Liver tumor (benign or cancerous).
Or, if you have any of the following:
- Chest pain (angina pectoris).
- Unexplained vaginal bleeding (until a diagnosis is reached by your doctor).

- Yellowing of the whites of the eyes or of the skin (jaundice) during pregnancy or during previous use of the pill.
- Known or suspected pregnancy.
Tell your health-care provider if you have ever had any of these conditions. Your health-care provider can recommend another method of birth control.

OTHER CONSIDERATIONS BEFORE TAKING ORAL CONTRACEPTIVES

Tell your health-care provider if you or any family member has ever had:
- Breast nodules, fibrocystic disease of the breast, an abnormal breast X ray or mammogram
- Diabetes
- Elevated cholesterol or triglycerides
- High blood pressure
- Migraine or other headaches or epilepsy
- Mental depression
- Gallbladder, heart, or kidney disease
- History of scanty or irregular menstrual periods
Women with any of these conditions should be checked often by their health-care provider if they choose to use oral contraceptives. Also, be sure to inform your doctor or health-care provider if you smoke or are on any medications.

RISKS OF TAKING ORAL CONTRACEPTIVES

1. *Risk of developing blood clots*
Blood clots and blockage of blood vessels are the most serious side effects of taking oral contraceptives and can be fatal. In particular, a clot in the legs can cause thrombophlebitis and a clot that travels to the lungs can cause a sudden blocking of the vessel carrying blood to the lungs. Rarely, clots occur in the blood vessels of the eye and may cause blindness, double vision, or impaired vision.

If you take oral contraceptives and need elective surgery, need to stay in bed for a prolonged illness, or have recently delivered a baby, you may be at risk of developing blood clots. You should consult your doctor about stopping oral contraceptives three to four weeks before surgery and not taking oral contraceptives for two weeks after surgery or during bed rest. You should also not take oral contraceptives soon after delivery of a baby or a midtrimester pregnancy termination. It is advisable to wait for at least four weeks after delivery if you are not breast-feeding. If you are breast-feeding, you should wait until you have weaned your child before using the pill. (See also the section on breast-feeding in General Precautions.)

2. *Heart attacks and strokes*
Oral contraceptives may increase the tendency to develop strokes (stoppage or rupture of blood vessels in the brain) and angina pectoris and heart attacks (blockage of blood vessels in the heart). Any of these conditions can cause death or serious disability.

Smoking greatly increases the possibility of suffering heart attacks and strokes. Furthermore, smoking and the use of oral contraceptives greatly increase the chances of developing and dying of heart disease.

3. *Gallbladder disease*
Oral-contraceptive users probably have a greater risk than nonusers of having gallbladder disease, although this risk may be related to pills containing high doses of estrogens.

4. *Liver tumors*
In rare cases, oral contraceptives can cause benign but dangerous liver tumors. These benign liver tumors can rupture and cause fatal internal bleeding. In addition, a possible but not definite association has been found with the pill and liver cancers in two studies in which a few women who developed these very rare cancers were found to have used oral contraceptives for long periods. However, liver cancers are extremely rare. The chance of developing liver cancer from using the pill is thus even rarer.

5. *Cancer of the reproductive organs*
There is, at present, no confirmed evidence that oral contraceptives increase the risk of cancer of the reproductive organs in human studies. Several studies have found no overall increase in the risk of developing breast cancer. However, women who use oral contraceptives and have a strong family history of breast cancer or who have breast nodules or abnormal mammograms should be closely followed by their doctors.

Some studies have found an increase in the incidence of cancer of the cervix in women who use oral contraceptives. However, this finding may be related to factors other than the use of oral contraceptives.

ESTIMATED RISK OF DEATH FROM A BIRTH-CONTROL METHOD OR PREGNANCY

All methods of birth control and pregnancy are associated with a risk of developing certain diseases which may lead to disability or death. An estimate of the number of deaths associated with different methods of birth control and pregnancy has been calculated and is shown in the following table.
[See table on top of next page.]
In the above table, the risk of death from any birth control method is less than the risk of childbirth, except for oral-contraceptive users over the age of 35 who smoke and pill

Continued on next page

Wyeth-Ayerst Laboratories—Cont.

users over the age of 40 even if they do not smoke. It can be seen in the table that for women aged 15 to 39, the risk of death was highest with pregnancy (7 to 26 deaths per 100,000 women, depending on age). Among pill users who do not smoke, the risk of death was always lower than that associated with pregnancy for any age group, except for those women over the age of 40, when the risk increases to 32 deaths per 100,000 women, compared to 28 associated with pregnancy at that age. However, for pill users who smoke and are over the age of 35, the estimated number of deaths exceeds those for other methods of birth control. If a woman is over the age of 40 and smokes, her estimated risk of death is four times higher (117/100,000 women) than the estimated risk associated with pregnancy (28/100,000 women) in that age group.

The suggestion that women over 40 who don't smoke should not take oral contraceptives is based on information from older high-dose pills and on less-selective use of pills than is practiced today. An Advisory Committee of the FDA discussed this issue in 1989 and recommended that the benefits of oral-contraceptive use by healthy, nonsmoking women over 40 years of age may outweigh the possible risks. However, all women, especially older women, are cautioned to use the lowest-dose pill that is effective.

WARNING SIGNALS

If any of these adverse effects occur while you are taking oral contraceptives, call your doctor immediately:

- Sharp chest pain, coughing of blood, or sudden shortness of breath (indicating a possible clot in the lung)
- Pain in the calf (indicating a possible clot in the leg)
- Crushing chest pain or heaviness in the chest (indicating a possible heart attack)
- Sudden severe headache or vomiting, dizziness or fainting, disturbances of vision or speech, weakness, or numbness in an arm or leg (indicating a possible stroke)
- Sudden partial or complete loss of vision (indicating a possible clot in the eye)
- Breast lumps (indicating possible breast cancer or fibrocystic disease of the breast; ask your doctor or health-care provider to show you how to examine your breasts)
- Severe pain or tenderness in the stomach area (indicating a possibly ruptured liver tumor)
- Difficulty in sleeping, weakness, lack of energy, fatigue, or change in mood (possibly indicating severe depression)
- Jaundice or a yellowing of the skin or eyeballs, accompanied frequently by fever, fatigue, loss of appetite, dark-colored urine, or light-colored bowel movements (indicating possible liver problems)

SIDE EFFECTS OF ORAL CONTRACEPTIVES

1. Vaginal bleeding

Irregular vaginal bleeding or spotting may occur while you are taking the pills. Irregular bleeding may vary from slight staining between menstrual periods to breakthrough bleeding which is a flow much like a regular period. Irregular bleeding occurs most often during the first few months of oral-contraceptive use, but may also occur after you have been taking the pill for some time. Such bleeding may be temporary and usually does not indicate any serious problems. It is important to continue taking your pills on schedule. If the bleeding occurs in more than one cycle or lasts for more than a few days, talk to your doctor or health-care provider.

2. Contact lenses

If you wear contact lenses and notice a change in vision or an inability to wear your lenses, contact your doctor or health-care provider.

3. Fluid retention

Oral contraceptives may cause edema (fluid retention) with swelling of the fingers or ankles and may raise your blood pressure. If you experience fluid retention, contact your doctor or health-care provider.

4. Melasma

A spotty darkening of the skin is possible, particularly of the face.

5. Other side effects

Other side effects may include change in appetite, headache, nervousness, depression, dizziness, loss of scalp hair, rash, and vaginal infections.

If any of these side effects bother you, call your doctor or health-care provider.

GENERAL PRECAUTIONS

1. Missed periods and use of oral contraceptives before or during early pregnancy

There may be times when you may not menstruate regularly after you have completed taking a cycle of pills. If you have taken your pills regularly and miss one menstrual period, continue taking your pills for the next cycle but be sure to inform your health care provider before doing so. If you have not taken the pills daily as instructed and missed a menstrual period, or if you missed two consecutive menstrual periods, you may be pregnant. Check with your health-care provider immediately to determine whether you are preg-

ANNUAL NUMBER OF BIRTH-RELATED OR METHOD-RELATED DEATHS ASSOCIATED WITH CONTROL OF FERTILITY PER 100,000 NONSTERILE WOMEN, BY FERTILITY CONTROL METHOD ACCORDING TO AGE						
Method of control and outcome	15–19	20–24	25–29	30–34	35–39	40–44
No fertility control methods*	7.0	7.4	9.1	14.8	25.7	28.2
Oral contraceptives nonsmoker**	0.3	0.5	0.9	1.9	13.8	31.6
Oral contraceptives smoker**	2.2	3.4	6.6	13.5	51.1	117.2
IUD**	0.8	0.8	1.0	1.0	1.4	1.4
Condom*	1.1	1.6	0.7	0.2	0.3	0.4
Diaphragm/ spermicide*	1.9	1.2	1.2	1.3	2.2	2.8
Periodic abstinence*	2.5	1.6	1.6	1.7	2.9	3.6

* Deaths are birth related
** Deaths are method related

nant. Do not continue to take oral contraceptives until you are sure you are not pregnant, but continue to use another method of contraception.

There is no conclusive evidence that oral-contraceptive use is associated with an increase in birth defects, when taken inadvertently during early pregnancy. Previously, a few studies had reported that oral contraceptives might be associated with birth defects, but these findings have not been confirmed. Nevertheless, oral contraceptives or any other drugs should not be used during pregnancy unless clearly necessary and prescribed by your doctor. You should check with your doctor about risks to your unborn child of any medication taken during pregnancy.

2. While breast-feeding

If you are breast-feeding, consult your doctor before starting oral contraceptives. Some of the drug will be passed on to the child in the milk. A few adverse effects on the child have been reported, including yellowing of the skin (jaundice) and breast enlargement. In addition, oral contraceptives may decrease the amount and quality of your milk. If possible, do not use oral contraceptives while breast-feeding. You should use another method of contraception since breast-feeding provides only partial protection from becoming pregnant, and this partial protection decreases significantly as you breast-feed for longer periods of time. You should consider starting oral contraceptives only after you have weaned your child completely.

3. Laboratory tests

If you are scheduled for any laboratory tests, tell your doctor you are taking birth-control pills. Certain blood tests may be affected by birth-control pills.

4. Drug interactions

Certain drugs may interact with birth-control pills to make them less effective in preventing pregnancy or cause an increase in breakthrough bleeding. Such drugs include rifampin, drugs used for epilepsy such as barbiturates (for example, phenobarbital) and phenytoin (Dilantin is one brand of this drug), phenylbutazone (Butazolidin is one brand), and possibly certain antibiotics. You may need to use an additional method of contraception during any cycle in which you take drugs that can make oral contraceptives less effective.

HOW TO TAKE THE PILL

This product (like all oral contraceptives) is intended to prevent pregnancy. It does not protect against transmission of HIV (AIDS) and other sexually transmitted diseases such as chlamydia, genital herpes, genital warts, gonorrhea, hepatitis B, and syphilis.

IMPORTANT POINTS TO REMEMBER

BEFORE YOU START TAKING YOUR PILLS:

1. BE SURE TO READ THESE DIRECTIONS:
Before you start taking your pills.
Anytime you are not sure what to do.
2. THE RIGHT WAY TO TAKE THE PILL IS TO TAKE ONE PILL EVERY DAY AT THE SAME TIME.
If you miss pills you could get pregnant. This includes starting the pack late. The more pills you miss, the more likely you are to get pregnant.
3. MANY WOMEN HAVE SPOTTING OR LIGHT BLEEDING, OR MAY FEEL SICK TO THEIR STOMACH DURING THE FIRST 1-3 PACKS OF PILLS.
If you feel sick to your stomach, do not stop taking the pill. The problem will usually go away. If it doesn't go away, check with your doctor or clinic.
4. MISSING PILLS CAN ALSO CAUSE SPOTTING OR LIGHT BLEEDING, even when you make up these missed pills.
On the days you take 2 pills to make up for missed pills, you could also feel a little sick to your stomach.
5. IF YOU HAVE VOMITING OR DIARRHEA, for any reason, or IF YOU TAKE SOME MEDICINES, including some antibiotics, your pills may not work as well. Use a back-

up method (such as condoms, foam, or sponge) until you check with your doctor or clinic.
6. IF YOU HAVE TROUBLE REMEMBERING TO TAKE THE PILL, talk to your doctor or clinic about how to make pill-taking easier or about using another method of birth control.
7. IF YOU HAVE ANY QUESTIONS OR ARE UNSURE ABOUT THE INFORMATION IN THIS LEAFLET, call your doctor or clinic.
NORDETTE®· 21, OVRAL®, LO/OVRAL®, NORDETTE®-28, OVRAL®-28, AND LO/OVRAL®-28

BEFORE YOU START TAKING YOUR PILLS

1. DECIDE WHAT TIME OF DAY YOU WANT TO TAKE YOUR PILL.
It is important to take it at about the same time every day.
2. LOOK AT YOUR PILL PACK TO SEE IF IT HAS 21 OR 28 PILLS:
The *21-pill pack* has 21 "active" white or light-orange pills (with hormones) to take for 3 weeks, followed by 1 week without pills.
The *28-pill pack* has 21 "active" white or light-orange pills (with hormones) to take for 3 weeks, followed by 1 week of reminder pink pills (without hormones).
3. ALSO FIND:
1) where on the pack to start taking pills, and
2) in what order to take the pills (follow the arrows).

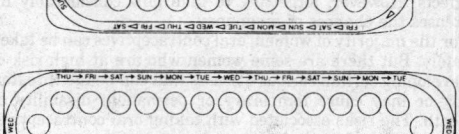

4. BE SURE YOU HAVE READY AT ALL TIMES: ANOTHER KIND OF BIRTH CONTROL (such as condoms, foams or sponge) to use as a back-up in case you miss pills. AN EXTRA, FULL PILL PACK.

WHEN TO START THE *FIRST* PACK OF PILLS

For the 21-day pill pack you have two choices of which day to start taking your first pack of pills. (See **DAY 1 START** or **SUNDAY START** directions below.) Decide with your doctor or clinic which is the best day for you. The 28-day pill pack accommodates a **SUNDAY START** only. For either pill pack pick a time of day which will be easy to remember.
DAY 1 START:
These instructions are for the 21-day pill pack only. The 28-day pill pack does not accommodate a **DAY 1 START** dosage regimen.
1. Take the first "active" white or light-orange pill of the first pack during the *first 24 hours of your period.*
2. You will not need to use a back-up method of birth control, since you are starting the pill at the beginning of your period.
SUNDAY START:
These instructions are for either the 21-day or the 28-day pill pack.
1. Take the first "active" white or light-orange pill of the first pack on the *Sunday after your period starts,* even if you are still bleeding. If your period begins on Sunday, start the pack that same day.
2. *Use another method of birth control* as a back-up method if you have sex anytime from the Sunday you start your first

pack until the next Sunday (7 days). Condoms, foam, or the sponge are good back-up methods of birth control.

WHAT TO DO DURING THE MONTH

1. TAKE ONE PILL AT THE SAME TIME EVERY DAY UNTIL THE PACK IS EMPTY.
Do not skip pills even if you are spotting or bleeding between monthly periods or feel sick to your stomach (nausea).
Do not skip pills even if you do not have sex very often.
2. WHEN YOU FINISH A PACK OR SWITCH YOUR BRAND OF PILLS:
21 pills: Wait 7 days to start the next pack. You will probably have your period during that week. Be sure that no more than 7 days pass between 21-day packs.
28 pills: Start the next pack on the day after your last "reminder" pill. Do not wait any days between packs.

WHAT TO DO IF YOU MISS PILLS

If you **MISS** 1 white or light-orange "active" pill:
1. Take it as soon as you remember. Take the next pill at your regular time. This means you take 2 pills in 1 day.
2. You do not need to use a back-up birth control method if you have sex.
If you **MISS 2** white or light-orange "active" pills in a row in **WEEK 1 or WEEK 2** of your pack:
1. Take 2 pills on the day you remember and 2 pills the next day.
2. Then take 1 pill a day until you finish the pack.
3. You MAY BECOME PREGNANT if you have sex in the *7 days* after you miss pills. You MUST use another birth control method (such as condoms, foam, or sponge) as a back-up for those 7 days.
If you **MISS 2** white or light-orange "active" pills in a row in **THE 3rd WEEK**:
The ***Day 1 Starter*** instructions are for the 21-day pill pack only. The 28-day pill pack does not accommodate a **DAY 1 START** dosage regimen. The ***Sunday Starter*** instructions are for either the 21-day or 28-day pill pack.
1. ***If you are a Day 1 Starter:***
THROW OUT the rest of the pill pack and start a new pack that same day.
If you are a Sunday Starter:
Keep taking 1 pill every day until Sunday.
On Sunday, THROW OUT the rest of the pack and start a new pack of pills that same day.
2. You may not have your period this month but this is expected. However, if you miss your period 2 months in a row, call your doctor or clinic because you might be pregnant.
3. You MAY BECOME PREGNANT if you have sex in the *7 days* after you miss pills. You MUST use another birth control method (such as condoms, foam, or sponge) as a back-up for those 7 days.
If you **MISS 3 OR MORE** white or light-orange "active" pills in a row (during the first 3 weeks):
The ***Day 1 Starter*** instructions are for the 21-day pill pack only. The 28-day pill pack does not accommodate a **DAY 1 START** dosage regimen. The ***Sunday Starter*** instructions are for either the 21-day or 28-day pill pack.
1. ***If you are a Day 1 Starter:***
THROW OUT the rest of the pill pack and start a new pack that same day.
If you are a Sunday Starter:
Keep taking 1 pill every day until Sunday.
On Sunday, THROW OUT the rest of the pack and start a new pack of pills that same day.
2. You may not have your period this month but this is expected. However, if you miss your period 2 months in a row, call your doctor or clinic because you might be pregnant.
3. You MAY BECOME PREGNANT if you have sex in the *7 days* after you miss pills. You MUST use another birth control method (such as condoms, foam, or sponge) as a back-up for those 7 days.

A REMINDER FOR THOSE ON 28-DAY PACKS:
If you forget any of the 7 pink "reminder" pills in Week 4:
THROW AWAY the pills you missed.
Keep taking 1 pill each day until the pack is empty.
You do not need a back-up method if you start your next pack on time.

FINALLY, IF YOU ARE STILL NOT SURE WHAT TO DO ABOUT THE PILLS YOU HAVE MISSED:
Use a BACK-UP METHOD anytime you have sex.
KEEP TAKING ONE PILL EACH DAY until you can reach your doctor or clinic.
OVRETTE®
Ovrette is administered on a continuous daily dosage schedule, one tablet each day, every day of the year. Take the first tablet on the first day of your menstrual period. Tablets should be taken at the same time every day, without interruption, whether bleeding occurs or not. If bleeding is prolonged (more than 8 days) or unusually heavy, you should contact your doctor.
Forgotten pills
The risk of pregnancy increases with each tablet missed. Therefore, it is very important that you take one tablet daily as directed. If you miss one tablet, take it as soon as you remember and also take your next tablet at the regular time. If you miss two tablets, take one of the missed tablets as soon as you remember, as well as your regular tablet for that day at the proper time. Furthermore, you should use another method of birth control in addition to taking Ovrette until you have taken fourteen days (2 weeks) of medication.
If more than two tablets have been missed, Ovrette should be discontinued immediately and another method of birth control used until the start of your next menstrual period. Then you may resume taking Ovrette.

Pregnancy due to pill failure
The incidence of pill failure resulting in pregnancy is approximately less than 1.0% if taken every day as directed, but more typical failure rates are less than 3.0%. If failure does occur, the risk to the fetus is minimal.
RISKS TO THE FETUS
If you do become pregnant while using oral contraceptives, the risk to the fetus is small, on the order of no more than one per thousand. You should, however, discuss the risks to the developing child with your doctor.
Pregnancy after stopping the pill
There may be some delay in becoming pregnant after you stop using oral contraceptives, especially if you had irregular menstrual cycles before you used oral contraceptives. It may be advisable to postpone conception until you begin menstruating regularly once you have stopped taking the pill and desire pregnancy.
There does not appear to be any increase in birth defects in newborn babies when pregnancy occurs soon after stopping the pill.
Overdosage
Serious ill effects have not been reported following ingestion of large doses of oral contraceptives by young children. Overdosage may cause nausea and withdrawal bleeding in females. In case of overdosage, contact your health-care provider or pharmacist.
Other information
Your health-care provider will take a medical and family history before prescribing oral contraceptives and will examine you. The physical examination may be delayed to another time if you request it and the health-care provider believes that it is appropriate to postpone it. You should be reexamined at least once a year. Be sure to inform your health-care provider if there is a family history of any of the conditions listed previously in this leaflet. Be sure to keep all appointments with your health-care provider, because this is a time to determine if there are early signs of side effects of oral-contraceptive use.
Do not use the drug for any condition other than the one for which it was prescribed. This drug has been prescribed specifically for you; do not give it to others who may want birth-control pills.
HEALTH BENEFITS FROM ORAL CONTRACEPTIVES
In addition to preventing pregnancy, use of oral contraceptives may provide certain benefits. They are:
- Menstrual cycles may become more regular
- Blood flow during menstruation may be lighter, and less iron may be lost. Therefore, anemia due to iron deficiency is less likely to occur.
- Pain or other symptoms during menstruation may be encountered less frequently
- Ovarian cysts may occur less frequently
- Ectopic (tubal) pregnancy may occur less frequently
- Noncancerous cysts or lumps in the breast may occur less frequently
- Acute pelvic inflammatory disease may occur less frequently
- Oral-contraceptive use may provide some protection against developing two forms of cancer: cancer of the ovaries and cancer of the lining of the uterus.

If you want more information about birth-control pills, ask your doctor or pharmacist. They have a more technical leaflet called the Professional Labeling which you may wish to read.

Shown in Product Identification Guide, page 340

LO/OVRAL®-28 ℞

[lōh-oh 'vral-28]
Tablets
(norgestrel and ethinyl estradiol tablets)

Patients should be counseled that this product does not protect against HIV infection (AIDS) and other sexually transmitted diseases.

DESCRIPTION
21 white LO/OVRAL tablets, each containing 0.3 mg of norgestrel (*dl*-13-beta-ethyl-17-alpha-ethinyl-17-beta-hydroxygon-4-en-3-one), a totally synthetic progestogen, and 0.03 mg of ethinyl estradiol (19-nor-17α-pregna-1,3,5(10)-trien-20-yne-3,17-diol), and 7 pink inert tablets. The inactive ingredients present are cellulose, D&C Red 30, lactose, magnesium stearate, and polacrilin potassium.

CLINICAL PHARMACOLOGY
See LO/OVRAL®.

INDICATIONS AND USAGE
See LO/OVRAL.

CONTRAINDICATIONS
See LO/OVRAL.

WARNINGS
See LO/OVRAL.

PRECAUTIONS
See LO/OVRAL.
Drug Interactions: See LO/OVRAL.
Carcinogenesis: See LO/OVRAL.
Pregnancy: See LO/OVRAL.
Nursing Mothers: See LO/OVRAL.
Information for the Patient: See LO/OVRAL.

ADVERSE REACTIONS
See LO/OVRAL.

OVERDOSAGE
See LO/OVRAL.

NONCONTRACEPTIVE HEALTH BENEFITS
See LO/OVRAL.

DOSAGE AND ADMINISTRATION
To achieve maximum contraceptive effectiveness, LO/OVRAL-28 must be taken exactly as directed and at intervals not exceeding 24 hours.
The dosage of LO/OVRAL-28 is one white tablet daily for 21 consecutive days followed by one pink inert tablet daily for 7 consecutive days according to prescribed schedule. It is recommended that tablets be taken at the same time each day, preferably after the evening meal or at bedtime.
During the first cycle of medication, the patient is instructed to begin taking LO/OVRAL-28 on the first Sunday after the onset of menstruation. If menstruation begins on a Sunday, the first tablet (white) is taken that day. One white tablet should be taken daily for 21 consecutive days followed by one pink inert tablet daily for 7 consecutive days. Withdrawal bleeding should usually occur within three days following discontinuation of white tablets. During the first cycle, contraceptive reliance should not be placed on LO/OVRAL-28 until a white tablet has been taken daily for 7 consecutive days. The possibility of ovulation and conception prior to initiation of medication should be considered.
The patient begins her next and all subsequent 28-day courses of tablets on the same day of the week (Sunday) on which she began her first course, following the same schedule: 21 days on white tablets—7 days on pink inert tablets. If in any cycle the patient starts tablets later than the proper day, she should protect herself by using another method of birth control until she has taken a white tablet daily for 7 consecutive days.
If spotting or breakthrough bleeding occurs, the patient is instructed to continue on the same regimen. This type of bleeding is usually transient and without significance; however, if the bleeding is persistent or prolonged, the patient is advised to consult her physician. Although the occurrence of pregnancy is highly unlikely if LO/OVRAL-28 is taken according to directions, if withdrawal bleeding does not occur, the possibility of pregnancy must be considered. If the patient has not adhered to the prescribed schedule (missed one or more tablets or started taking them on a day later than she should have), the probability of pregnancy should be considered at the time of the first missed period and appropriate diagnostic measures taken before the medication is resumed. If the patient has adhered to the prescribed regimen and misses two consecutive periods, pregnancy should be ruled out before continuing the contraceptive regimen.
For additional patient instructions regarding missed pills, see the "WHAT TO DO IF YOU MISS PILLS" section in the **DETAILED PATIENT LABELING** for LO/OVRAL.
Any time the patient misses two or more white tablets, she should also use another method of contraception until she has taken a white tablet daily for seven consecutive days. If the patient misses one or more pink tablets, she is still protected against pregnancy **provided** she begins taking white tablets again on the proper day.
If breakthrough bleeding occurs following missed white tablets, it will usually be transient and of no consequence. While there is little likelihood of ovulation occurring if only one or two white tablets are missed, the possibility of ovulation increases with each successive day that scheduled white tablets are missed.
In the nonlactating mother, LO/OVRAL-28 may be initiated postpartum, for contraception. When the tablets are administered in the postpartum period, the increased risk of thromboembolic disease associated with the postpartum

Continued on next page

Wyeth-Ayerst Laboratories—Cont.

period must be considered (see "Contraindications", "Warnings", and "Precautions" concerning thromboembolic disease). It is to be noted that early resumption of ovulation may occur if Parlodel® (bromocriptine mesylate) has been used for the prevention of lactation.

HOW SUPPLIED

LO/OVRAL®-28 Tablets (0.3 mg norgestrel and 0.03 mg ethinyl estradiol) are available in packages of 6 PILPAK® dispensers, each containing 28 tablets as follows:
21 active tablets, NDC 0008-0078, white, round tablet marked "WYETH" and "78".
7 inert tablets, NDC 0008-0486, pink, round tablet marked "WYETH" and "486".
ALSO AVAILABLE:
LO/OVRAL®-28 Tablets (0.3 mg norgestrel and 0.03 mg ethinyl estradiol) are available in packages of 12 PILPAK® dispensers for clinic use only, each containing 28 tablets as follows:
21 active tablets, NDC 0008-0078, white, round tablet marked "WYETH" and "78".
7 inert tablets, NDC 0008-0486, pink, round tablet marked "WYETH" and "486".

References available upon request.
Brief Summary Patient Package Insert: See LO/OVRAL.
DETAILED PATIENT LABELING: See LO/OVRAL.

HOW TO TAKE THE PILL

For Lo/Ovral-28 PILPAK® Dispenser, See LO/OVRAL.
For Lo/Ovral-28 Clinic Pilpak®, See below.
HOW TO TAKE THE PILL
This product (like all oral contraceptives) is intended to prevent pregnancy. It does not protect against transmission of HIV (AIDS) and other sexually transmitted diseases such as chlamydia, genital herpes, genital warts, gonorrhea, hepatitis B, and syphilis.

IMPORTANT POINTS TO REMEMBER

BEFORE YOU START TAKING YOUR PILLS:
1. BE SURE TO READ THESE DIRECTIONS:
Before you start taking your pills.
Anytime you are not sure what to do.
2. THE RIGHT WAY TO TAKE THE PILL IS TO TAKE ONE PILL EVERY DAY AT THE SAME TIME.
If you miss pills you could get pregnant. This includes starting the pack late. The more pills you miss, the more likely you are to get pregnant.
3. MANY WOMEN HAVE SPOTTING OR LIGHT BLEEDING, OR MAY FEEL SICK TO THEIR STOMACH DURING THE FIRST 1–3 PACKS OF PILLS.
If you feel sick to your stomach, do not stop taking the pill. The problem will usually go away. If it doesn't go away, check with your doctor or clinic.
4. MISSING PILLS CAN ALSO CAUSE SPOTTING OR LIGHT BLEEDING, even when you make up these missed pills.
On the days you take 2 pills to make up for missed pills, you could also feel a little sick to your stomach.
5. IF YOU HAVE VOMITING OR DIARRHEA, for any reason, or IF YOU TAKE SOME MEDICINES, including some antibiotics, your pills may not work as well. Use a back-up method (such as condoms, foam, or sponge) until you check with your doctor or clinic.
6. IF YOU HAVE TROUBLE REMEMBERING TO TAKE THE PILL, talk to your doctor or clinic about how to make pill-taking easier or about using another method of birth control.
7. IF YOU HAVE ANY QUESTIONS OR ARE UNSURE ABOUT THE INFORMATION IN THIS LEAFLET, call your doctor or clinic.

NORDETTE®-21, OVRAL®, LO/OVRAL®, NORDETTE®-28, OVRAL®-28, AND LO/OVRAL®-28

BEFORE YOU START TAKING YOUR PILLS

1. DECIDE WHAT TIME OF DAY YOU WANT TO TAKE YOUR PILL.
It is important to take it at about the same time every day.
2. LOOK AT YOUR PILL PACK TO SEE IF IT HAS 21 OR 28 PILLS:
The *21-pill pack* has 21 "active" white or light-orange pills (with hormones) to take for 3 weeks, followed by 1 week without pills.
The *28-pill pack* has 21 "active" white or light-orange pills (with hormones) to take for 3 weeks, followed by 1 week of reminder pink pills (without hormones).

3. ALSO FIND:
1) where on the pack to start taking pills,
2) in what order to take the pills (follow the arrows), and
3) the week numbers as shown in the picture below.

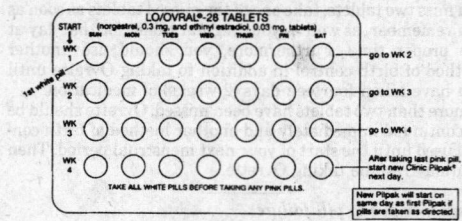

4. BE SURE YOU HAVE READY AT ALL TIMES:
ANOTHER KIND OF BIRTH CONTROL (such as condoms, foam or sponge) to use as a back-up in case you miss pills.
AN EXTRA, FULL PILL PACK.

WHEN TO START THE *FIRST* PACK OF PILLS:

For the 21-day pill pack you have two choices of which day to start taking your first pack of pills. (See **DAY 1 START** or **SUNDAY START** directions below.) Decide with your doctor or clinic which is the best day for you. The 28-day pill pack accommodates a **SUNDAY START** only. For either pill pack pick a time of day which will be easy to remember.
DAY 1 START:
These instructions are for the 21-day pill pack only. The 28-day pill pack does not accommodate a **DAY 1 START** dosage regimen.
1. Take the first "active" white or light-orange pill of the first pack during the *first 24 hours of your period*.
2. You will not need to use a back-up method of birth control, since you are starting the pill at the beginning of your period.
SUNDAY START:
These instructions are for either the 21-day or the 28-day pill pack.
1. Take the first "active" white or light-orange pill of the first pack on the *Sunday after your period starts*, even if you are still bleeding. If your period begins on Sunday, start the pack that same day.
2. *Use another method of birth control* as a back-up method if you have sex anytime from the Sunday you start your first pack until the next Sunday (7 days). Condoms, foam, or the sponge are good back-up methods of birth control.

WHAT TO DO DURING THE MONTH:

1. TAKE ONE PILL AT THE SAME TIME EVERY DAY UNTIL THE PACK IS EMPTY.
Do not skip pills even if you are spotting or bleeding between monthly periods or feel sick to your stomach (nausea).
Do not skip pills even if you do not have sex very often.
2. WHEN YOU FINISH A PACK OR SWITCH YOUR BRAND OF PILLS:
21 pills: Wait 7 days to start the next pack. You will probably have your period during that week. Be sure that no more than 7 days pass between 21-day packs.
28 pills: Start the next pack on the day after your last "reminder" pill. Do not wait any days between packs.

WHAT TO DO IF YOU MISS PILLS

If yoy **MISS 1** white or light-orange "active" pill:
1. Take it as soon as you remember. Take the next pill at your regular time. This means you take 2 pills in 1 day.
2. You do not need to use a back-up birth control method if you have sex.
If you **MISS 2** white or light-orange "active" pills in a row in **WEEK 1 OR WEEK 2** of your pack:
1. Take 2 pills on the day you remember and 2 pills the next day.
2. Then take 1 pill a day until you finish the pack.
3. You MAY BECOME PREGNANT if you have sex in the 7 *days* after you miss pills. You MUST use another birth control method (such as condoms, foam, or sponge) as a back-up for those 7 days.
If you **MISS 2** white or light-orange "active" pills in a row in **THE 3rd WEEK:**
The **Day 1 Starter** instructions are for the 21-day pill pack only. The 28-day pill pack does not accommodate a **DAY 1 START** dosage regimen. The **Sunday Starter** instructions are for either the 21-day or 28-day pill pack.
1. *If you are a Day 1 Starter:*
THROW OUT the rest of the pill pack and start a new pack that same day.
If you are a Sunday Starter:
Keep taking 1 pill every day until Sunday.
On Sunday, THROW OUT the rest of the pack and start a new pack of pills that same day.

2. You may not have your period this month but this is expected.
However, if you miss your period 2 months in a row, call your doctor or clinic because you might be pregnant.
3. You MAY BECOME PREGNANT if you have sex in the 7 *days* after you miss pills. You MUST use another birth control method (such as condoms, foam, or sponge) as a back-up for those 7 days.
If you **MISS 3 OR MORE** white or light-orange "active" pills in a row (during the first 3 weeks):
The **Day 1 Starter** instructions are for the 21-day pill pack only. The 28-day pill pack does not accommodate a **DAY 1 START** dosage regimen. The **Sunday Starter** instructions are for either the 21-day or 28-day pill pack.
1. **If you are a Day 1 Starter:**
THROW OUT the rest of the pill pack and start a new pack that same day.
If you are a Sunday Starter:
Keep taking 1 pill every day until Sunday.
On Sunday, THROW OUT the rest of the pack and start a new pack of pills that same day.
2. You may not have your period this month but this is expected.
However, if you miss your period 2 months in a row, call your doctor or clinic because you might be pregnant.
3. You MAY BECOME PREGNANT if you have sex in the 7 *days* after you miss pills. You MUST use another birth control method (such as condoms, foam, or sponge) as a back-up for those 7 days.

A REMINDER FOR THOSE ON 28-DAY PACKS:

If your forget any of the 7 pink "reminder" pills in Week 4:
THROW AWAY the pills you missed.
Keep taking 1 pill each day until the pack is empty.
You do not need a back-up method if you start your next pack on time.

FINALLY, IF YOU ARE STILL NOT SURE WHAT TO DO ABOUT THE PILLS YOU HAVE MISSED:

Use a BACK-UP METHOD anytime you have sex.
KEEP TAKING ONE PILL EACH DAY until you can reach your doctor or clinic.
OVRETTE®
Ovrette is administered on a continuous daily dosage schedule, one tablet each day, every day of the year. Take the first tablet on the first day of your menstrual period. Tablets should be taken at the same time every day without interruption, whether bleeding occurs or not. If bleeding is prolonged (more than 8 days) or unusually heavy, you should contact your doctor.
Forgotten pills
The risk of pregnancy increases with each tablet missed. Therefore, it is very important that you take one tablet daily as directed. If you miss one tablet, take it as soon as you remember and also take your next tablet at the regular time. If you miss two tablets, take one of the missed tablets as soon as you remember, as well as your regular tablet for that day at the proper time. Furthermore, you should use another method of birth control in addition to taking Ovrette until you have taken fourteen days (2 weeks) of medication.
If more than two tablets have been missed, Ovrette should be discontinued immediately and another method of birth control used until the start of your next menstrual period. Then you may resume taking Ovrette.

Pregnancy due to pill failure
The incidence of pill failure resulting in pregnancy is approximately less than 1.0% if taken every day as directed, but more typical failure rates are less than 3.0%. If failure does occur, the risk to the fetus is minimal.
RISKS TO THE FETUS
If you do become pregnant while using oral contraceptives, the risk to the fetus is small, on the order of no more than one per thousand. You should, however, discuss the risks to the developing child with your doctor.
Pregnancy after stopping the pill
There may be some delay in becoming pregnant after you stop using oral contraceptives, especially if you had irregular menstrual cycles before you used oral contraceptives. It may be advisable to postpone conception until you begin menstruating regularly once you have stopped taking the pill and desire pregnancy.
There does not appear to be any increase in birth defects in newborn babies when pregnancy occurs soon after stopping the pill.
Overdosage
Serious ill effects have not been reported following ingestion of large doses of oral contraceptives by young children. Overdosage may cause nausea and withdrawal bleeding in females. In case of overdosage, contact your health-care provider or pharmacist.
Other information
Your health-care provider will take a medical and family history before prescribing oral contraceptives and will examine you. The physical examination may be delayed to another time if you request it and the health-care provider be-

lieves that it is appropriate to postpone it. You should be reexamined at least once a year. Be sure to inform your health-care provider if there is a family history of any of the conditions listed previously in this leaflet. Be sure to keep all appointments with your health-care provider, because this is a time to determine if there are early signs of side effects of oral-contraceptive use.

Do not use the drug for any condition other than the one for which it was prescribed. This drug has been prescribed specifically for you; do not give it to others who may want birth-control pills.

HEALTH BENEFITS FROM ORAL CONTRACEPTIVES: See Lo/OVRAL.

Shown in Product Identification Guide, page 340

MAZANOR® Ⓒ℞
[maz 'a-nor]
(mazindol)

DESCRIPTION

Mazanor (mazindol) is an imidazoisoindole anorectic agent. It is chemically designated as 5-p-chloro-phenyl-5-hydroxy-2,3-dihydro-5H-imidazo (2,1-a) isoindole, a tautomeric form of 2-[2'-(p-chlorobenzoyl) phenyl]-2-imidazoline. Mazanor tablets contain 1 mg mazindol. The inactive ingredients present are calcium sulfate, cellulose, lactose, magnesium stearate, povidone, and talc.

HOW SUPPLIED

Mazanor® (mazindol) Tablets are available in the following dosage strength in bottles of 30 tablets:

1 mg, NDC 0008-0071-03, white, round, scored tablet marked "WYETH" and "71".

Keep tightly closed.
Store below 25° C (77° F).
Dispense in tight container.

For prescribing information, write to Professional Service, Wyeth-Ayerst Laboratories, P.O. Box 8299, Philadelphia, PA 19101, or contact your local Wyeth-Ayerst representative.

MEPERGAN® Ⓒ℞
[mep 'er-gan]
(meperidine HCl and promethazine HCl) Injection

DESCRIPTION

This product is available in concentration providing 25 mg each of meperidine hydrochloride and promethazine hydrochloride per mL with 0.1 mg edetate disodium, 0.04 mg calcium chloride, and not more than 0.75 mg sodium formaldehyde sulfoxylate, 0.25 mg sodium metabisulfite, and 5 mg phenol with sodium acetate buffer.

ACTIONS

Meperidine hydrochloride is a narcotic analgesic with multiple actions qualitatively similar to those of morphine. Phenergan®, promethazine HCl, is a phenothiazine derivative that has several different pharmacologic properties including antihistaminic, sedative, and antiemetic actions.

INDICATIONS

As a preanesthetic medication when analgesia and sedation are indicated. As an adjunct to local and general anesthesia.

CONTRAINDICATIONS

Hypersensitivity to meperidine or promethazine.

Under no circumstances should Mepergan be given by intra-arterial injection, due to the likelihood of severe arteriospasm and the possibility of resultant gangrene (see "Warnings").

Mepergan should not be given by the subcutaneous route; evidence of chemical irritation has been noted, and necrotic lesions have resulted on rare occasions following subcutaneous injection. The preferred parenteral route of administration is by deep intramuscular injection.

Meperidine is contraindicated in patients who are receiving monoamine oxidase inhibitors (MAOI) or those who have received such agents within 14 days. Therapeutic doses of meperidine have inconsistently precipitated unpredictable, severe, and occasionally fatal reactions in patients who have received such agents within 14 days. The mechanism of these reactions is unclear. Some have been characterized by coma, severe respiratory depression, cyanosis, and hypotension and have resembled the syndrome of acute narcotic overdose. In other reactions the predominant manifestations have been hyperexcitability, convulsions, tachycardia, hyperpyrexia, and hypertension. Although it is not known that other narcotics are free of the risk of such reactions, virtually all of the reported reactions have occurred with meperidine. If a narcotic is needed in such patients, a sensitivity test should be performed in which repeated, small, incremental doses of morphine are administered over the course of several hours while the patient's condition and vital signs are under careful observation.

(Intravenous hydrocortisone or prednisolone have been used to treat severe reactions, with the addition of intravenous chlorpromazine in those cases exhibiting hypertension and hyperpyrexia. The usefulness and safety of narcotic antagonists in the treatment of these reactions is unknown.)

WARNINGS

Mepergan Injection contains sodium metabisulfite, a sulfite that may cause allergic-type reactions, including anaphylactic symptoms and life-threatening or less severe asthmatic episodes, in certain susceptible people. The overall prevalence of sulfite sensitivity in the general population is unknown and probably low. Sulfite sensitivity is seen more frequently in asthmatic than in nonasthmatic people.

Tolerance and Addiction Liability

Warning—may be habit-forming

DRUG DEPENDENCE

Meperidine can produce drug dependence of the morphine type and therefore has the potential for being abused. Psychic dependence, physical dependence, and tolerance may develop upon repeated administration of meperidine, and it should be prescribed and administered with the same degree of caution appropriate to the use of morphine. Like other narcotics, meperidine is subject to the provisions of the Federal narcotic laws.

INTERACTION WITH OTHER CENTRAL NERVOUS SYSTEM DEPRESSANTS

Meperidine should be used with great caution and in reduced dosage in patients who are concurrently receiving other narcotic analgesics, general anesthetics, phenothiazines, other tranquilizers, sedative-hypnotics, tricyclic antidepressants, and other CNS depressants (including alcohol). Respiratory depression, hypotension, and profound sedation or coma may result.

The sedative action of promethazine hydrochloride is additive to the sedative effects of central nervous system depressants; therefore, agents such as alcohol, barbiturates, and narcotic analgesics should either be eliminated or given in reduced dosage in the presence of promethazine hydrochloride. When given concomitantly with promethazine hydrochloride, the dose of barbiturates should be reduced by at least one-half and the dose of analgesic depressants, such as morphine or meperidine, should be reduced by one-quarter to one-half.

HEAD INJURY AND INCREASED INTRACRANIAL PRESSURE

The respiratory-depressant effects of meperidine and its capacity to elevate cerebrospinal-fluid pressure may be markedly exaggerated in the presence of head injury, other intracranial lesions, or a preexisting increase in intracranial pressure. Furthermore, narcotics produce adverse reactions which may obscure the clinical course of patients with head injuries. In such patients, meperidine must be used with extreme caution and only if its use is deemed essential.

INADVERTENT INTRA-ARTERIAL INJECTION

Due to the close proximity of arteries and veins in the areas most commonly used for intravenous injection, extreme care should be exercised to avoid perivascular extravasation or inadvertent intra-arterial injection of Mepergan. Reports compatible with inadvertent intra-arterial injection suggest that pain, severe chemical irritation, severe spasm of distal vessels, and resultant gangrene requiring amputation is likely under such circumstances. Intravenous injection was intended in all the cases reported, but perivascular extravasation or arterial placement of the needle is now suspect. There is no proven successful management of this condition after it occurs, although sympathetic block and heparinization are commonly employed during the acute management because of the results of animal experiments with other known arteriolar irritants. Aspiration of dark blood does not preclude intra-arterial needle placement, because blood is discolored upon contact with promethazine. Use of syringes with rigid plungers or of small bore needles might obscure typical arterial backflow if this is relied upon alone.

INTRAVENOUS USE

If necessary, meperidine may be given intravenously, but the injection should be given very slowly, preferably in the form of a diluted solution. Rapid intravenous injection of narcotic analgesics, including meperidine, increases the incidence of adverse reactions; severe respiratory depression, apnea, hypotension, peripheral circulatory collapse, and cardiac arrest have occurred. Meperidine should not be administered intravenously unless a narcotic antagonist and the facilities for assisted or controlled respiration are immediately available. When meperidine is given parenterally, especially intravenously, the patient should be lying down.

When used intravenously, Mepergan should be given at a rate not to exceed 1 mL (25 mg of each component) per minute. When administering any irritant drug intravenously, it is usually preferable to inject it through the tubing of an intravenous infusion set that is known to be functioning satisfactorily. In the event that a patient complains of pain during intended intravenous injection of Mepergan, the injection should immediately be stopped to provide for evaluation of possible arterial placement or perivascular extravasation.

ASTHMA AND OTHER RESPIRATORY CONDITIONS

Meperidine should be used with extreme caution in patients having an acute asthmatic attack, patients with chronic obstructive pulmonary disease or cor pulmonale, patients having a substantially decreased respiratory reserve, and patients with preexisting respiratory depression, hypoxia, or hypercapnia. In such patients, even usual therapeutic doses of narcotics may decrease respiratory drive while simultaneously increasing airway resistance to the point of apnea.

HYPOTENSIVE EFFECT

The administration of meperidine may result in severe hypotension in an individual whose ability to maintain his blood pressure has already been compromised by a depleted blood volume or concurrent administration of drugs such as the phenothiazines or certain anesthetics.

USAGE IN AMBULATORY PATIENTS

Meperidine may impair the mental and/or physical abilities required for the performance of potentially hazardous tasks, such as driving a car or operating machinery. The patient should be cautioned accordingly.

Meperidine, like other narcotics, may produce orthostatic hypotension in ambulatory patients.

USAGE IN PREGNANCY AND LACTATION

Meperidine should not be used in pregnant women prior to the labor period, unless in the judgment of the physician the potential benefits outweigh the possible hazards, because safe use in pregnancy prior to labor has not been established relative to possible adverse effects on fetal development.

When used as an obstetrical analgesic, meperidine crosses the placental barrier and can produce respiratory depression in the newborn; resuscitation may be required (see "Overdosage").

Meperidine appears in the milk of nursing mothers receiving the drug.

PRECAUTIONS

SUPRAVENTRICULAR TACHYCARDIAS

Meperidine should be used with caution in patients with atrial flutter and other supraventricular tachycardias because of a possible vagolytic action which may produce a significant increase in the ventricular response rate.

CONVULSIONS

Meperidine may aggravate preexisting convulsions in patients with convulsive disorders. If dosage is escalated substantially above recommended levels because of tolerance development, convulsions may occur in individuals without a history of convulsive disorders.

ACUTE ABDOMINAL CONDITIONS

The administration of meperidine or other narcotics may obscure the diagnosis or clinical course in patients with acute abdominal conditions.

SPECIAL-RISK PATIENTS

Meperidine should be given with caution, and the initial dose should be reduced in certain patients, such as the elderly or debilitated, and those with severe impairment of hepatic or renal function, hypothyroidism, Addison's disease, and prostatic hypertrophy or urethral stricture.

Antiemetics may mask the symptoms of an unrecognized disease and thereby interfere with diagnosis.

Patients in pain who have received inadequate or no analgesia have been noted to develop "athetoid-like" movements of the upper extremities following the parenteral administration of promethazine. These symptoms usually disappear upon adequate control of the pain.

Ambulatory patients should be cautioned against driving automobiles or operating dangerous machinery until it is known that they do not become drowsy or dizzy from promethazine hydrochloride therapy.

ADVERSE REACTIONS

The major hazards of meperidine, as with other narcotic analgesics, are respiratory depression and, to a lesser degree, circulatory depression; respiratory arrest, shock, and cardiac arrest have occurred.

The most frequently observed adverse reactions include light-headedness, dizziness, sedation, nausea, vomiting, and sweating. These effects seem to be more prominent in ambulatory patients and in those who are not experiencing severe pain. In such individuals, lower doses are advisable. Some adverse reactions in ambulatory patients may be alleviated if the patient lies down.

Other adverse reactions include:

CENTRAL NERVOUS SYSTEM

Euphoria, dysphoria, weakness, headache, agitation, tremor, uncoordinated muscle movements, transient hallucinations and disorientation, visual disturbances and, rarely, extrapyramidal reactions.

GASTROINTESTINAL

Dry mouth, constipation, biliary-tract spasm.

CARDIOVASCULAR

Flushing of the face, tachycardia, bradycardia, palpitation, faintness, syncope.

Continued on next page

Wyeth-Ayerst Laboratories—Cont.

Cardiovascular effects from promethazine have been rare. Minor increases in blood pressure and occasional mild hypotension have been reported. Venous thrombosis at the injection site has been reported. Intra-arterial injection of Mepergan may result in gangrene of the affected extremity (see "Warnings").

GENITOURINARY

Urinary retention.

ALLERGIC

Pruritus, urticaria, other skin rashes, wheal and flare over the vein with IV injection.

Photosensitivity, although extremely rare, has been reported. Occurrence of photosensitivity may be a contraindication to further treatment with promethazine or related drugs.

OTHER

Pain at injection site; local tissue irritation, induration, and possible tissue necrosis, particularly when injection is repeated at same site; antidiuretic effect.

Patients may occasionally complain of autonomic reactions, such as dryness of the mouth, blurring of vision and, rarely, dizziness following the use of promethazine.

Very rare cases have been reported where patients receiving promethazine have developed leukopenia. In one instance agranulocytosis has been reported. In nearly every instance reported, other toxic agents known to have caused these conditions have been associated with the administration of promethazine.

DOSAGE AND ADMINISTRATION

Parenteral drug products should be inspected visually for particulate matter and discoloration prior to administration, whenever solution and container permit.

WARNING—BARBITURATES ARE NOT CHEMICALLY COMPATIBLE IN SOLUTION WITH MEPERGAN (MEPERIDINE HYDROCHLORIDE AND PROMETHAZINE HYDROCHLORIDE) AND SHOULD NOT BE MIXED IN THE SAME SYRINGE.

Mepergan is usually administered intramuscularly. However, in certain specific situations, the intravenous route may be employed. INADVERTENT INTRA-ARTERIAL INJECTION CAN RESULT IN GANGRENE OF THE AFFECTED EXTREMITY (see "Warnings"). SUBCUTANEOUS ADMINISTRATION IS CONTRAINDICATED, AS IT MAY RESULT IN TISSUE NECROSIS (see "Contraindications"). INJECTION INTO OR NEAR PERIPHERAL NERVES MAY RESULT IN PERMANENT NEUROLOGICAL DEFICIT.

When used intravenously, the rate should not be greater than 1 mL of Mepergan (25 mg of each component) per minute; it is preferable to inject through the tubing of an intravenous infusion set that is known to be functioning satisfactorily.

The TUBEX® BLUNT POINTE™ Sterile Cartridge Unit is suitable for substances to be administered intravenously only. It is intended for use with injection sets specifically manufactured as "needle-less" injection systems. TUBEX® BLUNT POINTE™ is compatible with Abbott's LifeShield® prepierced reseal injection site, Baxter's InterLink® Injection Site, and B. Braun Medical's SafSite® Reflux Valve, Consult manufacturer's recommendations regarding "Directions for Use" of the "needle-less" system. It is also intended for admixture with, and convenient administration of various medicaments when using Drug Vial Adapters for "needle-less" injection systems.

The TUBEX® Sterile Cartridge-Needle Unit is suitable for substances to be administered intravenously or intramuscularly.

The TUBEX® Sterile Cartridge-Needle Unit is designed for single-dose use. VIALS should be used when required doses are fractions of a milliliter, as indicated below.

ADULT DOSE: 1 to 2 mL (25 to 50 mg of each component) per single injection, which can be repeated every 3 to 4 hours.

CHILDREN 12 YEARS OF AGE AND UNDER: 0.5 mg of each component per pound of body weight. The dosage may be repeated every 3 to 4 hours as necessary.

For preanesthetic medication the usual adult dose is 2 mL (50 mg of each component) intramuscularly with or without appropriate atropine-like drug. Atropine sulfate, 0.3 to 0.4 mg, or scopolamine hydrobromide, 0.25 to 0.4 mg, in sterile solution may be mixed in the same syringe with Mepergan. Repeat doses of 50 mg or less of both promethazine and meperidine may be administered by either route at 3- to 4-hour intervals, as necessary. As an adjunct to local or general anesthesia, the usual dose is 2 mL (50 mg each of meperidine and promethazine).

OVERDOSAGE

SYMPTOMS

Serious overdose with meperidine is characterized by respiratory depression (a decrease in respiratory rate and/or tidal volume, Cheyne-Stokes respiration, cyanosis), extreme somnolence progressing to stupor or coma, skeletal muscle flaccidity, cold and clammy skin, and sometimes bradycardia and hypotension. In severe overdosage, particularly by the intravenous route, apnea, circulatory collapse, cardiac arrest, and death may occur.

TREATMENT

Primary attention should be given to the reestablishment of adequate respiratory exchange through provision of a patent airway and institution of assisted or controlled ventilation. The narcotic antagonist, naloxone hydrochloride, is a specific antidote against respiratory depression which may result from overdosage or unusual sensitivity to narcotics, including meperidine. The usual initial adult dose of naloxone is 0.4 to 2.0 mg, administered intravenously. If the desired degree of counteraction and improvement in respiratory functions is not obtained, this dosage can be repeated at two- to three-minute intervals while resuscitation efforts continue. If 10 mg of naloxone have been administered without an improvement in the clinical situation, the diagnosis of Mepergan overdose should be questioned.

An antagonist should not be administered in absence of clinically significant respiratory or cardiovascular depression. Oxygen, intravenous fluids, vasopressors, and other supportive measures should be employed as indicated.

NOTE: In an individual physically dependent on narcotics, the administration of the usual dose of a narcotic antagonist will precipitate an acute withdrawal syndrome. The severity of this syndrome will depend on the degree of physical dependence and the dose of antagonist administered. The use of narcotic antagonists in such individuals should be avoided if possible. If a narcotic antagonist must be used to treat serious respiratory depression in the physically dependent patient, the antagonist should be administered with extreme care and only one-tenth to one-fifth the usual initial dose administered.

Attempted suicides with promethazine have resulted in deep sedation, coma, rarely convulsions and cardiorespiratory symptoms compatible with the depth of sedation present. Extrapyramidal reactions may be treated with anticholinergic antiparkinson agents, diphenhydramine, or barbiturates.

If severe hypotension occurs, levarterenol or phenylephrine may be indicated. Epinephrine is probably best avoided, since it has been suggested that promethazine overdosage could produce a partial alpha-adrenergic blockade.

A paradoxical reaction, characterized by hyperexcitability and nightmares, has been reported in children receiving large single doses of promethazine.

HOW SUPPLIED

Mepergan® (meperidine HCl and promethazine HCl) Injection is available in TUBEX® BLUNT POINTE™ Sterile Cartridge Units and Sterile Cartridge-Needle Units, in boxes of 10 TUBEX in TAMP-R-TEL® tamper-resistant packages as follows:

NDC 0008-0235-50, 2 mL size Blunt Pointe™

NDC 0008-0235-01, 2 mL size (22 gauge x 1-¼inch needle).

Mepergan (meperidine HCl and promethazine HCl) Injection is also available in vials as follows:

NDC 0008-0234, 10 mL vial.

Do not use if solution is discolored or contains a precipitate.
Protect from light
Use carton to protect contents from light
Store at room temperature, approximately 25° C (77° F)

MYSOLINE® ℞

[mī'sō-lēn]
(primidone)
Anticonvulsant

CAUTION: Federal law prohibits dispensing without prescription.

DESCRIPTION

Chemical name: 5-ethyldihydro-5-phenyl-4,6 (1H, 5H) pyrimidinedione.

Structural formula:

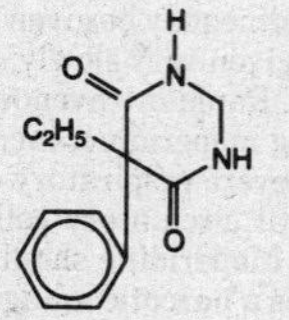

Mysoline is a white, crystalline, highly stable substance, M.P. 279–284°C. It is poorly soluble in water (60 mg per 100 mL at 37°C) and in most organic solvents. It possesses no acidic properties, in contrast to its barbiturate analog.

Mysoline 50 mg and 250 mg tablets contain the following inactive ingredients: Microcrystalline Cellulose, NF; Lactose, USP; Methylcellulose, USP; Sodium Starch Glycolate, NF; Talc, USP; Sodium Lauryl Sulfate, NF; Magnesium Stearate, NF; Water, USP, Purified.

Mysoline 250 mg tablets also contain Yellow Iron Oxide, NF.

Mysoline suspension contains these inactive ingredients: Ammonia Solution, Diluted; Citric Acid, USP; D&C Yellow No. 10; FD&C Yellow No. 6; Magnesium Aluminum Silicate; Methylparaben, NF; Propylparaben, NF; Saccharin Sodium, NF; Sodium Alginate; Sodium Citrate; Sodium Hypochlorite Solution, USP; Sorbic Acid, NF; Sorbitan Monolaurate; Water, USP, Purified; Flavors.

ACTIONS

Mysoline raises electro- or chemoshock seizure thresholds or alters seizure patterns in experimental animals. The mechanism(s) of primidone's antiepileptic action is not known.

Primidone *per se* has anticonvulsant activity as do its two metabolites, phenobarbital and phenylethylmalonamide (PEMA). In addition to its anticonvulsant activity, PEMA potentiates the anticonvulsant activity of phenobarbital in experimental animals.

INDICATIONS

Mysoline, used alone or concomitantly with other anticonvulsants, is indicated in the control of grand mal, psychomotor, and focal epileptic seizures. It may control grand mal seizures refractory to other anticonvulsant therapy.

CONTRAINDICATIONS

Primidone is contraindicated in: 1) patients with porphyria and 2) patients who are hypersensitive to phenobarbital (see ACTIONS).

WARNINGS

The abrupt withdrawal of antiepileptic medication may precipitate status epilepticus.

The therapeutic efficacy of a dosage regimen takes several weeks before it can be assessed.

USAGE IN PREGNANCY

The effects of Mysoline in human pregnancy and nursing infants are unknown.

Recent reports suggest an association between the use of anticonvulsant drugs by women with epilepsy and an elevated incidence of birth defects in children born to these women. Data are more extensive with respect to diphenylhydantoin and phenobarbital, but these are also the most commonly prescribed anticonvulsants; less systematic or anecdotal reports suggest a possible similar association with the use of all known anticonvulsant drugs.

The reports suggesting an elevated incidence of birth defects in children of drug-treated epileptic women cannot be regarded as adequate to prove a definite cause-and-effect relationship. There are intrinsic methodologic problems in obtaining adequate data on drug teratogenicity in humans; the possibility also exists that other factors leading to birth defects, e.g., genetic factors or the epileptic condition itself, may be more important than drug therapy. The majority of mothers on anticonvulsant medication deliver normal infants. It is important to note that anticonvulsant drugs should not be discontinued in patients in whom the drug is administered to prevent major seizures because of the strong possibility of precipitating status epilepticus with attendant hypoxia and threat to life. In individual cases where the severity and frequency of the seizure disorders are such that the removal of medication does not pose a serious threat to the patient, discontinuation of the drug may be considered prior to and during pregnancy, although it cannot be said with any confidence that even minor seizures do not pose some hazard to the developing embryo or fetus.

The prescribing physician will wish to weigh these considerations in treating or counseling epileptic women of childbearing potential.

Neonatal hemorrhage, with a coagulation defect resembling vitamin K deficiency, has been described in newborns whose mothers were taking primidone and other anticonvulsants. Pregnant women under anticonvulsant therapy should receive prophylactic vitamin K_1 therapy for one month prior to, and during, delivery.

PRECAUTIONS

The total daily dosage should not exceed 2 g. Since Mysoline therapy generally extends over prolonged periods, a complete blood count and a sequential multiple analysis-12 (SMA-12) test should be made every six months.

IN NURSING MOTHERS

There is evidence that in mothers treated with primidone, the drug appears in the milk in substantial quantities. Since tests for the presence of primidone in biological fluids are too complex to be carried out in the average clinical laboratory, it is suggested that the presence of undue somnolence and drowsiness in nursing newborns of Mysoline-treated mothers be taken as an indication that nursing should be discontinued.

ADVERSE REACTIONS

The most frequently occurring early side effects are ataxia and vertigo. These tend to disappear with continued therapy, or with reduction of initial dosage. Occasionally, the following have been reported: nausea, anorexia, vomiting, fatigue, hyperirritability, emotional disturbances, sexual impotency,

diplopia, nystagmus, drowsiness, and morbilliform skin eruptions. Granulocytopenia, agranulocytosis, and red-cell hypoplasia and aplasia, have been reported rarely. These and, occasionally, other persistent or severe side effects may necessitate withdrawal of the drug. Megaloblastic anemia may occur as a rare idiosyncrasy to Mysoline and to other anticonvulsants. The anemia responds to folic acid without necessity of discontinuing medication.

DOSAGE AND ADMINISTRATION
ADULT DOSAGE
Patients 8 years of age and older who have received no previous treatment may be started on Mysoline according to the following regimen using either 50 mg or scored 250 mg Mysoline tablets.

Days 1 to 3: 100 to 125 mg at bedtime
Days 4 to 6: 100 to 125 mg b.i.d.
Days 7 to 9: 100 to 125 mg t.i.d.
Day 10 to maintenance: 250 mg t.i.d.

For most adults and children 8 years of age and over, the usual maintenance dosage is three to four 250 mg Mysoline tablets daily in divided doses (250 mg t.i.d. or q.i.d.). If required, an increase to five or six 250 mg tablets daily may be made but daily doses should not exceed 500 mg q.i.d.

INITIAL: ADULTS AND CHILDREN OVER 8

KEY: · = 50 mg tablet   ● = 250 mg tablet

DAY	1	2	3	4	5	6
AM				··	··	
NOON						
PM	··	··	··	··	··	··

DAY	7	8	9	10	11	12
AM	··	··	··	●		
NOON	··	··	··	●	Adjust to	
PM	··	··	··	●	Maintenance	

Dosage should be individualized to provide maximum benefit. In some cases, serum blood level determinations of primidone may be necessary for optimal dosage adjustment. The clinically effective serum level for primidone is between 5 to 12 μg/mL.

IN PATIENTS ALREADY RECEIVING OTHER ANTICONVULSANTS
Mysoline should be started at 100 to 125 mg at bedtime and gradually increased to maintenance level as the other drug is gradually decreased. This regimen should be continued until satisfactory dosage level is achieved for the combination, or the other medication is completely withdrawn. When therapy with Mysoline alone is the objective, the transition from concomitant therapy should not be completed in less than two weeks.

PEDIATRIC DOSAGE
For children under 8 years of age, the following regimen may be used:

Days 1 to 3: 50 mg at bedtime
Days 4 to 6: 50 mg b.i.d.
Days 7 to 9: 100 mg b.i.d.
Day 10 to maintenance: 125 mg t.i.d. to 250 mg t.i.d.

For children under 8 years of age, the usual maintenance dosage is 125 to 250 mg three times daily or, 10 to 25 mg/kg/day in divided doses.

HOW SUPPLIED
MYSOLINE TABLETS
Each square-shaped, scored, yellow tablet, identified by "MYSOLINE 250" and an embossed M, contains 250 mg of primidone, in bottles of 100 (NDC 0046-0430-81) and 1,000 (NDC 0046-0430-91).

Also available in a unit-dose package of 100 (NDC 0046-0430-99).

Each square-shaped, scored, white tablet, identified by "MYSOLINE 50 " and an embossed M, contains 50 mg of primidone, in bottles of 100 (NDC 0046-0431-81) and 500 (NDC 0046-0431-85).

The appearance of these tablets is a trademark of Wyeth-Ayerst Laboratories.

MYSOLINE SUSPENSION
Each 5 mL (teaspoonful) contains 250 mg of primidone, in bottles of 8 fluid ounces (NDC 0046-3850-08).

Store at room temperature, approximately 25° C (77° F).
Dispense in a tight, light-resistant container as defined in the U.S.P.

Shown in Product Identification Guide, page 340

NAPRELAN®   ℞
(naproxen sodium)
CONTROLLED RELEASE TABLETS
Equivalent to 375 mg and 500 mg naproxen

DESCRIPTION
Naprelan contains naproxen sodium, a member of the arylacetic acid group of nonsteroidal anti-inflammatory drugs (NSAIDs).

Naprelan uses the proprietary IPDAS™ (Intestinal Protective Drug Absorption System) technology. It is a rapidly disintegrating tablet system combining an immediate release component and a sustained release component of microparticles that are widely dispersed, allowing absorption of the active ingredient throughout the gastrointestinal (GI) tract, maintaining blood levels over 24 hours.

The chemical name for naproxen sodium is 2-naphthaleneacetic acid, 6-methoxy-α-methyl-sodium salt, (S)- with the following structural formula:

CH₃
CHCOONa

CH₃O
Naproxen sodium

Molecular Formula: Molecular Weight:
$C_{14}H_{13}NaO_3$ 252.24

Naproxen sodium is an odorless crystalline powder, white to creamy in color. It is soluble in methanol and water.

Naprelan contains 412.5 mg or 550 mg of naproxen sodium, equivalent to 375 mg and 500 mg of naproxen and 37.5 mg and 50 mg sodium respectively. Each Naprelan tablet also contains the following inactive ingredients: ammonio methacrylate copolymer Type A, ammonio methacrylate copolymer Type B, citric acid, crospovidone, magnesium stearate, methacrylic acid copolymer Type A, microcrystalline cellulose, povidone, and talc. The tablet coating contains hydroxypropyl methylcellulose, polyethylene glycol, and titanium dioxide.

CLINICAL PHARMACOLOGY
Naproxen is a nonsteroidal anti-inflammatory drug (NSAID), with analgesic and antipyretic properties. As with other NSAIDs, its mode of action is not fully understood; however, its ability to inhibit prostaglandin synthesis may be involved in the anti-inflammatory effect.

PHARMACOKINETICS
Although naproxen itself is well absorbed, the sodium salt form is more rapidly absorbed resulting in higher peak plasma levels for a given dose. Approximately 30% of the total naproxen sodium dose in Naprelan is present in the dosage form as an immediate release component. The remaining naproxen sodium is coated as microparticles to provide sustained release properties. After oral administration, plasma levels of naproxen are detected within 30 minutes of dosing, with peak plasma levels occurring approximately 5 hours after dosing. The observed terminal elimination half-life of naproxen from both immediate release naproxen sodium and Naprelan is approximately 15 hours. Steady state levels of naproxen are achieved in 3 days and the degree of naproxen accumulation in the blood is consistent with this.

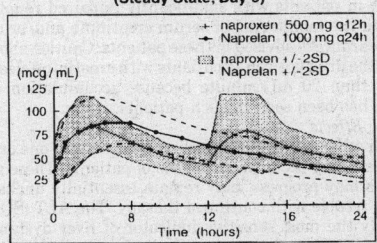

Plasma Naproxen Concentrations
Mean of 24 Subjects (+/-2SD)
(Steady State, Day 5)

Pharmacokinetic Parameters at Steady State Day 5 (Mean of 24 Subjects)

Parameter (units)	naproxen 500 mg Q12h/5 days (1000 mg)			Naprelan 2 x 500 mg tablets (1000 mg) Q24h/5 days		
	Mean	SD	Range	Mean	SD	Range
AUC 0-24 (mcgxh/mL)	1446	168	1167–1858	1448	145	1173–1774
C_{max} (mcg/mL)	95	13	71–117	94	13	74–127
C_{avg} (mcg/mL)	60	7	49–77	60	6	49–74
C_{min} (mcg/mL)	36	9	13–51	33	7	23–48
T_{max} (hrs)	3	1	1–4	5	2	2–10

Absorption
Naproxen itself is rapidly and completely absorbed from the GI tract with an *in vivo* bioavailability of 95%. Based on the pharmacokinetic profile, the absorption phase of Naprelan occurs in the first 4–6 hours after administration. This coincides with disintegration of the tablet in the stomach, the transit of the sustained release microparticles through the small intestine and into the proximal large intestine. An *in vivo* imaging study has been performed in healthy volunteers which confirms rapid disintegration of the tablet matrix and dispersion of the microparticles.

The absorption rate from the sustained release particulate component of Naprelan is slower than that for conventional naproxen sodium tablets. It is this prolongation of drug absorption processes which maintains plasma levels and allows for once daily dosing.

Food Effects
No significant food effects were observed when twenty-four subjects were given a single dose of Naprelan 500 mg either after an overnight fast or 30 minutes after a meal. In common with conventional naproxen and naproxen sodium formulations, food causes a slight decrease in the rate of naproxen absorption following Naprelan administration.

Distribution
Naproxen has a volume of distribution of 0.16 L/kg. At therapeutic levels naproxen is greater than 99% albumin-bound. At doses of naproxen greater than 500 mg/day there is a less than proportional increase in plasma levels due to an increase in clearance caused by saturation of plasma protein binding at higher doses. However the concentration of unbound naproxen continues to increase proportionally to dose. Naprelan exhibits similar dose proportional characteristics.

Metabolism
Naproxen is extensively metabolized to 6-0-desmethyl naproxen and both parent and metabolites do not induce metabolizing enzymes.

Elimination
The elimination half-life of Naprelan and conventional naproxen is approximately 15 hours. Steady state conditions are attained after 2–3 doses of Naprelan. Most of the drug is excreted in the urine, primarily as unchanged naproxen (less than 1%), 6-0-desmethyl naproxen (less than 1%) and their glucuronide or other conjugates (66–92%). A small amount (< 5%) of the drug is excreted in the feces. The rate of excretion has been found to coincide closely with the rate of clearance from the plasma. In patients with renal failure metabolites may accumulate.

Special Populations
Pediatric Use
No pediatric studies have been performed with Naprelan, thus safety of Naprelan in pediatric populations has not been established.

Renal Insufficiency
Naproxen pharmacokinetics have not been determined in subjects with renal insufficiency. Given that naproxen is metabolized and conjugates are primarily excreted by the kidneys, the potential exists for naproxen metabolites to accumulate in the presence of renal insufficiency.

CLINICAL STUDIES
RHEUMATOID ARTHRITIS
The use of Naprelan for the management of the signs and symptoms of rheumatoid arthritis was assessed in a 12 week double-blind, randomized, placebo and active-controlled study in 348 patients. Two Naprelan 500 mg tablets (1000 mg) once daily and naproxen 500 mg tablets twice daily (1000 mg) were more effective than placebo. Clinical effectiveness was demonstrated at one week and continued for the duration of the study.

OSTEOARTHRITIS
The use of Naprelan for the management of the signs and symptoms of osteoarthritis of the knee was assessed in a 12 week double-blind, placebo and active-controlled study in 347 patients. Two Naprelan 500 mg tablets (1000 mg) once daily and naproxen 500 mg tablets twice daily (1000 mg) were more effective than placebo. Clinical effectiveness was demonstrated at one week and continued for the duration of the study.

ANALGESIA
The onset of the analgesic effect of Naprelan was seen within 30 minutes in a pharmacokinetic/pharmacodynamic study of patients with pain following oral surgery. In controlled clinical trials, naproxen has been used in combination with gold, D-penicillamine, methotrexate and corticosteroids. Its use in combination with salicylate is not recommended because there is evidence that aspirin increases the rate of excretion of naproxen and data are inadequate to demonstrate that naproxen and aspirin produce greater improvement over that achieved with aspirin alone. In addition, as with other NSAIDs the combination may result in higher frequency of adverse events than demonstrated for either product alone.

Continued on next page

Wyeth-Ayerst Laboratories—Cont.

SPECIAL STUDIES

In a double-blind randomized, parallel group study, 19 subjects received either two Naprelan 500 mg tablets (1000 mg) once daily or naproxen 500 mg tablets (1000 mg) twice daily for 7 days. Mucosal biopsy scores and endoscope scores were lower in the subjects who received Naprelan. In another double-blind, randomized, crossover study, 23 subjects received two Naprelan 500 mg tablets (1000 mg) once daily, naproxen 500 mg tablets (1000 mg) twice daily and aspirin 650 mg four times daily (2600 mg) for 7 days each. There were significantly fewer duodenal erosions seen with Naprelan than with either naproxen or aspirin. There were significantly fewer gastric erosions with both Naprelan and naproxen than with aspirin.

The clinical significance of these findings is unknown.

INDIVIDUALIZATION OF DOSAGE

RHEUMATOID ARTHRITIS, OSTEOARTHRITIS, AND ANKYLOSING SPONDYLITIS

Naprelan like other NSAIDs shows considerable variation in response. The recommended starting dose of Naprelan in adults is two Naprelan 375 mg tablets (750 mg) once daily, or two Naprelan 500 mg tablets (1000 mg) once daily. Patients already taking naproxen 250 mg, 375 mg or 500 mg twice daily (morning and evening) may have their total daily dose replaced with Naprelan as a single daily dose.

During long-term administration, the dose of Naprelan may be adjusted up or down depending on the clinical response of the patient.

In patients who tolerate lower doses of Naprelan well, the dose may be increased to three Naprelan 500 mg tablets (1500 mg) once daily for limited periods when a higher level of anti-inflammatory/analgesic activity is required. When treating patients, especially at the higher dose levels, the physician should observe sufficient increased clinical benefit to offset the potential increased risk. (See CLINICAL PHARMACOLOGY). The lowest effective dose should be sought and used in every patient.

Symptomatic improvement in arthritis usually begins within one week; however, treatment for two weeks may be required to achieve a therapeutic benefit. A lower dose should be considered in patients with renal or hepatic impairment or in elderly patients (see PRECAUTIONS). Studies indicate that although total plasma concentration of naproxen is unchanged, the unbound plasma fraction of naproxen is increased in the elderly. Caution is advised when high doses are required and some adjustment of dosage may be required in elderly patients. As with other drugs used in the elderly it is prudent to use the lowest effective dose.

ANALGESIA, DYSMENORRHEA, BURSITIS, AND TENDINITIS

The recommended starting dose is two Naprelan 500 mg tablets (1000 mg) once daily. For patients requiring greater analgesic benefit, three Naprelan 500 mg tablets (1500 mg) may be used for a limited period. Thereafter, the total daily dose should not exceed two Naprelan 500 mg tablets (1000 mg).

ACUTE GOUT

The recommended dose on the first day is two or three Naprelan 500 mg tablets (1000–1500 mg) once daily, followed by two Naprelan 500 mg tablets (1000 mg) once daily, until the attack has subsided.

INDICATIONS AND USAGE

Naprelan is indicated for the treatment of rheumatoid arthritis, osteoarthritis, ankylosing spondylitis, tendinitis, bursitis, and acute gout. It is also indicated in the relief of mild to moderate pain and the treatment of primary dysmenorrhea.

CONTRAINDICATIONS

All naproxen products are contraindicated in patients who have had allergic reactions to prescription as well as to over-the-counter products containing naproxen. Anaphylactoid reactions may occur in patients without previous known exposure or hypersensitivity to aspirin, naproxen, or other NSAIDs, or in individuals with a history of angioedema, urticaria, bronchospastic reactivity (e.g., asthma), and nasal polyps. Anaphylactoid reactions, like anaphylaxis, may have a fatal outcome. Therefore, careful questioning of patients for such things as asthma, nasal polyps, urticaria, and hypotension associated with NSAIDs before starting therapy is important. In addition, if such symptoms occur during therapy, treatment with Naprelan should be discontinued.

WARNINGS

RISK OF GI ULCERATION, BLEEDING AND PERFORATION WITH NSAID THERAPY

Serious GI toxicity, such as bleeding, ulceration, and perforation, can occur at any time, with or without warning symptoms, in patients treated chronically with NSAID therapy. Although minor upper GI problems, such as dyspepsia, are common, usually developing early in therapy, physicians should remain alert for ulcerations and bleeding in patients treated chronically with NSAIDs even in the absence of previous GI tract symptoms. In patients observed in clinical trials with naproxen of several months to two years duration, symptomatic upper GI ulcers, gross bleeding or perforation appear to occur in approximately 1% of patients treated for 3–6 months, and in about 2–4% of patients treated for one year. Physicians should inform patients about the signs and/or symptoms of serious GI toxicity and what steps to take if they occur.

Studies to date with all naproxen products have not identified any subset of patients not at risk of developing peptic ulceration and bleeding or any differences between different naproxen products in their propensity to cause peptic ulceration and bleeding. Except for a prior history of serious GI events and other risk factors known to be associated with peptic ulcer disease, such as alcoholism, smoking etc., no risk factors (e.g., age, sex) have been associated with increased risk. Elderly or debilitated patients seem to tolerate ulceration or bleeding less well than other individuals and most spontaneous reports of fatal GI events are in this population. Studies to date are inconclusive concerning the relative risk of various NSAIDs in causing such reactions. High doses of any NSAID probably carry a greater risk of these reactions, although controlled clinical trials showing this do not exist in most cases. In considering the use of relatively large doses (within the recommended dosage range), sufficient benefit should be anticipated to offset the potential increased risk of GI toxicity.

PRECAUTIONS

GENERAL

NAPRELAN SHOULD NOT BE USED CONCOMITANTLY WITH OTHER NAPROXEN PRODUCTS SINCE THEY ALL CIRCULATE IN THE PLASMA AS THE NAPROXEN ANION. The antipyretic and anti-inflammatory activities of the drug may reduce fever and inflammation, thus diminishing their utility as diagnostic signs.

Because of adverse eye findings in animal studies with drugs of this class, it is recommended that ophthalmic studies be carried out if any change or disturbance in vision occurs.

Renal Effects

As with other NSAIDs, long term administration of naproxen to animals has resulted in renal papillary necrosis and other abnormal renal pathology. In humans, there have been reports of acute interstitial nephritis, hematuria, proteinuria, and occasionally nephrotic syndrome associated with naproxen-containing products and other NSAIDs since they have been marketed.

A second form of renal toxicity has been seen in patients taking naproxen as well as other NSAIDs. In patients with prerenal conditions with reduction in renal blood flow or blood volume, renal prostaglandins have a supportive role in the maintenance of renal perfusion. Administration of a NSAID may cause a dose-dependent reduction in prostaglandin formation and may precipitate overt renal decompensation. Patients at greatest risk of this reaction are those with impaired renal function, heart failure, liver dysfunction, diuretic use, and the elderly. Discontinuation of NSAID therapy is typically followed by recovery to the pretreatment state.

Naproxen and its metabolites are eliminated primarily by the kidneys, therefore the drug should be used with great caution in patients with significantly impaired renal function and the monitoring of serum creatinine and/or creatinine clearance is advised in these patients. Caution should be used if the drug is given to patients with creatinine clearance of less than 20 mL/minute because accumulation of naproxen has been seen in such patients.

Hepatic Effects

As with other NSAIDs, borderline elevations of one or more liver tests may occur in up to 15% of patients. These abnormalities may progress, may remain essentially unchanged, or may resolve with continued therapy. The ALT (SGPT) is probably the most sensitive indicator of liver dysfunction. Meaningful (3 times the upper limit of normal) elevations of ALT (SGPT) or AST (SGOT) occurred in controlled clinical trials in less than 1% of patients. A patient with symptoms and/or signs suggesting liver dysfunction, or in whom an abnormal liver test has occurred, should be evaluated for evidence of the development of more severe hepatic reaction while on therapy with naproxen. Severe hepatic reactions, including jaundice and cases of fatal hepatitis have been reported with naproxen as with other NSAIDs. Although such reactions are rare, if abnormal liver tests persist or worsen, if clinical signs and symptoms consistent with liver disease develop, or if systemic manifestations occur (e.g. eosinophilia, rash, fever, etc.), naproxen should be discontinued. Chronic alcoholic liver disease and probably other diseases with decreased or abnormal plasma proteins (albumin) reduce the total plasma concentration of naproxen, but the plasma concentration of unbound naproxen is increased. Caution is advised when high doses are required and some adjustment of dosage may be required in these patients. It is prudent to use the lowest effective dose.

Fluid Retention and Edema

Peripheral edema has been observed in some patients receiving naproxen. Naprelan (naproxen sodium) tablets contain 37.5 mg or 50 mg of sodium (1.5 mEq or 2.0 mEq respectively). This should be considered in patients whose overall intake of sodium must be severely restricted. For these reasons, Naprelan should be used with caution in patients with fluid retention, hypertension or heart failure.

INFORMATION FOR PATIENTS

Naprelan, like other drugs of its class, is not free of side effects. This formulation of naproxen can cause discomfort and, rarely, there are more serious side effects, such as GI bleeding, which may result in hospitalization and even fatal outcomes. NSAIDs are often essential agents in the management of arthritis and have a major role in the treatment of pain but they also may be commonly employed for conditions which are less serious. Physicians may wish to discuss with their patients the potential risks (see WARNINGS, PRECAUTIONS, and ADVERSE REACTIONS) and likely benefits of Naprelan treatment. Caution should be exercised by patients whose activities require alertness if they experience drowsiness, dizziness, vertigo or depression during therapy with naproxen.

LABORATORY TESTS

Because serious GI tract ulceration and bleeding can occur without warning symptoms, physicians should follow patients chronically treated with Naprelan for the signs and symptoms of ulceration and bleeding, and should inform them of the importance of this follow-up and what they should do if certain signs and symptoms do appear. Patients with initial hemoglobin values of 10 grams or less who are to receive long-term therapy should have hemoglobin values determined periodically. (See WARNINGS—RISK OF GI ULCERATION, BLEEDING AND PERFORATION WITH NSAID THERAPY).

DRUG INTERACTIONS

The use of NSAIDs in patients who are receiving ACE inhibitors may potentiate renal disease states (See PRECAUTIONS—*Renal Effects*). *In vitro* studies have shown that naproxen anion, because of its affinity for protein, may displace from their binding site other drugs which are also albumin-bound (see CLINICAL PHARMACOLOGY—PHARMACOKINETICS).

Theoretically, the naproxen anion itself could likewise be displaced. Short-term controlled studies failed to show that taking the drug significantly affects prothrombin times when administered to individuals on coumarin-type anticoagulants. Caution is advised nonetheless, since interactions have been seen with other nonsteroidal agents of this class. Similarly, patients receiving the drug and a hydantoin, sulfonamide or sulfonylurea should be observed for signs of toxicity to these drugs.

Concomitant administration of naproxen and aspirin is not recommended because naproxen is displaced from its binding sites during the concomitant administration of aspirin, resulting in lower plasma concentrations and peak plasma levels.

The natriuretic effect of furosemide has been reported to be inhibited by some drugs of this class. Inhibition of renal lithium clearance leading to increases in plasma lithium concentrations has also been reported. Naproxen and other NSAIDs can reduce the antihypertensive effect of propranolol and other beta-blockers.

Probenecid given concurrently increases naproxen anion plasma levels and extends its plasma half-life significantly. Caution should be used if naproxen is administered concomitantly with methotrexate. Naproxen, naproxen sodium and other NSAIDs have been reported to reduce the tubular secretion of methotrexate in an animal model, possibly increasing the toxicity of methotrexate.

DRUG/LABORATORY TEST INTERACTIONS

Naproxen may decrease platelet aggregation and prolong bleeding time. This effect should be kept in mind when bleeding times are determined. The administration of naproxen may result in increased urinary values for 17-ketogenic steroids because of an interaction between the drug and/or its metabolites with m-dinitrobenzene used in this assay. Although 17-hydroxy-corticosteroid measurements (Porter-Silber test) do not appear to be artifactually altered, it is suggested that therapy with naproxen be temporarily discontinued 72 hours before adrenal function tests are performed if the Porter-Silber test is to be used.

Naproxen may interfere with some urinary assays of 5-hydroxyindoleacetic acid (5HIAA).

CARCINOGENESIS

A two year study was performed in rats to evaluate the carcinogenic potential of naproxen at doses of 8 mg/kg/day, 16 mg/kg/day, and 24 mg/kg/day (50 mg/m², 100 mg/m², and 150 mg/m²). The maximum dose used was 0.28 times the systemic exposure to humans at the recommended dose. No evidence of tumorigenicity was found.

PREGNANCY
Teratogenic Effects: Pregnancy Category B
Reproduction studies have been performed in rats at 20 mg/kg/day (125 mg/m^2/day, 0.23 times the human systemic exposure) rabbits at 20 mg/kg/day (220 mg/m^2/day, 0.27 times the human systemic exposure) and mice at 170 mg/kg/day (510 mg/m^2/day, 0.28 times the human systemic exposure) with no evidence of impaired fertility or harm to the fetus due to the drug. There are no adequate and well-controlled studies in pregnant women. Because animal reproduction studies are not always predictive of human response, Naprelan should be used during pregnancy only if the potential benefits justify the potential risks to the fetus.
Nonteratogenic Effects
There is some evidence to suggest that when inhibitors of prostaglandin synthesis are used to delay preterm labor there is an increased risk of neonatal complications such as necrotizing enterocolitis, patent ductus arteriosus, and intracranial hemorrhage. Naproxen treatment given in the late pregnancy to delay parturition has been associated with persistent pulmonary hypertension, renal dysfunction, and abnormal prostaglandin E levels in preterm infants. Because of the known effect of drugs of this class on the human fetal cardiovascular system (closure of ductus arteriosus), use during third trimester should be avoided.
NURSING MOTHERS
The naproxen anion has been found in the milk of lactating women at a concentration of approximately 1% of that found in the plasma. Because of the possible adverse effects of prostaglandin-inhibiting drugs on neonates, use in nursing mothers should be avoided.
PEDIATRIC USE
No pediatric studies have been performed with Naprelan, thus safety of Naprelan in pediatric populations has not been established.

ADVERSE REACTIONS
As with all drugs in this class, the frequency and severity of adverse events depends on several factors: the dose of the drug and duration of treatment; the age, the sex, physical condition of the patient; any concurrent medical diagnoses or individual risk factors.
The following adverse reactions are divided into three parts based on frequency and whether or not the possibility exists of a causal relationship between drug usage and these adverse events. In those reactions listed as "Probable Causal Relationship" there is at least one case for each adverse reaction where there is evidence to suggest that there is a causal relationship between drug usage and the reported event.
The adverse reactions reported were based on the results from two double-blind controlled clinical trials of three months duration with an additional nine month open-label extension. A total of 542 patients received Naprelan either in the double-blind period or in the nine month open-label extension. Of these 542 patients, 232 received Naprelan, 167 were initially treated with Naprosyn and 143 were initially treated with placebo. Adverse reactions reported by patients who received Naprelan are shown by body system. Those adverse reactions observed with naproxen but not reported in controlled trials with Naprelan are italicized.
The most frequent adverse events from the double-blind and open-label clinical trials were headache (15%), followed by dyspepsia (14%), and flu syndrome (10%). The incidence of other adverse events occurring in 3%–9% of the patients are marked with an asterisk.
Those reactions occurring in less than 3% of the patients are unmarked.
INCIDENCE GREATER THAN 1% (PROBABLE CAUSAL RELATIONSHIP)
Body as a Whole—Pain (back)*, pain*, infection*, fever, injury (accident), asthenia, pain chest, headache (15%), flu syndrome (10%).
Gastrointestinal—Nausea*, diarrhea*, constipation*, abdominal pain*, flatulence, gastritis, vomiting, dysphagia, dyspepsia (14%), *heartburn*, stomatitis.*
Hematologic—Anemia, ecchymosis.
Respiratory—Pharyngitis*, rhinitis*, sinusitis*, bronchitis, cough increased.
Renal—Urinary tract infection*, cystitis.
Dermatologic—Skin rash*, *skin eruptions*, ecchymoses*, purpura.*
Metabolic and Nutrition—Peripheral edema, hyperglycemia.
Central Nervous System—Dizziness, paresthesia, insomnia, *drowsiness*, lightheadedness.*
Cardiovascular—Hypertension, *edema*, dyspnea*, palpitations.*
Musculoskeletal—Cramps (leg), myalgia, arthralgia, joint disorder, tendon disorder.
Special Senses—*Tinnitus*, hearing disturbances, visual disturbances.*
General—*Thirst.*
INCIDENCE LESS THAN 1% (PROBABLE CAUSAL RELATIONSHIP)
Body as a Whole—Abscess, monilia, neck rigid, pain neck, abdomen enlarged, carcinoma, cellulitis, edema general, LE syndrome, malaise, mucous membrane disorder, allergic reaction, pain pelvic.
Gastrointestinal—Anorexia, cholecystitis, cholelithiasis, eructation, GI hemorrhage, rectal hemorrhage, stomatitis aphthous, stomatitis ulcer, ulcer mouth, ulcer stomach, periodontal abscess, cardiospasm, colitis, esophagitis, gastroenteritis, GI disorder, rectal disorder, tooth disorder, hepatosplenomegaly, liver function abnormality, melena, ulcer esophagus, *hematemesis, jaundice, pancreatitis, necrosis.*
Renal—Dysmenorrhea, dysuria, kidney function abnormality, nocturia, prostate disorder, pyelonephritis, carcinoma breast, urinary incontinence, kidney calculus, kidney failure, menorrhagia, metrorrhagia, neoplasm breast, nephrosclerosis, hematuria, pain kidney, pyuria, urine abnormal, urinary frequency, urinary retention, uterine spasm, vaginitis, *glomerular nephritis, hyperkalemia, interstitial nephritis, nephrotic syndrome, renal disease, renal failure, renal papillary necrosis.*
Hematologic—Leukopenia, bleeding time increased, eosinophilia, abnormal RBC, abnormal WBC, thrombocytopenia, *agranulocytosis, granulocytopenia.*
Central Nervous System—Depression, anxiety, hypertonia, nervousness, neuralgia, neuritis, vertigo, amnesia, confusion, co-ordination, abnormal diplopia, emotional lability, hematoma subdural, paralysis, *dream abnormalities, inability to concentrate, muscle weakness.*
Dermatologic: Angiodermatitis, herpes simplex, dry skin, sweating, ulcer skin, acne, alopecia, dermatitis contact, eczema, herpes zoster, nail disorder, skin necrosis, subcutaneous nodule, pruritis, urticaria, neoplasm skin, *photosensitive dermatitis, photosensitivity reactions resembling porphyria cutaneous tarda, epidermolysis bullosa.*
Special Senses—Amblyopia scleritis, cataract, conjunctivitis, deaf, ear disorder, keratoconjunctivitis, lacrimation disorder, otitis media, pain eye.
Cardiovascular—Angina pectoris, coronary artery disease, myocardial infarction, deep thrombophlebitis, vasodilation, vascular anomaly, arrhythmia, bundle branch block, abnormal ECG, heart failure right, hemorrhage, migraine, aortic stenosis, syncope, tachycardia, *congestive heart failure.*
Respiratory—Asthma, dyspnea, lung edema, laryngitis, lung disorder, epistaxis, pneumonia, respiratory distress, respiratory disorder, *eosinophilic pneumonitis.*
Musculoskeletal—Myasthenia, bone disorder, spontaneous bone fracture, fibrotendinitis, bone pain, ptosis, spasm general, bursitis.
Metabolic and Nutrition—Creatinine increase, glucosuria, hypercholesteremia, albuminuria, alkalosis, BUN increased, dehydration, edema, glucose tolerance decrease, hyperuricemia, hypokalemia, SGOT increase, SGPT increase, weight decrease.
General—*Anaphylactoid reactions, angioneurotic edema, menstrual disorders, hypoglycemia, pyrexia (chills and fevers).*
INCIDENCE LESS THAN 1% (CAUSAL RELATIONSHIP UNKNOWN)
Other adverse reactions listed in the naproxen package label, but not reported by those who received Naprelan are shown in italics. These observations are being listed as alerting information to the physician.
Hematologic—*Aplastic anemia, hemolytic anemia.*
Central Nervous System: *Aseptic meningitis, cognitive dysfunction.*
Dermatologic—*Epidermal necrolysis, erythema multiforme, Stevens-Johnson syndrome.*
Gastrointestinal—*Non-peptic GI ulceration, ulcerative stomatitis.*
Cardiovascular—*Vasculitis.*

OVERDOSAGE
Significant naproxen overdosage may be characterized by drowsiness, heartburn, indigestion, nausea, or vomiting. Because naproxen sodium may be rapidly absorbed, high and early blood levels should be anticipated. A few patients have experienced seizures, but it is not clear whether or not these were drug-related. It is not known what dose of the drug would be life threatening. The oral LD_{50} of the drug is 500 mg/kg in rats, 1200 mg/kg in mice, 4000 mg/kg in hamsters and greater than 1000 mg/kg in dogs.
Should a patient ingest a large number of tablets, accidentally or purposefully, the stomach may be emptied and usual supportive measures employed. In animals 0.5 g/kg of activated charcoal was effective in reducing plasma levels of naproxen. Hemodialysis does not decrease the plasma concentration of naproxen because of the high degree of its protein binding.

DOSAGE AND ADMINISTRATION
RHEUMATOID ARTHRITIS, OSTEOARTHRITIS, AND ANKYLOSING SPONDYLITIS
The usual daily dose of Naprelan is two Naprelan 375 mg tablets (750 mg) once daily, or two Naprelan 500 mg tablets (1000 mg) once a day. Both larger and smaller doses may be required in individual patients (see **Individualization of Dosage**). Regardless of indication, the dosage should be individualized to achieve effective dose and minimize adverse events, however the maximum daily dose is three Naprelan 500 mg once daily.
MANAGEMENT OF PAIN, PRIMARY DYSMENORRHEA, AND ACUTE TENDINITIS AND BURSITIS
The recommended starting dose is two Naprelan 500 mg tablets (1000 mg) once daily. For patients requiring greater analgesic benefit, three Naprelan 500 mg tablets (1500 mg) may be used for a limited period. Thereafter, the total daily dose should not exceed two Naprelan 500 mg tablets (1000 mg).
ACUTE GOUT
The recommended dose on the first day is two to three Naprelan 500 mg tablets (1000–1500 mg) once daily, followed by two Naprelan 500 mg tablets (1000 mg) once daily, until the attack has subsided.

HOW SUPPLIED
Naprelan® (naproxen sodium) Controlled Release Tablets are available as follows:
Naprelan 375: white, capsule-shaped tablet with "W" on one side and "901" on the reverse; in bottles of 100; NDC 0008-0901-03. Each tablet contains 412.5 mg naproxen sodium equivalent to 375 mg naproxen.
Naprelan 500: white, capsule-shaped tablet with "W" on one side and "902" on the reverse; in bottles of 75; NDC 0008-0902-02. Each tablet contains 550 mg naproxen sodium equivalent to 500 mg naproxen.
Caution: Federal law prohibits dispensing without prescription.
US Patent Pending.
Store at controlled room temperature, 20°–25° C (68°–77° F).
Dispense in a well-closed container.
Manufactured for
Wyeth Laboratories Inc.
A Wyeth-Ayerst Company
Philadelphia, PA 19101
by
élan pharma ltd.
Athlone, Ireland
Shown in Product Identification Guide, page 340

NORDETTE®–21 ℞
[nor-det'-21]
TABLETS
(levonorgestrel and ethinyl estradiol tablets)

Patients should be counseled that this product does not protect against HIV infection (AIDS) and other sexually transmitted diseases.

DESCRIPTION
ORAL CONTRACEPTIVE
Each Nordette tablet contains 0.15 mg of levonorgestrel (d(-)-13 beta-ethyl-17-alpha-ethinyl-17-beta-hydroxygon-4-en-3-one), a totally synthetic progestogen, and 0.03 mg of ethinyl estradiol (19-nor-17α-pregna-1,3,5 (10)-trien-20-yne-3,17-diol). The inactive ingredients present are cellulose, FD&C Yellow 6, lactose, magnesium stearate, and polacrilin potassium.

CLINICAL PHARMACOLOGY
Combination oral contraceptives act by suppression of gonadotropins. Although the primary mechanism of this action is inhibition of ovulation, other alterations include changes in the cervical mucus (which increase the difficulty of sperm entry into the uterus) and the endometrium (which reduce the likelihood of implantation).

INDICATIONS AND USAGE
Oral contraceptives are indicated for the prevention of pregnancy in women who elect to use this product as a method of contraception.
Oral contraceptives are highly effective. Table I lists the typical accidental pregnancy rates for users of combination oral contraceptives and other methods of contraception. The efficacy of these contraceptive methods, except sterilization and the IUD, depends upon the reliability with which they are used. Correct and consistent use of methods can result in lower failure rates.

TABLE I: LOWEST EXPECTED AND TYPICAL FAILURE RATES DURING THE FIRST YEAR OF CONTINUOUS USE OF A METHOD
% of Women Experiencing an Accidental Pregnancy in the First Year of Continuous Use

Method	Lowest Expected*	Typical**
(No Contraception)	(85)	(85)
Oral contraceptives		3
combined	0.1	N/A***
progestin only	0.5	N/A***
Diaphragm with spermicidal cream or jelly	6	18

Continued on next page

Wyeth-Ayerst Laboratories—Cont.

Spermicides alone (foams and vaginal suppositories)	3	21
Vaginal Sponge		
nulliparous	6	18
multiparous	9	28
DEPO-PROVERA® (injectable progestogen)	0.3	0.3
NORPLANT® SYSTEM (implants)	0.2#	0.2#
IUD		3
progesterone	2	N/A***
copper T 380A	0.8	N/A***
Condom without spermicides	2	12
Periodic abstinence (all methods)	1–9	20
Female sterilization	0.2	0.4
Male sterilization	0.1	0.15

Adapted from J. Trussell et al., Table 1, Studies in Family Planning, 21(1). Jan.–Feb. 1990.

* The authors' best guess of the percentage of women expected to experience an accidental pregnancy among couples who initiate a method (not necessarily for the first time) and who use it consistently and correctly during the first year if they do not stop use for any other reason.

** This term represents "typical" couples who initiate use of a method (not necessarily for the first time), who experience an accidental pregnancy during the first year if they do not stop use for any other reason.

*** N/A—Data not available

This data is based on NORPLANT® SYSTEM clinical trials.

CONTRAINDICATIONS

Oral contraceptives should not be used in women with any of the following conditions:

- Thrombophlebitis or thromboembolic disorders.
- A past history of deep-vein thrombophlebitis or thromboembolic disorders.
- Cerebral-vascular or coronary-artery disease.
- Known or suspected carcinoma of the breast.
- Carcinoma of the endometrium or other known or suspected estrogen-dependent neoplasia.
- Undiagnosed abnormal genital bleeding.
- Cholestatic jaundice of pregnancy or jaundice with prior pill use.
- Hepatic adenomas or carcinomas.
- Known or suspected pregnancy.

WARNINGS

Cigarette smoking increases the risk of serious cardiovascular side effects from oral-contraceptive use. This risk increases with age and with heavy smoking (15 or more cigarettes per day) and is quite marked in women over 35 years of age. Women who use oral contraceptives should be strongly advised not to smoke.

The use of oral contraceptives is associated with increased risks of several serious conditions including myocardial infarction, thromboembolism, stroke, hepatic neoplasia, gallbladder disease, and hypertension, although the risk of serious morbidity or mortality is very small in healthy women without underlying risk factors. The risk of morbidity and mortality increases significantly in the presence of other underlying risk factors such as hypertension, hyperlipidemias, obesity, and diabetes.

Practitioners prescribing oral contraceptives should be familiar with the following information relating to these risks.

The information contained in this package insert is based principally on studies carried out in patients who used oral contraceptives with higher formulations of estrogens and progestogens than those in common use today. The effect of long-term use of the oral contraceptives with lower formulations of both estrogens and progestogens remains to be determined.

Throughout this labeling, epidemiological studies reported are of two types: retrospective or case control studies and prospective or cohort studies. Case control studies provide a measure of the relative risk of disease, namely, a ratio of the incidence of a disease among oral-contraceptive users to that among nonusers. The relative risk does not provide information on the actual clinical occurrence of a disease. Cohort studies provide a measure of attributable risk, which is the difference in the incidence of disease between oral-contraceptive users and nonusers. The attributable risk does provide information about the actual occurrence of a disease in the population. For further information, the reader is referred to a text on epidemiological methods.

1. THROMBOEMBOLIC DISORDERS AND OTHER VASCULAR PROBLEMS

a. *Myocardial infarction*

An increased risk of myocardial infarction has been attributed to oral-contraceptive use. This risk is primarily in smokers or women with other underlying risk factors for coronary-artery disease such as hypertension, hypercholesterolemia, morbid obesity, and diabetes. The relative risk of heart attack for current oral-contraceptive users has been estimated to be two to six. The risk is very low under the age of 30.

Smoking in combination with oral-contraceptive use has been shown to contribute substantially to the incidence of myocardial infarctions in women in their mid-thirties or older with smoking accounting for the majority of excess cases. Mortality rates associated with circulatory disease have been shown to increase substantially in smokers over the age of 35 and nonsmokers over the age of 40 (Table II) among women who use oral contraceptives.

CIRCULATORY DISEASE MORTALITY RATES PER 100,000 WOMAN YEARS BY AGE, SMOKING STATUS AND ORAL-CONTRACEPTIVE USE

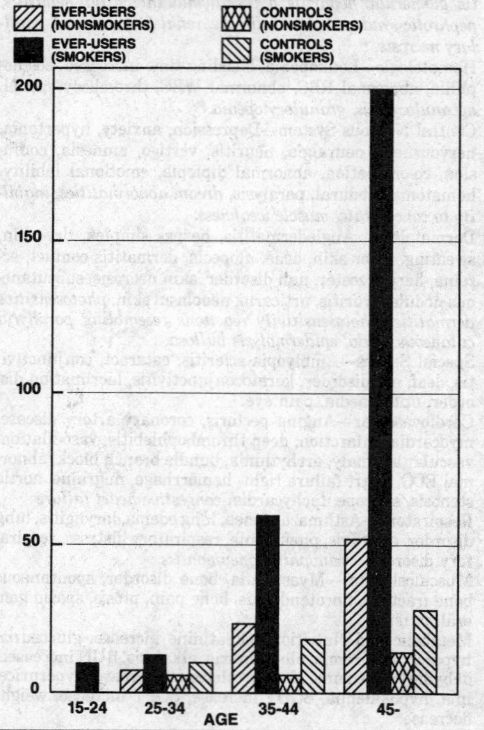

TABLE II. (Adapted from P.M. Layde and V. Beral, Lancet. 1:541–546, 1981.)

Oral contraceptives may compound the effects of well-known risk factors, such as hypertension, diabetes, hyperlipidemias, age, and obesity. In particular, some progestogens are known to decrease HDL cholesterol and cause glucose intolerance, while estrogens may create a state of hyperinsulinism. Oral contraceptives have been shown to increase blood pressure among users (see section 9 in "Warnings"). Similar effects on risk factors have been associated with an increased risk of heart disease. Oral contraceptives must be used with caution in women with cardiovascular disease risk factors.

b. *Thromboembolism*

An increased risk of thromboembolic and thrombotic disease associated with the use of oral contraceptives is well established. Case control studies have found the relative risk of users compared to nonusers to be 3 for the first episode of superficial venous thrombosis, 4 to 11 for deep vein thrombosis or pulmonary embolism, and 1.5 to 6 for women with predisposing conditions for venous thromboembolic disease. Cohort studies have shown the relative risk to be somewhat lower, about 3 for new cases and about 4.5 for new cases requiring hospitalization. The risk of thromboembolic disease due to oral contraceptives is not related to length of use and disappears after pill use is stopped.

A two- to four-fold increase in relative risk of postoperative thromboembolic complications has been reported with the use of oral contraceptives. The relative risk of venous thrombosis in women who have predisposing conditions is twice that of women without such medical conditions. If feasible, oral contraceptives should be discontinued at least four weeks prior to and for two weeks after elective surgery of a type associated with an increase in risk of thromboembolism and during and following prolonged immobilization. Since the immediate postpartum period is also associated with an increased risk of thromboembolism, oral contraceptives should be started no earlier than four to six weeks after delivery in women who elect not to breast feed, or a midtrimester pregnancy termination.

c. *Cerebrovascular diseases*

Oral contraceptives have been shown to increase both the relative and attributable risks of cerebrovascular events (thrombotic and hemorrhagic strokes), although, in general, the risk is greatest among older (>35 years), hypertensive women who also smoke. Hypertension was found to be a risk factor for both users and nonusers, for both types of strokes, while smoking interacted to increase the risk for hemorrhagic strokes.

In a large study, the relative risk of thrombotic strokes has been shown to range from 3 for normotensive users to 14 for users with severe hypertension. The relative risk of hemorrhagic stroke is reported to be 1.2 for nonsmokers who used oral contraceptives, 2.6 for smokers who did not use oral contraceptives, 7.6 for smokers who used oral contraceptives, 1.8 for normotensive users and 25.7 for users with severe hypertension. The attributable risk is also greater in older women.

d. *Dose-related risk of vascular disease from oral contraceptives*

A positive association has been observed between the amount of estrogen and progestogen in oral contraceptives and the risk of vascular disease. A decline in serum high-density lipoproteins (HDL) has been reported with many progestational agents. A decline in serum high-density lipoproteins has been associated with an increased incidence of ischemic heart disease. Because estrogens increase HDL cholesterol, the net effect of an oral contraceptive depends on a balance achieved between doses of estrogen and progestogen and the nature and absolute amount of progestogen used in the contraceptive. The amount of both hormones should be considered in the choice of an oral contraceptive.

Minimizing exposure to estrogen and progestogen is in keeping with good principles of therapeutics. For any particular estrogen/progestogen combination, the dosage regimen prescribed should be one which contains the least amount of estrogen and progestogen that is compatible with a low failure rate and the needs of the individual patient. New acceptors of oral-contraceptive agents should be started on preparations containing less than 50 mcg of estrogen.

e. *Persistence of risk of vascular disease*

There are two studies which have shown persistence of risk of vascular disease for ever-users of oral contraceptives. In a study in the United States, the risk of developing myocardial infarction after discontinuing oral contraceptives persists for at least 9 years for women 40 to 49 years who had used oral contraceptives for five or more years, but this increased risk was not demonstrated in other age groups. In another study in Great Britain, the risk of developing cerebrovascular disease persisted for at least 6 years after discontinuation of oral contraceptives, although excess risk was very small. However, both studies were performed with oral contraceptive formulations containing 50 micrograms or higher of estrogens.

2. ESTIMATES OF MORTALITY FROM CONTRACEPTIVE USE

One study gathered data from a variety of sources which have estimated the mortality rate associated with different methods of contraception at different ages (Table III). These estimates include the combined risk of death associated with contraceptive methods plus the risk attributable to pregnancy in the event of method failure. Each method of contraception has its specific benefits and risks. The study concluded that with the exception of oral-contraceptive users 35 and older who smoke and 40 and older who do not smoke, mortality associated with all methods of birth control is less than that associated with childbirth. The observation of a possible increase in risk of mortality with age for oral-contraceptive users is based on data gathered in the 1970's—but not reported until 1983. However, current clinical practice involves the use of lower estrogen dose formulations combined with careful restriction of oral-contraceptive use to women who do not have the various risk factors listed in this labeling.

Because of these changes in practice and, also, because of some limited new data which suggest that the risk of cardiovascular disease with the use of oral contraceptives may now be less than previously observed, the Fertility and Maternal Health Drugs Advisory Committee was asked to review the topic in 1989. The Committee concluded that although cardiovascular-disease risks may be increased with oral-contraceptive use after age 40 in healthy nonsmoking women (even with the newer low-dose formulations), there are greater potential health risks associated with pregnancy in older women and with the alternative surgical and medical procedures which may be necessary if such women do not have access to effective and acceptable means of contraception. Therefore, the Committee recommended that the benefits of oral-contraceptive use by healthy nonsmoking women over 40 may outweigh the possible risks. Of course, older women, as all women who take oral contraceptives, should take the lowest possible dose formulation that is effective.

[See table at top of next page.]

3. CARCINOMA OF THE REPRODUCTIVE ORGANS

Numerous epidemiological studies have been performed on the incidence of breast, endometrial, ovarian, and cervical cancer in women using oral contraceptives. The overwhelming evidence in the literature suggests that the use of oral contraceptives is not associated with an increase in the risk of developing breast cancer, regardless of the age and parity

of first use or with most of the marketed brands and doses. The Cancer and Steroid Hormone (CASH) study also showed no latent effect on the risk of breast cancer for at least a decade following long-term use. A few studies have shown a slightly increased relative risk of developing breast cancer, although the methodology of these studies, which included differences in examination of users and nonusers and differences in age at start of use, has been questioned.

Some studies suggest that oral-contraceptive use has been associated with an increase in the risk of cervical intraepithelial neoplasia in some populations of women. However, there continues to be controversy about the extent to which such findings may be due to differences in sexual behavior and other factors.

In spite of many studies of the relationship between oral-contraceptive use and breast and cervical cancers, a cause-and-effect relationship has not been established.

4. HEPATIC NEOPLASIA

Benign hepatic adenomas are associated with oral-contraceptive use, although the incidence of benign tumors is rare in the United States. Indirect calculations have estimated the attributable risk to be in the range of 3.3 cases/100,000 for users, a risk that increases after four or more years of use. Rupture of rare, benign, hepatic adenomas may cause death through intra-abdominal hemorrhage.

Studies from Britain have shown an increased risk of developing hepatocellular carcinoma in long-term (>8 years) oral-contraceptive users. However, these cancers are extremely rare in the U.S. and the attributable risk (the excess incidence) of liver cancers in oral-contraceptive users approaches less than one per million users.

5. OCULAR LESIONS

There have been clincial case reports of retinal thrombosis associated with the use of oral contraceptives. Oral contraceptives should be discontinued if there is unexplained partial or complete loss of vision; onset of proptosis or diplopia; papilledema; or retinal vascular lesions. Appropriate diagnostic and therapeutic measures should be undertaken immediately.

6. ORAL-CONTRACEPTIVE USE BEFORE OR DURING EARLY PREGNANCY

Extensive epidemiological studies have revealed no increased risk of birth defects in women who have used oral contraceptives prior to pregnancy. Studies also do not suggest a teratogenic effect, particularly insofar as cardiac anomalies and limb-reduction defects are concerned, when taken inadvertently during early pregnancy.

The administration of oral contraceptives to induce withdrawal bleeding should not be used as a test for pregnancy. Oral contraceptives should not be used during pregnancy to treat threatened or habitual abortion.

It is recommended that for any patient who has missed two consecutive periods, pregnancy should be ruled out before continuing oral-contraceptive use. If the patient has not adhered to the prescribed schedule, the possibility of pregnancy should be considered at the time of the first missed period. Oral-contraceptive use should be discontinued until pregnancy is confirmed.

7. GALLBLADDER DISEASE

Earlier studies have reported an increased lifetime relative risk of gallbladder surgery in users of oral contraceptives and estrogens. More recent studies, however, have shown that the relative risk of developing gallbladder disease among oral-contraceptive users may be minimal. The recent findings of minimal risk may be related to the use of oral-contraceptive formulations containing lower hormonal doses of estrogens and progestogens.

8. CARBOHYDRATE AND LIPID METABOLIC EFFECTS

Oral contraceptives have been shown to cause glucose intolerance in a significant percentage of users. Oral contraceptives containing greater than 75 micrograms of estrogens cause hyperinsulinism, while lower doses of estrogen cause less glucose intolerance. Progestogens increase insulin secretion and create insulin resistance, this effect varying with different progestational agents. However, in the nondiabetic woman, oral contraceptives appear to have no effect on fasting blood glucose. Because of these demonstrated effects, prediabetic and diabetic women should be carefully observed while taking oral contraceptives.

A small proportion of women will have persistent hypertriglyceridemia while on the pill. As discussed earlier (see Warnings 1a and 1d), changes in serum triglycerides and lipoprotein levels have been reported in oral-contraceptive users.

9. ELEVATED BLOOD PRESSURE

An increase in blood pressure has been reported in women taking oral contraceptives, and this increase is more likely in older oral-contraceptive users and with continued use. Data from the Royal College of General Practitioners and subsequent randomized trials have shown that the incidence of hypertension increases with increasing quantities of progestogens.

Women with a history of hypertension or hypertension-related diseases, or renal disease should be encouraged to use another method of contraception. If women with hypertension elect to use oral contraceptives, they should be monitored closely, and if significant elevation of blood pressure occurs, oral contraceptives should be discontinued. For most women, elevated blood pressure will return to normal after stopping oral contraceptives, and there is no difference in the occurrence of hypertension among ever- and never-users.

TABLE III—ANNUAL NUMBER OF BIRTH-RELATED OR METHOD-RELATED DEATHS ASSOCIATED WITH CONTROL OF FERTILITY PER 100,000 NONSTERILE WOMEN, BY FERTILITY-CONTROL METHOD ACCORDING TO AGE

Method of control and outcome	15–19	20–24	25–29	30–34	35–39	40–44
No fertility-control methods*	7.0	7.4	9.1	14.8	25.7	28.2
Oral contraceptives nonsmoker**	0.3	0.5	0.9	1.9	13.8	31.6
Oral contraceptives smoker**	2.2	3.4	6.6	13.5	51.1	117.2
IUD**	0.8	0.8	1.0	1.0	1.4	1.4
Condom*	1.1	1.6	0.7	0.2	0.3	0.4
Diaphragm/spermicide*	1.9	1.2	1.2	1.3	2.2	2.8
Periodic abstinence*	2.5	1.6	1.6	1.7	2.9	3.6

* Deaths are birth related

** Deaths are method related

Adapted from H.W. Ory, Family Planning Perspectives, 15:57–63, 1983.

10. HEADACHE

The onset or exacerbation of migraine or development of headache with a new pattern that is recurrent, persistent, or severe requires discontinuation of oral contraceptives and evaluation of the cause.

11. BLEEDING IRREGULARITIES

Breakthrough bleeding and spotting are sometimes encountered in patients on oral contraceptives, especially during the first three months of use. The type and dose of progestogen may be important. Non-hormonal causes should be considered and adequate diagnostic measures taken to rule out malignancy or pregnancy in the event of breakthrough bleeding, as in the case of any abnormal vaginal bleeding. If pathology has been excluded, time or a change to another formulation may solve the problem. In the event of amenorrhea, pregnancy should be ruled out.

Some women may encounter post-pill amenorrhea or oligomenorrhea, especially when such a condition was preexistent.

PRECAUTIONS

Patients should be counseled that this product does not protect against HIV infection (AIDS) and other sexually transmitted diseases.

1. PHYSICAL EXAMINATION AND FOLLOW-UP

A periodic history and physical examination is appropriate for all women, including women using oral contraceptives. The physical examination, however, may be deferred until after initiation of oral contraceptives if requested by the woman and judged appropriate by the clinician. The physical examination should include special reference to blood pressure, breasts, abdomen and pelvic organs, including cervical cytology, and relevant laboratory tests. In case of undiagnosed, persistent or recurrent abnormal vaginal bleeding, appropriate diagnostic measures should be conducted to rule out malignancy. Women with a strong family history of breast cancer or who have breast nodules should be monitored with particular care.

2. LIPID DISORDERS

Women who are being treated for hyperlipidemias should be followed closely if they elect to use oral contraceptives. Some progestogens may elevate LDL levels and may render the control of hyperlipidemias more difficult. (See "Warnings," 1d.).

3. LIVER FUNCTION

If jaundice develops in any woman receiving such drugs, the medication should be discontinued. Steroid hormones may be poorly metabolized in patients with impaired liver function.

4. FLUID RETENTION

Oral contraceptives may cause some degree of fluid retention. They should be prescribed with caution, and only with careful monitoring, in patients with conditions which might be aggravated by fluid retention.

5. EMOTIONAL DISORDERS

Patients becoming significantly depressed while taking oral contraceptives should stop the medication and use an alternate method of contraception in an attempt to determine whether the symptom is drug related.

Women with a history of depression should be carefully observed and the drug discontinued if depression recurs to a serious degree.

6. CONTACT LENSES

Contact-lens wearers who develop visual changes or changes in lens tolerance should be assessed by an ophthalmologist.

7. DRUG INTERACTIONS

Reduced efficacy and increased incidence of breakthrough bleeding and menstrual irregularities have been associated with concomitant use of rifampin. A similar assocation, though less marked, has been suggested with barbiturates, phenylbutazone, phenytoin sodium, and possibly with griseofulvin, ampicillin and tetracyclines.

8. INTERACTIONS WITH LABORATORY TESTS

Certain endocrine- and liver-function tests and blood components may be affected by oral contraceptives:

a. Increased prothrombin and factors VII, VIII, IX, and X; decreased antithrombin 3; increased norepinephrine-induced platelet aggregability.
b. Increased thyroid-binding globulin (TBG) leading to increased circulating total thyroid hormone, as measured by protein-bound iodine (PBI), T4 by column or by radioimmunoassay. Free T3 resin uptake is decreased, reflecting the elevated TBG; free T4 concentration is unaltered.
c. Other binding proteins may be elevated in serum.
d. Sex-binding globulins are increased and result in elevated levels of total circulating sex steroids and corticoids; however, free or biologically active levels remain unchanged.
e. Triglycerides may be increased.
f. Glucose tolerance may be decreased.
g. Serum folate levels may be depressed by oral contraceptive therapy. This may be of clinical significance if a woman becomes pregnant shortly after discontinuing oral contraceptives.

9. CARCINOGENESIS

See "Warnings" section.

10. PREGNANCY

Pregnancy Category X. See Contraindications and Warnings sections.

11. NURSING MOTHERS

Small amounts of oral-contraceptive steroids have been identified in the milk of nursing mothers, and a few adverse effects on the child have been reported, including jaundice and breast enlargement. In addition, oral contraceptives given in the postpartum period may interfere with lactation by decreasing the quantity and quality of breast milk. If possible, the nursing mother should be advised not to use oral contraceptives but to use other forms of contraception until she has completely weaned her child.

INFORMATION FOR THE PATIENT

See LO/OVRAL.

ADVERSE REACTIONS

An increased risk of the following serious adverse reactions has been associated with the use of oral contraceptives (see "Warnings" section):

Thrombophlebitis.
Arterial thromboembolism.
Pulmonary embolism.
Myocardial infarction.
Cerebral hemorrhage.
Cerebral thrombosis.
Hypertension.
Gallbladder disease.
Hepatic adenomas or benign liver tumors.

There is evidence of an association between the following conditions and the use of oral contraceptives, although additional confirmatory studies are needed:

Mesenteric thrombosis.
Retinal thrombosis

The following adverse reactions have been reported in patients receiving oral contraceptives and are believed to be drug-related:

Nausea.
Vomiting.
Gastrointestinal symptoms (such as abdominal cramps and bloating).
Breakthrough bleeding.
Spotting.
Change in menstrual flow.
Amenorrhea.

Continued on next page

Wyeth-Ayerst Laboratories—Cont.

Temporary infertility after discontinuation of treatment.
Edema.
Melasma which may persist.
Breast changes: tenderness, enlargement, secretion.
Change in weight (increase or decrease).
Change in cervical erosion and secretion.
Diminution in lactation when given immediately postpartum.
Cholestatic jaundice.
Migraine.
Rash (allergic).
Mental depression.
Reduced tolerance to carbohydrates.
Vaginal candidiasis.
Change in corneal curvature (steepening).
Intolerance to contact lenses.

The following adverse reactions have been reported in users of oral contraceptives, and the association has been neither confirmed nor refuted:

Congenital anomalies.
Premenstrual syndrome.
Cataracts.
Optic neuritis.
Changes in appetite.
Cystitis-like syndrome.
Headache.
Nervousness.
Dizziness.
Hirsutism.
Loss of scalp hair.
Erythema multiforme.
Erythema nodosum.
Hemorrhagic eruption.
Vaginitis.
Porphyria.
Impaired renal function.
Hemolytic uremic syndrome.
Budd-Chiari syndrome.
Acne.
Changes in libido.
Colitis.
Sickle-cell disease.
Cerebral-vascular disease with mitral valve prolapse.
Lupus-like syndromes.

OVERDOSAGE

Serious ill effects have not been reported following acute ingestion of large doses of oral contraceptives by young children. Overdosage may cause nausea, and withdrawal bleeding may occur in females.

NONCONTRACEPTIVE HEALTH BENEFITS

The following noncontraceptive health benefits related to the use of oral contraceptives are supported by epidemiological studies which largely utilized oral-contraceptive formulations containing doses exceeding 0.035 mg of ethinyl estradiol or 0.05 mg of mestranol.

Effects on menses:
- Increased menstrual cycle regularity
- Decreased blood loss and decreased incidence of iron deficiency anemia
- Decreased incidence of dysmenorrhea

Effects related to inhibition of ovulation:
- Decreased incidence of functional ovarian cysts
- Decreased incidence of ectopic pregnancies

Effects from long-term use:
- Decreased incidence of fibroadenomas and fibrocystic disease of the breast
- Decreased incidence of acute pelvic inflammatory disease
- Decreased incidence of endometrial cancer
- Decreased incidence of ovarian cancer

DOSAGE AND ADMINISTRATION

To achieve maximum contraceptive effectiveness, Nordette-21 must be taken exactly as directed and at intervals not exceeding 24 hours.

The dosage of Nordette-21 is one tablet daily for 21 consecutive days per menstrual cycle according to prescribed schedule. Tablets are then discontinued for 7 days (three weeks on, one week off).

It is recommended that Nordette-21 tablets be taken at the same time each day, preferably after the evening meal or at bedtime.

During the first cycle of medication, the patient is instructed to take one Nordette-21 tablet daily for twenty-one consecutive days, beginning on the first day (Day 1 Start) of her menstrual cycle or on the Sunday after her period begins (Sunday Start). (The first day of menstruation is day one.) The tablets are then discontinued for one week (7 days). Withdrawal bleeding should usually occur within 3 days following discontinuation of Nordette-21. (For Day 1 Start: If Nordette-21 is first taken later than the first day of the first menstrual cycle of medication or postpartum, contraceptive reliance should not be placed on Nordette-21 until after the first seven consecutive days of administration. For Sunday Start: Contraceptive reliance should not be placed on Nordette-21 until after the first seven consecutive days of administration. The possibility of ovulation and conception prior to initiation of medication should be considered.)

The patient begins her next and all subsequent 21-day courses of Nordette-21 tablets on the same day of the week that she began her first course, following the same schedule: 21 days on—7 days off. She begins taking her tablets on the 8th day after discontinuance regardless of whether or not a menstrual period has occurred or is still in progress. Any time a new cycle of Nordette-21 is started later than the 8th day, the patient should be protected by another means of contraception until she has taken a tablet daily for seven consecutive days.

If spotting or breakthrough bleeding occurs, the patient is instructed to continue on the same regimen. This type of bleeding is usually transient and without significance; however, if the bleeding is persistent or prolonged the patient is advised to consult her physician. Although the occurrence of pregnancy is highly unlikely if Nordette-21 is taken according to directions, if withdrawal bleeding does not occur, the possibility of pregnancy must be considered. If the patient has not adhered to the prescribed schedule (missed one or more tablets or started taking them on a day later than she should have) the probability of pregnancy should be considered at the time of the first missed period and appropriate diagnostic measures taken before the medication is resumed. If the patient has adhered to the prescribed regimen and misses two consecutive periods, pregnancy should be ruled out before continuing the contraceptive regimen.

For additional patient instructions regarding missed pills, see the "WHAT TO DO IF YOU MISS PILLS" section in the **DETAILED PATIENT LABELING** for LO/OVRAL.

Any time the patient misses one or two tablets she should also use another method of contraception until she has taken a tablet daily for seven consecutive days. If breakthrough bleeding occurs following missed tablets, it will usually be transient and of no consequence. While there is little likelihood of ovulation occurring if only one or two tablets are missed, the possibility of ovulation increases with each successive day that scheduled tablets are missed.

In the nonlactating mother, Nordette-21 may be initiated postpartum, for contraception. When the tablets are administered in the postpartum period, the increased risk of thromboembolic disease associated with the postpartum period must be considered (see "Contraindications," "Warnings," and "Precautions" concerning thromboembolic disease). It is to be noted that early resumption of ovulation may occur if Parlodel® (bromocriptine mesylate) has been used for the prevention of lactation.

HOW SUPPLIED

Nordette®-21 Tablets (0.15 mg levonorgestrel and 0.03 mg ethinyl estradiol) are available in 6 PILPAK® dispensers of 21 tablets each as follows: NDC 0008-0075, light-orange, round tablet marked "WYETH" and "75".

References available upon request.

Brief Summary Patient Package Insert: See Lo/Ovral.
DETAILED PATIENT LABELING: See Lo/Ovral.

Shown in Product Identification Guide, page 340

NORDETTE®-28 ℞

[nor-det '-28]
TABLETS
(levonorgestrel and ethinyl estradiol tablets)

Patients should be counseled that this product does not protect against HIV infection (AIDS) and other sexually transmitted diseases.

DESCRIPTION

21 light-orange Nordette tablets, each containing 0.15 mg of levonorgestrel (*d* (-)-13 beta-ethyl -17-alpha-ethinyl-17-beta-hydroxygon-4-en-3-one), a totally synthetic progestogen, and 0.03 mg of ethinyl estradiol (19-nor-17α-pregna-1,3,5 (10)-trien-20-yne-3,17-diol), and 7 pink inert tablets. The inactive ingredients present are cellulose, D&C Red 30, FD&C Yellow 6, lactose, magnesium stearate, and polacrilin potassium.

CLINICAL PHARMACOLOGY
See NORDETTE®-21

INDICATIONS AND USAGE
See NORDETTE-21

CONTRAINDICATIONS
See NORDETTE-21

WARNINGS
See NORDETTE-21

PRECAUTIONS
See NORDETTE-21
Drug Interactions: See NORDETTE-21
Carcinogenesis: See NORDETTE-21
Nursing Mothers: See NORDETTE-21
Information for the Patient: See LO/OVRAL.

ADVERSE REACTIONS
See NORDETTE-21

OVERDOSAGE
See NORDETTE-21

NONCONTRACEPTIVE HEALTH BENEFITS
See NORDETTE-21

DOSAGE AND ADMINISTRATION

To achieve maximum contraceptive effectiveness, Nordette-28 must be taken exactly as directed and at intervals not exceeding 24 hours.

The dosage of Nordette-28 is one light-orange tablet daily for 21 consecutive days, followed by one pink inert tablet daily for 7 consecutive days, according to prescribed schedule.

It is recommended that tablets be taken at the same time each day, preferably after the evening meal or at bedtime.

During the first cycle of medication, the patient is instructed to begin taking Nordette-28 on the first Sunday after the onset of menstruation. If menstruation begins on a Sunday, the first tablet (light-orange) is taken that day. One light-orange tablet should be taken daily for 21 consecutive days, followed by one pink inert tablet daily for 7 consecutive days. Withdrawal bleeding should usually occur within three days following discontinuation of light-orange tablets. During the first cycle, contraceptive reliance should not be placed on Nordette-28 until a light-orange tablet has been taken daily for 7 consecutive days. The possibility of ovulation and conception prior to initiation of medication should be considered.

The patient begins her next and all subsequent 28-day courses of tablets on the same day of the week (Sunday) on which she began her first course, following the same schedule: 21 days on light-orange tablets—7 days on pink inert tablets. If in any cycle the patient starts tablets later than the proper day, she should protect herself by using another method of birth control until she has taken a light-orange tablet daily for 7 consecutive days.

If spotting or breakthrough bleeding occurs, the patient is instructed to continue on the same regimen. This type of bleeding is usually transient and without significance; however, if the bleeding is persistent or prolonged, the patient is advised to consult her physician. Although the occurrence of pregnancy is highly unlikely if Nordette-28 is taken according to directions, if withdrawal bleeding does not occur, the possibility of pregnancy must be considered. If the patient has not adhered to the prescribed schedule (missed one or more tablets or started taking them on a day later than she should have), the probability of pregnancy should be considered at the time of the first missed period and appropriate diagnostic measures taken before the medication is resumed. If the patient has adhered to the prescribed regimen and misses two consecutive periods, pregnancy should be ruled out before continuing the contraceptive regimen.

For additional patient instructions regarding missed pills, see the "WHAT TO DO IF YOU MISS PILLS" section in the **DETAILED PATIENT LABELING** for LO/OVRAL.

Any time the patient misses two or more light-orange tablets, she should also use another method of contraception until she has taken a light-orange tablet daily for seven consecutive days. If the patient misses one or more pink tablets, she is still protected against pregnancy **provided** she begins taking light-orange tablets again on the proper day.

If breakthrough bleeding occurs following missed light-orange tablets, it will usually be transient and of no consequence. While there is little likelihood of ovulation occurring if only one or two light-orange tablets are missed, the possibility of ovulation increases with each successive day that scheduled light-orange tablets are missed.

In the nonlactating mother, Nordette-28 may be initiated postpartum, for contraception. When the tablets are administered in the postpartum period, the increased risk of thromboembolic disease associated with the postpartum period must be considered (see "Contraindications", "Warnings", and "Precautions" concerning thromboembolic disease). It is to be noted that early resumption of ovulation may occur if Parlodel® (bromocriptine mesylate) has been used for the prevention of lactation.

HOW SUPPLIED

Nordette®-28 Tablets (0.15 mg levonorgestrel and 0.03 mg ethinyl estradiol) are available in 6 PILPAK® dispensers, each containing 28 tablets as follows:
21 active tablets, NDC 0008-2533, light-orange, round tablet marked "WYETH" and "75".
7 inert tablets, NDC 0008-0486, pink, round tablet marked "WYETH" and "486".

ALSO AVAILABLE:
Nordette®-28 Tablets (0.15 mg levonorgestrel and 0.03 mg ethinyl estradiol) are available in packages of 12 PILPAK® dispensers for clinic use only, each containing 28 tablets as follows:

21 active tablets, NDC 0008-2533, light-orange, round tablet marked "WYETH" and "75".
7 inert tablets, NDC 0008-0486, pink, round tablet marked "WYETH" and "486".

References available upon request.
Brief Summary Patient Package Insert: See LO/OVRAL.
DETAILED PATIENT LABELING: See LO/OVRAL.
HOW TO TAKE THE PILL
For Nordette-28 PILPAK® Dispenser, See LO/OVRAL.
For Nordette-28 Clinic Pilpak®, See below.
HOW TO TAKE THE PILL
This product (like all oral contraceptives) is intended to prevent pregnancy. It does not protect against transmission of HIV (AIDS) and other sexually transmitted diseases such as chlamydia, genital herpes, genital warts, gonorrhea, hepatitis B, and syphilis.

IMPORTANT POINTS TO REMEMBER

BEFORE YOU START TAKING YOUR PILLS:
1. BE SURE TO READ THESE DIRECTIONS:
Before you start taking your pills.
Anytime you are not sure what to do.
2. THE RIGHT WAY TO TAKE THE PILL IS TO TAKE ONE EVERY DAY AT THE SAME TIME.
If you miss pills you could get pregnant. This includes starting the pack late. The more pills you miss, the more likely you are to get pregnant.
3. MANY WOMEN HAVE SPOTTING OR LIGHT BLEEDING, OR MAY FEEL SICK TO THEIR STOMACH DURING THE FIRST 1–3 PACKS OF PILLS.
If you feel sick to your stomach, do not stop taking the pill. The problem will usually go away. If it does not go away, check with your doctor or clinic.
4. MISSING PILLS CAN ALSO CAUSE SPOTTING OR LIGHT BLEEDING, even when you make up these pills.
On the days you take 2 pills to make up for missed pills, you could also feel a little sick to your stomach.
5. IF YOU HAVE VOMITING OR DIARRHEA, for any reason, or IF YOU TAKE SOME MEDICINES, including some antibiotics, your pills may not work as well. Use a back-up method (such as condoms, foam, or sponge) until you check with your doctor or clinic.
6. IF YOU HAVE TROUBLE REMEMBERING TO TAKE THE PILL, talk to your doctor or clinic about how to make pill-taking easier or about using another method of birth control.
7. IF YOU HAVE QUESTIONS OR ARE UNSURE ABOUT THE INFORMATION IN THIS LEAFLET, call your doctor or clinic.
NORDETTE®-21, OVRAL®, LO/OVRAL®, NORDETTE® -28, OVRAL®-28, AND LO/OVRAL®-28

BEFORE YOU START TAKING YOUR PILLS

1. DECIDE WHAT TIME OF DAY YOU WANT TO TAKE YOUR PILL
It is important to take it at about the same time every day.
2. LOOK AT YOUR PILL PACK TO SEE IF IT HAS 21 OR 28 PILLS:
The *21-pill pack* has 21 "active" white or light-orange pills (with hormones) to take for 3 weeks, followed by 1 week without pills.
The *28-pill pack* has 21 "active" white or light-orange pills (with hormones) to take for 3 weeks, followed by 1 week of reminder pink pills (without hormones).
3. ALSO FIND:
1) where on the pack to start taking the pills,
2) in what order to take the pills (follow the arrows), and
3) the week numbers as shown in the picture below.

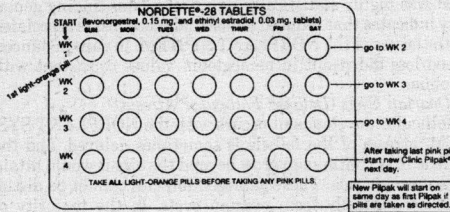

4. BE SURE YOU HAVE READY AT ALL TIMES.
ANOTHER KIND OF BIRTH CONTROL (such as condoms, foam or sponge) to use as a back-up in case you miss pills.
AND EXTRA, FULL PILL PACK

WHEN YOU START THE *FIRST* PACK OF PILLS:

For the 21-day pill pack you have two choices of which day to start taking your first pack of pills. (See **DAY 1 START** or **SUNDAY START** directions below.) Decide with your doctor or clinic which is the best day for you. The 28-day pill pack accommodates a **SUNDAY START** only. For either pill pack pick a time of day which will be easy to remember.
DAY 1 START:
These instructions are for the 21-day pill pack only. The 28-day pill pack does not accommodate a **DAY 1 START** dosage regimen.
1. Take the first "active" white or light-orange pill on the first pack during the *first 24 hours of your period*.
2. You will not need to use a back-up method of birth control, since you are starting the pill at the beginning of your period.
SUNDAY START:
These instructions are for either the 21-day or the 28-day pill pack.
1. Take the first "active" white or light-orange pill of the first pack on the *Sunday after your period starts*, even if you are still bleeding. If your period begins on Sunday, start the pack that same day.
2. *Use another method of birth control* as a back-up method if you have sex anytime from the Sunday you start you first pack until the next Sunday (7 days). Condoms, foam, or the sponge are good back-up methods of birth control.

WHAT TO DO DURING THE MONTH:

1. **TAKE ONE PILL AT THE SAME TIME EVERY DAY UNTIL THE PACK IS EMPTY.**
Do not skip pills even if you are spotting or bleeding between monthly periods or feel sick to your stomach (nausea).
Do not skip pills even if you do not have sex very often.
2. **WHEN YOU FINISH A PACK OR SWITCH YOUR BRAND OF PILLS:**
21 pills: Wait 7 days to start the next pack. You will probably have your period during that week. Be sure that no more than 7 days pass between 21-day packs.
28 pills: Start the next pack on the day after your last "reminder" pill.
Do not wait any days between packs.

WHAT TO DO IF YOU MISS PILLS

If you **MISS 1** white or light-orange "active" pill:
1. Take it as soon as you remember. Take the pill at your regular time. This means you take 2 pills in 1 day.
2. You do not need to use a back-up birth control method if you have sex.
If you **MISS 2** white or light-orange "active" pills in a row in **WEEK 1 OR WEEK 2** of your pack:
1. Take 2 pills on the day you remember and 2 pills the next day.
2. Then take 1 pill a day until you finish the pack.
3. You MAY BECOME PREGNANT if you have sex in the 7 days after you miss pills. You MUST use another birth control method (such as condoms, foam, or sponge) as a back-up for those 7 days.
If you **MISS 2** white or light-orange "active" pills in a row in **THE 3rd WEEK:**
The *Day 1 Starter* instructions are for the 21-day pill pack only. The 28-day pill pack does not accommodate a **DAY 1 START** dosage regimen. The *Sunday Starter* instructions are for either the 21-day or 28-day pill pack.
1. *If you are a Day 1 Starter:*
THROW OUT the rest of the pill pack and start a new pack that same day.
If you are a Sunday Starter:
Keep taking 1 pill every day until Sunday.
On Sunday, THROW OUT the rest of the pack and start a new pack of pills that same day.
2. You may not have your period this month but this is expected. However, if you miss your period 2 months in a row, call your doctor or clinic because you might be pregnant.
3. You MAY BECOME PREGNANT if you have sex in the 7 days after you miss pills. You MUST use another method (such as condoms, foam, or sponge) as a back-up for those 7 days.
If you **MISS 3 OR MORE** white or light-orange "active" pills in a row (during the first 3 weeks):
The *Day 1 Starter* instructions are for the 21-day pill pack only. The 28-day pill pack does not accommodate a **DAY 1 START** dosage regimen. The *Sunday Starter* instructions are for either the 21-day or 28-day pill pack.
1. *If you are a Day 1 Starter*
THROW OUT the rest of the pill pack and start a new pack that same day.

If you are a Sunday Starter
Keep taking 1 pill every day until Sunday.
On Sunday, THROW OUT the rest of the pack and start a new pack of pills that same day.
2. You may not have your period this month but this is expected. However, if you miss your period 2 months in a row, call your doctor or clinic because you might be pregnant.
3. You MAY BECOME PREGNANT if you have sex in the 7 days after you miss pills. You MUST use another birth control method (such as condoms, foam, or sponge) as a back-up for those 7 days.

A REMINDER FOR THOSE ON 28-DAY PACKS:

If you forget any of the 7 pink "reminder" pills in Week 4:
THROW AWAY the pills you missed.
Keep taking 1 pill each day until the pack is empty.
You do not need a back-up method if you start your next pack on time.

FINALLY, IF YOU ARE STILL NOT SURE WHAT TO DO ABOUT THE PILLS YOU HAVE MISSED:

Use a BACK-UP METHOD anytime you have sex.
KEEP TAKING ONE PILL EACH DAY until you can reach your doctor or clinic.
OVRETTE®
Ovrette is administered on a continuous daily dosage schedule, one tablet daily each day, every day of the year. Take the first tablet on the first day of your menstrual period, Tablets should be taken at the same time every day, without interruption, whether bleeding occurs or not. If bleeding is prolonged (more than 8 days) or unusually heavy, you should contact your doctor.
Forgotten pills
The risk of pregnancy increases with each tablet missed. Therefore, it is very important that you take one tablet daily as directed. If you miss one tablet, take it as soon as you remember and also take your next tablet at the regular time. If you miss two tablets, take one of the missed tablets as soon as you remember, as well as your regular tablet for that day at the proper time. Furthermore, you should use another method of birth control in addition to taking Ovrette until you have taken fourteen days (2 weeks) of medication. If more than two tablets have been missed, Ovrette should be discontinued immediately and another method of birth control used until the start of your next menstrual period. Then you may resume taking Ovrette.

Pregnancy due to pill failure
The incidence of pill failure resulting in pregnancy is approximately less than 1.0% if taken every day as directed, but more typical failure rates are less than 3.0%. If failure does occur, the risk to the fetus is minimal.
RISKS TO THE FETUS
If you do become pregnant while using oral contraceptives, the risk to the fetus is small, on the order of no more than one per thousand. You should, however, discuss the risks to the developing child with your doctor.
Pregnancy after stopping the pill
There may be some delay in becoming pregnant after you stop using oral contraceptives, especially if you had irregular menstrual cycles before you used oral contraceptives. It may be advisable to postpone conception until you begin menstruating regularly once you have stopped taking the pill and desire pregnancy.
There does not appear to be any increase in birth defects in newborn babies when pregnancy occurs soon after stopping the pill.
Overdosage
Serious ill effects have not been reported following ingestion of large doses of oral contraceptives by young children. Overdosage may cause nausea and withdrawal bleeding in females. In case of overdosage, contact your health-care provider or pharmacist.
Other information
Your health-care provider will take a medical and family history before prescibing oral contraceptives and will examine you. The physical examination may be delayed to another time if you request it and the health-care provider believes that it is appropriate to postpone it. You should be reexamined at least once a year. Be sure to inform your health-care provider if there is a family history of any of the conditions listed previously in this leaflet. Be sure to keep all appointments with your health-care provider, because this is a time to determine if there are early signs of side effects of oral-contraceptive use.
Do not use the drug for any condition other than the one for which it was prescribed. This drug has been prescribed specifically for you; do not give it to others who may want birth-control pills.

HEALTH BENEFITS FROM ORAL CONTRACEPTIVES: See LO/OVRAL.

Shown in Product Identification Guide, page 340

Continued on next page

Wyeth-Ayerst Laboratories—Cont.

NORPLANT® SYSTEM   ℞
(levonorgestrel implants)

Patients should be counseled that this product does not protect against HIV infection (AIDS) and other sexually transmitted diseases.
Prescribing Information

DESCRIPTION

The NORPLANT SYSTEM kit contains levonorgestrel implants, a set of six flexible closed capsules made of silicone rubber tubing (Silastic®, dimethylsiloxane/methylvinylsiloxane copolymer), each containing 36 mg of the progestin levonorgestrel contained in an insertion kit to facilitate implantation. The capsules are sealed with Silastic (polydimethylsiloxane) adhesive and sterilized. Each capsule is 2.4 mm in diameter and 34 mm in length. The capsules are inserted in a superficial plane beneath the skin of the upper arm. Information contained herewith regarding safety and efficacy was derived from studies which used two slightly different Silastic tubing formulations. The formulation being used in the NORPLANT SYSTEM has slightly higher release rates of levonorgestrel and at least comparable efficacy.
Evidence indicates that the dose of levonorgestrel provided by the NORPLANT SYSTEM is initially about 85 mcg/day followed by a decline to about 50 mcg/day by 9 months and to about 35 mcg/day by 18 months with a further decline thereafter to about 30 mcg/day. The NORPLANT SYSTEM is a progestin-only product and does not contain estrogen.
Levonorgestrel, (d(-)-13-beta-ethyl-17-alpha-ethinyl-17-beta-hydroxygon-4-en-3-one), the active ingredient in the NORPLANT SYSTEM, has a molecular weight of 312.46 and the following structural formula:

Levonorgestrel

CLINICAL PHARMACOLOGY

Levonorgestrel is a totally synthetic and biologically active progestin which exhibits no significant estrogenic activity and is highly progestational. The absolute configuration conforms to that of D-natural steroids. Levonorgestrel is not subjected to a "first-pass" effect and is virtually 100% bioavailable. Plasma concentrations average approximately 0.30 ng/mL over 5 years but are highly variable as a function of individual metabolism and body weight.
Diffusion of levonorgestrel through the wall of each capsule provides a continuous low dose of the progestin. Resulting blood levels are substantially below those generally observed among users of combination oral contraceptives containing the progestins norgestrel or levonorgestrel. Because of the range of variability in blood levels and variation in individual response, blood levels alone are not predictive of the risk of pregnancy in an individual woman.
At least two mechanisms are active in preventing pregnancy: ovulation inhibition and thickening of the cervical mucus. Other mechanisms may add to these contraceptive effects.
Levonorgestrel concentrations among women show considerable variation depending on individual clearance rates, body weight, and possibly other factors. Levonorgestrel concentrations reach a maximum, or near maximum, within 24 hours after placement with mean values of 1600 ± 1100 pg/mL. They decline rapidly over the first month partially due to a circulating protein, SHBG, that binds levonorgestrel and which is depressed by the presence of levonorgestrel. At 3 months, mean levels decline to values of around 400 pg/mL while concentrations normalized to a 60 kg body weight were 327 ± 119 (SD) pg/mL at 12 months with further decline by 1.4 pg/mL/month to reach 258 ± 95 (SD) pg/mL at 60 months. Concentrations decreased with increasing body weight by a mean of 3.3 pg/mL/kg. After capsule removal, mean concentrations drop to below 100 pg/mL by 96 hours and to below assay sensitivity (50 pg/mL) by 5 to 14 days. Fertility rates return to levels comparable to those seen in the general population of women using no method of contraception. Circulating concentrations can be used to forecast the risk of pregnancy only in a general statistical sense. Mean concentrations associated with pregnancy have been 210 ± 60 (SD) pg/mL. However, in clinical studies, 20 percent of women had one or more values below 200 pg/mL but an average annual gross pregnancy rate of less than 1.0 per 100 women through 5 years.
Although lipoprotein levels were altered in several clinical studies with the NORPLANT SYSTEM, the long-term clinical effects of these changes have not been determined. A decrease in total cholesterol levels has been reported in all lipoprotein studies and reached statistical significance in several. Both increases and decreases in high-density lipoprotein (HDL) levels have been reported in clinical trials. No statistically significant increases have been reported in the ratio of total cholesterol to HDL-cholesterol. Low-density lipoprotein (LDL) levels decreased during NORPLANT SYSTEM use. Triglyceride levels also decreased from pretreatment values.

INDICATIONS AND USAGE

The NORPLANT SYSTEM is indicated for the prevention of pregnancy and is a long-term (up to 5 years) reversible contraceptive system. The capsules should be removed by the end of the 5th year. New capsules may be inserted at that time if continuing contraceptive protection is desired.
In multicenter trials with the NORPLANT SYSTEM, involving 2470 women, the relationship between body weight and efficacy was investigated. Tabulated below is the pregnancy experience as a function of body weight. Because NORPLANT SYSTEM is a long-term method of contraception, this is reported over five years of use.
[See Table 1 below.]
Typically, pregnancy rates with contraceptive methods are reported for only the first year of use as shown below. The efficacy of these contraceptive methods, except the IUD and sterilization, depends in part on the reliability of use. The efficacy of the NORPLANT SYSTEM does not depend on patient compliance. However, no contraceptive method is 100% effective.

TABLE 2
Lowest Expected and Typical Failure Rates (%)
During the First Year of Use of a Contraceptive Method

Method	Lowest Expected	Typical
NORPLANT SYSTEM (6 capsules)	0.09	0.09
Male Sterilization	0.1	0.15
Female Sterilization	0.4	0.4
DEPO-PROVERA® (injectable progestogen)	0.3	0.3
Oral contraceptives		3
Combined	0.1	NA
Progestin only	0.5	NA
IUD		
Progesterone	1.5	2.0
Copper T 380A	0.6	0.8
Condom (male) without spermicide	3	12
(female) without spermicide	5	21
Cervical Cap		
Nulliparous women	9	18
Parous women	26	36
Diaphragm with spermicidal cream or jelly	6	18
Spermicides alone (foam, creams, jellies, and vaginal suppositories)	6	21
Periodic abstinence (all methods)	1–9*	20
Withdrawal	4	19
No contraception (planned pregnancy)	85	85

NA—not available
* Depending on method (calendar, ovulation, symptothermal, post-ovulation) Adapted from Hatcher, RA et al. *Contraceptive Technology*, 16th Revised Edition. New York, NY: Irvington Publishers, 1994.

NORPLANT SYSTEM gross annual discontinuation and continuation rates are summarized in Table 3.
[See Table 3 below.]

CONTRAINDICATIONS

1. Active thrombophlebitis or thromboembolic disorders. There is insufficient information regarding women who have had previous thromboembolic disease.
2. Undiagnosed abnormal genital bleeding.
3. Known or suspected pregnancy.
4. Acute liver disease; benign or malignant liver tumors.
5. Known or suspected carcinoma of the breast.
6. History of idiopathic intracranial hypertension.
7. Hypersensitivity to levonorgestrel or any of the other components of the NORPLANT SYSTEM.

WARNINGS

A. WARNINGS BASED ON EXPERIENCE WITH THE NORPLANT SYSTEM
1. Bleeding Irregularities
Most women can expect some variation in menstrual bleeding patterns. Irregular menstrual bleeding, intermenstrual spotting, prolonged episodes of bleeding and spotting, and amenorrhea occur in some women. Irregular bleeding patterns associated with the NORPLANT SYSTEM could mask symptoms of cervical or endometrial cancer. Overall, these irregularities diminish with continuing use. Since some NORPLANT SYSTEM users experience periods of amenorrhea, missed menstrual periods cannot serve as the only means of identifying early pregnancy. Pregnancy tests should be performed whenever a pregnancy is suspected. Six (6) weeks or more of amenorrhea after a pattern of regular menses may signal pregnancy. If pregnancy occurs, the capsules must be removed.
Although bleeding irregularities have occurred in clinical trials, proportionately more women had increases rather than decreases in hemoglobin concentrations, a difference that was highly statistically significant. This finding generally indicates that reduced menstrual blood loss is associated with the use of the NORPLANT SYSTEM. In rare instances, blood loss did result in hemoglobin values consistent with anemia.
2. Ovarian Cysts (Delayed Follicular Atresia)
If follicular development occurs with the NORPLANT SYSTEM, atresia of the follicle is sometimes delayed, and the follicle may continue to grow beyond the size it would attain in a normal cycle. These enlarged follicles can be distinguished clinically from ovarian cysts. In the majority of women, enlarged follicles will spontaneously disappear and should not require surgery. Rarely, they may twist or rupture, sometimes causing abdominal pain, and surgical intervention may be required.
3. Ectopic Pregnancies
Ectopic pregnancies have occurred among NORPLANT SYSTEM users, although clinical studies have shown no

TABLE 1
Annual and Five-Year Cumulative Pregnancy Rates
Per 100 Users by Weight Class

Weight class	year 1	year 2	year 3	year 4	year 5	Cumulative
<50 kg (<110 lbs)	0.2	0	0	0	0	0.2
50–59 kg (110–130 lbs)	0.2	0.5	0.4	2.0	0.4	3.4
60–69 kg (131–153 lbs)	0.4	0.5	1.6	1.7	0.8	5.0
≥70 kg (≥154 lbs)	0	1.1	5.1	2.5	0	8.5
All	0.2	0.5	1.2	1.6	0.4	3.9

TABLE 3
Annual and Five-Year Cumulative Rates
per 100 Users

	year 1	year 2	year 3	year 4	year 5	Cumulative
Pregnancy	0.2	0.5	1.2	1.6	0.4	3.9
Bleeding Irregularities	9.1	7.9	4.9	3.3	2.9	25.1
Medical (excl. bleeding irreg.)	6.0	5.6	4.1	4.0	5.1	22.4
Personal	4.6	7.7	11.7	10.7	11.7	38.7
Continuation	81.0	77.4	79.2	76.7	77.6	29.5

increase in the rate of ectopic pregnancies per year among NORPLANT SYSTEM users as compared with users of no method or of IUDs. The incidence among NORPLANT SYSTEM users was 1.3 per 1000 woman-years, a rate significantly below the rate that has been estimated for noncontraceptive users in the United States (2.7 to 3.0 per 1000 woman-years). The risk of ectopic pregnancy may increase with the duration of NORPLANT SYSTEM use and possibly with increased weight of the user. Physicians should be alert to the possibility of an ectopic pregnancy among women using the NORPLANT SYSTEM who become pregnant or complain of lower-abdominal pain. Any patient who presents with lower-abdominal pain must be evaluated to rule out ectopic pregnancy.

4. *Foreign-body Carcinogenesis*
Rarely, cancers have occurred at the site of foreign-body intrusions or old scars. None has been reported in NORPLANT SYSTEM clinical trials. In rodents, which are highly susceptible to such cancers, the incidence decreases with decreasing size of the foreign body. Because of the resistance of human beings to these cancers and because of the small size of the capsules, the risk to users of the NORPLANT SYSTEM is judged to be minimal.

5. *Thromboembolic Disorders and Other Vascular Problems*
An increased risk of thromboembolic and thrombotic disease (pulmonary embolism, superficial venous thrombosis, and deep-vein thrombosis) has been found to be associated with the use of combination oral contraceptives. The relative risk has been estimated to be 4- to 11-fold higher for users than for nonusers. There have also been post-marketing reports of these events coincident with NORPLANT SYSTEM use. The reports of thrombophlebitis and superficial phlebitis have more commonly occurred in the arm of insertion. Some of these cases have been associated with trauma to that arm.
Cerebrovascular Disorders: Combination oral contraceptives have been shown to increase both the relative and attributable risks of cerebrovascular events (thrombotic and hemorrhagic strokes), although, in general, the risk is greatest among older (> 35 years) hypertensive women who also smoke. Hypertension was found to be a risk factor for both users and nonusers for both types of strokes, while smoking interacted to increase the risk for hemorrhagic strokes. There have been post-marketing reports of stroke coincident with NORPLANT SYSTEM use.
Myocardial Infarction: An increased risk of myocardial infarction has been attributed to combination oral-contraceptive use. This is thought to be primarily thrombotic in origin and is related to the estrogen component of combination oral contraceptives. This increased risk occurs primarily in smokers or in women with other underlying risk factors for coronary-artery disease, such as family history of coronary-artery disease, hypertension, hypercholesterolemia, morbid obesity, and diabetes. The current relative risk of heart attack for combination oral-contraceptive users has been estimated as 2 to 6 times the risk for nonusers. The absolute risk is very low for women under 30 years of age.
Studies indicate a significant trend toward higher rates of myocardial infarctions and strokes with increasing doses of progestin in combination oral contraceptives. However, a recent study showed no increased risk of myocardial infarction associated with the past use of levonorgestrel-containing combination oral contraceptives. There have been post-marketing reports of myocardial infarction coincident with NORPLANT SYSTEM use.
Patients who develop active thrombophlebitis or thromboembolic disease should have the NORPLANT SYSTEM capsules removed. Removal should also be considered in women who will be subjected to prolonged immobilization due to surgery or other illnesses.

6. *Use Before or During Early Pregnancy*
Extensive epidemiological studies have revealed no increased risk of birth defects in women who have used oral contraceptives prior to pregnancy. Studies also do not suggest a teratogenic effect, particularly insofar as cardiac anomalies and limb-reduction defects are concerned, when taken inadvertently during early pregnancy. There is no evidence suggesting that the risk associated with NORPLANT SYSTEM use is different.
There have been rare reports of congenital anomalies in offspring of women who were using the NORPLANT SYSTEM inadvertently during early pregnancy. A cause and effect relationship is not believed to exist.

7. *Idiopathic Intracranial Hypertension*
Idiopathic intracranial hypertension (pseudotumor cerebri, benign intracranial hypertension) is a disorder of unknown etiology which is seen most commonly in obese females of reproductive age. There have been reports of idiopathic intracranial hypertension in NORPLANT SYSTEM users. A cardinal sign of idiopathic intracranial hypertension is papilledema; early symptoms may include headache (associated with a change in frequency, pattern, severity, or persistence; of particular importance are those headaches that are unremitting in nature) and visual disturbances. Patients with these symptoms, particularly obese patients or those with recent weight gain, should be screened for papilledema and, if present, the patient should be referred to a neurologist for further diagnosis and care. NORPLANT SYSTEM should be removed from patients experiencing this disorder.

B. WARNINGS BASED ON EXPERIENCE WITH COMBINATION (PROGESTIN PLUS ESTROGEN) ORAL CONTRACEPTIVES

1. *Cigarette Smoking*
Cigarette smoking increases the risk of serious cardiovascular side effects from the use of combination oral contraceptives. This risk increases with age and with heavy smoking (15 or more cigarettes per day) and is quite marked in women over 35 years old. While this is believed to be an estrogen-related effect, it is not known whether a similar risk exists with progestin-only methods such as the NORPLANT SYSTEM; however, women who use the NORPLANT SYSTEM should be advised not to smoke.

2. *Elevated Blood Pressure*
Increased blood pressure has been reported in users of combination oral contraceptives. The prevalence of elevated blood pressure increases with long exposure. Although there were no statistically significant trends among NORPLANT SYSTEM users in clinical trials, physicians should be aware of the possibility of elevated blood pressure with the NORPLANT SYSTEM.

3. *Carcinoma*
Numerous epidemiological studies have been performed to determine the incidence of breast, endometrial, ovarian, and cervical cancer in women using combination oral contraceptives. Recent evidence in the literature suggests that use of combination oral contraceptives is not associated with an increased risk of developing breast cancer in the overall population of users. The Cancer and Steroid Hormone (CASH) study also showed no latent effect on the risk of breast cancer for at least a decade following long-term use. However, some of these same recent studies have shown an increased relative risk of breast cancer in certain subgroups of combination oral-contraceptive users, although no consistent pattern of findings has been identified. This information should be considered when prescribing the NORPLANT SYSTEM.
Some studies suggest that combination oral-contraceptive use has been associated with an increase in the risk of cervical intraepithelial neoplasia in some populations of women. However, there continues to be controversy about the extent to which such findings may be due to differences in sexual behavior and other factors. In spite of many studies of the relationship between combination oral-contraceptive use and breast and cervical cancers, a cause-and-effect relationship has not been established.
Evidence indicates that combination oral contraceptives may decrease the risk of ovarian and endometrial cancer. Irregular bleeding patterns associated with the NORPLANT SYSTEM could mask symptoms of cervical or endometrial cancer.

4. *Hepatic Tumors*
Hepatic adenomas have been found to be associated with the use of combination oral contraceptives with an estimated incidence of about 3 occurrences per 100,000 users per year, a risk that increases after 4 or more years of use. Although benign, hepatic adenomas may rupture and cause death through intra-abdominal hemorrhage. The contribution of the progestin component of oral contraceptives to the development of hepatic adenomas is not known.

5. *Ocular Lesions*
There have been clinical case reports of retinal thrombosis associated with the use of oral contraceptives. Although it is believed that this adverse reaction is related to the estrogen component of oral contraceptives, the NORPLANT SYSTEM capsules should be removed if there is unexplained partial or complete loss of vision; onset of proptosis or diplopia; papilledema; or retinal vascular lesions. Appropriate diagnostic and therapeutic measures should be undertaken immediately.

6. *Gallbladder Disease*
Earlier studies have reported an increased lifetime relative risk of gallbladder surgery in users of oral contraceptives and estrogens. More recent studies, however, have shown that the relative risk of developing gallbladder disease among oral-contraceptive users may be minimal. The recent findings of minimal risk may be related to the use of oral-contraceptive formulations containing lower hormonal doses of estrogens and progestins. The association of this risk with use of the NORPLANT SYSTEM progestin-only method is not known.

PRECAUTIONS

GENERAL

Patients should be counseled that this product does not protect against HIV infection (AIDS) and other sexually transmitted diseases.

1. *Physical Examination and Follow-Up*
A complete medical history and physical examination should be taken prior to the implantation or reimplantation of NORPLANT SYSTEM capsules and at least annually during its use. These physical examinations should include special reference to the implant site, blood pressure, breasts, abdomen and pelvic organs, including cervical cytology and relevant laboratory tests. In case of undiagnosed, persistent or recurrent abnormal vaginal bleeding, appropriate diagnostic measures should be conducted to rule out malignancy. Women with a strong family history of breast cancer or who have breast nodules should be monitored with particular care.

2. *Carbohydrate Metabolism*
An altered glucose tolerance characterized by decreased insulin sensitivity following glucose loading has been found in some users of combination and progestin-only oral contraceptives. The effects of the NORPLANT SYSTEM on carbohydrate metabolism appear to be minimal. In a study in which pretreatment serum-glucose levels were compared with levels after 1 and 2 years of NORPLANT SYSTEM use, no statistically significant differences in mean serum-glucose levels were evident 2 hours after glucose loading. The clinical significance of these findings is unknown, but diabetic patients should be carefully observed while using the NORPLANT SYSTEM.
Women who are being treated for hyperlipidemias should be followed closely if they elect to use the NORPLANT SYSTEM. Some progestins may elevate LDL levels and may render the control of hyperlipidemias more difficult. (See "Warnings," A.5.)

3. *Liver Function*
If jaundice develops in any women while using the NORPLANT SYSTEM, consideration should be given to removing the capsules. Steroid hormones may be poorly metabolized in patients with impaired liver function.

4. *Fluid Retention*
Steroid contraceptives may cause some degree of fluid retention. They should be prescribed with caution, and only with careful monitoring, in patients with conditions which might be aggravated by fluid retention.

5. *Emotional Disorders*
Consideration should be given to removing NORPLANT SYSTEM capsules in women who become significantly depressed since the symptom may be drug-related. Women with a history of depression should be carefully observed and removal considered if depression recurs to a serious degree.

6. *Contact Lenses*
Contact-lens wearers who develop visual changes or changes in lens tolerance should be assessed by an ophthalmologist.

7. *Autoimmune Disease*
Autoimmune diseases such as scleroderma, systemic lupus erythematosus and rheumatoid arthritis occur in the general population and more frequently among women of childbearing age. There have been rare reports of various autoimmune diseases, including the above, in NORPLANT SYSTEM users; however, the rate of reporting is significantly less than the expected incidence for these diseases. Studies have raised the possibility of developing antibodies against silicone-containing devices; however, the specificity and clinical relevance of these antibodies are unknown. While it is believed that the occurrence of autoimmune disease among NORPLANT SYSTEM users is coincidental, health-care providers should be alert to the earliest manifestations.

8. *Insertion and Removal*
To be sure that the woman is not pregnant at the time of capsule placement and to assure contraceptive effectiveness during the first cycle of use, it is advisable that insertion be done during the first 7 days of the menstrual cycle or immediately following an abortion. However, NORPLANT SYSTEM capsules may be inserted at any time during the cycle provided pregnancy has been excluded and a nonhormonal contraceptive method is used for at least 7 days following insertion. Insertion is not recommended before 6 weeks post-partum in breast-feeding women.
Insertion and removal are not difficult procedures but instructions must be followed closely. It is strongly advised that all health-care professionals who insert and remove NORPLANT SYSTEM capsules be instructed in the procedures before they attempt them. A proper insertion just under the skin will facilitate removals. Proper NORPLANT SYSTEM insertion and removal should result in minimal scarring. If the capsules are placed too deeply, they can be harder to remove. There have been infrequent reports of the use of general anesthesia during the removal procedure; it is generally not required. Before initiating the removal procedure, all NORPLANT SYSTEM capsules should be located via palpation. If all six capsules cannot be palpated, they may be localized via ultrasound (7 MHz), X ray, or compression mammography. If all capsules cannot be removed at the first attempt, removal should be attempted later when the site has healed. Bruising may occur at the implant site during insertion or removal. Other cutaneous reactions that have been reported include blistering, ulcerations and sloughing. There have been reports of arm pain, numbness and tingling following these procedures. In some women, hyperpigmentation occurs over the implantation site but is usually reversible following removal. See detailed Insertion and Removal Instructions below.

Continued on next page

Wyeth-Ayerst Laboratories—Cont.

9. Infections

Infection at the implant site, including cellulitis, has been uncommon. Attention to aseptic technique and proper insertion and removal of the NORPLANT SYSTEM capsules reduces the possibility of infection. If infection occurs, suitable treatment should be instituted. If infection persists, the capsules should be removed.

10. Capsule Expulsion and Displacement

Expulsion of capsules was uncommon. It occurred more frequently when placement of the capsules was extremely shallow, too close to the incision, or when infection was present. Replacement of an expelled capsule must be accomplished using a new sterile capsule. If infection is present, it should be treated and cured before replacement. Contraceptive efficacy may be inadequate with fewer than 6 capsules.

There have been reports of capsule displacement (i.e., movement) most of which involve minor changes in the positioning of the capsules. However, infrequent reports of significant displacement (a few to several inches) have been received. Some reports have been associated with pain or discomfort. In the event that capsule movement occurs, the removal technique may need to be modified, such as additional incisions or visits.

11. Provisions for Removal

Women should be advised that the capsules will be removed at any time for any reason. The removal should be done on such request or at the end of 5 years of usage by personnel instructed in the removal technique.

Upon removal, NORPLANT SYSTEM capsules should be disposed of in accordance with Center for Disease Control Guidelines for the handling of biohazardous waste.

DRUG INTERACTIONS

Reduced efficacy (pregnancy) has been reported for NORPLANT SYSTEM users taking phenytoin and carbamazepine. These drugs may increase the metabolism of levonorgestrel through induction of microsomal liver enzymes. NORPLANT SYSTEM users should be warned of the possibility of decreased efficacy with the use of the drugs exhibiting enzyme-inducing activity such as those noted above and rifampicin. For women receiving long-term therapy with hepatic enzyme inducers, another method of contraception should be considered.

DRUG/LABORATORY TEST INTERACTIONS

Certain endocrine tests may be affected by NORPLANT SYSTEM use:
1. Sex-hormone-binding globulin concentrations are decreased.
2. Thyroxine concentrations may be slightly decreased and triiodothyronine uptake increased.

CARCINOGENESIS

See "Warnings" section.

PREGNANCY

Pregnancy Category X. See "Warnings" section.

NURSING MOTHERS

Steroids are not considered the contraceptives of first choice for breast-feeding women. Levonorgestrel has been identified in the breast milk. The health of breast-fed infants whose mothers began using the NORPLANT SYSTEM during the 5th to 7th week postpartum was evaluated: no significant effects were observed on the growth or development of infants who were followed to 12 months of age. No data are available on use in breast-feeding mothers earlier than this after parturition.

INFORMATION FOR THE PATIENT

See Patient Labeling.

Two copies of the Patient Labeling are included to help describe the characteristics of the NORPLANT SYSTEM to the patient. One copy should be provided to the patient. Patients should also be advised that the Prescribing Information is available to them at their request. It is recommended that propective users be fully informed about the risks and benefits associated with use of the NORPLANT SYSTEM, with other forms of contraception, and with no contraception at all. It is also recommended that prospective users be fully informed about the insertion and removal procedures. Health-care providers may wish to obtain informed consent from all patients in light of the techniques involved with insertion and removal.

ADVERSE REACTIONS

The following adverse reactions have been associated with the NORPLANT SYSTEM during the first year of use. They include:

Many bleeding days or prolonged bleeding	27.6%
Spotting	17.1%
Amenorrhea	9.4%
Irregular (onsets of) bleeding	7.6%
Frequent bleeding onsets	7.0%
Scanty bleeding	5.2%
Pain or itching near implant site (usually transient)	3.7%

Infection at implant site	0.7%

In addition, removal difficulties have been reported with a frequency of 6.2%, which is based on 849 removals occurring through 5 years of use.

Clinical studies comparing NORPLANT® SYSTEM users with other contraceptive method users suggest that the following adverse reactions occurring during the first year are probably associated with NORPLANT SYSTEM use. These reactions have also been reported post-marketing:

Headache
Nervousness, Anxiety
Nausea/Vomiting
Dizziness
Adnexal enlargement
Dermatitis/Rash
Acne
Change of appetite
Mastalgia
Weight gain
Hirsutism, hypertrichosis, and scalp-hair loss

In addition, the following adverse reactions have been reported with a frequency of 5% or greater during the first year and are possibly related to NORPLANT SYSTEM use:

Breast discharge
Cervicitis
Musculoskeletal pain
Abdominal discomfort
Leukorrhea
Vaginitis

The following adverse reactions have been reported post-marketing with an incidence of less than 1% and are possibly related to NORPLANT SYSTEM use:

Emotional lability
Idiopathic intracranial hypertension (IIH, pseudotumor cerebri, benign intracranial hypertension)
Dysmenorrhea
Migraine
Arm pain
Numbness
Tingling
Depression

The following adverse reactions have been reported post-marketing with an incidence of less than 1%. These events occurred under circumstances where a causal relationship to the NORPLANT SYSTEM is unknown. These reactions are listed as information for physicians:

Congenital anomalies
Pulmonary embolism
Superficial venous thrombosis
Deep-vein thrombosis
Myocardial infarction
Thrombotic thrombocytopenic purpura (TTP)
Stroke
Pruritus
Urticaria
Asthenia (fatigue/weakness)

OVERDOSAGE

Overdosage can result if more than six capsules of the NORPLANT SYSTEM are in situ. All implanted NORPLANT SYSTEM capsules should be removed before inserting a new set of NORPLANT SYSTEM capsules. Overdosage may cause fluid retention with its associated effects and uterine bleeding irregularities.

DOSAGE AND ADMINISTRATION

The NORPLANT SYSTEM consists of six Silastic® capsules, each containing 36 mg of the progestin, levonorgestrel. The total administered (implanted) dose is 216 mg. Implantation of all six capsules should be performed during the first 7 days of the onset of menses by a health-care professional instructed in the NORPLANT SYSTEM insertion technique. Insertion is subdermal in the midportion of the upper arm about 8 to 10 cm above the elbow crease. Distribution should be in a fanlike pattern, about 15 degrees apart, for a total of 75 degrees. Proper insertion will facilitate later removal. (See section on Insertion/Removal.)

HOW SUPPLIED

The NORPLANT SYSTEM Kit includes the following items:
1 NORPLANT SYSTEM (levonorgestrel implants), a set of six implants (capsules)
1 NORPLANT SYSTEM trocar
1 Scalpel
1 Forceps
1 Syringe
2 Syringe needles
1 Package of skin closures
3 Packages of gauze sponges
1 Stretch bandage
1 Surgical drape (fenestrated)
2 Surgical drapes

Store at room temperature away from excess heat and moisture.

Note: The indented statement below is required by the Federal government's Clean Air Act for all products containing or manufactured with chlorofluorocarbons (CFC's).

> **WARNING:** Manufactured with dichlorodifluoromethane, a substance which harms public health and environment by destroying ozone in the upper atmosphere.

A notice similar to the above WARNING has been placed in the patient information leaflet of this product pursuant to EPA regulations.

Dichlorodifluoromethane is a chemical used in the sterilization process of the NORPLANT SYSTEM and is not contained in the product itself.

NDC 0008-2564-01

References available upon request.

INSTRUCTIONS FOR INSERTION AND REMOVAL

The NORPLANT SYSTEM consists of six levonorgestrel-releasing capsules that are inserted subdermally in the medial aspect of the upper arm.

The NORPLANT SYSTEM provides up to 5 years of effective contraceptive protection.

The basis for successful use and subsequent removal of NORPLANT SYSTEM capsules is a correct and carefully performed subdermal insertion of the six capsules. It is recommended that health-care professionals performing insertions or removals of NORPLANT SYSTEM capsules avail themselves of instruction and supervision in the proper technique prior to attempting these procedures. During insertion, special attention should be given to the following:
—asepsis.
—correct subdermal placement of the capsules.
—careful technique to minimize tissue trauma.

This will help to avoid infections and excessive scarring at the insertion area and will help keep the capsules from being inserted too deeply in the tissue. If the capsules are placed too deeply, they will be more difficult to remove than correctly placed subdermal capsules.

INSERTION PROCEDURE

Insertion should be performed within seven days from the onset of menses. However, NORPLANT SYSTEM capsules may be inserted at any time during the cycle provided pregnancy has been excluded and a nonhormonal contraceptive method is used for at least 7 days following insertion. It is recommended that a complete history and physical examination, including a gynecologic examination, be performed before the insertion of NORPLANT SYSTEM capsules. Determine if the subject has any allergies to the antiseptic or anesthetic to be used or contraindications to progestin-only contraception. If none are found, the capsules are inserted using the procedure outlined below.

One NORPLANT SYSTEM set consists of six capsules in a sterile pouch. The insertion is performed under aseptic conditions using a trocar to place the capsules under the skin.

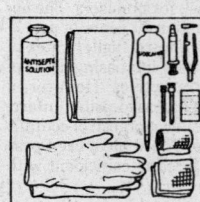

Figure 1: The following equipment is recommended for the insertion:
—an examining table for the patient to lie on.
—sterile surgical drapes, sterile gloves (free of talc), antiseptic solution.
—local anesthetic, needles, and syringe.
—#11 scalpel, #10 trocar, forceps.
—skin closure, sterile gauze, and compresses.

The plastic cover and tray are NOT STERILE.

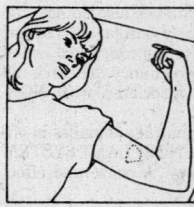

Figure 2: Have the patient lie on her back on the examination table with her left arm (if the patient is left-handed, the right arm) flexed at the elbow and externally rotated so that her hand is lying by her head. The capsules will be inserted subdermally through a small 2-mm incision and positioned in a fanlike manner with the fan opening towards the shoulder.

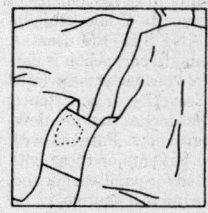

Figure 3: Prep the patient's upper arm with antiseptic solution; cover the arm above and below the insertion area with a sterile cloth. The optimal insertion area is in the inside of the upper arm about 8 to 10 cm above the elbow crease.

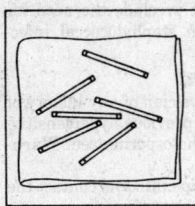

Figure 4: Open the sterile NOR-PLANT SYSTEM package carefully by pulling apart the sheets of the pouch, allowing the capsules to fall onto a sterile drape. Count the six capsules.

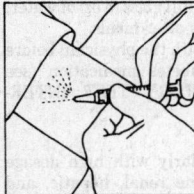

Figure 5: After determining the absence of known allergies to the anesthetic agent or related drugs, fill a 5-mL syringe with the local anesthetic. Since blood loss is minimal with this procedure, use of epinephrine-containing anesthetics is not considered necessary. Anesthetize the insertion area by first inserting the needle under the skin and injecting a small amount of anesthetic. Then anesthetize six areas about 4 to 4.5 cm long, to mimic the fanlike position of the implanted capsules.

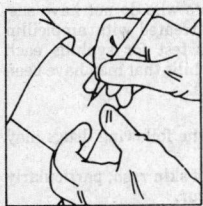

Figure 6: Use the scalpel to make a small incision (about 2 mm) just through the dermis of the skin.
Alternatively, the trocar may be inserted directly through the skin without making an incision with the scalpel. The bevel of the trocar should always face up during the insertion.

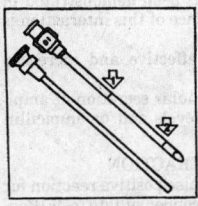

Figure 7: The trocar has two marks on it. The first mark is closer to the hub and indicates how far the trocar should be introduced under the skin before the loading of each capsule. The second mark is close to the tip and indicates how much of the trocar should remain under the skin following the insertion of each implant.

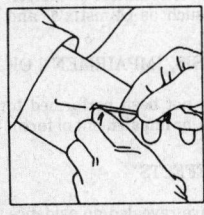

Figure 8: Insert the tip of the trocar through the incision beneath the skin at a shallow angle. Once the trocar is inserted, it should be oriented with the the bevel up toward the skin to keep the capsules in a superficial plane. It is important to keep the trocar subdermal by tenting the skin with the trocar, as failure to do so may result in deep placement of the capsules and could make removal more difficult.
Advance the trocar gently under the skin to the first mark near the hub of the trocar. The tip of the trocar is now at a distance of about 4 to 4.5 cm from the incision.
Do not force the trocar, and if resistance is felt, try another direction.

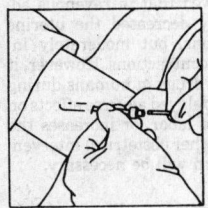

Figure 9: When the trocar has been inserted the appropriate distance, remove the obturator and load the first capsule into the trocar using the thumb and forefinger.

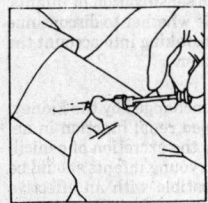

Figure 10: Gently advance the capsule with the obturator towards the tip of the trocar until you feel resistance. Never force the obturator.

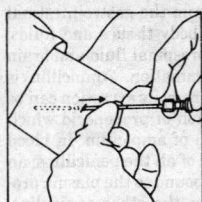

Figure 11: Hold the obturator steady, and bring the trocar back until it touches the handle of the obturator.

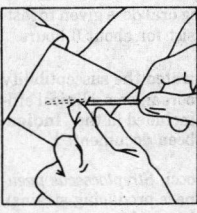

Figure 12: The capsule should have been released under the skin when the mark close to the tip of the trocar is visible in the incision. Release of the capsule can be checked by palpation. It is important to keep the obturator steady and not to push the capsule into the tissue.

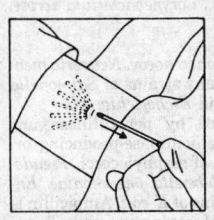

Figure 13: Do not remove the trocar from the incision until all capsules have been inserted. The trocar is withdrawn only to the mark close to its tip. Each succeeding capsule is always inserted next to the previous one, to form a fanlike shape. Fix the position of the previous capsule with the forefinger and and middle finger of the free hand, and advance the trocar along the tips of the fingers. This will ensure a suitable distance of about 15 degrees between capsules and keep the trocar from puncturing any of the previously inserted capsules.
Leave a distance of about 5 mm between the incision and the tips of the capsules. This will help avoid spontaneous expulsions. The correct position of the capsules can be ensured by feeling them with the fingers after the insertion has been completed.

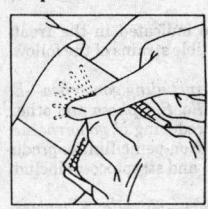

Figure 14: After placement of the sixth capsule, a sterile gauze may be used to apply pressure briefly to the insertion site to ensure hemostasis. Palpate the distal ends of the capsules to make sure that all six have been properly placed.

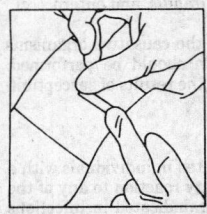

Figure 15: Press the edges of the incision together, and close the incision with a skin closure. Suturing the incision should not be necessary.

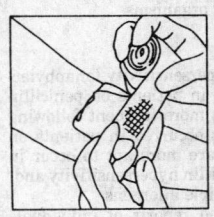

Figure 16: Cover the insertion area with a dry compress, and wrap gauze around the arm to ensure hemostasis.
Observe the patient for a few minutes for signs of syncope or bleeding from the incision before she is discharged.
Advise the patient to keep the insertion area dry and avoid heavy lifting for 2 to 3 days. The gauze may be removed after 1 day, and the butterfly bandage as soon as the incision has healed, i.e., normally in 3 days.

REMOVAL PROCEDURE

Described below is a removal procedure which was developed and used during the clinical trials for the NORPLANT SYSTEM. As with many surgical procedures, variations of the technique have appeared and some have been published. No one particular procedure routinely appears to have any advantage over another.
It is recommended that removals be prescheduled so that preparations for carrying out the procedure can be facilitated.
Removal of the capsules should be performed very gently and will usually take more time than insertion. Capsules are sometimes nicked, cut, or broken during removal. The incidence of overall removal difficulties, including damage to capsules, has been 13.2 percent. Less than half of these removal difficulties have caused inconvenience to the patient. If the removal of some of the capsules proves difficult, have the patient return for another visit. The remaining capsule(s) will be easier to remove after the area is healed. It may be appropriate to seek consultation or provide referral for patients in whom initial attempts at capsule removal prove difficult. If contraception is still desired, a barrier method should be advised until all capsules are removed. The position of the patient and the asepsis are the same as for insertion.

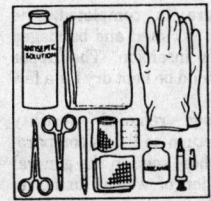

Figure 17: The following equipment is needed for the removal:
—an examining table for the patient to lie on.
—sterile surgical drapes, sterile gloves (free of talc), antiseptic solution.
—local anesthetic, needles, and syringe.
—#11 scalpel, forceps (straight and curved mosquito).
—skin closure, sterile gauze, and compresses.

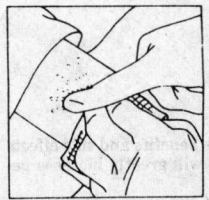

Figure 18: Palpate the capsules to make sure that all six capsules have been located, marking their position with a sterile marker. If all six capsules cannot be palpated, they may be localized via ultrasound (7 MHz), X ray, or compression mammography.

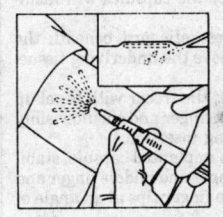

Figure 19: Once all six capsules are located, apply a small amount of local anesthetic *under* the capsule ends nearest the original incision site. This will serve to raise the ends of the capsules. Anesthetic injected over the capsules will obscure them and make removal more difficult. Additional small amounts of the anesthetic can be used for the removal of each of the capsules, if required.

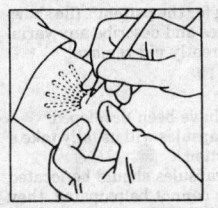

Figure 20: Make a 4-mm incision with the scalpel close to the ends of the capsules. Do not make a large incision.

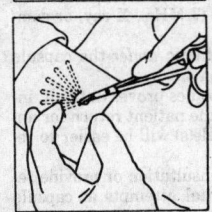

Figure 21: Push each capsule gently towards the incision with the fingers. When the tip is visible or near to the incision, grasp it with a mosquito forceps.

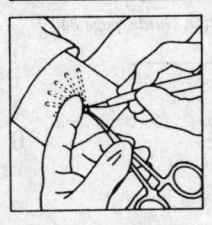

Figure 22: Use the scalpel, forceps, or gauze to very gently open the tissue sheath that has formed around the capsule.

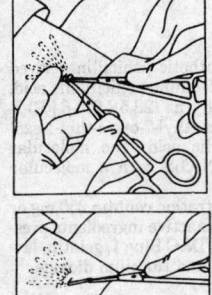

Figures 23 and 24: Remove the capsule from the incision with the second forceps.

Continued on next page

Wyeth-Ayerst Laboratories—Cont.

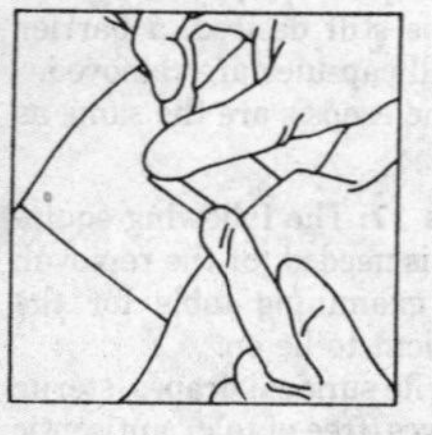

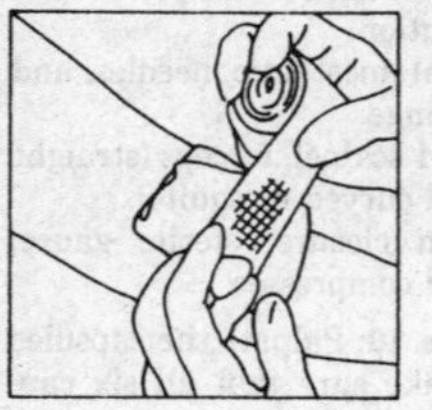

Figures 25 and 26: After the procedure is completed, the incision is closed and bandaged as with insertion. The upper arm should be kept dry for a few days.

Following removal, fertility rates return to levels comparable to those seen in the general population of women using no method of contraception, and a pregnancy may occur at any time.

HINTS

Insertion

—Counselling of the patient on the benefits and side effects of the method prior to insertion will greatly increase patient satisfaction.
—Correct subdermal placement of the capsules will facilitate removal.
—Before insertion, apply the anesthetic just beneath the skin so as to raise the dermis above the underlying tissue.
—Never force the trocar.
—To ensure subdermal placement, the trocar with bevel up should be supported by the index finger and should visibly raise the skin at all times during insertion.
—To avoid damaging the previous implanted capsule, stabilize the capsule with your forefinger and middle finger and advance the trocar alongside the finger tips at an angle of 15 degrees.
—After insertion, make a drawing for the patient's file showing the location of the 6 capsules and describe any variations in placement. This will greatly aid removal.

Removal

—Alternate removal techniques have been developed.
—The removal of the implanted capsules will usually take a little more time than the insertion.
—Before initiating removal, all capsules should be located by palpation. If all six capsules cannot be palpated, they may be localized via ultrasound (7 MHz), X ray, or compression mammography.
—Before removal, apply the anesthetic *under* the capsule ends nearest the original incision site.
—If the removal of some of the capsules proves difficult, interrupt the procedure and have the patient return for another visit. The remaining capsule(s) will be easier to remove after the area is healed.
—It may be appropriate to seek consultation or provide referral for patients in whom initial attempts at capsule removal prove difficult.

Shown in Product Identification Guide, page 340

OMNIPEN® ℞

[om 'nī-pen]
(ampicillin)
CAPSULES

DESCRIPTION

Omnipen (ampicillin) is a semisynthetic penicillin derived from the basic penicillin nucleus, 6-amino-penicillanic acid. Ampicillin is designated chemically as (2S,5R,6R)-6-[(R)-2-Amino-2-phenylacetamido] -3,3- dimethyl-7-oxo-4-thia-1-aza -bicyclo [3.2.0] heptane-2-carboxylic acid. The molecular formula for ampicillin is $C_{16}H_{19}N_3O_4S$ with a molecular weight of 349.40.

Omnipen capsules for oral administration contain 250 mg or 500 mg ampicillin anhydrous. The inactive ingredients present are D&C Red 22, D&C Red 28, FD&C Blue 1, gelatin, lactose, methylcellulose, stearic acid, and titanium dioxide.

CLINICAL PHARMACOLOGY

Ampicillin is bactericidal at low concentrations and is clinically effective not only against the gram-positive organisms usually susceptible to penicillin G, but also against a variety of gram-negative organisms. It is stable in the presence of gastric acid and is well absorbed from the gastrointestinal tract. It diffuses readily into most body tissues and fluids; however, penetration into the cerebrospinal fluid and brain occurs only with meningeal inflammation. Ampicillin is excreted largely unchanged in the urine; its excretion can be delayed by concurrent administration of probenecid which inhibits the renal tubular secretion of ampicillin. In blood serum, ampicillin is the least bound of all the penicillins; an average of about 20% of the drug is bound to the plasma proteins as compared to 60 to 90% for the other penicillins. Blood serum levels of approximately 2 mcg/mL are attained within 1 to 2 hours following a 250 mg oral dose given to fasting adults. Detectable amounts persist for about 6 hours.

MICROBIOLOGY

While *in vitro* studies have demonstrated the susceptibility of most strains of the following microorganisms, clinical efficacy for infections other than those included in the "**Indications and Usage**" section has not been documented.

Gram-Positive

Alpha- and beta-hemolytic streptococci, *Streptococcus pneumoniae,* staphylococci (non-penicillinase-producing strains), *Bacillus anthracis, Clostridium* sp., *Corynebacterium xerose,* and most strains of enterococci.

Gram-Negative

Hemophilus influenzae, Neisseria gonorrhoeae, Neisseria meningitidis, Proteus mirabilis, and many strains of *Salmonella* (including *S. typhosa*), *Shigella,* and *Escherichia coli.*

NOTE: Ampicillin is inactivated by penicillinase and therefore is ineffective against penicillinase-producing organisms including certain strains of staphylococci, *Pseudomonas aeruginosa, P. vulgaris, Klebsiella pneumoniae, Enterobacter aerogenes,* and some strains of *E. coli.* Ampicillin is not active against Rickettsia, Mycoplasma, and "large viruses" (Miyagawanella).

Testing for Susceptibility

The invading organism should be cultured and its susceptibility demonstrated as a guide to therapy. If the Kirby-Bauer method of disc susceptibility is used, a 10 mcg ampicillin disc should be used to determine the relative *in vitro* susceptibility.

INDICATIONS AND USAGE

Omnipen (ampicillin) Capsules are indicated in the treatment of infections caused by susceptible strains of the following microorganisms:

Infections of the genitourinary tract including gonorrhea—E. coli, P. mirabilis, enterococci, *Shigella, S. typhosa* and other *Salmonella,* and non-penicillinase-producing *N. gonorrhoeae.*

Infections of the respiratory tract—Non-penicillinase-producing *H. influenzae* and staphylococci, and streptococci including *Streptococcus pneumoniae.*

Infections of the gastrointestinal tract—Shigella, S. typhosa and other *Salmonella, E. coli, P. mirabilis,* and enterococci.

Meningitis—N. meningitidis.

Bacteriology studies to determine the causative organisms and their sensitivity to ampicillin should be performed. Therapy may be instituted prior to the results of susceptibility testing.

CONTRAINDICATIONS

The use of this drug is contraindicated in individuals with a history of a previous hypersensitivity reaction to any of the penicillins. Ampicillin is also contraindicated in infections caused by penicillinase-producing organisms.

WARNINGS

Serious and occasionally fatal hypersensitivity (anaphylactic) reactions have been reported in patients on penicillin therapy. Although anaphylaxis is more frequent following parenteral administration, it has occurred in patients on oral penicillins. These reactions are more apt to occur in individuals with a history of penicillin hypersensitivity and/or a history of sensitivity to multiple allergens.

There have been well-documented reports of individuals with a history of penicillin hypersensitivity who experienced severe hypersensitivity reactions when treated with cephalosporins. Before initiating therapy with any penicillin, careful inquiry should be made concerning previous hypersensitivity reactions to penicillins, cephalosporins, or other allergens. If an allergic reaction occurs, the drug should be discontinued and appropriate therapy should be instituted.

Serious anaphylactoid reactions require immediate emergency treatment with epinephrine. Oxygen, intravenous steroids, and airway management, including intubation, should also be administered as indicated.

PRECAUTIONS

GENERAL

Prolonged use of antibiotics may promote the overgrowth of nonsusceptible organisms, including fungi. Should superinfection occur, appropriate measures should be taken.

Patients with gonorrhea who also have syphilis should be given additional appropriate parenteral penicillin treatment.

Treatment with ampicillin does not preclude the need for surgical procedures, particularly in staphylococcal infections.

INFORMATION FOR THE PATIENT

1. The patient should inform the physician of any history of sensitivity to allergens, including previous hypersensitivity reactions to penicillins and cephalosporins (see "**Warnings**").
2. The patient should discontinue ampicillin and contact the physician immediately if any side effect occurs (see "**Warnings**").
3. Ampicillin should be taken with a full glass (8 oz) of water, one-half hour before or two hours after meals.
4. Diabetic patients should consult with the physician before changing diet or dosage of diabetes medication (see "**Precautions**—DRUG/LABORATORY TEST INTERACTION").

LABORATORY TESTS

In prolonged therapy, and particularly with high dosage regimens, periodic evaluation of the renal, hepatic, and hematopoietic systems is recommended.

In streptococcal infections, therapy must be sufficient to eliminate the organism (10 days minimum); otherwise, the sequelae of streptococcal disease may occur. Cultures should be taken following completion of treatment to determine whether streptococci have been eradicated.

Cases of gonococcal infection with a suspected lesion of syphilis should have dark-field examinations ruling out syphilis before receiving ampicillin. Patients who do not have suspected lesions of syphilis and are treated with ampicillin should have a follow-up serologic test for syphilis each month for four months to detect syphilis that may have been masked by treatment for gonorrhea.

DRUG INTERACTIONS

When administered concurrently, the following drugs may interact with ampicillin:

Allopurinol—Increased possibility of skin rash, particularly in hyperuricemic patients, may occur.

Bacteriostatic antibiotics—Chloramphenicol, erythromycins, sulfonamides, or tetracyclines may interfere with the bactericidal effect of penicillins. This has been demonstrated *in vitro;* however, the clinical significance of this interaction is not well-documented.

Oral contraceptives—May be less effective and increased breakthrough bleeding may occur.

Probenecid—May decrease renal tubular secretion of ampicillin resulting in increased blood levels and/or ampicillin toxicity.

DRUG/LABORATORY TEST INTERACTION

After treatment with ampicillin, a false-positive reaction for glucose in the urine may occur with copper sulfate tests (Benedict's solution, Fehling's solution, or Clinitest® tablets) but not with enzyme based tests such as Clinistix® and TesTape®.

CARCINOGENESIS, MUTAGENESIS, IMPAIRMENT OF FERTILITY

Long-term studies in animals have not been performed to evalute carcinogenesis, mutagenesis, or impairment of fertility in males or females.

PREGNANCY: TERATOGENIC EFFECTS
CATEGORY B

Reproduction studies in animals have revealed no evidence of impaired fertility or harm to the fetus due to penicillin. There are, however, no adequate and well-controlled studies in pregnant women. Because animal reproduction studies are not always predictive of human response, penicillin should be used during pregnancy only if clearly needed.

LABOR AND DELIVERY

Oral ampicillin-class antibiotics are poorly absorbed during labor. Studies in guinea pigs showed that intravenous administration of ampicillin slightly decreased the uterine tone and frequency of contractions, but moderately increased the height and duration of contractions. However, it is not known whether use of these drugs in humans during labor or delivery has immediate or delayed adverse effects on the fetus, prolongs the duration of labor, or increases the likelihood that forceps delivery or other obstetrical intervention or resuscitation of the newborn will be necessary.

NURSING MOTHERS

Ampicillin-class antibiotics are excreted in milk. Ampicillin use by nursing mothers may lead to sensitization of infants; therefore, a decision should be made whether to discontinue nursing or to discontinue ampicillin, taking into account the importance of the drug to the mother.

PEDIATRIC USE

Penicillins are excreted primarily unchanged by the kidney; therefore, the incompletely developed renal function in neonates and young infants will delay the excretion of penicillin. Administration to neonates and young infants should be limited to the lowest dosage compatible with an effective therapeutic regimen (see "**Dosage and Administration**").

ADVERSE REACTIONS

As with other penicillins, it may be expected that untoward reactions will be essentially limited to sensitivity phenomena. They are more likely to occur in individuals who have previously demonstrated hypersensitivity to penicillins and in those with a history of allergy, asthma, hay fever, or urticaria.

The following adverse reactions have been reported as associated with the use of ampicillin:

Gastrointestinal: glossitis, stomatitis, nausea, vomiting, enterocolitis, pseudomembranous colitis, and diarrhea. These reactions are usually associated with oral dosage forms of the drug.

Hypersensitivity Reactions: an erythematous, mildly pruritic, maculopapular skin rash has been reported fairly frequently. The rash, which usually does not develop within the first week of therapy, may cover the entire body including the soles, palms, and oral mucosa. The eruption usually disappears in three to seven days. Other hypersensitivity reactions that have been reported are: skin rash, pruritus, urticaria, erythema multiforme, and an occasional case of exfoliative dermatitis. Anaphylaxis is the most serious reaction experienced and has usually been associated with the parenteral dosage form of the drug.

NOTE: Urticaria, other skin rashes, and serum sickness-like reactions may be controlled with antihistamines and, if necessary, systemic corticosteroids. Whenever such reactions occur, ampicillin should be discontinued, unless, in the opinion of the physician, the condition being treated is life-threatening and amenable only to ampicillin therapy. Serious anaphylactic reactions require emergency measures (see "**Warnings**").

Liver: A moderate elevation in the serum glutamic-oxaloacetic transaminase (SGOT) has been noted, but the significance of this finding is unknown.

Hemic and Lymphatic Systems: Anemia, thrombocytopenia, thrombocytopenic purpura, eosinophilia, leukopenia, and agranulocytosis have been reported during therapy with penicillins. These reactions are usually reversible on discontinuation of therapy and are believed to be hypersensitivity phenomena.

Other adverse reactions that have been reported with the use of ampicillin are laryngeal stridor and high fever. An occasional patient may complain of sore mouth or tongue as with any oral penicillin preparation.

OVERDOSAGE

In case of overdosage, discontinue medication, treat symptomatically and institute supportive measures as required. In patients with renal function impairment, ampicillin-class antibiotics can be removed by hemodialysis but not by peritoneal dialysis.

DOSAGE AND ADMINISTRATION

Adults and children weighing over 20 kg:

For genitourinary- or gastrointestinal-tract infections other than gonorrhea in men and women—the usual dose is 500 mg q.i.d in equally spaced doses (i.e., 500 mg every 6 hours); larger doses may be required for severe or chronic infections.

For the treatment of gonorrhea in both men and women—a single oral dose of 3.5 grams of ampicillin with 1 gram of probenecid administered simultaneously is recommended. Physicians are cautioned to use no less than the above recommended dosage for the treatment of gonorrhea. Follow-up cultures should be obtained from the original site(s) of infection 7 to 14 days after therapy. In women, it is also desirable to obtain culture test-of-cure from both the endocervical and anal canals. Prolonged intensive therapy is needed for complications such as prostatitis and epididymitis.

For respiratory-tract infections—the usual dose is 250 mg q.i.d. in equally spaced doses (i.e., 250 mg every 6 hours).

Children weighing 20 kg or less:

For genitourinary- or gastrointestinal-tract infections—the usual dose is 100 mg/kg/day total, administered q.i.d. in equally divided and spaced doses (i.e., every 6 hours).

For respiratory infections—the usual dose is 50 mg/kg/day total, administered in equally divided and spaced doses three to four times daily (i.e., every 8 to every 6 hours).

Doses for children should not exceed doses recommended for adults.

In all patients, irrespective of age and weight: Larger doses may be required for severe or chronic infections. Although ampicillin is resistant to degradation by gastric acid, it should be administered at least one-half hour before or two hours after meals for maximal absorption. Except for the single-dose regimen for gonorrhea referred to above, therapy should be continued for a minimum of 48 to 72 hours after the patient becomes asymptomatic or evidence of bacterial eradication has been obtained. In infections caused by hemolytic strains of streptococci, a minimum of 10 days' treatment is recommended to guard against the risk of rheumatic fever or glomerulonephritis (see "**Precautions**—LABORATORY TESTS").

In the treatment of chronic urinary or gastrointestinal infections, frequent bacteriologic and clinical appraisal is necessary during therapy and may be necessary for several months afterwards. Stubborn infections may require treatment for several weeks. Smaller doses than those indicated above should not be used.

HOW SUPPLIED

Omnipen® (ampicillin) Capsules contain 250 mg or 500 mg ampicillin anhydrous and are available as follows:

250 mg, violet and pink capsule marked "WYETH" and "53", in bottles of 500 capsules (NDC 0008-0053-05).

500 mg, violet and pink capsule marked "WYETH" and "309", in bottles of 100 (NDC 0008-0309-03) and 500 capsules (NDC 0008-0309-06).

Keep tightly closed.

Dispense in a tight container.

Store at room temperature, approximately 25° C (77° F).

Shown in Product Identification Guide, page 340

OMNIPEN® ℞

[om ′nĭ-pen]

(ampicillin)

for ORAL SUSPENSION

DESCRIPTION

Omnipen (ampicillin) is a semisynthetic penicillin derived from the basic penicillin nucleus, 6-amino-penicillanic acid. Ampicillin is designated chemically as (2S, 5R, 6R)-6-[(R)-2-Amino -2- phenylacetamido] -3,3- dimethyl -7- oxo -4- thia-1-aza-bicyclo [3.2.0]heptane-2-carboxylic acid. The molecular formula for ampicillin is $C_{16}H_{19}N_3O_4S$ with a molecular weight of 349.40.

Omnipen for oral suspension is a powder which when reconstituted as directed yields a suspension of 125 mg or 250 mg ampicillin per 5 mL. The inactive ingredients present are artificial flavors, colloidal silicon dioxide, methylparaben, propylparaben, sodium benzoate, sodium citrate, sucrose, and water. Each dosage strength of suspension also contains the following:

125 mg per 5 mL—carboxymethylcellulose sodium, FD&C Blue 1, FD&C Red 40, FD&C Yellow 6, and natural flavors;

250 mg per 5 mL—D&C Red 28.

CLINICAL PHARMACOLOGY

Ampicillin is bactericidal at low concentrations and is clinically effective not only against the gram-positive organisms usually susceptible to penicillin G, but also against a variety of gram-negative organisms. It is stable in the presence of gastric acid and is well absorbed from the gastrointestinal tract. It diffuses readily into most body tissues and fluids; however, penetration into the cerebrospinal fluid and brain occurs only with meningeal inflammation.

Ampicillin is excreted largely unchanged in the urine; its excretion can be delayed by concurrent administration of probenecid which inhibits the renal tubular secretion of ampicillin. In blood serum, ampicillin is the least bound of all the penicillins; an average of about 20% of the drug is bound to the plasma proteins as compared to 60 to 90% for the other penicillins. Blood serum levels of approximately 2 mcg/mL are attained within 1 to 2 hours following a 250 mg oral dose given to fasting adults. Detectable amounts persist for about 6 hours.

MICROBIOLOGY

While *in vitro* studies have demonstrated the susceptibility of most strains of the following microorganisms, clinical efficacy for infections other than those included in the "**Indications and Usage**" section has not been documented.

Gram-Positive

Alpha- and beta-hemolytic streptococci, *Streptococcus pneumoniae*, staphylococci (non-penicillinase-producing), *Bacillus anthracis*, *Clostridium* sp., *Corynebacterium xerose*, and most strains of enterococci.

Gram-Negative

Hemophilus influenzae, *Neisseria gonorrhoeae*, *Neisseria meningitidis*, *Proteus mirabilis*, and many strains of Salmonella (including *S. typhosa*), Shigella, and *Escherichia coli*.

NOTE: Ampicillin is inactivated by penicillinase and therefore is ineffective against penicillinase-producing organisms including certain strains of staphylococci, *Pseudomonas aeruginosa*, *P. vulgaris*, *Klebsiella pneumoniae*, *Enterobacter aerogenes*, and some strains of *E. coli*. Ampicillin is not active against Rickettsia, Mycoplasma, and "large viruses" (Miyagawanella).

Testing for Susceptibility

The invading organism should be cultured and its susceptibility demonstrated as a guide to therapy. If the Kirby-Bauer method of disc susceptibility is used, a 10 mcg ampicillin disc should be used to determine the relative *in vitro* susceptibility.

INDICATIONS AND USAGE

Omnipen (ampicillin) for Oral Suspension is indicated in the treatment of infections caused by susceptible strains of the following microorganisms:

Infections of the genitourinary tract including gonorrhea—E. coli, P. mirabilis, enterococci, *Shigella, S. typhosa* and other *Salmonella,* and non-penicillinase-producing *N. gonorrhoeae.*

Infections of the respiratory tract—Non-penicillinase-producing *H. influenzae* and staphylococci, and streptococci including *Streptococcus pneumoniae.*

Infections of the gastrointestinal tract—Shigella, S. typhosa and other *Salmonella, E. coli, P. mirabilis* and enterococci.

Meningitis—N. meningitidis.

Bacteriology studies to determine the causative organisms and their sensitivity to ampicillin should be performed. Therapy may be instituted prior to the results of susceptibility testing.

CONTRAINDICATIONS

The use of this drug is contraindicated in individuals with a history of previous hypersensitivity reaction to any of the penicillins. Ampicillin is also contraindicated in infections caused by penicillinase-producing organisms.

WARNINGS

Serious and occasionally fatal hypersensitivity (anaphylactic) reactions have been reported in patients on penicillin therapy. Although anaphylaxis is more frequent following parenteral therapy, it has occurred in patients on oral penicillins. These reactions are more apt to occur in individuals with a history of sensitivity to multiple allergens.

There have been well-documented reports of individuals with a history of penicillin hypersensitivity who experienced severe reactions when treated with cephalosporins. Before initiating therapy with any penicillin, careful inquiry should be made concerning previous hypersensitivity reactions to penicillins, cephalosporins, or other allergens. If an allergic reaction occurs, the drug should be discontinued and appropriate therapy instituted.

Serious anaphylactoid reactions require immediate emergency treatment with epinephrine. Oxygen, intravenous steroids, and airway management, including intubation, should also be administered as indicated.

PRECAUTIONS

GENERAL

Prolonged use of antibiotics may promote the overgrowth of nonsusceptible organisms, including fungi. Should superinfection occur, appropriate measures should be taken.

Patients with gonorrhea who also have syphilis should be given additional appropriate parenteral penicillin treatment.

Treatment with ampicillin does not preclude the need for surgical procedures, particularly in staphylococcal infections.

INFORMATION FOR THE PATIENT

1. The patient should inform the physician of any history of sensitivity to allergens, including previous hypersensitivity reactions to penicillins and cephalosporins (see "**Warnings**").
2. The patient should discontinue ampicillin and contact the physician immediately if any side effect occurs (see "**Warnings**").
3. Ampicillin should be taken with a full glass (8 oz.) of water, one-half hour before or two hours after meals.
4. Diabetic patients should consult with the physician before changing diet or dosage of diabetes medication (see "**Precautions**—DRUG/LABORATORY TEST INTERACTION").

LABORATORY TESTS

In prolonged therapy, and particularly with high dosage regimens, periodic evaluation of the renal, hepatic, and hematopoietic systems is recommended.

In streptococcal infections, therapy must be sufficient to eliminate the organism (10 days minimum); otherwise the sequelae of streptococcal disease may occur. Cultures should be taken following completion of treatment to determine whether streptococci have been eradicated.

Cases of gonococcal infection with a suspected lesion of syphilis should have darkfield examination ruling out syphilis before receiving ampicillin. Patients who do not have suspected lesions of syphilis and are treated with ampicillin should have a follow-up serologic test for syphilis each month for four months to detect syphilis that may have been masked by treatment or gonorrhea.

DRUG INTERACTIONS

When administered concurrently, the following drugs may interact with ampicillin:

Allopurinol—Increased possibility of skin rash, particularly in hyperuricemic patients, may occur.

Bacteriostatic antibiotics—Chloramphenicol, erythromycins, sulfonamides, or tetracyclines may interfere with the bactericidal effect of penicillins. This has been demonstrated *in vitro*; however, the clinical significance of this interaction is not well-documented.

Oral contraceptives—May be less effective and increased breakthrough bleeding may occur.

Probenecid—May decrease renal tubular secretion of ampicillin resulting in increased blood levels and/or ampicillin toxicity.

Continued on next page

Wyeth-Ayerst Laboratories—Cont.

DRUG/LABORATORY TEST INTERACTION
After treatment with ampicillin, a false-positive reaction for glucose in the urine may occur with copper sulfate tests (Benedict's solution, Fehling's solution, or Clinitest® tablets) but not with enzyme based tests such as Clinistix® and TesTape®.

CARCINOGENESIS, MUTAGENESIS, IMPAIRMENT OF FERTILITY
Long-term studies in animals have not been performed to evaluate carcinogenesis, mutagenesis, or impairment of fertility in males or females.

PREGNANCY: TERATOGENIC EFFECTS
CATEGORY B
Reproduction studies in animals have revealed no evidence of impaired fertility or harm to the fetus due to penicillin. There are, however, no adequate and well-controlled studies in pregnant women. Because animal reproduction studies are not always predictive of human response, penicillin should be used during pregnancy only if clearly needed.

LABOR AND DELIVERY
Oral ampicillin-class antibiotics are poorly absorbed during labor. Studies in guinea pigs showed that intravenous administration of ampicillin slightly decreased the uterine tone and frequency of contractions, but moderately increased the height and duration of contractions. However, it is not known whether use of these drugs in humans during labor or delivery has immediate or delayed adverse effects on the fetus, prolongs the duration of labor, or increases the likelihood that forceps delivery or other obstetrical intervention or resuscitation of the newborn will be necessary.

NURSING MOTHERS
Ampicillin-class antibiotics are excreted in milk. Ampicillin use by nursing mothers may lead to sensitization of infants; therefore, a decision should be made whether to discontinue nursing or to discontinue ampicillin, taking into account the importance of the drug to the mother.

PEDIATRIC USE
Penicillins are excreted primarily unchanged by the kidney; therefore, the incompletely developed renal function in neonates and young infants will delay the excretion of penicillin. Administration to neonates and young infants should be limited to the lowest dosage compatible with an effective therapeutic regimen (see **"Dosage and Administration"**).

ADVERSE REACTIONS

As with other penicillins, it may be expected that untoward reactions will be essentially limited to sensitivity phenomena. They are more likely to occur in individuals who have previously demonstrated hypersensitivity to penicillins and in those with a history of allergy, asthma, hay fever, or urticaria.

The following adverse reactions have been reported as associated with the use of ampicillin:

Gastrointestinal—glossitis, stomatitis, nausea, vomiting, enterocolitis, pseudomembranous colitis, and diarrhea. These reactions are usually associated with oral-dosage forms of the drug.

Hypersensitivity Reactions —an erythematous, mildly pruritic, maculopapular rash has been reported fairly frequently. The rash, which usually does not develop within the first week of therapy, may cover the entire body, including the soles, palms, and oral mucosa. The eruption usually disappears in three to seven days. Other hypersensitivity reactions that have been reported are: skin rash, pruritis, urticaria, erythema multiforme, and an occasional case of exfoliative dermatitis. Anaphylaxis is the most serious reaction experienced and has usually been associated with the parenteral dosage form of the drug.

NOTE: Urticaria, other skin rashes, and serum-sickness-like reactions may be controlled by antihistamines and, if necessary, systemic corticosteroids. Whenever such reactions occur, ampicillin should be discontinued unless, in the opinion of the physician, the condition being treated is life-threatening and amenable only to the ampicillin therapy. Serious anaphylactic reactions require emergency measures (see **WARNINGS**).

Liver—A moderate elevation in serum glutamic-oxaloacetic transaminase (SGOT) has been noted, but the significance of this finding is unknown.

Hemic and Lymphatic Systems—Anemia, thrombocytopenia, thrombocytopenic purpura, eosinophilia, leukopenia, and agranulocytosis have been reported during therapy with penicillins. These reactions are usually reversible on discontinuation of therapy and are believed to be hypersensitivity phenomena.

Other adverse reactions that have been reported with the use of ampicillin are laryngeal stridor and high fever. An occasional patient may complain of sore mouth or tongue as with any oral penicillin preparation.

OVERDOSAGE

In case of overdosage, discontinue medication, treat symptomatically and institute supportive measures as required. In patients with renal function impairment, ampicillin-class antibiotics can be removed by hemodialysis but not by peritoneal dialysis.

DOSAGE AND ADMINISTRATION

Adults and children weighing over 20 kg:

For genitourinary- or gastrointestinal-tract infections other than gonorrhea in men and women—the usual dose is 500 mg q.i.d. in equally spaced doses (i.e., 500 mg every 6 hours); larger doses may be required for severe or chronic infections.

For the treatment of gonorrhea in both men and women—a single oral dose of 3.5 grams of ampicillin with 1 gram of probenecid administered simultaneously is recommended. Physicians are cautioned to use no less than the above recommended dosage for the treatment of gonorrhea. Follow-up cultures should be obtained from the original site(s) of infection 7 to 14 days after therapy. In women, it is also desirable to obtain culture test-of-cure from both the endocervical and anal canals. Prolonged intensive therapy is needed for complications such as prostatitis and epididymitis.

For respiratory-tract infections—the usual dose is 250 mg q.i.d. in equally spaced doses (i.e., 250 mg every 6 hours).

Children weighing 20 kg or less:

For genitourinary- or gastrointestinal-tract infections—the usual dose is 100 mg/kg/day total, administered q.i.d. in equally divided and spaced doses (i.e., every 6 hours).

For respiratory infections—the usual dose is 50 mg/kg/day total, administered in equally divided and spaced doses three to four times daily (i.e., every 8 to every 6 hours).

Doses for children should not exceed doses recommended for adults.

In all patients, irrespective of age and weight: Larger doses may be required for severe or chronic infections. Although ampicillin is resistant to degradation by gastric acid, it should be administered at least one-half hour before or two hours after meals for maximal absorption. Except for the single-dose regimen for gonorrhea referred to above, therapy should be continued for a minimum of 48 to 72 hours after the patient becomes asymptomatic or evidence of bacterial eradication has been obtained. In infections caused by hemolytic strains of streptococci, a minimum of 10 days' treatment is recommended to guard against the risk of rheumatic fever or glomerulonephritis (see **"Precautions**—LABORATORY TESTS").

In the treatment of chronic urinary or gastrointestinal infections, frequent bacteriologic and clinical appraisal is necessary during therapy and may be necessary for several months afterwards. Stubborn infections may require treatment for several weeks. Smaller doses than those indicated above should not be used.

HOW SUPPLIED

Omnipen® (ampicillin) for Oral Suspension, is available in the following dosage strengths as a powder, which when reconstituted as directed yields a palatable suspension:

125 mg per 5 mL, NDC 0008-0054, white powder in bottles to make 100 mL, 150 mL, or 200 mL of salmon-colored suspension.

250 mg per 5 mL, NDC 0008-0055, white powder in bottles to make 100 mL, 150 mL, or 200 mL of pink suspension.

Store at room temperature [approximately 25° C (77° F)] before reconstitution.

Shake well before using.

Keep tightly closed.

When stored in refrigerator discard unused portion after 14 days, or when stored at room temperature discard unused portion after 7 days (250 mg per 5 mL).

When stored in refrigerator discard unused portion after 14 days (125 mg per 5 mL).

ORUDIS® ℞
[ō''roo'dĭs]
(ketoprofen)
Capsules

ORUVAIL® ℞
[or'ü văl]
(ketoprofen)
Extended-Release
Capsules

DESCRIPTION

Ketoprofen is a nonsteroidal anti-inflammatory drug. The chemical name for ketoprofen is 2-(3-benzoylphenyl)-propionic acid with the following structural formula:

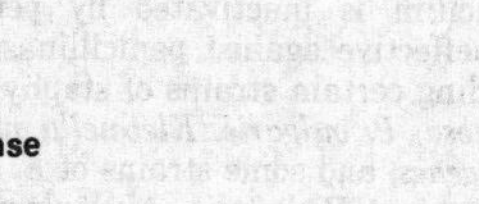

Its empirical formula is $C_{16}H_{14}O_3$, with a molecular weight of 254.29. It has a pKa of 5.94 in methanol:water (3:1) and an n-octanol:water partition coefficient of 0.97 (buffer pH 7.4).

Ketoprofen is a white or off-white, odorless, nonhygroscopic, fine to granular powder, melting at about 95° C. It is freely soluble in ethanol, chloroform, acetone, ether and soluble in benzene and strong alkali, but practically insoluble in water at 20° C.

Orudis capsules contain 25 mg, 50 mg, or 75 mg of ketoprofen for oral administration. The inactive ingredients present are D&C Yellow 10, FD&C Blue 1, FD&C Yellow 6, gelatin, lactose, magnesium stearate, and titanium dioxide. The 25 mg dosage strength also contains D&C Red 28 and FD&C Red 40.

Each Oruvail 100 mg, 150 mg, or 200 mg capsule contains ketoprofen in the form of hundreds of coated pellets. The dissolution of the pellets is pH dependent with optimum dissolution occurring at pH 6.5–7.5. There is no dissolution at pH 1.

In addition to the active ingredient, each 100 mg, 150 mg, or 200 mg capsule of Oruvail contains the following inactive ingredients: D&C Red 22, D&C Red 28, FD&C Blue 1, ethyl cellulose, gelatin, shellac, silicon dioxide, sodium lauryl sulfate, starch, sucrose, talc, titanium dioxide, and other proprietary ingredients. The 100 and 150 mg capsules also contain D&C Yellow 10 and FD&C Green 3.

CLINICAL PHARMACOLOGY

Ketoprofen is a nonsteroidal anti-inflammatory drug with analgesic and antipyretic properties.

The anti-inflammatory, analgesic, and antipyretic properties of ketoprofen have been demonstrated in classical animal and *in vitro* test systems. In anti-inflammatory models ketoprofen has been shown to have inhibitory effects on prostaglandin and leukotriene synthesis, to have antibradykinin activity, as well as to have lysosomal membrane-stabilizing action. However, its mode of action, like that of other nonsteroidal anti-inflammatory drugs, is not fully understood.

PHARMACODYNAMICS

Ketoprofen is a racemate with only the S enantiomer possessing pharmacological activity. The enantiomers have similar concentration time curves and do not appear to interact with one another.

An analgesic effect-concentration relationship for ketoprofen was established in an oral surgery pain study with Orudis. The effect-site rate constant (k_{e0}) was estimated to be 0.9 $hour^{-1}$ (95% confidence limits: 0 to 2.1), and the concentration (Ce_{50}) of ketoprofen that produced one-half the maximum PID (pain intensity difference) was 0.3 μg/mL (95% confidence limits: 0.1 to 0.5). Thirty-three (33) to 68% of patients had an onset of action (as measured by reporting some pain relief) within 30 minutes following a single oral dose in postoperative pain and dysmenorrhea studies. Pain relief (as measured by remedication) persisted for up to 6 hours in 26 to 72% of patients in these studies.

PHARMACOKINETICS

GENERAL
Orudis and Oruvail capsules both contain ketoprofen. They differ only in their release characteristics. Orudis capsules release drug in the stomach whereas the pellets in Oruvail capsules are designed to resist dissolution in the low pH of gastric fluid but release drug at a controlled rate in the higher pH environment of the small intestine (see **"DESCRIPTION"**).

Irrespective of the pattern of release, the systemic availability (F_s) when either oral formulation is compared with IV administration is approximately 90% in humans. For 75 to 200 mg single doses, the area under the curve has been shown to be dose proportional. The figure depicts the plasma time curves associated with both products.

Ketoprofen is >99% bound to plasma proteins, mainly to albumin.

Separate sections follow which delineate differences between Orudis and Oruvail capsules.

ABSORPTION
Orudis capsules—Ketoprofen is rapidly and well-absorbed, with peak plasma levels occurring within 0.5 to 2 hours.

Oruvail capsules—Ketoprofen is also well-absorbed from this dosage form, although an observable increase in plasma levels does not occur until approximately 2 to 3 hours after taking the formulation. Peak plasma levels are usually reached 6 to 7 hours after dosing. (See Figure and Table, below).

When ketoprofen is administered with food, its total bioavailability (AUC) is not altered; however, the rate of absorption from either dosage form is slowed.

Orudis capsules—Food intake reduces C_{max} by approximately one-half and increases the mean time to peak concentration (t_{max}) from 1.2 hours for fasting subjects (range, 0.5 to 3 hours) to 2.0 hours for fed subjects (range, 0.75 to 3 hours). The fluctuation of plasma peaks may also be influenced by circadian changes in the absorption process.

Concomitant administration of magnesium hydroxide and aluminum hydroxide does not interfere with absorption of ketoprofen from Orudis capsules.

Oruvail capsules—Administration of Oruvail with a high-fat meal causes a delay of about 2 hours in reaching the C_{max}; neither the total bioavailability (AUC) nor the C_{max} is af-

fected. Circardian changes in the absorption process have not been studied.

The administration of antacids or other drugs which may raise stomach pH would not be expected to change the rate or extent of absorption of ketoprofen from Oruvail capsules.

MULTIPLE DOSING

Steady-state concentrations of ketoprofen are attained within 24 hours after commencing treatment with Orudis or Oruvail capsules. In studies with healthy male volunteers, trough levels at 24 hours following administration of Oruvail 200 mg capsules were 0.4 mg/L compared with 0.07 mg/L at 24 hours following administration of Orudis 50 mg capsules QID (12 hours) or 0.13 mg/L following administration of Orudis 75 mg capsules TID for 12 hours. Thus, relative to the peak plasma concentration, the accumulation of ketoprofen after multiple doses of Oruvail or Orudis capsules is minimal.

The figure below shows a reduction in peak height and area after the second 50 mg dose. This is probably due to a combination of food effects, circadian effects, and plasma sampling times. It is unclear to what extent each factor contributes to the loss of peak height and area.

The shaded area represents ±1 standard deviation (S.D.) around the mean for Orudis or Oruvail.

KETOPROFEN PLASMA CONCENTRATIONS IN SUBJECTS RECEIVING 200 MG OF ORUVAIL ONCE A DAY (QD), OR ORUDIS 50 MG EVERY 4 HOURS FOR 16 HOURS

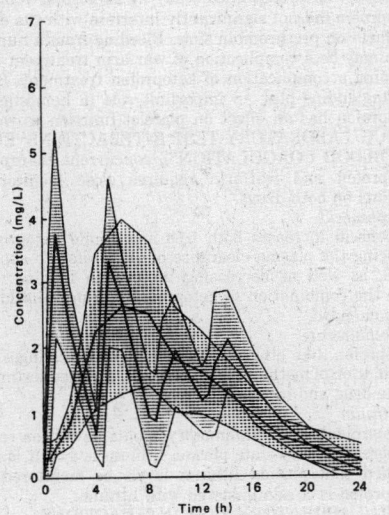

COMPARISON OF PHARMACOKINETIC PARAMETERS# FOR ORUDIS AND ORUVAIL

Kinetic Parameters	Orudis (4×50 mg)	Oruvail (1×200 mg)
Extent of oral absorption (bioavailability) F_s (%)	~90	~90
Peak plasma levels C_{max} (mg/L)		
Fasted	3.9±1.3	3.1±1.2
Fed	2.4±1.0	3.4±1.3
Time to peak concentration t_{max} (h)		
Fasted	1.2±0.6	6.8±2.1
Fed	2.0±0.8	9.2±2.6
Area under plasma concentration-time curve AUC_{0-24h} (mg·h/L)		
Fasted	32.1±7.2	30.1±7.9
Fed	36.6±8.1	31.3±8.1
Oral-dose clearance CL/F (L/h)	6.9±0.8	6.8±1.8
Half-life $t_{1/2}$ (h) [See footnote 1]	2.1±1.2	5.4±2.2

#Values expressed are mean ± standard deviation
[1] In the case of Oruvail, absorption is slowed, intrinsic clearance is unchanged, but because the rate of elimination is dependent on absorption, the half-life is prolonged.

METABOLISM

The metabolic fate of ketoprofen is glucuronide conjugation to form an unstable acyl-glucuronide. The glucuronic acid moiety can be converted back to the parent compound. Thus, the metabolite serves as a potential reservoir for parent drug, and this may be important in persons with renal insufficiency, whereby the conjugate may accumulate in the serum and undergo deconjugation back to the parent drug (see "SPECIAL POPULATIONS: Renally impaired").The conjugates are reported to appear only in trace amounts in plasma in healthy adults, but are higher in elderly subjects—presumably because of reduced renal clearance. It has been demonstrated that in elderly subjects following multiple doses (50 mg every 6 h), the ratio of conjugated to parent ketoprofen AUC was 30% and 3%, respectively for the S & R enantiomers.

There are no known active metabolites of ketoprofen. Ketoprofen has been shown not to induce drug-metabolizing enzymes.

ELIMINATION

The plasma clearance of ketoprofen is approximately 0.08 L/kg/h with a V_d of 0.1 L/kg after IV administration. The elimination half-life of ketoprofen has been reported to be 2.05±0.58 h (Mean ± S.D.) following IV administration, from 2 to 4 h following administration of Orudis capsules, and 5.4±2.2 h after administration of Oruvail 200 mg capsules. In cases of slow drug absorption, the elimination rate is dependent on the absorption rate and thus $t_{1/2}$ relative to an IV dose appears prolonged.

After a single 200 mg dose of Oruvail, the plasma levels decline slowly, and average 0.4 mg/L after 24 hours (see Figure above).

In a 24-hour period, approximately 80% of an administered dose of ketoprofen is excreted in the urine, primarily as the glucuronide metabolite.

Enterohepatic recirculation of the drug has been postulated, although biliary levels have never been measured to confirm this.

SPECIAL POPULATIONS

Elderly: Clearance and unbound fraction

The plasma and renal clearance of ketoprofen is reduced in the elderly (mean age, 73 years) compared to a younger normal population (mean age, 27 years). Hence, ketoprofen peak concentration and AUC increase with increasing age. In addition, there is a corresponding increase in unbound fraction with increasing age. Data from one trial suggest that the increase is greater in women than in men. It has not been determined whether age-related changes in absorption among the elderly contribute to the changes in bioavailability of ketoprofen.

Orudis capsules—In a study conducted with young and elderly men and women, results for subjects older than 75 years of age showed that free drug AUC increased by 40% and C_{max} increased by 60% as compared with estimates of the same parameters in young subjects (those younger than 35 years of age; see "INDIVIDUALIZATION OF DOSAGE").

Also in the elderly, the ratio of intrinsic clearance/availability decreased by 35% and plasma half-life was prolonged by 26%. This reduction is thought to be due to a decrease in hepatic extraction associated with aging.

Oruvail capsules—The effects of age and gender on ketoprofen disposition were investigated in 2 small studies in which elderly male and female subjects received Oruvail 200 mg capsules. The results were compared with those from another study conducted in healthy young men.

Compared to the younger subject group, the elimination half-life in the elderly was prolonged by 54% and total drug C_{max} and AUC were 40% and 70% higher, respectively. Plasma concentrations in the elderly after single doses and at steady state were essentially the same. Thus, no drug accumulation occurs.

In comparison to younger subjects taking the immediate-release formulation (Orudis), there was a decrease of 16% and 25% in total drug C_{max} and AUC, respectively, among the elderly. Free drug data are not available for Oruvail.

Renally impaired

Studies of the effects of renal-function impairment have been small. They indicate a decrease in clearance in patients with impaired renal function. In 23 patients with renal impairment, free ketoprofen peak concentration was not significantly elevated, but free ketoprofen clearance was reduced from 15 L/kg/h for normal subjects to 7 L/kg/h in patients with mildly impaired renal function, and to 4 L/kg/h in patients with moderately to severely impaired renal function. The elimination $t_{1/2}$ was prolonged from 1.6 hours in normal subjects to approximately 3 hours in patients with mild renal impairment, and to approximately 5 to 9 hours in patients with moderately to severely impaired renal function.

No studies have been conducted in patients with renal impairment taking Oruvail capsules (see "INDIVIDUALIZATION OF DOSAGE").

Hepatically impaired

For patients with alcoholic cirrhosis, no significant changes in the kinetic disposition of Oruvail capsules were observed relative to age-matched normal subjects: the plasma clearance of drug was 0.07 L/kg/h in 26 hepatically impaired patients. The elimination half-life was comparable to that observed for normal subjects. However, the unbound (biologically active) fraction was approximately doubled, probably due to hypoalbuminemia and high variability which was observed in the pharmacokinetics for cirrhotic patients. Therefore, these patients should be carefully monitored and daily doses of ketoprofen kept at the minimum providing the desired therapeutic effect.

No studies have been conducted in patients with heptic impairment taking Oruvail capsules (see "INDIVIDUALIZATION OF DOSAGE").

CLINICAL TRIALS

RHEUMATOID ARTHRITIS AND OSTEOARTHRITIS

The efficacy of ketoprofen has been demonstrated in patients with rheumatoid arthritis and osteoarthritis. Using standard assessments of therapeutic response, there were no detectable differences in effectiveness or in the incidence of adverse events in crossover comparison of Orudis and Oruvail. In other trials, ketoprofen demonstrated effectiveness comparable to aspirin, ibuprofen, naproxen, piroxicam, diclofenac and indomethacin. In some of these studies there were more dropouts due to gastrointestinal side effects among patients on ketoprofen than among patients on other NSAIDs.

In studies with patients with rheumatoid arthritis, ketoprofen was administered in combination with gold salts, antimalarials, low-dose methotrexate, d-penicillamine, and/or corticosteroids with results comparable to those seen with control nonsteroidal drugs.

MANAGEMENT OF PAIN

The effectiveness of Orudis as a general-purpose analgesic has been studied in standard pain models which have shown the effectiveness of doses of 25 to 150 mg. Doses of 25 mg were superior to placebo. Doses larger than 25 mg generally could not be shown to be significantly more effective, but there was a tendency toward faster onset and greater duration of action with 50 mg, and, in the case of dysmenorrhea, a significantly greater effect overall with 75 mg. Doses greater than 50 to 75 mg did not have increased analgesic effect. Studies in postoperative pain have shown that Orudis in doses of 25 to 100 mg was comparable to 650 mg of acetaminophen with 60 mg of codeine, or 650 mg of acetaminophen with 10 mg of oxycodone. Ketoprofen tended to be somewhat slower in onset; peak pain relief was about the same and the duration of the effect tended to be 1 to 2 hours longer, particularly with the higher doses of ketoprofen.

The use of Oruvail in patients with acute pain is not recommended, since, in comparison to Orudis, Oruvail would be expected to have a delayed analgesic response due to its extended-release characteristics.

INDIVIDUALIZATION OF DOSAGE

The recommended starting dose of ketoprofen in otherwise healthy patients is Orudis, 75 mg three times or 50 mg four times a day, or Oruvail, 200 mg administered once a day. Smaller doses of Orudis or Oruvail should be utilized initially in small individuals or in debilitated or elderly patients. The recommended maximum daily dose of ketoprofen is 300 mg/day for Orudis or 200 mg/day for Oruvail. Concomitant use of Orudis and Oruvail is not recommended. If minor side effects appear, they may disappear at a lower dose which may still have an adequate therapeutic effect. If well tolerated but not optimally effective, the dosage may be increased. Individual patients may show a better response to 300 mg of Orudis daily as compared to 200 mg, although in well-controlled clinical trials patients on 300 mg did not show greater mean effectiveness. They did, however, show an increased frequency of upper- and lower-GI distress and headaches. It is of interest that women also had an increased frequency of these adverse effects compared to men. When treating patients with 300 mg/day, the physician should observe sufficient increased clinical benefit to offset potential increased risk.

In patients with mildly impaired renal function, the maximum recommended total daily dose of Orudis or Oruvail is 150 mg. In patients with a more severe renal impairment (GFR less than 25 mL/min/1.73 m^2 or end-stage renal impairment), the maximum total daily dose of Orudis or Oruvail should not exceed 100 mg.

In elderly patients, renal function may be reduced with apparently normal serum creatinine and/or BUN levels. Therefore, it is recommended that the initial dosage of Orudis or Oruvail should be reduced for patients over 75 years of age.

Continued on next page

Wyeth-Ayerst Laboratories—Cont.

It is recommended that for patients with impaired liver function and serum albumin concentration less than 3.5 g/dL, the maximum initial total daily dose of Orudis or Oruvail should be 100 mg. All patients with metabolic impairment, particularly those with both hypoalbuminemia and reduced renal function, may have increased levels of free (biologically active) ketoprofen and should be closely monitored. The dosage may be increased to the range recommended for the general population, if necessary, only after good individual tolerance has been ascertained.

Because hypoalbuminemia and reduced renal function both increase the fraction of free drug (biologically active form), patients who have both conditions may be at greater risk of adverse effects. Therefore, it is recommended that such patients also be started on lower doses of Orudis or Oruvail and closely monitored.

As with other nonsteroidal anti-inflammatory drugs, the predominant adverse effects of ketoprofen are gastrointestinal. To attempt to minimize these effects, physicians may wish to prescribe that Orudis or Oruvail be taken with antacids, food, or milk. Although food delays the absorption of both formulations (see "CLINICAL PHARMACOLOGY"), in most of the clinical trials ketoprofen was taken with food or milk.

Physicians may want to make specific recommendations to patients about when they should take Orudis or Oruvail in relation to food and/or what patients should do if they experience minor GI symptoms associated with either formulation.

INDICATIONS AND USAGE

Orudis or Oruvail are indicated for the management of the signs and symptoms of rheumatoid arthritis and osteoarthritis. Oruvail is not recommended for treatment of acute pain because of its extended-release characteristics (see "PHARMACOKINETICS").

Orudis is indicated for the management of pain. Orudis is also indicated for treatment of primary dysmenorrhea.

CONTRAINDICATIONS

Ketoprofen is contraindicated in patients who have shown hypersensitivity to it. Ketoprofen should not be given to patients in whom aspirin or other nonsteroidal anti-inflammatory drugs induce asthma, urticaria, or other allergic-type reactions, because severe, rarely fatal, anaphylactic reactions to ketoprofen have been reported in such patients.

WARNINGS

RISK OF GI ULCERATION, BLEEDING, AND PERFORATION WITH NSAID THERAPY

Serious gastrointestinal toxicity, such as bleeding, ulceration, and perforation, can occur at any time with or without warning symptoms, in patients treated chronically with NSAID therapy. Although minor upper-gastrointestinal problems, such as dyspepsia, are common, usually developing early in therapy, physicians should remain alert for ulceration and bleeding in patients treated chronically with NSAIDs even in the absence of previous GI-tract symptoms. In patients observed in clinical trials of several months to two years' duration, symptomatic upper-GI ulcers, gross bleeding, or perforation appear to occur in approximately 1% of patients treated for 3 to 6 months, and in about 2–4% of patients treated for one year. Physicians should inform patients about the signs and/or symptoms of serious GI toxicity and what steps to take if they occur.

Studies to date have not identified any subset of patients not at risk of developing peptic ulceration and bleeding. Except for a prior history of serious GI events and other risk factors known to be associated with peptic ulcer disease, such as alcoholism, smoking, etc., no other risk factors (e.g., age, sex) have been associated with increased risk. Elderly or debilitated patients seem to tolerate ulceration or bleeding less well than other individuals, and most spontaneous reports of fatal GI events are in this population. Studies to date are inconclusive concerning the relative risk of various NSAIDs in causing such reactions. High doses of any NSAID probably carry a greater risk of these reactions, although controlled clinical trials showing this do not exist in most cases. In considering the use of relatively large doses (within the recommended dosage range), sufficient benefit should be anticipated to offset the potential increased risk of GI toxicity.

GENERAL PRECAUTIONS

Ketoprofen and other nonsteroidal anti-inflammatory drugs cause nephritis in mice and rats associated with chronic administration. Rare cases of interstitial nephritis or nephrotic syndrome have been reported in humans with ketoprofen since it has been marketed.

A second form of renal toxicity has been seen in patients with conditions leading to a reduction in renal blood flow or blood volume, where renal prostaglandins have a supportive role in the maintenance of renal blood flow. In these patients, administration of a nonsteroidal anti-inflammatory

drug results in a dose-dependent decrease in prostaglandin synthesis and, secondarily, in renal blood flow which may precipitate overt renal failure. Patients at greatest risk of this reaction are those with impaired renal function, heart failure, liver dysfunction, those taking diuretics, and the elderly. Discontinuation of nonsteroidal anti-inflammatory drug therapy is typically followed by recovery to the pretreatment state.

Since ketoprofen is primarily eliminated by the kidneys and its pharmacokinetics are altered by renal failure (see "CLINICAL PHARMACOLOGY"), patients with significantly impaired renal function should be closely monitored, and a reduction of dosage should be anticipated to avoid accumulation of ketoprofen and/or its metabolites (see "INDIVIDUALIZATION OF DOSAGE").

As with other nonsteroidal anti-inflammatory drugs, borderline elevations of one or more liver function tests may occur in up to 15% of patients. These abnormalities may progress, may remain essentially unchanged, or may disappear with continued therapy. The ALT (SGPT) test is probably the most sensitive indicator of liver dysfunction. Meaningful (3 times the upper limit of normal) elevations of ALT or AST (SGOT) occurred in controlled clinical trials in less than 1% of patients. A patient with symptoms and/or signs suggesting liver dysfunction, or in whom an abnormal liver test has occurred, should be evaluated for evidence of the development of a more severe hepatic reaction while on therapy with ketoprofen. Serious hepatic reactions, including jaundice, have been reported from post-marketing experience with ketoprofen as well as with other nonsteroidal anti-inflammatory drugs.

In patients with chronic liver disease with reduced serum albumin levels, ketoprofen's pharmacokinetics are altered (see "CLINICAL PHARMACOLOGY"). Such patients should be closely monitored, and a reduction of dosage should be anticipated to avoid high blood levels of ketoprofen and/or its metabolites (see "INDIVIDUALIZATION OF DOSAGE").

If steroid dosage is reduced or eliminated during therapy, it should be reduced slowly and the patients observed closely for any evidence of adverse effects, including adrenal insufficiency and exacerbation of symptoms of arthritis.

Anemia is commonly observed in rheumatoid arthritis and is sometimes aggravated by nonsteroidal anti-inflammatory drugs, which may produce fluid retention or significant gastrointestinal blood loss in some patients. Patients on long-term treatment with NSAIDs, including Orudis or Oruvail, should have their hemoglobin or hematocrit checked if they develop signs or symptoms of anemia.

Peripheral edema has been observed in approximately 2% of patients taking ketoprofen. Therefore, as with other nonsteroidal anti-inflammatory drugs, ketoprofen should be used with caution in patients with fluid retention, hypertension, or heart failure.

INFORMATION FOR PATIENTS

Orudis or Oruvail contain ketoprofen. Like other drugs of its class, ketoprofen is not free of side effects. The side effects of these drugs can cause discomfort and, rarely, there are more serious side effects, such as gastrointestinal bleeding, which may result in hospitalization and even fatal outcomes.

NSAIDs are often essential agents in the management of arthritis and have a major role in the treatment of pain, but they also may be commonly employed for conditions which are less serious. Physicians may wish to discuss with their patients the potential risks (see "WARNINGS," "GENERAL PRECAUTIONS," and "ADVERSE REACTIONS" sections) and likely benefits of NSAID treatment, particularly when the drugs are used for less serious conditions where treatment without NSAIDs may represent an acceptable alternative to both the patient and physician.

Because aspirin causes an increase in the level of unbound ketoprofen, patients should be advised not to take aspirin while taking ketoprofen (see "DRUG INTERACTIONS"). It is possible that minor adverse symptoms of gastric intolerance may be prevented by administering Orudis with antacids, food, or milk. Oruvail has not been studied with antacids. Because food and milk do affect the rate but not the extent of absorption (see "CLINICAL PHARMACOLOGY"), physicians may want to make specific recommendations to patients about when they should take ketoprofen in relation to food and/or what patients should do if they experience minor GI symptoms associated with ketoprofen therapy.

LABORATORY TESTS

Because serious GI-tract ulceration and bleeding can occur without warning symptoms, physicians should follow chronically treated patients for the signs and symptoms of ulceration and bleeding and should inform them of the importance of this follow-up (see "WARNINGS—RISK OF GI ULCERATION, BLEEDING, AND PERFORATION WITH NSAID THERAPY").

DRUG INTERACTIONS

The following drug interactions were studied with ketoprofen doses of 200 mg/day. The possibility of increased interaction should be kept in mind when Orudis doses greater

than 50 mg as a single dose or 200 mg of ketoprofen per day are used concomitantly with highly bound drugs.

1. *Antacids*

Concomitant administration of magnesium hydroxide and aluminum hydroxide does not interfere with the rate or extent of the absorption of ketoprofen administered as Orudis.

2. *Aspirin*

Ketoprofen does not alter aspirin absorption; however, in a study of 12 normal subjects, concurrent administration of aspirin decreased ketoprofen protein binding and increased ketoprofen plasma clearance from 0.07 L/kg/h without aspirin to 0.11 L/kg/h with aspirin. The clinical significance of these changes has not been adequately studied. Therefore, concurrent use of aspirin and ketoprofen is not recommended.

3. *Diuretic*

Hydrochlorothiazide, given concomitantly with ketoprofen, produces a reduction in urinary potassium and chloride excretion compared to hydrochlorothiazide alone. Patients taking diuretics are at greater risk of developing renal failure secondary to a decrease in renal blood flow caused by prostaglandin inhibition (see "GENERAL PRECAUTIONS").

4. *Digoxin*

In a study in 12 patients with congestive heart failure where ketoprofen and digoxin were concomitantly administered, ketoprofen did not alter the serum levels of digoxin.

5. *Warfarin*

In a short-term controlled study in 14 normal volunteers, ketoprofen did not significantly interfere with the effect of warfarin on prothrombin time. Bleeding from a number of sites may be a complication of warfarin treatment and GI bleeding a complication of ketoprofen treatment. Because prostaglandins play an important role in hemostasis and ketoprofen has an effect on platelet function as well (see "DRUG/LABORATORY TEST INTERACTIONS: EFFECT ON BLOOD COAGULATION"), concurrent therapy with ketoprofen and warfarin requires close monitoring of patients on both drugs.

6. *Probenecid*

Probenecid increases both free and bound ketoprofen by reducing the plasma clearance of ketoprofen to about one-third, as well as decreasing its protein binding. Therefore, the combination of ketoprofen and probenecid is not recommended.

7. *Methotrexate*

Ketoprofen, like other NSAIDs, may cause changes in the elimination of methotrexate leading to elevated serum levels of the drug and increased toxicity.

8. *Lithium*

Nonsteroidal anti-inflammatory agents have been reported to increase steady-state plasma lithium levels. It is recommended that plasma lithium levels be monitored when ketoprofen is co-administered with lithium.

DRUG/LABORATORY TEST INTERACTIONS: EFFECT ON BLOOD COAGULATION

Ketoprofen decreases platelet adhesion and aggregation. Therefore, it can prolong bleeding time by approximately 3 to 4 minutes from baseline values. There is no significant change in platelet count, prothrombin time, partial thromboplastin time, or thrombin time.

CARCINOGENESIS, MUTAGENESIS, IMPAIRMENT OF FERTILITY

Chronic oral toxicity studies in mice (up to 32 mg/kg/day; 96 mg/m²/day) did not indicate a carcinogenic potential for ketoprofen. The maximum recommended human therapeutic dose is 300 mg/day for a 60 kg patient with a body surface area of 1.6 m², which is 5 mg/kg/day or 185 mg/m²/day. Thus the mice were treated at 0.5 times the maximum human daily dose based on surface area.

A 2-year carcinogenicity study in rats, using doses up to 6.0 mg/kg/day (36 mg/m²/day), showed no evidence of tumorigenic potential. All groups were treated for 104 weeks except the females receiving 6.0 mg/kg/day (36 mg/m²/day) where the drug treatment was terminated in week 81 because of low survival; the remaining rats were sacrificed after week 87. Their survival in the groups treated for 104 weeks was within 6% of the control group. An earlier 2-year study with doses up to 12.5 mg/kg/day (75 mg/m²/day) also showed no evidence of tumorigenicity, but the survival rate was low and the study was therefore judged inconclusive. Ketoprofen did not show mutagenic potential in the Ames Test. Ketoprofen administered to male rats (up to 9 mg/kg/day; or 54 mg/m²/day) had no significant effect on reproductive performance or fertility. In female rats administered 6 or 9 mg/kg/day (36 or 54 mg/m²/day), a decrease in the number of implantation sites has been noted. The dosages of 36 mg/m²/day in rats represent 0.2 times the maximum recommended human dose of 185 mg/m²/day (see above).

Abnormal spermatogenesis or inhibition of spermatogenesis developed in rats and dogs at high doses, and a decrease in the weight of the testes occurred in dogs and baboons at high doses.

TERATOGENIC EFFECTS: PREGNANCY CATEGORY B

In teratology studies ketoprofen administered to mice at doses up to 12 mg/kg/day (36 mg/m^2/day) and rats at doses up to 9 mg/kg/day (54 mg/m^2/day), the approximate equivalent of 0.2 times the maximum recommended therapeutic dose of 185 mg/m^2/day, showed no teratogenic or embryotoxic effects. In separate studies in rabbits, maternally toxic doses were associated with embryotoxicity but not teratogenicity.

There are no adequate and well-controlled studies in pregnant women. Because animal teratology studies are not always predictive of the human response, ketoprofen should be used during pregnancy only if the potential benefit justifies the risk.

LABOR AND DELIVERY

The effects of ketoprofen on labor and delivery in pregnant women are unknown. Studies in rats have shown ketoprofen at doses of 6 mg/kg (36 mg/m^2/day, approximately equal to 0.2 times the maximum recommended human dose) prolongs pregnancy when given before the onset of labor. Because of the known effects of prostaglandin-inhibiting drugs on the fetal cardiovascular system (closure of ductus arteriosus), use of ketoprofen during late pregnancy should be avoided.

NURSING MOTHERS

Data on secretion in human milk after ingestion of ketoprofen do not exist. In rats, ketoprofen at doses of 9 mg/kg (54 mg/m^2/day; approximately 0.3 times the maximum human therapeutic dose) did not affect perinatal development. Upon administration to lactating dogs, the milk concentration of ketoprofen was found to be 4 to 5% of the plasma drug level. As with other drugs that are excreted in milk, ketoprofen is not recommended for use in nursing mothers.

PEDIATRIC USE

Ketoprofen is not recommended for use in pediatric patients, because its safety and effectiveness have not been studied in the pediatric population.

ADVERSE REACTIONS

The incidence of common adverse reactions (above 1%) was obtained from a population of 835 Orudis-treated patients in double-blind trials lasting from 4 to 54 weeks and in 622 Oruvail-treated (200 mg/day) patients in trials lasting from 4 to 16 weeks.

Minor gastrointestinal side effects predominated; upper gastrointestinal symptoms were more common than lower gastrointestinal symptoms. In crossover trials in 321 patients with rheumatoid arthritis or osteoarthritis, there was no difference in either upper or lower gastrointestinal symptoms between patients treated with 200 mg of Oruvail once a day or 75 mg of Orudis TID (225 mg/day). Peptic ulcer or GI bleeding occurred in controlled clinical trials in less than 1% of 1,076 patients; however, in open label continuation studies in 1,292 patients the rate was greater than 2%.

The incidence of peptic ulceration in patients on NSAIDs is dependent on many risk factors including age, sex, smoking, alcohol use, diet, stress, concomitant drugs such as aspirin and corticosteroids, as well as the dose and duration of treatment with NSAIDs (see "**WARNINGS**").

Gastrointestinal reactions were followed in frequency by central nervous system side effects, such as headache, dizziness, or drowsiness. The incidence of some adverse reactions appears to be dose-related (see "**DOSAGE AND ADMINISTRATION**"). Rare adverse reactions (incidence less than 1%) were collected from foreign reports to manufacturers and regulatory agencies, publications, and U.S. clinical trials.

Reactions are listed below under body system, then by incidence or number of cases in decreasing incidence.

INCIDENCE GREATER THAN 1% (PROBABLE CAUSAL RELATIONSHIP)

Digestive: Dyspepsia (11%), nausea*, abdominal pain*, diarrhea*, constipation*, flatulence*, anorexia, vomiting, stomatitis.

Nervous System: Headache*, dizziness, CNS inhibition (i.e., pooled reports of somnolence, malaise, depression, etc.) or excitation (i.e., insomnia, nervousness, dreams, etc.)*.

Special Senses: Tinnitus, visual disturbance.

Skin and Appendages: Rash.

Urogenital: Impairment of renal function (edema, increased BUN)*, signs or symptoms of urinary-tract irritation.

*Adverse events occurring in 3 to 9% of patients.

INCIDENCE LESS THAN 1% (PROBABLE CAUSAL RELATIONSHIP)

Body as a Whole: Chills, facial edema, infection, pain, allergic reaction, anaphylaxis.

Cardiovascular: Hypertension, palpitation, tachycardia, congestive heart failure, peripheral vascular disease, vasodilation.

Digestive: Appetite increased, dry mouth, eructation, gastritis, rectal hemorrhage, melena, fecal occult blood, salivation, peptic ulcer, gastrointestinal perforation, hematemesis, intestinal ulceration.

Hemic: Hypocoagulability, agranulocytosis, anemia, hemolysis, purpura, thrombocytopenia.

Metabolic and Nutritional: Thirst, weight gain, weight loss, hepatic dysfunction, hyponatremia.

Musculoskeletal: Myalgia.

Nervous System: Amnesia, confusion, impotence, migraine, paresthesia, vertigo.

Respiratory: Dyspnea, hemoptysis, epistaxis, pharyngitis, rhinitis, bronchospasm, laryngeal edema.

Skin and Appendages: Alopecia, eczema, pruritus, purpuric rash, sweating, urticaria, bullous rash, exfoliative dermatitis, photosensitivity, skin discoloration, onycholysis.

Special Senses: Conjunctivitis, conjunctivitis sicca, eye pain, hearing impairment, retinal hemorrhage and pigmentation change, taste perversion.

Urogenital: Menometrorrhagia, hematuria, renal failure, interstitial nephritis, nephrotic syndrome.

INCIDENCE LESS THAN 1% (CAUSAL RELATIONSHIP UNKNOWN)

The following rare adverse reactions, whose causal relationship to ketoprofen is uncertain, are being listed to serve as alerting information to the physician.

Body as a Whole: Septicemia, shock.

Cardiovascular: Arrhythmias, myocardial infarction.

Digestive: Buccal necrosis, ulcerative colitis, microvesicular steatosis, jaundice, pancreatitis.

Endocrine: Diabetes mellitus (aggravated).

Nervous System: Dysphoria, hallucination, libido disturbance, nightmares, personality disorder, aseptic meningitis.

Urogenital: Acute tubulopathy, gynecomastia.

OVERDOSAGE

Signs and symptoms following acute NSAID overdose are usually limited to lethargy, drowsiness, nausea, vomiting, and epigastric pain, which are generally reversible with supportive care. Respiratory depression, coma, or convulsions have occurred following large ketoprofen overdoses. Gastrointestinal bleeding, hypotension, hypertension, or acute renal failure may occur, but are rare.

Patients should be managed by symptomatic and supportive care following an NSAID overdose. There are no specific antidotes. Gut decontamination may be indicated in patients with symptoms seen within 4 hours (longer for sustained-release products) or following a large overdose (5 to 10 times the usual dose). This should be accomplished via emesis and/or activated charcoal (60 to 100 g in adults, 1 to 2 g/kg in children) with a saline cathartic or sorbitol added to the first dose. Forced diuresis, alkalinization of the urine, hemodialysis or hemoperfusion would probably not be useful due to ketoprofen's high protein binding.

Case reports include twenty-six overdoses: 6 were in children, 16 in adolescents, and 4 in adults. Five of these patients had minor symptoms (vomiting in 4, drowsiness in 1 child). A 12-year-old girl had tonic-clonic convulsions 1–2 hours after ingesting an unknown quantity of ketoprofen and 1 or 2 tablets of acetaminophen with hydrocodone. Her ketoprofen level was 1128 mg/L (56 times the upper therapeutic level of 20 mg/L) 3–4 hours post ingestion. Full recovery ensued 18 hours after ingestion following management with intubation, diazepam, and activated charcoal. A 45-year-old woman ingested twelve 200 mg Oruvail and 375 mL vodka, was treated with emesis and supportive measures 2 hours after ingestion, and recovered completely with her only complaint being mild epigastric pain.

DOSAGE AND ADMINISTRATION

RHEUMATOID ARTHRITIS AND OSTEOARTHRITIS

The recommended starting dose of ketoprofen in otherwise healthy patients is for Orudis 75 mg three times or 50 mg four times a day, or for Oruvail 200 mg administered once a day. Smaller doses of Orudis or Oruvail should be utilized initially in small individuals, in debilitated or elderly patients. The recommended maximum daily dose of ketoprofen is 300 mg/day for Orudis or 200 mg/day for Oruvail (see "**INDIVIDUALIZATION OF DOSAGE**").

Dosages higher than 300 mg/day of Orudis or 200 mg/day of Oruvail are not recommended because they have not been studied.

Concomitant use of Orudis and Oruvail is not recommended. Relatively smaller people may need smaller doses (See "**INDIVIDUALIZATION OF DOSAGE**".)

MANAGEMENT OF PAIN AND DYSMENORRHEA

The usual dose of Orudis recommended for mild-to-moderate pain and dysmenorrhea is 25 to 50 mg every 6 to 8 hours as necessary. A smaller dose should be utilized initially in small individuals, in debilitated or elderly patients, or in patients with renal or liver disease (see "**GENERAL PRECAUTIONS**"). A larger dose may be tried if the patient's response to a previous dose was less than satisfactory, but doses above 75 mg have not been shown to give added analgesia. Daily doses above 300 mg are not recommended because they have not been adequately studied. Because of its typical nonsteroidal anti-inflammatory drug-side-effect profile, including as its principal adverse effect GI side effects (see "**WARNINGS**" and "**ADVERSE REACTIONS**"), higher doses of Orudis should be used with caution and patients receiving them observed carefully (see "**INDIVIDUALIZATION OF DOSAGE**"l).

Oruvail is not recommended for use in treating acute pain because of its extended-release characteristics.

HOW SUPPLIED

Orudis® (ketoprofen) Capsules are available as follows:

25 mg, NDC 0008-4186, dark-green and red capsule marked "WYETH 4186" on one side and "ORUDIS 25" on the reverse side, in bottles of 100 capsules.

50 mg, NDC 0008-4181, dark-green and light-green capsule marked "WYETH 4181" on one side and "ORUDIS 50" on the reverse side, in bottles of 100 capsules.

75 mg, NDC 0008-4187, dark-green and white capsule marked "WYETH 4187" on one side and "ORUDIS 75" on the reverse side, in bottles of 100 and 500 capsules, and in Redipak® cartons of 100, each containing 10 blister strips of 10 capsules.

Oruvail® (ketoprofen) Extended-Release Capsules are available as follows:

100 mg, NDC 0008-0821, opaque pink and dark-green capsule marked with two radial bands and "ORUVAIL 100" in bottles of 100 capsules and in Redipak® cartons each containing 10 blister strips of 10 capsules.

150 mg, NDC 0008-0822, opaque pink and light-green capsule marked with two radial bands and "ORUVAIL 150" in bottles of 100 capsules and in Redipak® cartons each containing 10 blister strips of 10 capsules.

200 mg, NDC 0008-0690, opaque pink and off-white capsule marked with two radial bands and "ORUVAIL 200" in bottles of 100 capsules and in Redipak® cartons of 100 each containing 10 blister strips of 10 capsules.

Keep tightly closed.

Store at room temperature, approximately 25° C (77° F).

Dispense in a tight container.

Oruvail capsules should be protected from direct light and excessive heat and humidity.

The appearance of these capsules is a trademark of Wyeth-Ayerst Laboratories.

Caution: Federal law prohibits dispensing without prescription.

By arrangement with Rhone-Poulenc Rorer France, Orudis Capsules manufactured and distributed by Wyeth Laboratories Inc.

Oruvail Capsules distributed by Wyeth Laboratories Inc.

Shown in Product Identification Guide, page 340

OVRAL® ℞

[oh 'vral]

TABLETS

(norgestrel and ethinyl estradiol tablets)

Patients should be counseled that this product does not protect against HIV infection (AIDS) and other sexually transmitted diseases.

DESCRIPTION

Each Ovral tablet contains 0.5 mg of norgestrel (*dl* -13-beta-ethyl-17-alpha-ethinyl -17- beta-hydroxygon -4- en -3- one), a totally synthetic progestogen, and 0.05 mg of ethinyl estradiol (19-nor-17α-pregna-1,3,5 (10)-trien-20-yne-3,17-diol). The inactive ingredients present are cellulose, lactose, magnesium stearate, and polacrilin potassium.

CLINICAL PHARMACOLOGY

See LO/OVRAL®.

INDICATIONS AND USAGE

Oral contraceptives are indicated for the prevention of pregnancy in women who elect to use this product as a method of contraception.

Oral contraceptives are highly effective. Table I lists the typical accidental pregnancy rates for users of combination oral contraceptives and other methods of contraception. The efficacy of these contraceptive methods, except sterilization and the IUD, depends upon the reliability with which they are used. Correct and consistent use of methods can result in lower failure rates.

TABLE I: LOWEST EXPECTED AND TYPICAL FAILURE RATES DURING THE FIRST YEAR OF CONTINUOUS USE OF A METHOD

% of Women Experiencing an Accidental Pregnancy in the First Year of Continuous Use

Method	Lowest Expected*	Typical**
(No Contraception)	(85)	(85)
Oral contraceptives		3
combined	0.1	N/A***
progestin only	0.5	N/A***
Diaphragm with spermicidal cream or jelly	6	18
Spermicides alone (foams and vaginal suppositories)	3	21

Continued on next page

Wyeth-Ayerst Laboratories—Cont.

Vaginal Sponge		
nulliparous	6	18
multiparous	9	28
DEPO-PROVERA®		
(injectable progestogen)	0.3	0.3
NORPLANT® SYSTEM (implants)	0.2#	0.2#
IUD		3
progesterone	2	N/A***
copper T 380A	0.8	N/A***
Condom without spermicides	2	12
Periodic abstinence		
(all methods)	1–9	20
Female sterilization	0.2	0.4
Male sterilization	0.1	0.15

Adapted from J. Trussell et al., Table 1, Studies in Family Planning, 21(1), Jan.–Feb. 1990.

 * The authors' best guess of the percentage of women expected to experience an accidental pregnancy among couples who initiate a method (not necessarily for the first time) and who use it consistently and correctly during the first year if they do not stop for any other reason.

 ** This term represents "typical" couples who initiate use of a method (not necessarily for the first time), who experience an accidental pregnancy during the first year if they do not stop use for any other reason.

 *** N/A—Data not available

 \# This data is based on NORPLANT® SYSTEM clinical trials.

CONTRAINDICATIONS
See LO/OVRAL.

WARNINGS
See LO/OVRAL.

PRECAUTIONS
See LO/OVRAL.

Drug Interactions: See LO/OVRAL
Carcinogenesis: See LO/OVRAL
Pregnancy: See LO/OVRAL
Nursing Mothers: See LO/OVRAL
Information For The Patient: See LO/OVRAL.

ADVERSE REACTIONS
See LO/OVRAL.

OVERDOSAGE
See LO/OVRAL.

NONCONTRACEPTIVE HEALTH BENEFITS
See LO/OVRAL.

DOSAGE AND ADMINISTRATION
To achieve maximum contraceptive effectiveness, Ovral must be taken exactly as directed and at intervals not exceeding 24 hours.

The dosage of Ovral is one tablet daily for 21 consecutive days per menstrual cycle according to prescribed schedule. Tablets are then discontinued for 7 days (three weeks on, one week off).

It is recommended that Ovral tablets be taken at the same time each day, preferably after the evening meal or at bedtime.

During the first cycle of medication, the patient is instructed to take one Ovral tablet daily for twenty-one consecutive days, beginning on the first day (Day 1 Start) of her menstrual cycle or on the Sunday after her period begins (Sunday Start). (The first day of menstruation is day one.) The tablets are then discontinued for one week (7 days). Withdrawal bleeding should usually occur within 3 days following discontinuation of Ovral. (For Day 1 Start: If Ovral is first taken later than the first day of the first menstrual cycle of medication or postpartum, contraceptive reliance should not be placed on Ovral until after the first seven consecutive days of administration. For Sunday Start: Contraceptive reliance should not be placed on Ovral until after the first seven consecutive days of administration. The possibility of ovulation and conception prior to initiation of medication should be considered.) The patient begins her next and all subsequent 21-day courses of Ovral tablets on the same day of the week that she began her first course, following the same schedule: 21 days on—7 days off. She begins taking her tablets on the 8th day after discontinuance, regardless of whether or not a menstrual period has occurred or is still in progress. Any time a new cycle of Ovral is started later than the 8th day, the patient should be protected by another means of contraception until she has taken a tablet daily for seven consecutive days.

If spotting or breakthrough bleeding occurs, the patient is instructed to continue on the same regimen. This type of bleeding is usually transient and without significance; however, if the bleeding is persistent or prolonged, the patient is advised to consult her physician. Although the occurrence of pregnancy is highly unlikely if Ovral is taken according to

directions, if withdrawal bleeding does not occur, the possibility of pregnancy must be considered. If the patient has not adhered to the prescribed schedule (missed one or more tablets or started taking them on a day later than she should have), the probability of pregnancy should be considered at the time of the first missed period and appropriate diagnostic measures taken before the medication is resumed. If the patient has adhered to the prescribed regimen and misses two consecutive periods, pregnancy should be ruled out before continuing the contraceptive regimen.

For additional patient instructions regarding missed pills, see the "WHAT TO DO IF YOU MISS PILLS" section in the **DETAILED PATIENT LABELING** for LO/OVRAL.

Any time the patient misses two or more tablets, she should also use another method of contraception until she has taken a tablet daily for seven consecutive days. If breakthrough bleeding occurs following missed tablets, it will usually be transient and of no consequence. While there is little likelihood of ovulation occurring if only one or two tablets are missed, the possibility of ovulation increases with each successive day that scheduled tablets are missed.

In the nonlactating mother, Ovral may be initiated postpartum, for contraception. When the tablets are administered in the postpartum period, the increased risk of thromboembolic disease associated with the postpartum period must be considered (see Contraindications, Warnings, and Precautions concerning thromboembolic disease). It is to be noted that early resumption of ovulation may occur if Parlodel® (bromocriptine mesylate) has been used for the prevention of lactation.

HOW SUPPLIED
Ovral® Tablets (0.5 mg norgestrel and 0.05 mg ethinyl estradiol), Wyeth®, are available in packages of 6 PILPAK® dispensers with 21 tablets each as follows: NDC 0008-0056-01, white, round tablet marked "WYETH" and "56".

References available upon request.
Brief Summary Patient Package Insert: See LO/OVRAL.
DETAILED PATIENT LABELING: See LO/OVRAL.
Shown in Product Identification Guide, page 340

OVRAL®-28
[oh 'vral-28]
Tablets
(norgestrel and ethinyl estradiol tablets)

℞

Patients should be counseled that this product does not protect against HIV infection (AIDS) and other sexually transmitted diseases.

DESCRIPTION
21 white Ovral tablets, each containing 0.5 mg of norgestrel (*dl*-13-beta-ethyl-17-alpha-ethinyl-17-beta-hydroxygon-4-en-3-one), a totally synthetic progestogen, and 0.05 mg of ethinyl estradiol (19-nor-17α-pregna-1,3,5 (10)-trien-20-yne-3,17-diol), and 7 pink inert tablets. The inactive ingredients present are cellulose, D&C Red 30, lactose, magnesium stearate, and polacrilin potassium.

CLINICAL PHARMACOLOGY
See LO/OVRAL®.

INDICATIONS AND USAGE
See OVRAL®.

CONTRAINDICATIONS
See LO/OVRAL.

WARNINGS
See LO/OVRAL.

PRECAUTIONS
See LO/OVRAL.
Drug Interactions: See LO/OVRAL.
Carcinogenesis: See LO/OVRAL.
Pregnancy: See LO/OVRAL.
Nursing Mothers: See LO/OVRAL.
Information for the Patient: See LO/OVRAL.

ADVERSE REACTIONS
See LO/OVRAL.

OVERDOSAGE
See LO/OVRAL.

NONCONTRACEPTIVE HEALTH BENEFITS
See LO/OVRAL.

DOSAGE AND ADMINISTRATION
To achieve maximum contraceptive effectiveness, Ovral-28 must be taken exactly as directed and at intervals not exceeding 24 hours.

The dosage of Ovral-28 is one white tablet daily for 21 consecutive days followed by one pink inert tablet daily for 7 consecutive days according to prescribed schedule.

It is recommended that OVRAL-28 tablets be taken at the same time each day, preferably after the evening meal or at bedtime. During the first cycle of medication, the patient is instructed to begin taking Ovral-28 on the first Sunday after

the onset of menstruation. If menstruation begins on a Sunday, the first tablet (white) is taken that day. One white tablet should be taken daily for 21 consecutive days followed by one pink inert tablet daily for 7 consecutive days. Withdrawal bleeding should usually occur within three days following discontinuation of white tablets. During the first cycle, contraceptive reliance should not be placed on Ovral-28 until a white tablet has been taken daily for 7 consecutive days. The possibility of ovulation and conception prior to initiation of medication should be considered.

The patient begins her next and all subsequent 28-day courses of tablets on the same day of the week (Sunday) on which she began her first course, following the same schedule: 21 days on white tablets—7 days on pink inert tablets. If in any cycle the patient starts tablets later than the proper day, she should protect herself by using another method of birth control until she has taken a white tablet daily for 7 consecutive days.

If spotting or breakthrough bleeding occurs, the patient is instructed to continue on the same regimen. This type of bleeding is usually transient and without significance; however, if the bleeding is persistent or prolonged, the patient is advised to consult her physician. Although the occurrence of pregnancy is highly unlikely if Ovral-28 is taken according to directions, if withdrawal bleeding does not occur, the possibility of pregnancy must be considered. If the patient has not adhered to the prescribed schedule (missed one or more tablets or started taking them on a day later than she should have), the probability of pregnancy should be considered at the time of the first missed period and appropriate diagnostic measures taken before the medication is resumed. If the patient has adhered to the prescribed regimen and misses two consecutive periods, pregnancy should be ruled out before continuing the contraceptive regimen.

For additional patient instructions regarding missed pills, see the "WHAT TO DO IF YOU MISS PILLS" section in the **DETAILED PATIENT LABELING** for LO/OVRAL.

Any time the patient misses two or more white tablets, she should also use another method of contraception until she has taken a white tablet daily for seven consecutive days. If the patient misses one or more pink tablets, she is still protected against pregnancy **provided** she begins taking white tablets again on the proper day.

If breakthrough bleeding occurs following missed white tablets, it will usually be transient and of no consequence. While there is little likelihood of ovulation occurring if only one or two white tablets are missed, the possibility of ovulation increases with each successive day that scheduled white tablets are missed.

In the nonlactating mother, Ovral-28 may be initiated postpartum, for contraception. When the tablets are administered in the postpartum period, the increased risk of thromboembolic disease associated with the postpartum period must be considered (see "Contraindications", "Warnings", and "Precautions" concerning thromboembolic disease). It is to be noted that early resumption of ovulation may occur if Parlodel® (bromocriptine mesylate) has been used for the prevention of lactation.

HOW SUPPLIED
Ovral®-28 Tablets (0.5 mg norgestrel and 0.05 mg ethinyl estradiol), are available in packages of 6 PILPAK® dispensers, each containing 28 tablets as follows:
21 active tablets, NDC 0008-0056, white, round tablet marked "WYETH" and "56".
7 inert tablets, NDC 0008-0445, pink, round tablet marked "WYETH" and "445".

References available upon request.
Brief Summary Patient Package Insert: See LO/OVRAL.
DETAILED PATIENT LABELING: See LO/OVRAL.
Shown in Product Identification Guide, page 340

OVRETTE®
[oh-vret ']
Tablets
(norgestrel tablets)

℞

Patients should be counseled that this product does not protect against HIV infection (AIDS) and other sexually transmitted diseases.
Each OVRETTE® tablet contains 0.075 mg of norgestrel (*dl*-13-beta-ethyl-17-alpha-ethinyl-17-beta-hydroxygon-4-en-3-one). The inactive ingredients present are cellulose, FD&C Yellow 5, lactose, magnesium stearate, and polacrilin potassium.

DESCRIPTION
Each OVRETTE tablet contains 0.075 mg of a single active steroid ingredient, norgestrel, a totally synthetic progestogen. The available data suggest that the *d* (-)enantiomeric form of norgestrel is the biologically active portion. This form amounts to 0.0375 mg per OVRETTE tablet.

CLINICAL PHARMACOLOGY

The primary mechanism through which OVRETTE prevents conception is not known, but progestogen-only contraceptives are known to alter the cervical mucus, exert a progestational effect on the endometrium, interfering with implantation, and, in some patients, suppress ovulation.

INDICATIONS AND USAGE

See LO/OVRAL®.

CONTRAINDICATIONS

See LO/OVRAL.

WARNINGS

See LO/OVRAL.

PRECAUTIONS

See LO/OVRAL.

INFORMATION FOR THE PATIENT

See LO/OVRAL.

DRUG INTERACTIONS

See LO/OVRAL.

CARCINOGENESIS

See LO/OVRAL.

PREGNANCY

See LO/OVRAL.

NURSING MOTHERS

See LO/OVRAL.

ADVERSE REACTIONS

See LO/OVRAL.

OVERDOSAGE

See LO/OVRAL.

DOSAGE AND ADMINISTRATION

To achieve maximum contraceptive effectiveness, OVRETTE must be taken exactly as directed and at intervals not exceeding 24 hours. OVRETTE is administered on a continuous daily dosage regimen starting on the first day of menstruation, i.e., one tablet each day, every day of the year. Tablets should be taken at the same time each day and continued daily, without interruption, whether bleeding occurs or not. The patient should be advised that, if prolonged bleeding occurs, she should consult her physician. In the nonlactating mother, OVRETTE may be initiated postpartum, for contraception. When the tablets are administered in the postpartum period, the increased risk of thromboembolic disease associated with the postpartum period must be considered (see "Contraindications," "Warnings," and "Precautions" concerning thromboembolic disease). It is to be noted that early resumption of ovulation may occur if Parlodel® (bromocriptine mesylate) has been used for the prevention of lactation.

The risk of pregnancy increases with each tablet missed. If the patient misses one tablet, she should be instructed to take it as soon as she remembers and to also take her next tablet at the regular time. If she misses two tablets, she should take one of the missed tablets as soon as she remembers, as well as taking her regular tablet for that day at the proper time. Furthermore, she should use a method of nonhormonal contraception in addition to taking OVRETTE until fourteen tablets have been taken. If more than 2 tablets have been missed, OVRETTE should be discontinued immediately and a method of nonhormonal contraception should be used until menses has appeared or pregnancy has been excluded. If menses does not appear within 45 days from the last period, a method of nonhormonal contraception should be substituted until the start of the next menstrual period or an appropriate diagnostic procedure is performed to rule out pregnancy.

HOW SUPPLIED

OVRETTE® Tablets (0.075 mg norgestrel) are available in packages of 6 PILPAK® dispensers with 28 tablets each as follows: NDC 0008-0062-01, yellow, round tablet marked "WYETH" and "62".

REFERENCES

Available upon request.
Brief Summary Patient Package Insert: See LO/OVRAL
DETAILED PATIENT LABELING: See LO/OVRAL.

PEN•VEE® K   ℞

[pen-vee-kay]
(penicillin V potassium)
TABLETS • FOR ORAL SOLUTION

DESCRIPTION

Penicillin V is the phenoxymethyl analog of penicillin G. Penicillin V potassium is the potassium salt of penicillin V. Pen•Vee K tablets contain penicillin V potassium equivalent to 250 mg (400,000 units) or 500 mg (800,000 units) penicillin V. The inactive ingredients present are carboxy-methylcellulose sodium, magnesium stearate, and stearic acid. The 250 mg dosage strength also contains lactose. Pen•Vee K for oral solution is a powder which when reconstituted as directed yields solution of penicillin V potassium equivalent to 125 mg (200,000 units) or 250 mg (400,000 units) penicillin V per 5 mL. The inactive ingredients present are artificial and natural flavors, citric acid, FD&C Red 40, saccharin sodium, sodium benzoate, sodium citrate, sodium propionate, sucrose, and water. The 250 mg per 5 mL dosage strength also contains edetate disodium and FD&C Yellow 6.

ACTION AND PHARMACOLOGY

Penicillin V exerts a bactericidal action against penicillin-sensitive microorganisms during the stage of active multiplication. It acts through the inhibition of biosynthesis of cell-wall mucopeptide. It is not active against the penicillinase-producing bacteria, which include many strains of staphylococci. The drug exerts high in vitro activity against staphylococci (except penicillinase-producing strains), streptococci (groups A, C, G, H, L, and M), and pneumococci. Other organisms sensitive in vitro to penicillin V are Corynebacterium diphtheriae, Bacillus anthracis, Clostridia, Actinomyces bovis, Streptobacillus moniliformis, Listeria monocytogenes, Leptospira, and Neisseria gonorrhoeae. Treponema pallidum is extremely sensitive.

The potassium salt of penicillin V has the distinct advantage over penicillin G in resistance to inactivation by gastric acid. It may be given with meals; however, blood levels are slightly higher when the drug is given on an empty stomach. Average blood levels are two to five times higher than the levels following the same dose of oral penicillin G and also show much less individual variation.

Once absorbed, penicillin V is about 80% bound to serum protein. Tissue levels are highest in the kidneys, with lesser amounts in the liver, skin, and intestines. Small amounts are found in all other body tissues and the cerebrospinal fluid. The drug is excreted as rapidly as it is absorbed in individuals with normal kidney function; however, recovery of the drug from the urine indicates that only about 25% of the dose given is absorbed. In neonates, young infants, and individuals with impaired kidney function, excretion is considerably delayed.

INDICATIONS

Penicillin V potassium is indicated in the treatment of mild to moderately severe infections due to penicillin G-sensitive microorganisms. Therapy should be guided by bacteriological studies (including sensitivity tests) and by clinical response.

Note: Severe pneumonia, empyema, bacteremia, pericarditis, meningitis, and arthritis should not be treated with penicillin V during the acute stage.

Indicated surgical procedures should be performed.

The following infections will usually respond to adequate dosage of penicillin V.

Streptococcal infections (without bacteremia). Mild-to-moderate infections of the upper respiratory tract, scarlet fever, and mild erysipelas.

Note: Streptococci in groups A, C, G, H, L, and M are very sensitive to penicillin. Other groups, including group D (enterococcus), are resistant.

Pneumococcal infections. Mild to moderately severe infections of the respiratory tract.

Staphylococcal infections—penicillin-G-sensitive. Mild infections of the skin and soft tissues.

Note: Reports indicate an increasing number of strains of staphylococci resistant to penicillin G, emphasizing the need for culture and sensitivity studies in treating suspected staphylococcal infections.

Fusospirochetosis (Vincent's gingivitis and pharyngitis)—Mild to moderately severe infections of the oropharynx usually respond to therapy with oral penicillin.

Note: Necessary dental care should be accomplished in infections involving the gum tissue.

Medical conditions in which oral penicillin therapy is indicated as prophylaxis:

For the prevention of recurrence following rheumatic fever and/or chorea: Prophylaxis with oral penicillin on a continuing basis has proven effective in preventing recurrence of these conditions.

Although no controlled clinical efficacy studies have been conducted, penicillin V has been suggested by the American Heart Association and the American Dental Association for use as an oral regimen for prophylaxis against bacterial endocarditis in patients who have congenital heart disease or rheumatic or other acquired valvular heart disease when they undergo dental procedures and surgical procedures of the upper respiratory tract.[1] Oral penicillin should not be used in those patients at particularly high risk for endocarditis (e.g., those with prosthetic heart valves or surgically constructed systemic-pulmonary shunts). Penicillin V should not be used as adjunctive prophylaxis for genitourinary instrumentation or surgery, lower-intestinal-tract surgery, sigmoidoscopy, and childbirth. Since it may happen that alpha hemolytic streptococci relatively resistant to penicillin may be found when patients are receiving continuous oral penicillin for secondary prevention of rheumatic fever, prophylactic agents other than penicillin may be chosen for these patients and prescribed in addition to their continuous rheumatic fever prophylactic regimen.

Note: When selecting antibiotics for the prevention of bacterial endocarditis, the physician or dentist should read the full joint statement of the American Heart Association and the American Dental Association.[1]

CONTRAINDICATIONS

A previous hypersensitivity reaction to any penicillin is a contraindication.

WARNINGS

Serious and occasionally fatal hypersensitivity (anaphylactoid) reactions have been reported in patients on penicillin therapy. Although anaphylaxis is more frequent following parenteral therapy, it has occurred in patients on oral penicillins. These reactions are more apt to occur in individuals with a history of sensitivity to multiple allergens.

There have been well-documented reports of individuals with a history of penicillin hypersensitivity reactions who have experienced severe hypersensitivity reactions when treated with a cephalosporin. Before therapy with a penicillin, careful inquiry should be made concerning previous hypersensitivity reactions to penicillins, cephalosporins, and other allergens. If an allergic reaction occurs, the drug should be discontinued and the patient treated with the usual agents, e.g., pressor amines, antihistamines, and corticosteroids.

PRECAUTIONS

Penicillin should be used with caution in individuals with histories of significant allergies and/or asthma.

The oral route of administration should not be relied upon in patients with severe illness, or with nausea, vomiting, gastric dilatation, cardiospasm, or intestinal hypermotility. Occasional patients will not absorb therapeutic amounts of orally administered penicillin.

In streptococcal infections, therapy must be sufficient to eliminate the organism (10-day minimum); otherwise the sequelae of streptococcal disease may occur. Cultures should be taken following completion of treatment to determine whether streptococci have been eradicated.

Prolonged use of antibiotics may promote the overgrowth of nonsusceptible organisms, including fungi. Should superinfection occur, appropriate measures should be taken.

ADVERSE REACTIONS

Although the incidence of reactions to oral penicillins has been reported with much less frequency than following parenteral therapy, it should be remembered that all degrees of hypersensitivity, including fatal anaphylaxis, have been reported with oral penicillin.

The most common reactions to oral penicillin are nausea, vomiting, epigastric distress, diarrhea, and black hairy tongue. The hypersensitivity reactions reported are skin eruptions (maculopapular to exfoliative dermatitis), urticaria and other serum-sicknesslike reactions, laryngeal edema, and anaphylaxis. Fever and eosinophilia may frequently be the only reaction observed. Hemolytic anemia, leukopenia, thrombocytopenia, neuropathy, and nephropathy are infrequent reactions and usually associated with high doses of parenteral penicillin.

DOSAGE AND ADMINISTRATION

The dosage of penicillin V should be determined according to the sensitivity of the causative microorganisms and the severity of infection, and adjusted to the clinical response of the patient.

The usual dosage recommendations for adults and children 12 years and over are as follows:

Streptococcal infections—mild to moderately severe—of the upper respiratory tract and including scarlet fever and erysipelas: 125 to 250 mg (200,000 to 400,000 units) every 6 to 8 hours for 10 days.

Pneumococcal infections—mild to moderately severe—of the respiratory tract, including otitis media: 250 to 500 mg (400,000 to 800,000 units) every 6 hours until the patient has been afebrile for at least 2 days.

Staphylococcal infections—mild infections of skin and soft tissue (culture and sensitivity tests should be performed): 250 to 500 mg (400,000 to 800,000 units) every 6 to 8 hours.

Fusospirochetosis (Vincent's infection) of the oropharynx. Mild to moderately severe infections: 250 to 500 mg (400,000 to 800,000 units) every 6 to 8 hours.

For the prevention of recurrence following rheumatic fever and/or chorea: 125 to 250 mg (200,000 to 400,000 units) twice daily on a continuing basis.

For prophylaxis against bacterial endocarditis[1] in patients with congenital heart disease or rheumatic or other acquired valvular heart disease when undergoing dental procedures or surgical procedures of the upper respiratory tract: 2.0 gram of penicillin V (1.0 gram for children under 60 lbs.) 1

Continued on next page

Wyeth-Ayerst Laboratories—Cont.

hour before the procedure, and then, 1.0 gram (500 mg for children under 60 lbs.) 6 hours later.

HOW SUPPLIED

Pen·Vee® K (penicillin V potassium) Tablets contain penicillin V potassium equivalent to 250 mg (400,000 units) or 500 mg (800,000 units) penicillin V. They are white, round, scored tablets supplied as follows:

250 mg (400,000 units), NDC 0008-0059, marked "WYETH" and "59", in bottles of 100 or 500 tablets, and in Redipak® cartons of 100 individually wrapped tablets.

500 mg (800,000 units), NDC 0008-0390, marked "WYETH" and "390", in bottles of 100 or 500 tablets, and in Redipak® cartons of 100 individually wrapped tablets.

Keep tightly closed.

Store at room temperature, approximately 25°C (77°F).

Dispense in tight container.

Pen·Vee® K (penicillin V potassium) for Oral Solution is available as a powder which when reconstituted as directed yields a palatable solution of penicillin V potassium equivalent to 125 mg (200,000 units) or 250 mg (400,000 units) penicillin V per 5 mL and is supplied as follows:

125 mg (200,000 units) per 5 mL, NDC 0008-0004, faint pink powder, in bottles to make 100 mL or 200 mL of red solution.

250 mg (400,000 units) per 5 mL, NDC 0008-0036, light peach-colored powder, in bottles to make 100 mL, 150 mL, or 200 mL of light-orange solution.

Keep tightly closed.

Store at room temperature [approximately 25°C (77°F)] before reconstitution.

After reconstitution, solution must be stored in a refrigerator.

Discard any unused portion after 14 days.

REFERENCE

1. American Heart Association, 1984. Prevention of bacterial endocarditis. Circulation 70(6):1123A–1127A.

Shown in Product Identification Guide, page 340

PEPTAVLON® ℞

[pĕp-tăv'lon]
(pentagastrin)
for subcutaneous injection

HOW SUPPLIED

Peptavlon (pentagastrin) is available in 2 mL ampuls. Each mL contains 0.25 mg (250 micrograms) pentagastrin. Cartons of 10 ampuls (NDC 0046-3290-10).

Refrigerate, 2°C to 8°C (36°F to 46°F), and protect from light.

Do not use if discolored.

For full prescribing information turn to the Diagnostic Product Information section of this edition of the PDR.

PHENERGAN® ℞

[fen'er-gan]
(promethazine HCl Injection, USP)
INJECTION

DESCRIPTION

Promethazine Hydrochloride Injection, USP is a sterile solution for deep intramuscular or intravenous administration. Promethazine HCl (10H-phenothiazine-10-ethanamine, N,N,α-trimethyl-, monohydrochloride) has a chemical formula of $C_{17}H_{21}ClN_2S$ and molecular weight of 320.87.

Each mL contains promethazine hydrochloride, either 25 mg or 50 mg, edetate disodium 0.1 mg, calcium chloride 0.04 mg, sodium metabisulfite 0.25 mg and phenol 5 mg in Water for Injection. pH 4.0–5.5; buffered with acetic acid-sodium acetate. Sealed under nitrogen.

Each mL of TUBEX® Sterile Cartridge Units contains either 25 or 50 mg promethazine hydrochloride with 0.1 mg edetate disodium, 0.04 mg calcium chloride, not more than 5 mg monothioglycerol and 5 mg phenol with sodium acetate-acetic acid buffer. Sealed under nitrogen.

ACTIONS

Promethazine hydrochloride, a phenothiazine derivative, possesses antihistaminic, sedative, antimotion-sickness, antiemetic, and anticholinergic effects. The duration of action is generally from four to six hours. The major side reaction of this drug is sedation. As an antihistamine, it acts by competitive antagonism but does not block the release of histamine. It antagonizes in varying degrees most but not all of the pharmacological effects of histamine.

INDICATIONS AND USAGE

The injectable form of promethazine hydrochloride is indicated for the following conditions:

1. Amelioration of allergic reactions to blood or plasma.
2. In anaphylaxis as an adjunct to epinephrine and other standard measures after the acute symptoms have been controlled.
3. For other uncomplicated allergic conditions of the immediate type when oral therapy is impossible or contraindicated.
4. Active treatment of motion sickness.
5. Preoperative, postoperative, and obstetric (during labor) sedation.
6. Prevention and control of nausea and vomiting associated with certain types of anesthesia and surgery.
7. As an adjunct to analgesics for the control of postoperative pain.
8. For sedation and relief of apprehension and to produce light sleep from which the patient can be easily aroused.
9. Intravenously in special surgical situations, such as repeated bronchoscopy, ophthalmic surgery, and poor-risk patients, with reduced amounts of meperidine or other narcotic analgesic as an adjunct to anesthesia and analgesia.

CONTRAINDICATIONS

Promethazine is contraindicated in comatose states, in patients who have received large amounts of central-nervous-system depressants (alcohol, sedative-hypnotics, including barbiturates, general anesthetics, narcotics, narcotic analgesics, tranquilizers, etc.), and in patients who have demonstrated an idiosyncrasy or hypersensitivity to promethazine. Under no circumstances should promethazine be given by intra-arterial injection due to the likelihood of severe arteriospasm and the possibility of resultant gangrene (see "WARNINGS").

Promethazine Injection should not be given by the subcutaneous route; evidence of chemical irritation has been noted, and necrotic lesions have resulted on rare occasions following subcutaneous injection. The preferred parenteral route of administration is by deep intramuscular injection.

WARNINGS

Promethazine HCl Injection (ampuls only) contains sodium metabisulfite, a sulfite that may cause allergic-type reactions, including anaphylactic symptoms and life-threatening or less severe asthmatic episodes, in certain susceptible people. The overall prevalence of sulfite sensitivity in the general population is unknown and probably low. Sulfite sensitivity is seen more frequently in asthmatic than in nonasthmatic people.

Promethazine may impair the mental and/or physical abilities required for the performance of potentially hazardous tasks, such as driving a vehicle or operating machinery. The concomitant use of alcohol, sedative-hypnotics (including barbiturates), general anesthetics, narcotics, narcotic analgesics, tranquilizers or other central-nervous-system depressants may have an additive sedative effect. Patients should be warned accordingly.

USAGE IN PREGNANCY

The safe use of promethazine has not been established with respect to the possible adverse effects upon fetal development. Therefore, the need for the use of this drug during pregnancy should be weighed against the possible but unknown hazards to the developing fetus.

USE IN CHILDREN

Excessively large dosages of antihistamines, including promethazine, in children may cause hallucinations, convulsions, and sudden death. In children who are acutely ill associated with dehydration, there is an increased susceptibility to dystonias with the use of promethazine hydrochloride injection.

CAUTION SHOULD BE EXERCISED WHEN ADMINISTERING PROMETHAZINE TO CHILDREN. ANTIEMETICS ARE NOT RECOMMENDED FOR TREATMENT OF UNCOMPLICATED VOMITING IN CHILDREN, AND THEIR USE SHOULD BE LIMITED TO PROLONGED VOMITING OF KNOWN ETIOLOGY. THE EXTRAPYRAMIDAL SYMPTOMS WHICH CAN OCCUR SECONDARY TO PROMETHAZINE ADMINISTRATION MAY BE CONFUSED WITH THE CNS SIGNS OF UNDIAGNOSED PRIMARY DISEASE, e.g., ENCEPHALOPATHY OR REYE'S SYNDROME. THE USE OF PROMETHAZINE SHOULD BE AVOIDED IN CHILDREN WHOSE SIGNS AND SYMPTOMS MAY SUGGEST REYE'S SYNDROME OR OTHER HEPATIC DISEASES.

USE IN THE ELDERLY (APPROXIMATELY 60 YEARS OR OLDER)

Since therapeutic requirements for sedative drugs tend to be less in elderly patients, the dosage of promethazine should be reduced for these patients.

OTHER CONSIDERATIONS

Drugs having anticholinergic properties should be used with caution in patients with asthmatic attack, narrow-angle glaucoma, prostatic hypertrophy, stenosing peptic ulcer, pyloroduodenal obstruction, and bladder-neck obstruction. Promethazine should be used with caution in patients with bone-marrow depression. Leukopenia and agranulocytosis have been reported, usually when promethazine has been used in association with other known toxic agents.

INADVERTENT INTRA-ARTERIAL INJECTION

Due to the close proximity of arteries and veins in the areas most commonly used for intravenous injection, extreme care should be exercised to avoid perivascular extravasation or inadvertent intra-arterial injection. Reports compatible with inadvertent intra-arterial injection of promethazine, usually in conjunction with other drugs intended for intravenous use, suggest that pain, severe chemical irritation, severe spasm of distal vessels, and resultant gangrene requiring amputation are likely under such circumstances. Intravenous injection was intended in all the cases reported, but perivascular extravasation or arterial placement of the needle is now suspect. There is no proven successful management of this condition after it occurs, although sympathetic block and heparinization are commonly employed during the acute management because of the results of animal experiments with other known arteriolar irritants. Aspiration of dark blood does not preclude intra-arterial needle placement, because blood is discolored upon contact with promethazine. Use of syringes with rigid plungers or of small bore needles might obscure typical arterial backflow if this is relied upon alone.

When used intravenously, promethazine hydrochloride should be given in a concentration no greater than 25 mg per mL and at a rate not to exceed 25 mg per minute. When administering any irritant drug intravenously, it is usually preferable to inject it through the tubing of an intravenous infusion set that is known to be functioning satisfactorily. In the event that a patient complains of pain during intended intravenous injection of promethazine, the injection should immediately be stopped to provide for evaluation of possible arterial placement or perivascular extravasation.

PRECAUTIONS

Promethazine may significantly affect the actions of other drugs. It may increase, prolong, or intensify the sedative action of central-nervous-system depressants, such as alcohol, sedative hypnotics (including barbiturates), general anesthetics, narcotics, narcotic analgesics, tranquilizers, etc. When given concomitantly with promethazine hydrochloride, the dose of barbiturates should be reduced by at least one-half, and the dose of narcotics should be reduced by one-quarter to one-half. Dosage must be individualized. Excessive amounts of promethazine relative to a narcotic may lead to restlessness and motor hyperactivity in the patient with pain; these symptoms usually disappear with adequate control of the pain. Promethazine should be used cautiously in persons with cardiovascular disease or impairment of liver function.

Although reversal of the vasopressor effect of epinephrine has not been reported with promethazine, the possibility should be considered in case of promethazine overdose.

ADVERSE REACTIONS

CNS EFFECTS

Drowsiness is the most prominent CNS effect of this drug. Extrapyramidal reactions may occur with high doses; this is almost always responsive to a reduction in dosage. Other reported reactions include dizziness, lassitude, tinnitus, incoordination, fatigue, blurred vision, euphoria, diplopia, nervousness, insomnia, tremors, convulsive seizures, oculogyric crises, excitation, catatonic-like states, and hysteria.

CARDIOVASCULAR EFFECTS

Tachycardia, bradycardia, faintness, dizziness, and increases and decreases in blood pressure have been reported following the use of promethazine hydrochloride injection. Venous thrombosis at the injection site has been reported. INTRA-ARTERIAL INJECTION MAY RESULT IN GANGRENE OF THE AFFECTED EXTREMITY ("see WARNINGS").

GASTROINTESTINAL

Nausea and vomiting have been reported, usually in association with surgical procedures and combination drug therapy.

ALLERGIC REACTIONS

These include urticaria, dermatitis, asthma, and photosensitivity. Angioneurotic edema has been reported.

OTHER REPORTED REACTIONS

Leukopenia and agranulocytosis, usually when promethazine has been used in association with other known toxic agents, have been reported. Thrombocytopenic purpura and jaundice of the obstructive type have been associated with the use of promethazine. The jaundice is usually reversible on discontinuation of the drug. Subcutaneous injection has resulted in tissue necrosis. Nasal stuffiness may occur. Dry mouth has been reported.

LABORATORY TESTS

The following laboratory tests may be affected in patients who are receiving therapy with promethazine hydrochloride:

Pregnancy Tests—Diagnostic pregnancy tests based on immunological reactions between HCG and anti-HCG may result in false-negative or false-positive interpretations.

Glucose Tolerance Test—An increase in glucose tolerance has been reported in patients receiving promethazine hydrochloride.

PARADOXICAL REACTIONS (OVERDOSAGE)
Hyperexcitability and abnormal movements, which have been reported in children following a single administration of promethazine, may be manifestations of relative overdosage, in which case, consideration should be given to the discontinuation of the promethazine and to the use of other drugs. Respiratory depression, nightmares, delirium, and agitated behavior have also been reported in some of these patients.

DRUG INTERACTIONS
NARCOTICS AND BARBITURATES
The CNS-depressant effects of narcotics and barbiturates are additive with promethazine hydrochloride.
MONOAMINE OXIDASE INHIBITORS (MAOI)
Drug interactions, including an increased incidence of extrapyramidal effects, have been reported when some MAOI and phenothiazines are used concomitantly. Although such a reaction has not been reported with promethazine, the possibility should be considered.

DOSAGE AND ADMINISTRATION
The preferred parenteral route of administration for promethazine hydrochloride is by deep intramuscular injection. The proper intravenous administration of this product is well tolerated, but use of this route is not without some hazard.
INADVERTENT INTRA-ARTERIAL INJECTION CAN RESULT IN GANGRENE OF THE AFFECTED EXTREMITY (see "Warnings"). SUBCUTANEOUS INJECTION IS CONTRAINDICATED, AS IT MAY RESULT IN TISSUE NECROSIS (see "Contraindications"). When used intravenously, promethazine hydrochloride should be given in concentration no greater than 25 mg/mL at a rate not to exceed 25 mg per minute; it is preferable to inject through the tubing of an intravenous infusion set that is known to be functioning satisfactorily.
The TUBEX® Sterile Cartridge-Needle Unit is suitable for substances to be administered intravenously or intramuscularly.
ALLERGIC CONDITIONS
The average adult dose is 25 mg. This dose may be repeated within two hours if necessary, but continued therapy, if indicated, should be via the oral route as soon as existing circumstances permit. After initiation of treatment, dosage should be adjusted to the smallest amount adequate to relieve symptoms. The average adult dose for amelioration of allergic reactions to blood or plasma is 25 mg.
SEDATION
In hospitalized adult patients, nighttime sedation may be achieved by a dose of 25 to 50 mg of promethazine hydrochloride.
PREOPERATIVE AND POSTOPERATIVE USE
As an adjunct to preoperative or postoperative medication, 25 to 50 mg of promethazine hydrochloride in adults may be combined with appropriately reduced doses of analgesics and atropine-like drugs as desired. Dosage of concomitant analgesic or hypnotic medication should be reduced accordingly.
NAUSEA AND VOMITING
For control of nausea and vomiting, the usual adult dose is 12.5 to 25 mg, not to be repeated more frequently than every four hours. When used for control of postoperative nausea and vomiting, the medication may be administered either intramuscularly or intravenously and dosage of analgesics and barbiturates reduced accordingly.
OBSTETRICS
Promethazine hydrochloride in doses of 50 mg will provide sedation and relieve apprehension in the early stages of labor. When labor is definitely established, 25 to 75 mg (average dose, 50 mg) promethazine hydrochloride may be given intramuscularly or intravenously with an appropriately reduced dose of any desired narcotic. Amnesic agents may be administered as necessary. If necessary, promethazine with a reduced dose of analgesic may be repeated once or twice at four-hour intervals in the course of a normal labor. A maximum total dose of 100 mg of promethazine may be administered during a 24-hour period to patients in labor.
CHILDREN
In children under the age of 12 years, the dosage should not exceed half that of the suggested adult dose. As an adjunct to premedication, the suggested dose is 0.5 mg per lb. of body weight in combination with an equal dose of narcotic or barbiturate and the appropriate dose of an atropine-like drug. Antiemetics should not be used in vomiting of unknown etiology in children.

MANAGEMENT OF OVERDOSAGE
Signs and symptoms of overdosage range from mild depression of the central nervous system and cardiovascular system to profound hypotension, respiratory depression, and unconsciousness. Stimulation may be evident, especially in children and geriatric patients. Atropine-like signs and symptoms—dry mouth, fixed, dilated pupils, flushing, etc., as well as gastrointestinal symptoms, may occur. The treatment of overdosage is essentially symptomatic and supportive. Early gastric lavage may be beneficial if promethazine has been taken orally. Centrally acting emetics are of little use.
Avoid analeptics, which may cause convulsions. Severe hypotension usually responds to the administration of levarterenol or phenylephrine. EPINEPHRINE SHOULD NOT BE USED, since its use in a patient with partial adrenergic blockade may further lower the blood pressure. Extrapyramidal reactions may be treated with anticholinergic antiparkinson agents, diphenhydramine, or barbiturates. Additional measures include oxygen and intravenous fluids. Limited experience with dialysis indicates that it is not helpful.
Parenteral drug products should be inspected visually for particulate matter and discoloration prior to administration, whenever solution and container permit.

HOW SUPPLIED
Phenergan® Injection (Promethazine HCl Injection, USP) is available as follows:
25 mg/mL, 1 mL ampuls packaged in 25s (*NDC* 0008-0063-01)
50 mg/mL, 1 mL ampuls packaged in 25s (*NDC* 0008-0746-01).
STORGE
Protect from light. Keep covered in carton until time of use
Store at controlled room temperature 15°–30°C (59°–86°F).
Do not use if soluton has developed color or contains a precipitate.
ALSO AVAILABLE
Phenergan® Injection (Promethazine HCl Injection, USP) is also available in TUBEX® Sterile Cartridge-Needle Units, either 25 or 50 mg per mL, in packages of 10 TUBEX (1 mL size), as follows:
25 mg per mL, NDC 0008-0416-01, 1 mL size (22 gauge × 1¼ inch needle).
50 mg per mL, NDC 0008-0417-01, 1 mL size (22 gauge × 1¼ inch needle).
Store at room temperature, between 15°C-25°C (59°F-77°F).
Protect from light.
Use carton to protect contents from light.
Do not use if solution is discolored or contains a precipitate.

PHENERGAN® ℞
[fen 'er-gan]
(promethazine hydrochloride)
Syrup Plain and
PHENERGAN® ℞
(promethazine hydrochloride)
Syrup Fortis

DESCRIPTION
Each teaspoon (5 mL) of Phenergan Syrup Plain contains 6.25 mg promethazine hydrochloride in a flavored syrup base with a pH between 4.7 and 5.2. Alcohol 7%. The inactive ingredients present are artificial and natural flavors, citric acid, D&C Red 33, D&C Yellow 10, FD&C Blue 1, FD&C Yellow 6, glycerin, saccharin sodium, sodium benzoate, sodium citrate, sodium propionate, water, and other ingredients.
Each teaspoon (5 mL) of Phenergan Syrup Fortis contains 25 mg promethazine hydrochloride in a flavored syrup base with a pH between 5.0 and 5.5. Alcohol 1.5%. The inactive ingredients present are artificial and natural flavors, citric acid, saccharin sodium, sodium benzoate, sodium propionate, water, and other ingredients.
Promethazine hydrochloride is a racemic compound; the empirical formula is $C_{17}H_{20}N_2S \cdot HCl$ and its molecular weight is 320.88.
Promethazine hydrochloride, a phenothiazine derivative, is designated chemically as N,N,α-trimethyl-10*H*-phenothiazine-10-ethanamine monohydrochloride with the following structural formula:

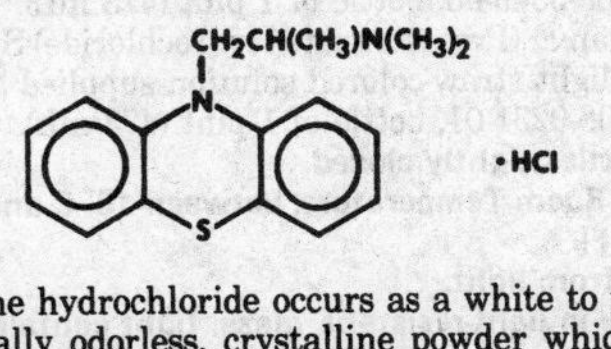

Promethazine hydrochloride occurs as a white to faint yellow, practically odorless, crystalline powder which slowly oxidizes and turns blue on prolonged exposure to air. It is soluble in water and freely soluble in alcohol.

CLINICAL PHARMACOLOGY
Promethazine is a phenothiazine derivative which differs structurally from the antipsychotic phenothiazines by the presence of a branched side chain and no ring substitution. It is thought that this configuration is responsible for its relative lack (1/10 that of chlorpromazine) of dopaminergic (CNS) action.
Promethazine is an H_1 receptor blocking agent. In addition to its antihistaminic action, it provides clinically useful sedative and antiemetic effects. In therapeutic dosage, promethazine produces no significant effects on the cardiovascular system.
Promethazine is well absorbed from the gastrointestinal tract. Clinical effects are apparent within 20 minutes after oral administration and generally last four to six hours, although they may persist as long as 12 hours. Promethazine is metabolized by the liver to a variety of compounds; the sulfoxides of promethazine and N-demethylpromethazine are the predominant metabolites appearing in the urine.

INDICATIONS AND USAGE
Phenergan is useful for:
Perennial and seasonal allergic rhinitis.
Vasomotor rhinitis.
Allergic conjunctivitis due to inhalant allergens and foods.
Mild, uncomplicated allergic skin manifestations of urticaria and angioedema.
Amelioration of allergic reactions to blood or plasma.
Dermographism.
Anaphylactic reactions, as adjunctive therapy to epinephrine and other standard measures, after the acute manifestations have been controlled.
Preoperative, postoperative, or obstetric sedation.
Prevention and control of nausea and vomiting associated with certain types of anesthesia and surgery.
Therapy adjunctive to meperidine or other analgesics for control of postoperative pain.
Sedation in both children and adults, as well as relief of apprehension and production of light sleep from which the patient can be easily aroused.
Active and prophylactic treatment of motion sickness.
Antiemetic therapy in postoperative patients.

CONTRAINDICATIONS
Promethazine is contraindicated in individuals known to be hypersensitive or to have had an idiosyncratic reaction to promethazine or to other phenothiazines.
Antihistamines are contraindicated for use in the treatment of lower respiratory tract symptoms including asthma.

WARNINGS
Promethazine may cause marked drowsiness. Ambulatory patients should be cautioned against such activities as driving or operating dangerous machinery until it is known that they do not become drowsy or dizzy from promethazine therapy.
The sedative action of promethazine hydrochloride is additive to the sedative effects of central nervous system depressants; therefore, agents such as alcohol, narcotic analgesics, sedatives, hypnotics, and tranquilizers should either be eliminated or given in reduced dosage in the presence of promethazine hydrochloride. When given concomitantly with promethazine hydrochloride, the dose of barbiturates should be reduced by at least one-half, and the dose of analgesic depressants, such as morphine or meperidine, should be reduced by one-quarter to one-half.
Promethazine may lower seizure threshold. This should be taken into consideration when administering to persons with known seizure disorders or when giving in combination with narcotics or local anesthetics which may also affect seizure threshold.
Sedative drugs or CNS depressants should be avoided in patients with a history of sleep apnea.
Antihistamines should be used with caution in patients with narrow-angle glaucoma, stenosing peptic ulcer, pyloroduodenal obstruction, and urinary bladder obstruction due to symptomatic prostatic hypertrophy and narrowing of the bladder neck.
Administration of promethazine has been associated with reported cholestatic jaundice.

PRECAUTIONS
GENERAL
Promethazine should be used cautiously in persons with cardiovascular disease or with impairment of liver function.
INFORMATION FOR PATIENTS
Phenergan may cause marked drowsiness or impair the mental and/or physical abilities required for the performance of potentially hazardous tasks, such as driving a vehicle or operating machinery. Ambulatory patients should be told to avoid engaging in such activities until it is known that they do not become drowsy or dizzy from Phenergan therapy. Children should be supervised to avoid potential harm in bike riding or in other hazardous activities.
The concomitant use of alcohol or other central nervous system depressants, including narcotic analgesics, sedatives, hypnotics, and tranquilizers, may have an additive effect and should be avoided or their dosage reduced.
Patients should be advised to report any involuntary muscle movements or unusual sensitivity to sunlight.
DRUG INTERACTIONS
The sedative action of promethazine is additive to the sedative effects of other central nervous system depressants, including alcohol, narcotic analgesics, sedatives, hypnotics, tricyclic antidepressants, and tranquilizers; therefore, these agents should be avoided or administered in reduced dosage to patients receiving promethazine.

Continued on next page

Wyeth-Ayerst Laboratories—Cont.

DRUG/LABORATORY TEST INTERACTIONS
The following laboratory tests may be affected in patients who are receiving therapy with promethazine hydrochloride:
Pregnancy Tests
Diagnostic pregnancy tests based on immunological reactions between HCG and anti-HCG may result in false-negative or false-positive interpretations.
Glucose Tolerance Test
An increase in blood glucose has been reported in patients receiving promethazine.
CARCINOGENESIS, MUTAGENESIS, IMPAIRMENT OF FERTILITY
Long-term animal studies have not been performed to assess the carcinogenic potential of promethazine, nor are there other animal or human data concerning carcinogenicity, mutagenicity, or impairment of fertility with this drug. Promethazine was nonmutagenic in the *Salmonella* test system of Ames.
PREGNANCY
Teratogenic Effects—Pregnancy Category C
Teratogenic effects have not been demonstrated in rat-feeding studies at doses of 6.25 and 12.5 mg/kg of promethazine. These doses are from approximately 2.1 to 4.2 times the maximum recommended total daily dose of promethazine for a 50-kg subject, depending upon the indication for which the drug is prescribed. Specific studies to test the action of the drug on parturition, lactation, and development of the animal neonate were not done, but a general preliminary study in rats indicated no effect on these parameters. Although antihistamines, including promethazine, have been found to produce fetal mortality in rodents, the pharmacological effects of histamine in the rodent do not parallel those in man. There are no adequate and well-controlled studies of promethazine in pregnant women. Phenergan should be used during pregnancy only if the potential benefit justifies the potential risk to the fetus.
Nonteratogenic Effects
Promethazine taken within two weeks of delivery may inhibit platelet aggregation in the newborn.
LABOR AND DELIVERY
Phenergan, in appropriate dosage form, may be used alone or as an adjunct to narcotic analgesics during labor and delivery. (See "Indications and Usage" and "Dosage and Administration.")
See also "Nonteratogenic Effects."
NURSING MOTHERS
It is not known whether promethazine is excreted in human milk. Caution should be exercised when promethazine is administered to a nursing woman.
PEDIATRIC USE
This product should not be used in children under 2 years of age because safety for such use has not been established.

ADVERSE REACTIONS

Nervous System—Sedation, sleepiness, occasional blurred vision, dryness of mouth, dizziness; rarely confusion, disorientation, and extrapyramidal symptoms such as oculogyric crisis, torticollis, and tongue protrusion (usually in association with parenteral injection or excessive dosage).
Cardiovascular—Increased or decreased blood pressure.
Dermatologic—Rash, rarely photosensitivity.
Hematologic—Rarely leukopenia, thrombocytopenia; agranulocytosis (1 case).
Gastrointestinal—Nausea and vomiting.

OVERDOSAGE

Signs and symptoms of overdosage with promethazine range from mild depression of the central nervous system and cardiovascular system to profound hypotension, respiratory depression, and unconsciousness.
Stimulation may be evident, especially in children and geriatric patients. Convulsions may rarely occur. A paradoxical reaction has been reported in children receiving single doses of 75 mg to 125 mg orally, characterized by hyperexcitability and nightmares.
Atropinelike signs and symptoms—dry mouth, fixed, dilated pupils, flushing, as well as gastrointestinal symptoms, may occur.
TREATMENT
Treatment of overdosage is essentially symptomatic and supportive. Only in cases of extreme overdosage or individual sensitivity do vital signs including respiration, pulse, blood pressure, temperature, and EKG need to be monitored. Activated charcoal orally or by lavage may be given, or sodium or magnesium sulfate orally as a cathartic. Attention should be given to the reestablishment of adequate respiratory exchange through provision of a patent airway and institution of assisted or controlled ventilation. Diazepam may be used to control convulsions. Acidosis and electrolyte losses should be corrected. Note that any depressant effects of promethazine are not reversed by naloxone. Avoid analeptics which may cause convulsions.
Severe hypotension usually responds to the administration of norepinephrine or phenylephrine. EPINEPHRINE SHOULD NOT BE USED, since its use in patients with partial adrenergic blockade may further lower the blood pressure.
Limited experience with dialysis indicates that it is not helpful.

DOSAGE AND ADMINISTRATION

ALLERGY
The average oral dose is 25 mg taken before retiring; however, 12.5 mg may be taken before meals and on retiring, if necessary. Children tolerate this product well. Single 25-mg doses at bedtime or 6.25 to 12.5 mg taken three times daily will usually suffice. After initiation of treatment in children or adults, dosage should be adjusted to the smallest amount adequate to relieve symptoms.
Phenergan Rectal Suppositories may be used if the oral route is not feasible, but oral therapy should be resumed as soon as possible if continued therapy is indicated.
The administration of promethazine hydrochloride in 25-mg doses will control minor transfusion reactions of an allergic nature.
MOTION SICKNESS
The average adult dose is 25 mg taken twice daily. The initial dose should be taken one-half to one hour before anticipated travel and be repeated 8 to 12 hours later, if necessary. On succeeding days of travel, it is recommended that 25 mg be given on arising and again before the evening meal. For children, Phenergan Tablets, Syrup, or Rectal Suppositories, 12.5 to 25 mg, twice daily, may be administered.
NAUSEA AND VOMITING
The average effective dose of Phenergan for the active therapy of nausea and vomiting in children or adults is 25 mg. When oral medication cannot be tolerated, the dose should be given parenterally (cf. Phenergan Injection) or by rectal suppository. 12.5- to 25-mg doses may be repeated, as necessary, at 4- to 6-hour intervals.
For nausea and vomiting in children, the usual dose is 0.5 mg per pound of body weight, and the dose should be adjusted to the age and weight of the patient and the severity of the condition being treated.
For prophylaxis of nausea and vomiting, as during surgery and the postoperative period, the average dose is 25 mg repeated at 4- to 6-hour intervals, as necessary.
SEDATION
This product relieves apprehension and induces a quiet sleep from which the patient can be easily aroused. Administration of 12.5 to 25 mg Phenergan by the oral route or by rectal suppository at bedtime will provide sedation in children. Adults usually require 25 to 50 mg for nighttime, presurgical, or obstetrical sedation.
PRE- AND POSTOPERATIVE USE
Phenergan in 12.5- to 25-mg doses for children and 50-mg doses for adults the night before surgery relieves apprehension and produces a quiet sleep.
For preoperative medication children require doses of 0.5 mg per pound of body weight in combination with an equal dose of meperidine and the appropriate dose of an atropinelike drug.
Usual adult dosage is 50 mg Phenergan with an equal amount of meperidine and the required amount of a belladonna alkaloid.
Postoperative sedation and adjunctive use with analgesics may be obtained by the administration of 12.5 to 25 mg in children and 25- to 50-mg doses in adults.
Phenergan Syrup Plain and Phenergan Syrup Fortis are not recommended for children under 2 years of age.

HOW SUPPLIED

Phenergan® (Promethazine Hydrochloride) Syrup Plain is a clear, green solution supplied as follows:
NDC 0008-0549-02, case of 24 bottles of 4 fl. oz. (118 mL).
NDC 0008-0549-03, bottle of 1 pint (473 mL).
Phenergan® (Promethazine Hydrochloride) Syrup Fortis is a clear, light straw-colored solution supplied as follows:
NDC 0008-0231-01, bottle of 1 pint (473 mL).
Keep bottles tightly closed.
Store at Room Temperature, between 15° C and 25° C (59° F and 77° F).
Protect from light.
Dispense in light-resistant, glass, tight containers.

PHENERGAN® ℞

[fen 'er-gan]
(promethazine HCl)
TABLETS •
SUPPOSITORIES

DESCRIPTION

Each tablet of Phenergan contains 12.5 mg, 25 mg, or 50 mg promethazine hydrochloride. The inactive ingredients present are lactose, magnesium stearate, and methylcellulose. Each dosage strength also contains the following:
12.5 mg—FD&C Yellow 6 and saccharin sodium;
25 mg—saccharin sodium;
50 mg—FD&C Red 40.
Each rectal suppository of Phenergan contains 12.5 mg, 25 mg, or 50 mg promethazine hydrochloride with ascorbyl palmitate, silicon dioxide, white wax, and cocoa butter.
Promethazine hydrochloride is a racemic compound; the empirical formula is $C_{17}H_{20}N_2S \cdot HCl$ and its molecular weight is 320.88.
Promethazine hydrochloride, a phenothiazine derivative, is designated chemically as N,N,α-trimethyl-10H-phenothiazine-10-ethanamine monohydrochloride.
Promethazine hydrochloride occurs as a white to faint yellow, practically odorless, crystalline powder which slowly oxidizes and turns blue on prolonged exposure to air. It is soluble in water and freely soluble in alcohol.

CLINICAL PHARMACOLOGY

Promethazine is a phenothiazine derivative which differs structurally from the antipsychotic phenothiazines by the presence of a branched side chain and no ring substitution. It is thought that this configuration is responsible for its relative lack ($\frac{1}{10}$ that of chlorpromazine) of dopaminergic (CNS) action.
Promethazine is an H_1 receptor blocking agent. In addition to its antihistaminic action, it provides clinically useful sedative and antiemetic effects. In therapeutic dosage, promethazine produces no significant effects on the cardiovascular system.
Promethazine is well absorbed from the gastrointestinal tract. Clinical effects are apparent within 20 minutes after oral administration and generally last four to six hours, although they may persist as long as 12 hours. Promethazine is metabolized by the liver to a variety of compounds; the sulfoxides of promethazine and N-demethylpromethazine are the predominant metabolites appearing in the urine.

INDICATIONS AND USAGE

Phenergan, either orally or by suppository, is useful for:
Perennial and seasonal allergic rhinitis.
Vasomotor rhinitis.
Allergic conjunctivitis due to inhalant allergens and foods.
Mild, uncomplicated allergic skin manifestations of urticaria and angioedema.
Amelioration of allergic reactions to blood or plasma.
Dermographism.
Anaphylactic reactions, as adjunctive therapy to epinephrine and other standard measures, after the acute manifestations have been controlled.
Preoperative, postoperative, or obstetric sedation.
Prevention and control of nausea and vomiting associated with certain types of anesthesia and surgery.
Therapy adjunctive to meperidine or other analgesics for control of postoperative pain.
Sedation in both children and adults, as well as relief of apprehension and production of light sleep from which the patient can be easily aroused.
Active and prophylactic treatment of motion sickness.
Antiemetic therapy in postoperative patients.

CONTRAINDICATIONS

Promethazine is contraindicated in individuals known to be hypersensitive or to have had an idiosyncratic reaction to promethazine or to other phenothiazines.
Antihistamines are contraindicated for use in the treatment of lower respiratory tract symptoms including asthma.

WARNINGS

Promethazine may cause marked drowsiness. Ambulatory patients should be cautioned against such activities as driving or operating dangerous machinery until it is known that they do not become drowsy or dizzy from promethazine therapy.
The sedative action of promethazine hydrochloride is additive to the sedative effects of central nervous system depressants; therefore, agents such as alcohol, narcotic analgesics, sedatives, hypnotics, and tranquilizers should either be eliminated or given in reduced dosage in the presence of promethazine hydrochloride. When given concomitantly with promethazine hydrochloride, the dose of barbiturates should be reduced by at least one-half, and the dose of analgesic depressants, such as morphine or meperidine, should be reduced by one-quarter to one-half.
Promethazine may lower seizure threshold. This should be taken into consideration when administering to persons with known seizure disorders or when giving in combination with narcotics and local anesthetics which may also affect seizure threshold.
Sedative drugs or CNS depressants should be avoided in patients with a history of sleep apnea.
Antihistamines should be used with caution in patients with narrow-angle glaucoma, stenosing peptic ulcer, pyloroduodenal obstruction, and urinary bladder obstruction due to symptomatic prostatic hypertrophy and narrowing of the bladder neck.
Administration of promethazine has been associated with reported cholestatic jaundice.

PRECAUTIONS

GENERAL

Promethazine should be used cautiously in persons with cardiovascular disease or with impairment of liver function.

INFORMATION FOR PATIENTS

Phenergan may cause marked drowsiness or impair the mental and/or physical abilities required for the performance of potentially hazardous tasks, such as driving a vehicle or operating machinery. Ambulatory patients should be told to avoid engaging in such activities until it is known that they do not become drowsy or dizzy from Phenergan therapy. Children should be supervised to avoid potential harm in bike riding or in other hazardous activities.

The concomitant use of alcohol or other central nervous system depressants, including narcotic analgesics, sedatives, hypnotics, and tranquilizers, may have an additive effect and should be avoided or their dosage reduced.

Patients should be advised to report any involuntary muscle movements or unusual sensitivity to sunlight.

DRUG INTERACTIONS

The sedative action of promethazine is additive to the sedative effects of other central nervous system depressants, including alcohol, narcotic analgesics, sedatives, hypnotics, tricyclic antidepressants, and tranquilizers; therefore, these agents should be avoided or administered in reduced dosage to patients receiving promethazine.

DRUG/LABORATORY TEST INTERACTIONS

The following laboratory tests may be affected in patients who are receiving therapy with promethazine hydrochloride:

Pregnancy Tests

Diagnostic pregnancy tests based on immunological reactions between HCG and anti-HCG may result in false-negative or false-positive interpretations.

Glucose Tolerance Test

An increase in blood glucose has been reported in patients receiving promethazine.

CARCINOGENESIS, MUTAGENESIS, IMPAIRMENT OF FERTILITY

Long-term animal studies have not been performed to assess the carcinogenic potential of promethazine, nor are there other animal or human data concerning carcinogenicity, mutagenicity, or impairment of fertility with this drug. Promethazine was nonmutagenic in the *Salmonella* test system of Ames.

PREGNANCY

Teratogenic Effects—Pregnancy Category C

Teratogenic effects have not been demonstrated in rat-feeding studies at doses of 6.25 and 12.5 mg/kg of promethazine. These doses are from approximately 2.1 to 4.2 times the maximum recommended total daily dose of promethazine for a 50-kg subject, depending upon the indication for which the drug is prescribed. Specific studies to test the action of the drug on parturition, lactation, and development of the animal neonate were not done, but a general preliminary study in rats indicated no effect on these parameters. Although antihistamines, including promethazine, have been found to produce fetal mortality in rodents, the pharmacological effects of histamine in the rodent do not parallel those in man. There are no adequate and well-controlled studies of promethazine in pregnant women. Phenergan should be used during pregnancy only if the potential benefit justifies the potential risk to the fetus.

Nonteratogenic Effects

Promethazine taken within two weeks of delivery may inhibit platelet aggregation in the newborn.

LABOR AND DELIVERY

Phenergan, in appropriate dosage form, may be used alone or as an adjunct to narcotic analgesics during labor and delivery. (See "Indications and Usage" and "Dosage and Administration.")

See also "Nonteratogenic Effects."

NURSING MOTHERS

It is not known whether promethazine is excreted in human milk. Caution should be exercised when promethazine is administered to a nursing woman.

PEDIATRIC USE

This product should not be used in children under 2 years of age because safety for such use has not been established.

ADVERSE REACTIONS

Nervous System—Sedation, sleepiness, occasional blurred vision, dryness of mouth, dizziness; rarely confusion, disorientation, and extrapyramidal symptoms such as oculogyric crisis, torticollis, and tongue protrusion (usually in association with parenteral injection or excessive dosage).

Cardiovascular—Increased or decreased blood pressure.

Dermatologic—Rash, rarely photosensitivity.

Hematologic—Rarely leukopenia, thrombocytopenia; agranulocytosis (1 case).

Gastrointestinal—Nausea and vomiting.

OVERDOSAGE

Signs and symptoms of overdosage with promethazine range from mild depression of the central nervous system and cardiovascular system to profound hypotension, respiratory depression, and unconsciousness.

Stimulation may be evident, especially in children and geriatric patients. Convulsions may rarely occur. A paradoxical reaction has been reported in children receiving single doses of 75 mg to 125 mg orally, characterized by hyperexcitability and nightmares.

Atropine-like signs and symptoms—dry mouth, fixed, dilated pupils, flushing, as well as gastrointestinal symptoms, may occur.

TREATMENT

Treatment of overdosage is essentially symptomatic and supportive. Only in cases of extreme overdosage or individual sensitivity do vital signs, including respiration, pulse, blood pressure, temperature, and EKG, need to be monitored. Activated charcoal orally or by lavage may be given, or sodium or magnesium sulfate orally as a cathartic. Attention should be given to the reestablishment of adequate respiratory exchange through provision of a patent airway and institution of assisted or controlled ventilation. Diazepam may be used to control convulsions. Acidosis and electrolyte losses should be corrected. Note that any depressant effects of promethazine are not reversed by naloxone. Avoid analeptics which may cause convulsions.

Severe hypotension usually responds to the administration of norepinephrine or phenylephrine. EPINEPHRINE SHOULD NOT BE USED, since its use in patients with partial adrenergic blockade may further lower the blood pressure.

Limited experience with dialysis indicates that it is not helpful.

DOSAGE AND ADMINISTRATION

ALLERGY

The average oral dose is 25 mg taken before retiring; however, 12.5 mg may be taken before meals and on retiring, if necessary. Children tolerate this product well. Single 25-mg doses at bedtime or 6.25 to 12.5 mg taken three times daily will usually suffice. After initiation of treatment in children or adults, dosage should be adjusted to the smallest amount adequate to relieve symptoms. The administration of promethazine hydrochloride in 25-mg doses will control minor transfusion reactions of an allergic nature.

MOTION SICKNESS

The average adult dose is 25 mg taken twice daily. The initial dose should be taken one-half to one hour before anticipated travel and be repeated 8 to 12 hours later, if necessary. On succeeding days of travel, it is recommended that 25 mg be given on arising and again before the evening meal. For children, Phenergan Tablets, Syrup, or Rectal Suppositories, 12.5 to 25 mg, twice daily, may be administered.

NAUSEA AND VOMITING

The average effective dose of Phenergan for the active therapy of nausea and vomiting in children or adults is 25 mg. When oral medication cannot be tolerated, the dose should be given parenterally (cf. Phenergan Injection) or by rectal suppository. 12.5- to 25-mg doses may be repeated, as necessary, at 4- to 6-hour intervals.

For nausea and vomiting in children, the usual dose is 0.5 mg per pound of body weight, and the dose should be adjusted to the age and weight of the patient and the severity of the condition being treated.

For prophylaxis of nausea and vomiting, as during surgery and the postoperative period, the average dose is 25 mg repeated at 4- to 6-hour intervals, as necessary.

SEDATION

This product relieves apprehension and induces a quiet sleep from which the patient can be easily aroused. Administration of 12.5 to 25 mg Phenergan by the oral route or by rectal suppository at bedtime will provide sedation in children. Adults usually require 25 to 50 mg for nighttime, presurgical, or obstetrical sedation.

PRE- AND POSTOPERATIVE USE

Phenergan in 12.5- to 25-mg doses for children and 50-mg doses for adults the night before surgery relieves apprehension and produces a quiet sleep.

For preoperative medication children require doses of 0.5 mg per pound of body weight in combination with an equal dose of meperidine and the appropriate dose of an atropine-like drug.

Usual adult dosage is 50 mg Phenergan with an equal amount of meperidine and the required amount of a belladonna alkaloid.

Postoperative sedation and adjunctive use with analgesics may be obtained by the administration of 12.5 to 25 mg in children and 25- to 50-mg doses in adults.

Phenergan Tablets and Phenergan Rectal Suppositories are not recommended for children under 2 years of age.

HOW SUPPLIED

Phenergan® (promethazine HCl) Tablets are available as follows:

12.5 mg, orange tablet with "WYETH" on one side and "19" on the scored reverse side.

NDC 0008-0019-01, bottle of 100 tablets.

25 mg, white tablet with "WYETH" and "27" on one side and scored on the reverse side.

NDC 0008-0027-02, bottle of 100 tablets.

NDC 0008-0027-07, Redipak® carton of 100 tablets (10 blister strips of 10).

50 mg, pink tablet with "WYETH" on one side and "227" on the other side.

NDC 0008-0227-01, bottle of 100 tablets.

Keep tightly closed.

Store at room temperature, between 15°C and 25°C (59°F and 77°F).

Protect from light.

Dispense in light-resistant, tight container.

Use carton to protect contents from light.

Phenergan® (promethazine HCl) Rectal Suppositories are available in boxes of 12 as follows:

12.5 mg, ivory, torpedo-shaped suppository wrapped in copper-colored foil, NDC 0008-0498-01.

25 mg, ivory, torpedo-shaped suppository wrapped in light-green foil, NDC 0008-0212-01.

50 mg, ivory, torpedo-shaped suppository wrapped in blue foil, NDC 0008-0229-01.

Store refrigerated between 2°–8°C (36°–46°F).

Dispense in well-closed container.

Shown in Product Identification Guide, page 340

PHENERGAN® Ⓒ ℞

[fen 'er-gan]

with codeine

(Warning—may be habit-forming)

(Promethazine Hydrochloride and Codeine Phosphate) Syrup

DESCRIPTION

Each teaspoon (5 mL) of Phenergan with codeine contains 10 mg codeine phosphate (Warning—may be habit-forming) and 6.25 mg promethazine hydrochloride in a flavored syrup base with a pH between 4.7 and 5.2. Alcohol 7%. The inactive ingredients present are artificial and natural flavors, citric acid, D&C Red 33, FD&C Blue 1, FD&C Yellow 6, glycerine, saccharin sodium, sodium benzoate, sodium citrate, sodium propionate, water, and other ingredients.

Codeine is one of the naturally occurring phenanthrene alkaloids of opium derived from the opium poppy; it is classified pharmacologically as a narcotic analgesic. Codeine phosphate may be chemically named as (5α,6α)-7, 8-didehydro-4, 5-epoxy-3-methoxy-17-methylmorphinan-6-ol phosphate (1:1) (salt) hemihydrate with the following structural formula:

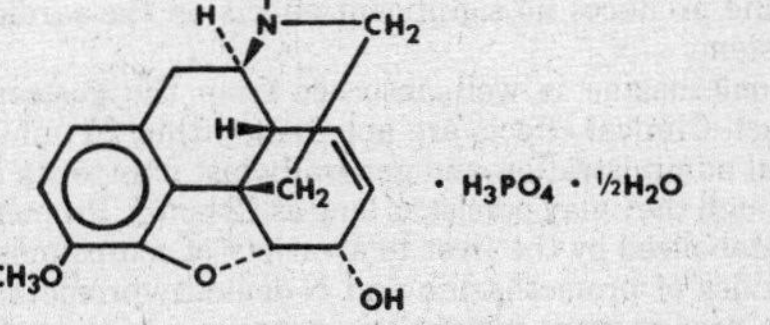

The phosphate salt of codeine occurs as white, needle-shaped crystals or white crystalline powder. Codeine phosphate is freely soluble in water and slightly soluble in alcohol, with a molecular weight of 406.37. The empirical formula is $C_{18}H_{21}NO_3 \cdot H_3PO_4 \cdot ½H_2O$, and the stereochemistry is 5α, 6α isomer as indicated in the structure.

Promethazine hydrochloride is a racemic compound; the empirical formula is $C_{17}H_{20}N_2S \cdot HCl$ and its molecular weight is 320.88.

Promethazine hydrochloride, a phenothiazine derivative, is designated chemically as N,N,α-trimethyl-10*H*-phenothiazine-10-ethanamine monohydrochloride with the following structural formula:

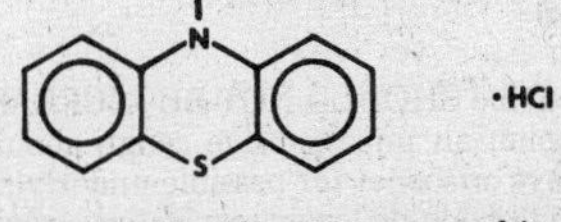

Promethazine hydrochloride occurs as a white to faint yellow, practically odorless, crystalline powder which slowly oxidizes and turns blue on prolonged exposure to air. It is soluble in water and freely soluble in alcohol.

CLINICAL PHARMACOLOGY

CODEINE

Narcotic analgesics, including codeine, exert their primary effects on the central nervous system and gastrointestinal tract. The analgesic effects of codeine are due to its central action; however, the precise sites of action have not been

Continued on next page

Wyeth-Ayerst Laboratories—Cont.

determined, and the mechanisms involved appear to be quite complex. Codeine resembles morphine both structurally and pharmacologically, but its actions at the doses of codeine used therapeutically are milder, with less sedation, respiratory depression, and gastrointestinal, urinary, and pupillary effects. Codeine produces an increase in biliary tract pressure, but less than morphine or meperidine. Codeine is less constipating than morphine.

Codeine has good antitussive activity, although less than that of morphine at equal doses. It is used in preference to morphine, because side effects are infrequent at the usual antitussive dose of codeine.

Codeine in oral therapeutic dosage does not usually exert major effects on the cardiovascular system.

Narcotic analgesics may cause nausea and vomiting by stimulating the chemoreceptor trigger zone (CTZ); however, they also depress the vomiting center, so that subsequent doses are unlikely to produce vomiting. Nausea is minimal after usual oral doses of codeine.

Narcotic analgesics cause histamine release, which appears to be responsible for wheals or urticaria sometimes seen at the site of injection on parenteral administration. Histamine release may also produce dilation of cutaneous blood vessels, with resultant flushing of the face and neck, pruritus, and sweating.

Codeine and its salts are well absorbed following both oral and parenteral administration. Codeine is about 2/3 as effective orally as parenterally. Codeine is metabolized primarily in the liver by enzymes of the endoplasmic reticulum, where it undergoes O-demethylation, N-demethylation, and partial conjugation with glucuronic acid. The drug is excreted primarily in the urine, largely as inactive metabolites and small amounts of free and conjugated morphine. Negligible amounts of codeine and its metabolites are found in the feces. Following oral or subcutaneous administration of codeine, the onset of analgesia occurs within 15 to 30 minutes and lasts for four to six hours.

The cough-depressing action, in animal studies, was observed to occur 15 minutes after oral administration of codeine, peak action at 45 to 60 minutes after ingestion. The duration of action, which is dose-dependent, usually did not exceed 3 hours.

PROMETHAZINE
Promethazine is a phenothiazine derivative which differs structurally from the antipsychotic phenothiazines by the presence of a branched side chain and no ring substitution. It is thought that this configuration is responsible for its lack (1/10 that of chlorpromazine) of dopaminergic (CNS) action. Promethazine is an H_1 receptor blocking agent. In addition to its antihistaminic action, it provides clinically useful sedative and antiemetic effects. In therapeutic dosages, promethazine produces no significant effects on the cardiovascular system.

Promethazine is well absorbed from the gastrointestinal tract. Clinical effects are apparent within 20 minutes after oral administration and generally last four to six hours, although they may persist as long as 12 hours. Promethazine is metabolized by the liver to a variety of compounds; the sulfoxides of promethazine and N-demethylpromethazine are the predominant metabolites appearing in the urine.

INDICATIONS AND USAGE
Phenergan with codeine is indicated for the temporary relief of coughs and upper respiratory symptoms associated with allergy or the common cold.

CONTRAINDICATIONS
Codeine is contraindicated in patients with a known hypersensitivity to the drug.

Promethazine is contraindicated in individuals known to be hypersensitive or to have had an idiosyncratic reaction to promethazine or to other phenothiazines.

Antihistamines and codeine are both contraindicated for use in the treatment of lower respiratory tract symptoms, including asthma.

WARNINGS
CODEINE
Dosage of codeine SHOULD NOT BE INCREASED if cough fails to respond; an unresponsive cough should be reevaluated in 5 days or sooner for possible underlying pathology, such as foreign body or lower respiratory tract disease.
Codeine may cause or aggravate constipation.
Respiratory depression leading to arrest, coma, and death has occurred with the use of codeine antitussives in young children, particularly in the under-one-year infants whose ability to deactivate the drug is not fully developed.
Administration of codeine may be accompanied by histamine release and should be used with caution in atopic children.
Head Injury and Increased Intracranial Pressure
The respiratory-depressant effects of narcotic analgesics and their capacity to elevate cerebrospinal fluid pressure may be markedly exaggerated in the presence of head injury, intra-

cranial lesions, or a preexisting increase in intracranial pressure. Narcotics may produce adverse reactions which may obscure the clinical course of patients with head injuries.
Asthma and Other Respiratory Conditions
Narcotic analgesics or cough suppressants, including codeine, should not be used in asthmatic patients (see "Contraindications"). Nor should they be used in acute febrile illness associated with productive cough or in chronic respiratory disease where interference with ability to clear the tracheobronchial tree of secretions would have a deleterious effect on the patient's respiratory function.
Hypotensive Effect
Codeine may produce orthostatic hypotension in ambulatory patients.
PROMETHAZINE
Promethazine may cause marked drowsiness. Ambulatory patients should be cautioned against such activities as driving or operating dangerous machinery until it is known that they do not become drowsy or dizzy from promethazine therapy.
The sedative action of promethazine hydrochloride is additive to the sedative effects of central nervous system depressants; therefore, agents such as alcohol, narcotic analgesics, sedatives, hypnotics, and tranquilizers should either be eliminated or given in reduced dosage in the presence of promethazine hydrochloride. When given concomitantly with promethazine hydrochloride, the dose of barbiturates should be reduced by at least one-half, and the dose of analgesic depressants, such as morphine or meperidine, should be reduced by one-quarter to one-half.
Promethazine may lower seizure threshold. This should be taken into consideration when administering to persons with known seizure disorders or when giving in combination with narcotics or local anesthetics which may also affect seizure threshold.
Sedative drugs or CNS depressants should be avoided in patients with a history of sleep apnea.
Antihistamines should be used with caution in patients with narrow-angle glaucoma, stenosing peptic ulcer, pyloroduodenal obstruction, and urinary bladder obstruction due to symptomatic prostatic hypertrophy and narrowing of the bladder neck.
Administration of promethazine has been associated with reported cholestatic jaundice.

PRECAUTIONS
Animal reproduction studies have not been conducted with the drug combination—promethazine and codeine. It is not known whether this drug combination can cause fetal harm when administered to a pregnant woman or can affect reproduction capacity. Phenergan with codeine should be given to a pregnant woman only if clearly needed.
GENERAL
Narcotic analgesics, including codeine, should be administered with caution and the initial dose reduced in patients with acute abdominal conditions, convulsive disorders, significant hepatic or renal impairment, fever, hypothyroidism, Addison's disease, ulcerative colitis, prostatic hypertrophy, in patients with recent gastrointestinal or urinary tract surgery, and in the very young or elderly or debilitated patients. Promethazine should be used cautiously in persons with cardiovascular disease or with impairment of liver function.
INFORMATION FOR PATIENTS
Phenergan with codeine may cause marked drowsiness or may impair the mental and/or physical abilities required for the performance of potentially hazardous tasks, such as driving a vehicle or operating machinery. Ambulatory patients should be told to avoid engaging in such activities until it is known that they do not become drowsy or dizzy from Phenergan with codeine therapy. Children should be supervised to avoid potential harm in bike riding or in other hazardous activities.
The concomitant use of alcohol or other central nervous system depressants, including narcotic analgesics, sedatives, hypnotics, and tranquilizers, may have an additive effect and should be avoided or their dosage reduced.
Patients should be advised to report any involuntary muscle movements or unusual sensitivity to sunlight.
Codeine, like other narcotic analgesics, may produce orthostatic hypotension in some ambulatory patients. Patients should be cautioned accordingly.
DRUG INTERACTIONS
CODEINE
In patients receiving MAO inhibitors, an initial small test dose is advisable to allow observation of any excessive narcotic effects or MAOI interaction.
PROMETHAZINE
The sedative action of promethazine is additive to the effects of other central nervous system depressants, including alcohol, narcotic analgesics, sedatives, hypnotics, tricyclic antidepressants, and tranquilizers; therefore, these agents should be avoided or administered in reduced dosage to patients receiving promethazine.
DRUG/LABORATORY TEST INTERACTIONS
Because narcotic analgesics may increase biliary tract pressure, with resultant increases in plasma amylase or lipase

levels, determination of these enzyme levels may be unreliable for 24 hours after a narcotic analgesic has been given. The following laboratory tests may be affected in patients who are receiving therapy with promethazine hydrochloride:
Pregnancy Tests
Diagnostic pregnancy tests based on immunological reactions between HCG and anti-HCG may result in false-negative or false-positive interpretations.
Glucose Tolerance Test
An increase in blood glucose has been reported in patients receiving promethazine.
CARCINOGENESIS, MUTAGENESIS, IMPAIRMENT OF FERTILITY
Long-term animal studies have not been performed to assess the carcinogenic potential of codeine or of promethazine, nor are there other animal or human data concerning carcinogenicity, mutagenicity, or impairment of fertility with these agents. Codeine has been reported to show no evidence of carcinogenicity or mutagenicity in a variety of test systems, including the micronucleus and sperm abnormality assays and the *Salmonella* assay. Promethazine was nonmutagenic in the *Salmonella* test system of Ames.
PREGNANCY
Teratogenic Effects —Pregnancy Category C
CODEINE
A study in rats and rabbits reported no teratogenic effect of codeine administered during the period of organogenesis in doses ranging from 5 to 120 mg/kg. In the rat, doses at the 120-mg/kg level, in the toxic range for the adult animal, were associated with an increase in embryo resorption at the time of implantation. In another study a single 100-mg/kg dose of codeine administered to pregnant mice reportedly resulted in delayed ossification in the offspring.
There are no studies in humans, and the significance of these findings to humans, if any, is not known.
PROMETHAZINE
Teratogenic effects have not been demonstrated in rat-feeding studies at doses of 6.25 and 12.5 mg/kg of promethazine. These doses are 8.3 and 16.7 times the maximum recommended total daily dose of promethazine for a 50-kg subject. Specific studies to test the action of the drug on parturition, lactation, and development of the animal neonate were not done, but a general preliminary study in rats indicated no effect on these parameters. Although antihistamines, including promethazine, have been found to produce fetal mortality in rodents, the pharmacological effects of histamine in the rodent do not parallel those in man. There are no adequate and well-controlled studies of promethazine in pregnant women.
Phenergan with codeine should be used during pregnancy only if the potential benefit justifies the potential risk to the fetus.
Nonteratogenic Effects
Dependence has been reported in newborns whose mothers took opiates regularly during pregnancy. Withdrawal signs include irritability, excessive crying, tremors, hyperreflexia, fever, vomiting, and diarrhea. Signs usually appear during the first few days of life.
Promethazine taken within two weeks of delivery may inhibit platelet aggregation in the newborn.
LABOR AND DELIVERY
Narcotic analgesics cross the placental barrier. The closer to delivery and the larger the dose used, the greater the possibility of respiratory depression in the newborn. Narcotic analgesics should be avoided during labor if delivery of a premature infant is anticipated. If the mother has received narcotic analgesics during labor, newborn infants should be observed closely for signs of respiratory depression. Resuscitation may be required (see "Overdosage"). The effect of codeine, if any, on the later growth, development, and functional maturation of the child is unknown.
See also "Nonteratogenic Effects."
NURSING MOTHERS
Some studies, but not others, have reported detectable amounts of codeine in breast milk. The levels are probably not clinically significant after usual therapeutic dosage. The possibility of clinically important amounts being excreted in breast milk in individuals abusing codeine should be considered.
It is not known whether promethazine is excreted in human milk.
Caution should be exercised when Phenergan with codeine is administered to a nursing woman.
PEDIATRIC USE
This product should not be used in children under 2 years of age because safety for such use has not been established.

ADVERSE REACTIONS
CODEINE
Nervous System —CNS depression, particularly respiratory depression, and to a lesser extent circulatory depression; light-headedness, dizziness, sedation, euphoria, dysphoria, headache, transient hallucination, disorientation, visual disturbances, and convulsions.

PHENERGAN WITH CODEINE

Adults	1 teaspoon (5 mL) every 4 to 6 hours, not to exceed 30.0 mL in 24 hours.
Children 6 years to under 12 years	$\frac{1}{2}$ to 1 teaspoon (2.5 to 5 mL) every 4 to 6 hours, not to exceed 30.0 mL in 24 hours.
Children under 6 years (weight: 18 kg or 40 lbs)	$\frac{1}{4}$ to $\frac{1}{2}$ teaspoon (1.25 to 2.5 mL) every 4 to 6 hours, not to exceed 9.0 mL in 24 hours.
Children under 6 years (weight: 16 kg or 35 lbs)	$\frac{1}{4}$ to $\frac{1}{2}$ teaspoon (1.25 to 2.5 mL) every 4 to 6 hours, not to exceed 8.0 mL in 24 hours.
Children under 6 years (weight: 14 kg or 30 lbs)	$\frac{1}{4}$ to $\frac{1}{2}$ teaspoon (1.25 to 2.5 mL) every 4 to 6 hours, not to exceed 7.0 mL in 24 hours.
Children under 6 years (weight: 12 kg or 25 lbs)	$\frac{1}{4}$ to $\frac{1}{2}$ teaspoon (1.25 to 2.5 mL) every 4 to 6 hours, not to exceed 6.0 mL in 24 hours.

Phenergan with codeine is not recommended for children under 2 years of age.

Cardiovascular—Tachycardia, bradycardia, palpitation, faintness, syncope, orthostatic hypotension (common to narcotic analgesics).

Gastrointestinal—Nausea, vomiting, constipation, and biliary tract spasm. Patients with chronic ulcerative colitis may experience increased colonic motility; in patients with acute ulcerative colitis, toxic dilation has been reported.

Genitourinary—Oliguria, urinary retention; antidiuretic effect has been reported (common to narcotic analgesics).

Allergic—Infrequent pruritus, giant urticaria, angioneurotic edema, and laryngeal edema.

Other—Flushing of the face, sweating and pruritus (due to opiate-induced histamine release); weakness.

PROMETHAZINE

Nervous System—Sedation, sleepiness, occasional blurred vision, dryness of mouth, dizziness; rarely confusion, disorientation, and extrapyramidal symptoms such as oculogyric crisis, torticollis, and tongue protrusion (usually in association with parenteral injection or excessive dosage).

Cardiovascular—Increased or decreased blood pressure.

Dermatologic—Rash, rarely photosensitivity.

Hematologic—Rarely leukopenia, thrombocytopenia; agranulocytosis (1 case).

Gastrointestinal—Nausea and vomiting.

DRUG ABUSE AND DEPENDENCE

CONTROLLED SUBSTANCE

Phenergan with codeine is a Schedule V Controlled Substance.

ABUSE

Codeine is known to be subject to abuse; however, the abuse potential of oral codeine appears to be quite low. Even parenteral codeine does not appear to offer the psychic effects sought by addicts to the same degree as heroin or morphine. However, codeine must be administered only under close supervision to patients with a history of drug abuse or dependence.

DEPENDENCE

Psychological dependence, physical dependence, and tolerance are known to occur with codeine.

OVERDOSAGE

CODEINE

Serious overdose with codeine is characterized by respiratory depression (a decrease in respiratory rate and/or tidal volume, Cheyne-Stokes respiration, cyanosis), extreme somnolence progressing to stupor or coma, skeletal muscle flaccidity, cold and clammy skin, and sometimes bradycardia and hypotension. The triad of coma, pinpoint pupils, and respiratory depression is strongly suggestive of opiate poisoning. In severe overdosage, particularly by the intravenous route, apnea, circulatory collapse, cardiac arrest, and death may occur. Promethazine is additive to the depressant effects of codeine.

It is difficult to determine what constitutes a standard toxic or lethal dose. However, the lethal oral dose of codeine in an adult is reported to be in the range of 0.5 to 1.0 gram. Infants and children are believed to be relatively more sensitive to opiates on a body-weight basis. Elderly patients are also comparatively intolerant to opiates.

PROMETHAZINE

Signs and symptoms of overdosage with promethazine range from mild depression of the central nervous system and cardiovascular system to profound hypotension, respiratory depression, and unconsciousness.

Stimulation may be evident, especially in children and geriatric patients. Convulsions may rarely occur. A paradoxical reaction has been reported in children receiving single doses of 75 mg to 125 mg orally, characterized by hyperexcitability and nightmares.

Atropine-like signs and symptoms—dry mouth, fixed, dilated pupils, flushing, as well as gastrointestinal symptoms, may occur.

TREATMENT

The treatment of overdosage with Phenergan with codeine is essentially symptomatic and supportive. Only in cases of extreme overdosage or individual sensitivity do vital signs including respiration, pulse, blood pressure, temperature, and EKG need to be monitored. Activated charcoal orally or

by lavage may be given, or sodium or magnesium sulfate orally as a cathartic. Attention should be given to the reestablishment of adequate respiratory exchange through provision of a patent airway and institution of assisted or controlled ventilation. The narcotic antagonist, naloxone hydrochloride, may be administered when significant respiratory depression occurs with Phenergan with codeine; any depressant effects of promethazine are not reversed with naloxone. Diazepam may be used to control convulsions. Avoid analeptics, which may cause convulsions. Acidosis and electrolyte losses should be corrected. A rise in temperature or pulmonary complications may signal the need for institution of antibiotic therapy.

Severe hypotension usually responds to the administration of norepinephrine or phenylephrine. EPINEPHRINE SHOULD NOT BE USED, since its use in a patient with partial adrenergic blockade may further lower the blood pressure.

Limited experience with dialysis indicates that it is not helpful.

DOSAGE AND ADMINISTRATION

The average effective dose is given in the following table: [See table above.]

HOW SUPPLIED

Phenergan® with codeine is a clear, purple solution supplied as follows:

NDC 0008-0550-02, case of 24 bottles of 4 fl. oz. (118 mL).
NDC 0008-0550-03, bottle of 1 pint (473 mL).

Keep tightly closed—Store at room temperature, between 15° C and 25° C (59° F and 77° F).

Protect from light.

Dispense in light-resistant, glass, tight container.

PHENERGAN®   ℞

[fen 'er-gan]

with dextromethorphan

(Promethazine Hydrochloride and Dextromethorphan Hydrobromide)

Syrup

DESCRIPTION

Each teaspoon (5 mL) of Phenergan with dextromethorphan contains 6.25 mg promethazine hydrochloride and 15 mg dextromethorphan hydrobromide in a flavored syrup base with a pH between 4.7 and 5.2. Alcohol 7%. The inactive ingredients present are artificial and natural flavors, citric acid, D&C Yellow 10, FD&C Yellow 6, glycerin, saccharin sodium, sodium benzoate, sodium citrate, sodium propionate, water, and other ingredients.

Promethazine hydrochloride is a racemic compound; the empirical formula is $C_{17}H_{20}N_2S \cdot HCl$ and its molecular weight is 320.88.

Promethazine hydrochloride, a phenothiazine derivative, is designated chemically as N,N,α-trimethyl-10*H*-phenothiazine-10-ethanamine monohydrochloride with the following structural formula:

$$CH_2CH(CH_3)N(CH_3)_2$$

Promethazine hydrochloride occurs as a white to faint yellow, practically odorless, crystalline powder which slowly oxidizes and turns blue on prolonged exposure to air. It is soluble in water and freely soluble in alcohol.

Dextromethorphan hydrobromide is a salt of the methyl ether of the dextrorotatory isomer of levorphanol, a narcotic analgesic. It is chemically named as 3-methoxy-17-methyl-9α, 13α, 14α-morphinan hydrobromide monohydrate with the following structural formula:

[See structure at top of next column.]

Dextromethorphan hydrobromide monohydrate occurs as white crystals, is sparingly soluble in water, and is freely soluble in alcohol. The empirical formula is $C_{18}H_{25}NO \cdot HBr \cdot H_2O$, and the molecular weight of the monohydrate is 370.33. Dextromethorphan HBr monohydrate is dextrorotatory with a specific rotation of +27.6 degrees in water (20 degrees C, sodium D-line).

CLINICAL PHARMACOLOGY

PROMETHAZINE

Promethazine is a phenothiazine derivative which differs structurally from the antipsychotic phenothiazines by the presence of a branched side chain and no ring substitution. It is thought that this configuration is responsible for its relative lack (1/10 that of chlorpromazine) of dopaminergic (CNS) action.

Promethazine is an H_1 receptor blocking agent. In addition to its antihistaminic action, it provides clinically useful sedative and antiemetic effects. In therapeutic dosages, promethazine produces no significant effects on the cardiovascular system.

Promethazine is well absorbed from the gastrointestinal tract. Clinical effects are apparent within 20 minutes after oral administration and generally last four to six hours, although they may persist as long as 12 hours. Promethazine is metabolized by the liver to a variety of compounds; the sulfoxides of promethazine and N-demethylpromethazine are the predominant metabolites appearing in the urine.

DEXTROMETHORPHAN

Dextromethorphan is an antitussive agent and, unlike the isomeric levorphanol, it has no analgesic or addictive properties.

The drug acts centrally and elevates the threshold for coughing. It is about equal to codeine in depressing the cough reflex. In therapeutic dosage dextromethorphan does not inhibit ciliary activity.

Dextromethorphan is rapidly absorbed from the gastrointestinal tract and exerts its effect in 15 to 30 minutes. The duration of action after oral administration is approximately three to six hours. Dextromethorphan is metabolized primarily by liver enzymes undergoing O-demethylation, N-demethylation, and partial conjugation with glucuronic acid and sulfate. In humans, (+)-3-hydroxy-N-methylmorphinan, (+)-3-hydroxymorphinan, and traces of unmetabolized drug were found in urine after oral administration.

INDICATIONS AND USAGE

Phenergan with dextromethorphan is indicated for the temporary relief of coughs and upper respiratory symptoms associated with allergy or the common cold.

CONTRAINDICATIONS

Promethazine is contraindicated in individuals known to be hypersensitive or to have had an idiosyncratic reaction to promethazine or to other phenothiazines.

Antihistamines are contraindicated for use in the treatment of lower respiratory tract symptoms, including asthma.

Dextromethorphan should not be used in patients receiving a monoamine oxidase inhibitor (MAOI).

WARNINGS

PROMETHAZINE

Promethazine may cause marked drowsiness. Ambulatory patients should be cautioned against such activities as driving or operating dangerous machinery until it is known that they do not become drowsy or dizzy from promethazine therapy.

The sedative action of promethazine hydrochloride is additive to the sedative effects of central nervous system depressants; therefore, agents such as alcohol, narcotic analgesics, sedatives, hypnotics, and tranquilizers should either be eliminated or given in reduced dosage in the presence of promethazine hydrochloride. When given concomitantly with promethazine hydrochloride, the dose of barbiturates should be reduced by at least one-half, and the dose of analgesic depressants, such as morphine or meperidine, should be reduced by one-quarter to one-half.

Promethazine may lower seizure threshold. This should be taken into consideration when administering to persons with known seizure disorders or when giving in combination with narcotics or local anesthetics which may also affect seizure threshold.

Sedative drugs or CNS depressants should be avoided in patients with a history of sleep apnea.

Antihistamines should be used with caution in patients with narrow-angle glaucoma, stenosing peptic ulcer, pyloroduodenal obstruction, and urinary bladder obstruction due to

Continued on next page

Wyeth-Ayerst Laboratories—Cont.

symptomatic prostatic hypertrophy and narrowing of the bladder neck.
Administration of promethazine has been associated with reported cholestatic jaundice.
DEXTROMETHORPHAN
Administration of dextromethorphan may be accompanied by histamine release and should be used with caution in atopic children.

PRECAUTIONS

Animal reproduction studies have not been conducted with the drug combination—promethazine and dextromethorphan. It is not known whether this drug combination can cause fetal harm when administered to a pregnant woman or can affect reproduction capacity. Phenergan with dextromethorphan should be given to a pregnant woman only if clearly needed.
GENERAL
Promethazine should be used cautiously in persons with cardiovascular disease or with impairment of liver function.
Dextromethorphan should be used with caution in sedated patients, in the debilitated, and in patients confined to the supine position.
INFORMATION FOR PATIENTS
Phenergan with dextromethorphan may cause marked drowsiness or impair the mental and/or physical abilities required for the performance of potentially hazardous tasks, such as driving a vehicle or operating machinery.
Ambulatory patients should be told to avoid engaging in such activities until it is known that they do not become drowsy or dizzy from Phenergan with dextromethorphan therapy. Children should be supervised to avoid potential harm in bike riding or in other hazardous activities.
The concomitant use of alcohol or other central nervous system depressants, including narcotic analgesics, sedatives, hypnotics, and tranquilizers, may have an additive effect and should be avoided or their dosage reduced.
Patients should be advised to report any involuntary muscle movements or unusual sensitivity to sunlight.
DRUG INTERACTIONS
The sedative action of promethazine is additive to the sedative effects of other central nervous system depressants, including alcohol, narcotic analgesics, sedatives, hypnotics, tricyclic antidepressants, and tranquilizers; therefore, these agents should be avoided or administered in reduced dosage to patients receiving promethazine.
DRUG/LABORATORY TEST INTERACTIONS
The following laboratory tests may be affected in patients who are receiving therapy with promethazine hydrochloride:
Pregnancy Tests
Diagnostic pregnancy tests based on immunological reactions between HCG and anti-HCG may result in false-negative or false-positive interpretations.
Glucose Tolerance Test
An increase in blood glucose has been reported in patients receiving promethazine.
CARCINOGENESIS, MUTAGENESIS, IMPAIRMENT OF FERTILITY
Long-term animal studies have not been performed to assess the carcinogenic potential of promethazine or of dextromethorphan. There are no animal or human data concerning the carcinogenicity, mutagenicity, or impairment of fertility with these drugs. Promethazine was nonmutagenic in the *Salmonella* test system of Ames.
PREGNANCY
Teratogenic Effects —Pregnancy Category C
Teratogenic effects have not been demonstrated in rat-feeding studies at doses of 6.25 and 12.5 mg/kg of promethazine. These doses are 8.3 and 16.7 times the maximum recommended total daily dose for a 50-kg subject. Specific studies to test the action of the drug on parturition, lactation, and development of the animal neonate were not done, but a general preliminary study in rats indicated no effect on these parameters. Although antihistamines, including promethazine, have been found to produce fetal mortality in rodents, the pharmacological effects of histamine in the rodent do not parallel those in man. There are no adequate and well-controlled studies of promethazine in pregnant women.
Phenergan with dextromethorphan should be used during pregnancy only if the potential benefit justifies the potential risk to the fetus.
Nonteratogenic Effects
Promethazine taken within two weeks of delivery may inhibit platelet aggregation in the newborn.
LABOR AND DELIVERY
See "Nonteratogenic Effects."
NURSING MOTHERS
It is not known whether promethazine or dextromethorphan is excreted in human milk. Caution should be exercised when Phenergan with dextromethorphan is administered to a nursing woman.
PEDIATRIC USE
This product should not be used in children under 2 years of age because safety for that use has not been established.

ADVERSE REACTIONS

PROMETHAZINE
Nervous System —Sedation, sleepiness, occasional blurred vision, dryness of mouth, dizziness; rarely confusion, disorientation, and extrapyramidal symptoms such as oculogyric crisis, torticollis, and tongue protrusion (usually in association with parenteral injection or excessive dosage).
Cardiovascular —Increased or decreased blood pressure.
Dermatologic —Rash, rarely photosensitivity.
Hematologic —Rarely leukopenia, thrombocytopenia; agranulocytosis (1 case).
Gastrointestinal —Nausea and vomiting.
DEXTROMETHORPHAN
Dextromethorphan hydrobromide occasionally causes slight drowsiness, dizziness, and gastrointestinal disturbances.

DRUG ABUSE AND DEPENDENCE

According to the WHO Expert Committee on Drug Dependence, dextromethorphan could produce very slight psychic dependence but no physical dependence.

OVERDOSAGE

PROMETHAZINE
Signs and symptoms of overdosage with promethazine range from mild depression of the central nervous system and cardiovascular system to profound hypotension, respiratory depression, and unconsciousness.
Stimulation may be evident, especially in children and geriatric patients. Convulsions may rarely occur. A paradoxical reaction has been reported in children receiving single doses of 75 mg to 125 mg orally, characterized by hyperexcitability and nightmares.
Atropine-like signs and symptoms—dry mouth, fixed, dilated pupils, flushing, as well as gastrointestinal symptoms, may occur.
DEXTROMETHORPHAN
Dextromethorphan may produce central excitement and mental confusion. Very high doses may produce respiratory depression. One case of toxic psychosis (hyperactivity, marked visual and auditory hallucinations) after ingestion of a single dose of 20 tablets (300 mg) of dextromethorphan has been reported.
TREATMENT
Treatment of overdosage with Phenergan with dextromethorphan is essentially symptomatic and supportive. Only in cases of extreme overdosage or individual sensitivity do vital signs including respiration, pulse, blood pressure, temperature, and EKG need to be monitored. Activated charcoal orally or by lavage may be given, or sodium or magnesium sulfate orally as a cathartic. Attention should be given to the reestablishment of adequate respiratory exchange through provision of a patent airway and institution of assisted or controlled ventilation. Diazepam may be used to control convulsions. Acidosis and electrolyte losses should be corrected. The antidotal efficacy of narcotic antagonists to dextromethorphan has not been established; note that any of the depressant effects of promethazine are not reversed by naloxone. Avoid analeptics, which may cause convulsions.
Severe hypotension usually responds to the administration of norepinephrine or phenylephrine. EPINEPHRINE SHOULD NOT BE USED, since its use in a patient with partial adrenergic blockade may further lower the blood pressure.
Limited experience with dialysis indicates that it is not helpful.

DOSAGE AND ADMINISTRATION

The average effective dose for adults is one teaspoon (5 mL) every 4 to 6 hours, not to exceed 30.0 mL in 24 hours. For children 6 years to under 12 years of age, the dose is one-half to one teaspoon (2.5 to 5.0 mL) every 4 to 6 hours, not to exceed 20.0 mL in 24 hours. For children 2 years to under 6 years of age, the dose is one-quarter to one-half teaspoon (1.25 to 2.5 mL) every 4 to 6 hours, not to exceed 10.0 mL in 24 hours.
Phenergan with dextromethorphan is not recommended for children under 2 years of age.

HOW SUPPLIED

Phenergan® with dextromethorphan (Promethazine Hydrochloride and Dextromethorphan Hydrobromide) Syrup is a clear, yellow solution supplied as follows:
NDC 0008-0548-02, case of 24 bottles of 4 fl. oz. (118 mL).
NDC 0008-0548-03, bottle of 1 pint (473 mL).
Keep bottles tightly closed and store at room temperature between 15° and 25°C (59° and 77°F).
Protect from light.
Dispense in light-resistant, glass, tight containers.

PHENERGAN® VC ℞

[fen'er-gan]
(Promethazine Hydrochloride and Phenylephrine Hydrochloride) Syrup

DESCRIPTION

Each teaspoon (5 mL) of Phenergan VC contains 6.25 mg promethazine hydrochloride and 5 mg phenylephrine hydrochloride in a flavored syrup base with a pH between 4.7 and 5.2. Alcohol 7%. The inactive ingredients present are artificial and natural flavors, citric acid, FD&C Yellow 6, glycerin, saccharin sodium, sodium benzoate, sodium citrate, sodium propionate, water, and other ingredients.
Promethazine hydrochloride is a racemic compound; the empirical formula is $C_{17}H_{20}N_2S \cdot HCl$ and its molecular weight is 320.88.
Promethazine hydrochloride, a phenothiazine derivative, is designated chemically as N,N,α-trimethyl-10*H*-phenothiazine-10-ethanamine monohydrochloride with the following structural formula:

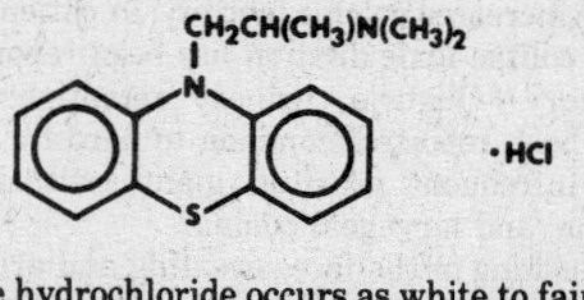

Promethazine hydrochloride occurs as white to faint yellow, practically odorless, crystalline powder which slowly oxidizes and turns blue on prolonged exposure to air. It is soluble in water and freely soluble in alcohol.
Phenylephrine hydrochloride is a sympathomimetic amine salt. It may be chemically named as 3-hydroxy-α-[(methylamino)methyl]-benzenemethanol hydrochloride and has the following chemical formula:

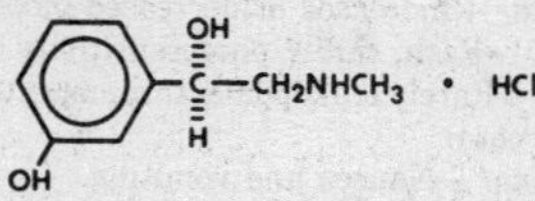

Phenylephrine hydrochloride occurs as white or nearly white crystals, having a bitter taste. It is freely soluble in water and alcohol, with a molecular weight of 203.67. The empirical formula is $C_9H_{13}NO_2 \cdot HCl$, and the stereochemistry is R-isomer as indicated in the structure; Specific Rotation—between −42° and −47.5°.
Phenylephrine hydrochloride is subject to oxidation and must be protected from light and air.

CLINICAL PHARMACOLOGY

PROMETHAZINE
Promethazine is a phenothiazine derivative which differs structurally from the antipsychotic phenothiazines by the presence of a branched side chain and no ring substitution. It is thought that this configuration is responsible for its relative lack (1/10 that of chlorpromazine) of dopaminergic (CNS) action.
Promethazine is an H_1 receptor blocking agent. In addition to its antihistaminic action, it provides clinically useful sedative and antiemetic effects. In therapeutic dosages, promethazine produces no significant effects on the cardiovascular system.
Promethazine is well absorbed from the gastrointestinal tract. Clinical effects are apparent within 20 minutes after oral administration and generally last four to six hours, although they may persist as long as 12 hours. Promethazine is metabolized by the liver to a variety of compounds; the sulfoxides of promethazine and N-demethylpromethazine are the predominant metabolites appearing in the urine.
PHENYLEPHRINE
Phenylephrine is a potent postsynaptic α-receptor agonist with little effect on β receptors of the heart. Phenylephrine has no effect on β-adrenergic receptors of the bronchi or peripheral blood vessels. A direct action at receptors accounts for the greater part of its effects, only a small part being due to its ability to release norepinephrine.
Therapeutic doses of phenylephrine mainly cause vasoconstriction. Phenylephrine increases resistance and, to a lesser extent, decreases capacitance of blood vessels. Total peripheral resistance is increased, resulting in increased systolic and diastolic blood pressure. Pulmonary arterial pressure is usually increased, and renal blood flow is usually decreased. Local vasoconstriction and hemostasis occur following topical application or infiltration of phenylephrine into tissues.
The main effect of phenylephrine on the heart is bradycardia; it produces a positive inotropic effect on the myocardium in doses greater than those usually used therapeutically. Rarely, the drug may increase the irritability of the heart, causing arrhythmias. Cardiac output is decreased slightly. Phenylephrine increases the work of the heart by increasing peripheral arterial resistance.
Phenylephrine has a mild central stimulant effect.
Following oral administration or topical application of phenylephrine to the mucosa, constriction of blood vessels in the

nasal mucosa relieves nasal congestion associated with allergy or head colds. Following oral administration, nasal decongestion may occur within 15 or 20 minutes and may persist for up to 4 hours.

Phenylephrine is irregularly absorbed from and readily metabolized in the gastrointestinal tract. Phenylephrine is metabolized in the liver and intestine by monoamine oxidase. The metabolites and their route and rate of excretion have not been identified. The pharmacologic action of phenylephrine is terminated at least partially by uptake of the drug into tissues.

INDICATIONS AND USAGE

Phenergan VC is indicated for the temporary relief of upper respiratory symptoms, including nasal congestion, associated with allergy or the common cold.

CONTRAINDICATIONS

Promethazine is contraindicated in individuals known to be hypersensitive or to have had an idiosyncratic reaction to promethazine or to other phenothiazines.

Antihistamines are contraindicated for use in the treatment of lower respiratory tract symptoms or asthma.

Phenylephrine is contraindicated in patients with hypertension or with peripheral vascular insufficiency (ischemia may result with risk of gangrene or thrombosis of compromised vascular beds). Phenylephrine should not be used in patients known to be hypersensitive to the drug or in those receiving a monoamine oxidase inhibitor (MAOI).

WARNINGS

PROMETHAZINE

Promethazine may cause marked drowsiness. Ambulatory patients should be cautioned against such activities as driving or operating dangerous machinery until it is known that they do not become drowsy or dizzy from promethazine therapy.

The sedative action of promethazine hydrochloride is additive to the sedative effects of central nervous system depressants; therefore, agents such as alcohol, narcotic analgesics, sedatives, hypnotics, and tranquilizers should either be eliminated or given in reduced dosage in the presence of promethazine hydrochloride. When given concomitantly with promethazine hydrochloride, the dose of barbiturates should be reduced by at least one-half, and the dose of analgesic depressants, such as morphine or meperidine, should be reduced by one-quarter to one-half.

Promethazine may lower seizure threshold. This should be taken into consideration when administering to persons with known seizure disorders or when giving in combination with narcotics or local anesthetics which may also affect seizure threshold.

Sedative drugs or CNS depressants should be avoided in patients with a history of sleep apnea.

Antihistamines should be used with caution in patients with narrow-angle glaucoma, stenosing peptic ulcer, pyloroduodenal obstruction, and urinary bladder obstruction due to symptomatic prostatic hypertrophy and narrowing of the bladder neck.

Administration of promethazine has been associated with reported cholestatic jaundice.

PHENYLEPHRINE

Because phenylephrine is an adrenergic agent, it should be given with caution to patients with thyroid diseases, diabetes mellitus, and heart diseases or those receiving tricyclic antidepressants.

Men with symptomatic, benign prostatic hypertrophy can experience urinary retention when given oral nasal decongestants.

Phenylephrine can cause a decrease in cardiac output, and extreme caution should be used when administering the drug, parenterally or orally, to patients with arteriosclerosis, to elderly individuals, and/or to patients with initially poor cerebral or coronary circulation.

Phenylephrine should be used with caution in patients taking diet preparations, such as amphetamines or phenylpropanolamine, because synergistic adrenergic effects could result in serious hypertensive response and possible stroke.

PRECAUTIONS

Animal reproduction studies have not been conducted with the drug combination—promethazine and phenylephrine. It is not known whether this drug combination can cause fetal harm when administered to a pregnant woman or can affect reproduction capacity. Phenergan VC should be given to a pregnant woman only if clearly needed.

GENERAL

Promethazine should be used cautiously in persons with cardiovascular disease or impairment of liver function.

Phenylephrine should be used with caution in patients with cardiovascular disease, particularly hypertension.

INFORMATION FOR PATIENTS

Phenergan VC may cause marked drowsiness or impair the mental and/or physical abilities required for the performance of potentially hazardous tasks, such as driving a vehicle or operating machinery. Ambulatory patients should be told to avoid engaging in such activities until it is known that

PHENERGAN VC

PHENYLEPHRINE

Drug	Effect
Phenylephrine with prior administration of monoamine oxidase inhibitors (MAOI).	Cardiac pressor response potentiated. May cause acute hypertensive crisis.
Phenylephrine with tricyclic antidepressants.	Pressor response increased.
Phenylephrine with ergot alkaloids.	Excessive rise in blood pressure.
Phenylephrine with bronchodilator sympathomimetic agents and with epinephrine or other sympathomimetics.	Tachycardia or other arrhythmias may occur.
Phenylephrine with prior administration of propranolol or other β-adrenergic blockers.	Cardiostimulating effects blocked.
Phenylephrine with atropine sulfate.	Reflex bradycardia blocked; pressor response enhanced.
Phenylephrine with prior administration of phentolamine or other α-adrenergic blockers.	Pressor response decreased.
Phenylephrine with diet preparations, such as amphetamines or phenylpropanolamine.	Synergistic adrenergic response.

they do not become drowsy or dizzy from Phenergan VC therapy. Children should be supervised to avoid potential harm in bike riding or other hazardous activities.

The concomitant use of alcohol or other central nervous system depressants, including narcotic analgesics, sedatives, hypnotics, and tranquilizers, may have an additive effect and should be avoided or their dosage reduced.

Patients should be advised to report any involuntary muscle movements or unusual sensitivity to sunlight.

DRUG INTERACTIONS
PROMETHAZINE

The sedative action of promethazine is additive to the sedative effects of other central nervous system depressants, including alcohol, narcotic analgesics, sedatives, hypnotics, tricyclic antidepressants, and tranquilizers; therefore, these agents should be avoided or administered in reduced dosage to patients receiving promethazine.

[See table above.]

DRUG/LABORATORY TEST INTERACTIONS

The following laboratory tests may be affected in patients who are receiving therapy with promethazine hydrochloride:

Pregnancy Tests

Diagnostic pregnancy tests based on immunological reactions between HCG and anti-HCG may result in false-negative or false-positive interpretations.

Glucose Tolerance Test

An increase in blood glucose has been reported in patients receiving promethazine.

CARCINOGENESIS, MUTAGENESIS, IMPAIRMENT OF FERTILITY
PROMETHAZINE

Long-term animal studies have not been performed to assess the carcinogenic potential of promethazine, nor are there other animal or human data concerning carcinogenicity, mutagenicity, or impairment of fertility with this drug. Promethazine was nonmutagenic in the *Salmonella* test system of Ames.

PHENYLEPHRINE

A study which followed the development of cancer in 143,574 patients over a four-year period indicated that in 11,981 patients who received phenylephrine (systemic or topical), there was no statistically significant association between the drug and cancer at any or all sites.

Long-term animal studies have not been performed to assess the carcinogenic potential of phenylephrine, nor are there other animal or human data concerning mutagenicity.

A study of the effects of adrenergic drugs on ovum transport in rabbits indicated that treatment with phenylephrine did not alter incidence of pregnancy; the number of implantations was significantly reduced when high doses of the drug were used.

PREGNANCY
Teratogenic Effects —Pregnancy Category C
PROMETHAZINE

Teratogenic effects have not been demonstrated in rat-feeding studies at doses of 6.25 and 12.5 mg/kg of promethazine. These doses are 8.3 and 16.7 times the maximum recommended total daily dose of promethazine for a 50-kg subject. Specific studies to test the action of the drug on parturition, lactation, and development of the animal neonate were not done, but a general preliminary study in rats indicated no effect on these parameters. Although antihistamines, including promethazine, have been found to produce fetal mortality in rodents, the pharmacologic effects of histamine in the rodent do not parallel those in man. There are no adequate and well-controlled studies of promethazine in pregnant women.

PHENYLEPHRINE

A study in rabbits indicated that continued moderate overexposure to phenylephrine (3 mg/day) during the second half of pregnancy (22nd day of gestation to delivery) may contribute to perinatal wastage, prematurity, premature labor, and possibly fetal anomalies; when phenylephrine (3 mg/day) was given to rabbits during the first half of pregnancy (3rd day after mating for seven days), a significant number gave birth to litters of low birth weight. Another study showed that phenylephrine was associated with anomalies of aortic arch and with ventricular septal defect in the chick embryo. Phenergan VC should be used during pregnancy only if the potential benefit justifies the potential risk to the fetus.

Nonteratogenic Effects

Promethazine taken within two weeks of delivery may inhibit platelet aggregation in the newborn.

LABOR AND DELIVERY

Administration of phenylephrine to patients in late pregnancy or labor may cause fetal anoxia or bradycardia by increasing contractility of the uterus and decreasing uterine blood flow.

See also "Nonteratogenic Effects."

NURSING MOTHERS

It is not known whether promethazine or phenylephrine is excreted in human milk.

Caution should be exercised when Phenergan VC is administered to a nursing woman.

PEDIATRIC USE

This product should not be used in children under 2 years of age because safety for such use has not been established.

ADVERSE REACTIONS
PROMETHAZINE

Nervous System —Sedation, sleepiness, occasional blurred vision, dryness of mouth, dizziness; rarely confusion, disorientation, and extrapyramidal symptoms such as oculogyric crisis, torticollis, and tongue protrusion (usually in association with parenteral injection or excessive dosage).

Cardiovascular —Increased or decreased blood pressure.

Dermatologic —Rash, rarely photosensitivity.

Hematologic —Rarely leukopenia, thrombocytopenia; agranulocytosis (1 case).

Gastrointestinal —Nausea and vomiting.

PHENYLEPHRINE

Nervous System —Restlessness, anxiety, nervousness, and dizziness.

Cardiovascular —Hypertension (see "Warnings").

Other —Precordial pain, respiratory distress, tremor, and weakness.

OVERDOSAGE
PROMETHAZINE

Signs and symptoms of overdosage with promethazine range from mild depression of the central nervous system and cardiovascular system to profound hypotension, respiratory depression, and unconsciousness.

Stimulation may be evident, especially in children and geriatric patients. Convulsions may rarely occur. A paradoxical reaction has been reported in children receiving single doses of 75 mg to 125 mg orally, characterized by hyperexcitability and nightmares.

Atropine-like signs and symptoms—dry mouth, fixed, dilated pupils, flushing, as well as gastrointestinal symptoms, may occur.

PHENYLEPHRINE

Signs and symptoms of overdosage with phenylephrine include hypertension, headache, convulsions, cerebral hemorrhage, and vomiting. Ventricular premature beats and short

Continued on next page

Wyeth-Ayerst Laboratories—Cont.

paroxysms of ventricular tachycardia may also occur. Headache may be a symptom of hypertension. Bradycardia may also be seen early in phenylephrine overdosage through stimulation of baroreceptors.

TREATMENT

Treatment of overdosage with Phenergan VC is essentially symptomatic and supportive. Only in cases of extreme overdosage or individual sensitivity do vital signs including respiration, pulse, blood pressure, temperature, and EKG need to be monitored. Activated charcoal orally or by lavage may be given, or sodium or magnesium sulfate orally as a cathartic. Attention should be given to the reestablishment of adequate respiratory exchange through provision of a patent airway and institution of assisted or controlled ventilation. Diazepam may be used to control convulsions. Acidosis and electrolyte losses should be corrected. Note that any depressant effects of promethazine are not reversed by naloxone. Avoid analeptics which may cause convulsions.

Severe hypotension usually responds to the administration of norepinephrine or phenylephrine. EPINEPHRINE SHOULD NOT BE USED, since its use in patients with partial adrenergic blockade may further lower the blood pressure.

Limited experience with dialysis indicates that it is not helpful.

DOSAGE AND ADMINISTRATION

The recommended adult dose is one teaspoon (5 mL) every 4 to 6 hours, not to exceed 30.0 mL in 24 hours. For children 6 years to under 12 years of age, the dose is one-half to one teaspoon (2.5 to 5.0 mL) repeated at 4- to 6-hour intervals, not to exceed 30.0 mL in 24 hours. For children 2 years to under 6 years of age, the dose is one-quarter to one-half teaspoon (1.25 to 2.5 mL) every 4 to 6 hours.

Phenergan VC is not recommended for children under 2 years of age.

HOW SUPPLIED

Phenergan® VC (Promethazine Hydrochloride and Phenylephrine Hydrochloride) Syrup, is a clear, orange-yellow solution supplied as follows:

NDC 0008-0551-02, case of 24 bottles of 4 fl. oz. (118 mL).

NDC 0008-0551-03, bottle of 1 pint (473 mL).

Keep bottles tightly closed and store at room temperature between 15° and 25°C (59° and 77°F).

Protect from light.

Dispense in light-resistant, glass, tight containers.

PHENERGAN® VC ℭ ℞

[fen 'er-gan]

with codeine

(Warning—may be habit-forming)

(Promethazine Hydrochloride, Phenylephrine Hydrochloride, and Codeine Phosphate) Syrup

DESCRIPTION

Each teaspoon (5 mL) of Phenergan VC with codeine contains 10 mg codeine phosphate (Warning—may be habit-forming), 6.25 mg promethazine hydrochloride, and 5 mg phenylephrine hydrochloride in a flavored syrup base with a pH between 4.7 and 5.2. Alcohol 7%. The inactive ingredients present are artificial and natural flavors, citric acid, D&C Red 33, FD&C Yellow 6, glycerin, saccharin sodium, sodium benzoate, sodium citrate, sodium propionate, water, and other ingredients.

Codeine is one of the naturally occurring phenanthrene alkaloids of opium derived from the opium poppy; it is classified pharmacologically as a narcotic analgesic. Codeine phosphate may be chemically named as (5α,6α)–7,8–didehydro–4,5–epoxy–3–methoxy–17–methylmorphinan–6–ol phosphate (1:1) (salt) hemihydrate with the following structural formula:

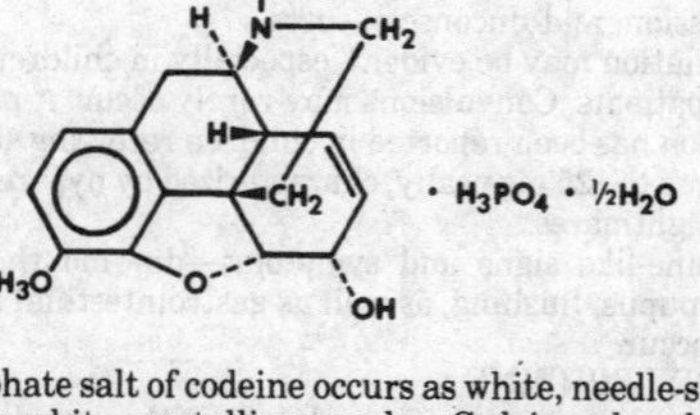

The phosphate salt of codeine occurs as white, needle-shaped crystals or white crystalline powder. Codeine phosphate is freely soluble in water and slightly soluble in alcohol, with a molecular weight of 406.37. The empirical formula is $C_{18}H_{21}NO_3 \cdot H_3PO_4 \cdot \frac{1}{2}H_2O$, and the stereochemistry is 5α, 6α isomer as indicated in the structure.

Promethazine hydrochloride is a racemic compound; the empirical formula is $C_{17}H_{20}N_2S \cdot HCl$ and its molecular weight is 320.88.

Promethazine hydrochloride, a phenothiazine derivative, is designated chemically as N,N,α-trimethyl-10*H*-phenothiazine-10-ethanamine monohydrochloride with the following structural formula:

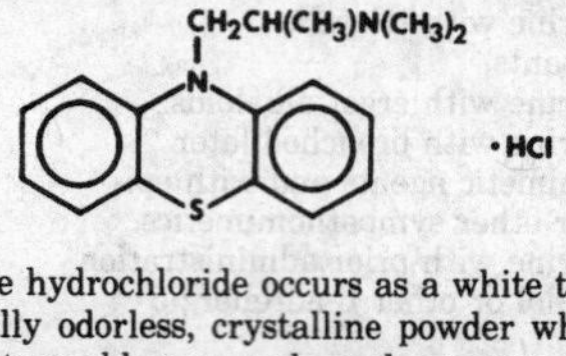

Promethazine hydrochloride occurs as a white to faint yellow, practically odorless, crystalline powder which slowly oxidizes and turns blue on prolonged exposure to air. It is soluble in water and freely soluble in alcohol.

Phenylephrine hydrochloride is a sympathomimetic amine salt. It may be chemically named as 3-hydroxy-α-[(methylamino)methyl]-benzenemethanol hydrochloride and has the following chemical formula:

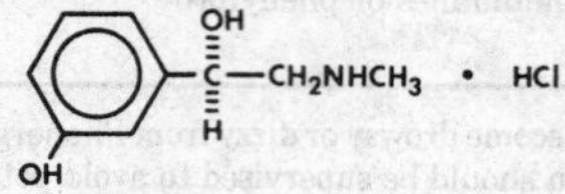

Phenylephrine hydrochloride occurs as white or nearly white crystals, having a bitter taste. It is freely soluble in water and alcohol, with a molecular weight of 203.67. The empirical formula is $C_9H_{13}NO_2 \cdot HCl$, and the stereochemistry is R-isomer as indicated in the structure; Specific Rotation—between −42° and −47.5°. Phenylephrine hydrochloride is subject to oxidation and must be protected from light and air.

CLINICAL PHARMACOLOGY

CODEINE: Narcotic analgesics, including codeine, exert their primary effects on the central nervous system and gastrointestinal tract. The analgesic effects of codeine are due to its central action; however, the precise sites of action have not been determined, and the mechanisms involved appear to be quite complex. Codeine resembles morphine both structurally and pharmacologically, but its actions at the doses of codeine used therapeutically are milder, with less sedation, respiratory depression, and gastrointestinal, urinary, and pupillary effects. Codeine produces an increase in biliary tract pressure, but less than morphine or meperidine. Codeine is less constipating than morphine.

Codeine has good antitussive activity, although less than that of morphine at equal doses. It is used in preference to morphine, because side effects are infrequent at the usual antitussive dose of codeine.

Codeine in oral therapeutic dosage does not usually exert major effects on the cardiovascular system.

Narcotic analgesics may cause nausea and vomiting by stimulating the chemoreceptor trigger zone (CTZ); however, they also depress the vomiting center, so that subsequent doses are unlikely to produce vomiting. Nausea is minimal after usual oral doses of codeine.

Narcotic analgesics cause histamine release, which appears to be responsible for wheals or urticaria sometimes seen at the site of injection on parenteral administration. Histamine release may also produce dilation of cutaneous blood vessels, with resultant flushing of the face and neck, pruritus, and sweating.

Codeine and its salts are well absorbed following both oral and parenteral administration. Codeine is about ⅔ as effective orally as parenterally. Codeine is metabolized primarily in the liver by enzymes of the endoplasmic reticulum, where it undergoes O-demethylation, N-demethylation, and partial conjugation with glucuronic acid. The drug is excreted primarily in the urine, largely as inactive metabolites and small amounts of free and conjugated morphine. Negligible amounts of codeine and its metabolites are found in the feces.

Following oral or subcutaneous administration of codeine, the onset of analgesia occurs within 15 to 30 minutes and lasts for four to six hours.

The cough-depressing action, in animal studies, was observed to occur 15 minutes after oral administration of codeine, peak action at 45 to 60 minutes after ingestion. The duration of action, which is dose-dependent, usually did not exceed 3 hours.

PROMETHAZINE: Promethazine is a phenothiazine derivative which differs structurally from the antipsychotic phenothiazines by the presence of a branched side chain and no ring substitution. It is thought that this configuration is responsible for its relative lack (1/10 that of chlorpromazine) of dopaminergic (CNS) action.

Promethazine is an H_1 receptor blocking agent. In addition to its antihistaminic action, it provides clinically useful sedative and antiemetic effects. In therapeutic dosages, promethazine produces no significant effects on the cardiovascular system.

Promethazine is well absorbed from the gastrointestinal tract. Clinical effects are apparent within 20 minutes after oral administration and generally last four to six hours, although they may persist as long as 12 hours. Promethazine is metabolized by the liver to a variety of compounds; the sulfoxides of promethazine and N-demethylpromethazine are the predominant metabolites appearing in the urine.

PHENYLEPHRINE: Phenylephrine is a potent postsynaptic α-receptor agonist with little effect on β receptors of the heart. Phenylephrine has no effect on β-adrenergic receptors of the bronchi or peripheral blood vessels. A direct action at receptors accounts for the greater part of its effects, only a small part being due to its ability to release norepinephrine.

Therapeutic doses of phenylephrine mainly cause vasoconstriction. Phenylephrine increases resistance and, to a lesser extent, decreases capacitance of blood vessels. Total peripheral resistance is increased, resulting in increased systolic and diastolic blood pressure. Pulmonary arterial pressure is usually increased, and renal blood flow is usually decreased. Local vasoconstriction and hemostasis occur following topical application or infiltration of phenylephrine into tissues.

The main effect of phenylephrine on the heart is bradycardia; it produces a positive inotropic effect on the myocardium in doses greater than those usually used therapeutically. Rarely, the drug may increase the irritability of the heart, causing arrhythmias. Cardiac output is decreased slightly. Phenylephrine increases the work of the heart by increasing peripheral arterial resistance.

Phenylephrine has a mild central stimulant effect.

Following oral administration or topical application of phenylephrine to the mucosa, constriction of blood vessels in the nasal mucosa relieves nasal congestion associated with allergy or head colds. Following oral administration, nasal decongestion may occur within 15 or 20 minutes and may persist for up to 4 hours.

Phenylephrine is irregularly absorbed from and readily metabolized in the gastrointestinal tract. Phenylephrine is metabolized in the liver and intestine by monoamine oxidase. The metabolites and their route and rate of excretion have not been identified. The pharmacologic action of phenylephrine is terminated at least partially by uptake of the drug into tissues.

INDICATIONS AND USAGE

Phenergan VC with codeine is indicated for the temporary relief of coughs and upper respiratory symptoms, including nasal congestion, associated with allergy or the common cold.

CONTRAINDICATIONS

Codeine is contraindicated in patients with a known hypersensitivity to the drug.

Promethazine is contraindicated in individuals known to be hypersensitive or to have had an idiosyncratic reaction to promethazine or to other phenothiazines.

Phenylephrine is contraindicated in patients with hypertension or with peripheral vascular insufficiency (ischemia may result with risk of gangrene or thrombosis of compromised vascular beds). Phenylephrine should not be used in patients known to be hypersensitive to the drug or in those receiving a monoamine oxidase inhibitor (MAOI).

Antihistamines and codeine are both contraindicated for use in the treatment of lower respiratory tract symptoms, including asthma.

WARNINGS

CODEINE: Dosage of codeine SHOULD NOT BE INCREASED if cough fails to respond; an unresponsive cough should be reevaluated in 5 days or sooner for possible underlying pathology, such as foreign body or lower respiratory tract disease.

Codeine may cause or aggravate constipation.

Respiratory depression leading to arrest, coma, and death has occurred with the use of codeine antitussives in young children, particularly in the under-one-year infants whose ability to deactivate the drug is not fully developed.

Administration of codeine may be accompanied by histamine release and should be used with caution in atopic children.

Head Injury and Increased Intracranial Pressure

The respiratory-depressant effects of narcotic analgesics and their capacity to elevate cerebrospinal fluid pressure may be markedly exaggerated in the presence of head injury, intracranial lesions, or a preexisting increase in intracranial pressure. Narcotics may produce adverse reactions which may obscure the clinical course of patients with head injuries.

Asthma and Other Respiratory Conditions

Narcotic analgesics or cough suppressants, including codeine, should not be used in asthmatic patients (see "Contraindications"). Nor should they be used in acute febrile illness associated with productive cough or in chronic respiratory disease where interference with ability to clear the tracheobronchial tree of secretions would have a deleterious effect on the patient's respiratory function.

PHENERGAN VC WITH CODEINE

PHENYLEPHRINE

Drug	Effect
Phenylephrine with prior administration of monoamine oxidase inhibitors (MAOI).	Cardiac pressor response potentiated. May cause acute hypertensive crisis.
Phenylephrine with tricyclic antidepressants.	Pressor response increased.
Phenylephrine with ergot alkaloids.	Excessive rise in blood pressure.
Phenylephrine with bronchodilator sympathomimetic agents and with epinephrine or other sympathomimetics.	Tachycardia or other arrhythmias may occur.
Phenylephrine with prior administration of propranolol or other β-adrenergic blockers.	Cardiostimulating effects blocked.
Phenylephrine with atropine sulfate.	Reflex bradycardia blocked; pressor response enhanced.
Phenylephrine with prior administration of phentolamine or other α-adrenergic blockers.	Pressor response decreased.
Phenylephrine with diet preparations, such as amphetamines or phenylpropanolamine.	Synergistic adrenergic response.

Hypotensive Effect
Codeine may produce orthostatic hypotension in ambulatory patients.
PROMETHAZINE: Promethazine may cause marked drowsiness. Ambulatory patients should be cautioned against such activities as driving or operating dangerous machinery until it is known that they do not become drowsy or dizzy from promethazine therapy.
The sedative action of promethazine hydrochloride is additive to the sedative effects of central nervous system depressants; therefore, agents such as alcohol, narcotic analgesics, sedatives, hypnotics, and tranquilizers should either be eliminated or given in reduced dosage in the presence of promethazine hydrochloride. When given concomitantly with promethazine hydrochloride, the dose of barbiturates should be reduced by at least one-half, and the dose of analgesic depressants, such as morphine or meperidine, should be reduced by one-quarter to one-half.
Promethazine may lower seizure threshold. This should be taken into consideration when administering to persons with known seizure disorders or when giving in combination with narcotics or local anesthetics which may also affect seizure threshold.
Sedative drugs or CNS depressants should be avoided in patients with a history of sleep apnea. Antihistamines should be used with caution in patients with narrow-angle glaucoma, stenosing peptic ulcer, pyloroduodenal obstruction, and urinary bladder obstruction due to symptomatic prostatic hypertrophy and narrowing of the bladder neck.
Administration of promethazine has been associated with reported cholestatic jaundice.
PHENYLEPHRINE: Because phenylephrine is an adrenergic agent, it should be given with caution to patients with thyroid diseases, diabetes mellitus, and heart diseases or those receiving tricyclic antidepressants.
Men with symptomatic, benign prostatic hypertrophy can experience urinary retention when given oral nasal decongestants.
Phenylephrine can cause a decrease in cardiac output, and extreme caution should be used when administering the drug, parenterally or orally, to patients with arteriosclerosis, to elderly individuals, and/or to patients with initially poor cerebral or coronary circulation.
Phenylephrine should be used with caution in patients taking diet preparations, such as amphetamines or phenylpropanolamine, because synergistic adrenergic effects could result in serious hypertensive response and possible stroke.

PRECAUTIONS

Animal reproduction studies have not been conducted with the drug combination—promethazine, phenylephrine, and codeine. It is not known whether this drug combination can cause fetal harm when administered to a pregnant woman or can affect reproduction capacity. Phenergan VC with codeine should be given to a pregnant woman only if clearly needed.
GENERAL
Narcotic analgesics, including codeine, should be administered with caution and the initial dose reduced in patients with acute abdominal conditions, convulsive disorders, significant hepatic or renal impairment, fever, hypothyroidism, Addison's disease, ulcerative colitis, prostatic hypertrophy, in patients with recent gastrointestinal or urinary tract surgery, and in the very young or elderly or debilitated patients.
Promethazine should be used cautiously in persons with cardiovascular disease or with impairment of liver function.
Phenylephrine should be used with caution in patients with cardiovascular disease, particularly hypertension.
INFORMATION FOR PATIENTS
Phenergan VC with codeine may cause marked drowsiness or impair the mental and/or physical abilities required for the performance of potentially hazardous tasks, such as driving a vehicle or operating machinery. Ambulatory patients should be told to avoid engaging in such activities until it is known that they do not become drowsy or dizzy from Phenergan VC with codeine therapy. Children should be supervised to avoid potential harm in bike riding or in other hazardous activities.
The concomitant use of alcohol or other central nervous system depressants, including narcotic analgesics, sedatives, hypnotics, and tranquilizers, may have an additive effect and should be avoided or their dosage reduced.
Patients should be advised to report any involuntary muscle movements or unusual sensitivity to sunlight.
Codeine, like other narcotic analgesics, may produce orthostatic hypotension in some ambulatory patients. Patients should be cautioned accordingly.
DRUG INTERACTIONS
CODEINE: In patients receiving MAO inhibitors, an initial small test dose is advisable to allow observation of any excessive narcotic effects or MAOI interaction.
PROMETHAZINE: The sedative action of promethazine is additive to the effects of other central nervous system depressants, including alcohol, narcotic analgesics, sedatives, hypnotics, tricyclic antidepressants, and tranquilizers; therefore, these agents should be avoided or administered in reduced dosage to patients receiving promethazine.
[See table above.]
DRUG/LABORATORY TEST INTERACTIONS
Because narcotic analgesics may increase biliary tract pressure, with resultant increases in plasma amylase or lipase levels, determination of these enzyme levels may be unreliable for 24 hours after a narcotic analgesic has been given.
The following laboratory tests may be affected in patients who are receiving therapy with promethazine hydrochloride:
Pregnancy Tests
Diagnostic pregnancy tests based on immunological reactions between HCG and anti-HCG may result in false-negative or false-positive interpretations.
Glucose Tolerance Test
An increase in blood glucose has been reported in patients receiving promethazine.
CARCINOGENESIS, MUTAGENESIS, IMPAIRMENT OF FERTILITY
CODEINE AND PROMETHAZINE
Long-term animal studies have not been performed to assess the carcinogenic potential of codeine or of promethazine, nor are there other animal or human data concerning carcinogenicity, mutagenicity, or impairment of fertility with these agents. Codeine has been reported to show no evidence of carcinogenicity or mutagenicity in a variety of test systems, including the micronucleus and sperm abnormality assays and the *Salmonella* assay. Promethazine was nonmutagenic in the *Salmonella* test system of Ames.
PHENYLEPHRINE
A study which followed the development of cancer in 143,574 patients over a four-year period indicated that in 11,981 patients who received phenylephrine (systemic or topical), there was no statistically significant association between the drug and cancer at any or all sites.
Long-term animal studies have not been performed to assess the carcinogenic potential of phenylephrine, nor are there other animal or human data concerning mutagenicity.
A study of the effects of adrenergic drugs on ovum transport in rabbits indicated that treatment with phenylephrine did not alter incidence of pregnancy; the number of implantations was significantly reduced when high doses of the drug were used.
PREGNANCY
Teratogenic Effects —Pregnancy Category C
CODEINE: A study in rats and rabbits reported no teratogenic effect of codeine administered during the period of organogenesis in doses ranging from 5 to 120 mg/kg. In the rat, doses at the 120-mg/kg level, in the toxic range for the adult animal, were associated with an increase in embryo resorption at the time of implantation. In another study a single 100-mg/kg dose of codeine administered to pregnant mice reportedly resulted in delayed ossification in the offspring.
There are no studies in humans, and the significance of these findings to humans, if any, is not known.
PROMETHAZINE: Teratogenic effects have not been demonstrated in rat-feeding studies at doses of 6.25 and 12.5 mg/kg of promethazine. These doses are 8.3 and 16.7 times the maximum recommended total daily dose for a 50-kg subject. Specific studies to test the action of the drug on parturition, lactation, and development of the animal neonate were not done, but a general preliminary study in rats indicated no effect on these parameters. Although antihistamines, including promethazine, have been found to produce fetal mortality in rodents, the pharmacological effects of histamine in the rodent do not parallel those in man. There are no adequate and well-controlled studies of promethazine in pregnant women.
PHENYLEPHRINE: A study in rabbits indicated that continued moderate overexposure to phenylephrine (3 mg/day) during the second half of pregnancy (22nd day of gestation to delivery) may contribute to perinatal wastage, prematurity, premature labor, and possibly fetal anomalies; when phenylephrine (3 mg/day) was given to rabbits during the first half of pregnancy (3rd day after mating for seven days), a significant number gave birth to litters of low birth weight. Another study showed that phenylephrine was associated with anomalies of aortic arch and with ventricular septal defect in the chick embryo.
Phenergan VC with codeine should be used during pregnancy only if the potential benefit justifies the potential risk to the fetus.
Nonteratogenic Effects
Dependence has been reported in newborns whose mothers took opiates regularly during pregnancy. Withdrawal signs include irritability, excessive crying, tremors, hyperreflexia, fever, vomiting, and diarrhea. Signs usually appear during the first few days of life.
Promethazine taken within two weeks of delivery may inhibit platelet aggregation in the newborn.
LABOR AND DELIVERY
Narcotic analgesics cross the placental barrier. The closer to delivery and the larger the dose used, the greater the possibility of respiratory depression in the newborn. Narcotic analgesics should be avoided during labor if delivery of a premature infant is anticipated. If the mother has received narcotic analgesics during labor, newborn infants should be observed closely for signs of respiratory depression. Resuscitation may be required (see "Overdosage"). The effect of codeine, if any, on the later growth, development, and functional maturation of the child is unknown.
Administration of phenylephrine to patients in late pregnancy or labor may cause fetal anoxia or bradycardia by increasing contractility of the uterus and decreasing uterine blood flow.
See also "Nonteratogenic Effects."
NURSING MOTHERS
Some studies, but not others, have reported detectable amounts of codeine in breast milk. The levels are probably not clinically significant after usual therapeutic dosage. The possibility of clinically important amounts being excreted in breast milk in individuals abusing codeine should be considered.
It is not known whether either phenylephrine or promethazine is excreted in human milk.
Caution should be exercised when Phenergan VC with codeine is administered to a nursing woman.
PEDIATRIC USE
This product should not be used in children under 2 years of age because safety for such use has not been established.

ADVERSE REACTIONS

CODEINE
Nervous System —CNS depression, particularly respiratory depression, and to a lesser extent circulatory depression; light-headedness, dizziness, sedation, euphoria, dysphoria, headache, transient hallucination, disorientation, visual disturbances, and convulsions.
Cardiovascular —Tachycardia, bradycardia, palpitation, faintness, syncope, orthostatic hypotension (common to narcotic analgesics).
Gastrointestinal —Nausea, vomiting, constipation, and biliary tract spasm. Patients with chronic ulcerative colitis may

Continued on next page

Wyeth-Ayerst Laboratories—Cont.

PHENERGAN VC WITH CODEINE

Adults	1 teaspoon (5 mL) every 4 to 6 hours, not to exceed 30.0 mL in 24 hours.
Children 6 years to under 12 years	½ to 1 teaspoon (2.5 to 5 mL) every 4 to 6 hours, not to exceed 30.0 mL in 24 hours.
Children under 6 years (weight: 18 kg or 40 lbs)	¼ to ½ teaspoon (1.25 to 2.5 mL) every 4 to 6 hours, not to exceed 9.0 mL in 24 hours.
Children under 6 years (weight: 16 kg or 35 lbs)	¼ to ½ teaspoon (1.25 to 2.5 mL) every 4 to 6 hours, not to exceed 8.0 mL in 24 hours.
Children under 6 years (weight: 14 kg or 30 lbs)	¼ to ½ teaspoon (1.25 to 2.5 mL) every 4 to 6 hours, not to exceed 7.0 mL in 24 hours.
Children under 6 years (weight: 12 kg or 25 lbs)	¼ to ½ teaspoon (1.25 to 2.5 mL) every 4 to 6 hours, not to exceed 6.0 mL in 24 hours.

Phenergan VC with codeine is not recommended for children under 2 years of age.

experience increased colonic motility; in patients with acute ulcerative colitis, toxic dilation has been reported.

Genitourinary—Oliguria, urinary retention; antidiuretic effect has been reported (common to narcotic analgesics).

Allergic—Infrequent pruritus, giant urticaria, angioneurotic edema, and laryngeal edema.

Other—Flushing of the face, sweating and pruritus (due to opiate-induced histamine release); weakness.

PROMETHAZINE

Nervous System—Sedation, sleepiness, occasional blurred vision, dryness of mouth, dizziness; rarely confusion, disorientation, and extrapyramidal symptoms such as oculogyric crisis, torticollis, and tongue protrusion (usually in association with parenteral injection or excessive dosage).

Cardiovascular—Increased or decreased blood pressure.

Dermatologic—Rash, rarely photosensitivity.

Hematologic—Rarely leukopenia, thrombocytopenia; agranulocytosis (1 case).

Gastrointestinal—Nausea and vomiting.

PHENYLEPHRINE

Nervous System—Restlessness, anxiety, nervousness, and dizziness.

Cardiovascular—Hypertension (see "Warnings").

Other—Precordial pain, respiratory distress, tremor, and weakness.

DRUG ABUSE AND DEPENDENCE

CONTROLLED SUBSTANCE

Phenergan VC with codeine is a Schedule V Controlled Substance.

ABUSE

Codeine is known to be subject to abuse; however, the abuse potential of oral codeine appears to be quite low. Even parenteral codeine does not appear to offer the psychic effects sought by addicts to the same degree as heroin or morphine. However, codeine must be administered only under close supervision to patients with a history of drug abuse or dependence.

DEPENDENCE

Psychological dependence, physical dependence, and tolerance are known to occur with codeine.

OVERDOSAGE

CODEINE: Serious overdose with codeine is characterized by respiratory depression (a decrease in respiratory rate and/or tidal volume, Cheyne-Stokes respiration, cyanosis), extreme somnolence progressing to stupor or coma, skeletal muscle flaccidity, cold and clammy skin, and sometimes bradycardia and hypotension. The triad of coma, pinpoint pupils, and respiratory depression is strongly suggestive of opiate poisoning. In severe overdosage, particularly by the intravenous route, apnea, circulatory collapse, cardiac arrest, and death may occur. Promethazine is additive to the depressant effects of codeine.

It is difficult to determine what constitutes a standard toxic or lethal dose. However, the lethal oral dose of codeine in an adult is reported to be in the range of 0.5 to 1.0 gram. Infants and children are believed to be relatively more sensitive to opiates on a body-weight basis. Elderly patients are also comparatively intolerant to opiates.

PROMETHAZINE: Signs and symptoms of overdosage with promethazine range from mild depression of the central nervous system and cardiovascular system to profound hypotension, respiratory depression, and unconsciousness.

Stimulation may be evident, especially in children and geriatric patients. Convulsions may rarely occur. A paradoxical reaction has been reported in children receiving single doses of 75 mg to 125 mg orally, characterized by hyperexcitability and nightmares.

Atropine-like signs and symptoms—dry mouth, fixed, dilated pupils, flushing, as well as gastrointestinal symptoms, may occur.

PHENYLEPHRINE: Signs and symptoms of overdosage with phenylephrine include hypertension, headache, convulsions, cerebral hemorrhage, and vomiting. Ventricular premature beats and short paroxysms of ventricular tachycardia may also occur. Headache may be a symptom of hypertension. Bradycardia may also be seen early in phenylephrine overdosage through stimulation of baroreceptors.

TREATMENT

Treatment of overdosage with Phenergan VC with codeine is essentially symptomatic and supportive. Only in cases of extreme overdosage or individual sensitivity do vital signs including respiration, pulse, blood pressure, temperature, and EKG need to be monitored. Activated charcoal orally or by lavage may be given, or sodium or magnesium sulfate orally as a cathartic. Attention should be given to the reestablishment of adequate respiratory exchange through provision of a patent airway and institution of assisted or controlled ventilation. The narcotic antagonist, naloxone hydrochloride, may be administered when significant respiratory depression occurs with Phenergan VC with codeine; any depressant effects of promethazine are not reversed by naloxone. Diazepam may be used to control convulsions. Avoid analeptics, which may cause convulsions. Acidosis and electrolyte losses should be corrected. A rise in temperature or pulmonary complications may signal the need for institution of antibiotic therapy.

Severe hypotension usually responds to the administration of norepinephrine or phenylephrine. EPINEPHRINE SHOULD NOT BE USED, since its use in a patient with partial adrenergic blockade may further lower the blood pressure.

Limited experience with dialysis indicates that it is not helpful.

DOSAGE AND ADMINISTRATION

The average effective dose is given in the following table:
[See table above.]

HOW SUPPLIED

Phenergan® VC with codeine is a clear, reddish-orange solution supplied as follows:

NDC 0008-0552-02, case of 24 bottles of 4 fl. oz. (118 mL).
NDC 0008-0552-03, bottle of 1 pint (473 mL).

Keep tightly closed—Stored at room temperature, between 15° C and 25° C (59° F and 77° F).

Protect from light.

Dispense in light-resistant, glass, tight container.

PLEGINE®   (II) ℞

[plěj-ēn']

(phendimetrazine tartrate tablets)
Anorexiant

CAUTION: Federal law prohibits dispensing without prescription.

DESCRIPTION

Chemical name: (+)-3,4-Dimethyl-2-phenylmorpholine Tartrate

Structural formula:

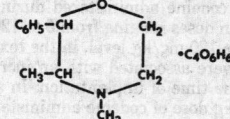

Plegine is the dextro isomer of phendimetrazine tartrate. Phendimetrazine tartrate is a white, odorless powder with a bitter taste. It is soluble in water, methanol, and ethanol. Plegine contains these inactive ingredients: D&C Yellow No. 10; FD&C Yellow No. 6; Lactose, NF; Magnesium Stearate, NF; Polyethylene Glycol 8000, NF.

HOW SUPPLIED

Plegine—Each scored tablet contains 35 mg phendimetrazine tartrate, in bottles of 100 (NDC 0046-0755-81).

Store at room temperature, approximately 25°C.

For prescribing information write to Professional Service, Wyeth-Ayerst Laboratories, P.O. Box 8299, Philadelphia, PA 19101, or contact your local Wyeth-Ayerst representative.

PMB® 200   ℞

Each tablet contains:

Premarin® (conjugated estrogens, USP)	0.45 mg
Meprobamate, USP	200 mg

PMB® 400

Each tablet contains:

Premarin® (conjugated estrogens, USP)	0.45 mg
Meprobamate, USP	400 mg

Caution: Federal law prohibits dispensing without prescription.

---

1. ESTROGENS HAVE BEEN REPORTED TO INCREASE THE RISK OF ENDOMETRIAL CARCINOMA.

Three independent, case-controlled studies have reported an increased risk of endometrial cancer in postmenopausal women exposed to exogenous estrogens for more than one year.[1-3] This risk was independent of the other known risk factors for endometrial cancer. These studies are further supported by the finding that incidence rates of endometrial cancer have increased sharply since 1969 in eight different areas of the United States with population-based cancer-reporting systems, an increase which may be related to the rapidly expanding use of estrogens during the last decade.[4]

The three case-controlled studies reported that the risk of endometrial cancer in estrogen users was about 4.5 to 13.9 times greater than in nonusers. The risk appears to depend on both duration of treatment[1] and on estrogen dose.[3] In view of these findings, when estrogens are used for the treatment of menopausal symptoms, the lowest dose that will control symptoms should be utilized and medication should be discontinued as soon as possible. When prolonged treatment is medically indicated, the patient should be reassessed, on at least a semi-annual basis to determine the need for continued therapy. Although the evidence must be considered preliminary, one study suggests that cyclic administration of low doses of estrogen may carry less risk than continuous administration.[3] It therefore appears prudent to utilize such a regimen.

Close clinical surveillance of all women taking estrogens is important. In all cases of undiagnosed persistent or recurring abnormal vaginal bleeding, adequate diagnostic measures should be undertaken to rule out malignancy.

There is no evidence at present that "natural" estrogens are more or less hazardous than "synthetic" estrogens at equi-estrogenic doses.

2. ESTROGENS SHOULD NOT BE USED DURING PREGNANCY.

The use of female sex hormones, both estrogens and progestogens, during early pregnancy may seriously damage the offspring. It has been shown that females exposed in utero to diethylstilbestrol, a nonsteroidal estrogen, have an increased risk of developing, in later life, a form of vaginal or cervical cancer that is ordinarily extremely rare.[5,6] This risk has been estimated as not greater than 4 per 1,000 exposures.[7] Furthermore, a high percentage of such exposed women (from 30% to 90%) have been found to have vaginal adenosis,[8-12] epithelial changes of the vagina and cervix. Although these changes are histologically benign, it is not known whether they are precursors of malignancy. Although similar data are not available with the use of other estrogens, it cannot be presumed they would not induce similar changes.

Several reports suggest an association between intrauterine exposure to female sex hormones and congenital anomalies, including congenital heart defects and limb-reduction defects.[13-16] One case-controlled study[16] estimated a 4.7-fold increased risk of limb-reduction defects in infants exposed in utero to sex hormones (oral contraceptives, hormone withdrawal tests for pregnancy, or attempted treatment for threatened abortion). Some of these exposures were very short and involved only a few days of treatment. The data suggest that the risk of limb-reduction defects in exposed fetuses is somewhat less than 1 per 1,000.

In the past, female sex hormones have been used during pregnancy in an attempt to treat threatened or habitual abortion. There is considerable evidence that estrogens are ineffective for these indications, and there is no evidence from well-controlled studies that progestogens are effective for these uses.

If PMB is used during pregnancy, or if the patient becomes pregnant while taking this drug, she should be apprised of the potential risks to the fetus, and the advisability of pregnancy continuation.

3. THIS FIXED-COMBINATION DRUG IS NOT INDICATED FOR INITIAL THERAPY.
In cases where estrogen given alone has not alleviated anxiety and tension existing as part of the menopausal symptom complex, therapy may then consist of separate administration of estrogen and meprobamate in order to determine the appropriate dosage of each drug for the patient. If this fixed combination represents the dosage so determined, its use may be more convenient in patient management. The treatment of such patients is not static, but must be re-evaluated as conditions in each patient warrant.

DESCRIPTION

PMB is a combination of Premarin® (conjugated estrogens, USP) and meprobamate, USP, a tranquilizing agent, in tablet form for oral administration.
Premarin (conjugated estrogens, USP) is a mixture of estrogens, obtained exclusively from natural sources, occurring as the sodium salts of water-soluble estrogen sulfates blended to represent the average composition of material derived from pregnant mares' urine. It contains estrone, equilin, and 17α-dihydroequilin, together with smaller amounts of 17α-estradiol, equilenin, and 17 α-dihydroequilenin as salts of their sulfate esters.
Meprobamate, USP, is the dicarbamic acid ester of 2-methyl-2-*n*-propyl-1,3-propanediol.
PMB 200: Each tablet contains 0.45 mg of Premarin® (conjugated estrogens, USP) and 200 mg Meprobamate, USP.
PMB 400: Each tablet contains 0.45 mg of Premarin® (conjugated estrogens, USP) and 400 mg Meprobamate, USP.
PMB Tablets contain the following inactive ingredients: calcium phosphate, calcium sulfate, carnauba wax, cellulose, lactose, magnesium stearate, methylcellulose, pharmaceutical glaze, sucrose, talc, titanium dioxide.
—PMB 200 Tablets also contain: D&C Yellow No. 10, FD&C Blue No. 1, FD&C Yellow No. 6.
—PMB 400 Tablets also contain: FD&C Blue No. 2, D&C Red No. 7, D&C Red No. 27.

CLINICAL PHARMACOLOGY

Estrogens are important in the development and maintenance of the female reproductive system and secondary sex characteristics. They promote growth and development of the vagina, uterus, and fallopian tubes, and enlargement of the breasts. Indirectly, they contribute to the shaping of the skeleton, maintenance of tone and elasticity of urogenital structures, changes in the epiphyses of the long bones that allow for the pubertal growth spurt and its termination, growth of axillary and pubic hair, and pigmentation of the nipples and genitals. Decline of estrogenic activity at the end of the menstrual cycle can bring on menstruation, although the cessation of progesterone secretion is the most important factor in the mature ovulatory cycle. However, in the preovulatory or nonovulatory cycle, estrogen is the primary determinant in the onset of menstruation. Estrogens also affect the release of pituitary gonadotropins.
The pharmacologic effects of conjugated estrogens are similar to those of endogenous estrogens. They are soluble in water and are well absorbed from the gastrointestinal tract.
In responsive tissues (female genital organs, breasts, hypothalamus, pituitary) estrogens enter the cell and are transported into the nucleus. As a result of estrogen action, specific RNA and protein synthesis occurs.
Metabolism and inactivation occur primarily in the liver. Some estrogens are excreted into the bile; however, they are reabsorbed from the intestine and returned to the liver through the portal venous system. Water-soluble estrogen conjugates are strongly acidic and are ionized in body fluids, which favor excretion through the kidneys since tubular reabsorption is minimal.
Meprobamate is used clinically for the reduction of anxiety and tension. The precise mechanism(s) of its action is not known. It is well absorbed from the gastrointestinal tract and has a physiological half-life of about 10 hours. It is excreted in the urine primarily as hydroxymeprobamate and as a glucuronide.
The combination of PREMARIN with meprobamate as provided in PMB relieves the underlying estrogen deficiency and affords tranquilizing activity to ameliorate the anxiety and tension not due to estrogen deficiency.

INDICATIONS AND USAGE

For the treatment of moderate-to-severe vasomotor symptoms of the menopause when anxiety and tension are part of the symptom complex and only in those cases in which the use of estrogens alone has not resulted in alleviation of such symptoms. PMB HAS NOT BEEN SHOWN TO BE EFFECTIVE FOR ANY PURPOSE DURING PREGNANCY AND ITS USE MAY CAUSE SEVERE HARM TO THE FETUS (SEE BOXED WARNING).

CONTRAINDICATIONS

Estrogens should not be used in women with any of the following conditions:
1. Known or suspected cancer of the breast except in appropriately selected patients being treated for metastatic disease.
2. Known or suspected estrogen-dependent neoplasia.
3. Known or suspected pregnancy (see Boxed Warning).
4. Undiagnosed abnormal genital bleeding.
5. Active thrombophlebitis or thromboembolic disorders.
6. A past history of thrombophlebitis, thrombosis, or thromboembolic disorders associated with previous estrogen use.
Meprobamate should not be used in patients with the following conditions:
1. A history of allergic or idiosyncratic reactions to meprobamate or related compounds such as carisoprodol, mebutamate, tybamate, or carbromal.
2. Acute intermittent porphyria.

WARNINGS

USAGE IN PREGNANCY AND LACTATION.
An increased risk of congenital malformations associated with the use of minor tranquilizers (meprobamate, chlordiazepoxide, and diazepam) during the first trimester of pregnancy has been suggested in several studies. Because use of these drugs is rarely a matter of urgency, their use during this period should almost always be avoided. The possibility that a woman of childbearing potential may be pregnant at the time of institution of therapy should be considered. Patients should be advised that if they become pregnant during therapy or intend to become pregnant they should communicate with their physicians about the desirability of discontinuing the drug.
Meprobamate passes the placental barrier. It is present both in umbilical cord blood at or near maternal plasma levels and in breast milk of lactating mothers at concentrations two to four times that of maternal plasma. When use of meprobamate is contemplated in breast-feeding patients, the drug's higher concentrations in breast milk as compared to maternal plasma levels should be considered.
USAGE IN CHILDREN
PMB is not intended for use in pediatric patients.
ASSOCIATED WITH ESTROGEN ADMINISTRATION
1. *Induction of malignant neoplasms:* Estrogens have been reported to increase the risk of endometrial carcinoma. (See Boxed Warning.) However, a recent, large, case-controlled study indicated no increase in risk of breast cancer in postmenopausal women.[18]
2. *Gallbladder disease:* A recent study has reported a 2- to 3-fold increase in the risk of surgically confirmed gallbladder disease in women receiving postmenopausal estrogens,[17] similar to the 2-fold increase previously noted in users of oral contraceptives.[19,24a]
3. *Effects similar to those caused by estrogen-progestogen oral contraceptives:* There are several serious adverse effects of oral contraceptives, most of which have not, up to now, been documented as consequences of postmenopausal estrogen therapy. This may reflect the comparatively low doses of estrogen used in postmenopausal women. It would be expected that the larger doses of estrogen used to treat prostatic or breast cancer are more likely to result in these adverse effects, and, in fact, it has been shown that there is an increased risk of thrombosis in men receiving estrogens for prostatic cancer.[20–23]
a. *Thromboembolic disease:* It is now well established that users of oral contraceptives have an increased risk of various thromboembolic and thrombotic vascular diseases, such as thrombophlebitis, pulmonary embolism, stroke, and myocardial infarction.[24–31] Cases of retinal thrombosis, mesenteric thrombosis, and optic neuritis have been reported in oral-contraceptive users. There is evidence that the risk of several of these adverse reactions is related to the dose of the drug.[32,33] An increased risk of postsurgery thromboembolic complications has also been reported in users of oral-contraceptives.[34,35] If feasible, estrogen should be discontinued at least 4 weeks before surgery of the type associated with an increased risk of thromboembolism, or during periods of prolonged immobilization.
While an increased rate of thromboembolic and thrombotic disease in postmenopausal users of estrogens has not been found,[17–24,25–36] this does not rule out the possibility that such an increase may be present or that subgroups of women who have underlying risk factors or who are receiving relatively large doses of estrogens may have increased risk. Therefore estrogens should not be used in persons with active thrombophlebitis or thromboembolic disorders, and they should not be used (except in treatment of malignancy) in persons with a history of such disorders in association with estrogen use. They should be used with caution in patients with cerebral vascular or coronary artery disease and only for those in whom estrogens are clearly needed.
Large doses of estrogen (5 mg conjugated estrogens per day), comparable to those used to treat cancer of the prostate and breast, have been shown in a large prospective clinical trial in men[37] to increase the risk of nonfatal myocardial infarction, pulmonary embolism, and thrombophlebitis. When estrogen doses of this size are used, any of the thromboembolic and thrombotic adverse effects associated with oral contraceptive use should be considered a clear risk.
b. *Hepatic adenoma:* Benign hepatic adenomas appear to be associated with the use of oral contraceptives.[38–40] Although benign, and rare, these may rupture and may cause death through intra-abdominal hemorrhage. Such lesions have not yet been reported in association with other estrogen or progestogen preparations but should be considered in estrogen users having abdominal pain and tenderness, abdominal mass, or hypovolemic shock. Hepatocellular carcinoma has also been reported in women taking estrogen-containing oral contraceptives.[39] The relationship of this malignancy to these drugs is not known at this time.
c. *Elevated blood pressure:* Women using oral contraceptives sometimes experience increased blood pressure which, in most cases, returns to normal on discontinuing the drug. There is now a report that this may occur with use of estrogens in the menopause[41] and blood pressure should be monitored with estrogen use, especially if high doses are used.
d. *Glucose tolerance:* A worsening of glucose tolerance has been observed in a significant percentage of patients on estrogen-containing oral contraceptives. For this reason, diabetic patients should be carefully observed while receiving estrogen.
4. *Hypercalcemia:* Administration of estrogens may lead to severe hypercalcemia in patients with breast cancer and bone metastases. If this occurs, the drug should be stopped and appropriate measures taken to reduce the serum calcium level.
ASSOCIATED WITH MEPROBAMATE ADMINISTRATION
1. *Drug Dependence:* Physical dependence, psychological dependence, and abuse have occurred. When chronic intoxication from prolonged use occurs, it usually involves ingestion of greater than recommended doses and is manifested by ataxia, slurred speech, and vertigo. Therefore, careful supervision of dose and amounts prescribed is advised, as well as avoidance of prolonged administration, especially for alcoholics and other patients with a known propensity for taking excessive quantities of drugs.
Sudden withdrawal of the drug after prolonged and excessive use may precipitate recurrence of pre-existing symptoms, such as anxiety, anorexia, or insomnia, or withdrawal reactions, such as vomiting, ataxia, tremors, muscle twitching, confusional states, hallucinosis, and, rarely, convulsive seizures. Such seizures are more likely to occur in persons with central nervous system damage or pre-existent or latent convulsive disorders. Onset of withdrawal symptoms occurs usually within 12 to 48 hours after discontinuation of meprobamate; symptoms usually cease within the next 12 to 48 hours.
When excessive dosage has continued for weeks or months, dosage should be reduced gradually over a period of one or two weeks rather than abruptly stopped. Alternatively, a short-acting barbiturate may be substituted, then gradually withdrawn.
2. *Potentially Hazardous Tasks:* Patients should be warned that this drug may impair the mental and/or physical abilities required for the performance of potentially hazardous tasks such as driving a motor vehicle or operating machinery.
3. *Additive Effects:* Since the effects of meprobamate and alcohol or meprobamate and other CNS depressants or psychotropic drugs may be additive, appropriate caution should be exercised with patients who take more than one of these agents simultaneously.

PRECAUTIONS

GENERAL PRECAUTIONS
Associated with Estrogen
1. A complete medical and family history should be taken prior to the initiation of any estrogen therapy. The pretreatment and periodic physical examinations should include special reference to blood pressure, breasts, abdomen, and pelvic organs, and should include a Papanicolaou smear. As a general rule, estrogen should not be prescribed for longer than one year without another physical examination being performed.
2. Fluid retention—Because estrogens may cause some degree of fluid retention, conditions which might be influenced by this factor such as asthma, epilepsy, migraine, and cardiac or renal dysfunction, require careful observation.
3. Certain patients may develop undesirable manifestations of excessive estrogenic stimulation, such as abnormal or excessive uterine bleeding, mastodynia, etc.
4. Prolonged administration of unopposed estrogen therapy has been reported to increase the risk of endometrial hyperplasia in some patients.
5. Oral contraceptives appear to be associated with an increased incidence of mental depression.[24a] Although it is not clear whether this is due to the estrogenic or progestogenic component of the contraceptive, patients with a history of depression should be carefully observed.

Continued on next page

Wyeth-Ayerst Laboratories—Cont.

6. Pre-existing uterine leiomyomata may increase in size during estrogen use.

7. The pathologist should be advised of estrogen therapy when relevant specimens are submitted.

8. Patients with a past history of jaundice during pregnancy have an increased risk of recurrence of jaundice while receiving estrogen-containing oral contraceptive therapy. If jaundice develops in any patient receiving estrogen, the medication should be discontinued while the cause is investigated.

9. Estrogens may be poorly metabolized in patients with impaired liver function and should be administered with caution in such patients.

10. Because estrogens influence the metabolism of calcium and phosphorus, they should be used with caution in patients with metabolic bone diseases that are associated with hypercalcemia or in patients with renal insufficiency.

11. Because of the effects of estrogens on epiphyseal closure, they should be used judiciously in young patients in whom bone growth is not complete.

Concomitant Progestin Use

The lowest effective dose appropriate for the specific indication should be utilized. Studies of the addition of a progestin for 7 or more days of a cycle of estrogen administration have reported a lowered incidence of endometrial hyperplasia. Morphological and biochemical studies of the endometrium suggest that 10 to 13 days of progestin are needed to provide maximal maturation of the endometrium and to eliminate any hyperplastic changes. Whether this will provide protection from endometrial carcinoma has not been clearly established. There are possible additional risks which may be associated with the inclusion of progestin in estrogen replacement regimens. If concomitant progestin therapy is used, potential risks may include adverse effects on carbohydrate and lipid metabolism. The choice of progestin and dosage may be important in minimizing these adverse effects.

Associated with Meprobamate

1. The lowest effective dose should be administered, particularly to debilitated patients, in order to preclude oversedation.

2. The possibility of suicide attempts should be considered and the least amount of drug feasible should be dispensed at any one time.

3. Meprobamate is metabolized in the liver and excreted by the kidney; to avoid its excess accumulation, caution should be exercised in administration to patients with compromised liver or kidney function.

4. Meprobamate occasionally may precipitate seizures in epileptic patients.

INFORMATION FOR PATIENTS

(See text which appears after the PHYSICIAN REFERENCES.)

DRUG/LABORATORY TEST INTERACTIONS

Certain endocrine and liver function tests may be affected by estrogen-containing oral contraceptives. The following similar changes may be expected with larger doses of estrogen.

a. Increased sulfobromophthalein retention.

b. Increased prothrombin and factors VII, VIII, IX, and X; decreased antithrombin 3; increased norepinephrine-induced platelet aggregability.

c. Increased thyroid binding globulin (TBG) leading to increased circulating total thyroid hormone, as measured by PBI, T_4 by column, or T_4 by radioimmunoassay. Free T_3 resin uptake is decreased, reflecting the elevated TBG; free T_4 concentration is unaltered.

d. Impaired glucose tolerance.

e. Decreased pregnanediol excretion.

f. Reduced response to metyrapone test.

g. Reduced serum folate concentration.

h. Increased serum triglyceride and phospholipid concentration.

MUTAGENESIS AND CARCINOGENESIS

Long-term, continuous administration of natural and synthetic estrogens in certain animal species increases the frequency of carcinomas of the breast, cervix, vagina, and liver. However in a recent, large, case-controlled study of postmenopausal women, there was no increase in risk of breast cancer with use of conjugated estrogens.[18]

PREGNANCY CATEGORY X

(See CONTRAINDICATIONS and Boxed Warning.)

NURSING MOTHERS

Because of the potential for serious adverse reactions in nursing infants from PMB, a decision should be made whether to discontinue nursing or to discontinue the drugs, taking into account the importance of the drug to the mother. (See WARNINGS section for information on use in pregnancy and lactation.)

PEDIATRIC USE

Safety and effectiveness in pediatric patients have not been established.

ADVERSE REACTIONS

ASSOCIATED WITH ESTROGEN ADMINISTRATION

(See WARNINGS regarding induction of neoplasia, adverse effects on the fetus, increased incidence of gallbladder disease, and adverse effects similar to those of oral contraceptives, including thromboembolism.) The following additional adverse reactions have been reported with estrogenic therapy, including oral contraceptives:

1. *Genitourinary system:* Breakthrough bleeding, spotting, change in menstrual flow; dysmenorrhea; premenstrual-like syndrome; amenorrhea during and after treatment; increase in size of uterine fibromyomata; vaginal candidiasis; change in cervical erosion and in degree of cervical secretion; cystitis-like syndrome.

2. *Breasts:* Tenderness, enlargement, secretion.

3. *Gastrointestinal:* Nausea, vomiting; abdominal cramps, bloating; cholestatic jaundice.

4. *Skin:* Chloasma or melasma which may persist when drug is discontinued; erythema multiforme; erythema nodosum; hemorrhagic eruption; loss of scalp hair; hirsutism.

5. *Eyes:* Steepening of corneal curvature; intolerance to contact lenses.

6. *CNS:* Headache, migraine, dizziness; mental depression; chorea.

7. *Miscellaneous:* Increase or decrease in weight; reduced carbohydrate tolerance; aggravation of porphyria; edema; changes in libido.

THE FOLLOWING HAVE BEEN REPORTED WITH MEPROBAMATE THERAPY

1. *Central Nervous System:* Drowsiness, ataxia, dizziness; slurred speech, headache, vertigo, weakness, paresthesias, impairment of visual accommodation, euphoria, overstimulation, paradoxical excitement, fast EEG activity.

2. *Gastrointestinal:* Nausea, vomiting, diarrhea.

3. *Cardiovascular:* Palpitations, tachycardia, various forms of arrhythmia, transient ECG changes, syncope; also, hypotensive crises (including one fatal case).

4. *Allergic or Idiosyncratic:* Allergic or idiosyncratic reactions are usually seen within the period of the first to fourth dose in patients having had no previous contact with the drug. Milder reactions are characterized by an itchy, urticarial, or erythematous maculopapular rash which may be generalized or confined to the groin. Other reactions have included leukopenia, acute nonthrombocytopenic purpura, petechiae, ecchymoses, eosinophilia, peripheral edema, adenopathy, fever, fixed drug eruption with cross reaction to carisoprodol, and cross sensitivity between meprobamate/mebutamate and meprobamate/carbromal.

More severe hypersensitivity reactions, rarely reported, include hyperpyrexia, chills, angioneurotic edema, bronchospasm, oliguria, and anuria. Also, anaphylaxis, erythema multiforme, exfoliative dermatitis, stomatitis, proctitis, Stevens-Johnson syndrome, and bullous dermatitis, including one fatal case of the latter, following administration of meprobamate in combination with prednisolone.

In case of allergic or idiosyncratic reactions to meprobamate, discontinue the drug and initiate appropriate symptomatic therapy, which may include epinephrine, antihistamines, and in severe cases corticosteroids. In evaluating possible allergic reactions, also consider allergy to excipients (information on excipients is available to physicians on request).

5. *Hematologic* (See also "*Allergic or Idiosyncratic.*"): —Agranulocytosis and aplastic anemia have been reported, although no causal relationship has been established. These cases rarely were fatal. Rare cases of thrombocytopenic purpura have been reported.

6. *Other:* Exacerbation of porphyric symptoms.

OVERDOSAGE

ACUTE OVERDOSAGE (ESTROGEN ALONE)

Numerous reports of ingestion of large doses of estrogen-containing oral contraceptives by young children indicate that acute serious ill effects do not occur. Overdosage of estrogen may cause nausea, and withdrawal bleeding may occur in females.

ACUTE SIMPLE OVERDOSAGE (MEPROBAMATE ALONE)

Death has been reported with ingestion of as little as 12 grams meprobamate and survival with as much as 40 grams.

BLOOD LEVELS

0.5 to 2.0 mg% represents the usual blood level range of meprobamate after therapeutic doses. The level may occasionally be as high as 3.0 mg%.

3 to 10 mg% usually corresponds to findings of mild-to-moderate symptoms of overdosage, such as stupor or light coma.

10 to 20 mg% usually corresponds to deeper coma, requiring more intensive treatment. Some fatalities occur.

At levels greater than 20 mg%, more fatalities than survivals can be expected.

ACUTE COMBINED (ALCOHOL OR OTHER CNS DEPRESSANTS OR PSYCHOTROPIC DRUGS)

Overdosage

Since effects can be additive, a history of ingestion of a low dose of meprobamate plus any of these compounds (or of a

relatively low blood or tissue level) cannot be used as a prognostic indicator.

In cases where excessive doses have been taken, sleep ensues rapidly and blood pressure, pulse, and respiratory rates are reduced to basal levels. Any drug remaining in the stomach should be removed and symptomatic therapy given. Should respiration or blood pressure become compromised, respiratory assistance, central nervous system stimulants, and pressor agents should be administered cautiously as indicated. Meprobamate is metabolized in the liver and excreted by the kidney. Diuresis, osmotic (mannitol) diuresis, peritoneal dialysis, and hemodialysis have been used successfully. Careful monitoring of urinary output is necessary and caution should be taken to avoid overhydration. Relapse and death, after initial recovery, have been attributed to incomplete gastric emptying and delayed absorption. Meprobamate can be measured in biological fluids by two methods: colorimetric[42] and gas chromatographic.[43]

DOSAGE AND ADMINISTRATION

GIVEN CYCLICALLY FOR SHORT-TERM USE ONLY

For the treatment of moderate-to-severe vasomotor symptoms of the menopause when anxiety and tension are part of the symptom complex and only in those cases in which the use of estrogens alone has not resulted in alleviation of such symptoms.

The lowest dose that will control symptoms should be chosen and medication should be discontinued as promptly as possible. The usual dosage of conjugated estrogen is 1.25 milligrams daily. The usual dosage of meprobamate is 1,200 to 1,600 milligrams daily.

Administration should be cyclic (eg, three weeks on and one week off).

Attempts to discontinue or taper medication should be made at three- to six-month intervals.

PMB® 200 & PMB® 400

The usual dosage is one tablet of either strength three times daily administered cyclically. Use of meprobamate during the rest period should be considered for those patients who may require continuing medication with tranquilizer. After the first few cycles of therapy, the patient's need for continuing the use of the meprobamate component should be reevaluated.

Daily dosage should be adjusted to individual requirements. The daily dosage should not exceed 6 tablets of PMB 200 per day or 4 tablets of PMB 400 per day.

Treated patients with an intact uterus should be monitored closely for signs of endometrial cancer and appropriate diagnostic measures should be taken to rule out malignancy in the event of persistent or recurring abnormal vaginal bleeding.

HOW SUPPLIED

PMB® 200 [Premarin (conjugated estrogens, USP) with Meprobamate, USP] Tablets

Each oblong *green* tablet contains 0.45 mg Premarin and 200 mg meprobamate, in bottles of 60 (NDC 0046-0880-60).

PMB® 400 [Premarin (conjugated estrogens, USP) with Meprobamate, USP] Tablets

Each oblong *pink* tablet contains 0.45 mg Premarin and 400 mg meprobamate, in bottles of 60 (NDC 0046-0881-60).

The appearance of these tablets is a trademark of Wyeth-Ayerst Laboratories.

Store at room temperature (approximately 25°C).

Dispense in a well-closed container as defined in the USP.

PHYSICIAN REFERENCES

1. Ziel, H. K., *et al.*: N. Engl. J. Med. *293*:1167–1170, 1975.
2. Smith, D. C., *et al.*: N. Engl. J. Med. *293*:1164–1167, 1975.
3. Mack, T. M., *et al.*: N. Engl. J. Med. *294*:1262–1267, 1976.
4. Weiss, N. S., *et al.*: N. Engl. J. Med. *294*:1259–1262, 1976.
5. Herbst, A. L., *et al.*: N. Engl. J. Med. *284*:878–881, 1971.
6. Greenwald, P., *et al.*: N. Engl. J. Med. *285*:390–392, 1971.
7. Lanier, A., *et al.*: Mayo Clin. Proc. *48*:793–799, 1973.
8. Herbst, A., *et al.*: Obstet. Gynecol. *40*:287–298, 1972.
9. Herbst, A., *et al.*: Am. J. Obstet. Gynecol. *118*:607–615, 1974.
10. Herbst, A., *et al.*: N. Engl. J. Med. *292*:334–339, 1975.
11. Stafl, A., *et al.*: Obstet. Gynecol. *43*:118–128, 1974.
12. Sherman, A. I., *et al.*: Obstet. Gynecol. *44*:531–545, 1974.
13. Gal, I., *et al.*: Nature *216*:83, 1967.
14. Levy, E. P., *et al.*: Lancet *1*:611, 1973.
15. Nora, J., *et al.*: Lancet *1*:941–942, 1973.
16. Janerich, D. T., *et al.*: N. Engl. J. Med. *291*:697–700, 1974.
17. Boston Collaborative Drug Surveillance Program: N. Engl. J. Med. *290*:15–19, 1974.
18. Kaufman, D.W., *et al.*: J.A.M.A. 252:63–67, 1984.
19. Boston Collaborative Drug Surveillance Program: Lancet *1*:1399–1404, 1973.

20. Daniel, D. G., *et al.*: Lancet *2*:287–289, 1967.
21. The Veterans Administration Cooperative Urological Research Group: J. Urol. *98*:516–522, 1967.
22. Bailar, J. C.: Lancet *2*:560, 1967.
23. Blackard, C., *et al.*: Cancer *26*:249–256, 1970.
24. Royal College of General Practitioners: J. R. Coll. Gen. Pract. *13*:267–279, 1967.
24a. Royal College of General Practitioners: Oral Contraceptives and Health, New York, Pitman Corp., 1974.
25. Inman, W. H. W., *et al.*: Br. Med. J. *2*:193–199, 1968.
26. Vessey, M. P., *et al.*: Br. Med. J. *2*:651–657, 1969.
27. Sartwell, P. E., *et al.*: Am. J. Epidemiol. *90*:365–380, 1969.
28. Collaborative Group for the Study of Stroke in Young Women: N. Engl. J. Med. *288*:871–878, 1973.
29. Collaborative Group for the Study of Stroke in Young Women: J.A.M.A. *231*:718–722, 1975.
30. Mann, J. I., *et al.*: Br. Med. J. *2*:245–248, 1975.
31. Mann, J. I., *et al.*: Br. Med. J. *2*:241–245, 1975.
32. Inman, W. H. W., *et al.*: Br. Med. J. *2*:203–209, 1970.
33. Stolley, P. D., *et al.*: Am. J. Epidemiol. *102*:197–208, 1975.
34. Vessey, M. P., *et al.*: Br. Med. J. *3*:123–126, 1970.
35. Greene, G. R., *et al.*: Am. J. Public Health *62*:680–685, 1972.
36. Rosenberg, L., *et al.*: N. Engl. J. Med. *294*:1256–1259, 1976.
37. Coronary Drug Project Research Group: J.A.M.A. *214*:1303–1313, 1970.
38. Baum, J., *et al.*: Lancet *2*:926–928, 1973.
39. Mays, E. T., *et al.*: J.A.M.A. *235*:730–732, 1976.
40. Edmondson, H. A., *et al.*: N. Engl. J. Med. *294*:470–472, 1976.
41. Pfeffer, R. I., *et al.*: Am. J. Epidemiol. *103*:445–456, 1976.
42. Hoffman, A. J., *et al.*: J. Am. Pharm. Assoc. *48*:740, 1959.
43. Douglas, J. F., *et al.*: Anal. Chem. *39*:956, 1967.

INFORMATION FOR THE PATIENT

What You Should Know About Estrogens

Estrogens are female hormones produced by the ovaries. The ovaries make several different kinds of estrogens. In addition, scientists have been able to make a variety of synthetic estrogens. As far as we know, all these estrogens have similar properties and, therefore, much the same usefulness, side effects, and risks. This leaflet is intended to help you understand what estrogens are used for, the risks involved in their use, and how to use them as safely as possible.

This leaflet includes the most important information about estrogens, but not all the information. If you want to know more, you should ask your doctor for more information, or you can ask your doctor or pharmacist to let you read the package insert prepared for the doctor.

Uses of Estrogen

THERE IS NO PROPER USE OF ESTROGENS IN A PREGNANT WOMAN

Estrogens are prescribed by doctors for a number of purposes, including:

1. To provide estrogen during a period of adjustment when a woman's ovaries stop producing a majority of her estrogens, in order to prevent certain uncomfortable symptoms of estrogen deficiency. (With the menopause, which generally occurs between the ages of 45 and 55, women produce a much smaller amount of estrogens.)
2. To prevent symptoms of estrogen deficiency when a woman's ovaries have been removed surgically before the natural menopause.
3. To prevent pregnancy. (Estrogens are given along with a progestogen, another female hormone; these combinations are called oral contraceptives, or birth control pills. Patient labeling is available to women taking oral contraceptives and they will not be discussed in this leaflet.)
4. To treat certain cancers in women and men.

Estrogens in the Menopause

In the natural course of their lives, all women eventually experience a decrease in estrogen production. This usually occurs between ages 45 and 55, but may occur earlier or later. Sometimes the ovaries may need to be removed before natural menopause by an operation, producing a "surgical menopause."

When the amount of estrogen in the blood begins to decrease, many women may develop typical symptoms: feelings of warmth in the face, neck, and chest or sudden intense episodes of heat and sweating throughout the body (called "hot flashes" or "hot flushes"). These symptoms are sometimes very uncomfortable. Some women may also develop changes in the vagina (called "atrophic vaginitis") that cause discomfort, especially during and after intercourse.

Estrogens can be prescribed to treat these symptoms of the menopause. It is estimated that considerably more than half of all women undergoing the menopause have only mild symptoms or no symptoms at all and therefore do not need estrogens. Other women may need estrogens for a few months, while their bodies adjust to lower estrogen levels.

Sometimes the need will be for periods longer than six months. In an attempt to avoid overstimulation of the uterus (womb), estrogens are usually given cyclically during each month of use, such as three weeks of pills followed by one week without pills.

Sometimes women experience nervous symptoms or depression during menopause. There is no evidence that estrogens are effective for such symptoms without associated vasomotor symptoms. In the absence of vasomotor symptoms, estrogens should not be used to treat nervous symptoms, although other treatment may be needed.

You may have heard that taking estrogens for long periods (years) after the menopause will keep your skin soft and supple and keep you feeling young. There is no evidence that this is so, however, and such long-term treatment carries important risks.

The Dangers of Estrogens

1. *Endometrial cancer.* There are reports that if estrogens are used in the postmenopausal period for more than a year, there is an increased risk of *endometrial cancer* (cancer of the lining of the uterus). Women taking estrogens have roughly 5- to 10-times as great a chance of getting this cancer as women who take no estrogens. To put this another way, while a postmenopausal woman not taking estrogens has 1 chance in 1,000 each year of getting endometrial cancer, a woman taking estrogens has 5 to 10 chances in 1,000 each year. For this reason *it is important to take estrogens only when they are really needed.*

The risk of this cancer is greater the longer estrogens are used and when larger doses are taken. Therefore, you should not take more estrogen than your doctor prescribes. *It is important to take the lowest dose of estrogen that will control symptoms and to take it only as long as it is needed.* If estrogens are needed for longer periods of time, your doctor will want to re-evaluate your need for estrogens at least every six months.

Women using estrogens should report any vaginal bleeding to their doctors; such bleeding may be of no importance, but it can be an early warning of endometrial cancer. If you have undiagnosed vaginal bleeding, you should not use estrogens until a diagnosis is made and you are certain there is no endometrial cancer.

NOTE: If you have had your uterus removed (total hysterectomy), there is no danger of developing endometrial cancer.

2. *Other possible cancers.* Estrogens can cause development of other tumors in animals, such as tumors of the breast, cervix, vagina, or liver, when given for a long time. At present there is no good evidence that women using estrogen in the menopause have an increased risk of such tumors, but there is no way yet to be sure they do not; and one study raises the possibility that use of estrogens in the menopause may increase the risk of breast cancer many years later. This is a further reason to use estrogens only when clearly needed. While you are taking estrogens, it is important that you go to your doctor at least once a year for a physical examination. Also, if members of your family have had breast cancer or if you have breast nodules or abnormal mammograms (breast X rays), your doctor may wish to carry out more frequent examinations of your breasts.

3. *Gallbladder disease.* Women who use estrogens after menopause are more likely to develop gallbladder disease needing surgery then women who do not use estrogens. Birth control pills have a similar effect.

4. *Abnormal blood clotting.* Oral contraceptives increase the risk of blood clotting in various parts of the body. This can result in a stroke (if the clot is in the brain), a heart attack (clot in a blood vessel of the heart), or a pulmonary embolus (a clot which forms in the legs or pelvis, then breaks off and travels to the lungs). Any of these can be fatal.

At this time, use of estrogens in the menopause is not known to cause such blood clotting, but this has not been fully studied and there could still prove to be such a risk. It is recommended that if you have had clotting in the legs or lungs, or a heart attack or stroke while you were using estrogens or birth control pills, you should not use estrogens (unless they are being used to treat cancer of the breast or prostate). If you have had a stroke or heart attack, or if you have angina pectoris, estrogens should be used with great caution and only if clearly needed (for example, if you have severe symptoms of the menopause).

Special Warning About Pregnancy

You should not receive estrogen if you are pregnant. If this should occur, there is a greater than usual chance that the developing child will be born with a birth defect, although the possibility remains fairly small. A female child may have an increased risk of developing cancer of the vagina or cervix later in life (in the teens or twenties). Every possible effort should be made to avoid exposure to estrogens during pregnancy. If exposure occurs, see your doctor.

Other Effects of Estrogens

In addition to the serious known risks of estrogens described above, estrogens have the following side effects and potential risks:

1. *Nausea and vomiting.* The most common side effect of estrogen therapy is nausea. Vomiting is less common.
2. *Effects on breasts.* Estrogens may cause breast tenderness or enlargement and may cause the breasts to secrete a liquid. These effects are not dangerous.
3. *Effects on the uterus.* Estrogens may cause benign fibroid tumors of the uterus to get larger.
4. *Effects on liver.* Women taking oral contraceptives develop, on rare occasions, a tumor of the liver which can rupture and bleed into the abdomen and may cause death. So far, these tumors have not been reported in women using estrogens in the menopause, but you should report any swelling or unusual pain or tenderness in the abdomen to your doctor immediately.

Women with a past history of jaundice (yellowing of the skin and white parts of the eyes) may get jaundice again during estrogen use. If this occurs, stop taking estrogens and see your doctor.

5. *Other effects.* Estrogens may cause excess fluids to be retained in the body. This may make some conditions worse, such as asthma, epilepsy, migraine, heart disease, or kidney disease.

Summary

Estrogens have important uses, but they have serious risks as well. You must decide, with your doctor, whether the risks are acceptable to you in view of the benefits of treatment. Except where your doctor has prescribed estrogens for use in special cases of cancer of the breast or prostate, you should not use estrogens if you have cancer of the breast or uterus, are pregnant, have undiagnosed abnormal vaginal bleeding, clotting in the legs or lungs, or have had a stroke, heart attack or angina, or clotting in the legs or lungs in the past while you were taking estrogens.

You can use estrogens as safely as possible by understanding that your doctor will require regular physical examinations while you are taking them and will try to discontinue the drug as soon as possible and use the smallest dose possible. Be alert for signs of trouble including:

1. Abnormal bleeding from the vagina.
2. Pains in the calves or chest or sudden shortness of breath, or coughing blood.
3. Severe headache, dizziness, faintness, or changes in vision.
4. Breast lumps (you should ask your doctor how to examine your own breasts).
5. Jaundice (yellowing of the skin).
6. Mental depression.

Your doctor has prescribed this drug for you and you alone. Do not give the drug to anyone else.

Shown in Product Identification Guide, page 340

PREMARIN® INTRAVENOUS   ℞
[*prĕm 'a-rĭn*]
(conjugated estrogens, USP)
for Injection
Specially prepared for Intravenous &
Intramuscular use

Caution: Federal law prohibits dispensing without prescription.

---

1. ESTROGENS HAVE BEEN REPORTED TO INCREASE THE RISK OF ENDOMETRIAL CARCINOMA.

Three independent, case-controlled studies have reported an increased risk of endometrial cancer in postmenopausal women exposed to exogenous estrogens for more than one year.[1–3] This risk was independent of the other known risk factors for endometrial cancer. These studies are further supported by the finding that incidence rates of endometrial cancer have increased sharply since 1969 in eight different areas of the United States with population-based cancer-reporting systems, an increase which may be related to the rapidly expanding use of estrogens during the last decade.[4]

The three case-controlled studies reported that the risk of endometrial cancer in estrogen users was about 4.5 to 13.9 times greater than in nonusers. The risk appears to depend on both duration of treatment[1] and on estrogen dose.[3] In view of these findings, when estrogens are used for the treatment of menopausal symptoms, the lowest dose that will control symptoms should be utilized and medication should be discontinued as soon as possible. When prolonged treatment is medically indicated, the patient should be reassessed, on at least a semi-annual basis, to determine the need for continued therapy. Although the evidence must be considered preliminary, one study suggests that cyclic administration of low doses of estrogen may carry less risk than continuous administration.[3] It therefore appears prudent to utilize such a regimen.

Continued on next page

Wyeth-Ayerst Laboratories—Cont.

Close clinical surveillance of all women taking estrogens is important. In all cases of undiagnosed persistent or recurring abnormal vaginal bleeding, adequate diagnostic measures should be undertaken to rule out malignancy.

There is no evidence at present that "natural" estrogens are more or less hazardous than "synthetic" estrogens at equiestrogenic doses.

2. ESTROGENS SHOULD NOT BE USED DURING PREGNANCY.

The use of female sex hormones, both estrogens and progestogens, during early pregnancy may seriously damage the offspring. It has been shown that females exposed *in utero* to diethylstilbestrol, a nonsteroidal estrogen, have an increased risk of developing, in later life, a form of vaginal or cervical cancer that is ordinarily extremely rare.[5,6] This risk has been estimated as not greater than 4 per 1,000 exposures.[7] Furthermore, a high percentage of such exposed women (from 30% to 90%) have been found to have vaginal adenosis,[8-12] epithelial changes of the vagina and cervix. Although these changes are histologically benign, it is not known whether they are precursors of malignancy. Although similar data are not available with the use of other estrogens, it cannot be presumed they would not induce similar changes.

Several reports suggest an association between intrauterine exposure to female sex hormones and congenital anomalies, including congenital heart defects and limb-reduction defects.[13-16] One case-controlled study[16] estimated a 4.7-fold increased risk of limb-reduction defects in infants exposed *in utero* to sex hormones (oral contraceptives, hormone withdrawal tests for pregnancy, or attempted treatment for threatened abortion). Some of these exposures were very short and involved only a few days of treatment. The data suggest that the risk of limb-reduction defects in exposed fetuses is somewhat less than 1 per 1,000.

In the past, female sex hormones have been used during pregnancy in an attempt to treat threatened or habitual abortion. There is considerable evidence that estrogens are ineffective for these indications, and there is no evidence from well-controlled studies that progestogens are effective for these uses.

If Premarin Intravenous (conjugated estrogens, USP) for injection is used during pregnancy, or if the patient becomes pregnant while taking this drug, she should be apprised of the potential risks to the fetus, and the advisability of pregnancy continuation.

DESCRIPTION

Each Secule® vial contains 25 mg of conjugated estrogens, USP, in a sterile lyophilized cake which also contains lactose 200 mg, sodium citrate 12.2 mg, and simethicone 0.2 mg. The pH is adjusted with sodium hydroxide or hydrochloric acid. A sterile diluent (5 mL) containing 2% benzyl alcohol in sterile water is provided for reconstitution. The reconstituted solution is suitable for intravenous or intramuscular injection.

Premarin (conjugated estrogens, USP) is a mixture of estrogens obtained exclusively from natural sources, occurring as the sodium salts of water-soluble estrogen sulfates blended to represent the average composition of material derived from pregnant mares' urine. It contains estrone, equilin, and 17 α-dihydroequilin, together with smaller amounts of 17 α-estradiol, equilenin, and 17 α-dihydroequilenin as salts of their sulfate esters.

CLINICAL PHARMACOLOGY

Estrogens are important in the development and maintenance of the female reproductive system and secondary sex characteristics. They promote growth and development of the vagina, uterus, and fallopian tubes, and enlargement of the breasts. Indirectly, they contribute to the shaping of the skeleton, maintenance of tone and elasticity of urogenital structures, changes in the epiphyses of the long bones that allow for the pubertal growth spurt and its termination, growth of axillary and pubic hair, and pigmentation of the nipples and genitals. Decline of estrogenic activity at the end of the menstrual cycle can bring on menstruation, although the cessation of progesterone secretion is the most important factor in the mature ovulatory cycle. However, in the preovulatory or nonovulatory cycle, estrogen is the primary determinant in the onset of menstruation. Estrogens also affect the release of pituitary gonadotropins.

The pharmacologic effects of conjugated estrogens are similar to those of endogenous estrogens. They are soluble in water and may be administered by intravenous or intramuscular injection.

In responsive tissues (female genital organs, breasts, hypothalamus, pituitary) estrogens enter the cell and are transported into the nucleus. As a result of estrogen action, specific RNA and protein synthesis occurs.

Metabolism and inactivation occur primarily in the liver. Some estrogens are excreted into the bile; however, they are reabsorbed from the intestine and returned to the liver through the portal venous system. Water-soluble estrogen conjugates are strongly acidic and, therefore, ionized in body fluids, which favor excretion through the kidneys since tubular reabsorption is minimal.

INDICATION

Premarin Intravenous (conjugated estrogens, USP) for injection is indicated in the treatment of abnormal uterine bleeding due to hormonal imbalance in the absence of organic pathology.

CONTRAINDICATIONS

Estrogens should not be used in women with any of the following conditions:

1. Known or suspected cancer of the breast, except in appropriately selected patients being treated for metastatic disease.
2. Known or suspected estrogen-dependent neoplasia.
3. Known or suspected pregnancy (see Boxed Warning).
4. Undiagnosed abnormal genital bleeding.
5. Active thrombophlebitis or thromboembolic disorders.
6. A past history of thrombophlebitis, thrombosis, or thromboembolic disorders associated with previous estrogen use (except when used in treatment of breast malignancy).

WARNINGS

1. *Induction of malignant neoplasms.* Long-term, continuous administration of natural and synthetic estrogens in certain animal species increases the frequency of carcinomas of the breast, cervix, vagina, and liver. There are now reports that estrogens increase the risk of carcinoma of the endometrium in humans (see Boxed Warning).

At the present time there is no satisfactory evidence that estrogens given to postmenopausal women increase the risk of cancer of the breast,[17] although a recent long-term follow-up of a single physician's practice has raised this possibility.[18] Because of the animal data, there is a need for caution in prescribing estrogens for women with a strong family history of breast cancer, or who have breast nodules, fibrocystic disease, or abnormal mammograms.

2. *Gallbladder disease.* A recent study has reported a 2- to 3-fold increase in the risk of surgically confirmed gallbladder disease in women receiving postmenopausal estrogens,[17] similar to the 2-fold increase previously noted in users of oral contraceptives.[19,24a]

3. *Effects similar to those caused by estrogen-progestogen oral contraceptives.* There are several serious adverse effects of oral contraceptives, most of which have not, up to now, been documented as consequences of postmenopausal estrogen therapy. This may reflect the comparatively low doses of estrogen used in postmenopausal women. It would be expected that the larger doses of estrogen used to treat prostatic or breast cancer are more likely to result in these adverse effects, and, in fact, it has been shown that there is an increased risk of thrombosis in men receiving estrogens for prostatic cancer.[20-23]

a. *Thromboembolic disease.* It is now well established that users of oral contraceptives have an increased risk of various thromboembolic and thrombotic vascular diseases, such as thrombophlebitis, pulmonary embolism, stroke, and myocardial infarction.[24-31] Cases of retinal thrombosis, mesenteric thrombosis, and optic neuritis have been reported in oral-contraceptive users. There is evidence that the risk of several of these adverse reactions is related to the dose of the drug.[32,33] An increased risk of postsurgery thromboembolic complications has also been reported in users of oral contraceptives.[34,35] If feasible, estrogen should be discontinued at least 4 weeks before surgery of the type associated with an increased risk of thromboembolism, or during periods of prolonged immobilization.

While an increased rate of thromboembolic and thrombotic disease in postmenopausal users of estrogens has not been found,[17-24,25-36] this does not rule out the possibility that such an increase may be present, or that subgroups of women who have underlying risk factors, or who are receiving relatively large doses of estrogens, may have increased risk. Therefore estrogens should not be used in persons with active thrombophlebitis or thromboembolic disorders, and they should not be used (except in treatment of malignancy) in persons with a history of such disorders in association with estrogen use. They should be used with caution in patients with cerebral vascular or coronary artery disease and only for those in whom estrogens are clearly needed.

Large doses of estrogen (5 mg conjugated estrogens per day), comparable to those used to treat cancer of the prostate and breast, have been shown in a large prospective clinical trial in men[37] to increase the risk of nonfatal myocardial infarction, pulmonary embolism, and thrombophlebitis. When estrogen doses of this size are used, any of the thromboembolic and thrombotic adverse effects associated with oral-contraceptive use should be considered a clear risk.

b. *Hepatic adenoma.* Benign hepatic adenomas appear to be associated with the use of oral contraceptives.[38-40] Although benign, and rare, these may rupture and may cause death through intra-abdominal hemorrhage. Such lesions have not yet been reported in association with other estrogen or progestogen preparations but should be considered in estrogen users having abdominal pain and tenderness, abdominal mass, or hypovolemic shock. Hepatocellular carcinoma has also been reported in women taking estrogen-containing oral contraceptives.[39] The relationship of this malignancy to these drugs is not known at this time.

c. *Elevated blood pressure.* Women using oral contraceptives sometimes experience increased blood pressure which, in most cases, returns to normal on discontinuing the drug. There is now a report that this may occur with use of estrogens in the menopause[41] and blood pressure should be monitored with estrogen use, especially if high doses are used.

d. *Glucose tolerance.* A worsening of glucose tolerance has been observed in a significant percentage of patients on estrogen-containing oral contraceptives. For this reason, diabetic patients should be carefully observed while receiving estrogen.

4. *Hypercalcemia.* Administration of estrogens may lead to severe hypercalcemia in patients with breast cancer and bone metastases. If this occurs, the drug should be stopped and appropriate measures taken to reduce the serum calcium level.

PRECAUTIONS

A. GENERAL PRECAUTIONS

1. A complete medical and family history should be taken prior to the initiation of any estrogen therapy. The pretreatment and periodic physical examinations should include special reference to blood pressure, breasts, abdomen, and pelvic organs, and should include a Papanicolaou smear. As a general rule, estrogen should not be prescribed for longer than one year without another physical examination being performed.

2. Fluid retention—Because estrogens may cause some degree of fluid retention, conditions which might be influenced by this factor such as asthma, epilepsy, migraine, and cardiac or renal dysfunction, require careful observation.

3. Certain patients may develop undesirable manifestations of excessive estrogenic stimulation, such as abnormal or excessive uterine bleeding, mastodynia, etc.

4. Oral contraceptives appear to be associated with an increased incidence of mental depression.[24a] Although it is not clear whether this is due to the estrogenic or progestogenic component of the contraceptive, patients with a history of depression should be carefully observed.

5. Preexisting uterine leiomyomata may increase in size during estrogen use.

6. The pathologist should be advised of estrogen therapy when relevant specimens are submitted.

7. Patients with a past history of jaundice during pregnancy have an increased risk of recurrence of jaundice while receiving estrogen-containing oral contraceptive therapy. If jaundice develops in any patient receiving estrogen, the medication should be discontinued while the cause is investigated.

8. Estrogens may be poorly metabolized in patients with impaired liver function and they should be administered with caution in such patients.

9. Because estrogens influence the metabolism of calcium and phosphorus, they should be used with caution in patients with metabolic bone diseases that are associated with hypercalcemia or in patients with renal insufficiency.

10. Because of the effects of estrogens on epiphyseal closure, they should be used judiciously in young patients in whom bone growth is not yet complete.

11. Certain endocrine and liver function tests may be affected by estrogen-containing oral contraceptives. The following similar changes may be expected with larger doses of estrogen:

a. Increased sulfobromophthalein retention.
b. Increased prothrombin and factors VII, VIII, IX, and X; decreased antithrombin 3; increased norepinephrine-induced platelet aggregability.
c. Increased thyroid binding globulin (TBG) leading to increased circulating total thyroid hormone, as measured by PBI, T4 by column, or T4 by radioimmunoassay. Free T3 resin uptake is decreased, reflecting the elevated TBG; free T4 concentration is unaltered.
d. Impaired glucose tolerance.
e. Decreased pregnanediol excretion.
f. Reduced response to metyrapone test.
g. Reduced serum folate concentration.
h. Increased serum triglyceride and phospholipid concentration.

B. INFORMATION FOR THE PATIENT

See text which appears after the PHYSICIAN REFERENCES.

C. PREGNANCY CATEGORY X
See CONTRAINDICATIONS and Boxed Warning.
D. NURSING MOTHERS
As a general principle, the administration of any drug to nursing mothers should be done only when clearly necessary, since many drugs are excreted in human milk.

ADVERSE REACTIONS

(See WARNINGS regarding induction of neoplasia, adverse effects on the fetus, increased incidence of gallbladder disease, and adverse effects similar to those of oral contraceptives, including thromboembolism.) The following additional adverse reactions have been reported with estrogenic therapy, including oral contraceptives:
1. *Genitourinary system:* Breakthrough bleeding, spotting, change in menstrual flow; dysmenorrhea; premenstrual-like syndrome; amenorrhea during and after treatment; increase in size of uterine fibromyomata; vaginal candidiasis; change in cervical erosion and in degree of cervical secretion; cystitis-like syndrome.
2. *Breasts:* Tenderness, enlargement, secretion.
3. *Gastrointestinal:* Nausea, vomiting; abdominal cramps, bloating; cholestatic jaundice.
4. *Skin:* Chloasma or melasma which may persist when drug is discontinued; erythema multiforme; erythema nodosum; hemorrhagic eruption; loss of scalp hair; hirsutism.
5. *Eyes:* Steepening of corneal curvature; intolerance to contact lenses.
6. *CNS:* Headache, migraine, dizziness; mental depression; chorea.
7. *Miscellaneous:* Increase or decrease in weight; reduced carbohydrate tolerance; aggravation of porphyria; edema; changes in libido.

ACUTE OVERDOSAGE

Numerous reports of ingestion of large doses of estrogen-containing oral contraceptives by young children indicate that acute serious ill effects do not occur. Overdosage of estrogen may cause nausea, and withdrawal bleeding may occur in females.

DOSAGE AND ADMINISTRATION

Abnormal uterine bleeding due to hormonal imbalance: One 25 mg injection, intravenously or intramuscularly. Intravenous use is preferred since more rapid response can be expected from this mode of administration.
Repeat in 6 to 12 hours if necessary. The use of Premarin Intravenous (conjugated estrogens, USP) for injection does not preclude the advisability of other appropriate measures. The usual precautionary measures governing intravenous administration should be adhered to. Injection should be made SLOWLY to obviate the occurrence of flushes.
Infusion of Premarin Intravenous (conjugated estrogens, USP) for injection with other agents is not generally recommended. In emergencies, however, when an infusion has already been started it may be expedient to make the injection into the tubing just distal to the infusion needle. If so used, compatibility of solutions must be considered.
Compatibility of solutions: Premarin Intravenous is compatible with normal saline, dextrose, and invert sugar solutions. IT IS NOT COMPATIBLE WITH PROTEIN HYDROLYSATE, ASCORBIC ACID, OR ANY SOLUTION WITH AN ACID pH.
Treated patients with an intact uterus should be monitored closely for signs of endometrial cancer, and appropriate diagnostic measures should be taken to rule out malignancy in the event of persistent or recurring abnormal vaginal bleeding.

Directions For Storage and Reconstitution

Storage before reconstitution: Store package in refrigerator, 2°–8°C (36°–46°F).
To reconstitute: First withdraw air from Secule® vial so as to facilitate introduction of sterile diluent. Then, flow the sterile diluent slowly against side of Secule® vial and agitate gently. DO NOT SHAKE VIOLENTLY.
Storage after reconstitution: It is common practice to utilize the reconstituted solution within a few hours. If it is necessary to keep the reconstituted solution for more than a few hours, store the reconstituted solution under refrigeration (2°–8°C). Under these conditions, the solution is stable for 60 days, and is suitable for use unless darkening or precipitation occurs.

HOW SUPPLIED

NDC 0046-0749-05—Each package provides: (1) One Secule® vial containing 25 mg of conjugated estrogens, USP, for injection (also lactose 200 mg, sodium citrate 12.2 mg, and simethicone 0.2 mg). The pH is adjusted with sodium hydroxide or hydrochloric acid. (2) One 5 mL ampul sterile diluent with 2% benzyl alcohol in sterile water. Premarin Intravenous (conjugated estrogens, USP) for injection is prepared by cryodesiccation.
SECULE®—Registered trademark to designate a vial containing an injectable preparation in dry form.

PHYSICIAN REFERENCES

1. Ziel, H. K., *et al.*: N. Engl. J. Med. *293* :1167–1170, 1975.
2. Smith, D. C., *et al.*: N. Engl. J. Med. *293* :1164–1167, 1975.
3. Mack, T. M., *et al.*: N. Engl. J. Med. *294* :1262–1267, 1976.
4. Weiss, N. S., *et al.*: N. Engl. J. Med. *294* :1259–1262, 1976.
5. Herbst, A. L., *et al.*: N. Engl. J. Med. *284* :878–881, 1971.
6. Greenwald, P., *et al.*: N. Engl. J. Med. *285* :390–392, 1971.
7. Lanier, A., *et al.*: Mayo Clin. Proc. *48* :793–799, 1973.
8. Herbst, A., *et al.*: Obstet. Gynecol. *40* :287–298, 1972.
9. Herbst, A., *et al.*: Am. J. Obstet. Gynecol. *118* :607–615, 1974.
10. Herbst, A., *et al.*: N. Engl. J. Med. *292* :334–339, 1975.
11. Stafl, A., *et al.*: Obstet. Gynecol. *43* :118–128, 1974.
12. Sherman, A. I., *et al.*: Obstet. Gynecol. *44* :531–545, 1974.
13. Gal, I., *et al.*: Nature *216* :83, 1967.
14. Levy, E. P., *et al.*: Lancet *1* :611, 1973.
15. Nora, J., *et al.*: Lancet *1* :941–942, 1973.
16. Janerich, D. T., *et al.*: N. Engl. J. Med. *291* :697–700, 1974.
17. Boston Collaborative Drug Surveillance Program: N. Engl. J. Med. *290* :15–19, 1974.
18. Hoover, R., *et al.*: N. Engl. J. Med. *295* :401–405, 1976.
19. Boston Collaborative Drug Surveillance Program: Lancet *1* :1399–1404, 1973.
20. Daniel, D. G., *et al.*: Lancet *2* :287–289, 1967.
21. The Veterans Administration Cooperative Urological Research Group: J. Urol. *98* :516–522, 1967.
22. Bailar, J. C.: Lancet *2* :560, 1967.
23. Blackard, C., *et al.*: Cancer *26* :249–256, 1970.
24. Royal College of General Practitioners: J. R. Coll. Gen. Pract. *13* :267–279, 1967.
24a. Royal College of General Practitioners: Oral Contraceptives and Health, New York, Pitman Corp., 1974.
25. Inman, W. H. W., *et al.*: Br. Med. J. *2* :193–199, 1968.
26. Vessey, M. P., *et al.*: Br. Med. J. *2* :651–657, 1969.
27. Sartwell, P. E., *et al.*: Am. J. Epidemiol. *90* :365–380, 1969.
28. Collaborative Group for the Study of Stroke in Young Women: N. Engl. J. Med. *288* :871–878, 1973.
29. Collaborative Group for the Study of Stroke in Young Women: J.A.M.A. *231* :718–722, 1975.
30. Mann, J. I., *et al.*: Br. Med. J. *2* :245–248, 1975.
31. Mann, J. I., *et al.*: Br. Med. J. *2* :241–245, 1975.
32. Inman, W. H. W., *et al.*: Br. Med. J. *2* :203–209, 1970.
33. Stolley, P. D., *et al.*: Am. J. Epidemiol. *102* :197–208, 1975.
34. Vessey, M. P., *et al.*: Br. Med. J. *3* :123–126, 1970.
35. Greene, G. R., *et al.*: Am. J. Public Health *62* :680–685, 1972.
36. Rosenberg, L., *et al.*: N. Engl. J. Med. *294* :1256–1259, 1976.
37. Coronary Drug Project Research Group: J.A.M.A. *214* :1303–1313, 1970.
38. Baum, J., *et al.*: Lancet *2* :926–928, 1973.
39. Mays, E. T., *et al.*: J.A.M.A. *235* :730–732, 1976.
40. Edmondson, H. A., *et al.*: N. Engl. J. Med. *294* :470–472, 1976.
41. Pfeffer, R. I., *et al.*: Am. J. Epidemiol. *103* :445–456, 1976.

INFORMATION FOR THE PATIENT

What You Should Know About Estrogens

Estrogens are female hormones produced by the ovaries. The ovaries make several different kinds of estrogens. In addition, scientists have been able to make a variety of synthetic estrogens. As far as we know, all these estrogens have similar properties and, therefore, much the same usefulness, side effects, and risks. This leaflet is intended to help you understand what estrogens are used for, the risks involved in their use, and how to use them as safely as possible.
This leaflet includes the most important information about estrogens, but not all the information. If you want to know more, you should ask your doctor for more information, or you can ask your doctor or pharmacist to let you read the package insert prepared for the doctor.

Uses of Estrogen

THERE IS NO PROPER USE OF ESTROGENS IN A PREGNANT WOMAN: Estrogens are prescribed by doctors for a number of purposes, including:
1. To provide estrogen during a period of adjustment when a woman's ovaries stop producing a majority of her estrogens, in order to prevent certain uncomfortable symptoms of estrogen deficiency. (With the menopause, which generally occurs between the ages of 45 and 55, women produce a much smaller amount of estrogens.)
2. To prevent symptoms of estrogen deficiency when a woman's ovaries have been removed surgically before the natural menopause.
3. To prevent pregnancy. (Estrogens are given along with a progestogen, another female hormone; these combinations are called oral contraceptives, or birth-control pills. Patient labeling is available to women taking oral contraceptives and they will not be discussed in this leaflet.)
4. To treat certain cancers in women and men.

Estrogens in the Menopause

In the natural course of their lives, all women eventually experience a decrease in estrogen production. This usually occurs between ages 45 and 55, but may occur earlier or later. Sometimes the ovaries may need to be removed before natural menopause by an operation, producing a "surgical menopause."
When the amount of estrogen in the blood begins to decrease, many women may develop typical symptoms: feelings of warmth in the face, neck, and chest, or sudden intense episodes of heat and sweating throughout the body (called "hot flashes" or "hot flushes"). These symptoms are sometimes very uncomfortable. Some women may also develop changes in the vagina (called "atrophic vaginitis") that cause discomfort, especially during and after intercourse.
Estrogens can be prescribed to treat these symptoms of the menopause. It is estimated that considerably more than half of all women undergoing the menopause have only mild symptoms or no symptoms at all and, therefore, do not need estrogens. Other women may need estrogens for a few months, while their bodies adjust to lower estrogen levels. Sometimes the need will be for periods longer than six months. In an attempt to avoid overstimulation of the uterus (womb), estrogens are usually given cyclically during each month of use, such as three weeks of pills followed by one week without pills.
Sometimes women experience nervous symptoms or depression during menopause. There is no evidence that estrogens are effective for such symptoms without associated vasomotor symptoms. In the absence of vasomotor symptoms, estrogens should not be used to treat nervous symptoms, although other treatment may be needed.
You may have heard that taking estrogens for long periods (years) after the menopause will keep your skin soft and supple and keep you feeling young. There is no evidence that this is so, however, and such long-term treatment carries important risks.

The Dangers of Estrogens

1. *Endometrial cancer.* There are reports that if estrogens are used in the postmenopausal period for more than a year, there is an increased risk of *endometrial cancer* (cancer of the lining of the uterus). Women taking estrogens have roughly 5- to 10-times as great a chance of getting this cancer as women who take no estrogens. To put this another way, while a postmenopausal woman not taking estrogens has 1 chance in 1,000 each year of getting endometrial cancer, a woman taking estrogens has 5 to 10 chances in 1,000 each year. For this reason *it is important to take estrogens only when they are really needed.*
The risk of this cancer is greater the longer estrogens are used and when larger doses are taken. Therefore, you should not take more estrogen than your doctor prescribes. *It is important to take the lowest dose of estrogen that will control symptoms and to take it only as long as it is needed.* If estrogens are needed for longer periods of time, your doctor will want to reevaluate your need for estrogens at least every six months.
Women using estrogens should report any vaginal bleeding to their doctors; such bleeding may be of no importance, but it can be an early warning of endometrial cancer. If you have undiagnosed vaginal bleeding, you should not use estrogens until a diagnosis is made and you are certain there is no endometrial cancer.
Note: If you have had your uterus removed (total hysterectomy), there is no danger of developing endometrial cancer.
2. *Other possible cancers.* Estrogens can cause development of other tumors in animals, such as tumors of the breast, cervix, vagina, or liver, when given for a long time. At present there is no good evidence that women using estrogen in the menopause have an increased risk of such tumors, but there is no way yet to be sure they do not; and one study raises the possibility that use of estrogens in the menopause may increase the risk of breast cancer many years later. This is a further reason to use estrogens only when clearly needed. While you are taking estrogens, it is important that you go to your doctor at least once a year for a physical examination. Also, if members of your family have had breast cancers, or if you have breast nodules, or abnormal mammograms (breast X rays), your doctor may wish to carry out more frequent examinations of your breasts.
3. *Gallbladder disease.* Women who use estrogens after menopause are more likely to develop gallbladder disease needing surgery than women who do not use estrogens. Birth-control pills have a similar effect.
4. *Abnormal blood clotting.* Oral contraceptives increase the risk of blood clotting in various parts of the body. This can result in a stroke (if the clot is in the brain), a heart attack (a clot in a blood vessel of the heart), or a pulmonary

Continued on next page

Wyeth-Ayerst Laboratories—Cont.

embolus (a clot which forms in the legs or pelvis, then breaks off and travels to the lungs). Any of these can be fatal.

At this time, use of estrogens in the menopause is not known to cause such blood clotting, but this has not been fully studied and there could still prove to be such a risk. It is recommended that if you have had clotting in the legs or lungs, or a heart attack or stroke, while you were using estrogens or birth-control pills, you should not use estrogens (unless they are being used to treat cancer of the breast or prostate). If you have had a stroke or heart attack, or if you have angina pectoris, estrogens should be used with great caution and only if clearly needed (for example, if you have severe symptoms of the menopause).

Special Warning About Pregnancy

You should not receive estrogen if you are pregnant. If this should occur, there is a greater than usual chance that the developing child will be born with a birth defect, although the possibility remains fairly small. A female child may have an increased risk of developing cancer of the vagina or cervix later in life (in the teens or twenties). Every possible effort should be made to avoid exposure to estrogens during pregnancy. If exposure occurs, see your doctor.

Other Effects of Estrogens

In addition to the serious known risks of estrogens described above, estrogens have the following side effects and potential risks:

1. *Nausea and vomiting.* The most common side effect of estrogen therapy is nausea. Vomiting is less common.
2. *Effects on breasts.* Estrogens may cause breast tenderness or enlargement and may cause the breasts to secrete a liquid. These effects are not dangerous.
3. *Effects on the uterus.* Estrogens may cause benign fibroid tumors of the uterus to get larger.
4. *Effects on liver.* Women taking oral contraceptives develop, on rare occasions, a tumor of the liver which can rupture and bleed into the abdomen and may cause death. So far, these tumors have not been reported in women using estrogens in the menopause, but you should report any swelling or unusual pain or tenderness in the abdomen to your doctor immediately.

Women with a past history of jaundice (yellowing of the skin and white parts of the eyes) may get jaundice again during estrogen use. If this occurs, stop taking estrogens and see your doctor.

5. *Other effects.* Estrogens may cause excess fluid to be retained in the body. This may make some conditions worse, such as asthma, epilepsy, migraine, heart disease, or kidney disease.

Summary

Estrogens have important uses, but they have serious risks as well. You must decide, with your doctor, whether the risks are acceptable to you in view of the benefits of treatment. Except where your doctor has prescribed estrogens for use in special cases of cancer of the breast or prostate, you should not use estrogens if you have cancer of the breast or uterus, are pregnant, have undiagnosed abnormal vaginal bleeding, clotting in the legs or lungs, or have had a stroke, heart attack or angina, or clotting in the legs or lungs in the past while you were taking estrogens.

You can use estrogens as safely as possible by understanding that your doctor will require regular physical examinations while you are taking them, will try to discontinue the drug as soon as possible, and use the smallest dose possible. Be alert for signs of trouble including:

1. Abnormal bleeding from the vagina.
2. Pains in the calves or chest, or sudden shortness of breath, or coughing blood.
3. Severe headache, dizziness, faintness, or changes in vision.
4. Breast lumps (you should ask your doctor how to examine your own breasts).
5. Jaundice (yellowing of the skin).
6. Mental depression.

Your doctor has prescribed this drug for you and you alone. Do not give the drug to anyone else.

HOW SUPPLIED

Premarin® (conjugated estrogens tablets, USP) tablets for oral administration.

Premarin® Vaginal Cream—Premarin® in a nonliquefying base, designed for vaginal use.

Premarin® with Methyltestosterone—a combination of Premarin® and methyltestosterone (an androgen) in tablet form for oral administration.

PMB® 200, 400—a combination of Premarin® and meprobamate (a tranquilizing agent) in tablet form for oral administration.

Premarin® Intravenous—Premarin® specially prepared for intravenous and intramuscular use.

PREMARIN®
[prĕm 'a-rĭn]
(conjugated estrogens tablets, USP)

℞

Caution: Federal law prohibits dispensing without prescription.

---

1. **ESTROGENS HAVE BEEN REPORTED TO INCREASE THE RISK OF ENDOMETRIAL CARCINOMA IN POSTMENOPAUSAL WOMEN.**

Close clinical surveillance of all women taking estrogens is important. Adequate diagnostic measures, including endometrial sampling when indicated, should be undertaken to rule out malignancy in all cases of undiagnosed persistent or recurring abnormal vaginal bleeding. There is currently no evidence that "natural" estrogens are more or less hazardous than "synthetic" estrogens at equiestrogenic doses.

2. **ESTROGENS SHOULD NOT BE USED DURING PREGNANCY.**

Estrogen therapy during pregnancy is associated with an increased risk of congenital defects in the reproductive organs of the male and female fetus, an increased risk of vaginal adenosis, squamous cell dysplasia of the uterine cervix, and vaginal cancer in the female later in life. The 1985 DES Task Force concluded that women who used DES during their pregnancies may subsequently experience an increased risk of breast cancer. However, a causal relationship is still unproven, and the observed level of risk is similar to that for a number of other breast-cancer risk factors.

There is no indication for estrogen therapy during pregnancy. Estrogens are ineffective for the prevention or treatment of threatened or habitual abortion.

DESCRIPTION

Premarin (conjugated estrogens tablets, USP) for oral administration contains a mixture of estrogens obtained exclusively from natural sources, occurring as the sodium salts of water-soluble estrogen sulfates blended to represent the average composition of material derived from pregnant mares' urine. It contains estrone, equilin, and 17 α-dihydroequilin, together with smaller amounts of 17 α-estradiol, equilenin, and 17 α-dihydroequilenin as salts of their sulfate esters. Tablets for oral administration are available in 0.3 mg, 0.625 mg, 0.9 mg, 1.25 mg, and 2.5 mg strengths of conjugated estrogens.

Premarin Tablets contain the following inactive ingredients: calcium phosphate tribasic, calcium sulfate, carnauba wax, cellulose, glyceryl monooleate, lactose, magnesium stearate, methylcellulose, pharmaceutical glaze, polyethylene glycol, stearic acid, sucrose, titanium dioxide.

—0.3 mg tablets also contain: D&C Yellow No. 10, FD&C Blue No. 1, FD&C Blue No. 2, FD&C Yellow No. 6, talc;
—0.625 mg tablets also contain: FD&C Blue No. 2, D&C Red No. 27, FD&C Red No. 40;
—0.9 mg tablets also contain: D&C Red No. 6, D&C Red No. 7, talc;
—1.25 mg tablets also contain: black iron oxide, D&C Yellow No. 10, FD&C Yellow No. 6, talc;
—2.5 mg tablets also contain: FD&C Blue No. 2, D&C Red No. 7, talc.

CLINICAL PHARMACOLOGY

Estrogens are important in the development and maintenance of the female reproductive system and secondary sex characteristics. They promote growth and development of the vagina, uterus, and fallopian tubes, and enlargement of the breasts. Indirectly, they contribute to the shaping of the skeleton, maintenance of tone and elasticity of urogenital structures, changes in the epiphyses of the long bones that allow for the pubertal growth spurt and its termination, growth of axillary and pubic hair, and pigmentation of the nipples and genitals. Decline of estrogenic activity at the end of the menstrual cycle can bring on menstruation, although the cessation of progesterone secretion is the most important factor in the mature ovulatory cycle. However, in the preovulatory or nonovulatory cycle, estrogen is the primary determinant in the onset of menstruation. Estrogens also affect the release of pituitary gonadotropins.

The pharmacologic effects of conjugated estrogens are similar to those of endogenous estrogens. They are soluble in water and are well absorbed from the gastrointestinal tract. In responsive tissues (female genital organs, breasts, hypothalamus, pituitary) estrogens enter the cell and are transported into the nucleus. As a result of estrogen action, specific RNA and protein synthesis occurs.

Metabolism and inactivation occur primarily in the liver. Some estrogens are excreted into the bile; however, they are reabsorbed from the intestine and returned to the liver through the portal venous system. Water-soluble estrogen conjugates are strongly acidic and are ionized in body fluids,

which favor excretion through the kidneys since tubular reabsorption is minimal.

INDICATIONS AND USAGE

Premarin (conjugated estrogens tablets, USP) is indicated in the treatment of:

1. Moderate to severe vasomotor symptoms associated with the menopause. There is no adequate evidence that estrogens are effective for nervous symptoms or depression which might occur during menopause and they should not be used to treat these conditions.
2. Atrophic vaginitis.
3. Osteoporosis (loss of bone mass). The mainstays of prevention and management of osteoporosis are estrogen and calcium; exercise and nutrition may be important adjuncts. Estrogen replacement therapy is the most effective single modality for the prevention of osteoporosis in women. Estrogen reduces bone resorption and retards or halts postmenopausal bone loss. Case-controlled studies have shown an approximately 60-percent reduction in hip and wrist fractures in women whose estrogen replacement was begun within a few years of menopause. Studies also suggest that estrogen reduces the rate of vertebral fractures. Even when started as late as 6 years after menopause, estrogen prevents further loss of bone mass but does not restore it to premenopausal levels. The lowest effective dose for prevention and treatment of osteoporosis should be utilized. (See "DOSAGE AND ADMINISTRATION.")

Women are at higher risk than men because they have less bone mass, and for several years following natural or induced menopause, the rate of bone mass decline is accelerated. Early menopause is one of the strongest predictors for the development of osteoporosis. White women are at higher risk than black women, and white men are at higher risk than black men. Women who are underweight also have osteoporosis more often than overweight women. Cigarette smoking may be an additional factor in increasing risk. Calcium deficiency has been implicated in the pathogenesis of the disease. Therefore, when not contraindicated, it is recommended that postmenopausal women receive an elemental calcium intake of 1000 to 1500 mg/day.

Immobilization and prolonged bed rest produce rapid bone loss, while weight-bearing exercise has been shown both to reduce bone loss and to increase bone mass. The optimal type and amount of physical activity that would prevent osteoporosis have not been established.

4. Hypoestrogenism due to hypogonadism, castration, or primary ovarian failure.
5. Breast cancer (for palliation only) in appropriately selected women and men with metastatic disease.
6. Advanced androgen-dependent carcinoma of the prostate (for palliation only).

CONTRAINDICATIONS

Estrogens should not be used in women (or men) with any of the following conditions:

1. Known or suspected pregnancy (see Boxed Warning). Estrogen may cause fetal harm when administered to a pregnant woman.
2. Known or suspected cancer of the breast except in appropriately selected patients being treated for metastatic disease.
3. Known or suspected estrogen-dependent neoplasia.
4. Undiagnosed abnormal genital bleeding.
5. Active thrombophlebitis or thromboembolic disorders.
6. Women on estrogen replacement therapy have not been reported to have an increased risk of thrombophlebitis and/or thromboembolic disease. However, there is insufficient information regarding women who have had previous thromboembolic disease.

Premarin Tablets should not be used in patients hypersensitive to their ingredients.

WARNINGS

1. *Induction of malignant neoplasms.* Some studies have suggested a possible increased incidence of breast cancer in those women on estrogen therapy taking higher doses for prolonged periods of time. The majority of studies, however, have not shown an association with the usual doses used for estrogen replacement therapy. Women on this therapy should have regular breast examinations and should be instructed in breast self-examination. The reported endometrial cancer risk among estrogen users was about 4-fold or greater than in nonusers and appears dependent on duration of treatment and on estrogen dose. There is no significant increased risk associated with the use of estrogens for less than one year. The greatest risk appears associated with prolonged use—five years or more. In one study, persistence of risk was demonstrated for 10 years after cessation of estrogen treatment. In another study, a significant decrease in the incidence of endometrial cancer occurred six months after estrogen withdrawal.

Estrogen therapy during pregnancy is associated with an increased risk of fetal congenital reproductive-tract disorders. In females there is an increased risk of vaginal adenosis, squamous-cell dysplasia of the cervix, and cancer later in life; in the male, urogenital abnormalities. Although some of

these changes are benign, it is not known whether they are precursors of malignancy.

2. *Gallbladder disease.* A recent study has reported a 2.5-fold increase in the risk of surgically confirmed gallbladder disease in women receiving postmenopausal estrogens.

3. *Cardiovascular disease.* Large doses of estrogen (5 mg conjugated estrogens per day), comparable to those used to treat cancer of the prostate and breast, have been shown in a large prospective clinical trial in men to increase the risk of nonfatal myocardial infarction, pulmonary embolism, and thrombophlebitis. It cannot necessarily be extrapolated from men to women. However, to avoid the theoretical cardiovascular risk caused by high estrogen doses, the doses for estrogen replacement therapy should not exceed the recommended dose.

4. *Elevated blood pressure.* There is no evidence that this may occur with use of estrogens in the menopause. However, blood pressure should be monitored with estrogen use, especially if high doses are used.

5. *Hypercalcemia.* Administration of estrogens may lead to severe hypercalcemia in patients with breast cancer and bone metastases. If this occurs, the drug should be stopped and appropriate measures taken to reduce the serum calcium level.

PRECAUTIONS

A. GENERAL

1. *Addition of a progestin.* Studies of the addition of a progestin for seven or more days of a cycle of estrogen administration have reported a lowered incidence of endometrial hyperplasia. Morphological and biochemical studies of endometrium suggest that 10 to 13 days of progestin are needed to provide maximal maturation of the endometrium and to eliminate any hyperplastic changes. Whether this will provide protection from endometrial carcinoma has not been clearly established. There are possible additional risks which may be associated with the inclusion of progestin in estrogen replacement regimens. The potential risks include adverse effects on carbohydrate and lipid metabolism. The choice of progestin and dosage may be important in minimizing these adverse effects.

2. *Physical examination.* A complete medical and family history should be taken prior to the initiation of any estrogen therapy. The pretreatment and periodic physical examinations should include special reference to blood pressure, breasts, abdomen, and pelvic organs, and should include a Papanicolaou smear. As a general rule, estrogen should not be prescribed for longer than one year without another physical examination being performed.

3. *Familial hyperlipoproteinemia.* Estrogen therapy may be associated with massive elevations of plasma triglycerides leading to pancreatitis and other complications in patients with familial defects of lipoprotein metabolism.

4. *Fluid retention.* Because estrogens may cause some degree of fluid retention, conditions which might be influenced by this factor, such as asthma, epilepsy, migraine, and cardiac or renal dysfunction, require careful observation.

5. *Uterine bleeding and mastodynia.* Certain patients may develop undesirable manifestations of estrogenic stimulation, such as abnormal uterine bleeding and mastodynia.

6. *Uterine fibroids.* Preexisting uterine leiomyomata may increase in size during prolonged high-dose estrogen use.

7. *Impaired liver function.* Estrogens may be poorly metabolized in patients with impaired liver function and should be administered with caution.

8. *Hypercalcemia and renal insufficiency.* Prolonged use of estrogens can alter the metabolism of calcium and phosphorus. Estrogens should be used with caution in patients with metabolic bone disease.

B. INFORMATION FOR THE PATIENT

See text of Patient Package Insert which appears after the "HOW SUPPLIED" section.

C. LABORATORY TESTS

Clinical response at the smallest dose should generally be the guide to estrogen administration for relief of symptoms for those indications in which symptoms are observable. However, for prevention and treatment of osteoporosis see "DOSAGE AND ADMINISTRATION" section. Tests used to measure adequacy of estrogen replacement therapy include serum estrone and estradiol levels and suppression of serum gonadotrophin levels.

D. DRUG/LABORATORY TEST INTERACTIONS

Some of these drug/laboratory test interactions have been observed only with estrogen-progestin combinations (oral contraceptives):

1. Increased prothrombin and factors VII, VIII, IX and X; decreased antithrombin 3; increased norepinephrine-induced platelet aggregability, decreased fibrinolysis.

2. Increased thyroid-binding globulin (TBG) leading to increased circulating total thyroid hormone, as measured by T4 levels determined either by column or by radioimmunoassay. Free T3 resin uptake is decreased, reflecting the elevated TBG; free T4 concentration is unaltered.

3. Impaired glucose tolerance.

4. Reduced response to metyrapone test.

5. Reduced serum folate concentration.

E. MUTAGENESIS AND CARCINOGENESIS

Long-term continuous administration of natural and synthetic estrogens in certain animal species increases the frequency of carcinomas of the breast, cervix, vagina, and liver.

F. PREGNANCY CATEGORY X

Estrogens should not be used during pregnancy. (See CONTRAINDICATIONS and Boxed Warning.)

G. NURSING MOTHERS

As a general principle, the administration of any drug to nursing mothers should be done only when clearly necessary since many drugs are excreted in human milk.

ADVERSE REACTIONS

(See "WARNINGS" regarding induction of neoplasia, adverse effects on the fetus, increased incidence of gallbladder disease.) The following additional adverse reactions have been reported with estrogen therapy.

1. *Genitourinary system.* Changes in vaginal bleeding pattern and abnormal withdrawal bleeding or flow. Breakthrough bleeding, spotting. Increase in size of uterine fibromyomata. Vaginal candidiasis. Change in amount of cervical secretion.

2. *Breasts.* Tenderness, enlargement.

3. *Gastrointestinal.* Nausea, vomiting; abdominal cramps, bloating; cholestatic jaundice, pancreatitis.

4. *Skin.* Chloasma or melasma that may persist when drug is discontinued; erythema multiforme; erythema nodosum; hemorrhagic eruption; loss of scalp hair; hirsutism.

5. *Eyes.* Steepening of corneal curvature; intolerance of contact lenses.

6. *CNS.* Headache, migraine, dizziness; mental depression; chorea.

7. *Miscellaneous.* Increase or decrease in weight; reduced carbohydrate tolerance; aggravation of porphyria; edema; changes in libido.

ACUTE OVERDOSAGE

Numerous reports of ingestion of large doses of estrogen-containing oral contraceptives by young children indicate that acute serious ill effects do not occur. Overdosage of estrogen may cause nausea and vomiting.

DOSAGE AND ADMINISTRATION

1. For treatment of moderate to severe vasomotor symptoms and atrophic vaginitis associated with the menopause. The lowest dose that will control symptoms should be chosen, and medication should be discontinued as promptly as possible.

Attempts to discontinue or taper medication should be made at 3-month to 6-month intervals.

USUAL DOSAGE RANGES

Vasomotor symptoms—1.25 mg daily. If the patient has not menstruated within the last two months or more, cyclic administration is started arbitrarily. If the patient is menstruating, cyclic (e.g., three weeks on and one week off) administration is started on day 5 of bleeding.

Atrophic vaginitis—0.3 mg to 1.25 mg or more daily, depending upon the tissue response of the individual patient. Administer cyclically.

2. Hypoestrogenism due to:

a. Female hypogonadism—2.5 mg to 7.5 mg daily, in divided doses for 20 days, followed by a rest period of 10 days' duration. If bleeding does not occur by the end of this period, the same dosage schedule is repeated. The number of courses of estrogen therapy necessary to produce bleeding may vary depending on the responsiveness of the endometrium.

If bleeding occurs before the end of the 10-day period, begin a 20-day estrogen-progestin cyclic regimen with Premarin, 2.5 mg to 7.5 mg daily in divided doses, for 20 days. During the last five days of estrogen therapy, give an oral progestin. If bleeding occurs before this regimen is concluded, therapy is discontinued and may be resumed on the fifth day of bleeding.

b. Female castration or primary ovarian failure— 1.25 mg daily, cyclically. Adjust dosage, upward or downward, according to severity of symptoms and response of the patient. For maintenance, adjust dosage to lowest level that will provide effective control.

3. Osteoporosis (loss of bone mass)—0.625 mg daily. Administration should be cyclic (e.g., three weeks on and one week off).

4. Advanced androgen-dependent carcinoma of the prostate, for palliation only—1.25 mg to 2.5 mg three times daily. The effectiveness of therapy can be judged by phosphatase determinations as well as by symptomatic improvement of the patient.

5. Breast cancer (for palliation only) in appropriately selected women and men with metastatic disease. Suggested dosage is 10 mg three times daily for a period of at least three months.

Treated patients with an intact uterus should be monitored closely for signs of endometrial cancer, and appropriate diagnostic measures should be taken to rule out malignancy in the event of persistent or recurring abnormal vaginal bleeding.

HOW SUPPLIED

Premarin® (conjugated estrogens tablets, USP)

—Each oval purple tablet contains 2.5 mg, in bottles of 100 (NDC 0046-0865-81) and 1,000 (NDC 0046-0865-91).

—Each oval yellow tablet contains 1.25 mg, in bottles of 100 (NDC 0046-0866-81); 1,000 (NDC 0046-0866-91); 5,000 (NDC 0046-0866-95); and Unit-Dose packages of 100 (NDC 0046-0866-99).

—Each oval white tablet contains 0.9 mg, in bottles of 100 (NDC 0046-0864-81).

—Each oval maroon tablet contains 0.625 mg, in bottles of 100 (NDC 0046-0867-81); 1,000 (NDC 0046-0867-91); 5,000 (NDC 0046-0867-95); and Unit-Dose packages of 100 (NDC 0046-0867-99).

—Each oval green tablet contains 0.3 mg, in bottles of 100 (NDC 0046-0868-81) and 1,000 (NDC 0046-0868-91).

The appearance of these tablets is a trademark of Wyeth-Ayerst Laboratories.

Store at room temperature (approximately 25° C).

Dispense in a well-closed container as defined in the USP.

INFORMATION FOR THE PATIENT

This leaflet describes when and how to use estrogens and the risks of estrogen treatment.

ESTROGEN DRUGS

Estrogens have several important uses but also some risks. You must decide, with your doctor, whether the risks of estrogens are acceptable in view of their benefits. If you decide to start taking estrogens, check with your doctor to make sure you are using the lowest possible effective dose. The length of treatment with estrogens will depend upon the reason for use. This should also be discussed with your doctor.

USES OF ESTROGEN

To reduce menopausal symptoms. Estrogens are hormones produced by the ovaries. The decrease in the amount of estrogen that occurs in all women, usually between ages 45 and 55, causes the menopause. Sometimes the ovaries are removed by an operation, causing "surgical menopause." When the amount of estrogen begins to decrease, some women develop very uncomfortable symptoms, such as feelings of warmth in the face, neck and chest or sudden intense episodes of heat and sweating ("hot flashes"). The use of drugs containing estrogens can help the body adjust to lower estrogen levels.

Most women have none or only mild menopausal symptoms and do not need estrogens. Other women may need estrogens for a few months while their bodies adjust to lower estrogen levels. The majority of women do not need estrogen replacement for longer than six months for these symptoms.

To prevent brittle bones. After age 40, and especially after menopause, some women develop osteoporosis. This is a thinning of the bones that makes them weaker and more likely to break, often leading to fractures of vertebrae, hip, and wrist bones. Taking estrogens after the menopause slows down bone loss and may prevent bones from breaking. Eating foods that are high in calcium (such as milk products) or taking calcium supplements (1,000 to 1,500 milligrams per day) and certain types of exercise may also help prevent osteoporosis. Since estrogen use is associated with some risk, its use in the prevention of osteoporosis should be confined to women who appear to be susceptible to this condition. The following characteristics are often present in women who are likely to develop osteoporosis: white race, thinness, and cigarette smoking.

Women who had their menopause by the surgical removal of their ovaries at a relatively young age are good candidates for estrogen replacement therapy to prevent osteoporosis.

To treat certain types of abnormal uterine bleeding due to hormonal imbalance.

To treat atrophic vaginitis (itching, burning, dryness in or around the vagina).

To treat certain cancers.

WHEN ESTROGENS SHOULD NOT BE USED

Estrogens should not be used:

During pregnancy. Although the possibility is fairly small, there is a greater risk of having a child born with a birth defect if you take estrogens during pregnancy. A male child may have an increased risk of developing abnormalities of the urinary system and sex organs. A female child may have an increased risk of developing cancer of the vagina or cervix in her teens or twenties. Estrogen is not effective in preventing miscarriage (abortion).

If you have had any heart or circulation problems. Estrogen therapy should be used only after consultation with your physician and only in recommended doses. Patients with a tendency for abnormal blood clotting should avoid estrogen use (see below).

If you have had cancer. Since estrogens increase the risk of certain cancers, you should not take estrogens if you have ever had cancer of the breast or uterus. In certain situations,

Continued on next page

Wyeth-Ayerst Laboratories—Cont.

your doctor may choose to use estrogen in the treatment of breast cancer.

When they are ineffective. Sometimes women experience nervous symptoms or depression during menopause. There is no evidence that estrogens are effective for such symptoms. You may have heard that taking estrogens for long periods (years) after menopause will keep your skin soft and supple and keep you feeling young. There is no evidence that this is so and such long-term treatment may carry serious risks.

DANGERS OF ESTROGENS

Cancer of the uterus. The risk of cancer of the uterus increases the longer estrogens are used and when larger doses are taken. One study showed that when estrogens are discontinued, this increased risk of cancer seems to fall off quickly. In another study, the persistence of risk was demonstrated for 10 years after stopping estrogen treatment. Because of this risk, *it is important to take the lowest dose of estrogen that will control your symptoms and to take it only as long as you need it.* There is a higher risk of cancer of the uterus if you are overweight, diabetic, or have high blood pressure.

If you have had your uterus removed (total hysterectomy), there is no danger of developing cancer of the uterus.

Cancer of the breast. The majority of studies have shown no association with the usual doses used for estrogen replacement therapy and breast cancer. Some studies have suggested a possible increased incidence of breast cancer in those women taking estrogens for prolonged periods of time and especially if higher doses are used.

Regular breast examinations by a health professional and self-examination are recommended for women receiving estrogen therapy, as they are for all women.

Gallbladder disease. Women who use estrogens after menopause are more likely to develop gallbladder disease needing surgery than women who do not use estrogens.

Abnormal blood clotting. Taking estrogens may increase the risk of blood clots. These clots can cause a stroke, heart attack or pulmonary embolus, any of which may be fatal.

SIDE EFFECTS

In addition to the risks listed above, the following side effects have been reported with estrogen use:

- Nausea and vomiting.
- Breast tenderness or enlargement.
- Enlargement of benign tumors of the uterus.
- Retention of excess fluid. This may make some conditions worsen, such as asthma, epilepsy, migraine, heart disease, or kidney disease.
- A spotty darkening of the skin, particularly on the face.

REDUCING RISK OF ESTROGEN USE

If you decide to take estrogens, you can reduce your risks by carefully monitoring your treatment.

See your doctor regularly. While you are taking estrogens, it is important that you visit your doctor at least once a year for a physical examination. If members of your family have had breast cancer or if you have ever had breast nodules or an abnormal mammogram (breast X ray), you may need to have more frequent breast examinations.

Reevaluate your need for estrogens. You and your doctor should reevaluate your need for estrogens at least every six months.

Be alert for signs of trouble. Report these or any other unusual side effects to your doctor immediately:

- Abnormal bleeding from the vagina.
- Pains in the calves or chest, a sudden shortness of breath or coughing blood (indicating possible clots in the legs, heart, or lungs).
- Severe headache, dizziness, faintness, or changes in vision, indicating possible clots in the brain or eye.
- Breast lumps.
- Yellowing of the skin.
- Pain, swelling, or tenderness in the abdomen.

OTHER INFORMATION

Some physicians may choose to prescribe another hormonal drug to be used in association with estrogen treatment. These drugs, progestins, have been reported to lower the frequency of occurrence of a possible precancerous condition of the uterine lining. Whether this will provide protection from uterine cancer has not been clearly established. There are possible additional risks that may be associated with the inclusion of a progestin in estrogen treatment. The possible risks include unfavorable effects on blood fats and sugars. The choice of progestin and its dosage may be important in minimizing these effects.

Your doctor has prescribed this drug for you and you alone. Do not give the drug to anyone else.

If you will be taking calcium supplements as part of the treatment to help prevent osteoporosis, check with your doctor about the amounts recommended.

Keep this and all drugs out of the reach of children. In case of overdose, call your doctor, hospital, or poison control center immediately.

This leaflet provides the most important information about estrogens. If you want to read more, ask your doctor or pharmacist to let you read the professional labeling.

HOW SUPPLIED

Premarin® (conjugated estrogens tablets, USP)—tablets for oral administration.

Each oval purple tablet contains 2.5 mg.
Each oval yellow tablet contains 1.25 mg.
Each oval white tablet contains 0.9 mg.
Each oval maroon tablet contains 0.625 mg.
Each oval green tablet contains 0.3 mg.
The appearance of these tablets is a trademark of Wyeth-Ayerst Laboratories.

Shown in Product Identification Guide, page 340

PREMARIN® ℞
[prĕm 'a-rin]
(conjugated estrogens)
VAGINAL CREAM
in a nonliquefying base

Caution: Federal law prohibits dispensing without prescription.

> 1. ESTROGENS HAVE BEEN REPORTED TO INCREASE THE RISK OF ENDOMETRIAL CARCINOMA.
>
> Three independent, case-controlled studies have reported an increased risk of endometrial cancer in postmenopausal women exposed to exogenous estrogens for more than one year.[1-3] This risk was independent of the other known risk factors for endometrial cancer. These studies are further supported by the finding that incidence rates of endometrial cancer have increased sharply since 1969 in eight different areas of the United States with population-based cancer-reporting systems, an increase which may be related to the rapidly expanding use of estrogens during the last decade.[4]
> The three case-controlled studies reported that the risk of endometrial cancer in estrogen users was about 4.5 to 13.9 times greater than in nonusers. The risk appears to depend on both duration of treatment[1] and on estrogen dose.[3] In view of these findings, when estrogens are used for the treatment of menopausal symptoms, the lowest dose that will control symptoms should be utilized and medication should be discontinued as soon as possible. When prolonged treatment is medically indicated, the patient should be reassessed, on at least a semi-annual basis, to determine the need for continued therapy. Although the evidence must be considered preliminary, one study suggests that cyclic administration of low doses of estrogen may carry less risk than continuous administration.[3] It therefore appears prudent to utilize such a regimen.
> Close clinical surveillance of all women taking estrogens is important. In all cases of undiagnosed persistent or recurring abnormal vaginal bleeding, adequate diagnostic measures should be undertaken to rule out malignancy.
> There is no evidence at present that "natural" estrogens are more or less hazardous than "synthetic" estrogens at equi-estrogenic doses.
> 2. ESTROGENS SHOULD NOT BE USED DURING PREGNANCY.
> The use of female sex hormones, both estrogens and progestogens, during early pregnancy may seriously damage the offspring. It has been shown that females exposed *in utero* to diethylstilbestrol, a nonsteroidal estrogen, have an increased risk of developing, in later life, a form of vaginal or cervical cancer that is ordinarily extremely rare.[5,6] This risk has been estimated as not greater than 4 per 1,000 exposures.[7] Furthermore, a high percentage of such exposed women (from 30% to 90%) have been found to have vaginal adenosis,[8-12] epithelial changes of the vagina and cervix. Although these changes are histologically benign, it is not known whether they are precursors of malignancy. Although similar data are not available with the use of other estrogens, it cannot be presumed they would not induce similar changes.
> Several reports suggest an association between intrauterine exposure to female sex hormones and congenital anomalies, including congenital heart defects and limb-reduction defects.[13-16] One case-controlled study[16] estimated a 4.7-fold increased risk of limb-reduction defects in infants exposed *in utero* to sex hormones (oral contraceptives, hormone withdrawal tests for pregnancy, or attempted treatment for threatened abortion). Some of these exposures were very short and involved only a few days of treatment. The data suggest that the risk of limb-reduction defects in exposed fetuses is somewhat less than 1 per 1,000.

> In the past, female sex hormones have been used during pregnancy in an attempt to treat threatened or habitual abortion. There is considerable evidence that estrogens are ineffective for these indications, and there is no evidence from well-controlled studies that progestogens are effective for these uses.
> If Premarin (conjugated estrogens) Vaginal Cream is used during pregnancy, or if the patient becomes pregnant while taking this drug, she should be apprised of the potential risks to the fetus, and the advisability of pregnancy continuation.

DESCRIPTION

Each gram of Premarin® (conjugated estrogens) Vaginal Cream contains 0.625 mg conjugated estrogens, USP, in a nonliquefying base containing cetyl esters wax, cetyl alcohol, white wax, glyceryl monostearate, propylene glycol monostearate, methyl stearate, benzyl alcohol, sodium lauryl sulfate, glycerin, and mineral oil. Premarin Vaginal Cream is applied intravaginally.

Premarin (conjugated estrogens) is a mixture of estrogens obtained exclusively from natural sources, occurring as the sodium salts of water-soluble estrogen sulfates blended to represent the average composition of material derived from pregnant mares' urine. It contains estrone, equilin, and 17 α-dihydroequilin, together with smaller amounts of 17 α-estradiol, equilenin, and 17 α-dihydroequilenin as salts of their sulfate esters.

CLINICAL PHARMACOLOGY

Estrogens are important in the development and maintenance of the female reproductive system and secondary sex characteristics. They promote growth and development of the vagina, uterus, and fallopian tubes, and enlargement of the breasts. Indirectly, they contribute to the shaping of the skeleton, maintenance of tone and elasticity of urogenital structures, changes in the epiphyses of the long bones that allow for the pubertal growth spurt and its termination, growth of axillary and pubic hair, and pigmentation of the nipples and genitals. Decline of estrogenic activity at the end of the menstrual cycle can bring on menstruation, although the cessation of progesterone secretion is the most important factor in the mature ovulatory cycle. However, in the preovulatory or nonovulatory cycle, estrogen is the primary determinant in the onset of menstruation. Estrogens also affect the release of pituitary gonadotropins.

The pharmacologic effects of conjugated estrogens are similar to those of endogenous estrogens. They are soluble in water and may be absorbed from mucosal surfaces after local administration.

In responsive tissues (female genital organs, breasts, hypothalamus, pituitary) estrogens enter the cell and are transported into the nucleus. As a result of estrogen action, specific RNA and protein synthesis occurs.

Metabolism and inactivation occur primarily in the liver. Some estrogens are excreted into the bile; however, they are reabsorbed from the intestine and returned to the liver through the portal venous system. Water-soluble estrogen conjugates are strongly acidic and, therefore, ionized in body fluids, which favor excretion through the kidneys since tubular reabsorption is minimal.

INDICATIONS AND USAGE

Premarin (conjugated estrogens) Vaginal Cream is indicated in the treatment of atrophic vaginitis and kraurosis vulvae. Premarin Vaginal Cream HAS NOT BEEN SHOWN TO BE EFFECTIVE FOR ANY PURPOSE DURING PREGNANCY AND ITS USE MAY CAUSE SEVERE HARM TO THE FETUS (SEE BOXED WARNING).

CONTRAINDICATIONS

Estrogens should not be used in women with any of the following conditions:
1. Known or suspected cancer of the breast except in appropriately selected patients being treated for metastatic disease.
2. Known or suspected estrogen-dependent neoplasia.
3. Known or suspected pregnancy (see Boxed Warning).
4. Undiagnosed abnormal genital bleeding.
5. Active thrombophlebitis or thromboembolic disorders.
6. A past history of thrombophlebitis, thrombosis, or thromboembolic disorders associated with previous estrogen use (except when used in treatment of breast malignancy). Premarin Vaginal Cream should not be used in patients hypersensitive to its ingredients.

WARNINGS

1. *Induction of malignant neoplasms.* Long-term, continuous administration of natural and synthetic estrogens in certain animal species increases the frequency of carcinomas of the breast, cervix, vagina, and liver. There are now reports that estrogens increase the risk of carcinoma of the endometrium in humans (see Boxed Warning).

At the present time there is no satisfactory evidence that estrogens given to postmenopausal women increase the risk of cancer of the breast,[17] although a recent long-term follow-up of a single physician's practice has raised this possibil-

ity.[18] Because of the animal data, there is a need for caution in prescribing estrogens for women with a strong family history of breast cancer or who have breast nodules, fibrocystic disease, or abnormal mammograms.

2. *Gallbladder disease.* A recent study has reported a 2- to 3-fold increase in the risk of surgically confirmed gallbladder disease in women receiving postmenopausal estrogens,[17] similar to the 2-fold increase previously noted in users of oral contraceptives.[19,24a]

3. *Effects similar to those caused by estrogen-progestogen oral contraceptives.* There are several serious adverse effects of oral contraceptives, most of which have not, up to now, been documented as consequences of postmenopausal estrogen therapy. This may reflect the comparatively low doses of estrogen used in postmenopausal women. It would be expected that the larger doses of estrogen used to treat prostatic or breast cancer are more likely to result in these adverse effects, and, in fact, it has been shown that there is an increased risk of thrombosis in men receiving estrogens for prostatic cancer.[20-23]

a. *Thromboembolic disease.* It is now well established that users of oral contraceptives have an increased risk of various thromboembolic and thrombotic vascular diseases, such as thrombophlebitis, pulmonary embolism, stroke, and myocardial infarction.[24-31] Cases of retinal thrombosis, mesenteric thrombosis, and optic neuritis have been reported in oral-contraceptive users. There is evidence that the risk of several of these adverse reactions is related to the dose of the drug.[32,33] An increased risk of postsurgery thromboembolic complications has also been reported in users of oral contraceptives.[34,35] If feasible, estrogen should be discontinued at least 4 weeks before surgery of the type associated with an increased risk of thromboembolism, or during periods of prolonged immobilization.

While an increased rate of thromboembolic and thrombotic disease in postmenopausal users of estrogens has not been found,[17-24,25-36] this does not rule out the possibility that such an increase may be present, or that subgroups of women who have underlying risk factors, or who are receiving relatively large doses of estrogens, may have increased risk. Therefore, estrogens should not be used in persons with active thrombophlebitis or thromboembolic disorders, and they should not be used (except in treatment of malignancy) in persons with a history of such disorders in association with estrogen use. They should be used with caution in patients with cerebral vascular or coronary artery disease and only for those in whom estrogens are clearly needed.

Large doses of estrogen (5 mg conjugated estrogens per day), comparable to those used to treat cancer of the prostate and breast, have been shown in a large prospective clinical trial in men[37] to increase the risk of nonfatal myocardial infarction, pulmonary embolism, and thrombophlebitis. When estrogen doses of this size are used, any of the thromboembolic and thrombotic adverse effects associated with oral-contraceptive use should be considered a clear risk.

b. *Hepatic adenoma.* Benign hepatic adenomas appear to be associated with the use of oral contraceptives.[38-40] Although benign, and rare, these may rupture and may cause death through intra-abdominal hemorrhage. Such lesions have not yet been reported in association with other estrogen or progestogen preparations but should be considered in estrogen users having abdominal pain and tenderness, abdominal mass, or hypovolemic shock. Hepatocellular carcinoma has also been reported in women taking estrogen-containing oral contraceptives.[39] The relationship of this malignancy to these drugs is not known at this time.

c. *Elevated blood pressure.* Women using oral contraceptives sometimes experience increased blood pressure which, in most cases, returns to normal on discontinuing the drug. There is now a report that this may occur with use of estrogens in the menopause[41] and blood pressure should be monitored with estrogen use, especially if high doses are used.

d. *Glucose tolerance.* A worsening of glucose tolerance has been observed in a significant percentage of patients on estrogen-containing oral contraceptives. For this reason, diabetic patients should be carefully observed while receiving estrogen.

4. *Hypercalcemia.* Administration of estrogens may lead to severe hypercalcemia in patients with breast cancer and bone metastases. If this occurs, the drug should be stopped and appropriate measures taken to reduce the serum calcium level.

PRECAUTIONS

A. GENERAL PRECAUTIONS.

1. A complete medical and family history should be taken prior to the initiation of any estrogen therapy. The pretreatment and periodic physical examinations should include special reference to blood pressure, breasts, abdomen, and pelvic organs, and should include a Papanicolaou smear. As a general rule, estrogens should not be prescribed for longer than one year without another physical examination being performed.

2. Fluid retention—Because estrogens may cause some degree of fluid retention, conditions which might be influenced by this factor, such as asthma, epilepsy, migraine, and cardiac or renal dysfunction, require careful observation.

3. Familial hyperlipoproteinemia—Estrogen therapy may be associated with massive elevations of plasma triglycerides leading to pancreatitis and other complications in patients with familial defects of lipoprotein metabolism.

4. Certain patients may develop undesirable manifestations of excessive estrogenic stimulation, such as abnormal or excessive uterine bleeding, mastodynia, etc.

5. Prolonged administration of unopposed estrogen therapy has been reported to increase the risk of endometrial hyperplasia in some patients.

6. Oral contraceptives appear to be associated with an increased incidence of mental depression.[24a] Although it is not clear whether this is due to the estrogenic or progestogenic component of the contraceptive, patients with a history of depression should be carefully observed.

7. Preexisting uterine leiomyomata may increase in size during estrogen use.

8. The pathologist should be advised of estrogen therapy when relevant specimens are submitted.

9. Patients with a past history of jaundice during pregnancy have an increased risk of recurrence of jaundice while receiving estrogen-containing oral-contraceptive therapy. If jaundice develops in any patient receiving estrogen, the medication should be discontinued while the cause is investigated.

10. Estrogens may be poorly metabolized in patients with impaired liver function and should be administered with caution in such patients.

11. Because estrogens influence the metabolism of calcium and phosphorus, they should be used with caution in patients with metabolic bone diseases that are associated with hypercalcemia or in patients with renal insufficiency.

12. Because of the effects of estrogens on epiphyseal closure, they should be used judiciously in young patients in whom bone growth is not complete.

CONCOMITANT PROGESTIN USE:

The lowest effective dose appropriate for the specific indication should be utilized. Studies of the addition of a progestin for 7 or more days of a cycle of estrogen administration have reported a lowered incidence of endometrial hyperplasia. Morphological and biochemical studies of the endometrium suggest that 10 to 13 days of progestin are needed to provide maximal maturation of the endometrium and to eliminate any hyperplastic changes. Whether this will provide protection from endometrial carcinoma has not been clearly established. There are possible additional risks which may be associated with the inclusion of progestin in estrogen replacement regimens. If concomitant progestin therapy is used, potential risks may include adverse effects on carbohydrate and lipid metabolism. The choice of progestin and dosage may be important in minimizing these adverse effects.

B. INFORMATION FOR PATIENTS

(See text which appears after the PHYSICIAN REFERENCES.)

C. DRUG/LABORATORY TEST INTERACTIONS

Certain endocrine and liver function tests may be affected by estrogen-containing oral contraceptives. The following similar changes may be expected with larger doses of estrogen:

a. Increased sulfobromophthalein retention.

b. Increased prothrombin and factors VII, VIII, IX, and X; decreased antithrombin 3; increased norepinephrine-induced platelet aggregability.

c. Increased thyroid binding globulin (TBG) leading to increased circulating total thyroid hormone, as measured by PBI, T_4 by column, or T_4 by radioimmunoassay. Free T_3 resin uptake is decreased, reflecting the elevated TBG; free T_4 concentration is unaltered.

d. Impaired glucose tolerance.

e. Decreased pregnanediol excretion.

f. Reduced response to metyrapone test.

g. Reduced serum folate concentration.

h. Increased serum triglyceride and phospholipid concentration.

D. CARCINOGENESIS, MUTAGENESIS, IMPAIRMENT OF FERTILITY

(See WARNINGS section for information on carcinogenesis.)

E. PREGNANCY CATEGORY X

(See CONTRAINDICATIONS and Boxed Warning.)

F. NURSING MOTHERS

It is not known whether this drug is excreted in human milk. Because many drugs are excreted in human milk and because of the potential for serious adverse reactions in nursing infants from estrogens, a decision should be made whether to discontinue nursing or to discontinue the drug, taking into account the importance of the drug to the mother.

G. PEDIATRIC USE

Safety and effectiveness in pediatric patients have not been established.

ADVERSE REACTIONS

(See WARNINGS regarding induction of neoplasia, adverse effects on the fetus, increased incidence of gallbladder disease, and adverse effects similar to those of oral contraceptives, including thromboembolism.) The following additional adverse reactions have been reported with estrogenic therapy, including oral contraceptives:

1. *Genitourinary system:* Breakthrough bleeding, spotting, change in menstrual flow; dysmenorrhea; premenstrual-like syndrome; amenorrhea during and after treatment; increase in size of uterine fibromyomata; vaginal candidiasis; change in cervical erosion and in degree of cervical secretion; cystitis-like syndrome.

2. *Breasts:* Tenderness, enlargement, secretion.

3. *Gastrointestinal:* Nausea, vomiting; abdominal cramps, bloating; cholestatic jaundice, pancreatitis.

4. *Skin:* Chloasma or melasma which may persist when drug is discontinued; erythema multiforme; erythema nodosum; hemorrhagic eruption; loss of scalp hair; hirsutism.

5. *Eyes:* Steepening of corneal curvature; intolerance to contact lenses.

6. *CNS:* Headache, migraine, dizziness; mental depression; chorea.

7. *Miscellaneous:* Increase or decrease in weight; reduced carbohydrate tolerance; aggravation of porphyria; edema; changes in libido.

OVERDOSAGE

Numerous reports of ingestion of large doses of estrogen-containing oral contraceptives by young children indicate that acute serious ill effects do not occur. Overdosage of estrogens may cause nausea, and withdrawal bleeding may occur in females.

DOSAGE AND ADMINISTRATION

Given cyclically for short-term use only:
For treatment of atrophic vaginitis, or kraurosis vulvae.
The lowest dose that will control symptoms should be chosen and medication should be discontinued as promptly as possible.
Administration should be cyclic (e.g., three weeks on and one week off).
Attempts to discontinue or taper medication should be made at three- to six-month intervals.

USUAL DOSAGE RANGE:
½ to 2 g daily, intravaginally, depending on the severity of the condition.
Treated patients with an intact uterus should be monitored closely for signs of endometrial cancer, and appropriate diagnostic measures should be taken to rule out malignancy in the event of persistent or recurring abnormal vaginal bleeding.

INSTRUCTIONS FOR USE OF GENTLE MEASURE™ APPLICATOR:
1. Remove cap from tube.
2. Screw nozzle end of applicator onto tube.
3. *Gently* squeeze tube from the *bottom* to force sufficient cream into the barrel to provide the prescribed dose. Use the marked stopping points on the applicator as a guideline to measure the correct dose.
4. Unscrew applicator from tube.
5. Lie on back with knees drawn up. To deliver medication, gently insert applicator deeply into vagina and press plunger downward to its original position.
TO CLEANSE: Pull plunger to remove it from barrel. Wash with mild soap and warm water.
DO NOT BOIL OR USE HOT WATER.

HOW SUPPLIED

Premarin (conjugated estrogens) Vaginal Cream—Each gram contains 0.625 mg conjugated estrogens, USP.
Combination package: Each contains Net Wt. 1½ oz (42.5 g) tube with one plastic applicator calibrated in ½ g increments to a maximum of 2 g (NDC 0046-0872-93).
Also Available—Refill package: Each contains Net Wt. 1½ oz (42.5 g) tube (NDC 0046-0872-01).
Store at room temperature (approximately 25° C).

PHYSICIAN REFERENCES

1. Ziel, H. K., *et al.*: N. Engl. J. Med. *293*:1167–1170, 1975.
2. Smith, D. C., *et al.*: N. Engl. J. Med. *293*:1164–1167, 1975.
3. Mack, T. M., *et al.*: N. Engl. J. Med *294*:1262–1267, 1976.
4. Weiss, N. S., *et al.*: N. Engl. J. Med. *294*:1259–1262, 1976.
5. Herbst, A. L., *et al.*: N. Engl. J. Med. *284*:878–881, 1971.
6. Greenwald, P., *et al.*: N. Engl. J. Med. *285*:390–392, 1971.
7. Lanier, A., *et al.*: Mayo Clin. Proc. *48*:793–799, 1973.
8. Herbst, A., *et al.*: Obstet. Gynecol. *40*:287–298, 1972.
9. Herbst, A., *et al.*: Am. J. Obstet. Gynecol. *118*:607–615, 1974.
10. Herbst, A., *et al.*: N. Engl. J. Med. *292*:334–339, 1975.
11. Stafl, A., *et al.*: Obstet. Gynecol. *43*:118–128, 1974.
12. Sherman, A. I., *et al.*: Obstet. Gynecol. *44*:531–545, 1974.
13. Gal, I., *et al.*: Nature *216*:83, 1967.
14. Levy, E. P., *et al.*: Lancet *1*:611, 1973.

Continued on next page

Wyeth-Ayerst Laboratories—Cont.

15. Nora, J., *et al.*: Lancet *1*:941–942, 1973.
16. Janerich, D. T., *et al.*: N. Engl. J. Med. *291*:697–700, 1974.
17. Boston Collaborative Drug Surveillance Program: N. Engl. J. Med. *290*:15–19, 1974.
18. Hoover, R., *et al.*: N. Engl. J. Med. *295*:401–405, 1976.
19. Boston Collaborative Drug Surveillance Program: Lancet *1*:1399–1404, 1973.
20. Daniel, D. G., *et al.*: Lancet *2*:287–289, 1967.
21. The Veterans Administration Cooperative Urological Research Group: J. Urol. *98*:516–522, 1967.
22. Bailar, J. C.: Lancet *2*:560, 1967.
23. Blackard, C., *et al.*: Cancer *26*:249–256, 1970.
24. Royal College of General Practitioners: J. R. Coll. Gen. Pract. *13*:267–279, 1967.

24a. Royal College of General Practitioners: Oral Contraceptives and Health, New York, Pitman Corp., 1974.

25. Inman, W. H. W., *et al.*: Br. Med. J. *2*:193–199, 1968.
26. Vessey, M. P., *et al.*: Br. Med. J. *2*:651–657, 1969.
27. Sartwell, P. E., *et al.*: Am. J. Epidemiol. *90*:365–380, 1969.
28. Collaborative Group for the Study of Stroke in Young Women: N. Engl. J. Med. *288*:871–878, 1973.
29. Collaborative Group for the Study of Stroke in Young Women: J.A.M.A. *231*:718–722, 1975.
30. Mann, J. I., *et al.*: Br. Med. J. *2*:245–248, 1975.
31. Mann, J. I., *et al.*: Br. Med. J. *2*:241–245, 1975.
32. Inman, W. H. W., *et al.*: Br. Med. J. *2*:203–209, 1970.
33. Stolley, P. D., *et al.*: Am. J. Epidemiol. *102*:197–208, 1975.
34. Vessey, M. P., *et al.*: Br. Med. J. *3*:123–126, 1970.
35. Greene, G. R., *et al.*: Am. J. Public Health *62*:680–685, 1972.
36. Rosenberg, L., *et al.*: N. Engl. J. Med. *294*:1256–1259, 1976.
37. Coronary Drug Project Research Group: J.A.M.A. *214*:1303–1313, 1970.
38. Baum, J., *et al.*: Lancet *2*:926–928, 1973.
39. Mays, E. T., *et al.*: J.A.M.A. *235*:730–732, 1976.
40. Edmondson, H. A., *et al.*: N. Engl. J. Med. *294*:470–472, 1976.
41. Pfeffer, R. I., *et al.*: Am. J. Epidemiol. *103*:445–456, 1976.

INFORMATION FOR THE PATIENT

WHAT YOU SHOULD KNOW ABOUT ESTROGENS

Estrogens are female hormones produced by the ovaries. The ovaries make several different kinds of estrogens. In addition, scientists have been able to make a variety of synthetic estrogens. As far as we know, all these estrogens have similar properties and, therefore, much the same usefulness, side effects, and risks. This leaflet is intended to help you understand what estrogens are used for, the risks involved in their use, and how to use them as safely as possible.

This leaflet includes the most important information about estrogens, but not all the information. If you want to know more, you should ask your doctor for more information or you can ask your doctor or pharmacist to let you read the package insert prepared for the doctor.

USES OF ESTROGEN

THERE IS NO PROPER USE OF ESTROGENS IN A PREGNANT WOMAN.

Estrogens are prescribed by doctors for a number of purposes, including:

1. To provide estrogen during a period of adjustment when a woman's ovaries stop producing a majority of her estrogens, in order to prevent certain uncomfortable symptoms of estrogen deficiency. (With the menopause, which generally occurs between the ages of 45 and 55, women produce a much smaller amount of estrogens.)
2. To prevent symptoms of estrogen deficiency when a woman's ovaries have been removed surgically before the natural menopause.
3. To prevent pregnancy. (Estrogens are given along with a progestogen, another female hormone; these combinations are called oral contraceptives, or birth-control pills. Patient labeling is available to women taking oral contraceptives and they will not be discussed in this leaflet.)
4. To treat certain cancers in women and men.

ESTROGENS IN THE MENOPAUSE

In the natural course of their lives, all women eventually experience a decrease in estrogen production. This usually occurs between ages 45 and 55, but may occur earlier or later. Sometimes the ovaries may need to be removed before natural menopause by an operation, producing a "surgical menopause."

When the amount of estrogen in the blood begins to decrease, many women may develop typical symptoms: feelings of warmth in the face, neck, and chest, or sudden intense episodes of heat and sweating throughout the body (called "hot flashes" or "hot flushes"). These symptoms are sometimes very uncomfortable. Some women may also develop changes in the vagina (called "atrophic vaginitis") that cause discomfort, especially during and after intercourse.

Estrogens can be prescribed to treat these symptoms of the menopause. It is estimated that considerably more than half of all women undergoing the menopause have only mild symptoms or no symptoms at all and, therefore, do not need estrogens. Other women may need estrogens for a few months, while their bodies adjust to lower estrogen levels. Sometimes the need will be for periods longer than six months. In an attempt to avoid overstimulation of the uterus (womb), estrogens are usually given cyclically during each month of use, such as three weeks of pills followed by one week without pills.

Sometimes women experience nervous symptoms or depression during menopause. There is no evidence that estrogens are effective for such symptoms without associated vasomotor symptoms. In the absence of vasomotor symptoms, estrogens should not be used to treat nervous symptoms, although other treatment may be needed.

You may have heard that taking estrogens for long periods (years) after the menopause will keep your skin soft and supple and keep you feeling young. There is no evidence that this is so, however, and such long-term treatment carries important risks.

THE DANGERS OF ESTROGENS

1. *Endometrial cancer.* There are reports that if estrogens are used in the postmenopausal period for more than a year, there is an increased risk of *endometrial cancer* (cancer of the lining of the uterus). Women taking estrogens have roughly 5- to 10-times as great a chance of getting this cancer as women who take no estrogens. To put this another way, while a postmenopausal woman not taking estrogens has 1 chance in 1,000 each year of getting endometrial cancer, a woman taking estrogens has 5 to 10 chances in 1,000 each year. For this reason *it is important to take estrogens only when they are really needed.*

The risk of this cancer is greater the longer estrogens are used and when larger doses are taken. Therefore, you should not take more estrogen than your doctor prescribes. *It is important to take the lowest dose of estrogen that will control symptoms and to take it only as long as it is needed.* If estrogens are needed for longer periods of time, your doctor will want to reevaluate your need for estrogens at least every six months.

Women using estrogens should report any vaginal bleeding to their doctors; such bleeding may be of no importance, but it can be an early warning of endometrial cancer. If you have undiagnosed vaginal bleeding, you should not use estrogens until a diagnosis is made and you are certain there is no endometrial cancer.

Note: If you have had your uterus removed (total hysterectomy), there is no danger of developing endometrial cancer.

2. *Other possible cancers.* Estrogens can cause development of other tumors in animals, such as tumors of the breast, cervix, vagina, or liver, when given for a long time. At present there is no good evidence that women using estrogen in the menopause have an increased risk of such tumors, but there is no way yet to be sure they do not; and one study raises the possibility that use of estrogens in the menopause may increase the risk of breast cancer many years later. This is a further reason to use estrogens only when clearly needed. While you are taking estrogens, it is important that you go to your doctor at least once a year for a physical examination. Also, if members of your family have had breast cancer or if you have breast nodules, or abnormal mammograms (breast X rays), your doctor may wish to carry out more frequent examinations of your breasts.

3. *Gallbladder disease.* Women who use estrogens after menopause are more likely to develop gallbladder disease needing surgery than women who do not use estrogens. Birth-control pills have a similar effect.

4. *Abnormal blood clotting.* Oral contraceptives increase the risk of blood clotting in various parts of the body. This can result in a stroke (if the clot is in the brain), a heart attack (a clot in a blood vessel of the heart), or a pulmonary embolus (a clot which forms in the legs or pelvis, then breaks off and travels to the lungs). Any of these can be fatal.

At this time, use of estrogens in the menopause is not known to cause such blood clotting, but this has not been fully studied and there could still prove to be such a risk. It is recommended that if you have had clotting in the legs or lungs, or a heart attack or stroke while you were using estrogens or birth-control pills, you should not use estrogens (unless they are being used to treat cancer of the breast or prostate). If you have had a stroke or heart attack, or if you have angina pectoris, estrogens should be used with great caution and only if clearly needed (for example, if you have severe symptoms of the menopause).

SPECIAL WARNING ABOUT PREGNANCY

You should not receive estrogen if you are pregnant. If this should occur, there is a greater than usual chance that the developing child will be born with a birth defect, although the possibility remains fairly small. A female child may have an increased risk of developing cancer of the vagina or cervix later in life (in the teens or twenties). Every possible effort should be made to avoid exposure to estrogens during pregnancy. If exposure occurs, see your doctor.

OTHER EFFECTS OF ESTROGENS

In addition to the serious known risks of estrogens described above, estrogens have the following side effects and potential risks:

1. *Nausea and vomiting.* The most common side effect of estrogen therapy is nausea. Vomiting is less common.
2. *Effects on breasts.* Estrogens may cause breast tenderness or enlargement and may cause the breasts to secrete a liquid. These effects are not dangerous.
3. *Effects on the uterus.* Estrogens may cause benign fibroid tumors of the uterus to get larger.
4. *Effects on liver.* Women taking oral contraceptives develop, on rare occasions, a tumor of the liver which can rupture and bleed into the abdomen and may cause death. So far, these tumors have not been reported in women using estrogens in the menopause, but you should report any swelling or unusual pain or tenderness in the abdomen to your doctor immediately.

Women with a past history of jaundice (yellowing of the skin and white parts of the eyes) may get jaundice again during estrogen use. If this occurs, stop taking estrogens and see your doctor.

5. *Other effects.* Estrogens may cause excess fluid to be retained in the body. This may make some conditions worse, such as asthma, epilepsy, migraine, heart disease, or kidney disease.

SUMMARY

Estrogens have important uses, but they have serious risks as well. You must decide, with your doctor, whether the risks are acceptable to you in view of the benefits of treatment. Except where your doctor has prescribed estrogens for use in special cases of cancer of the breast or prostate, you should not use estrogens if you have cancer of the breast or uterus, are pregnant, have undiagnosed abnormal vaginal bleeding, clotting in the legs or lungs, or have had a stroke, heart attack or angina, or clotting in the legs or lungs in the past while you were taking estrogens.

You can use estrogens as safely as possible by understanding that your doctor will require regular physical examinations while you are taking them, will try to discontinue the drug as soon as possible, and use the smallest dose possible. Be alert for signs of trouble including:

1. Abnormal bleeding from the vagina.
2. Pains in the calves or chest, sudden shortness of breath, or coughing blood.
3. Severe headache, dizziness, faintness, or changes in vision.
4. Breast lumps (you should ask your doctor how to examine your own breasts).
5. Jaundice (yellowing of the skin).
6. Mental depression.

Your doctor has prescribed this drug for you and you alone. Do not give the drug to anyone else.

HOW SUPPLIED

Premarin (conjugated estrogens) Vaginal Cream—Each gram contains 0.625 mg conjugated estrogens, USP.

Combination package: Each contains Net Wt. 1½ oz (42.5 g) tube with one plastic applicator calibrated in ½ g increments to a maximum of 2 g (NDC 0046-0872-93).

Also Available—Refill package: Each contains Net Wt. 1½ oz (42.5 g) tube (NDC 0046-0872-01).

Store at room temperature (approximately 25° C).

INSTRUCTIONS FOR USE OF PREMARIN®
(conjugated estrogens)
VAGINAL CREAM Gentle Measure™ APPLICATOR:

The Gentle Measure Applicator has been specifically designed for comfortable, easy use.

1. Remove cap from tube.
2. Screw nozzle end of applicator onto tube.
3. *Gently* squeeze tube from the *bottom* to force sufficient cream into the barrel to provide the prescribed dose. Use the marked stopping points on the applicator as a guideline to measure the correct dose.
4. Unscrew applicator from tube.
5. Lie on back with knees drawn up. To deliver medication, gently insert applicator deeply into vagina and press plunger downward to its original position.

TO CLEANSE: Pull plunger to remove it from barrel. Wash with mild soap and warm water.

DO NOT BOIL OR USE HOT WATER.

Shown in Product Identification Guide, page 340

PREMPHASE® ℞

(conjugated estrogens/medroxyprogesterone acetate tablets)

Caution: Federal law prohibits dispensing without prescription.

ESTROGENS HAVE BEEN REPORTED TO INCREASE THE RISK OF ENDOMETRIAL CARCINOMA IN POST-MENOPAUSAL WOMEN. THIS FINDING REFERS TO ESTROGENS GIVEN WITHOUT PROGESTIN.
Progestins taken with estrogen drugs significantly reduce but do not eliminate this risk. Close clinical surveillance of all women taking estrogens is important. Adequate diagnostic measures, including endometrial sampling when indicated, should be undertaken to rule out malignancy in all cases of undiagnosed persistent or recurring abnormal vaginal bleeding. There is no evidence that "natural" estrogens are more or less hazardous than "synthetic" estrogens at equiestrogenic doses.
ESTROGENS/PROGESTINS SHOULD NOT BE USED DURING PREGNANCY.
There is no indication for estrogen therapy during pregnancy or during the immediate postpartum period. Estrogen therapy during pregnancy is associated with an increased risk of congenital defects in the reproductive organs of the fetus, and possibly other birth defects. Estrogens are not indicated for the prevention of postpartum breast engorgement.
Studies of women who received diethylstilbestrol (DES) during pregnancy have shown that female offspring have an increased risk of vaginal adenosis, squamous cell dysplasia of the uterine cervix, and clear cell vaginal cancer later in life; male offspring have an increased risk of urogenital abnormalities and possibly testicular cancer later in life. The 1985 DES Task Force concluded that use of DES during pregnancy is associated with subsequent increased risk of breast cancer in the mothers, although a causal relationship remains unproven and the observed level of excess risk is similar to that for a number of other breast cancer risk factors.
Several reports also suggest an association between intrauterine exposure to progestational drugs in the first trimester of pregnancy and genital abnormalities in male and female fetuses. The risk of hypospadias, 5 to 8 per 1000 male births in the general population, may be approximately doubled with exposure to these drugs. There are insufficient data to quantify the risk to exposed female fetuses; some of these drugs induce mild virilization of the external genitalia of the female fetus. If the patient is exposed to PREMPHASE® (conjugated estrogens/medroxyprogesterone acetate) during pregnancy, or if she becomes pregnant while taking these drugs, she should be apprised of the potential risks to the fetus.
Estrogens are ineffective for the prevention or treatment of threatened or habitual abortion. There is no adequate evidence that progestational agents are effective in preventing habitual abortion when such drugs are given during the first trimester of pregnancy. Furthermore, in the vast majority of women, the cause of abortion is a defective ovum, which progestational agents could not be expected to influence. In addition, the use of progestational agents with their uterine-relaxant properties, in patients with fertilized defective ova, may cause a delay in spontaneous abortion.

DESCRIPTION

PREMPHASE therapy consists of two separate tablets, a maroon Premarin® tablet containing 0.625 mg of conjugated estrogens which is taken orally on days 1 through 14 and a light-blue tablet containing 0.625 mg of the conjugated estrogens found in Premarin tablets and 5 mg of medroxyprogesterone acetate (MPA) which is taken orally on days 15 through 28.
The conjugated estrogens found in Premarin tablets are a mixture of sodium estrone sulfate and sodium equilin sulfate. It contains as concomitant components sodium sulfate conjugates 17α-dihydroequilin, 17α-estradiol and 17β-dihydroequilin.
Medroxyprogesterone acetate, a derivative of progesterone, is a white to off-white, odorless, crystalline powder, stable in air, melting between 200° C and 210° C. It is freely soluble in chloroform, soluble in acetone and in dioxane, sparingly soluble in alcohol and methanol, slightly soluble in ether, and insoluble in water. The chemical name for MPA is pregn-4-ene-3,20-dione, 17-(acetyloxy)-6-methyl-,(6α).
Each Premarin tablet for oral administration contains 0.625 mg of conjugated estrogens and the following inactive ingredients: calcium phosphate tribasic, calcium sulfate, carnauba wax, cellulose, glyceryl monooleate, lactose, magnesium stearate, methylcellulose, pharmaceutical glaze, polyethylene glycol, stearic acid, sucrose, titanium dioxide, FD&C Blue No. 2, D&C Red No. 27, FD&C Red No. 40.
Each light-blue tablet for oral administration contains 0.625 mg of the conjugated estrogens found in Premarin and 5 mg of medroxyprogesterone acetate and the following inactive ingredients: calcium phosphate tribasic, calcium sulfate, carnauba wax, cellulose, glyceryl monooleate, lactose, mag-

INCIDENCE OF ENDOMETRIAL HYPERPLASIA AFTER ONE YEAR OF TREATMENT

Patient	Dose Groups	
	PREMPHASE 0.625 mg/5 mg	Premarin 0.625 mg
Total number of patients	279	283
No. (%) of patients with biopsies		
● all focal and non-focal hyperplasia	3 (1)*	57 (20)
● excluding focal cystic hyperplasia	1 (<1)*	25 (8)

*Significant (p < 0.001) in comparison with Premarin alone (0.625 mg).

MEAN PERCENT CHANGE FROM BASELINE LIPID PROFILE VALUES AFTER ONE YEAR OF TREATMENT

Lipid Parameter	Dose Groups	
	PREMPHASE 0.625 mg/5 mg	Premarin 0.625 mg
Total Cholesterol	-3.5*,†	0.2
HDL-C	4.4*,†	14.1*
HDL$_2$-C	30.3*,†	70.8*
LDL-C	-8.7*	-7.7*
Triglycerides	27.5*,†	39.4*

*Significantly (p ≤ 0.05) different from baseline value.
†Significantly (p ≤ 0.05) different from Premarin alone.

nesium stearate, methylcellulose, pharmaceutical glaze, polyethylene glycol, sucrose, povidone, titanium dioxide, FD&C Blue No. 2.

CLINICAL PHARMACOLOGY

Estrogens are important in the development and maintenance of the female reproductive system and secondary sex characteristics. By a direct action, they cause growth and development of the uterus, fallopian tubes, and vagina. With other hormones, such as pituitary hormones and progesterone, they cause enlargement of the breasts through promotion of ductal growth, stromal development, and the accretion of fat. Estrogens are intricately involved with other hormones, especially progesterone, in the processes of the ovulatory menstrual cycle and pregnancy and affect the release of pituitary gonadotropins. They also contribute to the shaping of the skeleton, maintenance of tone and elasticity of urogenital structures, changes in the epiphyses of the long bones that allow for the pubertal growth spurt and its termination, and pigmentation of the nipples and genitals.
The use of unopposed estrogen therapy has been associated with an increased risk of endometrial hyperplasia, a possible precursor of endometrial adenocarcinoma. The results of clinical studies indicate that the addition of a progestin to an estrogen replacement regimen for more than 10 days per cycle reduces the incidence of endometrial hyperplasia and the attendant risk of adenocarcinoma in women with intact uteri. The addition of a progestin to an estrogen replacement regimen has not been shown to interfere with the efficacy of estrogen replacement therapy for its approved indications. Data from a large clinical trial indicate that MPA administered in the recommended dose to women receiving Premarin 0.625 mg reduces the incidence of hyperplastic changes and hence reduces the risk of developing adenocarcinoma. This is the clinical rationale for PREMPHASE.
The following table summarizes the incidence of endometrial hyperplasia after 1 year of treatment with the combined regimens.
[See first table above.]

INFORMATION REGARDING LIPID EFFECTS

The results of a clinical trial conducted in a 97% Caucasian population at low risk for cardiovascular disease show that PREMPHASE increases HDL-C and the HDL$_2$-C subfraction significantly less than Premarin alone, but decreases LDL-C comparably with Premarin alone. Total Cholesterol concentrations were significantly lower after 1 year of treatment than at baseline.
The following table summarizes mean percent changes from baseline lipid parameter values after 1 year of treatment with the combined regimens.
[See second table above.]
The pharmacologic effects of the administered conjugated estrogens are similar to those of endogenous estrogens. In responsive tissue (female genital organs, breasts, hypothalamus, pituitary) estrogens enter the cell and are transported into the nucleus. As a result of the estrogen action, specific RNA and protein synthesis occurs.
Androgenic and anabolic effects of MPA have been noted, but the drug is apparently devoid of significant estrogenic activity. Parenterally administered MPA inhibits gonadotropin production, which in turn prevents follicular maturation and ovulation, although available data indicate that this

does not occur when the usually recommended oral dosage is given as single daily doses. MPA may achieve its beneficial effect on the endometrium in part by decreasing nuclear estradiol receptors and suppression of epithelial DNA synthesis in endometrial tissue.

PHARMACOKINETICS

ABSORPTION

Conjugated estrogens are soluble in water and are well absorbed from the gastrointestinal tract after release from the drug formulation. However, PREMPHASE contains a modified-release formulation of conjugated estrogens that slowly releases estrogens over several hours. Maximum plasma concentrations of the various conjugated and unconjugated estrogens are attained within 4 to 10 hours after dose administration. MPA is rapidly absorbed from the gastrointestinal tract, and maximum MPA plasma concentrations are attained within 2 to 4 hours after dose administration.

DISTRIBUTION

The conjugated estrogens bind mainly to albumin, but the unconjugated estrogens bind to both albumin and sex-hormone-binding globulin (SHBG). The apparent terminal-phase disposition half-life ($t_{1/2}$) of the various estrogens is prolonged by the slow absorption from PREMPHASE and ranges from 10 to 24 hours. MPA is approximately 90% bound to plasma proteins but does not bind to SHBG. MPA has a $t_{1/2}$ of 46 hours.

METABOLISM

Metabolism and inactivation of estrogens occur primarily in the liver. Some estrogens are excreted into the bile; however, they are reabsorbed from the intestine and returned to the liver through the portal venous system. Metabolism and elimination of MPA occurs primarily in the liver via hydroxylation, with subsequent conjugation and elimination in the urine.

EXCRETION

Water-soluble estrogen conjugates are strongly acidic and are ionized in body fluids, which favor excretion through the kidneys since tubular reabsorption is minimal. Most metabolites of MPA are excreted as glucuronide conjugates with only minor amounts excreted as sulfates.

DRUG-DRUG INTERACTIONS

Coadministration of conjugated estrogens with MPA does not affect the pharmacokinetic profile of MPA; similarly, MPA does not affect the pharmacokinetic profile of the conjugated or unconjugated estrogens.

FOOD-DRUG INTERACTIONS

A single dose study in twenty healthy, postmenopausal women was conducted to investigate any potential drug interaction when PREMPHASE is administered with a high fat breakfast.
Administration with food decreased total estrone C_{max} by 18% and increased total equilin C_{max} by 38% compared to the fasting state, with no other effect on the rate or extent or absorption of other conjugated or unconjugated estrogens. Administration with food approximately doubles MPA C_{max} and increases MPA AUC by approximately 20%.
TABLE 1 summarizes the pharmacokinetic parameters estimated for unconjugated and conjugated estrogens, and med-

Continued on next page

Wyeth-Ayerst Laboratories—Cont.

roxyprogesterone acetate from a single dose bioequivalence study involving 51 postmenopausal women.

[See Table 1 below.]

INDICATIONS AND USAGE

PREMPHASE therapy is indicated in women with an intact uterus for the:

1. Treatment of moderate to severe vasomotor symptoms associated with the menopause. There is no adequate evidence that estrogens are effective for nervous symptoms or depression which might occur during menopause and they should not be used to treat these conditions.
2. Treatment of vulvar and vaginal atrophy.
3. Prevention of osteoporosis.

Since estrogen administration is associated with risks as well as benefits, selection of patients ideally should be based on prospective identification of risk factors for developing osteoporosis. Unfortunately, there is no certain way to identify those women who will develop osteoporotic fractures. Most prospective studies of efficacy for this indication have been carried out in white menopausal women, without stratification by other risk factors, and tend to show a universally salutary effect on bone. Thus, patient selection must be individualized based on the balance of risks and benefits.

Estrogen replacement therapy reduces bone resorption and retards or halts postmenopausal bone loss. Case-control studies have shown an approximately 60% reduction in hip and wrist fractures in women whose estrogen replacement was begun within a few years of menopause. Studies also suggest that estrogen reduces the rate of vertebral fractures. Even when started as late as 6 years after menopause, estrogen may prevent further loss of bone mass for as long as the treatment is continued. When estrogen therapy is discontinued, bone mass declines at a rate comparable to that in the immediate postmenopausal period. There is no evidence that estrogen replacement therapy restores bone mass to premenopausal levels.

At skeletal maturity there are sex and race differences in both the total amount of bone present and its density, in favor of men and blacks. Thus, women are at higher risk than men because they start with less bone mass and, for several years following natural or induced menopause, the rate of bone mass decline is accelerated. White and Asian women are at higher risk than black women.

Early menopause is one of the strongest predictors for the development of osteoporosis. In addition, other factors affecting the skeleton which are associated with osteoporosis include genetic factors (small build, family history), endocrine factors (nulliparity, thyrotoxicosis, hyperparathyroidism, Cushing's syndrome, hyperprolactinemia, type I diabetes), lifestyle (cigarette smoking, alcohol abuse, sedentary exercise habits) and nutrition (below average body weight, dietary calcium intake).

The mainstays of prevention and management of osteoporosis are estrogen, an adequate lifetime calcium intake, and exercise. Postmenopausal women absorb dietary calcium less efficiently than premenopausal women and require an average of 1500 mg/day of elemental calcium to remain in neutral calcium balance. By comparison, premenopausal women require about 1000 mg/day and the average calcium intake in the USA is 400–600 mg/day. Therefore, when not contraindicated, calcium supplementation may be helpful. Weight-bearing exercise and nutrition may be important adjuncts to the prevention and management of osteoporosis. Immobilization and prolonged bed rest produce rapid bone loss, while weight-bearing exercise has been shown both to reduce bone loss and to increase bone mass. The optimal type and amount of physical activity that would prevent osteoporosis have not been established; however, in two studies an hour of walking and running exercises twice or three times weekly significantly increased lumbar spine bone mass.

CONTRAINDICATIONS

Estrogens/progestins combined should not be used in women under any of the following conditions or circumstances:

1. Known or suspected pregnancy, including use for missed abortion or as a diagnostic test for pregnancy (see Boxed Warning). Estrogen or progestin may cause fetal harm when administered to a pregnant woman.
2. Known or suspected cancer of the breast.
3. Known or suspected estrogen-dependent neoplasia.
4. Undiagnosed abnormal genital bleeding.
5. Active or past history of thrombophlebitis, thromboembolic disorders, or stroke.
6. Liver dysfunction or disease.

PREMPHASE therapy should not be used in patients hypersensitive to the ingredients contained in the tablets.

WARNINGS

ALL WARNINGS BELOW PERTAIN TO THE USE OF THIS COMBINATION PRODUCT.

Based on experience with estrogens and/or progestins:

1. *Induction of malignant neoplasms*

Breast cancer. Some studies have reported a moderately increased risk of breast cancer (relative risk of 1.3 to 2.0) in those women on estrogen replacement therapy taking higher doses, or in those taking lower doses for prolonged periods of time, especially in excess of 10 years. The majority of studies, however, have not shown an association in women who have ever used estrogen replacement therapy.

The effect of added progestins on the risk of breast cancer is unknown, although a moderately increased risk in those taking combination estrogen/progestin therapy has been reported. Other studies have not shown this relationship. In a one year clinical trial of PREMPRO™, PREMPHASE and Premarin alone, 5 new cases of breast cancer were detected among 1377 women who received the combination treatments, while no new cases were detected among 347 women who received Premarin alone. The overall incidence of breast cancer in this clinical trial does not exceed that expected in the general population.

In the three year clinical Postmenopausal Estrogen Progestin Intervention (PEPI) trial of 875 women to assess differences among placebo, unopposed Premarin, and three different combination hormone therapy regimens, one (1) new case of breast cancer was detected in the placebo group (n=174), one in the Premarin alone group (n=175), none in the continuous Premarin plus medroxyprogesterone acetate group (n=174) and two (2) in the continuous Premarin plus cyclic medroxyprogesterone acetate group (n=174).

Women on hormone replacement therapy should have regular breast examinations and should be instructed in breast self-examination, and women over the age of 50 should have regular mammograms.

Endometrial cancer. The reported endometrial cancer risk among users of unopposed estrogen was about 2- to 12-fold greater than in nonusers and appears dependent on duration of treatment and on estrogen dose. There is no significant increased risk associated with the use of estrogens for less than one year. The greatest risk appears associated with prolonged use, with increased risks of 15- to 24-fold for five years or more. In three studies, persistence of risk was demonstrated for 8 to over 15 years after cessation of estrogen treatment. In one study, a significant decrease in the incidence of endometrial cancer occurred six months after estrogen withdrawal.

A large clinical trial has demonstrated that when MPA is administered with Premarin, there is a markedly reduced incidence of endometrial hyperplasia, a possible precursor of endometrial cancer. Endometrial hyperplasia has been reported in a large clinical trial to occur at a rate of approximately 1% or less with PREMPHASE. Studies have also demonstrated a reduced risk of endometrial cancer when a progestin is administered with estrogen replacement therapy. In the large clinical trial described above, only a single case of endometrial cancer was reported to occur among women taking combination Premarin/MPA therapy.

Clinical surveillance of all women taking estrogen/progestin combinations is important. Adequate diagnostic measures, including endometrial sampling when indicated, should be undertaken to rule out malignancy in all cases of undiagnosed persistent or recurring abnormal vaginal bleeding.

2. *Cardiovascular disease.* Large doses of estrogens (5 mg conjugated estrogens per day), comparable to those used to treat cancer of the prostate and breast, have been shown in a large prospective clinical trial in men to increase the risk of nonfatal myocardial infarction, pulmonary embolism, and thrombophlebitis. These risks cannot necessarily be extrapolated from men to women or from unopposed estrogen to combination estrogen/progestin therapy. However, to avoid the theoretical cardiovascular risk to women caused by high estrogen doses, the dose for estrogen replacement therapy should not exceed the lowest effective dose.

3. *Effects during pregnancy.* Use in pregnancy is not recommended. See Boxed Warning.

4. *Gallbladder disease.* Two studies have reported a 2- to 4-fold increase in the risk of surgically confirmed gallbladder disease in women receiving postmenopausal estrogens. In a large clinical trial, 5 of 1029 subjects taking Premarin/Cycrin® at doses comparable to PREMPHASE developed cholecystitis with cholelithiasis that required cholecystectomy.

5. *Elevated blood pressure.* Occasional blood pressure increases during estrogen replacement therapy have been attributed to idiosyncratic reactions to estrogens. More often, blood pressure has remained the same or has dropped. One study showed that postmenopausal estrogen users had higher blood pressure than nonusers. In a large clinical trial, transient elevations from baseline of 40 mm Hg or more systolic and 20 mm Hg or more diastolic were reported in less than 2% and 4% of postmenopausal subjects, respectively. Two other studies showed slightly lower blood pressure among estrogen users compared to nonusers. Postmenopausal estrogen use does not increase the risk of stroke. Nonetheless, blood pressure should be monitored at regular intervals with estrogen use.

TABLE 1. PHARMACOKINETIC PARAMETERS FOR UNCONJUGATED AND CONJUGATED ESTROGENS, AND MEDROXYPROGESTERONE ACETATE

Pharmacokinetic Profile of Unconjugated Estrogens
Following a Dose of 2 × 0.625 mg CE/5 mg MPA Combination Tablets

Drug	C_{max} (pg/mL) ±SD	t_{max} (h) ±SD	$t_{1/2}$ (h) ±SD	AUC (pg•h/mL) ±SD
estrone	124 ±53	10.0 ±3.5	62.2 ±85.2	6303 ±2542
baseline-adjusted estrone	104 ±51	10.0 ±3.5	26.0 ±25.9	3136 ±1598
equilin	54 ±23	8.9 ±3.0	15.5 ±8.2	1179 ±540

Pharmacokinetic Profile of Conjugated Estrogens
Following a Dose of 2 × 0.625 mg CE/5 mg MPA Combination Tablets

Drug	C_{max} (ng/mL) ±SD	t_{max} (h) ±SD	$t_{1/2}$ (h) ±SD	AUC (ng•h/mL) ±SD
total estrone	6.3 ±3.0	9.1 ±2.6	23.6 ±8.4	151 ±63
baseline-adjusted total estrone	6.2 ±3.0	9.1 ±2.6	20.6 ±7.3	139 ±56
total equilin	4.2 ±2.2	7.0 ±2.5	17.2 ±22.6	72 ±36

Pharmacokinetic Profile of MPA
Following a Dose of 2 × 0.625 mg CE/5 mg MPA Combination Tablets

Drug	C_{max} (ng/mL) ±SD	t_{max} (h) ±SD	$t_{1/2}$ (h) ±SD	Cl/F (L/h/kg) ±SD
medroxyprogesterone acetate	4.8 ±1.5	2.4 ±1.2	46.3 ±18.0	1.6 ±0.5

C_{max} = peak plasma concentration
t_{max} = time peak concentration occurs
$t_{1/2}$ = terminal-phase disposition half-life $(0.693/\lambda_z)$
AUC = total area under the curve
Cl/F = apparent oral clearance

6. *Hypercalcemia.* Administration of estrogens may lead to severe hypercalcemia in patients with breast cancer and bone metastases. If this occurs, the drugs should be stopped and appropriate measures taken to reduce the serum calcium level.

7. *Thromboembolic disorders.* The physician should be alert to the earliest manifestations of thrombotic disorders (thrombophlebitis, cerebrovascular disorders, pulmonary embolism, and retinal thrombosis). Should any of these occur or be suspected, the drugs should be discontinued immediately.

8. *Visual abnormalities.* Discontinue medication pending examination if there is sudden partial or complete loss of vision, or a sudden onset of proptosis, diplopia, or migraine. If examination reveals papilledema or retinal vascular lesions, medication should be withdrawn.

PRECAUTIONS
GENERAL
Based on experience with estrogens and/or progestins:

1. *Cardiovascular risk.* A causal relationship between estrogen replacement therapy and reduction of cardiovascular disease in postmenopausal women has not been proven. Furthermore, the effect of added progestins on this putative benefit is not yet known.

In recent years many published studies have suggested that there may be a cause-effect relationship between postmenopausal oral estrogen replacement therapy *without added progestins* and a decrease in cardiovascular disease in women. Although most of the observational studies which assessed this statistical association have reported a 20% to 50% reduction in coronary heart disease risk and associated mortality in estrogen takers, the following should be considered when interpreting these reports.

Because only one of these studies was randomized and it was too small to yield statistically significant results, all relevant studies were subject to selection bias. Thus, the apparently reduced risk of coronary artery disease cannot be attributed with certainty to estrogen replacement therapy. It may instead have been caused by life-style and medical characteristics of the women studied with the result that healthier women were selected for estrogen therapy. In general, treated women were of higher socioeconomic and educational status, more slender, more physically active, more likely to have undergone surgical menopause, and less likely to have diabetes than the untreated women. Although some studies attempted to control for these selection factors, it is common for properly designed randomized trials to fail to confirm benefits suggested by less rigorous study designs. Thus, ongoing and future large-scale randomized trials may fail to confirm this apparent benefit.

Current medical practice often includes the use of concomitant progestin therapy in women with intact uteri. While the effects of added progestins on the risk of ischemic heart disease are not known, medroxyprogesterone acetate at the dose in PREMPHASE attenuates much of the favorable effect of conjugated estrogens on HDL levels, although it maintains the favorable effect of conjugated estrogens on LDL levels (see **Clinical Pharmacology**).

While the effects of added progestins on the risk of breast cancer are also unknown, available epidemiologic evidence suggests that progestins do not reduce, and may enhance, the moderately increased breast cancer risk that has been reported with prolonged estrogen replacement therapy (see **Warnings**).

The safety data regarding PREMPHASE were obtained primarily from clinical trials and epidemiologic studies of postmenopausal Caucasian women, who were at generally low risk for cardiovascular disease and higher than average risk for osteoporosis. The safety profile of PREMPHASE derived from these study populations cannot necessarily be extrapolated to other populations of diverse racial and/or demographic composition. When considering prescribing PREMPHASE, physicians are advised to weigh the potential benefits and risks of therapy as applicable to each individual patient.

2. *Use in hysterectomized women.* Existing data do not support the use of the combination of estrogen and progestin in postmenopausal women without a uterus. There are possible risks which may be associated with the inclusion of progestin in estrogen replacement regimens. The potential risks include some deterioration in glucose tolerance, as reported in a large clinical trial of PREMPHASE, and less favorable effects on lipid metabolism as compared to the lipid effects of Premarin alone (see **Clinical Pharmacology**).

3. *Physical examination.* A complete medical and family history should be taken prior to the initiation of any estrogen/progestin therapy. The pretreatment and periodic physical examinations should include special reference to blood pressure, breasts, abdomen, and pelvic organs, and should include a Papanicolaou smear. As a general rule, estrogen should not be prescribed for longer than one year without another physical examination being performed.

4. *Fluid retention.* Because estrogens/progestins may cause some degree of fluid retention, conditions which might be influenced by this factor, such as asthma, epilepsy, migraine,

and cardiac or renal dysfunction, require careful observation.

5. *Uterine bleeding.* Certain patients may develop abnormal uterine bleeding. In cases of undiagnosed abnormal uterine bleeding, adequate diagnostic measures are indicated. (See **Warnings**.)

6. The pathologist should be advised of estrogen/progestin therapy when relevant specimens are submitted.

Based on experience with estrogens:

1. *Familial hyperlipoproteinemia.* Estrogen therapy may be associated with massive elevations of plasma triglycerides leading to pancreatitis and other complications in patients with familial defects of lipoprotein metabolism.

2. *Hypercoagulability.* Some studies have shown that women taking estrogen replacement therapy have hypercoagulability primarily related to decreased antithrombin activity. This effect appears dose- and duration-dependent and is less pronounced than that associated with oral contraceptive use. Also, postmenopausal women tend to have changes in levels of coagulation parameters at baseline compared to premenopausal women. There is some suggestion that low-dose mestranol may increase the risk of thromboembolism in postmenopausal women, although the majority of studies (of primarily conjugated estrogens users) report no such increase. There is insufficient information on hypercoagulability in women who have had previous thromboembolic disease. In a large clinical trial of PREMPHASE, factors VII and X concentrations and plasminogen activity increased by 8%, 13%, and 14% over baseline, respectively, and antithrombin III activity decreased approximately 1% from baseline.

3. *Mastodynia.* Certain patients may develop undesirable manifestations of estrogenic stimulation such as mastodynia. In a large clinical trial of PREMPHASE, approximately one third of the subjects reported breast pain during treatment with PREMPHASE, versus 12% for Premarin alone.

Based on experience with progestins:

1. *Lipoprotein metabolism.* See **Clinical Pharmacology**.

2. *Impaired glucose tolerance.* See **Use in hysterectomized women**, above.

3. *Depression.* Patients who have a history of depression should be observed and the drugs discontinued if the depression recurs to a serious degree.

INFORMATION FOR THE PATIENT
See text of Patient Package Insert which appears after the **How Supplied** section.

DRUG/LABORATORY TEST INTERACTIONS
1. Accelerated prothrombin time, partial thromboplastin time, and platelet aggregation time; increased platelet count; increased factors II, VII antigen, VIII coagulant activity, IX, X, XII, VII-X complex, II-VII-X complex, and beta-thromboglobulin; decreased levels of anti-factor Xa and antithrombin III, decreased antithrombin III activity; increased levels of fibrinogen and fibrinogen activity; increased plasminogen antigen and activity.

2. Increased thyroid-binding globulin (TBG) leading to increased circulating total thyroid hormone, as measured by protein-bound iodine (PBI), T_4 levels (by column or by radioimmunoassay) or T_3 levels by radioimmunoassay. T_3 resin uptake is decreased, reflecting the elevated TBG. Free T_4 and free T_3 concentrations are unaltered.

3. Other binding proteins may be elevated in serum, i.e., corticosteroid binding globulin (CBG), sex hormone-binding globulin (SHBG), leading to increased circulating corticosteroids and sex steroids respectively. Free or biologically active hormone concentrations are unchanged. Other plasma proteins may be increased (angiotensinogen/renin substrate, alpha-1-antitrypsin, ceruloplasmin).

4. Increased plasma HDL and HDL-2 subfraction concentrations, reduced LDL cholesterol concentration, increased triglyceride levels.

5. Impaired glucose tolerance. For this reason, diabetic patients should be carefully observed while receiving estrogen/progestin therapy.

6. Reduced response to metyrapone test.

7. Reduced serum folate concentration.

8. Aminoglutethimide administered concomitantly with MPA may significantly depress the bioavailability of MPA.

CARCINOGENESIS, MUTAGENESIS, AND IMPAIRMENT OF FERTILITY
Long term continuous administration of natural and synthetic estrogens in certain animal species increases the frequency of carcinomas of the breasts, uterus, cervix, vagina, testis, and liver. (See **Contraindications** and **Warnings**.)

In a two-year oral study of MPA in which female rats were exposed to dosages of up to 5000 µg/kg/day in their diets (50 times higher—based on AUC values—than the level observed experimentally in women taking 10 mg of MPA), a dose-related increase in pancreatic islet cell tumors (adenomas and carcinomas) occurred. Pancreatic tumor incidence was increased at 1000 and 5000 µg/kg/day, but not at 200 µg/kg/day.

A decreased incidence of spontaneous mammary gland tumors was observed in all three MPA-treated groups, compared to controls, in the two-year rat study. The mechanism

for the decreased incidence of mammary gland tumors observed in the MPA-treated rats may be linked to the significant decrease in serum prolactin concentration observed in rats.

Beagle dogs treated with MPA developed mammary nodules, some of which were malignant. Although nodules occasionally appeared in control animals, they were intermittent in nature, whereas the nodules in the drug-treated animals were larger, more numerous, persistent, and there were some breast malignancies with metastases. It is known that progestogens stimulate synthesis and release of growth hormone in dogs. The growth hormone, along with the progestogen, stimulates mammary growth and tumors. In contrast, growth hormone in humans is not increased, nor does growth hormone have any significant mammotrophic role. Therefore, the MPA-induced increase of mammary tumors in dogs probably has no significance to humans. No pancreatic tumors occurred in dogs.

PREGNANCY CATEGORY X
Estrogens/progestins should not be used during pregnancy. See **Contraindications** and Boxed Warning.

NURSING MOTHERS
As a general principle, the administration of any drug to nursing mothers should be done only when clearly necessary since many drugs are excreted in human milk. Estrogen administration to nursing mothers has been shown to decrease the quantity and quality of the milk. Detectable amounts of progestin have been identified in the milk of mothers receiving the drug. The effect of this on the nursing infant has not been determined.

ADVERSE REACTIONS
(See **Warnings** regarding induction of neoplasia, adverse effects on the fetus, increased incidence of gallbladder disease, elevated blood pressure, thromboembolic disorders, cardiovascular disease, visual abnormalities, and hypercalcemia and **Precautions** for cardiovascular disease.)

The following adverse reactions have been reported with estrogen and/or progestin therapy:

Genitourinary system. Changes in vaginal bleeding pattern and abnormal withdrawal bleeding or flow, breakthrough bleeding, spotting, change in amount of cervical secretion, premenstrual-like syndrome, cystitis-like syndrome, increase in size of uterine leiomyomata, vaginal candidiasis, amenorrhea, changes in cervical erosion.

Breasts. Tenderness, enlargement, galactorrhea.

Gastrointestinal. Nausea, cholestatic jaundice, changes in appetite, vomiting, abdominal cramps, bloating, increased incidence of gallbladder disease, pancreatitis.

Skin. Chloasma or melasma that may persist when drug is discontinued, erythema multiforme, erythema nodosum, hemorrhagic eruption, loss of scalp hair, hirsutism, itching, urticaria, pruritus, generalized rash, rash (allergic) with and without pruritus, acne.

Cardiovascular. In susceptible individuals, change in blood pressure, thrombophlebitis, pulmonary embolism, cerebral thrombosis and embolism.

CNS. Headache, dizziness, mental depression, nervousness, migraine, chorea, insomnia, somnolence.

Eyes. Neuro-ocular lesions, e.g., retinal thrombosis and optic neuritis. Steepening of corneal curvature, intolerance of contact lenses.

Miscellaneous. Increase or decrease in weight, edema, changes in libido, fatigue, backache, reduced carbohydrate tolerance, aggravation of porphyria, pyrexia, anaphylactoid reactions, anaphylaxis.

ACUTE OVERDOSAGE
Serious ill effects have not been reported following acute ingestion of large doses of estrogen/progestin-containing oral contraceptives by young children. Overdosage may cause nausea and vomiting, and withdrawal bleeding may occur in females.

DOSAGE AND ADMINISTRATION
PREMPHASE® therapy consists of two separate tablets; one maroon 0.625 mg Premarin® tablet taken daily on days 1 through 14 and one light-blue tablet, containing 0.625 mg conjugated estrogens and 5 mg of medroxyprogesterone acetate, taken on days 15 through 28.

1. For treatment of moderate to severe vasomotor symptoms and vulvar and vaginal atrophy associated with menopause. Patients should be reevaluated at 3-month to 6-month intervals to determine if treatment for symptoms is still necessary.

2. For prevention of osteoporosis. Treated patients with an intact uterus should be monitored closely for signs of endometrial cancer, and appropriate diagnostic measures should be taken to rule out malignancy in the event of persistent or recurring abnormal vaginal bleeding.

HOW SUPPLIED
PREMPHASE® therapy consists of two separate tablets; one maroon Premarin® tablet taken daily on days 1

Continued on next page

Wyeth-Ayerst Laboratories—Cont.

through 14 and one light-blue tablet taken on days 15 through 28.

Each carton contains 2 blister cards. One blister card contains 14 oval, maroon Premarin tablets containing 0.625 mg of conjugated estrogens for oral administration. The second blister card contains 14 oval, light-blue tablets which contain 0.625 mg of the conjugated estrogens found in Premarin tablets and 5 mg of medroxyprogesterone acetate for oral administration.

The appearance of Premarin® tablets is a trademark of Wyeth-Ayerst Laboratories. The appearance of the conjugated estrogens/medroxyprogesterone acetate combination tablets is a registered trademark.

Store at room temperature, 20° C–25° C (68° F–77° F).

INFORMATION FOR THE PATIENT

> ESTROGENS INCREASE THE RISK OF CANCER OF THE UTERUS IN WOMEN WHO HAVE HAD THEIR MENOPAUSE ("CHANGE OF LIFE"). THIS FINDING REFERS TO ESTROGENS GIVEN WITHOUT PROGESTIN.
>
> Progestin drugs taken with estrogen-containing drugs significantly reduce but do not eliminate this risk. If you use any estrogen-containing drug, it is important to visit your doctor regularly and report any unusual vaginal bleeding right away. Vaginal bleeding after menopause may be a warning sign of uterine cancer. Your doctor should evaluate any unusual vaginal bleeding to find out the cause.
>
> **ESTROGENS/PROGESTINS SHOULD NOT BE USED DURING PREGNANCY.**
>
> Estrogens and progestins do not prevent miscarriage (spontaneous abortion) and are not needed in the days following childbirth. If you take estrogens during pregnancy your unborn child has a greater than usual chance of having birth defects. The risk of developing these defects is small, but clearly larger than the risk in children whose mothers did not take estrogens during pregnancy. These birth defects may affect the baby's urinary system and sex organs. Daughters born to mothers who took DES (an estrogen drug) have a higher than usual chance of developing cancer of the vagina or cervix when they become teenagers or young adults. Sons may have a higher than usual chance of developing cancer of the testicles when they become teenagers or young adults.
>
> There is an increased risk of birth defects in children whose mothers take this drug during the first four months of pregnancy. Several reports suggest an association between mothers who take these drugs in the first trimester of pregnancy and genital abnormalities in male and female babies. The risk to the male baby is the possibility of being born with a condition in which the opening of the penis is on the underside rather than the tip of the penis (hypospadias). Hypospadias occurs in about 5 to 8 per 1,000 male births and is about doubled with exposure to these drugs. There is not enough information to quantify the risk to exposed female fetuses. However, enlargement of the clitoris and fusion of the labia may occur, although rarely.
>
> Therefore, since drugs of this type may induce mild masculinization of the external genitalia of the female fetus, as well as hypospadias in the male fetus, it is wise to avoid using the drug during the first trimester of pregnancy. These drugs have been used as a test for pregnancy, but such use is no longer considered safe because of possible damage to a developing baby. Also, more rapid methods for testing for pregnancy are now available. If you take PREMPHASE and later find you were pregnant when you took it, be sure to discuss this with your doctor as soon as possible.

Your physician has prescribed PREMPHASE, a combination of two hormones, an estrogen and a progestin. This leaflet describes the major benefits and risks of your treatment, as well as how and when treatment should be taken.

PREMPHASE replaces the hormones in your body which naturally decrease at menopause. The hormone combination you will be taking has been shown to provide the benefits of estrogen replacement therapy while lowering the frequency of a possible precancerous condition of the uterine lining. This therapy is not intended for women who have had a hysterectomy (surgical removal of the uterus).

Estrogens have several important uses but also some risks. You must decide, with your doctor, whether the risks of estrogens are acceptable when weighed against their benefits. The length of treatment with estrogens can vary from woman to woman. Check with your doctor to make sure you are using the lowest possible effective dose.

With PREMPHASE therapy several menstrual-like bleeding patterns may occur. These may range from absence of bleeding to irregular bleeding. If bleeding occurs, it is frequently light spotting or moderate menstrual-like bleeding, but it may be heavy. If you experience vaginal bleeding while taking PREMPHASE, you should discuss your bleeding pattern with your doctor and set up an appropriate schedule for follow-up care.

USES OF ESTROGEN

To reduce moderate to severe menopausal symptoms. Estrogens are hormones produced by the ovaries of normal women. When a woman is between the ages of 45 and 55, the ovaries normally stop making estrogens. This leads to a drop in body estrogen levels that causes the "change of life" or menopause (the end of monthly menstrual periods). A sudden drop in estrogen levels also occurs if both ovaries are removed during an operation before natural menopause takes place. This is referred to as "surgical menopause."

When the estrogen levels begin dropping, some women develop very uncomfortable symptoms, such as feelings of warmth in the face, neck, and chest, or sudden intense episodes of heat and sweating ("hot flashes" or "hot flushes"). Using estrogen drugs can help the body adjust to lower estrogen levels and reduce these symptoms. In some women the symptoms are mild; in others they can be severe. These symptoms may last only a few months or longer. Taking PREMPHASE can alleviate these symptoms. If you are not taking hormones for other reasons, such as the prevention of osteoporosis, you should take PREMPHASE only as long as you need it for relief from your menopausal symptoms.

To prevent thinning of bones. Osteoporosis is a thinning of the bones that makes them weaker and allows them to break more easily. The bones of the spine, wrists, and hips break most often in osteoporosis. Both men and women start to lose bone mass after about age 40, but women lose bone mass faster after the menopause. Using estrogens after the menopause slows down bone thinning and may prevent bones from breaking. Lifelong adequate calcium intake, either from diet (such as dairy products) or from calcium supplements (to reach a total daily intake of 1000 milligrams per day before menopause or 1500 milligrams per day after menopause), may help to prevent osteoporosis. Regular weight-bearing exercise (like walking and running for an hour, two or three times a week) may also help to prevent osteoporosis. Before you change your calcium intake or exercise habits, it is important to discuss these lifestyle changes with your doctor to find out if they are safe for you.

Since estrogen use has some risks, only women who are likely to develop osteoporosis should use estrogens for prevention. Women who are likely to develop osteoporosis often have the following characteristics:

- White or Asian race
- Small, slim body frame
- Cigarette-smoking habit
- Family history of osteoporosis (in a mother, sister, or aunt)
- Early menopause either natural or because of surgical removal of ovaries ("surgical menopause")

To treat vulvar and vaginal atrophy (itching, burning, dryness in or around the vagina, difficulty or burning on urination) associated with menopause.

WHO SHOULD NOT USE ESTROGENS

During pregnancy (see Boxed Warning). If you think you may be pregnant, do not use any form of estrogen-containing drug. Using estrogens while you are pregnant may cause your unborn child to have birth defects. Estrogens do not prevent miscarriage.

If you have unusual vaginal bleeding which has not been evaluated by your doctor (see Boxed Warning). Unusual vaginal bleeding can be a warning sign of cancer of the uterus, especially if it happens after menopause. Your doctor must find out the cause of the bleeding so that he or she can recommend the proper treatment. Taking estrogens without visiting your doctor can cause you serious harm if your vaginal bleeding is caused by cancer of the uterus.

If you have had cancer. Since estrogens increase the risk of certain types of cancer, you should not use estrogens if you have ever had cancer of the breast or uterus.

If you have any circulation problems. Estrogen drugs should not be used except in unusually special situations in which your doctor decides that you need estrogen therapy so much that the risks are acceptable. Women with abnormal blood clotting conditions should avoid estrogen use (see **Risks of Estrogens and/or Progestins**).

When they do not work. During menopause, some women develop nervous symptoms or depression. Estrogens do not relieve these symptoms. You may have heard that taking estrogens for years after menopause will keep your skin soft and supple and keep you feeling young. There is no evidence for these claims and such long-term estrogen use may have serious risks.

After childbirth or when breastfeeding a baby. Estrogen should not be used to try to stop the breast from filling with milk after a baby is born. Such treatment may increase the risk of developing blood clots (see **Risks of Estrogens and/or Progestins**).

If you are breastfeeding, you should avoid using any drugs because many drugs pass through to the baby in the milk. While nursing a baby, you should take drugs only on the advice of your health-care provider.

RISKS OF ESTROGENS AND/OR PROGESTINS

Cancer of the uterus. The risk of cancer of the uterus increases when estrogens are used alone, the longer they are used, and when larger doses are taken. There is a higher risk of cancer of the uterus if you are overweight, diabetic, or have high blood pressure. The hormone combination you will be taking contains estrogen and progestin. This combination has been shown to provide the benefits of estrogen replacement therapy for the **Uses of Estrogen** listed above, while reducing the risk of a precancerous condition of the uterine lining (see **Other Information,** below).

However, additional risks may be associated with the inclusion of a progestin in estrogen treatment. The possible risks include less favorable effects on blood fats as compared to Premarin alone, unfavorable effects on blood sugars, and a possible increase in breast cancer risk (see *Cancer of the breast,* below). Usually, the smaller the dose and the shorter the duration of treatment, the more these effects are minimized. Check with your doctor to make sure you are using the lowest effective dose and only for as long as you need it. If you have had your uterus removed, there is no risk of developing cancer of the uterus and no benefit to be gained by using a combination estrogen/progestin product.

Cancer of the breast. Most studies have not shown a higher risk of breast cancer in women who have ever used estrogens. However, some studies have reported that breast cancer developed more often (up to twice the usual rate) in women who used estrogens for long periods of time (especially more than 10 years), or who used high doses for shorter time periods. The effects of added progestin on the risk of breast cancer are unknown. Some studies have reported a somewhat increased risk, even higher than the possible risk associated with estrogens alone. Others have not. Regular breast examinations by a health professional and monthly self-examination are recommended for all women. Regular mammograms are recommended for all women over 50 years of age.

Gallbladder disease. Women who use estrogens after menopause are more likely to develop gallbladder disease needing surgery than women who do not use estrogens.

Inflammation of the pancreas. Women with high triglyceride levels may have an increased risk of developing inflammation of the pancreas.

Abnormal blood clotting. Taking estrogens may cause changes in your blood clotting system. These changes allow the blood to clot more easily, possibly allowing clots to form in your bloodstream. If blood clots do form in your bloodstream, they can cut off the blood supply to vital organs, causing serious problems. These problems may include a stroke (by cutting off blood to the brain), a heart attack (by cutting off blood to the heart), a pulmonary embolus (by cutting off blood to the lungs), or other problems. Any of these conditions may cause death or serious long-term disability. However, most studies of low-dose estrogen use by women do not show an increased risk of these complications.

Excess calcium in the blood. Taking estrogens may lead to severe hypercalcemia in women with breast and/or bone cancer.

During pregnancy. There is an increased risk of birth defects in children whose mothers take this drug during the first four months of pregnancy. Several reports suggest an association between mothers who take these drugs in the first trimester of pregnancy and genital abnormalities in male and female babies. The risk to the male baby is the possibility of being born with a condition in which the opening of the penis is on the underside rather than the tip of the penis (hypospadias). Hypospadias occurs in about 5 to 8 per 1,000 male births and is about doubled with exposure to these drugs. There is not enough information to quantify the risk to exposed female fetuses. However, enlargement of the clitoris and fusion of the labia may occur, although rarely.

Therefore, since drugs of this type may induce mild masculinization of the external genitalia of the female fetus, as well as hypospadias in the male fetus, it is wise to avoid using the drug during the first trimester of pregnancy. These drugs have been used as a test for pregnancy, but such use is no longer considered safe because of possible damage to a developing baby. Also, more rapid methods for testing for pregnancy are now available. If you take PREMPHASE and later find you were pregnant when you took it, be sure to discuss this with your doctor as soon as possible.

SIDE EFFECTS WITH ESTROGENS AND/OR PROGESTINS

In addition to the risks listed above, the following side effects have been reported with estrogen and/or progestin use:

- Nausea, vomiting, pain, cramps, swelling, or tenderness in the abdomen.
- Yellowing of the skin and/or whites of the eyes.
- Breast tenderness or enlargement.
- Enlargement of benign tumors ("fibroids") of the uterus.

- Irregular bleeding or spotting.
- Change in amount of cervical secretion.
- Vaginal yeast infections.
- Retention of excess fluid. This may make some conditions worsen, such as asthma, epilepsy, migraine, heart disease, or kidney disease.
- A spotty darkening of the skin, particularly on the face; reddening of the skin; skin rashes.
- Worsening of porphyria.
- Headache, migraines, dizziness, faintness, or changes in vision (including intolerance to contact lenses).
- Mental depression.
- Involuntary muscle spasms.
- Hair loss or abnormal hairiness.
- Increase or decrease in weight.
- Changes in sex drive.
- Possible changes in blood sugar.

REDUCING THE RISKS OF ESTROGEN/PROGESTIN

If you decide to take an estrogen/progestin combination, you can reduce your risks by carefully monitoring your treatment.

See your doctor regularly. While you are taking PREMPHASE, it is important to visit your doctor at least once a year for a checkup. If you develop vaginal bleeding while taking estrogens, you may need further evaluation. If members of your family have had breast cancer or if you have ever had breast lumps or an abnormal mammogram (breast X ray), you may need to have more frequent breast examinations.

Reassess your need for treatment. You and your doctor should reevaluate whether or not you still need estrogens at least every six months.

Be alert for signs of trouble. If any of these warning signals (or any other unusual symptoms) happen while you are using estrogen/progestin, call your doctor immediately:

- Abnormal bleeding from the vagina (possible uterine abnormality).
- Pains in the calves or chest, a sudden shortness of breath or coughing blood (indicating possible clots in the legs, heart, or lungs).
- Severe headache or vomiting, dizziness, faintness, or changes in vision or speech, weakness or numbness of an arm or leg (indicating possible clots in the brain or eye).
- Breast lumps (possible breast cancer; ask your doctor or health professional to show you how to examine your breasts monthly).
- Yellowing of the skin and/or whites of the eyes (possible liver problems).
- Pain, swelling, or tenderness in the abdomen (possible gallbladder problem).

OTHER INFORMATION

1. Estrogens increase the risk of developing a condition (endometrial hyperplasia) that may lead to cancer of the lining of the uterus. Taking progestins, another hormonal drug, with estrogens lowers the risk of developing this condition. Therefore, since your uterus has not been removed, your doctor has prescribed PREMPHASE, which includes both a progestin and estrogens.

You should know, however, that taking estrogens *with* progestins may have unhealthy effects on blood sugar, which might make a diabetic condition worse.

Additional risks include a possible further increase in breast cancer risk which may be associated with long-term estrogen use.

Some research has shown that estrogens taken *without* progestins may protect women against developing heart disease. However, this is not certain. The protection shown may have been caused by the characteristics of the estrogen-treated women and not by the estrogen treatment itself. In general, treated women were slimmer, more physically active, and were less likely to have diabetes than the untreated women. These characteristics are known to protect against heart disease.

You are cautioned to discuss very carefully with your doctor or health-care provider all the possible risks and benefits of long-term estrogen and progestin treatment as they affect you personally.

2. Your doctor has prescribed this drug for you and you alone. Do not give the drug to anyone else.
3. If you will be taking calcium supplements as part of the treatment to help prevent osteoporosis, check with your doctor about the amounts recommended.
4. Keep this and all drugs out of the reach of children. In case of overdose, call your doctor, hospital, or poison control center immediately.
5. This leaflet provides the most important information about PREMPHASE. If you want to read more, ask your doctor or pharmacist to let you read the professional labeling. The professional labeling is also published in a book called *The Physicians' Desk Reference*, which is available in bookstores and public libraries.

HOW SUPPLIED

Your doctor has prescribed PREMPHASE®, a combination of two separate tablets; one maroon Premarin® tablet taken daily on days 1 through 14 and one light-blue tablet taken on days 15 through 28.

Each carton contains 2 blister cards. One blister card contains 14 oval, maroon Premarin® tablets containing 0.625 mg of conjugated estrogens for oral administration. The second blister card contains 14 oval, light-blue tablets which contain 0.625 mg of the conjugated estrogens found in Premarin tablets and 5 mg of medroxyprogesterone acetate for oral administration.

The appearance of Premarin® tablets is a trademark of Wyeth-Ayerst Laboratories. The appearance of the conjugated estrogens/medroxyprogesterone acetate combination tablets is a registered trademark.

Store at room temperature, 20° C–25° C (68° F–77° F).

Shown in Product Identification Guide, page 341

PREMPRO™ ℞

(conjugated estrogens/medroxyprogesterone acetate tablets)

Caution: Federal law prohibits dispensing without prescription.

ESTROGENS HAVE BEEN REPORTED TO INCREASE THE RISK OF ENDOMETRIAL CARCINOMA IN POSTMENOPAUSAL WOMEN. THIS FINDING REFERS TO ESTROGENS GIVEN WITHOUT PROGESTIN.

Progestins taken with estrogen drugs significantly reduce but do not eliminate this risk. Close clinical surveillance of all women taking estrogens is important. Adequate diagnostic measures, including endometrial sampling when indicated, should be undertaken to rule out malignancy in all cases of undiagnosed persistent or recurring abnormal vaginal bleeding. There is no evidence that "natural" estrogens are more or less hazardous than "synthetic" estrogens at equiestrogenic doses.

ESTROGENS/PROGESTINS SHOULD NOT BE USED DURING PREGNANCY.

There is no indication for estrogen therapy during pregnancy or during the immediate postpartum period. Estrogen therapy during pregnancy is associated with an increased risk of congenital defects in the reproductive organs of the fetus, and possibly other birth defects. Estrogens are not indicated for the prevention of postpartum breast engorgement.

Studies of women who received diethylstilbestrol (DES) during pregnancy have shown that female offspring have an increased risk of vaginal adenosis, squamous cell dysplasia of the uterine cervix, and clear cell vaginal cancer later in life; male offspring have an increased risk of urogenital abnormalities and possibly testicular cancer later in life. The 1985 DES Task Force concluded that use of DES during pregnancy is associated with subsequent increased risk of breast cancer in the mothers, although a causal relationship remains unproven and the observed level of excess risk is similar to that for a number of other breast cancer risk factors.

Several reports also suggest an association between intrauterine exposure to progestational drugs in the first trimester of pregnancy and genital abnormalities in male and female fetuses. The risk of hypospadias, 5 to 8 per 1000 male births in the general population, may be approximately doubled with exposure to these drugs. There are insufficient data to quantify the risk to exposed female fetuses; some of these drugs induce mild virilization of the external genitalia of the female fetus. If the patient is exposed to PREMPRO™ (conjugated estrogens/medroxyprogesterone acetate) during pregnancy, or if she becomes pregnant while taking these drugs, she should be apprised of the potential risks to the fetus.

Estrogens are ineffective for the prevention or treatment of threatened or habitual abortion. There is no adequate evidence that progestational agents are effective in preventing habitual abortion when such drugs are given during the first trimester of pregnancy. Furthermore, in the vast majority of women, the cause of abortion is a defective ovum, which progestational agents could not be expected to influence. In addition, the use of progestational agents with their uterine-relaxant properties, in patients with fertilized defective ova, may cause a delay in spontaneous abortion.

DESCRIPTION

PREMPRO therapy consists of a single tablet containing 0.625 mg of the conjugated estrogens found in Premarin® tablets and 2.5 mg of medroxyprogesterone acetate (MPA) for oral administration.

The conjugated estrogens found in Premarin tablets are a mixture of sodium estrone sulfate and sodium equilin sulfate. They contain as concomitant components sodium sulfate conjugates 17α-dihydroequilin, 17α-estradiol and 17β-dihydroequilin.

Medroxyprogesterone acetate is a derivative of progesterone. It is a white to off-white, odorless, crystalline powder, stable in air, melting between 200° C and 210° C. It is freely soluble in chloroform, soluble in acetone and in dioxane, sparingly soluble in alcohol and in methanol, slightly soluble in ether, and insoluble in water. The chemical name for MPA is pregn-4-ene-3,20-dione, 17-(acetyloxy)-6-methyl-, (6α)-.

Each peach tablet for oral administration contains 0.625 mg conjugated estrogens, 2.5 mg of medroxyprogesterone acetate and the following inactive ingredients: calcium phosphate tribasic, calcium sulfate, carnauba wax, cellulose, glyceryl monooleate, lactose, magnesium stearate, methylcellulose, pharmaceutical glaze, polyethylene glycol, sucrose, povidone, titanium dioxide, red ferric oxide.

CLINICAL PHARMACOLOGY

Estrogens are important in the development and maintenance of the female reproductive system and secondary sex characteristics. By a direct action, they cause growth and development of the uterus, fallopian tubes, and vagina. With other hormones, such as pituitary hormones and progesterone, they cause enlargement of the breasts through promotion of ductal growth, stromal development, and the accretion of fat. Estrogens are intricately involved with other hormones, especially progesterone, in the processes of the ovulatory menstrual cycle and pregnancy and affect the release of pituitary gonadotropins. They also contribute to the shaping of the skeleton, maintenance of tone and elasticity of urogenital structures, changes in the epiphyses of the long bones that allow for the pubertal growth spurt and its termination, and pigmentation of the nipples and genitals.

The use of unopposed estrogen therapy has been associated with an increased risk of endometrial hyperplasia, a possible precursor of endometrial adenocarcinoma. The results of clinical studies indicate that the addition of a progestin to an estrogen replacement regimen for more than 10 days per cycle reduces the incidence of endometrial hyperplasia and the attendant risk of adenocarcinoma in women with intact uteri. The addition of a progestin to an estrogen replacement regimen has not been shown to interfere with the efficacy of estrogen replacement therapy for its approved indications. Data from a large clinical trial indicate that MPA administered in the recommended dose to women receiving Premarin 0.625 mg reduces the incidence of hyperplastic changes and hence reduces the risk of developing adenocarcinoma. This is the clinical rationale for PREMPRO.

The following table summarizes the incidence of endometrial hyperplasia after 1 year of treatment with the combined regimens.

[See table below.]

In a one-year clinical trial of 340 women using PREMPRO, the incidence of amenorrhea increased over time. Sixteen to twenty percent of the patients experienced amenorrhea during the entire 13 cycles of the study. The following describes cumulative amenorrhea which is defined as amenorrhea continuing from a given cycle to the end of the study. Of 278 women who completed the study, the incidence of cumulative amenorrhea from cycle 9 through 13 was 49%. Based on analysis of all enrolled patients, the incidence of cumulative amenorrhea in cycles 9 through 13 was 40%. This includes 59 dropouts; of the 59 dropouts 9 discontinued for reasons relating to bleeding and 16 had amenor-

INCIDENCE OF ENDOMETRIAL HYPERPLASIA
AFTER ONE YEAR OF TREATMENT

	Dose Groups	
Patient	PREMPRO 0.625 mg/2.5 mg	Premarin 0.625 mg
Total number of patients	279	283
No. (%) of patients with biopsies		
• all focal and non-focal hyperplasia	2 (<1)*	57 (20)
• excluding focal cystic hyperplasia	2 (<1)*	25 (8)

*Significant ($p < 0.001$) in comparison with Premarin alone (0.625 mg).

Continued on next page

Wyeth-Ayerst Laboratories—Cont.

rhea throughout the period of their participation in the study.
[See graph below.]

INFORMATION REGARDING LIPID EFFECTS

The results of a clinical trial conducted in a 97% Caucasian population at low risk for cardiovascular disease show that PREMPRO increases HDL-C and the HDL_2-C subfraction significantly less than Premarin alone, but decreases LDL-C comparably with Premarin alone. Total Cholesterol concentrations were significantly lower after 1 year of treatment than at baseline.

The following table summarizes mean percent changes from baseline lipid parameter values after 1 year of treatment with the combined regimens.
[See table above.]

The pharmacologic effects of the administered conjugated estrogens are similar to those of endogenous estrogens. In responsive tissue (female genital organs, breasts, hypothalamus, pituitary) estrogens enter the cell and are transported into the nucleus. As a result of the estrogen action, specific RNA and protein synthesis occurs.

Androgenic and anabolic effects of MPA have been noted, but the drug is apparently devoid of significant estrogenic activity. Parenterally administered MPA inhibits gonadotropin production, which in turn prevents follicular maturation and ovulation, although available data indicate that this does not occur when the usually recommended oral dosage is given as single daily doses. MPA may achieve its beneficial effect on the endometrium in part by decreasing nuclear estradiol receptors and suppression of epithelial DNA synthesis in endometrial tissue.

PHARMACOKINETICS

ABSORPTION

Conjugated estrogens are soluble in water and are well absorbed from the gastrointestinal tract after release from the drug formulation. However, PREMPRO contains a modified-release formulation of conjugated estrogens that slowly releases estrogens over several hours. Maximum plasma concentrations of the various conjugated and unconjugated estrogens are attained within 4 to 10 hours after dose administration. MPA is rapidly absorbed from the gastrointestinal tract, and maximum MPA plasma concentrations are attained within 2 to 4 hours after dose administration.

DISTRIBUTION

The conjugated estrogens bind mainly to albumin, but the unconjugated estrogens bind to both albumin and sex-hormone-binding globulin (SHBG). The apparent terminal-phase disposition half-life ($t_{1/2}$) of the various estrogens is prolonged by the slow absorption from PREMPRO and ranges from 10 to 24 hours. MPA is approximately 90% bound to plasma proteins but does not bind to SHBG. MPA has a mean $t_{1/2}$ of 38 hours.

METABOLISM

Metabolism and inactivation of estrogens occur primarily in the liver. Some estrogens are excreted into the bile; however, they are reabsorbed from the intestine and returned to the liver through the portal venous system. Metabolism and elimination of MPA occurs primarily in the liver via hydroxylation, with subsequent conjugation and elimination in the urine.

EXCRETION

Water-soluble estrogen conjugates are strongly acidic and are ionized in body fluids, which favor excretion through the kidneys since tubular reabsorption is minimal. Most metabolites of MPA are excreted as glucuronide conjugates with only minor amounts excreted as sulfates.

DRUG-DRUG INTERACTIONS

Coadministration of conjugated estrogens with MPA does not affect the pharmacokinetic profile of MPA; similarly, MPA does not affect the pharmacokinetic profile of the conjugated or unconjugated estrogens.

FOOD-DRUG INTERACTIONS

A single dose study in twenty healthy, postmenopausal women was conducted to investigate any potential drug interaction when PREMPRO is administered with a high fat breakfast.

Administration with food decreased the C_{max} of total estrone by 34% compared to the fasting state, with no other effect on the rate or extent of absorption of other conjugated or unconjugated estrogens. Administration with food approximately doubles MPA C_{max} and increases MPA AUC by approximately 30%.

TABLE 1 summarizes the pharmacokinetic parameters estimated for unconjugated and conjugated estrogens, and medroxyprogesterone acetate from a single dose bioequivalence study involving 54 healthy, postmenopausal women.
[See Table 1 at top of next page.]

INDICATIONS AND USAGE

PREMPRO therapy is indicated in women with an intact uterus for the:

1. Treatment of moderate to severe vasomotor symptoms associated with the menopause. There is no adequate evidence that estrogens are effective for nervous symptoms or depression which might occur during menopause and they should not be used to treat these conditions.
2. Treatment of vulvar and vaginal atrophy.
3. Prevention of osteoporosis.

Since estrogen administration is associated with risks as well as benefits, selection of patients ideally should be based on prospective identification of risk factors for developing osteoporosis. Unfortunately, there is no certain way to identify those women who will develop osteoporotic fractures. Most prospective studies of efficacy for this indication have been carried out in white menopausal women, without stratification by other risk factors, and tend to show a universally

salutary effect on bone. Thus, patient selection must be individualized based on the balance of risks and benefits.

Estrogen replacement therapy reduces bone resorption and retards or halts postmenopausal bone loss. Case-control studies have shown an approximately 60% reduction in hip and wrist fractures in women whose estrogen replacement was begun within a few years of menopause. Studies also suggest that estrogen reduces the rate of vertebral fractures. Even when started as late as 6 years after menopause, estrogen may prevent further loss of bone mass for as long as the treatment is continued. When estrogen therapy is discontinued, bone mass declines at a rate comparable to that in the immediate postmenopausal period. There is no evidence that estrogen replacement therapy restores bone mass to premenopausal levels.

At skeletal maturity there are sex and race differences in both the total amount of bone present and its density, in favor of men and blacks. Thus, women are at higher risk than men because they start with less bone mass and, for several years following natural or induced menopause, the rate of bone mass decline is accelerated. White and Asian women are at higher risk than black women.

Early menopause is one of the strongest predictors for the development of osteoporosis. In addition, other factors affecting the skeleton which are associated with osteoporosis include genetic factors (small build, family history), endocrine factors (nulliparity, thyrotoxicosis, hyperparathyroidism, Cushing's syndrome, hyperprolactinemia, type I diabetes), lifestyle (cigarette smoking, alcohol abuse, sedentary exercise habits) and nutrition (below average body weight, dietary calcium intake).

The mainstays of prevention and management of osteoporosis are estrogen, an adequate lifetime calcium intake, and exercise. Postmenopausal women absorb dietary calcium less efficiently than premenopausal women and require an average of 1500 mg/day of elemental calcium to remain in neutral calcium balance. By comparison, premenopausal women require about 1000 mg/day and the average calcium intake in the USA is 400–600 mg/day. Therefore, when not contraindicated, calcium supplementation may be helpful. Weight-bearing exercise and nutrition may be important adjuncts to the prevention and management of osteoporosis. Immobilization and prolonged bed rest produce rapid bone loss, while weight-bearing exercise has been shown both to reduce bone loss and to increase bone mass. The optimal type and amount of physical activity that would prevent osteoporosis have not been established; however, in two studies an hour of walking and running exercises twice or three times weekly significantly increased lumbar spine bone mass.

CONTRAINDICATIONS

Estrogens/progestins combined should not be used in women under any of the following conditions or circumstances:

1. Known or suspected pregnancy, including use for missed abortion or as a diagnostic test for pregnancy (see Boxed Warning). Estrogen or progestin may cause fetal harm when administered to a pregnant woman.
2. Known or suspected cancer of the breast.
3. Known or suspected estrogen-dependent neoplasia.
4. Undiagnosed abnormal genital bleeding.
5. Active or past history of thrombophlebitis, thromboembolic disorders, or stroke.
6. Liver dysfunction or disease.

PREMPRO therapy should not be used in patients hypersensitive to the ingredients contained in the tablets.

WARNINGS

ALL WARNINGS BELOW PERTAIN TO THE USE OF THIS COMBINATION PRODUCT.
Based on experience with estrogens and/or progestins:

1. *Induction of malignant neoplasms*
Breast cancer. Some studies have reported a moderately increased risk of breast cancer (relative risk of 1.3 to 2.0) in those women on estrogen replacement therapy taking higher doses, or in those taking lower doses for prolonged periods of time, especially in excess of 10 years. The majority of studies, however, have not shown an association in women who have ever used estrogen replacement therapy.

MEAN PERCENT CHANGE FROM BASELINE LIPID PROFILE VALUES AFTER ONE YEAR OF TREATMENT

	Dose Groups	
Lipid Parameter	PREMPRO 0.625 mg/2.5 mg	Premarin 0.625 mg
Total Cholesterol	-4.7*,†	0.2
HDL-C	3.5*,†	14.1*
HDL_2-C	34.7*,†	70.8*
LDL-C	-10.3*	-7.7*
Triglycerides	24.1*,†	39.4*

* Significantly (p ≤ 0.05) different from baseline value.
† Significantly (p ≤ 0.05) different from Premarin alone.

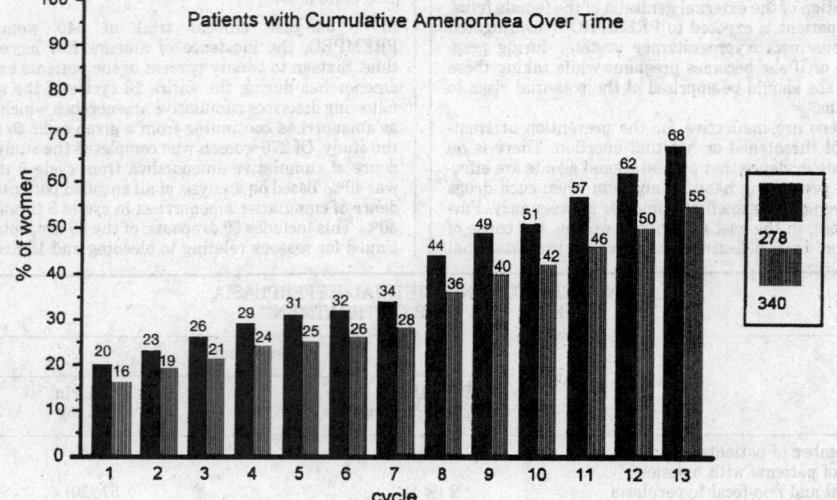

Figure 1. Cumulative amenorrhea

The effect of added progestins on the risk of breast cancer is unknown, although a moderately increased risk in those taking combination estrogen/progestin therapy has been reported. Other studies have not shown this relationship. In a one year clinical trial of PREMPRO, PREMPHASE® and Premarin alone, 5 new cases of breast cancer were detected among 1377 women who received the combination treatments, while no new cases were detected among 347 women who received Premarin alone. The overall incidence of breast cancer in this clinical trial does not exceed that expected in the general population.

In the three year clinical Postmenopausal Estrogen Progestin Intervention (PEPI) trial of 875 women to assess differences among placebo, unopposed Premarin, and three different combination hormone therapy regimens, one (1) new case of breast cancer was detected in the placebo group (n=174), one in the Premarin alone group (n=175), none in the continuous Premarin plus continuous medroxyprogesterone acetate group (n=174), and two (2) in the continuous Premarin plus cyclic medroxyprogesterone acetate group (n=174).

Women on hormone replacement therapy should have regular breast examinations and should be instructed in breast self-examination, and women over the age of 50 should have regular mammograms.

Endometrial cancer. The reported endometrial cancer risk among users of unopposed estrogen was about 2- to 12-fold greater than in nonusers and appears dependent on duration of treatment and on estrogen dose. There is no significant increased risk associated with the use of estrogens for less than one year. The greatest risk appears associated with prolonged use, with increased risks of 15- to 24-fold for five years or more. In three studies, persistence of risk was demonstrated for 8 to over 15 years after cessation of estrogen treatment. In one study, a significant decrease in the incidence of endometrial cancer occurred six months after estrogen withdrawal.

A large clinical trial has demonstrated that when MPA is administered with Premarin, there is a markedly reduced incidence of endometrial hyperplasia, a possible precursor of endometrial cancer. Endometrial hyperplasia has been reported in a large clinical trial to occur at a rate of approximately 1% or less with PREMPRO. Studies have also demonstrated a reduced risk of endometrial cancer when a progestin is administered with estrogen replacement therapy. In the large clinical trial described above, only a single case of endometrial cancer was reported to occur among women taking combination Premarin/MPA therapy.

Clinical surveillance of all women taking estrogen/progestin combinations is important. Adequate diagnostic measures, including endometrial sampling when indicated, should be undertaken to rule out malignancy in all cases of undiagnosed persistent or recurring abnormal vaginal bleeding.

2. *Cardiovascular disease.* Large doses of estrogens (5 mg conjugated estrogens per day), comparable to those used to treat cancer of the prostate and breast, have been shown in a large prospective clinical trial in men to increase the risk of nonfatal myocardial infarction, pulmonary embolism, and thrombophlebitis. These risks cannot necessarily be extrapolated from men to women or from unopposed estrogen to combination estrogen/progestin therapy. However, to avoid the theoretical cardiovascular risk to women caused by high estrogen doses, the dose for estrogen replacement therapy should not exceed the lowest effective dose.

3. *Effects during pregnancy.* Use in pregnancy is not recommended. See Boxed Warning.

4. *Gallbladder disease.* Two studies have reported a 2- to 4-fold increase in the risk of surgically confirmed gallbladder disease in women receiving postmenopausal estrogens. In a large clinical trial, 5 of 1029 subjects taking Premarin/Cycrin® at doses comparable to PREMPRO developed cholecystitis with cholelithiasis that required cholecystectomy.

5. *Elevated blood pressure.* Occasional blood pressure increases during estrogen replacement therapy have been attributed to idiosyncratic reactions to estrogens. More often, blood pressure has remained the same or has dropped. One study showed that postmenopausal estrogen users have higher blood pressure than nonusers. In a large clinical trial, transient elevations from baseline of 40 mm Hg or more systolic and 20 mm Hg or more diastolic were reported in less than 2% and 4% of postmenopausal subjects, respectively. Two other studies showed slightly lower blood pressure among estrogen users compared to nonusers. Postmenopausal estrogen use does not increase the risk of stroke. Nonetheless, blood pressure should be monitored at regular intervals with estrogen use.

6. *Hypercalcemia.* Administration of estrogens may lead to severe hypercalcemia in patients with breast cancer and bone metastases. If this occurs, the drugs should be stopped and appropriate measures taken to reduce the serum calcium level.

7. *Thromboembolic disorders.* The physician should be alert to the earliest manifestations of thrombotic disorders (thrombophlebitis, cerebrovascular disorders, pulmonary embolism, and retinal thrombosis). Should any of these occur

TABLE 1. PHARMACOKINETIC PARAMETERS FOR UNCONJUGATED AND CONJUGATED ESTROGENS, AND MEDROXYPROGESTERONE ACETATE

Pharmacokinetic Profile of Unconjugated Estrogens Following a Dose of 2 × 0.625 mg CE/2.5 mg MPA Combination Tablets

Drug	C_{max} (pg/mL) ±SD	t_{max} (h) ±SD	$t_{1/2}$ (h) ±SD	AUC (pg•h/mL) ±SD
estrone	175 ±41	7.6 ±1.8	31.6 ±7.4	5358 ±1840
baseline-adjusted estrone	159 ±41	7.6 ±1.8	16.9 ±5.8	3313 ±1310
equilin	71 ±22	5.8 ±2.0	9.9 ±3.5	951 ±413

Pharmacokinetic Profile of Conjugated Estrogens Following a Dose of 2 × 0.625 mg CE/2.5 mg MPA Combination Tablets

Drug	C_{max} (ng/mL) ±SD	t_{max} (h) ±SD	$t_{1/2}$ (h) ±SD	AUC (ng•h/mL) ±SD
total estrone	6.6 ±2.5	6.1 ±1.7	20.7 ±7.0	116 ±68
baseline-adjusted total estrone	6.4 ±2.5	6.1 ±1.7	15.4 ±5.2	100 ±57
total equilin	5.1 ±2.3	4.6 ±1.6	11.4 ±2.9	50 ±35

Pharmacokinetic Profile of MPA Following a Dose of 2 × 0.625 mg CE/2.5 mg MPA Combination Tablets

Drug	C_{max} (ng/mL) ±SD	t_{max} (h) ±SD	$t_{1/2}$ (h) ±SD	Cl/F (L/h/kg) ±SD
medroxyprogesterone acetate	1.5 ±0.6	2.8 ±1.5	37.6 ±11.2	2.3 ±0.7

C_{max} = peak plasma concentration
t_{max} = time peak concentration occurs
$t_{1/2}$ = terminal-phase disposition half-life $(0.693/\lambda_z)$
AUC = total area under the curve
Cl/F = apparent oral clearance

or be suspected, the drugs should be discontinued immediately.

8. *Visual abnormalities.* Discontinue medication pending examination if there is sudden partial or complete loss of vision, or a sudden onset of proptosis, diplopia, or migraine. If examination reveals papilledema or retinal vascular lesions, medication should be withdrawn.

PRECAUTIONS
GENERAL
Based on experience with estrogens and/or progestins:

1. *Cardiovascular risk.* A causal relationship between estrogen replacement therapy and reduction of cardiovascular disease in postmenopausal women has not been proven. Furthermore, the effect of added progestins on this putative benefit is not yet known.

In recent years many published studies have suggested that there may be a cause-effect relationship between postmenopausal oral estrogen replacement therapy *without added progestins* and a decrease in cardiovascular disease in women. Although most of the observational studies which assessed this statistical association have reported a 20% to 50% reduction in coronary heart disease risk and associated mortality in estrogen takers, the following should be considered when interpreting these reports.

Because only one of these studies was randomized and it was too small to yield statistically significant results, all relevant studies were subject to selection bias. Thus, the apparently reduced risk of coronary artery disease cannot be attributed with certainty to estrogen replacement therapy. It may instead have been caused by life-style and medical characteristics of the women studied with the result that healthier women were selected for estrogen therapy. In general, treated women were of higher socioeconomic and educational status, more slender, more physically active, less likely to have undergone surgical menopause, and less likely to have diabetes than the untreated women. Although some studies attempted to control for these selection factors, it is common for properly designed randomized trials to fail to confirm benefits suggested by less rigorous study designs. Thus, ongoing and future large-scale randomized trials may fail to confirm this apparent benefit.

Current medical practice often includes the use of concomitant progestin therapy in women with intact uteri. While the effects of added progestins on the risk of ischemic heart disease are not known, medroxyprogesterone acetate at the dose in PREMPRO attenuates much of the favorable effect of conjugated estrogens on HDL levels, although it maintains the favorable effect of conjugated estrogens on LDL levels (see **Clinical Pharmacology**).

While the effects of added progestins on the risk of breast cancer are also unknown, available epidemiologic evidence suggests that progestins do not reduce, and may enhance, the moderately increased breast cancer risk that has been reported with prolonged estrogen replacement therapy (see **Warnings**).

The safety data regarding PREMPRO were obtained primarily from clinical trials and epidemiologic studies of postmenopausal Caucasian women, who were at generally low risk for cardiovascular disease and higher than average risk for osteoporosis. The safety profile of PREMPRO derived from these study populations cannot necessarily be extrapolated to other populations of diverse racial and/or demographic composition. When considering prescribing PREMPRO, physicians are advised to weigh the potential benefits and risks of therapy as applicable to each individual patient.

2. *Use in hysterectomized women.* Existing data do not support the use of the combination of estrogen and progestin in postmenopausal women without a uterus. There are possible risks which may be associated with the inclusion of progestin in estrogen replacement regimens. The potential risks include some deterioration in glucose tolerance, as reported in a large clinical trial of PREMPRO, and less favorable effects on lipid metabolism as compared to the lipid effects of Premarin alone (see **Clinical Pharmacology**).

3. *Physical examination.* A complete medical and family history should be taken prior to the initiation of any estrogen/progestin therapy. The pretreatment and periodic physical examinations should include special reference to blood pressure, breasts, abdomen, and pelvic organs, and should include a Papanicolaou smear. As a general rule, estrogen should not be prescribed for longer than one year without another physical examination being performed.

4. *Fluid retention.* Because estrogens/progestins may cause some degree of fluid retention, conditions which might be influenced by this factor, such as asthma, epilepsy, migraine, and cardiac or renal dysfunction, require careful observation.

5. *Uterine bleeding.* Certain patients may develop abnormal uterine bleeding. In cases of undiagnosed abnormal uterine bleeding, adequate diagnostic measures are indicated. (See **Warnings.**)

6. The pathologist should be advised of estrogen/progestin therapy when relevant specimens are submitted.

Based on experience with estrogens:

1. *Familial hyperlipoproteinemia.* Estrogen therapy may be associated with massive elevations of plasma triglycerides

Continued on next page

Wyeth-Ayerst Laboratories—Cont.

leading to pancreatitis and other complications in patients with familial defects of lipoprotein metabolism.

2. *Hypercoagulability.* Some studies have shown that women taking estrogen replacement therapy have hypercoagulability primarily related to decreased antithrombin activity. This effect appears dose- and duration-dependent and is less pronounced than that associated with oral contraceptive use. Also, postmenopausal women tend to have changes in levels of coagulation parameters at baseline compared to premenopausal women. There is some suggestion that low-dose mestranol may increase the risk of thromboembolism in postmenopausal women, although the majority of studies (of primarily conjugated estrogens users) report no such increase. There is insufficient information on hypercoagulability in women who have had previous thromboembolic disease. In a large clinical trial of PREMPRO, factors VII and X concentrations and plasminogen activity increased by 20%, 13%, and 14% over baseline, respectively, and antithrombin III activity decreased approximately 5% from baseline.

3. *Mastodynia.* Certain patients may develop undesirable manifestations of estrogenic stimulation such as mastodynia. In a large clinical trial of PREMPRO, approximately one third of the subjects reported breast pain during treatment with PREMPRO, versus 12% for Premarin® alone.
Based on experience with progestins:

1. *Lipoprotein metabolism.* See **Clinical Pharmacology.**
2. *Impaired glucose tolerance.* See *Use in hysterectomized women,* above.
3. *Depression.* Patients who have a history of depression should be observed and the drugs discontinued if the depression recurs to a serious degree.

INFORMATION FOR THE PATIENT
See text of Patient Package Insert which appears after the **How Supplied** section.

DRUG/LABORATORY TEST INTERACTIONS
1. Accelerated prothrombin time, partial thromboplastin time, and platelet aggregation time; increased platelet count; increased factors II, VII antigen, VIII coagulant activity, IX, X, XII, VII-X complex, II-VII-X complex, and beta-thromboglobulin; decreased levels of anti-factor Xa and antithrombin III, decreased antithrombin III activity; increased levels of fibrinogen and fibrinogen activity; increased plasminogen antigen and activity.
2. Increased thyroid-binding globulin (TBG) leading to increased circulating total thyroid hormone, as measured by protein-bound iodine (PBI), T_4 levels (by column or by radioimmunoassay) or T_3 levels by radioimmunoassay, T_3 resin uptake is decreased, reflecting the elevated TBG. Free T_4 and free T_3 concentrations are unaltered.
3. Other binding proteins may be elevated in serum, i.e., corticosteroid binding globulin (CBG), sex hormone-binding globulin (SHBG), leading to increased circulating corticosteroids and sex steroids respectively. Free or biologically active hormone concentrations are unchanged. Other plasma proteins may be increased (angiotensinogen/renin substrate, alpha-1-antitrypsin, ceruloplasmin).
4. Increased plasma HDL and HDL-2 subfraction concentrations, reduced LDL cholesterol concentration, increased triglyceride levels.
5. Impaired glucose tolerance. For this reason, diabetic patients should be carefully observed while receiving estrogen/progestin therapy.
6. Reduced response to metyrapone test.
7. Reduced serum folate concentration.
8. Aminoglutethimide administered concomitantly with MPA may significantly depress the bioavailability of MPA.

CARCINOGENESIS, MUTAGENESIS, AND IMPAIRMENT OF FERTILITY
Long term continuous administration of natural and synthetic estrogens in certain animal species increases the frequency of carcinomas of the breasts, uterus, cervix, vagina, testis, and liver. (See **Contraindications** and **Warnings.**)
In a two-year oral study of MPA in which female rats were exposed to dosages of up to 5000 µg/kg/day in their diets (50 times higher—based on AUC values—than the level observed experimentally in women taking 10 mg of MPA), a dose-related increase in pancreatic islet cell tumors (adenomas and carcinomas) occurred. Pancreatic tumor incidence was increased at 1000 and 5000 µg/kg/day, but not at 200 µg/kg/day.
A decreased incidence of spontaneous mammary gland tumors was observed in all three MPA-treated groups, compared to controls, in the two-year rat study. The mechanism for the decreased incidence of mammary gland tumors observed in the MPA-treated rats may be linked to the significant decrease in serum prolactin concentration observed in rats.
Beagle dogs treated with MPA developed mammary nodules, some of which were malignant. Although nodules occasionally appeared in control animals, they were intermittent in nature, whereas the nodules in the drug-treated animals

were larger, more numerous, persistent, and there were some breast malignancies with metastases. It is known that progestogens stimulate synthesis and release of growth hormone in dogs. The growth hormone, along with the progestogen, stimulates mammary growth and tumors. In contrast, growth hormone in humans is not increased, nor does growth hormone have any significant mammotrophic role. Therefore, the MPA-induced increase of mammary tumors in dogs probably has no significance to humans. No pancreatic tumors occurred in dogs.

PREGNANCY CATEGORY X
Estrogens/progestins should not be used during pregnancy. See **Contraindications** and Boxed Warning.

NURSING MOTHERS
As a general principle, the administration of any drug to nursing mothers should be done only when clearly necessary since many drugs are excreted in human milk. Estrogen administration to nursing mothers has been shown to decrease the quantity and quality of the milk. Detectable amounts of progestin have been identified in the milk of mothers receiving the drug. The effect of this on the nursing infant has not been determined.

ADVERSE REACTIONS
(See **Warnings** regarding induction of neoplasia, adverse effects on the fetus, increased incidence of gallbladder disease, elevated blood pressure, thromboembolic disorders, cardiovascular disease, visual abnormalities, and hypercalcemia and **Precautions** for cardiovascular disease.)
The following adverse reactions have been reported with estrogen and/or progestin therapy:
Genitourinary system. Changes in vaginal bleeding pattern and abnormal withdrawal bleeding or flow, breakthrough bleeding, spotting, change in amount of cervical secretion, premenstrual-like syndrome, cystitis-like syndrome, increase in size of uterine leiomyomata, vaginal candidiasis, amenorrhea, changes in cervical erosion.
Breasts. Tenderness, enlargement, galactorrhea.
Gastrointestinal. Nausea, cholestatic jaundice, changes in appetite, vomiting, abdominal cramps, bloating, increased incidence of gallbladder disease, pancreatitis.
Skin. Chloasma or melasma that may persist when drug is discontinued, erythema multiforme, erythema nodosum, hemorrhagic eruption, loss of scalp hair, hirsutism, itching, urticaria, pruritus, generalized rash, rash (allergic) with and without pruritus, acne.
Cardiovascular. In susceptible individuals, change in blood pressure, thrombophlebitis, pulmonary embolism, cerebral thrombosis and embolism.
CNS. Headache, dizziness, mental depression, nervousness, migraine, chorea, insomnia, somnolence.
Eyes. Neuro-ocular lesions, e.g., retinal thrombosis and optic neuritis. Steepening of corneal curvature, intolerance of contact lenses.
Miscellaneous. Increase or decrease in weight, edema, changes in libido, fatigue, backache, reduced carbohydrate tolerance, aggravation of porphyria, pyrexia, anaphylactoid reactions, anaphylaxis.

ACUTE OVERDOSAGE
Serious ill effects have not been reported following acute ingestion of large doses of estrogen/progestin-containing oral contraceptives by young children. Overdosage may cause nausea and vomiting, and withdrawal bleeding may occur in females.

DOSAGE AND ADMINISTRATION
PREMPRO therapy consists of a single tablet to be taken once daily.
1. For treatment of moderate to severe vasomotor symptoms and vulvar and vaginal atrophy associated with menopause—PREMPRO 0.625 mg/2.5 mg daily. Patients should be reevaluated at 3-month to 6-month intervals to determine if treatment for symptoms is still necessary.
2. For prevention of osteoporosis—PREMPRO 0.625 mg/2.5 mg daily. Treated patients with an intact uterus should be monitored closely for signs of endometrial cancer, and appropriate diagnostic measures should be taken to rule out malignancy in the event of persistent or recurring abnormal vaginal bleeding.

HOW SUPPLIED
PREMPRO™ therapy consists of a single tablet to be taken once daily.
Each carton contains 2 blister cards. Each blister card contains 14 oval, peach tablets containing 0.625 mg of the conjugated estrogens found in Premarin® tablets and 2.5 mg of medroxyprogesterone acetate for oral administration.
The appearance of PREMPRO™ tablets is a trademark of Wyeth-Ayerst Laboratories.
Store at room temperature, 20° C–25° C (68° F–77° F).

INFORMATION FOR THE PATIENT

ESTROGENS INCREASE THE RISK OF CANCER OF THE UTERUS IN WOMEN WHO HAVE HAD THEIR MENOPAUSE ("CHANGE OF LIFE"). THIS FIND-

ING REFERS TO ESTROGENS GIVEN WITHOUT PROGESTIN.
Progestin drugs taken with estrogen-containing drugs significantly reduce but do not eliminate this risk. If you use any estrogen-containing drug, it is important to visit your doctor regularly and report any unusual vaginal bleeding right away. Vaginal bleeding after menopause may be a warning sign of uterine cancer. Your doctor should evaluate any unusual vaginal bleeding to find out the cause.

ESTROGENS/PROGESTINS SHOULD NOT BE USED DURING PREGNANCY.
Estrogens and progestins do not prevent miscarriage (spontaneous abortion) and are not needed in the days following childbirth. If you take estrogens during pregnancy your unborn child has a greater than usual chance of having birth defects. The risk of developing these defects is small, but clearly larger than the risk in children whose mothers did not take estrogens during pregnancy. These birth defects may affect the baby's urinary system and sex organs. Daughters born to mothers who took DES (an estrogen drug) have a higher than usual chance of developing cancer of the vagina or cervix when they become teenagers or young adults. Sons may have a higher than usual chance of developing cancer of the testicles when they become teenagers or young adults.
There is an increased risk of birth defects in children whose mothers take this drug during the first four months of pregnancy. Several reports suggest an association between mothers who take these drugs in the first trimester of pregnancy and genital abnormalities in male and female babies. The risk to the male baby is the possibility of being born with a condition in which the opening of the penis is on the underside rather than the tip of the penis (hypospadias). Hypospadias occurs in about 5 to 8 per 1,000 male births and is about doubled with exposure to these drugs. There is not enough information to quantify the risk to exposed female fetuses. However, enlargement of the clitoris and fusion of the labia may occur, although rarely.
Therefore, since drugs of this type may induce mild masculinization of the external genitalia of the female fetus, as well as hypospadias in the male fetus, it is wise to avoid using the drug during the first trimester of pregnancy. These drugs have been used as a test for pregnancy, but such use is no longer considered safe because of possible damage to a developing baby. Also, more rapid methods for testing for pregnancy are now available. If you take PREMPRO and later find you were pregnant when you took it, be sure to discuss this with your doctor as soon as possible.

Your physician has prescribed PREMPRO, a combination of two hormones, an estrogen and a progestin. This leaflet describes the major benefits and risks of your treatment, as well as how and when treatment should be taken.
PREMPRO replaces the hormones in your body which naturally decrease at menopause. The hormone combination you will be taking has been shown to provide the benefits of estrogen replacement therapy while lowering the frequency of a possible precancerous condition of the uterine lining. This therapy is not intended for women who have had a hysterectomy (surgical removal of the uterus).
Estrogens have several important uses but also some risks. You must decide, with your doctor, whether the risks of estrogens are acceptable when weighed against their benefits. The length of treatment with estrogens can vary from woman to woman. Check with your doctor to make sure you are using the lowest possible effective dose.
With PREMPRO therapy several menstrual-like bleeding patterns may occur. These may range from absence of bleeding to irregular bleeding. If bleeding occurs, it is frequently light spotting or moderate menstrual-like bleeding, but it may be heavy. If you experience vaginal bleeding while taking PREMPRO, you should discuss your bleeding pattern with your doctor and set up an appropriate schedule for follow-up care.

USES OF ESTROGEN
To reduce moderate to severe menopausal symptoms. Estrogens are hormones produced by the ovaries of normal women. When a woman is between the ages of 45 and 55, the ovaries normally stop making estrogens. This leads to a drop in body estrogen levels that causes the "change of life" or menopause (the end of monthly menstrual periods). A sudden drop in estrogen levels also occurs if both ovaries are removed during an operation before natural menopause takes place. This is referred to as "surgical menopause."
When the estrogen levels begin dropping, some women develop very uncomfortable symptoms, such as feelings of warmth in the face, neck, and chest, or sudden intense episodes of heat and sweating ("hot flashes" or "hot flushes"). Using estrogen drugs can help the body adjust to lower estrogen levels and reduce these symptoms. In some women the symptoms are mild; in others they can be severe. These

symptoms may last only a few months or longer. Taking PREMPRO can alleviate these symptoms. If you are not taking hormones for other reasons, such as the prevention of osteoporosis, you should take PREMPRO only as long as you need it for relief from your menopausal symptoms.

To prevent thinning of bones. Osteoporosis is a thinning of the bones that makes them weaker and allows them to break more easily. The bones of the spine, wrists, and hips break most often in osteoporosis. Both men and women start to lose bone mass after about age 40, but women lose bone mass faster after the menopause. Using estrogens after the menopause slows down bone thinning and may prevent bones from breaking. Lifelong adequate calcium intake, either from diet (such as dairy products) or from calcium supplements (to reach a total daily intake of 1000 milligrams per day before menopause or 1500 milligrams per day after menopause), may help to prevent osteoporosis. Regular weight-bearing exercise (like walking and running for an hour, two or three times a week) may also help to prevent osteoporosis. Before you change your calcium intake or exercise habits, it is important to discuss these lifestyle changes with your doctor to find out if they are safe for you.

Since estrogen use has some risks, only women who are likely to develop osteoporosis should use estrogens for prevention. Women who are likely to develop osteoporosis often have the following characteristics:
* White or Asian race
* Small, slim body frame
* Cigarette-smoking habit
* Family history of osteoporosis (in a mother, sister, or aunt)
* Early menopause either natural or because of surgical removal of ovaries ("surgical menopause")

To treat vulvar and vaginal atrophy (itching, burning, dryness in or around the vagina, difficulty or burning on urination) associated with menopause.

WHO SHOULD NOT USE ESTROGENS

During pregnancy (see Boxed Warning). If you think you may be pregnant, do not use any form of estrogen-containing drug. Using estrogens while you are pregnant may cause your unborn child to have birth defects. Estrogens do not prevent miscarriage.

If you have unusual vaginal bleeding which has not been evaluated by your doctor (see Boxed Warning). Unusual vaginal bleeding can be a warning sign of cancer of the uterus, especially if it happens after menopause. Your doctor must find out the cause of the bleeding so that he or she can recommend the proper treatment. Taking estrogens without visiting your doctor can cause you serious harm if your vaginal bleeding is caused by cancer of the uterus.

If you have had cancer. Since estrogens increase the risk of certain types of cancer, you should not use estrogens if you have ever had cancer of the breast or uterus.

If you have any circulation problems. Estrogen drugs should not be used except in unusually special situations in which your doctor decides that you need estrogen therapy so much that the risks are acceptable. Women with abnormal blood clotting conditions should avoid estrogen use (see **Risks of Estrogens and/or Progestins**).

When they do not work. During menopause, some women develop nervous symptoms or depression. Estrogens do not relieve these symptoms. You may have heard that taking estrogens for years after menopause will keep your skin soft and supple and keep you feeling young. There is no evidence for these claims and such long-term estrogen use may have serious risks.

After childbirth or when breastfeeding a baby. Estrogen should not be used to try to stop the breast from filling with milk after a baby is born. Such treatment may increase the risk of developing blood clots (see **Risks of Estrogens and/or Progestins**).

If you are breastfeeding, you should avoid using any drugs because many drugs pass through to the baby in the milk. While nursing a baby, you should take drugs only on the advice of your health-care provider.

RISKS OF ESTROGENS AND/OR PROGESTINS

Cancer of the uterus. The risk of cancer of the uterus increases when estrogens are used alone, the longer they are used, and when larger doses are taken. There is a higher risk of cancer of the uterus if you are overweight, diabetic, or have high blood pressure. The hormone combination you will be taking contains estrogen and progestin. This combination has been shown to provide the benefits of estrogen replacement therapy for the **Uses of Estrogen** listed above, while reducing the risk of a precancerous condition of the uterine lining (see **Other Information,** below).

However, additional risks may be associated with the inclusion of a progestin in estrogen treatment. The possible risks include less favorable effects on blood fats as compared to Premarin alone, unfavorable effects on blood sugars, and a possible increase in breast cancer risk (see *Cancer of the breast,* below). Usually, the smaller the dose and the shorter the duration of treatment, the more these effects are minimized. Check with your doctor to make sure you are using the lowest effective dose and only for as long as you need it.

If you have had your uterus removed, there is no risk of developing cancer of the uterus and no benefit to be gained by using a combination estrogen/progestin product.

Cancer of the breast. Most studies have not shown a higher risk of breast cancer in women who have ever used estrogens. However, some studies have reported that breast cancer developed more often (up to twice the usual rate) in women who used estrogens for long periods of time (especially more than 10 years), or who used high doses for shorter time periods. The effects of added progestin on the risk of breast cancer are unknown. Some studies have reported a somewhat increased risk, even higher than the possible risk associated with estrogens alone. Others have not. Regular breast examinations by a health professional and monthly self-examination are recommended for all women. Regular mammograms are recommended for all women over 50 years of age.

Gallbladder disease. Women who use estrogens after menopause are more likely to develop gallbladder disease needing surgery than women who do not use estrogens.

Inflammation of the pancreas. Women with high triglyceride levels may have an increased risk of developing inflammation of the pancreas.

Abnormal blood clotting. Taking estrogens may cause changes in your blood clotting system. These changes allow the blood to clot more easily, possibly allowing clots to form in your bloodstream. If blood clots do form in your bloodstream, they can cut off the blood supply to vital organs, causing serious problems. These problems may include a stroke (by cutting off blood to the brain), a heart attack (by cutting off blood to the heart), a pulmonary embolus (by cutting off blood to the lungs), or other problems. Any of these conditions may cause death or serious long-term disability. However, most studies of low-dose estrogen use by women do not show an increased risk of these complications.

Excess calcium in the blood. Taking estrogens may lead to severe hypercalcemia in women with breast and/or bone cancer.

During pregnancy. There is an increased risk of birth defects in children whose mothers take this drug during the first four months of pregnancy. Several reports suggest an association between mothers who take these drugs in the first trimester of pregnancy and genital abnormalities in male and female babies. The risk to the male baby is the possibility of being born with a condition in which the opening of the penis is on the underside rather than the tip of the penis (hypospadias). Hypospadias occurs in about 5 to 8 per 1,000 male births and is about doubled with exposure to these drugs. There is not enough information to quantify the risk to exposed female fetuses. However, enlargement of the clitoris and fusion of the labia may occur, although rarely. Therefore, since drugs of this type may induce mild masculinization of the external genitalia of the female fetus, as well as hypospadias in the male fetus, it is wise to avoid using the drug during the first trimester of pregnancy. These drugs have been used as a test for pregnancy, but such use is no longer considered safe because of possible damage to a developing baby. Also, more rapid methods for testing for pregnancy are now available. If you take PREMPRO and later find you were pregnant when you took it, be sure to discuss this with your doctor as soon as possible.

SIDE EFFECTS WITH ESTROGENS AND/OR PROGESTINS

In addition to the risks listed above, the following side effects have been reported with estrogen and/or progestin use:
* Nausea, vomiting, pain, cramps, swelling, or tenderness in the abdomen.
* Yellowing of the skin and/or whites of the eyes.
* Breast tenderness or enlargement.
* Enlargement of benign tumors ("fibroids") of the uterus.
* Irregular bleeding or spotting.
* Change in amount of cervical secretion.
* Vaginal yeast infections.
* Retention of excess fluid. This may make some conditions worsen, such as asthma, epilepsy, migraine, heart disease, or kidney disease.
* A spotty darkening of the skin, particularly on the face; reddening of the skin; skin rashes.
* Worsening of porphyria.
* Headache, migraines, dizziness, faintness, or changes in vision (including intolerance to contact lenses).
* Mental depression.
* Involuntary muscle spasms.
* Hair loss or abnormal hairiness.
* Increase or decrease in weight.
* Changes in sex drive.
* Possible changes in blood sugar.

REDUCING THE RISKS OF ESTROGEN/PROGESTIN

If you decide to take an estrogen/progestin combination, you can reduce your risks by carefully monitoring your treatment.

See your doctor regularly. While you are taking PREMPRO, it is important to visit your doctor at least once a

year for a checkup. If you develop vaginal bleeding while taking estrogens, you may need further evaluation. If members of your family have had breast cancer or if you have ever had breast lumps or an abnormal mammogram (breast X ray), you may need to have more frequent breast examinations.

Reassess your need for treatment. You and your doctor should reevaluate whether or not you still need estrogens at least every six months.

Be alert for signs of trouble. If any of these warning signals (or any other unusual symptoms) happen while you are using estrogen/progestin, call your doctor immediately:
* Abnormal bleeding from the vagina (possible uterine abnormality).
* Pains in the calves or chest, a sudden shortness of breath or coughing blood (indicating possible clots in the legs, heart, or lungs).
* Severe headache or vomiting, dizziness, faintness, or changes in vision or speech, weakness or numbness of an arm or leg (indicating possible clots in the brain or eye).
* Breast lumps (possible breast cancer; ask your doctor or health professional to show you how to examine your breasts monthly).
* Yellowing of the skin and/or whites of the eyes (possible liver problems).
* Pain, swelling, or tenderness in the abdomen (possible gallbladder problem).

OTHER INFORMATION

1. Estrogens increase the risk of developing a condition (endometrial hyperplasia) that may lead to cancer of the lining of the uterus. Taking progestins, another hormonal drug, with estrogens lowers the risk of developing this condition. Therefore, since your uterus has not been removed, your doctor has prescribed PREMPRO, which includes both a progestin and estrogens.

You should know, however, that taking estrogens *with* progestins may have unhealthy effects on blood sugar, which might make a diabetic condition worse. Additional risks include a possible further increase in breast cancer risk which may be associated with long-term estrogen use.

Some research has shown that estrogens taken *without* progestins may protect women against developing heart disease. However, this is not certain. The protection shown may have been caused by the characteristics of the estrogen-treated women and not by the estrogen treatment itself. In general, treated women were slimmer, more physically active, and were less likely to have diabetes than the untreated women. These characteristics are known to protect against heart disease.

You are cautioned to discuss very carefully with your doctor or health-care provider all the possible risks and benefits of long-term estrogen and progestin treatment as they affect you personally.

2. Your doctor has prescribed this drug for you and you alone. Do not give the drug to anyone else.

3. If you will be taking calcium supplements as part of the treatment to help prevent osteoporosis, check with your doctor about the amounts recommended.

4. Keep this and all drugs out of the reach of children. In case of overdose, call your doctor, hospital, or poison control center immediately.

5. This leaflet provides the most important information about PREMPRO. If you want to read more, ask your doctor or pharmacist to let you read the professional labeling. The professional labeling is also published in a book called *The Physicians' Desk Reference,* which is available in bookstores and public libraries.

HOW SUPPLIED

Your doctor has prescribed PREMPRO™, a combination of the conjugated estrogens found in Premarin® tablets and medroxyprogesterone acetate (MPA). PREMPRO therapy consists of a single peach tablet to be taken once daily.

Each carton contains (2) blister cards. Each blister card contains 14 oval, peach tablets containing 0.625 mg of the conjugated estrogens found in Premarin tablets and 2.5 mg of medroxyprogesterone acetate for oral administration.

The appearance of PREMPRO™ tablets is a trademark of Wyeth-Ayerst Laboratories.

Store at room temperature, 20° C–25° C (68° F–77° F).

Shown in Product Identification Guide, page 341

PROTOPAM® CHLORIDE   ℞
(pralidoxime chloride)
Lyophilized Powder for Injection

Caution: Federal law prohibits dispensing without prescription.

DESCRIPTION

Chemical name: 2-formyl-1-methylpyridinium chloride oxime. Available in the United States as Protopam Chloride,

Continued on next page

pralidoxime chloride is frequently referred to as 2-PAM Chloride.
Structural formula:

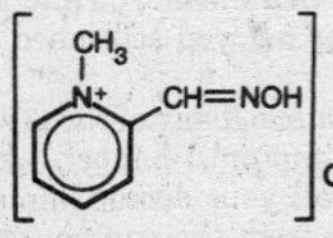

Pralidoxime chloride occurs as an odorless, white, nonhygroscopic, crystalline powder which is soluble in water to the extent of 1 g in less than 1 mL. Stable in air, it melts between 215° and 225°C, with decomposition.
The specific activity of the drug resides in the 2-formyl-1-methylpyridinium ion and is independent of the particular salt employed. The chloride is preferred because of physiologic compatibility, excellent water solubility at all temperatures, and high potency per gram, due to its low (173) molecular weight.
Pralidoxime chloride is a cholinesterase reactivator.
Protopam Chloride for intravenous injection or infusion is prepared by cryodesiccation. Each vial contains 1 g of sterile pralidoxime chloride, and NaOH to adjust pH, to be reconstituted with 20 mL of Sterile Water for Injection, USP. The pH of the reconstituted solution is 3.5 to 4.5. Intramuscular or subcutaneous injection may be used when intravenous injection is not feasible.

CLINICAL PHARMACOLOGY

The principal action of pralidoxime is to reactivate cholinesterase (mainly outside of the central nervous system) which has been inactivated by phosphorylation due to an organophosphate pesticide or related compound. The destruction of accumulated acetylcholine can then proceed, and neuromuscular junctions will again function normally. Pralidoxime also slows the process of "aging" of phosphorylated cholinesterase to a nonreactivatable form, and detoxifies certain organophosphates by direct chemical reaction. The drug has its most critical effect in relieving paralysis of the muscles of respiration. Because pralidoxime is less effective in relieving depression of the respiratory center, atropine is always required concomitantly to block the effect of accumulated acetylcholine at this site. Pralidoxime relieves muscarinic signs and symptoms, salivation, bronchospasm, etc., but this action is relatively unimportant since atropine is adequate for this purpose.
Pralidoxime is distributed throughout the extracellular water; it is not bound to plasma protein. The drug is rapidly excreted in the urine partly unchanged, and partly as a metabolite produced by the liver. Consequently, pralidoxime is relatively short acting, and repeated doses may be needed, especially where there is any evidence of continuing absorption of the poison.
The minimum therapeutic concentration of pralidoxime in plasma is 4 μg/mL; this level is reached in about 16 minutes after a single injection of 600 mg Protopam Chloride. The apparent half-life of Protopam Chloride is 74 to 77 minutes.
It has been reported[1] that the supplemental use of oxime cholinesterase reactivators (such as pralidoxime) reduces the incidence and severity of developmental defects in chick embryos exposed to such known teratogens as parathion, bidrin, carbachol, and neostigmine. This protective effect of the oximes was shown to be dose related.

INDICATIONS AND USAGE

Protopam is indicated as an antidote: (1) in the treatment of poisoning due to those pesticides and chemicals of the organophosphate class which have anticholinesterase activity and (2) in the control of overdosage by anticholinesterase drugs used in the treatment of myasthenia gravis.
The principal indications for the use of pralidoxime are muscle weakness and respiratory depression. In severe poisoning, respiratory depression may be due to muscle weakness.

CONTRAINDICATIONS

There are no known absolute contraindications for the use of Protopam. Relative contraindications include known hypersensitivity to the drug and other situations in which the risk of its use clearly outweighs possible benefit (see "**Precautions**").

WARNINGS

Protopam is not effective in the treatment of poisoning due to phosphorus, inorganic phosphates, or organophosphates not having anticholinesterase activity
Protopam is **not** indicated as an antidote for intoxication by pesticides of the carbamate class since it may increase the toxicity of carbaryl.

PRECAUTIONS

GENERAL
Pralidoxime has been very well tolerated in most cases, but it must be remembered that the desperate condition of the organophosphate-poisoned patient will generally mask such minor signs and symptoms as have been noted in normal subjects.
Intravenous administration of Protopam should be carried out slowly and, preferably, by infusion, since certain side effects, such as tachycardia, laryngospasm, and muscle rigidity, have been attributed in a few cases to a too-rapid rate of injection. (See "**Dosage and Administration**".)
Protopam should be used with great caution in treating organophosphate overdosage in cases of myasthenia gravis since it may precipitate a myasthenic crisis.
Because pralidoxime is excreted in the urine, a decrease in renal function will result in increased blood levels of the drug. Thus, the dosage of pralidoxime should be reduced in the presence of renal insufficiency.
LABORATORY TESTS
Treatment of organophosphate poisoning should be instituted without waiting for the results of laboratory tests. Red blood cell, plasma cholinesterase, and urinary paranitrophenol measurements (in the case of parathion exposure) may be helpful in confirming the diagnosis and following the course of the illness. A reduction in red blood cell cholinesterase concentration to below 50% of normal has been seen only with organophosphate ester poisoning.
DRUG INTERACTIONS
When atropine and pralidoxime are used together, the signs of atropinization (flushing, mydriasis, tachycardia, dryness of the mouth and nose) may occur earlier than might be expected when atropine is used alone. This is especially true if the total dose of atropine has been large and the administration of pralidoxime has been delayed.[2–4]
The following precautions should be kept in mind in the treatment of anticholinesterase poisoning, although they do not bear directly on the use of pralidoxime: since barbiturates are potentiated by the anticholinesterases, they should be used cautiously in the treatment of convulsions; morphine, theophylline, aminophylline, succinylcholine, reserpine, and phenothiazine-type tranquilizers should be avoided in patients with organophosphate poisoning.
CARCINOGENESIS, MUTAGENESIS, IMPAIRMENT OF FERTILITY
Since pralidoxime chloride is indicated for short-term emergency use only, no investigations of its potential for carcinogenesis, mutagenesis, or impairment of fertility have been conducted by the manufacturer, or reported in the literature.
PREGNANCY
Teratogenic Effects —Pregnancy Category C:
Animal reproduction studies have not been conducted with pralidoxime. It is also not known whether pralidoxime can cause fetal harm when administered to a pregnant woman or can affect reproduction capacity. Pralidoxime should be given to a pregnant woman only if clearly needed.
NURSING MOTHERS
It is not known whether this drug is excreted in human milk. Because many drugs are excreted in human milk, caution should be exercised when pralidoxime is administered to a nursing woman.
PEDIATRIC USE
Safety and effectiveness in pediatric patients have not been estabished.

ADVERSE REACTIONS

Forty to 60 minutes after intramuscular injection, mild to moderate pain may be experienced at the site of injection.
Pralidoxime may cause blurred vision, diplopia and impaired accommodation, dizziness, headache, drowsiness, nausea, tachycardia, increased systolic and diastolic blood pressure, hyperventilation, and muscular weakness when given parenterally to normal volunteers who have not been exposed to anticholinesterase poisons. In patients, it is very difficult to differentiate the toxic effects produced by atropine or the organophosphate compounds from those of the drug.
Elevations in SGOT and/or SGPT enzyme levels were observed in 1 of 6 normal volunteers given 1200 mg of pralidoxime chloride intramuscularly, and in 4 of 6 volunteers given 1800 mg intramuscularly. Levels returned to normal in about 2 weeks. Transient elevations in creatine phosphokinase were observed in all normal volunteers given the drug.
A single intramuscular injection of 330 mg in 1 mL in rabbits caused myonecrosis, inflammation, and hemorrhage.
When atropine and pralidoxime are used together, the signs of atropinization may occur earlier than might be expected when atropine is used alone. This is especially true if the total dose of atropine has been large and the administration of pralidoxime has been delayed.[2–4] Excitement and manic behavior immediately following recovery of consciousness have been reported in several cases. However, similar behavior has occurred in cases of organophosphate poisoning that were not treated with pralidoxime.[3,5,6]

DRUG ABUSE AND DEPENDENCE

Pralidoxime chloride is not subject to abuse and possesses no known potential for dependence.

OVERDOSAGE

MANIFESTATIONS OF OVERDOSAGE
Observed in normal subjects only: dizziness, blurred vision, diplopia, headache, impaired accommodation, nausea, slight tachycardia. In therapy it has been difficult to differentiate side effects due to the drug from those due to the effects of the poison.
TREATMENT OF OVERDOSAGE
Artificial respiration and other supportive therapy should be administered as needed.
ACUTE TOXICITY
IV—man TDLo: 14 mg/kg (toxic effects: CNS)
IV—rat LD50: 96 mg/kg
IM—rat LD50: 150 mg/kg
ORAL—mouse LD50: 4100 mg/kg
IP—mouse LD50: 155 mg/kg
IV—mouse LD50: 90 mg/kg
IM—mouse LD50: 180 mg/kg
IV—rabbit LD50: 95 mg/kg
IM—guinea pig LD50: 168 mg/kg

DOSAGE AND ADMINISTRATION

ORGANOPHOSPHATE POISONING
"Pralidoxime is most effective if administered immediately after poisoning. Generally, little is accomplished if the drug is given more than 36 hours after termination of exposure. When the poison has been ingested, however, exposure may continue for some time due to slow absorption from the lower bowel, and fatal relapses have been reported after initial improvement. Continued administration for several days may be useful in such patients. Close supervision of the patient is indicated for at least 48 to 72 hours. If dermal exposure has occurred, clothing should be removed and the hair and skin washed thoroughly with sodium bicarbonate or alcohol as soon as possible. Diazepam may be given cautiously if convulsions are not controlled by atropine."[7]
Severe poisoning (coma, cyanosis, respiratory depression) requires intensive management. This includes the removal of secretions, airway management, the correction of acidosis, and hypoxemia.
Atropine should be given as soon as possible after hypoxemia is improved. Atropine should not be given in the presence of significant hypoxia due to the risk of atropine-induced ventricular fibrillation. In adults, atropine may be given intravenously in doses of 2 to 4 mg. This should be repeated at 5- to 10-minute intervals until full atropinization (secretions are inhibited) or signs of atropine toxicity appear (delirium, hyperthermia, muscle twitching).
Some degree of atropinization should be maintained for at least 48 hours, and until any depressed blood cholinesterase activity is reversed.
Morphine, theophylline, aminophylline, and succinylcholine are contraindicated. Tranquilizers of the reserpine or phenothiazine type are to be avoided.
After the effects of atropine become apparent, Protopam may be administered.
PROTOPAM CHLORIDE INJECTION
Parenteral drug products should be inspected visually for particulate matter and discoloration prior to administration, whenever solution and container permit.
Discard unused solution after a dose has been withdrawn.
In adults, inject an initial dose of 1 to 2 g of Protopam, preferably as an infusion in 100 mL of saline, over a 15- to 30-minute period. If this is not practical or if pulmonary edema is present, the dose should be given slowly by intravenous injection as a 5 percent solution in water over not less than five minutes. After about an hour, a second dose of 1 to 2 g will be indicated if muscle weakness has not been relieved. Additional doses may be given cautiously if muscle weakness persists.
Too-rapid administration may result in temporary worsening of cholinergic manifestations. Injection rate should not exceed 200 mg/minute. If intravenous administration is not feasible, intramuscular or subcutaneous injection should be used.
In severe cases, especially after ingestion of the posion, it may be desirable to monitor the effect of therapy electrocardiographically because of the possibility of heart block due to the anticholinesterase. Where the poison has been ingested, it is particularly important to take into account the likelihood of continuing absorption from the lower bowel since this constitutes new exposure. In such cases, additional doses of Protopam (pralidoxime) may be needed every three to eight hours. In effect, the patient should be "titrated" with Protopam as long as signs of poisoning recur. As in all cases of organophosphate poisoning, care should be taken to keep the patient under observation for at least 24 hours.
If convulsions interfere with respiration, they may be controlled by the slow intravenous injection of diazepam, up to 20 mg in adults.
ANTICHOLINESTERASE OVERDOSAGE
As an antagonist to such anticholinesterases as neostigmine, pyridostigmine, and ambenonium, which are used in the treatment of myasthenia gravis, Protopam may be given in a

dosage of 1 to 2 g intravenously followed by increments of 250 mg every five minutes.

HOW SUPPLIED

NDC 0046-0374-06—*Hospital Package:* This contains six 20 mL vials of 1 g each of sterile Protopam Chloride (pralidoxime chloride) white to off-white porous cake*, without diluent or syringe. Solution may be prepared by adding 20 mL of Sterile Water for Injection, USP. These are single-dose vials for intravenous injection or for intravenous infusion after further dilution with physiologic saline. Intramuscular or subcutaneous injection may be used when intravenous injection is not feasible.

---

*When necessary, sodium hydroxide is added during processing to adjust the pH.

Store at room temperature (approximately 25°C).

ANIMAL PHARMACOLOGY AND TOXICOLOGY

The following table lists chemical and trade or generic names of pesticides, chemicals, and drugs against which Protopam (usually administered in conjunction with atropine) has been found to have antidotal activity on the basis of animal experiments. All compounds listed are organophosphates having anticholinesterase activity. A great many additional substances are in industrial use but have been omitted because of lack of special information.

AAT—see PARATHION

AFLIX®—see FORMOTHION

ALKRON®—See PARATHION

AMERICAN CYANAMID 3422—see PARATHION

AMITON—diethyl-S-(2-diethylaminoethyl)phosphorothiolate

ANTHIO®—see FORMOTHION

APHAMITE—see PARATHION

ARMIN—ethyl-4-nitrophenylethylphosphonate

AZINPHOS-METHYL—dimethyl-S-(4-oxo-1,2,3,-benzotriazin-3 (4H)-ylmethyl) phosphorodithioate

MORPHOTHION—dimethyl-S-2-keto-2-(N-morpholyl)ethyl-phosphorodithioate

NEGUVON®—see TRICHLOROFON

NIRAN®—see PARATHION

NITROSTIGMINE—see PARATHION

O,O-DIETHYL-O-p-NITROPHENYL PHOSPHOROTHIOATE—see PARATHION

O,O-DIETHYL-O-p-NITROPHENYLTHIO PHOSPHATE—see PARATHION

OR 1191—see PHOSPHAMIDON

OS 1836—see VINYLPHOS

OXYDEMETONMETHYL—dimethyl-S-2-(ethylsulfinyl) ethyl phosphorothiolate

PARAOXON—diethyl (4-nitrophenyl) phosphate

PARATHION—diethyl (4-nitrophenyl) phosphorothionate

PENPHOS—see PARATHION

PHENCAPTON—diethyl-S-(2,5-dichlorophenylmercaptomethyl) phosphorodithioate

PHOSDRIN®—see MEVINPHOS

PHOS-KIL—see PARATHION

PHOSPHAMIDON—1-chloro-1-diethylcarbamoyl-1-propen-2-yl-dimethylphosphate

PHOSPHOLINE IODIDE®—see echothiophate iodide

PHOSPHOROTHIOIC ACID, O,O-DIETHYL-O-p-NITROPHENYL ESTER—see PARATHION

PLANTHION—see PARATHION

QUELETOX—see FENTHION

RHODIATOX®—see PARATHION

RUELENE®—4-tert-butyl-2-chlorophenylmethyl-N-methylphosphoroamidate

SARIN—isopropyl-methylphosphonofluoridate

SHELL OS 1836—see VINYLPHOS

SHELL 2046—see MEVINPHOS

SNP—see PARATHION

SOMAN—pinacolyl-methylphosphonofluoridate

SYSTOX®—diethyl-(2-ethylmercaptoethyl) phosphorothionate

TEP—see TEPP

TEPP—tetraethylpyro phosphate

THIOPHOS®—see PARATHION

TIGUVON—see FENTHION

TRICHLOROFON—dimethyl-1-hydroxy-2,2,2-trichloroethylphosphonate

VAPONA®—see DICHLORVOS

VAPOPHOS—see PARATHION

VINYLPHOS—diethyl-2-chloro-vinylphosphate

PROTOPAM appears to be ineffective, or marginally effective, against poisoning by:
CIODRIN® (alpha-methylbenzyl-3[dimethoxyphosphinyloxy]-ciscrotonate)
DIMEFOX (tetramethylphosphorodiamidic fluoride)
DIMETHOATE (dimethyl-S-[N-methylcarbamoylmethyl]-phosphorodithioate)
METHYL DIAZINON (dimethyl-[2-isopropyl-4-methyl-pyrimidyl]-phosphorothionate)
METHYL PHENCAPTON (dimethyl-S-[2,5-dichlorophenyl-mercaptomethyl]phosphorodithioate)
PHORATE (diethyl-S-ethylmercaptomethylphosphorodithioate)
SCHRADAN (octamethylpyrophosphoramide)
WEPSYN® (5-amino-1-[bis-(dimethylamino) phosphinyl]-3-phenyl-1,2,4-triazole).
The use of Protopam should, nevertheless, be considered in any life-threatening situation resulting from poisoning by these compounds, since the limited and arbitrary conditions of pharmacologic screening do not always accurately reflect the usefulness of Protopam in the clinical situation.

CLINICAL STUDIES

The use of Protopam (pralidoxime) has been reported in the treatment of human cases of poisoning by the following substances:
Azodrin
Diazinon
Dichlorvos (DDVP) with chlordane
Disulfoton
EPN
Isoflurophate
Malathion
Metasystox I® and Fenthion
Methyldemeton
Methylparathion
Mevinphos
Parathion
Parathion and Mevinphos
Phosphamidon
Sarin
Systox®
TEPP
Of these cases, over 100 were due to parathion, about a dozen each to malathion, diazinon, and mevinphos, and a few to each of the other compounds.

REFERENCES

1. LANDAUER, W.: Cholinomimetic teratogens. V. The effect of oximes and related cholinesterase reactivators, *Teratology 15* :33 (Feb) 1977.
2. MOLLER, K.O., JENSEN-HOLM, J., and LAUSEN, H.H.: *Ugeskr. Laeg. 123* :501, 1961.
3. NAMBA, T., NOLTE, C.T., JACKREL, J. and GROB, D.: Poisoning due to organophosphate insecticides. Acute and chronic manifestations, *Amer. J. Med. 50* :475 (Apr), 1971.
4. ARENA, J.M.: Poisoning, Toxicology Symptoms, Treatments, ed. 4, Springfield, IL, Charles C. Thomas, 1979, p. 133.
5. BRACHFELD, J., and ZAVON, M.R.: Organic phosphate (Phosdrin®) intoxication. Report of a case and the results of treatment with 2-PAM, *Arch. Environ. Health 11* :859, 1965.
6. HAYES, W.J., Jr.: Toxicology of Pesticides, Baltimore, The Williams & Wilkins Company, 1975, p. 416.
7. AMA Department of Drugs: AMA Drug Evaluations, ed. 4, Chicago, American Medical Association, 1980, p. 1455.

REDUX™   © ℞

[*ree 'duks*]
(dexfenfluramine hydrochloride capsules)

DESCRIPTION

Redux (dexfenfluramine hydrochloride capsules), an anti-obesity drug, is a serotonin reuptake inhibitor and releasing agent. Redux is available for oral administration in white, opaque, hard-gelatin capsules. The active ingredient is dexfenfluramine hydrochloride. Each capsule contains 15 mg dexfenfluramine hydrochloride. Inactive ingredients include: lactose, gelatin capsule, corn starch, microcrystalline cellulose, talc, titanium dioxide, magnesium stearate, colloidal silicon dioxide, and edible ink.

Dexfenfluramine hydrochloride, a white to off-white crystalline powder, is designated chemically as (S)-N-ethyl-α-methyl-3-(trifluoromethyl) benzene-ethanamine hydrochloride and has a molecular weight of 267.7. Its empirical formula is $C_{12}H_{16}F_3N{\bullet}HCl$ and its structural formula is:

Dexfenfluramine hydrochloride is freely soluble in water, alcohol, chloroform, and methanol. The pK_a of dexfenfluramine hydrochloride is 10.

CLINICAL PHARMACOLOGY

Pharmacologic Actions

The action of Redux in treating obesity is primarily via decreased caloric intake associated with increased serotonin levels in brain synapses. Redux is a serotonin reuptake inhibitor and releasing agent. *In vitro* studies have confirmed the dual serotoninergic mechanism of action of dexfenfluramine by demonstrating that the drug inhibits serotonin reuptake by axon terminals and causes the release of serotonin from synaptosomes. In animals, the reduced caloric intake and the loss in body weight elicited by dexfenfluramine is associated with release of serotonin from presynaptic axon terminals in the brain, inhibition of neuronal serotonin reuptake, and, therefore, an increase of serotonin receptor activation. This results in an enhancement of serotoninergic transmission in the centers of feeding behavior, located in the ventromedial nucleus of the hypothalamus. In rats, enhanced serotoninergic transmission induced by dexfenfluramine selectively suppressed appetite for carbohydrates which resulted in reduction of food consumption when the dietary carbohydrate to protein ratio was high. Unlike amphetamines and other serotonin-active agonists and antagonists, dexfenfluramine neither enhances nor suppresses dopamine-mediated neurotransmission.

In clinical trials, Redux treatment in conjunction with a reduced-calorie diet is associated with a reduction in appetite and may slow gastric emptying. These and other actions may contribute to the reduction in caloric consumption associated with Redux. In one clinical trial, Redux was shown to preferentially decrease carbohydrate consumption at meals and to manage carbohydrate craving between meals by decreasing the consumption of snack foods with a high carbohydrate content in patients who frequently snack on such foods.

Pharmacokinetics and Metabolism

Systemic Bioavailability

Dexfenfluramine is completely absorbed after oral dosing, with a systemic bioavailability of about 68% because of first pass metabolism by the liver. In studies in which patients received a single 30-mg oral dose of dexfenfluramine, mean peak plasma concentrations of dexfenfluramine ranged between 11 and 41 ng/mL in individual patients after 1.5 to 8.0 hours. The average terminal elimination half-life of plasma dexfenfluramine ranged from 17 to 20 hours, and the average total body clearance of dexfenfluramine was 691.9 mL/min. In man, following doses of 15 mg Redux twice a day for 15 days, mean maximal plasma dexfenfluramine concentrations ranging from 15 to 92 ng/mL were observed, and steady-state plasma levels were achieved 8 days after the initial dose. The average steady-state plasma concentrations were somewhat lower than predicted by single-dose pharmacokinetics and the average time to steady-state was longer

Continued on next page

Wyeth-Ayerst Laboratories—Cont.

than the predicted 4 to 5 days. The major active metabolite, *d*-norfenfluramine, accumulated to maximal plasma concentrations of about 26 ng/mL, with steady-state plasma levels occurring at about 9 days. The *d*-norfenfluramine plasma half-life is estimated to be 32 hours. After reaching steady-state levels, there was no evidence of increasing concentrations of dexfenfluramine or *d*-norfenfluramine in plasma during 12 months of dosing. Following administration of single 30-mg, 40-mg, and 60-mg doses of dexfenfluramine to healthy volunteers, dexfenfluramine C_{max} values of 25 ng/mL, 33 ng/mL, and 51 ng/mL and area-under-the-curve$_{0\text{-}t}$ values of 144 ng·hr/mL, 191 ng·hr/mL, and 275 ng·hr/mL, respectively, were found. In a dose response study of Redux involving obese patients treated for 12 weeks, dexfenfluramine C_{min} values of 24 ng/mL at a dose of 15 mg twice daily and 58 ng/mL at a dose of 30 mg twice daily were observed. These data suggest that plasma concentrations of dexfenfluramine increase in proportion to the administered dose.

Protein Binding and Distribution

At a dexfenfluramine plasma concentration of 100 ng/mL, 36% is bound to plasma proteins. Dexfenfluramine is distributed into body tissue in non-obese subjects, with a volume of distribution of 839 L.

Metabolism

Dexfenfluramine is metabolized in the liver. The first steps in the metabolism of dexfenfluramine are dealkylation, resulting in formation of the active metabolite, *d*-norfenfluramine and deamination to an inactive *d*-hydroxy derivative. In a study of drug metabolism using radiolabeled dexfenfluramine, levofenfluramine and *d,l*-fenfluramine in two healthy subjects, 92% of the administered radioactivity was found in urine and 1% in feces over 6 days. Fenfluramine accounted for 7% to 19% and norfenfluramine accounted for 4% to 11% of the urine radioactivity. Other metabolites (inactive) included 1-(m-trifluoromethylphenyl)-1,2-propane diol (21 to 38%), m-trifluoromethyl benzoic acid (7 to 22%), m-trifluoromethyl hippuric acid (<1 to 11%), and 1-(m-trifluoromethylphenyl)-propan-2-ol (2 to 4%).

Renal Disease and Liver Disease

Specific studies in patients with renal and hepatic impairment have not been conducted.

Obese Patients

In obese patients who received a single 30-mg dose, a mean peak plasma dexfenfluramine concentration of about 22.3 ng/mL is reached after about 5.2 hours. In a parallel-group, multiple-dose pharmacokinetic study of dexfenfluramine (15 mg twice daily) there were no significant differences in steady-state pharmacokinetic parameters between obese and non-obese subjects.

Age

The pharmacokinetics of a single 30-mg dose of Redux in eight elderly patients, ranging from 66 to 83 years of age, have been examined in one study. The mean maximal plasma concentration was 21.8 ng/mL, and ranged from 9.7 to 33.0 ng/mL in individual patients. Time to maximal plasma concentration was about 5 hours and ranged from 3 hours to 10 hours. Area-under-the-curve to infinity was 615 ng·hr/mL and ranged from 16 to 1205 ng·hr/mL. Mean (±SD) steady-state plasma concentrations of dexfenfluramine and *d*-norfenfluramine after six months of treatment (15 mg twice daily) in 18 obese patients over 60 years old were 27.3 (±16.3) ng/mL and 14.0 (±7.4) ng/mL, respectively, compared to values of 24.1 (±15.9) and 15.6 (±11.2), respectively, in 268 patients under 60 years old. In a cohort of these patients followed through 12 months of treatment (15 mg twice daily) mean (±SD) steady-state plasma concentrations of dexfenfluramine and *d*-norfenfluramine in 17 obese patients over 60 years old were 32.9 (±16.8) ng/mL and 18.0 (±8.0) ng/mL, respectively, compared to values of 23.9 (±12.9) and 14.4 (±8.2), respectively, in 186 obese patients under 60 years old.

Clinical Studies

Observational epidemiologic studies have established a relationship between obesity and the risks for cardiovascular disease, non-insulin dependent diabetes mellitus (NIDDM), certain forms of cancer, gallstones, certain respiratory disorders, and an increase in overall mortality. These studies suggest that weight loss, if maintained, may produce health benefits for some patients with chronic obesity who may also be at risk for other diseases.

The long-term effects of Redux on the morbidity and mortality associated with obesity have not been established. Short-term (<4 months), placebo-controlled, double-blind studies have provided evidence that Redux does not adversely affect glycemia, lipid profile, or blood pressure control in obese patients. Some short-term studies have suggested that weight loss with Redux may be associated with a reduction in hyperglycemia in obese diabetic patients, a reduction in blood pressure in obese hypertensive patients, and improvement in the lipid profile in obese hyperlipidemic patients.

Redux has been shown to be effective in reducing excess body weight in obese patients. In 16 of 17 double-blind, placebo-controlled trials, of various treatment durations and with different design features, where all patients were on reduced-calorie diets, Redux-treated patients lost statistically significantly more weight on average than those treated with placebo. In these studies, weight loss was evident within 4 weeks of initiating treatment, even in some patients where reduced-calorie diet alone had failed to induce a significant weight loss.

In the INDEX study, a one-year, double-blind, placebo-controlled trial of obese patients, Redux, in conjunction with a reduced-calorie diet, produced a significant reduction in weight during the first 4 to 6 months. This response was maintained during continuation of therapy (up to 12 months of treatment). The percentage of patients who achieved various levels of weight loss at 1 year are shown below:

Percentage of Patients Losing Weight at One Year

	≥ 15% loss		≥ 10% loss		≥ 5% loss	
	Redux	Pbo	Redux	Pbo	Redux	Pbo
Completers* (Redux n=297/ Placebo n=262)	29%	16%	52%	30%	72%	50%
All patients ** (Redux n=463/ Placebo n=467)	21%	10%	40%	21%	64%	43%

* Data for patients who completed the entire 12-month period of the trial.

** Data for all patients who received study drug and who had any post-baseline measurement; for those patients who discontinued treatment before 12 months, the last observed data is carried-forward through the end of the study and analyzed with data from those patients who completed the trial.

Based on another analysis of the INDEX study, among all patients who were treated with Redux and identified as initial responders (*i.e.*, lost at least 4 pounds in the first 4 weeks of therapy), 60% went on to lose ≥10% of their initial body weight by the end of 1 year of treatment. Among Redux-treated patients, 78% were identified as initial responders. At the end of 1 year, the mean weight loss for the initial responders was 22 pounds, while the non-responders had a mean weight loss of 6 pounds.

Among obese patients who had been successful in losing weight by dieting alone (*i.e.*, lost at least 10 pounds in the prior year), the addition of Redux to the regimen resulted in the further loss of 26% of initial excess weight, while successful dieters who received placebo lost only 7% of initial excess weight.

INDICATIONS AND USAGE

Redux is indicated for the management of obesity including weight loss and maintenance of weight loss in patients on a reduced calorie diet. Redux is recommended for obese patients with an initial body mass index ≥30 kg/m², or ≥27 kg/m² in the presence of other risk factors (*e.g.*, hypertension, diabetes, hyperlipidemia).

The safety and effectiveness of Redux beyond 1 year have not been determined at this time.

Below is a chart of Body Mass Index (BMI) based on various heights and weights.

BMI is calculated by taking the patient's weight, in kg, divided by the patient's height, in meters, squared. Metric conversions are as follows: pounds ÷ 2.2 = kg; inches × 0.0254 = meters.

BODY MASS INDEX (BMI), kg/m²

	Height (feet, inches)					
Weight (pounds)	5'0"	5'3"	5'6"	5'9"	6'0"	6'3"
140	27	25	23	21	19	18
150	29	27	24	22	20	19
160	31	28	26	24	22	20
170	33	30	28	25	23	21
180	35	32	29	27	25	23
190	37	34	31	28	26	24
200	39	36	32	30	27	25
210	41	37	34	31	29	26
220	43	39	36	33	30	28
230	45	41	37	34	31	29
240	47	43	39	36	33	30
250	49	44	40	37	34	31

Patients with BMI values ≥30 may be candidates for Redux therapy.

Patients with BMI values of 27-29 may be candidates for Redux therapy if they also have a concomitant risk factor (*e.g.*, hypertension, diabetes, hyperlipidemia).

CONTRAINDICATIONS

Redux is contraindicated in patients with diagnosed pulmonary hypertension (see **WARNINGS**).

Redux is contraindicated in patients receiving monoamine oxidase inhibitors (see **PRECAUTIONS**—***Drug Interactions***).

Redux is contraindicated in patients with hypersensitivity to dexfenfluramine, fenfluramine, or related compounds.

WARNINGS

Primary Pulmonary Hypertension

A 2-year, international (5 country), case-control (epidemiological) study identified 95 primary pulmonary hypertension (PPH) cases; 20 of these had been exposed to anorexigens in the past, and 9 of the 20 had been exposed to anorexigens for longer than three months. In this study, the use of anorexigens for longer than 3 months was associated with an increase in the risk of developing PPH (odds ratio = 9.1, 95% confidence interval = 2.6–31.5). This increased risk of PPH was concentrated in persons who had used the drugs within the preceding year; there was no significant increase in risk for persons who had taken the drugs more than 1 year ago or for persons who had used these agents for 3 months or less. In the general population, the yearly occurrence of PPH is estimated to be about 1–2 cases per 1,000,000 persons. Therefore, the case-control study indicated an estimated risk associated with the long-term use of anorexigen drugs of about 18 cases per million persons exposed per year. According to the case-control study, obesity itself (body mass index ≥ 30 kg/m²) was also associated with an increase of about two-fold in the risk of developing PPH. PPH is a serious condition; the 4-year survival rate has been reported to be 55%.

The initial symptom of pulmonary hypertension is generally dyspnea. Other initial symptoms include: angina pectoris, syncope, or lower extremity edema. *Patients should be advised to report immediately any deterioration in exercise tolerance. Treatment should be discontinued in patients who develop new, unexplained symptoms of dyspnea, angina pectoris, syncope, or lower extremity edema. These patients should be evaluated for the etiology of these symptoms and the possible presence of pulmonary hypertension.*

Neurochemical Findings in Animals

Dexfenfluramine and its active metabolite *d*-norfenfluramine are believed to reduce food intake through interactions with the serotoninergic neurotransmitter system. In animals, doses of dexfenfluramine that result in brain concentrations approximately 10 times those observed in humans produce prolonged reductions (weeks to months) in brain serotonin concentrations following cessation of dexfenfluramine treatment. These reductions in brain serotonin concentrations are accompanied by correlate observations of diminished visualization of serotoninergic neurons by immunohistochemical techniques and decreased numbers of serotonin transporters. Some investigators have interpreted these results as surrogate indicators of neurotoxicity; others have interpreted these results as an extension of the pharmacology of serotonin reuptake inhibitors. Resolution of differences in the interpretation of the animal findings may occur with further research.

Changes in brain serotonin concentrations following acute, high-dose dexfenfluramine administration have been noted in all animal species and with all routes of drug administration tested. Prolonged reductions in brain serotonin concentrations in rats have been observed following acute, but not escalating, dose regimens. In mice, 2 years of drug administration at a dose producing at least 12 times the human brain level of dexfenfluramine produced no change in brain serotonin concentrations or serotonin transporter number. Changes in brain serotonin concentrations generally have been found to be reversible; however, the dose and brain concentration of dexfenfluramine and *d*-norfenfluramine may affect reversibility. Persistent reductions in brain serotonin concentrations and neuronal serotonin immunoreactivity were observed in three squirrel monkeys 14–17 months after a 4-day, 10 mg/kg/day subcutaneous dose regimen of dexfenfluramine; the effects of lower doses or different dose regimens were not reported in this study. In a separate study, other squirrel monkeys given this high-dose regimen achieved brain concentrations of dexfenfluramine approximately 35 times those of obese patients taking normal therapeutic doses.

Studies employing experimental techniques that are independent of serotonin content (*e.g.*, retrograde transport, silver staining, glial fibrillary acidic protein content) could not detect neuronal damage at doses of dexfenfluramine in animals producing decreased brain serotonin concentrations. The observed neurochemical changes were not associated with persistent changes in animal behavior.

The relevance of the animal findings to humans is not known.

Miscellaneous

Organic causes of obesity (*e.g.*, hypothyroidism) should be excluded before prescribing Redux.

Redux should be used with caution in patients with glaucoma.

PRECAUTIONS

General

Because of Redux's potential to produce mild-to-moderate drowsiness, the patient's individual response should be assessed before engaging in activities requiring alertness. Redux may potentiate the sedative effects of alcohol or other drugs with CNS action.

If the patient develops any symptoms of intolerance, e.g., nausea and vomiting, the dosage should be reduced, or the drug discontinued.

Misuse Potential

As with any weight-loss agent, the potential exists for misuse of Redux in inappropriate patient populations (e.g., patients with anorexia nervosa or bulimia). See **INDICATIONS AND USAGE** for recommended prescribing guidelines.

Information for Patients

Patients should be informed that false-positive urine drug tests for amphetamines have been observed for up to 24 hours following a 30-mg dose (2 capsules) of Redux. See **Drug/Laboratory Test Interactions**.

Combination Therapy

The safety and efficacy of dexfenfluramine in combination with other weight-loss agents have not been studied; therefore, concomitant use is not recommended.

Use in Patients with Concomitant Illness

Weight loss has been associated with a reduction in hyperglycemia in obese diabetic patients, a reduction of blood pressure in obese hypertensive patients, and an improvement in the lipid profile in obese hyperlipidemic patients. Therefore, when Redux™ (dexfenfluramine hydrochloride capsules) is used for the management of obesity associated with hypertension, diabetes, or dyslipidemia, there may be changes in these conditions and the medications used to treat them should be monitored, and adjusted, if necessary.

Drug Interactions

In patients receiving nonselective monoamine oxidase inhibitors (MAOIs) (e.g., selegiline hydrochloride) in combination with serotoninergic agents (e.g., fluoxetine, fluvoxamine, paroxetine, sertraline, venlafaxine), there have been reports of serious, sometimes fatal, reactions. Because Redux is a serotonin releaser and reuptake inhibitor, Redux should not be used concomitantly with a MAO inhibitor (see **CONTRA-INDICATIONS**).

At least 14 days should elapse between discontinuation of a MAO inhibitor and initiation of treatment with Redux. At least 3 weeks should elapse between discontinuation of Redux and initiation of treatment with a MAO inhibitor.

A rare, but serious, constellation of symptoms, termed "serotonin syndrome," has been reported with the concomitant use of selective serotonin reuptake inhibitors (SSRIs) and agents for migraine therapy, such as Imitrex® (sumatriptan succinate) and dihydroergotamine. The syndrome requires immediate medical attention and may include one or more of the following symptoms: excitement, hypomania, restlessness, loss of consciousness, confusion, disorientation, anxiety, agitation, motor weakness, myoclonus, tremor, hemiballismus, hyperreflexia, ataxia, dysarthria, incoordination, hyperthermia, shivering, pupillary dilation, diaphoresis, emesis, and tachycardia.

Redux should not be administered with other serotoninergic agents. The appropriate interval between administration of these agents and Redux has not been established.

The use of dexfenfluramine with other CNS-active drugs has not been systematically evaluated; consequently, caution is advised if dexfenfluramine and such drugs are prescribed concurrently.

Drug/Laboratory Test Interactions

False-positive urine drug tests for amphetamines by ELISA have been observed for up to 24 hours following a 30-mg dose (2 capsules) of Redux. Patients should be informed of this possible false-positive laboratory finding when undergoing urine drug screenings. Gas chromatography/mass spectroscopy can distinguish false-positive urine drug tests caused by dexfenfluramine from true-positive drug tests. See *Information for Patients.*

Carcinogenesis, Mutagenesis, Impairment of Fertility

Carcinogenicity studies in rats and mice have not shown a carcinogenic potential for dexfenfluramine at doses up to 12 mg/kg and 27 mg/kg, respectively. These doses are 4.8 and 5.8 times the daily human dose (calculated on a body surface area [mg/m^2] basis). When given to pregnant rats, dexfenfluramine caused a significant reduction in the number of fetuses and live young.

Dexfenfluramine has no detectable mutagenic activity as determined by the Ames test, gene conversion-DNA repair test, evaluation of the clastogenic effect on cultures of human lymphocytes, mouse lymphoma cell mutation test, and the micronucleus test in the mouse.

Pregnancy

Teratogenic Effects—Pregnancy Category C

Dexfenfluramine produced dose-related effects on reproduction and fertility in rats. In a three-generation fertility and reproduction study, administration of dexfenfluramine to female rats at 2.5 and 5 times the human daily dose (calculated on a body surface area [mg/m^2] basis) caused significant reductions in body weight and weight gain throughout pregnancy; the number of placental implantations and fetuses was reduced, there was a reduced number of live young, and delayed ossification was seen in the fetuses. No significant treatment-related adverse effects or abnormalities were observed in second- and third-generation rats. Teratogenicity studies were conducted in rats and rabbits. Neither study showed any treatment-related embryotoxicity or teratogenicity at doses up to 10 times the daily human dose (calculated on a body surface area [mg/m^2] basis). There are no adequate and well-controlled studies of Redux in pregnant women. Redux is not recommended for pregnant women.

Nursing Mothers

Dexfenfluramine is excreted in rat milk. It is not known whether dexfenfluramine is excreted in human milk. Therefore, dexfenfluramine should not be administered to a nursing woman.

Use in Other Populations

Pediatric Use

Safety and effectiveness of Redux in pediatric patients have not been established.

Geriatric Use

As with all CNS-active medications, caution should be exercised in treating elderly patients with Redux. Clinical studies of Redux did not include sufficient numbers of patients aged 65 or older to determine whether they respond differently than younger patients. Pharmacokinetics in elderly patients are discussed in **CLINICAL PHARMACOLOGY.**

ADVERSE REACTIONS

Commonly Observed

The most commonly observed, treatment-emergent adverse events associated with the use of Redux in double-blind, placebo-controlled clinical trials were diarrhea (17.5%), dry mouth (12.5%), and somnolence (7.1%). These and other commonly observed adverse reactions were generally mild and transient. (Commonly observed is defined as incidence of 5% or greater and incidence in dexfenfluramine group at least twice that of placebo group, as derived from the table below.)

Associated with Discontinuation of Treatment

Seven percent of the 1159 patients who received dexfenfluramine in double-blind, placebo-controlled clinical trials discontinued treatment because of an adverse event. The most common adverse events resulting in discontinuation included asthenia, insomnia, headache, and depression. Five percent of the 1138 placebo-treated patients discontinued because of an adverse event.

Incidence in Controlled Clinical Trials

The following table lists treatment-emergent adverse events from several double-blind, placebo-controlled trials that occurred at a frequency of 2% or more among patients treated with Redux and occurred at least as frequently as the placebo group, regardless of relationship to study medication.

[See table above.]

TREATMENT-EMERGENT ADVERSE EVENTS FROM PLACEBO-CONTROLLED CLINICAL TRIALS

ADVERSE EVENT	PERCENT OF REDUX-TREATED PATIENTS (15 mg twice daily) (n=1159)	PERCENT OF PLACEBO-TREATED PATIENTS (n=1138)
BODY AS A WHOLE		
Headache	16.1	15.5
Asthenia	15.8	10.7
Abdominal Pain	6.7	6.0
Chills	2.9	1.2
Accidental Injury	2.8	2.3
GASTROINTESTINAL SYSTEM		
Diarrhea	17.5	7.3
Vomiting	3.2	2.9
METABOLIC/NUTRITIONAL SYSTEM		
Thirst	2.8	1.1
NERVOUS SYSTEM		
Insomnia	19.9	18.6
Dry Mouth	12.5	5.0
Somnolence	7.1	3.4
Dizziness	5.5	4.0
Depression	4.7	3.6
Vertigo	3.1	1.7
Emotional Lability	3.1	2.7
Abnormal Dreams	2.0	1.4
Thinking Abnormal	2.0	1.1
RESPIRATORY SYSTEM		
Pharyngitis	6.1	5.6
Cough Increased	3.6	3.0
Bronchitis	3.4	1.8
SKIN/APPENDAGES		
Rash	2.3	2.2
UROGENITAL SYSTEM		
Urinary Frequency	2.8	1.1
Polyuria	2.1	1.0

Patients may experience more than one type of adverse event. Only events that occurred at a frequency of 2% or more in dexfenfluramine-treated patients and were at least as frequent as in placebo-treated patients are included.

Other Events Observed in Controlled Clinical Trials

The events below are classified within body system categories and enumerated in order of decreasing frequency using the following definitions. Frequent adverse events are those occurring in more than 1/100 patients but were not described above because the frequency in dexfenfluramine-treated patients was less than that in placebo-treated patients or they occurred at a rate less than 2%. Infrequent adverse events are those occurring in 1/100 to 1/1000 patients, while rare adverse events are those occurring in only one patient during placebo-controlled clinical trials.

Body as a whole—Frequent: infection, flu syndrome, pain, back pain, fever, allergic reaction. *Infrequent:* malaise, neck pain, chest pain, generalized edema, stress, face edema, neoplasm, pelvic pain. *Rare:* adenoma, immune system disorder, neck rigidity, suicide attempt.

Cardiovascular system—Frequent: hypertension, angina pectoris, palpitation, vasodilation, migraine. *Infrequent:* cardiovascular disorder, tachycardia, postural hypotension, hypotension, peripheral vascular disorder, syncope, arrhythmia, extrasystoles, hemorrhage, thrombophlebitis, varicose vein. *Rare:* heart block, pulmonary embolus, thrombosis.

Gastrointestinal system—Frequent: constipation, nausea, dyspepsia, increased appetite, rectal disorder, gastritis, gastroenteritis, flatulence. *Infrequent:* colitis, eructation, gastrointestinal hemorrhage, enteritis, peptic ulcer, hepatitis, hepatomegaly. *Rare:* appendicitis, cholelithiasis, fecal incontinence, melena, mouth ulceration, pancreatitis, rectal hemorrhage, sialoadenitis.

Endocrine—Infrequent: goiter, diabetes mellitus, thyroid disorder. *Rare:* hypothyroidism.

Hemic and lymphatic system—Infrequent: anemia, lymphedema. *Rare:* coagulation disorder, lymphadenopathy, polycythemia, thrombocythemia.

Metabolic and nutritional—Infrequent: edema, gout, hypoglycemia, hypokalemia. *Rare:* hyperglycemia, hyperkalemia, hyperlipemia, hyperuricemia.

Musculoskeletal system—Frequent: arthralgia, myalgia, arthritis. *Infrequent:* leg cramps, joint disorder, bone disorder, tenosynovitis, myasthenia, rheumatoid arthritis. *Rare:* bursitis, tetany.

Nervous system—Frequent: nervousness, anxiety, increased libido, hypertonia, paresthesia. *Infrequent:* tremor, amnesia, euphoria, decreased libido, incoordination, neuralgia, speech disorder, ataxia, hypokinesia, sleep disorder, abnormal gait, agitation, confusion, depersonalization, diplopia, hostility, hyperesthesia, hyperkinesia, peripheral neuritis. *Rare:* apathy, dementia, hallucinations, hypotonia, neuritis, neurosis, paralysis.

Continued on next page

Wyeth-Ayerst Laboratories—Cont.

Respiratory system—Frequent: rhinitis, sinusitis. *Infrequent:* asthma, dyspnea, epistaxis, laryngitis. *Rare:* apnea, hyperventilation.
Skin and appendages—Frequent: sweating, alopecia, urticaria, pruritus. *Infrequent:* skin disorder, fungal dermatitis, hirsutism, eczema, psoriasis. *Rare:* skin hypertrophy.
Special senses—Frequent: taste perversion, amblyopia. *Infrequent:* abnormal vision, conjunctivitis, eye disorder, glaucoma, tinnitus, vestibular disorder, dry eyes, mydriasis. *Rare:* abnormality of accommodation, anisocoria, lacrimation disorder, miosis, parosmia, retinal disorder.
Urogenital system—Frequent: menstrual disorder, urinary tract infection, nocturia, dysmenorrhea. *Infrequent:* amenorrhea, dysuria, oliguria, albuminuria, breast pain, kidney calculus, kidney pain. *Rare:* spontaneous abortion, threatened abortion, breast neoplasm, endometrial disorder, female lactation, hematuria, impotence, mastitis, nephritis, prostatic disorder, testis disorder, urinary incontinence, urinary retention, uterine hemorrhage.

In controlled clinical trials, there has been no consistent pattern of laboratory abnormalities in patients treated with dexfenfluramine.

Post-introduction Reports
Voluntary reports of adverse events temporally associated with dexfenfluramine that have been received since market introduction in countries other than the US, for which the association with the drug is unknown, and which are not included in descriptions of adverse events elsewhere in this labeling, include the following:
Body as a whole—anaphylaxis, congenital anomaly, eventration, hypothermia, laryngeal edema, peritonitis, reaction aggravation, retroperitoneal fibrosis, scleroderma, sudden death.
Cardiovascular system—pulmonary hypertension (see **WARNINGS**), atrial fibrillation, cardiomyopathy, cerebral vasculitis, ECG abnormal, heart arrest, heart failure, myocardial infarction, myocarditis, shock, tachycardia, ventricular fibrillation, ventricular tachycardia.
Digestive system—dysphagia, gastrointestinal disorder, tongue disorder.
Endocrine system—diabetic coma.
Gastrointestinal system—hepatic failure, jaundice, liver damage.
Hemic and lymphatic system—agranulocytosis, antinuclear antibody present, bone marrow depression, ecchymosis, hemolytic anemia, pancytopenia.
Metabolic and nutritional—dehydration, elevated lipases, increased prolactin, thyroid disease, weight increase.
Musculoskeletal—myopathy.
Nervous system—antisocial reaction, apathy, cerebellar ataxia, cerebrovascular accident (including cerebral hemorrhage, cerebral infarction, cerebral ischemia and cochlear infarction), choreoathetosis, convulsions, decreased reflexes, delirium, drug dependence, dyslexia, encephalopathy, grand mal convulsions, Guillain-Barré syndrome, hemiplegia, hypoesthesia, manic-depressive psychosis, manic reaction, memory loss, meningism, meningitis, neuropathy, papilledema, paraplegia, personality disorder, reflexes increased, retrobulbar neuritis, schizophrenic reaction, stupor, subdural hematoma, twitch, withdrawal syndrome.
Respiratory system—pulmonary hypertension (see **WARNINGS**), diffuse interstitial pneumonitis, dyspnea, hiccup, lung edema.
Skin and appendages—angioedema, bullous eruption, erythema multiforme, lower extremity purpura, purpura annularis telangiectodes, Stevens-Johnson syndrome (erythema multiforme major).
Special senses—ophthalmoplegia, photophobia, transitory deafness, visual field defects.
Urogenital system—breast enlargement, carcinoma (breast), carcinoma (cervix), ejaculation abnormal, gynecomastia, hypomenorrhea, kidney failure, placenta previa, urinary tract disorder.

Adverse Events Occurring After Discontinuation
In controlled clinical trials and/or in post-marketing reports, symptoms have been reported within a few days after discontinuation of Redux. These include one or more of the following: abdominal pain, anxiety, asthenia, delusion, depression, diarrhea, dizziness, hypertension, insomnia, nausea and vomiting.

DRUG ABUSE AND DEPENDENCE

Controlled Substance Class
Dexfenfluramine is a controlled substance in Schedule IV.
Abuse and Physical and Psychological Dependence
Dexfenfluramine is not an amphetamine or a stimulant. There is no evidence of addictive or drug-seeking behavior in pre-marketing clinical studies. Dexfenfluramine was inactive in rat and monkey self-administration, drug-discrimination, and place-preference models of abuse potential.

OVERDOSAGE

Human Experience
Post-marketing experience in Europe over 10 years (August 1984 through December 1994) in an estimated 10 million patients provided reports of 66 instances of overdose (maximum dose per body mass of 54 mg/kg, maximum total dose of 1800 mg), including eight children 6 years of age or under. Three deaths have occurred in association with dexfenfluramine overdosage. One patient with a history of suicide attempts ingested 1800 mg dexfenfluramine and 20 to 30 capsules of Tranxene (clorazepate), one patient was found dead, assumed to have consumed approximately 1500 mg of dexfenfluramine, and the third patient consumed dexfenfluramine (quantity unknown) and several other drugs in an apparent suicide. The second patient had post-mortem levels of dexfenfluramine of 3300 ng/mL, and positive levels for amphetamines and cannabinoids. The exact causes of death were unknown. In 23 other cases of dexfenfluramine overdose, plasma drug levels were determined; the maximum reported plasma drug level for dexfenfluramine was 778 ng/mL (with *d*-norfenfluramine 37 ng/mL); the maximum *d*-norfenfluramine level was 371 ng/mL (with dexfenfluramine 483 ng/mL).
Symptoms associated with overdosage consisted mainly of agitation, drowsiness, mydriasis, sweating, shivering, nausea, and vomiting.
Other symptoms observed with dexfenfluramine overdose and not noted under **ADVERSE REACTIONS** include cold sensation, excitation, nystagmus, garrulousness, delusions, bladder tenesmus, chattering teeth, abnormal reflexes, facial myoclonus, trismus, tonic-clonic seizures, impairment of consciousness, coma (stage 2–4), sinus bradycardia, repolarization abnormalities, right anterior hemiblock, polypnea, diffuse bronchial rales, and flushing.
Animal Experience
Significant acute toxicity occurred at oral doses greater than 40, 70, and 75 mg/kg in rats, mice, and guinea pigs, respectively. A dose of 40 mg/kg is approximately 31 times greater than the effective anorectic dose in rats.
Management of Overdose
General supportive measures for oral drug overdose should be instituted. Measures that have been used in dexfenfluramine overdose cases include aspiration of gastric contents, gastric lavage with activated charcoal, osmotic diuresis, forced acid diuresis, and careful monitoring of CNS or repiratory depression. The effectiveness of dialysis is not known. Patients should be followed closely until there is no further evidence of drug-related CNS effects. No specific therapy for dexfenfluramine overdose is known.

DOSAGE AND ADMINISTRATION

The usual dosage is one 15-mg capsule twice daily, with meals. Doses above 30 mg per day are not recommended.
Analysis of numerous variables has indicated that about 60% of patients who lose at least 4 pounds in the first 4 weeks of treatment with Redux in combination with a reduced-calorie diet lose at least 10% of their initial body weight by the end of 1 year of treatment. If a patient has not lost at least 4 pounds in the first 4 weeks of treatment, the physician should consider reevaluation of therapy which may include discontinuation of Redux.
The safety and effectiveness of Redux beyond 1 year have not been determined at this time.
Infrequently, symptoms (*e.g.,* abdominal pain, anxiety, asthenia, delusion, depression, diarrhea, dizziness, hypertension, insomnia, nausea and vomiting) have occurred within several days following cessation of Redux. If the physician notes such symptoms, clinical judgment should guide the treatment, which may include tapering the dose (15 mg once daily) for 2 weeks prior to complete discontinuation.

HOW SUPPLIED

Redux™ (dexfenfluramine hydrochloride capsules) 15 mg, is supplied in number 3, white, opaque, hard-gelatin capsules. Each capsule is marked with "REDUX" and three black vertical bands. Redux is provided as follows:
HDPE bottles containing:
60 capsules per package (NDC 0008-0904-01)
Store at room temperature, between 15°C and 30°C (59°F and 86°F).
CAUTION: Federal law prohibits dispensing without prescription.
Address medical inquiries to:
Wyeth-Ayerst Laboratories
1-610-688-4400
Redux™ is a trademark of ORSEM (SERVIER).
Manufactured for and distributed by:
Wyeth Laboratories Inc.
A Wyeth-Ayerst Company
Philadelphia, PA 19101
Under license from:
Interneuron Pharmaceuticals, Inc.
Lexington, MA 02173
8A0551
Shown in Product Identification Guide, page 341

SECTRAL® ℞

[sek'tral]
(acebutolol hydrochloride)
Capsules

DESCRIPTION

Sectral (acebutolol HCl) is a selective, hydrophilic beta-adrenoreceptor blocking agent with mild intrinsic sympathomimetic activity for use in treating patients with hypertension and ventricular arrhythmias. It is marketed in capsule form for oral administration. Sectral capsules are provided in two dosage strengths which contain 200 or 400 mg of acebutolol as the hydrochloride salt. The inactive ingredients present are D&C Red 22, FD&C Blue 1, FD&C Yellow 6, gelatin, povidone, starch, stearic acid, and titanium dioxide. The 200 mg dosage strength also contains D&C Red 28 and the 400 mg dosage strength also contains FD&C Red 40.
Acebutolol HCl has the following structural formula:

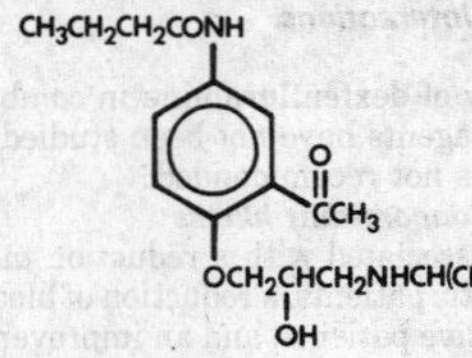

$C_{18}H_{28}N_2O_4 \cdot HCl$ M.W. 372.9

Acebutolol HCl is a white or slightly off-white powder freely soluble in water, and less soluble in alcohol. Chemically it is defined as the hydrochloride salt of Butanamide, N-[3-acetyl-4-[2-hydroxy-3-[(1-methylethyl)amino]propoxy]phenyl]-, (±)- or (±)-3'-Acetyl-4'-[2-hydroxy -3- (isopropylamino) propoxy] butyranilide.

CLINICAL PHARMACOLOGY

Sectral is a cardioselective, β-adrenoreceptor blocking agent, which possesses mild intrinsic sympathomimetic activity (ISA) in its therapeutically effective dose range.
PHARMACODYNAMICS
β_1-cardioselectivity has been demonstrated in experimental animal studies. In anesthetized dogs and cats, Sectral is more potent in antagonizing isoproterenol-induced tachycardia (β_1) than in antagonizing isoproterenol-induced vasodilatation (β_2). In guinea pigs and cats, it is more potent in antagonizing this tachycardia than in antagonizing isoproterenol-induced bronchodilatation (β_2). ISA of Sectral has been demonstrated in catecholamine-depleted rats by tachycardia induced by intravenous administration of this agent. A membrane-stabilizing effect has been detected in animals, but only with high concentrations of Sectral.
Clinical studies have demonstrated β_1-blocking activity at the recommended doses by: a) reduction in the resting heart rate and decrease in exercise-induced tachycardia; b) reduction in cardiac output at rest and after exercise; c) reduction of systolic and diastolic blood pressures at rest and postexercise; d) inhibition of isoproterenol-induced tachycardia.
The β_1-selectivity of Sectral has also been demonstrated on the basis of the following vascular and bronchial effects:
Vascular Effects: Sectral has less antagonistic effects on peripheral vascular β_2-receptors at rest and after epinephrine stimulation than nonselective β-antagonists.
Bronchial Effects: In single-dose studies in asthmatics examining effects of various beta-blockers on pulmonary function, low doses of acebutolol produce less evidence of bronchoconstriction and less reduction of beta$_2$ agonist, bronchodilating effects, than nonselective agents like propranolol but more than atenolol.
ISA has been observed with Sectral in man, as shown by a slightly smaller (about 3 beats per minute) decrease in resting heart rate when compared to equivalent β-blocking doses of propranolol, metoprolol or atenolol. Chronic therapy with Sectral induced no significant alteration in the blood lipid profile.
Sectral has been shown to delay AV conduction time and to increase the refractoriness of the AV node without significantly affecting sinus node recovery time, atrial refractory period, or the HV conduction time. The membrane-stabilizing effect of Sectral is not manifest at the doses used clinically.
Significant reductions in resting and exercise heart rates and systolic blood pressures have been observed 1.5 hours after Sectral administration with maximal effects occurring between 3 and 8 hours postdosing in normal volunteers. Sectral has demonstrated a significant effect on exercise-induced tachycardia 24 to 30 hours after drug administration.
There are significant correlations between plasma levels of acebutolol and both the reduction in resting heart rate and the percent of β-blockade of exercise-induced tachycardia.
The antihypertensive effect of Sectral has been shown in double-blind controlled studies to be superior to placebo and similar to propranolol and hydrochlorothiazide. In addition, patients responding to Sectral administered twice daily had

a similar response whether the dosage regimen was changed to once daily administration or continued on a b.i.d. regimen. Most patients responded to 400 to 800 mg per day in divided doses.

The antiarrhythmic effect of Sectral was compared with placebo, propranolol, and quinidine. Compared with placebo, Sectral significantly reduced mean total ventricular ectopic beats (VEB), paired VEB, multiform VEB, R-on-T beats, and ventricular tachycardia (VT). Both Sectral and propranolol significantly reduced mean total and paired VEB and VT. Sectral and quinidine significantly reduced resting total and complex VEB; the antiarrhythmic efficacy of Sectral was also observed during exercise.

PHARMACOKINETICS AND METABOLISM

Sectral is well absorbed from the GI tract. It is subject to extensive first-pass hepatic biotransformation, with an absolute bioavailability of approximately 40% for the parent compound. The major metabolite, an N-acetyl derivative (diacetolol), is pharmacologically active. This metabolite is equipotent to Sectral and in cats is more cardioselective than Sectral; therefore, this first-pass phenomenon does not attenuate the therapeutic effect of Sectral. Food intake does not have a significant effect on the area under the plasma concentration-time curve (AUC) of Sectral although the rate of absorption and peak concentration decreased slightly.

The plasma elimination half-life of Sectral is approximately 3 to 4 hours, while that of its metabolite, diacetolol, is 8 to 13 hours. The time to reach peak concentration for Sectral is 2.5 hours and for diacetolol, after oral administration of Sectral, 3.5 hours.

Within the single oral dose range of 200 to 400 mg, the kinetics are dose proportional. However, this linearity is not seen at higher doses, probably due to saturation of hepatic biotransformation sites. In addition, after multiple dosing the lack of linearity is also seen by AUC increases of approximately 100% as compared to single oral dosing. Elimination via renal excretion is approximately 30% to 40% and by non-renal mechanisms 50% to 60%, which includes excretion into the bile and direct passage through the intestinal wall. Sectral has a low binding affinity for plasma proteins (about 26%). Sectral and its metabolite, diacetolol, are relatively hydrophilic and, therefore, only minimal quantities have been detected in the cerebrospinal fluid (CSF).

Drug interaction studies with tolbutamide and warfarin indicated no influence on the therapeutic effects of these compounds. Digoxin and hydrochlorothiazide plasma levels were not affected by concomitant Sectral administration. The kinetics of Sectral were not significantly altered by concomitant administration of hydrochlorothiazide, hydralazine, sulfinpyrazone, or oral contraceptives.

In patients with renal impairment, there is no effect on the elimination half-life of Sectral, but there is decreased elimination of the metabolite, diacetolol, resulting in a two- to three-fold increase in its half-life. For this reason, the drug should be administered with caution in patients with renal insufficiency (see "Precautions"). Sectral and its major metabolite are dialyzable.

Sectral crosses the placental barrier and is secreted in breast milk.

In geriatric patients, the bioavailability of Sectral and its metabolite is increased, approximately two-fold, probably due to decreases in the first-pass metabolism and renal function in the elderly.

INDICATIONS AND USAGE

HYPERTENSION

Sectral is indicated for the management of hypertension in adults. It may be used alone or in combination with other antihypertensive agents, especially thiazide-type diuretics.

VENTRICULAR ARRHYTHMIAS

Sectral is indicated in the management of ventricular premature beats; it reduces the total number of premature beats, as well as the number of paired and multiform ventricular ectopic beats, and R-on-T beats.

CONTRAINDICATIONS

Sectral is contraindicated in: 1) persistently severe bradycardia; 2) second- and third-degree heart block; 3) overt cardiac failure; and 4) cardiogenic shock. (See "WARNINGS.")

WARNINGS

CARDIAC FAILURE

Sympathetic stimulation may be essential for support of the circulation in individuals with diminished myocardial contractility, and its inhibition by β-adrenergic receptor blockade may precipitate more severe failure. Although β-blockers should be avoided in overt cardiac failure, Sectral can be used with caution in patients with a history of heart failure who are controlled with digitalis and/or diuretics. Both digitalis and Sectral impair AV conduction. If cardiac failure persists, therapy with Sectral should be withdrawn.

IN PATIENTS WITHOUT A HISTORY OF CARDIAC FAILURE

In patients with aortic or mitral valve disease or compromised left ventricular function, continued depression of the myocardium with β-blocking agents over a period of time may lead to cardiac failure. At the first signs of failure, pa-

tients should be digitalized and/or be given a diuretic and the response observed closely. If cardiac failure continues despite adequate digitalization and/or diuretic, Sectral therapy should be withdrawn.

EXACERBATION OF ISCHEMIC HEART DISEASE FOLLOWING ABRUPT WITHDRAWAL

Following abrupt cessation of therapy with certain β-blocking agents in patients with coronary artery disease, exacerbation of angina pectoris and, in some cases, myocardial infarction and death have been reported. Therefore, such patients should be cautioned against interruption of therapy without a physician's advice. Even in the absence of overt ischemic heart disease, when discontinuation of Sectral is planned, the patient should be carefully observed, and should be advised to limit physical activity to a minimum while Sectral is gradually withdrawn over a period of about two weeks. (If therapy with an alternative β-blocker is desired, the patient may be transferred directly to comparable doses of another agent without interruption of β-blocking therapy.) If an exacerbation of angina pectoris occurs, antianginal therapy should be restarted immediately in full doses and the patient hospitalized until his condition stabilizes.

PERIPHERAL VASCULAR DISEASE

Treatment with β-antagonists reduces cardiac output and can precipitate or aggravate the symptoms of arterial insufficiency in patients with peripheral or mesenteric vascular disease. Caution should be exercised with such patients, and they should be observed closely for evidence of progression of arterial obstruction.

BRONCHOSPASTIC DISEASES

PATIENTS WITH BRONCHOSPASTIC DISEASE SHOULD, IN GENERAL, NOT RECEIVE A β-BLOCKER. Because of its relative β_1-selectivity, however, low doses of Sectral may be used with caution in patients with bronchospastic disease who do not respond to, or who cannot tolerate, alternative treatment. Since β_1-selectivity is not absolute and is dose-dependent, the lowest possible dose of Sectral should be used initially, preferably in divided doses to avoid the higher plasma levels associated with the longer dose-interval. A bronchodilator, such as a theophylline or a β_2-stimulant, should be made available in advance with instructions concerning its use.

ANESTHESIA AND MAJOR SURGERY

The necessity, or desirability, of withdrawal of a β-blocking therapy prior to major surgery is controversial. β-adrenergic receptor blockade impairs the ability of the heart to respond to β-adrenergically mediated reflex stimuli. While this might be of benefit in preventing arrhythmic response, the risk of excessive myocardial depression during general anesthesia may be enhanced and difficulty in restarting and maintaining the heart beat has been reported with beta-blockers. If treatment is continued, particular care should be taken when using anesthetic agents which depress the myocardium, such as ether, cyclopropane and trichlorethylene, and it is prudent to use the lowest possible dose of Sectral. Sectral, like other β-blockers, is a competitive inhibitor of β-receptor agonists, and its effect on the heart can be reversed by cautious administration of such agents (e.g., dobutamine or isoproterenol—see "Overdose").

Manifestations of excessive vagal tone (e.g., profound bradycardia, hypotension) may be corrected with atropine 1 to 3 mg IV in divided doses.

DIABETES AND HYPOGLYCEMIA

β-blockers may potentiate insulin-induced hypoglycemia and mask some of its manifestations such as tachycardia; however, dizziness and sweating are usually not significantly affected. Diabetic patients should be warned of the possibility of masked hypoglycemia.

THYROTOXICOSIS

β-adrenergic blockade may mask certain clinical signs (tachycardia) of hyperthyroidism. Abrupt withdrawal of β-blockade may precipitate a thyroid storm; therefore, patients suspected of developing thyrotoxicosis from whom Sectral therapy is to be withdrawn should be monitored closely.

PRECAUTIONS

IMPAIRED RENAL OR HEPATIC FUNCTION

Studies on the effect of acebutolol in patients with renal insufficiency have not been performed in the U.S. Foreign published experience shows that acebutolol has been used successfully in chronic renal insufficiency. Acebutolol is excreted through the GI tract, but the active metabolite, diacetolol, is eliminated predominantly by the kidney. There is a linear relationship between renal clearance of diacetolol and creatinine clearance. Therefore, the daily dose of acebutolol should be reduced by 50% when the creatinine clearance is less than 50 mL/min and by 75% when it is less than 25 mL/min. Sectral should be used cautiously in patients with impaired hepatic function.

Sectral has been used successfully and without problems in elderly patients in the U.S. clinical trials without specific adjustment of dosage. However, elderly patients may require lower maintenance doses because the bioavailability of both Sectral and its metabolite are approximately doubled in this age group.

INFORMATION FOR PATIENTS

Patients, especially those with evidence of coronary artery disease, should be warned against interruption or discontinuation of Sectral therapy without a physician's supervision. Although cardiac failure rarely occurs in properly selected patients, those being treated with β-adrenergic blocking agents should be advised to consult a physician if they develop signs or symptoms suggestive of impending CHF, or unexplained respiratory symptoms.

Patients should also be warned of possible severe hypertensive reactions from concomitant use of α-adrenergic stimulants, such as the nasal decongestants commonly used in OTC cold preparations and nasal drops.

CLINICAL LABORATORY FINDINGS

Sectral, like other β-blockers, has been associated with the development of antinuclear antibodies (ANA). In prospective clinical trials, patients receiving Sectral had a dose-dependent increase in the development of positive ANA titers, and the overall incidence was higher than that observed with propranolol. Symptoms (generally persistent arthralgias and myalgias) related to this laboratory abnormality were infrequent (less than 1% with both drugs). Symptoms and ANA titers were reversible upon discontinuation of treatment.

DRUG INTERACTIONS

Catecholamine-depleting drugs, such as reserpine, may have an additive effect when given with β-blocking agents. Patients treated with Sectral plus catecholamine depletors should, therefore, be observed closely for evidence of marked bradycardia or hypotension which may present as vertigo, syncope/presyncope, or orthostatic changes in blood pressure without compensatory tachycardia. Exaggerated hypertensive responses have been reported from the combined use of β-adrenergic antagonists and α-adrenergic stimulants, including those contained in proprietary cold remedies and vasoconstrictive nasal drops. Patients receiving β-blockers should be warned of this potential hazard.

Blunting of the antihypertensive effect of beta-adrenoceptor blocking agents by nonsteroidal anti-inflammatory drugs has been reported.

No significant interactions with digoxin, hydrochlorothiazide, hydralazine, sulfinpyrazone, oral contraceptives, tolbutamide, or warfarin have been observed.

CARCINOGENESIS, MUTAGENESIS, IMPAIRMENT OF FERTILITY

Chronic oral toxicity studies in rats and mice, employing dose levels as high as 300 mg/kg/day, which is equivalent to 15 times the maximum recommended (60 kg) human dose, did not indicate a carcinogenic potential for Sectral. Diacetolol, the major metabolite of Sectral in man, was without carcinogenic potential in rats when tested at doses as high as 1800 mg/kg/day. Sectral and diacetolol were also shown to be devoid of mutagenic potential in the Ames Test. Sectral, administered orally to two generations of male and female rats at doses of up to 240 mg/kg/day (equivalent to 12 times the maximum recommended therapeutic dose in a 60-kg human) and diacetolol, administered to two generations of male and female rats at doses of up to 1000 mg/kg/day, had no significant impact on reproductive performance or fertility.

PREGNANCY

Teratogenic Effects:

Pregnancy Category B: Reproduction studies have been performed with Sectral in rats (up to 630 mg/kg/day) and rabbits (up to 135 mg/kg/day). These doses are equivalent to approximately 31.5 and 6.8 times the maximum recommended therapeutic dose in a 60-kg human, respectively. The compound was not teratogenic in either species. In the rabbit, however, doses of 135 mg/kg/day caused slight fetal growth retardation; this effect was considered to be a result of maternal toxicity, as evidenced by reduced food intake, a lowered rate of body weight gain, and mortality. Studies have also been performed in these species with diacetolol (at doses of up to 450 mg/kg/day in rabbits and up to 1800 mg/kg/day in rats). Other than a significant elevation in postimplantation loss with 450 mg/kg/day diacetolol, a level at which food consumption and body weight gain were reduced in rabbit dams and a nonstatistically significant increase in incidence of bilateral cataract in rat fetuses from dams treated with 1800 mg/kg/day diacetolol, there was no evidence of harm to the fetus. There are no adequate and well-controlled trials in pregnant women. Because animal teratology studies are not always predictive of the human response, Sectral should be used during pregnancy only if the potential benefit justifies the risk to the fetus.

Nonteratogenic Effects:

Studies in humans have shown that both acebutolol and diacetolol cross the placenta. Neonates of mothers who have received acebutolol during pregnancy have reduced birth weight, decreased blood pressure, and decreased heart rate. In the newborn the elimination half-life of acebutolol was 6 to 14 hours, while the half-life of diacetolol was 24 to 30 hours for the first 24 hours after birth, followed by a half-life

Continued on next page

Wyeth-Ayerst Laboratories—Cont.

of 12 to 16 hours. Adequate facilities for monitoring these infants at birth should be available.

LABOR AND DELIVERY

The effect of Sectral on labor and delivery in pregnant women is unknown. Studies in animals have not shown any effect of Sectral on the usual course of labor and delivery.

NURSING MOTHERS

Acebutolol and diacetolol also appear in breast milk with a milk:plasma ratio of 7.1 and 12.2, respectively. Use in nursing mothers is not recommended.

PEDIATRIC USE

Safety and effectiveness in pediatric patients have not been established.

ADVERSE REACTIONS

Sectral is well tolerated in properly selected patients. Most adverse reactions have been mild, not required discontinuation of therapy, and tended to decrease as duration of treatment increases.

The following table shows the frequency of treatment-related side effects derived from controlled clinical trials in patients with hypertension, angina pectoris, and arrhythmia. These patients received Sectral, propranolol, or hydrochlorothiazide as monotherapy, or placebo.

[See table at right.]

The following selected (potentially important) side effects were seen in up to 2% of Sectral patients:

Cardiovascular: hypotension, bradycardia, heart failure.
Central Nervous System: anxiety, hyper/hypoesthesia, impotence.
Dermatological: pruritus.
Gastrointestinal: vomiting, abdominal pain.
Genitourinary: dysuria, nocturia.
Liver and Biliary System: A small number of cases of liver abnormalities (increased SGOT, SGPT, LDH) have been reported in association with acebutolol therapy. In some cases increased bilirubin or alkaline phosphatase, fever, malaise, dark urine, anorexia, nausea, headache, and/or other symptoms have been reported. In some of the reported cases, the symptoms and signs were confirmed by rechallenge with acebutolol. The abnormalities were reversible upon cessation of acebutolol therapy.
Musculoskeletal: back pain, joint pain.
Respiratory: pharyngitis, wheezing.
Special Senses: conjunctivitis, dry eye, eye pain.
Autoimmune: In extremely rare instances, systemic lupus erythematosus has been reported.

The incidence of drug-related adverse effects (volunteered and solicited) according to Sectral dose is shown below. (Data from 266 hypertensive patients treated for 3 months on a constant dose.)

Body System	400 mg/day (N = 132)	800 mg/day (N = 63)	1200 mg/day (N = 71)
Cardiovascular	5%	2%	1%
Gastrointestinal	3%	3%	7%
Musculoskeletal	2%	3%	4%
Central Nervous System	9%	13%	17%
Respiratory	1%	5%	6%
Skin	1%	2%	1%
Special Senses	2%	2%	6%
Genitourinary	2%	3%	1%

POTENTIAL ADVERSE EFFECTS

In addition, certain adverse effects not listed above have been reported with other β-blocking agents and should also be considered as potential adverse effects of Sectral.

Central Nervous System: Reversible mental depression progressing to catatonia (an acute syndrome characterized by disorientation for time and place), short-term memory loss, emotional lability, slightly clouded sensorium, and decreased performance (neuropsychometrics).
Cardiovascular: Intensification of AV block (see "Contraindications").
Allergic: Erythematous rash, fever combined with aching and sore throat, laryngospasm, and respiratory distress.
Hematologic: Agranulocytosis, nonthrombocytopenic, and thrombocytopenic purpura.
Gastrointestinal: Mesenteric arterial thrombosis and ischemic colitis.
Miscellaneous: Reversible alopecia and Peyronie's disease. The oculomucocutaneous syndrome associated with the β-blocker practolol has not been reported with Sectral during investigational use and extensive foreign clinical experience.

OVERDOSAGE

No specific information on emergency treatment of overdosage is available for Sectral. However, overdosage with other β-blocking agents has been accompanied by extreme brady-

cardia, advanced atrioventricular block, intraventricular conduction defects, hypotension, severe congestive heart failure, seizures, and in susceptible patients, bronchospasm and hypoglycemia. Although specific information on the emergency treatment of Sectral overdose is not available, on the basis of the pharmacological actions and the observations in treating overdoses with other β-blockers, the following general measures should be considered:

1. Empty stomach by emesis or lavage.
2. Bradycardia: IV atropine (1 to 3 mg in divided doses). If antivagal response is inadequate, administer isoproterenol cautiously since larger than usual doses of isoproterenol may be required.
3. Persistent hypotension in spite of correction of bradycardia: Administer vasopressor (e.g., epinephrine, levarterenol, dopamine, or dobutamine) with frequent monitoring of blood pressure and pulse rate.
4. Bronchospasm: A theophylline derivative, such as aminophylline and/or parenteral β_2-stimulant, such as terbutaline.
5. Cardiac failure: Digitalize the patient and/or administer a diuretic. It has been reported that glucagon is useful in this situation.

Sectral is dialyzable.

DOSAGE AND ADMINISTRATION

HYPERTENSION

The initial dosage of Sectral in uncomplicated mild-to-moderate hypertension is 400 mg. This can be given as a single daily dose, but in occasional patients twice daily dosing may be required for adequate 24-hour blood-pressure control. An optimal response is usually achieved with dosages of 400 to 800 mg per day, although some patients have been maintained on as little as 200 mg per day. Patients with more severe hypertension or who have demonstrated inadequate control may respond to a total of 1200 mg daily (administered b.i.d.), or to the addition of a second antihypertensive agent. Beta-1 selectivity diminishes as dosage is increased.

VENTRICULAR ARRHYTHMIA

The usual initial dose of Sectral is 400 mg daily given as 200 mg b.i.d. Dosage should be increased gradually until an optimal clinical response is obtained, generally at 600 to 1200 mg per day. If treatment is to be discontinued, the dosage should be reduced gradually over a period of about two weeks.

USE IN OLDER PATIENTS

Older patients have an approximately 2-fold increase in bioavailability and may require lower maintenance doses. Doses above 800 mg/day should be avoided in the elderly.

HOW SUPPLIED

Sectral® (acebutolol HCl) is available in the following dosage strengths:

200 mg, opaque purple and orange capsule marked "WYETH 4177" and "Sectral 200"
NDC 0008-4177-01, in bottles of 100 capsules.
NDC 0008-4177-04, in Redipak® cartons of 100 capsules (10 blister strips of 10).
Keep tightly closed
Store at room temperature, approximately 25° C (77°F)

TOTAL VOLUNTEERED AND ELICITED (U.S. STUDIES)

Body System/ Adverse Reaction	SECTRAL (N = 1002) %	Propranolol (N =424) %	Hydrochloro- thiazide (N = 178) %	Placebo (N = 314) %
Cardiovascular				
Chest Pain	2	4	4	1
Edema	2	2	4	1
Central Nervous System				
Depression	2	1	3	1
Dizziness	6	7	12	2
Fatigue	11	17	10	4
Headache	6	9	13	4
Insomnia	3	6	5	1
Abnormal dreams	2	3	0	1
Dermatologic				
Rash	2	2	4	1
Gastrointestinal				
Constipation	4	2	7	0
Diarrhea	4	5	5	1
Dyspepsia	4	6	3	1
Flatulence	3	4	7	1
Nausea	4	6	3	0
Genitourinary				
Micturition (frequency)	3	1	9	< 1
Musculoskeletal				
Arthralgia	2	1	3	2
Myalgia	2	1	4	0
Respiratory				
Cough	1	1	2	0
Dyspnea	4	6	4	2
Rhinitis	2	1	4	< 1
Special Senses				
Abnormal Vision	2	2	3	0

Protect from light
Dispense in a light-resistant, tight container
Use carton to protect contents from light
400 mg, opaque brown and orange capsule marked "WYETH 4179" and "Sectral 400"
NDC 0008-4179-01, in bottles of 100 capsules.
Keep tightly closed
Store at room temperature, approximately 25°C (77°F)
Dispense in a tight container
The appearance of these capsules is a trademark of Wyeth-Ayerst Laboratories.

by arrangement with Rhone-Poulenc Rorer France

Shown in Product Identification Guide, page 341

SERAX® ℮ ℞

[*ser 'aks*]
(oxazepam)
CAPSULES ● TABLETS

DESCRIPTION

Serax is the first of a chemically new series of compounds, the 3-hydroxybenzodiazepinones. A new therapeutic agent providing versatility and flexibility in control of common emotional disturbances, this product exerts prompt action in a wide variety of disorders associated with anxiety, tension, agitation, and irritability, and anxiety associated with depression. In tolerance and toxicity studies on several animal species, this product reveals significantly greater safety factors than related compounds (chlordiazepoxide and diazepam) and manifests a wide separation of effective doses and doses inducing side effects.

Serax capsules contain 10 mg, 15 mg, or 30 mg oxazepam. The inactive ingredients present are gelatin, lactose, titanium dioxide, and other ingredients. Each dosage strength also contains the following:
10 mg—D&C Red 22, D&C Red 28, and FD&C Blue 1;
15 mg—FD&C Red 40 and FD&C Yellow 6;
30 mg—D&C Red 28, FD&C Red 40, and FD&C Blue 1.
Serax tablets contain 15 mg oxazepam. The inactive ingredients present are FD&C Yellow 5, lactose, magnesium stearate, methylcellulose, and polacrilin potassium.
Serax is 7-chloro-1,3,-dihydro-3-hydroxy-5-phenyl-$2H$-1,4-benzodiazepin-2-one, a white crystalline powder with a molecular weight of 286.7.

CLINICAL PHARMACOLOGY

Pharmacokinetic testing in twelve volunteers demonstrated that when given as a single 30 mg dose, the capsule, tablet, and suspension were equivalent in extent of absorption. For the capsule and tablet, peak plasma levels averaged 450 ng/mL and were observed to occur about 3 hours after dosing. The mean elimination half-life for oxazepam was approximately 8.2 hours (range 5.7 to 10.9 hours).
This product has a single, major inactive metabolite in man, a glucuronide excreted in the urine.

ANIMAL PHARMACOLOGY AND TOXICOLOGY

In mice, Serax exerts an anticonvulsant (anti-Metrazol®) activity at 50-percent-effective doses of about 0.6 mg/kg orally. (Such anticonvulsant activity of benzodiazepines correlates with their tranquilizing properties.) To produce ataxia (rotabar test) and sedation (abolition of spontaneous motor activity), the 50-percent-effective doses of this product are greater than 5 mg/kg orally. Thus, about ten times the therapeutic (anticonvulsant) dose must be given before ataxia ensues, indicating a wide separation of effective doses and doses inducing side effects.

In evaluation of antianxiety activity of compounds, conflict behavioral tests in rats differentiate continuous response for food in the presence of anxiety-provoking stress (shock) from drug-induced motor incoordination. This product shows significant separation of doses required to relieve anxiety and doses producing sedation or ataxia. Ataxia-producing doses exceed those of related CNS-acting drugs.

Acute oral LD_{50} in mice is greater than 5000 mg/kg, compared to 800 mg/kg for a related compound (chlordiazepoxide).

Subacute toxicity studies in dogs for four weeks at 480 mg/kg daily showed no specific changes; at 960 mg/kg two out of eight died with evidence of circulatory collapse. This wide margin of safety is significant compared to chlordiazepoxide HCl, which showed nonspecific changes in six dogs at 80 mg/kg. On chlordiazepoxide, two out of six died with evidence of circulatory collapse at 127 mg/kg, and six out of six died at 200 mg/kg daily. Chronic toxicity studies of Serax in dogs at 120 mg/kg/day for 52 weeks produced no toxic manifestation.

Fatty metamorphosis of the liver has been noted in six-week toxicity studies in rats given this product at 0.5% of the diet. Such accumulations of fat are considered reversible, as there is no liver necrosis or fibrosis.

Breeding studies in rats through two successive litters did not produce fetal abnormality.

Oxazepam has not been adequately evaluated for mutagenic activity.

In a carcinogenicity study, oxazepam was administered with diet to rats for two years. Male rats receiving 30 times the maximum human dose showed a statistical increase, when compared to controls, in benign thyroid follicular cell tumors, testicular interstitial cell adenomas, and prostatic adenomas. An earlier published study reported that mice fed dietary dosages of 35 or 100 times the human daily dose of oxazepam for 9 months developed a dose-related increase in liver adenomas.[1] In an independent analysis of some of the microscopic slides from this mouse study several of these tumors were classified as liver carcinomas. At this time, there is no evidence that clinical use of oxazepam is associated with tumors.

INDICATIONS

Serax (oxazepam) is indicated for the management of anxiety disorders or for the short-term relief of the symptoms of anxiety. Anxiety or tension associated with the stress of everyday life usually does not require treatment with an anxiolytic.

Anxiety associated with depression is also responsive to Serax therapy.

This product has been found particularly useful in the management of anxiety, tension, agitation, and irritability in older patients.

Alcoholics with acute tremulousness, inebriation, or with anxiety associated with alcohol withdrawal are responsive to therapy.

The effectiveness of Serax in long-term use, that is, more than 4 months, has not been assessed by systematic clinical studies. The physician should reassess periodically the usefulness of the drug for the individual patient.

CONTRAINDICATIONS

History of previous hypersensitivity reaction to oxazepam. Oxazepam is not indicated in psychoses.

WARNINGS

As with other CNS-acting drugs, patients should be cautioned against driving automobiles or operating dangerous machinery until it is known that they do not become drowsy or dizzy on oxazepam therapy.

Patients should be warned that the effects of alcohol or other CNS-depressant drugs may be additive to those of Serax, possibly requiring adjustment of dosage or elimination of such agents.

PHYSICAL AND PSYCHOLOGICAL DEPENDENCE

Withdrawal symptoms, similar in character to those noted with barbiturates and alcohol (convulsions, tremor, abdominal and muscle cramps, vomiting, and sweating), have occurred following abrupt discontinuance of oxazepam. The more severe withdrawal symptoms have usually been limited to those patients who received excessive doses over an extended period of time. Generally milder withdrawal symptoms (e.g., dysphoria and insomnia) have been reported following abrupt discontinuance of benzodiazepines taken continuously at therapeutic levels for several months. Consequently, after extended therapy, abrupt discontinuation should generally be avoided and a gradual dosage-tapering schedule followed. Addiction-prone individuals (such as drug addicts or alcoholics) should be under careful surveillance when receiving oxazepam or other psychotropic agents because of the predisposition of such patients to habituation and dependence.

SERAX (oxazepam)

USUAL DOSE

Mild-to-moderate anxiety, with associated tension, irritability, agitation, or related symptoms of functional origin or secondary to organic disease.	10 to 15 mg, 3 or 4 times daily
Severe anxiety syndromes, agitation, or anxiety associated with depression.	15 to 30 mg, 3 or 4 times daily
Older patients with anxiety, tension, irritability, and agitation.	Initial dosage: 10 mg, 3 times daily. If necessary, increase cautiously to 15 mg, 3 or 4 times daily
Alcoholics with acute inebriation, tremulousness, or anxiety on withdrawal.	15 to 30 mg, 3 or 4 times daily

USE IN PREGNANCY

An increased risk of congenital malformations associated with the use of minor tranquilizers (chlordiazepoxide, diazepam, and meprobamate) during the first trimester of pregnancy has been suggested in several studies. Serax, a benzodiazepine derivative, has not been studied adequately to determine whether it, too, may be associated with an increased risk of fetal abnormality. Because use of these drugs is rarely a matter of urgency, their use during this period should almost always be avoided. The possibility that a woman of childbearing potential may be pregnant at the time of institution of therapy should be considered. Patients should be advised that if they become pregnant during therapy or intend to become pregnant they should communicate with their physician about the desirability of discontinuing the drug.

PRECAUTIONS

Although hypotension has occurred only rarely, oxazepam should be administered with caution to patients in whom a drop in blood pressure might lead to cardiac complications. This is particularly true in the elderly patient.

Serax 15 mg tablets, *but none of the other available dosage forms of this product,* contain FD&C Yellow 5 (tartrazine) which may cause allergic-type reactions (including bronchial asthma) in certain susceptible individuals. Although the overall incidence of FD&C Yellow 5 (tartrazine) sensitivity in the general population is low, it is frequently seen in patients who also have aspirin hypersensitivity.

INFORMATION FOR PATIENTS

To assure the safe and effective use of Serax (oxazepam), patients should be informed that, since benzodiazepines may produce psychological and physical dependence, it is advisable that they consult with their physician before either increasing the dose or abruptly discontinuing this drug.

ADVERSE REACTIONS

The necessity for discontinuation of therapy due to undesirable effects has been rare. Transient, mild drowsiness is commonly seen in the first few days of therapy. If it persists, the dosage should be reduced. In few instances, dizziness, vertigo, headache, and rarely syncope have occurred either alone or together with drowsiness. Mild paradoxical reactions, i.e., excitement, stimulation of affect, have been reported in psychiatric patients; these reactions may be secondary to relief of anxiety and usually appear in the first two weeks of therapy.

Other side effects occurring during oxazepam therapy include rare instances of minor diffuse skin rashes—morbilliform, urticarial, and maculopapular—nausea, lethargy, edema, slurred speech, tremor, and altered libido. Such side effects have been infrequent and are generally controlled with reduction of dosage.

Although rare, leukopenia and hepatic dysfunction including jaundice have been reported during therapy. Periodic blood counts and liver-function tests are advisable.

Ataxia with oxazepam has been reported in rare instances and does not appear to be specifically related to dose or age.

Although the following side reactions have not as yet been reported with oxazepam, they have occurred with related compounds (chlordiazepoxide and diazepam): paradoxical excitation with severe rage reactions, hallucinations, menstrual irregularities, change in EEG pattern, blood dyscrasias including agranulocytosis, blurred vision, diplopia, incontinence, stupor, disorientation, fever, and euphoria.

Transient amnesia or memory impairment has been reported in association with the use of benzodiazepines.

Overdosage

In the management of overdosage with any drug, it should be born in mind that multiple agents may have been taken.

SYMPTOMS

Overdosage of benzodiazepines is usually manifested by varying degrees of central nervous system depression ranging from drowsiness to coma. In mild cases, symptoms include drowsiness, mental confusion and lethargy. In more serious cases, and especially when other drugs or alcohol were ingested, symptoms may include ataxia, hypotonia, hypotension, hypnotic state, stage one (1) to three (3) coma, and very rarely, death.

MANAGEMENT

Induced vomiting and/or gastric lavage should be undertaken, followed by general supportive care, monitoring of vital signs, and close observation of the patient. Hypotension, though unlikely, usually may be controlled with norepinephrine bitartrate injection. The value of dialysis has not been adequately determined for oxazepam.

The benzodiazepine antagonist flumazenil may be used in hospitalized patients as an adjunct to, not as a substitute for, proper management of benzodiazepine overdose. **The prescriber should be aware of a risk of seizure in association with flumazenil treatment, particularly in long-term benzodiazepine users and in cyclic antidepressant overdose.** The complete flumazenil package insert including **"Contraindications," "Warnings,"** and **"Precautions"** should be consulted prior to use.

DOSAGE AND ADMINISTRATION

Because of the flexibility of this product and the range of emotional disturbances responsive to it, dosage should be individualized for maximum beneficial effects.

[See table above.]

This product is not indicated in children under 6 years of age. Absolute dosage for children 6 to 12 years of age is not established.

HOW SUPPLIED

Serax® (oxazepam) Capsules and Tablets are available in the following dosage strengths:

10 mg, NDC 0008-0051, white and pink capsule banded with Wyeth logo and marked "SERAX", "10", and "51", in bottles of 100 and 500 capsules, and in Redipak® cartons of 25 capsules.

15 mg, NDC 0008-0006, white and red capsule banded with Wyeth logo and marked "SERAX", "15", and "6", in bottles of 100 and 500 capsules, and in Redipak cartons of 25 capsules.

30 mg, NDC 0008-0052, white and maroon capsule banded with Wyeth logo and marked "SERAX", "30", and "52", in bottles of 100 and 500 capsules, and in Redipak cartons of 25 capsules.

15 mg, NDC 0008-0317, yellow, five-sided tablet with a raised "S" and a "15" on one side and "WYETH" and "317" on reverse side, in bottles of 100 tablets.

The appearance of SERAX capsules and tablets is a trademark of Wyeth-Ayerst Laboratories.

Store at room temperature, approximately 25°C (77°F).
Keep tightly closed.
Dispense in tight container.

REFERENCE

1. FOX, KA.; LAHCEN, R.B.: Liver-cell Adenomas and Peliosis Hepatis in Mice Associated with Oxazepam. Res. Commun. Chem. Pathol. Pharmacol. *8*:481–488, 1974.

Shown in Product Identification Guide, page 341

SURMONTIL® ℞
[sir 'mon "til]
(trimipramine maleate)

DESCRIPTION

Surmontil (trimipramine maleate) is 5-(3-dimethylamino-2-methylpropyl)-10,11-dihydro-5H-dibenz (b,f) azepine acid maleate (racemic form).

[See structure on top of next page.]

Continued on next page

Wyeth-Ayerst Laboratories—Cont.

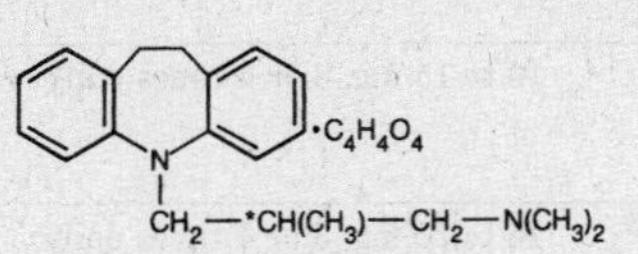

MOLECULAR FORMULA: $C_{20}H_{26}N_2 \cdot C_4H_4O_4$

MOLECULAR WEIGHT: 410.5

Surmontil capsules contain trimipramine maleate equivalent to 25 mg, 50 mg, or 100 mg of trimipramine as the base. The inactive ingredients present are FD&C Blue 1, gelatin, lactose, magnesium stearate, and titanium dioxide. The 25 mg dosage strength also contains D&C Yellow 10 and FD&C Yellow 6; the 50 mg dosage strength also contains D&C Red 28, FD&C Red 40, and FD&C Yellow 6.

Trimipramine maleate is prepared as a racemic mixture which can be resolved into levorotatory and dextrorotatory isomers. The asymmetric center responsible for optical isomerism is marked in the formula by an asterisk. Trimipramine maleate is an almost odorless, white or slightly cream-colored, crystalline substance, melting at 140–144°C. It is very slightly soluble in ether and water, is slightly soluble in ethyl alcohol and acetone, and freely soluble in chloroform and methanol at 20°C.

CLINICAL PHARMACOLOGY

Surmontil is an antidepressant with an anxiety-reducing sedative component to its action. The mode of action of Surmontil on the central nervous system is not known. However, unlike amphetamine-type compounds it does not act primarily by stimulation of the central nervous system. It does not act by inhibition of the monoamine oxidase system.

INDICATIONS AND USAGE

Surmontil is indicated for the relief of symptoms of depression. Endogenous depression is more likely to be alleviated than other depressive states. In studies with neurotic outpatients, the drug appeared to be equivalent to amitriptyline in the less-depressed patients but somewhat less effective than amitriptyline in the more severely depressed patients. In hospitalized depressed patients, trimipramine and imipramine were equally effective in relieving depression.

CONTRAINDICATIONS

Surmontil is contraindicated in cases of known hypersensitivity to the drug. The possibility of cross-sensitivity to other dibenzazepine compounds should be kept in mind. Surmontil should not be given in conjunction with drugs of the monoamine oxidase inhibitor class (e.g., tranylcypromine, isocarboxazid or phenelzine sulfate). The concomitant use of monoamine oxidase inhibitors (MAOI) and tricyclic compounds similar to Surmontil has caused severe hyperpyretic reactions, convulsive crises, and death in some patients. At least two weeks should elapse after cessation of therapy with MAOI before instituting therapy with Surmontil. Initial dosage should be low and increased gradually with caution and careful observation of the patient. The drug is contraindicated during the acute recovery period after a myocardial infarction.

WARNINGS

GENERAL CONSIDERATION FOR USE

Extreme caution should be used when this drug is given to patients with any evidence of cardiovascular disease because of the possibility of conduction defects, arrhythmias, myocardial infarction, strokes, and tachycardia.

Caution is advised in patients with increased intraocular pressure, history of urinary retention, or history of narrow-angle glaucoma because of the drug's anticholinergic properties; hyperthyroid patients or those on thyroid medication because of the possibility of cardiovascular toxicity; patients with a history of seizure disorder, because this drug has been shown to lower the seizure threshold; patients receiving guanethidine or similar agents, since Surmontil may block the pharmacologic effects of these drugs.

Since the drug may impair the mental and/or physical abilities required for the performance of potentially hazardous tasks, such as operating an automobile or machinery, the patient should be cautioned accordingly.

PRECAUTIONS

GENERAL

The possibility of suicide is inherent in any severely depressed patient and persists until a significant remission occurs. When a patient with a serious suicidal potential is not hospitalized, the prescription should be for the smallest amount feasible.

In schizophrenic patients activation of the psychosis may occur and require reduction of dosage or the addition of a major tranquilizer to the therapeutic regime.

Manic or hypomanic episodes may occur in some patients, in particular those with cyclic-type disorders. In some cases therapy with Surmontil must be discontinued until the episode is relieved, after which therapy may be reinstituted at lower dosages if still required.

Concurrent administration of Surmontil and electroshock therapy may increase the hazards of therapy. Such treatment should be limited to those patients for whom it is essential. When possible, discontinue the drug for several days prior to elective surgery.

Surmontil should be used with caution in patients with impaired liver function.

Chronic animal studies showed occasional occurrence of hepatic congestion, fatty infiltration, or increased serum liver enzymes at the highest dose of 60 mg/kg/day.

Both elevation and lowering of blood sugar have been reported with tricyclic antidepressants.

DRUG INTERACTIONS

Cimetidine

There is evidence that cimetidine inhibits the elimination of tricyclic antidepressants. Downward adjustment of Surmontil dosage may be required if cimetidine therapy is initiated; upward adjustment if cimetidine therapy is discontinued.

Alcohol

Patients should be warned that the concomitant use of alcoholic beverages may be associated with exaggerated effects.

Catecholamines/Anticholinergics

It has been reported that tricyclic antidepressants can potentiate the effects of catecholamines. Similarly, atropinelike effects may be more pronounced in patients receiving anticholinergic therapy. Therefore, particular care should be exercised when it is necessary to administer tricyclic antidepressants with sympathomimetic amines, local decongestants, local anesthetics containing epinephrine, atropine or drugs with an anticholinergic effect. In resistant cases of depression in adults, a dose of 2.5 mg/kg/day may have to be exceeded. If a higher dose is needed, ECG monitoring should be maintained during the initiation of therapy and at appropriate intervals during stabilization of dose.

Drugs Metabolized by P450 2D6

The biochemical activity of the drug metabolizing isozyme cytochrome P450 2D6 (debrisoquin hydroxylase) is reduced in a subset of the caucasian population (about 7–10% of caucasians are so called "poor metabolizers"); reliable estimates of the prevalence of reduced P450 2D6 isozyme activity among Asian, African, and other populations are not yet available. Poor metabolizers have higher than expected plasma concentrations of tricyclic antidepressants (TCAs) when given usual doses. Depending on the fraction of drug metabolized by P450 2D6, the increase in plasma concentration may be small, or quite large (8 fold increase in plasma AUC of the TCA).

In addition, certain drugs inhibit the activity of this isozyme and make normal metabolizers resemble poor metabolizers. An individual who is stable on a given dose of TCA may become abruptly toxic when given one of these inhibiting drugs as concomitant therapy. The drugs that inhibit cytochrome P450 2D6 include some that are not metabolized by the enzyme (quinidine; cimetidine) and many that are substrates for P450 2D6 (many other antidepressants, phenothiazines, and the Type 1C antiarrhythmics propafenone and flecainide). While all the selective serotonin reuptake inhibitors (SSRIs), e.g., fluoxetine, sertraline, and paroxetine, inhibit P450 2D6, they may vary in the extent of inhibition. The extent to which SSRI TCA interactions may pose clinical problems will depend on the degree of inhibition and the pharmacokinetics of the SSRI involved. Nevertheless, caution is indicated in the co-administration of TCAs with any of the SSRIs and also in switching from one class to the other. Of particular importance, sufficient time must elapse before initiating TCA treatment in a patient being withdrawn from fluoxetine, given the long half-life of the parent and active metabolite (at least 5 weeks may be necessary).

Concomitant use of tricyclic antidepressants with drugs that can inhibit cytochrome P450 2D6 may require lower doses than usually prescribed for either the tricyclic antidepressant or the other drug.

Furthermore, whenever one of these other drugs is withdrawn from co-therapy, an increased dose of tricyclic antidepressant may be required. It is desirable to monitor TCA plasma levels whenever a TCA is going to be co-administered with another drug known to be an inhibitor of P450 2D6.

CARCINOGENESIS, MUTAGENESIS, IMPAIRMENT OF FERTILTIY

Semen studies in man (four schizophrenics and nine normal volunteers) revealed no significant changes in sperm morphology. It is recognized that drugs having a parasympathetic effect, including tricyclic antidepressants, may alter the ejaculatory response.

Chronic animal studies showed occasional evidence of degeneration of seminiferous tubules at the highest dose of 60 mg/kg/day.

PREGNANCY

Teratogenic Effects—Pregnancy Category C

Surmontil has shown evidence of embryo-toxicity and/or increased incidence of major anomalies in rats or rabbits at doses 20 times the human dose. There are no adequate and well-controlled studies in pregnant women. Surmontil should be used during pregnancy only if the potential benefit justifies the potential risk to the fetus.

PEDIATRIC USE

This drug is not recommended for use in children, since safety and effectiveness in the pediatric age group have not been established.

ADVERSE REACTIONS

Note: The pharmacological similarities among the tricyclic antidepressants require that each of the reactions be considered when Surmontil is administered. Some of the adverse reactions included in this listing have not in fact been reported with Surmontil.

CARDIOVASCULAR

Hypotension, hypertension, tachycardia, palpitation, myocardial infarction, arrhythmias, heart block, stroke.

PSYCHIATRIC

Confusional states (especially the elderly) with hallucinations, disorientation, delusions; anxiety, restlessness, agitation; insomnia and nightmares; hypomania; exacerbation of psychosis.

NEUROLOGICAL

Numbness, tingling, paresthesias of extremities; incoordination, ataxia, tremors; peripheral neuropathy; extrapyramidal symptoms; seizures, alterations in EEG patterns; tinnitus; syndrome of inappropriate ADH (antidiuretic hormone) secretion.

ANTICHOLINERGIC

Dry mouth and, rarely, associated sublingual adenitis; blurred vision, disturbances of accommodation, mydriasis, constipation, paralytic ileus; urinary retention, delayed micturition, dilation of the urinary tract.

ALLERGIC

Skin rash, petechiae, urticaria, itching, photosensitization, edema of face and tongue.

HEMATOLOGIC

Bone-marrow depression including agranulocytosis, eosinophilia; purpura; thrombocytopenia. Leukocyte and differential counts should be performed in any patient who develops fever and sore throat during therapy; the drug should be discontinued if there is evidence of pathological neutrophil depression.

GASTROINTESTINAL

Nausea and vomiting, anorexia, epigastric distress, diarrhea, peculiar taste, stomatitis, abdominal cramps, black tongue.

ENDOCRINE

Gynecomastia in the male; breast enlargement and galactorrhea in the female; increased or decreased libido, impotence; testicular swelling; elevation or depression of blood-sugar levels.

OTHER

Jaundice (simulating obstructive); altered liver function; weight gain or loss; perspiration; flushing; urinary frequency; drowsiness, dizziness, weakness, and fatigue; headache; parotid swelling; alopecia.

WITHDRAWAL SYMPTOMS

Though not indicative of addiction, abrupt cessation of treatment after prolonged therapy may produce nausea, headache, and malaise.

DOSAGE AND ADMINISTRATION

Dosage should be initiated at a low level and increased gradually, noting carefully the clinical response and any evidence of intolerance.

Lower dosages are recommended for elderly patients and adolescents. Lower dosages are also recommended for outpatients as compared to hospitalized patients who will be under close supervision. It is not possible to prescribe a single dosage schedule of Surmontil that will be therapeutically effective in all patients. The physical psychodynamic factors contributing to depressive symptomatology are very complex; spontaneous remissions or exacerbations of depressive symptoms may occur with or without drug therapy. Consequently, the recommended dosage regimens are furnished as a guide which may be modified by factors such as the age of the patient, chronicity and severity of the disease, medical condition of the patient, and degree of psychotherapeutic support.

Most antidepressant drugs have a lag period of ten days to four weeks before a therapeutic response is noted. Increasing the dose will not shorten this period but rather increase the incidence of adverse reactions.

USUAL ADULT DOSE

Outpatients and Office Patients—Initially, 75 mg/day in divided doses, increased to 150 mg/day. Dosages over 200 mg/day are not recommended. Maintenance therapy is in the range of 50 to 150 mg/day. For convenient therapy and to facilitate patient compliance, the total dosage requirement may be given at bedtime.

Hospitalized Patients—Initially, 100 mg/day in divided doses. This may be increased gradually in a few days to 200 mg/day, depending upon individual response and tolerance. If improvement does not occur in 2 to 3 weeks, the dose may be increased to the maximum recommended dose of 250 to 300 mg/day.

Adolescent and Geriatric Patients—Initially, a dose of 50 mg/day is recommended, with gradual increments up to 100 mg/day, depending upon patient response and tolerance.

Maintenance—Following remission, maintenance medication may be required for a longer period of time, at the lowest dose that will maintain remission. Maintenance therapy is preferably administered as a single dose at bedtime. To minimize relapse, maintenance therapy should be continued for about three months.

OVERDOSAGE

SIGNS AND SYMPTOMS

The response of the patient to toxic overdosage of tricyclic antidepressants may vary in severity and is conditioned by factors such as age, amount ingested, amount absorbed, interval between ingestion and start of treatment. Surmontil is not recommended for infants or young children. Should accidental ingestion occur in any amount, it should be regarded as serious and potentially fatal.

CNS abnormalities may include drowsiness, stupor, coma, ataxia, restlessness, agitation, hyperactive reflexes, muscle rigidity, athetoid and choreiform movements, and convulsions. Cardiac abnormalities may include arrhythmia, tachycardia, ECG evidence of impaired conduction, and signs of congestive failure. Other symptoms may include respiratory depression, cyanosis, hypotension, shock, vomiting, hyperpyrexia, mydriasis, and diaphoresis.

Treatment is supportive and symptomatic as no specific antidote is known. Depending upon need the following measures can be considered:

1. Surmontil is not recommended for use in infants and children. Hospitalization with continuous cardiac monitoring for up to 4 days is recommended for children who have ingested Surmontil in any amount. This is based on the reported greater sensitivity of children to acute overdosage with tricyclic antidepressants.
2. Blood and urine levels may not reflect the severity of the poisoning and are mostly of diagnostic value.
3. CNS involvement, respiratory depression, or cardiac arrhythmia can occur suddenly; hospitalization and close observation are necessary, even when the amount ingested is thought to be small or initial toxicity appears slight. Patients with any alteration of ECG should have continuous cardiac monitoring for at least 72 hours and be observed until well after the cardiac status has returned to normal; relapses may occur after apparent recovery.
4. The slow intravenous administration of physostigmine salicylate has been reported to reverse most of the cardiovascular and CNS effects of overdosage with tricyclic antidepressants. In adults, 1 to 3 mg has been reported to be effective. In children, start with 0.5 mg and repeat at 5-minute intervals to determine the minimum effective dose; do not exceed 2.0 mg. Avoid rapid injection, to reduce the possibility of physostigmine-induced convulsions. Because of the short duration of action of physostigmine, it may be necessary to repeat doses at 30- to 60-minute intervals as necessary.
5. In the alert patient, empty the stomach rapidly by induced emesis, followed by lavage. In the obtunded patient, secure the airway with a cuffed endotracheal tube before beginning lavage (do not induce emesis). Instillation of activated-charcoal slurry may help reduce absorption of trimipramine.
6. Minimize external stimulation to reduce the tendency to convulsions. If anticonvulsants are necessary, diazepam, short-acting barbiturates, paraldehyde, or methocarbamol may be useful. Do not use barbiturates if MAO inhibitors have been taken recently.
7. Maintain adequate respiratory exchange. Do not use respiratory stimulants.
8. Shock should be treated with supportive measures, such as intravenous fluids, oxygen, and corticosteroids. Digitalis may increase conduction abnormalities and further irritate an already sensitized myocardium. If congestive heart failure necessitates rapid digitalization, particular care must be exercised.
9. Hyperpyrexia should be controlled by whatever external means available, including ice packs and cooling sponge baths if necessary.
10. Hemodialysis, peritoneal dialysis, exchange transfusions, and forced diuresis have been generally reported as ineffective in tricyclic poisoning.

HOW SUPPLIED

Surmontil® (trimipramine maleate) Capsules are available in the following dosage strengths:
25 mg, NDC 0008-4132, opaque blue and yellow capsule marked "WYETH" and "4132", in bottles of 100 capsules.
50 mg, NDC 0008-4133, opaque blue and orange capsule marked "WYETH" and "4133", in bottles of 100 capsules and in Redipak cartons of 100 capsules (10 blister strips of 10).
100 mg, NDC 0008-4158, opaque blue and white capsule marked "WYETH" and "4158", in bottles of 100 capsules.

Store at room temperature, approximately 25°C (77°F).
Keep bottles tightly closed.
Dispense in tight container.
Protect capsules packaged in blister strips from moisture.
The appearance of these capsules is a trademark of Wyeth-Ayerst Laboratories.

by arrangement with Rhone-Poulenc Rorer France

Shown in Product Identification Guide, page 341

SYNALGOS®-DC   ℞

[sĭn 'al "gŏs]
Capsules

DESCRIPTION

Each Synalgos-DC capsule contains 16 mg drocode (dihydrocodeine) bitartrate (Warning—may be habit-forming), 356.4 mg aspirin, and 30 mg caffeine.
The inactive ingredients present are alginic acid, cellulose, D&C Red 28, FD&C Blue 1, gelatin, iron oxides, stearic acid, and titanium dioxide.

HOW SUPPLIED

Synalgos®-DC Capsules are supplied in bottles of 100 and 500 capsules as follows:
NDC 0008-4191, blue and gray capsule marked "WYETH" and "4191".
Store at room temperature (approximately 25°C).
Keep tightly closed.
Dispense in tight container.
For prescribing information write to Professional Service, Wyeth-Ayerst Laboratories, P.O. Box 8299, Philadelphia, PA 19101, or contact your local Wyeth-Ayerst representative.

TRECATOR®-SC   ℞

[trek "ă 'tŏre]
(ethionamide)
Sugar-Coated Tablets

DESCRIPTION

Trecator-SC (ethionamide) is used in the treatment of tuberculosis. The chemical name for ethionamide is 2-ethylthioisonicotinamide with the following structural formula:

Ethionamide is a yellow, crystalline, nonhygroscopic compound with a faint-to-moderate sulfide odor. It is practically insoluble in water and ether but soluble in methanol and ethanol. It melts at about 162°C and is stable at ordinary temperatures and humidities.
Trecator-SC tablets contain 250 mg of ethionamide. The inactive ingredients present are acacia, calcium carbonate, carnauba wax, confectioners' sugar, FD&C Yellow 6, gelatin, lactose, magnesium stearate, methylcellulose, pharmaceutical glaze, polacrilin potassium, povidone, sodium benzoate, sucrose, talc, titanium dioxide, and white wax.

ACTION

Bacteriostatic against *Mycobacterium tuberculosis*.

INDICATIONS

Failure after adequate treatment with primary drugs (i.e., isoniazid, streptomycin, aminosalicylic acid) in any form of active tuberculosis. Ethionamide should only be given with other effective antituberculous agents.

CONTRAINDICATIONS

Severe hypersensitivity.
Severe hepatic damage.

WARNING

USE IN PREGNANCY

Teratogenic effects have been demonstrated in animals (rabbits, rats) receiving doses in excess of those recommended in humans. Use of the drug should be avoided during pregnancy or in women of childbearing potential unless the benefits outweigh its possible hazard.

USE IN CHILDREN

Optimum dosage for children has not been established. This, however, does not preclude use of the drug when its use is crucial to therapy.

PRECAUTIONS

Pretreatment examinations should include *in vitro* susceptibility tests of recent cultures of *M. tuberculosis* from the patient as measured against ethionamide and the usual primary antituberculous drugs.
Determinations of serum transaminase (SGOT, SGPT) should be made prior to and every 2 to 4 weeks during therapy.

In patients with diabetes mellitus, management may be more difficult and hepatitis occurs more frequently.
Ethionamide may intensify the adverse effects of the other antituberculous drugs administered concomitantly. Convulsions have been reported, and special care should be taken, particularly when ethionamide is administered with cycloserine.

ADVERSE REACTIONS

The most common side effect is gastrointestinal intolerance. Other adverse effects similar to those seen with isoniazid have been reported: peripheral neuritis, optic neuritis, psychic disturbances (including mental depression), postural hypotension, skin rashes, thrombocytopenia, pellagralike syndrome, jaundice and/or hepatitis, increased difficulty in management of diabetes mellitus, stomatitis, gynecomastia, and impotence.

DOSAGE AND ADMINISTRATION

Ethionamide should be administered with at least one other effective antituberculous drug.
Average Adult Dose: 0.5 gram to 1.0 gram/day in divided doses.
Concomitant administration of pyridoxine is recommended.

HOW SUPPLIED

Trecator®-SC (ethionamide) Tablets are supplied in bottles of 100 tablets as follows:
250 mg, NDC 0008-4130, orange, sugar-coated tablet marked "WYETH" and "4130".
Store at room temperature, approximately 25°C (77°F)
Keep tightly closed
Dispense in tight container

TRIPHASIL®-21   ℞

[tri-fa 'sil]
Tablets
(levonorgestrel and ethinyl estradiol tablets—triphasic regimen)

Patients should be counseled that this product does not protect against HIV infection (AIDS) and other sexually transmitted diseases.

DESCRIPTION

Each Triphasil cycle of 21 tablets consists of three different drug phases as follows: Phase 1 comprised of 6 brown tablets, each containing 0.050 mg of levonorgestrel (d(-)-13 beta-ethyl-17-alpha-ethinyl-17-beta-hydroxygon-4-en-3-one), a totally synthetic progestogen, and 0.030 mg of ethinyl estradiol (19-nor-17α-pregna-1,3,5(10)-trien -20- yne-3,17-diol); phase 2 comprised of 5 white tablets, each containing 0.075 mg levonorgestrel and 0.040 mg ethinyl estradiol; and phase 3 comprised of 10 light-yellow tablets, each containing 0.125 mg levonorgestrel and 0.030 mg ethinyl estradiol. The inactive ingredients present are cellulose, iron oxides, lactose, magnesium stearate, polacrilin potassium, polyethylene glycol, titanium dioxide, and hydroxypropyl methylcellulose.

Levonorgestrel

Ethinyl Estradiol

CLINICAL PHARMACOLOGY

Combination oral contraceptives act by suppression of gonadotropins. Although the primary mechanism of this action is inhibition of ovulation, other alterations include changes in the cervical mucus (which increase the difficulty of sperm entry into the uterus) and the endometrium (which reduce the likelihood of implantation).

INDICATIONS AND USAGE

Oral contraceptives are indicated for the prevention of pregnancy in women who elect to use this product as a method of contraception.
Oral contraceptives are highly effective. Table I lists the typical accidental pregnancy rates for users of combination oral contraceptives and other methods of contraception. The efficacy of these contraceptive methods, except sterilization and the IUD, depends upon the reliability with which they are used. Correct and consistent use of methods can result in lower failure rates.

Continued on next page

Wyeth-Ayerst Laboratories—Cont.

TABLE I: LOWEST EXPECTED AND TYPICAL FAILURE RATES DURING THE FIRST YEAR OF CONTINUOUS USE OF A METHOD

% of Women Experiencing an Accidental Pregnancy in the First Year of Continuous Use

Method	Lowest Expected*	Typical**
(No Contraception)	(85)	(85)
Oral contraceptives		3
combined	0.1	N/A***
progestin only	0.5	N/A***
Diaphragm with spermicidal cream or jelly	6	18
Spermicides alone (foams and vaginal suppositories)	3	21
Vaginal Sponge		
nulliparous	6	18
multiparous	9	28
DEPO-PROVERA® (injectable progestogen)	0.3	0.3
NORPLANT® SYSTEM (implants)	0.2#	0.2#
IUD		3
progesterone	2	N/A***
copper T 380A	0.8	N/A***
Condom without spermicides	2	12
Periodic abstinence (all methods)	1–9	20
Female sterilization	0.2	0.4
Male sterilization	0.1	0.15

Adapted from J. Trussell et al., Table 1, Studies in Family Planning, *21(1)*: Jan.–Feb. 1990.

* The authors' best guess of the percentage of women expected to experience an accidental pregnancy among couples who initiate a method (not necessarily for the first time) and who use it consistently and correctly during the first year if they do not stop use for any other reason.

** This term represents "typical" couples who initiate use of a method (not necessarily for the first time), who experience an accidental pregnancy during the first year if they do not stop use for any other reason.

*** N/A—Data not available.

#This data is based on Norplant System clinical trials.

CONTRAINDICATIONS

Oral contraceptives should not be used in women with any of the following conditions:

Thrombophlebitis or thromboembolic disorders.

A past history of deep-vein thrombophlebitis or thromboembolic disorders.

Cerebral-vascular or coronary-artery disease.

Known or suspected carcinoma of the breast.

Carcinoma of the endometrium or other known or suspected estrogen-dependent neoplasia.

Undiagnosed abnormal genital bleeding.

Cholestatic jaundice of pregnancy or jaundice with prior pill use.

Hepatic adenomas or carcinomas.

Known or suspected pregnancy.

WARNINGS

Cigarette smoking increases the risk of serious cardiovascular side effects from oral-contraceptive use. This risk increases with age and with heavy smoking (15 or more cigarettes per day) and is quite marked in women over 35 years of age. Women who use oral contraceptives should be strongly advised not to smoke.

The use of oral contraceptives is associated with increased risks of several serious conditions including myocardial infarction, thromboembolism, stroke, hepatic neoplasia, gallbladder disease, and hypertension, although the risk of serious morbidity or mortality is very small in healthy women without underlying factors. The risk of morbidity and mortality increases significantly in the presence of other underlying risk factors such as hypertension, hyperlipidemias, obesity, and diabetes.

Practitioners prescribing oral contraceptives should be familiar with the following information relating to these risks.

The information contained in this package insert is based principally on studies carried out in patients who used oral contraceptives with higher formulations of estrogens and progestogens than those in common use today. The effect of long-term use of the oral contraceptives with lower formulations of both estrogens and progestogens remains to be determined.

Throughout this labeling, epidemiological studies reported are of two types: retrospective or case control studies and prospective or cohort studies. Case control studies provide a measure of the relative risk of disease, namely, a ratio of the incidence of a disease among oral-contraceptive users to that among nonusers. The relative risk does not provide information on the actual clinical occurrence of a disease. Cohort studies provide a measure of attributable risk, which is the difference in the incidence of disease between oral-contraceptive users and nonusers. The attributable risk does provide information about the actual occurrence of a disease in the population. For further information, the reader is referred to a text on epidemiological methods.

1. THROMBOEMBOLIC DISORDERS AND OTHER VASCULAR PROBLEMS

a. *Myocardial infarction*

An increased risk of myocardial infarction has been attributed to oral-contraceptive use. This risk is primarily in smokers or women with other underlying risk factors for coronary-artery disease such as hypertension, hypercholesterolemia, morbid obesity, and diabetes. The relative risk of heart attack for current oral-contraceptive users has been estimated to be two to six. The risk is very low under the age of 30.

Smoking in combination with oral-contraceptive use has been shown to contribute substantially to the incidence of myocardial infarctions in women in their mid-thirties or older with smoking accounting for the majority of excess cases. Mortality rates associated with circulatory disease have been shown to increase substantially in smokers over the age of 35 and nonsmokers over the age of 40 (Table II) among women who use oral contraceptives.

CIRCULATORY DISEASE MORTALITY RATES PER 100,000 WOMEN YEARS BY AGE, SMOKING STATUS AND ORAL-CONTRACEPTIVE USE

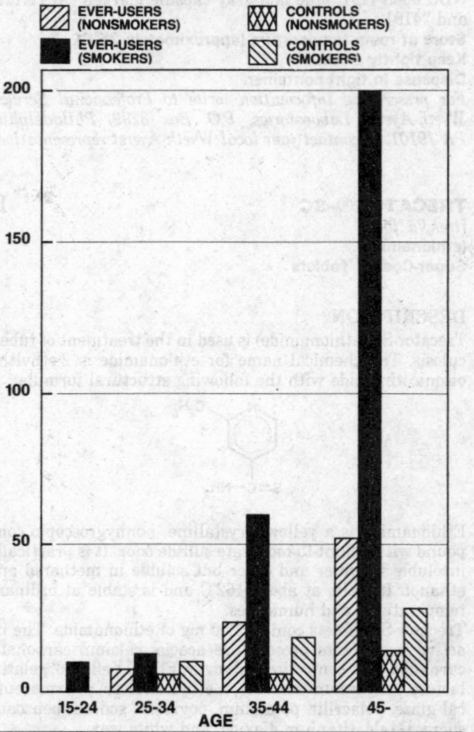

TABLE II. (Adapted from P.M. Layde and V. Beral, Lancet, 1:541–546, 1981.)

Oral contraceptives may compound the effects of well-known risk factors, such as hypertension, diabetes, hyperlipidemias, age, and obesity. In particular, some progestogens are known to decrease HDL cholesterol and cause glucose intolerance, while estrogens may create a state of hyperinsulinism. Oral contraceptives have been shown to increase blood pressure among users (see section 9 in "Warnings"). Similar effects on risk factors have been associated with an increased risk of heart disease. Oral contraceptives must be used with caution in women with cardiovascular disease risk factors.

b. *Thromboembolism*

An increased risk of thromboembolic and thrombotic disease associated with the use of oral contraceptives is well established. Case control studies have found the relative risk of users compared to nonusers to be 3 for the first episode of superficial venous thrombosis, 4 to 11 for deep-vein thrombosis or pulmonary embolism, and 1.5 to 6 for women with predisposing conditions for venous thromboembolic disease. Cohort studies have shown the relative risk to be somewhat lower, about 3 for new cases and about 4.5 for new cases requiring hospitalization. The risk of thromboembolic disease due to oral contraceptives is not related to length of use and disappears after pill use is stopped.

A two- to four-fold increase in relative risk of postoperative thromboembolic complications has been reported with the use of oral contraceptives. The relative risk of venous thrombosis in women who have predisposing conditions is twice that of women without such medical conditions. If feasible, oral contraceptives should be discontinued at least four weeks prior to and for two weeks after elective surgery of a type associated with an increase in risk of thromboembolism and during and following prolonged immobilization. Since the immediate postpartum period is also associated with an increased risk of thromboembolism, oral contraceptives should be started no earlier than four to six weeks after delivery in women who elect not to breast-feed, or a midtrimester pregnancy termination.

c. *Cerebrovascular diseases*

Oral contraceptives have been shown to increase both the relative and attributable risks of cerebrovascular events (thrombotic and hemorrhagic strokes), although, in general, the risk is greatest among older (> 35 years), hypertensive women who also smoke. Hypertension was found to be a risk factor for both users and nonusers, for both types of strokes, while smoking interacted to increase the risk for hemorrhagic strokes.

In a large study, the relative risk of thrombotic strokes has been shown to range from 3 for normotensive users to 14 for users with severe hypertension. The relative risk of hemorrhagic stroke is reported to be 1.2 for nonsmokers who used oral contraceptives, 2.6 for smokers who did not use oral contraceptives, 7.6 for smokers who used oral contraceptives, 1.8 for normotensive users, and 25.7 for users with severe hypertension. The attributable risk is also greater in older women.

d. *Dose-related risk of vascular disease from oral contraceptives*

A positive association has been observed between the amount of estrogen and progestogen in oral contraceptives and the risk of vascular disease. A decline in serum high-density lipoproteins (HDL) has been reported with many progestational agents. A decline in serum high-density lipoproteins has been associated with an increased incidence of ischemic heart disease. Because estrogens increase HDL cholesterol, the net effect of an oral contraceptive depends on a balance achieved between doses of estrogen and progestogen and the nature and absolute amount of progestogen used in the contraceptive. The amount of both hormones should be considered in the choice of an oral contraceptive.

Minimizing exposure to estrogen and progestogen is in keeping with good principles of therapeutics. For any particular estrogen/progestogen combination, the dosage regimen prescribed should be one which contains the least amount of estrogen and progestogen that is compatible with a low failure rate and the needs of the individual patient. New acceptors of oral-contraceptive agents should be started on preparations containing less than 50 mcg of estrogen.

e. *Persistence of risk of vascular disease*

There are two studies which have shown persistence of risk of vascular disease for ever-users of oral contraceptives. In a study in the United States, the risk of developing myocardial infarction after discontinuing oral contraceptives persists for at least 9 years for women 40 to 49 years who had used oral contraceptives for five or more years, but this increased risk was not demonstrated in other age groups. In another study in Great Britain, the risk of developing cerebrovascular disease persisted for at least 6 years after discontinuation of oral contraceptives, although excess risk was very small. However, both studies were performed with oral- contraceptive formulations containing 50 micrograms or higher of estrogens.

2. ESTIMATES OF MORTALITY FROM CONTRACEPTIVE USE

One study gathered data from a variety of sources which have estimated the mortality rate associated with different methods of contraception at different ages (Table III). These estimates include the combined risk of death associated with contraceptive methods plus the risk attributable to pregnancy in the event of method failure. Each method of contraception has its specific benefits and risks. The study concluded that with the exception of oral-contraceptive users 35 and older who smoke and 40 and older who do not smoke, mortality associated with all methods of birth control is less than that associated with childbirth. The observation of a possible increase in risk of mortality with age for oral-contraceptive users is based on data gathered in the 1970's—but not reported until 1983. However, current clinical practice involves the use of lower estrogen dose formulations combined with careful restriction of oral-contraceptive use to women who do not have the various risk factors listed in this labeling.

Because of these changes in practice and, also, because of some limited new data which suggest that the risk of cardiovascular disease with the use of oral contraceptives may now be less than previously observed, the Fertility and Maternal Health Drugs Advisory Committee was asked to review the topic in 1989. The Committee concluded that although cardiovascular-disease risks may be increased with oral-contraceptive use after age 40 in healthy nonsmoking women (even with the newer low-dose formulations), there are greater potential health risks associated with pregnancy in older women and with the alternative surgical and medical procedures which may be necessary if such women do not have access to effective and acceptable means of contraception.

Therefore, the Committee recommended that the benefits of oral-contraceptive use by healthy nonsmoking women over

40 may outweigh the possible risks. Of course, older women, as all women who take oral contraceptives, should take the lowest possible dose formulation that is effective.

[See Table III at right.]

3. CARCINOMA OF THE REPRODUCTIVE ORGANS

Numerous epidemiological studies have been performed on the incidence of breast, endometrial, ovarian, and cervical cancer in women using oral contraceptives. The overwhelming evidence in the literature suggests that the use of oral contraceptives is not associated with an increase in the risk of developing breast cancer, regardless of the age and parity of first use or with most of the marketed brands and doses. The Cancer and Steroid Hormone (CASH) study also showed no latent effect on the risk of breast cancer for at least a decade following long-term use. A few studies have shown a slightly increased relative risk of developing breast cancer, although the methodology of these studies, which included differences in examination of users and nonusers and differences in age at start of use, has been questioned.

Some studies suggest that oral-contraceptive use has been associated with an increase in the risk of cervical intraepithelial neoplasia in some populations of women. However, there continues to be controversy about the extent to which such findings may be due to differences in sexual behavior and other factors.

In spite of many studies of the relationship between oral-contraceptive use and breast and cervical cancers, a cause-and-effect relationship has not been established.

4. HEPATIC NEOPLASIA

Benign hepatic adenomas are associated with oral-contraceptive use, although the incidence of benign tumors is rare in the United States. Indirect calculations have estimated the attributable risk to be in the range of 3.3 cases/100,000 for users, a risk that increases after four or more years of use. Rupture of rare, benign, hepatic adenomas may cause death through intra-abdominal hemorrhage.

Studies from Britain have shown an increased risk of developing hepatocellular carcinoma in long-term (>8 years) oral-contraceptive users. However, these cancers are extremely rare in the U.S., and the attributable risk (the excess incidence) of liver cancers in oral-contraceptive users approaches less than one per million users.

5. OCULAR LESIONS

There have been clincial case reports of retinal thrombosis associated with the use of oral contraceptives. Oral contraceptives should be discontinued if there is unexplained partial or complete loss of vision; onset of proptosis or diplopia; papilledema; or retinal vascular lesions. Appropriate diagnostic and therapeutic measures should be undertaken immediately.

6. ORAL-CONTRACEPTIVE USE BEFORE OR DURING EARLY PREGNANCY

Extensive epidemiological studies have revealed no increased risk of birth defects in women who have used oral contraceptives prior to pregnancy. Studies also do not suggest a teratogenic effect, particularly insofar as cardiac anomalies and limb-reduction defects are concerned, when taken inadvertently during early pregnancy.

The administration of oral contraceptives to induce withdrawal bleeding should not be used as a test for pregnancy. Oral contraceptives should not be used during pregnancy to treat threatened or habitual abortion.

It is recommended that for any patient who has missed two consecutive periods, pregnancy should be ruled out before continuing oral-contraceptive use. If the patient has not adhered to the prescribed schedule, the possibility of pregnancy should be considered at the time of the first missed period. Oral-contraceptive use should be discontinued if pregnancy is confirmed.

7. GALLBLADDER DISEASE

Earlier studies have reported an increased lifetime relative risk of gallbladder surgery in users of oral contraceptives and estrogens. More recent studies, however, have shown that the relative risk of developing gallbladder disease among oral-contraceptive users may be minimal. The recent findings of minimal risk may be related to the use of oral-contraceptive formulations containing lower hormonal doses of estrogens and progestogens.

8. CARBOHYDRATE AND LIPID METABOLIC EFFECTS

Oral contraceptives have been shown to cause glucose intolerance in a significant percentage of users. Oral contraceptives containing greater than 75 micrograms of estrogens cause hyperinsulinism, while lower doses of estrogen cause less glucose intolerance. Progestogens increase insulin secretion and create insulin resistance, this effect varying with different progestational agents. However, in the nondiabetic woman, oral contraceptives appear to have no effect on fasting blood glucose. Because of these demonstrated effects, prediabetic and diabetic women should be carefully observed while taking oral contraceptives.

A small proportion of women will have persistent hypertriglyceridemia while on the pill. As discussed earlier (see "WARNINGS" 1a. and 1d.), changes in serum triglycerides and lipoprotein levels have been reported in oral-contraceptive users.

TABLE III—ANNUAL NUMBER OF BIRTH-RELATED OR METHOD-RELATED DEATHS ASSOCIATED WITH CONTROL OF FERTILITY PER 100,000 NONSTERILE WOMEN, BY FERTILITY-CONTROL METHOD ACCORDING TO AGE

Method of control and outcome	15–19	20–24	25–29	30–34	35–39	40–44
No fertility-control methods*	7.0	7.4	9.1	14.8	25.7	28.2
Oral contraceptives nonsmoker**	0.3	0.5	0.9	1.9	13.8	31.6
Oral contraceptives smoker**	2.2	3.4	6.6	13.5	51.1	117.2
IUD**	0.8	0.8	1.0	1.0	1.4	1.4
Condom*	1.1	1.6	0.7	0.2	0.3	0.4
Diaphragm/ spermicide*	1.9	1.2	1.2	1.3	2.2	2.8
Periodic abstinence*	2.5	1.6	1.6	1.7	2.9	3.6

* Deaths are birth related

** Deaths are method related

Adapted from H.W. Ory, Family Planning Perspectives, 15:57–63, 1983.

9. ELEVATED BLOOD PRESSURE

An increase in blood pressure has been reported in women taking oral contraceptives, and this increase is more likely in older oral-contraceptive users and with continued use. Data from the Royal College of General Practitioners and subsequent randomized trials have shown that the incidence of hypertension increases with increasing quantities of progestations.

Women with a history of hypertension or hypertension-related diseases, or renal disease, should be encouraged to use another method of contraception. If women with hypertension elect to use oral contraceptives, they should be monitored closely, and if significant elevation of blood pressure occurs, oral contraceptives should be discontinued. For most women, elevated blood pressure will return to normal after stopping oral contraceptives, and there is no difference in the occurrence of hypertension between ever- and never-users.

10. HEADACHE

The onset or exacerbation of migraine or development of headache with a new pattern that is recurrent, persistent, or severe requires discontinuation of oral contraceptives and evaluation of the cause.

11. BLEEDING IRREGULARITIES

Breakthrough bleeding and spotting are sometimes encountered in patients on oral contraceptives, especially during the first three months of use. The type and dose of progestogen may be important. Nonhormonal causes should be considered and adequate diagnostic measures taken to rule out malignancy or pregnancy in the event of breakthrough bleeding, as in the case of any abnormal vaginal bleeding. If pathology has been excluded, time or a change to another formulation may solve the problem. In the event of amenorrhea, pregnancy should be ruled out.

Some women may encounter post-pill amenorrhea or oligomenorrhea, especially when such a condition was preexistent.

PRECAUTIONS

Patients should be counseled that this product does not protect against HIV infection (AIDS) and other sexually transmitted diseases.

1. PHYSICAL EXAMINATION AND FOLLOW-UP

A periodic history and physical examination is appropriate for all women, including women using oral contraceptives. The physical examination, however, may be deferred until after initiation of oral contraceptives if requested by the woman and judged appropriate by the clinician. The physical examination should include special reference to blood pressure, breasts, abdomen and pelvic organs, including cervical cytology, and relevant laboratory tests. In case of undiagnosed, persistent or recurrent abnormal vaginal bleeding, appropriate diagnostic measures should be conducted to rule out malignancy. Women with a strong family history of breast cancer or who have breast nodules should be monitored with particular care.

2. LIPID DISORDERS

Women who are being treated for hyperlipidemias should be followed closely if they elect to use oral contraceptives. Some progestogens may elevate LDL levels and may render the control of hyperlipidemias more difficult. (See "Warnings," 1d.)

3. LIVER FUNCTION

If jaundice develops in any woman receiving such drugs, the medication should be discontinued. Steroid hormones may be poorly metabolized in patients with impaired liver function.

4. FLUID RETENTION

Oral contraceptives may cause some degree of fluid retention. They should be prescribed with caution, and only with careful monitoring, in patients with conditions which might be aggravated by fluid retention.

5. EMOTIONAL DISORDERS

Patients becoming significantly depressed while taking oral contraceptives should stop the medication and use an alternate method of contraception in an attempt to determine whether the symptom is drug related.

Women with a history of depression should be carefully observed and the drug discontinued if depression recurs to a serious degree.

6. CONTACT LENSES

Contact-lens wearers who develop visual changes or changes in lens tolerance should be assessed by an ophthalmologist.

7. DRUG INTERACTIONS

Reduced efficacy and increased incidence of breakthrough bleeding and menstrual irregularities have been associated with concomitant use of rifampin. A similar association, though less marked, has been suggested with barbiturates, phenylbutazone, phenytoin sodium, and possibly with griseofulvin, ampicillin, and tetracyclines.

8. INTERACTIONS WITH LABORATORY TESTS

Certain endocrine- and liver-function tests and blood components may be affected by oral contraceptives:

a. Increased prothrombin and factors VII, VIII, IX, and X; decreased antithrombin 3; increased norepinephrine-induced platelet aggregability.
b. Increased thyroid-binding globulin (TBG) leading to increased circulating total thyroid hormone, as measured by protein-bound iodine (PBI), T4 by column or by radioimmunoassay. Free T3 resin uptake is decreased, reflecting the elevated TBG; free T4 concentration is unaltered.
c. Other binding proteins may be elevated in serum.
d. Sex-binding globulins are increased and result in elevated levels of total circulating sex steroids and corticoids; however, free or biologically active levels remain unchanged.
e. Triglycerides may be increased.
f. Glucose tolerance may be decreased.
g. Serum folate levels may be depressed by oral-contraceptive therapy. This may be of clinical significance if a woman becomes pregnant shortly after discontinuing oral contraceptives.

9. CARCINOGENESIS

See "Warnings" section.

10. PREGNANCY

Pregnancy Category X. See "Contraindications" and "Warnings" sections.

11. NURSING MOTHERS

Small amounts of oral-contraceptive steroids have been identified in the milk of nursing mothers, and a few adverse effects on the child have been reported, including jaundice and breast enlargement. In addition, oral contraceptives given in the postpartum period may interfere with lactation by decreasing the quantity and quality of breast milk. If possible, the nursing mother should be advised not to use oral contraceptives but to use other forms of contraception until she has completely weaned her child.

INFORMATION FOR THE PATIENT

See Patient Labeling Printed Below.

ADVERSE REACTIONS

An increased risk of the following serious adverse reactions has been associated with the use of oral contraceptives (see "Warnings" section):

Thrombophlebitis.
Arterial thromboembolism.
Pulmonary embolism.
Myocardial infarction.
Cerebral hemorrhage.
Cerebral thrombosis.
Hypertension.
Gallbladder disease.
Hepatic adenomas or benign liver tumors.

There is evidence of an association between the following conditions and the use of oral contraceptives, although additional confirmatory studies are needed:

Continued on next page

Wyeth-Ayerst Laboratories—Cont.

Mesenteric thrombosis.

Retinal thrombosis.

The following adverse reactions have been reported in patients receiving oral contraceptives and are believed to be drug-related:

Nausea

Vomiting

Gastrointestinal symptoms (such as abdominal cramps and bloating).

Breakthrough bleeding.

Spotting.

Change in menstrual flow.

Amenorrhea.

Temporary infertility after discontinuation of treatment.

Edema.

Melasma which may persist.

Breast changes: tenderness, enlargement, secretion.

Change in weight (increase or decrease).

Change in cervical erosion and cervical secretion.

Diminution in lactation when given immediately postpartum.

Cholestatic jaundice.

Migraine.

Rash (allergic).

Mental depression.

Reduced tolerance to carbohydrates.

Vaginal candidiasis.

Change in corneal curvature (steepening).

Intolerance to contact lenses.

The following adverse reactions have been reported in users of oral contraceptives, and the association has been neither confirmed nor refuted:

Congenital anomalies.

Premenstrual syndrome.

Cataracts.

Optic neuritis.

Changes in appetite.

Cystitis-like syndrome.

Headache.

Nervousness.

Dizziness.

Hirsutism.

Loss of scalp hair.

Erythema multiforme.

Erythema nodosum.

Hemorrhagic eruption.

Vaginitis.

Porphyria.

Impaired renal function.

Hemolytic uremic syndrome.

Budd-Chiari syndrome.

Acne.

Changes in libido.

Colitis.

Sickle-cell disease.

Cerebral-vascular disease with mitral valve prolapse.

Lupus-like syndromes.

OVERDOSAGE

Serious ill effects have not been reported following acute ingestion of large doses of oral contraceptives by young children. Overdosage may cause nausea, and withdrawal bleeding may occur in females.

NONCONTRACEPTIVE HEALTH BENEFITS

The following noncontraceptive health benefits related to the use of oral contraceptives are supported by epidemiological studies which largely utilized oral-contraceptive formulations containing doses exceeding 0.035 mg of ethinyl estradiol or 0.05 mg of mestranol.

Effects on menses:

Increased menstrual cycle regularity.

Decreased blood loss and decreased incidence of iron-deficiency anemia.

Decreased incidence of dysmenorrhea.

Effects related to inhibition of ovulation:

Decreased incidence of functional ovarian cysts.

Decreased incidence of ectopic pregnancies.

Effects from long-term use:

Decreased incidence of fibroadenomas and fibrocystic disease of the breast.

Decreased incidence of acute pelvic inflammatory disease.

Decreased incidence of endometrial cancer.

Decreased incidence of ovarian cancer.

DOSAGE AND ADMINISTRATION

To achieve maximum contraceptive effectiveness, Triphasil-21 Tablets (levonorgestrel and ethinyl estradiol tablets—triphasic regimen) must be taken exactly as directed and at intervals not exceeding 24 hours.

Triphasil-21 Tablets are a three-phase preparation. The dosage of Triphasil-21 Tablets is one tablet daily for 21 consecutive days per menstrual cycle in the following order: 6 brown tablets (phase 1), followed by 5 white tablets (phase 2), and then followed by the last 10 light-yellow tablets (phase 3), according to the prescribed schedule. Tablets are then dis-

continued for 7 days (three weeks on, one week off). It is recommended that Triphasil-21 Tablets be taken at the same time each day, preferably after the evening meal or at bedtime. During the first cycle of medication, the patient should be instructed to take one Triphasil-21 Tablet daily in the order of 6 brown, 5 white and finally, 10 light-yellow tablets for twenty-one (21) consecutive days, beginning on day one (1) of her menstrual cycle. (The first day of menstruation is day one.) The tablets are then discontinued for one week (7 days). Withdrawal bleeding usually occurs within 3 days following discontinuation of Triphasil-21 Tablets. (If Triphasil-21 Tablets are first taken later than the first day of the first menstrual cycle of medication or postpartum, contraceptive reliance should not be placed on Triphasil-21 Tablets until after the first 7 consecutive days of administration. The possibility of ovulation and conception prior to initiation of medication should be considered.)

When switching from another oral contraceptive, Triphasil-21 Tablets should be started on the first day of bleeding following the last tablet taken of the previous oral contraceptive.

The patient begins her next and all subsequent 21-day courses of Triphasil-21 Tablets on the same day of the week that she began her first course, following the same schedule: 21 days on—7 days off. She begins taking her brown tablets on the 8th day after discontinuance regardless of whether or not a menstrual period has occurred or is still in progress. Any time the next cycle of Triphasil-21 Tablets is started later than the 8th day, the patient should be protected by another means of contraception until she has taken a tablet daily for seven consecutive days.

If spotting or breakthrough bleeding occurs, the patient is instructed to continue on the same regimen. This type of bleeding is usually transient and without significance; however, if the bleeding is persistent or prolonged, the patient is advised to consult her physician. Although the occurrence of pregnancy is highly unlikely if Triphasil-21 Tablets are taken according to directions, if withdrawal bleeding does not occur, the possibility of pregnancy must be considered. If the patient has not adhered to the prescribed schedule (missed one or more tablets or started taking them on a day later than she should have), the probability of pregnancy should be considered at the time of the first missed period and appropriate diagnostic measures taken before the medication is resumed. If the patient has adhered to the prescribed regimen and misses two consecutive periods, pregnancy should be ruled out before continuing the contraceptive regimen.

The risk of pregnancy increases with each tablet missed. For additional patient instructions regarding missed pills, see the "WHAT TO DO IF YOU MISS PILLS" section in the DETAILED PATIENT LABELING below. If breakthrough bleeding occurs following missed tablets, it will usually be transient and of no consequence.

In the nonlactating mother, Triphasil-21 may be initiated postpartum, for contraception. When the tablets are administered in the postpartum period, the increased risk of thromboembolic disease associated with the postpartum period must be considered (See "Contraindications", "Warnings", and "Precautions" concerning thromboembolic disease). It is to be noted that early resumption of ovulation may occur if Parlodel® (bromocriptine mesylate) has been used for the prevention of lactation.

HOW SUPPLIED

Triphasil®-21 Tablets (levonorgestrel and ethinyl estradiol tablets—triphasic regimen) NDC 0008-2535, are available in packages of 3 dial dispensers. Each cycle contains 21 round, coated tablets as follows:

NDC 0008-0641, six brown tablets marked "   " and "641", each containing 0.050 mg levonorgestrel and 0.030 mg ethinyl estradiol;

NDC 0008-0642, five white to off-white tablets marked "   " and "642", each containing 0.075 mg levonorgestrel and 0.040 mg ethinyl estradiol; and

NDC 0008-0643, ten light-yellow tablets marked "   " and "643", each containing 0.125 mg levonorgestrel and 0.030 mg ethinyl estradiol.

References available upon request.

Brief Summary Patient Package Insert

This product (like all oral contraceptives) is intended to prevent pregnancy. It does not protect against HIV infection (AIDS) and other sexually transmitted diseases.

Oral contraceptives, also known as "birth-control pills" or "the pill," are taken to prevent pregnancy, and when taken correctly, have a failure rate of less than 1.0% per year when used without missing any pills. The typical failure rate of large numbers of pill users is less than 3.0% per year when women who miss pills are included. For most women oral contraceptives are also free of serious or unpleasant side effects. However, forgetting to take pills considerably increases the chances of pregnancy.

For the majority of women, oral contraceptives can be taken safely. But there are some women who are at high risk of developing certain serious diseases that can be life-threaten-

ing or may cause temporary or permanent disability or death. The risks associated with taking oral contraceptives increase significantly if you:

• smoke.

• have high blood pressure, diabetes, high cholesterol.

• have or have had clotting disorders, heart attack, stroke, angina pectoris, cancer of the breast or sex organs, jaundice or malignant or benign liver tumors.

You should not take the pill if you suspect you are pregnant or have unexplained vaginal bleeding.

> **Cigarette smoking increases the risk of serious adverse effects on the heart and blood vessels from oral-contraceptive use. This risk increases with age and with heavy smoking (15 or more cigarettes per day) and is quite marked in women over 35 years of age. Women who use oral contraceptives should not smoke.**

Most side effects of the pill are not serious. The most common such effects are nausea, vomiting, bleeding between menstrual periods, weight gain, breast tenderness, and difficulty wearing contact lenses. These side effects, especially nausea and vomiting, may subside within the first three months of use.

The serious side effects of the pill occur very infrequently, especially if you are in good health and do not smoke. However, you should know that the following medical conditions have been associated with or made worse by the pill:

1. Blood clots in the legs (thrombophlebitis), lungs (pulmonary embolism), stoppage or rupture of a blood vessel in the brain (stroke), blockage of blood vessels in the heart (heart attack and angina pectoris) or other organs of the body. As mentioned above, smoking increases the risk of heart attacks and strokes and subsequent serious medical consequences.

2. Liver tumors, which may rupture and cause severe bleeding. A possible but not definite association has been found with the pill and liver cancer. However, liver cancers are extremely rare. The chance of developing liver cancer from using the pill is thus even rarer.

3. High blood pressure, although blood pressure usually returns to normal when the pill is stopped.

The symptoms associated with these serious side effects are discussed in the detailed leaflet given to you with your supply of pills. Notify your doctor or health-care provider if you notice any unusual physical disturbances while taking the pill. In addition, drugs such as rifampin, as well as some anticonvulsants and some antibiotics, may decrease oral-contraceptive effectiveness.

Studies to date of women taking the pill have not shown an increase in the incidence of cancer of the breast or cervix. There is, however, insufficient evidence to rule out the possibility that pills may cause such cancers.

Taking the pill provides some important noncontraceptive benefits. These include less painful menstruation, less menstrual blood loss and anemia, fewer pelvic infections, and fewer cancers of the ovary and the lining of the uterus.

Be sure to discuss any medical condition you may have with your health care provider. Your health-care provider will take a medical and family history before prescribing oral contraceptives and will examine you. The physical examination may be delayed to another time if you request it and the health-care provider believes that it is appropriate to postpone it. You should be reexamined at least once a year while taking oral contraceptives. The detailed patient information leaflet gives you further information which you should read and discuss with your health-care provider.

DETAILED PATIENT LABELING

This product (like all oral contraceptives) is intended to prevent pregnancy. It does not protect against HIV infection (AIDS) and other sexually transmitted diseases.

INTRODUCTION

Any woman who considers using oral contraceptives (the birth control pill or the pill) should understand the benefits and risks of using this form of birth control. This leaflet will give you much of the information you will need to make this decision and will also help you determine if you are at risk of developing any of the serious side effects of the pill. It will tell you how to use the pill properly so that it will be as effective as possible. However, this leaflet is not a replacement for a careful discussion between you and your health-care provider. You should discuss the information provided in this leaflet with him or her, both when you first start taking the pill and during your revisits. You should also follow your health-care provider's advice with regard to regular check-ups while you are on the pill.

EFFECTIVENESS OF ORAL CONTRACEPTIVES

Oral contraceptives or "birth-control pills" or "the pill" are used to prevent pregnancy and are more effective than other nonsurgical methods of birth control. When they are taken correctly, the chance of becoming pregnant is less than 1.0% when used perfectly, without missing any pills. Typical failure rates are actually 3.0% per year. The chance of becoming

pregnant increases with each missed pill during the menstrual cycle.
In comparison, typical failure rates for other nonsurgical methods of birth control during the first year of use are as follows:
IUD: 3%.
DEPO-PROVERA® (injectable progestogen): 0.3%.
NORPLANT® SYSTEM (implants): 0.2%.
Diaphragm with spermicides: 18%.
Spermicides alone: 21%.
Vaginal sponge: 18 to 28%.
Condom alone: 12%.
Periodic abstinence: 20%.
No methods: 85%.

WHO SHOULD NOT TAKE ORAL CONTRACEPTIVES

Cigarette smoking increases the risk of serious adverse effects on the heart and blood vessels from oral-contraceptive use. This risk increases with age and with heavy smoking (15 or more cigarettes per day) and is quite marked in women over 35 years of age. Women who use oral contraceptives should not smoke.

Some women should not use the pill. For example, you should not take the pill if you are pregnant or think you may be pregnant. You should also not use the pill if you have any of the following conditions:
- Heart attack or stroke.
- Blood clots in the legs (thrombophlebitis), lungs (pulmonary embolism), or eyes.
- Blood clots in the deep veins of your legs.
- Known or suspected breast cancer or cancer of the lining of the uterus, cervix, or vagina.
- Liver tumor (benign or cancerous).

Or, if you have any of the following:
- Chest pain (angina pectoris).
- Unexplained vaginal bleeding (until a diagnosis is reached by your doctor).
- Yellowing of the whites of the eyes or of the skin (jaundice) during pregnancy or during previous use of the pill.
- Known or suspected pregnancy.

Tell your health-care provider if you have ever had any of these conditions. Your health-care provider can recommend another method of birth control.

OTHER CONSIDERATIONS BEFORE TAKING ORAL CONTRACEPTIVES

Tell your health-care provider if you or any family member has ever had:
- Breast nodules, fibrocystic disease of the breast, an abnormal breast X-ray or mammogram.
- Diabetes.
- Elevated cholesterol or triglycerides.
- High blood pressure.
- Migraine or other headaches or epilepsy.
- Mental depression.
- Gallbladder, heart or kidney disease.
- History of scanty or irregular menstrual periods.

Women with any of these conditions should be checked often by their health-care provider if they choose to use oral contraceptives. Also, be sure to inform your doctor or health-care provider if you smoke or are on any medications.

RISKS OF TAKING ORAL CONTRACEPTIVES

1. *Risk of developing blood clots*
Blood clots and blockage of blood vessels are the most serious side effects of taking oral contraceptives and can be fatal. In particular, a clot in the legs can cause thrombophlebitis and a clot that travels to the lungs can cause a sudden blocking of the vessel carrying blood to the lungs. Rarely, clots occur in the blood vessels of the eye and may cause blindness, double vision, or impaired vision.
If you take oral contraceptives and need elective surgery, need to stay in bed for a prolonged illness, or have recently delivered a baby, you may be at risk of developing blood clots. You should consult your doctor about stopping oral contraceptives three to four weeks before surgery and not taking oral contraceptives for two weeks after surgery or during bed rest. You should also not take oral contraceptives soon after delivery of a baby or a midtrimester pregnancy termination. It is advisable to wait for at least four weeks after delivery if you are not breast-feeding. If you are breast-feeding, you should wait until you have weaned your child before using the pill. (See also the section on breast-feeding in General Precautions.)

2. *Heart attacks and strokes*
Oral contraceptives may increase the tendency to develop strokes (stoppage or rupture of blood vessels in the brain) and angina pectoris and heart attacks (blockage of blood vessels in the heart). Any of these conditions can cause death or serious disability.
Smoking greatly increases the possibility of suffering heart attacks and strokes. Furthermore, smoking and the use of oral contraceptives greatly increase the chances of developing and dying of heart disease.

ANNUAL NUMBER OF BIRTH-RELATED OR METHOD-RELATED DEATHS ASSOCIATED WITH CONTROL OF FERTILITY PER 100,000 NONSTERILE WOMEN, BY FERTILITY-CONTROL METHOD ACCORDING TO AGE

Method of control and outcome	15–19	20–24	25–29	30–34	35–39	40–44
No fertility-control methods*	7.0	7.4	9.1	14.8	25.7	28.2
Oral contraceptives nonsmoker**	0.3	0.5	0.9	1.9	13.8	31.6
Oral contraceptives smoker**	2.2	3.4	6.6	13.5	51.1	117.2
IUD**	0.8	0.8	1.0	1.0	1.4	1.4
Condom*	1.1	1.6	0.7	0.2	0.3	0.4
Diaphragm/spermicide*	1.9	1.2	1.2	1.3	2.2	2.8
Periodic abstinence*	2.5	1.6	1.6	1.7	2.9	3.6

* Deaths are birth related
** Deaths are method related

3. *Gallbladder disease*
Oral-contraceptive users probably have a greater risk than nonusers of having gallbladder disease, although this risk may be related to pills containing high doses of estrogens.

4. *Liver tumors*
In rare cases, oral contraceptives can cause benign but dangerous liver tumors. These benign liver tumors can rupture and cause fatal internal bleeding. In addition, a possible but not definite association has been found with the pill and liver cancers in two studies in which a few women who developed these very rare cancers were found to have used oral contraceptives for long periods. However, liver cancers are extremely rare. The chance of developing liver cancer from using the pill is thus even rarer.

5. *Cancer of the reproductive organs*
There is, at present, no confirmed evidence that oral contraceptives increase in the risk of cancer of the reproductive organs in human studies. Several studies have found no overall increase in the risk of developing breast cancer. However, women who use oral contraceptives and have a strong family history of breast cancer or who have breast nodules or abnormal mammograms should be closely followed by their doctors.
Some studies have found an increase in the incidence of cancer of the cervix in women who use oral contraceptives. However, this finding may be related to factors other than the use of oral contraceptives.

ESTIMATED RISK OF DEATH FROM A BIRTH-CONTROL METHOD OR PREGNANCY

All methods of birth control and pregnancy are associated with a risk of developing certain diseases which may lead to disability or death. An estimate of the number of deaths associated with different methods of birth control and pregnancy has been calculated and is shown in the following table.
[See table above.]
In the above table, the risk of death from any birth-control method is less than the risk of childbirth, except for oral-contraceptive users over the age of 35 who smoke and pill users over the age of 40 even if they do not smoke. It can be seen in the table that for women aged 15 to 39, the risk of death was highest with pregnancy (7 to 26 deaths per 100,000 women, depending on age). Among pill users who do not smoke, the risk of death was always lower than that associated with pregnancy for any age group, except for those women over the age of 40, when the risk increases to 32 deaths per 100,000 women, compared to 28 associated with pregnancy at that age. However, for pill users who smoke and are over the age of 35, the estimated number of deaths exceeds those for other methods of birth control. If a woman is over the age of 40 and smokes, her estimated risk of death is four times higher (117/100,000 women) than the estimated risk associated with pregnancy (28/100,000 women) in that age group.
The suggestion that women over 40 who don't smoke should not take oral contraceptives is based on information from older high-dose pills and on less-selective use of pills than is practiced today. An Advisory Committee of the FDA discussed this issue in 1989 and recommended that the benefits of oral-contraceptive use by healthy, nonsmoking women over 40 years of age may outweigh the possible risks. However, all women, especially older women, are cautioned to use the lowest-dose pill that is effective.

WARNING SIGNALS

If any of these adverse effects occur while you are taking oral contraceptives, call your doctor immediately:
- Sharp chest pain, coughing of blood, or sudden shortness of breath (indicating a possible clot in the lung).
- Pain in the calf (indicating a possible clot in the leg).
- Crushing chest pain or heaviness in the chest (indicating a possible heart attack).
- Sudden severe headache or vomiting, dizziness or fainting, disturbances of vision or speech, weakness, or numbness in an arm or leg (indicating a possible stroke).
- Sudden partial or complete loss of vision (indicating a possible clot in the eye).
- Breast lumps (indicating possible breast cancer or fibrocystic disease of the breast; ask your doctor or health care provider to show you how to examine your breasts).
- Severe pain or tenderness in the stomach area (indicating a possibly ruptured liver tumor).
- Difficulty in sleeping, weakness, lack of energy, fatigue, or change in mood (possibly indicating severe depression).
- Jaundice or a yellowing of the skin or eyeballs, accompanied frequently by fever, fatigue, loss of appetite, dark colored urine, or light-colored bowel movements (indicating possible liver problems).

SIDE EFFECTS OF ORAL CONTRACEPTIVES

1. *Vaginal bleeding*
Irregular vaginal bleeding or spotting may occur while you are taking the pills. Irregular bleeding may vary from slight staining between menstrual periods to breakthrough bleeding which is a flow much like a regular period. Irregular bleeding occurs most often during the first few months of oral-contraceptive use, but may also occur after you have been taking the pill for some time. Such bleeding may be temporary and usually does not indicate any serious problems. It is important to continue taking your pills on schedule. If the bleeding occurs in more than one cycle or lasts for more than a few days, talk to your doctor or health-care provider.

2. *Contact lenses*
If you wear contact lenses and notice a change in vision or an inability to wear your lenses, contact your doctor or health-care provider.

3. *Fluid retention*
Oral contraceptives may cause edema (fluid retention) with swelling of the fingers or ankles and may raise your blood pressure. If you experience fluid retention, contact your doctor or health-care provider.

4. *Melasma*
A spotty darkening of the skin is possible, particularly of the face.

5. *Other side effects*
Other side effects may include change in appetite, headache, nervousness, depression, dizziness, loss of scalp hair, rash, and vaginal infections.
If any of these side effects bother you, call your doctor or health-care provider.

GENERAL PRECAUTIONS

1. *Missed periods and use of oral contraceptives before or during early pregnancy*
There may be times when you may not menstruate regularly after you have completed taking a cycle of pills. If you have taken your pills regularly and miss one menstrual period, continue taking your pills for the next cycle but be sure to inform your health-care provider before doing so. If you have not taken the pills daily as instructed and missed a menstrual period, or if you missed two consecutive menstrual periods, you may be pregnant. Check with your health-care provider immediately to determine whether you are pregnant. Do not continue to take oral contraceptives until you are sure you are not pregnant, but continue to use another method of contraception.
There is no conclusive evidence that oral-contraceptive use is associated with an increase in birth defects when taken inadvertently during early pregnancy. Previously, a few studies had reported that oral contraceptives might be associated with birth defects, but these studies have not been confirmed. Nevertheless, oral contraceptives or any other drugs should not be used during pregnancy unless clearly necessary and prescribed by your doctor. You should check with your doctor about risks to your unborn child of any medication taken during pregnancy.

Continued on next page

Wyeth-Ayerst Laboratories—Cont.

2. *While breast-feeding*

If you are breast-feeding, consult your doctor before starting oral contraceptives. Some of the drug will be passed on to the child in the milk. A few adverse effects on the child have been reported, including yellowing of the skin (jaundice) and breast enlargement. In addition, oral contraceptives may decrease the amount and quality of your milk. If possible, do not use oral contraceptives while breast-feeding. You should use another method of contraception since breast-feeding provides only partial protection from becoming pregnant, and this partial protection decreases significantly as you breast-feed for longer periods of time. You should consider starting oral contraceptives only after you have weaned your child completely.

3. *Laboratory tests*

If you are scheduled for any laboratory tests, tell your doctor you are taking birth-control pills. Certain blood tests may be affected by birth-control pills.

4. *Drug interactions*

Certain drugs may interact with birth-control pills to make them less effective in preventing pregnancy or cause an increase in breakthrough bleeding. Such drugs include rifampin, drugs used for epilepsy such as barbiturates (for example, phenobarbital) and phenytoin (Dilantin is one brand of this drug), phenylbutazone (Butazolidin is one brand), and possibly certain antibiotics. You may need to use an additional method of contraception during any cycle in which you take drugs that can make oral contraceptives less effective.

HOW TO TAKE THE PILL

This product (like all oral contraceptives) is intended to prevent pregnancy. It does not protect against transmission of HIV (AIDS) and other sexually transmitted diseases such as chlamydia, genital herpes, genital warts, gonorrhea, hepatitis B, and syphilis.

IMPORTANT POINTS TO REMEMBER

BEFORE YOU START TAKING YOUR PILLS:

1. BE SURE TO READ THESE DIRECTIONS:
Before you start taking your pills.
Anytime you are not sure what to do.

2. THE RIGHT WAY TO TAKE THE PILL IS TO TAKE ONE PILL EVERY DAY AT THE SAME TIME.
If you miss pills you could get pregnant. This includes starting the pack late. The more pills you miss, the more likely you are to get pregnant.

3. MANY WOMEN HAVE SPOTTING OR LIGHT BLEEDING, OR MAY FEEL SICK TO THEIR STOMACH DURING THE FIRST 1–3 PACKS OF PILLS.
If you feel sick to your stomach, do not stop taking the pill. The problem will usually go away. If it doesn't go away, check with your doctor or clinic.

4. MISSING PILLS CAN ALSO CAUSE SPOTTING OR LIGHT BLEEDING, even when you make up these missed pills.
On the days you take 2 pills to make up for missed pills, you could also feel a little sick to your stomach.

5. IF YOU HAVE VOMITING OR DIARRHEA, for any reason, or IF YOU TAKE SOME MEDICINES, including some antibiotics, your pills may not work as well.
Use a back-up method (such as condoms, foam, or sponge) until you check with your doctor or clinic.

6. IF YOU HAVE TROUBLE REMEMBERING TO TAKE THE PILL, talk to your doctor or clinic about how to make pill-taking easier or about using another method of birth control.

7. IF YOU HAVE ANY QUESTIONS OR ARE UNSURE ABOUT THE INFORMATION IN THIS LEAFLET, call your doctor or clinic.

***BEFORE* YOU START TAKING YOUR PILLS**

1. DECIDE WHAT TIME OF DAY YOU WANT TO TAKE YOUR PILL. It is important to take it at about the same time every day.

2. LOOK AT YOUR PILL PACK TO SEE IF IT HAS 21 OR 28 PILLS:
The *21-pill pack* has 21 "active" brown, white or light-yellow pills (with hormones) to take for 3 weeks, followed by 1 week without pills.
The *28-pill pack* has 21 "active" brown, white or light-yellow pills (with hormones) to take for 3 weeks, followed by 1 week of reminder light-green pills (without hormones).

3. ALSO FIND:
1) where on the pack to start taking pills, and
2) in what order to take the pills (follow the arrows).

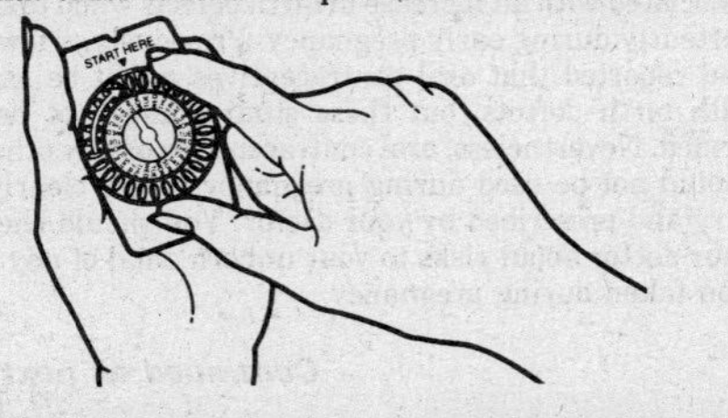

4. BE SURE YOU HAVE READY AT ALL TIMES:
ANOTHER KIND OF BIRTH CONTROL (such as condoms, foam or sponge) to use as a back-up in case you miss pills.
AN EXTRA, FULL PILL PACK.

WHEN TO START THE *FIRST* PACK OF PILLS:

You have a choice of which day to start taking your first pack of pills. Decide with your doctor or clinic which is the best day for you. Pick a time of day which will be easy to remember.

DAY 1 START:

1. Take the first "active" brown pill of the first pack during the *first 24 hours of your period.*
2. You will not need to use a back-up method of birth control, since you are starting the pill at the beginning of your period.

SUNDAY START:

1. Take the first "active" brown pill of the first pack on the *Sunday after your period starts,* even if you are still bleeding. If your period begins on Sunday, start the pack that same day.
2. *Use another method of birth control* as a back-up method if you have sex anytime from the Sunday you start your first pack until the next Sunday (7 days). Condoms, foam, or the sponge are good back-up methods of birth control.

WHAT TO DO DURING THE MONTH:

1. TAKE ONE PILL AT THE SAME TIME EVERY DAY UNTIL THE PACK IS EMPTY.
Do not skip pills even if you are spotting or bleeding between monthly periods or feel sick to your stomach (nausea).
Do not skip pills even if you do not have sex very often.

2. WHEN YOU FINISH A PACK OR SWITCH YOUR BRAND OF PILLS:
21 pills: Wait 7 days to start the next pack. You will probably have your period during that week. Be sure that no more than 7 days pass between 21-day packs.
28 pills: Start the next pack on the day after your last "reminder" pill. Do not wait any days between packs.

WHAT TO DO IF YOU MISS PILLS

If you **MISS 1** brown, white or light-yellow "active" pill:
1. Take it as soon as you remember. Take the next pill at your regular time. This means you take 2 pills in 1 day.
2. You do not need to use a back-up birth-control method if you have sex.

If you **MISS 2** brown, white or light-yellow "active" pills in a row in **WEEK 1 OR WEEK 2** of your pack:
1. Take 2 pills on the day you remember and 2 pills the next day.
2. Then take 1 pill a day until you finish the pack.
3. You MAY BECOME PREGNANT if you have sex in the 7 *days* after you miss pills. You MUST use another birth-control method (such as condoms, foam, or sponge) as a back-up for those 7 days.

If you **MISS 2** brown, white or light-yellow "active" pills in a row in **THE 3rd WEEK:**
1. ***If you are a Day 1 Starter:***
THROW OUT the rest of the pill pack and start a new pack that same day.
If you are a Sunday Starter:
Keep taking 1 pill every day until Sunday.
On Sunday, THROW OUT the rest of the pack and start a new pack of pills that same day.
2. You may not have your period this month but this is expected. However, if you miss your period 2 months in a row, call your doctor or clinic because you might be pregnant.
3. You MAY BECOME PREGNANT if you have sex in the 7 *days* after you miss pills. You MUST use another birth-control method (such as condoms, foam, or sponge) as a back-up for those 7 days.

If you **MISS 3 OR MORE** brown, white or light-yellow "active" pills in a row (during the first 3 weeks):
1. ***If you are a Day 1 Starter:***
THROW OUT the rest of the pill pack and start a new pack that same day.
If you are a Sunday Starter:
Keep taking 1 pill every day until Sunday.
On Sunday, THROW OUT the rest of the pack and start a new pack of pills that same day.
2. You may not have your period this month but this is expected. However, if you miss your period 2 months in a row, call your doctor or clinic because you might be pregnant.
3. You MAY BECOME PREGNANT if you have sex in the 7 *days* after you miss pills. You MUST use another birth control method (such as condoms, foam, or sponge) as a back-up for those 7 days.

A REMINDER FOR THOSE ON 28-DAY PACKS:

If you forget any of the 7 light-green "reminder" pills in Week 4:
THROW AWAY the pills you missed.
Keep taking 1 pill each day until the pack is empty.
You do not need a back-up method if you start your next pack on time.

FINALLY, IF YOU ARE STILL NOT SURE WHAT TO DO ABOUT THE PILLS YOU HAVE MISSED:

Use a BACK-UP METHOD anytime you have sex.
KEEP TAKING ONE PILL EACH DAY until you can reach your doctor or clinic.

Pregnancy due to pill failure

The incidence of pill failure resulting in pregnancy is approximately less than 1.0% if taken every day as directed, but more typical failure rates are less than 3.0%. If failure does occur, the risk to the fetus is minimal.

RISKS TO THE FETUS

If you do become pregnant while using oral contraceptives, the risk to the fetus is small, on the order of no more than one per thousand. You should, however, discuss the risks to the developing child with your doctor.

Pregnancy after stopping the pill

There may be some delay in becoming pregnant after you stop using oral contraceptives, especially if you had irregular menstrual cycles before you used oral contraceptives. It may be advisable to postpone conception until you begin menstruating regularly once you have stopped taking the pill and desire pregnancy.

There does not appear to be any increase in birth defects in newborn babies when pregnancy occurs soon after stopping the pill.

Overdosage

Serious ill effects have not been reported following ingestion of large doses of oral contraceptives by young children. Overdosage may cause nausea and withdrawal bleeding in females. In case of overdosage, contact your health-care provider or pharmacist.

Other information

Your health-care provider will take a medical and family history before prescribing oral contraceptives and will examine you. The physical examination may be delayed to another time if you request it and the health-care provider believes that it is appropriate to postpone it. You should be reexamined at least once a year. Be sure to inform your health-care provider if there is a family history of any of the conditions listed previously in this leaflet. Be sure to keep all appointments with your health-care provider, because this is a time to determine if there are early signs of side effects of oral-contraceptive use.

Do not use the drug for any condition other than the one for which it was prescribed. This drug has been prescribed specifically for you; do not give it to others who may want birth-control pills.

HEALTH BENEFITS FROM ORAL CONTRACEPTIVES

In addition to preventing pregnancy, use of oral contraceptives may provide certain benefits. They are:

- Menstrual cycles may become more regular.
- Blood flow during menstruation may be lighter and less iron may be lost. Therefore, anemia due to iron deficiency is less likely to occur.
- Pain or other symptoms during menstruation may be encountered less frequently.
- Ovarian cysts may occur less frequently.
- Ectopic (tubal) pregnancy may occur less frequently.
- Noncancerous cysts or lumps in the breast may occur less frequently.
- Acute pelvic inflammatory disease may occur less frequently.
- Oral-contraceptive use may provide some protection against developing two forms of cancer: cancer of the ovaries and cancer of the lining of the uterus.

If you want more information about birth-control pills, ask your doctor or pharmacist. They have a more technical leaflet called the Professional Labeling which you may wish to read.

Shown in Product Identification Guide, page 341

TRIPHASIL®-28 ℞

[*tri-fa 'sil*]

Tablets

(levonorgestrel and ethinyl estradiol tablets—triphasic regimen)

Patients should be counseled that this product does not protect against HIV infection (AIDS) and other sexually transmitted diseases.

DESCRIPTION

Each Triphasil cycle of 28 tablets consists of three different drug phases as follows: Phase 1 comprised of 6 brown tablets, each containing 0.050 mg of levonorgestrel (d(-)-13beta-ethy l -17- alpha-ethinyl- 17 -beta-hydroxygon-4-en-3-one), a totally synthetic progestogen, and 0.030 mg of ethinyl estradiol (19- nor- 17α-pregna -1,3,5(10)- trien -20- yne- 3,17 -diol); phase 2 comprised of 5 white tablets, each containing 0.075 mg levonorgestrel and 0.040 mg ethinyl estradiol; and phase 3 comprised of 10 light-yellow tablets, each containing 0.125 mg levonorgestrel and 0.030 mg ethinyl estradiol; then followed by 7 light-green inert tablets. The inactive ingredients present are cellulose, FD&C Blue 1, iron oxides, lactose, mag-

nesium stearate, polacrilin potassium, polyethylene glycol, titanium dioxide, and hydroxypropyl methylcellulose.

Levonorgestrel

Ethinyl Estradiol

CLINICAL PHARMACOLOGY
See Triphasil®-21.

INDICATIONS AND USAGE
See Triphasil-21.

CONTRAINDICATIONS
See Triphasil-21.

WARNINGS
See Triphasil-21.

PRECAUTIONS
See Triphasil-21.

DRUG INTERACTIONS
See Triphasil-21.

CARCINOGENESIS
See Triphasil-21.

PREGNANCY
See Triphasil-21.

NURSING MOTHERS
See Triphasil-21.

INFORMATION FOR THE PATIENT
See Triphasil-21.

ADVERSE REACTIONS
See Triphasil-21.

OVERDOSAGE
See Triphasil-21.

NONCONTRACEPTIVE HEALTH BENEFITS
See Triphasil-21.

DOSAGE AND ADMINISTRATION
To achieve maximum contraceptive effectiveness, Triphasil-28 Tablets (levonorgestrel and ethinyl estradiol tablets—triphasic regimen) must be taken exactly as directed and at intervals not exceeding 24 hours.

Triphasil-28 Tablets are a three-phase preparation plus 7 inert tablets. The dosage of Triphasil-28 Tablets is **one tablet daily** for 28 consecutive days in the following order: 6 brown tablets (phase 1), followed by 5 white tablets (phase 2), followed by 10 light-yellow tablets (phase 3), plus 7 light-green inert tablets, according to the prescribed schedule.

It is recommended that Triphasil-28 Tablets be taken at the same time each day, preferably after the evening meal or at bedtime. During the first cycle of medication, the patient should be instructed to take one Triphasil-28 Tablet daily in the order of 6 brown, 5 white, 10 light-yellow tablets, and then 7 light-green inert tablets for twenty-eight (28) consecutive days, beginning on day one (1) of her menstrual cycle. (The first day of menstruation is day one.) Withdrawal bleeding usually occurs within 3 days following the last light-yellow tablet. (If Triphasil-28 Tablets are first taken later than the first day of the first menstrual cycle of medication or postpartum, contraceptive reliance should not be placed on Triphasil-28 Tablets until after the first 7 consecutive days of administration. The possibility of ovulation and conception prior to initiation of medication should be considered.)

When switching from another oral contraceptive, Triphasil-28 Tablets should be started on the first day of bleeding following the last active tablet taken of the previous oral contraceptive.

The patient begins her next and all subsequent 28-day courses of Triphasil-28 Tablets on the same day of the week that she began her first course, following the same schedule. She begins taking her brown tablets on the next day after ingestion of the last light-green tablet, regardless of whether or not a menstrual period has occurred or is still in progress. Any time a subsequent cycle of Triphasil-28 Tablets is started later than the next day, the patient should be protected by another means of contraception until she has taken a tablet daily for seven consecutive days.

If spotting or breakthrough bleeding occurs, the patient is instructed to continue on the same regimen. This type of bleeding is usually transient and without significance; however, if the bleeding is persistent or prolonged, the patient is advised to consult her physician. Although the occurrence of pregnancy is highly unlikely if Triphasil-28 Tablets are taken according to directions, if withdrawal bleeding does not occur, the possibility of pregnancy must be considered. If the patient has not adhered to the prescribed schedule (missed one or more tablets or started taking them on a day later than she should have), the probability of pregnancy should be considered at the time of the first missed period and appropriate diagnostic measures taken before the medication is resumed. If the patient has adhered to the prescribed regimen and misses two consecutive periods, pregnancy should be ruled out before continuing the contraceptive regimen.

The risk of pregnancy increases with each active (brown, white, or light-yellow) tablet missed. For additional patient instructions regarding missed pills, see the "WHAT TO DO IF YOU MISS PILLS" section in the DETAILED PATIENT LABELING below. If breakthrough bleeding occurs following missed active tablets, it will usually be transient and of no consequence. If the patient misses one or more light-green tablets, she is still protected against pregnancy **provided** she begins taking brown tablets again on the proper day.

In the nonlactating mother, Triphasil-28 may be initiated postpartum, for contraception. When the tablets are administered in the postpartum period, the increased risk of thromboembolic disease associated with the postpartum period must be considered (See "Contraindications", "Warnings", and "Precautions" concerning thromboembolic disease). It is to be noted that early resumption of ovulation may occur if Parlodel® (bromocriptine mesylate) has been used for the prevention of lactation.

HOW SUPPLIED
Triphasil®-28 Tablets (levonorgestrel and ethinyl estradiol tablets—triphasic regimen), NDC 0008-2536, are available in packages of 3 dial dispensers. Each cycle contains 28 round, coated tablets as follows:

NDC 0008-0641, six brown tablets marked "**w**" and "641", each containing 0.050 mg levonorgestrel and 0.030 mg ethinyl estradiol;

NDC 0008-0642, five white to off-white tablets marked "**w**" and "642", each containing 0.075 mg levonorgestrel and 0.040 mg ethinyl estradiol;

NDC 0008-0643, ten light-yellow tablets marked "**w**" and "643", each containing 0.125 mg levonorgestrel and 0.030 mg ethinyl estradiol; and

NDC 0008-0650, seven light-green inert tablets marked "**w**" and "650".

ALSO AVAILABLE:
Triphasil®-28 Tablets (levonorgestrel and ethinyl estradiol tablets—triphasic regimen), NDC 0008-2536, are available in packages of 12 Pilpak® dispensers for clinic use only. Each cycle contains 28 round, coated tablets as follows:

NDC 0008-0641, six brown tablets marked "**w**" and "641", each containing 0.050 mg levonorgestrel and 0.030 mg ethinyl estradiol;

NDC 0008-0642, five white to off-white tablets marked "**w**" and "642", each containing 0.075 mg levonorgestrel and 0.040 mg ethinyl estradiol;

NDC 0008-0643, ten light-yellow tablets marked "**w**" and "643", each containing 0.125 mg levonorgestrel and 0.030 mg ethinyl estradiol; and

NDC 0008-0650, seven light-green inert tablets marked "**w**" and "650".

REFERENCES
Available upon request.
Brief Summary Patient Package Insert: See Triphasil-21.
DETAILED PATIENT LABELING: See Triphasil-21.

HOW TO TAKE THE PILL
For Triphasil-28 Dial Dispenser: See Triphasil-21.
For Triphasil-28 Clinic Pilpak®, See below.
HOW TO TAKE THE PILL
This product (like all oral contraceptives) is intended to prevent pregnancy. It does not protect against transmission of HIV (AIDS) and other sexually transmitted diseases such as chlamydia, genital herpes, genital warts, gonorrhea, hepatitis B, and syphilis.

IMPORTANT POINTS TO REMEMBER
BEFORE YOU START TAKING YOUR PILLS:
1. BE SURE TO READ THESE DIRECTIONS:
Before you start taking your pills.
Anytime you are not sure what to do.
2. THE RIGHT WAY TO TAKE THE PILL IS TO TAKE ONE PILL EVERY DAY AT THE SAME TIME.
If you miss pills you could get pregnant. This includes starting the pack late. The more pills you miss, the more likely you are to get pregnant.
3. MANY WOMEN HAVE SPOTTING OR LIGHT BLEEDING, OR MAY FEEL SICK TO THEIR STOMACH DURING THE FIRST 1–3 PACKS OF PILLS.

If you feel sick to your stomach, do not stop taking the pill. The problem will usually go away. If it doesn't go away, check with your doctor or clinic.
4. MISSING PILLS CAN ALSO CAUSE SPOTTING OR LIGHT BLEEDING, even when you make up these missed pills.
On the days you take 2 pills to make up for missed pills, you could also feel a little sick to your stomach.
5. IF YOU HAVE VOMITING OR DIARRHEA, for any reason, or IF YOU TAKE SOME MEDICINES, including some antibiotics, your pills may not work as well.
Use a back-up method (such as condoms, foam, or sponge) until you check with your doctor or clinic.
6. IF YOU HAVE TROUBLE REMEMBERING TO TAKE THE PILL, talk to your doctor or clinic about how to make pill-taking easier or about using another method of birth control.
7. IF YOU HAVE ANY QUESTIONS OR ARE UNSURE ABOUT THE INFORMATION IN THIS LEAFLET, call your doctor or clinic.

BEFORE YOU START TAKING YOUR PILLS
1. DECIDE WHAT TIME OF DAY YOU WANT TO TAKE YOUR PILL.
It is important to take it about the same time every day.
2. LOOK AT YOUR PILL PACK TO SEE IF IT HAS 21 OR 28 PILLS:
The *21-pill pack* has 21 "active" brown, white or light-yellow pills (with hormones) to take for 3 weeks, followed by 1 week without pills.
The *28-pill pack* has 21 "active" brown, white or light-yellow pills (with hormones) to take for 3 weeks, followed by 1 week of reminder light-green pills (without hormones).
3. ALSO FIND:
1) where on the pack to start taking pills.
2) in what order to take the pills (follow the arrows), and
3) the week numbers as shown in the picture below.

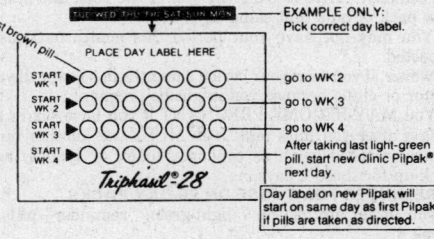

4. BE SURE YOU HAVE READY AT ALL TIMES:
ANOTHER KIND OF BIRTH CONTROL (such as condoms, foam or sponge) to use as a back-up in case you miss pills.
AN EXTRA, FULL PILL PACK.

WHEN TO START THE *FIRST* PACK OF PILLS
You have a choice of which day to start taking your first pack of pills. Decide with your doctor or clinic which is the best day for you. Pick a time of day which will be easy to remember.
DAY 1 START:
1. Take the first "active" brown pill of the first pack during the *first 24 hours of your period.*
2. You will not need to use a back-up method of birth control, since you are starting the pill at the beginning of your period.
SUNDAY START:
1. Take the first "active" brown pill of the first pack on the *Sunday after your period starts,* even if you are still bleeding. If your period begins on Sunday, start the pack that same day.
2. *Use another method of birth control* as a back-up method if you have sex anytime from the Sunday you start your first pack until the next Sunday (7 days). Condoms, foam or the sponge are good back-up methods of birth control.

WHAT TO DO DURING THE MONTH
1. TAKE ONE PILL AT THE SAME TIME EVERY DAY UNTIL THE PACK IS EMPTY.
Do not skip pills even if you are spotting or bleeding between monthly periods or feel sick to your stomach (nausea).
Do not skip pills even if you do not have sex very often.
2. WHEN YOU FINISH A PACK OR SWITCH YOUR BRAND OF PILLS:
21 pills: Wait 7 days to start the next pack. You will probably have your period during that week. Be sure that no more than 7 days pass between 21-day packs.
28 pills: Start the next pack on the day after your last "reminder" pill. Do not wait any days between packs.

WHAT TO DO IF YOU MISS PILLS
If you **MISS 1** brown, white or light-yellow "active" pill:
1. Take it as soon as you remember. Take the next pill at your regular time. This means you take 2 pills in 1 day.

Continued on next page

Wyeth-Ayerst Laboratories—Cont.

2. You do not need to use a back-up birth-control method if you have sex.

If you **MISS 2** brown, white or light-yellow "active" pills in a row in **WEEK 1 OR WEEK 2** of your pack:

1. Take 2 pills on the day you remember and 2 pills the next day.

2. Then take 1 pill a day until you finish the pack.

3. You MAY BECOME PREGNANT if you have sex in the 7 *days* after you miss pills. You MUST use another birth-control method (such as condoms, foam, or sponge) as a back-up for those 7 days.

If you **MISS 2** brown, white or light-yellow "active" pills in a row in **THE 3rd WEEK:**

1. *If you are a Day 1 Starter.*

THROW OUT the rest of the pill pack and start a new pack that same day.

If you are a Sunday Starter:

Keep taking 1 pill every day until Sunday.

On Sunday, THROW OUT the rest of the pack and start a new pack of pills that same day.

2. You may not have your period this month but this is expected.

However, if you miss your period 2 months in a row, call your doctor or clinic because you might be pregnant.

3. You MAY BECOME PREGNANT if you have sex in the 7 *days* after you miss pills. You MUST use another birth-control method (such as condoms, foam, or sponge) as a back-up for those 7 days.

If you **MISS 3 OR MORE** brown, white or light-yellow "active" pills in a row (during the first 3 weeks):

1. *If you are a Day 1 Starter:*

THROW OUT the rest of the pill pack and start a new pack that same day.

If you are a Sunday Starter:

Keep taking 1 pill every day until Sunday.

On Sunday, THROW OUT the rest of the pack and start a new pack of pills that same day.

2. You may not have your period this month but this is expected.

However, if you miss your period 2 months in a row, call your doctor or clinic because you might be pregnant.

3. You MAY BECOME PREGNANT if you have sex in the 7 *days* after you miss pills. You MUST use another birth-control method (such as condoms, foam, or sponge) as a back-up for those 7 days.

A REMINDER FOR THOSE ON 28-DAY PACKS

If you forget any of the 7 light-green "reminder" pills in Week 4:

THROW AWAY the pills you missed.

Keep taking 1 pill each day until the pack is empty.

You do not need a back-up method if you start your next pack on time.

FINALLY, IF YOU ARE STILL NOT SURE WHAT TO DO ABOUT THE PILLS YOU HAVE MISSED

Use a BACK-UP METHOD anytime you have sex.

KEEP TAKING ONE PILL EACH DAY until you can reach your doctor or clinic.

Pregnancy due to pill failure

The incidence of pill failure resulting in pregnancy is approximately less than 1.0% if taken every day as directed, but more typical failure rates are less than 3.0%. If failure does occur, the risk to the fetus is minimal.

RISKS TO THE FETUS

If you do become pregnant while using oral contraceptives, the risk to the fetus is small, on the order of no more than one per thousand. You should, however, discuss the risks to the developing child with your doctor.

Pregnancy after stopping the pill

There may be some delay in becoming pregnant after you stop using oral contraceptives, especially if you had irregular menstrual cycles before you used oral contraceptives. It may be advisable to postpone conception until you begin menstruating regularly once you have stopped taking the pill and desire pregnancy.

There does not appear to be any increase in birth defects in newborn babies when pregnancy occurs soon after stopping the pill.

Overdosage

Serious ill effects have not been reported following ingestion of large doses of oral contraceptives by young children. Overdosage may cause nausea and withdrawal bleeding in females. In case of overdosage, contact your health-care provider or pharmacist.

Other information

Your health-care provider will take a medical and family history before prescribing oral contraceptives and will examine you. The physical examination may be delayed to another time if you request it and the health-care provider believes that it is appropriate to postpone it. You should be reexamined at least once a year. Be sure to inform your health-care provider if there is a family history of any of the conditions listed previously in this leaflet. Be sure to keep all appointments with your health-care provider, because this is

a time to determine if there are early signs of side effects of oral-contraceptive use.

Do not use the drug for any condition other than the one for which it was prescribed. This drug has been prescribed specifically for you; do not give it to others who may want birth-control pills.

HEALTH BENEFITS FROM ORAL CONTRACEPTIVES: See Triphasil-21.

Shown in Product Identification Guide, page 341

TUBEX® Closed Injection System
[tū 'beks]

The TUBEX® closed injection system delivers injectable medication in accurately machine-measured doses with each sterile, prefilled cartridge-needle unit permanently identified up to the moment of injection. Precisely calibrated single-use cartridge-needle units eliminate cross contamination and minimize dosage errors. Super-sharp, siliconized needles minimize penetration pressure. Medication is easily delivered via the TUBEX Injector.

TUBEX sterile cartridge-needle units are ready for instant use, fit easily into the physician's bag, and are readily stored and inventoried in the office.

TAMP-R-TEL® (tamper-resistant package) — a clear, sturdy plastic package for all TUBEX narcotics and barbiturates — adds a new dimension to the handling and record keeping of these controlled drugs. In TAMP-R-TEL, each TUBEX sterile cartridge-needle unit is locked into an individual slot within the package by its own end-lock tab, which is easily broken to release the unit for use. Once the end-lock tab is broken, it is almost impossible to replace it. TAMP-R-TEL thus enhances package integrity, discourages pilferage and facilitates "at a glance" drug count.

The following products are currently available in TUBEX closed injection system. *For prescribing information on products listed, write to Professional Service, Wyeth-Ayerst Laboratories, P.O. Box 8299, Philadelphia, PA 19101, or contact your local Wyeth-Ayerst representative.*

Product and Needle Size Units Per Pkg	NDC 0008-
NARCOTICS in TAMP-R-TEL® **(tamper-resistant package)**	
CODEINE PHOSPHATE, USP Ⓒ●	
30 mg ($^1/_2$ gr.) (25 G × $^5/_8$″) 10—1 mL	0728-01
30 mg ($^1/_2$ gr.) 10 TUBEX® BLUNT POINTE™ Sterile Cartridge Units—1 mL in TAMP-R-TEL®	0728-50
60 mg (1 gr.) (25 G × $^5/_8$″) 10—1 mL	0729-01
60 mg (1 gr.) 10 TUBEX® BLUNT POINTE™ Sterile Cartridge Units—1 mL in TAMP-R-TEL®	0729-50
HYDROMORPHONE HYDROCHLORIDE, USP Ⓒ●	
1 mg ($^1/_{60}$ gr.) (22 G × $^1/_4$″) 10—1 mL fill in 2 mL	0387-03
1 mg ($^1/_{60}$ gr.) 10 TUBEX® BLUNT POINTE™ Sterile Cartridge Units—1 mL fill in 2 mL in TAMP-R-TEL®	0387-50
2 mg ($^1/_{30}$ gr.) (22 G × $^1/_4$″) 10—1 mL fill in 2 mL	0295-01
2 mg ($^1/_{30}$ gr.) 10 TUBEX® BLUNT POINTE™ Sterile Cartridge Units—1 mL fill in 2 mL in TAMP-R-TEL®	0295-50
4 mg ($^1/_{15}$ gr.) (22 G × $^1/_4$″) 10—1 mL fill in 2 mL	0296-01
4 mg ($^1/_{15}$ gr.) 10 TUBEX® BLUNT POINTE™ Sterile Cartridge Units—1 mL fill in 2 mL in TAMP-R-TEL®	0296-50
MEPERGAN® (Meperidine HCl and Promethazine HCl) 25 mg each/mL Ⓒ● (22 G × $^1/_4$″) 10—2 mL	0235-01
10 TUBEX® BLUNT POINTE™ Sterile Cartridge Units in TAMP-R-TEL®	0235-50

MEPERIDINE HYDROCHLORIDE, USP Ⓒ●	
25 mg (22 G × $^1/_4$″) 10—1 mL fill in 2 mL	0601-02
25 mg 10 TUBEX® BLUNT POINTE™ Sterile Cartridge Units—1 mL fill in 2 mL	0601-50
50 mg (22 G × $^1/_4$″) 10—1 mL fill in 2 mL	0602-02
50 mg 10 TUBEX® BLUNT POINTE™ Sterile Cartridge Units—1 mL fill in 2 mL in TAMP-R-TEL®	0602-50
75 mg (22 G × $^1/_4$″) 10—1 mL fill in 2 mL	0605-02
75 mg 10 TUBEX® BLUNT POINTE™ Sterile Cartridge Units—1 mL fill in 2 mL in TAMP-R-TEL®	0605-50
100 mg (22 G × $^1/_4$″) 10—1 mL fill in 2 mL	0613-02
100 mg 10 TUBEX® BLUNT POINTE™ Sterile Cartridge Units—1 mL fill in 2 mL in TAMP-R-TEL®	0613-50
MORPHINE SULFATE, USP Ⓒ●	
2 mg ($^1/_{30}$ gr.) (25 G × $^5/_8$″) 10—1 mL	0649-01
2 mg ($^1/_{30}$ gr.) 10 TUBEX® BLUNT POINTE™ Sterile Cartridge Units—2 mL in TAMP-R-TEL®	0649-50
4 mg ($^1/_{15}$ gr.) (25 G × $^5/_8$″) 10—1 mL	0653-01
4 mg ($^1/_{15}$ gr.) 10 TUBEX® BLUNT POINTE™ Sterile Cartridge Units—1 mL in TAMP-R-TEL®	0653-50
8 mg ($^1/_8$ gr.) (25 G × $^5/_8$″) 10—1 mL fill in 2 mL	0655-01
8 mg ($^1/_8$ gr.) (22 G × $^1/_4$″) 10—1 mL fill in 2 mL	0655-03
8 mg ($^1/_8$ gr.) 10 TUBEX® BLUNT POINTE™ Sterile Cartridge Units—1 mL fill in 2 mL in TAMP-R-TEL®	0655-50
10 mg ($^1/_6$ gr.) (22 G × $^1/_4$″) 10—1 mL fill in 1 mL	0656-01
10 mg ($^1/_6$ gr.) 10 TUBEX® BLUNT POINTE™ Sterile Cartridge Units—1 mL fill in 2 mL in TAMP-R-TEL®	0656-50
15 mg ($^1/_4$ gr.) (22 G × $^1/_4$″) 10—1 mL fill in 2 mL	0657-01
15 mg ($^1/_4$ gr.) 10 TUBEX® BLUNT POINTE™ Sterile Cartridge Units—1 mL fill in 2 mL in TAMP-R-TEL®	0657-50
BARBITURATES in TAMP-R-TEL® **PENTOBARBITAL SODIUM, USP** Ⓒ●	
100 mg ($1^1/_2$ gr.) (22 G × $^1/_4$″) 10—2 mL	0303-02
100 mg ($1^1/_2$ gr.) 10 TUBEX® BLUNT POINTE™ Sterile Cartridge Units—2 mL in TAMP-R-TEL®	0303-50
PHENOBARBITAL SODIUM, USP Ⓒ	
30 mg ($^1/_2$ gr.) (22 G × $^1/_4$″) 10—1 mL	0499-01
30 mg ($^1/_2$ gr.) 10 TUBEX® BLUNT POINTE™ Sterile Cartridge Units—1 mL in TAMP-R-TEL®	0499-50

60 mg (1 gr.) (22 G × 1¼″)
10—1 mL ... 0747-01

60 mg (1 gr.)
10 TUBEX® BLUNT POINTE™ Sterile
Cartridge Units—1 mL
in TAMP-R-TEL® ... 0747-50

130 mg (2 gr.) (22 G × 1¼″)
10—1 mL ... 0304-01

130 mg (2 gr.)
10 TUBEX® BLUNT POINTE™ Sterile
Cartridge Units—1 mL
in TAMP-R-TEL® ... 0304-50

SECOBARBITAL SODIUM, USP Ⓒ●
100 mg (1½ gr.) (22 G × 1¼″)
10—2 mL ... 0305-02

100 mg (1½ gr.)
10 TUBEX® BLUNT POINTE™ Sterile
Cartridge Units—2 mL
in TAMP-R-TEL® ... 0305-50

● Narcotic order blank required.

ANTIBIOTICS
BICILLIN® C-R (Penicillin G Benzathine and Penicillin G
Procaine Suspension) 300,000 U each/mL
600,000 U (20 G × 1¼″)
10—1 mL ... 0026-17

1,200,000 U (20 G × 1¼″)
10—2 mL ... 0026-16

2,400,000 U (18 G × 2″)
10—4 mL ... 0026-22
(disposable syringe)

BICILLIN C-R 900/300
(900,000 units Penicillin G Benzathine and 300,000 units
Penicillin G Procaine in suspension)
1,200,000 U (20 G × 1¼″)
10—2 mL ... 0079-01

BICILLIN LONG-ACTING (Sterile Penicillin G Benzathine
Suspension)
600,000 U (20 G × 1¼″)
10—1 mL ... 0021-08

1,200,000 U (20 G × 1¼″)
10—2 mL ... 0021-07

2,400,000 U (18 G × 2″)
10—4 mL ... 0021-12
(disposable syringe)

WYCILLIN® (Sterile Penicillin G Procaine Suspension)
600,000 U (20 G × 1¼″)
10—1 mL ... 0018-10

1,200,000 U (20 G × 1¼″)
10—2 mL ... 0018-08

2,400,000 U (18 G × 2″)
10—4 mL ... 0018-12
(disposable syringe)

BIOLOGICALS
FluShield®
INFLUENZA VIRUS VACCINE
Trivalent, Types A and B
(chromatograph- and filtered-purified subvirion antigen)
1996-1997 Formula
(25 G × 5/8″)
10—0.5 mL ... 0849-02

VITAMINS
THIAMINE HYDROCHLORIDE, USP
100 mg (22 G × 1¼″)
10—1 mL fill in 2 mL ... 0302-01

CARDIOVASCULAR AGENTS
DIGOXIN, USP
0.25 mg (22 G × 1¼″)
10—1 mL ... 0480-02

0.5 mg (22 G × 1¼″)
10—2 mL ... 0480-01

EPINEPHRINE, USP (1:1000)
(25 G × 5/8″)
10—1 mL ... 0263-01

HEPARIN SODIUM, USP
1,000 USP units (22 G × 1¼″)
10—1 mL ... 0275-01

1,000 USP units
10 TUBEX® BLUNT POINTE™ Sterile
Cartridge Units—1 mL
in TAMP-R-TEL® ... 0275-50

2,500 USP units (25 G × 5/8″)
10—1 mL ... 0482-01

5,000 USP units (25 G × 5/8″)
10—0.5 mL ... 0277-02

5,000 USP units (25 G × 5/8″)
50—0.5 mL ... 0277-03

5,000 USP units (25 G × 5/8″)
10—1.0 mL ... 0278-02

7,500 USP units (25 G × 5/8″)
10—1 mL ... 0293-01

10,000 USP units (25 G × 5/8″)
10—1 mL ... 0277-01

20,000 USP units (25 G × 5/8″)
10—1 mL ... 0276-01

SPECIAL AGENTS
ATIVAN® (Lorazepam) Ⓒ

1 mg/ 0.5 mL (22 G × 1¼″)
10—0.5 mL fill in 1 mL ... 0581-07

1 mg/0.5 mL (22 G × 1¼″)
10—0.5 mL fill in 1 mL in TAMP-R-TEL® ... 0581-05

2 mg/mL (22 G × 1¼″)
10—1 mL fill in 2 mL ... 0581-02

2 mg/mL (22 G × 1¼″)
10—1 mL fill in 2 mL
in TAMP-R-TEL® ... 0581-06

2 mg/mL
10 TUBEX® BLUNT POINTE™ Sterile
Cartridge Units—1 mL fill
in 2 mL ... 0581-52

2 mg/mL
10 TUBEX® BLUNT POINTE™ Sterile
Cartridge Units—1 mL fill
in 2 mL in TAMP-R-TEL® ... 0581-53

4 mg/mL (22 G × 1¼″)
10—1 mL fill in 2 mL ... 0570-02

4 mg/mL (22 G × 1¼″)
10—1 mL fill in 2 mL
in TAMP-R-TEL® ... 0570-05

4 mg/mL
10 TUBEX® BLUNT POINTE™ Sterile
Cartridge Units—1 mL fill
in 2 mL ... 0570-50

4 mg/mL
10 TUBEX® BLUNT POINTE™ Sterile
Cartridge Units—1 mL fill in 2 mL
in TAMP-R-TEL® ... 0570-51

DIMENHYDRINATE, USP
50 mg (22 G × 1¼″)
10—1 mL ... 0485-01

DIPHENHYDRAMINE HYDROCHLORIDE, USP
50 mg (22 G × 1¼″)
10—1 mL ... 0384-01

HEPARIN FLUSH 2.5 mL KITS
25 USP units
(25 G × 5/8″)
30 Kits ... 2528-02
Each Unit of Use Kit contains:
One 2.5 mL size (25 G × 5/8″) TUBEX Heparin Lock Flush
Solution, USP, 10 USP units per mL and two 2.5 mL size (25
G × 5/8″) TUBEX Bacteriostatic Sodium Chloride Injection,
USP.

HEPARIN FLUSH 2.5 mL KITS
25 USP units per TUBEX® BLUNT POINTE™ Sterile
Cartridge Unit
30 Kits ... 2528-51
Each Unit of Use Kit contains:
One TUBEX BLUNT POINTE (2.5 mL) Heparin Lock Flush
Solution, USP, 25 USP units heparin sodium per TUBEX
BLUNT POINTE or 10 USP units per mL. Two TUBEX
BLUNT POINTE (2.5 mL) Bacteriostatic Sodium Chloride
Injection, USP.

250 USP units
(25 G × 5/8″)
30 Kits ... 2529-02
Each Unit of Use Kit contains:
One 2.5 mL size (25 G × 5/8″) TUBEX Heparin Lock Flush
Solution, USP, 100 USP units per mL and two 2.5 mL size (25
G × 5/8″) TUBEX Bacteriostatic Sodium Chloride Injection,
USP.

250 USP units per TUBEX® BLUNT POINTE™ Sterile
Cartridge Unit
30 Kits ... 2529-51
Each Unit of Use Kit contains:
One TUBEX BLUNT POINTE (2.5 mL) Heparin Lock Flush
Solution, USP, 250 USP units heparin sodium per TUBEX
BLUNT POINTE or 100 USP units per mL. Two TUBEX
BLUNT POINTE (2.5 mL) Bacteriostatic Sodium Chloride
Injection, USP.

HEPARIN FLUSH KITS
10 USP units
(25 G × 5/8″)
50 Kits ... 2528-01
Each Unit of Use Kit contains:
One 1 mL size (25 G × 5/8″) TUBEX Heparin Lock Flush
Solution, USP, 10 USP units per mL and two 2.5 mL size (25
G × 5/8″) TUBEX Bacteriostatic Sodium Chloride Injection,
USP.

10 USP units per TUBEX® BLUNT POINTE™ Sterile
Cartridge Unit
50 Kits ... 2528-50
Each Unit of Use Kit contains:
One 1 mL size TUBEX BLUNT POINTE Heparin Lock Flush
Solution, USP, 10 USP units per mL and two 2.5 mL size
TUBEX BLUNT POINTE Bacteriostatic Sodium Chloride
Injection, USP.

100 USP units
(25 G × 5/8″)
50 Kits ... 2529-01
Each Unit of Use Kit contains:
One 1 mL size (25 G × 5/8″) TUBEX Heparin Lock Flush
Solution, USP, 100 USP units per mL and two 2.5 mL size (25
G × 5/8″) TUBEX Bacteriostatic Sodium Chloride Injection,
USP.

100 USP units per TUBEX® BLUNT POINTE™ Sterile
Cartridge Unit
50 Kits ... 2529-50
Each Unit of Use Kit contains:
One 1 mL size TUBEX BLUNT POINTE Heparin Lock Flush
Solution, USP, 100 USP units per mL and two 2.5 mL size
TUBEX BLUNT POINTE Bacteriostatic Sodium Chloride
Injection, USP.

HEPARIN FLUSH 1 mL KITS
10 USP units
(25 G × 5/8″)
50 Kits ... 2528-03
Each Unit of Use Kit contains:
One 1 mL size (25 G × 5/8″) TUBEX Heparin Lock Flush
Solution, USP, 10 USP units per mL and two 1 mL size (25 G
× 5/8″) TUBEX Bacteriostatic Sodium Chloride Injection,
USP.

10 USP units per TUBEX® BLUNT POINTE™ Sterile
Cartridge Unit
50 Kits ... 2528-52
Each Unit of Use Kit contains:
One 1 mL size TUBEX BLUNT POINTE Heparin Lock Flush
Solution, USP, 10 USP units per mL and two 1 mL size
TUBEX BLUNT POINTE Bacteriostatic Sodium Chloride
Injection, USP.

100 USP units
(25 G × 5/8″)
50 Kits ... 2529-03
Each Unit of Use Kit contains:
One 1 mL size (25 G × 5/8″) TUBEX Heparin Lock Flush
Solution, USP, 100 USP units per mL and two 1 mL size (25 G
× 5/8″) TUBEX Bacteriostatic Sodium Chloride Injection,
USP.

Continued on next page

Wyeth-Ayerst Laboratories—Cont.

100 USP units per TUBEX® BLUNT POINTE™ Sterile Cartridge Unit

50 Kits	2529-52

Each Unit of Use Kit contains:
One 1 mL size TUBEX BLUNT POINTE Heparin Lock Flush Solution, USP, 100 USP units per mL and two 1 mL size TUBEX BLUNT POINTE Bacteriostatic Sodium Chloride Injection, USP.

HEPARIN LOCK FLUSH Solution, USP

10 USP units per mL (25 G × ⁵/₈″)	
50—1 mL	0523-01
100 USP units per mL (25 G × ⁵/₈″)	
50—1 mL	0487-01
10 USP units per mL—25 USP units per TUBEX (25 G × ⁵/₈″)	
50—2.5 mL	0523-02
100 USP units per mL—250 USP units per TUBEX (25 G × ⁵/₈″)	
50—2.5 mL	0487-03
10 USP units per mL 50 TUBEX® BLUNT POINTE™ Sterile Cartridge Units—1 mL	0523-50
100 USP units per mL 50 TUBEX® BLUNT POINTE™ Sterile Cartridge Units—1 mL	0487-50
10 USP units per mL—25 USP units per TUBEX 50 TUBEX® BLUNT POINTE™ Sterile Cartridge Units—2.5 mL	0523-51
100 USP units per mL—250 USP units per TUBEX 50 TUBEX® BLUNT POINTE™ Sterile Cartridge Units—2.5 mL	0487-51

PHENERGAN® (Promethazine HCl)

25 mg (22 G × 1¹/₄″)	
10—1 mL	0416-01
25 mg 10 TUBEX® BLUNT POINTE™ Sterile Cartridge Units—1 mL	0416-50
50 mg (22 G × 1¹/₄″)	
10—1 mL	0417-01

PROCHLORPERAZINE EDISYLATE, USP

5 mg (22 G × 1¹/₄″)	
10—1 mL	0542-01
10 mg (22 G × 1¹/₄″)	
10—2 mL	0542-02

SODIUM CHLORIDE, USP (Bacteriostatic)

(25 G × ⁵/₈″)	
50—1 mL	0333-08
50 TUBEX® BLUNT POINTE™ Sterile Cartridge Units—1 mL	0333-51
(22 G × 1¹/₄″)	
50—2.5 mL	0333-05
(25 G × ⁵/₈″)	
50—2.5 mL	0333-02
50 TUBEX® BLUNT POINTE™ Sterile Cartridge Units—2.5 mL	0333-50

Shown in Product Identification Guide, page 341
PLEASE NOTE: THE WYETH-AYERST METAL TUBEX HYPODERMIC SYRINGE AND TUBEX FAST-TRAK SYRINGE HAVE BEEN DISCONTINUED AND REPLACED BY THE TUBEX INJECTOR. EXCHANGE OF THESE DISCONTINUED SYRINGES IS AVAILABLE, FREE OF CHARGE, FROM YOUR WYETH-AYERST AND/OR ELKINS-SINN SALES REPRESENTATIVE, OR FROM WYETH-AYERST DIRECTLY. FOR LOADING AND UNLOADING INFORMATION OF THESE DISCONTINUED SYRINGES, CONTACT THE MEDICAL AFFAIRS DEPARTMENT, AT WYETH-AYERST LABORATORIES, P.O. BOX 8299, PHILADELPHIA, PA 19101.

TUBEX® Injector
NOTE: The TUBEX® Injector is reusable: do not discard.

TUBEX® Sterile Cartridge-Needle Unit

DIRECTIONS FOR USE:

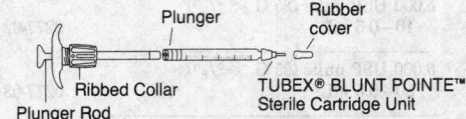

Ribbed Collar / Plunger Rod / Plunger / TUBEX® Sterile Cartridge-Needle Unit

TUBEX® BLUNT POINTE™ Sterile Cartridge Unit

DIRECTIONS FOR USE:

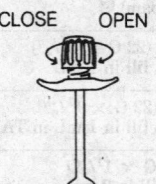

Plunger / Rubber cover / Ribbed Collar / Plunger Rod / TUBEX® BLUNT POINTE™ Sterile Cartridge Unit

TUBEX® BLUNT POINTE™ Sterile Cartridge Unit is intended for use with injection sets specifically manufactured as "needle-less" injection systems. TUBEX® BLUNT POINTE™ Sterile Cartridge Unit is compatible with Abbott's LifeShield® prepierced reseal injection site, Baxter's Interlink® Injection Site and B. Braun Medical's SafSite® Reflux Valve. Consult manufacturer's recommendations regarding "Directions for Use" of the "needle-less" system.

To load a TUBEX® Sterile Cartridge-Needle Unit into the TUBEX® Injector
1. Turn the ribbed collar to the "OPEN" position until it stops.

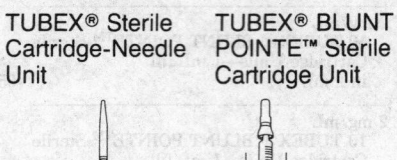

CLOSE   OPEN

2. Hold the Injector with the open end up and fully insert the TUBEX® Sterile Cartridge Unit.
Firmly tighten the ribbed collar in the direction of the "CLOSE" arrow.

TUBEX® Sterile Cartridge-Needle Unit   TUBEX® BLUNT POINTE™ Sterile Cartridge Unit

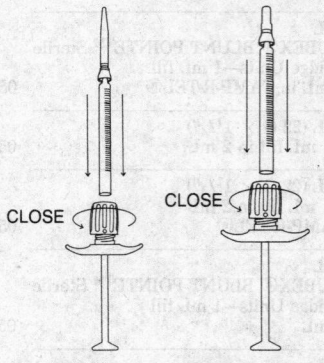

CLOSE   CLOSE

3. Thread the plunger rod into the plunger of the TUBEX® Sterile Cartridge Unit until slight resistance is felt.

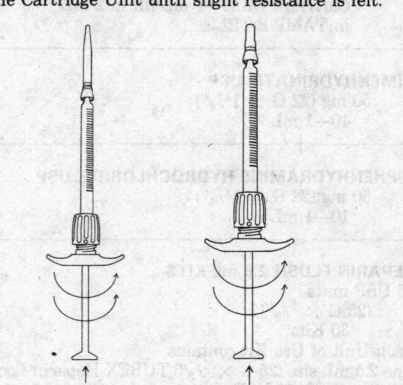

The Injector is now ready for use in the usual manner.

[See Figure at top of next column.]

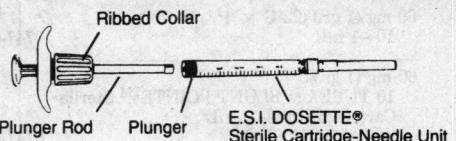

Ribbed Collar / Plunger Rod / Plunger / E.S.I. DOSETTE® Sterile Cartridge-Needle Unit

To load an E.S.I. DOSETTE® Sterile Cartridge-Needle Unit into the TUBEX® Injector
1. Turn the ribbed collar to the "OPEN" position until it stops.

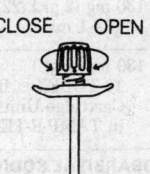

CLOSE   OPEN

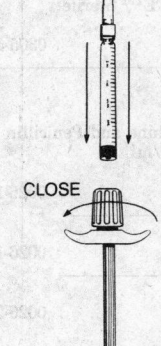

2. Hold the Injector with the open end up and fully insert the DOSETTE® Sterile Cartridge-Needle Unit. Firmly tighten the ribbed collar in the direction of the "CLOSE" arrow.

3. Thread the plunger rod into the plunger of the DOSETTE® Sterile Cartridge-Needle Unit until slight resistance is felt.

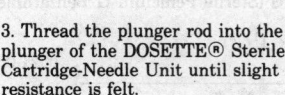

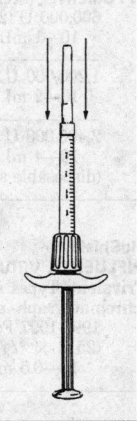

4. Engage the needle-cap assembly by pulling the cap down over the silver cartridge hub. The needle is fully engaged when the silver hub is completely covered.
The Injector is now ready for use in the usual manner.

To administer TUBEX®/DOSETTE® Sterile Cartridge-Needle Unit
Method of administration is the same as with conventional syringe. Remove needle cover by grasping it securely; twist and pull. Introduce needle into patient, aspirate by pulling back slightly on the plunger, and inject.

To administer TUBEX® BLUNT POINTE™ Sterile Cartridge Units
"Needle-less" IV set administration is similar to administration with conventional syringes. Remove rubber cover by grasping it securely; twist and pull. For B. Braun Medical's SafSite® Reflux Valves, aseptically swab

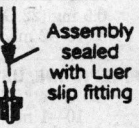

Assembly sealed with Luer slip fitting

the luer slip fitting of the BLUNT POINTE™ sterile cartridge tip assembly with a sterile, individually wrapped, saturated 70% Isopropyl Alcohol swab. This action will remove the lubricant coating from the tip to facilitate a tight seal. Introduce TUBEX® BLUNT POINTE™ Sterile Cartridge Unit into the "needle-less" IV set as per manufacturer's "Directions for Use."

To remove the empty TUBEX®/DOSETTE® Cartridge Unit and dispose into a vertical disposal container
1. Do not recap the needle/point. Disengage the plunger rod.

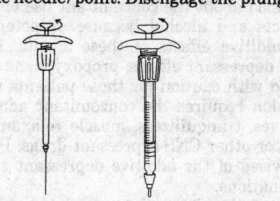

2. Hold the Injector, needle/point pointing down, over a verticle disposal container and loosen the ribbed collar. TUBEX®/DOSETTE® Cartridge Unit will drop into the container.

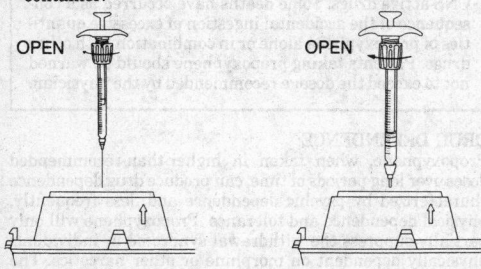

3. Discard the cover.

To remove the empty TUBEX®/DOSETTE® Cartridge Unit and dispose into a horizontal (mailbox) disposal container
1. Do not recap the needle/point. Disengage the plunger rod.
2. Open the horizontal (mailbox) disposal container. Insert TUBEX®/DOSETTE® Cartridge Unit, needle/point pointing down, halfway into container. Close the container lid on cartridge. Loosen ribbed collar; TUBEX®/DOSETTE® Cartridge Unit will drop into the container.

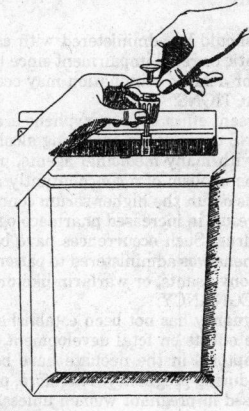

3. Discard the cover.
The TUBEX® Injector is reusable and should not be discarded.
Used TUBEX®/DOSETTE® Cartridge Units should not be employed for successive injections or as multiple-dose containers. They are intended to be used only once and discarded. **NOTE:** Any graduated markings on TUBEX®/DOSETTE® Sterile Cartridge Units are to be used only as a guide in mixing, withdrawing, or administering measured doses.
Wyeth-Ayerst does not recommend and will not accept responsibility for the use of any cartridge-needle units or needleless system other than TUBEX® or E.S.I. DOSETTE® Cartridge Units in the TUBEX® Injector.
The ESI DOSETTE® cartridge holder has been discontinued. For instructions of its use, contact Medical Affairs, Wyeth-Ayerst Laboratories, P.O. Box 8299, Phila., PA 19101.
Shown in Product Identification Guide, page 341

TYPHOID VACCINE
USP   ℞

DESCRIPTION
Typhoid Vaccine, USP is a saline suspension containing not more than 1000 million Salmonella typhosa (Ty-2-strain) organisms per mL. After growing on veal infusion agar (containing 0.5 percent sodium chloride, 2 percent peptone, and 5 percent agar), the bacteria are washed off the medium, suspended in buffered sodium chloride injection, and killed by a combination of phenol and heat. Phenol (0.5 percent) is added to the final vaccine as preservative. Typhoid Vaccine, USP is tested for safety, potency, and purity and standardized according to F.D.A. Additional Standards for Bacterial Vaccines, 21 C.F.R. 620.10-620.15.

INDICATIONS
Typhoid Vaccine, USP is indicated for active immunization against typhoid fever. Based on data obtained from field studies, it has been estimated that typhoid vaccine is 70% or more effective in preventing typhoid fever, depending in part on the degree of exposure.
Routine immunization against typhoid is no longer recommended for persons residing in the United States. Selective immunization is indicated in the following situations:
1. Intimate exposure to a known typhoid carrier, as would occur with continued household contact.
2. Foreign travel to areas where typhoid fever is endemic.
Although at one time typhoid immunization was suggested for persons attending summer camps or for residents of areas where flooding has occurred, there are no data to support continuation of such practices.[1,2]

CONTRAINDICATIONS
Administration should be postponed in the presence of acute respiratory or other active infection.
A severe systemic or allergic reaction following a prior dose is a contraindication to further use.[3]

PRECAUTIONS
A sterile syringe and needle should be used for each patient to prevent transmission of hepatitis B virus and other infectious agents from one person to another.
Specific information concerning use of typhoid vaccine during pregnancy is not available. However, as with other inactivated bacterial vaccines, its use is not contraindicated during pregnancy unless the intended recipient has manifested significant systemic or allergic reactions following administration of prior doses. Use of typhoid vaccine during pregnancy should be individualized to reflect actual need.
Before the injection of any biological, the physician should take all precautions known for prevention of allergic or any other side reactions. This should include: A review of the patient's history regarding possible sensitivity; the ready availability of epinephrine 1:1000 and other appropriate agents used for control of immediate allergic reactions; and a knowledge of the recent literature pertaining to use of the biological concerned.

REACTIONS
Most recipients of typhoid vaccine experience some degree of local and systemic response, usually beginning within 24 hours of administration and persisting for one or two days. Local reactions are usually manifested by erythema, induration, and tenderness and should be expected in all those injected intracutaneously.
Systemic manifestations may include malaise, headache, myalgia, and elevated temperature.

DOSAGE
PRIMARY IMMUNIZATION
1. Adults and children over 10 years of age:
Two doses of 0.5 mL each, administered subcutaneously, at an interval of four or more weeks.
2. Children less than 10 years of age:
Two doses of 0.25 mL, each administered subcutaneously, at an interval of four or more weeks.
In instances where there is insufficient time for two doses administered at the specified intervals, three doses of the appropriate volume may be given at weekly intervals.
BOOSTER DOSES
1. Adults and children over 10 years of age:
0.5 mL, administered subcutaneously, or 0.1 mL, injected intracutaneously (intradermally).
2. Children 6 months to 10 years of age:
0.25 mL, administered subcutaneously, or 0.1 mL, intracutaneously (intradermally)
Under conditions of continued or repeated exposure, a booster dose should be given at least every three years. In instances where an interval of more than three years has elapsed since primary immunization or the last booster dose, a single booster dose is considered sufficient; it is not necessary to repeat the primary immunizing series.

ADMINISTRATION
Shake vial vigorously before withdrawing each dose.
Before injection, the rubber diaphragm of the vial and the skin over the site to be injected should be cleansed and prepared with a suitable germicide.
After insertion of the needle, aspirate to help avoid inadvertent injection into a blood vessel.

HOW SUPPLIED
Typhoid Vaccine, USP is supplied in vials of 5 mL and 10 mL, each containing 8 units per mL.

REFERENCES
1. Recommendations of the Public Health Service Advisory Committee on Immunization Practices—Typhoid Vaccine. Morbidity and Mortality Weekly Report 27 (No. 27): 231, 1978.
2. Report of the Committee on Infectious Diseases, American Academy of Pediatrics, 1982 (Red Book).
3. Recommendations of the Public Health Service Advisory Committee on Immunization Practices—General Recommendations on Immunization. Morbidity and Mortality Weekly Report 29 (No.7): 76, 1980.
Manufactured by: Wyeth Laboratories Inc., Marietta, PA 17547.

UNIPEN®
[*ū 'ni-pen*]   ℞
(nafcillin sodium) as the monohydrate
CAPSULES

DESCRIPTION
Unipen is a semisynthetic penicillin developed by Wyeth-Ayerst research. Although primarily designed as an anti-staphylococcal penicillin, in limited clinical trials it has been shown to be effective in the treatment of infections caused by pneumococci and Group A beta-hemolytic streptococci. Because of this wide gram-positive spectrum, this product is particularly suitable for *Initial Therapy* in severe or potentially severe infections before definitive culture results are known and in which staphylococci are suspected.
This product is readily soluble and can be conveniently administered in both oral and parenteral dosage forms. It is resistant to inactivation by staphylococcal penicillinase. Following intramuscular administration in humans, it rapidly appears in the plasma, penetrates body tissues in high concentration, and diffuses well into pleural, pericardial, and synovial fluids.
Unipen capsules contain nafcillin sodium as the monohydrate equivalent to 250 mg nafcillin. The inactive ingredients present are calcium carbonate, D&C Yellow 10, FD&C Blue 1, FD&C Yellow 6, gelatin, mineral oil, and titanium dioxide.
Unipen tablets contain nafcillin sodium as the monohydrate equivalent to 500 mg nafcillin. The inactive ingredients present are calcium carbonate, cellulose, hydroxypropyl methylcellulose, lactose, magnesium stearate, polacrilin potassium, starch, and talc.
NOTE: Unipen contains 2.9 milliequivalents of sodium per gram of nafcillin as the sodium salt.

HOW SUPPLIED
FOR ORAL ADMINISTRATION
Capsules
Supplied as capsules containing nafcillin sodium as the monohydrate equivalent to 250 mg nafcillin, buffered with calcium carbonate, as follows:
NDC 0008-0057-03, green and yellow capsule marked "WYETH" and "57", in bottles of 100 capsules.
Store at room temperature, approx. 25° C (77° F).
Keep tightly closed.
Dispense in tight container.
The appearance of these capsules is a trademark of Wyeth-Ayerst Laboratories.

BIBLIOGRAPHY
A bibliography is available upon request.

WYANOIDS® Relief Factor   OTC
[*wi 'a-noids*]
Hemorrhoidal Suppositories

(See PDR For Nonprescription Drugs)

WYCILLIN®   ℞
[*wi-sil 'in*]
(penicillin G procaine suspension)
INJECTION

FOR DEEP INTRAMUSCULAR INJECTION ONLY

DESCRIPTION
This product is designed to provide a stable aqueous suspension of penicillin G procaine, ready for immediate use. This eliminates the necessity for addition of any diluent, required for the usual dry formulation of injectable penicillin.
Each Tubex Sterile Cartridge-Needle Unit, 1,200,000 units (2 mL size) or 600,000 units (1 mL size), or disposable syringe, 2,400,000 units (4 mL size), contains penicillin G procaine in a stabilized aqueous suspension with sodium citrate buffer; and as w/v, approximately 0.5% lecithin, 0.5% carboxy-

Continued on next page

Wyeth-Ayerst Laboratories—Cont.

methylcellulose, 0.5% povidone, 0.1% methylparaben, and 0.01% propylparaben.
Wycillin must be stored in a refrigerator. Keep from freezing. This will prevent deterioration and assure that no significant loss of potency occurs within the expiration date.
Wycillin suspension in the TUBEX and disposable syringe formulations is viscous and opaque. Read **"Contraindications," "Warnings," "Precautions,"** and **"Dosage and Administration"** sections prior to use.

HOW SUPPLIED

Wycillin® (penicillin G procaine suspension) is supplied in packages of 10 TUBEX® Sterile Cartridge-Needle Units (20 gauge × $1^1/_4$ inch needle), as follows:
1 mL size, containing 600,000 units per TUBEX, NDC 0008-0018-10.
2 mL size, containing 1,200,000 units per TUBEX, NDC 0008-0018-08.
Store in a refrigerator.
Keep from freezing.
ALSO AVAILABLE:
Wycillin (penicillin G procaine suspension) is also available in packages of 10 disposable syringes as follows:
4 mL size, containing 2,400,000 units per syringe (18 gauge × 2 inch needle), NDC 0008-0018-12.
For prescribing information write to Professional Service, Wyeth-Ayerst Laboratories, P.O. Box 8299, Philadelphia, PA 19101, or contact your local Wyeth-Ayerst representative.

WYDASE® ℞

[*wi-dās*]
(hyaluronidase)

DESCRIPTION

Wydase, a protein enzyme, is a preparation of highly purified bovine testicular hyaluronidase. The exact chemical structure of this enzyme is unknown. Wydase is available in two dosage forms:
WYDASE LYOPHILIZED
Hyaluronidase, dehydrated in the frozen state under high vacuum, with lactose and thimerosal (mercury derivative), is supplied as a sterile, white, odorless, amorphous solid and is to be reconstituted with Sodium Chloride Injection, USP, before use, usually in the proportion of one mL per 150 USP units of hyaluronidase (Wydase Lyophilized).
Each vial of 1,500 USP units contains 1.0 mg thimerosal (mercury derivative), added as a preservative, and 13.3 mg lactose. Each vial of 150 USP units contains 0.075 mg thimerosal (mercury derivative), added as a preservative, and 2.66 mg lactose.
WYDASE STABILIZED SOLUTION
A hyaluronidase injection solution ready for use, colorless and odorless, containing 150 USP units of hyaluronidase per mL with 8.5 mg sodium chloride, 1 mg edetate disodium, 0.4 mg calcium chloride, monobasic sodium phosphate buffer, and not more than 0.1 mg thimerosal (mercury derivative).
The USP and the NF hyaluronidase units are the equivalent to the turbidity-reducing (TR) unit and to the International Unit.

HOW SUPPLIED

Wydase® Lyophilized is supplied as follows:
150 USP (TR) units of hyaluronidase
NDC 0008-0121-01, 1 mL vial, as single vials.
Not Recommended for IV Use.
Store at controlled room temperature in a dry place. Store sterile reconstituted solution below 30°C (86°F). Use within 24 hours.
Following reconstitution, store vial in upright position.
1,500 USP (TR) units of hyaluronidase
NDC 0008-0149-01, 10 mL vial, as single vials.
Not Recommended for IV Use.
Store at controlled room temperature in a dry place. Store sterile reconstituted solution below 30°C (86°F). Use within 14 days.
Following reconstitution, store vial in upright position.
Wydase® Stabilized Solution is supplied as follows:
150 USP (TR) units of hyaluronidase per mL
NDC 0008-0170-01, 1 mL vial, as single vials.
NDC 0008-0170-02, 10 mL vial, as single vials.
Not Recommended for IV Use.
Store in a refrigerator.
Do not use if solution is discolored or contains a precipitate.
For prescribing information write to Professional Service, Wyeth-Ayerst Laboratories, P.O. Box 8299, Philadelphia, PA 19101, or contact your local Wyeth-Ayerst representative.

WYGESIC® Ⓒ ℞

[*wi-je'zik*]
(propoxyphene HCl and acetaminophen)
Tablets

DESCRIPTION

Wygesic tablets contain 65 mg propoxyphene HCl and 650 mg acetaminophen. The inactive ingredients present are cellulose, D&C Yellow 10, FD&C Blue 1, FD&C Yellow 6, hydrogenated vegetable oil, hydroxypropyl methylcellulose, methylcellulose, polacrilin potassium, polyethylene glycol, and titanium dioxide.
Propoxyphene hydrochloride is an odorless white crystalline powder with a bitter taste. It is freely soluble in water. Chemically, it is [S-(R*,S*)]-α[2-(dimethylamino)-1-methylethyl]-α-phenylbenzeneethanol, propanoate (ester), hydrochloride, which can be represented by the following structural formula:

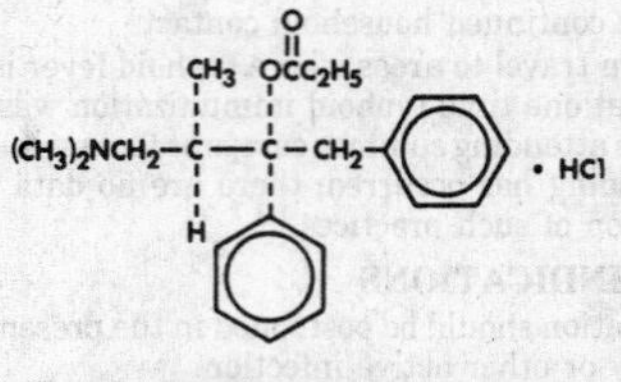

Acetaminophen is a white, crystalline powder, possessing a slightly bitter taste. It is soluble in boiling water and freely soluble in alcohol. Chemically, it is N-Acetyl-p-aminophenol, which can be presented by the following structural formula:

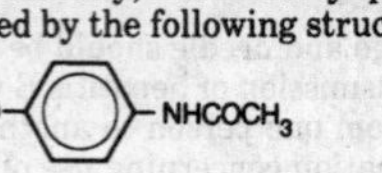

CLINICAL PHARMACOLOGY

Propoxyphene is a centrally acting narcotic analgesic agent. Equimolar doses of propoxyphene hydrochloride provide similar plasma concentrations. Following administration of 65, 130, or 195 mg of propoxyphene hydrochloride, the bioavailability of propoxyphene is equivalent to that of 100, 200, or 300 mg respectively of propoxyphene napsylate. Peak plasma concentrations of propoxyphene are reached in 2 to $2^1/_2$ hours. After a 65 mg oral dose of propoxyphene hydrochloride, peak plasma levels of 0.05 to 0.1 mcg/mL are achieved.
Repeated doses of propoxyphene at 6-hour intervals lead to increasing plasma concentrations, with a plateau after the ninth dose at 48 hours.
Propoxyphene is metabolized in the liver to yield norpropoxyphene. Propoxyphene has a half-life of 6 to 12 hours, whereas that of norpropoxyphene is 30 to 36 hours.
Norpropoxyphene has substantially less central nervous system depressant effect than propoxyphene, but a greater local anesthetic effect, which is similar to that of amitriptyline and antiarrhythmic agents, such as lidocaine and quinidine.
In animal studies in which propoxyphene and norpropoxyphene were continuously infused in large amounts, intracardiac conduction time (P-R and QRS intervals) was prolonged. Any intracardiac conduction delay attributable to high concentrations of norpropoxyphene may be of relatively long duration.
ACTIONS
Propoxyphene is a mild narcotic analgesic structurally related to methadone. The potency of propoxyphene hydrochloride is from two-thirds to equal that of codeine.
Propoxyphene hydrochloride and acetaminophen provide the analgesic activity of propoxyphene napsylate and the antipyretic-analgesic activity of acetaminophen.
The combination of propoxyphene and acetaminophen produces greater analgesia than that produced by either propoxyphene or acetaminophen alone.

INDICATIONS

Wygesic is indicated for the relief of mild-to-moderate pain, either when pain is present alone or when it is accompanied by fever.

CONTRAINDICATIONS

Hypersensitivity to propoxyphene or to acetaminophen.

WARNINGS

Do not prescribe propoxyphene for patients who are suicidal or addiction-prone.
Prescribe propoxyphene with caution for patients taking tranquilizers or antidepressant drugs and patients who use alcohol in excess.
Tell your patients not to exceed the recommended dose and to limit their intake of alcohol.
Propoxyphene products in excessive doses, either alone or in combination with other CNS depressants, including alcohol, are a major cause of drug-related deaths. Fatalities within the first hour of overdosage are not uncommon. In a survey of deaths due to overdosage conducted in 1975, in approximately 20% of the fatal cases, death occurred within the first hour (5% occurred within 15 minutes). Propoxyphene should not be taken in doses higher than those recommended by the physician. The judicious prescribing of propoxyphene is essential to the safe use of this drug. With patients who are depressed or suicidal, consideration should be given to the use of nonnarcotic analgesics. Patients should be cautioned about the concomitant use of propoxyphene products and alcohol because of potentially serious CNS-additive effects of these agents. Because of its added depressant effects, propoxyphene should be prescribed with caution for those patients whose medical condition requires the concomitant administration of sedatives, tranquilizers, muscle relaxants, antidepressants, or other CNS-depressant drugs. Patients should be advised of the additive depressant effects of these combinations.
Many of the propoxyphene-related deaths have occurred in patients with previous histories of emotional disturbances or suicidal ideation or attempts as well as histories of misuse of tranquilizers, alcohol, and other CNS-active drugs. Some deaths have occurred as a consequence of the accidental ingestion of excessive quantities of propoxyphene alone or in combination with other drugs. Patients taking propoxyphene should be warned not to exceed the dosage recommended by the physician.

DRUG DEPENDENCE:
Propoxyphene, when taken in higher-than-recommended doses over long periods of time, can produce drug dependence characterized by psychic dependence and, less frequently, physical dependence and tolerance. Propoxyphene will only partially suppress the withdrawal syndrome in individuals physically dependent on morphine or other narcotics. The abuse liability of propoxyphene is qualitatively similar to that of codeine although quantitatively less, and propoxyphene should be prescribed with the same degree of caution appropriate to the use of codeine.
USAGE IN AMBULATORY PATIENTS:
Propoxyphene may impair the mental and/or physical abilities required for the performance of potentially hazardous tasks, such as driving a car or operating machinery. The patient should be cautioned accordingly.

PRECAUTIONS

GENERAL:
Propoxyphene should be administered with caution to patients with hepatic or renal impairment since higher serum concentrations or delayed elimination may occur.
DRUG INTERACTIONS:
The CNS-depressant effect of propoxyphene is additive with that of other CNS depressants, including alcohol.
As is the case with many medicinal agents, propoxyphene may slow the metabolism of a concomitantly administered drug. Should this occur, the higher serum concentrations of that drug may result in increased pharmacologic or adverse effects of that drug. Such occurrences have been reported when propoxyphene was administered to patients on antidepressants, anticonvulsants, or warfarin-like drugs.
USAGE IN PREGNANCY:
Safe use in pregnancy has not been established relative to possible adverse effects on fetal development. Instances of withdrawal symptoms in the neonate have been reported following usage during pregnancy. Therefore, propoxyphene should not be used in pregnant women unless, in the judgment of the physician, the potential benefits outweigh the possible hazards.
USAGE IN NURSING MOTHERS:
Low levels of propoxyphene have been detected in human milk. In postpartum studies involving nursing mothers who were given propoxyphene, no adverse effects were noted in infants receiving mother's milk.
USAGE IN CHILDREN:
Propoxyphene is not recommended for use in children, because documented clinical experience has been insufficient to establish safety and a suitable dosage regimen in the pediatric age group.
A Patient Information Sheet is available for this product. See text following "How Supplied" section below.

ADVERSE REACTIONS

In a survey conducted in hospitalized patients, less than 1% of patients taking propoxyphene hydrochloride at recommended doses experienced side effects. The most frequently reported have been dizziness, sedation, nausea, and vomiting. Some of these adverse reactions may be alleviated if the patient lies down.
Other adverse reactions include constipation, abdominal pain, skin rashes, light-headedness, headache, weakness, euphoria, dysphoria, and minor visual disturbances.
Liver dysfunction has been reported in association with both active components of propoxyphene and acetaminophen tablets.

Propoxyphene therapy has been associated with abnormal liver-function tests and, more rarely, with instances of reversible jaundice.

Hepatic necrosis may result from acute overdoses of acetaminophen (see "Management of Overdosage"). In chronic ethanol abusers, this has been reported rarely with short-term use of acetaminophen doses of 2.5 to 10 g/day. Fatalities have occurred.

MANAGEMENT OF OVERDOSAGE

In all cases of suspected overdosage, call your regional Poison Control Center to obtain the most up-to-date information about the treatment of overdosage. This recommendation is made because, in general, information regarding the treatment of overdosage may change more rapidly than do package inserts.

Initial consideration should be given to the management of the CNS effects of propoxyphene overdosage. Resuscitative measures should be initiated promptly.

SYMPTOMS OF PROPOXYPHENE OVERDOSAGE:

The manifestations of acute overdosage with propoxyphene are those of narcotic overdosage. The patient is usually somnolent, but may be stuporous or comatose and convulsing. Respiratory depression is characteristic. The ventilatory rate and/or tidal volume is decreased, which results in cyanosis and hypoxia. Pupils, initially pinpoint, may become dilated as hypoxia increases. Cheyne-Stokes respiration and apnea may occur. Blood pressure and heart rate are usually normal initially, but blood pressure falls and cardiac performance deteriorates, which ultimately results in pulmonary edema and circulatory collapse unless the respiratory depression is corrected and adequate ventilation is restored promptly. Cardiac arrhythmias and conduction delay may be present. A combined respiratory-metabolic acidosis occurs, owing to retained CO_2 (hypercapnea) and to lactic acid formed during anaerobic glycolysis. Acidosis may be severe if large amounts of salicylates have also been ingested. Death may occur.

TREATMENT OF PROPOXYPHENE OVERDOSAGE:

Attention should be directed first to establishing a patent airway and to restoring ventilation. Mechanically assisted ventilation, with or without oxygen, may be required, and positive-pressure respiration may be desirable if pulmonary edema is present.

The narcotic antagonist naloxone hydrochloride will markedly reduce the degree of respiratory depression, and 0.4 to 2 mg should be administered promptly, preferably intravenously. If the desired degree of counteraction with improvement in respiratory function is not obtained, naloxone should be repeated at 2- to 3-minute intervals. The duration of action of the antagonist may be brief. If no response is observed after 10 mg of naloxone have been administered, the diagnosis of propoxyphene toxicity should be questioned. Naloxone hydrochloride may also be administered by continuous intravenous infusion.

TREATMENT OF PROPOXYPHENE OVERDOSAGE IN CHILDREN:

The usual initial dose of naloxone in children is 0.01 mg/kg body weight given intravenously. If this dose does not result in the desired degree of clinical improvement, a subsequent increased dose of 0.1 mg/kg body weight may be administered. If an IV route of administration is not available, naloxone may be administered IM or subcutaneously in divided doses. If necessary, naloxone can be diluted with sterile water for injection.

Blood gases, pH, and electrolytes should be monitored in order that acidosis and any electrolyte disturbance present may be corrected promptly. Acidosis, hypoxia, and generalized CNS depression predispose to the development of cardiac arrhythmias. Ventricular fibrillation or cardiac arrest may occur and necessitate the full complement of cardiopulmonary resuscitation (CPR) measures. Respiratory acidosis rapidly subsides as ventilation is restored and hypercapnea eliminated, but lactic acidosis may require intravenous bicarbonate for prompt correction.

Electrocardiographic monitoring is essential. Prompt correction of hypoxia, acidosis, and electrolyte disturbance (when present) will help prevent these cardiac complications and will increase the effectiveness of agents administered to restore normal cardiac function.

In addition to the use of a narcotic antagonist, the patient may require careful titration with an anticonvulsant to control convulsions. Analeptic drugs (for example, caffeine or amphetamine) should not be used because of their tendency to precipitate convulsions.

General supportive measures, in addition to oxygen, include, when necessary, intravenous fluids, vasopressor-inotropic compounds, and, when infection is likely, anti-infective agents. Gastric lavage may be useful, and activated charcoal can adsorb a significant amount of ingested propoxyphene. Dialysis is of little value in poisoning due to propoxyphene. Efforts should be made to determine whether other agents, such as alcohol, barbiturates, tranquilizers, or other CNS depressants, were also ingested, since these increase CNS depression as well as cause specific toxic effects.

SYMPTOMS OF ACETAMINOPHEN OVERDOSAGE:

Shortly after oral ingestion of an overdosage of acetaminophen and for the next 24 hours, anorexia, nausea, vomiting, and abdominal pain have been noted. The patient may then present no symptoms, but evidence of liver dysfunction may be apparent during the next 24 to 48 hours, with elevated serum transaminase and lactic dehydrogenase levels, an increase in serum bilirubin concentrations, and a prolonged prothrombin time. Death from hepatic failure may result 3 to 7 days after overdosage.

Acute renal failure may accompany the hepatic dysfunction and has been noted in patients who do not exhibit signs of fulminant hepatic failure. Typically, renal impairment is more apparent 6 to 9 days after ingestion of the overdose.

TREATMENT OF ACETAMINOPHEN OVERDOSAGE:

Acetaminophen in massive overdosage may cause hepatic toxicity in some patients. In all cases of suspected overdose, you may wish to call your regional poison center for assistance in diagnosis and for directions in the use of N-acetylcysteine as an antidote.

In adults, hepatic toxicity has rarely been reported with acute overdoses of less than 10 g and fatalities with less than 15 g. Importantly, young children seem to be more resistant than adults to the hepatotoxic effect of an acetaminophen overdose. Despite this, the measures outlined below should be initiated in any adult or child suspected of having ingested an acetaminophen overdose. Clinical and laboratory evidence of hepatic toxicity may not be apparent until 48 to 72 hours postingestion. Early symptoms following a potentially hepatotoxic overdose may include: nausea, vomiting, diaphoresis, and general malaise.

The stomach should be emptied promptly by lavage or by induction of emesis with syrup of ipecac. Patients' estimates of the quantity of a drug ingested are notoriously unreliable. Therefore, if an acetaminophen overdose is suspected, a serum acetaminophen assay should be obtained as early as possible, but no sooner than four hours following ingestion. Liver-function studies should be obtained initially and repeated at 24-hour intervals.

The antidote, N-acetylcysteine, should be administered as early as possible, preferably within 16 hours of the overdose ingestion for optimal results, but in any case, within 24 hours. Following recovery, there are no residual, structural or functional hepatic abnormalities.

ANIMAL TOXICOLOGY:

The acute lethal doses of the hydrochloride and napsylate salts of propoxyphene were determined in 4 species. The results shown in Figure 1 indicate that on a molar basis, the napsylate salt is less toxic than the hydrochloride. This may be due to the relative insolubility and retarded absorption of propoxyphene napsylate.

FIGURE 1
ACUTE ORAL TOXICITY OF PROPOXYPHENE
LD_{50} (mg/kg)=SE
LD_{50} (mMole/kg)

Species	Propoxyphene Hydrochloride	Propoxyphene Napsylate
Mouse	282 ± 39	915 ± 163
	0.75	1.62
Rat	230 ± 44	647 ± 95
	0.61	1.14
Rabbit	ca. 82	>183
	0.22	>0.32
Dog	ca. 100	>183
	0.27	>0.32

Some indication of the relative insolubility and retarded absorption of propoxyphene napsylate was obtained by measuring plasma propoxyphene levels in 2 groups of 4 dogs following oral administration of equimolar doses of the 2 salts. Although none of the animals in this experiment died, 3 of the 4 dogs given propoxyphene hydrochloride exhibited convulsive seizures during the time interval corresponding to the peak plasma levels. The 4 animals receiving the napsylate salt were ataxic but not acutely ill.

DOSAGE AND ADMINISTRATION

The product is given orally. The usual dose is 65 mg propoxyphene HCl and 650 mg acetaminophen every 4 hours as needed for pain. The maximum recommended dose of propoxyphene HCl is 390 mg per day.

Consideration should be given to a reduced total daily dosage in patients with hepatic or renal impairment.

HOW SUPPLIED

Wygesic® (propoxyphene HCl and acetaminophen) Tablets, 65 mg propoxyphene and 650 mg acetaminophen, are available as follows:

NDC 0008-0085, green, capsule-shaped, scored, film-coated tablet marked "WYETH" and "85", in bottles of 100 and 500 tablets, and in REDIPAK® cartons of 100 tablets (10 blister strips of 10).

Keep tightly closed.
Protect from light.
Store at controlled room temperature, 20°-25°C (68°-77°F).
Dispense in tight, light-resistant container as defined in the USP.

PATIENT INFORMATION

Summary

Products containing propoxyphene are used to relieve pain. LIMIT YOUR INTAKE OF ALCOHOL WHILE TAKING THIS DRUG. Make sure your doctor knows if you are taking tranquilizers, sleep aids, antidepressants, antihistamines, or any other drugs that make you sleepy. Combining propoxyphene with alcohol or these drugs in excessive doses is dangerous.

Use care while driving a car or using machines until you see how the drug affects you, because propoxyphene can make you sleepy. Do not take more of the drug than your doctor prescribed. Dependence has occurred when patients have taken propoxyphene for a long period of time at doses greater than recommended.

The rest of this leaflet gives you more information about propoxyphene. Please read it and keep it for further use.

Uses for Propoxyphene

Products containing propoxyphene are used for the relief of mild to moderate pain. Products which contain propoxyphene plus acetaminophen are prescribed for the relief of pain or pain associated with fever.

Before taking Propoxyphene

Make sure your doctor knows if you have ever had an allergic reaction to propoxyphene or acetaminophen.

The effect of propoxyphene in children under 12 has not been studied. Therefore, use of the drug in this age group is not recommended.

How to take Propoxyphene

Follow your doctor's directions exactly. Do not increase the amount you take without your doctor's approval. If you miss a dose of the drug, do not take twice as much the next time.

Pregnancy

Do not take propoxyphene during pregnancy unless your doctor knows you are pregnant and specifically recommends its use. Cases of temporary dependence in the newborn have occurred when the mother has taken propoxyphene consistently in the weeks before delivery. As a general principle, no drug should be taken during pregnancy unless it is clearly necessary.

General Caution

Heavy use of alcohol with propoxyphene is hazardous and may lead to overdosage symptoms (see "Overdosage" below); THEREFORE, LIMIT YOUR INTAKE OF ALCOHOL WHILE TAKING PROPOXYPHENE.

Combinations of excessive doses of propoxyphene, alcohol, and tranquilizers are dangerous. Make sure your doctor knows if you are taking tranquilizers, sleep aids, antidepressant drugs, antihistamines, or any other drugs that make you sleepy. The use of these drugs with propoxyphene increases their sedative effects and may lead to overdosage symptoms, including death (see "Overdosage" below).

Propoxyphene may cause drowsiness or impair your mental and/or physical abilities; therefore, use caution when driving a vehicle or operating dangerous machinery. DO NOT perform any hazardous task until you have seen your response to this drug.

Propoxyphene may increase the concentration in the body of medications such as anticoagulants ("blood thinners"), antidepressants, or drugs used for epilepsy. The result may be excessive or adverse effects of these medications. Make sure your doctor knows if you are taking any of these medications.

Dependence

You can become dependent on propoxyphene if you take it in higher than recommended doses over a long period of time. Dependence is a feeling of need for the drug and a feeling that you cannot perform normally without it.

Overdosage

An overdosage of propoxyphene, alone or in combination with other drugs, including alcohol, may cause weakness, difficulty in breathing, confusion, anxiety, and more severe drowsiness and dizziness. Extreme overdosage may lead to unconsciousness and death.

If the propoxyphene product contains acetaminophen, the overdosage symptoms include nausea, vomiting, lack of appetite, and abdominal pain. Liver damage may occur.

In any suspected overdosage situation, contact your doctor or nearest hospital emergency room. GET EMERGENCY HELP IMMEDIATELY. KEEP THIS AND ALL DRUGS OUT OF THE REACH OF CHILDREN.

Possible Side Effects

When propoxyphene is taken as directed, side effects are infrequent. Among those reported are drowsiness, dizziness, nausea, and vomiting. If these effects occur, it may help if you lie down and rest.

Less frequently reported side effects are constipation, abdominal pain, skin rashes, light-headedness, headache,

Continued on next page

Wyeth-Ayerst Laboratories—Cont.

weakness, minor visual disturbances, and feelings of elation or discomfort.

If side effects occur and concern you, contact your doctor.

Other Information

The safe and effective use of propoxyphene depends on your taking it exactly as directed. This drug has been prescribed specifically for you and your present condition. Do not give this drug to others who may have similar symptoms. Do not use it for any other reason.

If you would like more information about propoxyphene, ask your doctor or pharmacist. They have a more technical leaflet (professional labeling) you may read.

Shown in Product Identification Guide, page 341

WYMOX®
[wi'moks]
(amoxicillin)
Capsules and Oral Suspension

℞

DESCRIPTION

Wymox (amoxicillin) is a semisynthetic penicillin, an analog of ampicillin, with a broad spectrum of bactericidal activity against many gram-positive and gram-negative microorganisms. Chemically, it is D-(-)-a-amino-p-hydroxybenzyl penicillin trihydrate.

Wymox capsules contain amoxicillin as the trihydrate equivalent to 250 mg or 500 mg amoxicillin. The inactive ingredients present are colloidal silicon dioxide, D&C Yellow 10, FD&C Blue 1, gelatin, iron oxide, magnesium stearate, sodium lauryl sulfate, and titanium dioxide.

Wymox oral suspension is a powder which when reconstituted as directed yields a suspension of amoxicillin trihydrate equivalent to 125 mg or 250 mg amoxicillin per 5 mL. The inactive ingredients present are artificial flavors, carboxymethylcellulose sodium, cellulose, citric acid, D&C Red 28, FD&C Red 40, mannitol, sodium citrate, sucrose, and water.

HOW SUPPLIED

Wymox® (amoxicillin) Capsules contain amoxicillin as the trihydrate equivalent to 250 mg or 500 mg amoxicillin and are supplied as follows:

250 mg, NDC 0008-0559, grey and green capsule marked "WYETH" and "559", in bottles of 100 and 500 capsules.

500 mg, NDC 0008-0560, grey and green capsule marked "WYETH" and "560", in bottles of 50 and 500 capsules.

Store at room temperature, approximately 25°C (77°F).
Keep tightly closed.
Protect from light.
Dispense in light-resistant, tight container.

Wymox® (amoxicillin) Oral Suspension is available as a pink powder which when reconstituted as directed yields a palatable, pink suspension of amoxicillin trihydrate equivalent to 125 mg or 250 mg amoxicillin per 5 mL and is supplied as follows:

125 mg per 5 mL, NDC 0008-0557, in bottles to make 100 mL or 150 mL.

250 mg per 5 mL, NDC 0008-0558, in bottles to make 100 mL or 150 mL.

Store at room temperature, [approximately 25°C (77°F)] before reconstitution.
Keep tightly closed.
Shake well before using.
Store under refrigeration. Discard any unused portion after 14 days.

For prescribing information write to Professional Service, Wyeth-Ayerst Laboratories, P.O. Box 8299, Philadelphia, PA 19101, or contact your local Wyeth-Ayerst representative.

Shown in Product Identification Guide, page 341

WYTENSIN®
[wi-ten'sin]
(guanabenz acetate)

℞

DESCRIPTION

Wytensin (guanabenz acetate), an antihypertensive agent for oral administration, is an aminoguanidine derivative, 2,6-dichlorobenzylideneaminoguanidine acetate, and its structural formula is:

It is an odorless, white to off-white, crystalline substance, sparingly soluble in water and soluble in alcohol, with a mo-

lecular weight of 291.14. Each tablet of Wytensin is equivalent to 4 mg or 8 mg of free guanabenz base. The inactive ingredients present are cellulose, iron oxide, lactose, and magnesium stearate. The 8 mg dosage strength also contains FD&C Blue 2.

Wytensin is available as 4 mg or 8 mg tablets for oral administration.

HOW SUPPLIED

Wytensin® (guanabenz acetate) Tablets are available in the following dosage strengths:

4 mg, NDC 0008-0073, orange, five-sided tablet with a raised "W"and a "4"under the "W" on one side and "WYETH 73" on reverse side, in bottles of 100 and 500 tablets and in Redipak® cartons of 100 tablets (10 blister strips of 10).

8 mg, NDC 0008-0074, gray, five-sided tablet with a raised "W" and an "8" under the "W" on one side and "WYETH 74" on scored reverse side, in bottles of 100 tablets.

The appearance of these tablets is a trademark of Wyeth-Ayerst Laboratories.

Keep tightly closed.
Store at room temperature, approximately 25°C (77°F).
Protect from light.
Dispense in light-resistant, tight container.

EDUCATIONAL MATERIAL

Films—Slides—Videos

The Wyeth-Ayerst Audiovisual Catalog, listing films, audiovisual, and slide programs available through the Wyeth-Ayerst Film Library or on loan through the local Wyeth-Ayerst representative, can be obtained by writing Professional Service, Wyeth-Ayerst Laboratories, P.O. Box 8299, Philadelphia, PA 19101.

Zeneca Pharmaceuticals
A Business Unit of Zeneca Inc.
WILMINGTON, DE 19850-5437 USA

For Medical Information Contact:
Generally:
Yvonne Graham, Manager Professional Services
(302) 886-2231

After Hours and Weekend Emergencies:
(302) 886-3000

ARIMIDEX®
anastrozole
TABLETS

℞

DESCRIPTION

ARIMIDEX® (anastrozole) tablets for oral administration contain 1 mg of anastrozole, a non-steroidal aromatase inhibitor. It is chemically described as 1,3-Benzenediacetonitrile, α, α, α', α'-tetramethyl-5-(1H-1,2,4-triazol-1-ylmethyl). Its molecular formula is $C_{17}H_{19}N_5$ and its structural formula is:

Anastrozole is an off-white powder with a molecular weight of 293.4. Anastrozole has moderate aqueous solubility (0.5 mg/mL at 25°C); solubility is independent of pH in the physiological range. Anastrozole is freely soluble in methanol, acetone, ethanol, and tetrahydrofuran, and very soluble in acetonitrile.

Each tablet contains as inactive ingredients: lactose, magnesium stearate, hydroxypropylmethylcellulose, polyethylene glycol, povidone, sodium starch glycolate, and titanium dioxide.

CLINICAL PHARMACOLOGY
Mechanism of Action

Many breast cancers have estrogen receptors and growth of these tumors can be stimulated by estrogens. In post-menopausal women, the principal source of circulating estrogen (primarily estradiol) is conversion of adrenally-generated androstenedione to estrone by aromatase in peripheral tissues, such as adipose tissue, with further conversion of estrone to estradiol. Many breast cancers also contain aromatase; the importance of tumor-generated estrogens is uncertain.

Treatment of breast cancer has included efforts to decrease estrogen levels by ovariectomy premenopausally and by use of antiestrogens and progestational agents both pre- and post-menopausally, and these interventions lead to decreased tumor mass or delayed progression of tumor growth in some women.

Anastrozole is a potent and selective non-steroidal aromatase inhibitor. It significantly lowers serum estradiol concentrations and has no detectable effect on formation of adrenal corticosteroids or aldosterone.

Pharmacokinetics

Inhibition of aromatase activity is primarily due to anastrozole, the parent drug. Studies with radiolabeled drug have demonstrated that orally administered anastrozole is well absorbed into the systemic circulation with 83 to 85% of the radiolabel recovered in urine and feces. Food does not affect the extent of absorption. Elimination of anastrozole is primarily via hepatic metabolism (approximately 85%) and to a lesser extent, renal excretion (approximately 11%), and anastrozole has a mean terminal elimination half-life of approximately 50 hours in postmenopausal women. The major circulating metabolite of anastrozole, triazole, lacks pharmacologic activity. The pharmacokinetic parameters are similar in patients and in healthy postmenopausal volunteers. The pharmacokinetics of anastrozole are linear over the dose range of 1 to 20 mg and do not change with repeated dosing. Consistent with the approximately 2-day terminal elimination half-life, plasma concentrations approach steady-state levels at about 7 days of once daily dosing and steady-state levels are approximately three- to four-fold higher than levels observed after a single dose of ARIMIDEX. Anastrozole is 40% bound to plasma proteins in the therapeutic range.

Metabolism and Excretion: Studies of postmenopausal women demonstrated that anastrozole is extensively metabolized with about 10% of the dose excreted in the urine as unchanged drug within 72 hours of dosing, and the remainder (about 60% of the dose) excreted in the urine as metabolites. Metabolism of anastrozole occurs by N-dealkylation, hydroxylation and glucuronidation. Three metabolites of anastrozole have been identified in human plasma and urine. The known metabolites are triazole, a glucuronide conjugate of hydroxy-anastrozole, and a glucuronide of anastrozole itself. Several minor (less than 5% of the radioactive dose) metabolites have not been identified.

Because renal elimination is not a significant pathway of elimination, total body clearance of anastrozole is unchanged even in severe (creatinine clearance less than 30 mL/min/1.73m²) renal impairment; dosing adjustment in patients with renal dysfunction is not necessary (see Special Populations and DOSAGE AND ADMINISTRATION sections). Dosage adjustment is also unnecessary in patients with stable hepatic cirrhosis (see Special Populations and DOSAGE AND ADMINISTRATION sections).

Special Populations

Geriatric: Anastrozole pharmacokinetics have been investigated in postmenopausal female volunteers and patients with breast cancer. No age related effects were seen over the range <50 to >80 years.

Race: Anastrozole pharmacokinetic differences due to race have not been studied.

Renal Insufficiency: Anastrozole pharmacokinetics have been investigated in subjects with renal insufficiency. Anastrozole renal clearance decreased proportionally with creatinine clearance and was approximately 50% lower in volunteers with severe renal impairment (creatinine clearance less than 30 mL/min/1.73m²) compared to controls. Since only about 10% of anastrozole is excreted unchanged in the urine, the reduction in renal clearance did not influence the total body clearance (see DOSAGE AND ADMINISTRATION).

Hepatic Insufficiency: Hepatic metabolism accounts for approximately 85% of anastrozole elimination. Anastrozole pharmacokinetics have been investigated in subjects with hepatic cirrhosis related to alcohol abuse. The apparent oral clearance (CL/F) of anastrozole was approximately 30% lower in subjects with stable hepatic cirrhosis than in control subjects with normal liver function. However, plasma anastrozole concentrations in the subjects with hepatic cirrhosis were within the range of concentrations seen in normal subjects across all clinical trials (see DOSAGE AND ADMINISTRATION), so that no dosage adjustment is needed.

Drug-Drug Interactions: Anastrozole inhibited reactions catalyzed by cytochrome P450 1A2, 2C8/9, and 3A4 in vitro with Ki values which were approximately 30 times higher than the mean steady-state C_{max} values observed following a 1-mg daily dose. Anastrozole had no inhibitory effect on reactions catalyzed by cytochrome P450 2A6 or 2D6 in vitro. Administration of a single 30 mg/kg or multiple 10 mg/kg doses of anastrozole to subjects had no effect on the clearance of antipyrine or urinary recovery of antipyrine metabolites. Based on these in vitro and in vivo results, it is unlikely that co-administration of ARIMIDEX 1 mg with other drugs will result in clinically significant inhibition of cytochrome P450 mediated metabolism.

Pharmacodynamics

Effect on Estradiol: Mean serum concentrations of estradiol were evaluated in multiple daily dosing trials with 0.5, 1, 3, 5, and 10 mg if ARIMIDEX in postmenopausal women with advanced breast cancer. Clinically significant suppression of serum estradiol was seen with all doses. Doses of 1 mg and higher resulted in suppression of mean serum concentrations of estradiol to the lower limit of detection (3.7 pmol/L). The recommended daily dose, ARIMIDEX 1 mg, reduced estradiol by approximately 70% within 24 hours and by approximately 80% after 14 days of daily dosing. Suppression of serum estradiol was maintained for up to 6 days after cessation of daily dosing with ARIMIDEX 1 mg.

Effect on Corticosteroids: In multiple daily dosing trials with 3, 5, and 10 mg, the selectivity of anastrozole was assessed by examining the effects on corticosteroid synthesis. For all doses, anastrozole did not effect cortisol or aldosterone secretion at baseline or in response to ACTH. No glucocorticoid or mineralocorticoid replacement therapy is necessary with anastrozole.

Other Endocrine Effects: In multiple daily dosing trials with 5 and 10 mg, thyroid stimulation hormone (TSH) was measured; there was no increase in TSH during the administration of ARIMIDEX. ARIMIDEX does not possess direct progestogenic, androgenic, or estrogenic activity in animals, but does perturb the circulating levels of progesterone, androgens, and estrogens.

Clinical Studies

Anastrozole was studied in two well-controlled clinical trials (0004, a North American study; 0005, a predominately European study) in postmenopausal women with advanced breast cancer who had disease progression following tamoxifen therapy for either advanced or early breast cancer. Some of the patients had also received previous cytotoxic treatment. Most patients were ER-positive; a smaller fraction were ER-unknown or ER-negative (the ER-negative patients were eligible only if they had had a positive response to tamoxifen). Eligible patients with measurable and non-measurable disease were randomized to receive either a single daily dose of 1 mg or 10 mg of ARIMIDEX or megestrol acetate 40 mg four times a day. The studies were double-blinded with respect to ARIMIDEX. Time to progression and objective response (only patients with measurable disease could be considered partial responders) rates were the primary efficacy variables. Objective response rates were calculated based on the Union Internationale Contre le Cancer (UICC) criteria. The rate of prolonged (more than 24 weeks) stable disease, the rate of progression, and survival were also calculated.

Both trials included over 375 patients; demographics and other baseline characteristics were similar for the three treatment groups in each trial. Patients in the 0005 trial had responded better to prior tamoxifen treatment. Of the patients entered who had prior tamoxifen therapy for advanced disease (58% in Trial 0004; 57% in Trial 0005), 18% of these patients in Trial 0004 and 42% in Trial 0005 were reported by the primary investigator to have responded. In Trial 0004, 81% of patients were ER-positive, 13% were ER-unknown, and 6% were ER-negative. In Trial 0005, 58% of patients were ER-positive, 37% were ER-unknown, and 5% were ER-negative. In Trial 0004, 60% of patients had measurable disease compared to 80% in Trial 0005. The sites of metastatic disease were similar among treatment groups for each trial. On average, 40% of the patients had soft tissue metastases, 60% had bone metastases, and 40% had visceral (15% liver) metastases.

As shown in the table below, similar results were observed among treatment groups and between the two trials. None of the within-trial differences were statistically significant.

	ARIMIDEX 1 mg	ARIMIDEX 10 mg	Megestrol Acetate 160 mg
Trial 0004 (N. America)	(n=128)	(n=130)	(n=128)
Median Follow-up (days)	179	182	176
Time to Progression (days)	170	143	151
Objective Response (all patients) (%)	10.2	5.4	5.5
Stable Disease for >24 weeks (%)	26.6	23.8	29.7
Progression (%)	48.4	50.0	51.6
Trial 0005 (Europe, Australia, S.Africa)	(n=135)	(n=118)	(n=125)
Median Follow-up (days)	192	185	182
Time to Progression (days)	132	156	120
Objective Response (all patients) (%)	10.4	12.7	10.4
Stable Disease for >24 weeks (%)	23.7	21.2	22.4
Progression (%)	58.5	50.8	56.0

Approximately ⅓ of the patients in each treatment group in both studies had either an objective response or stabilization of their disease for greater than 24 weeks. Among the 263 patients who received ARIMIDEX 1 mg, there were 6 complete responders and 21 partial responders. In patients who had an objective response, over 60% of the patients responded for greater than 6 months and over 15% responded for greater than 12 months.

To compare the three treatments, hazard ratios for time to progression (ratio of the likelihood of progression for two treatments over the period of study) and odds ratios for response rates, together with their confidence intervals, were calculated for the pooled studies. These show that, in general, the three treatments were similar in efficacy, but that confidence intervals were fairly wide. There is, in these data, no indication that ARIMIDEX 10 mg is superior to ARIMIDEX 1 mg. For time to progression for the ARIMIDEX 1 mg comparison to megestrol acetate, the hazard ratio (ARIMIDEX/megestrol acetate) was 0.97 [0.75, 1.24] ($p=0.76$); for ARIMIDEX 10 mg compared to megestrol acetate, the hazard ratio was 0.92 [0.71, 1.19] ($p=0.47$). The odds ratio and confidence intervals of the comparison between each dose of ARIMIDEX and megestrol acetate for objective response rate demonstrate that both ARIMIDEX 1 mg and ARIMIDEX 10 mg were similar in efficacy to the comparator. For the ARIMIDEX 1 mg comparison to megestrol acetate, the odds ratio (ARIMIDEX/megestrol acetate) was 1.32 [0.66, 2.65] ($p=0.37$); for the ARIMIDEX 10 mg comparison to megestrol acetate, the odds ratio was 1.15 [0.55, 2.36] ($p=0.68$). There were too few deaths occurring across treatment groups of both trials to draw conclusions on overall survival differences.

There were no differences in response seen between women over or under 65. There were too few non-white patients studied to draw conclusions about racial differences in response rates.

INDICATIONS AND USAGE

ARIMIDEX is indicated for the treatment of advanced breast cancer in postmenopausal women with disease progression following tamoxifen therapy.

Patients with ER-negative disease and patients who did not respond to previous tamoxifen therapy rarely responded to ARIMIDEX.

CONTRAINDICATIONS

None known.

WARNINGS

ARIMIDEX can cause fetal harm when administered to a pregnant woman. Anastrozole has been found to cross the placenta following oral administration of 0.1 mg/kg in rats and rabbits (about ¾ and 1.5 times the recommended human dose, respectively, on a mg/m^2 basis. Studies in both rats and rabbits at doses equal to or greater than 0.1 and 0.02 mg/kg/day, respectively (about ¾ and ⅓, respectively, the recommended human dose on a mg/m^2 basis), administration during the period of organogenesis showed that anastrozole increased pregnancy loss (increased pre- and/or post-implantation loss, increased resorption, and decreased numbers of live fetuses); effects were dose-related in rats. Placental weights were significantly increased in rats at doses of 0.1 mg/kg/day or more.

Evidence of fetotoxicity, including delayed fetal development (i.e., incomplete ossification and depressed fetal body weights), was observed in rats administered doses of 1 mg/kg/day (which produced plasma anastrozole C_{ssmax} and $AUC_{0-24\ hr}$ that were 19 times and 9 times higher than the respective values found in healthy post-menopausal humans at the recommended dose). There was no evidence of teratogenicity in rats administered doses up to 1.0 mg/kg/day. In rabbits, anastrozole caused pregnancy failure at doses equal to or greater than 1.0 mg/kg/day (about 16 times the recommended human dose on a mg/m^2 basis); there was no evidence of teratogenicity in rabbits administered 0.2 mg/kg/day (about 3 times the recommended human dose on a mg/m^2 basis).

There are no adequate and well-controlled studies in pregnant women using ARIMIDEX. If ARIMIDEX is used during pregnancy or if the patient becomes pregnant while receiving this drug, the patient should be apprised of the potential hazard to the fetus or potential risk for loss of the pregnancy.

PRECAUTIONS

General: Before starting treatment with ARIMIDEX, pregnancy must be excluded (see WARNINGS).

ARIMIDEX should be administered under the supervision of a qualified physician experienced in the use of anticancer agents.

Laboratory Tests: Three-fold elevations of mean serum gamma glutamyl transferase (GT) levels have been observed among patients with liver metastases receiving ARIMIDEX or megestrol acetate. These changes were likely related to the progression of liver metastases in these patients, although other contributing factors could not be ruled out.

Drug Interactions: (See CLINICAL PHARMACOLOGY)

Anastrozole inhibited *in vitro* metabolic reactions catalyzed by cytochromes P450 1A2, 2C8/9, and 3A4 but only at relatively high concentrations. Anastrozole did not inhibit P450 2A6 or the polymorphic P450 2D6 in human liver microsomes. Anastrozole did not alter the pharmacokinetics of antipyrine. Although there have been no formal interaction studies other than with antipyrine, based on these *in vivo* and *in vitro* studies, it is unlikely that co-administration of a 1-mg dose of ARIMIDEX with other drugs will result in clinically significant drug inhibition of cytochrome P450-mediated metabolism of the other drugs.

Drug/Laboratory Test Interactions: No clinically significant changes in the results of clinical laboratory tests have been observed.

Carcinogenesis: No long-term animal studies have been conducted to assess the carcinogenic potential of ARIMIDEX.

Mutagenesis: ARIMIDEX has not been shown to be mutagenic in *in vitro* tests (Ames and E. coli bacterial tests, CHO-K1 gene mutation assay) or clastogenic either *in vitro* (chromosome aberrations in human lymphocytes) or *in vivo* (micronucleus test in rats).

Impairment of Fertility: Studies to investigate the effect of ARIMIDEX on fertility have not been conducted; however, chronic studies indicated hypertrophy of the ovaries and the presence of follicular cysts in rats administered doses equal to or greater than 1 mg/kg/day (which produced plasma anastrozole C_{ssmax} and $AUC_{0-24\ hr}$ than were 19 and 9 times higher than the respective values found in healthy post-menopausal humans at the recommended dose). In addition, hyperplastic uteri were observed in chronic studies of female dogs administered doses equal to or greater than 1 mg/kg/day (which produced plasma anastrozole C_{ssmax} and $AUC_{0-24\ hr}$ that were 22 times and 16 times higher than the respective values found in post-menopausal humans at the recommended dose). It is not known whether these effects on the reproductive organs of animals are associated with impaired fertility in humans.

Pregnancy: Pregnancy Category D: (See WARNINGS).

Nursing Mothers: It is not known if anastrozole is excreted in human milk. Because many drugs are excreted in human milk, caution should be exercised when ARIMIDEX is administered to a nursing woman (see WARNINGS and PRECAUTIONS).

Pediatric Use: The safety and efficacy of ARIMIDEX in pediatric patients have not been established.

Geriatric Use: Fifty percent of patients in studies 0004 and 0005 were 65 or older. Response rates and time to progression were similar for the over 65 and younger patients.

ADVERSE REACTIONS

ARIMIDEX was generally well tolerated in two well-controlled clinical trials (i.e., Trials 0004 and 0005), with less than 3.3% of the ARIMIDEX-treated patients and 4.0% of the megestrol acetate-treated patients withdrawing due to an adverse event.

The principal adverse event more common with ARIMIDEX than megestrol acetate was diarrhea. Adverse events reported in greater than 5% of the patients in any of the treatment groups in these two well-controlled clinical trials, regardless of causality, are presented below:

Number (n) and Percentage of Patients with Adverse Event †

Adverse Event	ARIMIDEX 1 mg (n=262) n	%	ARIMIDEX 10 mg (n=246) n	%	Megestrol Acetate 160 mg (n=253) n	%
Asthenia	42	(16.0)	33	(13.4)	47	(18.6)
Nausea	41	(15.6)	48	(19.5)	28	(11.1)
Headache	34	(13.0)	44	(17.9)	24	(9.5)
Hot Flushes	32	(12.2)	29	(10.6)	21	(8.3)
Pain	28	(10.7)	38	(15.4)	29	(11.5)
Back Pain	28	(10.7)	26	(10.6)	19	(7.5)
Dyspnea	24	(9.2)	27	(11.0)	53	(20.9)
Vomiting	24	(9.2)	26	(10.6)	16	(6.3)
Cough Increased	22	(8.4)	18	(7.3)	19	(7.5)
Diarrhea	22	(8.4)	18	(7.3)	7	(2.8)
Constipation	18	(6.9)	18	(7.3)	21	(8.3)
Abdominal Pain	18	(6.9)	14	(5.7)	18	(7.1)
Anorexia	18	(6.9)	19	(7.7)	11	(4.3)
Bone Pain	17	(6.5)	26	(11.8)	19	(7.5)
Pharyngitis	16	(6.1)	23	(9.3)	15	(5.9)
Dizziness	16	(6.1)	12	(4.9)	15	(5.9)
Rash	15	(5.7)	15	(6.1)	19	(7.5)
Dry Mouth	15	(5.7)	11	(4.5)	13	(5.1)

Continued on next page

Zeneca Pharmaceuticals—Cont.

Peripheral						
Edema	14	(5.3)	21	(8.5)	28	(11.1)
Pelvic Pain	14	(5.3)	17	(6.9)	13	(5.1)
Depression	14	(5.3)	6	(2.4)	5	(2.0)
Chest Pain	13	(5.0)	18	(7.3)	13	(5.1)
Paresthesia	12	(4.6)	15	(6.1)	9	(3.6)
Vaginal						
Hemorrhage	6	(2.3)	4	(1.6)	13	(5.1)
Weight Gain	4	(1.5)	9	(3.7)	30	(11.9)
Sweating	4	(1.5)	3	(1.2)	16	(6.3)
Increased						
Appetite	0	(0)	1	(0.4)	13	(5.1)

† A patient may have more than one adverse event.

Other less frequent (2% to 5%) adverse experiences reported in patients receiving ARIMIDEX 1 mg in either Trial 0004 or Trial 0005 are listed below. These adverse experiences are listed by body system and are in order of decreasing frequency within each body system regardless of assessed causality.

Body as a Whole: Flu syndrome; fever; neck pain; malaise; accidental injury; infection
Cardiovascular: Hypertension; thrombophlebitis
Hepatic: Gamma GT increased; SGOT increased; SGPT increased
Hematologic: Anemia; leukopenia
Metabolic and Nutritional: Alkaline phosphatase increased; weight loss
Mean serum total cholesterol levels increased by 0.5 mmol/L among patients receiving ARIMIDEX. Increases in LDL cholesterol have been shown to contribute to these changes.
Musculoskeletal: Myalgia; arthralgia; pathological fracture
Nervous: Somnolence; confusion; insomnia; anxiety; nervousness
Respiratory: Sinusitis; bronchitis; rhinitis
Skin and Appendages: Hair thinning; pruritus
Urogenital: Urinary tract infection; breast pain
The incidences of the following adverse event groups, potentially causally related to one or both of the therapies because of their pharmacology, were statistically analyzed: weight gain, edema, thromboembolic disease, gastrointestinal disturbance, hot flushes, and vaginal dryness. These six groups, and the adverse events captured in the groups, were prospectively defined. The results are shown in the table below.

Number (n) and Percentage of Patients

	ARIMIDEX 1 mg (n=262)		ARIMIDEX 10 mg (n=246)		Megestrol Acetate 160 mg (n=253)	
Adverse Event Group	n	%	n	%	n	%
Gastrointestinal Disturbance	77	(29.4)	81	(32.9)	54	(21.3)
Hot Flushes	33	(12.6)	29	(11.8)	35	(13.8)
Edema	19	(7.3)	28	(11.4)	35	(13.8)
Thomboembolic Disease	9	(3.4)	4	(1.6)	12	(4.7)
Vaginal Dryness	5	(1.9)	3	(1.2)	2	(0.8)
Weight Gain	4	(1.5)	10	(4.1)	30	(11.9)

More patients treated with megestrol acetate reported weight gain as an adverse event compared to patients treated with ARIMIDEX 1 mg ($p<0.0001$). Other differences were not statistically significant.
An examination of the magnitude of change in weight in all patients was also conducted. Thirty-four percent (87/253) of the patients treated with megestrol acetate experienced weight gain of 5% or more and 11% (27/253) of the patients treated with megestrol acetate experienced weight gain of 10% or more. Among patients treated with ARIMIDEX 1 mg, 13 % (33/262) experienced weight gain of 5% or more and 3% (6/262) experienced weight gain of 10% or more. On average, this 5 to 10% weight gain represented between 6 and 12 pounds.
No patients receiving ARIMIDEX or megestrol acetate discontinued treatment due to drug-related weight gain.

OVERDOSAGE

Clinical trials have been conducted with ARIMIDEX, up to 60 mg in a single dose given to healthy male volunteers and up to 10 mg daily given to postmenopausal women with advanced breast cancer; these dosages were well tolerated. A single dose of ARIMIDEX that results in life-threatening symptoms has not been established. In rats, lethality was observed after single oral doses that were greater than 100 mg/kg (about 800 times the recommended human dose on a mg/m^2 basis) and was associated with severe irritation to the stomach (necrosis, gastritis, ulceration, and hemorrhage). There is no specific antidote to overdosage and treatment must be symptomatic. In the management of an overdose, consider that multiple agents may have been taken. Vomiting may be induced if the patient is alert. Dialysis may be helpful because ARIMIDEX is not highly protein bound. General supportive care, including frequent monitoring of vital signs and close observation of the patient, is indicated.

DOSAGE AND ADMINISTRATION

The dose of ARIMIDEX is one 1-mg tablet taken once a day. Patients treated with ARIMIDEX do not require glucocorticoid or mineralocorticoid replacement therapy.
Patients with Hepatic Impairment: (See CLINICAL PHARMACOLOGY) Hepatic metabolism accounts for approximately 85% of anastrozole elimination. Although clearance of anastrozole was decreased in patients with cirrhosis due to alcohol abuse, plasma anastrozole concentrations stayed in the usual range seen in patients without liver disease. Therefore, no changes in dose are recommended for patients with mild-to-moderate hepatic impairment, although patients should be monitored for side effects. ARIMIDEX has not been studied in patients with severe hepatic impairment.
Patients with Renal Impairment: No changes in dose are necessary for patients with renal impairment.

HOW SUPPLIED

White, biconvex, film-coated tablets containing 1 mg of anastrozole. The tablets are impressed on one side with a logo consisting of a letter "A" (upper case) with an arrowhead attached to the foot of the extended right leg of the "A" and on the reverse with the tablet strength marking "Adx 1". These tablets are supplied in bottles of 30 tablets (NDC 0310-0201-30)
Store at controlled room temperature, 20°–25°C (68°–77°F) [see USP].
ZENECA Pharmaceuticals
A Business Unit of Zeneca Inc.
Wilmington, Delaware 19850-5437
64076-01 Rev C 01/96
Shown in Product Identification Guide, page 341

CASODEX® ℞
bicalutamide tablets

DESCRIPTION

CASODEX® (bicalutamide) Tablets for oral administration contain 50 mg of bicalutamide, a non-steroidal antiandrogen with no other known endocrine activity. The chemical name is propanamide, N-[4-cyano-3-(trifluoromethyl)phenyl]-3-[(4-fluorophenyl)sulfonyl]-2-hydroxy-2-methyl-,(+−). The structural and empirical formulas are:

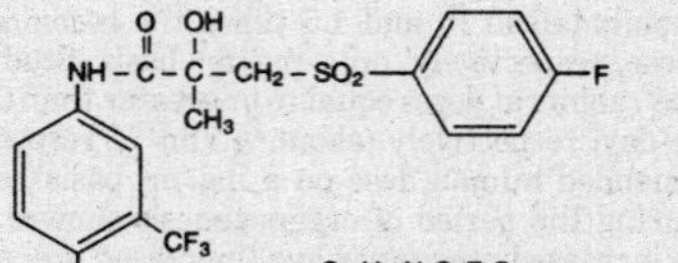

$C_{18}H_{14}N_2O_4F_4S$

Bicalutamide has a molecular weight of 430.37. The pKa' is approximately 12. Bicalutamide is a fine white to off-white powder which is practically insoluble in water at 37°C (5 mg per 1000 mL), slightly soluble in chloroform and absolute ethanol, sparingly soluble in methanol, and soluble in acetone and tetrahydrofuran.
CASODEX is a racemate with its antiandrogenic activity being almost exclusively exhibited by the R-enantiomer of bicalutamide; the S-enantiomer is essentially inactive.
The inactive ingredients of CASODEX Tablets are lactose, magnesium stearate, methylhydroxypropylcellulose, polyethylene glycol, polyvidone, sodium starch glycollate, and titanium dioxide.

CLINICAL PHARMACOLOGY

Mechanism of Action: CASODEX is a non-steroidal antiandrogen. It competitively inhibits the action of androgens by binding to cytosol androgen receptors in the target tissue. Prostatic carcinoma is known to be androgen sensitive and responds to treatment that counteracts the effect of androgen and/or removes the source of androgen.
In clinical trials with CASODEX as a single agent for prostate cancer, rises in serum testosterone and estradiol have been noted. When CASODEX is combined with luteinizing hormone-releasing hormone (LHRH) analogue therapy, CASODEX does not affect the suppression of serum testosterone induced by the LHRH analogue.
Pharmacokinetics
Absorption: Bicalutamide is well-absorbed following oral administration, although the absolute bioavailability is unknown. Co-administration of bicalutamide with food has no clinically significant effect on rate or extent of absorption.
Distribution: Bicalutamide is highly protein-bound (96%). See Drug-Drug Interactions below.
Metabolism/Elimination: Bicalutamide undergoes stereospecific metabolism. The S (inactive) isomer is metabolized primarily by glucuronidation. The R (active) isomer also undergoes glucuronidation but is predominantly oxidized to an inactive metabolite followed by glucuronidation. Both the parent and metabolite glucuronides are eliminated in the urine and feces. The S-enantiomer is rapidly cleared relative to the R-enantiomer, with the R-enantiomer accounting for about 99% of total steady-state plasma levels.
Special Populations
Geriatric: In two studies in patients given 50 or 150 mg daily, no significant relationship between age and steady-state levels of total bicalutamide or the acitve R-enantiomer has been shown.
Hepatic Insufficiency: No clinically significant difference in the pharmacokinetics of either enantiomer of bicalutamide was noted in patients with mild-to-moderate hepatic disease as compared to healthy controls. Patients with severe liver disease have significantly longer half-life values for the R-enantiomer.
Renal Insufficiency: Renal impairment (as measured by creatinine clearance) had no significant effect on the elimination of total bicalutamide or the active R-enantiomer.
Women, Pediatrics: Because of the mechanism of action and the indication, bicalutamide has not been studied in women or pediatric subjects.
Drug-Drug Interactions: Clinical studies have not shown any drug interactions between bicalutamide and LHRH analogues (goserelin or leuprolide). There is no evidence that bicalutamide induces hepatic enzymes. *In vitro* protein-binding studies have shown that bicalutamide can displace coumarin anticoagulants from binding sites. Prothrombin times should be closely monitored in patients already receiving coumarin anticoagulants who are started on CASODEX.
Pharmacokinetics of the active enantiomer of CASODEX in normal males and patients with prostate cancer are presented in Table 1

Table 1

Parameter	Mean	CV%	95% Confidence Interval
Normal Males (n=30)			
Apparent Oral Clearance (L/hr)	0.320	32.1	0.281–0.358
Single Dose Peak Concentration (μg/mL)	0.768	23.2	0.702–0.835
Single Dose Time to Peak Concentration (hours)	31.3	46.5	25.9–36.7
Half-Life (days)	5.8	39.5	4.9–6.7
Patients with Prostate Cancer (n=40)			
C_{SS} (μg/mL)	8.939	39.2	7.817–10.06

CV = Coefficient of Variation
C_{SS} = Mean Steady-State Concentration

Clinical Studies
In a large multicenter, double-blind, controlled clinical trial, 813 patients with previously untreated advanced prostate cancer were randomized to receive CASODEX 50 mg once daily (404 patients) or flutamide 250 mg (409 patients) three times a day, each in combination with LHRH analogues (either goserelin acetate implant or leuprolide acetate depot). At a median follow-up of 95 weeks, time to treatment failure with CASODEX-LHRH analogue therapy was not dissimilar when compared to flutamide-LHRH analogue therapy.
At the same timepoint, 130 (32%) patients treated with CASODEX-LHRH analogue therapy and 145 (35%) patients treated with flutamide-LHRH analogue therapy had died.
Quality of life was assessed with self-administered patient questionnaires on pain, social functioning, emotional wellbeing, vitality, activity limitation, bed disability, overall health, physical capacity, general symptoms, and treatment related symptoms. Assessment of the Quality of Life questionnaires did not indicate consistent significant differences between the two treatment groups.

INDICATIONS AND USAGE

CASODEX is indicated for use in combination therapy with a luteinizing hormone-releasing hormone (LHRH) analogue for the treatment of advanced prostate cancer.

CONTRAINDICATIONS

CASODEX is contraindicated in any patient who has shown a hypersensitivity reaction to the drug or any of the tablet's components.
CASODEX may cause fetal harm when administered to pregnant women. The male offspring of rats receiving doses of 10 mg/kg/day (plasma drug concentrations in rats equal to approximately ⅔ human therapeutic concentrations*)

and above were observed to have reduced anogenital distance and hypospadias in reproductive toxicology studies. These pharmacological effects have been observed with other antiandrogens. No other teratogenic effects were observed in rabbits receiving doses up to 200 mg/kg/day (approximately 1/3 human therapeutic concentrations*) or rats receiving doses up to 250 mg/kg/day (approximately 2 times human therapeutic concentrations*). CASODEX is contraindicated in women who are, or may become pregnant. If this drug is used during pregnancy, or if the patient becomes pregnant while taking this drug, the patient should be apprised of the potential hazard to the fetus.

WARNINGS

In clinical trials with CASODEX as a single agent for prostate cancer, gynecomastia and breast pain have been reported in up to 38% and 39% of patients, respectively.

PRECAUTIONS

CASODEX should be used with caution in patients with moderate-to-severe hepatic impairment. CASODEX is extensively metabolized by the liver. Limited data in subjects with severe hepatic impairment suggest that excretion of CASODEX may be delayed and could lead to further accumulation. Periodic liver function tests should be considered for patients on long-term therapy.

Information for Patients: Patients should be informed that therapy with CASODEX and the LHRH analogue should be initiated concomitantly, and that they should not interrupt or stop taking these medications without consulting their physician. Treatment with CASODEX should be started at the same time as treatment with an LHRH analogue.

Laboratory Tests: Regular assessments of serum Prostate Specific Antigen (PSA) may be helpful in monitoring the patient's response. If PSA levels rise during CASODEX therapy, the patient should be evaluated for clinical progression. For patients who have objective progression of disease together with an elevated PSA, a treatment-free period of antiandrogen, while continuing the LHRH analogue, may be considered.

Since transaminase abnormalities and, rarely, jaundice have been reported with the use of CASODEX, periodic liver function tests should be considered. If clinically indicated, eg, when the patient has jaundice or laboratory evidence of liver injury in the absence of liver metastases, CASODEX therapy should be discontinued. If transaminases increase over 2 times the upper limit of normal, treatment should be discontinued. Abnormalities are usually reversible upon discontinuation.

Drug Interactions: *In vitro* studies have shown CASODEX can displace coumarin anticoagulants, such as warfarin, from their protein-binding sites. It is recommended that if CASODEX is started in patients already receiving coumarin anticoagulants, prothrombin times should be closely monitored and adjustment of the anticoagulant dose may be necessary (see CLINICAL PHARMACOLOGY, Drug-Drug Interactions).

Carcinogenesis, Mutagenesis, Impairment of Fertility: Two-year oral carcinogenicity studies were conducted in both male and female rats and mice at doses of 5, 15 or 75 mg/kg/day of bicalutamide. A variety of tumor target organ effects were identified and were attributed to the antiandrogenicity of bicalutamide, namely, testicular benign interstitial (Leydig) cell tumors in male rats at all dose levels (the steady-state plasma concentration with the 5 mg/kg/day dose is approximately 2/3 human therapeutic concentrations*) and uterine adenocarcinoma in female rats at 75 mg/kg/day (approximately 1 1/2 times the human therapeutic concentrations*). There is no evidence of Leydig cell hyperplasia in patients; uterine tumors are not relevant to the indicated patient population.

A small increase in the incidence of hepatocellular carcinoma in male mice given 75 mg/kg/day of bicalutamide (approximately 4 times human therapeutic concentrations*) and an increased incidence of benign thyroid follicular cell adenomas in rats given 5 mg/kg/day (approximately 2/3 human therapeutic concentrations*) and above were recorded. These neoplastic changes were progressions of non-neoplastic changes related to hepatic enzyme induction observed in animal toxicity studies. Enzyme induction has not been observed following bicalutamide administration in man. There were no tumorigenic effects suggestive of genotoxic carcinogenesis.

A comprehensive battery of both *in vitro* and *in vivo* genotoxicity tests (yeast gene conversion, Ames, *E. coli*, CHO/HGPRT, human lymphocyte cytogenetic, mouse micronucleus, and rat bone marrow cytogenetic tests) has demonstrated that CASODEX does not have genotoxic activity.

Administration of CASODEX may lead to inhibition of spermatogenesis. The long-term effects of CASODEX on male fertility have not been studied.

In male rats dosed at 250 mg/kg/day (approximately 2 times human therapeutic concentrations*), the precoital interval and time to successful mating were increased in the first pairing but no effects on fertility following successful mating were seen. These effects were reversed by 7 weeks after the end of an 11-week period of dosing.

No effects on female rats dosed at 10, 50 and 250 mg/kg/day (approximately 2/3, 1 and 2 times human therapeutic concentrations, respectively*) or their female offspring were observed. Administration of bicalutamide to pregnant females resulted in feminization of the male offspring leading to hypospadias at all dose levels. Affected male offspring were also impotent.

*Based on a maximum dose of 50 mg/day of bicalutamide for an average 70 kg patient.

Pregnancy: Pregnancy Category X (see CONTRAINDICATIONS).

Nursing Mothers: It is not known whether this drug is excreted in human milk. Because many drugs are excreted in human milk, caution should be exercised when CASODEX is administered to a nursing woman.

Pediatric Use: Safety and effectiveness of CASODEX in pediatric patients have not been established.

ADVERSE REACTIONS

In patients with advanced prostate cancer treated with CASODEX in combination with an LHRH analogue, the most frequent adverse experience was hot flashes (49%).

Diarrhea was the adverse event most frequently leading to treatment withdrawal: 6% of the patients treated with flutamide-LHRH analogue and 0.5% of the patients treated with CASODEX-LHRH analogue.

In the multicenter, double-blind, controlled clinical trial comparing CASODEX 50 mg once daily with flutamide 250 mg three times a day, each in combination with an LHRH analogue, the following adverse experiences with an incidence of 5% or greater, regardless of causality, have been reported.

Table 2
Incidence of Adverse Events
(≥5% in Either Treatment Group)
Regardless of Causality

Adverse Event	Treatment Group Number of Patients (%)			
	CASODEX Plus LHRH Analogue (n=401)		Flutamide Plus LHRH Analogue (n=407)	
Body as a Whole				
Pain (General)	109	(27)	93	(23)
Back Pain	62	(15)	68	(17)
Asthenia	60	(15)	69	(17)
Pelvic Pain	52	(13)	46	(11)
Infection	41	(10)	35	(9)
Abdominal Pain	33	(8)	31	(8)
Chest Pain	24	(6)	20	(5)
Headache	17	(4)	20	(5)
Flu Syndrome	16	(4)	20	(5)
Cardiovascular				
Hot Flashes	196	(49)	202	(50)
Hypertension	21	(5)	18	(4)
Digestive				
Constipation	67	(17)	50	(12)
Nausea	44	(11)	45	(11)
Diarrhea	40	(10)	98	(24)
Increased Liver Enzyme Test†	25	(6)	40	(10)
Flatulence	22	(5)	16	(4)
Vomiting	12	(3)	20	(5)
Hemic and Lymphatic				
Anemia††	29	(7)	35	(9)
Metabolic and Nutritional				
Peripheral Edema	34	(8)	28	(7)
Hyperglycemia	20	(5)	16	(4)
Weight Loss	16	(4)	20	(5)
Musculoskeletal				
Bone Pain	18	(4)	26	(6)
Nervous System				
Dizziness	30	(7)	27	(7)
Paresthesia	24	(6)	27	(7)
Insomnia	19	(5)	30	(7)
Respiratory System				
Dyspnea	30	(7)	24	(6)
Skin and Appendages				
Rash	25	(6)	20	(5)
Sweating	23	(6)	18	(4)
Urogenital				
Nocturia	35	(9)	43	(11)
Hematuria	30	(7)	20	(5)
Urinary Tract Infection	26	(6)	24	(6)
Impotence	20	(5)	29	(7)
Gynecomastia	19	(5)	23	(6)
Urinary Incontinence	9	(2)	20	(5)

† Increased liver enzyme test includes increases in AST, ALT or both.

†† Anemia includes anemia, hypochromic- and iron deficiency anemia.

Other less frequent (greater than or equal to 2%, but less than 5%) adverse experiences reported in the CASODEX-LHRH analogue treatment group are listed below by body system and are in order of decreasing frequency within each body system regardless of causality. Some of these are commonly reported in elderly patients.

Body as a Whole: Edema; Neoplasm; Fever; Neck pain; Chills; Sepsis

Cardiovascular: Angina pectoris; Congestive heart failure

Digestive: Anorexia; Dyspepsia; Rectal hemorrhage; Dry mouth; Melena

Endocrine: Breast pain; Diabetes mellitus

Metabolic and Nutritional: Alkaline phosphatase increased; Weight gain; Creatinine increased; Dehydration; Gout

Musculoskeletal: Myasthenia; Arthritis; Myalgia; Leg cramps; Pathological fracture

Nervous: Anxiety; Depression; Libido decreased; Hypertonia; Confusion; Neuropathy; Somnolence; Nervousness

Respiratory: Cough increased; Pharyngitis; Bronchitis; Pneumonia; Rhinitis; Lung disorder

Skin and Appendages: Dry skin; Pruritus; Alopecia, Injection site reaction

Urogenital: Urinary frequency; Urination impaired; Dysuria; Urinary retention; Urinary urgency

Abnormal Laboratory Test Values: Laboratory abnormalities including elevated AST, ALT, bilirubin, BUN, and creatinine and decreased hemoglobin and white cell count have been reported in both CASODEX-LHRH analogue treated and flutamide-LHRH analogue treated patients. Increased liver enzyme tests and decreases in hemoglobin were reported less frequently with CASODEX-LHRH analogue therapy. Other changes were reported with similar incidences in both treatment groups.

OVERDOSAGE

In animal studies, CASODEX demonstrated a low acute toxicity. Doses greater than 2000 mg/kg would be necessary to produce significant mortality in mice and rats.

Long-term clinical trials have been conducted with dosages up to 200 mg of CASODEX daily and these dosages have been well tolerated. A single dose of CASODEX that results in symptoms of an overdose considered to be life-threatening has not been established.

There is no specific antidote; treatment of an overdose should be symptomatic.

In the management of an overdose with CASODEX, vomiting may be induced if the patient is alert. It should be remembered that, in this patient population, multiple drugs may have been taken. Dialysis is not likely to be helpful since CASODEX is highly protein bound and is extensively metabolized. General supportive care, including frequent monitoring of vital signs and close observation of the patient, is indicated.

DOSAGE AND ADMINISTRATION

The recommended dose for CASODEX therapy in combination with an LHRH analogue is one 50 mg tablet once daily (morning or evening), with or without food. It is recommended that CASODEX be taken at the same time each day. Treatment with CASODEX should be started at the same time as treatment with an LHRH analogue.

Dosage Adjustment in Renal Impairment: No dosage adjustment is necessary for patients with renal impairment (See CLINICAL PHARMACOLOGY, Special Populations, Renal Insufficiency).

HOW SUPPLIED

50 mg Tablet. (NDC 0310-0705) White, film-coated tablets (identified on one side with "CDX50" and on the reverse with the "CASODEX logo") are supplied in unit dose blisters of 30 tablets per carton (0310-0705-39), bottles of 30 tablets (0310-0705-30) and bottles of 100 tablets (0310-0705-10).

Store at controlled room temperature, 20°–25°C (68°–77°F).

Made in Germany.

Manufactured for
ZENECA Pharmaceuticals
A Business Unit of Zeneca Inc.
Wilmington, Delaware 19850-5437 USA
by Zeneca GmbH, Plankstadt, Germany
64066-02 Rev F 10/95

Shown in Product Identification Guide, page 341

Continued on next page

Zeneca Pharmaceuticals—Cont.

CEFOTAN® ℞

[cef'o-tan]

cefotetan disodium for injection

For Intravenous or Intramuscular Use

CEFOTAN® ℞

cefotetan injection

In GALAXY® Plastic Container (PL 2040)

For Intravenous Use Only

DESCRIPTION

CEFOTAN (cefotetan disodium for injection) and CEFOTAN (cefotetan injection) in Galaxy®* plastic container (PL 2040) as cefotetan disodium are sterile, semisynthetic, broad-spectrum, beta-lactamase resistant, cephalosporin (cephamycin) antibiotics for parenteral administration. It is the disodium salt of [6R-(6α,7α)] -7- [[[4-(2-amino-1-carboxy-2-oxoethylidene)-1,3-dithietan-2-yl]carbonyl]amino]-7-methoxy-3-[[(1-methyl-1*H*-tetrazol-5-yl)thio]methyl]-8-oxo-5-thia-1-azabicyclo[4.2.0]oct-2-ene-2-carboxylic acid. Its molecular formula is $C_{17}H_{15}N_7Na_2O_8S_4$ with a molecular weight of 619.57.

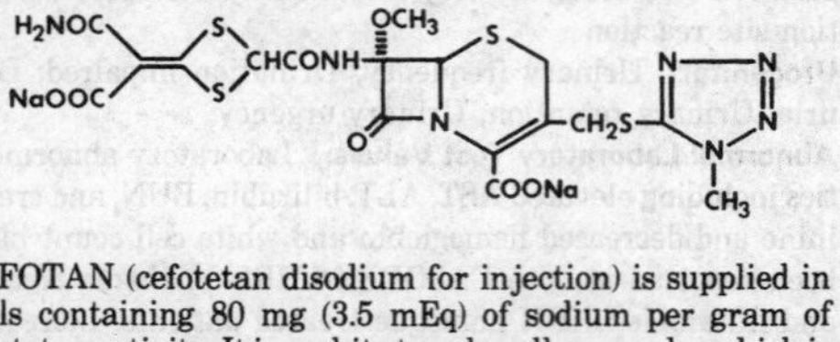

CEFOTAN (cefotetan disodium for injection) is supplied in vials containing 80 mg (3.5 mEq) of sodium per gram of cefotetan activity. It is a white to pale yellow powder which is very soluble in water. Reconstituted solutions of CEFOTAN (cefotetan disodium for injection) are intended for intravenous and intramuscular administration. The solution varies from colorless to yellow depending on the concentration. The pH of freshly reconstituted solutions is usually between 4.5 to 6.5.

CEFOTAN in the ADD-Vantage Vial† is intended for intravenous use only after dilution with the appropriate volume of ADD-Vantage diluent solution.

CEFOTAN is available in two vial strengths. Each CEFOTAN 1 g vial contains cefotetan disodium equivalent to 1 g cefotetan activity. Each CEFOTAN 2 g vial contains cefotetan disodium equivalent to 2 g cefotetan activity.

CEFOTAN (cefotetan injection) in the Galaxy® plastic container (PL 2040) is a frozen, iso-osmotic, sterile, nonpyrogenic premixed 50 mL solution containing 1 g or 2 g cefotetan as cefotetan disodium. Dextrose, USP has been added to adjust the osmolality to 300 mOsmol/kg (approximately 1.9 g and 1.1 g to the 1 g and 2 g dosages, respectively); sodium bicarbonate has been added to convert cefotetan free acid to the sodium salt. The pH has been adjusted between 4 and 6.5 with sodium bicarbonate and may have been adjusted with hydrochloric acid. CEFOTAN (cefotetan injection) in the Galaxy® plastic container (PL 2040) contains 80 mg (3.5 mEq) of sodium per gram of cefotetan activity. After thawing to room temperature, the solution is intended for intravenous use only.

This Galaxy® container is fabricated from a specially designed multilayer plastic (PL 2040). Solutions are in contact with the polyethylene layer of this container and can leach out certain chemical components of the plastic in very small amounts within the expiration dating period. The suitability of the plastic has been confirmed in tests in animals according to the USP biological tests for plastic containers as well as by tissue culture toxicity.

CLINICAL PHARMACOLOGY

High plasma levels of cefotetan are attained after intravenous and intramuscular administration of single doses to normal volunteers.

PLASMA CONCENTRATIONS AFTER 1 GRAM IV[a] OR IM DOSE
Mean Plasma Concentration (μg/mL)
Time After Injection

Route	15 min	30 min	1h	2h	4h	8h	12h
IV	92	158	103	72	42	18	9
IM	34	56	71	68	47	20	9

[a]30-minute infusion

PLASMA CONCENTRATIONS AFTER 2 GRAM IV[a] OR IM DOSE
Mean Plasma Concentration (μg/mL)
Time After Injection

Route	5 min	10 min	1h	3h	5h	9h	12h
IV	237	223	135	74	48	22	12[b]
IM	—	20	75	91	69	33	19

[a] Injected over 3 minutes
[b] Concentrations estimated from regression line

The plasma elimination half-life of cefotetan is 3 to 4.6 hours after either intravenous or intramuscular administration.

Repeated administration of CEFOTAN does not result in accumulation of the drug in normal subjects.

Cefotetan is 88% plasma protein bound.

No active metabolites of cefotetan have been detected; however, small amounts (less than 7%) of cefotetan in plasma and urine may be converted to its tautomer, which has antimicrobial activity similar to the parent drug.

In normal patients, from 51% to 81% of an administered dose of CEFOTAN is excreted unchanged by the kidneys over a 24 hour period, which results in high and prolonged urinary concentrations. Following intravenous doses of 1 gram and 2 grams, urinary concentrations are highest during the first hour and reach concentrations of approximately 1700 and 3500 μg/mL respectively.

In volunteers with reduced renal function, the plasma half-life of cefotetan is prolonged. The mean terminal half-life increases with declining renal function, from approximately 4 hours in volunteers with normal renal function to about 10 hours in those with moderate renal impairment. There is a linear correlation between the systemic clearance of cefotetan and creatinine clearance. When renal function is impaired, a reduced dosing schedule based on creatinine clearance must be used. (see DOSAGE AND ADMINISTRATION).

Therapeutic levels of cefotetan are achieved in many body tissues and fluids including:

skin	ureter
muscle	bladder
fat	maxillary sinus mucosa
myometrium	tonsil
endometrium	bile
cervix	peritoneal fluid
ovary	umbilical cord serum
kidney	amniotic fluid

Microbiology

The bactericidal action of cefotetan results from inhibition of cell wall synthesis. Cefotetan has *in vitro* activity against a wide range of aerobic and anaerobic gram-positive and gram-negative organisms. The methoxy group in the 7-alpha position provides cefotetan with a high degree of stability in the presence of beta-lactamases including both penicillinases and cephalosporinase of gram-negative bacteria.

Cefotetan has been shown to be active against most strains of the following organisms **both *in vitro* and in clinical infections** (see INDICATIONS AND USAGE).

Gram-Negative Aerobes
Escherichia coli
Haemophilus influenzae (including ampicillin-resistant strains)
Klebsiella species (including *K. pneumoniae)*
Morganella morganii
Neisseria gonorrhoeae (nonpenicillinase-producing strains)
Proteus mirabilis
Proteus vulgaris
Providencia rettgeri
Serratia marcescens

NOTE: Approximately one-half of the usually clinically significant strains of *Enterobacter* species (e.g., *E. aerogenes* and *E. cloacae*) are resistant to cefotetan. Most strains of *Pseudomonas aeruginosa* and *Acinetobacter* species are resistant to cefotetan.

Gram-Positive Aerobes
Staphylococcus aureus (including penicillinase- and nonpenicillinase-producing strains)
Staphylococcus epidermidis
Streptococcus agalactiae (group B beta-hemolytic streptococcus)
Streptococcus pneumoniae
Streptococcus pyogenes

NOTE: Methicillin-resistant staphylococci are resistant to cephalosporins. Some strains of *Staphylococcus epidermidis* and most strains of enterococci, e.g., *Enterococcus faecalis* (formerly *Streptococcus faecalis*) are resistant to cefotetan.

Anaerobes
Prevotella bivia (formerly *Bacteroides bivius*)
Prevotella disiens (formerly *Bacteroides disiens)*
Bacteroides fragilis
Prevotella melaninogenica (formerly Bacteroides melaninogenicus)
Bacteroides vulgatus
Fusobacterium species
Gram-positive bacilli (including *Clostridium* species; see WARNINGS)

NOTE: Most strains of *C. difficile* are resistant (see WARNINGS).

Peptococcus niger
Peptostreptococcus species

NOTE: Many strains of *B. distasonis, B. ovatus* and *B. thetaiotaomicron* are resistant to cefotetan *in vitro*. However, the therapeutic utility of cefotetan against these organisms cannot be accurately predicted on the basis of *in vitro* susceptibility tests alone.

The following *in vitro* data are available but their clinical significance is unknown. Cefotetan has been shown to be active *in vitro* against most strains of the following organisms:

Gram-Negative Aerobes
Citrobacter species (including *C. diversus* and *C. freundii*)
Klebsiella oxytoca
Moraxella (Branhamella) catarrhalis
Neisseria gonorrhoeae (penicillinase-producing strains)
Salmonella species
Serratia species
Shigella species
Yersinia enterocolitica

Anaerobes
Porphyromonas asaccharolytica (formerly *Bacteroides asaccharolyticus)*
Prevotella oralis (formerly *Bacteroides oralis)*
Bacteroides splanchnicus
Clostridium difficile (see WARNINGS)
Propionibacterium species
Veillonella species

Susceptibility Tests

Dilution Techniques: Quantitative methods are used to determine antimicrobial minimal inhibitory concentrations (MIC's). These MIC's provide estimates of the susceptibility of bacteria to antimicrobial compounds. The MICs should be determined using a standardized procedure. Standardized procedures are based on a dilution method[1] (broth or agar) or equivalent with standardized inoculum concentrations and standardized concentrations or cefotetan powder. The MIC values should be interpreted according to the following criteria:

MIC (μg/mL)	Interpretation
≤16	Susceptible (S)
32	Intermediate (I)
≥64	Resistant (R)

A report of 'Susceptible' indicates that the pathogen is likely to be inhibited if the antimicrobial compound in the blood reaches the concentrations usually achievable. A report of 'Intermediate' indicates that the result should be considered equivocal, and if the microorganism is not fully susceptible to alternative, clinically feasible drugs, the test should be repeated. This category implies possible clinical applicability in body sites where the drug is physiologically concentrated or in situations where high dosage of drug can be used. This category also provides a buffer zone which prevents small uncontrolled technical factors from causing major discrepancies in interpretation. A report of 'Resistant' indicates that the pathogen is not likely to be inhibited if the antimicrobial compound in the blood reaches the concentrations usually achievable; other therapy should be selected.

Standardized susceptibility test procedures require the use of laboratory control microorganisms to control the technical aspects of the laboratory procedures. Standard cefotetan powder should provide the following MIC values:

Microorganism	MIC (μg/mL)
E. coli ATCC 25922	0.06–0.25
S. aureus ATCC 29213	4–16

Diffusion Techniques: Quantitative methods that require measurement of zone diameters also provide reproducible estimates of the susceptibility of bacteria to antimicrobial compounds. One such standardized procedure[2] requires the use of the standardized inoculum concentrations. This procedure uses paper disks impregnated with 30 μg cefotetan to test the susceptibility of microorganisms to cefotetan.

Reports from the laboratory providing results of the standard single-disk susceptibility test with a 30 μg cefotetan disk should be interpreted according to the following criteria:

Zone Diameter (mm)	Interpretation
≥16	Susceptible (S)
13–15	Intermediate (I)
≤12	Resistant (R)

Interpretation should be as stated above for results using dilution techniques. Interpretation involves correlation of the diameter obtained in the disk test with the MIC for cefotetan.

As with standardized dilution techniques, diffusion methods require the use of laboratory control microorganisms that are used to control the technical aspects of the laboratory procedures. For the diffusion technique, the 30 μg cefotetan disk should provide the following zone diameters in these laboratory test quality control strains.

Microorganism	Zone Diameter (mm)
E. coli ATCC 25922	28–34
S. aureus ATCC 25923	17–23

Anaerobic Techniques: For anaerobic bacteria, the susceptibility to cefotetan as MIC's can be determined by standardized test methods[3]. The MIC values obtained should be interpreted according to the following criteria:

MIC (µg/mL)	Interpretation
≤ 16	Susceptible (S)
32	Intermediate (I)
≥ 64	Resistant (R)

Interpretation is identical to that stated above for results using dilution techniques.

As with other susceptibility techniques, the use of laboratory control microorganisms is required to control the technical aspects of the laboratory standardized procedures. Standardized cefotetan powder should provide the following MIC values:

Microorganism	MIC (µg/mL)
Bacteroides fragilis ATCC 25285	4–16
Bacteroides thetaiotaomicron ATCC 29741	32–128
Eubacterium lentum ATCC 43055	32–128

INDICATIONS AND USAGE

Treatment
CEFOTAN is indicated for the therapeutic treatment of the following infections when caused by susceptible strains of the designated organisms:

Urinary Tract Infections caused by *E. coli, Klebsiella* spp (including *K. pneumoniae*), *Proteus mirabilis* and *Proteus* spp (which may include the organisms now called *Proteus vulgaris, Providencia rettgeri*, and *Morganella morganii*).

Lower Respiratory Tract Infections caused by *Streptococcus pneumoniae, Staphylococcus aureus* (penicillinase- and non-penicillinase-producing strains), *Haemophilus influenzae* (including ampicillin- resistant strains), *Klebsiella* species (including *K. pneumoniae*), *E. coli, Proteus mirabilis*, and *Serratia marcescens**.

Skin and Skin Structure Infections due to *Staphylococcus aureus* (penicillinase- and nonpenicillinase-producing strains), *Staphylococcus epidermidis, Streptococcus pyogenes, Streptococcus* species (excluding enterococci), *Escherichia coli, Klebsiella pneumoniae, Peptococcus niger*, Peptostreptococcus* species.

Gynecologic Infections caused by *Staphylococcus aureus*, (including penicillinase- and nonpenicillinase-producing strains), *Staphylococcus epidermidis, Streptococcus* species (excluding enterococci), *Streptococcus agalactiae, E. coli, Proteus mirabilis, Neisseria gonorrhoeae*, Bacteroides species (excluding *B. distasonis, B. ovatus, B. thetaiotaomicron*), *Fusobacterium* species*, and gram-positive anaerobic cocci (including *Peptococcus niger* and *Peptostreptococcus* species).

Cefotetan, like other cephalosporins, has no activity against *Chlamydia trachomatis*. Therefore, when cephalosporins are used in the treatment of pelvic inflammatory disease, and *C. trachomatis* is one of the suspected pathogens, appropriate antichlamydial coverage should be added.

Intra-abdominal Infections caused by *E. coli, Klebsiella* species (including *K. pneumoniae*), *Streptococcus* species (excluding enterococci), *Bacteroides* species (excluding *B. distasonis, B. ovatus, B. thetaiotaomicron*) and *Clostridium* species*.

Bone and Joint Infections caused by *Staphylococcus aureus.**
*Efficacy for this organism in this organ system was studied in fewer than ten infections.

Specimens for bacteriological examination should be obtained in order to isolate and identify causative organisms and to determine their susceptibilities to cefotetan. Therapy may be instituted before results of susceptibility studies are known; however, once these results become available, the antibiotic treatment should be adjusted accordingly.

In cases of confirmed or suspected gram-positive or gram-negative sepsis or in patients with other serious infections in which the causative organism has not been identified, it is possible to use CEFOTAN concomitantly with an aminoglycoside. Cefotetan combinations with aminoglycosides have been shown to be synergistic *in vitro* against many Enterobacteriaceae and also some other gram-negative bacteria. The dosage recommended in the labeling of both antibiotics may be given and depends on the severity of the infection and the patient's condition.

NOTE: Increases in serum creatinine have occurred when CEFOTAN was given alone. If CEFOTAN and an aminoglycoside are used concomitantly, renal function should be carefully monitored, because nephrotoxicity may be potentiated.

Prophylaxis
The preoperative administration of CEFOTAN may reduce the incidence of certain postoperative infections in patients undergoing surgical procedures that are classified as clean contaminated or potentially contaminated (e.g., cesarean section, abdominal or vaginal hysterectomy, transurethral surgery, biliary tract surgery, and gastrointestinal surgery). If there are signs and symptoms of infection, specimens for culture should be obtained for identification of the causative organism so that appropriate therapeutic measures may be initiated.

CONTRAINDICATIONS
CEFOTAN is contraindicated in patients with known allergy to the cephalosporin group of antibiotics.

WARNINGS
BEFORE THERAPY WITH CEFOTAN IS INSTITUTED, CAREFUL INQUIRY SHOULD BE MADE TO DETERMINE WHETHER THE PATIENT HAS HAD PREVIOUS HYPERSENSITIVITY REACTIONS TO CEFOTETAN, CEPHALOSPORINS, PENICILLINS, OR OTHER DRUGS. IF THIS PRODUCT IS TO BE GIVEN TO PENICILLIN-SENSITIVE PATIENTS, CAUTION SHOULD BE EXERCISED BECAUSE CROSS-HYPERSENSITIVITY AMONG BETA-LACTAM ANTIBIOTICS HAS BEEN CLEARLY DOCUMENTED AND MAY OCCUR IN UP TO 10% OF PATIENTS WITH A HISTORY OF PENICILLIN ALLERGY. IF AN ALLERGIC REACTION TO CEFOTAN OCCURS, DISCONTINUE THE DRUG. SERIOUS ACUTE HYPERSENSITIVITY REACTIONS MAY REQUIRE TREATMENT WITH EPINEPHRINE AND OTHER EMERGENCY MEASURES, INCLUDING OXYGEN, INTRAVENOUS FLUIDS, INTRAVENOUS ANTIHISTAMINES, CORTICOSTEROIDS, PRESSOR AMINES, AND AIRWAY MANAGEMENT, AS CLINICALLY INDICATED.

Pseudomembranous colitis has been reported with nearly all antibacterial agents, including cefotetan, and may range in severity from mild to life-threatening. Therefore, it is important to consider this diagnosis in patients who present with diarrhea subsequent to the administration of antibacterial agents.

Treatment with antibacterial agents alters the normal flora of the colon and may permit overgrowth of clostridia. Studies indicate that a toxin produced by *Clostridium difficile* is a primary cause of "antibiotic-associated colitis".

After the diagnosis of pseudomembranous colitis has been established, appropriate therapeutic measures should be initiated. Mild cases of pseudomembranous colitis usually respond to drug discontinuation alone. In moderate to severe cases, consideration should be given to management with fluids and electrolytes, protein supplementation, and treatment with an antibacterial drug clinically effective against *Clostridium difficile* colitis. (See ADVERSE REACTIONS.)

In common with many other broad-spectrum antibiotics, CEFOTAN may be associated with a fall in prothrombin activity and, possibly, subsequent bleeding. Those at increased risk include patients with renal or hepatobiliary impairment or poor nutritional state, the elderly, and patients with cancer. Prothrombin time should be monitored and exogenous vitamin K administered as indicated.

Hemolytic anemia has been reported for cephalosporin-class antibiotics. Severe cases of hemolytic anemia, including fatalities, have been reported in association with the administration of CEFOTAN. Such reports are uncommon. If a patient develops a hematologic abnormality subsequent to the administration of cefotetan, a diagnosis of drug-induced hemolytic anemia should be considered.

PRECAUTIONS
General: As with other broad-spectrum antibiotics, prolonged use of CEFOTAN may result in overgrowth of nonsusceptible organisms. Careful observation of the patient is essential. If superinfection does occur during therapy, appropriate measures should be taken.

CEFOTAN should be used with caution in individuals with a history of gastrointestinal disease, particularly colitis.

Information for Patients: As with some other cephalosporins, a disulfiram-like reaction characterized by flushing, sweating, headache, and tachycardia may occur when alcohol (beer, wine, etc.) is ingested within 72 hours after CEFOTAN administration. Patients should be cautioned about the ingestion of alcoholic beverages following the administration of CEFOTAN.

Drug Interactions: Increases in serum creatinine have occurred when CEFOTAN was given alone. If CEFOTAN and an aminoglycoside are used concomitantly, renal function should be carefully monitored, because nephrotoxicity may be potentiated.

Drug/Laboratory Test Interactions: The administration of CEFOTAN may result in a false positive reaction for glucose in the urine using Clinitest®‡, Benedict's solution, or Fehling's solution. It is recommended that glucose tests based on enzymatic glucose oxidase be used.

As with other cephalosporins, high concentrations of cefotetan may interfere with measurement of serum and urine creatinine levels by Jaffe′ reaction and produce false increases in the levels of creatinine reported.

Carcinogenesis, Mutagenesis, Impairment of Fertility: Although long-term studies in animals have not been performed to evaluate carcinogenic potential, no mutagenic potential of cefotetan was found in standard laboratory tests. Cefotetan has adverse effects on the testes of prepubertal rats. Subcutaneous administration of 500 mg/kg/day (approximately 8-16 times the usual adult human dose) on days 6-35 of life (thought to be developmentally analogous to late childhood and prepuberty in humans) resulted in reduced testicular weight and seminiferous tubule degeneration in 10 of 10 animals. Affected cells included spermatogonia and spermatocytes; Sertoli and Leydig cells were unaffected. Incidence and severity of lesions were dose-dependent; at 120

mg/kg/day (approximately 2-4 times the usual human dose) only 1 of 10 treated animals was affected, and the degree of degeneration was mild.

Similar lesions have been observed in experiments of comparable design with other methylthiotetrazole-containing antibiotics and impaired fertility has been reported, particularly at high dose levels. No testicular effects were observed in 7-week-old rats treated with up to 1000 mg/kg/day SC for 5 weeks, or in infant dogs (3 weeks old) that received up to 300 mg/kg/day IV for 5 weeks. The relevance of these findings to humans is unknown.

Pregnancy: Teratogenic Effects. Pregnancy Category B: Reproduction studies have been performed in rats and monkeys at doses up to 20 times the human dose and have revealed no evidence of impaired fertility or harm to the fetus due to cefotetan. There are, however, no adequate and well-controlled studies in pregnant women. Because animal reproductive studies are not always predictive of human response, this drug should be used during pregnancy only if clearly needed.

Nursing Mothers: Cefotetan is excreted in human milk in very low concentrations. Caution should be exercised when cefotetan is administered to a nursing woman.

Pediatric Use: Safety and effectiveness in children have not been established.

ADVERSE REACTIONS
In clinical studies, the following adverse effects were considered related to CEFOTAN therapy. Those appearing in italics have been reported during postmarketing experience.

Gastrointestinal symptoms occurred in 1.5% of patients, the most frequent were diarrhea (1 in 80) and nausea (1 in 700); *pseudomembranous colitis*. Onset of pseudomembranous colitis symptoms may occur during or after antibiotic treatment or surgical prophylaxis. (See **WARNINGS**.)

Hematologic laboratory abnormalities occurred in 1.4% of patients and included eosinophilia (1 in 200), positive direct Coombs' test (1 in 250), and thrombocytosis (1 in 300); *agranulocytosis, hemolytic anemia, leukopenia, thrombocytopenia, and prolonged prothrombin time with or without bleeding.*

Hepatic enzyme elevations occurred in 1.2% of patients and included a rise in ALT (SGPT) (1 in 150), AST (SGOT) (1 in 300), alkaline phosphatase (1 in 700), and LDH (1 in 700).

Hypersensitivity reactions were reported in 1.2% of patients and included rash (1 in 150) and itching (1 in 700); *anaphylactic reactions and urticaria.*

Local effects were reported in less than 1% of patients and included phlebitis at the site of injection (1 in 300), and discomfort (1 in 500).

Renal: *Elevations in BUN and serum creatinine have been reported.*

Urogenital: *Nephrotoxicity has rarely been reported.*

Miscellaneous: *Fever*

In addition to the adverse reactions listed above which have been observed in patients treated with cefotetan, the following adverse reactions and altered laboratory tests have been reported for cephalosporin-class antibiotics: pruritus, Stevens-Johnson syndrome, erythema multiforme, toxic epidermal necrolysis, vomiting, abdominal pain, colitis, superinfection, vaginitis including vaginal candidiasis, renal dysfunction, toxic nephropathy, hepatic dysfunction including cholestasis, aplastic anemia, hemorrhage, elevated bilirubin, pancytopenia, and neutropenia.

Several cephalosporins have been implicated in triggering seizures, particularly in patients with renal impairment, when the dosage was not reduced. (See DOSAGE AND ADMINISTRATION and OVERDOSAGE.) If seizures associated with drug therapy occur, the drug should be discontinued. Anticonvulsant therapy can be given if clinically indicated.

OVERDOSAGE
Information on overdosage with CEFOTAN in humans is not available. If overdosage should occur, it should be treated symptomatically and hemodialysis considered, particularly if renal function is compromised.

DOSAGE AND ADMINISTRATION
Treatment
Cefotetan injection in Galaxy® plastic container should not be used for intramuscular administration.

CEFOTAN in the ADD-Vantage Vial is intended for intravenous infusion only, after dilution with the appropriate volume of ADD-Vantage diluent solution.

The usual adult dosage is 1 or 2 grams of CEFOTAN (cefotetan disodium for injection) administered intravenously or intramuscularly or CEFOTAN (cefotetan injection) in the Galaxy® plastic container (PL 2040) administered intravenously every 12 hours for 5 to 10 days. Proper dosage and route of administration should be determined by the condition of the patient, severity of the infection, and susceptibility of the causative organism.

[See first table on top of next page.]

Continued on next page

Zeneca Pharmaceuticals—Cont.

General Guidelines for Dosage of CEFOTAN

Type of Infection	Daily Dose	Frequency and Route
Urinary Tract	1–4 grams	500 mg every 12 hours IV or IM 1 or 2 g every 24 hours IV or IM 1 or 2 g every 12 hours IV or IM
Skin & Skin Structure		
Mild–Moderate[a]	2 grams	2 g every 24 hours IV 1 g every 12 hours IV or IM
Severe	4 grams	2 g every 12 hours IV
Other Sites	2–4 grams	1 or 2 g every 12 hours IV or IM
Severe	4 grams	2 g every 12 hours IV
Life-Threatening	6 grams[b]	3 g every 12 hours IV

[a] *Klebsiella pneumoniae* skin and skin structure infections should be treated with 1 or 2 grams every 12 hours IV or IM.
[b] Maximum daily dosage should not exceed 6 grams.

DOSAGE GUIDELINES FOR PATIENTS WITH IMPAIRED RENAL FUNCTION

Creatinine Clearance mL/min	Dose	Frequency
>30	Usual Recommended Dosage*	Every 12 hours
10–30	Usual Recommended Dosage*	Every 24 hours
<10	Usual Recommended Dosage*	Every 48 hours

*Dose determined by the type and severity of infection, and susceptibility of the causative organism.

If *Chlamydia trachomatis* is a suspected pathogen in gynecologic infections, appropriate antichlamydial coverage should be added, since cefotetan has no activity against this organism.

Prophylaxis:
To prevent postoperative infection in clean contaminated or potentially contaminated surgery in adults, the recommended dosage is 1 or 2 g of CEFOTAN administered once, intravenously, 30 to 60 minutes prior to surgery. In patients undergoing cesarean section, the dose should be administered as soon as the umbilical cord is clamped.

Impaired Renal Function:
When renal function is impaired, a reduced dosage schedule must be employed. The following dosage guidelines may be used.
[See second table above.]
Alternatively, the dosing interval may remain constant at 12 hour intervals, but the dose reduced to one-half the usual recommended dose for patients with a creatinine clearance of 10-30 mL/min, and one-quarter the usual recommended dose for patients with a creatinine clearance of less than 10 mL/min.
When only serum creatinine levels are available, creatinine clearance may be calculated from the following formula. The serum creatinine level should represent a steady state of renal function.

Males:
$$\frac{\text{Weight (kg)} \times (140 - \text{age})}{72 \times \text{serum creatinine (mg/100 mL)}}$$

Females: $0.9 \times$ value for males

Cefotetan is dialyzable and it is recommended that for patients undergoing intermittent hemodialysis, one-quarter of the usual recommended dose be given every 24 hours on days between dialysis and one-half the usual recommended dose on the day of dialysis.

CEFOTETAN DISODIUM FOR INJECTION

Preparation of Solution From Cefotetan Disodium For Injection
For Intravenous Use: Reconstitute with Sterile Water for Injection. Shake to dissolve and let stand until clear.

Vial Size	Amount of Diluent Added (mL)	Approximate Withdrawable Vol (mL)	Approximate Average Concentration (mg/mL)
1 gram	10	10.5	95
2 gram	10–20	11–21	182–95

Infusion bottles (100 mL) may be reconstituted with 50 to 100 mL of Dextrose Injection 5% or Sodium Chloride Injection 0.9%.
NOTE: ADD-VANTAGE VIALS ARE NOT TO BE USED IN THIS MANNER
For ADD-Vantage Vials: ADD-Vantage Vials of CEFOTAN are to be reconstituted only with Sodium Chloride Injection 0.9% or Dextrose Injection 5% in the 50 mL, 100 mL or 250 mL Flexible Diluent Containers. CEFOTAN supplied in single-use ADD-Vantage Vials should be prepared as directed.
Directions for Use of CEFOTAN (cefotetan disodium for injection) in ADD-Vantage Vials:
To Open Diluent Container: Peel overwrap from the corner and remove container. Some opacity of the plastic due to moisture absorption during the sterilization process may be observed. This is normal and does not affect the solution quality or safety. The opacity will diminish gradually.

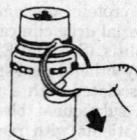

Figure 1

To Assemble ADD-Vantage Vial and Flexible Diluent Container: (Use Aseptic Technique)
1. Remove the protective covers from the top of the vial and the vial port on the diluent container as follows:
   a. To remove the breakaway vial cap, swing the pull ring over the top of the vial and pull down far enough to start the opening (See Figure 1), then pull straight up to remove the cap. (See Figure 2.) **NOTE:** Once the breakaway cap has been removed, do not access vial with syringe.

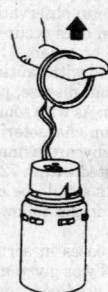

Figure 2

   b. To remove the vial port cover, grasp the tab on the pull ring, pull up to break the three tie strings, then pull back to remove the cover. (See Figure 3.)

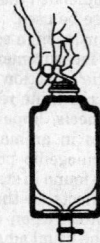

Figure 3

2. Screw the vial into the vial port until it will go no further. THE VIAL MUST BE SCREWED IN TIGHTLY TO ASSURE A SEAL. This occurs approximately 1/2 turn (180°) after the first audible click. (See Figure 4.) The clicking sound does not assure a seal; the vial must be turned as far as it will go. **NOTE: ONCE VIAL IS SEATED, DO NOT ATTEMPT TO REMOVE.** (See Figure 4.)

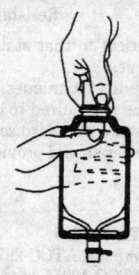

Figure 4

3. Recheck the vial to assure that it is tight by trying to turn it further in the direction of assembly.
4. Label appropriately.
To Prepare Admixture:
1. Squeeze the bottom of the diluent container gently to inflate the portion of the container surrounding the end of the drug vial.
2. With the other hand, push the drug vial down into the container telescoping the walls of the container. Grasp the inner cap of the vial through the walls of the container. (See Figure 5.)

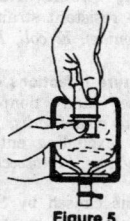

Figure 5

3. Pull the inner cap from the drug vial. (See Figure 6.) Verify that the rubber stopper has been pulled out and invert the system several times, allowing the drug and diluent to mix.

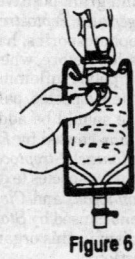

Figure 6

4. Mix contents thoroughly and use within the specified time.
Preparation For Administration: (Use Aseptic Technique)
1. Confirm the activation and admixture of vial contents.
2. Check for leaks by squeezing container firmly. If leaks are found, discard unit as sterility may be impaired.
3. Close flow control clamp of administration set.
4. Remove cover from outlet port at bottom of container.
5. Insert piercing pin of administration set into port with a twisting motion until the pin is firmly seated. **NOTE:** See full directions on administration set carton.
6. Lift the free end of the hanger loop on the bottom of the vial, breaking the two tie strings. Bend the loop outward to lock it in the upright position, then suspend container from hanger.
7. Squeeze and release drip chamber to establish proper fluid level in chamber.
8. Open flow control clamp and clear air from set. Close clamp.
9. Attach set to venipuncture device. If device is not indwelling, prime and make venipuncture.
10. Regulate rate of administration with flow control clamp.
WARNING: Do not use flexible container in series connections.

For Intramuscular Use: Reconstitute with Sterile Water for Injection; Bacteriostatic Water for Injection; Sodium Chloride Injection 0.9%, USP; 0.5% Lidocaine HCl; or 1% Lidocaine HCl. Shake to dissolve and let stand until clear.

Vial Size	Amount of Diluent Added (mL)	Approximate Withdrawable Vol (mL)	Average Concentration (mg/mL)
1 gram	2	2.5	400
2 gram	3	4	500

Intravenous Administration:
The intravenous route is preferable for patients with bacteremia, bacterial septicemia, or other severe or life-threatening infections, or for patients who may be poor risks because of lowered resistance resulting from such debilitating conditions as malnutrition, trauma, surgery, diabetes, heart failure, or malignancy, particularly if shock is present or impending.
For intermittent intravenous administration, a solution containing 1 gram or 2 grams of CEFOTAN (cefotetan disodium for injection) in Sterile Water for Injection can be injected over a period of three to five minutes. Using an infusion system, the solution may also be given over a longer period of time through the tubing system by which the patient may be receiving other intravenous solutions. Butterfly® or scalp vein- type needles are preferred for this type of infusion. However, during infusion of the solution containing CEFOTAN (cefotetan disodium for injection), it is advisable to discontinue temporarily the administration of other solutions at the same site.
NOTE: Solutions of CEFOTAN must not be admixed with solutions containing aminoglycosides. If CEFOTAN and aminoglycosides are to be administered to the same patient, they must be administered separately and not as a mixed injection.
Intramuscular Administration:
As with all intramuscular preparations, (cefotetan disodium for injection) should be injected well within the body of a relatively large muscle such as the upper outer quadrant of the buttock (i.e., gluteus maximus); aspiration is necessary to avoid inadvertent injection into a blood vessel.
CEFOTETAN INJECTION
Directions for Use of CEFOTAN (cefotetan injection) in Galaxy® Plastic Container (PL2040)
CEFOTAN (cefotetan injection) in Galaxy® plastic container (PL 2040) is for intravenous administration only.
Storage: Store in a freezer capable of maintaining a temperature of -20°C/-4°F.
Thawing of Plastic Container: Thaw frozen container at room temperature (25°C/77°F) or in a refrigerator (5°C/41°F).
[DO NOT FORCE THAW BY IMMERSION IN WATER BATHS OR BY MICROWAVE IRRADIATION.]
Check for minute leaks by squeezing container firmly. If leaks are detected, discard solution as sterility may be impaired.
The container should be visually inspected. Components of the solution may precipitate in the frozen state and will dissolve upon reaching room temperature with little or no agitation. Potency is not affected. Agitate after solution has reached room temperature. If after visual inspection the solution remains cloudy or if an insoluble precipitate is noted or if any seals or outlet ports are not intact, the container should be discarded.
Preparation of Intravenous Use (Use aseptic technique):
1. Suspend container from eyelet support.
2. Remove protector from outlet port at bottom of container.
3. Attach administration set. Refer to complete directions accompanying set.

Caution: Do not use plastic containers in series connections. Such use could result in air embolism due to residual air being drawn from the primary container before administration of the fluid from the secondary container is complete.
Intravenous Administration:
The intravenous route is preferable for patients with bacteremia, bacterial septicemia, or other severe or life threatening infections, or for patients who may be poor risks because of lowered resistance resulting from such debilitating conditions as malnutrition, trauma, surgery, diabetes, heart failure, or malignancy, particularly if shock is present or impending.
Using an infusion system, CEFOTAN (cefotetan injection) in Galaxy® plastic container (PL 2040) should be given over 20 to 60 minutes through the tubing system by which the patient may be receiving other intravenous solutions. Butterfly® or scalp vein-type needles are preferred for this type of infusion. However, during infusion of the solution containing CEFOTAN (cefotetan injection) in Galaxy® plastic container (PL 2040), it is advisable to discontinue temporarily the administration of other solutions at the same site.
Compatibility and Stability of CEFOTAN Products:
Frozen samples should be thawed at room temperature before use. After the periods mentioned below, any unused solutions or frozen material should be discarded. **DO NOT REFREEZE.**
NOTE: Solutions of CEFOTAN must not be admixed-with solutions containing aminoglycosides. If CEFOTAN and aminoglycosides are to be administered to the same patient, they must be administered separately and not as a mixed injection. **DO NOT ADD SUPPLEMENTARY MEDICATION.**
CEFOTETAN DISODIUM FOR INJECTION
CEFOTAN (cefotetan disodium for injection) reconstituted as described above (PREPARATION OF SOLUTION) maintains satisfactory potency for 24 hours at room temperature (25°C/77°F), for 96 hours under refrigeration (5°C/41°F), and for at least 1 week in the frozen state (-20°C/-4°F). After reconstitution and subsequent storage in disposable glass or plastic syringes, CEFOTAN (cefotetan disodium for injection) is stable for 24 hours at room temperature and 96 hours under refrigeration.
ADD-Vantage Vials:
Ordinarily, ADD-Vantage Vials should be reconstituted only when it is certain that the patient is ready to receive the drug. However, ADD-Vantage Vials of CEFOTAN reconstituted as described in Preparation of Solution, for ADD-Vantage Vials, maintains satisfactory potency for 24 hours at room temperature (25°C/77°F).
(DO NOT REFRIGERATE OR FREEZE CEFOTAN IN ADD-VANTAGE VIALS.)
CEFOTETAN INJECTION
The thawed solution in Galaxy® plastic container (PL 2040) remains chemically stable for 48 hours at room temperature (25°C/77°F) or for 21 days under refrigeration (5°C/41°F).
NOTE: Parenteral drug products should be inspected visually for particulate matter and discoloration prior to administration whenever solution and container permit.

HOW SUPPLIED

CEFOTAN (cefotetan disodium for injection) is a dry, white to pale yellow powder supplied in vials containing cefotetan disodium equivalent to 1 g and 2 g cefotetan activity for intravenous and intramuscular administration. The vials should not be stored at temperatures above 22° C (72° F) and should be protected from light.
1 g ADD-Vantage Vial (NDC 0310-0376-31)
2 g ADD-Vantage Vial (NDC 0310-0377-32)
1 g Vial (NDC 0310-0376-10)
2 g Vial (NDC 0310-0377-20)
1 g Piggyback Vial (NDC 0310-0376-11)
2 g Piggyback Vial (NDC 0310-0377-21)
CEFOTAN is also available as a 10 g pharmacy bulk package.
10g in 100 mL Vial (NDC 0310-0375-10)
CEFOTAN (cefotetan injection) is supplied as a frozen, iso-osmotic, premixed solution in single dose Galaxy® plastic containers (PL 2040) as follows:
1 g in 50 mL plastic container (NDC 0310-0378-51)
2 g in 50 mL plastic container (NDC 0310-0379-51)
Store containers at or below -20°C/-4°F. **[See DIRECTIONS FOR USE OF CEFOTAN (cefotetan injection) IN GALAXY® PLASTIC CONTAINER (PL 2040)].**

REFERENCES

1. National Committee for Clinical Laboratory Standards. Methods for Dilution Antimicrobial Susceptibility Tests for Bacteria that Grow Aerobically—Third Edition. Approved Standard NCCLS Document M7-A3, Vol. 13, No. 25, NCCLS, Villanova, PA, December, 1993.
2. National Committee for Clinical Laboratory Standards. Performance Standards for antimicrobial Disk Susceptibility Tests—Fifth Edition. Approved Standard NCCLS Document M2-A5, Vol. 13, No. 24, NCCLS, Villanova, PA, December 1993.
3. National Committee for Clinical Laboratory Standards. Methods for Antimicrobial Susceptibility Testing of Anaerobic Bacteria—Third Edition. Approved Standard NCCLS Document M11-A3, Vol 13, No. 26, NCCLS, Villanova, PA, December 1993.
*Galaxy® is a registered trademark of Baxter Healthcare Corporation.
†ADD-Vantage is a registered trademark of Abbott Laboratories Inc.
‡ Clinitest® is a registered trademark of Ames Division, Miles Laboratories, Inc.
CEFOTAN® (cefotetan injection) in Galaxy® plastic container (PL 2040) is manufactured by Baxter Healthcare Corporation, Deerfield, Illinois 60015 USA for Zeneca Pharmaceuticals.
CEFOTAN® (cefotetan disodium for injection) is manufactured by SmithKline Beecham Corporation for:
Zeneca Pharmaceuticals
A Business Unit of Zeneca Inc.
Wilmington, Delaware 19850-5437
Rev E 1/96 SIC 64065-01
Shown in Product Identification Guide, page 341

DIPRIVAN® 1% ℞
INJECTABLE EMULSION
10 mg/mL propofol
FOR I.V. ADMINISTRATION
Formerly DIPRIVAN® (propofol) Injection
PROFESSIONAL INFORMATION BROCHURE

DESCRIPTION

DIPRIVAN® Injectable Emulsion is a sterile, nonpyrogenic emulsion containing 10 mg/mL of propofol suitable for intravenous administration. Propofol is chemically described as 2,6-diisopropylphenol and has a molecular weight of 178.27. The structural and molecular formulas are:

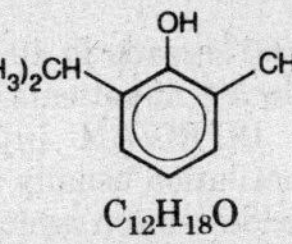

$C_{12}H_{18}O$

Propofol is very slightly soluble in water and, thus, is formulated in a white, oil-in-water emulsion. The pKa is 11. The octanol/water partition coefficient for propofol 6761:1 at a pH of 6-8.5. In addition to the active component, propofol, the formulation also contains soybean oil (100 mg/mL), glycerol (22.5 mg/mL), egg lecithin (12 mg/mL), and disodium edetate (0.005%); with sodium hydroxide to adjust pH. The DIPRIVAN Injectable Emulsion is isotonic and has a pH of 7-8.5.
STRICT ASEPTIC TECHNIQUE MUST ALWAYS BE MAINTAINED DURING HANDLING. DIPRIVAN INJECTABLE EMULSION IS A SINGLE-USE PARENTERAL PRODUCT WHICH CONTAINS 0.005% DISODIUM EDETATE TO RETARD THE RATE OF GROWTH OF MICROORGANISMS IN THE EVENT OF ACCIDENTAL EXTRINSIC CONTAMINATION. HOWEVER, DIPRIVAN INJECTABLE EMULSION CAN STILL SUPPORT THE GROWTH OF MICROORGANISMS AS IT IS NOT AN ANTIMICROBIALLY PRESERVED PRODUCT UNDER USP STANDARDS. ACCORDINGLY, STRICT ASEPTIC TECHNIQUE MUST STILL BE ADHERED TO. DO NOT USE IF CONTAMINATION IS SUSPECTED. DISCARD UNUSED PORTIONS AS DIRECTED WITHIN THE REQUIRED TIME LIMITS (SEE DOSAGE AND ADMINISTRATION, HANDLING PROCEDURES). THERE HAVE BEEN REPORTS IN WHICH FAILURE TO USE ASEPTIC TECHNIQUE WHEN HANDLING DIPRIVAN INJECTABLE EMULSION WAS ASSOCIATED WITH MICROBIAL CONTAMINATION OF THE PRODUCT AND WITH FEVER, INFECTION/SEPSIS, OTHER LIFE-THREATENING ILLNESS, AND/OR DEATH.

CLINICAL PHARMACOLOGY

General
DIPRIVAN Injectable Emulsion is an intravenous sedative-hypnotic agent for use in the induction and maintenance of anesthesia or sedation. Intravenous injection of a therapeutic dose of propofol produces hypnosis rapidly with minimal excitation, usually within 40 seconds from the start of an injection (the time for one arm-brain circulation). As with other rapidly acting intravenous anesthetic agents, the half-time of the blood-brain equilibration is approximately 1 to 3 minutes, and this accounts for the rapid induction of anesthesia.
Pharmacodynamics
Pharmacodynamic properties of propofol are dependent upon the therapeutic blood propofol concentrations. Steady state propofol blood concentrations are generally proportional to infusion rates, especially within an individual patient. Undesirable side effects such as cardiorespiratory depression are likely to occur at higher blood concentrations which result from bolus dosing or rapid increase in infusion rate. An adequate interval (3 to 5 minutes) must be allowed between clinical dosage adjustments in order to assess drug effects.
The hemodynamic effects of DIPRIVAN Injectable Emulsion during induction of anesthesia vary. If spontaneous ventilation is maintained, the major cardiovascular effects are arterial hypotension (sometimes greater than a 30% decrease) with little or no change in heart rate and no appreciable decrease in cardiac output. If ventilation is assisted or controlled (positive pressure ventilation), the degree and incidence of decrease in cardiac output are accentuated. Addition of a potent opioid (e.g., fentanyl) when used as a premedicant further decreases cardiac output and respiratory drive.
If anesthesia is continued by infusion of DIPRIVAN Injectable Emulsion, the stimulation of endotracheal intubation and surgery may return arterial pressure towards normal. However, cardiac output may remain depressed. Comparative clinical studies have shown that the hemodynamic effects of DIPRIVAN Injectable Emulsion during induction of anesthesia are generally more pronounced than with other IV induction agents traditionally used for this purpose.
Clinical and preclinical studies suggest that DIPRIVAN Injectable Emulsion is rarely associated with elevation of plasma histamine levels.
Induction of anesthesia with DIPRIVAN Injectable Emulsion is frequently associated with apnea in both adults and children. In 1573 adult patients who received DIPRIVAN Injectable Emulsion (2 to 2.5 mg/kg), apnea lasted less than 30 seconds in 7% of patients, 30-60 seconds in 24% of patients, and more than 60 seconds in 12% of patients. In the 213 pediatric patients between the ages of 3 and 12 years assessable for apnea who received DIPRIVAN Injectable Emulsion (1 to 3.6 mg/kg), apnea lasted less than 30 seconds

Continued on next page

Zeneca Pharmaceuticals—Cont.

in 12% of patients, 30-60 seconds in 10% of patients, and more than 60 seconds in 5% of patients.

During maintenance, DIPRIVAN Injectable Emulsion causes a decrease in ventilation usually associated with an increase in carbon dioxide tension which may be marked depending upon the rate of administration and other concurrent medications (e.g., opioids, sedatives, etc.).

During monitored anesthesia care (MAC) sedation, attention must be given to the cardiorespiratory effects of DIPRIVAN Injectable Emulsion. Hypotension, oxyhemoglobin desaturation, apnea, airway obstruction, and/or oxygen desaturation can occur, especially following a rapid bolus of DIPRIVAN Injectable Emulsion. During initiation of MAC sedation, slow infusion or slow injection techniques are preferable over rapid bolus administration, and during maintenance of MAC sedation, a variable rate infusion is preferable over intermittent bolus administration in order to minimize undesirable cardiorespiratory effects. In the elderly, debilitated, or ASA III/IV patients, rapid (single or repeated) bolus dose administration should not be used for MAC sedation. (See WARNINGS.) DIPRIVAN Injectable Emulsion is not recommended for MAC Sedation in children because safety and effectiveness have not been established.

Clinical studies in humans and studies in animals show that DIPRIVAN Injectable Emulsion does not suppress the adrenal response to ACTH. Preliminary findings in patients with normal intraocular pressure indicate that DIPRIVAN Injectable Emulsion anesthesia produces a decrease in intraocular pressure which may be associated with a concomitant decrease in systemic vascular resistance.

Animal studies and limited experience in susceptible patients have not indicated any propensity of DIPRIVAN Injectable Emulsion to induce malignant hyperthermia.

Studies to date indicate that DIPRIVAN Injectable Emulsion when used in combination with hypocarbia increases cerebrovascular resistance and decreases cerebral blood flow, cerebral metabolic oxygen consumption, and intracranial pressure. DIPRIVAN Injectable Emulsion does not affect cerebrovascular reactivity to changes in arterial carbon dioxide tension. (see Clinical Trials—Neuroanesthesia).

Hemosiderin deposits have been observed in the livers of dogs receiving DIPRIVAN Injectable Emulsion containing 0.005% disodium edetate over a four week period; the clinical significance is unknown.

Pharmacokinetics

The proper use of DIPRIVAN Injectable Emulsion requires an understanding of the disposition and elimination characteristics of propofol.

The pharmacokinetics of propofol are well described by a three compartment linear model with compartments representing the plasma, rapidly equilibrating tissues, and slowly equilibrating tissues.

Following an IV bolus dose, there is rapid equilibration between the plasma and the highly perfused tissue of the brain, thus accounting for the rapid onset of anesthesia. Plasma levels initially decline rapidly as a result of both rapid distribution and high metabolic clearance. Distribution accounts for about half of this decline following a bolus of propofol. However, distribution is not constant over time, but decreases as body tissues equilibrate with plasma and become saturated. The rate at which equilibration occurs is a function of the rate and duration of the infusion. When equilibration occurs there is no longer a net transfer of propofol between tissues and plasma.

Discontinuation of the recommended doses of DIPRIVAN Injectable Emulsion after the maintenance of anesthesia for approximately one-hour, or for sedation in the ICU for one-day, results in a prompt decrease in blood propofol concentrations and rapid awakening. Longer infusions (10 days of ICU sedation) result in accumulation of significant tissue stores of propofol, such that the reduction in circulating propofol is slowed and the time to awakening is increased.

By daily titration of DIPRIVAN Injectable Emulsion dosage to achieve only the minimum effective therapeutic concentration, rapid awakening within 10 to 15 minutes will occur even after long term administration. If, however, higher than necessary infusion levels have been maintained for a long time, propofol will be redistributed from fat and muscle to the plasma, and this return of propofol from peripheral tissues will slow recovery.

The figure below illustrates the fall of plasma propofol levels following ICU sedation infusions of various durations.

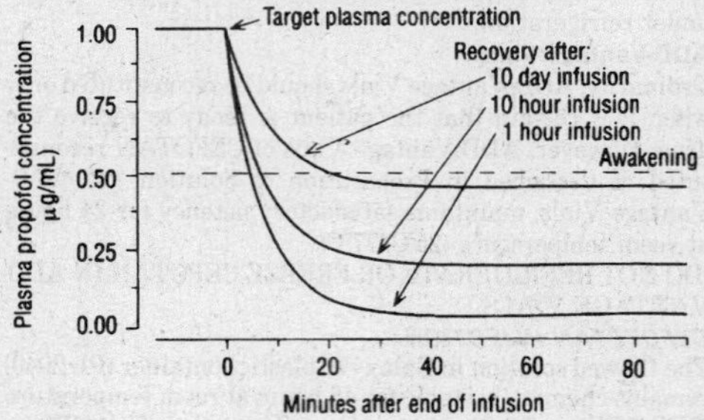

The large contribution of distribution (about 50%) to the fall of propofol plasma levels following brief infusions means that after very long infusions (at steady state), about half the initial rate will maintain the same plasma levels. Failure to reduce the infusion rate in patients receiving DIPRIVAN Injectable Emulsion for extended periods may result in excessively high blood concentrations of the drug. Thus, titration to clinical response and daily evaluation of sedation levels are important during use of DIPRIVAN Injectable Emulsion infusion for ICU sedation, especially of long duration.

Adults: Propofol clearance ranges from 23-50 mL/kg/min (1.6 to 3.4 L/min in 70 kg adults). It is chiefly eliminated by hepatic conjugation to inactive metabolites which are excreted by the kidney. A glucuronide conjugate accounts for about 50% of the administered dose. Propofol has a steady state volume of distribution (10-day infusion) approaching 60 L/kg in healthy adults. A difference in pharmacokinetics due to gender has not been observed. The terminal half-life of propofol after a 10-day infusion is 1 to 3 days.

Geriatrics: With increasing patient age, the dose of propofol needed to achieve a defined anesthetic endpoint (dose-requirement) decreases. This does not appear to be an age-related change of pharmacodynamics or brain sensitivity, as measured by EEG burst suppression. With increasing patient age pharmacokinetic changes are such that for a given IV bolus dose, higher peak plasma concentrations occur, which can explain the decreased dose requirement. These higher peak plasma concentrations in the elderly can predispose patients to cardiorespiratory effects including hypotension, apnea, airway obstruction and/or oxygen desaturation. The higher plasma levels reflect an age-related decrease in volume of distribution and reduced intercompartmental clearance. Lower doses are thus recommended for initiation and maintenance of sedation/anesthesia in elderly patients. (See CLINICAL PHARMACOLOGY—Individualization of Dosage.)

Pediatrics: The pharmacokinetics of propofol were studied in 53 children between the ages of 3 and 12 years who received DIPRIVAN Injectable Emulsion for periods of approximately 1–2 hours. The observed distribution and clearance of propofol in these children was similar to adults.

Organ Failure: The pharmacokinetics of propofol do not appear to be different in people with chronic hepatic cirrhosis or chronic renal impairment compared to adults with normal hepatic and renal function. The effects of acute hepatic or renal failure on the pharmacokinetics of propofol have not been studied.

Clinical Trials

Anesthesia and Monitored Anesthesia Care (MAC) Sedation

DIPRIVAN Injectable Emulsion was compared to intravenous and inhalational anesthetic or sedative agents in 91 trials involving a total of 5,135 patients. Of these 3,354 received DIPRIVAN Injectable Emulsion and comprised the overall safety database for anesthesia and MAC sedation. Fifty-five of these trials, 20 for anesthesia induction and 35 for induction and maintenance of anesthesia or MAC sedation, were carried out in the US or Canada and provided the basis for dosage recommendations and the adverse event profile during anesthesia or MAC sedation.

Pediatric Anesthesia

DIPRIVAN Injectable Emulsion was compared to standard anesthetic agents in 12 clinical trials involving 534 patients receiving DIPRIVAN Injectable Emulsion. Of these, 349 were from US/Canadian clinical trials and comprised the overall safety database for Pediatric Anesthesia.

TABLE 1. PEDIATRIC ANESTHESIA CLINICAL TRIALS
Patients Receiving DIPRIVAN Injectable Emulsion
Median and (Range)

	Induction Only	Induction and Maintenance
Number of Patients*	243	105
Induction Bolus Dosages	2.5 mg/kg (1–3.5)	3 mg/kg (2–3.6)
Injection Duration	20 sec (6–45)	
Maintenance Dosage	—	181 µg/kg/min (107–418)
Maintenance Duration	—	78 min (29–268)

*Body weight not recorded for one patient.

Neuroanesthesia

DIPRIVAN Injectable Emulsion was studied in 50 patients undergoing craniotomy for supratentorial tumors in two clinical trials. The mean lesion size (anterior/posterior and lateral) was 31 mm and 32 mm in one trial and 55 mm and 42 mm in the other trial respectively. [See Table 2 below.]

In ten of these patients, DIPRIVAN Injectable Emulsion was administered by infusion in a controlled clinical trial to evaluate the effect of DIPRIVAN Injectable Emulsion on cerebrospinal fluid pressure (CSFP). The mean arterial pressure was maintained relatively constant over 25 minutes with a change from baseline of -4% ± 17% (mean ± SD), whereas the percent change in cerebrospinal fluid pressure (CSFP) was -46% ± 14%. As CSFP is an indirect measure of intracranial pressure (ICP), when given by infusion or slow bolus, DIPRIVAN Injectable Emulsion, in combination with hypocarbia, is capable of decreasing ICP independent of changes in arterial pressure.

TABLE 2. NEUROANESTHESIA CLINICAL TRIALS
Patients Receiving DIPRIVAN Injectable Emulsion Median and (Range)

Patient Type	No. of Patients	Induction Bolus Dosages (mg/kg)	Maintenance Dosage (µg/kg/min)	Maintenance Duration (min)
Craniotomy patients	50	1.36 (0.9–6.9)	146 (68–425)	285 (48–622)

Intensive Care Unit (ICU) Sedation

DIPRIVAN Injectable Emulsion was compared to benzodiazepines and/or opioids in 14 clinical trials involving a total of 550 ICU patients. Of these, 302 received DIPRIVAN Injectable Emulsion and comprise the overall safety database for ICU sedation. Six of these studies were carried out in the US or Canada and provide the basis for dosage recommendations and the adverse event profile.

Information from 193 literature reports of DIPRIVAN Injectable Emulsion used for ICU sedation in over 950 patients and information from the clinical trials are summarized below: [See Table 3 at top of next page.]

Cardiac Anesthesia

DIPRIVAN Injectable Emulsion was evaluated in 5 clinical trials conducted in the US and Canada, involving a total of 569 patients undergoing coronary artery bypass graft (CABG). Of these, 301 patients received DIPRIVAN Injectable Emulsion. They comprise the safety database for cardiac anesthesia and provide the basis for dosage recommendations in this patient population, in conjunction with reports in the published literature.

Individualization of Dosage

General: STRICT ASEPTIC TECHNIQUE MUST ALWAYS BE MAINTAINED DURING HANDLING. DIPRIVAN INJECTABLE EMULSION IS A SINGLE-USE PARENTERAL PRODUCT WHICH CONTAINS 0.005% DISODIUM EDETATE TO RETARD THE RATE OF GROWTH OF MICROORGANISMS IN THE EVENT OF ACCIDENTAL EXTRINSIC CONTAMINATION. HOWEVER, DIPRIVAN INJECTABLE EMULSION CAN STILL SUPPORT THE GROWTH OF MICROORGANISMS AS IT IS NOT AN ANTIMICROBIALLY PRESERVED PRODUCT UNDER USP STANDARDS. ACCORDINGLY, STRICT ASEPTIC TECHNIQUE MUST STILL BE ADHERED TO. DO NOT USE IF CONTAMINATION IS SUSPECTED. DISCARD UNUSED PORTIONS AS DIRECTED WITHIN THE REQUIRED TIME LIMITS (SEE DOSAGE AND ADMINISTRATION, HANDLING PROCEDURES). THERE HAVE BEEN REPORTS IN WHICH FAILURE TO USE ASEPTIC TECHNIQUE WHEN HANDLING DIPRIVAN INJECTABLE EMULSION WAS ASSOCIATED WITH MICROBIAL CONTAMINATION OF THE PRODUCT AND WITH FEVER, INFECTION/SEPSIS, OTHER LIFE-THREATENING ILLNESS, AND/OR DEATH.

Propofol blood concentrations at steady state are generally proportional to infusion rates, especially in individual patients. Undesirable effects such as cardiorespiratory depression are likely to occur at higher blood concentrations which result from bolus dosing or rapid increases in the infusion rate. An adequate interval (3 to 5 minutes) must be allowed between clinical dosage adjustments in order to assess drug effects.

When administering DIPRIVAN Injectable Emulsion by infusion, syringe pumps or volumetric pumps are recommended to provide controlled infusion rates. When infusing DIPRIVAN Injectable Emulsion to patients undergoing magnetic resonance imaging, metered control devices may be utilized if mechanical pumps are impractical.

Changes in vital signs (increases in pulse rate, blood pressure, sweating and/or tearing) that indicate a response to surgical stimulation or lightening of anesthesia may be controlled by the administration of DIPRIVAN Injectable Emulsion 25 mg (2.5 mL) to 50 mg (5 mL) incremental boluses and/or by increasing the infusion rate.

For minor surgical procedures (e.g., body surface) nitrous oxide (60%-70%) can be combined with a variable rate DIPRIVAN Injectable Emulsion infusion to provide satisfactory anesthesia. With more stimulating surgical procedures (e.g., intra-abdominal), or if supplementation with nitrous oxide is not provided, administration rate(s) of DIPRIVAN Injectable Emulsion and/or opioids should be increased in order to provide adequate anesthesia.
Infusion rates should always be titrated downward in the absence of clinical signs of light anesthesia until a mild response to surgical stimulation is obtained in order to avoid administration of DIPRIVAN Injectable Emulsion at rates higher than are clinically necessary. Generally, rates of 50 to 100 μg/kg/min in adults, should be achieved during maintenance in order to optimize recovery times.
Other drugs that cause CNS depression (hypnotics/sedatives, inhalational anesthetics, and opioids) can increase CNS depression induced by propofol. Morphine premedication (0.15 mg/kg) with nitrous oxide 67% in oxygen has been shown to decrease the necessary propofol injection maintenance infusion rate and therapeutic blood concentrations when compared to nonnarcotic (lorazepam) premedication.

Induction of General Anesthesia:

Adult Patients: Most adult patients under 55 years of age and classified ASA I/II require 2 to 2.5 mg/kg of DIPRIVAN Injectable Emulsion for induction when unpremedicated or when premedicated with oral benzodiazepines or intramuscular opioids. For induction, DIPRIVAN Injectable Emulsion should be titrated (approximately 40 mg every 10 seconds) against the response of the patient until the clinical signs show the onset of anesthesia. As with other sedative-hypnotic agents, the amount of intravenous opioid and/or benzodiazepine premedication will influence the response of the patient to an induction dose of DIPRIVAN Injectable Emulsion.

Elderly, Debilitated, or ASA III/IV Patients: It is important to be familiar and experienced with the intravenous use of DIPRIVAN Injectable Emulsion before treating elderly, debilitated, or ASA III/IV patients. Due to the reduced clearance and higher blood concentrations, most of these patients require approximately 1 to 1.5 mg/kg (approximately 20 mg every 10 seconds) of DIPRIVAN Injectable Emulsion for induction of anesthesia according to their condition and responses. A rapid bolus should not be used, as this will increase the likelihood of undesirable cardiorespiratory depression including hypotension, apnea, airway obstruction, and/or oxygen desaturation. (See DOSAGE AND ADMINISTRATION.)

Neurosurgical Patients: Slower induction is recommended using boluses of 20 mg every 10 seconds. Slower boluses or infusions of DIPRIVAN Injectable Emulsion for induction of anesthesia, titrated to clinical responses, will generally result in reduced induction dosage requirements (1 to 2 mg/kg). (See PRECAUTIONS and DOSAGE AND ADMINISTRATION.)

Cardiac Anesthesia: DIPRIVAN Injectable Emulsion has been well-studied in patients with coronary artery disease, but experience in patients with hemodynamically significant valvular or congenital heart disease is limited. As with other anesthetic and sedative-hypnotic agents, DIPRIVAN Injectable Emulsion in healthy patients causes a decrease in blood pressure that is secondary to decreases in preload (ventricular filling volume at the end of the diastole) and afterload (arterial resistance at the beginning of the systole). The magnitude of these changes is proportional to the blood and effect site concentrations achieved. These concentrations depend upon the dose and speed of the induction and maintenance infusion rates.
In addition, lower heart rates are observed during maintenance with DIPRIVAN Injectable Emulsion, possibly due to reduction of the sympathetic activity and/or resetting of the baroreceptor reflexes. Therefore, anticholinergic agents should be administered when increases in vagal tone are anticipated.

TABLE 3. ICU SEDATION CLINICAL TRIALS AND LITERATURE
Patients receiving DIPRIVAN Injectable Emulsion Median and (Range)

ICU Patient Type	Number of Patients: Trials	Number of Patients: Literature	Sedation Dose: μg/kg/min	Sedation Dose: mg/kg/h	Sedation Duration: Hours
Post-CABG	41	—	11	0.66	10
			(0.1–30)	(0.006–1.8)	(2–14)
	—	334	(5–100)	(0.3–6)	(4–24)
Post-Surgical	60	—	20	1.2	18
			(6–53)	(0.4–3.2)	(0.3–187)
	—	142	(23–82)	(1.4–4.9)	(6–96)
Neuro/Head Trauma	7	—	25	1.5	168
			(13–37)	(0.8–2.2)	(112–282)
	—	184	(8.3–87)	(0.5–5.2)	(8 hr–5 days)
Medical	49	—	41	2.5	72
			(9–131)	(0.5–7.9)	(0.4–337)
	—	76	(3.3–62)	(0.2–3.7)	(4–96)
Special Patients					
ARDS/Resp. Failure	—	56	(10–142)	(0.6–8.5)	(1 hr–8 days)
COPD/Asthma	—	49	(17–75)	(1–4.5)	(1–8 days)
Status Epilepticus	—	15	(25–167)	(1.5–10)	(1–21 days)
Tetanus	—	11	(5–100)	(0.3–6)	(1–25 days)

Trials (Individual patients from clinical studies)
Literature (Individual patients from published reports)
CABG (Coronary Artery Bypass Graft)
ARDS (Adult Respiratory Distress Syndrome)

As with other anesthetic agents, DIPRIVAN Injectable Emulsion reduces myocardial oxygen consumption. Further studies are needed to confirm and delineate the extent of these effects on the myocardium and the coronary vascular system.
Morphine premedication (0.15 mg/kg) with nitrous oxide 67% in oxygen has been shown to decrease the necessary DIPRIVAN Injectable Emulsion maintenance infusion rates and therapeutic blood concentrations when compared to nonnarcotic (lorazepam) premedication. The rate of DIPRIVAN Injectable Emulsion administration should be determined based on the patient's premedication and adjusted according to clinical responses.
A rapid bolus induction should be avoided. A slow rate of approximately 20 mg every 10 seconds until induction onset (0.5 to 1.5 mg/kg) should be used. In order to assure adequate anesthesia, when DIPRIVAN Injectable Emulsion is used as the primary agent, maintenance infusion rates should not be less than 100 μg/kg/min and should be supplemented with analgesic levels of continuous opioid administration. When an opioid is used as the primary agent, DIPRIVAN Injectable Emulsion maintenance rates should not be less than 50 μg/kg/min, and care should be taken to ensure amnesia with concomitant benzodiazepines. Higher doses of DIPRIVAN Injectable Emulsion will reduce the opioid requirements (see Table 4). When DIPRIVAN Injectable Emulsion is used as the primary anesthetic, it should not be administered with the high-dose opioid technique as this may increase the likelihood of hypotension (see PRECAUTIONS - Cardiac Anesthesia).
[See Table 4 below.]

Maintenance of General Anesthesia

In adults, anesthesia can be maintained by administering DIPRIVAN Injectable Emulsion by infusion or intermittent IV bolus injection. The patient's clinical response will determine the infusion rate or the amount and frequency of incremental injections.

Continuous Infusion: DIPRIVAN Injectable Emulsion 100 to 200 μg/kg/min administered in a variable rate infusion with 60%-70% nitrous oxide and oxygen provides anesthesia for patients undergoing general surgery. Maintenance by infusion of DIPRIVAN Injectable Emulsion should immediately follow the induction dose in order to provide satisfactory or continuous anesthesia during the induction phase. During this initial period following the induction dose, higher rates of infusion are generally required (150 to 200 μg/kg/min) for the first 10 to 15 minutes. Infusion rates should subsequently be decreased 30%-50% during the first half-hour of maintenance.
Other drugs that cause CNS depression (hypnotics/sedatives, inhalational anesthetics, and opioids) can increase the CNS depression induced by propofol.

Intermittent Bolus: Increments of DIPRIVAN Injectable Emulsion 25 mg (2.5 mL) to 50 mg (5 mL) may be administered with nitrous oxide in adult patients undergoing general surgery. The incremental boluses should be administered when changes in vital signs indicate a response to surgical stimulation or light anesthesia.
DIPRIVAN Injectable Emulsion has been used with a variety of agents commonly used in anesthesia such as atropine, scopolamine, glycopyrrolate, diazepam, depolarizing and nondepolarizing muscle relaxants, and opioid analgesics, as well as with inhalational and regional anesthetic agents.
In the elderly, debilitated, or ASA III/IV patients, rapid bolus doses should not be used, as this will increase cardiorespiratory effects including hypotension, apnea, airway obstruction, and/or oxygen desaturation.

Pediatric Anesthesia:

Induction of General Anesthesia: Most pediatric patients 3 years of age or older and classified ASA I or II require 2.5 to 3.5 mg/kg of DIPRIVAN Injectable Emulsion for induction when unpremedicated or when lightly premedicated with oral benzodiazepines or intramuscular opioids. Within this dosage range, younger children may require larger induction doses than older children. As with other sedative-hypnotic agents, the amount of intravenous opioid and/or benzodiazepine premedication will influence the response of the patient to an induction dose of DIPRIVAN Injectable Emulsion. In addition, a lower dosage is recommended for children classified ASA III or IV. Attention should be paid to minimize pain on injection when administering DIPRIVAN Injectable Emulsion to pediatric patients. Rapid boluses of DIPRIVAN Injectable Emulsion may be administered if small veins are pretreated with lidocaine or when antecubital or larger veins are utilized (See PRECAUTIONS—General).
DIPRIVAN Injectable Emulsion administered in a variable rate infusion with nitrous oxide 60%-70% provides satisfactory anesthesia for most pediatric patients 3 years of age or older, ASA I or II, undergoing general anesthesia.

Maintenance of General Anesthesia: Maintenance by infusion of DIPRIVAN Injectable Emulsion at a rate of 200–300 μg/kg/min should immediately follow the induction dose. Following the first half-hour of maintenance, if clinical signs of light anesthesia are not present, the infusion rate should be decreased; during this period, infusion rates of 125–150 μg/kg/min are typically needed. However, younger children (5 years of age or less) may require larger maintenance infusion rates than older children.

Monitored Anesthesia Care (MAC) Sedation in Adults: When DIPRIVAN Injectable Emulsion is administered for MAC sedation, rates of administration should be individualized and titrated to clinical response. In most patients, the rates of DIPRIVAN Injectable Emulsion administration will be in the range of 25–75 μg/kg/min.
During initiation of MAC sedation, slow infusion or slow injection techniques are preferable over rapid bolus administration. During maintenance of MAC sedation, a variable rate infusion is preferable over intermittent bolus dose administration. In the elderly, debilitated, or ASA III/IV patients, rapid (single or repeated) bolus dose administration

Continued on next page

Table 4. Cardiac Anesthesia Techniques

Primary Agent	Rate	Secondary Agent/Rate
		(Following Induction with Primary Agent)
Diprivan Injectable Emulsion		OPIOID[a]/0.05–0.075 μg/kg/min (no bolus)
Preinduction anxiolysis	25 μg/kg/min	
Induction	0.5–1.5 mg/kg over 60 sec	
Maintenance (Titrated to Clinical Response)	100–150 μg/kg/min	
OPIOID[b]		Diprivan Injectable Emulsion/50–100 μg/kg/min (no bolus)
Induction	25–50 μg/kg	
Maintenance	0.2–0.3 μg/kg/min	

[a] OPIOID is defined in terms of fentanyl equivalents, i.e.,
1 μg of fentanyl = 5 μg of alfentanil (for bolus)
= 10 μg of alfentanil (for maintenance)
or
= 0.1 μg of sufentanil
[b] Care should be taken to ensure amnesia with concomitant benzodiazepine therapy

Zeneca Pharmaceuticals—Cont.

should not be used for MAC sedation. (See WARNINGS.) **A rapid bolus injection can result in undesirable cardiorespiratory depression including hypotension, apnea, airway obstruction, and/or oxygen desaturation.**

Initiation of MAC Sedation: For initiation of MAC sedation, either an infusion or a slow injection method may be utilized while closely monitoring cardiorespiratory function. With the infusion method, sedation may be initiated by infusing DIPRIVAN Injectable Emulsion at 100 to 150 µg/kg/min (6 to 9 mg/kg/h) for a period of 3 to 5 minutes and titrating to the desired level of sedation while closely monitoring respiratory function. With the slow injection method for initiation, patients will require approximately 0.5 mg/kg administered over 3 to 5 minutes and titrated to clinical responses. When DIPRIVAN Injectable Emulsion is administered slowly over 3 to 5 minutes, most patients will be adequately sedated and the peak drug effect can be achieved while minimizing undesirable cardiorespiratory effects occurring at high plasma levels.

In the elderly, debilitated, or ASA III/IV patients, rapid (single or repeated) bolus dose administration should not be used for MAC sedation. (See WARNINGS.) The rate of administration should be over 3–5 minutes and the dosage of DIPRIVAN Injectable Emulsion should be reduced to approximately 80% of the usual adult dosage in these patients according to their condition, responses, and changes in vital signs. (See DOSAGE AND ADMINISTRATION.)

Maintenance of MAC Sedation: For maintenance of sedation, a variable rate infusion method is preferable over an intermittent bolus dose method. With the variable rate infusion method, patients will generally require maintenance rates of 25 to 75 µg/kg/min (1.5 to 4.5 mg/kg/h) during the first 10 to 15 minutes of sedation maintenance. Infusion rates should subsequently be decreased over time to 25 to 50 µg/kg/min and adjusted to clinical responses. In titrating to clinical effect, allow approximately 2 minutes for onset of peak drug effect.

Infusion rates should always be titrated downward in the absence of clinical signs of light sedation until mild responses to stimulation are obtained in order to avoid sedative administration of DIPRIVAN Injectable Emulsion at rates higher than are clinically necessary.

If the intermittent bolus dose method is used, increments of DIPRIVAN Injectable Emulsion 10 mg (1 mL) or 20 mg (2 mL) can be administered and titrated to desired level of sedation. With the intermittent bolus method of sedation maintenance there is the potential for respiratory depression, transient increases in sedation depth, and/or prolongation of recovery.

In the elderly, debilitated, or ASA III/IV patients, rapid (single or repeated) bolus dose administration should not be used for MAC sedation. (See WARNINGS.) The rate of administration and the dosage of DIPRIVAN Injectable Emulsion should be reduced to approximately 80% of the usual adult dosage in these patients according to their condition, responses, and changes in vital signs. (See DOSAGE AND ADMINISTRATION.)

DIPRIVAN Injectable Emulsion can be administered as the sole agent for maintenance of MAC sedation during surgical/diagnostic procedures. When DIPRIVAN Injectable Emulsion sedation is supplemented with opioid and/or benzodiazepine medications, these agents increase the sedative and respiratory effects of DIPRIVAN Injectable Emulsion and may also result in a slower recovery profile. (See PRECAUTIONS, Drug Interactions.)

ICU Sedation: (See WARNINGS and DOSAGE AND ADMINISTRATION, Handling Procedures.) For intubated, mechanically ventilated adult patients, Intensive Care Unit (ICU) sedation should be initiated slowly with a continuous infusion in order to titrate to desired clinical effect and minimize hypotension. (See DOSAGE AND ADMINISTRATION.)

Across all 6 US/Canadian clinical studies, the mean infusion maintenance rate for all DIPRIVAN Injectable Emulsion patients was 27 ± 21 µg/kg/min. The maintenance infusion rates required to maintain adequate sedation ranged from 2.8 µg/kg/min to 130 µg/kg/min. The infusion rate was lower in patients over 55 years of age (approximately 20 µg/kg/min) compared to patients under 55 years of age (approximately 38 µg/kg/min). In these studies, morphine or fentanyl was used as needed for analgesia.

Most adult ICU patients recovering from the effects of general anesthesia or deep sedation will require maintenance rates of 5 to 50 µg/kg/min (0.3 to 3 mg/kg/h) individualized and titrated to clinical response. (See DOSAGE AND ADMINISTRATION.) With medical ICU patients or patients who have recovered from the effects of general anesthesia or deep sedation, the rate of administration of 50 µg/kg/min or higher may be required to achieve adequate sedation. These higher rates of administration may increase the likelihood of patients developing hypotension.

Although there are reports of reduced analgesic requirements, most patients received opioids for analgesia during maintenance of ICU sedation. Some patients also received benzodiazepines and/or neuromuscular blocking agents. During long-term maintenance of sedation, some ICU patients were awakened once or twice every 24 hours for assessment of neurologic or respiratory function. (See Clinical Trials, Table 3.)

In post-CABG (coronary artery bypass graft) patients, the maintenance rate of propofol administration was usually low (median 11 µg/kg/min) due to the intraoperative administration of high opioid doses. Patients receiving DIPRIVAN Injectable Emulsion required 35% less nitroprusside than midazolam patients; this difference was statistically significant (P < 0.05). During initiation of sedation in Post-CABG patients, a 15% to 20% decrease in blood pressure was seen in the first 60 minutes. It was not possible to determine cardiovascular effects in patients with severely compromised ventricular function (See Clinical Trials, Table 3).

In Medical or Postsurgical ICU studies comparing DIPRIVAN Injectable Emulsion to benzodiazepine infusion or bolus, there were no apparent differences in maintenance of adequate sedation, mean arterial pressure, or laboratory findings. Like the comparators, DIPRIVAN Injectable Emulsion reduced blood cortisol during sedation while maintaining responsivity to challenges with adrenocorticotropic hormone (ACTH). Case reports from the published literature generally reflect that DIPRIVAN Injectable Emulsion has been used safely in patients with a history of porphyria or malignant hyperthermia.

In hemodynamically stable head trauma patients ranging in age from 19-43 years, adequate sedation was maintained with DIPRIVAN Injectable Emulsion or morphine (N=7 in each group). There were no apparent differences in adequacy of sedation, intracranial pressure, cerebral perfusion pressure, or neurologic recovery between the treatment groups. In literature reports from Neurosurgical ICU and severely head-injured patients DIPRIVAN Injectable Emulsion infusion with or without diuretics and hyperventilation controlled intracranial pressure while maintaining cerebral perfusion pressure. In some patients, bolus doses resulted in decreased blood pressure and compromised cerebral perfusion pressure. (See Clinical Trials, Table 3.)

DIPRIVAN Injectable Emulsion was found to be effective in status epilepticus which was refractory to the standard anticonvulsant therapies. For these patients as well as for ARDS/respiratory failure and tetanus patients, sedation maintenance dosages were generally higher than those for other critically ill patient populations. (See Clinical Trials, Table 3.)

Abrupt discontinuation of DIPRIVAN Injectable Emulsion prior to weaning or for daily evaluation of sedation levels should be avoided. This may result in rapid awakening with associated anxiety, agitation, and resistance to mechanical ventilation. Infusions of DIPRIVAN Injectable Emulsion should be adjusted to maintain a light level of sedation through the weaning process or evaluation of sedation level. (See PRECAUTIONS.)

INDICATIONS AND USAGE

DIPRIVAN Injectable Emulsion is an IV sedative-hypnotic agent that can be used for both induction and/or maintenance of anesthesia as part of a balanced anesthetic technique for inpatient and outpatient surgery in adults and in children 3 years of age or older.

DIPRIVAN Injectable Emulsion, when administered intravenously as directed, can be used to initiate and maintain monitored anesthesia care (MAC) sedation during diagnostic procedures in adults. DIPRIVAN Injectable Emulsion may also be used for MAC sedation in conjunction with local/regional anesthesia in patients undergoing surgical procedures. (See PRECAUTIONS.)

DIPRIVAN Injectable Emulsion should only be administered to intubated, mechanically ventilated adult patients in the Intensive Care Unit (ICU) to provide continuous sedation and control of stress responses. In this setting, DIPRIVAN Injectable Emulsion should be administered only by persons skilled in the medical management of critically ill patients and trained in cardiovascular resuscitation and airway management.

DIPRIVAN Injectable Emulsion is not recommended for obstetrics, including cesarean section deliveries. DIPRIVAN Injectable Emulsion crosses the placenta, and as with other general anesthetic agents, the administration of DIPRIVAN Injectable Emulsion may be associated with neonatal depression. (See PRECAUTIONS.)

DIPRIVAN Injectable Emulsion is not recommended for use in nursing mothers because DIPRIVAN Injectable Emulsion has been reported to be excreted in human milk and the effects of oral absorption of small amounts of propofol are not known. (See PRECAUTIONS.)

DIPRIVAN Injectable Emulsion is not recommended for anesthesia in children below the age of 3 years because safety and effectiveness have not been established. DIPRIVAN Injectable Emulsion is not recommended for MAC sedation in children because safety and effectiveness

have not been established. DIPRIVAN Injectable Emulsion is not recommended for pediatric ICU sedation because safety and effectiveness have not been established.

CONTRAINDICATIONS

DIPRIVAN Injectable Emulsion is contraindicated in patients with a known hypersensitivity to DIPRIVAN Injectable Emulsion or its components, or when general anesthesia or sedation are contraindicated.

WARNINGS

For general anesthesia or monitored anesthesia care (MAC) sedation, DIPRIVAN Injectable Emulsion should be administered only by persons trained in the administration of general anesthesia and not involved in the conduct of the surgical/diagnostic procedure. Patients should be continuously monitored, and facilities for maintenance of a patent airway, artificial ventilation, and oxygen enrichment and circulatory resuscitation must be immediately available.

For sedation of intubated, mechanically ventilated adult patients in the Intensive Care Unit (ICU), DIPRIVAN Injectable Emulsion should be administered only by persons skilled in the management of critically ill patients and trained in cardiovascular resuscitation and airway management.

In the elderly, debilitated, or ASA III/IV patients, rapid (single or repeated) bolus administration should not be used during general anesthesia or MAC sedation in order to minimize undesirable cardiorespiratory depression, including hypotension, apnea, airway obstruction, and/or oxygen desaturation.

MAC sedation patients should be continuously monitored by persons not involved in the conduct of the surgical or diagnostic procedure; oxygen supplementation should be immediately available and provided where clinically indicated; and oxygen saturation should be monitored in all patients. Patients should be continuously monitored for early signs of hypotension, apnea, airway obstruction, and/or oxygen desaturation. These cardiorespiratory effects are more likely to occur following rapid initiation (loading) boluses or during supplemental maintenance boluses, especially in the elderly, debilitated, or ASA III/IV patients.

DIPRIVAN Injectable Emulsion should not be coadministered through the same IV catheter with blood or plasma because compatibility has not been established. *In vitro* tests have shown that aggregates of the globular component of the emulsion vehicle have occurred with blood/plasma/serum from humans and animals. The clinical significance is not known.

STRICT ASEPTIC TECHNIQUE MUST ALWAYS BE MAINTAINED DURING HANDLING. DIPRIVAN INJECTABLE EMULSION IS A SINGLE-USE PARENTERAL PRODUCT WHICH CONTAINS 0.005% DISODIUM EDETATE TO RETARD THE RATE OF GROWTH OF MICROORGANISMS IN THE EVENT OF ACCIDENTAL EXTRINSIC CONTAMINATION. HOWEVER, DIPRIVAN INJECTABLE EMULSION CAN STILL SUPPORT THE GROWTH OF MICROORGANISMS AS IT IS NOT AN ANTIMICROBIALLY PRESERVED PRODUCT UNDER USP STANDARDS. ACCORDINGLY, STRICT ASEPTIC TECHNIQUE MUST STILL BE ADHERED TO. DO NOT USE IF CONTAMINATION IS SUSPECTED. DISCARD UNUSED PORTIONS AS DIRECTED WITHIN THE REQUIRED TIME LIMITS (SEE DOSAGE AND ADMINISTRATION, HANDLING PROCEDURES). THERE HAVE BEEN REPORTS IN WHICH FAILURE TO USE ASEPTIC TECHNIQUE WHEN HANDLING DIPRIVAN INJECTABLE EMULSION WAS ASSOCIATED WITH MICROBIAL CONTAMINATION OF THE PRODUCT AND WITH FEVER, INFECTION/SEPSIS, OTHER LIFE-THREATENING ILLNESS, AND/OR DEATH.

PRECAUTIONS

General: A lower induction dose and a slower maintenance rate of administration should be used in elderly, debilitated, or ASA III/IV patients. (See CLINICAL PHARMACOLOGY —Individualization of Dosage.) Patients should be continuously monitored for early signs of significant hypotension and/or bradycardia. Treatment may include increasing the rate of intravenous fluid, elevation of lower extremities, use of pressor agents, or administration of atropine. Apnea often occurs during induction and may persist for more than 60 seconds. Ventilatory support may be required. Because DIPRIVAN Injectable Emulsion is an emulsion, caution should be exercised in patients with disorders of lipid metabolism such as primary hyperlipoproteinemia, diabetic hyperlipemia, and pancreatitis.

The clinical criteria for discharge from the recovery/day surgery area established for each institution should be satisfied before discharge of the patient from the care of the anesthesiologist.

When DIPRIVAN Injectable Emulsion is administered to an epileptic patient, there may be a risk of seizure during the recovery phase.

In adults and children, attention should be paid to minimize pain on administration of DIPRIVAN Injectable Emulsion. Transient local pain can be minimized if the larger veins of the forearm or antecubital fossa are used. Pain during intravenous injection may also be reduced by prior injection of IV

lidocaine (1 mL of a 1% solution). Pain on injection occurred frequently in pediatric patients (45%) when a small vein of the hand was utilized without lidocaine pretreatment. With lidocaine pretreatment or when antecubital veins were utilized, pain was minimal (incidence less than 10%) and well tolerated.

Venous sequelae (phlebitis or thrombosis) have been reported rarely (<1%). In two well-controlled clinical studies using dedicated intravenous catheters, no instances of venous sequelae were observed up to 14 days following induction.

Intra-arterial Injection in animals did not induce local tissue effects. Accidental intra-arterial injection has been reported in patients, and, other than pain, there were no major sequelae.

Intentional Injection into subcutaneous or perivascular tissues of animals caused minimal tissue reaction. During the post-marketing period, there have been rare reports of local pain, swelling, blisters, and/or tissue necrosis following accidental extravasation of DIPRIVAN Injectable Emulsion. Perioperative myoclonia, rarely including convulsions and opisthotonos, has occurred in temporal relationship in cases in which DIPRIVAN Injectable Emulsion has been administered.

Clinical features of anaphylaxis, which may include angioedema, bronchospasm, erythema, and hypotension, occur rarely following DIPRIVAN Injectable Emulsion administration, although use of other drugs in most instances makes the relationship to DIPRIVAN Injectable Emulsion unclear. There have been rare reports of pulmonary edema in temporal relationship to the administration of DIPRIVAN Injectable Emulsion, although a causal relationship is unknown.

DIPRIVAN Injectable Emulsion has no vagolytic activity. Reports of bradycardia, asystole, and rarely, cardiac arrest have been associated with DIPRIVAN Injectable Emulsion. The intravenous administration of anticholinergic agents (e.g., atropine or glycopyrrolate) should be considered to modify potential increases in vagal tone due to concomitant agents (e.g., succinylcholine) or surgical stimuli.

Intensive Care Unit Sedation: (See WARNINGS and DOSAGE AND ADMINISTRATION, Handling Procedures.)
The administration of DIPRIVAN Injectable Emulsion should be initiated as a continuous infusion and changes in the rate of administration made slowly (>5 min) in order to minimize hypotension and avoid acute overdosage. (See CLINICAL PHARMACOLOGY—Individualization of Dosage.)

Patients should be monitored for early signs of significant hypotension and/or cardiovascular depression, which may be profound. These effects are responsive to discontinuation of DIPRIVAN Injectable Emulsion, IV fluid administration, and/or vasopressor therapy.

As with other sedative medications, there is wide interpatient variability in DIPRIVAN Injectable Emulsion dosage requirements, and these requirements may change with time.

Failure to reduce the infusion rate in patients receiving DIPRIVAN Injectable Emulsion for extended periods may result in excessively high blood concentrations of the drug. Thus, titration to clinical response and daily evaluation of sedation levels are important during use of DIPRIVAN Injectable Emulsion infusion for ICU sedation, especially of long duration.

Opioids and paralytic agents should be discontinued and respiratory function optimized prior to weaning patients from mechanical ventilation. Infusions of DIPRIVAN Injectable Emulsion should be adjusted to maintain a light level of sedation prior to weaning patients from mechanical ventilatory support. Throughout the weaning process, this level of sedation may be maintained in the absence of respiratory depression. Because of the rapid clearance of DIPRIVAN Injectable Emulsion, abrupt discontinuation of a patient's infusion may result in rapid awakening of the patient with associated anxiety, agitation, and resistance to mechanical ventilation, making weaning from mechanical ventilation difficult. It is therefore recommended that administration of DIPRIVAN Injectable Emulsion be continued in order to maintain a light level of sedation throughout the weaning process until 10–15 minutes prior to extubation, at which time the infusion can be discontinued.

Since DIPRIVAN Injectable Emulsion is formulated in an oil-in-water emulsion, elevations in serum triglycerides may occur when DIPRIVAN Injectable Emulsion is administered for extended periods of time. Patients at risk of hyperlipidemia should be monitored for increases in serum triglycerides or serum turbidity. Administration of DIPRIVAN Injectable Emulsion should be adjusted if fat is being inadequately cleared from the body. A reduction in the quantity of concurrently administered lipids is indicated to compensate for the amount of lipid infused as part of the DIPRIVAN Injectable Emulsion formulation; 1 mL of DIPRIVAN Injectable Emulsion contains approximately 0.1 g of fat (1.1 kcal). In patients who are predisposed to zinc deficiency, such as those with burns, diarrhea, and/or major sepsis, the need for

supplemental zinc should be considered during prolonged therapy with DIPRIVAN Injectable Emulsion.
EDTA is a strong chelator of trace metals—including zinc. Calcium disodium edetate has been used in gram quantities to treat heavy metal toxicity. When used in this manner it is possible that as much as 10 mg of elemental zinc can be lost per day via this mechanism. Although with DIPRIVAN Injectable Emulsion there are no reports of decreased zinc levels or zinc deficiency-related adverse events, DIPRIVAN Injectable Emulsion should not be infused for longer than 5 days without providing a drug holiday to safely replace estimated or measured urine zinc losses.

At high doses (2–3 grams per day), EDTA has been reported, on rare occasions, to be toxic to the renal tubules. Studies to date, in patients with normal or impaired renal function have not shown any alteration in renal function with DIPRIVAN Injectable Emulsion containing 0.005% disodium edetate. In patients at risk for renal impairment, urinalysis and urine sediment should be checked before initiation of sedation and then be monitored on alternate days during sedation.

The long-term administration of DIPRIVAN Injectable Emulsion to patients with renal failure and/or hepatic insufficiency has not been evaluated.
Neurosurgical Anesthesia: When DIPRIVAN Injectable Emulsion is used in patients with increased intracranial pressure or impaired cerebral circulation, significant decreases in mean arterial pressure should be avoided because of the resultant decreases in cerebral perfusion pressure. To avoid significant hypotension and decreases in cerebral perfusion pressure, an infusion or slow bolus of approximately 20 mg every 10 seconds should be utilized instead of rapid, more frequent, and/or larger boluses of DIPRIVAN Injectable Emulsion. Slower induction titrated to clinical responses, will generally result in reduced induction dosage requirements (1 to 2 mg/kg). When increased ICP is suspected, hyperventilation and hypocarbia should accompany the administration of DIPRIVAN Injectable Emulsion. (See DOSAGE AND ADMINISTRATION.)

Cardiac Anesthesia:
Slower rates of administration should be utilized in premedicated patients, geriatric patients, patients with recent fluid shifts, or patients who are hemodynamically unstable. Any fluid deficits should be corrected prior to administration of DIPRIVAN Injectable Emulsion. In those patients where additional fluid therapy may be contraindicated, other measures, e.g., elevation of lower extremities, or use of pressor agents, may be useful to offset the hypotension which is associated with the induction of anesthesia with DIPRIVAN Injectable Emulsion.

Information for Patients: Patients should be advised that performance of activities requiring mental alertness, such as operating a motor vehicle, or hazardous machinery or signing legal documents may be impaired for some time after general anesthesia or sedation.

Drug Interactions: The induction dose requirements of DIPRIVAN Injectable Emulsion may be reduced in patients with intramuscular or intravenous premedication, particularly with narcotics (e.g., morphine, meperidine, and fentanyl, etc.) and combinations of opioids and sedatives (e.g., benzodiazepines, barbiturates, chloral hydrate, droperidol, etc.). These agents may increase the anesthetic or sedative effects of DIPRIVAN Injectable Emulsion and may also result in more pronounced decreases in systolic, diastolic, and mean arterial pressures and cardiac output.

During maintenance of anesthesia or sedation, the rate of DIPRIVAN Injectable Emulsion administration should be adjusted according to the desired level of anesthesia or sedation and may be reduced in the presence of supplemental analgesic agents (e.g., nitrous oxide or opioids). The concurrent administration of potent inhalational agents (e.g., isoflurane, enflurane, and halothane) during maintenance with DIPRIVAN Injectable Emulsion has not been extensively evaluated. These inhalational agents can also be expected to increase the anesthetic or sedative and cardiorespiratory effects of DIPRIVAN Injectable Emulsion.

DIPRIVAN Injectable Emulsion does not cause a clinically significant change in onset, intensity or duration of action of the commonly used neuromuscular blocking agents (e.g., succinylcholine and nondepolarizing muscle relaxants).

No significant adverse interactions with commonly used premedications or drugs used during anesthesia or sedation (including a range of muscle relaxants, inhalational agents, analgesic agents, and local anesthetic agents) have been observed.

Carcinogenesis, Mutagenesis, Impairment of Fertility: Animal carcinogenicity studies have not been performed with propofol.

In vitro and *in vivo* animal tests failed to show any potential for mutagenicity by propofol. Tests for mutagenicity included the Ames (using *Salmonella* sp) mutation test, gene mutation/gene conversion using *Saccharomyces cerevisiae, in vitro* cytogenetic studies in Chinese hamsters, and a mouse micronucleus test.

Studies in female rats at intravenous doses up to 15 mg/kg/day (6 times the maximum recommended human induction

dose) for 2 weeks before pregnancy to day 7 of gestation did not show impaired fertility. Male fertility in rats was not affected in a dominant lethal study at intravenous doses up to 15 mg/kg/day for 5 days.

Pregnancy Category B: Reproduction studies have been performed in rats and rabbits at intravenous doses of 15 mg/kg/day (6 times the recommended human induction dose) and have revealed no evidence of impaired fertility or harm to the fetus due to propofol. Propofol, however, has been shown to cause maternal deaths in rats and rabbits and decreased pup survival during the lactating period in dams treated with 15 mg/kg/day (or 6 times the recommended human induction dose). The pharmacological activity (anesthesia) of the drug on the mother is probably responsible for the adverse effects seen in the offspring. There are, however, no adequate and well-controlled studies in pregnant women. Because animal reproduction studies are not always predictive of human responses, this drug should be used during pregnancy only if clearly needed.

Labor and Delivery: DIPRIVAN Injectable Emulsion is not recommended for obstetrics, including cesarean section deliveries. DIPRIVAN Injectable Emulsion crosses the placenta, and as with other general anesthetic agents, the administration of DIPRIVAN Injectable Emulsion may be associated with neonatal depression.

Nursing Mothers: DIPRIVAN Injectable Emulsion is not recommended for use in nursing mothers because DIPRIVAN Injectable Emulsion has been reported to be excreted in human milk and the effects of oral absorption of small amounts of propofol are not known.

Pediatrics: DIPRIVAN Injectable Emulsion is not recommended for use in pediatric patients for ICU or MAC sedation. In addition, DIPRIVAN Injectable Emulsion is not recommended for general anesthesia for children below the age of 3 years because safety and effectiveness have not been established.

Although no causal relationship has been established, serious adverse events (including fatalities) have been reported in children given DIPRIVAN Injectable Emulsion for ICU sedation. These events were seen most often in children with respiratory tract infections given doses in excess of those recommended for adults.

ADVERSE REACTIONS
General
Adverse event information is derived from controlled clinical trials and worldwide marketing experience. In the description below, rates of the more common events represent US/Canadian clinical study results. Less frequent events are also derived from publications and marketing experience in over 8 million patients; there are insufficient data to support an accurate estimate of their incidence rates. These studies were conducted using a variety of premedicants, varying lengths of surgical/diagnostic procedures, and various other anesthetic/sedative agents. Most adverse events were mild and transient.

Anesthesia and MAC Sedation in Adults
The following estimates of adverse events for DIPRIVAN Injectable Emulsion include data from clinical trials in general anesthesia/MAC sedation (N=2889 adult patients). The adverse events listed below as probably causally related are those events in which the actual incidence rate in patients treated with DIPRIVAN Injectable Emulsion was greater than the comparator incidence rate in these trials. Therefore, incidence rates for anesthesia and MAC sedation in adults generally represent estimates of the percentage of clinical trial patients which appeared to have probable causal relationship.

The adverse experience profile from reports of 150 patients in the MAC sedation clinical trials is similar to the profile established with DIPRIVAN Injectable Emulsion during anesthesia (see below). During MAC sedation clinical trials, significant respiratory events included cough, upper airway obstruction, apnea, hypoventilation, and dyspnea.

Anesthesia in Children
Generally the adverse experience profile from reports of 349 DIPRIVAN Injectable Emulsion pediatric patients between the ages of 3 and 12 years in the US/Canadian anesthesia clinical trials is similar to the profile established with DIPRIVAN Injectable Emulsion during anesthesia in adults (see Pediatric percentages [Peds %] below). Although not reported as an adverse event in clinical trials, apnea is frequently observed in pediatric patients.

ICU Sedation in Adults
The following estimates of adverse events include data from clinical trials in ICU sedation (N=159) patients. Probably related incidence rates for ICU sedation were determined by individual case report form review. Probable causality was based upon an apparent dose response relationship and/or positive responses to rechallenge. In many instances the presence of concomitant disease and concomitant therapy made the causal relationship unknown. Therefore, incidence rates for ICU sedation generally represent estimates of the

Continued on next page

Zeneca Pharmaceuticals—Cont.

percentage of clinical trial patients which appeared to have a probable causal relationship.
[See table below.]

DRUG ABUSE AND DEPENDENCE

Rare cases of self-administration of DIPRIVAN Injectable Emulsion by health care professionals have been reported, including some fatalities. DIPRIVAN Injectable Emulsion should be managed to prevent the risk of diversion, including restriction of access and accounting procedures as appropriate to the clinical setting.

OVERDOSAGE

If overdosage occurs, DIPRIVAN Injectable Emulsion administration should be discontinued immediately. Overdosage is likely to cause cardiorespiratory depression. Respiratory depression should be treated by artificial ventilation with oxygen. Cardiovascular depression may require repositioning of the patient by raising the patient's legs, increasing the flow rate of intravenous fluids and administering pressor agents and/or anticholinergic agents.

DOSAGE AND ADMINISTRATION

Dosage and rate of administration should be individualized and titrated to the desired effect, according to clinically rele-

vant factors, including preinduction and concomitant medications, age, ASA physical classification, and level of debilitation of the patient.

The following is abbreviated dosage and administration information which is only intended as a general guide in the use of DIPRIVAN Injectable Emulsion. Prior to administering DIPRIVAN Injectable Emulsion, it is imperative that the physician review and be completely familiar with the specific dosage and administration information detailed in the CLINICAL PHARMACOLOGY—Individualization of Dosage section.

In the elderly, debilitated , or ASA III/IV patients, rapid bolus doses should not be the method of administration. (See WARNINGS.)

Intensive Care Unit Sedation:
STRICT ASEPTIC TECHNIQUE MUST ALWAYS BE MAINTAINED DURING HANDLING. DIPRIVAN INJECTABLE EMULSION IS A SINGLE-USE PARENTERAL PRODUCT WHICH CONTAINS 0.005% DISODIUM EDETATE TO RETARD THE RATE OF GROWTH OF MICROORGANISMS IN THE EVENT OF ACCIDENTAL EXTRINSIC CONTAMINATION. HOWEVER, DIPRIVAN INJECTABLE EMULSION CAN STILL SUPPORT THE GROWTH OF MICROORGANISMS AS IT IS NOT AN ANTIMICROBIALLY PRESERVED PRODUCT UNDER USP STANDARDS. ACCORDINGLY, STRICT ASEPTIC TECHNIQUE MUST STILL BE ADHERED TO. DO NOT USE IF CONTAMINATION IS SUSPECTED.

(see DOSAGE AND ADMINISTRATION, Handling Procedures.) DIPRIVAN Injectable Emulsion should be individualized according to the patient's condition and response, blood lipid profile, and vital signs. (See PRECAUTIONS–ICU Sedation.) For intubated, mechanically ventilated adult patients, Intensive Care Unit (ICU) sedation should be initiated slowly with a continuous infusion in order to titrate to desired clinical effect and minimize hypotension. When indicated, initiation of sedation should begin at 5 μg/kg/min (0.3 mg/kg/h). The infusion rate should be increased by increments of 5 to 10 μg/kg/min (0.3 to 0.6 mg/kg/h) until the desired level of sedation is achieved. A minimum period of 5 minutes between adjustments should be allowed for onset of peak drug effect. Most adult patients require maintenance rates of 5 to 50 μg/kg/min (0.3 to 3 mg/kg/h) or higher. Dosages of DIPRIVAN Injectable Emulsion should be reduced in patients who have received large dosages of narcotics. Conversely, the DIPRIVAN Injectable Emulsion dosage requirement may be reduced by adequate management of pain with analgesic agents. As with other sedative medications, there is interpatient variability in dosage requirements, and these requirements may change with time. (See DOSAGE GUIDE.) EVALUATION OF LEVEL OF SEDATION AND ASSESSMENT OF CNS FUNCTION SHOULD BE CARRIED OUT DAILY THROUGHOUT MAINTENANCE TO DETERMINE THE MINIMUM DOSE OF DIPRIVAN INJECTABLE EMULSION REQUIRED FOR SEDATION (See CLINICAL TRIALS, ICU Sedation). Bolus administration of 10 or 20 mg should only be used to rapidly increase depth of sedation in patients where hypotension is not likely to occur. Patients with compromised myocardial function, intravascular volume depletion, or abnormally low vascular tone (e.g. sepsis) may be more susceptible to hypotension. (See PRECAUTIONS.)

EDTA is a strong chelator of trace metals—including zinc. Calcium disodium edetate has been used in gram quantities to treat heavy metal toxicity. When used in this manner it is possible that as much as 10 mg of elemental zinc can be lost per day via this mechanism. Although with DIPRIVAN Injectable Emulsion there are no reports of decreased zinc levels or zinc deficiency-related adverse events, DIPRIVAN Injectable Emulsion should not be infused for longer than 5 days without providing a drug holiday to safely replace estimated or measured urine zinc losses.

At high doses (2–3 grams per day), EDTA has been reported, on rare occasions, to be toxic to the renal tubules. Studies to-date, in patients with normal or impaired renal function have not shown any alteration in renal function with DIPRIVAN Injectable Emulsion containing 0.005% disodium edetate. In patients at risk for renal impairment, urinalysis and urine sediment should be checked before initiation of sedation and then monitored on alternate days during sedation.

SUMMARY OF DOSAGE GUIDELINES—Dosages and rates of administration in the following table should be individualized and titrated to clinical response. Safety and dose requirements in pediatric patients have only been established for induction and maintenance of anesthesia. For complete dosage information, see CLINICAL PHARMACOLOGY—Individualization of Dosage.

Incidence greater than 1%—Probably Causally Related

	Anesthesia/MAC Sedation	ICU Sedation
Cardiovascular:	Bradycardia Hypotension* [Peds: 17%] [Hypertension Peds: 8%] (see also CLINICAL PHARMACOLOGY)	Bradycardia, Decreased Cardiac Output, Hypotension 26%
Central Nervous System:	Movement* [Peds: 17%]	
Injection Site:	Burning/Stinging or Pain, 17.6% [Peds: 10%]	
Metabolic/Nutritional:		Hyperlipemia*
Respiratory	Apnea (see also CLINICAL PHARMACOLOGY)	Respiratory Acidosis During Weaning*
Skin and Appendages:	Rash [Peds: 5%]	

Events without an * or % had an incidence of 1%–3%
*Incidence of events 3% to 10%

Incidence less than 1%—Probably Causally Related

	Anesthesia/MAC Sedation	ICU Sedation
Body as a Whole:	Anaphylaxis/Anaphylactoid Reaction Perinatal Disorder	
Cardiovascular:	Premature Atrial Contractions Syncope	
Central Nervous System:	Hypertonia/Dystonia, Paresthesia	Agitation
Digestive:	Hypersalivation	
Musculoskeletal:	Myalgia	
Respiratory:	Wheezing	Decreased Lung Function
Skin and Appendages:	Flushing, Pruritus	
Special Senses:	Amblyopia	
Urogenital:	Cloudy Urine	Green Urine

Incidence less than 1%—Causal Relationship Unknown

	Anesthesia/MAC Sedation	ICU Sedation
Body as a Whole:	Asthenia, Awareness, Chest Pain Extremities Pain, Fever, Increased Drug Effect, Neck Rigidity/Stiffness, Trunk Pain	Fever, Sepsis, Trunk Pain Whole Body Weakness
Cardiovascular:	Arrhythmia, Atrial Fibrillation, Atrioventricular Heart Block, Bigeminy, Bleeding, Bundle Branch Block, Cardiac Arrest, ECG Abnormal, Edema Extrasystole, Heart Block, Hypertension, Myocardial Infarction, Myocardial Ischemia, Premature Ventricular Contractions, ST Segment Depression, Supraventricular Tachycardia, Tachycardia, Ventricular Fibrillation	Arrhythmia, Atrial Fibrillation, Bigeminy, Cardiac Arrest, Extrasystole, Right Heart Failure, Ventricular Tachycardia
Central Nervous System:	Abnormal Dreams, Agitation, Amorous Behavior, Anxiety, Bucking/Jerking/Thrashing, Chills/Shivering, Clonic/Myoclonic Movement, Combativeness, Confusion, Delirium, Depression, Dizziness, Emotional Lability, Euphoria, Fatigue, Hallucinations, Headache, Hypotonia, Hysteria, Insomnia, Moaning, Neuropathy, Opisthotonos, Rigidity, Seizures, Somnolence, Tremor, Twitching	Chills/Shivering, Intracranial Hypertension Seizures, Somnolence, Thinking Abnormal
Digestive:	Cramping, Diarrhea, Dry Mouth, Enlarged Parotid, Nausea, Swallowing, Vomiting	Ileus, Liver Function Abnormal
Hematologic/Lymphatic:	Coagulation Disorder, Leukocytosis	
Injection Site:	Hives/Itching, Phlebitis, Redness/Discoloration	
Metabolic/Nutritional:	Hyperkalemia, Hyperlipemia	BUN Increased, Creatinine Increased, Dehydration, Hyperglycemia, Metabolic Acidosis, Osmolality Increased
Respiratory:	Bronchospasm, Burning in Throat, Cough Dyspnea, Hiccough, Hyperventilation, Hypoventilation, Hypoxia, Laryngospasm, Pharyngitis, Sneezing, Tachypnea, Upper Airway Obstruction	Hypoxia
Skin and Appendages	Conjunctival Hyperemia, Diaphoresis, Urticaria	Rash
Special Senses:	Diplopia, Ear Pain, Eye Pain, Nystagmus, Taste Perversion, Tinnitus	
Urogenital:	Oliguria, Urine Retention	Kidney Failure

INDICATION	DOSAGE AND ADMINISTRATION

Induction of General Anesthesia

Healthy Adults Less Than 55 Years of Age:
40 mg every 10 seconds until induction onset (2 to 2.5 mg/kg).
Elderly, Debilitated, or ASA III/IV Patients:
20 mg every 10 seconds until induction onset (1 to 1.5 mg/kg).
Cardiac Anesthesia:
20 mg every 10 seconds until induction onset (0.5 to 1.5 mg/kg).
Neurosurgical Patients:
20 mg every 10 seconds until induction onset (1 to 2 mg/kg).
Pediatric—healthy, 3 years of age or older:
2.5 to 3.5 mg/kg administered over 20–30 seconds.

Maintenance of General Anesthesia: Infusion

Healthy Adults Less Than 55 Years of Age:
100 to 200 μg/kg/min (6 to 12 mg/kg/h).
Elderly, Debilitated, ASA III/IV Patients:
50 to 100 μg/kg/min (3 to 6 mg/kg/h).
Cardiac Anesthesia: Most patients require:
Primary DIPRIVAN Injectable Emulsion with Secondary Opioid—100–150 μg/kg/min
Low-Dose DIPRIVAN Injectable Emulsion with Primary Opioid— 50–100 μg/kg/min (See CLINICAL PHARMACOLOGY, Table 4)
Neurosurgical Patients:
100 to 200 μg/kg/min (6 to 12 mg/kg/h).
Pediatric—healthy, 3 years of age or older:
125 to 300 μg/kg/min (7.5 to 18 mg/kg/h)

Maintenance of General Anesthesia: Intermittent Bolus

Healthy Adults Less Than 55 Years of Age: Increments of 20 to 50 mg as needed.

Initiation of MAC Sedation

Healthy Adults Less Than 55 Years of Age: Slow infusion or slow injection techniques are recommended to avoid apnea or hypotension. Most patients require an infusion of 100 to 150 μg/kg/min (6 to 9 mg/kg/h) for 3 to 5 minutes or a slow injection of 0.5 mg/kg over 3 to 5 minutes followed immediately by a maintenance infusion.

Elderly, Debilitated, Neurosurgical, or ASA III/IV Patients: Most patients require dosages similar to healthy adults. Rapid boluses are to be avoided (See WARNINGS.)

Maintenance of MAC Sedation

Healthy Adults Less Than 55 Years of Age: A variable rate infusion technique is preferable over an intermittent bolus technique. Most patients require an infusion of 25 to 75 μg/kg/min (1.5 to 4.5 mg/kg/h) or incremental bolus doses of 10 mg or 20 mg.

In Elderly, Debilitated, Neurosurgical, or ASA III/IV Patients: Most patients require 80% of the usual adult dose. A rapid (single or repeated) bolus dose should not be used. (See WARNINGS.)

Initiation and Maintenance of ICU Sedation in Intubated, Mechanically Ventilated

Adult Patients—Because of the lingering effects of previous anesthetic or sedative agents, in most patients the initial infusion should be 5 μg/kg/min (0.3 mg/kg/h) for at least 5 minutes. Subsequent increments of 5 to 10 μg/kg/min (0.3 to 0.6 mg/kg/h) over 5 to 10 minutes may be used until desired level of sedation is achieved. Maintenance rates of 5 to 50 μg/kg/min (0.3 to 3 mg/kg/h) or higher may be required. **Evaluation of level of sedation and assessment of CNS function should be carried out daily throughout maintenance to determine the minimum dose of DIPRIVAN Injectable Emulsion required for sedation.**

The tubing and any unused portions of DIPRIVAN Injectable Emulsion should be discarded after 12 hours because DIPRIVAN Injectable Emulsion contains no preservatives and is capable of supporting growth of microorganisms. (See WARNINGS, and DOSAGE AND ADMINISTRATION.)

Compatibility and Stability: DIPRIVAN Injectable Emulsion should not be mixed with other therapeutic agents prior to administration.

Dilution Prior to Administration: When DIPRIVAN Injectable Emulsion is diluted prior to administration, it should only be diluted with 5% Dextrose Injection, USP, and it should not be diluted to a concentration less than 2 mg/mL because it is an emulsion. In diluted form it has been shown to be more stable when in contact with glass than with plastic (95% potency after 2 hours of running infusion in plastic).

Administration with Other Fluids: Compatibility of DIPRIVAN Injectable Emulsion with the coadministration of blood/serum/plasma has not been established. (See WARNINGS.) DIPRIVAN Injectable Emulsion has been shown to be compatible when administered with the following intravenous fluids.

– 5% Dextrose Injection, USP
– Lactated Ringers Injection, USP
– Lactated Ringers and 5% Dextrose Injection
– 5% Dextrose and 0.45% Sodium Chloride Injection, USP
– 5% Dextrose and 0.2% Sodium Chloride Injection, USP

Assembly Instructions for Pre-Filled Syringe

1. Remove the Luer connector from packaging.
2. Remove glass syringe barrel from tray and check for cracks or leaks. Shake. Remove the blue plastic cover. Disinfect the rubber stopper using alcohol swab provided in package. Allow to dry.
3. Pull off needle cover from Luer connector. The bevel of the needle spike is slightly bent (c-tip) to prevent potential coring.
4. Stand the syringe barrel vertically on a hard surface and push Luer connector on to syringe barrel so needle penetrates rubber seal and connector slides over the blue seal until firmly seated. (Fig. 1)

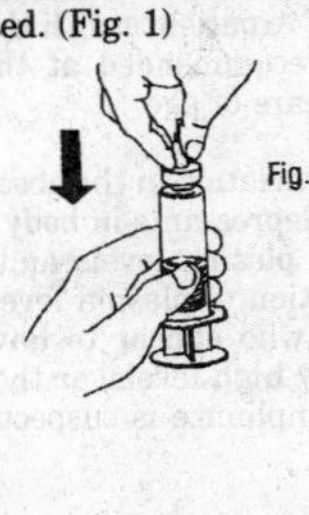

Fig.1

5. Add plunger rod by screwing clockwise. CAUTION: the rod must be fully screwed on, otherwise it may detach which could result in siphoning of the syringe contents. (Fig. 2)

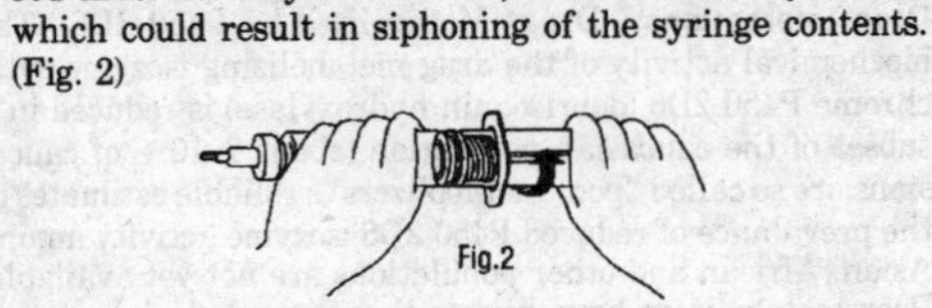

Fig.2

6. Unscrew Luer cover remove excess nitrogen gas from the syringe (a small nitrogen gas bubble may remain). Assemble administration line and connect syringe.

Handling Procedures

General

Parenteral drug products should be inspected visually for particulate matter and discoloration prior to administration whenever solution and container permit.

Clinical experience with the use of in-line filters and DIPRIVAN Injectable Emulsion during anesthesia or ICU/MAC sedation is limited. DIPRIVAN Injectable Emulsion should only be administered through a filter with a pore size of 5 microns or greater unless it has been demonstrated that the filter does not restrict the flow of DIPRIVAN Injectable Emulsion and/or cause the breakdown of the emulsion. Filters should be used with caution and where clinically appropriate. Continuous monitoring is necessary due to the potential for restricted flow and/or breakdown of the emulsion. Do not use if there is evidence of separation of the phases of the emulsion.

Rare cases of self-administration of DIPRIVAN Injectable Emulsion, by health care professionals have been reported, including some fatalities (See DRUG ABUSE AND DEPENDENCE).

STRICT ASEPTIC TECHNIQUE MUST ALWAYS BE MAINTAINED DURING HANDLING. DIPRIVAN INJECTABLE EMULSION IS A SINGLE-USE PARENTERAL PRODUCT; WHICH CONTAINS 0.005% DISODIUM EDETATE TO RETARD THE RATE OF GROWTH OF MICROORGANISMS IN THE EVENT OF ACCIDENTAL EXTRINSIC CONTAMINATION. HOWEVER, DIPRIVAN INJECTABLE EMULSION CAN STILL SUPPORT THE GROWTH OF MICROORGANISMS AS IT IS NOT AN ANTIMICROBIALLY PRESERVED PRODUCT UNDER USP STANDARDS. ACCORDINGLY, STRICT ASEPTIC TECHNIQUE MUST STILL BE ADHERED TO. DO NOT USE IF CONTAMINATION IS SUSPECTED. DISCARD UNUSED PORTIONS AS DIRECTED WITHIN THE REQUIRED TIME LIMITS (SEE DOSAGE AND ADMINISTRATION, HANDLING PROCEDURES). THERE HAVE BEEN REPORTS IN WHICH FAILURE TO USE ASEPTIC TECHNIQUE WHEN HANDLING DIPRIVAN INJECTABLE EMULSION WAS ASSOCIATED WITH MICROBIAL CONTAMINATION OF THE PRODUCT AND WITH FEVER, INFECTION/SEPSIS, OTHER LIFE-THREATENING ILLNESS, AND/OR DEATH.

Guideline for Aseptic Technique for General Anesthesia/MAC Sedation

DIPRIVAN Injectable Emulsion should be prepared for use just prior to initiation of each individual anesthetic/sedative procedure. The ampule neck surface, or vial/pre-filled syringe rubber stopper should be disinfected using 70% isopropyl alcohol. DIPRIVAN Injectable Emulsion should be drawn into sterile syringes immediately after ampules or vials are opened. When withdrawing DIPRIVAN Injectable Emulsion from vials, a sterile vent spike should be used. The syringe(s) should be labeled with appropriate information including the date and time the ampule or vial was opened. Administration should commence promptly and be completed within 6 hours after the ampules, vials, or pre-filled syringes have been opened.

DIPRIVAN Injectable Emulsion should be prepared for single patient use only. Any unused portions of DIPRIVAN Injectable Emulsion, reservoirs, dedicated administration tubing and/or solutions containing DIPRIVAN Injectable Emulsion must be discarded at the end of the anesthetic procedure or at 6 hours, whichever occurs sooner. The IV line should be flushed every 6 hours and at the end of the anesthetic procedure to remove residual DIPRIVAN Injectable Emulsion.

Guidelines for Aseptic Technique for ICU Sedation

When DIPRIVAN Injectable Emulsion is administered directly from the vial, strict aseptic techniques must be followed. The vial rubber stopper should be disinfected using 70% isopropyl alcohol. A sterile vent spike and sterile tubing must be used for administration of DIPRIVAN Injectable Emulsion. As with other lipid emulsions, the number of IV line manipulations should be minimized. Administration should commence promptly and must be completed within 12 hours after the vial has been spiked. The tubing and any unused portions of DIPRIVAN Injectable Emulsion must be discarded after 12 hours.

If DIPRIVAN Injectable Emulsion is transferred to a syringe or other container prior to administration, the handling procedures for General anesthesia/MAC sedation should be followed, and the product should be discarded and administration lines changed after 6 hours.

HOW SUPPLIED

DIPRIVAN Injectable Emulsion is available in ready to use 20 mL ampules, 50 mL infusion vials, 100 mL infusion vials, and 50 mL pre-filled syringes containing 10 mg/mL of propofol.

20 mL ampules (NDC 0310-0300-20)
50 mL infusion vials (NDC 0310-0300-50)
100 mL infusion vials (NDC 0310-0300-11)
50 mL pre-filled syringes (NDC 0310-0300-54)

Propofol undergoes oxidative degradation, in the presence of oxygen, and is therefore packaged under nitrogen to eliminate this degradation path.

Store between 4°–22°C (40°–72° F). Refrigeration is not recommended. Shake well before use.

Manufactured for:
ZENECA
Pharmaceuticals
A Business Unit of Zeneca Inc.
Wilmington, Delaware 19850-5437
64090-01 Rev D 06/96

Shown in Product Identification Guide, page 341

ELAVIL® ℞
(AMITRIPTYLINE HCl)
Tablets and Injection

DESCRIPTION

Amitriptyline HCl is 3-(10,11-dihydro-5*H*-dibenzo [*a,d*] cycloheptene-5-ylidene)-*N,N*-dimethyl-1-propanamine hydrochloride. Its empirical formula is $C_{20}H_{23}N \bullet HCl$ and its structural formula is:

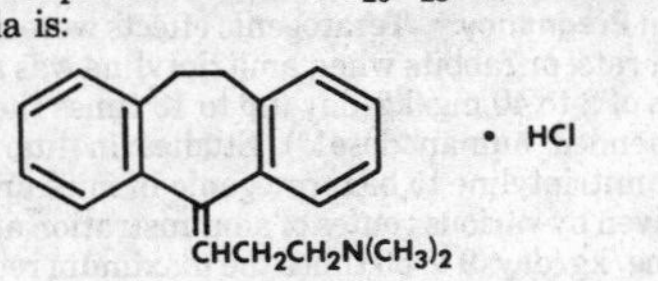

Amitriptyline HCl, a dibenzocycloheptadiene derivative, has a molecular weight of 313.87. It is a white, odorless, crystalline compound which is freely soluble in water.

ELAVIL* (Amitriptyline HCl) is supplied as 10 mg, 25 mg, 50 mg, 75 mg, 100 mg, and 150 mg tablets and as a sterile solution for intramuscular use. Inactive ingredients of the tablets are calcium phosphate, cellulose, colloidal silicon dioxide, hydroxypropyl cellulose, hydroxypropyl methylcellulose, lactose, magnesium stearate, starch, stearic acid, talc, and titanium dioxide. Tablets ELAVIL 10 mg also contain FD&C Blue 1. Tablets ELAVIL 25 mg also contain D&C Yellow 10, FD&C Blue 1, and FD&C Yellow 6. Tablets ELAVIL 50 mg also contain D&C Yellow 10, FD&C Yellow 6 and iron oxide. Tablets ELAVIL 75 mg also contain FD&C Yellow 6. Tablets ELAVIL 100 mg also contain FD&C Blue 2 and FD&C Red 40. Tablets ELAVIL 150 mg also contain FD&C Blue 2 and FD&C Yellow 6. Each milliliter of the sterile solution contains:

Amitriptyline hydrochloride	10 mg
Dextrose	44 mg
Water for Injection, q.s	1 mL
Added as preservatives:	
Methylparabel	1.5 mg
Propylparaben	0.2 mg

ACTIONS

ELAVIL is an antidepressant with sedative effects. Its mechanism of action in man is not known. It is not a monoamine oxidase inhibitor and it does not act primarily by stimulation of the central nervous system.

Amitriptyline inhibits the membrane pump mechanism responsible for uptake of norepinephrine and serotonin in adrenergic and serotonergic neurons. Pharmacologically this action may potentiate or prolong neuronal activity since reuptake of this biogenic amines is important physiologically in terminating transmitting activity. This interference with the reuptake of norepinephrine and/or serotonin is believed by some to underlie the antidepressant activity of amitriptyline.

INDICATIONS

For the relief of symptoms of depression. Endogenous depression is more likely to be alleviated than are other depressive states.

CONTRAINDICATIONS

ELAVIL is contraindicated in patients who have shown prior hypersensitivity to it.

It should not be given concomitantly with monoamine oxidase inhibitors. Hyperpyretic crises, severe convulsions, and deaths have occurred in patients receiving tricyclic antidepressant and monoamine oxidase inhibiting drugs simulta-

Continued on next page

Zeneca Pharmaceuticals—Cont.

neously. When it is desired to replace a monoamine oxidase inhibitor with ELAVIL, a minimum of 14 days should be allowed to elapse after the former is discontinued. ELAVIL should then be initiated cautiously with gradual increase in dosage until optimum response is achieved.

This drug is not recommended for use during the acute recovery phase following myocardial infarction.

WARNINGS

ELAVIL may block the antihypertensive action of guanethidine or similarly acting compounds.

It should be used with caution in patients with a history of seizures and, because of its atropine-like action, in patients with a history of urinary retention, angle-closure glaucoma or increased intraocular pressure. In patients with angle-closure glaucoma, even average doses may precipitate an attack.

Patients with cardiovascular disorders should be watched closely. Tricyclic antidepressant drugs, including ELAVIL, particularly when given in high doses, have been reported to produce arrhythmias, sinus tachycardia, and prolongation of the conduction time. Myocardial infarction and stroke have been reported with drugs of this class.

Close supervision is required when ELAVIL is given to hyperthyroid patients or those receiving thyroid medication. ELAVIL may enhance the response to alcohol and the effects of barbituates and other CNS depressants. In patients who may use alcohol excessively, it should be borne in mind that the potentiation may increase the danger inherent in any suicide attempt or overdosage. Delirium has been reported with concurrent administration of amitriptyline and disulfiram.

Usage in Pregnancy: Teratogenic effects were not observed in mice, rats, or rabbits when amitriptyline was given orally at doses of 2 to 40 mg/kg/day (up to 13 times the maximum recommended human dose**). Studies in literature have shown amitriptyline to be teratogenic in mice and hamsters when given by various routes of administration at doses of 28 to 100 mg/kg/day (9 to 33 times the maximum recommended human dose), producing multiple malformations. Another study in the rat reported that an oral dose of 25 mg/kg/day (8 times the maximum recommended human dose) produced delays in ossification of fetal vertebral bodies without other signs of embryotoxicity. In rabbits, an oral dose of 60 mg/kg/day (20 times the maximum recommended human dose) was reported to cause incomplete ossification of the cranial bones.

Amitriptyline has been shown to cross the placenta. Although a causal relationship has not been established, there have been a few reports of adverse events, including CNS effects, limb deformities, or developmental delay, in infants whose mothers had taken amitriptyline during pregnancy. There are no adequate and well-controlled studies in pregnant women. ELAVIL should be used during pregnancy only if the potential benefit to the mother justifies the potential risk to the fetus.

Nursing Mothers: Amitriptyline is excreted into breast milk. In one report in which a patient received amitriptyline 100 mg/day while nursing her infant, levels of 83–141 ng/mL were detected in the mother's serum. Levels of 135–151 ng/mL were found in the breast milk, but no trace of the drug could be detected in the infant's serum.

Because of the potential for serious adverse reactions in nursing infants from amitriptyline, a decision should be made whether to discontinue nursing or to discontinue the drug taking into account the importance of the drug to the mother.

Usage in Children: In view of the lack of experience with the use of this drug in children, it is not recommended at the present time for patients under 12 years of age.

PRECAUTIONS

Schizophrenic patients may develop increased symptoms of psychosis; patients with paranoid symptomatology may have an exaggeration of such symptoms. Depressed patients, particularly those with known manic-depressive illness, may experience a shift to mania or hypomania. In these circumstances the dose of amitriptyline may be reduced or a major tranquilizer such as perphenazine may be administered concurrently.

The possibility of suicide in depressed patients remains until significant remission occurs. Potentially suicidal patients should not have access to large quantities of this drug. Prescriptions should be written for the smallest amount feasible.

Concurrent administration of ELAVIL and electroshock therapy may increase the hazards associated with such therapy. Such treatment should be limited to patients for whom it is essential.

When possible, the drug should be discontinued several days before elective surgery.

Both elevation and lowering of blood sugar levels have been reported.

ELAVIL should be used with caution in patients with impared liver function.

Drug Interactions: Drugs Metabolized by P450 2D6—The biochemical activity of the drug metabolizing isozyme cytochrome P450 2D6 (debrisoquin hydroxylase) is reduced in a subset of the caucasian population (about 7–10% of caucasians are so called "poor metabolizers"); reliable estimates of the prevalance of reduced P450 2D6 isozyme activity among Asian, African and other populations are not yet available. Poor metabolizers have higher than expected plasma concentrations of tricyclic antidepressants (TCAs) when given usual doses. Depending on the fraction of drug metabolized by P450 2D6, the increase in plasma concentration may be small, or quite large (8-fold increase in plasma AUC of the TCA).

In addition, certain drugs inhibit the activity of this isozyme and make normal metabolizers resemble poor metabolizers. An individual who is stable on a given dose of TCA may become abruptly toxic when given one of these inhibiting drugs as concomitant therapy. The drugs that inhibit cytochrome P450 2D6 include some that are not metabolized by the enzyme (quinidine; cimetidine) and many that are substrates for P450 2D6 (many other antidepressants, phenothiazines, and the Type 1C antiarrhythmics propafenone and flecainidine). While all the selective serotonin reuptake inhibitors (SSRIs), e.g., fluoxetine, sertraline, and paroxetine, inhibit P450 2D6, they may vary in the extent of inhibition. The extent to which SSRI-TCA interactions may pose clinical problems will depend on the degree of inhibition and the pharmacokinetics of the SSRI involved. Nevertheless, caution is indicated in the coadministration of TCAs with any of the SSRIs and also in switching from one class to the other. Of particular importance, sufficient time must elapse before initiating TCA treatment in a patient being withdrawn from fluoxetine, given the long half-life of the parent and active metabolite (at least 5 weeks may be necessary).

Concomitant use of tricyclic antidepressants with drugs that can inhibit cytochrome P450 2D6 may require lower doses than usually prescribed for either the tricyclic antidepressant or the other drug. Furthermore, whenever one of these other drugs is withdrawn from co-therapy, an increased dose of tricyclic antidepressant may be required. It is desirable to monitor TCA plasma levels whenever a TCA is going to be coadministered with another drug known to be an inhibitor of P450 2D6.

Monoamine oxidase inhibitors—see CONTRAINDICATIONS section. Guanethidine or similarly acting compounds; thyroid medication; alcohol, barbiturates and other CNS depressants; and disulfiram—see WARNINGS section. When ELAVIL is given with anticholinergic agents or sympathomimetic drugs, including epinephrine combined with local anesthetics, close supervision and careful adjustment of dosages are required.

Hyperpyrexia has been reported when ELAVIL is administered with anticholinergic agents or with neuroleptic drugs, particularly during hot weather.

Paralytic ileus may occur in patients taking tricyclic antidepressants in combination with anticholinergic-type drugs. Cimetidine is reported to reduce hepatic metabolism of certain tricyclic antidepressants, thereby delaying elimination and increasing steady-state concentrations of these drugs. Clinically significant effects have been reported with the tricyclic antidepressants when used concomitantly with cimetidine. Increases in plasma levels of tricyclic antidepressants, and in the frequency and severity of side effects, particularly anticholinergic, have been reported when cimetidine was added to the drug regimen. Discontinuation of cimetidine in well-controlled patients receiving tricyclic antidepressants and cimetidine may decrease the plasma levels and efficacy of the antidepressants.

Caution is advised if patients receive large doses of ethchlorvynol concurrently. Transient delirium has been reported in patients who were treated with one gram of ethchlorvynol and 75–150 mg of ELAVIL.

Information for Patients: While on therapy with ELAVIL, patients should be advised as to the possible impairment of mental and/or physical abilities required for performance of hazardous tasks, such as operating machinery or driving a motor vehicle.

ADVERSE REACTIONS

Within each category the following adverse reactions are listed in order of decreasing severity. Included in the listing are a few adverse reactions which have not been reported with this specific drug. However, pharmacological similarities among the tricyclic antidepressant drugs require that each of the reactions be considered when amitriptyline is administered.

Cardiovascular: Myocardial infarction; stroke; nonspecific ECG changes and changes in AV conduction; heart block; arrhythmias; hypotension, particularly orthostatic hypotension; syncope; hypertension; tachycardia; palpitation.

CNS and Neuromuscular: Coma; seizures; hallucinations; delusions; confusional states; disorientation; incoordination; ataxia; tremors; peripheral neuropathy; numbness, tingling, and paresthesias of the extremities; extrapyramidal symp-

toms including abnormal involuntary movements and tardive dyskinesia; dysarthria; disturbed concentration; excitement; anxiety; insomnia; restlessness; nightmares; drowsiness; dizziness; weakness; fatigue; headache; syndrome of inappropriate ADH (antidiuretic hormone) secretion; tinnitus; alteration in EEG patterns.

Anticholinergic: Paralytic ileus; hyperpyrexia; urinary retention; dilatation of the urinary tract; constipation; blurred vision, disturbance of accommodation, increased ocular pressure, mydriasis; dry mouth.

Allergic: Skin rash; urticaria, photosensitization; edema of face and tongue.

Hematologic: Bone marrow depression including agranulocytosis, leukopenia, thrombocytopenia; purpura; eosinophilia.

Gastrointestinal: Rarely hepatitis (including altered liver function and jaundice); nausea; epigastric distress; vomiting; anorexia; stomatitis, peculiar taste; diarrhea; parotid swelling; black tongue.

Endocrine: Testicular swelling and gynecomastia in the male; breast enlargement and galactorrhea in the female; increased or decreased libido; impotence; elevation and lowering of blood sugar levels.

Other: Alopecia; edema; weight gain or loss; urinary frequency; increased perspiration.

Withdrawal Symptoms: After prolonged administration, abrupt cessation of treatment may produce nausea, headache, and malaise. Gradual dosage reduction has been reported to produce, within two weeks, transient symptoms including irritability, restlessness, and dream and sleep disturbance.

These symptoms are not indicative of addiction. Rare instances have been reported of mania or hypomania occurring within 2–7 days following cessation of chronic therapy with tricyclic antidepressants.

Causal Relationship Unknown: Other reactions, reported under circumstances where a causal relationship could not be established, are listed to serve as alerting information to physicians:

Body as a Whole: Lupus-like syndrome (migratory arthritis, positive ANA and rheumatoid factor).

Digestive: Hepatic failure, ageusia.

DOSAGE AND ADMINISTRATION

Oral Dosage

Dosage should be initiated at a low level and increased gradually, noting carefully the clinical response and any evidence of intolerance.

Initial Dosage for Adults: For outpatients 75 mg of amitriptyline HCl a day in divided doses is usually satisfactory. If necessary, this may be increased to a total of 150 mg per day. Increases are made preferably in the late afternoon and/or bedtime doses. A sedative effect may be apparent before the antidepressant effect is noted, but an adequate therapeutic effect may take as long as 30 days to develop.

An alternate method of initiating therapy in outpatients is to begin with 50 to 100 mg amitriptyline HCl at bedtime. This may be increased by 25 or 50 mg as necessary in the bedtime dose to a total of 150 mg per day.

Hospitalized patients may require 100 mg a day initially. This can be increased gradually to 200 mg a day if necessary. A small number of hospitalized patients may need as much as 300 mg a day.

Adolescent and Elderly Patients: In general, lower dosages are recommended for these patients. Ten mg 3 times a day with 20 mg at bedtime may be satisfactory in adolescent and elderly patients who do not tolerate higher dosages.

Maintenance: The usual maintenance dosage of amitriptyline HCl is 50 to 100 mg per day. In some patients 40 mg per day is sufficient. For maintenance therapy the total daily dosage may be given in a single dose preferably at bedtime. When satisfactory improvement has been reached, dosage should be reduced to the lowest amount that will maintain relief of symptoms. It is appropriate to continue maintenance therapy 3 months or longer to lessen the possibility of relapse.

Intramuscular Dosage

Initially, 20 to 30 mg (2 to 3 mL) four times a day.

When ELAVIL Injection is administered intramuscularly, the effects may appear more rapidly than with oral administration.

When ELAVIL Injection is used for initial therapy in patients unable or unwilling to take ELAVIL Tablets, the tablets should replace the injection as soon as possible.

Usage in Children

In view of the lack of experience with the use of this drug in children, it is not recommended at the present time for patients under 12 years of age.

Plasma Levels

Because of the wide variation in the absorption and distribution of tricyclic antidepressants in body fluids, it is difficult to directly correlate plasma levels and therapeutic effect. However, determination of plasma levels may be useful in identifying patients who appear to have toxic effects and may have excessively high levels, or those in whom lack of absorption or noncompliance is suspected. Adjustments in

dosage should be made according to the patient's clinical response and not on the basis of plasma levels.***

OVERDOSAGE

Deaths may occur from overdosage with this class of drugs. Multiple drug ingestion (including alcohol) is common in deliberate tricyclic antidepressant overdosage. As the management is complex and changing, it is recommended that the physician contact a poison control center for current information on treatment. Signs and symptoms of toxicity develop rapidly after tricyclic antidepressant overdose, therefore, hospital monitoring is required as soon as possible.

Manifestations: Critical manifestations of overdose include: cardiac dysrhythmias, severe hypotension, convulsions, and CNS depression, including coma. Changes in the electrocardiogram, particularly in QRS axis or width, are clinically significant indicators of tricyclic antidepressant toxicity.

Other signs of overdose may include: impaired myocardial contractility, confusion; disturbed concentration, transient visual hallucinations, dilated pupils, disorders of ocular motility, agitation, hyperactive reflexes, polyradiculoneuropathy, stupor, drowsiness, muscle rigidity, vomiting, hypothermia, hyperpyrexia, or any of the symptoms listed under ADVERSE REACTIONS.

Management:

General: Obtain an ECG and immediately initiate cardiac monitoring. Protect the patient's airway, establish an intravenous line and initiate gastric decontamination. A minimum of six hours of observation with cardiac monitoring and observation for signs of CNS or respiratory depression, hypotension, cardiac dysrhythmias and/or conduction blocks, and seizures is necessary. If signs of toxicity occur at any time during the period, extended monitoring is required. There are case reports of patients succumbing to fatal dysrhythmias late after overdose; these patients had clinical evidence of significant poisoning prior to death and most received inadequate gastrointestinal decontamination. Monitoring of plasma drug levels should not guide management of the patient.

Gastrointestinal Decontamination: All patients suspected of tricyclic antidepressant overdose should receive gastrointestinal decontamination. This should include large volume gastric lavage followed by activated charcoal. If consciousness is impaired, the airway should be secured prior to lavage. Emesis is contraindicated.

Cardiovascular: A maximal limb-lead QRS duration of ≥0.10 seconds may be the best indication of the severity of the overdose. Intravenous sodium bicarbonate should be used to maintain the serum pH in the range of 7.45 to 7.55. If the pH response is inadequate, hyperventilation may also be used. Concomitant use of hyperventilation and sodium bicarbonate should be done with extreme caution, with frequent pH monitoring. A pH >7.60 or a $pCO_2 < 20$ mm Hg is undesirable. Dysrhythmias unresponsive to sodium bicarbonate therapy/hyperventilation may respond to lidocaine, bretylium or phenytoin. Type 1A and 1C antiarrhyghmics are generally contraindicated (e.g., quinidine, disopyramide, and procainamide).

In rare instances, hemoperfusion may be beneficial in acute refractory cardiovascular instability in patients with acute toxicity. However, hemodialysis, peritoneal dialysis, exchange tranfusions, and forced diuresis generally have been reported as ineffective in tricyclic antidepressant poisoning.

CNS: In patients with CNS depression, early intubation is advised because of the potential for abrupt deterioration. Seizures should be controlled with benzodiazepines, or if these are ineffective, other anticonvulsants, (e.g., phenobarbital, phenytoin). Physostiqmine is not recommended except to treat life-threatening symptoms that have been unresponsive to other therapies, and then only in consultation with a poison control center.

Psychiatric Follow-up: Since overdosage is often deliberate, patients may attempt suicide by other means during the recovery phase. Psychiatric referral may be appropriate.

Pediatric Managment: The principles of management of pediatric and adult overdosages are similar. It is strongly recommended that the physician contact the local poison control center for specific pediatric treatment.

HOW SUPPLIED

Tablets ELAVIL, 10 mg, are blue, round, film coated tablets, identified with "40" debossed on one side and "ELAVIL" on the other side. They are supplied as follows:

NDC 0310-0040-10 bottles of 100
NDC 0310-0040-34 bottles of 1000

Tablets ELAVIL, 25 mg, are yellow, round, film coated tablets, identified with "45" debossed on one side and "ELAVIL" on the other side. They are supplied as follows:

NDC 0310-0045-10 bottles of 100
NDC 0310-0045-39 unit dose packages of 100
NDC 0310-0045-34 bottles of 1000
NDC 0310-0045-50 bottles of 5000

Tablets ELAVIL, 50 mg, are beige, round, film coated tablets, identified with "41" debossed on one side and "ELAVIL" on the other side. They are supplied as follows:

NDC 0310-0041-10 bottles of 100
NDC 0310-0041-39 unit dose packages of 100
NDC 0310-0041-34 bottles of 1000

Tablets ELAVIL, 75 mg, are orange, round, film coated tablets, identified with "42" debossed on one side and "ELAVIL" on the other side. They are supplied as follows:

NDC 0310-0042-10 bottles of 100

Tablets ELAVIL, 100 mg, are mauve, round, film coated tablets, identified with "43" debossed on one side and "ELAVIL" on the other side. They are supplied as follows:

NDC 0310-0043-10 bottles of 100

Tablets ELAVIL, 150 mg, are blue, capsule shaped, film coated tablets, identified with "47" debossed on one side and "ELAVIL" on the other side. They are supplied as follows:

NDC 0310-0047-30 bottles of 30
NDC 0310-0047-10 bottles of 100

Injection ELAVIL, 10 mg/mL, is a clear, colorless solution, and is supplied as follows:

NDC 0310-0049-10 in 10 mL vials

Storage: Store Tablets ELAVIL in a well-closed container. Avoid storage at temperatures above 30°C (86°F). In addition, Tablets ELAVIL 10 mg must be protected from light and stored in a well-closed, light-resistant container.

Protect ELAVIL Injection from freezing and avoid storage above 30°C (86°F).

METABOLISM

Studies in man following oral administration of ^{14}C-labeled drug indicated at amitriptyline is rapidly absorbed and metabolized. Radioactivity of the plasma was practically negligible, although significant amounts of radioactivity appeared in the urine by 4 to 6 hours and one-half to one-third of the drug was excreted within 24 hours.

Amitriptyline is metabolized by N-demethylation and bridge hydroxulation in man, rabbit, and rat. Virtually the entire dose is excreted as glucuronide or sulfate conjugate of metabolites, with little unchanged drug appearing in the urine. Other metabolic pathways may be involved.

REFERENCES

Ayd FJ Jr: Amitriptyline (ELAVIL) therapy for depressive reactions. Psychosomatics 1960;1:320–325.

Diamond S: Human metabolizer of amitriptyline tagged with carbon 14. Curr Ther Res, Mar 1965, pp 170–175.

Dorfman W: Clinical experiences with amitriptyline (ELAVIL): A preliminary report. Psychosomatics 1960;1:153–155.

Fallette JM, Stasney CR, Mintz AA: Amitriptyline poisoning treated with physostigmine. South Med J 1970;63:1492–1493.

Hollister LE, Overall JE, Johnson M, et al: Controlled comparison of amitriptyline, imipramine and placebo in hospitalized depressed patients. J Nerve Ment Dis 1964:139:370–375.

Hordern A, Burt CG, Holt NF: Depressive states: A pharmacotherapeutic study, Springfield study. Springfield, Ill, Charles C. Thomas, 1965.

Klerman GL, Cole JO: Clinical pharmacology of imipramine and related antidepressant compounds. Int J Psychiatry 1976;3:267–304.

McConaghy N, Joffe AD, Kingston WR, et al: Correlation of clinical features of depressed out-patients with response to amitriptyline and protiptyline. Br J Psychiatry 1968;114:103–106.

McDonald IM, Perkins M, Marjerrison G, et al: A controlled comparison of amitriptyline and electroconvulsive therapy in the treatment of depression. Am J Psychiatry 1966;122:1427–1431.

Slovis T, Ott J, Teitelbaum, et al: Physostigmine therapy in acute tricyclic antidepressant poisoning. Clin Toxicol 1971;4:451–459.

Symposium on depression with special studies of a new antidepressant amitriptyline. Dis Nerv Syst, (Sect 2) May 1961, pp 5–56.

*Registered trademark of ZENECA Inc.
**Based on a maximum recommended amitripyline dose of 150 mg/day or 3 mg/kg/day for a 50 kg patient.
***Hollister LE: JAMA 1979;241:2350–2533.

Manufactured for:
ZENECA Pharmaceuticals
A Business Unit of Zeneca Inc.
Wilmington, Delaware 19850-5437
by MERCK & Co., Inc., West Point, PA 19486, USA
64059-01 Rev I 05/96

Shown in Product Identification Guide, page 341

HIBICLENS® Antiseptic/Antimicrobial OTC
[hi'bi-klenz]
Skin Cleanser
(chlorhexidine gluconate)

DESCRIPTION

HIBICLENS is an antiseptic antimicrobial skin cleanser possessing bactericidal activities. HIBICLENS contains 4% w/v HIBITANE® (chlorhexidine gluconate), a chemically unique hexamethylenebis biguanide with inactive ingredients: Fragrance, isopropyl alcohol 4%, purified water, Red 40, and other ingredients, in a mild, sudsing base adjusted to pH 5.0–6.5 for optimal activity and stability as well as compatibility with the normal pH of the skin.

ACTION

HIBICLENS is bactericidal on contact. It has antiseptic activity and a persistent antimicrobial effect with rapid bactericidal activity against a wide range of microorganisms, including gram-positive bacteria, and gram-negative bacteria such as *Pseudomonas aeruginosa.* The effectiveness of HIBICLENS is not signficantly reduced by the presence of organic matter, such as blood.[1]

In a study[2] simulating surgical use, the immediate bactericidal effect of HIBICLENS after a single six-minute scrub resulted in a 99.9% reduction in resident bacterial flora, with a reduction of 99.98% after the eleventh scrub. Reductions on surgically gloved hands were maintained over the six-hour test period.

HIBICLENS displays persistent antimicrobial action. In one study[2], 93% of a radiolabeled formulation of HIBICLENS remained present on uncovered skin after five hours.

HIBICLENS prevents skin infection thereby reducing the risk of cross-infection.

INDICATIONS

HIBICLENS is indicated for use as a surgical scrub, as a health-care personnel handwash, for patient preoperative showering and bathing, as a patient preoperative skin preparation, and as a skin wound cleanser and general skin cleanser.

SAFETY

The extensive use of chlorhexidine gluconate for over 20 years outside the United States has produced no evidence of absorption of the compound through intact skin. The potential for producing skin reactions is extremely low. HIBICLENS can be used many times a day without causing irritation, dryness, or discomfort. Experimental studies indicate that when used for cleaning superficial wounds, HIBICLENS will neither cause additional tissue injury nor delay healing.

WARNINGS

FOR EXTERNAL USE ONLY. KEEP OUT OF EYES, EARS AND MOUTH. HIBICLENS SHOULD NOT BE USED AS A PREOPERATIVE SKIN PREPARATION OF THE FACE OR HEAD. MISUSE OF HIBICLENS HAS BEEN REPORTED TO CAUSE SERIOUS AND PERMANENT EYE INJURY WHEN IT HAS BEEN PERMITTED TO ENTER AND REMAIN IN THE EYE DURING SURGICAL PROCEDURES. IF HIBICLENS SHOULD CONTACT THESE AREAS, RINSE OUT PROMPTLY AND THOROUGHLY WITH WATER.

Avoid contact with meninges. HIBICLENS should not be used by persons who have a sensitivity to it or its components. Chlorhexidine gluconate has been reported to cause deafness when instilled in the middle ear through perforated ear drums. Irritation, sensitization and generalized allergic reactions have been reported with chlorhexidine-containing products, especially in the genital areas. If adverse reactions occur, discontinue use immediately and if severe, contact a physician. Keep this and all drugs out of the reach of children. In case of accidental ingestion, seek professional assistance or contact a Poison Control Center immediately.

Accidental ingestion: Chlorhexidine gluconate taken orally is poorly absorbed. Treat with gastric lavage using milk, egg white, gelatin or mild soap. Employ supportive measures as appropriate.

Avoid excessive heat (above 104°F).

DIRECTIONS FOR USE

Skin Wound and General skin Cleansing

Wounds which involve more than the superficial layers of the skin should not be routinely treated with HIBICLENS. HIBICLENS should not be used for repeated general skin cleansing of large body areas except in those patients whose underlying condition makes it necessary to reduce the bacterial population of the skin. To use, thoroughly rinse the area to be cleansed with water. Apply the minimum amount of HIBICLENS necessary to cover the skin or wound area and wash gently. Rinse again thoroughly.

Preoperative Skin Preparation

Apply HIBICLENS liberally to surgical site and swab for at least two minutes. Dry with a sterile towel. Repeat procedure for an additional two minutes and dry with a sterile towel.

Preoperative Showering and Whole-Body bathing

The patient should be instructed to wash the entire body, including the scalp, on two consecutive occasions immediately prior to surgery. Each procedure should consist of two consecutive thorough applications of HIBICLENS followed by thorough rinsing. If the patient's condition allows, showering is recommended for whole-body bathing. The recommended procedure is: Wet the body, including hair. Wash the

Continued on next page

Zeneca Pharmaceuticals—Cont.

Operation	Water Level	Temperature	Time (Min)	Supplies/100 lb
Break	Low	180°F	20	1.5 lb oxalic acid
Flush	High	Cold	1	—
Emulsify	Low	160°F	5	18 oz emulsifier
Flush	High	Cold	1	—
Bleach	Low	180°F	20	2 lb alkali builder and 1 lb organic bleach
Rinse	High	Cold	1	—
Antichlor	High	Cold	2	4 oz antichlor
Rinse	High	Cold	1	—
Rinse	High	Cold	1	—
Sour	Low	Cold	4	2 oz rust removing sour

hair using 25 mL of HIBICLENS and the body with another 25 mL of HIBICLENS. Rinse. Repeat. Rinse thoroughly after second application.

HEALTH-CARE PERSONNEL USE
SURGICAL HAND SCRUB
Directions for use of HIBICLENS Liquid: Wet hands and forearms with water. Scrub for 3 minutes with about 5 mL of HIBICLENS and a wet brush, paying particular attention to the nails, cuticles, and interdigital spaces. A separate nail cleaner may be used. Rinse thoroughly. Wash for an additional 3 minutes with 5 mL of HIBICLENS and rinse under running water. Dry thoroughly.

Personnel Hand Wash
Wet hands with warm water. (Avoid using very cold or very hot water.) Dispense about 5 mL of HIBICLENS into cupped hands. Wash for 15 seconds. (Do not use excessive pressure to produce additional lather.) Rinse thoroughly with warm water. Dry thoroughly.

Directions for use of HIBICLENS® Sponge/Brush: Open package and remove nail cleaner. Wet hands. Use nail cleaner under fingernails and to clean cuticles. Wet hands and forearms to the elbow with warm water. (Avoid using very cold or very hot water.) Wet sponge side of sponge/brush. Squeeze and pump immediately to work up adequate lather. Apply lather to hands and forearms using *sponge* side of the product. *Start 3 minute scrub* by using the brush side of the product to scrub *only* nails, cuticles, and interdigital areas. Use sponge side for scrubbing hands and forearms. (Avoid using brush on these more sensitive areas.) Rinse thoroughly with warm water. Scrub for an additional 3 minutes *using sponge side* only. To produce additional lather, add a small amount of water and pump the sponge. (While scrubbing, do not use excessive pressure to produce lather—a small amount of lather is all that is required to adequately cleanse skin with HIBICLENS.) Rinse and dry thoroughly, blotting hands and forearms with a soft sterile towel.

IMPORTANT LAUNDERING ADVICE FOR HOSPITAL STAFF AND OTHER USERS OF ANTISEPTIC PATIENT SKIN PREPARATIONS CONTAINING CHLORHEXIDINE GLUCONATE
Chlorhexidine gluconate is a unique agent that most closely fits the definition of an ideal antimicrobial agent, having (among others) one of the most important characteristics of persistent activity. This persistence is due to chlorhexidine gluconate binding to the protein of the skin and, thus, being available for residual activity over a relatively long period of time.

Chlorhexidine gluconate, however, binds not only to protein of the skin, but also to many fabrics, particularly cotton. Thus, special laundering procedures should be considered when such products contact these fabrics. As a result of such contact, chlorhexidine gluconate may become adsorbed onto the fabric and not be removed by washing. If sufficient available chlorine is present during the washing procedure, a fast brown stain may develop due to a chemical reaction between chlorhexidine gluconate and chlorine.

SUGGESTED LAUNDERING PROCEDURES TO LIMIT STAINING
1. **Not Aging.** Avoid allowing the product to age (set) on unwashed linens.
2. **Flushing and Washing.** A flush operation as the initial step in the wash process is helpful in the laundering of linen exposed to chlorhexidine gluconate. Such flushing is also important in the laundering of linen which contains organic materials such as blood or pus. For best results, warm water flushes (90°–100°F) are recommended. After a number of initial flushings followed by a washing with a low alkaline/nonchlorine detergent, most articles which come in contact with chlorhexidine gluconate should have an acceptable level of whiteness. If a rewash process using bleach is necessary to achieve a greater degree of whiteness, the bleach used should be a nonchlorine bleach.
3. **Not Using Chlorine Bleach.** Modern laundering methods often make the use of chlorine bleach unnecessary. It is worthwhile trying to wash without chlorine to ascertain if the resulting degree of whiteness is acceptable. Omission of chlorine from the laundering process can extend the useful life of cotton articles since oxidizing bleaches such as chlorine may cause some damage to cellulose even when used in low concentration.
4. **Changing to a Peroxide-Type Bleach, Such as Sodium Perborate, Sodium Percarbonate or Hydrogen Peroxide.** This should eliminate the reaction which could occur with the use of chlorine bleaches. If a chlorine bleach must be used, a concentration of less than 7 ppm available chlorine (¹⁄₁₀ the normal bleach level) is suggested to minimize possible staining.

A NOTE ON LAUNDERING OF PERSONAL CLOTHING
The laundering procedures set forth above using low alkaline, nonchlorinated laundry detergents are also applicable to laundering of uniforms and lab coats. Commercially available laundry detergents which do not contain chlorine include Borax, Borateem, Dreft, Oxydol, and Ivory Snow. These products, however, will not remove stains previously set into the fabric.

RECLAMATION OF STAINED LINENS
For those linens which previously have been stained due to the chemical reaction between chlorhexidine gluconate and chlorine, the following laundering procedure may be helpful in reducing the visible stain:

[See table above.]

HOW SUPPLIED
For general handwashing locations: pocket-size, 15 mL foil Packettes; plastic disposable bottles of 4 oz and 8 oz with dispenser caps; and 16 oz filled globes. *For surgical scrub areas:* disposable, unit-of-use 22 mL impregnated Sponge/Brushes with nail cleaner; plastic disposable bottles of 32 oz and 1 gal. The 32-oz bottle is designed for a special foot-operated wall dispenser. A hand-operated wall dispenser is available for the 16-oz globe. Hand pumps are available for 16 oz, 32 oz, and 1 gal sizes. Liquid: NDC 0310-0575. Sponge/Brush: NDC 0310-0577.

REFERENCES
1. Lowbury, EJL and Lilly, HA: The effect of blood on disinfection of surgeons' hands, Brit. J. Surg. 61:19–21 (Jan.) 1974.
2. Peterson AF, Rosenberg A, Alatary SD: Comparative evaluation of surgical scrub preparations, Surg. Gynecol. Obstet. 146:63–65 (Jan.) 1978.
Zeneca Pharmaceuticals
A Business Unit of Zeneca Inc.
Wilmington, DE 19850-5437 USA
Shown in Product Identification Guide, pages 341 and 342

HIBISTAT® Germicidal Hand Rinse OTC
HIBISTAT® TOWELETTE
Germicidal Handwipe
[hi'bi-stat]
(chlorhexidine gluconate)

DESCRIPTION
HIBISTAT is a germicidal hand rinse which provides rapid bactericidal action and has a persistent antimicrobial effect against a wide range of microorganisms. HIBISTAT is a clear, colorless liquid containing 0.5% w/w HIBITANE® (chlorhexidine gluconate) with inactive ingredients: emollients, isopropyl alcohol 70%, purified water.

INDICATIONS
HIBISTAT is indicated for health-care personnel use as a germicidal hand rinse. HIBISTAT is for hand hygiene on physically clean hands. It is used in those situations where hands are physically clean, but in need of degerming, when routine handwashing is not convenient or desirable. HIBISTAT provides rapid germicidal action and has a persistent effect.
HIBISTAT should be used in-between patients and procedures where there are no sinks available or continued return to the sink area is inconvenient. HIBISTAT can be used as an alternative to detergent-based products when hands are physically clean. Also, HIBISTAT is an effective germicidal hand rinse following a soap and water handwash.

WARNINGS
Flammable. This product is alcohol based. Alcohol is extremely flammable. It should be kept away from flame or devices which may generate an electrical spark.
FOR EXTERNAL USE ONLY. KEEP OUT OF EYES, EARS AND MOUTH. HIBISTAT SHOULD NOT BE USED AS A PREOPERATIVE SKIN PREPARATION OF THE FACE OR HEAD. MISUSE OF CHLORHEXIDINE-CONTAINING PRODUCTS HAS BEEN REPORTED TO CAUSE SERIOUS AND PERMANENT EYE INJURY WHEN IT HAS BEEN PERMITTED TO ENTER AND REMAIN IN THE EYE DURING SURGICAL PROCEDURES. IF HIBISTAT SHOULD CONTACT THESE AREAS, RINSE OUT PROMPTLY AND THOROUGHLY WITH WATER. Avoid contact with meninges. HIBISTAT should not be used by persons who have a sensitivity to it or its components. Chlorhexidine gluconate has been reported to cause deafness when instilled in the middle ear through perforated ear drums. Irritation, sensitization, and generalized allergic reactions have been reported with chlorhexidine-containing products, especially in the genital areas. If adverse reactions occur, discontinue use immediately and if severe, contact a physician. Keep this and all drugs out of the reach of children. In case of accidental ingestion, seek professional assistance or contact a Poison Control Center immediately. Avoid excessive heat (above 104°F).
Accidental ingestion: Chlorhexidine gluconate taken orally is poorly absorbed. Treat with gastric lavage using milk, egg white, gelatin or mild soap avoiding pulmonary aspiration. Do not use apomorphine. Assist respiration if necessary and keep patient warm. Intravenous levulose can accelerate alcohol metabolism. In severe cases, hemodialysis or peritoneal dialysis may be appropriate.

DIRECTIONS FOR USE
HIBISTAT Towelette: Rub hands vigorously with HIBISTAT Towelette for approximately 15 seconds, paying particular attention to nails and interdigital spaces. HIBISTAT dries rapidly in use. No water or towel drying are necessary. The emollients contained in the HIBISTAT Towelette protect the hands from the potential drying effect of alcohol.
HIBISTAT Liquid: Dispense about 5 mL of HIBISTAT into cupped hands and rub vigorously until dry (about 15 seconds), paying particular attention to nails and interdigital spaces. HIBISTAT dries rapidly in use. No water or toweling are necessary. The emollients contained in HIBISTAT protect the hands from the potential drying effect of alcohol.

LAUNDERING
Chlorhexidine gluconate chemically reacts with chlorine to form a brown stain on fabric. Fabric which has come in contact with chlorhexidine gluconate should be rinsed well and washed without the addition of chlorine products. If bleach is desired, only nonchlorine bleach should be used. Full laundering instructions are packed with each case of HIBISTAT. (Please see HIBICLENS® for full laundering instructions.)

HOW SUPPLIED
In plastic disposable bottles of 4 oz and 8 oz with flip-top cap, and in disposable towelettes containing 5 mL, packaged 50 towelettes to a carton.
NDC 0310-0585 (bottles)
NDC 0310-0587 (towelettes)
Manufactured For:
Zeneca Pharmaceuticals
A Business Unit of Zeneca Inc.
Wilmington, DE 19850-5437 USA
by ACCUPAC, Inc
Shown in Product Identification Guide, page 342

KADIAN™ C II ℞
Morphine Sulfate Sustained Release
KADIAN™ 20 mg Capsules
KADIAN™ 50 mg Capsules
KADIAN™ 100 mg Capsules

Warning: May be habit forming

DESCRIPTION
KADIAN™ capsules 20, 50 and 100 mg contain identical polymer coated sustained release pellets of morphine sulfate for oral administration.
Chemically, morphine sulfate is 7,8-didehydro-4,5 α-epoxy-17-methyl-morphinan-3,6 α-diol sulfate (2:1) (salt) pentahydrate and has the following structural formula:

Morphine sulfate is an odorless, white, crystalline powder with a bitter taste and a molecular weight of 758 (as the sulfate). It has a solubility of 1 in 21 parts of water and 1 in 1000 parts of alcohol, but is practically insoluble in chloroform or ether. The octanol:water partition coefficient of morphine is 1.42 at physiologic pH and the pK_b is 7.9 for the tertiary nitrogen (mostly ionized at pH 7.4).

Each KADIAN™ Sustained Release Capsule contains either 20, 50 or 100 mg of Morphine Sulfate USP and the following inactive ingredients common to all strengths: Hydroxypropyl Methylcellulose, Ethylcellulose, Methacrylic Acid Copolymer, Polyethylene Glycol, Diethyl Phthalate, Talc, Black Ink SW-9009, Corn Starch and Sucrose.

CLINICAL PHARMACOLOGY

Morphine is a natural product that is the prototype for the class of natural and synthetic opioid analgesics. Opioids produce a wide spectrum of pharmacologic effects including analgesia, dysphoria, euphoria, somnolence, respiratory depression, diminished gastrointestinal motility, altered circulatory dynamics, histamine release and physical dependence.

Morphine produces both its therapeutic and its adverse effects by interaction with one or more classes of specific opioid receptors located throughout the body. Morphine acts as a pure agonist, binding with and activating opioid receptors at sites in the peri-aqueductal and peri-ventricular grey matter, the ventro-medial medulla and the spinal cord to produce analgesia.

Effects on the Central Nervous System

The principal therapeutic actions of morphine are analgesia, sedation and alterations of mood. Opioids of this class do not usually eliminate pain, but they do reduce the perception of pain by the central nervous system.

Morphine produces respiratory depression by reducing the responsiveness of the brain stem respiratory centers to increases in carbon dioxide tension (or to direct electrical stimulation).

Morphine depresses the cough reflex by direct effect on the cough center in the medulla. Antitussive effects may occur with doses lower than those usually required for analgesia.

Morphine causes miosis, even in total darkness, and little tolerance develops to this effect. Pinpoint pupils are a sign of opioid overdose but are not pathognomonic (e.g. pontine lesions of hemorrhagic or ischemic origins may produce similar findings). Marked mydriasis rather than miosis may be seen due to severe hypoxia in overdose situations.

Effects on the Gastrointestinal Tract

Gastric, biliary and pancreatic secretions are decreased by morphine. Morphine causes a reduction in motility associated with an increase in tone in the antrum of the stomach and duodenum. Digestion of food in the small intestine is delayed and propulsive contractions are decreased. Propulsive peristaltic waves in the colon are decreased, while tone is increased to the point of spasm. The end result is constipation. Morphine can cause a marked increase in biliary tract pressure as a result of spasm of the sphincter of Oddi.

Effects on the Cardiovascular System

Morphine produces peripheral vasodilation which may result in orthostatic hypotension or syncope. Release of histamine may be induced by morphine and can contribute to opioid-induced hypotension. Manifestations of histamine release and/or peripheral vasodilation may include pruritus, flushing, red eyes and sweating.

Pharmacodynamics

The relationship between the blood level of morphine and the analgesic response will depend on the patient's age, state of health, medical condition, and the extent of previous opioid treatment.

A minimum effective concentration (MEC) of morphine for pain relief has been reported as 27.2 ± 14.5 ng/mL (mean $\pm$ SD) in cancer patients treated with morphine solution. These results compare with the MEC for plasma morphine reported as 14.7 ± 4.8 ng/mL (mean $\pm$ SD) in patients with postoperative pain. The high degree of variation is of clinical significance as it may result in either under-dosing or over-dosing if the dosage is not adjusted to the patients clinical status and analgesic response (see **PRECAUTIONS** and **DOSAGE AND ADMINISTRATION**).

For opioid-tolerant patients the situation is much more complex. Some patients will become rapidly tolerant to the analgesic effects of morphine, and will require high daily oral morphine doses for adequate pain control. Since the development of tolerance to both the therapeutic and adverse effects of opioids is highly individualized, the dose of morphine should be individualized to the patient's condition and should not be based on an arbitrary choice of a dose or blood level to be achieved.

Table 1: Mean pharmacokinetic parameters (% coefficient variation) resulting from a fasting single dose study in normal volunteers and a multiple dose study in patients with cancer pain.

Regimen/ Dosage Form	AUC[#, +] (ng.h/mL)	C_{max}[+] (ng/mL)	T_{max} (h)	C_{min}[+] (ng/mL)	Fluctuation[*]
Single Dose (n=24)					
KADIAN™ Capsule	271.0 (19.4)	15.6 (24.4)	8.6 (41.1)	na [^]	na
Controlled-Release Tablet	304.3 (19.1)	30.5 (32.1)	2.5 (52.6)	na	na
Morphine Solution	362.4 (42.6)	64.4 (38.2)	0.9 (55.8)	na	na
Multiple Dose (n=24)					
KADIAN™ Capsule q24h	500.9 (38.6)	37.3 (37.7)	10.3 (32.2)	9.9 (52.3)	3.0 (45.5)
Controlled-Release Tablet q12h	457.3 (40.2)	36.9 (42.0)	4.4 (53.0)	7.6 (60.3)	4.1 (51.5)

\# For single dose AUC = AUC_{0-48h}, for multiple dose AUC = AUC_{0-24h} at steady state
\+ For single dose parameter normalized to 100 mg, for multiple dose parameter normalized to 100 mg per 24 hours.
* Steady-state fluctuation in plasma concentrations = $C_{max}-C_{min}/C_{min}$
^ Not applicable

Pharmacokinetics

KADIAN™ capsules contain polymer coated sustained release pellets of morphine sulfate that release morphine significantly more slowly than from morphine sulfate tablets and shorter-acting controlled-release oral morphine sulfate preparations. KADIAN™ activity is primarily due to morphine. One metabolite, morphine-6-glucuronide, has been shown to have analgesic activity, but poorly crosses the blood-brain barrier.

Following oral administration, the extent of absorption is essentially the same for immediate or sustained release formulations, although the time to peak blood level (T_{max}) will be longer and the C_{max} will be lower for formulations that delay the release of morphine in the gastrointestinal tract. Elimination of morphine is primarily via hepatic metabolism to glucuronide metabolites (55 to 65%) which are then renally excreted. The terminal half-life of morphine is 2 to 4 hours, however, a longer term half-life of about 15 hours has been reported in studies where blood has been sampled up to 48 hours.

The single-dose pharmacokinetics of KADIAN™ are linear over the dosage range of 30 to 100 mg. The single dose and multiple dose pharmacokinetic parameters of KADIAN™ in normal volunteers are summarized in Table 1.

[See Table 1 above.]

Absorption

Following the administration of oral morphine solution, approximately 50% of the morphine absorbed reaches the systemic circulation within 30 minutes. However, following the administration of an equal amount of KADIAN™ to healthy volunteers, this occurs, on average, after 8 hours. As with most forms of oral morphine, because of pre-systemic elimination, only about 20 to 40% of the administered dose reaches the systemic circulation.

Food Effects: While concurrent administration of food slows the rate of absorption of KADIAN™, the extent of absorption is not affected and KADIAN™ can be administered without regard to meals.

Steady State: When KADIAN™ is given on a fixed dosing regimen to patients with chronic pain due to malignancy, steady state is achieved in about two days. At steady state, KADIAN™ will have a significantly lower C_{max} and a higher C_{min} than equivalent doses of oral morphine solution and some other controlled-release preparations (see Graph 1).

Graph 1 (Study # MOB-1/90): Mean steady state plasma morphine concentrations for KADIAN™ (twice a day), controlled-release morphine tablet (twice a day) and oral morphine solution (every 4 hours); plasma concentrations are normalized to 100 mg every 24 hours. (n=24).

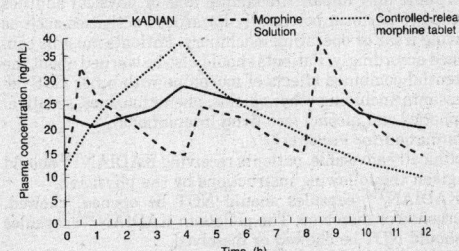

When given once-daily (every 24 hours) to 24 patients with malignancy, KADIAN™ had a similar C_{max} and higher C_{min} at steady state in clinical usage, when compared to twice-daily (every 12 hours) controlled-release morphine tablets (MS Contin®), given at an equivalent total daily dosage (see Graph 2 and Table 1). Drug-disease interactions are frequently seen in the older and more gravely ill patients, and may result in both altered absorption and reduced clearance as compared to normal volunteers (see **Geriatric, Hepatic Failure,** and **Renal Insufficiency** sections).

Graph 2 (Study # MOR-9/92): Dose normalized mean steady state plasma morphine concentrations for KADIAN™ (once a day), and an equivalent dose of a 12-hour, controlled-release morphine tablet given twice a day. Plasma concentrations are normalized to 100 mg every 24 hours. (n=24).

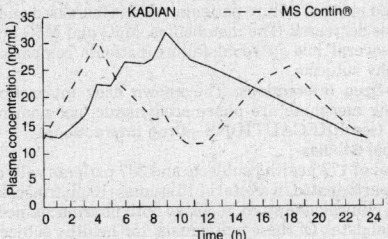

Distribution

Once absorbed, morphine is distributed to skeletal muscle, kidneys, liver, intestinal tract, lungs, spleen and brain.

The volume of distribution of morphine is approximately 3 to 4 L/kg. Morphine is 30 to 35% reversibly bound to plasma proteins.

Although the primary site of action of morphine is in the CNS, only small quantities pass the blood-brain barrier. Morphine also crosses the placental membranes (see **PRECAUTIONS—Pregnancy**) and has been found in breast milk (see **PRECAUTIONS—Nursing Mothers**)

Metabolism

The major pathway of the detoxification of morphine is conjugation, either with D-glucuronic acid in the liver to produce glucuronides or with sulfuric acid to give morphine-3-etheral sulfate. Although a small fraction (less than 5%) of morphine is demethylated, for all practical purposes, virtually all morphine is converted to glucuronide metabolites including morphine-3-glucuronide, M3G (about 50%) and morphine-6-glucuronide, M6G (about 5 to 15%). Studies in healthy subjects and cancer patients have shown that the glucuronide metabolite to morphine mean molar ratios (based on AUC) are similar after both single doses and at steady state for KADIAN™, 12-hour controlled-release morphine sulfate tablets and morphine sulfate solution M3G has no significant analgesic activity. M6G has been shown to have opioid agonist and analgesic activity in humans.

Excretion

Approximately 10% of morphine dose is excreted unchanged in the urine. Most of the dose is excreted in the urine as M3G and M6G. A small amount of the glucuronide metabolites is excreted in the bile and there is some minor enterohepatic cycling. Seven to 10% of administered morphine is excreted in the feces.

The mean adult plasma clearance is about 20-30 mL/minute/kg. The effective terminal half- life of morphine after IV administration is reported to be approximately 2.0 hours. Longer plasma sampling in some studies suggests a longer terminal half-life of morphine of about 15 hours.

Special Populations

Geriatric: The elderly may have increased sensitivity to morphine and may achieve higher and more variable serum levels than younger patients. In adults, the duration of analgesia increases progressively with age, though the degree of analgesia remains unchanged. KADIAN™ pharmacokinetics have not been investigated in elderly patients (>65 years) although such patients were included in the clinical studies.

Nursing Mothers: Morphine is excreted in the maternal milk, and the milk to plasma morphine AUC ratio is about 2.5:1. The amount of morphine received by the infant depends on the maternal plasma concentration, amount of

Continued on next page

Zeneca Pharmaceuticals—Cont.

milk ingested by the infant, and the extent of first pass metabolism.

Pediatric: Infants under 1 month of age have a prolonged elimination half-life and decreased clearance relative to older infants and children. The clearance of morphine and its elimination half-life begin to approach adult values by the second month of life. Children old enough to take capsules should have pharmacokinetic parameters similar to adults, dosed on a per kilogram basis (see **PRECAUTIONS—Pediatric Use**).

Gender: No meaningful differences between male and female patients were demonstrated in the analysis of the pharmacokinetic data from clinical studies.

Race: Pharmacokinetic differences due to race may exist. Chinese subjects given intravenous morphine in one study had a higher clearance when compared to caucasian subjects $(1852 \pm 116$ mL/min versus 1495 ± 80 mL/min).

Hepatic Failure: The pharmacokinetics of morphine were found to be significantly altered in individuals with alcoholic cirrhosis. The clearance was found to decrease with a corresponding increase in half-life. The M3G and M6G to morphine plasma AUC ratios also decreased in these patients indicating a decrease in metabolic activity.

Renal Insufficiency: The pharmacokinetics of morphine are altered in renal failure patients. AUC is increased and clearance is decreased. The metabolites, M3G and M6G accumulate several fold in renal failure patients compared with healthy subjects.

Drug-Drug Interactions: The known drug interactions involving morphine are pharmacodynamic, not pharmacokinetic (see **PRECAUTIONS—Drug Interactions**).

Clinical Studies

A total of 177 healthy subjects and 337 patients with cancer pain participated in a total of 15 studies (10 pharmacokinetic and 6 clinical; one study reported both pharmacokinetic and clinical data). Of these individuals, 158 healthy subjects and 268 patients received KADIAN™. In the controlled clinical studies patients were followed for a median duration of 7 days and in the open label studies patients were followed for up to 12-24 months. KADIAN™ was compared to oral morphine solution and to either MS Contin® or to a 12-hour controlled-release morphine tablet bioequivalent to MS Contin® using trial designs that followed the clinical and pharmacokinetic performance of each treatment in cancer patients receiving chronic opioid therapy.

In two controlled studies, patients with moderate to severe cancer pain were titrated with immediate-release morphine (IRM) solution or tablets to a stable total daily dose of morphine for at least three consecutive days, then randomized to KADIAN™ or 12-hour controlled-release morphine for seven days of observation. KADIAN™ given once a day proved similar to the same total dose of morphine given in divided doses in a 12-hour dosage form, with respect to pain relief, use of rescue medication, patient and investigator global assessment, and quality of sleep. Individual patient differences in the pattern of pain control emphasize the need to individualize both dose and dosing interval (see **DOSAGE AND ADMINISTRATION**).

INDICATIONS AND USAGE

KADIAN™ is indicated for the management of moderate to severe pain where treatment with an opioid analgesic is indicated for more than a few days (see **CLINICAL PHARMACOLOGY; Clinical Studies**).

KADIAN™ was developed for use in patients with chronic pain who require repeated dosing with a potent opioid analgesic, and has been tested in patients with pain due to malignant conditions. KADIAN™ has not been tested as an analgesic for the treatment of acute pain or in the postoperative setting and is not recommended for such use.

CONTRAINDICATIONS

KADIAN™ is contraindicated in patients with a known hypersensitivity to morphine, morphine salts or any of the capsule components.

KADIAN™ is contraindicated in patients with respiratory depression in the absence of resuscitative equipment, and in patients with acute or severe bronchial asthma.

KADIAN™ is contraindicated in any patient who has or is suspected of having paralytic ileus.

WARNINGS
(See also **CLINICAL PHARMACOLOGY**)

Impaired Respiration

Respiratory depression is the chief hazard of all morphine preparations. Respiratory depression occurs more frequently in elderly and debilitated patients, and those suffering from conditions accompanied by hypoxia, hypercapnia, or upper airway obstruction (when even moderate therapeutic doses may significantly decrease pulmonary ventilation).

Morphine should be used with extreme caution in patients with chronic obstructive pulmonary disease or cor pulmonale, and in patients having a substantially decreased respiratory reserve (e.g. severe kyphoscoliosis), hypoxia, hyper-

capnia, or pre-existing respiratory depression. In such patients, even usual therapeutic doses of morphine may increase airway resistance and decrease respiratory drive to the point of apnea.

Head Injury and Increased Intracranial Pressure

The respiratory depressant effects of morphine with carbon dioxide retention and secondary elevation of cerebrospinal fluid pressure may be markedly exaggerated in the presence of head injury, other intracranial lesions, or a pre-existing increase in intracranial pressure. Morphine produces effects which may obscure neurologic signs of further increases in pressure in patients with head injuries. Morphine should only be administered under such circumstances when considered essential and then with extreme care.

Hypotensive Effect

KADIAN™, like all opioid analgesics, may cause severe hypotension in an individual whose ability to maintain blood pressure has already been compromised by a reduced blood volume, or a concurrent administration of drugs such as phenothiazines or general anesthetics. (see also **PRECAUTIONS—Drug Interactions**). KADIAN™ may produce orthostatic hypotension and syncope in ambulatory patients. KADIAN™, like all opioid analgesics, should be administered with caution to patients in circulatory shock, as vasodilation produced by the drug may further reduce cardiac output and blood pressure.

Gastrointestinal Obstruction

KADIAN™ should not be given to patients with gastrointestinal obstruction, particularly paralytic ileus, as there is a risk of the product remaining in the stomach for an extended period and the subsequent release of a bolus of morphine when normal gut motility is restored. As with other solid morphine formulations diarrhea may reduce morphine absorption.

PRECAUTIONS
(See also **CLINICAL PHARMACOLOGY**)

General

KADIAN™ is intended for use in patients who require continuous treatment with a potent opioid analgesic. As with any potent opioid, it is critical to adjust the dosing regimen for KADIAN™ for each patient, taking into account the patient's prior analgesic treatment experience. Although it is clearly impossible to enumerate every consideration that is important to the selection of the initial dose of KADIAN™, attention should be given to the points under **DOSAGE AND ADMINISTRATION**.

Cordotomy

Patients taking KADIAN™ who are scheduled for cordotomy or other interruption of pain transmission pathways should have KADIAN™ ceased 24 hours prior to the procedure and the pain controlled by parenteral short-acting opioids. In addition, the post-procedure titration of analgesics for such patients should be individualized to avoid either oversedation or withdrawal syndromes.

Use in Pancreatic/Biliary Tract Disease

KADIAN™ may cause spasm of the sphincter of Oddi and should be used with caution in patients with biliary tract disease, including acute pancreatitis. Opioids may cause increases in the serum amylase level.

Special risk groups

KADIAN™ should be administered with caution, and in reduced dosages in elderly or debilitated patients; patients with severe renal or hepatic insufficiency; patients with Addison's disease; myxedema; hypothyroidism; prostatic hypertrophy or urethral stricture.

Caution should also be exercised in the administration of KADIAN™ to patients with CNS depression, toxic psychosis, acute alcoholism and delirium tremens, and convulsive disorders.

Driving and operating machinery

Morphine may impair the mental and/or physical abilities needed to perform potentially hazardous activities such as driving a car or operating machinery. Patients must be cautioned accordingly. Patients should also be warned about the potential combined effects of morphine with other CNS depressants, including other opioids, phenothiazines, sedative/hypnotics and alcohol (see **Drug Interactions**).

Information for Patients

If clinically advisable, patients receiving KADIAN™ should be given the following instructions by the physician:

1. KADIAN™ capsules should NOT be opened, chewed, crushed or dissolved. The pellets in KADIAN™ capsules should NOT be chewed or dissolved.
2. The dose of KADIAN™ should not be adjusted without consulting the physician.
3. Morphine may impair mental and/or physical ability required for the performance of potentially hazardous tasks (e.g. driving, operating machinery). Patients started on KADIAN™ or whose dose has been changed should refrain from dangerous activity until it is established that they are not adversely affected.
4. Morphine should not be taken with alcohol or other CNS depressants (sleeping medication, tranquilizers) because additive effects including CNS depression may occur. A

physician should be consulted if other medications are currently being used or are prescribed for future use.
5. Women of childbearing potential who become or are planning to become pregnant, should consult a physician.
6. Upon completion of therapy, it may be appropriate to taper the morphine dose, rather than abruptly discontinuing it.
7. While psychological dependence ("addiction") to morphine used in the treatment of pain is very rare, morphine is one of a class of drugs known to be abused and should be handled accordingly.
8. As with other opioids, patients taking KADIAN™ should be advised that severe constipation could occur and appropriate laxatives, stool softeners and other appropriate treatments should be initiated from the beginning of opioid therapy.

Drug Interactions

<u>CNS Depressants:</u> Morphine should be used with great caution and in reduced dosage in patients who are concurrently receiving other central nervous system (CNS) depressants including sedatives, hypnotics, general anesthetics, antiemetics, phenothiazines, other tranquilizers and alcohol because of the risk of respiratory depression, hypotension and profound sedation or coma. When such combined therapy is contemplated, the initial dose of one or both agents should be reduced by at least 50%.

<u>Muscle Relaxants:</u> Morphine may enhance the neuromuscular blocking action of skeletal relaxants and produce an increased degree of respiratory depression.

<u>Mixed Agonist/Antagonist Opioid Analgesics:</u> From a theoretical perspective, mixed agonist/antagonist analgesics (i.e. pentazocine, nalbuphine and butorphanol) should NOT be administered to patients who have received or are receiving a course of therapy with a pure opioid agonist analgesic. In these patients, mixed agonist/antagonist analgesics may reduce the analgesic effect and/or may precipitate withdrawal symptoms.

<u>Monoamine Oxidase Inhibitors (MAOIs):</u> MAOIs have been reported to intensify the effects of at least one opioid drug causing anxiety, confusion and significant depression of respiration or coma. We do not recommend the use of KADIAN™ in patients taking MAOIs or within 14 days of stopping such treatment.

<u>Cimetidine:</u> There is an isolated report of confusion and severe respiratory depression when a hemodialysis patient was concurrently administered morphine and cimetidine.

<u>Diuretics:</u> Morphine can reduce the efficacy of diuretics by inducing the release of antidiuretic hormone. Morphine may also lead to acute retention of urine by causing spasm of the sphincter of the bladder, particularly in men with prostatism.

<u>Food:</u> The bioavailability of KADIAN™ is not significantly affected by food. KADIAN Capsules should be swallowed whole. The capsules, as well as the pellets contained in the capsules, however, must not be crushed, chewed, or mixed with food due to risk of overdose (see **DOSAGE AND ADMINISTRATION**, and **INFORMATION FOR PATIENTS**).

Carcinogenicity/Mutagenicity/Impairment of Fertility

Long-term studies in animals to evaluate the carcinogenic potential of morphine have not been conducted. There are no reports of carcinogenic effects in humans.

In vitro studies have reported that morphine is non-mutagenic in the Ames test with *Salmonella*, and induces chromosomal aberrations in human leukocytes and lethal mutation induction in *Drosophila*. Morphine was found to be mutagenic *in vitro* in human T-cells, increasing the DNA fragmentation. *In vivo*, morphine was mutagenic in the mouse micronucleus test and induced chromosomal aberrations in spermatids and murine lymphocytes.

Chronic opioid abusers (e.g., heroin abusers) and their offspring display higher rates of chromosomal damage. However, the rates of chromosomal abnormalities were similar in nonexposed individuals and in heroin users enrolled in long term opioid maintenance programs.

Pregnancy

Teratogenic effects (Pregnancy Category C)

Teratogenic effects of morphine have been reported in the animal literature. High parental doses during the second trimester were teratogenic in neurological, soft and skeletal tissue. The abnormalities included encephalopathy and axial skeletal fusions. These doses were often maternally toxic and were 0.3 to 3-fold the maximum recommended human dose (MRHD) on a mg/m² basis. The relative contribution of morphine-induced maternal hypoxia and malnutrition, each of which can be teratogenic, has not been clearly defined. Treatment of male rats with approximately 3-fold the MRHD for 10 days prior to mating decreased litter size and viability.

Nonteratogenic effects

Morphine given subcutaneously, at non-maternally toxic doses, to rats during the third trimester with approximately 0.15-fold the MRHD caused reversible reductions in brain and spinal cord volume, and testes size and body weight in the offspring, and decreased fertility in female offspring. The offspring of rats and hamsters treated orally or intraperito-

neally throughout pregnancy with 0.04- to 0.3-fold the MRHD of morphine have demonstrated delayed growth, motor and sexual maturation and decreased male fertility. Chronic morphine exposure of fetal animals resulted in mild withdrawal, altered reflex and motor skill development, and altered responsiveness to morphine that persisted into adulthood.

There are no well-controlled studies of chronic *in utero* exposure to morphine sulfate in human subjects. However, uncontrolled retrospective studies of human neonates chronically exposed to other opioids *in utero*, demonstrated reduced brain volume which normalized over the first month of life. Infants born to opioid-abusing mothers are more often small for gestational age, have a decreased ventilatory response to CO_2 and increased risk of sudden infant death syndrome.

Morphine should only be used during pregnancy if the need for strong opioid analgesia justifies the potential risk to the fetus.

Labor and Delivery

KADIAN™ is not recommended for use in women during and immediately prior to labor, where shorter acting analgesics or other analgesic techniques are more appropriate. Occasionally, opioid analgesics may prolong labor through actions which temporarily reduce the strength, duration and frequency of uterine contractions. However this effect is not consistent and may be offset by an increased rate of cervical dilatation which tends to shorten labor.

Neonates whose mothers received opioid analgesics during labor should be observed closely for signs of respiratory depression. A specific opioid antagonist, such as naloxone or nalmefene, should be available for reversal of opioid-induced respiratory depression in the neonate.

Neonatal Withdrawal Syndrome

Chronic maternal use of opiates or opioids during pregnancy coexposes the fetus. The newborn may experience subsequent neonatal withdrawal syndrome (NWS). Manifestations of NWS include irritability, hyperactivity, abnormal sleep pattern, high-pitched cry, tremor, vomiting, diarrhea, weight loss, and failure to gain weight. The onset, duration, and severity of the disorder differ based on such factors as the addictive drug used, time and amount of mothers last dose, and rate of elimination of the drug from the newborn. Approaches to the treatment of this syndrome have included supportive care and, when indicated, drugs such as paragoric or phenobarbital.

Nursing Mothers

Low levels of morphine sulfate have been detected in human milk. Withdrawal symptoms can occur in breast-feeding infants when maternal administration of morphine sulfate is stopped. Because of the potential for adverse reactions in nursing infants from KADIAN™, a decision should be made whether to discontinue nursing or discontinue the drug, taking into account the importance of the drug to the mother.

Pediatric Use

There are studies from the literature reporting the safe and effective use of both immediate and sustained release oral morphine preparations for analgesia in children who were dosed on a per kilogram basis. The safety of KADIAN™ has not been directly investigated in patients below the age of 18 years and both the dosage form and range of doses available are not suitable for the treatment of very small children or those who are not old enough to take capsules safely.

ADVERSE REACTIONS

Serious adverse reactions that may be associated with KADIAN™ therapy in clinical use are those observed with other opioid analgesics and include: respiratory depression, respiratory arrest, circulatory depression, cardiac arrest, hypotension, and/or shock (see **OVERDOSAGE, WARNINGS**).

The less severe adverse events seen on initiation of therapy with KADIAN™ are also typical opioid side effects. These events are dose dependent, and their frequency depends on the clinical setting, the patient's level of opioid tolerance, and host factors specific to the individual. They should be expected and managed as a part of opioid analgesia. The most frequent of these include drowsiness, dizziness, constipation and nausea. In many cases, the frequency of these events during initiation of therapy may be minimized by careful individualization of starting dosage, slow titration, and the avoidance of large rapid swings in plasma concentrations of the opioid. Many of these adverse events, will cease or decrease as KADIAN™ therapy is continued and some degree of tolerance is developed, but others may be expected to remain troublesome throughout therapy.

Management of Excessive Drowsiness

Most patients receiving morphine will experience initial drowsiness. This usually disappears within 3–5 days and is not a cause of concern unless it is excessive, or accompanied by unsteadiness or confusion. Dizziness and unsteadiness may be associated with postural hypotension, particularly in elderly or debilitated patients, and has been associated with syncope and falls in non-tolerant patients started on opiods. Excessive or persistent sedation should be investigated. Factors to be considered should include: concurrent sedative medications, the presence of hepatic or renal insufficiency, hypoxia or hypercapnia due to exacerbated respiratory failure, intolerance to the dose used (especially in older patients), disease severity and the patient's general condition. The dosage should be adjusted according to individual needs, but additional care should be used in the selection of initial doses for the elderly patient, the cachectic or gravely ill patient, or in patients not already familiar with opioid analgesic medications to prevent excessive sedation at the onset of treatment.

Management of Nausea and Vomiting

Nausea and vomiting is common after single doses of morphine or as an early undesirable effect of chronic opioid therapy. The prescription of a suitable antiemetic should be considered, with the awareness that sedation may result (see **Drug Interactions**). The frequency of nausea and vomiting usually decreases within a week or so but may persist due to opioid-induced gastric stasis. Metoclopramide is often useful in such patients.

Management of Constipation

Virtually all patients suffer from constipation while taking opioids on a chronic basis. Some patients, particularly elderly, debilitated or bedridden patients may become impacted. Tolerance does not usually develop for the constipating effects of opioids. Patients must be cautioned accordingly and laxatives, softeners and other appropriate treatments should be used prophylactically from the beginning of opioid therapy.

Adverse Events Probably Related to KADIAN™ Administration

In controlled clinical trials in patients with chronic cancer pain the most common adverse events reported by patients at least once during therapy were drowsiness (9%), constipation (9%), nausea (7%), dizziness (6%), and anxiety (6%).

Other less common side effects expected from morphine or seen in less than 3% of patients in the clinical trials were:

Body as a Whole: Asthenia, accidental injury, fever, pain, chest pain, headache, diaphoresis, chills, flu syndrome, back pain, malaise, withdrawal sydrome

Cardiovascular: Tachycardia, atrial fibrillation, hypotension, hypertension, pallor, facial flushing, palpitations, bradycardia, syncope

Central Nervous System: Confusion, dry mouth, anxiety, abnormal thinking, abnormal dreams, lethargy, depression, tremor, loss of concentration, insomnia, amnesia, paresthesia, agitation, vertigo, foot drop, ataxia, hypesthesia, slurred speech, hallucinations, vasodilation, euphoria, apathy, seizures, myoclonus

Endocrine: Hypoatrenia due to inappropriate ADH secretion, gynecomastia

Gastrointestinal: Vomiting, anorexia, dysphagia, dyspepsia, diarrhea, abdominal pain, stomach atony disorder, gastroesophageal reflux, delayed gastric emptying, biliary colic

Hemic & Lymphatic: Anemia, leukopenia, thrombocytopenia

Metabolic & Nutritional: Peripheral edema, hyponatremia, edema

Musculoskeletal: Back pain, bone pain, arthralgia

Respiratory: Hiccup, rhinitis, atelectasis, asthma, hypoxia, dyspnea, respiratory insufficiency, voice alteration, depressed cough reflex, non-cardiogenic pulmonary edema

Skin and Appendages: Rash, decubitis ulcer, pruritus, skin flush

Special Senses: Amblyopia, conjunctivitis, miosis, blurred vision, nystagmus, diplopia

Urogenital: Urinary abnormality, amenorrhea, urinary retention, urinary hesitancy, reduced libido, reduced potency, prolonged labor

DRUG ABUSE AND DEPENDENCE

Morphine is the prototype of opioid agonist drugs, and may be subject to misuse, abuse and addiction. Addiction to opioids prescribed for pain management is rare, but requests for opioids from patients addicted to opioids are common and physicians should take appropriate care in prescribing this controlled substance.

Opioid analgesics may cause physical dependence. Physical dependence results in withdrawal symptoms in patients who abruptly discontinue the drug. Withdrawal also may be precipitated through the administration of drugs with opioid antagonist activity, e.g. naloxone, nalmefene, or mixed agonist/antagonist analgesics (pentazocine, butorphanol, nalbuphine), (see also **OVERDOSAGE**).

Physical dependence usually does not occur to a clinically significant degree until after several weeks of continued opioid usage. Tolerance, in which increasingly large doses are required in order to produce the same degree of analgesia, is initially manifested by a shortened duration of analgesic effect, and subsequently, by decreases in the intensity of analgesia.

In chronic pain patients, and in opioid-tolerant cancer patients, the administration of KADIAN™ should be guided by the degree of tolerance manifested. Physical dependence, per se, is not ordinarily a concern when one is dealing with a patient in pain, and fear of tolerance should not deter using adequate doses to adequately relieve pain.

If morphine is abruptly discontinued an abstinence syndrome may occur. This is usually mild and is characterized by rhinitis, myalgia, abdominal cramping and occasional diarrhea. Most observable symptoms disappear in 5–14 days without treatment; however, there may be a phase of secondary or chronic abstinence which may last for 2–6 months characterized by insomnia, irritability and muscular aches.

If treatment of physical dependence of patients taking morphine is necessary, the patient may be detoxified by gradual reduction of the dose. Gastrointestinal disturbances or dehydration should be treated with supportive care.

KADIAN™ has no role in the management of opioid addiction.

OVERDOSAGE

Symptoms

Acute overdosage with morphine is manifested by respiratory depression, somnolence progressing to stupor or coma, skeletal muscle flaccidity, cold and clammy skin, constricted pupils, and, sometimes, pulmonary edema, bradycardia, hypotension and death. Marked mydriasis rather than miosis may be seen due to severe hypoxia in overdose situations.

Treatment

Primary attention should be given to the re-establishment of a patent airway and institution of assisted or controlled ventilation. Gastric contents may need to be emptied to remove unabsorbed drug when a sustained release formulation such as KADIAN™ has been taken. Care should be taken to secure the airway before attempting treatment by gastric emptying or activated charcoal.

The pure opioid antagonists, naloxone or nalmefene, are specific antidotes to respiratory depression which results from opioid overdose. Since the duration of reversal would be expected to be less than the duration of action of KADIAN™, the patient must be carefully monitored until spontaneous respiration is reliably re-established. KADIAN™ will continue to release and add to the morphine load for up to 24 hours after administration and the management of an overdose should be monitored accordingly. If the response to opioid antagonists is suboptimal or not sustained, additional antagonist should be given as directed by the manufacturer of the product.

Opioid antagonists should not be administered in the absence of clinically significant respiratory or circulatory depression secondary to morphine overdose. Such agents should be administered cautiously to persons who are known, or suspected to be physically dependent on KADIAN™. In such cases, an abrupt or complete reversal of opioid effects may precipitate an acute abstinence syndrome.

Opioid Tolerant Individuals: In an individual physically dependent on opioids, administration of the usual dose of the antagonist will precipitate an acute withdrawal. The severity of the withdrawal produced will depend on the degree of physical dependence and the dose of the antagonist administered. Use of an opioid antagonist should be reserved for cases where such treatment is clearly needed. If it is necessary to treat serious respiratory depression in the physically dependent patient, administration of the antagonist should be begun with care and by titration with smaller than usual doses.

Supportive measures (including oxygen, vasopressors) should be employed in the management of circulatory shock and pulmonary edema as indicated. Cardiac arrest or arrhythmias may require cardiac massage or defibrillation.

DOSAGE AND ADMINISTRATION

KADIAN™ CAPSULES SHOULD BE SWALLOWED WHOLE.

THE CAPSULES SHOULD NOT BE OPENED, CHEWED, CRUSHED, DISSOLVED, OR MIXED WITH FOOD. THE PELLETS IN KADIAN™ CAPSULES SHOULD NOT BE CHEWED, CRUSHED OR DISSOLVED.

TAKING BROKEN, CHEWED OR CRUSHED KADIAN™ CAPSULES WILL LEAD TO THE RAPID RELEASE AND ABSORPTION OF A POTENTIALLY TOXIC DOSE OF MORPHINE.

The sustained release nature of KADIAN™ allows it to be administered on <u>either</u> a once-a-day or twice-a-day schedule.

KADIAN™ produces analgesia similar to that produced by conventional immediate-release and controlled-release formulations for the same total daily dose of morphine. However, peak and trough blood levels depend on the release characteristics of each specific formulation, and other oral morphines may not be therapeutically equivalent to KADIAN™ for an individual patient.

KADIAN™ capsules have the same extent of absorption (AUC) as immediate-release oral formulations and controlled-release oral formulations of morphine sulfate. However, key pharmacokinetic parameters (e.g. C_{max}, T_{max}) for KADIAN™ are significantly different from other controlled-release oral formulations.

As with any potent opioid drug product, it is critical to adjust the dosing regimen for each patient individually, taking into

Continued on next page

Zeneca Pharmaceuticals—Cont.

account the patient's prior analgesic treatment experience. In the selection of the initial dose of KADIAN™, attention should be given to:

1) the total daily dose, potency and kind of opioid the patient has been taking previously;
2) the reliability of the relative potency estimate used to calculate the equivalent dose of morphine needed;
3) the patient's degree of opioid tolerance;
4) the general condition and medical status of the patient;
5) concurrent medication;
6) the type and severity of the patient's pain.

The following dosing recommendations, therefore, can only be considered suggested approaches to what is actually a series of clinical decisions over time in the management of the pain of an individual patient.

Conversion from Other Oral Morphine Formulations to KADIAN™

Patients on other oral morphine formulations may be converted to KADIAN™ by administering one-half of the patient's total daily oral morphine dose as KADIAN™ capsules every 12 hours (twice-a-day) or by administering the total daily oral morphine dose as KADIAN™ capsules every 24 hours (once-a-day). KADIAN™ should not be given more frequently than every 12 hours.

Conversion from Parenteral Morphine or Other Parenteral or Oral Opioids to KADIAN™

KADIAN™ can be administered to patients previously receiving treatment with parenteral morphine or other opioids. While there are useful tables of oral and parenteral equivalents in cancer analgesia, there is substantial interpatient variation in the relative potency of different opioid drugs and formulations. For these reasons, it is better to underestimate the patient's 24 hour oral morphine requirement and provide rescue medication, than to overestimate and manage an adverse event. The following general points should be considered:

Parenteral to oral morphine ratio: It may take anywhere from 2–6 mg of oral morphine to provide analgesia equivalent to 1 mg of parenteral morphine. A dose of oral morphine three times the daily parenteral morphine requirement may be sufficient in chronic use settings.

Other parenteral or oral opioids to oral morphine sulfate: Physicians are advised to refer to published relative potency data, keeping in mind that such ratios are only approximate. In general, it is safest to give half of the estimated daily morphine demand as the initial dose, and to manage inadequate analgesia by supplementation with immediate-release morphine. (See discussion which follows.)

The first dose of KADIAN™ may be taken with the last dose of any immediate-release (short-acting) opioid medication due to the long delay until the peak effect after administration of KADIAN™.

Use of KADIAN™ as the First Opioid Analgesic

There has been no evaluation of KADIAN™ as an initial opioid analgesic in the management of pain. Because it may be more difficult to titrate a patient to adequate analgesia using a sustained-release morphine, it is ordinarily advisable to begin treatment using an immediate-release morphine formulation.

Individualization of Dosage

The best use of opioid analgesics in the management of chronic malignant and non-malignant pain is challenging, and is well described in materials published by the World Health Organization and the Agency for Health Care Policy and Research which are available from Zeneca Pharmaceuticals upon request. KADIAN™ is a third step drug which is most useful when the patient requires a constant level of opioid analgesia as a "floor" or "platform" from which to manage breakthrough pain. When a patient has reached the point where comfort cannot be provided with a combination of non-opioid medications (NSAIDs and acetaminophen) and intermittent use of moderate or strong opioids, the patient's total opioid therapy should be converted into a 24 hour oral morphine equivalent.

KADIAN™ should be started by administering one-half of the estimated total daily oral morphine dose every 12 hours (twice-a-day) or by administering the total daily oral morphine dose every 24 hours (once-a-day). The dose should be titrated no more frequently than every-other-day to allow the patients to stabilize before escalating the dose. If breakthrough pain occurs, the dose may be supplemented with a small dose (less than 20% of the total daily dose) of a short-acting analgesic. Patients who are excessively sedated after a once-a-day dose or who regularly experience inadequate analgesia before the next dose should be switched to twice-a-day dosing.

Patients who do not have a proven tolerance to opioids should be started only on the 20 mg strength, and usually should be increased at a rate not greater than 20 mg every-other-day. Most patients will rapidly develop some degree of tolerance, requiring dosage adjustment until they have achieved their individual best balance between baseline analgesia and opioid side effects such as confusion, sedation and constipation. No guidance can be given as to the recommended maximal dose, especially in patients with chronic pain of malignancy. In such cases the total dose of KADIAN™ should be advanced until the desired therapeutic endpoint is reached or clinically significant opioid-related adverse reactions intervene.

Considerations in the Adjustment of Dosing Regimens

If signs of excessive opioid effects are observed early in the dosing interval, the next dose should be reduced. If this adjustment leads to inadequate analgesia, that is, if breakthrough pain occurs when KADIAN™ is administered on an every 24 hours dosing regimen, consideration should be given to dosing every 12 hours. If breakthrough pain occurs on a 12 hour dosing regimen a supplemental dose of a short-acting analgesic may be given. As experience is gained, adjustments in both dose and dosing interval can be made to obtain an appropriate balance between pain relief and opioid side effects. To avoid accumulation the dosing interval of KADIAN™ should not be reduced below 12 hours.

Conversion from KADIAN™ to Other Controlled-Release Oral Morphine Formulations

KADIAN™ is not bioequivalent to other controlled-release morphine preparations. Although for a given dose the same total amount of morphine is available from KADIAN™ as from morphine solution or controlled-release morphine tablets, the slower release of morphine from KADIAN™ results in reduced maximum and increased minimum plasma morphine concentrations than with shorter acting morphine products. Conversion from KADIAN™ to the same total daily dose of controlled-release morphine preparations may lead to either excessive sedation at peak or inadequate analgesia at trough and close observation and appropriate dosage adjustments are recommended.

Conversion from KADIAN™ to Parenteral Opioids

When converting a patient from KADIAN™ to parenteral opioids, it is best to calculate an equivalent parenteral dose, and then initiate treatment at half of this calculated value. For example, to estimate the required 24 hour dose of parenteral morphine for a patient taking KADIAN™, one would take the 24 hour KADIAN™ dose, divide by an oral to parenteral conversion ratio of 3, divide the estimated 24 hour parenteral dose into six divided doses (for a four hour dosing interval), then halve this dose as an initial trial.

For example, to estimate the required parenteral morphine dose for a patient taking 360 mg of KADIAN™ a day, divide the 360 mg daily oral morphine dose by a conversion ratio of 1 mg of parenteral morphine for every 3 mg of oral morphine. The estimated 120 mg daily parenteral requirement is then divided into six 20 mg doses, and half of this, or 10 mg, is then given every 4 hours as an initial trial dose.

This approach is likely to require a dosage increase in the first 24 hours for many patients, but is recommended because it is less likely to cause overdose than trying to establish an equivalent dose without titration.

Opioid analgesic agents may not effectively relieve dysesthetic pain, post-herpetic neuralgia, stabbing pains, activity-related pain, and some forms of headache. This does not mean that patients suffering from these types of pain should not be given an adequate trial of opioid analgesics. However, such patients may need to be promptly evaluated for other types of pain therapy.

Safety and Handling

KADIAN™ consists of closed hard gelatin capsules containing polymer coated morphine sulfate pellets that pose no known handling risk to health care workers. Oral morphine products are not known to be associated with a high risk of diversion, but all strong opioids are liable to diversion and misuse both by the general public and health care workers, and should be handled accordingly.

HOW SUPPLIED

KADIAN™ capsules contain white to off-white or tan colored polymer coated sustained release pellets of morphine sulfate and are available in three dose strengths:

20 mg size 4 capsule, clear cap imprinted KADIAN and clear body imprinted 20 mg. Capsules are supplied in: bottles of 60 (NDC 0310-342-60), 100 (NDC 0310-342-10), and 500 (NDC 0310-342-50), and unit dose packages of 100 (NDC 0310-342-39).

50 mg size 2 capsule, clear cap imprinted KADIAN and clear body imprinted with 50 mg. Capsules are supplied in: bottles of 60 (NDC 0310-345-60), 100 (NDC 0310-345-10), and 500 (NDC 0310-345-50), and unit dose packages of 100 (NDC 0310-345-39).

100 mg size 0 capsule, clear cap imprinted KADIAN and clear body imprinted with 100 mg. Capsules are supplied in: bottles of 60 (NDC 0310-341-60), and 100 (NDC 0310-341-10), and unit dose packages of 100 (NDC 0310-341-39).

Store capsules at controlled room temperature 15° to 30°C (59° to 86°F). Protect from light and moisture.

Dispense in sealed, tamper-evident, childproof, light-resistant container.

CAUTION

DEA Order Form Required.

Federal law prohibits dispensing without prescription.

KADIAN™ is a trademark of F.H. Faulding & Co. Limited
MS Contin® is a registered trademark of The Purdue Frederick Company
Manufactured for:
Zeneca Pharmaceuticals
A Business Unit of Zeneca Inc.
Wilmington, Delaware 19850-5437 USA
By: Purepac Pharmaceutical Co.
Elizabeth, New Jersey 07207
Rev G 07/96 SIC 64093-01

MERREM® I.V. ℞

(meropenem for injection)
For Intravenous Use Only

DESCRIPTION

MERREM® I.V. (meropenem for injection) is a sterile, pyrogen-free, synthetic, broad-spectrum, carbapenem antibiotic for intravenous administration. It is (4R,5S,6S)-3-[[(3S,5S)-5-(Dimethylcarbamoyl)-3-pyrrolidinyl]thio]-6-[(1R)-1-hydroxyethyl]-4-methyl-7-oxo-1-azabicyclo[3.2.0]hept-2-ene-2-carboxylic acid trihydrate. Its empirical formula is $C_{17}H_{25}N_3O_5S \bullet 3H_2O$ with a molecular weight of 437.52. Its structural formula is:

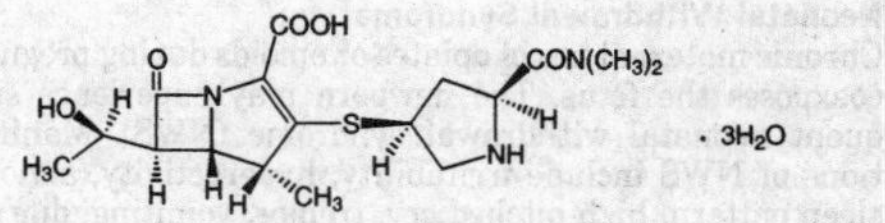

MERREM I.V. is a white to pale yellow crystalline powder. The solution varies from colorless to yellow depending on the concentration. The pH of freshly constituted solutions is between 7.3 and 8.3. Meropenem is soluble in 5% monobasic potassium phosphate solution, sparingly soluble in water, very slightly soluble in hydrated ethanol, and practically insoluble in acetone or ether.

When constituted as instructed (See **DOSAGE AND ADMINISTRATION; PREPARATION OF SOLUTION**), each 1 g MERREM I.V. vial will deliver 1 g of meropenem and 90.2 mg of sodium as sodium carbonate (3.92 mEq). Each 500 mg MERREM I.V. vial will deliver 500 mg meropenem and 45.1 mg of sodium as sodium carbonate (1.96 mEq).

MERREM I.V. in the ADD-Vantage† vial is intended for intravenous use only after dilution with the appropriate volume of diluent solution in the Abbott ADD-Vantage® diluent container (See **DOSAGE AND ADMINISTRATION-PREPARATION OF SOLUTION**). MERREM I.V. in the ADD-Vantage vial is available in two strengths. Each 1 g ADD-Vantage vial of MERREM I.V. will deliver 90.2 mg of sodium as sodium carbonate (3.92 mEq), and each 500 mg ADD-Vantage vial will deliver 45.1 mg of sodium as sodium carbonate (1.96 mEq).

CLINICAL PHARMACOLOGY

At the end of a 30-minute intravenous infusion of a single dose of MERREM I.V. in normal volunteers, mean peak plasma concentrations are approximately 23 µg/mL (range 14–26) for the 500 mg dose and 49 µg/mL (range 39–58) for the 1 g dose. A 5-minute intravenous bolus injection of MERREM I.V. in normal volunteers results in mean peak plasma concentrations of approximately 45 µg/mL (range 18–65) for the 500 mg dose and 112 µg/mL (range 83–140) for the 1 g dose.

Following intravenous doses of 500 mg, mean plasma concentrations of meropenem usually decline to approximately 1 µg/mL at 6 hours after administration.

In subjects with normal renal function, the elimination half-life of MERREM I.V. is approximately 1 hour. Approximately 70% of the intravenously administered dose is recovered as unchanged meropenem in the urine over 12 hours, after which little further urinary excretion is detectable. Urinary concentrations of meropenem in excess of 10 µg/mL are maintained for up to 5 hours after a 500 mg dose. No accumulation of meropenem in plasma or urine was observed with regimens using 500 mg administered every 8 hours or 1 g administered every 6 hours in volunteers with normal renal function.

Plasma protein binding of meropenem is approximately 2%.

There is one metabolite which is microbiologically inactive.

Meropenem penetrates well into most body fluids and tissues including cerebrospinal fluid, achieving concentrations matching or exceeding those required to inhibit most susceptible bacteria. After a single intravenous dose of MERREM I.V., the highest mean concentrations of meropenem were

found in tissues and fluids at 1 hour (0.5 to 1.5 hours) after the start of infusion, except where indicated in the tissues and fluids listed in the table below.

[See table at right.]

The pharmacokinetics of MERREM I.V. in pediatric patients 2 years of age or older are essentially similar to those in adults. The elimination half-life for meropenem was approximately 1.5 hours in pediatric patients of age 3 months to 2 years. The pharmacokinetics are linear over the dose range from 10 to 40 mg/kg.

Pharmacokinetic studies with MERREM I.V. in patients with renal insufficiency have shown that the plasma clearance of meropenem correlates with creatinine clearance. Dosage adjustments are necessary in subjects with renal impairment. (See **DOSAGE AND ADMINISTRATION - Use in Adults with Renal Impairment.**) A pharmacokinetic study with MERREM I.V. in elderly patients with renal insufficiency has shown a reduction in plasma clearance of meropenem that correlates with age-associated reduction in creatinine clearance.

Meropenem I.V. is hemodialyzable. However, there is no information on the usefulness of hemodialysis to treat overdosage. (See **OVERDOSAGE.**)

A pharmacokinetic study with MERREM I.V. in patients with hepatic impairment has shown no effects of liver disease on the pharmacokinetics of meropenem.

MICROBIOLOGY

The bactericidal activity of meropenem results from the inhibition of cell wall synthesis. Meropenem readily penetrates the cell wall of most gram-positive and gram-negative bacteria to reach penicillin-binding-protein (PBP) targets. Its strongest affinities are toward PBPs 2, 3 and 4 of *Escherichia coli* and *Pseudomonas aeruginosa*; and PBPs 1, 2 and 4 of *Staphylococcus aureus*. Bactericidal concentrations (defined as a 3 $\log_{10}$ reduction in cell counts within 12 to 24 hours) are typically 1–2 times the bacteriostatic concentrations of meropenem, with the exception of *Listeria monocytogenes*, against which lethal activity is not observed.

Meropenem has significant stability to hydrolysis by β-lactamases of most categories, both penicillinases and cephalosporinases produced by gram-positive and gram-negative bacteria, with the exception of metallo-β-lactamases. Meropenem should not be used to treat methicillin-resistant staphylococci. Cross-resistance is sometimes observed with strains resistant to other carbapenems.

In vitro tests show meropenem to act synergistically with aminoglycoside antibiotics against some isolates of *Pseudomonas aeruginosa*.

Meropenem has been shown to be active against most strains of the following microorganisms, both *in vitro* and in clinical infections as described in the **INDICATIONS AND USAGE** section.

Gram-Positive Aerobes
Streptococcus pneumoniae (excluding penicillin-resistant strains)
Viridans group streptococci
NOTE: Penicillin-resistant strains had meropenem MIC90 values of 1 or 2 µg/mL, which is above the 0.12 µg/mL susceptible breakpoint for this species.

Gram-Negative Aerobes
Escherichia coli
Haemophilus influenzae (β-lactamase and non-β-lactamase-producing)
Klebsiella pneumoniae
Neisseria meningitidis
Pseudomonas aeruginosa

Anaerobes
Bacteroides fragilis
Bacteroides thetaiotaomicron
Peptostreptococcus species
The following *in vitro* data are available, **but their clinical significance is unknown.**

Meropenem exhibits *in vitro* minimum inhibitory concentrations (MICs) of 0.12 µg/mL against most (≥ 90%) strains of *Streptococcus pneumoniae*, 0.5 µg/mL or less against most (≥ 90%) of *Haemophilus influenzae*, and 4 µg/mL or less against most (≥ 90%) strains of the other microorganisms in the following list; however, the safety and effectiveness of meropenem in treating clinical infections due to these microorganisms have not been established in adequate and well-controlled clinical trials.

Gram-Positive Aerobes
Staphylococcus aureus (β-lactamase and non β-lactamase producing)
Staphylococcus epidermidis (β-lactamase and non β-lactamase-producing)
NOTE: Staphylococci which are resistant to methicillin/oxacillin must be considered resistant to meropenem.

Gram-Negative Aerobes
Acinetobacter species
Aeromonas hydrophila
Campylobacter jejuni
Citrobacter diversus

Citrobacter freundii
Enterobacter cloacae
Haemophilus influenzae (ampicillin-resistant, non-β-lactamase producing strains [BLNAR strains])
Hafnia alvei
Klebsiella oxytoca
Moraxella catarrhalis (β-lactamase and non-β-lactamase-producing strains)
Morganella morganii
Pasteurella multocida
Proteus mirabilis
Proteus vulgaris
Salmonella species
Serratia marcescens
Shigella species
Yersinia enterocolitica
Anaerobes
Bacteroides distasonis
Bacteroides ovatus
Bacteroides uniformis
Bacteroides ureolyticus
Bacteroides vulgatus
Clostridium difficile
Clostridium perfringens
Eubacterium lentum
Fusobacterium species
Prevotella bivia
Prevotella intermedia
Prevotella melaninogenica
Porphyromonas asaccharolytica
Propionibacterium acnes

SUSCEPTIBILITY TESTS

Dilution Techniques:
Quantitative methods are used to determine antimicrobial minimal inhibitory concentrations (MICs). These MICs provide estimates of the susceptibility of bacteria to antimicrobial compounds. The MIC's should be determined using a standardized procedure. Standardized procedures are based on a dilution method[1] (broth or agar) or equivalent with standardized inoculum concentrations and standardized concentrations of meropenem powder. The MIC values should be interpreted according to the following criteria for indicated aerobic organisms other than *Haemophilus* species and streptococci:

MIC (µg/mL)	Interpretation
≤ 4	(S) Susceptible
8	(I) Intermediate
≥ 16	(R) Resistant

Haemophilus Test Media (HTM) and the following interpretive criteria should be used when testing *Haemophilus* species:

MIC (µg/mL)	Interpretation
≤ 0.5	(S) Susceptible

The current absence of resistant strains precludes defining any categories other than "Susceptible". Strains yielding results suggestive of a "Nonsusceptible" category should be submitted to a reference laboratory for further testing.
The following criteria should be used when testing streptococci and *Streptococcus pneumoniae*:

When testing *S. pneumoniae*:

MIC (µg/mL)	Interpretation
≤ 0.12	(S) Susceptible

When testing viridans group streptococci:

MIC (µg/mL)	Interpretation
≤ 0.5	(S) Susceptible

The current absence of resistant strains precludes defining any categories other than "Susceptible". Strains yielding results suggestive of a "Nonsusceptible" category should be submitted to a reference laboratory for further testing.

A report of 'Susceptible' indicates that the pathogen is likely to be inhibited if the antimicrobial compound in the blood reaches the concentrations usually achievable. A report of 'Intermediate' indicates that the result should be considered equivocal, and, if the microorganism is not fully susceptible to alternative, clinically feasible drugs, the test should be repeated. This category implies possible clinical applicability in body sites where the drug is physiologically concentrated or in situations where high dosage of drug can be used. This category also provides a buffer zone which prevents small uncontrolled technical factors from causing major discrepancies in interpretation. A report of 'Resistant' indicates that the pathogen is not likely to be inhibited if the antimicrobial compound in the blood reaches the concentrations usually achievable; other therapy should be selected.

Standardized susceptibility test procedures require the use of laboratory control microorganisms to control the technical aspects of the laboratory procedures. Standard meropenem powder should provide the following MIC values:

Microorganism	ATCC	MIC (µg/mL)
Enterococcus faecalis	29212	2.0–8.0
Escherichia coli	25922	0.008–0.06
Haemophilus influenzae	49247	0.06–0.25
Pseudomonas aeruginosa	27853	0.25–1.0
Streptococcus pneumoniae	49619	0.06–0.25

Diffusion Techniques:
Quantitative methods that require measurement of zone diameters also provide reproducible estimates of the susceptibility of bacteria to antimicrobial compounds. One such standardized procedure[2] requires the use of standardized inoculum concentrations. This procedure uses paper disks impregnated with 10-µg of meropenem to test the susceptibility of microorganisms to meropenem.

Reports from the laboratory providing results of the standard single-disk susceptibility test with a 10-µg disk should be interpreted according to the following criteria for indicated aerobic organisms other than *Haemophilus* species and streptococci:

Zone Diameter (mm)	Interpretation
≥ 16	(S) Susceptible
14–15	(I) Intermediate
≤ 13	(R) Resistant

Haemophilus Test Media and the following criteria should be used when testing *Haemophilus* species:

Zone Diameter (mm)	Interpretation
≥ 20	(S) Susceptible

The current absence of resistant strains precludes defining any categories other than "Susceptible". Strains yielding

Meropenem Concentrations in Selected Tissues (Highest Concentrations Reported)

Tissue	I.V. Dose (g)	Number of Samples	Mean [µg/mL or µg/(g)][***]	Range [µg/mL or µg/(g)]
Endometrium	0.5	7	4.2	1.7–10.2
Myometrium	0.5	15	3.8	0.4–8.1
Ovary	0.5	8	2.8	0.8–4.8
Cervix	0.5	2	7.0	5.4–8.5
Fallopian tube	0.5	9	1.7	0.3–3.4
Skin	0.5	22	3.3	0.5–12.6
Skin	1.0	10	5.3	1.3–16.7
Colon	1.0	2	2.6	2.5–2.7
Bile	1.0	7	14.6 (3 h)	4.0–25.7
Gallbladder	1.0	1	—	3.9
Interstitial fluid	1.0	5	26.3	20.9–37.4
Peritoneal fluid	1.0	9	30.2	7.4–54.6
Lung	1.0	2	4.8 (2 h)	1.4–8.2
Bronchial mucosa	1.0	7	4.5	1.3–11.1
Muscle	1.0	2	6.1 (2 h)	5.3–6.9
Fascia	1.0	9	8.8	1.5–20
Heart valves	1.0	7	9.7	6.4–12.1
Myocardium	1.0	10	15.5	5.2–25.5
CSF (inflamed)	20 mg/kg[*]	8	1.1 (2 h)	0.2–10.8
	40 mg/kg[**]	5	3.3 (3 h)	0.9–6.5
CSF (uninflamed)	1.0	4	0.2 (2 h)	0.1–0.3

[*]in pediatric patients of age 5 months to 8 years
[**]in pediatric patients of age 1 month to 15 years
[***]at 1 hour unless otherwise noted

Continued on next page

Zeneca Pharmaceuticals—Cont.

results suggestive of a "Nonsusceptible" category should be submitted to a reference laboratory for further testing. *Streptococcus pneumoniae* isolates should be tested using 1 μg/mL oxacillin disk. Isolates with oxacillin zone sizes of ≥ 20 mm are susceptible (MIC ≤ 0.06 μg/mL) to penicillin and can be considered susceptible to meropenem for approved indications, and meropenem need not be tested. A meropenem MIC should be determined on isolates of *S. pneumoniae* with oxacillin zone sizes of ≤ 19 mm. The disk test does not distinguish penicillin intermediate strains (i.e., MICs = 0.12–1.0 μg/mL) from strains that are penicillin resistant (i.e., MICs ≥ 2 μg/mL). Viridans group streptococci should be tested for meropenem susceptibility using an MIC method. Reliable disk diffusion tests for meropenem do not yet exist for testing streptococci.

Interpretation should be as stated above for results using dilution techniques. Interpretation involves correlation of the diameter obtained in the disk test with the MIC for meropenem.

As with standardized dilution techniques, diffusion methods require the use of laboratory control microorganisms that are used to control the technical aspects of the laboratory procedures. For the diffusion technique, the 10-μg meropenem disk should provide the following zone diameters in these laboratory test quality control strains:

Microorganism	ATCC	Zone Diameter (mm)
Escherichia coli	25922	28–34
Haemophilus influenzae	49247	20–28
Pseudomonas aeruginosa	27853	27–33

Anaerobic Techniques:

for anaerobic bacteria, susceptibility to meropenem as MICs can be determined by standardized test methods.[3] The MIC values obtained should be interpreted according to the following criteria:

MIC (μg/mL)	Interpretation
≤ 4	(S) Susceptible
8	(I) Intermediate
≥ 16	(R) Resistant

Interpretation is identical to that stated above for results using dilution techniques.

As with other susceptibility techniques, the use of laboratory control microorganisms is required to control the technical aspects of the laboratory standardized procedures. Standardized meropenem powder should provide the following MIC values:

Microorganism	ATCC	MIC (μg/mL)
Bacteroides fragilis	25285	0.06–0.25
Bacteroides thetaiotaomicron	29741	0.125–0.5

INDICATIONS AND USAGE

MERREM I.V. is indicated as single agent therapy for the treatment of the following infections when caused by susceptible strains of the designated microorganisms:

Intra-abdominal Infections

Complicated appendicitis and peritonitis caused by viridans group streptococci, *Escherichia coli*, *Klebsiella pneumoniae*, *Pseudomonas aeruginosa*, *Bacteroides fragilis*, *B. thetaiotaomicron*, and *Peptostreptococcus* species.

Bacterial Meningitis (pediatric patients ≥ 3 months only)

Bacterial meningitis caused by *Streptococcus pneumoniae*‡, *Haemophilus influenzae* (β-lactamase and non-β-lactamase-producing strains), and *Neisseria meningitidis*.

‡Penicillin-resistant strains have not been studied in clinical trials.

MERREM I.V. has been found to be effective in eliminating concurrent bacteremia in association with bacteria meningitis.

For information regarding use in pediatric patients (3 months of age and older) See **PRECAUTIONS - Pediatrics**, **ADVERSE REACTIONS**, and **DOSAGE AND ADMINISTRATION** sections.

Appropriate cultures should usually be performed before initiating antimicrobial treatment in order to isolate and identify the organisms causing infection and determine their susceptibility to MERREM I.V.

MERREM I.V. is useful as presumptive therapy in the indicated condition (i.e., intra-abdominal infections) prior to the identification of the causative organisms because of its broad spectrum of bactericidal activity.

Antimicrobial therapy should be adjusted, if appropriate, once the results of culture(s) and antimicrobial susceptibility testing are known.

CONTRAINDICATIONS

MERREM I.V. is contraindicated in patients with known hypersensitivity to any component of this product or to other drugs in the same class or in patients who have demonstrated anaphylactic reactions to β-lactams.

WARNINGS

SERIOUS AND OCCASIONALLY FATAL HYPERSENSITIVITY (ANAPHYLACTIC) REACTIONS HAVE BEEN REPORTED IN PATIENTS RECEIVING THERAPY WITH β-LACTAMS. THESE REACTIONS ARE MORE LIKELY TO OCCUR IN INDIVIDUALS WITH A HISTORY OF SENSITIVITY TO MULTIPLE ALLERGENS.

THERE HAVE BEEN REPORTS OF INDIVIDUALS WITH A HISTORY OF PENICILLIN HYPERSENSITIVITY WHO HAVE EXPERIENCED SEVERE HYPERSENSITIVITY REACTIONS WHEN TREATED WITH ANOTHER β-LACTAM. BEFORE INITIATING THERAPY WITH MERREM I.V., CAREFUL INQUIRY SHOULD BE MADE CONCERNING PREVIOUS HYPERSENSITIVITY REACTIONS TO PENICILLINS, CEPHALOSPORINS, OTHER β-LACTAMS, AND OTHER ALLERGENS. IF AN ALLERGIC REACTION TO MERREM I.V. OCCURS, DISCONTINUE THE DRUG IMMEDIATELY. **SERIOUS ANAPHYLACTIC REACTIONS REQUIRE IMMEDIATE EMERGENCY TREATMENT WITH EPINEPHRINE, OXYGEN, INTRAVENOUS STEROIDS, AND AIRWAY MANAGEMENT, INCLUDING INTUBATION. OTHER THERAPY MAY ALSO BE ADMINISTERED AS INDICATED.**

Seizures and other CNS adverse experiences have been reported during treatment with MERREM I.V. (See **PRECAUTIONS** and **ADVERSE REACTIONS**.)

Pseudomembranous colitis has been reported with nearly all antibacterial agents, including meropenem, and may range in severity from mild to life-threatening. Therefore, it is important to consider this diagnosis in patients who present with diarrhea subsequent to the administration of antibacterial agents.

Treatment with antibacterial agents alters the normal flora of the colon and may permit overgrowth of clostridia. Studies indicate that a toxin produced by *Clostridium difficile* is a primary cause of "antibiotic-associated colitis".

After the diagnosis of pseudomembranous colitis has been established, appropriate therapeutic measures should be initiated. Mild cases of pseudomembranous colitis usually respond to drug discontinuation alone. In moderate-to-severe cases, consideration should be given to management with fluids and electrolytes, protein supplementation, and treatment with an antibacterial drug clinically effective against *Clostridium difficile* colitis.

PRECAUTIONS

General: Seizures and other CNS adverse experiences have been reported during treatment with MERREM I.V. These adverse experiences have occurred most commonly in patients with CNS disorders (e.g., brain lesions or history of seizures) or with bacterial meningitis and/or compromised renal function.

During the initial clinical investigations, 2038 immunocompetent adult patients were treated for infections outside the CNS with MERREM I.V. (500 mg or 1000 mg q 8 hours). Overall seizures, whether drug related or not, occurred in 0.5% of the meropenem-treated patients. All meropenem-treated patients with seizures had pre-existing contributing factors. Among these are included prior history of seizures or CNS abnormality and concomitant medications with seizure potential. Dosage adjustment is recommended in patients with advanced age and/or reduced renal function. (See **DOSAGE AND ADMINISTRATION - Use in Adults with Renal Impairment.**)

Close adherence to the recommended dosage regimens is urged, especially in patients with known factors that predispose to convulsive activity. Anticonvulsant therapy should be continued in patients with known seizure disorders. If focal tremors, myoclonus, or seizures occur, patients should be evaluated neurologically, placed on anticonvulsant therapy if not already instituted, and the dosage of MERREM I.V. re-examined to determine whether it should be decreased or the antibiotic discontinued.

In patients with renal dysfunction, thrombocytopenia has been observed but no clinical bleeding reported. (See **DOSAGE AND ADMINISTRATION - Use in Adults with Renal Impairment.**)

There is inadequate information regarding the use of MERREM I.V. in patients on hemodilysis.

As with other broad-spectrum antibiotics, prolonged use of meropenem may result in overgrowth of nonsusceptible organisms. Repeated evaluation of the patient is essential. If superinfection does occur during therapy, appropriate measures should be taken.

Laboratory Tests: While MERREM I.V. possesses the characteristic low toxicity of the beta-lactam group of antibiotics, periodic assessment of organ system functions, including renal, hepatic, and hematopoietic, is advisable during prolonged therapy.

Drug Interactions: Probenecid competes with meropenem for active tubular secretion and thus inhibits the renal excretion of meropenem. This led to statistically significant increases in the elimination half-life (38%) and in the extent of systemic exposure (56%). Therefore, the coadministration of probenecid with meropenem is not recommended.

Other than probenecid, no specific drug interaction studies were conducted.

Carcinogenesis, Mutagenesis, Impairment of Fertility:

Carcinogenesis: Carcinogenesis studies have not been performed.

Mutagenesis: Genetic toxicity studies were performed with meropenem using the bacterial reverse mutation test, the Chinese hamster ovary HGPRT assay, cultured human lymphocytes cytogenic assay, and the mouse micronucleus test. There was no evidence of mutagenic potential found in any of these tests.

Impairment of fertility: Reproductive studies were performed with meropenem in rats at doses up to 1000 mg/kg/day, and cynomolgus monkeys at doses up to 360 mg/kg/day (on the basis of AUC comparisons, approximately 1.8 times and 3.7 times, respectively, to the human exposure at the usual dose of 1 g every 8 hours). There was no reproductive toxicity seen.

Pregnancy Category B: Reproductive studies have been performed with meropenem in rats at doses of up to 1000 mg/kg/day, and cynomolgus monkeys at doses of up to 360 mg/kg/day (on the basis of AUC comparisons, approximately 1.8 times and 3.7 times respectively, to the human exposure at the usual dose of 1 g every 8 hours). These studies revealed no evidence of impaired fertility or harm to the fetus due to meropenem, although there were slight changes in fetal body weight at doses of 250 mg/kg/day (on the basis of AUC comparisons, 0.4 times the human exposure at a dose of 1 g every 8 hours) and above in rats. There are, however, no adequate and well-controlled studies in pregnant women. Because animal reproduction studies are not always predictive of human response, this drug should be used during pregnancy only if clearly needed.

Pediatrics: The safety and effectiveness of MERREM I.V. have been established for pediatric patients ≥ 3 months of age. Use of MERREM I.V. in pediatric patients with bacterial meningitis is supported by evidence from adequate and well-controlled studies in the pediatric population. Use of MERREM I.V. in pediatric patients with intra-abdominal infections is supported by evidence from adequate and well-controlled studies with adults with additional data from pediatric pharmacokinetics studies and controlled clinical trials in pediatric patients. (See **CLINICAL PHARMACOLOGY, INDICATIONS AND USAGE, ADVERSE REACTIONS, DOSAGE AND ADMINISTRATION**, and **CLINICAL STUDIES** sections.)

Nursing Mothers: It is not known whether this drug is excreted in human milk. Because many drugs are excreted in human milk, caution should be exercised when MERREM I.V. is administered to a nursing woman.

ADVERSE REACTIONS

Adult Patients:

During the initial clinical investigations, 2038 immunocompetent adult patients were treated for infections outside the CNS with MERREM I.V. (500 mg or 1000 mg q 8 hours). Deaths in 3 patients were assessed as possibly related to meropenem; 28 (1.4%) patients had meropenem discontinued because of adverse events. Many patients in these trials were severely ill and had multiple background diseases, physiological impairments and were receiving multiple other drug therapies. In the seriously ill population, it was not possible to determine the relationship between observed adverse events and therapy with MERREM I.V.

The following adverse reaction frequencies were derived from the clinical trials in the 2038 patients treated with MERREM I.V.

Local Adverse Reactions

Local adverse reactions that were reported irrespective of the relationship to therapy with MERREM I.V. were as follows:

Inflammation at the injection site	3.0%
Phlebitis/thrombophlebitis	1.2%
Injection site reaction	1.1%
Pain at the injection site	0.4%
Edema at the injection site	0.2%

Systemic Adverse Reactions

Systemic adverse clinical reactions that were reported irrespective of the relationship to MERREM I.V. occurring in greater than 1.0% of the patients with diarrhea (5.0%), nausea/vomiting (3.9%), headache (2.8%), rash (1.7%), pruritus (1.6%), apnea (1.2%), and constipation (1.2%).

Additional adverse systemic clinical reactions that were reported irrespective of relationship to therapy with MERREM I.V. and occurring in less than 1.0% but greater than 0.1% of the patients are listed below within each body system in order of decreasing frequency:

Bleeding events [gastrointestinal hemorrhage, melena, epistaxis, and hemoperitoneum] occurred in 0.7% of meropenem patients.

Body as a Whole: pain, abdominal pain, chest pain, sepsis, shock, fever, abdominal enlargement, back pain, hepatic failure

Cardiovascular: heart failure, heart arrest, tachycardia, hypertension, myocardial infarction, pulmonary embolus, bradycardia, hypotension, syncope

Digestive: oral moniliasis, anorexia, cholestatic jaundice/jaundice, flatulence, ileus

Hemic/lymphatic: anemia

Metabolic/nutritional: peripheral edema, hypoxia

Nervous system: insomnia, agitation/delirium, confusion, dizziness, seizure (See **PRECAUTIONS**), nervousness, paresthesia, hallucinations, somnolence, anxiety, depression

Respiratory: respiratory disorder, dyspnea

Skin and Appendages: urticaria, sweating

Urogenital system: dysuria, kidney failure

Adverse Laboratory Changes

Adverse laboratory changes that were reported irrespective of relationship to MERREM I.V. occurring in greater than 0.2% of the patients were as follows:

Hepatic: increased SGPT (ALT), SGOT (AST), alkaline phosphatase, LDH, and bilirubin

Hematologic: increased platelets, increased eosinophils, prolonged prothrombin time, prolonged partial thromboplastin time, decreased platelets, positive direct or indirect Coombs test, decreased hemoglobin, decreased hematocrit, decreased WBC, shortened prothrombin time and shortened partial thromboplastin time.

Renal: increased creatinine and increased BUN

NOTE: It is not known if the safety profile of MERREM I.V. is changed in patients with varying degrees of renal impairment.

Urinalysis: presence of urine red blood cells

Pediatric Patients:

Clinical Adverse Reactions

MERREM I.V. was studied in 417 pediatric patients (≥ 3 months to <13 years of age) with serious bacterial infections at dosages of 10 to 20 mg/kg every 8 hours. The types of clinical adverse events seen in these patients are similar to the adults, with the most common adverse events reported as possibly, probably or definitely related to MERREM I.V. and their rates of occurrence as follows:

Diarrhea	4.3%
Rash	1.4%
Vomiting	1.0%

MERREM I.V. was studied in 198 pediatric patients (≥ 3 months to <17 years of age) with meningitis at a dosage of 40 mg/kg every 8 hours. The types of clinical adverse events seen in these patients are similar to the adults, with the most common adverse events reported as possibly, probably, or definitely related to MERREM I.V. and their rates of occurrence as follows:

Rash (mostly diaper area moniliasis)	3.5%
Diarrhea	3.5%
Oral Moniliasis	2.0%
Glossitis	1.0%

In the meningitis studies the rates of seizure activity during therapy were comparable between patients with no CNS abnormalities who received meropenem and those who received comparator agents (either cefotaxime or ceftriaxone). In the MERREM I.V. treated group, 12/15 patients with seizures had late onset seizures (defined as occurring on day 3 or later) versus 7/20 in the comparator arm.

Adverse Laboratory Changes:

Laboratory abnormalities seen in the pediatric-aged patients in both the pediatric and the meningitis studies are similar to those reported in adult patients.

There is no experience in pediatric patients with renal impairment.

Post-marketing Experience:

No post-marketing experience is available.

OVERDOSAGE

In mice and rats, large intravenous doses of meropenem (2200-4000 mg/kg) have been associated with ataxia, dyspnea, convulsions, and mortalities.

Intentional overdosing of MERREM I.V. is unlikely, although accidental overdosing might occur if large doses are given to patients with reduced renal function. The largest dose of meropenem administered in clinical trials has been 2 g given intravenously every 8 hours. At this dosage, no adverse pharmacological effects or increased safety risks have been observed.

No specific information is available for the treatment of MERREM I.V. overdosage. In the event of an overdose, MERREM I.V. should be discontinued and general supportive treatment given until renal elimination takes place. Meropenem and its metabolite are readily dialyzable and effectively removed by hemodialysis; however, no information is available on the use of hemodialysis to treat overdosage.

CLINICAL STUDIES

Intra-abdominal:

One controlled clinical study of complicated intra-abdominal infection was performed in the United States where meropenem was compared to clindamycin/tobramycin. Three controlled clinical studies of complicated intra-abdominal infec-

Treatment Arm	No. evaluable/ No. enrolled (%)	Microbiologic Eradication Rate	Clinical Cure Rate	Outcome
meropenem	146/516 (28%)	98/146 (67%)	101/146 (69%)	
imipenem	65/220 (30%)	40/65 (62%)	42/65 (65%)	Meropenem equivalent to control
cefotaxime/ metronidazole	26/85 (30%)	22/26 (85%)	22/26 (85%)	Meropenem not equivalent to control
clindamycin/ tobramycin	50/212 (24%)	38/50 (76%)	38/50 (76%)	Meropenem equivalent to control

tions were performed in Europe; meropenem was compared to imipenem (two trials) and cefotaxime/metronidazole (one trial).

Using strict evaluability criteria and microbiologic eradication and clinical cures at follow-up which occurred 7 or more days after completion of therapy, the following presumptive microbiologic eradication/clinical cure rates and statistical findings were obtained: [See table above.]

The finding that meropenem was not statistically equivalent of cefotaxim/metronidazole may have been due to uneven assignment of more seriously ill patients to the meropenem arm. Currently there is no additional information available to further interpret this observation.

Bacterial Meningitis:

Four hundred forty-six patients (397 pediatric patients ≥ 3 months to < 17 years of age) were enrolled in 4 separate clinical trials and randomized to treatment with meropenem (n=225) at a dose of 40 mg/kg q 8 hours or a comparator drug, i.e., cefotaxime (n=187) or ceftriaxone (n=34), at the approved dosing regimens. A comparable number of patients were found to be clinically evaluable (ranging from 61–68%) and with a similar distribution of pathogens isolated on initial CSF culture.

Patients were defined as clinically not cured if any one of the following three criteria were met:

1. At the 5–7 week post-completion of therapy visit, the patient had any one of the following: moderate to severe motor, behavior or development deficits, hearing loss of >60 decibels in one or both ears, or blindness.
2. During therapy the patient's clinical status necessitated the addition of other antibiotics.
3. Either during or post-therapy, the patient developed a large subdural effusion needing surgical drainage, or a cerebral abscess, or a bacteriologic relapse.

Using the definition, the following efficacy rates were obtained, per organism. The values represent the number of patients clinically cured/number of clinically evaluable patients, with the percent cure in parentheses.

MICROORGANISM	MERREM I.V.	COMPARATOR
S. pneumoniae	17/24 (71)	19/30 (63)
H. influenzae (+)	8/10 (80)	6/6 (100)
H. influenzae (-/NT)	44/59 (75)	44/60 (73)
N. meningitidis	30/35 (86)	35/39 (90)
TOTAL (including others)	102/131 (78)	108/140 (77)

(+) β-lactamase-producing; (-/NT) non-β-lactamase-producing or not tested

Sequelae were the most common reason patients were assessed as clinically not cured.

Five patients were found to be bacteriologically not cured, 3 in the comparator group (1 relapse and 2 patients with cerebral abscesses) and 2 in the meropenem group (1 relapse and 1 with continued growth of *Pseudomonas aeruginosa*).

The adverse events seen were comparable between the two treatment groups both in type and frequency. The meropenem group did have a statistically higher number of patients with transient elevation of liver enzymes. (See **ADVERSE REACTIONS**.) Rates of seizure activity during therapy were comparable between patients with no CNS abnormalities who received meropenem and those who received comparator agents. In the MERREM I.V. treated group, 12/15 patients with seizures had late onset seizures (defined as occurring on day 3 or later) versus 7/20 in the comparator arm.

With respect to hearing loss, 263 of the 271 evaluable patients had at least one hearing test performed post-therapy. The following table shows the degree of hearing loss between the meropenem-treated patients and the comparator-treated patients.

Degree of Hearing Loss (in one or both ears)	Meropenem n=128	Comparator n=135
No loss	61%	56%
20–40 decibels	20%	24%
>40–60 decibels	8%	7%
>60 decibels	9%	10%

DOSAGE AND ADMINISTRATION

Adults: One gram (1 g) by intravenous administration every 8 hours. MERREM I.V. should be given by intravenous infusion, over approximately 15 to 30 minutes or as an intravenous bolus injection (5 to 20 mL) over approximately 3–5 minutes.

Use in Adults with Renal Impairment: Dosage should be reduced in patients with creatinine clearance less than 51 mL/min. (See dosing table below.)

Recommended MERREM I.V. Dosage Schedule for Adults With Impaired Renal Function

Creatinine Clearance (mL/min)	Dose (dependent on type of infection)	Dosing Interval
26–50	recommended dose (1000 mg)	every 12 hours
10–25	one-half recommended dose	every 12 hours
<10	one-half recommended dose	every 24 hours

When only serum creatinine is available, the following formula (Cockcroft and Gault equation)[4] may be used to estimate creatinine clearance.

Males: Creatinine Clearance (mL/min) =

$$\frac{\text{Weight (kg)} \times (140 - \text{age})}{72 \times \text{serum creatinine (mg/dL)}}$$

Females: $0.85 \times$ above value

There is inadequate information regarding the use of MERREM I.V. in patients on hemodialysis.

There is no experience with peritoneal dialysis.

Use in Adults With Hepatic Insufficiency: No dosage adjustment is necessary in patients with impaired hepatic function.

Use in Elderly Patients: No dosage adjustment is required for elderly patients with creatinine clearance values above 50 mL/min.

Use in Pediatric Patients: For pediatric patients from 3 months of age and older, the MERREM I.V. dose is 20 or 40 mg/kg every 8 hours (maximum dose is 2 g every 8 hours), depending on the type of infection (intra-abdominal or meningitis). (See Dosing Table Below.) Pediatric patients weighing over 50 kg should be administered MERREM I.V. at a dose of 1 g every 8 hours for intra-abdominal infections and 2 g every 8 hours for meningitis. MERREM I.V. should be given as intravenous infusion over approximately 15 to 30 minutes or as an intravenous bolus injection (5 to 20 mL) over approximately 3–5 minutes.

Recommended MERREM I.V. Dosage Schedule for Pediatrics With Normal Renal Function

Type of Infection	Dose (mg/kg)	Dosing Interval
Intra-abdominal	20	every 8 hours
Meningitis	40	every 8 hours

There is no experience in pediatric patients with renal impairment.

PREPARATION OF SOLUTION

For Intravenous Bolus Administration

Constitute injection vials (500 mg/20 mL and 1 g/30 mL) with sterile Water for Injection (See table below.) Shake to dissolve and let stand until clear.

Vial Size	Amount of Diluent Added (mL)	Approximate Withdrawable Volume (mL)	Approximate Average Concentration (mg/mL)
500 mg/20 mL	10	10	50
1 g/30 mL	20	20	50

Continued on next page

Zeneca Pharmaceuticals—Cont.

For Infusion

Infusion vials (500 mg/100 mL and 1 g/100 mL) may be directly constituted with a compatible infusion fluid. (See **COMPATIBILITY AND STABILITY**). Alternatively, an injection vial may be constituted, then the resulting solution added to an I.V. container and further diluted with an appropriate infusion fluid. (See **COMPATIBILITY AND STABILITY**).

NOTE: ADD-VANTAGE VIALS ARE NOT TO BE USED IN THIS MANNER.

For ADD-Vantage Vials

ADD-Vantage vials of MERREM I.V. are to be constituted only with Sodium Chloride Injection 0.45%, Sodium Chloride Injection 0.9% or Dextrose Injection 5% in the 50, 100, and 250 mL Abbott ADD-Vantage® flexible diluent containers. MERREM I.V. supplied in single-use ADD-Vantage vials should be prepared as directed.

DIRECTIONS FOR USE OF MERREM I.V. (meropenem for injection) IN ADD-VANTAGE VIALS:

To Open Diluent Container: Peel overwrap from the corner and remove from container. Some opacity of the plastic due to moisture absorption during the sterilization process may be observed. This is normal and does not affect the solution quality or safety. The opacity will diminish gradually.

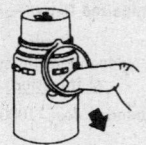

Figure 1

To Assemble ADD-Vantage Vial and Flexible Diluent Container: (Use Aseptic Technique)
1. Remove the protective covers from the top of the vial and the vial port on the diluent container as follows:
   a. To remove the breakaway vial cap, swing the pull ring over the top of the vial and pull down far enough to start the opening (See Figure 1), then pull straight up to remove the cap. (See Figure 2.)
   NOTE: Once the breakaway cap has been removed, do not access vial with syringe.

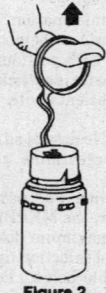

Figure 2

   b. To remove the vial port cover, grasp the tab on the pull ring, pull up to break the three tie strings, then pull back to remove the cover. (See Figure 3.)

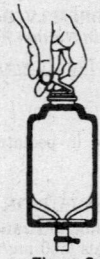

Figure 3

2. Screw the vial into the vial port until it will go no further. THE VIAL MUST BE SCREWED IN TIGHTLY TO ASSURE A SEAL. This occurs approximately $1/2$ turn (180°) after the first audible click. (See Figure 4.) The clicking sound does not assure a seal; the vial must be turned as far as it will go.
   NOTE: ONCE VIAL IS SEATED, DO NOT ATTEMPT TO REMOVE.
   [See Figure at top of next column.]

3. Recheck the vial to assure that it is tight by trying to turn it further in the direction of assembly.
4. Label appropriately.

To Prepare Admixture:
1. Squeeze the bottom of the diluent container gently to in-

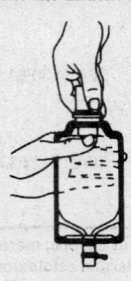

Figure 4

flate the portion of the container surrounding the end of the drug vial.
2. With the other hand, push the drug vial down into the container telescoping the walls of the container. Grasp the inner cap of the vial through the walls of the container. (See Figure 5.)

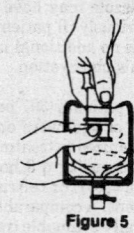

Figure 5

3. Pull the inner cap from the drug vial. (See Figure 6.) Verify that the rubber stopper has been pulled out and invert the system several times, allowing the drug and diluent to mix.

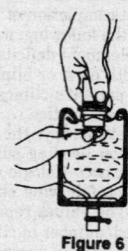

Figure 6

4. Mix contents thoroughly and use within the specified time.

Preparation For Administration: (Use Aseptic Technique)
1. Confirm the activation and admixture of vial contents.
2. Check for leaks by squeezing container firmly. If leaks are found, discard unit as sterility may be impaired.
3. Close flow control clamp of administration set.
4. Remove cover from outlet port at bottom of container.
5. Insert piercing pin of administration set into port with a twisting motion until the pin is firmly seated.
   NOTE: See full directions on administration set carton.
6. Lift the free end of the hanger loop on the bottom of the vial, breaking the two tie strings. Bend the loop outward to lock it in the upright position, then suspend container from hanger.
7. Squeeze and release drip chamber to establish proper fluid level in chamber.
8. Open flow control clamp and clear air from set. Close clamp.
9. Attach set to venipuncture device. If device is not indwelling, prime and make venipuncture.
10. Regulate rate of administration with flow control clamp.
WARNING: Do not use flexible container in series connections.

COMPATIBILITY AND STABILITY

Compatibility of MERREM I.V. with other drugs has not been established. MERREM I.V. should not be mixed with or physically added to solutions containing other drugs. Freshly prepared solutions of MERREM I.V. should be used whenever possible. However, constituted solutions of MERREM I.V. maintain satisfactory potency at controlled room temperature 15–25°C (59–77°F) or under refrigeration at 4°C (39°F) as described below. Solutions of intravenous MERREM I.V. should not be frozen.

Intravenous Bolus Administration

MERREM I.V. injection vials constituted with sterile Water for Injection for bolus administration (up to 50 mg/mL of MERREM I.V.) may be stored for up to 2 hours at controlled room temperature 15–25°C (59–77°F) or for up to 12 hours at 4°C (39°F).

Intravenous Infusion Administration

Stability in Infusion Vials: MERREM I.V. infusion vials constituted with Sodium Chloride Injection 0.9% (MERREM I.V. concentrations ranging from 2.5 to 50 mg/mL) are stable for up to 2 hours at controlled room temperature 15–25°C (55–77°F) or for up to 18 hours at 4°C (39°F). Infusion vials of MERREM I.V. constituted with Dextrose Injection 5% (MERREM I.V. concentrations ranging from 2.5 to 50 mg/mL) are stable for up to 1 hour at controlled room temperature 15–25°C (59–77°F) or for up to 8 hours at 4°C (39°F).

Stability in Plastic I.V. Bags: Solutions prepared for infusion (MERREM I.V. concentrations ranging from 1 to 20 mg/mL) may be stored in plastic intravenous bags with diluents as shown below:

	Number of Hours Stable at Controlled Room Temperature 15–25°C (59–77°F)	Number of Hours Stable at 4°C (39°F)
Sodium Chloride Injection 0.9%	4	24
Dextrose Injection 5.0%	1	4
Dextrose Injection 10.0%	1	2
Dextrose and Sodium Chloride Injection 5.0%/0.9%	1	2
Dextrose and Sodium Chloride Injection 5.0%/0.2%	1	4
Potassium Chloride in Dextrose Injection 0.15%/5.0%	1	6
Sodium Bicarbonate in Dextrose Injection 0.02%/5.0%	1	6
Dextrose Injection 5.0% in Normosol®-M	1	8
Dextrose Injection 5.0% in Ringers Lactate Injection	1	4
Dextrose and Sodium Chloride Injection 2.5%/0.45%	3	12
Mannitol Injection 2.5%	2	16
Ringers Injection	4	24
Ringers Lactate Injection	4	12
Sodium Lactate Injection 1/6 N	2	24
Sodium Bicarbonate Injection 5.0%	1	4

Stability in Baxter Minibag Plus: Solutions of MERREM I.V. (MERREM I.V. concentrations ranging from 2.5 to 20 mg/mL) in Baxter Minibag Plus bags with Sodium Chloride Injection 0.9% may be stored for up to 4 hours at controlled room temperatures 15–25°C (59–77°F) or for up to 24 hours at 4°C (39°F). Solutions of MERREM I.V. (MERREM I.V. concentrations ranging from 2.5 to 20 mg/mL) in Baxter Minibag Plus bags with Dextrose Injection 5.0% may be stored up to 1 hour at controlled room temperatures 15–25°C (59–77°F) or for up to 6 hours at 4°C (39°F).

Stability in Plastic Syringes, Tubing and Intravenous Infusion Sets: Solutions of MERREM I.V. (MERREM I.V. concentrations ranging from 1 to 20 mg/mL) in Water for Injection or Sodium Chloride Injection 0.9% (for up to 4 hours) or in Dextrose Injection 5.0% (for up to 2 hours) at controlled room temperatures 15–25°C (59–77°F) are stable in plastic syringes, plastic tubing, drip chambers, and volume control devices of common intravenous infusion sets.

ADD-Vantage Vials: ADD-Vantage vials diluted in Sodium Chloride Injection 0.45% (MERREM I.V. concentrations ranging from 5 to 20 mg/mL) may be stored for up to 6 hours at controlled room temperature 15–25°C (59–77°F) or for 24 hours at 4°C (39°F). ADD-Vantage vials diluted in Sodium Chloride Injection 0.9% (MERREM I.V. concentrations ranging from 1–20 mg/mL) may be stored for up to 4 hours at controlled room temperature 15–25°C (59–77°F) or for 24 hours at 4°C (39°F). ADD-Vantage vials diluted with Dextrose Injection 5.0% (MERREM I.V. concentrations ranging from 1–20 mg/mL) may be stored for up to 1 hour at controlled room temperature 15–25°C (59–77°F) or for 8 hours at 4°C (39°F).

NOTE: Parenteral drug products should be inspected visually for particulate matter and discoloration prior to administration, whenever solution and container permit.

HOW SUPPLIED

MERREM I.V. is supplied in 20 mL and 30 mL injection vials containing sufficient meropenem to deliver 500 mg or 1 g for intravenous administration, respectively. MERREM I.V. is supplied in 100 mL infusion vials containing sufficient meropenem to deliver 500 mg or 1 g for intravenous administration. The dry powder should be stored at controlled room temperature 20–25°C (68–77°F) [see USP].

MERREM I.V. is also supplied as ADD-Vantage Vials containing sufficient meropenem to deliver 500 mg or 1 g for intravenous administration.

500 mg/20 mL Injection Vial (NDC 0310-0325-20)
500 mg/100 mL Infusion Vial (NDC 0310-0325-11)
1 g/30 mL Injection Vial (NDC 0310-0321-30)
1 g/100 mL Infusion Vial (NDC 0310-0321-11)

500 mg/15 mL ADD-Vantage (NDC 0310-0325-15)
1 g/15 mL ADD-Vantage (NDC 0310-0321-15)

REFERENCES

1. National Committee for Clinical Laboratory Standards. Methods for Dilution Antimicrobial Susceptibility Tests for Bacteria that Grow Aerobically — Third Edition. Approved Standard NCCLS Document M7-A3, Vol. 13, No. 25, NCCLS, Villanova, PA, December, 1993.
2. National Committee for Clinical Laboratory Standards. Performance Standards for Antimicrobial Disk Susceptibility Tests — Fifth Edition. Approved Standard NCCLS Document M2-A5, Vol. 13, No. 24, NCCLS, Villanova, PA. December 1993.
3. National Committee for Clinical Laboratory Standards. Methods for Antimicrobial Susceptibility Testing of Anaerobic Bacteria – Third Edition. Approved Standard NCCLS Document M11-A3, Vol. 13, No. 26, NCCLS, Villanova, PA. December 1993.
4. Cockcroft DW, Gault MH. Prediction of creatinine clearance from serum creatinine. Nephron. 1976; 16.31-41.

†ADD-Vantage is a registered trademark of Abbott Laboratories Inc.

MERREM® (meropenem for injection) is manufactured by:
Sumitomo Pharmaceuticals Co. Ltd
Oita Works
Tsurusaki 2200
Oita-shi
Oita
Japan

Manufactured for:
Zeneca Pharmaceuticals
A business unit of Zeneca Inc.
Wilmington, DE 19850-5437
Rev F 07/96 SIC 64041-00

NOLVADEX® ℞

[nol 'va-dex]
tamoxifen citrate

DESCRIPTION

NOLVADEX® (tamoxifen citrate) Tablets, a nonsteroidal antiestrogen, are for oral administration. NOLVADEX Tablets are available as:

10 mg Tablets. Each tablet contains 15.2 mg of tamoxifen citrate which is equivalent to 10 mg of tamoxifen.

20 mg Tablets. Each tablet contains 30.4 mg of tamoxifen citrate which is equivalent to 20 mg of tamoxifen.

Inactive Ingredients: carboxymethylcellulose calcium, magnesium stearate, mannitol and starch.

Chemically, NOLVADEX is the trans-isomer of a triphenylethylene derivative. The chemical name is (Z)2-[4-(1,2-diphenyl-1-butenyl) phenoxy]-N, N-dimethylethanamine 2-hydroxy-1,2,3-propanetricarboxylate (1:1). The structural and empirical formulas are:

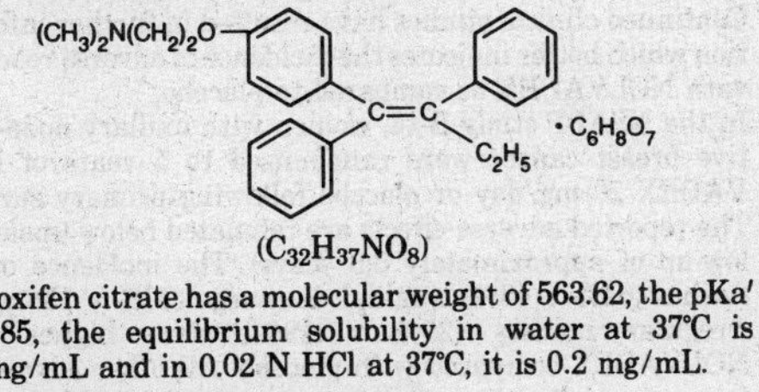

($C_{32}H_{37}NO_8$)

Tamoxifen citrate has a molecular weight of 563.62, the pKa′ is 8.85, the equilibrium solubility in water at 37°C is 0.5 mg/mL and in 0.02 N HCl at 37°C, it is 0.2 mg/mL.

CLINICAL PHARMACOLOGY

NOLVADEX is a nonsteroidal agent which has demonstrated potent antiestrogenic properties in animal test systems. The antiestrogenic effects may be related to its ability to compete with estrogen for binding sites in target tissues such as breast. Tamoxifen inhibits the induction of rat mammary carcinoma induced by dimethylbenzanthracene (DMBA) and causes the regression of already established DMBA-induced tumors. In this rat model, tamoxifen appears to exert its antitumor effects by binding the estrogen receptors.

In cytosols derived from human breast adenocarcinomas, tamoxifen competes with estradiol for estrogen receptor protein.

Tamoxifen is extensively metabolized after oral administration. Studies in women receiving 20 mg of ^{14}C tamoxifen have shown that approximately 65% of the administered dose was excreted from the body over a period of 2 weeks with fecal excretion as the primary route of elimination. The drug was excreted mainly as polar conjugates, with unchanged drug and unconjugated metabolites accounting for less than 30% of the total fecal radioactivity.

N-desmethyl tamoxifen was the major metabolite found in patients' plasma. The biological activity of N-desmethyl tamoxifen appears to be similar to tamoxifen. 4-Hydroxytamoxifen and a side chain primary alcohol derivative of tamoxifen have been identified as minor metabolities in plasma.

Following a single oral dose of 20 mg tamoxifen, an average peak plasma concentration of 40 ng/mL (range 35 to 45 ng/mL) occurred approximately 5 hours after dosing. The decline in plasma concentrations of tamoxifen is biphasic with a terminal elimination half-life of about 5 to 7 days. The average peak plasma concentration for N-desmethyl tamoxifen is 15 ng/mL (range 10 to 20 ng/mL). Chronic administration of 10 mg tamoxifen given twice daily for three months to patients results in average steady-state plasma concentrations of 120 ng/mL (range 67–183 ng/mL) for tamoxifen and 336 ng/mL (range 148–654 ng/mL) for N-desmethyl tamoxifen. The average steady-state plasma concentrations of tamoxifen and N-desmethyl tamoxifen after administration of 20 mg tamoxifen once daily for three months are 122 ng/mL (range 71–183 ng/mL) and 353 ng/mL (range 152–706 ng/mL), respectively. After initiation of therapy, steady state concentrations for tamoxifen are achieved in about 4 weeks and steady state concentrations for N-desmethyl tamoxifen are achieved in about 8 weeks, suggesting a half-life of approximately 14 days for this metabolite.

In a 3-month crossover steady-state bioavailability study with NOLVADEX 10 mg twice a day versus NOLVADEX 20 mg given once daily, the results deomonstrated that NOLVADEX 20 mg taken once daily has comparable bioavailability to NOLVADEX 10 mg taken twice a day.

Clinical Studies: The Early Breast Cancer Trialists' Collaborative Group (EBCTCG) conducted worldwide overviews of systemic adjuvant therapy for early breast cancer in 1985 and again in 1990. In 1992, 10-year outcome data were reported for 29,892 women in 40 randomized trials of adjuvant tamoxifen using doses of 20–40 mg/day for 1–5+ years (median 2 years). Fifty-one percent were entered into trials comparing tamoxifen to no adjuvant therapy and 49% were entered into trials of tamoxifen in combination with chemotherapy vs. the same chemotherapy alone. Twenty-nine percent were <50 years of age and 71% were ≥50 years. Fifty-seven percent were node-positive and 43% were node-negative. Fifty percent of the tumors were estrogen receptor (ER) positive (≥10 fmol/mg), 18% were ER poor (<10 fmol/mg), and 32% were ER unknown.

The overall recurrence-free survival at 10 years of follow-up was 51.2% for tamoxifen versus 44.7% for control (logrank 2p <0.00001). Overall survival at 10 years was 58.8% for tamoxifen versus 52.6% for control (logrank 2p <0.00001). Both the absolute risk of relapse and the absolute benefit of treatment with tamoxifen were greater in women with positive nodes than in women with negative nodes. In women with positive nodes, 10-year recurrence-free survival was 41.9% for tamoxifen versus 33.1% for control (logrank 1p <0.00001). Ten-year survival was 50.4% for tamoxifen versus 42.2% for control (logrank 1p <0.00001). In women with negative nodes, recurrence-free survival was 68.1% for tamoxifen versus 63.1% for control (logrank 1p <0.00001). Survival at 10 years was 74.5% for tamoxifen versus 71.0% for control (logrank 1p = 0.0002).

The reduction in the annual odds of recurrence with tamoxifen was 12% in women <50 years of age versus 29% in women ≥50 years. Similarly, the reduction in the annual odds of death was 6% versus 20%. The reduction in the annual odds of recurrence with tamoxifen was significantly greater in ER positive (32%) than in ER poor (13%) tumors (1p <0.00001). The reduction in recurrence and mortality was greater in those studies that used tamoxifen for longer (≥2 years) rather than shorter (<2 years) periods. There was no indication that doses greater than 20 mg per day were more effective.

Two studies (Hubay and NSABP B-09) demonstrated an improved disease-free survival following radical or modified radical mastectomy in postmenopausal women or women 50 years of age or older with surgically curable breast cancer with positive axillary nodes when NOLVADEX was added to adjuvant cytotoxic chemotherapy. In the Hubay study, NOLVADEX was added to "low-dose" CMF (cyclophosphamide, methotrexate and fluorouracil). In the NSABP B-09 study, NOLVADEX was added to melphalan [L-phenylalanine mustard (P)] and fluorouracil (F).

In the Hubay study, patients with a positive (more than 3 fmol) estrogen receptor were more likely to benefit. In the NSABP B-09 study in women age 50–59 years, only women with both estrogen and progesterone receptor levels 10 fmol or greater clearly benefited, while there was a nonstatistically significant trend toward adverse effect in women with both estrogen and progesterone receptor levels less than 10 fmol. In women age 60–70 years, there was a trend toward a beneficial effect of NOLVADEX without any clear relationship to estrogen or progesterone receptor status.

Three prospective studies (ECOG-1178, Toronto, NATO) using NOLVADEX adjuvantly as a single agent demonstrated an improved disease-free survival following total mastectomy and axillary dissection for postmenopausal women with positive axillary nodes compared to placebo/no treatment controls. The NATO study also demonstrated an overall survival benefit.

NSABP B-14, a prospective, double-blind, randomized study, evaluated NOLVADEX versus placebo in the treatment of women with axillary node-negative, estrogen-receptor positive (≥ 10 fmol/mg cytosol protein) breast cancer (as adjuvant therapy, following total mastectomy and axillary dissection, or segmental resection, axillary dissection, and breast radiation). After five years of treatment, a significant improvement in disease-free survival was demonstrated in women receiving NOLVADEX. This benefit was apparent both in women under age 50 and in women at or beyond age 50. In this trial women who received tamoxifen for five years and were disease-free at the end of this 5-year period were offered an additional five years of NOLVADEX, or placebo in a double-blind randomized scheme. With four years of follow-up after this rerandomization, 92% of the women that received five years of NOLVADEX followed by placebo are alive and disease-free, compared to 86% of the women scheduled to receive 10 years of NOLVADEX. This difference was not statistically significant. One additional randomized study (NATO) demonstrated improved disease-free survival for NOLVADEX compared to no adjuvant therapy following total mastectomy and axillary dissection in postmenopausal women with axillary node-negative breast cancer. In this study, the benefits of NOLVADEX appeared to be independent of estrogen receptor status.

Three prospective, randomized studies (Ingle, Pritchard, Buchanan) compared NOLVADEX to ovarian ablation (oophorectomy or ovarian irradiation) in premenopausal women with advanced breast cancer. Although the objective response rate, time to treatment failure, and survival were similar with both treatments, the limited patient accrual prevented a demonstration of equivalence. In an overview analysis of survival data from the three studies, the hazard ratio for death (NOLVADEX/ovarian ablation) was 1.00 with two-sided 95% confidence intervals of 0.73 to 1.37. Elevated serum and plasma estrogens have been observed in premenopausal women receiving NOLVADEX. However, the data from the randomized studies do not suggest an adverse effect. A limited number of premenopausal patients with disease progression during NOLVADEX therapy responded to subsequent ovarian ablation.

In a large randomized trial in Sweden of adjuvant NOLVADEX 40 mg/day for 2–5 years, the incidence of second primary breast tumors was reduced in the tamoxifen arm (p<0.05). In the NSABP B-14 trial in which patients were randomized to NOLVADEX 20 mg/day for 5 years versus placebo, the incidence of second primary breast cancers is also reduced.

Published results from 122 patients (119 evaluable) and case reports in 16 patients (13 evaluable) treated with NOLVADEX have shown that NOLVADEX is effective for the palliative treatment of male breast cancer. Sixty-six of these 132 evaluable patients responded to NOLVADEX which constitutes a 50% objective response rate.

INDICATIONS AND USAGE

Adjuvant Therapy: NOLVADEX is indicated for the treatment of axillary node-negative breast cancer in women following total mastectomy or segmental mastectomy, axillary dissection, and breast irradiation. Data are insufficient to predict which women are most likely to benefit and to determine if NOLVADEX provides any benefit in women with tumors less than 1 cm.

NOLVADEX is indicated for the treatment of node-positive breast cancer in postmenopausal women following total mastectomy, or segmental mastectomy, axillary dissection, and breast irradiation. In some NOLVADEX adjuvant studies, most of the benefit to date has been in the subgroup with 4 or more positive axillary nodes.

The estrogen and progesterone receptor values may help to predict whether adjuvant NOLVADEX therapy is likely to be beneficial.

Therapy for Advanced Disease: NOLVADEX is effective in the treatment of metastatic breast cancer in women and men. In premenopausal women with metastatic breast cancer, NOLVADEX is an alternative to oophorectomy or ovarian irradiation. Available evidence indicates that patients whose tumors are estrogen receptor positive are more likely to benefit from NOLVADEX therapy.

CONTRAINDICATIONS

NOLVADEX is contraindicated in patients with known hypersensitivity to the drug.

WARNINGS

Visual disturbance including corneal changes, cataracts and retinopathy have been reported in patients receiving NOLVADEX.

As with other additive hormonal therapy (estrogens and androgens), hypercalcemia has been reported in some breast cancer patients with bone metastases within a few weeks of starting treatment with NOLVADEX. If hypercalcemia does occur, appropriate measures should be taken and, if severe, NOLVADEX should be discontinued.

An increased incidence of endometrial changes including hyperplasia, polyps, and endometrial cancer has been reported in association with NOLVADEX treatment. The incidence and pattern of this increase suggest that the un-

Continued on next page

Zeneca Pharmaceuticals—Cont.

derlying mechanism is related to the estrogenic properties of NOLVADEX. Any patients receiving or having previously received NOLVADEX who report abnormal vaginal bleeding should be promptly evaluated.

In a large randomized trial in Sweden of adjuvant NOLVADEX 40 mg/day for 2–5 years, an increased incidence of uterine cancer was noted. Twenty three of 1,372 patients randomized to receive NOLVADEX versus 4 of 1,357 patients randomized to the observation group developed cancer of the uterus [RR = 5.6 (1.9–16.2), $p < .001$]. One of the patients with cancer of the uterus who was randomized to receive NOLVADEX never took the drug. After approximately 6.8 years of follow-up in the NSABP B-14 trial, 15 of 1,419 women randomized to receive NOLVADEX 20 mg/day for 5 years developed uterine cancer and 2 of the 1,424 women randomized to receive placebo, who subsequently were treated with NOLVADEX, also developed uterine cancer. Most of the uterine cancers were diagnosed at an early stage, but deaths from uterine cancer have been reported. Patients receiving NOLVADEX should have routine gynecological care and they should promptly inform their physician if they experience any menstrual irregularities, abnormal vaginal bleeding, change in vaginal discharge, or pelvic pain or pressure.

NOLVADEX has been associated with changes in liver enzyme levels, and on rare occasions, a spectrum of more severe liver abnormalities including fatty liver, cholestasis, hepatitis and hepatic necrosis. A few of these serious cases included fatalities. In most reported cases the relationship to NOLVADEX is uncertain. However, some positive rechallenges and dechallenges have been reported.

In the Swedish trial using adjuvant NOLVADEX 40 mg/day for 2–5 years, 3 cases of liver cancer have been reported in the NOLVADEX-treated group versus 1 case in the observation group. In other clinical trials evaluating NOLVADEX, no other cases of liver cancer have been reported to date.

Data from the NSABP B-14 study show no increase in other (non-uterine) cancers among patients receiving NOLVADEX. However, a number of second primary tumors, occurring at sites other than the endometrium, have been reported following the treatment of breast cancer with NOLVADEX in clinical trials. Whether an increased risk for other (non-uterine) cancers is associated with NOLVADEX is still uncertain and continues to be evaluated.

Pregnancy Category D: NOLVADEX may cause fetal harm when administered to a pregnant woman. Women should be advised not to become pregnant while taking NOLVADEX and should use barrier or nonhormonal contraceptive measures if sexually active. Effects on reproductive functions are expected from the antiestrogenic properties of the drug. In reproductive studies in rats at dose levels equal to or below the human dose, nonteratogenic developmental skeletal changes were seen and were found reversible. In addition, in fertility studies in rats and in teratology studies in rabbits using doses at or below those used in humans, a lower incidence of embryo implantation and a higher incidence of fetal death or retarded in utero growth were observed, with slower learning behavior in some rat pups when compared to historical controls. Several pregnant marmosets were dosed during organogenesis or in the last half of pregnancy. No deformations were seen and, although the dose was high enough to terminate pregnancy in some animals, those that did maintain pregnancy showed no evidence of teratogenic malformations.

In rodent models of fetal reproductive tract development, tamoxifen (at doses 0.3 to 2.4-fold the human maximum recommended dose on a mg/m^2 basis) caused changes in both sexes that are similar to those caused by estradiol, ethynylestradiol and diethylstilbestrol. Although the clinical relevance of these changes is unknown, some of these changes, especially vaginal adenosis, are similar to those seen in young women who were exposed to diethylstilbestrol in utero and who have a 1 in 1000 risk of developing clear-cell adenocarcinoma of the vagina or cervix. To date, in utero exposure to tamoxifen has not been shown to cause vaginal adenosis, or clear-cell adenocarcinoma of the vagina or cervix, in young women. However, only a small number of young women have been exposed to tamoxifen in utero, and a smaller number have been followed long enough (to age 15–20) to determine whether vaginal or cervical neoplasia could occur as a result of this exposure.

There are no adequate and well controlled trials of tamoxifen in pregnant women. There have been a small number of reports of vaginal bleeding, spontaneous abortions, birth defects, and fetal deaths in pregnant women. If this drug is used during pregnancy, or the patient becomes pregnant while taking this drug, or within approximately two months after discontinuing therapy, the patient should be apprised of the potential risks to the fetus including the potential long term risk of a DES-like syndrome.

PRECAUTIONS

General: Decreases in platelet counts, usually to 50,000–100,000/mm^3, infrequently lower, have been occasionally reported in patients taking NOLVADEX for breast cancer. In patients with significant thrombocytopenia, rare hemorrhagic episodes have occurred, but it is uncertain if these episodes are due to NOLVADEX therapy. Leukopenia has been observed, sometimes in association with anemia and/or thrombocytopenia. There have been rare reports of neutropenia and pancytopenia in patients receiving NOLVADEX; this can sometimes be severe.

Information for Patients: Women taking or having previously taken NOLVADEX should be instructed to report abnormal vaginal bleeding which should be promptly investigated.

Laboratory Tests: Periodic complete blood counts, including platelet counts, and periodic liver function tests should be obtained.

Drug Interactions: When NOLVADEX is used in combination with coumarin-type anticoagulants, a significant increase in anticoagulant effect may occur. Where such coadministration exists, careful monitoring of the patient's prothrombin time is recommended.

There is an increased risk of thromboembolic events occurring when cytotoxic agents are used in combination with NOLVADEX.

Tamoxifen, N-desmethyl tamoxifen and 4-Hydroxytamoxifen have been found to be potent inhibitors of hepatic cytochrome p-450 mixed function oxidases. The effect of tamoxifen on metabolism and excretion of other antineoplastic drugs, such as cyclophosphamide and other drugs that require mixed function oxidases for activation, is not known.

One patient receiving NOLVADEX with concomitant phenobarbital exhibited a steady state serum level of tamoxifen lower than that observed for other patients (ie, 26 ng/mL vs. mean value of 122 ng/mL). However, the clinical significance of this finding is not known.

Concomitant bromocriptine therapy has been shown to elevate serum tamoxifen and N-desmethyltamoxifen.

Drug/Laboratory Testing Interactions: During postmarketing surveillance, T_4 elevations were reported for a few postmenopausal patients which may be explained by increases in thyroid-binding globulin. These elevations were not accompanied by clinical hyperthyroidism.

Variations in the karyopyknotic index on vaginal smears and various degrees of estrogen effect on Pap smears have been infrequently seen in postmenopausal patients given NOLVADEX.

In the postmarketing experience with NOLVADEX, infrequent cases of hyperlipidemias have been reported. Periodic monitoring of plasma triglycerides and cholesterol may be indicated in patients with pre-existing hyperlipidemias.

Carcinogenesis: A conventional carcinogenesis study in rats, (doses of 5, 20, and 35 mg/kg/day for up to 2 years) revealed hepatocellular carcinoma at all doses, and the incidence of these tumors was significantly greater among rats given 20 or 35 mg/kg/day (69%) than those given 5 mg/kg/day (14%). The incidence of these tumors in rats given 5 mg/kg/day (29.5 mg/m^2) was significantly greater than in controls.

In addition, preliminary data from 2 independent reports of 6-month studies in rats reveal liver tumors which in one study are classified as malignant. (See WARNINGS.)

Endocrine changes in immature and mature mice were investigated in a 13-month study. Granulosa cell ovarian tumors and interstitial cell testicular tumors were found in mice receiving NOLVADEX, but not in the controls.

Mutagenesis: Although no genotoxic potential was found in a conventional battery of in vivo and in vitro tests with pro- and eukaryotic test systems with drug metabolizing systems present, increased levels of DNA adducts have been found in the livers of rats exposed to tamoxifen. Tamoxifen also has been found to increase levels of micronucleus formation in vitro in human lymphoblastoid cell line (MCL-5). Based on these findings, tamoxifen is genotoxic in rodent and human MCL-5 cells.

Impairment of Fertility: Fertility in female rats was decreased following administration of 0.04 mg/kg for two weeks prior to mating through day 7 of pregnancy. There was a decreased number of implantations, and all fetuses were found dead.

Following administration to rats of 0.16 mg/kg from days 7–17 of pregnancy, there were increased numbers of fetal deaths. Administration of 0.125 mg/kg to rabbits during days 6–18 of pregnancy resulted in abortion or premature delivery. Fetal deaths occurred at higher doses. There were no teratogenic changes in either rat or rabbit segment II studies. Several pregnant marmosets were dosed with 10 mg/kg/day either during organogenesis or in the last half of pregnancy. No deformations were seen, and although the dose was high enough to terminate pregnancy in some animals, those that did maintain pregnancy showed no evidence of teratogenic malformations. Rats given 0.16 mg/kg from day 17 of pregnancy to 1 day before weaning demonstrated increased numbers of dead pups at parturition. It was reported that some rat pups showed slower learning behavior, but this did not achieve statistical significance in one study, and in another study where significance was reported, this was obtained by comparing dosed animals with controls of another study.

The recommended daily human dose of 20–40 mg corresponds to 0.4–0.8 mg/kg for an average 50 kg woman.

Pregnancy Category D: See WARNINGS.

Nursing Mothers: It is not known whether this drug is excreted in human milk. Because many drugs are excreted in human milk and because of the potential for serious adverse reactions in nursing infants from NOLVADEX, a decision should be made whether to discontinue nursing or to discontinue the drug, taking into account the importance of the drug to the mother.

Pediatric Use: The safety and efficacy of NOLVADEX in pediatric patients have not been established.

ADVERSE REACTIONS

Adverse reactions to NOLVADEX are relatively mild and rarely severe enough to require discontinuation of treatment.

In patients treated with NOLVADEX for metastatic breast cancer, the most frequent adverse reactions to NOLVADEX are hot flashes and nausea and/or vomiting. These may occur in up to one-fourth of patients.

Less frequently reported adverse reactions are vaginal bleeding, vaginal discharge, menstrual irregularities and skin rash. Usually these have not been of sufficient severity to require dosage reduction or discontinuation of treatment.

Increased bone and tumor pain and, also, local disease flare have occurred, which are sometimes associated with a good tumor response. Patients with increased bone pain may require additional analgesics. Patients with soft tissue disease may have sudden increases in the size of preexisting lesions, sometimes associated with marked erythema within and surrounding the lesions and/or the development of new lesions. When they occur, the bone pain or disease flare are seen shortly after starting NOLVADEX and generally subside rapidly.

Other adverse reactions which are seen infrequently are hypercalcemia, peripheral edema, distaste for food, pruritus vulvae, depression, dizziness, light-headedness, headache, hair thinning and/or partial hair loss, and vaginal dryness.

NOLVADEX has been associated with changes in liver enzyme levels, and on rare occasions, a spectrum of more severe liver abnormalities including fatty liver, cholestasis, hepatitis and hepatic necrosis. A few of these serious cases included fatalities. In most reported cases the relationship to NOLVADEX is uncertain. However, some positive rechallenges and dechallenges have been reported.

There have been a few reports of endometriosis and uterine fibroids in women receiving NOLVADEX. The underlying mechanism may be due to the partial estrogenic effect of NOLVADEX. Ovarian cysts have been observed in a small number of premenopausal patients with advanced breast cancer who have been treated with NOLVADEX.

Continued clinical studies have resulted in further information which better indicates the incidence of adverse reactions with NOLVADEX as compared to placebo.

In the NSABP study B-14, women with axillary node-negative breast cancer were randomized to 5 years of NOLVADEX 20 mg/day or placebo following primary surgery. The reported adverse effects are tabulated below (mean follow-up of approximately 6.8 years). The incidence of hot flashes (64% v 48%), vaginal discharge (30% v 15%), and irregular menses (25% v 19%) were higher with NOLVADEX compared with placebo. All other adverse effects occurred with similar frequency in the two treatment groups, with the exception of thrombotic events which although rare, were more common with NOLVADEX than with placebo. Two of the patients treated with NOLVADEX who had thrombotic events died.

NSABP B-14 STUDY

Adverse Effect	% of Women NOLVADEX (n=1424)	Placebo (n=1440)
Hot Flashes	63.9	47.6
Weight Gain (>5%)	38.1	40.1
Fluid Retention	32.4	29.7
Vaginal Discharge	29.6	15.2
Nausea	25.7	23.9
Irregular Menses	24.6	18.8
Weight Loss (>5%)	22.6	18.0
Skin Changes	18.7	15.3
Increased BUN	18.1	20.2
Diarrhea	11.2	14.0
Increased SGOT	4.8	2.8
Increased Alkaline Phosphatase	3.0	4.6
Vomiting	2.1	1.7
Increased Bilirubin	1.8	1.2
Increased Creatinine	1.7	1.0
Thrombocytopenia*	1.5	1.2
Leukopenia**	0.4	1.1

Thrombotic Events		
Deep Vein Thrombosis	0.8	0.3
Pulmonary Embolism	0.4	0.1
Superficial Phlebitis	0.3	0.0

*Defined as a platelet count of $< 100{,}000/mm^3$
**Defined as a white blood cell count of $< 3000/mm^3$

In the Eastern Cooperative Oncology Group (ECOG) adjuvant breast cancer trial, NOLVADEX or placebo was administered for 2 years to women following mastectomy. When compared to placebo, NOLVADEX showed a significantly higher incidence of hot flashes (19% versus 8% for placebo). The incidence of all other adverse reactions was similar in the 2 treatment groups with the exception of thrombocytopenia where the incidence for NOLVADEX was 10% versus 3% for placebo, an observation of borderline statistical significance.
The other adverse reactions reported equally in the ECOG study for NOLVADEX and placebo include abnormal renal function tests, fatigue, dyspnea, anorexia, cough, and abdominal cramps. A relationship of these reactions to the administration of NOLVADEX has not been demonstrated since the frequency was not significantly different from that reported in placebo treated women.
In other adjuvant studies, Toronto and NOLVADEX Adjuvant Trial Organization (NATO), women received either NOLVADEX or no therapy. In the Toronto study, hot flashes and nausea and/or vomiting were observed in 29% and 19% of patients, respectively, for NOLVADEX versus 1% and 0% in the untreated group. In the NATO trial, hot flashes, nausea and/or vomiting and vaginal bleeding were reported in 2.8%, 2.1%, and 2.0% of women, respectively, for NOLVADEX versus 0.2% for each in the untreated group.
The following table summarizes the incidence of adverse reactions reported at a frequency of 2% or greater from clinical trials (Ingle, Pritchard, Buchanan) which compared NOLVADEX therapy to ovarian ablation in premenopausal patients with metastatic breast cancer.

	NOLVADEX All Effects Number of Women (%)		OVARIAN ABLATION All Effects Number of Women (%)	
Adverse Reactions*	n=104		n=100	
Flush	34	(32.7)	46	(46)
Amenorrhea	17	(16.3)	69	(69)
Altered Menses	13	(12.5)	5	(5)
Oligomenorrhea	9	(8.7)	1	(1)
Bone Pain	6	(5.7)	6	(6)
Menstrual Disorder	6	(5.7)	4	(4)
Nausea	5	(4.8)	4	(4)
Cough/Coughing	4	(3.8)	1	(1)
Edema	4	(3.8)	1	(1)
Fatigue	4	(3.8)	1	(1)
Musculoskeletal Pain	3	(2.8)	0	(0)
Pain	3	(2.8)	4	(4)
Ovarian Cyst(s)	3	(2.8)	2	(2)
Depression	2	(1.9)	2	(2)
Abdominal Cramps	1	(1)	2	(2)
Anorexia	1	(1)	2	(2)

*Some women had more than one adverse reaction.

NOLVADEX is well tolerated in males with breast cancer. Reports from the literature and case reports suggest that the safety profile of NOLVADEX in males is similar to that seen in women. Loss of libido and impotence have resulted in discontinuation of tamoxifen therapy in male patients. Also, in oligospermic males treated with tamoxifen, LH, FSH, testosterone and estrogen levels were elevated. No significant clinical changes were reported.

OVERDOSAGE

Signs observed at the highest doses following studies to determine LD_{50} in animals were respiratory difficulties and convulsions.
Acute overdosage in humans has not been reported. In a study of advanced metastatic cancer patients which specifically determined the maximum tolerated dose of NOLVADEX in evaluating the use of very high doses to reverse multidrug resistance, acute neurotoxicity manifested by tremor, hyperreflexia, unsteady gait and dizziness were noted. These symptoms occurred within 3–5 days of beginning NOLVADEX and cleared within 2–5 days after stopping therapy. No permanent neurologic toxicity was noted. One patient experienced a seizure several days after NOLVADEX was discontinued and neurotoxic symptoms had resolved. The causal relationship of the seizure to NOLVADEX therapy is unknown. Doses given in these patients were all greater than 400 mg/m^2 loading dose, followed by maintenance doses of 150 mg/m^2 of NOLVADEX given twice a day.
In the same study, prolongation of the QT interval on the electrocardiogram was noted when patients were given doses higher than 250 mg/m^2 loading dose, followed by maintenance doses of 80 mg/m^2 of NOLVADEX given twice a day. For a woman with a body surface area of 1.5 m^2 the minimal loading dose and maintenance doses given at which neurological symptoms and QT changes occurred were at least 6 fold higher in respect to the maximum recommended dose.
No specific treatment for overdosage is known; treatment must be symptomatic.

DOSAGE AND ADMINISTRATION

For patients with breast cancer, the recommended daily dose is 20–40 mg. Dosages greater than 20 mg per day should be given in divided doses (morning and evening).
In three single agent adjuvant studies in women, one 10 mg NOLVADEX tablet was administered two (ECOG and NATO) or three (Toronto) times a day for two years. In the EBCTCG 1990 overview, the reduction in recurrence and mortality was greater in those studies that used tamoxifen for two years or longer than in those that used tamoxifen for less than two years. There was no indication that doses greater than 20 mg per day were more effective. In B-14, the NSABP adjuvant study in women with node-negative breast cancer, one 10 mg NOLVADEX tablet was given twice a day for at least five years. Results of the B-14 study suggest that continuation of therapy beyond five years does not provide additional benefit (see CLINICAL PHARMACOLOGY). The optimal duration of adjuvant NOLVADEX therapy remains to be determined.

HOW SUPPLIED

10 mg Tablets containing tamoxifen as the citrate in an amount equivalent to 10 mg of tamoxifen (round, biconvex, uncoated, white tablet identified with NOLVADEX 600 debossed on one side and a cameo debossed on the other side) are supplied in bottles of 60 tablets and 250 tablets. NDC 0310-0600.
20 mg Tablets containing tamoxifen as the citrate in an amount equivalent to 20 mg of tamoxifen (round, biconvex, uncoated, white tablet identified with NOLVADEX 604 debossed on one side and a cameo debossed on the other side) are supplied in bottles of 30 tablets. NDC 0310-0604.
Store at controlled room temperature, 20–25° C (68–77° F) [see USP].
ZENECA Pharmaceuticals
A Business Unit of ZENECA Inc.
Wilmington, DE 19850-5437 USA
SIC 64100-00 Rev O 03/96
Shown in Product Identification Guide, page 342

SORBITRATE® ℞

[*sorb'i-trate*]
(Isosorbide Dinitrate)

DESCRIPTION

Isosorbide dinitrate (ISDN) is 1,4:3,6-dianhydro-D-glucitol 2,5-dinitrate, an organic nitrate whose structural formula is:

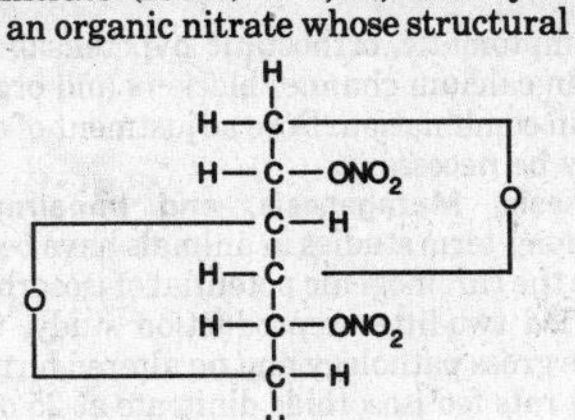

and whose molecular weight is 236.14. The organic nitrates are vasodilators, active on both arteries and veins.
Isosorbide dinitrate is a white, crystalline, odorless compound which is stable in air and in solution, has a melting point of 70°C and has an optical rotation of +134° (c = 1.0, alcohol, 20°C). Isosorbide dinitrate is freely soluble in organic solvents such as acetone, alcohol, and ether; but is only sparingly soluble in water.
SORBITRATE is available as:

SORBITRATE® SUBLINGUAL

2.5 mg Sublingual Tablet. Each tablet contains 2.5 mg of isosorbide dinitrate. Inactive Ingredients: corn starch, lactose (hydrous), magnesium stearate, pregelatinized starch.
5 mg Sublingual Tablet. Each tablet contains 5 mg of isosorbide dinitrate. Inactive Ingredients: corn starch, lactose (hydrous), magnesium stearate, pregelatinized starch, Red 7.

SORBITRATE® CHEWABLE

5 mg Chewable Tablet. Each tablet contains 5 mg of isosorbide dinitrate. Inactive Ingredients: Blue 1, confectioner's sugar, corn starch, flavor, hydrogenated vegetable oil, magnesium stearate, mannitol, povidone, Yellow 10.
10 mg Chewable Tablet. Each tablet contains 10 mg of isosorbide dinitrate. Inactive Ingredients: confectioner's sugar, corn starch, flavor, hydrogenated vegetable oil, magnesium stearate, mannitol, povidone, Yellow 10.

SORBITRATE® ORAL

5 mg Oral Tablet. Each tablet contains 5 mg of isosorbide dinitrate. Inactive Ingredients: Blue 1, corn starch, lactose (hydrous), magnesium stearate, pregelatinized starch, Yellow 10.
10 mg Oral Tablet. Each tablet contains 10 mg of isosorbide dinitrate. Inactive Ingredients: corn starch, lactose (hydrous), magnesium stearate, pregelatinized starch, Yellow 10.
20 mg Oral Tablet. Each tablet contains 20 mg of isosorbide dinitrate. Inactive Ingredients: Blue 1, corn starch, lactose (hydrous), magnesium stearate, pregelatinized starch.
30 mg Oral Tablet. Each tablet contains 30 mg of isosorbide dinitrate. Inactive Ingredients: corn starch, lactose (hydrous), magnesium stearate, pregelatinized starch.
40 mg Oral Tablet. Each tablet contains 40 mg of isosorbide dinitrate. Inactive Ingredients: Blue 1, corn starch, lactose (hydrous), magnesium stearate, pregelatinized starch.

CLINICAL PHARMACOLOGY

The principal pharmacological action of isosorbide dinitrate is relaxation of vascular smooth muscle and consequent dilatation of peripheral arteries and veins, especially the latter. Dilatation of the veins promotes peripheral pooling of blood and decreases venous return to the heart, thereby reducing left ventricular end-diastolic pressure and pulmonary capillary wedge pressure (preload). Arteriolar relaxation reduces systemic vascular resistance, systolic arterial pressure, and mean arterial pressure (afterload). Dilatation of the coronary arteries also occurs. The relative importance of preload reduction, afterload reduction, and coronary dilatation remains undefined.
Dosing regimens for most chronically used drugs are designed to provide plasma concentrations that are continuously greater than a minimally effective concentration. This strategy is inappropriate for organic nitrates. Several well-controlled clinical trials have used exercise testing to assess the anti-anginal efficacy of continuously-delivered nitrates. In the large majority of these trials, active agents were no more effective than placebo after 24 hours (or less) of continuous therapy. Attempts to overcome nitrate tolerance by dose escalation, even to doses far in excess of those used acutely, have consistently failed. Only after nitrates have been absent from the body for several hours has their anti-anginal efficacy been restored.
Pharmacokinetics: Once absorbed, the distribution volume of isosorbide dinitrate is 2–4 L/kg, and this volume is cleared at the rate of 2–4 L/min, so ISDN's half-life in serum is about an hour. Since the clearance exceeds hepatic blood flow, considerable extrahepatic metabolism must also occur. Clearance is effected primarily by denitration to the 2-mononitrate (15%–25%) and the 5-mononitrate (75%–85%).
Both metabolites have biological activity, especially the 5-mononitrate. With an overall half-life of about 5 hours, the 5-mononitrate is cleared from the serum by denitration to isosorbide; glucuronidation to the 5-mononitrate glucuronide; and denitration/hydration to sorbitol. The 2-mononitrate has been less well studied, but it appears to participate in the same metabolic pathways, with a half-life of about 2 hours.
The daily dose-free interval sufficient to avoid tolerance to organic nitrates has not been well defined. Studies of nitroglycerin (an organic nitrate with a very short half-life) have shown that daily dose-free intervals of 10–12 hours are usually sufficient to minimize tolerance. Daily dose-free intervals that have succeeded in avoiding tolerance during trials of moderate doses (eg, 30 mg) of immediate-release ISDN have generally been somewhat longer (at least 14 hours), but this is consistent with the longer half-lives of ISDN and its active metabolites.
Few well-controlled clinical trials of organic nitrates have been designed to detect rebound or withdrawal effects. In one such trial, however, subjects receiving nitrogylcerin had *less* exercise tolerance at the end of the daily dose-free interval than the parallel group receiving placebo. The incidence, magnitude, and clinical significance of similar phenomena in patients receiving ISDN have not been studied.
Bioavailability of ISDN after single sublingual doses is 40%–50%. Multiple-dose studies of sublingual ISDN pharmacokinetics have not been reported; multiple-dose studies of ingested ISDN have observed progressive increases in bioavailability during chronic therapy. Serum levels of ISDN reach their maxima 10–15 minutes after sublingual dosing.
Absorption of isosorbide dinitrate after oral dosing is nearly complete, but bioavailability is highly varible (10%–90%), with extensive first-pass metabolism in the liver. Serum levels reach their maxima about an hour after ingestion. The average bioavailability of ISDN is about 25%; most studies have observed progressive increases in bioavailability during chronic therapy.
The absorption kinetics of chewable isosorbide dinitrate tablets have not been studied. Absorption of ingested ISDN is known to be nearly complete, although bioavailability is highly variable. Ingested ISDN undergoes extensive first-

Continued on next page

Zeneca Pharmaceuticals—Cont.

pass metabolism in the liver; it is not known what portion of this first-pass effect is avoided by buccal absorption of the chewable formulation.

Kinetic studies of absorption of immediate-release formulations of ISDN have found highly variable bioavailability with extensive first-pass metabolism in the liver. Most such studies have observed progressive increases in bioavailability during chronic therapy.

Clinical Trials: In a controlled trial in which 0.4 mg of sublingual nitroglycerin took 1.9 minutes to begin to produce an anti-anginal effect, 5 mg of sublingual ISDN took 3.4 minutes to begin to produce a similar effect. In the same trial, the anti-anginal effect of the sublingual nitrogylcerin was evident for about an hour, while that of the sublingual ISDN lasted about 2 hours.

In other controlled trials, the anti-anginal efficacy of sublingual ISDN has persisted for periods ranging from 30 minutes up to 4 hours.

Multiple-dose trials of sublingual ISDN have not been reported. Multiple-dose trials of ingested formulations of ISDN have shown that ISDN's anti-anginal efficacy is substantially attenuated by tolerance unless the daily regimen does not include at least one interdosing interval of at least 14 hours. The daily interdosing interval necessary in any chronic regimen using sublingual ISDN is not known.

In clinical trials, immediate-release oral isosorbide dinitrate has been administered in a variety of regimens, with total daily doses ranging from 30 mg to 480 mg.

Controlled trials of single oral doses of isosorbide dinitrate have demonstrated effective reductions in exercise-related angina for up to 8 hours. Anti-anginal activity is present about 1 hour after dosing.

Most controlled trials of multiple-dose oral ISDN taken every 12 hours (or more frequently) for several weeks have shown statistically significant anti-anginal efficacy for only 2 hours after dosing. Once-daily regimens, and regimens with at least one daily interval of at least 14 hours (eg, a regimen providing doses at 0800, 1400 and 1800) have shown efficacy after the first dose of each day that was similar to that shown in the single-dose studies cited above.

In controlled trials in which sublingual nitroglycerin took 1½–2 minutes to begin to produce an anti-anginal effect, chewable ISDN tablets took 2½–3 minutes to begin to produce a similar effect. In these same trials, the anti-anginal effect of sublingual nitroglycerin was evident for about 1–1½ hours, while that of chewable ISDN lasted about an hour longer.

Clinical trials of chewable ISDN have used doses of 5 and 10 mg. It is not known whether lower doses would be equally effective.

Multiple-dose trials of chewable ISDN have not been reported. Multiple-dose trials of ingested formulations of ISDN have shown that ISDN's anti-anginal efficacy is substantially attenuated by tolerance unless the daily regimen does not include at least one interdosing interval of at least 14 hours. The daily interdosing interval necessary in any chronic regimen using chewable ISDN is, because of the rapid onset of action of this formulation, probably somewhat longer.

From large, well-controlled studies of other nitrates, it is reasonable to believe that the maximal achievable daily duration of anti-anginal effect from isosorbide dinitrate is about 12 hours. No dosing regimen for isosorbide dinitrate has, however, ever actually been shown to achieve this duration of effect. In the absence of data from multiple-dose trials, and considering the capacity of organic nitrates to induce tolerance, it is not reasonable to assume that multiple sublingual ISDN tablets taken during the course of a day will all have similar effects.

INDICATIONS AND USAGE

SORBITRATE sublingual tablets and chewable tablets are indicated for the prevention and treatment of angina pectoris due to coronary artery disease. However, because the onset of action of these tablets is significantly slower than that of sublingual nitroglycerin, they are not the drug of first choice for abortion of an acute anginal episode.

SORBITRATE oral tablets are indicated for the prevention of angina pectoris due to coronary artery disease. The onset of action of immediate release oral isosorbide dinitrate is not sufficiently rapid for this product to be useful in aborting an acute anginal episode.

CONTRAINDICATIONS

Allergic reactions to organic nitrates are extremely rare, but they do occur. Isosorbide dinitrate is contraindicated in patients who are allergic to it or other nitrates.

WARNINGS

The benefits of isosorbide dinitrate in patients with acute myocardial infarction or congestive heart failure have not been established. If one elects to use isosorbide dinitrate in these conditions, careful clinical or hemodynamic monitoring must be used to avoid the hazards of hypotension and tachycardia. Because the effects of oral and chewable ISDN tablets are so difficult to terminate rapidly, this formulation is not recommended in these settings.

PRECAUTIONS

General: Severe hypotension, particularly with upright posture, may occur with even small doses of isosorbide dinitrate. This drug should therefore be used with caution in patients who may be volume depleted or who, for whatever reason (eg, diuretics), are already hypotensive. Hypotension induced by isosorbide dinitrate may be accompanied by paradoxical bradycardia and increased angina pectoris.

Nitrate therapy may aggravate the angina caused by hypertrophic cardiomyopathy.

As tolerance to isosorbide dinitrate develops, the effect of sublingual nitroglycerin on exercise tolerance, allthough still observable, is somewhat blunted.

In industrial workers who have had long-term exposure to unknown (presumably high) doses of organic nitrates, tolerance clearly occurs. Chest pain, acute myocardial infarction, and even sudden death have occurred during temporary withdrawal of nitrates from these workers, demonstrating the existence of true physical dependence.

Some clinical trials in angina patients have provided nitroglycerin for about 12 continuous hours of every 24-hour day. During the daily dose-free intervals in some of these trials, anginal attacks have been more easily provoked than before treatment, and patients have demonstrated hemodynamic rebound and decreased exercise tolerance. The importance of these observations to the routine, clinical use of isosorbide dinitrate is not known. It may be prudent to gradually withdraw patients from ISDN when the therapy is being terminated, rather than stopping the drug abruptly.

Information for Patients: Patients should be told that the anti-anginal efficacy of isosorbide dinitrate is strongly related to its dosing regimen, so the prescribed schedule of dosing should be followed carefully. In particular, daily headaches sometimes accompany treatment with isosorbide dinitrate. In patients who get these headaches, the headaches are a marker of the activity of the drug. Patients should resist the temptation to avoid headaches by altering the schedule of their treatment with isosorbide dinitrate, since loss of headache may be associated with simultaneous loss of anti-anginal efficacy. Aspirin and/or acetaminophen, on the other hand, often successfully relieve isosorbide dinitrate-induced headaches with no deleterious effect on isosorbide dinitrate's anti-anginal efficacy.

Treatment with isosorbide dinitrate may be associated with lightheadedness on standing, especially just after rising from a recumbent or seated position. This effect may be more frequent in patients who have also consumed alcohol.

DRUG INTERACTIONS

The vasodilating effects of isosorbide dinitrate may be additive with those of other vasodilators. Alcohol, in particular, has been found to exhibit additive effects of this variety.

ISDN acts directly on vascular smooth muscle; therefore, any other agent that acts on vascular smooth muscle can be expected to have decreased or increased effect depending on the agents.

Marked symptomatic, orthostatic hypotension has been reported when calcium channel blockers and organic nitrates were used in combination. Dose adjustment of either class of agents may be necessary.

Carcinogenesis, Mutagenesis, and Impairment of Fertility: No long-term studies in animals have been performed to evaluate the carcinogenic potential of isosorbide dinitrate. In a modified two-litter reproduction study, there was no remarkable gross pathology and no altered fertility or gestation among rats fed isosorbide dinitrate at 25 or 100 mg/kg/day.

Pregnancy: Pregnancy Category C: At oral doses 35 and 150 times the maximum recommended human daily dose, isosorbide dinitrate has been shown to cause a dose-related increase in embryotoxicity (increase in mummified pups) in rabbits. There are no adequate, well-controlled studies in pregnant women. Isosorbide dinitrate should be used during pregnancy only if the potential benefit justifies the potential risk to the fetus.

Nursing Mothers: It is not known whether isosorbide dinitrate is excreted is human milk. Because many drugs are excreted in human milk, caution should be exercised when isosorbide dinitrate is administered to a nursing woman.

Pediatric Use: Safety and effectiveness in children have not been established.

ADVERSE REACTIONS

Adverse reactions to isosorbide dinitrate are generally dose-related, and almost all of these reactions are the result of isosorbide dinitrate's activity as a vasodilator. Headache, which may be severe and persistent, is the most commonly reported side effect. Headache may be recurrent with each daily dose, especially at higher doses. Cutaneous vasodilation with flushing may occur. Transient episodes of lightheadedness, dizziness, and weakness, as well as other signs of cerebral ischemia associated with postural hypotension, may also occur. Hypotension occurs infrequently, but in some patients it may be severe enough to warrant discontinuation of therapy. (See OVERDOSAGE.)

Syncope, crescendo angina, and rebound hypertension have been reported but are uncommon.

Extremely rarely, ordinary doses of organic nitrates have caused methemoglobinemia in normal seeming patients. Methemoglobinemia is so infrequent at these doses that further discussion of its diagnosis and treatment is deferred. (See OVERDOSAGE.)

Data are not available to allow estimation of the frequency of adverse reactions during treatment with SORBITRATE tablets.

OVERDOSAGE

Hemodynamic Effects: The ill effects of isosorbide dinitrate overdose are generally the results of isosorbide dinitrate's capacity to induce vasodilatation, venous pooling, reduced cardiac output, and hypotension. These hemodynamic changes may have protean manifestations, including increased intracranial pressure, with any or all of the following: persistent throbbing headache, confusion, and moderate fever; vertigo; palpitations; visual disturbances; nausea and vomiting (possibly with colic and even bloody diarrhea); syncope (especially in the upright posture); initial hyperpnea; air hunger; and dyspnea, later followed by slow breathing and/or reduced ventilatory effort; diaphoresis, with the skin either flushed or cold and clammy; heart block and bradycardia; paralysis; coma; seizures; and death.

Laboratory determinations of serum levels of isosorbide dinitrate and its metabolites are not widely available, and such determinations have, in any event, not established role in the management of isosorbide dinitrate overdose.

There are no data suggesting what dose of isosorbide dinitrate is likely to be life-threatening in humans. In rats, the median acute lethal dose (LD_{50}) was found to be 1100 mg/kg (approximately 500 times the recommended therapeutic dose in humans).

No data are available to suggest physiological maneuvers (eg, maneuvers to change the pH of the urine) that might accelerate elimination of isosorbide dinitrate and its active metabolites. Similarly, it is not known which—if any—of these substances can usefully be removed from the body by hemodialysis.

No specific antagonist to the vasodilator effects of isosorbide dinitrate is known, and no intervention has been subject to controlled study as a therapy of isosorbide dinitrate overdose. Because the hypotension associated with isosorbide dinitrate overdose is the result of venodilatation and arterial hypovolemia, prudent therapy in this situation should be directed toward increase in central fluid volume. Passive elevation of the patient's legs and passive movement of extremities may be sufficient, but intravenous infusion of normal saline or similar fluid may also be necessary.

The use epinephrine or other arterial vasoconstrictors in this setting is likely to do more harm than good.

In patients with renal disease or congestive heart failure, therapy resulting in central volume expansion is not without hazard. Treatment of isosorbide dinitrate overdose in these patients may be subtle and difficult, and invasive monitoring may be required.

Methemoglobinemia: Nitrate ions liberated during metabolism of isosorbide dinitrate can oxidize hemoglobin into methemoglobin. Even in patients totally without cytochrome b_5 reductase activity, however, and even assuming that the nitrate moieties of isosorbide dinitrate are quantitatively applied to oxidation of hemoglobin, about 1 mg/kg of isosorbide dinitrate should be required before any of these patients manifests clinically significant ($\geq 10\%$) methemoglobinemia. In patients with normal reductase function, significant production of methemoglobin should require even larger doses of isosorbide dinitrate. In one study in which 36 patients received 2–4 weeks of continuous nitroglycerin therapy at 3.1 to 4.4 mg/hr (equivalent, in total administered dose of nitrate ions, to 4.8–6.9 mg of bioavailable isosorbide dinitrate per hour), the average methemoglobin level measured was 0.2%; this was comparable to that observed in parallel patients who received placebo.

Notwithstanding these observations, there are case reports of significant methemoglobinemia in association with moderate overdoses of organic nitrates. None of the affected patients had been thought to be unusually susceptible.

Methemoglobin levels are available from most clinical laboratories. The diagnosis should be suspected in patients who exhibit signs of impaired oxygen delivery despite adequate cardiac output and adequate arterial pO_2. Classically, methemoglobinemic blood is described as chocolate brown, without color change on exposure to air.

When methemoglobinemia is diagnosed, the treatment of choice is methylene blue, 1–2 mg/kg intravenously.

DOSAGE AND ADMINISTRATION

As noted above (**CLINICAL PHARMACOLOGY**), multiple studies with ISDN and other nitrates have shown that maintenance of continuous 24-hour plasma levels results in refractory tolerance. Every dosing regimen for ISDN must provide a daily dose-free interval to minimize the develop-

ment of this tolerance. To achieve the necessary nitrate-free interval with immediate-release oral ISDN, it appears that at least one of the daily dose-free intervals must be at least 14 hours long. In the case of sublingual and chewable tablets, it is probably true that one of the daily dose-free intervals must be somewhat longer than 14 hours.

As also noted above (**CLINICAL PHARMACOLOGY**), the effects of the second and later doses have been smaller and shorter-lasting than the effects of the first.

Large controlled studies with other nitrates suggest that no dosing regimen with SORBITRATE Tablets should be expected to provide more than about 12 hours of continuous anti-anginal efficacy per day.

A patient anticipating activity likely to cause angina should take one SORBITRATE Chewable Tablet, 5 mg, about 15 minutes before the activity is expected to begin. SORBITRATE Sublingual Tablet, 2.5 mg to 5 mg, may be used to abort an acute anginal episode, but this use is recommended only in patients who fail to respond to sublingual nitroglycerin.

In clinical trials, immediate-release oral isosorbide dinitrate has been administered in a variety of regimens, with total daily doses ranging from 30 mg to 480 mg.

As with all titratable drugs, it is important to administer the minimum dose that produces the desired effect. The usual starting dose of SORBITRATE Oral Tablets is 5 mg to 20 mg, two or three times daily. For maintenance therapy, 10 mg to 40 mg, two to three times daily is recommended. Some patients may require higher doses. A daily dose-free interval of at least 14 hours is advisable to minimize tolerance. The optimal interval will vary with the individual patient, dose and regimen.

HOW SUPPLIED

SORBITRATE® Sublingual

2.5 mg Sublingual Tablets. (NDC-0310-0853) White, round tablets (identified front "S", reverse "853") are supplied in bottles of 100.

5 mg Sublingual Tablets. (NDC-0310-0760) Pink, round tablets (identified front "S", reverse "760") are supplied in bottles of 100

SORBITRATE® Chewable

5 mg Chewable Tablets. (NDC-0310-0810) Green, round, scored tablets (identified front "S", reverse "810") are supplied in bottles of 100 and 500.

10 mg Chewable Tablets. (NDC-0310-0815) Yellow, round, scored tablets (identified front "S", reverse "815") are supplied in bottles of 100.

SORBITRATE Oral

5 mg Oral Tablets. (NDC-0310-0770) Green, oval-shaped, scored tablets (identified front "S", reverse "770") are supplied in bottles of 100 and 500 and Unit Dose 100.

10 mg Oral Tablets. (NDC-0310-0780) Yellow, oval-shaped, scored tablets (identified front "S", reverse "780") are supplied in bottles of 100, 500 and Unit Dose 100.

20 mg Oral Tablets. (NDC-0310-0820) Blue, oval-shaped, scored tablets (identified front "S", reverse "820") are supplied in bottles of 100 and Unit Dose 100.

30 mg Oral Tablets. (NDC-0310-0773) White, oval-shaped, scored tablets (identified front "S", reverse "773") are supplied in bottles of 100 and Unit Dose 100.

40 mg Oral Tablets. (NDC-0310-0774) Light Blue, oval-shaped, scored tablets (identified front "S", reverse "774") are supplied in bottles of 100 and Unit Dose 100.

Avoid storage at temperatures above 25°C (77°F).

Zeneca Pharmaceuticals
A Business Unit of Zeneca Inc.
Wilmington, DE 19850-5437

Rev N 08/95 SIC No. 64027-07

Shown in Product Identification Guide, page 342

SULAR® ℞

(Nisoldipine)
Extended Release Tablets
For Oral Use

DESCRIPTION

SULAR® (nisoldipine) is an extended release tablet dosage form of the dihydropyridine calcium channel blocker nisoldipine. Nisoldipine is 3,5-pyridinedicarboxylic acid, 1,4-dihydro-2,6-dimethyl-4-(2-nitrophenyl)-, methyl 2-methylpropyl ester, $C_{20}H_{24}N_2O_6$, and has the structural formula:

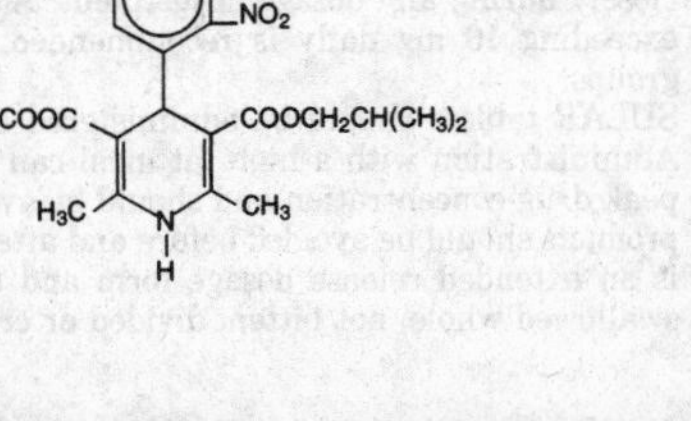

Nisoldipine is a yellow crystalline substance, practically insoluble in water but soluble in ethanol. It has a molecular weight of 388.4. SULAR tablets consist of an external coat and an internal core. Both coat and core contain nisoldipine, the coat as a slow release formulation and the core as a fast release formulation. SULAR tablets contain either 10, 20, 30 or 40 mg of nisoldipine for once-a-day oral administration.

Inert ingredients in the formulation are: hydroxypropylcellulose, lactose, corn starch, crospovidone, microcrystalline cellulose, sodium lauryl sulfate, povidone and magnesium stearate. The inert ingredients in the film coating are: hydroxypropylmethylcellulose, polyethylene glycol, ferric oxide, and titanium dioxide.

CLINICAL PHARMACOLOGY

Mechanism of Action

Nisoldipine is a member of the dihydropyridine class of calcium channel antagonists (calcium ion antagonists or slow channel blockers) that inhibit the transmembrane influx of calcium into vascular smooth muscle and cardiac muscle. It reversibly competes with other dihydropyridines for binding to the calcium channel. Because the contractile process of vascular smooth muscle is dependent upon the movement of extracellular calcium into the muscle through specific ion channels, inhibition of the calcium channel results in dilation of the arterioles. *In vitro* studies show that the effects of nisoldipine on contractile processes are selective, with greater potency on vascular smooth muscle than on cardiac muscle. Although, like other dihydropyridine calcium channel blockers, nisoldipine has negative inotropic effects *in vitro*, studies conducted in intact anesthetized animals have shown that the vasodilating effect occurs at doses lower than those that affect cardiac contractility.

The effect of nisoldipine on blood pressure is principally a consequence of a dose-related decrease of peripheral vascular resistance. While nisoldipine, like other dihydropyridines, exhibits a mild diuretic effect, most of the antihypertensive activity is attributed to its effect on peripheral vascular resistance.

Pharmacokinetics and Metabolism

Nisoldipine pharmacokinetics are independent of the dose in the range of 20 to 60 mg, with plasma concentrations proportional to dose. Nisoldipine accumulation, during multiple dosing, is predictable from a single dose.

Nisoldipine is relatively well absorbed into the systemic circulation with 87% of the radiolabeled drug recovered in urine and feces. The absolute bioavailability of nisoldipine is about 5%. Nisoldipine's low bioavailability is due, in part, to pre-systemic metabolism in the gut wall, and this metabolism decreases from the proximal to the distal parts of the intestine. Food with a high fat content has a pronounced effect on the release of of nisoldipine from the coat-core formulation and results in a significant increase in peak concentration (C_{max}) by up to 300%. Total exposure, however, is decreased about 25%, presumably because more of the drug is released proximally. This effect appears to be specific for nisoldipine in the controlled release formulation, as a less pronounced food effect was seen with the immediate release tablet. Concomitant intake of a high fat meal with SULAR should be avoided.

Maximal plasma concentrations of nisoldipine are reached 6 to 12 hours after dosing. The terminal elimination half-life (reflecting post absorption clearance of nisoldipine) ranges from 7 to 12 hours. C_{max} and AUC increase by factors of approximately 1.3 and 1.5, respectively, from first dose to steady state. After oral administration, the concentration of (+) nisoldipine, the active enantiomer, is about 6 times higher than the (−) inactive enantiomer. The plasma protein binding of nisoldipine is very high, with less than 1% unbound over the plasma concentration range of 100 ng/mL to 10 mcg/mL.

Nisoldipine is highly metabolized; 5 major urinary metabolites have been identified. Although 60–80% of an oral dose undergoes urinary excretion, only traces of unchanged nisoldipine are found in urine. The major biotransformation pathway appears to be the hydroxylation of the isobutyl ester. A hydroxylated derivative of the side chain, present in plasma at concentrations approximately equal to the parent compound, appears to be the only active metabolite, and has about 10% of the activity of the parent compound. Cytochrome P_{450} enzymes are believed to play a major role in the metabolism of nisoldipine. The particular isoenzyme system responsible for its metabolism has not been identified, but other dihydropyridines are metabolized by cytochrome P_{450} IIIA4. Nisoldipine should not be administered with grapefruit juice as this has been shown, in a study of 12 subjects, to interfere with nisoldipine metabolism, resulting in a mean increase in C_{max} of about 3-fold (ranging up to about 7-fold) and AUC of almost 2-fold (ranging up to about 5-fold). A similar phenomenon has been seen with several other dihydropyridine calcium channel blockers.

Special Populations

Renal dysfunction: Because renal elimination is not an important pathway, bioavailability and pharmacokinetics of SULAR were not significantly different in patients with various degrees of renal impairment. Dosing adjustments in patients with mild to moderate renal impairment are not necessary.

Geriatric: Elderly patients have been found to have 2 to 3 fold higher plasma concentrations (C_{max} and AUC) than young subjects. This should be reflected in more cautious dosing (See DOSAGE AND ADMINISTRATION).

Hepatic Insufficiency: In patients with liver cirrhosis given 10 mg SULAR, plasma concentrations of the parent compound were 4 to 5 times higher than those in healthy young subjects. Lower starting and maintenance doses should be used in cirrhotic patients (See DOSAGE AND ADMINISTRATION).

Gender and Race: The effect of gender or race on the pharmacokinetics of nisoldipine has not been investigated.

Disease States: Hypertension does not significantly alter the pharmacokinetics of nisoldipine.

Pharmacodynamics

Hemodynamic Effects

Administration of a single dose of nisoldipine leads to decreased systemic vascular resistance and blood pressure with a transient increase in heart rate. The change in heart rate is greater with immediate release nisoldipine preparations. The effect on blood pressure is directly related to the initial degree of elevation above normal. Chronic administration of nisoldipine results in a sustained decrease in vascular resistance and small increases in stroke index and left ventricular ejection fraction. A study of the immediate release formulation showed no effect of nisoldipine on the renin-angiotensin-aldosterone system or on plasma norepinephrine concentration in normals. Changes in blood pressure in hypertensive patients given SULAR were dose related over the range of 10–60 mg/day.

Nisoldipine does not appear to have significant negative inotropic activity in intact animals or humans, and did not lead to worsening of clinical heart failure in three small studies of patients with asymptomatic and symptomatic left ventricular dysfunction. There is little information, however, in patients with severe congestive heart failure, and all calcium channel blockers should be used with caution in any patient with heart failure.

Electropyhysiologic Effects

Nisoldipine has no clinically important chronotropic effects. Except for mild shortening of sinus cycle, SA conduction time and AH intervals, single oral doses up to 20 mg of immediate release nisoldipine did not significantly change other conduction parameters. Similar electrophysiologic effects were seen with single iv doses, which could be blunted in patients pre-treated with beta-blockers. Dose and plasma level related flattening or inversion of T-waves have been observed in a few small studies. Such reports were concentrated in patients receiving rapidly increased high doses in one study; the phenomenon has not been a cause of safety concern in large clinical trials.

Clinical Studies In Hypertension

The antihypertensive efficacy of SULAR was studied in 5 double-blind, placebo-controlled, randomized studies, in which over 600 patients were treated with SULAR as monotherapy and about 300 with placebo; 4 of the five studies compared 2 or 3 fixed doses while the fifth allowed titration from 10–40 mg. Once daily administration of SULAR produced sustained reductions in systolic and diastolic blood pressures over the 24 hour dosing interval in both supine and standing positions. The mean placebo-subtracted reductions in supine systolic and diastolic blood pressure at trough, 24 hours post-dose, in these studies, are shown below. Changes in standing blood pressure were similar:

MEAN SUPINE TROUGH SYSTOLIC AND DIASTOLIC BLOOD PRESSURE CHANGES (mm Hg)

SULAR Dose (mg/day)	10 mg	20 mg	30 mg	40 mg	60 mg	10–40 mg titrated
Systolic	8	11	11	14	15	15
Diastolic	3	5	7	7	10	8

In patients receiving atenolol, supine blood pressure reductions with SULAR at 20, 40 and 60 mg once daily were 12/6, 19/8 and 22/10 mm Hg, respectively. The sustained antihypertensive effect of SULAR was demonstrated by 24 hour blood pressure monitoring and examination of peak and trough effects. The trough/peak ratios ranged from 70 to 100% for diastolic and systolic blood pressure. The mean change in heart rate in these studies was less than one beat per minute. In 4 of the 5 studies, patients received initial doses of 20–30 mg SULAR without incident (excessive effects on blood pressure or heart rate). The fifth study started patients on lower doses of SULAR.

Patient race and gender did not influence the blood pressure lowering effect of SULAR. Despite the higher plasma concentration of nisoldipine in the elderly, there was no consis-

Continued on next page

Zeneca Pharmaceuticals—Cont.

tent difference in their blood pressure response except that the 10 mg dose was somewhat more effective than in nonelderly patients. No postural effect on blood pressure was apparent and there was no evidence of tolerance to the antihypertensive effect of SULAR in patients treated for up to one year.

INDICATIONS AND USAGE

SULAR is indicated for the treatment of hypertension. It may be used alone or in combination with other antihypertensive agents.

CONTRAINDICATIONS

SULAR is contraindicated in patients with known hypersensitivity to dihydropyridine calcium channel blockers.

WARNINGS

Increased angina and/or myocardial infarction in patients with coronary artery disease: Rarely, patients, particularly those with severe obstructive coronary artery disease, have developed increased frequency, duration and/or severity of angina, or acute myocardial infarction on starting calcium channel blocker therapy or at the time of dosage increase. The mechanism of this effect has not been established. In controlled studies of SULAR in patients with angina this was seen about 1.5% of the time in patients given nisoldipine, compared with 0.9% in patients given placebo.

PRECAUTIONS

General

Hypotension: Because nisoldipine, like other vasodilators, decreases peripheral vascular resistance, careful monitoring of blood pressure during the initial administration and titration of SULAR is recommended. Close observation is especially important for patients already taking medications that are known to lower blood pressure. Although in most patients the hypotensive effect of SULAR is modest and well tolerated, occasional patients have had excessive and poorly tolerated hypotension. These responses have usually occurred during initial titration or at the time of subsequent upward dosage adjustment.

Congestive Heart Failure: Although acute hemodynamic studies of nisoldipine in patients with NYHA Class II–IV heart failure have not demonstrated negative inotropic effects, safety of SULAR in patients with heart failure has not been established. Caution therefore should be exercised when using SULAR in patients with heart failure or compromised ventricular function, particularly in combination with a beta-blocker.

Patients with Hepatic Impairment: Because nisoldipine is extensively metabolized by the liver and, in patients with cirrhosis, it reaches blood concentrations about 5 times those in normals, SULAR should be administered cautiously in patients with severe hepatic dysfunction (See DOSAGE AND ADMINISTRATION).

Information for Patients: SULAR is an extended release tablet and should be swallowed whole. Tablets should not be chewed, divided or crushed. SULAR should not be administered with a high fat meal. Grapefruit juice, which has been shown to increase significantly the bioavailability of nisoldipine and other dihydropyridine type calcium channel blockers, should not be taken with SULAR.

Laboratory Tests: SULAR is not known to interfere with the interpretation of laboratory tests.

Drug Interactions: A 30 to 45% increase in AUC and C_{max} of nisoldipine was observed with concomitant administration of cimetidine 400 mg twice daily. Ranitidine 150 mg twice daily did not interact significantly with nisoldipine (AUC was decreased by 15–20%). No pharmacodynamic effects of either histamine H_2 receptor antagonist were observed.

Pharmacokinetic interactions between nisoldipine and beta-blockers (atenolol, propranolol) were variable and not significant. Propranolol attenuated the heart rate increase following administration of immediate release nisoldipine. The blood pressure effect of SULAR tended to be greater in patients on atenolol than in patients on no other anithypertensive therapy.

Quinidine at 648 mg bid decreased the bioavailability (AUC) of nisoldipine by 26%, but not the peak concentration. The immediate release, but not the coat-core formulation of nisoldipine increased plasma quinidine concentrations by about 20%. This interaction was not accompanied by ECG changes and its clinical significance is not known.

No significant interactions were found between nisoldipine and warfarin or digoxin.

Carcinogenesis, Mutagenesis, Impairment of Fertility: Dietary administration of nisoldipine to male and female rats for up to 24 months (mean doses up to 82 and 111 mg/kg/day, 16 and 19 times the maximum recommended human dose {MRHD} on a mg/m^2 basis, respectively) and female mice for up to 21 months (mean doses of up to 217 mg/kg/day, 20 times the MRHD on a mg/m^2 basis) revealed no evidence of tumorigenic effect of nisoldipine. In male mice receiving a mean dose of 163 mg nisolipine/kg/day (16 times the MRHD of 60 mg/day on a mg/m^2 basis), an increased frequency of stomach papilloma, but still within the historical range, was observed. No evidence of stomach neoplasia was observed at lower doses (up to 58 mg/kg/day). Nisoldipine was negative when tested in a battery of genotoxicity assays including the Ames test and the CHO/HGRPT assay for mutagenicity and the *in vivo* mouse micronucleus test and *in vitro* CHO cell test for clastogenicity.

When administered to male and female rats at doses of up to 30 mg/kg/day (about 5 times the MRHD on a mg/m^2 basis) nisoldipine had no effect on fertility.

Pregnancy Category C: Nisoldipine was neither teratogenic nor fetotoxic at doses that were not maternally toxic. Nisoldipine was fetotoxic but not teratogenic in rats and rabbits at doses resulting in maternal toxicity (reduced maternal body weight gain). In pregnant rats, increased fetal resporption (post-implantation loss) was observed at 100 mg/kg/day and decreased fetal weight was observed at both 30 and 100 mg/kg/day. These doses are, respectively, about 5 and 16 times the MRHD when compared on a mg/m^2 basis. In pregnant rabbits, decreased fetal and placental weights were observed at a dose of 30 mg/kg/day, about 10 times the MRHD when compared on a mg/m^2 basis. In a study in which pregnant monkeys (both treated and control) had high rates of abortion and mortality, the only surviving fetus from a group exposed to a maternal dose of 100 mg nisoldipine/kg/day (about 30 times the MRHD when compared on a mg/m^2 basis) presented with forelimb and vertebral abnormalities not previously seen in control monkeys of the same strain. There are no adequate and well controlled studies in pregnant women. SULAR should be used in pregnancy only if the potential benefit justifies the potential risk to the fetus.

Nursing Mothers: It is not known whether nisoldipine is excreted in human milk. Because many drugs are excreted in human milk, a decision should be made to discontinue nursing, or to discontinue SULAR, taking into account the importance of the drug to the mother.

ADVERSE EXPERIENCES

More than 6000 patients world-wide have received nisoldipine in clinical trials for the treatment of hypertension, either as the immediate release or the SULAR extended release formulation. Of about 1,500 patients who received SULAR in hypertension studies, about 55% were exposed for at least 2 months and about one third were exposed for over 6 months, the great majority at doses of 20 to 60 mg daily.

SULAR is generally well-tolerated. In the U.S. clinical trials of SULAR in hypertension, 10.9% of the 921 SULAR patients discontinued treatment due to adverse events compared with 2.9% of 280 placebo patients. The frequency of discontinuations due to adverse experiences was related to dose, with a 5.4% discontinuation rate at 10 mg daily and a 10.9% discontinuation rate at 60 mg daily.

The most frequently occurring adverse experiences with SULAR are those related to its vasodilator properties; these are generally mild and only occasionally lead to patient withdrawal from treatment. The table below, from U.S. placebo-controlled parallel dose response trials of SULAR using doses from 10–60 mg once daily in patients with hypertension, lists all of the adverse events, regardless of the causal relationship to SULAR, for which the overall incidence on SULAR was both >1% and greater with SULAR than with placebo.

Adverse Event	Nisoldipine (%) (n=663)	Placebo (%) (n=280)
Peripheral Edema	22	10
Headache	22	15
Dizziness	5	4
Pharyngitis	5	4
Vasodilation	4	2
Sinusitis	3	2
Palpitation	3	1
Chest Pain	2	1
Nausea	2	1
Rash	2	1

Only peripheral edema and possibly dizziness appear to be dose related.

Adverse Event		SULAR				
	Placebo	10 mg	20 mg	30 mg	40 mg	60 mg
(Rates in %)	N=280	N=30	N=170	N=105	N=139	N=137
Peripheral Edema	10	7	15	20	27	29
Dizziness	4	7	3	3	4	10

The common adverse events occurred at about the same rate in men as in women, and at a similar rate in patients over age 65 as in those under that age, except that headache was much less common in older patients. Except for peripheral edema and vasodilation, which were more common in whites, adverse event rates were similar in blacks and whites.

The following adverse events occurred in ≤1% of all patients treated for hypertension in U.S. and foreign clinical trials, or with unspecified incidence in other studies. Although a causal relationship of SULAR to these events cannot be established, they are listed to alert the physician to a possible relationship with SULAR treatment.

Body As A Whole: cellulitis, chills, facial edema, fever, flu syndrome, malaise

Cardiovascular: atrial fibrillation, cerebrovascular accident, congestive heart failure, first degree AV block, hypertension, hypotension, jugular venous distension, migraine, myocardial infarction, postural hypotension, ventricular extrasystoles, supraventricular tachycardia, syncope, systolic ejection murmur, T wave abnormalities on ECG (flattening, inversion, nonspecific changes), venous insufficiency

Digestive: abnormal liver function tests, anorexia, colitis, diarrhea, dry mouth, dyspepsia, dysphagia, flatulence, gastritis, gastrointestinal hemorrhage, gingival hyperplasia, glossitis, hepatomegaly, increased appetite, melena, mouth ulceration

Endocrine: diabetes mellitus, thyroiditis

Hemic and Lymphatic: anemia, ecchymoses, leukopenia, petechiae

Metabolic and Nutritional: gout, hypokalemia, increased serum creatine kinase, increased nonprotein nitrogen, weight gain, weight loss

Musculoskeletal: arthralgia, arthritis, leg cramps, myalgia, myasthenia, myositis, tenosynovitis

Nervous: abnormal dreams, abnormal thinking and confusion, amnesia, anxiety, ataxia, cerebral ischemia, decreased libido, depression, hypesthesia, hypertonia, insomnia, nervousness, paresthesia, somnolence, tremor, vertigo

Respiratory: asthma, dyspnea, end inspiratory wheeze and fine rales, epistaxis, increased cough, laryngitis, pharyngitis, pleural effusion, rhinitis, sinusitis

Skin and Appendages: acne, alopecia, dry skin, exfoliative dermatitis, fungal dermatitis, herpes simplex, herpes zoster, maculopapular rash, pruritus, pustular rash, skin discoloration, skin ulcer, sweating, urticaria

Special senses: abnormal vision, amblyopia, blepharitis, conjunctivitis, ear pain, glaucoma, itchy eyes, keratoconjunctivitis, otitis media, retinal detachment, tinnitus, watery eyes, taste disturbance, temporary unilateral loss of vision, vitreous floater, watery eyes

Urogenital: dysuria, hematuria, impotence, nocturia, urinary frequency, increased BUN and serum creatinine, vaginal hemorrhage, vaginitis.

In addition to experience with SULAR, there is extensive experience with the immediate release formulation of nisoldipine. Adverse events were generally similar to those seen with SULAR. Unusual events observed with immediate release nisoldipine but not observed with SULAR, were one case each of angioedema and photosensitivity. Spontaneous reports from postmarketing experience with the immediate release formulation of nisoldipine have not revealed any additional adverse events not identified in the above listings.

OVERDOSAGE

There is no experience with nisoldipine overdosage. Generally, overdosage with other dihydropyridines leading to pronounced hypotension calls for active cardiovascular support including monitoring of cardiovascular and respiratory function, elevation of extremities, judicious use of calcium infusion, pressor agents and fluids. Clearance of nisoldipine would be expected to be slowed in patients with impaired liver function. Since nisoldipine is highly protein bound, dialysis is not likely to be of any benefit; however, plasmapheresis may be beneficial.

DOSAGE AND ADMINISTRATION

The dosage of SULAR must be adjusted to each patient's needs. Therapy usually should be initiated with 20 mg orally once daily, then increased by 10 mg per week or longer intervals, to attain adequate control of blood pressure. Usual maintenance dosage is 20 to 40 mg once daily. Blood pressure response increases over the 10–60 mg daily dose range but adverse event rates also increase. Doses beyond 60 mg once daily are not recommended. SULAR has been used safely with diuretics, ACE inhibitors, and beta-blocking agents.

Patients over age 65, or patients with impaired liver function are expected to develop higher plasma concentrations of nisoldipine. Their blood pressure should be monitored closely during any dosage adjustment. A starting dose not exceeding 10 mg daily is recommended in these patient groups.

SULAR tablets should be administered orally once daily. Administration with a high fat meal can lead to excessive peak drug concentration and should be avoided. Grapefruit products should be avoided before and after dosing. SULAR is an extended release dosage form and tablets should be swallowed whole, not bitten, divided or crushed.

HOW SUPPLIED

SULAR extended release tablets are supplied at 10 mg, 20 mg, 30 mg, and 40 mg round film coated tablets. The different strengths can be identified as follows:

Strength	Color	Markings
10 mg	Oyster	891 on one side and ZENECA 10 on the other side.
20 mg	Yellow Cream	892 on one side and ZENECA 20 on the other side.
30 mg	Mustard	893 on one side and ZENECA 30 on the other side.
40 mg	Burnt Orange	894 on one side and ZENECA 40 on the other side.

SULAR Tablets are supplied in:

	Strength	NDC Code
Bottles of 100	10 mg	0310-0891-10
	20 mg	0310-0892-10
	30 mg	0310-0893-10
	40 mg	0310-0894-10
Unit Dose Packages of 100	10 mg	0310-0891-39
	20 mg	0310-0892-39
	30 mg	0310-0893-39

The tablets should be protected from light and moisture and stored below 86°F (30°C). Dispense in tight, light-resistant containers.

Manufactured AG for
ZENECA Pharmaceuticals
A Business Unit of Zeneca Inc.
Wilmington, Delaware 19850-5437
By Bayer AG
Made in Germany
64088-01 Rev D 02/96

Shown in Product Identification Guide, page 342

TENORETIC® (atenolol and chlorthalidone) ℞

[ten"o-ret'ic]

DESCRIPTION

TENORETIC® (atenolol and chlorthalidone) is for the treatment of hypertension. It combines the antihypertensive activity of two agents: a $beta_1$-selective (cardioselective) hydrophilic blocking agent (atenolol, TENORMIN®) and a monosulfonamyl diuretic (chlorthalidone). Atenolol is Benzeneacetamide, 4-[2'-hydroxy-3'-[(1-methylethyl) amino] propoxy].-.

$C_{14}H_{22}N_2O_3$

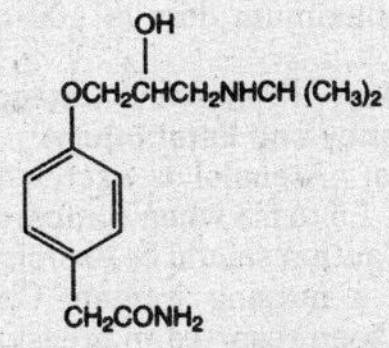
OH
OCH2CHCH2NHCH (CH3)2
CH2CONH2

Atenolol (free base) is a relatively polar hydrophilic compound with a water solubility of 26.5 mg/mL at 37°C. It is freely soluble in 1N HCl (300 mg/mL at 25°C) and less soluble in chloroform (3 mg/mL at 25°C).

Chlorthalidone is 2-Chloro-5-(1-hydroxy-3-oxo-1-isoindolinyl) benzene sulfonamide:

$C_{14}H_{11}ClN_2O_4S$

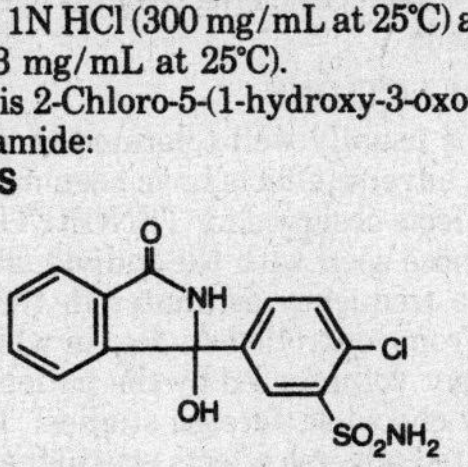
O
NH
Cl
OH
SO2NH2

Chlorthalidone has a water solubility of 12 mg/100 mL at 20°C.

Each TENORETIC 100 Tablet contains:
Atenolol (TENORMIN®) .... 100 mg
Chlorthalidone .... 25 mg

Each TENORETIC 50 Tablet contains:
Atenolol (TENORMIN®) .... 50 mg
Chlorthalidone .... 25 mg

Inactive ingredients: magnesium stearate, microcrystalline cellulose, povidone, sodium starch glycolate.

CLINICAL PHARMACOLOGY

TENORETIC

Atenolol and chlorthalidone have been used singly and concomitantly for the treatment of hypertension. The antihypertensive effects of these agents are additive, and studies have shown that there is no interference with bioavailability when these agents are given together in the single combination tablet. Therefore, this combination provides a convenient formulation for the concomitant administration of these two entities. In patients with more severe hypertension, TENORETIC may be administered with other antihypertensives such as vasodilators.

Atenolol

Atenolol is a $beta_1$-selective (cardioselective) beta-adrenergic receptor blocking agent without membrane stabilizing or intrinsic sympathomimetic (partial agonist) activities. This preferential effect is not absolute, however, and at higher doses, atenolol inhibits $beta_2$-adrenoreceptors, chiefly located in the bronchial and vascular musculature.

Pharmacodynamics: In standard animal or human pharmacological tests, beta-adrenoreceptor blocking activity of atenolol has been demonstrated by: (1) reduction in resting and exercise heart rates and cardiac output, (2) reduction of systolic and diastolic blood pressure at rest and on exercise, (3) inhibition of isoproterenol induced tachycardia and (4) reduction in reflex orthostatic tachycardia.

A significant beta-blocking effect of atenolol, as measured by reduction of exercise tachycardia, is apparent within one hour following oral administration of a single dose. This effect is maximal at about 2 to 4 hours and persists for at least 24 hours. The effect at 24 hours is dose related and also bears a linear relationship to the logarithm of plasma atenolol concentration. However, as has been shown for all beta-blocking agents, the antihypertensive effect does not appear to be related to plasma level.

In normal subjects, the $beta_1$-selectivity of atenolol has been shown by its reduced ability to reverse the $beta_2$-mediated vasodilating effect of isoproterenol as compared to equivalent beta-blocking doses of propranolol. In asthmatic patients, a dose of atenolol producing a greater effect on resting heart rate than propranolol resulted in much less increase in airway resistance. In a placebo controlled comparison of approximately equipotent oral doses of several beta blockers, atenolol produced a significantly smaller decrease of FEV_1 than nonselective beta blockers, such as propranolol and unlike those agents did not inhibit bronchodilation in response to isoproterenol.

Consistent with its negative chronotropic effect due to beta blockade of the SA node, atenolol increases sinus cycle length and sinus node recovery time. Conduction in the AV node is also prolonged. Atenolol is devoid of membrane stabilizing activity, and increasing the dose well beyond that producing beta blockade does not further depress myocardial contractility. Several studies have demonstrated a moderate (approximately 10%) increase in stroke volume at rest and exercise.

In controlled clinical trials, atenolol given as a single daily dose, was an effective antihypertensive agent providing 24-hour reduction of blood pressure. Atenolol has been studied in combination with thiazide-type diuretics and the blood pressure effects of the combination are approximately additive. Atenolol is also compatible with methyldopa, hydralazine and prazosin, the combination resulting in a larger fall in blood pressure than with the single agents. The dose range of atenolol is narrow, and increasing the dose beyond 100 mg once daily is not associated with increased antihypertensive effect. The mechanisms of the antihypertensive effects of beta-blocking agents have not been established. Several mechanisms have been proposed and include: (1) competitive antagonism of catecholamines at peripheral (especially cardiac) adrenergic neuron sites, leading to decreased cardiac output, (2) a central effect leading to reduced sympathetic outflow to the periphery and (3) suppression of renin activity. The results from long-term studies have not shown any diminution of the antihypertensive efficacy of atenolol with prolonged use.

Pharmacokinetics and Metabolism: In man, absorption of an oral dose is rapid and consistent but incomplete. Approximately 50% of an oral dose is absorbed from the gastrointestinal tract, the remainder being excreted unchanged in the feces. Peak blood levels are reached between 2 and 4 hours after ingestion. Unlike propranolol or metoprolol, but like nadolol, hydrophilic atenolol undergoes little or no metabolism by the liver, and the absorbed portion is eliminated primarily by renal excretion. Atenolol also differs from propranolol in that only a small amount (6–16%) is bound to proteins in the plasma. This kinetic profile results in relatively consistent plasma drug levels with about a fourfold interpatient variation. There is no information as to the pharmacokinetic effect of atenolol on chlorthalidone.

The elimination half-life of atenolol is approximately 6 to 7 hours and there is no alteration of the kinetic profile of the drug by chronic administration. Following doses of 50 mg or 100 mg, both beta-blocking and antihypertensive effects persist for at least 24 hours. When renal function is impaired, elimination of atenolol is closely related to the glomerular filtration rate; but significant accumulation does not occur until the creatinine clearance falls below 35 mL/min/1.73m^2 (see circular for atenolol [TENORMIN®]).

Chlorthalidone

Chlorthalidone is a monosulfonamyl diuretic which differs chemically from thiazide diuretics in that a double ring system is incorporated in its structure. It is an oral diuretic with prolonged action and low toxicity. The diuretic effect of the drug occurs within 2 hours of an oral dose. It produces diuresis with greatly increased secretion of sodium and chloride.

At maximal therapeutic dosage, chlorthalidone is approximately equal in its diuretic effect to comparable maximal therapeutic doses of benzothiadiazine diuretics. The site of action appears to be the cortical diluting segment of the ascending limb of Henle's loop of the nephron.

INDICATIONS AND USAGE

TENORETIC is indicated in the treatment of hypertension. This fixed dose combination drug is not indicated for initial therapy of hypertension. If the fixed dose combination represents the dose appropriate to the individual patient's needs, it may be more convenient than the separate components.

CONTRAINDICATIONS

TENORETIC is contraindicated in patients with: sinus bradycardia; heart block greater than first degree; cardiogenic shock; overt cardiac failure (see WARNINGS); anuria; hypersensitivity to this product or to sulfonamide-derived drugs.

WARNINGS

Cardiac Failure: Sympathetic stimulation is necessary in supporting circulatory function in congestive heart failure, and beta blockade carries the potential hazard of further depressing myocardial contractility and precipitating more severe failure. In patients who have congestive heart failure controlled by digitalis and/or diuretics, TENORETIC should be administered cautiously. Both digitalis and atenolol slow AV conduction.

IN PATIENTS WITHOUT A HISTORY OF CARDIAC FAILURE, continued depression of the myocardium with beta-blocking agents over a period of time can, in some cases, lead to cardiac failure. At the first sign or symptom of impending cardiac failure, patients receiving TENORETIC should be digitalized and/or be given additional diuretic therapy. Observe the patient closely. If cardiac failure continues despite adequate digitalization and diuretic therapy, TENORETIC therapy should be withdrawn.

Renal and Hepatic Disease and Electrolyte Disturbances: Since atenolol is excreted via the kidneys, TENORETIC should be used with caution in patients with impaired renal function.

In patients with renal disease, thiazides may precipitate azotemia. Since cumultive effects may develop in the presence of impaired renal function, if progressive renal impairment becomes evident, TENORETIC should be discontinued.

In patients with impaired hepatic function or progressive liver disease, minor alterations in fluid and electrolyte balance may precipitate hepatic coma. TENORETIC should be used with caution in these patients.

Ischemic Heart Disease: Following abrupt cessation of therapy with certain beta-blocking agents in patients with coronary artery disease, exacerbations of angina pectoris and, in some cases, myocardial infarction have been reported. Therefore, such patients should be cautioned against interruption of therapy without the physician's advice. Even in the absence of overt angina pectoris, when discontinuation of TENORETIC is planned, the patient should be carefully observed and should be advised to limit physical activity to a minimum. TENORETIC should be reinstated if withdrawal symptoms occur. Because coronary artery disease is common and may be unrecognized, it may be prudent not to discontinue TENORETIC therapy abruptly even in patients treated only for hypertension.

Concomitant Use of Calcium Channel Blockers: Bradycardia and heart block can occur and the left ventricular end diastolic pressure can rise when beta blockers are administered with verapamil or diltiazem. Patients with pre-existing conduction abnormalities or left ventricular dysfunction are particularly susceptible (see PRECAUTIONS).

Bronchospastic Diseases: PATIENTS WITH BRONCHOSPASTIC DISEASE SHOULD, IN GENERAL, NOT RECEIVE BETA BLOCKERS. Because of its relative $beta_1$-selectivity, however, TENORETIC may be used with caution in patients with bronchospastic disease who do not respond to or cannot tolerate, other antihypertensive treatment. Since $beta_1$-selectivity is not absolute, the lowest possible dose of TENORETIC should be used and a $beta_2$-stimulating agent (bronchodilator) should be made available. If dosage must be increased, dividing the dose should be considered in order to achieve lower peak blood levels.

Anesthesia and Major Surgery: It is not advisable to withdraw beta-adrenoreceptor blocking drugs prior to surgery in the majority of patients. However, care should be taken when using anesthetic agents such as those which may depress the myocardium. Vagal dominance, if it occurs, may be corrected with atropine (1–2 mg IV).

Beta blockers are competitive inhibitors of beta-receptor agonists and their effects on the heart can be reversed by administration of such agents; eg, dobutamine or isoproterenol with caution (see section on Overdosage).

Metabolic and Endocrine Effects: TENORETIC may be used with caution in diabetic patients. Beta blockers may

Continued on next page

Zeneca Pharmaceuticals—Cont.

mask tachycardia occurring with hypoglycemia, but other manifestations such as dizziness and sweating may not be significantly affected. At recommended doses atenolol does not potentiate insulin-induced hypoglycemia and, unlike nonselective beta blockers, does not delay recovery of blood glucose to normal levels.

Insulin requirements in diabetic patients may be increased, decreased or unchanged; latent diabetes mellitus may become manifest during chlorthalidone administration.

Beta-adrenergic blockade may mask certain clinical signs (eg, tachycardia) of hyperthyroidism. Abrupt withdrawal of beta blockade might precipitate a thyroid storm; therefore, patients suspected of developing thyrotoxicosis from whom TENORETIC therapy is to be withdrawn should be monitored closely.

Because calcium excretion is decreased by thiazides, TENORETIC should be discontinued before carrying out tests for parathyroid function. Pathologic changes in the parathyroid glands, with hypercalcemia and hypophosphatemia, have been observed in a few patients on prolonged thiazide therapy; however, the common complications of hyperparathyroidism such as renal lithiasis, bone resorption, and peptic ulceration have not been seen.

Hyperuricemia may occur, or acute gout may be precipitated in certain patients receiving thiazide therapy.

Pregnancy and Fetal Injury: Atenolol can cause fetal harm when administered to a pregnant woman. Atenolol crosses the placental barrier and appears in cord blood. Administration of atenolol, starting in the second trimester of pregnancy, has been associated with the birth of infants that are small for gestational age. No studies have been performed on the use of atenolol in the first trimester and the possibility of fetal injury cannot be excluded. If this drug is used during pregnancy, or if the patient becomes pregnant while taking this drug, the patient should be apprised of the potential hazard to the fetus.

TENORETIC was studied for teratogenic potential in the rat and rabbit. Doses of atenolol/chlorthalidone of 8/2, 80/20, and 240/60 mg/kg/day were administered orally to pregnant rats with no evidence of embryofetotoxicity observed. Two studies were conducted in rabbits. In the first study, pregnant rabbits were dosed with 8/2, 80/20, and 160/40 mg/kg/day of atenolol/chlorthalidone. No teratogenic effects were noted, but embryonic resorptions were observed at all dose levels (ranging from approximately 5 times to 100 times the maximum recommended human dose*). In the second rabbit study, doses of atenolol/chlorthalidone were 4/1, 8/2, and 20/5 mg/kg/day. No teratogenic or embryotoxic effects were demonstrated.

Atenolol—Atenolol has been shown to produce a dose-related increase in embryo/fetal resorptions in rats at doses equal to or greater than 50 mg/kg/day or 25 or more times the maximum recommended human antihypertensive dose.* Although similar effects were not seen in rabbits, the compound was not evaluated in rabbits at doses above 25 mg/kg/day or 12.5 times the maximum recommended human antihypertensive dose.*

*Based on the maximum dose of 100 mg/day in a 50 kg patient.

Chlorthalidone—Thiazides cross the placental barrier and appear in cord blood. The use of chlorthalidone and related drugs in pregnant women requires that the anticipated benefits of the drug be weighed against possible hazards to the fetus. These hazards include fetal or neonatal jaundice, thrombocytopenia and possibly other adverse reactions which have occurred in the adult.

PRECAUTIONS

General: TENORETIC may aggravate peripheral arterial circulatory disorders.

Electrolyte and Fluid Balance Status: Periodic determination of serum electrolytes to detect possible electrolyte imbalance should be performed at appropriate intervals.

Patients should be observed for clinical signs of fluid or electrolyte imbalance; ie, hyponatremia, hypochloremic alkalosis, and hypokalemia. Serum and urine electrolyte determinations are particularly important when the patient is vomiting excessively or receiving parenteral fluids. Warning signs or symptoms of fluid and electrolyte imbalance include dryness of the mouth, thirst, weakness, lethargy, drowsiness, restlessness, muscle pains or cramps, muscular fatigue, hypotension, oliguria, tachycardia, and gastrointestinal disturbances such as nausea and vomiting.

Measurement of potassium levels is appropriate especially in elderly patients, those receiving digitalis preparations for cardiac failure, patients whose dietary intake of potassium is abnormally low, or those suffering from gastrointestinal complaints.

Hypokalemia may develop especially with brisk diuresis, when severe cirrhosis is present, or during concomitant use of corticosteroids or ACTH.

Interference with adequate oral electrolyte intake will also contribute to hypokalemia. Hypokalemia can sensitize or exaggerate the response of the heart to the toxic effects of digitalis (eg, increased ventricular irritability). Hypokalemia may be avoided or treated by use of potassium supplements or foods with a high potassium content.

Any chloride deficit during thiazide therapy is generally mild and usually does not require specific treatment except under extraordinary circumstances (as in liver disease or renal disease). Dilutional hyponatremia may occur in edematous patients in hot weather; appropriate therapy is water restriction rather than administration of salt except in rare instances when the hyponatremia is life-threatening. In actual salt depletion, appropriate replacement is the therapy of choice.

Drug Interactions: TENORETIC may potentiate the action of other antihypertensive agents used concomitantly. Patients treated with TENORETIC plus a catecholamine depletor (eg, reserpine) should be closely observed for evidence of hypotension and/or marked bradycardia which may produce vertigo, syncope or postural hypotension.

Calcium channel blockers may also have an additive effect when given with TENORETIC. (See WARNINGS.)

Thiazides may decrease arterial responsiveness to norepinephrine. This diminution is not sufficient to preclude the therapeutic effectiveness of norepinephrine. Thiazides may increase the responsiveness to tubocurarine.

Lithium generally should not be given with diuretics because they reduce its renal clearance and add a high risk of lithium toxicity. Read circulars for lithium preparations before use of such preparations with TENORETIC.

Beta blockers may exacerbate the rebound hypertension which can follow the withdrawal of cloridine. If the two drugs are coadministered, the beta blocker should be withdrawn several days before the gradual withdrawal of clonidine. If replacing clonidine by beta-blocker therapy, the introduction of beta blockers should be delayed for several days after clonidine administration has stopped.

While taking beta blockers, patients with a history of anaphylactic reaction to a variety of allergens may have a more severe reaction on repeated challenge, either accidental, diagnostic or therapeutic. Such patients may be unresponsive to the usual doses of epinephrine used to treat the allergic reaction.

Other Precautions: In patients receiving thiazides, sensitivity reactions may occur with or without a history of allergy or bronchial asthma. The possible exacerbation or activation of systemic lupus erythematosus has been reported. The antihypertensive effects of thiazides may be enhanced in the postsympathectomy patient.

Carcinogenesis, Mutagenesis, Impairment of Fertility: Two long-term (maximum dosing duration of 18 or 24 months) rat studies and one long-term (maximum dosing duration of 18 months) mouse study, each employing dose levels as high as 300 mg/kg/day or 150 times the maximum recommended human antihypertensive dose,* did not indicate a carcinogenic potential of atenolol. A third (24 month) rat study, employing doses of 500 and 1,500 mg/kg/day (250 and 750 times the maximum recommended human antihypertensive dose*) resulted in increased incidences of benign adrenal medullary tumors in males and females, mammary fibroadenomas in females, and anterior pituitary adenomas and thyroid parafollicular cell carcinomas in males. No evidence of a mutagenic potential of atenolol was uncovered in the dominant lethal test (mouse), in vivo cytogenetics test (Chinese hamster) or Ames test (*S typhimurium*).

Fertility of male or female rats (evaluated at dose levels as high as 200 mg/kg/day or 100 times the maximum recommended human dose*) was unaffected by atenolol administration.

Animal Toxicology: Six month oral administration studies were conducted in rats and dogs using TENORETIC doses up to 12.5 mg/kg/day (atenolol/chlorthalidone 10/2.5 mg/kg/day—approximately five times the maximum recommended human antihypertensive dose*). There were no functional or morphological abnormalities resulting from dosing either compound alone or together other than minor changes in heart rate, blood pressure and urine chemistry which were attributed to the known pharmacologic properties of atenolol and/or chlorthalidone.

Chronic studies of atenolol performed in animals have revealed the occurrence of vacuolation of epithelial cells of Brunner's glands in the duodenum of both male and female dogs at all tested dose levels (starting at 15 mg/kg/day or 7.5 times the maximum recommended human antihypertensive dose*) and increased incidence of atrial degeneration of hearts of male rats at 300 but not 150 mg atenolol/kg/day (150 and 75 times the maximum recommended human antihypertensive dose*, respectively).

*Based on the maximum dose of 100 mg/day in a 50 kg patient.

Use in Pregnancy: Pregnancy Category D. See WARNINGS—Pregnancy and Fetal Injury.

Nursing Mothers: Atenolol is excreted in human breast milk at a ratio of 1.5 to 6.8 when compared to the concentration in plasma. Caution should be exercised when atenolol is administered to a nursing woman. Clinically significant bradycardia has been reported in breast fed infants. Premature infants, or infants with impaired renal function, may be more likely to develop adverse effects.

Pediatric Use: Safety and effectiveness in children have not been established.

ADVERSE REACTIONS

TENORETIC is usually well tolerated in properly selected patients. Most adverse effects have been mild and transient. The adverse effects observed for TENORETIC are essentially the same as those seen with the individual components.

Atenolol: The frequency estimates in the following table were derived from controlled studies in which adverse reactions were either volunteered by the patient (US studies) or elicited, eg, by checklist (foreign studies). The reported frequency of elicited adverse effects was higher for both atenolol and placebo-treated patients than when these reactions were volunteered. Where frequency of adverse effects for atenolol and placebo is similar, causal relationship to atenolol is uncertain.

[See table at left.]

	Volunteered (US Studies)		Total—Volunteered and Elicited (Foreign + US Studies)	
	Atenolol n=164 %	Placebo n=206 %	Atenolol n=399 %	Placebo n=407 %
CARDIOVASCULAR				
Bradycardia	3	0	3	0
Cold Extremities	0	0.5	12	5
Postural Hypotension	2	1	4	5
Leg Pain	0	0.5	3	1
CENTRAL NERVOUS SYSTEM/ NEUROMUSCULAR				
Dizziness	4	1	13	6
Vertigo	2	0.5	2	0.2
Light-Headedness	1	0	3	0.7
Tiredness	0.6	0.5	26	13
Fatigue	3	1	6	5
Lethargy	1	0	3	0.7
Drowsiness	0.6	0	2	0.5
Depression	0.6	0.5	12	9
Dreaming	0	0	3	1
GASTROINTESTINAL				
Diarrhea	2	0	3	2
Nausea	4	1	3	1
RESPIRATORY (see Warnings)				
Wheeziness	0	0	3	3
Dyspnea	0.6	1	6	4

During postmarketing experience, the following have been reported in temporal relationship to the use of the drug: elevated liver enzymes and/or billirubin, hallucinations, headache, impotence, Peyronie's disease, postural hypotension which may be associated with syncope, psoriasiform rash or exacerbation of psoriasis, psychoses, purpura, reversible alopecia, thrombocytopenia and visual disturbances. TENORETIC, like other beta blockers, has been associated with the development of antinuclear antibodies (ANA) and lupus syndrome.

Chlorthalidone: Cardiovascular: orthostatic hypotension; Gastrointestinal: anorexia, gastric irritation, vomiting, cramping, constipation, jaundice (intrahepatic cholestatic jaundice), pancreatitis; CNS: vertigo, paresthesias, xanthop-

sia; Hematologic: leukopenia, agranulocytosis, thrombocytopenia, aplastic anemia; Hypersensitivity: purpura, photosensitivity, rash, urticaria, necrotizing angiitis (vasculitis) (cutaneous vasculitis), Lyell's syndrome (toxic epidermal necrolysis); Miscellaneous: hyperglycemia, glycosuria, hyperuricemia, muscle spasm, weakness, restlessness. Clinical trials of TENORETIC conducted in the United States (89 patients treated with TENORETIC) revealed no new or unexpected adverse effects.

POTENTIAL ADVERSE EFFECTS: In addition, a variety of adverse effects not observed in clinical trials with atenolol but reported with other beta-adrenergic blocking agents should be considered potential adverse effects of atenolol. Nervous System: Reversible mental depression progressing to catatonia; an acute reversible syndrome characterized by disorientation for time and place, short-term memory loss, emotional lability, slightly clouded sensorium, decreased performance on neuropsychometrics; Cardiovascular: Intensification of AV block (see CONTRAINDICATIONS); Gastrointestinal: Mesenteric arterial thrombosis, ischemic colitis; Hematologic: Agranulocytosis; Allergic: Erythematous rash, fever combined with aching and sore throat, laryngospasm and respiratory distress; Other: Raynaud's phenomenon.

MISCELLANEOUS: There have been reports of skin rashes and/or dry eyes associated with the use of beta-adrenergic blocking drugs. The reported incidence is small, and, in most cases, the symptoms have cleared when treatment was withdrawn. Discontinuance of the drug should be considered if any such reaction is not otherwise explicable. Patients should be closely monitored following cessation of therapy. (See DOSAGE AND ADMINISTRATION.)

The oculomucocutaneous syndrome associated with the beta blocker practolol has not been reported with atenolol (TENORMIN). Furthermore, a number of patients who had previously demonstrated established practolol reactions were transferred to atenolol (TENORMIN) therapy with subsequent resolution or quiescence of the reaction.

Clinical Laboratory Test Findings: Clinically important changes in standard laboratory parameters were rarely associated with the administration of TENORETIC. The changes in laboratory parameters were not progressive and usually were not associated with clinical manifestations. The most common changes were increases in uric acid and decreases in serum potassium.

OVERDOSAGE

No specific information is available with regard to overdosage and TENORETIC in humans. Treatment should be symptomatic and supportive and directed to the removal of any unabsorbed drug by induced emesis, or administration or activated charcoal. Atenolol can be removed from the general circulation by hemodialysis. Further consideration should be given to dehydration, electrolyte imbalance and hypotension by established procedures.

Atenolol: Overdosage with atenolol has been reported with patients surviving acute doses as high as 5 g. One death was reported in a man who may have taken as much as 10 g acutely.

The predominant symptoms reported following atenolol overdose are lethargy, disorder of respiratory drive, wheezing, sinus pause, and bradycardia. Additionally, common effects associated with overdosage of any beta-adrenergic blocking agent are congestive heart failure, hypotension, bronchospasm, and/or hypoglycemia. Other treatment modalities should be employed at the physician's discretion and may include:

BRADYCARDIA: Atropine 1–2 mg intravenously. If there is no response to vagal blockade, give isoproterenol cautiously. In refractory cases, a transvenous cardiac pacemaker may be indicated. Glucagon in a 10 mg intravenous bolus has been reported to be useful. If required, this may be repeated or followed by an intravenous infusion of glucagon 1–10 mg/h depending on response.

HEART BLOCK (SECOND OR THIRD DEGREE): Isoproterenol or transvenous pacemaker.

CONGESTIVE HEART FAILURE: Digitalize the patient and administer a diuretic. Glucagon has been reported to be useful.

HYPOTENSION: Vasopressors such as dopamine or norepinephrine (levarterenol). Monitor blood pressure continuously.

BRONCHOSPASM: A $beta_2$-stimulant such as isoproterenol or terbutaline and/or aminophylline.

HYPOGLYCEMIA: Intravenous glucose.

ELECTROLYTE DISTURBANCE: Monitor electrolyte levels and renal function. Institute measures to maintain hydration and electrolytes.

Based on the severity of symptoms, management may require intensive support care and facilities for applying cardiac and respiratory support.

Chlorthalidone: Symptoms of chlorthalidone overdose include nausea, weakness, dizziness and disturbances of electrolyte balance.

DOSAGE AND ADMINISTRATION

DOSAGE MUST BE INDIVIDUALIZED (See INDICATIONS AND USAGE)

Chlorthalidone is usually given at a dose of 25 mg daily; the usual initial dose of atenolol is 50 mg daily. Therefore, the initial dose should be one TENORETIC 50 tablet given once a day. If an optimal response is not achieved, the dosage should be increased to one TENORETIC 100 tablet given once a day. When necessary, another antihypertensive agent may be added gradually beginning with 50 percent of the usual recommended starting dose to avoid an excessive fall in blood pressure.

Since atenolol is excreted via the kidneys, dosage should be adjusted in cases of severe impairment of renal function. No significant accumulation of atenolol occurs until creatinine clearance falls below 35 mL/min/1.73m^2 (normal range is 100–150 mL/min/1.73m^2); therefore, the following maximum dosages are recommended for patients with renal impairment.

Creatinine Clearance (mL/min/1.73m^2)	Atenolol Elimination Half-life (hrs)	Maximum Dosage
15–35	16–27	50 mg daily
< 15	> 27	50 mg every other day

HOW SUPPLIED

TENORETIC 50 Tablets (atenolol 50 mg and chlorthalidone 25 mg), NDC 0310-0115, (white, round, biconvex, uncoated tablets with TENORETIC on one side and 115 on the other side, bisected) are supplied in bottles of 100 tablets.

TENORETIC 100 Tablets (atenolol 100 mg and chlorthalidone 25 mg), NDC 0310-0117, (white, round, biconvex, uncoated tablets with TENORETIC on one side and 117 on the other side) are supplied in bottles of 100 tablets.

Store at controlled room temperature, 15°–30°C (59°–86°F).

Dispense in well-closed, light-resistant containers.

Manufactured by IPR Pharmaceuticals Inc.

Distributed by:

ZENECA Pharmaceuticals

A Business Unit of Zeneca Inc.

Wilmington, Delaware 19850-5437 USA

64049-03 Rev Y 09/95

Shown in Product Identification Guide, page 342

TENORMIN® Tablets ℞
TENORMIN® I.V. Injection
[*ten-or'min*]
(atenolol)

DESCRIPTION

TENORMIN (atenolol), a synthetic, $beta_1$-selective (cardioselective) adrenoreceptor blocking agent, may be chemically described as benzeneacetamide, 4-[2'-hydroxy-3'-[(1-methylethyl)amino]propoxy]-. The molecular and structural formulas are:

$C_{14}H_{22}N_2O_3$

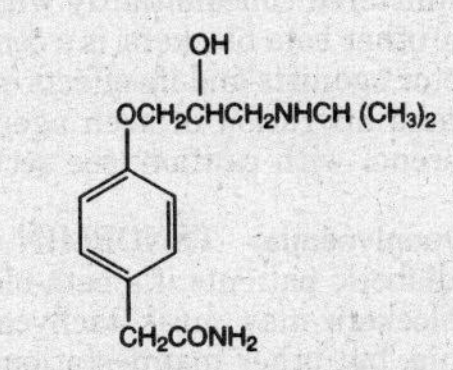

Atenolol (free base) has a molecular weight of 266. It is a relatively polar hydrophilic compound with a water solubility of 26.5 mg/mL at 37°C and a log partition coefficient (octanol/water) of 0.23. It is freely soluble in 1N HCl (300 mg/mL at 25°C) and less soluble in chloroform (3 mg/mL at 25°C).

TENORMIN is available as 25, 50 and 100 mg tablets for oral administration. TENORMIN for parenteral administration is available as TENORMIN I.V. Injection containing 5 mg atenolol in 10 mL sterile, isotonic, citrate-buffered, aqueous solution. The pH of the solution is 5.5–6.5.

Inactive Ingredients: TENORMIN Tablets: Magnesium stearate, microcrystalline cellulose, povidone, sodium starch glycolate. TENORMIN I.V. Injection: Sodium chloride for isotonicity and citric acid and sodium hydroxide to adjust pH.

CLINICAL PHARMACOLOGY

TENORMIN is a $beta_1$-selective (cardioselective) beta-adrenergic receptor blocking agent without membrane stabilizing or intrinsic sympathomimetic (partial agonist) activities. This preferential effect is not absolute, however, and at higher doses, TENORMIN inhibits $beta_2$-adrenoreceptors, chiefly located in the bronchial and vascular musculature.

Pharmacokinetics and Metabolism: In man, absorption of an oral dose is rapid and consistent but incomplete. Approximately 50% of an oral dose is absorbed from the gastrointestinal tract, the remainder being excreted unchanged in the feces. Peak blood levels are reached between two (2) and four (4) hours after ingestion. Unlike propranolol or metoprolol, but like nadolol, TENORMIN undergoes little or no metabolism by the liver, and the absorbed portion is eliminated primarily by renal excretion. Over 85% of an intravenous dose is excreted in urine within 24 hours compared with approximately 50% for an oral dose. TENORMIN also differs from propranolol in that only a small amount (6%–16%) is bound to proteins in the plasma. This kinetic profile results in relatively consistent plasma drug levels with about a fourfold interpatient variation.

The elimination half-life of oral TENORMIN is approximately 6 to 7 hours, and there is no alteration of the kinetic profile of the drug by chronic administration. Following intravenous administration, peak plasma levels are reached within 5 minutes. Declines from peak levels are rapid (5- to 10-fold) during the first 7 hours; thereafter, plasma levels decay with a half-life similar to that of orally administered drug. Following oral doses of 50 mg or 100 mg, both beta-blocking and antihypertensive effects persist for at least 24 hours. When renal function is impaired, elimination of TENORMIN is closely related to the glomerular filtration rate; significant accumulation occurs when the creatinine clearance falls below 35 mL/min/1.73m^2. (See DOSAGE AND ADMINISTRATION).

Pharmacodynamics: In standard animal or human pharmacological tests, beta-adrenoreceptor blocking activity of TENORMIN has been demonstrated by: (1) reduction in resting and exercise heart rate and cardiac output, (2) reduction of systolic and diastolic blood pressure at rest and on exercise, (3) inhibition of isoproterenol induced tachycardia, and (4) reduction in reflex orthostatic tachycardia.

A significant beta-blocking effect of TENORMIN, as measured by reduction of exercise tachycardia, is apparent within one hour following oral administration of a single dose. This effect is maximal at about 2 to 4 hours, and persists for at least 24 hours. Maximum reduction in exercise tachycardia occurs within 5 minutes of an intravenous dose. For both orally and intravenously administered drug, the duration of action is dose related and also bears a linear relationship to the logarithm of plasma TENORMIN concentration. The effect on exercise tachycardia of a single 10 mg intravenous dose is largely dissipated by 12 hours, whereas beta-blocking activity of single oral doses of 50 mg and 100 mg is still evident beyond 24 hours following administration. However, as has been shown for all beta-blocking agents, the antihypertensive effect does not appear to be related to plasma level.

In normal subjects, the $beta_1$-selectivity of TENORMIN has been shown by its reduced ability to reverse the $beta_2$-mediated vasodilating effect of isoproterenol as compared to equivalent beta-blocking doses of propranolol. In asthmatic patients, a dose of TENORMIN producing a greater effect on resting heart rate than propranolol resulted in much less increase in airway resistance. In a placebo controlled comparison of approximately equipotent oral doses of several beta blockers, TENORMIN produced a significantly smaller decrease of FEV_1 than nonselective beta blockers such as propranolol and, unlike those agents, did not inhibit bronchodilation in response to isoproterenol.

Consistent with its negative chronotropic effect due to beta blockade of the SA node, TENORMIN increases sinus cycle length and sinus node recovery time. Conduction in the AV node is also prolonged. TENORMIN is devoid of membrane stabilizing activity, and increasing the dose well beyond that producing beta blockade does not further depress myocardial contractility. Several studies have demonstrated a moderate (approximately 10%) increase in stroke volume at rest and during exercise.

In controlled clinical trials, TENORMIN, given as a single daily oral dose, was an effective antihypertensive agent providing 24-hour reduction of blood pressure. TENORMIN has been studied in combination with thiazide-type diuretics, and the blood pressure effects of the combination are approximately additive. TENORMIN is also compatible with methyldopa, hydralazine, and prazosin, each combination resulting in a larger fall in blood pressure than with the single agents. The dose range of TENORMIN is narrow and increasing the dose beyond 100 mg once daily is not associated with increased antihypertensive effect. The mechanisms of the antihypertensive effects of beta-blocking agents have not been established. Several possible mechanisms have been proposed and include: (1) competitive antagonism of catecholamines at peripheral (especially cardiac) adrenergic neuron sites, leading to decreased cardiac output, (2) a central effect leading to reduced sympathetic outflow to the periphery, and (3) suppression of renin activity. The results from long-term studies have not shown any diminution of the antihypertensive efficacy of TENORMIN with prolonged use.

By blocking the positive chronotropic and inotropic effects of catecholamines and by decreasing blood pressure, atenolol generally reduces the oxygen requirements of the heart at

Continued on next page

Zeneca Pharmaceuticals—Cont.

any given level of effort, making it useful for many patients in the long-term management of angina pectoris. On the other hand, atenolol can increase oxygen requirements by increasing left ventricular fiber length and end diastolic pressure, particularly in patients with heart failure.

In a multicenter clinical trial (ISIS-1) conducted in 16,027 patients with suspected myocardial infarction, patients presenting within 12 hours (mean = 5 hours) after the onset of pain were randomized to either conventional therapy plus TENORMIN (n = 8,037), or conventional therapy alone (n = 7,990). Patients with a heart rate of <50 bpm or systolic blood pressure <100 mm Hg, or with other contraindications to beta blockade, were excluded. Thirty-eight percent of each group were treated within 4 hours of onset of pain. The mean time from onset of pain to entry was 5.0 ± 2.7 hours in both groups. Patients in the TENORMIN group were to receive TENORMIN I.V. Injection 5–10 mg given over 5 minutes plus TENORMIN Tablets 50 mg every 12 hours orally on the first study day (the first oral dose administered about 15 minutes after the IV dose) followed by either TENORMIN Tablets 100 mg once daily or TENORMIN Tablets 50 mg twice daily on days 2–7. The groups were similar in demographic and medical history characteristics and in electrocardiographic evidence of myocardial infarction, bundle branch block, and first degree atrioventricular block at entry.

During the treatment period (days 0–7), the vascular mortality rates were 3.89% in the TENORMIN group (313 deaths) and 4.57% in the control group (365 deaths). This absolute difference in rates, 0.68%, is statistically significant at the P <0.05 level. The absolute difference translates into a proportional reduction of 15% (3.89-4.57/4.57 = −0.15). The 95% confidence limits are 1%–27%. Most of the difference was attributed to mortality in days 0-1 (TENORMIN—121 deaths; control—171 deaths).

Despite the large size of the ISIS-1 trial, it is not possible to identify clearly subgroups of patients most likely or least likely to benefit from early treatment with atenolol. Good clinical judgment suggests, however, that patients who are dependent on sympathetic stimulation for maintenance of adequate cardiac output and blood pressure are not good candidates for beta blockade. Indeed, the trial protocol reflected that judgment by excluding patients with blood pressure consistently below 100 mm Hg systolic. The overall results of the study are compatible with the possibility that patients with borderline blood pressure (less than 120 mm Hg systolic), especially if over 60 years of age, are less likely to benefit.

The mechanism through which atenolol improves survival in patients with definite or suspected acute myocardial infarction is unknown, as is the case for other beta blockers in the postinfarction setting. Atenolol, in addition to its effects on survival, has shown other clinical benefits including reduced frequency of ventricular premature beats, reduced chest pain, and reduced enzyme elevation.

INDICATIONS AND USAGE

Hypertension: TENORMIN is indicated in the management of hypertension. It may be used alone or concomitantly with other antihypertensive agents, particularly with a thiazide-type diuretic.

Angina Pectoris Due to Coronary Atherosclerosis: TENORMIN is indicated for the long-term management of patients with angina pectoris.

Acute Myocardial Infarction: TENORMIN is indicated in the management of hemodynamically stable patients with definite or suspected acute myocardial infarction to reduce cardiovascular mortality. Treatment can be initiated as soon as the patient's clinical condition allows. (See DOSAGE AND ADMINISTRATION, CONTRAINDICATIONS, AND WARNINGS.) In general, there is no basis for treating patients like those who were excluded from the ISIS-1 trial (blood pressure less than 100 mm Hg systolic, heart rate less than 50 bpm) or have other reasons to avoid beta blockade. As noted above, some subgroups (eg, elderly patients with systolic blood pressure below 120 mm Hg) seemed less likely to benefit.

CONTRAINDICATIONS

TENORMIN is contraindicated in sinus bradycardia, heart block greater than first degree, cardiogenic shock, and overt cardiac failure. (See WARNINGS.)

WARNINGS

Cardiac Failure: Sympathetic stimulation is necessary in supporting circulatory function in congestive heart failure, and beta blockade carries the potential hazard of further depressing myocardial contractility and precipitating more severe failure. In patients who have congestive heart failure controlled by digitalis and/or diuretics, TENORMIN should be administered cautiously. Both digitalis and atenolol slow AV conduction.

In patients with acute myocardial infarction, cardiac failure which is not promptly and effectively controlled by 80 mg of intravenous furosemide or equivalent therapy is a contraindication to beta-blocker treatment.

In Patients Without a History of Cardiac Failure: Continued depression of the myocardium with beta-blocking agents over a period of time can, in some cases, lead to cardiac failure. At the first sign or symptom of impending cardiac failure, patients should be fully digitalized and/or be given a diuretic and the response observed closely. If cardiac failure continues despite adequate digitalization and diuresis, TENORMIN should be withdrawn. (SEE DOSAGE AND ADMINISTRATION.)

> **Cessation of Therapy with TENORMIN:** Patients with coronary artery disease, who are being treated with TENORMIN, should be advised against abrupt discontinuation of therapy. Severe exacerbation of angina and the occurrence of myocardial infarction and ventricular arrhythmias have been reported in angina patients following the abrupt discontinuation of therapy with beta blockers. The last two complications may occur with or without preceding exacerbation of the angina pectoris. As with other beta blockers, when discontinuation of TENORMIN is planned, the patients should be carefully observed and advised to limit physical activity to a minimum. If the angina worsens or acute coronary insufficiency develops, it is recommenced that TENORMIN be promptly reinstituted, at least temporarily. Because coronary artery disease is common and may be unrecognized, it may be prudent not to discontinue TENORMIN therapy abruptly even in patients treated only for hypertension. (See DOSAGE AND ADMINISTRATION.)

Concomitant Use of Calcium Channel Blockers: Bradycardia and heart block can occur and the left ventricular end diastolic pressure can rise when beta blockers are administered with verapamil or diltiazem. Patients with pre-existing conduction abnormalities or left ventricular dysfunction are particularly susceptible. (See PRECAUTIONS.)

Bronchospastic Diseases: PATIENTS WITH BRONCHOSPASTIC DISEASE SHOULD, IN GENERAL, NOT RECEIVE BETA BLOCKERS. Because of its relative $beta_1$ selectivity, however, TENORMIN may be used with caution in patients with bronchospastic disease who do not respond to, or cannot tolerate, other antihypertensive treatment. Since $beta_1$ selectivity is not absolute, the lowest possible dose of TENORMIN should be used with therapy initiated at 50 mg and a $beta_2$-stimulating agent (bronchodilator) should be made available. If dosage must be increased, dividing the dose should be considered in order to achieve lower peak blood levels.

Anesthesia and Major Surgery: It is not advisable to withdraw beta-adrenoreceptor blocking drugs prior to surgery in the majority of patients. However, care should be taken when using anesthetic agents such as those which may depress the myocardium. Vagal dominance, if it occurs, may be corrected with atropine (1-2 mg IV).

Additionally, caution should be used when TENORMIN I.V. Injection is administered concomitantly with such agents. TENORMIN, like other beta blockers, is a competitive inhibitor of beta-receptor agonists and its effects on the heart can be reversed by administration of such agents: eg, dobutamine or isoproterenol with caution (see section on OVERDOSAGE).

Diabetes and Hypoglycemia: TENORMIN should be used with caution in diabetic patients if a beta-blocking agent is required. Beta blockers may mask tachycardia occurring with hypoglycemia, but other manifestations such as dizziness and sweating may not be significantly affected. At recommended doses TENORMIN does not potentiate insulin-induced hypoglycemia and, unlike nonselective beta blockers, does not delay recovery of blood glucose to normal levels.

Thyrotoxicosis: Beta-adrenergic blockade may mask certain clinical signs (eg, tachycardia) of hyperthyroidism. Patients suspected of having thyroid disease should be monitored closely when adminstering TENORMIN I.V. Injection. Abrupt withdrawal of beta blockade might precipitate a thyroid storm; therefore, patients suspected of developing thyrotoxicosis from whom TENORMIN therapy is to be withdrawn should be monitored closely. (See DOSAGE AND ADMINISTRATION.)

Pregnancy and Fetal Injury: Atenolol can cause fetal harm when administered to a pregnant woman. Atenolol crosses the placental barrier and appears in cord blood. Administration of atenolol, starting in the second trimester of pregnancy, has been associated with the birth of infants that are small for gestational age. No studies have been performed on the use of atenolol in the first trimester and the possibility of fetal injury cannot be excluded. If this drug is used during pregnancy, or if the patient becomes pregnant while taking this drug, the patient should be apprised of the potential hazard to the fetus.

Atenolol has been shown to produce a dose-related increase in embryo/fetal resorptions in rats at doses equal to or greater than 50 mg/kg/day or 25 or more times the maximum recommended human antihypertensive dose*. Although similar effects were not seen in rabbits, the compound was not evaluated in rabbits at doses above 25 mg/kg/day or 12.5 times the maximum recommended human antihypertensive dose*.

*Based on the maximum dose of 100 mg/day in a 50 kg patient.

PRECAUTIONS

General: Patients already on a beta blocker must be evaluated carefully before TENORMIN is administered. Initial and subsequent TENORMIN dosages can be adjusted downward depending on clinical observations including pulse and blood pressure. TENORMIN may aggravate peripheral arterial circulatory disorders.

Impaired Renal Function: The drug should be used with caution in patients with impaired renal function. (See DOSAGE AND ADMINISTRATION.)

Drug Interactions: Catecholamine-depleting drugs (eg, reserpine) may have an additive effect when given with beta-blocking agents. Patients treated with TENORMIN plus a catecholamine depletor should therefore be closely observed for evidence of hypotension and/or marked bradycardia which may produce vertigo, syncope or postural hypotension.

Calcium channel blockers may also have an additive effect when given with TENORMIN (See WARNINGS.).

Beta blockers may exacerbate the rebound hypertension which can follow the withdrawal of clonidine. If the two drugs are coadministered, the beta blocker should be withdrawn several days before the gradual withdrawal of clonidine. If replacing clonidine by beta-blocker therapy, the introduction of beta blockers should be delayed for several days after clonidine administration has stopped.

Caution should be exercised with TENORMIN I.V. Injection when given in close proximity with drugs that may also have a depressant effect on myocardial contractility. On rare occasions, concomitant use of intravenous beta blockers and intravenous verapamil has resulted in serious adverse reactions, especially in patients with severe cardiomyopathy, congestive heart failure, or recent myocardial infarction.

Information on concurrent usage of atenolol and aspirin is limited. Data from several studies, ie, TIMI-II, ISIS-2, currently do not suggest any clinical interaction between aspirin and beta blockers in the acute myocardial infarction setting.

While taking beta blockers, patients with a history of anaphylactic reaction to a variety of allergens may have a more severe reaction on repeated challenge, either accidental, diagnostic or therapeutic. Such patients may be unresponsive to the usual doses of epinephrine used to treat the allergic reaction.

Carcinogenesis, Mutagenesis, Impairment of Fertility: Two long-term (maximum dosing duration of 18 or 24 months) rat studies and one long-term (maximum dosing duration of 18 months) mouse study, each employing dose levels as high as 300 mg/kg/day or 150 times the maximum recommended human antihypertensive dose,* did not indicate a carcinogenic potential of atenolol. A third (24 month) rat study, employing doses of 500 and 1,500 mg/kg/day (250 and 750 times the maximum recommended human antihypertensive dose*) resulted in increased incidences of benign adrenal medullary tumors in males and females, mammary fibroadenomas in females, and anterior pituitary adenomas and thyroid parafollicular cell carcinomas in males. No evidence of a mutagenic potential of atenolol was uncovered in the dominant lethal test (mouse), in vivo cytogenetics test (Chinese hamster) or Ames test (*S typhimurium*).

Fertility of male or female rats (evaluated at dose levels as high as 200 mg/kg/day or 100 times the maximum recommended human dose*) was unaffected by atenolol administration.

Animal Toxicology: Chronic studies employing oral atenolol performed in animals have revealed the occurrence of vacuolation of epithelial cells of Brunner's glands in the duodenum of both male and female dogs at all tested dose levels of atenolol (starting at 15 mg/kg/day or 7.5 times the maximum recommended human antihypertensive dose*) and increased incidence of atrial degeneration of hearts of male rats at 300 but not 150 mg atenolol/kg/day (150 and 75 times the maximum recommended human antihypertensive dose,* respectively).

*Based on the maximum dose of 100 mg/day in a 50 kg patient.

Usage in Pregnancy: Pregnancy Category D: See WARNINGS—Pregnancy and Fetal Injury.

Nursing Mothers: Atenolol is excreted in human breast milk at a ratio of 1.5 to 6.8 when compared to the concentration in plasma. Caution should be exercised when TENORMIN is administered to a nursing woman. Clinically significant bradycardia has been reported in breast fed infants. Premature infants, or infants with impaired renal function, may be more likely to develop adverse effects.

Pediatric Use: Safety and effectiveness in children have not been established.

ADVERSE REACTIONS

Most adverse effects have been mild and transient. The frequency estimates in the following table were derived from controlled studies in hypertensive patients in which adverse reactions were either volunteered by the patient (US studies) or elicited, eg, by checklist (foreign studies). The reported frequency of elicited adverse effects was higher for both TENORMIN and placebo-treated patients than when these reactions were volunteered. Where frequency of adverse effects of TENORMIN and placebo is similar, causal relationship to TENORMIN is uncertain.
[See first table at right.]

Acute Myocardial Infarction: In a series of investigations in the treatment of acute myocardial infarction, bradycardia and hypotension occurred more commonly, as expected for any beta blocker, in atenolol-treated patients than in control patients. However, these usually responded to atropine and/or to withholding further dosage of atenolol. The incidence of heart failure was not increased by atenolol. Inotropic agents were infrequently used. The reported frequency of these and other events occurring during these investigations is given in the following table.

In a study of 477 patients, the following adverse events were reported during either intravenous and/or oral atenolol administration:
[See second table at right.]

In the subsequent International Study of Infarct Survival (ISIS-1) including over 16,000 patients of whom 8,037 were randomized to receive TENORMIN treatment, the dosage of intravenous and subsequent oral TENORMIN was either discontinued or reduced for the following reasons:
[See third table at right.]

During postmarketing experience with TENORMIN, the following have been reported in temporal relationship to the use of the drug: elevated liver enzymes and/or bilirubin, hallucinations, headache, impotence, Peyronie's disease, postural hypotension which may be associated with syncope, psoriasiform rash or exacerbation of psoriasis, psychoses, purpura, reversible alopecia, thrombocytopenia and visual disturbances. TENORMIN, like other beta blockers, has been associated with the development of antinuclear antibodies (ANA) and lupus syndrome.

POTENTIAL ADVERSE EFFECTS

In addition, a variety of adverse effects have been reported with other beta-adrenergic blocking agents, and may be considered potential adverse effects of TENORMIN.

Hematologic: Agranulocytosis.
Allergic: Fever, combined with aching and sore throat, laryngospasm, and respiratory distress.
Central Nervous System: Reversible mental depression progressing to catatonia; an acute reversible syndrome characterized by disorientation of time and place; short-term memory loss; emotional lability with slightly clouded sensorium; and decreased performance on neuropsychometrics.
Gastrointestinal: Mesenteric arterial thrombosis, ischemic colitis.
Other: Erythematous rash, Raynaud's phenomenon.
Miscellaneous: There have been reports of skin rashes and/or dry eyes associated with the use of beta-adrenergic blocking drugs. The reported incidence is small, and in most cases, the symptoms have cleared when treatment was withdrawn. Discontinuance of the drug should be considered if any such reaction is not otherwise explicable. Patients should be closely monitored following cessation of therapy. (See DOSAGE AND ADMINISTRATION.)

The oculomucocutaneous syndrome associated with the beta blocker practolol has not been reported with TENORMIN. Furthermore, a number of patients who had previously demonstrated established practolol reactions were transferred to TENORMIN therapy with subsequent resolution or quiescence of the reaction.

OVERDOSAGE

Overdosage with TENORMIN has been reported with patients surviving acute doses as high as 5 g. One death was reported in a man who may have taken as much as 10 g acutely.

The predominant symptoms reported following TENORMIN overdose are lethargy, disorder of respiratory drive, wheezing, sinus pause and bradycardia. Additionally, common effects associated with overdosage of any beta-adrenergic blocking agent and which might also be expected in TENORMIN overdose are congestive heart failure, hypotension, bronchospasm and/or hypoglycemia.

Treatment of overdose should be directed to the removal of any unabsorbed drug by induced emesis, gastric lavage, or administration of activated charcoal. TENORMIN can be removed from the general circulation by hemodialysis. Other treatment modalities should be employed at the physician's discretion and may include:

BRADYCARDIA: Atropine intravenously. If there is no response to vagal blockade, give isoproterenol cautiously. In refractory cases, a transvenous cardiac pacemaker may be indicated.

	Volunteered (US Studies)		Total—Volunteered and Elicited (Foreign + US Studies)	
	Atenolol (n = 164) %	Placebo (n = 206) %	Atenolol (n = 399) %	Placebo (n = 407) %
CARDIOVASCULAR				
Bradycardia	3	0	3	0
Cold Extremities	0	0.5	12	5
Postural Hypotension	2	1	4	5
Leg Pain	0	0.5	3	1
CENTRAL NERVOUS SYSTEM/NEUROMUSCULAR				
Dizziness	4	1	13	6
Vertigo	2	0.5	2	0.2
Light-headedness	1	0	3	0.7
Tiredness	0.6	0.5	26	13
Fatigue	3	1	6	5
Lethargy	1	0	3	0.7
Drowsiness	0.6	0	2	0.5
Depression	0.6	0.5	12	9
Dreaming	0	0	3	1
GASTROINTESTINAL				
Diarrhea	2	0	3	2
Nausea	4	1	3	1
RESPIRATORY (see WARNINGS)				
Wheeziness	0	0	3	3
Dyspnea	0.6	1	6	4

	Conventional Therapy Plus Atenolol (n=244)		Conventional Therapy Alone (n=233)	
Bradycardia	43	(18%)	24	(10%)
Hypotension	60	(25%)	34	(15%)
Bronchospasm	3	(1.2%)	2	(0.9%)
Heart Failure	46	(19%)	56	(24%)
Heart Block	11	(4.5%)	10	(4.3%)
BBB + Major Axis Deviation	16	(6.6%)	28	(12%)
Supraventricular Tachycardia	28	(11.5%)	45	(19%)
Atrial Fibrillation	12	(5%)	29	(11%)
Atrial Flutter	4	(1.6%)	7	(3%)
Ventricular Tachycardia	39	(16%)	52	(22%)
Cardiac Reinfarction	0	(0%)	6	(2.6%)
Total Cardiac Arrests	4	(1.6%)	16	(6.9%)
Nonfatal Cardiac Arrests	4	(1.6%)	12	(5.1%)
Deaths	7	(2.9%)	16	(6.9%)
Cardiogenic Shock	1	(0.4%)	4	(1.7%)
Development of Ventricular Septal Defect	0	(0%)	2	(0.9%)
Development of Mitral Regurgitation	0	(0%)	2	(0.9%)
Renal Failure	1	(0.4%)	0	(0%)
Pulmonary Emboli	3	(1.2%)	0	(0%)

Reasons for Reduced Dosage	IV Atenolol Reduced Dose (<5 mg)*		Oral Partial Dose	
Hypotension/Bradycardia	105	(1.3%)	1168	(14.5%)
Cardiogenic Shock	4	(.04%)	35	(.44%)
Reinfarction	0	(0%)	5	(.06%)
Cardiac Arrest	5	(.06%)	28	(.34%)
Heart Block (> first degree)	5	(.06%)	143	(1.7%)
Cardiac Failure	1	(.01%)	233	(2.9%)
Arrhythmias	3	(.04%)	22	(.27%)
Bronchospasm	1	(.01%)	50	(.62%)

*Full dosage was 10 mg and some patients received less than 10 mg but more than 5 mg.

HEART BLOCK (SECOND OR THIRD DEGREE): Isoproterenol or transvenous cardiac pacemaker.
CARDIAC FAILURE: Digitalize the patient and administer a diuretic. Glucagon has been reported to be useful.
HYPOTENSION: Vasopressors such as dopamine or norepinephrine (levarterenol). Monitor blood pressure continuously.
BRONCHOSPASM: A beta$_2$ stimulant such as isoproterenol or terbutaline and/or aminophylline.
HYPOGLYCEMIA: Intravenous glucose.
Based on the severity of symptoms, management may require intensive support care and facilities for applying cardiac and respiratory support.

DOSAGE AND ADMINISTRATION

Hypertension: The initial dose of TENORMIN is 50 mg given as one tablet a day either alone or added to diuretic therapy. The full effect of this dose will usually be seen within one to two weeks. If an optimal response is not achieved, the dosage should be increased to TENORMIN 100 mg given as one tablet a day. Increasing the dosage beyond 100 mg a day is unlikely to produce any further benefit. TENORMIN may be used alone or concomitantly with other antihypertensive agents including thiazide-type diuretics, hydralazine, prazosin, and alpha-methyldopa.

Angina Pectoris: The initial dose of TENORMIN is 50 mg given as one tablet a day. If an optimal response is not achieved within one week, the dosage should be increased to TENORMIN 100 mg given as one tablet a day. Some patients may require a dosage of 200 mg once a day for optimal effect. Twenty-four hour control with once daily dosing is achieved by giving doses larger than necessary to achieve an immediate maximum effect. The maximum early effect on exercise tolerance occurs with doses of 50 to 100 mg, but at these doses the effect at 24 hours is attenuated, averaging about 50% to 75% of that observed with once a day oral doses of 200 mg.

Acute Myocardial Infarction: In patients with definite or suspected acute myocardial infarction, treatment with TENORMIN I.V. Injection should be initiated as soon as

Continued on next page

Zeneca Pharmaceuticals—Cont.

possible after the patient's arrival in the hospital and after eligibility is established. Such treatment should be initiated in a coronary care or similar unit immediately after the patient's hemodynamic condition has stabilized. Treatment should begin with the intravenous administration of 5 mg TENORMIN over 5 minutes followed by another 5 mg intravenous injection 10 minutes later. TENORMIN I.V. Injection should be administered under carefully controlled conditions including monitoring of blood pressure, heart rate, and electrocardiogram. Dilutions of TENORMIN I.V. Injection in Dextrose Injection USP, Sodium Chloride Injection USP, or Sodium Chloride and Dextrose Injection may be used. These admixtures are stable for 48 hours if they are not used immediately.

In patients who tolerate the full intravenous dose (10 mg), TENORMIN Tablets 50 mg should be initiated 10 minutes after the last intravenous dose followed by another 50 mg oral dose 12 hours later. Thereafter, TENORMIN can be given orally either 100 mg once daily or 50 mg twice a day for a further 6–9 days or until discharge from the hospital. If bradycardia or hypotension requiring treatment or any other untoward effects occur, TENORMIN should be discontinued. (See full prescribing information prior to initiating therapy with TENORMIN tablets.)

Data from other beta blocker trials suggest that if there is any question concerning the use of IV beta blocker or clinical estimate that there is a contraindication, the IV beta blocker may be eliminated and patients fulfilling the safety criteria may be given TENORMIN Tablets 50 mg twice daily or 100 mg once a day for at least seven days (if the IV dosing is excluded).

Although the demonstration of efficacy of TENORMIN is based entirely on data from the first seven postinfarction days, data from other beta blocker trials suggest that treatment with beta blockers that are effective in the postinfarction setting may be continued for one to three years if there are no contraindications.

TENORMIN is an additional treatment to standard coronary care unit therapy.

Elderly Patients or Patients with Renal Impairment: TENORMIN is excreted by the kidneys; consequently dosage should be adjusted in cases of severe impairment of renal function. Some reduction in dosage may also be appropriate for the elderly, since decreased kidney function is a physiologic consequence of aging. Atenolol excretion would be expected to decrease with advancing age.

No significant accumulation of TENORMIN occurs until creatinine clearance falls below 35 mL/min/1.73 m^2. Accumulation of atenolol and prolongation of its half-life were studied in subjects with creatinine clearance between 5 and 105 mL/min. Peak plasma levels were significantly increased in subjects with creatinine clearances below 30 mL/min.

The following maximum oral dosages are recommended for elderly, renally-impaired patients and for patients with renal impairment due to other causes:

Creatinine Clearance (mL/min/1.73m^2)	Atenolol Elimination Half-Life (h)	Maximum Dosage
15–35	16–27	50 mg daily
<15	>27	25 mg daily

Some renally-impaired or elderly patients being treated for hypertension may require a lower starting dose of TENORMIN: 25 mg given as one tablet a day. If this 25 mg dose is used, assessment of efficacy must be made carefully. This should include measurement of blood pressure just prior to the next dose ("trough" blood pressure) to ensure that the treatment effect is present for a full 24 hours.

Although a similar dosage reduction may be considered for elderly and/or renally-impaired patients being treated for indications other than hypertension, data are not available for these patient populations.

Patients on hemodialysis should be given 25 mg or 50 mg after each dialysis; this should be done under hospital supervision as marked falls in blood pressure can occur.

Cessation of Therapy in Patients with Angina Pectoris: If withdrawal of TENORMIN therapy is planned, it should be achieved gradually and patients should be carefully observed and advised to limit physical activity to a minimum.

Parenteral drug products should be inspected visually for particulate matter and discoloration prior to administration, whenever solution and container permit.

HOW SUPPLIED

TENORMIN Tablets: Tablets of 25 mg atenolol, NDC 0310-0107 (round, flat, uncoated white tablets identified with "T" debossed on one side and 107 debossed on the other side) are supplied in bottles of 100 tablets.

Tablets of 50 mg atenolol, NDC 0310-0105 (round, flat, uncoated white tablets identified with "TENORMIN" debossed on one side and 105 debossed on the other side, bisected) are supplied in bottles of 100 tablets and 1000 tablets, and unit dose packages of 100 tablets.

Tablets of 100 mg atenolol, NDC 0310-0101 (round, flat, uncoated white tablets identified with "TENORMIN" debossed on one side and 101 debossed on the other side) are supplied in bottles of 100 tablets and unit dose packages of 100 tablets.

Store at controlled room temperature, 15°–30°C (59°–86°F). Dispense in well-closed, light resistant containers.

TENORMIN I.V. Injection:

TENORMIN I.V. Injection, NDC 0310-0108, is supplied as 5 mg atenolol in 10 mL ampules of isotonic citrate-buffered aqueous solution.

Protect from light. Keep ampules in outer packaging until time of use. Store at room temperature.

Manufactured by: IPR Pharmaceuticals Inc.
Distributed by: Zeneca Pharmaceuticals
A Business Unit of Zeneca Inc.
Wilmington, Delaware 19850-5437 USA
64028-07 Rev F 09/95

Shown in Product Identification Guide, page 342

ZESTORETIC® ℞

[zes 'tor-etic]

LISINOPRIL/HYDROCHLOROTHIAZIDE

> **USE IN PREGNANCY**
>
> **When used in pregnancy during the second and third trimesters, ACE inhibitors can cause injury and even death to the developing fetus.** When pregnancy is detected, ZESTORETIC should be discontinued as soon as possible. See WARNINGS, Pregnancy, Lisinopril, Fetal/Neonatal Morbidity and Mortality.

DESCRIPTION

ZESTORETIC® (Lisinopril and Hydrochlorothiazide) combines an angiotensin converting enzyme inhibitor, lisinopril, and a diuretic, hydrochlorothiazide.

Lisinopril, a synthetic peptide derivative, is an oral long-acting angiotensin converting enzyme inhibitor. It is chemically described as (S)-1-[N^2-(1-carboxy-3-phenylpropyl)-L-lysyl]-L-proline dihydrate. Its empirical formula is $C_{21}H_{31}N_3O_5 \cdot 2H_2O$ and its structural formula is:

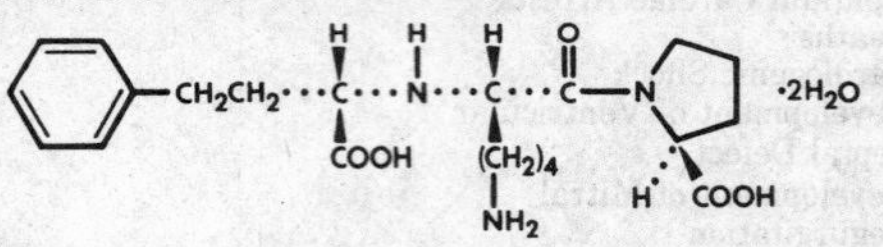

Lisinopril is a white to off-white, crystalline powder, with a molecular weight of 441.53. It is soluble in water, sparingly soluble in methanol, and practically insoluble in ethanol.

Hydrochlorothiazide is 6-chloro-3,4-dihydro-2H-1,2,4-benzothiadiazine-7-sulfonamide 1,1-dioxide. Its empirical formula is $C_7H_8ClN_3O_4S_2$ and its structural formula is:

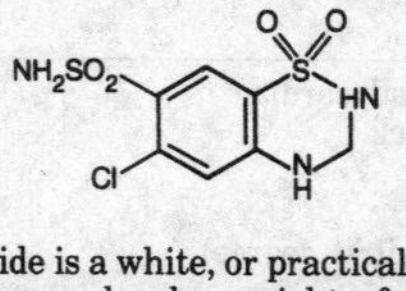

Hydrochlorothiazide is a white, or practically white, crystalline powder with a molecular weight of 297.72, which is slightly soluble in water, but freely soluble in sodium hydroxide solution.

ZESTORETIC is available for oral use in three tablet combinations of lisinopril with hydrochlorothiazide: ZESTORETIC 10-12.5 containing 10 mg lisinopril and 12.5 mg hydrochlorothiazide; ZESTORETIC 20-12.5 containing 20 mg lisinopril and 12.5 mg hydrochlorothiazide; and, ZESTORETIC 20–25 containing 20 mg lisinopril and 25 mg hydrochlorothiazide.

Inactive Ingredients:

10–12.5 Tablets—calcium phosphate, magnesium stearate, mannitol, red ferric oxide, starch, yellow ferric oxide.

20-12.5 Tablets—calcium phosphate, magnesium stearate, mannitol, starch.

20-25 Tablets—calcium phosphate, magnesium stearate, mannitol, red ferric oxide, starch, yellow ferric oxide.

CLINICAL PHARMACOLOGY

Lisinopril and Hydrochlorothiazide

As a result of its diuretic effects, hydrochlorothiazide increases plasma renin activity, increases aldosterone secretion, and decreases serum potassium. Administration of lisinopril blocks the renin-angiotensin aldosterone axis and tends to reverse the potassium loss associated with the diuretic.

In clinical studies, the extent of blood pressure reduction seen with the combination of lisinopril and hydrochlorothiazide was approximately additive. The ZESTORETIC 10–12.5 combination worked equally well in black and white patients. The ZESTORETIC 20–12.5 and ZESTORETIC 20–25 combinations appeared somewhat less effective in black patients, but relatively few black patients were studied. In most patients, the antihypertensive effect of ZESTORETIC was sustained for at least 24 hours.

In a randomized, controlled comparison, the mean antihypertensive effects of ZESTORETIC 20-12.5 and ZESTORETIC 20-25 were similar, suggesting that many patients who respond adequately to the latter combination may be controlled with ZESTORETIC 20-12.5. (See DOSAGE AND ADMINISTRATION.)

Concomitant administration of lisinopril and hydrochlorothiazide has little or no effect on the bioavailability of either drug. The combination tablet is bioequivalent to concomitant administration of the separate entities.

Lisinopril

Mechanism of Action: Lisinopril inhibits angiotensin-converting enzyme (ACE) in human subjects and animals. ACE is a peptidyl dipeptidase that catalyzes the conversion of angiotensin I to the vasoconstrictor substance, angiotensin II. Angiotensin II also stimulates aldosterone secretion by the adrenal cortex. Inhibition of ACE results in decreased plasma angiotensin II which leads to decreased vasopressor activity and to decreased aldosterone secretion. The latter decrease may result in a small increase of serum potassium. Removal of angiotensin II negative feedback on renin secretion leads to increased plasma renin activity. In hypertensive patients with normal renal function treated with lisinopril alone for up to 24 weeks, the mean increase in serum potassium was less than 0.1 mEq/L; however, approximately 15 percent of patients had increases greater than 0.5 mEq/L and approximately six percent had a decrease greater than 0.5 mEq/L. In the same study, patients treated with lisinopril plus a thiazide diuretic showed essentially no change in serum potassium. (See PRECAUTIONS.)

ACE is identical to kininase, an enzyme that degrades bradykinin. Whether increased levels of bradykinin, a potent vasodepressor peptide, play a role in the therapeutic effects of lisinopril remains to be elucidated.

While the mechanism through which lisinopril lowers blood pressure is believed to be primarily suppression of the renin-angiotensin-aldosterone system, lisinopril is antihypertensive even in patients with low-renin hypertension. Although lisinopril was antihypertensive in all races studied, black hypertensive patients (usually a low-renin hypertensive population) had a smaller average response to lisinopril monotherapy than non-black patients.

Pharmacokinetics and Metabolism: Following oral administration of lisinopril, peak serum concentrations occur within about 7 hours. Declining serum concentrations exhibit a prolonged terminal phase which does not contribute to drug accumulation. This terminal phase probably represents saturable binding to ACE and is not proportional to dose. Lisinopril does not appear to be bound to other serum proteins.

Lisinopril does not undergo metabolism and is excreted unchanged entirely in the urine. Based on urinary recovery, the mean extent of absorption of lisinopril is approximately 25 percent, with large intersubject variability (6%–60%) at all doses tested (5–80 mg). Lisinopril absorption is not influenced by the presence of food in the gastrointestinal tract.

Upon multiple dosing, lisinopril exhibits an effective half-life of accumulation of 12 hours.

Impaired renal function decreases elimination of lisinopril, which is excreted principally through the kidneys, but this decrease becomes clinically important only when the glomerular filtration rate is below 30 mL/min. Above this glomerular filtration rate, the elimination half-life is little changed. With greater impairment, however, peak and trough lisinopril levels increase, time to peak concentration increases and time to attain steady state is prolonged. Older patients, on average, have (approximately doubled) higher blood levels and area under the plasma concentration time curve (AUC) than younger patients. (See DOSAGE AND ADMINISTRATION.) Lisinopril can be removed by hemodialysis.

Studies in rats indicate that lisinopril crosses the blood-brain barrier poorly. Multiple doses of lisinopril in rats do not result in accumulation in any tissues. However, milk of lactating rats contains radioactivity following administration of ^{14}C lisinopril. By whole body autoradiography, radioactivity was found in the placenta following administration of labeled drug to pregnant rats, but none was found in the fetuses.

Pharmacodynamics: Administration of lisinopril to patients with hypertension results in a reduction of supine and standing blood pressure to about the same extent with no compensatory tachycardia. Symptomatic postural hypotension is usually not observed although it can occur and should be anticipated in volume and/or salt-depleted patients. (See WARNINGS.)

In most patients studied, onset of antihypertensive activity was seen at one hour after oral administration of an individ-

ual dose of lisinopril, with peak reduction of blood pressure achieved by six hours.

In some patients achievement of optimal blood pressure reduction may require two to four weeks of therapy.

At recommended single daily doses, antihypertensive effects have been maintained for at least 24 hours, after dosing, although the effect at 24 hours was substantially smaller than the effect six hours after dosing.

The antihypertensive effects of lisinopril have continued during long term therapy. Abrupt withdrawal of lisinopril has not been associated with a rapid increase in blood pressure; nor with a significant overshoot of pretreatment blood pressure.

In hemodynamic studies in patients with essential hypertension, blood pressure reduction was accompanied by a reduction in peripheral arterial resistance with little or no change in cardiac output and in heart rate. In a study in nine hypertensive patients, following administration of lisinopril, there was an increase in mean renal blood flow that was not significant. Data from several small studies are inconsistent with respect to the effect of lisinopril on glomerular filtration rate in hypertensive patients with normal renal function, but suggest that changes, if any, are not large.

In patients with renovascular hypertension lisinopril has been shown to be well tolerated and effective in controlling blood pressure. (See PRECAUTIONS.)

Hydrochlorothiazide

The mechanism of the antihypertensive effect of thiazides is unknown. Thiazides do not usually affect normal blood pressure.

Hydrochlorothiazide is a diuretic and antihypertensive. It affects the distal renal tubular mechanism of electrolyte reabsorption. Hydrochlorothiazide increases excretion of sodium and chloride in approximately equivalent amounts. Natriuresis may be accompanied by some loss of potassium and bicarbonate.

After oral use diuresis begins within two hours, peaks in about four hours and lasts about 6 to 12 hours.

Hydrochlorothiazide is not metabolized but is eliminated rapidly by the kidney. When plasma levels have been followed for at least 24 hours, the plasma half-life has been observed to vary between 5.6 and 14.8 hours. At least 61 percent of the oral dose is eliminated unchanged within 24 hours. Hydrochlorothiazide crosses the placental but not the blood-brain barrier.

INDICATIONS AND USAGE

ZESTORETIC is indicated for the treatment of hypertension. These fixed-dose combinations are not indicated for initial therapy (see DOSAGE AND ADMINISTRATION).

In using ZESTORETIC, consideration should be given to the fact that an angiotensin converting enzyme inhibitor, captopril, has caused agranulocytosis, particularly in patients with renal impairment or collagen vascular disease, and that available data are insufficient to show that lisinopril does not have a similar risk. (See WARNINGS.)

In considering the use of ZESTORETIC, it should be noted that ACE inhibitors have been associated with a higher rate of angioedema in black than in nonblack patients (see WARNINGS, Lisinopril, Angioedema).

CONTRAINDICATIONS

ZESTORETIC is contraindicated in patients who are hypersensitive to any component of this product and in patients with a history of angioedema related to previous treatment with an angiotensin converting enzyme inhibitor. Because of the hydrochlorothiazide component, this product is contraindicated in patients with anuria or hypersensitivity to other sulfonamide-derived drugs.

WARNINGS

Lisinopril

Anaphylactoid and Possibly Related Reactions: Presumably because angiotensin-converting enzyme inhibitors affect the metabolism of eicosanoids and polypeptides, including endogenous bradykinin, patients receiving ACE inhibitors (including ZESTORETIC) may be subject to a variety of adverse reactions, some of them serious.

Angioedema: Angioedema of the face, extremities, lips, tongue, glottis and/or larynx has been reported rarely in patients treated with angiotensin converting enzyme inhibitors, including lisinopril. This may occur at any time during treatment. ACE inhibitors have been associated with a higher rate of angioedema in black than in nonblack patients. ZESTORETIC should be promptly discontinued and the appropriate therapy and monitoring should be provided until complete and sustained resolution of signs and symptoms has occurred. In instances where swelling has been confined to the face and lips the condition has generally resolved without treatment, although antihistamines have been useful in relieving symptoms. Angioedema associated with laryngeal edema may be fatal. **Where there is involvement of the tongue, glottis or larynx, likely to cause airway obstruction, subcutaneous epinephrine solution 1:1000 (0.3 mL to 0.5 mL) and/or measures necessary to ensure a patent airway should be promptly provided. (See ADVERSE REACTIONS.)**

Patients with a history or angioedema unrelated to ACE inhibitor therapy may be at increased risk of angioedema while receiving an ACE inhibitor (see also INDICATIONS AND USAGE and CONTRAINDICATIONS).

Anaphylactoid Reactions During Desensitization: Two patients undergoing desensitizing treatment with hymenoptra venom while receiving ACE inhibitors sustained life-threatening anaphylactoid reactions. In the same patients, these reactions were avoided when ACE inhibitors were temporarily withheld, but they reappeared upon inadvertent rechallenge.

Anaphylactoid Reactions During Membrane Exposure: Thiazide-containing combination products are not recommended in patients with severe renal dysfunction. Sudden and potentially life-threatening anaphylactoid reactions have been reported in some patients dialyzed with high-flux membranes (eg, AN69¶) and treated concomitantly with an ACE inhibitor. In such patients, dialysis must be stopped immediately, and aggressive therapy for anaphylactoid reactions be initiated. Symptoms have not been relieved by antihistamines in these situations. In these patients, consideration should be given to using a different type of dialysis membrane or a different class of antihypertensive agent. Anaphylactoid reactions have also been reported in patients undergoing low-density lipoprotein apheresis with dextran sulfate absorption (a procedure dependent upon devices not approved in the United States.)

Hypotension and Related Effects: Excessive hypotension was rarely seen in uncomplicated hypertensive patients but is a possible consequence of lisinopril use in salt/volume-depleted persons such as those treated vigorously with diuretics or patients on dialysis. (See PRECAUTIONS, Drug Interactions and ADVERSE REACTIONS.)

Syncope has been reported in 0.8 percent of patients receiving ZESTORETIC. In patients with hypertension receiving lisinopril alone, the incidence of syncope was 0.1 percent. The overall incidence of syncope may be reduced by proper titration of the individual components. (See PRECAUTIONS, Drug Interactions, ADVERSE REACTIONS and DOSAGE AND ADMINISTRATION.)

In patients with severe congestive heart failure, with or without associated renal insufficiency, excessive hypotension has been observed and may be associated with oliguria and/or progressive azotemia, and rarely with acute renal failure and/or death. Because of the potential fall in blood pressure in these patients, therapy should be started under very close medical supervision. Such patients should be followed closely for the first two weeks of treatment and whenever the dose of lisinopril and/or diuretic is increased. Similar considerations apply to patients with ischemic heart or cerebrovascular disease in whom an excessive fall in blood pressure could result in a myocardial infarction or cerebrovascular accident.

If hypotension occurs, the patient should be placed in supine position and, if necessary, receive an intravenous infusion of normal saline. A transient hypotensive response is not a contraindication to further doses which usually can be given without difficulty once the blood pressure has increased after volume expansion.

Leukopenia/Neutropenia/Agranulocytosis: Another angiotensin converting enzyme inhibitor, captopril, has been shown to cause agranulocytosis and bone marrow depression, rarely in uncomplicated patients but more frequently in patients with renal impairment, especially if they also have a collagen vascular disease. Available data from clinical trials of lisinopril are insufficient to show that lisinopril does not cause agranulocytosis at similar rates. Marketing experience has revealed rare cases of leukopenia/neutropenia and bone marrow depression in which a causal relationship to lisinopril cannot be excluded. Periodic monitoring of white blood cell counts in patients with collagen vascular disease and renal disease should be considered.

Hepatic Failure: Rarely, ACE inhibitors have been associated with a syndrome that starts with cholestatic jaundice and progresses to fulminant hepatic necrosis and (sometimes) death. The mechanism of this syndrome is not understood. Patients receiving ACE inhibitors who develop jaundice or marked elevations of hepatic enzymes should discontinue the ACE inhibitor and receive appropriate medical follow-up.

Pregnancy

Lisinopril and Hydrochlorothiazide: Teratogenicity studies were conducted in mice and rats with up to 90 mg/kg/day of lisinopril (56 times the maximum recommended human dose) in combination with 10 mg/kg/day of hydrochlorothiazide (2.5 times the maximum recommended human dose). Maternal or fetotoxic effects were not seen in mice with the combination. In rats decreased maternal weight gain and decreased fetal weight occurred down to $^{3}/_{10}$ mg/kg/day (the lowest dose tested). Associated with the decreased fetal weight was a delay in fetal ossification. The decreased fetal weight and delay in fetal ossification were not seen in saline-supplemented animals given 90/10 mg/kg/day.

When used in pregnancy during the second and third trimesters, ACE inhibitors can cause injury and even death to the developing fetus. When pregnancy is detected ZESTORETIC should be discontinued as soon as possible. (See Lisinopril, Fetal/Neonatal Morbidity and Mortality below.)

Lisinopril

Fetal/Neonatal Morbidity and Mortality: ACE inhibitors can cause fetal and neonatal morbidity and death when administered to pregnant women. Several dozen cases have been reported in the world literature. When pregnancy is detected, ACE inhibitor therapy should be discontinued as soon as possible.

The use of ACE inhibitors during the second and third trimesters of pregnancy has been associated with fetal and neonatal injury, including hypotension, neonatal skull hypoplasia, anuria, reversible or irreversible renal failure, and death. Oligohydramnios has also been reported, presumably resulting from decreased fetal renal function; oligohydramnios in this setting has been associated with fetal limb contractures, craniofacial deformation, and hypoplastic lung development. Prematurity, intrauterine growth retardation, and patent ductus arteriosus have also been reported, although it is not clear whether these occurrences were due to the ACE-inhibitor exposure.

These adverse effects do not appear to have resulted from intrauterine ACE-inhibitor exposure that has been limited to the first trimester. Mothers whose embryos and fetuses are exposed to ACE inhibitors only during the first trimester should be so informed. Nonetheless, when patients become pregnant, physicians should make every effort to discontinue the use of ZESTORETIC as soon as possible.

Rarely (probably less often than once in every thousand pregnancies), no alternative to ACE inhibitors will be found. In these rare cases, the mothers should be apprised of the potential hazards to their fetuses, and serial ultrasound examinations should be performed to assess the intraamniotic environment.

If oligohydramnios is observed, ZESTORETIC should be discontinued unless it is considered lifesaving for the mother. Contraction stress testing (CST), a nonstress test (NST), or biophysical profiling (BPP) may be appropriate, depending upon the week of pregnancy. Patients and physicians should be aware, however, that oligohydramnios may not appear until after the fetus has sustained irreversible injury.

Infants with histories of in utero exposure to ACE inhibitors should be closely observed for hypotension, oliguria, and hyperkalemia. If oliguria occurs, attention should be directed toward support of blood pressure and renal perfusion. Exchange transfusion or dialysis may be required as means of reversing hypotension and/or substituting for disordered renal function. Lisinopril, which crosses the placenta, has been removed from neonatal circulation by peritoneal dialysis with some clinical benefit, and theoretically may be removed by exchange transfusion, although there is no experience with the latter procedure.

No teratogenic effects of lisinopril were seen in studies of pregnant rats, mice, and rabbits. On a mg/kg basis, the doses used were up to 625 times (in mice), 188 times (in rats), 0.6 times (in rabbits) the maximum recommended human dose.

Hydrochlorothiazide

Teratogenic Effects: Reproduction studies in the rabbit, the mouse and the rat at doses up to 100 mg/kg/day (50 times the human dose) showed no evidence of external abnormalities of the fetus due to hydrochlorothiazide. Hydrochlorothiazide given in a two-litter study in rats at doses of 4–5.6 mg/kg/day (approximately 1–2 times the usual daily human dose) did not impair fertility or produce birth abnormalities in the offspring. Thiazides cross the placental barrier and appear in cord blood.

Nonteratogenic Effects: These may include fetal or neonatal jaundice, thrombocytopenia, and possibly other adverse reactions have occurred in the adult.

Hydrochlorothiazide

Thiazides should be used with caution in severe renal disease. In patients with renal disease, thiazides may precipitate azotemia. Cumulative effects of the drug may develop in patients with impaired renal function.

Thiazides should be used with caution in patients with impaired hepatic function or progressive liver disease, since minor alterations of fluid and electrolyte balance may precipitate hepatic coma.

Sensitivity reactions may occur in patients with or without a history of allergy or bronchial asthma.

The possibility of exacerbation or activation of systemic lupus erythematosus has been reported.

Lithium generally should not be given with thiazides. (See PRECAUTIONS, Drug Interactions, Lisinopril and Hydrochlorothiazide.)

PRECAUTIONS

General

Lisinopril

Impaired Renal Function: As a consequence of inhibiting the renin-angiotensin-aldosterone system, changes in renal function may be anticipated in susceptible individuals. In patients with severe congestive heart failure whose renal

Continued on next page

Zeneca Pharmaceuticals—Cont.

function may depend on the activity of the renin-angiotensin-aldosterone system, treatment with angiotensin converting enzyme inhibitors, including lisinopril, may be associated with oliguria and/or progressive azotemia and rarely with acute renal failure and/or death.

In hypertensive patients with unilateral or bilateral renal artery stenosis, increases in blood urea nitrogen and serum creatinine may occur. Experience with another angiotensin converting enzyme inhibitor suggests that these increases are usually reversible upon discontinuation of lisinopril and/or diuretic therapy. In such patients renal function should be monitored during the first few weeks of therapy.

Some hypertensive patients with no apparent pre-existing renal vascular disease have developed increases in blood urea and serum creatinine, usually minor and transient, especially when lisinopril has been given concomitantly with a diuretic. This is more likely to occur in patients with pre-existing renal impairment. Dosage reduction of lisinopril and/or discontinuation of the diuretic may be required.

Evaluation of the hypertensive patient should always include assessment of renal function. (See DOSAGE and ADMINISTRATION.)

Hyperkalemia: In clinical trials hyperkalemia (serum potassium greater than 5.7 mEq/L) occurred in approximately 1.4 percent of hypertensive patients treated with lisinopril plus hydrochlorothiazide. In most cases these were isolated values which resolved despite continued therapy. Hyperkalemia was not a cause of discontinuation of therapy. Risk factors for the development of hyperkalemia include renal insufficiency, diabetes mellitus, and the concomitant use of potassium-sparing diuretics, potassium supplements and/or potassium-containing salt substitutes, which should be used cautiously if at all with ZESTORETIC. (See Drug Interactions.)

Cough: Presumably due to the inhibition of the degradation of endogenous bradykinin, persistent nonproductive cough has been reported with all ACE inhibitors, almost always resolving after discontinuation of therapy. ACE inhibitor-induced cough should be considered in the differential diagnosis of cough.

Surgery/Anesthesia: In patients undergoing major surgery or during anesthesia with agents that produce hypotension, lisinopril may block angiotensin II formation secondary to compensatory renin release. If hypotension occurs and is considered to be due to this mechanism, it can be corrected by volume expansion.

Hydrochlorothiazide

Periodic determination of serum electrolytes to detect possible electrolyte imbalance should be performed at appropriate intervals.

All patients receiving thiazide therapy should be observed for clinical signs of fluid or electrolyte imbalance: namely, hyponatremia, hypochloremic alkalosis, and hypokalemia. Serum and urine electrolyte determinations are particularly important when the patient is vomiting excessively or receiving parenteral fluids. Warning signs or symptoms of fluid and electrolyte imbalance, irrespective of cause, include dryness of mouth, thirst, weakness, lethargy, drowsiness, restlessness, confusion, seizures, muscle pains or cramps, muscular fatigue hypotension, oliguria, tachycardia, and gastrointestinal disturbances such as nausea and vomiting.

Hypokalemia may develop, especially with brisk diuresis, when severe cirrhosis is present, or after prolonged therapy. Interference with adequate oral electrolyte intake will also contribute to hypokalemia. Hypokalemia may cause cardiac arrhythmia and may also sensitize or exaggerate the response of the heart to the toxic effects of digitalis (eg, increased ventricular irritability). Because lisinopril reduces the production of aldosterone, concomitant therapy with lisinopril attenuates the diuretic-induced potassium loss. (See Drug Interactions, Agents Increasing Serum Potassium.)

Although any chloride deficit is generally mild and usually does not require specific treatment, except under extraordinary circumstances (as in liver disease or renal disease), chloride replacement may be required in the treatment of metabolic alkalosis.

Dilutional hyponatremia may occur in edematous patients in hot weather; appropriate therapy is water restriction, rather than administration of salt except in rare instances when the hyponatremia is life-threatening. In actual salt depletion, appropriate replacement is the therapy of choice.

Hyperuricemia may occur or frank gout may be precipitated in certain patients receiving thiazide therapy.

In diabetic patients dosage adjustments of insulin or oral hypoglycemic agents may be required. Hyperglycemia may occur with thiazide diuretics. Thus latent diabetes mellitus may become manifest during thiazide therapy.

The antihypertensive effects of the drug may be enhanced in the postsympathectomy patient.

If progressive renal impairment becomes evident consider withholding or discontinuing diuretic therapy.

Thiazides have been shown to increase the urinary excretion of magnesium; this may result in hypomagnesemia.

Thiazides may decrease urinary calcium excretion. Thiazides may cause intermittent and slight elevation of serum calcium in the absence of known disorders of calcium metabolism. Marked hypercalcemia may be evidence of hidden hyperparathyroidism. Thiazides should be discontinued before carrying out tests for parathyroid function.

Increases in cholesterol and triglyceride levels may be associated with thiazide diuretic therapy.

Information for Patients

Angioedema: Angioedema, including laryngeal edema, may occur at any time during treatment with angiotensin converting enzyme inhibitors, including ZESTORETIC. Patients should be so advised and told to report immediately any signs or symptoms suggesting angioedema (swelling of face, extremities, eyes, lips, tongue, difficulty in swallowing or breathing) and to take no more drug until they have consulted with the prescribing physician.

Symptomatic Hypotension: Patients should be cautioned to report lightheadedness especially during the first few days of therapy. If actual syncope occurs, the patients should be told to discontinue the drug until they have consulted with the prescribing physician.

All patients should be cautioned that excessive perspiration and dehydration may lead to an excessive fall in blood pressure because of reduction in fluid volume. Other causes of volume depletion such as vomiting or diarrhea may also lead to a fall in blood pressure; patients should be advised to consult with their physician.

Hyperkalemia: Patients should be told not to use salt substitutes containing potassium without consulting their physician.

Leukopenia/Neutropenia: Patients should be told to report promptly any indication of infection (eg, sore throat, fever) which may be a sign of leukopenia/neutropenia.

Pregnancy: Female patients of childbearing age should be told about the consequences of second- and third-trimester exposure to ACE inhibitors, and they should also be told that these consequences do not appear to have resulted from intrauterine ACE-inhibitor exposure that has been limited to the first trimester. These patients should be asked to report pregnancies to their physicians as soon as possible.

NOTE: As with many other drugs, certain advice to patients being treated with ZESTORETIC is warranted. This information is intended to aid in the safe and effective use of this medication. It is not a disclosure of all possible adverse or intended effects.

Drug Interactions

Lisinopril

Hypotension—Patients on Diuretic Therapy: Patients on diuretics and especially those in whom diuretic therapy was recently instituted, may occasionally experience an excessive reduction of blood pressure after initiation of therapy with lisinopril. The possibility of hypotensive effects with lisinopril can be minimized by either discontinuing the diuretic or increasing the salt intake prior to initiation of treatment with lisinopril. If it is necessary to continue the diuretic, initiate therapy with lisinopril at a dose of 5 mg daily, and provide close medical supervision after the initial dose for at least two hours and until blood pressure has stabilized for at least an additional hour. (See WARNINGS, and DOSAGE AND ADMINISTRATION.) When a diuretic is added to the therapy of a patient receiving lisinopril, an additional antihypertensive effect is usually observed. (See DOSAGE AND ADMINISTRATION.)

Indomethacin: In a study in 36 patients with mild to moderate hypertension where the antihypertensive effects of lisinopril alone were compared to lisinopril given concomitantly with indomethacin, the use of indomethacin was associated with a reduced effect, although the difference between the two regimens was not significant.

Other Agents: Lisinopril has been used concomitantly with nitrates and/or digoxin without evidence of clinically significant adverse interactions. No meaningful clinically important pharmacokinetic interactions occurred when lisinopril was used concomitantly with propranolol, digoxin, or hydrochlorothiazide. The presence of food in the stomach does not alter the bioavailability of lisinopril.

Agents Increasing Serum Potassium: Lisinopril attenuates potassium loss caused by thiazide-type diuretics. Use of lisinopril with potassium-sparing diuretics (eg, spironolactone, triamterene, or amiloride), potassium supplements, or potassium-containing salt substitutes may lead to significant increases in serum potassium. Therefore, if concomitant use of these agents is indicated, because of demonstrated hypokalemia, they should be used with caution and with frequent monitoring of serum potassium.

Lithium: Lithium toxicity has been reported in patients receiving lithium concomitantly with drugs which cause elimination of sodium, including ACE inhibitors. Lithium toxicity was usually reversible upon discontinuation of lithium and the ACE inhibitor. It is recommended that serum lithium levels be monitored frequently if lisinopril is administered concomitantly with lithium.

Hydrochlorothiazide

When administered concurrently the following drugs may interact with thiazide diuretics.

Alcohol, barbiturates, or narcotics—potentiation of orthostatic hypotension may occur.

Antidiabetic drugs (oral agents and insulin)—dosage adjustment of the antidiabetic drug may be required.

Other antihypertensive drugs—additive effect or potentiation.

Cholestyramine and colestipol resins- Absorbtion of hydrochlorothiazide is impaired in the presence of anionic exchange resins. Single doses of either cholestyramine or colestipol resins bind the hydrochlorothiazide and reduce its absorption from the gastrointestinal tract by up to 85 and 43 percent, respectively.

Corticosteroids, ACTH—intensified electrolyte depletion, particularly hypokalemia.

Pressor amines (eg, norepinephrine)—possible decreased response to pressor amines but not sufficient to preclude their use.

Skeletal muscle relaxants, nondepolarizing (eg, tubocurarine)—possible increased responsiveness to the muscle relaxant.

Lithium—should not generally be given with diuretics. Diuretic agents reduce the renal clearance of lithium and add a high risk of lithium toxicity. Refer to the package insert for lithium preparations before use of such preparations with ZESTORETIC.

Non-Steroidal Anti-inflammatory Drugs—In some patients, the administration of a non-steroidal anti-inflammatory agent can reduce the diuretic, natriuretic, and antihypertensive effects of loop, potassium-sparing and thiazide diuretics. Therefore, when ZESTORETIC and non-steroidal anti-inflammatory agents are used concomitantly, the patient should be observed closely to determine if the desired effect of ZESTORETIC is obtained.

Carcinogenesis, Mutagenesis, Impairment of Fertility

Lisinopril and Hydrochlorothiazide: Lisinopril in combination with hydrochlorothiazide was not mutagenic in a microbial mutagen test using *Salmonella typhimurium* (Ames test) or *Escherichia coli* with or without metabolic activation or in a forward mutation assay using Chinese hamster lung cells. Lisinopril and hydrochlorothiazide did not produce DNA single strand breaks in an *in vitro* alkaline elution rat hepatocyte assay. In addition, it did not produce increases in chromosomal aberrations in an *in vitro* test in Chinese hamster ovary cells or in an *in vivo* study in mouse bone marrow.

Lisinopril: There was no evidence of a tumorigenic effect when lisinopril was administered for 105 weeks to male and female rats at doses up to 90 mg/kg/day (about 56 or 9 times* the maximum daily human dose, based on body weight and body surface area respectively). There was no evidence of carcinogenicity when lisinopril was administered for 92 weeks to (male and female) mice at doses up to 135 mg/kg/day (about 84 times* the maximum recommended daily human dose). This dose was 6.8 times the maximum human dose based on body surface area in mice.

*Calculations assume a human weight of 50 kg and human body surface area of 1.62 m^2.

Lisinopril was not mutagenic in the Ames microbial mutagen test with or without metabolic activation. It was also negative in a forward mutation assay using Chinese hamster lung cells. Lisinopril did not produce single strand DNA breaks in an *in vitro* alkaline elution rat hepatocyte assay. In addition, lisinopril did not produce increases in chromosomal aberrations in an *in vitro* test in Chinese hamster ovary cells or in an *in vivo* study in mouse bone marrow.

There were no adverse effects on reproductive performance in male and female rats treated with up to 300 mg/kg/day of lisinopril. This dose is 188 times and 30 times the maximum daily human dose based on mg/kg and mg/m^2, respectively.

Hydrochlorothiazide: Two-year feeding studies in mice and rats conducted under the auspices of the National Toxicology Program (NTP) uncovered no evidence of a carcinogenic potential of hydrochlorothiazide in female mice (at doses of up to approximately 600 mg/kg/day) or in male and female rats (at doses of up to approximately 100 mg/kg/day). These doses are 150 times and 12 times for mice and 25 times and 4 times for rats the maximum human daily dose based on mg/kg and mg/m^2, respectively. The NTP, however, found equivocal evidence for hepatocarcinogenicity in male mice.

Hydrochlorothiazide was not genotoxic *in vitro* in the Ames mutagenicity assay of *Salmonella typhimurium* strains TA 98, TA 100, TA 1535, TA 1537, and TA 1538 and in the Chinese Hamster Ovary (CHO) test for chromosomal aberrations, or *in vivo* in assays using mouse germinal cell chromosomes. Chinese hamster bone marrow chromosomes, and the *Drosophila* sex-linked recessive lethal trait gene. Positive test results were obtained only in the *in vitro* CHO Sister Chromatid Exchange (clastogenicity) and in the Mouse Lymphoma Cell (mutagenicity) assays, using concentrations of hydrochlorothiazide from 43 to 1300 μg/mL, and in the

Aspergillus nidulans nondisjunction assay at an unspecified concentration.

Hydrochlorothiazide had no adverse effects on the fertility of mice and rats of either sex in studies wherein these species were exposed, via their diet, to doses of up to 100 and 4 mg/kg, respectively, prior to conception and throughout gestation. In mice this dose is 25 times and 2 times the maximum daily human dose based on mg/kg and mg/m^2, respectively. In rats this dose is 1 times and 0.2 times the maximum daily human dose based on mg/kg and mg/m^2, respectively.

Pregnancy

Pregnancy Categories C (first trimester) and D (second and third trimesters). See WARNINGS, Pregnancy, Lisinopril, Fetal/Neonatal Morbidity and Mortality.

Nursing Mothers

It is not known whether lisinopril is excreted in human milk. However, milk of lactating rats contains radioactivity following administration of ^{14}C lisinopril. In another study, lisinopril was present in rat milk at levels similar to plasma levels in the dams. Thiazides do appear in human milk. Because of the potential for serious adverse reactions in nursing infants from ACE inhibitors and hydrochlorothiazide, a decision should be made whether to discontinue nursing and/or discontinue ZESTORETIC, taking into account the importance of the drug to the mother.

Pediatric Use

Safety and effectiveness in children have not been established.

ADVERSE REACTIONS

ZESTORETIC has been evaluated for safety in 930 patients including 100 patients treated for 50 weeks or more.

In clinical trials with ZESTORETIC no adverse experiences peculiar to this combination drug have been observed. Adverse experiences that have occurred have been limited to those that have been previously reported with lisinopril or hydrochlorothiazide.

The most frequent clinical adverse experiences in controlled trials (including open label extensions) with any combination of lisinopril and hydrochlorothiazide were: dizziness (7.5%), headache (5.2%), cough (3.9%), fatigue (3.7%) and orthostatic effects (3.2%) all of which were more common than in placebo-treated patients. Generally, adverse experiences were mild and transient in nature, but see WARNINGS regarding angioedema and excessive hypotension or syncope. Discontinuation of therapy due to adverse effects was required in 4.4% of patients principally because of dizziness, cough, fatigue and muscle cramps.

Adverse experiences occurring in greater than one percent of patients treated with lisinopril plus hydrochlorothiazide in controlled clinical trials are shown below.

Percent of Patients in Controlled Studies

	Lisinopril and Hydrochlorothiazide (n=930) Incidence (discontinuation)		Placebo (n=207) Incidence
Dizziness	7.5	(0.8)	1.9
Headache	5.2	(0.3)	1.9
Cough	3.9	(0.6)	1.0
Fatigue	3.7	(0.4)	1.0
Orthostatic Effects	3.2	(0.1)	1.0
Diarrhea	2.5	(0.2)	2.4
Nausea	2.2	(0.1)	2.4
Upper Respiratory Infection	2.2	(0.0)	0.0
Muscle Cramps	2.0	(0.4)	0.5
Asthenia	1.8	(0.2)	1.0
Paresthesia	1.5	(0.1)	0.0
Hypotension	1.4	(0.3)	0.5
Vomiting	1.4	(0.1)	0.5
Dyspepsia	1.3	(0.0)	0.0
Rash	1.2	(0.1)	0.5
Impotence	1.2	(0.3)	0.0

Clinical adverse experiences occurring in 0.3% to 1.0% of patients in controlled trials included:

Body as a Whole: Chest pain, abdominal pain, syncope, chest discomfort, fever, trauma, virus infection. **Cardiovascular:** Palpitation, orthostatic hypotension. **Digestive:** Gastrointestinal cramps, dry mouth, constipation, heartburn. **Musculoskeletal:** Back pain, shoulder pain, knee pain, back strain, myalgia, foot pain. **Nervous/Psychiatric:** Decreased libido, vertigo, depression, somnolence. **Respiratory:** Common cold, nasal congestion, influenza, bronchitis, pharyngeal pain, dyspnea, pulmonary congestion, chronic sinusitis, allergic rhinitis, pharyngeal discomfort. **Skin:** Flushing, pruritus, skin inflammation, diaphoresis. **Special Senses:** Blurred vision, tinnitus, otalgia. **Urogenital:** Urinary tract infection.

Angioedema: Angioedema of the face, extremities, lips, tongue, glottis and/or larynx has been reported rarely. (See WARNINGS.)

Hypotension: In clinical trials, adverse effects relating to hypotension occurred as follows: hypotension (1.4%), orthostatic hypotension (0.5%), other orthostatic effects (3.2%). In addition syncope occurred in 0.8% of patients. (See WARNINGS.)

Cough: See PRECAUTIONS-Cough.

Clinical Laboratory Test Findings

Serum Electrolytes: (See PRECAUTIONS.)

Creatinine, Blood Urea Nitrogen: Minor reversible increases in blood urea nitrogen and serum creatinine were observed in patients with essential hypertension treated with ZESTORETIC. More marked increases have also been reported and were more likely to occur in patients with renal artery stenosis. (See PRECAUTIONS.)

Serum Uric Acid, Glucose, Magnesium, Cholesterol, Triglycerides and Calcium: (See PRECAUTIONS).

Hemoglobin and Hematocrit: Small decreases in hemoglobin and hematocrit (mean decreases of approximately 0.5 g% and 1.5 vol%, respectively) occurred frequently in hypertensive patients treated with ZESTORETIC but were rarely of clinical importance unless another cause of anemia coexisted. In clinical trials, 0.4% of patients discontinued therapy due to anemia.

Liver Function Tests: Rarely, elevations of liver enzymes and/or serum bilirubin have occurred. (See WARNINGS, Hepatic Failure.)

Other adverse reactions that have been reported with the individual components are listed below:

Lisinopril—In clinical trials adverse reactions which occurred with lisinopril were also seen with ZESTORETIC. In addition, and since lisinopril has been marketed, the following adverse reactions have been reported with lisinopril and should be considered potential adverse reactions for ZESTORETIC: **Body as a Whole:** Anaphylactoid reactions (see WARNINGS, Anaphylactoid Reactions During Membrane Exposure), malaise, edema, facial edema, pain, pelvic pain, flank pain, chills; **Cardiovascular:** Cardiac arrest, myocardial infarction or cerebrovascular accident, possibly secondary to excessive hypotension in high risk patients (see WARNINGS, Hypotension), pulmonary embolism and infarction, worsening of heart failure, arrhythmias (including tachycardia, ventricular tachycardia, atrial tachycardia, atrial fibrillation, bradycardia, and premature ventricular contractions), angina pectoris, transient ischemic attacks, paroxysmal nocturnal dyspnea, decreased blood pressure, peripheral edema, vasculitis; **Digestive:** Pancreatitis, hepatitis (hepatocellular or cholestatic jaundice) (see WARNINGS, Hepatic Failure), gastritis, anorexia, flatulence, increased salivation; **Endocrine:** Diabetes mellitus; **Hematologic:** Rare cases of bone marrow depression, hemolytic anemia, leukopenia/Neutropenia, and thrombocytopenia, have been reported in which a casual relationship to lisinopril can not be excluded; **Metabolic:** Gout, weight loss, dehydration, fluid overload, weight gain; **Musculoskeletal:** Arthritis, arthralgia, neck pain, hip pain, joint pain, leg pain, arm pain, lumbago; **Nervous System/Psychiatric:** Ataxia, memory impairment, tremor, insomnia, stroke, nervousness, confusion, peripheral neuropathy (eg, paresthesia, dysesthesia), spasm, hypersomnia, irritability; **Respiratory:** Malignant lung neoplasms, hemoptysis, pulmonary edema, pulmonary infiltrates, bronchospasm, asthma, pleural effusion, pneumonia, wheezing, orthopnea, painful respiration, epistaxis, laryngitis, sinusitis, pharyngitis, rhinitis, rhinorrhea, chest sound abnormalities; **Skin:** Urticaria, alopecia, herpes zoster, photosensitivity, skin lesions, skin infections, pemphigus, erythema, rare cases of other severe skin reactions including toxic epidermal necrolysis and Stevens-Johnson syndrome, (causal relationship has not been established); **Special Senses:** Visual loss, diplopia, photophobia, taste alteration; **Urogenital:** Acute renal failure, oliguria, anuria, uremia, progressive azotemia, renal dysfunction (see PRECAUTIONS and DOSAGE AND ADMINISTRATION), pyelonephritis, dysuria, breast pain.

Miscellaneous: A symptom complex has been reported which may include a positive ANA, an elevated erythrocyte sedimentation rate, arthralgia/arthritis, myalgia, fever, vasculitis, eosinophilia and leukocytosis. Rash, photosensitivity or other dermatological manifestations may occur alone or in combination with these symptoms.

Fetal/Neonatal Morbidity and Mortality

See WARNINGS—Pregnancy, Lisinopril, Fetal/Neonatal Morbidity and Mortality.

Hydrochlorothiazide—Body as a Whole: Weakness **Digestive:** Anorexia, gastric irritation, cramping, jaundice (intrahepatic cholestatic jaundice) (see WARNINGS, Hepatic Failure), pancreatitis, sialoadenitis, constipation; **Hematologic:** Leukopenia, agranulocytosis, thrombocytopenia, aplastic anemia, hemolytic anemia; **Musculoskeletal:** Muscle spasm; **Nervous System/Psychiatric:** Restlessness; **Renal:** Renal failure, renal dysfunction, interstitial nephritis (see WARNINGS): **Skin:** Erythema multiforme including Stevens-Johnson syndrome, exfoliative dermatitis including toxic epidermal necrolysis, alopecia; **Special Senses:** Xanthopsia; **Hypersensitivity:** Purpura, photosensitivity, urticaria, necrotizing angitis (vasculitis and cutaneous vasculitis), respiratory distress including pneumonitis and pulmonary edema, anaphylactic reactions.

OVERDOSAGE

No specific information is available on the treatment of overdosage with ZESTORETIC. Treatment is symptomatic and supportive. Therapy with ZESTORETIC should be discontinued and the patient observed closely. Suggested measures include induction of emesis and/or gastric lavage, and correction of dehydration, electrolyte imbalance and hypotension by established procedures.

Lisinopril: Following a single oral dose of 20 g/kg no lethality occurred in rats and death occurred in one of 20 mice receiving the same dose. The most likely manifestation of overdosage would be hypotension, for which the usual treatment would be intravenous infusion of normal saline solution.

Lisinopril can be removed by hemodialysis.

Hydrochlorothiazide: Oral administration of a single oral dose of 10 g/kg to mice and rats was not lethal. The most common signs and symptoms observed are those caused by electrolyte depletion (hypokalemia, hypochloremia, hyponatremia) and dehydration resulting from excessive diuresis. If digitalis has also been administered, hypokalemia may accentuate cardiac arrhythmias.

DOSAGE AND ADMINISTRATION

Lisinopril monotherapy is an effective treatment of hypertension in once-daily doses of 10-80 mg, while hydrochlorothiazide monotherapy is effective in doses of 25-100 mg. In clinical trials of lisinopril/hydrochlorothiazide combination therapy using lisinopril doses of 10-80 mg and hydrochlorothiazide doses of 6.25-50 mg, the antihypertensive response rates generally increased with increasing dose of either component.

The side effects (see WARNINGS) of lisinopril are generally rare and apparently independent of dose; those of hydrochlorothiazide are a mixture of dose-dependent phenomena (primarily hypokalemia) and dose-independent phenomena (eg., pancreatitis), the former much more common than the latter. Therapy with any combination of lisinopril and hydrochlorothiazide may be associated with either or both dose-independent or dose-dependent side effects, but addition of lisinopril in clinical trials blunted the hypokalemia normally seen with diuretics.

To minimize dose-dependent side effects, it is usually appropriate to begin combination therapy only after a patient has failed to achieve the desired effect with monotherapy.

Dose Titration Guided by Clinical Effect: A patient whose blood pressure is not adequately controlled with either lisinopril or hydrochlorothiazide monotherapy may be switched to lisinopril/HCTZ 10/12.5 or lisinopril/HCTZ 20/12.5, depending on current monotherapy dose. Further increases of either or both components should depend on clinical response with blood pressure measured at the interdosing interval to ensure that there is an adequate antihypertensive effect at that time. The hydrochlorothiazide dose should generally not be increased until 2-3 weeks have elapsed. After addition of the diuretic it may be possible to reduce the dose of lisinopril. Patients whose blood pressures are adequately controlled with 25 mg of daily hydrochlorothiazide, but who experience significant potassium loss with this regimen may achieve similar or greater blood-pressure control without electrolyte disturbance if they are switched to lisinopril/HCTZ 10/12.5.

In patients who are currrently being treated with a diuretic, symptomatic hypotension occasionally may occur following the initial dose of lisinopril. The diuretic should, if possible, be discontinued for two to three days before beginning therapy with lisinopril to reduce the likelihood of hypotension. (See WARNINGS.) If the patient's blood pressure is not controlled with lisinopril alone, diuretic therapy may be resumed.

If the diuretic cannot be discontinued, an initial dose of 5 mg of lisinopril should be used under medical supervision for at least two hours and until blood pressure has stabilized for at least an additional hour. (See WARNINGS AND PRECAUTIONS, Drug Interactions.)

Concomitant administration of ZESTORETIC with potassium supplements, potassium salt substitutes or potassium-sparing diuretics may lead to increases of serum potassium. (See PRECAUTIONS.)

Replacement Therapy: The combination may be substituted for the titrated individual components.

Use in Elderly: In general, blood pressure response and adverse experiences were similar in younger and older patients given ZESTORETIC. However, in a multiple dose pharmacokinetic study in elderly versus young patients using the lisinopril/hydrochlorothiazide combination, area under the plasma concentration time curve (AUC) increased approximately 120% for lisinopril and approximately 80% for hydrochlorothiazide in older patients. Therefore, dosage adjustments in elderly patients should be made with particular caution.

Use in Renal Impairment: Regimens of therapy with lisinopril/HCTZ need not take account of renal function as long as

Continued on next page

Zeneca Pharmaceuticals—Cont.

the patient's creatinine clearance is >30 mL/min/1.7m^2 (serum creatinine roughly ≤ 3 mg/dL or 265 μmol/L). In patients with more severe renal impairment, loop diuretics are preferred to thiazides, so lisinopril/HCTZ is not recommended (see WARNINGS, Anaphylactoid Reactions During Membrane Exposure).

HOW SUPPLIED

ZESTORETIC 10-12.5 Tablets (NDC 0310-0141) Peach, round, biconvex, uncoated tablets identified with "141" debossed on one side and "ZESTORETIC" on the other side are supplied in bottles of 100 tablets.

ZESTORETIC 20-12.5 Tablets (NDC 0310-0142) White, round, biconvex, uncoated tablets identified with "142" debossed on one side and "ZESTORETIC" on the other side are supplied in bottles of 100 tablets.

ZESTORETIC 20-25 Tablets (NDC 0310-0145) Peach, round, biconvex, uncoated tablets identified with "145" debossed on one side and "ZESTORETIC" on the other side are supplied in bottles of 100 tablets.

Store at controlled room temperature, 15°-30° C (59°-86° F). Protect from excessive light and humidity.

¶Registered trademark of Hospal Ltd.

Manufactured by: IPR Pharmaceuticals Inc.

Distributed by:

ZENECA PHARMACEUTICALS

A Business Unit of Zeneca Inc.

Wilmington, DE 19850-5437

SIC 64084-00 Rev H 11/95

Shown in Product Identification Guide, page 342

ONCE-DAILY

ZESTRIL® LISINOPRIL ℞

> **USE IN PREGNANCY**
>
> **When used in pregnancy during the second and third trimesters, ACE inhibitors can cause injury and even death to the developing fetus.** When pregnancy is detected, ZESTRIL should be discontinued as soon as possible. See WARNINGS, Fetal/Neonatal Morbidity and Mortality.

DESCRIPTION

Lisinopril is an oral long-acting angiotensin converting enzyme inhibitor. Lisinopril, a synthetic peptide derivative, is chemically described as (S)-1-[N^2-(1-Carboxy-3-phenylpropyl)-L-lysyl]-L-proline dihydrate. Its empirical formula is $C_{21}H_{31}N_3O_5 \cdot 2H_2O$ and its structural formula is:

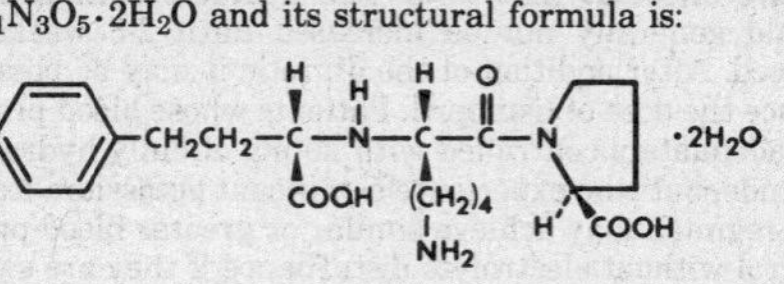

Lisinopril is a white to off-white, crystalline powder, with a molecular weight of 441.53. It is soluble in water and sparingly soluble in methanol and practically insoluble in ethanol.

ZESTRIL is supplied as 2.5 mg, 5 mg, 10 mg, 20 mg and 40 mg tablets for oral administration.

Inactive Ingredients:

2.5 mg tablets—calcium phosphate, magnesium stearate, mannitol, starch.

5, 10 and 20 mg tablets—calcium phosphate, magnesium stearate, mannitol, red ferric oxide, starch.

40 mg tablets—calcium phosphate, magnesium stearate, mannitol, starch, yellow ferric oxide.

CLINICAL PHARMACOLOGY

Mechanism of Action: Lisinopril inhibits angiotensin converting enzyme (ACE) in human subjects and animals. ACE is a peptidyl dipeptidase that catalyzes the conversion of angiotensin I to the vasoconstrictor substance, angiotensin II. Angiotensin II also stimulates aldosterone secretion by the adrenal cortex. The beneficial effects of lisinopril in hypertension and heart failure appear to result primarily from suppression of the renin-angiotensin-aldosterone system. Inhibition of ACE results in decreased plasma angiotensin II which leads to decreased vasopressor activity and to decreased aldosterone secretion. The latter decrease may result in a small increase of serum potassium. In hypertensive patients with normal renal function treated with ZESTRIL alone for up to 24 weeks, the mean increase in serum potassium was approximately 0.1 mEq/L; however, approximately 15% of patients had increases greater than 0.5 mEq/L and approximately 6% had a decrease greater than 0.5 mEq/L. In the same study, patients treated with ZESTRIL and hydrochlorothiazide for up to 24 weeks had a mean decrease in serum potassium of 0.1 mEq/L; approximately 4% of patients had increases greater than 0.5 mEq/L and approximately 12% had a decrease greater than 0.5 mEq/L. (See PRECAUTIONS.) Removal of angiotensin II negative feedback on renin secretion leads to increased plasma renin activity.

ACE is identical to kininase, an enzyme that degrades bradykinin. Whether increased levels of bradykinin, a potent vasodepressor peptide, play a role in the therapeutic effects of ZESTRIL remains to be elucidated.

While the mechanism through which ZESTRIL lowers blood pressure is believed to be primarily suppression of the renin-angiotensin-aldosterone system, ZESTRIL is antihypertensive even in patients with low-renin hypertension. Although ZESTRIL was antihypertensive in all races studied, black hypertensive patients (usually a low-renin hypertensive population) had a smaller average response to monotherapy than nonblack patients.

Concomitant administration of ZESTRIL and hydrochlorothiazide further reduced blood pressure in black and nonblack patients and any racial differences in blood pressure response were no longer evident.

Pharmacokinetics and Metabolism: Following oral administration of ZESTRIL, peak serum concentrations of lisinopril occur within about 7 hours, although there was a trend to a small delay in time taken to reach peak serum concentrations in acute myocardial infarction patients. Declining serum concentrations exhibit a prolonged terminal phase which does not contribute to drug accumulation. This terminal phase probably represents saturable binding to ACE and is not proportional to dose.

Lisinopril does not appear to be bound to other serum proteins. Lisinopril does not undergo metabolism and is excreted unchanged entirely in the urine. Based on urinary recovery, the mean extent of absorption of lisinopril is approximately 25%, with large intersubject variability (6%-60%) at all doses tested (5-80 mg). Lisinopril absorption is not influenced by the presence of food in the gastrointestinal tract. The absolute bioavailability of lisinopril is reduced to 16% in patients with stable NYHA Class II-IV congestive heart failure, and the volume of distribution appears to be slightly smaller than that in normal subjects. The oral bioavailability of lisinopril in patients with acute myocardial infarction is similar to that in healthy volunteers.

Upon multiple dosing, lisinopril exhibits an effective half-life of accumulation of 12 hours.

Impaired renal function decreases elimination of lisinopril, which is excreted principally through the kidneys, but this decrease becomes clinically important only when the glomerular filtration rate is below 30 mL/min. Above this glomerular filtration rate, the elimination half-life is little changed. With greater impairment, however, peak and trough lisinopril levels increase, time to peak concentration increases and time to attain steady state is prolonged. Older patients, on average, have (approximately doubled) higher blood levels and the area under the plasma concentration time curve (AUC) than younger patients. (See DOSAGE AND ADMINISTRATION.) Lisinopril can be removed by hemodialysis.

Studies in rats indicate that lisinopril crosses the blood-brain barrier poorly. Multiple doses of lisinopril in rats do not result in accumulation in any tissues. Milk of lactating rats contains radioactivity following administration of ^{14}C lisinopril. By whole body autoradiography, radioactivity was found in the placenta following administration of labeled drug to pregnant rats, but none was found in the fetuses.

Pharmacodynamics and Clinical Effects

Hypertension: Administration of ZESTRIL to patients with hypertension results in a reduction of both supine and standing blood pressure to about the same extent with no compensatory tachycardia. Symptomatic postural hypotension is usually not observed although it can occur and should be anticipated in volume and/or salt-depleted patients. (See WARNINGS.) When given together with thiazide-type diuretics, the blood pressure lowering effects of the two drugs are approximately additive.

In most patients studied, onset of antihypertensive activity was seen at one hour after oral administration of an individual dose of ZESTRIL, with peak reduction of blood pressure achieved by 6 hours. Although an antihypertensive effect was observed 24 hours after dosing with recommended single daily doses, the effect was more consistent and the mean effect was considerably larger in some studies with doses of 20 mg or more than with lower doses. However, at all doses studied, the mean antihypertensive effect was substantially smaller 24 hours after dosing than it was 6 hours after dosing.

In some patients achievement of optimal blood pressure reduction may require two to four weeks of therapy.

The antihypertensive effects of ZESTRIL are maintained during long-term therapy. Abrupt withdrawal of ZESTRIL has not been associated with a rapid increase in blood pressure, or a significant increase in blood pressure compared to pretreatment levels.

Two dose-response studies utilizing a once daily regimen were conducted in 438 mild to moderate hypertensive patients not on a diuretic. Blood pressure was measured 24 hours after dosing. An antihypertensive effect of ZESTRIL was seen with 5 mg in some patients. However, in both studies blood pressure reduction occurred sooner and was greater in patients treated with 10, 20 or 80 mg of ZESTRIL. In controlled clinical studies, ZESTRIL 20-80 mg has been compared in patients with mild to moderate hypertension to hydrochlorothiazide 12.5-50 mg and with atenolol 50-200 mg; and in patients with moderate to severe hypertension to metoprolol 100-200 mg. It was superior to hydrochlorothiazide in effects on systolic and diastolic pressure in a population that was ¾ caucasian. ZESTRIL was approximately equivalent to atenolol and metoprolol in effects on diastolic blood pressure, and had somewhat greater effects on systolic blood pressure.

ZESTRIL had similar effectiveness and adverse effects in younger and older (>65 years) patients. It was less effective in blacks than in caucasians.

In hemodynamic studies in patients with essential hypertension, blood pressure reduction was accompanied by a reduction in peripheral arterial resistance with little or no change in cardiac output and in heart rate. In a study in nine hypertensive patients, following administration of ZESTRIL, there was an increase in mean renal blood flow that was not significant. Data from several small studies are inconsistent with respect to the effect of lisinopril on glomerular filtration rate in hypertensive patients with normal renal function, but suggest that changes, if any, are not large.

In patients with renovascular hypertension ZESTRIL has been shown to be well tolerated and effective in controlling blood pressure. (See PRECAUTIONS.)

Heart Failure: During baseline-controlled clinical trials, in patients receiving digitalis and diuretics, single doses of ZESTRIL resulted in decreases in pulmonary capillary wedge pressure, systemic vascular resistance and blood pressure accompanied by an increase in cardiac output and no change in heart rate.

In two placebo controlled, 12-week clinical studies, ZESTRIL as adjunctive therapy to digitalis and diuretics improved the following signs and symptoms due to congestive heart failure: edema, rales, paroxysmal nocturnal dyspnea and jugular venous distention. In one of the studies, beneficial response was also noted for: orthopnea, presence of third heart sound and the number of patients classified as NYHA Class III and IV. Exercise tolerance was also improved in this study. The effect of lisinopril on mortality in patients with heart failure has not been evaluated.

Acute Myocardial Infarction: The Gruppo Italiano per lo Studio della Sopravvienza nell'Infarto Miocardico (GISSI-3) study was a multicenter, controlled, randomized, unblinded clinical trial conducted in 19,394 patients with acute myocardial infarction admitted to a coronary care unit. It was designed to examine the effects of short-term (6 week) treatment with lisinopril, nitrates, their combination, or no therapy on short-term (6 week) mortality and on longer-term death and markedly impaired cardiac function. Patients presenting within 24 hours of the onset of symptoms who were hemodynamically stable were randomized, in a 2×2 factorial design, to six weeks of either 1) ZESTRIL alone (n=4841), 2) nitrates alone (n=4869), 3) ZESTRIL plus nitrates (n=4841), or 4) open control (n=4843). All patients received routine therapies, including thrombolytics (72%), aspirin (84%), and a beta-blocker (31%), as appropriate, normally utilized in acute myocardial infarction (MI) patients.

The protocol excluded patients with hypotension (systolic blood pressure ≤ 100 mmHg), severe heart failure, cardiogenic shock, and renal dysfunction (serum creatinine >2 mg/dL and/or proteinuria >500 mg/24h). Doses of ZESTRIL were adjusted as necessary according to protocol (see DOSAGE AND ADMINISTRATION).

Study treatment was withdrawn at six weeks except where clinical conditions indicated continuation of treatment.

The primary outcomes of the trial were the overall mortality at 6 weeks and a combined endpoint at 6 months after the myocardial infarction, consisting of a number of patients who died, had late (day 4) clinical congestive heart failure, or had extensive left ventricular damage defined as ejection fraction $\leq 35\%$ or an akinetic-dyskinetic [A-D] score $\geq 45\%$. Patients receiving ZESTRIL (n=9646), alone or with nitrates, had an 11% lower risk of death (2p [two-tailed] =0.04) compared to patients receiving no ZESTRIL (n=9672) (6.4% vs. 7.2%, respectively) at six weeks. Although patients randomized to receive ZESTRIL for up to six weeks also fared numerically better on the combined endpoint at 6 months, the open nature of the assessment of heart failure, substantial loss to follow-up echocardiography, and substantial excess use of lisinopril between 6 weeks and 6 months in the group randomized to 6 weeks of lisinopril, preclude any conclusion about this endpoint.

Patients with acute myocardial infarction, treated with ZESTRIL, had a higher (9.0% versus 3.7%) incidence of persistent hypotension (systolic blood pressure <90 mmHg for more than 1 hour) and renal dysfunction (2.4% versus 1.1%) in-hospital and at six weeks (increasing creatinine concentration to over 3 mg/dL or a doubling or more of the baseline

serum creatinine concentration). See ADVERSE REACTIONS—Acute Myocardial infarction.

INDICATIONS AND USAGE

Hypertension: ZESTRIL is indicated for the treatment of hypertension. It may be used alone as initial therapy or concomitantly with other classes of antihypertensive agents.

Heart Failure: ZESTRIL is indicated as adjunctive therapy in the management of heart failure in patients who are not responding adequately to diuretics and digitalis.

Acute Myocardial Infarction: ZESTRIL is indicated for the treatment of hemodynamically stable patients within 24 hours of acute myocardial infarction, to improve survival. Patients should receive, as appropriate, the standard recommended treatments such as thrombolytics, aspirin and betablockers.

In using ZESTRIL, consideration should be given to the fact that another angiotensin converting enzyme inhibitor, captopril, has caused agranulocytosis, particularly in patients with renal impairment or collagen vascular disease, and that available data are insufficient to show that ZESTRIL does not have a similar risk. (See WARNINGS.)

In considering the use of ZESTRIL, it should be noted that in controlled trials ACE inhibitors have an effect on blood pressure that is less in black patients than in nonblacks. In addition, ACE inhibitors have been associated with a higher rate of angioedema in black than in nonblack patients (see WARNINGS, Angioedema).

CONTRAINDICATIONS

ZESTRIL is contraindicated in patients who are hypersensitive to this product and in patients with a history of angioedema related to previous treatment with an angiotensin converting enzyme inhibitor.

WARNINGS

Anaphylactoid and Possibly Related Reactions: Presumably because angiotensin-converting enzyme inhibitors affect the metabolism of eicosanoids and polypeptides, including endogenous bradykinin, patients receiving ACE inhibitors (including ZESTRIL) may be subject to a variety of adverse reactions, some of them serious.

Angioedema: Angioedema of the face, extremities, lips, tongue, glottis and/or larynx has been reported in patients treated with angiotensin converting enzyme inhibitors, including ZESTRIL. This may occur at any time during treatment. ACE inhibitors have been associated with a higher rate of angioedema in black than in nonblack patients. ZESTRIL should be promptly discontinued and appropriate therapy and monitoring should be provided until complete and sustained resolution of signs and symptoms has occurred. In instances where swelling has been confined to the face and lips the condition has generally resolved without treatment, although antihistamines have been useful in relieving symptoms. Angioedema associated with laryngeal edema may be fatal. **Where there is involvement of the tongue, glottis or larynx, likely to cause airway obstruction, appropriate therapy, e.g., subcutaneous epinephrine solution 1:1000 (0.3 mL to 0.5 mL) and/or measures necessary to ensure a patent airway should be promptly provided. (See ADVERSE REACTIONS.)**

Patients with a history of angioedema unrelated to ACE inhibitor therapy may be at increased risk of angioedema while receiving an ACE inhibitor. (See also INDICATIONS AND USAGE and CONTRAINDICATIONS.)

Anaphylactoid Reactions During Desensitization: Two patients undergoing desensitizing treatment with hymenoptera venom while receiving ACE inhibitors sustained life-threatening anaphylactoid reactions. In the same patients, these reactions were avoided when ACE inhibitors were temporarily withheld, but they reappeared upon inadvertent rechallenge.

Anaphylactoid Reactions During Membrane Exposure: Sudden and potentially life-threatening anaphylactoid reactions have been reported in some patients dialyzed with high-flux membranes (e.g., AN69¶) and treated concomitantly with an ACE inhibitor. In such patients, dialysis must be stopped immediately, and aggressive therapy for anaphylactoid reactions be initiated. Symptoms have not been relieved by antihistamines in these situations. In these patients, consideration should be given to using a different type of dialysis membrane or a different class of antihypertensive agent. Anaphylactoid reactions have also been reported in patients undergoing low-density lipoprotein apheresis with dextran sulfate absorption (a procedure dependent upon devices not approved in the United States.)

Hypotension: Excessive hypotension is rare in patients with uncomplicated hypertension treated with ZESTRIL alone.

Patients with heart failure given ZESTRIL commonly have some reduction in blood pressure, with peak blood pressure reduction occurring 6 to 8 hours post dose, but discontinuation of therapy because of continuing symptomatic hypotension usually is not necessary when dosing instructions are followed; caution should be observed when initiating therapy. (See DOSAGE AND ADMINISTRATION.)

Patients at risk of excessive hypotension, sometimes associated with oliguria and/or progressive azotemia, and rarely with acute renal failure and/or death, include those with the following conditions or characteristics: heart failure with systolic blood pressure below 100 mmHg, hyponatremia, high dose diuretic therapy, recent intensive diuresis or increase in diuretic dose, renal dialysis, or severe volume and/or salt depletion of any etiology. It may be advisable to eliminate the diuretic (except in patients with heart failure), reduce the diuretic dose or increase salt intake cautiously before initiating therapy with ZESTRIL in patients at risk for excessive hypotension who are able to tolerate such adjustments. (See PRECAUTIONS, Drug Interactions and ADVERSE REACTIONS.)

Patients with acute myocardial infarction in the GISSI-3 trial had a higher (9.0% versus 3.7%) incidence of persistent hypotension (systolic blood pressure <90 mmHg for more than 1 hour) when treated with ZESTRIL. Treatment with ZESTRIL must not be initiated in acute myocardial infarction patients at risk of further serious hemodynamic deterioration after treatment with a vasodilator (systolic blood pressure of 100 mmHg or lower) or cardiogenic shock.

In patients at risk of excessive hypotension, therapy should be started under very close medical supervision and such patients should be followed closely for the first two weeks of treatment and whenever the dose of ZESTRIL and/or diuretic is increased. Similar considerations may apply to patients with ischemic heart or cerebrovascular disease, or in patients with acute myocardial infarction, in whom an excessive fall in blood pressure could result in a myocardial infarction or cerebrovascular accident.

If excessive hypotension occurs, the patient should be placed in the supine position and, if necessary, receive an intravenous infusion of normal saline. A transient hypotensive response is not a contraindication to further doses of ZESTRIL which usually can be given without difficulty once the blood pressure has stabilized. If symptomatic hypotension develops, a dose reduction or discontinuation of ZESTRIL or concomitant diuretic may be necessary.

Leukopenia/Neutropenia/Agranulocytosis: Another angiotensin converting enzyme inhibitor, captopril, has been shown to cause agranulocytosis and bone marrow depression, rarely in uncomplicated patients but more frequently in patients with renal impairment especially if they also have a collagen vascular disease. Available data from clinical trials of ZESTRIL are insufficient to show that ZESTRIL does not cause agranulocytosis at similar rates. Marketing experience has revealed rare cases of leukopenia/neutropenia and bone marrow depression in which a causal relationship to lisinopril cannot be excluded. Periodic monitoring of white blood cell counts in patients with collagen vascular disease and renal disease should be considered.

Hepatic Failure: Rarely, ACE inhibitors have been associated with a syndrome that starts with cholestatic jaundice and progresses to fulminant hepatic necrosis and (sometimes) death. The machanism of this syndrome is not understood. Patients receiving ACE inhibitors who develop jaundice or marked elevations of hepatic enzymes should discontinue the ACE inhibitor and receive appropriate medical follow-up.

Fetal/Neonatal Morbidity and Mortality: ACE inhibitors can cause fetal and neonatal morbidity and death when administered to pregnant women. Several dozen cases have been reported in the world literature. When pregnancy is detected, ACE inhibitors should be discontinued as soon as possible.

The use of ACE inhibitors during the second and third trimesters of pregnancy has been associated with fetal and neonatal injury, including hypotension, neonatal skull hypoplasia, anuria, reversible or irreversible renal failure, and death. Oligohydramnios has also been reported, presumably resulting from decreased fetal renal function; oligohydramnios in this setting has been associated with fetal limb contractures, craniofacial deformation, and hypoplastic lung development. Prematurity, intrauterine growth retardation, and patent ductus arteriosus have also been reported, although it is not clear whether these occurrences were due to the ACE-inhibitor exposure.

These adverse effects do not appear to have resulted from intrauterine ACE-inhibitor exposure that has been limited to the first trimester. Mothers whose embryos and fetuses are exposed to ACE inhibitors only during the first trimester should be so informed. Nonetheless, when patients become pregnant, physicians should make every effort to discontinue the use of ZESTRIL as soon as possible.

Rarely (probably less often than once in every thousand pregnancies), no alternative to ACE inhibitors will be found. In these rare cases, the mothers should be apprised of the potential hazards to their fetuses, and serial ultrasound examinations should be performed to assess the intraamniotic environment.

If oligohydramnios is observed, ZESTRIL should be discontinued unless it is considered lifesaving for the mother. Contraction stress testing (CST), a nonstress test (NST), or biophysical profiling (BPP) may be appropriate, depending upon the week of pregnancy. Patients and physicians should be aware, however, that oligohydramnios may not appear until after the fetus has sustained irreversible injury.

Infants with histories of *in utero* exposure to ACE inhibitors should be closely observed for hypotension, oliguria, and hyperkaliemia. If oliguria occurs, attention should be directed toward support of blood pressure and renal perfusion. Exchange transfusion or dialysis may be required as means of reversing hypotension and/or substituting for disordered renal function. Lisinopril, which crosses the placenta, has been removed from neonatal circulation by peritoneal dialysis with some clinical benefit, and theoretically may be removed by exchange transfusion, although there is no experience with the latter procedure.

No teratogenic effects of lisinopril were seen in studies of pregnant rats, mice, and rabbits. On a mg/kg basis, the doses used were up to 625 times (in mice), 188 times (in rats), and 0.6 times (in rabbits) the maximum recommended human dose.

PRECAUTIONS

General

Impaired Renal Function: As a consequence of inhibiting the renin-angiotensin-aldosterone system, changes in renal function may be anticipated in susceptible individuals. In patients with severe congestive heart failure whose renal function may depend on the activity of the renin-angiotensin-aldosterone system, treatment with angiotensin converting enzyme inhibitors, including ZESTRIL, may be associated with oliguria and/or progressive azotemia and rarely with acute renal failure and/or death.

In hypertensive patients with unilateral or bilateral renal artery stenosis, increases in blood urea nitrogen and serum creatinine may occur. Experience with another angiotensin converting enzyme inhibitor suggests that these increases are usually reversible upon discontinuation of ZESTRIL and/or diuretic therapy. In such patients, renal function should be monitored during the first few weeks of therapy.

Some patients with hypertension or heart failure with no apparent preexisting renal vascular disease have developed increases in blood urea nitrogen and serum creatinine, usually minor and transient, especially when ZESTRIL has been given concomitantly with a diuretic. This is more likely to occur in patients with pre-existing renal impairment. Dosage reduction and/or discontinuation of the diuretic and/or ZESTRIL may be required.

Patients with acute myocardial infarction in the GISSI-3 trial, treated with ZESTRIL had a higher (2.4% versus 1.1%) incidence of renal dysfunction in-hospital and at six weeks (increasing creatinine concentration to over 3 mg/dL or a doubling or more of the baseline serum creatinine concentration). In acute myocardial infarction, treatment with ZESTRIL should be initiated with caution in patients with evidence of renal dysfunction, defined as serum creatinine concentration exceeding 2 mg/dL. If renal dysfunction develops during treatment with ZESTRIL (serum creatinine concentration exceeding 3 mg/dL or a doubling from the pretreatment value) then the physician should consider withdrawal of ZESTRIL.

Evaluation of patients with hypertension, heart failure, or myocardial infarction should always include assessment of renal function. (See DOSAGE AND ADMINISTRATION.)

Hyperkalemia: In clinical trials hyperkalemia (serum potassium greater than 5.7 mEq/L) occurred in approximately 2.2% of hypertensive patients and 4.8% of patients with heart failure. In most cases these were isolated values which resolved despite continued therapy. Hyperkalemia was a cause of discontinuation of therapy in approximately 0.1% of hypertensive patients; 0.6% of patients with heart failure and 0.1% of patients with myocardial infarction. Risk factors for the development of hyperkalemia include renal insufficiency, diabetes mellitus, and the concomitant use of potassium-sparing diuretics, potassium supplements and/or potassium-containing salt substitutes, which should be used cautiously, if at all, with ZESTRIL. (See Drug Interactions.)

Cough: Presumably due to the inhibition of the degradation of endogenous bradykinin, persistent nonproductive cough has been reported with all ACE inhibitors, almost always resolving after discontinuation of therapy. ACE inhibitor-induced cough should be considered in the differential diagnosis of cough.

Surgery/Anesthesia: In patients undergoing major surgery or during anesthesia with agents that produce hypotension, ZESTRIL may block angiotensin II formation secondary to compensatory renin release. If hypotension occurs and is considered to be due to this mechanism, it can be corrected by volume expansion.

Information for Patients

Angioedema: Angioedema, including laryngeal edema, may occur at any time during treatment with angiotensin converting enzyme inhibitors, including ZESTRIL. Patients should be so advised and told to report immediately any signs or symptoms suggesting angioedema (swelling of face, extremities, eyes, lips, tongue, difficulty in swallowing or

Continued on next page

Zeneca Pharmaceuticals—Cont.

breathing) and to take no more drug until they have consulted with the prescribing physician.

Symptomatic Hypotension: Patients should be cautioned to report lightheadedness especially during the first few days of therapy. If actual syncope occurs, the patient should be told to discontinue the drug until they have consulted with the prescribing physician.

All patients should be cautioned that excessive perspiration and dehydration may lead to an excessive fall in blood pressure because of reduction in fluid volume. Other causes of volume depletion such as vomiting or diarrhea may also lead to a fall in blood pressure; patients should be advised to consult with their physician.

Hyperkalemia: Patients should be told not to use salt substitutes containing potassium without consulting their physician.

Leukopenia/Neutropenia: Patients should be told to report promptly any indication of infection (e.g., sore throat, fever) which may be a sign of leukopenia/neutropenia.

Pregnancy: Female patients of childbearing age should be told about the consequences of second- and third-trimester exposure to ACE inhibitors, and they should also be told that these consequences do not appear to have resulted from intrauterine ACE-inhibitor exposure that has been limited to the first trimester. These patients should be asked to report pregnancies to their physicians as soon as possible.

NOTE: As with many other drugs, certain advice to patients being treated with ZESTRIL is warranted. This information is intended to aid in the safe and effective use of this medication. It is not a disclosure of all possible adverse or intended effects.

Drug Interactions

Hypotension—Patients on Diuretic Therapy: Patients on diuretics and especially those in whom diuretic therapy was recently instituted, may occasionally experience an excessive reduction of blood pressure after initiation of therapy with ZESTRIL. The possibility of hypotensive effects with ZESTRIL can be minimized by either discontinuing the diuretic or increasing the salt intake prior to initiation of treatment with ZESTRIL. If it is necessary to continue the diuretic, initiate therapy with ZESTRIL at a dose of 5 mg daily, and provide close medical supervision after the initial dose until blood pressure has stabilized. (See WARNINGS, and DOSAGE AND ADMINISTRATION.) When a diuretic is added to the therapy of a patient receiving ZESTRIL, an additional antihypertensive effect is usually observed. Studies with ACE inhibitors in combination with diuretics indicate that the dose of the ACE inhibitor can be reduced when it is given with a diuretic. (See DOSAGE AND ADMINISTRATION.)

Indomethacin: In a study in 36 patients with mild to moderate hypertension where the antihypertensive effects of ZESTRIL alone were compared to ZESTRIL given concomitantly with indomethacin was asso-

ciated with a reduced effect, although the difference between the two regimens was not significant.

Other Agents: ZESTRIL has been used concomitantly with nitrates and/or digoxin without evidence of clinically significant adverse interactions. This included post myocardial infarction patients who were receiving intravenous or transdermal nitroglycerin. No clinically important pharmacokinetic interactions occurred when ZESTRIL was used concomitantly with propranolol or hydrochlorothiazide. The presence of food in the stomach does not alter the bioavailability of ZESTRIL.

Agents Increasing Serum Potassium: ZESTRIL attenuates potassium loss caused by thiazide-type diuretics. Use of ZESTRIL with potassium-sparing diuretics (e.g., spironolactone, triamterene or amiloride), potassium supplements, or potassium-containing salt substitutes may lead to significant increases in serum potassium. Therefore, if concomitant use of these agents is indicated because of demonstrated hypokalemia, they should be used with caution and with frequent monitoring of serum potassium. Potassium sparing agents should generally not be used in patients with heart failure who are receiving ZESTRIL.

Lithium: Lithium toxicity has been reported in patients receiving lithium concomitantly with drugs which cause elimination of sodium, including ACE inhibitors. Lithium toxicity was usually reversible upon discontinuation of lithium and the ACE inhibitor. It is recommended that serum lithium levels be monitored frequently if ZESTRIL is administered concomitantly with lithium.

Carcinogenesis, Mutagenesis, Impairment of Fertility: There was no evidence of a tumorigenic effect when lisinopril was administered for 105 weeks to male and female rats at doses up to 90 mg/kg/day (about 56 or 9 times* the maximum recommended daily human dose, based on body weight and body surface area, respectively). There was no evidence of carcinogenicity when lisinopril was administered for 92 weeks to (male and female) mice at doses up to 135 mg/kg/day (about 84 times* the maximum recommended daily human dose). This dose was 6.8 times the maximum human dose based on body surface area in mice.

*Calculations assume a human weight of 50 kg and human body surface area of 1.62 m².

Lisinopril was not mutagenic in the Ames microbial mutagen test with or without metabolic activation. It was also negative in a forward mutation assay using Chinese hamster lung cells. Lisinopril did not produce single strand DNA breaks in an *in vitro* alkaline elution rat hepatocyte assay. In addition, lisinopril did not produce increases in chromosomal aberrations in an *in vitro* test in Chinese hamster ovary cells or in an *in vivo* study in mouse bone marrow. There were no adverse effects on reproductive performance in male and female rats treated with up to 300 mg/kg/day of lisinopril. This dose is 188 times and 30 times the maximum human dose when based on mg/kg and mg/m², respectively.

Pregnancy

Pregnancy Categories C (first trimester) and D (second and third trimesters). See WARNINGS, Fetal/Neonatal Morbidity and Mortality.

Nursing Mothers: Milk of lactating rats contains radioactivity following administration of ¹⁴C lisinopril. It is not known whether this drug is excreted in human milk. Because many drugs are excreted in human milk and because of the potential for serious adverse reactions in nursing infants from ACE inhibitors, a decision should be made whether to discontinue nursing and/or discontinue ZESTRIL, taking into account the importance of the drug to the mother.

Pediatric Use: Safety and effectiveness in children have not been established.

ADVERSE REACTIONS

ZESTRIL has been found to be generally well tolerated in controlled clinical trials involving 1969 patients with hypertension or heart failure. For the most part, adverse experiences were mild and transient.

Hypertension:

In clinical trials in patients with hypertension treated with ZESTRIL, discontinuation of therapy due to clinical adverse experiences occurred in 5.7% of patients. The overall frequency of adverse experiences could not be related to total daily dosage within the recommended therapeutic dosage range.

For adverse experiences occurring in greater than 1% of patients with hypertension treated with ZESTRIL or ZESTRIL plus hydrochlothiazide in controlled clinical trials, and more frequently with ZESTRIL and/or ZESTRIL plus hydrochlorothiazide than placebo, comparative incidence data are listed in the table below:

[See table at bottom left.]

Heart Failure:

In patients with heart failure treated with ZESTRIL for up to four years, discontinuation of therapy due to clinical adverse experiences occurred in 11.0% of patients. In controlled studies in patients with heart failure, therapy was discontinued in 8.1% of patients treated with ZESTRIL for 12 weeks, compared to 7.7% of patients treated with placebo for 12 weeks.

The following table lists those adverse experiences which occurred in greater than 1% of patients with heart failure treated with ZESTRIL or placebo for up to 12 weeks in controlled clinical trials, and more frequently on ZESTRIL than placebo.

	Controlled Trials			
	ZESTRIL (n=407) Incidence (discontinuation) 12 weeks		Placebo (n=155) Incidence (discontinuation) 12 weeks	
Body as a Whole				
Chest Pain	3.4	(0.2)	1.3	(0.0)
Abdominal Pain	2.2	(0.7)	1.9	(0.0)
Cardiovascular				
Hypotension	4.4	(1.7)	0.6	(0.6)
Digestive				
Diarrhea	3.7	(0.5)	1.9	(0.0)
Nervous/Psychiatric				
Dizziness	11.8	(1.2)	4.5	(1.3)
Headache	4.4	(0.2)	3.9	(0.0)
Respiratory				
Upper Respiratory Infection	1.5	(0.0)	1.3	(0.0)
Skin				
Rash	1.7	(0.5)	0.6	(0.6)

Also observed at >1% with ZESTRIL but more frequent or as frequent on placebo than ZESTRIL in controlled trials were asthenia, angina pectoris, nausea, dyspnea, cough, and pruritus.

Worsening of heart failure, anorexia, increased salivation, muscle cramps, back pain, myalgia, depression, chest sound abnormalities, and pulmonary edema were also seen in controlled clinical trials, but were more common on placebo than ZESTRIL.

Acute Myocardial Infarction: In the GISSI-3 trial, in patients treated with ZESTRIL for six weeks following acute myocardial infarction, discontinuation of therapy occurred in 17.6% of patients.

Patients treated with ZESTRIL had a sigificantly higher incidence of hypotension and renal dysfunction compared with patients not taking ZESTRIL.

In the GISSI-3 trial, hypotension (9.7%), renal dysfunction (2.0%), cough (0.5%), post infarction angina (0.3%), skin rash and generalized edema (0.01%), and angioedema (0.01%) resulted in withdrawal of treatment. In elderly patients treated with ZESTRIL, discontinuation due to renal dysfunction was 4.2%.

Other clinical adverse experiences occurring in 0.3% to 1.0% of patients with hypertension or heart failure treated with ZESTRIL in controlled clinical trials and rarer, serious, pos-

PERCENT OF PATIENTS IN CONTROLLED STUDIES

	ZESTRIL (n=1349) Incidence (discontinuation)		ZESTRIL/Hydrochlorothiazide (n=629) Incidence (discontinuation)		PLACEBO (n=207) Incidence (discontinuation)	
Body as a Whole						
Fatigue	2.5	(0.3)	4.0	(0.5)	1.0	(0.0)
Asthenia	1.3	(0.5)	2.1	(0.2)	1.0	(0.0)
Orthostatic Effects	1.2	(0.0)	3.5	(0.2)	1.0	(0.0)
Cardiovascular						
Hypotension	1.2	(0.5)	1.6	(0.5)	0.5	(0.5)
Digestive						
Diarrhea	2.7	(0.2)	2.7	(0.3)	2.4	(0.0)
Nausea	2.0	(0.4)	2.5	(0.2)	2.4	(0.0)
Vomiting	1.1	(0.2)	1.4	(0.1)	0.5	(0.0)
Dyspepsia	0.9	(0.0)	1.9	(0.0)	0.0	(0.0)
Musculoskeletal						
Muscle Cramps	0.5	(0.0)	2.9	(0.8)	0.5	(0.0)
Nervous/Psychiatric						
Headache	5.7	(0.2)	4.5	(0.5)	1.9	(0.0)
Dizziness	5.4	(0.4)	9.2	(1.0)	1.9	(0.0)
Paresthesia	0.8	(0.1)	2.1	(0.2)	0.0	(0.0)
Decreased Libido	0.4	(0.1)	1.3	(0.1)	0.0	(0.0)
Vertigo	0.2	(0.1)	1.1	(0.2)	0.0	(0.0)
Respiratory						
Cough	3.5	(0.7)	4.6	(0.8)	1.0	(0.0)
Upper Respiratory Infection	2.1	(0.1)	2.7	(0.1)	0.0	(0.0)
Common Cold	1.1	(0.1)	1.3	(0.1)	0.0	(0.0)
Nasal Congestion	0.4	(0.1)	1.3	(0.1)	0.0	(0.0)
Influenza	0.3	(0.1)	1.1	(0.1)	0.0	(0.0)
Skin						
Rash	1.3	(0.4)	1.6	(0.2)	0.5	(0.5)
Urogenital						
Impotence	1.0	(0.4)	1.6	(0.5)	0.0	(0.0)

Chest pain and back pain were also seen, but were more common on placebo than ZESTRIL.

sibly drug-related events reported in uncontrolled studies or marketing experience are listed below, and within each category are in order of decreasing severity:

Body as a Whole: Anaphylactoid reactions (see WARNINGS, Anaphylactoid Reactions During Membrane Exposure), syncope, orthostatic effects, chest discomfort, pain, pelvic pain, flank pain, edema, facial edema, virus infection, fever, chills, malaise.

Cardiovascular: Cardiac arrest; myocardial infarction or cerebrovascular accident possibly secondary to excessive hypotension in high risk patients (see WARNINGS, Hypotension); pulmonary embolism and infarction, arrhythmias (including ventricular tachycardia, atrial tachycardia, atrial fibrillation, bradycardia and premature ventricular contractions), palpitations, transient ischemic attacks, paroxysmal nocturnal dyspnea, orthostatic hypotension, decreased blood pressure, peripheral edema, vasculitis.

Digestive: Pancreatitis, hepatitis (hepatocellular or cholestatic jaundice) (see WARNINGS, Hepatic Failure), vomiting, gastritis, dyspepsia, heartburn, gastrointestinal cramps, constipation, flatulence, dry mouth.

Hematologic: Rare cases of bone marrow depression, hemolytic anemia, leukopenia/neutropenia and thrombocytopenia.

Endocrine: Diabetes mellitus.

Metabolic: Weight loss, dehydration, fluid overload, gout, weight gain.

Musculoskeletal: Arthritis, arthralgia, neck pain, hip pain, low back pain, joint pain, leg pain, knee pain, shoulder pain, arm pain, lumbago.

Nervous System/Psychiatric: Stroke, ataxia, memory impairment, tremor, peripheral neuropathy (e.g., dysesthesia), spasm, paresthesia, confusion, insomnia, somnolence, hypersomnia, irritability and nervousness.

Respiratory System: Malignant lung neoplasms, hemoptysis, pulmonary infiltrates, bronchospasm, asthma, pleural effusion, pneumonia, bronchitis, wheezing, orthopnea, painful respiration, epistaxis, laryngitis, sinusitis, pharyngeal pain, pharyngitis, rhinitis, rhinorrhea.

Skin: Urticaria, alopecia, herpes zoster, photosensitivity, skin lesions, skin infections, pemphigus, erythema, flushing, diaphoresis. Other severe skin reactions have been reported rarely, including toxic epidermal necrolysis and Stevens-Johnson syndrome; causal relationship has not been established.

Special Senses: Visual loss, diplopia, blurred vision, tinnitus, photophobia, taste alteration.

Urogenital System: Acute renal failure, oliguria, anuria, uremia, progressive azotemia, renal dysfunction. (see PRECAUTIONS and DOSAGE AND ADMINISTRATION), pyelonephritis, dysuria, urinary tract infection, breast pain.

Miscellaneous: A symptom complex has been reported which may include a positive ANA, an elevated erythrocyte sedimentation rate, arthralgia/arthritis, myalgia, fever, vasculitis, eosinophilia and leukocytosis. Rash, photosensitivity or other dermatological manifestations may occur alone or in combination with these symptoms.

ANGIOEDEMA: Angioedema has been reported in patients receiving ZESTRIL (0.1%). Angioedema associated with laryngeal edema may be fatal. If angioedema of the face, extremities, lips, tongue, glottis and/or larynx occurs, treatment with ZESTRIL should be discontinued and appropriate therapy instituted immediately. (See WARNINGS.)

HYPOTENSION: In hypertensive patients, hypotension occurred in 1.2% and syncope occurred in 0.1% of patients. Hypotension or syncope was a cause of discontinuation of therapy in 0.5% of hypertensive patients. In patients with heart failure, hypotension occurred in 5.3% and syncope occurred in 1.8% of patients. These adverse experiences were causes for discontinuation of therapy in 1.8% of these patients. In patients treated with ZESTRIL for six weeks after acute myocardial infarction, hypotension (systolic blood pressure ≤100 mmHg) resulted in discontinuation of therapy in 9.7% of the patients. (See WARNINGS.)

Fetal/Neonatal Morbidity and Mortality: See WARNINGS, Fetal/Neonatal Morbidity and Mortality.

Cough: See PRECAUTIONS—Cough

Clinical Laboratory Test Findings

Serum Electrolytes: Hyperkalemia (See PRECAUTIONS), hyponatremia.

Creatinine, Blood Urea Nitrogen: Minor increases in blood urea nitrogen and serum creatinine, reversible upon discontinuation of therapy, were observed in about 2.0% of patients with essential hypertension treated with ZESTRIL alone. Increases were more common in patients receiving concomitant diuretics and in patients with renal artery stenosis. (See PRECAUTIONS.) Reversible minor increases in blood urea nitrogen and serum creatinine were observed in approximately 11.6% of patients with heart failure on concomitant diuretic therapy. Frequently, these abnormalities resolved when the dosage of the diuretic was decreased.

Hemoglobin and Hematocrit: Small decreases in hemoglobin and hematocrit (mean decreases of approximately 0.4 g% and 1.3 vol%, respectively) occurred frequently in patients treated with ZESTRIL but were rarely of clinical importance in patients without some other cause of anemia. In clinical trials, less than 0.1% of patients discontinued therapy due to anemia.

Liver Function Tests: Rarely, elevations of liver enzymes and/or serum bilirubin have occurred. (See WARNINGS, Hepatic Failure.)

In hypertensive patients, 2.0% discontinued therapy due to laboratory adverse experiences, principally elevations in blood urea nitrogen (0.6%), serum creatinine (0.5%) and serum potassium (0.4%).

In the heart failure trials, 3.4% of patients discontinued therapy due to laboratory adverse experiences; 1.8% due to elevations in blood urea nitrogen and/or creatinine and 0.6% due to elevations in serum potassium.

In the myocardial infarction trial, 2.0% of patients receiving ZESTRIL discontinued therapy due to renal dysfunction (increasing creatinine concentration to over 3 mg/dL or a doubling or more of the baseline serum creatinine concentration); less than 1.0% of patients discontinued therapy due to other laboratory adverse experiences: 0.1% with hyperkalemia and less than 0.1% with hepatic enzyme alterations.

OVERDOSAGE

Following a single oral dose of 20 g/kg no lethality occurred in rats, and death occurred in one of 20 mice receiving the same dose. The most likely manifestation of overdosage would be hypotension, for which the usual treatment would be intravenous infusion of normal saline solution.

Lisinopril can be removed by hemodialysis.

DOSAGE AND ADMINISTRATION

Hypertension

Initial Therapy: In patients with uncomplicated essential hypertension not on diuretic therapy, the recommended initial dose is 10 mg once a day. Dosage should be adjusted according to blood pressure response. The usual dosage range is 20 to 40 mg per day administered in a single daily dose. The antihypertensive effect may diminish toward the end of the dosing interval regardless of the administered dose, but most commonly with a dose of 10 mg daily. This can be evaluated by measuring blood pressure just prior to dosing to determine whether satisfactory control is being maintained for 24 hours. If it is not, an increase in dose should be considered. Doses up to 80 mg have been used but do not appear to give greater effect. If blood pressure is not controlled with ZESTRIL alone, a low dose of a diuretic may be added. Hydrochlorothiazide, 12.5 mg has been shown to provide an additive effect. After the addition of a diuretic, it may be possible to reduce the dose of ZESTRIL.

Diuretic Treated Patients: In hypertensive patients who are currently being treated with a diuretic, symptomatic hypotension may occur occasionally following the initial dose of ZESTRIL. The diuretic should be discontinued, if possible, for two to three days before beginning therapy with ZESTRIL to reduce the likelihood of hypotension. (See WARNINGS.) The dosage of ZESTRIL should be adjusted according to blood pressure response. If the patient's blood pressure is not controlled with ZESTRIL alone, diuretic therapy may be resumed as described above.

If the diuretic cannot be discontinued, an initial dose of 5 mg should be used under medical supervision for at least two hours and until blood pressure has stabilized for at least an additional hour. (See WARNINGS and PRECAUTIONS, Drug Interactions.)

Concomitant administration of ZESTRIL with potassium supplements, potassium salt substitutes, or potassium-sparing diuretics may lead to increases of serum potassium. (See PRECAUTIONS.)

Dosage Adjustment in Renal Impairment: The usual dose of ZESTRIL (10 mg) is recommended for patients with creatinine clearance >30 mL/min (serum creatinine of up to approximately 3 mg/dL). For patients with creatinine clearance ≥10 mL/min ≤30 mL/min (serum creatinine ≥3 mg/dL), the first dose is 5 mg once daily. For patients with creatinine clearance <10 mL/min (usually on hemodialysis) the recommended initial dose is 2.5 mg. The dosage may be titrated upward until blood pressure is controlled or to a maximum of 40 mg daily.

Renal Status	Creatinine Clearance mL/min	Initial Dose mg/day
Normal Renal Function to Mild Impairment	>30	10
Moderate to Severe Impairment	≥10 ≤30	5
Dialysis Patients*	<10	2.5**

* See WARNINGS, Anaphylactoid Reactions During Membrane Exposure.

** Dosage interval should be adjusted depending on the blood pressure response.

Heart Failure

ZESTRIL is indicated as adjunctive therapy with diuretics and digitalis. The recommended starting dose is 5 mg once a day. When initiating treatment with lisinopril in patients with heart failure, the initial dose should be administered under medical observation, especially in those patients with low blood pressure (systolic blood pressure below 100 mmHg). The mean peak blood pressure lowering occurs six to eight hours after dosing. Observation should continue until blood pressure is stable. The concomitant diuretic dose should be reduced, if possible, to help minimize hypovolemia which may contribute to hypotension. (See WARNINGS and PRECAUTIONS, Drug Interactions.) The appearance of hypotension after the initial dose of ZESTRIL does not preclude subsequent careful dose titration with the drug, following effective management of the hypotension.

The usual effective dosage range is 5 to 20 mg per day administered as a single daily dose.

Dosage Adjustment in Patients with Heart Failure and Renal Impairment or Hyponatremia: In patients with heart failure who have hyponatremia (serum sodium <130 mEq/L) or moderate to severe renal impairment (creatinine clearance ≤30 mL/min or serum creatinine >3 mg/dL), therapy with ZESTRIL should be initiated at a dose of 2.5 mg once a day under close medical supervision. (See WARNINGS and PRECAUTIONS, Drug Interactions.).

Acute Myocardial Infarction: In hemodynamically stable patients within 24 hours of the onset of symptoms of acute myocardial infarction, the first dose of ZESTRIL is 5 mg given orally, followed by 5 mg after 24 hours, 10 mg after 48 hours and then 10 mg of ZESTRIL once daily. Dosing should continue for six weeks. Patients should receive, as appropriate, the standard recommended treatments such as thrombolytics, aspirin, and beta-blockers.

Patients with a low systolic blood pressure (≤120 mmHg) when treatment is started or during the first 3 days after the infarct should be given a lower 2.5 mg oral dose of ZESTRIL (see WARNINGS). If hypotension occurs (systolic blood pressure ≤100 mmHg) a daily maintenance dose of 5 mg may be given with temporary reductions to 2.5 mg if needed. If prolonged hypotension occurs (systolic blood pressure <90 mmHg for more than 1 hour) ZESTRIL should be withdrawn. For patients who develop symptoms of heart failure, see DOSAGE AND ADMINISTRATION, Heart Failure.

Dosgae Adjustment in Patients With Myocardial Infarction with Renal Impairment: In acute myocardial infarction, treatment with ZESTRIL should be initiated with caution in patients with evidence of renal dysfunction, defined as serum creatinine concentration exceeding 2 mg/dL. No evaluation of dosing adjustments in myocardial infarction patients with severe renal impairment has been performed.

Use in Elderly: In general, blood pressure response and adverse experiences were similar in younger and older patients given similar doses of ZESTRIL. Pharmacokinetic studies, however, indicate that maximum blood levels and area under the plasma concentration time curve (AUC) are doubled in older patients, so that dosage adjustments should be made with particular caution.

HOW SUPPLIED

2.5 mg Tablets (NDC 0310-0135) white, oval, biconvex, uncoated tablets identifed as "ZESTRIL 2½" on one side and "135" on the other side are supplied in bottles of 100 tablets. ZESTRIL 2.5 mg tablets ar manufactured by Zeneca Pharmaceuticals.

5 mg Tablets (NDC 0310-0130) pink, capsule-shaped, biconvex, bisected, uncoated tablets, identified "ZESTRIL" on one side, and "130" on the other side are supplied in bottles of 100 tablets and 1000 tablets, and unit dose packages of 100 tablets.

10 mg Tablets (NDC 0310-0131) pink, round, biconvex, uncoated tablets identified "ZESTRIL 10" debossed on one side, and "131" debossed on the other side are supplied in bottles of 100 tablets, 1000 tablets, 3000 tablets, and unit dose packages of 100 tablets.

20 mg Tablets (NDC 0310-0132) red, round, biconvex, uncoated tablets identified "ZESTRIL 20" debossed on one side, and "132" debossed on the other side are supplied in bottles of 100 tablets, 1000 tablets, 3000 tablets, and unit dose packages of 100 tablets.

40 mg Tablets (NDC 0310-0134) yellow, round, biconvex, uncoated tablets identified "ZESTRIL 40" debossed on one side, and "134" debossed on the other side are supplied in bottles of 100 tablets.

Store at controlled room temperature, 15°C to 30°C (59°F to 86°F). Protect from moisture, freezing and excessive heat. Dispense in a tight container.

¶Registered trademark of Hospal Ltd.

Manufactured by: IPR Pharmaceuticals Inc.

Distributed by:

ZENECA Pharmaceuticals

A Business Unit of Zeneca Inc.

Wilmington, Delaware 19850-5437

64094-00 Rev G 11/95

Shown in Product Identification Guide, page 342

Continued on next page

Zeneca Pharmaceuticals—Cont.

ZOLADEX® 3.6 mg ℞
GOSERELIN ACETATE IMPLANT
Equivalent to 3.6 mg goserelin

DESCRIPTION

ZOLADEX® (goserelin acetate implant), contains a potent synthetic decapeptide analogue of luteinizing hormone-releasing hormone (LHRH), also known as a gonadotropin releasing hormone (GnRH) agonist analogue. Goserelin acetate is chemically described as an acetate salt of [D-Ser(Bu^t)^6,Azgly^{10}]LHRH. Its chemical structure is pyro-Glu-His-Trp-Ser-Tyr-D-Ser(Bu^t)-Leu-Arg-Pro-Azgly-NH$_2$ acetate [$C_{59}H_{84}N_{18}O_{14} \cdot (C_2H_4O_2)_x$ where x = 1 to 2.4].

Goserelin acetate is an off-white powder with a molecular weight of 1269 Daltons (free base). It is freely soluble in glacial acetic acid. It is soluble in water, 0.1M hydrochloric acid, 0.1M sodium hydroxide, dimethylformamide and dimethyl sulfoxide. Goserelin acetate is practically insoluble in acetone, chloroform and ether.

ZOLADEX is supplied as a sterile, biodegradable product containing goserelin acetate equivalent to 3.6 mg of goserelin. ZOLADEX is designed for subcutaneous injection with continuous release over a 28-day period. Goserelin acetate is dispersed in a matrix of D,L-lactic and glycolic acids copolymer (13.3–14.3 mg/dose) containing less than 2.5% acetic acid and up to 15% goserelin-related substances and presented as a sterile, white to cream colored 1-mm diameter cylinder, preloaded in a special single use syringe with a 16-gauge needle and overwrapped in a sealed, light and moisture proof, aluminum foil laminate pouch containing a desiccant capsule. Studies of the D,L-lactic and glycolic acids copolymer have indicated that it is completely biodegradable and has no demonstrable antigenic potential.

CLINICAL PHARMACOLOGY

Mechanism of Action: ZOLADEX is a synthetic decapeptide analogue of LHRH. ZOLADEX acts as a potent inhibitor of pituitary gonadotropin secretion when administered in the biodegradable formulation.

Following initial administration in males, ZOLADEX causes an initial increase in serum luteinizing hormone (LH) and follicle stimulating hormone (FSH) levels with subsequent increases in serum levels of testosterone. Chronic administration of ZOLADEX leads to sustained suppression of pituitary gonadotropins, and serum levels of testosterone consequently fall into the range normally seen in surgically castrated men approximately 2–4 weeks after initiation of therapy. This leads to accessory sex organ regression. In animal and in in vitro studies, administration of goserelin resulted in the regression or inhibition of growth of the hormonally sensitive dimethylbenzanthracene (DMBA)-induced rat mammary tumor and Dunning R3327 prostate tumor. In clinical trials with follow-up of more than 2 years, suppression of serum testosterone to castrate levels has been maintained for the duration of therapy.

In females, a similar down-regulation of the pituitary gland by chronic exposure to ZOLADEX leads to suppression of gonadotropin secretion, a decrease in serum estradiol to levels consistent with the postmenopausal state, and would be expected to lead to a reduction of ovarian size and function, reduction in the size of the uterus and mammary gland, as well as a regression of sex hormone-responsive tumors, if present. Serum estradiol is suppressed to levels similar to those observed in postmenopausal women within 3 weeks following initial administration; however, after suppression was attained, isolated elevations of estradiol were seen in 10% of the patients enrolled in clinical trials. Serum LH and FSH are suppressed to follicular phase levels within four weeks after initial administration of drug and are usually maintained at that range with continued use of ZOLADEX. In 5% or less of women treated with ZOLADEX, FSH and LH levels may not be suppressed to follicular phase levels on day 28 post treatment with use of a single 3.6 mg depot injection. In certain individuals, suppression of any of these hormones to such levels may not be achieved with ZOLADEX. Estradiol, LH and FSH levels return to pretreatment values within 12 weeks following the last implant administration in all but rare cases.

Pharmacokinetics: The pharmacokinetics of ZOLADEX have been determined in both male and female healthy volunteers and patients. In these studies, ZOLADEX was administered as a single 250 μg (aqueous solution) dose and as a single or multiple 3.6 mg depot dose by subcutaneous route. The absorption of radiolabeled drug was rapid, and the peak blood radioactivity levels occurred between 0.5 and 1.0 hour after dosing. The pharmacokinetic parameter estimates of ZOLADEX after administration of 3.6 mg depot for 2 months in males and females are presented in the following table. [See table below.]

Parameters (Units)	Males n=7	Females n=9
Peak Plasma Concentration (ng/mL)	2.84 ± 1.81	1.46 ±0.82
Time to Peak Concentration (days)	12–15	8–22
Area Under the Curve (0–28 days) (ng.h/mL)	27.8 ± 15.3	18.5 ± 10.3
Systemic Clearance (mL/min)	110.5 ± 47.5	163.9 ± 71.0
*Apparent Volume of Distribution (L)	44.1 ± 13.6	20.3 ± 4.1
*Elimination Half-life (h)	4.2 ± 1.1	2.3 ± 0.6

*The apparent volume of distribution and the elimination half-life were determined after subcutaneous administration of 250 μg aqueous solution of goserelin.

Pharmacokinetic data were obtained using a nonspecific RIA method.

Goserelin is released from the depot at a much slower rate initially for the first 8 days, and then there is more rapid and continuous release for the remainder of the 28-day dosing period. Despite the change in the releasing rate of goserelin, administration of ZOLADEX every 28 days resulted in testosterone levels that were suppressed to and maintained in the range normally seen in surgically castrated men.

When ZOLADEX 3.6 mg depot was used for treating male and female patients with normal renal and hepatic function, there was no significant evidence of drug accumulation. However, in clinical trials the minimum serum levels of a few patients were increased. These levels can be attributed to interpatient variation.

Distribution: The apparent volumes of distribution determined after subcutaneous administration of 250 μg aqueous solution of goserelin were 44.1 and 20.3 liters for males and females, respectively. The plasma protein binding of goserelin obtained from one sample was found to be 27.3%.

Metabolism: Metabolism of goserelin, by hydrolysis of the C-terminal amino acids, is the major clearance mechanism. The major circulating component in serum appeared to be 1–7 fragment, and the major component presented in urine of one healthy male volunteer was 5–10 fragment. The metabolism of goserelin in humans yields a similar but narrow profile of metabolites to that found in other species. All metabolites found in humans have also been found in toxicology species.

Excretion: Clearance of goserelin following subcutaneous administration of the solution formulation of goserelin is very rapid and occurs via a combination of hepatic metabolism and urinary excretion. More than 90% of a subcutaneous radiolabeled solution formulation dose of goserelin is excreted in urine. Approximately 20% of the dose in urine is accounted for by unchanged goserelin. The total body clearance of goserelin (administered subcutaneously as a 3.6 mg depot) was significantly ($p < 0.05$) greater (163.9 versus 110.5 mL/min) in females compared to males.

Special Populations: In clinical trials with the solution formulation of goserelin, male patients with impaired renal function (creatinine clearance < 20 mL/min) had a total body clearance and serum elimination half-life of 31.5 mL/min and 12.1 hours, respectively, compared to 133 mL/min and 4.2 hours for subjects with normal renal function (creatinine clearance > 70 mL/min). In females, the effects of reduced goserelin clearance due to impaired renal function on drug efficacy and toxicity are unknown. The total body clearances and serum elimination half-lives were similar between normal and hepatic impaired patients receiving 250 μg solution formation of goserelin. Pharmacokinetic studies using the aqueous formulation of goserelin in patients with renal and hepatic impairment do not indicate a need for dose adjustment with the use of the depot formulation.

Drug-Drug Interactions: No formal drug-drug interaction studies have been performed.

Clinical Studies—Endometriosis: In controlled clinical studies using the 3.6 mg formulation every 28 days for 6 months, ZOLADEX was shown to be as effective as danazol therapy in relieving clinical symptoms (dysmenorrhea, dyspareunia and pelvic pain) and signs (pelvic tenderness, pelvic induration) of endometriosis and decreasing the size of endometrial lesions as determined by laparoscopy. In one study comparing ZOLADEX with danazol (800 mg/day), 63% of ZOLADEX-treated patients and 42% of danazol-treated patients had a greater than or equal to 50% reduction in the extent of endometrial lesions. In the second study comparing ZOLADEX with danazol (600 mg/day), 62% of ZOLADEX-treated and 51% of danazol-treated patients had a greater than or equal to 50% reduction in the extent of endometrial lesions. The clinical significance of a decrease in endometriotic lesions is not known at this time; and in addition, laparoscopic staging of endometriosis does not necessarily correlate with severity of symptoms.

In these two studies, ZOLADEX led to amenorrhea in 92% and 80%, respectively, of all treated women within 8 weeks after initial administration. Menses usually resumed within 8 weeks following completion of therapy.

Within 4 weeks following initial administration, clinical symptoms were significantly reduced, and at the end of treatment were, on average, reduced by approximately 84%.

During the first two months of ZOLADEX use, some women experience vaginal bleeding of variable duration and intensity. In all likelihood, this bleeding represents estrogen withdrawal bleeding, and is expected to stop spontaneously.

This is insufficient evidence to determine whether pregnancy rates are enhanced or adversely affected by the use of ZOLADEX.

Clinical Studies—Breast Cancer: The Southwest Oncology Group conducted a prospective, randomized clinical trial (SWOG-8692 [INT-0075]) in premenopausal women with advanced estrogen receptor positive or progesterone receptor positive breast cancer which compared ZOLADEX with oophorectomy. On the basis of interim data from 124 women, the best objective response (CR+PR) for the ZOLADEX group is 22% versus 12% for the oophorectomy group. The median time to treatment failure is 6.7 months for patients treated with ZOLADEX and 5.5 months for patients treated with oophorectomy. The median survival time for the ZOLADEX arm is 33.2 months and for the oophorectomy arm is 33.6 months.

Subjective responses based on measures of pain control and performance status were observed with both treatments; 48% of the women in the ZOLADEX treatment group and 50% in the oophorectomy group had subjective responses. In the clinical trial (SWOG-8692 [INT 0075]), the mean post treatment estradinol level was reported as 17.8 pg/mL. (The mean estradiol level in post-menopausal women as reported in the literature is 13 pg/mL). During the conduct of the clinical trial, women whose estradiol levels were not reduced to the postmenopausal range, received two ZOLADEX depots, thus, increasing the dose of ZOLADEX from 3.6 mg to 7.2 mg.

Findings were similar in uncontrolled clinical trials involving patients with hormone receptor positive and negative breast cancer. Premenopausal women with estrogen receptor (ER) status of positive, negative, or unknown participated in the uncontrolled (Phase II and Trial 2302) clinical trials. Objective tumor responses were seen regardless of ER status, as shown in the following table.

OBJECTIVE RESPONSE BY ER STATUS

	CR + PR/Total No. (%)			
ER status	Phase II (N=228)		Trial 2302 (N=159)	
Positive	43/119	(36)	31/86	(36)
Negative	6/33	(18)	3/26	(10)
Unknown	20/76	(26)	18/44	(41)

INDICATIONS AND USAGE

Prostatic Carcinoma: ZOLADEX is indicated in the palliative treatment of advanced carcinoma of the prostate. ZOLADEX offers an alternative treatment of prostatic cancer when orchiectomy or estrogen administration are either not indicated or unacceptable to the patient.

In controlled studies of patients with advanced prostatic cancer comparing ZOLADEX to orchiectomy, the long-term endocrine responses and objective responses were similar between the two treatment arms. Additionally, duration of survival was similar between the two treatment arms in a major comparative trial.

Endometriosis: ZOLADEX is indicated for the management of endometriosis, including pain relief and reduction of endometriotic lesions for the duration of therapy. Experience with ZOLADEX for the management of endometriosis has been limited to women 18 years of age and older treated for 6 months.

Advanced Breast Cancer: ZOLADEX is indicated for use in the palliative treatment of advanced breast cancer in pre- and perimenopausal women.

The estrogen and progesterone receptor values may help to predict whether ZOLADEX therapy is likely to be beneficial. (See CLINICAL PHARMACOLOGY.)

CONTRAINDICATIONS

ZOLADEX is contraindicated in those patients who have a known hypersensitivity to LHRH, LHRH agonist analogues or any of the components in ZOLADEX.

ZOLADEX is contraindicated in women being treated for endometriosis who are or may become pregnant while receiving the drug. ZOLADEX can cause fetal harm when administered to a pregnant women. Effects on reproductive function, as a result of antigonadotrophic properties of the drug, are expected to occur on chronic administration.

Effective nonhormonal contraception must be used by all premenopausal women during ZOLADEX therapy and for

12 weeks following discontinuation of therapy. There are no adequate and well-controlled studies in pregnant women using ZOLADEX. If this drug is used during pregnancy, or the patient being treated for endometriosis becomes pregnant while taking this drug, the patient should be apprised of the potential hazard to the fetus or potential risk for loss of the pregnancy. Women of childbearing potential should be advised to avoid becoming pregnant.

For a description of findings in animal reproductive toxicity studies, see WARNINGS.

ZOLADEX is contraindicated in women who are breast feeding (see Nursing Mothers Section).

WARNINGS

Before starting treatment with Zoladex, pregnancy must be excluded. Safe use of Zoladex in pregnancy has not been established. ZOLADEX can cause fetal harm when administered to a pregnant woman. ZOLADEX has been found to cross the placenta following subcutaneous administration of 50 and 1000 μg/kg in rats and rabbits, respectively. Studies in both rats and rabbits at doses equal to or greater than 2 and 20 μg/kg/day, respectively (about $\frac{1}{10}$ and 2 times the daily maximum recommended human dose, respectively, on a mg/m^2 basis), administered during the period of organogenesis, have confirmed that ZOLADEX will increase pregnancy loss, and is embryotoxic/fetotoxic (characterized by increased preimplantation loss, increased resorption and an increase in umbilical hernia in rats at a dose of ≥ 10 μg/kg/day [about $\frac{1}{2}$ the recommended human dose on a mg/m^2 basis]); effects were dose-related. In additional reproduction studies in rats, ZOLADEX was found to decrease fetus and pup survival.

There are no adequate and well-controlled studies in pregnant women using ZOLADEX. Women of childbearing potential should be advised to avoid becoming pregnant.

When used every 28 days, ZOLADEX usually inhibits ovulation and stops menstruation. Contraception is not ensured, however, by taking ZOLADEX. During treatment, pregnancy must be avoided by the use of nonhormonal methods of contraception. If ZOLADEX is used during pregnancy in a patient with advanced breast cancer or the patient becomes pregnant while receiving this drug, the patient must be apprised of the potential risk for loss of the pregnancy due to possible hormonal imbalance as a result of the expected pharmacologic action of ZOLADEX treatment.

Following the last ZOLADEX injection, nonhormonal methods of contraception must be continued until the return of menses or for at least 12 weeks. (See CONTRAINDICATIONS.)

Prostate and Breast Cancer: Initially, ZOLADEX, like other LHRH agonists, causes transient increases in serum levels of testosterone in men with prostate cancer, and estrogen in women with breast cancer. Transient worsening of symptoms, or the occurrence of additional signs and symptoms of prostate or breast cancer, may occasionally develop during the first few weeks of ZOLADEX treatment. A small number of patients may experience a temporary increase in bone pain, which can be managed symtomatically. As with other LHRH agonists, isolated cases of ureteral obstruction and spinal cord compression have been observed in patients with prostate cancer. If spinal cord compression or renal impairment develops, standard treatment of these complications should be instituted. For extreme cases in prostate cancer patients, an immediate orchiectomy should be considered.

As with other LHRH agonists or hormonal therapies (antiestrogens, estrogens, etc.), hypercalcemia has been reported in some prostate and breast cancer patients with bone metastases after starting treatment with ZOLADEX. If hypercalcemia does occur, appropriate treatment measures should be initiated.

PRECAUTIONS

General: Hypersensitivity, antibody formation and acute anaphylactic reactions have been reported with other LHRH agonist analogues. Currently, no anaphylactic reactions have been reported with the use of ZOLADEX.

Of 115 women worldwide treated with ZOLADEX and tested for development of binding to goserelin following treatment with ZOLADEX, one patient showed low-titer binding to goserelin. On further testing of this patient's plasma obtained following treatment, her goserelin binding component was found not to be precipitated with rabbit antihuman immunoglobulin polyvalent sera. These findings suggest the possibility of antibody formation.

Information for Patients

Males: The use of ZOLADEX in patients at particular risk of developing ureteral obstruction or spinal cord compression should be considered carefully and the patients monitored closely during the first month of therapy. Patients with ureteral obstruction or spinal cord compression should have appropriate treatment prior to initiation of ZOLADEX therapy.

Females: Patients must be made aware of the following information:

1. Since menstruation should stop with effective doses of ZOLADEX the patient should notify her physician if regular menstruation persists. Patients missing one or more successive doses of ZOLADEX may experience breakthrough menstrual bleeding.
2. ZOLADEX should not be prescribed if the patient is pregnant, breast feeding, lactating, has nondiagnosed abnormal vaginal bleeding, or is allergic to any of the components of ZOLADEX.
3. Use of ZOLADEX in pregnancy is contraindicated in women being treated for endometriosis. Therefore, a nonhormonal method of contraception should be used during treatment. Patients should be advised that if they miss one or more successive doses of ZOLADEX, breakthrough menstrual bleeding or ovulation may occur with the potential for conception. If a patient becomes pregnant during treatment for endometriosis, ZOLADEX treatment should be discontinued and the patient should be advised of the possible risks to the pregnancy and fetus. (See CONTRAINDICATIONS.)
   For patients being treated for advanced breast cancer, see WARNINGS.
4. Those adverse events occurring most frequently in clinical studies with ZOLADEX are associated with hypoestrogenism; of these the most frequently reported are hot flashes (flushes), headaches, vaginal dryness, emotional lability, change in libido, depression, sweating and change in breast size.
5. As with other LHRH agonist analogues, treatment with ZOLADEX induces a hypoestrogenic state which results in a loss of bone mineral density (BMD) over the course of treatment, some of which may not be reversible. In patients with a history of prior treatment that may have resulted in bone mineral density loss and/or in patients with major risk factors for decreased bone mineral density such as chronic alcohol abuse and/or tobacco abuse, significant family history of osteoporosis, or chronic use of drugs that can reduce bone density such as anticonvulsants or corticosteroids, ZOLADEX therapy may pose an additional risk. In these patients the risks and benefits must be weighed carefully before therapy with ZOLADEX is instituted.
6. Currently, there are no clinical data on the effects of retreatment or treatment of benign gynecological conditions with ZOLADEX for periods in excess of 6 months.
7. As with other hormonal interventions that disrupt the pituitary-gonadal axis, some patients may have delayed return to menses. The rare patient, however, may experience persistent amenorrhea.

Drug Interactions: No formal drug-drug interaction studies have been performed. No confirmed interactions have been reported between ZOLADEX and other drugs.

Drug/Laboratory Test Interactions: Administration of ZOLADEX in therapeutic doses results in suppression of the pituitary-gonadal system. Because of this suppression, diagnostic tests of pituitary-gonadotropic and gonadal functions conducted during treatment and until the resumption of menses may show results which are misleading. Normal function is usually restored within 12 weeks after treatment is discontinued.

Carcinogenesis, Mutagenesis, Impairment of Fertility: Subcutaneous implant of ZOLADEX in male and female rats once every 4 weeks for 1 year and recovery for 23 weeks at doses of about 80 and 150 μg/kg (males) and 50 and 100 μg/kg (females) daily (about 3 to 9 times the recommended human dose on a mg/m^2 basis) resulted in an increased incidence of pituitary adenomas. An increased incidence of pituitary adenomas was also observed following subcutaneous implant of ZOLADEX in rats at similar dose levels for a period of 72 weeks in males and 101 weeks in females. The relevance of the rat pituitary adenomas to humans has not been established. Subcutaneous implants of ZOLADEX every 3 weeks for 2 years delivered to mice at doses of up 2400 μg/kg/day (about 70 times the recommended human dose on a mg/m^2 basis) resulted in an increased incidence of histocytic sarcoma of the vertebral column and femur.

Mutagenicity tests using bacterial and mammalian systems for point mutations and cytogenetic effects have provided no evidence for mutagenic potential.

Administration of goserelin led to changes that were consistent with gonadal suppression in both male and female rats as a result of its endocrine action. In male rats administered 500–1000 μg/kg/day (about 30–60 times the recommended human dose on a mg/m^2 basis), a decrease in weight and atrophic histological changes were observed in the testes, epididymis, seminal vesicle and prostate gland with complete suppression of spermatogenesis. In female rats administered 50–1000 μg/kg/day (about 3–60 times the recommended daily human dose on a mg/m^2 basis), suppression of ovarian function led to decreased size and weight of ovaries and secondary sex organs; follicular development was arrested at the antral stage and the corpora lutea were reduced in size and number. Except for the testes, almost complete histologic reversal of these effects in males and females was observed several weeks after dosing was stopped; however, fertility and general reproductive performance were reduced in those that became pregnant after goserelin was discontinued. Fertile matings occurred within 2 weeks after cessation of dosing, even though total recovery of reproductive function may not have occurred before mating took place; and, the ovulation rate, the corresponding implantation rate, and number of live fetuses were reduced.

Based on histological examination, drug effects on reproductive organs were reversible in male and female dogs administered 107–214 μg/kg/day ZOLADEX (about 20–40 times the recommended daily human dose on a mg/m^2 basis) when drug treatment was stopped after continuous administration for 1 year.

Pregnancy: Pregnancy Category X for treatment of endometrosis. See CONTRAINDICATIONS section. **Pregnancy Category D** for treatment of advanced breast cancer in pre- and perimenopausal women. See WARNINGS section.

Nursing Mothers: ZOLADEX has been shown to be excreted in the milk of lactating rats. It is not known if this drug is excreted in human milk. Because many drugs are excreted in human milk, and because of the potential for serious adverse reactions from ZOLADEX in nursing infants, mothers should discontinue nursing prior to taking the drug.

Pediatric Use: The safety and efficacy of ZOLADEX in pediatric patients have not been established.

ADVERSE REACTIONS

Males: ZOLADEX has been found to be generally well tolerated in clinical trials. Adverse reactions reported in these trials were rarely severe enough to result in the patients' withdrawal from ZOLADEX treatment. As seen with other hormonal therapies, the most commonly observed adverse events during ZOLADEX therapy were due to the expected physiological effects from decreased testosterone levels. These included hot flashes, sexual dysfunction and decreased erections.

Initially, ZOLADEX, like other LHRH agonists, causes transient increases in serum levels of testosterone. A small percentage of patients experienced a temporary worsening of signs and symptoms (see WARNINGS section), usually manifested by an increase in cancer-related pain which was managed symptomatically. Isolated cases of exacerbation of disease symptoms, either ureteral obstruction or spinal cord compression, occurred at similar rates in controlled clinical trials with both ZOLADEX and orchiectomy. The relationship of these events to therapy is uncertain.

In the controlled clinical trials of ZOLADEX versus orchiectomy, the following events were reported as adverse reactions in greater than 5% of the patients.

	TREATMENT RECEIVED	
ADVERSE EVENT	ZOLADEX (n=242) %	ORCHIECTOMY (n=254) %
Hot Flashes	62	53
Sexual Dysfunction	21	15
Decreased Erections	18	16
Lower Urinary Tract Symptoms	13	8
Lethargy	8	4
Pain (worsened in the first 30 days)	8	3
Edema	7	8
Upper Respiratory Infection	7	2
Rash	6	1
Sweating	6	4
Anorexia	5	2
Chronic Obstructive Pulmonary Disease	5	3
Congestive Heart Failure	5	1
Dizziness	5	4
Insomnia	5	1
Nausea	5	2
Complications of Surgery	0	18†

†Complications related to surgery were reported in 18% of the orchiectomy patients, while only 3% of ZOLADEX patients reported adverse reactions at the injection site. The surgical complications included scrotal infection (5.9%), groin pain (4.7%), wound seepage (3.1%), scrotal hematoma (2.8%), incisional discomfort (1.6%) and skin necrosis (1.2%).

The following additional adverse reactions were reported in greater than 1% but less than 5% of the patients treated with ZOLADEX: CARDIOVASCULAR—arrhythmia, cerebrovascular accident, hypertension, myocardial infarction, peripheral vascular disorder, chest pain; CENTRAL NERVOUS SYSTEM—anxiety, depression, headache; GASTROINTESTINAL—constipation, diarrhea, ulcer, vomiting; HEMATOLOGIC—anemia; METABOLIC/NUTRITIONAL—gout, hyperglycemia, weight increase; MISCELLANEOUS—chills, fever; UROGENITAL—renal insuf-

Continued on next page

Zeneca Pharmaceuticals—Cont.

ficiency, urinary obstruction, urinary tract infection, breast swelling and tenderness.

Females: As would be expected with a drug that results in hypoestrogenism, the most frequently reported adverse reactions were those related to this effect.

Endometriosis: In controlled clinical trials comparing ZOLADEX every 28 days and danazol daily for the treatment of endometriosis, the following events were reported at a frequency of 5% or greater:

	TREATMENT RECEIVED	
ADVERSE EVENT	ZOLADEX (n=411) %	DANAZOL (n=207) %
Hot Flushes	96	67
Vaginitis	75	43
Headache	75	63
Emotional Lability	60	56
Libido Decreased	61	44
Sweating	45	30
Depression	54	48
Acne	42	55
Breast Atrophy	33	42
Seborrhea	26	52
Peripheral Edema	21	34
Breast Enlargement	18	15
Pelvic Symptoms	18	23
Pain	17	16
Dyspareunia	14	5
Libido Increased	12	19
Infection	13	11
Asthenia	11	13
Nausea	8	14
Hirsutism	7	15
Insomnia	11	4
Breast Pain	7	4
Abdominal Pain	7	7
Back Pain	7	13
Flu Syndrome	5	5
Dizziness	6	4
Application Site Reaction	6	—
Voice Alterations	3	8
Pharyngitis	5	2
Hair Disorders	4	11
Myalgia	3	11
Nervousness	3	5
Weight Gain	3	23
Leg Cramps	2	6
Increased Appetite	2	5
Pruritis	2	6
Hypertonia	1	10

The following adverse events not already listed above were reported at a frequency of 1% or greater, regardless of causality, in ZOLADEX-treated women from all clinical trials: WHOLE BODY—allergic reaction, chest pain, fever, malaise; CARDIOVASCULAR—hemorrhage, hypertension, migraine, palpitations, tachycardia; DIGESTIVE—anorexia, constipation, diarrhea, dry mouth, dyspepsia, flatulence; HEMATOLOGIC—ecchymosis; METABOLIC AND NUTRITIONAL—edema; MUSCULOSKELETAL—arthralgia, joint disorder; CNS—anxiety, paresthesia, somnolence, thinking abnormal; RESPIRATORY—bronchitis, cough increased, epistaxis, rhinitis; sinusitis; SKIN—alopecia, dry skin, rash, skin discoloration; SPECIAL SENSES—amblyopia, dry eyes; UROGENITAL—dysmenorrhea, urinary frequency, urinary tract infection, vaginal hemorrhage.

Changes in Bone Mineral Density: After 6 months of ZOLADEX treatment, 109 female patients treated with ZOLADEX showed an average 4.3% decrease of vertebral trabecular bone mineral density (BMD) as compared to pretreatment values. BMD was measured by dual-photon absorptiometry or dual energy x-ray absorptiometry. Sixty-six of these patients were assessed for BMD loss 6 months after the completion (posttherapy) of the 6-month therapy period. Data from these patients showed an average 2.4% BMD loss compared to pretreatment values. Twenty-eight of the 109 patients were assessed for BMD at 12 months posttherapy. Data from these patients showed an average decrease of 2.5% in BMD compared to pretreatment values. These data suggest a possibility of partial reversibility.

Changes in Laboratory Values During Treatment

Plasma Enzymes: Elevation of liver enzymes (AST, ALT) have been reported in female patients exposed to ZOLADEX (representing less than 1% of all patients).

Lipids: In a controlled trial, ZOLADEX therapy resulted in a minor, but statistically significant effect on serum lipids. In patients treated for endometriosis at 6 months following initiation of therapy, danazol treatment resulted in a mean increase in LDL cholesterol of 33.3 mg/dL and a decrease in HDL cholesterol of 21.3 mg/dL compared to increases of 21.3 and 2.7 mg/dL in LDL cholesterol and HDL cholesterol, respectively, for ZOLADEX-treated patients. Triglycerides increased by 8.0 mg/dL in ZOLADEX-treated patients compared to a decrease of 8.9 mg/dL in danazol-treated patients. In patients treated for endometriosis, ZOLADEX increased total cholesterol and LDL cholesterol during 6 months of treatment. However, ZOLADEX therapy resulted in HDL cholesterol levels which were significantly higher relative to danazol therapy. At the end of 6 months of treatment, HDL cholesterol fractions (HDL_2 and HDL_3) were decreased by 13.5 and 7.7 mg/dL, respectively, for danazol-treated patients compared to treatment increases of 1.9 and 0.8 mg/dL, respectively, for ZOLADEX treated patients.

Breast Cancer: The adverse event profile for women with advanced breast cancer treated with ZOLADEX is consistent with the profile described above for women treated with ZOLADEX for endometriosis. In a controlled clinical trial (SWOG-8692) comparing ZOLADEX with oophorectomy in premenopausal and perimenopausal women with advanced breast cancer, the following events were reported at a frequency of 5% or greater in either treatment group regardless of casuality.

	TREATMENT RECEIVED	
ADVERSE EVENT	ZOLADEX (n=57) % of Pts.	OOPHORECTOMY (n=55) % of Pts.
Hot Flashes	70	47
Tumor Flare	23	4
Nausea	11	7
Edema	5	0
Malaise/Fatigue/Lethargy	5	2
Vomiting	4	7

In the Phase II clinical trial program in 333 pre- and perimenopausal women with advanced breast cancer, hot flashes were reported in 75.9% of patients and decreased libido was noted in 47.7% of patients. These two adverse events reflect the pharmacological actions of ZOLADEX. Injection site reactions were reported in less than 1% of patients.

OVERDOSAGE

The pharmacologic properties of ZOLADEX and its mode of administration make accidental or intentional overdosage unlikely. There is no experience of overdosage from clinical trials. Animal studies indicate that no increased pharmacologic effect occurred at higher doses or more frequent administration. Subcutaneous doses of the drug as high as 1 mg/kg/day in rats and dogs did not produce any nonendocrine related sequelae; this dose is greater than 400 times that proposed for human use. If overdosage occurs, it should be managed symptomatically.

DOSAGE AND ADMINISTRATION

ZOLADEX, at a dose of 3.6 mg, should be administered subcutaneously every 28 days into the upper abdominal wall using an aseptic technique under the supervision of a physician.

While a delay of a few days is permissible, every effort should be made to adhere to the 28-day schedule.

For the management of advanced prostate cancer and breast cancer, Zoladex is intended for long-term administration unless clinically inappropriate.

For the management of endometriosis, the recommended duration of administration is 6 months.

Currently, there are no clinical data on the effect of treatment of benign gynecological conditions with ZOLADEX for periods in excess of 6 months.

Retreatment cannot be recommended for the management of endometriosis since safety data for retreatment are not available. If the symptoms of endometriosis recur after a course of therapy, and further treatment with ZOLADEX is contemplated, consideration should be given to monitoring bone mineral density.

No dosage adjustment is necessary for patients with renal or hepatic impairment.

Administration Technique: The proper method of administration of ZOLADEX is described in the instructions that follow.

1. The package should be inspected for damage prior to opening. If the package is damaged, the syringe should not be used. Do not remove the sterile syringe from the package until immediately before use. Examine the syringe for damage, and check that ZOLADEX is visible in the translucent chamber.
2. Clean an area of the upper abdominal wall with an alcohol swab. (A local anesthetic may be used in the normal fashion at the option of the administrator or patient.)
3. Grasp red plastic safety clip tab, pull out and away from needle, and discard immediately. Then remove needle cover.
4. Using an aseptic technique, stretch or pinch the patient's skin with one hand, and grip the syringe barrel. Insert the hypodermic needle into the subcutaneous tissue.

   NOTE: The ZOLADEX syringe cannot be used for aspiration. If the hypodermic needle penetrates a large vessel, blood will be seen instantly in the syringe chamber. If a vessel is penetrated, withdraw the needle and inject with a new syringe elsewhere.
5. Change the direction of the needle so it parallels the abdominal wall. Push the needle in until the barrel hub touches the patient's skin. Withdraw the needle one centimeter to create a space to discharge ZOLADEX. Fully depress the plunger to discharge ZOLADEX.
6. Withdraw the needle. Then bandage the site. Confirm discharge of ZOLADEX by ensuring tip of the plunger is visible within the tip of the needle. Dispose of the used needle and syringe in a safe manner.

   NOTE: In the unlikely event of the need to surgically remove ZOLADEX, it may be localized by ultrasound.

HOW SUPPLIED

ZOLADEX is supplied as a sterile and totally biodegradable D,L-lactic and glycolic acids copolymer (13.3–14.3 mg/dose) impregnated with goserelin acetate equivalent to 3.6 mg of goserelin in a disposable syringe device fitted with a 16 gauge hypodermic needle (NDC 0310-0960). The unit is sterile and comes in a sealed, light and moisture proof, aluminum foil laminate pouch containing a desiccant capsule. Store at room temperature (do not exceed 25°C).

Made in the United Kingdom
Manufactured for
ZENECA
Pharmaceuticals
A Business Unit of Zeneca Inc.
Wilmington, Delaware 19850–5437
by Zeneca Limited, Macclesfield, England
64067-01 Rev X 12/95

Shown in Product Identification Guide, pages 342

ZOLADEX® 3-MONTH ℞

GOSERELIN ACETATE IMPLANT 10.8 mg
Equivalent to 10.8 mg goserelin

FOR USE IN MEN WITH PROSTATE CANCER

DESCRIPTION

ZOLADEX® (goserelin acetate implant), contains a potent synthetic decapeptide analogue of luteinizing hormone-releasing hormone (LHRH), also known as a gonadotropin releasing hormone (GnRH) agonist analogue. Goserelin acetate is chemically described as an acetate salt of [D-Ser(Bu^t)^6,Azgly^{10}]LHRH. Its chemical structure is pyro-Glu-His-Trp-Ser-Tyr-D-Ser(Bu^t)-Leu-Arg-Pro-Azgly-NH_2 acetate [$C_{59}H_{84}N_{18}O_{14} \cdot (C_2H_4O_2)_x$ where x = 1 to 2.4].

Goserelin acetate is an off-white powder with a molecular weight of 1269 Daltons (free base). It is freely soluble in glacial acetic acid. It is soluble in water, 0.1M hydrochloric acid, 0.1M sodium hydroxide, dimethylformamide and dimethyl sulfoxide. Goserelin acetate is practically insoluble in acetone, chloroform and ether.

ZOLADEX 10.8 mg implant is supplied as a sterile, biodegradable product containing goserelin acetate equivalent to 10.8 mg of goserelin. ZOLADEX is designed for subcutaneous implantation with continuous release over a 12-week period. Goserelin acetate is dispersed in a matrix of D,L-lactic and glycolic acids copolymer (12.82–14.76 mg/dose) containing less than 2% acetic acid and up to 10% goserelin-related substances and presented as a sterile, white to cream colored 1.5 mm diameter cylinder, preloaded in a special single–use syringe with a 14–gauge needle and overwrapped in a sealed, light–and moisture proof, aluminum foil laminate pouch containing a desiccant capsule.

Studies of the D,L-lactic and glycolic acids copolymer have indicated that it is completely biodegradable and has no demonstrable antigenic potential.

ZOLADEX is also supplied as a sterile, biodegradable product containing goserelin acetate equivalent to 3.6 mg of goserelin designed for administration every 28 days.

CLINICAL PHARMACOLOGY

Mechanism of Action: ZOLADEX is a synthetic decapeptide analogue of LHRH. ZOLADEX acts as a potent inhibitor of pituitary gonadotropin secretion when administered in the biodegradable formulation.

Following initial administration, ZOLADEX causes an initial increase in serum–luteinizing hormone (LH) and follicle–stimulating hormone (FSH) levels with subsequent increases in serum levels of testosterone. Chronic administration of ZOLADEX leads to sustained suppression of pituitary gonadotropins, and serum levels of testosterone consequently fall into the range normally seen in surgically castrated men approximately 21 days after initiation of therapy. This leads to accessory sex organ regression.

In animal and in *in vitro* studies, administration of goserelin resulted in the regression or inhibition of growth of the hormonally sensitive dimethylbenzanthracene (DMBA)-induced rat mammary tumor and Dunning R3327 prostate tumor.

In clinical trials using ZOLADEX 3.6 mg with follow-up of more than 2 years, suppression of serum testosterone to castrate levels has been maintained for the duration of therapy.

Pharmacokinetics: The pharmacokinetics of goserelin have been determined in healthy male volunteers and prostate cancer patients using an RIA method, which has been shown to be specific for goserelin in the presence of its metabolites.

Serum goserelin concentrations in prostate cancer patients administered three 3.6 mg depots followed by one 10.8 mg depot are displayed in Figure 1. The profiles for both formulations are primarily dependent upon the rate of drug release from the depots. For the 3.6 mg depot, mean concentrations gradually rise to reach a peak of about 3 ng/mL at around 15 days after administration and then decline to approximately 0.5 ng/mL by the end of the treatment period. For the 10.8 mg depot, mean concentrations increase to reach a peak of about 8 ng/mL within the first 24 hours and then decline rapidly up to Day 4. Thereafter, mean concentrations remain relatively stable in the range of about 0.3 to 1 ng/mL up to the end of the treatment period.

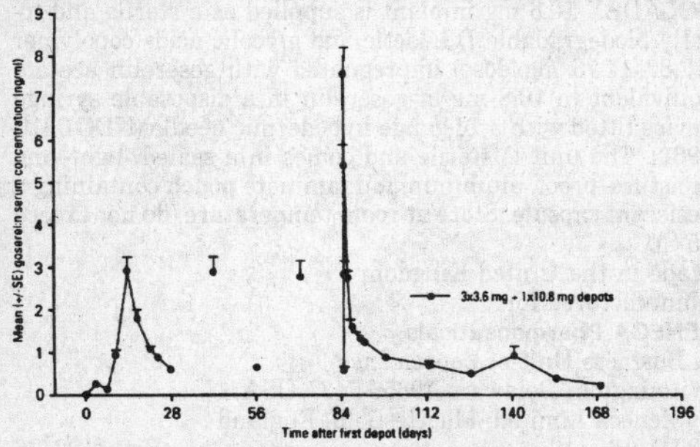

Figure 1: Goserelin serum concentrations during dosing three ZOLADEX 3.6 mg depots (0, 28, 56 days) then one ZOLADEX 10.8 mg depot (84 days) to prostate cancer patients.

Absorption: The absorption of radiolabelled drug was rapid following administration as a single 250 μg (aqueous solution) dose to volunteers by the subcutaneous route. The pharmacokinetics of goserelin following administration of a ZOLADEX 10.8 mg depot to patients with prostate cancer are determined by the release of drug from the depot; representative data are summarized in Table 1.

Release of goserelin from the depot was relatively rapid shortly after administration resulting in a peak concentration being observed 2 hours after dosing. Sustained release of goserelin produced a reasonably stable systemic exposure from Day 4 until the end of the 12-week dosing interval. This overall profile resulted in testosterone levels that were suppressed to and maintained within the range normally observed in surgically castrated men (0–1.73 nmol/L or 0–50 ng/dL), over the dosing interval in approximately 91% (145/160) of patients studied. In 6 of 15 patients that escaped from castrate range, serum testosterone levels were maintained below 2.0 nmol/L (58 ng/dL) and in only one of the 15 patients did the depot completely fail to maintain serum testosterone levels to within the recognized castrate range over a 336-day period (4 depot injections). In the 8 additional patients, a transient escape was followed 14 days later by a level within the castrate range. There is no clinically significant accumulation of goserelin following administration of four depots administered at 12-week intervals.

Distribution: The plasma protein-binding of goserelin is low (<30%).

Metabolism/Elimination: Clearance of goserelin following subcutaneous administration of the solution formulation of goserelin is very rapid and occurs via a combination of hepatic metabolism and urinary excretion. The metabolism of goserelin in humans yields a similar but narrow profile of metabolites to that found in other species. All the human metabolites have also been found in the toxicology species. The major component in serum was the 1–7 fragment formed by hydrolysis of the C-terminal amino acids.

Excretion: More than 90% of a subcutaneous radiolabelled solution formulation dose of goserelin is excreted in urine. Approximately 20% of the dose recovered in urine is accounted for by unchanged goserelin.

Special Populations

Renal Insufficiency: In clinical trials with the solution formulation of goserelin, subjects with impaired renal function (creatinine clearance less than 20 mL/min) had a serum elimination half-life of 12.1 hours compared to 4.2 hours for subjects with normal renal function (creatinine clearance greater than 70 mL/min). However, there was no evidence for any accumulation of goserelin on multiple dosing of the ZOLADEX 10.8 mg depot to subjects with impaired renal function. There was no evidence for any increase in incidence of adverse events in renally impaired patients administered the 10.8 mg depot. These data indicate that there is no need for any dosage adjustment when administering ZOLADEX 10.8 mg to subjects with impaired renal function.

Hepatic Insufficiency: The clearance and half-life of goserelin administered as an aqueous solution are not affected by hepatic impairment. These data indicate that there is no need for any dosage adjustment when administering ZOLADEX 10.8 mg to subjects with impaired hepatic function.

Geriatric: There is no need for any dosage adjustment when administering ZOLADEX 10.8 mg to geriatric patients.

Body Weight: A decline of approximately 1 to 2.5% in the AUC after administration of a 10.8 mg depot was observed with a kilogram increase in body weight. In obese patients who have not responded clinically, testosterone levels should be monitored closely.

Drug-Drug Interactions: No formal drug-drug interaction studies have been performed.

Table 1

Goserelin pharmacokinetic parameters for the 10.8 mg depot

Parameter	n	Mean	SE	95% Cl Lower	95% Cl Upper
Systemic clearance (mL/min)	41	121	6.6	108	134
C_{max} (ng/mL)	41	8.85	0.44	7.96	9.74
T_{max} (h)	41	1.80	0.05	1.70	1.92
C_{min} (ng/mL)	44	0.37	0.03	0.30	0.43
Elimination Half-life (h) ¶	7	4.16	0.40	3.12	5.20

¶ = determined after subcutaneous administration of 250 μg aqueous solution of goserelin.
SE = standard error of the mean
95% Cl = 95% confidence interval

Clinical Studies: In two controlled clinical trials, 160 patients with advanced prostate cancer were randomized to receive either one 3.6 mg ZOLADEX implant every four weeks or a single 10.8 mg ZOLADEX implant every 12 weeks. Mean serum testosterone suppression was similar between the two arms. PSA falls at three months were 94% in patients who received the 10.8 mg implant and 92.5% in patients that received three 3.6 mg implants.

Periodic monitoring of serum testosterone levels should be considered if the anticipated clinical or biochemical response to treatment has not been achieved. A clinical outcome similar to that produced with the use of the 3.6 mg implant administered every 28 days is predicted with ZOLADEX 10.8 mg implant administered every 12 weeks (84 days). Total testosterone was measured by the DPC Coat-A-Count radioimmunoassay method which, as defined by the manufacturers, is highly specific and accurate. Acceptable variability of approximately 20% at low testosterone levels has been demonstrated in the clinical studies performed with the ZOLADEX 10.8 mg depot.

INDICATIONS AND USAGE

Prostatic Carcinoma: ZOLADEX is indicated in the palliative treatment of advanced carcinoma of the prostate. ZOLADEX offers an alternative treatment of prostatic cancer when orchiectomy or estrogen administration are either not indicated or unacceptable to the patient.

In controlled studies of patients with advanced prostatic cancer comparing ZOLADEX 3.6 mg to orchiectomy, the long-term endocrine responses and objective responses were similar between the two treatment arms. Additionally, duration of survival was similar between the two treatment arms in a major comparative trial.

In controlled studies of patients with advanced prostatic cancer, ZOLADEX 10.8 mg implant produced pharmacodynamically similar effect in terms of suppression of serum testosterone to that achieved with ZOLADEX 3.6 mg implant. Clinical outcome similar to that produced with the use of the ZOLADEX 3.6 mg implant administered every 28 days is predicted with the ZOLADEX 10.8 mg implant administered every 12 weeks.

CONTRAINDICATIONS

A report of an anaphylactic reaction to synthetic GnRH (Factrel) has been reported in the medical literature. ZOLADEX is contraindicated in those patients who have a known hypersensitivity to LHRH, LHRH agonist analogues or any of the components in ZOLADEX.

ZOLADEX 10.8 mg implant is not indicated in women as the data are insufficient to support reliable suppression of serum estradiol. For female patients requiring treatment with goserelin, refer to the prescribing information for ZOLADEX 3.6 mg implant.

ZOLADEX is contraindicated in women who are or may become pregnant while receiving the drug. In studies in rats and rabbits, ZOLADEX increased preimplantation loss, resorptions, and abortions (see Pregnancy section). In rats and dogs, ZOLADEX suppressed ovarian function, decreased ovarian weight and size, and led to atrophic changes in secondary sex organs. Further evidence suggests that fertility was reduced in female rats that became pregnant after ZOLADEX was stopped. These effects are an expected consequence of the hormonal alterations produced by ZOLADEX in humans. If a patient becomes pregnant during treatment, the drug must be discontinued and the patient must be apprised of the potential risk for loss of the pregnancy due to possible hormonal imbalance as a result of the expected pharmacologic action of ZOLADEX treatment. In animal studies, there was no evidence that ZOLADEX possessed the potential to cause teratogenicity in rabbits; however, in rats the incidence of umbilical hernia was significantly increased with treatment. (See Pregnancy, Teratogenic Effects.)

WARNINGS

Initially, ZOLADEX, like other LHRH agonists, causes transient increases in serum levels of testosterone. Transient worsening of symptoms, or the occurrence of additional signs and symptoms of prostatic cancer, may occasionally develop during the first few weeks of ZOLADEX treatment. A small number of patients may experience a temporary increase in bone pain, which can be managed symptomatically. As with other LHRH agonists, isolated cases of ureteral obstruction and spinal cord compression have been observed. If spinal cord compression or renal impairment develops, standard treatment of these complications should be instituted, and in extreme cases an immediate orchiectomy considered.

PRECAUTIONS

General: Hypersensitivity, antibody formation and acute anaphylactic reactions have been reported with other LHRH agonist analogues. Currently, no anaphylactic reactions have been reported with the use of ZOLADEX (Data on file, Zeneca Pharmaceuticals).

Of 115 women worldwide treated with ZOLADEX 3.6 mg and tested for development of binding to goserelin following treatment with ZOLADEX, one patient showed low-titer binding to goserelin. On further testing of this patient's plasma obtained following treatment, her goserelin binding component was found not to be precipitated with rabbit antihuman immunoglobulin polyvalent sera. These findings suggest the possibility of anitbody formation.

Information for Patients: The use of ZOLADEX in patients at particular risk of developing ureteral obstruction or spinal cord compression should be considered carefully and the patients monitored closely during the first month of therapy. Patients with ureteral obstruction or spinal cord compression should have appropriate treatment prior to initiation of ZOLADEX therapy.

Drug Interactions: No drug interaction studies with other drugs have been conducted with ZOLADEX. No confirmed interactions have been reported between ZOLADEX and other drugs.

Drug/Laboratory Test Interactions: Administration of ZOLADEX in therapeutic doses results in suppression of the pituitary-gonadal system. Because of this suppression, diagnostic tests of pituitary-gonadotropic and gonadal functions conducted during treatment may show results which are misleading.

Carcinogenesis, Mutagenesis, Impairment of Fertility: Subcutaneous implant of ZOLADEX in male and female rats once every 4 weeks for 1 year and recovery for 23 weeks at doses of about 80 and 150 μg/kg (males) and 50 and 100 μg/kg (females) daily (about 3 to 9 times the recommended human dose on a mg/m^2 basis) resulted in an increased incidence of pituitary adenomas. An increased incidence of pituitary adenomas was also observed following subcutaneous implant of ZOLADEX in rats at similar dose levels for a period of 72 weeks in males and 101 weeks in females. The relevance of the rat pituitary adenomas to humans has not been established. Subcutaneous implants of ZOLADEX every 3 weeks for 2 years delivered to mice at doses of up 2400 μg/kg/day (about 70 times the recommended human dose on a mg/m^2 basis) resulted in an increased incidence of histiocytic sarcoma of the vertebral column and femur.

Mutagenicity tests using bacterial and mammalian systems for point mutations and cytogenetic effects have provided no evidence for mutagenic potential.

Administration of goserelin led to changes that were consistent with gonadal suppression in both male and female rats as a result of its endocrine action. In male rats administered 500–1000 μg/kg/day (about 30–60 times the recommended human dose on a mg/m^2 basis), a decrease in weight and atrophic histological changes were observed in the testes, epididymis, seminal vesicle and prostate gland with complete suppression of spermatogenesis. In female rats administered 50–1000 μg/ky/day (about 3–60 times the recommended daily human dose on a mg/m^2 basis), suppression of ovarian function led to decreased size and weight of ovaries and secondary sex organs; follicular development was arrested at the antral stage and the corpora lutea were reduced in size and number. Except for the testes, almost complete histologic reversal of these effects in males and females was observed several weeks after dosing was stopped; however, fertility and general reproductive performance were reduced in those that became pregnant after goserelin was discontinued. Fertile matings occurred within 2 weeks after cessation

Continued on next page

Zeneca Pharmaceuticals—Cont.

of dosing, even though total recovery of reproductive function may not have occurred before mating took place; and, the ovulation rate, the corresponding implantation rate, and number of live fetuses were reduced.

Based on histological examination, drug effects on reproductive organs seem to be completely reversible in male and female dogs when drug treatment was stopped after continuous administration for 1 year at 100 times the recommended monthly dose.

Pregnancy, Teratogenic Effects: Pregnancy Category X. See CONTRAINDICATIONS section. ZOLADEX 10.8 mg is not indicated in women as the data are insufficient to support reliable suppression of serum estradiol. Studies in both rats and rabbits at doses of 2, 10, 20, and 50 µg/kg/day and 20, 250, and 1,000 µg/kg/day, respectively (about $^1/_{10}$ to 3 times and 2 to 100 times the daily maximum recommended human dose, respectively, on a mg/m² basis), administered during the period of organogenesis, have confirmed that ZOLADEX will increase pregnancy loss in a dose-related manner. While there was no evidence that ZOLADEX possessed the potential to cause teratogenicity in rabbits, in rats the incidence of umbilical hernia was significantly increased at doses greater than 10 mg/kg/day (about $^1/_2$ the recommended dose on a mg/m² basis).

Nursing Mothers: It is not known if this drug is excreted in human milk. Many drugs are excreted in human milk and there is a potential for serious adverse reactions in nursing infants of mothers receiving ZOLADEX (See CONTRAINDICATIONS).

Pediatric Use: Safety and efficacy of ZOLADEX in pediatric patients have not been established.

ADVERSE REACTIONS

As with other endocrine therapies, hypercalcemia (increased calcium) has rarely been reported in cancer patients with bone metastases following initiation of treatment with ZOLADEX or other LHRH agonists.

ZOLADEX has been found to be generally well tolerated in clinical trials. Adverse reactions reported in these trials were rarely severe enough to result in the patients' withdrawal from ZOLADEX treatment. As seen with other hormonal therapies, the most commonly observed adverse events during ZOLADEX therapy were due to the expected physiological effects from decreased testosterone levels. These included hot flashes, sexual dysfunction and decreased erections.

Initially, ZOLADEX, like other LHRH agonists, causes transient increases in serum levels of testosterone. A small percentage of patients experienced a temporary worsening of signs and symptoms (see WARNINGS section), usually manifested by an increase in cancer-related pain which was managed symptomatically. Isolated cases of exacerbation of disease symptoms, either ureteral obstruction or spinal cord compression, occurred at similar rates in controlled clinical trials with both ZOLADEX and orchiectomy. The relationship of these events to therapy is uncertain.

Two controlled clinical trials using ZOLADEX 10.8 mg versus ZOLADEX 3.6 mg were conducted. During a comparative phase, patients were randomized to receive either a single 10.8 mg implant or three consecutive 3.6 mg implants every 4 weeks over weeks 0–12. During this phase, the only adverse event reported in greater than 5% of patients was hot flashes, with an incidence of 47% in the ZOLADEX 10.8 mg group and 48% in the ZOLADEX 3.6 mg group.

From weeks 12–48 all patients were treated with a 10.8 mg implant every 12 weeks. During this noncomparative phase, the following adverse events were reported in greater than 5% of patients:

Adverse Event	ZOLADEX 10.8 mg (n=157) %
Hot Flashes	64
Pain (General)	14
Gynecomastia	8
Pelvic Pain	6
Bone Pain	6
Asthenia	5

The following adverse events were reported in greater than 1%, but less than 5% of patients treated with ZOLADEX 10.8 mg implant every 12 weeks. Some of these are commonly reported in elderly patients.

WHOLE BODY—Abdominal pain, Back pain, Flu syndrome, Headache, Sepsis, Aggravation reaction
CARDIOVASCULAR—Angina pectoris, Cerebral ischemia, Cerebrovascular accident, Heart failure, Pulmonary embolus, Varicose veins

DIGESTIVE—Diarrhea, Hematemesis
ENDOCRINE—Diabetes mellitus
HEMATOLOGIC—Anemia
METABOLIC—Peripheral edema
NERVOUS SYSTEM—Dizziness, Paresthesis, Urinary retention
RESPIRATORY—Cough increased, Dyspnea, Pneumonia
SKIN—Herpes simplex, Pruritus
UROGENITAL—Bladder neoplasm, Breast pain, Hematuria, Impotence, Urinary frequency, Urinary incontinence, Urinary tract disorder, Urinary tract infection, Urination impaired.

The following adverse events not already listed above were reported in patients receiving ZOLADEX 3.6 mg in other clinical trials. Inclusion does not necessarily represent a causal relationship to ZOLADEX 10.8 mg.

WHOLE BODY—Allergic reaction, Chills, Fever, Infection, Injection site reaction, Lethargy, Malaise
CARDIOVASCULAR—Arrhythmia, Chest pain, Hemorrhage, Hypertension, Migraine, Myocardial infarction, Palpitations, Peripheral vascular disorder, Tachycardia
DIGESTIVE—Anorexia, Constipation, Dry mouth, Dyspepsia, Flatulence, Increased appetite, Nausea, Ulcer, Vomiting
HEMATOLOGIC—Ecchymosis
METABOLIC—Edema, Gout, Hyperglycemia, Weight increase
MUSCULOSKELETAL—Arthraliga, Hypertonia, Joint disorder, Leg cramps, Myalgia, Osteoporosis
NERVOUS SYSTEM—Anxiety, Depression, Emotional lability, Headache, Insomnia, Nervousness, Somnolence, Thinking abnormal
RESPIRATORY—Bronchitis, Chronic obstructive pulmonary disease, Epistaxis, Rhinitis, Sinusitis, Upper respiratory infection, Voice alterations
SKIN—Acne, Alopecia, Dry skin, Hair disorders, Rash, Seborrhea, Skin discoloration, Sweating
SPECIAL SENSES—Amblyopia, Dry eyes
UROGENITAL—Breast tenderness, Decreased erections, Renal insufficiency, Sexual dysfunction, Urinary obstruction

Changes in Laboratory Values During Treatment

Plasma Enzymes: Elevation of liver enzymes (AST, ALT) have been reported in female patients exposed to ZOLADEX 3.6 mg (representing less than 1% of all patients). There was no other evidence of abnormal liver function. Causality between these changes and ZOLADEX have not been established.

Lipids: In a controlled trial in females, ZOLADEX 3.6 mg implant therapy resulted in a minor, but statistically significant effect on serum lipids (ie, increases in LDL cholesterol of 21.3 mg/dL, increases in HDL cholesterol of 2.7 mg/dL; and triglycerides increased by 8.0 mg/dL).

OVERDOSAGE

The pharmacologic properties of ZOLADEX and its mode of administration make accidental or intentional overdosage unlikely. There is no experience of overdosage from clinical trials. Animal studies indicate that no increased pharmacologic effect occurred at higher doses or more frequent administration. Subcutaneous doses of the drug as high as 1 mg/kg/day in rats and dogs did not produce any nonendocrine related sequelae; this dose is greater than 400 times that proposed for human use. If overdosage occurs, it should be managed symptomatically.

DOSAGE AND ADMINISTRATION

ZOLADEX, at a dose of 10.8 mg, should be administered subcutaneously every 12 weeks into the upper abdominal wall using an aseptic technique under the supervision of a physician.

While a delay of a few days is permissible, every effort should be made to adhere to the 12-week schedule.

For the management of advanced prostate cancer, ZOLADEX is intended for long-term administration unless clinically inappropriate.

No dosage adjustment is necessary for patients with renal or hepatic impairment.

ZOLADEX 10.8 mg implant is not indicated in women as the data are insufficient to support reliable suppression of serum estradiol. For female patients requiring treatment with goserelin, refer to the prescribing information for ZOLADEX 3.6 mg implant.

Administration Technique: The proper method of administration of ZOLADEX is described in the instructions that follow.

1. The package should be inspected for damage prior to opening. If the package is damaged, the syringe should not be used. Do not remove the sterile syringe from the package until immediately before use. Examine the syringe for damage, and check that ZOLADEX is visible in the translucent chamber.
2. Clean an area of the upper abdominal wall with an alcohol swab. (A local anesthetic may be used in the normal fashion at the option of the administrator or patient.)
3. Grasp blue plastic safety clip tab, pull out and away from

needle, and discard immediately. Then remove needle cover.
4. Using an aseptic technique, stretch or pinch the patient's skin with one hand, and grip the syringe barrel. Insert the hypodermic needle into the subcutaneous tissue.
   NOTE: The ZOLADEX syringe cannot be used for aspiration. If the hypodermic needle penetrates a large vessel, blood will seen be instantly in the syringe chamber. If a vessel is penetrated, withdraw the needle and inject with a new syringe elsewhere.
5. Change the direction of the needle so it parallels the abdominal wall. Push the needle in until the barrel hub touches the patient's skin. Withdraw the needle one centimeter to create a space to discharge ZOLADEX. Fully depress the plunger to discharge ZOLADEX.
6. Withdraw the needle. Then bandage the site. Confirm discharge of ZOLADEX by ensuring tip of the plunger is visible within the tip of the needle. Dispose of the used needle and syringe in a safe manner.
   NOTE: In the unlikely event of the need to surgically remove ZOLADEX, it may be localized by ultrasound.

HOW SUPPLIED

ZOLADEX 10.8 mg implant is supplied as a sterile and totally biodegradable D,L-lactic and glycolic acids copolymer (12.82–14.76 mg/dose) impregnated with goserelin acetate equivalent to 10.8 mg of goserelin in a disposable syringe device fitted with a 14-gauge hypodermic needle (NDC 0310-0961). The unit is sterile and comes in a sealed, light–and moisture–proof, aluminum foil laminate pouch containing a desiccant capsule. Store at room temperature (do not exceed 25°C).

Made in the United Kingdom
Manufactured for
ZENECA Pharmaceuticals
A Business Unit of Zeneca Inc.
Wilmington, Delaware 19850-5437 USA
by Zeneca Limited, Macclesfield, England
63941-01   Rev B 02/96
Shown in Product Identification Guide, page 342

Bristol-Myers Squibb Oncology/ Immunology Division
A Bristol-Myers Squibb Company
P.O. BOX 4500
PRINCETON, NJ 08543-4500

For Medical Information Contact:
Generally:
Bristol-Myers Squibb Drug Information Department
P.O. Box 4500
Princeton, NJ 08543-4500
(800) 426-7644
Adverse Drug Experiences
and Product Defects Reporting call
during business hours only:
(609) 252-3737

Sales and Ordering:
Orders may be placed by:
1. Calling the following toll-free number between 8:30 AM–6:00 PM EST:
   Continental U.S.: (800) 631-5244
   Alaska-Hawaii: (800) 631-5244
2. Mail orders and all inquiries should be sent to:
   Bristol-Myers Squibb Oncology Division
   Attn: Customer Service
   P.O. Box 5250
   Princeton, NJ 08543-5250
3. Faxing your purchase orders to:
   (800) 523-2965
4. Transmitting computer-to-computer on the NWDA and UCS formats through Ordernet Services use: DEA #PE0048579

VIDEX®   ℞
(didanosine)
VIDEX® (didanosine) Chewable/Dispersible Buffered Tablets
VIDEX® (didanosine) Buffered Powder for Oral Solution
VIDEX® (didanosine) Pediatric Powder for Oral Solution
CAUTION: FEDERAL LAW PROHIBITS DISPENSING WITHOUT PRESCRIPTION.

WARNING
PANCREATITIS, WHICH HAS BEEN FATAL IN SOME CASES, IS THE MAJOR CLINICAL TOXICITY ASSOCIATED WITH VIDEX® (didanosine) THERAPY. PANCREATITIS MUST BE CONSIDERED WHENEVER A

PATIENT RECEIVING VIDEX DEVELOPS ABDOMINAL PAIN AND NAUSEA, VOMITING, OR ELEVATED BIOCHEMICAL MARKERS. UNDER THESE CIRCUMSTANCES, VIDEX USE SHOULD BE SUSPENDED UNTIL THE DIAGNOSIS OF PANCREATITIS IS EXCLUDED (SEE "WARNINGS").

DESCRIPTION

VIDEX® (didanosine) is the brand name for didanosine [formerly called dideoxyinosine (ddI)], a synthetic purine nucleoside analogue active against the Human Immunodeficiency Virus (HIV). VIDEX Chewable/Dispersible Buffered Tablets are available for oral administration in strengths of 25, 50, 100, or 150 mg of didanosine. Each tablet is buffered with calcium carbonate and magnesium hydroxide. VIDEX tablets also contain aspartame, sorbitol, microcrystalline cellulose, polyplasdone, mandarin-orange flavor, and magnesium stearate.

VIDEX Buffered Powder for Oral Solution is supplied for oral administration in single-dose packets containing 100, 167, or 250 mg of didanosine. Packets of each product strength also contain a citrate-phosphate buffer (composed of dibasic sodium phosphate, sodium citrate, and citric acid) and sucrose.

VIDEX Pediatric Powder for Oral Solution is supplied for oral administration in 4- or 8-ounce glass bottles containing 2 or 4 grams of didanosine, respectively.

The chemical name for didanosine is 2',3'-dideoxyinosine. The structural formula is:

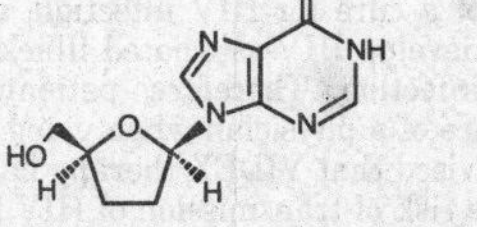

Didanosine is a white crystalline powder with the molecular formula $C_{10}H_{12}N_4O_3$ and a molecular weight of 236.2. The aqueous solubility of didanosine at 25°C and pH of approximately 6 is 27.3 mg/mL. Didanosine is unstable in acidic solutions. For example, at pH <3 and 37°C, 10 percent of didanosine decomposes to hypoxanthine in less than 2 minutes.

MICROBIOLOGY

Mechanism of Action

Didanosine is a synthetic nucleoside analogue of the naturally occurring nucleoside deoxyadenosine in which the 3'-hydroxyl (OH) group is replaced by hydrogen. Intracellularly, didanosine is converted by cellular enzymes to the active metabolite, dideoxyadenosine 5'-triphosphate (ddATP). Dideoxyadenosine 5'-triphosphate inhibits the activity of HIV-1 reverse transcriptase both by competing with the natural substrate, deoxyadenosine 5'-triphosphate (dATP), and by its incorporation into viral DNA. The lack of a 3'-OH group in the incorporated nucleoside analogue prevents the formation of the 5' to 3' phosphodiester linkage essential for DNA chain elongation and, therefore, the viral DNA growth is terminated.

***In Vitro* HIV Susceptibility**

The *in vitro* anti-HIV-1 activity of didanosine was evaluated in a variety of HIV-1 infected lymphoblastic cell lines and monocyte/macrophage cell cultures. Didanosine has shown antiviral activity against laboratory and clinical isolates of HIV-1. The concentration of drug necessary to inhibit viral replication by 50 percent (IC_{50}) ranged from 2.5 to 10 μM (1 μM = 0.24 μ/mL) in lymphoblastic cell lines and 0.01 to 0.1 μM in monocyte/macrophage cell cultures. The relationship between *in vitro* susceptibility of HIV to didanosine and the inhibition of HIV replication in humans has not been established.

Drug Resistance

HIV-1 isolates with reduced sensitivity to didanosine have been selected *in vitro* and were also obtained from patients treated with didanosine. Genetic analysis of these isolates showed a predominant mutation at Leu 74 (Leu 74 Val) and another mutation at Met 184 (Met 184 Val) in the Pol gene that encodes for the reverse transcriptase.

Cross-resistance

The potential for cross-resistance between reverse transcriptase inhibitors and protease inhibitors is low because of the different enzyme targets involved. Mutations in the reverse transcriptase gene at both codons 74 and 184 are associated with cross-resistance to zalcitabine. Lamivudine-resistant isolates containing only the Met 184 Val mutation have been recovered and these isolates showed a 4- to 8-fold decrease in didanosine sensitivity. HIV-1 isolates with multidrug resistance mutations to zidovudine, didanosine, zalcitabine, stavudine and lamivudine have been reported (2/39 patients) following combination therapy with zidovudine and didanosine for 2 years. Multidrug resistance was dependent on five mutations (Ala 62 Val, Val 75 Ile, Phe 77 Leu, Phe 116 Tyr and Gln 151 Met) in the reverse transcriptase gene. Of these, the mutation at codon position 151 (Q151M) played a significant role in the development of viable virus with a multidrug resistance phenotype.

Animal Toxicology

Evidence of a dose-limiting skeletal muscle toxicity has been observed in mice and rats (but not in dogs) following long-term (greater than 90 days) dosing with didanosine at doses that were approximately 1.2 to 12 times the estimated human exposure. The relationship of this finding to the potential of VIDEX (didanosine) to cause myopathy in humans is unclear. However, human myopathy has been associated with administration of other nucleoside analogues.

Pharmacokinetics

Didanosine pharmacokinetics were evaluated in 69 patients with AIDS or AIDS-Related Complex, Patients received a 60 minute IV infusion of didanosine once or twice a day for 2 weeks; total daily doses ranged from 0.8 mg/kg to 33 mg/kg. Oral doses equivalent to twice the IV doses were administered for an additional 4 weeks. Oral doses were administered as a lyophilized formulation similar in composition to VIDEX Pediatric Powder for Oral Solution.

Absorption: Although there was significant variability between patients, C_{MAX} and AUC increased in proportion to dose over the range of doses administered in clinical practice. The absolute bioavailablity of didanosine was 33±14% at doses of 7 mg/kg or less. Because didanosine degrades rapidly at acidic pH, VIDEX Chewable/Dispersible Tablets and VIDEX Buffered Powder for Oral Solution contain buffering agents. VIDEX (didanosine) Pediatric Powder for Oral Solution must be administered with antacids. (see "DOSAGE AND ADMINISTRATION")

Administration of nonmarketed chewable/dispersible buffered didanosine tablets 30 minutes or 1 hour before a meal did not result in any significant changes in bioavailability, compared to administration under fasting conditions (n=10, asymptomatic HIV postive patients). When the tablets were administered 1 or 2 hours after a meal, C_{MAX} and AUC were decreased by approximately 55%, which was comparable to the decreases observed when the formulation was administered immediately after a meal. (see "DOSAGE AND ADMINISTRATION")

Distribution: The steady state volume of distribution following IV administration was 0.81±0.22 L/kg. *In vitro*, didanosine is less than 5 percent bound to human plasma proteins. The concentration of didanosine in cerebrospinal fluid samples (n=5) collected 1 hour after IV infusion averaged 21 percent of the simultaneous plasma concentration.

Elimination: Following IV administration, total clearance was approximately 11.8±3.1 mL/min/kg. Following oral administration, elimination half-life was 1.5±0.6 hours. There was no evidence of accumulation of didanosine after either IV or oral dosing; steady-state pharmacokinetic parameters did not differ significantly from values obtained after single dose.

Metabolism: The metabolism of didanosine has not been evaluated in man. When ^{14}C-radiolabeled didanosine was administered to dogs as a single IV or oral dose, extensive metabolism occurred. The major metabolite identified in the urine, allantoin, represented approximately 61 percent of the administered radiolabel after oral administration. Three putative metabolites tentatively identified in the urine were hypoxanthine, xanthine, and uric acid. A similar metabolic profile was observed in rat plasma after oral administration of ^{14}C-radiolabeled didanosine to male and female rats. The metabolic fate of the dideoxyribose moiety, released subsequent to enzymatic or chemical hydrolysis of the glycosidic bond, has not been determined. Based upon data from animal studies, it is presumed that the metabolism of didanosine in man will occur by the same pathways responsible for the elimination of endogenous purines.

The intracellular half-life of ddATP, the metabolite presumed to be responsible for the antiretroviral activity of didanosine, is reported to be 8 to 24 hours *in vitro*. The half-life of intracellular ddATP *in vivo* has not been measured.

Excretion: Renal clearance was approximately 6.4±2.4 mL/min/kg following either IV or oral administration. Active tubular secretion in addition to glomerular filtration is responsible for the renal elimination of didanosine. Urinary recovery of didanosine after a single dose was 55±17 percent and 20±8 percent of the dose following IV and oral administration, respectively.

Special Populations

Renal Impairment: Didanosine pharmacokinetics were compared between HIV positive patients with normal renal function (n=6) and patients with severe renal impairment. Patients with severe renal impairment had creatinine clearances less than 10 mL/min/1.73 m² and were maintained on CAPD (n=5) or hemodialysis (n=6). Total body clearance following IV administeration was 3.3±0.8 mL/min/kg in patients with severe renal impairment and 13.0±1.6 mL/min/kg in patients with normal renal function. The mean elimination half-life following oral administration of didanosine increased from approximately 1.5 hours in patients with normal renal function to approximately 4 hours in patients with severe renal impairment. The absolute bioavailability of didanosine was not affected in patients with renal impairment. Following oral administration, didanosine was not detectable in peritoneal dialysate fluid; recovery in hemodialysate ranged from 0.6 to 7.4% of the dose over a 3–4 hour dialysis period. Approximately 35% of the didanosine present in the body at the start of dialysis was eliminated during the hemodialysis session. (see "DOSAGE AND ADMINISTRATION") The effect of mild to moderate renal impairment on didanosine pharmacokinetics has not been studied.

Hepatic Impairment: The effect of hepatic impairment on didanosine pharmacokinetics has not been studied.

Pediatric Patients: For pharmacokinetic properties of didanosine in pediatric patients, see "**PRECAUTIONS, Pediatric Use.**"

INDICATIONS AND USAGE

Videx is indicated for the treatment of HIV infection when antiretroviral therapy is warranted.

This indication is based on the results of four randomized, double-blind controlled clinical trials. (see "Description of Clinical Data" and "PRECAUTIONS, Pediatric Use")

The duration of clinical benefit from antiretroviral therapy may be limited. Alteration in antiretroviral therapy should be considered if disease progression occurs while receiving VIDEX.

Description of Clinical Data

Controlled Clinical Trial ACTG 175

ACTG 175 was a randomized, double-blind, controlled trial that compared ZDV 200 mg TID; VIDEX 200 mg BID; ZDV + VIDEX; and ZDV + ddC 0.75 mg TID. A total of 2467 HIV-infected adults with baseline CD4 counts of 200–500 cells/mm³ (mean=352) and no prior AIDS-defining event enrolled with the following demographics: male (82%), Caucasian (70%), mean age of 35 years, asymptomatic HIV infection (81%) and prior antiretroviral use (57%, mean duration = 89.5 weeks). The overall mean duration of study treatment was 99 weeks.

Results: The incidence of AIDS-defining events or death is shown in the following table:

[See table above.]

Table 1
First AIDS-defining Event or Death and Death Only by Study Arm and Antiretroviral Experience

Antiretroviral Experience	Event	ZDV	VIDEX	ZDV + VIDEX	ZDV + ddC
Overall	n	619	620	613	615
	AIDS/Death	96 (16%)	71 (11%)	65 (11%)	76 (12%)
	Death Only	54 (9%)	29 (5%)	31 (5%)	40 (7%)
Naive	n	269	268	263	267
	AIDS/Death	32 (12%)	23 (9%)	20 (8%)	16 (6%)
	Death Only	18 (7%)	11 (4%)	11 (4%)	9 (3%)
Experienced	n	350	352	350	348
	AIDS/Death	64 (18%)	48 (14%)	45 (13%)	60 (17%)
	Death Only	36 (10%)	18 (5%)	20 (6%)	31 (9%)

Controlled Clinical Trial ACTG 116A

ACTG 116A was a randomized, double-blind, controlled trial that compared high and recommended doses of VIDEX to zidovudine in patients who had received up to 16 weeks of zidovudine therapy. 617 HIV-infected adults enrolled with the following demographics: male (92%), Caucasian (73%), mean age of 36 years, median CD4 cell count of 130 cells/mm³, symptomatic HIV infection (67%) or AIDS (26%) and median duration of prior antiretroviral use of 8 weeks. The median duration of study treatment was 60 weeks.

Results: In the three treatment groups, the time until development of a first new AIDS-defining event or death was similar. Patients randomized to zidovudine had longer survival times than patients randomized to VIDEX recommended dose with mortality rates of 26% and 21% for VIDEX recommended dose and zidovudine, respectively.

Continued on next page

Bristol-Myers Squibb Oncology—Cont.

Controlled Clinical Trial ACTG 116B/117

ACTG 116B/117 was a randomized, double-blind, controlled clinical trial that compared high and recommended doses of VIDEX (didanosine) to zidovudine in patients who had tolerated four months or greater of prior zidovudine therapy. 913 HIV-infected adults enrolled with the following demographics: male (96%), Caucasian (82%), mean age of 37 years, median CD4 cell count of 95 cells/mm^3, symptomatic HIV infection (60%) or AIDS (30%) and median duration of prior antiretroviral use of 59.4 weeks. The median duration of study treatment was 49.7 weeks.

Results: Subjects randomized to the currently recommended dose of VIDEX had a lower rate of progression to a new AIDS-defining event or death compared to those randomized to ZDV (32% vs. 41%, respectively). Survival rates were similar for the two treatment groups.

CONTRAINDICATION

VIDEX is contraindicated in patients with previously demonstrated clinically significant hypersensitivity to any of the components of the formulations.

WARNINGS

1. Pancreatitis

PANCREATITIS, WHICH HAS BEEN FATAL IN SOME CASES, IS THE MAJOR CLINICAL TOXICITY ASSOCIATED WITH VIDEX THERAPY. PANCREATITIS MUST BE CONSIDERED WHENEVER A PATIENT RECEIVING VIDEX DEVELOPS ABDOMINAL PAIN AND NAUSEA, VOMITING, OR ELEVATED AMYLAPSE OR LIPASE AND VIDEX USE SHOULD BE SUSPENDED UNTIL THE DIAGNOSIS OF PANCREATITIS IS EXCLUDED.

When treatment with other drugs known to cause pancreatic toxicity is required (for example, IV pentamidine), suspension of VIDEX (didanosine) is recommended. In patients with risk factors for pancreatitis, such as a history of pancreatitis, alcohol consumption, or elevated triglycerides, VIDEX should be used with extreme caution and only if clearly indicated. Patients with advanced HIV infection are at increased risk of pancreatitis and should be followed closely. Patients with renal impairment may be at greater risk for pancreatitis if treated without dose adjustment.

The incidence of pancreatitis rises with increasing doses of VIDEX. The incidences of pancreatitis, AND THE RELATIONSHIP TO VIDEX DOSE AND ZIDOVUDINE, for the ACTG 175, 116B/117 and 116A trials are described in the table below: [See Table 2 below.]

In phase I studies, the frequency of pancreatitis was dose related and occurred 8/91 (9%) of patients who received < 12.5 mg/kg/day and in 21/79 (27%) of patients who received > 12.5 mg/kg/day.

In pediatric studies, pancreatitis occurred in 2 of 60 (3%) patients treated at entry doses below 300 mg/m^2/day and in 5 of 38 (13%) patients treated at higher doses. In pediatric patients with symptoms similar to those described above, VIDEX use should be suspended until the diagnosis of pancreatitis is excluded.

2. Liver Failure

Hepatitis, which in some instances was fulminant or associated with lactic acidosis, has been reported postmarketing.

3. Retinal depigmentation and vision

Retinal changes and optic neuritis have been reported in several pediatric patients who received VIDEX at and above the recommended dose. Retinal depigmentation and optic neuritis have been reported in several adult patients. Children receiving VIDEX should undergo dilated retinal examination every 6 months or if a change in vision occurs. Periodic retinal examinations should be considered for adult patients receiving VIDEX. (See "**ADVERSE REACTIONS.**")

PRECAUTIONS

General

Patients receiving VIDEX or any other antiretroviral therapy may continue to develop opportunistic infections and other complications of HIV infection, and therefore should remain under close clinical observation by physicians experienced in the treatment of patients with associated HIV diseases.

To avoid a reduction in the bioavailability of didanosine, VIDEX should be administered at least 30 minutes before a meal.

Patients with Phenylketonuria: VIDEX (didanosine) Chewable/ Dispersible Buffered Tablets contain the following quantities of phenylalanine:

Table 3

	All Strengths
Phenylalanine per 2-tablet dose	73 mg
Phenylalanine per tablet	36.5 mg

Patients on Sodium-Restricted Diets: VIDEX Buffered Powder for Oral Solution: Each single-dose packet of VIDEX Buffered Powder for Oral Solution contains 1380 mg sodium.

Patients With Renal Impairment: Patients with renal impairment (serum creatinine > 1.5 mg/dL or creatinine clearance < 60 mL/min) may be at greater risk of toxicity from VIDEX due to decreased drug clearance. The clearance of didanosine is reduced in patients with severe renal insufficiency (Clcr 10 mL/min/1.73 m^2) (see "**CLINICAL PHARMACOLOGY**" section). A dose reduction is recommended in these patients (see "**DOSAGE AND ADMINISTRATION**" section). The magnesium content of each buffered tablet of VIDEX is 8.6 mEq. This may present an excessive load of magnesium to patients with significant renal impairment, particularly after prolonged dosing.

Patients With Hepatic Impairment: Patients with hepatic impairment may be at greater risk for toxicity related to VIDEX treatment due to altered metabolism; a dose reduction may be necessary.

Hyperuricemia: VIDEX has been associated with asymptomatic hyperuricemia; treatment suspension may be necessary if clinical measures aimed at reducing uric acid levels fail.

Diarrhea: VIDEX Buffered Powder for Oral Solution was associated with diarrhea in 34 percent of patients in the phase 1 adult studies (see "**ADVERSE REACTIONS**"). If diarrhea develops in a patient receiving VIDEX Buffered Powder for Oral Solution, a trial of VIDEX Chewable/Dispersible Buffered Tablets should be considered.

Pediatric Use

Results from Controlled Clinical Trial ACTG 152

ACTG 152 was a randomized, double-blind, controlled trial that compared ZDV 180 mg/m^2 q6h; VIDEX 120 mg/m^2 q12h; and ZDV (120 mg/m^{2}q6h) + VIDEX (90 mg/m^2 q12h). A total of 831 HIV-infected pediatric patients were enrolled with the following demographics: male (50%), racial minority groups (86%), mean age of 3.8 years (54% were < 30 months of age), perinatally acquired infection (90%), naive to antiretroviral treatment (89%). The overall median duration of study treatment was 20 months.

Results: The incidence of clinical progression or death is shown in the following table:

Table 4
Clinical Progression or Death and Death Only by Study Arm

	Treatment		
Event	ZDV N=276	VIDEX (didanosine) N=281	VIDEX+ZDV N=274
Disease Progression† or Death	74 (27%)	54 (19%)	48 (18%)
Death Only	31 (11%)	20 (7%)	23 (8%)

†Disease Progression was defined as any of the following weight growth failure, brain growth failure, ≥2 opportunistic infections or malignancy.

Pharmacokinetic Properties in Pediatric Patients

The pharmacokinetics of didanosine have been evaluated in two pediatric studies. In the first study, 20 patients received a single IV dose ranging from 40 to 90 mg/m^2, and multiple, twice-daily oral doses of 80 to 180 mg/m^2 didanosine. In the second study, 47 patients received a single IV dose, followed by multiple, three-times-daily oral doses ranging from 20 to 180 mg/m^2. The average (+ SD) age of the patients enrolled in both studies was 7.5 (+ 4.9) years, and ranged from 0.7 to 18.9 years. Fourteen patients were older than 12 years of age. In both studies, a lyophilized formulation similar in composition to VIDEX Pediatric Powder for Oral Solution was administered orally. The C_{MAX} and AUC values, increased in proportion to dose after IV and oral administration, although a significant variability among patients was noted. Using data from both studies, the average (+ SD) elimination half-life after an oral dose was 0.8 (+ 0.3) hours. Absolute bioavailability averaged 25 (+ 20) percent after a single dose. Urinary recovery and renal clearance values, obtained only in the first study, averaged 18 (+ 10) percent and 240 (+ 90) mL/min/m^2, respectively, after a single oral dose. There was no evidence of accumulation of didanosine after the administration of oral doses for an average of 26 days. The volume of distribution after IV administration averaged 28 (+ 15) L/m^2. The average total body clearance following a single IV dose was 516 (+ 184) mL/min/m^2. Total body clearance was independent of age, and was similar to the value obtained in adult patients (446 + 116 mL/min/m^2) administered at doses ranging from 15 to 839 mg/m^2. In cerebrospinal fluid samples collected from 7 patients, at times ranging from 1.5 to 3.5 hr after a single IV or PO dose, the concentration of didanosine (range: 0.04 to 0.12 μg/mL) corresponded to 12 to 85 percent (average: 46 percent) of the concentration in a simultaneous plasma sample.

Table 2
Number (%) of Patients with Pancreatitis
(ACTG 175, 116B/117 and 116A Trial Data)

	High Dose VIDEX			Recommended VIDEX Dose			Zidovudine	
	116A	116B/117	175	116A	116B/117	175	116A	116B/117
N	207	311	620	196	298	619	208	304
Pancreatitis	18 (9%)*	31 (10%)*	7 (1%)	14 (7%)	17 (6%)	1 (<1%)	7 (3%)	6 (2%)

*Two fatalities occurred in this group.

Information for Patients

VIDEX is not a cure for HIV infection, and patients may continue to develop HIV-associated illnesses, including opportunistic infection. Therefore, patients should remain under the care of a physician when using VIDEX. Patients should be advised that VIDEX therapy has not been shown to reduce the risk of transmission of HIV to others through sexual contact or blood contamination.

Patients should be informed that the major toxicity of VIDEX is pancreatitis, which has been fatal in some patients. Patients should also be aware that peripheral neuropathy may develop. Patients should be counseled that these toxicities occur with greatest frequency in patients with a history of these events, and that dose modification and/or discontinuation of VIDEX may be required if toxicity develops. They should be cautioned about the use of other medications that may exacerbate the VIDEX toxicity, including alcohol.

Drug Interactions

Coadministration of VIDEX with drugs that are known to cause pancreatitis may increase the risk of this toxicity (see "WARNINGS") and should be done with extreme caution and only if clearly indicated. Neuropathy has occurred more frequently in patients with a history of neuropathy or neurotoxic drug therapy and these patients may be at increased risk of neuropathy during VIDEX therapy (see "**ADVERSE REACTIONS**").

Drug interaction studies have demonstrated that there are no clinically significant interactions with VIDEX and the following: ketoconazole, ranitidine, loperamide, metoclopramide and rifabutin. Drugs whose absorption can be affected by the level of acidity in the stomach (e.g., ketoconazole, dapsone), should be administered at least 2 hours prior to dosing with VIDEX. A study in 4 patients revealed that concomitant administration of ganciclovir does not significantly affect the pharmacokinetics of didanosine. There is no evidence that VIDEX potentiates the myelosuppressive effects of ganciclovir or zidovudine.

As with other products containing or mixed with magnesium and/or aluminum antacid components, VIDEX Chewable/ Dispersible Buffered Tablets or VIDEX Pediatric Powder for Oral Solution should not be administered with a prescription antibiotic containing any form of tetracycline.

Plasma concentrations of some quinolone antibiotics are decreased when administered with antacids containing magnesium or aluminum. Therefore, doses of quinolone antibiotics should not be administered within 2 hours of taking VIDEX Chewable/Dispersible Buffered Tablets or Pediatric Powder for Oral Solution. Concomitant administration of antacids containing magnesium or aluminum with VIDEX Chewable/ Dispersible Buffered Tablets or Pediatric Powder for Oral Solution may potentiate adverse effects associated with the antacid components.

Carcinogenesis and Mutagenesis

Lifetime carcinogenicity studies were conducted in mice and rats for 22 and 24 months, respectively. In the mouse study, initial doses of 120, 800 and 1200 mg/kg/day for each sex, were lowered after 8 months to 120, 210 and 210 mg/kg/day for females and 120, 300 and 600 mg/kg/day for males. The two higher doses exceeded the maximally tolerated dose in females and the high dose exceeded the maximally tolerated dose in males. The low dose in females represented 0.68-fold maximum human exposure and the intermediate dose in males represented 1.7-fold maximum human exposure. In the rat study, initial doses were 100, 250, and 1000 mg/kg/

day, and the high dose was lowered to 500 mg/kg/day after 18 months. The upper dose in male and female rats represented 3-fold maximum human exposure.

Didanosine induced no significant increase in neoplastic lesions in mice or rats at maximally tolerated doses.

No evidence of mutagenicity (with or without metabolic activation) was observed in Ames *Salmonella* mutagenicity assays or in a mutagenicity assay conducted with *Escherichia coli* tester strain WP2 uvrA where only a slight increase in revertants was observed with didanosine. In a mammalian cell gene mutation assay conducted in L5178Y/TK+/− mouse lymphoma cells, didanosine was weakly positive both in the absence and presence of metabolic activation at concentrations of approximately 2000 μg/mL and above. In an *in vitro* cytogenetic study performed in cultured human peripheral lymphocytes, high concentrations of didanosine ($\geq$ 500 μg/mL) elevated the frequency of cells bearing chromosome aberrations. Another *in vitro* mammalian cell chromosome aberration study using Chinese Hamster Lung cells revealed that didanosine produces chromosome aberrations at $\geq$500 μg/mL after 48 hours of exposure. However, no significant elevations in the frequency of cells with chromosome aberrations were seen at didanosine concentrations up to 250 μg/mL. In a BALB/c 3T3 *in vitro* transformation assay, didanosine was considered positive only at concentrations of 3000 μg/mL and above. No evidence of genotoxicity was observed in rat and mouse micronucleus assays.

The results from the genotoxicity studies suggest that didanosine is not mutagenic at biologically and pharmacologically relevant doses. At significantly elevated doses *in vitro*, the genotoxic effects of didanosine are similar in magnitude to those seen with natural DNA nucleosides.

Pregnancy, Reproduction and Fertility

Pregnancy Category B. Reproduction studies have been performed in rats and rabbits at doses up to 12 and 14.2 times the estimated human exposure (based upon plasma levels), respectively, and have revealed no evidence of impaired fertility or harm to the fetus due to didanosine. At approximately 12 times the estimated human exposure, didanosine was slightly toxic to female rats and their pups during mid and late lactation. These rats showed reduced food intake and body weight gains but the physical and functional development of the offspring was not impaired and there were no major changes in the F2 generation. A study in rats showed that didanosine and/or its metabolites are transferred to the fetus through the placenta. There are no adequate and well-controlled studies in pregnant women. Because animal reproduction studies are not always predictive of human response, this drug should be used during pregnancy only if clearly needed.

Nursing Mothers

A study in rats showed that following oral administration, didanosine and/or its metabolites were excreted into the milk of lactating rats. Although it is not known if didanosine is excreted in human milk, there is the potential for adverse effects from didanosine in nursing infants. Mothers should be instructed to discontinue nursing if they are receiving didanosine. This instruction is consistent with the Centers for Disease Control recommendation that HIV-infected mothers not breast feed their infants to avoid risking postnatal transmission of HIV infection.

ADVERSE REACTIONS

THE MAJOR TOXICITY OF VIDEX (didanosine) IS PANCREATITIS. OTHER IMPORTANT TOXICITIES INCLUDE LIVER FAILURE AND RETINAL CHANGES (see "WARNINGS").

Adults: Clinical adverse events that occurred in at least 5 percent of adult patients in the ACTG 116B/117 or 116A clinical trials are provided in Table 5. The types of adverse events reported to occur in the ACTG 175 trial in VIDEX-treated patients were generally similar to those events reported in other controlled clinical trials, although the incidence of adverse events was generally lower in all treatment groups in this population with less advanced HIV disease. Adverse events reported to occur in patients treated with VIDEX + ZDV combination therapy in the ACTG 175 clinical trial were generally similar to those reported in patients treated with either individual drug.

Table 5
Clinical Adverse Events: Cumulative Incidence ≥5% at VIDEX Recommended Dose (ACTG 116B/117 and 116A)

	Percent of Patients			
	Recommended VIDEX Dose		Zidovudine	
Adverse Events	116A N=197	116B/117 N=298	116A N=212	116B/117 N=304
Diarrhea	19	28	15	21
Neuropathy (all grades)	17	20	14	12
Chills/Fever	9	12	12	11
Rash/Pruritus	7	9	8	5
Abdominal Pain	13	7	8	8
Asthenia	4	7	8	9
Headache	6	7	12	7
Pain	6	7	6	3
Nausea & Vomiting	7	7	14	6
Pancreatitis	7	6	3	2

The cumulative incidences of serious laboratory abnormalities in clinical trials ACTG 116B/117 and 116 A are listed in Table 6. The types of serious laboratory abnormalities reported in the ACTG 175 trial in VIDEX-treated patients were generally similar to those reported in other controlled clinical trials. Serious laboratory abnormalities reported in patients treated with VIDEX + ZDV combination therapy in the ACTG 175 clinical trial were generally similar to those reported in patients treated with either individual drug.

Table 6
ACTG 116B/117 and 116A Clinical Trials: Cumulative Incidences of Serious Laboratory Abnormalities

	Percent of Patients			
Lab Tests	Recommended VIDEX Dose		Zidovudine	
(Seriously Abnormal Level)	116A N=197	116B/117 N=298	116A N=212	116B/117 N=304
Hemoglobin (<8.0 g/dL)	6	3	8	5
Leukopenia (<2000/mL)	13	16	26	22
Granulocytopenia (<750/mL)	6	8	19	15
Thrombocytopenia (<50,000/mL)	2	2	4	3
SGOT (AST) (>5 × ULN)	9	7	4	6
SGPT (ALT) (>5 × ULN)	9	6	6	6
Alkaline phosphatase (>5 × ULN)	4	1	1	1
Bilirubin (>2.6 × ULN)	1	1	1	1
Amylase (≥1.4 ×ULN)	17	15	12	5
Uric Acid (>12 mg/dL)	3	2	1	1

Peripheral neuropathy occurs in patients treated with VIDEX and the frequency appears to be dose related. In phase I studies, neuropathy occurred in 31/91 (34%) patients who received < 12.5 mg/kg/day and in 40/79 (51%) patients who received > 12.5 mg/kg/day. See Table 5 for incidence in controlled trials.

Patients should be monitored for the development of a neuropathy that is usually characterized by numbness, tingling or pain in the feet or hands. Neuropathy has occurred more frequently in patients with a history of neuropathy or neurotoxic drug therapy and these patients may be at increased risk of neuropathy during VIDEX therapy.

Other adverse events that have been reported in controlled clinical trials and have been received as part of ongoing surveillance include:

Body as a Whole—anaphylactoid reaction.
Digestive Disorders— anorexia, dyspepsia and flatulence.
Exocrine Gland Disorders—sialoadenitis, parotid gland enlargement, dry mouth and dry eyes.
Metabolic Disorders—hypoglycemia and hyperglycemia.
Musculoskeletal Disorders—arthralgia and myopathy.

Rare cases of rhabdomyolysis associated with VIDEX use have been reported. A few of these cases were complicated by acute renal failure, which required hemodialysis.

Retinal depigmentation and optic neuritis have been reported in several adult patients.

Reports of hepatitis, diabetes mellitus, myalgia (with or without increases in creatine phosphokinase), and alopecia have been received post-marketing.

Pediatric Patients: Adverse events reported to occur in the pediatric patients in the ACTG 152 trial were generally similar to those reported in adults.

In pediatric phase I studies, pancreatitis occurred in 2 of 60 (3 percent) patients treated at entry doses below 300 mg/m²/day and in 5 of 38 (13 percent) patients treated at higher doses.

Retinal changes and optic neuritis have been reported in several pediatric patients who received VIDEX (didanosine) at and above the recommended dose.

Serious laboratory abnormalities experienced by the pediatric patients in the ACTG 152 clinical trial are listed in Table 7.

Table 7
Pediatric Patient Serious Laboratory Abnormalities in ACTG 152 (Cumulative Incidences)

	Percent of Patients		
Laboratory Test Seriously Abnormal Level	VIDEX N=281	VIDEX +ZDV N=274	ZDV N=276
Hemoglobin (<7.5 g/dL)	5	7	10
Leukopenia (<2000/mL)	<1	<1	1
Granulocytopenia (<500/mL)	11	16	27
Thrombocytopenia (<50,000/mL)	6	7	7
SGOT (AST) (≥5 × ULN)	14	10	16
SGPT (ALT) (≥10 × ULN)	5	2	7
Alkaline Phosphatase (≥2 × ULN)	7	9	10
Bilirubin (≥2.6 × ULN)	6	3	4
Amylase (≥3.1 × ULN)	5	6	7
Creatine Kinase (≥5.1 × ULN)	6	8	8
Uric Acid (≥3.5 × ULN)	<1	<1	<1

OVERDOSAGE

There is no known antidote for VIDEX overdosage. In phase 1 studies, in which VIDEX was initially administered at doses ten times the currently recommended dose, toxicities included: pancreatitis, peripheral neuropathy, diarrhea, hyperuricemia and hepatic dysfunction. Didanosine is not dialyzable by peritoneal dialysis, although there is some clearance by hemodialysis (see "Pharmacokinetics" subsection of "CLINICAL PHARMACOLOGY" section).

DOSAGE AND ADMINISTRATION

Dosage:
Adults: The dosing interval should be 12 hours. **All VIDEX formulations should be administered at least 30 minutes before a meal. Adult patients should take 2 tablets at each dose so that adequate buffering is provided to prevent gastric acid degradation of didanosine.** The recommended starting dose in adults is dependent on weight as outlined in the table below:

Table 8
Adult Dosing

Patient Weight	VIDEX Tablets	VIDEX Buffered Powder
≥ 60 kg	200 mg BID	250 mg BID
< 60 kg	125 mg BID	167 mg BID

Pediatric Patients: The recommended dosing interval is 12 hours. **All VIDEX formulations should be administered at least 30 minutes before a meal.** The recommended dose of VIDEX monotherapy in pediatric patients is 120 mg/m² BID.

Dose Adjustment:
Clinical signs suggestive of pancreatitis should prompt dose suspension and careful evaluation of the possibility of pancreatitis. Only after pancreatitis has been ruled out should dosing be resumed.

Patients who have presented symptoms of neuropathy may tolerate a reduced dose of VIDEX after resolution of these symptoms upon drug discontinuation.

Although there are insufficient data to recommend a specific dose adjustment of VIDEX in patients with mild or moderate renal impairment, a dose reduction should be considered. In anuric patients requiring dialysis, it is recommended that one fourth of the total daily dose of VIDEX be administered once a day (see "CLINICAL PHARMACOLOGY" section). There are insufficient data to recommend a specific dose adjustment of VIDEX in patients with hepatic impairment, but an adjustment in the dose in these patients should also be considered.

Continued on next page

Bristol-Myers Squibb Oncology—Cont.

Method of Preparation:
VIDEX Chewable/Dispersible Buffered Tablets
Adult Dosing: Two tablets should be thoroughly chewed, manually crushed, or dispersed in at least 1 ounce of water prior to consumption. To disperse tablets, add 2 tablets to at least 1 ounce of drinking water. Stir until a uniform dispersion forms, and drink the entire dispersion immediately. If additional flavoring is desired, the dispersion may be diluted with one ounce of clear apple juice. Stir the further diluted dispersion just prior to consumption. The dispersion with clear apple juice is stable at room temperature, 62–73°F (17–23°C), for up to one hour.
VIDEX Buffered Powder for Oral Solution
1. Open packet carefully and pour contents into a container with approximately 4 ounces of drinking water. Do not mix with fruit juice or other acid-containing liquid.
2. Stir until the powder completely dissolves (approximately 2 to 3 minutes).
3. Drink the entire solution immediately.

VIDEX Pediatric Powder for Oral Solution
Prior to dispensing, the pharmacist must constitute dry powder with Purified Water, USP, to an initial concentration of 20 mg/mL and immediately mix the resulting solution with antacid to a final concentration of 10 mg/mL as follows:
20 mg/mL Initial Solution: Constitute the product to 20 mg/mL by adding 100 mL or 200 mL of Purified Water, USP, to the 2 g or 4 g of VIDEX powder, respectively, in the product bottle.
10 mg/mL Final Admixture: 1. Immediately mix one part of the 20 mg/mL initial solution with one part of either Mylanta® Double Strength Liquid (Mylanta® is a registered trademark of Stuart Pharmaceuticals, Division of ICI Americas, Inc. Mylanta® Double Strength, formerly Mylanta® II, is distributed by Johnson & Johnson/Merck, Consumer Pharmaceuticals Company, Fort Washington, PA 19034 [USA]), Extra Strength Maalox® Plus Suspension, or Maalox® TC Suspension (Maalox® is a registered trademark of William H. Rorer Inc., Unit of Rhone-Poulenc) for a final dispensing concentration of 10 mg VIDEX per mL. For patient home use, the admixture should be dispensed in appropriately sized, flint-glass bottles with child-resistant closures. This admixture is stable for 30 days under refrigeration, 36° to 46° F (2° to 8° C).
2. Instruct the patient to shake the admixture thoroughly prior to use and to store the tightly closed container in the refrigerator, 36° to 46° F (2° to 8° C), up to 30 days.

HOW SUPPLIED

VIDEX® (didanosine) Chewable/Dispersible Buffered Tablets are round, off white to light orange/yellow with a mottled appearance; orange-flavored, tablets embossed with "VIDEX" on one side and the product strength on the other. The tablets are available in the following strengths of VIDEX: 25, 50, 100, or 150 mg. Sixty tablets are packaged in bottles with child-resistant closures.
The tablets should be stored in tightly closed bottles at 59° to 86° F (15° to 30° C). If dispersed in water, the dose may be held for up to 1 hour at ambient temperature.
VIDEX Buffered Powder for Oral Solution is supplied in single-dose, child-resistant foil packets in the following strengths of VIDEX (didanosine): 100, 167, or 250 mg. Each product strength provides a sweetened, buffered solution of VIDEX.
The packets should be stored at 59° to 86° F (15° to 30° C). After dissolving in water, the solution may be stored at ambient room temperature for up to 4 hours.
VIDEX Pediatric Powder for Oral Solution is supplied in 4- and 8-ounce glass bottles containing 2 g or 4 g of VIDEX, respectively.
The bottles of powder should be stored at 59° to 86° F (15° to 30° C). The VIDEX admixture may be stored up to 30 days in a refrigerator, 36° to 46° F (2° to 8° C). Discard any unused portion after 30 days.
The NDC numbers for the previously described VIDEX products are:

Table 9

NDC NO.	Packaging Information	Product Strength
VIDEX® Chewable/Dispersible Buffered Tablets		
0087-6650-01	60 tablets/bottle	25 mg/tablet
0087-6651-01	60 tablets/bottle	50 mg/tablet
0087-6652-01	60 tablets/bottle	100 mg/tablet
0087-6653-01	60 tablets/bottle	150 mg/tablet
VIDEX® Buffered Powder for Oral Solution		
0087-6614-43	One single-dose foil packet*	100 mg/packet
0087-6615-43	One single-dose foil packet*	167 mg/packet
0087-6616-43	One single-dose foil packet*	250 mg/packet
VIDEX® Pediatric Powder for Oral Solution		
0087-6632-41	One bottle per carton	2 g/bottle
0087-6633-41	One bottle per carton	4 g/bottle

*Packaged as 30 packets per carton.

US Patent No.: 4,861,759

HANDLING AND DISPOSAL

Spill, Leak and Disposal Procedure
Avoid generating dust during clean-up of powdered products; use wet mop or damp sponge. Clean surface with soap and water as necessary. Containerize larger spills.
There is no single preferred method of disposal of containerized waste. Disposal options include incineration, landfill, or sewer as dictated by specific circumstances and relevant national, state, and local regulations.
BRISTOL-MYERS SQUIBB
Immunology
Bristol-Myers Squibb Company
Princeton, NJ 08543
U.S.A.
F8-B001-7-96 P9691-01
Revised July 1996
Shown in Product Identification Guide, page 308

Pharmanex, Inc.
625 COCHRAN STREET
SIMI VALLEY, CA 93065

Direct Inquiries to:
Michael Chang, Ph.D or
Janet Thompson, Ph.D
(805) 582-9300
FAX: (805) 582-9301

Medical Emergency Contact:
Michael Chang, Ph.D.
(805) 582-9300
FAX: (805) 582-9301

BIO-GINKGO™ 27/7 and BIO-GINKGO™ 24/6 OTC
[*bī'ō-gĭng'ko*]
Ginkgo biloba leaf Extract
60 mg tablets
Dietary Supplement

DESCRIPTION

The supplemental use of Ginkgo leaves was first mentioned in an ancient Chinese materia medica published in 2800 B.C.; modern scientific research into the benefits and active constituents of Ginkgo began in the late 1950s. Twenty years of research led to the development of a standardized, concentrated extract from the leaves. Today, *Ginkgo biloba* extract (GBE) is one of the most widely used botanicals in the world and the focus of extensive scientific research, including over 300 published studies and reports to its credit.
BIO-GINKGO is an all-natural extract of *Ginkgo biloba* leaf. Pharmanex employs on-site harvest management and testing to ensure that only fresh, clean leaves of the highest quality are procured. BIO-GINKGO extract is manufactured to high quality standards using a 23 step extraction and washing process requiring approximately 50 pounds of leaves to yield just one pound of extract. BIO-GINKGO is available in two formulations:
(1)BIO-GINKGO 27/7 (≥27% ginkgo flavone glycosides and ≥7% terpene lactones); contains significantly greater levels of the identified active constituents than the standard formulation.
(2)BIO-GINKGO 24/6 (24% ginkgo flavone glycosides and 6% terpene lactones).
BIO-GINKGO extract is stringently analyzed by HPLC method of assure achievement of proper levels of flavonoid glycosides (as measured by the percentage of Ksempferol, Quercetin and Isorhamnetin content), and for terpene lactone content, as measured by the percentage of ginkgolide A,B, C and bilobalide content. Each batch of BIO-GINKGO extract is tested against fifteen additional quality criteria ranging from heavy metal content to bacteria units per gram.
BIO-GINKGO 24/6 and 27/7 are supplied in 60 mg easy-to-swallow tablets and sold as Dietary Supplements for oral administration. Tables are coated (gold colored coating for BIO-GINKGO 24/6 and green colored coating for BIO-GINKGO 27/7) for ease of swallowing. Inactive ingredients include: lactose amhydrous, microcrystalline cellulose, corn starch, sodium starch glycolate, Opadry yellow or green, colloidal silicon dioxide, magnesium stearate, Opadry clear.

BENEFITS OF GINKGO BILOBA EXTRACT (GBE)

The extensive body of scientific studies have elucidated the following benefits of GBE in the body:
Circulation
GBE helps maintain normal circulation in the body, including the brain and the extremities (legs, feet, arms, hands) without a "borrowing" effect from adjacent areas of normal flow. It also helps promote efficient circulation by helping maintain the tone and elasticity of both large blood vessels (arteries) and smaller blood vessels (capillaries).
Terpene lactones, which are specific to GBE, inhibit platelet activating factor (PAF). In particular, ginkgolide B has been shown to bind to PAF receptors.
Improves memory and enhances mental function
After eight to twelve weeks of supplementation, GBE has been reported in studies to increase the rate at which information is transmitted at the nerve cell level resulting from its ability to increase blood flow to the brain and Central Nervous System (CNS).
Antioxidant Activity
GBE is reported to have potent antioxidant properties. Antioxidants appear to help combat free radicals which are considered to be a key factor in the cell and tissue damage associated with the aging process. Free radicals may be produced from chemical, physical or emotional stresses on the body. The brain and CNS have a high lipid content in the brain cells' membranes. Free radicals may attack the lipids in cell membranes and may from lipid peroxides, which are known to damage membrane integrity with a gradual loss of semipermeability. Antioxidants appear to help block the formation of lipid peroxides.

RECOMMENDED USE

For dietary supplement use: take one 60 mg tablet twice per day, in the morning and evening, with fluid after a meal; swallow tablets without chewing them.
For optimal results, take BIO-GINKGO 24/6 or 27/7 as a dietary supplement daily. Users should allow up to 12 weeks for optimum benefits to manifest themselves, although some people notice benefits in as little as two to three weeks.

CONTRAINDICATIONS

—Hypersensitivity to Ginkgo biloba preparations.
—No known drug interactions; contact your doctor if you are taking a prescription medicine.
—Pregnancy and lactation: Use only on the advise of your physician.
—Keep out of reach of children. Inadequate information is available on the use of GBE in children under the age of 18 years old.

ADVERSE EFFECTS/TOXICOLOGY

GBE appears to be well tolerated. There have not been any reports of significant adverse reactions to GBE at the prescribed dosages or in patients ingesting as much as 600 mg of the extract in one dose.
The mild adverse reactions that have been reported include mild gastrointestinal discomfort in less than 1% of persons in studies conducted, as well as rare reports of allergic skin reactions. Some people may experience a mild, transient headache for the first two or three days of use.

TOXICITY/OVERDOSAGE

Both the acute and chronic toxicity level is very low for ginkgo extracts studied: the LD_{50} for oral administration to mice is 7,725 mg/kg body weight. Very large doses in humans may cause restlessness, diarrhea, nausea, vomiting, and other unpleasant effects, usually of a relatively mild nature. If these occur, cease taking the product or reduce the dosage.

HOW SUPPLIED

Tablets of BIO-GINKGO 27/7 and 24/6 are 60 mg each supplied in packages of 40 count and boxed in a plastic-aluminum foil pack, BIO-GINKGO 27/7 and 24/6 can be purchased throughout the United States at major drug, grocery and discount retail outlets in the dietary supplement category: natural products section. Ask the store Pharmacist for more details.
Storage: Store in a dry, cool place. Avoid excessive heat. Protect from light.
Shelf Life: Expiration date is imprinted on bottom of box and on each blister pack.
The statements in the Physicians' Desk Reference regarding BIO-GINKGO have not been evaluated by the Food and Drug Administration. This product is not intended to diagnose, treat, cure or prevent any disease.

EDUCATION MATERIALS

For more information and a booklet about BIO-GINKGO and PHARMANEX, INC. products, call toll free 1-800-780-5180. For retail availability, or to talk to someone directly, please dial 1-805-582-9300 (FAX: 1-805-582-9301). For specific health-related questions about BIO-GINKGO, call the Natural Products Hotline at 1-800-247-5169, 9:00 am to 5:00 pm, Mountain Time. Visit our website and access information directly from the Internet: http://www.pharmanex.com
Shown in Product Identification Guide, page 329

CHOLESTIN™ OTC
[*kō lĕs'tĭn*]
600 mg capsules
Dietary Supplement

DESCRIPTION
CHOLESTIN is a natural, dietary supplement for use by adults concerned about maintaining healthy cholesterol levels, and should be used as part of a program including a healthy low fat diet and regular exercise. The key ingredients in CHOLESTIN have been used for centuries in China, and are produced today through modern fermentation techniques to assure consistent product quality and potency. In numerous foreign human clinical trials involving a significant number of human subjects, CHOLESTIN (including a more concentrated product) has been reported to have a positive influence on maintaining normal levels of blood lipids, including: human serum total cholesterol (TC) levels, serum triglyceride (TG) levels, low density lipoprotein cholesterol (LDL-c) levels, and high density lipoprotein (HDL-c) levels after continual supplementation for 4 to 8 weeks. These benefits were observed throughout the period of supplementation.
CHOLESTIN is prepared from premium rice fermented with *Moascus purpureus* Went yeast and contains the natural fermentation by-products produced by the yeast. These natural by-products include a mixture of substances which resemble known HMG-CoA reductase inhibitors, plus unsaturated fatty acids, amino acids and naturally-occurring red pigment.
CHOLESTIN capsules are supplied in 600 mg easy to swallow clear capsules for oral administration; the clear gelatin capsules are USP quality and designed to disintegrate within 30 minutes after ingestion.

RECOMMENDED USE
Dietary supplementation with CHOLESTIN is recommended for healthy adult males and post-menopausal women concerned about maintaining desirable cholesterol levels, and for whom their physician has determined that dietary supplementation rather than medical treatment is appropriate. CHOLESTIN is intended for use as part of a multiple cholesterol maintenance program that includes a healthy diet that is restricted in saturated fat and cholesterol, and other appropriate measures including regular exercise. CHOLESTIN is not recommended for treating a disease.
As a dietary supplement it is recommended that two 600 mg capsules of CHOLESTIN be taken twice per day (2 capsules with or shortly after the morning meal and 2 capsules with or shortly after the evening meal). Do not take more than 4 capsules in any 24 hour period.

WARNINGS
- DO NOT USE this product if you are pregnant, can become pregnant, or are breast feeding.
- CHOLESTIN is for adult use only. Cholestin is not to be used in anyone under 20 years of age.
- DO NOT TAKE CHOLESTIN concurrently with any other drug without prior consultation with your doctor.
- Ingredients in CHOLESTIN (HMG-CoA reductase inhibitors e.g., lovastatin) have been associated with some rare but serious side effects, including serious diseases of the liver and skeletal muscle.
- DO NOT TAKE CHOLESTIN if:
  - You are at risk for liver disease, have active liver disease or any history of liver disease;
  - You consume substantial amounts of alcohol (more than 3 drinks per day);
  - You have a serious infection;
  - You have undergone an organ transplantation;
  - You have a serious disease or physical disorder or have recently undergone major surgery.
- Immediately discontinue use of CHOLESTIN if you experience any unexplained muscle pain, tenderness or weakness, especially if accompanied by flu symptoms.
- CHOLESTIN should be taken with a meal to minimize the risk of digestive tract discomfort.

Keep out of the reach of children.

OVERDOSAGE
The tolerance limit of mice to CHOLESTIN is 16 grams per kg, which is equivalent to 533 times the level recommended for use as dietary supplement. Rats continuously force-fed CHOLESTIN for four months showed no abnormalities in all testing parameters and pathological examinations, and showed no differences to the control group.
Based on foreign clinical studies, no adverse effects were observed during the eight week study period. A small number of individuals reported slight discomfort in the digestive tract.
Until further experience is obtained, no specific treatment of overconsumption of CHOLESTIN can be recommended.

HOW SUPPLIED
Capsules of CHOLESTIN 600 mg each are supplied in packages of 48 or 80 count. The deep purple-red powder is enclosed in an easy-to-swallow clear gelatin capsule, and boxed in plastic-aluminum foil blister packs. CHOLESTIN can be purchased throughout the United States at major drug, grocery and mass merchandiser chains in the dietary supplement category: natural healthcare products section. Ask your Pharmacist for more details.
Storage: Store in a dry, cool place. Avoid excessive heat. Protect from light.
Shelf Life: Expiration date is imprinted on bottom of box and each blister pack.
The statement in the Physicians' Desk Reference regarding CHOLESTIN have not been evaluated by the Food and Drug Administration. This product is not intended to diagnose, treat, cure or prevent any disease.

EDUCATION MATERIALS
For more information and a booklet about CHOLESTIN and other PHARMANEX, INC products, call toll free 1-800-780-5180. For retail availability, or to talk to someone directly, please dial 1-805-582-9300 (FAX: 1-805-582-9301). For specific health-related questions about CHOLESTIN, call the Natural Products Hotline at 1-800-247-5169, 9:00 am to 5:00 pm, Mountain Time. Visit our website and access information directly from the Internet: http://www.pharmanex.com

Shown in Product Identification Guide, page 329

CORDYMAX Cs-4™ OTC
Cordyceps sinensis
[*kord'ə-măk sē ēs fŏr, kord' ə-seps sĭ-nĕn-sĭs*]
525 mg capsules
Dietary Supplement

DESCRIPTION
Cordyceps sinensis (Berk) Sacc, is one of the most valued natural products in Traditional Chinese Medicine and is prized as a potent tonic to promote general well-being. Cs-4 is an all natural fermentation product whereby the isolated principle active component of natural *Cordyceps sinensis,* the fungus *Paecilomyces heptali* Chen, is grown on a proprietary blend of natural nutrients. In a biotechnologically aseptic environment, Pharmanex uses a proprietary deep-layer fermentation process that simulates the natural high altitude (greater than 14,000 feet) environment of the Tibetan plateau which is an optimal environment for the growth of *Cordyceps sinensis.*
Cs-4 most closely resembles the natural Cordyceps product in its scientifically-supported effects, and has an official monograph approved by the Chinese Ministry of Health distinguishing it as the first Traditional Chinese Medicine that has gone through pharmacology, toxicology and human studies in China. Cs-4 is standardized by HPLC method which ensures a potent and consistent product.
Cs-4 promotes a broad spectrum of health promoting functions, including the maintenance of normal, healthy lung function and general quality of life, including symptoms of tiredness and fatigue, by increased energizing effects and vigor. Cs-4 is not reported to stimulate the Central Nervous System or exhibit gastrointestinal tract effects.
CordyMax Cs-4 capsules are supplied in 525 mg easy-to-swallow clear gelatin capsules as a Dietary Supplement. The principle components of Cs-4 are adenosine, adenine, uracil, uridine, mannitol, beta-sitosterol, oligosaccharides, polysaccharides, eighteen common amino acids and the following vitamins and minerals: zinc, potassium, manganese, phosphorus, selenium, vitamin B-1, vitamin B-2 and vitamin E. Clear gelatin capsules are USP quality and are designed to disintegrate within 30 minutes after ingestion.

RECOMMENDED USE
As a dietary supplement: take two 525 mg capsules, three times per day with water and food.

USUAL DURATION OF USE
The effects of CordyMax Cs-4 are gradual; while mild effects are evident within a week, the most significant benefits take 3 to 6 weeks. Cs-4 has been taken as a daily dietary supplement by many people for years.

CONTRAINDICATIONS
None identified based on foreign human studies.

ADVERSE EFFECTS
Some subjects in human foreign studies showed a very slight sensation of thirst and one subject showed slight stomach discomfort; these effects were considered quite tolerable with the subjects. With the exception of one case of allergic skin reaction, no other adverse effects have been reported from clinicians and hospital records in China since the initial introduction of Cs-4 in 1989. Cs-4 has no reported CNS or GI effects.

WARNINGS
CordyMax Cs-4 has not been evaluated in children and should not be used by anyone under 18 years of age. CordyMax Cs-4 should not be used by pregnant or lactating women without advice from a physician.

OVERDOSAGE/TOXICITY
No incidence of toxic reaction has been reported.
Acute toxicity studies: The LD_{50} for oral administration to mice showed no death as 80 g/kg body weight.

HOW SUPPLIED
Capsules of CordyMax Cs-4™ 525 mg each are supplied in packages of 64 or 112 count. The dark brown powder is enclosed in an easy-to-swallow clear gelatin capsules, and boxed in plastic-aluminum foil blister packs. CordyMax Cs-4 can be purchased throughout the United States at major drug, grocery and discount stores in the dietary supplement category: natural products section. Ask the Pharmacist for more details.
Storage: Store in a dry, cool place, Avoid excessive heat. Protect from light.
Shelf Life: Expiration date is imprinted on bottom of box and each foil blister pack.
The statements in the Physicians' Desk Reference regarding CordyMax Cs-4 have not been evaluated by the Food and Drug Administration. This product is not intended to diagnose, treat, cure or prevent any disease.

EDUCATION MATERIALS
For more information and a booklet about CordyMax Cs-4 and other PHARMANEX INC. products, please call toll free at 1-800-780-5180. To speak with someone directly, call 1-805-582-9300 (FAX: 1-805-582-9301). For specific health-related questions about CordyMax Cs-4, call the Natural Products Hotline at 1-800-247-5169. Visit our website and access information directly from the Internet at http://www.pharmanex.com.

TĒGREEN 97™ OTC
[*tē'grēn 97*]
250 mg capsules
Dietary Supplement

DESCRIPTION
TĒGREEN 97 is a green tea polyphenol extract derived from the leaves of the tea plant *Camellia sinensis.* The composition of TĒGREEN 97 is similar to the natural profile of the fresh leaf, which is rich in the flavonol group of polyphenols known as catechins, as well as lesser amounts of proanthocyanidins, chlorophyll and caffeine. The major components of interest are the polyphenosis, which have been scientifically-demonstrated to have superior free radical scavenging and antioxidant properties.
The term polyphenol denotes the presence of multiple rings. The major polyphenols in green tea, and the most significant of all tea components, are the catechins faction: epicatechin (EC), epigallocatechin (EGC), epicatechin gallate (ECG), epigallocatechin gallate (EGCg), and proanthocyanidins. Of these factions, gallocatechins, especially ECG and EGCg appear to have the greatest capacity to quench free radicals.
The chemical composition of green tea leaves varies with climate, season, horticultural practices, and age of the leaf (position of the leaf on the harvested shoot). TĒGREEN 97 is produced from high quality green tea leaves and processed through proprietary manufacturing methods to consistently provide a product with a high concentration of polyphenols (97%). Over two-thirds of the polyphenols in TĒGREEN 97 are the important catechins faction as determined by HPLC method:

TEGREEN 97 Polyphenolic Profile

Total polyphenols	≥97%	
Catechins faction	≥65%	
L-EGCg	≥40%	(-)-epigallocatechin gallate
L-ECG	≥10%	(-)-epicatechin gallate
L-EGC	≥10%	(-)-epigallocatechin
L-EC	≥5%	(-)-epicatechin

Others: proanthocyanidines, lignans and phenolic acids
Minimal amounts of caffeine ≤2.5%

TĒGREEN 97 capsules are supplied in 250 mg small, easy-to-swallow clear gelatin capsules as a Dietary Supplement for oral administration. The deep green color of TĒGREEN 97's raw material result from the unique, mild extraction and purification process that allows for the retention of the natural chlorophyll found in fresh green tea leaves. Capsules are USP quality and are designed to disintegrate within 30 minutes after ingestion.

SCIENTIFIC SUPPORT
The ingestion of green tea polyphenols covers a very broad spectrum of functions promoting general well-being. In large scale epidemiological studies in Asia (totaling more than 100,000 people for study periods up to 10 years), daily consumption of more than four cups of a green tea beverage has been associated with significant overall health maintenance of subjects, even after adjustments were made for age, smoking, alcohol consumption and relative body weight.

Continued on next page

Pharmanex—Cont.

The polyphenols in green tea offer antioxidant benefits by combatting free radicals which are involved in damaging cells, including DNA. Free radicals may form inside the body through exposure to dietary, occupational and/or environmental toxins. Upon ingestion, concentrations of green tea polyphenols can be easily detected in blood, urine and feces, suggesting that polyphenols are efficiently absorbed and are available to tissues and cells.

A number of science-based experiments indicate that green tea polyphenols (especially EGCg) may help:
(1) block the formation of some potentially toxic compounds, such as nitrosamines
(2) suppress the activation of free radicals
(3) detoxify or trap free radicals
(4) inhibit spontaneous and photo-enhanced lipid peroxidation

In addition to exerting antioxidant activity on its own, green tea polyphenols may increase the activity of antioxidant and detoxifying enzymes such as glutathione peroxidase, glutathione reductase, glutathione S-transferase, catalase, and quinone reductase in certain cells and tissues.

RECOMMENDED USE

As a dietary supplement: Take one 250 mg capsule daily, which includes ≥ 160 mg of catechins, of which ≥ 100 mg is EGCg. TĒGREEN 97 can be taken any time of the day, but should be taken with water and food. Each capsule provides the amount of green tea polyphenols typically found in four cups of high quality green tea, with only small amounts of caffeine.

To achieve the health related benefits of a green tea regimen, one may need to consume an amount of green tea or green tea polyphenols equivalent to the amount consumed in the positive population studies—approximately three to four cups per day.

CONTRAINDICATIONS

For adults only, keep out of reach of children. Pregnant or lactating women should use only on the advise of a physician.

ADVERSE EFFECTS

The polyphenol content in green tea is not known to be associated with any significant side effects or toxicity. Since TĒGREEN 97 contains only small amounts of caffeine (≤ 2.5%), it may not produce the stimulant effect caused by the consumption of caffeine containing beverages in some people.

HOW SUPPLIED

TĒGREEN 97 capsules are supplied in 250 mg small, easy-to-swallow clear gelatin capsules in packages of 30 count and boxed in plastic-aluminum foil blister packs. TĒGREEN 97 can be purchased throughout the United States at major drug, grocery and discount stores in the dietary supplement category: natural products section. Ask the Pharmacist for more details.

Storage: Store in a dry, cool place. Avoid excessive heat. Protect from light.

Shelf Life: Expiration date is imprinted on bottom of box and each foil blister pack.

The statements in the Physicians' Desk Reference regarding TĒGREEN 97 have not been evaluated by the Food and Drug Administration. This product is not intended to diagnose, treat, cure or prevent any disease.

EDUCATION MATERIALS

For more information and a booklet about TĒGREEN 97 and PHARMANEX, INC products call toll free 1-800-780-5180. For retail availability, or to talk to someone directly, please dial 1-805-582-9300 (FAX: 1-805-582-9301). For specific health-related questions about TĒGREEN 97, call the Natural Products Hotline at 1-800-247-5169 from 9:00am to 5:00 pm Mountain Time. Visit our website and access information directly from the Internet: http://www.pharmanex.com

SECTION 6

DIAGNOSTIC PRODUCT INFORMATION

This section is made possible through the courtesy of the manufacturers whose products appear on the following pages. The information concerning each product has been prepared, edited, and approved by the medical department, medical director, and/or medical counsel of each manufacturer.

When a product appearing in PHYSICIANS' DESK REFERENCE has an official package circular, its description must be in full compliance with Food & Drug Administration regulations pertaining to labeling for prescription drugs. These regulations require that in PDR "indications, effects, dosages, routes, methods, and frequency and duration of administration, and any relevant warnings, hazards, contraindications, side effects, and precautions" must be *"same in language and emphasis"* as the approved labeling for the product. The FDA regards the words *"same in language and emphasis"* as requiring VERBATIM use of the approved labeling providing such information. Furthermore, information that is emphasized in the approved labeling by the use of type set in a box, or in capitals, boldface, or italics, must be given the same emphasis in PDR.

For products that do not have official package circulars, the publisher has emphasized the necessity of describing such products comprehensively, so that physicians can have access to all information essential for intelligent and informed decision-making.

The product descriptions in PHYSICIANS' DESK REFERENCE include all information made available to PDR by the manufacturer. The publisher does not warrant or guarantee any product, and does not perform any independent analysis of the information provided. Inclusion of a product in PDR does not represent an endorsement, and the publisher does not necessarily advocate the use of any product listed.

This edition of PHYSICIANS' DESK REFERENCE contains the latest information available when the book went to press. As new drugs are released and new research data and clinical findings become available throughout the year, the information in the PDR database is revised accordingly. These revisions are published twice annually in the PDR Supplements and are then incorporated in the following edition of the book. To be certain that you have the most current data, always consult the supplements or the latest edition before administering any product described in the following pages.

Connaught Laboratories, Inc.

A Pasteur Mérieux Company
SWIFTWATER, PA 18370

For Medical Information Contact:
Generally:
Medical Affairs
(800) VACCINE
(800) 822-2463
Adverse Drug Experiences:
Medical Director
(717) 839-7187
(800) 835-3592

Sales and Ordering:
Connaught Laboratories, Inc.
Customer Service
(800) VACCINE
(800) 822-2463
(717) 839-7187

MONO-VACC® TEST (O.T.) ℞
[*mon ʹō-vak*]
TUBERCULIN, OLD,
Multiple Puncture Device

DESCRIPTION
The Tuberculin, Old, Mono-Vacc® Test (O.T.) is a sterile, multiple puncture intradermal test for the detection of tuberculin sensitivity. It provides a convenient and reliable method for determining tuberculin sensitivity of individuals in tuberculosis screening programs or for office or clinical use.
The Mono-Vacc® Test (O.T.) unit consists of a sterile, disposable, multi-puncture plastic scarifier with liquid old tuberculin on the points. No preservative has been added. A plastic cap provides an airtight seal over the points assuring sterility of the points and tuberculin until the unit is used.
Tuberculin color variation may occur between different lots without alteration of potency or stability.
The preloaded test unit is disposable.

HOW SUPPLIED
Tamperproof.
Box of 25 tests.

MUMPS SKIN TEST ANTIGEN, USP ℞
MSTA™

NOT FOR IMMUNIZATION, DIAGNOSIS, OR TREATMENT
NOT FOR DIAGNOSIS OF IMMUNITY TO MUMPS
Caution: Federal (U.S.A.) law prohibits dispensing without prescription.

DESCRIPTION
MSTA™, Mumps Skin Test Antigen, is a sterile suspension of killed mumps virus for intradermal use. It is prepared from the extraembryonic fluid of the virus-infected chicken embryo and is concentrated and purified by differential centrifugation. The virus is killed with formaldehyde solution, 1:1000, and is then diluted with isotonic sodium chloride solution. The resultant product contains approximately 0.012 molar glycine and less than 1:8,000 formaldehyde solution. Thimerosal (mercury derivative) 1:10,000 is added as a preservative. Each ml of the skin test antigen contains 40 complement-fixing units. This product after shaking is slightly opalescent in color.

CLINICAL PHARMACOLOGY
Information is available concerning the pharmacologic mode of action of skin test antigen.[1] Skin testing is a widely employed and readily available method of clinically assessing the cellular immune response. A positive skin-test reaction indicates previous antigenic exposure. T-cell competence, an intact inflammatory response, and is an assessment of the cellular integrity of the immune response.
Skin testing with MSTA detects delayed-hypersensitivity.[2] Since most of the population (except for the very young) have had contact or infection with mumps virus,[3] they usually demonstrate a delayed-hypersensitivity reaction to Mumps Skin Test Antigen if an adequate cellular immune system exists.[4]
A single masked placebo-controlled study involving 90 cancer subjects was performed using Mumps Skin Test Antigen (MSTA), Tetanus Toxoid Fluid, Mixed Respiratory Vaccine, Dermatophyton O, staphage lysate and PPD (Tubersol®). The injection sites were read at 48 and 72 hours. The number of positive reactors to MSTA was greater than the number of positive subjects receiving the other antigens. None of the patients experienced any sloughing, necrosis, abscess formation, or painful lymphadenopathy as a result of the MSTA skin test. This study demonstrated that MSTA evoked a positive delayed-hypersensitivity (DH) reaction in immunocompetent individuals. The frequency of reactions in subjects with an impaired immune system was reduced. The sensitivity of MSTA has been demonstrated by the fact that: 1) in all instances when any of the other test antigens were positive, MSTA was also positive; and 2) several subjects showed a DH reaction to MSTA but not show a DH reaction to the other antigen.[2]

INDICATIONS AND USAGE
MSTA, Mumps Skin Test Antigen, is indicated when detection of a delayed-hypersensitivity (DH) reaction is desired. MSTA has not been tested in persons immunized with live mumps vaccine; therefore, its safety and efficacy in this population group has not been established.

CONTRAINDICATIONS
MUMPS VIRUS FOR THE PREPARATION OF MUMPS SKIN TEST ANTIGEN IS PROPAGATED IN EGGS. THEREFORE, THIS PRODUCT SHOULD NOT BE ADMINISTERED TO ANYONE WITH A HISTORY OF HYPERSENSITIVITY (ALLERGY), ESPECIALLY ANAPHYLACTIC REACTIONS TO EGGS OR EGG PRODUCTS. IT IS ALSO A CONTRAINDICATION TO ADMINISTER MSTA TO INDIVIDUALS KNOWN TO BE SENSITIVE TO THIMEROSAL. IN ANY CASE, EPINEPHRINE INJECTION (1:1000) MUST BE IMMEDIATELY AVAILABLE TO COMBAT UNEXPECTED ANAPHYLACTIC OR OTHER ALLERGIC REACTIONS.

WARNINGS
Neurologic complications, such as encephalopathies or peripherial-nervous systems disorders, or anaphylactic reactions have followed the administration of almost all biologics, although these have not been reported after the injection of Mumps Skin Test Antigen.

PRECAUTIONS
GENERAL
Epinephrine Injection (1:1000) must be immediately available to combat unexpected anaphylactic or other allergic reactions.
A separate sterile syringe and needle or a sterile disposable unit should be used for each individual patient to prevent transmission of hepatitis or other infectious agents from one person to another.
The antigen must be given intradermally. If it is injected subcutaneously, no reaction or an unreliable reaction may occur.
PREGNANCY
REPRODUCTIVE STUDIES—PREGNANCY CATEGORY C
Animal reproduction studies have not been conducted with Mumps Skin Test Antigen. It is not known whether Mumps Skin Test Antigen can cause fetal harm when administered to a pregnant woman or can affect reproduction capacity. Mumps Skin Test Antigen should be given to a pregnant woman only if clearly needed. There are no carefully done studies available on the effect of the drug on later growth, development, and functional maturation of the child.
USAGE IN NURSING MOTHERS
It is not known whether this drug is excreted in human milk. Because many drugs are excreted in human milk, caution should be exercised when Mumps Skin Test Antigen is administered to a nursing woman.
PEDIATRIC USE
Safety and effectiveness in children have not been established.
USAGE IN YOUNG ADULTS
Safety and effectiveness have not been established in young adults who have been immunized with live mumps vaccine.

ADVERSE REACTIONS
Local reactions may include tenderness, pruritis, vesiculation and rash. Sloughing, necrosis, abscess formation, or regional lymphadenopathy may be associated with unusually large DH reactions. Adverse reactions may include nausea, anorexia, headache, unsteadiness, drowsiness, sweating, sensation of warmth and lymphadenopathy. None of these reactions were noted in the clinical study.[2]
Epinephrine Injection (1:1000) must be immediately available to combat unexpected anaphylactic and other allergic reactions.

DOSAGE AND ADMINISTRATION
Parenteral drug products should be inspected visually for extraneous particulate matter and/or discoloration prior to administration.
SHAKE VIAL WELL before withdrawing each dose.
A separate sterile syringe and needle or a sterile disposable unit should be used for each individual patient to prevent transmission of hepatitis or other infectious agents from one person to another.
An injection of 0.1 ml of the antigen is made on the inner surface of the forearm. Before injection, the skin over the site to be injected should be cleansed with a suitable germicide. Care should be taken to inject the test antigen intradermally.
Interpretation of Reactions—The reaction should be examined in 48 to 72 hours. A mean diameter (i.e., the longest width plus the longest length, divided by 2) of induration of 5 mm or more indicates a positive DH reaction to the antigen. A negative reaction, if the test dose has been given correctly, usually indicates either anergy or nonsensitivity. Pseudopositive reactions may develop in persons highly sensitive to egg protein.

HOW SUPPLIED
Vial, 1 ml (10 tests)
STORAGE
Store between 2°–8°C (35°–46°F). DO NOT FREEZE.

REFERENCES
1. Holborow, E.J., et al: Immunology in Medicine. Second Edition, pp 19 and 121. Grune & Stratton, 1983
2. Unpublished data available from Connaught Laboratories, Inc., compiled 1983
3. Petersdorf, R.G.: Mumps, in Harrison's Principles of Internal Medicine, Ed. 7 (edited by M. M. Wintrobe, G. W. Thorn, R. D. Adams, E. Braunwald, K. J. Isselbacher, and R.G. Petersdorf) p 985. New York: McGraw-Hill Book Company, 1974
4. Dempster, G.: Mumps in Textbook of Virology, Ed.5 (edited by A.J. Rhodes and C.E. Van Rooyen) p 461 Baltimore: The Williams & Wilkins Co., 1968

CONNAUGHT® is a trademark owned by Connaught Laboratories.
Manufactured by:
CONNAUGHT LABORATORIES, INC.
Swiftwater, Pennsylvania 18370, U.S.A.
Product information as of August, 1984

0639

TUBERSOL® ℞
[*tū ʹ-bur-sŏl*]
TUBERCULIN PURIFIED PROTEIN DERIVATIVE (MANTOUX)
Diagnostic Antigen

DESCRIPTION
Tuberculin PPD (Mantoux)—Tubersol® for intracutaneous (Mantoux) tuberculin testing is available in stabilized solutions bio-equivalent to 5 U.S. units (TU) PPD-S per test dose (0.1 ml) and stabilized solutions diluted to a calculated bioequivalence of 1 TU and 250 TU strengths per test dose (0.1 ml).
Tubersol® is prepared by the Connaught Laboratories Limited from a large Master Batch, Connaught Tuberculin (CT68), which has been obtained from a human strain of *Mycobacterium tuberculosis* grown on a protein-free synthetic medium. The use of a standard preparation derived from a single batch (CT68) has been recommended[2] in order to eliminate batch to batch variation by the same manufacturer.
Tubersol is a sterile isotonic solution of Tuberculin in phosphate buffered saline containing Tween 80 (0.0005%) as a stabilizer. Phenol 0.28% is added as a preservative.[3,4,5]
Independent studies conducted by the U.S. Public Health Service in humans have determined the amount of CT68 in stabilized solution necessary to produce bio-equivalency with Tuberculin PPD-S (in phosphate buffer without Tween 80) using 5 U.S. units (TU) Tuberculin PPD-S as the standard.
Prior to release, each successive lot is tested for potency in sensitized guinea pigs in comparison with the House Standard prepared from Batch CT68 and with the U.S. Standard Tuberculin PPD-S distributed by the Office of Biologics, Food and Drug Administration, Bethesda, Maryland, U.S.A.[6]

CLINICAL PHARMACOLOGY
Intracutaneous tuberculin testing is an accepted aid in the diagnosis of tuberculosis infection.
The reaction to intracutaneously injected tuberculin is a delayed (cellular) hypersensitivity reaction. The reaction which characteristically shows a delayed course, reaching its peak more than 24 hours after administration, consists of induration due to cell infiltration and occasionally vesiculation and necrosis. Clinically, a delayed hypersensitivity reaction to tuberculin is a manifestation of previous infection with *M. tuberculosis* or a variety of non-tuberculosis bacteria. In most cases sensitization is induced by natural mycobacterial infection or by vaccination with BCG Vaccine.
The sensitization following infection with mycobacteria occurs primarily in the regional lymph nodes. Small lymphocytes (T lymphocytes) proliferate in response to the antigenic stimulus to give rise to specifically sensitized lymphocytes. After several weeks, these lymphocytes enter the blood stream and circulate for long periods of time. Subsequent restimulation of these sensitized lymphocytes with the same or a similar antigen, such as the intradermal injection of tuberculin, evokes a local reaction mediated by these cells. The tuberculin reaction is characterized by the early predominance of mononuclear cells (small and medium sized lymphocytes and monocytes). Only a small proportion of these cells appear to be lymphocytes sensitized to tuberculin.

Most cells are brought into the reaction through the release of biologically active substances by sensitized lymphocytes. An increase in vascular permeability leading to erythema and edema also occurs in tuberculin reactions.
Characteristically, delayed hypersensitivity reactions to tuberculin begin at 5 to 6 hours, are maximal at 48 to 72 hours and subside over a period of days. In those who are elderly or those who are being tested for the first time reactions may develop slowly and may not peak until after 72 hours. Immediate hypersensitivity reactions to tuberculin or to constituents of the diluent can also occur.
Not all infected persons will have a delayed hypersensitivity reaction to a tuberculin test. A large number of factors has been reported to cause a decreased ability to respond to the tuberculin test in the presence of tuberculous infection including viral infections (measles, mumps, chickenpox), live virus vaccinations (measles, mumps, polio), overwhelming tuberculosis, other bacterial infections, drugs (corticosteroids and many other immunosuppressive agents), and malignancy.[7]

INDICATIONS AND USAGE

Tubersol is indicated as an aid in the detection of infection with *Mycobacterium tuberculosis.*
For the initial intracutaneous (Mantoux) tuberculin test it is customary to use 5 U.S. units (TU) per test dose of 0.1 ml. The 1 TU per test dose (0.1 ml) preparation is used for individuals suspected of being highly sensitized since larger initial doses may result in severe skin reactions. The preparation containing **250 TU per test dose (0.1 ml), should be used exclusively for the testing of individuals who fail to react to a previous injection of 5 TU and under no circumstance is it to be used for the initial injection.**

CONTRAINDICATIONS

Tubersol should not be administered to known tuberculin positive reactors because of the severity of reactions (eg. vesiculation, ulceration or necrosis) that may occur at the test site in highly sensitive persons.

WARNINGS

Tuberson 250 TU per test dose (0.1 ml) is not, under any circumstances, to be used for the initial injection.
Avoid injecting Tubersol subcutaneously. Of this occurs, no local reaction will develop, but a general febrile reaction and/or acute inflammation around old tuberculosis lesions may occur in highly sensitive individuals.

PRECAUTIONS

a) General
A separate **sterile** syringe and needle must be used for each individual injection to prevent possibility of transmission of viral hepatitis or other infectious agents from one person to another.
The possibility of allergic reactions in individuals sensitive to the components of the product should be borne in mind. Epinephrine Hydrochloride Solution (1:1000) should be readily available for use in case an anaphylactic or acute hypersensitivity reaction occurs.
Failure to store and handle Tubersol as recommended will result in a loss of potency and inaccurate test results.

b) Information For Patients
Reactivity to the test may be depressed or suppressed for as long as 5 to 6 weeks in individuals who have received concurrent or recent immunization with certain virus vaccines (measles, influenza), who have had viral infections (rubeola, influenza, mumps and probably others) or who are receiving corticosteroids or immunosuppressive agents.
In those who are elderly or being tested for the first time reactions may develop slowly and may not peak until after 72 hours.
Vesiculation, ulceration or necrosis may appear at the test site in highly sensitive persons. Pain, pruritus and discomfort at the test site may also occur.

c) Laboratory Tests
Since a positive tuberculin reaction (10 mm or more) does not necessarily indicate the presence of active tuberculous disease, individuals showing such positive tuberculin reactions should be subjected to other diagnostic procedures, such as X-ray examination of the chest and microbiological examination of the sputum.
In the case of doubtful tuberculin reactions (5 to 9 mm) to 5 TU, the possibility should not be excluded that the skin sensitivity is due to previous contact with atypical mycobacteria or previous BCG vaccination. In the absence of signs of tuberculous disease, differential diagnosis by means of intracutaneous skin tests with PPD's derived from atypical mycobacteria may be indicated.

d) Drug Interactions
Reactivity to the test may be depressed or suppressed in individuals who are receiving corticosteroids or immunosuppressive agents.
Reactivity to PPD may be temporarily depressed by certain live virus vaccines (measles, mumps, rubella). Therefore, if a tuberculin test is to be performed, it should be administered either before or simultaneously with the injection of measles, mumps and rubella vaccines in combined form or as separate antigens.

e) Carcinogenesis, Mutagenesis, Impairment of Fertility
The product is not used for extended treatment over a long period of time.

f) Pregnancy Category C (Tuberculin)
Animal reproduction studies have not been conducted with Tubersol. It is also not known whether Tubersol can cause fetal harm when administered to a pregnant woman or can affect reproduction capacity. Tubersol should be given to a pregnant woman only if clearly needed.
However, the risk of unrecognized tuberculosis and the close post partum contact between a mother with active disease and an infant leaves the infant in grave danger of tuberculosis and complications such as tuberculous meningitis. Therefore, the prescribing physician will want to consider if the potential benefits outweigh the possible risks for performing the tuberculin test on a pregnant woman or a woman of childbearing age, particularly in certain high risk populations.

ADVERSE REACTIONS

In highly sensitized individuals, strongly positive reactions including vesiculation, ulceration or necrosis may occur at the test site. Cold packs or topical steroid preparations may be employed for symptomatic relief of the associated pain, pruritus and discomfort.
Strongly positive reactions may result in scarring at the test site.
Immediate erythematous or other reactions may occur at the injection site. The reason(s) for these infrequent occurrences are presently unknown.

DOSAGE AND ADMINISTRATION

The Test: The Mantoux test is performed by intracutaneously injecting, with a syringe and needle, 0.1 ml of Tubersol. It is customary to use 5 TU per test dose. The 1 TU per test dose preparation is used for individuals suspected of being highly sensitized since larger initial doses may result in severe skin reactions. **The preparation containing 250 TU per test dose should be used exclusively for the testing of individuals who fail to react to a previous injection of 5 TU and under no circumstances is it to be used for the initial injection.**
The result is read 48 to 72 hours after administration and induration only is considered in interpreting the test.
Method of Administration: The following procedure is recommended for performing the Mantoux test:

1. The site of the test is the flexor surface of the forearm about 4 inches below the bend of the elbow.
2. The skin of the forearm is first cleansed with alcohol and allowed to dry.
3. The test dose (0.1 ml) of Tuberculin PPD is administered with a 1 ml syringe calibrated in tenths and fitted with a short, one-half inch, 26 or 27 gauge needle.
4. Disposable sterile syringes and needles may be used. Glass syringes and needles should be sterilized by autoclaving (121°C for 30 minutes), by boiling or by the use of dry heat. Do not sterilize by means of alcohol.
5. The rubber cap of the vial should be wiped with a sterile piece of cotton moistened with alcohol and allowed to dry. The needle is then inserted gently through the cap and the required amount of the Tuberculin PPD is drawn into the syringe.
6. The point of the needle is inserted into the most superficial layers of the skin with the needle bevel pointing upward. If the intracutaneous injection is performed properly, a definite white bleb will rise at the needle point, about 10 mm (3/8″) in diameter. This will disappear within minutes. No dressing is required.

In the event of a subcutaneous injection (i.e. no bleb formed), the test should be repeated immediately at another site.
Tubersol is a stabilized solution of Tuberculin PPD. Data indicate that Tubersol will remain stable for at least four weeks when prefilled into syringes and stored between 2° and 8°C.[4] However, in order to avoid possible contamination of the product this practice is not recommended.
Parenteral drug products should be inspected visually for particulate matter and discoloration prior to administration, whenever solutions and container permit.
Interpretation of the Test: The test should be read 48 to 72 hours after administration of Tubersol. Sensitivity is indicated by induration, usually accompanied by erythema. The widest diameter of distinctly palpable induration should be recorded in millimeters (mm). Presence of edema and necrosis should also be recorded.
A positive reaction indicates a sensitivity to tuberculin, which may be the result of a previous infection with mycobacteria. This infection, likely due to *Mycobacterium tuberculosis,* may have occurred years ago or may be of recent origin. Reactions should be interpreted as follows:
Positive Reaction—Any palpable induration measuring 10 mm or more is considered a positive reaction. In the case of tuberculosis suspects or close contacts of individuals with tuberculosis an induration of 5 mm or even smaller should be interpreted as a positive reaction and appropriate additional follow-up measures initiated.
Doubtful Reaction—Induration measuring 5 to 9 mm indicates a doubtful reaction. Retesting is indicated using a different site and 5 TU per test dose.
The possibility should not be excluded that the skin sensitivity is due to previous contact with atypical mycobacteria or previous BCG vaccination.
Negative Reaction—Induration of less than 5 mm is considered negative. An individual who does not show a positive reaction to either 1 TU or 5 TU on the first test may be retetested with 5 TU and if still found negative further testing with 0.1 ml containing 250 TU of Tuberculin PPD (Mantoux) is suggested. If the latter test is employed, it may be given in the other forearm.
An individual who does not show a positive reaction to an initial injection of either 1 TU and 5 TU or 5 TU alone, and to a subsequent injection of 250 TU of Tuberculin PPD may be considered as tuberculin negative.
Booster Effect—Infection of an individual with tubercle bacilli or other mycobacteria results in a delayed hypersensitivity response to tuberculin which is demonstrated by the skin test. The delayed hypersensitivity response may gradually wane over a period of years. If a person receives a tuberculin test at this time (after several years) the response may be a reaction that is not significant. The stimulus of the test may boost or increase the size of the reaction to a second test, sometimes causing an apparent conversion or development of sensitivity. The booster effect can be seen on a second test done as soon as a week after the initial stimulating test and can persist for a year, and perhaps longer. When routine periodic tuberculin testing of adults is done, two stage testing should be used to minimize the likelihood of interpreting a boosted reaction as a conversion,[7,8]
Since a positive tuberculin reaction does not necessarily indicate the presence of active tuberculosis disease, individuals showing a positive tuberculin reaction should be subjected to other diagnostic procedures.
Those individuals giving a positive tuberculin reaction may or may not show evidence of tuberculosis disease. Chest X-ray examination and microbiological examination of the sputum in these cases are recommended as a means of determining the presence or absence of pulmonary tuberculosis.

HOW SUPPLIED

Tubersol bioequivalent to 5 U.S. units (TU) PPD-S per test dose (0.1 ml) is available in 1 ml and 5 ml vials.
Tubersol 1 TU and 250 TU per test dose (0.1 ml) are available in 1 ml vials. Tubersol solutions are ready for immediate use without any further dilution.

Storage
Tubersol should be stored between 2° and 8°C (35° and 46°F).[5,9] Tuberculin solutions can be adversely affected by exposure to light. The product should be stored in the dark except when doses are actually being withdrawn from vial.[10]
A vial of Tuberculin PPD which has been opened and in use for one month should be discarded because oxidation and degradation may have reduced the potency.[11]

REFERENCES

1. Landi, S.: Preparation, purification, and stability of tuberculin. Appl. Microbiol. **11**: 408–412, 1963.
2. Canadian Tuberculosis and Respiratory Disease Association: Classification and reporting of tuberculosis in Canada, Ottawa, the Association, 1972 p. 42.
3. Landi, S., Held, H. R., Hauschild, A. H. W., Hilsheimer, R.: Adsorption of tuberculin PPD to glass and plastic surfaces. Bull. WHO **35**: 593–602, 1966.
4. Landi, S., Held, H. R., Tseng, M. D.: Disparity of potency between stabilized and nonstabilized dilute tuberculin solutions. Am. Rev. Respir. Dis. **104**: 385–393, 1971.
5. Landi, S., Held, H. R.: Stability of dilute solutions of tuberculin purified protein derivative. Tubercle **59**: 121–133, 1978.
6. U.S. Code of Federal Regulations, Title 21, Part 650, Subpart B—tuberculin, 144–146, April 1, 1981.
7. The Tuberculin Skin Test. Am. Rev. Respir. Dis. **124**: 356–363, 1981.
8. American Thoracic Society: Diagnostic Standards and Classification of Tuberculosis and Other Mycobacterial Diseases (14th ed.), 1980. Am. Rev. Respir. Dis. **123**: 343–358, 1981.
9. Landi, S., Held, H. R.: Stability of dilute solution of tuberculin purified protein derivative at extreme temperatures. J. Biol. Stand. **9**: 195–199, 1981.
10. Landi, S., Held, H. R.: Effect of light on tuberculin purified protein derivative solutions. Am. Rev. Respir. Dis. **111**: 52–61, 1975.
11. Landi, S., Held, H. R.: Effect of oxidation on the stability of tuberculin purified protein derivative (PPD) In: International Symposium on Tuberculins and BCG Vaccine. Basel: International Association of Biological Standardization, 1983. (Developments in Biological Standardization) In press.

Continued on next page

Connaught Laboratories—Cont.

Manufactured by:
CONNAUGHT
LABORATORIES LIMITED
A POSTEUR MÉRIEUX COMPANY
WILLOWDALE, ONTARIO, CANADA
Distributed by:
CONNAUGHT LABORATORIES INC.
Swiftwater, Pennsylvania 18370,
U.S.A.
01-686 CLI

Ferring Laboratories, Inc.
400 RELLA BLVD, SUITE 201
SUFFERN, NY 10901-4249

ACTHREL® ℞
(corticorelin ovine triflutate for injection)
For intravenous injection only
DIAGNOSTIC USE ONLY

DESCRIPTION
ACTHREL® (corticorelin ovine triflutate for injection) is a sterile, nonpyrogenic, lyophilized white cake powder, containing corticorelin ovine triflutate, a trifluoroacetate salt of a synthetic peptide that is used for the determination of pituitary corticotroph responsiveness. Corticorelin ovine has an amino acid sequence identical to ovine corticotropin releasing hormone (oCRH). Corticorelin ovine is an analogue of the naturally occurring human CRH (hCRH) peptide. Both peptides are potent stimulators of adrenocorticotropic hormone (ACTH) release from the anterior pituitary. ACTH stimulates cortisol production from the adrenal cortex. The structural formula for corticorelin ovine triflutate is described below:

Ser-Gln-Glu-Pro-Pro-Ile-Ser-Leu-Asp-Leu-Thr-Phe-His-Leu-Leu-Arg-Glu-Val-Leu-Glu-Met-Thr-Lys-Ala-Asp-Gln-Leu-Ala-Gln-Gln-Ala-His-Ser-Asn-Arg-Lys-Leu-Leu-Asp-Ile-Ala-NH_2 • xCF_3COOH

whereas $x=4-8$.

The empirical formula of corticorelin ovine is $C_{205}H_{339}N_{59}O_{63}S$ with a molecular weight of 4670.35 Daltons.

ACTHREL® for Injection is available in vials containing 100 mcg corticorelin ovine (as the trifluoroacetate), 0.88 mg ascorbic acid, 10 mg lactose, and 20 mg albumin human, USP. Trace amounts of chloride ion may be present from the manufacturing process. The preparation is intended for intravenous administration.

CLINICAL PHARMACOLOGY
Pharmacodynamics: In normal subjects, intravenous administration of corticorelin results in a rapid and sustained increase of plasma ACTH levels and a near parallel increase of plasma cortisol. In addition, intravenous administration of corticorelin to normal subjects causes a concomitant and prolonged release of the related proopiomelanocortin peptides β- and γ-lipotropins and β-endorphin. A number of dose-response studies have been performed on normal subjects using a range of corticorelin doses. In one study, doses of corticorelin ranging from 0.001 to 30 mcg/kg body weight were administered to 29 healthy volunteers. Blood samples were taken over a 2-hour period for determination of plasma ACTH and cortisol concentrations. There was a direct dose-dependent relationship that was more pronounced for ACTH than for cortisol. The threshold dose was 0.03 mcg/kg, the half-maximal dose was 0.3–1.0 mcg/kg and the maximally effective dose was 3–10 mcg/kg.

Plasma ACTH levels in normal subjects increased 2 minutes after injection of corticorelin doses of ≥ 0.3 mcg/kg and reached peak levels after 10–15 minutes. Plasma cortisol levels increased within 10 minutes and reached peak levels at 30 to 60 minutes. As the dose of corticorelin was increased, the rises in plasma ACTH and cortisol were more sustained, showing a biphasic response with a second lower peak at 2–3 hours after injection. Similar results were found in another study using 0.3, 3.0, and 30 mcg/kg doses. The duration of mean plasma ACTH increase after injection of 0.3, 3.0, and 30 mcg/kg was 4, 7, and 8 hours, respectively. The effect on plasma cortisol was similar, but more prolonged. Because there are differences in basal levels and peak response levels following a.m. or p.m. administration, it is recommended that subsequent evaluations in the same patient using the corticorelin stimulation test be carried out at the same time of day as the original evaluation.

Baseline ACTH and cortisol levels are usually higher in the morning. Pooled ACTH values from normal unstressed subjects (n=119) were 25 ± 7 pg/mL in the a.m. and 10 ± 3 in the p.m.; similar pooled cortisol values (n=170) were 11 ± 3 mcg/dL in the a.m. and 4 ± 2 mcg/dL in the p.m. The normal unstressed person has about seven to ten secretory episodes of ACTH each day. Most of them occur in the early morning hours and are responsible for the morning plasma cortisol surge. The following figure shows the daily circadian rhythm of ACTH and cortisol secretions in a normal unstressed person.

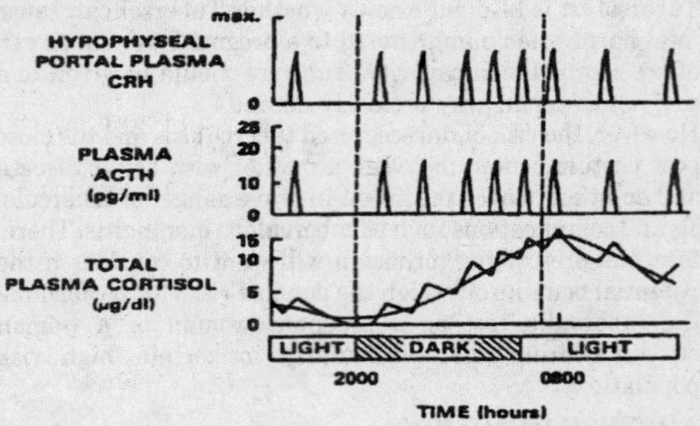

Insulin, plasma renin activity, prolactin, and growth hormone release are not affected by corticorelin administration in humans.

Continuous 24-hour infusion of corticorelin (0.5, 1.0 and 3.0 mcg/kg/hr) increased plasma ACTH concentrations to a plateau of 15–20 pg/mL by the third hour and urinary-free cortisol reaches 173±43 mcg/dL, by 24 hours, comparable to those levels observed in patients with major depression, but less than levels noted in Cushing's disease. Continuous infusion did not abolish the circadian rhythm of plasma ACTH and cortisol, but did appear to desensitize the corticotroph.

Intermittent doses of corticorelin (25 mcg every 4 hours for 72 hours), however, continued to elicit the expected ACTH and cortisol responses.

Intravenous administration of 1 mcg/kg corticorelin in combination with 10 pressor units intramuscular vasopressin had a synergistic effect on ACTH and a less marked synergistic effect on cortisol secretion.

The basal and peak response levels of ACTH and cortisol to a 1 mcg/kg or 100 mcg dose of corticorelin administered to normal volunteers in the morning and the evening are given below. These values were obtained by combining the results from 9 clinical trials conducted in the a.m. and 4 clinical trials conducted in the p.m.

The following table is to be used only as a general guide.

Basal Concentrations and Peak Responses of ACTH and Cortisol in Normal Subjects after 1 mcg/kg or 100 mcg of ACTHREL®

Time of Day	No. of Subjects	ACTH Concentration mean (range) pg/mL		Cortisol Concentration mean (range) mcg/dL	
		Basal	Peak	Basal	Peak
a.m.	143	28 (16–65)	68 (39–114)	11 (8–13)	21 (17–25)
p.m.	70	9 (8–13)	30 (25–42)	4 (2–6)	16 (15–18)

Pharmacokinetics: Following a single intravenous injection of 1 mcg/kg of corticorelin to normal men, the disappearance of immunoreactive corticorelin (IR-corticorelin) from plasma follows a biexponential decay curve. Plasma half-lives for IR-corticorelin are 11.6±1.5 minutes (mean ± SE) for the fast component and 73±8 minutes for the slow component. The mean volume of distribution for IR-corticorelin is 6.2±0.5 L with an approximate metabolic clearance rate of 95±11 L/m²/day. Graded intravenous doses of corticorelin (0.01, 0.03, 0.1, 0.3, 1, 3, 10, 30 mcg/kg) produced a linear increase in plasma IR-corticorelin.

Corticorelin does not appear to be bound specifically by a circulating plasma protein.

INDICATIONS AND USAGE
ACTHREL® is indicated for use in differentiating pituitary and ectopic production of ACTH in patients with ACTH-dependent Cushing's syndrome.

Differential Diagnosis: There are two forms of Cushing's syndrome:

(a) ACTH-dependent (83%), in which hypercortisolism is due either to pituitary hypersecretion of ACTH (Cushing's disease) resulting from an adenoma (40%, usually microadenomas) or nonadenomatous hyperplasia, possibly of hypothalamic origin (28%), or for hypercortisolism that is secondary to ectopic secretion of ACTH (15%) and,

(b) ACTH-independent (17%), in which hypercortisolism is due to autonomous cortisol secretion by an adrenal tumor (9% adenomas, 8% carcinomas).

After the establishment of hypercortisolism consistent with the presence of Cushing's syndrome, and following the elimination of autonomous adrenal hyperfunction as its cause, the corticorelin test is used to aid in establishing the source of excessive ACTH secretion.

The corticorelin stimulation test helps to differentiate between the etiologies of ACTH-dependent hypercortisolism as follows:

1. High basal plasma ACTH plus high basal plasma cortisol (20–40 mcg/dL). ACTHREL® injection (1 mcg/kg) results in:
   a. Increased plasma ACTH levels
   b. Increased plasma cortisol levels
   Diagnosis: Cushing's disease (ACTH of pituitary origin)
2. High basal plasma ACTH (may be very high) plus high basal plasma cortisol (20–40 mcg/dL).
   ACTHREL® injection (1 mcg/kg) results in:
   a. Little or no response of plasma ACTH levels
   b. Little or no response of plasma cortisol levels
   Diagnosis: Ectopic ACTH syndrome

Test Methodology: To evaluate the status of the pituitary-adrenal axis in the differentiation of a pituitary source from an ectopic source of excessive ACTH secretion, a corticorelin test procedure requires a minimum of five blood samples.

Procedure

1. Venous blood samples should be drawn 15 minutes before and immediately prior to ACTHREL® administration. The ACTH baseline is obtained by averaging the values of the two samples.
2. Administer ACTHREL® as an intravenous infusion over a 30 to 60 second interval at a dose of 1 mcg/kg body weight. Higher dosages are not recommended (see **PRECAUTIONS** and **ADVERSE REACTIONS**).
3. Draw venous blood samples at 15, 30, and 60 minutes after administration.
4. Blood samples should be handled as recommended by the laboratory that will determine their ACTH content. It is extremely important to recognize that the reliability of the corticorelin stimulation test is directly related to the inter-assay and intra-assay variability of the laboratory performing the assay.

Cortisol determinations may be performed on the same blood samples for the same time points as outlined above. The blood sample handling precautions noted for ACTH should be followed for cortisol.

Interpretation of Test Results: The interpretation of the ACTH and cortisol responses following ACTHREL® administration requires a knowledge of the clinical status of the individual patient, understanding of hypothalamic-pituitary-adrenal physiology, and familiarity with the normal hormonal ranges and the standards used by the laboratory that performs the ACTH and cortisol assays.

Cushing's Disease

The results of challenge with corticorelin injection have been reported in approximately 300 patients with Cushing's disease. Although the ACTH and cortisol responses were variable, a hyper-response to corticorelin was seen in a majority of patients, despite high basal cortisol levels. This response pattern indicates an impairment of the negative feedback of cortisol on the pituitary. Patients with pituitary-dependent Cushing's disease tested with corticorelin do not show the negative correlation between basal and stimulated levels of ACTH and cortisol that is found in normal subjects. A positive correlation between basal ACTH levels and maximum ACTH increments after corticorelin administration has been found in Cushing's disease patients.

Ectopic ACTH Secretion

Patients with Cushing's syndrome due to ectopic ACTH secretion (N=32) were found to have very high basal levels of ACTH and cortisol, which were not further stimulated by corticorelin. However, there have been rare instances of patients with ectopic sources of ACTH that have responded to the corticorelin test.

SUMMARY OF ACTH RESPONSES IN PATIENTS WITH HIGH BASAL CORTISOL

	High ACTH Response	Low ACTH Response
High Basal ACTH	Cushing's Disease	Ectopic ACTH Secretion

CUSHING'S DISEASE ACTH RESPONSES
(mean of 181 patients)
Basal ACTH 63 ±72 pg/mL (mean ±SD)
Peak ACTH 189 ±262 pg/mL (mean ±SD)
Mean of individual change from baseline +227%

ECTOPIC ACTH SECRETION RESPONSES
(mean for 31 patients)
Basal ACTH 266 ±464 pg/mL (mean ±SD)
Peak ACTH 276 ±466 pg/mL (mean ±SD)
Mean of individual change from baseline +15%

False negative responses to the corticorelin test in Cushing's disease patients occur approximately 5 to 10% of the time, which may lead the clinician to an incorrect diagnosis of ectopic production of ACTH at that frequency. (See **INDICATIONS AND USAGE, Differential Diagnosis**).

PRECAUTIONS

General: The severity of adverse effects to a corticorelin injection appear to be dose-dependent. Dosages above 1 mcg/kg are not recommended. While few adverse effects have been observed at the 1 mcg/kg or 100 mcg dose, higher doses have been associated with transient tachycardia, decreased blood pressure, loss of consciousness, and asystole (see **ADVERSE REACTIONS**). These symptoms can be substantially reduced by administering the drug as a 30-second intravenous infusion instead of a bolus injection. At a dose of 200 mcg corticorelin, 4 of 60 volunteers and patients with disturbances of the hypothalamic-pituitary-adrenal (HPA) axis were reported to have had decreased blood pressures. One patient had a severe hypotensive reaction with asystole. Three other patients had an "absence-like" loss of consciousness lasting approximately 5 minutes. In subsequent investigations by the same investigators over a 3-year period using 100 mcg of corticorelin, one patient in approximately 150 to 200 experienced a severe drop in blood pressure and loss of sinus rhythm after receiving 55 mcg of corticorelin, which may have been due to interaction with heparin. (See **Drug Interactions**).

Drug Interactions: The plasma ACTH response to corticorelin injection is inhibited or blunted in normal subjects pretreated with dexamethasone. The use of a heparin solution to maintain i.v. cannula patency during the corticorelin test is not recommended. A possible interaction between corticorelin and heparin may have been responsible for a major hypotensive reaction that occurred after corticorelin administration. (See **ADVERSE REACTIONS**).

Carcinogenesis, Mutagenesis, Impairment of Fertility: Animal studies have not been conducted with corticorelin to evaluate carcinogenic potential, mutagenicity, or effect on fertility.

Pregnancy (Pregnancy Category C): Animal reproduction studies have not been conducted with corticorelin. It is also not known whether corticorelin can cause fetal harm when administered to a pregnant woman or can affect reproductive capacity. ACTHREL® should be given to a pregnant woman only if clearly needed.

Nursing Mothers: It is not known whether corticorelin is secreted in human milk. Because many drugs are excreted in human milk, caution should be exercised when ACTHREL® is administered to a nursing woman.

PEDIATRIC USE

Only a few tests have been performed on children. Dosages were 1 mcg/kg body weight. Patient studies have involved only children with multiple hypothalamic and/or pituitary hormone deficiencies, or tumors. Only two studies with normal pediatric subjects have been conducted. No differences in response to the corticorelin test have been reported in the children studied.

ADVERSE REACTIONS

Adverse effects reported with 1 mcg/kg or 100 mcg/patient include flushing of the face, neck, and upper chest (16%; 45/276), beginning almost immediately and lasting 3 to 5 minutes. Recipients have also reported an urge to take a deep breath (6%; 3/49), which occurs with a timing similar to, but less frequently than, that of flushing. Higher doses (≥ 3 mcg/kg) are associated with more prolonged flushing, tachycardia, hypotension, dyspnea, and "chest compression" or tightness. In addition, at doses of ≥ 5 mcg/kg, significant increases in heart rate and decreases in blood pressure were observed. The cardiovascular effects occurred 2–3 minutes after injection and lasted for 30–60 minutes. The facial flushing was more prolonged, lasting up to 4 hours in some subjects. All signs and symptoms could be reduced by administering the drug as a 30-second infusion instead of by bolus injection.

Total doses of up to 200 mcg of corticorelin were administered as a bolus injection to 60 men and women, including both healthy normal subjects and patients with endocrine disorders. In most cases, only minor adverse effects, such as transient flushing and feelings of dyspnea, were noted. However, a few patients with disorders of the pituitary-adrenal axis had major symptoms. One patient had a more precipitous fall in blood pressure and pulse rate and developed asystole, which required resuscitation. In two patients with Cushing's disease and in one with secondary adrenal insufficiency, an "absence-like" loss of consciousness occurred, which started within a few seconds after the injection of corticorelin and lasted from 10 seconds to 5 minutes. This was accompanied by a slight fall in blood pressure. (See **PRECAUTIONS** and **DRUG INTERACTIONS**.)

OVERDOSAGE

Symptoms of overdose include severe facial flushing, cardiovascular changes and dyspnea. In the event of toxic overdose (see **ADVERSE REACTIONS**), adverse effects should be treated symptomatically.

DOSAGE AND ADMINISTRATION

Dosage: A single intravenous dose of ACTHREL® at 1 mcg/kg is recommended for the testing of pituitary corticotrophin function. A dose of 1 mcg/kg is the lowest dose that produces maximal cortisol responses and significant (though apparently sub-maximal) ACTH responses. Doses above 1 mcg/kg are not recommended (see **PRECAUTIONS** and **ADVERSE REACTIONS**).

At a dose of 1 mcg/kg, the ACTH and cortisol responses to ACTHREL® are prolonged and remain elevated for up to 2 hours. The maximum increment in plasma ACTH occurs between 15 and 60 minutes after ACTHREL® administration, whereas the maximum increment in plasma cortisol occurs between 30 and 120 minutes. In a clinical study of 30 normal healthy men, the peak plasma ACTH and cortisol responses to ACTHREL® administration in the early afternoon occurred at 42 ±29 minutes and 65 ±26 minutes (average ±SD), respectively. If a repeat evaluation using the corticorelin stimulation test with ACTHREL® is needed, it is recommended that the repeat test be carried out at the same time of day as the original test because there are differences in basal levels and peak response levels following a.m. or p.m. administration to normal humans.

Administration: ACTHREL® is to be reconstituted aseptically with 2 mL of Sodium Chloride Injection, USP (0.9% sodium chloride at the time of use by injecting 2 mL of the saline diluent into the lyophilized drug product cake. To avoid bubble formation, DO NOT SHAKE the vial; instead, roll the vial to dissolve the drug product. The sterile solution containing 50 mcg corticorelin ovine triflutate/mL is then ready for injection by the intravenous route. The dosage to be administered is determined by the patient's weight (1 mcg corticorelin ovine triflutate /kg). Some of the adverse effects can be reduced by administering the drug as an infusion over 30 seconds instead of as a bolus injection.

Parenteral drug products should be inspected visually for particulate matter and discoloration prior to administration, whenever solution and container permit.

HOW SUPPLIED

ACTHREL® is supplied as a sterile, nonpyrogenic, lyophilized, white cake containing 100 mcg corticorelin ovine (as the trifluoroacetate), 0.88 mg ascorbic acid, 10 mg lactose, and 20 mg human albumin. Trace amounts of chloride ion may be present from the manufacturing process. The package provides a single-dose, rubber-capped, 5-mL, brown-glass vial (NDC 55566-0301-1) containing 100 mcg corticorelin ovine (as the trifluoroacetate). ACTHREL® is stable in the lyophilized form when stored frozen at −20°C to −15°C (−4°F to +5°F) and protected from light. The reconstituted solution should be used immediately. Discard unused reconstituted solution.

Manufactured for:
Ferring Laboratories, Inc.
Suffern, New York 10901
By:
Ben Venue Laboratories, Inc.
Bedford, OH 44146

"Caution: Federal law prohibits dispensing without a prescription"

1996 FERRING LABORATORIES, INC.
5/96
DC-125

SECRETIN–FERRING ℞

[si-krē'tin]
secretin
For diagnostic use in pancreatic dysfunction

DESCRIPTION

Secretin is a gastrointestinal peptide hormone that was first extracted from porcine duodenum by Jorpes & Mutt (1961). The heptacosa-peptide was subsequently sequenced and synthesized by Mutt, Bodansky and their co-workers at the Karolinska Institute. Secretin-Ferring is a highly purified naturally occurring porcine hormone with a potency of not less than 3000 clinical units (CU) per mg peptide. Secretin is chemically defined as follows:

Mol.Wt. 3055.5
Empirical Formula: $C_{130}H_{220}N_{44}O_{41}$
Structural Formula: H-His-Ser-Asp-Gly-Thr-Phe-Thr-Ser-Glu-Leu-Ser-Arg-Leu-Arg-Asp-Ser-Ala-Arg-Leu-Gln-Arg-Leu-Leu-Gln-Gly-Leu-Val-NH_2

Secretin-Ferring contains 75 CU of lyophilized, sterile purified secretin, 1 mg of L-cysteine hydrochloride, and 20 mg of mannitol per vial. When reconstituted in 7.5 ml of Sodium Chloride Injection USP, each mL of solution contains 10 CU secretin for intravenous use. The pH of the reconstituted solution has a range of 2.5-5.0

CLINICAL PHARMACOLOGY

The primary action of secretin is to increase the volume and bicarbonate content of secreted pancreatic juices. The standard unit of activity used for Secretin-Ferring is the clinical unit defined by Jorpes & Mutt in 1966. In a study of 6 healthy subjects the $t(^1/_2)$ for secretin approximated 4 minutes with a clearance rate of 540 mL/min (Kolts and McGuigan, 1977).

Normal ranges for pancreatic secretory response to intravenous secretin in patients with defined pancreatic diseases have been shown to vary. The variation is related to the secretin product used as well as inter-investigator differences in operative technique. However, it has been demonstrated that properly performed tests with secretin will identify pancreatic disease (Gutierrez and Baron, 1972, Lagerlöf et al., 1967).

The pancreatic secretory responses to secretin in normal subjects and patients with well-documented pancreatitis are shown in Table 1 (Gutierrez and Baron, 1972).

[See Table 1 below.]

The values obtained for Table 1 are derived from a single study by investigators skilled in performing the secretin test and are to be taken only as guidelines. These results should not be generalized to results of secretin testing conducted in other laboratories. However, a volume response of less than 2.0 mL/kg/hr, bicarbonate concentration of less than 90 mEq/liter and bicarbonate output of less than 0.2 mEq/kg/hr are consistent with impaired pancreatic function. A physician or institution planning to perform secretin testing for diagnosis of pancreatic disease should begin by assessing enough normal subjects (≥ 5) to develop proficiency in proper technique and to generate normal response ranges for the three commonly assessed parameters of pancreatic exocrine response to Secretin-Ferring.

Proper technique for carrying out the secretin test of pancreatic function is described in DOSAGE AND ADMINISTRATION.

Secretin-Ferring administered intravenously stimulates gastrin release in patients with gastrinoma (Zollinger-Ellison syndrome), whereas no or only small changes in serum gastrin concentrations occur in normal subjects. Secretin-Ferring may produce a small decrease in serum gastrin levels in patients with duodenal ulcer disease. This gastrin response is the basis for the use of Secretin-Ferring as a provocative test in the evaluation of patients in whom gastrinoma is a diagnostic consideration. Accepted technique for carrying out the secretin provocation test is detailed in DOSAGE AND ADMINISTRATION.

INDICATIONS AND USAGE

Secretin-Ferring (secretin) is indicated for:
(1) Diagnosis of pancreatic exocrine disease.
(2) As an adjunct in obtaining desquamated pancreatic cells for cytopathologic examination.
(3) Diagnosis of gastrinoma (Zollinger-Ellison syndrome).

CONTRAINDICATIONS

Patients suffering from acute pancreatitis should not receive Secretin-Ferring until the attack has subsided.

WARNINGS

Because of a potential allergic reaction to secretin, patients should receive an initial intravenous test dose of 0.1-1.0 CU. If no allergic reaction is noted after one minute the recommended dose may be injected slowly over 1 minute. A test dose is especially important in patients with a history of atopic allergy and/or asthma. Appropriate measures for the treatment of acute hypersensitivity reactions should be immediately available.

PRECAUTIONS

GENERAL: Patients who have undergone vagotomy, or are receiving anticholinergics at the time of secretin testing,

Table 1

	Normal male subjects (10)[a]	Chronic Pancreatitis (5)
Volume secreted (mL/kg/hr)	3.6±0.8[b]	1.1± 0.6
HCO_3 content (mEq/L)	114± 20	71±33
HCO_3 output (mEq/kg/hr)	0.436± 0.141	0.105±0.093

[a] number of subjects.
[b] x ±S.D.

Continued on next page

Ferring Laboratories—Cont.

or who have inflammatory bowel disease may be hyporesponsive to secretin stimulation. This response does not indicate pancreatic disease. A greater than normal volume response to secretin stimulation, which can mask coexisting pancreatic disease, is occasionally encountered in patients with alcoholic or other liver disease.
DRUG/LABORATORY TEST INTERACTION: The concomitant use of anticholinergic agents may make patients hyporesponsive (false positive).
CARCINOGENESIS, MUTAGENESIS, IMPAIRMENT OF FERTILITY: Long-term studies in animals have not been performed to evaluate the carcinogenic, mutagenic potential or possible impairment of fertility effects of secretin.
PREGNANCY (CATEGORY C): Animal reproduction studies have not been conducted with Secretin-Ferring. It is also not known whether Secretin-Ferring can cause fetal harm when administered to a pregnant woman or can affect reproductive capacity. Secretin-Ferring should be given to a pregnant woman for diagnosis of gastrinoma (Zollinger-Ellison syndrome) only if clearly needed. Insofar as fluoroscopic guidance is usually necessary to position the double-lumen tube used in the pancreatic function test, this test should be postponed until after delivery.
NURSING MOTHERS: It is not known whether secretin is excreted in human milk. Because many drugs are excreted in human milk, caution is advised when Secretin-Ferring is administered to a nursing woman. Further, normal values for pancreatic secretory response to Secretin-Ferring and for serum gastrin response have not been established for nursing women.
PEDIATRIC USE: Safety and effectiveness in children have not been established.

ADVERSE REACTIONS

No adverse reactions to Secretin-Ferring have been reported.

DOSAGE AND ADMINISTRATION

Secretin-Ferring should be prepared immediately prior to use. The contents of a vial are dissolved in 7.5 mL of Sodium Chloride Injection USP, to yield a concentration of 10 CU per mL. Avoid vigorous shaking. Discard any unused portion after reconstitution.
The reconstituted drug product should be inspected visually prior to administration. If particulate matter or discoloration are seen, the product should be discarded.

DOSAGE

PANCREATIC FUNCTION TESTING AND PROCEDURE FOR OBTAINING DESQUAMATED PANCREATIC CELLS FOR CYTOPATHOLOGY: 1 CU per kg body weight by slow intravenous injection over 1 minute.
DIAGNOSIS OF GASTRINOMA (Zollinger-Ellison syndrome): 2 CU per kg body weight by slow intravenous injection over 1 minute.

ADMINISTRATION

1. PANCREATIC FUNCTION TESTING: A Dreiling type, radioopaque, double-lumen tube is passed through the mouth following a 12-15 hour fast. The proximal lumen of the tube is placed in the gastric antrum and the distal lumen just beyond the papilla of Vater with the aid of fluoroscopic guidance. The positioning of the tube must be confirmed and the tube secured prior to secretin testing. A negative pressure of 25-40 mm Hg is applied to both lumens and maintained throughout the test. Interruption of suction at 1 minute intervals improves the reliability of fluid collections. When uncontaminated duodenal contents are obtained - i.e., when these secretions are clear, although possibly bile stained, and have a pH of ≥ 6.0 - a baseline sample of duodenal fluids is collected for 2 consecutive 10 minute periods. Subsequent to the baseline collections, Secretin-Ferring at a dose of 1 CU/kg of body weight is injected intravenously in approximately 1 minute. Duodenal fluid is then collected for 60 minutes after secretin administration. The aspirate is fractioned into four collection periods, the first two at 10 minute intervals, and the last two at 20 minute intervals. The duodenal lumen of the tube is cleared with an injection of air after collection of each fraction. Wide variations in volume of the aspirate will be indicative of incomplete aspiration or contamination. Each fraction of duodenal fluid is to be chilled and subsequently analyzed for volume and bicarbonate concentration.
2. PROCEDURE FOR OBTAINING DESQUAMATED PANCREATIC CELLS FOR CYTOPATHOLOGY: A duodenal aspirate obtained as under Pancreatic Function Testing is submitted for cytopathological examination.
3. SECRETIN TESTING FOR GASTRINOMA (Zollinger-Ellison syndrome). The patient should have fasted for at least 12 hours prior to beginning the test. Prior to injection of Secretin-Ferring, two blood samples are drawn for determination of fasting serum gastrin levels (baseline values). Subsequently, 2 CU of Secretin-Ferring per kg of body weight are administered intravenously over 1 minute; post-injection blood samples are collected after 1,2,5,10 and 30 minutes for determination of serum gastrin concentrations.
Gastrinoma is strongly indicated in patients with elevated fasting serum gastrin concentrations in the 120-500 pg/mL range (determined by RIA using an antibody to gastrin similar to that prepared by Rehfeld) and in patients who show an increase in serum gastrin concentration of more than 110 pg per mL over basal level.

HOW SUPPLIED

Secretin-Ferring is supplied as a lyophilized sterile powder in 10 mL vials (NDC 55566-1075-1) containing 75 CU. The unreconstituted product should be stored at −20°C (freezer). However, the biological activity of Secretin-Ferring will not be significantly decreased by storage at temperatures up to 25°C for up to 3 weeks. Expiration date is marked on the label.
Caution: Federal (USA) law prohibits dispensing without prescription.

REFERENCES

Jorpes, E., and Mutt, V.: On the biological activity and amino acid composition of secretin. Acta Chem Scand 15 (1961) 1790–1791.
Jorpes, E., and Mutt V.: On the biological assay of secretin. The reference standard. Acta Physiol Scand 66 (1966) 316–325.
Kolts, B.E. and Mc Guigan, J.E.: Radioimmunoassay Measurement of Secretin Half-Life in Man. Gastroenterol. 72 (1977) 55–60.
Lagerlöf, H.O., et al.: A secretin test with high doses of secretin and correction for incomplete recovery of duodenal juice. Gastroenterol 52 (1967) 67–77.
Gutierrez, L.V., and Baron, J.H.: A comparison of Boots and GIH secretin as stimuli of pancreatic secretion in human subjects with or without chronic pancreatitis. Gut 13 (1972) 721–725.
Manufactured for
FERRING LABORATORIES, INC.
Suffern, N.Y. 10901
By:
Ferring AB
Malmö, Sweden
DC-120 Rev. 06/88

THYREL® TRH ℞

(protirelin)
Injection
FOR INTRAVENOUS ADMINISTRATION

DESCRIPTION

Chemically, Thyrel® TRH (protirelin) is identified as 5-oxo-L-prolyl-L-histidyl-L-proline amide. It is a synthetic tripeptide that is believed to be structurally identical to the naturally-occurring thyrotropin-releasing hormone produced by the hypothalamus. The CAS Registry Number is 24305-27-9. The structural formula is:

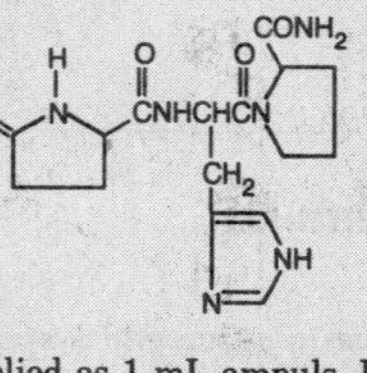

Thyrel TRH is supplied as 1 mL ampuls. Each ampul contains 500 μg protirelin in a sterile non-pyrogenic isotonic saline solution having a pH of approximately 6.5. In addition, each ampul contains sodium chloride 9.0 mg, Water for Injection, hydrochloric acid and sodium hydroxide as needed to adjust pH. Thyrel TRH is intended for intravenous administration.

CLINICAL PHARMACOLOGY

Pharmacologically, Thyrel TRH increases the release of the thyroid stimulating hormone (TSH) from the anterior pituitary. Prolactin release is also increased. It has recently been observed that approximately 65% of acromegalic patients tested respond with a rise in circulating growth hormone levels; the clinical significance is as yet not clear. Following intravenous administration, the mean plasma half-life of protirelin in normal subjects is approximately five minutes. TSH levels rise rapidly and reach a peak at 20 to 30 minutes. The decline in TSH levels takes place more slowly, approaching baseline levels after approximately three hours.

INDICATIONS AND USAGE

Thyrel TRH is indicated as an adjunctive agent in the diagnostic assessment of thyroid function. As an adjunct to other diagnostic procedures, testing with Thyrel® TRH (protirelin) may yield useful information in patients with pituitary or hypothalamic dysfunction.
Thyrel TRH is indicated as an adjunct to evaluate the effectiveness of thyrotropin suppression with a particular dose of T_4 in patients with nodular or diffuse goiter. A normal TSH baseline value and a minimal difference between the 30 minute and baseline response to Thyrel TRH injection would indicate adequate suppression of the pituitary secretion of TSH.
Thyrel TRH may be used, adjunctively, for adjustment of thyroid hormone dosage given to patients with primary hypothyroidism. A normal or slightly blunted TSH response, thirty minutes following Thyrel TRH injection, would indicate adequate replacement therapy.

CONTRAINDICATIONS

Thyrel TRH is contraindicated in patients with a known hypersensitivity to the drug.

WARNINGS

Transient changes in blood pressure, either increases or decreases, frequently occur immediately following administration of Thyrel TRH. Blood pressure should therefore be measured before Thyrel TRH is administered and at frequent intervals during the first 15 minutes after its administration. Increases in systolic pressure (usually less than 30 mm Hg) and/or increases in diastolic pressure (usually less than 20 mm Hg) have been observed more frequently than decreases in pressure. These changes have not ordinarily persisted for more than 15 minutes nor have they required therapy. More severe degrees of hypertension or hypotension with or without syncope have been reported in a few patients. To minimize the incidence and/or severity of hypotension, the patient should be supine before, during, and after Thyrel TRH administration. If a clinically important change in blood pressure occurs, monitoring of blood pressure should be continued until it returns to baseline levels.
Thyrel TRH should not be administered to patients in whom marked, rapid changes in blood pressure would be dangerous unless the potential benefit clearly outweighs the potential risk.

PRECAUTIONS

Thyroid hormones reduce the TSH response to Thyrel® TRH. Accordingly, patients in whom Thyrel TRH is to be used diagnostically should be taken off liothyronine (T_3) approximately seven days prior to testing and should be taken off thyroid medications containing levothyroxine (T_4), e.g., desiccated thyroid, thyroglobulin, or liotrix, at least 14 days before testing. Hormone therapy is NOT to be discontinued when the test is used to evaluate the effectiveness of thyroid suppression with a particular dose of T_4 in patients with nodular or diffuse goiter, or for adjustment of thyroid hormone dosage given to patients with primary hypothyroidism.
Chronic administration of levodopa has been reported to inhibit the TSH response to Thyrel TRH.
It is not advisable to withdraw maintenance doses of adrenocortical drugs used in the therapy of known hypopituitarism. Several published reports have shown that prolonged treatment with glucocorticoids at physiologic doses has no significant effect on the TSH response to thyrotropin releasing hormone, but that the administration of pharmacologic doses of steroids reduces the TSH response. Therapeutic doses of acetylsalicylic acid (2 to 3.6 g/day) have been reported to inhibit the TSH response to protirelin. The ingestion of acetylsalicylic acid caused the peak level of TSH to decrease approximately 30% as compared to values obtained without acetylsalicylic acid administration. In both cases, the TSH peak occurred 30 minutes post-administration of protirelin.

Carcinogenesis, Mutagenesis, Impairment of Fertility
Long-term animal studies have not been performed to evaluate the carcinogenic potential of protirelin. Studies to determine potential effects concerning mutagenesis or impairment of fertility have also not been performed.

Pregnancy (Category C)
Protirelin has been shown to increase the number of resorptions in rabbits, but not in rats, when given in doses $1^1/_2$ and 6 times the human dose. There are no adequate and well-controlled studies in pregnant women. Thyrel TRH should be used during pregnancy only if the potential benefit justifies the potential risk to the fetus.

Nursing Mothers
It is not known whether this drug is excreted in human milk. Because many drugs are excreted in human milk, caution should be exercised when Thyrel® TRH is administered to a nursing woman.

ADVERSE REACTIONS

Side effects have been reported in about 50% of the patients tested with Thyrel TRH. Generally, the side effects are minor, have occurred promptly, and have persisted for only a few minutes following injection.

Cardiovascular reactions:
Marked changes in blood pressure, including both hypertension and hypotension with or without syncope, have been reported in a small number of patients.

Endocrine reaction:
Breast enlargement and leakage in lactating women for up to two or three days.

Other reactions:

Headaches, sometimes severe, and transient amaurosis in patients with pituitary tumors. Rarely, convulsions may occur in patients with predisposing conditions, e.g. epilepsy, brain damage. Nausea; urge to urinate; flushed sensation; lightheadedness; bad taste in mouth; abdominal discomfort; and dry mouth. Less frequently reported were: anxiety; sweating; tightness in the throat; pressure in the chest; tingling sensation; drowsiness; and allergic reactions.

Pituitary apoplexy requiring acute neurosurgical intervention has been reported infrequently for patients with pituitary macroadenomas following the acute administration of protirelin injection in the setting of combined anterior pituitary function testing in conjunction with LHRH and insulin.

DOSAGE AND ADMINISTRATION

Thyrel TRH is intended for intravenous administration with the patient in the supine position. The drug is administered as a bolus over a period of 15 to 30 seconds, with the patient remaining supine until all scheduled post injection blood samples have been taken. Blood pressure should be measured before Thyrel TRH is administered and at frequent intervals during the first 15 minutes thereafter (see **WARNINGS**). Have the patient urinate before injecting Thyrel TRH.

Dosage:

Adults: 500 μg. Doses between 200 and 500 μg have been used. 500 μg is considered the optimum dose to give the maximum response in the greatest number of patients. Doses greater than 500 μg are unlikely to elicit a greater TSH response.

Children age 6 to 16 years: 7 μg/kg body weight up to a dose of 500 μg.

Infants and children up to 6 years: Experience is limited in this age group; doses of 7 μg/kg have been administered.

One blood sample for TSH assay should be drawn immediately prior to the injection of Thyrel® TRH, and a second sample should be obtained 30 minutes after injection.

The TSH response to Thyrel TRH is reduced by repetitive administration of the drug. Accordingly, if the Thyrel TRH test is repeated, an interval of seven days before testing is recommended.

Elevated serum lipids may interfere with the TSH assay. Thus, fasting (except in patients with hypopituitarism) or a low-fat meal is recommended prior to the test.

INTERPRETATION OF TEST RESULTS

Interpretation of the TSH response to Thyrel TRH requires an understanding of thyroid-pituitary-hypothalamic physiology and knowledge of the clinical status of the individual patient.

Because the TSH test results may vary with the laboratory, the physician should be familiar with the TSH assay method used and the normal range for the laboratory performing the assay. TSH response 30 minutes after Thyrel TRH administration in normal subjects and in patients with hyperthyroidism and hypothyroidism are presented in Figure 1. The diagnoses were established prior to the administration of Thyrel TRH on the basis of the clinical history, physical examination, and the results of other thyroid and/or pituitary function tests.

[See Figure 1 at top of next column.]

Among the normal euthyroid subjects, women and children were found to have higher levels of TSH at 30 minutes than men.

Among the patients with hyperthyroidism or primary (thyroidal), secondary (pituitary), or tertiary (hypothalamic) hypothyroidism, no significant differences in TSH levels by age or sex were found.

Normal: Baseline TSH levels of less than 10 microunits/mL (μU/mL) were observed in 97% of euthyroid normal subjects tested. Thirty minutes after Thyrel TRH, the serum TSH increased by 2.0 μU/mL or more in 95% of euthyroid subjects.

Hyperthyroidism: All hyperthyroid patients tested had baseline TSH levels of less than 10 μU/mL and a rise of less than 2 μU/mL 30 minutes after Thyrel® TRH.

Primary (thyroidal) hypothyroidism: The diagnosis of primary hypothyroidism is frequently supported by finding clearly elevated baseline TSH levels; 93% of patients tested had levels above 10 μU/mL. Thyrel TRH administration to these patients generally would not be expected to yield additional useful information. Ninety-four percent of patients with primary hypothyroidism given Thyrel® TRH in clinical trials responded with a rise in TSH of 2.0 μU/mL or greater. Since this response is also found in normal subjects, Thyrel TRH testing does not differentiate primary hypothyroidism from normal.

Figure 1

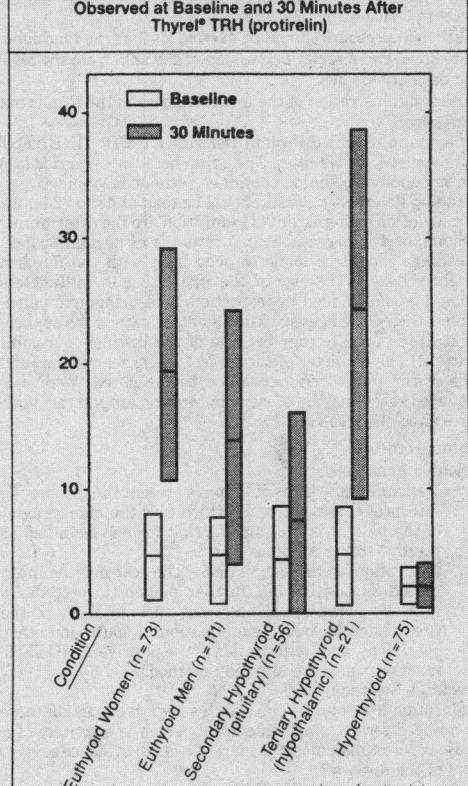

Mean ± One Standard Deviation of TSH Levels (μU/mL) Observed at Baseline and 30 Minutes After Thyrel® TRH (protirelin)

□ Baseline
■ 30 Minutes

(n = number of patients)

Table 1

Characterization Based on Serum TSH Levels at Baseline and 30 Minutes after Thyrel® TRH (protirelin)

	Baseline (Serum TSH (μU/mL)	Change of Serum TSH (μU/mL) at 30 minutes
Euthyroidism (normal thyroid function)	10 or less (usually 6 or less; 20% have <1.5 μU/mL)	2 or more (usually 6 to 30)
Hyperthyroidism	10 or less (usually 4 or less)	less than 2
Primary Hypothyroidism (thyroidal)	more than 10 (usually 15 to 100)	2 or more (usually 20 or more)
Secondary Hypothyroidism (pituitary)	10 or less (usually 6 or less)	less than 2 (59%) 2 to 50 (41%)
Tertiary Hypothyroidism (hypothalamic)	10 or less (often less than 2)	2 or more

Secondary (pituitary) and tertiary (hypothalamic) hypothyroidism. In the presence of clinical and other laboratory evidence of hypothyroidism, the finding of a baseline TSH level less than 10 μU/mL should suggest secondary or tertiary hypothyroidism. In this situation, a response to Thyrel TRH of less than 2 μU/mL suggests secondary hypothyroidism since this response was observed in about 60% of patients with secondary hypothyroidism and only approximately 5% of patients with tertiary hypothyroidism. A TSH response to Thyrel TRH greater than 2 μU/mL is not helpful in differentiating between secondary and tertiary hypothyroidism since this response was noted in about 40% of the former and about 95% of the latter.

Establishing the diagnosis of secondary or tertiary hypothyroidism requires a careful history and physical examination along with appropriate tests of anterior pituitary and/or target gland function. The Thyrel® TRH test should not be used as the only laboratory determinant for establishing these diagnoses.

HOW SUPPLIED

As 1 mL ampuls – boxes of 5 (NDC 55566-0081-5). Each mL contains Thyrel TRH 0.50 mg (500 μg), sodium chloride 9.0 mg for isotonicity, hydrochloric acid and sodium hydroxide as needed to adjust pH.

Store at controlled room temperature (59° to 86°F).

Caution: Federal law prohibits dispensing without a prescription.

Manufacturer for:
FERRING LABORATORIES, INC.
Suffern, NY 10901
By: Akorn Manufacturing, Inc.
Decatur, IL 62525
DC-115C   Rev. 10/95

Lederle Laboratories
A Division of American Cyanamid Co.
ONE CYANAMID PLAZA
WAYNE, NJ 07470

PPD TINE TEST®   ℞
[tīne tĕst]
Tuberculin, Purified Protein Derivative

DESCRIPTION

The Tuberculin, Purified Protein Derivative (PPD) TINE TEST is a simple, multiple-puncture, disposable intradermal test device for the detection of tuberculin reactivity. These convenient devices are especially useful in mass tuberculosis screening programs.

Each test unit consists of a stainless steel disc attached to a light blue plastic handle. Projecting from the disc are four triangular-shaped prongs (tines) which are 2 mm long and approximately 4 mm apart. The tines have been mechanically dipped into a concentrated solution of PPD. The PPD concentrate is prepared by the Seibert Process[1,2] and is stabilized with 7% acacia (gum arabic), 30% dextrose, and 5% glycerol. The glycerol also acts as a humectant preventing the film on the tines from becoming brittle-dry. The final PPD concentrate is standardized against U.S. Standard PPD. Following dipping, the tines are capped and sterilized with ethylene oxide. No preservative has been added. The unit is disposable and there is no need for syringes, needles, and other equipment necessary for the standard intradermal tests.

PPD TINE TEST units have been standardized by clinical evaluation in human subjects to give reactions equivalent to or more potent than 5 TU (US tuberculin units) of standard PPD administered intradermally in the Mantoux test. However, all multiple-puncture-type devices must be regarded as screening tools, and other appropriate diagnostic procedures such as the Mantoux test should be utilized for retesting individuals with positive reactions.

CLINICAL PHARMACOLOGY

Tuberculin deposited in the skin of tuberculin reactive individuals reacts with sensitized lymphocytes to effect the release of mediators of cellular hypersensitivity. Some of these mediators (eg, skin reactive factor) induce an inflammatory response in the skin causing the induration and erythema characteristic of a "positive" reaction.[3,4]

INDICATIONS AND USAGE

Tuberculin, Purified Protein Derivative (PPD) TINE TEST is indicated to detect tuberculin-sensitive individuals. PPD TINE TEST units are also useful in programs to determine priorities for additional testing (eg, chest X-rays) and in epidemiological surveys to identify those areas having high levels of infection.

Data obtained from clinical studies with a total of 3,062 volunteer subjects (males and females), ranging in age from 4 to 96 years, of which 47.5% (1,443) were Mantoux positive, clearly demonstrates that PPD TINE TEST, when used as a screening test to determine tuberculin reactivity, is associated with very little, if any, adverse reactivity. Other than the skin test reaction itself, slight vesiculation and slight ulceration were the only adverse experiences reported. The slight to mild vesiculation was equally divided between the two tests (TINE TEST, 54/3,062, 1.78%; and PPD-T Mantoux, 55/3,062, 1.81%). The slight ulceration observed with one subject at 72 hours was associated with the TINE TEST site. Of the subjects classified as positive or intermediate by PPD-T Mantoux, 93.8% were classified similarly with the TINE TEST. The results of the clinical trials revealed a 72-hour false positive rate of 10.9% and a false negative rate of 6.2%.

In clinical studies of more than 1,800 PPD-S Mantoux positive subjects, only 6.3% gave negative PPD TINE TEST reactions at 72 hours; of more than 1,900 PPD TINE TEST positive tests, less than 11% gave negative Mantoux results.

The frequency of repeated tuberculin tests depends on risk of exposure of the individual and on the prevalence of tuberculosis in the population group. The repeated testing of uninfected individuals does not sensitize to tuberculin. Among individuals with waning sensitivity to homologous or heterologous mycobacterial antigens, however, the stimulus of a

Continued on next page

Lederle—Cont.

tuberculin test may "boost" or increase the size of the reaction to a second test, even causing an apparent development of sensitivity in some cases.[3]

Tuberculin testing should be done with caution in individuals with active tuberculosis. (See **PRECAUTIONS**.)

CONTRAINDICATIONS

There are no known contraindications for use of Tuberculin, Purified Protein Derivative (PPD) TINE TEST. See **PRECAUTIONS** for information regarding special care to be exercised for safe and effective use.

WARNINGS

There are no known serious adverse reactions or potential safety hazards associated with the use of Tuberculin, Purified Protein Derivative (PPD) TINE TEST. However, as with the use of any biological product, the possibility of anaphylactic reaction should be considered. See **PRECAUTIONS** for information regarding special care to be exercised for safe and effective use.

PRECAUTIONS

Tuberculin testing should be done with caution in individuals with active tuberculosis. Although activation of quiescent lesions is rare, if a patient has a history of occurrence of vesiculation and necrosis with a previous tuberculin test by any method, tuberculin testing should be avoided.

Although clinical allergy to acacia is very rare, this product contains some acacia as stabilizer and should be used with caution in patients with known allergy to this component. In these instances remedial measures for anaphylactoid reactions, including epinephrine injection (1:1,000), must be available for immediate use.

Reactivity to the test may be suppressed in patients who are receiving corticosteroids or immunosuppressive agents, or those who have recently been immunized with live virus vaccines such as measles, mumps, rubella, polio. If tuberculin skin testing is indicated it should be done preceding, or at the time of such immunization, and read 48 to 72 hours later. If the test is not administered in the time suggested, an interval of 4 to 6 weeks should be allowed between tuberculin skin testing and immunization with live virus vaccines to prevent suppression of tuberculin reactivity.[5]

With a positive reaction further diagnostic procedures must be considered. These may include X-ray of the chest, microbiological examinations of sputa and other specimens, and confirmation of the positive TINE TEST reaction (except vesiculation reactions) using the Mantoux method. In general, the TINE TEST does not need to be repeated.

Antituberculous chemotherapy should not be instituted solely on the basis of a single positive TINE TEST.

When vesiculation occurs, the reaction is to be interpreted as strongly positive and a repeat test by the Mantoux method must not be attempted. Similar or more severe vesiculation with or without necrosis is likely to occur.

Pregnancy Category C. Animal reproduction studies have not been conducted with Tuberculin, Purified Protein Derivative (PPD) TINE TEST. It is also not known whether PPD TINE TEST can cause fetal harm when administered to a pregnant woman or affect reproduction capacity. Tuberculin, Purified Protein Derivative (PPD) TINE TEST should be given to a pregnant woman only if clearly needed. During pregnancy, known positive reactors may demonstrate a negative response to a PPD TINE TEST.

Tuberculin, Purified Protein Derivative (PPD) TINE TEST units must never be reused. The units should be discarded into an impenetrable sharps container without recapping.

ADVERSE REACTIONS

Vesiculation (positive reaction), ulceration, or necrosis may occur at the test site in highly sensitive persons. Pain, pruritus, and discomfort at the test site may be relieved by cold packs or by topical glucocorticoid ointment or cream. Transient bleeding may be observed at a puncture site and is of no significance.

DOSAGE AND ADMINISTRATION

PPD TINE TEST units have been standardized by clinical evaluation in human subjects to give reactions equivalent to or more potent than 5 TU (US tuberculin units) of standard PPD administered intradermally in the Mantoux test. However, all multiple puncture-type devices must be regarded as screening tools and other appropriate diagnostic procedures, such as the Mantoux test, should be utilized for retesting reactors.

The volar surface of the upper one-third of the forearm, over a muscle belly, is the preferred site. Hairy areas, and areas without adequate subcutaneous tissue, eg, concavities over a tendon or bone, should be avoided.

Alcohol, acetone, ether, or soap and water may be used to cleanse the skin. The area must be clean and thoroughly dry before application of the PPD TINE TEST.

Expose the four coated tines by removing the protective cap while holding the plastic handle. Grasp the patient's forearm firmly, since the sharp momentary sting may cause the pa-

tient to jerk his or her arm, resulting in scratching. Stretch the skin of the forearm tightly and apply the disc with the other hand. **Hold at least one second.** Release tension grip on forearm. Withdraw tine unit.

Sufficient pressure should be exerted so that the four puncture sites, and circular depression of the skin from the plastic base are visible.

After administration of the test, local care of the skin is not necessary.

Tuberculin, Purified Protein Derivative (PPD) TINE TEST units *must never be reused.* The units should be discarded into an impenetrable sharps container without recapping.

Reading Reactions: Tests should be read at 48 to 72 hours. Vesiculation or the extent of induration are the determining factors; erythema without induration is of no significance. Readings should be made in good light with the forearm slightly flexed. The size of the induration in millimeters should be determined by inspection, measuring, and palpation with gentle finger stroking. Identification of the application site is usually easy because of the distinct four-point pattern. The diameter of the largest single reaction around one of the puncture sites should be measured. With pronounced reactions, the areas of induration around the puncture sites may coalesce.

Interpretation:

Positive Reactions

A. Vesiculation. If vesiculation is present the test may be interpreted as positive, in which case the management of the patient is the same as that for one classified as positive to the Mantoux test.[3]

B. Induration, 2 mm or greater. The test may be interpreted as positive but further diagnostic procedures must be considered. These may include X-ray of the chest, microbiological examination of sputa and other specimens, and confirmation of the positive TINE TEST reaction using the Mantoux method.

Negative Reaction

Induration less than 2 mm. With a negative reaction there is no need for retesting unless the person is a contact of a patient with tuberculosis or there is clinical evidence suggestive of the disease.[3]

Induration indicator cards illustrating typical reactions are enclosed.

HOW SUPPLIED

Tuberculin, Purified Protein Derivative (PPD) TINE TEST is supplied as follows:

NDC 0005-2720–25   25 individual tests
NDC 0005-2720–28   100 individual tests

STORAGE

STORE AT CONTROLLED ROOM TEMPERATURE 15°C TO 30°C (59°F TO 86°F).
DO NOT REFRIGERATE.

REFERENCES

1. Seibert FB. Isolation and properties of purified protein derivative of tuberculin. *Am Rev Tuberc.* 1934;30:713–720.
2. Seibert FB, Glenn JF. Tuberculin purified protein derivative—preparation and analysis of a large quantity for standard. *Amer Rev Tuberc.* 1941;44:9–25.
3. Comstock CW, Daniel TM, Snider DE Jr, et al. The tuberculin skin test.*Amer Rev Resp Dis.* 1981;124:356–363.
4. Freeman BA. *Burrows Textbook of Microbiology.* 22nd ed. Philadelphia, Pa: W. B. Saunders Company; 1985: 295–299.
5. American Academy of Pediatrics. *Report of the Committee on Infectious Diseases.* 21st ed. Elk Grove Village, Ill: American Academy of Pediatrics. 1988:429–447.

Manufactured by:
LEDERLE LABORATORIES DIVISION
American Cyanamid Company
Pearl River, NY 10965

Shown in Product Identification Guide, page 321

TUBERCULIN, OLD, TINE TEST®   ℞
[*too-ber-cu-lĭn*]

DESCRIPTION

The Tuberculin, Old, TINE TEST is a sterile, simple, multiple-puncture, disposable intradermal test device for the detection of tuberculin reactivity. These convenient devices are especially useful in mass tuberculosis screening programs.

Each test unit consists of a stainless steel disc attached to a white plastic handle. Projecting from the disc are four triangular-shaped prongs (tines) which are 2 mm long and approximately 4 mm apart. The tines have been mechanically dipped into a solution of Old Tuberculin, containing 7% acacia (gum arabic) and 8.5% lactose as stabilizers, and then dried. The entire unit has been sterilized by Cobalt 60 irradiation. No preservative has been added. The unit is disposable

and there is no need for syringes, needles, and other equipment necessary for the standard intradermal tests.

Tuberculin, Old, TINE TEST units have been standardized by clinical evaluation in human subjects to give reactions equivalent to or more potent than 5 TU (US tuberculin units) of standard Old Tuberculin administered intradermally in the Mantoux test. However, all multiple-puncture-type devices must be regarded as screening tools, and other appropriate diagnostic procedures, such as the Mantoux test, should be utilized for retesting individuals with positive reactions.

CLINICAL PHARMACOLOGY

Tuberculin deposited in the skin of tuberculin reactive individuals reacts with sensitized lymphocytes to effect the release of mediators of cellular hypersensitivity. Some of these mediators (eg, skin reactive factor) induce an inflammatory response in the skin causing the induration and erythema characteristic of a "positive" reaction.[1,2]

INDICATIONS AND USAGE

Tuberculin, Old, TINE TEST is indicated to detect tuberculin-sensitive individuals. Tuberculin, Old, TINE TEST units are also useful in programs to determine priorities for additional testing (eg, chest X-rays) and in epidemiological surveys to identify those areas having high levels of infection. In clinical studies covering various geographical areas of the US and all age groups, with a total of 30,588 test subjects, there were 911 (4%) false positive reactors among 26,236 subjects who were Mantoux negative, and 342 (8%) false negative reactors among 4,352 subjects who were Mantoux positive.

The frequency of repeated tuberculin tests depends on risk of exposure of the individual and on the prevalence of tuberculosis in the population group. The repeated testing of uninfected individuals does not sensitize to tuberculin. Among individuals with waning sensitivity to homologous or heterologous mycobacterial antigens, however, the stimulus of a tuberculin test may "boost" or increase the size of the reaction to a second test, even causing an apparent development of sensitivity in some cases.[1]

Tuberculin testing should be done with caution in individuals with active tuberculosis (see **PRECAUTIONS**).

CONTRAINDICATIONS

There are no known contraindications for use of Tuberculin, Old, TINE TEST. See **PRECAUTIONS** for information regarding special care to be exercised for safe and effective use.

WARNINGS

There are no known serious adverse reactions or potential safety hazards associated with the use of Tuberculin, Old, TINE TEST. However, as with the use of any biological product, the possibility of anaphylactic reaction should be considered. See **PRECAUTIONS** for information regarding special care to be exercised for safe and effective use.

PRECAUTIONS

Tuberculin testing should be done with caution in individuals with active tuberculosis. Although activation of quiescent lesions is rare, if a patient has a history of occurrence of vesiculation and necrosis with a previous tuberculin test by any method, tuberculin testing should be avoided.

Although clinical allergy to acacia is very rare, this product contains some acacia as stabilizer and should be used with caution in patients with known allergy to this component. In these instances, remedial measures for anaphylactoid reactions, including epinephrine injection (1:1000), must be available for immediate use.

Reactivity to the test may be suppressed in patients who are receiving corticosteroids or immunosuppressive agents, or those who have recently been immunized with live virus vaccines such as measles, mumps, rubella, polio. If tuberculin skin testing is indicated it should be done preceding, or at the time of such immunization, and read 48 to 72 hours later. If the test is not administered in the time suggested, an interval of 4 to 6 weeks should be allowed between tuberculin skin testing and immunization with live virus vaccines to prevent suppression of tuberculin reactivity.[3]

With a positive reaction further diagnostic procedures must be considered. These may include X-ray of the chest, microbiological examinations of sputa and other specimens, and confirmation of the positive TINE TEST reaction (except vesiculation reactions) using the Mantoux method. In general, the TINE TEST does not need to be repeated.

Antituberculous chemotherapy should not be instituted solely on the basis of a single positive TINE TEST.

When vesiculation occurs, the reaction is to be interpreted as strongly positive and a repeat test by the Mantoux method must not be attempted. Similar or more severe vesiculation with or without necrosis is likely to occur.

Pregnancy Category C: Animal reproduction studies have not been conducted with Tuberculin, Old, TINE TEST. It is also not known whether Tuberculin, Old, TINE TEST can cause fetal harm when administered to a pregnant woman or affect reproduction capacity. Tuberculin, Old, TINE TEST should be given to a pregnant woman only if clearly needed.

During pregnancy, known positive reactors may demonstrate a negative response to a Tuberculin, Old, TINE TEST. Tuberculin, Old, TINE TEST units must never be reused. The units should be discarded into an impenetrable sharps container without recapping.

ADVERSE REACTIONS

Vesiculation (positive reaction), ulceration, or necrosis may occur at the test site in highly sensitive persons. Pain, pruritus, and discomfort at the test site may be relieved by cold packs or by topical glucocorticoid ointment or cream. Transient bleeding may be observed at a puncture site and is of no significance.

DOSAGE AND ADMINISTRATION

Tuberculin, Old, TINE TEST units have been standardized by clinical evaluation in human subjects to give reactions equivalent to or more potent than 5 TU (US tuberculin units) of standard Old Tuberculin administered intradermally in the Mantoux test. However, all multiple-puncture-type devices must be regarded as screening tools, and other appropriate diagnostic procedures, such as the Mantoux test, should be utilized for retesting reactors.

The volar surface of the upper one-third of the forearm, over a muscle belly, is the preferred site. Hairy areas, and areas without adequate subcutaneous tissue, eg, concavities over a tendon or bone, should be avoided.

Alcohol, acetone, ether, or soap and water may be used to cleanse the skin. The area must be clean and thoroughly dry before application of the Tuberculin, Old, TINE TEST.

Expose the four coated tines by removing the protective cap while holding the plastic handle. Grasp the patient's forearm firmly, since the sharp momentary sting may cause the patient to jerk his or her arm, resulting in scratching. Stretch the skin of the forearm tightly and apply the disc with the other hand. **Hold at least one second.** Release tension grip on forearm. Withdraw tine unit.

Sufficient pressure should be exerted so that the four puncture sites, and circular depression of the skin from the plastic base are visible.

After administration of the test, local care of the skin is not necessary.

Tuberculin, Old, TINE TEST units *must never be reused.* The units should be discarded into an impenetrable sharps container without recapping.

Reading Reactions: Tests should be read at 48 to 72 hours. Vesiculation or the extent of induration are the determining factors; erythema without induration is of no significance. Readings should be made in good light with the forearm slightly flexed. The size of the induration in millimeters should be determined by inspection, measuring, and palpation with gentle finger stroking. Identification of the application site is usually easy because of the distinct four-point pattern. The diameter of the largest single reaction around one of the puncture sites should be measured. With pronounced reactions, the areas of induration around the puncture sites may coalesce.

INTERPRETATION

Positive Reactions:

A. Vesiculation.   If vesiculation is present, the test may be interpreted as positive, in which case the management of the patient is the same as that for one classified as positive to the Mantoux test.[1]

B. Induration, 2 mm or greater.   The test may be interpreted as positive but further diagnostic procedures must be considered. These may include X-ray of the chest, microbiological examination of sputa and other specimens, and confirmation of the positive TINE TEST reaction using the Mantoux method.

Negative Reaction:

Induration less than 2 mm. With a negative reaction there is no need for retesting unless the person is a contact of a patient with tuberculosis or there is clinical evidence suggestive of the disease.[1]

Induration indicator cards illustrating typical reactions are enclosed.

HOW SUPPLIED

Tuberculin, Old, TINE TEST is supplied as follows:

NDC 0005-2722-25 25 individual tests
NDC 0005-2722-28 100 individual tests
NDC 0005-2722-34 250 individual tests

STORAGE

STORE AT CONTROLLED ROOM TEMPERATURE 15°C–30°C (59°F–86°F). DO NOT REFRIGERATE.

REFERENCES

1. Comstock GW, Daniel TM, Snider DE Jr, et al. The tuberculin skin test. *Am Rev Respir Dis.* 1981;124:356–363.
2. Freeman BA. *Burrows Textbook of Microbiology*, 22nd ed. Philadelphia, Pa: W. B. Saunders Company; 1985: 295–299.
3. *American Academy of Pediatrics. Report of the Committee on Infectious Diseases.* 21st ed. Elk Grove Village, Ill: American Academy of Pediatrics; 1988:429–447.

Manufactured by:
LEDERLE LABORATORIES DIVISION
American Cyanamid Company
Pearl River, NY 10965

Shown in Product Identification Guide, page 321

Serono Laboratories, Inc.
100 LONGWATER CIRCLE
NORWELL, MA 02061

GEREF®   ℞
(sermorelin acetate for injection)
For intravenous injection only
FOR DIAGNOSTIC USE ONLY

DESCRIPTION

Geref® (sermorelin acetate for injection) is a sterile, non-pyrogenic, lyophilized preparation containing 50 mcg sermorelin (as the acetate), 5 mg mannitol, 0.66 mg monobasic sodium phosphate, and 0.04 mg dibasic sodium phosphate. Sermorelin acetate is an acetate salt of a synthetic, 29-amino acid polypeptide that is the amino-terminal segment of the naturally occurring human growth hormone-releasing hormone (GHRH or GRH) consisting of 44 amino acid residues. The structural formula for sermorelin acetate is presented below:

Tyr-Ala-Asp-Ala-Ile-Phe-Thr-Asn-Ser-Tyr-
Arg-Lys-Val-Leu-Gly-Gln-Leu-Ser-Ala-Arg-
Lys-Leu-Leu-Gln-Asp-Ile-Met-Ser-Arg-NH$_2$·(C$_2$H$_4$O$_2$)$_{3-6}$

The free base of sermorelin has the empirical formula $C_{149}H_{246}N_{44}O_{42}S_1$ and a molecular weight of 3,358 daltons. Sermorelin appears to be equivalent to GRH (1-44) in its ability to stimulate growth hormone secretion in humans. It has also been called GRH (1-29) and GHRH (1-29).

CLINICAL PHARMACOLOGY

Sermorelin increases plasma growth hormone (GH) concentrations by direct stimulation of the pituitary gland to release GH.

Because baseline GH levels are generally very low (< 4 ng/mL), provocative tests may be useful in determining the functional GH-secreting capability of the pituitary somatotroph. Adults and children with normal responses to standard provocative tests of GH secretion were used to define the range of normal plasma GH-level responses to Geref®. It was found that the absolute peak GH level following Geref® infusion and the time elapsed from infusion to that peak are appropriate measures to evaluate the response to GH infusion. Doses of Geref® used in children and adults in these studies ranged from 0.3 to 6.06 mcg/kg with a majority of patients receiving 1 mcg/kg. Based on these studies and published reports, 1 mcg/kg was chosen as the recommended dose for diagnostic purposes.

A total of 71 Geref® injection tests were performed on 47 boys and 24 girls who showed normal responses to standard, indirect provocative tests such as clonidine, L-dopa, and arginine. The GH peak plasma response to Geref® was 28 ± 15 ng/mL (average ± S.D.) and the time to this peak was 30 ± 27 minutes (average ± S.D.).

Of all children who had GH responses of > 7 ng/mL to standard provocative tests, 96% also had responses to Geref® of > 7 ng/mL. In 77 patients who failed to respond to standard provocative tests, mean GH peak responses to Geref® were significantly lower compared to the mean GH peak response of normal control children. However, 53% of the children who failed to respond to standard tests had a GH response to Geref® of more than 7 ng/mL, suggesting that clinical GH deficiency is frequently not due to somatotroph failure.

The following figure shows the time course of average plasma GH-level responses to Geref® injection in normal children and those with subnormal responses to standard provocative tests, i.e., growth hormone-deficient (GHD) children.

[See Figure at top of next column.]

In 14 published reports that utilized different forms of GRH including GRH (1-44), GRH (1-40), and formulations of GRH (1-29) other than Geref®, 167 normal young adults of both sexes, 19 to 40 years old, were tested with approximately 1 mcg/kg GRH peptide. The data derived from pooling these results are similar to the results obtained from 14 normal male adults, 19 to 30 years old tested with Geref®:

ADULT VOLUNTEERS

Source	N	Age Range	Range of Mean Peak GH (ng/mL)	Mean Peak GH (ng/mL)
14 Studies	167	19–40	10–41	22
Geref®	14	19–30	—	24

In adults, time to peak GH response to Geref® was 35 ± 29 minutes (average ± S.D.).

Preliminary studies have demonstrated a decline in GH responsiveness to GRH with age in persons over 40 years old,

---

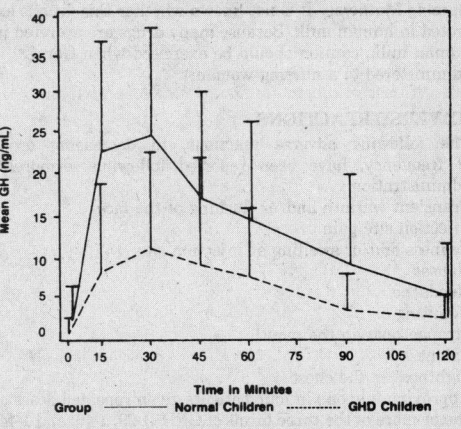

Mean (& SD) of GH Response to Geref® in Normal and GHD Children

Time in Minutes
Group —— Normal Children ········ GHD Children

but the normal range of GH response to Geref® in older adults has not been established.

INDICATIONS AND USAGE

Geref® as a single intravenous injection is indicated for evaluating the ability of the somatotroph of the pituitary gland to secrete growth hormone (GH). A normal plasma GH response to Geref® demonstrates that the somatotroph is intact. However, a normal response does not exclude GH deficiency because this deficiency is frequently the result of hypothalamic dysfunction in the presence of an intact somatotroph. The Geref® stimulation test is most easily interpreted when there is a subnormal response to conventional provocative testing and a normal response to Geref®. Such findings suggest that hypothalamic dysfunction is the cause for the growth hormone deficiency. When both conventional and Geref® testing result in subnormal GH responses, the site of dysfunction cannot be determined with certainty because some patients with GH deficiency due to hypothalamic dysfunction require repeated Geref® administration before demonstrating a normal response.

The Geref® test has not been found useful in the diagnosis of acromegaly.

CONTRAINDICATIONS

Geref® is contraindicated in patients hypersensitive to sermorelin acetate or any of the excipients.

WARNINGS

Although hypersensitivity reactions have been observed with other polypeptide hormones, to date no such reactions have been reported following the administration of a single dose of Geref®. Antibody formation has been reported in humans after chronic subcutaneous administration of large doses of sermorelin (see Adverse Reactions section).

PRECAUTIONS

Drug Interactions: The Geref® test should not be conducted in the presence of drugs that directly affect the pituitary secretion of somatotropin. These include preparations that contain or release somatostatin, insulin, glucocorticoids, or cyclooxygenase inhibitors such as aspirin or indomethacin. Somatotropin levels may be transiently elevated by clonidine, levodopa, and insulin-induced hypoglycemia. Response to Geref® may be blunted in patients who are receiving muscarinic antagonists (atropine) or who are hypothyroid or being treated with antithyroid medications such as propylthiouracil. Obesity, hyperglycemia, and elevated plasma fatty acids generally are associated with subnormal GH responses to Geref®. Exogenous growth hormone therapy should be discontinued at least one week before administering the Geref® test.

Carcinogensis, Mutagenesis, Impairment of Fertility: There have been no long-term studies performed in animals to assess the carcinogenic potential of Geref®. Geref® was not mutagenic in *in vitro* or *in vivo* genetic toxicology studies.

Pregnancy Category C: Sermorelin acetate has been shown to produce minor variations in fetuses of rats and rabbits when given in subcutaneous doses of 50, 150, and 500 mcg/kg. In the rat teratology study, external malformations (thin tail) were observed in the higher dose groups, and there was an increase in minor skeletal variants at the high dose. Some visceral malformations (hydroureter) were observed in all treatment groups, with the incidence greatest in the high-dose group. In rabbits, minor skeletal anomalies were significantly greater in the treated animals than in the controls. There are no adequate and well-controlled studies in pregnant women. Geref® should be used during pregnancy only if the potential benefit justifies the potential risk to the fetus.

Continued on next page

Serono Laboratories—Cont.

Nursing Mothers: It is not known whether this drug is excreted in human milk. Because many drugs are excreted in human milk, caution should be exercised when Geref® is administered to a nursing woman.

ADVERSE REACTIONS

The following adverse reactions, in decreasing order of frequency, have been reported following sermorelin administration:

Transient warmth and/or flushing of the face
Injection site pain
Redness and/or swelling at injection site
Nausea
Headache
Vomiting
Strange taste in the mouth
Paleness
Tightness in the chest

Approximately one in four patients given repeated doses of one or more of the three forms of GRH (1-29, 1-40, and 1-44) has developed antibodies to GRH. The clinical significance of these antibodies is unknown. One patient who developed antibodies to GRH (1-44) also experienced an allergic reaction described as severe redness, swelling, and urticaria at the injection sites. No long-lasting effects from this reaction were reported. No symptomatic allergic reactions to GRH (1-29) have been reported.

OVERDOSAGE

Changes of heart rate and blood pressure have been reported with the various GRH peptides in intravenous doses exceeding 10 mcg/kg. Cardiovascular collapse is a conceivable, but as of yet, unreported, complication of overdosage with GRH (1-29).

DOSAGE AND ADMINISTRATION

Geref® dosage should be individualized for each patient according to his/her weight. It is recommended that Geref® be administered in a single intravenous dose of 1.0 mcg/kg body weight in the morning following an overnight fast.

DIRECTIONS

Children (or subjects less than 50 kg)
1) Reconstitute the contents of one 50 mcg ampule of Geref® with a minimum of 0.5 mL of the accompanying sterile diluent.
2) Venous blood samples for growth hormone determinations should be drawn 15 minutes before and immediately prior to Geref® administration.
3) Administer a bolus of 1 mcg/kg body weight Geref® intravenously followed by a 3 mL normal saline flush.
4) Draw venous blood samples for growth hormone determinations at 15, 30, 45, and 60 minutes after Geref® administration.

Adults (or subjects over 50 kg)
1) Determine the number of ampules needed, based on a dose of 1 mcg/kg body weight.
2) Reconstitute the contents of each ampule with a minimum of 0.5 mL of the accompanying sterile diluent.
3) Follow steps 2–4 above.

Parenteral drug products should be inspected visually for particulate matter and discoloration prior to administration, whenever solution and container permit. The drug should be discarded if not dissolved or if the reconstituted solution is cloudy or discolored.

HOW SUPPLIED

Geref® is supplied in sterile, nonpyrogenic, lyophilized form in ampules containing 50 mcg sermorelin (as the acetate). The following package combination is available:
NDC 44087-4050-1
1 ampule containing 50 mcg sermorelin (as the acetate) and 1 vial containing 2 mL 0.9% Sodium Chloride Injection, USP
The lyophilized product must be stored refrigerated (2°–8°C/36°–46°F). Use immediately after reconstitution. Discard unused material.

Caution: Federal law prohibits dispensing without prescription.
References available on request.

Manufactured for:
SERONO LABORATORIES, INC.
Randolph, MA 02368 USA
by: Laboratoires Serono, SA
Aubonne, Switzerland
© SERONO LABORATORIES, INC. 1991, 1993

Wyeth-Ayerst Laboratories
**Division of American Home
Products Corporation
P.O. BOX 8299
PHILADELPHIA, PA 19101**

FACTREL®   ℞
[fắc 'trel]
**(gonadorelin hydrochloride)
Synthetic Luteinizing Hormone Releasing
Hormone (LH-RH)
DIAGNOSTIC USE ONLY**

Caution: Federal law prohibits dispensing without prescription.

DESCRIPTION

An agent for use in evaluating hypothalamic-pituitary gonadotropic function. FACTREL (gonadorelin hydrochloride) injectable is available as a sterile lyophilized powder for reconstitution and administration by subcutaneous or intravenous routes.

Chemical Name: 5-oxo-L-prolyl-L-histidyl-L-tryptophyl-L-seryl-L-tyrosyl-glycyl-L-leucyl-L-arginyl-L-prolyl glycinamide hydrochloride
[See chemical structure below.]
FACTREL is $C_{55}H_{75}N_{17}O_{13}HCl$, as the mono- or dihydrochloride, or their mixture. The gonadorelin base has a molecular weight of 1182.33. It is a white powder, soluble in alcohol and water, hygroscopic and moisture-sensitive, and stable at room temperature. The synthetic decapeptide, FACTREL, has a chemical composition and structure identical to the natural hormone, identified from porcine or ovine hypothalami.
Each SECULE® vial of FACTREL contains 100 or 500 mcg gonadorelin as the hydrochloride, with 100 mg lactose, USP. Each ampul of sterile diluent contains 2% benzyl alcohol in sterile water.

CLINICAL PHARMACOLOGY

FACTREL has been shown to have gonadotropin-releasing effects upon the anterior pituitary. The range for normal baseline LH levels, as determined from the literature, is 5–25 mIU/mL in postpubertal males, and postpubertal and premenopausal females. The standard used is the Second International Reference Preparation—HMC. This range may not correspond in each laboratory performing the assay since the concentration of LH in normal individuals varies with different assay methods. The normal responses to FACTREL analyzed from the results of clinical studies included:
(1) LH peak (mIU/mL)
(highest LH value post-FACTREL administration)
(2) Maximum LH increase (mIU/mL)
(peak LH value—LH baseline value)
(3) LH percent response
$$\frac{\text{peak LH—baseline LH}}{\text{baseline LH}} \times 100\%$$
(4) Time to peak (minutes)
(time required to reach LH peak value)
Normal adult subjects were shown to have these LH responses following FACTREL administration by subcutaneous or intravenous routes.
I.   MALE ADULTS:
A) Subcutaneous Administration
The results are based on 18 tests in males between the ages of 18–42 years, inclusive:
(1) LH peak: mean 60.3 ± 26.2 mIU/mL
100% ≥ 24.0 mIU/mL
90% ≥ 32.8 mIU/mL
(2) Maximum LH increase: mean 46.7 ± 20.8 mIU/mL
100% ≥ 12.3 mIU/mL
90% ≥ 20.9 mIU/mL

(3) LH percent response: mean $437 \pm 243\%$
range: 66–1853%
90% ≥ 188%
(4) Time to peak: mean 34 ± 13 min
B) Intravenous Administration
The results are based on 26 tests in males between the ages of 19–58 years, inclusive:
(1) LH peak: mean 63.8 ± 40.3 mIU/mL
100% ≥ 12.6 mIU/mL
90% ≥ 26.0 mIU/mL
(2) Maximum LH increase: mean 51.3 ± 35.2 mIU/mL
100% ≥ 7.4 mIU/mL
90% ≥ 14.8 mIU/mL
(3) LH percent response: mean $481 \pm 184\%$
range: 67–2139%
90% ≥ 142%
(4) Time to peak: mean 27 ± 14 min
In males older than 50 years, the LH baseline and peak levels tend to be higher; however, the maximum LH increases do not differ in regard to age.
II. FEMALE ADULTS:
A) Subcutaneous Administration
The results are based on 38 tests in females between the ages of 19–36 years, inclusive:
(1) LH peak: mean 67.9 ± 27.5 mIU/mL
100% ≥ 12.5 mIU/mL
90% ≥ 39.0 mIU/mL
(2) Maximum LH increase: mean 52.8 ± 26.4 mIU/mL
100% ≥ 7.5 mIU/mL
90% ≥ 23.8 mIU/mL
(3) LH percent response: mean $374 \pm 221\%$
range: 108–981%
90% ≥ 185%
(4) Time to peak: mean 71.5 ± 49.6 min
B) Intravenous Administration
The results are based on 31 tests in females between the ages of 20–35 years, inclusive:
(1) LH peak: mean 57.6 ± 36.7 mIU/mL
100% ≥ 20.0 mIU/mL
90% ≥ 24.6 mIU/mL
(2) Maximum LH increase: mean 44.5 ± 31.8 mIU/mL
100% ≥ 7.5 mIU/mL
90% ≥ 16.2 mIU/mL
(3) LH percent response: mean $356 \pm 282\%$
range: 60–1300%
90% ≥ 142%
(4) Time to peak: mean 36 ± 24 min
The FACTREL tests on which the normal female responses are based were performed in the early follicular phase of the menstrual cycle (Days 1–7).

In menopausal and postmenopausal females, the baseline LH levels are elevated and the maximum LH increases are exaggerated when compared with the premenopausal levels. Patients with clinically diagnosed or suspected pituitary and/or hypothalamic dysfunction were often shown to have subnormal or no LH responses following FACTREL administration. For example, in clinical tests of 6 patients with known postpubertal panhypopituitarism, and 11 patients with Prader-Willi syndrome, 100% showed subnormal responses or no rise in LH. Subnormal responses to the FACTREL test also were observed in 21 (95%) of 22 patients with prepubertal panhypopituitarism. In 19 patients with Sheehan's syndrome, 16 (84%) had a subnormal response. In the FACTREL test in 44 patients with Kallmann's syndrome, 33 (77%) had subnormal LH responses.

INDICATIONS AND USAGE

FACTREL as a single injection is indicated for evaluating the functional capacity and response of the gonadotropes of the anterior pituitary. This single-injection test does not measure pituitary gonadotropic reserve, for which more prolonged or repeated administration may be required. The LH response is useful in testing patients with suspected go-

Structural Formula:

nadotropin deficiency, whether due to the hypothalamus alone or in combination with anterior pituitary failure. FACTREL is also indicated for evaluating residual gonadotropic function of the pituitary following removal of a pituitary tumor by surgery and/or irradiation. In clinical studies to date, however, the single-injection test has not been useful in differentiating pituitary disorders from hypothalamic disorders. The FACTREL test can be performed concomitantly with other post-treatment evaluations. The results of the FACTREL test complement the clinical examination and other laboratory tests used to confirm or substantiate hypogonadotropic hypogonadism.

In cases where there is a normal response, it indicates the presence of functional pituitary gonadotropes. The single-injection test does not measure pituitary gonadotropic reserve.

CONTRAINDICATIONS
Hypersensitivity to gonadorelin hydrochloride or any of the components.

PRECAUTIONS
A. GENERAL
Although allergic and hypersensitivity reactions have been observed with other polypeptide hormones, and rarely with multiple doses of FACTREL, to date no such reactions have been reported following the administration of a single 100 mcg dose of FACTREL.

Antibody formation has been reported rarely after chronic administration of large doses of FACTREL.

B. DRUG INTERACTIONS
The FACTREL test should be conducted in the absence of other drugs which directly affect the pituitary secretion of the gonadotropins. These would include a variety of preparations which contain androgens, estrogens, progestins, or glucocorticoids. The gonadotropin levels may be transiently elevated by spironolactone, minimally elevated by levodopa, and suppressed by oral contraceptives and digoxin. The response to FACTREL may be blunted by phenothiazines and dopamine antagonists which cause a rise in prolactin.

C. CARCINOGENESIS, MUTAGENESIS, IMPAIRMENT OF FERTILITY
Repetitive, high doses of FACTREL may cause luteolysis and inhibition of spermatogenesis. No long-term animal studies have been done to evaluate carcinogenic potential.

D. PREGNANCY CATEGORY B.
Reproduction studies have been performed in mice, rats, and rabbits at doses up to 50 times the human dose, and have revealed no evidence of harm to the fetus due to FACTREL. There are, however, no adequate and well-controlled studies in pregnant women. Because animal reproduction studies are not always predictive of human response, this drug should be used during pregnancy only if clearly needed. Appropriate precautions should be taken because the effects of LH-RH on the fetus and developing offspring have not been adequately evaluated.

Nursing Mothers: It is not known whether this drug is excreted in human milk. Because many drugs are excreted in human milk, caution should be exercised when FACTREL is administered to a nursing woman.

Pediatric Use: Safety and effectiveness in pediatric patients have not been established.

ADVERSE REACTIONS
Systemic effects have been reported rarely following administration of 100 mcg of FACTREL.
CNS: headache, light-headedness.
GI: nausea, abdominal discomfort.
Dermatologic: local swelling, occasionally with pain and pruritis, at the injection site may occur following subcutaneous administration; local and generalized skin rash have been noted after chronic subcutaneous administration.
Cardiovascular: flushing.

Rare instances of hypersensitivity reaction (bronchospasm, tachycardia, flushing, urticaria, induration at injection site) and anaphylactic reactions have been reported following multiple-dose administration.

There has been a report of pituitary apoplexy and sudden blindness following gonadotropin-releasing hormone administration to a patient with a gonadotropin-secreting adenoma.

OVERDOSAGE
FACTREL has been administered parenterally in doses up to 3 mg b.i.d. for 28 days without any signs or symptoms of overdosage. In case of overdosage or idiosyncrasy, symptomatic treatment should be administered as required.

DOSAGE AND ADMINISTRATION
Parenteral drug products should be inspected visually for particulate matter and discoloration prior to administration, whenever solution and container permit.
Adults: 100 mcg dose, subcutaneously or intravenously. In females for whom the phase of the menstrual cycle can be established, the test should be performed in the early follicular phase (Days 1–7).

TEST METHODOLOGY
To determine the status of the gonadotropin secretory capacity of the anterior pituitary, a test procedure requiring seven venous blood samples for LH is recommended.

PROCEDURE:
1. Venous blood samples should be drawn at -15 minutes and immediately prior to FACTREL administration. The LH baseline is obtained by averaging the LH values of the two samples.
2. Administer a bolus of 100 mcg of FACTREL subcutaneously or intravenously.
3. Draw venous blood samples at 15, 30, 45, 60, and 120 minutes after administration.
4. Blood samples should be handled as recommended by the laboratory that will determine the LH content. It must be emphasized that the reliability of the test is directly related to the inter-assay and intra-assay reliability of the laboratory performing the assay.

INTERPRETATION OF TEST RESULTS
Interpretation of the LH response to FACTREL requires an understanding of the hypothalamic-pituitary physiology, knowledge of the clinical status of the individual patient, and familiarity with the normal ranges and the standards used in the laboratory performing the LH assays.

Figures 1 through 4 represent the LH response curves after FACTREL administration in normal subjects. The normal LH response curves were established between the 10th percentile (B line) and 90th percentile (A line) of all LH responses in normal subjects analyzed from the results of clinical studies. LH values are reported in units of mIU/mL and time is displayed in minutes. Individual patient responses should be plotted on the appropriate curve. A subnormal response in patients is defined as three or more LH values which fall below the B line of the normal LH response curve. In cases where there is a blunted or borderline response, the FACTREL test should be repeated.

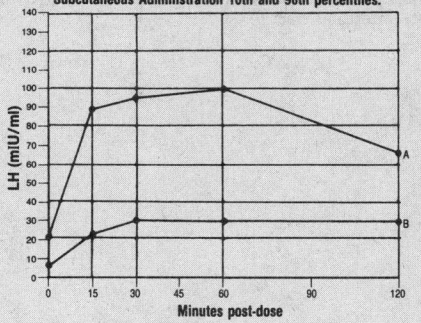

Fig. 1
Normal Male LH Response After FACTREL 100 mcg.
Subcutaneous Administration 10th and 90th percentiles.

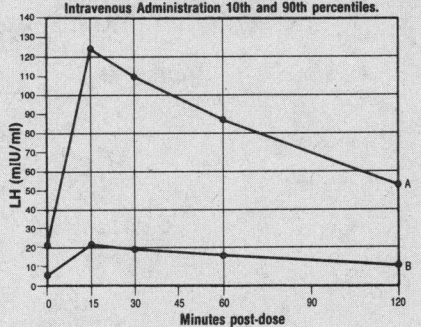

Fig. 2
Normal Male LH Response After FACTREL 100 mcg.
Intravenous Administration 10th and 90th percentiles.

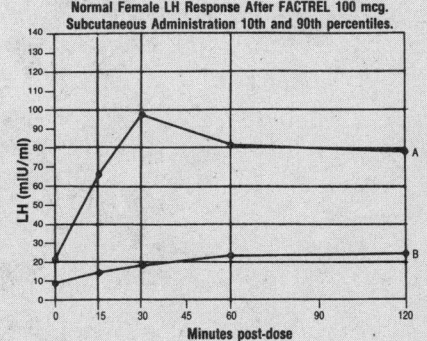

Fig. 3
Normal Female LH Response After FACTREL 100 mcg.
Subcutaneous Administration 10th and 90th percentiles.

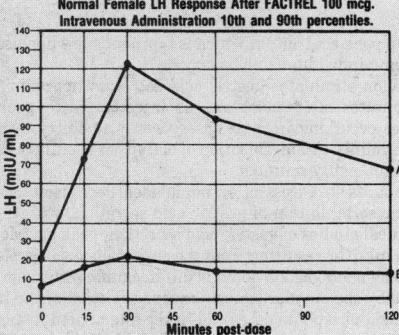

Fig. 4
Normal Female LH Response After FACTREL 100 mcg.
Intravenous Administration 10th and 90th percentiles.

The FACTREL test complements the clinical assessment of patients with a variety of endocrine disorders involving the hypothalamic-pituitary axis. In cases where there is a normal response, it indicates the presence of functional pituitary gonadotropes. The single-injection test does not determine the pathophysiological cause for the subnormal response and does not measure pituitary gonadotropic reserve.

HOW SUPPLIED
LYOPHILIZED POWDER—
in single-dose Secule® vials containing 100 mcg (NDC 0046-0507-05) and 500 mcg (NDC 0046-0509-05) gonadorelin as the hydrochloride with 100 mg lactose, USP. Each Secule® vial is accompanied by one ampul containing 2 mL sterile diluent of 2% benzyl alcohol in sterile water.

DIRECTIONS
Store at room temperature (approximately 25°C).
Reconstitute 100 mcg Secule® vial with 1.0 mL of the accompanying sterile diluent.
Reconstitute 500 mcg Secule® vial with 2.0 mL of the accompanying sterile diluent.
Prepare solution immediately before use.
After reconstitution, store at room temperature and use within 1 day.
Discard unused reconstituted solution and diluent.
Secule®—Registered trademark to designate a vial containing an injectable preparation in dry form.

PEPTAVLON®   ℞
[pĕp-tăv′lon]
(pentagastrin)
for subcutaneous injection

Caution: Federal law prohibits dispensing without prescription.

DESCRIPTION
Peptavlon (pentagastrin) is a diagnostic agent for evaluation of gastric acid secretory function.
Chemical name: N-t-butyloxycarbonyl-B-alanyl-L-tryptophyl-L-methionyl-L-aspartyl-L-phenylalanyl amide.
Structural formula:

$$N—(CH_3)_3COC—\beta Ala—Trp—Met—Asp—Phe—NH_2$$

Pentagastrin is a synthetic pentapeptide containing the carboxyl terminal tetrapeptide, the active portion found in all natural gastrins. Pentagastrin is a colorless crystalline solid. It is soluble in dimethylformamide and dimethylsulfoxide; it is almost insoluble in water, ethanol, ether, benzene, chloroform, and ethyl acetate. Peptavlon is sterile and nonpyrogenic.

Each mL of injection contains 0.25 mg (250 mcg) pentagastrin. Peptavlon also contains 8.8 mg sodium chloride and Water for Injection, USP. The pH is adjusted with ammonium hydroxide and/or hydrochloric acid. Peptavlon is available in 2 mL ampules for subcutaneous administration.

CLINICAL PHARMACOLOGY
Peptavlon (pentagastrin) contains the C-terminal tetrapeptide responsible for the actions of the natural gastrins and, therefore, acts as a physiologic gastric acid secretagogue. The recommended dose of 6 mcg/kg subcutaneously pro-

Continued on next page

Consult 1997 supplements and future editions for revisions

Wyeth-Ayerst Laboratories—Cont.

duces a peak acid output which is reproducible when used in the same individual.

Peptavlon stimulates gastric acid secretion approximately ten minutes after subcutaneous injection, with peak responses occurring in most cases twenty to thirty minutes after administration. Duration of activity is usually between sixty and eighty minutes.

In amounts in excess of recommended dose, pentagastrin may cause inhibition of gastric acid secretion.

In clinical studies of gastric acid secretion, peak gastric output in mEq/hr resulting from the subcutaneous injection of 6 mcg/kg pentagastrin does not differ significantly from that caused by the standard subcutaneous injection of the histamine acid phosphate dose used in the augmented histamine test (40 mcg/kg). For example, in 25 normal volunteers, pentagastrin produced an average peak acid output of 28.4 mEq/hr, compared with 24.7 mEq/hr by histamine. In 45 patients with duodenal ulcer, or suspected duodenal ulcer, pentagastrin produced an average peak gastric acid output of 39.7 mEq/hr, compared with 33.7 mEq/hr by histamine. In 18 patients with gastric ulcer, or suspected gastric ulcer, pentagastrin produced an average peak acid output of 17.4 mEq/hr, compared with 19.4 mEq/hr by histamine. The overall mean for peak acid secretion by pentagastrin was 24.8 mEq/hr, compared with 22.6 mEq/hr by histamine. No biochemical abnormality which might indicate specific organ toxicity has been encountered following the administration of pentagastrin.

INDICATIONS AND USAGE

Peptavlon is used as a diagnostic agent to evaluate gastric acid secretory function. It is useful in testing for:

Anacidity: as a diagnostic aid in patients with suspected pernicious anemia, atrophic gastritis, or gastric carcinoma.

Hypersecretion: as a diagnostic aid in patients with suspected duodenal ulcer or postoperative stomal ulcer, and for the diagnosis of Zollinger-Ellison tumor.

Peptavlon (pentagastrin) is also useful in determining the adequacy of acid-reducing operations for peptic ulcer.

CONTRAINDICATIONS

Hypersensitivity or idiosyncrasy to pentagastrin.

WARNINGS

In amounts in excess of the recommended dose, pentagastrin may cause inhibition of gastric acid secretion.

PRECAUTIONS

Use with caution in patients with pancreatic, hepatic, or biliary disease. Like gastrin, pentagastrin could, in some cases, have the physiologic effect of stimulating pancreatic enzyme and bicarbonate secretion, as well as biliary flow.

CARCINOGENESIS, MUTAGENESIS, IMPAIRMENT OF FERTILITY

Long-term studies in animals to evaluate carcinogenic potential and studies to evaluate the mutagenic potential or effect on fertility have not been conducted.

PREGNANCY: TERATOGENIC EFFECTS

Pregnancy Category C—Animal reproduction studies have not been conducted with Peptavlon. It is also not known whether Peptavlon can cause fetal harm when administered to a pregnant woman or can affect reproduction capacity. Peptavlon should be given to a pregnant woman only if clearly needed.

NURSING MOTHERS

It is not known whether this drug is excreted in human milk. Because many drugs are excreted in human milk, caution should be exercised when Peptavlon is administered to a nursing woman.

PEDIATRIC USE

Safety and effectiveness in children have not been established.

ADVERSE REACTIONS

Pentagastrin causes fewer and less severe cardiovascular and other adverse reactions than histamine or betazole. The majority of reactions to pentagastrin are related to the gastrointestinal tract.

The following reactions associated with the use of pentagastrin have been reported.

Gastrointestinal: Abdominal pain, desire to defecate, nausea, vomiting, borborygmi, blood-tinged mucus

Cardiovascular: Flushing, tachycardia

Central Nervous System: Dizziness, faintness or light-headedness, drowsiness, sinking feeling, transient blurring of vision, tiredness, headache

Allergic and Hypersensitivity Reactions: May occur in some patients.

Miscellaneous: Shortness of breath, heavy sensation in arms and legs, tingling in fingers, chills, sweating, generalized burning sensation, warmth, pain at site of injection, bile in collected specimens

OVERDOSAGE

In case of overdosage or idiosyncrasy, symptomatic treatment should be administered as required.

DOSAGE AND ADMINISTRATION

Adults: 6 mcg/kg subcutaneously. Effect begins in about ten minutes; peak response usually occurs in twenty to thirty minutes. (For discussion of the test and explicit directions, consult Baron, JH: Gastric Function Tests, in Wastell, C: *Chronic Duodenal Ulcer,* New York, Appleton-Century-Crofts, 1972, pp 82–114.)

Parenteral drug products should be inspected visually for particulate matter and discoloration prior to administration, whenever solution and container permit.

HOW SUPPLIED

Peptavlon (pentagastrin) is available in 2 mL ampuls. Each mL contains 0.25 mg (250 micrograms) pentagastrin. Cartons of 10 ampuls (NDC 0046-3290-10).

Refrigerate, 2°C to 8°C (36°F to 46°F), and protect from light. Do not use if discolored.

POISON CONTROL CENTERS

Many of the centers listed below are certified by the American Association of Poison Control Centers. To receive certification, each center has to meet certain criteria. It must, for example, serve a large geographic area; it must be open 24 hours a day and provide direct-dial or toll-free access; it must be supervised by a medical director; and it must have registered pharmacists or nurses available to answer questions from the public. Certified centers are marked by an asterisk after the name.

The centers have a wide variety of toxicology resources, including a computerized database of some 750,000 substances maintained by MICROMEDEX, INC., an affiliate of PDR. Staff members are trained to resolve toxic situations in the home of the caller, though hospital referrals are given in some instances. The centers also offer a range of educational services to both the public and healthcare professionals. In some states, these larger centers exist side by side with smaller centers offering a more limited range of services.

Within each state, centers are listed alphabetically by city. Telephone numbers designated "TTY" are teletype lines for the hearing-impaired. "TDD" numbers reach a telecommunication device for the deaf.

ALABAMA

BIRMINGHAM
Regional Poison Control Center
Children's Hospital of Alabama (*)
1600 7th Ave. South
Birmingham, AL 35233-1711
Business: 205-939-9720
Emergency: 205-933-4050
205-939-9201
800-292-6678 (AL)
Fax: 205-939-9245

TUSCALOOSA
Alabama Poison Control
Systems, Inc. (*)
408 A. Paul Bryant Dr. East
Tuscaloosa, AL 35401
Business: 205-345-0600
Emergency: 205-345-0600
800-462-0800 (AL)
Fax: 205-759-7994

ALASKA

ANCHORAGE
Anchorage Poison Center
Providence Hospital
P.O. Box 196604
3200 Providence Dr.
Anchorage, AK 99519-6604
Business: 907-562-2211
ext. 3633
Emergency: 907-261-3193
800-478-3193
(AK)
Fax: 907-261-3645

FAIRBANKS
Fairbanks Poison
Control Center
1650 Cowles St.
Fairbanks, AK 99701
Business: 907-456-7182
Emergency: 907-456-7182
Fax: 907-458-5553

ARIZONA

PHOENIX
Samaritan Regional
Poison Center (*)
Good Samaritan
Medical Center
1111 East McDowell Rd.
Phoenix, AZ 85006
Business: 602-495-4884
Emergency: 602-253-3334
Fax: 602-256-7579

TUCSON
Arizona Poison & Drug
Information Center (*)
University of Arizona
Arizona Health Sciences Center
1501 North Campbell Ave.
#1156
Tucson, AZ 85724
Emergency: 520-626-6016
800-362-0101 (AZ)
Fax: 520-626-2720

ARKANSAS

LITTLE ROCK
Arkansas Poison and Drug
Information Center
College of Pharmacy - UAMS
4301 West Markham St.
Slot 522-2
Little Rock, AR 72205
Business: 501-661-6161
Emergency: 800-376-4766 (AR)

CALIFORNIA

FRESNO
Central California Regional
Poison Control Center (*)
Valley Children's Hospital
3151 North Millbrook
Fresno, CA 93703
Business: 209-241-6040
Emergency: 209-445-1222
800-346-5922
(Central CA)
Fax: 209-241-6050

LOS ANGELES
Los Angeles County Regional
Drug & Poison Information
Center (*)
LAC & USC Medical Center
1200 North State St.
Los Angeles, CA 90033
Business: 213-226-7741
Emergency: 213-222-3212
800-777-6476
Fax: 213-226-4194

SACRAMENTO
UC Davis Medical Center
Regional Poison Control Center (*)
2315 Stockton Blvd.
Sacramento, CA 95817
Business: 916-734-3415
Emergency: 916-734-3692
800-342-9293
(N. CA only)
Fax: 916-734-7796

SAN DIEGO
San Diego Regional
Poison Center (*)
UCSD Medical Center
200 West Arbor Dr.
San Diego, CA 92103-8925
Business: 619-543-3666
Emergency: 619-543-6000
800-876-4766
(San Diego
and Imperial
counties only)
Fax: 619-692-1867

SAN FRANCISCO
San Francisco Bay Area
Regional Poison Control Center (*)
SF General Hospital
1001 Potrero Ave., Bldg. 80
San Francisco, CA 94110
Business: 415-206-5524
Emergency: 800-523-2222
Fax: 415-821-8513

COLORADO

DENVER
Rocky Mountain Poison and
Drug Center (*)
8802 East 9th Ave. Bldg. 752
Denver, CO 80220
Business: 303-739-1100
Emergency: 303-629-1123
TTY: 303-739-1127
Fax: 303-739-1119

CONNECTICUT

FARMINGTON
Connecticut Poison Control
Center (*)
University of Connecticut
Health Center
263 Farmington Ave.
Farmington, CT 06032
Business: 203-679-3473
Emergency: 800-343-2722 (CT)
TTY: 203-679-4346
Fax: 203-679-1623

DISTRICT OF COLUMBIA

WASHINGTON, DC
National Capital Poison Center (*)
3201 New Mexico Ave., NW
Suite 310
Washington, DC 20016
Business: 202-362-3867
Emergency: 202-625-3333
TTY: 202-362-8563
Fax: 202-362-8377

FLORIDA

JACKSONVILLE
Florida Poison Information
Center of Jacksonville
655 W. 8th St.
Jacksonville, FL 32209
Emergency: 904-549-4480
Fax: 904-549-4063

MIAMI
Florida Poison Information
Center of Miami
P.O. Box 016960, R-131
Miami, FL 33101
Emergency: 305-585-5253
Fax: 305-242-9762

TAMPA
Florida Poison Information
and Toxicology
Resource Center (*)
Tampa General Hospital
P.O. Box 1289
Tampa, FL 33601
Emergency: 813-253-4444
800-282-3171 (FL)
Fax: 813-253-4443

GEORGIA

ATLANTA
Georgia Poison Center (*)
Grady Health System
80 Butler St. SE
P.O. Box 26066
Atlanta, GA 30335-3801
Emergency: 404-616-9000
800-282-5846 (GA)
Fax: 404-616-6657

MACON
Regional Poison Control Center
Medical Center
of Central Georgia
777 Hemlock St.
Macon, GA 31201
Poison Ctr: 912-633-1427
Fax: 912-633-5082

ILLINOIS

CHICAGO
Chicago & NE Illinois Regional
Poison Control Center
Rush-Presbyterian-
St. Luke's Medical Center
1653 West Congress Pkwy.
Chicago, IL 60612
Business: 312-942-7064
Emergency: 312-942-5969
800-942-5969 (IL)
Fax: 312-942-4260

URBANA
ASPCA/National Animal Poison
Control Center (*)
1717 Philo Rd., Suite 36
Urbana, IL 61801
Business: 217-333-2053
800-548-2423
(24-hour
subscribers)
Fax: 217-244-1580

INDIANA

INDIANAPOLIS
Indiana Poison Center (*)
Methodist Hospital of Indiana
1701 North Senate Blvd.
P.O. Box 1367
Indianapolis, IN 46206-1367
Emergency: 317-929-2323
800-382-9097 (IN)
TTY: 317-929-2336
Fax: 317-929-2337

IOWA

DES MOINES
Variety Club Poison and Drug
Information Center
Iowa Methodist Medical Center
1200 Pleasant St.
Des Moines, IA 50309
Business: 515-241-6254
Emergency: 800-362-2327 (IA)
Fax: 515-241-5085

IOWA CITY
Poison Control Center (*)
University of Iowa Hospitals
and Clinics
200 Hawkins Dr.
Iowa City, IA 52242
Business: 319-356-2577
Emergency: 800-272-6477
(IA only)

KANSAS

KANSAS CITY
Mid-America Poison Control
Center
University of Kansas Medical
Center
3901 Rainbow Blvd.
Room B-400
Kansas City, KS 66160-7231
Business & 913-588-6633
Emergency: 800-332-6633 (KS)
Fax: 913-588-2350

TOPEKA
Stormont-Vail Regional Medical
Center
Emergency Department
1500 West 10th
Topeka, KS 66604
Business: 913-354-6000
Emergency: 913-354-6100
Fax: 913-354-5004

KENTUCKY

LOUISVILLE
Kentucky Regional
Poison Center (*)
Kosair Children's Hospital
Medical Towers S., Suite 572
P.O. Box 35070
Louisville, KY 40232-5070
Business: 502-629-7264
Emergency: 502-629-7275
502-589-8222
800-722-5725 (KY)
Fax: 502-629-7277

LOUISIANA

MONROE
Louisiana Drug and Poison
Information Center (*)
Northeast Louisiana University
School of Pharmacy
Monroe, LA 71209-6430
Business: 318-342-1710
Emergency: 800-256-9822 (LA)
Fax: 318-342-1744

MAINE

PORTLAND
Maine Poison Center (*)
Maine Medical Center
22 Bramhall St.
Portland, ME 04102
Business: 207-871-2950
Emergency: 800-442-6305 (ME)
Fax: 207-871-6226

MARYLAND

BALTIMORE
Maryland Poison Center (*)
University of Maryland
School of Pharmacy
20 North Pine St.
Baltimore, MD 21201
Business: 410-706-7604
Emergency: 410-706-7701
800-492-2414
(MD only)
TTY: 410-706-1858
Fax: 410-706-7184

MASSACHUSETTS

BOSTON
Massachusetts Poison Control
System (*)
300 Longwood Ave.
Boston, MA 02115
Emergency: 617-232-2120
800-682-9211
TTY: 617-355-6089
Fax: 617-738-0032

MICHIGAN

DETROIT
Poison Control Center (*)
Children's Hospital of Michigan
Harper Professional
Office Bldg., Suite 425
Detroit, MI 48201
Business: 313-745-5335
Emergency: 313-745-5711
Fax: 313-745-5493

GRAND RAPIDS
Blodgett Regional Poison Center (*)
Blodgett Memorial
Medical Center
1840 Wealthy St. SE
Grand Rapids, MI 49506
Business: 616-774-5329
Emergency: 800-764-7661 (MI)
Fax: 616-774-7204

MINNESOTA

MINNEAPOLIS
Hennepin Regional
Poison Center (*)
Hennepin County Medical Center
701 Park Ave.
Minneapolis, MN 55415
Business: 612-347-3144
Emergency: 612-347-3141
TTY: 612-904-4691
Fax: 612-904-4289

Minnesota Regional
Poison Center (*)
8100 34th Ave. South
Box 1309
Minneapolis, MN 55440
Business: 612-851-8100
Emergency: 612-221-2113
Fax: 612-851-8166

MISSISSIPPI

HATTIESBURG
Poison Center
Forrest General Hospital
400 South 28th Ave.
Hattiesburg, MS 39401
Business: 601-288-4221
Emergency: 601-288-4235

JACKSON
Mississippi Regional Poison
Control (*)
University of Mississippi
Medical Center
2500 North State St.
Jackson, MS 39216
Business: 601-984-1675
Emergency: 601-354-7660
Fax: 601-984-1676

MISSOURI

KANSAS CITY
Poison Control Center (*)
Children's Mercy Hospital
2401 Gillham Rd.
Kansas City, MO 64108
Business: 816-234-3053
Emergency: 816-234-3430
Fax: 816-234-3421

ST. LOUIS
Cardinal Glennon Children's
Hospital
Regional Poison Center (*)
1465 South Grand Blvd.
St. Louis, MO 63104
Emergency: 314-772-5200
800-366-8888
Fax: 314-577-5355

MONTANA

DENVER, CO
Rocky Mountain Poison and
Drug Center (*)
8802 E. 9th Ave.
Denver, CO 80220
Emergency: 303-629-1123
800-525-5042 (MT)
Fax: 303-739-1119

NEBRASKA

OMAHA
The Poison Center (*)
Children's Memorial Hospital
8301 Dodge St.
Omaha, NE 68114
Emergency: 402-390-5555
      (Omaha)
      800-955-9119
      (NE, WY)
Fax: 404-354-3049

NEVADA

LAS VEGAS
Poison Center
Humana Medical Center
3186 Maryland Pkwy.
Las Vegas, NV 89109
Emergency: 800-446-6179 (NV)

RENO
Poison Center
Washoe Medical Center
77 Pringle Way
Reno, NV 89520
Business: 702-328-4129
Emergency: 702-328-4100
Fax: 702-328-5555

NEW HAMPSHIRE

LEBANON
New Hampshire Poison
Information Center (*)
Dartmouth-Hitchcock Medical
Center
1 Medical Center Dr.
Lebanon, NH 03756
Emergency: 603-650-5000
      (ask for
      Poison Center)
      800-562-8236
      (NH only)
Fax: 603-650-8986

NEW JERSEY

NEWARK
New Jersey Poison Information
and Education System
Newark Beth Israel
Medical Center
201 Lyons Ave.
Newark, NJ 07112
Emergency: POISON-1
      (800-764-7661)
TTY: POISON-1
      (800-764-7661)
Fax: 201-705-8098

PHILLIPSBURG
Warren Hospital
Poison Control Center
185 Roseberry St.
Phillipsburg, NJ 08865
Business: 908-859-6768
Emergency: 908-859-6767
      800-962-1253 (NJ)
Fax: 908-859-6812

NEW MEXICO

ALBUQUERQUE
New Mexico Poison & Drug
Information Center
University of New Mexico
Albuquerque, NM 87131-1076
Emergency: 505-843-2551
      800-432-6866 (NM)
Fax: 505-277-5892

NEW YORK

BUFFALO
Western New York Regional
Poison Control Center
Children's Hospital of Buffalo
219 Bryant St.
Buffalo, NY 14222
Business: 716-878-7657
Emergency: 716-878-7654
      800-888-7655
      (NY & W. PA only)

MINEOLA
L.I. Regional Poison Control
Center (*)
Winthrop University Hospital
259 First St.
Mineola, NY 11501
Emergency: 516-542-2323
TTY: 516-747-3323
Fax: 516-739-2070

NEW YORK
New York City Poison Control
Center (*)
NYC Dept. of Health
455 First Ave., Room 123
New York, NY 10016
Business: 212-447-8154
Emergency: 212-340-4494
      212-POISONS
      (212-764-7667)
TTD: 212-689-9014
Fax: 212-447-8223

NORTH TARRYTOWN
Hudson Valley
Poison Center
Phelps Memorial Hospital
701 N. Broadway
North Tarrytown, NY 10591
Emergency: 914-353-1000
      800-336-6997
Fax: 914-353-1050

ROCHESTER
Finger Lakes Regional Poison
Control Center (*)
University of Rochester
Medical Center
601 Elmwood Ave.
Rochester, NY 14642
Business: 716-273-4155
Emergency: 716-275-3232
      800-333-0542 (NY)
Fax: 716-244-1677

SYRACUSE
Central NY Poison
Control Center
SUNY Health
Science Center
750 East Adams St.
Syracuse, NY 13210
Business: 315-464-7073
Emergency: 315-476-4766
      800-252-5655 (NY)
Fax: 315-464-7077

NORTH CAROLINA

ASHEVILLE
Western North Carolina Poison
Control Center (*)
Memorial Mission Hospital
509 Biltmore Ave.
Asheville, NC 28801
Emergency: 704-255-4490
      800-542-4225 (NC)
Fax: 704-255-4467

CHARLOTTE
Carolinas Poison Center (*)
P.O. Box 32861
Charlotte, NC 28232-2861
Business: 704-355-3054
Emergency: 704-355-4000
      (Charlotte area)
      800-848-6946

NORTH DAKOTA

FARGO
North Dakota Poison
Information Center (*)
Meritcare Medical Center
720 North 4th St.
Fargo, ND 58122
Business: 701-234-6062
Emergency: 701-234-5575
      800-732-2200 (ND)
Fax: 701-234-5090

OHIO

AKRON
Akron Regional Poison Control
Center
Children's Hospital
Medical Center
1 Perkins Square
Akron, OH 44308
Business: 330-258-3066
Emergency: 330-379-8562
      800-362-9922 (OH)
TTY: 330-379-8446
Fax: 330-379-8447

CINCINNATI
Regional Poison Control System
Cincinnati Drug and
Poison Information Center (*)
University of Cincinnati
College of Medicine
P.O. Box 670144
Cincinnati, OH 45267-0144
Emergency: 513-558-5111
      800-872-5111 (OH)
Fax: 513-558-5301

CLEVELAND
Greater Cleveland Poison
Control Center (*)
11100 Euclid Ave.
Cleveland, OH 44106
Emergency: 216-231-4455
      888-231-4455
Fax: 216-844-3242

COLUMBUS
Central Ohio Poison Center (*)
700 Children's Dr.
Columbus, OH 43205-2696
Business: 614-722-2635
Emergency: 614-228-1323
      800-682-7625
TTY: 614-228-2272
Fax: 614-221-2672

Greater Dayton Area Hospital
Association (*) at Central Ohio
Poison Center
700 Children's Dr.
Columbus, OH 43205
Business: 614-722-2635
Emergency: 513-222-2227
      800-762-0727 (OH)

TOLEDO
Poison Information Center of
NW Ohio (*)
Medical College of
Ohio Hospital
3000 Arlington Ave.
Toledo, OH 43614
Business: 419-381-3898
Emergency: 419-381-3897
      800-589-3897 (OH)
Fax: 419-381-2818

ZANESVILLE
Drug Information/Poison
Control Center (*)
Bethesda Hospital
2951 Maple Ave.
Zanesville, OH 43701
Business: 614-454-4246
Emergency: 614-454-4221
      614-454-4000
      800-686-4221 (OH)
Fax: 614-454-4059

OKLAHOMA

OKLAHOMA CITY
Oklahoma Poison
Control Center (*)
University of Oklahoma and
Children's Hospital
of Oklahoma
940 Northeast 13th St.
Oklahoma City, OK 73104
Emergency: 405-271-5454
      (Bus.)
      800-522-4611
      (Bus.) (OK)
TTD: 405-271-1122
Fax: 405-271-1816

OREGON

PORTLAND
Oregon Poison Center (*)
Oregon Health Sciences
University
3181 SW Sam Jackson Park Rd.
Portland, OR 97201
Emergency: 503-494-8968
      800-452-7165 (OR)
Fax: 503-494-4980

PENNSYLVANIA

HERSHEY
Central Pennsylvania Poison
Center (*)
University Hospital, Milton
S. Hershey Medical Center
P.O. Box 850
Hershey, PA 17033
Emergency: 800-521-6110
Fax: 717-531-6932

LANCASTER
Poison Control Center (*)
St. Joseph Hospital and Health
Care Center
250 College Ave.
Lancaster, PA 17604
Business: 717-299-4546
Emergency: 717-291-8111
Fax: 717-291-8346

PHILADELPHIA
The Poison Control Center (*)
3600 Market St.
Room 220
Philadelphia, PA 19104-2641
Business: 215-590-2003
Emergency: 215-386-2100
      800-722-7112
Fax: 215-590-4419

PITTSBURGH
Pittsburgh Poison Center (*)
Children's Hospital of Pittsburgh
3705 Fifth Ave.
Pittsburgh, PA 15213
Business: 412-692-5600
Emergency: 412-681-6669
Fax: 412-692-7497

RHODE ISLAND

PROVIDENCE
Rhode Island Poison Center (*)
Rhode Island Hospital
593 Eddy St.
Providence, RI 02903
Emergency: 401-444-5727
Fax: 401-444-8062

SOUTH CAROLINA

COLUMBIA
Palmetto Poison Center (*)
College of Pharmacy
University of South Carolina
Columbia, SC 29208
Business: 803-777-7909
Emergency: 803-777-1117
      800-922-1117 (SC)
Fax: 803-777-6127

SOUTH DAKOTA

ABERDEEN
Poison Control Center
St. Luke's Midland Regional
Medical Center
305 South State St.
Aberdeen, SD 57401
Business: 605-622-5000
Emergency: 605-622-5100
      800-592-1889
      (SD, MN, ND, WY)

RAPID CITY
Rapid City Regional
Poison Center
835 Fairmont Blvd.
P.O. Box 6000
Rapid City, SD 57709
Business &
Emergency: 605-341-3333

SIOUX FALLS
McKennan Poison Center
McKennan Hospital
800 East 21st St.
P.O. Box 5045
Sioux Falls, SD 57117-5045
Business: 605-322-8305
Emergency: 605-322-3894
      800-843-0505
      (IA, MN, NE, ND)
      800-952-0123 (SD)
Fax: 605-322-8378

TENNESSEE

MEMPHIS
Southern Poison Center (*)
847 Monroe Ave.
Suite 230
Memphis, TN 38163
Business: 901-448-6800
Emergency: 901-528-6048
      800-288-9999
      (TN only)
Fax: 901-448-5419

NASHVILLE
Middle Tennessee
Poison Center (*)
501 Oxford House
1161 21st Ave. S.
Nashville, TN 37232
Business: 615-936-0760
Emergency: 615-936-2034
      800-288-9999
      (TN)
TTD: 615-936-2047
Fax: 615-936-2046

TEXAS

DALLAS
North Texas Poison Center
Texas Poison Center Network (*)
Parkland Memorial Hospital
5201 Harry Hines Blvd.
P.O. Box 35926
Dallas, TX 75235
Business: 214-590-6625
Emergency: 800-Poison-1
      (800-764-7661)
Fax: 214-590-5008

EL PASO
West Texas Regional Poison
Center (*)
4815 Alameda Ave.
El Paso, TX 79905
Business: 915-521-7661
Emergency: 800-764-7661
      (800-POISON-1)
Fax: 915-521-7978

GALVESTON
Southeast Texas
Poison Center (*)
University of Texas
Medical Branch
Trauma Center
Room 3-112
Galveston, TX 77555-1175
Emergency: 409-765-1420
      800-764-7661
      (TX only)
Fax: 409-772-3917

TEMPLE
Drug Information Center
Scott and White Memorial
Hospital
2401 South 31st St.
Temple, TX 76508
Business: 817-724-4636
Fax: 817-724-1731

UTAH

SALT LAKE CITY
Utah Poison Control Center (*)
410 Chipeta Way
Suite 230
Salt Lake City, UT 84108
Emergency: 801-581-2151
      800-456-7707
      (UT)
Fax: 801-581-4199

VERMONT

BURLINGTON
Vermont Poison Center (*)
Fletcher Allen Health Care
111 Colchester Ave.
Burlington, VT 05401
Business: 802-656-2721
Emergency: 802-658-3456
Fax: 802-656-4802

VIRGINIA

CHARLOTTESVILLE
Blue Ridge Poison Center
Blue Ridge Hospital
Box 67
Charlottesville, VA 22901
Emergency: 804-924-5543
      800-451-1428
Fax: 804-971-8657

RICHMOND
Virginia Poison Center
Virginia Commonwealth
University
P.O. Box 980522
Richmond, VA 23298-0522
Emergency: 804-828-9123
Fax: 804-828-5291

WASHINGTON

SEATTLE
Washington Poison Center (*)
155 NE 100th St., Suite 400
Seattle, WA 98125-8012
Business: 206-517-2351
Emergency: 206-526-2121
      800-732-6985 (WA)
TTY: 206-517-2394
      800-572-0638 (WA)
Fax: 206-526-8490

WEST VIRGINIA

CHARLESTON
West Virginia Poison Center (*)
West Virginia University
3110 MacCorkle Ave. SE
Charleston, WV 25304
Business: 304-347-1212
Emergency: 304-348-4211
      800-642-3625 (WV)
Fax: 304-348-9560

PARKERSBURG
Poison Center
St. Joseph's Hospital Center
19th St. and Murdoch Ave.
Parkersburg, WV 26101
Emergency: 304-424-4222
Fax: 304-424-4766

WISCONSIN

MADISON
Poison Control Center (*)
University of Wisconsin
Hospital and Clinics
600 Highland Ave.
E5/238
Madison, WI 53792
Business: 608-262-7537
Emergency: 608-262-3702
      800-815-8855 (WI)

MILWAUKEE
Children's Hospital
Poison Center
Children's Hospital of
Wisconsin
9000 W. Wisconsin Ave.
P.O. Box 1997
Milwaukee, WI 53201
Business: 414-266-2000
Emergency: 414-266-2222
      800-815-8855 (WI)
Fax: 414-266-2820

DISCONTINUED PRODUCTS

Listed alphabetically by manufacturer below are products withdrawn from the market by their suppliers. In some instances, marketing privileges may have been transferred to another company.

To double-check on current availability, please consult the Brand and Generic Name Index in the front of the book.

ABANA PHARMACEUTICALS, INC.
Nasabid

ADAMS LABORATORIES, INC.
Deconsal C Expectorant
Deconsal Pediatric Capsules
Deconsal Pediatric Suspension
Humibid DM Pediatric Capsules

ADVANCED NUTRITIONAL TECHNOLOGY, INC.
Pediavit Drops
Sof C 500

BOCK PHARMACAL CO.
Emetrol Solution–Cherry
Emetrol Solution–Lemon-Mint

BOEHRINGER MANNHEIM THERAPEUTICS
Anexsia 5/500
Anexsia 7.5/650

BRISTOL-MYERS SQUIBB CO.
Vagistat-1

CENTRAL PHARMACEUTICALS, INC.
Cenocort-A 40 Sterile Suspension
Cenocort Forte Sterile Suspension
Codimal-A Injectable
Dexacen L.A.-8 Sterile Suspension
Dexacen-4 Injectable
Niferex Daily Tablets
Niferex Forte Elixir
Rep-Pred 40 Sterile Suspension
Rep-Pred 80 Sterile Suspension
Rubesol-1000 Injectable
Theoclear L.A.-130 Capsules
Theoclear L.A.-260 Capsules

CHIRON THERAPEUTICS
Acetylcysteine Solution, USP
Cerubidine
Doxorubicin HCl for Injection, USP
Doxorubicin HCl Injection, USP
Etoposide Injection
Leucovorin Calcium for Injection
Methotrexate Sodium Injection, USP
Mitomycin for Injection, USP
Sterile Cytarabine, USP
Sterile Vinblastine Sulfate, USP

DEY LABORATORIES
Isoetharine Inhalation Solution, USP

DURAMED
Aspirin 15gr Delayed Release Tablets

ELKINS-SINN, INC.
Tobramycin Sulfate Injection

ICN PHARMACEUTICALS, INC.
Android 10 Tablets
Android 25 Tablets
Oreton Methyl

KNOLL LABORATORIES
SSD RP Cream
Travase Ointment

LEDERLE LABORATORIES
Maxzide and Maxzide 25 MG Tablets

3M PHARMACEUTICALS
Duo-Medihaler with adaptor
Duo-Medihaler refill
Tambocor 50mg unit dose blister strips
Tambocor 100mg unit dose blister strips

MCNEIL CONSUMER PRODUCTS
Chemet
Rx Nicotrol

MCNEIL PHARMACEUTICAL
Paraflex

OCLASSEN PHARMACEUTICALS
Micanol 1% Anthralin Cream, USP

PERSŌN & COVEY, INC.
Solbar PF 15 Cream

A.H. ROBINS
Donnatal No. 2 Tablets
Exna Tablets
Robitet 250 Hydrochloride Robicaps
Robitet 500 Hydrochloride Robicaps

ROCHE LABORATORIES INC.
Arfonad Ampuls
Azo Gantanol Tablets
Azo Gantrisin Tablets
Brevicon 21-Day Tablets
Brevicon 28-Day Tablets
Femstat Prefill Vaginal Cream 2%
Femstat Vaginal Cream 2%
Konakion Injection
Lidex Cream 0.05%
Lidex Gel 0.05%
Lidex Ointment 0.05%
Lidex Topical Solution 0.05%
Lidex-E Cream 0.05%
Norinyl 1+35 21-Day Tablets
Norinyl 1+35 28-Day Tablets
Norinyl 1+50 21-Day Tablets
Norinyl 1+50 28-day Tablets
Nor QD Tablets
Provocholine for Inhalation
Solatene Capsules
Synalar Creams 0.025%, 0.01%
Synalar Ointment 0.025%
Synalar Topical Solution 0.01%
Synarel Nasal Solution for Central Precocious Puberty
Synarel Nasal Solution for Endometriosis
Synemol Cream 0.025%
Tri-Norinyl 21-Day Tablets
Tri-Norinyl 28-Day tablets
Valrelease Capsules

ROCHE PRODUCTS INC.
Endep Tablets
Libritabs Tablets
Quarzan Capsules

ROXANE LABORATORIES, INC.
Amitriptyline Hydrochloride Tablets
Chloral Hydrate Syrup, USP
Chloral Hydrate Capsules, USP
Imipramine Hydrochloride Tablets, USP

SANDOZ PHARMACEUTICALS CORPORATION
Eldepryl Tablets
Hydergine Sublingual Tablets 0.5mg, 100's
Hydergine Sublingual Tablets 1mg, 100's
Klorvess Effervescent Tablets

SMITHKLINE BEECHAM PHARMACEUTICALS
Vontrol

U.S. PHARMACEUTICAL CORPORATION
Isovex Capsules

UPSHER-SMITH LABORATORIES, INC.
Niacin-Rx
Niacor-B_3 Tablets

WAKEFIELD PHARMACEUTICALS, INC.
Hem Fe Capsules
Oncet Capsules

WESTWOOD-SQUIBB PHARMACEUTICALS INC.
Mycostatin Ointment

WYETH-AYERST LABORATORIES
Children's Advil Suspension
Aludrox
Bonamil Infant Formula
Cyanocobalamin Injection
Diphtheria and Tetanus Toxoids Adsorbed, Ultrafined, Pediatric
Largon Injection
Nursoy Infant Formula
Omnipen-N Injection
Oxytocin Injection, USP
SMA Infant Formula
Tetanus and Diphtheria Toxoids Adsorbed for Adult Use, Ultrafined
Tetanus Toxoid Fluid, Purified, Ultrafined
Tetanus Toxoid Adsorbed, aluminum phosphate adsorbed, Ultrafined
Thiosulfil Forte
Unipen Injection

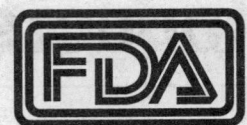

U.S. FOOD AND DRUG ADMINISTRATION

Professional and Consumer Information Numbers

Medical Product Reporting Programs

MedWatch (24 hour service) **800-332-1088**
Reporting of problems with drugs, devices, biologics (except vaccines), medical foods, dietary supplements.

Vaccine Adverse Event Reporting (24 hour service) **800-822-7967**
Reporting of vaccine-related problems.

Mandatory Medical Device Reporting **301-594-3886**
Reporting required from User facilities regarding device-related deaths and serious injuries.

Veterinary Adverse Drug Reaction Program (7:30 a.m. to 4:00 p.m., eastern time) **301-594-1751**
Reporting of adverse drug events in animals (collect calls accepted).

Medical Advertising Information (24 hour service) **800-238-7332**
Inquiries from health professionals regarding product promotion.

Information for Health Professionals

Drug Information Branch **301-827-4573**
Information on human drugs including hormones.

Center for Devices and Radiological Health **301-443-4190**
Automated request for information on medical devices and radiation-emitting products.

Office of Health Affairs Medicine Staff **301-443-5470**
Information for health professionals on FDA activities.

General Information

General Consumer Inquiries **301-443-3170**
Consumer information on regulated products/issues.

Freedom of Information **301-443-6310**
Request for publicly available FDA documents.

Office of Public Affairs **301-443-1130**
Interviews/press inquiries on FDA activities.

Breast Implant Inquiries (24 hour service) **800-532-4440**
Prerecorded message/request information.

Seafood Hotline (24 hour service) **800-332-4010**
Prerecorded message/request information (English/Spanish).

All numbers accessible 8:00 a.m. to 4:30 p.m. eastern time, except where otherwise noted.

VACCINE ADVERSE EVENT REPORTING SYSTEM
24 Hour Toll-free information line 1-800-822-7967
P.O. Box 1100, Rockville, MD 20849-1100
PATIENT IDENTITY KEPT CONFIDENTIAL

VAERS

Patient Name:

Last ____ First ____ M.I.

Address
_____
_____
_____

City ____ State ____ Zip

Telephone no. (____)_____

Vaccine administered by (Name):

Responsible
Physician _____
Facility Name/Address
_____
_____
_____

City ____ State ____ Zip

Telephone no. (____)_____

Form completed by (Name):

Relation ☐ Vaccine Provider ☐ Patient/Parent
to Patient ☐ Manufacturer ☐ Other
Address *(if different from patient or provider)*
_____
_____
_____

City ____ State ____ Zip

Telephone no. (____)_____

| 1. State | 2. County where administered | 3. Date of birth __/__/__ mm dd yy | 4. Patient age | 5. Sex ☐ M ☐ F | 6. Date form completed __/__/__ mm dd yy |

7. Describe adverse event(s) (symptoms, signs, time course) and treatment, if any

8. Check all appropriate:
☐ Patient died (date ___/___/___)
  mm dd yy
☐ Life threatening illness
☐ Required emergency room/doctor visit
☐ Required hospitalization (_____days)
☐ Resulted in prolongation of hospitalization
☐ Resulted in permanent disability
☐ None of the above

9. Patient recovered ☐ YES ☐ NO ☐ UNKNOWN

10. Date of vaccination __/__/__ mm dd yy Time ____ AM PM

11. Adverse event onset __/__/__ mm dd yy Time ____ AM PM

12. Relevant diagnostic tests/laboratory data

13. Enter all vaccines given on date listed in no. 10

	Vaccine (type)	Manufacturer	Lot number	Route/Site	No. Previous doses
a.					
b.					
c.					
d.					

14. Any other vaccinations within 4 weeks prior to the date listed in no. 10

	Vaccine (type)	Manufacturer	Lot number	Route/Site	No. Previous doses	Date given
a.						
b.						

15. Vaccinated at:
☐ Private doctor's office/hospital ☐ Military clinic/hospital
☐ Public health clinic/hospital ☐ Other/unknown

16. Vaccine purchased with:
☐ Private funds ☐ Military funds
☐ Public funds ☐ Other /unknown

17. Other medications

18. Illness at time of vaccination (specify)

19. Pre-existing physician-diagnosed allergies, birth defects, medical conditions (specify)

20. Have you reported this adverse event previously?
☐ No ☐ To health department
☐ To doctor ☐ To manufacturer

Only for children 5 and under

22. Birth weight _____ lb. _____ oz.

23. No. of brothers and sisters

21. Adverse event following prior vaccination (check all applicable, specify)

	Adverse Event	Onset Age	Type Vaccine	Dose no. in series
☐ In patient				
☐ In brother or sister				

Only for reports submitted by manufacturer/immunization project

24. Mfr. / imm. proj. report no.

25. Date received by mfr. / imm. proj.

26. 15 day report? ☐ Yes ☐ No

27. Report type ☐ Initial ☐ Follow-Up

Form VAERS -1

Vaccine Adverse Event Reporting System

Health care providers and manufacturers are required by law (42 USC 300aa-25) to report reactions to vaccines listed in the Vaccine Injury Table. Reports for reactions to other vaccines are voluntary except when required as a condition of immunization grant awards.

The form appears overleaf and may be photocopied for submission.

DIRECTIONS FOR COMPLETING FORM
(Additional pages may be attached if more space is needed.)

GENERAL

- Use a separate form for each patient. Complete the form to the best of your abilities. Items 3, 4, 7, 8, 10, 11, and 13 are considered essential and should be completed whenever possible. Parents/Guardians may need to consult the facility where the vaccine was administered for some of the information (such as manufacturer, lot number or laboratory data.)
- Refer to the Reportable Events Table (RET) for events mandated for reporting by law. Reporting for other serious events felt to be related but not on the RET is encouraged.
- Health care providers other than the vaccine administrator (VA) treating a patient for a suspected adverse event should notify the VA and provide the information about the adverse event to allow the VA to complete the form to meet the VA's legal responsibility.
- These data will be used to increase understanding of adverse events following vaccination and will become part of CDC Privacy Act System 09-20-0136, "Epidemiologic Studies and Surveillance of Disease Problems". Information identifying the person who received the vaccine or that person's legal representative will not be made available to the public, but may be available to the vaccinee or legal representative.
- Postage will be paid by addressee. Forms may be photocopied (must be front & back on same sheet).

SPECIFIC INSTRUCTIONS

Form Completed By: To be used by parents/guardians, vaccine manufacturers/distributors, vaccine administrators, and/or the person completing the form on behalf of the patient or the health professional who administered the vaccine.

Item 7: Describe the suspected adverse event. Such things as temperature, local and general signs and symptoms, time course, duration of symptoms diagnosis, treatment and recovery should be noted.

Item 9: Check "YES" if the patient's health condition is the same as it was prior to the vaccine, "NO" if the patient has not returned to the pre-vaccination state of health, or "UNKNOWN" if the patient's condition is not known.

Item 10: Give dates and times as specifically as you can remember. If you do not know the exact time, please
and 11: indicate "AM" or "PM" when possible if this information is known. If more than one adverse event, give the onset date and time for the most serious event.

Item 12: Include "negative" or "normal" results of any relevant tests performed as well as abnormal findings.

Item 13: List ONLY those vaccines given on the day listed in Item 10.

Item 14: List any other vaccines that the patient received within 4 weeks prior to the date listed in Item 10.

Item 16: This section refers to how the person who gave the vaccine purchased it, not to the patient's insurance.

Item 17: List any prescription or non-prescription medications the patient was taking when the vaccine(s) was given.

Item 18: List any short term illnesses the patient had on the date the vaccine(s) was given (i.e., cold, flu, ear infection).

Item 19: List any pre-existing physician-diagnosed allergies, birth defects, medical conditions (including developmental and/or neurologic disorders) for the patient.

Item 21: List any suspected adverse events the patient, or the patient's brothers or sisters, may have had to previous vaccinations. If more than one brother or sister, or if the patient has reacted to more than one prior vaccine, use additional pages to explain completely. For the onset age of a patient, provide the age in months if less than two years old.

Item 26: This space is for manufacturers' use only.

TABLE OF REPORTABLE EVENTS FOLLOWING VACCINATION

Vaccine/Toxoid	Event	Interval from Vaccination
DTP, DTaP, DTP-HiB, P, DT, Td, TT.	A. Anaphylaxis or anaphylactic shock	7 days
	B. Encephalopathy (or encephalitis)	7 days
	C. Any sequela (including death) of above events	No limit
	D. Events described in manufacturer's package insert as contraindications to additional doses of vaccine	See package insert
Measles & mumps in any combination; MMR, MR, M.	A. Anaphylaxis or anaphylactic shock	7 days
	B. Encephalopathy (or encephalitis)	15 days
	C. Residual seizure disorder	15 days
	D. Any sequela (including death) of above events	No limit
	E. Events described in manufacturer's package insert as contraindications to additional doses of vaccine	See package insert
Rubella in any combination; MMR, MR, R.	A. Chronic arthritis	42 days
	B. Anaphylaxis or anaphylactic shock	7 days
	C. Encephalopathy (or encephalitis)	15 days
	D. Residual seizure disorder	15 days
	E. Any sequela (including death) of above events	No limit
	F. Events described in manufacturer's package insert as contraindications to additional doses of vaccine	See package insert
Oral Polio (OPV)	A. Paralytic polio	
	—in a non-immunodeficient recipient	30 days
	—in an immunodeficient recipient	6 months
	—in a vaccine-associated community case	No limit
	B. Any sequela (including death) of above events	No limit
	C. Events described in manufacturer's package insert as contraindications to additional doses of vaccine	See package insert
Inactivated Polio (IPV)	A. Anaphylaxis or anaphylactic shock	7 days
	D. Any sequela (including death) of the above events	No limit
	E. Events described in manufacturer's package insert as contraindications to additional doses of vaccine	See package insert

The Reportable Events Table (RET) reflects what is reportable by law (42 USC 300aa-25) to the Vaccine Adverse Event Reporting System (VAERS) including conditions found in the manufacturers package insert. In addition, individuals are encouraged to report **ANY** clinically significant or unexpected events (even if you are not certain the vaccine caused the event) for **ANY** vaccine, whether or not it is listed on the RET. Manufacturers are also required by regulation (21CFR 600.80) to report to the VAERS program all adverse events made known to them for any vaccine.

Effective March 1995. Revised 21 May 1996.

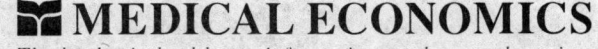

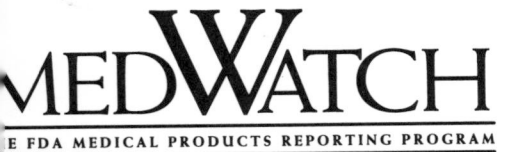

For **VOLUNTARY** reporting
by health professionals of adverse
events and product problems

Page ____ of ____

Form Approved: OMB No. 0910-0291 Expires: 4/30/96
See OMB statement on reverse

FDA Use Only

Triage unit
sequence #

A. Patient information

| 1. Patient identifier | 2. Age at time of event:
or _____
Date of birth: | 3. **Sex** ☐ female ☐ male | 4. **Weight** ____ lbs
or
____ kgs |

In confidence

B. Adverse event or product problem

☐ **Adverse event**   and/or   ☐ **Product problem** (e.g., defects/malfunctions)

Outcomes attributed to adverse event
(check all that apply)

☐ death _____ (mo/day/yr)
☐ life-threatening
☐ hospitalization – initial or prolonged

☐ disability
☐ congenital anomaly
☐ required intervention to prevent permanent impairment/damage
☐ other: _____

| 3. Date of event (mo/day/yr) | 4. Date of this report (mo/day/yr) |

5. Describe event or problem

6. Relevant tests/laboratory data, including dates

7. Other relevant history, including preexisting medical conditions (e.g., allergies, race, pregnancy, smoking and alcohol use, hepatic/renal dysfunction, etc.)

C. Suspect medication(s)

1. **Name** (give labeled strength & mfr/labeler, if known)

#1 _____

#2 _____

| 2. **Dose, frequency & route used**
#1
#2 | 3. **Therapy dates** (if unknown, give duration) from/to (or best estimate)
#1
#2 |

| 4. **Diagnosis for use** (indication)
#1
#2 | 5. **Event abated after use stopped or dose reduced**
#1 ☐ yes ☐ no ☐ doesn't apply
#2 ☐ yes ☐ no ☐ doesn't apply |

| 6. **Lot #** (if known)
#1
#2 | 7. **Exp. date** (if known)
#1
#2 | 8. **Event reappeared after reintroduction**
#1 ☐ yes ☐ no ☐ doesn't apply
#2 ☐ yes ☐ no ☐ doesn't apply |

9. **NDC #** (for product problems only) ____ – ____

10. **Concomitant medical products** and therapy dates (exclude treatment of event)

D. Suspect medical device

1. **Brand name**

2. **Type of device**

| 3. **Manufacturer name & address** | 4. **Operator of device**
☐ health professional
☐ lay user/patient
☐ other: _____ |

5. **Expiration date** (mo/day/yr)

6. model # _____
catalog # _____
serial # _____
lot # _____
other #

7. **If implanted, give date** (mo/day/yr)

8. **If explanted, give date** (mo/day/yr)

9. **Device available for evaluation?**   (Do not send to FDA)
☐ yes   ☐ no   ☐ returned to manufacturer on _____ (mo/day/yr)

10. **Concomitant medical products** and therapy dates (exclude treatment of event)

E. Reporter (see confidentiality section on back)

| 1. **Name & address** | phone # |

| 2. **Health professional?** ☐ yes ☐ no | 3. **Occupation** | 4. **Also reported to** ☐ manufacturer ☐ user facility ☐ distributor |

5. If you do NOT want your identity disclosed to the manufacturer, place an " X " in this box. ☐

Mail to: MEDWATCH
5600 Fishers Lane
Rockville, MD 20852-9787

or FAX to:
1-800-FDA-0178

FDA Form 3500 1/96   **Submission of a report does not constitute an admission that medical personnel or the product caused or contributed to the event.**

ADVICE ABOUT VOLUNTARY REPORTING

Report experiences with:

- medications (drugs or biologics)
- medical devices (including in-vitro diagnostics)
- special nutritional products (dietary supplements, medical foods, infant formulas)
- other products regulated by FDA

Report SERIOUS adverse events. An event is serious when the patient outcome is:

- death
- life-threatening (real risk of dying)
- hospitalization (initial or prolonged)
- disability (significant, persistent or permanent)
- congenital anomaly
- required intervention to prevent permanent impairment or damage

Report even if:

- you're not certain the product caused the event
- you don't have all the details

Report product problems – quality, performance or safety concerns such as:

- suspected contamination
- questionable stability
- defective components
- poor packaging or labeling
- therapeutic failures

How to report:

- just fill in the sections that apply to your report
- use section C for all products except medical devices
- attach additional blank pages if needed
- use a separate form for each patient
- report either to FDA or the manufacturer (or both)

Important numbers:

- 1-800-FDA-0178 to FAX report
- 1-800-FDA-7737 to report by modem
- 1-800-FDA-1088 to report by phone or for more information
- 1-800-822-7967 for a VAERS form for vaccines

If your report involves a serious adverse event with a device and it occurred in a facility outside a doctor's office, that facility may be legally required to report to FDA and/or the manufacturer. Please notify the person in that facility who would handle such reporting.

Confidentiality: The patient's identity is held in strict confidence by FDA and protected to the fullest extent of the law. The reporter's identity, including the identity of a self-reporter, may be shared with the manufacturer unless requested otherwise. However, FDA will not disclose the reporter's identity in response to a request from the public, pursuant to the Freedom of Information Act.

FDA Form 3500-back   **Please Use Address Provided Below – Just Fold In Thirds, Tape and Mail**

Department of Health and Human Services

Public Health Service
Food and Drug Administration
Rockville, MD 20857

Official Business
Penalty for Private Use $300

NO POSTAGE
NECESSARY
IF MAILED
IN THE
UNITED STATES
OR APO/FPO

BUSINESS REPLY MAIL
FIRST CLASS MAIL   PERMIT NO. 946   ROCKVILLE, MD

POSTAGE WILL BE PAID BY FOOD AND DRUG ADMINISTRATION

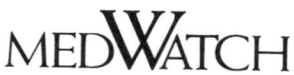

The FDA Medical Products Reporting Program
Food and Drug Administration
5600 Fishers Lane
Rockville, MD 20852-9787